Sleisenger and Fordtran's

GASTROINTESTINAL and LIVER DISEASE

PATHOPHYSIOLOGY | DIAGNOSIS | MANAGEMENT

EDITORS

RAYMOND T. CHUNG, MD
Professor of Medicine
Harvard Medical School
Zhou Family Endowed Chair
Chief, Gastroenterology, Hepatology and Endoscopy
Mass General Brigham
Associate Member, Broad Institute
Boston, Massachusetts

DAVID T. RUBIN, MD
Joseph B. Kirsner Professor of Medicine
Chief, Section of Gastroenterology, Hepatology, and Nutrition
Department of Medicine
University of Chicago
Chicago, Illinois

C. MEL WILCOX, MD, MSPH
Chief of Gastroenterology and Hepatology
Director, Pancreatology
Digestive Health Institute
Chair, US Pancreatic Disease Study Group
Orlando Health
Orlando, Florida

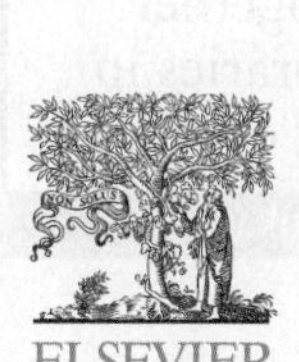

ELSEVIER

Elsevier
1600 John F. Kennedy Blvd.
Ste 1800
Philadelphia, PA 19103-2899

SLEISENGER AND FORDTRAN'S GASTROINTESTINAL AND LIVER DISEASE,
TWELFTH EDITION

ISBN: 978-0-443-11657-5
Volume 1: 978-0-443-11704-6
Volume 2: 978-0-443-11705-3

Notice

Practitioners and researchers must always rely on their own experience and knowledge in evaluating and using any information, methods, compounds or experiments described herein. Because of rapid advances in the medical sciences, in particular, independent verification of diagnoses and drug dosages should be made. To the fullest extent of the law, no responsibility is assumed by Elsevier, authors, editors or contributors for any injury and/or damage to persons or property as a matter of products liability, negligence or otherwise, or from any use or operation of any methods, products, instructions, or ideas contained in the material herein.

Executive Content Strategist: Nancy Anastasi Duffy
Content Development Manager: Meghan Andress
Senior Content Development Specialist: Kevin Travers
Publishing Services Manager: Catherine Jackson
Senior Project Manager: Cindy Thoms
Senior Book Designer: Patrick Ferguson

Printed in Canada

Last digit is the print number: 9 8 7 6 5 4 3 2 1

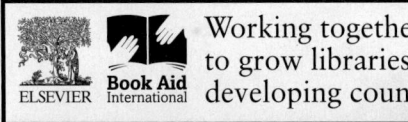

Contributors

Nezam H. Afdhal, MD, DSc
Chief of Gastroenterology and Hepatology
Beth Israel Deaconess Medical Center
Charlotte and Irving Rabb Professor of Medicine
Harvard Medical School
Boston, Massachusetts, United States

Rakesh Aggarwal MD, DM
Professor, Department of Gastroenterology
Sanjay Gandhi Postgraduate Institute of Medical Sciences
Lucknow, UP, India

Sameer Al Diffalha, MD
Associate Professor of Pathology
University of Alabama at Birmingham
Birmingham, Alabama, United States

Jaime Almandoz, MD, MBA, FTOS
Associate Professor of Internal Medicine
Endocrinology
University of Texas Southwestern
Dallas, Texas, United States

Taymeyah Al-Toubah, MPH
Senior Research Project Manager GI Oncology
H. Lee Moffitt Cancer Center
Tampa, Florida, United States

Amin Amin, MB, ChB
Assistant Professor, Internal Medicine: Digestive and Liver Diseases
University of Texas Southwestern
Dallas, Texas, United States

Ashwin N. Ananthakrishnan, MD, MPH
Director of the MGH Crohn's and Colitis Center
Associate Professor of Medicine
Harvard Medical School Division of Gastroenterology
Massachusetts General Hospital
Boston, Massachusetts, United States

Karin L. Andersson, MD, MPH
Assistant Professor of Medicine, Harvard Medical School
Hepatologist, Division of Gastroenterology
Massachusetts General Hospital
Boston, Massachusetts, United States

Louis J. Aronne, MD
Sanford I. Weill Professor of Metabolic Research
Department of Medicine
Weill Cornell Medicine
New York, New York, United States

Jordan E. Axelrad, MD, MPH
Director, Clinical and Translational Research
Inflammatory Bowel Disease Center
NYU Langone Health
Associate Professor
Division of Gastroenterology
NYU Grossman School of Medicine
New York, New York, United States

Fernando Azpiroz, MD, PhD
Chief, Department of Gastroenterology
University Hospital Vall d'Hebron
Professor of Medicine
Universitat Autònoma de Barcelona
Barcelona, Spain

William Balistreri, MD
Pediatric Liver Care Center
Gastroenterology, Hepatology, and Nutrition
Cincinnati Children's Hospital Medical Center
Cincinnati, Ohio, United States

Ji Young Bang, MD, MPH
Director of Clinical Research, Digestive Health Institute
Orlando Health
Orlando, Florida, United States

S. George Barreto, FRACS, PhD
Consultant, HPB and Liver Transplant Unit
Flinders Medical Centre
Deputy Director, Medical Program (MD)
Coordinator | MD Advanced Studies
College of Medicine and Public Health
Flinders University
Bedford Park South Africa

Lee M. Bass, MD
Professor of Pediatrics
Gastroenterology, Hepatology, and Nutrition
Ann and Robert H. Lurie Children's Hospital of Chicago
Chicago, Illinois, United States

Alex S. Befeler, MD
Professor of Internal Medicine and Medical Director Liver Transplantation
Division of Gastroenterology and Hepatology
Saint Louis University
St. Louis, Missouri, United States

Daniel Behin, MD
Assistant Professor of Medicine
Montefiore Medical Center
New York, New York, United States

Mark Benson, MD
Professor of Medicine
Section of Gastroenterology and Hepatology
University of Wisconsin School of Medicine and Public Health
Madison, Wisconsin, United States

Adil E. Bharucha, MBBS, MD
Professor of Medicine
Division of Gastroenterology and Hepatology
Mayo Clinic
Rochester, Minnesota, United States

Divya B. Bhatt, MD, MA
Assistant Professor of Medicine Digestive and Liver Diseases
University of Texas Southwestern Medical Center
Assistant Professor of Gastroenterology
Veterans Affairs North Texas Health Care System
Dallas, Texas, United States

Taft P. Bhuket, MD
Associate Clinical Professor of Medicine
Division of Gastroenterology
University of California, San Francisco
San Francisco, California, United States;
Chief of Gastroenterology and Hepatology, Director of Endoscopy
Alameda Health System
Oakland, California, United States

Yangzom D. Bhutia, DVM, PhD
Assistant Professor, Cell Biology and Biochemistry
Texas Tech University Health Sciences Center
Lubbock, Texas, United States

J. Andrew Bird, MD
Professor, Pediatrics, Division of Allergy and Immunology
University of Texas Southwestern Medical Center
Director, Food Allergy Center
Children's Medical Center
Dallas, Texas, United States

Diego V. Bohórquez, PhD
Associate Professor
Departments of Medicine and Neurobiology
Duke University Medical Center
Durham, North Carolina, United States

Shoma Bommena, MD, MS
Fellow in Gastroenterology and Hepatology, Internal Medicine
University of Arizona College of Medicine
Tucson, Arizona, United States

Jan Bornschein, MD
Nuffield Department of Experimental Medicine
Oxford, United Kingdom

Christopher L. Bowlus, MD
Professor and Chief
Division of Gastroenterology and Hepatology
University of California Davis
Sacramento, California, United States

Lawrence J. Brandt, MD
Professor of Medicine and Surgery
Albert Einstein College of Medicine
Emeritus Chief, Division of Gastroenterology
Montefiore Medical Center
Bronx, New York, United States

Robert Scott Bresalier, MD
Professor of Medicine
Lydia and Birdie J Resoft Distinguished Professor in GI Oncology
Gastroenterology, Hepatology, and Nutrition
The University of Texas MD Anderson Cancer Center
Houston, Texas, United States

Stuart M. Brierley, PhD
Professor, NHMRC Investigator Leadership Fellow
Hopwood Centre for Neurobiology, Lifelong Health Theme
South Australian Health and Medical Research Institute (SAHMRI)
Adelaide, Australia

Simon J.H. Brookes, PhD
Professor, Human Physiology
College of Medicine, Flinders University
Adelaide, South Australia, Australia

Alan L. Buchman, MD, MSPH
Professor of Clinical Surgery
University of Illinois at Chicago
Director, Gastroenterology
Chicago, Illinois, United States,
Elevance Health
Intestinal Rehabilitation and Transplant Center
Indianapolis, Indiana, United States

Callie B. Burgin, MD
Assistant Professor of Clinical Dermatology
Dermatology, Indiana University School of Medicine
Indianapolis, Indiana, United States

Ezra Burstein, MD, PhD
Professor, Departments of Internal Medicine and Molecular Biology
UT Southwestern Medical Center
Dallas, Texas, United States

Allison M. Bush, MD, MPH
Gastroenterology
Uniformed Services University
Bethesda, Maryland, United States

James P. Callaway, MD
Assistant Professor, Department of Gastroenterology
University of Alabama at Birmingham
Birmingham, Alabama, United States

David J. Cangemi, MD
Consultant, Gastroenterology and Hepatology
Mayo Clinic
Jacksonville, Florida, United States

Dustin A. Carlson, MD, MS
Assistant Professor of Medicine
Northwestern University Feinberg School of Medicine
Chicago, Illinois, United States

Andres F. Carrion, MD
Gastroenterologist and Hepatologist
GastroMed
Miami, Florida, United States

Amanda K. Cartee, MD
Assistant Professor, Gastroenterology and Hepatology
University of Alabama at Birmingham
Birmingham, Alabama, United States

Francis K.L. Chan, MBChB(Hons), MD, DSc
Professor of Medicine
Department of Medicine and Therapeutics
Chinese University of Hong Kong
Hong Kong, China

Michael R. Charlton, MD
Professor of Medicine
Chief of Hepatology
Director, Center for Liver Diseases
Medical Director, Transplantation Institute
University of Chicago
Chicago, Illinois, United States

Ellie Chen, MD
Division of Gastroenterology
University of California, Los Angeles
Los Angeles, California, United States

Alice Cheng, MD, PhD
Assistant Professor of Medicine
University of Chicago
Chicago, Illinois, United States

Shivakumar Chitturi, MD
Associate Professor
Australian National University
Senior Staff Hepatologist
The Canberra Hospital
Australian Capital Territory, Australia

Daniel C. Chung, MD
Professor of Medicine
Harvard Medical School
Division of Gastroenterology
Massachusetts General Hospital
Medical Co-Director
Center for Cancer Risk Analysis
Massachusetts General Hospital Cancer Center
Boston, Massachusetts, United States

Raymond T. Chung, MD
Professor of Medicine
Harvard Medical School
Zhou Family Endowed Chair
Chief, Gastroenterology, Hepatology and Endoscopy
Mass General Brigham
Associate Member, Broad Institute
Boston, Massachusetts, United States

Gregory A. Coté, MD, MS
Division Head, Professor, Department of Medicine
Division of Gastroenterology and Hepatology
Oregon Health & Science University
Portland, Oregon, United States

Cary C. Cotton, MD, MPH
Assistant Professor of Medicine
Department of Medicine
Division of Gastroenterology and Hepatology
UNC School of Medicine
Chapel Hill, North Carolina, United States

Marc Roger Couturier, PhD, D(ABMM)
Professor, ARUP Laboratories
University of Utah
Salt Lake City, Utah, United States

Brian G. Czito, MD
Professor, Radiation Oncology
Duke University Medical Center
Durham, North Carolina, United States

Sushila Dalal, MD
Associate Professor of Medicine
Section of Gastroenterology, Hepatology, and Nutrition
University of Chicago
Chicago, Illinois, United States

Paul A. Dawson, PhD
Professor Pediatrics
Gastroenterology, Hepatology, and Nutrition
Emory University
Atlanta, Georgia, United States

Jose Debes, MD, PhD, MS
Professor, Division of Infectious Diseases and International Medicine
Department of Medicine
University of Minnesota
Minneapolis, Minnesota, United States

Roshani J. Desai, MD
Assistant Professor, Gastroenterology and Hepatology
Saint Louis University
Saint Louis, Missouri, United States

Jill K. Deutsch, MD
Assistant Professor, Department of Internal Medicine
Section of Digestive Diseases
Yale New Haven Hospital
Yale University School of Medicine
New Haven, Connecticut, United States

Kenneth R. DeVault, MD
Professor of Medicine and Chair
Mayo Clinic College of Medicine
Jacksonville, Florida, United States

John K. DiBaise, MD
Professor of Medicine
Division of Gastroenterology and Hepatology
Mayo Clinic
Scottsdale, Arizona, United States

Philip G. Dinning, PhD
Senior Hospital Scientist
Department of Gastroenterology and Surgery
Professor, College of Medicine and Public Health
Flinders Medical Centre
Adelaide, South Australia, Australia

Michael Dougan, MD, PhD
Associate Professor of Medicine
Harvard Medical School
Division of Gastroenterology, Hepatology and Endoscopy
Mass General Brigham
Boston, Massachusetts, United States

Douglas A. Drossman, MD
Professor Emeritus of Medicine and Psychiatry
Division of Digestive Disease and Nutrition
University of North Carolina
President, Center for Education and Practice of Biopsychosocial Care
Chapel Hill, North Carolina, United States
President, Drossman Gastroenterology PLLC
Durham, North Carolina, United States

Kerry B. Dunbar, MD, PhD
Section Chief, VA Gastroenterology Section
Department of Medicine—Gastroenterology and Hepatology
VA North Texas Healthcare System—Dallas VA Medical Center
Associate Professor of Medicine
Department of Medicine—Division of Gastroenterology and Hepatology
University of Texas Southwestern Medical School
Dallas, Texas, United States

Steven A. Edmundowicz, MD
Professor of Medicine
Interim Director, Division of Gastroenterology and Hepatology
University of Colorado Anschutz Medical Campus
Aurora, Colorado, United States

Adam Edwards, MD, MS
Assistant Professor, Department of Medicine
University of Alabama at Birmingham
Birmingham, Alabama, United States

David E. Elliott, MD, PhD
University of Iowa Carver College of Medicine
Department of Internal Medicine
Division of Gastroenterology and Hepatology
Iowa City VAHCS, Department of Internal Medicine
Veterans Administration Health Care System
Iowa City, Iowa, United States

B. Joseph Elmunzer, MD, MSc
Peter B. Cotton Professor of Medicine and Endoscopic Innovation
Division of Gastroenterology and Hepatology
Medical University of South Carolina, Charleston
Charleston, South Carolina, United States

Charles O. Elson, MD
Professor of Medicine and Microbiology
Vice Chair for Research in the Department of Medicine
Basil I. Hirschowitz Chair in Gastroenterology
University of Alabama at Birmingham
Birmingham, Alabama, United States

Swathi Eluri, MD, MSCR
Assistant Professor of Medicine
Division of Gastroenterology and Hepatology
University of North Carolina School of Medicine
Chapel Hill, North Carolina, United States

Jill E. Elwing, MD
Assistant Professor of Medicine
Division of Gastroenterology
John T. Milliken Department of Medicine
Washington University in St. Louis
St. Louis, Missouri, United States

Michael B. Fallon, MD
Chair, Professor of Medicine
Gastroenterology, Hepatology, and Nutrition
University of Arizona
Vice Chair, Department of Internal Medicine
University of Arizona—Phoenix
Phoenix, Arizona, United States

Jordan J. Feld, MD, MPH
Professor of Medicine
University of Toronto
Research Director
Toronto Centre for Liver Disease
Senior Scientist
Sandra Rotman Centre for Global Health
Toronto General Hospital
Toronto, Ontario, Canada

Marc Fenster, MD
Division of Gastroenterology
Montefiore Medical Center
Albert Einstein College of Medicine
Bronx, New York, United States

Nielsen Fernandez-Becker, MD
Clinical Associate Professor of Medicine
Division of Gastroenterology and Hepatology
Stanford University
Redwood City, California, United States

Paul Feuerstadt, MD
Attending Physician, Gastroenterology
Gastroenterology Center of Connecticut
Hamden, Connecticut
Associate Clinical Professor of Medicine, Gastroenterology
Yale University School of Medicine
New Haven, Connecticut, United States

Peter Fickert, Prof
Division of Gastroenterology and Hepatology
Medical University of Graz
Graz, Austria

David R. Flum, MD, MPH, FACS
Professor of Surgery
University of Washington,
Seattle, Washington, United States

Lawrence S. Friedman, MD
Professor of Medicine, Harvard Medical School
Professor of Medicine, Tufts University School of Medicine
The Anton R. Fried, MD
Chair, Department of Medicine
Newton-Wellesley Hospital
Newton, Massachusetts Assistant Chief of Medicine
Massachusetts General Hospital
Boston, Massachusetts, United States

Vadivel Ganapathy, PhD
Professor, Cell Biology and Biochemistry
Texas Tech University Health Sciences Center
Lubbock, Texas, United States

Marc G. Ghany, MD, MHSc
Senior Investigator, Liver Diseases Branch
National Institute of Diabetes and Digestive and Kidney Diseases
National Institutes of Health
Bethesda, Maryland, United States

Pere Ginès, MD, PhD
Chairman, Liver Unit, Hospital Clinic Barcelona
Full Professor of Medicine, University of Barcelona
Principal Investigator
Institut d'Investigacions Biomediques August Pi i Sunyer (IDIBAPS)
Barcelona, Spain

Robert E. Glasgow, MD
Professor and Vice Chairman, Surgery
University of Utah
Salt Lake City, Utah, United States

Amit Goel, MBBS, MD, DNB, DM
Professor and Head, Hepatology
Sanjay Gandhi Postgraduate Institute of Medical Sciences
Lucknow, Uttar Pradesh, India

Amanda R. Gomez, MD, MPH
Assistant Professor
Division of Gastroenterology, Hepatology, and Nutrition
Ann & Robert H. Lurie Children's Hospital of Chicago
Chicago, Illinois, United States

Alex J. Gooding, MD, PhD
Medical Resident, Radiation Oncology
Duke University
Durham, North Carolina, United States

Gregory J. Gores, MD
Professor of Medicine
Division of Gastroenterology and Hepatology
Mayo Clinic
Rochester, Minnesota, United States

Peter H.R. Green, MD
Phyllis and Ivan Seidenberg Professor of Medicine
Columbia University Medical Center
New York, New York, United States

Drew Gunnells, MD, FACS
Assistant Professor, GI Surgery
University of Alabama at Birgmingham
Birmingham, Alabama, United States

Malika Gupta, MBBS
Associate Professor of Pediatrics
Department of Pediatrics
University of Texas Southwestern
Dallas, Texas, United States

C. Prakash Gyawali, MD, MRCP
Professor of Medicine
Division of Gastroenterology
Department of Medicine
Washington University in St. Louis
St. Louis, Missouri, United States

Hazem Hammad, MD
Assistant Professor of Medicine
Division of Gastroenterology and Hepatology
University of Colorado Anschutz Medical Campus
Aurora, Colorado, United States

Heinz F. Hammer, MD
Associate Professor of Medicine
Department of Internal Medicine
Medical University
Graz, Austria

David J. Hass, MD
Associate Clinical Professor of Medicine
Division of Digestive Diseases
Yale University School of Medicine
New Haven, Connecticut, United States

Asif Hitawala, MBBS
Liver Disease Branch
NIH/NIDDK
Bethesda, Maryland, United States

Thanh P. Ho, MD
Assistant Professor of Oncology
Department of Oncology
Mayo Clinic
Rochester, Minnesota, United States

David M. Hockenbery, MD
Member, Clinical Research
Fred Hutchinson Cancer Research Center
Professor of Medicine
Division of Gastroenterology
University of Washington
Seattle, Washington, United States

Christoph Högenauer, MD
Associate Professor of Medicine
Department of Internal Medicine
Medical University of Graz
Graz, Austria

Jacinta A. Holmes, MBBS, PhD
Division of Gastroenterology
Massachusetts General Hospital
Boston, Massachusetts, United States
Gastroenterology, St. Vincent's Hospital
University of Melbourne
Fitzroy, Victoria, Australia

Amy E. Hosmer, MD
Clinical Assistant Professor, Medicine
Digestive Health Institute
University Hospitals of Cleveland
Cleveland, Ohio, United States

Colin W. Howden, MD
Professor Emeritus, Hyman Professor of Medicine
Division of Gastroenterology
University of Tennessee Health Science Center
Memphis, Tennessee, United States

Bridget Hron, MD, MMSc
Assistant Professor, Pediatrics
Harvard Medical School
Associate Director, Center for Nutrition
Boston Children's Hospital
Boston, Massachusetts, United States

Christine Hsu, MD
NIH-NIDDK, Liver Disease Branch
National Institute of Digestive and Diabetes and Kidney Diseases
Bethesda, Maryland, United States

Sohail Z. Husain, MD
Professor of Pediatrics
Division of Gastroenterology, Hepatology, and Nutrition
Stanford University School of Medicine
Stanford, California, United States

Neil Hyman, MD
Chief, Section of Colon and Rectal Surgery
Co-Director Digestive Disease Center
Department of Surgery
University of Chicago Medicine
Chicago, Illinois, United States

Sumera I. Ilyas, MBBS
Assistant Professor of Medicine
Division of Gastroenterology and Hepatology
Mayo Clinic
Rochester, Minnesota, United States

M. Nedim Ince, MD
University of Iowa Carver College of Medicine
Department of Internal Medicine
Division of Gastroenterology and Hepatology
Iowa City VAHCS, Department of Internal Medicine
Veterans Administration Health Care System
Department of Internal Medicine
Veterans Administration Health Care System
Iowa City, Iowa, United States

Johanna C. Iturrino Moreda, MD
Assistant Professor of Medicine
Harvard Medical School
Beth Israel Deaconess Medical Center
Boston, Massachusetts, United States

Harry L.A. Janssen, MD, PhD
Professor of Medicine, Gastroenterology and Hepatology
University of Toronto
Toronto, Ontario, Canada
Professor of Medicine, Gastroenterology and Hepatology
Erasmus MC University Medical Center
Rotterdam, Netherlands

Dennis M. Jensen, MD
Professor of Medicine, Gastrointestinal
David Geffen School of Medicine at UCLA
Staff Physician, Medicine-Gastrointestinal
VA Greater Los Angeles Healthcare System
Key Investigator, Director
Human Studies Core and Gastrointestinal Hemostasis Research Unit
CURE Digestive Diseases Research Center
Los Angeles, California, United States

D. Rohan Jeyarajah, MD
Chair of Surgery, Assistant Chair of Clinical Sciences, Head of Surgery
TCU and UNTHSC School of Medicine
Fort Worth, Texas, United States
Director, Gastrointestinal Services, Methodist Richardson Medical Center
Director, HPB/UGI Fellowship
Associate Program Director, General Surgery Residency Program
Methodist Richardson Medical Center
Richardson, Texas, United States

Adrià Juanola, PhD
Clinician, Liver Unit
Hospital Clínic de Barcelona
Institut d'Investigacions Biomèdiques August Pi i Sunyer (IDIBAPS)
Barcelona, Spain

Patrick S. Kamath, MD
Professor of Medicine, Division of Gastroenterology and Hepatology
Consultant, Gastroenterology and Hepatology
Mayo Clinic College of Medicine and Science
Rochester, Minnesota, United States

Nuray Kanbur, MD
Professor of Pediatrics
University of Ottawa
Ottawa, Ontario, Canada

Gilaad G. Kaplan, MD, MPH
Professor of Medicine
University of Calgary
Calgary, Alberta, Canada

Jennifer Katz, MD
Assistant Professor of Medicine
Division of Gastroenterology
Montefiore Medical Center
Bronx, New York, United States

David A. Katzka, MD
Professor of and Consultant in Medicine, Gastroenterology
Mayo Clinic
Rochester, Minnesota, United States

Debra K. Katzman, MD, FRCPC
Professor of Pediatrics, Department of Pediatrics
The Hospital for Sick Children and University of Toronto
Toronto, Ontario, Canada

Jonathan D. Kaunitz, MD
Professor of Medicine and Surgery
UCLA School of Medicine
Attending Gastroenterologist
West Los Angeles Veterans Affairs Medical Center
Los Angeles, California, United States

Laurie Keefer, PhD
Professor Medicine and Psychiatry
Icahn School of Medicine at Mount Sinai
New York, New York, United States

Ciarán P. Kelly, MD
Professor of Medicine, Gastroenterology
Harvard Medical School
J Thomas Lamont Professor of Gastroenterology
Beth Israel Deaconess Medical Center
Boston, Massachusetts, United States

Sahil Khanna, MBBS, MS
Associate Professor of Medicine
Gastroenterology and Hepatology
Mayo Clinic
Rochester, Minnesota, United States

Arthur Yu-shin Kim, MD
Associate Professor of Medicine
Harvard Medical School
Division of Infectious Diseases
Massachusetts General Hospital
Boston, Massachusetts, United States

Kenneth L. Koch, MD
Professor of Medicine, Department of Medicine
Section on Gastroenterology and Hepatology
Wake Forest University School of Medicine
Winston-Salem, North Carolina, United States

Kris V. Kowdley, MD
Director
Liver Institute Northwest
Seattle, Washington, United States

Braden Kuo, MD
Director of the MGH Center for Neurointestinal Health
Gastroenterology
Massachusetts General Hospital
Boston, Massachusetts, United States

Brian E. Lacy, MD, PhD
Professor of Medicine
Division of Gastroenterology
Mayo Clinic
Jacksonville, Florida, United States

Anne M. Larson, MD
Clinical Professor of Medicine
Division of Gastroenterology/Hepatology
University of Washington
Seattle, Washington, United States

Ivan S.F. Lau, MB, BCh, BAO
Clinical Lecturer, Medicine and Therapeutics
The Chinese University of Hong Kong
Sha Tin, Hong Kong

James Y.W. Lau, MD
Professor of Surgery
Department of Surgery
The Chinese University of Hong Kong
Director
Endoscopy Centre
Prince of Wales Hospital
Hong Kong, China

Benjamin Lebwohl, MD, MS
Associate Professor of Medicine and Epidemiology
Columbia University Medical Center
New York, New York, United States

Peter J. Lee, MBChB
Assistant Professor of Clinical Medicine
Gastroenterology, Hepatology and Nutrition
The Ohio State University Wexner Medical Center
Columbus, Ohio, United States

William M. Lee, MD
Professor, Internal Medicine
UT Southwestern Medical Center at Dallas
Dallas, Texas, United States

Anthony J. Lembo, MD
Vice Chair of Research
Digestive Disease and Surgery Institute
Cleveland Clinic
Cleveland, Ohio, United States

Cynthia Levy, MD
Professor of Medicine
Division of Digestive Health and Liver Diseases
University of Miami
Miami, Florida, United States

Blair Lewis, MD
Medical Director, Carnegie Hill Endoscopy
Clinical Professor of Medicine
Mount Sinai Medical Center
New York, New York, United States

James H. Lewis, MD
Professor of Medicine, Director of Hepatology
Division of Gastroenterology
Georgetown University Medical Center
Washington, DC, United States

Rodger A. Liddle, MD
Professor of Medicine
Department of Medicine
Duke University Medical Center
Durham, North Carolina, United States

Steven D. Lidofsky, MD, PhD
Professor of Medicine, University of Vermont
Director of Hepatology, University of Vermont Medical Center
Burlington, Vermont, United States

Cara L. Mack, MD
Chief Professor of Pediatrics
Division of Gastroenterology
Medical College of Wisconsin, Children's
Milwaukee, Wisconsin, United States

Matthias Maiwald, MD, PhD
Senior Consultant in Microbiology
Department of Pathology and Laboratory Medicine
KK Women's and Children's Hospital, Singapore
Adjunct Associate Professor
Department of Microbiology and Immunology
Yong Loo Lin School of Medicine, National University of Singapore
Adjunct Associate Professor
Duke-NUS Graduate Medical School
Singapore, Singapore

Lawrence A. Mark, MD, PhD
Associate Professor of Clinical Dermatology
Department of Dermatology
Indiana University School of Medicine
Indianapolis, Indiana, United States

Paul Martin, MD, FRCP, FRCPI
Hepatologist, Karsh Division of Gastroenterology and Hepatology
Cedars Sinai
Los Angeles, California, United States

Joel B. Mason, MD
Professor of Medicine and Nutrition
Divisions of Gastroenterology and Clinical Nutrition
Tufts University
Director, Vitamins and Carcinogenesis Laboratory
USDA Human Nutrition Research Center at Tufts University
Boston, Massachusetts, United States

Blaine A. Mathison, BS, M(ASCP)
Technical Director of Parasitology
Technical Operations, Infectious Diseases
ARUP Laboratories
Salt Lake City, Utah, United States

Jeffrey B. Matthews, MD
Dallas B. Phemister Professor and Chairman
Department of Surgery
The University of Chicago Medicine
Chicago, Illinois, United States

Marlyn J. Mayo, MD
Professor of Internal Medicine
University of Texas Southwestern
Dallas, Texas, United States

Craig J. McClain, MD
Professor of Medicine and Pharmacology and Toxicology
Vice President for Health Affairs and Research
University of Louisville
Director, Gastroenterology
Robley Rex VA Medical Center
Louisville, Kentucky, United States

Stephen A. McClave, MD
Professor and Director of Clinical Nutrition
Department of Medicine
University of Louisville School of Medicine
Louisville, Kentucky, United States

Megha S. Mehta, MD
Assistant Professor of Pediatrics
University of Texas Southwestern Medical Center
Dallas, Texas, United States

Joanna M.P. Melia, MD
Assistant Professor of Medicine
Johns Hopkins University School of Medicine
Baltimore, Maryland, United States

Dejan Micic, MD
Associate Professor of Medicine
Division Chief, Division of Gastroenterology and Nutrition
Loyola University Medical Center
Maywood, Illinois, United States

Frederick H. Millham, MD, MBA
Surgeon-in-Chief, Surgery
South Shore Hospital
Weymouth, Massachusetts
Associate Professor of Surgery (Part Time)
Harvard Medical School
Boston, Massachusetts, United States

Ginat W. Mirowski, DMD, MD
Adjunct Associate Professor
Department of Oral Pathology, Medicine, and Radiology
Indiana University School of Dentistry
Adjunct Clinical Associate Professor
Department of Dermatology
Indiana University School of Medicine
Indianapolis, Indiana, United States

Daniel S. Mishkin, MD, CM
Physician, Gastroenterology
Atrius Health
Lecturer, Harvard Medical School
Boston, Massachusetts, United States

John Magaña Morton, MD, MPH, MHA
Medical Director of Bariatric and Minimally Invasive Surgery
Department of Surgery
Yale School of Medicine
New Haven, Connecticut, United States

Baha Moshiree, MD, MSci
Professor of Medicine, Gastroenterology
Atrium Health, Wake Forest Medical University
Charlotte, North Carolina, United States

William Conan Mustain, MD
Associate Professor of Surgery
Division of Colon and Rectal Surgery
University of Arkansas for Medical Sciences
Little Rock, Arkansas, United States

Mayur Narkhede, MD
Assistant Professor, Department of Internal Medicine
Division of Hematology/Oncology
University of Alabama at Birmingham
Birmingham, Alabama, United States

Rohit Nathani, MBBS
Gestroenterology Fellows
Department of Internal Medicine
The University of Iowa
Iowa City, Iowa, United States

Filipe Gaio Nery, MD
Physician, Departamento de Anestesiologia
Cuidados Intensivos e Emergência
Centro Hospitalar do Porto–Hospital Santo António
Porto, Researcher, EPIUnit, Instituto de Saúde Pública
Universidade do Porto, Porto
Researcher, Ciências Médicas
Instituto de Ciências Biomédicas de Abel Salazar
Porto, Portugal

Siew C. Ng, MBBS (Lond), PhD (Lond)
Professor of Medicine
Department of Medicine and Therapeutics
State Key Laboratory of Digestive Disease
LKS Institute of Health Science
The Chinese University of Hong Kong
Hong Kong, China

Nhi T. Nguyen, MS
Graduate Student, Cell Biology and Biochemistry
Texas Tech University Health Sciences Center
Lubbock, Texas, United States

Long H. Nguyen, MD, MS
Assistant Professor of Medicine
Massachusetts General Hospital and Harvard Medical School
Boston, Massachusetts, United States

Mark L. Norris, BSc (Hon), MD
Professor of Pediatrics, Pediatrics
Children's Hospital of Eastern Ontario
University of Ottawa
Ottawa, Ontario, Canada

Mazen Noureddin, MD, MHSc
Professor of Medicine
Lynda K. and David M. Underwood Center for Digestive Disorders
Houston Methodist Hospital
Houston, Texas, United States

Kinga S. Olortegui, MD, MS
Assistant Professor of Surgery
The University of Chicago Medicine
Chicago, Illinois, United States

Endashaw Omer, MD, MPH, AGAF, FACG, PNS
Associate Professor of Internal Medicine
University of Louisville
Associate Professor of Internal Medicine
VA Medical Center
Lousville, Kentucky, United States

Babak J. Orandi, MD, PhD, MSc, FACS, ABOM Diplomate
Associate Professor of Surgery and Medicine
Departments of Surgery and Medicine
New York University
New York, New York, United States

Tamas Ordog, MD
Professor of Physiology
Department of Physiology and Biomedical Engineering and Division of Gastroenterology and Hepatology
Department of Medicine
Mayo Clinic
Rochester, Minnesota, United States

Stephen J. Pandol, MD
Professor, Medicine
Cedars-Sinai Medical Center
Los Angeles, California, United States

Georgios I. Papachristou, MD, PhD
Professor of Medicine, Gastroenterology
Ohio State University
Powell, Ohio, United States

Darrell S. Pardi, MD, MS
Chair, Division of Gastroenterology and Hepatology
Professor of Medicine
Mayo Clinic
Rochester, Minnesota, United States

Parth Patel, MD
Washington Regional Gastroenterology
Washington Regional/UAMS Internal Medicine Residency GME Faculty
Fayetteville, Arkansas, United States

Mythili Pathipati, AB, MD
Gastroenterology
Massachusetts General Hospital
Boston, Massachusetts, United States

Mark R. Pedersen, MD
Assistant Professor, Internal Medicine, Digestive and Liver Disease
University of Texas Southwestern Medical Center
Dallas, Texas, United States

Vyjeyanthi S. Periyakoil, MD
Director, Palliative Care Education and Training
Department of Medicine
Stanford University School of Medicine
Stanford, California, United States

Patrick R. Pfau, MD
Professor, Chief of Clinical Gastroenterology
Section of Gastroenterology and Hepatology
University of Wisconsin School of Medicine and Public Health
Madison, Wisconsin, United States

Anna Evans Phillips, MD, MS
Assistant Professor of Medicine
Department of Medicine
Division of Gastroenterology, Hepatology, and Nutrition
University of Pittsburgh School of Medicine
Pittsburgh, Pennsylvania, United States

Elisa Pose, MD, PhD
Hepatologist, Liver Unit, Hospital Clínic de Barcelona
Institut d'Investigacions Biomèdiques August Pi i Sunyer (IDIBAPS)
Centro de Investigación Biomédica en Red de Enfermedades Hepáticas y Digestivas (CIBEReHD)
Barcelona, Spain

Daniel S. Pratt, MD
Director, Autoimmune and Cholestatic Liver Center
Division of Gastroenterology
Massachusetts General Hospital
Assistant Professor of Medicine
Harvard Medical School
Boston, Massachusetts, United States

David O. Prichard, MB, BCh, PhD
Gastroenterologist
Gastroenterology and Hepatology
Mayo Clinic
Rochester, Minnesota

Michael Quante, Prof
Universitätsklinikum Freiburg
Klinik für Innere Medizin II
Gastrointestinale Onkologie
Freiburg, Germany

Balakrishnan S. Ramakrishna, MBBS, MD, DM, PhD
Director, Institute of Gastroenterology
SRM Institutes for Medical Science
Chennai, Tamil Nadu, India

Mrinalini C. Rao, PhD
Professor, Department of Physiology and Biophysics
Division of Gastroenterology and Hepatology
University of Illinois at Chicago
Chicago, Illinois, United States

Satish S.C. Rao, MD, PhD
Professor of Medicine
Harold J. Harrison, MD Distinguished University Chair in Gastroenterology, Medicine-Gastroenterology/Hepatology
Augusta University
Augusta, Georgia, United States

Christopher K. Rayner, MBBS, PhD
Professor, Adelaide Medical School, University of Adelaide
Consultant Gastroenterologist
Department of Gastroenterology and Hepatology
Royal Adelaide Hospital
Adelaide, South Australia, Australia

Miguel D. Regueiro, MD
Chair and Professor of Medicine
Department of Gastroenterology and Hepatology
Cleveland Clinic, Digestive Disease and Surgery Institute
Cleveland, Ohio, United States

John F. Reinus, MD
Professor of Medicine
Department of Medicine
Albert Einstein College of Medicine
Medical Director of Liver Transplantation
Montefiore-Einstein Center for Transplantation
Montefiore Medical Center
Bronx, New York, United States

David A. Relman, MD
Thomas C. and Joan M. Merigan Professor, Departments of Medicine and Microbiology and Immunology
Stanford University, Stanford, California
Chief of Infectious Diseases
Veterans Affairs Palo Alto Health Care System
Palo Alto, California, United States

Joel E. Richter, MD
Professor and Director, Division of Digestive Diseases and Nutrition
University of South Florida
Director, Joy McCann Culverhouse Center for Swallowing Disorders
University of South Florida
Tampa, Florida, United States

Mary E. Rinella, MD
Professor of Medicine
University of Chicago
Chicago, Illinois, United States

Eve A. Roberts, MD, PhD
Professor Emerita, Pediatrics, Medicine, and Pharmacology and Toxicology
University of Toronto
Adjunct Scientist, Genetics and Genome Biology Program
Hospital for Sick Children Research Institute
Associate, Division of Gastroenterology, Hepatology, and Nutrition
The Hospital for Sick Children
Toronto, Ontario, Canada
Associate Fellow, History of Science and Technology Program
University of King's College
Halifax, Nova Scotia, Canada

Matthew L. Roberts, MD
Associate Professor of Surgery
Department of Surgery
University of Arkansas for Medical Sciences
Little Rock, Arkansas, United States

Stephanie Romutis, MD
Clinical Assistant Professor of Medicine, Gastroenterology
University of Pittsburgh Medical Center
Clinical Assistant Professor of Medicine, Gastroenterology
VA Pittsburgh Medical Center
Pittsburgh, Pennsylvania, United States

Marc E. Rothenberg, MD, PhD
Professor of Pediatrics, Allergy & Immunology
Cincinnati Children's Hospital Medical Center
Cincinnati, Ohio, United States

Jayanta Roy-Chowdhury, MBBS
Professor, Departments of Medicine and Genetics
Director, Genetic Engineering and Gene Therapy Core Facility
Albert Einstein College of Medicine
New York, New York, United States

Namita Roy-Chowdhury, PhD
Professor, Departments of Medicine and Genetics
Albert Einstein College of Medicine
New York, New York, United States

David T. Rubin, MD
Joseph B. Kirsner Professor of Medicine
Chief, Section of Gastroenterology, Hepatology, and Nutrition
Department of Medicine
University of Chicago
Chicago, Illinois, United States

Gustavo A. Rubio, MD
Associate Medical Director
Colon and Rectal Surgery
Jackson Health System,
Miami, Florida, United States

Jayashree Sarathy, PhD
Professor, Department of Biological Sciences
Director of Graduate Programs, Biological Sciences
Benedictine University
Lisle, Illinois
Visiting Research Professor
Department of Physiology and Biophysics
University of Illinois at Chicago
Chicago, Illinois, United States

Jessica B. Sarthi, PhD
Research Scientist, Pediatrics, Gastroenterology, Hepatology and Nutrition
Palo Alto, California, United States

Thomas J. Savides, MD
Professor of Clinical Medicine
Division of Gastroenterology
University of California San Diego
La Jolla, California, United States

Gregory S. Sayuk, MD, MPH
Professor of Medicine and Psychiatry, Gastroenterology Division
Washington University in St. Louis School of Medicine
Staff Physician, Gastroenterology Section
St. Louis Veterans Affairs Medical Center
St. Louis, Missouri, United States

Zachary M. Sellers, MD, PhD
Assistant Professor of Pediatrics
Pediatrics - Gastroenterology
Stanford University
Palo Alto, California, United States

Vijay H. Shah, MD
Carol M. Gatton Professor of Medicine, Physiology, and Cancer Cell Biology
Kinney Executive Dean of Research,
Chair Department of Medicine
Mayo Clinic College of Medicine and Science
Rochester, Minnesota, United States

Nicholas J. Shaheen, MD, MPH
Professor of Medicine
University of North Carolina
Chapel Hill, North Carolina, United States

Jordan M. Shapiro, MD, MS
Staff Physician, Gastro Health and Nutrition
Houston, Texas, United States

Angela Shih, MD
Assistant in Pathology, Pathology
Massachusetts General Hospital
Assistant Professor, Harvard Medical School
Boston, Massachusetts, United States

Stuti Girish Shroff, MBBS, PhD
Department of Pathology
Mass General Hospital
Mass General Brigham
Watertown, Massachusetts, United States

Vikesh Singh, MD, MSc
Professor of Medicine, Division of Gastroenterology
Director of Endoscopy, Director of Pancreatology
Johns Hopkins University School of Medicine
Baltimore, Maryland, United States

Maria H. Sjogren, MD, MPH
Senior Hepatologist, Department of Medicine
Walter Reed National Medical Center
Bethesda, Maryland, United States

Valeriya Skorobogatko, MD
Resident Appointee
Department of Dermatology
Indiana University School of Medicine
Indianapolis, Indiana, United States

Adam Slivka, MD, PhD
Professor, Medicine
University of Pittsburgh Medical Center
Pittsburgh, Pennsylvania, United States

Phillip D. Smith, MD
Professor of Medicine and Microbiology
University of Alabama at Birmingham
Birmingham, Alabama, United States

Kjetil Soreide, MD, PhD, FRCS (Edin), FACS, FEBS (Hon)
Consultant Surgeon (HPB Unit), Karolinska Institutet
Karolinska University Hospital
Stockholm, Sweden
General and HPB Surgeon, Dept of Gastrointestinal Surgery
Stavanger University Hospital
Professor of Surgery, Department of Clinical Medicine
University of Bergen
Bergen, Norway

Milan J. Sonneveld, MD, PhD
Gastroenterology and Hepatology
Erasmus University Medical Center
Rotterdam, Netherlands

James E. Squires, MD, MS
Associate Professor, Department of Pediatrics
Associate Director of Hepatology
UPMC Children's Hospital of Pittsburgh
Pittsburgh, Pennsylvania, United States

Neil H. Stollman, MD
Associate Clinical Professor, Department of Medicine
Division of Gastroenterology
University of California San Francisco
San Francisco, California
Chief Division of Gastroenterology
Alta Bates Summit Medical Center
Oakland, California, United States

R. Todd Stravitz, MD
Professor of Medicine, Internal Medicine
Virginia Commonwealth University
Richmond, Virginia, United States

Sarah E. Streett, MD
Clinical Associate Professor
Director IBD Education
Division of Gastroenterology and Hepatology
Stanford University
Redwood City, California, United States

Jonathan R. Strosberg, MD
Professor, Gastrointestinal Oncology
Moffitt Cancer Center
Tampa, Florida, United States

Frederick J. Suchy, MD
Senior Research Strategist
Children's Hospital Colorado
Professor of Pediatrics and Associate Dean for Child Health Research, Pediatrics
University of Colorado School of Medicine
Aurora, Colorado, United States

Shelby Sullivan, MD
Director of the Metabolic and Bariatric Program
Division of Gastroenterology and Hepatology
Center for Digestive Health
Dartmouth-Hitchcock Health
Lebanon, New Hampshire

Shahnaz Sultan, MD, MHSc
Doctor of Medicine
University of Minnesota
Minneapolis, Minnesota, United States

Hidekazu Suzuki, MD, PhD
Associate Professor
Division of Gastroenterology and Hepatology
Department of Internal Medicine
Keio University School of Medicine
Tokyo, Japan

Gyongyi Szabo, MD, PhD
Mitchell T. Rabkin, MD Chair, Chief Academic Officer
Beth Israel Deaconess Medical Center and Beth Israel Lahey Health
Faculty Dean for Academic Affairs
Harvard Medical School
Boston, Massachusetts, United States

Nicholas J. Talley, MD, PhD
Pro Vice-Chancellor and Professor, Distinguished Laureate Professor
Faculty of Health and Medicine
University of Newcastle, Australia
Newcastle, New South Wales, Australia

Narci C. Teoh, MD
Professor of Medicine, Australian National University
Senior Staff Hepatologist
The Canberra Hospital
Australian Capital Territory, Australia

June Tome, MD
Gastroenterology and Hepatology
Mayo Clinic
Rochester, Minnesota, United States

Clara Y. Tow, BA, MD
Assistant Professor of Medicine, Internal Medicine/Hepatology
Montefiore Medical Center
Albert Einstein College of Medicine
Bronx, New York, United States

Shannan Tujios, MD
Associate Professor, Internal Medicine
University of Texas Southwestern Medical Center
Dallas, Texas, United States

Kiran Turaga, MD, MPH
Associate Professor
Department of Surgery
The University of Chicago
Chicago, Illinois, United States

Konstantin Umanskiy, MD
Professor of Surgery
University of Chicago
Chicago, Illinois, United States

Michael F. Vaezi, MD, PhD, MS
Professor of Medicine and Otolaryngology
Clinical Director, Division of Gastroenterology and Hepatology
Vanderbilt University Medical Center
Nashville, Tennessee, United States

Dominique Charles Valla, MD
Professor Emeritus of Hepatology, Liver Unit
Hôpital Beaujon, APHP, Clichy-la-Garenne
France
CRI, UMR1149
Inserm and Université de Paris
Paris, France

Shyam M. Varadarajulu, MD
President, Digestive Health Institute
Orlando Health
Winter Park, Florida, United States

Christopher Vélez, MD
Associate Program Director, Advanced Fellowship in Functional and Gastrointestinal Motility Disorders
Center for Neurointestinal Health
Division of Gastroenterology, Department of Medicine
Massachusetts General Hospital
Assistant Professor, Harvard Medical School
Boston, Massachusetts, United States

Axel von Herbay, MD
Professor of Pathology, Faculty of Medicine
University of Heidelberg
Heidelberg Hans Pathologie
Hamburg, Germany

Nikita Wadhwani, MBBS
Resident Physician, General Surgery
University of Alabama at Birmingham
Birmingham, Alabama, United States

David Q.-H. Wang, MD, PhD,[†]
Professor of Medicine, Departments of Medicine and Genetics
Director, Molecular Biology and Next Generation Technology Core
Marion Bessin Liver Research Center
Albert Einstein College of Medicine
Bronx, New York, United States

Sachin Wani, MD
Professor of Medicine, Division of Gastroenterology and Hepatology
Katy O and Paul M Rady Endowed Chair in Esophageal Cancer Research
Executive Director, Katy O and Paul M Rady Esophageal and Gastric Center of Excellence
University of Colorado Anschutz Medical Campus
Aurora, Colorado, United States

Frederick Weber, MD
Clinical Professor, Division of Gastroenterology and Hepatology
University of Alabama Birmingham
Birmingham, Alabama, United States

Barry K. Wershil, MD
Professor, Pediatrics
Northwestern University Feinberg School of Medicine
Chief, Division of Gastroenterology, Hepatology, and Nutrition, Pediatrics
Ann & Robert H. Lurie Children's Hospital of Chicago
Chicago, Illinois, United States

David C. Whitcomb, MD, PhD
Professor, Medicine, Cell Biology and Molecular Physiology, and Human Genetics
University of Pittsburgh and UPMC
Pittsburgh, Pennsylvania, United States

C. Mel Wilcox, MD, MSPH
Chief of Gastroenterology and Hepatology
Director, Pancreatology
Digestive Health Institute
Chair, US Pancreatic Disease Study Group
Orlando Health
Orlando, Florida, United States

Christopher G. Willett, MD
Mark W. Dewhirst Distinguished Professor and Chairman, Radiation Oncology
Duke University
Durham, North Carolina, United States

John A. Windsor, BSc, MD, FRACS, FACS, FRCSEd, FRSNZ
Professor of Surgery and Director of the Surgical and Translational Research Centre
University of Auckland
Honorary Consultant HBP/Upper GI Surgeon
Auckland City Hospital
Auckland, New Zealand

Simin Zhang, MD
Division of Rheumatology, Allergy and Immunology
Department of Internal Medicine
University of Cincinnati College of Medicine
Cincinnati Children's Hospital Medical Center
Cincinnati, Ohio, United States

Irene Y. Zhang, MD, MPH
General Surgery Resident, Department of Surgery
University of Washington
Seattle, Washington, United States

Foreword

We are honored to present the Foreword to the twelfth edition of *Sleisenger and Fordtran's Gastrointestinal and Liver Disease*. For over five decades, this textbook has stood as a foundational reference for clinicians, educators, and researchers in gastroenterology and hepatology. When first published in 1973, by Drs. Marvin H. Sleisenger and John S. Fordtran, the book was heralded for its groundbreaking inclusion of detailed discussions of the pathophysiologic basis of diseases. Each subsequent edition has reflected the dynamic evolution of our field, and this latest volume continues that tradition with a renewed commitment to scientific rigor, clinical relevance, and global inclusivity.

This edition is especially meaningful as we pay tribute to the late Dr. Mark Feldman, whose visionary leadership and editorial excellence helped shape this work into the gold standard it is today. Mark served as an associate editor of the fifth edition and co-editor of the sixth through eleventh editions; sadly, he passed away on March 5, 2024. His contributions to academic medicine and gastroenterology were profound—his scholarship, mentorship, and editorial voice elevated the quality of this text and inspired generations of physicians. A master "tablemaker" with a talent for stylistic clarity and consistency, Mark left an indelible stamp on this book. We are grateful to the editors for allowing the dedication of this edition to his memory and for honoring his enduring legacy.

As we were preparing this Foreword, we also learned of the passing, on February 23, 2025, of the legendary John S. Fordtran, founding co-editor of this textbook and a superb writer, editor, researcher, and educator. As noted in his obituary, John was "more than a brilliant doctor. He was a mentor, a storyteller, a man of integrity, and a rock of quiet strength and humility. He lived a life…marked by kindness and an unshakable love for those around him."*

On a positive note, we are delighted to pass the torch to three outstanding new editors, each of whom served as an associate editor of the eleventh edition. Dr. Raymond T. Chung, a global authority in hepatology, brings deep insight into liver disease and translational research; Dr. David T. Rubin, a pioneer in inflammatory bowel disease and precision medicine, provides a forward-looking perspective on innovation and patient-centered care, and Dr. C. Mel Wilcox, a respected clinician, interventional endoscopist, and educator, contributes a wealth of experience in gastrointestinal disorders and academic leadership. Their collective vision has enriched this edition in both scope and depth, and they have assembled an international array of outstanding authors who are foremost authorities in their fields.

This twelfth edition arrives at a time of remarkable progress in gastroenterology and hepatology. Advances in artificial intelligence and machine learning are transforming diagnostic imaging and endoscopic interpretation. The expansion of multi-omics technologies—genomics, proteomics, and metabolomics—is enabling personalized approaches to complex diseases such as inflammatory bowel disease, colorectal cancer, and metabolic dysfunction-associated steatotic liver disease. Novel biologic agents and small molecules are reshaping therapeutic strategies, while research in intestinal microbiota, gut-brain interactions, and autoimmune mechanisms continues to uncover new pathways of disease pathogenesis and new opportunities for treatment (and new complications of such treatments).

In addition to scientific and clinical advancements, this edition expands coverage of critical issues that shape the practice of medicine today. Areas such as health equity, digital health, palliative care, and the impact of climate change on gastrointestinal health are thoughtfully incorporated, reflecting the broader context in which we care for patients.

This classic textbook remains steadfast in its commitment to the principles that have defined it since its inception: scientific excellence, clinical utility, and educational clarity. We are confident that this edition will continue to serve as a trusted companion for all who seek to understand and improve the care of patients with gastrointestinal and liver diseases.

Lawrence S. Friedman, MD
Newton, MA
Lawrence J. Brandt, MD
Bronx, NY
Former Editors of *Sleisenger and Fordtran's Gastrointestinal and Liver Disease*

*https://obits.dallasnews.com/us/obituaries/dallasmorningnews/name/john-fordtran-obituary?id=57732653, accessed August 15, 2025

The Sleisenger and Fordtran Editors

Mark Feldman, MD

Editions 5-11

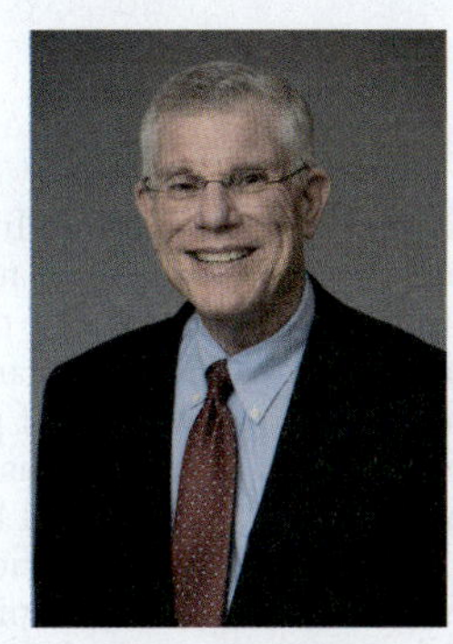

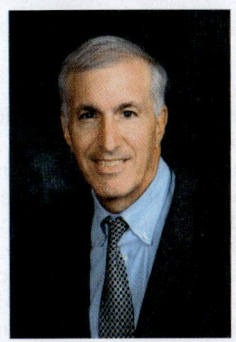

Lawrence S. Friedman, MD

Editions 7-11

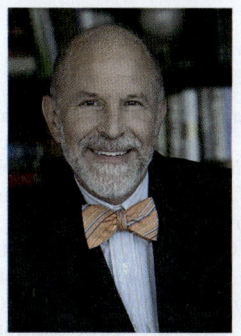

Lawrence J. Brandt, MD

Editions 8-11

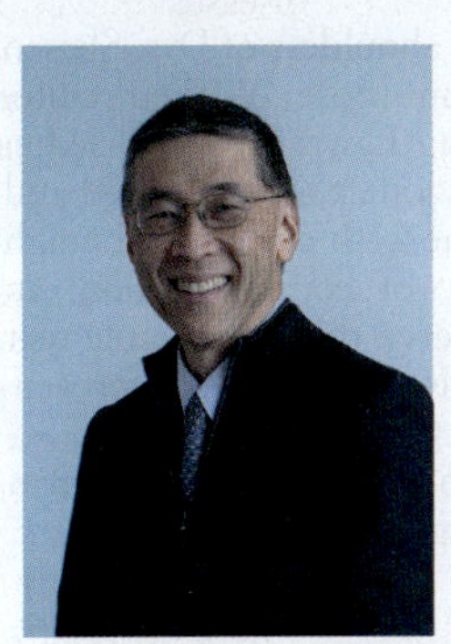

Raymond T. Chung, MD

Editions 11, 12

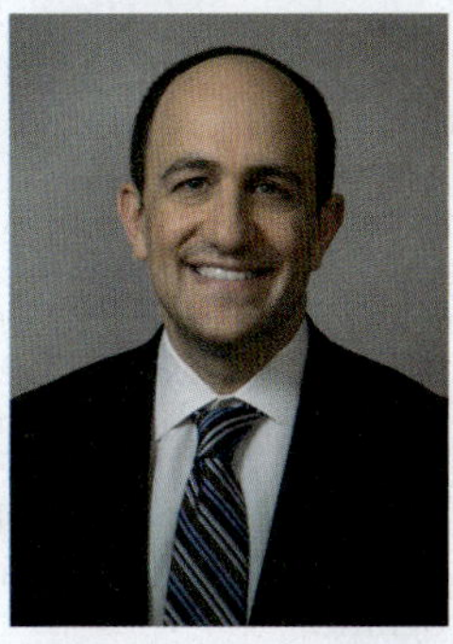

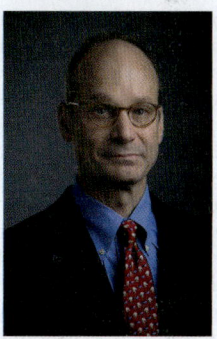

David T. Rubin, MD

Editions 11, 12

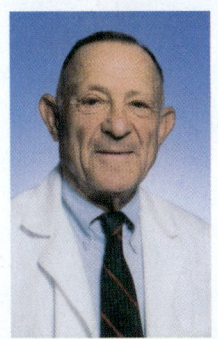

C. Mel Wilcox, MD

Editions 11, 12

Marvin H. Sleisenger, MD

Editions 1-7

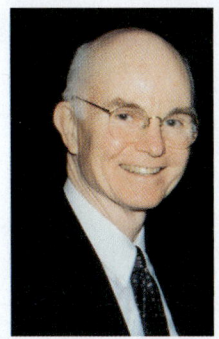

John S. Fordtran, MD

Editions 1-5

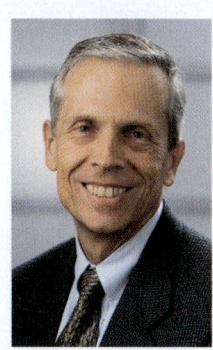

Bruce F. Scharschmidt, MD

Editions 5-6

Preface

Over a half century ago, Drs. Marvin H. Sleisenger and John S. Fordtran embarked on a project to develop a textbook that incorporated pathophysiologic principles underpinning digestive diseases. Their project, the original edition of the textbook that now bears their names, was both novel and extremely well received. Of course, the ultimate testament to the success of their approach has been manifest as international recognition and the publication of ten more editions of this now classic text.

With this, the 12th edition of *Sleisenger & Fordtran's Gastrointestinal and Liver Disease: Pathophysiology/Diagnosis/Management*, we are pleased to honor the approach developed by Drs. Sleisenger and Fordtran by providing updates on the diagnosis and treatment of chronic hepatitis B and C, including curative treatments for HCV; evolution in the management of *Helicobacter pylori* infection and its complications; improvements in techniques for screening and surveillance of gastrointestinal cancer; new approaches to the recognition and treatment of Barrett esophagus; the remarkable expansion and increased incidence and prevalence of IBD across the globe; the development of many advanced therapies, mechanistic targets, and new strategies for the management of IBD; improvements in endoscopic management of pancreaticobiliary disorders and gastrointestinal bleeding; enhanced understanding of the gut microbiome and its role in the pathophysiology of nearly all GI and hepatic disorders (and many non-GI disorders, too!); the rapid pace of our understanding of disorders of gut-brain interaction and their expanding treatment options; recognition of the increasing array of autoimmune diseases affecting the entire GI tract and liver; and continued advances in transplantation of solid organs, including liver, pancreas, and small intestine. In recognition of more recent trends in medicine, we introduce new chapters to describe the GI and hepatic complications of the immune checkpoint inhibitors that have revolutionized cancer therapy; advances in our understanding of the benefits of palliative care applied to GI and hepatology; and, in the aftermath of the COVID-19 pandemic, recognition of the short- and long-term consequences of coronavirus infection. In many of the chapters throughout the text, the possible application of rapid advances in artificial intelligence to the management of GI disorders, particularly in the areas of diagnosis and prognosis, has been introduced. In addition to topical breadth, we have continued the S and F tradition of including diverse authors from around the world, including rising stars in their disciplines.

We are proud to stand on the shoulders of Drs. Sleisenger and Fordtran, and more directly on those of their editorial descendants, Drs. Mark Feldman, Lawrence S. Friedman, and Lawrence J. Brandt. In their wisdom, they mentored and "broke us in" as Associate Editors for the 11th edition and taught us the art of precision writing, clarity of communication, and most importantly stewardship to preserve this remarkable text. As we assume the Editorship of the 12th edition, we are forever grateful for their guidance and trust.

Regretfully, one of those mentors, Dr. Mark Feldman, passed away on March 5, 2024, at the age of 76. We miss Mark greatly. We dedicate the 12th edition to his memory.

Raymond T. Chung
David T. Rubin
C. Mel Wilcox

Acknowledgments

The editors of the 12th edition of *Sleisenger & Fordtran's Gastrointestinal and Liver Disease* express their gratitude to the more than 240 authors from North America, Europe, Asia, and Australia who contributed their deep knowledge and experience to this book. We are indebted to the talented staff at Elsevier, particularly Kevin Travers and Nancy Duffy who assembled the book. Special thanks to Cindy Thoms, who oversaw the highly professional production of the book. We thank our predecessors and mentors Drs. Lawrence Friedman and Lawrence Brandt for their thoughtful Foreword, but more importantly for teaching us the fine art of editing. We remember and fondly acknowledge the mentorship and contributions of our third predecessor, Dr. Mark Feldman, who passed away in 2024. We are thankful for the love and support of our spouses: Rebecca Rubin, and Diane Abraczinskas. Finally, we thank our caregiver and scientist readers who will use this updated edition to improve the care and outcomes of those who suffer from digestive illnesses.

Contents

VOLUME 2

PART X
Liver

PART XI
Small and Large Intestine

Video Contents

Abbreviation List

AASLD American Association for the Study of Liver Diseases
ACG American College of Gastroenterology
ACTH Corticotropin
AE Angioectasia
AFP Alpha fetoprotein
AGA American Gastroenterological Association
AIDS Acquired immunodeficiency syndrome
ACLF Acute on chronic liver failure
ALD Alcohol-associated liver disease
ALF Acute liver failure
ALT Alanine aminotransferase
AMA Antimitochondrial antibodies
ANA Antinuclear antibodies
ANCA Antineutrophil cytoplasmic antibodies
APACHE Acute physiology and chronic health examination
APC Argon plasma coagulation
ASGE American Society for Gastrointestinal Endoscopy
AST Aspartate aminotransferase
ATP Adenosine triphosphate
BICAP Bipolar electrocoagulation
BMI Body mass index
BRBPR Bright red blood per rectum
CBC Complete blood count
CCK Cholecystokinin
CEA Carcinoembryonic antigen
CDI *Clostridioides difficile* infection
CF Cystic fibrosis
CFTR Cystic fibrosis transmembrane conductance regulator
CMV Cytomegalovirus
CNS Central nervous system
CO_2 Carbon dioxide
COVID-19 Coronavirus disease 2019
COX Cyclooxygenase
CT Computed tomography
CTA Computed tomography angiography
CTP Child-Turcotte-Pugh score
DAA Direct-acting antiviral agent
DIC Disseminated intravascular coagulation
DILI Drug-induced liver injury
DNA Deoxyribonucleic acid
DU Duodenal ulcer
DVT Deep vein thrombosis
EBV Epstein-Barr virus
EGD Esophagogastroduodenoscopy
EGF Epidermal growth factor
EMG Electromyography
ERCP Endoscopic retrograde cholangiopancreatography
ESR Erythrocyte sedimentation rate
EUS Endoscopic ultrasonography
FDA U.S. Food and Drug Administration
FIB-4 Fibrosis-4 index
FNA Fine-needle aspiration
GAVE Gastric antral vascular ectasia
GERD Gastroesophageal reflux disease
GGTP Gamma glutamyl transpeptidase
GI Gastrointestinal
GIST GI stromal tumor
GU Gastric ulcer
H&E Hematoxylin and eosin
H2RA Histamine-2 receptor antagonist
HAV Hepatitis A virus
HBV Hepatitis B virus
HCC Hepatocellular carcinoma
HCG Human chorionic gonadotropin
HCV Hepatitis C virus
HDL High-density lipoprotein
HDV Hepatitis D virus
HELLP Hemolysis, elevated liver enzymes, low platelets
HEV Hepatitis E virus
Hgb Hemoglobin
HHT Hereditary hemorrhagic telangiectasia
HIV Human immunodeficiency virus
HLA Human leukocyte antigen
HPV Human papillomavirus
HSV Herpes simplex virus
Hp *Helicobacter pylori*
IBD Inflammatory bowel disease
IBS Irritable bowel syndrome
ICI Immune checkpoint inhibitor
ICU Intensive care unit
IMA Inferior mesenteric artery
IMT Intestinal microbiota transplantation
INR International normalized ratio
IV Intravenous
IVIG Intravenous immunoglobulin
LDH Lactate dehydrogenase
LDL Low-density lipoprotein
LGI Lower gastrointestinal
LGIB Lower gastrointestinal bleed

LLQ Left lower quadrant
LT Liver transplantation
LUQ Left upper quadrant
MASLD Metabolic dysfunction-associated liver disease
MASH Metabolic dysfunction-associated steatohepatitis
MELD Model for end-stage liver disease
MEN Multiple endocrine neoplasia
MHC Major histocompatibility complex
MRA Magnetic resonance angiography
MRCP Magnetic resonance cholangiopancreatography
MRI Magnetic resonance imaging
NG Nasogastric
NPO Nil per os (nothing by mouth)
NSAID(s) Nonsteroidal anti-inflammatory drug(s)
O_2 Oxygen
PBC Primary biliary cholangitis
PCR Polymerase chain reaction
PET Positron emission tomography
PPI Proton pump inhibitor
PSC Primary sclerosing cholangitis
PSE Portosystemic encephalopathy
PUD Peptic ulcer disease
RA Rheumatoid arthritis
RLQ Right lower quadrant
RNA Ribonucleic acid
RUQ Right upper quadrant
SBO Small bowel obstruction
SBP Spontaneous bacterial peritonitis
SIBO Small intestinal bacterial overgrowth
SLE Systemic lupus erythematosus
SOD Sphincter of Oddi dysfunction
TB Tuberculosis
TG Triglyceride(s)
TIPS Transjugular intrahepatic portosystemic shunt
TNF Tumor necrosis factor
TNM Tumor node metastasis
TPN Total parenteral nutrition
UC Ulcerative colitis
UDCA Ursodeoxycholic acid
UGI Upper gastrointestinal
UGIB Upper gastrointestinal bleed
UGIS Upper gastrointestinal series
UNOS United Network for Organ Sharing
US Ultrasonography
USA United States of America
VLDL Very-low-density lipoprotein
WBC White blood cell
WHO World Health Organization
ZES Zollinger-Ellison syndrome

PART I

Biology of the Gastrointestinal Tract

1 Cellular Growth and Neoplasia

Ezra Burstein

IN THIS CHAPTER

Normal cellular proliferation and differentiation are essential to tissue homeostasis in all organs, including the digestive tract. The neoplastic process involves a fundamental disruption of these mechanisms, which can give rise to local tumor formation and metastasis with the additional acquisition of other hallmarks of cancer. As a group, malignancies of the GI tract are the leading cause of cancer-associated mortality, and it is therefore essential to understand the underlying biology that gives rise to tumor formation. This chapter reviews mechanisms of normal cellular growth and the fundamental molecular alterations that facilitate malignant transformation. The basic concepts discussed in this chapter provide the framework for the discussion of specific GI neoplasms in later chapters.

MECHANISMS OF NORMAL TISSUE HOMEOSTASIS

Cellular Proliferation

Tissue homeostasis is maintained by the delicate balance of cellular proliferation and differentiation, which provide new cellular elements to replace dying cells as part of normal tissue function or during tissue repair. At a fundamental level, neoplasia arises when cell proliferation escapes the homeostatic mechanisms that maintain this process in balance with senescence and programmed cell death. Cell proliferation occurs as cells divide, a process that occurs through an orderly set of steps referred to as the cell cycle (Fig. 1.1). In preparation for cell division, there is a period of biosynthetic activity called the *G_1 phase* that is typically associated with an increase of cell size. This phase is followed by a precise duplication of the genome, designated as the *S phase* of the cycle. After an intervening gap period designated as the *G_2 phase*, mitosis occurs during the *M phase*.

The commitment to proceed to DNA replication occurs at the G_1/S checkpoint or restriction (R) point. Cells may exit this cycle of active proliferation before reaching the R point and enter a quiescent phase known as G_0. Cells can subsequently reenter the cell cycle from the G_0 state (see Fig. 1.1). Another checkpoint exists at the boundary between the G_2 and M phases. The G_2/M checkpoint ensures that mitosis does not proceed prior to the repair of any damaged DNA after genome replication. Impaired function of these checkpoints is frequently observed in cancers.

Regulation of cell cycle progression is achieved principally by a set of proteins known as cyclins and cyclin-dependent kinases (CDKs). These proteins are expressed in specific parts of the cell cycle and regulate the G_1/S and G_2/M checkpoints. During the G_1 phase, cyclins D and E are most active.[1] Overexpression of cyclin D1 in fibroblasts results in more rapid entry of cells into the S phase, and, consistent with a role in cancer, cyclin D1 is frequently overexpressed in a number of GI and non-GI malignancies.[2] During the S phase, cyclin A is predominantly expressed, and by the G_2 phase, cyclin B is the main regulator (see Fig. 1.1).

Each cyclin forms a complex with a CDK and functions as a catalyst for CDK activity in a cell cycle–dependent fashion (see Fig. 1.1). The cyclin-CDK complexes regulate cell cycle progression through phosphorylation of key target proteins. For example, cyclin D1–dependent progression from G_1 to S phase is the result of cyclin D1/CDK4 phosphorylation of the tumor suppression pRb, the product of the retinoblastoma gene, as well as the Rb family members p130 and p107.[3] These proteins sequester E2F transcription factors that promote the expression of factors required for S phase, and their phosphorylation by CDK4 leads to their functional inhibition. Thus loss of Rb expression

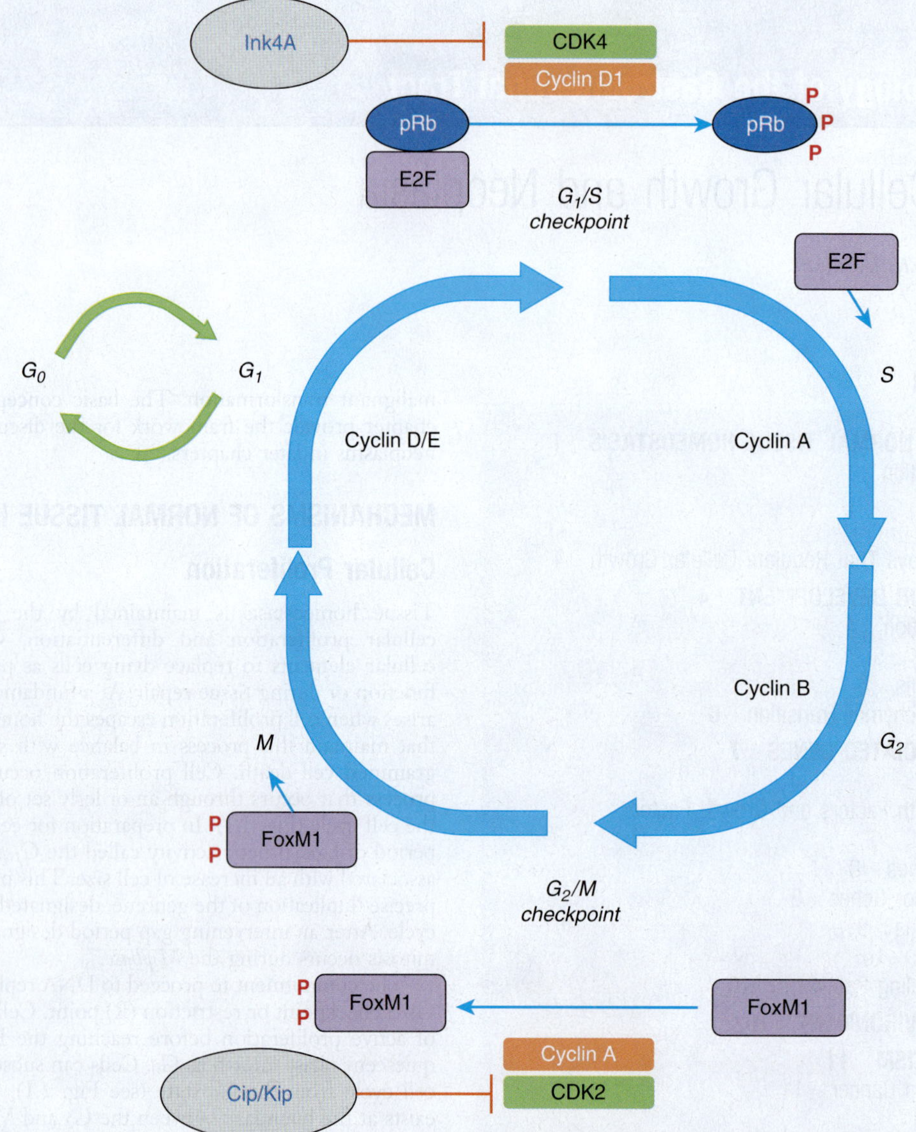

Fig. 1.1 Regulation of the cell cycle by (cycs), cyclin-dependent kinases (CDKs), and CDK inhibitors. In the normal cell cycle, DNA synthesis (in which chromosomal DNA is duplicated) occurs in the S phase, whereas mitosis (in which nuclei first divide to form a pair of new nuclei, followed by actual cellular division to form a pair of daughter cells) takes place in the M phase. The S and M phases are separated by two gap phases: the G_1 phase after mitosis and before DNA synthesis, and the G_2 phase following the S phase. During these gap phases, the cell is synthesizing proteins and metabolites, increasing its mass, and preparing for the S and M phase. Cell cycle progression is regulated primarily at two points, the *G_2/M* and *G_1/S* checkpoints, through the coordinated activities of cyclins and CDKs, which, in turn, are negatively regulated by CDK inhibitors (*Ink4* and *Cip/Kip* families). *CDK4*, Cyclin-dependent kinase 4; *P*, phosphate group.

also accomplishes more rapid progression to S phase and is another genetic lesion seen in many tumors. An analogous circuit is found in the G_2/M transition, where cyclin A/CDK2 mediates the activation of another transcriptional regulator, FoxM1, required for the expression of factors involved in mitosis.[4]

The cell cycle is also regulated by multiple CDK inhibitors, which are classified into various classes and are referred by multiple names.[5] CDK4 and CDK6 are inhibited by members of the Ink4 family of inhibitors known as p16^{INK4a} (encoded by the *Cdkn2a* gene), p15^{INK4b} (*Cdkn2b*), p18^{INK4c} (*Cdkn2c*), and p19$_{INK4d}$ (*Cdkn2d*).[6] Thus these factors also impinge on cyclin D1/CDK4 regulation of pRb, and consequent E2F activity and S phase entry. p16^{INK4a} loss in cancer results in greater activation of CDK4 and is frequently inactivated in GI cancers, a finding consistent with its function as a tumor suppressor gene.[7,8] Members of the Cip/Kip family of CDK inhibitors are known as p21^{Cip1} (*Cdkn1a*), p27^{Kip1} (*Cdkn1b*), and p57^{Kip2} (*Cdkn1c*) and are more promiscuous and interfere with multiple cyclin/CDK complexes, including CDK2. Altogether, it is clear that alterations in the normal regulation of cell cycle progression are commonly encountered in cancer.

Apoptosis

Apoptosis is a form of cell death that is genetically programmed and executed by specific proteases known as caspases.[9] Similar to other protease cascades, such as the coagulation system, caspases become active upon cleavage of an inactive pro-form, typically through the action of another caspase or as a result of focal accumulation of inactive caspases. Apoptosis is an important mechanism that counterbalances cell proliferation; thus escape from normal apoptotic mechanisms plays a critical role in oncogenesis. Morphologically, apoptosis is characterized by distinctive features that include chromatin compaction, condensation of the cytoplasm, nuclear fragmentation, and marked alterations at the plasma membrane, resulting in compacted apoptotic bodies that are eventually phagocytosed and eliminated. Nonneoplastic pathologies in the GI tract and the liver can be associated with increased apoptotic cell death, including drug-induced enteropathies and GI involvement in graft-versus-host disease.[10,11]

Apoptosis may be triggered by internal or external stimuli. Internal stimuli of apoptosis may include nutrient deprivation, hypoxia, DNA damage, or other stressors, including specific toxins, chemical signals, and pathogens. Apoptosis routinely occurs during normal development to facilitate tissue patterning. Similarly, a number of stress situations, including tissue inflammation, can trigger apoptosis. Apoptosis may also be stimulated by specific cell surface receptors belonging to the tumor necrosis factor receptor superfamily, including tumor necrosis factor R1 and Fas, which are referred to as death receptors (Fig. 1.2).

At the intracellular level, the last common event in all forms of apoptosis is the activation of so-called executioner caspases, caspase-3 and -7, which mediate the cleavage of a large number of downstream targets that eventually precipitate cell death. Proapoptotic signals frequently converge at the level of the mitochondria, where they destabilize the mitochondrial membrane and collapse the electrical gradient required for aerobic respiration (see Fig. 1.2). Besides the effects that mitochondrial disruption causes on cellular energetics, this process leads to the release into the cytosol of proteins normally present in the intermembrane space of the mitochondria, including cytochrome *c*, a component of the respiratory chain. In the cytosol, cytochrome *c* helps in the assembly of a multiprotein complex known as the apoptosome, which contains Apaf1 and facilitates the activation of caspase-9, a direct activator of caspase-3 and -7. On the other hand, death receptors activate executioner caspases through receptor-initiated intracellular signaling events that result in the upstream activation of caspase-8.

The mitochondrial membrane permeabilization events that lead to apoptosome formation are controlled by proteins of the Bcl-2 family. On the one hand, Bax and Bak help form the mitochondrial membrane pore, whereas Bcl-2, Bcl-xL, and Mcl-1 inhibit pore formation. The stoichiometric ratio between proapoptotic and antiapoptotic members of the Bcl-2 family can determine the balance between cell survival and cell death.[12] In cancer, alterations in the balance of proapoptotic and antiapoptotic factors, including member of the Bcl-2 family, are common events.

Apoptosis is associated with a contraction of the cell into a so-called apoptotic body, which is phagocytosed by other tissue-resident cells, typically macrophages. As such, it causes limited if any tissue inflammation and has been referred to as a form of "silent death." In contrast, over the last 2 decades, multiple specific death pathways associated with tissue inflammation have been reported.[13,14] These programs are biochemically and morphologically distinct from apoptosis and are associated with the release of cellular contents into the tissue environment. One such program is called necroptosis and is executed by the activation of the kinases RIP1 and RIP3, which activate a pseudokinase known as MLKL, which, upon phosphorylation, results in MLKL aggregation at the plasma membrane and formation of a transmembrane pore that precipitates this form of cell death. Cell surface receptors belonging to the tumor necrosis factor receptor superfamily, such as TNFR1, sit upstream of this pathway as well as classical apoptosis. While necroptosis is thought to be a component of tissue injury in inflammation, disruption of necroptosis in oncogenesis is beginning to be appreciated.[15] Another related form of cell death is called pyroptosis and results from extensive activation of caspase-1, a protease that acts downstream of the inflammasome. Like necroptosis, cell death is eventually triggered by the formation of pores at the plasma membrane through cleavage and activation of gasdermin D. A number of other forms of cell death triggered by particular stresses continue to be described, including iron-dependent cell death or ferroptosis, among many emerging programs.[16]

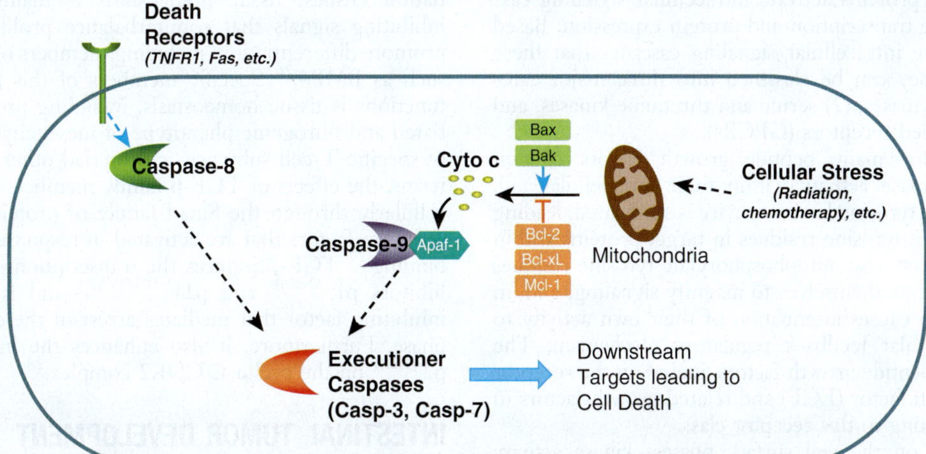

Fig. 1.2 Apoptosis (programmed cell death) counterbalances cellular proliferation to regulate overall tissue growth. A complex interplay of proapoptotic and antiapoptotic molecules results in downstream activation of caspases that mediate cell death. Some of these signals are initiated through cellular stress that can destabilize mitochondrial membranes, and some are initiated through death receptors, including *TNFR1* and *Fas*. The mitochondrial step is regulated by the interplay between proapoptotic *(Bax, Bak)* and antiapoptotic *(Bcl-2, Bcl-xL)* molecules. Upon mitochondrial permeabilization, cytochrome *c* release promotes the formation of the apoptosome complex (*Apaf1*, *caspase-9*, and *cytochrome c*). Activation of caspase-8 (downstream of death receptor) or of caspase-9 (as a result of apoptosome formation) leads to activation of executioner caspases (3 and 7) that are responsible for targeting downstream targets that are responsible for cell death.

Senescence

Senescence is the process by which cells permanently lose their ability to divide. Senescence may occur in response to the stress induced by the activation of oncogenes or DNA damage or after a fixed number of cellular divisions (replicative senescence). Associated with the exit from the cell cycle, senescence is associated with a secretory phenotype that includes a variety of proinflammatory factors. As a physiologic event, senescence limits dysregulated or excessive proliferation. However, when dysregulated, senescence can also contribute to aging and depletion of stem cells.[17] During carcinogenesis, senescence is frequently bypassed or lost.

Replicative senescence is triggered by the shortening of telomeres, repetitive sequences at the end of chromosomes that protect genomic integrity. Telomeres shorten with each cell division, and when they reach a critically short length, they initiate DNA damage signaling and cellular senescence. This phenomenon can be routinely seen in vitro when primary cells undergo repeated rounds of replication, eventually acquiring critically short telomeres.[18] To prevent senescence from being triggered by sustained replication, cancer cells activate the telomerase enzyme, which adds additional telomeres to the end of chromosomes, an enzyme present during development but not in normal adult tissues.[19]

Signaling Pathways That Regulate Cellular Growth

Cellular proliferation is achieved through transition of cells from G_0 arrest into the active cell cycle (see Fig. 1.1). Although progression through the cell cycle is controlled by the regulatory mechanisms just described, overall proliferation is also modulated by external stimuli. Growth factors that bind to specific transmembrane receptors on the cell surface are especially important. Moreover, acting through transmembrane cell surface receptors, extracellular matrix and cell-cell adhesion molecules (i.e., integrins, cadherins, selectins, and proteoglycans) can also have a significant impact on cell proliferation. Alterations in cell-matrix or cell-cell interactions are particularly important in contributing to the invasive phenotype of malignant cells.

After ligand binding, the cytoplasmic tails of these transmembrane receptor proteins activate intracellular signaling cascades that alter gene transcription and protein expression. Based on the nature of the intracellular signaling cascades that these receptors initiate, they can be classified into three major categories: (1) tyrosine kinases, (2) serine and threonine kinases, and (3) G protein–coupled receptors (GPCRs).

The receptors for many peptide growth factors contain intrinsic tyrosine kinase activity within their intracellular tail. After ligand binding, tyrosine kinase activity is stimulated, leading to phosphorylation of tyrosine residues in target proteins within the cell. Most receptors also autophosphorylate tyrosine residues present in the receptors themselves to magnify signaling, and, in some cases, this also causes attenuation of their own activity to affect an intramolecular feedback regulatory mechanism. The receptors for many peptide growth factors, including the receptor for epidermal growth factor (EGF) and related growth factors in the EGF family, belong to this receptor class.

Other receptors on the cell surface possess kinase activity directed toward serine or threonine residues rather than tyrosine. These receptors also phosphorylate a variety of cellular proteins, leading to a cascade of biological responses. Multiple sites of serine and threonine phosphorylation are present on many growth factor receptors, including the tyrosine kinase receptors, suggesting the existence of significant interactions among various receptors present on a single cell.[20] The transforming growth factor (TGF)-α receptor complex is one important example of a serine-threonine kinase–containing transmembrane receptor.

Many receptors are members of the so-called 7-membrane-spanning receptor family. These receptors are coupled to guanine nucleotide binding proteins, also known as G proteins, and thus the receptors are referred to as GPCRs. G proteins undergo a conformational change that is dependent on the presence of guanosine phosphates.[21] Activation of G proteins can trigger a variety of intracellular signals, including stimulation of phospholipase C and the generation of phosphoinositides (most importantly, inositol 1,4,5-triphosphate) and diacylglycerol through hydrolysis of membrane phospholipids, as well as the modulation of the second messengers, cyclic adenosine monophosphate and guanosine monophosphate.[22] Somatostatin receptors exemplify a GPCR prevalent in the GI tract.

Binding of growth factors and cytokines to cell surface receptors typically produces alterations in a variety of cellular functions that influence growth. These functions include ion transport, nutrient uptake, and protein synthesis. However, the ligand-receptor interaction must ultimately modify one or more of the homeostatic mechanisms discussed to affect cellular proliferation.

The Wnt pathway is one important example of a signaling pathway that regulates a diverse number of homeostatic mechanisms to control proliferation of intestinal epithelial cells (Fig. 1.3). Evolutionarily conserved among several species, Wnt signaling, as a rule, regulates proliferation in the stem cell niche and is essential for epithelial homeostasis in the GI tract. From a signaling perspective, its actions are largely the result of the accumulation of β-catenin in the nucleus, where it binds with the transcription factor Tcf-4 to activate a set of target genes.[23] In normal cells, β-catenin is largely associated with adherens junctions, and the cytoplasmic pool of this protein is rapidly degraded through a phosphorylation and ubiquitination pathway. This is mediated by the so-called destruction complex, which includes the tumor suppressor APC. When secreted Wnt ligands bind to cell surface receptors of the Frizzled family, the constitutive degradation of β-catenin is inhibited, which results in the nuclear accumulation of this factor, and the subsequent transcriptional activation of genes that promote cell proliferation. Inhibition of the Wnt signal in mice can be achieved by deletion of Tcf-4 or overexpression of the Wnt inhibitor Dickkopf1, which results in dramatic hypoproliferation of the intestinal epithelium.[24,25] Wnt signaling is most active in the base of the crypt, and as differentiation ensues, tissue homeostasis is maintained by growth-inhibiting signals that counterbalance proliferative signals and promote differentiation, including members of the TGF-β family such as BMP4.[26] Specific members of this family have unique functions is tissue homeostasis, including promoting a differentiated and fibrogenic phenotype of mesenchymal cells, induction of specific T-cell subtypes, and myriad other activities. In broad terms, the effects of TGF-β family members are mediated intracellularly through the Smad family of proteins, which are transcription factors that are activated in response to ligand-receptor binding.[27] TGF-β induces the transcription of the cell cycle inhibitors $p15^{INK4b}$ and $p21^{CIP1/WAF1}$ and is a potent growth-inhibiting factor that mediates arrest of the cell cycle at the G_1 phase. Furthermore, it also enhances the inhibitory activity of $p27^{KIP1}$ on the cyclin E/CDK2 complex.[28]

INTESTINAL TUMOR DEVELOPMENT

Multistep Formation

Multiple sequential genetic alterations are required for the transformation of normal intestinal epithelium to neoplasia. This multistep nature of tumorigenesis is most directly illustrated by the changes that accrue in the development of colonic neoplasia (see Chapter 129). The progression from normal epithelium through adenomatous polyps to malignant neoplasia is paralleled by the accumulation of genetic alterations that change key

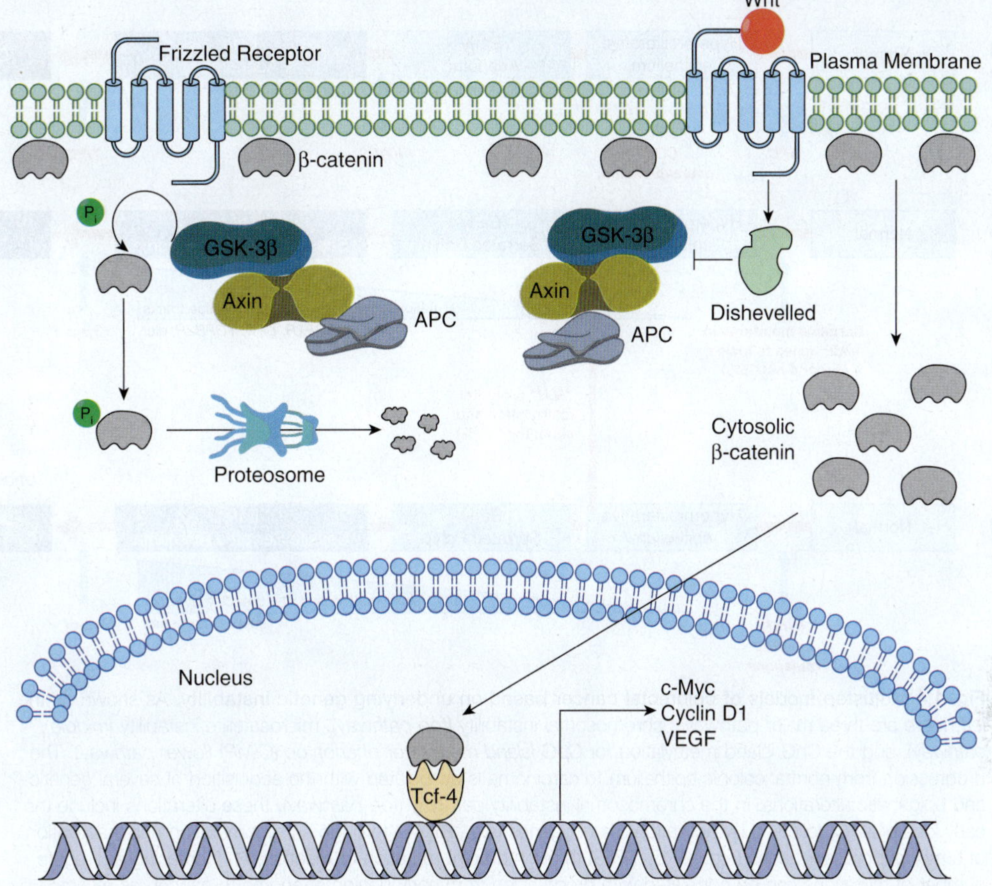

Fig. 1.3 The Wnt signaling pathway is an important regulator of intestinal epithelial cell proliferation and tumorigenesis. In the absence of a Wnt signal (*left top*), cytosolic β-catenin is regulated by the destruction complex, consisting of *APC*, *Axin*, and glycogen synthase kinase-3β (*GSK-3β*). The destruction complex phosphorylates α-catenin and targets it for degradation via the ubiquitin-proteosome pathway. In the presence of an active Wnt signal (*right top*), β-catenin degradation is prevented and the protein is stabilized, leading to excess cytoplasmic β-catenin that is translocated to the nucleus. Nuclear β-catenin interacts with the *Tcf-4* transcription factor to regulate the expression of many key target genes. *APC*, Adenomatous polyposis coli; *P*, phosphate group; *Ub*, ubiquitin; *VEGF*, vascular endothelial growth factor.

pathways that control proliferation and tissue homeostasis. Studies on the molecular pathogenesis of colon cancer have served as a paradigm for the elucidation of genetic alterations in other GI cancers, including gastric and pancreatic cancer.

Genomic instability is observed in almost all cancers in the GI tract. This genetically unstable environment promotes the accumulation of the multiple alterations that characterize GI cancers. Instability of the genome may result from several mechanisms, including changes in the genome DNA sequence or through modifications of the nucleotides to alter their functionality, a process called epigenetic change. In colon cancer, there are now three well-recognized forms of genetic/epigenetic instability that promote carcinogenesis (Fig. 1.4), and they have been termed *chromosomal instability*, *microsatellite instability* (MSI), and *CpG island methylator phenotype* (CIMP).[29,30] Chromosomal instability refers to alterations in chromosomal structure resulting in large chromosomal deletions, duplications, and translocations, which in aggregate result in a state of aneuploidy. In contrast, MSI refers to frequent alterations in tracts of repetitive DNA sequences (referred to microsatellite DNA), and cells with MSI are often diploid or near-diploid on a chromosomal level (see later discussion on DNA repair). CIMP refers to the accumulation of an epigenetic modification, methylation of guanine residues in so-called CpG-islands, areas rich in cytidine and guanine in gene promoter sites. This modification has a potent effect on gene transcription and results in gene silencing. Other forms of epigenetic change involve the chemical modification of the histone proteins that are required for the assembly of the nucleosome and that control chromatin compaction and DNA access. Although mutations in histones themselves are rare in cancer, mutations in the enzymes that modify histones are emerging as an important group of tumor-associated mutations. It is important to note that involvements by these pathways are not mutually exclusive.

Clonal Expansion

Clonal expansion is essential to tumor development.[31] The acquisition of a mutation that may provide a growth or survival advantage to a cell is followed by a clonal expansion of these mutated cells. As this population grows, and particularly with the acquisition of genetic/epigenetic instability, a second round of clonal expansion occurs as a cell within this population sustains still another genetic alteration that further enhances its growth properties. This iterative process of selection, with accumulating genetic alterations, results in malignancy. Because of the nature of the clonal expansion process, once frank malignancy has developed, it is often the case that multiple clones are present in the

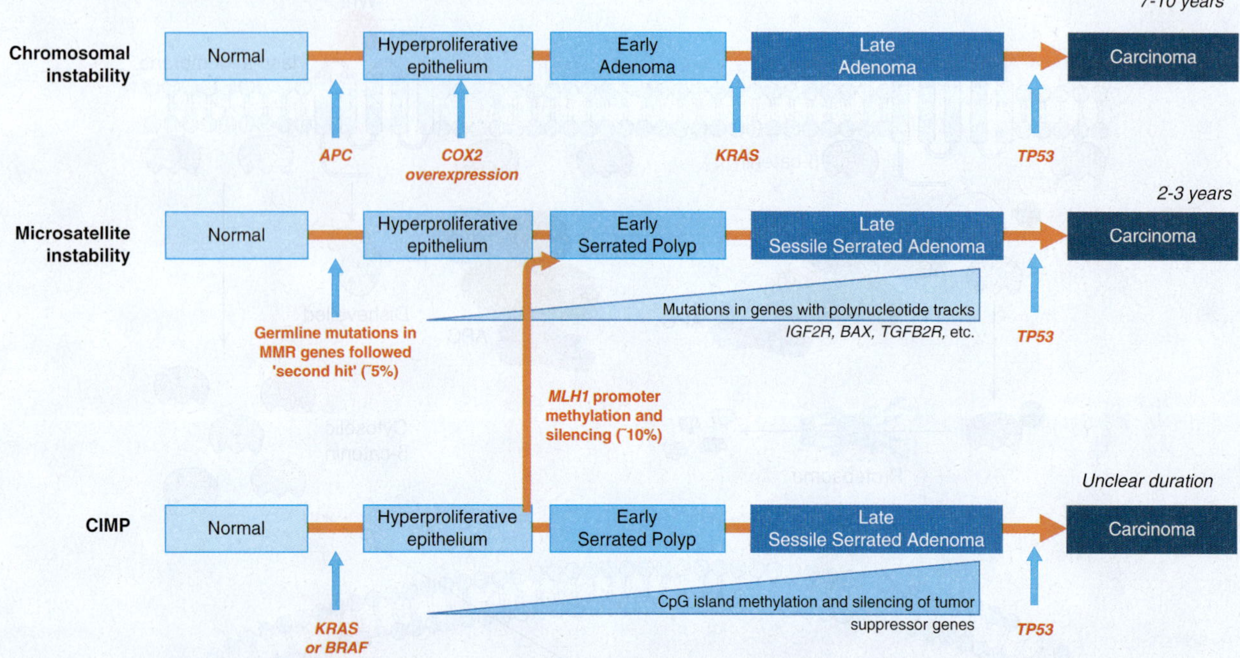

Fig. 1.4 Multistep models of colorectal cancer based on underlying genetic instability. As shown on the *left*, there are three major pathways: chromosomal instability (*top pathway*), microsatellite instability (*middle pathway*), and the CpG island methylation, or *CpG island methylator phenotype (CIMP)* (*lower pathway*). The progression from normal colonic epithelium to carcinoma is associated with the acquisition of several genetic and epigenetic alterations. In the chromosomal instability pathway (*top pathway*), these alterations include the early loss of *APC*, followed by activation of oncogenes (e.g., *KRAS*) through a point mutation and inactivation of tumor suppressor genes (e.g., *APC, TP53*) through a point mutation or deletion. An increasing aggregate number of mutations can be correlated with progression from early benign adenoma to cancer, as reflected by analysis of polyps by size. In the microsatellite instability model (*middle pathway*), mutations in DNA mismatch repair (*MMR*) genes create a mutator phenotype in which mutations accumulate in specific target genes (see the section on DNA mismatch repair). Tumors develop much more rapidly through this pathway than through the chromosomal instability pathway (2–3 years compared to 7–10 years). Germline mutations in *MMR* genes account for 5% of all colorectal tumors. In the *CIMP* pathway (*lower pathway*), the initiating event is hypothesized to be a *BRAF* or *KRAS* activating mutation that somehow triggers extensive CpG island methylation, particularly of gene promoters, resulting in gene silencing. Among the potential gene targets is *MLH1*, a component of the MMR pathway, and when silenced as part of the *CIMP* pathway, the tumor evolves along a similar molecular as microsatellite unstable cancers (MSI-H). Sporadic *MLH1* methylation and silencing accounts for nearly 10% of sporadic colorectal cancers. Alternatively, serrated adenomas arising in the *CIMP* pathway can undergo a pathway similar to that of chromosomal instability to become microsatellite stable tumors.

same tumor, with a different catalog of mutations harbored among various cancer cells. Referred to as *tumor heterogeneity*, this ongoing process may give certain cells selection advantages.[32] Metastasis may be facilitated by the evolution of a subset of tumor cells that acquire the capability of traversing the circulatory or lymphatic systems and thriving in a new environment.

Cancer Stem Cells

Recognition of tumor heterogeneity has led to the *cancer stem cell (CSC) hypothesis*, which asserts that there exists a subset of tumor cells that have stem cell–like properties. CSCs are believed to be the tumor-initiating cells from which clonal expansion occurs. Moreover, it is hypothesized that the eradication of these cells is a key therapeutic goal because failure to do so may result in relapse of disease. Within this CSC hypothesis, there are two models.[33] The first is a hierarchical model in which CSCs serve as progenitors for all cells in a given tumor, whereas other cells have limited long-term reproductive potential. The basic evidence for this model is the finding that only cells with specific surface markers can repopulate the tumor in xenotransplantation experiments. In the GI tract, analysis of putative CSCs demonstrates transcriptional programs and markers shared with normal intestinal stem cells, such as Lgr5 and EphB2, which identify and purify colon CSCs.[34] The second stochastic model posits that each cancer cell has the same potential to be a CSC, but this determination is stochastically based on internal factors in addition to external environmental cues. Recent studies in this area have identified that CSCs do not need to be rare or quiescent, as may be the case for adult stem cells in many normal tissues, and that there is substantial plasticity within a tumor that may determine the nature of the stem cell population.[35,36]

Epithelial-Mesenchymal Transition

It has been noted that within tumors of epithelial origin, some cells acquire features of mesenchymal cells. A similar process occurs during normal embryogenesis, when polarized epithelial cells no longer recognize the boundaries imposed by adjacent epithelial cells or their basement membrane and adopt features of migratory mesenchymal cells. This phenomenon, designated *epithelial-mesenchymal transition* (EMT), endows cells with the ability to move through tissue planes that normally serve as boundaries for epithelial cells, such as the basement membrane, a dense matrix of collagen, glycoproteins, and proteoglycans. The transmigration of tumor cells through the basement membrane likely involves the production of key proteolytic activities. Alternatively, the tumor cell may produce factors capable of activating proenzymes present in the extracellular matrix. For example, the tumor may produce urokinase, itself a protease, or plasminogen activator. Having gained access to the interstitial stromal compartment, tumor cells can then enter lymphatic and blood vessels and metastasize.

In addition to these properties, it has been recognized that cells that undergo EMT acquire not only invasive features but also CSC-like features.[37]

One key feature of EMT is the loss of adherens junctions that normally maintain epithelial cell-cell interactions. The molecular correlate of this phenomenon is the loss of expression of E-cadherin, a critical component of the adherens junction.[38] Mutations in E-cadherin are common in many GI cancers, particularly gastric cancer, where germline mutations in E-cadherin are also linked to hereditary diffuse gastric cancer.

NEOPLASIA-ASSOCIATED GENES

Genes that become altered during the neoplastic process belong to two distinct groups: (1) oncogenes, which actively confer a growth-promoting property, or (2) tumor suppressor genes, the products of which normally restrain growth or proliferation. An important category within tumor suppressor genes includes DNA repair genes, which prevent accumulation of new mutations. Activation of oncogenes or inactivation of tumor suppressor genes contributes to malignant transformation. Although most of these genes encode for proteins, many cancer-promoting genes that harbor oncogenic and tumor-suppressive functions do not encode for proteins but rather for RNAs that modulate genomic function, so-called noncoding RNAs.

Oncogenes

According to the Catalog of Somatic Mutations in Cancer (COSMIC),[39] there are close to 80 oncogenes with strong evidence of involvement in cancer. Genes that encode a normal cellular protein, whose function may promote the neoplastic process (e.g., antiapoptotic function and cell proliferation stimulation), may function as oncogenes when they are expressed at inappropriately high levels. A typical mechanism for this phenomenon is gene amplification, when tumors acquire multiple copies of a normal gene resulting in a dosage effect that leads to increased gene expression.

In other cases, a variety of mutations may lead to inappropriately high activity of a normal gene, leading to cancer-promoting activities. Point mutations or large gene rearrangements resulting in fusion proteins are examples of mutations that can lead to oncogene activation. For example, several genes that encode tyrosine kinase–containing growth factor receptors become oncogenes after a mutation results in unregulated tyrosine kinase activity that is no longer dependent on the presence of the appropriate ligand (e.g., EGF). Because of their tumor-promoting activity, these mutations tend to be recurrent among specific cancer classes. The normal cellular genes from which the oncogenes derive are designated *proto-oncogenes.* Most of these genes are widely expressed in many different types of tumor cells.

Finally, another source of oncogenes are virally encoded proteins that may affect cellular growth or survival.[40] These factors, while evolved to favor the viral cycle, may in some instances favor neoplastic development and this is the reason why specific viruses are associated with increased cancer risk. In addition, in the case of retroviruses, the ability of the viral genome to insert itself in the genome of the host can lead to disruptions in the expression of genes in the vicinity of insertion sites, which at times, may have oncogenic activities.

The proteins encoded by oncogenes may affect any of the hallmarks of cancer, such as stimulate growth factor pathways, promote tumor invasion, prevent cell death, or have other tumor-promoting actions. With regards to promoting growth factor pathways, oncogenes may encode for (1) growth factors or their receptors or for (2) intracellular signal transduction molecules downstream of the receptor itself, including transcription factors that mediate the actions of the growth factor at the level of the nucleus.

Oncogenic Growth Factors and Growth Factor Receptors

The transforming effects of enhanced expression of a variety of growth factors have been demonstrated both in vitro and in vivo. Cancer cells may engage in autocrine signaling to promote their growth or coax the adjacent stroma to hypersecrete such growth-stimulating factors. More frequently, a variety of receptors are upregulated in expression or dysregulated leading to constitutive action. Among them, are receptor tyrosine kinases of the EGF receptor family (ERBB1-4), which are frequently upregulated in a variety of GI cancers. Other examples of activated receptors that can act as oncogenes include c-MET and c-KIT.[41,42]

Signal Transduction–Related Oncogenes

Intermediate steps that effectively translate ligand-receptor binding to an intracellular signal are essential in mediating functional responses of the cell. Mutations in genes that encode key proteins that participate in signal transduction can also lead to cellular transformation (Fig. 1.5). In this regard, the largest family of oncogenes encodes proteins with protein kinase activity. Many members of this large oncogene group are expressed by neoplasms of the GI tract, and these include the Src nonreceptor tyrosine kinase that associates with the inner surface of the plasma membrane.

G proteins regulate signaling of the large family of GPCRs through the exchange of guanosine triphosphate with guanosine diphosphate. Like G proteins, members of the *RAS* family of genes, also regulate cellular function in a GTP/GDP-dependent fashion and are among the most commonly detected oncogenes in GI tract cancers. The RAS family contains three genes: *H-RAS*, *K-RAS*, and *N-RAS*. These factors are essential to transduce signals from various growth receptor signaling cascades and point mutations that result in activating amino acid substitutions at critical hot spot positions convert the normal gene into an oncogene.

To date, almost all *RAS* mutations in GI malignancies occur in the *K-RAS* oncogene. The highest mutation frequency is found in tumors of the exocrine pancreas (>90%).[43] *RAS* genes activated through point mutation have been identified in approximately 50% of colonic cancers as well as a subset of serrated tumors (see Fig. 1.4).[44]

Most oncogenic mutations in *ras* cause biochemical changes that maintain it in the active, guanosine triphosphate (GTP)–bound state by reducing guanosine triphosphatase activity or by destabilizing the inactive guanosine diphosphate–bound form. However, several *RAS* mutants retain significant guanosine triphosphatase activity; therefore other mechanisms that convert *RAS* to a transforming protein may be involved.[45] The most

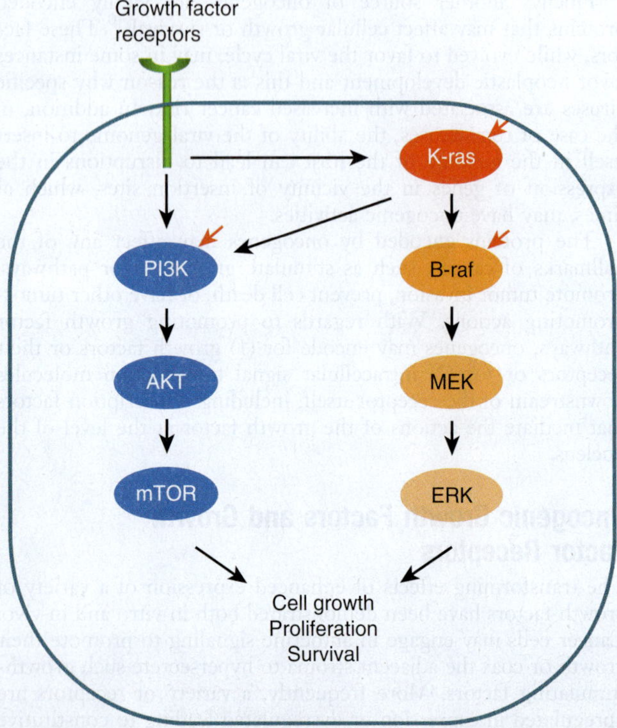

Fig. 1.5 Signal transduction downstream of growth factor receptors, where *K-RAS* plays a major role. Oncogenic *K-RAS* can activate multiple signaling pathways. Molecules that are frequently mutated in colorectal cancer are noted by a *red arrow* and include *K-RAS* (40%), *B-RAF* (10%), and PI3K (15%). *AKT*, Cellular homolog of v-Akt oncogene; *ERK*, extracellular signal-regulated kinase; *MEK*, MAPK/ERK kinase; *mTOR*, mammalian target of rapamycin; *PI3K*; phosphoinositide-3 kinase.

common mutations in *K-RAS* are highly prevalent among many tumor types and have been the focus of multiple attempts at developing specific inhibitors. When this proved to be exceedingly challenging, a consensus emerged that *K-RAS* was undruggable; however, this concept has been recently challenged and specific inhibitors of mutated *K-RAS* are in active clinical testing for various tumors.[46]

A functional consequence of RAS activation is the phosphorylation and activation of key downstream serine/threonine kinases. One important target of RAS is B-RAF. In colon cancers without an identifiable *K-RAS* mutation, 20% possess an activating *B-RAF* mutation,[47] consistent with the concept that the activation of an oncogenic pathway can be achieved through an alteration in any of several sequential components of a particular pathway (see Fig. 1.5).

Nuclear Oncogenes

Many cellular oncogenes encode proteins that localize to the nucleus. In essence, these nuclear oncogene products are the final mediators of signal transduction pathways that are also affected by cytoplasmic and plasma membrane–bound oncoproteins, because they act as transcription factors that regulate expression of certain genes that enhance cellular proliferation and suppress normal differentiation.

The role of nuclear oncogenes is illustrated by the Myc family. The c-Myc protein product is involved in critical cellular functions like proliferation, differentiation, apoptosis, transformation, and transcriptional activation of key genes.[48] Frequently, c-Myc is overexpressed or amplified in many GI cancers. It has been found

TABLE 1.1 Mutations Associated with Hereditary Gastrointestinal Cancer Syndromes

Disorder	Gene(s) Mutated
FAP, AFAP, Gardner syndrome	*APC*
Lynch syndrome (HNPCC)	*MLH1, MSH2, PMS2, MSH6, EPCAM* (through disruption of the neighboring *MSH2* gene)
MAP	*MUTYH*
Peutz-Jeghers syndrome	*STK11*
Cowden's disease	*PTEN*
Juvenile polyposis	*SMAD4, BMPR1A*
Hereditary diffuse gastric cancer	*CDH1*
Hereditary pancreatic cancer	*ATM, BRCA1, BRCA2, PALB2, PALLD, CDKN2A, PRSS1, SPINK1, PRSS2, CTRC, CFTR*
MEN1	*Menin*

AFAP, Attenuated FAP; *APC*, adenomatous polyposis coli; *FAP*, familial adenomatous polyposis; *HNPCC*, hereditary nonpolyposis colorectal cancer; *MAP*, MUTYH-associated polyposis; *MEN1*, multiple endocrine neoplasia, type 1; *MUTYH*, mutY homolog.

to be a transcriptional target of the β-catenin/Tcf-4 complex in colorectal cancers (see Fig. 1.3), which may explain the overexpression of c-Myc observed in this cancer type.[49]

Tumor Suppressor Genes

Mutations of tumor suppressor genes are associated with all GI cancers, and a number of these genes and their products have been identified and characterized (Table 1.1). Unlike gain-of-function mutations, which are characteristic of oncogenes, mutations in tumor suppressor genes are loss-of-function mutations and are therefore biallelic.

Initial recognition of the existence of tumor suppressor genes was derived from genetic analyses of cancer-prone families. In the GI tract, hereditary colon cancer, gastric cancer, and pancreatic cancer syndromes are the best described and are discussed elsewhere in this text (see Chapters 56, 59, and 128). In these syndromes, there is a marked increase in risk for a particular tumor in the absence of other predisposing environmental factors. Tumors arise typically at a younger age than they do in the general population, and multiple primary tumors may develop within the target tissue.

From a genetic standpoint, cancer genetic syndromes most often have an autosomal dominant mode of Mendelian inheritance. Based on observations in hereditary retinoblastoma, Knudson proposed the "two-hit" hypothesis,[50] which explains the relationship between sporadic and familial forms of cancer. Whereas sporadic tumors are initiated by somatic biallelic inactivating mutations of a tumor suppressor gene, tumors in familial cancer syndromes are accelerated by the inheritance of a monoallelic mutation of a tumor suppressor gene present in all cells in affected family members. When this germline mutation is followed by a somatic mutation in the remaining normal allele of the tumor suppressor gene, this gives rise to the development of a neoplastic clone that eventually gives rise to a tumor (Fig. 1.6). Because of the germline mutation, the barrier to full inactivation of the tumor suppressor is diminished substantially because only one additional hit is required, leading to the younger age of onset and the potential for tumor multiplicity that accompanies these syndromes.

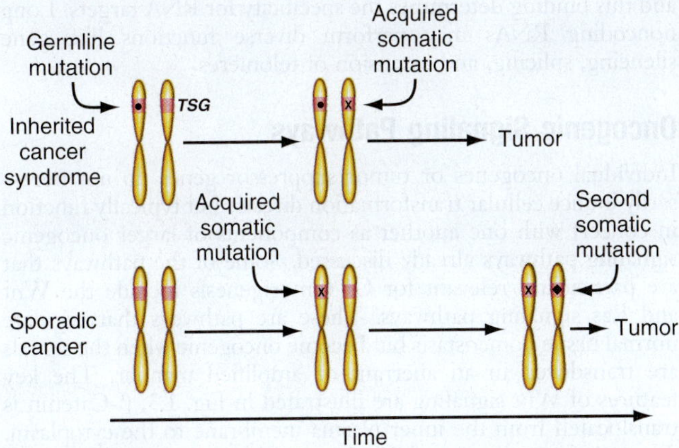

Fig. 1.6 Knudson's two-hit hypothesis. In an inherited cancer syndrome, one chromosome has an inactive tumor suppressor gene (TSG) locus because of a germline mutation. The counterpart TSG on the remaining paired chromosome is subsequently inactivated by a somatic mutation, leading to tumor formation. In contrast, in a sporadic cancer, the two alleles of the TSG need to become inactivated through two independent somatic mutations, an event that is less likely to occur within a single cell.

Although this two-hit model has been generally observed, there are exceptions. Some tumor suppressors may function to increase cancer risk when only one allele is mutated. Moreover, some cancer genetic syndromes display somatic recessive mode of inheritance because genetic risk is conferred only when biallelic inactivating mutations are present. Another important feature of tumor suppressor genes is that they do not function identically in every tissue type. Consequently, the inactivation of a particular tumor suppressor gene is tumorigenic only in certain tissues. For example, the tumor suppressor genes *RB1* and *VHL* play crucial roles in retinoblastomas and renal cell cancer, respectively, but are rarely mutated in GI malignancies. Tumor suppressor genes shown to have a critical role in the pathogenesis of GI malignancies, *APC*, *TP53*, and *SMAD4*, are described later. Furthermore, we will discuss DNA repair pathways that, when lost, can give rise to neoplasia and therefore function as tumor suppressor factors.

Adenomatous Polyposis Coli Gene

Genetic linkage analysis revealed markers on chromosome 5q21 that were tightly linked to polyp development in affected members of kindreds with familial adenomatous polyposis (FAP) and Gardner's syndrome.[51] Further work led to the identification of the gene responsible for FAP, the *APC* gene.[52–54] The full spectrum of adenomatous polyposis syndromes attributable to *APC* is discussed in detail in Chapter 128. Somatic mutations in *APC* have also been found in most sporadic colon polyps and cancers.[55,56] Mutations in *APC* are characteristically identified in the earliest adenomas, indicating that *APC* plays a critical role as the gatekeeper in the multistep progression from normal epithelial cell to colon cancer (see Fig. 1.4).

The *APC* gene comprises 15 exons and encodes a predicted protein of 2843 amino acids, or approximately 310 kDa. Most germline and somatic *APC* gene mutations result in a premature stop codon and therefore a truncated *APC* protein product and loss of function. As discussed earlier, *APC* is a negative regulator of the Wnt signaling pathway and its inactivation results in a state that resembles constitutive activation of Wnt. Intracellularly, this is manifested by the stabilization of β-catenin, which mediates the transcriptional effects of Wnt activation and the subsequent oncogenic phenotype (see Fig. 1.3). Interestingly, another mechanism to achieve this signaling outcome is mutations in β-catenin itself that render the protein impervious to *APC*-dependent degradation.

TP53 Gene

This is the most commonly mutated gene in human cancer,[57] and point mutations in *TP53* are found with high frequency in all cancers of the GI tract.[58] In fact, point mutations in *TP53* have been identified in as many as 50% to 70% of sporadic colon cancers (see Fig. 1.4). Interestingly, these mutations arise relatively late in the oncogenic process as the gene is mutated in only a small subset of colonic adenomas.[59]

Named for a 53-kDa–sized encoded protein, p53 is a nuclear phosphoprotein that plays a key role in cell cycle regulation and apoptosis.[58] In the nucleus, p53 functions as a transcription factor that can be induced by conditions of cellular stress, such as ionizing radiation, growth factor withdrawal, or cytotoxic therapy. Induction of p53 arrests cells at the G_1 phase to facilitate DNA repair, senescence, or trigger apoptosis. These responses are mediated in part by its transcriptional targets such as the $p21^{CIP1/WAF1}$ inhibitor of the cell cycle or the proapoptotic gene, *PUMA*.[60] Interestingly, it is often the case that *TP53* mutations occur as the combination of a genomic deletion encompassing one allele, together with a missense mutation in the second allele that targets specific hotspots within the protein. Recent evidence indicates that the genomic deletions function not only by removing *TP53* but through the loss of adjacent genes with tumor-suppressive activities.[61] Furthermore, the second type of mutations, resulting in specific missense mutations, are thought to contribute gain-of-function tumorigenic activities.[62] In addition to the *TP53* point mutations in sporadic cancers, germline *TP53* mutations have been observed in the Li-Fraumeni syndrome, an autosomal dominant familial disorder in which breast carcinoma, soft tissue sarcoma, osteosarcoma, leukemia, brain tumor, colon cancer, and adrenocortical carcinoma can develop in affected persons.[63]

SMAD4 Gene

SMAD4 is a tumor suppressor gene located on chromosome 18q and is deleted or mutated in most pancreatic adenocarcinomas and a subset of colon cancers. Smad4, the protein encoded by this gene, is an essential intracellular mediator of factors belonging to the TGF-β superfamily. Smad4 functions as a transcription factor and is an obligate partner of other members of the Smad protein family.[64] Mutant Smad4 lacks these properties and, among other effects, leads to loss of TGF-β inhibition of proliferation. Germline mutations in *SMAD4* result in the juvenile polyposis syndrome (see Chapter 128).

DNA Repair Genes

DNA replication itself and various types of DNA damaging agents can introduce errors into the genome. These errors include spontaneous mismatching of nucleotides during normal DNA replication, oxidative damage of nucleotides, and complete double-strand breaks. Therefore a variety of cellular mechanisms have evolved to prevent or correct DNA errors. One type of error that develops during replication may occur in repetitive mononucleotide or dinucleotide stretches of DNA, so-called microsatellite regions.[65] These repetitive regions are prone to DNA mismatches, which if not resolved, can result in short insertions or deletions. The cellular machinery devoted to correct these errors is referred to as the mismatch repair system. The enzymes bind mismatched DNA, cut the DNA strand with the mismatched nucleotide, unwind the DNA fragment, fill in the gap with the correct nucleotide, and finally reseal the remaining nick. The family of DNA mismatch repair genes includes two basic molecular components, a mismatch recognition complex composed of MSH2 and MSH6, and an excision inducing complex composed of MLH1 and PMS2. Mutations in any of these genes result in defective mismatch repair, and when one allele is inherited due to a germline mutation, they give rise to Lynch syndrome, also known as *hereditary nonpolyposis colorectal cancer*.[66,67] Complete loss of a mismatch repair factor leads to very high rates of DNA mutations, and mismatch repair defective tumors accumulate a high burden of cancer somatic mutations, typically over 2000 somatic mutations, resulting in a large number of tumor-specific neoantigens.[68] Affected cells are called *replication error positive*, in contrast to the replication error–negative phenotype.[69,70] Because microsatellite DNA sequences are primarily affected by this type of genetic instability, the tumor cells display insertions or deletions in these stretches of DNA when compared to nontumor tissue, a phenomenon referred to as MSI. Mechanistically, the absence of DNA repair does not directly cause cancer but creates a milieu that permits accumulation of mutations in a variety of genes that contain repetitive DNA sequences, such as the TGF-β type II receptor, IGF type II receptor, BAX, and E2F-4, among others.

Loss of mismatch repair genes represents an important mechanism for the accumulation of mutations within a tumor (see Fig. 1.4). While 5% of colon cancers are due to Lynch syndrome, that is, germline mutations in the mismatch repair system, twice as many tumors (10%) display similar molecular characteristics without a germline mutation in any of the mismatch repair genes. These tumors are most often driven by somatic loss of function in this system, most often as a result of silencing of *MLH1* gene expression as a result of an epigenetic change in the promoter region of this gene, a process called DNA methylation. *MLH1* promoter hypermethylation is most often observed in lesions that are serrated adenomas by histology and that also carry *B-RAF* mutations (see Fig. 1.4). Finally, it has been recognized that another mechanism that can lead to a state of high mutation burden is the loss of exonuclease proofreading activity of the replicative DNA polymerases involved in copying DNA during replication and endoded by the *POLE* and *POLD1* genes.[71]

Another important DNA repair pathway involved in carcinogenesis is mediated by the *MUTYH* gene. It encodes a DNA glycosylase that participates in the repair of oxidized guanine nucleotides, such as 8-oxoguanine residues, that may inappropriately pair with adenines, ultimately leading to somatic G:C→T:A mutations if uncorrected. Biallelic mutations in *MUTYH* results in an adenomatous polyposis syndrome that resembles FAP, except that its mode of inheritance is autosomal recessive (see Chapter 128).[72,73] Interestingly, G:C→T:A mutations in the *APC* gene were almost universally found in the polyps of patients with germline MUTYH mutations, indicating that there are important similarities in the molecular pathogenesis of polyps in the MUTYH and FAP syndromes.

Noncoding RNAs

Our genomes harbor a variety of genes whose products are RNAs that do not encode for a protein. The RNA products, termed *noncoding RNAs*, consist of a broad category of active RNA molecules that can mediate a variety of effects. The categories of noncoding RNAs are rapidly expanding and include so-called microRNAs and long noncoding RNAs, which are frequently dysregulated in cancers. The microRNAs play a critical role in silencing of other RNA transcripts via RNA degradation or translational inhibition and typically regulate dozens of target RNAs at a time. Their biogenesis involves conventional gene transcription, followed by processing of the resulting RNA by a variety of nuclease cleavage events, resulting ultimately in the generation of small interfering RNAs (siRNAs) by the protein Dicer. These siRNAs bind to complementary mRNA sequences, and this binding determines the specificity for RNA targets. Long noncoding RNAs may perform diverse functions like gene silencing, splicing, and extension of telomeres.

Oncogenic Signaling Pathways

Individual oncogenes or tumor suppressor genes do not necessarily induce cellular transformation directly but typically function in concert with one another as components of larger oncogenic signaling pathways already discussed. Some of the pathways that are particularly relevant for GI tumorigenesis include the Wnt and Ras signaling pathways. These are pathways that regulate normal tissue homeostasis but become oncogenic when the signals are transduced in an aberrant or amplified manner. The key features of Wnt signaling are illustrated in Fig. 1.3. β-Catenin is translocated from the inner plasma membrane to the cytoplasm. There, it forms a macromolecular complex with the APC protein Axin and glycogen synthase kinase-3β. Phosphorylation of β-catenin by glycogen synthase kinase-3β triggers its degradation. In the presence of an active Wnt signal, β-catenin is stabilized and enters the nucleus, where it interacts with the transcription factor Tcf-4 to upregulate a number of key target genes, including *c-Myc*, *cyclin D1*, and *vascular endothelial growth factor (VEGF)*. As discussed earlier, Wnt signaling is essential for regulating proliferation of normal intestinal epithelium, and dysregulated Wnt signaling is an almost universal feature of all colorectal cancers. The latter can result from a mutation in the *APC*, *Axin*, or *β-catenin* genes, although alterations in the *APC* tumor suppressor gene are the most common. An alteration in just one of these components is sufficient to activate the entire pathway. Thus it is essential to consider individual genetic alterations in the context of the overall signaling pathway in which they function.

Because pathways are typically not linear, additional levels of complexity arise. There is frequent overlap among pathways, and the distinction between pathways can be somewhat arbitrary. For example, mutations in the *K-RAS* oncogene result in activation of multiple distinct signaling pathways, including Raf/ERK/MAPK, PI3K/Akt, and nuclear factor-κB, all of which play an important role in tumorigenesis (see Fig. 1.5). Crosstalk between these effector pathways serves to modulate the cellular responses further. For example, Akt, a target of PI3K, can phosphorylate Raf and thereby regulate signaling through the MAPK pathway.[74] Finally, each of these signaling pathways regulates multiple biological processes related to tumorigenesis,[75] including cell cycle progression, apoptosis, senescence, angiogenesis, and invasion.

Another pathway that plays a particularly important role in GI tumors is the cyclooxygenase-2 (COX-2) pathway. The enzyme COX-2 is a key regulator of prostaglandin synthesis that is induced in inflammation and neoplasia. Although no mutations of COX-2 have been described, an overexpression of COX-2 in colonic adenomas and cancers is associated with tumor progression and angiogenesis (see Fig. 1.4), primarily through induction of prostaglandin E_2 synthesis. Inhibition of COX-2 with a variety of agents (aspirin, nonsteroidal antiinflammatory drugs, or COX-2 selective inhibitors such as celecoxib) is associated with a reduced risk of colorectal adenomas and cancer.[76]

TUMOR MICROENVIRONMENT

Cancer is ultimately a complex tissue consisting not only of neoplastic cells harboring a number of genetic lesions, as outlined previously, but the composite of a number of cellular components that endow the tumor with all of its properties. Indeed, the contribution of nonneoplastic cells to the behavior and evolution of a tumor is increasingly recognized. Cellular elements with recognized contributions to the behavior of the tumor include its mesenchymal cells, its vasculature, a variety of immune cells recruited to the tumor and particularly in tumors of the intestinal tract, and tumor-associated microbiota that contribute significantly to the tumor microenvironment. In addition, these elements acting in concert lead to a metabolic environment, such as the oxygen and nutrient supply of the tumor, that often plays a significant role in the evolution of the tumor at the primary site and its potential for distant metastasis.

TUMOR METABOLISM

Tumor cells exhibit abnormal metabolic profiles to facilitate their growth and anabolic needs. Observations in 1924 from Nobel Laureate Otto Heinrich Warburg revealed that tumor cells displayed dramatic increases in aerobic glycolysis and diminished mitochondrial respiration. This metabolic state, known as the *Warburg effect,* has been validated and is a hallmark feature of most malignancies.[77] It is becoming increasingly clear that integration of the genetic lesions that characterize cancer formation is responsible for the changes in cellular metabolism that accompany cellular transformation. Many of the genes implicated in GI cancers (*p53, K-RAS, PI3K, mTOR, HIF,* and *Myc*) can in fact regulate metabolic pathways. Moreover, germline mutations in metabolic regulators (e.g., subunits of succinate dehydrogenase) that are not classical oncogenes or tumor suppressor genes have been associated with a high risk of tumorigenesis (pheochromocytoma and paraganglioma).[78,79] The selection advantage of increased glycolysis in cancer cells may include greater tolerance to hypoxic environments and shunting of metabolic byproducts (e.g., lactate) to other biosynthetic pathways. These altered metabolic pathways are promising new targets for therapy.

Inflammation and Cancer

Immune cells recruited to the tumor microenvironment can result in a variety of effects. On the one hand, tumor immune surveillance is well recognized, and immunosuppressed states increase the risk of cancer development. On the other hand, a number of cellular elements of hematopoietic origin can promote primary tumor growth, prevent effective immune surveillance, or promote the acquisition of features of neoplastic cells that facilitate metastasis. Myeloid cells with immature characteristics, so-called myeloid-derived suppressor cells, are an important example of this phenomenon.[80]

In addition, a number of chronic inflammatory conditions increase the site-specific risk of cancer; examples of this include ulcerative colitis (see Chapter 117), chronic gastritis (see Chapter 54), chronic pancreatitis (see Chapter 61), Barrett's esophagus (see Chapter 49), and chronic viral hepatitis (see Chapters 81 and 82). The influences of inflammation on the development of neoplasia are multifaceted and complex. Cytokines produced by inflammatory cells can lead to activation of antiapoptotic and pro-proliferative signals in tumor cells mediated by transcription factors such as nuclear factor-κB and STAT3.[81,82] Immune cells may also promote remodeling of the vascular network and promote angiogenesis (discussed later). Inflammation may also induce DNA damage from cytokine-stimulated production of reactive oxygen species.

Microbiome

The human body possesses more than 100 trillion microbes, and the largest concentration of these organisms is present in the GI tract. The interaction between these organisms and the host is an area of great interest, particularly for a broad range of autoimmune, metabolic, and neoplastic disorders.[83] Interestingly, colonic tumors are associated with specific subsets of bacteria, and the tumor-associated microbial species have the capacity of inducing colonic tumors in specified animal models.[84] *Fusobacterium nucleatum,* an organism typically found in the oral cavity, is an example of this behavior as it can be found in association with colon tumors and, when introduced into colon cancer models driven by germline *APC* mutations, can drive colon tumorigenesis.[85]

BIOLOGICAL FEATURES OF TUMOR METASTASIS

The establishment of distant metastases requires multiple processes, many of which involve alterations in interactions between tumor cells and normal host cells. To metastasize, a cell or group of cells must detach from the primary tumor, gain access to the lymphatic or vascular space, adhere to the endothelial surface at a distant site, penetrate the vessel wall to invade the second tissue site, and finally proliferate as a second tumor focus. Angiogenesis is necessary for the proliferation of the primary tumor and tumor metastases. Tumor cells must also overcome host immune cell killing. As a result, few circulating tumor cells (<0.01%) successfully initiate metastatic foci. A "survival of the fittest" view of metastasis has been proposed, in which selective competition favors metastasis of a subpopulation of cells from the primary site.[86] In favor of this view is the fact that the mutational landscape of the primary and distant tumor sites are often distinct, indicating that only specific tumor clones acquire the ability to metastasize.

Angiogenesis and Lymphangiogenesis

Angiogenesis is essential to sustain continued growth of the primary tumor. If new vessels are not developed as the primary tumor expands, cells most distant from available vessels are deprived of an adequate source of nutrition and oxygen, and central necrosis occurs. Neovascularization is also an important permissive factor in facilitating metastatic dissemination of tumors.[87] A number of protein growth factors produced by malignant tumor cells and stromal cells have been found to be potent stimuli of angiogenesis, including VEGF-A, basic fibroblast growth factor, and TGF-β. VEGF-A is perhaps the most critical factor that is upregulated in most tumor types, including colorectal cancer. Multiple genetic pathways implicated in GI carcinogenesis modulate *VEGF-A* expression, including Wnt and mutant *RAS.*[88]

Angiogenesis occurs in an ordered series of events. Endothelial cells in the parent vessel are stimulated to degrade the endothelial basement membrane, migrate into the perivascular stroma, and initiate a capillary sprout. The sprout develops into a tubular structure that, in turn, develops into a capillary network. In vitro models that recapitulate the early events of angiogenesis indicate that this process involves a balance between proteases and protease inhibitors in a manner similar to that during tumor invasion. Indeed, functional parallels between tumor invasion and angiogenesis are evident in their mutual requirement for cellular motility, basement membrane proteolysis, and cell growth.

In addition to angiogenesis, lymphangiogenesis plays an important role in tumor metastasis. Some important clues into the molecular basis of tumor lymphangiogenesis have been obtained. VEGF-C or VEGF-D bind to the VEGF receptor-3 on lymphatic endothelial cells to stimulate formation of new lymphatic vessels.[89] This results in the development of new lymphatic channels within the tumor mass and, consequently, enhanced dissemination of tumor cells to regional lymph nodes.[90]

ENVIRONMENTAL INFLUENCES

Fundamentally, cancer is a genetic disorder, and genetic mutation is the common denominator of agents or mechanisms that contribute to the development of neoplasia. Environmental factors play an important role in tumorigenesis insofar as they affect the progression of the underlying genetic lesions.

Chemical Carcinogenesis

Many compounds that have carcinogenic potential often require metabolic modification by host enzymes, a process called metabolic activation. The initial compound, the procarcinogen, is converted by host enzymes to an electrophilic derivative, which then chemically modifies DNA. Mutations result from errors that occur during DNA replication as a result of distorted base pairs. Factors that influence the potency of any chemical carcinogen include the equilibrium between activation of the procarcinogen and deactivation or degradation of the carcinogen.[91] Deactivation typically occurs through a conjugation reaction, usually in the liver.

These principles are exemplified by experimental colonic carcinomas that arise in rodents fed cycasin, a glucosylated compound present in the cycad nut. The glucose residue of cycasin is cleaved in the rat liver by α-glucosidase to form methylazoxymethanol, which is subsequently deformylated by enzymes in the liver and colon to give rise to methyldiazonium, a carcinogen. These same metabolites are formed through hepatic enzymatic modification of the compound dimethylhydrazine and result in colon cancer in the rat.

In humans, regular tobacco use is strongly associated with a higher risk of multiple GI cancers, including pancreatic and colon cancer. Among active smokers with long-term tobacco use, the risk for pancreatic cancer can be elevated twofold. Multiple carcinogenic agents, including arsenic, benzene, and ethylene oxide, have been identified in cigarettes, but the chemicals linked specifically to the development of pancreatic or colon cancer have not yet been defined.

Dietary Factors

Chemical mutagenesis may be especially important in the development of cancers within the GI tract and related organs. The mucosal surfaces from which most primary cancers in the GI tract develop are exposed to a complex mixture of dietary constituents that are potential carcinogens or procarcinogens. The frequency of contamination of food with aflatoxins, a fungal metabolite, parallels the incidence of hepatocellular carcinoma in various areas of the world.[92] Studies demonstrating that aflatoxins cause mutations in the *TP53* gene in hepatocellular carcinoma have provided a compelling link between genes and the environment.[92]

Nitrates present in many foods appear to be additional dietary constituents that may act as procarcinogens in the GI tract. Diet-derived nitrates can be converted by bacterial action in a hypochlorhydric stomach to nitrites and subsequently to mutagenic nitrosamines.[93] These events may underlie the documented correlation between dietary intake of foods high in nitrates and the incidence of gastric cancer in different populations.

Other dietary factors may modulate the biological potency of dietary procarcinogens. Variations in the relative and absolute amounts of dietary fats may lead to alterations in the composition of the colonic microflora and their metabolic characteristics, resulting in modulation of the production of enzymes that convert dietary constituents into potentially mutagenic compounds. Changes in dietary fiber content can alter the transit time of luminal contents in the bowel, thereby changing the duration of exposure of the mucosa to potential mutagens. Bile salt content may be an additional luminal factor that can modulate the biological effect of procarcinogens. Deconjugated bile salts may promote carcinogenesis through mucosal injury and enhanced epithelial proliferation.

These mechanisms could explain well-documented correlations between the intake of various dietary constituents and the incidence of colorectal cancer in certain populations (see Chapter 129). Populations that have a high fiber intake and resulting fast colonic transit times generally exhibit a lower incidence of colorectal cancer than populations with low fiber intake and delayed transit. The incidence of colorectal cancer in Japanese immigrants to the United States who consume a Western diet is much higher than that of native Japanese who consume a traditional Japanese diet.[94]

MOLECULAR MEDICINE: CURRENT AND FUTURE APPROACHES IN GASTROINTESTINAL ONCOLOGY

Next-Generation Sequencing

DNA sequencing relies on polymerase-mediated strand synthesis and the detection of the incorporated nucleotides throughout the successive steps of the chemical reaction, by a variety of physicochemical methods. The ability to monitor billions of reactions simultaneously, so-called massively parallel sequencing, along with the ability to computationally assemble short sequence reads into a continuous long read, have revolutionized sequencing technologies. These new approaches, often referred to as next-generation sequencing (NGS), are finding their way into the clinical care of patients with cancer in a variety of settings.[95] First, sequencing of germline DNA is increasingly used to define if a patient may have a cancer genetic syndrome. Second, these technologies can be applied to determine the mutational landscape of a tumor to guide treatment decisions.

The extent of DNA sequencing may involve the entire genome. Whole-genome sequencing uses DNA from a defined source without any step of enrichment or selection. Another method is to subject the sample to preliminary step of enrichment, where areas of interest are extracted from the sample, using hybridization methods and primer libraries, with the goal of decreasing the complexity of the sample and increasing the number of reads possible during the sequencing reaction. With greater number of reads available, so-called reading depth, the accuracy of sequencing increases and the cost is also reduced. The most common enrichment method is to focus on the areas of the genome known to harbor genes, collectively referred to as the exome, which corresponds to about 1% of the entire genome. For certain applications, subsets of genes from the entire exome may be the only ones enriched for sequencing, and this is the basis for NGS-based diagnostic tests that focus on gene panels relevant to cancer. Because NGS involves short reads that are computationally assembled into predicted long reads, this technology is insensitive to gene inversions, large insertions, or generally copy number variants that affect one allele.

Cancer and Tumor Genomics

As genetic information is obtained from sequencing analysis, understanding the potential impact of the genetic changes observed becomes an important challenge. *Single-nucleotide variants* refer to changes in a single base pair of the genetic code compared to a reference sequence. *Nonsense mutations* refer to the introduction of a premature stop codon. Single-nucleotide variants at splice-acceptor or donor sites may result in exon loss or misexpression of intronic sequences. These types of changes are relatively easy to interpret and adjudicate. Missense changes are those that result in a change in the amino acid encoded by the codon. Given the normal genetic variation present in the human population, understanding whether these changes are deleterious can be quite difficult to accomplish. When the effect of such variants is not known, these are referred to as "variants of unknown significance." Important limitations of exome sequencing at the present time include variants of unknown significance adjudication, detection of copy number variants and large rearrangements, and the potential for intronic or promoter mutations not detectable by exome capture strategies.

Molecular Diagnostics

Genetic testing is a powerful tool to identify high-risk families and define the cancer risk for individual family members. Today, sequencing panels that assess most of the genes associated with familial cancer syndromes are commercially available. Application of genetic testing must take into consideration the sensitivity and specificity of the assay as well as issues of patient confidentiality and potential impact on health and life insurance. Because these tests rely on target enrichment, it is important to be aware of their potential limitations. For these reasons, genetic counseling is an essential component of the genetic testing process.

In addition to genetic germline testing, molecular phenotyping of tumors for the purpose of guiding therapeutic decisions is important. To detect tumors due to defects in mismatch repair, testing for MSI can be performed on archived colon tumor samples.[96] In addition, loss of immunohistochemical staining for any of the four proteins required for mismatch repair (MLH1, PMS2, MSH2, and MSH6) may provide similar information. Studies have demonstrated that the MSI status of a colon tumor is predictive of the response to 5-fluorouracil–based chemotherapy.[97,98] More recently, it has been shown that mismatch repair–deficient tumors, due to their high burden of somatic mutations and tumor neoantigens, are highly responsive to immune checkpoint inhibition therapy.[99]

Therapies that target specific signaling pathways are likely to increase as our molecular understanding of GI cancers increases. Antibodies that target EGF receptors and block the EGF receptor signaling pathway have proved therapeutic benefit in colorectal cancer. However, their benefit has been shown only in cancers lacking activating mutations in *K-RAS*. Testing for *K-RAS* mutations in colorectal cancers is now the standard of care before the administration of such targeted therapy. In addition, small molecule tyrosine kinase inhibitors of the *c-KIT* oncogene now constitute routine treatment of GI stromal tumors (see Chapter 42).[100] Molecular techniques may also find a role in the staging of disease. For example, capture of small numbers of circulating tumor cells prior to the discovery of metastasis may yield prognostic and therapeutic benefits.[101] Finally, as more tests for genetic markers become available, monitoring for disease recurrence after surgery may become another important application.

Full references for this chapter can be found on https://ebooks.health.elsevier.com.

2 Mucosal Immunology and Inflammation

Charles O. Elson, Phillip D. Smith

IN THIS CHAPTER

Mucosal immunity refers to immune responses that occur at mucosal sites. The demands on the mucosal immune system are quite distinct from their systemic counterparts. At mucosal sites, the "outside world" is typically separated from the inner world by a single layer of epithelium. The mucosal immune system exists at a number of sites, including the intestinal tract, respiratory tract (especially the upper respiratory tract), urogenital tract, mammary glands, eyes, and ears. Each of these sites encounters a distinctive array of environmental stimuli and has evolved its own set of cell populations. Nevertheless, these different compartments can interact and share some cell populations and together form a common mucosal immune system. This chapter focuses on the intestinal mucosal immune system.[1]

The intestinal mucosa forms the largest compartment of the mucosal immune system and is unique in several aspects.[2] Relative to other mucosal sites, the intestine contains billions to trillions of microorganisms, including bacteria, fungi, and viruses. These organisms and their products, along with ingested food, represent an enormous antigenic load that must be tolerated to maintain mucosal homeostasis. This unusual environment and the demands associated with it have resulted in the development of a distinct immune system composed of inductive lymphoid follicles named *gut-associated lymphoid tissue* (GALT) and effector cells distributed in the epithelium [intraepithelial lymphocytes (IELs)] and in the lamina propria (LP) as mononuclear cells (LPMCs). Collectively, these cells comprise the largest number of cells in the immune system.

The specific characteristics and peculiarities of the mucosal immune cells reflect the unique milieu in which the cells function. To maintain mucosal homeostasis in the intestinal mucosa, one of the most important tasks of the immune system is to differentiate potentially harmful antigens such as pathogenic bacteria and toxins from products that may benefit the body such as molecules derived from food or commensal bacteria. To achieve homeostasis, cells, immunoglobulins (Igs), and secreted mediators function in a coordinated fashion. In contrast to the systemic immune system, whose focus is to act quickly within seconds of encountering a foreign antigen, the mucosal immune system is poised to respond but is predominantly tolerant, rejecting harmful antigens but allowing beneficial/harmless ones to persist without evoking harmful immune responses such as allergic reactions or inflammation.

Billions of activated plasma cells, memory T cells, memory B cells, macrophages, and dendritic cells (DCs) reside in the LP, but significant active inflammation is not present. This phenomenon has been called *controlled or physiologic inflammation* (Fig. 2.1). Importantly, entry of immune cells into the LP and cell activation is antigen-driven. Thus germ-free mice have few immune cells in their LP, but within hours to days after colonization with normal intestinal commensals, a massive influx and activation of cells occurs. A similar process begins in human neonates, whose intestine is colonized at birth, initiating the development of the mucosal immune system and stimulating innate and adaptive systemic immunity. The microbiota expands and changes in infancy, resulting in trillions of gut bacteria that are in communication with host cells in every GI organ and have profound effects on the intestinal vascular, nervous, and immune systems. Composition of the commensal microbiota during early childhood and adulthood is impacted by modern life influences, including birth by cesarean section rather than vaginal delivery, frequent exposure to antibiotics and diet.[52] Humans have coevolved with their microbiota and have developed multiple mechanisms of response, including intestinal epithelial cells (IECs) and innate, adaptive, and regulatory immune components.[24]

An abnormal composition of gut microbiota has been implicated in multiple metabolic and immune diseases, including IBD. Many, if not most, of the gene variants conferring susceptibility to IBD are linked to cells and functions involved in each of the components that regulate host-microbiota interactions.[25] The microbiota itself is the subject of Chapter 3. Despite the persistence of the antigenic drive of the intestinal microbiota, intestinal lymphocyte effector cells fail to develop into aggressive inflammation-producing cells. Bacteria or their products play a role in this persistent state of suspended activation[3] contributing to the control of inflammation in the intestinal mucosa.

IMMUNOGLOBULINS OF THE MUCOSAL SURFACE

IgA, an immunoregulatory antibody: Secretory IgA (SIgA) is the hallmark Ig in mucosal immune responses (Fig. 2.2). IgG is the most abundant isotype in the systemic immune system, whereas IgA is the most abundant antibody in mucosal secretions. Given the numbers of IgA^+ plasma cells and the 3–5 g of IgA produced daily in humans, IgA is the most abundant antibody in the body.

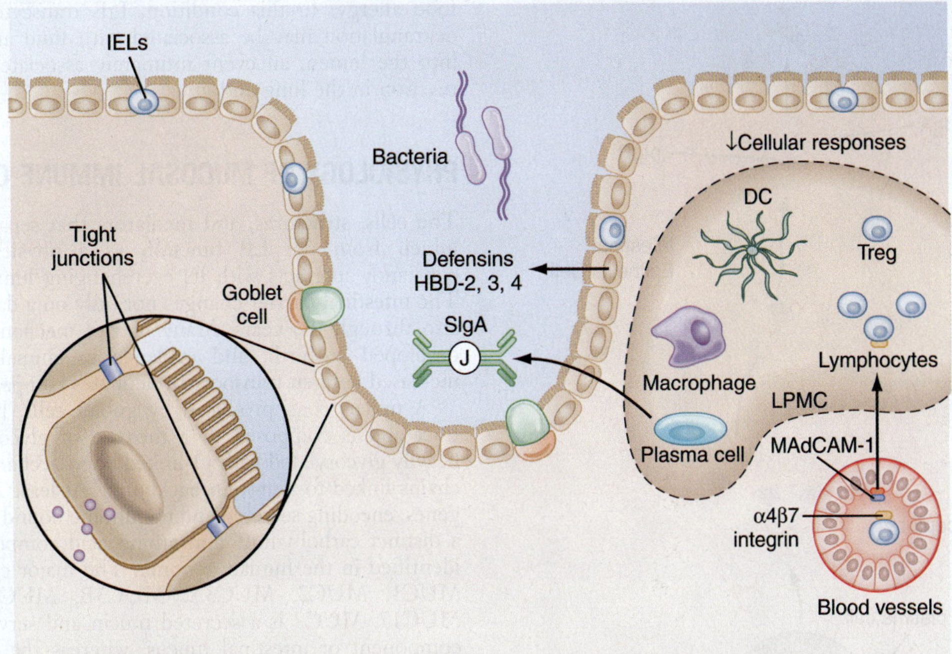

Fig. 2.1 Mechanisms for dampening mucosal immune responses. The intestine uses a number of distinct mechanisms to dampen mucosal immune responses. The major source of antigen in the intestine is the commensal bacterial flora, but both innate and adaptive responses control local responses. Physical barriers like mucins secreted by goblet cells and tight junctions between epithelial cells prevent invasion by luminal flora *(circle inset)*. Defensins like HBD-2, -3, and -4 are thought to maintain sterility of the crypt, whereas secretory immunoglobulin A produced by local plasma cells prevents attachment and invasion by luminal bacteria, thereby reducing antigenic load. Even with antigenic challenge, intestinal lymphocytes, macrophages, and dendritic cells are programmed to not respond as a consequence of decreased expression of pattern recognition receptors (e.g., Toll-like receptors) and a decrease in the ability of lymphocytes to be activated through their antigen receptor. Egress of circulating lymphocytes from blood vessels such as high endothelial venules is directed by the integrin α4β7, which recognizes the addressin MAdCAM-1, is also shown. *DC*, Dendritic cell; *HBD*, human β-defensin; *IELs*, intraepithelial lymphocytes; *LPMC*, lamina propria mononuclear cells; *MAdCAM*, mucosal addressin cell adhesion molecule; *SIgA*, secretory immunoglobulin A, a dimer with a connecting J chain; *Treg*, T regulatory cells (formerly known as *suppressor T cells*).

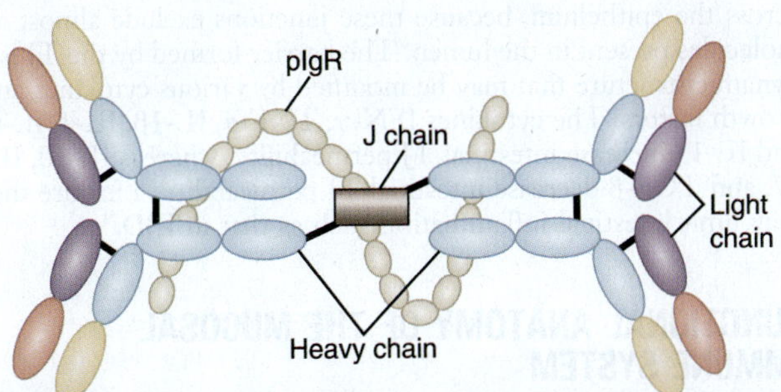

Fig. 2.2 Secretory immunoglobulin (Ig)A complex. Two IgA molecules are linked by a J chain and stabilized by polymeric Ig receptor (pIgR) to form dimeric secretory IgA. In humans there are two IgA subclasses, IgA1 and IgA2. IgA1 is predominant in serum and in milk.[79] Both subclasses are glycoslylated (not shown) but in different patterns that confer different effector functions.[80]

SIgA is a dimeric form of IgA produced by plasma cells in the LP and transported into the gut lumen through the intestinal epithelium by a specialized pathway (Fig. 2.3). Two IgA molecules (homodimers) are bound together by J chain (produced by plasma cells). Subsequently, the homodimer binds to a highly specialized glycoprotein, the *polymeric Ig receptor* (pIgR), a 55-kD glycoprotein produced by epithelial cells. The pIgR is expressed on the basolateral membrane of the IEC and binds only to dimeric IgA or IgM (also polymerized with J chain). Once bound to the pIgR on the IEC, SIgA is actively transported within vesicles to the apical membrane of the IEC. The vesicle fuses with the apical membrane, and a portion of the pIgR (secretory component) coupled to the IgA complex is released into the intestinal lumen. Within the lumen, secretory component serves to protect the SIgA dimer from degradation by luminal proteases and gastric acid.[4]

SIgA binds to mucus, enhancing its ability to bind and trap microbes and microbial products. In this and other ways, SIgA mediates the host microbiota interaction in the intestine.[77] In addition to its unique form, SIgA is also unusual in that it is anti-inflammatory in nature. It does not bind classical complement components but rather binds luminal bacterial antigens, preventing their uptake by epithelium and promoting their agglutination and subsequent removal. This process, referred to as "immune exclusion," includes agglutination, entrapment, and clearance of antigen due to specific interaction with the secreted antibody, as opposed to nonspecific mechanisms of exclusion exerted by the epithelium (e.g., mucus production, proteolytic digestion, defensin secretion). SIgA also may exert specific protective immunity against certain pathogens via more direct

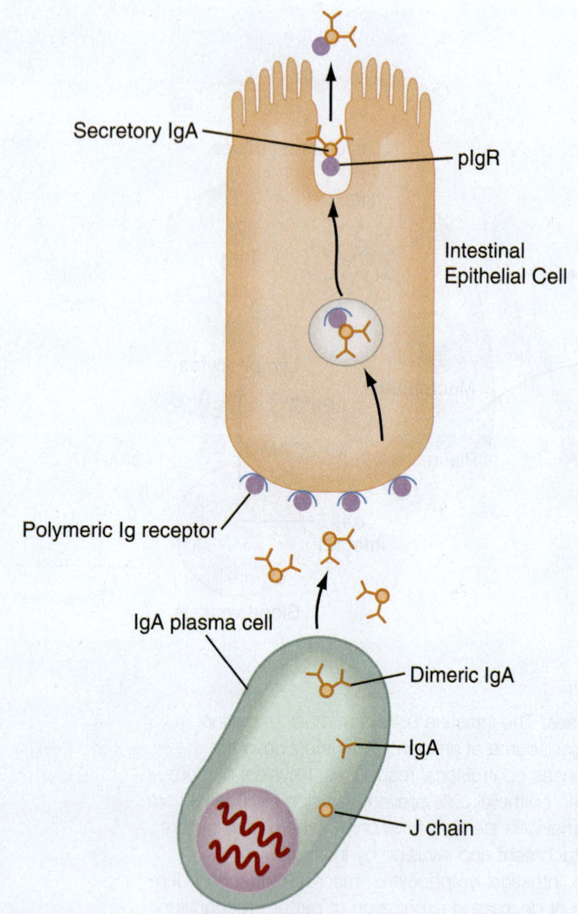

Fig. 2.3 Assembly and secretion of dimeric immunoglobulin A (*IgA*). IgA and J chain produced by IgA-committed plasma cells (*bottom*) dimerize to form polymeric IgA, which covalently binds to membrane-bound polymeric Ig receptor produced by intestinal epithelial cells (*top*). This complex is internalized, transported to the apical surface of epithelial cell, and secreted into the lumen. *pIgR*, Polymeric immunoglobulin receptor.

mechanisms such as the suppression of bacterial virulence, as well as nonantigen specific binding to bacterial glycan residues on free or bound pIgR, or the SIgA complex. M cells in Peyer patches (discussed later) selectively bind SIgA and SIgA immune complexes, and uptake of antigen-IgA complexes via M cells is a potential mechanism to dampen local inflammatory responses.

IgM is another antibody capable of binding the pIgR. Like IgA, IgM uses J chain produced by plasma cells to form polymers—in the case of IgM, a pentamer. pIgR binds to the Fc portion of the antibody formed during polymerization. The ability of IgM to bind pIgR may be important in patients with IgA deficiency, where secretory IgM compensates for the absence of IgA in the lumen.

SIgA is the major antibody isotype produced in the mucosa, but IgG is present in the mucosa as well. The neonatal Fc receptor (FcR_N) expressed by IECs can serve as a bidirectional transporter of IgG and is important in control of certain neonatal infections and IgG metabolism. In patients with IBD, marked increases in IgG within the LP and lumen have been detected.[5]

IgE production may play an important role in the intestinal response to helminths and in food allergy (see Chapter 11). CD23 (low-affinity IgE Fc receptor) has been reported to be expressed by gut epithelial cells, and one model has suggested that it may facilitate antigen uptake and resultant mast cell degranulation in food allergy. In this condition, IgE transcytosis and mast cell degranulation may be associated with fluid and electrolyte loss into the lumen, an event intimately associated with an allergic reaction in the lung and gut.

PHYSIOLOGY OF MUCOSAL IMMUNE CELLS

The cells, structures, and mediators that separate the intestinal lumen from the LP function as a physical barrier, which constantly interacts with its everchanging luminal environment. The intestinal barrier changes not only on a day-to-day basis but also through the years. Many barrier mechanisms are not fully developed at birth, and evidence in animal studies supports increased antigen transport in neonates compared to adults.

A mucus coat, produced by goblet cells, lines the intestinal tract and is composed of a mixture of glycoproteins (mucins) heavily glycosylated with O-linked oligosaccharides and *N*-glycan chains linked to a protein backbone.[6] At least 21 different mucin genes, encoding secreted and membrane bound mucins, each with a distinct carbohydrate and amino acid composition, have been identified in the human genome. The major colonic mucins are MUC1, MUC2, MUC3A, MUC3B, MUC4, MUC13, and MUC17. MUC2 is a secreted mucin and serves as the primary component of intestinal mucus, whereas the other mucins are membrane bound. The membrane-bound mucins participate in processes such as cell signaling, adhesion, growth, and immune modulation. Mucus protects the intestinal epithelium by several mechanisms, including its stickiness and competitive binding of its glycoprotein receptors to decrease microorganism penetration. In the colon there are two mucus layers, a loose outer layer containing bacteria and a dense inner layer devoid of bacteria.[7] The mucus stream also moves luminal contents away from epithelial cells. Further, intestinal infection and inflammation are associated with disruption or dysfunction of the mucus barrier, which may be accompanied by altered innate and adaptive host immune responses to the microbiota.

Below the mucus layer, the epithelium acts as a physical barrier that normally prevents antigen penetration through epithelial cells (the transcellular route) and through intercellular spaces (the paracellular route), the latter regulated by tight junction (TJ) complexes (e.g., zona occludens), and the subjunctional space. TJs have the greater role in preventing macromolecular diffusion across the epithelium, because these junctions exclude almost all molecules present in the lumen. The barrier formed by the TJ is a dynamic structure that may be modified by various cytokines and growth factors. The cytokines IFN-γ, TNF-α, IL-1β, IL-4, IL-6, and IL-13 increase intestinal TJ permeability, whereas IL-10, IL-17, and TGF-β decrease intestinal TJ permeability, a feature that may limit intestinal inflammation such as that in IBD.[9]

FUNCTIONAL ANATOMY OF THE MUCOSAL IMMUNE SYSTEM

Several key features of the mucosal immune system facilitate the maintenance of homeostasis and clearance of pathogens. The mucosal immune system is comprised of inductive and effector compartments. Peyer patches and other lymphoid follicles comprise the inductive compartment and are known as GALT. Lymphoid cells in the epithelium (IELs) and the LP [LP lymphocytes (LPLs)] are innate and antigen-experienced memory cells, and comprise the effector compartment. Cell populations and the immune response in the epithelium, subepithelium, LP, Peyer patches, and mesenteric lymph nodes (MLNs) may differ substantially. Cells residing in these compartments differ not only topographically but also phenotypically and functionally.

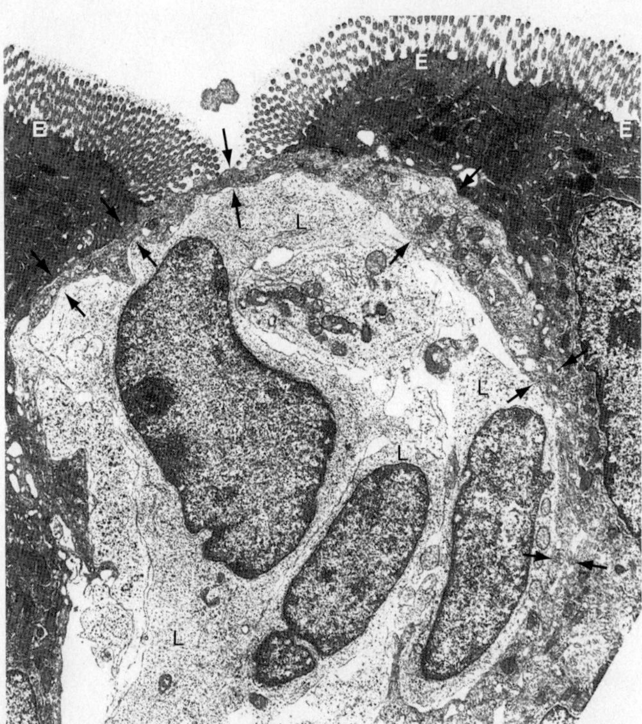

Fig. 2.4 M cell. Transmission electron micrograph from noncolumnar region of a Peyer patch epithelium shows a cross-sectional view of a microfold (M) cell, as well as associated microvillus-covered intestinal epithelial cells and at least 3 lymphoid cells *(L)*. Note the attenuated cytoplasm of the M cell *(between arrows)* that bridges the surface between microvillus-covered epithelial cells, forming tight junctions with them and producing a barrier between lymphoid cells and the intestinal lumen (×9600). *B*, B cell; *E*, intestinal epithelial cell. (From Owen RL, Jones AL. Epithelial cell specialization within human Peyer's patches: an ultrastructural study of intestinal lymphoid follicles. *Gastroenterology*. 1974;66:189–203.)

Peyer Patches and M Cells

The follicle-associated epithelium (FAE) is a specialized epithelium overlying the Peyer patch and isolated lymphoid follicles. The M (microfold) cells in the FAE, in contrast to the adjacent absorptive epithelium, have few microvilli, a limited mucin overlayer, a thin elongated cytoplasm, and a shape that forms a pocket surrounding subepithelial lymphocytes, macrophages, T cells, B cells, and DCs (Fig. 2.4). M cells are highly specialized for phagocytosis and transcytosis, and are capable of taking up large particulate antigens from the lumen and transporting them intact into the subepithelial space.[10] These cells contain few lysosomes, and thus little or no processing of antigen occurs. The apical surface of M cells expresses several unique lectin-like molecules that help promote binding to specific pathogens such as poliovirus, *Shigella flexneri*, and *Listeria monocytogenes*. Antigens that bind to the M cell and are transported to the underlying Peyer patches, or to adjacent epithelial cells in the case of *S. flexneri* or *L. monocytogenes*, generally elicit a positive (SIgA) response.[38] Thus M cells appear to be critical for the initial positive aspects of mucosal immunity. However, certain pathogens or their toxins may exploit M cells and use M cell transcytosis to penetrate the intestinal mucosa.

The M cell is a conduit to Peyer patches and lymphoid follicles. Antigens transcytosed across the M cell and into the subepithelial pocket are taken up by macrophages and DCs and carried into the Peyer patch. Once antigens enter the Peyer patch, TGF-β-secreting T cells promote B cell isotype switching to IgA. Induction of M cell differentiation from conventional epithelial cells is dependent on direct contact between the epithelium and Peyer patch lymphocytes,[10] mediated, at least in part, by the stromal RANKL activating TRAF6 and by lymphotoxin. M cells are not present in B cell–deficient animals, which lack Peyer patches nor are they present in mice lacking the TRAF6 gene. Peyer patches have T cell–dependent areas and B cell–dependent/germinal centers typical of lymph nodes but only efferent lymphatics.

After activation in the Peyer patch, lymphocytes are induced to express α4β7 integrin that provides a homing signal for mucosal sites where the endothelial ligand is MadCAM-1.[11,12] Lymphocytes exit the Peyer patch, traffic to the MLN, and then the thoracic duct, into the main intestinal lymphatic drainage system, which empties into the circulation (Fig. 2.5). There, mucosally activated cells circulate in the bloodstream to exit in high endothelial venules in various mucosal sites. B cells can reenter Peyer's patches germinal centers where further Ig mutation and affinity maturation occurs.[81] Cells bearing α4β7 molecules exit in the LP, where they then undergo terminal differentiation. Chemokines and their receptors (discussed later) as well as adhesion molecules and ligands help direct this trafficking pattern.

Intestinal Epithelial Cells

The intestinal epithelium is composed of a single layer of columnar cells that separates the luminal contents from the subepithelial LP. IECs originate from self-renewing $Lgr5^+$ stem cells at the base of the crypt in close proximity to Wnt factor-producing stromal cells, referred to as the stem cell zone.[51] Epithelial stem cells migrate up the villus and differentiate into absorptive or secretory epithelial cells, goblet cells, Paneth cells, enteroendocrine cells, Tuft cells, and M cells. The canonical Wnt/β-catenin pathway proteins regulate cell proliferation and the noncanonical pathway proteins regulate cell migration, thereby contributing to the maintenance of the intestinal epithelial population; mutations in the Wnt/β-catenin pathway disrupts homeostasis and are associated with the adenomatosis polyposis syndrome and the initiation of colon cancer.[35] Under normal circumstances, IECs have a 4-5 day life cycle before being sloughed into the lumen and replaced by newly arrived epithelial cells that differentiate as they migrate up the villus.

In addition to its role in selective absorption and secretion (see Chapter 103), the intestinal epithelium plays a fundamental role in mucosal immunity, despite epithelial cells being non-hematopoietic cells. The immune function of IECs is reflected in the wide array of regulatory and cytokine genes identified in the epithelium during conditions of homeostasis and pathogen challenge.[42] The role of the epithelium in mucosal immunity includes barrier function, pathogen recognition, recruitment of innate immune cells, and modulation of adaptive immune cells. The epithelial barrier is critical for maintaining mucosal homeostasis and deterring the entry of commensal microbiota, enteric pathogens, and foreign antigens. Barrier function is aided by soluble antimicrobial proteins such as α-defensins produced by Paneth cells (see below), β-defensins produced by epithelial cells, and mucus produced by goblet cells. The integrity of the barrier is maintained by both the epithelial cells and their intercellular TJs, which occlude the intercellular space and regulate solute transport. TJ proteins on the lateral epithelial cell surface are composed of claudins, zonal occludens, and other occludens, the function of which is facilitated by lateral adherens junctions and desmosomes.[8] TJs are the target of some pathogenic bacteria, including *Clostridioides difficile*, *Bacteroides fragilis*, and *Vibrio cholerae*. Mouse studies indicate that subepithelial DC extensions (dendrites) express junctional proteins, and can penetrate the junctional space and take up luminal bacteria.[35]

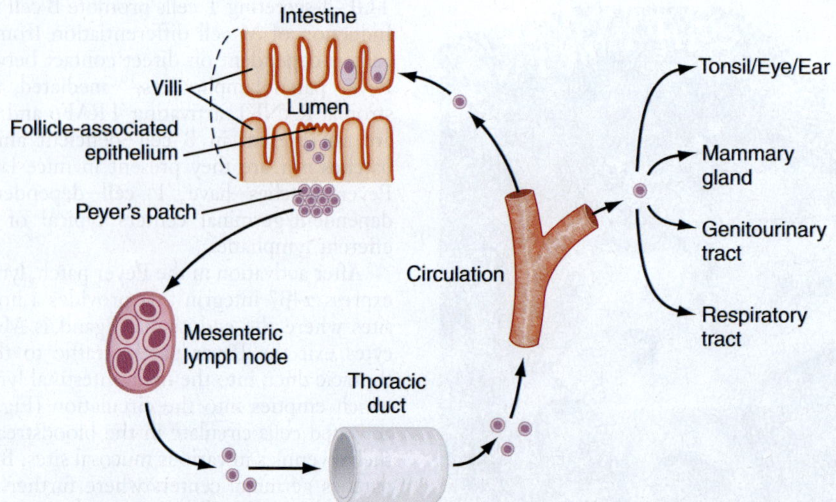

Fig. 2.5 Mucosal lymphocyte migration. Following antigenic stimulation, T and B lymphocytes migrate from the intestine (Peyer patch) to the draining mesenteric lymph nodes, where they further differentiate and then reach the systemic circulation via the thoracic duct. Cells bearing appropriate mucosal addressin then selectively home to mucosal surfaces that constitute the common mucosa-associated lymphoid tissue, including the intestinal immune system.

The polarized intestinal epithelium expresses an array of receptors that facilitate microbe recognition. Toll-like receptors (TLRs) 1–9, which detect conserved microbe and pathogen-associated molecular patterns (PAMPs; see below), are expressed by human IECs, although TLR4 is expressed constitutively at low levels. The cells also express nucleotide-binding oligomerization domain-containing proteins 1 and 2 (NOD1,2), which detect components of bacterial peptidoglycans. The signaling pathways linked to these receptors, including NF-κB, induce the expression of inflammatory cytokines and chemokines.[36] Epithelial cell sialic acid, histo-blood group antigens, heat shock cognate proteins, and cell-surface integrins may serve as attachment molecules and/or coreceptors for viruses such as rotavirus.[49] Finally, neonatal Fc receptor (FcRn) bidirectionally transports IgG across epithelial cells, delivering Ig-bound antigen to the mucosal immune system. Through these receptor and attachment mechanisms, luminal pathogens induce a wide array of proinflammatory cytokines and chemokines that recruit LP immune cells,[44] thereby augmenting epithelial cell-induced inflammatory responses. IECs also appear to play a key role in mucosal homeostasis through microbiota-induced release of epithelial cell thymic stromal lymphopoietin, which drives tolerogenic DCs that release IL-10 and the IgA regulatory cytokine IL-6.[40] The pleotropic function of IECs is further reflected in the cells' expression of major histocompatibility complex (MHC) class I and II molecules, supporting antigen presentation to $CD8^+$ T cells and $CD4^+$ T cells, respectively. In addition to the direct microbe stimulation of epithelial cells, luminal microbes and antigens are presented to subepithelial immune cells by specialized follicle-associated M cells, goblet cell-associated passages (GAPs) (see below) and TJ-penetrating DC dendrites (see above). Thus through multiple mechanisms, the functionally versatile intestinal epithelium plays a key role in the induction of innate and adaptive mucosal responses to luminal antigens.

Paneth Cells

Paneth cells are a secretory population derived from epithelial stem cells and reside in the base of the crypts in the small intestine.[10] These cells can readily be identified on stains due to the large eosinophilic granules that occupy most of their cytoplasm (see Chapter 100). These granules contain high concentrations of antimicrobial peptides, including α-defensins, lysozyme, C-type lectins, and phospholipase-A2. They secrete these antimicrobial peptides into the lumen of the crypt, thus keeping it relatively sterile. Defensins are released upon stimulation by various bacterial ligands, including endotoxin, which induce Paneth cells via TLRs and nuclear oligomerization domain 2 (NOD2). Paneth cells colocalize with stem cells at the base of crypts and have been shown to provide important factors preserving stem cell function in addition to the antimicrobial peptides. Paneth cell development is regulated by transcription factors in the WNT pathway and the NOD signaling cascade such as the transcription factor MATH-1. A transcriptional repressor, GFI-1, is important in Paneth cell development by suppressing a proenteroendocrine cell transcription factor, neurogenin-3 (NEUROG3). Decreased numbers of Paneth cells and of defensins 5 and 6 are associated with ileal Crohn disease. Because of their highly secretory nature with strong synthesis of various molecules, Paneth cells are dependent on the unfolded protein response to maintain intracellular homeostasis. Interference with the unfolded protein response in mice has led to ileitis.[13,14]

Goblet Cells

Goblet cells are a secretory type of epithelial cell that is specialized in the production of mucins and other molecules. Two types of mucin layers are present in the gut. One is an unattached or loose layer, which is characteristic of the small intestine. The second mucus layer, which is attached and impenetrable to bacteria, is present in the distal colon. In addition to their physical properties, mucins interact with antimicrobial peptides to maintain a high concentration of the latter close to the epithelium. A variety of cytokines increase MUC2 expression, including IL-1β, IL-4, IL-6, IL-13, and TNF-α. Several metalloproteinases, including ADAM-10 and ADAM-17, as well as meprin-23, are involved in the release of mucin proteins into the intestinal lumen. Goblet cells also selectively produce trefoil factor-3 (TFF-3), which can influence mucus viscosity and is important in epithelial repair after injury. Mice deficient in TFF-3 are highly susceptible to dextran sulfate sodium (DSS) colitis due to an inability to heal the lesions. Innate immune cells also interact with goblet cells increasing their number by stimulating enterocytes to differentiate into goblet cells. ILC2-derived IL-13 and ILC3-derived IL-22 have been implicated in increasing goblet cell hyperplasia and mucin production.

Goblet cells also serve to transmit antigen across the epithelial layer through goblet-associated antigen passages (GAPs). This function is achieved through an acetylcholine-dependent endocytic event in which soluble cargo is delivered by transcytosis across the cell, a pathway separate from that of mucin secretion.[45] Soluble antigens and bacteria have been shown to cross goblet cells and be presented to subjacent CD103^{+} CX3CR1— tolerogenic DCs. CD103^{+} DCs then migrate to the MLN where they induce antigen-specific T regulatory (Treg) cells. Thus GAPs appear to contribute to the maintenance of intestinal homeostasis.[27]

Tuft Cells

Tuft cells are a type of epithelial cell that is infrequent in the normal intestine but are increased in number during parasite infection. Tuft cells are identified by a distinct morphology, characterized by microvilli projecting from the apical membrane, and a distinguishing genotype, characterized by ATOH1 and Neurog 3 expression. Tuft cells express genes associated with taste receptors (see Chapter 4) and are able to discern helminths in the intestinal lumen via these chemosensors. Tuft cells produce the cytokine IL-25, which activates type 2 innate lymphoid cells (ILC2) to produce IL-13 that in turn stimulates mucin production and helps clear the parasite. ILC2-produced IL-13 provides a positive feedback loop by increasing the number of tuft cells.[15,16]

Recognition of Pathogen-Associated Molecular Patterns by Pattern Recognition Receptors

Classical antigen-presenting cells (APCs) in the systemic immune system possess the innate capacity to recognize highly conserved PAMPs on bacteria and viruses. Receptors for PAMPs are expressed on both the APC surface, including TLR1-2 (senses peptidoglycan), TLR6-2 (triacylated lipoproteins), TLR4 [lipopolysaccharide (LPS)] and TLR5 (flagellin), and intracellularly, including TLR3 (dsRNA), TLR7 (ssRNA), TLR8 (G-rich oligonucleotides) and TLR9 (CpG oligonucleotide), and the nucleotide-binding oligomerization domains 1 and 2 (NOD1,2; bacterial peptidoglycan derivatives).[53] Although IECs are exposed to large numbers of luminal bacteria, they retain the ability to recognize many components of these bacteria. IEC proinflammatory responses are downregulated in the normal setting. For example, IECs do not respond to bacteria LPS due to the absence of TLR4, the LPS receptor. However, the expression of other pattern recognition receptors (PRRs) is maintained, including expression of TLR5. TLR5 is expressed basolaterally and is positioned to identify organisms such as *Salmonella* species that have invaded the epithelial layer.[17] After invasion and engagement of TLR5, the intestinal epithelium is induced to secrete a broad array of cytokines and chemokines that attract inflammatory cells to the local environment to control the spread of infection.

Intracellular NOD1 and NOD2 have been shown to contribute to intestinal inflammation. About 25% of Crohn disease patients have mutations in the NOD2/CARD15 gene, interfering with their ability to mount an appropriate immune response to bacterial stimuli (see Chapter 117). In addition, TLRs that are normally weakly expressed by IECs are expressed at higher levels on IECs from patients with IBD. Expression of different TLRs by IECs, as well as their contribution to innate and adaptive T and B cell responses in both intestinal inflammation and homeostasis, has been demonstrated in several murine models.

In contrast, some bacteria induce anti-inflammatory cytokine production (e.g., IL-10) and increase expression of peroxisome proliferator—activated receptor-γ by IECs. Furthermore, other bacterial products (e.g., from *Bacteroides thetaiotaomicron*) help promote the barrier and IEC differentiation.

ANTIGEN PRESENTATION IN THE GUT

Effective immune responses to antigenic proteins require the help of T lymphocytes. This in turn depends on the antigen being presented by APCs that internalize, digest, and couple a small fragment of the antigen to a surface MHC heterodimer that eventually interacts with either CD4^{+} T-cell receptor (TCR) (MHC class II) or CD8^{+} TCR (MHC class I). Multiple cells in the intestinal mucosa can act as APCs, including DCs, macrophages, epithelial cells, and B cells. The ability of these cells to present antigen to CD4 T cells depends on the expression of class II MHC molecules on their surface, which are present on the epithelium of the normal small intestine but to a lesser extent colonocytes in both humans and rodents. In vitro studies have demonstrated that isolated enterocytes from rat and human small intestine can present antigens to previously primed T cells, raising the possibility that the intestinal IECs may present peptides to T cells that are localized below the epithelium. Thus IECs are capable of both antigen processing and presentation in the appropriate context to cells within the LP. Interestingly, bidirectional lymphocyte-epithelial crosstalk exists in the LP, and LPLs promote mucosal barrier function via Notch-1 signaling and induction of IEC differentiation, polarization, and barrier function. Importantly, increased expression of MHC class II molecules by IECs has been reported in IBD, which likely increases the potential of IECs to activate lymphocytes. In the setting of epithelial cell injury or loss, as in Crohn disease, microbe-epithelial cell—DC crosstalk is replaced by a microbe—stromal cell—DC crosstalk in which luminal microbes induce a potent inflammatory response by subepithelial stromal cells.[39]

Interestingly, drugs used to treat IBD (e.g., 5-aminosalicylate preparations) may reduce IEC MHC class II expression. In addition to MHC class II expression, IECs in normal subjects and IBD patients express a variety of costimulatory molecules required for T-cell activation (see Fig. 2.6). These molecules include intercellular adhesion molecule (ICAM)-1, which binds to leukocyte function associated antigen (LFA)-l on the T cell and ICOS ligand and PD-L1. CD86 (B7-2), which binds to CD28 and CTLA-4, is expressed by IECs in ulcerative colitis. Interestingly, unique expression of these costimulatory molecules by IECs may be involved in the distinct regulation of mucosal responses. Small intestinal IECs do not express CD80 (B7-1), and thus activation of naïve T cells by IECs is improbable. However, increased expression during intestinal inflammation may serve to augment T-cell stimulation. Understanding antigen presentation by IECs has important clinical implications, exemplified by the critical role of epithelial MHC class II expression in the initiation of lethal graft-versus-host-disease (GVHD) in a mouse model and the prevention of GVHD by therapeutically neutralizing macrophage p12/23p40, which regulates ileal epithelial MHC class II expression.[47]

MHC class I and nonclassical class I molecules are also expressed by IECs. Thus antigen presentation to certain T cell populations is possible and has been reported by several groups. Specifically, CD1d expressed on human IECs is able to present antigen (in a complex with CEACAM5) to CD8^{+} T cells. CD1d-restricted natural killer T (NKT) cells, effector memory cells that share characteristics of innate and adaptive lymphocytes, are among the earliest responders in immune reactions and affect activation of other immune cell lineages such as natural killer (NK) cells, T cells, and B cells. NKT cells participate in immune

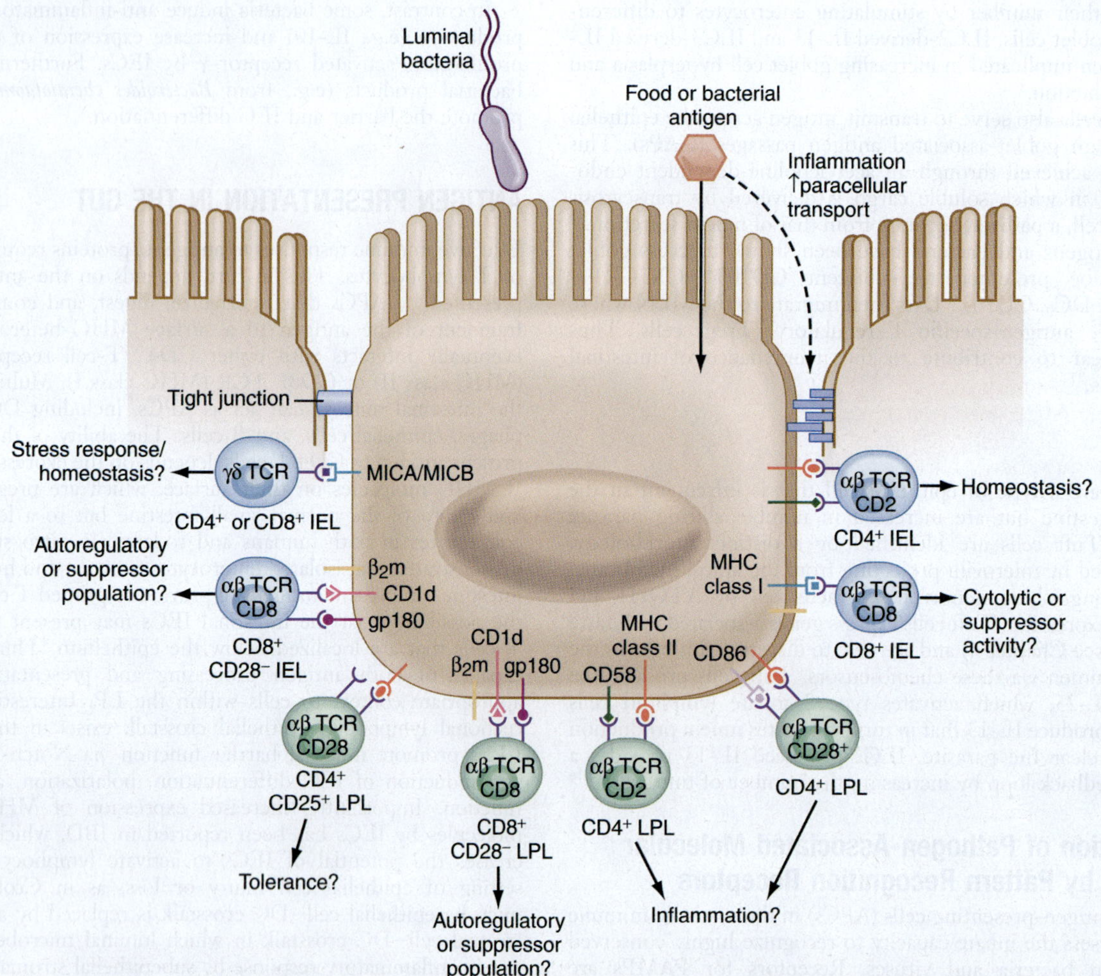

Fig. 2.6 A normal intestinal epithelial cell (IEC). The IEC is shown to express classic MHC molecules (classes I and II) that have the potential to present conventional antigen to local T-cell populations and a broad array of nonclassic class I molecules [e.g., CD1d, MICA/MICB, and β2m (shown in the figure) and MR-1, ULBP, and HLA-E], which have the potential to present unconventional antigens to unique T-cell populations. In addition, alternate pathways of activation appear to be functional in the intestine (e.g., activation via a CD58-CD2 interaction), and classic costimulatory molecules are not expressed on IECs, although CD86 may be induced in patients with UC. Other members of the B7 family are expressed, such as PO-L1 (CD274) and ICOS-L (CD275), and may play a role in local T-cell activation. β2 microglobulin (β2m) associates with MHC class I, CD1d, HLA-E, HLA-G, and FcRn. *β2m*, β2 microglobulin; *gp180*, membrane glycoprotein 180 (a CD8 ligand); *IEL*, intraepithelial lymphocyte; *LPL*, lamina propria lymphocyte; *MHC*, major histocompatibility complex; *MICA/MICB*, MHC class I-related chains A and B; *TCR*, T-cell receptor.

responses in infectious, malignant, and immune-mediated diseases. Other nonclassical class I molecules are expressed by IECs. The role of MICA, a stress-induced MHC-related molecule expressed on normal IECs and recognized by the NKG2D-activating receptor on $CD8^+$ T cells, T cells, and NK cells, may be of specific importance, since Crohn disease patients have increased numbers of $CD4^+NKG2D^+$ T cells with a Th1 cytokine profile in the intestinal mucosa.

In humans, IECs activate $CD8^+$ Treg cells that are involved in local tolerance and interaction with $CD8^+$ IECs. The role of IECs in the regulation of mucosal immunity is best demonstrated in studies with IBD tissues. IECs derived from IBD patients, in contrast to those derived from normal subjects, stimulate $CD4^+$ T cells *in vitro* rather than regulatory $CD8^+$ cells. Furthermore, oral antigen administration does not result in tolerance in IBD patients but causes active immunity.

EFFECTOR COMPARTMENTS WITHIN THE GUT IMMUNE SYSTEM

Two lymphocyte populations, IELs and LPLs, reside in the intestinal mucosa. The compartmentalization of these two distinct cell populations correlates with their ability to respond to distinct microenvironmental cues.[80]

Intraepithelial Lymphocytes

IELs form one of the main branches of the intestinal immune system, balancing protective immunity with support of epithelial barrier integrity. In the small intestine, IELs are more than 98% T cells and mostly $CD8^+$, including $CD8^+\alpha$ T cells, as well as $CD4^+CD8^+$ double-positive, and $CD4^-CD8^-$ double-negative cells. IELs contain T cells expressing the γδ TCR. Roughly half of murine small bowel IELs express the $\gamma\delta$ TCR, whereas both the murine and human large intestine contain primarily $\alpha\beta$ $CD4^+$ or $\alpha\beta$ $CD8^+$ T cells similar to those present in the systemic immune system.

Based on their phenotype, IELs are classified into two subsets: *induced IELs* (iIELs),[82] including TCR$\alpha\beta$ T cells selected in the thymus by conventional MHC class I and II, and *natural IELs* (*nIELs*), including TCR$\alpha\beta$ $CD8^+\alpha\alpha$, TCR$\gamma\delta$ double-positive, and TCR$\gamma\delta$ double-negative cells.[18] Both iIEL and nIEL are cytolytic, killing via granzyme or by engagement of Fas, and secrete Th1 cytokines. However, iIELs can transfer protection against a variety of pathogenic organisms, whereas nIELs are unable to transfer immunologic protection, and do not possess immunologic memory. This difference may be due to nIEL activation by IECs in situ by nonclassical MHC molecules rather than by the polymorphic MHC-expressed molecules on professional APCs that activate iIELs. Both IEL subsets express NK cell molecules. IELs express a variety of activation markers and are $CD45RO^+$ (memory cells). IELs also express the integrin or CD103, which is induced by TGF-β and binds to E-cadherin on IECs. Isolated, IELs are difficult to activate through their TCR and barely proliferate, even in response to potent stimuli, and may be activated by alternative pathways (e.g., via CD2).

A broad spectrum of cytokines are produced by IELs, including IFN-γ, TNF-α, IL-2, IL-4, IL-6, IL-10, TGF-β, keratinocyte growth factor, and IL-17, with important effects on intestinal barrier function and local immune responses.

Functionally, IELs kill epithelial cells that have undergone stress due to infection, transformation, or invasion by other cells. IELs have been proposed to suppress local immune cells, although the evidence that they actually function in luminal antigen recognition is weak. IELs do not traffic in and out of the epithelium. Rather, epithelial cells move over the IELs as the epithelial cells move from the crypt to the villus surface. IELs appear to serve as beneficial sentinels for epithelial integrity but can be pathogenic, that is, IELs cause cytolysis of stressed epithelial cells contributing to the mucosal damage in celiac disease.

Lamina Propria Lymphocytes and Mononuclear Cells

The LP is the major effector site in gut mucosa, containing an abundance of antigen-experienced memory T cells and B cells. Clearly, the mucosal LP operates under a distinct set of rules compared to the systemic immune system, reflected in its functional anatomy (no organized structure) and its responses and regulation. Highly specialized cells mediate these effects, some detected only in the LP.

LP mononuclear cells (LPMCs) are a heterogeneous group of cells[80] (see Fig. 2.1). A prevalent cell type is the IgA^+ plasma cell but more than 50% of LPMCs are T cells and B cells in addition to macrophages and DCs. In contrast to IELs, LPLs express the mucosal addressin α4β7, but similar to IELs, LPLs express an activated memory phenotype and proliferate poorly in response to engagement of the TCR. Alternate pathways of LPL activation are mainly through CD2 and CD28.

In the healthy mucosa, LPMCs do not respond to antigen stimulation via the TCR and have an increased tendency to undergo apoptosis if activated inappropriately, dampening responses to normal luminal contents. The mechanism underlying the increased apoptosis may relate to engagement of the death receptor Fas and its ligand on activated LPLs, and the imbalance between the intracellular anti- and proapoptotic factors, Bcl2 and Bax. Defects in this proapoptotic balance have been reported in Crohn disease.

Together, the above-described mechanisms and others contribute to *controlled/physiologic inflammation*, which characterizes healthy intestinal mucosa. When regulatory mechanisms are disrupted, *uncontrolled inflammation* occurs, as in the mucosa of patients with IBD.

T-Cell Differentiation

In GALT (see Fig. 2.5), B and T lymphocytes interact with antigen. Activation and maturation of T lymphocytes from naïve Th0 cells to distinct Th subpopulations is strongly influenced by the microenvironment, particularly the microbiota, and by responses to pathogens.[19] Viral infections induce CD4 Th1 cells, whereas parasitic colonization induces the $CD4^+$ Th2 subset. $CD4^+$ Th17 effector cells respond to extracellular bacteria and fungi. The microbiota shapes the mucosal T-cell response. For example, in mice, the commensal known as segmented filamentous bacteria (*Candidatus arthromitus*) selectively induces Th17 CD4 cells.

DCs, professional APCs within the GALT, and their secreted mediators skew T lymphocytes to one of several effector cells. Th1 cells secreting IL-2, IFN-γ, and TNF-α develop when DCs secrete IL-12, which induces activation and phosphorylation of the transcription factor STAT-4 (signal transducer and activator of transcription factor 4). STAT-4 in turn induces IFN-γ expression and production. IFN-γ induces activation of STAT-1, and consequently of T-bet (T box expressed in T cells), which is the master transcription factor that induces Th1 cytokine and IL-12 receptor β2 production, while simultaneously suppressing Th2 cytokine production. Thus a cycle promoting Th1 and suppressing Th2 responses is created. Activation of T-bet is possibly an essential step for Th1-mediated mucosal diseases, such as those seen in some patients with Crohn disease. Another important Th1-promoting cytokine is IL-18. IL-18 mediates its effects on T cells through augmentation of IL-12Rβ2 chain expression, AP-1(c-fos/c-jun)-dependent transactivation of the IFN-γ promoter, and activation of NF-κB (nuclear factor κB).

In contrast, when IL-4 is secreted by DCs or other mucosal cells, Th2 cytokine production (IL-4, IL-5, IL-6, IL-9, IL-10, IL-13) occurs by the activation of STAT-6 followed by activation of the master transcription factor GATA-3. GATA-3 is capable of promoting the expression of several Th2 cytokines, including IL-4, IL-5, and IL-13. In addition to IL-4, IL-13 also plays an important role in Th2 development and IgE synthesis in an IL-4-independent fashion. These cytokines appear to contribute to the development of food allergies (see Chapter 10). IL-5 induces B cells expressing surface IgA to differentiate into IgA-producing plasma cells. IL-6 causes a marked increase in IgA secretion, with little effect on either IgM or IgG synthesis.

A third important LP CD4 subset is Th17 cells. The Th1-polarizing cytokine IL-12, composed of the p40 and p35 subunits, has similarities with the Th17-polarizing cytokine IL-23, composed of p40 and a unique p19 subunit. The possibility that some of the inflammatory activity previously attributed to an IL-12–driven Th1 pathway might actually be an IL-23-driven Th17 pathway was supported by studies showing that intestinal inflammation was still possible when IL-12 was inhibited, and that inhibition of IL-23, rather than IL12, ameliorated inflammation. In IBD, the expression of both IL-12 and IL-23 is increased, and inhibition of the common p40 subunit of IL-12 and IL-23, and of IL-23p19 is beneficial in the clinical treatment of both Crohn disease and ulcerative colitis patients. Th17 cells express retinoid-related orphan receptor-γt (RORγt), which is the master transcription factor for these cells. In addition to RORγt, human Th17 cells express IL-23R, CCR6, and CD161, whereas they lack CXCR3, a chemokine receptor characteristic of Th1 cells. The main effector cytokines secreted by Th17 cells are IL-17A, IL-17F, IL-21, IL-22, IL-26, TNF-α, and the chemokine CCL20. Human Th17 cells differentiate under the influence of IL-1β, IL-6, IL-21, IL-23, and TGF-β. In humans, not all Th17 cells produce IL-22, and a Th22 subset of CD4 helper T cells that produces IL-22, but not IL-17 has been identified. IL-17 promotes recruitment and activation of neutrophils, whereas IL-22 promotes mucosal healing through epithelial proliferation, increased epithelial antimicrobial peptide and mucus production.

Regulatory T cells (Tregs) are abundant in the intestine and, similar to CD4 effector cells, are also comprised of subsets, which are distributed unevenly along the length of the bowel, reflecting the different microenvironment.[26] The major Treg subset expresses the transcription factor, Foxp3. Foxp3$^+$ Tregs are generated in the thymus (tTreg) and are also called "natural Tregs." Foxp3$^+$ Tregs also can be generated in the periphery from naïve CD4 T cells and are termed "peripheral Tregs" (pTreg) or induced Tregs. A subset of pTregs is present in colonic mucosa in humans and mice and express the transcription factor RORγt, typical of Th17 cells. Interestingly, the Foxp3$^+$ RORγt$^+$ Treg cells are induced in suckling mice by the microbiota, which is taken up via goblet-associated passages.[27] Foxp3–T regulatory 1 cells (Tr1) are also present in gut mucosa in fairly high abundance and selectively produce high amounts of IL-10. Foxp3$^+$ Tregs produce TGF-β only or TGF-β plus IL-10 as their inhibitory effector cytokines.

Certain microbiota or their products can induce the different types of Tregs in mice. For example, the polysaccharide A component of *B. fragilis* selectively induces Foxp3$^+$ IL-10$^+$ CD4 T cells.[28,29] An assortment of microbiota *Clostridia* has been shown to induce Foxp3$^+$ Tregs in mouse colonic mucosa,[30] and this effect is at least partially due to the production of short-chain fatty acids (SCFAs; acetate, propionate, and butyrate) that these organisms produce during fermentation. SCFAs have genome-encoded receptors on innate and adaptive immune cells in mice, which tend to dampen immune responses. Humans have the same SCFA receptors and presumably have similar Treg responses to the SCFA.[31–34] SCFAs such as butyrate, rather than glucose, are the major nutritional fuel of enterocytes. Thus the depletion of bacteria producing SCFA, which has been identified in IBD, could have multiple detrimental effects, both on the epithelium and on Treg function. In mice, deficiency of the effector cytokines of Tregs, such as TGF-β and IL-10, results in colitis. Deficiency of IL-10 and/or its receptor, by inactivating mutations in humans, results in early onset IBD.[35] Tregs and their effector cytokines are thus crucial for maintaining homeostasis in the intestine by controlling pathogenic innate and adaptive responses.

The biology of T-cell lineages in the LP is complex, related in part to the plasticity of these cell populations. Under specific circumstances, Th17 cells may become Th1 cells. Moreover, regulatory Foxp3$^+$ cells expressing Th17 cytokines and having potent suppressor activity *in vitro* were recently identified in humans. These findings suggest that a degree of plasticity *in vivo* exists in all known T-cell subsets, reflected in their capacity to produce specific cytokines depending on the microenvironment. Th17 cells play a homeostatic role in gut mucosa,[20] which may explain the failure of anti–IL-17A monoclonal antibody therapy in active Crohn disease. Addressing the complexity of the LP milieu with its vast amounts of mediators and effectors, including the microbiota, will likely contribute to better designed therapeutic strategies to modify intestinal inflammation.

Innate Lymphoid Cells

The recently identified innate lymphoid cells (ILCs) produce T helper (Th) cell–associated cytokines but do not express a TCR or cell-surface markers that are associated with other immune cell lineages. Thus ILCs are lineage marker-negative, and their immune response is not antigen-specific. ILCs are effectors of innate immunity and regulators of tissue modeling. ILCs have several subpopulations with distinct cytokine expression patterns that resemble the helper T-cell subsets Th1, Th2, and Th17.[21]

Group 1 ILCs include ILC1 cells and NK cells. ILC1 cells express the transcription factor T-bet and respond to IL-12 by producing IFN-γ. They differ from NK cells in that—they do not express the NK cell markers CD16 and CD94, and lack perforin and granzyme B. ILC1 cells are increased in the inflamed intestine of Crohn disease patients, suggesting a role for ILC1 cells in the pathogenesis of intestinal inflammation.

Group 2 ILCs include ILC2 cells, which are also termed *natural helper cells*, *nuocytes*, and *innate helper 2*. Their transcription factors are retinoic acid receptor-related orphan receptor-α and GATA3, and they have key roles in anthelminthic responses and allergic lung inflammation.

Group 3 ILCs include ILC3 and lymphoid tissue inducer cells. Some cells of this group express the NK cell-activating receptor NKp46, which depends on the transcription factor RORγt, and lack the cytotoxic effectors perforin and granzyme. Group 3 ILCs express IL-22 but not IFN-γ or TNF. A subset of ILC3 express MHC class II and serve to regulate adaptive CD4$^+$ T-cell responses to microbiota antigens.[22] The contribution of ILCs to mucosal homeostasis and intestinal inflammation is a subject of intensive research. In this connection, mouse studies indicate that prior to weaning and the development of adaptive T-cell responses, ILC3 cells modulate the expansion of some bacterial species, especially those with inflammatory potential, and through IL-22 release regulate IEC lipid metabolism, impacting both bacterial commensalism and metabolic homeostasis.[38]

Dendritic Cells

DCs play a central role in tolerance and immunity in the intestinal mucosa. DCs continuously migrate within lymphoid tissues and present self-antigens, likely from dying apoptotic cells to maintain self-tolerance, as well as non–self-antigens. In the LP of the mouse distal small intestine, DCs express the chemokine receptor CX3CR1 and form transepithelial dendrites that allow direct sampling of luminal antigen. IECs expressing CCL25 (the ligand for CCR9 and CCR10) may attract DCs to the small intestinal mucosa, whereas CCL28 (the ligand for CCR3 and CCR10) attracts DCs to colonic mucosa.

DCs process internalized antigens more slowly than macrophages, possibly contributing to local tolerance. Tolerance induction by DCs is associated with (1) their degree of maturation at the time of antigen presentation to T cells (immature DCs activate Tregs), (2) downregulation of costimulatory molecules CD80 and CD86, (3) production of the suppressive cytokines IL-10, TGF-β, and IFN-α, and (4) interaction with the costimulatory molecule CD200. A newly described cell (called Thetis cells) with transcriptional features of DCs and medullary thymus epithelial cells emerges with regulatory T cells shortly after birth, potentially augmenting tolerance to self-antigens and commensal microbiota.[48] Murine CD103$^+$ DCs are able to perform all stages of antigen processing, including uptake, transportation, and presentation of bacterial antigens. In the mouse LP, CD103$^+$ DCs share the burden of immunosurveillance with CX3CR1$^+$ macrophages, and impaired function of these subpopulations may contribute to the development of IBD.

Macrophages

Among all body tissues, macrophages are most numerous in the gastrointestinal mucosa, residing in high numbers throughout the LP. In this critical location, macrophages protect against pathogens and noxious substances that breach the epithelium, contribute to tolerance to commensal bacteria and food antigens, and maintain tissue homeostasis by scavenging apoptotic and dead cells. Intestinal macrophages mediate these innate functions through powerful phagocytic and bactericidal capabilities.

Innate cell responses to microbes are initiated within minutes, and are directed toward PAMPs, the conserved carbohydrate, lipid, and nucleic acid molecules present on microbes. Macrophages recognize PAMPs through predetermined repertoires of PRRs that include the prototypic germline-encoded transmembrane TLRs and cytosolic sensors, including nucleotide-binding oligomerization domain (NOD)-like receptors. The predetermined nature of PRRs facilitates rapid innate responses to microbial antigens but limits the diversity of ligands to which macrophages can respond.

After infancy, intestinal macrophages are derived from and replenished by circulating monocytes, which recruit to the LP.[50] In the gut LP, however, macrophages display a unique innate receptor phenotype with very limited proinflammatory capabilities, termed *inflammation anergy*, despite the presence of potent phagocytic and bacteriocidal activity. Three important features contribute to the inflammation anergy. First, intestinal macrophages in healthy mucosa do not express the receptors for LPS (CD14), IgA (CD89), IgG (CD16, 32, and 64), CR3 (CD11b/CD18), CR4 (CD11c/CD18), growth factor receptors for IL-2 (CD25) and IL-3 (CD123), the integrin LFA-1 (CD11a), and TREM-1. Intestinal macrophages also express very low levels of chemokine receptors CCR5 and CXCR4, the coreceptors for R5 and X4 HIV-1. The mechanism by which the expression of these receptors is suppressed is not known, but since monocytes, the source of intestinal macrophages, express the receptors, local factors likely contribute to this unique phenotype, possibly through the induction of epigenetic regulation, as newly recruited monocytes take up residence in the LP. Still, intestinal macrophages express some receptors involved in the recognition of, and interaction with, potentially harmful microbes, notably TLR1 and TLR3–9, as well as TGF-β RI and RII, which mediate recruitment and active Smad signaling. The unique receptor phenotype of intestinal macrophages has profound functional implications. For example, the absence of CD14 is consistent with the inability of intestinal macrophages to recognize LPS, a feature well suited to macrophages residing in a microenvironment potentially rich in immunostimulatory LPS.[41]

The second contribution to the inflammation anergy characteristic of intestinal macrophages is dysregulated NF-κB signaling.[54] LP stromal cell factors, particularly TGF-β, potently downregulate monocyte TRIF, MyD88, and TRAF6 proteins, leading to the inability of monocytes newly recruited into the LP to phosphorylate NF-κB p65. Intestinal macrophages also express increased levels of mRNA for a suppressor of cytokine signaling (SOCS1), which promotes the degradation of MAL (MyD88 adaptor-like protein), and increased levels of sterile Armadillo motif-containing protein (SARM), which inhibits TRIF signaling. MyD88 is a critical element in the NF-κB activation pathway for all TLRs, except TLR3, and TRIF mediates TLR3-induced regulated on activation, normal T cell expressed and secreted (RANTES) and IFN-γ production, as well as TLR4-mediated MyD88-independent signaling. In addition, intestinal macrophages are unable to activate NF-κB through mitogen-activated protein kinase pathways involving phosphorylated(p) p38, p-ERK, or p-JNK, pathways dependent on TRAF6. These dysregulations lead to the marked inability of intestinal macrophages to activate NF-κB and thus release of NF-κB pathway-dependent proinflammatory cytokines.

The third mechanistic component of inflammation anergy is active TGF-β signaling.[55] Intestinal macrophage TGF-β RI and RII are activated by local stromal TGF-β to induce the Smad signal cascade. Smad4, a key component of the cascade, associates with the phosphorylated heterodimeric Smad2/3 complex and then translocates into the nucleus, initiating gene transcription for IκBα, which sequesters NF-κB in the cytoplasm. In contrast to blood monocytes, intestinal macrophages do not express the pathway inhibitor Smad7, causing a constitutive expression of IκBα and blockade of NF-κB signal transduction, thereby inhibiting NF-κB-mediated responses.

Together, these overlapping mechanisms, induced mainly by stromal TGF-β, cause profound inflammation anergy in human resident intestinal macrophages. Recent studies also indicate that stimulus-exposed intestinal macrophages do not polarize into classical and alternatively activated (M1, M2) macrophages characteristic of mouse tissue macrophages. In the setting of infection or a disrupted epithelium, immunostimulatory microbes and microbial products that breach the epithelium are rapidly phagocytosed by intestinal macrophages that provide potent, but noninflammatory, host defense. Similarly, intestinal macrophages clear apoptotic cells and debris in a noninflammatory manner. RNA sequencing has revealed transcriptional and functional heterogeneity among mucosal macrophages, driven in part by the gut microbiota.[46] Thus intestinal macrophages play a fundamental role in promoting the absence, or near absence, of inflammation that characterizes healthy human intestinal mucosa.

Oral Tolerance

An essential aspect of the highly regulated mucosal immune system is oral tolerance, which refers to the antigen-specific nonresponse to orally administrated antigens. This phenomenon, also observed at other mucosal surfaces, is termed *mucosal tolerance*.[83,84] The immune system tightly regulates the response to the vast array of antigens introduced via the oral route, particularly those that avoid complete digestion. Remarkably, up to 2% of dietary proteins enter the draining enteric vasculature fully intact. Oral tolerance ensures nonresponse to these antigens. The ability of the intestinal mucosal immune system to discriminate between harmful, harmless, or beneficial antigens and to generate a differential immune response toward each type of antigen has been investigated extensively in animal models and is present in humans.[23] Disruption of oral tolerance/mucosal tolerance may result in food allergies, celiac disease, and IBDs and has been implicated in systemic immune-mediated diseases. Oral tolerance as a therapeutic modality has been tested clinically in autoimmune diseases and although ineffective, efforts to improve the therapy continue.[85]

An important distinction between oral tolerance to food antigens and mucosal tolerance to the microbiota is that—the former attenuates intestinal and systemic immune responses, whereas the latter attenuates only mucosal immune responses.[150] Various factors that influence the induction of oral tolerance include the host's age, genetic factors, nature of the antigen, and the form and dose of the tolerogen. Digestion plays a significant role in oral tolerance, as large macromolecules are broken down, rendering potentially immunogenic substances nonimmunogenic or tolerogenic.

Achieving oral tolerance in neonates is challenging, likely due to the relatively permeable intestinal barrier and the immaturity of the mucosal immune system. However, oral tolerance can be induced within 3 months of age, suppressing many previous antibody responses to food antigens. The limited neonatal diet may further protect infants from mounting a vigorous response to food antigens. Interestingly, the intestinal microbiota influences the development of oral tolerance, possibly through a modulation of cytokine responses, enhancing intestinal barrier function, suppressing inflammation, and secreting metabolites that inhibit inflammatory cytokine production. Continuous exposure to microbial molecules such as LPS during pregnancy and early infancy has been associated with a lower prevalence of atopy and asthma in children.

The nature and form of the antigen also impact tolerance induction. Protein antigens are the most tolerogenic compared with carbohydrates and lipids. Soluble forms of antigens, such as ovalbumin, are more tolerogenic than aggregated forms. The site of antigen sampling and prior sensitization to antigens through an extraintestinal route can affect tolerance induction.

The dose of administered antigen is also critical to the form of oral tolerance generated. In mouse models, high antigen doses may lead to clonal deletion or anergy of T cells, while low doses of antigen activate regulatory/suppressor T cells. Regulatory T cells (Treg) of both CD4 and CD8 lineages may have a role in oral tolerance, although depletion of CD8 T cells in mice does not affect induction of oral tolerance. CD4$^+$ Treg cells appear to be activated in the Peyer patch and secrete TGF-β, which is a potent suppressor of T and B cell responses, while promoting the production of IgA by inducing a genetic switch from IgM to IgA in B cells. Production of TGF-β and IL-10 by Treg cells elicited by low-dose antigen administration helps explain an associated phenomenon of oral tolerance termed *bystander suppression*. Oral tolerance is antigen-specific, but the effector arm is antigen nonspecific. When an irrelevant (bystander) antigen is coadministered systemically with the tolerogen, suppression of T and B cell responses to the irrelevant antigen also will occur (hence bystander suppression), because secreted TGF-β and IL-10 can suppress the response to the coadministered antigen. T regulatory 1 cells (Tr1), which produce only IL-10, a potent immunosuppressive cytokine, may also participate in bystander suppression and oral tolerance. In mice, the deletion of CD4$^+$ Treg cell activity results in IBD, whereas its expansion ameliorates murine colitis. In IBD patients, the number of Treg cells is generally greater than in controls, and a peripheral-to-intestinal shift has been suggested. Whether the failure of these cells to protect against IBD is due to an intrinsic defect or microenvironmental effects is not yet known.

Antigen-specific CD8$^+$ T cells may play a role in oral tolerance, and the regulation of mucosal immune responses. CD8$^+$CD28$^-$ T cells with regulatory activity, induced by IECs, may control intestinal inflammation. The number of such cells is significantly reduced in the LP of patients with IBD, suggesting a role for these epithelial-induced T regulatory cells in the control of intestinal inflammation.

Finally, the cell serving as the APC, as well as by the site of antigen uptake, influence oral tolerance. In mice, orally administered reovirus type III is taken up by M cells expressing reovirus type III–specific receptors (see Fig. 2.2). This induces an active IgA response. In contrast, reovirus I infects IECs and induces tolerance. Thus whether a specific antigen enters the mucosa through M cells or IECs may dictate the type of immune response generated (IgA vs. tolerance). Notably, certain oral vaccines, like poliovirus, effectively stimulate active immunity in the gut by binding to M cells.

Chemokine Role in Homeostasis and Inflammation

Many of the chemokines secreted in the GALT are produced by IECs, evidence for epithelial cell participation in regulating intestinal immune responses. Of the chemokines secreted, those produced by IECs have the capacity to attract inflammatory cells such as lymphocytes, macrophages, and DCs, thus contributing to normal mucosal homeostasis (Table 2.1). The production of most of these chemokines is increased during infection and inflammation.

The chemokine CCL5 RANTES is secreted predominantly by macrophages but can also be produced by human IECs. RANTES may have a role in innate, as well as adaptive mucosal immunity, and increased RANTES expression has been demonstrated in the mucosa of patients with ulcerative colitis. The CXC chemokines, including monokine induced by interferon-γ (MIG, CXCL9), IFN-γ-inducible protein 10 (IP-10, CXCL10), a chemokine that appears to promote Th1 responses, and IFN-γ-inducible T cell α-chemoattractant (ITAC, CXCL11) are constitutively expressed by lymphocytes, endothelial cells, and human colonic IECs. Their

TABLE 2.1 Chemokines, Their Receptors, Cells That Produce Them, and Target Cell(s)

Chemokine	Receptor	Produced By	Target Cell	References
CCL5 (RANTES)		IEC Mφ	T cells Eosinophils Leukocytes	[57]
CXCL9 (MIG)	CXCR3	Colon IECs Endothelial cells Lymphocytes	Th1 CXCR3$^+$ NK DC	[58,59]
CXCL10 (IP10)	CXCR3	Colon IECs Endothelial cells Lymphocytes	Th1 CXCR3$^+$	[58,59]
CXCL11 (ITAC)	CXCR3	Colon IECs Endothelial cells Lymphocytes	Th1 XCXR3$^+$	[58,59]
CCL25 (TECK)	CCR9	IEC	CD8$^+$ E7	[60–63]
CX3CL1 (Fractalkine)	CX3CR1	IEC	CD8>CD4 monocytes NK cells	[64–66,71]
CCL28 (MEC)	CCR3 CCR10	Colon IEC	CD4 Tm eosinophils	[71]
CCL22 (MDC)	CCR4	Colon IEC	CD4 Th1	[67]
CCL20 (MIP3α)	CCR6	IEC	DCs CD4 Tm	[68–70]
CXCL12	CXCR4 CXCR7	IEC	CD4 Th1 CD45RO$^+$ Plasma cells	[72–76]
CXCL8 (IL-8)	CXCR1>CXCR2	IEC Mφ Neutrophils	Neutrophils	[77]

DC, Dendritic cell; *IEC*, intestinal epithelial cell; *Mφ*, macrophage; *NK*, natural killer.

expression and polarized basolateral secretion increase after IFN-γ stimulation. CXC chemokines attract Th1 cells expressing high levels of CXCR3, contribute to NK T cell chemotaxis and increased cytolytic responses, and activate subsets of DCs.

In contrast to the inflammation-related CXCR3 receptor, a tissue-specific chemokine receptor, CCR9, is constitutively expressed on small intestinal IELs and LPLs. Its ligand, the chemokine thymus-expressed chemokine (TECK, CCL25) is differentially expressed in the jejunal and ileal epithelium, where decreasing levels of expression from the crypt up to the villous have been reported. CCL25 expression by IECs has been shown to be increased in the inflamed small intestine of patients with Crohn disease, with increased CCR9 expression by peripheral blood lymphocytes and decreased expression by LPLs.

Fractalkine (CX3CL1) is a unique chemokine expressed by IECs that combines the properties of chemokines and adhesion molecules. CX3CL1 attracts NK cells, monocytes, $CD8^+$ T lymphocytes, and to a lesser extent $CD4^+$ T lymphocytes, which express the specific receptor CX3CR1. Its expression is increased in Crohn disease, specifically in the basolateral aspect of IECs.

Macrophage-derived chemokine (MDC, CCL22) is constitutively expressed and secreted by colonic IECs and attracts $CCR4^+$ Th2 cytokine-producing lymphocytes. Polarized basolateral secretion of MDC/CCL22 from stimulated colonic IEC lines has been reported. The specific recruitment of lymphocytes that preferentially secrete anti-inflammatory cytokines supports an important role for the intestinal epithelium in orchestrating normal mucosal homeostasis and adds to the accumulating evidence that these cells possess the ability to regulate mucosal immune responses.

The chemokine macrophage inflammatory protein-3α (MIP3, CCL20) is unique in its ability to specifically attract immature DCs as well as memory $CD4^+$ T lymphocytes. CCL20 is also expressed and produced by human small intestinal ECs (mainly in the FAE) and by colonic IECs and may be the mediator of lymphocyte adhesion to the α4β7 ligand MAdCAM-1. MIP3α expression and secretion is increased in colonic IECs derived from IBD patients. Mucosal memory T cells, as well as IECs, express CCR6, the cognate receptor for MIP3α.

Mucosal defenses, including microbiota itself, provide protection from intestinal pathogens. The microbiota competes with, and provides resistance to, colonization by transient bacteria and pathogens in food and water. Some enteric pathogens induce host inflammation that, in turn, kills anaerobes in the gut, thus opening a niche for the aerotolerant pathogen. Certain bacteria are pathogens because they have evolved mechanisms to breach the mucosal barrier. In healthy mucosa, resident macrophages potently phagocytose and kill such microbes in a noninflammatory manner, but in disease conditions, the mechanism(s) responsible for inflammation anergy are disrupted allowing the macrophages to retain the proinflammatory profile of their monocyte progenitors. However, once IECs are invaded, they produce large amounts of chemokines such as IL-8, which attract neutrophils and monocytes from the blood into the gut at the site of infection. Such phagocytes are inflammatory and produce more chemokines, as well as other cytokines, rapidly acquiring a critical mass and killing the invading bacteria, thus resolving the infection.

Full references for this chapter can be found at https://ebooks.health.elsevier.com.

3 The Enteric Microbiota

Alice Cheng, Sushila Dalal

IN THIS CHAPTER

CHARACTERISTICS OF THE HUMAN INTESTINAL MICROBIOME

The intestinal microbiome[1] is a diverse ecosystem comprising bacteria, archaea, fungi, and viruses that profoundly impacts human physiology and disease (Box 3.1). The intestinal microbiota has been known and used to modulate human health since antiquity,[1] but we have only begun to understand composition and mechanism with the advances of next-generation sequencing (NGS) and associated bioinformatic tools (Box 3.2). From these studies, we have learned that the composition of the intestinal microbiota varies significantly among individuals such that there is no universal "healthy" microbiota in terms of microbial membership. This variation reflects differences in the relative abundance of the 55 dominant phyla: Bacteroidetes, Firmicutes, Proteobacteria, Actinobacteria, and Verrucomicrobia.[2,3] In contrast to composition, microbial genes and functional properties are conserved among individuals,[4] including central metabolic pathways and metabolism of carbohydrates and proteins.[5] Still, there remain significant interindividual differences in the microbial functions such as drug metabolism, pathogenicity islands, and nutrient transporters.[5] Several external factors further shape the healthy intestinal microbiome (Fig. 3.1) with diet having the most prominent effects, followed by age and medications.

Spatial and Anatomic Variation of the Microbiome

The microbiota composition varies along the gastrointestinal (GI) tract, from mouth to anus through its longitudinal and radial axes.[6] There are several factors that determine the localization of bacteria within different niches in the intestine, including oxidation-reduction potential, chemical and nutrient gradients, host-immune activity, and the mucus layer (Fig. 3.2).[7] The highest bacterial density, perhaps due to increased nutrient availability and slower transit, is in the colon that typically harbors 10^{11-12} colony-forming units (cfu) per gram fecal matter of intestinal contents or 10^{13-14} bacterial cells when scaled to the total colonic contents[8,9] (see Fig. 3.1). In contrast, the high concentration of bile acids, acidity, and relatively rapid transit through the small intestine contribute to lower abundance and diversity of microbiota as typical duodenal colonization is $10^{4-5} \times 10^3$ cfu/g of contents in the distal ileum and 10^{8-9} cfu/g of contents in the duodenal aspirate.[9,10] Additionally, there is a radial gradient of bacterial colonization within the lumen due to mucin, antimicrobial peptides, and oxygen tension. Mucin is the primary microbial barrier in the colon, which harbors an epithelial-adjacent layer of dense mucin mostly devoid of bacteria and a loose, microbially colonized outer layer.[11] In contrast, the small intestine harbors a single, incomplete mucus layer, and secreted host antimicrobial peptides and lectins, such as REGIIIγ, are thought to be the main defense against luminal microbes.[12,13] In both small and large intestines, the radial distribution of oxygen from the mucosa to the lumen accounts for differences in microbial membership, genetics, and function that reflect the effect of oxygen availability. In general greater numbers of Bacteroides and Clostridia phyla populate the intestinal lumen, and Proteobacteria and Actinobacteria phyla tend to associate more closely with the mucosa.[14]

Given the variation in spatial microbial distribution, we may not capture the complete contribution to phenotype with stool sampling alone. A more regionally targeted sampling approach is needed to understand the microbial effects in regulating host metabolism, digestion and absorption, local immune systems, and

BOX 3.1 Glossary of Terms Used to Describe Relationships Among Individual Organisms Within the Microbiota and Between the Microbiota and Host

Allochthonous: Organisms found in a place other than their origin.

Autochthonous: Organisms that are indigenous to their present location.

Commensal: Strictly speaking, the term *commensal* (derived from *cum mensa*, "to share a table") describes a relationship between two organisms in which one organism benefits and the other is unaffected. In most instances, however, the term *commensal* is used to describe the in situ microbes colonizing a particular niche without doing harm but may include organisms that provide a benefit to each other or to the host.

Microbiome: The microorganisms, their genomes (i.e., genes), and the surrounding environmental conditions.[198]

Microbiota: The population of microorganisms (bacteria, archaea, lower and higher eukaryotes, and viruses) organisms in a particular niche.[199]

Pathobiont: Usually refers to an organism that is a potential pathogen but only causes disease under a given set of circumstances such as when the microbiome is perturbed. An example is *Clostridioides difficile*, which can be carried in the intestine of healthy individuals but usually only causes a problem after antibiotic treatment.

Pathogen: Any pathologic (disease-causing) organism.

Pharmabiotic: Any biological entity mined from human microbiota and with a proven biological effect. These entities could include live or dead microbes, cell wall components, purified proteins or lipids, individual metabolites (e.g., neurotransmitters), or active enzymes.

Prebiotic: A nondigestible compound that, through its metabolization by microorganisms in the intestine, modulates functional capacity of the microbial community, thus conferring a beneficial physiological effect on the host.[200]

Probiotic: Live microorganisms that when administered in adequate amounts confer a health benefit on the host.

Symbiont: Any organism participating in a symbiotic (mutually beneficial) relationship.

Synbiotic: A nondigestible compound that contains both prebiotics and probiotics and combines nutrients appropriate to stimulate the specific beneficial microbe in the synbiotic.

in causing or contributing to diseases such as IBD, IBS, food allergy, celiac disease, and colon cancer.[14]

Temporal Changes in the Intestinal Microbiome

A healthy stable microbiome configuration changes over an individual's lifetime. At birth, infant microbiomes are dominated by *Bifidobacterium* and *Lactobacillus* species, which are the primary consumers of human milk sugars and proteins.[15] However, antibiotics during early childhood or the peripartum period[16,17] can shift the balance toward *Escherichia*, *Klebsiella*, and *Enterococcal* species.[16–19] After weaning and introduction of solid foods, the infant microbiome becomes superseded by adult microbial species from the *Bacteroides*, *Clostridial*, and *Lachnospiraceae* genera although there can be variation across age and geography.[15] Overall, the microbiome configuration remains relatively stable through adulthood though species diversity and metabolic output wane with age.[2,20] While there is significant interpersonal variation of microbiome configuration[21] for any healthy individual, their daily configuration remains stable and resilient unless disrupted by major perturbations such as significant dietary shifts, antibiotics, or pathogen infections (Fig. 3.1).[22]

Nonbacterial Members of the Intestinal Microbiome

GI fungi comprise the *mycobiome* that consists of a relatively small portion of the intestinal microbiota. However, metagenomic sequencing likely underestimates population abundance[23,24] and the immunomodulatory, ecologic, and metabolic impact of fungi are understudied and underappreciated. *Candida* is the most prevalent fungal genus[25,26] with *Candida albicans*, *Candida tropicalis*, *Candida glabrata*, and *Candida parapsilosis* predominantly found in humans.[23] As with bacterial species, mycobiome membership is highly influenced by the environment[27] and diet.[28] The competitive relationship of bacteria and fungi is evident from the overgrowth of fungi following the use of antibiotics,[27,29] and the overgrowth of the mycobiome can drive downstream inflammatory signaling impacting diverse conditions such as IBD and allergic airway responses[30–32] (see Chapter 117).[33]

The gut *virome* mostly comprises bacteriophages, which are viruses that infect and lyse bacterial cells. Bacteriophages have high strain selectivity and can precisely deplete susceptible strains to change the composition of intestinal bacterial communities.[34] Similar to bacteria, the gut virome varies among individuals but is relatively stable within individuals and responds to dietary changes.[35–37] Bacteriophages can directly affect the immune system by stimulating the macrophage production of inflammatory cytokines, such as IL1-beta and interferon,[38,39] and enhancing DNA vaccine potency.[40] The effects of bacteriophages on bacteria can be exploited therapeutically and may represent a novel and important mode of treatment; these are currently being developed and deployed against multidrug-resistant bacteria.[41]

Eukaryotic viruses can also influence the immune system[42] and in particular, Norovirus and SARS-CoV-2 have been shown to restructure the human gut microbiota and immune response.[43,44] Viruses in turn can influence the host by affecting other members of the microbiota, but much work is needed to identify such trans-kingdom interactions, including better annotated databases of viral DNA sequences and techniques to deeply characterize viruses.

FACTORS IMPACTING MICROBIOME STRUCTURE AND RESILIENCE

Early Life

Multiple factors can influence the infant microbiome to shape future health and immunity. Early development of the intestinal microbiome is critical in educating the mucosal[45,46] and systemic immune response.[47–49] The majority of intestinal colonization occurs with birth, and birth modality is one of the initial determinants of colonizing organisms. Mode of delivery and feeding can highly impact microbiota configuration[50,51]; however, it is not clear how strongly the above interventions and changes in the microbiota impact health outcomes and thus this remains a major topic of investigation. By far, the strongest early-life impact is with antibiotic exposure, in which infant exposure to broad spectrum antibiotics has been linked to a higher risk of conditions such as asthma, type I diabetes, and obesity later in life.[52]

Sex

Women harbor higher levels of microbiota diversity and functional richness than men,[2] and a decreased abundance of *Bacteroides* and *Prevotella* species.[53] Preclinical studies have observed that the differential effects can be attributed to how the microbiota tunes androgen receptor activity.[54,55]

BOX 3.2 Techniques to Assess Microbiota Composition and Functionality

MICROBIOTA COMPOSITION

Microbial Culture

Early studies dissecting the microbiota composition were technologically limited by culture-based techniques, which in turn relied on specialized growth media under varying conditions to identify specific microbes. This restricted our ability to identify only a small subset of organisms for which established culture conditions had been described and which accounted for 5%–15% of the intestinal bacteria we know to constitute the microbiome today.[201,202] As a result, locations with limited diversity were often considered sterile given the inability to culture their resident bacteria. Today, however, nearly all locations in the body have been described to have characteristic resident microbes[84,203,204] as a result of culture-independent sequence-based identification methodologies. Sequencing-based data have also improved our ability to culture bacteria previously considered to be unculturable. We are now able to culture a significant proportion of an individual's fecal microbiota, using various culturing conditions,[205,206] which has allowed us to determine the relevance of microbial compositional changes and the interactions and impact of individual or groups of bacteria on host phenotypes using models such as germ-free mice.

Microscopy

Early methods included scanning and transmission electron microscopy of intestinal tissue, which provided estimates of diversity based on morphology and high-resolution images of individual bacteria but did not allow bacterial identification.[207,208] The use of general stains, such as the Gram stain, provides resolution beyond morphology but also is insufficient for identification. Fluorescence microscopy provides the opportunity to identify bacteria by fluorescence in situ hybridization to microbe-specific 16S rRNA.[209] The increased availability of sequencing data has allowed the development of more precise fluorescence in situ hybridization probes and carries the advantage of not requiring culture. The fixation methods are compatible with preserving mucus, and the use of multiple probes simultaneously allows detection of several bacteria within a sample.[210,211] In addition, it is one of the primary tools to define the biogeography of microbes within the intestine and the interaction of bacteria with the host at the mucosal surface. The advances in fluorophores, imaging, and computational tools have significantly improved our ability to visualize microbes both in vivo and in vitro. Conventional fluorescent probes require oxygen limiting their utility in vivo, but new tools using "click" chemistry allow tagging of bacteria with oxygen-independent fluorescent tags for in vivo tracking.[212]

Next-Generation Sequencing. The early culture-independent compositional tools used denaturing gradient gel electrophoresis to separate different-sized bands that represented distinct taxonomic groups.[7] However, with the advent of next-generation sequencing technologies (e.g., Illumina, 454, Ion Torrent, SOLiD, etc.), marker-based (16S rRNA gene) and shotgun sequencing of all genes within a community have superseded denaturing gradient gel electrophoresis, especially given the declining cost of sequencing. The marker-based approach takes advantage of the conservation of DNA sequence in the gene encoding the 16S rRNA subunit that is found in all microbes. Interceding variable regions are targeted for amplification by polymerase chain reaction, allowing a simultaneous identification of different taxa within a sample. However, marker-based sequencing is limited in its ability to identify taxa beyond the genus level given the small amplicon sizes. Third-generation sequencing technologies, such as single-molecule real-time sequencing, have emerged, which will likely supersede the current methodologies, given their potential to generate read lengths (continuous sequence from a single piece of DNA) of 10 kb.[201]

Microbial Function. Compositional data are limited in the ability to provide insight into host-microbe interactions; hence it is important to move beyond detailing which microorganisms are present to determining their role, function, and effects of their metabolic products on the intestinal microbial community and the host. This is especially important given that core microbial functions appear to be conserved despite compositional heterogeneity among human populations.

Metagenomics. Often referred to as whole genome sequencing, or shotgun sequencing, metagenomics allows the characterization of all genes in a microbial community and provides the broad functional potential of a community. It cannot, however, provide the specific functionality under a given set of conditions.

Metatranscriptomics

Transcriptomic approaches like RNAseq provide a snapshot of gene-expression profiles of microbial communities under a given condition. These data can be used to further infer differential expression of metabolic pathways using analysis tools such as HUMAnN3.[213]

Metaproteomics and Metabolomics. Metaproteomics provides a comprehensive characterization of proteins, whereas metabolomics provides a comprehensive characterization of small molecules and metabolites, each from microbial communities. Both approaches allow the characterization of the overall metabolic state of complex communities resulting from differential gene expression among communities or the same community under different conditions. For proteomics, proteins can either be directly separated based on hydrophobicity, charge, or both, using liquid chromatography (LC) or digested to peptides via proteases such as trypsin prior to chromatographic separation followed by mass spectrometry (MS) for the parent peptide and tandem MS-MS for fragmentation information. The biggest challenge currently is the downstream bioinformatics processing because a predicted protein database needs to be constructed from metagenomic information to assign the obtained peptide sequence information to the proteins. Alternatively, the vast diversity of small molecules, and differences in properties and concentrations, require that multiple methods be used to cover the vast array of metabolites; these include separation using LC, gas chromatography, high-pressure LC, ultra-pressure LC, coupled to MS, and proton nuclear magnetic resonance spectroscopy (^{1}H-NMR).[214] Metabolomics can be done in a targeted or nontargeted manner and downstream processing using statistical methods allows an identification of discriminative features. One of the challenges that remains is the accurate identification of metabolites in MS spectra, though there has been significant progress with multiple spectral databases such as HMDB, METLIN, and ChemSpider, all of which are being constantly updated.

Modeling Microbes In Vitro and In Vivo

Organoids. Organoids are derived from tissue stem cells or pluripotent stem cells and can be maintained in culture, wherein they maintain their polarity and recapitulate the composition and organization of cells, thus representing an ideal in vitro system to study host-microbe interactions in the context of specific diseases. There are several methods used to study host-microbe dynamics, including coculture; exposing an organoid-derived monolayer to microbes/microbial products; and microinjection, which is especially relevant for studying luminal interactions as well as modeling anaerobic microbes.[215]

Germ-Free Mice. Although humans are the ideal biological system to study microbes, animal models are needed to help deconstruct complex interactions and delineate mechanisms underlying host-microbiome interactions. Conventional mouse models provide conceptual knowledge, but they are limited in their translatability and ability to study defined colonization states. Germ-free and gnotobiotic (previously germ-free mice but now colonized with defined microbial associations) animal models allow modeling of individual microbes as well as complex communities from mice or other species (human; humanized mice) to study microbe-microbe and microbe-host interactions. Recapitulating phenotypic features of disease states following transfer of microbial communities allows for the identification of microbe-driven phenotypes. They are also ideal for studying the effects of host, environment, and dietary factors on the microbiome in a controlled setting. In regard to translatability, humanized mice faithfully recapitulate the structure and function of human microbial communities[216] and represent a readily translatable preclinical model.

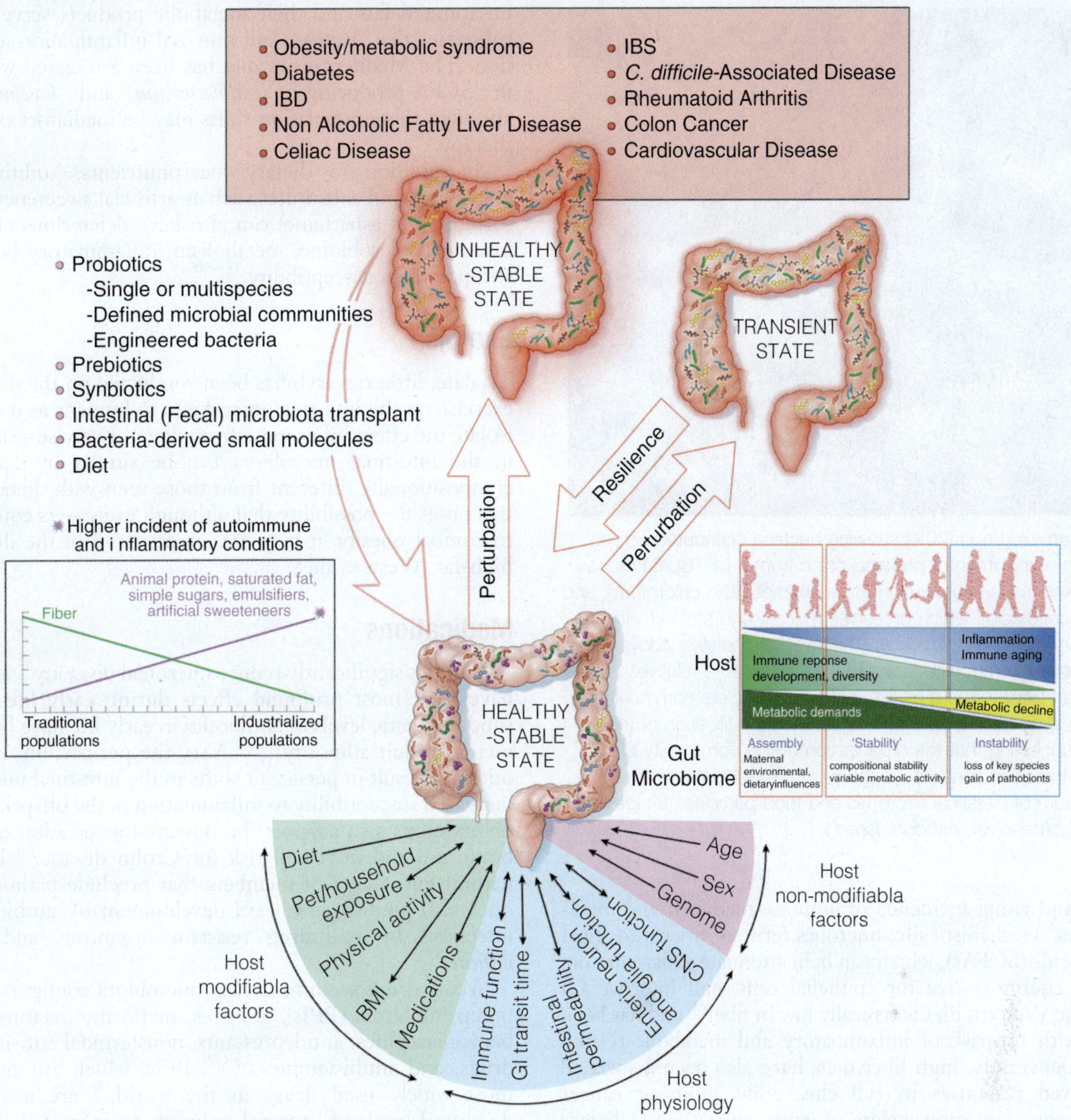

Fig. 3.1 Characteristics of intestinal microbiota. The figure outlines the modifiable and nonmodifiable host factors influencing the intestinal microbiota, the reciprocal interactions between intestinal microbiota and host physiology, the resilience of the microbiome, as well as the consequence of deleterious shifts in the microbiome and the potential mechanisms to manipulate the microbiome.

Genetics

The intestinal microbiota composition in monozygotic twins is more similar to one another than those of dizygotic twins, which suggests a role for host genes in selecting for certain microbial taxa.[56] Some of these associations have been uncovered such as *FUT2* polymorphisms,[57] variants in immunity-related genes, and genes that alter bile acid levels.[2] However, heritability appears to shape 10% or less of the microbial taxa[58] and phyla abundances are more highly influenced by environmental factors. Furthermore, heritability may be the result of intragenerational transfer of key bacteria; for example, Christensenellaceae, which co-occurs with other heritable taxa, is enriched in lean individuals and is itself associated with leanness.[58]

Geography and Diet

Intestinal microbiota composition varies significantly with geography, which represents combined effects of cultural, dietary, and environmental factors. For example, the microbiota composition of individuals living in industrialized settings of the United States and Western Europe is distinct and less diverse compared to agrarian and nonindustrialized areas such as Malawi, Tanzania, Burkina Faso, or the Amazon.[15,59–61] In particular, residents of nonurban settings have a greater proportion of the genera *Prevotella*, *Treponema*, and a lower proportion of Bacteroides phyla.[59,62]

Functionally, the industrialized microbiome is more adapted to digest the high protein, simple carbohydrate Western diet. Western microbiota harbor greater numbers of metabolic pathways and genes aimed at metabolism of amino acids and simple sugars when compared to nonindustrialized microbiota.[63] Conversely, nonindustrialized microbiomes harbor a greater number of metabolic pathways for the digestion of dietary fibers typically found in native berries, seeds, tubers, corms, and rhizomes.[59,64,65,15] Thus dietary fibers are thought to be a driving force between this agrarian and the industrial divide,[35] where rapid industrialization has been associated with transformation of

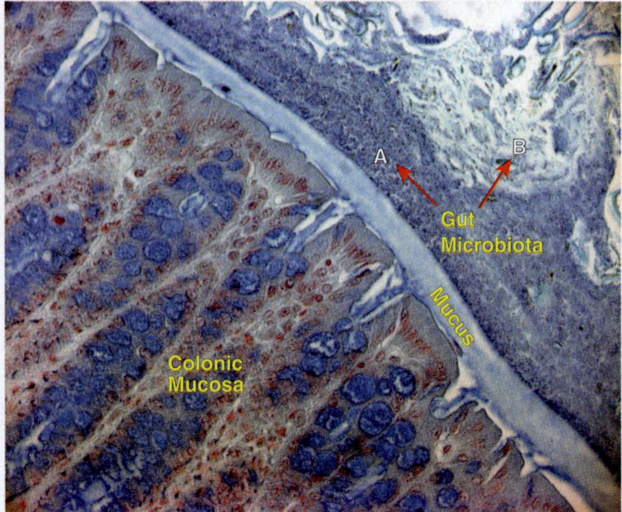

Fig. 3.2 Photomicrograph (20×) showing bacteria distributed across the mucosa in a specimen of proximal colon from a C57BL/6J mouse. Tissue was fixed in Carnoy solution (60% ethanol, 30% chloroform, and 10% glacial acetic acid), which preserves mucus, and stained with Alcian blue, which highlights mucus. The layer immediately above the colonic mucus is the mucosa-associated microbiota—a relatively stable community that likely forms a biofilm matrix that confers community stability, even after colonic lavage. There is faint stratification of the microbiota, suggesting that the organization of this community is not random. The transition zone above the mucosa-associated microbiota zone is a mixture of intestinal microbes and food particles. *(Image courtesy Dr. Lev Lichtenstein, Ashdod, Israel.)*

microbiota and rising incidence of immune-mediated and metabolic diseases. Mechanistically, microbes ferment fiber into short chain fatty acids (SCFAs), which can help attenuate inflammation, serve as an energy source for epithelial cells, and improve GI transit.[66] The Western diet is typically low in fiber[66] and has been associated with the risk of inflammatory and metabolic-related diseases.[66] Conversely, high fiber diets have also been associated with improved responses to cell checkpoint inhibitor cancer immunotherapy and suppression of graft versus host disease (GVHD).[67,68] Many studies are underway to further elucidate microbial digestion of dietary fibers and their impact on human health and disease.[69] In such, these dietary interventions and substrates will constitute the next wave of microbiome investigation and therapy.[69,70,22]

Ketogenic diet—High protein, high fat diets are known to worsen cardiovascular disease, but we are just beginning to understand their impact on the health of the microbiome. In preclinical and clinical studies, a high-protein diet results in increased microbial density and colitogenic potential.[71] Adherence to extremes of high protein, high fat diets can generate ketone bodies, which actively suppress members of the human gut microbiota and proinflammatory T-cell populations.[72] However, it is not known if these changes translate into long-term gut health or disease.

Enteral nutrition—The mechanisms by which enteral nutrition modulates inflammation are not well understood. Enteral nutrition biases the microbiome toward proinflammatory members of Firmicutes and Proteobacteria phyla,[73,74] yet seems to decrease inflammation and improve mucosal healing.[75] How enteral nutrition mediates these changes and modulates inflammation is not well understood and presents an opportunity for future investigation.

Mediterranean diet—The Mediterranean diet is rich in unsaturated fats that have anti-inflammatory properties. These unsaturated fats and their metabolic products serve as reducing substrates that decrease gut mucosal inflammation and oxygenation. The Mediterranean diet has been associated with increases in SCFA-producing *Faecalibacterium* and *Roseburia* species, although these population shifts may be mediators or markers of therapy.[76,77]

In addition to dietary macronutrients, additives such as emulsifiers and substitutes such as artificial sweeteners (sucralose, sorbitol, and aspartame) can also have deleterious effects on the intestinal microbiome, metabolism, inflammatory bowel disease, and pathogen susceptibility.[78–80]

Exercise

To date, little research has been conducted on the direct effect of exercise on the intestinal microbiota in humans as it is difficult to isolate the effects of exercise from diet.[81] Exercise-related changes in the intestinal microbiota can be similar in magnitude but compositionally different from those seen with dietary change;[82] this raises the possibility that although exercise is commonly used to combat obesity, it may not attenuate all of the ill effects of a high-fat, Western diet.

Medications

Antibiotics significantly reduce microbial diversity[83] and appear to have their most profound effects during early life where even subtherapeutic levels of antibiotics in early life have been found to increase adult adiposity.[84,85] Also, the peripartum use of antibiotics can result in persistent shifts in the intestinal microbiota and increased susceptibility to inflammation in the offspring;[16,17] these observations also support the observed association of early antibiotic use and increased risk for Crohn disease.[86] By depleting natural microbiota of members that preclude pathogens, antibiotics also predispose toward development of antibiotic resistant infections by multidrug resistant organisms and *Clostridium difficile*.[87]

Many drugs seem to impact microbiota configuration: proton pump inhibitors (PPIs), laxatives, metformin, statins, hormones, benzodiazepines, antidepressants, nonsteroidal anti-inflammatory drugs, and antihistamines.[2,88,89] PPIs, which are among the 10 most widely used drugs in the world,[90] are associated with decreased levels of bacterial richness, an increased abundance of oral microbes, and the presence of potential pathogens in the intestine.[90]

Other Lifestyle Factors

Habits such as smoking or alcohol consumption, as well as psychological stress,[91] have been associated with changes in the intestinal microbiota. The adverse effects of smoking on microbial diversity can be indirectly inferred from the increase in diversity observed after smoking cessation.[35,92] Household contacts also can have an effect on the microbiota composition. Individuals in the same household share skin microbiota and, interestingly, household pets significantly increase sharing of skin microbiota among household contacts.[93]

THE EFFECT OF HOST-INTESTINAL MICROBIOME INTERACTIONS ON HOST PHYSIOLOGY

Interactions between humans and their intestinal microbes are bidirectional: reciprocal signaling occurs between the microbiota and the immune system, the GI tract, and even the nervous system. The mechanisms by which microbial metabolites influence host physiology remains an active area of study. The intestinal microbiota metabolizes tryptophan into several bioactive molecules that act as ligands for aryl hydrocarbon receptor (AhR) and serotonin receptor 4. Microbiota-derived AhR ligands have been found to be protective against peripheral and central nervous inflammation with potential impact on diseases such as IBD, multiple sclerosis, and neuropsychiatric disorders.[94] Intestinal microbes also produce metabolites that mimic human *N*-acyl amides that interact with G protein-coupled receptors (GPCRs) to regulate GI physiology.[95] GPCRs that interact with human *N*-acyl amides have been implicated in diseases such as diabetes, obesity, cancer, and IBD. These are only two cases of a wide array of microbial metabolites that directly influence host physiology.

INTERACTIONS BETWEEN THE INTESTINAL MICROBIOME AND THE IMMUNE SYSTEM

The intestinal microbiome shapes the maturation of the immune system, and the immune system, in turn, can modulate the composition of the microbiota and its proinflammatory potential. Epithelial and dendritic cells represent the first line of contact with the intestinal microbiota. Host cells use pattern recognition receptors, such as Toll-like receptors (TLRs), NOD-like receptors, and C-type lectins, to recognize microorganism-associated molecular patterns on the surface of both commensal microbes and pathogens. Intestinal microbes generate immune tolerance to survive in the intestine.[96] Microbes also produce a rich array of other immunomodulatory molecules, including CpG (cytosine phosphodiesterase guanine) DNA, which acts on TLR9 receptors; ATP, which acts on specific sensors (P2X and P2Y) to promote the generation of intestinal Th17 cells and immunomodulatory SCFAs.[97–99]

The host-immune system, in turn, helps contain and shape the composition of the intestinal microbiota. Epithelial cells produce antibacterial proteins, such as α-defensins, which limit contact between bacteria and the epithelial cells.[13] Disturbances of host-microbe signaling have been linked with aberrant expansion of some components of the microbiota that may adversely influence the inflammatory response and risk of disease.[100] Defects at various levels, including specific TLRs and transcription factors involved in innate immunity, can result in the emergence of "colitogenic" microbes and promulgation of innate and adaptive immune responses.[101–104]

Notably, the mycobiome is a powerful immune stimulus. Fungal glycoprotein cell walls are potent activators of innate immunity via TLRs 2 and 4, complement, and dectin-1 receptors, which mediate the secretion of inflammatory cytokines IL17, IL22, and NF-κB.[23] Fungal immune activation has been implicated in multiple diseases, including IBD, GVHD, and hepatitis B.[105]

INTERACTIONS BETWEEN THE INTESTINAL MICROBIOME AND THE GASTROINTESTINAL TRANSIT

The key functions of the GI tract that facilitate digestion and absorption of nutrients include motility, secretion, and sensation. GI transit time varies within and between populations worldwide.[106] However, variation in transit time can be associated with diverse disease states, including infections, inflammatory conditions, and functional disorders such as IBS with constipation or diarrhea.[107] GI transit is an example of the bidirectional interactions between the intestinal microbiome and the GI tract. Thus transplanting a complex fecal microbial community from a healthy human into a germ-free mouse stimulates production of the neurotransmitter serotonin and significantly shortens GI transit time, suggesting a role for intestinal microbes in modulating GI transit. Alternatively, increasing or decreasing GI transit time using medications such as polyethylene glycol or loperamide in humanized mice (ex-germ-free mice colonized with human bacteria) significantly changes the intestinal microbial community,[107] and similar alterations in intestinal microbiota composition and function have been reported in patients with diarrhea and constipation.[108,109] Some examples of microbial mediators that affect GI transit time include lipopolysaccharide, which can influence enteric neuronal survival, and SCFAs, which can stimulate intestinal synthesis of serotonin, which, in turn, plays an important role in GI motility, secretion, and sensation.[110] It is not surprising that the magnitude of impact on GI transit depends considerably on the diet the humanized mouse is fed,[110] given that diet can affect downstream mediators such as SCFAs. In addition to transit, the intestinal microbiome can also influence sensation in the GI tract as evidenced by the development of visceral hypersensitivity following the transfer of microbiota from patients with IBS to germ-free rats. In addition to the disruption of the intestinal microbiota in early life,[111] a correlation has been described between visceral hypersensitivity and expansion of *Escherichia coli*. The intestinal microbiome plays an important role in maintaining the epithelial barrier as well as fluid and electrolyte transport. Specific members of the intestinal microbiota can alter the expression of tight junction proteins in the epithelium, and microbial metabolites, such as butyrate, play an important role in maintaining the epithelial barrier. Microbial deconjugation and metabolism of bile acids can alter the pool of bile acids such as chenodeoxycholic acid and deoxycholic acid, which act as secretagogues in the colon.

THE MICROBIOME-GUT-BRAIN AXIS

The influence of our intestinal microbes extends far beyond the GI tract. The brain and intestinal tract communicate bidirectionally via a complex interaction of the nervous system, circulatory system, and immune system.[112] Microbial metabolites, such as SCFAs, secondary bile acid metabolites, and tryptophan metabolites, can interact directly with the enteroendocrine cells or enterochromaffin cells of the enteric nervous system to activate the vagus nerve and communicate with the CNS, while others may cross the intestinal barrier in the circulatory system and directly access the CNS through the blood-brain barrier.[113] Microbial associated molecular patterns, such as lipopolysaccharide or TLR ligands, can activate immune cell cytokine release, which can then affect the CNS directly.[112]

The intestinal microbiome has an impact on the development of the nervous system, affecting everything from the formation of the blood-brain barrier to myelination to neurogenesis.[114] Epidemiological studies have shown that maternal infections and inflammation can increase autism spectrum disorder (ASD) and schizophrenia risk in offspring.[115]

These findings have spurred interest in the relationship between the intestinal microbiome and mental health in humans, including links with ASDs, anxiety disorders, depression, pain sensitivity, learning, and memory.[116,117] The intestinal microbiota of ASD patients differs from typically developing (TD) patients, with a higher ratio of Bacteroidetes to Firmicutes in ASD patients.[118] Probiotic treatment with *Lactobacillus* and *Bifidobacterium* of ASD mice or humans have reported improvements in symptoms such as mood, anxiety, sleep, and depression.[119,120] Altered microbiomes as compared to healthy individuals have also been described in patients with major depressive disorder. Therapies used to treat depression, such as selective serotonin reuptake inhibitors, serotonin and norepinephrine reuptake inhibitors, and tricyclic antidepressant have been found to affect microbial diversities and may be involved in patients' response to treatment.[121]

THE ROLE OF THE INTESTINAL MICROBIOME IN HUMAN DISEASE

Metabolic Function

Obesity (see Chapter 8): A number of lines of evidence point to a link between the intestinal microbiome and obesity. There is an abundance of observational data showing changes in microbiota composition at multiple taxonomic levels and decreased microbial diversity in obesity. The experimental data in support of the link between the microbiome and obesity include the lack of diet-induced obesity in germ-free mice and the greater weight gain following colonization of germ-free mice with intestinal microbiota from an obese human twin than from the lean twin.[122] Several putative mechanisms supporting a role for the intestinal microbiome in obesity and diabetes have been proposed such as increased energy harvest by microbial glycoside hydrolases, decreased muscle fatty acid oxidation mediated by a decrease in activated protein kinase, increased hepatic lipogenesis, alteration of satiety hormones, and induction of chronic low-grade inflammation. The intestinal microbiome decreases *fiaf* gene expression, which allows for more lipoprotein lipase activity and subsequently more white adipose tissue fat storage.[123] Microbial metabolites induce microRNA 181 family expression in diet-induced obese mice and humans, leading to decreased energy expenditure and increased body weight.[124] The small intestinal microbiome plays an important role in lipid digestion and absorption and may contribute to obesity.[125]

Type 2 diabetes (T2D): Similar to obesity, there are observational and experimental data supporting a role for the intestinal microbiome in T2D. In a pilot human study, fecal microbiome transplants (FMTs) from lean donors improved insulin sensitivity and increased microbial diversity and butyrate-producing bacteria in obese recipients.[126,127] The intestinal microbiome is also an important determinant of glycemic responses to different dietary nutrients,[128] which further supports its role both as a determinant and a therapeutic target in T2D. Potential mechanisms by which an altered microbiome may affect metabolism, insulin resistance and T2D include the modification of inflammatory cytokines, alterations in intestinal permeability leading to increased exposure to microbial components, effects on glycogen synthesis and gluconeogenesis related genes, and alterations in fatty acid synthesis and oxidation.[129]

Metabolic dysfunction associated liver disease (MASLD) (see Chapter 89): MASLD, previously known as nonalcoholic fatty liver disease (NAFLD), is hepatic steatosis in the setting of at least another cardiometabolic condition such as T2D or obesity. The role of the gut microbiome and its associate metabolites in MASLD have been established through multiple lines of evidence. Dysbiosis, evidence by decreased microbial diversity and an altered ratio of Firmicutes to Bacteroidetes phyla has been noted and is associated with disruption in the intestinal barrier, with increased exposure of bacteria and their metabolic products to the liver, which can trigger inflammation.[130] Dysregulated microbial metabolites such as SCFAs, bile acids, tryptophan metabolites, and ethanol, have been linked to MASLD and hepatocellular carcinoma development.[123,131] Additionally, microbial components, such as flagellin, lipopolysaccharide, peptidoglycan, and polysaccharide A, have been found to contribute to disease.[130] Gene variants and gene expression associated with MASLD also shape the composition and function of the gut microbiota. In the turn, the intestinal microbiota and its metabolites can cause epigenetic change associated with the development of MASLD.[130] Gut microbial signatures have also been associated with risk of MASLD, MASH, and hepatocellular carcinoma.

Inflammatory Diseases

IBD (see Chapters 117 and 118): The role of the intestinal microbiome in IBD has been extensively studied. Genetic studies link IBD with host polymorphisms in genes that function as bacterial sensors, such as nucleotide-binding oligomerization domain-containing protein 2 (*NOD2*) and *TLR4*,[84] suggesting an etiologic role for the intestinal microbiome. This relationship is further supported by improvement in subsets of patients with IBD after antibiotic treatment.[132] Furthermore, a meta-analysis has found that exposure to antibiotics increases the odds of being newly diagnosed with Crohn disease.[133] The absence of inflammation in susceptible germ-free animals suggests that the intestinal microbiome is an important component of IBD pathogenesis. There is significant heterogeneity among the described intestinal microbiota changes in patients with IBD, which is expected, given that IBD is a multifactorial disease and several contributing factors, such as genetics, early life exposure, and diet, are also known to influence the intestinal microbiota composition. A reduction in alpha diversity is seen as a consistent trend, but relative increase in the abundance of *Enterobacteriaceae*, including *E. coli* and *Fusobacterium*, have also been described in patients with IBD. While significant interindividual variation in bacterial genus and species exists about individual patients, metagenomic and metabolomic studies suggest that functional outcomes of microbial changes in IBD patients may have the most impact on disease activity. Patients with active IBD have decreased abundance *Roseburia* species and *Faecalibacterium prausnitzii*, both of which produce butyrate. Butyrate inhibits inflammation through an enhanced number of Treg cells, inhibition of proinflammatory cytokines, and stimulation of anti-inflammatory cytokines. Therefore a lack of microbial butyrate production is linked to higher levels of intestinal inflammation.[134] Decreased conversion of primary to secondary bile acids due to decreased levels of *F. prausnitzii* and *E. coli* also occurs in IBD and may be another mechanism by which dysbiosis contributes to inflammation. Secondary bile acids act through TGR4 to exert anti-inflammatory changes in intestinal epithelium.[135]

Celiac disease (see Chapter 109): Celiac disease is an immune-mediated condition triggered by gluten in genetically susceptible individuals.[136] However, while 30%–45% of the population carries the genetic risk alleles (HLA DQ2 and DQ8), only about 1% of the population develops celiac disease.[137] Therefore environmental triggers of celiac disease have been implicated. Viral infection with adenovirus, enterovirus, hepatitis C virus, and rotavirus has been associated with increased celiac disease incidence.[138] Treatment of HLA DQ8 transgenic mice with reovirus strain T1L prior to feeding with gliadin, a derivative of gluten, leads to the development of antibodies directed again gluten and intestinal inflammation in response to gluten.[139] Reovirus infection does also occur in humans, often during early childhood, when food, including gluten containing wheat is introduced, and when children are most susceptible to develop celiac disease. Celiac disease patients also have higher levels of reovirus antibodies than controls, which establishes the possibility that there may be a link between reovirus infection and celiac disease in humans as well. Subsequent studies have found that reoviruses can lead to loss of tolerance to food antigens through a suppression of Treg cell conversion and a stimulation of inflammatory Th1 response to the food antigen.[140] Most recently, the intestinal single-celled protist *Tritrichomonas arnold* from the class Parabasalia is found to prevent viral mediated loss of tolerance by modifying dendritic cells to promote Treg cell development and limit inflammatory Th1 cell responses.[141] Human stool samples from celiac patients do have less Parabasalia than the stool of healthy controls.

The oral microbiome of patients with celiac disease and those with refractory celiac also differs from healthy controls and contains higher salivary glutenase activity.[142] While the significance of these changes in the oral microbiome are unclear, the increased microbial metabolism of gluten in the mouth may lead to changes in gluten processing and presentation to the immune system in the intestine.

Cancer

Colorectal cancer (CRC; see Chapter 127): The intestinal microbiome may trigger carcinogenesis, either directly (by producing carcinogenic molecules) or indirectly (by creating a proinflammatory microenvironment).[143] Meta-analysis of sequencing data from CRC patient fecal metagenomes has found an enrichment of oral bacteria such as *Peptostreptococcus anaerobius*, *Porphyromonas asaccharolytica*, *Solobacterium moorei*, and *Prevotella intermedia* in the stool.[144,145] Colon bacteria enriched in CRC patients include *Bacteroides fragilis*, *E. coli*, *Streptococcus gallolyticus, and Morganella morganii*.[146] Transfer of fecal microbiota from CRC patients into germ-free mice does enhance colon cell proliferation and accelerates carcinogen induce colon tumorogenesis.[147] Mechanisms by which bacteria may promote CRC include the microbial production of genotoxins that cause DNA mutagenesis, modification of oncogene signaling cascades through pathobiont interaction with cell surface receptions, promotion of immune evasion, interaction with host gene or epigenetic change, conjugation of bile into carcinogenic secondary bile acids, and promotion of inflammation.[148]

Disorders of the Gut-Brain Interaction

A role for intestinal bacteria in disorders of the gut-brain interaction, such as IBS, has been proposed based on compositional changes in the microbiota and their role in modulating host physiology, including GI transit, epithelial barrier function, intestinal secretion, visceral sensation, and modulation of the gut-brain axis (see Chapter 124). There is no consistent "IBS-microbiota" pattern, but there appears to be a decrease in microbial diversity and alterations at different taxonomic levels.[149,150] Several microbial metabolites such as SCFAs, hydrogen sulfide, methane, tryptamine, and bile acids have demonstrated effects on host physiology.[149] Microbiota-targeted therapies are widely used in functional GI disorders. Many patients note worsened symptoms after ingesting certain foods. The low FODMAP (fermentable oligosaccharides, disaccharides, monosaccharides, and polyols) diet has been shown to improve symptoms in patient with IBS as compared to baseline diet or other dietary interventions. Gut microbial metabolism of high FODMAP foods may lead to GI symptoms through increased intestinal pressure and serotonin release.[151] Limited data suggest that intestinal microbial profiles, such as those with more Firmicutes and less Bacteroidetes, may lead to a higher chance of response to the low FODMAP diet.[152] Dietary consumption of a diet high in ultra-processed food is also associated with an increased incidence of IBS.[153]

The available data suggest improvement in global symptoms such as bloating and flatulence when considering all probiotics[154] but do not provide support for a therapeutic action of any specific probiotic, prebiotic, or synbiotic (see Chapter 132). FMT has also been used to treat patients with IBS-D, albeit with varied results.[155] As with other diseases, more rigorous trials need to be performed before the role of FMT for IBS, if any, can be determined.

THE ROLE OF THE INTESTINAL MICROBIOME IN MODULATION OF DRUG RESPONSE

The intestinal microbiome is an important factor in the observed interindividual differences in therapeutic responses and adverse events to medications. Intestinal microbiota-encoded genes not only enhance the metabolic capabilities of the host[156] but also play a role in the biotransformation of luminal compounds including medications.[157] The plasticity of the microbiome makes it an even more relevant factor because, in contrast to genes, the microbiome is modifiable. The microbiome has been identified as having a role in determining response to medications, mediating the effect of medications, and metabolism of certain medications, thereby affecting their efficacy or adverse effects.[158] Although several such interactions have been identified, some are described in animal models and hence need to be confirmed in humans and validated across different cohorts. Secondary bile acids and coprostanol, which are a result of microbial metabolism, may be predictive of response to statins.[159] The intestinal microbiome composition determines response to immune checkpoint inhibitor therapies. Melanoma patients with positive response to cell checkpoint inhibitor anti-PD-1 therapy were found to have higher alpha diversity and functional differences, including upregulation of anabolic pathways in their oral and fecal microbiome as compared to nonresponders. Transfer of the microbiome of anti-PD-1 responders to germ-free mice results in increased responsiveness of the micro and the anti-PD-1 therapy.[160,161] Furthermore, FMT from anti-PD-1 responder melanoma patients to patients refractory to therapy was able to overcome therapy resistance in 30% of patients.[162,163]

In addition, the intestinal microbiome may also be responsible in part for the antidiabetic effects of metformin.[164] The intestinal microbiome may also explain the interindividual differences in response to the common analgesic acetaminophen,[165] given that *p*-cresol produced by certain bacteria (e.g., *Clostridioides* genera) can compete with acetaminophen as a substrate for Sulfotransferase Family 1A Member 1, a human liver enzyme (SULT1A1),[165] and lead to a buildup of *N*-acetyl-*p*-benzoquinone imine, which, in turn, leads to hepatotoxicity. The chemotherapeutic agent irinotecan (CPT-11) used in treatment of colon and pancreatic cancer is inactivated in the liver, but the inactive metabolites can be transformed into active drug by bacterial β-glucuronidases, which in turn results in diarrhea, a significant side effect that may necessitate discontinuation of the drug in some patients.[166] A targeted inhibition of such bacterial enzymes can significantly improve compliance with chemotherapeutic regimens without affecting efficacy. These examples represent just the tip of the iceberg and given the immense metabolic potential of the intestinal microbiota,[167] it likely plays an important role in the biotransformation and response of most therapeutic agents.

THERAPEUTIC MODULATION OF THE INTESTINAL MICROBIOME

The intestinal microbiome is an important area of study as it represents a modifiable factor in pathophysiology of disease and response to medications. There are several approaches currently used to modulate the microbiome (see Fig. 3.1) ranging from an ecosystem approach as in IMT, use of selected bacterial strains alone or in combination with probiotics, stimulation of specific bacterial community functions through prebiotics, and combination approaches as with synbiotics and diet. IMT has had the most significant impact in the management of acute conditions as *Clostridioides difficile* infection (CDI), which is now the most common health care–associated infection in the United States.[168,169] There are several mechanisms that contribute to the effectiveness of IMT in CDI, including an increase in secondary bile acid production, restoration of microbial diversity and filling of open nutritional niches, and changes in microbial community structure with an increase in butyrate producers. Overall, the response rate of IMT in RCDI ranges from 80% to 95%[170] and in a meta-analysis (observational studies), the primary cure rate was

91.2% and the overall recurrence rate was 5.5%.[171] Patients who have received allogeneic stem cell transplant for malignancy and develop GVHD have been found to have a less diverse microbiome with few anaerobes.[172] IMT has success with patients with steroid dependent or steroid refractory GVHD and is under further study. IMT has also been successful in reducing multidrug-resistant organism colonization. A randomized controlled trial of IMT in renal transplant recipients showed that eight out of nine IMT-treated patients were MDRO culture negative at the end of the study, and the time to recurrent MDRO infection was longer in the treatment group.[173] Pilot studies in patients colonized with vancomycin-resistant *Enterococcus* (VRE) show that IMT may be beneficial in the decontamination of VRE.[174,175] However, long-term benefit in more chronic conditions, such as inflammatory bowel disease or disorders of the gut-brain interaction, has remained a challenge.

Stool substitutes are currently being studied and may replace IMT in the near future. IMT does carry a risk of transmission of pathogens or transfer or microbes that may be associated with an increased risk of certain diseases or may be pro-oncogenic. Furthermore, IMT donor fecal material is limited in quantity and uniformity. The US Food and Drug Administration has recently created a new designation called "Live biotherapeutic products (LBPs)" to refer to live bacterial products that go through the regulatory process of a drug. Vowst (Seres Therapeutics, Boston, USA) is an oral encapsulated therapy composed of live purified *Firmicutes* spores approved for the prevention of recurrent CDI[176] and Rebyota (Ferring Pharmaceuticals, Saint-Prex, Switzerland) is a live microbial suspension given rectally for prevention of recurrent *C. difficile*.[177]

In contrast, probiotics are live microbial products that confer a health benefit but are not regulated as drug therapies. Although there are trends that support benefits for certain probiotic strains or formulations in diarrheal states, necrotizing enterocolitis, IBD, and IBS,[178,179] there are major shortcomings in relation to clinical studies of probiotics, making it difficult to derive a clinically useful message (see Chapter 130). The microbial consortia approach appears to be more promising with studies showing that defined consortia of commensal bacteria containing the *Clostridium* cluster XIVa species, *Blautia producta* and *Clostridium bolteae* can restore colonization resistance against VRE[180]; consortia of commensal bacteria within the Clostridiales order can confer resistance to *Listeria monocytogenes*[181]; and consortia containing *Clostridium scindens* can restore colonization resistance against *C. difficile*.[182] The identification of specific microbial mediators and improved understanding of the mechanism underlying the effects of intestinal bacteria will help develop the next generation of more targeted probiotics, including genetically engineered commensal/probiotic organisms to deliver vaccines or therapeutic molecules.[183,184] Prebiotics were initially designed to boost certain beneficial bacteria such as *Lactobacilli* and *Bifidobacteria*; however, this approach has since evolved to focus on the overall functionality of the microbial community and its effect on host function; as a result, this group is no longer restricted to specific oligosaccharides but includes a wide array of dietary ingredients. A *synbiotic* refers to the combination of a prebiotic with a probiotic, which in theory should amplify the benefits of the probiotic and this has in fact been seen in a large study of infants for the prevention of sepsis.[185] The safety record of microbiota-targeted therapies has been good[186,187]; however, the data lack the rigor that one associates with drug safety monitoring.[188] The intestinal microbiota is also a rich source of a relatively new class of therapeutics often referred to as pharmabiotics, which includes the exopolysaccharide coat[189,190] and pili[191] of certain bifidobacteria; antibacterial molecules, known as bacteriocins; antibacterial phages; and even bacterial DNA, which has been demonstrated to exert anti-inflammatory activity.[192–197]

FUTURE DIRECTIONS

We need metrics to define and measure a healthy microbiome. Since there is no clear healthy microbiome configuration from a strain cataloging, sequencing perspective, we need to develop metabolic or transcriptomic measurements that better measure microbiome functional outputs such as metabolite production and immune modulation. Furthermore, as we expand our understanding of microbial metabolic pathways and the interaction of microbial metabolites with host physiology, we will be able to develop more precise interventions using an integrated systems biology approach, potentially tailored to an individual's microbiome.

We continue to map the contribution of microorganisms other than bacteria, such as fungi, bacteriophages, and parasites and the interkingdom signaling among the microorganisms and the host, which will could be crucial for effective manipulation of the microbiome.

To better realize the full potential of the intestinal microbiome, we still face significant challenges in the form of heterogeneity in collection, sequencing, and analysis of samples, differences in species and strains of bacteria used in interventions, reliance on association of specific microbes with disease states, and lack of recognition of the microbiome as an important biological variable in clinical studies and drug trials.

Acknowledgments

The authors gratefully acknowledge the important and valuable contributions of the authors of previous editions, Eugene Chang, MD and Purna Kashyap, MBBS.

Full references for this chapter can be found on https://ebooks.health.elsevier.com.

4 Gut Sensory Transduction

Diego V. Bohórquez, Rodger A. Liddle

IN THIS CHAPTER

The GI tract relies on hormones and neurotransmitters to integrate signals arising in the lumen with whole-body homeostasis. For instance, satiety in the brain is, to a great extent, induced by the presence of food in the gut. This process begins with ingestion of nutrients that stimulate sensory cells in the intestinal epithelium that modulate food intake via the release of specific chemical messengers. Classic studies established enteroendocrine cells as the source of hormone peptides that regulate appetite. Recent discoveries have shown that some enteroendocrine cells, known as neuropod cells, synapse directly with nerves to regulate appetitive choices. GI hormones and neurotransmitters are intimately involved with every aspect of the digestive process, including ingestion and absorption of nutrients. It is not surprising therefore that these transmitters are essential for life.[1,2] In this chapter, the critical role of the regulatory transmitters in GI function is analyzed by covering the following aspects: their synthesis and secretion from sensory epithelial cells, how food or other GI luminal factors trigger their release, the most representative members, and their importance in the context of disease.

HORMONES AND NEUROTRANSMITTERS

The sensory cells of the GI epithelium, enteroendocrine cells and neuropod cells, as well as neurons of the enteric nervous system are the main producers of chemical messengers, which are released in the form of hormones or neurotransmitters. Enteroendocrine and neuropod cells reside in the intestinal mucosa as single cells that are scattered among more numerous enterocytes—the absorptive cells of the gut. These sensory epithelial cells are oriented with their apical surface open to the lumen, where they are exposed to food and other contents within the gut lumen. Upon stimulation, enteroendocrine cells release from their basolateral surface hormones, which enter the paracellular space where they are taken up into the blood. In contrast, neuropod cells detect nutrients and rapidly release neurotransmitters that activate specific vagal nodose neurons. Below the mucosal epithelium are found enteric neurons, and even though villi and crypts are richly innervated, enteric neurons are not believed to be directly exposed to nutrients in the lumen of the gut.

Defining Hormones and Neurotransmitters

Criteria exist for determining if a candidate transmitter is a true hormone or a neurotransmitter. The first hormone to be discovered was secretin, when it was shown that injection of intestinal extracts into the blood stimulated pancreatic secretion.[3] Since then, the following criteria have been established to prove that a substance functions as a hormone. *First*, the stimulation of one organ must cause distant response by acting through the blood. *Second*, the response must be independent of neural stimulation. *Third*, no response should occur in the absence of the secretory organ. And *fourth*, the response should be reproducible by applying pure amounts of the candidate hormone onto the target tissue. There are more than 30 GI hormones that meet these criteria, and their singularities are discussed in "The Transmitters" section of this chapter.

Demonstrating that a chemical is a neurotransmitter is perhaps more challenging, the following criteria are agreed to define a neurotransmitter. *First*, the candidate molecule must be present within a presynaptic neuron. *Second*, the transmitter must be released in response to presynaptic depolarization. And, *third*, specific candidate-receptors must be present on the postsynaptic cell.

Hormones are commonly thought to reside exclusively in the endocrine system and neurotransmitters in the nervous system. However, these concepts were proposed when no technologies existed to visualize a single cell communicating with its surroundings. Today, it is becoming clearer that both systems are closely and synergistically related. Indeed, some cells exert both endocrine and neural actions. For example, peripheral sensory cells, such as taste cells of the tongue and solitary chemosensory olfactory cells of the nose, are known as paraneurons and can release both hormones in the bloodstream and neurotransmitters at synaptic connections.[4] In the intestinal epithelium, enteroendocrine and neuropod cells perform these functions.[5,6] Moreover, one transmitter can act both as a hormone or neurotransmitter depending on its location. For instance, upon the ingestion of food, cholecystokinin (CCK) is typically released from enteroendocrine cells into the bloodstream to act as a hormone. However, CCK is also abundant in nerves of the GI tract and brain, where it is released at synaptic terminals to act as a neurotransmitter. This conservation of transmitters allows the same messenger to have different physiologic actions at different locations and is made possible by the manner in which the transmitter is delivered to its target tissues.

Modes of Transmitter Release

Transmitters from sensory epithelial cells can be released onto their targets in the following manner: endocrine, paracrine, autocrine, or through synaptic neurotransmission (Fig. 4.1).

Endocrine

This type of communication occurs when transmitters are secreted into the bloodstream. The most common endocrine transmitters are peptides, lipids, and monoamines, and are collectively known as *hormones*. In the GI tract the most common type of hormone is in the peptide form (e.g., peptide YY, gastrin, and secretin). Hormones bind to specific receptors on the surface of target cells at remote sites and regulate metabolic processes.[7]

Paracrine

In contrast to endocrine mechanisms used to reach distant targets through the blood, signaling cells of the GI tract can also produce transmitters that act on neighboring cells. This process is known as *paracrine signaling* and is typical of enteroendocrine cells that produce somatostatin.[8] Paracrine transmitters are secreted locally and cannot diffuse far. They bind to receptors on nearby cells to exert their biological actions. Once released, the transmitter is rapidly taken up by the target cell, catabolized by extracellular

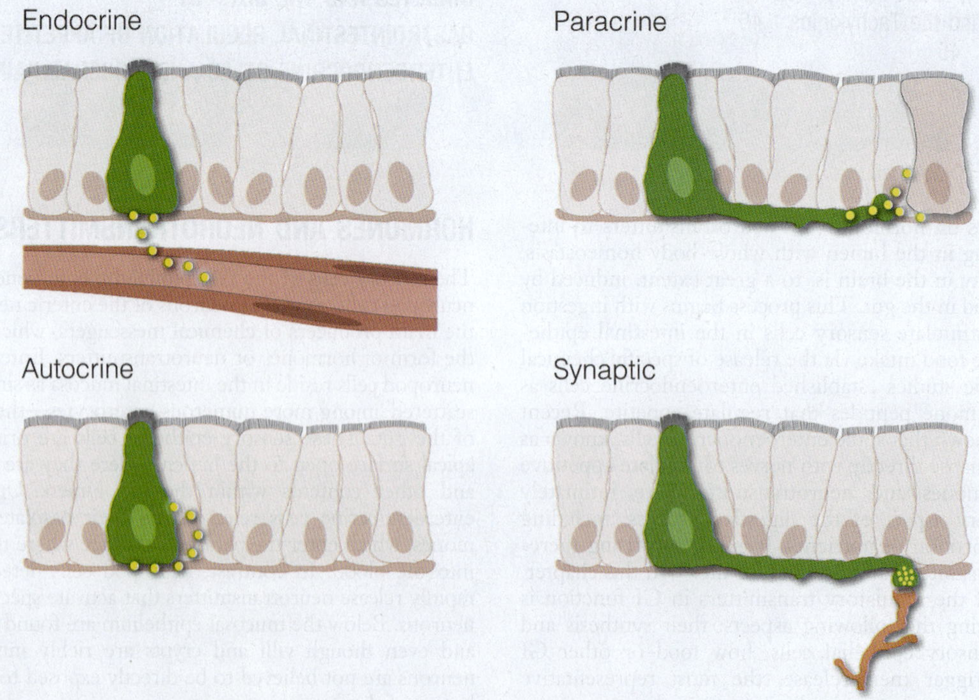

Fig. 4.1 Modes of transmitter release. Transmitters can be secreted from chemosensory cells and neurons through the following mechanisms: endocrine (into the blood), paracrine (locally into the paracellular space acting on nearby cells), autocrine (locally into the paracellular space acting on the releasing cell), or synaptic (neurotransmission).

enzymes, or become adherent to extracellular matrix, thus limiting the transmitter's ability to act at distant sites. Because paracrine signals act locally, their onset of action is generally rapid and can be terminated abruptly. By comparison, endocrine signaling takes much longer, and termination of signaling requires clearance of hormone from the circulation. Paracrine transmitters can be peptides (e.g., somatostatin) or monoamines (e.g., histamine).

Autocrine

Some cells possess cell surface receptors for their own messengers. In this way, when a messenger is released, it can act on the same secreting cell. This mode of transmission is known as *autocrine* and has been demonstrated for several growth factors. Autocrine signaling has been implicated in the growth of certain cancers, including colorectal cancer (see Chapter 1).[9]

Neurotransmission

In the GI epithelium, this is the domain of neuropod cells. These sensory epithelial cells form synapses with nerves throughout the GI tract. Neurotransmission is also the domain of enteric neurons. Together, they form the enteric nervous system which is a complex network of nerve cells that must communicate efficiently to regulate numerous GI functions (Fig. 4.2). When neurons of the GI tract are activated, signals in the form of neurotransmitters are released at specific synapses on target cell. In this way, they influence the function of other neurons, muscle cells, epithelial and secretory cells, and other specialized cells of the GI tract, such as enteric glia. Neurotransmitters are critical for the processes of digestion, including the coordination of gut motility and secretion. Although the GI tract secretes a variety of neurotransmitters, the most common are peptides such as vasoactive intestinal polypeptide (VIP), or small molecules, such as acetylcholine and norepinephrine. Other molecules, such as nitric oxide (NO), can simply diffuse across the synaptic cleft to exert an effect on the postsynaptic cell. Some nerves release peptides or neurotransmitters directly into the blood. This process is called *neurocrine signaling* and may be used to cause systemic effects depending on the transmitter released.

The major hormones and neurotransmitters of the GI tract are listed in Box 4.1. Their actions depend on specific receptors located on target tissues. For instance, the specificity of neurotransmitter action is dependent on the precise location at which the nerve synapses with the target cell. Adjusting their synthesis, catabolism, or secretion regulates the transmitter concentration within the releasing cell. Once secreted, the concentration of a transmitter can be quickly modulated by catabolism or, in the case of neurotransmitters, reuptake into the secretory neuron. Many peptide transmitters have very short half-lives of 2–5 minutes. This allows for rapid initiation and termination of signaling.

TRANSDUCING SIGNALS FROM THE GI LUMEN

The process of nutrient sensing involves the activation of cell-surface receptors that trigger the release of transmitters. The transmitters then either enter the bloodstream or activate sensory afferent nerves. Enteroendocrine cells interact with nerves indirectly. Through paracrine or endocrine signals, they influence distant receptors in target cells. However, recent discoveries show that enteroendocrine cells also connect with nerves—these are known as neuropod cells.[204,205] Neuropod cells express pre-, post-, and transsynaptic proteins and connect to sensory neurons through synapses (Fig. 4.3). Recent studies show that these connections have broad applications, from appetitive decisions to mood and anxiety. Some key components involved in the transduction of signals from the lumen of the gut to the rest of the body are described in the following sections.

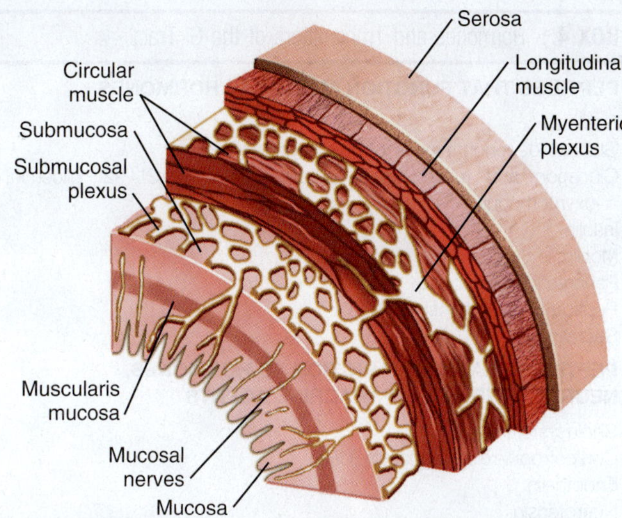

Fig. 4.2 Organization of the enteric nervous system. The enteric nervous system is composed of two major plexuses, one submucosal and one located between the circular and longitudinal smooth muscle layers. These neurons receive and coordinate neural transmission from the GI tract and central nervous system.

Recognizing Signals Through Cell Surface Receptors

GI epithelial cells recognize molecules in the lumen using membrane bound receptors. When activated, receptors transduce signals from the outside of the cell into the cytoplasm. Although the process is rather complex, there are key checkpoints at which the signaling cascade can be regulated. Some of these checkpoints occur at the moment of receptor activation, desensitization, internalization, and/or resensitization. Because of their regulatory potential, these are attractive targets for therapeutic intervention.

Receptors are grouped into major families depending on their structures and signaling mechanisms. The major families of cell surface receptors include G protein–coupled receptors (GPCRs), enzyme-coupled receptors, and ion channels. The following are some of the main aspects of each receptor family.

G Protein–Coupled Receptors

GPCRs are typified by their seven transmembrane domains. They are the most common family of protein receptors and have broad physiological applications, ranging from sensing light in the retina to allow vision to sensing nutrients in the GI tract to regulate food intake. When stimulated by a specific ligand, GPCRs undergo conformational changes leading to their association with a *G protein*—hence their name. These G proteins are bound to the intracellular surface of the cell membrane[10,11] and are composed of three distinct subunits—α, β, and γ. It is the *Gα subunit* that confers the name of the G protein (Table 4.1). For instance, G proteins that stimulate an effector (e.g., adenylate cyclase) are classified as Gs (for stimulatory), whereas those that inhibit an effector are called Gi (for inhibitory).[12–14] When the G protein acts on the *effector*, this causes a rapid increase in the intracellular concentrations of a *second messenger* (e.g., cyclic AMP or calcium). The second messenger then changes the activity of one or more protein kinases to catalyze the phosphorylation of an existing protein and ultimately modify the physiological activity.

BOX 4.1 Hormones and Transmitters of the GI Tract

PEPTIDES THAT FUNCTION MAINLY AS HORMONES

Gastrin
Glucose-dependent insulinotropic peptide (GIP)
Glucagon and related gene products (GLP-1, GLP-2, glicentin, oxyntomodulin)
Insulin
Motilin
Pancreatic polypeptide
Peptide tyrosine tyrosine (PYY)
Secretin

PEPTIDES THAT MAY FUNCTION AS HORMONES, NEUROPEPTIDES, OR PARACRINE AGENTS

Cholecystokinin (CCK)
Corticotropin-releasing factor (CRF)
Endothelin
Neurotensin
Somatostatin

PEPTIDES THAT ACT PRINCIPALLY AS NEUROPEPTIDES

Calcitonin gene-related peptide (CGRP)
Dynorphin and related gene products
Enkephalin and related gene products
Galanin
Gastrin-releasing peptide (GRP)
Neuromedin U
Neuropeptide Y
Peptide histidine isoleucine (PHI) or peptide histidine methionine (PHM)
Pituitary adenylate cyclase–activating peptide (PACAP)
Substance P and other tachykinins (neurokinin A, neurokinin B)
Thyrotropin-releasing hormone (TRH)
Vasoactive intestinal peptide (VIP)

PEPTIDES THAT ACT AS GROWTH FACTORS

Epidermal growth factor
Fibroblast growth factor
Insulin-like factors
Nerve growth factor
Platelet-derived growth factor
Transforming growth factor-β
Vascular endothelial growth factor

PEPTIDES THAT ACT AS INFLAMMATORY MEDIATORS

Interferons
Interleukins
Lymphokines
Monokines
Tumor necrosis factor-α

PEPTIDES THAT ACT ON NEURONS

Cholecystokinin
Gastrin
Motilin

NONPEPTIDE TRANSMITTERS PRODUCED IN THE GUT

Acetylcholine
Adenosine triphosphate (ATP)
Dopamine
γ-Aminobutyric acid (GABA)
Histamine
5-Hydroxytryptamine (5-HT, serotonin)
Nitric oxide
Norepinephrine
Prostaglandins and other eicosanoids

NEWLY RECOGNIZED HORMONES OR NEUROPEPTIDES

Amylin
Ghrelin
Guanylin and uroguanylin
Leptin

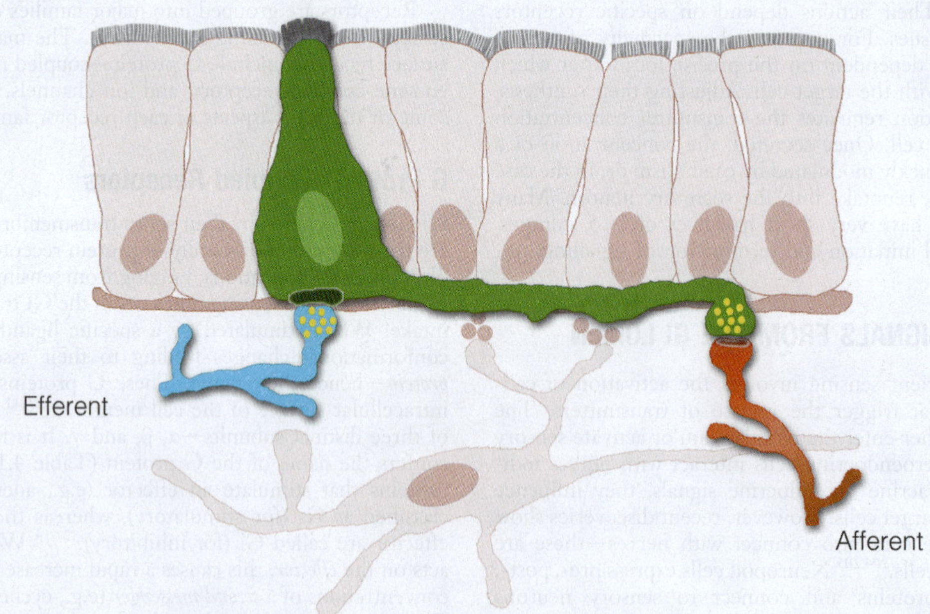

Fig. 4.3 Neuropod cells. Enteroendocrine cells that connect to neurons are known as neuropod cells and are capable of sending and possibly receiving neuronal signals.

TABLE 4.1 Classification of G Protein α Subunits and Their Signaling Pathways

Class	Signaling
Gαs	Adenylate cyclase, calcium channels
Gαi and Gαo	Adenylate cyclase, cyclic guanosine monophosphate, phosphodiesterase, c-Src, STAT 3
Gαq	Phospholipase C-β
Gα12 and Gα13	Sodium-hydrogen exchange

In general, the GPCR signaling mechanism involves the following events. When the **ligand** or first messenger binds to the receptor, the receptor changes its conformation and binds to the **G protein** complex. In the resting state, the G protein complex does not interact with the receptor. However, once bound, there is a molecular substitution in the **Gα subunit**—a guanosine diphosphate (GDP) is replaced by a guanosine triphosphate (GTP). This replacement causes the activation of the Gα subunit. The active Gα subunit then separates from the β and γ subunits, and moves laterally in the membrane to activate an **effector**. Working through different Gα subunits, the activity of an effector can be up- or downregulated. When the interaction is completed, the GTP bound to the Gα subunit is hydrolyzed back to GDP and dissociated from Gα. In this way, Gα moves back to reunite with the other two subunits. The effector then induces an increase in the intracellular concentration of a **second messenger**. The two most common second messengers are cyclic adenosine monophosphate (cAMP) and calcium. The mechanisms involving each second messenger are briefly outlined as follows.

Signaling Through Cyclic Adenosine Monophosphate (cAMP)

This second messenger is a classic downstream effector of β adrenergic receptors, a family of GPCRs that have been well characterized. These receptors are coupled to Gαs and activate adenylyl cyclase, which catalyzes the conversion of adenosine triphosphate (ATP) to cAMP. High concentrations of cAMP then modify the activity of protein kinase A (PKA) that ultimately modulates rate-limiting enzymes involved in important physiological functions. For instance, modulation of glycogen phosphorylase increases the conversion of glycogen to glucose-1 phosphate, leading to a rise in blood glucose levels.

Signaling Through Calcium (Ca^{2+})

GPCRs associated with Gαq subunits use Ca^{2+} as a second messenger. An increase in intracellular concentrations of Ca^{2+} can result from the activation of voltage-gated Ca^{2+} channels, ligand gated Ca^{2+} channels, or the release of cytosolic Ca^{2+} activated by membrane phospholipids. The latter is triggered by activation of GPCRs associated with Gαq. When active, Gαq moves along the cell membrane to activate the enzyme phospholipase C (PLC)-β. PLC-β then cleaves the membrane phospholipid phosphatidyl inositol bisphosphate into *diacylglycerol* and inositol 1,4,5-trisphosphate (*IP_3*), generating two potential signaling molecules. *Diacylglycerol* in the presence of Ca^{2+} activates protein kinase C. In addition, a rise in Ca^{2+} levels from internal stores can also activate Ca^{2+}–calmodulin kinase. In this way, two different kinases are activated: Ca^{2+}–calmodulin kinase by increasing cytosolic Ca^{2+} and protein kinase C by the action of diacylglycerol and Ca^{2+}. These kinases then catalyze the phosphorylation of target proteins within the cell. Following receptor activation, **IP_3** moves from the plasma membrane into the cytoplasm to bind IP_3 receptors located on the endoplasmic reticulum and mitochondria. IP_3 receptor binding causes release of Ca^{2+} from intracellular organelles to further increase cytoplasmic Ca^{2+} concentrations. Ultimately, Ca^{2+} cytoplasmic concentrations are restored to normal by active transport out of the cell or by reuptake into intracellular Ca^{2+} stores.

If the cell is overstimulated, a process of adaptation occurs to prevent the cell from overresponding. Attenuation of signaling occurs through either ligand-induced receptor *desensitization* or receptor *internalization*. The receptor is desensitized by means of phosphorylation. Phosphorylation can also further label the receptor for internalization, which is accomplished by activation of specific receptor kinases and the recruitment of arrestin-like molecules that uncouple the receptor from the G protein.[15] Uncoupling and subsequent receptor internalization ends signaling and eventually restores cell responsiveness.

Enzyme-Coupled Receptors

The most representative of the enzyme-coupled receptors are the tyrosine kinase receptor family. These receptors are primarily targets of growth factors, such as epidermal growth factor. These receptors are unique in that they are both a receptor and a tyrosine kinase. When activated, the receptors catalyze the transfer of phosphate from ATP to the target proteins. Enzyme-coupled receptors are composed of three domains: a ligand-binding extracellular domain, a transmembrane domain, and a cytoplasmic domain. The cytoplasmic domain contains a protein tyrosine kinase region and substrate region for agonist-activated receptor phosphorylation. In this way, phosphorylation from other kinases or autophosphorylation can modulate the activity of the tyrosine kinase receptor.[16] In general, receptor tyrosine kinases exist in the cell membrane as monomers. However, with ligand binding, these receptors dimerize, autophosphorylate, and initiate other intracellular signal transduction pathways that ultimately modulate physiological function.[17] Receptor tyrosine kinases are further discussed in Chapter 1 in relation to cellular growth and neoplasia.[18]

There are several other types of enzyme-coupled receptors, including receptor guanylate cyclases, nonreceptor tyrosine kinases, receptor tyrosine phosphatases, and receptor serine/threonine kinases. Although these receptors act through different enzymes, the signaling principles are similar to those of tyrosine kinase receptors.

Ion Channel–Coupled Receptors

Ion channel–coupled receptors are involved in rapid signaling between cells. This type of receptors is important in tissues where electrical impulses drive signaling, such as nerve cells and muscle. For instance, in neurons, ion channels open or close in response to a relatively small number of neurotransmitters and allow the flow of particular ions across the plasma membrane. The kinetics of the flow depend on the concentrations inside and outside the cell. This flow of ions regulates the excitability of the target cell to ultimately trigger processes, such as neurotransmission, muscle contraction, electrolyte and fluid secretion, or hormone release.

An example of this type of receptor is the transient receptor potential cation channel M5, or better known as TRPM5. This ion-channel receptor is activated by elevated intracellular Ca^{2+} concentrations and is a key component in the transduction of the taste signals bitter, sweet, and umami.[19] Moreover, it has been recently shown to mediate the release of opioids and hormones, such as CCK, from enteroendocrine cells.[20] Thus ion channel–coupled receptors can be attractive targets to modulate the function of sensory cells in the epithelium of the GI tract.

Mechanosensors

Mechanotransduction is the ability of a cell to convert a mechanical stimulus, such as pressure or shear force, into an electrochemical signal. In sensory cells, mechanical signals cause the release of hormones or neurotransmitters. In nonsensory cells, mechanical signals regulate cell growth, differentiation, transformation, secretion, and survival. All cells of the intestinal epithelia respond to mechanical stimuli but only specialized sensory cells, such as enteroendocrine cells, relay signals via hormones and neurotransmitters. Many types of membrane proteins are involved in mechanotransduction, including specialized cytoskeletal proteins, tight junction molecules, GPCRs, kinases, and ion channels. In intestinal epithelia, force is rapidly transduced by mechanically activated ion channels. Piezo proteins are a family of ion channels that are gated by mechanical force.[206] In sensory epithelial cells, such as enterochromaffin cells, mechanical stimulation causes the release of serotonin from enterochromaffin cells and have been implicated in the pathogenesis of irritable bowel syndrome (IBS). In model systems, pharmacologic blockade or genetic deletion of Piezo2 channels reduced stretch-induced intracellular calcium signaling, serotonin release, and intestinal secretion.[207]

NUTRIENT CHEMOSENSING

Sugars

Appetitive decisions are only transiently reinforced by the aroma or taste of nutrients. Instead, nutrients must enter the intestine for food preferences to be reinforced. In the case of sugar, animals can distinguish it from noncaloric sweeteners even in the absence of sweet taste signaling from the tongue. In recent years, it was discovered that neuropod cells guide an animal's preference for sugar over sweetener.[208] Sugars are both sweet and nutritive. To sort these properties in sugars, neuropod cells use a distinct set of molecular receptors and neurotransmitters. They detect sweetness through the taste receptor, Tas1r3, and the glucose molecule using the sodium glucose transporter 1. When their Tas1r3 receptor is activated, neuropod cells release the neurotransmitter ATP. Instead, when the glucose molecule enters the cell through the sodium glucose transporter 1, the cell releases glutamate. In this way, neuropod cells convey the sweetness and nutritive value of sugar to distinct vagal neurons so the message can be carried to the brain (Fig. 4.4).

When intestinal neuropod cells are silenced, a mouse is unable to distinguish a sugar solution from a noncaloric sweetener. This same effect is replicated when the neuropod cell's glutamatergic neurotransmission is pharmacologically inhibited. The effect is analogous to silencing retinal cone cells to render the animal color blind. An animal's consumption of sweetener or water is significantly increased when paired with stimulation of intestinal neuropod cells. Stimulating neuropod cells increases the reward value of the stimuli. This observation shows that appetitive choices are guided by nutrient sensing in the gut epithelium.

Lipids

Lipids in the intestinal lumen are potent inducers of satiety and modulators of whole-body metabolism. Although the mechanisms are not completely understood, specific lipids are recognized by cell surface receptors, which activate the release of several hormones, including CCK, peptide YY, and glucagon-like peptide-1 (GLP-1). The lipids can be in the form of triglycerides or free fatty acids of various chain lengths. Different lipids are recognized by different receptors. For instance, the Gq coupled GPCRs 40 (i.e., FFAR1) and 120 respond to medium- and long-chain fatty acids; whereas the $G\alpha_i$ coupled GPR41 (i.e., FFAR3) and GPR43 (i.e., FFAR2) bind to short-chain fatty acids of 2–5 carbons.[21] It is possible that some GPCRs respond to lipids in the lumen of the gut. Other non-GPCRs are also involved in lipid sensing, such as the immunoglobulin-like domain containing receptor (ILDR). ILDR is expressed in CCK cells and is activated by the combination of fatty acids and lipoproteins suggesting that fatty acids must be absorbed to stimulate CCK secretion. Although the specific location of most nutrient receptors has yet to be determined, it may be that at least some lipids need to be digested and absorbed prior to activating hormone release. This hypothesis is supported by studies, in which the infusion of lipid in the intestine triggers hormone secretion but only if chylomicrons, lipoprotein particles formed from absorbed lipids, are allowed to form.[22]

Some lipid-generated sensory signals appear to travel through afferent fibers of the vagus nerve. For instance, infusion lipids into the duodenum increases brown fat temperature, and this effect is abolished if lipids are infused along with tetracaine—a potent local anesthetic used to block vagal afferents activation.[23] Signals traveling through afferent nerves or the bloodstream ultimately induce homeostatic changes (e.g., satiety, body temperature, and GI motility) in response to the presence of nutrients in the GI lumen.

Proteins and Amino Acids

Proteins can also be potent stimulants of GI hormone secretion. Most proteins stimulate hormone secretion only when digested to peptones and amino acids (AAs). Recently, enteroendocrine cells have been found to express several classes of AA receptors that mediate hormone secretion. For instance, the calcium sensing receptor (CaSR), which was originally identified for its ability to detect and respond to extracellular Ca^{2+} and regulate calcium homeostasis in the kidney and parathyroid gland,[24] also recognizes L-AAs and di- and tri-peptides.[25] A clear role for CaSR has been established in the regulation of L-AA-stimulated gastrin and gastric acid secretion.[26,27] The aromatic AAs phenylalanine and tryptophan are the most potent AAs for stimulating CaSR and are also the most potent for stimulating CCK secretion. The discovery of CaSR in CCK cells and its link to secretion support its physiological importance as a nutrient sensor in the GI tract. Besides CCK, CaSR appears to also mediate the secretion of glucose-dependent insulinotropic polypeptide (GIP), GLP-1, and peptide YY (PYY).[28–30]

Another AA sensing receptor closely related to CaSR is the GPCR, GPRC6A. GPRC6A responds to basic AAs and is expressed in taste cells and enteroendocrine cells of the distal small intestine where it mediates the secretion of GLP-1.[31] Genetic deletion of GPRC6A leads to diet-induced obesity, implying that this receptor is important for metabolic regulation.[32] Finally, the taste receptors, T1R1/T1R3, also recognize acidic AAs and do not appear to be restricted to taste cells of the tongue but instead are distributed in chemosensory cells throughout the body. Together, CaSR, GPFC6A, and T1R1/T1R3 respond to all of the 20 L-AAs and represent a comprehensive mechanism to sense AA nutrient stimuli.

Partially digested protein in the form of peptones can also stimulate hormone secretion. The GPCR GPR93 is not only a lysophosphatidic acid receptor but is also activated by peptone.[33] GPR93 is expressed in enterocytes and enteroendocrine cells, where its activation has been coupled to CCK secretion.[34] Thus GPR93 may be the mechanism by which peptone stimulates CCK release following a meal.

Some intact proteins stimulate hormone secretion indirectly through a class of endogenous luminally active hormone releasing factors, including luminal CCK-releasing factor (LCRF)[35] and diazepam binding inhibitor (DBI).[36] The most potent proteins are those that compete for trypsin binding and allow the endogenous releasing factor to escape proteolytic digestion within the gut lumen.

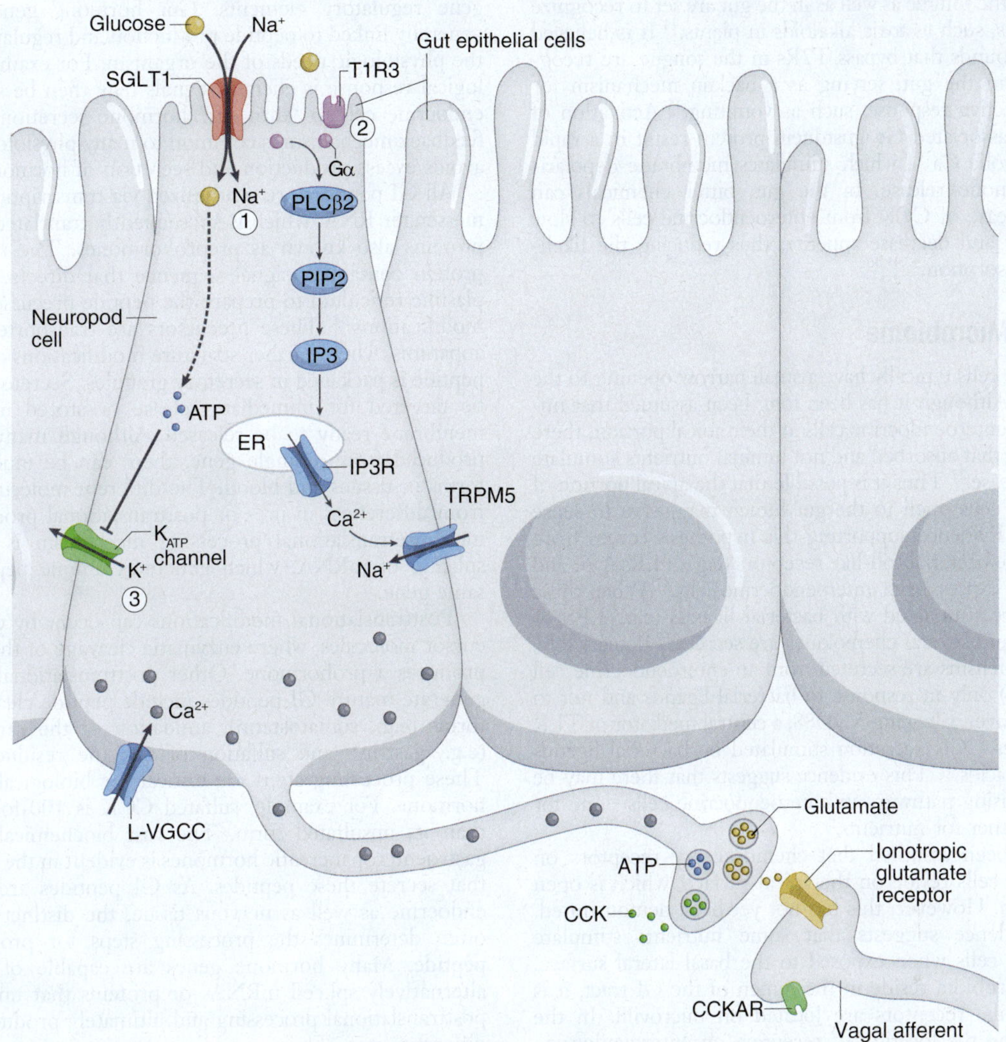

Fig. 4.4 Sensing sugar in the gut epithelium. In the GI epithelium, the neurotransducers are neuropod cells. These sensory epithelial cells form synapses with nerves throughout the GI tract and can signal to the brain. In the case of sugar, neuropods signal its presence in the gut using the neurotransmitter glutamate. They detect glucose in a meal using the sodium glucose transporter 1 (SGLT1). When glucose enters neuropod cells through SGLT1, they release glutamate to activate a specific population of vagal nodose neurons. In contrast, when neuropod cells detect a sweetener (e.g., sucralose) using the sweet taste receptor Tas1r3, they release the neurotransmitter ATP. This ability of neuropod cells to sort in seconds the properties of nutrients is essential for an animal to guide an animal's appetitive choices, such as the ability to seek and consume the most prevalent carbohydrate in nature—glucose. (From Liu WW, Bohórquez DV. The neural basis of sugar preference. *Nat Rev Neurosci*. 2022;23(10):584–595.)

Tastants

Sensing tastants in various foods is important to regulate pleasure, reward, food intake, and other important metabolic functions. The GI tract detects chemicals and toxins through specific receptors expressed by specialized chemosensory cells. These cells are best characterized in the tongue, where they are concentrated in taste buds. Taste receptor cells can detect chemicals that give rise to the five different flavors: sweet, salty, sour, bitter, and umami—the savory taste of soy sauce. Although this is an active area of research, only the sensing mechanisms for sweet, bitter, and umami flavors are well understood. These three flavors are mediated by the activation of two families of GPCRs: taste-1 receptors (T1Rs) and taste-2 receptors (T2Rs). In humans, there are 30 T2R proteins and three T1Rs, named T1R1, T1R2, and T1R3.[37–39]

Sweet and *umami* flavors are recognized by T1Rs. In the tongue, T1R1 and T1R2 are expressed in separate taste receptor cells, but always along with T1R3. In this way, the receptors form heterodimers that allow the detection of sweet ligands in the case of T1R2 + T1R3, and umami in the case of T1R1 + T1R3.[40] T1Rs are also expressed in enteroendocrine cells.[41] Here, the binding of glucose to T1R2 + T1R3 receptors in enteroendocrine cells in the gut lumen leads to secretion of incretin hormones, such as GLP-1. GLP-1 ultimately modulates a wide variety of functions, including insulin secretion, nutrient absorption, and gut motility.[42] Consequently, gut-expressed taste signaling has become an active area of research to develop therapies for diet-related disorders, such as type 2 diabetes.[43]

Bitter perception functions as a warning signal against the ingestion of toxic substances through direct taste aversion, induction of the pharyngeal gag reflex, and nausea. The wide array of

T2Rs present in the tongue as well as in the gut are set to recognize bitter compounds, such as toxic alkaloids in plants.[44] It is believed that bitter compounds that bypass T2Rs in the tongue are recognized by T2Rs in the gut, serving as a backup mechanism for inducing a protective response, such as vomiting.[45] Activation of T2Rs and their associated Gα-gustducin protein result in a rapid increase in cytosolic Ca^{2+}, which stimulates membrane depolarization and hormone release. In the gut, bitter chemicals can stimulate the release of CCK from enteroendocrine cells to slow gastric emptying and decrease appetite, thus reducing the likelihood of toxin absorption.[42,45,46]

Sensing the Microbiome

Enteroendocrine cells typically have a small narrow opening to the luminal surface. Although it has been long been assumed that nutrients stimulate enteroendocrine cells at their apical portion, there are some reports that absorbed and not luminal nutrients stimulate gut hormone release.[22] Thus it is possible that the apical portion of enteroendocrine cells open to the gut lumen may serve to sense bacterial inputs. Evidence supporting this hypothesis comes from the fact that some bacterial toll-like receptors (e.g., TLRs 4, 5, and 9) are exclusively expressed in enteroendocrine cells.[47] When these specific TLRs are stimulated with bacterial ligands (e.g., LPS or flagellin), CCK and several chemokines are secreted. Remarkably, cytokines and defensins are secreted from an enteroendocrine cell line (i.e., STC-1) only in response to bacterial ligands and not to fatty acids. Moreover, silencing MyD88, a central mediator of TLR signaling, reduces CCK secretion stimulated by bacterial ligands but not by fatty acids.[47] This evidence suggests that there may be two different sensing pathways in enteroendocrine cells—one for bacteria and another for nutrients.

It has long been assumed that chemosensory receptors on enteroendocrine cells reside on the apical surface, which is open to the gut lumen. However, this has not yet been demonstrated, and recent evidence suggests that some nutrients stimulate enteroendocrine cells when exposed to the basal lateral surface. Because gut microbiota reside in the lumen of the GI tract, it is likely that toll-like receptors are located on microvilli. In the future, elucidating the location of receptors on enteroendocrine cells may facilitate the design of drugs to target specific receptors and modulate the secretion of hormones involved in appetite regulation and insulin secretion.

Other Factors Stimulating Transmitter Release

There is evidence that GI hormones can be released by certain nonnutrient factors present in the lumen of the gut. CCK was the first hormone shown to be regulated by an intraluminal releasing factor.[35,48] LCRF was purified from intestinal washings and shown to stimulate CCK release when instilled into the lumen of animals. Other luminal factors causing the release of CCK are the diazepam-binding inhibitor and the pancreatic monitor peptide.[36,49] It has been proposed that a secretin-releasing factor regulates secretin secretion in an acid-sensitive way.[50] The pancreatic secretory trypsin inhibitor, better known as *monitor peptide*, is an endogenous trypsin inhibitor produced by pancreatic acinar cells.[51] When secreted into the duodenum, monitor peptide directly stimulates CCK secretion from I cells. These proteins act directly on enteroendocrine cells, most likely through cell surface receptors. The existence of these releasing factors highlights the existence of underappreciated bioactive molecules within the lumen of the gut.

THE TRANSMITTERS

The same factors that stimulate transmitter release simultaneously modulate the expression of specific transmitter genes through gene regulatory elements. Gut hormone gene expression is generally linked to peptide production and regulated according to the physiologic needs of the organism. For example, once a biological response is elicited, signals may then be sent back to the endocrine cell to "turn off" hormone secretion. This negative feedback mechanism is common to many physiologic systems and avoids excess production and secretion of hormones.

All GI peptides are synthesized via transcription of DNA into messenger RNA, which is subsequently translated into precursor proteins also known as preprohormones. The newly translated protein contains a signal sequence that directs it to the endoplasmic reticulum to prepare the peptide precursor for structural modifications.[52] These precursors are transported to the Golgi apparatus, where further structure modifications occur before the peptide is packaged in secretory granules. Secretory granules may be targeted for immediate release or stored near the plasma membrane ready to be released. Although many hormones are produced from a single gene, there can be multiple molecular forms in tissues and blood. The different molecular forms result from differences in pre- or posttranslational processing. A common pretranslational processing mechanism is the alternative splicing of mRNA, which generates unique peptides from the same gene.

Posttranslational modifications can occur by cleavage of precursor molecules, where enzymatic cleavage of the signal peptide produces a prohormone. Other posttranslational processes that generate mature GI peptides include peptide cleavage to smaller forms (e.g., somatostatin), amidation of the carboxyl terminus (e.g., gastrin), and sulfation of tyrosine residues (e.g., CCK). These processing steps are critical for biological activity of the hormone. For example, sulfated CCK is 100-fold more potent than its unsulfated form. The vast biochemical complexity of gastroenteropancreatic hormones is evident in the different tissues that secrete these peptides. As GI peptides are secreted from endocrine as well as nervous tissue, the distinct tissue involved often determines the processing steps for production of the peptide. Many hormone genes are capable of manufacturing alternatively spliced mRNAs or proteins that undergo different posttranslational processing and ultimately produce hormones of different sizes. These modifications are important for receptor binding, signal transduction, and consequent cellular responses.[53] As follows, we outline the major characteristics of GI transmitters, including neuropeptides, neurotransmitters, and other transmitters.

Gut Neuropeptides

It was previously believed that a single enteroendocrine cell (EEC) produced only one hormone. However, with transcriptomic profiling of purified EECs, it is now known that EECs produce multiple types of peptide hormones and neurotransmitters.[3,54,55] Therefore the categorization of EECs by the hormones they produce is not as straightforward as the traditional single letter nomenclature implied. It is also evident that stimulation of a single EEC can cause the release of multiple transmitters and thereby exert a variety of physiological responses. We summarize the major biological actions of the major transmitters from the gut in the following sections.

Gastrin

As discussed in more detail in Chapter 51, gastrin is the major hormone that stimulates gastric acid secretion. Subsequently, gastrin was found to have growth-promoting effects on the gastric mucosa and possibly some cancers.[56] Human gastrin is the product of a single gene located on chromosome 17. The active hormone is generated from a precursor peptide called preprogastrin. Human preprogastrin contains 101 AAs, but is processed by sequential enzymatic cleavage to the two major forms of gastrin: G_{34} and G_{17} and some small forms. The common feature of all gastrins is an amidated tetrapeptide (Try-Met-Asp-Phe-NH_2) carboxyl terminus, which imparts full biological activity. A nonamidated form of gastrin known as *glycine-extended gastrin* is produced by colonic mucosa. Glycine-extended gastrin has been shown in animal models to stimulate proliferation of normal colonic mucosa and enhance the development of colorectal cancer. It is not known whether local production of this form of gastrin contributes to human colon carcinogenesis, and the receptor for glycine-extended gastrin has not been identified.[57,58]

Most gastrin is produced in endocrine cells of the gastric antrum.[59] Much smaller amounts of gastrin are produced in other regions of the GI tract, including the proximal stomach, duodenum, jejunum, ileum, colon, and pancreas. Gastrin also has been found outside the GI tract, including in the brain, adrenal gland, respiratory tract, and reproductive organs, although its biological role in these sites is unknown.

The receptors for gastrin and CCK are related and constitute the so-called gastrin-CCK receptor family. The CCK-1 and CCK-2 (previously known as CCK-A and -B) receptor complementary DNAs were cloned from the pancreas and brain, respectively, after which it was recognized that the CCK-2 receptor is identical to the gastrin receptor of the stomach.[51]

The CCK-1 receptor is present in the gallbladder and, in most species, in the pancreas. The CCK-1 receptor has a 1000-fold higher affinity for CCK than for gastrin. The CCK-1 and CCK-2 gastrin receptors have greater than 50% sequence homology and respond differently to various receptor antagonists and to gastrin.

Gastrin is released from specialized endocrine cells (G cells) into the circulation in response to a meal. The specific components of a meal that stimulate gastrin release include protein, peptides, and AAs. Gastrin release is profoundly influenced by the pH of the stomach. Fasting and increased gastric acidity inhibit gastrin release, whereas a high gastric pH is a strong stimulus for its secretion.

Hypergastrinemia occurs in pathologic states associated with decreased acid production, such as atrophic gastritis. Serum gastrin levels can also become elevated in patients on prolonged acid-suppressive medications, such as histamine receptor antagonists and proton pump inhibitors. Hypergastrinemia in these conditions is caused by stimulation of gastrin production by the alkaline pH environment. Another important but far less common cause of hypergastrinemia is a gastrin-producing tumor, also known as Zollinger-Ellison syndrome (see Chapter 51).

Cholecystokinin

CCK is a peptide transmitter produced primarily by enteroendocrine cells of the proximal small intestine and is secreted into the blood following ingestion of a meal. Circulating CCK binds to specific CCK-1 receptors on the gallbladder, pancreas, smooth muscle of the stomach, and peripheral nerves to stimulate gallbladder contraction and pancreatic secretion, regulate gastric emptying and bowel motility, and induce satiety.[51] These effects serve to coordinate the ingestion, digestion, and absorption of dietary nutrients. Ingested fat and protein are the major food components that stimulate CCK release.

CCK was originally identified as a 33-AA peptide. However, since its discovery, larger and smaller forms of CCK have been isolated from blood, intestine, and brain. All forms of CCK are produced from a single gene by posttranslational processing of a preprohormone. Forms of CCK ranging in size from CCK-58 to -8 have similar biological activities.[60]

CCK is the major hormonal regulator of gallbladder contraction. It also plays an important role in regulating meal-stimulated pancreatic secretion (see Chapter 58). In many species, this latter effect is mediated directly through receptors on pancreatic acinar cells, but in humans, in whom pancreatic CCK-1 receptors are less abundant, CCK appears to stimulate pancreatic secretion indirectly through enteropancreatic neurons that possess CCK-1 receptors. In some species, CCK has trophic effects on the pancreas, although its potential role in human pancreatic neoplasia is speculative. CCK also has been shown to delay gastric emptying.[61] This action may be important in coordinating the delivery of food from the stomach to the intestine. CCK has been proposed as a major mediator of satiety and food intake, an effect that is particularly noticeable when food is in the stomach or intestine. CCK inhibits gastric acid secretion by binding to CCK-1 receptors on somatostatin (D) cells in the antrum and oxyntic mucosa. Somatostatin acts locally to inhibit gastrin release from adjacent G cells and directly inhibits acid secretion from parietal cells.[62]

Clinically, CCK has been used together with secretin to stimulate pancreatic secretion for pancreatic function testing. It is also used radiographically or scintigraphically to evaluate gallbladder contractility. There are no known diseases of CCK excess. Low CCK levels have been reported in individuals with celiac disease who have reduced intestinal mucosal surface area and in those with bulimia nervosa.[63,64] Elevated levels of CCK have been reported in some patients with chronic pancreatitis (see Chapter 61), presumably because of reduced pancreatic enzyme secretion and interruption of negative feedback regulation of CCK release.[65]

Secretin

The first hormone, secretin, was discovered when it was observed that intestinal extracts, when injected intravenously into dogs, caused pancreatic secretion.[66] Secretin is released by acid in the duodenum and stimulates pancreatic fluid and bicarbonate secretion, leading to neutralization of acidic chyme in the intestine (see Chapter 56). Secretin also inhibits gastric acid secretion (see Chapter 51) and intestinal motility.

Human secretin is a 27-AA peptide and, similar to many other GI peptides, is amidated at the carboxyl terminus. It is the founding member of the secretin-glucagon-VIP family of structurally related GI hormones. Secretin is most abundant in enteroendocrine cells of the small intestine but appears to be expressed in nearly all EECs.[67]

The secretin receptor is a member of a large family of GPCRs that is structurally similar to receptors for glucagon, calcitonin, parathyroid hormone, pituitary adenylate cyclase–activating peptide (PACAP), and VIP.

One of the major physiological actions of secretin is stimulation of pancreatic fluid and bicarbonate secretion (see Chapter 56). Pancreatic bicarbonate, on reaching the duodenum, neutralizes gastric acid and raises the duodenal pH, thereby "turning off" secretin release (negative feedback). It has been suggested that acid-stimulated secretin release is regulated by an endogenous intestinal secretin-releasing factor.[68] This peptide stimulates secretin release until the flow of pancreatic proteases is sufficient to degrade the releasing factor and terminate secretin release.

Although the primary action of secretin is to produce pancreatic fluid and bicarbonate secretion, it is also an enterogastrone, a substance that is released when fat is present in the GI lumen and that inhibits gastric acid secretion. In physiologic concentrations, secretin inhibits gastrin release, gastric acid secretion, and gastric motility.[69] The most common clinical application of secretin is to provoke gastrin release for the diagnosis of gastrin-secreting tumors,[70] as discussed in Chapter 34.

Vasoactive Intestinal Polypeptide

VIP is a neuromodulator that has broad significance in intestinal physiology. VIP is a potent vasodilator that increases blood flow in the GI tract and causes smooth muscle relaxation and epithelial cell secretion.[71,72] As a chemical messenger, VIP is released from nerve terminals and acts locally on cells bearing VIP receptors. VIP belongs to a family of GI peptides, including secretin and glucagon, that are structurally related. The VIP receptor is a GPCR that stimulates intracellular cAMP generation.

Like other GI peptides, VIP is synthesized as a precursor molecule that is cleaved to an active peptide of 28 AAs. VIP is expressed primarily in neurons of the peripheral-enteric and central nervous systems and is released along with other peptides, including primarily PHI and/or PHM (see Box 4.1).[73]

VIP is an important neurotransmitter throughout the central and peripheral nervous systems.[74] Because of its wide distribution, VIP has effects on many organ systems; most notably, in the GI tract, VIP stimulates fluid and electrolyte secretion from intestinal epithelium and bile duct cholangiocytes.[75,76]

VIP, along with NO, is a primary component of non-adrenergic, noncholinergic nerve transmission in the gut.[77] GI smooth muscle exhibits a basal tone, or sustained tension, caused by rhythmic depolarizations of the smooth muscle membrane potential. VIP serves as an inhibitory transmitter of this rhythmic activity, causing membrane hyperpolarization and subsequent relaxation of GI smooth muscle. Accordingly, VIP is an important neuromodulator of sphincters of the GI tract, including the lower esophageal sphincter and sphincter of Oddi. In certain pathologic conditions, such as achalasia and Hirschsprung disease, the lack of VIP innervation is believed to play a major role in defective esophageal relaxation and bowel dysmotility, respectively.[78,79]

Unlike GI endocrine cells that line the mucosa of the gut, VIP is produced and released from neurons and it is likely that most measurable VIP in serum is of neuronal origin. Normally, serum VIP levels are low and do not appreciably change with a meal. However, in pancreatic cholera, also known as Verner-Morrison syndrome and manifested by watery diarrhea, hypokalemia, and achlorhydria,[80] VIP levels can be extraordinarily high.[76] VIP-secreting tumors usually produce a voluminous diarrhea[81] (see Chapter 34).

Glucagon

Glucagon is synthesized and released from pancreatic alpha cells and from intestinal endocrine cells of the ileum and colon. Pancreatic glucagon is a 29-AA peptide that regulates glucose homeostasis via gluconeogenesis, glycogenolysis, and lipolysis and is counterregulatory to insulin. The gene for glucagon encodes not only preproglucagon but also GLPs. This precursor peptide consists of a signal peptide, a glucagon-related polypeptide, glucagon, and GLP-1 and GLP-2. Tissue-specific peptide processing occurs through prohormone convertases that produce glucagon in the pancreas and GLP-1 and GLP-2 in the intestine (Fig. 4.5).[82,83]

Glucagon and GLP-1 regulate glucose homeostasis.[84] Glucagon is released from the endocrine pancreas in response to a meal and binds to GPCRs on skeletal muscle and the liver to exert its glucoregulatory effects. GLP-1 stimulates insulin secretion and augments the insulin-releasing effects of glucose on the pancreatic beta cell (see later, "Enteroinsular Axis"). GLP-1 analogs have been developed for the treatment of type 2 diabetes mellitus. A long-acting human GLP-1 analog improves beta cell function and can lower body weight in patients with type 2 diabetes.[85,86] GLP-2

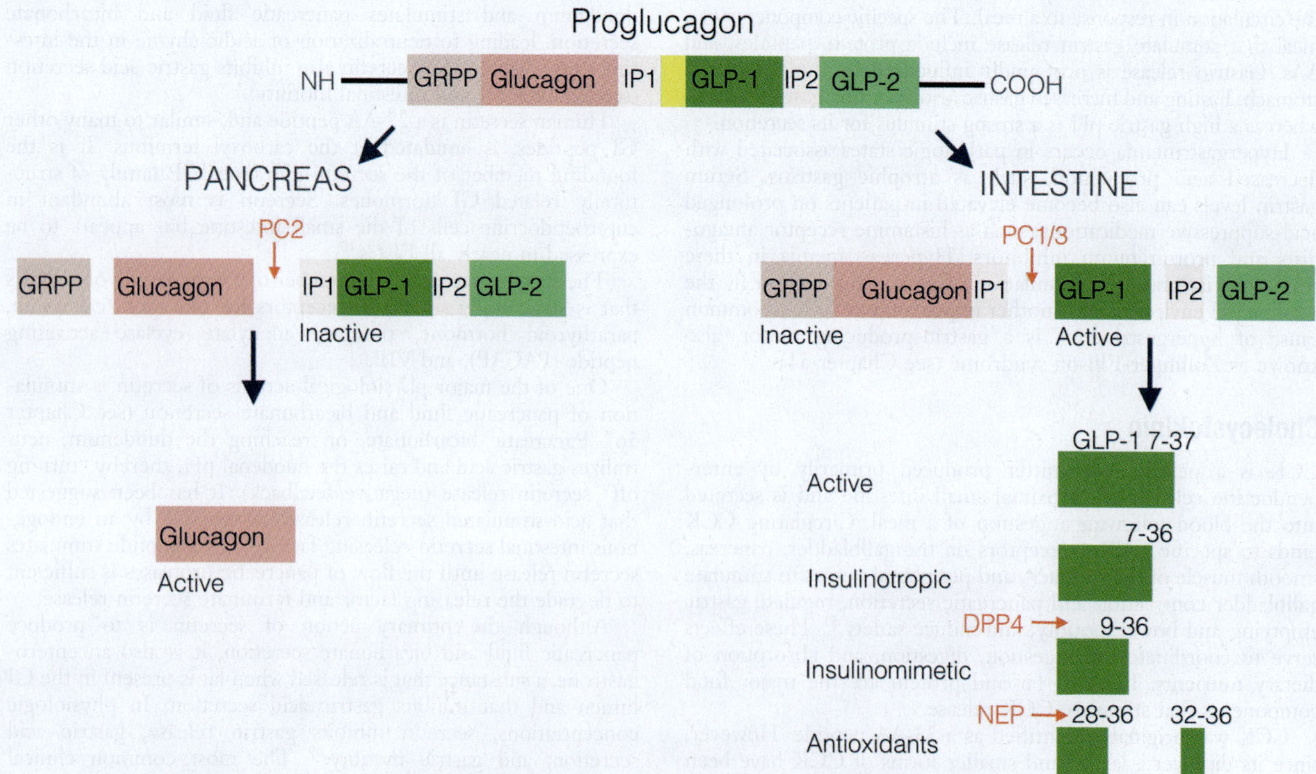

Fig. 4.5 Posttranslational processing of glucagon. The glucagon gene is transcribed and translated into proglucagon, a precursor peptide that undergoes enzymatic cleavage (*yellow box*). The product of the cleavage depends on the type of enzyme. For instance, PC2 expressed in the pancreas cleaves proglucagon into active glucagon; whereas, PC1/3 expressed in the intestine cleaves proglucagon into a peptide fragment that gives rise to glucagon-like peptide-1 (*GLP-1*) and glucagon-like peptide-2 (*GLP-2*). In the intestine, GLP-1 is further processed into smaller fragments with different bioactive functions. Some of the enzymes involved in the process are dipeptidyl peptidase-4 (*DPP4*) and neutral endopeptidase (*NEP*).

is an intestinal growth factor that increases villus height, stimulates intestinal crypt proliferation, and prevents enterocyte apoptosis. Based on these actions, GLP-2 agonists are used for the treatment of short bowel syndrome.

Glucose-Dependent Insulinotropic Polypeptide

GIP was discovered because of its ability to inhibit gastric acid secretion (enterogastrone effect) and was originally termed *gastric inhibitory polypeptide*. It was subsequently shown that the effects on gastric acid secretion occur only at very high concentrations that are above the physiologic range. However, GIP has a potent effect on insulin release that (like GLP-1) potentiates glucose-stimulated insulin secretion.[87] Based on this action, GIP was redefined as glucose-dependent insulinotropic polypeptide.

GIP is a 42-AA peptide produced by cells in the mucosa of the small intestine. GIP is released into the blood in response to ingestion of glucose or fat. In the presence of elevated blood glucose levels, GIP binds to its receptor on pancreatic beta cells, activating adenylate cyclase and other pathways that increase intracellular calcium concentrations, leading to insulin secretion. Importantly; however, the effects on insulin secretion occur only if hyperglycemia exists; GIP does not stimulate insulin release under normoglycemic conditions.

GIP receptors are also expressed on adipocytes, through which GIP augments triglyceride storage, which may contribute to fat accumulation. Based on the insulinotropic properties of GIP, coupled with its effects on adipocytes, it has been proposed that GIP may play a role in obesity and development of insulin resistance associated with type 2 diabetes mellitus.[88] Consistent with this proposal was the experimental finding that mice lacking the GIP receptor do not gain weight when placed on a high-fat diet.[89] It remains to be seen whether GIP antagonists can be used to treat obesity. In rare circumstances, receptors for GIP may be aberrantly expressed in the adrenal cortex, resulting in food-dependent Cushing syndrome.[90,91]

Pancreatic Polypeptide Family

Originally isolated during the preparation of insulin, pancreatic polypeptide (PP) is the founding member of the PP family.[92] The PP family of peptides includes neuropeptide Y (NPY) and PYY, which were discovered because of the presence of a C-terminal tyrosine amide.[93,94] PP is stored and secreted from specialized pancreatic endocrine cells (PP cells),[95] whereas NPY is a principal neurotransmitter found in the central and peripheral nervous systems.[96] PYY has been localized to enteroendocrine cells throughout the GI tract but is found in greatest concentrations in the ileum and colon, where it is produced in the same cells that synthesize GLPs.[97]

The PP-PYY-NPY family of peptides functions as endocrine, paracrine, and neurocrine transmitters in the regulation of a number of actions that result from binding to one of five receptor subtypes.[98] PP inhibits pancreatic exocrine secretion, gallbladder contraction, and gut motility.[99] PYY inhibits vagally stimulated gastric acid secretion and other motor and secretory functions.[100] An abbreviated form of PYY lacking the first two AAs of the normally produced 36-AA peptide, PYY_{3-36}, has been shown to reduce food intake when administered to humans, indicating that intestinally released peptide may play a role in regulating meal size.[101] Many PYY cells possess neuropods that run along the basal surface of adjacent enterocytes, which possess Y1 and Y2 PYY receptor subtypes. It is likely that locally released PYY exerts a colonic antisecretory effect.[102] NPY is one of the most abundant peptides in the central nervous system and, in contrast to PYY_{3-36}, is a potent stimulant of food intake.[103] Peripherally, NPY affects vascular and GI smooth muscle function.[104]

Substance P and the Tachykinins

Substance P belongs to the tachykinin family of peptides, which includes neurokinin A and neurokinin B. The tachykinins are found throughout the peripheral and central nervous systems and are important mediators of neuropathic inflammation.[105] Tachykinins, as a group, are encoded by two genes that produce preprotachykinin A and preprotachykinin B. Common to both is a well-conserved C-terminal pentapeptide. Transcriptional and translational processing produce substance P, neurokinin A, and/or neurokinin B, which are regulated in large part by alternative splicing. These peptides function primarily as neuropeptides. Substance P is a neurotransmitter of primary sensory afferent neurons and binds to specific receptors in lamina I of the spinal cord.[106] Three receptors for this family of peptides have been identified—NK-1, NK-2, and NK-3.[107] Substance P is the primary ligand for the NK-1 receptor, neurokinin A for the NK-2 receptor, and neurokinin B for the NK-3 receptor. However, all these peptides can bind and signal through all three receptor subtypes.

Substance P has been implicated as a primary mediator of neurogenic inflammation. In the intestine, *Clostridium difficile*–initiated experimental colitis results from toxin-induced release of substance P and consequent activation of the NK-1 receptor.[108] These inflammatory sequelae can be blocked by substance P receptor antagonists. Substance P receptors are more abundant in the intestine of patients with ulcerative colitis and Crohn's disease.[109]

Somatostatin

This is a 14-AA cyclic peptide that was initially identified as an inhibitor of growth hormone secretion. Since its discovery, it has been found in almost every organ in the body and throughout the GI tract. In the gut, somatostatin is produced by D cells in the gastric and intestinal mucosa and islets of the pancreas, as well as enteric neurons.[110] Somatostatin has a number of pharmacologic effects that are mostly inhibitory.

In the stomach, somatostatin plays an important role in regulating gastric acid secretion.[111] In the antrum, D cells are open to the lumen, where they are directly exposed to acid. A low gastric pH stimulates D cells that lie near gastrin-producing cells to secrete somatostatin and inhibit gastrin release (see Chapter 51). Reduced gastrin secretion decreases the stimulus for acid production and the pH of the stomach contents rises. Thus some of the inhibitory effects of gastric acid on gastrin release (see earlier, "Gastrin") are mediated by somatostatin.

Somatostatin release is also influenced by mechanical stimulation, dietary components of a meal, including protein, fat, and glucose, and other hormones and neurotransmitters.[112] Muscarinic stimulation appears to be the most important neural stimulus to somatostatin secretion.

At least five somatostatin receptors have been identified that account for divergent pharmacologic properties.[113] For example, receptor subtypes 2 and 3 couple to inhibitory G proteins but receptor subtype 1 does not. In addition, only somatostatin receptor subtype 3 inhibits adenylate cyclase. The inhibitory effects of somatostatin are mediated by a decrease in cAMP, Ca^{2+} channel inhibition, or K^+ channel opening.

In the gut, somatostatin has broad inhibitory actions. In addition to effects on gastric acid, somatostatin reduces pepsinogen secretion. Somatostatin profoundly inhibits pancreatic enzyme, fluid, and bicarbonate secretion and reduces bile flow.[114] The effects of somatostatin on gut motility are largely inhibitory, with the exception that it stimulates the migrating motor complex (MMC), possibly through effects on motilin. Somatostatin also reduces intestinal transport of nutrients and fluid, reduces splanchnic blood flow, and has inhibitory effects on tissue growth and proliferation.[115,116]

Because of its varied physiologic effects, somatostatin has several clinically important pharmacologic uses. Many endocrine cells possess somatostatin receptors and are sensitive to inhibitory regulation. Therefore somatostatin and more recently developed somatostatin analogs are used to treat conditions of hormone excess produced by endocrine tumors, such as acromegaly, carcinoid tumors, and islet cell tumors (including gastrinomas).[117] Its ability to reduce splanchnic blood flow and portal venous pressure has led to somatostatin analogs being used in treating esophageal variceal bleeding (see Chapter 94).[118] The inhibitory effects on secretion have been exploited by using somatostatin analogs to treat some forms of diarrhea and reduce fluid output from pancreatic fistulas. Many endocrine tumors express abundant somatostatin receptors, making it possible to use radiolabeled somatostatin analogs, such as octreotide, to localize even small tumors throughout the body.

Motilin

Motilin is a 22-AA peptide produced by endocrine cells of the duodenal epithelium.[119] Motilin is not released by the stimulation of food but instead is secreted into the blood in a periodic and recurrent pattern that is synchronized with the MMC under fasting conditions. Elevations in blood motilin levels regulate the phase III contractions that initiate in the antroduodenal region and progress toward the distal gut.

Motilin binds to specific receptors on smooth muscle cells of the esophagus, stomach, and small and large intestines through which it exerts propulsive activity.[120] Agonists to the motilin receptor, such as erythromycin, have pronounced effects on GI motility, which occasionally produce undesired side effects of abdominal cramping and diarrhea.[121] However, motilin agonists may be useful to treat conditions of impaired gastric and intestinal motility and are being investigated for the treatment of constipation-predominant IBS.[122]

Leptin

Leptin is a 167-AA protein that is secreted primarily from adipocytes. Blood leptin levels reflect total body fat stores.[123] Its primary action appears to be to reduce food intake. Leptin is a member of the cytokine family of signaling molecules. Five different forms of leptin receptors have been reported.[124] A short form of the receptor appears to transport leptin from the blood across the blood-brain barrier, where it has access to the hypothalamus. A long form of the leptin receptor is located in hypothalamic nuclei, where leptin binds and activates the Janus kinase signal transduction and translation system (JAK STAT).[125] Small amounts of leptin are produced by the chief cells of the stomach and by the placenta, and are present in breast milk.

Peripheral administration of leptin reduces food intake. However, this effect is reduced as animals become obese. Interestingly, when injected into the central nervous system, obese animals respond normally to leptin and reduce food intake, suggesting that leptin "resistance" in obesity occurs at the level of the leptin receptor that transports leptin across the blood–brain barrier.[126] Leptin's ability to reduce food intake occurs within the brain by decreasing NPY (a potent stimulant of food intake) and by increasing α-melanocyte-stimulating hormone (α-MSH), an inhibitor of food intake.[127] Peripherally, leptin acts synergistically with CCK to reduce meal size.[128] In obese rats lacking the leptin receptor, the synergistic effects of leptin plus CCK to reduce meal size are lost but could be restored with genetic reconstitution of the leptin receptor in the brain.[129] One might expect loss of leptin-CCK synergy on meal size in those rare cases of human obesity caused by leptin receptor defects or even with leptin resistance.

Blood levels of leptin increase as obesity develops and leptin appears to reflect total fat content.[130] At the cellular level, large adipocytes produce more leptin than small adipocytes. Because of its effects on food intake, it was initially thought that exogenous leptin could be used therapeutically to treat obesity. However, only a very modest effect on weight loss has been demonstrated in clinical trials. Leptin deficiency has been reported as a cause of obesity in a few families, but this condition is extremely rare.[131,132] Mutation of the leptin receptor has been described as a cause of obesity in at least one family.[133]

Ghrelin

Ghrelin is a 28-AA peptide produced by the stomach and is the natural ligand for the growth hormone secretagogue receptor.[134] When administered centrally or peripherally, ghrelin stimulates growth hormone secretion, increases food intake, and produces weight gain.[135,136] Circulating ghrelin levels increase during periods of fasting or under conditions associated with negative energy balance, such as starvation or anorexia. In contrast, ghrelin levels are low after eating and in obesity. Ghrelin appears to play a central role in the neurohormonal regulation of food intake and energy homeostasis.

The gastric fundus is the most abundant source of ghrelin, although lower amounts of ghrelin are found in the intestine, pancreas, pituitary, kidney, and placenta. Ghrelin is produced by distinctive endocrine cells known as P/D1 cells[137,138] that are of two types, open and closed. The open type is exposed to the lumen of the stomach, where it comes into contact with gastric contents, whereas the closed type lies near the capillary network of the lamina propria.[139] Both cell types secrete hormone into the bloodstream. Based on its structure, ghrelin is a member of the motilin family of peptides and, like motilin, ghrelin stimulates gastric contraction and enhances stomach emptying.

The observations that circulating ghrelin levels increase sharply before a meal and fall abruptly after a meal suggest that it serves as a signal for initiation of feeding. The effects of food on plasma ghrelin levels can be reproduced by ingestion of glucose and appear to be unrelated to the physical effects of a meal on gastric distention. Circulating ghrelin levels are low in states of positive energy balance such as obesity and are inversely correlated with body mass index.[140,141] Conversely, ghrelin levels are high in fasting, cachexia, and anorexia. Importantly, weight loss increases circulating ghrelin levels.[142]

Ghrelin released from the stomach acts on the vagus nerve to exert its effects on feeding. However, it is also active when delivered to the central nervous system, and in this location, ghrelin activates NPY and agouti-related protein-producing neurons in the arcuate nucleus of the hypothalamus, which are involved in the regulation of feeding.[136,143]

Gastric bypass patients do not demonstrate the premeal increase in plasma ghrelin that is seen in normal individuals.[144] This lack of ghrelin release may be one of the mechanisms contributing to the overall effectiveness of gastric bypass surgery for inducing weight loss.

Prader-Willi syndrome is a congenital obesity syndrome characterized by severe hyperphagia, growth hormone deficiency, and hypogonadism. Although obesity is ordinarily associated with low ghrelin levels, patients with Prader-Willi syndrome have high circulating ghrelin levels that do not decline after a meal.[145,146] The levels of ghrelin in this syndrome are similar to those that can stimulate appetite and increase food intake in individuals receiving infusions of exogenous ghrelin, suggesting that abnormal ghrelin secretion may be responsible for the hyperphagia in Prader-Willi syndrome.[147]

NEUROTRANSMITTERS

A limited number of transmitters have been described in neurotransmission throughout the GI tract. Even though their distribution is widespread, neurotransmitters confer specific and time limited actions at precise sites by virtue of their local release and reuptake or inactivation.

Acetylcholine

Acetylcholine is synthesized in cholinergic neurons and is the principal regulator of GI motility and pancreatic secretion. Acetylcholine is stored in nerve terminals and released by nerve depolarization. Released acetylcholine binds to postsynaptic muscarinic and/or nicotinic receptors. Nicotinic acetylcholine receptors belong to a family of ligand-gated ion channels and are homopentamers or heteropentamers composed of α, β, γ, δ, and ε subunits.[148] The α subunit is believed to be the mediator of postsynaptic membrane depolarization following acetylcholine receptor binding. Muscarinic receptors belong to the heptahelical GPCR family. There are five known muscarinic cholinergic receptors (M1 to M5). Muscarinic receptors can be further classified based on receptor signal transduction, with M1, M3, and M5 stimulating adenylate cyclase and M2 and M4 inhibiting this enzyme. Acetylcholine is degraded by the enzyme acetylcholinesterase, and the products may be recycled through high-affinity transporters on the nerve terminal.

Catecholamines

The primary catecholamine neurotransmitters of the enteric nervous system include norepinephrine and dopamine. Norepinephrine is synthesized from tyrosine and released from postganglionic sympathetic nerve terminals that innervate enteric ganglia and blood vessels. Tyrosine is converted to dopa by tyrosine hydroxylase. Dopa is initially converted into dopamine by dopa decarboxylase and packaged into secretory granules. Norepinephrine is formed from dopamine by the action of dopamine β-hydroxylase in the secretory granule. After an appropriate stimulus, norepinephrine-containing secretory granules are released from nerve terminals and bind to adrenergic receptors.

Adrenergic receptors are G protein–coupled, have seven typical membrane-spanning domains, and are of two basic types, α and β. α-Adrenergic receptors are further classified into α1A, α1B, α2A, α2B, α2C, and α2D. Similarly, β receptors include β1, β2, and β3. Adrenergic receptors are known to signal through various G proteins, resulting in stimulation or inhibition of adenylate cyclase and other effector systems. Norepinephrine signaling is terminated by intracellular monoamine oxidase or by rapid reuptake by an amine transporter. The actions of adrenergic receptor stimulation regulate smooth muscle contraction, intestinal blood flow, and GI secretion.

Dopamine

Dopamine is an important mediator of GI secretion, absorption, and motility and is the predominant catecholamine neurotransmitter of the central and peripheral nervous systems. In the central nervous system, dopamine regulates food intake, emotions, and endocrine responses and, peripherally, controls hormone secretion, vascular tone, and GI motility. Characterization of dopamine in the GI tract has been challenging for several reasons. First, dopamine can produce inhibitory and excitatory effects on GI motility.[149] In general, the excitatory response, which is mediated by presynaptic receptors, occurs at a lower agonist concentration than the inhibitory effect, which is mediated by postsynaptic receptors. Second, localization of dopamine receptors has been hampered by identification of dopamine receptors in locations that appear to be species specific.[150] Third, studies of dopamine in GI tract motility have often used pharmacologic amounts of this agonist. Therefore the interpretation of results has been confounded by the ability of dopamine to activate adrenergic receptors at high doses.

Classically, dopamine was thought to act via two distinct receptor subtypes, type 1 and type 2. Molecular cloning has now demonstrated five dopamine receptor subtypes, each with a unique molecular structure and gene locus.[151] Dopamine receptors are integral membrane GPCRs, and each receptor subtype has a specific pharmacologic profile when exposed to agonists and antagonists. After release from the nerve terminal, dopamine is cleared from the synaptic cleft by a specific dopamine transporter.

Serotonin

Serotonin has long been known to play a role in GI neurotransmission.[152] The GI tract contains more than 95% of the total body serotonin, and serotonin is important in various processes, including epithelial secretion, bowel motility, nausea, and emesis.[152] Serotonin is synthesized from tryptophan, an essential AA, and is converted to its active form in nerve terminals. Secreted serotonin is inactivated in the synaptic cleft by reuptake via a serotonin-specific transporter. Most plasma serotonin is derived from the gut, where it is found in mucosal enterochromaffin cells and the enteric nervous system. Serotonin mediates its effects by binding to a specific receptor. There are seven different serotonin receptor subtypes found on enteric neurons, enterochromaffin cells, and GI smooth muscle (5-HT1 to 5-HT7).

The actions of serotonin are complex (Fig. 4.6).[153] It can cause smooth muscle contraction through stimulation of cholinergic nerves or relaxation by stimulating inhibitory NO-containing neurons.[154] Serotonin released from mucosal cells stimulates sensory neurons, initiating a peristaltic reflex and secretion (via 5-HT4 receptors), and modulates sensation through activation of 5-HT3 receptors.[156] The myenteric plexus contains serotoninergic interneurons that project to the submucosal plexus and ganglia extrinsic to the bowel wall. Extrinsic neurons activated by serotonin participate in bowel sensation and may be responsible for abdominal pain, nausea, and symptoms associated with IBS. Intrinsic neurons activated by serotonin are primary components of the peristaltic and secretory reflexes responsible for normal GI function. Serotonin also may activate vagal afferent pathways and, in the central nervous system, modulates appetite, mood, and sexual function. Because of these diverse effects, it is not surprising that selective serotonin reuptake inhibitor drugs, commonly used to treat depression and anxiety, have prominent GI side effects when compared with placebo treatment.

Serotonin and its receptor have been implicated in the pathogenesis of motility disorders of the GI tract.[154] Characterization of specific serotonin receptor subtypes has led to the development of selective agonists and antagonists for the treatment of IBS and chronic constipation and diarrhea. For example, 5-HT3 receptor antagonists, which reduce intestinal secretion, are used to treat diarrhea-predominant IBS. 5-HT4 receptor agonists elicit prokinetic effects and are used to treat constipation-predominant IBS and other motility disorders.[155,156]

Serotonin can also be enzymatically converted to melatonin by serotonin *N*-acetyltransferase.[157] Other than the pineal gland, the GI tract is the major source of the body's melatonin. Melatonin is produced in enterochromaffin cells and released into the blood after ingestion of a meal. A number of actions on the GI tract have been described for melatonin, including reducing gastric acid and pepsin secretion, inducing smooth muscle relaxation, and preventing epithelial injury through an antioxidant effect.[158] It has been proposed that melatonin released after a meal may contribute to postprandial somnolence.[159]

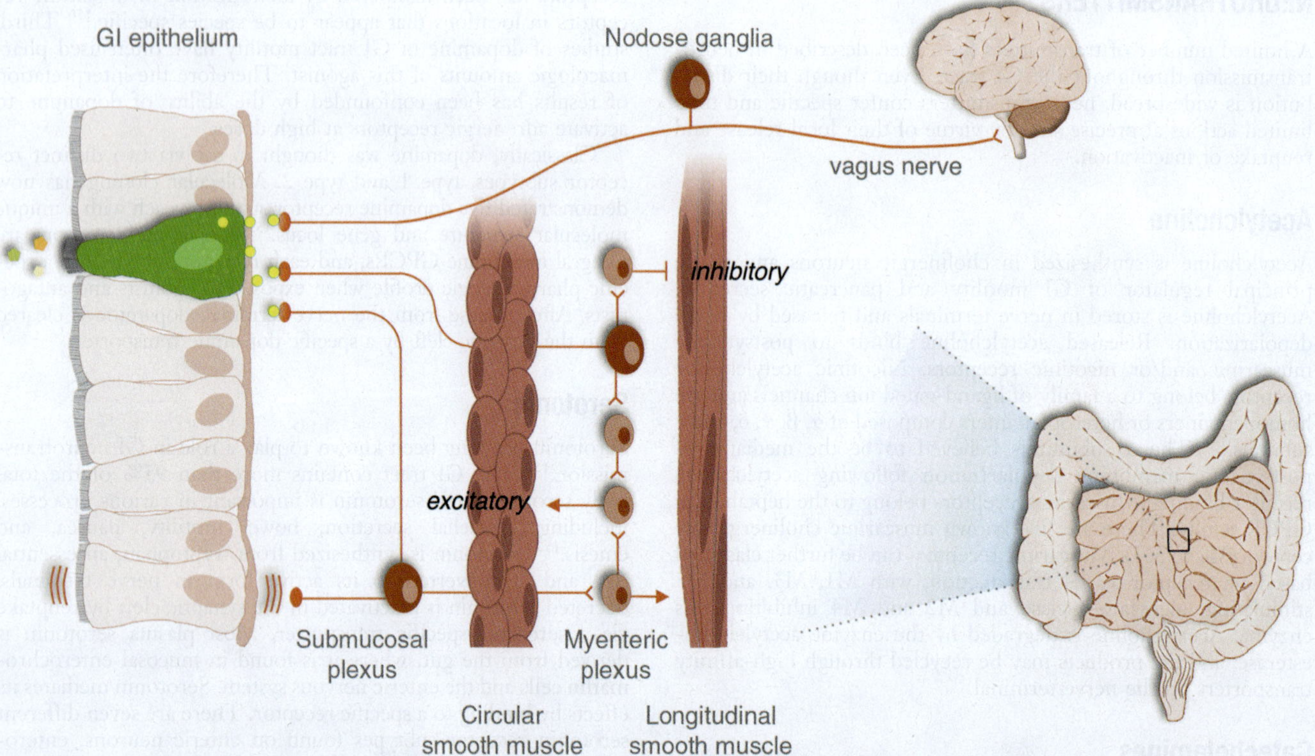

Fig. 4.6 Serotonin in the enteric nervous system. About 90% of the body's serotonin is produced by enterochromaffin cells (*green*) of the intestinal epithelium. Enterochromaffin cells are sensory cells that release serotonin (5-hydroxytryptamine, 5-HT), in response to GI luminal contents. Released 5-HT stimulates afferent fibers of the vagus nerve, which carry sensory information to the brain. The cell bodies of these vagal neurons are clustered in the nodose ganglia. In addition, 5-HT can also stimulate nerve fibers from neurons in the submucosal plexus or myenteric plexus. The information integrated at these plexuses regulates the excitation or inhibition of both the circular and/or the longitudinal smooth muscle. The synchronous contraction of these two layers of smooth muscle facilitates the churning and propulsion of chyme (partly digested food).

Histamine

In the GI tract, histamine is best known for its central role in regulating gastric acid secretion (see Chapter 51) and intestinal motility. Histamine is produced by enterochromaffin-like cells of the stomach and intestine, as well as enteric nerves. Histamine is synthesized from L-histidine by histidine decarboxylase and activates three GPCR subtypes. H1 receptors are found on smooth muscle and vascular endothelial cells and are linked to PLC activation. As such, the H1 receptor mediates many of the allergic responses induced by histamine. H2 receptors are present on gastric parietal cells, smooth muscle, and cardiac myocytes. H2 receptor binding stimulates Gs (G proteins that stimulate adenylate cyclase) and activates adenylate cyclase. H3 receptors are present in the central nervous system and enterochromaffin cells of the GI tract. These receptors signal through Gi and inhibit adenylate cyclase.[160] Histamine can also interact with the *N*-methyl-D-aspartate (NMDA) receptor and enhance activity of NMDA-bearing neurons independently of the three known histamine receptor subtypes.

Unlike other neurotransmitters, there is no known transporter responsible for termination of histamine's action. However, histamine is metabolized to telemethylhistamine by histamine *N*-methyltransferase and is then degraded to telemethylimidazoleacetic acid by monoamine oxidase B and an aldehyde dehydrogenase.

Nitric Oxide

NO is a unique chemical messenger produced from L-arginine by the enzyme nitric oxide synthase (NOS).[161] Three types of NOS are known. Types I and III are also known as endothelial NOS and neuronal NOS, respectively, and are constitutively active. Small changes in NOS activity can occur through elevations in intracellular calcium. The inducible form of NOS (type II) is apparent only when cells become activated by specific inflammatory cytokines. This form of NOS can produce large amounts of NO and is calcium independent. NOS is often colocalized with VIP and PACAP in neurons of the enteric nervous system.[162]

NO, being an unstable gas, has a relatively short half-life. Unlike most neurotransmitters and hormones, NO does not act via a membrane-bound receptor. Instead, NO readily diffuses into adjacent cells to activate guanylate cyclase directly (Fig. 4.7). NO activity is terminated by its oxidation to nitrate and nitrite. Many enteric nerves use NO to signal neighboring cells and induce epithelial secretion, vasodilation, or muscle relaxation. NO is also produced by macrophages and neutrophils to help kill invading organisms.[163]

CANNABINOIDS AND OTHER CHEMICAL TRANSMITTERS

Cannabinoids

There are three categories of cannabinoids: synthetic, phytocannabinoids found in plants, and endocannabinoids. Endocannabinoids, in particular, have similar functions to neurotransmitters, in that they participate in synaptic

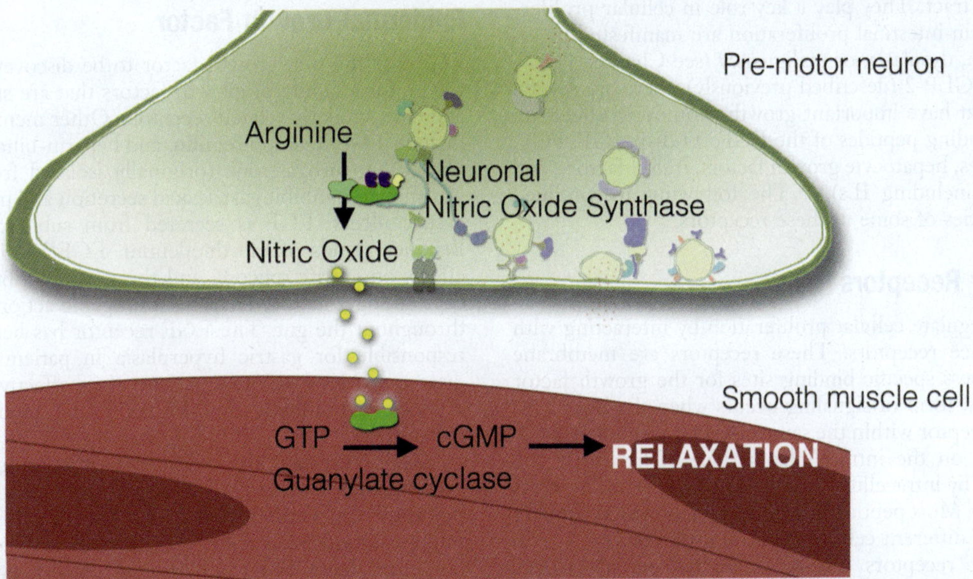

Fig. 4.7 Relaxing smooth muscle tone through nitric oxide (NO). NO, synthesized from arginine by nitric oxide synthase, diffuses across the plasma membrane into smooth muscle cells. NO binds to and activates guanylyl cyclase, which converts guanosine triphosphate to cGMP. cGMP causes smooth muscle relaxation. (Modified from Alberts B, Bray D, Lewis J, et al, eds. *Molecular Biology of the Cell*. 4th ed. New York: Garland Science; 2002:831.)

transmission.[164] In contrast to typical neurotransmitters, however, the flow of endocannabinoid signaling is retrograde to conventional neurontransmitters.[165] Because of their lipophilic nature, endocannabinoids are membrane-bound molecules thought to be enriched in postsynaptic neurons. Thus when released, endocannabinoids move from postsynapses to act on presynaptic cannabinoid receptors and depress presynaptic function.[166] In this manner, endocannabinoid signaling helps postsynaptic neurons regulate the secretion of transmitters from the sensory cell.

There are several types of endocannabinoid ligands, including arachidonoylethanolamide (anandamide), 2-arachidonoyl, 2-arachidonyl glyceryl ether (Noladin ether), *N*-arachidonoyl-dopamine, virodhamine, and lysophosphatidylinositol. Endocannabinoids, as well as other cannabinoids, modulate metabolism and behavior by acting on the GPCR cannabinoid receptors CB1 and CB2. Both receptors are distributed throughout the body, although CB1 is primarily found in neurons and epithelial chemosensory cells and CB2 is mainly present in cells of the immune system.

In the GI tract, CB1 receptors are also involved in counteracting proinflammatory responses and preventing the development of colitis.[167] In addition to activating classical cannabinoid receptors, endocannabinoids can also stimulate GPCRs, such as GPR119. Importantly, GPR119 is a receptor found in enteroendocrine cells of the small intestine, and its activation by endocannabinoids triggers the release of satiety-inducing hormones, such as CCK and peptide YY.[167] These findings have made the field of GI endocannabinoid research an active area for the development of therapeutic treatments.

Adenosine

Adenosine is an endogenous nucleoside that acts through any of four GPCR subtypes.[168] Adenosine causes relaxation of intestinal smooth muscle and stimulates intestinal secretion. Adenosine can also cause peripheral vasodilation and activation of nociceptors that participate in neural pain pathways.

Cytokines

Cytokines are a group of polypeptides produced by various immunomodulatory cells and are involved in cell proliferation, immunity, and inflammation. Cytokines are induced by specific stimuli, such as toxins produced by pathogens, and often elicit a complex response involving other cellular mediators to eradicate the foreign substance. Cytokines may be categorized as interleukins (ILs), tumor necrosis factors (TNFs), lymphotoxins, interferons, colony-stimulating factors (CSFs), and others.[169] ILs can be further subtyped into at least 35 separate substances, IL-1 to IL-35. There are two TNFs, TNF-α and TNF-β, which are also known as lymphotoxin-α. Interferons are produced during viral or bacterial infection and come in two varieties, interferon-α (also known as leukocyte-derived interferon or interferon-β) and interferon-γ. Interferon-α is produced by T lymphocytes and has been used clinically for the treatment of viral hepatitis (see Chapters 81 and 82). The major CSFs are granulocyte mononuclear phagocyte CSF, mononuclear phagocyte CSF, and granulocyte CSF. These agents are used for chemotherapy-induced neutropenia and marrow support after bone marrow transplantation. Chemokines initiate and propagate inflammation and are of two groups, CXC (α chemokines) and CC (β chemokines). Other cytokines, such as transforming growth factor-β (TGF)-β and platelet-derived growth factor (PDGF), have proliferative effects.

THE IMPORTANCE OF HORMONES AND NEUROTRANSMITTERS

Growth and Abnormal Growth of the Gut

Growth of GI tissues is a balance between cellular proliferation and senescence. Many factors participate in maintenance of the GI mucosa. Nutrients and other luminal factors stimulate growth of the intestinal mucosa and are necessary to maintain normal digestive and absorptive functions. Hormones and transmitters serve as secondary messengers that are normally secreted in response to food ingestion and mediate many of the nutrient effects on the GI tract. They play a key role in cellular proliferation. Alterations in intestinal proliferation are manifested by atrophy, hyperplasia, dysplasia, or malignancy (see Chapter 1).

In addition to GLP-2 (described previously), there are several growth factors that have important growth promoting effects on the GI tract, including peptides of the EGF, TGF-β, IGF, FGF, and PDGF families, hepatocyte growth factors, trefoil factors, and many cytokines (including ILs).[170] The following are outlined important properties of some of these receptors.

Growth Factor Receptors

Growth factors regulate cellular proliferation by interacting with specific cell surface receptors. These receptors are membrane proteins that possess specific binding sites for the growth factor ligand. An unusual form of signaling occurs when the ligand interacts with its receptor within the same cell. For example, PDGF receptors present on the intracellular surface of fibroblast cell lines are activated by intracellular ligand. This process is known as *intracrine signaling*. Most peptide growth factors, however, interact with receptors on different cells to regulate proliferation.

Growth factor receptors can be single polypeptide chains containing one membrane-spanning region, such as the receptor for EGF, or they may be composed of two subunit heterodimers, with one subunit containing a transmembrane domain and the other residing intracellularly but covalently bound to the transmembrane subunit. Heterodimers may also dimerize to form a receptor composed of four subunits (e.g., IGF receptor). Binding of the ligand to its receptor usually causes aggregation of two or more receptors and activation of intrinsic tyrosine kinase activity. Growth factor receptors also can autophosphorylate when bound to a ligand. In addition, receptor tyrosine kinase activity may phosphorylate other intracellular proteins important in signal transduction. Autophosphorylation attenuates the receptor's kinase activity and often leads to downregulation and internalization of the receptor. Mutation of the receptor at its autophosphorylation site may lead to constitutive receptor activity and cellular transformation. Growth factor receptors may couple to various intracellular signaling pathways, including adenylate cyclase, PLC, calcium-calmodulin protein kinases, MAP kinase, and nuclear transcription factors. Thus growth factors play important and varied roles in most cells of the GI tract. It is not surprising, therefore, that mutations in growth factor receptors or downstream signaling proteins can lead to unregulated cell growth and neoplasia (see Chapter 1).

An important action of growth factors is their ability to modulate the expression of transacting transcription factors that can regulate expression of many other genes.[171] Early response genes such as jun and fos are activated rapidly after ligand binding and control the expression of many other genes involved in cellular proliferation. Other important transcriptional factors include c-myc and nuclear factor κB (NF-κB). The latter is found in the cytoplasm in an inactive form and, following ligand binding, translocates to the nucleus, where it activates other transcription factors. NF-κB is a key target for strategies to regulate cellular proliferation and inflammation. In its phosphorylated form Rb-1, originally identified in retinoblastoma, is an inhibitor of cellular proliferation that complexes with the transcription factor p53. Dephosphorylation of Rb-1 releases p53, which activates other genes leading to cellular proliferation.

Almost all growth factors of the GI tract exert paracrine effects. However, many growth factors also possess autocrine and even intracrine actions. It has become apparent that growth factors and other signaling molecules secreted into the lumen of the gut can have important local biological actions. Distant effects of growth factors found in the circulation may be important for growth of certain types of cancers, particularly lung and colon cancer.

Epidermal Growth Factor

EGF was the first growth factor to be discovered. It is the prototype for a family of growth factors that are structurally related and have similarly related receptors. Other members of the family include TGF-α, amphiregulin, and heparin-binding EGF. EGF is identical to urogastrone (originally isolated from urine), which was shown to inhibit gastric acid secretion and promote healing of gastric ulcers. EGF is secreted from submaxillary glands and Brunner glands of the duodenum. EGF has important trophic effects on gastric mucosa, and the wide distribution of EGF receptors suggests that EGF has mitogenic actions on various cells throughout the gut. The EGF receptor has been reported to be responsible for gastric hyperplasia in patients with Ménétrier disease.[172] Moreover, two patients were effectively treated with a monoclonal antibody that blocks ligand binding to the EGF receptor.[173]

EGF receptors are considered important targets for the experimental treatment of human cancer based on the evidence that they play a critical role in the growth and survival of certain tumors. Monoclonal antibodies, as well as small tyrosine kinase inhibitors have been undergoing clinical evaluation for the treatment of human tumors.[174]

Transforming Growth Factor-α

TGF-α is produced by most epithelial cells of the GI tract and acts through the EGF receptor. Therefore it shares trophic properties with EGF. It is believed to play a key role in gastric reconstitution after mucosal injury. Moreover, it appears to be important in intestinal neoplasia because most gastric and colon cancers produce TGF-α (see Chapters 56 and 129).

Transforming Growth Factor-β

A family of TGF-β peptides exerts various biological actions, including stimulation of proliferation, differentiation, embryonic development, and formation of extracellular matrix.[175] In contrast with the TGF-α receptor, there are three distinct TGF-β receptors.[176] TGF-β modulates cell growth and proliferation in nearly all cell types and can enhance its own production from cells. It is likely that TGF-β plays a critical role in inflammation and tissue repair. TGF-β augments collagen production by recruitment of fibroblasts through its chemoattractant properties. This action can have beneficial or deleterious effects, depending on its site of deposition and abundance. For example, TGF-β may play a key role in the development of adhesions following surgery.[177]

Insulin-Like Growth Factors

Alternative splicing of the insulin gene produces two structurally related peptides, IGF I and IGF II.[178] IGFs signal through at least three different IGF receptors. The IGF I receptor is a tyrosine kinase, and the IGF II receptor is identical to the mannose 6-phosphate receptor. Although the exact function of IGFs in the GI tract is not clearly understood, they have potent mitogenic activity in intestinal epithelium. IGF II appears to be critical for embryonic development.

Fibroblast Growth Factor and Platelet-Derived Growth Factor

At least seven related FGFs have been identified.[179] These peptides have mitogenic effects on various cell types, including mesenchymal cells, and likely play an important role in organogenesis and neovascularization.[180] Although not unique to the GI tract, PDGF is one of the most thoroughly studied growth factors.

It is important for fibroblast growth, and its receptor is expressed in the liver and throughout the GI tract, where it appears to promote wound healing.

Trefoil Factors

Trefoil factors (pS2, spasmolysin, and intestinal trefoil factor, also known as TTF1, 2, and 3, respectively) are a family of proteins expressed throughout the GI tract.[181] They share a common structure, having six cysteine residues and three disulfide bonds, creating a cloverleaf appearance that stabilizes the peptide within the gut lumen. The pS2 peptide is produced in the gastric mucosa, spasmolysin is found in the antrum and pancreas, and intestinal trefoil factor is produced throughout the small and large intestines. These peptides are produced by mucous neck cells in the stomach or goblet cells in the intestine and are secreted onto the mucosal surface of the gut. It is likely that trefoil factors act on the apical surface of the epithelial cells, where they have growth-promoting properties on the GI mucosa.

Other peptides signaling through GPCRs may also have growth-promoting effects. Three important examples include gastrin, CCK, and gastrin-releasing peptide. Gastrin stimulates the growth of enterochromaffin-like cells of the stomach and induces proliferation of the oxyntic mucosa containing parietal cells.[182] Gastrin binds to CCK-2 receptors of the stomach and activates PLC and Ras pathways, which ultimately results in activation of protein kinase C and MAP kinase, respectively. MAP kinase, which can also be activated by tyrosine kinase receptors typical of growth factors, causes the phosphorylation of transcription factors that are involved in cellular proliferation. In some cells, cAMP and PKA exert synergistic effects on cellular growth through activation of nuclear transcription factors such as cAMP-responsive element binding (protein). However, in other cells, cAMP antagonizes proliferation. Therefore depending on the cell type, the effects of growth factors, such as EGF, IGF, and PDGF may be enhanced by hormones that stimulate cAMP production. Certain colon cancer cells possess CCK-2 receptors and respond to the proliferative effects of gastrin. Moreover, gastrin may be produced by some colon cancers, enabling it to exert an autocrine effect to promote cancer growth.[183] Whether circulating gastrin initiates colon cancer development is unknown.

DIABETES AND THE GUT

GI hormones play an important role in the regulation of insulin secretion and glucose homeostasis. These hormones control processes that facilitate the digestion and absorption of nutrients, as well as disposal of nutrients that have reached the bloodstream. In particular, gut peptides control postprandial glucose levels through three different mechanisms: (1) stimulation of insulin secretion from pancreatic beta cells; (2) inhibition of hepatic gluconeogenesis by suppression of glucagon secretion; and (3) delaying the delivery of carbohydrates to the small intestine by inhibiting gastric emptying.[184] Each of these actions reduces the blood glucose excursions that normally occur after eating.

Approximately 50% of the insulin released after a meal is the result of GI hormones that potentiate insulin secretion.[185] This interaction is known as the enteroinsular axis and the gut peptides that stimulate insulin release are known as incretins. The major incretins are GLP-1 and GIP. GLP-1 not only stimulates insulin secretion but also increases beta cell mass, inhibits glucagon secretion, and delays gastric emptying. GIP stimulates insulin secretion when glucose levels are elevated and decreases glucagon-stimulated hepatic glucose production.[186] Thus on ingestion of a meal, glucose, as it is absorbed, stimulates GLP-1 and GIP secretion. Circulating glucose then stimulates beta cell production of insulin, and this effect is substantially augmented by incretins acting in conjunction with glucose to increase insulin levels.

Postprandial hyperglycemia may also be controlled by delaying the delivery of food from the stomach to the small intestine, allowing the rise in insulin to keep pace with the rate of glucose absorption. Several gut hormones that delay gastric emptying have been shown to reduce postprandial glucose levels (Box 4.2).[184] Amylin (islet amyloid polypeptide) is a 37-AA peptide synthesized primarily in the beta cells of the pancreatic islets together with insulin. Although it was originally recognized for its ability to form amyloid deposits in association with beta cell loss, it has more recently been found to suppress glucagon secretion, delay gastric emptying, and induce satiety.[187] Insulin resistance in obese patients is associated with increased levels of both insulin and amylin.

Type 2 diabetes mellitus is characterized by high circulating insulin levels and insulin resistance. In addition, insulin levels do not increase appropriately after a meal and significant hyperglycemia occurs, which is consistent with an impaired incretin effect. GIP secretion is preserved in type 2 diabetes; however the insulinotropic effect of GIP is reduced.[188] Although the precise cause is unknown, the defect in GIP-stimulated insulin release is most pronounced in the late phase of insulin secretion. In contrast to GIP, GLP-1 secretion is reduced in insulin-resistant type 2 diabetics. The lower GLP-1 levels are caused by impaired secretion rather than increased degradation of the hormone.[189] Unlike GIP, the insulin response to infusion of GLP-1 is preserved, indicating that the beta cell can respond normally to this incretin hormone. These observations paved the way for GLP-1 administration as a viable treatment for the hyperglycemia associated with diabetes.[190] The growing evidence that beta cell failure may develop in type 2 diabetes supports the use of incretin hormones, such as GLP-1, or agents that delay GLP-1 degradation by the enzyme dipeptidyl peptidase-4 to enhance beta cell function.[191,192] Several GLP-1-based incretin analogs are now used clinically for the treatment of diabetes while dual GLP-1/GIP drugs are under investigation.[193,209]

BOX 4.2 GI Peptides That Regulate Postprandial Blood Glucose Levels

STIMULATE INSULIN RELEASE

Glucagon-like peptide-1
Glucose-dependent insulinotropic peptide
Gastrin releasing peptide
Cholecystokinin (potentiates amino acid–stimulated insulin release)
Gastrin (in presence of amino acids)
Vasoactive intestinal peptide (potentiates glucose-stimulated insulin release)
Pituitary adenylate cyclase–activating peptide (potentiates glucose-stimulated insulin release)
Motilin

DELAY GASTRIC EMPTYING

Cholecystokinin
Glucagon-like peptide-1
Amylin
Secretin

INHIBIT GLUCAGON RELEASE

Amylin
Glucagon-like peptide-1
Increase Beta Cell Proliferation and Survival
Glucagon-like peptide-1
Glucose-dependent insulinotropic peptide

GASTROINTESTINAL REGULATION OF APPETITE

Some GI hormones control the size of an ingested meal and are known as satiety signals. Satiety hormones share several qualities.[195] First, they decrease meal size. Second, blocking their endogenous activity leads to increased meal size. Third, reduction of food intake is not the result of an aversion to food. Fourth, secretion of the hormone is caused by ingestion of food that normally causes cessation of eating (Table 4.2). Most satiety signals interact with specific receptors on nerves leading from the GI tract to the hindbrain. The discovery that enteroendocrine cells synapse to nerves raises the possibility that satiety signals are initially regulated by neurotransmission signals and subsequently reinforced by hormonal signals.[54,196] Other sensory systems, such as taste, integrate both mechanisms to accomplish short- and long-term sensory signaling.

CCK is one of the most extensively studied satiety hormones. In a time- and dose-dependent manner, CCK reduces food intake in animals and humans,[197] an effect that is mediated by CCK-1 receptors residing on vagus nerve endings.[198] The effect of CCK on food intake is a proven physiologic action because administration of a CCK receptor antagonist induces hunger and results in larger meal sizes. CCK also delays the rate at which food empties from the stomach, which may explain why the satiety actions of CCK are most apparent when the stomach is distended. Together, these findings indicate that CCK provides a signal for terminating a meal.

GLP-1 is produced by enteroendocrine cells in the ileum and colon and is released in response to food in the intestine. Although the primary action of GLP-1 is to stimulate insulin secretion, it also delays gastric emptying. Moreover, infusion of GLP-1 increases satiety and produces feelings of fullness, thereby reducing food intake without causing aversion.[199] GLP-1 receptors are found in the periventricular nucleus, dorsal medial hypothalamus, and arcuate nucleus of the hypothalamus, which are important areas in the regulation of hunger. Like CCK, central administration of GLP-1 suppresses food intake.

PYY is also produced by enteroendocrine cells of the ileum and colon. Two forms of PYY are released into the circulation, PYY_{1-36} and PYY_{3-36}. PYY_{1-36} binds to all subtypes of the NPY family of receptors, whereas PYY_{3-36} has strong affinity for the Y2 receptor. When administered to animals, PYY_{3-36} causes a reduction in food intake, and mice lacking the Y2 receptor are resistant to the anorexigenic effects of PYY_{3-36}, indicating that PYY_{3-36} signals satiety through this receptor.[200] PYY_{3-36} has been shown in humans to decrease hunger scores and caloric intake.[201] Interestingly, most of the GI peptide receptors involved in satiety are also found in the brain, where they mediate similar satiety effects. This may represent conservation of peptide signals that serve similar purposes.

Leptin is referred to as an adiposity signal because it is released into the blood in proportion to the amount of body fat and is considered a long-term regulator of energy balance. Together with CCK, leptin reduces food intake and produces a greater reduction in body weight than either agent alone.[128] Therefore it appears that long-term regulators of energy balance can affect short-term regulators through a decrease in meal size, which may promote weight reduction.

Hunger and initiation of a meal are intimately related. Ghrelin is intriguing because it is the only known circulating GI hormone that has orexigenic effects.[144] Produced by the stomach, ghrelin levels increase abruptly before the onset of a meal and decrease rapidly after eating, suggesting that it signals initiation of a meal. Consistent with this role are studies demonstrating that administration of antighrelin antibodies or a ghrelin receptor antagonist suppresses food intake.[202] It is not known if ghrelin is responsible for the hunger pains and audible bowel sounds that occur in people who are hungry.

Bariatric surgery, in particular Roux-en-Y gastric bypass, is the most effective procedure for long-term weight loss in morbid obesity. Although it had been assumed that weight loss accompanying this procedure was the result of reduced gastric capacity and calorie malabsorption, recent evidence of reduced ghrelin release and exaggerated PYY release after a meal has suggested that hormonal factors may contribute to reduced calorie intake.[203]

TABLE 4.2 GI Peptides That Regulate Satiety and Food Intake

Reduce Food Intake	Increase Food Intake
Cholecystokinin (CCK)	Ghrelin
Glucagon-like peptide-1	
Peptide tyrosine tyrosine (PYY_{3-36})	
Gastrin-releasing peptide	
Amylin	
Apolipoprotein A-IV	
Somatostatin	

ENTEROENDOCRINE CELLS AND VISCERAL PAIN

Visceral pain is a major contributor to morbidity in IBS. The pathophysiological basis of IBS is unknown, and treatments have been largely symptomatic. Guanylyl cyclase-C (GUCY2C) is a receptor/enzyme complex located on the apical surface of gut epithelial cells that mediates intestinal fluid secretion normally stimulated by the intraluminal peptides guanylin and uroguanylin. Synthetic GUCY2C agonists, such as linaclotide and plecanatide, have been developed to treat constipation-predominant IBS. Interestingly, these agents not only stimulate intestinal fluid secretion but also ameliorate visceral pain. GUCY2C activation increases intracellular cGMP, and it was assumed that secreted cGMP desensitized sensory nerve firing. However, it was recently demonstrated in a mouse model that GUCY2C is expressed in neuropod cells (EECs that synapse with neurons) and mediates linaclotide-induced reduction in visceral pain through an EEC-dependent mechanism.[210] Although the transmitter released from EECs is unknown, this observation suggests that it might be possible to dissociate the secretory and analgesic effects of GUCY2C agonism as a method to treat visceral pain without stimulating intestinal fluid secretion.

Full references for this chapter can be found at ebooks.health.elsevier.com.

5 Biopsychosocial Issues in Gastroenterology

Laurie Keefer, Douglas A. Drossman

IN THIS CHAPTER

This chapter presents an overview of the biopsychosocial (BPS) model of digestive disease and its critical role in managing gastrointestinal (GI) conditions in their psychological, behavioral, and sociocultural context.[1] Practicing gastroenterology from the BPS model requires a commitment to understanding a patient's underlying GI anatomy, physiological function, and the psychosocial "influencers" that (1) predispose an individual to the development of a GI condition or a flare-up, (2) impact one's clinical and symptomatic response, and (3) effect care management. The BPS model of digestive disorders forms the basis of integrated care models[2] that increasingly demonstrate improved care quality and reduced health system costs in boths disorder of gut-brain interactions (DGBIs), including IBS[3] and IBD.[4,5] The brain-gut axis serves as the neuroanatomical and neurophysiological substrate for the BPS model of digestive disorders, and patient-centered care serves as the basis for optimizing the patient-provider relationship. These factors will be central to the content in this chapter.

This chapter is divided into three sections. First, illustrated through Case 1, a complex case of abdominal pain, we demonstrate the value offered to both the patient and provider when shifting from a biomedical approach to the BPS framework. In "The Gut-Brain-Microbiome Axis" section, we describe the various components of the BPS model that drive symptom experience in our patients. Specifically, we consider factors that influence (1) vulnerability toward the development, exacerbation, or severity of a GI condition, and (2) how one's behavioral response to a GI diagnosis, symptoms, treatment, and the health care system impacts care and outcomes. In "Clinical Implications of the Biopsychosocial Model. How to "Treating to Target" by Understanding Your Patient's Biopsychosocial Context" section, we apply what we have learned in "The Gut-Brain-Microbiome Axis" section to patient management—including the importance of communication skills that foster a strong doctor-patient relationship, the role of central neuromodulation[6] and the basis for a referral for brain-gut behavior therapy.[7]

THE VALUE OF THE BIOPSYCHOSOCIAL MODEL IN DIGESTIVE DISEASE

In the practice of medicine, feeling confused, even stuck, when discrepancies exist between what we observe and what we expect is common, especially when we must diagnose and care for a patient who has symptoms that do not match our biomedical understanding of their disease state. Failure to find a specific structural cause for medical symptoms is the rule rather than the exception in ambulatory care, with as many as 30% of primary care visits and up to 66% of specialty care visits being attributed to syndromes without an organic cause.[8]

The Biomedical Model

In Western civilization, the traditional understanding of *illness* (the personal experience of ill health or bodily dysfunction, as determined by current or previous disease as well as psychosocial, family, and cultural influences) and *disease* (abnormalities in structure and function of organs and tissues)[9] has been termed the *biomedical model.*[1,10]

The biomedical model adheres to two basic premises:

1) A medical disorder can be linearly reduced to a single cause (reductionism). Once the cause is identified, it can be modified and ultimately cured. Although this approach may seem to work for certain problems—like acute infectious diseases, it does not work for chronic infections such as tuberculosis or HIV, for which host factors also play a role in the clinical expression. The biomedical model is incompatible with chronic digestive disorders, all of which have genetic,

environmental, and psychosocial contributions to their phenotypic expression.

2) A medical disorder can be dichotomized as *organic*, a condition with objectively defined structural abnormalities, or as *functional*, with symptoms having no specifically identifiable structure. This is the mind-body dualism that presumes distinguishing medical (organic) from psychological (functional) illness and relegates functional disorders to conditions with no cause or treatment. Mind-body dualism has not been supported in gastroenterology—we have seen the "organification" of functional GI and motility disorders.[11] We have increasingly recognized the functional and psychological aspects of organic GI diseases.[12]

The limitations of the biomedical model[13] are well illustrated by the following case history, also depicted through video 5.1.

CASE #1

Ms. L, a 42-year-old woman, presents to her new physician with a 20-year history of mid to lower abdominal pain with nausea and occasional vomiting. She states, "I can't live with this pain anymore." Her bowel function is normal, and her weight is stable. She cannot work, believes the symptoms have taken over her life, and perceives no control over her symptoms or any ability to decrease them. She has a history of postinfection IBS, converting from IBS-D to IBS-C associated with depression, and she experienced sexual and physical abuse as a child. She now requests narcotics for pain relief because "that is the only thing that works." She would like her physician to expeditiously "find the cause of the pain and remove it." The medical record shows frequent emergency room visits and several hospital admissions where extensive diagnostic studies are negative. Studies included upper GI series with small bowel follow-through, upper endoscopy, colonoscopy, video capsule study, CT of the abdomen and pelvis, pelvic United States, and laparoscopy). Medical treatments for the pain, including acid blockers, secretagogues for constipation, and antispasmodics, were ineffective. She refuses neuromodulators, stating she does not have a psychiatric problem. Over time, increasing doses of narcotics are given for pain relief. A prior cholecystectomy due to a low ejection fraction and a hysterectomy for presumed endometriosis did not relieve the pain. On this occasion, an exploratory laparotomy was done with no meaningful findings. Postprocedure the patient required increasing doses of opioids. On this visit, the patient requests narcotic pain medication for relief and to be admitted for further diagnostic studies. The doctor suggests the patient go off narcotics and use antidepressants, but the patient assertively refuses. To view a simulation of this clinical encounter, see video 5.1

A consulting psychiatrist is then consulted who confirmed a diagnosis of major depression and post-traumatic stress disorder (PTSD) from the history of abuse but cautions that the need to exclude other medical diseases. At the end of the visit, the physician recommends that no further studies are needed, and the patient should see a psychologist for therapy. The patient requests to go to another medical facility.

This case of a patient with a severe DGBI[14,15] can be challenging when approached from the biomedical model. In addition to difficulties in diagnosis and management, strong feelings may arise that are maladaptive to the patient-provider relationship.[16] First, the provider and patient approach the problem dualistically. With no evidence of a structural (organic) diagnosis to explain the symptoms for over 20 years, the patient insists that further diagnostic studies be done to "find and fix" the problem. The provider, limited in their ability to communicate the origins or current extent of the symptoms, recommends antidepressants and to go off narcotics. However, without appropriate communication skills, the patients interpret the recommendations from a dualistic perspective and strongly refuse.

DGBI CLINICAL PEARL: MAKE AN EARLY, POSITIVE DIAGNOSIS

The significance of medical providers accepting that there will be a high prevalence of functional somatic syndromes in their practice has positive implications for the health care system and the patient. In a head-to-head randomized trial of more than 300 primary care patients followed over 1 year, the group who received a confident, "positive diagnosis" of IBS versus the group who received a diagnosis only after all other potential organic causes had been excluded ("exclusion diagnosis") were just as satisfied with their care and were more likely to have been started on an appropriate medical treatment. The patients with a positive diagnosis also had lower health care costs. Interestingly, in the entire sample of 300 patients, there was no "conversion" of diagnosis to organic conditions such as IBD, celiac disease, or cancer.[17] Indeed, it is now part of the American College of Gastroenterology IBS Guidelines to provide a positive diagnosis to reduce treatment delays and unnecessary diagnostic costs.[18]

In Case 1, we can positively diagnose the patient with post-infection IBS that later transitions to *centrally mediated abdominal pain syndrome (CAPS)*,[19] 1 of 37 adult DGBIs[20] that comprise over 40% of a gastroenterologist's practice (see Chapter 13). Added to this is the use of opioids leading to opioid-induced constipation and narcotic bowel syndrome.[21] Mutual acceptance of these diagnoses is the key to beginning a proper plan of care. Because DGBI do not fit into a biomedical construct, they are often considered psychosomatic,[13] this viewpoint increases the risk that unneeded and costly diagnostic tests will be ordered.

The biomedical model also influences the attitudes and satisfaction of the provider—despite the high prevalence of DGBI in outpatient gastroenterology practice, 20% of surveyed US gastroenterology fellows feel frustrated when seeing patients with DGBI, with as many as 40% of 3rd-year GI fellows indicating they do not want to see DGBIs in their outpatient practice. Frustration and stigmatizing attitudes were further tied to discomfort with understanding the cause of nonorganic symptoms, modeling of dismissive attitudes by attending gastroenterologists, and trainee lack of training and confidence in the use of advanced communication skills, neuromodulators, or brain-gut behavior therapies.[22]

Notable psychosocial features contributing to this patient's illness are evident—major loss, depression, an abuse history with post-traumatic stress disorder (PTSD), and catastrophic thinking—yet the patient minimizes these features. The patient views psychosocial factors as separate from, and often less important than, a specific medical disease, and the physician feels unable to address the psychological aspects of care. This avoidance on both the patient and provider results in a referral to a psychiatrist. In turn, the psychiatrist notes the psychological features but raises concern about whether a medical diagnosis has been overlooked or, consistent with the medical model, assigns a psychiatric diagnosis that does not necessarily inform the presenting problem. These viewpoints deflect attention from the relevant diagnoses and proper management, so the process of seeking a diagnosis continues.

A related feature in this case is impairment in the interaction between the physician and patient; their goals and expectations for care are at odds. Whereas the patient wants a quick fix, the physician sees her condition as chronic and ultimately requiring psychological intervention. In response, the patient requests referral to another facility, a response that might have been

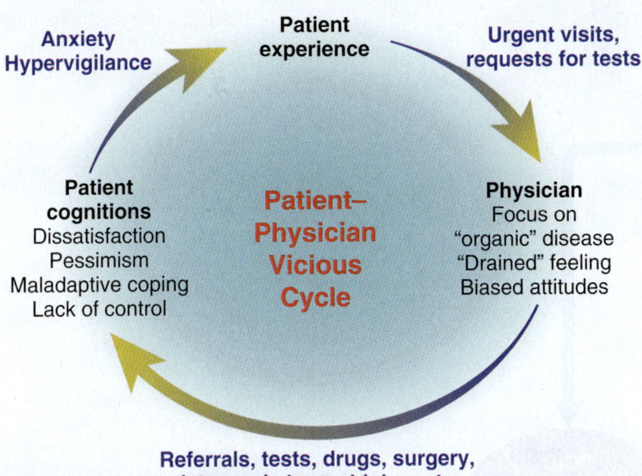

Fig. 5.1 Patient-physician vicious cycle. The vicious cycle relates to three components: (1) functional-organic dichotomy in which the diagnosis of a functional GI disorder is not recognized, and the effort is directed toward further tests to identify an organic disease; (2) limited ability to identify and address underlying psychosocial factors that contribute to the illness; and (3) an impaired patient-physician relationship, with a lack of shared decision-making about diagnosis and treatment. As indicated in this diagram, the risk of the vicious cycle is for increased testing, high health care costs, many referrals, and mutual dissatisfaction in care until the cycle is broken. (Adapted from Longstreth GF, Drossman DA. Severe irritable bowel and functional abdominal pain syndromes: managing the patient and health care costs. *Clin Gastroenterol Hepatol*. 2005;3:397–400.)

avoided if the physician had used communication skills that focused on education and negotiation of a mutual plan of care.[23]

This "vicious cycle" of ineffective care (Fig. 5.1) results from the limitations imposed by the biomedical model. The cycle occurs not only for patients with DGBIs but also for those with structural disorders such as IBD, for which pain and diarrhea are not explained by the degree of inflammation seen in laboratory values or through endoscopy,[12] and symptoms like pain, fatigue, and disability persist well after endoscopic remission has been achieved.[24] Again, the exception is the rule with respect to mismatch between inflammation and GI symptoms, with 40%-60% of patients with IBD exhibiting IBS-type symptoms while their IBD is in remission.[25] The reality is that (1) most patient's symptoms are incompletely explained by structural abnormalities; (2) psychosocial factors predispose individuals to the onset and perpetuation of illness and disease, contributing to the illness experience and strongly influencing the clinical outcome; and (3) successful application of this understanding and proper management requires an effective physician-patient relationship.

The Biopsychosocial Model

The *BPS model*[26] proposes that illness and disease result not from a single cause but from simultaneously interacting systems at the cellular, tissue, organism, interpersonal, and environmental levels. Furthermore, psychosocial factors have direct physiologic and pathologic consequences, and vice versa. For example, change at the subcellular level (e.g., HIV infection, genetic, or environmental susceptibility to IBD) has the potential to affect organ function, the person, the family, and society. Similarly, a change at the interpersonal level, such as the death of a spouse, can affect psychological status, cellular immunity, and ultimately disease susceptibility.[27] The BPS model also explains why the clinical expression of biological substrates (e.g., alterations in oncogenes) and associated responses to treatment vary among patients.

Fig. 5.2, the BPS for chronic digestive disorders, sets the stage for "The Gut-Brain-Microbiome Axis" section. Below, we will explore how early life factors can not only increase one's risk of developing a GI condition but can also influence an individual's later psychosocial environment, physiologic functioning, and disease (pathologic) expression via reciprocal interactions within the gut-brain (enteric nervous system [NS]-CNS) axis.

THE GUT-BRAIN-MICROBIOME AXIS

The gut-brain-microbiome axis is the neuroanatomic and neurophysiological substrate for the BPS model, and several factors inform one's vulnerability and response to GI symptoms.

We have divided this section into two parts. In "Risk and Vulnerability to the *Development, Exacerbation, and/or Severity* of Chronic Digestive Conditions" section, we will focus on early development, physiologic conditioning, and intergenerational transmission of illness behavior as well as the impact of early life adversity on both vulnerability and response to GI disorders. In "Early Development" section, we will also consider how these early risk/vulnerability factors ultimately drive one's *response* to their GI symptoms and conditions later on in life—we will focus on the link between stress and the GI tract, as well as the impact of psychological comorbidity and maladaptive cognitive-affective processes on symptom response. We will also discuss how symptom response is a target of DGBI treatment, including central neuromodulators and brain-gut behavior therapies across the spectrum of digestive disorders.[7]

Risk and Vulnerability to the *Development, Exacerbation, and/or Severity* of Chronic Digestive Conditions

Early Development

No other organ system is as closely connected to the brain as the GI system. As shown in Fig. 5.3, the development of the NS in the embryo begins with the neural crest. Over time the neural crest grows and differentiates into the forebrain, midbrain, and spinal cord. From the future spinal cord, spinal ganglia migrate into the early gut to become the future enteric NS (ENS).

In other words, the brain-gut axis is a neuroanatomic substrate that is "hardwired" before birth as a complex integrated circuitry network that communicates information between the CNS and myenteric plexus[28] to the end-organ structures. The GBA is a bidirectional system in which thoughts, feelings, and memories lead to neurotransmitter release (the software) that affects sensory, motor, endocrine, autonomic, immune, and inflammatory function.[29,30] Gut microbiota also engages in a similar bidirectional communication network with the brain via neural, endocrine, and immune pathways. Growing evidence supports the significance of the microbiome in the onset and maintenance of behavioral disorders, including anxiety, depression, and cognitive disorders as well as chronic visceral pain.[31] Dysregulation of the gut-brain-microbiome axis explains GI motility disturbances, abdominal pain, and other unpleasant GI sensations (e.g., nausea, fullness, and rectal hypersensitivity) and can be considered the primary underlying pathophysiology for disorders of gut-brain interaction (DGBI).[32] This will be described in more detail later in the chapter.

At or perhaps even before birth, a person's genetic composition and interactions with the environment begin to affect later behaviors and susceptibility to illness. Growing evidence has also pointed to the role of the early life environment in the

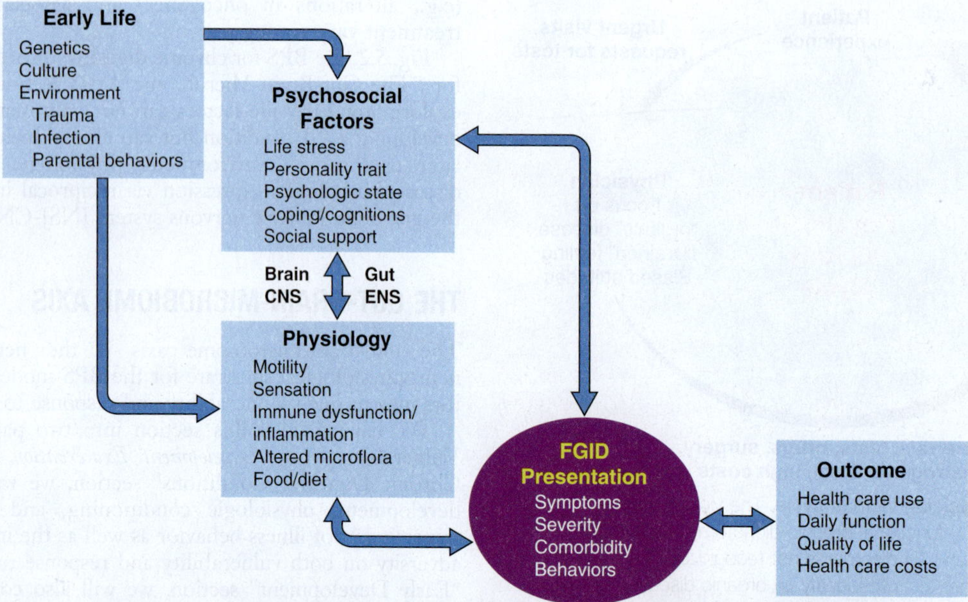

Fig. 5.2 The biopsychosocial conceptual model. Although the figure highlights functional GI diseases disorder of gut-brain interactions (*DGBIs*), it is applicable to all digestive disorders. Early life factors (e.g., genetic predisposition, early learning, and cultural milieu) can influence an individual's later psychosocial environment, physiologic functioning, and disease (pathologic) expression via reciprocal interactions within the gut-brain (CNS–enteric nervous system [*ENS*]) axis. The product of this gut-brain interaction will affect symptom experience and behavior and ultimately the clinical outcome. (Adapted from Van Oudenhove L, Crowell MD, Drossman DA, et al. Biopsychosocial aspects of functional gastrointestinal disorders. *Gastroenterology*. 2016;150:1355–1367, with permission from the Rome Foundation.)

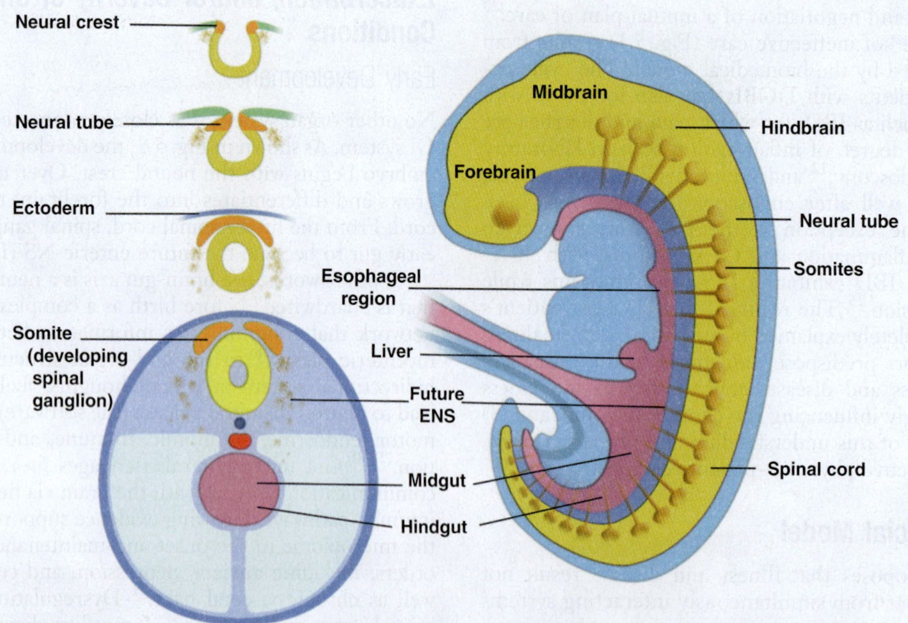

Fig. 5.3 Connection between the brain and nerves of the GI system. This figure shows the development of the nervous system in the embryo beginning with the neural crest. Over time, the neural crest grows and differentiates into the forebrain, midbrain, and spinal cord. From the future spinal cord, spinal ganglia migrate from the cord into the early gut to become the future enteric nervous system (*ENS*). Therefore the ENS, spinal cord, and CNS are "hardwired." No other organ system is as closely connected to the brain as the GI system. This helps explain the clinical observation of the close relationship between psychosocial features and gut functioning, the gut-brain axis. (From Van Oudenhove L, Crowell MD, Drossman DA, et al. Biopsychosocial aspects of functional gastrointestinal disorders. *Gastroenterology*. 2016;150:1355–1367, with permission from the Rome Foundation.)

susceptibility to inflammatory bowel disease[33] and to shared genomics between one's genetic susceptibility to developing IBS, chronic pain disorders, anxiety, and/or depression.[34]

Physiologic Conditioning

Early (and even later in life) conditioning experiences may also influence physiologic functioning and the development of psychophysiological disorders. Psychophysiological reactions involve psychologically induced alterations in the function of target organs, without structural change. They are often viewed as physiologic concomitants of emotions such as anger or fear, although the person is not always aware of these emotions. Persistence of an altered physiologic state or an enhanced physiologic response to psychological stimuli is considered a psychophysiologic disorder by some researchers. Visceral functions, such as secretion of digestive juices and motility of the gallbladder, stomach, and intestine, can be classically conditioned[35] even by family interaction. *Classical conditioning*, as described by Pavlov, involves linking an unconditioned stimulus (sound of a bell) with a conditioned stimulus (food) that elicits a conditioned response (salivation). After several trials, the unconditioned stimulus can produce the conditioned response.

It has been demonstrated that fear of benign GI sensations can be acquired through classical conditioning, a finding that has implications for newer behavioral treatments that incorporate exposure-based techniques (see later).[36] In the first study of its kind, 52 healthy participants with no history of GI symptoms were randomized to either a condition in which a nonpainful esophageal balloon distention preceded a painful one (experimental) or to a condition in which the painful condition was administered but *not* paired with the benign balloon distension (control). The experimental groups demonstrated higher pain expectancy, augmented skin conductance response, and a potentiated startle reflex in response to benign balloon distention but fortunately were able to be deconditioned through an extinction paradigm after the experiment was completed.[37]

By contrast, *operant conditioning* involves development of a desired response through motivation and reinforcement. Playing basketball is an example; accuracy improves through practice, and the correct behavior is reinforced by the reward of scoring a basket—operant conditioning can explain illness behavior as below. Operant learning, or learning based on reinforcement, may be impaired in patients with chronic pain conditions, including IBS and fibromyalgia.[38] Experimental and brain imaging studies identifying connections among memory, learning, cognition, and visceral pain as potential targets for intervention are an exciting area of research with strong implications for brain-gut behavior therapies.[39,40]

Parenting and Intergenerational Transmission of Illness Behavior

Operant conditioning is also the primary form of learning in childhood, and parents can play a significant role in reinforcing illness behavior. Well-designed studies have supported the role of early modeling of symptom experience and behavior in the clinical expression of GI symptoms and disorders, mediated by parental distress levels and maladaptive coping.[41–43] Furthermore, early familial attention toward GI symptoms[44] can influence health behaviors and health care–seeking behaviors, the costs and consequences of which are often carried into adulthood.[45]

CASE #2

A young child, Johnny, wakes up on the day of a school examination with anxiety and "flight-fight" symptoms of tachycardia, diaphoresis, abdominal cramps, and diarrhea. The parent keeps the child home because of a "tummy-ache" and allows him to stay in bed and watch television. The teacher says that he can make up a test when he returns to school. Several days later, when the child is encouraged to go back to school, the symptoms recur.

EXAMPLE OF OPERANT CONDITIONING IN THE TRANSMISSION OF ILLNESS BEHAVIOR

In Case 2 (Johnny), the parent focused on the abdominal discomfort as an illness that required absence from school rather than as a physiologic response to a distressing situation. Staying home allowed the child to avoid the feared situation without addressing the determinants of the fear. Repetition of the feared situation led to a conditionally enhanced psychophysiological symptom response and altered the child's perception of these symptoms as an illness, leading to health care–seeking behaviors later in life (illness modeling).[46] Indeed, children whose mothers reinforce illness behavior have been found to experience more severe stomach aches and more school absences than other children.[47]

In two studies,[35,48] patients with IBS who sought health care recalled more parental attention toward their illnesses than those with IBS who did not seek health care; they stayed home from school and saw physicians more often and received more gifts and privileges. Using a validated symptom provocation test[49] to evaluate the significance of parental solicitousness on abdominal pain complaints, parents were asked to show positive or sympathetic responses to their children's pain complaints; when they did, the frequency of the child's pain complaints was higher than when parents were instructed to ignore or distract the child from the same complaints.[50]

It may be possible to remediate parental behaviors and prevent the development or exacerbation of GI complaints. In a large clinical trial of children with functional abdominal pain (now termed recurrent abdominal pain), 200 children and their parents were randomly assigned to cognitive-behavioral therapy (CBT) targeting the parents' responses to their children's pain complaints and coping strategies or to an educational control condition. Changes in parents' cognitions about their child's pain emerged as a mediator of positive outcomes, thereby demonstrating that a parent's cognitions affect a child's DGBIs[51]; this was later replicated in IBD.[52]

Finally, certain GI disorders may be influenced by learning difficulties or emotionally challenging interactions that occur early in life. Disorders of anorectal function (e.g., dyssynergic defecation and encopresis) may have resulted from painful defecation or difficulties relating to bowel training[53] and can be treated by reconditioning through anorectal biofeedback.[54] Encopretic children may withhold stool out of fear of the toilet, to struggle for control, or to receive attention from parents and may require behavior therapy.[55]

Race, Ethnicity, Culture, Family, and Society

Social and cultural belief systems modify how a patient experiences illness and interacts with the health care system.[56] This issue has become more relevant as medical education and health care systems have become global,[57] and there has been an increased emphasis on mitigating race, ethnicity, and socioeconomic disparities within the United States and other Westernized health systems.

There are well-known disparities in time to an IBD diagnosis,[58] access and response to medical and surgical treatment,[59–61] and a serious lack of racial/ethnic representation in clinical trials[62] and/or inadequate reporting of race and ethnicity in research.[63] Furthermore, there are disparities in perceived degree of disability,[64] perceived stress,[65] and use of mental health care[66] in IBD, although these have all been noted across the spectrum of digestive disorders.

Food and diet, often altered by a GI diagnosis, are also major determinants of health and symptom severity that may manifest differently by culture and geographic region. Diet may influence the intestinal microbiota, host immune function, and influence treatment recommendations. Similarly, food-related quality of life in response to dietary restrictions required for management of disease can be substantially influenced by culture, particularly amongst Southeast Asians.[67]

Racial, ethnic, socioeconomic, and cultural influences directly impact the patient's experience of GI illness. To reduce known disparities in care and improve patient outcomes, providers are expected to practice within a culturally competent framework—this begins with inquiring about the patient's understanding of the onset, beliefs about cause, clinical course, and desired or expected treatment of an illness and treatment response.

Examples of how cultural factors have previously influenced care of GI patients are described in Box 5.1, albeit much of the research in this area has not been updated to reflect current practice and is likely subject to reinterpretation.

Early Life Adversity, Abuse, and Trauma

Adverse childhood experiences (ACEs) directly influence health and well-being throughout the lifespan. These are believed to be cumulative in their risk—the more ACEs, the more impact on health. ACEs often include physical, emotional, and sexual abuse but can also include physical and emotional neglect and household dysfunction, including domestic violence, mental illness or substance abuse, incarceration, or divorce. ACEs are associated with a twofold increase in the onset of IBS, with as many as 50% of people living with IBS reporting more than two early adverse life events.[73,74]

Adverse community environments such as poverty, discrimination, lack of economic mobility or social capital, poor-quality housing or affordability, and community violence also contribute to poorer health outcomes, although these have not specifically been studied in GI. Trauma-informed care is of increasing interest in gastroenterology given the high prevalence of trauma in our patient population coupled with the nature of our invasive tests and procedures.[75] Perhaps the most robust research in early life adversity among patients living with digestive disorders comes from studies of childhood sexual and physical abuse.

Childhood Abuse

Childhood sexual and physical abuse can have physical and emotional consequences, thereby affecting the development or severity of DGBIs as well as extraintestinal manifestations.[76] Newer research suggests that low resilience, or the inability to recover and adapt to stressful life events (stress hyper-responsiveness), along with low social support, including not having a trusted adult to confide in, could be two potential pathways through which early life adversity increases one's risk for IBS.[77]

Compared with patients without a history of abuse, patients seen in a referral gastroenterology practice with a history of sexual or physical abuse reported 70% more severe pain ($P < .0001$) and 40% greater psychological distress ($P < .0001$), spent over 2.5 times more days in bed in the previous 3 months (11.9 vs. 4.5 days; $P < .0007$), had almost twice as poor daily function ($P < .0001$), saw physicians more often (8.7 vs. 6.7 visits over 6 months; $P < .03$), and even underwent more surgical procedures (4.9 vs. 3.8 procedures; $P < .04$) unrelated to the GI diagnosis.[78] Higher symptom severity and treatment seeking can explain the higher association of abuse histories with GI illness in referral centers and specialty groups when compared with primary care.[79–81] Part of trauma-informed gastroenterology care includes asking and acknowledging abuse history in the GI setting.[75]

Several possible mechanisms help explain the relationship between a history of abuse and poor outcome.[80,82] These mechanisms include (1) susceptibility to developing psychological conditions that increase the perception of visceral signals or their noxiousness (central hypervigilance and somatization); (2) development of psychophysiological (e.g., autonomic, humoral, and immunologic) responses that alter intestinal motor or sensory function or promote inflammation[83]; (3) development of peripheral or central sensitization from increased motility or physical trauma (visceral hyperalgesia or allodynia); (4) an abnormal appraisal of and behavioral response to physical sensations of

BOX 5.1 Examples of Previous Cross-Cultural Research in DGBI

Illnesses in which the diagnosis is not well related to structural or physiologic disease markers are influenced by cultural factors that must be understood to be managed properly. From a global perspective, 70%–90% of all self-recognized illnesses are managed outside traditional medical facilities, often with self-help groups or religious practitioners providing a substantial portion of the care.[68] Cognitive processing of bodily feelings has a powerful cultural element, depending on how one believes the body works; some groups perceive certain symptoms to be more dangerous and threatening than do other groups. In some nonliterate societies, individuals freely describe hallucinations that are fully accepted by others in the community.[69] In fact, the meaning of the hallucinations, not their presence, is the focus of interest, particularly when reported by those in a position of power. Conversely, in Western societies, the emphasis is on rationality and control, and hallucinations produce fear and may be viewed as a manifestation of psychosis until proved otherwise.

Cultural factors influence how symptoms are communicated. In qualitative ethnographic studies conducted in New York City in the mid-20th century, [69,70] first- and second-generation Jewish and Italian patients were observed to embellish the description of pain by reporting more symptoms in more bodily locations and with more dysfunction and greater emotional expression than did other white immigrants. By contrast, the Irish tended to minimize the description of the pain, and the "Old Americans" (Protestants) were stoic. These behaviors related to family attitudes and mores surrounding illness can either reinforce or extinguish attention drawing symptom reporting. Whereas Italians were satisfied to hear that the pain was not a serious problem, the Jewish patients needed to understand the meaning of the pain and its future consequences. In a cross-European survey of patients with IBD, Southern European patients (i.e., from Italy and Portugal) reported more and greater degrees of worry and concern about their IBD than did their Northern European counterparts.[71]

Cultural differences in explanatory models between physicians and patients may distort communication and produce misunderstandings or negative perceptions. For example, there is no word in Spanish to define the concept of "bloating," a symptom commonly reported in English-speaking countries.[57] In China, communicating psychological distress is stigmatizing,[68] so when a person is in distress, reporting physical symptoms (somatization) is more acceptable.[72]

perceived threat (response bias); and (5) development of maladaptive coping styles that lead to increased illness behavior and health care seeking (e.g., catastrophizing). Physiologically, in patients with IBS and a history of abuse, rectal distention produces more pain reporting with greater activation of the dorsal anterior cingulate cortex (ACC) (see later),[14] compared with patients with IBS and no history of abuse; the pain and activation of the brain subside after treatment.[84]

A history of abuse in a patient with IBS leads to greater dorsal ACC activation and reporting of pain with rectal distention than either condition alone.[14] Early life adversity has also been linked to alterations in core brain networks associated with emotion regulation and salience, likely in a sex-dependent manner.[85] With clinical recovery, CNS activity returns to normal (i.e., reduced midcingulate cortex [MCC] and increased insular activation).[84,86] Similarly, other emotional trauma, such as social pain (due to major loss and social disruption), activates the same areas of the brain (dorsal ACC and insula), again indicating the close association between a patient's psychosocial state and pain.[87]

See Drossman DA. Abuse, trauma, and GI illness: is there a link? *Am J Gastroenterol.* 2011;106:15–25 (Video 5.2)

Finally, a report of the Institute of Medicine's studies on Persian Gulf War veterans[88] portrays a strong relationship between the deployment of soldiers to a war zone (with traumatic exposure to injury, mutilation, and dead bodies) and the ensuing development of medical and psychological symptoms and syndromes. In fact, clusters of several medical symptoms were noted, such as "Gulf War Syndrome," including IBS, chronic fatigue, and chemical sensitivity syndrome, in addition to PTSD and cognitive impairments. The psychological effects of abuse or wartime exposure may disrupt central pain modulation systems and brain circuits at the interface of emotion and pain.[14] These changes lead to a lowering of sensation thresholds, with a loss of the brain's ability to filter bodily sensations. The result is increased physical and psychological symptoms and more intense pain and syndromes (e.g., IBS, fibromyalgia, headache, and widespread body pain), a condition that has been variably described as somatization, comorbidity, or extraintestinal functional GI symptoms.[88]

As we saw in this section, the physiological and psychological effects of early life adversity and trauma include the prolonged and cumulative impact of physical and psychological stress on the mind and body. The negative effects of stressful life events on a person's vulnerability to GI disorders, as well as the severity with which they experience them, require the physician to address them in the care of all GI patients; sometimes it is sufficient to acknowledge that adverse life events do not usually *improve* one's health. Prospective studies have demonstrated that the experience of stressful life events is associated with IBS symptom exacerbation[89] and frequent health care seeking among adults with IBS.[57] In a study of wearables (devices that can sense disease activation) in ulcerative colitis, longitudinally evaluated perceived stress was associated with systemic inflammation and symptoms with associated changes in heart rate variability, a measure of stress on the gut-brain axis, preceding both symptomatic and inflammatory flares.[90] We will go into more detail in the next section as to the impact that one's *response* to stress has on the regulation of the gut-brain axis.

We have now covered the BPS factors affecting *vulnerability* to the development or severity of GI disorders. These vulnerabilities are carried throughout the lifespan and overlap with the next section, factors affecting one's *response* to GI sensations, symptoms, and conditions. One thing to keep in mind about chronic diseases is that the factors that may have started out the condition are not always the same factors that maintain them. A good example of this is postinfection IBS that we will also discuss below.

Factors Affecting One's Response to GI Symptoms: The Bidirectional Connection Among Stress, Psychological Distress, Mood, and the Digestive Tract

The product of the interacting effects of brain and GI tract relates to the clinical expression of illness and disease—namely, the symptom experience and subsequent illness-related behaviors. The meaning of illness, the perceived effect of alterations in body image (e.g., having a colostomy), social acceptability, the degree of functional impairment and its implications at work and at home, and the likelihood of surgery or untimely death must all be dealt with by the patient. How well the patient adapts, known as their psychological and physical resilience,[91] in addition to the quality of the physician's involvement and expertise, is crucial to the patient's psychological well-being and clinical course. Some chronically ill patients regress and become dependent, adopting a disability role. Their continued symptoms, restricted activity, and health care needs tax family, friends, and health care providers, all of whom may feel helpless to provide enough emotional or medical assistance. Other patients resist help to avoid acknowledging their imposed dependence. The family must then deal with feelings of guilt and anger, the expressions of which, although unavoidable, are not usually socially permitted. Often the physician carries the burden of the feelings of the patient and family and must reconcile the two. In most cases, the problems are worked out, and the patient establishes a pattern of coping. If the patient has limited capacity to cope psychologically with the illness, the disorder is particularly incapacitating, or the interpersonal family relationships are unstable, additional efforts by the physician and ancillary personnel (e.g., psychological counselors, social workers, and peer support groups) will be required.

The Stress Response and the Gut-Brain Axis

Stress can influence one's vulnerability to the onset or exacerbation and affect one's response to normal digestive processes. For example, healthy individuals commonly report abdominal discomfort or a change in bowel function when upset or distressed.[92] Only a subset of people actually seek treatment for these stress-mediated GI symptoms—indeed, severity of symptom reporting is almost always taken into account by clinicians who manage patients—assessment of the types and levels of stress (why are you seeking care now?) is recommended to implement proper care.[93]

DEFINING STRESS AND COPING FROM A STIMULUS-RESPONSE FRAMEWORK

Any influence on one's steady state that requires adjustment or adaptation can be considered stress, but the term is nonspecific and encompasses both the stimulus and its effects. The stimulus can be a biological event such as infection, a social event such as a change of residence, or even a disturbing thought. Stress can be desirable or undesirable. Some stimuli, such as pain, sex, or threat of injury, often elicit a predictable response in animals and humans. By contrast, life events have more varied effects, depending on the individual's personal interpretation of the event. A divorce might be considered a positive experience for one person and a disappointment for another. A stimulus can produce a variety of responses in different persons or in the same person at different times. The effect may not be observed or may be a psychological response (anxiety and depression), a physiologic change (diarrhea and diaphoresis), the onset of disease (asthma and colitis), or any combination of these. A person's interpretation of events as stressful or not and his or her response to stress depend on prior experience, attitudes, coping mechanisms, personality, culture, and biological factors, including susceptibility to disease.

In humans, Beaumont,[94] Wolf,[95] and Engel[96] observed changes in the color of the mucosa and secretory activity of a gastric pouch or fistula in response to psychological and physical stimuli. Gastric hyperemia and increased motility and secretion were linked to feelings of anger, intense pleasure, or aggressive behavior toward others. Conversely, mucosal pallor and decreased secretion and motor activity accompanied fear or depression, states of withdrawal (i.e., giving-up behavior), or disengagement from others. Complicated cognitive tasks produce high-amplitude, high-velocity esophageal contractions,[97] a reduction in Phase II intestinal motor activity,[98] and prolongation of Phase III activity of the migrating myoelectric complex[99] in the small intestine (see Chapter 101). Experimentally induced anger increases motor and spike potential activity in the colon and is greater in patients with DGBIs.[100] Physical or psychological stress also lowers the pain threshold, more so in patients with IBS than others.[101]

In both animal models and human studies, stress affects the mucosa to enhance proinflammatory cytokine production and mast cell activation and degranulation, particularly near enteric neurons, thereby leading to visceral sensitization.[102] Stress also enhances mucosal permeability due to weakening of tight junctions, with an increase in bacterial translocation into the intestinal wall.[103–105] Acute stress triggers the hypothalamic-pituitary axis, leading to increases in cortisol levels and activation of the autonomic NS, with increases in proinflammatory cytokines such as TNF-α, interleukin (IL)-6, and interferon-γ.[106,107] Stress can lead to a change in intestinal microflora composition, with a shift from "good" to "bad" bacteria. These changes, along with an altered immune response, can result in inflammation and susceptibility to both IBS (particularly postinfection IBS) and IBD.[108] Conversely, alteration of the intestinal microflora can reciprocate back via the gut-brain axis to affect CNS functioning, including mood, learning, and memory.[109]

A useful model highlighting the reciprocal relationship between stress and altered immunity is the condition known as postinfection IBS, which develops in about 10% of patients after a bout of infectious enteritis.[110] In a 2018 Rome Foundation Working Team report, postinfection IBS was reported to involve changes in the intestinal microbiome as well as epithelial, serotonergic, and immune system factors,[110] supporting early views of the pathogenesis of postinfection IBS as an inflammation-induced altered mucosal immune response that sensitizes visceral afferent nerves in a setting of emotional distress.[111] In postinfection or mucosal injury (as in the case of IBD and IBS), the CNS amplification of the visceral signals that occur in psychologically distressed persons is believed to raise the afferent signals to conscious awareness, thereby leading to enhanced perception of symptoms.[112] Both enterochromaffin cell hyperplasia (with increased production of 5-hydroxytryptamine [HT]) and depression are equally important predictors of the development of postinfection IBS (risk ratio, 3.8 and 3.2, respectively).[113]

Role of Neurotransmitters

As noted previously, the richly innervated nerve plexuses and neuroendocrine associations of the CNS and ENS provide the hardwiring for the gut-brain axis. Mediation of these activities involves neurotransmitters and neuropeptides commonly found in the CNS and intestine. Depending on their locations, these substances have integrated activities on both GI function and human behavior. This observation is not surprising because the hardwiring between brain and gut is established from an anlage that begins as one unit (neural tube) and then differentiates with the growing organism into the "big brain" and the "little brain" in the gut.

For example, the stress hormone corticotropin-releasing factor (CRF) has central stress-modulatory effects yet different intestinal physiologic effects. CRF produces gastric stasis and an increase in the colonic transit rate in response to psychologically aversive stimuli[114] and can increase visceral hypersensitivity[115] and alter immune functioning[29]; therefore CRF may play a role in stress-induced exacerbations of IBS (see Chapter 124),[116] cyclic vomiting syndrome (see Chapter 16),[117] and other stress-mediated disorders.

Peptides may be secreted at nerve endings as neurotransmitters or directly from cell walls and thus have local or paracrine effects. Several key neurotransmitters act within the gut-brain axis.[28,118] Acetylcholine is the main mediator of the parasympathetic system and drives motility in the enteric system; disturbances of this activity can lead to constipation and gastroparesis. Biological amines, such as serotonin, norepinephrine (NE), and dopamine, act in the periphery to mediate the effects of the sympathetic NS to regulate the balance between constipation and diarrhea and centrally to modulate mood, emotional behavior, and pain. Calcitonin gene-related peptide (CGRP), bradykinins, and tachykinins (e.g., substance P) are involved in visceral hyperalgesia and pain syndromes. The opioid system can raise the threshold for pain and impair peristalsis and secretion; centrally, it may paradoxically produce hyperalgesia.[119]

These associations have relevance in terms of treatment. Chronic GI pain is modulated by the gate control system of the gut-brain axis (see also Chapter 13). Therefore because certain areas of the brain have the capability to up or downregulate incoming visceral signals, neurotransmitters common to both brain and gut (e.g., noradrenergic and serotonergic neurotransmitters) can be used to attempt to reduce the painful experience. A Rome Foundation Working Team Report[6] has recommended the use of central neuromodulators (previously identified as antidepressants, antipsychotics, and other psychotropics, as used in psychiatry) for treatment of chronic GI pain or other GI functions via this gut-brain axis pain control mechanism and their possible central effects on neurogenesis (see later).[6]

Hypothalamic-Pituitary-Adrenal Axis

The principal mediators of the stress-immune response include CRF and the locus coeruleus-NE (LC-NE) systems in the CNS. These systems are influenced by numerous positive and negative feedback systems that allow behavioral and peripheral adaptations to stress.[120] The peripheral limb of the CRF system is the hypothalamic-pituitary-adrenal (HPA) axis, a negative feedback system involved in psychoneuroimmune regulation. In the HPA system, inflammatory cytokines, primarily TNF-α, IL-1, and IL-6, liberated during inflammation, as well as multiple neural inputs from other regions within the hypothalamus and other brain regions, including the amygdala and medial prefrontal cortex, stimulate the paraventricular nucleus of the hypothalamus to secrete CRF. CRF stimulates the pituitary gland to release adrenocorticotropic hormone (ACTH, or corticotropin), which, in turn, stimulates the adrenal glands to release glucocorticoids. Finally, the glucocorticoids suppress inflammation and cytokine production, thereby completing the negative feedback loop.[121] Catecholamines can increase proinflammatory cytokines. The parasympathetic system in general has an anti-inflammatory effect. HPA activation may also be due to reduction in negative feedback loops (e.g., downregulation of glucocorticoid receptors in the hippocampus, as shown in early life stress in animal models).[122,123]

CRF is recognized to be important via central and peripheral pathways in stress-related modulation of GI motor and sensory function[114] and may be involved in the generation or maintenance of pain-related symptoms that are sensitive to modulation by psychological stress.[107] Disruptions in the HPA system can lead to behavioral and systemic disorders as a result of increased (e.g., Cushing syndrome, depression, susceptibility to infection) or decreased (e.g., adrenal insufficiency, RA, chronic fatigue syndrome, and PTSD) HPA axis reactivity.[120]

IBD may also be affected through this stress-mediated system.[124] Not only does disease activation have genetic and infectious contributions, but phenotypic expression may also be influenced by gut-brain pathways, including the autonomic NS and HPA axis, proinflammatory GI CRF, the intestinal barrier, and luminal bacteria, all of which are mediated by the CNS. Growing evidence in IBD also suggests that disease activation is influenced by psychosocial vulnerabilities, including perceived stress, maladaptive coping, and psychiatric comorbidities.[124–126]

Co-Occurring Depression and Anxiety in GI Disorders

Psychiatric diagnoses are definable collections of psychological symptoms and behaviors (Axis I). Gastroenterologists usually see these conditions as a factor concomitant with the presenting GI disorder, and there may be a genetic basis to this.[34] This co-occurrence of a psychiatric diagnosis in patients with a medical disorder (comorbidity) is more commonly seen in referral than primary practices,[127] and the psychiatric diagnosis aggravates the clinical presentation and outcome of the medical disorder.

Anxiety and depression are the most commonly noted psychiatric disorders in DGBI and IBD; people living with IBS are 3× more likely than healthy controls to report symptoms of anxiety and depression,[128] with highest rates in younger females. In IBD, one in four and one in three patients experience depression or anxiety, respectively.[129] Depression presents as more severe among people with IBS, likely due to higher psychological contribution to disease state.[128] Suicidal ideation has been estimated to be present in 15%–38% of patients with IBS and has been linked to hopelessness associated with symptom severity, interference with life, and inadequacy of treatment.[130] The incidence of suicide in IBD is also increasingly reported.[131,132] Depression and anxiety are often amenable to psychopharmacologic or psychological treatments.[79,130,133]

When present, psychological distress can lower one's pain threshold,[101] is a comorbid factor in the development of post-infection IBS and dyspepsia,[134] and influences symptom severity, health care seeking, utilization of services, and clinical outcome in DGBI.[133] In IBD, depression can increase rates of clinical flare, surgery, hospitalizations, steroid use, and opioid use and cost the health system up to 5× as much to manage.[135]

While there is some evidence that psychological symptoms may precede the onset of a GI condition (IBD, IBS, etc), for the most part, it is more common that psychological symptoms occur after diagnosis, in response to symptoms, low quality of life, and impaired self-management skills. In IBD, psychological distress occurs within the first 2 years of diagnosis[24] and may represent a failure of treatment to include whole person care,[136] whereas development of these conditions in DGBI may be more contributory to shared vulnerability (Box 5.2).

Certain psychiatric disorders and personality traits adversely affect the illness presentation to the point of interfering with family interactions, socialization, and interactions with physicians. The *Diagnostic and Statistical Manual of Mental Disorders* (DSM)-5 has discarded the concept of "somatization" in favor of *somatic symptom disorder* (SSD; *DSM5 300.82*). In this diagnostic category, somatic symptoms may or may not be medically unexplained but are distressing, disabling, and associated with excessive and disproportionate thoughts, feelings, and behaviors for more than 6 months.[139,140] Other disorders in this category include *factitious disorder* (*DSM5 300.19*), which is characterized by falsification of symptoms and deceptive behaviors related to these symptoms and possibly *Munchausen syndrome*, in which a patient surreptitiously simulates illness (e.g., ingesting laxatives, causing GI bleeding, and feigning symptoms of medical illness) to obtain certain effects

BOX 5.2 The Depression-Inflammation Link

Many behavioral features (e.g., fever, fatigue, anorexia, and depression) of chronic inflammatory diseases, including IBD, cancer, infection, and other catabolic conditions, produce what has been called "sickness behavior," and this process is associated with peripheral cytokine activation that produces central effects.[137,138] Depressed patients with increased inflammatory biomarkers have been found to be less likely to respond to treatment, and in several studies, antidepressant therapy has been associated with decreased inflammatory responses within the body. Preliminary data from patients with inflammatory disorders as well as from medically healthy depressed patients suggest that inhibiting proinflammatory cytokines or their signaling pathways may improve a patient's depressed mood and increase the response to treatment with conventional antidepressant medications.[6]

(e.g., to receive narcotics or operations and procedures) (see Chapter 23). Also included is *borderline personality disorder* (*DSM5 301.83*), in which the individual demonstrates unstable and intense (e.g., overly dependent) interpersonal relationships, experiences marked shifts in mood, and exhibits impulsive (e.g., suicidal, self-mutilating, and sexual) behaviors.[141] For patients with these disorders, it is important for the care provider to maintain clear boundaries of medical care (e.g., not to order studies solely based on the patient's requests), to be clear on time constraints, and to avoid unwanted emotional interactions.

CONNECTING THE DOTS BETWEEN EARLY LIFE AND LATER SYMPTOM RESPONSE

An association between psychological distress and the illness may not be evident to the patient. When patients with IBS who saw a physician were compared with those who had not seen a physician, the former group reported greater psychological difficulties but also denied the role of these difficulties in their illnesses.[141]

As we described above, this behavioral response may have developed through operant conditioning in early life. Johnny from Case 2, who reported somatic symptoms when distressed, may not have recognized or communicated the association of symptoms with the stressful antecedents because these antecedents were not acknowledged or attended to within his family. The ability to become consciously aware of one's own feelings is believed to be a cognitive skill that goes through a developmental process similar to that described by Piaget for other cognitive functions.[27] This development, however, may be suppressed in oppressive family environments and appears to be associated with somatization.

Amplification of Visceral Signals

Various types of stimuli can amplify ascending visceral pathways. It is important to note that visceral pain perception does not necessarily map directly to the degree or intensity of peripheral afferent input but rather is amplified through cognitive and affective circuits at the level of the brain and through descending modulatory pathways. For example, negative affectivity, including neuroticism and somatization, affects the processing and modulation of visceral pain in a variety of health conditions.[142] Cognitively, distraction and expectancy can both mitigate the experience of visceral pain perception.[143] Dysfunction of this visceral pain neuromatrix will allow physiological (nonnoxious) stimuli to be perceived as painful or unpleasant, a phenomenon known as *visceral hypersensitivity*. The persistence of such pain over time forms the basis for a conceptual model of DGBI.

Furthermore, as pain becomes more severe, central mechanisms begin to play a larger role in symptom experience.[15]

Visceral signals in the gut can be amplified in several ways prior to ascending via the gut-brain axis. These processes are interrelated and can vary among patients. Sensitization of primary afferent pathways can occur in response to infection, trauma, and other factors that cause inflammation, as well as dysmotility from repeated distension.[144] Mucosal biopsies in patients with IBS indicate neuroplastic remodeling as well as release of proteases that affect the response properties of the primary afferents, thereby leading to hypersensitivity.[145] Enteric infection, along with psychological distress, as discussed earlier, reflects gut-brain mechanisms that lead to postinfection IBS and dyspepsia.[146] Epithelial immune activation is associated with increased expression of mucosal inflammatory cytokines and enhanced release of neuropeptides (e.g., substance P, CGRP) from primary sensory nerve endings (see earlier[147]). Stress-mediated mast cell degranulation, particularly near enteric neurons, is associated with sensitization of afferent neurons,[102] epithelial permeability increases in response to stress and appears to be mediated via mast cell degranulation products, including CRF and proteases.[148,149]

Transmission to the CNS

Fig. 5.4 shows ascending afferent pathways from the colon. After the first-order visceral neurons are stimulated, they project to the spinal cord, where they synapse with second-order neurons and ascend to the thalamus and midbrain. Of the several supraspinal pathways (spinothalamic, spinoreticular, and spinomesencephalic), the spinothalamic tract shown on the right in Fig. 5.4 terminates in the medial thalamus and projects as third-order neurons to the primary somatosensory cortex. This pathway is important for sensory discrimination and localization of visceral and somatic stimuli (i.e., determining the location and intensity of pain). The spinoreticular tract (middle pathway) conducts sensory information from the spinal cord to the brainstem (reticular formation). This region is involved mainly in the affective and motivational properties of visceral stimulation, that is, the emotional component of pain. The reticulothalamic tract projects from the reticular formation to the medial thalamus on the left and then to the cingulate cortex. The cingulate cortex (see Fig. 5.3) is divided into components that include the perigenual ACC (pACC), which is involved in affect; the MCC, which is involved with behavioral response modification; and the insula, which is associated with reception of incoming visceral signals. These areas are involved in processing noxious visceral and somatic information. This multicomponent integration of nociceptive information, dispersed to the somatotypic-intensity area (lateral sensory cortex) and to the emotional or motivational-affective area of the medial cortex, explains variability in the experience and reporting of pain.

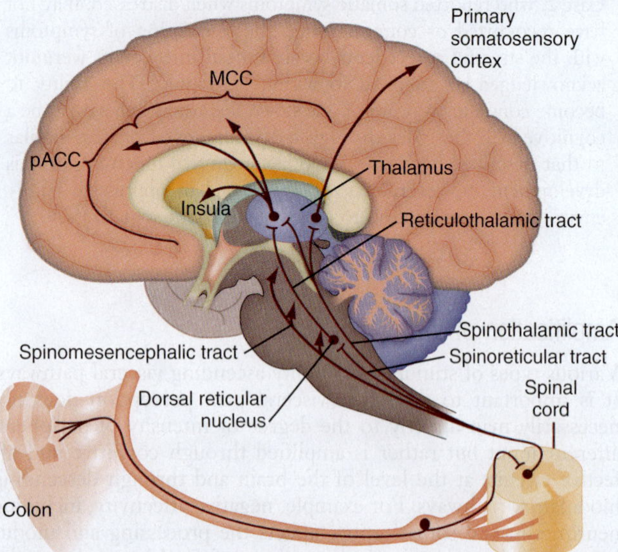

Fig. 5.4 Visceral pain transmission to the CNS. This figure shows the ascending visceral pathways from the intestine to somatosensory and limbic structures in the brain via spinal and midbrain pathways. *MCC*, Midcingulate cortex; *pACC*, perigenual anterior cingulate cortex. (From Drossman DA. Functional abdominal pain syndrome. *Clin Gastroenterol Hepatol*. 2004;2:353–365.)

This conceptual scheme of pain modulation through sensory and motivational-affective components has been supported by studies with PET imaging using radiolabeled oxygen.[150] In healthy subjects who immerse their hands in hot (47°C) water, hypnotic suggestion can make the experience painful or pleasant. Notably, no differences are observed between the two groups in somatosensory cortical activation, but in hypnotized subjects who experience the hand immersion as painful, activation of the ACC is higher. The hypnotic suggestion differentiates the functioning of these two pain systems. The suggestion of unpleasantness is specifically encoded in the anterior midcingulate portion of the ACC, an area involved with negative perceptions of fear and unpleasantness and associated with functional pain syndromes (see later).

Central Amplification

The circuits involved in pain modulation and emotional status involve overlapping brain regions (anterior insular cortex, ACC, medial prefrontal regions, and amygdala), and this overlap may be the basis for the emotional characterizations of pain in GI patients.[84,151,152] The brain circuitry involved in hypervigilance, increased attention to threats, and maladaptive coping in individuals with anxiety has been well described.[153] Increased activity in hypervigilance-associated brain networks leads to the modulation of sensory input; therefore these networks represent a likely pathway by which pain circuits become dysregulated.[154]

In a 2022 systematic review of 348 studies of risk and protective factors for the development and persistence of painful disorders of gut-brain interaction, female sex, history of gastroenteritis (infection), abuse, stress, psychological disorders, somatic symptoms and poor sleep were the strongest risk factors for both children and adults with pain predominant DGBIs.[155] Interestingly, protective factors for adults included social support and optimism.[155]

Fig. 5.5 illustrates this association for functional and structural GI disorders. For most patients with mild-to-moderate symptoms, environmental and bowel-related factors (e.g., intestinal infection, inflammation or injury, diet, and hormonal factors) can lead to afferent excitation and up-regulation of afferent neuronal activity. Patients with moderate-to-severe symptoms also have impaired central modulation of pain as a result of various psychosocial factors, with decreased central inhibitory effects on afferent signals at the level of the spinal cord (disinhibition). In effect, the more severe and constant the pain and the more it is associated with other comorbid symptoms, the more likely the pain is predominantly centrally mediated. Fig. 5.6 demonstrates the concept of central sensitization.

Visceral sensitization relates to the up-regulation of neural signals within first-order ENS neurons occurring at the gut mucosa level (e.g., altered mucosal immune activation, mast cell degranulation, and cytokine release in the gut submucosa). *Central sensitization* relates to CNS up-regulation. Repeated stimulation of the first-order neurons leads to sensitization of spinal circuits, thereby increasing the signal originating from the dorsal horn

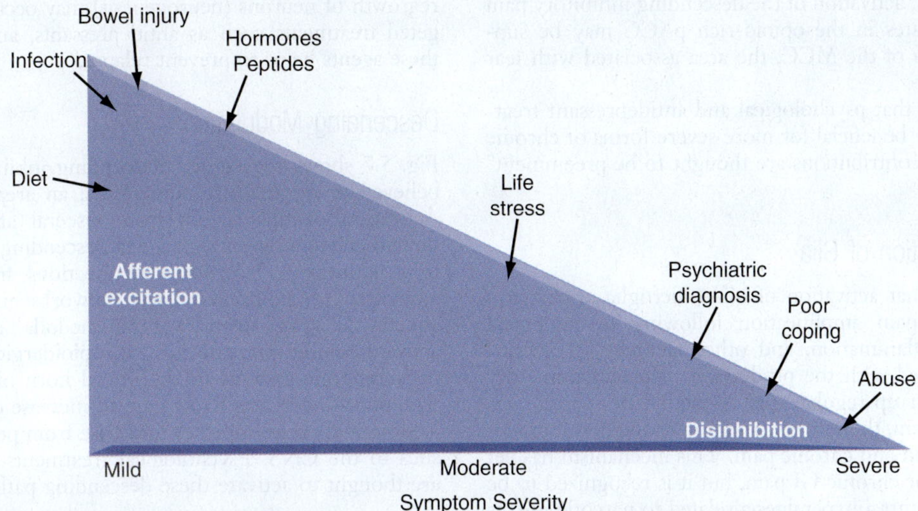

Fig. 5.5 Gut-brain influences on symptom severity. This figure conceptualizes gut-brain influences on symptom severity (*horizontal axis*). With mild-to-moderate symptoms, gut-related factors (e.g., infection, inflammation, bowel injury, hormones, and peptides) lead to afferent excitation and up-regulation of afferent neuronal activity. For the smaller group of patients with moderate to severe symptoms, central modulation of pain is impaired, leading to decreased central inhibitory effects on afferent signals at the level of the spinal cord (disinhibition). Factors that contribute to this effect may include life stress and abuse, comorbid psychiatric diagnoses, and poor coping. Knowing the purported site of action (intestine, brain, or both) can help in determining the treatment approach, such as whether to use medications that target the intestine or brain. (Adapted from Drossman DA. The biopsychosocial continuum in visceral pain. In: Pasricha PJ, Willis D, Gehhart GF, eds. *Chronic abdominal and visceral pain: theory and practice*. New York: Informa Healthcare; 2006.)

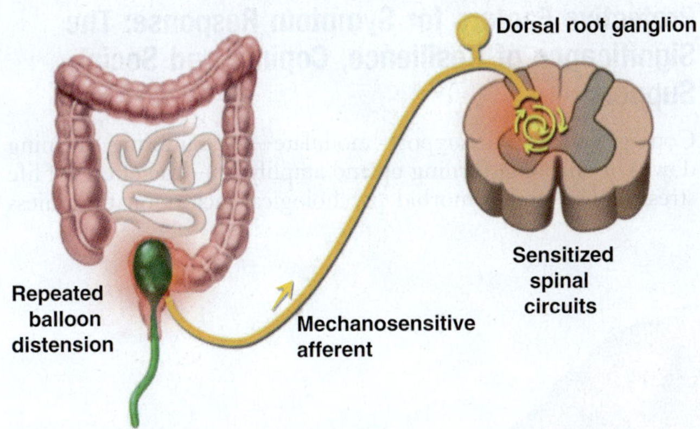

Fig. 5.6 Central sensitization relates to CNS up-regulation. Repeated stimulation of the first-order neuron leads to sensitization of spinal circuits, thereby increasing the signal originating from the dorsal horn synapse and then via second-order neurons to the brain. Central sensitization may also be enhanced at the level of the brain through connections from centers subsuming stress-related activation. The result is enhanced pain or other types of GI dysfunction that originate from gut to brain through these ascending augmented pathways. (From Van Oudenhove L, Crowell MD, Drossman DA, et al. Biopsychosocial aspects of functional gastrointestinal disorders. *Gastroenterology*. 2016;150:1355–1367, with permission from the Rome Foundation.)

synapse and then via second-order neurons to the brain. Central sensitization may also be enhanced at the level of the brain through connections from centers that subsume stress-related activation. The result is enhanced pain or other types of GI dysfunction that originate from gut through these ascending augmented pathways to the brain.

Knowing the severity of the disorder and the purported site of action (i.e., intestine, brain, or both) can help when choosing an approach to treatment (see later). When peripheral influences on severity predominate, medications, surgery, or other modalities that act on the intestine are the primary treatment considerations. As pain becomes more severe, however, behavioral and psychopharmacologic treatments must be added.[19] Pharmacologic recommendations are discussed later. Five classes of brain-gut behavior therapy hold the most promise for centrally mediated pain conditions, including self-management training, CBT, mindfulness/acceptance-based therapies, and gut-directed hypnotherapy. These are typically administered individually by a health psychologist or other mental health provider familiar with GI physiology, always in conjunction with medical treatment and a strong patient-provider relationship.[7]

Fear Conditioning

Brain imaging studies have shown preferential activation of various sites in the brain's limbic system as a result of psychological distress, rectal distension, and other stimuli compared with control subjects. The ACC, which is involved in the motivational and affective components of the limbic (medial) pain system, is dysfunctional in patients with IBS and other chronic painful conditions such as fibromyalgia.[156,157] The pACC, an area rich in opioids and associated with emotional encoding and down-regulation of pain, and the dorsal ACC (also called the *rostral* or *anterior MCC*) may be activated to varying degrees in response to painful stimuli. The dorsal ACC, along with the amygdala, is associated with unpleasantness, fear, and an increase in responses to motor pain.[158] When PET and functional MRI are used to evaluate the response of the ACC to rectal distention or to the anticipation of distension, patients with IBS display preferential activation of the MCC and less activation of the pACC than controls.[86,156] In IBS, activation of the descending inhibitory pain pathway that originates in the opioid-rich pACC may be supplanted by activation of the MCC, the area associated with fear and unpleasantness.

The data suggest that psychological and antidepressant treatments are potentially beneficial for more severe forms of chronic pain in which CNS contributions are thought to be preeminent[6] (see later).

Spinal Cord Activation of Glia

Evidence indicates that activation of glia (microglia, astrocytes) may also enhance pain amplification following psychological stress, peripheral inflammation, and other factors.[159–161] Glial activation is associated with the production of proinflammatory cytokines, which can up-regulate the *N*-methyl-D-aspartate receptor signaling system, thereby contributing to the development of central sensitization and chronic pain. This mechanism has yet to be fully studied for chronic GI pain, but it is recognized to be the mechanism for central hyperalgesia related to narcotic use, as in narcotic bowel syndrome (see Chapter 13).[119]

Structural Changes

Growing evidence suggests that severe stress, psychiatric disorders, and chronic pain—separately or in combination—are neurodegenerative disorders much like Alzheimer disease and Parkinson disease; functional MRI studies using voxel-based morphometry have shown significant losses of cortical neuron density in key areas of the brain associated with these conditions. These changes are reported to involve the ACC and orbitofrontal cortex in major depression and bipolar disorder[162]; the hippocampus in PTSD and sexual and physical abuse[163]; the ACC, posterior cingulate cortex, and ventromedial prefrontal cortex in chronic somatic pain[164]; and the dorsal ACC in IBS[88] and painful chronic pancreatitis.[165] One hypothesis is that these structural changes are the result of degenerative effects of stress mediators on the CNS that fatigue central control mechanisms and produce central sensitization. The changes may play a role in the transition of intermittent visceral pain conditions such as IBS into more chronic and persistent pain over many years, as in *CAPS*.[19] Notably, there is evidence that regrowth of neurons (neurogenesis) may occur with centrally targeted treatments such as antidepressants, and prolonged use of these agents helps to prevent relapse.[6]

Descending Modulation

Fig. 5.7 shows the central descending inhibitory system that is believed to originate in the pACC, an area rich in opioids.[166] Activation of this region from visceral afferent activity may downregulate afferent signals via descending corticofugal inhibitory pathways. Descending connections from the ACC and amygdala to pontomedullary networks—including the periaqueductal gray, rostral ventral medulla, and raphe nuclei—activate inhibitory pathways via opioidergic, serotonergic, and noradrenergic systems to the dorsal horn of the spinal cord.[167] The dorsal horn acts like a gate to increase or decrease the projection of afferent impulses that arise from peripheral nociceptive sites to the CNS. Psychological treatments and antidepressants are thought to activate these descending pathways.

Cytokines and the Brain

Stress may have proinflammatory effects, but intestinal inflammation may also affect behavior reciprocally via activation of cytokines. Inflammation may be a common mechanism for disease even in the brain. Inflammation can affect neurotransmitter metabolism, neuroendocrine function, and neural plasticity in the brain, and there is increasing evidence that major depression and other psychiatric disorders may be mediated by inflammatory factors in GI conditions.[24]Release of inflammatory cytokines from glial cells in the dorsal horn up-regulates pain pathways and can produce narcotic hyperalgesia and narcotic bowel syndrome.[119]

Protective Factors for Symptom Response: The Significance of Resilience, Coping, and Social Support

Coping and social support modulate—by buffering (turning down) or enabling (turning up and amplifying)—the effects of life stress, abuse, and comorbid psychological factors on the illness

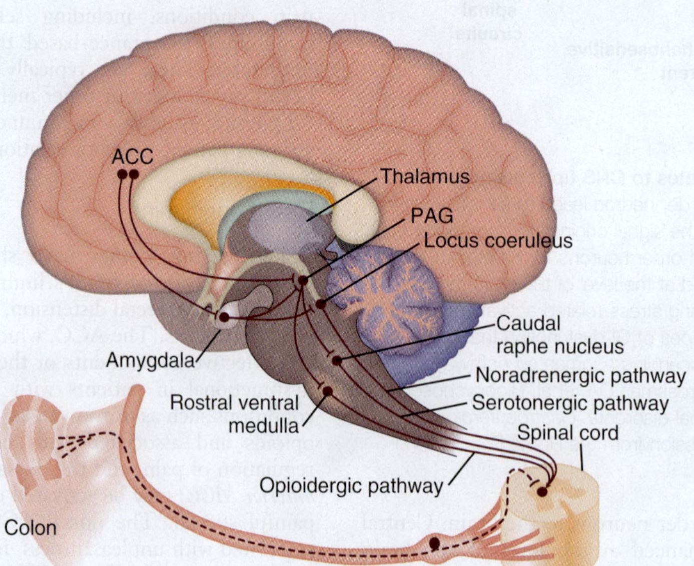

Fig. 5.7 Descending transmission of pain regulatory signals. This figure demonstrates the corticofugal descending inhibitory pathways from the CNS to the spinal cord. The descending pathway is consistent with the gate control theory of pain modulation. *ACC*, Anterior cingulate cortex; *PAG*, periaqueductal gray. (From Drossman DA. Functional abdominal pain syndrome. *Clin Gastroenterol Hepatol*. 2004;2:353–365.)

and its outcome. Coping has been defined as "efforts, both action-oriented and intrapsychic, to manage (i.e., master, tolerate, minimize) environmental and internal demands and conflicts that tax or exceed a person's resources."[168] Flexibility in coping strategies based on the stressor (problem-focused coping when the problem has a solution, emotion-focused coping when the problem does not have a solution) is a critical aspect of adjustment to illness.[169] There is some evidence that patients with functional GI disorders may exhibit inflexibility in coping style, leading to negative affect and high symptom reporting.[170–172] Patients with Crohn's disease who score low on avoidance-based coping strategies (distraction, numbing, diversion) are least likely to relapse.[173] Alternative, disease acceptance, optimism, and psychological resilience have been associated with improved outcomes, including less anxiety, lower disease activity, and reduced surgeries. [174] For GI diagnoses of all types, a maladaptive emotional coping style, specifically catastrophizing, along with the perceived inability to decrease symptoms, is associated with higher pain scores, more physician visits, and poorer functioning over the subsequent one-year period.[175] Catastrophizing is also associated with more difficult interpersonal relationships,[89] predicts postoperative pain,[176] and contributes to greater worry and suffering in patients with IBS.[177] Efforts made through psychological treatments to improve a person's appraisal of the stress of illness and their ability to manage symptoms are likely to improve health status and outcome.[79]

Social support through family, religious, and community organizations and other social networks can have similar benefits in reducing the impact of stressors on physical and mental illness, thereby improving the ability to cope with the illness.[178,179] Negative social relationships in particular are most strongly related to poor health outcomes.[180] Patients who perceive social support from their health care provider are also likely to see more improved symptoms and quality of life.[181]

In a study of more than 200 patients with high risk IBD, a multidisciplinary program that included nursing, social work, nutrition, and clinical pharmacy and was designed to foster resilience and community led to improved outcomes over time, including higher resilience and reductions in unplanned care, opioid, and steroid use—more importantly, this study demonstrated that a positive psychology/resilience-based approach to gastroenterology may be an earlier way to incorporate integrated care by nonmental health professionals [182] in both IBD and IBS.[183]

CLINICAL IMPLICATIONS OF THE BIOPSYCHOSOCIAL MODEL. HOW TO "TREATING TO TARGET" BY UNDERSTANDING YOUR PATIENT'S BIOPSYCHOSOCIAL CONTEXT

The physician should obtain, organize, and integrate psychosocial information to achieve optimal care. The recommendations offered here are particularly useful for patients who have chronic illness or major psychosocial difficulties.[184]

History Taking

The physician's dialogue with the patient is the most important asset for enhancing the physician-patient relationship, developing a diagnosis, and formulating treatment and is often underused. Consider the information obtained in the following office interview:

Physician (looking at chart)*:* "How can I help you?"
Patient (pauses, looks pensive)*:* "I developed a flare-up of my *Crohn's* ... pain, nausea, and vomiting, when I came back from vacation."
Physician (interrupting)*:* "Was the pain like what you had before?"
Patient: "Yes, well almost, I think."
Physician (looks up)*:* "Was it made worse by food?"
Patient: "Yes."
Physician (leaning forward)*:* "Did you have fever? or diarrhea?"
Patient (looks down)*:* "Well yes, I think. ... I didn't take my temperature."
Physician: "So you had fever and diarrhea?"
Patient: "Uh no, well, they were a little loose ... I guess."

In this exchange, some relevant information was not elicited, and because of the interruptions and leading questions, the accuracy of the information after the first question is uncertain. Furthermore, the nonverbal communication did not facilitate an effective physician-patient interaction.

The medical history should be obtained through a patient-centered, nondirective interview during which the patient is encouraged to tell the story in his or her own way so that the events contributing to the illness unfold naturally. Open-ended questions are used initially to generate hypotheses, and additional information is obtained with facilitating expressions—"Yes?," "Can you tell me more?"—repeating the patient's previous statements, head nodding, or even silent pauses with an expectant look can facilitate history taking. Avoid closed-ended (yes-no) questions at first, although they can be used later to characterize the symptoms further. Refrain from using multiple-choice or leading questions, because the patient's desire to comply may bias the responses.

The traditional medical and social histories should not be separated but elicited together so that the medical problem is described in the context of the psychosocial events surrounding the illness. The setting of symptom onset or exacerbation should always be obtained. At all times, the questions should communicate the physician's willingness to address the biological and psychological aspects of the illness:

Physician (concerned, looking at patient)*:* "How can I help you?"
Patient (pauses)*:* "I developed a flare-up of my Crohn's ... the pain, nausea, and vomiting, when I came back from vacation."
Physician: "Yes?"
Patient: "I was about to start my new position as floor supervisor and thought I'd take a vacation to get prepared, and then all this happened."
Physician (pauses)*:* "Oh, I see."
Patient (continues): "I started getting that cramping feeling right here [points to lower abdomen], and then it got worse after eating. So I knew I'd be obstructed again if I didn't get in to see you."
Physician: "Hmm. Any other symptoms?"
Patient: "Well, I felt warm, but didn't take my temperature."
Physician: "What was your bowel pattern like?"
Patient: "They started getting loose when I was on vacation. Now they're slowing down. I haven't gone today."

The number of verbal exchanges is the same, yet the patient offers more information. The clinical features are clearer, and additional information about an association of symptoms with beginning a new job situation is obtained. This interview method also encourages patient self-awareness and allows consideration of possible behavioral treatments (e.g., stress reduction techniques, job change, and counseling) that may ameliorate future flare-ups of the patient's symptoms.

The historical information should be obtained from the perspective of the patient's understanding of the illness. Important questions to ask include:

"What do you think is causing this problem?"

"Why are you coming to see me now?"
"What type of treatment do you think you should receive?"
"What do you fear most about your illness?"

Additional information on methods to improve history taking and communication skills is found in Table 5.1.[184]

Evaluating the Data

The physician must assess the relative influences of the biological, psychological, and social dimensions on the illness. Determining whether psychosocial or biological processes are operative in an illness is unnecessary and possibly countertherapeutic. Usually, both are important, and treatment is based on determining which is identifiable and remediable. A negative medical evaluation is not sufficient for making a psychosocial diagnosis. Box 5.3 lists several questions to consider in the assessment and evaluation of the patient.

Diagnostic Decision-Making

Deciding which tests to order will depend on their clinical usefulness. A number of questions should be considered: Is a test safe and cost-effective? Will the results make a difference in treatment? Patients who are persistent in their requests for further studies or who challenge their physician's competence may tempt the physician to schedule unneeded studies or surgery out of uncertainty or out of feeling that he or she needs to do something. This temptation can be avoided by basing decisions on the objective evaluation of data (e.g., blood in the stool, fever, and abnormal serum chemistry values) rather than solely on the patient's illness behavior.

The case of Ms. L (Case #1), the patient with persistent and unexplained abdominal pain, is an example familiar to the gastroenterologist. The urge to work up a patient with chronic abdominal pain must be tempered by the evidence that an adequate initial evaluation considerably reduces the likelihood of

TABLE 5.1 Nonverbal and Verbal Factors That Facilitate or Inhibit Communication

Factor	Facilitate	Inhibit
Nonverbal		
Clinical environment	Private, comfortable	Noisy, physical barriers
Eye contact	Frequent	Infrequent or constant
Listening	Actively listening; questions relate to what the patient says	Distracted or preoccupied (e.g., typing)
Body posture	Direct, open, relaxed	Body turned, arms folded
Head nodding	Well timed	Infrequent or excessive
Body proximity	Close enough to touch	Too close or too distant
Facial expression	Shows interest and understanding	Preoccupied, bored, disapproving
Voice	Gentle	Harsh, rushed
Touching	Helpful if well timed and used to communicate empathy	Insincere if inappropriate or improperly timed
Synchrony (arms, legs)	Concordant	Discordant
Verbal		
Question forms	Open-ended to generate hypotheses	Rigid or stereotyped style
	Closed-ended to test hypotheses	Multiple choice or leading questions ("You didn't … did you?")
	Uses the patient's words	Uses unfamiliar words or jargon
	Facilitates patient discussion by "echoing" and affirmative gestures	Interruptions, undue control of conversation
	Uses summarizing statements	Not done
Question/interview style	Nonjudgmental	Judgmental
	Follows lead of patient's prior comments (patient centered)	Follows own preset style or agenda
	Uses a narrative thread	Unorganized
	Uses silence appropriately	Interrupts or uses too much silence
	Reassures and encourages appropriately	Reassures or encourages prematurely or in an unwarranted manner
	Communicates empathy	Does not provide or not sincere
Recommendations	Elicits feedback and negotiates	Does not elicit feedback; directly states views
Asks/provides medical information	Appropriate to the clinical issues	Asks too many biomedical questions and provides too detailed information
Asks/provides psychosocial information	Elicits in a sensitive and nonthreatening manner	Ignores psychosocial data or asks intrusive or probing questions
Humor	Uses humor when appropriate and facilitative	Uses no or inappropriate humor

BOX 5.3 Questions to Consider in the Clinical Evaluation of the Patient

Does the patient have acute or chronic illness?
What is the patient's life history of illness?
Why is the patient coming for medical care now?
What are the patient's perceptions and expectations?
Does the patient exhibit abnormal illness behavior?
What is the impact of the illness on the patient?
Is there a concurrent psychiatric diagnosis?
Are there cultural or ethnic influences?
How does the family interact around the illness?
What are the patient's other psychosocial resources?
How extensive should the evaluation be?
Should the patient be referred to a psychiatric consultant?

finding an overlooked cause later. Here, the clinical approach is not medical diagnosis but psychosocial assessment and treatment of the chronic pain.[19] Factors associated with or exacerbating chronic pain symptoms include: (1) a recent disruption in the family or social environment (e.g., child leaving home, argument); (2) major loss or anniversaries of losses (e.g., death of a family member or friend, hysterectomy, interference with the outcome of pregnancy); (3) history of sexual or physical abuse; (4) onset or worsening of depression or other psychiatric diagnosis; and (5) a hidden agenda (e.g., narcotic-seeking behavior, laxative abuse, pending litigation, disability). Although consultation and treatment with a mental health provider may be needed, it is important that the physician continue to be involved in the patient's care and be vigilant about the development of new findings.[185]

At times, decisions must be made with incomplete or nonspecific information. Particularly for chronic symptoms, when studies are unrevealing and the patient is clinically stable, it is wise to tolerate the uncertainty in diagnosis and observe the patient for new developments over a period of time. Experienced physicians usually make diagnostic and treatment decisions based on the degree of change in the condition over weeks or months, rather than on one or two occasions.

Consultation with a psychiatrist or health psychologist should be considered when additional psychological data could clarify the illness or improve patient care.[185] Examples include: (1) identification of a psychiatric diagnosis for which specific treatment (e.g., psychopharmacologic agents) may be beneficial; (2) serious impairment of the patient's level of psychosocial functioning (e.g., inability to work); or (3) consideration of invasive diagnostic or therapeutic strategies on the basis of the patient's complaints, without clear indications from the medical data.

Treatment Approach

Establishing a Therapeutic Relationship

The physician can establish a therapeutic relationship with a patient through good communication skills that are implemented by using specific guidelines: (1) allowing the patient to complete his or her opening statement; (2) eliciting concerns and establishing a rapport; (3) using a combination of open-ended and closed-ended questions to gather and clarify information; (4) identifying and responding to the patient's personal situation, beliefs, and values; (5) using language the patient can understand to explain diagnosis and treatment plans; (6) checking for the patient's understanding; (7) encouraging the patient to participate in decisions and exploring the patient's willingness and ability to follow care plans; (8) asking for other concerns the patient might have; and (9) discussing follow-up activities expected of the patient before closing the visit.[186] This strategy must be individualized because patients vary in the degree of negotiation and participation they require. Overall, the physician must be nonjudgmental, show interest in the patient's well-being, and be prepared to exercise effective communication skills.[184] For a review on how to establish a therapeutic patient-centered collaborative relationship, go to video 5.3

Eliciting, Evaluating, and Communicating the Role of Psychosocial Factors

Fear of disapproval and lack of trust often prevent a patient from sharing intimate thoughts and feelings, an obstacle that a good physician-patient relationship can overcome. When the patient is unwilling or unable to accept the role of psychosocial factors in illness, the physician can still obtain such information indirectly by inference and should not attempt to provide the patient with insight. If the patient asks whether the problem is just "in my head," the physician should explain that illness is rarely either mental or physical; that understanding all factors, including the patient's feelings, is important; and that many chronic conditions are associated with depression or unrealistic fears. Consistent with the BPS model of illness, discussing psychosocial and biological factors in terms of causation (e.g., by stating, "It is common for stress to cause your problems") or exclusion (e.g., by stating, "The workup is negative; it must be stress") is not helpful. The following interview illustrates the way in which a patient's chronic pain can be understood by discussion of the brain-gut axis: Video 5.4

Providing Reassurance

A patient's fears and concerns require reassurance. If the reassurance is premature, inadequate, or inappropriate, it will be perceived as insincere or as a lack of thoroughness by the physician. The physician should respond to the patient's needs and requests empathically but not succumb to pressure to do anything that would not be in the patient's best interest. For example, disability may be a disincentive to helping the patient re-establish wellness and return to gainful employment. If the patient does not qualify for disability, the physician should be clear about it.

Recognizing the Patient's Adaptations to Chronic Illness

Illness is associated with certain "benefits" for the patient, such as increased attention and support, release from usual responsibilities, and possibly social and financial compensation. For some patients, more may be lost by giving up the state of illness than gained by wellness, and improvement may be slow. The patient can be helped by improving his or her psychosocial adjustment to the illness (e.g., improving coping strategies).

Reinforcing Healthy Behaviors

Sometimes, complaints of physical distress are a maladaptive effort to communicate emotional distress or receive attention. The physician may unwittingly reinforce this behavior in several ways: (1) paying a great deal of attention to the patient's complaints to the exclusion of other aspects; (2) acting on each complaint by ordering diagnostic studies or giving a prescriptive medication; or (3) assuming total responsibility for the patient's well-being. The patient learns to keep the physician's interest by reporting symptoms rather than by trying to improve, thereby perpetuating the cycle of symptom recitation and passive interaction.

To encourage a patient to take more responsibility for their care and have a heightened sense of control, the physician may offer a choice among several treatments or help design a self-management program. The physician should limit discussion about symptoms to what is needed to satisfy medical concerns and focus instead on adaptations to the illness rather than the cure. I often find it best not to ask about the patient's symptom (e.g., "How is your pain?") because the question puts my attention on the fact that the patient is having symptoms. Rather, I ask about the symptoms in the context of the patient's health-promoting behaviors (e.g., "What are you doing to manage your pain?").

Central Neuromodulation

Psychopharmacologic agents act on neurotransmitter receptors in the brain-gut regulatory pathways that target serotonergic, noradrenergic, dopaminergic, and opioidergic receptor sites and produce various effects that include: (1) reducing visceral afferent signaling arising from painful GI conditions; (2) treating GI pain by facilitating central downregulating pathways; (3) depending on the agent, modifying diarrhea or constipation; (4) reducing anxiety, depression, nausea, and loss of appetite; and (5) in higher doses, treating major depression or other psychiatric disorders.[6,159] For a video on how to explain the rationale for neuromodulator treatment go to video 5.5

With the publication of Rome IV,[187] the Rome Foundation has established new definitional guidelines that relabel agents working both in the brain and gut as "gut-brain neuromodulators."[6] This term includes the primarily *central neuromodulators* (e.g., antidepressants, antipsychotics, azapirones, and other centrally acting agents) and the primarily *peripheral neuromodulators*, including serotonergic, chloride channel, delta ligand agents, and others (not discussed in this section). It is believed that this new terminology will improve understanding of their pharmacologic value, reduce stigma, and likely improve treatment adherence when treating patients with GI disorders.

The major classes of the antidepressant-type central neuromodulators used for treating GI disorders include the tricyclic antidepressants (TCAs) (e.g., amitriptyline, imipramine, desipramine, and nortriptyline), the selective serotonin reuptake inhibitors (SSRIs) (e.g., fluoxetine, sertraline, citalopram, escitalopram, and paroxetine), the serotonin and norepinephrine reuptake inhibitors (SNRIs) (e.g., duloxetine, venlafaxine, desvenlafaxine, and milnacipran), and the noradrenergic and specific serotonin agents (tetracyclics) (e.g., mirtazapine and mianserin). The antianxiety agents include benzodiazepines (e.g., lorazepam and clonazepam) and the azapirones (e.g., buspirone). The newer atypical antipsychotics (e.g., quetiapine, olanzapine, and aripiprazole) are used as augmenting agents in addition to having antianxiety effects. More detailed discussion of the pharmacology, clinical actions, and side effects of these agents for treating GI disorders can be found elsewhere.[6,159] For a review of the classes of neuromodulators, their pharmacology, and the treatment approach as discussed below, go to video 5.6

Tricyclic Antidepressants

The TCAs can reduce chronic pain[188,189] through peripheral and central mechanisms, including activation of corticofugal pain inhibitory pathways by noradrenergic and serotonergic activation, reducing afferent signaling in the gut, and, in higher doses, treating psychiatric comorbidity such as anxiety and depression. Their noradrenergic and anticholinergic effects also reduce intestinal transit rate and can therefore help patients with diarrhea. The usual starting dose is 25–50 mg, and the dose can be increased as needed to 100 mg on average. TCAs can also treat major and secondary depressive symptoms when used in full antidepressant doses ($\geq$150 mg/day). Their antihistaminic and anticholinergic side effects may lead to nonadherence because of constipation, orthostasis, or dry mouth and eyes. However, the secondary amine TCAs (desipramine, nortriptyline) have less activation on cholinergic and histaminic receptors and produce fewer of these side effects than the tertiary amines (TCAs; amitriptyline, imipramine).

Selective Serotonin Reuptake Inhibitors

Due to their lack of noradrenergic effect, SSRIs are not considered helpful for painful GI symptoms. However, they are often used in full doses to reduce concurrent anxiety, major depression, panic disorder, and other high-anxiety traits (e.g., obsessive-compulsive disorder, PTSD, and social phobia). Because of their dominant serotonergic effect, SSRIs can produce diarrhea and even anxiety at the initiation of treatment.

Serotonin and Norepinephrine Reuptake Inhibitors

The SNRIs are particularly helpful for treating painful conditions because they have dominant noradrenergic and serotonergic action like the TCAs and are approved for diabetic pain, fibromyalgia, and other somatic pain syndromes. They may also be used off-label for visceral pain conditions and do not have the antihistaminic or anticholinergic side effects of TCAs or SSRIs. Nausea is the predominant side effect, which can be ameliorated if taken with meals. Duloxetine is usually started at 30 mg/day and increased to 60 or even 90 mg after several weeks, if needed. Venlafaxine needs to be used in higher doses (over 150 mg/day) for treating painful conditions due to the lack of noradrenergic effect in lower doses. Milnacipran (50–100 mg twice daily) is not marketed as an antidepressant but for treatment of somatic painful conditions.

Tetracyclic Agents

Mirtazapine has complex serotonergic and noradrenergic properties leading to multiple effects in addition to treating depression. Its 5-HT_3 antagonist action is probably responsible for its antiemetic properties and antidiarrheal effects, and its antihistaminic action is helpful for sedation. It is also an appetite stimulant (weight gain is a side effect) and can be used for the treatment of anxiety. The dose ranges from 7.5 to 30 mg usually taken at night due to its sedation effect.

Antianxiety Agents

The benzodiazepines are frequently used to ameliorate acute anxiety, particularly if the anxiety is associated with stress-induced flare-ups of bowel disturbance. Their potential benefit should be balanced with the long-term risks of sedation, drug interactions, habituation, and rebound after withdrawal, and they are not recommended for chronic use. Buspirone is a nonbenzodiazepine azapirone that is used for generalized anxiety disorder and, because of its 5-HT_1 action, has been recommended for treating functional dyspepsia (in doses of 15–30 mg twice daily) due to its effect on fundic relaxation.

Atypical Antipsychotic Agents

Although originally developed for treating schizophrenia and bipolar disorder, in low doses the atypical antipsychotics have profound antianxiety effects, and some agents (e.g., quetiapine and olanzapine) have sedation effects, whereas others (e.g., aripiprazole and brexpiprazole) are more activating but may produce akathisia. They can be used for patients with GI disorders to augment the effect of an antidepressant for chronic pain, just as they are used to augment the treatment of depression (see later). The dose may be one-half to one-third of that used for treating major psychiatric disorders.

Opioids

Opioids have no role in treating patients with chronic pain or a psychosocial disturbance because of their potential for abuse, dependency, and narcotic bowel syndrome.[21,190] Patients in whom narcotic bowel syndrome develops need to be identified and can be treated successfully with detoxification (see Chapter 13).[191] The following video addresses how the provider can respond to the patient urgently requesting to be prescribed opioids: Video 5.7

Augmentation Treatment

When a single agent is unsuccessful, treatment can be enhanced by using low-dose drug combinations to achieve synergistic effects. The concept of augmentation involves activation of different receptor sites in the brain to enhance the therapeutic effect.[6,159] This approach also minimizes side effects when a single agent is pushed to higher doses. Augmentation can be accomplished by adding an antidepressant, peripheral neuromodulator agent for treating pain (e.g., gabapentin), or a regulator of bowel symptoms (e.g., alosetron and lubiprostone) (see Chapters 17 and 20). Another central neuromodulator that can be added is buspirone.[192,193] A low-dose atypical antipsychotic (e.g., quetiapine) can be added to a TCA or SNRI to augment pain control, reduce anxiety, and enhance sleep.[194]

Prevention of Relapse

Prevention of relapse relates to the concept that continued treatment with a neuromodulator beyond the period of achieving clinical benefit will reduce the likelihood of relapse or recurrence.[195] This is supported through evidence that continued antidepressant treatment may be associated with reversal of the clinical disorder through neurogenesis.[196,197] To reduce the likelihood of relapse when treating DGBIs, we empirically recommend that treatment be continued for 6–12 months after a treatment response.

Pharmacogenomic Testing

Pharmacogenomics examines the variability of the expression of individual genes relevant to disease susceptibility, as well as drug response, at cellular, tissue, individual, or population levels. Genetic polymorphisms may also influence the response to medications through their effect on drug metabolism.[198] Pharmacogenomic measurement of almost all central neuromodulators is available, and their use is growing, particularly in the management of chronic pain.[199] Therefore pharmacogenomic testing may be of value for selecting an optimal neuromodulator, optimizing benefit and reducing toxicity, or augmenting treatment by using several medications for which drug interactions should be avoided.[200]

Brain-Gut Behavior Therapies

A 2022 Rome Foundation Working Team Report made up of experts in the field of psychogastroenterology decided to rename psychological interventions that have been shown to be effective in the management of DGBI, and to a lesser extent IBD as brain-gut behavior therapies to reflect their adaptation to GI-specific concerns, their treatment targets of reduced GI symptoms and improved GI-related quality of life and to de-stigmatize their use among patients.[7] The following video demonstrates how a BGBT provider explains the rationale of these treatments to a patient who is reluctant to commit: Video 5.8

BGBTs are clinician-administered, highly personalized nonpharmacologic approaches focused on remediating GI symptoms and GI-specific quality of life. Five classes of BGBT have been identified; the specific brain-gut target, as well as the modality, type of provider and patient preference, will influence choice of intervention.[7] Below we briefly describe each of the classes and their targets:

Self-management training: Often nurse led, disease self-management programs are based in self-efficacy theory—that having education about one's condition and to feel supported and empowered to manage it will drive symptom relief and quality of life. Self-management training includes skills to promote a healthy lifestyle, including sleep, exercise, nutrition, and stress, and has been shown to positively affect outcome in both DGBI [201] and IBD.[202] Self-management programs can be delivered flexibly, with evidence for their success in group settings, over the telephone, in the form of self-help workbooks, and even more recently through online support.[203]

Cognitive behavior therapy (CBT): CBT is a brief, skills-based, collaborative therapy that seeks to remediate maladaptive thoughts and coping styles known to amplify GI symptoms.[204] Some of the most common targets in CBT for IBS include hyperarousal, visceral anxiety/symptom-specific fear, and pain catastrophizing.[205] CBT can be administered to individuals or in groups,[206,207] via the internet,[208,209] and has been shown to be effective in as few as four sessions.[210] CBT has been shown to be effective in a range of digestive disorders, including teenagers[211,212] and adults with IBD.[213] In fact CBT is one of the most well-tested BGBTs for DGBIs, with more than 30 randomized controlled trials (RCTs) also supporting its use in groups, online, and with reduced therapist contact. Contextually based CBT approaches including acceptance and commitment therapy and mindfulness-based cognitive therapy have also been tested in both DGBI and IBS[214] and IBD[215] with positive results. Efforts to understand potential mediators and moderators of outcomes are underway.[216]

Mindfulness-based stress reduction has shown effectiveness for a wide range of psychological and medical conditions, including DGBI[217] and IBD,[218] and is rooted in the belief that being grounded in the moment, accepting pain as inevitable, can reduce suffering and stress and improve emotion regulation. Mindfulness has shown promise in group settings and can be delivered by nonmental health providers.

Gut-directed hypnosis is a heightened state of awareness and mental focus, often induced by deep relaxation, that allows for gut-specific healing suggestions to enter the brain without resistance. Data from studies in different centers support the use of hypnosis as an effective, viable treatment option in IBS that improves symptoms and quality of life and reduces stress and anxiety[219,220]; the beneficial effects of hypnosis have been shown to persist at long-term follow-up.[221] Gut-directed hypnotherapy can be successfully delivered via groups [222] and video calls,[223] and digital options are emerging on the market as well. Hypnosis has also shown success in reducing inflammatory markers in stool acquired during sigmoidoscopy[224] and prolonging clinical remission in patients with IBD.[225]

Clinician-Related Issues

A patient's psychosocial difficulties may affect the clinician's attitudes and behaviors[16] and, if not recognized, may adversely affect the patient's care. Physicians are uncomfortable making decisions in the face of diagnostic uncertainty,[226] because the assumption is that more knowledge will make the illness more treatable. Nevertheless, many clinical treatments are undertaken for symptoms or psychosocial concerns that are not based on a specific diagnosis, particularly for patients with unexplained complaints who demand a diagnosis or for those who are thought to be litigious. The physician risks excessive diagnostic testing or unneeded or harmful treatments in such patients (sometimes called "furor medicus").[227] Alternatively, the physician may not believe that the complaints are legitimate and may then exhibit behaviors (e.g., referring the patient to a psychiatrist) that the patient will recognize as rejection.

Some patients and physicians experience interpersonal conflicts. The patient, feeling helpless and out of control, may behave in ways the physician interprets as dependent and demanding; these feelings may lead to blame or stigmatization by the physician. The physician must understand that these behaviors are part of the patient's maladaptive communication style and should not be perceived as personal. Some patients develop psychosocial adaptations to chronic illness (e.g., family attention, control through the illness behaviors, disability) that delay ultimate improvement, and these patients may not acknowledge the physician's efforts. In these situations, treatment is best refocused from efforts to cure to efforts to improve daily function, despite continued symptoms. Gratification can be obtained from the personal effort rather than from the patient's expressions of gratitude. Finally, each physician must set personal limits in time and energy on the care of patients who are particularly challenging. Limiting the length of office visits, allocating part of the patient's care to other health care workers, and, when necessary, saying "no" to the patient are all important methods of achieving a balance between the physician's personal needs and benefit to the patient.

Full references for this chapter can be found on https://ebooks.health.elsevier.com.

PART II Nutrition in Gastroenterology

6 Nutritional Principles and Assessment of the Gastroenterology Patient

Joel B. Mason, Bridget Hron

IN THIS CHAPTER

Diligent attention to patients' nutritional needs can have a major positive impact on medical outcomes. This is particularly true in GI and liver disease because many of these conditions, in addition to altering nutrient metabolism and requirements, are prone to interfering with ingestion and assimilation of nutrients. Nutritional management, however, often continues to be an inadequately or incorrectly addressed component of patient care.

Inadequate or misdirected attention to nutritional issues is due, in part, to failure to distinguish patients who stand to benefit from nutritional care from those whose outcomes will not respond to nutritional intervention. The fact that many clinical trials have failed to demonstrate a benefit of nutritional support in hospitalized patients is often because such a distinction has not been made. The major aim of this chapter is to provide the scientific principles and practical tools necessary to recognize patients who will benefit from focused attention to their nutritional needs and to provide the guidance necessary to develop a suitable nutritional plan for these individuals.

Over or underfeeding a patient can be detrimental to clinical outcomes, so developing a nutritional plan most appropriately begins by determining the patient's estimated caloric and protein needs.

BASIC NUTRITIONAL CONCEPTS

Energy Stores

Endogenous energy stores are oxidized continuously for fuel. Triglyceride (TG) present in adipose tissue is the body's major fuel reserve and is critical for survival during periods of starvation (Table 6.1; values for 70 kg man are shown). The high energy density and hydrophobic nature of TGs make them five-fold better fuel per unit mass than glycogen. TGs liberate 9.3 kcal/g when oxidized and are stored compactly as oil inside the fat cell. In comparison, glycogen produces only 4.1 kcal/g on oxidation and is stored intracellularly as a gel, containing approximately 2 g of water per gram of glycogen. Adipose tissue cannot provide fuel for certain tissues like bone marrow, erythrocytes, leukocytes, renal medulla, the lens and retina, and peripheral nerves, which cannot oxidize lipids and require glucose for their energy supply. During endurance exercise, glycogen and TGs in muscle tissue provide an important source of fuel for working muscles.

Energy Metabolism

Energy is required continuously for normal organ function, maintenance of metabolic homeostasis, heat production, and performance of mechanical work. Daily total energy expenditure (TEE) has three components: resting energy expenditure (REE) ($\approx$70% of TEE); the energy expenditure of physical activity ($\approx$20% of TEE); and the thermic effect of feeding ($\approx$10% of TEE), which is the temporary increase in energy expenditure that accompanies enteral ingestion or parenteral administration of nutrients. Although the latter two components of TEE should be considered when estimating caloric needs for ambulatory individuals, in acutely ill, hospitalized patients, the energy expended in physical activity is typically ignored, and the energy expended in the thermic effect of feeding is built into the predictive equations that follow.

Resting Energy Expenditure

REE represents energy expenditure while a person lies quietly awake in an interprandial state; under these conditions, about 1 kcal/kg body weight is consumed per hour in healthy adults. Energy requirements of specific tissues differ dramatically (Table 6.2). The liver, intestine, brain, kidneys, and heart constitute roughly 10% of total body weight but account for about 75% of REE. In contrast, skeletal muscle at rest consumes some 20% of REE but represents approximately 40% of body weight. Adipose tissue consumes less than 5% of REE but usually accounts for greater than 20% of body weight.

An accurate assessment of REE is best obtained by indirect calorimetry, in which in vivo energy expenditure is estimated by measuring carbon dioxide production and oxygen consumption while the subject is at rest. Although indirect calorimetry is considered a gold standard for determining REE, obtaining such a measurement is not always practical and, in most instances, is unnecessary. Instead, one of several empiric equations can be used to estimate resting energy requirements (Table 6.3).[1–5] The Harris-Benedict and Mifflin equations are designed for use in adults, whereas the WHO formulas include equations for both children and adults. These equations are generally accurate in healthy subjects but are inaccurate, for example, in persons who are at extremes in weight because of anomalous body composition, which is in these settings where determination by indirect calorimetry is useful.[5] In the setting of acute illness, the predictive equations are usually adequate, although it is necessary to insert correction factors of one type or another since inflammation and metabolic stress greatly influence energy expenditure. Protein-energy malnutrition (PEM) and hypocaloric feeding without superimposed illness each decrease REE to values 10% −15% below those expected for actual body size, whereas acute illness or trauma predictably increases energy expenditure (see later).

Energy Expenditure of Physical Activity

The effect of physical activity on energy expenditure depends on the intensity and duration of daily activities. Highly trained athletes can increase their TEE 10- to 20-fold during athletic events. The activity factors shown in Table 6.4, each expressed as a multiple of REE, can be used to estimate TEE in active patients. The energy expended during a particular physical activity is equal to (REE per hour)×(activity factor)×(duration of activity in hours). TEE represents the summation of energy expended during all daily activities, including rest periods.

Thermic Effect of Feeding

Eating or infusing nutrients increases metabolic rate. Dietary protein causes the greatest stimulation of metabolic rate, followed

TABLE 6.1 Endogenous Fuel Stores in a 70-kg Man

		Mass	
Tissue	**Fuel Source**	**Grams**	**Kilocalories**
Adipose	Triglyceride	13,000	121,000
Liver	Protein	300	1200
	Glycogen	100	400
	Triglyceride	50	450
Muscle	Protein	6000	24,000
	Glycogen	400	1600
	Triglyceride	250	2250
Blood	Glucose	3	12
	Triglyceride	4	37
	Free fatty acids	0.5	5

TABLE 6.2 Resting Energy Requirements of Various Tissues in a 70-kg Man

	Tissue Mass		Energy Consumed		
Tissue	**Grams**	**Percentage Body Weight**	**Kcal/Day**	**Kcal/g Tissue/Day**	**Percentage REE**
Liver	1550	2.2	445	0.28	19
GI tract	2000	3.0	300	0.15	13
Brain	1400	2.0	420	0.30	18
Kidneys	300	0.4	360	1.27	15
Heart	300	0.4	235	0.80	10
Skeletal muscle	28,000	40.0	400	0.014	18
Adipose	15,000	21.0	80	0.005	4

REE, Resting energy expenditure.

TABLE 6.3 Commonly Used Formulas for Calculating Resting Energy Expenditure

Harris–Benedict Equation		
Men	$66 + (13.7 \times W) + (5 \times H) - (6.8 \times A)$	
Women	$665 + (9.6 \times W) + (1.8 \times H) - (4.7 \times A)$	
Mifflin Equation Men	$(10 \times W) + (6.25 \times H) - (5 \times A) + 5$	
Women	$(10 \times W) + (6.25 \times H) - (5 \times A) - 161$	
World Health Organization Formula		
Age (year)	**Male**	**Female**
0–3	$(60.9 \times W) - 54$	$(60.1 \times W) - 51$
3–10	$(22.7 \times W) - 495$	$(22.5 \times W) + 499$
10–18	$(17.5 \times W) + 651$	$(12.2 \times W) + 746$
18–30	$(15.3 \times W) + 679$	$(14.7 \times W) + 996$
30–60	$(11.2 \times W) + 879$	$(8.7 \times W) + 829$
>60	$(13.5 \times W) + 987$	$(10.5 \times W) + 596$

Calculated as kilocalories per day.
A, Age in years; *H*, height in centimeters; *W*, weight in kilograms.

TABLE 6.4 Relative Thermic Effect of Various Levels of Physical Activity

Activity Level	Examples	Activity Factor
Resting		1.0
Very light	Standing, driving, typing	1.1–2.0
Light	Walking 2–3 mi/h, shopping, light housekeeping	2.1–4.0
Moderate	Walking 3–4 mi/h, biking, gardening, scrubbing floors	4.1–6.0
Heavy	Running, swimming, climbing, basketball	6.1–10.0

Adapted from Alpers DA, Stenson WF, Bier DM. *Manual of Nutritional Therapeutics*. Boston: Little, Brown; 1995.

by carbohydrate and then fat. A meal containing all these nutrients usually increases metabolic rate by 5%–10% of ingested or infused calories.

Recommended Energy Intake in Hospitalized Patients

In arriving at a nutritional plan for hospitalized patients, it is usually not necessary to obtain actual measurements of energy expenditure with a bedside indirect calorimeter. A number of simple formulas can be used instead and make up in practical value what they lack in accuracy. A few examples follow.

Methods Incorporating Metabolic Stress Factors. Metabolic stress (i.e., any injury or illness that incites some degree of systemic inflammation) will increase the metabolic rate through a variety of mechanisms (see later). The increase in energy expenditure is roughly proportional to the magnitude of the stress.[6] Thus the total daily energy requirement of an acutely ill patient can be estimated by multiplying the predicted REE (as determined by the Harris-Benedict or WHO equations) by a stress factor:

$$\text{TEE} = \text{REE} \times \text{Stress factor}$$

Table 6.5 delineates metabolic stress factors that accompany some common conditions and clinical scenarios in inpatients. Because the Mifflin equation was not designed to be used to estimate TEE with stress factors, it is not recommended in this context. In acutely ill hospitalized patients, it is not usually necessary to include an activity factor.

An alternative and simple formula for adult inpatients, although accompanied by some further loss in accuracy, is

- 20–25 kcal/kg of actual body weight (ABW)/day for unstressed or mildly stressed patients
- 25–30 kcal/ABW/day for moderately stressed patients
- 30–35 kcal/ABW/day for severely stressed patients

In using this formula, adjustments are necessary when the ABW is a misleading reflection of lean body mass. An adjusted ideal body weight (IBW) should be substituted for ABW in obese individuals who are more than 30% heavier than their IBW (desirable body weights appear in Table 6.6). Using an adjusted IBW helps prevent an overestimation of energy requirements[6] and is calculated as follows:

$$\text{Adjusted IBW} = \text{IBW} + 0.5\ (\text{ABW} - \text{IBW})$$

In patients with large artifactual increases in weight due to extracellular fluid retention (e.g., ascites), the IBW should be used to estimate energy requirements rather than the ABW.

TABLE 6.5 Metabolic Stress Factors for Estimating Total Energy Expenditure in Hospitalized Patients

Injury or Illness	Relative Stress Factor[a]
Second- or third-degree burns, >40% BSA	1.6–2.0
Multiple trauma	1.5–1.7
Second- or third-degree burns, 20%–40% BSA	1.4–1.5
Severe infections	1.3–1.4
Acute pancreatitis	1.1–1.2
Second- or third-degree burns, 10%–20% BSA	1.2–1.4
Long bone fracture	1.2
Peritonitis	1.2
Uncomplicated postoperative state	1.1

[a]A stress factor of 1.0 is assumed for healthy controls.
BSA, Body surface area.
From Psota T, Chen KY. Measuring energy expenditure in clinical populations: rewards and challenges. *Eur J Clin Nutr*. 2013;67:436–442.

Method Without a Stress Factor. The most accurate and extensively validated equation for predicting daily energy expenditure in ill patients is one that does not incorporate a stress factor; it does, however, require knowledge of the minute ventilation, so its use is restricted to patients on mechanical ventilation.[4] This formula (often referred to as the "Penn State Equation") is

$$\text{TEE} = (\text{REE calculated by Mifflin equation} \times 0.96) + (T_{\max} \times 167) + (V_e \times 31) - 6212$$

$T_{\max}$ is the maximum temperature in Celsius over the past 24 hours; V_e is expired minute ventilation in liters.

Table 6.7 describes a simple alternative method for estimating total daily energy requirements in hospitalized patients; it is based on body mass index (BMI).[7] It lacks the extensive validation of the prior algorithm as well as some of its accuracy, but it does not require knowledge of minute ventilation, is straightforward and consequently has some genuine utilitarian value. Common sense has to be applied when using an inexact means such as this to estimate energy expenditure in hospitalized individuals, because illness commonly interjects artifacts into these calculations (e.g., ascites and anasarca).

Caloric Delivery and Avoidance of Hyperglycemia. Over the past two decades, the trend has generally been toward a more conservative approach to caloric delivery in acutely ill patients. One reason for this conservatism is that acute illness and its management often exacerbate preexisting diabetes or produce *de novo* glucose intolerance. As a result, hyperglycemia is a frequent consequence of enteral, and especially parenteral, nutrition. The issue seems to be particularly germane for ICU patients, in whom even modest hyperglycemia results in worse clinical outcomes, usually of an infectious nature. High-quality clinical trials in surgical ICU (SICU)[8] and medical ICU (MICU)[9] patients have found that morbidity is substantially and significantly reduced in those randomized to intensive insulin therapy who maintained serum glucose levels below 111 mg/dL, compared with those whose glucose values were maintained below 215 mg/dL. Mortality was also significantly lower among SICU patients randomized to receive tight glucose control, although in the MICU study, such reductions in mortality caused by tight glucose control were only realized in those who resided in the MICU greater than 3 days. Similarly, in a clinical trial of pediatric ICU patients, secondary infections, length of PICU stay, and mortality were all

TABLE 6.6 Desirable Weight in Relation to Height for Men and Women 25 Years or Older

Men, Medium Frame			Women, Medium Frame		
	Weight (lb)			Weight (lb)	
Height (ft/inches)	**Range**	**Midpoint**	**Height (ft/inches)**	**Range**	**Midpoint**
5′1″	113–124	118.5	4′8″	93–104	98.5
5′2″	116–128	122	4′9″	95–107	101
5′3″	119–131	125	4′10″	98–110	104
5′4″	122–134	128	4′11″	101–113	107
5′5″	125–138	131.5	5′0″	104–116	110
5′6″	129–142	135.5	5′1″	107–119	113
5′7″	133–147	140	5′2″	110–123	116.5
5′8″	137–151	144	5′3″	113–127	120
5′9″	141–155	148	5′4″	117–132	124.5
5′10″	145–160	153	5′5″	121–136	128.5
5′11″	149–165	157	5′6″	125–140	132.5
6′0″	153–170	161.5	5′7″	129–144	136.5
6′1″	157–175	166	5′8″	133–148	140.5
6′2″	162–180	171	5′9″	137–152	144.5
6′3″	167–185	176	5′10″	141–156	148.5

Corrected to nude weights and heights by assuming 1-inch heel for men, 2-inch heel for women, and indoor clothing weight of 5 and 3 lbs for men and women, respectively.

Data from Metropolitan Life Insurance Company. New height standards for men and women. *Stat Bull*. 1959;40:1–4.

TABLE 6.7 Estimated Energy Requirements for Hospitalized Patients Based on Body Mass Index

Body Mass Index (kg/m²)	Energy Requirements (kcal/kg/day)[a]
<15	35–40
15–19	30–35
20–29	20–25
≥30	15–20

[a]These values are recommended for critically ill patients and all obese patients; add 20% of the total calories when estimating energy requirements in noncritically ill patients.

The lower range within each body mass index (BMI) category should be considered in calculating energy requirements for insulin-resistant or critically ill patients to decrease the risk of hyperglycemia and infection associated with overfeeding.

reduced by intensive age-specific glucose control.[10] These observations are almost certainly the clinical expression of the numerous mechanistic impairments that acute hyperglycemia produces in the innate immune system.[11]

The clinical benefits of tight glucose control in the ICU, however, have not always been reproducible[12] and come at the cost of more frequent hypoglycemic episodes,[8–10,12] so the issue of *how tight* glucose control should be remains controversial. Extremely tight control, with a target range of 81–108 mg/dL, produced a 13-fold greater risk of hypoglycemia and a significantly greater mortality in a large multicenter trial of ICU patients[13] and is, therefore, excessive. An expert panel recommended instituting protocols to keep blood sugar levels at 150 mg/dL or lower in ICU patients, preferably by use of a continuous infusion of insulin, with monitoring every 1–2 hours so that appropriate adjustments can be made and blood sugar values less than 70 mg/dL are avoided.[14] The results of a meta-analysis of 29 trials in critically ill patients recapitulate the previously observed discrepancies between SICU and MICU patients.[15] Overall, the relative risk of septicemia was reduced approximately 25% in those randomized to tight glucose control, although this salutary effect was largely attributable to the SICU patients, in whom reduction in septicemia was almost 50%; no benefit was observed in MICU patients, nor were differences in overall mortality evident in any of the categories of critically ill patients.

The question of appropriate caloric delivery to critically ill overweight and obese patients, who nowadays account for a burgeoning proportion of patients cared for in ICUs, is a controversial issue. A popular nutritional approach to such patients is so-called hypocaloric feeding, in which only 60%–70% of the estimated energy requirement (or 11–14 kcal/kg of ABW) is delivered in conjunction with 2–2.5 g of protein/kg of IBW per day, the latter minimizing the risk of producing net protein catabolism and loss of lean body mass. The purported advantages of hypocaloric feeding include improved glycemic control and prevention of metabolic complications like hypercapnia and hypertriglyceridemia. Reduction in fat mass and weight is another consequence of hypocaloric feeding but should never be a primary objective in feeding obese ICU patients. Systematic reviews that have examined the use of hypocaloric feeding in obese ICU patients and which have examined important endpoints such as mortality, length of stay, duration of mechanical ventilation, and infectious complications have not yet been able to arrive at a consistent consensus either supporting net benefits or risks of hypocaloric, compared to normocaloric, nutrition support.[16] Thus the matter remains an unsettled one.

Proteins

Twenty different amino acids (AAs) are commonly found in human proteins. Some AAs (histidine, isoleucine, leucine, lysine, methionine, phenylalanine, threonine, tryptophan, valine, and possibly arginine) are considered essential (alternatively: "indispensable") because their carbon skeletons cannot be synthesized by the body. Other AAs (glycine, alanine, serine, cysteine, tyrosine, glutamine, glutamic acid, asparagine, and aspartic acid) are nonessential in most circumstances because they can be made from endogenous precursors or essential AAs. In disease states and in preterm infants, intracellular and/or plasma concentrations of certain nonessential AAs are often very low and thought of as "conditionally essential" AAs. For many years, supplemental glutamine was included in TPN to compensate for cellular depletion of this AA during critical illness. However, rigorously conducted clinical trials have shown no benefit associated with administration of supplemental IV glutamine.[17–19] In a randomized placebo-controlled multicenter, multinational trial of critically ill adults with multiorgan failure, glutamine supplementation was even associated with an increase in mortality.[18] Evidently, repletion of a conditionally essential AA during acute illness does not necessarily convey a benefit. However, there continues to be interest in defining clinical scenarios in critical illness (e.g., premature infants), in which supplementation with conditionally essential AAs might improve clinical outcomes.[20] Arginine, cysteine, glycine, glutamine, proline, and tyrosine are AAs that fall into this category.

The body of an average 75-kg man contains about 12 kg of protein. Unlike fat and carbohydrate, there is no storage depot for protein, so excess intake is catabolized, and the nitrogen component is excreted. Inadequate protein intake causes net nitrogen losses, and because no depot form of protein exists, there is an obligatory net loss of functioning protein. The US recommended daily allowance (RDA) of protein has been established at 0.8 g/kg/day, which reflects a mean calculated requirement of 0.6 g/kg/day plus an added factor to take into account the biological variance in requirement observed in a healthy population. Intravenously administered AAs are as effective in maintaining nitrogen balance as oral protein of the same AA composition.

An individual's protein requirement is affected by several factors, such as the amount of nonprotein calories provided, overall energy requirements, protein quality, and the patient's nutritional status (Table 6.8). Protein requirements increase when calorie intake does not meet energy needs. The magnitude of this increase is directly proportional to the deficit in energy supply. Therefore nitrogen balance reflects both protein intake and energy balance. Correcting a negative nitrogen balance can sometimes be achieved merely by increasing caloric delivery if the total amount of calories has been inadequate.

As metabolic stress (and with it, metabolic rate) increases, nitrogen excretion increases proportionately; quantitatively, the relationship is approximately 2 mg nitrogen (N)/kcal of REE. In part, this increase is explained by the fact that in metabolic stress, a larger proportion of the total substrate oxidized for energy is from protein. This has two important implications for managing the nutritional needs of ill patients. The first is that illness, by increasing catabolism and metabolic rate, increases the absolute requirement for protein (see Table 6.8) and does so in a manner that is roughly proportional to the degree of stress. Second, because a greater proportion of energy substrate in acute illness comes from protein, nitrogen balance is more readily achieved if a larger proportion of the total calories is from protein. In healthy adults, as little as 10% of total calories has to come from protein to maintain health, whereas in the ill patient, nitrogen balance is achieved more easily if 15%–25% of total calories are delivered as protein.

Protein requirements are also determined by the adequacy of essential AAs in the protein source. Inadequate amounts of an essential AA result in inefficient uptake, so proteins of low biologic quality increase the protein requirement. In normal adults, approximately 15%–20% of total protein requirements should be in the form of essential AAs.

Additional protein delivery is needed to compensate for excess loss in specific patient populations (e.g., patients with burn injuries, open wounds, protein-losing enteropathy, and nephrotic syndrome). Delivering less protein than is needed is often a necessary compromise in patients with acute kidney failure who are not adequately dialyzed; in this situation, the rise in azotemia is directly proportional to protein delivery. Once adequate dialysis is available, protein delivery should be increased to the actual projected need, including additional protein to compensate for losses resulting from dialysis (see Table 6.8). Most patients with hepatic encephalopathy respond to simple pharmacologic measures and, therefore, do not require protein restriction; those who do not respond may benefit from a modest protein restriction ($\approx$0.6 g/kg/day).

TABLE 6.8 Recommended Daily Protein Intake

Clinical Condition	Daily Protein Requirement (g/kg IBW)
Normal	0.80
Metabolic stress	1.0–1.6
Hemodialysis	1.2–1.4
Peritoneal dialysis	1.3–1.5

Additional protein requirements are needed to compensate for excess protein loss in specific patient populations (e.g., patients with burn injuries, open wounds, protein-losing enteropathy, or nephropathy). Lower protein intake may be necessary for patients with renal insufficiency not treated by dialysis and certain patients with liver disease and hepatic encephalopathy.

IBW, Ideal body weight.

Nitrogen Balance

Nitrogen (N) balance is commonly used as a proxy measure of protein balance (i.e., whether the quantity of protein [or AAs] taken in is sufficient to prevent any net loss of protein). N balance is calculated as the difference between N intake and N losses in urine, stool, skin, and body fluids. In the clinical setting, it can be conveniently calculated as follows for adults:

$$\text{N balance} = (\text{Grams of N administered as nutrition}) - (\text{Urinary urea N}[g] + 4)$$

Every 6.25 g of administered protein (or AAs) contains approximately 1 g of N. The additional 4 g of N loss incorporated into the equation accounts for the insensible losses from the other abovementioned sources, and because urinary urea N only accounts for approximately 80% of total urinary nitrogen. N balance is a suitable surrogate for protein balance, because ~98% of total body N is in protein, regardless of one's health.

A positive N balance (i.e., intake > loss) represents anabolism and a net increase in total body protein, whereas a negative N balance represents net protein catabolism. For example, a negative N balance of 1 g/day represents a 6.25 g/day loss of body protein, equivalent to a 30 g/day loss of hydrated lean tissue. In practice, N balance studies tend to be artificially positive because of overestimation of dietary N intake and underestimation of losses due to incomplete urine collections and unmeasured outputs. It is best to wait at least 4 days after a substantial change in protein delivery before N balance is determined, because a labile N pool exists, and this tends to dampen and retard changes that otherwise would be observed as a result of altered protein intake.

Carbohydrates

Complete digestion of the principal dietary digestible carbohydrates—starch, sucrose, and lactose—generates monosaccharides (glucose, fructose, and galactose). In addition, 5–20 g of indigestible carbohydrates (soluble and insoluble fibers) are typically consumed daily. All cells can generate energy (adenosine triphosphate) by metabolizing glucose to three-carbon compounds via glycolysis or to carbon dioxide and water via glycolysis and the tricarboxylic acid (TCA) cycle.

There is no absolute dietary requirement for carbohydrate; glucose can be synthesized endogenously from either AAs or glycerol. Regardless, carbohydrate is an important fuel because of the interactions between carbohydrate and protein metabolism. Carbohydrate intake stimulates insulin secretion, which inhibits muscle protein breakdown, stimulates muscle protein synthesis, and decreases endogenous glucose production from AAs. In addition, glucose is the required or preferred fuel for red and white blood cells, the renal medulla, eye tissues, peripheral nerves, and the brain. However, once glucose requirements for these tissues are met (≈150 g/day), the protein-sparing effects of carbohydrate and fat are similar.[21]

Lipids

Lipids consist of TGs, sterols, and phospholipids. These compounds serve as sources of energy; precursors for steroid hormone, prostaglandin, thromboxane, and leukotriene synthesis; structural components of cell membranes; and carriers of essential nutrients. Dietary lipids are composed mainly of TGs, which contain saturated and unsaturated long-chain fatty acids (FAs) of 16–18 carbons. Use of fat as a fuel requires hydrolysis of endogenous or exogenous TGs and cellular uptake of released FAs (see Chapter 104). Long-chain FAs are delivered across the outer and inner mitochondrial membranes by a carnitine-dependent transport system. Once inside the mitochondria, FAs are degraded by beta oxidation to acetyl coenzyme A, which then enters the TCA cycle. Therefore the ability to use fat as a fuel depends on normally functioning mitochondria. A decrease in the abundance or function of mitochondria associated with aging[22] or deconditioning favors the use of carbohydrate as fuel.[23]

Essential Fatty Acids

Humans lack the desaturase enzyme needed to produce the *n*-3 (double bond between carbons 3 and 4) and *n*-6 (double bond between carbons 6 and 7) FA series. Therefore linoleic acid (C18:2, *n*-6) and linolenic acid (C18:3, *n*-3) are essential FAs and should constitute at least 2% and 0.5%, respectively, of the daily caloric intake to prevent a deficiency state. Before the advent of parenteral nutrition, essential FA deficiency (EFAD) was only recognized in infants and manifested as a scaly rash with a specific alteration in the plasma FA profile (see later). Adults were thought not to be susceptible to EFAD because of sufficient essential FA stores in adipose tissue. However, an abnormal FA profile in conjunction with a clinical syndrome of EFAD is now known to sometimes occur in adults with severe short bowel syndrome who are on long-term TPN that lacks parenteral lipids.[24] Adults who have moderate-to-severe fat malabsorption (fractional fat excretion >20%) from other causes and who are not TPN-dependent also frequently display a biochemical profile of EFAD,[25] although whether such a biochemical state carries adverse clinical consequences is unclear. Moreover, TPN lacking any source of fat may lead to EFAD in adults if no exogenous source of EFAs is available. The plasma pattern of EFAD may be observed as early as 10 days after glucose-based TPN is started and before the onset of any clinical features. In this situation, EFAD is probably due to the increase in plasma insulin concentrations caused by TPN, because insulin inhibits lipolysis and, therefore, the release of endogenous essential FAs. The biochemical diagnosis of EFAD is defined as an absolute and relative deficiency in the two EFAs in the plasma FA profile. The full clinical EFAD syndrome includes alopecia, scaly dermatitis, capillary fragility, poor wound healing, increased susceptibility to infection, fatty liver, and growth retardation in infants and children.

Major Minerals

Major minerals are inorganic nutrients that are required in large (>100 mg/day) quantities and are important for ionic equilibrium, water balance, and normal cell function. Malnutrition and nutritional repletion can have dramatic effects on major mineral balance. Evaluation of macromineral deficiency and the RDA of minerals for healthy adults are shown in Table 6.9.

MICRONUTRIENTS

Micronutrients (vitamins and trace minerals) are a diverse array of dietary components necessary to sustain health. The physiologic roles of micronutrients are as varied as their composition. Some are used in enzymes as coenzymes or prosthetic groups, others as biochemical substrates or hormones; in some cases, their functions are not well defined. The average daily dietary intake for each micronutrient required to sustain normal physiologic operations is measured in milligrams or smaller quantities. In this way, micronutrients are distinguished from macronutrients (carbohydrates, fats, and proteins) and macrominerals (calcium, magnesium, and phosphorus).

TABLE 6.9 Major Mineral Requirements and Assessment of Deficiency

				Laboratory Evaluation	
Mineral	**Enteral**	**Parenteral (mmol)**	**Symptoms or Signs of Deficiency**	**Test**	**Comment**
Calcium	1000–1200 mg	5–15	Metabolic bone disease, tetany, arrhythmias	24-h urinary calcium Dual-energy radiation absorptiometry	Reflects recent intake Reflects bone calcium content
Magnesium	300–400 mg	5–15	Weakness, twitching, tetany, arrhythmias, hypocalcemia	Serum magnesium Urinary magnesium	May not reflect body stores May not reflect body stores
Phosphorus	800–1200 mg	20–60	Weakness, fatigue, leukocyte and platelet dysfunction, hemolytic anemia, cardiac failure, decreased oxygenation	Plasma phosphorus	May not reflect body stores
Potassium	2–5 g	60–100	Weakness, paresthesias, arrhythmias	Serum potassium	May not reflect body stores
Sodium	0.5–5 g	60–150	Hypovolemia, weakness	Urinary sodium	May not reflect body stores; clinical evaluation is best

An individual's dietary requirement for any given micronutrient is determined by many factors, including its bioavailability, the amount needed to sustain its normal physiologic functions, a person's sex and age, any diseases or drugs that affect the nutrient's metabolism, and certain lifestyle habits like smoking and alcohol use. The US National Academy of Sciences Food and Nutrition Board regularly updates dietary guidelines that define the quantity of each micronutrient that is "adequate to meet the known nutrient needs of practically all healthy persons." These RDAs underwent revision between 1998 and 2001, and the values for adults appear in Tables 6.10 and 6.11. An RDA takes into account the biologic variability in the population, so RDAs are set two standard deviations (SDs) above the mean requirement; this allows the requirements of 97.5% of the population to be met. Thus ingestion of quantities that are somewhat less than the RDA is often sufficient to meet the needs of a particular individual. A "tolerable upper limit," which is "the maximal daily level of oral intake that is likely to pose no adverse health risks," has been established for most micronutrients (see Tables 6.10 and 6.11). Present recommendations for how much of each micronutrient is needed in individuals on TPN are based on far less data than were available for development of the RDAs. Nevertheless, it is important to have guidelines, and Table 6.12 provides such recommendations.

TABLE 6.10 Salient Features of Vitamins

Vitamin	Deficiency (RDA)[a]	Toxicity (TUL)[b]	Assessment of Status
A	Follicular hyperkeratosis and night blindness are early indicators. Conjunctival xerosis, degeneration of the cornea (keratomalacia), and dedifferentiation of rapidly proliferating epithelia are later indications of deficiency. Bitot spots (focal areas of the conjunctiva or cornea with foamy appearance) are an indication of xerosis. Blindness caused by corneal destruction and retinal dysfunction may ensue. Increased susceptibility to infection is also a consequence (1 µg of retinol is equivalent to 3.33 IU of vitamin A; F, 700 µg; M, 900 µg).	In adults, >150,000 µg may cause acute toxicity: fatal intracranial hypertension, skin exfoliation, and hepatocellular injury. Chronic toxicity may occur with habitual daily intake of >10,000 µg: alopecia, ataxia, bone and muscle pain, dermatitis, cheilitis, conjunctivitis, pseudotumor cerebri, hepatic fibrosis, hyperlipidemia, and hyperostosis are common. Single large doses of vitamin A (30,000 µg) or habitual intake of >4500 µg/day during early pregnancy can be teratogenic. Excessive intake of carotenoids causes a benign condition characterized by yellowish discoloration of the skin (3000 µg).	Retinol concentration in the plasma, as well as vitamin A concentrations in milk and tears, are reasonably accurate measures of status. Toxicity is best assessed by elevated levels of retinyl esters in plasma. A quantitative measure of dark adaptation for night vision and electroretinography are useful functional tests.
D	Deficiency results in decreased mineralization of newly formed bone, a condition called *rickets* in childhood and *osteomalacia* in adults. Deficiency also contributes to osteoporosis in later life and is common following gastric bypass procedures. Expansion of epiphyseal growth plates and replacement of normal bone with unmineralized bone matrix are the cardinal features of rickets; the latter feature also characterizes osteomalacia. Deformity of bone and pathologic fractures result. Decreased serum concentrations of calcium and phosphate may occur (1 µg is equivalent to 40 IU; 15 µg, ages 19–70; 20 µg, ages >70).	Excess amounts result in abnormally high concentrations of calcium and phosphate in the serum; metastatic calcifications, renal damage, and altered mentation may occur (100 µg for ages >9).	Serum concentration of the major circulating metabolite, 25-hydroxyvitamin D, is an excellent indicator of systemic status except in advanced kidney disease (stages 4–5), in which impairment of renal 1-hydroxylation results in dissociation of the mono- and dihydroxy vitamin concentrations; measuring the serum concentration of 1,25-dihydroxyvitamin D is then necessary.
E	Deficiency caused by dietary inadequacy is rare in developed countries. Usually seen in premature infants, individuals with fat malabsorption, and individuals with abetalipoproteinemia. RBC fragility occurs and can produce hemolytic anemia. Neuronal degeneration produces peripheral neuropathies, ophthalmoplegia, and destruction of the posterior columns of the spinal cord. Neurologic disease is frequently irreversible if deficiency is not corrected early enough. May contribute to hemolytic anemia and retrolental fibroplasia in premature infants. Has been reported to suppress cell-mediated immunity (15 mg).	Depressed levels of vitamin K-dependent procoagulants, potentiation of oral anticoagulants, and impaired leukocyte function have been reported. Doses of 800 mg/day have been reported to increase slightly the incidence of hemorrhagic stroke (1000 mg).	Plasma or serum concentration of alpha-tocopherol is used most commonly. Additional accuracy is obtained by expressing this value per mg of total plasma lipid. The RBC peroxide hemolysis test is not entirely specific but is a useful measure of the susceptibility of cell membranes to oxidation.

Continued

TABLE 6.10 Salient Features of Vitamins—cont'd

Vitamin	Deficiency (RDA)[a]	Toxicity (TUL)[b]	Assessment of Status
K	Deficiency syndrome is uncommon except in breast-fed newborns (in whom it may cause "hemorrhagic disease of the newborn"), adults who have fat malabsorption or are taking drugs that interfere with vitamin K metabolism (e.g., warfarin, phenytoin, broad-spectrum antibiotics), and individuals taking large doses of vitamin E and anticoagulant drugs. Excessive hemorrhage is the usual manifestation (F, 90 μg; M, 120 μg).	Rapid IV infusion of vitamin K_1 has been associated with dyspnea, flushing, and cardiovascular collapse; this is likely related to the dispersing agents in the dissolution solvent. Supplementation may interfere with warfarin-based anticoagulation. Pregnant women taking large amounts of the provitamin menadione may deliver infants with hemolytic anemia, hyperbilirubinemia, and kernicterus (TUL not established).	Prothrombin time is typically used as a measure of functional vitamin K status; it is neither sensitive nor specific for vitamin K deficiency. Determination of fasting plasma vitamin K is an accurate indicator. Undercarboxylated plasma prothrombin is also an accurate metric, but only for detecting the deficient state, and is less widely available.
Thiamine (vitamin B_1)	Classic deficiency syndrome (beriberi) remains endemic in Asian populations consuming polished rice diet. Globally, alcoholism, chronic renal dialysis, and persistent nausea and vomiting after bariatric surgery are common precipitants. High carbohydrate intake increases the need for B_1. Mild deficiency commonly produces irritability, fatigue, and headaches. More pronounced deficiency can produce peripheral neuropathy, cardiovascular and cerebral dysfunction. Cardiovascular involvement (wet beriberi) includes heart failure and low peripheral vascular resistance. Cerebral disease includes nystagmus, ophthalmoplegia, and ataxia (Wernicke encephalopathy), as well as hallucinations, impaired short-term memory, and confabulation (Korsakoff psychosis). Deficiency syndrome responds within 24 h to parenteral thiamine but is partially or wholly irreversible after a certain stage (F, 1.1 mg; M, 1.2 mg).	Excess intake is largely excreted in the urine, although parenteral doses of >400 mg/day are reported to cause lethargy, ataxia, and reduced tone of the GI tract (TUL not established).	The most effective measure of vitamin B_1 status is the RBC transketolase activity coefficient, which measures enzyme activity before and after addition of exogenous TPP; RBCs from a deficient individual express a substantial increase in enzyme activity with addition of TPP. Thiamine concentrations in the blood or urine are also measured.
Riboflavin (vitamin B_2)	Deficiency is usually seen in conjunction with deficiencies of other B vitamins. Isolated deficiency of riboflavin produces hyperemia and edema of nasopharyngeal mucosa, cheilosis, angular stomatitis, glossitis, seborrheic dermatitis, and normochromic, normocytic anemia (F, 1.1 mg; M, 1.3 mg).	Toxicity has not been reported in humans (TUL not established).	Most common method of assessment is determining the activity coefficient of glutathione reductase in RBCs (the test is invalid for individuals with glucose-6-phosphate dehydrogenase deficiency). Measurements of blood and urine concentrations are less desirable methods.
Niacin (vitamin B_3)	Pellagra is the classic deficiency syndrome and is often seen in populations in which corn is the major source of energy. Still endemic in parts of China, Africa, and India. Diarrhea, dementia (or associated symptoms of anxiety or insomnia), and a pigmented dermatitis that develops in sun-exposed areas are typical features. Glossitis, stomatitis, vaginitis, vertigo, and burning dysesthesias are early signs. Occasionally occurs in carcinoid syndrome, because tryptophan is diverted to other synthetic pathways (F, 14 mg; M, 16 mg).	Human toxicity is known largely through studies examining hypolipidemic effects; includes flushing, hyperglycemia, hepatocellular injury, and hyperuricemia (35 mg).	Assessment of status is problematic; blood levels of the vitamin are not reliable. Measurement of urinary excretion of the niacin metabolites *N*-methylnicotinamide and 2-pyridone are thought to be the most effective means of assessment.

6

TABLE 6.10 Salient Features of Vitamins—cont'd

Vitamin	Deficiency (RDA)[a]	Toxicity (TUL)[b]	Assessment of Status
Pantothenic acid (vitamin B_5)	Deficiency is rare; reported only as a result of feeding semisynthetic diets or consumption of an antagonist such as calcium homopantothenate, which has been used to treat Alzheimer disease. Experimental isolated deficiency in humans produces fatigue, abdominal pain and vomiting, insomnia, and paresthesias of the extremities (5 mg).	Diarrhea is reported to occur with doses exceeding 10 g/day (TUL not established).	Whole blood and urine concentrations of pantothenic acid are indicators of status; serum levels are not thought to be accurate.
Pyridoxine (vitamin B_6)	Deficiency is usually seen in conjunction with other water-soluble vitamin deficiencies. Stomatitis, angular cheilosis, glossitis, irritability, depression, and confusion occur in moderate to severe depletion; normochromic, normocytic anemia has been reported in severe deficiency. Abnormal EEGs and, in infants, convulsions also have been reported. Isoniazid, cycloserine, penicillamine, ethanol, and theophylline are drugs that can inhibit B_6 metabolism (ages 19–50, 1.3 mg; >50 year, 1.5 mg for women, 1.7 mg for men).	Chronic use with doses exceeding 200 mg/day (in adults) may cause peripheral neuropathies and photosensitivity (100 mg).	Many useful laboratory methods of assessment exist. Plasma or erythrocyte PLP levels are most common. Urinary excretion of xanthurenic acid after an oral tryptophan load or activity indices of RBC aminotransferases (ALT and AST) all are functional measures of B_6-dependent enzyme activity.
Biotin (vitamin B_7)	Isolated deficiency is rare. Deficiency in humans has been produced experimentally by dietary inadequacy, prolonged administration of TPN that lacks the vitamin, and ingestion of large quantities of raw egg white, which contains avidin, a protein that binds biotin with such high affinity that it renders it bio-unavailable. Alterations in mental status, myalgias, hyperesthesias, and anorexia occur. Later, seborrheic dermatitis and alopecia develop. Biotin deficiency is usually accompanied by lactic acidosis and organic aciduria (30 μg).	Toxicity has not been reported in humans, with doses as high as 60 mg/day in children (TUL not established).	Plasma and urine concentrations of biotin are diminished in the deficient state. Elevated urine concentrations of methyl citrate, 3-methylcrotonylglycine, and 3-hydroxyisovalerate are also observed in deficiency.
Folate (vitamin B_9)	Women of childbearing age are the most likely to develop deficiency. The classic deficiency syndrome is a megaloblastic anemia. Hematopoietic cells in the bone marrow become enlarged and have immature nuclei, reflecting ineffective DNA synthesis. The peripheral blood smear demonstrates macro-ovalocytes and polymorphonuclear leukocytes with an average of more than 3.5 nuclear lobes. Megaloblastic changes in other rapidly proliferating epithelia (e.g., oral mucosa, GI tract) produce glossitis and diarrhea, respectively. Sulfasalazine and diphenytoin inhibit absorption, predisposing to deficiency. Habitually low intake may increase the risk of colorectal cancer. (400 μg of dietary folate equivalent [DFE]; 1 μg folic acid = 1 μg DFE; 1 μg food folate = 0.6 μg DFE).	Daily dosage >1000 μg may partially correct the anemia of B_{12} deficiency and therefore mask (and perhaps exacerbate) the associated neuropathy. Large doses are reported to lower seizure threshold in individuals prone to seizures. Parenteral administration is rarely reported to cause allergic phenomena from dispersion agents (1000 μg).	Serum folate levels reflect short-term folate balance, whereas RBC folate is a better reflection of tissue status. Serum homocysteine levels rise early in deficiency but are nonspecific because B_{12} or B_6 deficiency, renal insufficiency, and older age may also cause elevations.

Continued

TABLE 6.10 Salient Features of Vitamins—cont'd

Vitamin	Deficiency (RDA)[a]	Toxicity (TUL)[b]	Assessment of Status
Cobalamin (vitamin B_{12})	Dietary inadequacy is a rare cause of deficiency, except in strict vegetarians. The vast majority of cases of deficiency arise from loss of intestinal absorption—a result of pernicious anemia, pancreatic insufficiency, atrophic gastritis, SIBO, or ileal disease. Megaloblastic anemia and megaloblastic changes in other epithelia (see "Folate") are the result of sustained depletion. Demyelination of peripheral nerves, the posterior and lateral columns of the spinal cord, and nerves within the brain may occur. Altered mentation, depression, and psychoses occur. Hematologic and neurologic complications may occur independently. Folate supplementation in doses exceeding 1000 μg/day may partly correct the anemia, thereby masking (or perhaps exacerbating) the neuropathic complications (2.4 μg).	A few allergic reactions have been reported from crystalline B_{12} preparations and are probably due to impurities, not the vitamin (TUL not established).	Serum or plasma concentrations are generally accurate. Subtle deficiency with neurologic complications is increasingly recognized among those ≥60 year of age, and can best be established by concurrently measuring the concentration of plasma B_{12} and (1) serum methylmalonic acid (MMA) or (2) holotranscobalamin II (holoTCII) because the latter are sensitive indicators of cellular deficiency. A low-normal plasma B_{12} of 200–350 pg/mL (=148–258 pmol/L) with an elevated MMA or decreased holoTCII should be considered a state of deficiency.
Ascorbic and dehydroascorbic acid (vitamin C)	Overt deficiency is uncommonly observed in developed countries. The classic deficiency syndrome is scurvy, characterized by fatigue, depression, and widespread abnormalities in connective tissues (e.g., inflamed gingivae, petechiae, perifollicular hemorrhages, impaired wound healing, coiled hairs, hyperkeratosis, and bleeding into body cavities). In infants, defects in ossification and bone growth may occur. Tobacco smoking lowers plasma and leukocyte vitamin C levels (F, 75 mg; M, 90 mg; the requirement for cigarette smokers is increased by 35 mg/day).	Quantities exceeding 500 mg/day (in adults) sometimes cause nausea and diarrhea. Acidification of the urine with vitamin C supplementation, and the potential for enhanced oxalate synthesis, have raised concerns regarding nephrolithiasis, but this has yet to be demonstrated. Supplementation with vitamin C may interfere with laboratory tests based on redox potential (e.g., fecal occult blood testing, serum cholesterol, serum glucose). Withdrawal from chronic ingestion of high doses of vitamin C supplements should occur gradually over 1 month because accommodation does seem to occur, raising a concern for rebound scurvy (2000 mg).	Plasma ascorbic acid concentration reflects recent dietary intake, whereas leukocyte levels more closely reflect tissue stores. Plasma levels in women are ≈20% higher than in men for any given dietary intake.

[a]*RDA*, Recommended daily allowance; established for female (F) and male (M) adults by the U.S. Food and Nutrition Board, 1999–2001 (updated in 2010 for vitamin D and calcium). In some cases, data are insufficient to establish an RDA, in which case the adequate intake (AI) established by the board is listed.
[b]*TUL*, Tolerable upper level; established for adults by the US Food and Nutrition Board, 1999–2001.
EEG, Electroencephalogram; *PLP*, pyridoxyl 5-phosphate; *RBC*, red blood cell; *TPP*, thiamine pyrophosphate.
Adapted from Goldman L, Ausiello D, Arend W, et al, eds. *Cecil Textbook of Medicine*. 23rd ed. Philadelphia: WB Saunders; 2014.

TABLE 6.11 Salient Features of Trace Minerals

Mineral	Deficiency (RDA)[a]	Toxicity (TUL)[b]	Assessment of Status
Chromium	Deficiency in humans is only described for patients on long-term TPN containing inadequate chromium. Hyperglycemia or impaired glucose tolerance is uniformly observed. Elevated plasma free fatty acid concentrations, neuropathy, encephalopathy, and abnormalities in nitrogen metabolism are also reported. Whether supplemental chromium may improve glucose tolerance in mildly glucose intolerant but otherwise healthy individuals remains controversial (F, 25 μg; M, 35 μg).	Toxicity after oral ingestion is uncommon and seems confined to gastric irritation. Airborne exposure may cause contact dermatitis, eczema, skin ulcers, and bronchogenic carcinoma (No TUL established).	Plasma or serum concentration of chromium is a crude indicator of chromium status; it appears to be meaningful when the value is markedly above or below the normal range.

TABLE 6.11 Salient Features of Trace Minerals—cont'd

Mineral	Deficiency (RDA)[a]	Toxicity (TUL)[b]	Assessment of Status
Copper	Dietary deficiency is rare; it has been observed in premature and low-birth-weight infants exclusively fed a cow's milk diet and in individuals on long-term TPN without copper. Clinical manifestations include depigmentation of skin and hair, neurologic disturbances, leukopenia and hypochromic, microcytic anemia, skeletal abnormalities, and poor wound healing. The anemia arises from impaired uptake of iron and is, therefore, a secondary form of iron deficiency anemia. The deficiency syndrome, except the anemia and leukopenia, is also observed in Menkes disease, a rare inherited condition associated with impaired copper uptake (900 μg).	Acute copper toxicity has been described after excessive oral intake and with absorption of copper salts applied to burned skin. Milder manifestations include nausea, vomiting, epigastric pain, and diarrhea; coma and hepatocellular injury may ensue in severe cases. Toxicity may be seen with doses as low as 70 μg/kg/day. Chronic toxicity is also described. Wilson disease is a rare inherited disease associated with abnormally low ceruloplasmin levels and accumulation of copper particularly in the liver and brain, eventually leading to damage of these two organs (10 mg).	Practical methods for detecting marginal deficiency are not available. Marked deficiency is reliably detected by diminished serum copper and ceruloplasmin concentrations, as well as low erythrocyte superoxide dismutase activity.
Fluoride	Intake of <0.1 mg/day in infants and 0.5 mg/day in children is associated with an increased incidence of dental caries. Optimal intake in adults is between 1.5 and 4.0 mg/day (F, 3 mg; M, 4.0 mg).	Acute ingestion of >30 mg/kg body weight of fluoride is likely to cause death. Excessive chronic intake (0.1 mg/kg/day) leads to mottling of the teeth (dental fluorosis), calcification of tendons and ligaments, and exostoses, and may increase brittleness of bones (10 mg).	Estimates of intake or clinical assessment are used because no reliable laboratory test exists.
Iodine	In the absence of supplementation, populations relying primarily on food from soils with low iodine content have endemic iodine deficiency. Maternal iodine deficiency leads to fetal deficiency, which produces spontaneous abortions, stillbirths, hypothyroidism, cretinism, and dwarfism. Rapid brain development continues through the second year, and permanent cognitive deficits may be induced by iodine deficiency during that period. In adults, compensatory hypertrophy of the thyroid (goiter) occurs, along with varying degrees of hypothyroidism (150 μg).	Large doses (>2 mg/day in adults) may induce hypothyroidism by blocking thyroid hormone synthesis. Supplementation with >100 μg/day to an individual who was formerly deficient occasionally induces hyperthyroidism (1.1 mg).	Urinary excretion of iodine is an effective laboratory means of assessment. The thyroid-stimulating hormone (TSH) level in the blood is an indirect, not entirely specific means of assessment. Iodine status of a population can be estimated by the prevalence of goiter.
Iron	Most common micronutrient deficiency in the world. Women of childbearing age constitute the highest risk group because of menstrual blood losses, pregnancy, and lactation. Hookworm infection is the most common cause worldwide. The classic deficiency syndrome is hypochromic microcytic anemia. Glossitis and koilonychia (spoon nails) are also observed. Easy fatigability often develops as an early symptom before appearance of anemia. In children, mild deficiency of insufficient severity to cause anemia is associated with behavioral disturbances and poor school performance (postmenopausal F, 8 mg; M, 8 mg; premenopausal F, 18 mg).	Iron overload typically occurs when habitual dietary intake is extremely high, intestinal absorption is excessive, repeated parenteral administration of iron occurs, or a combination of these factors exists. Excessive iron stores usually accumulate in reticuloendothelial tissues and cause little damage (hemosiderosis). If overload continues, iron will eventually begin to accumulate in tissues such as hepatic parenchyma, pancreas, heart, and synovium, damaging these tissues (hemochromatosis). Hereditary hemochromatosis arises as a result of homozygosity of a common recessive trait. Excessive intestinal absorption of iron is observed in homozygotes (45 mg).	Negative iron balance initially leads to depletion of iron stores in the bone marrow; bone marrow biopsy and the concentration of serum ferritin are accurate and early indicators of such depletion. As deficiency becomes more severe, serum iron (SI) decreases and total iron binding capacity (TIBC) increases; an iron saturation (= SI/TIBC) of <16% suggests iron deficiency. Microcytosis, hypochromia, and anemia ensue in latter stages of the deficient state. Elevated levels of serum ferritin or an iron saturation >60% raises suspicion of iron overload, although systemic inflammation elevates serum ferritin level regardless of iron status.

Continued

TABLE 6.11 Salient Features of Trace Minerals—cont'd

Mineral	Deficiency (RDA)[a]	Toxicity (TUL)[b]	Assessment of Status
Manganese	Manganese deficiency has not been conclusively demonstrated in humans. It is said to cause hypocholesterolemia, weight loss, hair and nail changes, dermatitis, and impaired synthesis of vitamin K–dependent proteins (F, 1.8 mg; M, 2.3 mg).	Toxicity by oral ingestion is unknown in humans. Toxic inhalation causes hallucinations, other alterations in mentation, and extrapyramidal movement disorders (11 mg).	Until the deficiency syndrome is better defined, an appropriate measure of status will be difficult to develop.
Molybdenum	Cases of human deficiency are extremely rare; caused by TPN lacking the element or by parenteral administration of sulfite. Reported to result in hyperoxypurinemia, hypouricemia, low urinary sulfate excretion, and CNS disturbances (45 μg).	Molybdenum has low toxicity; occupational exposures and high dietary intake are linked to hyperuricemia and gout in epidemiologic studies (2 mg).	No effective clinically available assessment exists. Rare cases of deficiency are associated with hypouricemia, hypermethionemia, and low levels of urinary sulfate with elevated excretion of sulfite, xanthine, and hypoxanthine.
Selenium	Deficiency is rare in North America but has been observed in individuals on long-term TPN lacking selenium. Such individuals have myalgias and/or cardiomyopathy. Populations in some regions of the world, most notably some parts of China, have marginal intake of selenium. It is in these regions of China that Keshan disease is endemic, a condition characterized by cardiomyopathy. Keshan disease can be prevented (but not treated) by selenium supplementation (55 μg).	Toxicity is associated with nausea, diarrhea, alterations in mental status, peripheral neuropathy, and loss of hair and nails; such symptoms were observed in adults who inadvertently consumed between 27 and 2400 mg (400 μg).	Erythrocyte glutathione peroxidase activity and plasma, or whole blood, selenium concentrations are the most commonly used methods of assessment. They are moderately accurate indicators of status.
Zinc	Deficiency of zinc has its most profound effect on rapidly proliferating tissues. Mild deficiency causes growth retardation in children. More severe deficiency is associated with growth arrest, teratogenicity, hypogonadism, and infertility, dysgeusia, poor wound healing, diarrhea, dermatitis on the extremities and around orifices, glossitis, alopecia, corneal clouding, loss of dark adaptation, and behavioral changes. Impaired cellular immunity also is observed. Excessive loss of GI secretions (e.g., through chronic diarrhea or fistulas) may precipitate deficiency. Acrodermatitis enteropathica is a rare recessively inherited disease in which intestinal absorption of zinc is impaired (F, 8 mg; M, 11 mg).	Acute zinc toxicity can usually be induced by ingestion of >200 mg of zinc in a single day (in adults). It is manifested by epigastric pain, nausea, vomiting, and diarrhea. Hyperpnea, diaphoresis, and weakness may follow inhalation of zinc fumes. Copper and zinc compete for intestinal absorption: chronic ingestion of >25 mg zinc/day may lead to copper deficiency. Chronic ingestion of >150 mg/day has been reported to cause gastric erosions, low high-density lipoprotein cholesterol levels, and impaired cellular immunity (40 mg).	There are no accurate indicators of zinc status available for routine clinical use. Plasma, erythrocyte, and hair zinc concentrations are frequently misleading. Acute illness, in particular, is known to diminish plasma zinc levels, in part by inducing a shift of zinc out of the plasma compartment and into the liver. Functional tests that determine dark adaptation, taste acuity, and rate of wound healing lack specificity.

[a]Recommended daily allowance (RDA) established for female (F) and male (M) adults by the US Food and Nutrition Board, 1999–2001. In some cases, insufficient data exist to establish an RDA, in which case the adequate intake (AI) established by the Board is listed.
[b]Tolerable upper level (TUL) established for adults by the US Food and Nutrition Board, 1999–2001.
Adapted from Goldman L, Ausiello D, Arend W, et al, eds. *Cecil Textbook of Medicine*. 22nd ed. Philadelphia: WB Saunders; 2004.

Vitamins

Vitamins are categorized as fat soluble (A, D, E, K) or water soluble (all others) (see Table 6.10). This categorization remains physiologically meaningful; none of the fat-soluble vitamins appear to serve as coenzymes, whereas almost all of the water-soluble vitamins appear to function in that role. Also, the absorption of fat-soluble vitamins is primarily through a micellar route, whereas the water-soluble vitamins are not absorbed in a lipophilic phase in the intestine (see Chapter 105).

Trace Minerals

Compelling evidence exists for the essential nature of 10 trace elements in humans: iron, zinc, copper, chromium, selenium, iodine, fluorine, manganese, molybdenum, and cobalt (see Table 6.11). The biochemical functions of trace elements have not been as well characterized as those of the vitamins, but most of their functions appear to be as components of prosthetic groups or as cofactors for enzymes.

Aside from iron, the trace mineral depletion clinicians are most likely to encounter is zinc deficiency. Zinc depletion is a

TABLE 6.12 Guidelines for Daily Administration of Parenteral Micronutrients in Adults and Children

Micronutrient	Adults	Children
Fat-soluble vitamins		
A	1000 μg (= 3300 IU)	700 μg
D	5 μg (= 200 IU)	10 μg
E	10 mg (= 10 IU)	7 mg
K	1 mg	200 μg
Water-soluble vitamins		
C	100 mg	80 mg
B_6	4 mg	1 mg
B_{12}	5 μg	1 μg
Biotin	60 μg	20 μg
Folate	400 μg	140 μg
Niacin	40 mg	17 mg
Pantothenic acid	15 mg	5 mg
Riboflavin	3.6 mg	1.4 mg
Thiamine	3 mg	1.2 mg
Trace elements		
Chromium	10–15 μg	0.2 μg/kg/day
Copper	0.5–1.5 mg	20 μg/kg/day
Iodine[a]	—	—
Iron	1–2 mg	1 mg/day
Manganese	0.1 mg	1 μg/kg/day
Molybdenum	15 μg	0.25 μg/kg/day
Selenium	100 μg	2 μg/kg/day
Zinc	2.5–4.0 mg	50 μg/kg/day

[a]Naturally occurring contamination of parenteral nutrition formulas appears to provide sufficient quantities of iodine.

Adult vitamin guidelines adapted from American Society of Parenteral and Enteral Nutrition (ASPEN). Board of Directors and the Clinical Guidelines Task Force. Guidelines for the use of parenteral and enteral nutrition in adult and pediatric patients. *J Parenter Enteral Nutr*. 2002;26:144. Children's values adapted from Greene HL, Hambidge KM, Schanler R, Tsang RC. Guidelines for the use of vitamins, trace elements, calcium, magnesium, and phosphorus in infants and children receiving total parenteral nutrition: report of the Subcommittee on Pediatric Parenteral Nutrient Requirements from the Committee on Clinical Practice Issues of the American Society for Clinical Nutrition. *Am J Clin Nutr*. 1988;48:1324–1342; *Am J Clin Nutr*. 1989;49:1332 and *Am J Clin Nutr*. 1989;50:560.

particularly germane issue to the gastroenterologist, because the GI tract is both the organ that effects absorption of the mineral as well as the major route of excretion. Chronically excessive losses of GI secretions, especially of the upper GI tract, such as the chronic diarrhea accompanying Crohn's or celiac disease, are known precipitants for zinc deficiency, and, in these settings, zinc requirements often increase several-fold.[26] Nevertheless, a biochemical diagnosis of zinc deficiency is problematic (as is true for many of the other essential trace minerals) because accurate laboratory assessment of zinc status is complicated by the very low concentrations of zinc in bodily fluids and tissues, a lack of correlation between serum and red blood cell levels with levels in the target tissues, and the reality that suitable functional tests have yet to be devised. Furthermore, in acute illness, a shift in zinc occurs from the serum compartment into the liver, further obscuring the diagnostic value of serum zinc levels.[27] It is often best to simply proceed with empiric zinc supplementation in patients whose clinical scenario puts them at high risk of zinc deficiency.

The content of Mn in TPN has been observed to vary from 0.01 to 2.2 mg/day, and multiple reports indicate that TPN solutions that deliver several-fold more manganese than what is recommended in Table 6.12 may lead to deposition of the mineral in the basal ganglia, with resulting extrapyramidal symptoms, seizures, or both.[28] Neurotoxicity to Mn has been observed in adults receiving >500 μg/day in TPN and in pediatric patients receiving >40 μg/kg/day. Because the content of manganese varies widely in the different trace element mixtures available for TPN compounding, health professionals need to be mindful of this issue as protocols for TPN mixtures are developed.

Physiologic and Pathophysiologic Factors Affecting Micronutrient Requirements

Age

An evolution of physiology continues throughout the life cycle, impacting on the requirements of certain micronutrients; as a result, specific RDAs for older adults have now been developed. The mean vitamin B_{12} status of most populations, for example, declines substantially with older age, in large part because of the high prevalence of atrophic gastritis and its resultant impairment of protein-bound (i.e., the form found in foodstuffs) vitamin B_{12} absorption.[29] Some 10%–15% of the older ambulatory population is thought to have significant vitamin B_{12} depletion, and neuropathic degeneration may occur in older individuals whose plasma vitamin B_{12} levels are in the low-normal range (150–300 pg/mL) even in the absence of hematologic manifestations. For this reason, the use of sensitive indicators of cellular depletion of vitamin B_{12} (e.g., serum methylmalonic acid levels in conjunction with serum levels of vitamin B_{12}) is now recommended for diagnosis.[30] Proton pump inhibitors and metformin, drugs commonly prescribed to elder adults, inhibit B_{12} absorption, thereby contributing to the issue. Some experts suggest that older adults should consume a portion of their vitamin B_{12} requirement in the crystalline form (i.e., as a supplement) rather than relying only on the naturally occurring protein-bound forms found in food. Compared with younger adults, elders require greater quantities of vitamins B_6 and D and calcium to maintain health, and these requirements are reflected in the new RDAs (see Tables 6.10 and 6.11).

Malabsorption and Maldigestion

Both fat- and water-soluble micronutrients are absorbed predominantly in the proximal small intestine, the only exception being vitamin B_{12}, which is absorbed in the ileum. Diffuse mucosal diseases that affect the proximal portion of the GI tract are, therefore, likely to result in multiple deficiencies. Even in the absence of proximal small intestinal disease, however, extensive ileal disease, SIBO, and chronic cholestasis may interfere with the maintenance of adequate intraluminal conjugated bile acid concentrations and thereby may impair absorption of fat-soluble vitamins.

Conditions that produce fat malabsorption are frequently associated with selective deficiencies of the fat-soluble vitamins. The early stages of many vitamin deficiencies are not apparent clinically and therefore may go undetected until progression of the deficiency has resulted in significant morbidity. This can be disastrous in conditions like spinocerebellar degeneration due to vitamin E deficiency, which often is irreversible.[31] Fat-soluble vitamin deficiencies are well-recognized complications of cystic fibrosis and congenital biliary atresia, in which fat malabsorption often is overt, but monitoring is also necessary in conditions associated with more subtle fat malabsorption, such as the latter stages of chronic cholestatic liver disease.[31]

Restitution of vitamin deficiencies can sometimes be difficult when severe fat malabsorption is present, and initial correction may require parenteral administration. In severe fat malabsorption, chemically modified forms of vitamins D and E that largely bypass the need for the lipophilic phase of intestinal absorption are commercially available for oral use and can be helpful. The polyethylene glycol succinate form of vitamin E (Nutr-E-Sol) is very effective in patients with severe fat malabsorption who cannot absorb conventional alpha-tocopherol.[32] Similarly, hydroxylated forms of vitamin D (1-hydroxyvitamin D [Hectorol] and 1,25-dihydroxyvitamin D [Rocaltrol]) can be used in patients resistant to the more conventional forms of vitamin D. Monitoring of serum calcium levels is indicated in the first few weeks of therapy with hydroxylated forms of vitamin D because they are considerably more potent than vitamin D_2 or D_3, and risk of vitamin D toxicity exists. In contrast, water-miscible preparations of fat-soluble vitamins, in which a conventional form of vitamin A or E is dissolved in polysorbate 80 (e.g., Aquasol-E and Aquasol-A), have not been proved to improve overall absorption.

Maldigestion usually results from chronic pancreatic insufficiency, which, if untreated, frequently causes fat malabsorption and deficiencies of fat-soluble vitamins. Vitamin B_{12} malabsorption also can be demonstrated in this setting, but clinical vitamin B_{12} deficiency is rare unless other conditions known to diminish its absorption are also present. Whether long-term administration of PPIs alone warrants occasional checks of vitamin B_{12} status is a matter of debate.[33,34] Regardless, malabsorption of vitamin B_{12} from atrophic gastritis or with PPIs is confined to dietary sources of vitamin B_{12}. Small supplemental doses of crystalline vitamin B_{12} are absorbed readily in both cases. Histamine-2 receptor antagonists also inhibit protein-bound vitamin B_{12} absorption, although the effect is less potent than with the PPIs.[35]

Many medications may adversely affect micronutrient status. The manner in which drug-nutrient interaction occurs varies; some of the more common mechanisms are described in Table 6.13. A comprehensive discussion of drug-nutrient interactions is beyond the scope of this chapter, and the reader is referred to other references for a detailed discourse on this topic.[36]

STARVATION

During periods of energy or protein deficit or both, an array of compensatory mechanisms serves to lessen the pathophysiologic impact of these deficiencies. These responses decrease the metabolic rate, maintain glucose homeostasis, conserve body nitrogen, and increase the uptake of adipose tissue TGs to meet energy needs. To appreciate how acute illness disrupts this compensatory scheme, it is first necessary to understand how the body adapts to starvation in the absence of underlying disease.

During the first 24 hours of fasting, the most readily available energy substrates (i.e., circulating glucose, FAs and TGs, and liver and muscle glycogen) are used as fuel sources. The sum of energy provided by these stores in a 70-kg man, however, is only about 5000 kJ (1200 kcal) and therefore is less than a full day's requirements. Hepatic glucose production and oxidation decrease, whereas whole-body lipolysis increases, the latter providing additional FAs and ketone bodies.[37] Oxidation of FAs released from adipose tissue TGs accounts for about 65% of the energy consumed during the first 24 hours of fasting.

During the first several days of starvation, obligate glucose-requiring tissues like the brain and blood cells, which collectively account for about 20% of total energy consumption, can use only glycolytic pathways to obtain energy. Because FAs cannot be converted to carbohydrate by these glycolytic tissues, they must use glucose or substrates that can be converted to glucose. Glucogenic AAs derived from skeletal muscle (chiefly alanine and glutamine) are a major source of substrate for this purpose. Approximately 15% of the REE is provided by oxidation of protein.[38] The relative contribution of gluconeogenesis to hepatic glucose production increases as the rate of hepatic glycogenolysis declines because the latter process becomes redundant; after 24 hours of fasting, only 15% of liver glycogen stores remain.

During short-term starvation (1–14 days), several adaptive responses appear that lessen the loss of lean mass. A decline in levels of plasma insulin, an increase in plasma epinephrine levels, and an increase in lipolytic sensitivity to catecholamines stimulate adipose tissue lipolysis.[39,40] The increase in FA delivery to the liver, in conjunction with an increase in the ratio of plasma glucagon-to-insulin concentrations, enhances the production of ketone bodies by the liver. A maximal rate of ketogenesis is reached by 3 days of starvation, and plasma ketone body concentration is increased 75-fold by 7 days. In contrast to FAs, ketone bodies can cross the blood–brain barrier and provide most of the brain's energy needs by 7 days of starvation.[41] The use of ketone bodies by the brain greatly diminishes glucose requirements and thus spares the need for muscle protein degradation to provide glucose precursors. If early protein breakdown rates were to continue throughout starvation, a potentially lethal amount of muscle protein would be catabolized in less than 3 weeks. Similarly, the heart, kidney, and skeletal muscle change their primary fuel substrate to FAs and ketone bodies. Other tissues like bone marrow, renal medulla, and peripheral nerves switch from full oxidation of glucose to anaerobic glycolysis, resulting in increased production of pyruvate and lactate. The latter two compounds can be converted back to glucose in the liver using energy derived from fat oxidation via the Cori cycle, and the resulting glucose is available for systemic consumption. This enables energy stored as fat to be used for glucose synthesis.

Whole-body glucose production decreases by greater than 50% during the first few days of fasting because of a marked reduction in hepatic glucose output. As fasting continues, the conversion of glutamine to glucose in the kidney represents almost 50% of total glucose production. Energy is conserved by a decrease in physical activity secondary to fatigue and a roughly 10% reduction in REE resulting from increased conversion of active thyroid hormone to its inactive form and suppressed sympathetic nervous system activity.

During long-term starvation (14–60 days), maximal adaptation is reflected by a plateau in lipid, carbohydrate, and protein metabolism. The body relies almost entirely on adipose tissue for its fuel, providing greater than 90% of daily energy requirements.[42]

TABLE 6.13 Interactions of Drugs on Micronutrient Status

Drug(s)	Nutrient	Mechanism(s)
Cholestyramine	Vitamin D, folate	Adsorbs nutrient, decreases absorption
Dextroamphetamine, fenfluramine, levodopa	Potentially all micronutrients	Induces anorexia
Isoniazid	Pyridoxine	Impairs uptake of vitamin B_6
NSAIDs	Iron	GI blood loss
Penicillamine	Zinc	Increases renal excretion
PPIs	Vitamin B_{12}	Modest bacterial overgrowth, decreases gastric acid/pepsin, impairs absorption
Sulfasalazine	Folate	Impairs absorption and inhibits folate-dependent enzymes

From Goldman L, Ausiello D, Arend W, et al, eds. *Cecil Textbook of Medicine*. 22nd ed. Philadelphia: WB Saunders; 2004.

Muscle protein breakdown decreases to less than 30 g/day, causing a marked decrease in urea nitrogen production and excretion. The decrease in osmotic load diminishes urine volume to 200 mL/day, thereby reducing fluid requirements. Total glucose production decreases to approximately 75 g/day, providing fuel for glycolytic tissues (40 g/day) and the brain (35 g/day) while maintaining a constant plasma glucose concentration. Energy expenditure decreases by 20%–25% at 30 days of fasting and remains relatively constant thereafter despite continued starvation.

The metabolic response to short- and long-term starvation differs somewhat between lean and obese persons. Obesity is associated with a blunted increase in lipolysis and decrease in glucose production compared with that in lean persons.[43,44] In addition, protein breakdown and nitrogen losses are less in obese persons, thereby helping conserve muscle protein.[45]

Events that mark the terminal phase of starvation have been studied chiefly in laboratory animals. Body fat mass, muscle protein, and the sizes of most organs are markedly decreased. The weight and protein content of the brain, however, remain relatively stable. During the final phase of starvation, body fat stores reach a critical level, energy derived from body fat decreases, and muscle protein catabolism is accelerated. Death commonly occurs when there is a 30%–50% loss of skeletal muscle protein.[46] In humans, it has been proposed that there are certain thresholds beyond which lethality is inevitable: depletion of total body protein between 30% and 50% and of fat stores between 70% and 95%, or reduction of BMI below 13 kg/m^2 for men and 11 kg/m^2 for women.[47,48]

MALNUTRITION

In the broadest sense, malnutrition implies a sustained imbalance between nutrient availability and nutrient requirements. This imbalance results in a pathophysiologic state in which intermediary metabolism, organ function, and body composition are variously altered. *Sustained* is an important element of this definition, because homeostatic mechanisms and nutrient reserves are usually adequate to compensate for any short-term imbalance.

Customarily, the term *malnutrition* is used to describe a state of inadequacy in protein, calories, or both and is more precisely called PEM or *protein-calorie malnutrition*. Occasionally, it is used to describe a state of excessive availability, such as a sustained excess of calories (e.g., obesity) or a vitamin (e.g., vitamin toxicity).

Protein-Energy Malnutrition

There are different pathways whereby PEM may evolve. Primary PEM is caused by inadequate intake of protein, calories, or both, or, less commonly, when the protein ingested is of such poor quality that one or more essential AAs becomes a limiting factor in the maintenance of normal protein metabolism. Secondary PEM is caused by illness or injury.

Acute illnesses and injuries increase bodily requirements for protein and energy substrate and impair digestion, absorption, and uptake of these nutrients in various ways. Consequently, secondary PEM usually arises from multiple factors. Illness and injury also commonly induce anorexia (see later for mechanisms), so primary and secondary factors often act in concert to create PEM in the setting of illness.

Illness or injury may directly interfere with nutrient assimilation; for example, extensive ileal disease or resection may directly produce fat malabsorption and a caloric deficit. The most common causes of secondary PEM, however, are the remarkable increases in protein catabolism and energy expenditure that occur as a result of a systemic inflammatory response. REE may increase as much as 80% above basal levels in a manner roughly proportional to the magnitude of the inflammatory response, which, in turn, is roughly proportional to the severity and acuity of the illness. Thus REE in patients with extensive second- and third-degree burns (the prototype for maximal physiologic stress) may approach twice normal; with sepsis, REE is about 1.5 times normal, and with a localized infection or fracture of a long bone, REE is 25% above normal.[6] Such stress factors can be used to construct a formula for predicting the caloric needs of ill individuals (see Table 6.5).

Protein catabolism during illness or injury also increases in proportion to the severity and acuity of the insult and, therefore, parallels the increase in energy consumption. The magnitude of increase in protein catabolism, however, is proportionately greater than that observed with energy consumption such that urinary urea N losses, which reflect the degree of protein catabolism in acute illness, are about 2.5 times the basal level with maximal stress.[6] This increase in catabolism results in a net loss of protein because the rate of synthesis usually does not rise in concert with the rise in catabolism.[49] No known storage form of protein exists in the body, so any net loss of protein represents a loss of functionally active tissue. A healthy adult typically loses about 12 g N/day in urine, and excretion may increase to as much as 30 g/day during critical illness. Because 1 g of urinary N represents the catabolism of approximately 30 g of lean mass, it follows that severe illness may produce a daily loss of up to about 0.5 kg of lean mass as a result of excess protein catabolism. Most of this loss comes from skeletal muscle, where the efflux of AAs increases two- to sixfold in critically ill patients.[50]

Mobilization of AAs from skeletal muscle appears to be an adaptive response. Once liberated, these AAs, in part, are deaminated and used for gluconeogenesis; they are also taken up by the liver and other visceral organs. The proteolysis of muscle under stress thus enables the body to shift AAs from skeletal muscle (the somatic protein compartment) to the visceral organs (the visceral protein compartment), the functions of which are more critical for immediate survival during illness. Nevertheless, with sustained stress, the limitations of this adaptive response become evident, and even the visceral protein compartment sustains a contraction in mass.[42]

Primary Versus Secondary Protein-Energy Malnutrition: A Body Compartment Perspective

The type of tissue lost as malnutrition evolves is critical in determining the pathologic ramifications of weight loss. Over 95% of energy expenditure resides in the lean body mass, which is the maintenance of this body compartment that is most critical for health. Lean body mass can be subdivided further into somatic and visceral protein compartments, blood and bone cells, and extracellular lean mass, such as plasma and bone matrix (Fig. 6.1). In total- or semi-starvation in otherwise healthy individuals, adipose tissue predominates as a primary energy source; thus fat mass contracts to a much greater degree proportional to the loss of lean mass.[42] Alterations in metabolism from injury or illness, however, produce a proportionately greater loss of muscle mass such that it matches or exceeds the loss in fat mass.[51] Although the lean mass lost in illness is preferentially from the somatic protein compartment, with sustained stress there also will be a significant contraction of the visceral protein compartment (Table 6.14). The metabolic forces associated with acute illness and injury are potent, and the restoration of muscle mass is unlikely with nutritional support unless the underlying inflammatory condition is corrected. There is increasing interest in attenuating or reversing net catabolism with the use of exogenous anabolic agents in conjunction with nutrition, although, to date, it remains unclear whether administration of β-hydroxymethylbutyrate, growth hormone, oxandrolone, propranolol, or other anabolic agents in acute illness improves clinical outcomes and outweighs

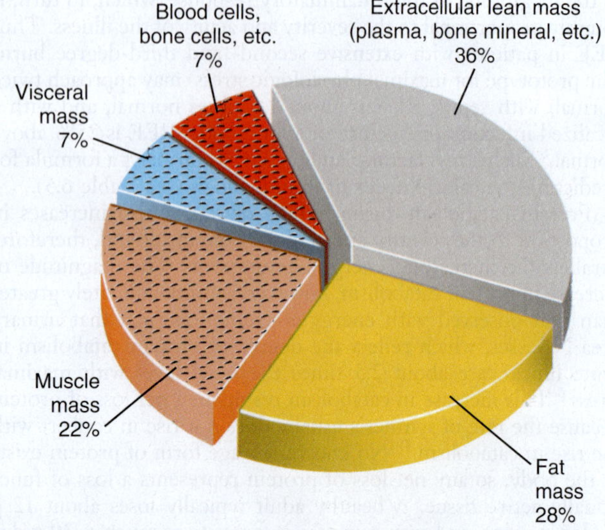

Fig. 6.1 Body composition analysis by weight in a healthy adult. Speckled segments and gray segment collectively represent lean body mass. Speckled segments alone represent body cell mass. (Adapted from Mason JB. Gastrointestinal cancer: nutritional support. In: Kelsen D, Daly J, Kern S, et al., eds. *Principles and Practice of Gastrointestinal Oncology*. Philadelphia: Lippincott Williams & Wilkins; 2002.)

TABLE 6.14 Body Compartment Wasting and Losses in Simple Starvation Versus Metabolic Stress

Parameter	Skeletal Muscle Wasting	Visceral Wasting	Loss of Fat Mass
Starvation	+	+/–[a]	+++
Metabolic stress	+++	++/–[a]	+++

[a]Relatively spared early in the process; can become pronounced with extended starvation or metabolic stress.

their potential side effects.[52] Another important ramification of the potency of the catabolic state associated with acute illness is that most of the weight gained with provision of nutritional support is the result of increases in fat mass and body water; only minor increases in lean mass are observed until the inflammatory focus is resolved.[53]

Cytokines are the most important mediators of alterations in energy and protein metabolism that accompany illness and injury. In a wide spectrum of systemic illnesses, increased secretion of interleukin (IL)-1β, tumor necrosis factor-α, IL-6, and interferon-γ has been observed to be associated with increased energy expenditure and protein catabolism, as well as the shift of AAs into the visceral compartments.[54–56] Such observations concur with in vitro studies in human cells and animal models that have shown remarkably potent effects of these cytokines (Table 6.15). In the wasting syndrome associated with cancer, proteolysis-inducing factor and zinc-α-2-glycoprotein ("lipid-mobilizing factor") are humoral mediators that appear to be unique to cancer cachexia, contributing to protein catabolism and loss of adipose tissue, respectively.[57] Promising data in animal models of cancer cachexia indicate that specific inhibitors of cancer-mediated protein catabolism can be designed that greatly reduce the morbidity and mortality associated with the cachexia produced by this disease.[58]

TABLE 6.15 Major Cytokines That Mediate Hypercatabolism and Hypermetabolism Associated With Metabolic Stress

Cytokine	Cell Sources	Metabolic Effects
IFN-γ	Lymphocytes, pulmonary macrophages	Increased monocyte respiratory burst
IL-1β	Monocytes/macrophages, neutrophils, lymphocytes, keratinocytes, Kupffer cells	Increased ACTH and cortisol levels Increased acute-phase protein synthesis Increased AA release from muscles Decreased insulin secretion Fever
IL-6	Monocytes/macrophages, keratinocytes, endothelial cells, fibroblasts, T cells, epithelial cells	Increased acute-phase protein synthesis Fever Decreased appetite
TNF-α	Monocytes/macrophages, lymphocytes, Kupffer cells, glial cells, endothelial cells, natural killer cells, mast cells	Decreased FFA synthesis Increased lipolysis Increased AA release from muscles Increased hepatic AA uptake Fever

AA, Amino acid; *FFA*, free fatty acid; *IFN*, interferon; *IL*, interleukin.
Adapted from Smith M, Lowry S. The hypercatabolic state. In: Shils M, Olson J, Shike M, Ross AC, eds. *Modern Nutrition in Health and Disease*. Baltimore: Williams & Wilkins; 1999:1555.

Protein-Energy Malnutrition in Children

Undernutrition in children differs from that in adults because it affects growth and development. Much of our prior understanding of undernutrition in children comes from observations made in developing nations where poverty, inadequate food supply, and unsanitary conditions lead to a high prevalence of PEM. However, it has been increasingly recognized that undernutrition is common in developed nations, disproportionately affecting children with underlying medical conditions and those with food insecurity. Anthropometrics can be used to define a child's malnutrition into mild, moderate, and severe categories based on *z*-score classification (Table 6.16).[59] The *z*-score measures the number of SDs away from the age- and sex-adjusted population mean that an individual's anthropometric value falls. A low weight-for-height *z*-score can be defined as acute malnutrition or "wasting." Chronic malnutrition can result in low height for age *z*-score, which is termed "stunting." A detailed physical exam is critical to confirm the diagnosis and assess for sequelae of malnutrition. The characteristics of the two severe forms of clinical PEM syndromes in children—kwashiorkor and marasmus—are outlined in Table 6.17.[60] Although these two syndromes are classified separately, in reality, clinical presentations in which they overlap often occur, and most children with malnutrition do not present with these extreme forms.

Kwashiorkor. The word *kwashiorkor*, from the Ga language of West Africa, means "disease of the displaced child" because it was commonly seen after weaning. The presence of peripheral edema distinguishes children with kwashiorkor from those with marasmus. Children with kwashiorkor also have characteristic skin and hair changes (see later). The abdomen is protuberant because of weakened abdominal muscles, intestinal distention, and hepatomegaly, but ascites is rare. The presence of ascites, therefore, should prompt the clinician to search for liver disease or

TABLE 6.16 Academy of Nutrition and Dietetics (AND) and American Society for Parenteral and Enteral Nutrition (ASPEN) Classification of Malnutrition in Children

	Mild Malnutrition	Moderate Malnutrition	Severe Malnutrition
PRIMARY INDICATORS WHEN SINGLE DATA POINT AVAILABLE			
Weight-for-height *z*-score	−1 to −1.9 *z*-score	−2 to −2.9 *z*-score	−3 to −3.9 *z*-score
BMI-for-age *z*-score	−1 to −1.9 *z*-score	−2 to −2.9 *z*-score	−3 to −3.9 *z*-score
Length/height-for-age *z*-score	No data	No data	<−3 *z*-score
Mid-upper arm circumference	≤−1 to −1.9 *z*-score	≤−2 to −2.9 *z*-score	≤−3 *z*-score
PRIMARY INDICATORS WHEN 2 OR MORE DATA POINTS AVAILABLE			
Weight gain velocity (<2 years of age)	<75% of the norm for expected weight gain	<50% of the norm for expected weight gain	<25% of the norm for expected weight gain
Weight loss (2–20 years of age)	5% usual body weight	7.5% usual body weight	10% usual body weight
Deceleration in weight for length/height *z*-score	Decline of 1 *z*-score	Decline of 2 *z*-scores	Decline of 3 *z*-scores
Inadequate nutrient intake	51%–75% estimated energy or protein need	26%–50% estimated energy or protein need	<25% estimated energy or protein need

For calculation of *z*-scores see https://peditools.org

Adapted from Becker P, Carney LN, Corkins MR, et al. Consensus statement of the Academy of Nutrition and Dietetics/American Society for Parenteral and Enteral Nutrition: indicators recommended for the identification and documentation of pediatric malnutrition (undernutrition). *Nutr Clin Pract.* 2015;30(1):147–161. https://doi.org/10.1177/0884533614557642. Epub 2014 Nov 24. PMID: 25422273).

TABLE 6.17 Features of Severe Protein-Energy Malnutrition Syndromes in Children

Parameter	Kwashiorkor	Marasmus
Appetite	Poor	Good
Edema	Present	Absent
Mood	Irritable when picked up, apathetic when alone	Alert
Weight for age (% expected)	60–80	<60
Weight for height	Normal or decreased	Markedly decreased

peritonitis. Children with kwashiorkor are typically lethargic and apathetic but become very irritable when held. Kwashiorkor most often occurs when a physiologic stress (e.g., infection) is superimposed on an already malnourished child. Because infection or other acute stress is usually present in kwashiorkor, the metabolic aberrations associated with secondary PEM are in play. A decrease in serum proteins, like albumin, is common, reflecting the acute-phase response.[61] Kwashiorkor is characterized by leaky cell membranes that permit movement of potassium and other intracellular ions into the extracellular space, causing water movement and edema.

Marasmus. Weight loss and marked depletion of subcutaneous fat and muscle mass are characteristic features of children with marasmus. Ribs, joints, and facial bones are prominent, and the skin is thin, loose, and lies in folds. In contrast to kwashiorkor, serum albumin levels are often normal, which, in turn, sustains normal oncotic pressure in the vascular compartment.

Contemporary studies of both adult and pediatric PEM in high-income countries typically focus on hospitalized patients with PEM, coexisting illness or injury, and overlapping features of kwashiorkor and marasmus. Children with malnutrition often require multidisciplinary evaluation to identify underlying contributing etiologies that inform personalized treatment approaches (Fig. 6.2). For example, a child with neurologic impairment may require evaluation by a speech language pathologist to identify aspiration, initiation of nutritional supplementation by registered dietitians, and placement and management of gastrostomy tube by pediatric gastroenterologists and surgeons, with critical input from the patient and their family.

Physiologic Impairments Caused by Protein-Energy Malnutrition

PEM adversely affects almost every organ system, although the brain usually is spared. Almost all adverse effects are reversible with nutritional restitution. The following discussion is not exhaustive; rather, it emphasizes impairments that commonly translate into overt morbidity or that are important in the diagnosis of PEM. The effects described reflect what occurs in primary PEM; superimposition of acute illness and secondary PEM often imposes more complexity.

System Effects

Gastrointestinal Tract. Although PEM alone produces adverse effects on GI structure and function, diminished stimulation of the GI tract by a lack of ingested nutrients has an independent effect. Thus sustained absence of nutrients passing through the intestine of healthy, nutritionally replete, parenterally fed individuals alone results in *functional* atrophy of the small intestinal mucosa, as evidenced by a loss of brush border enzymes and diminished integrity of the epithelial barrier. Villus atrophy may also be observed with a lack of intestinal stimulation, but in the absence of PEM, the degree of *structural* atrophy is minor.[62]

The structural and functional deterioration of the intestinal tract, pancreas, and liver as a result of PEM is described best in children. Marked blunting of the intestinal villi is seen and is usually associated with loss of some or all of the brush border hydrolases. Gastric and pancreatic secretions are reduced in volume and contain decreased concentrations of acid and digestive enzymes, respectively. The volume of bile and the concentrations of conjugated bile acids in bile are reduced. Increased numbers of facultative and anaerobic bacteria are found in the upper small

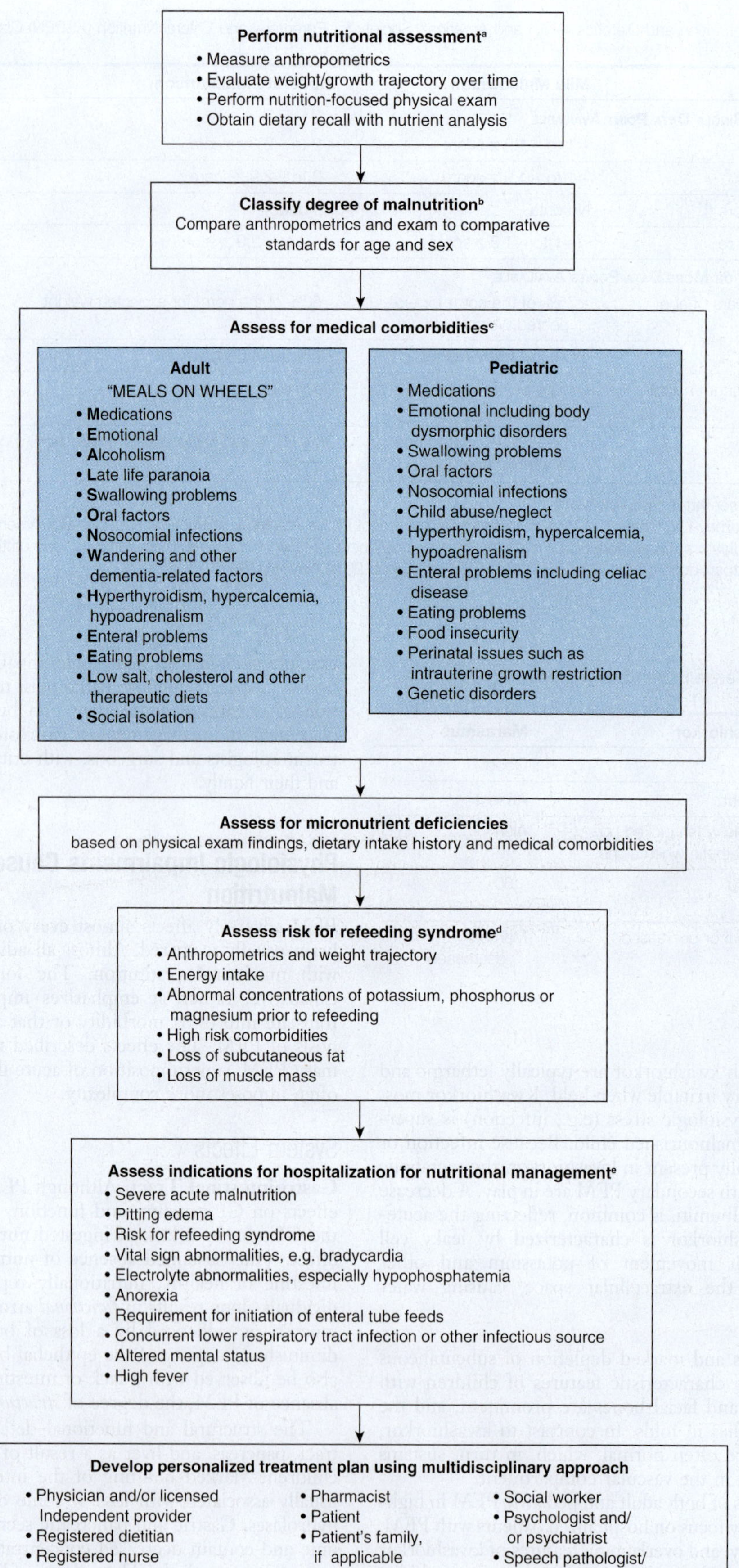

Fig. 6.2 Practical approach to the initial assessment and management of the adult or pediatric patient with malnutrition.

intestine, probably explaining the increased proportion of free bile acids in the intestinal lumen. Malabsorption of carbohydrates, fats, and fat- and water-soluble vitamins may occur, and the degree of steatorrhea is proportional to the severity of the PEM, creating a vicious cycle of further malnutrition. The abdominal protuberance sometimes seen in advanced malnutrition is thought to arise in part from intestinal hypomotility and gas distention.

Cardiovascular System. Moderate to severe PEM produces quantitative and qualitative declines in the cardiac muscle. Myocardial mass is diminished, although proportionately less than the loss in body weight. Myofibrillar atrophy, edema, and (less commonly) patchy necrosis and infiltration with chronic inflammatory cells are seen in the myocardium; these structural changes are associated with impaired myocardial performance. A decrease in stroke volume, cardiac output, and maximal work capacity may be observed and are most evident under conditions of increased demand. Such functional impairments are sometimes accompanied by bradycardia and, in conjunction with the factors noted, can lead to low blood pressure.

Immune System. The immune system is the most vulnerable to PEM, which explains why several functions of immunity are used diagnostically as indicators of malnutrition (e.g., total lymphocyte count and delayed skin hypersensitivity). The functional integrity of T lymphocytes, polymorphonuclear leukocytes, and complement is uniformly blunted, whereas impaired B lymphocyte production of antibodies is variably affected. A moderately to severely malnourished patient is an immunocompromised individual. Malnutrition leads to increased susceptibility to infection, which, in turn, promotes development of PEM, so a vicious cycle is created.

Respiratory System. The diaphragm and other respiratory muscles undergo structural and functional atrophy, diminishing inspiratory and expiratory pressures and vital capacity. These changes in muscular performance, in conjunction with blunted ventilatory drive, impair the ability to sustain ventilation in the severely malnourished individual. In patients with a tracheostomy, adherence of bacteria to the tracheal epithelium correlates with the severity of PEM, exacerbating other compromises in the immune system described earlier.

Endocrine System. Although alterations in hormones are common in PEM, many of the changes can be perceived as serving adaptive functions. The inadequate intake of food leads to a decrease in the availability of circulating glucose and AAs, low circulating levels of insulin, and increased levels of growth hormone. These alterations, in conjunction with the decreased levels of somatomedins and increased levels of cortisol in PEM, promote skeletal muscle catabolism and at the same time enhance incorporation of the liberated AAs into visceral organs. Urea synthesis is inhibited, decreasing nitrogen loss and enhancing reutilization of AAs. Enhancement of lipolysis and gluconeogenesis provides a substrate for energy needs.

Serum levels of triiodothyronine (T_3) and thyroxine (T_4) are commonly decreased in conjunction with increased concentrations of reverse T_3, resembling the pattern observed in the euthyroid sick syndrome. The decreased concentration of T_3 may play a role in decreasing REE and the protein catabolic rate observed in primary PEM.

Primary gonadal dysfunction is common in adults with moderate-to-severe PEM and results in impaired reproductive potential. Decreased circulating levels of testosterone in men and estrogen in women are evident, and amenorrhea is common. Delayed puberty or loss of menstrual periods most often occurs when lean body mass drops below a critical threshold. These changes can also be considered physiologic adaptations, because ensuring immediate survival is more critical than the need for sexual maturation in the child or reproduction in the adult.

Other Effects

Wound Healing. Well-nourished individuals lay down more collagen at the site of a surgical wound than those with even mild malnutrition. Nutritional repletion of the malnourished patient before surgery leads to better wound healing than if nutritional needs are only addressed postoperatively.

Skin. Undernutrition often causes dry, thin, and wrinkled skin, with atrophy of the basal layers of the epidermis and hyperkeratosis. Severe malnutrition may cause considerable depletion of skin protein and collagen. Patients with kwashiorkor experience sequential skin changes in different areas. Hyperpigmentation occurs first, followed by cracking and stripping of superficial layers, leaving behind hypopigmented, thin, and atrophic epidermis that is friable and easily macerated.

Hair. Scalp hair becomes thin and sparse and is easily pulled out. In contrast, the eyelashes become long and luxuriant, and there may be excessive lanugo in children. The hair of children with kwashiorkor develops hypopigmentation, with reddish-brown, gray, or blond discoloration. Adults may lose axillary and pubic hair.

Kidneys. Renal mass and function are often well preserved during undernutrition. When malnutrition is severe, however, there are decreases in kidney weight, glomerular filtration rate, ability to excrete acid and sodium, and ability to concentrate urine. Mild proteinuria also may occur.

Bone Marrow. Severe undernutrition suppresses bone marrow red blood cell and white blood cell production, leading to anemia, leukopenia, and lymphocytopenia.

NUTRITIONAL ASSESSMENT TECHNIQUES

The purpose of nutritional assessment is to identify PEM and other nutritional deficits even when they are not readily discernible. PEM can be subtle, but most cases are detected when a systematic nutritional assessment is performed. An example of subtle but clinically significant PEM is found in Child-Turcotte-Pugh class A patients with alcoholic cirrhosis. These individuals usually appear well-nourished. Indeed, one criterion to determine class A status is a normal serum albumin level, but studies of whole-body nitrogen by in vivo neutron activation analysis have demonstrated that more than half of these class A individuals have less than 80% of expected total body protein,[63] the threshold level below which patients have increased morbidity associated with malnutrition.[64]

In otherwise healthy people and in those who are chronically ill, PEM is usually defined by comparing an anthropometric measurement (e.g., weight for height) to established normative standards (see Tables 6.6 and 6.16). In contrast, there is no gold standard to define and measure PEM in the acutely ill patient, because most parameters used to assess PEM in otherwise healthy persons are altered by illness; weight and the concentration of serum proteins are prime examples.

Despite the inaccuracies inherent in assessing PEM in acutely ill individuals, the usefulness of nutritional assessment in this setting has been repeatedly demonstrated. Acutely ill patients who are malnourished sustain higher rates of malnutrition-related morbidity. Thus the presence of PEM has a predictive value. Even more importantly, identifying malnourished patients and then providing appropriate nutritional intervention is likely to improve clinical outcome.[65–69] Meta-analyses have underscored the importance of performing objective nutritional assessments to categorize inpatients, because individuals who are well-nourished or mildly malnourished seem to realize little benefit from intensive nutritional support.[70–72]

A comprehensive nutritional assessment requires a history, physical examination, evaluation of anthropometrics or functional measures of nutritional status, and a panel of laboratory blood tests. Some of the more commonly used assessment tools are weight, height, and other anthropometric measures (e.g., skinfold thickness and mid-arm measurements); functional measures (e.g., hand grip strength or skin testing for evidence of anergy); serum protein concentrations (e.g., albumin or prealbumin); complete blood count, including absolute lymphocyte count; and 24-hour urinary creatinine and blood urea nitrogen levels. Less readily available measures of body composition, such as bioelectrical impedance and total body potassium, can be helpful in the appropriate setting. Some of these measures lack a high degree of specificity but continue to be useful in clinical care because of their prognostic significance. Because no single parameter is sufficiently sensitive or specific to assess PEM, these tools are most effective when used in combination.

Importantly, if the clinician is undertaking a nutritional assessment solely to determine whether a patient falls into a category of moderate-to-severe PEM (and thus one who would benefit from intensive nutritional support), far less than comprehensive assessment will usually suffice; such simple means of categorization are provided in the following sections.

History

Weight Loss

How much weight has been lost, and over what time period? Unintentional weight loss associated with illness is the single most practical predictor of a clinically significant degree of PEM. It is useful to quantify such loss by determining whether the patient has sustained a mild (<5%), moderate (5%–10%), or severe (>10%) degree of loss over the preceding 6 months. Because acute illness incites a disproportionately large loss of lean mass, it is not surprising that 10% unintentional loss in body weight concurs with a 15%–20% decrease in total body protein.[64] This degree of unintentional loss is an important threshold because it is associated with impaired physiology, a poor clinical outcome, and extended hospitalization[73–75]; it also defines those individuals who will likely benefit from intensive nutritional support. Determining the magnitude of weight loss by history, however, has limited accuracy: one study found that one-third of patients with true weight loss go undetected by history, and one-quarter of those who had been weight-stable are miscategorized as having undergone weight loss.[76] Furthermore, the nutritional significance of changes in body weight can be confounded by changes in hydration status and extracellular fluid accumulation. Because weight loss is an imperfect indicator of PEM, it is useful to obtain other historical clues that can contribute to the identification of these patients (see later).

Food Intake

Has there been a change in habitual diet pattern (number, size, and contents of meals)? What is the reason for altered food intake (e.g., change in appetite, mental status or mood, ability to prepare meals, ability to chew or swallow, GI symptoms)?

Evidence of Malabsorption

Are there signs, symptoms, or both consistent with malabsorption?

Evidence of Specific Nutrient Deficiencies. Are there signs, symptoms, or both of specific nutrient deficiencies, including macrominerals, micronutrients, and water? (See Tables 6.9–6.11.)

Influence of Disease on Nutrient Requirements. Is the nature of the patient's underlying illness one that is likely to increase nutrient needs or nutrient losses?

Functional Status. Has the patient's ability to perform daily activities that determine consumption of wholesome meals changed? Can the patient still shop and prepare meals? Have finances interfered with the ability of the patient to purchase food?

Physical Examination

Hydration Status

The patient should be evaluated for signs of dehydration (e.g., hypotension, tachycardia, postural changes in blood pressure and pulse, mucosal xerosis, decreased axillary sweat, dry skin). Conversely, excess body fluid (e.g., edema or ascites) can mask underlying loss of lean mass.

Tissue Depletion

A general loss of adipose tissue can be assumed if there are well-defined bony, muscular, and venous outlines and loose skinfolds. A fold of skin pinched between the forefinger and thumb can reveal the adequacy of subcutaneous fat. The presence of hollowness in the cheeks, buttocks, and perianal area suggests body fat loss. Examination of the temporalis, interosseous, and quadriceps muscles should be done to judge muscle wasting.

Muscle Function

Strength testing of individual muscle groups can be performed to determine if there is generalized or localized muscle weakness (see: fist grip dynamometry [FGD]). Myocardial function can be evaluated, and respiratory muscle function can be assessed with spirometry.

Specific Nutrient Deficiencies

Rapidly proliferating tissues (e.g., oral mucosa, hair, skin, GI epithelium, and bone marrow) are often more sensitive to nutrient deficiencies than tissues that turn over more slowly (e.g., heart, skeletal muscle, and brain [see Tables 6.9–6.11]).

Anthropometry

Anthropometric techniques are those in which a quantitative measure of the size, weight, or volume of a body part is used to assess protein and calorie status. Historically, one of the most commonly used anthropometric parameters has been weight for height. This is a useful parameter when neither the patient nor family can provide reliable historical information, but it is less desirable than a history of unintentional weight loss since it relies on a normative standard established in a large control population, and inter-individual variability in the population limits this method's accuracy for correctly predicting PEM in one individual. Table 6.6 displays the 1959 Metropolitan Life Insurance Company "desirable body weights" that were established with prospective mortality data. The 1959 table remains preferable to the 1983 tables largely because of concerns that the latter did not include an adequate sampling of certain segments of the population and was, therefore, biased. In the context of the Metropolitan table, desirable weight for height is defined as that figure associated with maximal longevity. In general, individuals whose weight is less than 85% of the standard can be considered to have a clinically significant degree of PEM. Of note is that desirable weights in this table are substantially less than average weights in North America.

TABLE 6.18 Classification of Nutritional Status by Body Mass Index in Adults

Body Mass Index (kg/m^2)	Nutritional Status
<16.0	Severely malnourished
16.0–16.9	Moderately malnourished
17.0–18.4	Mildly malnourished
18.5–24.9	Normal
25.0–29.9	Overweight
30.0–34.9	Obese (class I)
35.0–39.9	Obese (class II)
≥40	Obese (class III)

BMI (Table 6.18), defined as weight (in kilograms) divided by height (in meters squared), has largely supplanted the use of weight for height, in part because it precludes the need to use normative data tables. BMIs outside the desirable range (18.5–24.9 kg/m^2) help identify patients at increased risk of adverse clinical outcomes. A BMI modestly above the desirable range has been shown to be predictive of adverse outcomes in the surgical management of many diseases[77–79] and in the medical management of conditions like alcoholic liver disease.[80] Similarly, a low BMI has been shown to be a robust independent risk factor in surgical and medical patients.[81] Extremely underweight adult patients (BMI <14 kg/m^2) are at high risk of death and should be strongly considered for admission to the hospital to initiate intensive nutritional support.

The BMI, like weight for height, is a surrogate and imperfect measure of body composition. A low BMI (<18.5 kg/m^2) is interpreted as an indication of PEM, and a high BMI (>24.9 kg/m^2) is interpreted as excessive adiposity. Although BMI is accurate in this regard for the vast majority of adults, it can be just as misleading as other measures that rely on body weight without a direct evaluation of body composition.[82] The individual with excessive fluid accumulation, where actual fat and body cell mass (BCM) are less than that implied by the BMI, and the muscle-bound athlete, where a high BMI is indicative of an extraordinarily large lean mass, are two examples of how the underlying assumptions inherent in the BMI are false. Sex and race are also confounding variables, although the differences are clinically irrelevant. More important are the remarkable changes in body composition that accompany development, making the interpretation of BMI in childhood and adolescence very complex.[83]

It should be apparent from this discussion that measurements of relevant body compartments (e.g., fat mass or fat-free mass [FFM]) can reveal important information about nutritional status that is often obscured by measurement of weight alone. Underwater (hydrostatic) weighing, dual-energy x-ray absorptiometry, air impedance plethysmography, total body potassium, isotopically labeled water dilution, in vivo neutron activation analysis, computed tomography, and magnetic resonance imaging are accurate noninvasive (or minimally invasive) techniques of measuring body compartments.[83–90] All are highly effective, but because of their expense, lack of accessibility, and impracticality, their use is largely relegated to the sphere of clinical research. A detailed understanding of these tools is beyond the scope of this chapter, but the primary use of each, with reference to detailed reviews, is outlined in Table 6.19.

In the clinical setting, simple but less accurate techniques are used to assess body compartments. An approximate measure of whole-body fat mass can be derived from assessing the thickness of subcutaneous fat, which in a normally proportioned adult contains roughly half of the body's adipose stores. The triceps and subscapular sites are used most commonly for this purpose, which is best to use the sum of the triceps and subscapular folds because sizable inter-individual differences exist in fat distribution. Furthermore, as total body fat changes, the subcutaneous fat at each site responds in a different manner. Similarly, mid-arm muscle circumference (MAMC) provides a measure of skeletal muscle mass. Table 6.20 contains guidelines for interpretation of skinfold and mid-arm muscle area based on data from the first two National Health and Nutrition Examination Surveys (NHANES I and II).[91]

TABLE 6.19 Advanced Techniques for Measurement of Body Compartments

Technique	Primary Use in Body Compartment Analysis
Air displacement plethysmography[91]	Proportion of body composed of FM, proportion of body composed of LM
CT[90]	Regional FM/LM
Dual-energy x-ray absorptiometry[92]	Absolute FM and LM; bone density
In vivo neutron activation analysis[95]	Total body protein, absolute FM, absolute LM
Isotopically labeled water and NaBr dilution[94]	TBW, ICW, ECW
MRI[96]	Regional FM/LM
Total body potassium[93]	Body cell mass
Underwater (hydrostatic) weighing[89]	Proportion of body composed of FM, proportion of body composed of LM

ECW, Extracellular water; *FM*, fat mass; *ICW*, intracellular water; *LM*, lean mass; *NaBr*, sodium bromide; *TBW*, total body water.

TABLE 6.20 Normative Standards for Upper Arm Muscle Area and Sum of Triceps and Subscapular Skinfolds

		Percentile		
Parameter	**Age**	**5th**	**50th**	**85th**
UPPER ARM MUSCLE AREA (CM^2)[a]				
Men	25–29	38	53	65
	45–49	37	55	66
	65–69	33	48	63
Women	25–29	20	30	38
	45–49	21	32	45
	65–69	22	35	46
SUM OF TRICEPS AND SUBSCAPULAR SKINFOLDS (MM)				
Men	25–29	12	24	41
	45–49	13	29	43
	65–69	12	27	42
Women	25–29	18	37	58
	45–49	21	46	68
	65–69	22	45	65

[a]Mid-upper arm muscle area (cm^2) is calculated as follows:

$$\text{For men: Area} = \frac{[\text{arm circumference} - \{\pi \times \text{triceps skinfold}\}]^2}{4\pi} - 10$$

$$\text{For women: Area} = \frac{[\text{arm circumference} - \{\pi \times \text{triceps skinfold}\}]^2}{4\pi} - 6.5$$

Adapted with permission from Frisancho AR. *Anthropometric Standards For The Assessment of Growth and Nutritional Status*. Ann Arbor, Michigan: University of Michigan Press; 1990.

Clinical use of skinfolds and appendicular muscle area has distinct weaknesses. As was true for the weight-for-height tables, there is considerable inter-individual variation in values, so these measurements are more useful in population studies than in an individual. Moreover, these measures are highly operator dependent.[92] Also, although the updated databases defining normative values no longer contain the race and age biases of older versions, correction factors for hydration and physical activity are still unavailable.

In practice, we have found the most useful clinical role for the measurement of skinfolds and muscle area is in tracking patients with serial measurements over time as a means of monitoring their recovery from disease or response to a clinical intervention. In this manner, the patient is being compared with themselves rather than with some normative value. In gastroenterology, the use of skinfolds and muscle area has been of particular value in the assessment and management of cirrhotic patients, because cirrhosis corrupts most other common measures of nutritional status. Abnormally low values for triceps skinfold and MAMC are independent predictors of mortality in patients with cirrhosis, and their incorporation into a Cox regression model improves the prognostic value of the Child-Turcotte Score.[93] Also, when patients with severe alcoholic hepatitis are treated with anabolic steroids, improvements in MAMC and other measures of the FFM correlate with a positive response to treatment.[94]

Interest continues in bioimpedance analysis as an inexpensive, relatively easy, noninvasive, and safe means of assessing FFM, BCM, and total body water. BCM is sometimes perceived as a more important measure of lean mass than FFM because it does not include nonliving lean mass (e.g., blood plasma and bone minerals [see Fig. 6.1]). Resistance to electrical flow through the body is measured, which is proportional to fat and bone mineral content because these body components have poor conductivity. Other components of the body are suffused with electrolyte-laden water that readily conducts an electric current, so calculations of total body water, FFM, and BCM can be made if one abides by some general assumptions that define the water content of each compartment. Its utility has been demonstrated, for example, for monitoring the FFM in outpatient renal dialysis and HIV-infected patients.[95,96] Acute illness, however, produces shifts in the amount and distribution of body water, rendering the technique largely worthless in the inpatient setting.[97] Furthermore, the algorithms used to calculate body composition contain assumptions about body water that can change with age, obesity, and disease state, so bioimpedance analysis must be revalidated within any population in which it is used.

Functional Measures of Protein-Calorie Status

Several techniques have been developed that exploit the fact that skeletal muscle function is impaired in PEM, although only one has acquired wide acceptance: FGD. FGD uses a handheld dynamometer to measure the maximal fist-grip force that can be elicited. When examined as a surrogate measure of total body protein in patients awaiting GI surgery, FGD correlated strongly with in vivo neutron activation analysis and with MAMC.[98] Similarly, FGD is excellent for detecting depleted BCM in cirrhotic patients,[99] a group in which it is notoriously difficult to perform nutritional assessment. As noted, valid indicators of moderate to severe PEM are strong predictors of clinical outcome in acutely ill patients, and FGD is effective in this regard. Preoperative patients whose fist-grip strength is less than 85% of age- and sex-corrected standards have a twofold increased risk of perioperative complications compared with those whose FGD is normal.[100] In patients undergoing surgery for GI cancers, FGD had superior sensitivity and specificity in predicting perioperative morbidity and mortality than a widely used discriminant analysis called the *prognostic nutritional index*.[101] FGD holds considerable promise for rapid and convenient assessment of protein-calorie status in both inpatients and outpatients, although the technique is limited by its requirement for an alert and cooperative patient.

Although PEM adversely affects the physiology of almost all organ systems, the immune system is particularly sensitive. Delayed hypersensitivity skin testing, which assesses the integrity of cell-mediated immunity, has been used most often in this regard. In critically ill patients, skin testing has value in predicting morbidity and mortality, but its interpretation is fraught with confounding variables such as older age, systemic infection, and major surgery, each of which independently depress reactivity. Furthermore, reactivity improves in an unpredictable manner with nutritional restitution, so it is not useful for monitoring patient progress.[102] The value of skin testing to assess nutritional status is used best as part of an array of parameters that collectively assess nutritional status (see later, "Discriminant Analyses of Protein-Calorie Status").

Biochemical Measures of Protein-Calorie Status

Serum Proteins

The serum concentrations of several proteins synthesized in the liver are used as indicators of protein-calorie status: albumin, prealbumin (transthyretin), transferrin, and retinol-binding protein (RBP) (Table 6.21). In the absence of concurrent illness or injury, a low concentration of any of these proteins strongly suggests the presence of PEM. Because the half-lives of prealbumin, transferrin, and RBP are considerably shorter than that of albumin, it follows that changes in nutritional status will be reflected more promptly in levels of these three proteins than in albumin.

However, a variety of nonnutritional factors can alter the serum concentration of these proteins, introducing the need for caution in their interpretation. Prealbumin levels are often elevated in chronic kidney disease or by glucocorticoid or oral contraceptive administration. The degree to which serum levels of all these proteins are decreased in cirrhosis increases incrementally with worsening grades of the Child classification, although even patients who are Child class A have a small decrease in albumin compared with healthy individuals.[103]

All these proteins behave as negative acute-phase reactants, that is, their serum concentrations drop in response to systemic inflammation, roughly proportional to the magnitude of the inflammatory response. This effect diminishes their reliability as indicators of PEM in the acutely ill patient, particularly when used as a sole metric of nutritional status. Nonetheless, with proper respect for their limited accuracy, they can still be useful. For example, prealbumin has been shown to be an efficient, rapid means of screening inpatients for PEM on hospital admission.[104]

Creatinine-Height Index

The amount of creatinine excreted in the urine over a 24-hour period, corrected for the patient's height, is an excellent means of assessing total skeletal muscle mass. The relationship holds because a relatively constant percentage ($\approx 2\%$) of muscle creatine is converted to creatinine each day. Values that are greater than 20% below sex- and height-adjusted normative values are indicative of moderate-to-severe PEM (Table 6.22). Updated normative creatinine-height index (CHI) values for children of ages 3–18 years are available.[105] In sick persons, the CHI tends to correlate with simple measures like unintentional weight loss, as well as with highly accurate measures of skeletal muscle like dual-energy x-ray absorptiometry.[106] In patients receiving prolonged mechanical ventilation, CHI is a strong independent risk factor concurring with the likelihood of successful weaning and survival.[107]

TABLE 6.21 Proteins Synthesized in the Liver and Used to Assess Nutritional Status

Serum Protein	Normal Value Mean ± SD (Range)[a]	Half-Life (Days)	Function	Comment[b]
Albumin	4.5 (3.5–5.0)	14–20	Maintains plasma oncotic pressure; carrier for small molecules	Serum levels altered by a variety of nonnutritional factors
Transferrin	2.3 (2.0–3.2)	8–9	Binds Fe^{2+} in plasma and transports it to bone marrow	Iron nutriture influences plasma level; increased during pregnancy, estrogen therapy, and acute hepatitis; reduced in protein-losing enteropathy and nephropathy, chronic infections, uremia, and acute catabolic states; often is measured indirectly as total iron-binding capacity
Transthyretin (prealbumin)	0.30 (0.2–0.5)	2–3	Binds T_3 and to a lesser extent T_4; is a carrier for RBP	Increased by corticosteroid, glucocorticoid, or oral contraceptive administration, in those with chronic kidney disease on dialysis; reduced in acute catabolic states, after surgery, in hyperthyroidism; serum level is determined by overall energy and nitrogen balance
Retinol-binding protein (RBP)	0.0372 ± 0.0073[c]	0.5	Transports vitamin A in plasma; binds noncovalently to prealbumin	Catabolized in the renal proximal tubular cell; with renal disease, RBP increases and its half-life is prolonged; low plasma levels in vitamin A deficiency, acute catabolic states, after surgery, and in hyperthyroidism

[a]Units are g/L. Normal range varies among centers; check local values.
[b]All the listed proteins are influenced by hydration and presence of hepatocellular dysfunction.
[c]Normal values are age- and sex-dependent. Table value is for pooled subjects.
SD, Standard deviation; T_3, triiodothyronine; T_4, thyroxine.
Adapted from Heymsfield S, Tighe A, Wang Z-M. Nutritional assessment by anthropometric and biochemical means. In: Shils M, Olson J, Shike M, eds. *Modern Nutrition in Health and Disease*. 8th ed. Philadelphia: Lea & Febiger; 1994:812.

TABLE 6.22 Normative Values for Daily Creatinine Excretion Based on Height

Men[a]		Women[b]	
Height (cm)	Ideal Creatinine (mg)	Height (cm)	Ideal Creatinine (mg)
157.5	1288	147.3	830
160.0	1325	149.9	851
162.6	1359	152.4	875
165.1	1386	154.9	900
167.6	1426	157.5	925
170.2	1467	160.0	949
172.7	1513	162.6	977
175.3	1555	165.1	1006
177.8	1596	167.6	1044
180.3	1642	170.2	1076
182.9	1691	172.7	1109
185.4	1739	175.3	1141
188.0	1785	177.8	1174
190.5	1831	180.3	1206
193.0	1891	182.9	1240

[a]Creatinine coefficient (men) = 23 mg/kg of ideal body weight.
[b]Creatinine coefficient (women) = 18 mg/kg of ideal body weight.
From Blackburn GL, Bistrian BR, Maini BS, et al. Nutritional and metabolic assessment of the hospitalized patient. *J Parenter Enteral Nutr*. 1977;1:11–22.

To avoid misleading results, potential confounders that must be considered include incomplete urine collection, abnormal or unstable renal function, excessive meat or milk ingestion immediately preceding or during the collection, and glucocorticoid administration, all of which can alter creatinine excretion independently of changes in muscle mass.

Discriminant Analyses of Protein-Calorie Status

As noted, many parameters used to measure PEM can also predict important clinical outcomes, although each parameter has its own limitations. Multifactorial indices that integrate combinations of these parameters have been developed through the use of discriminant analyses. By combining several parameters, the goal has been to arrive at a more accurate determination of whether a patient has a substantial degree of PEM and to optimize the ability to predict that patients will have adverse clinical outcomes due to PEM. Various indices have been developed for use in acutely hospitalized patients; for instance, the prognostic nutritional index (which incorporates serum albumin, transferrin, delayed skin hypersensitivity, and triceps skinfold) predicts the likelihood of postoperative complications and mortality in patients undergoing GI surgery,[108] and the Geriatric Nutritional Risk Index (which incorporates serum albumin and % IBW) predicts the likelihood of infectious complications and mortality among elderly inpatients.[109] Since readily available metrics of PEM in the acute care setting are heavily influenced by disease severity, these indices should not be considered accurate measures of the degree of malnutrition; more properly, they are best considered predictors of morbid and mortal events due to PEM.

Two more recent additions to this list of indices for the acute care setting are the Nutrition Risk Score-2002 and the NUTRIC score.[110] As is true of the older indices, their use has been designed and validated for a specific type of patient, namely, ICU patients. Some studies examining the utility of the NRS-2002 and NUTRIC scores have shown that these indices can discriminate those patients who genuinely benefit from intensive nutritional support from those who will not.[111–113]

The algorithm in Fig. 6.2 outlines a structured approach to determining the likelihood and magnitude of malnutrition in a patient, comorbidities that should be taken into consideration when formulating a nutritional plan, additional features of the patient's presentation that will help define some of the directions the plan should take, and those individuals who may need to be involved to carry out an effective plan. Practically, not all items in this algorithm will be readily available and integrated into the development of each patient's plan, but there remains great value in keeping the sequence of steps in mind as well as the considerations outlined in each box.

Rapid Screening Tools for Assessment of Targeted Populations

Assessing nutritional status with inexpensive, rapid, and convenient means that are accurate in identifying patients with PEM is of great value, particularly when large numbers of people need to be evaluated. Two such tools have been developed and extensively validated: the subjective global assessment (SGA) and the Mini-Nutritional Assessment (MNA).

Subjective Global Assessment

SGA was initially intended for use in surgical inpatients as a means of assessing nutritional status and predicting postoperative infections (Box 6.1); for the latter, it was found to be a better predictor than serum albumin concentration, delayed skin hypersensitivity, MAMC, CHI, and the prognostic nutritional index.[114] A focused history and physical examination are used to categorize patients as well nourished (category A), having mild or moderate malnutrition (category B), or having severe malnutrition (category C). Despite the subjective nature of some of its components, there is excellent agreement among independent observers.[115] The SGA has been shown to be reliable, even in the hands of first-year medical and surgical residents,[116] and has been validated as a predictor of clinical outcomes in chronically institutionalized older adults and patients with a variety of medical conditions.[117–119]

Mini-Nutritional Assessment

The MNA was developed as a rapidly administered screen to detect PEM in geriatric populations. A combination of history, limited physical examination, and simple anthropometrics (BMI, arm- and calf-circumference) can be obtained in a few minutes. Subjects receive a score that classifies them as being nourished, malnourished, or at risk of malnutrition. The MNA is a valid means of detecting PEM in older adults who are generally healthy and ambulatory, as well as those who are frail and institutionalized[120,121]; in the chronically institutionalized, it possesses considerable predictive value in projecting future morbidity.[122] One disadvantage of the MNA is that it does not screen for overweight or obesity. Other screening tools designed for geriatric populations, such as the Nutrition Screening Initiative, have the ability to screen for under- and overnutrition but have not been as extensively validated as the MNA.[123]

BOX 6.1 Subjective Global Assessment of Nutritional Status

HISTORY

Weight change:

Loss in past 6 months: amount = _________ kg;
% loss = _________

Change in past 2 weeks: _________ Increase _________
No change _________ Decrease

Dietary intake change:

No change _______ Change _______
Duration = _______ weeks

Dietary status:

_________ Suboptimal solid diet
_________ Hypocaloric liquids
_________ Starvation

Gastrointestinal symptoms (that have persisted for >2 weeks):

_______ None _______ Nausea _______ Vomiting _______
Diarrhea _______ Anorexia

Functional capacity:

_________ No dysfunction _________
Dysfunction Duration = _________ weeks

Type:

_________ Working suboptimally
_________ Ambulatory but not working
_________ Bedridden

Effect of disease on nutritional requirements:

Primary diagnosis: _________
Metabolic demand: ________ Low stress ________
Moderate stress ________ High stress ________

PHYSICAL EXAMINATION (NORMAL, MODERATE, OR SEVERE)

_________ Loss of subcutaneous fat (triceps, chest)
_________ Muscle wasting (quadriceps, deltoids)
_________ Ankle or sacral edema
_________ Ascites

SGA RATING

*The ranks of A, B, and C in the SGA are assigned on the basis of subjective weighting. A patient with weight loss and muscle wasting who is currently eating well and gaining weight is classified as well nourished. A patient with moderate weight loss (between 5% and 10%), continued compromise in food intake, continued weight loss, progressive functional impairment, and moderate stress due to illness is classified as moderately malnourished. A patient with severe weight loss (>10%), poor nutrient intake, progressive functional impairment, and muscle wasting is usually classified as having severe malnutrition.

A = Well nourished
B = Mild or moderate malnutrition
C = Severe malnutrition

AGGRESSIVE NUTRITIONAL SUPPORT IN THE HOSPITALIZED PATIENT

The chapter that follows provides descriptions of appropriate approaches to nutritional management of specific GI and hepatic diseases. As a means of introduction, however, it is first worth considering under what circumstances clinical observations indicate that "aggressive nutritional support" (defined as using whatever means necessary and practical to meet the patient's nutritional needs) truly benefits the acutely ill patient. In practice, any acutely ill patient who has moderate-to-severe malnutrition and is unlikely to be able to meet his or her own nutritional needs within 48 hours is a strong candidate for aggressive nutritional support. Another common indication for aggressive nutritional support is when a well-nourished or mildly malnourished inpatient is judged to be unlikely to meet at least 80% of his or her projected calorie or protein goals for the coming 10 days. To date, there is insufficient evidence-based science to prove efficacy for this latter indication, although common sense would suggest it to be true.

Catabolic forces that accompany acute illness make it difficult to correct nutritional deficits. In those with a high degree of sustained metabolic stress, nutritional support generally will not lead to an increase in the protein compartment of the body. Moreover, a gain in weight may not occur, and when it does, much of the initial gain is from water and an expanded fat mass.[124] Despite these limitations, even in the absence of weight gain or increases in serum protein levels, a course of nutritional support for an appropriate patient can improve physiologic functions and clinical outcomes.[125]

The following three sections cite some clinical scenarios particularly relevant to gastroenterology for which compelling clinical research upholds that aggressive nutritional support provides benefit to the hospitalized patient.

Malnourished Patients Undergoing Major Surgery

Nutritional support can be beneficial for moderately to severely malnourished patients who are scheduled to undergo major surgery. Aggressive nutritional support for 7 or more days before surgery reduces perioperative complications and sometimes mortality in malnourished patients.[65–72,126–128] In the Veterans Affairs TPN Cooperative Study,[65] which encompassed almost 500 subjects about to undergo major abdominal or thoracic surgery, patients who were categorized as severely malnourished and randomized to receive preoperative TPN realized an almost 90% decrease in noninfectious perioperative complications. No benefits were observed in mildly malnourished or well-nourished individuals. In trials of moderately to severely malnourished patients, preoperative nutrition support generally conveys sizeable benefits: a trial that enrolled 90 patients with gastric or colorectal cancers undergoing surgery demonstrated a 35% decline in overall complications and a significant reduction in mortality.[128] The observation that the benefits of preoperative nutritional support are confined to those with a substantial degree of malnutrition is the same conclusion reached by meta-analyses.[70,71] Deferring aggressive nutritional support until after surgery does not appear to have the same ability to diminish perioperative complications.[129]

Provision of nutrients via an enteral approach is also beneficial. There have been fewer trials done of preoperative enteral support than of preoperative TPN, but it appears that preoperative enteral support confers the same nutritional[130] and clinical[131] benefits as TPN. As with TPN, postoperative enteral nutrition in the absence of aggressive preoperative support is less likely to convey benefit to the patient.[132]

Patients Hospitalized with Decompensated Alcohol-Associated Liver Disease

The prevalence of moderate-to-severe PEM is so high in patients admitted for acute alcoholic hepatitis and other forms of decompensated alcoholic liver disease[63] that it is best to assume all such patients are malnourished. Furthermore, patients with acute alcoholic hepatitis usually fall far short of their nutritional needs when allowed to eat freely. Clinical trials have demonstrated that the rates of morbidity, mortality, and the speed of recovery are improved with prompt institution of enteral or parenteral nutrition in these patients.[66–68,133]

Patients Undergoing Radiation Therapy

The usefulness of aggressive nutrition support in patients undergoing radiation therapy has been studied most extensively in those who have head and neck and esophageal cancers. There is now reasonable evidence in these patients that placement of a PEG tube and administration of supplemental tube feedings during and after the course of radiation therapy prevents further deterioration of nutritional status.[134,135] In patients with head and neck cancers, supplemental PEG feedings have also been shown to improve quality of life. Although improvements in survival or decreased morbidity have not yet been demonstrated, improved quality of life alone may warrant its use in this setting.

Full references for this chapter can be found at https://ebooks.health.elsevier.com.

7 Nutritional Management

Endashaw Omer, Stephen A. McClave

IN THIS CHAPTER

NUTRITION IN SPECIFIC DISEASE STATES

Nutritional assessment and directed nutritional therapy are important in the treatment of many GI diseases. Familiarity with appropriate nutritional intervention is imperative to obtaining good clinical outcomes. The preceding chapter reviewed nutritional assessment, and this chapter will give an overview of nutritional concerns in common GI disorders and treatment of nutritional deficiencies by parenteral nutrition (PN) and enteral nutrition (EN).

Intestinal Failure

Intestinal failure (IF) describes a state of insufficient intestinal capacity to fulfill nutritional demands, resulting in dependency on the use of PN,[1] although the definition of IF has been revised by multiple sources. The reduction of the gut's absorptive function that does not require any intravenous supplementation to maintain health and/or growth can be considered intestinal insufficiency.[2] The European Society for Clinical Nutrition and Metabolism (ESPEN) is the first scientific society to issue a formal definition for IF. In the ESPEN definition, two criteria must be present: a "decreased absorption of macronutrients and/or water and electrolytes due to a loss of gut function" and the "need for parenteral support."[3] IF is further functionally classified into types I, II, and III. Type I IF is acute, short-term, and due to a self-limiting condition such as ileus following abdominal surgery, which may require a brief period of nutritional support.[4] Type II IF results from a prolonged acute condition, often in metabolically unstable patients who require IV supplementation over periods of weeks or months, and may be reversible or irreversible.[4] Type II IF patients may recover fully or progress to type III IF, which is a chronic state of IF requiring long-term nutritional support, typically in the form of home PN (HPN).[5] Etiologies include Crohn disease (CD) (see Chapter 117), radiation enteritis (see Chapter 39), intestinal obstruction (see Chapter 125), dysmotility (see Chapters 101, 102, and 126), intestinal trauma, congenital disorders (see Chapter 100), intestinal fistulae (see Chapters 29 and 115), and vascular complications (see Chapter 120).[1]

Short bowel syndrome (SBS) resulting in intestinal malabsorption and associated with a functional small intestine length of less than 200 cm is a common cause of IF (see Chapter 120). After extensive intestinal resection, three clinical stages have been described. The first stage occurs during the first few weeks after resection and is characterized by significant fluid and electrolyte shifts that require copious amounts of IV fluids to prevent dehydration. During the second stage, which may last for up to 2 years, there is both structural adaptation (increase in size and absorptive surface as a result of cellular hyperplasia) and functional adaptation (slowing of bowel transit to allow increased time for absorption). The third stage is a stable phase during which no further improvement or adaptive changes occur.[6] Nutritional management of SBS depends on the length and segment of small intestine removed, because the intestine has the ability to adapt and increase its absorptive function over time. Initially, PPIs are used to reduce gastric hypersecretion, and anticholinergic agents and opioids are used to slow intestinal transit. Patients may require larger doses of anticholinergics than are usually recommended, because absorption of oral medication may be limited. PN is usually required during stage 1 to meet nutritional needs.

During stage 2, oral feedings are advanced, and the volume of PN is reduced as oral feedings are increasingly tolerated. Patients should eat small, frequent meals—avoiding simple sugars, fiber, and nutrient-poor foods—and separate the times of fluid and solid food ingestion. Lactose is usually well tolerated, unless the proximal jejunum is resected. Dietary intake should be increased by at least 50% because most stable adult SBS patients absorb only half to two-thirds as many calories as normal. Such a polyphagic diet is best tolerated when consumed as five to six meals throughout the day.[7] Diarrhea may result from oral feedings and may limit weaning from PN. While percutaneous endoscopic gastrostomy (PEG) placement in the management of SBS is controversial, enteral tube feeding administered continuously over 12–24 hours is usually better tolerated than intermittent bolus feeding because of greater nutrient absorption and less osmotic diarrhea. EN is usually slowly advanced while PN is isocalorically decreased over several months, with frequent monitoring of tolerance as determined by the development of symptoms, amounts of food and fluid intake, stool and urine output, body weight, hydration status, and micronutrient levels.[8]

Following extensive resection of the small intestine, three distinct clinical types of SBS can be identified. In type I SBS, patients have only jejunum remaining with an end jejunostomy and no colon. These patients experience massive fluid losses, show little signs of adaptation over time, and are more likely to be PN dependent. In type II SBS, patients have variable length of jejunum connected in series with some portion of colon. Clinically they show greater signs of adaptation and demonstrate slow deterioration of nutritional status over time without parenteral support. Finally, in type III SBS, intestinal rehabilitation of the remaining small intestine is most likely to be successful (meaning the patient can resume intake of adequate oral nutrition) because the colon has been preserved and is in continuity with the small intestine and the ileocecal valve is maintained.[9] Production of glucagon-like peptide (GLP)-1 by the remnant of terminal ileum has a trophic effect and stimulates SB adaptation, as a result of which these patients rarely need EN or PN. Clinical factors useful in predicting the success of intestinal rehabilitation include the presence of residual disease in the remnant bowel, bowel length, the degree to which adaptation has occurred, and the duration of time on PN. Intestinal autonomy is defined by the ability of an SBS patient to live without PN and may be expected if a patient has 70–90 cm of small bowel and an intact colon, or 130–150 cm of small bowel with no colon. Through the period of adaptation, intestinal autonomy may be achieved more readily for calories than for fluid and electrolytes. Citrulline, a nonprotein amino acid produced by intestinal mucosa, has been proposed as a predictor of permanent versus transient IF.[7] In one study, a plasma citrulline level of below 20 μmol/L identified patients destined to have permanent IF, with positive and negative predictive values of 95% and 86%, respectively.[10]

Patients with severe SBS (<200 cm small bowel remaining) usually require a glucose-electrolyte oral rehydration solution (ORS). Ingestion of an ORS containing glucose with a sodium concentration of at least 90 mmol/L aids in water absorption by making use of sodium-glucose cotransporters in the jejunum (see Chapter 103). Between 2 and 3 L of an ORS solution should be sipped throughout the day. Hypoosmolar fluids should be avoided, as their absorption is dependent mostly on passive diffusion. Hyperosmolar fluids also should be avoided in patients with SBS, because they lead to fluid shifts into the bowel lumen, worsening diarrhea.[7] If a patient has had a partial ileal resection (resection of <100 cm) and has an intact colon, the bile-binding resin cholestyramine can be used to reduce bile salt-induced diarrhea. In patients with a limited amount of ileum remaining (>100 cm of ileum resected) and an intact colon, however, cholestyramine can increase diarrhea by depleting the bile salt pool. In general, fat restriction should not be used for SBS type I patients who do not have a colon, but it may be beneficial in reducing diarrhea for SBS types II and III, in which some length of colon remains.[11] Even in these latter types, however, fat restriction may not change the volume of diarrhea and polyphagia is made more difficult without the ingestion of calorically dense fatty foods. Vitamin B_{12} injections should be administered monthly if more than 50–60 cm of terminal ileum has been resected. The somatostatin analog octreotide has been shown to prolong small intestinal transit time and decrease GI secretions, but its use remains controversial because it is also associated with gallstone formation and decreased splanchnic protein synthesis and has not been shown to eliminate the need for PN.[12–15]

The use of growth hormone and glutamine to promote small intestinal mucosal hypertrophy and improve absorption is controversial. A single randomized controlled trial (RCT) demonstrated decreased PN volume, calories, and number of infusions with this approach, although the effects were short-lived, and measured parameters returned to baseline after cessation of therapy.[16,17] Use of a GLP-2 analog has been shown to be a trophic stimulator of small intestinal mucosa, resulting in improved absorption. Teduglutide, a GLP-2 analog, was shown in an RCT to significantly reduce the volume and number of days of PN for patients with IF and resulted in weaning from PN dependency in a small percentage of patients (see Chapter 106).[18]

Pancreatitis

Nutritional therapy in the management of acute pancreatitis (AP) has undergone a significant paradigm shift from previous practices. Historically, patients with AP were kept NPO to avoid the potential risk of further stimulating exocrine pancreatic secretion and worsening inflammation. Moderately severe and severe AP elicit an intense systemic inflammatory response resulting in a catabolic state, increasing caloric and nutritional requirements.[19] Reduced intestinal vascular perfusion in AP may result in gut mucosal damage. Subsequently, intestinal permeability increases, which may enable the translocation of bacteria from the bowel lumen to the portal circulation and mesenteric lymphatics.[20,21] This could result in organ failure, sepsis, and secondary infection of pancreatic and peripancreatic necrosis.[22] Early nutrition, particularly EN, mitigates these effects by several mechanisms: replenishing caloric losses, increasing splanchnic blood flow to preserve the integrity of the bowel mucosa, and stimulating intestinal motility. Over the past two decades there has been a shift toward early EN in AP patients, but also in all critically ill patients. Data on early feeding (initiated within 24–36 hours of admission) in AP have demonstrated lower risk of multiorgan failure (MOF), operative interventions, systemic infections, septic complications, and even mortality compared with what had been standard therapy (no EN/PN) or delayed EN.[23] The PYTHON (Early versus On-Demand Nasoenteric Tube Feeding in Acute Pancreatitis) study, an RCT in which patients were allocated to receive EN within 24 hours through a nasojejunal (NJ) catheter or be given an on-demand oral diet over the first 4 days (and then only start EN if the oral diet were not tolerated), seemed to refute these results. Outcomes showed that rates of major infection or death were no different between groups,[24] although only 20% of patients in this study were admitted to the ICU, and less than 8% had severe AP (defined by persistent MOF > 48 hours). The key issue in nutritional therapy is severity of the systemic inflammatory response syndrome (SIRS). If the SIRS response is severe enough to require admission to the ICU (especially if the patient is placed on mechanical ventilation), an NG/NJ tube should be placed and EN initiated within 24–36 hours of admission. If the SIRS response is minimal and the patient can be managed on the hospital wards, then oral diet should be offered as tolerated and EN considered only when there is failure to advance the diet after 4 days. Early initiation and advancement of EN should be performed with caution pending adequate resuscitation, as hemodynamically unstable patients requiring inotropic support may be at an increased risk of nonocclusive mesenteric ischemia (see Chapter 118).[25]

Two meta-analyses comparing EN with PN in severe AP have shown a significant 2-fold reduction in the risk of systemic and pancreatic infectious complications, and a 2.5-fold reduction in the risk of death in patients receiving EN.[26,27] In an American Gastroenterological Association (AGA) technical review of 12 RCTs, EN reduced the risk of infected peripancreatic necrosis [OR 0.28, 95% confidence interval (CI) 0.15–0.51], single-organ failure (OR 0.25, 95% CI, 0.10–0.62), and MOF (OR 0.41, 95% CI, 0.27–0.63)[28] compared with PN. Stratifying patients with severe AP from those with mild-to-moderate disease helps triage patients needing admission to the ICU, adequate hydration, treatment for early organ failure, and provision of early EN.[29] Moreover, three RCTs comparing gastric with jejunal feeding in severe AP showed no significant difference in the levels of infusion between groups with regard to tolerance or clinical outcome.[30,31]

The most recent guidelines from the AGA,[32] Acute Pancreatitis Task Force on Quality,[33] and a quality indicator expert panel[34] recommend initiating enteral feeding within 24–72 hours of admission. One meta-analysis of 7 RCTs with 691 patients demonstrated that initiating enteral feeding within 24 hours of admission compared with delayed enteral feeding (>24 hours) or PN was associated with a decrease in multiple organ failure [OR, 0.4 (95% CI, 0.2–0.79); $P = .008$].[35] In general, patients tolerating oral nutrition should be placed on a low-fat soft or solid diet.[36] If patients are unable to tolerate an oral diet within 72 hours, they should be started on nasoenteral nutrition (i.e., nasogastric or NJ).[37,38] Patients who cannot tolerate enteral feeding due to paralytic ileus, obstruction, or other causes should be started on PN within 72 hours.

Nutritional management in chronic pancreatitis (CP) remains challenging. As well-designed RCTs are scarce, in large part, recommendations can only be based on low-level evidence studies or expert opinion. For now, the consumption of a balanced diet remains the cornerstone recommendation for prevention, whereas more goal-directed interventions are indicated for specific nutrient deficiencies. Patients with CP often have weight loss associated with hypermetabolism, and their nutrient intake can be further compromised by abdominal pain, malabsorption, and diabetes.[39,40] Jejunal feeding in such patients has been used to improve weight as well as to reduce abdominal pain, GI side effects, and narcotic use.[41]

Oxidative stress has been implicated in the pathophysiology of CP and antioxidant supplementation with selenium, ascorbic acid, β-carotene, α-tocopherol, and methionine has been shown to provide pain relief in patients with CP.[42]

In a randomized, placebo-controlled trial of antioxidants used to treat the pain of CP, although therapy significantly raised blood levels of antioxidants, it did not have any beneficial effect on pain or quality of life of the 92 patients' studied.[43]

These findings refute another RCT of 127 patients with CP who were treated with antioxidant supplementation that found 32% of patients became pain free in the antioxidant group compared with 13% in the placebo group.[42] There was also a reduction in the number of painful days per month as well as the number of analgesic tablets used per month.[42] It should be noted that in this study, the mean patient age was 30 years and only slightly over a quarter had alcohol as the etiology for CP. Taken altogether, it would seem that elderly patients with alcohol as the etiology for their CP are less likely to benefit from antioxidant therapy than younger patients with a nonalcoholic etiology. Patients with CP should consume small, frequent meals and avoid foods that are difficult to digest (e.g., legumes). Fat restriction is no longer recommended. In patients with weight loss, medium-chain triglycerides (MCTs) may be useful to provide extra calories without causing steatorrhea. MCTs have no taste or smell, however, may be poorly tolerated because they can cause cramps, nausea, and diarrhea.[39,44] Fat-soluble vitamins, vitamin B_{12}, and calcium should be replaced as clinically indicated. A recent metanalysis of RCTs showed no significant pain reduction or change in quality of life in CP patients with use of antioxidants. However, further studies may identify a subgroup where they are more useful.[45]

Crohn Disease

CD (see Chapter 115) may be associated with malnutrition secondary to anorexia, malabsorption, increased intestinal losses, and the catabolic effects of systemic inflammation.[46] Deficiencies of magnesium, selenium, potassium, zinc, iron, and vitamin B_{12} are common.[47] Vitamin D deficiency is seen in about 50% of patients with CD. Besides a role in osteoporosis, vitamin D has also been implicated in the pathogenesis of CD, as it may downregulate TNF-α-related genes.[48–51] Although dietary therapy in IBD [with such commercial diets as the Colitis 5-Step, Atkins, South Beach, Specific Carbohydrate, CD exclusion diet (CDED), or the Maker's Diet] has been proposed to help reduce symptoms, few well-designed placebo-controlled studies exist. The use of EN, however, is an important component of IBD therapy for patients who cannot eat. RCTs in Asia comparing whole-day or half-day use of oral enteral formulas versus ad lib oral diets have shown significant improvement in IBD symptoms with EN.[52]

ESPEN 2020 guideline emphasized that here is no "IBD diet" that can be generally recommended to promote remission in IBD patients with active disease.[53] Although glucocorticoid therapy has been shown to be more effective than EN for inducing clinical remission of CD in adults,[54] EN in children is just as effective as glucocorticoids in inducing clinical remission. An enteral formula with transforming growth factor-β is marketed specifically for IBD, but there is no robust evidence to recommend its use at this time.[55]

CDED is built on the concept that Western diet promotes proinflammatory microbiome and mucosal barrier dysfunction. This diet excludes gluten, dairy products, animal fat, emulsifiers, and canned or processed foods. Dietary therapy involving partial enteral nutrition (PEN) with an exclusion diet seems to lead to high remission rates in early mild-to-moderate luminal CD in children and young adults.[56] An RCT showed that the combination CDED plus PEN induced sustained remission in a significantly higher proportion of patients than exclusive EN and produced changes in the fecal microbiome associated with remission.[57]

Among hospitalized patients with active CD, no significant differences in improvement have been shown in patients randomized to receive EN or PN.[58,59] Use of PN to achieve remission is problematic, as symptoms invariably recur once PN is stopped and an oral diet is resumed. The use of PN in IBD should be restricted to patients who have not responded to medications or in whom EN cannot be delivered. Bowel rest is not necessary to achieve remission in CD. Malnutrition is an independent risk factor for postoperative complications. The ESPEN 2020 guideline recommends the Enhanced Recovery After Surgery protocol for use in elective surgeries and additional nutrition in the form of EN or PN for optimization of postoperative outcomes in emergency settings.[60] There are a paucity of high-quality studies, however, that specifically address the issue of nutritional support to prevent postoperative complications in CD patients. One meta-analysis showed that CD patients who received preoperative EN or PN were 74% less likely to have postoperative complications compared with standard of care without EN or PN (20.0% vs. 61.3%, respectively).[61] A separate metaanalysis showed that in selected patients, preoperative PN resulted in improved nutritional status, fewer postoperative complications, and reduced disease severity.[62]

Eosinophilic Esophagitis

Dietary therapy for eosinophilic esophagitis is aimed at avoiding the potential allergens in food. An allergy testing guided diet has been tried with variable results with data limited to single-arm observational studies. Therefore diet limitation based on IgE mediated testing is not currently recommended.[63]

Elemental diet is efficacious with histologic and clinical response but difficult to adhere to and maintain.[64,65] Elimination diet involves avoiding common food triggers. Six food elimination diet (SFED) simultaneously, empirically eliminates six most common food groups: wheat, dairy/cow's milk, egg, nuts, soy, and seafood/shellfish.[66] The diet involves eliminating the six aforementioned foods for 6–8 weeks followed by endoscopy with biopsies. If successful, reintroduce 1–2 food groups in 6–8-week intervals followed by an endoscopy each time. The diet is costly and time consuming, and thus limited to highly motivated patients despite its efficacy. There are variations to the SFED like a single food elimination diet, a two food elimination diet, a four food elimination diet, and a step-up diet.[67,68]

Liver Disease

Malnutrition is common in advanced liver disease patients, with a prevalence of 50%–90% in those with cirrhosis, depending on the methods used for nutritional assessment.[69] Malnutrition leads to more complications (e.g., ascites and hepatorenal syndrome) and has been shown to be an independent predictor of survival. Among patients with cirrhosis and portal hypertension who are malnourished, the crude in-hospital mortality rate is 14.1%, compared with 7.5% in those who are not malnourished.[70,71] Malnutrition is one of the factors, if not the most important, contributing to frailty and sarcopenia. Frailty is common in patients with liver cirrhosis and is associated with a higher mortality irrespective of other cirrhosis-related complications.[72] Among patients with cirrhosis in the ambulatory setting, the reported prevalence of frailty has ranged from 17% to 43%.[73–75] Among hospitalized patients with cirrhosis, the prevalence of frailty is as high as 38% for inpatients with hepatic encephalopathy (HE) (and 18% for those without HE) when measured as disability using the ADL tool.[76,77] Sarcopenia is also common in adults with cirrhosis, affecting 30%–70% of patients with end-stage liver disease.[78]

Nutritional deficiencies among patients with liver disease result from many different factors acting in combination: malabsorption, altered metabolism, decreased nutrient storage, increased nutrient requirements, and decreased dietary intake resulting from anorexia, altered taste, and dietary restrictions. The etiology of anorexia is multifactorial and includes mechanical compression of the stomach by ascites as well as alterations in inflammatory and appetite mediators (e.g., increases in TNF-α and leptin).[69] Patients with cirrhosis have been found to have dysgeusia, which can result from magnesium and/or zinc deficiency.[79] Restriction of dietary sodium and protein (though not recommended) to manage ascites and HE, respectively, can further lead to reduced food variety and poor oral intake. In addition, patients with alcoholic cirrhosis often substitute alcohol for nutrient-rich foods. Decreased bile salt production results in an intolerance to high-fat foods and the development of fat-soluble vitamin malabsorption, especially in patients with cholestatic liver disease. Nutrient absorption may be further compromised by hypoalbuminemia, which results in edema of the small intestine. Moreover, some patients with alcoholic cirrhosis have CP, with a resultant maldigestion of protein and fats.

Portosystemic shunting can cause nutrients to bypass the liver, preventing them from being metabolized. Gluconeogenesis and protein catabolism are upregulated, glycogenolysis is downregulated, and insulin resistance occurs, leading to a depletion of muscle mass and fat mass because of their use as energy sources. Patients with cirrhosis have increased protein needs, and limiting their protein intake to prevent HE will only further accelerate protein-calorie malnutrition.[69] It has been shown that diets with a normal protein intake are well tolerated and do not worsen HE (see Chapter 96).[80] Patients should be fed according to their protein needs, and portosystemic encephalopathy treated with medications if it develops. Despite the high prevalence of insulin resistance among cirrhotic patients, carbohydrate restriction is not recommended to prevent the hypoglycemia associated with impaired glycogen synthesis and hepatic stores. The branched-chain amino acids (BCAAs) valine, leucine, and isoleucine are used preferentially as a protein source by patients in liver failure because they are metabolized by the muscle, kidney, adipose, and brain tissue. In contrast, the aromatic amino acids (AAAs) tyrosine, phenylalanine, and methionine are metabolized and deaminated solely by the liver. Normal serum AA concentrations are altered in cirrhosis, with a rise in AAAs and a fall in BCAAs. It is postulated that the rise in concentration of AAAs precipitates HE because they act as false neurotransmitters. In the past, BCAA supplementation has been shown to reduce hyperammonemia, because the metabolism of BCAAs by skeletal muscle supplies carbon skeletons for the formation of α-ketoglutarate, which combines with two ammonia molecules to become glutamine.[69,81] Newer guidelines suggest that use of a formulation enriched in BCAAs should not be expected to improve patient outcomes compared with standard whole-protein formulations in critically ill patients with liver disease. Outpatient RCTs suggest that long-term nutrition supplementation with oral BCAA granules may be useful in slowing progression of hepatic disease and prolonging event-free survival.[82–84] Patients with HE already receiving antibiotics and lactulose derive no further improvement in outcome (mental status or coma grade) by adding BCAAs to their therapy.[82–84]

Micronutrient deficiencies can occur in patients with cirrhosis. Water-soluble vitamin (vitamin B complex and C) deficiencies can occur in both alcohol-associated and nonalcohol-associated liver disease. Thiamine deficiency can lead to Wernicke encephalopathy and Korsakoff dementia, not only in alcoholics, but also in patients with HCV-related cirrhosis. As a result, thiamine supplementation is recommended in all patients with cirrhosis.[85] Decreased levels of folate and vitamin B_6 have been reported in HCV infection.[69] Fat-soluble vitamin deficiencies occur more frequently with cholestatic than parenchymal liver disease. Vitamin A deficiency has been reported in cirrhosis and is considered a risk factor for cancer, including HCC.[85] Vitamin D levels are low in patients with liver disease and fall as liver disease progresses,[86–88] as a result of which there is a high prevalence of osteoporosis in both cholestatic and noncholestatic liver diseases. Use of immunosuppressives, including glucocorticoids, as part of the treatment regimen for autoimmune hepatitis and following liver transplantation increases the risk for metabolic bone disease. Other risk factors for osteoporosis in patients with chronic liver disease (CLD) include advanced age, low BMI, hypogonadism, estrogen deficiency, low calcium intake, excessive alcohol use, tobacco use, and physical inactivity.[89] Vitamin E deficiency has been reported in both cholestatic and alcohol-associated liver disease, and low levels may facilitate progression of fatty liver to steatohepatitis. Zinc deficiency is also associated with liver disease, especially alcohol-associated liver disease, and may lead to anorexia, altered taste and smell, immune dysfunction, altered protein metabolism,[90] HE, and impaired glucose tolerance. Zinc supplementation improves glucose metabolism, but data for improvement in HE are conflicting.[85] Because copper and manganese are excreted into bile, these trace elements should be decreased or omitted from PN formulas in patients with cirrhosis or cholestatic liver disease.[90]

Coffee consumption has been linked with lower rates of both CLD and adverse clinical outcomes. A large observational study showed compared to noncoffee drinkers, coffee drinkers of any type had lower adjusted HRs of CLD (HR 0.79, 95% CI, 0.72–0.86), CLD or steatosis (HR 0.80, 95% CI, 0.75–0.86), death from CLD (HR 0.51, 95% CI, 0.39–0.67), and HCC (HR 0.80, 95% CI, 0.54–1.19).[91]

EN is preferred over PN in patients with cirrhosis who require nutritional support, because liver function can worsen, and patients with ascites may not be able to tolerate the large fluid volumes associated with PN.[85] Excess dextrose and glucose can lead to steatosis, and patients receiving long-term PN can develop cholestasis, fibrosis, and cirrhosis.[90] There is an increased risk for catheter sepsis secondary to immune dysfunction and increased intestinal permeability.[92,93] Lack of liver glycogen stores and reduced capacity for gluconeogenesis can lead to hypoglycemia and reductions in lean body mass during prolonged NPO periods. For these reasons, cirrhotic patients should not go more than 3 hours without eating, and a bedtime snack should be ingested. Patients with liver disease complicated by severe malnutrition have been shown to have more infections, longer ICU stays, and longer hospitalizations after liver transplantation, but there currently are no RCTs to show that preoperative nutritional support improves clinical outcomes of liver transplantation.[94,95] Early postoperative EN has been shown to reduce the incidence of sepsis, and postoperative PN has been shown to reduce the length of ICU stay.[96,97] Two randomized studies using a symbiotic (prebiotic and probiotic) regimen given enterally after liver transplantation have shown a reduction in bacterial infections.[98,99]

Diverticular Disease

Patients with diverticular disease (see Chapter 123) are often provided with incorrect nutritional information. Patients are told to avoid nuts, corn or foods/fruits that contain seeds because of fear that the hard, small particles may lodge in a diverticulum and precipitate diverticulitis, despite evidence showing no harm.[100–102]

Identified risk factors for incident diverticulitis fall into several broad categories—diet, lifestyle, medications, and genetics.[103] A prudent dietary pattern (high in fiber from fruits, vegetables, whole grains and legumes and low in red meat and sweets) and a vegetarian diet are associated with decreased risk of incident diverticulitis.[104] A number of previous retrospective and epidemiologic studies have suggested benefit from fiber in preventing symptomatic diverticular disease, but no well-designed RCTs support this practice.[105] Fiber intake should be at least 25 g/day and provided as insoluble fiber, such as that contained in wheat bran, bran muffins, and fiber-based cereals. A fiber supplement is not a replacement for a high-quality diet. The use of probiotics has had some success in treating and preventing diverticulitis.[106] The most frequently investigated probiotics studied to date have been different strains of Lactobacilli. A systematic review of 11 studies on probiotics in the treatment of diverticular disease showed regression or reduction of symptoms in a majority of the 764 patients evaluated.[108] However, high-quality data on the prevention of complications and recurrence are scant and currently the AGA guidelines recommend against the use of probiotics after uncomplicated diverticulitis.[108] There is insufficient evidence to support the use of any probiotic or cyclic rifaximin to prevent diverticulitis.[109,110] Obesity and physical inactivity have been shown to increase risk of symptomatic diverticular disease in both men and women.[111–114]

Dumping Syndrome

Dumping syndrome, which occurs when food passes too rapidly into the small intestine, can occur after gastrectomy, vagotomy, or esophageal surgery, and is increasingly being seen with the growing popularity of bariatric surgery (see Chapter 9). Two types of dumping syndrome are recognized. *Early dumping syndrome* occurs within 30 minutes of a meal and is characterized by abdominal pain, diarrhea, borborygmi, bloating, nausea, and vasomotor symptoms including flushing, sweating, tachycardia, hypotension, and syncope. This syndrome results from shifting of fluids out of the intravascular space and into the hyperosmolar environment of the duodenal lumen, as well as from enhanced release of GI hormones caused by a high carbohydrate load entering the small intestine. These hormones, including enteroglucagon, pancreatic polypeptide, peptide YY, vasoactive intestinal polypeptide, and neurotensin, have been implicated in the etiology of the vasomotor symptoms by causing systemic and splanchnic vasodilation.[115,116] *Late dumping syndrome* occurs 1–3 hours after a meal and is characterized by hypoglycemia, sweating, hunger, fatigue, and syncope and is thought to be related to hypoglycemia from the rapid (earlier) increase in insulin via GLP-1 in response to the excessive carbohydrate load in the jejunum. Dumping syndrome is diagnosed by clinical assessment and a modified oral glucose tolerance test.[115] Nutritional therapy for dumping syndrome is described later in this chapter.

Cancer

Protein-calorie malnutrition is a common problem for cancer patients. At presentation, the frequency of weight loss associated with cancer varies based on tumor type: 31%–40% in patients with sarcomas, breast, and hematologic cancers; 54%–64% in patients with colon, prostate, and lung cancers; and over 80% in patients with pancreatic and gastric cancers.[117] Malnutrition is not only affected by the type of cancer, but also by the specific antitumor therapy regimen and patient characteristics (age, gender, and comorbidities such as diabetes and GI disorders).[118] Malnutrition has been associated with reduced effectiveness of anticancer therapies, leading to longer duration of treatment and hospital stays, increased cost, and increased morbidity and mortality. The etiology of malnutrition in cancer patients is multifactorial and includes cancer cachexia (which is caused by tumor-induced metabolic abnormalities), impaired caloric intake, maldigestion, malabsorption, and GI toxicity from the cancer therapies themselves. Important mediators of cancer cachexia are thought to include proteolysis-inducing factor and lipid-mobilizing factor, which are produced by tumors, as well as alterations in the balance of neurohormones like neuropeptide Y (appetite stimulating) and proopiomelanocortin (anorexigenic stimulating). Proteolysis-inducing factor leads to decreased protein synthesis, increased protein degradation, and an increase in proinflammatory cytokines (interleukin-6 and interleukin-8). Lipid-mobilizing factor has been shown to increase lipolysis, leading to decreased body fat and weight, independent of caloric intake.[119]

Most practitioners start a dietary regimen for cancer patients by modifying the amount of food and pattern of eating (i.e., small, frequent meals), using additional foods or supplements, or changing the formulation of the food (liquids, pureed foods, etc.). Appetite stimulation with glucocorticoids and megestrol acetate has been used successfully in cancer patients with mild malnutrition.[120] Although both agents lead to improved appetite and weight gain, use of megestrol acetate is associated with a higher risk of DVT.[121,122] Routine use of nutritional support in non-malnourished cancer patients who are undergoing chemotherapy, radiation, or surgery is not recommended unless they are unable to ingest or to absorb adequate nutrients for a prolonged period of time, in which case studies have shown an improvement in weight and nitrogen balance, but not survival.[123] EN has been used successfully in patients with head and neck cancer (HNC) to prevent weight loss, reduce hospitalizations, and reduce interruptions in chemotherapy and radiotherapy, although dependence on PEG feedings may delay return of swallowing function and PO intake. Routine use of PN during chemotherapy has not been shown to decrease toxicity, improve tumor response, or decrease mortality.[123] PN has been found beneficial in patients who have developed severe GI mucositis after bone marrow or hematopoietic stem cell transplantation.[124] In hematopoietic stem cell transplant patients, EN compared with PN is associated with increased morbidity, diarrhea, and hyperglycemia and delayed time to engraftment but less weight and body fat loss.[123] Use of PN support in the cancer patient should be restricted to those patients with a reasonable life expectancy and a sufficient quality of life (Karnofsky score >50), who are not expected to maintain their nutritional needs for a prolonged period (see Chapter 133).

Obesity

Obesity is the second leading cause of preventable death, due to its association with type 2 diabetes, hypertension, coronary artery disease, cerebrovascular disease, obstructive sleep apnea, cancer, osteoarthritis, and depression.[125] Despite abundant adipose tissue, obese critically ill patients should receive early and timely nutrition therapy. Nutritional assessment of critically ill obese patients can be difficult. Current equations to estimate energy expenditure are invalid in this population, so indirect calorimetry remains the gold standard (see Chapter 6). In an obese patient with glucose intolerance or diabetes, the concentrated glucose solution in PN can lead to hyperglycemia, which in critically ill patients has been shown to increase the risk for nosocomial infection, weaken the immune response, delay wound healing, and increase overall mortality. During metabolic stress, protein breakdown leads to gluconeogenesis. Several studies have suggested that high protein hypocaloric feeding [2 g protein/kg ideal body weight (IBW)/day and 65%–70% of caloric requirements], also known as *permissive underfeeding*, is advantageous over standard nutritional regimens because oxidation of endogenous lipid stores supplies the energy source while protein supplementation is used to promote protein anabolism; this approach, however, is still debated. With permissive underfeeding, hyperglycemia is seen less often, and weight loss may occur with maintenance of lean body mass.[125] In critically ill obese patients, the American Society for Parenteral and Enteral Nutrition recommends 11–14 kcal/kg actual body weight per day for BMI 30–50 and 22–25 kcal/kg IBW/day for BMI greater than 50. The recommended dose of protein is 2 g/kg IBW for BMI of 30–40, and 2.5 g/kg IBW for BMI $\geq$ 40.[92]

The United States Preventive Service Task Force recommends that all adults be screened for obesity, and those with a BMI of 30 kg/m^2 or higher be offered a referral to intensive multicomponent behavioral interventions. Bariatric surgery is recommended for individuals with a BMI greater than 40 kg/m^2 and for those with a BMI greater than 35 kg/m^2 who have obesity-related comorbidities (see Chapter 8). Micronutrient deficiencies, particularly iron and vitamin D, are commonly present in obese patients and should be corrected preoperatively. After bariatric surgery, patients are sequentially advanced from a clear liquid diet to a solid diet, and postoperative nutritional guidance by a dedicated bariatric dietician is highly encouraged. In patients with Roux-en-Y gastric bypass, limitation in oral intake is necessary because of the small size of the gastric pouch. The shorter the length of the common channel in the Roux-en-Y gastric bypass, the more likely there will be micronutrient and macronutrient deficiencies.[126] The laparoscopic adjustable gastric band, which is least likely to cause nutritional problems, is gradually being phased out because of its high rate of complications requiring removal in greater than 40% of cases. The vertical sleeve gastrectomy is being increasingly utilized because of its less disruptive effect on GI physiology and its effective impact on weight reduction and decreased risk of diabetes. Not only is understanding a patient's postsurgical anatomy important, but also a basic knowledge of the various sites of nutrient absorption is essential to prevent and diagnose nutrient deficiencies (Table 7.1). Postbariatric surgery nutritional deficiencies can be divided into three types: protein-calorie malnutrition, vitamin and mineral deficiencies, and dehydration. Lifelong vitamin supplementation is started shortly after hospital discharge to prevent the development of nutritional deficiencies, which can develop gradually and may take years to manifest.[125]

Deterioration of nutritional status can occur postoperatively for a variety of reasons, including gastrojejunal anastomotic strictures and an excessively long segment of bypassed biliopancreatic limb. Micronutrient deficiencies can lead to anemia (iron, copper, zinc, folate, and vitamins B_{12}, A, and E), metabolic bone disease (calcium, vitamin D), encephalopathy (thiamine), polyneuropathy and myopathy (thiamine, copper, vitamins B_{12} and E), visual disturbance (thiamine, vitamins A and E), and rash (zinc, essential fatty acids, vitamin A) (see Chapter 105).[126] Iron, folate, calcium, and vitamin B_{12} deficiencies can occur after Roux-en-Y gastric bypass. After biliopancreatic diversion, zinc, sodium, chloride, magnesium, and fat-soluble vitamin deficiencies can occur. Dehydration is common after bariatric surgery, especially in warm weather and after vigorous exercise. The patient's ability to drink large amounts of fluid is restricted because of the reduced size of the stomach. Approximately 2 L of fluid intake is usually recommended per day, though the amount can vary depending on the specific patient and his or her daily activity.[125]

TABLE 7.1 Sites of Nutrient Absorption in the Stomach and Small Intestine

Site	Nutrient
Stomach	Water, ethyl alcohol, copper, iodide, fluoride, molybdenum
Duodenum	Calcium, iron, phosphorus, magnesium, copper, selenium, thiamin, riboflavin, niacin, biotin, folate; vitamins A, D, E, K
Jejunum	Dipeptides, tripeptides, amino acids, calcium, phosphorus, magnesium, iron, zinc, chromium, manganese, molybdenum, thiamin, riboflavin, niacin, pantothenic acid, biotin, folate; vitamins B_6, C, A, D, E, K
Ileum	Folate, magnesium; vitamins B_{12}, C, D

Data from Kaafarani HM, Shikora SA. Nutritional support of the obese and critically ill obese patient. *Surg Clin North Am*. 2011;91:837–855, viii–ix, Ret with permission.

For those not meeting criteria to undergo bariatric surgery or with an unsatisfactory response to lifestyle changes, pharmacotherapy is an option. According to the 2013 joint guidelines from the American College of Cardiology, the American Heart Association, and the Obesity Society for the management of overweight and obesity in adults, and the Endocrine Society's clinical practice guidelines on the pharmacologic management of obesity, pharmacotherapy for obesity should be considered if patients have a BMI of $\geq$30 kg/m^2 or a BMI of $\geq$27 kg/m^2 with weight-related comorbidities, such as hypertension, dyslipidemia, type 2 diabetes, or obstructive sleep apnea.[127,128] There are five main antiobesity medications (AOMs) for long-term use: semaglutide 2.4 mg, liraglutide 3.0 mg, phentermine-topiramate ER and naltrexone-bupropion ER and orlistat (see Chapter 8).

In November 2022 the AGA issued a new clinical practice guideline on pharmacological interventions for adults with obesity.[43] Authors developed this guideline in response to the underuse of AOMs relative to mounting evidence from RCTs for the agents' efficacy and to the increasing prevalence of obesity and related health conditions. In particular, the guideline advances those evidence-based recommendations from the ACC/AHA/TOS, the AACE/ACE, and the Endocrine Society. In obese or overweight adults who have an inadequate response to lifestyle interventions alone, long-term pharmacological therapy is recommended, with multiple effective and safe treatment options. The AGA recommends four drugs—semaglutide 2.4 mg, liraglutide 3.0 mg, phentermine-topiramate ER and naltrexone-bupropion ER—approved for long-term use were deemed to have a moderate or large magnitude of weight loss and small or notsubstantial harms, and hence a balance favoring their utilization. Furthermore, each of the four drugs used adjunctively with lifestyle interventions is likely to result in a high proportion of patients achieving 5% and 10% TBWL, which has a significant favorable effect on long-term health outcomes.[129] Orlistat is recommended by AACE/ACE as well.[130,131] Four drugs are currently available in the United States for short-term weight loss: phentermine, benzphetamine, diethylpropion, and phendimetrazine.

Phentermine has a relatively low cost and a low addiction potential and has shown efficacy and safety, and is thus widely prescribed. It is a schedule IV-controlled substance and classified as an adrenergic agonist that functions to increase resting energy expenditure and suppress appetite. As monotherapy, it is indicated for short-term use (3 months), as there are no long-term safety trials. When combined with topiramate ER, phentermine may be used long term. Orlistat promotes weight loss via an inhibition of pancreatic and gastric lipases, thus preventing the absorption of fat. Orlistat also has the added benefit of lowering serum glucose and improving insulin sensitivity.[132] Two agents—bupropion (a dopamine and norepinephrine reuptake inhibitor) and naltrexone (an opioid antagonist)—were FDA approved separately for the treatment of opioid dependence and alcohol use disorder. Together, naltrexone/bupropion affects the arcuate nucleus of the hypothalamus and the mesolimbic dopamine reward circuit, acting to regulate appetite and food cravings. Liraglutide was approved by the FDA for chronic weight management and treatment of type 2 diabetes. It mimics GLP-1, which is released in response to food intake, and acts to reduce hunger, decrease food intake, and delay gastric emptying.[133] In June 2021 the FDA approved semaglutide injection 2.4 mg subcutaneously once weekly as an adjunct to a reduced calorie diet and increased physical activity for chronic weight management in patients with a BMI of at least 27 kg/m^2 who have at least 1 weight-related complication or a BMI of at least 30 kg/m^2.[129]

The FDA is expected to approve another GIP1 agonist, Tirzepatide, which provided substantial and sustained reductions in body weight in a 72-week trial in participants with obesity. The mean percentage change in weight at Week 72 was −15.0% (95% CI, −15.9 to −14.2) with 5-mg weekly doses of tirzepatide, −19.5% (95% CI, −20.4 to −18.5) with 10-mg doses, and −20.9% (95% CI, −21.8 to −19.9) with 15-mg doses and −3.1% (95% CI, −4.3 to −1.9) with placebo ($P < .001$ for all comparisons with placebo).[134]

Critical Illness

Determination of nutritional risk in critically ill patients is important, as it emphasizes the fact that risk from a nutritional standpoint is twofolds, driven both by deteriorating nutritional status and disease severity. While patients with higher nutritional risk tend to have greater degrees of GI intolerance resulting in more difficulty in complying with the prescribed EN regimen, they are more likely to show improved outcomes from nutritional interventions than those with lower nutritional risk. American Society for Parenteral and Enteral Nutrition guidelines for nutritional therapy in the critically ill adult patient recommend that all patients admitted to the ICU undergo an initial nutritional risk screening. While the concept of nutritional risk is very important, use of the tools to determine such risk (the Nutritional Risk Screening 2002 or NRS-2002 and the Nutrition Risk in the Critically Ill or NUTRIC Score) is problematic. Patients determined to be at high nutritional risk (NRS-2002 >5 or NUTRIC score ≥5) should have EN started early within 24–36 hours of admission to the ICU. Advancement to goal should take 3–4 days to minimize the chance for overfeeding, as exogenous feeds are additive to endogenous gluconeogenesis by the liver; GI intolerance is monitored; electrolytes are scrutinized for evidence of refeeding syndrome; hypotensive patients on vasopressive agents are stabilized; and the process of autophagy is supported.[135,136] Getting to the protein goal sooner (1.2–2.0 g/kg/day) is more important than getting to the caloric goal (20–25 kcal/kg/day). Efforts to provide a goal of approximately 80% of estimated or calculated goal energy requirements should be made to achieve the clinical benefit of EN over the first week of hospitalization while avoiding risk of overfeeding. Although trophic feeds provide the nonnutritional benefit of feeding by preventing mucosal atrophy and maintaining intestinal integrity in low-to-moderate risk patients, they are insufficient to achieve the usual endpoints sought for EN therapy in high-risk patients. More than 50%−60% of goal energy is required to prevent increases in intestinal permeability and systemic infection in burn and bone-marrow transplant patients,[137] to promote faster return of cognitive function in head injury patients,[138] and to reduce mortality in high-risk hospitalized patients.[139] Likewise, a prospective study of high-risk surgery patients (NRS-2002 ≥5) who received sufficient preoperative nutrition therapy (>10 kcal/kg/day for 7 days) had significant reductions in nosocomial infections and overall complications compared with patients who received insufficient therapy.[140]

Once EN has commenced, patients should be monitored daily for tolerance. Inappropriate interruption of EN should be avoided, with NPO orders surrounding the time of tests and procedures kept to a minimum to avoid propagation of ileus and prevention of inadequate nutrient delivery. Gastric residual volumes (GRVs) should not be used as part of routine care to monitor ICU patients on EN, as GRVs do not correlate with the incidence of pneumonia, regurgitation, or aspiration, and are a poor surrogate marker for gastric emptying. EN protocols should be designed and implemented to increase the overall percentage of goal calories provided, with consideration for a volume-based feeding protocol to clearly define the daily goal volume of EN to be infused. Appropriate adjustments to protocol should be made in the setting of hemodynamic compromise or instability. In this scenario, EN should be withheld if vasopressive therapy is being initiated. Initiation or re-initiation of EN may be considered with caution once the patient is fully resuscitated and stable for 24–36 hours and pressor support has begun to be withdrawn. Critically ill patients are at increased risk for subclinical ischemia/reperfusion injury to the intestine, but data show that ischemic bowel is a very rare complication of EN, and that patients on stable low doses of vasopressors or even multiple vasopressors had lower ICU and hospital mortalities when EN was used than when it was withheld.[141]

In patients at low nutritional risk, PN should not be used until after the first 7 days following ICU admission if the patient cannot maintain volitional intake and early EN is not feasible.[92] If EN is not feasible in patients at high nutritional risk, it is appropriate to initiate PN as soon as possible after hospital admission, once resuscitation has been performed.[92,142] In any critically ill patient, regardless of risk, who is already on EN tube feeding but receiving less than 60% of the prescribed goal regimen, addition of supplemental PN should be withheld until after 7days from admission. This was a strong recommendation of ASPEN's 2021 guideline on critical illness nutrition.[136] As tolerance to EN improves, the amount of PN energy should be reduced and finally discontinued when the patient is receiving more than 60% of target energy requirements from EN.

In all ICU patients who require PN, high protein hypocaloric PN should be considered initially over the first week, with provision of 80% of energy requirements (20 kcal/kg actual body weight/day). Compared with eucaloric PN, permissive underfeeding has been shown to reduce the incidence of hyperglycemia, infections, ICU and hospital lengths of stay, and duration of mechanical ventilation.[92,143,144]

A recent large (>3000 patients) French multicenter trial titled *Low Versus Standard Calorie and Protein Feeding in Ventilated Adults with Shock: a Randomised, Controlled, Multicentre, Open-label, Parallel-group Trial (NUTRIREA-3)* showed that compared with standard calorie and protein targets, early calorie and protein restriction did not decrease mortality but was associated with faster recovery and fewer complications.[145]

A combination of antioxidant vitamins (including vitamins E and C) and trace minerals (including selenium, zinc, and copper) should be given enterally or parenterally to all critically ill patients receiving nutrition support, as these may reduce mortality for patients with burns, trauma, and critical illness requiring mechanical ventilation.[92,142]

NUTRITIONAL THERAPY

Enteral Nutrition

EN supports both the structural and functional integrity of the GI tract. EN sustains structural integrity by maintaining mucosal mass and villus height, stimulating epithelial cell proliferation, promoting the production of brush-border enzymes, and maintaining the secretory immunoglobulin (Ig)A-producing immunocytes, which make up the gut-associated lymphoid tissue. EN also maintains the functional integrity of the GI tract by maintaining tight junctions between the intraepithelial cells, sustaining a thick mucus layer, stimulating blood flow, and inducing the production and release of various trophic endogenous agents, including gastrin, CCK, bombesin, and bile salts. The provision of EN supports the role of the commensal microbiome and helps prevent the emergence of a virulent pathobiome in response to critical illness.[146]

In those patients who will not or cannot eat because of some dysfunction of the GI tract, a feeding tube is necessary to provide EN. The radiologist, gastroenterologist, or surgeon usually places these enteral access devices. This can be done at the bedside, fluoroscopically, endoscopically, or in the operating room, depending on the specific device and the expertise available.[147]

Nasoenteric Tube Access

The use of small bowel feedings to prevent tube-feeding aspiration events is a complicated and contentious issue. Small bowel feeding is recommended for critically ill patients determined to be at high risk of aspiration or those shown to be intolerant to gastric feeding.[92,148] Bedside nasoenteric tube (NET) placement (Fig. 7.1) is the most common enteral access technique used in the hospital and long-term care environments. Use of a commercial tube with an electromagnetic GPS imaging system greatly facilitates postpyloric placement of an NET. Alternatively, the endoscopic over-the-guidewire NET (ENET) technique can be used when placement under direct visualization is desired (Fig. 7.2). A bridle can be used to secure the ENET once it is placed (Fig. 7.3). For bedside NET placement, typically, an 8–12 Fr NG tube is lubricated and passed into the stomach with the patient's head flexed; the patient ingests sips of water to assist in passage of the tube.[149] Bedside auscultation to confirm proper position of the NG tube is problematic, and with the exception of those patients in whom tube placement was achieved using the electromagnetic GPS imaging system, every patient should have a bedside plain film to confirm proper positioning of the NG or NJ tube before initiating feedings; patient's mental status does not change this recommendation. Surprisingly, the success rate for spontaneous small bowel placement is greater for unweighted than weighted feeding tubes when placement is at the bedside (92% vs. 56%), and, in fact, the weighted tip may actually be an impediment to the tube's spontaneous passage.[150]

NJ feeding tubes can be placed endoscopically at the bedside with the patient moderately sedated. In the "drag-and-pull" method, a suture is attached to the end of an NJ tube and used to drag the tube into position in the small intestine with a grasping forceps. Because it is often difficult to release the suture from the grasping forceps, and also to remove the endoscope without removing the adjacent NJ tube, a hemoclip can be used to drag the tube and then clip it to the small intestine. A second common technique, the "over-the-guidewire" technique, requires the use of a 5-mm neonatal gastroscope passed through the nares to place a guidewire into the small intestine. The endoscope is removed, and the guidewire is left in place. A feeding tube is then passed over the guidewire and into position in the small intestine, with a success rate of 90%–100%.[151–153] A similar version of this technique uses a pediatric colonoscope passed through the mouth down into the small bowel. A guidewire is passed out into the bowel lumen, the scope is withdrawn, and the wire transferred out through the nose before final placement of the tube over the wire.[154,155]

NETs should be used in patients who will require EN via NG or NJ access for less than 1 month. Patients who have experienced repeated early failure to keep NETs in place or those anticipated to require a longer duration of feeding beyond 1 month should receive more durable enteral access, such as a PEG, direct percutaneous endoscopic jejunostomy (DPEJ), a combination percutaneous endoscopic gastrojejunostomy (PEGJ), surgical gastrostomy, or surgical jejunostomy.

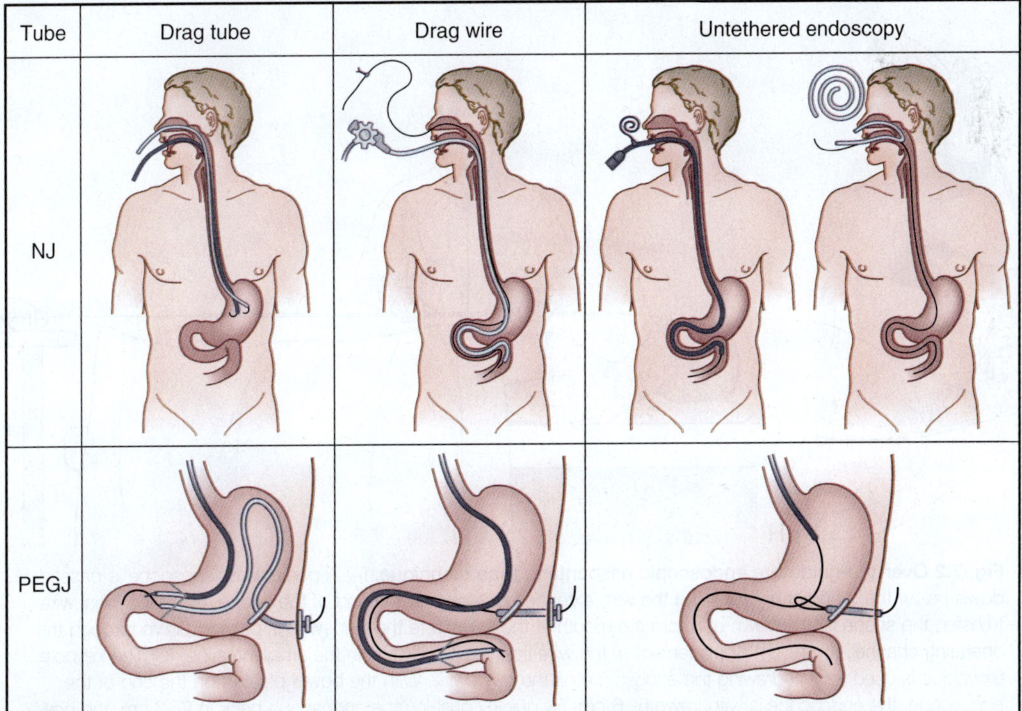

Fig. 7.1 Prioritizing techniques for enteral access. Dragging a tube into place increases the chance for proximal displacement when the scope is withdrawn. Dragging a wire is better, but torsion on the wire still impedes endoscopy. "Untethered" endoscopy technique allows placement of a wire and then delivery of the tube over the wire directly into the small intestine without the need to drag either into place using the endoscope. *NJ*, Nasojejunal; *PEGJ*, percutaneous endoscopic gastrojejunostomy. (*Source*: Reprinted with permission from Chandrasekhara V, Kochman M. *Techniques in Gastrointestinal Endoscopy*. Elsevier.)

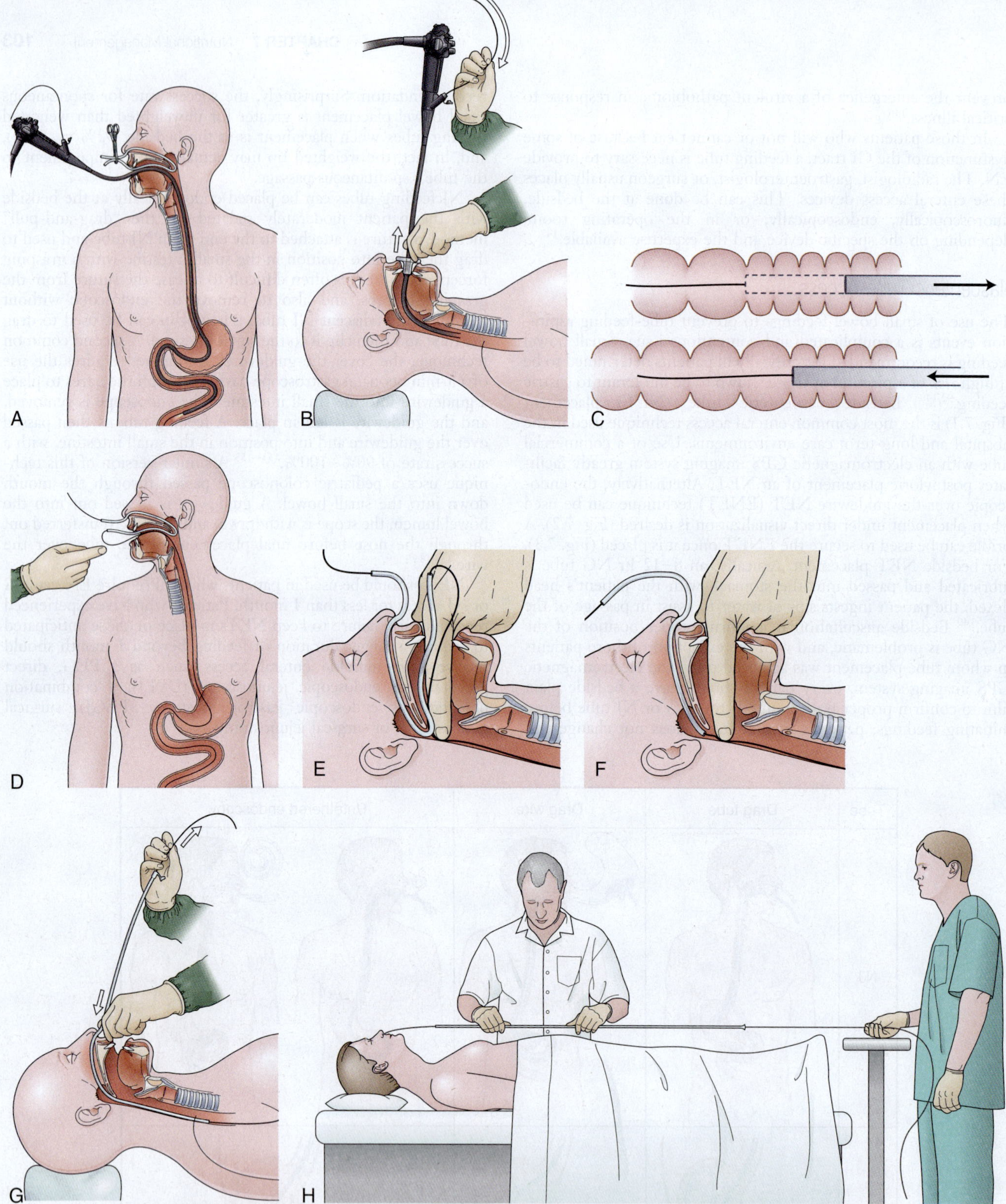

Fig. 7.2 Over-the-guidewire endoscopic nasoenteric tube technique. (A) A pediatric colonoscope is passed down below the ligament of Treitz and the wire extended out beyond the end of the scope. (B) In the initial wire transfer, the scope is withdrawn out from the mouth at the same rate the guidewire is passed down through the operating channel, to prevent displacement of the wire tip from its position in the small intestine. (C) The keyhole technique is used for withdrawing the endoscope off the guidewire. With the bowel pleated on the end of the endoscope, the endoscope is withdrawn 5–6 cm. By quickly pushing the endoscope back in 2–3 cm, the bowel comes off the endoscope one to two folds at a time. (D) With the wire protruding out through the mouth, the tip of the wire is then passed through the oronasal transfer tube. (E and F) The index finger is then used to pin the wire against the posterior pharyngeal wall while traction is placed on the wire protruding out through the nose, pulling on the wire until the wire is straight and tension is felt against the finger in the posterior pharynx. (G) In one technique for the final wire transfer, the feeding tube is passed over the wire down through the nares at the exact same rate that the wire is withdrawn out from the distal end of the feeding tube, again to avoid displacing the wire tip. (H) In an alternative technique for the final wire transfer, an assistant pins the wire to a "point in space" (using a bedside table), and the tube is then slid over the fixed wire into final position. (*Source*: Reprinted with permission from Chandrasekhara V, Kochman M. *Techniques in Gastrointestinal Endoscopy*. Elsevier.)

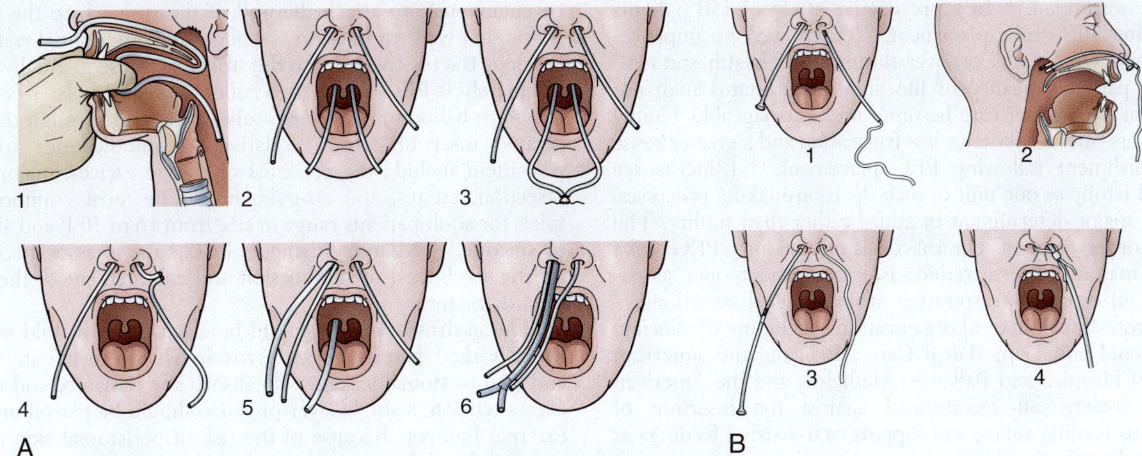

Fig. 7.3 Bridle technique for securing endoscopic nasoenteric tube. (A) Using two 5-Fr neonatal feeding tubes or (B) a commercial devising using 2 flexible sticks with magnetic ends. (*Source*: Reprinted with permission from Chandrasekhara V, Kochman M. *Techniques in Gastrointestinal Endoscopy*. Elsevier.)

Percutaneous Endoscopic Enteral Access

Insertion of a percutaneous enteral access tube usually requires the use of moderate or deep sedation and can be performed in the endoscopy suite, in the operating room, or at the bedside. In comparison to nasoenteric access, percutaneous enteral access has been shown to be more reliable, allowing patients to receive more calories daily because of a reduction in tube dysfunction.[156]

Indications for Percutaneous Access Devices

Percutaneous access devices, such as a PEG, are indicated for patients who will be unable to maintain sufficient nutritional intake for more than 1 month, despite a functional GI tract. While certain patient populations such as those patients with a stroke may see tremendous benefit from PEG placement as a bridge to return of swallowing function and oral intake, in other populations such as patients with advanced dementia or end-stage malignancy, benefit is more limited.[157–162] In high-risk patients, a high mortality after PEG is usually not a result of the procedure itself, but a reflection of the patient's comorbidities and moribund status. In addition to providing access for nutrition, PEG tubes may be placed for hydration and administration of medications as well as for gastric decompression. Some of the more common medical indications for PEG placement are described below.

Cancer

Patients with HNC are at high risk for malnutrition stemming from dysphagia from the tumor itself or from required antitumor therapies. Approximately 50% of patients with HNC require alternative means of nutritional support.[163] EN support via PEG has been shown to reduce the number of hospitalizations required from dehydration and malnutrition, prevent weight loss, and avoid treatment interruptions.[164] Tumor implantation at the ostomy site from dragging the PEG tube past the exophytic tumor mass is rare. In a retrospective case series of 304 patients receiving PEG tubes for HNC, only two developed stomal-site metastases (0.92%).[165] PEG placement in HNC is controversial only in that return of swallowing function and resumption of oral intake may be delayed by dependence on the PEG feedings. In patients with malignant bowel obstruction, a PEG tube can also be safely and effectively used for intestinal decompression. Such a "venting" PEG obviates the need for an NG tube, relieves symptoms of nausea and vomiting, and can allow end-of-life patients to be discharged from the hospital tolerating some degree of an oral soft diet.[166]

Use of EN or PN in advanced unresectable cancer is controversial. The Karnofsky Performance Scale Index can be used to assess quality of life in individual patients (see Chapter 132). Use of EN or PN may provide improved energy and psychological benefit in cases of advanced unresectable malignancies and should be considered if the patient has a Karnofsky score greater than 50 or if the initiation of either route of nutritional therapy allows the treatment regimen to be completed.[167] Ultimately, treatment strategies should reflect the preferences and values of the patient, as patient autonomy is paramount. The final decision to place a PEG may be based on cultural, personal, family, spiritual, and religious beliefs, and may not always be supported by scientific facts.

Stroke

Data support the use of PEG tubes in patients with stroke-related dysphagia, as a bridge to return of swallowing function and oral intake. A recent large meta-analysis of heterogeneous studies showed a rate of recovery was not uniformly reported and ranged from 30% to 87% in 3 months.[168] Compared with NG feeding, early PEG placement was found to be associated with a lower incidence of ventilator-associated pneumonia.[169] In a Cochrane meta-analysis, PEG feeding compared with NG tube feeding was associated with a reduction in treatment failures, and a higher overall rate of delivery of feeds. Following severe acute stroke, the decision to initiate tube feeding should be weighed based on choice, necessity, and comfort.[170]

Dementia

Despite widespread use, the benefit gained from PEG placement in patients with dementia remains unclear. In a prospective cohort study of more than 36,000 nursing home residents with recent onset of dysphagia, neither insertion of a PEG tube nor the timing of that insertion affected survival.[171] The most common reasons for PEG placement in patients with dementia include reduction in risk of aspiration, maintenance of skin integrity with prevention of pressure sores, improvement in quality of life, and prolongation of survival. The likelihood that these benefits will be achieved by PEG placement is limited. When patients with dementia are changed from hand feeding by staff or family members to PEG tube feeding, they are deprived of taste, touch, nurturing, and social interaction.[172] Over 70% of patients with dementia who have feeding tubes need to be restrained.[159] Risk of developing pressure ulcers in nursing home residents with PEG tube placement may actually increase because of decreased mobility and the need to be restrained.[162] In a prospective study of 150 patients followed after PEG-tube placement, 70% showed no improvement in functional status or overall subjective health status.[173] While the patient's quality of life and health status may not directly improve, his/her care becomes more manageable. Family and caregivers often experience less frustration and a greater sense of accomplishment following PEG placement.[173] Ethicists see patient and family as one unit in such decision-making processes. Justice is a major determinant in ethics rather than futility. The latter is cornerstone of clinical decision-making. PEG tube placement may do little to reduce aspiration pneumonia, as patients are still capable of aspirating oropharyngeal secretions.[174] Multiple professional medical organizations, including the Society for Post-Acute and Long-Term Care Medicine, the American Academy of Hospice and Palliative Medicine, and the American Geriatrics Society, all recommend against the insertion of percutaneous feeding tubes, and support oral-assisted feedings as the preferred method.

Percutaneous Endoscopic Gastrostomy

PEG was developed by Ponsky and Gauderer in the early 1980s.[175] The procedure involves placement of a PEG tube after endoscopic transillumination of the abdominal wall to choose an appropriate gastrostomy site (Fig. 7.4). If there is no transillumination or discreet indentation of a probing finger seen, the procedure should not be performed. The use of prophylactic IV antibiotics before the procedure is important to prevent peristomal infections after the procedure.[176,177] An antibiotic with optimal skin coverage, such as IV cefazolin (1 g), should be administered 30 minutes prior to the procedure.

Placement of a PEG tube can be accomplished by either the Ponsky (Pull) or Sachs-Vine (Push) technique, depending on physician preference, as both are equally effective.[178] A third technique [Russell (Introducer)] may be indicated in cases of an exophytic oropharyngeal or esophageal cancer, recent oropharyngeal incisions from a head and neck surgical procedure, or a tight esophageal stricture that impedes passage of the scope or PEG tube.[179] With the Russell technique, T-fasteners are placed percutaneously to attach the wall of the stomach to the anterior abdominal wall, an incision is made in the abdominal wall, and a fistulous tract is created into the stomach and sequentially dilated. Ultimately, a PEG tube with a balloon internal bolster (similar in design to balloon replacement tubes) is passed through the newly created insertion site.[180] Relative contraindications for PEG placement include the presence of gastric varices, major gastric resection, ascites, and coagulopathy. The most common PEG tubes for adult patients range in size from 16 to 20 F and are made of silicone.[181] A larger diameter PEG tube is associated with a greater likelihood of side torsion and enlargement of the stomal tract diameter.

The gastrostomy site should be cleansed with mild soap and water, rather than hydrogen peroxide which can irritate the skin and lead to stomal leakage. To absorb any moisture and to avoid excess tension, a single layer of gauze should be placed under the external bumper. Because of the risk of peristomal skin maceration and breakdown, occlusive dressings should not be used.

Replacement PEG tubes are broadly divided into two categories, replacement gastrostomy tubes and low-profile devices. Replacement gastrostomy tubes usually have a balloon-type internal bolster (Fig. 7.5). These balloon tubes can be inserted blindly through the gastrostomy site into the gastric lumen. The balloon is inflated to serve as the internal bolster. Because of balloon breakage, the tube often requires replacement within 3–6 months. There are also replacement PEG tubes with a distensible internal bumper. The internal bumper is stretched with a stylet and pushed blindly through the gastrostomy site; the stylet is then removed, allowing the internal bolster to assume its previous shape. Low-profile gastrostomy devices (Fig. 7.6) provide skin-level access to the gastric lumen and may be particularly useful for disoriented patients who may habitually tug at their bedclothes and pull out their tube connections. Low-profile PEG tubes come in predetermined stem lengths, and the gastrostomy tract length must be measured to choose the correct device. To access the low-profile device for feeding or gastric decompression, a separate access tube must be used to engage a valve in the top of the device.

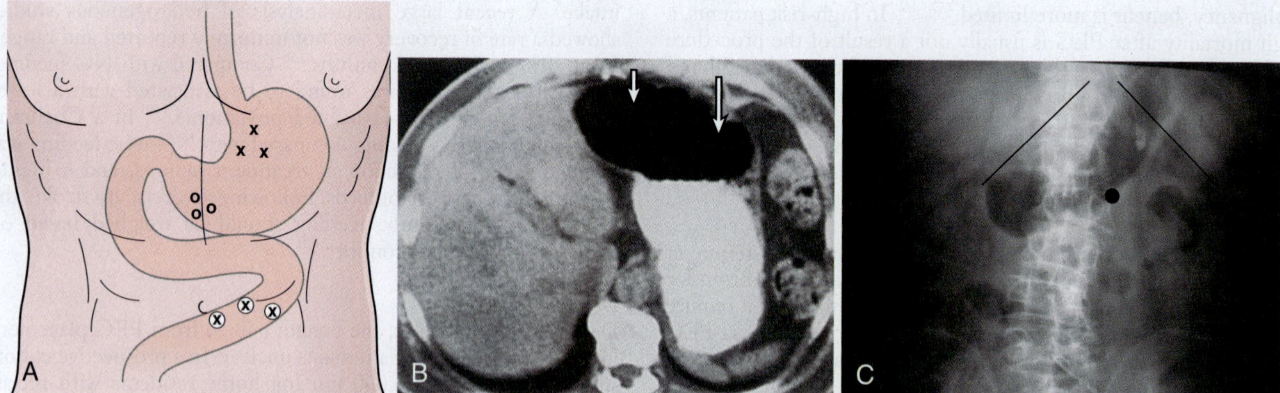

Fig. 7.4 Steps to localize percutaneous endoscopic gastrostomy (PEG), percutaneous endoscopic gastrojejunostomy (PEGJ), and direct percutaneous endoscopic jejunostomy (DPEJ) sites. (A) The traditional PEG site is marked by the *x* in the left upper quadrant. Better placement is above the umbilicus, close to the midline, or slightly to the patient's right of the midline position (*circles*). The PEG then is in the gastric antrum, which is ideal should conversion to a PEGJ be required later. *X with circles* show the tremendous variability in the site for DPEJ placement, which can occur anywhere from the left costal margin down to the left iliac crest. (B) CT scan shows that the PEG site slightly above or to the patient's right of the umbilicus coincides with the area with the most direct, perpendicular, and shortest tract in the gastric antrum. Traditional sites in the LUQ have a longer, more tangential tract into the midbody or even lower fundus. (C) Placing a coin in the umbilicus (*dark circle*) and injecting 500 mL of air through the NG tube before PEG placement helps identify the gastric antrum, easing selection of the PEG site. (*Source*: Reprinted with permission from Chandrasekhara V, Kochman M. *Techniques in Gastrointestinal Endoscopy*. Elsevier.)

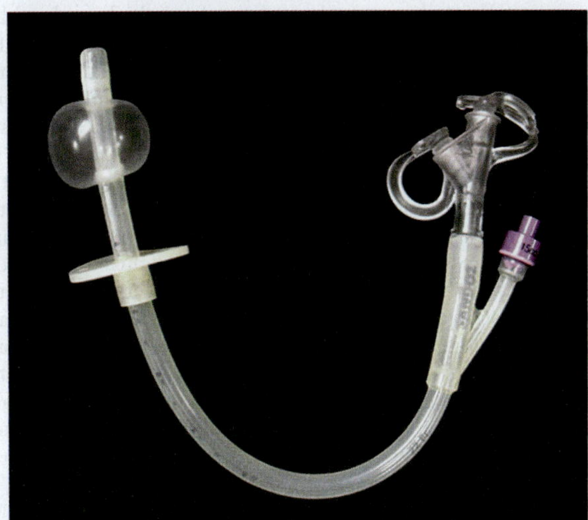

Fig. 7.5 Replacement gastrostomy tube.

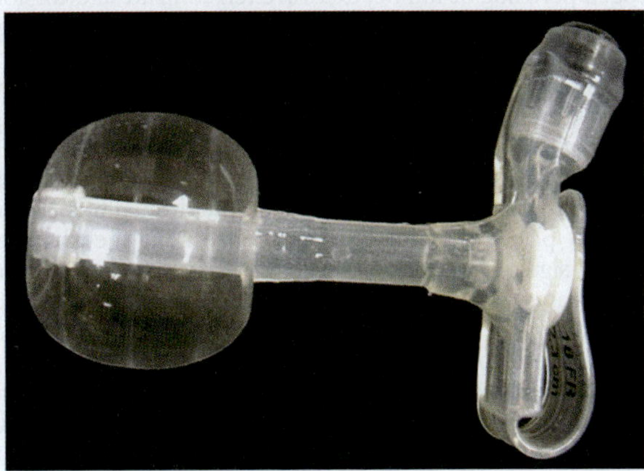

Fig. 7.6 Low-profile percutaneous endoscopic gastrostomy device.

Percutaneous Endoscopic Gastrojejunostomy

For patients for whom small bowel feedings are desired, endoscopic percutaneous access to the small intestine may be obtained by one of two ways. The first way involves a PEGJ, where a PEG is placed in the standard fashion, after which various techniques may be used to place a jejunal feeding tube through the PEG into the small intestine.[151,182,183] The second way involves a direct PEG (DPEJ), where a small diameter gastrostomy tube is placed directly into the proximal jejunum, using a variation of the Ponsky Pull technique.

Three common techniques are used for PEGJ placement. With the Kirby technique (Fig. 7.7), a guidewire passed through the PEG is grabbed by an extralong 320 cm biopsy forceps and dragged down into the proximal jejunum. The scope is withdrawn back to the proximal stomach above the PEG site holding the wire in place with the forceps. A 9 or 12 Fr J-tube is then passed through the existing PEG over the guidewire and into position in the small intestine (Figs. 7.8 and 7.9). The average longevity of this tube system is about 120 days.[182] With the Johlin technique (Fig. 7.10), a wire polypectomy snare is inserted through the gastrostomy tube into the stomach and the endoscope is then passed through the open snare and advanced as far as possible down into the proximal jejunum. A standard 0.035-in flexible-tip guidewire is passed through the endoscopic channel and passed out further into the small bowel. The endoscope is then slowly withdrawn back to the proximal stomach. The guidewire is

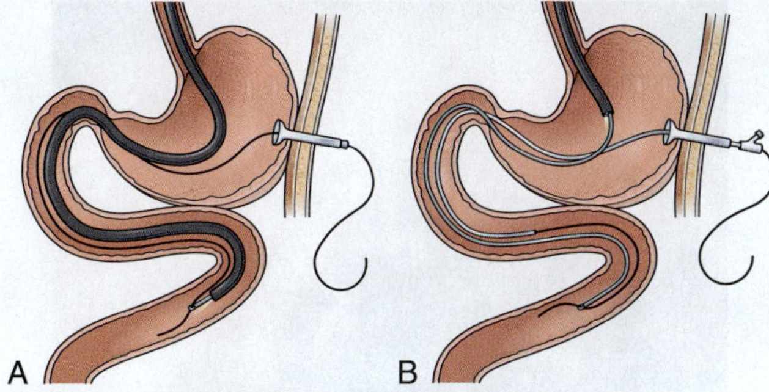

Fig. 7.7 Over-the-guidewire percutaneous endoscopic gastrojejunostomy technique, also known as the Kirby technique. (A) A single-stranded guidewire passed through a valve seated in the percutaneous endoscopic gastrostomy is grasped by a biopsy forceps passed down through a pediatric endoscope. The biopsy forceps is pushed outward through the end of the scope, holding the wire in place below the ligament of Treitz. (B) The endoscope is then withdrawn back into the stomach as the biopsy forceps is pushed outward through the end of the scope, holding the wire in place below the ligament of Treitz. Once the scope has been withdrawn back into the proximal stomach, the jejunal extension tube is passed over the wire until the distal end strikes the biopsy forceps at the end of the wire. (*Source*: Reprinted with permission from Chandrasekhara V, Kochman M. *Techniques in Gastrointestinal Endoscopy*. Elsevier.)

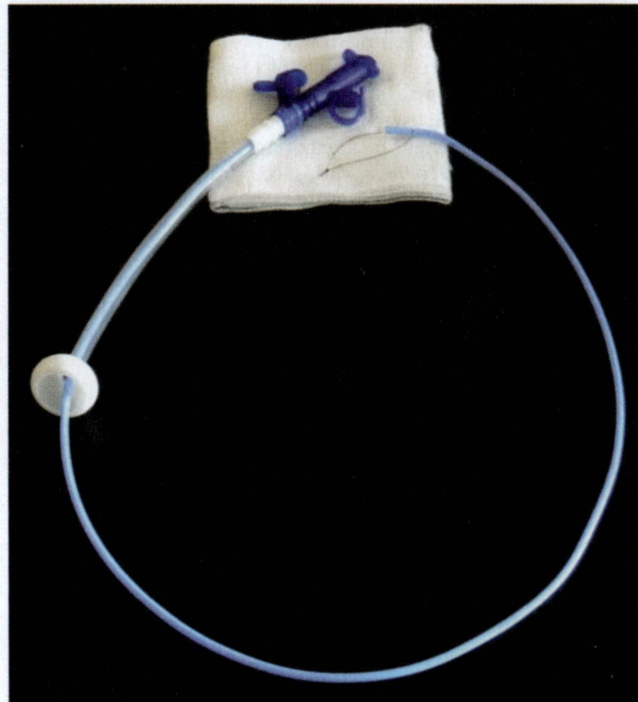

Fig. 7.8 Gastrojejunostomy (or percutaneous endoscopic gastrojejunostomy) feeding tube. A suture at the end of the jejunal feeding tube aids in its placement and can be secured to the jejunal wall using a hemoclip.

withdrawn out through the gastrostomy tube forming a wire loop. Pulling on the end of the wire exiting the endoscope helps determine the proximal end of the wire loop which can then be brought out through the PEG. The J-tube is threaded over the wire until its proximal end is seated in the gastrostomy tube, and the guidewire is then removed. A one-piece PEGJ system is

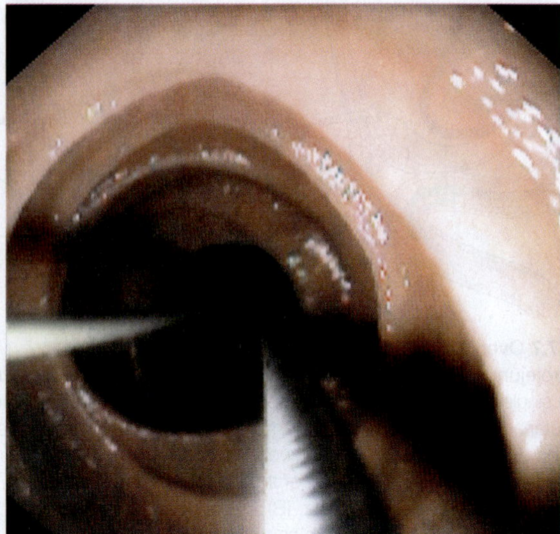

Fig. 7.9 Percutaneous endoscopic gastrojejunostomy showing over-the-guidewire placement technique.

available and generally used as a replacement device passed through a mature stomal tract. This tube can be passed over a guidewire during endoscopy using a variation of the Kirby technique. The internal bolster on this system is a balloon.

Direct Percutaneous Jejunostomy

DPEJ involves the direct placement of a small diameter 14–16 Fr PEG tube into the small intestine using a modified Ponsky Pull technique and a pediatric colonoscope to reach a puncture position beyond the ligament of Treitz (Fig. 7.11). Technical success rates vary from 68% to 98%, with success rates higher in patients with lower BMI or altered surgical anatomy (such as Billroth I and II procedures where the duodenum and proximal jejunum are brought out into the peritoneal space).[184–187] Successful placement is facilitated by having an experienced 2-person team (1 as "scope person", 1 as "skin person"), avoiding insufflation of the stomach, looking for transillumination immediately after passing below the ligament of Treitz, and using a 22-ga spinal needle to puncture the small bowel. Snaring the 22-ga sounding needle helps hold the small bowel in place while the trocar can be passed at the same angle and site. Once the snare is transferred to the trocar, the rest of the procedure is virtually identical to the Ponsky Pull technique for PEG placement. The Sachs-Vine Push and the Russel Introducer techniques should not be used for this procedure. Management of the DPEJ tube is likewise similar to that of PEG tubes.

Complications

Most post-PEG complications arise from a patient's comorbidities, such as poor wound healing, aspiration, or coagulopathy. To reduce the risk of aspiration, caregivers should raise the head of the patient's bed 30–45 degrees during feeding and for 1 hour afterward.[148] One common complication of PEG is peristomal wound infection.[188] Risk factors for peristomal infection include diabetes, obesity, malnutrition, chronic glucocorticoid use, small incisions at the PEG insertion site, lack of antibiotic prophylaxis, and excessive pressure of the external bumper on the PEG site.[189] Excessive tightening of the PEG tube external bolster against the abdominal wall can cause buried bumper syndrome (BBS) (Fig. 7.12), which in turn can lead to mucosal ulceration, bleeding, stomal leakage, peristomal infection, and even necrotizing fasciitis.[190] To minimize the chance for BBS, the external bolster of the PEG tube should be maintained up against the skin (without indentation) for 4 days postplacement, after which it should be carefully moved back 1 cm from the anterior abdominal wall.[190] Peristomal wound infections are often treated for 7 days with an oral antibiotic such as cephalexin to cover skin-related microorganisms. The infected area should also have daily topical cleansing with mild soap and water.

Yeast colonization of the silicone PEG can lead to degradation and loss of tube integrity, requiring timely replacement.[191] Clogged PEG tubes may be cleared by flushing with warm water, soft drinks, or a slurry of pancreatic enzymes mixed in a bicarbonate solution.[192] Mechanical declogging with a wire, specimen brush, endoscopic cleaning brush, or commercially available corkscrew declogging device may be required in some cases. Excessive growth of granulation tissue around the PEG tract represents an exuberant response to the wound injury. Topical silver nitrate can be applied to compress, cauterize, and remove excess granulation tissue at the gastrostomy site.[193]

Other common complications include peristomal leakage, fever, ileus, cutaneous ulceration, and tube dislodgement.[194–196] Leakage around the gastrostomy site is a common and under-recognized problem. Risk factors for peristomal leakage include the use of glucocorticoids, chemotherapy, excessive cleaning with hydrogen peroxide or iodine, excessive tension and side-torsion of the tube, and the absence of an external bumper. Leakage of gastric acid or bile around the PEG tube can cause erythema and skin breakdown that is often mistaken for infection. Treatment includes keeping the site dry with frequent dressing changes, topical zinc oxide, maintaining the external bumper 1 cm from the skin, stabilizing the gastrostomy tube with a vertical clamping device, and the use of PPIs.[93,189] Pneumoperitoneum is common after PEG placement and is of no concern in the absence of peritoneal signs. Any signs of peritoneal irritation should prompt an investigation with a contrast study through the PEG tube to determine the presence or absence of a leak. Confirmation of a leak should lead to surgical exploration.[197]

Major complications are rare and include intra-abdominal bleeding or hematoma formation, peritonitis, necrotizing fasciitis, gastric or colonic perforation, and hepatogastric, gastrocolic, and colocutaneous fistula formation. A colocutaneous fistula results from inadvertent placement of a percutaneous feeding tube through the colon before it enters the stomach. While sometimes acute, the usual presentation is more chronic and may be suspected if stool is seen around the PEG tube or the patient develops "diarrhea" immediately upon feeding through the PEG tube.

If a PEG tube becomes dislodged within 7 days of placement, the patient should be brought back to the endoscopy suite and a new PEG placed through the same site on the anterior abdominal wall. It is not necessary (or perhaps even possible) to pass through the same exact site in the gastric wall, because if close to the original site, cinching of the new bolsters and the cross configuration of the muscular layers of the gastric wall help seal the original entry tract. Such patients may benefit from a short course of a broad-spectrum antibiotic. If the PEG tube becomes dislodged more than 4 weeks after placement, the tract should be mature enough to blindly replace the PEG tube at the bedside without fluoroscopic or endoscopic monitoring. Proper placement should be confirmed with a contrast radiologic study through the PEG tube prior to using the tube for feedings.

With PEGJ tubes, the jejunal tube may migrate in a retrograde direction or become kinked so that it no longer functions. More than 50% of PEGJ tubes require reintervention within 6 months.[198] Tube migration occurs most commonly in patients who have persistent vomiting or in cases where the J-tube has been placed improperly.[182,199] Other factors for tube migration include failure to cut the PEG tube down to a short enough length (<10 cm), shortened length of the jejunal tube, and placement of the PEG tube too high in the body or fundus,

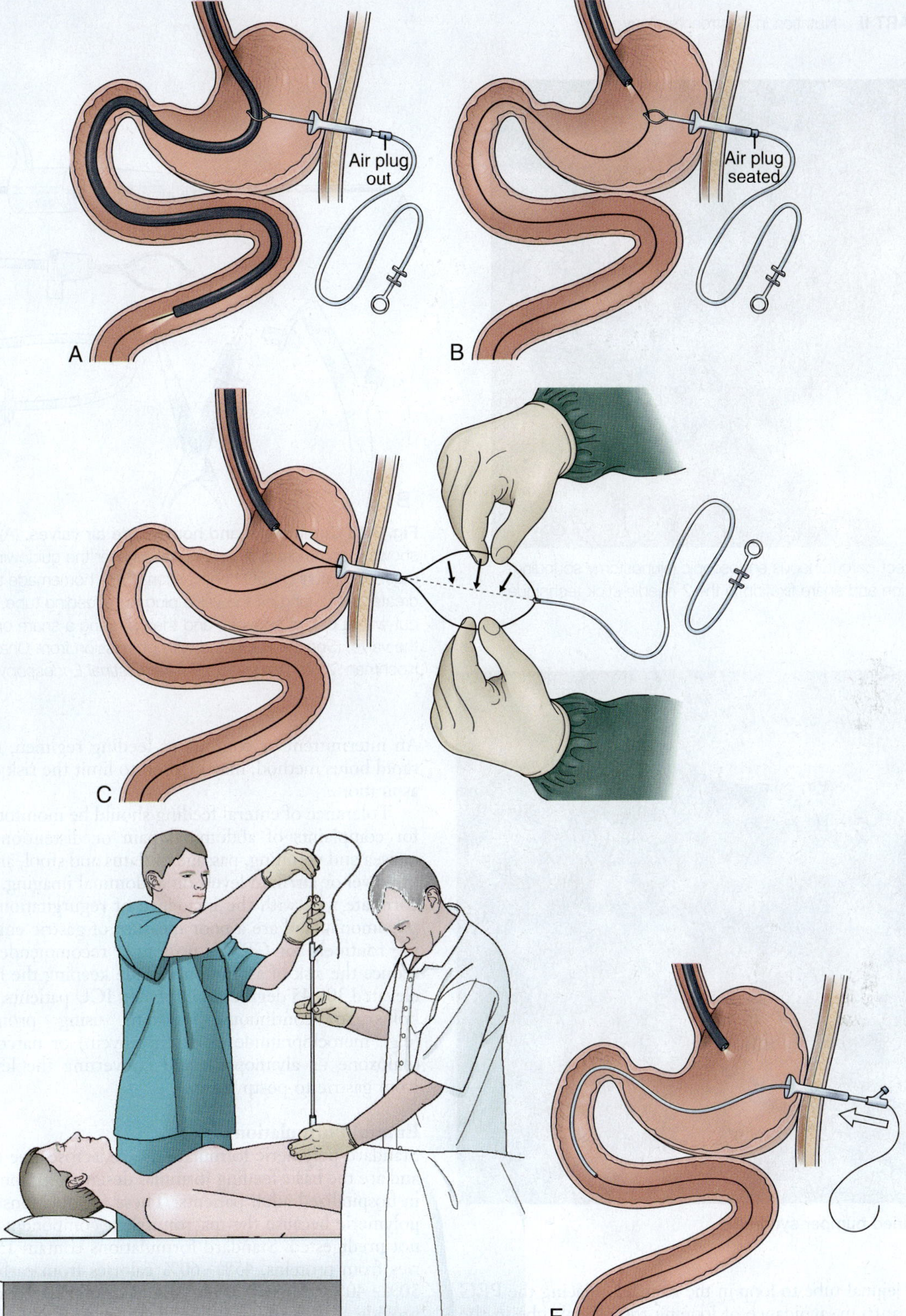

Fig. 7.10 Through-the-snare percutaneous endoscopic gastrojejunostomy technique, also known as the Johlin technique. (A) After initial placement of the percutaneous endoscopic gastrostomy (PEG), the PEG tube is cut down short to approximately 10 cm, and then a snare placed through a homemade or commercial air valve (Fig. 7.13) is passed into the stomach. A pediatric colonoscope is passed into the stomach, through the snare, and then down into the small intestine below the ligament of Treitz, after which the wire is extended beyond the end of the scope. (B) Using careful wire transfer technique, the endoscope is withdrawn back to the proximal stomach, keeping the tip of the wire in place below the ligament of Treitz. The air plug may be seated to allow observation of the snare within the stomach. (C) The snare is then closed on the wire, which is pulled out through the PEG. While the assistant holds the wire loop coming out from the PEG, the operator pulls on the wire extruding from the operating channel of the scope, to indicate which side of the wire loop represents the proximal end of the wire. The loop is then pulled out through the PEG. (D) An assistant provides a "point in space" to secure or fix the guidewire as the operator passes the jejunal tube down through the PEG. (E) The jejunal extension tube is passed down into final position, with the tip located well below the ligament of Treitz. (*Source*: Reprinted with permission from Chandrasekhara V, Kochman M. *Techniques in Gastrointestinal Endoscopy*. Elsevier.)

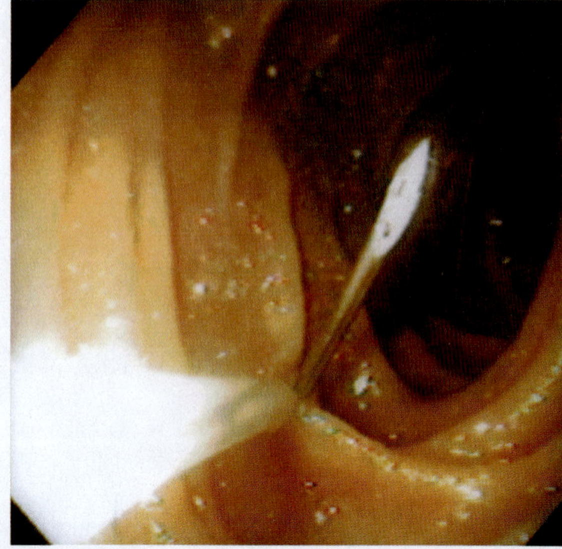

Fig. 7.11 Direct percutaneous endoscopic jejunostomy sounding-needle insertion and snare fixation in the 2-needle stick technique.

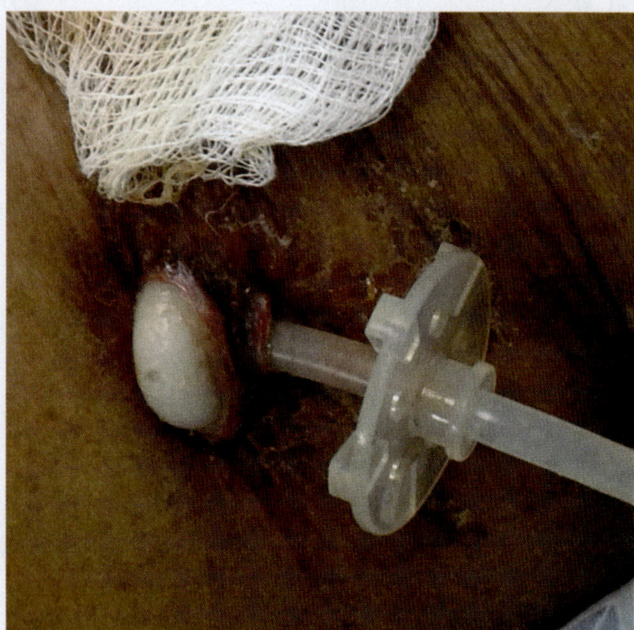

Fig. 7.12 Buried bumper syndrome.

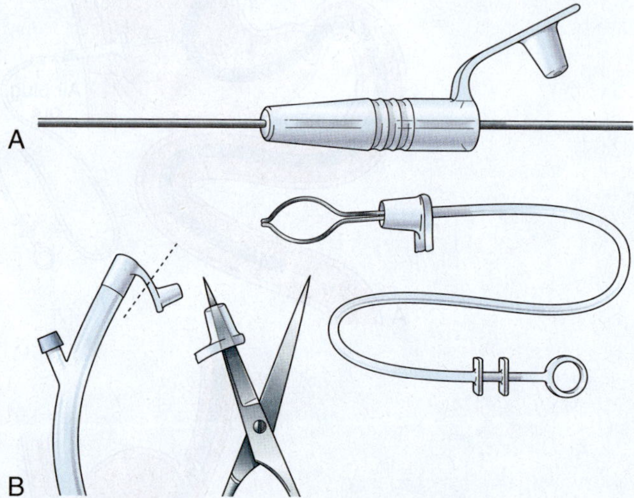

Fig. 7.13 Commercial and homemade air valves. (A) The top figure shows a commercial air valve passed over the guidewire, which is used most often during PEGJ conversion. (B) A homemade air valve may be created by cutting off the valve plug on a feeding tube, coring the valve out with a pair of scissors, and then passing a snare or wire through the valve. (*Source*: Reprinted with permission from Chandrasekhara V, Kochman M. *Techniques in Gastrointestinal Endoscopy*. Elsevier.)

causing the jejunal tube to loop in the stomach. Placing the PEG tube in the antrum, avoidance of looping the jejunal tube in the stomach, and securing the distal end of the jejunal tube with a hemoclip can prevent proximal migration.[189]

Enteral Feeding

Patients may receive their tube feedings by bolus, intermittent, or continuous methods. Bolus feeding delivery allows a relatively large volume of tube feeding (200–400 mL) to be delivered over a short period of time by a syringe. Intermittent feedings are delivered over a few hours by pump or by gravity drip using a bedside pole. Continuous feedings are usually delivered over 12–24 hours by a mechanical pump. Patients who receive small bowel feedings are almost always fed using continuous feedings. An intermittent or continuous feeding regimen, rather than the rapid bolus method, may be used to limit the risk of tube-feeding aspiration.

Tolerance of enteral feeding should be monitored by assessing for complaints of abdominal pain or distention, symptoms of nausea and vomiting, passage of flatus and stool, and dilated loops of bowel or air/fluid levels on abdominal imaging. GRV does not correlate well with the incidence of regurgitation, aspiration, or pneumonia, and are a poor measure of gastric emptying. Checking routinely for GRV is no longer recommended. Measures to reduce the risk of aspiration include keeping the head of the bed elevated 30–45 degrees in intubated ICU patients, changing from bolus to continuous infusion, using promotility drugs (e.g., metoclopramide or erythromycin) or narcotic antagonists (naloxone or alvimopan), and converting the level of infusion from gastric to postpyloric.

Enteral Formulations

Standard polymeric formulations are lactose-free and gluten-free and are the basic feeding formulas designed for long-term EN use in hospitalized adult patients. These formulations are denoted as polymeric because the macronutrient components are intact and not predigested. Standard formulations contain 15%–20% calories from proteins, 45%–60% calories from carbohydrates, and 30%–40% calories from fats. Generally, these formulations provide 1 kcal/mL, although they may be concentrated to 1.5–2.0 kcal/mL. As the calorie content per milliliter volume of tube feeding increases, the free water content of the formula decreases and the osmolarity increases. Most enteral formulas contain close to 80% free water. Formulas that are higher in protein are designated as high-nitrogen formulas.

Elemental formulas contain protein in the form of free amino acids and are nearly fat-free (i.e., less than 2%–3% of the caloric content is fat). Semielemental formulas contain protein in the form of small chain peptides, predominantly of 3–5 amino acids in length. Protein absorption is more efficient, as the small peptide chains can be transported across the intestinal wall intact by a single active transporter, rather than requiring a separate transporter for each amino acid (see Chapter 104). Fat is in the form of

MCT, which can be absorbed directly into the portal vein without lipase, colipase, or bile salt transportation (see Chapter 102). The semielemental small peptide/MCT oil formulations have largely supplanted the original elemental formulas, and are designed for patients with limited digestive capacity. While physiologic studies support greater absorption of the semielemental formulas than intact polymeric formulas in situations of compromised bowel function, clinical RCTs show little difference in outcome parameters.

Specialty organ-specific or disease-specific formulations are designed for patients with certain disease processes, such as diabetes, renal failure, hepatic failure, pulmonary disease, severe stress, or trauma. There is little or no data to show that these specialty formulations improve survival, or give any advantage with regard to clinical outcomes, compared with standard polymeric formulas when used for their intended disease states. Inadvertent use occurs usually for reasons involving their electrolyte profile, being low in potassium and phosphorus (renal formulas) or sodium (hepatic formulas). Protein should not be restricted in patients with either hepatic or renal failure.

Immune modulating formulas are supplemented with arginine, glutamine, omega-3 fatty acids, antioxidants, and nucleotides, substances shown to be important in immune modulation. Arginine is needed for cell growth and proliferation, wound healing, nitric oxide production, and lymphocyte differentiation. Arginine requirements increase in critical illness, and supplementation may facilitate wound healing.[200] Fish oil may help in reducing systemic inflammation. Patients most likely to show a benefit from arginine-fish oil, immune-enhancing formulas include those undergoing elective GI surgery and those postoperative patients in the surgical ICU requiring EN therapy. Use of immune modulating formulas in these patients reduces infectious complications, antibiotic needs, duration of mechanical ventilation, multiple organ dysfunction, and hospital stay.[201] While use of such formulas in a medical ICU patient is safe, current data show lack of efficacy in changing clinical outcomes. Similarly, use of a fish oil, antioxidant-containing, antiinflammatory formula in patients with acute lung injury or acute respiratory distress syndrome cannot be recommended for reasons of safety and lack of efficacy.

Complications of Enteral Feeding

GI side effects of tube feedings are reported in 15%–30% of patients, and include nausea, vomiting, abdominal distention, abdominal cramping, and diarrhea. Diarrhea is most commonly due to medications and less often to *Clostridioides difficile* enterocolitis (see Chapter 114). Medications can be altered from tablet to liquid form for easy instillation through the feeding tube, by dissolution in a sorbitol base (a known cathartic). Magnesium-containing medications, hypertonic medications, and promotility agents may also promote diarrhea. High-osmolarity EN formulations, even with an osmolarity as high as 600–700 mOsm/L, are rarely a cause of diarrhea. In a patient with new-onset diarrhea who was previously tolerant to an enteral formula, the patient should be assessed for medication-induced and infectious etiologies prior to changing the formula. There are no data to support dilution of the enteral formulation to improve GI tolerance. For patients with compromised bowel function, use of the semielemental formulas may improve absorption and reduce diarrhea. Soluble fiber supplementation or use of a commercial mixed soluble/insoluble fiber formula may improve diarrhea as well.[202,203]

Metabolic complications are less common with EN than with PN feeding. Dehydration and fluid shifts may occur with formulas of high concentration, especially if insufficient water is supplied. Hyperglycemia may occur with high rates of carbohydrate delivery in patients with glucose intolerance. Medication delivery may also be affected by concurrent tube feeding. Phenytoin administration is affected, because the drug binds to the enteral formula and forms a phenytoin-tube feeding complex that adheres to the wall of the feeding tube.[204] Ciprofloxacin has also been shown to bind with tube feedings, reducing its absorption. Vitamin K, present in many enteral formulas, will make a patient more resistant to the effects of warfarin.

Parenteral Nutrition

For patients with IF, nutrients can be delivered intravenously via PN. PN delivers a solution comprising macronutrients (carbohydrates, proteins, and lipids), micronutrients (vitamins, minerals, and trace elements), water, electrolytes, and medications. Carbohydrates are delivered as dextrose, proteins as amino acids, and lipids as IV fat emulsions (IVFEs). When all three macronutrients are combined into a single solution, it is referred to as a *total nutrient admixture* or *3-in-1 solution*. When IVFEs are given separately, the PN formula is referred to as a *2-in-1 solution*. Nutrients can be delivered into a central vein (central PN) or a peripheral vein (PPN). Use of PPN is restricted or prohibited in most hospital settings, because of the likelihood for abuse of the indications for PPN, and for sclerosing the veins despite keeping the osmolarity below 800–900 mOsm/L (which in turn leads to short-term duration of therapy of usually 12–36 hours). PN is usually delivered over 12–24 hours. A PN solution is six times more concentrated than blood (1800–2400 mOsm/L) and generally consists of approximately 30–50 g/L of protein and 1000–1200 kcal/L.

Parenteral Nutrition Formulation

To create a PN formula, one must first determine the caloric and protein needs of the patient, which are based on a prior nutritional assessment (see Chapter 5).[205] Protein and calorie needs increase with increasing metabolic stress, except in the critically ill. Each component of PN has a defined caloric content, with protein = 4 kcal/g, carbohydrate (dextrose) = 3.4 kcal/g, and IVFE = 10 kcal/g (9 kcal/g from fat, 1 kcal/g from emulsifier). Protein needs vary in the range of 1.2–2.0 g/kg/day depending on the level of metabolic stress. Protein should not be restricted, even in patients with severe HE or renal failure with azotemia requiring imminent dialysis. Fat is usually provided at 1 g/kg/day, but may need to be reduced or restricted for patients with hypertriglyceridemia (>400 mg/dL). Despite fat restriction, a minimal amount of fat is still given, usually 10% of estimated fat calories (or 500 mL of 20% Intralipid per week), to prevent essential fatty acid deficiency. The remainder of a patient's daily energy requirements is administered in the form of dextrose. To prevent hyperglycemia and refeeding syndrome (see later under Metabolic Complications), the amount of dextrose should initially not exceed 200 g. Dextrose should be titrated over the course of several days to the goal amount. Water is added to meet the patient's daily volume needs, with fluid volume restricted in patients with fluid overload, cardiopulmonary disease, or renal failure. Overall water requirements are estimated at 25–35 mL/kg/day.

Once the macronutrient components of a PN formula have been defined, electrolytes, trace elements, multivitamins, and medications like insulin, heparin, and PPIs or H2Bs can be added. Any of the components can be increased or decreased based on a patient's laboratory values and comorbid disease processes. For patients in an unmonitored non-ICU setting, potassium in the PN formula should not exceed 10 mEq/h. The amount of calcium and phosphorus in the PN solution must also be monitored, owing to the risk of precipitation of calcium-phosphate crystals. In general, the calcium-phosphorus sum [(mEq of calcium + mmol of phosphorus)/L] should be less than 45 to prevent precipitation. Vitamins and trace elements are added using preset solutions, but additional supplementation can be added based on documented needs. Because copper and manganese are excreted in bile, these minerals should be withheld in patients with cholestasis. Selenium should be decreased in patients with renal insufficiency, whereas zinc should be increased in patients with diarrhea, high output fistulas, or large wounds.[206] Moderate glycemic control is recommended, keeping serum glucose levels between 110 and 150 mg/dL by sliding scale coverage or addition of insulin to the solution.[92] A sample stepwise approach to writing a central PN order is shown in Box 7.1.

Administration

At initiation, the PN formula should be infused over 24 hours and later cycled over 12 hours. Patients with glucose intolerance or those at risk for refeeding syndrome (see later discussion of metabolic complications) should have their PN infused at 25% of their daily caloric needs for the first 24 hours. This ratio may be increased to full caloric needs over the following 48–72 hours, with monitoring of serum levels of glucose, magnesium, potassium, and phosphate, as well as fluid tolerance.[207] PN is infused via a large central vein. The port or lumen of the catheter utilized for PN must be used solely for PN infusion. Use of the PN port or lumen for blood drawing or infusion of other solutions increases the risk of catheter infection.

Laboratory Testing

Following PN initiation, certain serologic values must be monitored. In the first few days following initiation of PN infusion, serum concentrations of electrolytes, magnesium, phosphorus, calcium, potassium, and blood urea nitrogen should be monitored closely. After stabilization, these values can be checked weekly. In the HPN patient on long-term infusion, checking these routine laboratory tests is decreased in frequency to once per month. Complete blood cell counts should be performed monthly. In other clinically relevant cases, serum zinc, selenium, copper, chromium, vitamin B_{12}, and vitamin B_6 levels may have to be monitored. Because iron is not a standard additive for PN solutions, patients who are PN-dependent require monitoring for the development of iron deficiency anemia.

BOX 7.1 Stepwise Approach to Writing a Parenteral Nutrition Order for a 70-kg Man

CALORIC CONTENTS OF NUTRIENT SUBSTANCES

Protein: 4 kcal/g
Fat: 10 kcal/g
Carbohydrates: 3.4 kcal/g

ESTIMATED DAILY NEEDS FOR THIS PATIENT

Calories: 25 kcal/kg = 1750 kcal
Protein: 1.2 g/kg = 84 g
Fluids: 30 mL/kg = 2100 mL

STEPS

1. Add protein (1.2 g/kg/day) to the PN mixture.
   84 g of protein needed
   1 g of protein = 4 kcal (total, 336 kcal)
   1750 kcal-326 kcal = 1424 kcal still required
2. Add lipids (1–1.5 g/kg/day).
   70 g fat = 700 kcal
   1424 residual calories-700 kcal = 724 kcal still required
3. Add carbohydrates (3–5 g/kg/day).
   724 kcal/3.4 kcal/g carbohydrate = 212.9 g
4. Make total volume.
   30 mL/kg = 2100 mL

ADDITIONAL ADDITIVES

Electrolytes, minerals, and vitamins
Drug additives: H_2RAs, insulin, and heparin

Metabolic Complications

Metabolic complications may develop as a consequence of the glucose, amino acid, lipid, vitamin, electrolyte, or mineral content of the PN solution.[208] Hyperglycemia is the most common complication and is directly related to PN dextrose content, the patient's insulin sensitivity, and the rate of PN infusion. Critically ill patients and those with preexisting glucose intolerance require the most aggressive serum glucose monitoring. Patients who develop hyperglycemia should first be maintained on a sliding scale of regular insulin. Of the total amount of sliding scale insulin required over 24 hours, two-thirds should be added to the next day's PN formula. Further adjustments in insulin dosing may be required on a daily basis, and some patients in the ICU may require a separate insulin drip. Failure to control blood glucose levels results in an increase of infectious complications, such as catheter sepsis. In some hospitalized patients, blood glucose control may be difficult even with an insulin drip, and permissive underfeeding can be performed. In these patients, the risk of hyperglycemia and its consequences is greater than the risk of temporarily underfeeding the patient.

Refeeding syndrome is a metabolic consequence of nutrition support resulting from sudden provision of a large amount of glucose calories to a patient who was previously malnourished. Prolonged NPO status (>7 days), low BMI, alcoholism and weight loss prior to admission are risk factors. With nutrient infusion, the metabolism of these patients rapidly becomes anabolic. Insulin production is increased, pushing potassium, phosphorus, magnesium, and thiamine into the intracellular space, with resultant hypokalemia, hypophosphatemia, and hypomagnesemia.[209] Sodium retention and large fluid shifts can also occur and may place the patient at risk of developing heart failure, in addition to neurologic sequelae.[210] Sudden shifts in serum electrolytes may precipitate cardiac dysrhythmias. To prevent refeeding syndrome, the initial caloric content should be limited and the macronutrients gradually titrated (particularly dextrose) from 25% up to 80% to 100% of energy goals over 3–4 days, while electrolytes are carefully monitored and corrected as needed. While refeeding syndrome may be precipitated by EN or PN, risk is greater with provision of EN.

Abnormal liver enzymes are common after initiation of PN and typically feature elevations of serum aminotransferase levels up to twice normal. Greater elevations in aminotransferase levels and associated hyperbilirubinemia warrant investigation. PN can lead to three types of PN-associated hepatobiliary disease: steatosis, cholestasis, and gallbladder sludge/stones. Other causes of underlying liver disease should be excluded. US of the RUQ helps to exclude dilated bile ducts, presence of a liver mass, cholelithiasis, or biliary sludge. Lack of enteral stimulation results in decreased CCK release, with impaired bile flow and gallbladder contractility. Gallbladder stasis can lead to development of gallstones or gallbladder sludge, resulting in both calculus and acalculous cholecystitis. PN-associated steatosis presents as a fatty infiltration of the liver that is especially prominent in the periportal areas. Patients with PN-associated steatosis have modest elevations of serum aminotransferases that usually occur within 2 weeks of starting PN and may return to normal with time. Most patients with PN-associated steatosis are asymptomatic; the condition appears to be secondary to overfeeding and may respond to a reduction in the patient's total daily caloric infusion.[211] PN-associated cholestasis is a condition of impaired bile secretion that occurs predominantly in children and presents as an elevation of alkaline phosphatase, GGT, and bilirubin. In a small percentage of patients on HPN, long-term PN-associated cholestasis may progress to cirrhosis and liver failure. Repeated episodes of catheter sepsis may contribute to the probability of PN-induced liver injury. Bacterial and fungal infections are associated with cholestasis. SIBO is another risk factor for liver disease, most likely caused by the production of alcohol through fermentation or hepatotoxins by anaerobic bacteria.[93]

Choline deficiency may play a role in the development of liver disease associated with long-term PN[212]; the lipid source also is believed to contribute to this complication. In the United States, until July 2016 when SMOF (soy, MCT, olive oil, and fish oil) was approved, the lipid content of the PN solution was soy-based and composed mainly of long-chain triglycerides (e.g., linoleic acid, an omega-6 fatty acid), which are proinflammatory. Phytosterols and stanols in this lipid source may be hepatotoxic in some patients. Unlike soy-based long-chain triglycerides, MCT oil and olive oil are essentially devoid of proinflammatory properties. Fish oil, which is rich in omega-3 fatty acids, has anti-inflammatory properties. IVFEs with medium-chain triglycerides, olive oil, and fish oil (SMOF) are available in most centers. Fish oils have been shown to be effective in reversing PN-induced liver disease in prospective and retrospective studies in children.[213] In an adult receiving PN who develops elevated liver biochemical tests, appropriate management strategies include cycling the PN regimen over 12–18 hours each day, performing indirect calorimetry to confirm energy requirements and readjusting to avoid overfeeding, and switching the soy-based intralipid IVFE to a mixture of lipids (SMOF containing soy, MCTs, olive, and fish oils).

Patients who develop significant complications with PN use may be candidates for small bowel transplantation (see Chapter 106). These complications include progressive liver failure, repeated catheter sepsis, or thrombosis of major venous systems that precludes obtaining central venous access. Current 5-year survival rates for patients receiving small bowel transplants are close to 50%,[214] but the 5-year survival rate of patients on HPN are still better than the 5-year survival rate for patients receiving small bowel transplants. Quality-of-life differences between HPN and small bowel transplantation are still being explored.

Vascular Access Devices

Anatomically, the subclavian and internal jugular veins provide the safest and easiest central venous access. Compared with other central venous access sites, the subclavian vein is often chosen for long-term access, because of reduced catheter-associated complications. Multilumen catheters allow for infusion of a number of fluids and medications at the same time, but risk of infection increases with an increasing number of lumens.[215,216] Single-lumen catheters are preferred unless multiple ports are necessary for patient management. If a multilumen catheter is used, one lumen should be designated for only PN use.[217]

There are three types of central venous catheters (CVCs) available for PN infusion: peripherally inserted central catheter (PICC), tunneled indwelling CVC (Hickman, Broviac, or Groshong catheters), and implantable vascular access device (IVAD) or "port." PICC lines have been used for PN infusion both in the hospital and at home. The PICC line is generally placed in an upper extremity, with the tip of the catheter positioned in a central vein at the junction of the superior vena cava and the right atrium. PICC lines are associated with a reduction in major insertion complications (e.g., pneumothorax) compared with previously standard centrally inserted catheters. PICC lines should only be utilized for patients with anticipated short-term needs for PN. PICC lines are not appropriate for long-term use as they only remain patent for a maximum of 1–2 months and may promote venous sclerosis.

Tunneled indwelling CVCs are commonly used when a catheter is required for longer than 1–3 months. Indwelling catheters are tunneled subcutaneously, creating a physical barrier to bacterial infection. They have a Dacron cuff to induce tissue ingrowth and local fibrosis, thereby anchoring the catheter; this prevents accidental dislodgement and is believed to prevent bacterial migration up the catheter.[218] The catheter tip should be positioned in the distal third of the subclavian vein. Implantable ports are placed subcutaneously, usually on the chest wall, and by eliminating the external catheter portion, daily heparin flushes are unnecessary. Implantable ports require a specialized access needle to allow blood drawing or fluid infusion and have a limited lifetime of punctures; they also require a more extensive procedure for bedside removal than tunneled catheters. Single-lumen PICC lines and implantable ports have a lower incidence of catheter-related bloodstream infections [(CRBSI) 0/1000 and 0.19/1000 catheter-days, respectively] compared with tunneled (0.64/1000 catheter-days) and nontunneled CVCs (0.87/1000 catheter-days). Single-lumen PICC lines and implantable ports also have been shown to have a longer failure-free duration because of fewer mechanical complications (13.9% and 9.7%, respectively) than nontunneled catheters (17.8%).[219] While PICC and IVAD are associated with fewer complications overall, tunneled single lumen catheters are preferred. PICC is placed for short term use, and neither are ethanol lock compatible.

Central Venous Catheter Complications

CVC complications occur in an incidence range of 1%–20%.[220] Complications of subclavian vein catheter placement include hemothorax, pneumothorax, brachial plexus injury, hematoma, and subcutaneous emphysema. Common long-term catheter complications include sepsis, thrombosis, and catheter occlusion. Catheter breakage, dislodgement, and air emboli also can occur.

Catheter infection generally occurs from touch contamination. The predominant organism isolated is coagulase-negative staphylococcus; other organisms include resistant strains of Gram-positive cocci (e.g., *Staphylococcus aureus*, *Enterococcus* species, *Streptococcus* species), Gram-negative bacilli (e.g., *Klebsiella pneumoniae*, *Escherichia coli*, *Enterobacter cloacae*), and fungi (e.g., *Candida parapsilosis*, *Candida albicans*, *Candida glabrata*).[221,222] The major mechanism of catheter contamination is tracking of organisms from the skin to the subcutaneous tissues and catheter tip. In the home setting, the more time spent teaching the patient about the care and operation of the central venous access device, the less likely the patient is to develop infectious complications.[223]

Diagnosing catheter infections can be difficult because the white blood cell count may not be elevated if a patient is immunocompromised, and peripheral blood cultures can be negative. Catheter tip culture is a much more sensitive method of documenting catheter infections. Generally, bacterial infections of catheters can be treated with the catheter in place, whereas fungal catheter infections and tunnel infections of the catheter tract require catheter removal for effective treatment. It is common for broad-spectrum antibiotic or antifungal treatment of catheter infections to be initiated once the diagnosis is suspected, and definitive therapy is introduced when the organism is identified. Culture from the catheter and a peripheral site should be obtained. If the peripheral site culture returns positive, echocardiogram should be done to assess seeding heart valves. If cultures are positive, antibiotic should be continued and deescalated based on sensitivity results. Most often, catheters can be salvaged unless the infection is caused by *Candida* spp., MRSA, pseudomonas or a polymicrobial disease. Antibiotic or ethanol lock therapy should be considered if the catheter is kept which improves salvage rate compared to systemic antibiotic use alone.[224] If the catheter is removed, it should be replaced after 48–96 hours following negative blood culture.[225,226]

Addition of heparin (1000 U/L) to each bag of PN solution can prevent subclinical thrombus formation to which bacteria or fungi can attach, thereby potentially reducing the risk of catheter sepsis.

Routine use of anticoagulant therapy to reduce the risk of catheter-related infection, however, is not recommended.[227] When treating CVC infections, importance is given to the actual contact time between the bacteria or fungus in the catheter and the antibiotic or antifungal agent. Locking the antibiotic into an infected line (at the end of each infusion) may help reduce central line colonization.[228] Others advocate flushing the catheter daily with pharmaceutical grade 50%–70% ethanol to sterilize the catheter and reduce infectious events.[229] The use of catheter locks has been shown to reduce the risk of CRBSI. Antibiotic lock therapy has been shown to decrease the incidence of recurrent CRBSI. Ethanol has both bactericidal and fungicidal properties, and has a low risk for causing antimicrobial resistance.. A recent metanalysis of RCTs showed that an ethanol lock significantly reduced the incidence of CRBSI.[230] Thus use of prophylactic antimicrobial and ethanol lock solutions is usually recommended for those who have a history of multiple CRBSIs but has not shown benefit when applied to all patients newly started on HPN. Of note, ethanol locks should only be used in silicone Hickman catheters and cannot be used in polyurethane catheters.[231]

Catheter-induced thrombosis occurs secondary to irritation of the blood vessel wall. The thrombus usually is composed of fibrin. Precipitation of medication in the catheter occurs less commonly. Symptoms of central vein thrombus formation include neck pain, neck swelling, anterior chest wall venous distention, and reduced catheter function. Flushing the CVC with saline has proved as beneficial as flushing with heparin for preventing catheter occlusion by a thrombus.[232] Treatment of fibrin thrombus formation requires a thrombolytic agent like streptokinase, given as a bolus or continuous infusion.[233] Medication or precipitate occlusions can be treated by instilling small amounts of sodium hydroxide or hydrochloric acid, depending on whether the drug is acidic or basic, respectively.[234]

Special Diets

Clear liquid diets supply fluid and energy in a form that creates a minimal amount of residue. They are meant to avoid the high osmolar delivery of nutrients to the GI tract, which would result in fluid shifts and associated nausea and diarrhea. Clear liquid diets generally contain an abundance of carbohydrates but little protein or fat and are thereby nutritionally inadequate to meet basic metabolic needs. Little evidence suggests that a clear liquid diet is better tolerated than any other diet in the postoperative period. Even in AP, clear liquids should be avoided, advancing directly to regular diet shorten hospital length of stay. Where possible, clear liquid diets should not be prescribed, as there is no physiologic rationale for their use, they tend to be high in sodium content, and their provision cannot be justified other than fulfilling a patient's personal wishes. In contrast, early EN feeding after abdominal or thoracic surgery may reduce postoperative complications, hospital length of stay, and mortality (although vomiting may be increased).[235,236]

Full liquid diets are indicated for patients who are unable to chew, swallow, or digest solids. They are largely milk-based and should not be used for lactose-intolerant patients. They contain a large amount of simple carbohydrates and should be used with caution in diabetic patients.

Low-fiber, low-residue diets are used for patients with GI strictures as well as those with gastroparesis and are presumed to reduce the risk of obstruction while prolonging transit time. Carbohydrate intake is reduced, and well-cooked vegetables, refined cereals, and breads are used instead. For gastroparesis, low fat intake is also recommended.

High-fiber diets include soluble and insoluble fibers, which have a wide range of metabolic and physiologic effects. They are used to reduce intraluminal colon pressures in patients with diverticulosis. They may also be useful in diabetes by delaying glucose absorption, and in cardiovascular disease by lowering serum cholesterol and serum triglyceride levels. Life-long high-fiber diets may help prevent colon cancer. A high-fiber diet emphasizes foods such as vegetables, fruits, legumes, and whole-grain breads and cereals.

A postgastrectomy or antidumping diet involves ingestion of small, frequent meals high in protein and fat, to deliver a lower osmolarity solution to the small intestine. Simple sugars are avoided to prevent their rapid absorption.[237] Fluid intake should be restricted and separated from solid food intake to avoid rapid gastric transit. High pectin-containing foods, such as bananas and oranges are included in this diet to slow gastric output.

Low-fat diets are used to minimize diarrhea and steatorrhea associated with fat malabsorption, especially in patients with pancreatic or biliary dysfunction. In CP, low fat diet reduces pancreatic enzyme secretion, renders endogenously secreted lipase unstable and makes pancreatic enzyme replacement therapy less effective and should thus be avoided in most patients. Only 20% of patients with CP might benefit from low fat diet due to intolerance (pain) on regular diet.[238,239] In those patients placed on a low-fat diet for a prolonged period of time, fat-soluble vitamins (A, D, E, and K) must be supplemented. MCT oil may be used to substitute for long-chain triglycerides. MCTs have 6–12-carbon fatty acid chains, high aqueous solubility, and do not require bile salts for absorption in the small intestine.[240] MCTs do not require chylomicron formation and are absorbed directly into the portal venous system. Unfortunately, most MCT-based products are not very palatable. Many MCT-based products such as regular flavored semielemental formula with MCT oil and small chain peptides can have a medicinal taste. Vanilla flavored versions of these formulas with or without flavor packets increase palatability.[241]

The nature of training for the gastroenterologist provides the skillset to perform as a clinical nutritionist. Appropriate knowledge and clinical applications of nutritional issues are important requirements for management of most patients with GI disorders. Having the skills to achieve enteral access, the ability to achieve GI tolerance to enteral feeding, and an understanding of metabolic effects of illness or injury is integral to good patient care.

Full references for this chapter can be found at https://ebooks.health.elsevier.com.

8 Obesity

Babak J. Orandi, Louis J. Aronne

IN THIS CHAPTER

DEFINITIONS AND EPIDEMIOLOGY

Obesity is a chronic disease defined as an excess of body fat or adipose tissue. Adiposity per se is difficult to measure expediently; therefore the use of body mass index (BMI) has become the internationally recognized metric to define obesity. BMI is calculated by measuring weight in kilograms and dividing it by height in meters squared. A normal BMI is between 18.5 and 24.9 kg/m^2, and a BMI between 25 and 29.9 kg/m^2 is defined as overweight (Table 8.1). Individuals with a BMI of 30–34.9 kg/m^2 have class I obesity. A BMI of 35–39.9 kg/m^2 is defined as class II obesity, and a BMI of 40 kg/m^2 or greater is categorized as class III obesity. Of note, the term "morbid obesity," previously used to denote a BMI consistent with class III obesity, has fallen out of favor[1]; in a similar vein, the field has moved to using person-first language to refer to people with overweight or obesity (rather than describing people as being "overweight" or "obese") to minimize stigma.[2]

There is a robust discussion in the literature about the limitations of BMI as a metric for obesity. Notably, BMI does not convey information about body composition (e.g., lean mass versus fat mass), location of adipose tissue (e.g., visceral versus subcutaneous), and it can vary dramatically between male and female individuals and across the age spectrum.[3] Special consideration must be given to individuals who have higher muscle mass and, therefore, have higher calculated BMI but who may be metabolically healthy. The converse must also be considered; for example, certain populations may develop metabolic disease at lower BMI levels, such as patients of Asian and South Asian descent. Indeed, there is significant heterogeneity in the prevalence of obesity across various Asian and South Asian subgroups, as well as what the implications are for the risk of comorbidity development[4–6]; accordingly, for these groups, there is a different BMI-based diagnostic criteria (Table 8.1).[7] BMI is further limited in its ability to precisely identify patients at increased risk for cardiometabolic complications of obesity.[8,9]

Despite the limitations of BMI, its ease of use and utility in screening have made it the generally accepted metric for obesity. Based on this metric, obesity is increasing in prevalence globally and is now recognized as an epidemic by the World Health Organization.[10] From 1975 to 2016, there were dramatic increases in the prevalence of obesity in every region of the world.[11] By 2030, it is predicted that 57.8% of adults will have overweight or obesity globally.[12] In the United States, 19 states and 2 territories already have an adult obesity prevalence of at least 35%.[13] Indeed, it is estimated that by 2030, 48.9% of U.S. adults will have obesity, with 24.2% having at least class II obesity. Women, non-Hispanic black adults, and low-income adults will be disproportionally affected.[14] It is likely that the coronavirus 2019 (COVID-19) pandemic accelerated these trends.[15,16]

The rapid increase in the prevalence of obesity has led to greater awareness of the importance of treating obesity. The coverage of doctors' visits for obesity care by the Centers for Medicare and Medicaid began in 2012,[17] and the American Medical Association classified obesity as a disease state in 2013.[18] The American Board of Obesity Medicine was established in 2011 to serve as a credentialing body for physicians obtaining certification in obesity medicine. Obesity medicine is one of the fastest growing subspecialties, with more than 8200 physicians certified as of 2024.[19]

Etiology of Obesity

There are two competing theories to explain the pathophysiology underlying the obesity epidemic: the energy balance model and the carbohydrate-insulin model.[20] In the former, obesity is thought to be the result of a net excess in calories. According to this model, weight gain occurs when calories consumed exceed calories burned, with the surplus stored in fat; conversely, weight loss occurs when calorie expenditure exceeds calorie consumption, leading to a reduction in fat.[21,22] Under this paradigm, all calories are equal, irrespective of their provenance or composition.

In the carbohydrate-insulin model, carbohydrates, particularly those with a high glycemic index (described later in this chapter), promote insulin secretion, leading to rapid deposition of calories into adipose tissue, thereby removing it from the bloodstream and effectively depriving the rest of the body the use of those energy sources. The consequence is increased hunger and overeating.[23,24] Under this paradigm, all calories are not considered equal, and their provenance matters; those derived from high glycemic index foods are particularly injurious in terms of weight gain. The interested reader is encouraged to review some of the excellent summaries of the competing theories that have been written.[21,25] Importantly, proponents of both models concede that obesity is multifactorial, with a number of contributions and complex interactions of the factors described below, as well as numerous related complications (Figure 8.1).

Dietary Factors

A number of changes to the human diet globally over the past century, particularly pronounced in Western countries, are strongly associated with obesity:

- Increase in calorie-dense processed and ultra-processed foods. Calorie-dense processed and ultra-processed foods are typically high in added sugars and unhealthy saturated and trans fats and low in fiber. The extensive processing they undergo leads to a higher concentration of calories per given volume.[26] The relatively large amounts of added fat and sugar lead to

TABLE 8.1 Categories of Obesity Based on Body Mass Index (BMI) and Their Associated Cardiometabolic Comorbidity Risk

Weight Category	WHO Organization BMI Criteria (kg/m²)	Cardiometabolic Comorbidity Risk	Modified BMI Criteria for Asian Populations (kg/m²)[a]	Cardiometabolic Comorbidity Risk
Underweight	<18.5	Low	<18.5	Low
Normal	18.5–24.9	Average	18.5–22.9	Average
Overweight	25.0–29.9	Increased	23–24.9	Increased
Class I obesity	30.0–34.9	Moderate	25.0–29.9	Moderate
Class II obesity	35.0–39.9	Severe	30.0–34.9	Severe
Class III obesity	>40.0	Very severe	>35.0	Very severe

[a]Seo MH, Lee WY, Kim SS, et al. 2018 Korean Society for the study of obesity guideline for the management of obesity in Korea. *J Obes Metab Syndr*. 2019;28(1):40–45.

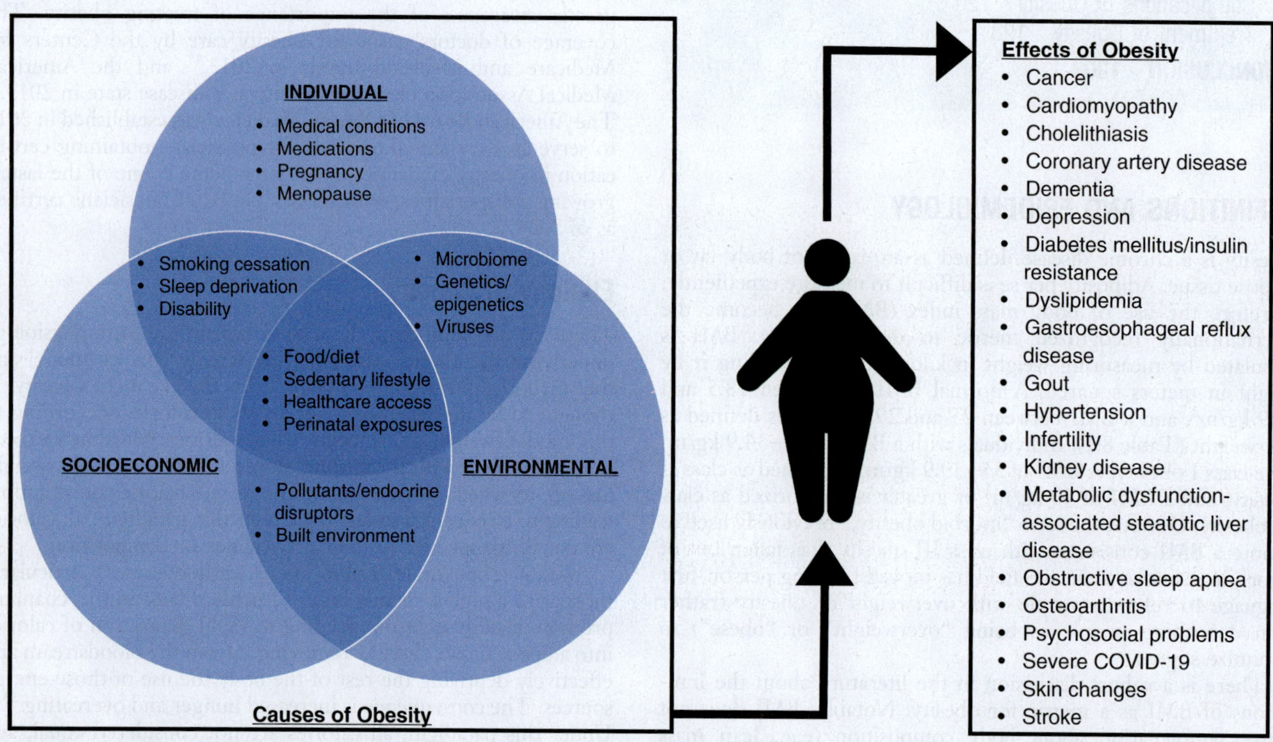

Fig. 8.1 Etiologies and effects of obesity.

hyperpalatable foods that are more pleasurable to eat, induce more cravings, and lead to increased calorie consumption and weight gain.[27,28] Indeed, these foods are associated with increased activity in the brain's hedonic reward-response areas.[29] A meta-analysis demonstrated increased BMI in those with diets higher in added sugars.[30] Similar findings have been reported with saturated fats and trans fats.[31] High-fiber diets promote satiety, regulate appetite, and enhance glycemic control; however, food processing tends to reduce the amount of fiber in food.[32] In a large, longitudinal cohort study, an increase per serving per day of highly processed foods led to significant weight gain over 4 years: 3.35 lb for french fries, 1.69 lb for potato chips, 1.00 lb for sugar-sweetened beverages, and 0.93 lb for processed meats. The opposite relationship was observed for unprocessed foods: −0.22 lb for vegetables, −0.37 lb for whole grains, −49 lb for fruits, and −0.57 lb for nuts.[33] Indeed, in a clinical trial of ad libitum unprocessed diet versus ultra-processed diet, participants were randomized to 2 weeks of one diet or the other, with crossover to the other arm after 2 weeks, all while being maintained in a metabolic unit.[34] The diets were matched for calories, macronutrients, energy density, fiber, sugar, sodium, and palatability as rated by participants. While in the ultra-processed diet arm of the study, participants consumed approximately 500 calories more per day and gained 0.9 kg over 2 weeks. During the unprocessed diet arm of the study, participants lost 0.9 kg the same time period.

- Increase in fast food consumption. Fast food items are particularly calorie-laden and on days of fast food consumption, people tend to consume more overall calories, fat, saturated fat, sodium, and carbonated beverages, and lower intake of salubrious foods and nutrients, such as fruits, vegetables, milk, and vitamins A and C.[35] For every fast food meal consumed per week, there is an associated 0.05 kg/m² increase in BMI over a 3-year period.[36] These findings are concerning because on any given day, 30% of U.S. adults consume fast food and fewer fast food restaurant meals have met American Heart Association nutrient criteria over time.[37,38]
- Increase in portion sizes. In general, portion sizes have increased over time, particularly during the 1970s and 1980s,

as evidenced by food advertisements that use larger size as a selling point, larger cupholders installed in more recently manufactured automobiles, and identical recipes in classic cookbooks having fewer servings in subsequent editions.[39] Numerous ready-to-eat products greatly exceed U.S. government recommendations. For example, cookie servings are 700% larger than recommended by the United States Department of Agriculture, and steaks are 224% larger.[39] Larger portion sizes are consistently associated with increased energy consumption "portion size effect," particularly from energy-dense foods.[40]

- Increase in sugar-sweetened beverage consumption. From 1977 to 2001, there was a 135% increase in energy consumed from sugar-sweetened beverages coupled with a 38% decrease in energy consumption in the form of milk, resulting in a net increase of 278 calories per person per day.[41] Sugar-sweetened beverage consumption is strongly associated with obesity and the development of type 2 diabetes, with increased consumption associated with greater weight gain and higher diabetes risk.[42,43] Encouragingly, national data have suggested declines in sugar-sweetened beverage consumption since the turn of the century.[44–47]

Physical Activity

A number of major medical societies and organizations recommend at least 150 minutes/week of moderate-intensity aerobic activity, 75 minutes/week of vigorous aerobic activity, or a combination of both, spread throughout the week, with at least 2 days of muscle-strengthening activities per week for adults.[48,49] Children and adolescents are recommended to get 60 minutes of daily moderate-to-vigorous intensity activity.[50,51] In recent decades, there have been significant declines in physical activity levels globally, with the declines particularly pronounced in developed countries. The global age-standardized prevalence of insufficient physical activity is 27.5% for adults; among adolescents ages 11–17, it is 81.0%.[52,53] A number of factors contribute to the decrease in physical activity. There has been a dramatic increase in screen time (television, video games, and computers) for both leisure and work.[54,55] The average U.S. adult now spends nearly 7 hours per day engaged in screen time.[56] Even after adjustment for age, smoking status, physical activity level, and diet, every 2-hour increase in television watching is associated with a 23% increase in the risk of obesity and a 14% increase in the risk of developing diabetes.[57] Occupational physical activity has also decreased, driven largely by decreases in manufacturing, mining, and logging jobs and an increase in health, education, leisure, and hospitality jobs. In 1960, 48% of all occupations required at least moderate-intensity physical activity; in 2008 only 20% did.[58] Increased suburban sprawl and widespread automobile ownership and use are associated with decreased physical activity, particularly walking.[59] The COVID-related lockdowns and subsequent increased shift to working from home have also led to decreases in physical activity.[60]

Genetics

A family history of obesity substantially increases an individual's likelihood of obesity. The biggest risk factor for obesity in a child is having a parent or first-degree relative with obesity. Having a first- or second-degree relative with type 2 diabetes is also an independent risk factor for insulin resistance. Although the risk of developing obesity has a strong genetic component—genetic associations are present in about 60%–70% of individuals with obesity—single gene defects are responsible for the obesity phenotype in fewer than 2% of cases.[61,62] The melanocortin-4 receptor (MC4R) gene, leptin gene, proopiomelanocortin (POMC) gene, and agouti gene all have significant effects on body fat and fat stores. Genetic abnormalities in MC4R may account for up to 6% of cases of early onset severe obesity in children.[63] Absence of leptin or ineffective or defective leptin receptors (LEPRs) is associated with severe obesity in rodents and humans.[64] Leptin has the dual effect of reducing food intake and increasing energy expenditure, both of which favor loss of body fat. The provision of leptin to leptin-deficient children reduced body weight and hunger, indicating the importance of leptin in normal-weight subjects.[65] Heterozygotes for leptin deficiency have low but detectable serum leptin levels and increased adiposity, indicating that low levels of leptin are associated with increased hunger and gain in body fat.[66] Although genetics accounts for approximately 10% of the intestinal microbial taxa, *Christensenellaceae* is a highly hereditable taxon associated with leanness. Testing for monogenic causes of obesity should be considered in the pediatric population when early onset or suspected syndromic obesity [obesity with additional phenotypic characteristics (e.g., developmental delay, intellectual disability, organ-specific anomalies, and dysmorphic features)] is noted.[67] Table 8.2 shows some of the genetic syndromes that frequently have obesity as a component of their clinical presentation.[68]

Perinatal Exposures

A variety of perinatal exposures have increasingly been implicated as risk factors for obesity in childhood and adulthood. For example, smoking during pregnancy is associated with a linear dose–response relationship (up to 15 cigarettes per day) to the

TABLE 8.2 Genetic Syndromes Associated with Obesity

Syndrome Name	Clinical Presentation	Genetic Mutation/Inheritance
Albright hereditary osteodystrophy/pseudohypoparathyroidism type Ia	Obesity, mental retardation, brachymetaphalangism, short stature	Missense, frameshift, nonsense, splice-site, deletions, insertions in GNAS1/GNAS. Autosomal dominant
Alström syndrome	Childhood obesity, insulin resistance and type 2 diabetes mellitus, blindness, hearing impairment	Frameshift, nonsense, missense in ALMS1. Autosomal recessive
Bardet-Biedl syndrome/Laurence-Moon-Bardet-Biedl syndrome	Obesity, retinitis pigmentosa, renal malformation, polydactyly, mental retardation, hypogonadism	Missense, nonsense, splice-site and frame-shift mutations in BBS1, BBS2. Autosomal recessive
Carpenter syndrome/acrocephalopolysyndactyly type II	Obesity, umbilical hernia, soft tissue syndactyly, congenital heart disease, mental retardation, hypogenitalism	Truncating, missense, nonsense mutations of RAB23. Autosomal recessive
Prader-Willi syndrome/Prader-Labhart-Willi	Obesity and hyperphagia, failure to thrive, hypotonia, genital hypoplasia, mental retardation, small hands and feet	Deletions, mutations, loss of paternal allele MKRN3/ZNF127/MAGEL2. Autosomal dominant, x-linked

From Kaur Y, de Souza RJ, Gibson WT, Meyre D. A systematic review of genetic syndromes with obesity. *Obes Rev*. 2017;18(6):603–634.

subsequent development of overweight and obesity in the offspring.[69] Children born to mothers who smoked during pregnancy are 50% more likely to develop overweight or obesity.[70]

Gestational diabetes has also been linked to an increased risk of childhood obesity. Children born to mothers diagnosed with diabetes tended to have a BMI 2.6 kg/m^2 higher than siblings born prior to the development of maternal diabetes.[71] In addition, the former had 3.7 higher odds of developing diabetes compared to the latter. Mechanisms proposed to explain these associations include fetal exposure to excessive insulin, inflammation, and altered adipokine profiles.[72] Children exposed to gestational diabetes before 26 weeks gestational age have increased hypothalamic activity in response to glucose, which is predictive of subsequent increased BMI.[73]

Maternal obesity and malnutrition during pregnancy have been linked with an increased risk of obesity in offspring, possibly through epigenetic changes that affect adipocyte differentiation and metabolism and/or alterations in the gut microbiome.[74] In a recent meta-analysis, maternal overweight in pregnancy was associated with an 89% increase in the odds of childhood obesity in offspring; maternal obesity in pregnancy was associated with a 264% increase in the odds of childhood obesity in offspring.[75]

In utero environmental exposures to so-called endocrine-disrupting chemicals may impact the development of sensitive neuroendocrine mechanisms and processes necessary for normal growth and development, leading to subsequent childhood and adulthood obesity[76]; however, the data are inconsistent, and a causative role for these agents and the subsequent development of obesity has not been established.[77]

Medical Conditions

A handful of relatively common medical conditions are recognized to lead to weight gain:

- Cushing's disease. Cushing's disease—the hyperproduction of endogenous glucocorticoids—results from a pituitary or ectopic tumor that secretes too much adrenocorticotropic hormone that leads to increased cortisol production (80%) or pathology of the adrenal gland or glands that leads to autonomous adrenal cortisol overproduction (20%).[78] Weight gain is a common feature, particularly abdominal weight gain. At an annual incidence of 1.6 cases per million person-years (versus an annual incidence for obesity of 17.2 per 1000 person-years for children with normal weight, 91.5 per 1000 person-years for children with overweight, and 28.1 per 1000 person-years for adults), Cushing's disease can be difficult to identify.[79–81] Guidelines are available to help direct screening for appropriate patients.[82]
- Hypothyroidism. While hypothyroidism may lead to some modest weight gain, a causal relationship between hypothyroidism and obesity is not entirely clear. Indeed, weight loss can lead to hypothyroidism.[83] Regardless, hypothyroidism is common in obesity, with approximately 14% of patients with obesity also having hypothyroidism.[84] Guidelines for screening are published elsewhere and begin with checking a serum thyroid-stimulating hormone level.[85]
- Polycystic ovarian syndrome. This is the most common endocrinological condition affecting women, with up to 18% of women affected.[86] Prevalence is highest in women with obesity, and the diagnosis is based on the revised Rotterdam Criteria. Women must have two of the following three present: oligo- or anovulation, clinical and/or biochemical signs of hyperandrogenism, and/or polycystic ovaries with the exclusion of other etiologies.[87] The directionality between PCOS and obesity is unclear (i.e., whether PCOS causes obesity or vice versa) and indeed most likely is bidirectional.[88] PCOS is discussed in greater detail later in this chapter.

Medication-Induced Weight Gain

Numerous classes of medications are well-known to cause weight gain through a variety of mechanisms, including enhancing appetite, decreasing metabolic rate, impairing glucose metabolism, and promoting fat storage. Over 20% of adults take an obesogenic medication.[89] Even if people taking these medications do not gain weight, the use of these medications can make it difficult to lose weight. These medications include allergy medications, antidepressants, antiepileptics, antihypertensives, antipsychotic agents, insulin and insulin secretagogues, cold remedies, contraceptive agents, and steroids (Cushing's syndrome) (Table 8.3).[90]

In addition to thoroughly reviewing patients' prescription medications, over-the-counter medications, and supplements, it is important to ask about other substance use, particularly cannabis products. These products are increasingly becoming decriminalized or legalized across the country, and patients may not be aware of the potential weight gain associated with them.[91,92]

TABLE 8.3 Medications Associated With Weight Gain and Potential Alternatives

Medication Class	Medications Associated with Weight Gain	Medications Associated with Less Weight Gain Are Weight Neutral and/or Induce Weight Loss
Allergy medications	Cetirizine, diphenhydramine, doxepin, fexofenadine, levocetirizine	Loratadine
Antidepressant agents	Amitriptyline, citalopram, fluoxetine (>1 year), mirtazapine, nortriptyline, paroxetine, sertraline (>1 year)	Bupropion, fluoxetine (<1 year), sertraline (<1 year)
Antidiabetic agents	Insulin, sulfonylureas, thiazolidinediones	DPP-4 inhibitors, GLP-1 receptor agonists, GLP-1/GIP receptor agonist, metformin, pramlintide, SGLT-2 inhibitors
Antiepileptic agents	Carbamazepine, gabapentin, pregabalin, valproate	Lamotrigine, levetiracetam, phenytoin, topiramate, zonisamide
Antihypertensive agents	Doxazosin, metoprolol, prazosin, propranolol, terazosin	Carvedilol, nebivolol
Antipsychotic agents	Clozapine, lithium, olanzapine, quetiapine, risperidone	Aripiprazole, ziprasidone
Cold remedies	Diphenhydramine	Use for as short of a duration as needed
Contraceptive agents	Depo-medroxyprogesterone acetate, combination oral contraceptive pills (older generation)	Copper IUD, low-dose combination oral contraceptive pill
Steroids	Glucocorticoids, progestins	Use lowest dose possible, NSAIDs, budesonide preparations, steroid inhalers

Smoking

Tobacco smokers tend to weigh less than nonsmokers.[93] While some have postulated that it may relate to decreased appetite and alterations in taste perception from smoking, studies have demonstrated no difference in caloric intake between smokers and nonsmokers[94]; however, smoking leads to a 10% increase in 24-hour energy expenditure, potentially through nicotine-induced sympathetic nervous system activation.[95] Accordingly, smoking cessation is associated with an average weight gain of 4.4 kg for men and 5.0 kg for women.[96] Concerns about weight gain can be a significant impediment to smoking cessation, and weight gain postsmoking cessation can lead to relapse.[97] Despite the risk of weight gain, smoking cessation should be strongly encouraged, since smoking is associated with the development of insulin resistance and truncal adiposity, both risk factors for metabolic syndrome.[98] Moreover, smoking cessation—even with subsequent weight gain—is associated with a significant reduction in the risk of cardiovascular disease and all-cause mortality compared to people who continue smoking.[99]

Microbiome

A growing body of evidence implicates alterations in the gut microbiome as a contributing factor to the obesity epidemic. Most of the body's bacteria reside in the colon; of the tens of trillions of bacteria in the colon, 80% belong to the *Firmicutes*, *Bacteroides*, and *Actinobacteria* phyla.[100,101] In individuals with obesity, there tends to be a predominance of *Firmicutes* and fewer *Bacteroides*, while the opposite is true in lean individuals.[102,103] The microbial profile associated with obesity leads to enhanced energy extraction from the diet, increased inflammation, and gene expression patterns that promote lipogenesis and fatty acid uptake.[104,105] Conversely, the microbial profile associated with leanness may enhance energy expenditure and reduce fat storage.[106] While there is growing evidence of a causal relationship between certain gut microbial profiles and obesity, interventions such as prebiotics, probiotics, and antibiotics to induce weight loss by altering the microbiome require additional study.

Poor Sleep

In recent years, poor sleep—both in terms of quantity and quality—has emerged as a potential risk factor for obesity, although much of the evidence is based on observational studies.[107,108] The increased prevalence of obesity in recent decades has coincided with a decline in sleep quality among both adults and children.[109,110] Poor sleep has been linked in a number of population-based studies to obesity and other metabolic and cardiovascular diseases. A study of over 138,000 people found that poor sleep was associated with a 14%, 23%, and 43% increase in the odds of obesity, myocardial infarction, and coronary artery disease.[111] A number of studies have suggested that the association between sleep and BMI follows a U-shaped curve, with BMI reaching a nadir around 7–8 hours of sleep per night.[112,113] These findings have been hypothesized to be related to serum leptin and ghrelin levels, two key appetite regulatory hormones, with the former being anorexic and the latter being orexigenic. In a study of patients who have sleep disorders, those with habitual sleep of 5 hours per night had 15.5% lower predicted serum leptin levels and 14.9% higher predicted ghrelin levels compared to those with habitual sleep of 8 hours per night.[112] This could imply that better sleep could lead to weight loss. In a study of 123 people with overweight and obesity undergoing caloric restriction, adequate sleep predicted greater fat mass loss[114]; however, further research is needed to determine if poor or inadequate sleep plays an etiologic role in the obesity epidemic.

PATHOPHYSIOLOGY OF OBESITY

Body weight and fat mass are subject to homeostatic control. The hypothalamus sits as the center of weight and appetite regulation. There are two bodies of neurons in the arcuate nucleus of the hypothalamus that integrate information from peripheral signals coming from adipocytes, the intestine, and the pancreas to regulate appetite and energy expenditure through thermogenesis.[115] One body of neurons expresses the orexigenic peptides neuropeptide Y and agouti-related peptide, each of which function to increase food intake and reduce energy expenditure. The other body of neurons expresses POMC and cocaine- and amphetamine-regulated transcript, which are anorexigenic peptides that lead to a reduction in appetite and increase in energy expenditure by activation of downstream pathways, such as activation of MC4R in the paraventricular nucleus of the hypothalamus.[116] In the disease of obesity, there is a disruption of this homeostasis as a result of impaired neurohormonal signaling. Damage to POMC neurons and concomitant inflammation have been associated with diet-induced obesity and resistance to weight-regulating hormones, including leptin and insulin.[117] This physiologic disruption is but one example of how the pathways regulating body weight are affected in the disease of obesity.

Intestinal peptides, including glucagon-like peptide (GLP), CCK, pancreatic polypeptide, and polypeptide YY, reduce food intake, whereas ghrelin, a small peptide produced in the stomach, stimulates food intake.[118] Metabolism of fatty acids in the brain may be another important control point. Oxidation of fatty acids modulates activity of 5′-adenosine monophosphate kinase, an enzyme that is activated or inhibited in relation to the ratio of adenosine monophosphate to adenosine triphosphate and is thought to be the underlying central point in the control system of food intake.[119]

PROGNOSIS OF OBESITY

Obesity has a tremendous impact on the physical, mental, and psychosocial aspects of the lives of those suffering from this disease. In a meta-analysis of 97 articles reporting on hazard ratios for all-cause mortality in relation to BMI categories, people with obesity of all classes relative to normal-weight individuals have higher all-cause mortality.[120] In one study, patients with class III obesity had reduced life expectancy by about 10 years, which is comparable to the effect of lifelong cigarette smoking.[121] A study using National Health and Nutrition Examination Survey data found that, compared with adults of normal weight, adults with class II and III obesity died 3.7 years earlier (all-cause mortality), and adults with class III obesity had cardiovascular disease–related deaths 5 years earlier.[122] In addition to the increased risk of mortality and the numerous complications described later in this chapter, increasing BMI is associated with worse health-related quality of life, greater impairments in activities, and diminished work productivity.[123]

Both primary and secondary prevention of obesity can improve life expectancy and comorbidities. Even modest weight loss of 5%–10% can lead to significant improvements in hypertension, hyperlipidemia, and glucose control; greater weight loss imparts further cardiometabolic benefits (Figure 8.2).[124] It is important to note that obesity should be considered a chronic and relapsing disease that requires ongoing treatment even after weight loss has occurred to prevent weight regain.

HISTORY, PHYSICAL EXAMINATION, AND LABORATORY EVALUATION OF PATIENTS WITH OBESITY

Eliciting a history in a patient with obesity is complicated because of the multifactorial nature of the disease, which can span an

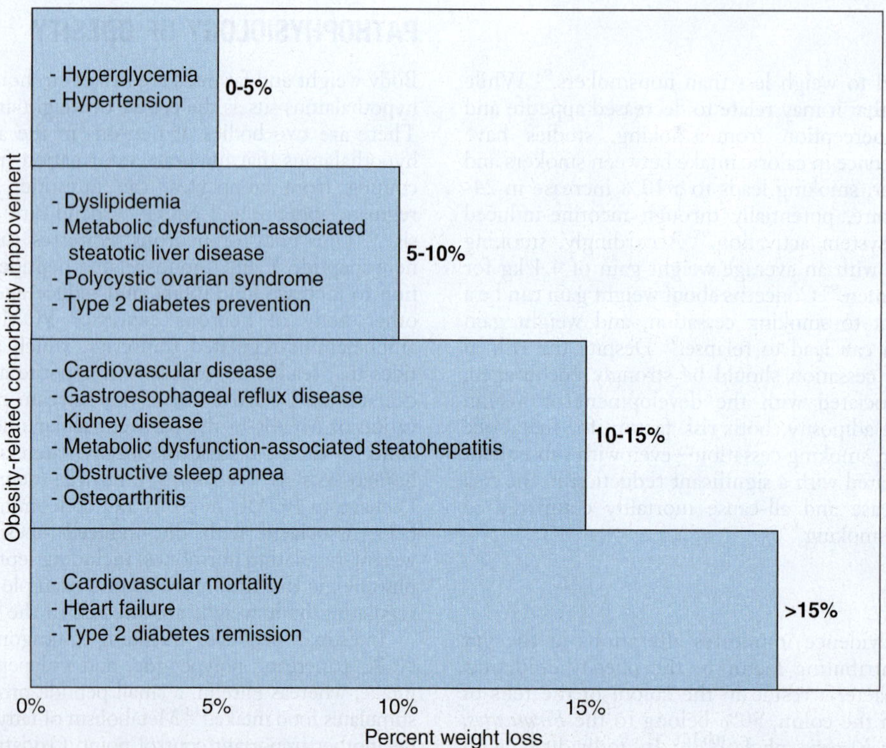

Fig. 8.2 Degree of weight loss associated with comorbidity improvement.

entire lifetime from in utero factors to job-related stressors and hormonal changes that occur as people progress through life. The history should address age of onset of obesity, minimum adult weight maintained for a year, and notable events associated with weight gain (e.g., cessation of smoking, pregnancy, menopause, and medication initiation/discontinuation). A history of psychiatric illness or of eating disorders such as anorexia, bulimia, or binge-eating disorder usually requires close follow-up with a mental health practitioner in addition to the obesity medicine specialist. The care of significant alcohol and substance abuse should take precedence over obesity treatment. A detailed history of smoking and smoking cessation should be included, because smoking cessation can result in weight gain or thwart attempts at weight loss; however, as mentioned, smoking cessation should be prioritized insomuch as the patient is willing. Eliciting a 24-hour dietary recall can be helpful in identifying areas for improvement and targets for intervention (e.g., focusing on eliminating sugar-sweetened beverages or using certain medications at a time of day when appetite is strongest or eating feels most out of control for a patient). A detailed history of a patient's current level of physical activity, including lifestyle and structured exercise, should be documented prior to initiating an exercise program. Finally, an assessment for sleep disorders, including snoring, sleep apnea, and daytime fatigue or morning headaches, should be obtained.

A comprehensive physical examination should be performed to evaluate causes of obesity, as well as the complications of this disease. Height and weight should be measured, and the BMI calculated to categorize the class of obesity. Waist circumference should be measured with the proper technique at the level directly above the iliac crests.[125] Blood pressure should be measured with an appropriately sized cuff to avoid mismeasurement by ill-fitting cuffs that are either too tight or too loose. Other findings to note include the presence of acanthosis nigricans and skin tags indicative of insulin resistance, violaceous striae, and dorsocervical fat pads indicative of hypercortisolism, and thyromegaly and delayed reflexes as signs of hypothyroidism. Obesity may be part of the clinical presentation of other endocrine disorders such as polycystic ovarian syndrome, Cushing syndrome, hypothyroidism, and acromegaly. Insulin resistance and hyperinsulinemia in the months or years before developing overt type 2 diabetes can lead to significant findings. Some findings, such as fungal skin infections, lower extremity edema, and foot deformities, may occur in patients with longstanding obesity.

Certain obesity complications may manifest only with laboratory and investigational testing. A hemoglobin A1c, fasting blood glucose, or 75 g oral glucose tolerance test should be considered to screen for type 2 diabetes.[126] A full lipid panel, including fractionated lipoprotein levels, may be helpful to assess for genetic disorders of lipid metabolism such as familial hypercholesterolemia. Hyperuricemia, hepatic steatosis, and cholestasis are often only discovered upon further laboratory testing. Therefore a complete laboratory evaluation should include blood glucose, uric acid, BUN, creatinine, ALT, AST, total and direct bilirubin, alkaline phosphatase, lipid panel, complete blood count, thyroid-stimulating hormone test, and urinalysis. Fasting serum insulin and glucose test values can be used to calculate homeostatic model assessment levels of insulin resistance by using an online calculator based on a well-validated equation to measure insulin resistance.[127] Measurements of body composition utilizing rapid, inexpensive methods such as bioelectrical impedance or dual-energy x-ray absorptiometry can provide more information on body fat percentage, sarcopenic obesity, and lean body mass and can be tracked longitudinally with a patient's course of treatment.[128]

Complications of Obesity

The complications of obesity are numerous. When overt complications of obesity are diagnosed, these conditions should be addressed concomitantly with medically supervised weight loss.

Cancer

The International Agency for Research on Cancer has determined that there are 13 cancers in which obesity plays a causal role in their development: esophageal, gastric, colon and rectum, liver, gallbladder, pancreas, postmenopausal breast, uterus, ovary, renal cell, meningioma, thyroid, and multiple myeloma.[129] In a prospective cohort of more than 900,000 adults in the United States, overweight and obesity accounted for 14% and 20% of all cancer deaths in men and women, respectively.[130]

The mechanisms underlying the relationship between obesity and cancer are complex. Adipose tissue produces hormones such as estrogen, insulin, and leptin, which can promote cancer cell growth and survival.[131] Chronic inflammation and insulin resistance, which are common in obesity, can promote cancer development.[129,132] Additionally, obesity can lead to changes in the metabolism of adipose tissue, which can contribute to cancer development.[133] Obesity treatment is associated with a significant reduction in the risk of cancer development. Indeed, treating obesity reduces the 10-year cumulative incidence of cancer development by 32% and cancer-related mortality by 48%.[134]

Cardiovascular Diseases

Obesity is a well-established risk factor for the development of cardiovascular diseases, specifically coronary artery disease, stroke, heart failure, arrhythmias, and sudden cardiac death.[135] The pathophysiological effects of obesity on the cardiovascular system are mediated by indirect (insulin resistance/diabetes, hypertension, dyslipidemia, and inflammation) and direct effects.[136] Increased circulating blood volume from enhanced sodium retention and sympathetic nervous system tone (see *Kidney Disease* section below) leads to maladaptive cardiac remodeling.[136,137] Pathological deposition of adipocytes in the myocardium leads to a proinflammatory local environment with subsequent fibrosis.[138–140]

Elevated BMI is thought to contribute to 16%–18% of ischemic heart disease age-standardized deaths.[141] Every 1 kg/m^2 increase in BMI confers a 5% and 7% increase in the risk of heart failure for men and for women.[142] Weight loss leads to significant reductions in the risks of cardiovascular disease and death, as well as improvements in heart failure.[143,144]

Diabetes Mellitus

Obesity is the strongest modifiable risk factor for type 2 diabetes mellitus, with risk of diabetes increasing dramatically with increased BMI.[145–147] A meta-analysis of prospective studies reported that the relative risk of developing diabetes for individuals with overweight was 2.9-fold higher than for individuals with normal BMI; the risk for people with obesity was 7.30-fold higher.[148]

In people with obesity, fasting and postprandial insulin concentrations are higher than in individuals without obesity. There are a variety of factors that cause this, including elevated free fatty acid levels that promote increased free fatty acid oxidation in muscle and liver and therefore decreased glucose utilization by muscle and liver, which triggers hepatic gluconeogenesis in response to elevated free fatty acids.[149] Adipocytes secrete a variety of pro-inflammatory hormones (e.g., leptin, IL-6, tumor necrosis factor), which increase free fatty acid levels; they also secrete adiponectin, a known insulin sensitizer, which is markedly reduced in the obese state.[150] As the insulin-producing beta cells of the pancreas decline in number and function as a result of hyperglycemia and oxidative stress, the balance of increasing insulin production to maintain normoglycemia becomes upset, leading to further hyperglycemia.[151,152]

Weight loss can reduce the risk of developing diabetes.[153–155] In general, losing 10% total body weight decreases the risk of diabetes by 80%.[156–158] It can also lead to significant improvements in glycemic parameters, a reduction in diabetes medications, and even regression of the disease.[159,160] In people with diabetes, 5%–10% total body weight loss led to 3.5-fold higher odds of reducing the hemoglobin A1c by 0.5%.[124] After bariatric surgery, 72% of patients achieved diabetes remission, with 30% maintaining that remission at 15 years of follow-up.[161,162] Therefore weight loss is part of the treatment guidelines in the American Diabetes Association guidelines and the American Association of Clinical Endocrinologists/American College of Endocrinology guidelines[163,164]; recent updates suggest that 10%–15% total body weight loss should be pursued for the potential of diabetes remission.[165]

Gallbladder Disease

The increased prevalence of cholelithiasis in patients with obesity has long been recognized. Most gallstones in Western countries are cholesterol stones (~75%),[166] which form when excess cholesterol in the bile leads to cholesterol crystal precipitation and subsequent stone formation.[167] Obesity's causal role in gallstone precipitation is through insulin resistance and hyperinsulinemia, which increases cholesterol synthesis in the liver and secretion into the gallbladder. Weight loss paradoxically is also implicated in the pathogenesis of cholelithiasis. This is because the flux of cholesterol mobilized from fat is increased throughout the biliary system.[168] Approximately 10%–25% of people with obesity develop gallstones within the first few months of a low-calorie diet; one-third of these patients will develop symptomatic cholelithiasis.[169] Excess weight loss of greater than 25% is a known risk factor.[170] Diets with moderate-to-high levels of fat prompt gallbladder contraction, thereby emptying its cholesterol content and perhaps reducing the increased risk of stone formation associated with weight loss. Similarly, the use of bile acids (e.g., ursodeoxycholic acid) may be advisable, as they reduce the risk of stone formation and need for cholecystectomy for symptomatic cholelithiasis.[171] See Chapters 67–69 for more details about gallbladder disease.

Gastroesophageal Reflux Disease

Overweight and obesity strongly contribute to the development of gastroesophageal reflux disease (GERD) through both mechanical and metabolic factors. Excess weight, particularly intra-abdominal weight, increases intra-abdominal pressure, leading to reflux of gastric contents into the esophagus.[172] Approximately 40% of individuals with class III obesity also have a hiatal hernia, which further contributes to GERD.[173] In addition to these mechanical factors, excess adiposity leads to a proinflammatory environment and disruptions in the normal levels of ghrelin, leptin, and adiponectin, leading to impaired lower esophageal sphincter function.[174] A number of studies have demonstrated that weight loss improves GERD, as measured by esophageal pH and by patient-reported symptoms.[175] Obesity is strongly associated with the development of Barrett's esophagus, a precursor lesion of esophageal adenocarcinoma.[176] Class III obesity is associated with a fivefold and threefold higher odds of esophageal adenocarcinoma and adenocarcinoma of the gastroesophageal junction.[177] See Chapter 48 for more detail about GERD.

Hypertension

The obese state is associated with perturbations in levels of leptin and insulin, as well as increased inflammation and oxidative stress, leading to activation of the renin-angiotensin-aldosterone system

(RAAS) and the sympathetic nervous system. The net effects are intravascular volume expansion, increased vascular tone with impaired vasodilation, ventricular hypertrophy with impaired diastolic relaxation, and renal dysfunction.[178,179]

In a nationally representative study, Must and colleagues demonstrated that 60%–70% of cases of hypertension were attributable to obesity.[180] The probability of someone with obesity also having hypertension is 35% higher than in someone without obesity.[181] Across a variety of obesity treatment modalities, weight loss reduces blood pressure and should be considered a mainstay of the treatment of hypertension.[182–186] On average, 1 kg of weight loss leads to a systolic blood pressure reduction of 1 mm Hg and a diastolic blood pressure reduction of 0.9 mm Hg.[187]

Infertility

Obesity adversely impacts fertility in both women and men. In women, obesity has been linked to menstrual dysfunction, anovulation, and PCOS, a common endocrine disorder with a global prevalence of 5%–15%.[188,189] Women with PCOS often have insulin resistance; the subsequent hyperinsulinemia stimulates excess androgen production by the ovaries, leading to acne, hirsutism, and male-pattern baldness.[189,190] Irregular menstrual cycles and anovulation make pregnancy difficult to achieve. Patients with PCOS undergoing fertility treatments often require higher doses of fertility drugs, are less likely to become pregnant, and risk complications like ovarian hyperstimulation syndrome.[190,191] Every 1 kg/m^2 increase in BMI above 29 kg/m^2 leads to a 4% lower likelihood of pregnancy in subfertile couples.[192] Women with PCOS who do achieve pregnancy are at higher risk of pregnancy complications (gestational diabetes, preeclampsia, spontaneous abortion, and preterm birth).[189]

In men, obesity is associated with lower testosterone levels, lower sperm quality, and diminished fertility.[193–195] Oxidative stress and inflammation in semen may impair sperm function and lead to heritable epigenetic changes and DNA damage.[196] Men with obesity are at greater risk of erectile dysfunction from hormonal and vascular alterations induced by excess adiposity.[197] Weight loss improves fertility in both women and men.[198–200]

Kidney Disease

The deleterious effects of obesity on the kidney are a result of complex physical, hormonal, hemodynamic, metabolic, and inflammatory factors that lead to direct and indirect injury, the latter mediated largely by diabetes and hypertension. There is epidemiologic evidence to suggest the majority of kidney injury occurs through these indirect effects of diabetes and hypertension and the subsequent development of diabetic and hypertensive nephropathy.[201] Compared to patients without obesity, patients with obesity have a 1.8-fold higher risk of chronic kidney disease[202]; class III obesity is associated with a sevenfold increase in the risk of end-stage kidney disease (ESKD).[203] Up to one-third of ESKD cases are thought to be related to excess weight.[204] Surgical and nonsurgical weight loss interventions are associated with significant improvements in albuminuria, proteinuria, hypertension, estimated glomerular filtration rate, and serum creatinine.[205–207]

The cascade of kidney injury pathways initiated by obesity is numerous, complex, and can lead to cycles of increasing injury (Fig. 8.3). The obese state is associated with increased extracellular and blood volume, which leads to glomerular hyperfiltration, afferent arteriolar vasodilation, and ultimately arteriosclerosis.[208] At the same time, RAAS activation causes efferent arteriolar vasoconstriction, increasing the pressure gradient and exacerbating injury.[209] RAAS activation also enhances renal sodium and water reabsorption, further increasing systemic and glomerular hypertension. RAAS activation also leads to upregulation in sodium-glucose-contransporter-2 (SGLT2) expression, which increases renal tubular glucose reabsorption, leading to hyperglycemia, which further increases SGLT2 expression; the hyperglycemic state contributes to hyperfiltration and inflammatory injury. Adipose tissue elaborates a number of proinflammatory cytokines (e.g., TNF-α and IL-6), leading to further inflammation, oxidative stress, and damage to the glomeruli of the kidney.[210,211] Obesity also leads to injurious hemodynamic changes. Increased intra-abdominal pressure causes compression of the renal parenchyma and renal vasculature, leading to intrarenal hypertension, which, in turn, leads to increased sodium and water

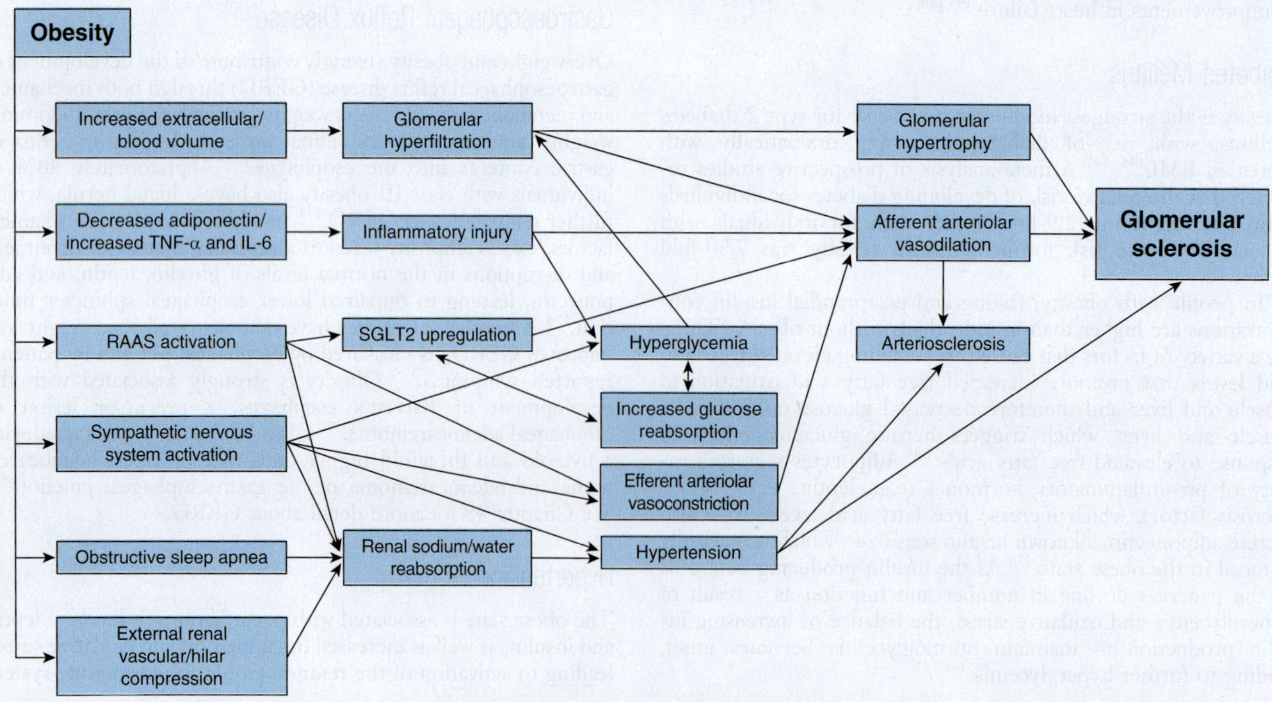

Fig. 8.3 Cycle of kidney injury associated with obesity.

reabsorption, further RAAS activation, and afferent arteriolar dilation.

It is worth noting that not only is obesity a major contributor to ESKD, but it also is a significant roadblock for patients to achieve kidney transplant eligibility.[212] This is important because kidney transplantation is the preferred treatment modality for ESKD and imparts a significant survival benefit for the recipient, even with higher risk transplants, and even in patients with high BMI.[213–216] To compound matters, many transplant candidates have a potential living donor who is ineligible to donate because of donor obesity and concerns for donors' long-term health.[217–219]

Lipid Derangements

The relationship between obesity and lipid derangements—including elevated triglycerides, low HDL cholesterol, and high LDL cholesterol, particularly the proatherogenic small dense LDL particles—has been well established in a number of large cohort studies.[220,221] Dyslipidemia is a major risk factor for the development of cardiovascular disease, and obesity contributes to this risk both through the increased risk of dyslipidemia and independently of it.[222] The underlying pathophysiology is complex, though insulin resistance is thought to play a major role.[223] Obesity management plays a major role in treating dyslipidemia, and a number of guidelines are available.[224,225] These include dietary changes, pharmacotherapy, and bariatric surgery, which have all been associated with subsequent improvements in lipid profiles.[226–230]

Liver Disease

Metabolic-dysfunction-associated steatotic liver disease (MASLD; previously nonalcoholic fatty liver disease but recently renamed[231,232]), and its more advanced form, metabolic-dysfunction-associated steatohepatitis (MASH, previously nonalcoholic steatohepatitis), are quite common. The global prevalence is estimated to be 30%, up 50% from 1990 to 2016.[233] This rapid increase in the prevalence is largely driven the obesity epidemic; these trends in MASLD/MASH have been demonstrated in a variety of populations, including children and adolescents.[234,235] Weight loss can lead to significant improvements and regression of MASLD/MASH.[144,236,237] See Chapter 89 for greater detail about MASLD/MASH.

Obstructive Sleep Apnea

Obstructive sleep apnea is characterized by repeated episodes of either partial or complete upper airway collapse, leading to hypoxia, hypercapnia, and sleep arousals.[238] These, in turn, lead to sympathetic nervous system activation, inflammation, and oxidative stress, increasing the risk of hypertension, diabetes, cardiovascular disease, and death.[239] Obesity is perhaps the most significant risk factor for the development of obstructive sleep apnea and results from fat deposition in the upper airway, thereby reducing airway diameter and increasing airway resistance.[240] The prevalence of obstructive sleep apnea has increased over time, mirroring the increased prevalence of obesity, and ranges from 79% to 83% in men and 43%–68% in women with class III obesity, compared to 7%–19% and 1%–9% for men and women with normal BMI.[241] Weight loss has been demonstrated to lead to improvements and remission in obstructive sleep apnea.[242]

Osteoarthritis

Osteoarthritis is a frequent complication of obesity that is thought to occur with increased mechanical stress on joint cartilage. This stress stimulates mechanoreceptors that lead to local inflammation and cartilage degradation[243]; however, osteoarthritis is also more common in nonweight-bearing joints of people with obesity than people without obesity, suggesting a systemic effect of excess weight.[244] Obesity is associated with 4.5-fold higher risk of osteoarthritis of the knee.[245] Obesity increases the risk of worse pain and functional outcomes and more complications after elective hip or knee arthroplasty.[246] Weight loss significantly reduces mechanical stress on the knee. For every 1 lb of weight loss, there is a four-fold reduction in the load exerted on the knee joint per step.[247] Weight loss reduces the risk of developing osteoarthritis and reduces the symptoms in those who already have it.[248–250]

Psychosocial Dysfunction

People with obesity frequently experience a number of adverse psychosocial conditions. Because psychosocial evaluations are a component of bariatric surgery evaluations, the prevalence has been particularly well-documented in the prebariatric surgery population: mood disorders (31.5%), disordered eating (50%), anxiety (24%), and substance use (10%).[251] A systematic review of reviews demonstrated that obesity is strongly inversely associated with general and obesity-specific health-related quality of life.[252] Children and adolescents with overweight or obesity, particularly females, experience significant psychosocial difficulties.[253] The direction of a causal relationship between depression and obesity is unclear and indeed may be bidirectional, though a preponderance of the evidence suggests that obesity may be more likely to lead to depression (than depression leading to obesity) through a variety of mechanisms, including stigma, teasing, functional impairment, poorer health-related quality of life, stress, and inflammation.[254] People with obesity frequently experience stigmatization, with significant mental health consequences.[255] The theoretical framework for weight-related stigmatization and its health consequences has been previously established.[256]

Treatment of Obesity

As mentioned earlier, even modest weight loss can lead to a significant reduction in the risk of metabolic complications of obesity.[124] In counseling patients and formulating therapeutic plans with patients, the approach to preventing and treating obesity should be viewed through a chronic disease lens, rather than as simply a cosmetic concern.[164] Diet and physical activity form the cornerstone for any weight loss treatment plan. In addition, whenever possible, concomitant medications that induce weight gain should be substituted with medications that are weight neutral or that can induce weight loss (Table 8.3). Of note, the surgical and endoscopic treatment of obesity is discussed in Chapter 9.

Treatment of Obesity: Dietary Approaches

In general, no dietary pattern of eating has been proven superior in clinical trials, and an internet search reveals many dozens of potential diets available. Adherence is perhaps the most important predictor of weight loss success, so the diet that any given patient likes and finds easiest to adhere to will likely produce the greatest weight loss for that particular patient.[257] Several of the most well-studied diets are discussed here, with the understanding that other certain diets, such as very low-calorie diets (<800 calories/day) and protein-sparing modified fasts, should be undertaken only with appropriate medical supervision. Regardless of the dietary approach pursued, it is important to emphasize the importance of minimizing—and ideally, eliminating—sugar-sweetened beverages and ultra-processed foods in the diet.

Varying Dietary Macronutrient Composition

A variety of diets have emerged that focus on varying the composition of macronutrients—fat, protein, and carbohydrates—in the diet. The effectiveness of these diets in weight loss depends upon individual preferences, adherence, and metabolic response. Proponents of the carbohydrate-insulin model often advocate for a low-carbohydrate diet, which tends to consist of 20–120 g of carbohydrates per day and can be higher in protein and lower in fat or vice versa. There is biological plausibility and some preliminary data to support the idea that a low-carbohydrate diet might be especially appropriate for patients with insulin resistance; however, that did not pan out in the larger Diet Intervention Examining the Factors Interacting with Treatment Success study.[258–260] A systematic review and meta-analysis found that low-carbohydrate diets were more effective in achieving weight loss compared to low-fat diets over a period of 6 months to 2 years.[261] Low-carbohydrate diets have been shown to induce greater satiety and lead to reductions in triglycerides and blood pressure.[262,263]

The ketogenic diet is the most extreme version of a low-carbohydrate diet, and energy intake is meant to consist of at least 70% fat to induce ketosis. Even in a calorie-restricted state, it can lead to appetite reductions.[264] A number of unpleasant side effects of the ketogenic diet have been reported, including cramping, weakness, halitosis, and constipation, and the diet may worsen hepatic steatosis and serum lipid levels, potentially increasing cardiovascular risk.[265]

Low-fat diets, which typically involve a reduction in the daily intake of fat to 30% of energy intake or less and an increase in carbohydrate intake, have been investigated for their impact on weight loss and overall health. A study comparing low-fat and low-carbohydrate diets found that both resulted in similar weight loss at 1 year.[260] Low-fat diets have shown benefits in reducing total and LDL cholesterol, as well as improving cardiovascular health.[266,267]

High-protein diets, characterized by increased intake of protein (at least 20% of energy intake from protein) at the expense of carbohydrates or fats, are associated with a higher thermic effect than carbohydrates or fats, leading to increased calorie expenditure on digestion.[268] Protein also enhances satiety and reduces appetite and helps mitigate the lean mass loss that accompanies weight loss.[269–271] It is important to note that long-term use of high-protein diets does require attention to several risks: kidney damage, osteoporosis, and stone formation.[272–274]

Low-Glycemic Index Diet

The glycemic index is a methodology of ranking a given food item's ability to impact serum blood glucose and represents the area under the glycemic-response curve of a particular food item compared to 50 g of glucose expressed as a percent.[275] Foods with values less than 55 are considered low-glycemic index foods, 56–69 are medium-glycemic index foods, and 70 or higher are high-glycemic index foods. A searchable database is available to identify the glycemic index of over 4000 food items.[276] The glycemic index was initially developed to help people with diabetes minimize dietary glycemic excursions. Some studies and meta-analyses have found the low-glycemic index diet to lead to decreases in hemoglobin A1c, fasting glucose, and BMI, particularly in people with diabetes, while others have found no difference in weight loss compared to other diets.[277–282] In an international study of patients across five continents, a high-glycemic index diet was associated with a 21% increase in the risk of a cardiovascular event or death and a 51% increase for those with preexisting cardiovascular disease compared to a low-glycemic index diet.[283]

Mediterranean Diet

For patients in whom cardiovascular health is a paramount concern, the Mediterranean diet can be suggested. While there is no single definition of a Mediterranean diet, these diets are high in fruits, vegetables, whole grains, beans, nuts, and seeds and use olive oil as an important source of monounsaturated fat. A Mediterranean diet allows moderate wine consumption. There are low-to-moderate amounts of fish, poultry, and dairy products, with little red meat. The Mediterranean diet is associated with reductions in overall mortality, cardiovascular mortality, and cancer incidence. In a randomized trial of 7447 adults at high risk for cardiovascular disease, the two groups assigned to the Mediterranean diet supplemented either with extra-virgin olive oil or mixed nuts had a 30% lower hazard of total cardiovascular events (stroke, myocardial infarction, and cardiovascular death) compared with a control group (counseled to eat a low-fat diet) over a median of 4.8 years of follow-up, an absolute reduction in risk of approximately 3 cardiovascular events per 1000 person-years.[284] Additional metaanalyses support these findings.[285,286] However, weight loss with the Mediterranean diet is similar to other comparator diets.[287]

Intermittent Energy Restriction

Based on the premise that fasting leads to a variety of beneficial metabolic changes such as normoglycemia, fatty acid mobilization, and glycogen depletion, a variety of intermittent energy-restriction diets have been proposed.[288] They are often divided into two broad categories: time-restricted feeding and intermittent fasting. The former refers to the practice of limiting energy intake to a window of 10 hours or less per day, and the latter refers to recurring, extended periods of little to no energy intake (typically 16–48 hours), followed by ad libitum energy intake.[289] Clinical trials and metaanalyses on intermittent energy restriction conclude that it is an alternative, though not superior, approach to chronic energy restriction for inducing weight loss, although some patients may demonstrate greater adherence.[290–292] The data are equivocal as to whether intermittent energy restriction mitigates the counter-regulatory mechanisms aimed at weight regain after diet-induced weight loss.[293]

Meal Replacement Diets

A structured way to induce a calorie deficit is through liquid meal replacement. Meal replacements can be used in some patients to achieve further weight loss. This approach can be used in the short term or as a partial liquid diet in the long term such as 1 or 2 meals replaced by low-calorie liquid (protein shake) and the remaining meals as energy-balanced meals.[294] A meta-analysis demonstrated a difference of −1.4 kg at 1-year of follow-up for patients on a meal replacement diet compared to other diets, with greater weight loss difference (−6.3 kg) for those who paired meal replacements with enhanced support from weight loss professionals.[295] A common use of low-calorie liquid is perioperatively around the time of bariatric surgery, but it can be done for longer periods if a patient is able to adhere to it.[296] A simple approach to induce weight loss can be a meal replacement program with calorie-controlled, individually packaged foods. Frozen low-calorie meals containing less than 400 kcal/package can be an especially convenient way to restrict calories.

Treatment of Obesity: Physical Activity

Physical activity guidelines have been described earlier in the chapter.[47,48] While those minimum guidelines confer numerous benefits independent of weight loss, including a dramatic reduction in mortality, they are generally insufficient for weight loss in the absence of calorie restriction.[297–300] However, physical activity is beneficial in promoting favorable body composition changes in the setting of weight loss. On average, for every 3–4 lb lost, 1 lb of fat-free mass is lost.[301] Physical activity, especially strength training and with adequate protein intake, can mitigate some of this muscle loss.[270,302]

Physical activity also plays a key role in weight loss maintenance. In contrast to the minimum recommendations—150 minutes/week of moderate-intensity aerobic activity, 75 minutes/

week of vigorous aerobic activity, or a combination of both, spread throughout the week, with at least 2 days of muscle-strengthening activities per week for adults[48,49]—recommendations to prevent weight regain include >250 minutes/week of moderate-intensity physical activity.[303] In a study of participants in the televised weight loss competition, "The Biggest Loser," at 6 years of follow-up, there was no difference in energy intake between those who maintained their weight loss and those who regained; however, those who maintained their weight loss had a 160% increase in their physical activity from baseline, compared to 34% for those who regained.[304]

Treatment of Obesity: Pharmacotherapy

In patients with an inadequate response to 6 months of lifestyle intervention and a BMI >30 kg/m^2 or >27 kg/m^2 with an obesity-related comorbidity (e.g., diabetes, hypertension, hyperlipidemia, and obstructive sleep apnea.), antiobesity medications (AOMs) should be considered.[164,305,306] In addition, AOMs can be used in patients who have previously undergone bariatric surgery (see Chapter 9) and would benefit from additional weight loss after reaching a plateau for further improvement in obesity-related comorbidities and/or weight regain after surgery.[307,308]

Ostensibly, the goal of pharmacotherapy is weight loss; more importantly, the goal is to improve obesity-related comorbidities. Patients seeking consultation for AOMs frequently inquire about the possibility of short-term medication use to "jump start" the weight loss process; however, obesity is a chronic disease that typically requires long-term treatment, and weight regain is typical following cessation of pharmacotherapy or any lifestyle intervention (and is frequently seen with weight loss procedures as well).[309–312] Additionally, patients and providers should be aware that pharmacotherapy is an adjunct to, and not a substitute for, lifestyle intervention and that maximal weight loss occurs when they are combined.

In selecting AOMs, there are a number of general considerations. First, AOMs that can simultaneously treat other concurrent health problems and induce weight loss are preferred to minimize polypharmacy and cost (e.g., topiramate for patients with frequent migraine headaches). Second, AOMs should be avoided that might exacerbate or be contraindicated with a patient's other medical problems (e.g., stimulants in the setting of anxiety disorder or uncontrolled hypertension). Third, cost is an important consideration as some AOMs, particularly GLP-1 agonists, can be prohibitively expensive. Fourth, more than one AOM may be required to achieve the desired weight loss. Fifth, AOMs are either classified as pregnancy category X or have not been sufficiently studied in pregnancy and lactation.[313] Women of childbearing potential should be counseled about this, and AOMs should generally be discontinued in women who are actively trying to conceive. Sixth, weight loss medication should not be given to a patient with a recent history of an eating disorder unless done with close coordination with the patient's psychiatrist to monitor for eating disorder relapse.

There are currently ten FDA-approved AOMs on the market, as well as a number of other medications that are used off-label for weight loss (Table 8.4).[314]

Diethylpropion, Benzphetamine, and Phendimetrazine

Diethylpropion, benzphetamine, and phendimetrazine are sympathomimetic amines approved for the short-term (typically less than or equal to 3 months) treatment of obesity. These drugs are amphetamine derivates and are infrequently prescribed in modern obesity medicine practice, particularly benzphetamine and phendimetrazine, as they are classified as schedule III agents by the U.S. Drug Enforcement Agency for their addictive potential.[315] Metaanalyses found that over an average of 17.6 and 8.9 weeks,

TABLE 8.4 List of FDA-Approved Antiobesity Medications and Medications Commonly Used Off-Label for Weight Loss

FDA-Approved Antiobesity Medications	Medications Commonly Used Off-Label for Weight Loss
Phentermine	Metformin
Benzphetamine	Bupropion
Phendimetrazine	Pramlintide
Diethylpropion	Sodium-glucose-transport-2 inhibitors
Orlistat	Topiramate
Phentermine-topiramate ER	Glucagon-like peptide-1 receptor agonists other than semaglutide/liraglutide
Bupropion-naltrexone	Naltrexone
Liraglutide 3.0 mg	Zonisamide
Setmelanotide	Lisdexamfetamine
Semaglutide 2.4 mg	
Tirzepatide	

patients treated with diethylpropion and benzphetamine had an average placebo-subtracted weight loss of 3.0 and 3.3 kg, respectively.[316,317] Phendimetrazine has a placebo-subtracted weight loss of 2.9 kg.[318]

While a few longer term studies have been performed with conflicting results,[319,320] the FDA indication for these drugs remains for short-term weight loss. They, along with phentermine (presented separately, also a sympathomimetic amine), received FDA approval well before current guidelines that require study of new agents in people with overweight/obesity for at least 1 year and have the following efficacy criteria: mean placebo-subtracted weight loss >5% of body weight or at least 35% of study participants losing >5% of total body weight.[321] Given more widespread recognition of obesity's chronic nature, these agents have largely fallen out of favor.

Phentermine/Topiramate ER

Like diethylpropion, benzphetamine, and phendimetrazine, phentermine is a centrally acting adrenergic agent approved for short-term use in obesity that works by suppressing appetite. Historically, it has been the most frequently prescribed AOM in the United States.[322] It is FDA-approved for the long-term treatment of obesity in conjunction with topiramate (marketed in a single capsule as Qsymia; Vivus, Inc.) in a controlled-release formulation. Marketed for migraine prophylaxis and epilepsy treatment, topiramate also centrally acts to reduce hunger. In combination, phentermine-topiramate ER has additive weight loss efficacy. Phentermine/topiramate ER is available in 4 doses: 3.75/23 mg (starting dose), 7.5/46 mg (lowest treatment dose), 11.25/69 mg, or 15/92 mg. The majority of patients start on 3.75/23 mg and progress to 7.5/46 mg, with higher doses used if the medication is well tolerated and maximal efficacy is required.

The 56-week EQUIP trial randomized 1267 participants with class II or higher obesity and without diabetes to placebo, 3.75/23, 7.5/46, 11.25/69, or 15/92 mg of phentermine/topiramate, all in addition to a calorie-reduced diet.[323] There was a stepwise increase in weight loss from placebo to increasing doses of phentermine/topiramate. Participants receiving 15/92 mg of phentermine/topiramate lost 10.9% of total body weight, compared to 1.6% for participants in the placebo arm. In the 15/92 mg arm, 66.7%, 47.2%, and 32.3% of participants lost at least 5%, 10%, and 15% of total body weight, compared to 17.3%,

7.4%, and 3.4% on placebo. The 15/92 mg group had improvements in systolic and diastolic blood pressure, serum fasting glucose, triglycerides, HDL, LDL, and total cholesterol compared to placebo. The 56-week CONQUER trial enrolled 2487 people with a BMI of 27–45 kg/m^2 and two or more comorbidities to placebo, 7.5/46, or 15/92 mg of phentermine/topiramate.[324] Weight loss and metabolic changes were similar to those seen in the EQUIP trial. The results of a 56-week extension of the CONQUER trial (the SEQUEL trial) included 676 people and led to long-term weight loss of −1.8%, −9.3%, and −10.5% for those receiving placebo, 7.5/46 mg, and 15/92 mg of phentermine/topiramate.[325] Amongst patients who were diabetes-free at baseline, those who received 7.5/46 mg had a 54% reduction in the likelihood of developing diabetes compared to placebo. Those who received 15/92 mg had a 76% reduction in diabetes development.

The FDA requires a Risk Evaluation and Mitigation Strategy to inform prescribers and females of reproductive potential about the increased risk of congenital malformation, specifically orofacial clefts, in infants exposed to phentermine/topiramate during the first trimester of pregnancy. The most common adverse events (AEs) with phentermine/topiramate ER include paresthesias, dizziness, dysgeusia, insomnia, constipation, and dry mouth. Medication interactions include an increased risk of malignant hypertension with monoamine oxidase (MAO) inhibitors and increased probability of rise in heart rate and blood pressure if used with other sympathomimetic amines. Some patients may benefit from just one component when the other component is contraindicated or its use is limited by side effects.

Orlistat

Until 2012, orlistat was the only FDA-approved drug for long-term use in weight loss; it is approved for ages 12 and up. A dosage of 60 mg three times daily is available over the counter, while 120 mg three times daily requires a prescription. Of note, the over-the-counter dose is FDA approved for BMI >25 kg/m^2. Orlistat's mechanism of action is through the inhibition of gastrointestinal lipases, thereby limiting enteral fat absorption by approximately 25% for the over-the-counter dose and 30% for the prescription-strength dose.[320] Paradoxically, orlistat can lead to decreased satiety, decreased fullness, and increased food consumption, thought to be mediated by increased gastric emptying and decreasing the anorexigenic hormones GLP-1, peptide YY, and cholecystokinin.[326]

Orlistat has been tested extensively in phase 3 randomized clinical trials.[327–336] In the longest duration clinical trial of an AOM published to date, orlistat 120 mg three times daily induced an average placebo-subtracted weight loss of 2.8 kg after 4 years compared to placebo.[335] In the orlistat arm, 72.8% and 41.0% lost at least 5% and 10% of total body weight, compared to 45.1% and 20.8% in the placebo arm. Among participants who completed the full 4 years of treatment, 52.8% versus 37.3% lost at least 5% total body weight in the orlistat versus placebo arm, and 26.2% versus 15.6% lost at least 10% total body weight in the orlistat versus placebo arm. In addition, there was a significant 37% reduction in the risk of progression to diabetes in the orlistat group compared to the placebo group (9.0% versus 6.2%). Treatment with orlistat leads to modest improvements in blood pressure and lipid profile parameters, with particularly helpful reductions in LDL, independent of weight loss.[337–340]

The most common side effects are fecal urgency, oily stool, and fecal incontinence, and these frequently limit its use as monotherapy in clinical practice, though clinical trial data suggest only a 3% absolute risk difference in discontinuation due to side effects compared with placebo.[341] Regardless, orlistat can be a helpful adjunct for patients experiencing constipation from other AOMs (e.g., naltrexone, bupropion-naltrexone, and GLP-1 agonists). Concurrent use of psyllium can be helpful in mitigating some of these side effects as well.[342] Orlistat can limit absorption of fat-soluble vitamins—A, D, E, and K—and may require oral supplementation to ameliorate this.[328,332] Vitamin supplementation should be taken at least 2 hours prior to or after the administration of orlistat. Perhaps the most widely studied FDA-approved AOM, orlistat, is infrequently used in clinical practice.

Naltrexone SR/Bupropion SR

Bupropion's primary mechanism of action is through dopamine and norepinephrine reuptake inhibition, thereby modulating the "reward pathway" that various foods can stimulate. Naltrexone is a pure opioid antagonist that blocks an opioid pathway that may slow weight loss. The most common AEs of naltrexone SR/bupropion SR are nausea, vomiting, constipation, headache, dizziness, insomnia, dry mouth, and an increased risk for seizure.

Four large phase III clinical trials, each 56 weeks in duration, established the efficacy of naltrexone SR/bupropion SR: Contrave Obesity Research (COR) I (n = 1742), COR II (n = 1496), COR-Behavioral Modification (COR-BMOD) (n = 793), and COR-Diabetes (n = 505).[343–346] Across these trials, total body weight loss ranged from 5.0% to 9.3% for participants receiving naltrexone SR/bupropion SR, compared to 1.1%–1.8% for participants in the placebo arm; 44.5%–66.4% of participants receiving naltrexone SR/bupropion SR achieved at least 5% total body weight loss, compared to 16.0%–42.5% of participants receiving placebo. The proportion of participants in the naltrexone SR/bupropion SR arm achieving 10% total body weight loss ranged from 18.5% to 41.5%, compared to 5.7%–20.2% of participants in the placebo arm.

As with phentermine/topiramate ER, patients can be prescribed the individual components of naltrexone SR/bupropion SR when one component is not tolerated or contraindicated. Of note, naltrexone can be useful for patients with concurrent alcohol use disorder, and bupropion can be helpful for patients who smoke.

Medication interactions of naltrexone SR/bupropion SR include MAO inhibitors (used during or within 14 days of administration), opioids, opioid agonists, and opioid partial agonists. Abrupt discontinuation of chronic use of alcohol, benzodiazepines, barbiturates, or antiepileptic drugs may further increase the risk for seizure. Naltrexone SR/bupropion SR should be avoided in patients with uncontrolled hypertension, history of seizures, or if there is a recent history of bulimia or anorexia nervosa. A recent history of bulimia with excessive vomiting may result in electrolyte abnormalities and predispose a person to seizures; that seizure risk increases further with the use of bupropion. Naltrexone should be avoided in patients requiring chronic opioid treatment and discontinued in anticipation of elective surgery to prevent poor postoperative pain control. The bupropion should be continued during the perioperative period.

Setmelanotide

A number of rare monogenic obesity syndromes impair MC4R signaling and lead to hyperphagia and childhood-onset severe obesity. Setmelanotide is an injectable MC4R agonist and is FDA-approved for patients 6 years of age and older who have POMC deficiency, proprotein convertase subtilisin/kexin type 1 deficiency, or LEPR deficiency.[347] Setmelanotide normalizes the MC4R pathway, leading to increased expenditure of energy, reduced hunger, and subsequent weight loss. In practice, this is a very rarely used medication in the everyday practice of obesity medicine, though there are ongoing clinical trials to determine setmelanotide's use for a number of other genetic causes of obesity [e.g., Bardet-Biedl syndrome and Alström syndrome (Table 8.2)].[348]

Glucagon-Like Peptide-1 Receptor Agonists

GLP-1 receptor agonists as a class of agents merit additional discussion. GLP-1 is an incretin hormone produced in the L-cells of the ileum in response to the presence of food and plays a key role in satiety and glucose metabolism, particularly by promoting pancreatic beta-cell glucose-dependent insulin secretion and inhibiting glucagon secretion from pancreatic alpha-cells.[349] In addition, GLP-1 receptor agonists bind to GLP-1 receptors in the arcuate nucleus of the hypothalamus. This activates the POMC/CART pathway and inhibits agouti-related peptide and neuropeptide Y, leading to reduced hunger, increased satiety, and weight loss.[350–352]

While all GLP-1 receptor agonists are approved for the treatment of type 2 diabetes mellitus (albiglutide, dulaglutide, exenatide, exenatide extended-release, liraglutide, lixisenatide, and semaglutide), only two are currently FDA-approved for weight loss—liraglutide and semaglutide—though the others are occasionally prescribed off-label for weight loss. Differing molecular structures and sizes across agents within this class lead to different profiles in terms of their effects on glycemic control, weight loss, side effects, and cardiovascular effects.[353] The most common side effects of GLP-1 receptor agonists are nausea, vomiting, diarrhea, constipation, and GERD.

It should be noted that all GLP-1 receptor agonists carry a black box warning regarding the association with medullary thyroid cancer in rodents. Several preclinical studies in rodents suggested this association, particularly with long-acting GLP-1 receptor analogs at supratherapeutic doses.[354,355] Human trials have not suggested that such an association exists.[356] A recent nested case-control study of patients in the French national health insurance system suggested there was an increased risk of medullary thyroid cancer in the first 1-3 years after GLP-1 receptor agonist use, though a number of major methodological issues have been raised.[357–359] The relevance to humans has not yet been determined. Regardless, these agents are contraindicated for patients with a personal or family history of medullary thyroid cancer or multiple endocrine neoplasia syndrome type 2.

Liraglutide 3.0 mg

Daily subcutaneous liraglutide 3.0 mg has been studied across a number of clinical trials (Table 8.5). In the largest of those, the Satiety and Clinical Adiposity—Liraglutide Evidence in individuals with and without diabetes (SCALE) obesity and prediabetes study, 3731 people with at least class I obesity or BMI >27 kg/m^2 with a nondiabetes obesity-related comorbidity were randomized to receive daily liraglutide 3.0 mg or placebo.[360] At 56 weeks, the average total body weight loss was 8.0% for participants in the treatment arm, compared with 2.6% for those in the placebo arm. In the treatment arm, 63.2%, 33.1%, and 14.4% lost at least 5%, 10%, and 15% of total body weight, compared with 27.1%, 10.6%, and 3.5% in the placebo arm. In terms of cardiometabolic benefits, the Liraglutide Effect and Action in Diabetes: Evaluation of Cardiovascular Outcome Results trial reported a 13% relative risk reduction in major adverse cardiovascular events (cardiovascular death, nonfatal myocardial infarction, and nonfatal stroke) compared to placebo, as well as a significant absolute decrease in hemoglobin A1c (−0.4%).[361]

Semaglutide 2.4 mg

Semaglutide is the result of modifications to a GLP-1 receptor analog that lead to resistance to enzymatic degradation, enhanced binding to albumin, and decreased wrong-site binding, giving it a half-life of 165 hours, rendering it suitable for once-weekly subcutaneous dosing.[350,351] The Semaglutide Treatment Effect in People with Obesity (STEP) series of clinical trials robustly established semaglutide's weight loss efficacy (Table 8.6).[229,362–368] In the largest trial of semaglutide for weight loss—STEP 1—1961 participants were randomized to receive semaglutide 2.4 mg subcutaneously weekly or placebo for 68 weeks.[229] The average total body weight loss in the treatment arm was 14.9% compared with 2.6% for participants in the placebo arm. In the semaglutide arm, 86.4%, 69.1%, 50.5%, and 32.0% of participants lost at least 5%, 10%, 15%, and 20% of total body weight, compared with 31.5%, 12.0%, 4.9%, and 1.7% in the participants receiving placebo. The Trial to Evaluate Cardiovascular and Other Long-term Outcomes with Semaglutide in Subjects with type 2 Diabetes (SUSTAIN-6) trial, conducted in individuals with type 2 diabetes and at high risk of cardiovascular disease, reported a 26% relative risk reduction in major adverse cardiovascular events compared with placebo.[369] A meta-analysis demonstrated significant improvements in hemoglobin A1c, systolic blood pressure, diastolic blood pressure, total cholesterol, HDL, LDL, and triglycerides for patients receiving semaglutide compared with placebo.[370] The Semaglutide Effects on Cardiovascular Outcomes in People with Overweight or Obesity trial evaluated the efficacy of semaglutide 2.4 mg versus placebo for prevention of major adverse cardiovascular events in over 17,000 people at least 45 years of age, BMI >27 kg/m^2, and established history of cardiovascular disease but without diabetes. Semaglutide 2.4 mg reduced the risk of major adverse cardiovascular events by 20%.[371]

Tirzepatide

The dual GLP-1 receptor agonist/glucose-dependent insulinotropic polypeptide (GIP) receptor agonist tirzepatide is approved by the FDA for both type 2 diabetes mellitus and for weight loss. In the phase 3 Study of Tirzepatide in Participants with Obesity or Overweight (SURMOUNT-1) clinical trial for weight loss, tirzepatide 15 mg subcutaneous weekly injection led to 22.5% total body weight loss versus 2.4% for participants receiving placebo.[228] By Week 72, 96.3%, 90.1%, 78.2%, 62.9%, and 39.7% of participants receiving tirzepatide lost at least 5%, 10%, 15%, 20%, and 25% total body weight, respectively, compared to 27.9%, 13.5%, 6.0%, 1.3%, and 0.3% of participants in the placebo arm.

Pharmacotherapy Pipeline

Numerous pharmacotherapy candidates are currently in the development pipeline. In a phase 2 clinical trial of retatrutide, an agent with GLP-1, GIP, and glucagon receptor agonism, participants receiving the 12 mg dose of retatrutide lost 24.2% total body weight, compared with 2.1% for participants in the placebo arm.[230] By Week 48, 100%, 93%, 83%, 63%, 48%, and 26% of participants receiving 12 mg of retatrutide lost at least 5%, 10%, 15%, 20%, 25%, and 30% total body weight, compared with 27%, 9%, 2%, 1%, 0%, and 0% of participants receiving placebo.

The oral daily nonpeptide GLP-1 receptor agonist orforglipron led to a 14.7% total body weight loss compared with 2.3% for patients receiving placebo in a phase 2 clinical trial.[372] By Week 36, 90%, 69%, and 48% of participants receiving 45 mg of orforglipron lost at least 5%, 10%, and 15% total body weight, compared to 24%, 9%, and 1% of participants receiving placebo.

A number of other promising agents for weight loss are in various stages of clinical trial development. Such agents include oral semaglutide; a combination of semaglutide and the amylin analog cagrilintide; an activin type II receptor monoclonal antibody that may lead to weight loss and simultaneous skeletal muscle growth; and a daily nonpeptide GLP-1 receptor agonist distinct from orforglipron.[373–376]

TABLE 8.5 Comparison of Liraglutide in Obesity Clinical Trials (Satiety and Clinical Adiposity—Liraglutide Evidence—SCALE Trials)

Trial	Study Population	Intervention	Study Duration	Sample Size	Percent Total Body Weight Loss	Weight Loss (kg)	Percent of Patients Achieving Weight Loss in Treatment Arm vs. Control Arm		
							5%	≥10%	≥15%
SCALE obesity and prediabetes[a]	Adults w/BMI >30 kg/m² or >27 kg/m² w/weight-related comorbidity without diabetes	Daily liraglutide 3.0 mg vs. placebo	56 weeks	3731	−8.0% vs. −2.6%	−8.4 vs. −2.8	63.2% vs. 27.1%	33.1% vs. 10.6%	14.4% vs. 3.5%
SCALE diabetes[b]	Adults w/BMI >30 kg/m² or >27 kg/m² w/ weight-related comorbidity with diabetes	Daily liraglutide 3.0 vs. 1.8 mg vs. placebo	56 weeks	846	−6.0% vs. −4.7% vs. −2.0%	6.4 vs. 5.0 vs. 2.2	54.3% vs. 40.4% vs. 21.4%	25.2% vs. 15.9% vs. 6.7%	NR
SCALE sleep apnoea[c]	Adults w/BMI >30 kg/m² with untreated moderate or severe OSA without diabetes	Daily liraglutide 3.0 mg vs. placebo	32 weeks	359	−5.7% vs. −1.6%	−6.7 vs. −1.9	46.3% vs. 18.5%	23.4% vs. 1.7%	NR
SCALE maintenance[d]	Adults w/BMI >30 kg/m² or >27 kg/m² w/ weight-related comorbidity without diabetes	Daily liraglutide 3.0 mg vs. placebo after 4−12 weeks of LCD and >5% total body weight loss	56 weeks	422	6.2% vs. 0.2% (after run-in period)	−6.0 vs. −0.1 (after run-in period)	50.5% vs. 21.8% (after run-in period)	26.1% vs. 6.3% (after run-in period)	NR
SCALE obesity and prediabetes[e]	Adults w/BMI >30 kg/m² or >27 kg/m² w/ weight-related comorbidity with prediabetes	Daily liraglutide 3.0 mg vs. placebo	160 weeks	2254	−6.1% vs. −1.9%	−6.5 vs. −2.0	49.6% vs. 23.7%	24.8% vs. 9.9%	11.0% vs. 3.1%
Liraglutide for adolescents with obesity[f]	Adolescents (12−17) w/BMI >95th percentile and >30 kg/m²	Daily liraglutide 3.0 mg vs. placebo	56 weeks	125	−2.6% vs. 2.4%	−2.3% vs. 2.2%	43.3% vs. 18.7%	26.1% vs. 8.1%	NR

[a]Pi-Sunyer X, et al. A randomized controlled trial of 3.0 mg of liraglutide in weight management. *N Engl J Med*. 2015;373(1):11–22.
[b]Davies MJ, et al. Efficacy of liraglutide for weight loss among patients with type 2 diabetes. The SCALE diabetes randomized clinical trial. *JAMA*. 2015;314(7):687−699.
[c]Blackman A, et al. Effect of liraglutide 3.0 mg in individuals with obesity and moderate or severe obstructive sleep apnoea: the SCALE Sleep Apnoea randomized clinical trial. *Int J Obes (Lond)*. 2016;40(8):1310−1319.
[d]Wadden TA, et al. Weight maintenance and additional weight loss with liraglutide after low calorie diet induced weight loss: the SCALE maintenance randomised study. *Int J Obes (Lond)*. 2013;37(11):1443−51.
[e]Le Roux CW, et al. 3 years of liraglutide versus placebo for type 2 diabetes risk reduction and weight management in individuals with prediabetes: a randomised, double blind trial. *Lancet*. 2017;389(10077):1399−1409.
[f]Kelly AS, et al. A randomized controlled trial of liraglutide for adolescents with obesity. *N Engl J Med*. 2020;382(22):2117−2128.
LCD, low calorie diet; *NR*, not reported; *OSA*, obstructive sleep apnea.

TABLE 8.6 Comparison of Semaglutide in Obesity Clinical Trials (Semaglutide Treatment Effect in People with Obesity [illegible])

STEP Trial	Study Population	Intervention	Study Duration	Sample Size	Percent Total Body Weight Loss	Weight Loss (kg)	Percent of Patients Achieving Weight Loss in Treatment Arm vs. Control Arm(s)			
							5%	≥10%	≥15%	≥20%
STEP 1[a]	Adults w/BMI >30 or >27 kg/m² w/>1 weight-related comorbidity without diabetes	Semaglutide 2.4 mg vs. placebo	68 weeks	1961	−14.9% vs. −2.4%	−15.3 vs. −2.6	86.4% vs. 31.5%	69.1% vs. 12.0%	50.5% vs. 4.9%	32.0% vs. 1.7%
STEP 2[b]	Adults w/BMI >27 kg/m² and w/diabetes	Weekly semaglutide 2.4 vs. 1.0 mg vs. placebo	68 weeks	1210	−9.6% vs. −7.0% vs. −3.4%	−9.7 vs. −6.9 vs. −3.5	68.8% vs. 57.1% vs. 28.5%	45.6% vs. 28.7% vs. 8.2%	25.8% vs. 13.7% vs. 3.2%	13.1% vs. 4.7% vs. 1.6%
STEP 3[c]	Adults w/BMI >30 or >27 kg/m² w/>1 weight-related comorbidity without diabetes	Weekly semaglutide 2.4 mg vs. placebo, both w/8-week low-calorie diet and 68-week intensive behavioral therapy	68 weeks	611	−16.0% vs. −5.7%	−16.8 vs. −6.2	86.6% vs. 47.5%	75.3% vs. 27.0%	55.8% vs. 13.2%	35.7% vs. 3.7%
STEP 4[d]	Adults w/BMI >30 or >27 kg/m² w/>1 weight-related comorbidity without diabetes	Weekly semaglutide 2.4 mg for all, w/randomization to 2.4 mg vs. placebo after 20 weeks	48 weeks (after 20 weeks run-in)	803	−7.9% vs. 6.9% (Weeks 20−68)	−7.1 vs. 6.1 (Weeks 20−68)	88.7% vs. 47.6% (Weeks 0−68)	79.0% vs. 20.4% (Weeks 0−68)	63.7% vs. 9.2% (Weeks 0−68)	38.6% vs. 4.8% (Weeks 0−68)
STEP 5[e]	Adults w/BMI >30 or >27 kg/m² w/>1 weight-related comorbidity without diabetes	Weekly semaglutide 2.4 mg vs. placebo	104 weeks	304	−15.2% vs. −2.6%	−16.1 vs. −3.2	77.1% vs. 34.4%	61.8% vs. 13.3%	52.1% vs. 7.0%	36.1% vs. 2.3%
STEP 6[f]	Adults w/BMI >35 kg/m² w/>1 weight-related comorbidity or >27 kg/m² w/>2 weight-related comorbidities	Weekly semaglutide 2.4 vs. 1.7 mg vs. placebo	68 weeks	401	−13.2% vs. −9.6% vs. −2.1%	−11.2 vs. −8.2 vs. −1.7	82.9% vs. 72.4% vs. 21.0%	60.6% vs. 41.8% vs. 5.0%	40.9% vs. 24.5% vs. 3.0%	19.7% vs. 11.2% vs. 2.0%
STEP 8[g]	Adults w/BMI >30 or >27 kg/m² w/>1 weight-related comorbidity without diabetes	Weekly semaglutide 2.4 mg vs. daily liraglutide 3.0 mg vs. placebo	68 weeks	388	−15.8% vs. −6.4% vs. −1.9%	−15.3 vs. −6.8	87.2% vs. 58.1% vs. 29.5%	70.9% vs. 25.6% vs. 15.4%	55.6% vs. 12.0% vs. 6.4%	38.5% vs. 6.0% 2.6%
STEP-TEENS[h]	Adolescents (12−17) w/BMI >95th or >85th percentile and >1 weight-related comorbidity	Weekly semaglutide 2.4 mg vs. placebo	68 weeks	201	−16.1% vs. 0.6%	−15.3 vs. 2.4	72.5% vs. 17.7%	61.8% vs. 8.1%	53.4% vs. 4.8%	37.4% vs. 3.2%

[a]Wilding JPH, Batterham RL, Calanna S, et al. Once-weekly semaglutide in adults with overweight or obesity. *N Engl J Med*. 2021;384(11):989−1002.

[b]Davies M, Faerch L, Jeppesen OK, et al. Semaglutide 2.4 mg once a week in adults with overweight or obesity, and type 2 diabetes (STEP 2): a randomised, double-blind, double-dummy, placebo-controlled, phase 3 trial. *Lancet*. 2021;397(10278):971−984.

[c]Wadden TA, Bailey TS, Billings LK, et al. Effect of subcutaneous semaglutide vs placebo as an adjunct to intensive behavioral therapy on body weight in adults with overweight or obesity: the STEP 3 randomized clinical trial. *JAMA*. 2021;325(14):1403−1413.

[d]Rubino D, Abrahamsson N, Davies M, et al. Effect of continued weekly subcutaneous semaglutide vs placebo on weight loss maintenance in adults with overweight or obesity: the STEP 4 randomized clinical trial. *JAMA*. 2021;325(14):1414−1425.

[e]Garvey WT, Batterham RL, Bhatta M, et al. Two-year effects of semaglutide in adults with overweight or obesity: the STEP 5 trial. *Nat Med*. 2022;28(10):2083−2091.

[f]Kadowaki T, Isendahl J, Khalid U, et al. Semaglutide once a week in adults with overweight or obesity, with or without type 2 diabetes in an east Asian population (STEP 6): a randomised, double-blind, double-dummy, placebo-controlled, phase 3a trial. *Lancet Diabetes Endocrinol*. 2022;10(3):193−206.

[g]Rubino DM, Greenway FL, Khalid U, et al. Effect of weekly subcutaneous semaglutide vs daily liraglutide on body weight in adults with overweight or obesity without diabetes: the STEP 8 randomized clinical trial. *JAMA*. 2022;327(2):138−150.

[h]Weghuber D, Barrett T, Barrientos-Perez M, et al. Once-weekly semaglutide in adolescents with obesity. *N Engl J Med*. 2022;387(24):2245−2257.

CONCLUSION

The disease of obesity has become a global epidemic and is a major cause of other noncommunicable diseases, including diabetes, cardiovascular disease, and cancer. Causes can be attributed to a combination of genetic, epigenetic, and environmental, and lifestyle phenomena. Current treatments range from dietary and behavioral interventions to pharmacologic and surgical therapies. Management of obesity is evolving, and obesity is now viewed as a multifactorial chronic disease that needs to involve a combination of medical therapies and, when appropriate, interventional procedures.

Full references for this chapter can be found at https://ebooks.health.elsevier.com.

9 Surgical and Endoscopic Treatment of Obesity

Shelby Sullivan, Steven A. Edmundowicz, John Magaña Morton

IN THIS CHAPTER

Severe obesity is the leading public health crisis of the industrialized world (see Chapter 8). The prevalence of obesity in the United States continues to rise at an alarming rate, with two-thirds of adults currently considered overweight, half of whom are obese.[1,2] The etiology of obesity is complex and only partially understood. Genetic, epigenetic, environmental, and psychological factors are all involved to varying degrees, but, conceptually, obesity is a disorder of energy imbalance wherein there is an increase in stored fat such that it compromises the patient's organ function, susceptibility to disease, and general health. Obesity has been shown to predispose to many diseases, including cardiovascular disease, diabetes mellitus, sleep apnea, and osteoarthritis (see Chapter 7).

Overweight is defined by a BMI greater than 25 kg/m^2; class I obesity, 30–34.9 kg/m^2; class II obesity 35–39.9 kg/m^2; class III obesity ≥40 kg/m^2; and super morbid obesity, greater than 50 kg/m^2. Rising rates of obesity are seen across the United States in men and women, and in all major racial, ethnic, and socioeconomic groups.[3,4] Severe obesity reduces life expectancy by 5–20 years, and for the first time in history, it is predicted that the current generation may have a shorter life expectancy than the last.[5]

Energy intake and expenditure are finely regulated by neural and hormonal mechanisms. Key players in energy regulation include insulin, leptin, ghrelin, and peptide YY. Insulin is a potent anabolic hormone with multiple synthetic and growth-promoting effects. Adipose cells secrete leptin, which reduces food intake and increases energy expenditure. Leptin's counterpart, ghrelin, is secreted by the fundus of the stomach and induces hunger while stimulating anabolism. Endocrine cells in the ileum and colon secrete peptide YY postprandially, and it is considered a signal of satiety.

Obesity is a complex disease with an array of root causes that vary for each patient. Weight loss may be achieved by behavioral, medical, endoscopic, and surgical methods. Combined with careful screening assessments and counseling, however, bariatric surgery is the most efficacious therapeutic option for an appropriate patient population.[6] Weight loss surgery has changed significantly since its inception in the 1950s. Today, with increased efforts by the American College of Surgeons and the American Society of Metabolic and Bariatric Surgery's new Metabolic and Bariatric Surgery Accreditation and Quality Improvement Program (MBSAQIP) to develop evidence-based recommendations, weight loss surgery has mortality rates comparable to routine general surgical procedures such as laparoscopic cholecystectomy or fundoplication.[7,8]

Experience of the surgeon and hospital can mitigate the risks associated with weight loss surgery. In the United States, a volume outcome effect has been recognized by the MBSAQIP and major insurers who require MBSAQIP accreditation.[9,10] Numerous criteria enable Bariatric Surgery Accreditation, but the primary current criteria are a surgeon's volume of greater than 25 cases and an annual hospital volume of greater than 50 stapled cases. The best demonstrated and most protective effect against complications is an accredited experienced surgeon and hospital.[9,11–14]

Roux-en-Y gastric bypass (RYGB) surgery induces sustained weight loss by altering metabolic processes through fundamental changes in appetite, energy regulation, satiety, and metabolism. Long-term follow-up studies have shown that RYGB positively affects patients' overall health by reversing some of the metabolic consequences of morbid obesity. RYGB is capable of reducing mortality by improving lipid levels, diabetes, hypertension, obstructive sleep apnea, and cardiovascular events such as myocardial infarction up to 12 years after the procedure and beyond.[15]

It has been shown that bariatric surgery is superior to medical therapy for weight loss, survival, and treatment of comorbidities.[16] The number of weight-loss operations is currently greater than 220,000 procedures annually with laparoscopic sleeve gastrectomy (SG) being the most commonly performed procedure.[17] The following discussion will include indications for surgery, preoperative evaluation, surgical techniques, outcomes, and peri- and postoperative complications.

EVALUATION AND SELECTION OF BARIATRIC SURGERY CANDIDATES

To qualify for bariatric surgery, patients must meet the 1991 NIH consensus criteria, which include having a BMI of 40 kg/m^2 or greater or a BMI of 35 kg/m^2 or greater with obesity-related comorbidities and at least 6 months of documented medically supervised weight loss attempts.[18] Given recent data, there are efforts to extend indications to include a BMI 30–35 kg/m^2 for patients with diabetes as noted in recent publications.[19] Obesity-related comorbidities include hypertension, diabetes mellitus, hyperlipidemia, GERD, arthritis, IBS, obstructive sleep apnea, and NASH. Substantial preoperative evaluation should attempt to discover potential occult comorbidities like coronary artery disease, sleep apnea, and obesity hypoventilation syndrome (Pickwickian syndrome). Because of the complexity of the preoperative evaluation, a multidisciplinary approach is necessary. The team should include a nutritionist, psychologists, anesthesiologists, bariatric surgeons, obesity medicine specialists and other subspecialists that can address any gastroenterologic-, cardiovascular-, pulmonary-, or endocrine-related issues. Family and social support should not be underestimated and also are an integral part of the team.[20] Additionally, patient education is paramount to successful outcomes after bariatric surgery. Educational sessions are mandatory with dieticians, specialized nurses, and the bariatric surgeon detailing pre- and postoperative diet and lifestyle modifications, as well as preparing patients for what to expect after surgery.

Some bariatric surgeons require patients to lose additional weight through diet and exercise between the time of the initial bariatric surgery consultation and the date of operation, particularly for patients with a risk of weight regain.[21] Preoperative weight loss is a method for "downstaging," in a fashion analogous to preoperative chemoradiation therapy for cancer. This additional required preoperative weight loss is not correlated with comorbidity resolution or complication rates.[21,22] However, it is associated with shorter operative times, a smaller liver, and greater weight loss at 1 year after the surgery. Therefore preoperative weight loss may be encouraged in all patients while balancing access to care so there is not a delay in treatment.[21]

Bariatric surgery candidates, in particular, benefit from preoperative nutrition evaluation and counseling. After surgery, patients are instructed to consume a progression of diets that start with full liquid, followed by pureed soft foods, and finally include regular-textured foods. Patients should also be reminded that bariatric surgery is a restrictive procedure, and therefore smaller, more frequent meals are most appropriate.[23]

Contraindications to bariatric surgery include psychiatric conditions such as schizophrenia, severe bipolar disorder, active substance abuse, recent major depression with hospitalization or suicide attempts, and developmental delay. Other contraindications include severe cardiac disease that would prohibit safe and effective anesthesia, severe coagulopathy, or inability to comply with rigorous postoperative nutritional requirements, including lifelong vitamin replacement. Age is not an absolute contraindication in patients with severe comorbidities and bariatric surgery is performed in patients older than age 65 or younger than age 18.[24]

Prior to surgery, patients should complete a screening process, including consultation with a surgeon, psychological evaluation, nutrition consultation, chest roentgenogram, electrocardiogram, and EGD.

A preoperative EGD is recommended by the European Association for Endoscopic Surgery to detect and treat any upper GI lesions that may cause postoperative complications or influence the decision of which type of bariatric surgery should be performed.[25] In a study of 272 gastric bypass patients who underwent preoperative EGD, 12% of patients had clinically significant preoperative findings that included erosive esophagitis (3.7%), Barrett esophagus (3.7%), gastric ulcer (2.9%), erosive gastritis (1.8%), duodenal ulcer (0.7%), and gastric carcinoid (0.3%); 1.1% had more than one lesion. Given that 12% of the patients who eventually underwent RYGB had clinically significant preoperative findings but that two-thirds of these patients had UGI symptoms, it is important to perform EGD preoperatively because the excluded distal stomach cannot be evaluated easily after a RYGB procedure.[26] In addition, preoperative screening for GERD is critical prior to a laparoscopic SG given that the greatest risk for postoperative GERD is preoperative GERD. Findings of severe reflux may guide the surgeon and patient alike in a procedure choice.[27]

Medical evaluations of cardiovascular disease, respiratory illness, and diabetes should be completed prior to surgery. Cardiovascular evaluation should include a recent history of chest pain and assessment of exercise tolerance. Patients with multiple risk factors such as a history of DVT or venous stasis disease may require temporary inferior vena cava filter placement prior to surgery to prevent venous thromboembolism.[28] It is also important to identify occult obstructive sleep apnea so that the anesthesiologist may anticipate periods of hypoxia in the immediate postoperative period when it may be compounded by narcotic pain medications and postoperative fluid shifts.[29] Additionally, diabetes must be well-controlled preoperatively to reduce the incidence of perioperative morbidity (e.g., wound infection).[29]

SURGICAL TREATMENTS FOR OBESITY

Gastric Bypass

After gastric bypass, both restrictive and hormonal mechanisms limit food intake and nutrient absorption. First performed by Mason and Ito in 1966, gastric bypass has since been modified twice: once in 1967 to incorporate a Roux limb rather than a loop gastrojejunostomy, and again in 1994 to be a primarily laparoscopic procedure.[30]

The laparoscopic approach is superior to the open approach and has considerably lower complication rates. Laparoscopic gastric bypass has reduced mortality rates and lowered rates of wound infection, pulmonary and thromboembolic complications, and incisional hernias, and has decreased the average hospitalization time to about 2 days.[31] There are many variations of laparoscopic RYGB techniques, but essential components include construction of a gastric pouch, attaching the pouch to the jejunum, and re-routing digestive enzymes such that they do not contact food until it reaches the jejunojejunostomy (Fig. 9.1A).[8]

At the time of surgery, care is taken to position the patient appropriately so as to facilitate intubation and prevent nerve compression and skin breakdown. To prevent postoperative nausea and vomiting, several strategies are employed, including IV hydration and small doses of glucocorticoid and ondansetron. An orogastric tube is placed to prevent gastric distension or aspiration. Prophylactic subcutaneous heparin (5000 units), sequential compression devices, and cefoxitin (2 g IV) should be administered prior to incision. In the operating room, endoscopes to enable evaluation of the stomach and deep intestine should be available.

Surgery is begun by placing an index trocar at 18 cm below the xiphoid in the midline after the Veress needle has been introduced to establish pneumoperitoneum. After remaining trocars are placed, laparoscopic exploration of the abdomen is conducted. The greater omentum is elevated, and the ligament of Treitz is identified. The jejunum is divided into biliopancreatic and Roux limbs at 20 cm distal to the ligament of Treitz. Next, the jejunojejunostomy is performed after a 75–150 cm Roux limb is passed toward the proximal gastric pouch, either through the transverse mesocolon (retrocolic) or in front of the colon (antecolic); the retrocolic method may either take a retrogastric or antegastric route. Any mesenteric defects between loops of bowel are potential hernia sites and, therefore, are closed with permanent running suture. The gastric pouch should be between 15 and 30 mL in size and is constructed based on the size of the lesser gastric curve. Finally, the gastrojejunostomy is constructed either through circular-stapled, linear-stapled, or hand-sewn techniques, and a surgical drain may be placed.

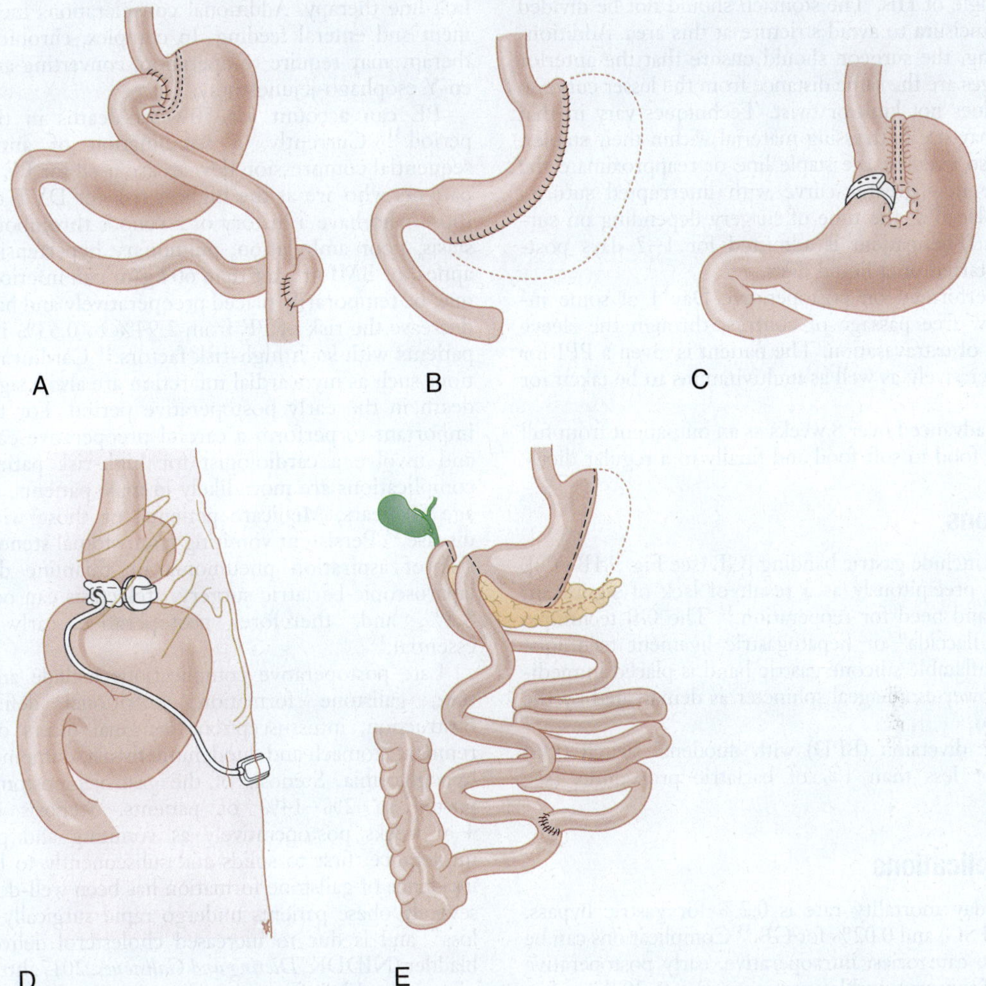

Fig. 9.1 Types of weight loss operations. (A) Roux-en-Y gastric bypass. (B) Gastric sleeve. (C) Vertical banded gastroplasty. (D) Laparoscopic adjustable gastric band. (E) Biliopancreatic diversion with duodenal switch. ((A–C) from the American Society for Bariatric Surgery. *The Story of Surgery for Obesity*. 2005. Available at https://asmbs.org.)

Potential pitfalls of the procedure include bleeding, inability of the Roux limb to reach the gastric pouch without tension, and unexpected anatomy such as malrotation, enlarged liver, excessive omentum, or thick abdominal wall. Though rare, unexpected findings during a laparoscopic gastric bypass may influence the operative course. These findings could include tenacious adhesions from previous surgery that require lysis, malrotation of the ligament of Treitz necessitating a mirror image approach to the technique, hernia findings that require a change in port placement, or a cirrhotic-appearing liver that may require biopsy or even aborting the case if varices or ascites is noted. A GIST that may not have been revealed with preoperative assessment may be resected in its entirety and the surgery completed as originally planned.

Sleeve Gastrectomy

The vertical SG (see Fig. 9.1E) involves removing about 80% of the stomach, with a resultant remaining sleeve that is lesser curve-based and is 28–32 Fr in diameter. It has been hypothesized that the tighter the sleeve, the more likely the possibility of a leak, which is the most common major complication after SG; other potential pitfalls may include bleeding or strictures. Care should be used while taking down the blood supply to the greater curvature of the stomach. An advanced bipolar cutting device or ultrasonic scalpel is used to seal the blood vessels. At the most proximal portion of the stomach, the short gastric vessels can be in close proximity to the spleen, and the surgeon must avoid excessive traction in this area to avoid a shear injury. A bougie (32–40 Fr) is used to guide the staple line along the sleeve. A tight sleeve, especially at the incisura, can lead to outflow obstruction and predispose to a more proximal leak. Many surgeons perform an intra-operative leak test with either air or methylene blue to evaluate the staple line. If the leak test is positive, then the staple line can be reinforced or oversewn in the areas of concern.

Patients are placed in the supine or split-leg position. Five trocars are used and placed at the surgeon's preference. The liver is then retracted to expose the stomach including the gastroesophageal junction. The gastrocolic ligament is then divided, and the vessels of the gastroepiploic arcade are cut using an advanced bipolar cutting device or the ultrasonic scalpel. Dissection is carried out along the greater curve of the stomach from 3 to 7 cm proximal to the pylorus up to the angle of His. The stomach is then freed from any posterior attachments within the lesser sac. Care should be taken to avoid injuring the splenic vein and artery during the dissection. A bougie (32–40 Fr) or endoscope is then passed into the stomach as a guide for stapling. The sleeve is then created with multiple staple loads from just proximal to the pylorus to the angle of His. The stomach should not be divided too close to the incisura to avoid stricture at this area. Additionally, when stapling, the surgeon should ensure that the anterior and posterior edges are the same distance from the lesser curve so that the sleeve does not kink or twist. Techniques vary in that some surgeons may use buttressing material within their staples. Surgeons may also oversew the staple line or reapproximate the omentum to the new greater curve with interrupted sutures. Drains may be placed at the time of surgery depending on surgeon preference. The patient is admitted for 1–2 days postoperatively and started on a liquid diet.

An UGI is performed on postoperative Day 1 at some institutions to show free passage of contrast through the sleeve without evidence of extravasation. The patient is given a PPI for 6 months postoperatively as well as multivitamins to be taken for life.

Diet is slowly advanced over 8 weeks as an outpatient from full liquids to pureed food to soft food and finally to a regular diet.

Other Operations

Other operations include gastric banding [GB (see Fig. 9.1B–C)]. GB has declined precipitously as a result of lack of significant treatment effect and need for reoperation.[32] The GB technique involves a "pars flaccida" or hepatogastric ligament technique whereby a soft, inflatable silicone gastric band is placed immediately below the lower esophageal sphincter as demarcated by the esophageal fat pad.

Biliopancreatic diversion (BPD) with duodenal switch (DS) now accounts for less than 1% of bariatric procedures (see Fig. 9.1D).

Surgical Complications

The average 30-day mortality rate is 0.2% for gastric bypass, 0.14% for vertical SG, and 0.02% for GB.[33] Complications can be divided into three categories: intraoperative, early postoperative (within 30 days of surgery), and late postoperative (>30 days after surgery). Significant progress has been made to monitor outcomes and develop evidence-based guidelines of criteria and benchmarks that determine safe practices. As mentioned, complication rates are directly related to the experience of the surgeon and hospital.

Complications of bariatric procedures include anastomotic leak or stenosis, pulmonary embolus (PE) and DVT, GI bleeding, nutritional deficiencies, wound complications, bowel obstructions, ulcers, hernias, and respiratory and cardiovascular complications. Among the different surgical procedures, the complication rates are proportional to the amount of weight loss produced by each operation. The odds of serious adverse events (AEs) at 1 year are as follows: SG, odds ratio (OR) = 3.22, 95% confidence interval CI: 2.64–3.92; RYGB, OR = 4.92, 95% CI: 4.38–5.54; BPD+DS, OR = 17.47, 95% CI: 14.19–21.52.[34]

Bowel ischemia may result from a twisted Roux limb or internal herniation that occurred during division of the mesentery.[35] Signs of intestinal ischemia are severe abdominal pain, hematochezia, and an acute abdomen.

Early postoperative complications are anastomotic leaks, pulmonary and cardiovascular complications including DVT and PE, and mortality. Anastomotic, gastric pouch, or duodenal leakage occurs with 2.2% of RYGB, 1.0% of vertical banded gastroplasty (VBG), and 1.8% of BPD.[33] Anastomotic leak, most commonly from the gastrojejunostomy or from the SG staple line, usually near the hiatus, is an independent risk factor for mortality.[36] It has been demonstrated that a surgeon's experience has significant influence on the leakage rate, with a rate of 1%–2% in experienced hands and up to 5% for surgeons earlier in their careers.[37] Leaks from SG occur infrequently but can be troublesome to treat. Drainage of leaks along with IV antibiotic therapy is first-line therapy. Additional considerations include stent placement and enteral feeding. In complex, chronic leaks, definitive therapy may require re-operation, converting an SG to a Roux-en-Y esophago-jejunostomy.[38]

PE can account for 50% of deaths in the perioperative period.[31] Currently, a combination of anticoagulants and sequential compression devices are used for PE prophylaxis. For patients who are at the highest risk for DVT or PE, including those who have a history of a venous thrombotic event, venous stasis, poor ambulation, pulmonary hypertension, severe sleep apnea, or BMI greater than 60 kg/m^2, an inferior vena cava filter may be temporarily placed preoperatively and has been shown to decrease the risk of PE from 2.94% to 0.63% in a series of 330 patients with such high-risk factors.[31] Cardiovascular complications such as myocardial infarction are also a significant cause of death in the early postoperative period. For this reason, it is important to perform a careful preoperative cardiac evaluation and involve a cardiologist for high-risk patients. Pulmonary complications are more likely in male patients, those older than age 50 years, Medicare patients, or those with chronic lung disease.[13] Persistent vomiting from stomal stenosis increases the risk of aspiration pneumonia or thiamine deficiency. After laparoscopic bariatric surgery, atelectasis can occur at a rate of 8.4%, and, therefore, postoperative early ambulation is essential.[35]

Late postoperative complications include anastomotic stricture, gallstone formation, nutritional deficiencies, bowel obstruction, intussusception, marginal ulcers or ulcers in the remnant stomach and duodenum, fistula, dumping syndrome, and hypoglycemia. Stenosis of the gastrojejunostomy has been reported in 2%–14% of patients. Stenosis often manifests 4–6 weeks postoperatively as vomiting and progressive food intolerance, first to solids and subsequently to liquids.[39] A high incidence of gallstone formation has been well-documented when severely obese patients undergo rapid surgically induced weight loss[40] and is due to increased cholesterol delivery to the gallbladder (NIDDK. *Dieting and Gallstones*. 2017. https://www.niddk.nih.gov/health-information/digestive-diseases/gallstones/dieting. Accessed April 4, 2019). Cholelithiasis develops in up to 38% of patients after RYGB. If a patient has gallstones preoperatively, the surgeon may elect to perform a concomitant cholecystectomy; this is less commonly performed with the laparoscopic approach because it is easier to do by open technique than laparoscopically.[41] Gallstone formation occurs secondary to a combination of vagus nerve damage, altered enteric nerve stimulation, decreased gallbladder emptying, and changes in calcium concentration and the bile salt/cholesterol ratio.[35] It has been shown in a double-blind randomized placebo-controlled trial that ursodiol at a daily dose of 600 mg for the first 6 months after surgery reduces the incidence of gallstones to 2%.[42] To reduce the incidence of cholelithiasis, a 6-month course of ursodiol is recommended for patients whose gallbladder is not removed prophylactically.[42] Nutritional deficiencies can be extensive, related to both the changes in anatomy and postoperative sequelae like persistent vomiting. Bowel obstruction occurs in 0.2%–7% of RYGB patients; the range varies depending on the surgical technique. For example, if the Roux limb is passed in a retrocolic fashion, there are three potential hernia sites: mesocolic, jejunal-jejunal, and between the colon and Roux limb.[20] Most bowel obstructions develop 6–24 months postoperatively, but they can occur earlier because of technical errors related to mesenteric defects. Bowel obstructions that occur early usually require bowel resection to prevent retrograde distention of the biliopancreatic limb and distal stomach, which could result in rupture of the distal gastric staple line and consequent peritonitis.[20] In later bowel obstructions, surgical intervention is only required after failure of NG decompression, IV fluid resuscitation, and NPO status. When intussusception occurs, it is usually years after surgery. Patients with the highest risk of developing intussusception are those who have lost more than 90% of their excess weight.[35]

Marginal ulcers are ulcers located in the jejunum near the anastomotic site. They are estimated to occur in 1%–16% of gastric bypass patients.[43,44] Perforated marginal ulcers occur in 1% of RYGB patients. Ulcer perforation is linked to smoking and use of NSAIDs or glucocorticoids.[45] The use of nonabsorbable sutures, as opposed to absorbable sutures, for the inner layer of the gastrojejunal anastomosis (GJA) is associated with increased ulcer incidence.[46] The presence of *Hp* also increases risk for marginal ulcers.[47] It is common practice for bariatric surgeons to use PPI therapy for 6 months postoperatively. If a marginal ulcer is recalcitrant to medical therapy, the possibility of a gastric-gastric fistula must be entertained, for which surgical correction is mandated. The remnant stomach maintains a pH of 2–3 and still responds to vagal and hormonal stimulation; therefore ulcers may also occur in the gastric remnant and duodenum years after surgery and independent of *Hp* status. Endoscopic evaluation of the gastric pouch is challenging given the divided stomach; thus unstable patients may require surgical exploration.[35] Fistulas occur rarely, and often concurrently with a marginal ulcer.[35] They form most commonly between the gastric pouch and gastric remnant and are due to a GI leak from the gastric pouch eroding into the gastric remnant.[48] Large, undiagnosed gastrogastric fistulas may result in weight regain.[20] Fistulas leading to weight regain require elective endoscopic or surgical repair.

Dumping syndrome can occur in up to 20% of RYGB patients[49]; it is classified as early or late depending on how soon it develops after a meal. Early dumping ensues 15–30 minutes after eating and is thought to be due to the rapid entry of hyperosmotic foods into the jejunum. It is due to rapid fluid shifts into the intestinal lumen with a meal which results in a parasympathetic response leading to a reduction in systemic vascular resistance, an effect called "splanchnic blood pooling."[50] Symptoms include cramping abdominal pain, voluminous diarrhea, bloating, dizziness, nausea, flushing, and tachycardia; symptoms result from hypovolemia and a subsequent sympathetic response.[35] Dumping syndrome is triggered by consumption of simple sugars, acidic foods, and nutrient-rich drinks such as Gatorade.[49] Foods high in protein and fiber should be consumed to avoid this uncomfortable syndrome; additional behavior modifications include smaller, frequent meals, lying down after meals, and avoidance of very hot and very cold foods[20] to reduce symptoms related to decreased systemic vascular resistance. Early dumping is usually self-limited and resolves between 7 and 12 weeks after surgery. Late dumping syndrome occurs 2–3 hours after a meal and is secondary to rapid glucose absorption, subsequent hyperglycemia, and release of glucagon-like peptide-1 and gastric inhibitory polypeptide. A relatively exaggerated insulin response ensues, leading to hypoglycemia and hypokalemia. Patients present with diaphoresis, weakness, fatigue, and dizziness.[49] The same modifications suggested for early dumping syndrome should also ameliorate the symptoms of late dumping syndrome.[35] Treatment includes dietary and medical interventions to control serum glucose levels.[35]

GI bleeding can occur postoperatively in 2.0% of RYGB, 0.7% of VBG, 0.3% of laparoscopic adjustable GB (LAGB) surgery, and 0.2% of BPD. In RYGB patients, postoperative dysphagia is not significantly worse than the patient's matched preoperative symptoms and can develop with food indiscretion, stricture formation, or other obstructions.[51]

Beyond the type of procedure, there are identified risk factors for complications after bariatric surgery including older age, male gender, greater BMI, comorbidities, and Medicare insurance status.[52–54] The increased risk for Medicare patients is beyond age, because eligibility for Medicare is disability, which may affect outcome. Although patients with the greatest number of risk factors carry the highest risk for surgery, they also may derive the most benefit from bariatric surgery, given the disease burden they carry.[14] Of note, complications may not affect long-term weight loss, which is the outcome that best predicts long-term mortality risk.[21]

Nutritional Deficiencies

Nutritional and vitamin deficiencies and electrolyte abnormalities occur in 16.9% of RYGB patients.[33] Patients who do not take daily vitamins postoperatively or patients who experience frequent vomiting are at increased risk of developing such deficiencies, most common of which are protein, iron, vitamin B_{12}, folate, calcium, and the fat-soluble vitamins A, D, E, and K.[55]

Prolonged vomiting may result in thiamine (vitamin B_1) deficiency, which can lead to Wernicke encephalopathy, a syndrome of confusion, ataxia, ophthalmoplegia, and impaired short-term memory (see Chapter 105). This neurologic deficit is preventable with appropriate administration of thiamine. If thiamine deficiency is suspected, the patient should be given IV or intramuscular thiamine immediately to increase the chances of symptom resolution.[56] Early treatment is imperative because persistent severe symptoms may not be reversible despite delayed administration of thiamine.

The parietal cells of the stomach produce intrinsic factor (IF), which is necessary for vitamin B_{12} absorption in the terminal ileum (see Chapter 106). Patients who undergo RYGB may develop B_{12} deficiency because RYGB separates the parietal cells in the fundus of the stomach from the smaller gastric pouch. There is, therefore, no contact between ingested food and IF until the intersection of the Roux limb in the jejunum.[57,58] In addition, the parietal cells of the stomach often cease to produce IF after RYGB, presumably because the fundus no longer has any contact with food.[59] Restrictive bariatric surgery does not cause vitamin B_{12} deficiency because the parietal cells in the fundus of the stomach remain in contact with the nutritive stream.[60]

Calcium, iron, and folate deficiency can occur because they are absorbed mainly in the duodenum and proximal jejunum. These segments of the digestive tract are commonly bypassed in gastric bypass surgery. Moreover, vitamin D is necessary for calcium absorption, and vitamin D deficiency further contributes to any calcium deficiency.[54]

Outcomes

The steep rise in bariatric surgery utilization can be attributed to its proved efficacy as a treatment for morbid obesity. Two meta-analysis have provided strong validation that bariatric surgery leads to successful weight loss and mortality reduction.[33] A meta-analysis by Buchwald that included 22,094 patients found the mean percentage of excess weight loss for all patients to be 61.2%.[6] Excess weight loss was highest for BPD with DS (70.1%) followed by VBG (68.2%), RYGB (61.6%), and lowest for LAGB (47.5%). A meta-analysis by Maggard found similar weight loss trends at 3 or more years postoperatively, with the greatest weight loss achieved after the malabsorptive procedures of BPD (53 kg) and RYGB (42 kg), and less weight loss after the restrictive LAGB (35 kg) and gastroplasty (32 kg).[6,33]

Such substantial weight loss is associated with a clear reduction in long-term mortality. A retrospective cohort study of 9949 RYGB patients matched to 9628 severely obese controls found that having RYGB surgery reduced the adjusted long-term mortality from any cause of death by 40%.[61] Among RYGB patients, mortality was decreased from coronary artery disease by 56%, from diabetes by 92%, and from cancer by 60%. In another study there was a 14% decrease in cancer incidence among patients who underwent RYGB. The biggest reductions in cancer incidence were seen among types of cancers that are considered obesity related: esophageal adenocarcinomas (2% reduction), colorectal (30% reduction), postmenopausal breast (4%), uterine corpus

(78%), non-Hodgkin lymphoma (27%), and multiple myeloma (54%).[62] The lower cancer risk of patients after RYGB is presumably due to weight loss, which has been shown in many studies to reduce cancer incidence. Furthermore, once obese patients lose weight, they may have easier access to needed health surveillance like Pap smears and colonoscopy. Finally, given that increased BMI leads to worse surgical oncologic outcomes, it may be surmised that with weight loss, a better surgical outcome may be anticipated.

Overall, bariatric surgery dramatically improves survival and decreases mortality from all disease-related causes of death. Only the rate of deaths not caused by disease (e.g., deaths resulting from accidents and suicide) increased after bariatric surgery and were 58% higher in RYGB patients.[60] One speculation as to why accidents and suicides were higher in the surgical group was the possibility of alcohol abuse. One study demonstrated altered alcohol metabolism after gastric bypass surgery, perhaps explaining a propensity for alcohol abuse.[63] A recent analysis found that due to increased rate of absorption of alcohol after RYGB, there was both an earlier and higher blood alcohol concentration. This concentration was high enough to be defined as a binge drinking episode, which is a risk factor for developing alcohol abuse.[64] One study of bariatric surgery candidates found that 9% reported suicide attempts and 19% reported alcohol abuse preoperatively.[40] There is concern that this vulnerable patient population has additional difficulty with the psychological adjustments to weight loss, which further supports the need for psychologic counseling before and after surgery.[65,66]

In addition to benefiting from decreased mortality, bariatric patients benefit from decreased morbidity. Severely obese patients suffer from more intense GI symptoms such as abdominal pain, heartburn, and sleep disturbances than do normal weight patients. Beyond the significant improvement in cardiac risk factors, weight loss surgery also provides enormous benefit for the many medical problems obesity causes. The reduction in GERD symptoms leads to significantly decreased medication use postoperatively for both PPIs (44% to 9%) and H2RAs (60%–10%). In fact, GERD resolution rates following RYGB are so robust that RYGB is a suggested treatment for recalcitrant GERD in severely obese patients.[50]

Recently, a number of clinical trials have demonstrated a dramatic effect of bariatric surgery on glycemic control in patients with type 2 diabetes, such that the need for medical therapy was decreased or eliminated. Moreover, in a prospective non-randomized case-matched Swedish trial, type 2 diabetes was significantly less likely to develop in obese participants who underwent a bariatric procedure than in their control counterparts.[67] Although this is not an indication that bariatric surgery should be used for the purpose of preventing development of type 2 diabetes in obese patients, nor serve as a replacement for medical therapy, it does suggest that the mechanisms by which bariatric surgery prevents progression from abnormalities in glucose metabolism to frank diabetes is an area that should be explored further.[66]

The effects of obesity are not merely physiologic. Administration of the SF36 survey shows that quality of life improves greatly after RYGB surgery. Preoperatively, severely obese patients score significantly lower than USA population norms in the categories of general health, vitality, physical functioning, bodily pain, and emotional and social functioning. As early as 3 months after RYGB, these same patients score no differently than U.S. norms in these categories.[68]

As bariatric surgery continues to grow, there is increasing recognition that obesity is a chronic and complex disease. As such, there likely will be variations to current therapy, gastric bypass being the most consistent across surgeons.[69] With such variation, there will be the potential for revision of previous surgeries. In fact, revisional surgery now accounts for 15% of total bariatric surgery. Current evaluation of revisional bariatric surgery outcomes indicates that morbidity is low and weight loss is adequate; however, revisional bariatric surgery morbidity is higher and weight loss is lower than morbidity with primary bariatric surgery.[70]

ENDOSCOPIC MANAGEMENT OF BARIATRIC SURGICAL COMPLICATIONS

Bariatric surgery is an effective means of treating obesity and its metabolic comorbidities, but these procedures are associated with significant complications that gastroenterologists must be able to recognize and address. Endoscopy plays a critical role in the diagnosis and management of many of these complications.

Ulceration

Ulceration at the GJA is a common late complication of RYGB. Incidence has varied widely in the literature, but a recent systematic review and administrative database study report incidence rates of 4.6%–6.28% of patients (Fig. 9.2).[71,72] GJA ulceration often develops in the first 3 months postoperatively but can occur at any time. Data from an administrative database showed an increase in the rate of surgical intervention for marginal ulceration over time from 6% at 1 year to 17% at 8 years, suggesting a higher morbidity from marginal ulcerations that occur many years later.[70] Patients typically present with epigastric pain, nausea, vomiting, food intolerance, overt or occult bleeding; however, up to 61% of patients are asymptomatic.[43] Moreover, ulcers can occur at any of the anastomoses created during a RYGB.

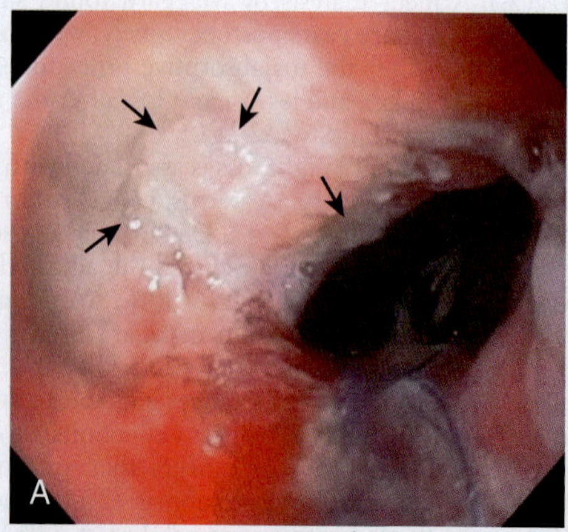

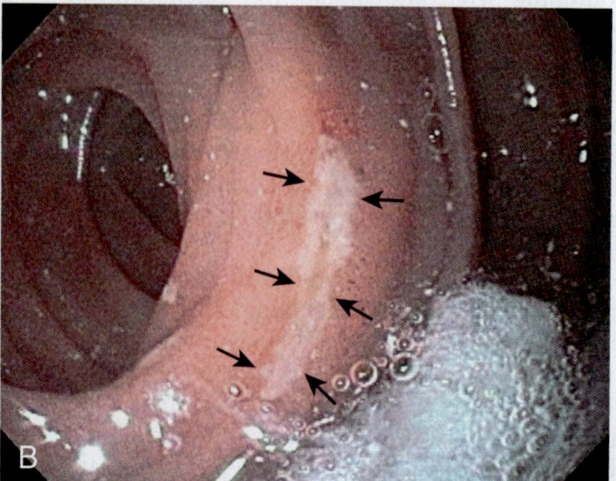

Fig. 9.2 (A) Anastomotic ulcer. (B) Jejunal ulcer. (Images courtesy Christopher C. Thompson, MD.)

Anastomotic ulcers may be due to small amounts of acid produced by the gastric pouch, ischemia, bile acid reflux, *Hp* infection, NSAIDs, smoking, alcohol, foreign bodies such as nonabsorbable sutures or staples, or tension on the Roux limb.[46,73–77] Gastrogastric fistula and staple line disruption also may result in ulceration from exposure to acid.

Evaluation for anastomotic ulceration may be performed with water-soluble contrast media (e.g., gastrografin) or careful endoscopy any time after surgery. Endoscopic evaluation should include the gastric pouch, GJA, and proximal Roux limb. This may be accomplished with a pediatric colonoscope, however a deep enteroscopy system is often necessary to reach the duodenum and excluded stomach. Size, depth, and potential etiologic factors should be noted for each ulcer. *Hp* fecal antigen testing may be the easiest and most accurate way to confirm the presence of *Hp*.[78]

Treatment of ulceration is multifaceted. In patients with RYGB, anastomotic ulcers should be treated with soluble PPI or capsules that are broken open, taken twice daily, and tapered over 6 months.[79] Sucralfate solution at 1 g four times daily should be used concurrently when possible; the tablet form of PPI does not appear to be as effective. Bile reflux can be treated with bile acid binders such as cholestyramine or colestipol. Smoking cessation is critical. Control of diabetes should be optimized. NSAIDs should be discontinued, if possible, or combined with PPI or PGE1 therapy if needed long term. *Hp* should be treated if active infection is found. Visible sutures or staples within the ulcer should be removed. Repeat upper endoscopy to check for healing is recommended at 2–3 months after initiation of medical therapy. If the ulcer fails to heal with maximal medical therapy, surgical revision has been the traditional next step in therapy.[70,80] Endoscopic therapy using an endoscopic suturing system to oversew and cover the ulceration has also been reported in a limited case series.[81]

Postoperative Gastrointestinal Bleeding

The incidence and type of GI bleeding after bariatric surgery is typically related to the type of surgery. UGI bleeding after bariatric surgery occurs more commonly after RYGB (1.5%–3.5% of cases[82–84]) than after LAGB, SG, and VBG. Bleeding can occur at multiple sites, including the pouch, anastomoses, staple lines, contiguous small intestine, excluded stomach, or bypassed small intestine. Additionally, patients can develop esophagitis with subsequent hemorrhage after bariatric surgery due to the altered anatomy. Early bleeding usually occurs within 24 hours postoperatively at the staple lines of the GJA, gastric remnant, or jejunojejunal anastomosis.[82,85] A significant proportion of early bleeding can be extraluminal and this should be considered if melena or hematemesis is not apparent; these patients may develop hemodynamic instability, oliguria, and abdominal distention without overt signs of GI blood loss. Late bleeding is often secondary to anastomotic ulceration; however, other sites of GI blood loss should also be considered including the remnant stomach.[86]

The esophagus, gastric pouch, and GJA are easily accessed with a standard upper endoscope. Bleeding in the excluded stomach or at the jejunojejunal anastomosis presents a more significant challenge. In these cases, device-assisted enteroscopy may be required. In cases of early bleeding, endoscopy carries a greater risk of perforation due to the immaturity of anastomoses and staple lines. If early endoscopy is performed, air insufflation should be minimized, or CO_2 insufflation should be used. Endoscopic therapy of bleeding is highly effective. As an alternative to thermal therapies, endoclips can be used in conjunction with epinephrine injection to minimize tissue injury at the site of bleeding (Fig. 9.3).[87–89] Electrocautery should be avoided at fresh staple lines. Hemostatic powders are another option, however, there are limited data on their use after bariatric surgery. Angiographic intervention can be considered, but the resulting ischemia is a concern in patients with new anastomoses.

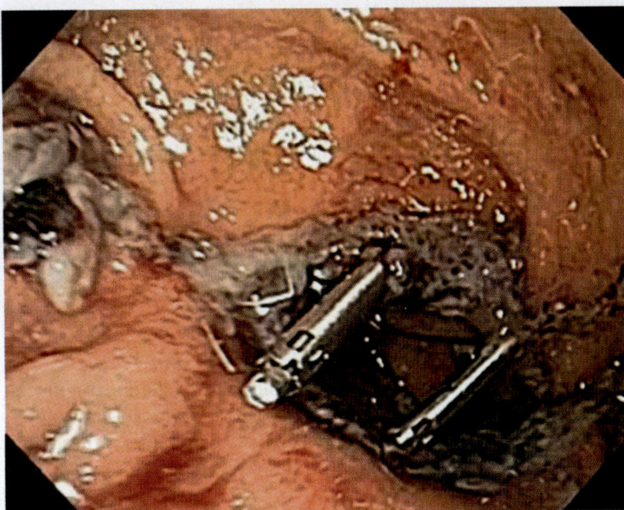

Fig. 9.3 Postoperative hemorrhage with hemostasis using endoscopic clips. (Images courtesy Christopher C. Thompson, MD.)

Stenosis

Stenosis is a common complication after bariatric surgery. Patients present with early satiety, nausea, vomiting, and dysphagia. Postprandial retrosternal or abdominal pain may also be present. In patients with history of RYGB, stenosis often occurs at the GJA, and rates of 1.5%–7.3%[90–93] are reported after laparoscopic RYGB. Most stenosis at the GJA develops 4–10 weeks after surgery. In cases of stricture formation incited by ulcer or foreign material, presentation may be delayed for months or years. Less common sites for stenosis after RYGB include the jejunojejunal anastomosis, sites of intestinal adhesions, and sites of passage through the mesocolon.

Endoscopy is an excellent diagnostic tool because the etiology (e.g., foreign body) can often be identified, and therapy applied concurrently. By definition, stomal stenosis is present if the standard 9.5 mm endoscope cannot traverse the anastomosis. Treatment of stomal stenosis can be performed with a through-the-scope (TTS) balloon, Savary dilator, or electrosurgical incision. Balloon dilation is the most commonly used technique and is successful in more than 90% of cases.[91,92] Some patients require two or three procedures, which can begin postoperatively when symptoms begin and be repeated every 2–3 weeks. The balloon catheter should be advanced beyond the GJA, with care to avoid entry into the blind limb; a guidewire and/or fluoroscopic imaging can be used when observation of catheter advancement is suboptimal, or resistance is encountered. Once the balloon is fully outside the endoscope, it can be inflated so that its midpoint applies radial pressure into the stricture for at least 60 seconds, or until the balloon "waist" disappears on fluoroscopy. Although 20 mm diameter has been reported to be successful, the smallest effective dilation is preferred (8–12 mm). A gradual approach to dilation over several sessions can reduce perforation risk (reported to be 2.1%–5%[91,92]) and decrease the possibility of overdilation with resultant weight regain. Suture material at the GJA may have to be removed to achieve successful dilation.[77]

Other types of bariatric surgery also may be complicated by stenosis. Patients with a history of LAGB may have obstruction as a result of edema or excess tissue at the level of the band. There may be a fibrous reaction to the band; in these cases, endoscopic dilation can be attempted if stenosis persists despite complete drainage of the band reservoir. Band removal, band replacement, or conversion to RYGB also may be considered if conservative measures are unsuccessful. Patients with history of SG may have stenosis at the gastroesophageal junction or at the incisura angularis. Serial endoscopic balloon dilation starting with a hydrostatic TTS balloon dilation can be attempted; pneumatic dilation at the site of the stricture has been reported as well.[77,94] Another approach to stenosis is temporary covered metal stent placement for up to 8 weeks. Ultimately, conversion to RYGB may be required.[93]

Foreign Body Complications

Foreign materials (e.g., sutures, staples, and bands) are placed during bariatric surgery. The foreign material, with its subsequent inflammatory response, may result in pain, ulceration, and obstruction. Implanted foreign bodies (e.g., bands and mesh) can also erode or migrate (Fig. 9.4).

Patients with chronic pain after bariatric surgery should undergo endoscopic examination with removal of visible retained foreign material. Foreign material has been associated with pain even when there is no adjacent visible inflammation. Traction on sutures or staples often reproduces pain. Ryou et al. demonstrated immediate symptomatic improvement in 71% of patients after foreign body removal.[95]

Leaks and Fistulae

A leak is caused by discontinuity of tissue apposition in the immediate postoperative period. The incidence of leak after bariatric surgery ranges from 1.7% to 2.6% after open RYGB, to 0.3% −4.2% after laparoscopic RYGB, and 0.7% to as high as 5.1% after SG.[95–100] A recent review of the MBSAQIP database revealed a leak incidence of 0.3% in 364,000 bariatric surgeries.[95] After RYGB, leaks can occur at several sites: the gastric pouch, GJA, jejunal stump, jejunojejunal anastomosis, excluded stomach, duodenal stump (in resectional bypass), and blind jejunal limb; all of these should be considered when a leak is suspected. The most common sites are the gastrojejunal (68%) or jejunojejunal (5%) anastomosis, or at gastric pouch staple lines (10%); an additional 14% involve multiple sites. Some leaks may be especially challenging to localize, such as those from the excluded stomach, because routine endoscopy and UGI series may be normal. Incidence of leak is highest in patients with divided RYGB. The risk of chronic gastrogastric fistula is highest when the pouch and excluded stomach are contiguous, as with the open surgical approach (Fig. 9.5). In patients with SG, most leaks occur in the proximal third of the stomach near the gastroesophageal junction (85.7%), while the remainder are found in the distal third.

Leaks are associated with a mortality rate of 3.3%–14%.[96] Other than PE, they are the most serious life-threatening complication of bariatric surgery. In addition to doubling the risk of mortality, leaks result in a sixfold increase in hospital stay. Patients who develop a leak are at increased risk for wound infection, sepsis, respiratory failure, renal failure, thromboembolism, internal hernia, and SBO.

Leaks often present without fever, leukocytosis, or pain. The most common reported sign of a leak is tachycardia,[97] present in 72%–92% of patients. Other symptoms and findings include nausea and vomiting (81%), fever (62%), and leukocytosis (48%), any of which demand a high suspicion for leak in patients after bariatric surgery. Objective findings include increased drain output, as well as elevated CRP greater than 22.9 mg/dL 2 days after surgery (sensitivity, 1.00). This differs from chronic gastrogastric fistulae, which have a more indolent course and typically manifest with acid reflux, abdominal discomfort, and weight regain. As gastric acid can flow into the pouch via a gastrogastric fistula, RYGB patients with heartburn, acid reflux, or anastomotic ulcer should be evaluated for fistula formation.[98]

As endoscopic management techniques for the bariatric surgery patient gain acceptance, they are being used earlier in the postoperative course. Dilation of distal stenoses should be performed. Exclusion techniques, such as stent placement, can occlude or bypass leaks. Leaks and fistulae also can be closed with clips, suturing devices, or sealants.

Stent placement to exclude the leak from the GI tract is the endoscopic technique supported by the most substantial body of evidence (Fig. 9.6). Stent placement allows the leak to heal while

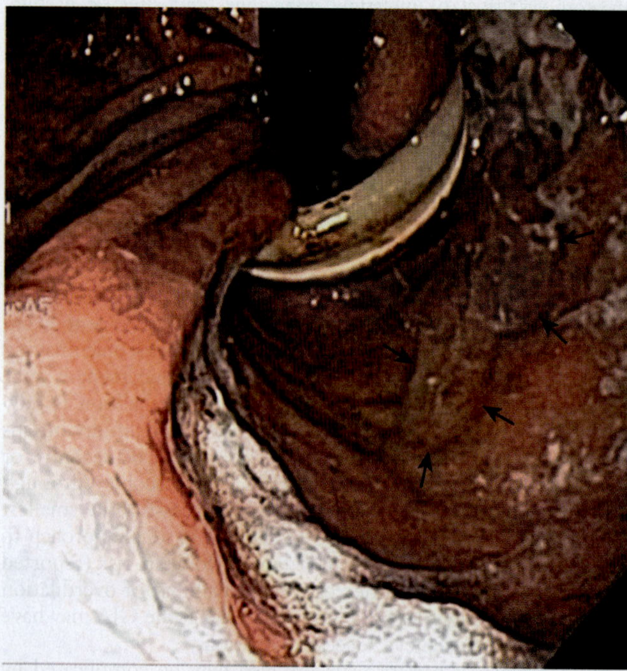

Fig. 9.4 Band erosion. (From El-Hayek K, Timratana P, Brethauer SA, Chand B. Complete endoscopic/transgastric retrieval of eroded gastric band: description of a novel technique and review of the literature. *SurgEndosc.* 2013;27:2974–2979.)

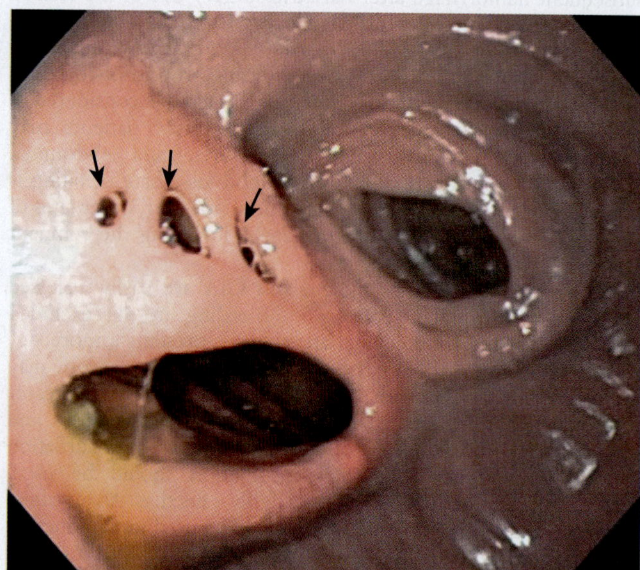

Fig. 9.5 Gastrogastric fistula. (Images courtesy Christopher C. Thompson, MD.)

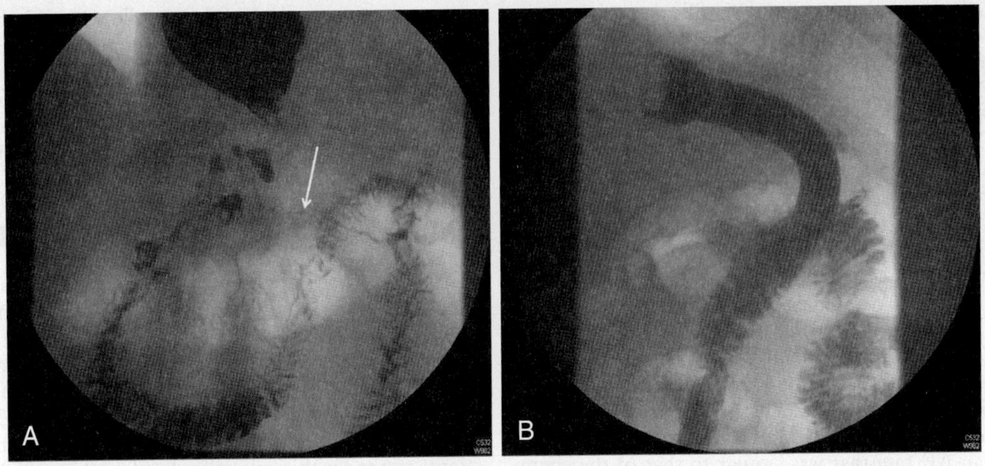

Fig. 9.6 (A) Gastrocutaneous leak (*arrow*). (B) Leak treated by stent placement. (Images courtesy Christopher C. Thompson, MD.)

enteral nutrition is resumed, potentially accelerating recovery and avoiding the need for parenteral nutrition. Peritoneal contamination is decreased, and improvement in abdominal pain may follow. Self-expanding metal stents have been used successfully, employing a forward-viewing endoscope and fluoroscopic guidance. A meta-analysis of stent placement for treatment of acute leaks after bariatric surgery by Puli et al. found a pooled proportion for successful leak closure, defined as radiologic evidence of leak closure after stent removal, of 87.8% (95% CI, 79.4% –94.2%).[99] Most leaks closed with one treatment, but re-stenting was reported in four of seven studies; 9% of patients had failure to respond and required revisional surgery. Stents were extracted between 4 and 8 weeks in the majority of studies. Stent migration was reported in 16.9% (95% CI, 9.3%–26.3%) of cases.

Endoscopic clips also have been used to close fistulae and leaks. Clips are used to approximate the tissue surrounding the defect to effect closure and, therefore, are best deployed perpendicular to the long axis of the defect. Thermal ablation or mechanical scraping of the tissue around the edges of the defect before clip deployment results in a more resilient seal. The Over-the-Scope Clip, Padlock (US Endoscopy) or OTSC (Ovesco Endoscopy AG, Tübingen, Germany), is a nitinol clip placed on a cap at the endoscope tip. A tissue anchor and twin grasper instrument are available and may be helpful in clip placement. Unlike clips inserted through the endoscope, which appose mucosa, the OTSCs can perform full-thickness apposition. Case series of GI tract fistula closure have shown success rates of 72% –91%.[98,101–104] Other small series have shown fibrin glue and various fistula plugs also to be effective.[105]

Pancreaticobiliary Disease

Endoscopic management of pancreatic and biliary disease with EUS and ERCP presents a unique challenge in patients with altered anatomy. Patients with LAGB, SG, and VBG are usually able to have successful EUS or ERCP with a side-viewing endoscope just as patients with normal anatomy. Unfortunately, rapid weight loss may induce a lithogenic state: nearly 50% of patients will develop gallstones or sludge after RYGB, and over 25% may undergo cholecystectomy. Patients with a history of RYGB and BPD+DS often require special tools and procedures to complete ERCP. While the papilla can be reached with balloon-assisted enteroscopy in most cases of RYGB, optimum alignment for cannulation and, if desired, placement of a protective pancreatic stent is not always possible. This has led to various approaches to access the diverted stomach and completion of ERCP with a side-viewing duodenoscope.[106,107] Prior to ERCP, preparation should include verification of need for ERCP as well as characterization of anatomy and pathology via cross-sectional imaging. Some patients have anatomy that is not amenable to a purely endoscopic approach, even via device-assisted enteroscopy. Typically, if surgery is planned, ERCP can be performed concurrently with laparoscopic assistance and access to the stomach. If surgery is not planned, then the options for accessing the major papilla to perform ERCP include laparoscopic-assisted ERCP, enteroscopy-assisted ERCP, direct biliary intervention by EUS, and the creation of a fistula between the gastric pouch and the bypassed stomach using EUS and a lumen-apposing fully covered metallic stent. EUS-directed transgastric ERCP is a transluminal approach to the bypassed stomach that can be completed in a single setting using a fully covered lumen-apposing metallic stent.[108,109]

Weight Regain and Dilated Gastrojejunal Anastomosis

Bariatric surgery is effective in achieving durable weight loss, but weight regain postoperatively is a potential problem; it reintroduces the risks of obesity-associated diseases and has significant impact on quality of life. Although initial weight loss after bariatric surgery is often dramatic, a weight plateau is typically achieved in 1–2 years. A recent analysis from the Veterans Affairs health care system followed 1787 patients after bariatric surgery with 81.9% follow-up at 10 years. The authors found that at 10 years after RYGB, 28.2% of patients had less than 20% total body weight loss (%TBWL), and 3.4% were within 5% of their baseline weight.[110] Given the large number of patients undergoing bariatric surgery, demand for therapy to address weight regain will continue to increase.

Weight regain after bariatric surgery is likely multifactorial. In a systematic review, these factors included nutritional noncompliance and grazing eating patterns, neuroendocrine-metabolic regulation, mental health issues (binge eating and substance abuse), physical inactivity, and anatomic issues.[111] After RYGB, weight regain can be seen with gastrogastric fistula, and it has been shown that larger pouch size and GJA diameter are associated with postoperative weight regain.[112,113] Similarly, weight gain can occur with SG, and in some cases is related to dilation of the sleeve.[114] Surgical revision to address these issues is problematic because complication rates are higher than with the primary procedures.[115,116] Medications have also been used to treat weight regain, however, in a retrospective analysis only one medication used off-label (topiramate) demonstrated significant weight loss, and only 56% of the entire cohort with inadequate weight loss or weight regain achieved 5% or more of their postsurgical total weight loss.[117] Endoluminal therapy for RYGB, however, has shown promise in effectively addressing weight regain with lower morbidity (Video 9.1). The advent of the new GLP-1 agonists may change the landscape for both primary weight loss and weight regain after bariatric surgery.[150] These new drugs can provide up to 20% TBWL which approaches that of bariatric surgery at 25%–35% TBWL. However, bariatric surgery has 20-year postoperative outcomes while the new antiobesity medications (AOMs) do not yet have longer-term follow-up data.

Transoral outlet reduction (TORe) has been studied on multiple platforms (Fig. 9.7). A randomized double-blinded trial compared TORe using the Bard EndoCinch with a sham procedure in 77 patients with GJA diameter wider than 20 mm.[118] GJA diameter was reduced to less than 10 mm in 89.6%, with no perforations and an AE rate that was similar to that of the sham group; 96% of revised patients had weight loss or stabilization in the following 6 months. Mean weight loss in the revised group was 3.9% compared with 0.2% in the sham group ($P = .014$) in an intent-to-treat analysis. The Apollo OverStitch Device (Apollo Endosurgery, Austin, TX) also has been shown to be effective at TORe by placing full-thickness sutures at the GJA.[119] A recent meta-analysis of three studies in patients who had weight regain after RYGB found that 77%–100% stopped gaining weight and that weight loss at 12 months was 5.83 ± 11 to 10.5 ± 12.5 kg.[120]

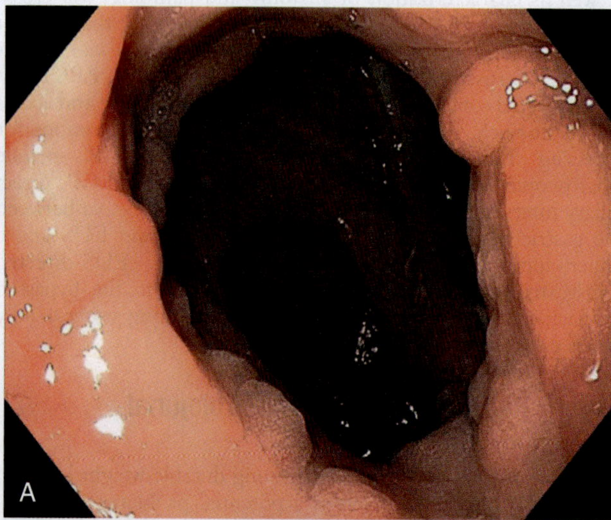

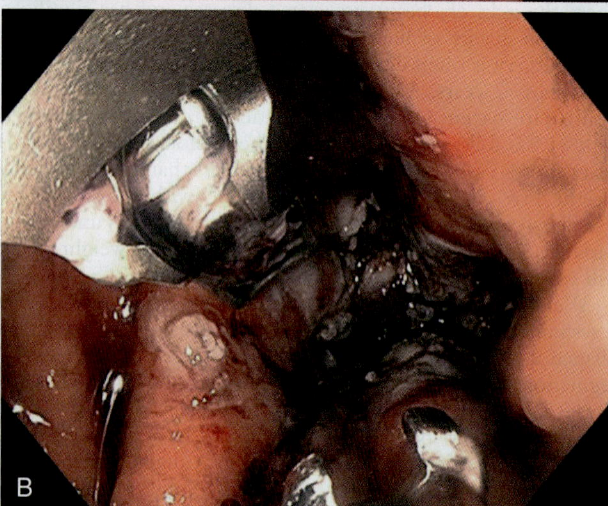

Fig. 9.7 Endoscopic suturing for dilated gastrojejunal anastomosis. Panel (A) before suturing and panel (B) after argon plasma coagulation and suturing with a purse-string technique. (Images courtesy Shelby Sullivan, MD.)

ENDOSCOPIC TREATMENTS FOR OBESITY

Endoscopic bariatric therapy (EBT) for the primary treatment of obesity has rapidly progressed in recent years with multiple devices approved by the FDA and many more therapies currently undergoing investigation. Although bariatric surgery is effective, patients are eligible only if they have obesity class III (BMI 40 kg/m^2) or obesity class II (BMI 35–39.9 kg/m^2) with significant associated comorbid illness. Not only do many patients not meet this criterion, but less than 2% of the population who meets this criterion undergoes bariatric surgery per year.[121] The reasons for the low surgical rates are likely multifactorial but highlight the need for additional treatment options. Lifestyle therapy should be considered the cornerstone for any obesity treatment plan but has limited effectiveness and durability on its own. Recent advances have also been made in obesity pharmacotherapy, and demonstrate modest improvement in weight loss over lifestyle therapy alone in randomized controlled trials.[122] Real-world clinical outcomes, however, may not demonstrate similar weight loss[123] or compliance with medication as seen in randomized controlled trials.[124]

EBTs approved to date have demonstrated significant weight loss compared with lifestyle therapy alone in multicenter randomized controlled trials, which will be reviewed in this section. Although weight loss is less than is seen with bariatric surgery, risk of serious AEs is also less than seen in bariatric surgery. Moreover, many of the devices have been approved for use in patients with a BMI between 30 and 40 kg/m^2, increasing treatment options in patients who would not qualify for bariatric surgery including the new AOMs.

EBTs can be divided into gastric therapies and small bowel therapies. Gastric therapies are devices or procedures that are placed or performed in the stomach. Small bowel therapies are devices or procedures that are placed or performed in the small bowel. Two distinguishing features of gastric and small bowel endoscopic bariatric therapies are their procedure or device placement location and weight loss-independent effects. Although no small bowel therapies have been approved yet by the FDA, data support both weight loss-dependent and weight loss-independent effects on metabolic outcomes. At this time, there are data to demonstrate weight loss-dependent effects on metabolic outcomes, but no data to suggest that gastric therapies have weight loss-independent effects on metabolic outcomes. As of the writing of this chapter, the only EBTs that have been approved by the FDA or are currently performed in the United States are gastric EBTs and they will be the focus of the remainder of this section.

Evaluation and Selection of Endoscopic Bariatric Therapy Candidates

In 2015, the ASGE published a position statement regarding EBTs in clinical practice.[125] The ASGE position statement recognized the clinical practice guidelines for the perioperative nutritional, metabolic, and nonsurgical support of bariatric patients undergoing bariatric surgery (updated in 2013 by the American Association of Clinical Endocrinologists, The Obesity Society, and the American Society for Metabolic and Bariatric Surgery[126]), but acknowledged that these guidelines may not be applicable to all EBTs. In contrast to bariatric surgical procedures,

EBTs are minimally invasive procedures, which may be short-term, reversible, or with minimal long-term changes to anatomy.

The reversibility, safety profile, and reduced risk of anesthesia have resulted in reduced preoperative evaluation criteria for device placement. At a minimum, the ASGE position statement recommended performing a medical history, physical exam, screening for obesity-related diseases, and commitment to lifestyle change, nutrition history, and routine laboratory testing.

Indications for EBTs vary based on the device and the study population used for FDA approval. In some cases, data on safety and efficacy are available for people outside of the FDA-labeled indications,[127,128] but any use outside FDA labeling is considered off-label use.

Endoscopic Bariatric Therapies Currently Performed in the United States

Four gastric EBTs have been approved by the FDA for the indication of weight loss; these include three intragastric balloons (IGBs) and one device for aspiration therapy. IGBs are space-occupying devices which are inflated in the stomach with either saline or nitrogen-mixed gas and removed endoscopically after 6 months. These devices promote weight loss through both taking up space in the stomach and, in the case of the fluid-filled balloons, also result in slowing of gastric emptying.[129] Other mechanisms may also promote satiety, but further research is needed in this area. Table 9.1 includes all of the currently approved IGB and their FDA indications.

Aspiration therapy is performed with a specialized endoscopically placed percutaneous gastrostomy tube with attachable components to facilitate removal of a portion of the gastric contents after a meal (Fig. 9.8). Patients not only remove a portion of the calories they consumed in the meal, but the device also promotes changes in eating behaviors, which result in decreased consumption of food at mealtime.[130]

One additional therapy, endoscopic sleeve gastroplasty, in which a series of sutures endoscopically placed in the gastric body changes the shape of the stomach to resemble a tube, is currently being performed in the United States. This therapy decreases gastric volume, resulting in satiety, and may also delay gastric emptying, although this has only been studied in four patients.[131] It is important to note that this procedure is not FDA approved, but is performed using a device which has 510(k) clearance from the FDA for the general purpose of tissue apposition in the GI tract.

Intragastric Balloons

Two of the currently FDA-approved IGBs are filled with saline and require endoscopic placement under direct visualization. The single fluid-filled balloon (Orbera Gastric Balloon, Apollo Endosurgery, Austin, TX) is delivered on a catheter, and is placed without a guidewire, similar to an orogastric tube. Once in the stomach, the balloon is filled with saline under direct visualization to a volume between 400 and 700 mL. After filling is complete, the catheter is pulled against the gastroesophageal junction to detach the balloon, and then removed out through the patient's mouth. After 6 months, a repeat endoscopy is performed during which a catheter containing a beveled needle is used to puncture the balloon, the needle is then removed, the catheter is advanced into the balloon, and the fluid is aspirated. Once the balloon is deflated, a 2-prong grasper is used to secure the balloon, and the balloon is pulled out through the patient's mouth.

The dual saline-filled IGB (ReShape Gastric Balloon, Apollo Endosurgery, Austin, TX) has recently been purchased by the same manufacturer as the single fluid-filled balloon but will no longer be manufactured. It is delivered into the body of the stomach over a guidewire placed during the initial portion of the endoscopy. Once in place, the guidewire is removed and the proximal balloon is filled with either 375 or 450 mL of saline mixed with methylene blue. Once the balloon inflation is complete, the balloon is sealed with 6 mL of mineral oil. The process is repeated for the distal balloon. Once completed, the catheter is pulled against the gastroesophageal junction to detach the balloons from the delivery catheter, which is then pulled out through the mouth. After 6 months, a repeat endoscopy is performed during which a catheter containing a nonbeveled needle is used to bore a hole in the balloon. The needle is retracted, the catheter is advanced into the balloon, and the fluid is aspirated. The process is repeated for the second balloon. Once both balloons are deflated, a 15-mm rat-tooth alligator forceps is used to rip a hole in each balloon and a hexagonal snare is used to secure the proximal tip of the device. The device is then pulled out through the patient's mouth.

The swallowable gas-filled IGBs (Obalon Balloon System, Obalon Therapeutics, Carlsbad, CA) each are swallowed in a capsule that is tethered to a catheter with a hydrophilic coating. Capsule transit into the stomach is verified by imaging with fluoroscopy or digital x-ray, and a pressure drop on the gas dispenser pressure sensor attached to the catheter outside of the patient's mouth indicates when the balloon is unfolding in the unconstrained space of the stomach. The valve regulating flow from the gas canister to the balloon is then opened and gas flows into the balloon to a final pressure of 9–13 kPa and volume of 250 mL. The catheter is then ejected off of the balloon with pressure from 1.5 mL of water injected into the catheter. This process is repeated at 2 and 8 weeks from the first balloon administration to administer all three balloons. Six months after the first balloon administration was performed, an endoscopic procedure is performed to remove the balloons. Each balloon is deflated with an injector needle attached to suction and then grasped with a 15-mm rat-tooth alligator forceps for removal out the mouth; the process is repeated for the remaining two balloons.

Aspiration Therapy Device

The implantable component of the aspiration therapy device (AspireAssist, Aspire Bariatrics, King of Prussia, PA) is a gastrostomy tube made of medical-grade silicone that is placed with standard pull PEG tube placement technique.[132] At the time of placement, an external pumper is placed, and the patient returns 1–2 weeks later for conversion of the external portion of the gastrostomy tube to a skin-port, which is used for aspirating. As with traditional PEG tube placement, patients should receive IV antibiotics 30 minutes before the procedure and should also have an additional 24 hours of oral antibiotic prophylaxis. As of April 2022, the Aspire Device has been removed from market due to economic constraints. (https://www.bariatricnews.net/post/aspire-bariatrics-withdraws-aspireassist-from-the-market-as-covid-takes-its-toll. Accessed May 2023).

Endoscopic Sleeve Gastroplasty

Endoscopic SG is performed using a suturing device fixed to the distal tip of the endoscope; currently the only marketed suturing device is the Overstitch (Apollo Endosurgery, Austin, TX). A standard upper endoscope is first used to evaluate the stomach and then place marks on the anterior and posterior walls of the stomach where sutures will be placed. The scope with the attached suturing device is inserted with or without an overtube into the stomach. Starting on the anterior wall in the distal gastric body adjacent to the incisura, tissue is grabbed with a tissue helix and pulled toward the scope to allow for the needle driver to pass the needle through the tissue. This process is repeated for 5–8 "bites" in a U- or Z-shape pattern, the needle is released from the needle exchange catheter, and a cinch is placed on the opposite end of the suture, bringing the tissue together between the needle and the cinch. Once desired tightening is achieved, the suture is

TABLE 9.1 FDA-Approved Intragastric Balloons

Device	Device Image	FDA Status
ReShape Dual Balloon System ReShape Medical, San Celemente, CA		Approved for BMI 30–40 kg/m² with 1 obesity related comorbidity
Orbera Intragastric Balloon, Apollo Endosurgery, Austin, TX	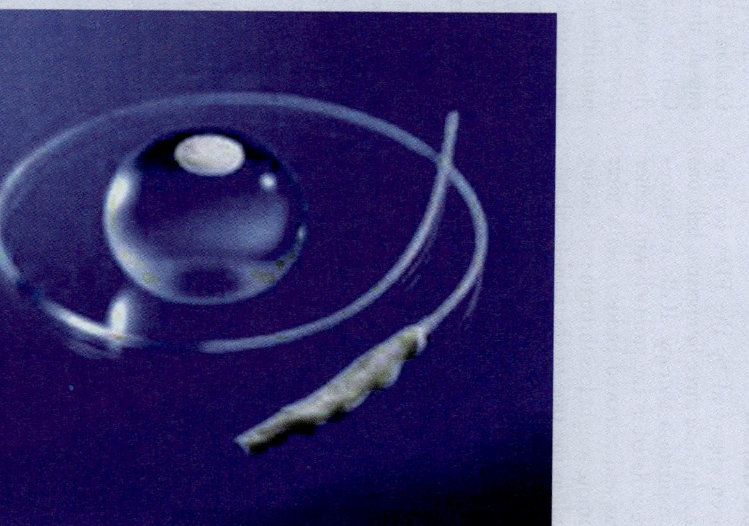	Approved for BMI 30–40 kg/m²

Obalon Balloon System, Obalon Therapeutics, Carlsbad, CA	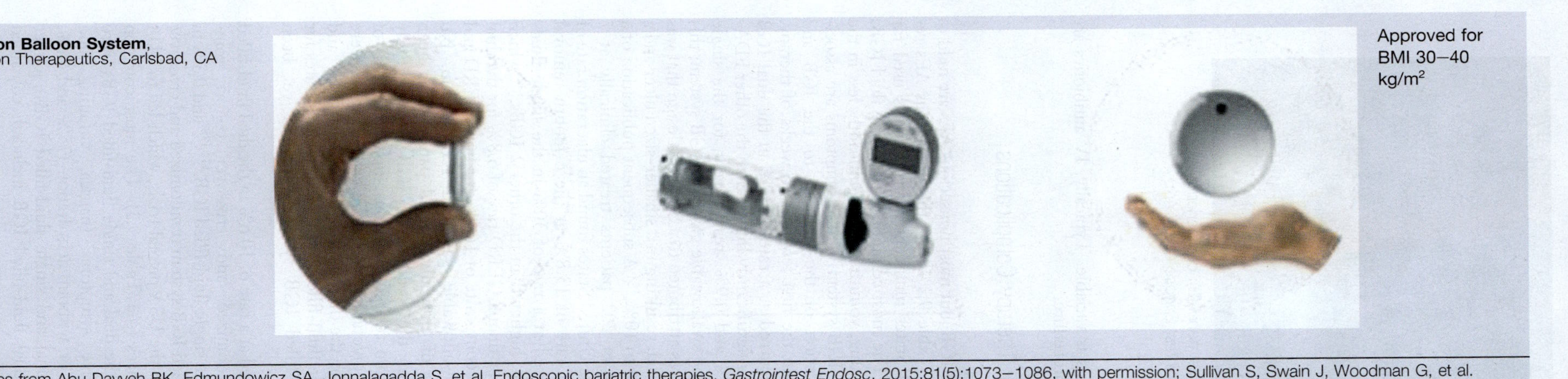	Approved for BMI 30–40 kg/m^2

Images from Abu Dayyeh BK, Edmundowicz SA, Jonnalagadda S, et al. Endoscopic bariatric therapies. *Gastrointest Endosc*. 2015;81(5):1073–1086, with permission; Sullivan S, Swain J, Woodman G, et al. Randomized sham-controlled trial of the 6-months swallowable gas-filled intragastric balloon system for weight loss. *Surg Obes Relat Dis*. 2018;14(12):1876–1889, with permission.

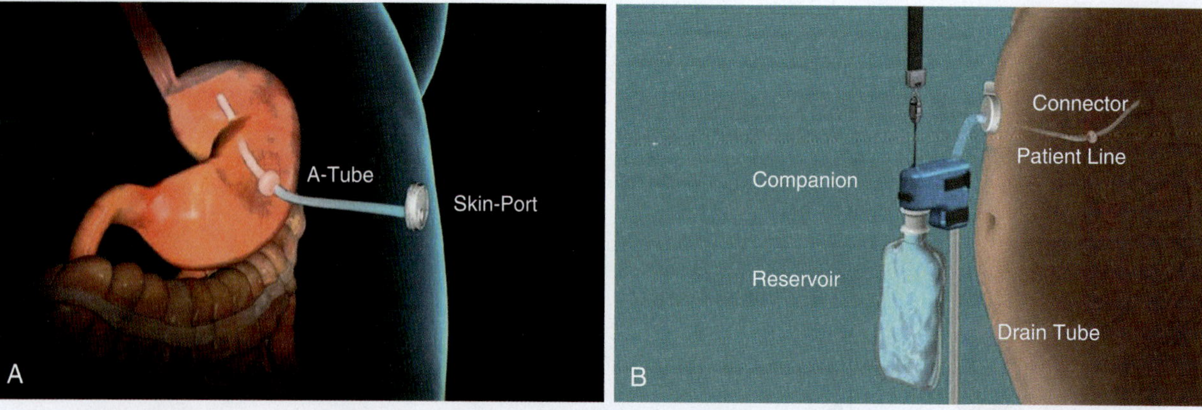

Fig. 9.8 Components of the AspireAssist System; panel (A): permanent components, panel (B): components only used during aspiration. (From Sullivan S. Aspiration therapy for obesity. *Gastrointest Endosc Clin N Am.* 2017;27(2):277–288, with permission.)

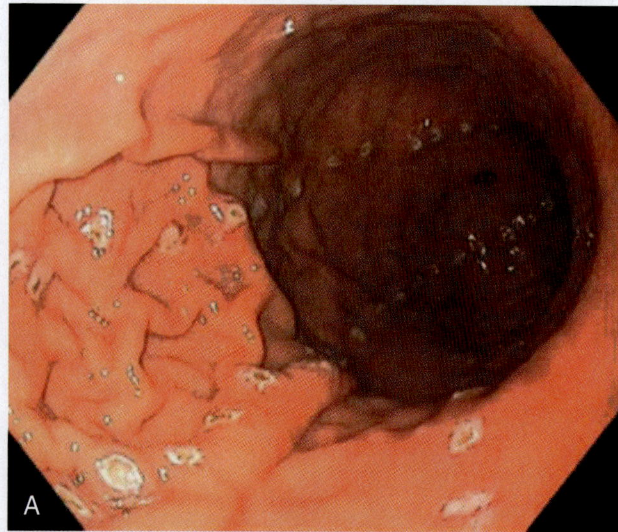

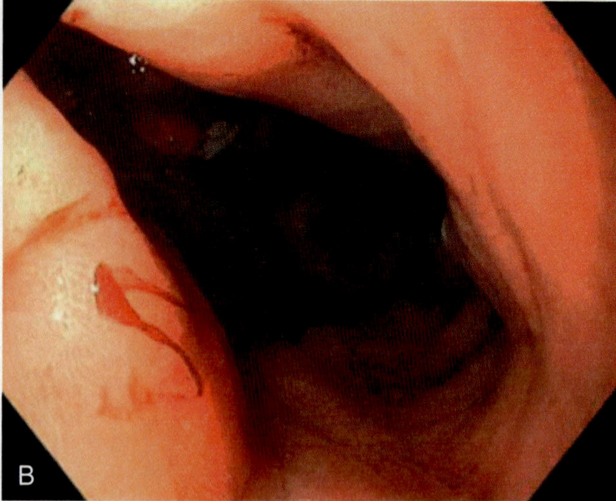

Fig. 9.9 Endoscopic sleeve gastroplasty. Panel (A): gastric body before the procedure, panel (B): gastric body after the procedure. (Courtesy Shelby Sullivan, MD.)

cut and the process is repeated moving proximally in the stomach until the proximal gastric body is reached (Fig. 9.9). Some practitioners place a second row of sutures to reinforce the first set of sutures placed, but this is variable. Typically, IV antibiotics are given at the time of procedure.

Endoscopic Bariatric Therapy Complications

Intragastric Balloons

AEs are common with IGB, but most nonserious AEs are mild to moderate in severity. Table 9.2 shows the nonserious AEs reported in the United States multicenter pivotal trials used for FDA approval.[133–136] The most common AEs for the fluid IGBs were nausea and vomiting; vomiting was significantly less in the swallowable gas-filled IGB system. These symptoms are associated with accommodation of the stomach to the IGB and generally resolve within the first few days to weeks of therapy. Gastric ulceration occurred at a rate of 35% in the dual IGB pivotal trial, which was significantly higher than the other FDA-approved IGBs at 0% and 0.9%, respectively, for the single fluid-filled IGB and the swallowable gas-filled IGB system; this difference, however, was attributed to a distal tip design that was modified during the trial, resulting in a smaller-sized ulcer and a reduction in incidence to 10%.[137] A subsequent publication of a retrospective analysis of 202 patients treated clinically at 7 different centers in the United States found an ulceration rate of 0.9% and an erosion rate of 13.8% at the 6-month removal period. GERD occurred at a rate of 30% in the single fluid-filled IGB pivotal trial, higher than the other 2 IGBs,[132] which was significantly higher than a GERD rate of 6.8% for the dual fluid-filled IGB and a composite of 16.9% for both GERD and dyspepsia for the swallowable gas-filled IGB system. No retrospective analysis of clinically treated patients has been published to date for the swallowable IGB system. Early removal rates (symptom-related and nonsymptom related) of the IGBs in the USA pivotal and USA clinical case series were 15%[136] and 6.4%[138] for the dual fluid-filled IGB, 18.8%[139] and 16.6%[140] for the single fluid-filled IGB. Early removal rates for the swallowable gas-filled IGB system have not yet been published.

Serious AEs occurred at a rate of 10.6% in the dual fluid-filled IGB (combined randomized and crossover cohort combined),[133,136] 10% in the single fluid-filled IGB,[132,138] and 0.3% in the swallowable gas-filled IGB system (randomized and crossover cohort combined)[134] in the USA pivotal trials, which led to FDA approval of these devices (see Table 9.2). The most common serious AEs for both the dual and single fluid-filled IGBs were due to accommodative symptoms (nausea, vomiting, and abdominal pain) with or without dehydration (75% and 71%, respectively, for the dual and single fluid-filled IGBs). Other serious AEs for the dual fluid-filled IGB included: contained

TABLE 9.2 Non-Serious Adverse Events in the Intragastric Balloon United States Multi-Center Trials

Adverse Event	ReShape (%)	Orbera (%)	Obalon (%)
Vomiting	86.7	86.8	17.3
Nausea	61.0	75.6	56.0
Abdominal pain	54.5	57.5	72.6
Gastric ulcer	35.2[a]	0	0.9
Dyspepsia	17.8	21.3	16.9[b]
Eructation	16.7	24.4	9.2
Abdominal discomfort	13.3	6.3	0
Abdominal distension	11.0	17.5	14.6
Erosive gastritis	9.1	0.6	7.1[c]
GERD	6.8	30.0	(See dyspepsia)
Erosive esophagitis	0.4	0.6	1.8
Constipation	5.3	0	2.7
Diarrhea	3.0	13.1	8.3

[a]After design modification of the distal tip of the ReShape Balloon, the ulcer rate decreased to 10%.
[b]Composite of dyspepsia and GERD.
[c]Composite of erythema, erosion, inflammation, or polyp.
From Sullivan S, Edmundowicz SA, Thompson CC. Endoscopic bariatric and metabolic therapies: new and emerging technologies. *Gastro.* 2017;152:1791–1801, with permission.

esophageal perforation, esophageal tear, UGI hemorrhage, gastric ulcers, pneumonia, and muscle pain. Other serious AEs for the single fluid-filled IGB included gastric outlet obstruction, gastric perforation with sepsis, aspiration pneumonia, and abdominal cramping with an IGB containing infected fluid. Only one serious AE occurred in the swallowable gas-filled IGB system pivotal trial, which was a bleeding ulcer in a patient on high-dose NSAIDs.

In the subsequent USA retrospective analysis of patients treated with the single fluid-filled IGB, nonserious AEs were not systematically recorded. However, 7% of patients were noted to have esophagitis after balloon removal (3% at baseline), 0.5% had an ulcer, and 0.5% had an esophageal tear. Overall, 8% of patients required outpatient IV fluids for dehydration after placement, 4% required hospitalization after IGB placement, and 1% required hospitalization after balloon removal.[139] Early IGB removals occurred in 16.6% of patients for nausea ($n = 11$), vomiting ($n = 19$), abdominal pain ($n = 4$), reflux ($n = 4$), a combination of symptoms ($n = 2$), and by patient request ($n = 13$). Additionally, in clinical series of the single fluid-filled IGB, one aspiration event was noted and one IGB deflation occurred, although this balloon passed out of the GI tract naturally. The most common nonserious AEs reported in the dual fluid-filled IGB were esophageal or gastric superficial tear on placement (8.4%) and removal ($n = 5$), nausea (73.8%), vomiting (49%), and post-procedure pain (25.2%). Early balloon removal was performed in 6.4% of patients for symptoms ($n = 10$), and spontaneous deflation occurred in 4 patients, 2 of whom required surgical removal of the balloon because it had migrated into the small intestine. An additional deflation was found on removal in a patient with a history of motor vehicle accident with blunt force trauma to the abdomen 1 week prior to removal.[137] One clinical registry of prospectively collected data has been published for the swallowable gas-filled IGB system including 1343 patients in the safety analysis. Nonserious AEs occurred in 14.22% of patients, the most common of which was abdominal pain (5.29%), nausea (4.69%), and vomiting (2.31%). Two serious AEs occurred, including dehydration requiring IV fluid administration in one patient (0.07%), and one gastric perforation treated with removal of the balloons and surgical repair of the perforation (0.07%).[141]

Although not seen in any of the pivotal trials or clinical registries, the FDA published an update to a letter to health care providers on June 4, 2018, which described 12 deaths from fluid-filled IGBs since its approval in the United States, with 7 of the 12 deaths occurring in the United States. Data on the root cause of these deaths are still unclear as of the writing of this chapter. Other events determined to be related to the fluid-filled IGBs, but not previously reported in the trials, included hyperinsufflation and pancreatitis. The rates of these AEs remains low, with a USA mortality rate from the dual and single fluid-filled IGB reported by the manufacturers as 0.06%[142] and 0.036%,[143] respectively. No reports of deaths attributable to the swallowable gas-filled IGB system have been reported in the United States as of the writing of this chapter.

Aspiration Therapy

Two randomized controlled trials have been performed in the United States comparing aspiration therapy and lifestyle therapy but only included one small single-center pilot study and one large multicenter trial. A previous version of the device with significant difference in the gastrostomy tube from the current gastrostomy tube was used in the pilot study and was associated with abdominal discomfort greater than 4 weeks after gastrostomy tube placement in all patients in the study (treatment group $n = 10$), which prompted a design change in the gastrostomy tube.[129] In the multicenter US trial (treatment group $n = 111$), peristomal granulation tissue was the most common AE at 40.5%. Other nonserious AEs that occurred in greater than 5% of patients included: abdominal pain less than 4 weeks after gastrostomy tube placement 37.8%; nausea/vomiting 17.1%; peristomal irritation 17.1%; intermittent abdominal discomfort 16.2%; possible or definite peristomal bacterial infection 13.5%; abdominal pain greater than 4 weeks after gastrostomy tube placement 8.1%; dyspepsia 6.3%; and peristomal inflammation 5.4%. Five serious AEs in four patients (3.6%) were reported including severe abdominal pain (two admissions in one subject), peritonitis, prepyloric ulcer, and a gastrostomy tube replacement due to a malfunction.[144]

Endoscopic Sleeve Gastroplasty

The first-in-man study with 3 study phases of procedure development included a total of 22 patients in the second phase (sites in the United States and Dominican Republic) and 77 patients in the third phase (sites in the United States, Dominican Republic, and Spain). AEs included "frequent" nausea, vomiting, and transient epigastric pain in the first week after the procedure, but no serious AEs were reported in either cohort.[145] Two large retrospective analyses ($n = 248$ and $n = 112$) which included sites both in the United States and outside of the USA and reporting AEs have been published.[146,147] Nonserious AEs were not systematically recorded in either study, but nausea, vomiting, and abdominal pain were described in a "large number of patients" in one series.[146] Five serious AEs (2%) occurred in the larger retrospective analysis including two perigastric inflammatory fluid collections treated with percutaneous drainage and antibiotics, extragastric hemorrhage due to splenic laceration, pulmonary embolism, and pneumoperitoneum/pneumothorax; the manuscript does not report on hospitalizations for accommodative symptoms.[145] In the second retrospective series, only three serious AEs occurred requiring hospitalization including two patients with bleeding (in one patient low-molecular-weight heparin and warfarin were started on Day 1 after the procedure) that required endoscopic therapy in one case. One perigastric fluid collection also occurred and managed with oral antibiotics as an outpatient.[146] The recent MERIT trial demonstrated 13% total body weight loss. (Dayyeh B, Bazerbachi F, Vargas E. Endoscopic sleeve gastroplasty for treatment of class 1 and 2 obesity (MERIT): a prospective, multicentre, randomised trial. *Lancet.* 2022;400(10350):441–451.

Nutritional Deficiencies

Nutritional deficiencies have not been reported as a consequence of IGBs or endoscopic sleeve gastroplasty. A pilot study for aspiration therapy reported on iron and vitamins D and B_{12}, with 4 of 10 subjects requiring iron supplementation, 3 of 10 subjects requiring vitamin D supplementation (due to low vitamin D at baseline), and 1 of 10 requiring B_{12} supplementation, which maintained normal concentrations of these micronutrients. Potassium supplements and PPI therapy were given to all subjects as part of the protocol[129]; this was not continued for the multicenter USA randomized controlled trial, and only 4 of 111 participants in the aspiration therapy group required supplementation during the first 52 weeks of the trial.[143]

Outcomes

Intragastric Balloons

Multicenter randomized controlled trials have been performed for all three FDA-approved IGBs. All of the studies used a moderate intensity lifestyle therapy (between 6 and 13 sessions) for the first 6 months; however, only two of the balloons, the dual fluid-filled IGB and the swallowable gas-filled IGB system, had a sham control group.[134,136] The effect of knowledge of group assignment in a weight loss device study has been shown to increase weight loss by approximately 40%.[148] This is consistent with weight loss differences seen in the active groups of the IGBs with randomized sham-controlled trial designs—the open label randomized controlled trial of the single fluid-filled IGB demonstrated 35%–40% more weight loss (Table 9.3). Moreover, clinical effectiveness data from both the dual fluid-filled IGB and single fluid IGB registries and the swallowable gas-filled IGB system registry demonstrate higher weight loss than was seen in the pivotal trials. In the dual fluid-filled IGB registry, 202 patients (age 47.8 ± 10.8 years, female 83.2%, BMI 36.7 ± 6.6 kg/m^2) underwent balloon placement. Weight loss was 11.4% ± 6.7% TBW at 6 months, but data were only available for 101 patients.[137] In the single fluid-filled IGB registry, 321 patients (age 48.1 ± 11.9 years, female 80%, BMI 37.6 ± 6.9 kg/m^2) underwent balloon placement. Weight loss was 11.8% ± 7.5% TBW at 6 months, but data were only available for 199 patients.[139] In the swallowable gas-filled IGB registry, 1387 patients initiated therapy, with 3.2% of patients excluded from the final analysis ($n = 36$ without a final weight and $n = 8$ with a starting BMI < 25 kg/m^2). A total of 1343 patients were included in the intention-to treat-analysis (age 45.7 ± 10.8 years, female 78.6%, BMI 35.4 ± 5.4 kg/m^2) which was defined as having at least 1 balloon for at least 1 day, and 82.1% of patients ($n = 1103$) were included in the completer analysis which was defined as a total of exactly 3 balloons administered for at least 20 weeks. Weight loss at 6 months was 9.9% ± 6.2% TBW in the completer analysis and 9.2% ± 6.3% TBW in the intention-to-treat analysis. An analysis including only the on-label population (BMI 30–40 kg/m^2 with 3 balloons for at least 20 weeks, $n = 787$) demonstrated weight loss of 10.0% ± 6.1% TBWL.[140]

Aspiration Therapy

Two randomized controlled trials in the United States have demonstrated weight loss superiority of aspiration therapy plus lifestyle therapy compared with lifestyle therapy alone. In a pilot study, 4 patients in the lifestyle therapy only group [age 45.3 ± 2.8 standard error of the mean (SEM) years, female 100%, BMI 39.3 ± 1.1 SEM kg/m^2] and 10 patients in the aspiration therapy plus lifestyle therapy only group (age 38.7 ± 2.3 SEM years, female 100%, BMI 42.0 ± 1.4 SEM kg/m^2) completed 1 year of therapy. The percentage of TBWL in the lifestyle therapy only group at 1 year was 5.9% ± 5.0% compared with 18.6% ± 2.3% in the aspiration therapy plus lifestyle ($P = .021$). Seven subjects in the aspiration therapy plus lifestyle therapy arm completed an additional year of therapy with 20.1% ± 3.5% TBWL at the end of year 2.[132]

In the PATHWAY Study, the modified intention-to treat-analysis included 60 patients in the lifestyle therapy only group (age 46.8 ± 11.6 years, female 88.3%, and BMI 40.9 ± 3.9 kg/m^2) and 111 patients in the aspiration therapy plus lifestyle therapy group (age 42.4 ± 10.0 years, female 86.5%, and BMI 42.0 ± 5.1 kg/m^2). The % TBWL in the lifestyle therapy only group compared with the aspiration therapy plus lifestyle therapy group was 3.5% ± 6.0% versus 12.1% ± 9.6% respectively, $P < .001$ for the modified intention-to-treat analysis; this compares with 4.9% ± 7.0% and 14.2% ± 9.8% for the lifestyle therapy only ($n = 31$) and aspiration therapy plus lifestyle therapy ($n = 82$) groups in the subjects that completed 1 year of therapy, $P < .001$.[143] A total of 55 subjects in the aspiration therapy plus lifestyle therapy group continued therapy beyond 1 year with 42, 22, and 15 subjects completing 2, 3, and 4 years of therapy with 15.3% ± 8.8%, 16.6% ± 10.5%, and 18.7% ± 11.7% TBWL, respectively.[149]

Endoscopic Sleeve Gastroplasty

Weight loss data from the first reported multicenter case series included 248 patients (age 44.5 ± 10 years, female 73%, BMI 37.8 ± 5.6 kg/m^2). Weight loss was 15.2% TBW (95% CI 14.2–16.3) at 6 months with 87% of patient follow-up and 18.6% TBW (95% CI 15.7–21.5) at 24 months with only 62% patient follow-up.[145] In the series by Sartoretto et al., 112 patients were included (age 45.1 ± 11.7 years, female 69%, and BMI 37.9 ± 6.7 kg/m^2). Weight loss was reported in 61.6% of the patients with 14.9% ± 6.1% TBW at 6 months.[146] Weight loss was also reported in a multiphase first-in-man series with USA patients included in phase 2 ($n = 22$, age 39.2 ± 1.2 years, female 91%, and BMI 34.3 ± 1.0 kg/m^2) and phase 3 ($n = 77$, age 41.3 ± 1.1 years, female 77%, and BMI 36.1 ± 0.6 kg/m^2).[144] Weight loss was reported in

TABLE 9.3 Subject Number, Body Mass Index, Percent Body Weight Loss, and Responder Rate for Modified Intention to Treat Randomized Cohorts (First 6 Months) of the United States Multi-Center Trials

	Number of Subjects		Body Mass Index (kg/m^2)		Percent Total Body Weight Loss		
Device	Control Group	Active Group	Control Group	Active Group	Control Group (%)	Active Group (%)	Active Group Responder Rate (%)[a]
Orbera	130	125	35.4 ± 2.7	35.2 ± 3.2	3.3 ± 5.0	10.2 ± 6.6	79.2
ReShape	139	187	35.4 ± 2.6	35.3 ± 2.8	3.3	6.8	48.8
Obalon	189	198	35.4 ± 2.7	35.1 ± 2.7	3.4 ± 5.0	6.6 ± 5.1	62.1

[a]Responder rate was defined as ≥5% total body weight loss for both Orbera and Obalon studies, but ≥25% excess weight loss for the ReShape study.
From Sullivan S, Edmundowicz SA, Thompson CC. Endoscopic bariatric and metabolic therapies: new and emerging technologies. *Gastro.* 2017;152:1791–1801, with permission.

91% of the phase 2 subjects with 17.3% ± 2.6% TBWL at 12 months and weight loss was reported in 57% of the phase 3 subjects with 17.4% ± 1.2% TBWL at 12 months. No randomized controlled trials of ESG have been performed to date.

Obesity in the United States is often unfairly stigmatized and attributed to careless eating habits or lack of exercise. In reality, causes of obesity are multifactorial, with issues that include genetics, physiology, socioeconomic status, level of education, access to healthful foods, and awareness of how food directly impacts health. The rapid growth of the obesity epidemic must be addressed in such a way as to achieve more immediate outcomes. Surgical treatment of morbid obesity is safer and more effective than ever. Bariatric surgery has become a routine component of general surgery training and currently represents the fastest-growing area in surgical training programs. Endoscopic bariatric therapies are new therapies with proven safety and effectiveness. Although these procedures, on average, produce less weight loss than bariatric surgery, they are also lower risk and provide important treatment options for patients with obesity. Moreover, endoscopic management of bariatric surgical complications continues to advance with more complications managed without the need for additional surgery. Health care providers must work together to optimally support and care for this population, whether patients are working independently to lose weight, considering weight loss endoscopic or surgical procedures, or have undergone weight loss endoscopic procedures or surgery. Weight-loss endoscopic procedures and surgery are most effective with proper patient selection and an appropriately trained procedural team. While risks exist, weight loss surgery and endoscopic bariatric therapies are potentially life-saving interventions in the right patients and in the right hands.

Full references for this chapter can be found at https://ebooks.health.elsevier.com.

10 Feeding and Eating Disorders

Debra K. Katzman, Nuray Kanbur, Mark L. Norris

IN THIS CHAPTER

Eating disorders (EDs) are mental disorders characterized by disturbances in body image, weight control, and/or dietary patterns. In the *Diagnostic and Statistical Manual of Mental Disorders*, 5th edition (DSM-5),[1] an updated and expanded section summarizes feeding and EDs that include (1) anorexia nervosa (AN); (2) bulimia nervosa (BN); (3) binge-eating disorder (BED); (4) avoidant/restrictive food intake disorder (ARFID); (5) pica; (6) rumination disorder; (7) other specified feeding or eating disorder (OSFED); and (8) unspecified feeding or eating disorder (USFED). This chapter provides a lifespan perspective with a focus on EDs seen in adults: AN, BN, and BED; other feeding and EDs, including pica, rumination disorder, and ARFID, are discussed only briefly. Although feeding and EDs are classified as mental disorders, their associated behaviors commonly result in and present with medical sequelae, many of which are gastrointestinal (GI). Because associated chronic undernutrition, overweight, and/or purging behaviors often result in medical complications that can be serious, chronic, and life threatening, individuals with feeding and EDs benefit from the ongoing care of a multidisciplinary treatment team. Indeed, AN and BN are among the mental disorders with the highest mortality.[2] Reviews suggest that GI complications are among the most prevalent experienced by patients with EDs.

EPIDEMIOLOGY

EDs have been described across diverse global settings, although epidemiologic data are best established for populations in North America and Europe. Most of the published epidemiologic data for feeding and EDs predate the revised diagnostic criteria published in the DSM-5. As expected, given the changes in DSM-5 that aimed to diminish the proportions of patients in residual categories, early studies suggest that the prevalence and incidence of AN, BN, and BED are higher, while proportional representation in the residual categories (previously ED not otherwise specified and now OSFED and USFED) have decreased.[3] A recent cross-sectional Canadian pediatric surveillance study reported the incidence of ARFID to be 2.02 per 100,000 patients.[276] Of note, few studies to date have investigated incidence and prevalence rates of pica, or rumination using the DSM-5.

A recent systematic review drawing upon DSM-5 feeding and ED populations suggests that the prevalence rate for AN ranges from 1.7% to 3.6%, with a point prevalence of 0.67%–1.2%.[4] Although BN has traditionally been more common than AN, the paucity of studies drawing upon DSM-5 populations has yet to establish this conclusively. BN has most commonly been assessed using point prevalence. Two separate studies reported near identical point prevalence rates for BN of 0.6% in girls and women.[4] A recent interview-based study revealed higher lifetime prevalence rates for BN compared with AN (2.6% vs. 0.8%, respectively).[5] Point prevalence rates for BED have ranged from 0.62% to 3.6% (female subjects only and males and female subjects combined, respectively).[4,6,7] Lifetime prevalence rates for OSFED are reported to be 0.3% in male subjects and 0.6% in female subjects,[4,8] with a point prevalence rate of 0% in male subjects and 2.4% in a sample of male and female subjects.[4,8] Lifetime prevalence rates for USFED range from 0.2% to 0.9% among male and female subjects.[8,9]

Relatively high prevalence rates are also reported for specific symptoms associated with disordered eating. In 2017 6% of school-going female adolescents in the United States reported vomiting or laxative use; 5.9% reported taking diet pills, powders, or liquids without a doctor's advice to lose weight or to prevent weight gain; and 17.4% reported fasting within the previous month to lose weight.[10] EDs occur across ethnically and socioeconomically diverse populations, but each of the EDs is more common in women than in men. Historically, boys and men have accounted for less than 10% of individuals with AN, 10% of those with BN, and 40% of those with BED.[11,12]

Studies have identified that approximately 14%[13,14] of children and adolescents admitted to adolescent inpatient ED programs and as many as 22.5% of individuals in a pediatric ED day treatment program met the DSM-5 diagnosis for ARFID; patients were younger, had longer duration of illness, were more likely to be male compared with those who had AN or BN, and were commonly diagnosed with comorbid psychiatric and/or medical symptoms.[13,14] Prevalence data on pica in the general population are unavailable and may vary widely in certain demographic strata. A recent systematic review of prevalence rates of DSM-5 feeding and EDs failed to identify any study that included pica or ARFID.[4] Whereas pica appears to be uncommon in healthy children in the United States, pica eating has been reported to be relatively more prevalent among U.S. children treated for sickle cell disease, adults with iron deficiency, institutionalized individuals, some school-age populations in Africa, and in some populations of pregnant women (e.g., in Africa).[15] The prevalence of rumination disorder is unknown, but it can occur in both children and adults.[15]

Finally, it is important to highlight the impact of the COVID-19 pandemic on EDs. The COVID-19 had a substantial increase in the number and severity of new and preexisting individuals suffering with EDs compared to prior years. There were reports showing an increase in new cases of EDs, a rise in individuals experiencing deteriorating symptoms, and an increase in hospital admissions and emergency room visits as a result of the COVID-19 pandemic.[277,278] A number of precipitating and perpetuating factors were thought to contribute to this surge of EDs, including an increase in mental health symptoms and disorders, disruption and restriction to routines, loss of connections with peers and family members, general social isolation, increase social media use, and public health mitigation strategies focusing on hand hygiene, social distancing, and mask wearing. The ongoing clinical burden of this surge is yet to be determined. However, the global surge in EDs has highlighted the need to capacity build in preparation should there be another global pandemic or crisis.[277,279,280]

CAUSATIVE FACTORS

Although incompletely understood, the cause of EDs is almost certainly multifactorial, with psychodevelopmental,[16] sociocultural,[17] and genetic[18] contributions to risk. Exposure to risk factors for dieting appears to elevate risk for AN and BN,[18,19] just as childhood exposure to negative comments about weight and shape elevate risk for BED.[20] Body dissatisfaction in a social context in which thinness,[21,22] self-efficacy, and control are valued may be an important means whereby dieting is initiated and disordered eating attitudes and behaviors ensue. Dietary restraint may precipitate a cycle of hunger, binge eating, and purging.[23] Among numerous risk correlates, childhood GI complaints have been found associated with earlier age of onset and greater severity of BN in a retrospective study,[24] and picky eating and digestive problems were found prospectively associated with AN in adolescence.[16]

It has been suggested that physiologic vulnerabilities may increase risk for an ED. Neurobiological targets have been identified as possibly playing a role in the pathogenesis of AN, BN, and BED. For decades, researchers have studied the psychobiology of EDs and the neurophysiologic correlates and determinants of energy intake, hunger, and satiety. Findings highlight the multifactorial and phenotypically diverse nature of eating behavior. For example, energy intake is influenced by complex interactions among signaling molecules from peripheral systems (e.g., GI peptides, vagal stimulation) and CNS neuropeptides and neuroamines. As is true of the search for obesity treatments, it is unlikely that single mechanisms will become the basis of therapeutic interventions for EDs. However, the greater our understanding of the physiology of ingestive behavior, the more likely we are to establish integrated therapy models in the future. There is a vast amount of literature on this topic, and what follows is simply a brief overview of the more commonly investigated mechanisms.

Satiety

Serotonin has long been a focus of attention for its possible role in disrupted satiety. There is substantial evidence that altered 5-hydroxytryptamine (5-HT, serotonin) functioning contributes to dysregulated appetite, mood, and impulse control in EDs and that such alteration persists after recovery from AN and BN, possibly reflecting premorbid vulnerability.[25,26] There also is evidence that cholecystokinin (CCK) levels are altered in ED populations. Findings for AN are inconsistent. Although there is some evidence that young women with AN have high levels of pre- and postprandial CCK that may impede treatment progress by contributing to postprandial nausea and vomiting,[27,28] other reports have shown decreased CCK compared with controls.[29] In patients with BN, there is consistent evidence for an impaired satiety response, characterized by a blunted postprandial CCK response as well as delayed gastric emptying.[30–32] In contrast, individuals with BED and obesity do not differ in postprandial CCK responses from those with obesity but no BED.[33] The relationships between CCK, binge eating, and BMI warrant further clarification. In patients with ARFID, fasting CCK levels were found to be higher than healthy controls, however this elevation was not related to BMI, subjective appetite measures or markers of disease.[281]

Peptide tyrosine (PYY), the intestinally derived anorexigen that elicits satiety, appears to be dysregulated in individuals with AN and BN, but not in those with BED. Young women with AN have demonstrated higher levels of PYY compared with controls, perhaps contributing to reduced food intake.[34,35] In individuals with BN, expected elevations in PYY after meals are blunted,[36,37] possibly playing a role in impaired satiety. A recent report found no differences between BED and non-BED groups in fasting levels and postprandial changes in PYY.[38] One study reported differences in levels of PYY between patients with AN, BN, and BED with levels being highest among patients with BED and lowest in those with AN.[282] The same study found levels of glucagon-like peptide 1 (GLP-1) to be increased in those with BED as compared to those with AN.[282] In another study that focused on comparisons between patients with ARFID, AN, and healthy controls, fasting and postprandial PYY did not differ between patients with ARFID or healthy controls.[283] Women with BN have been found to secrete abnormally low levels of the GI satiety peptides GLP-1 and pancreatic polypeptide, which is thought to be a consequence of the adaptation to large meals in the form of enlarged gastric capacity and reduced muscle tone in the gastric wall. Attenuated secretion of these GI satiety polypeptides may play a role in maintaining bulimic behavior.[39]

Appetite

The orexigenic peptide ghrelin is of interest in EDs because it is the only known GI hormone that stimulates appetite and promotes food intake.[40] Ghrelin influences secretion of growth hormone, induces adiposity, and is implicated in signaling the hypothalamic nuclei involved in energy homeostasis. Gastric secretion of ghrelin is stimulated by a combination of neural (vagus nerve), mechanical (distension), chemical (osmolarity;

caloric content and macronutrient composition of the meal) and hormonal (insulin) factors with unknown priority.[41] Consistent findings in the literature examining ghrelin in patients with AN have shown that (1) circulating basal levels of ghrelin are elevated, a likely consequence of prolonged starvation[40,42,43]; (2) growth hormone and appetite responses to ghrelin are blunted, suggesting ghrelin resistance or altered ghrelin sensitivity[41,44,45]; and (3) ghrelin levels return to normal after partial weight recovery, suggesting a physiologic effect to compensate for lack of nutritional intake and energy stores.[40,46] More recently, a randomized, double-blind, placebo-controlled trial using a ghrelin agonist in 22 outpatients with AN revealed that those treated with a ghrelin agonist demonstrated significantly decreased gastric emptying time, and a trend of greater weight gain after 4 weeks.[47]

Plasma levels of ghrelin are normal or elevated in individuals with BN, which suggests that abnormal eating behaviors, including binge eating and purging, may influence ghrelin secretion[36,37]; there is a postprandial blunted response (i.e., reduced suppression of ghrelin) in these patients.[48] The relationship between elevated ghrelin and binge eating in patients with BN requires further exploration.[46] Investigations of ghrelin functioning in individuals with BED have reported lower circulating levels of pre- and postprandial ghrelin, possibly reflecting downregulation in response to chronic overeating and smaller decreases in ghrelin after eating.[38] Des-acyl- and acyl-ghrelin were found to be higher in patients with AN compared to patients with BED, who had significantly lower levels of both.[282] Another group found that both fasting and postprandial ghrelin was elevated in patients with AN compared with both ARFID and healthy controls.[283]

Energy Storage

Leptin and adiponectin are hormonal signals associated with longer term regulation of body fat stores. Leptin is also directly implicated in satiety through its binding to the ventral medial nucleus of the hypothalamus, an area termed the *satiety center*. Leptin and adiponectin are both altered in patients with EDs. A number of studies have found evidence for hyperadiponectinemia and hypoleptinemia in populations of underweight AN with reversal following restoration of weight[49,50]; increased adiponectin levels may act protectively to support energy homeostasis during food deprivation. Individuals with BN also exhibit decreased plasma levels of leptin and increased levels of total plasma-adiponectin, which are inversely correlated with longer duration of illness and increased severity of symptoms.[51,52] The mechanism of altered leptin functioning in BN is unclear because blunted postprandial leptin levels are not observed in individuals with BED.[33] Interestingly, fasting leptin levels have been found to be significantly higher at discharge in patients with AN who had fair (BMI >18) versus poor outcomes (BMI <18); outcomes correlated with early weight loss after discharge, suggesting the potential utility of leptin as a biomarker of early weight relapse.[284]

There are other mechanisms of interest, including neuropeptide Y, peptides glucagon-like peptide-2, orexins A and B, the endocannabinoids, resistin (adipose tissue-specific secretory factor), and brain-derived neurotrophic factor, but more research is necessary to elucidate their roles in the pathophysiology of EDs. One high priority for research is clarifying whether observed psychobiological abnormalities are antecedents or consequences of disturbed eating behavior that return to normal after recovery; this information could shed light on cause and possible treatment targets. Patients often report intense discomfort after eating; as a reason, they continue to restrict intake. The discomfort may be dismissed as perceptual or psychological in the absence of any medical findings to support the symptoms, but there may be disruptions in CNS or peripheral signals contributing to this and other reported symptoms.

Intestinal Microbiota

Recent research suggests that the intestinal microbiota is likely to play an important role in the cause, progression, and treatment of EDs. The intestinal microbiota is necessary for normal physiology and this is underscored by the role of the intestinal microbiome in metabolic diseases. The intestinal microbiota can be conceptualized as a community of microorganisms, including bacteria, archaea, fungi, parasites, and viruses, found within the human GI tract (see Chapter 3).[274] The composition of an individual's intestinal microbiota is unique, and the relationships that the microbiota has with human health and disease is influenced by a number of host factors, including, but not limited to, genetics, nutrition, health and nutritional status, age, sex, geography, and exposures.[275] Although studies involving the microbiota and EDs are limited, emerging research suggests that patients with EDs have an altered intestinal microbiota[285–287] (dysbiosis) and this alteration persists even after short-term renourishment.[275,285,288] Dysbiosis has been thought to alter the gut–brain axis and to have an impact on appetite control and brain function that may contribute to the development of an ED. It is also thought that abnormal feeding behaviors and psychological stress feedback to the intestinal ecosystem, influencing physiological, cognitive, and social functioning. This relatively new area of study requires further exploration to help understand how intestinal microbes impact the human host with respect to the etiology of EDs and how the intestinal microbiota changes over the course of the illness. Understanding the role of the intestinal ecosystem in EDs could facilitate the development of novel microbiome-targeted treatments that may facilitate weight restoration, improve GI tolerance during refeeding, and help ameliorate mental health distress via the brain-gut-microbiota axis,[275] ultimately to improve the outcome of EDs.

ONSET AND COURSE

AN and BN most commonly have their onset in adolescence,[53,289] and BED usually manifests in the early 20s,[54] but EDs can occur throughout most of the life span and appear to be increasing in frequency in middle-aged and older women.[55,56] Diagnostic migration from one ED category to another is common.[57,290] ARFID most commonly has its onset in the early years but can continue into adulthood.[1] Pica has been described in both children and adults, but little is known about the courses of pica and rumination disorder.[15]

Lifetime comorbidity of AN, BN, and BED with other psychiatric disorders has been reported as high at 56.2%, 94.5%, and 63.6%, respectively.[58] Mortality associated with AN and BN combined is five times higher than expected and is one of the highest mortality rates among mental disorders.[2] Some data support the chronicity of AN, reporting that slightly less than half of survivors with AN make a full recovery, with 60% attaining a normal weight and 47% regaining normal eating behavior; 34% improve but only achieve partial recovery, whereas 21% follow a chronic course.[59] Other data suggest that recovery rates for AN may be more favorable than previously believed,[58] with a large twin cohort study reporting a 5-year clinical recovery rate of 66.8%.[60] In contrast, after a 5-year follow-up of 216 patients with BN and EDNOS, 74% and 78% of patients, respectively, were still in recovery.[61] In a 6-year longitudinal study of patients with BED, 43% of individuals continued to be symptomatic.[62] A recently published 22-year longitudinal study of patients with AN and BN demonstrated that the presence and persistence of binge-eating and purging behaviors were poor prognostic indicators to overall recovery and that comorbidity with depression at initial assessment strongly predicted the continuation of AN at the 22-year mark.[63]

In summary, despite decades of studies that have investigated potential treatment modalities for the EDs, up to 50% of treated individuals continue to be symptomatic in follow-up.[64]

EVALUATION

A substantial percentage of individuals with an ED in the United States do not receive specific treatment for this problem.[58] Despite clear diagnostic criteria for EDs, clinical detection is often problematic, and up to 50% of cases may go unrecognized in clinical settings. Moreover, individuals with EDs are often reluctant to disclose their symptoms.[65] Although individuals with AN are underweight by definition, this can be easily missed in clinical settings. Even when noted on evaluation, the medical seriousness of low weight frequently is unappreciated.[66] When an ED is suspected or confirmed, patients may decline or avoid medical or mental health care and a feature of AN can be denial of the medical seriousness of symptoms.[11] Therefore ascertainment of concerns about body shape, weight, fatness, and weight gain or loss can be especially challenging when patients are unable or unwilling to recognize or to disclose them.[67] Given that many individuals with EDs initially present in primary care or medical subspecialty settings, recognition of clinical signs and symptoms across diverse health care settings will facilitate appropriate referrals and make diagnostic evaluation and treatment plans more efficient. One study has reported that individuals with BN are more likely to seek help for their GI complaints before seeking treatment for their ED.[68] Familiarity with the diagnostic features and GI complications of EDs will help the clinician identify the most appropriate interventions, including the full spectrum of treatment resources available for a comprehensive treatment plan.

When an ED is suspected, a directed clinical interview about restrictive or binge eating and inappropriate compensatory measures to control weight (Box 10.1) is essential in determining the scope and severity of symptoms that underlie specific GI complaints and pose medical risk. Accurate and timely diagnosis of EDs is challenging for several reasons. First, patients may be unreliable reporters of their history, and BN and BED may be present without any abnormal physical findings, as may pica and rumination disorder. In addition, some dietary modifications and exercise behaviors certainly are appropriate, and discerning pathologic behavior that is consistent with a clinically significant ED can be difficult. There is considerable overlap in symptoms among the EDs; diagnostic specificity, however, is critical to effective management.

Given the frequent reluctance of patients to recognize or to disclose symptoms of an ED, targeted history taking may be essential to making a prompt diagnosis. In some cases, an ED may not be suspected or the diagnosis confirmed until physical findings suggestive of purging are detected, a suggestive pattern is noticed in weight changes, and/or there is difficulty gaining weight notwithstanding appropriate nutritional treatment and exclusion of other potential causes for low weight.

BOX 10.1 Behaviors Used to Compensate for Excessive Food Intake or to Prevent Weight Gain

PURGING BEHAVIORS

- Diuretic abuse
- Laxative and/or enema abuse
- Self-induced vomiting (including syrup of ipecac abuse)

NONPURGING BEHAVIORS

- Excessive physical activity
- Fasting, skipping meals, restrictive-eating pattern
- Inappropriate withholding or underdosing of insulin (among individuals with diabetes mellitus)
- Stimulant abuse (e.g., caffeine, ephedra, methylphenidate, cocaine)

DIAGNOSIS OF SPECIFIC FEEDING AND EATING DISORDERS

Anorexia Nervosa

AN is characterized by a significantly low weight (the weight that is less than minimally normal), fear of gaining weight (despite being thin), and a disturbance in the way body shape or weight is perceived (e.g., a denial of the medical seriousness of being underweight or feeling fat despite emaciation).[1] It is not uncommon for an individual with AN to deny or minimize fear of weight gain at initial evaluation (and sometimes an apparent absence of this fear persists).[69] Even if a patient does not admit or disclose an intense fear of weight gain, evidence of continuing behaviors that undermine weight gain (e.g., restrictive eating, purging, excessive exercising) may be used to establish this criterion. Individuals with AN typically restrict their food selections and caloric intake, but about half of those with AN also routinely binge eat and/or engage in inappropriate purging behaviors, such as self-induced vomiting or laxative use, to prevent weight gain (Box. 10.1). AN is further divided into two subtypes: restricting type (those who primarily control their weight through dieting, fasting, or exercising) and binge-eating/purging type (those who routinely purge calories to control weight and/or routinely binge eat).[1] In middle-aged and older women, new-onset AN may present in conjunction with difficulty making life transitions and fear of aging.[56] The diagnosis of AN may be delayed when patients present to a GI specialty practice without disclosing their concerns and behaviors relating to weight. Presentation with GI complaints, even if related to real symptoms or disease, can sometimes prove to be a "red herring," drawing attention away from and delaying diagnosis of an ED. One study of 20 consecutive patients who presented to a GI practice and ultimately were diagnosed with an ED found the diagnosis of an ED was delayed for an average of 13 months after presentation. Notably, all patients stated a desire to gain weight and denied attempts to lose weight via exercise, purging, or dietary restriction.[70] Individuals with AN are not always able or willing to frame their difficulty maintaining a healthy weight as intentional, so diagnosis may initially be unsuspected and delayed.

Bulimia Nervosa

The clinical hallmark of BN is recurrent binge eating accompanied by inappropriate compensatory behaviors to control weight or to purge calories consumed during a binge (see Box 10.1). On average, these behaviors must occur once each week for at least 3 months to meet diagnostic criteria.[1] Moreover, intrinsic to the diagnosis of BN is the excessive influence of weight and/or shape on self-image. Individuals with BN have poor self-image that is often anchored to their weight. It is not unusual for individuals with AN or BN to weigh themselves daily, even several times each day, and to experience fluctuations in self-esteem and mood based on the result.

By definition, *binge eating* is consumption of an unusually large amount of food during a "discrete period of time" (i.e., not overeating or "grazing" all day), accompanied by the feeling that the eating cannot be controlled.[1] Many patients describe an emotional numbing during the period of eating; for some, this state appears to motivate the bingeing. Most clinicians are familiar with self-induced vomiting as the primary purging behavior, but individuals with BN may also use alternative or additional means to prevent weight gain, including abuse of laxatives and/or enemas, diuretics, stimulants (including methylphenidate, cocaine, over-the-counter "natural" supplements, and caffeine), underdosing of insulin (for those with diabetes mellitus), fasting or restrictive eating, and excessive exercise (see Box 10.1). In adolescents with celiac disease, intentional consumption of gluten to promote weight loss has also been reported.[71] Whereas most individuals with BN use compensatory behaviors that include purging, those who only use excessive physical activity or fasting are more challenging to identify. As with overeating and dieting, it is frequently difficult to determine the line between culturally normative and pathologic behavior with excessive exercise. Generally, clinical suspicion should be raised when an individual continues to exercise despite an injury or illness, or if he or she is exercising routinely in excess of what a coach is advising for the team.

It is recommended that clinicians ask about purging behaviors if an ED is suspected. Although it is not certain that a patient will respond candidly, individuals are more likely than not to eventually disclose information about symptoms when asked.[65] Some patients report feeling relieved when clinicians pose such questions if they previously had not been able to discuss their symptoms. On occasion, however, patients report learning about techniques from clinicians' questions, so it is advisable for clinicians to provide a psychoeducational context for the questions (e.g., by conveying serious physical consequences associated with the behavior) and to avoid introducing information about a dangerous behavior (e.g., underdosing insulin), using appropriate discretion based upon the clinical context. Patients also benefit from learning that treatment is available and effective, and from feeling understood by their clinicians.

Whereas purging and other behaviors aimed at neutralizing or decreasing calorie intake and modifying weight can pose medical risks when chronic, some of them pose more immediate and potentially lethal consequences. Patients should be educated about these acute life-threatening risks, and steps should be taken to eradicate such behaviors immediately. For example, because of the serious neurotoxicity, cardiotoxicity, and risk of death associated with repeated ingestion of syrup of ipecac,[72] its ongoing use is a clinical emergency and may require immediate hospitalization. Many patients are unaware of the serious risk associated with syrup of ipecac use. Similarly, ephedra, now banned in the United States, poses risk of stroke or adverse cardiac events even in young adults.[73] Some ephedra-free supplements marketed as weight-loss agents may also be proarrhythmic and pose medical risks.[74] Although patients find it difficult to abstain from purging behaviors, they may be willing to substitute less immediately harmful behaviors while treatment is initiated.

Binge-Eating Disorder

BED is characterized by recurrent and persistent binge eating. To meet diagnostic criteria, binge episodes should occur at least weekly, on average, over a duration of 3 or more months. Unlike BN, BED is not associated with recurrent inappropriate compensatory behaviors to prevent weight gain. BED is distinguished from nonpathologic overeating by several possible associated symptoms, including rapid eating, eating irrespective of hunger, or satiety eating alone because of shame, and negative feelings after a binge.[1] Apart from overweight or obesity, which is common in BED, BED patients frequently present without any specifically associated physical findings. Although in some cases binge eating associated with BED may cause or perpetuate weight gain, many with BED develop symptoms only after they have become overweight. Individuals with BED are frequently distressed enough about their symptoms to seek medical help, although they may present seeking a solution to their weight gain rather than their binge eating. A substantial percentage of patients who seek weight loss treatment will have comorbid BED. Therefore medical subspecialists are likely to encounter these patients before they have been diagnosed with BED.

Avoidant/Restrictive Food Intake Disorder

ARFID was first introduced into the DSM-5 as a rearticulation of the DSM-IV's diagnosis Feeding Disorder of Infancy and Early Childhood.[83] ARFID is a diagnosis that occurs across the life span. The signature feature of ARFID is a disturbance in eating or feeding that yields significant nutritional or psychosocial compromise and/or requires special feeding measures (e.g., dietary supplements to correct a nutritional deficiency or enteral feeding to supply calories). Patients with ARFID do not have evidence of disturbance in the way in which they experience their body weight, shape or size. ARFID can be comorbid with other mental health disorders, including anxiety, obsessive-compulsive disorder, autism spectrum disorder, attention-deficit hyperactivity disorder, and learning disabilities. The nutritional deficits associated with ARFID may have an adverse impact on growth, development, and learning.[1,84] It is important to note that the diagnosis of ARFID covers a range of different clinical presentations. Recent studies suggest that ARFID is a heterogeneous diagnosis with three distinct classes: Acute medical (AM) class is distinct for increased likelihood of weight loss, a shorter length of illness (<12 months), medical hospitalization, and heart rate <60 beats per minute; Lack of Appetite (LOA) class is distinct for failure to gain weight and faltering growth; and Sensory class is distinct for avoiding certain foods and refusing to eat because of sensory characteristics of the food. A mixed group AM/LOA was noted to have characteristics of both AM and LOA classes.

Pica

Pica is a disorder characterized by recurrent and persistent ingestion of nonnutritive, nonfood substances, such as chalk, paper, paint chips, or laundry starch, for at least a month. Pica eating that is developmentally normal (e.g., an infant eating dirt) does not warrant a diagnosis of pica, although it may require clinical intervention. Pica eating behaviors is not part of a socially normative or culturally sanctioned practice. Pica can occur with another mental disorder or medical condition, and in such cases may warrant independent clinical attention.

Rumination Disorder

The hallmark of rumination disorder is repeated and persistent (over at least 1 month) effortless, voluntary regurgitation that is not solely attributable to a medical condition. Gastric contents that are brought up are sometimes spit out, rechewed or reswallowed. Regurgitation is sometimes used for self-soothing or self-stimulation. The prevalence of rumination disorder is unknown, but it can occur in both children and adults.[15] Rumination disorder is superseded by a diagnosis of AN or BN, although the behavior may be superimposed on other symptoms.

OTHER SPECIFIED FEEDING OR EATING DISORDER AND UNSPECIFIED FEEDING OR EATING DISORDER

OSFED and USFED comprise presentations that fall short of criteria for one of the major feeding or EDs, but are nonetheless clinically important because of distress or impairment, including serious medical consequences.

OSFED is used when the reason for not meeting full syndrome criteria is specified. A variety of ways a patient can present with clinically significant symptoms that do not meet the threshold for one or more diagnostic criteria include several named symptom presentations with provisional descriptions. These include atypical AN, subthreshold BN, subthreshold BED, night-eating syndrome (NES), and purging disorder (PD).[1] Three of the OSFED variants are characterized by failure to meet full syndrome criteria for AN, BN, or BED in the presence of the other criteria, as well as clinically significant distress or impairment. Atypical AN is characterized by a fear of fatness and body image disturbance in the absence of low weight. Patients with atypical AN meet all criteria for AN except that despite significant weight loss, weight is in the normal or above normal range.[1] For example, some individuals with a history of obesity lose a substantial amount of weight (e.g., following gastric bypass surgery) and while still in a normal weight range also manifest an extreme fear of weight gain and body image disturbance.[1] Since the patient's weight is in the normal range for age and height, the ED symptoms may be underestimated by health care providers and as a result, the diagnosis of atypical AN could be missed or a longer time to diagnose compared to AN.[291] However, the medical complications associated with atypical AN are similar and as serious to those observed in patients with AN, including bradycardia, hypotension, the electrolyte disturbances, reduced GFR, and refeeding syndrome as well as affecting many organ systems. In some cases, AM complications could even be more severe and the severity of weight loss appears to be a significant predictor of medical instability[292] in atypical AN. In atypical AN, the weight loss history, including longer duration of weight loss, rapid weight loss, and greater weight loss are associated with increased disease severity regardless of the current weight status.[292] Further, reduced bone mineral density (BMD) has been described in atypical AN as a long-term medical complication. Studies demonstrated patients with atypical AN have higher BMD than patients with typical AN but lower than healthy controls.[293–295] One study in adolescents with atypical AN estimated a 34.2% lifetime risk of low BMD.[296]

Subthreshold BN and BED are also OSFED variants. They are each characterized by meeting all criteria for BN or BED, respectively, except for frequency or duration. An individual with recurrent binge eating that occurs monthly but not weekly, in the presence of all other diagnostic criteria for either BN or BED, would meet criteria for OSFED if clinical impairment and/or distress were present.

Two other notable OSFED variants are NES and PD. First described in 1955,[75] NES is characterized by recurrent bouts of evening or nocturnal overeating—but not necessarily bingeing—without associated inappropriate compensatory behaviors to prevent weight gain. There has been no clear consensus on core criteria for NES, although investigators have proposed morning anorexia, evening hyperphagia (e.g., consuming a disproportionately large number of calories in the evening or after dinner), and sleep disturbance (operationalized in various ways, including difficulty falling or staying asleep). Some have proposed the additional criterion of eating in relation to sleep disturbance, such as during a nighttime awakening.[76] Given the insufficient research on operational criteria, prevalence, course, and differentiation from other EDs, NES still lacks a formal definition.[77] In the DSM-5, NES is described by recurrent evening or nighttime eating an individual is aware of, and not due to a medical, pharmacologic, or social contextual cause. As with other OSFED variants, the condition must be associated with clinically significant impairment or distress and cannot be better described by a different ED like BED or BN.[1] In one study, NES in obese study participants was associated with an average of 3.6 awakenings/night compared with just 0.3 awakenings/night for matched controls. Available data suggest that individuals with NES consume considerably fewer calories during their nocturnal eating episode compared with the usual intake of a binge associated with BN or BED.[78] NES can also occur in nonobese individuals[79] but is more common in the obese and may contribute to poor outcome in weight-loss treatment programs.[78,80]

PD, another OSFED variant, is characterized by recurrent purging symptoms in the absence of clinically significant binge-pattern eating. Like the other EDs, PD is more common among women than men, but peak onset (at age 20) appears to be later than for BN.[81] Lifetime prevalence of PD has been estimated as 1.1%–5.3% of young adult women. Course, outcome, and treatment strategies for PD require further research.[82]

USFED applies to patients with a clinical presentation in which symptoms characteristic of a feeding or ED cause clinically significant distress or impairment but do not meet the full criteria for any of the disorders. Further research of this group is necessary to ensure that these individuals are identified and not overlooked and treatment options are available.

Differential Diagnosis

Differential diagnosis of the EDs includes evaluation and exclusion of medical causes of weight loss, weight gain, anorexia, hyperphagia, vomiting, and other associated symptoms. These considerations are especially germane in cases of atypical presentations, or early- or late-onset EDs.[56] Occasionally, EDs can be mistaken for a medical condition, or a medical condition can be misdiagnosed as an ED. Individuals with a medical condition that is associated with loss of weight or appetite, however, will often express concern over their weight loss and changes in their body weight, shape, and size, whereas this is not the case in individuals with AN. Individuals with ARFID may express concern or distress about their poor appetite or nutrition. Medical causes of appetite and/or weight loss include hyperthyroidism, Addison disease, diabetes mellitus, malignancy, IBD, malabsorption, immunodeficiency, infectious diseases (e.g., TB, HIV), collagen vascular disease, substance abuse, mood and anxiety disorders, dementia, delirium, and psychosis (see Chapters 33 and 35). Food allergy or intolerance, as well as other GI diseases that can cause discomfort with eating should be excluded in patients with presentations consistent with ARFID.[1] Illnesses associated with weight gain include hypothyroidism, Cushing disease, and organic brain disease.

The differential diagnosis of hyperphagia is broad and includes Prader-Willi syndrome, dementia (including Alzheimer disease), and intracranial lesions. Hyperphagia has also been associated with the use of certain medications, particularly many of the psychotropic agents (e.g., lithium, valproate, tricyclic antidepressants, mirtazapine, conventional, and atypical antipsychotic agents), pregnancy,[85] and poststarvation refeeding.[86] The regurgitation associated with BN, rumination disorder, and PD (and sometimes AN) is volitional and is therefore distinctive from GERD or vomiting with nausea.[15]

Psychiatric illnesses associated with loss of appetite and weight loss include major depression, anxiety, and substance use disorders. Moreover, comorbid psychiatric illness is common among those with EDs[58] and frequently complicates their diagnosis and treatment. Thus identification of excessive concern with weight and food intake, unrealistic or inappropriate weight goals, or resistance to attempts to restore normal weight and/or limit excessive exercise can be helpful in distinguishing AN from another psychiatric illness or revealing the presence of an underlying comorbid ED. Because individuals with BN, BED, OSFED, and USFED can have an unremarkable physical examination on presentation, the diagnosis may remain obscure until the patient discloses his or her symptoms, or until the clinician suspects an ED based on other elements of the clinical history or course (weight fluctuations, menstrual irregularities).

Even though a *transdiagnostic* approach to treatment of EDs has been proposed, in which management focuses on common maintaining mechanisms across the EDs,[87] there is evidence of differential response to treatment across the EDs, and it is desirable to establish a clear diagnosis to optimize treatment effectiveness. Although there is a great deal of phenomenologic overlap among the EDs and individuals do cross over from one diagnostic category to another (Table 10.1),[57] categories are mutually exclusive according to the DSM-5 diagnostic criteria.[1] The exception to this rule is pica, which can co-occur with another ED. Generally, a diagnosis of AN will take precedence over all other feeding and ED diagnoses, and BN will supersede all other diagnoses with the exception of AN. A low weight criterion distinguishes AN from BN in some cases. Individuals who are substantially underweight and otherwise meet criteria for AN most likely should be classified as having AN even if bingeing, purging, or both are present. AN and ARFID both present with nutritional compromise, although in ARFID this can manifest as either low weight, not meeting weight expectations, faltering growth, or a nutritional deficiency, and individuals with ARFID lack body image disturbance and fear of fatness. Individuals with BED or BN can also have symptom overlap. BN is distinguished by recurrent purging and other behaviors directed at neutralizing excessive calorie intake so as to prevent weight gain, as well as an excessive concern with weight. Regurgitation associated with rumination disorder can be difficult to differentiate from purging associated with BN. Although the so-called vomiting associated with rumination disorder is volitional, it is also effortless in contrast to the purging that typifies BN, so is not by definition "vomiting." Patients and occasionally health care providers often mistake the two occurrences. Unlike AN and BN, rumination disorder is not associated with either body image disturbance or excessive weight or shape concerns.

OSFED and USFED diagnoses are reserved for individuals who do not meet full syndrome criteria for one of the major feeding or EDs, but nonetheless have associated clinically significant impairment or distress. For example, a normal or overweight individual who has an intense fear of weight gain and body image disturbance does not meet criteria for AN but rather for "atypical anorexia." Individuals who are of normal weight and have recurrent purging, but no bingeing, would likely be classified as having PD. Normal or overweight individuals with recurrent nighttime overeating but neither binge eating nor purging would likely be given a diagnosis of NES.

Nutritional, Medical, and Laboratory Evaluation

In addition to excluding medical and psychiatric causes of weight and appetite change, medical evaluation for confirmed or suspected EDs includes obtaining a full history of the patient's eating behaviors and symptoms with attention to the number of calories ingested daily, purging behaviors [e.g., vomiting or laxative use, diuretics, diet pills, ipecac, complementary, and alternative medications (see Chapter 132)], and exercise patterns. Often, medical evaluation will be guided by an assessment of nutritional status that includes determining appropriateness of weight for height, age, and gender.

TABLE 10.1 Distinguishing Features of Feeding and Eating Disorders

Feeding or Eating Disorder	Physical Signs Included in Diagnostic Criteria	Restrictive-Pattern Eating	Binge-Pattern Eating	Purging and Other Behaviors to Control Weight or Neutralize Effects of Caloric Intake	Excess Concern With Body Image or Weight
AN	Significantly underweight	Typically	May occur	Purging may occur in up to one-half of patients	Yes
ARFID	Significantly underweight or other nutritional deficiency	Typically may include not eating enough, avoidance of certain kinds of food due to sensory features, fear of food due to a traumatic eating experience (e.g., gagging, choking), or being indifferent to food	No	No	No
BED	None (patients are frequently overweight or obese)	No	Must occur an average of once per week for at least 3 months	No	Yes
BN	None (patients are generally normal weight or overweight)	May occur as behavior to control weight	Must occur an average of once per week for at least 3 months	Must occur an average of once per week to meet diagnostic criteria	Yes
Pica	No	No	No	No	No
Rumination disorder	No	No	No	Voluntary regurgitation occurs but is not intended to purge calories	No

AN, Anorexia nervosa; *ARFID,* avoidant/restrictive food intake disorder; *BED,* binge-eating disorder; *BN,* bulimia nervosa.
Data from American Psychiatric Association. *Diagnostic and Statistical Manual of Mental Disorders*. 5th ed. Arlington, VA: American Psychiatric Association; 2013.

Nutritional Evaluation

A detailed dietary history that includes an individual's 24-hour dietary recall can provide insight into caloric intake and quality of nutrition. The clinician should also explore the patient's beliefs about (and attitudes and behaviors toward) eating, food, weight, and health. The types of foods and beverages consumed to reduce hunger (e.g., caffeinated coffee, tea, diet soda), portion sizes, diet products used, calorie and fat intake, low-fat or fat-free foods consumed, and foods the individual considers forbidden (or bad) and safe (or good) should be assessed. Some individuals report undiagnosed food allergies, gluten sensitivity, or lactose intolerance; such concerns should be investigated as clinically indicated. The clinician should ask about vegetarianism and the patient's reasons for becoming a vegetarian.

Individuals with an ED may weigh themselves frequently, sometimes several times each day. People with AN may wear large, baggy clothing as a consequence of their body image distress, or to hide their weight loss from others. For individuals who binge, there may be disappearance of large quantities of food. For those who purge, they may exhibit frequent trips to the bathroom, especially after meals.

Individuals with EDs may display a number of behaviors and food rituals, including cutting food into tiny pieces and moving it around their plate, chewing food and spitting it out, taking small bites, eating the same foods daily, and taking a long time to complete meals. It is not uncommon for individuals with EDs to cook for others but not eat any of the food prepared.

A history of ingesting nonfood substances is essential in evaluating pica and will often require collateral history from a parent or caregiver. Avoidance of eating, as seen in patients with ARFID, can be associated with a history or fear of aversive consequences of eating (e.g., precipitated by a history of vomiting or a "traumatic" GI or other medical study).[1]

Special Considerations in the Determination of Weight and Weight Status

There are several established means for evaluating the nutritional status of patients with EDs in the office, central to which is measuring weight and height and calculating the BMI (see Chapter 6). Assessment of the appropriateness of weight for height is a key factor intrinsic to determining the urgency of medical and psychiatric care. For patients with AN, it is critical to not rely on self-reported weight, given the strong possibility of an inaccurate report. Individuals with AN may sometimes go to great lengths to conceal their low weights; some "water-load" prior to a clinical encounter, some attach or hide weights to one's body, and others layer loose and bulky clothing to create the illusion of being of normal weight. Assessment of weight, therefore, should factor in the possibility that a patient may wish to conceal a low weight or weight loss. Clinicians should consider having a scale in a private area (e.g., not in a hallway) and a clear and consistent protocol for weighing patients with AN. This might include asking patients to void prior to being weighed, change into a hospital gown, and remove heavy jewelry. When patients have a history of consuming water prior to an appointment to increase their measured weight, it may be helpful to check a urine specific gravity and electrolytes; hyponatremia may occur in individuals with excessive water intake or those who water-load.[88–90]

Standard means of evaluating the appropriateness of weight for height in adults includes the use of BMI, which is calculated using the following equation:

$$\text{BMI} = \frac{\text{Weight(in kg)}}{\text{Height(in m)}^2}$$

Although BMI may not be an appropriate standard to determine the health of weight status in all individuals (e.g., those who have relatively high lean muscle mass, certain ethnic groups),[91] BMI is generally considered a first-line assessment measure for most men and women aged 18 or older. BMI of 18.5–24.9 kg/m^2 for men and women is considered normal; BMI of 17.5 kg/m^2 or less meets the underweight criterion for AN in the ICD-10 (International Classification of Diseases 10)[11,92]; BMI of 25–29.9 kg/m^2 is consistent with overweight; and BMI over 30 kg/m^2 reflects obesity.[93]

Interpreting the severity of a low weight in adults will incorporate both the absolute BMI criterion (e.g., BMI < 15 kg/m^2 is given by the DSM-5 for extreme severity)[1] and the clinical context that includes both weight history and medical complications. BMI is calculated using the same formula for children and adolescents, and should be interpreted relative to other children of the same sex and age. BMI under 18 years of age is either expressed as a BMI percentile (underweight: less than the 5th percentile)[297] or as BMI Z scores (thinness: <-2 standard deviation)[298] for assessing low weight. However, it should be noted that BMI changes in adolescents are related to sexual development, rather than chronological age. Chronic undernutrition can delay sexual development and the pubertal growth spurt which confounds comparisons of BMI.

A number of other methods are routinely used to calculate percent of expected body weight for adults. One of the more widely used equations to calculate expected body weight in adults is as follows:

$$\text{Expected body weight} = \left(\frac{\text{Patient weight}}{\text{Expected weight for height and gender}}\right) \times 100$$

Although this is a linear equation (compared with the quadratic equation for BMI) and may be less useful at extreme heights, it is straightforward to calculate. Moreover, this formula may be conceptually easier for patients and families to understand, especially in setting weight goals or limits. A weight within the range from 90% to 110% of expected body weight will likely be considered normal and is a good place to begin for setting weight gain goals for patients with AN. Within this range, the goal will be refined by clinical history (including the patient's history of baseline, minimal, and maximal weights), whether and when menses return, and medical parameters like reversal of bone loss. For patients who are overweight or obese (>110% or >120% expected body weight, respectively), it may not always be realistic or desirable to set weight goals within the "normal BMI range."

For children and adolescents with AN, BN, or ARFID, the treatment goal weight (TGW) should be contextualized primarily according to growth history (weight, height, and pubertal stage), changes in body weight and height, energy intake and expenditure, and the extent to which the individual is thought to be malnourished.[299,300] Accurate, plotted measurements on growth charts help the clinician to understand individual premorbid physical growth trajectories. Age at pubertal onset, current pubertal stage, (if applicable) age at menarche and the weight at which menstrual periods ceased (menstrual threshold weight) should also be considered on an individual basis for setting a TGW. For patients with atypical AN, determination of TGW should be individualized and based on the individuals previous growth trajectory. For adolescents who were previously above the 95th percentile BMI, it is recommended that health care providers use the patient's vital signs and menstrual history to guide TGW; if vital signs and menses stabilize before reaching the patient's premorbid weight, additional weight gain may not be necessary.[301]

Patients who are severely nutritionally compromised may require inpatient care for both efficacy and safety of weight management. For underweight patients without this degree of compromise, the primary goals of nutritional management are increasing caloric intake to regain weight, ensuring adequate intake and balance of macro- and micronutrients, and reestablishing a dietary pattern of 3 meals and 1–3 snacks daily. In such cases, consultation with experienced ED practitioners regarding optimal refeeding and treatment support strategies should be strongly considered. Patients may also be supplemented with calcium (if dietary intake is inadequate), vitamin D, and/or multivitamins. Some patients may require additional dietary guidance, adjustments, and supplementation because many restrict not only calories but specific foods or food groups as well. For patients with BN, BED, and subthreshold BN and BED encompassed by OSFED, dietary intervention includes moderating excessive caloric intake and establishing a pattern of eating that is less vulnerable to emotional cues and excessive hunger. Many patients with EDs are quite knowledgeable about nutrition and commonly wish to avoid meeting with a dietitian, but information from a nutritional assessment is invaluable to the treatment team. Even well-informed patients are likely to benefit from reinforcement of more healthful and diverse food choices, meal patterns, and appropriate intake.

A thorough nutritional assessment should also include an evaluation of the fluid intake. Some patients may drink excessively to help them feel full and suppress appetite, to induce vomiting, or to water load prior to getting weighed in an effort to falsely increase their weight. Other patients may restrict their fluid intake to avoid feeling full or bloated.[302]

Medical Evaluation

The goal of the medical evaluation is to obtain information that will be helpful in formulating a diagnosis, evaluating the acute and long-term medical and psychiatric consequences of the feeding or ED, and determining a comprehensive treatment plan. Medical evaluation includes a clinical history with special attention to weight loss, weight fluctuations, and any bingeing, purging, or other inappropriate behaviors that affect or aim to control weight (see Box 10.1). Symptoms of medical complications of undernutrition, overnutrition, bingeing, purging, and excessive exercise, should be assessed, and a complete menstrual history should be clarified.

Physical examination includes a comprehensive assessment of potential complications of low, excessive, or unusual dietary intake, as well as nutritional deficiencies, underweight, overweight, excessive exercise, and purging behaviors. If an ED is suspected, physical examination may reveal signs that confirm nutritional compromise (e.g., bradycardia, hypotension, hypothermia, lanugo hair, breast tissue atrophy, muscle wasting, peripheral neuropathy) or suggest chronic purging [e.g., Russell sign (excoriation on the dorsum of the hand incurred during self-induced vomiting from chronic scraping against the central incisors)], hypoactive or hyperactive bowel sounds, an attenuated gag reflex,[94] tooth enamel erosion (perimolysis),[95] or parotid hypertrophy.[96]

Medical complications of behaviors associated with all feeding and EDs are potentially serious and too numerous to review in detail here; selected complications are listed in Table 10.2. Complications that are common and/or associated with serious morbidity should be actively sought on physical examination and laboratory studies so that appropriate interventions can be initiated. Examples of important and common findings include abnormal vital signs (e.g., hypotension, orthostatic changes in blood pressure and/or heart rate, bradycardia, hypothermia), low weight or overweight, dental pathology (e.g., perimolysis, dental caries, or both),[96–98] and osteopenia or osteoporosis.[99] Cardiac complications can be lethal and include prolonged QT interval, QT dispersion, ventricular arrhythmias, and cardiac syncope.[100,101] Neurologic findings in AN include cortical atrophy and increased cerebral ventricular size.[102] Endocrinologic abnormalities include menstrual disorders, low serum estradiol levels, low serum testosterone levels, hypercortisolism, and euthyroid sick syndrome, with resultant hypotension and cold intolerance.[103] Heavy metal toxicity is a potentially serious complication of pica.[5,104]

Intentional omission of insulin by individuals with type 1 diabetes for the sole purpose of inducing weight loss can also pose considerable risk. Similarly, some individuals with type 2 diabetes intentionally omit oral hypoglycemic agents, resulting in poor glycemic control and weight loss. Clinical signs that should raise suspicion include poor glycemic control, recurrent episodes of diabetic ketoacidosis, missed clinical appointments, poor self-esteem, and dietary manipulation.[105] The diagnosis of both an ED and diabetes, coupled with intentional omission of insulin use, is associated with higher glycosylated hemoglobin levels, increased episodes of hypoglycemia and resulting hospitalizations for diabetic ketoacidosis, growth retardation and pubertal delay in adolescence, and increased microvascular complications.[106,107]

Reported complications of ED during pregnancy include miscarriage, inadequate weight gain of the mother, intrauterine growth restriction, premature delivery, infants with low birth weight, and low Apgar scores, and perinatal death.[108–111]

Laboratory Evaluation

Laboratory evaluation should be done at the time of the initial assessment to rule out other medical illnesses and assess for acute metabolic derangement. Not uncommonly a malnourished individual with AN will have normal laboratory results, although those who actively binge and purge may exhibit a number of metabolic abnormalities.[107] Laboratory investigations should be performed during nutritional rehabilitation to monitor for a variety of serious and life-threatening metabolic, cardiovascular, and neurologic abnormalities that can occur as a result of refeeding (see Chapters 6 and 7).[112]

The choice of laboratory studies to evaluate medical complications of EDs will depend on the clinical history, presentation, and degree of malnutrition. For patients with AN, a complete blood cell count is recommended during initial assessment to assess for anemia, neutropenia, leukopenia, and thrombocytopenia.[303,304] A retrospective study of 67 patients with AN found that 27% had anemia, 17% had neutropenia, 36% had leukopenia, and 10% had thrombocytopenia.[113]

It is useful to obtain serum electrolyte levels for individuals in whom AN or BN is suspected or confirmed. Hypokalemia occurred in 4.6% of a large number of outpatients with EDs in one study[114] and in 6.8% of individuals with BN in another moderately-sized cohort[115]; in the latter study hypokalemia was significantly more common in patients with BN than in those without it. Although assessment for hypokalemia may not identify occult cases of BN, it will help identify and monitor individuals at risk for cardiac arrhythmias secondary to their ED. Hypochloremia, hypomagnesemia, hyponatremia, hypernatremia, and hypophosphatemia are also seen in patients with EDs.[106,107,115–117] For patients with AN, a serum glucose determination is recommended to identify hypoglycemia, which can be severe in this population.[118] Although hyperamylasemia is seen in 25%–60% of patients with BN, laboratory analysis of serum amylase is generally not clinically useful for detecting BN or gaging the severity of bingeing and purging symptoms.[119] An elevated serum amylase level in a patient with AN or BN often reflects increased salivary isoamylase activity,[119,120] but pancreatitis should be considered when clinically appropriate, given its occurrence in this patient population. Renal and liver biochemical testing and urinalysis should also be considered. If pica is suspected, testing serum for evidence of heavy metal toxicity (e.g., lead, mercury, copper, and zinc) is appropriate.

TABLE 10.2 Selected Clinical Features and Complications of Behaviors in Patients With Eating Disorders[a]

	Clinical Feature or Complication	
System Affected	**Associated With Weight Loss and Food Restriction or Binge Eating in Anorexia Nervosa or OSFED/USFED**	**Associated With Purging or Refeeding Behaviors in Anorexia Nervosa, Bulimia Nervosa, or OSFED/USFED**
Cardiovascular	Arrhythmia Bradycardia Chest pain Decreased cardiac size Diminished exercise capacity Dyspnea Edema Heart failure Hypotension Mitral valve prolapse Orthostasis Palpitations Prolonged QT interval QT dispersion Syncope	Cardiomyopathy (with ipecac use) Chest pain Edema Orthostasis Palpitations Prolonged QT interval Syncope Ventricular arrhythmia
Dermatologic	Acrocyanosis Brittle hair and nails Dry skin Hair loss Hypercarotenemia Lanugo	Russell's sign (knuckle lesions from repeated scraping against incisors)
Endocrine and metabolic	Amenorrhea and oligomenorrhea Euthyroid sick syndrome Hypercholesterolemia Hypocalcemia Hypoglycemia Hypomagnesemia Hyponatremia Hypophosphatemia Hypothermia Low serum estradiol, low serum testosterone levels Osteopenia, osteoporosis Pubertal delay, arrested growth	Amenorrhea and oligomenorrhea Hypercholesterolemia Hyperphosphatemia Hypochloremia Hypoglycemia Hypokalemia Hypomagnesemia Hyponatremia Hypophosphatemia Metabolic acidosis Metabolic alkalosis Secondary hyperaldosteronism
Gastrointestinal[b]	Acute gastric dilatation, necrosis, and perforation Anorectal dysfunction Constipation Delayed gastric emptying Early satiety Elevated liver enzyme levels Elevated serum amylase levels GERD Hepatic injury Hepatomegaly Pancreatitis Prolonged whole-gut transit time Rectal prolapse Slow colonic transit Superior mesenteric artery syndrome	Abdominal pain Acute gastric dilatation Barrett esophagus Bloating Constipation Delayed gastric emptying Diarrhea Dysphagia Elevated liver enzyme levels Elevated serum amylase levels Esophageal bleeding Esophageal ulcers, erosions, stricture Gastric necrosis, and perforation GERD Mallory-Weiss tear Hematemesis Pancreatitis Prolonged intestinal transit time Rectal bleeding Rectal prolapse
General	Irritability/mood changes	Irritability/mood changes Weight fluctuations
Genitourinary and reproductive	Acute kidney injury Amenorrhea Atrophic vaginitis Breast atrophy Infertility Pregnancy complications (including low birth weight, premature birth, and perinatal death); kidney stones in mother	Abnormal menses Azotemia Pregnancy complications (including low birth weight infant)
Hematologic	Anemia Leukopenia Neutropenia Thrombocytopenia	

Continued

TABLE 10.2 Selected Clinical Features and Complications of Behaviors in Patients With Eating Disorders[a]—cont'd

System Affected	Clinical Feature or Complication: Associated With Weight Loss and Food Restriction or Binge Eating in Anorexia Nervosa or OSFED/USFED	Clinical Feature or Complication: Associated With Purging or Refeeding Behaviors in Anorexia Nervosa, Bulimia Nervosa, or OSFED/USFED
Neurologic	Cognitive changes Cortical atrophy Delirium (in refeeding syndrome) Peripheral neuropathy Ventricular enlargement	Stroke (associated with ephedra use) Neuropathy (with ipecac use) Reduced or absent gag reflex
Oral, pharyngeal	Cheilosis Halitosis	Angular cheilitis Dental enamel erosion and caries Parotid gland enlargement Perimolysis Pharyngeal and soft palatal trauma Sialadenosis Vocal fold pathology

[a]Specific complications of pica, rumination disorder, and ARFID (avoidant/restrictive food intake disorder) not included.
[b]Gastrointestinal complications associated with binge-pattern eating in any of the eating disorders are not all listed but include weight gain, acute gastric dilatation, gastric rupture, GERD, increased gastric capacity, and increased stool volume.
OSFED, Other specified feeding or eating disorder; *USFED,* unspecified feeding or eating disorder.

In women with amenorrhea, evaluation of the cause is suggested, even if it is presumed to be related to decreased pulsatility of gonadotropin-releasing hormone secondary to weight loss.[103] Menstrual irregularities are common among women with EDs, but women with symptomatic EDs may continue to menstruate at presentation,[121] and women with AN can become pregnant[122]; a quantitative β-human chorionic gonadotropin and possibly a serum prolactin level are, therefore, recommended. Additional studies, such as follicle-stimulating hormone to evaluate ovarian function or neuroimaging studies to exclude a pituitary lesion, may be indicated in some clinical scenarios.

Thyroid function is commonly abnormal in patients with AN and BN and the most frequent finding is "low T3 syndrome" with normal thyroxine (T4) and TSH levels and decreased triiodothyronine (T3) levels.[305,306] Hypothyroidism in AN may be a physiologic response to starvation and a protective mechanism for energy conservation.[307] Thus it should not be taken as an indication to treat these patients with thyroid hormone.

Bone densitometry using dual-energy x-ray absorptiometry scans of the hip and spine are useful in identifying bone loss and can be repeated after a year to assess further bone loss if disease continues. Osteopenia and osteoporosis may be present in as many as 90% and 40%, respectively, of women with AN and are associated with risk of fractures and kyphosis.[99,123]

A baseline electrocardiogram is also recommended and can identify corrected QT (QTc) prolongation (patients with AN)[124] and prolongation of the QTc interval even in the absence of hypokalemia (patients with BN and EDNOS).[125] Some antipsychotic agents and tricyclic antidepressants can cause QTc prolongation, which can lead to torsades de pointes and sudden death. As such, careful selection of psychotropic medications and identification of a patient's risk for QTc prolongation should be explored and monitored. This population is also at risk of cardiac arrhythmias due to hypokalemia from purging. Ipecac abuse may result in potentially fatal cardiotoxicity, cardiomyopathy, and arrhythmias.[126]

GASTROINTESTINAL ABNORMALITIES ASSOCIATED WITH EATING DISORDERS

GI signs and symptoms are common in those with EDs (Box 10.2; also see Table 10.2). It has been asserted that the most dramatic changes in bodily function caused by AN are in the GI tract.[127] There is also evidence that many individuals with EDs present with a GI complaint *prior to* diagnosis of or seeking treatment for an ED.[128] Cross-sectional studies of hospital inpatients with EDs have suggested that 78%–98% have concurrent GI symptoms.[129–133] In addition, research has suggested that GI abnormalities associated with EDs may be related to the duration or presence of active ED symptoms.[134,135] GI findings associated with EDs are listed in Table 10.2.

BOX 10.2 Common Gastrointestinal Symptoms in Patients With Eating Disorders

- Abdominal pain
- Belching
- Bloating
- Borborygmi
- Changes in appetite
- Constipation
- Diarrhea
- Dyschezia
- Flatulence
- Nausea

Functional Gastrointestinal Disorders

GI symptoms have been shown to be more common in dieters (specifically, abdominal pain, bloating, and diarrhea)[136] and in those with binge eating (nausea, vomiting, and bloating) than in normal controls.[137] A large study of obese individuals with GI symptoms found a strong association between BED and abdominal pain and bloating after adjusting for BMI.[138] One study of 101 consecutive women admitted to an inpatient EDs program found that 98% had functional GI disorders (FGIDs) including IBS (52%), functional heartburn (51%), abdominal bloating (31%), constipation (24%), functional dysphagia (23%), and anorectal pain (22%). Overall, 52% of these women met criteria for $\geq$3 FGIDs.[133] Another study found that the presence of IBS, but not other FGIDs, in ED patients was strongly related to disordered eating and psychological feelings.[139] Janssen's group[140] suggested that once a FGID is established in a patient with an ED, psychological and physiologic factors will strengthen each other such that FGIDs and FGID symptoms could persist independent of the current status of the ED.

Esophageal Symptoms

Esophageal symptoms are commonly reported in patients with EDs. Esophageal dysfunction can be obscured by bulimic symptoms[94,141] and can be misdiagnosed as AN.[142] In a case-control study of 23 patients (11 restricting type and 12 binge eating/purging type), 15 patients complained of regurgitation (6 restrictors, 9 purgers), 14 complained of heartburn (6 restrictors, 8 purgers), and 4 complained of dysphagia (3 restrictors, 1 purger).[143] Abnormal esophageal motor activity has also been reported in patients with AN and BN.[144,145] Mild esophagitis is common (e.g., 22% of a case series of 37 consecutive patients) in patients with chronic BN, but more serious esophageal disease is rare.[146,147] Barrett's esophagus, Mallory-Weiss tears, and GERD have been reported in association with the chronic vomiting seen with BN.[148] Esophageal rupture is a potentially life-threatening risk that may complicate chronic vomiting.[149] Spontaneous perforation of the esophagus commonly results from a sudden increase in intra-abdominal pressure combined with relatively negative intrathoracic pressure caused by straining or vomiting (Boerhaave syndrome).

Liver Abnormalities

Elevated serum transaminase levels, hypoglycemia, and impaired coagulation (in the absence of other liver pathology) have been demonstrated in multiple studies of patients with AN.[150] In one study, elevated liver biochemical test results were documented in 4.1% of 879 patients presenting for treatment of an ED.[151] A probable cause that was distinct from the ED was identified in 47% of the study participants. In the remaining 53% of subjects, there was no other cause identified for the elevated liver enzymes other than the ED. Elevated liver enzymes have been reported in underweight and normal-weight study participants. Study results suggest that abnormal liver biochemical tests are neither a specific nor a common marker for an ED; other possible causes should be excluded before attributing these abnormalities to the ED.[151] Elevated liver biochemical test results and hepatomegaly may also be observed with initiation of refeeding in AN.[149,151] In cases where levels of indirect bilirubin are elevated in malnourished patients, other diagnoses (e.g., Gilbert syndrome) should also be considered. There are several case reports of severe liver dysfunction or damage in patients with AN attributed to malnutrition and associated hypoperfusion.[152–154] Finally, severe steatosis resulting in fatal hepatic failure has been reported in a patient with severe AN.[155]

Pancreas Complications

Acute pancreatitis has been reported in patients with AN and BN[156–158] and can also be associated with refeeding in AN.[159]

Superior Mesenteric Artery Syndrome

Superior mesenteric artery (SMA) syndrome is a rare disorder that can complicate AN. It results from severe weight loss with resultant collapse of the angle at which the SMA arises from the aorta and through which the duodenum passes; reduction of the angle results in compression of the third part of the duodenum by the SMA (see Chapter 36).[160] Because it manifests with vomiting, a concurrent diagnosis can be missed if this symptom is attributed to the ED.[161]

Gastric Motility

A recent systematic review revealed that controlled studies involving patients with AN were more likely to demonstrate delays in gastric motility, gastric emptying, and intestinal transit than comparator groups.[150] Similarly, delayed whole-gut transit time and delayed gastric emptying have also been reported in patients with BN.[30,119,127,162,163]

Numerous studies also have found abnormal gastric function in patients with EDs, including delayed gastric emptying in patients with AN and BN as mentioned earlier,[30,127,162–164] but also diminished gastric relaxation (BN),[165] bradygastria (AN and BN),[134] and higher gastric capacity (BN).[135] Physiologic sequelae of disordered eating, such as contracted or expanded gastric capacity, altered gastric motility, delayed large bowel transit (through reflex pathways),[166] and blunted postprandial CCK release, may perpetuate symptoms that exacerbate the excessive body image concern driving abnormal eating patterns.[30] There is evidence that subjective reports of GI symptoms do not correlate well with physiologic data in patients with EDs.[167]

Constipation

Prominent among GI symptoms in patients with AN, BN, and ARFID is constipation. In a study of 28 inpatients with an ED, 100% of patients with AN and 67% of patients with BN had constipation.[132] Constipation in AN and BN is thought to be the result of poor nutrition, decreased gut motility, dehydration, and hypokalemia due to purging behavior, such as vomiting or laxative abuse. In one study, children and adolescents with ARFID presented with one or more medical signs or symptoms, with constipation being the most common.[276] Nausea, vomiting, gastric fullness, bloating, diarrhea, decreased appetite, and early satiety are commonly seen in patients with AN, and bloating, flatulence, decreased appetite, abdominal pain, borborygmi, and nausea are commonly reported in patients with BN. In one study of 43 inpatients with severe BN, 74% reported bloating, 63% reported constipation, and 47% reported nausea; borborygmi and abdominal pain were also more frequent than in the comparison group of healthy controls.[130] Rectal bleeding and rectal prolapse have been reported in patients with AN and BN.[168,169]

Medications and Dietary Supplements

Clinicians should be aware of the many products readily available to patients with EDs that are frequently used as a means to control or reduce weight and that may also directly or indirectly contribute to GI symptoms. These products can result in significant GI symptoms and associated toxicities. Laxative abuse remains common among patients with EDs, particularly among those with BN. Neims et al. found that the lifetime occurrence of laxative use in patients with BN was 14.94%.[170] Other reports suggest that the prevalence of laxative abuse among patients with BN ranges from 10% to 60%. Laxatives are not an effective weight-reducing strategy, because they do not act in the small intestine where most absorption occurs; caloric absorption is decreased only by about 12% even with extreme laxative use. The most frequently abused group of laxatives is the stimulant class; side effects and toxicity include constipation, cathartic colon, GI bleeding, rectal prolapse, dehydration, and electrolyte abnormalities. Besides misuse of stimulant-type laxatives, patients have also been known to misuse bulk-producing laxatives, surfactants, hyperosmotic laxatives, and saline laxatives.

Ipecac is an emetic that is used to induce vomiting. In a suburban ED clinic, Greenfeld et al. found that 7.6% of patients had reported using ipecac; 4.7% experimented with it briefly; 3.1% used it chronically; and 1.1% used it regularly.[171] Steffen et al. reported that 18% of outpatients being treated for bulimic symptoms presented using ipecac at some point in their life.[172] Although ipecac is used infrequently, it can have lethal consequences, including cardiomyopathy.

There are also many complementary and alternative medications and dietary supplements marketed for their potential laxative and weight-loss properties (see Chapter 131). Patients with EDs should be screened for the use of diet pills, laxatives, diuretics, ipecac, and other substances and educated about the consequences associated with misuse of these products.

Other Life-Threatening Gastrointestinal Complications

In rare cases, catastrophic complications have been described in case reports of patients with EDs, including acute gastric dilation, gastric emphysema, gastric necrosis, gastric rupture, duodenal obstruction, necrotizing colitis, and perforation; occult GI bleeding (attributed to transient intestinal ischemia in the setting of endurance running) has also been reported.[156,173–182] In such cases, both help-seeking and diagnosis may be delayed or complicated by an undisclosed or unrecognized ED.[156,173,183]

Gastrointestinal Complications in Other Feeding and Eating Disorders

GI complications reported in association with pica include bezoar, pancreatitis, stercoral perforation, and constipation.[184,185] Esophageal perforation has been reported in rumination disorder.[186]

MANAGEMENT OF EATING DISORDERS IN THE ADULT

The primary goal of treatment for all EDs is the normalization of eating attitudes and behaviors, cessation of ED symptoms, and, where indicated, rehabilitation (and regulation) of weight. Active weight rehabilitation is a cornerstone of treatment for AN. As essential as weight gain is to reduce or reverse the medical and cognitive sequelae of severe undernutrition, it is one of the great challenges to successful treatment of restrictive EDs.

Optimally, management of patients with EDs includes integration of mental health, nutrition, and primary care (see Fig. 10.1). Occasionally, depending on severity of ED symptoms and degree of malnutrition, medical subspecialty consultation and care are helpful. Multidisciplinary management is desirable for several reasons. First, patients are at risk of medical, psychological, and nutritional complications of their disease. Second, patients commonly selectively avoid care essential to their ultimate recovery. For example, a patient may wish to avoid detection of an injury so that she or he can continue to participate in a team sport; another may find it difficult to undergo the psychological work necessary to address antecedents of his or her illness; or another may wish to bypass active weight management. Conversely, a patient may attempt to pursue relief for specific medical complications to the exclusion of appropriate psychological or nutritional therapies.

It is often helpful, if not essential, to establish a treatment agreement at the outset of care for a patient with an ED. This is particularly relevant in patients for whom the severity of their symptoms may compromise medical and psychological health to a degree that hospital-level care will be likely necessary during the course of treatment. A treatment agreement allows caregivers to establish initial treatment goals and criteria for which they may wish to adjust the level of intensity of care. This will allow transparency of expectations for the patient, facilitate a rapid response to emerging crises, and help avoid splitting among team members during the course of care. A treatment agreement also clarifies for patients the contingencies for treatment nonadherence or poor health. As part of the initiation of care, patients should be asked to give permission for open communication among the members of the clinical team. If a patient cannot agree to this, it signals potential difficulties in providing coordinated care, and the lack of agreement should be reconciled. Depending

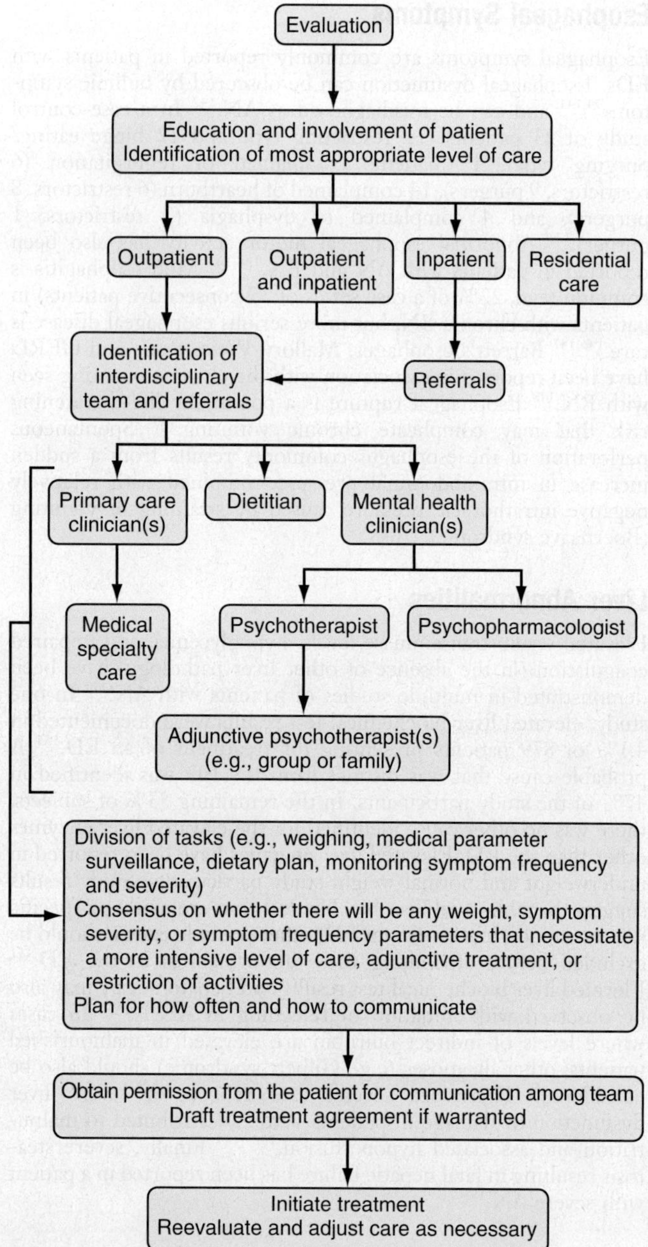

Fig. 10.1 Algorithm for team management of adult patients with an eating disorder.

on the patient's age and circumstances, a plan for how and what information will be shared with parents should also be established.

Psychiatric Treatment

Clinicians evaluating clinical trial data on the treatment of EDs should bear in mind that diagnostic criteria have recently been revised, and the diagnostic categories BN and BED now encompass individuals with lower frequency and shorter duration of behavioral symptoms than when these disorders were studied previously in clinical trials. Few clinical trial data are available on diagnostically heterogeneous groups. Indeed, there are limited data to guide treatment decisions for the large proportion of individuals with EDs who were formerly diagnosed as EDNOS (now OSFED and USFED). Preliminary data, however, suggest that enhanced cognitive behavioral therapy (CBT-E) may be effective in normal and overweight adults with a broad spectrum of eating pathology, including those formerly in the EDNOS category.[187]

In adult patients, psychiatric treatment for the EDs AN, BN, BED, and OSFED generally begins with psychotherapy. In many cases, pharmacotherapy is useful as an adjunctive treatment for BN and BED. Active weight management is indicated for AN. Usually, psychotherapy can be used to support weight management goals, although optimally it should be coordinated with the efforts of the dietitian and primary care clinician on the team. Regardless of the mode of psychotherapy chosen, specific behavioral strategies directed at establishing normal eating patterns and drawing the patient's attention to triggers for abnormal patterns can augment treatment. Among these, patients are encouraged to identify and avoid emotion-, schedule-, and food-related triggers to episodes of bingeing and to plan three regular meals and two between-meal snacks to prevent excessive hunger. A food journal that can be reviewed in treatment sessions may also allow patients to better identify relationships among psychosocial stressors, hunger, and symptoms and may provide a concrete framework from which to relate symptoms to other psychological concerns. Specific empirical data to guide treatment of pica, rumination disorder, or ARFID in adult patients are lacking. Two randomized controlled trials (RCTs) evaluating a nutritional intervention for pica did not support this approach, and there are no published RCTs on the treatment of rumination disorder.[15] Enhanced supervision or modification of the home environment may be important to prevent ingestion of toxic substances in individuals with intellectual disability who manifest pica eating.[15] Behavioral approaches to address avoidance associated with ARFID may also be helpful.[188]

Psychotherapeutic Options

A variety of psychotherapies have established efficacy for the EDs. Cognitive behavioral therapy (CBT) and interpersonal therapy (IPT) have received a great deal of research attention for the treatment of EDs. CBT is a structured, manual-based approach that addresses the relationships among thoughts, feelings, and behaviors. IPT is another short-term therapy focused on present-day interpersonal events and roles in relationships. The choice of psychotherapeutic modality will be guided by the diagnosis, medical and psychiatric comorbidities, desirability of targeting the ED symptoms versus broadening the therapeutic goals, treatment history, patient strengths and preferences, and availability of care. Initial recommendations should be evidence-based when possible, but clinical judgment is important to identify individual needs and situations where alternative treatment choices are appropriate.[190] Psychotherapies that have been examined with modest efficacy in treating adults with AN include CBT (eating focused and broadly focused), focal psychodynamic psychotherapy, IPT, Maudsley Model of AN Treatment for Adults (MANTRA), and specialist supportive clinical management.[308] CBT for AN is a structured, manual-based approach that focuses on changing weight-related behaviors, thoughts and feelings about food and weight by challenging cognitive distortions.[309–314] A study that compared CBT, IPT, and nonspecific supportive clinical management in the treatment of underweight outpatients with AN found that the supportive treatment produced better global outcomes than IPT, and, over 20 weeks, was superior to CBT in its impact on global functioning.[200] The efficacy of CBT for underweight individuals remains unclear, but it appears useful as a posthospitalization treatment for AN, contributing to improved outcomes and relapse prevention in adults after weight restoration.[201] Factors consistently predicting treatment outcome have not been identified.[191] In addition, some preliminary evidence suggests that CBT-ED (more formalized, manual-based version of CBT for EDs) may be effective for AN.[202] It has also been adapted for use with adolescents[315,316] and for use with patients who required a higher level of care.[313] MANTRA is a treatment based on flexible delivery of the workbook and consists of 20 sessions.[317–319] Available evidence has shown that family-based therapy (FBT) is effective in adolescents.[195,196] FBT positions parents as key members of the treatment team who facilitate normal adolescent growth and development by releasing adolescents from the diagnosis of ED. It is now considered first-line outpatient treatment for adolescents, particularly those who are younger and have a shorter duration of illness.[197] FBT may be considered for young adults who are living with their families and where the patient and their families are prepared to engage in this treatment.[198,199]

A number of treatments for BN have strong empirical support. CBT and IPT have been found effective, with CBT superior at reducing behavioral symptoms.[192] CBT led to faster improvement in symptoms, with better outcomes at the end of treatment, but at follow-up assessment there were no differences between CBT and IPT.[203] All guidelines recommend CBT (16–20 sessions over 4–5 months) as the first-line treatment of choice for BN,[189,190,192] but not all patients respond to CBT. In cases where there is minimal or no response to CBT alone by 6 weeks of treatment, a serotonin reuptake inhibitor (e.g., 60 mg fluoxetine daily) can be prescribed.[308] The combination of CBT plus high-dose fluoxetine (60 mg daily) is associated with somewhat better responses than fluoxetine alone.[320] For this reason, initial treatment could also include a combination of CBT and an SSRI (e.g., high-dose fluoxetine). Evidence for psychotherapies other than CBT is more limited; however, some clinicians incorporate other psychotherapeutic approaches, such as interpersonal or psychodynamic therapies into treatment.[321–325] CBT and IPT can be delivered in a group format as well as individually.[204,205] Other promising treatment options with preliminary empirical support include dialectical behavior therapy (DBT, an approach developed for borderline personality disorder that focuses on helping patients develop skills to regulate affect[206]) and a manual-based, guided self-change approach.[207] Although DBT skills training has not been well studied in patients with BN, these skills may be useful in individuals with co-occurring psychiatric disorders for which DBT would be indicated.[326–328] For a subset of patients, self-help or guided self-help with an evidence-based CBT manual[208] is an appropriate starting point for treatment in a stepped-care approach[190] or if other treatments are unavailable.[209] A variety of factors have been shown to be associated with treatment outcome in BN, but two emerge consistently: severity (higher frequency of binge eating) and duration of illness are associated with poorer outcomes.[192]

As with BN, some individuals with BED will benefit from an evidence-based self-help program as a first step in treatment or if other treatments are unavailable.[189,190,209] Studies have found that self-help intervention delivered in a variety of ways (with varying levels of professional or peer support) leads to better outcomes compared with control groups, with reductions in binge eating, binge days, and psychological features associated with BED.[193]

The American Psychiatric Association[308] recommends that patients with BED be treated with ED-focused CBT or IPT, in either individual or group formats. CBT is the most widely studied psychotherapy for BED[329] with evidence supporting its efficacy for behavioral and psychological symptoms, whether it is delivered in an individual or group format. IPT, individual or group, also appears to be effective in reducing binge eating.[330,331] Group IPT and adapted DBT are options to consider if CBT is not a good match for the individual or is unavailable. In one study, IPT was found to lead to similar abstinence rates as CBT at 1-year follow-up.[211] DBT has shown promising results, with a recovery rate of 56% at 6 months after treatment in one RCT.[212] It is important to note that treatments for BED do not usually result in weight loss, but their benefit may be in preventing further weight gain.[193]

A systematic review and meta-analysis of third-wave therapies (conceptualized as targeting the function or awareness of cognitions and emotions) identified 13 RCTs, the majority of which focused on BED.[213] Although large prepost symptom improvements were observed for all included treatments (DBT, schema therapy, acceptance and commitment therapy, mindfulness-based interventions, and compassion-focused therapy), none were generally superior to either CBT or other active comparisons.[214] As a result, the authors concluded that until further evidence becomes available, CBT should remain as the treatment of choice for both BN and BED.[214] Weight loss may be identified as a primary or secondary treatment goal for individuals with BED because of comorbid obesity. Models of binge eating have proposed that dietary restriction is an antecedent to binge eating, so there has been debate about the optimal means and order of addressing concurrent binge eating and obesity. Most data, however, have shown that a variety of weight-loss approaches do not exacerbate binge eating and may help reduce symptoms; one prospective study found no evidence that a reduced-calorie diet precipitated binge eating in women with obesity.[215] Behavioral weight-loss treatment (BWLT)[216] and very low-calorie diets[217,218] have been found effective for reducing symptoms of BED. At 2-year follow-up, IPT and CBT-guided self-help appear more effective in achieving remission from binge eating in BED than BWLT.[219] Another study, however, reported comparable longer term (6-year) outcomes between BWLT and CBT for patients with BED and obesity.[220] Adding exercise to treatment for BED is associated with greater decreases in binge eating and BMI.[221] Although a number of studies have found that treating binge eating does not translate to weight loss, some studies have found that reductions in binge eating can assist in modest weight loss among those with BED, especially when complete remission is achieved.[222]

Across all diagnoses and treatments, there has been little attention to differential outcomes by socioeconomic factors. Future studies to explore whether treatment efficacy differs by gender, age, race, ethnicity, socioeconomic status, or cultural group are warranted.[191,192] Given the frequent psychiatric comorbidity associated with EDs, as well as psychosocial risk correlates, some patients with an ED will benefit from psychodynamic psychotherapy and a flexible and eclectic approach depending on patient capabilities, goals, treatment history, and other psychosocial considerations.

Pharmacotherapy

Pharmacologic management has an adjunctive role for the treatment of BN and BED. Of the numerous agents that have been studied, only fluoxetine and lisdexamfetamine have the U.S. FDA approval for BN and BED, respectively. There is insufficient empiric support for efficacy of any agent in treating the primary symptoms of AN. Similarly, there are no clinical trial data to support recommendations for pharmacologic management of pica, rumination disorder, ARFID, OSFED, or USFED. Finally, there are no adequate available clinical trial data to support recommendations for pharmacologic management of EDs in children and adolescents.[223]

Among a variety of agents evaluated for treatment of the primary symptoms of AN, several have been studied; of these none have accumulated sufficient evidence to result in recommendations for routine clinical use. Although some data have suggested that olanzapine may be beneficial in promoting clinical improvement in AN, a recent meta-analysis failed to demonstrate superiority of atypical antipsychotics in achieving either significant increases in BMI or significant decreases in eating pathology.[224]

Given the lack of data supporting efficacy and safety in patients with AN, no pharmacologic agents can currently be recommended to promote weight gain in this patient population. Pharmacologic agents associated with weight gain for other indications should be used judiciously and with a candid discussion with the patient about the anticipated risks and benefits of appetite and weight changes. If such an agent is selected, symptoms should be monitored carefully to look for onset, recurrence, or increase in bingeing or purging behaviors.

Fluoxetine has not been found effective for treating the primary symptoms of AN in underweight patients[225] and has unclear benefit in stabilizing weight-recovered patients with AN.[226,227] Comorbid psychiatric illness is common among these patients and may improve with pharmacologic management, but depressive symptoms in severely underweight patients may not respond as well to antidepressant medication as in normal-weight patients.

Notwithstanding the very limited role for psychotropic medications in the management of AN, patients will likely need to optimize their calcium and vitamin D supplementation if dietary sources are inadequate.[103] Although oral contraceptive agents may mitigate some of the symptoms of hypoestrogenemia associated with AN, they do not protect against bone loss in this population,[228,229] an observation that has been attributed to the insulin-like growth factor-1 suppressive effects of oral estrogen or the dose or form of estrogen in oral pills. One study showed that estrogen administered as the 17β-estradiol transdermal patch to older girls with AN (bone age $\geq$15 years) or as small but increasing doses of oral ethinyl estradiol to younger girls (bone age $<$15 years, in whom growth was not complete) caused an increase in spine and hip BMD compared with placebo. However, complete catch-up in BMD did not occur with any of these measures.[230] It is useful for clinicians to bear in mind that for medical stabilization, and probably also as a prerequisite to developing the psychological insight necessary for recovery, weight restoration is the treatment of choice for underweight individuals with AN. Conservative use of pharmacologic agents for low BMD in adolescents at greatest risk may be considered.[230]

In contrast to the limitations of medication management for AN, a number of medications have established short-term modest efficacy for the treatment of BN, although remission rates are low.[231,232] CBT has better efficacy than medication to reduce the symptoms associated with BN, but there is some support for augmenting psychotherapy with medication, and this is fairly routine clinical practice. It is optimal to use pharmacotherapy as an adjunct to (rather than a substitute for) psychotherapy, but this approach may not be available or beneficial to all patients. Some evidence supports treatment with fluoxetine (60 mg/day) alone in a primary care setting.[233] Fluoxetine has also been found superior to placebo for treating bulimic symptoms in patients who have not responded adequately to CBT or IPT.[234]

Desipramine and imipramine (both at conventional antidepressant dosages as tolerated) have demonstrated efficacy in symptom reduction but are not as well-tolerated in patients with BN.[235] Topiramate has shown efficacy in reduction of binge and purge symptoms in two short-term RCTs in individuals with BN.[236–238] Other agents that have demonstrated at least some efficacy (but with less data available) include trazodone,[239] ondansetron (in patients with severe BN),[240] and other SSRIs, including sertraline, fluvoxamine, and citalopram.[232] A number of studies have investigated the efficacy of naltrexone in treating bulimic symptoms,[235] but only at higher doses was it superior to placebo in reducing symptoms in patients who had previously not responded to alternative pharmacotherapy.[241] Monitoring of liver biochemical test results is essential when this drug is used. Other medications with efficacy are relatively contraindicated for those with BN, given their potential adverse effects. Bupropion was associated with a higher than expected seizure risk during a clinical trial,[242] and there have been case reports of spontaneous hypertensive crises in patients with BN who were taking monoamine oxidase inhibitors.[243] Although fluvoxamine has shown some efficacy for BN relapse prevention in one RCT,[244] another RCT combining fluvoxamine with stepped-care psychotherapy not only did not show efficacy of this agent but also reported grand mal seizures in some participants on the active drug.[245]

Similar to BN, antidepressants have generally been shown to reduce binge eating and be well-tolerated in patients with BED. A variety of SSRIs (e.g., fluoxetine, citalopram, sertraline, and fluvoxamine), as well as serotonin-norepinephrine reuptake inhibitors (e.g., duloxetine for individuals with comorbid depression) have demonstrated some degree of efficacy.[232] In addition, many individuals with BED will have a cooccurring disorder that would warrant antidepressant treatment in its own right.[352] To date, there is insufficient information to recommend one antidepressant or class of antidepressants over another. Thus selection of an antidepressant should be based on tolerability, side effect profile, and potential for drug-drug interactions. In addition, for patients who have purging behaviors or a history of purging behaviors, bupropion is contraindicated, given the increased risk of seizures observed in individuals with BN in early clinical trials of high-dose immediate release bupropion.[353,354] To date, medications targeting weight management have shown mixed results for BED. Although orlistat (a lipase inhibitor) demonstrated a decrease in weight in patients with BED enrolled in a 24-week RCT, no change in binge frequency was documented when compared to placebo.[246] A more recent study in patients with BED also failed to demonstrate any reduction in binge episodes when compared to placebo.[247] Although topiramate has demonstrated some efficacy in reducing binge symptoms and weight in patients with BED, side effects and high attrition rates limit the generalizability of the findings for this population.[232]

In early 2015, lisdexamfetamine, a prodrug of dextroamphetamine, was approved for the treatment of moderate and severe BED in adults. Studies have been associated with modest short-term effects in BED.[333–337] Further, continued treatment with lisdexamfetamine was associated with less risk of relapse than when lisdexamfetamine was discontinued.[338] Physicians considering the use of stimulant medications for the treatment of BED should closely monitor heart rate, blood pressure, and general cardiovascular health in these patients. Caution is needed if it is used in individuals with hypertension or cardiac disease and more frequent monitoring of vital signs may be warranted. The possibility of stimulant misuse or dependence should also be considered before deciding on treatment with lisdexamfetamine as well as during treatment.

Nutritional Rehabilitation

Severely malnourished adult patients—especially those <70% −75% of expected body weight—may require inpatient care for nutritional rehabilitation. Patients with AN are at particularly high risk for refeeding syndrome, which can occur with any means of refeeding, including oral, enteral, and parenteral routes (see Chapter 6). Refeeding syndrome describes the clinical and metabolic derangements that occur during refeeding a malnourished patient. This is a serious complication that can present with a range of clinical symptoms, including rhabdomyolysis, hemolytic anemia, seizure, cardiac arrhythmias, cardiac failure or arrest, delirium, coma, and death; this can occur days to weeks after initiation of nutritional rehabilitation.[339,340] The hallmark biochemical marker of refeeding syndrome is hypophosphatemia [also known as refeeding hypophosphatemia (RH)]. Other electrolyte changes can also occur, including hypokalemia and hypomagnesemia. Although there is no universally accepted definition for refeeding syndrome,[341] the American Society for Parenteral and Enteral Nutrition has proposed a definition that includes criteria for stratification which should occur within 5 days of the reintroduction of nutrition: decrease in serum phosphorus, potassium, or magnesium levels by 10%−20% (mild), 20%−30% (moderate), or >30% (severe) and/or organ dysfunction resulting from a decrease in any of these and/or due to thiamin deficiency[342] Studies have shown that the degree of RH is correlated with lower weight [lower percent of expected body weight on admission to hospital and expressed as percent of median body mass index (%mBMI)] as opposed to the introduction of low- or high-calorie nutrition. Patient who are <70% mBMI have the highest risk for developing RH.[343] In addition, studies have also suggested that the magnitude of weight loss prior to admission among moderately malnourished patients with AN and atypical AN was associated with hypophosphatemia.[292,344,345] Further, studies exploring the best possible nutritional intervention in hospitalized patients with AN have shifted from the "start low and go slow" approach to higher energy refeeding, starting between 1400 and 2400 kcal/day.[344,346–350] Higher calorie refeeding, starting at 2000 kcal/day, has been shown to be safe and effective in restoring medical stability and reducing hospital stays without increasing risk for RH.

Currently, it is recommended that serum electrolytes, including phosphorus, magnesium, potassium, and calcium levels be monitored closely (e.g., daily after feeding begins) until stabilized (APA guidelines). Heart rate, respiratory rate, lower extremity edema, and signs of heart failure should also be evaluated daily for at least a week and then intermittently at longer intervals as the patient stabilizes. Cardiac telemetry should be used to monitor heart rhythm so that supplementation and other appropriate measures can be instituted if RH or other signs of refeeding syndrome develop. Delirium may occur in the second week of refeeding or later and may last for several weeks.[256–259]

Some experimental data have suggested that a healthful dieting intervention may be helpful in reducing bulimic symptoms,[260] but conventionally, weight-loss treatment has been discouraged in patients with BN, because dieting can stimulate bingeing and purging. BED is common in individuals who present for obesity surgery with some, but not all, symptoms of the full clinical syndrome.

Medical Management of Gastrointestinal Symptoms

Individuals with EDs are likely to have concurrent GI symptoms for which consultation may be sought. In some cases, behaviors associated with EDs result in serious GI complications. In other cases, GI symptoms may be mild and not correlate with underlying pathology but may compromise efforts to nutritionally rehabilitate the patient. Given that the restrictive eating, binge-pattern eating, and purging behaviors may underlie or exacerbate some of the GI symptoms, concurrent management of the ED is integral to preventing worsening of the GI manifestations of illness. Careful differential diagnosis is also necessary to avoid misattribution of symptoms to a feeding or ED and to detect primary GI pathology that may be obscured by one.

Subjective reports of GI symptoms may not reliably indicate pathology[146,261]; moreover, they may be mediated by affect[123] or body image concerns.[114] When patients complain of bloating and constipation, it is useful to determine to what extent these complaints stem from fear of gaining weight or reflect decreased GI motility.

A number of studies have evaluated improvement in GI function after nutritional rehabilitation. These studies have yielded mixed results, however, and conclusions have been limited by small sample sizes and nonrandomized designs. In one study, gastric emptying improved in patients with restricting-type AN but did not improve in patients with binge eating/purging–type AN after a 22-week treatment period of increasing dietary intake and CBT.[146] Self-reported GI symptom scores improved after treatment in this same study but remained abnormal and did not correlate with gastric emptying as evaluated by US examination.[146] Another study of a mixed sample of adolescents and adults with AN did not demonstrate significant improvement in gastric emptying after weight gain ($N = 6$) despite normalization of heart rate and blood pressure.[262] Other studies have suggested that nutritional rehabilitation is associated with improved gastric emptying in inpatients with AN, but it is unclear whether such improvement is related to refeeding per se or to weight gain.[263] Constipation is a frequent complaint of patients with AN and BN and may have multiple causes. Colonic transit appears to be delayed in patients with constipation and AN, but returns to normal within 3–4 weeks of refeeding in hospitalized patients with AN.[127,264] In one study, however, anorectal dysfunction in patients with AN with severe constipation did not significantly improve with refeeding. The investigators suggested that abnormal defecatory perception thresholds and expulsion dynamics in AN may have contributed to the patients' unremitting constipation.[264] From 10% to 60% of patients with AN[265] and BN[266] abuse laxatives, most commonly of the stimulant class.[267] Some patients use laxatives as their chief method of purging and may gradually escalate their daily dose to very large amounts. Although the relationship of laxative abuse to colonic dysfunction remains controversial (see Chapter 130),[268–270] it has been observed that patients with chronic laxative abuse complain of constipation while tapering off their laxatives. Rectal prolapse has been described with AN and BN and is thought to be linked to constipation, laxative use, excessive exercise, and increased intra-abdominal pressure upon self-induced vomiting.[138,162] Other medical concerns associated with laxative abuse include electrolyte and acid/base changes that can involve the renal and cardiovascular systems and may become life-threatening. The renin-aldosterone system becomes activated upon fluid loss, which leads to edema and acute weight gain when the laxative is discontinued. This can reinforce further laxative abuse when a patient feels bloated or experiences weight gain.[267]

Delayed intestinal transit and its associated clinical symptoms present a particularly interesting clinical challenge in patients with AN and BN. Existing data suggest that reestablishing regular food intake or weight gain will improve delayed gastric emptying and slowed colonic transit, although this may not be sufficient to restore normal GI function. Patients may resist active weight management or cessation of their disordered pattern of eating despite having a serious ED and associated GI complications. This resistance may be exacerbated by early satiety, abdominal pain, bloating, or constipation, all of which may reinforce the patient's excessive concern with weight or conviction that his or her diet has to be further restricted. Management of symptoms is further complicated by subjective symptom reports that do not correlate consistently with pathology; some complaints may be mediated by psychiatric symptoms or illness, including depression, anxiety, or distorted body image.

Because refeeding and establishing normal and healthful dietary patterns are both treatment goals and likely to improve symptoms, careful nutritional rehabilitation is a reasonable and conservative initial step in managing suspected delayed gastric emptying and slow colonic transit for inpatients with AN or BN. Patients are likely to benefit from the support and reassurance that many of the GI symptoms commonly associated with EDs (e.g., bloating, constipation, nausea, vomiting, diarrhea) will improve as eating and weight return to normal. Additional management strategies include dietary changes to reduce bloating, such as promoting smaller, more frequent meals; encouraging consumption of liquids earlier in the meal; and possibly initially providing a percentage of calories (no more than 25%–50%) in liquid form.[72,116]

Various prokinetic agents have been used to manage delayed gastric emptying in AN, although existing data do not support a recommendation for their use for gastric motility complaints in AN.[271]

Some clinicians have reservations about prescribing laxatives to treat the constipation that follows laxative abuse. Although it does not make sense to reproduce purging behavior using cathartics to treat constipation in this situation, some patients will benefit from a thoughtful bowel regimen to reduce discomfort and bloating. Increasing fluid intake, dietary fiber, and adding stool softeners and bulk-forming agents are often reasonable and conservative first-line treatments. Osmotic laxatives may be necessary for symptom relief in some cases.[272] Management of constipation may require anorectal retraining if it is due to anorectal dysfunction (see Chapters 20, 130, and 131).[264]

Some patients may benefit from symptomatic relief of GERD and esophagitis with antacids or H2RAs; PPIs may be required for relief of more severe symptoms.[72] Although such treatment may be appropriate clinically, the underlying cause and exacerbation of the GI complaint should be made clear to the patient and, when related to the ED, actively addressed in psychotherapeutic treatment. Functional GI disorders, including irritable bowel syndrome and functional dyspepsia, have been found to improve after nutritional and psychiatric treatment of EDs.[351]

Mild elevations of serum aminotransferase levels in AN secondary to malnutrition will likely remit with weight restoration. Elevated serum levels of liver enzymes in severely ill patients may be an indication of refeeding syndrome or reflect AN-related hypoperfusion and require emergent evaluation and intervention.[72,175]

Although many GI symptoms related to restrictive eating, binge-pattern eating, or purging can be managed conservatively, some GI complaints will require further diagnostic evaluation. Anecdotal reports of catastrophic GI complications of EDs, as well as primary GI illness that arises coincidentally with an ED or mimics an ED, suggest that complaints should be evaluated in their specific clinical context. SMA syndrome can clinically manifest with nausea, vomiting, epigastric abdominal pain, or nonspecific GI complaints and can be missed if this symptom is attributed to the ED alone. Further, SMA can hinder weight restoration in those with AN. There are case reports of ED-related gastric emphysema resulting from gastric muscular atrophy, "occlusion" of the gastroesophageal junction, and delayed gastric emptying.[273] Acute gastric dilatation is a rare complication of AN binge/purge subtype that results from decreased gastric motility and delayed gastric emptying[178]; it may be unsuspected in the absence of a clinical history of binge eating.[169] If acute gastric dilatation is confirmed in the setting of refeeding or in the presence of a history of an ED with binge eating, urgent NG decompression and fluid resuscitation are necessary because gastric necrosis, perforation, shock, and death can occur if treatment is delayed.[178] In some cases, laparotomy may be necessary.[133,136,169]

More clinical trial data to clarify treatment strategies for GI complaints associated with the feeding and EDs are warranted. However, management of GI symptoms in patients with an ED can be guided by several key considerations. Primary GI illness should be excluded and where appropriate, consideration that a feeding or ED may be obscuring or mimicking a primary GI illness. If functional GI symptoms appear to be associated with an ED, nutritional rehabilitation in combination with psychotherapeutic care should be considered as an initial step. Nutritional rehabilitation in AN will often require inpatient care and monitoring for serious potential complications, such as refeeding syndrome and acute gastric dilation. During treatment of an ED, resistance to weight gain, to eating normally, and to cessation of bingeing and purging is common, so the possibility that body image or emotional symptoms can result in medical GI complaints should be considered in the treatment plan.

CONCLUSION

Feeding and EDs are mental disorders that can lead to serious, chronic, and life-threatening medical complications, particularly GI issues. GI complications are highly prevalent among patients with EDs ranging from mild to severe. These complications underscore the necessity for a multidisciplinary treatment approach involving medical, nutritional, and psychological support for individuals with EDs.

Full references for this chapter can be found at ebooks.health.elsevier.com.

11 Food Allergies

Malika Gupta, J. Andrew Bird

IN THIS CHAPTER

The first recorded account of food allergy is attributed to Hippocrates, but it was not until 1921 that Prausnitz's classic experiment initiated scientific investigation of food allergy and established the immunologic basis of allergic reactions.[1] In his experiment, Prausnitz injected serum from his fish-allergic patient, Küstner, into his own skin; the next day he injected fish extract into the same areas and into control sites. A positive local reaction (Prausnitz-Küstner test) proved sensitivity could be transferred by a factor in serum (immunoglobulin (Ig)E antibodies) from an allergic to a nonallergic individual. In 1950 Loveless demonstrated that the patient's history and presence of food-specific IgE antibodies were often insufficient to diagnose food allergy in the first blinded placebo-controlled food trial of patients with milk allergy.[2] In the 3 decades that followed, standardized protocols were developed to evaluate food allergy, and the double-blind placebo-controlled oral food challenge emerged as the accepted standard for the diagnosis of food allergy.[3]

DEFINITIONS

Terminology used by investigators in the field of food allergy differs slightly in different parts of the world. The following represents current terminology in the United States.[4] An *adverse food reaction* is a generic term indicating any untoward reaction that occurs following ingestion of a food or food additive. Adverse food reactions may be further classified broadly as immune-mediated (food allergy or food hypersensitivity) or nonimmune mediated (food intolerance). *Food intolerances* comprise most adverse food reactions and are categorized as *enzymatic*, *pharmacologic*, or *idiopathic*. Secondary lactase deficiency is an enzymatic intolerance secondary to injury of the small intestine [e.g., following an infection that affects the gastrointestinal (GI) tract] (see Chapter 106), whereas most other enzyme deficiencies are rare inborn errors of metabolism and thus primarily affect infants and children. Pharmacologic food intolerances are present in individuals who are abnormally reactive to substances like vasoactive amines, which are normally present in some foods (e.g., tyramine in aged cheeses). Confirmed adverse food reactions for which the physiologic mechanism is not known are generally classified as idiopathic intolerances. Food allergies are usually characterized as IgE-mediated "immediate" or non-IgE-mediated "delayed"; the latter are presumed to be cell-mediated.

PREVALENCE

About 8% of children and between 2% and 10% of the overall US population have food allergies.[4,5] The prevalence of food allergies is greatest in the first few years of life and decreases over the first decade. The most common food allergens in young children include peanut (2.2%), cow's milk (1.9%), shellfish (1.3%), tree nuts (1.2%), egg (0.9%), finned fish (0.6%), wheat (0.5%), soy (0.5%), and sesame (0.2%).[6] Other than peanut, tree nuts, finned fish, and shellfish, most childhood food allergies are outgrown by the end of the first decade. Most children who develop cow's milk, egg, and/or peanut allergy do so in the first 2 or 3 years of life.[7] Peanut, tree nut, sesame seed, finned fish, and shellfish allergies tend to be lifelong, but about 20% of young children with peanut allergy develop clinical tolerance.[4] Food allergies may persist after childhood into adulthood or develop in adulthood, with the most common food allergies in adults consisting of shellfish (2%), peanut (0.6%), tree nuts (0.4%), and finned fish (0.4%).[8] About 5% of the population per European studies experiences limited oropharyngeal symptoms (e.g., itching and/or tingling of the lips, tongue, roof of the mouth, and throat) to raw fruits and vegetables. Most of these reactions occur in adolescents and adults who have seasonal allergic rhinitis and are due to cross-reactivity between homologous proteins in pollens (e.g., birch or ragweed pollens) and certain fruits and vegetables (e.g., raw apples, plums, cherry, kiwi, hazelnut, melons, and bananas), respectively (pollen-food allergy syndrome or oral allergy syndrome).[9,10] The prevalence of food allergies appears to be increasing.[11] Studies from the United States and United Kingdom indicate that the prevalence of peanut allergy has more than doubled in young children in a little over a decade.[12,13] In addition, children with atopic disorders have a higher prevalence of food allergies; for example, 35%–40% of children with moderate-to-severe atopic dermatitis have IgE-mediated food allergy.[14]

PATHOGENESIS

Unlike the systemic immune system, which recognizes relatively small quantities of antigen and mounts a brisk inflammatory response to neutralize potential pathogens, the mucosal immune system regularly encounters enormous quantities of antigen and generally functions to suppress immune reactivity to harmless foreign antigens (e.g., food proteins, commensal organisms), only mounting a brisk protective response to dangerous pathogens when appropriate (see Chapter 2). The GI tract is the largest reservoir of immune cells in the body, and the gut-associated lymphoid tissue (GALT), a component of the mucosal immune system, lies juxtaposed to the external environment; it acts to differentiate organisms and foreign proteins that are potentially harmful from those that are not, and to keep the commensal microbiota compartmentalized.[15] The mucosal immune system is separated from the intestinal lumen by a single layer of columnar epithelial cells that secrete a number of factors that contribute to barrier function, including mucins, antimicrobial peptides, and trefoil factors. The epithelial cells also transport antibodies, particularly IgA, into the intestinal lumen, where they contribute to barrier function by excluding the uptake of antigens or microbes. Just beneath this cell layer is the lamina propria of the mucosa, which is densely populated by resident immune cells, including $CD4^+$ and $CD8^+$ T-effector and regulatory T (Treg) cells, antibody-secreting B cells, and mononuclear phagocytes [macrophages and dendritic cells (DCs)]. These scattered immune cells make up the effector sites of the mucosal immune system and function to recognize and clear pathogenic challenges from the environment. Peyer patches and isolated lymphoid follicles are situated within the intestinal mucosa, and with nearby mesenteric lymph nodes (MLN) form inductive sites where antigen-specific cellular and humoral immune responses are first generated. Specialized epithelial cells (M cells) overlie Peyer patches and contribute to the selective uptake of particulate antigens into this site. In contrast, soluble antigens are primarily taken up across the epithelial cells lining the villi and are carried into the MLNs. Lack of reactivity to our commensal flora is in part achieved by a specialized regulatory environment that may also shape the immune response to antigens derived from the diet. Antigen-presenting cells and macrophages of the intestinal mucosa are hyporesponsive to many microbial ligands[16] and secrete high levels of immunoregulatory cytokines like interleukin (IL)-10.[17] Both innate (natural killer cells, polymorphonuclear leukocytes, macrophages, epithelial cells, and Toll-like receptors) and adaptive immune responses [intraepithelial and lamina propria lymphocytes, Peyer patches, secretory IgA (sIgA), and cytokines] provide an active barrier to foreign antigens. Developmental immaturity of various components of the intestinal barrier and immune system reduces the efficiency of the infant mucosal barrier; the activity of various enzymes is suboptimal in the newborn period, and the sIgA system is not fully mature until 4 years of age. This immature state of the mucosal barrier may play a role in the increased prevalence of GI infections and food allergies seen in the first few years of life. Studies have also shown that alteration of the physiologic barrier function (e.g., gastric acidity) can lead to increased IgE sensitization in children and adults.[18]

A highly efficient GI mucosal barrier has evolved that provides an enormous surface area for processing and absorbing ingested food and discharging waste products.[19] This barrier uses physiologic and immunologic barriers to prevent penetration of foreign antigens (Box 11.1). The physiologic barrier is composed of epithelial cells joined by tight junctions and covered with a thick mucus layer that traps particles, bacteria, and viruses; trefoil factors [TFFs; protease-resistant proteins secreted by mucus-secreting cells of the stomach (TFF1, TFF2) and intestine (TFF3)] that help strengthen and promote restoration of the barrier; and luminal and brush-border enzymes, bile salts, and extremes of pH—all of which serve to destroy pathogens and render antigens nonimmunogenic. Despite the evolution of this complex mucosal barrier, about 2% of ingested food antigens are absorbed and transported through the normal mature intestine and throughout the body in an immunologically intact form.[15] In an elegant series of experiments performed more than 75 years ago, Walzer et al. used sera from food-allergic patients to passively sensitize volunteers and demonstrate that immunologically intact antigens cross the mucosal barrier and disseminate rapidly throughout the body.[20,21] Increased gastric acidity and the presence of food in the intestine decrease antigen absorption, whereas hypochlorhydria (e.g., H_2B- and PPI-induced) and ingestion of alcohol increase antigen absorption.[22] These immunologically intact proteins typically do not provoke adverse reactions because most individuals have developed tolerance, but in a sensitized individual, allergic reactions will occur. Although more common in the developing GALT of young children, it is clear that cellular and IgE-mediated allergic responses to foods can develop at any age.

BOX 11.1 Physiologic and Immunologic Barriers of the Gastrointestinal Tract

PHYSIOLOGIC BARRIERS

- Block penetration of ingested antigens
  - Epithelial cells—single cell layer of columnar epithelium
  - Glycocalyx—coating of complex glycoprotein and mucins that traps particles
  - Intestinal microvillus membrane structure—prevents penetration
  - Tight junctions joining adjacent enterocytes—prevent penetration even of small peptides
  - Intestinal peristalsis—flushes trapped particles out in the stool
- Break down ingested antigens
  - Salivary amylases and mastication
  - Gastric acid and pepsins
  - Pancreatic enzymes
  - Intestinal enzymes
  - Intestinal epithelial cell lysozyme activity

IMMUNOLOGIC BARRIERS

- Block penetration of ingested antigens
  - Antigen-specific sIgA in intestinal lumen
- Clear antigens penetrating the gastrointestinal barrier
  - Serum antigen-specific IgA and IgG
- Reticuloendothelial system

As already noted, the dominant response in GALT is suppression, or tolerance. As first described in 1911 by Osborne and Wells,[23] antigens ingested via the oral route induce a systemic nonresponsiveness that has been termed *oral tolerance*. Antigens first ingested and then injected in an attempt to immunize an animal could not elicit an immune response. Similar findings have been demonstrated in humans following feeding and immunization with a neoantigen, keyhole limpet hemocyanin.[24] Oral tolerance was shown to be an active regulatory response by the demonstration that this nonresponsive state could be induced in naïve mice through the transfer of T cells. MLNs are essential for development of oral tolerance, and surgical or immunologic ablation of MLNs prevents development of oral tolerance.[25,26] Trafficking of immune cells to the intestine and from the intestine to the MLNs is regulated by expression of chemotactic cytokines (chemokines) and chemokine receptors. Expression of chemokine receptor CCR7 on DCs, which take up antigen from the intestine, is necessary for their migration from the lamina propria to MLNs, and is necessary for development of oral tolerance.[26] Transfer of DCs derived from the intestinal lamina propria can induce tolerance in naïve animals (Fig. 11.1).[27]

$CD103^+$ DCs isolated from the MLNs of mice and humans preferentially induce generation of gut-homing $CD4^+$ $Foxp3^+$ Tregs from naïve T cells. These $CD103^+$ cells express high levels of the enzyme RALDH2, a retinal dehydrogenase that converts retinal to retinoic acid. Both intestinal homing activity and regulatory activity of the responder T cells are dependent on retinoic acid derived from $CD103^+$ DCs. An important source of the precursor for retinoic acid comes from the diet in the form of vitamin A.[28] In addition to the DC signals to naïve T cells, stromal cells of the MLN also express high levels of retinoic acid-generating enzymes and are important for the imprinting of factors, such as *intestinal homing potential*.[29]

Evidence now indicates that the commensal bowel flora (microbiota) play a major role in shaping the mucosal immune

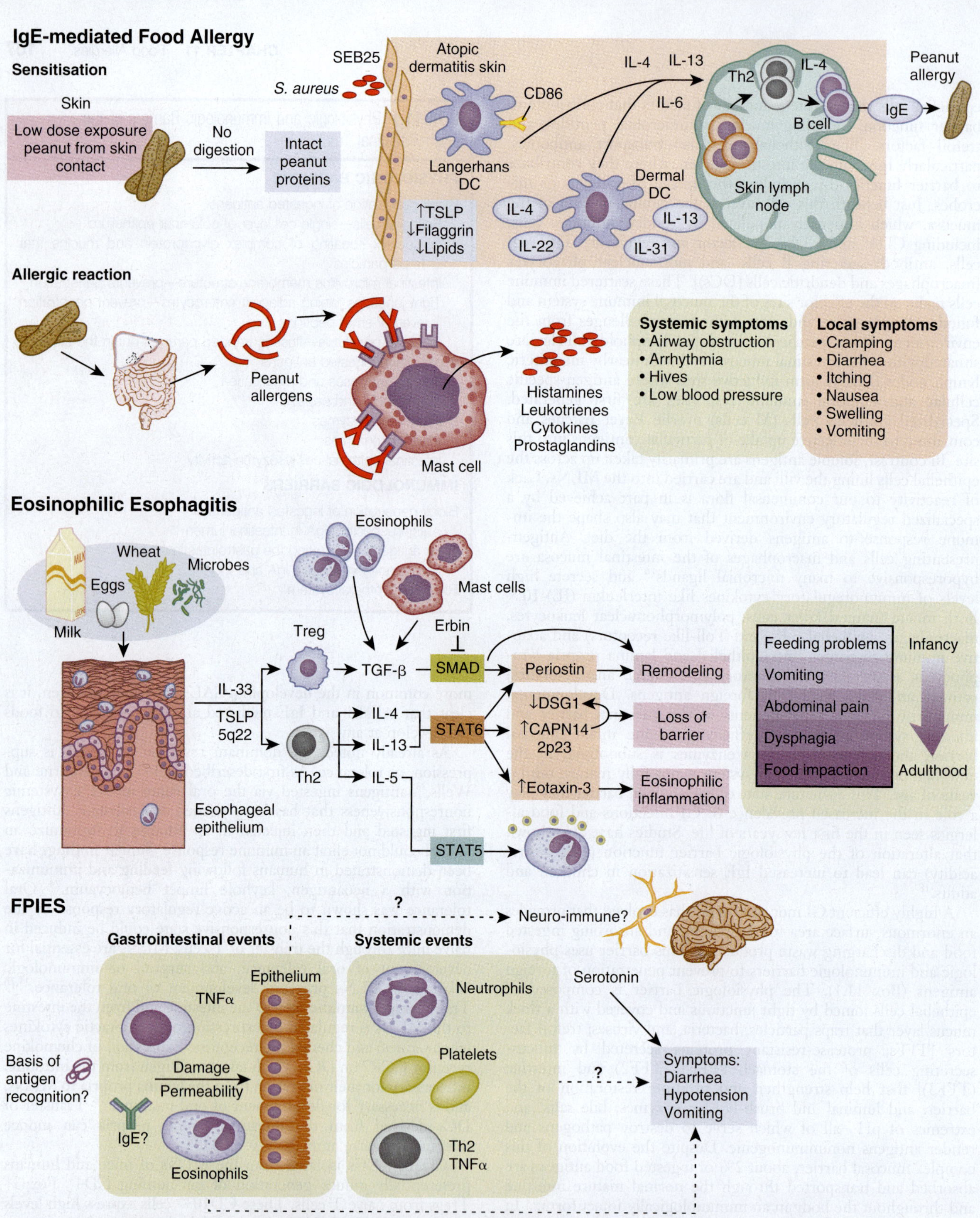

Fig. 11.1 Pathophysiology of food allergy. Immunoreactivity to foods may occur through IgE, non-IgE, and mixed mechanisms. Sensitization to food allergens in IgE-mediated disease occurs primarily through exposure through inflamed skin. Upon reexposure to allergen an immediate, IgE-mediated reaction may ensue, resulting in anaphylaxis. Eosinophilic esophagitis has been shown to result from the production of proatopy cytokines, such as interleukin-33 and TSLP activating T-regulatory and T-helper type 2 cells, to promote secretion of cytokines resulting in esophageal barrier disruption, tissue remodeling, and eosinophilic inflammation. Mechanisms underlying the development of FPIES are less understood. This figure depicts the variety of associated findings reported in FPIES patients though a unifying mechanism of disease pathogenesis is lacking. Eosinophils, plasma cells, and CD4+ T cells have been documented but their relevance in disease pathogenesis has not been established. Serotonin has been implicated in triggering symptoms of FPIES though it is not clear if it is a peripheral trigger of reactions or is restricted to central control of the vomiting reflex. *FPIES*, Food protein–induced enterocolitis syndrome; *IL*, interleukin; *TNF-α*; tumor necrosis factor-α; *TSLP*, thymic stromal lymphopoietin.

response. It has now been shown that there are approximately the same number of bacterial cells in the human body as there are human cells.[30] The number of bacteria in a 70 kg "reference man" is estimated at 3.8×10^{13}. The typical concentration of bacteria in the colon is estimated at 10^{11}/mL with a rounded up order of magnitude of 10^{14}.[30] An individual's microbiota is to some measure established in the first 24 hours after birth and depends on maternal flora, genetics, and local environment, including whether birth is by cesarean section or vaginal delivery (see Chapter 3). The intestinal microbiota is relatively stable throughout life after reaching the adult pattern somewhere after the first year of life.[31] In a recent study, mice with food allergy were found to have a specific intestinal microbiota capable of transferring disease susceptibility, suggesting that disease-associated microbiota may play a pathogenic role in the development of food allergy.[32] Studies in which lactating mothers and their offspring were fed *Lactobacillus* suggest that probiotics may be beneficial in preventing some atopic disorders, such as eczema,[33] but results from other studies are not consistent with this conclusion.

Intestinal epithelial cells (IECs) may also play a central regulatory role in determining the rate and pattern of uptake of ingested antigens. Studies in sensitized rats have indicated that intestinal antigen transport proceeds in two phases.[34] In the first phase, transepithelial transport occurs via endosomes, is antigen specific and mast cell independent, and occurs 10 times faster in sensitized rats compared with nonsensitized control animals. Antigen-specific IgE antibodies bound to the mucosal surface of IECs via Fc epsilon (Fcε)RII are responsible for this accelerated allergen entry. In the second phase, paracellular transport predominates. Loosening of the tight junctions occurs as a result of factors released by mast cells that are activated in the first phase. Whereas the first antigen-specific pathway involves antibody, the second nonspecific pathway most likely involves cytokines. Consistent with this concept, IECs express receptors for a number of cytokines (IL-1, IL-2, IL-6, IL-10, IL-12, IL-15, granulocyte-monocyte colony-stimulating factor, and interferon-γ) and have been shown to be functionally altered by exposure to these cytokines.

Oral tolerance of humoral and cellular immunity has been demonstrated in rodents and humans. Feeding of keyhole limpet hemocyanin to human volunteers resulted in T-cell tolerance but priming of B cells at both mucosal and systemic sites.[35,36] Failure of human infants to develop oral tolerance, or the breakdown of oral tolerance in older individuals, results in development of food allergy. Young infants are more prone to develop food-allergic reactions because of the immaturity of their immunologic system and, to some extent, their GI tract (see Box 11.1). Exclusive breast-feeding promotes development of oral tolerance and may prevent some food allergies and atopic dermatitis.[37] The protective effect of breast milk appears to be due to several factors, including decreased content of foreign proteins, the presence of sIgA (which provides passive protection against foreign protein and pathogens), and the presence of soluble factors (e.g., prolactin), which may induce earlier maturation of the intestinal barrier and the infant's immune response. The antibacterial activity of breast milk is well established, but the ability of breast milk sIgA to prevent food antigen penetration is less clear. Low concentrations of food-specific IgG, IgM, and IgA antibodies are commonly found in the serum of normal persons. Food protein-specific IgG antibodies tend to rise in the first months following introduction of a food, and then generally decline even though the food protein continues to be ingested.[38] Persons with various inflammatory bowel disorders (e.g., celiac disease [CD], food allergy) frequently have high levels of food-specific IgG and IgM antibodies, although there is no evidence these antibodies are pathogenic. Antigen-specific T cell proliferation in vitro alone does not represent a marker of immunopathogenicity but simply reflects response to antigen exposure.

In genetically predisposed individuals, antigen presentation leads to excessive Th2 responsiveness (i.e., lymphocytes that secrete IL-4, IL-5, IL-10, and IL-13), resulting in increased IgE production and expression of FcεI receptors on a variety of cells.[39] These IgE antibodies bind high-affinity FcεI receptors on mast cells, basophils, and DCs, as well as low-affinity FcεII (CD23) receptors on macrophages, monocytes, lymphocytes, eosinophils, and platelets. When food allergens penetrate mucosal barriers and reach IgE antibodies bound to mast cells or basophils, the cells are activated, and mediators (e.g., histamine, prostaglandins, leukotrienes) are released that induce vasodilation, smooth muscle contraction, and mucus secretion, which lead to symptoms of immediate hypersensitivity. These activated mast cells also may release a variety of cytokines (e.g., IL-4, IL-5, IL-6, TNF-α, platelet-activating factor), which may induce the IgE-mediated late-phase inflammation. Various symptoms have been associated with IgE-mediated allergic reactions: generalized (shock); cutaneous (urticaria, angioedema, pruritic morbilliform rash); oral (lip, tongue, and palatal pruritus and edema); GI (vomiting, diarrhea); and upper and lower respiratory (nasal congestion, laryngeal edema, and wheezing associated with ocular pruritus and tearing). A rise in the plasma histamine level has been associated with development of these symptoms after blinded food challenges.[40] In IgE-mediated GI reactions, endoscopic observation has revealed local vasodilation, edema, mucus secretion, and petechial hemorrhage.[41] Cell-mediated hypersensitivity reactions are believed responsible for eosinophilic esophagitis (EoE) and eosinophilic gastroenteritis (EG) (see Chapter 30). Activated T cells secrete IL-5 and other cytokines, attracting eosinophils, and inducing the inflammatory response that causes delayed onset of symptoms.[42] Expansion studies of T cells from biopsy specimens of milk-induced EoE patients have revealed large numbers of $CD4^+$ Th2 cells.[43]

In summary, the GI tract processes ingested food into a form that can be absorbed and used for energy and cell growth. During this process, nonimmunologic and immunologic mechanisms help destroy or block foreign antigens (e.g., bacteria, viruses, parasites, and food proteins) from entering the body proper. Despite this elegant barrier, antigenically intact food proteins enter the circulation, but in the normal host are largely ignored by the immune system, which has become "tolerized" to these nonpathogenic substances.

CLINICAL FEATURES

A number of GI food hypersensitivity disorders have been described (Box 11.2). Clinically, these disorders are generally divided into two main categories: IgE-mediated and non-IgE (cell)-mediated hypersensitivities. A number of other disorders may result in symptoms similar to food-allergic reactions, and these must be excluded during evaluation (Box 11.3).

Long before IgE antibodies were identified, studies of food hypersensitivity focused on radiologic changes associated with immediate hypersensitivity reactions. In one of the first of these reports, hypertonicity of the transverse and pelvic colon and hypotonicity of the cecum and ascending colon were noted following feeding of wheat to an allergic patient.[44] In a later report, fluoroscopy was used to compare barium contrast studies with and without food allergens in 12 food-allergic children[45]; gastric hypotonia and retention of the allergen test meal, prominent pylorospasm, and increased or decreased peristaltic activity of the intestines were noted.

In the late 1930s the rigid gastroscope was used to observe reactions in the stomachs of allergic patients. One study evaluated patients with GI food allergy or wheezing exacerbated by food ingestion and control subjects.[46] Thirty minutes after a food allergen was placed on the gastric mucosa, patients with GI food

BOX 11.2 Gastrointestinal Food Hypersensitivities

IMMUNOGLOBULIN E-MEDIATED FOOD HYPERSENSITIVITIES

GI allergy
Infantile colic (minor subset)
Pollen-food allergy (oral allergy syndrome)

MIXED IMMUNOGLOBULIN E- AND NONIMMUNOGLOBULIN E-MEDIATED HYPERSENSITIVITIES

Eosinophilic esophagitis
Eosinophilic gastritis
Eosinophilic gastroenteritis
Allergic eosinophilic proctocolitis

NONIMMUNOGLOBULIN E-MEDIATED FOOD HYPERSENSITIVITIES

Dietary protein–induced enteropathy
- Celiac disease
- Dermatitis herpetiformis

Food protein–induced enterocolitis syndrome

MECHANISM UNKNOWN

Cow's milk-induced occult GI blood loss and iron deficiency anemia of infancy
GERD
Infantile colic (subset)
IBD

BOX 11.3 Disorders That Must Be Differentiated From Food Hypersensitivities

BACTERIAL INFECTIONS AND DISORDERS THAT MAY CAUSE ADVERSE FOOD REACTIONS

Enterotoxigenic bacteria
- *Vibrio cholerae, toxigenic Escherichia coli, Clostridioides difficile*

Metabolic disorders
- Acrodermatitis enteropathica
- Hypo- or abetalipoproteinemia
- Primary carbohydrate malabsorption: lactase deficiency, sucrase deficiency
- Transient fructose and/or sorbitol malabsorption

Postinfection malabsorption (secondary disaccharidase deficiency, villus atrophy, bile salt deconjugation)
- Bacterial: *Shigella*, *C. difficile*
- Parasitic: *Giardia*, *Cryptosporidium*
- Viral: *Rotavirus*

ANATOMIC ABNORMALITIES

Hirschsprung disease (especially with enterocolitis)
Ileal stenosis
Intestinal lymphangiectasia
Short bowel syndrome

OTHER DISORDERS

Chronic nonspecific diarrhea of infancy
Cystic fibrosis
IBD
Tumors
- Neuroblastoma
- ZES (gastrinoma)

allergy had markedly hyperemic and edematous patches with thick gray mucus and scattered petechiae at these sites, similar to those reported earlier by Walzer in passively sensitized intestinal mucosal sites.[22] Only mild hyperemia of the gastric mucosa was noted in patients with wheezing provoked by food ingestion. Subsequent studies confirmed these earlier observations and established an IgE-mediated mechanism for the reactions.[41] Compared with normal controls, food-specific IgE antibodies and increased numbers of intestinal mast cells were demonstrated prior to challenge in food-allergic patients, and significant decreases in stainable mast cells and tissue histamine content were shown following a positive food challenge.

Immunoglobulin E-Mediated Disorders

The IgE-mediated food-induced GI allergic responses comprise two major symptom complexes: pollen-food allergy (oral allergy) syndrome and GI allergy. These disorders are distinguished by their rapid onset, usually within minutes to 1 hour of ingesting the offending food. Simple laboratory tests that detect food-specific IgE antibodies, such as prick skin tests and in vitro tests of serum food-specific IgE antibodies [e.g., ImmunoCAP (ThermoFisher Scientific, Waltham, MA)], are often useful in determining which foods are responsible for the patient's symptoms.[4]

Pollen-Food Allergy Syndrome

The pollen-food allergy syndrome (oral allergy syndrome) is a form of immediate contact hypersensitivity confined predominantly to the oropharynx and rarely involving other target organs.[29] Symptoms are most commonly associated with ingestion of various fresh (uncooked) fruits and vegetables and include the rapid onset of pruritus of the lips, tongue, palate, and throat, with or without angioedema generally followed by rapid resolution of symptoms. Symptoms result from local IgE-mediated reactions to conserved homologous proteins (structurally similar sequences of amino acids that remained unchanged through evolution) that are heat labile (i.e., readily destroyed by cooking) and shared by certain fruits, vegetables, and some plant pollens.[47] Patients with seasonal allergic rhinitis (hay fever) due to ragweed or birch pollen sensitivity are often afflicted with this syndrome. In up to 50% of patients with ragweed-induced allergic rhinitis, ingestion of melons (e.g., watermelon, cantaloupe, honeydew) and bananas will provoke oral symptoms,[4] whereas in birch pollen-allergic patients, symptoms may develop following ingestion of raw potatoes, carrots, celery, apples, hazelnuts, and kiwi. Diagnosis is based on a classic history and positive prick skin tests (i.e., "prick and prick": pricking the fresh fruit or vegetable with a needle and then pricking the skin of the patient) with the implicated fresh fruits or vegetables.

Gastrointestinal Allergy

GI allergy is a relatively common form of IgE-mediated hypersensitivity that generally accompanies allergic manifestations in other target organs (e.g., skin, airway) and results in a variety of symptoms.[4] Symptoms typically develop within minutes to 2 hours of consuming a food and consist of nausea, abdominal pain, cramps, vomiting, and/or diarrhea. Diagnosis is established by clinical history, evidence of food-specific IgE antibodies (positive skin prick tests or serum food-specific IgE antibodies), resolution of symptoms following complete elimination of the suspected food, and recurrence of symptoms following oral food challenges. GI allergy is common in IgE-mediated food allergies, with more than 50% of children experiencing abdominal symptoms during double-blind placebo-controlled oral food challenges.[48]

Mixed Immunoglobulin E- and Nonimmunoglobulin E-Mediated Disorders

EoE, EG, and allergic eosinophilic proctocolitis (AEP) may be caused by IgE- and/or non-IgE-mediated food allergies and are characterized by eosinophilic infiltration of the esophagus, stomach, and/or colonic walls with peripheral eosinophilia in up to 50% of patients (see Chapter 30 for a more complete discussion).[4,14] In the esophagus, basal hyperplasia and papillary lengthening are seen. The eosinophilic infiltrate may involve the mucosal, muscular, and/or serosal layers of the stomach or small intestine. Eosinophilic invasion of the muscular layer leads to thickening and rigidity, which may manifest as obstruction, whereas infiltration of the serosa commonly results in eosinophilic ascites. In most children with EoE-EG, food-induced IgE- and non-IgE-mediated reactions have been implicated in pathogenesis.[49,50] Patients with IgE-mediated food-induced symptoms generally have atopic disease (atopic dermatitis, allergic rhinitis, and/or asthma), elevated serum IgE concentrations, positive skin prick tests to various foods and inhalants, peripheral blood eosinophilia, iron deficiency anemia, and hypoalbuminemia.

Eosinophilic Esophagitis

EoE occurs predominantly in young children, especially boys, and manifests with reflux or vomiting, irritability, food refusal, early satiety, and failure to thrive; this contrasts with the adult presentation of reflux, epigastric or chest pain, dysphagia, and food impaction.[4,51] Food-induced EoE was first demonstrated in a group of 10 children with postprandial abdominal pain, early satiety or food refusal, vomiting or retching, failure to thrive, and refractoriness to standard medical therapy (4 of 10 had undergone Nissen fundoplication).[52] After 6–8 weeks of an amino acid–based formula (Neocate) plus corn and apples, symptoms completely resolved in eight patients and were markedly improved in two others. Esophageal biopsies revealed a marked reduction or clearing of the eosinophilic infiltrate and significant improvements in basal zone hyperplasia and length of the vascular papillae. Symptoms could be reproduced with the introduction of certain foods. In some children, pulmonary and esophageal inflammation appear to be associated, and some report seasonal esophageal symptoms.[51] EoE has increased in prevalence over the past decade, an observation some authors believe may be explained by the increased early use of antacids and prokinetic agents in young infants with symptoms of reflux. Because murine models of food-induced anaphylaxis require use of antacids for sensitization,[53] it is thought that antireflux medications may further compromise the young infant's intestinal barrier function. In a cohort study of 152 adults using H_2RAs or PPIs for 3 months, 10% of patients experienced an increase in food-specific IgE and 15% developed denovo IgE to specific foods.[54]

Diagnosis of EoE is based on a suggestive history, demonstration of an eosinophilic infiltrate in the esophageal mucosa [>15 eosinophils/high-power field (×40)], and the absence of other causes contributing to the symptoms and the eosinophilic infiltrate.[56] Multiple biopsies are necessary because of the potential patchiness of the lesions; a single esophageal biopsy specimen has a sensitivity of 55%, whereas taking five biopsy specimens increases sensitivity to 100%. Esophagoscopy may reveal mucosal rings (trachealization, feline esophagus), furrowing, ulcerations, whitish papules (which represent eosinophilic abscesses), or strictures, but endoscopic findings are normal in at least one-third of patients with EoE. There is some evidence to suggest that atopy patch testing may be useful in identifying foods responsible for the allergic inflammation, but further studies are necessary to confirm these early reports.[4] Elimination of suspect foods for 6–10 weeks should lead to resolution and normalization of esophageal histology, although clinical symptoms should improve substantially in 3–6 weeks.[55,57] Challenges consist of reintroducing the suspected food allergen and evaluating for recurrence of symptoms and/or eosinophilic infiltrate on biopsy. If food allergens are not identified as provoking agents, oral glucocorticoids are generally required to alleviate symptoms. Symptoms usually respond to glucocorticoid therapy, although recurrence is frequent when they are discontinued.[58] Topical glucocorticoid therapy with swallowed fluticasone spray or viscous budesonide has been shown to induce remission in 50%–80% of patients, but esophageal candidiasis may occur in up to 20% of patients using this form of treatment.[4,59] If exacerbations recur, a daily regimen of low-dose prednisone or prednisolone or prednisone every other day may be successful in suppressing symptoms.[51] The use of PPIs is now recommended as a first-line treatment for EoE.[56] PPIs act both by suppressing acid production and by their antiinflammatory effects.[60] In May 2022 the U.S. Food and Drug Administration (FDA) approved the use of dupilumab to treat EoE in patients 12 years of age and older and weighing at least 40 kg. Dupilumab is a biological therapy that inhibits IL-4 receptor alpha, the common binding site for IL-4 and IL-13, the two key cytokines driving type 2 inflammatory responses in EoE. In a three-part, phase 3 trial[61] of patients ages 12 years or older, there was an improvement in histological remission and symptom score in patients receiving 300 mg dupilumab subcutaneously weekly compared to controls. The most common side effects included injection site reactions, upper respiratory tract infections, arthralgia, and herpes viral infections among others. Reports of conditions, such as seronegative arthritis, enthesitis/enthesopathy, iridocyclitis, and psoriasis associated with dupilumab use, have led to concerns about the skewing of the immune response from Th2 to alternate cytokine pathways.[62] As such, the long-term safety of this drug compared to some of the other commonly used therapies for EoE is yet to be established.

Eosinophilic Gastroenteritis

EG manifests with abdominal pain, nausea, vomiting, diarrhea, and weight loss.[63] Generalized edema secondary to hypoalbuminemia may occur in some infants and young children with marked protein-losing enteropathy, often in the presence of minimal GI symptoms.[64] Rarely EG may manifest as pyloric stenosis in infants with outlet obstruction and postprandial projectile emesis.[65]

The immunopathogenesis of EG is not known but is believed to primarily involve cell-mediated mechanisms. A subset of patients has exacerbations of symptoms following ingestion of food to which they have specific IgE antibodies, but most reactions do not appear to involve this mechanism. Peripheral blood T cells from all EG patients evaluated, compared with normal controls, have been shown to secrete excessive amounts of the Th2 cytokines IL-4 and IL-5 in vitro, and T cells expanded from duodenal biopsies of EG patients express Th2 cytokines in vitro following antigen stimulation.[43]

The diagnosis of EG is dependent on a suggestive history, GI biopsy specimens that demonstrate a prominent eosinophilic infiltration, and peripheral eosinophilia, which occurs in about 50% of patients. Lesions are not uniform, so multiple biopsies are often necessary.[63] Allergy skin testing may be helpful in some cases to identify causative foods, but often a therapeutic trial of an elemental diet for 6–10 weeks is necessary to determine whether food allergy is provoking the disorder. In a study of children with EG and protein-losing enteropathy, institution of an amino acid–based formula therapy brought about resolution of symptoms and normalization of intestinal histology.[64] As with EoE, if no sensitization is found, a trial of glucocorticoids is recommended, although relapses frequently occur when they are discontinued. The long-term prognosis of this disorder is not well characterized. In a series of children with EG and protein-losing enteropathy, follow-up for 2.5–5.5 years revealed the persistence of food-responsive disease.

Allergic Eosinophilic Proctocolitis

AEP generally presents in the first few months of life and is most often due to cow's milk or soy protein hypersensitivity. Over half of reported cases now occur in breast-fed infants because of food antigens passed in maternal breast milk.[4,66] Affected infants usually appear healthy, often have formed stools, and are generally evaluated because of the presence of gross or occult blood in their stools. Blood loss is typically minor but can occasionally produce anemia. AEP in infancy has been identified as a potential risk factor for development of a functional GI disorder after the age of 4 years.[67] Lesions are generally confined to the distal large bowel and consist of mucosal edema, with infiltration of eosinophils into the epithelium and lamina propria. In severe cases with crypt destruction, neutrophils are also prominent. The immunologic mechanism underlying this disorder is unknown but is believed to involve a cell-mediated reaction. Because there is no evidence that IgE antibodies are involved in this disorder, skin prick testing or evaluation of food-specific IgE antibodies is not helpful. Diagnosis can be established when elimination of the responsible allergen leads to resolution of hematochezia. Dramatic improvement is usually seen within 72 hours of appropriate food allergen elimination, but complete clearing and resolution of mucosal lesions may take up to a month. Reintroduction of the allergen leads to recurrence of symptoms within several hours to days. Sigmoidoscopic findings vary and range from areas of patchy mucosal injection to severe friability, with small aphthoid ulcerations and bleeding. Colonic biopsy reveals a prominent eosinophilic infiltrate in the crypt epithelia and lamina propria. Children with cow's milk and soy protein–induced proctocolitis usually outgrow their protein sensitivity (i.e., become clinically tolerant within 6 months to 2 years of allergen avoidance), but refractory cases are occasionally seen.[66]

Infantile Colic

Infantile colic is an ill-defined syndrome of paroxysmal fussiness characterized by inconsolable agonized crying, drawing up of the legs, abdominal distention, and excessive gas. It generally develops in the first 2–4 weeks of life and persists through the third to fourth months of life. Various psychosocial and dietary factors have been implicated in the cause of infantile colic, but trials in bottle-fed and breast-fed infants have suggested that IgE-mediated hypersensitivity may be a pathogenic factor in 10% –15% of colicky infants. The fecal microbiota in infants with colic has been compared with that of control infants.[68] It was shown that microbiota diversity gradually increased after birth only in the control group and, that in the first weeks, the microbiota diversity of the colic group was significantly lower than that of the control group. At age 1 or 2 weeks, the earliest ages with significant differences, Proteobacteria were significantly increased, whereas *bifidobacteria* and *lactobacilli* were significantly reduced in infants with colic. Moreover, the colic phenotype correlated positively with specific groups of Proteobacteria, including *Escherichia*, *Klebsiella*, *Serratia*, *Vibrio*, *Yersinia*, and *Pseudomonas*. Diagnosis of food-induced colic is established by implementing several brief trials of hypoallergenic formula. In infants with food allergen–induced colic, symptoms are generally short-lived, so prolonged restricted diets are generally unnecessary.

Nonimmunoglobulin E-Mediated Disorders

Some GI food-allergic disorders are clearly not IgE-mediated and are believed to be due to different abnormal antigen processing and/or cell-mediated mechanisms; in these disorders, tests for evidence of food-specific IgE antibodies are of no value to identify the responsible food. Non-IgE-mediated hypersensitivities may be divided into two syndromes: food protein–induced enterocolitis and dietary protein–induced enteropathy.[4]

Food Protein–Induced Enterocolitis Syndrome

Food protein–induced enterocolitis syndrome (FPIES) is a disorder that may present with either chronic or acute symptoms. Chronic FPIES is a disorder that has only been reported in young infants less than 4 months of age fed with cow's milk or soy infant formula; presentation is with protracted vomiting and diarrhea that not infrequently results in dehydration and failure to thrive.[4,69] About one-third of infants with severe diarrhea develop acidosis and transient methemoglobinemia. Diagnosis is confirmed with resolution of the symptoms within days after elimination of the offending food. An acute FPIES reaction develops with reintroduction of the offending food (see subsequently) and symptoms include vomiting in the 1- to 4-hour period after ingestion with or without diarrhea in 24 hours (usually 5–10 hours).[70] Without a confirmatory challenge, the diagnosis of chronic FPIES remains presumptive.

Acute FPIES typically presents in the first year of life with repetitive, protracted vomiting that begins approximately 1–4 hours after food ingestion. Vomiting is accompanied by lethargy and pallor, and diarrhea may develop within 24 hours of ingestion.[72] Cow's milk and soy are the most common triggers, but solids, such as rice, oat, egg, wheat, peanut, tree nuts, chicken, turkey, and fish, have also been reported to provoke acute FPIES.[71,72] Breast-fed babies almost never develop symptoms while breast-feeding, but they may be sensitized through food proteins passed in the breast milk and experience a reaction to the first few feedings of the whole food.[72] FPIES in adults rarely has been reported, and finned fish, shellfish (e.g., shrimp, crab, lobster), and egg are the most commonly identified culprits in this age group.[2]

Stools obtained following an acute episode frequently contain occult blood, mucus, leukocytes, and increased carbohydrate content.[72] Stools from infants with chronic FPIES may reveal occult blood, neutrophils, eosinophils, Charcot-Leyden crystals, and/or reducing substances.[72] Jejunal biopsies reveal flattened villi, edema, and increased numbers of intraepithelial lymphocytes, eosinophils, and plasma cells producing IgM and IgA, with a decrease in intact mast cells, suggesting degranulation.[73]

The immunopathogenesis of this syndrome is not completely understood. Studies have indicated that the disorder may be caused by lower expression of type 1 transforming growth factor-β receptors than type 2 receptors, suggesting differential contributions of each receptor to the diverse biological activities of transforming growth factor-β in the intestinal epithelium. Symptomatic FPIES challenges have been associated with significant elevation in IL-17 family markers (IL-17A, IL-22, IL-17C, and CCL20), T-cell activation (IL-2), and innate inflammatory markers (IL-8, oncostatin M, leukemia inhibitory factor, TNF-alpha, IL-10, and IL-6).[74] Dietary avoidance recommendations are generally based on experience with coreactive foods (e.g., if reactive to rice, avoid oats; if reactive to cow's milk, avoid soy milk) (Table 11.1), and oral food challenges are often necessary to expand the diet and confirm whether or not tolerance has developed to a previously identified trigger.

A consensus approach to conducting an oral food challenge for FPIES diagnosis is lacking though a commonly used method consists of administering 0.03–0.6 g/kg body weight without exceeding 3 g of protein of the suspected protein allergen, while monitoring the peripheral blood white cell count. In conjunction with a positive food challenge, the absolute neutrophil count in the peripheral blood may increase at least 3500 cells/mm^3 within

TABLE 11.1 Common Food Coallergies in Children With Food Protein–Induced Enterocolitis Syndrome[66]

FPIES To	Clinical Cross-Reactivity/ Co-Allergy	Observed Occurrence (%)
Cow's milk	Soy	<30–40
	Any solid food	<16
Grains: rice, oats, etc.	Other grains (including rice)	About 50
Legumes	Soy	<80
Poultry	Other poultry	<40
	Cow's milk	<30–40
Solid food (any)	Another solid food	<44
	Cow's milk or soy	<25
Soy	Any solid food	<16

FPIES, Food protein–induced enterocolitis syndrome.

4–6 hours of developing symptoms, and neutrophils and eosinophils may be found in the stools. It has been reported that as many as 15% of food antigen challenges may lead to profuse vomiting, dehydration, and hypotension, so they must be performed under medical supervision.[75]

Food Protein–Induced Enteropathy

Food protein–induced enteropathy (excluding CD) frequently manifests in the first several months of life with diarrhea (mild-to-moderate steatorrhea in ≈80%) and poor weight gain.[66,76] Symptoms include protracted diarrhea, vomiting in up to two-thirds of patients, failure to thrive, and malabsorption demonstrated by the presence of reducing substances in the stools, increased fecal fat, and abnormal D-xylose absorption. Cow's milk sensitivity is the most frequent cause of this syndrome, but it has also been associated with sensitivities to soy, egg, wheat, rice, chicken, and fish. The diagnosis is established by identifying and excluding the responsible allergen from the diet, which should result in symptom resolution within several days to weeks. On endoscopy, patchy villus atrophy is evident, and biopsy reveals a prominent mononuclear round cell infiltrate and a small number of eosinophils, similar to CD but generally much less extensive. Colitic features like mucus per rectum and gross or microscopic hematochezia are usually absent, but anemia occurs in about 40% of affected infants, and protein loss occurs in most. Complete resolution of the intestinal lesions may require 6–18 months of allergen avoidance. Unlike CD, loss of protein sensitivity and clinical reactivity frequently occurs, but the natural history of this disorder has not been well studied.

Celiac Disease

CD is a more extensive enteropathy leading to malabsorption (see Chapter 109). Total villus atrophy and an extensive cellular infiltrate are associated with sensitivity to gliadin, the alcohol-soluble portion of gluten found in wheat, rye, and barley. CD is strongly associated with human leukocyte antigen-DQ2 (α1*0501, β1*0201), which is present in more than 90% of CD patients.[77] The incidence of CD has been reported as 1 in 141 in the United States[78] and appears to have been increasing in the past decade.[79] The striking increase in CD in Sweden compared with genetically similar Denmark,[80] and the variation in prevalence associated with changes in patterns of gluten feeding in Sweden, strongly implicate environmental factors (e.g., feeding practices) in the cause of this disorder.[81] The intestinal inflammation in CD is precipitated by exposure to gliadin and is associated with increased mucosal activity of tissue transglutaminase (TTG), which deamidates gliadin in an ordered and specific fashion, creating epitopes that bind efficiently to DQ2 and are recognized by T cells.[82]

Initial symptoms may include diarrhea or steatorrhea, abdominal distention and flatulence, weight loss, and occasionally nausea and vomiting. Oral ulcers and other extraintestinal symptoms secondary to malabsorption are not uncommon. Villus atrophy of the small bowel is a characteristic feature of CD patients who are ingesting gluten. IgA antibodies to gluten are present in more than 80% of adults and children with untreated CD.[83] In addition, patients generally have increased IgG antibodies to a variety of foods, presumably the result of increased food antigen absorption. Diagnosis has been dependent on demonstrating biopsy evidence of villus atrophy and an inflammatory infiltrate, resolution of biopsy findings after 6–12 weeks of gluten elimination, and recurrence of biopsy changes following gluten challenge. Revised diagnostic criteria have been proposed that require greater dependency on serologic studies. Quantitation of IgA TTG antibodies may be used for screening in children older than 2 years. Total IgA should also be measured if there is a possibility of IgA deficiency or both IgA- and IgG-based testing may be performed, for example, IgG-deamidated gliadin peptides and IgG TTG.[84] Diagnosis of CD, however, still requires an intestinal biopsy showing clear-cut evidence of villus atrophy while on a gluten-containing diet plus resolution of symptoms on a gluten-free diet, with serologic follow-up showing disappearance of the antibodies to confirm the diagnosis.[85] Once the diagnosis of CD is established, lifelong elimination of gluten-containing foods is necessary to control symptoms and possibly avoid the increased risk of GI malignancy.[85]

Dermatitis Herpetiformis

Dermatitis herpetiformis is a chronic blistering skin disorder associated with a gluten-sensitive enteropathy. It is characterized by a chronic, intensely pruritic, papulovesicular rash symmetrically distributed over the extensor surfaces and buttocks.[86,87] The histology of the intestinal lesion is almost identical to that seen in CD, although villus atrophy and the inflammatory infiltrate are generally milder, and T cell lines isolated from intestinal biopsy specimens of dermatitis herpetiformis patients produce significantly more IL-4 than T cell lines isolated from CD patients.[88] Although many patients have minimal or no GI complaints, small bowel biopsy generally confirms intestinal involvement. Elimination of gluten from the diet generally leads to resolution of skin symptoms and normalization of intestinal findings over several months. Administration of sulfones, the mainstay of therapy, leads to rapid resolution of skin symptoms, but has almost no effect on intestinal symptoms.

Other Gastrointestinal Disorders

Several other GI disorders have been suggested to be caused by food protein hypersensitivity. Ingestion of pasteurized whole cow's milk by infants younger than age 6 months may lead to occult GI blood loss and occasionally to iron deficiency anemia.[89] Substitution of heat-processed infant formula (including cow's milk-derived formulas) for whole cow's milk generally leads to resolution of symptoms within 3 days. GERD in young infants may be the result of food-induced EoE. In a study of 204 infants younger than 1 year of age with GERD (diagnosed by 24-hour esophageal pH testing and esophageal biopsy),[90] 42% were diagnosed with cow's milk-induced reflux by blinded milk challenges. These infants experienced resolution of GERD and normalization of pH studies once cow's milk was eliminated from the diet.[91] Constipation also has been reported to be caused by milk allergy,[92] although the underlying mechanism is unclear. Circumstantial evidence suggests a possible role of food allergy in

IBD (Crohn disease and UC), but convincing evidence of an immunopathogenic role remains to be established.

DIAGNOSIS

The diagnosis of food allergy is a clinical exercise involving a careful history, physical examination, and selective laboratory studies.[4] In some cases, the medical history may be useful in diagnosing food allergy (e.g., acute anaphylaxis after isolated ingestion of peanuts). Fewer than 50% of reported food-allergic reactions, however, can be verified by a double-blind placebo-controlled food challenge. Information useful in establishing that a food-allergic reaction has occurred and in constructing an appropriate oral food challenge includes the following: (1) food presumed to have provoked the reaction; (2) quantity of the suspected food ingested; (3) length of time between ingestion and symptom development; (4) type of symptoms provoked; and (5) whether similar symptoms developed on other occasions when the food was eaten. Although any food may induce an allergic reaction, a few foods are responsible for the vast majority of reactions (Box 11.4).

Fig. 11.2 depicts a standard approach for evaluating and managing adverse food reactions. If an IgE-mediated disorder is suspected, selected skin prick tests or quantification of food-specific IgE antibodies (e.g., ImmunoCAP) followed by an appropriate exclusion diet and blinded food challenge are warranted. Testing should be limited to the food(s) suspected of triggering the reaction because clinically irrelevant results are common and may lead to overly restrictive diets.[93] If a non-IgE-mediated GI hypersensitivity disorder is suspected, laboratory and endoscopic studies (± oral food challenges) are required to arrive at the correct diagnosis (see earlier). Table 11.2 compares the main features of 4 non-IgE-mediated food-allergic disorders. An exclusion diet eliminating all foods suspected by history and/or skin testing (for IgE-mediated disorders) should be conducted for 1–2 weeks in suspected IgE-mediated disorders, food-induced enterocolitis, and benign eosinophilic proctocolitis. Exclusion diets may have to be extended for as long as 12 weeks in other suspected GI hypersensitivity disorders (e.g., food protein–induced enteropathy, EoE, or EG) and may require use of elemental diets (e.g., Vivonex, Neocate, or EleCare) to exclude all antigens. If no improvement is noted and dietary compliance is ensured, it is unlikely food allergy is involved. Before undertaking blinded food challenges (single- or double-blind) in patients with non-IgE-mediated food allergies, suspect foods should be eliminated from the diet for 7–14 days before challenge and even longer if sequelae of the reaction persist for more than 14 days. Prescribing elimination diets, like prescribing medications, may have adverse effects (e.g., malnutrition or eating disorders) and should not be done in the absence of evidence that they are likely to be beneficial.

BOX 11.4 Foods Responsible for Most Immunoglobulin E-Mediated Food Hypersensitivity Disorders in Children*

- Peanuts
- Cow's milk
- Shellfish
- Tree nuts
- Egg
- Fish
- Wheat
- Soy
- Sesame

*Listed in order of overall prevalence.

Adapted from Gupta RS, Warren CM, Smith BM, et al. The public health impact of parent-reported childhood food allergies in the United States. *Pediatrics*. 2018;142(6):e20181235.

PREVENTION

Theories regarding the prevention of IgE-mediated food allergy have changed over the past several decades. In the 1970s it was suggested that premature introduction of cereal grains into the infant diet contributed to a perceived growing incidence of CD. In the 1980s and 1990s expert opinion suggested delayed introduction of allergenic solids might curb a growing incidence of IgE-mediated food allergy; however, the incidence of IgE-mediated food allergies seems to have, in fact, accelerated following this advice. It is likely that a number of factors have contributed to the recent rise in the incidence of food allergy, and several observational studies supported by a prospective, randomized controlled trial have now shown that early introduction of allergen into the diet of infants predisposed to development of allergic disease promotes a tolerogenic response rather than food allergy.[94]

The leading hypothesis surrounding the development of food allergy in infants predisposed to an allergic phenotype has been termed the dual allergen exposure hypothesis.[95] Murine models have shown that application of allergen to inflamed skin before introduction of allergen through the oral route promotes Th2 skewing and sensitization, whereas introduction of allergen to the GI mucosa through oral ingestion early in life promotes a tolerogenic response. Observational studies in humans have also supported findings from these murine experiments and prompted a randomized controlled trial, the LEAP trial (*L*earning *E*arly *A*bout *P*eanut allergy).

In the LEAP trial, infants 4–11 months of age without peanut allergy but with a high risk of developing peanut allergy (i.e., severe eczema and/or egg allergy) were divided into a group with evidence of sensitization to peanut and another without evidence of sensitization to peanut.[86] They were then randomly assigned to peanut avoidance or ingestion of at least 6 g of peanut protein divided into three or more servings per week for 60 months. All children were challenged to peanut at 60 months, and investigators were able to show an 81% reduction in risk of development of peanut allergy in those who ingested at least 6 g of peanut protein per week. The protective response was maintained after 12 months of peanut avoidance for the cohort that ingested peanut.[96] These striking data led to a change in guidelines from the National Institute of Allergy and Infectious Diseases, which recommended the early introduction of peanut but with prior testing to detect IgE-sensitization in infants at highest risk of developing a peanut allergy (severe eczema and/or an egg allergy).[97] However a consensus statement[98] advocates for early introduction (around 6 months; and no earlier than 4 months) of all allergenic foods (peanut, egg, cow's milk, soy, wheat, tree nuts, sesame, fish, and shellfish) irrespective of the risk level of an infant to develop a food allergy. Testing to detect sensitization via a SPT or a specific IgE test is not recommended. However, if directed by family preference, testing for food sensitization is performed, then infants with positive testing should undergo a supervised feeding test to the sensitized food in the allergist's office. Of note, only age-appropriate forms of nuts, and cooked forms of eggs are recommended when introducing these foods in an infant's diet for safety reasons. While introduction of dairy foods (cheese, yogurt) is encouraged, inclusion of direct cow's milk in an infant's diet is not recommended before the age of 12 months for other reasons. It is also important to assess developmental readiness of the infant prior to food introduction and introduce some common complementary foods prior to introduction of the highly allergenic foods.

While data on early introduction of allergenic foods to prevent allergy are most compelling for peanut and hen's egg,[99,100] the

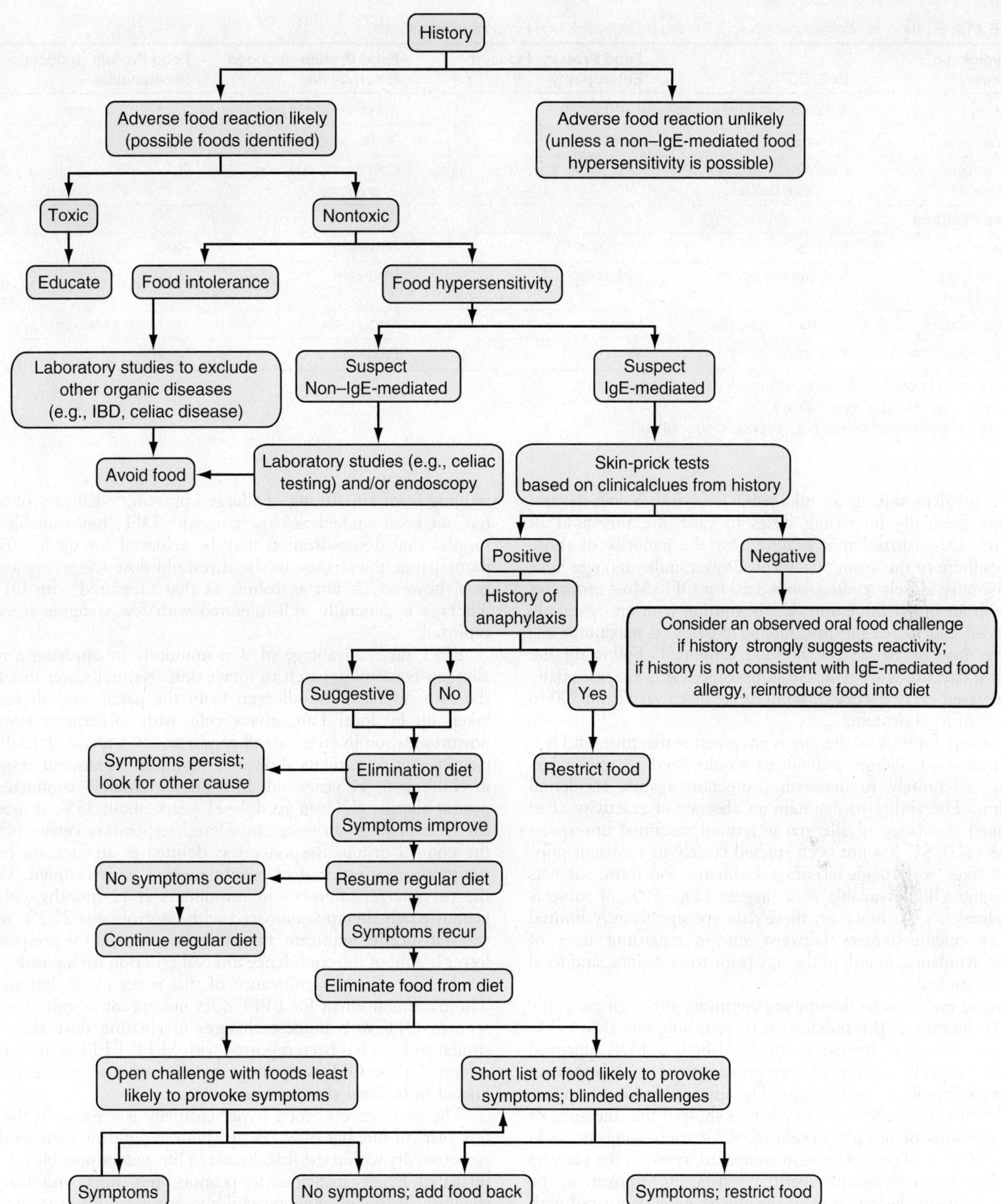

Fig. 11.2 **Algorithm for the evaluation and management of adverse food reactions.** *IgE*, Immunoglobulin E.

consensus statement notes that "there are no data showing harm" in the early introduction of other allergenic foods and therefore, recommends introducing these around 6 months of age.

TREATMENT AND NATURAL HISTORY

Once the diagnosis of food hypersensitivity is established, strict elimination of the offending allergen is the overarching standard of care and the only proved therapy for most foods (except for peanut in certain age groups; details below). Patients must be taught to scrutinize food labels to detect potential sources of hidden food allergens.[4] Drugs like H_1 and H_2 antihistamines and glucocorticoids can modify symptoms to food allergens but may have minimal efficacy or unacceptable side effects. Epinephrine must be available at all times and is required for treatment of anaphylaxis. Various immunotherapeutic approaches are now being studied for the treatment of IgE-mediated food allergies [e.g., oral immunotherapy (OIT), sublingual immunotherapy (SLIT), and epicutaneous immunotherapy (EPIT)].[101]

TABLE 11.2 Features of Nonimmunoglobulin E-Mediated Gastrointestinal Food Hypersensitivities

Epidemiologic Features	EoE, EG	Food Protein–Induced Enteropathy	Food Protein–Induced Enterocolitis	Food Protein–Induced Proctocolitis
Age of onset	1 month and older	1–18 month	2 weeks–9 months	1 week–3 months
Duration	≥1 year	18–36 months	9–36 months	6–18 months
Food proteins implicated	Cow's milk, egg, soy, wheat, barley	Cow's milk, soy, wheat, barley	Cow's milk, soy, rice, and oats	Cow's milk, soy, breast milk[a]
Clinical Features				
Diarrhea	Minimal	Moderate	Severe	Rare
Failure to thrive or weight loss	Moderate-to-severe	Moderate	Moderate	None
Hematochezia	Minimal-to-moderate	Moderate	Moderate	Moderate-to-severe
Vomiting/regurgitation	Prominent[b]	Variable	Prominent	None

[a]Food proteins in breast milk (most often cow's milk or egg protein).
[b]Retching or gastroesophageal reflux.
EG, Eosinophilic gastroenteritis; *EoE*, eosinophilic esophagitis.

OIT involves mixing an allergenic food into a vehicle and ingesting gradually increasing doses to raise the threshold of reactivity. Desensitization is achieved for the majority of those able to adhere to the dosing protocol. Peanut, milk, and egg have been the most closely studied foods used for OIT. Most protocols start with an initial escalation day, beginning with an extremely small dose and increasing in doubling doses to a maximum cumulative dose of 10–25 mg of food protein.[102] Following the escalation day, doses are typically administered at home once daily and increased every 2 weeks. Maintenance doses vary from 300 to 4000 mg of food protein.

The ideal duration of therapy is unknown at this time, and it is likely that most allergic individuals would need to remain on therapy indefinitely to maintain protection against accidental ingestion. The ability to maintain an absence of reactivity after prolonged avoidance of allergen is termed sustained unresponsiveness (SU). SU has not been studied closely in sufficient population sizes to provide accurate estimates for most subjects undergoing OIT. Available data suggest 13%–50% of subjects may achieve SU[102]; however, these data are significantly limited based on inconsistencies between studies regarding time of allergen avoidance, length of therapy prior to avoidance, and food allergens studied.

Adverse reactions to therapy are common, although generally mild. At the time of this publication there is only one U.S. FDA-approved therapy on the market. In 2020, the U.S. FDA approved the use of a specific peanut allergen powder to be used for peanut OIT in patients 4–17 years of age. The approval followed a phase 3 trial[103] in peanut allergic children that showed the tolerance of larger amounts of peanut protein (67% of study subjects could tolerate 600 mg of peanut protein compared to 4% in the placebo group) and lower symptom severity upon peanut exposure at the exit challenge in the group receiving this therapy compared with the control group (moderate symptoms were 25% vs. 59%, and severe symptoms were 5% vs. 11%, respectively, in study versus control groups). There is growing evidence in support of earlier initiation of OIT resulting in potentially improved efficacy and tolerability.[104,105]

SLIT involves placing small amounts of allergen solubilized in a liquid medium under the tongue where it is typically held for 2 minutes and then swallowed. The desensitization approaches studied with SLIT use a similar buildup protocol to those used with OIT with daily dosing and progressively larger doses given every 1–2 weeks. SLIT starting doses are typically in microgram quantities and maintenance doses are typically 100-fold smaller than maintenance doses achieved with OIT, with maximum doses ranging from 1 to 10 mg of allergen protein.[102] Efficacy of SLIT has not been studied as closely as with OIT, but available data suggest that desensitization may be achieved for up to 70% of participants; the change in the threshold dose triggering a reaction, however, is not as robust as that measured with OIT.[102] Therapy is generally well-tolerated with few systemic reactions reported.

EPIT takes advantage of skin immunity by applying a novel allergen-containing patch to intact skin. Natural water loss from the skin displaces the allergen from the patch, and allergen is taken up by local Langerhans cells with subsequent systemic downregulation in effector cell responses.[102] A phase 2b trial[106] in peanut-allergic patients showed a significant treatment response in children 6–11 years old. In a phase 3 trial,[107] conducted on peanut allergic children aged 4–11 years, about 35% of those in the treatment group were considered responders versus 14% in the control group. Response was defined as an increase in the symptom eliciting dose of peanut protein posttreatment. While the percentage difference in responders at 12 months with the peanut-patch therapy compared with controls was 21.7% which was statistically significant, the study did not meet the prespecified lower bound of the confidence interval criterion for a positive trial result. The clinical significance of this is yet to be determined. The treatment effect for EPIT does not appear as robust as that seen in OIT with modest changes in eliciting dose threshold, similar to what has been reported with SLIT. EPIT is more easily tolerated than OIT with the most common adverse event reported to be local skin reactions.

The prevalence of food hypersensitivity is greatest in the first few years of life, but most young children outgrow their food hypersensitivity within the first decade of life, except possibly for IgE-mediated hypersensitivities to peanuts, tree nuts, and fish and shellfish.[4] Although younger children are more likely to outgrow food hypersensitivity, older children and adults may also lose their food hypersensitivity (i.e., develop clinical tolerance and be able to ingest the food without symptoms) if the responsible food allergen can be identified and eliminated from the diet for a period of time.[14]

Current research in this field is providing new information regarding the pathogenesis of these disorders and should lead to development of new diagnostic and therapeutic algorithms. In the interim, specific food hypersensitivities must be diagnosed carefully, and patients must be educated to avoid ingesting the responsible food allergens.

Full references for this chapter can be found at ebooks.health.elsevier.com.

PART III Symptoms and Signs

12 Acute Abdominal Pain

Frederick H. Millham

IN THIS CHAPTER

Abdominal pain is a ubiquitous problem. It is estimated that as many as a quarter of all adults suffer from intermittent abdominal pain.[1] Acute abdominal pain is among the most frequent complaints that cause patients to visit an emergency department. In 2019, of 150 million emergency department visits in the United States, 13.1 million were due to abdominal pain, accounting for 9% of all emergency department visits that year.[2] As many as 40% of these patients have nonspecific findings.[3] Of the remainder for whom a specific diagnosis is ascertainable, most are found to have surgical disorders that warrant further evaluation and intervention.[3] In a small number, life-threatening pathologies are present. However, the peculiarities of nociception in the human gut can make distinguishing life-threatening disease from more banal pathology a challenge in real time. Moreover, the ongoing COVID-19 pandemic appears to have had an impact on the incidence of acute abdominal pain. Whereas during the first pandemic surge, at least, overall emergency department visits for acute abdominal pain may have decreased,[4,5] due primarily to a drop in admissions for nonspecific abdominal pain, it appears that the virus can, itself, cause abdominal pain,[6,7] and in some cases COVID-related abdominal pain may be a marker of severe disease.[8] Therefore, in the post-COVID world, it is more important than ever that acute abdominal pain be seriously and efficiently evaluated. Accurate diagnosis as soon as possible after presentation is critical so that the treatment of patients who are seriously ill is not delayed and resources are not overutilized on patients with a self-limited disorder. Evaluation must also account for changing presentation over time. It is not uncommon for life-threatening pathology to present with abdominal findings that evolve from reassuring to distressing over time. The evaluation of acute abdominal pain, therefore, must not only be nuanced but also ongoing.

ANATOMY AND PHYSIOLOGY OF ABDOMINAL NOCICEPTION

A little over 100 years ago, in a slim tome entitled *Early Diagnosis of the Acute Abdomen*, a work still popular today in its 22nd edition, British surgeon Zachary Cope stressed the importance of understanding the anatomy, embryology, and physiology of the GI tract to enable accurate diagnosis of diseases presenting with abdominal pain.[9] Despite the development of panels of laboratory tests and sophisticated axial imaging, this advice remains true a century later.

The unique neuroanatomy of the abdominal viscera contributes to three distinct types of pain: visceral, somatic-parietal, and referred. Visceral pain is usually vague in both onset and localization and perceived as a dull sensation in the abdominal midline. Somatic-parietal pain is more intense, sharp, and well localized. Referred pain is perceived at a point distant from the inciting pathology and may be perceived to be outside the abdomen entirely. Following Cope's advice, we can see how the anatomy, embryology, and physiology of the GI tract and its innervation can inform our understanding of abdominal pain.

Despite the fact that the abdominal contents (as well as those of the thorax and pelvis) are not primarily represented on the sensory homunculus of the parietal lobe of the brain, we are able to perceive and usually localize noxious stimuli from these areas.[10] Understanding the pathways pain signals take to get to the brain and how they originate is essential to understanding abdominal pain. Over the past decades, significant progress has been made in the understanding of the neuroanatomy underlying syndromes causing abdominal pain.[1,11]

The Enteric Nervous System

The GI tract has its own intrinsic "nervous system," the enteric nervous system (ENS), comprising an intricate and poorly understood network of interconnected neurons, glial cells, and ganglia in the submucosal plexus (Meissner's plexus) and intramuscular myenteric plexus (Auerbach's plexus). The ENS can function autonomously.[12] It employs a large menu of neurotransmitters exchanged among a diverse population of neurons.[13] It controls and coordinates peristaltic contraction, blood flow, and glandular secretion[1] (Fig. 12.1). While it is not, at present, thought to transduce painful stimuli, the ENS interacts with, and modulates the output of, sensory afferent fibers of the central nervous system, which are responsible for pain.[1,11] Similarly, crosstalk among visceral sensory afferent nerves and elements of the ENS is well documented.[14] The ENS participates in neuronal inflammation via complex interactions with neuroglial cells and enteric nerve endings.[15] In addition to its role in control of local GI function, the ENS also appears to interact with the gut microbiome.[16] These interactions may modulate pain signaling from the gut, including in the setting of irritable bowel syndrome and other cases of acute and chronic abdominal pain. Intriguingly, it is possible that the development and health of the ENS itself depend upon the development and health of the gut microbiome.[17,18]

While the ENS is increasingly recognized for its role in modulation of the perception of abdominal pain (nociception), the central nervous system transduces, transmits, and brings to conscious perception the nociceptive stimuli arising in the GI tract.

Visceral Sensory Innervation of the Gastrointestinal Tract

To understand the unique characteristics of the central innervation of the gut, we must start with its embryology. The gut develops as a midline structure and begins receiving innervation at the fourth to fifth week of gestation.[19] As a midline structure, afferent fibers from any given section of the GI tract enter the spinal cord bilaterally. This innervation is completed by the seventh to eighth week while the GI tract elongates. During this period, the developing GI tract is entirely herniated in the extraperitoneal yolk sac.[20] The gut returns to the peritoneal cavity and rotates to its final configuration at Week 10. Due to the timing of the gut afferent innervation, by the time of its internalization and rotation, the gut's sensory innervation has already been "plugged into" the CNS as a midline structure from top to bottom (see Fig. 12.1).

The histology of the visceral afferent nerves is also relevant to the understanding of visceral pain. There are three classes of human sensory nerves, based on conduction velocity, which is itself a function of fiber size and degree of myelination.[21] The nerves innervating the gut are smaller and more primitive than those innervating the skin and soft tissues. These visceral nerves are of two types: thin and unmyelinated C fibers, which transmit at 0.2–2 m/s, and slightly larger, thinly myelinated Aδ fibers, which conduct impulses at 5–30 m/s. Somatic sensory nerves, involved in skin touch sensation, are Aβ, large, and heavily myelinated. These fibers conduct impulses at 16–100 m/s.[21] These high-speed fibers of the somatic nervous system are not typically found innervating the GI tract, though recently Aβ nerve fibers have been found innervating the mesentery. Despite this new finding, it is generally true that visceral innervation derives from fine, relatively slowly conducting, unmyelinated, or lightly myelinated fibers (Fig. 12.2). They are also much fewer in number, meaning that not only are the signals slowly transmitted but each nerve also covers a relatively large area, resulting in poor discrimination.

These visceral afferent nerves innervate the GI tract by two pathways (Fig. 12.3). The first, associated with the parasympathetic innervation of the abdomen, is based on the vagus nerve, which innervates most of the foregut and midgut, and the pelvic parasympathetic plexus, which innervates the rectum and lower genitourinary tract.[22] Though we think of the vagus as a motor neuron, as many as 80% of human vagal fibers are afferent, having their cell bodies in the nodose ganglia or the jugular ganglia.[11]

The second pathway of abdominal visceral innervation is via spinal somatic afferents. In the past, these nerves have been described as "sympathetic" because their fibers travel along with sympathetic efferent nerves originating from the sympathetic ganglia. However, these nerves have their cell bodies in the dorsal root ganglia, like the somatic sensory afferents; therefore it is more appropriate to refer to these fibers as spinal visceral afferent nerves.[11]

Much of the vexing nature of visceral pain is explained by the anatomy of spinal visceral afferent nerves. As described above, spinal visceral afferent nerves for any given location often arise from either of the bilateral dorsal root ganglia. Just as the brain interprets stereo sound that is equal in each ear as midline, so too are pain signals arriving to both sides of the spinal cord are interpreted as coming from the midline. Additionally only 5%–15% of sensory afferent fibers entering the spinal cord arise in the viscera.[11] Relative to the somatic afferent nerves, there are very few visceral afferent nerves that cover at least as much territory. This relative paucity of nerve fibers per unit of tissue contributes to the poor geographic discrimination of visceral pain by the CNS.

Neuroanatomy of Referred Pain

Axons of spinal afferent fibers may also innervate different organs. This is known to be particularly true in the case of the lower colon and bladder as well as the colon and uterus.[23,24] This phenomenon, known as "dichotomization," may further add to poor discrimination and perhaps organ-to-organ pain referral.[11] The degree to which dichotomization contributes to referred pain remains a matter of debate.

Better understood is the mechanism behind referral of pain from the viscera to seemingly distant somatic dermatomes. First proposed by Ruch, in 1947, as "convergence-projection," second-order spinal afferent nerve fibers (spinothalmic tract) frequently receive input from visceral and somatic fibers often innervating structures that were adjacent embryologically but end up widely separated in the fully developed individual.[25] Common clinical examples of convergence are seen in Kehr's sign, where patients with splenic rupture experience sudden, severe, pain in the left shoulder.[26,27] In this case, the visceral afferent fibers of the left hemidiaphragm and somatic afferents from the left shoulder converge upon second-order spinothalamic tract nerves assigned to the sixth cervical dermatome (Fig. 12.4). Another example is the common presentation of pain caused by biliary colic masquerading as angina pectoris. In this case, two sets of spinal afferent nerves are convergent on a common second order spinothalamic tract neuron in the thoracic spinal cord. Atypical anginal pain referred to the jaw and neck likely results from convergence of vagal afferent nerves with somatic afferents arising from the second cervical spinal segment via intermediary pathways in the nucleus of the solitary tract.[28]

Understanding the wiring diagram of the ENS and the visceral afferent nervous systems gives us some understanding of abdominal pain, but it is insufficient. To gain the most complete understanding, we must understand gut receptors and their signaling. There has been, perhaps, no area of visceral pain research where more progress has been made over the past decade than gut receptor biology.[11] Researchers have defined as many as 13 different types of nerve endings or receptors in the GI tract.[29] There are four functional groups of receptors, within which are specialized structures, whose function is a matter of current research. Visceral nerve endings can be functionally grouped into

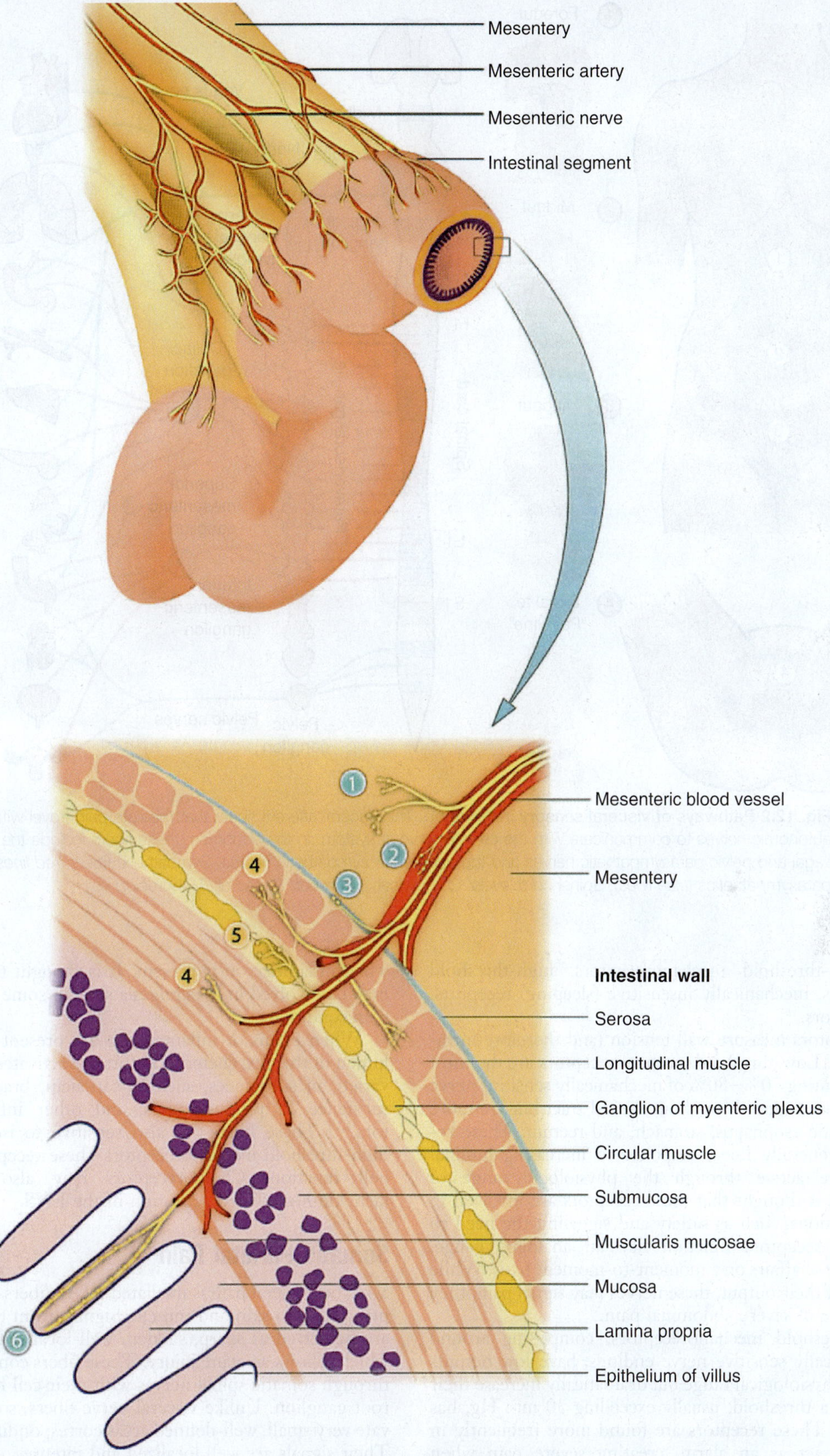

Fig. 12.1 Sensory innervation of the GI tract. The distribution of afferent sensory nerve endings in the intestinal wall is shown, as follows: (1) mesenteric blood vessels, (2) mesentery, (3) serosa, (4) intramuscular arrays (vagus nerves only), (5) intraganglionic laminar endings (vagus and pelvic nerves only), (6) mucosa. The principal contributors to nociception are 1, 2, 3, and 6. (Modified from Knowles CH, Aziz Q. Basic and clinical aspects of gastrointestinal pain. *Pain*. 2009;141:191-209.)

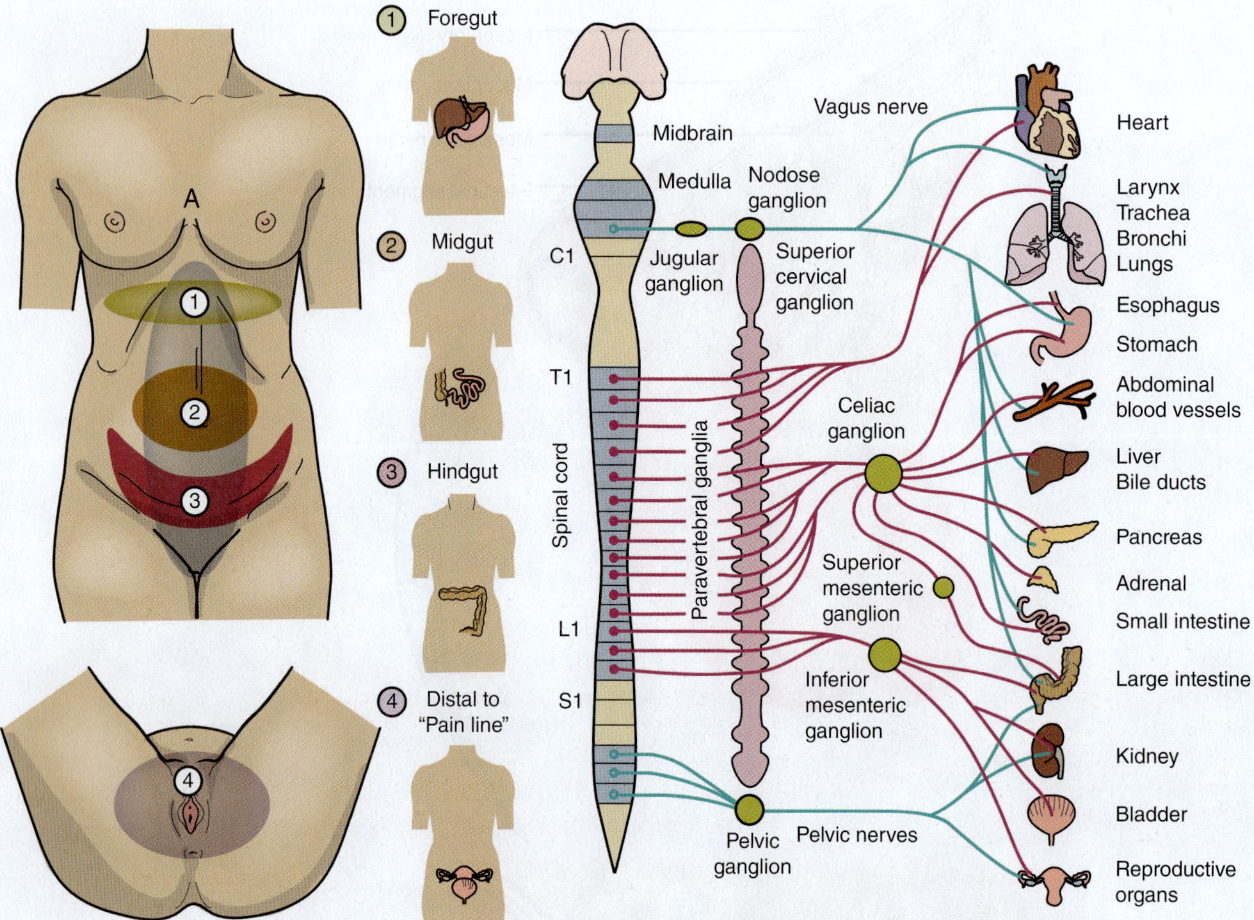

Fig. 12.2 Pathways of visceral sensory innervation. The visceral afferent fibers that mediate pain travel with autonomic nerves to communicate with the central nervous system. In the abdomen, these fibers include the vagal and pelvic parasympathetic nerves and thoracolumbar sympathetic nerves. Sympathetic fibers (*red lines*); parasympathetics (*blue lines*). Spinal cord levels: *C*, Cervical; *L*, lumbar; *S*, sacral; *T*, thoracic.

four types: low-threshold mechanoreceptors, high-threshold mechanoreceptors, mechanically insensitive (sleeping) receptors, and chemoreceptors.

Mechanoreceptors measure wall tension (and therefore intraluminal pressure). Low-threshold mechanoreceptors are the most common, representing 70%–80% of mechanically sensitive nerve endings.[11] They are found throughout the GI tract but are more concentrated in the esophagus, stomach, and rectum. These receptors have a generally linear response to increasing luminal pressure and are active through the physiologic range of 0–30 mm Hg. It is thought that these receptors are involved in routine GI sensations, such as satiety and signaling the need to defecate. These receptors function like an analogue gauge, signaling the state of affairs on a moment-to-moment basis. While at the high end of their output, these nerves may signal pain, they are not the source of severe abdominal pain.

The high-threshold mechanoreceptors, comprising around 20% of mechanically sensitive nerve endings, have low outputs throughout the physiological range but dramatically increase their firing rate when a threshold, usually exceeding 30 mm Hg, has been exceeded.[11] These receptors are found more frequently in the midgut and act as an alarm, creating severe pain when abnormally high intraluminal pressures are present.

The third type of mechanoreceptor is the mechanically-insensitive or "sleeping" receptor. These structures have no signal output under normal conditions but gain mechano-sensitivity when inflammation is present. It is thought that these receptors may be involved in hyperalgesia seen in some chronic abdominal pain conditions.[11]

When toxins or inflammation are present within the wall or lumen of the gut, chemoreceptors are activated. There are a wide variety of substances, such as capsaicin, bradykinin, histamine, substance P, prostaglandins, and other inflammatory mediators.[1,14] These fibers are also sensitive to ischemia.[11] Like the high-threshold mechanoreceptors, these receptors have an alarm bell function. Chemoreceptors may also be involved in tachykinin-mediated activation of the ENS.

Somatic-Parietal Pain

Somatic-parietal pain is mediated by Aδ fibers that are distributed principally to skin and muscle. Signals from this neural pathway are perceived as sharp, sudden, well-localized pain, such as that which follows an acute injury. These fibers convey pain sensations through somatic spinal nerves with their cell bodies in the dorsal root ganglion. Unlike visceral nerve fibers, somatic fibers innervate very small, well-defined areas corresponding to a dermatome. Their signals are well localized and intense.

Somatic-parietal pain arising from noxious stimulation of the parietal peritoneum is more intense and more precisely localized than visceral pain. An example of this difference occurs in acute appendicitis, in which early vague periumbilical visceral pain

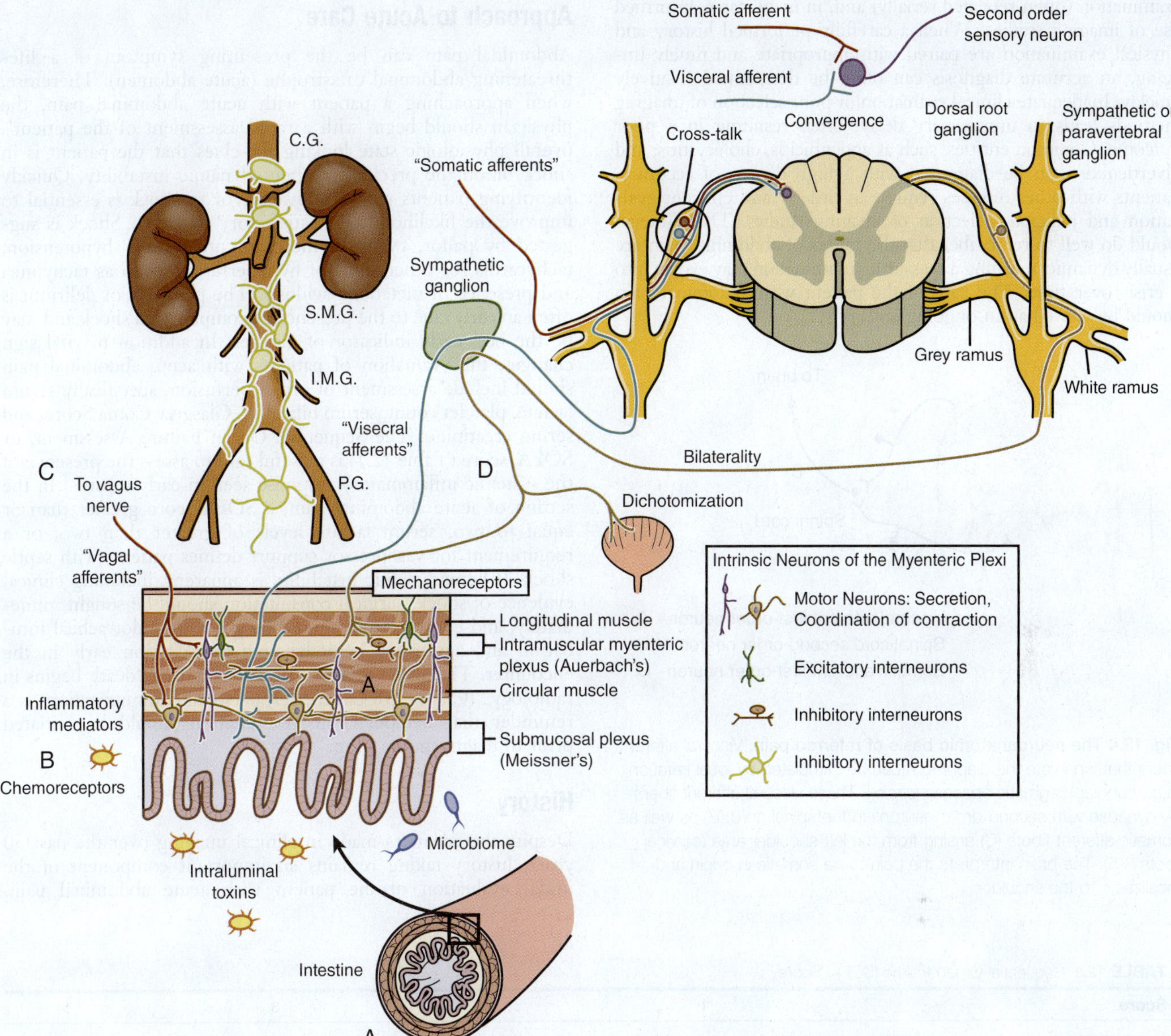

Fig. 12.3 Localization of visceral pain. Pain arising from organ areas depicted in 1, 2, and 3 is felt in the epigastrium, midabdomen, and hypogastrium, respectively, as shown in (A). The *arrow* in (A) indicates biliary pain that is referred to the right scapular area.

originating within the appendix is followed by localized somatic-parietal pain at McBurney's point that is produced by inflammatory involvement of the parietal peritoneum adjacent to the appendix. Somatic-parietal abdominal pain is usually aggravated by movement or vibration. It is this characteristic that results in the finding of rebound tenderness, characteristic of peritonitis. The nerve impulses that mediate such pain travel in somatic sensory spinal nerves that correspond to the cutaneous dermatomes of the skin from the sixth thoracic (T6) to first lumbar (L1) vertebral segment. Because these nerve fibers do not cross the midline at the spinal cord, lateralization of parietal pain is much more precise than in visceral pain.

Reflexive responses (e.g., involuntary guarding, abdominal rigidity) are mediated by spinal reflex arcs involving somatic-parietal pain pathways. Afferent pain impulses are modified by inhibitory mechanisms at the level of the spinal cord. Somatic Aδ fibers mediate touch, vibration, and proprioception in a dermatomal distribution that matches the visceral innervation of the injured viscera and synapse with inhibitory interneurons of the substantia gelatinosa in the spinal cord. In addition, inhibitory neurons that originate in the mesencephalon, periventricular gray matter, and caudate nucleus descend within the spinal cord to modulate afferent pain pathways. These inhibitory mechanisms allow cerebral influences to modify afferent pain impulses.[30] The experience or awareness of pain can be modified through a process known as attentional analgesia.[31] This phenomenon may explain the common situation, best expressed by Cope—the "curious and widely known fact that many who are taken with abdominal pain in the daytime, endure until evening before they feel compelled to send for the doctor"[9] (see Chapter 13).

EVALUATION

Effective evaluation of any patient with acute abdominal pain requires careful but expeditious history taking and physical examination (often repeated serially) and, in many cases, informed use of imaging studies. When a carefully performed history and physical examination are paired with appropriate and timely imaging, an accurate diagnosis can often be determined relatively quickly. Inadequate clinical evaluation or poor selection of imaging methods leads to unnecessary delay, often resulting in a poor outcome. Common entities, such as appendicitis, cholecystitis, and diverticulitis, can be diagnosed with a high degree of accuracy; patients with other diseases require an orderly and efficient evaluation and judicious selection of imaging studies. The clinician would do well to remember that the causes of abdominal pain are usually dynamic, meaning a reassuring examination may evolve into a crisis over time. The care of the patient with abdominal pain should be viewed as an ongoing enterprise.

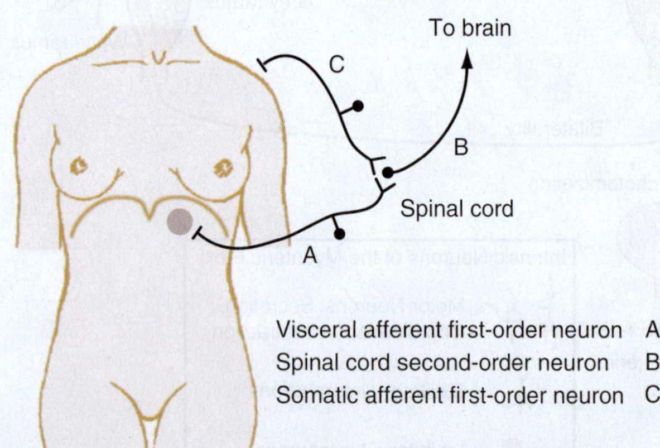

Fig. 12.4 The neuroanatomic basis of referred pain. Visceral afferent fibers that innervate the diaphragm can be stimulated by local irritation [e.g., subdiaphragmatic abscess (*circle*)]. These visceral afferent fibers (A) synapse with second-order neurons in the spinal cord (B) as well as somatic afferent fibers (C) arising from the left shoulder area (cervical roots 3-5). The brain interprets the pain to be somatic in origin and localizes it to the shoulder.

Approach to Acute Care

Abdominal pain can be the presenting symptom of a life-threatening abdominal catastrophe (acute abdomen). Therefore, when approaching a patient with acute abdominal pain, the physician should begin with a rapid assessment of the patient's overall physiologic state looking for clues that the patient is in shock or on the precipice of hemodynamic instability. Quickly identifying patients who are unstable or in shock is essential to improve the likelihood of a satisfactory outcome. Shock is suggested by pallor, cyanosis, mottling, prostration, hypotension, tachycardia, or other signs of hypoperfusion, such as tachypnea and presence of metabolic acidosis. The presence of delirium is often an early clue to the presence of compensated shock and may be the best early indicator of disaster. In addition to vital sign changes, the evaluation of patients with acute abdominal pain should include assessment of organ perfusion, specifically serum lactate, platelet count, serum bilirubin, Glasgow Coma Score, and serum creatinine. The Sequential Organ Failure Assessment, or SOFA, score (Table 12.1) is a useful tool to assess the presence of the systemic inflammatory response seen in early sepsis.[32] In the setting of acute abdominal pain, a SOFA score greater than or equal to two, serum lactate levels of greater than two, or a requirement for vasopressor support defines patients with septic shock. If hemodynamic instability is apparent, including clinical evidence of shock, surgical consultation should be sought immediately, and consideration should be given to endotracheal intubation and aggressive hemodynamic resuscitation early in the encounter. The adage in acute care surgery that "death begins in radiology" (Charlie McCabe, MD, personal communication) is a reminder that hemodynamic resuscitation should be initiated prior to diagnostic imaging.

History

Despite the advances made in clinical imaging over the past 50 years, history taking remains an important component of the initial evaluation of the patient with acute abdominal pain.

TABLE 12.1 Sequential Organ Failure (SOFA) Score

Score		1	2	3	4
Organ system	Units				
Respiratory					
PaO_2/FiO_2	mm Hg	<400	<300	<200[a]	<100[a]
Coagulation					
Platelets	000/mm^3	<150	<100	<50	<20
Liver					
Bilirubin	mg/dL	1.2–1.9	2.0–5.9	6.0–11.9	≥12
	µmol/L	20–32	33–101	102–204	>204
CNS					
Glasgow coma scale		13–14	10–12	6–9	<6
Renal					
Creatinine	mg/dL	1.2–1.9	2.0–3.4	3.5–4.9	>5
	µmol/L	110–170	171–299	300–440	>440
Urine output	mL/day	–	–	<500	<200

[a]Or requiring respiratory support.

SOFA score = sum of individual Organ System scores. Sepsis should be suspected if the SOFA score is greater than 2 in the setting of acute abdominal pain. Septic shock is defined as a SOFA score greater than 2 and serum lactate level greater than 2 mmol/L or if a vasopressor is required in the setting of infection.

Adapted From Singer M, Deutschman CS, Seymour CW, et al. The third international consensus definitions for sepsis and septic shock (Sepsis-3). *JAMA*. 2016;315:801–810.

TABLE 12.2 Comparison of Common Causes of Acute Abdominal Pain

Cause	Onset	Location	Character	Descriptor	Radiation	Intensity
Appendicitis	Gradual	Periumbilical area early; RLQ late	Diffuse early; localized later	Aching	None	++
Cholecystitis	Acute	Mid-epigastrium, RUQ, right scapula	Localized	Constricting	Scapula	++
Pancreatitis	Acute	Epigastrium, T10-L2 area of the back	Localized	Boring	Midback	++ to +++
Diverticulitis	Gradual	LLQ	Localized	Aching	None	++ to +++
Perforated peptic ulcer	Sudden	Epigastrium	Localized early, diffuse later	Burning	None	+++
SBO	Gradual	Periumbilical area	Diffuse	Cramping	None	++
Mesenteric ischemia, infarction	Sudden	Periumbilical area	Diffuse	Agonizing	None	+++
Ruptured abdominal aortic aneurysm	Sudden	Abdomen, back, flank	Diffuse	Tearing	None	+++
Gastroenteritis	Gradual	Periumbilical area	Diffuse	Spasmodic	None	+ to ++
Pelvic inflammatory disease	Gradual	Either LQ, pelvis	Localized	Aching	Upper thigh	++
Ruptured ectopic pregnancy	Sudden	Either LQ, pelvis	Localized	Sharp	None	++

+, mild; ++, moderate; +++, severe; *LQ*, Lower quadrant; *SBO*, small bowel obstruction.

Characteristic features of pain associated with various common causes of acute abdominal pain are shown in Table 12.2. Attention to these features can lead to a rapid clinical diagnosis or exclusion of important diseases in the differential, thereby enhancing the reliability and effectiveness of subsequent diagnostic testing.

Chronology

The time courses of several common causes of acute abdominal pain are diagrammed in Fig. 12.5. The rapidity of onset of pain is often a measure of the severity of the underlying disorder. Pain that is sudden in onset, severe, and generalized is likely to be the result of an intra-abdominal catastrophe, such as a perforated viscus, mesenteric infarction, or ruptured aneurysm. Affected patients usually recall the exact moment of onset of their pain. Progression is an important temporal factor in abdominal pain. In some disorders (e.g., gastroenteritis), pain is self-limited, whereas in others (e.g., appendicitis), pain is progressive. Pain associated with obstruction has a repeating crescendo-decrescendo pattern that may be diagnostic, particularly when it occurs in association with nausea and vomiting. The duration of abdominal pain is also important. Patients who seek evaluation of abdominal pain that has been present for an extended period (e.g., weeks) are less likely to have an acute life-threatening illness than patients who present within hours to days of the onset of their symptoms.

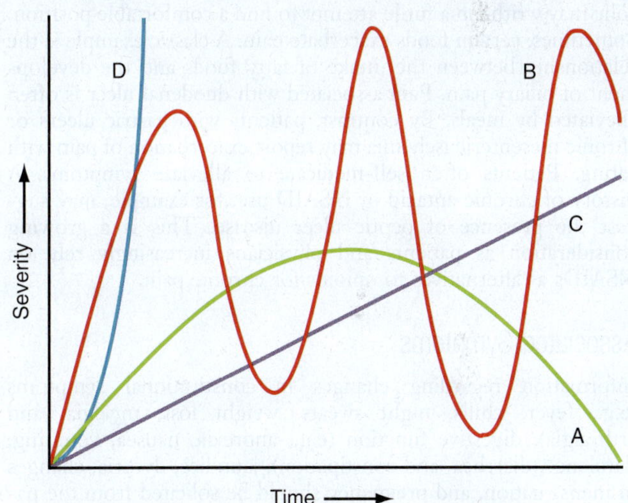

Fig. 12.5 Patterns of acute abdominal pain. (A) Many causes of abdominal pain subside spontaneously with time (e.g., gastroenteritis). (B) Some pain is colicky (i.e., the pain progresses and remits over time); examples include intestinal, renal, and biliary pain (colic). The time course may vary widely from minutes in intestinal and renal pain to days, weeks, or even months in biliary pain. (C) Commonly, acute abdominal pain is progressive, as in acute appendicitis or diverticulitis. (D) Certain conditions have a catastrophic onset, such as a ruptured abdominal aortic aneurysm (AAA).

Location

The location of abdominal pain provides a clue to interpreting the cause. As noted earlier, a given noxious stimulus may result in a combination of visceral, somatic-parietal, and referred pain, thereby creating confusion in interpretation unless the neuroanatomic pathways are considered. For example, the pain of diaphragmatic irritation from a left-sided subphrenic abscess may be referred to the shoulder and misinterpreted as pain from ischemic heart disease (Fig. 12.4). Pain radiating to the back from pancreatic or biliary pathology may be conflated with musculoskeletal processes, thereby delaying treatment. Changes in location may represent progression from visceral to localized parietal peritoneal irritation, as with appendicitis, or represent the development of diffuse peritoneal irritation, as with a perforated ulcer.

Intensity and Character

Acute abdominal pain usually follows one of three patterns. Pain that is prostrating, and physically incapacitates the sufferer is usually due to a severe life-threatening disease, such as a perforated viscus, ruptured aneurysm, or severe pancreatitis. In this situation, somatic-parietal pain is the driving theme. By contrast, patients with obstruction of a hollow viscus, as in intestinal obstruction, renal colic, or biliary pain, present with gradual onset of cramping pain that follows a sinusoidal pattern of intense pain alternating with periods of relief, suggesting periodic stimulation of high-threshold mechanoreceptors, with intervals of quiet. Nausea and vomiting are characteristic symptoms associated with this group of disorders; its presence should always suggest the obstruction of a smooth muscle-lined structure. The obstructed viscus need not be the intestine for nausea or vomiting to occur, as with obstructing ureteral stones. The third pattern is of gradually increasing discomfort, usually vague and poorly localized at the start but becoming more localized as the pain intensifies. This picture is usually due to inflammation, beginning with signals from visceral chemoreceptors, followed by somatic-parietal pain from parietal peritoneal inflammation, as with acute appendicitis or diverticulitis. Some disorders, such as acute cholecystitis, may start out as colicky pain but evolve into a constant pain as cystic duct obstruction leads to gallbladder inflammation and eventual irritation of the adjacent parietal peritoneum. The clinician should be cautious in assigning too much importance to a patient's description of the pain; exceptions are common, and a given descriptor may be attributable to several conditions. Symptoms in the elderly can be subtle despite the presence of life-threatening pathology, making this group particularly challenging.

Aggravating and Alleviating Factors

The relationship of pain to positional changes, meals, bowel movements, and stress may yield important diagnostic clues. Patients with peritonitis lie motionless, whereas those with renal colic may writhe in a futile attempt to find a comfortable position. Sometimes, certain foods exacerbate pain. A classic example is the relationship between the intake of fatty foods and the development of biliary pain. Pain associated with duodenal ulcer is often alleviated by meals. By contrast, patients with gastric ulcers or chronic mesenteric ischemia may report exacerbation of pain with eating. Patients often self-medicate to alleviate symptoms. A history of chronic antacid or NSAID use, for example, may suggest the presence of peptic ulcer disease. This is a growing consideration as patients and physicians increasingly rely on NSAIDs as alternatives to opioids for chronic pain.

Associated Symptoms

Information regarding changes in constitutional symptoms (e.g., fever, chills, night sweats, weight loss, myalgia, and arthralgia), digestive function (e.g., anorexia, nausea, vomiting, flatulence, diarrhea, and constipation), jaundice, dysuria, changes in menstruation, and pregnancy should be solicited from the patient. A careful review of these symptoms may reveal important diagnostic information. Clear vomitus suggests gastric outlet obstruction, whereas feculent vomitus suggests more distal small bowel or colonic obstruction. A constellation of findings may indicate a particular disease entity.

Past Medical History

A careful review of the patient's other medical problems often sheds light on the presentation of acute abdominal pain. Previous experience with similar symptoms suggests a recurrent problem. Patients with a history of partial small bowel obstruction (SBO), renal calculi, or pelvic inflammatory disease are likely to have recurrences. A patient whose presentation suggests intestinal obstruction, and who has no prior surgical history, deserves special attention because of the likelihood of surgical pathology, such as a hernia or neoplasm. Patients with a systemic illness, such as scleroderma, systemic lupus erythematosus (SLE), nephrotic syndrome, porphyria, or sickle cell disease, often have abdominal pain as a manifestation of the underlying disorder. Abdominal pain may also arise as a side effect of a medication taken for another disease.

Physical Examination

The physical examination of the patient with acute abdominal pain begins with an assessment of the patient's appearance and assessment for signs of delirium, sepsis, or shock, as described earlier. The patient's ability to converse, breathing pattern, position in bed, posture, degree of discomfort, and facial expression should be noted. A patient lying still in bed in the fetal position and reluctant to move or speak, with a distressed facial expression, is likely to have peritonitis. A patient who writhes and frequently changes position has purely visceral pain, as in intestinal obstruction or gastroenteritis. Tachypnea may be a sign of metabolic acidosis caused by shock. Atrial fibrillation noted on physical examination or an electrocardiogram may suggest mesenteric arterial embolus. All patients should undergo a careful systematic examination regardless of the differential diagnosis suggested by the history.

Abdominal Examination

Examination of the abdomen is central to evaluating a patient with acute abdominal pain and should begin with careful inspection. The entire abdomen, from the nipple line to the thighs, should be exposed. Obese patients should be asked whether the degree of protrusion of the abdominal wall is greater than usual. Asthenic patients may feel themselves to be distended but have relatively little apparent abdominal protrusion. Assessment for the presence of bowel sounds and their character should precede any maneuvers that will disturb the abdominal contents. Before concluding that an abdomen is silent, the examiner should listen for at least 2 minutes and in more than one quadrant of the abdomen. Experienced listeners may distinguish the high-pitched churning of a mechanical SBO from the hollow sounds of toxic megacolon (like dripping in a cavern). Nevertheless, some studies have cast doubt on the reliability of bowel sound assessment in patients with SBO and other conditions, as well as whether bowel sounds are even a reliable measure of intestinal peristalsis. Clinicians should avoid basing clinical decisions too heavily on assessment of bowel sounds.[33,34] Auscultation may, however, be a good way to assess tenderness. When listening with the stethoscope, the astute clinician may begin to palpate the abdomen with the head of the stethoscope while carefully watching the patient's facial expression. If tenderness is detected, an assessment for rebound tenderness should be carried out next to look for evidence of peritonitis. Rebound tenderness may be elicited by jarring the patient's bed or stretcher or by finger percussion. Palpation is performed next. If pain is emanating from one particular region, that area should be palpated last to detect involuntary guarding and muscular rigidity. Patients with a rigid abdomen rarely reveal any additional findings (e.g., a mass) on physical examination. Because these patients usually have a surgical emergency, abdominal examination should be done more completely once the patient is under anesthesia, just before laparotomy. In some cases, this practice can help with the planning of incisions.

Genital, Rectal, and Pelvic Examinations

The pelvic organs and external genitalia may be examined in patients with acute abdominal pain. The rectum and vagina provide additional avenues for a gentle palpation of pelvic viscera. Gynecologic pathology should be excluded in all women with acute abdominal pain. In the crowded post-COVID emergency department, such examination may be impractical.

Laboratory Data

The history and physical examination findings generally are not sufficient to establish a firm diagnosis in a patient with acute abdominal pain. All patients with acute abdominal pain should have a CBC, with a differential count, and urinalysis. Determination of serum electrolyte, blood urea nitrogen, creatinine, and glucose levels is useful for assessing the patient's fluid and acid-base status, renal function, and metabolic state and should be done for every patient with acute abdominal pain who presents to an emergency department. Urine or serum pregnancy testing must be performed in all women of reproductive age with abdominal pain. Liver biochemical tests and serum amylase or lipase levels should be ordered for patients with upper abdominal pain or with jaundice.

Leukocytosis, particularly when associated with band forms, is an important finding. Metabolic acidosis, an elevated serum lactate level, or depressed bicarbonate levels are associated with tissue hypoperfusion and shock. Patients who manifest these findings are likely to require urgent surgical intervention or intensive care.

Imaging Studies

CT

The development of high-speed helical CT has revolutionized the evaluation of acute abdominal pain. In many conditions, such as appendicitis, CT can almost eliminate diagnostic uncertainty. In the pre-CT era, history taking and physical examination alone had a specificity of approximately 80%; by contrast, the sensitivity and specificity of CT for acute appendicitis are 94% and 95%, respectively. A negative CT in the setting of acute abdominal pain has considerable value in excluding common disorders.

Although arguments against routine CT have been raised.[35] CT imaging has become an increasing part of the evaluation in all patients with acute abdominal pain.[36] Advances in technology have improved the quality of axial imaging while reducing exposure to ionizing radiation.[37] In a study undertaken in real time, Pandharipande et al. showed that in the evaluation of abdominal pain, axial imaging resulted in a change in diagnosis in approximately 50% of cases.[38] CT can be performed in a number of ways, and the most efficacious method must be chosen in any given clinical setting. For example, a patient with suspected renal colic should have a limited, noncontrast-enhanced, and renal calculus protocol CT; obtaining a standard oral and IV contrast CT, in this case, may obfuscate rather than illuminate the pathology. Alternatively, a patient in whom arterial occlusive disease is suspected should undergo CT arteriography using a bolus IV contrast technique. A radiologist should be consulted regarding the selection of the most appropriate CT study in a given patient. Second, some diseases, such as acute cholecystitis and cholangitis, are not optimally imaged by CT. A patient with RUQ pain who is suspected of having either of these diagnoses should undergo US of the RUQ as the primary diagnostic test. Third, as noted earlier, a patient who is unstable or exhibits signs of shock should be evaluated by a surgeon before any imaging study is considered. In a patient with suspected trauma or hemoperitoneum, the *f*ocused *a*bdominal *s*onogram for *t*rauma (FAST; see later), which can be done at the bedside in the emergency department, is a preferable approach. The presence of shock and fluid in the abdomen is an indication for immediate laparotomy, and further diagnostic maneuvers, including CT, add little value to the patient's care.

A final consideration regarding the role of CT in evaluating acute abdominal pain is radiation exposure. Particularly for patients younger than 35 years of age and those who have required multiple examinations, abdominal CT may increase the lifetime risk of cancer.[35] Additionally, unless a life-threatening condition is suspected, CT is best avoided in a pregnant patient, in whom MRI is a suitable alternative.[39]

US

FAST is a rapid, reliable, bedside test to detect fluid in the abdominal cavity. Although its main usefulness is for the evaluation of injured persons, this examination also aids in the diagnosis of any condition that results in free intraperitoneal fluid; imaging of the aorta can be added, allowing a rapid assessment for aortic aneurysm. Point-of-care abdominal US has become a routine and highly reliable part of the evaluation of acute abdominal pain.[40]

Other Diagnostic Tests

Other diagnostic imaging modalities such as MRI and radionuclide scanning [e.g., ^{99m}Tc-labeled hydroxyl iminodiacetic acid (HIDA) scan] and endoscopy usually take a secondary role in the evaluation of the patient with acute abdominal pain. Use of these tests is generally guided by the results of CT or US. Angiography may be useful not only for establishing a diagnosis of visceral ischemia but also for delivering therapy, either thrombolytic infusion or stenting, aimed at improving or reestablishing blood flow. Diagnostic peritoneal lavage, although seldom used now, is useful when a patient is too unstable from a cardiopulmonary standpoint to tolerate imaging studies. The finding of leukocytes in the lavage effluent in an unstable patient may, in extreme circumstances, constitute sufficient grounds for laparotomy. In a patient who is unstable and deteriorating and has signs of an acute abdomen, laparotomy as a diagnostic maneuver should be considered if imaging is felt to be prohibitively risky. An overall approach to the patient with acute abdominal pain is illustrated in Fig. 12.6.

CAUSES

Acute abdominal pain is usually defined as pain of less than 1 week in duration. Patients usually seek attention within the first 24–48 hours, although some may endure longer periods of abdominal discomfort. The most common reason for a patient to seek emergency department evaluation of abdominal pain is so-called nonspecific abdominal pain; between 25% and 50% of all patients who visit an emergency department for abdominal pain will have no specific disease identified. The distribution of the causes of abdominal pain in patients who present to an emergency department is shown in Table 12.3.

Acute Appendicitis

Among the most common disorders causing abdominal pain and one seen throughout the lifespan, appendicitis is emerging as a more nuanced and complex condition than was previously understood. The appendix is one of the most important of the GI-associated lymphatic tissues and appears to be a key moderator between intestinal microbiota and the immune function of the GI tract.[41] Furthermore, it appears that appendicitis is comprised of two distinct syndromes, complicated appendicitis (CA), and uncomplicated appendicitis (UA), which have differing clinical trajectories[42–44] and may even have different etiologies.[41]

CA, associated with perforation and/or abscess, occurs in the setting of bacterial breach of the appendicular mucosal lining, most typically by *Fusobacterium nucleatum/necrophorum*,[45–47] and infection of lymphoid tissue by *Bacteroides* species with abscess and necrosis/perforation.[41] In contrast, UA is associated with local reaction within the appendix lamina propria by lymphocytes producing antibody responses to previously sensitizing bacterial antigens, where infection/inflammation does not spread beyond the immediate submucosal zone.[41] Studies of gene expression in UA and CA suggest different immunological responses to each, including the tantalizing suggestion of a viral etiology for some cases of UA.[48]

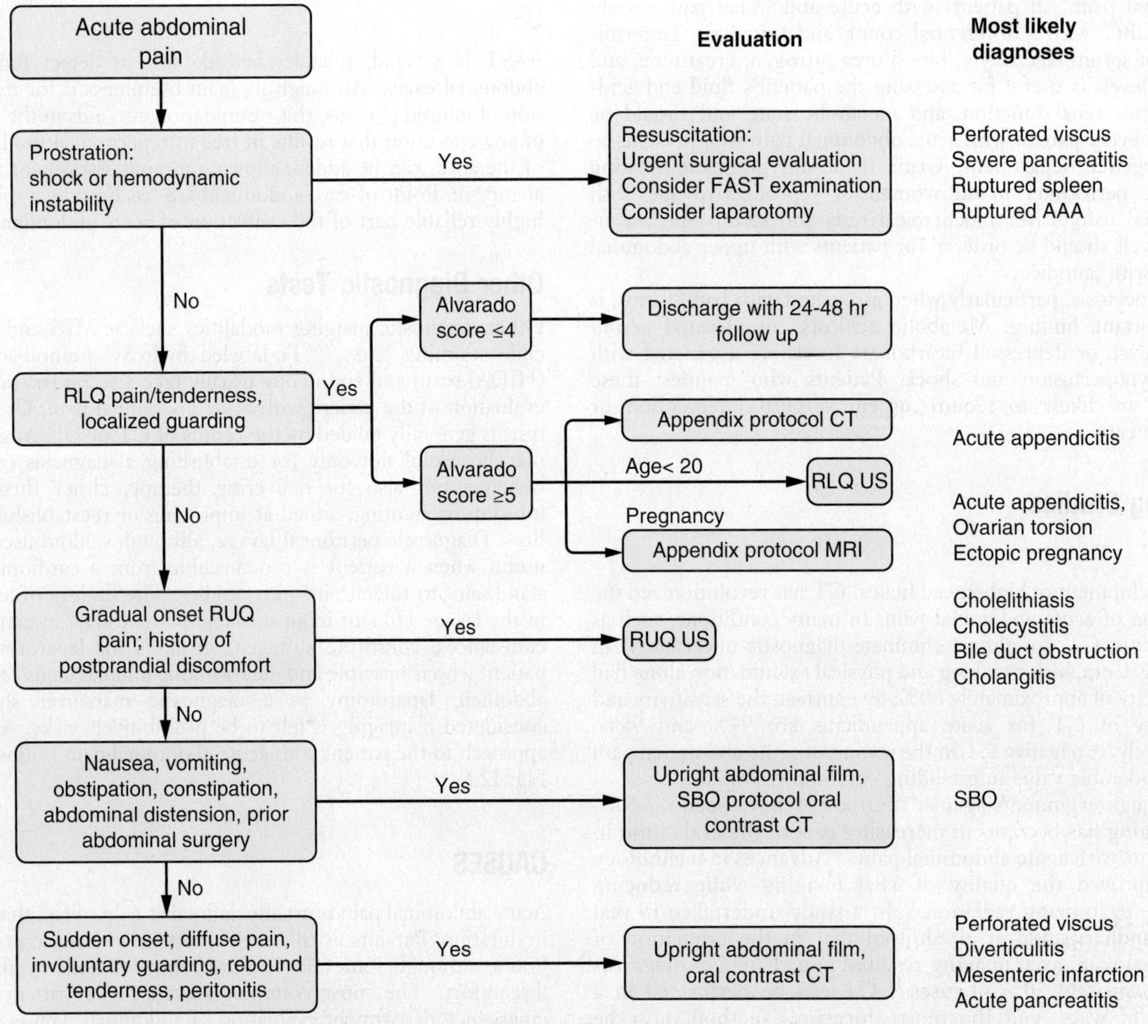

Fig. 12.6 An approach to the urgent evaluation of abdominal pain. Specific complaints and physical examination findings are coupled with appropriate imaging. For LLQ pain, the most likely diagnosis is diverticulitis. *AAA*, Abdominal aortic aneurysm; *FAST*, focused abdominal sonogram for trauma.

TABLE 12.3 Causes of Acute Abdominal Pain in Patients Presenting to an Emergency Department

Cause	%
Nonspecific abdominal pain	35
Appendicitis	17
Bowel obstruction	15
Urologic disease	6
Biliary disease	5
Diverticular disease	4
Pancreatitis	2
Medical illness	1
Other	15

From Irvin TT. Causes of abdominal pain in 1190 patients admitted to a British surgical service. *Br J Surg*. 1989;76:1121–1125.

Distinguishing UA from CA on clinical grounds alone may be impossible.[49] Both typically begin with prodromal symptoms of anorexia, nausea, and vague periumbilical pain. Within 6–8 hours, the pain migrates to the right lower quadrant (RLQ), and peritoneal signs develop. In UA, a low-grade fever to 38°C and mild leukocytosis are usually present. Systemic findings, such as fever and more prominent leukocytosis, are associated with CA formation. Common features of the history, physical examination, and WBC count in patients with appendicitis have been combined into a predictive tool known as the *Alvarado score* (Table 12.4).[50] For men, a score of four or less accurately excludes appendicitis; the score is less useful in women and children.[51] Generally, higher *Alvarado scores* correlate with a higher risk of CA. Atypical presentations of acute appendicitis, however, are common, and a diagnosis of acute appendicitis should not be rejected simply on the basis of the patient's history and physical examination alone. In children, mesenteric adenitis (or lymphadenitis) is frequently mistaken for acute appendicitis but is often preceded by a sore throat and is self-limited. Mesenteric adenitis may also be caused by *Yersinia enterocolitica* (see Chapter 112).

Plain abdominal films have no role in the diagnosis of acute appendicitis. US is becoming a first line diagnostic test for appendicitis, as it spares patients exposure to ionizing radiation. US has a much lower sensitivity, 78%, but has a specificity of 95%, approaching that of CT.[52] Use of CT dramatically improves the accuracy of diagnosis in patients with acute appendicitis. An appendix diameter greater than 10 mm is generally considered

TABLE 12.4 The Alvarado Score for Predicting Acute Appendicitis

Feature	Points
Migration of pain	1
Anorexia	1
Nausea	1
Tenderness in RLQ	2
Rebound tenderness	1
Elevated temperature	1
Leukocytosis	2
Left WBC shift	1
Sum	10

A score of 5–6 is suggestive of appendicitis; a score of 7–8 indicates probable appendicitis; and a score of 9–10 indicates that appendicitis is likely. Patients with scores greater than or equal to 5 should be evaluated by a surgeon or undergo an imaging study to look for appendicitis.

From Alvarado A. A practical score for the early diagnosis of acute appendicitis. *Ann Emerg Med*. 1986;15:557–564.

TABLE 12.5 Tokyo Criteria for the Diagnosis of Acute Cholecystitis

A. Local signs of inflammation
Murphy sign RUQ mass, tenderness, or pain
B. Systemic signs of inflammation
Fever Elevated C-reactive protein Elevated WBC count
C. Imaging findings characteristic of cholecystitis
Definite Diagnosis:
One item in A and one item in B or C, when acute cholecystitis is suspected clinically

Adapted from Hirota J, Takada T, Kawarada Y, et al. Diagnostic criteria and severity assessment of acute cholecystitis: Tokyo Guidelines. *Hepatobiliary Pancreat Surg*. 2007;14:78–82.

diagnostic of appendicitis, although the normal range for the diameter of the appendix may extend to nearly 13 mm,[53] the size range of "normal" and "pathological" appendices overlaps, meaning diameter alone does not establish the diagnosis.[54] Other CT signs of acute appendicitis include periappendiceal fat inflammation, the presence of fluid in the RLQ, and failure of contrast dye to fill the appendix.[55] The addition of CT has reduced the negative appendectomy rate to about 5%.[56] CT also allows the clinician to distinguish UA from CA. Concretions or fecaliths are present in as many as 25% of patients with appendicitis.[57] Because fecaliths are associated with failure of nonoperative management, this finding should be regarded as representing CA.

Because CT entails radiation exposure, some authorities advocate avoiding CT in children and adolescents, in whom a higher degree of diagnostic uncertainty is tolerated in favor of lower radiation exposure (see Chapter 122). In this setting, US of the appendix has a sensitivity of as high as 0.95% for UC.[58] In a pregnant patient for whom radiation exposure is also a significant concern, MRI has become the imaging method of choice, with a sensitivity and specificity of 92% and 97%, respectively, values approaching those of CT.[59]

Acute Biliary Disease

Biliary disease accounts for approximately 7% of visits to an emergency department for abdominal pain and 14%–21% of admissions for patients over 65 years of age.[60,61] Affected patients generally present at some point on the spectrum between biliary pain (biliary colic) and acute cholecystitis. Biliary pain is a syndrome of RUQ or epigastric pain, usually postprandial, caused by transient obstruction of the cystic duct by a gallstone; it is self-limited, generally lasting less than 6 hours. Acute cholecystitis is, in most cases, caused by persistent obstruction of the cystic duct by a gallstone. The pain of acute cholecystitis is almost indistinguishable from that of biliary pain, except that it is persistent. The pain usually is a dull ache that is localized to the RUQ or epigastrium with radiation around the back to the right scapula. Nausea, vomiting, and low-grade fever are common. On examination, RUQ tenderness, guarding, and Murphy sign (inspiratory arrest on palpation of the RUQ) are typical. The WBC count is usually mildly elevated but may be normal. Mild elevations in serum total bilirubin and alkaline phosphatase (ALP) levels are common.

Risk factors for gall stone formation, and therefore cholecystitis, are female sex, Native American ancestry, and pregnancy. Individuals from Asia and sub-Saharan Africa have lower risk.[62]

The role of gallstones in the etiology of biliary pain and acute cholecystitis makes US of the RUQ the key diagnostic test. Demonstration of gallstones may suggest biliary pain, whereas the finding of stones with gallbladder wall thickening, pericholecystic fluid, and pain on compression of the gallbladder with the US probe (sonographic Murphy sign) is essentially diagnostic of acute cholecystitis and has replaced hepatobiliary scintigraphy (e.g., HIDA scan) in the diagnosis of acute cholecystitis.[63] US, while sensitive for the presence of stones, with sensitivity 97% and specificity 99%, for the detection of acute cholecystitis, has poorer sensitivity (83.8%) though equivalent specificity (98.6%).[64] Consideration of imaging findings in the context of the physical examination and laboratory findings is essential for accurate diagnosis. The Tokyo consensus criteria for the diagnosis of acute cholecystitis are shown in Table 12.5. Patients with acute cholecystitis are best managed with cholecystectomy within 24 hours.[65] Patients who are older, tachycardic and have ultrasonographic evidence of gallbladder wall thickening, particularly those with a WBC count greater than 11,000/mm^3, are at higher risk for gangrenous cholecystitis and may require emergent open cholecystectomy.[66–68]

Patients who present with RUQ pain, jaundice, and signs of sepsis should be suspected of having obstruction of the bile duct by a gallstone. RUQ pain, fever and chills, and jaundice (Charcot triad) are suggestive of ascending cholangitis.[69] Elevation of ALP has been shown in multivariate models to predict choledocholithiasis.[70] However, serum ALP may be elevated in severe cholecystitis as well.[66] This measure may be a helpful adjunct, but by itself is not a reliable indicator of choledocholithiasis. Patients suffering from ascending cholangitis often require IV fluids, antibiotics, and bile duct drainages, usually by endoscopy (see Chapters 67-69 and 72).

Small Bowel Obstruction

Intestinal obstruction is a common cause of abdominal pain in both the developed and developing world and occurs in patients of all ages.[61] In pediatric patients, intussusception, congenital malformations, such as malrotation and Meckel diverticulum, are the most common causes.[71] In adults, about three-quarters of cases are caused by postoperative adhesions.[72,73] For patients with no history of abdominal surgery, malignancy and strictures cause approximately 25% of SBOs each.[74] Congenital adhesions are present in about 20%, the remaining 30% are equally divided among benign tumors, intussusceptions, foreign body impactions, internal hernias, and heterotopic tissue. SBO is characterized by sudden cramping, and periumbilical abdominal pain. Nausea and vomiting occur soon after the onset of pain and provide temporary relief of discomfort. Physical examination reveals an acutely ill, restless patient. Fever, tachycardia, and signs of volume contraction, including orthostatic hypotension, are common. Abdominal distention is usual but may be difficult to discern in the setting of obesity or in those with proximal obstructions. Although auscultation in patients with SBO is frequently thought to be characterized by hyperactive bowel sounds and audible rushes, these signs are unreliable.[33,34] Physical examination may be unremarkable even in the presence of visceral distress. Peritoneal signs should be considered a sign of intestinal ischemia or perforation. Leukocytosis and lactic acidosis also suggest intestinal ischemia or infarction. Any of these findings should prompt immediate surgical evaluation.

Plain abdominal radiographs are of little use in the diagnosis of SBO.[75] CT scan is the most useful screening test for suspected SBO. The presence of reduced bowel wall enhancement in the setting of other findings, such as nausea, vomiting, and obstipation, significantly increases the probability of strangulation; a lack of free abdominal fluid significantly decreases the probability of strangulation.[72,73,76,77] Other findings, such as a transition point, are not reliable predictors of ischemia or the need for intervention.[73]

In patients with SBO who have reassuring physical examinations and laboratory findings, initial treatment includes bowel rest, IV fluid hydration, nasogastric decompression, and close observation.[78] For patients with SBO who are admitted for a trial of nonoperative management, many centers administer 120 mL of dilute water-soluble contrast material (WSC) by mouth or nasogastric tube. The appearance of the contrast in the cecum within 24 hours predicts resolution of obstruction.[79] Use of WSC to confirm resolution of SBO may reduce overall length of hospital stay[80] and may result in more expeditious surgical intervention in some settings.[81] Surgery is required for patients who fail conservative management or have evidence of complete obstruction, especially if ischemia is suspected, but, overall, patients with adhesive SBO require surgery in fewer than 20% of cases (see Chapter 125).[82]

Acute Diverticulitis

Acute diverticulitis is a common disease. Approximately 80% of affected patients are older than 50 years of age.[83] The overall incidence of the disease has increased by as much as 50%, with an even greater increase in younger persons.[84,85] There is a poorly understood relationship between obesity and diverticular disease.[86] As obesity is increasingly prevalent in Western society, one expects the prevalence of diverticular disease will also increase in the near future. Patients with diverticulitis usually present with constant, dull LLQ pain and fever. They may complain of constipation or obstipation and are usually found to have a leukocytosis. Physical examination demonstrates LLQ tenderness and, in some cases, an LLQ mass. Localized peritoneal signs are frequent. In severe cases, generalized peritonitis may be present, making differentiation from other causes of a perforated viscus difficult. CT is reliable in confirming the diagnosis, with a sensitivity of 97%,[87–89] and should be performed routinely in the emergency evaluation of patients with diverticulitis.

Acute diverticulitis presents as a spectrum of disease from mild abdominal discomfort to gross fecal peritonitis, which is an acute surgical emergency. The severity of diverticulitis, as determined by CT, is best described using the Hinchey grading system (see Table 123.1 in Chapter 123). Patients with mild disease and no CT findings of perforation, in the absence of limiting comorbid disease, can generally be treated as outpatients. Those with Hinchey grade I diverticulitis (localized pericolic abscess or inflammation) frequently require hospitalization for IV antibiotics. Patients with Hinchey grade II diverticulitis (pelvic, intra-abdominal, or retroperitoneal abscess) should undergo CT-guided drainage of the abscess and receive a course of broad-spectrum IV antibiotics. Patients with Hinchey grades III (generalized purulent peritonitis) and IV (generalized fecal peritonitis) diverticulitis frequently require emergency surgery (see Chapter 123). Despite the descriptive utility of grading systems for diverticulitis, there is little evidence to support their predictive value in deciding between surgical and medical management.[90] Patients presenting with significant abdominal pain or tenderness benefit from early surgical consultation.

Acute Pancreatitis

Hospital admissions for acute pancreatitis in the United States are increasing.[91] Acute pancreatitis typically begins as acute pain in the epigastrium that is constant, unrelenting, and frequently described as boring through to the back or left scapular region. Fever, anorexia, nausea, and vomiting are typical. Patients with pancreatitis are usually more comfortable sitting upright, leaning forward slightly. Physical examination reveals an acutely ill patient in considerable distress. Patients are usually tachycardic and tachypneic. Abdominal examination reveals hypoactive bowel sounds and marked tenderness to percussion and palpation in the epigastrium. Abdominal rigidity is a variable finding. In rare patients, flank or periumbilical ecchymoses (Grey-Turner or Cullen sign, respectively) develop in the setting of pancreatic necrosis with hemorrhage. Extremities are often cool and cyanotic, reflecting underperfusion. WBC counts of 12,000–20,000/mm^3 are common. Elevated serum and urine amylase levels are usually present within the first few hours of pain; serum lipase is also elevated. Depending on the cause and severity of pancreatitis, serum electrolyte, calcium, and blood glucose levels and liver biochemical test and arterial blood gas results may be abnormal. US is useful for identifying gallstones as a potential cause of pancreatitis.

Although most cases of acute pancreatitis are self-limited, as many as 20% of patients have severe disease with local or systemic complications, including hypovolemia and shock, renal failure, liver failure, and hypocalcemia.[92] Overall mortality rate for acute pancreatitis is approximately 1%.[93] Because pancreatitis can be a treacherous disease, severe disease often disguised in a relatively benign appearing syndrome, a number of prognostic physiologic scales have been developed to estimate of the severity of acute pancreatitis and to forecast clinical deterioration; none are perfect.[94] The most enduring, the Ranson score, first published in 1974, remains useful and widely used, not to estimate risk of complication but as a checklist for the early assessment of patients with acute pancreatitis.[95] The Ranson score consists of five early and six late factors that indicate severe pancreatitis. A simpler bedside index of the severity of acute pancreatitis, consisting of blood urea nitrogen greater than 25 mg/dL, impaired mental status, systemic inflammatory response syndrome, age older than 60 years, and pleural effusion, has also proved useful.[96]

The Atlanta classification system for acute pancreatitis has great utility for bedside classification of the anatomic presentations pancreatitis may assume: interstitial edematous pancreatitis, necrotizing pancreatitis, acute pancreatic fluid collection, pancreatic pseudocyst, acute necrotic collection, or walled off necrosis.[97] Patients without organ failure or local or systemic complications are classified as *mild* and may be treated expectantly. *Moderately severe acute pancreatitis* is typified by organ failure of less than 48 hours' duration. When organ failure persists for longer than this time, or affects multiple organ systems, *severe acute pancreatitis* is present. Patients in this last group usually require multidisciplinary care in an intensive care unit. A minority of patients with severe acute pancreatitis present with a profound intra-abdominal catastrophe, usually caused by thrombosis of the middle colic artery or right colic artery, which travel in proximity to the head of the pancreas, with resulting colonic infarction. This process may not be seen clearly on CT obtained early in the course of disease and should be suspected in any case marked by rapid hemodynamic collapse. Such patients require immediate laparotomy (see Chapter 60).

Perforated Peptic Ulcer

The incidence and morbidity related to peptic ulcer disease have declined over the past two decades, now accounting for as few as 42 hospitalizations per 100,000 population,[98] with an estimated overall global prevalence rate of 99/100,000 in 2019, improved from a rate of 143 in 1990.[99] The epidemiology of PUD is changing (see Chapter 55). The incidence of *Helicobacter pylori* (Hp) infection has decreased dramatically since the late 1990s.[100] Improved therapies, including PPIs, eradication of Hp (see Chapter 54), and endoscopic methods for control of hemorrhage (see Chapter 21), have reduced the number of patients with PUD who require surgical intervention,[101] although the frequency of complicated disease has increased in older adults, in whom morbidity and mortality related to surgery are also increased.[102] The author's anecdotal experience suggests that the switch from opioids to NSAIDs in response to the epidemic of opioid use disorder has resulted in an increasing frequency of perforated PUD in younger patients.

Patients with a perforated peptic ulcer typically present with the sudden onset of severe diffuse abdominal pain. These patients may be able to specify the precise moment of the onset of symptoms. In the usual case, the afflicted patient presents acutely with excruciating abdominal pain, often without prodromal symptoms. Abdominal examination reveals peritonitis, with rebound tenderness, guarding, and abdominal muscular rigidity. In such cases, distinguishing perforated ulcer from other causes of a perforated viscus (e.g., perforated colonic diverticulum and perforated appendicitis) may not be possible. Older or debilitated patients may present with less dramatic symptoms, with perforation identified by the presence of free intraperitoneal air on an upright abdominal film or CT.

A perforated peptic ulcer should be suspected in any patient with the sudden onset of severe abdominal pain who presents with abdominal rigidity and free intraperitoneal air. Pneumoperitoneum is detected on an abdominal film in 75% of patients (Fig. 12.7). In equivocal cases, CT of the abdomen usually suggests the diagnosis by demonstrating edema in the region of the gastric antrum and duodenum, associated with extraluminal air. CT may not be diagnostic, however, and patients with diffuse peritonitis or hemodynamic collapse should be explored surgically. Laparotomy is acceptable as the primary diagnostic maneuver in such patients. Endoscopy is not advisable when the diagnosis of a perforated peptic ulcer is suspected; insufflation of the stomach can convert a sealed perforation into a free perforation. Survival following emergency surgery for complications of PUD is surprisingly poor. Implementation of evidence-based practice modeled on the *Surviving Sepsis Guidelines* in Denmark reduced the 30-day mortality rate from 30% to 25% in patients with a perforated peptic ulcer.[103] The 2-year mortality rate in these patients was over 40% (see also Chapter 55).

Acute Mesenteric Ischemia

Acute mesenteric ischemia can result from occlusion of a mesenteric vessel as a result of an embolus, which may emanate from an atheroma of the aorta or cardiac mural thrombus, or primary thrombosis of a mesenteric vessel, usually at a site of atherosclerotic stenosis. Embolic occlusion had accounted for up to 50% of cases of mesenteric ischemia in the 1980s but, because of advances in the management of risk factors for embolization, it accounts for no more than one-third of cases currently.[104] Visceral embolism most commonly affects the superior mesenteric artery, presumably because of the less acute angle of the superior mesenteric artery origin from the abdominal aorta.[105] Atherosclerotic stenosis of the mesenteric vessels can result in primary arterial thrombosis. Patients usually have a history of atherosclerotic disease, particularly in the coronary or cerebrovascular circulation. Nonocclusive mesenteric ischemia results from inadequate visceral perfusion and can also lead to intestinal ischemia and infarction; such cases are usually consequent to critical illnesses like cardiogenic or septic shock. Nonocclusive mesenteric ischemia, also referred to as "low-flow" mesenteric ischemia, accounts for as many as 14% of cases, and an equal number of cases of mesenteric ischemia result from venous thrombosis, usually associated with a thrombophilia, and focal segmental ischemia of the small intestine[106] (see Chapter 120). Because most cases of mesenteric ischemia occur in patients with significant cardiovascular comorbidities, outcomes are poor.[107] Perioperative mortality is over 50% and has improved little in the past 20 years.[104]

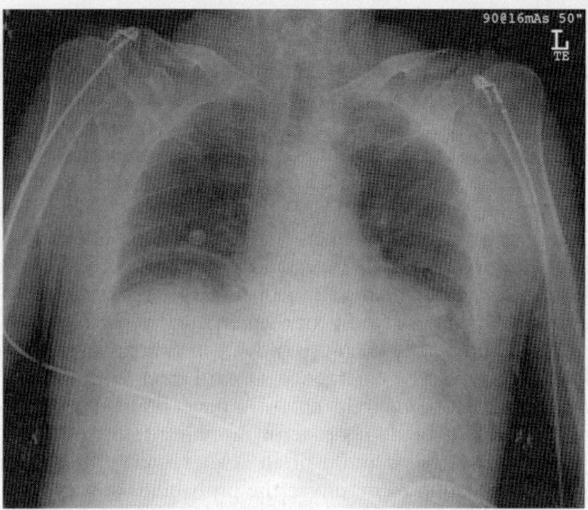

Fig. 12.7 Upright chest film of an 80-year-old man with the acute onset of severe epigastric pain demonstrating free intra-abdominal air under the right hemidiaphragm. The patient has pneumoperitoneum as a result of a perforated viscus. At surgery, perforation of an anterior duodenal ulcer was found.

The hallmark of the diagnosis of acute mesenteric ischemia is the abrupt onset of intense cramping epigastric and periumbilical pain out of proportion to the findings on abdominal examination. Other symptoms may include diarrhea, vomiting, bloating, and melena. On physical examination, most patients appear acutely ill, but the presentation may be subtle. Shock is present in about 25% of cases.

CT angiography is the best initial diagnostic test for suspected acute mesenteric ischemia. Mesenteric angiography may be useful for determining the cause of intestinal ischemia and defining the extent of vascular disease; however, CT has largely replaced formal angiography in these cases. Patients with acute embolic or thrombotic intestinal ischemia should be referred to immediate revascularization and bowel resection.[108] Patients with nonocclusive mesenteric ischemia are best managed by treatment of the underlying shock state. For patients with persistent symptoms, laparotomy for resection of infarcted intestine may be necessary. Transcatheter vasodilator therapy may be helpful for patients who are found to have vasospasm on visceral arteriography (see Chapter 120).

Abdominal Aortic Aneurysm

Rupture of an abdominal aortic aneurysm (AAA) is heralded by the sudden onset of acute, severe abdominal pain localized to the midabdomen or paravertebral or flank areas. The pain is tearing in nature and associated with prostration, lightheadedness, and diaphoresis. If the patient survives transit to the hospital, shock is the most common presentation. Physical examination reveals a pulsatile, tender abdominal mass in about 90% of cases. The classic triad of hypotension, a pulsatile mass, and abdominal pain is present in 75% of cases and mandates immediate surgical intervention.[109] In patients with a suggestive history, emergency department US is a reliable method for the diagnosis of AAA in patients in shock and is sufficient evidence for emergency surgical intervention. Endovascular methods for repair of an AAA have resulted in improved outcomes, although the short-term mortality rate is 40%.[110] Patients with suspected rupture of an AAA require urgent vascular surgery consultation to maximize the probability of survival.

Abdominal Compartment Syndrome

Although not usually presenting as acute abdominal pain, abdominal compartment syndrome (ACS) warrants consideration in any patient with an abdominal emergency. First reported in the setting of massive intra-abdominal trauma, ACS, defined as pathologic elevation of intra-abdominal pressure, is now recognized as a frequent complication of many severe disease processes.[111] The peritoneal cavity normally has a pressure of 5–7 mm Hg; it may be higher in obese persons.[112] Elevated intra-abdominal pressure may develop in patients who survive massive volume resuscitation with resulting visceral edema or who have a disease like severe pancreatitis that can cause visceral or retroperitoneal edema. Intra-abdominal hypertension (IAH) is defined as abdominal pressure of 12 mm Hg or higher.[113] Elevation of intra-abdominal pressure that compromises visceral perfusion defines ACS. The kidney is particularly prone to underperfusion in this setting, and renal failure may be the first sign of ACS.[113]

Primary ACS is defined as ACS that arises from pathology within the peritoneal cavity, such as gastric distention or edema from acute pancreatitis. More common is secondary ACS, in which massive bowel wall edema secondary to shock is responsible for IAH. A third form, tertiary ACS, or recurrent ACS, results from overzealous attempts at abdominal wound closure after management of primary or secondary ACS. Risk factors for ACS are listed in Box 12.1.

Intra-abdominal pressure can be measured simply by connecting a transducer to a urinary catheter, with the zero-reference point at the midaxillary line in a supine patient. An international consensus conference has established a grading scheme for ACS, shown in Table 12.6, based on the measured bladder pressure.[74] A normal value for bladder pressure is less than 7 mm Hg. Grade I ACS is defined as a pressure of 12–15 mm Hg, grade II as 16–20 mm Hg, grade III as 21–25 mm Hg, and grade IV as greater than 25 mm Hg. Nonsurgical options for treating low-grade ACS include gastric decompression, sedation, neuromuscular blockade, and placing the patient in a reverse Trendelenburg position while allowing the hips to remain in a neutral position, and diuretics. In a patient with high-grade ACS, particularly when renal or respiratory function is compromised, laparotomy with creation of an open abdomen is most effective.[114] Management of the open abdomen requires specific surgical expertise usually found in referral medical centers. Fortunately, the frequency of ACS has declined substantially in the 2000s, owing to increased awareness of the syndrome and advances in resuscitation.[115]

BOX 12.1 Risk Factors for Intra-abdominal Hypertension and Abdominal Compartment Syndrome

Abdominal surgery, especially with tight fascial closures
Acidosis (pH < 7.2)
Acute pancreatitis
Bacteremia
Coagulopathy (platelets <55,000/mm^3, or activated partial thromboplastin)
Time twice normal or higher, or prothrombin time <50% (INR > 1.5)
"Damage-control" laparotomy
Distended abdomen
Gastroparesis, gastric distention, or ileus
Hemoperitoneum/pneumoperitoneum
High BMI (>30 kg/m^2)
Hypothermia (core temperature <33°C)
Intra-abdominal infection/abscess
Intra-abdominal or retroperitoneal tumor
Laparoscopy with excessive inflation pressures
Liver dysfunction/cirrhosis with ascites
Major burns
Major trauma
Massive fluid resuscitation (>5 L of colloid or crystalloid/24 hours)
Massive incisional hernia repair
Mechanical ventilation
Multiple transfusions (>10 U of packed red blood cells/24 hours)
Peritoneal dialysis
Peritonitis
Pneumonia
Prone positioning
Sepsis
Use of positive end-expiratory pressure (PEEP) or the presence of "auto-PEEP"
Volvulus

Modified from Malbrain MNG, Cheatham M, Kirkpatrick A, et al. Results from the international conference of experts on intra-abdominal hypertension and abdominal compartment syndrome. I. Definitions. *Intensive Care Med.* 2006;32:1722–1732.

TABLE 12.6 Grading System for Intra-abdominal Hypertension[a]

Grade	Bladder Pressure (mm Hg)
Normal	<12
1	12–15
2	16–20
3	21–25
4	>25

[a]Abdominal compartment syndrome is present if intra-abdominal hypertension is accompanied by organ dysfunction.
Modified from Carr JA. Abdominal compartment syndrome: a decade of progress. *J Am Coll Surg*. 2013;216:135–146.

Other Intra-abdominal Causes

Other intra-abdominal causes of acute abdominal pain include gynecologic conditions (e.g., endometritis, acute salpingitis with or without tubo-ovarian abscess, ovarian cysts or torsion, and ectopic pregnancy); SBP (Chapter 95); functional dyspepsia (Chapter 15); infectious gastroenteritis (Chapters 112–114); viral hepatitis and other liver infections (Chapters 80–86); pyelonephritis; cystitis; mesenteric lymphadenitis; IBD (Chapters 117 and 118); and other bowel disorders, such as IBS (Chapter 124) and intestinal pseudo-obstruction (Chapter 126). Vascular compromise of an epiploic appendage due to axial torsion can result in epiploic appendagitis.[116] This syndrome can imitate appendicitis, diverticulitis, or other pathologies but has a self-limited natural history and usually requires only symptomatic management with NSAIDs.[116] The diagnosis is best confirmed by demonstration of an inflamed ovoid fatty mass adjacent to a noninflamed segment of the colon on CT.[117]

Extra-abdominal and Systemic Causes

Acute abdominal pain may arise from disorders involving extra-abdominal organs and systemic illnesses. Examples are listed in Box 12.2. Surgical intervention for patients with acute abdominal pain arising from an extra-abdominal or systemic illness is seldom required except in cases of pneumothorax, empyema, and esophageal perforation. Esophageal perforation may be iatrogenic, result from blunt or penetrating trauma, or occur spontaneously (Boerhaave syndrome; see Chapter 47).

BOX 12.2 Extra-abdominal and Systemic Causes of Acute Abdominal Pain

Cardiac
Endocarditis
Heart failure
Myocardial ischemia and infarction
Myocarditis
Thoracic
Empyema
Esophageal rupture (Boerhaave syndrome)
Esophageal spasm
Esophagitis
Pleurodynia (Bornholm disease)
Pneumonitis
Pneumothorax
Pulmonary embolism and infarction
Hematologic
Acute leukemia
Hemolytic anemia
Henoch-Schönlein purpura
Sickle cell disease
Metabolic
Acute adrenal insufficiency (Addison disease)
Diabetes mellitus (especially with ketoacidosis)
Hyperlipidemia
Hyperparathyroidism
Hypersensitivity reactions (e.g., to insect bites, reptile venoms)
Lead poisoning
Porphyria
Toxins
Uremia
Infections
Herpes zoster
Osteomyelitis
Syphilis
Typhoid fever
Nerologic
Abdominal epilepsy
Radiculopathy, spinal cord or peripheral nerve tumors, degenerative
Arthritis of the spine, herniated vertebral disk
Tabes dorsalis
Miscellaneous
Angioedema
Familial Mediterranean fever
Heat stroke
Muscle contusion, hematoma, and tumor
Narcotic withdrawal
Psychiatric disorders

Angioedema is characterized by acute, self-limited edema of the dermis, subcutaneous tissue, mucosa, and submucosa. The edema may affect the skin of the face, usually around the mouth, tongue, throat, extremities, and genitalia. Involvement of the GI tract may cause acute episodes of colicky pain, sometimes accompanied by nausea, vomiting, and diarrhea. Mast-cell mediated angioedema, often caused by allergic reactions to foods, drugs, or insect stings, is characterized by urticaria, flushing, pruritus, throat tightness, bronchospasm, and hypotension. Bradykinin-induced angioedema is not associated with these symptoms, has a more prolonged course, and is less clearly associated with an identifiable trigger, although angiotensin-converting enzyme inhibitor therapy is a known cause. Bowel wall angioedema can be seen in patients on angiotensin-converting enzyme inhibitors and in those with hereditary or acquired deficiency or dysfunction of C1 inhibitor and can be visualized on abdominal US or CT. Treatment of an attack depends on the acuity and severity and may include airway and hemodynamic support, discontinuation of potential triggers, antihistamines, glucocorticoids, and, in cases of hereditary angioedema, use of purified C1 inhibitor concentrate, a kallikrein inhibitor, and a bradykinin B2 receptor antagonist.

Special Circumstances

Extremes of Age

Evaluation of acute abdominal pain in patients at the extremes of age is a challenge. Historical information and physical examination findings are often difficult to elicit or are unreliable. Similarly, laboratory data may be misleadingly normal in the face of serious intra-abdominal pathology. For these reasons, patients at the extremes of age are often diagnosed late in the course of the disease, thereby resulting in increased morbidity. For example, the perforation rate for appendicitis in the general population averages 10% but exceeds 50% in infants. The presentation of acute abdominal conditions is highly variable in these populations, and a high index of suspicion is required. A carefully obtained history, thorough physical examination, and high index of suspicion are the most useful diagnostic aids.

In the pediatric population, the causes of acute abdominal pain vary with age. In infancy, intussusception, pyelonephritis, gastroesophageal reflux, Meckel diverticulitis, and bacterial or viral enteritis are common. In children, Meckel diverticulitis, cystitis, pneumonitis, enteritis, mesenteric lymphadenitis, and IBD are prevalent. In adolescents, pelvic inflammatory disease, IBD, and the common adult causes of acute abdominal pain predominate. In children of all ages, two of the most common causes of pain are acute appendicitis and abdominal trauma secondary to child abuse.

In the older adult population, biliary tract disease accounts for almost 25% of cases of acute abdominal pain and is followed in frequency by nonspecific abdominal pain, malignancy, intestinal obstruction, complicated PUD, and incarcerated hernia. Appendicitis, although rare in older patients, usually manifests late in its course and is associated with high morbidity and mortality rates.

Pregnancy

The gravid woman with acute abdominal pain presents a difficult diagnostic dilemma. Acute appendicitis and cholecystitis develop in pregnant women at the same rates as in their nonpregnant counterparts. A number of additional diagnoses, such as placental abruption and pain related to tension on the broad ligament, must be distinguished from nonobstetric diagnoses. The risk of radiation injury to the developing fetus must be considered when imaging studies are planned.

Surgery in pregnancy is not rare; approximately 1 in 500 pregnancies will be associated with a nonobstetrical general surgical intervention.[118] Primary consideration is given to the health of the mother. Emergency interventions during pregnancy carry a risk of fetal loss that varies with gestational age and the type of intervention. The middle 3 months of gestation are preferable for abdominal surgical intervention; this period presents the lowest risk for teratogenicity and spontaneous labor.[119]

Appendicitis occurs in about 1 in 2000 pregnancies and is equally distributed among the three trimesters. In later stages of pregnancy, the appendix may be displaced cephalad, with consequent displacement of the signs of peritoneal irritation away from McBurney point. US or, in challenging cases, MRI may be useful for establishing a diagnosis in this setting. Biliary tract disease is also common during pregnancy. Open or laparoscopic management of these diseases is safe but is associated with adverse obstetrical outcomes in approximately 5% of cases, which is not a statistically significant rate compared to patients not having surgery.[120]

Immunocompromised Hosts

In addition to diseases like appendicitis and cholecystitis that occur in the general population, a number of diseases unique to immunocompromised hosts may manifest with acute abdominal pain: neutropenic enterocolitis, drug-induced pancreatitis, graft-versus-host disease, pneumatosis intestinalis, and cytomegalovirus (CMV) and fungal infections (see Chapter 34). Patients infected with HIV can present a particular challenge (see Chapter 33). When advanced, HIV infection is associated with a number of other diseases that may present as acute abdominal pain. One of the most common abdominal disorders seen in immunocompromised persons in the developing world is primary peritonitis (see Chapter 37). Affected patients have suppurative peritonitis without a definable source. Spontaneous intestinal perforation, usually secondary to CMV infection, is also common in patients with advanced HIV infection. TB peritonitis is a consideration in patients from areas where TB is common.[121] Immunocompromised patients may lack the definitive signs of an acute abdominal crisis usually seen in immunocompetent persons; elevated temperature, peritoneal signs, and leukocytosis may be absent in these cases.

PHARMACOLOGIC MANAGEMENT

An unfortunate practice in the care of patients with acute abdominal pain is to delay administration of narcotics pending definitive surgical assessment. Sir Zachary Cope declared, "Morphine does little or nothing to stop serious intra-abdominal disease, but it puts an efficient screen in front of the symptoms."[9] The practice of delaying relief of pain in a suffering patient, however, does not appear to withstand careful clinical scrutiny. Six studies in which early administration of analgesia was compared with administration of placebo in patients with acute abdominal pain have shown that patients who receive analgesics are more comfortable and do not experience a delay in diagnosis.[9,122]

Patients with an acute abdominal process frequently require antibiotic treatment for peritonitis. When appropriate, antibiotic therapy aimed at the likely causative pathogens should be given as soon as a putative diagnosis is reached, but little benefit is derived from treating an immunocompetent patient with broad-spectrum antibiotics before a likely source is identified. Patients who are immunocompromised or neutropenic, however, should receive broad-spectrum antibiotics early in the course of management for acute abdominal pain.

Full references for this chapter can be found at https://ebooks.health.elsevier.com.

13 Chronic Abdominal Pain

Jill E. Elwing, Gregory S. Sayuk

IN THIS CHAPTER

INTRODUCTION

Abdominal pain often represents a challenging complaint for the clinician to evaluate. Though often benign and self-limited, abdominal pain can potentially reflect serious, life-threatening conditions (see Chapter 12). Chronic abdominal pain may result from both functional etiologies (disorders of gut-brain interaction, DGBI) and structural (organic) disorders. The differential diagnosis is broad, with several diagnoses considered in this chapter and elsewhere in this textbook (Box 13.1). The evaluation of chronic abdominal pain requires a familiarity with the key historical elements and symptom constellation to recognize DGBI, as well as an appropriate balance of indicated diagnostic testing without excessive or repeated evaluations. This chapter focuses on neuromuscular etiologies of chronic abdominal pain as well as recognized DGBI causes of chronic abdominal pain, including centrally mediated abdominal pain syndrome (CAPS) and narcotic bowel syndrome (NBS). The effective management of chronic abdominal pain requires a multimodal approach and takes into consideration our understanding of these disorders in the context of a biopsychosocial model.

DEFINITION AND CLINICAL APPROACH

Abdominal pain is considered chronic when it has been occurring constantly or intermittently for at least 6 months, acute when it has been occurring for no more than several days, and subacute when it has been occurring for more than several days but less than 6 months.

As in acute abdominal pain (see Chapter 12), in chronic abdominal pain the clinician must remain diligent and complete a thorough evaluation, including history, physical exam, and necessary tests to delineate a correct diagnosis, both avoiding overtesting and missing diagnoses that require a more urgent evaluation to prevent significant morbidity. Historical aspects of interest include the character, location, duration, radiation, intensity of pain, as well as any palliating or provoking factors. Associated symptoms, including weight loss, nausea, vomiting, and change in bowel habits should be elicited. Given the relatively symmetrical bilateral innervation of the abdominal organs, visceral pain emanating from the digestive tract has long been recognized to be perceived in the midline but is often diffuse and poorly localized.[1] Referred pain is ordinarily located in the cutaneous dermatomes with the same spinal cord level as the affected visceral inputs.[2] Previous medications, medical conditions, surgeries, and family history are important as they provide potential clues regarding the etiology of chronic abdominal pain. A history of other somatic disorders, psychiatric conditions, and prior trauma may support a DGBI diagnosis. Red flag features, such as weight loss, anemia, GI bleeding, nocturnal pain, and night sweats, alternatively, raise concern for a potential organic or structural etiology.

A thorough physical exam of the abdominal viscera and abdominal wall is helpful to assess findings supportive of a structural disorder. The abdominal examination should employ a combination of inspection, auscultation, percussion, and palpation. In a patient with an acute abdominal pain presentation in the context of a chronic abdominal pain history, the most critical step is to ascertain whether a process mandating immediate surgical intervention may have developed. In patients with chronic abdominal pain, alarm findings on examination include peritoneal signs such as rebound tenderness or guarding and abdominal bruit in the setting of mesenteric vascular disease. Consideration for a secondary acute process in the setting of chronic abdominal pain may be raised in a patient with worsening, new, recurrent abdominal pain, especially in the background of a concerning physical examination. Although additional clues on physical examination are not entirely specific, the "closed eyes" sign may be encountered in patients with CAPS (see below). Similarly, Carnett's sign and the hover sign (also detailed below) may be seen in persons with pain emanating from the abdominal wall.

A number of diagnostic evaluations, such as blood tests, stool tests, imaging studies (e.g., abdominal ultrasound or computed tomography scan), or endoscopic procedures (such as a colonoscopy or upper endoscopy), may be useful in the evaluation of chronic abdominal pain in the appropriate setting. The history and physical findings should direct diagnostic testing in patients with chronic abdominal pain; excessive testing can be costly and result in unnecessary anxiety and even lead to unnecessary interventions such as surgery. The indications for these radiologic investigations and their potential for clarifying an individual clinical situation differ. Endoscopic and radiologic testing in the context of specific disorders is discussed in detail elsewhere in this textbook.

CHRONIC ABDOMINAL WALL PAIN

Anterior Cutaneous Nerve Entrapment and Myofascial Pain Syndromes

Chronic abdominal wall pain (CAWP), including anterior cutaneous nerve entrapment syndrome (ACNES) and myofascial pain syndrome (MFPS), are relatively common conditions likely to account for approximately 10% of all chronic abdominal pain visits in the outpatient setting.[3,4] However, despite their relatively common prevalence, widespread recognition of CAWP is lacking, resulting in delays in diagnosis, costly testing and trials of medications, and at times unnecessary surgical intervention.[5–8] CAWP is more common in the middle decades (40–50 years of age) and more prevalent in women than men (4:1 ratio).[9] Comorbid conditions include other chronic functional pain disorders such as fibromyalgia, low back pain, and irritable bowel syndrome (IBS). A triggering event can be identified in less than half of cases, such as surgery, injury, obesity, or pregnancy.[9]

ACNES is hypothesized to result from the entrapment of a cutaneous branch of a sensory nerve that is derived from a neurovascular bundle emanating from spinal levels T7 to T12 at the anatomic point where the nerve makes a 90-degree turn into the rectus sheath, with subsequent ischemia and resultant somatic pain (Fig. 13.1).[10] Three distinct entrapment mechanisms may occur, including: (1) enlargement of the abdomen causing herniation through the fibrous ring, trapping of the nerve, and corresponding vasa nervorum, resulting in ischemia and pain; (2) enlargement of the abdomen and stretching or lengthening of the nerve results in pain; (3) alternatively, pain may result from entrapment within a scar postoperatively.[6,10]

Abdominal MFPS is thought to arise from focally tender points in taut bands of skeletal muscle (the "trigger point"). MFPSs often are more diffuse and associated with additional pain sites, including the back and neck. Causative factors include trauma, degenerative disk disease, osteoarthritis, over- or underuse, and can be exacerbated by psychological distress.[9]

Clinical features of CAWP include a lack of relationship to eating or bowel movements. Pain is often in the upper abdomen and exacerbated by exercise or external pressure.[11] Physical findings include focal pain, localizing pain on palpation, and pain at or near an abdominal scar. To meet the criteria of CAWP, patients must satisfy one criterion in each of the following categories: Category 1 is a point of maximal tenderness localized by one fingertip or pain at the site of tenderness that is constant in nature; Category 2 is superficial tenderness, maximum tenderness 2 cm or less, or tenderness increased by tensing the abdominal wall muscles (the Carnett test).[6] The Carnett test includes a maneuver where the patient is asked to raise their head or legs to tense the abdominal wall musculature while the clinician holds pressure at the site of tenderness. A positive Carnett's sign, worsening pain during contraction, has a 78% sensitivity and 88% specificity for an abdominal wall source.[12] In the case of MFPS, a trigger point can be identified using a single finger to palpate a tender area in the central portion of a muscle belly, which may elicit a "jump sign,"[13] the jerking away, or crying out as the myofascial trigger point is detected. The patient often guards the affected area from the examiner's hands "hover sign."[3]

Conservative measures, including reassurance, topical anesthetics, and neuromodulators, often are initially recommended, but success rates are variable.[11] When the diagnostic criteria suggest abdominal wall pain, trigger point injection may be considered for diagnostic and therapeutic benefits. A retrospective survey-based study with up to 12 months of follow-up found ultrasound-guided trigger-point injection resulted in significant symptom improvement in one-third of patients, with those not responding having a higher degree of somatization.[14] In a series of 137 patients who met criteria for CAWP and subsequently benefited from injection therapy, the diagnosis remained unchanged in 97% of these cases after a mean follow-up of 4 years.[11] Through inexpensive approaches such as the Carnett test and

BOX 13.1 Differential Diagnosis of Chronic or Recurrent Abdominal Pain

STRUCTURAL (OR ORGANIC) DISORDERS

Inflammatory

Appendicitis (Chapter 122)
Celiac disease and gluten sensitivity (Chapter 109)
Diverticular disease (Chapter 123)
Eosinophilic gastroenteritis (Chapter 30)
Epiploic appendagitis
IBD (Chapters 117 and 118)
Pelvic inflammatory diseases
PSC (Chapter 70)
Sclerosing mesenteritis (Chapter 37)

Vascular

Celiac artery syndrome (Chapter 36)
Mesenteric ischemia (Chapter 120)
Superior mesenteric artery syndrome (Chapter 16)

Metabolic

Diabetic neuropathy
Lead poisoning
Porphyria (Chapter 79)

Neuromuscular

Anterior cutaneous nerve entrapment syndrome
Myofascial pain syndrome
Slipping rib syndrome
Thoracic nerve radiculopathy

Other

Abdominal adhesions (Chapter 125)
Abdominal migraine (Chapter 16)
Abdominal neoplasms (Chapters 41–43, 50, 56, 62, 71, 98, 127–129)
Anaphylaxis (Chapter 11)
Angioedema (Chapter 12)
Cannabinoid hyperemesis syndrome (Chapter 16)
Chronic pancreatitis (Chapter 61)
Cyclic vomiting syndrome (Chapter 16)
Ehlers-Danlos syndrome
Endometriosis (Chapter 130)
Familial Mediterranean fever (Chapter 35)
Gallstones (Chapter 67)
Hernias (Chapter 27)
Intestinal malrotation (Chapter 100)
Intestinal obstruction (Chapter 125)
Lactose intolerance (Chapter 106)
Neurogenic abdominal pain (abdominal migraine, abdominal epilepsy) (Chapters 16 and 35)
PUD (Chapter 55)
Small intestinal and pelvic lipomatosis (Chapter 37)

FUNCTIONAL GI DISORDERS

Biliary pain (gallbladder or SOD) (Chapter 65)
Centrally mediated abdominal pain syndrome
Functional (nonulcer) dyspepsia (Chapter 15)
Gastroparesis (Chapter 52)
IBS (Chapter 124)
Levator ani syndrome (Chapter 131)
Narcotic bowel syndrome/opioid-induced GI hyperalgesia

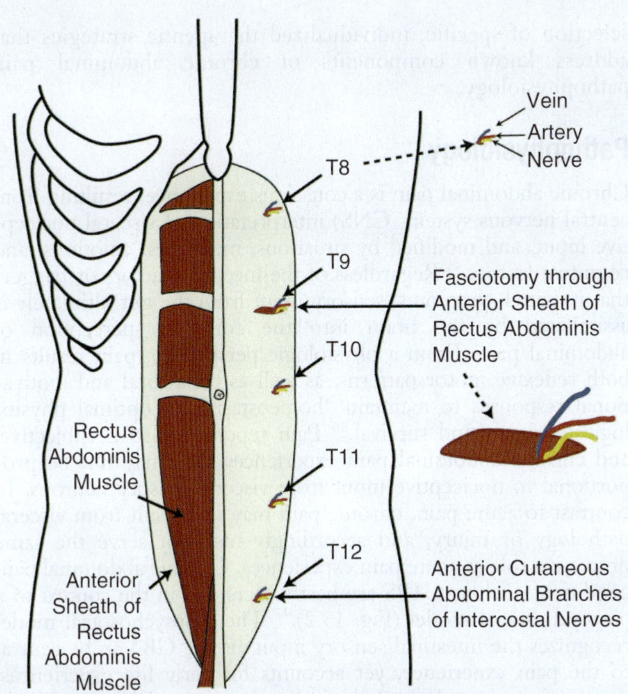

Fig. 13.1 Abdominal innervation and musculature relevant to the pathology and treatment of anterior cutaneous nerve entrapment syndrome (ACNES).[7] (From Lindsetmo RO, Stulberg J. Chronic abdominal wall pain—a diagnostic challenge for the surgeon. *Am J Surg*. 2009;198(1):129–134.)

trigger point injection, a diagnosis of CAWP can be firmly established, resulting in reduced health-care utilization and cost.[11,15] In highly selected cases, nerve resection surgery may be considered for refractory ACNES.[16–18] A retrospective observational study[17] and a double-blind, randomized, controlled trial[18] showed long-term benefits from anterior neurectomy in patients with symptoms refractory to conservative therapy. In the cases of myofascial pain, additional techniques, such as dry needling, acupuncture, and massage, may also be beneficial therapeutic modalities.[19]

Slipping Rib Syndrome and "Rib Tip Syndrome"

Slipping rib syndrome (SRS), or Cyriax syndrome, is a rare condition that causes unilateral pain in the upper abdomen or lower chest.[20] Like CAWP, unnecessary treatments for visceral causes of upper abdominal pain can occur without a good history and physical exam. This condition is seen in women to a greater degree than men, can be seen in all ages, and occurs equally on the left and right upper abdomen.[21–24]

The etiology is thought to be related to hypermobility of costal cartilage related to congenital laxity or trauma resulting in the cartilage of the lower (8th to 10th) false ribs to slip out of place, causing pain and discomfort in the upper abdomen or lower chest. The cartilage tips fall behind the superior adjacent rib during contraction of the abdominal musculature; pain results from the impingement of branches of the intercostal nerve and localized tissue inflammation.[25] Symptoms of SRS can include sharp, stabbing pain in the upper abdomen or lower chest, pain that worsens with deep breathing or coughing, and tenderness to palpation. The pain is unilateral and sharp, often lancinating in the subcostal region. A more protracted aching sensation may follow the acute pain. Diagnosis can be made through the "hooking maneuver," which entails pressure being placed under the costal margin and pulling the entire ribcage superiorly and anteriorly, eliciting pain and often an audible pop or click.[22] Dynamic ultrasound has been used to confirm the subluxation of the ribs during the hooking maneuver (87% sensitivity), Valsalva, or abdominal crunch (sensitivity of 54% and 13%, respectively).[26] Treatment for SRS usually involves reassurance that the condition is benign, pain management, and avoiding activities that aggravate the condition. Over-the-counter pain relievers, such as ibuprofen or acetaminophen, may help alleviate symptoms. In more severe cases, costochondral nerve blockade (a response to which supports the diagnosis) may be necessary. Rarely, surgical intervention is considered and could include rib or cartilage resection or rib plating.[27–30]

In persons with thoracic hyperkyphosis and kyphoscoliosis, "rib tip syndrome" (costo-iliac impingement) may cause pain resembling that of SRS. The condition can be successfully treated with a weighted back support device that centers the body over the legs (kypho-orthosis) and physical therapy.[31]

Thoracic Nerve Radiculopathy

Thoracic nerve radiculopathy can cause abdominal pain due to the disease of nerves in the thoracic spine region, including neuropathy related to back and spine disorders, diabetes mellitus, and herpes zoster infection.[32,33] The location and severity of the pain will depend upon the affected nerve; for example, T7 and T8 are more likely to be felt in the upper abdomen, whereas compression of T10 through T12 is more common to result in lower abdominal pain. History and physical examination will help make the diagnosis with neuropathic features of pain being reported, such as burning, numbness, tingling, or shooting sensations. Attention to the possibility of systemic disease and abnormal neurologic and dermatologic findings is part of the diagnostic key. Neurology consultation with electromyographic evaluation has been helpful to rule in thoracic nerve disease as a cause of abdominal pain.[34] Treatment for thoracic nerve radiculopathy often includes conservative measures such as physical therapy, antiinflammatory and pain medications, and alternative therapies such as massage or acupuncture, and surgery.[35]

CENTRALLY MEDIATED ABDOMINAL PAIN SYNDROME (CAPS)

Introduction

CAPS is a DGBI that manifests with chronic, continuous, or frequently recurrent abdominal symptoms, typically pain-predominant.[36] CAPS previously has been recognized by several other names, including functional abdominal pain syndrome (Rome III), chronic idiopathic abdominal pain, and chronic functional pain.[37] The pain experiences of CAPS are often severe and associated with considerable negative impact on affected patients' health-related quality of life, interpersonal relationships, and work productivity. Given the anatomical localization of CAPS pain experiences to the abdominal region, CAPS often is attributed to gastrointestinal origin by patients and providers alike. However, by definition structural or physiological GI abnormalities are not etiopathologic in CAPS.[38] Rather, as the condition name implies, CAPS is recognized to derive from derangements in pain signaling and processing at the level of the gut-brain axis (GBA). The severity and chronicity of CAPS pain experiences often leads to the pursuit of multiple uninformative diagnostic tests and even surgical interventions.[39] Though the pain experience with CAPS may be qualitatively similar to that associated with other painful DGBI, the primary pain complaint in the absence of additional GI symptoms or associated features delineates CAPS from other DGBI. CAPS is however often associated with other functional somatic syndromes (FSS) such as fibromyalgia as well as psychiatric comorbidities.

Epidemiology

CAPS is a less common diagnosis as compared to other DGBI, such as IBS or functional dyspepsia (FD). Prevalence estimates of functional abdominal pain (CAPS predecessor diagnosis) suggest that 0.5%–2.1% of adults are affected by the condition.[40] Like other DGBI, CAPS appears to be up to twice as common in women, and peaks in prevalence in the fourth decade of life, decreasing thereafter with age. However given that CAPS is a newer entity (first described in Rome IV in 2016), less is known about the epidemiology of CAPS relative to other DGBI. The majority of CAPS patients are high utilizers of the health-care system, with frequent physician visits, imaging and endoscopic investigations, and surgical interventions. CAPS patients also miss a greater number of workdays due to illness compared to those without abdominal pain symptoms.[41–43]

Etiology

Historically, the literature and previous research relating to chronic abdominal pain has centered on descriptive reports of symptomatic features rather than the neurobiology and mechanistic basis of the disorder. However, in recent years, the field has evolved to advance our understanding of the biologic basis of chronic abdominal pain.[44] More sophisticated insight into the molecular and neurologic pathways responsible for chronic abdominal pain is essential to the ultimate identification of biology-based subgroups with the goal an informed selection of specific, individualized therapeutic strategies that address known components of chronic abdominal pain pathophysiology.

Pathophysiology

Chronic abdominal pain is a conscious experience, resulting from central nervous system (CNS) interpretation of visceral nociceptive input, and modified by situations, memories, emotions, and cognitive factors.[45] Regardless of the inceptive factors or triggers that initiated symptoms, sensory input from the gut ultimately is assimilated by the brain into the conscious perception of abdominal pain. From a physiologic perspective, pain results in both reflexive motor patterns, as well as behavioral and motivational responses to maintain "homeostasis," or optimal physiological balance and survival.[46] Pain reporting also is subjective, and chronic abdominal pain experiences thus may not be proportional to nociceptive input from visceral sensory neurons. In contrast to acute pain, chronic pain may not result from visceral pathology or injury, and accordingly may not serve the same protective role as acute pain experiences. Chronic abdominal pain conditions such as CAPS are best understood in the context of a biopsychosocial model (Fig. 13.2).[47] The biopsychosocial model recognizes the intestinal sensory input via the GBA to be central to the pain experience, yet accounts for early life experiences, genetic factors, and psychological and experiential influences in the generation of chronic abdominal pain symptoms (see also Chapter 5).

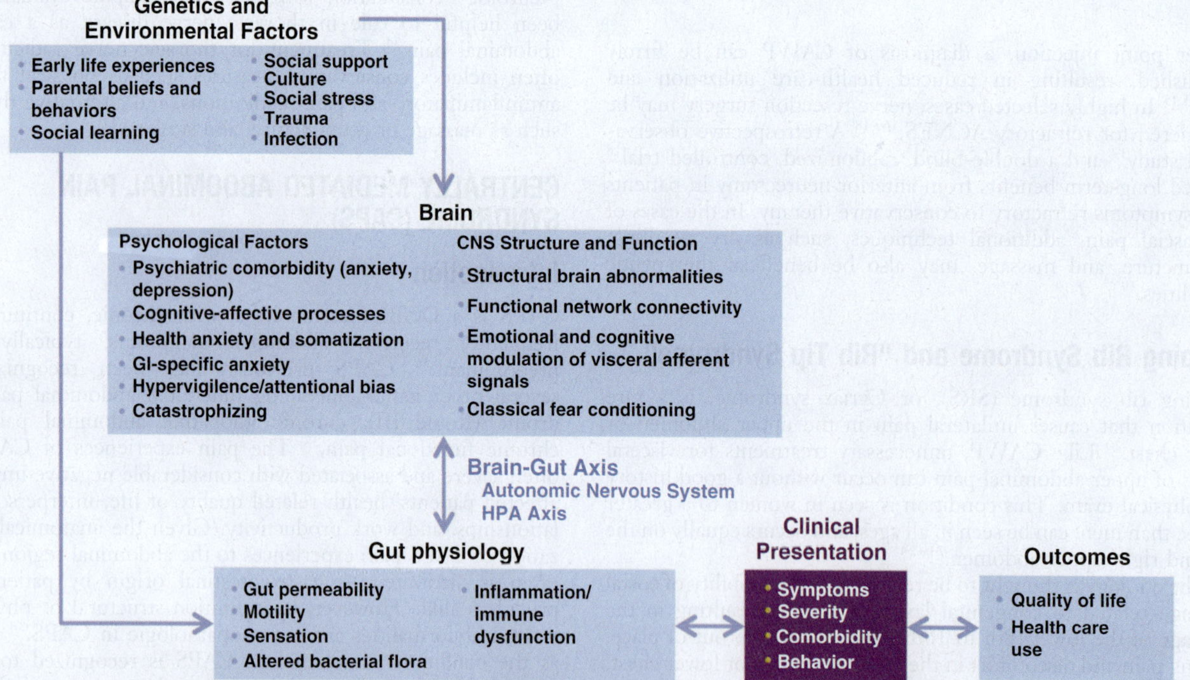

Fig. 13.2 Biopsychosocial model of centrally mediated abdominal pain syndrome (CAPS). The biopsychosocial model of illness recognizes the importance of early life factors (e.g., genetic, environmental, trauma) as risk factors to the development of CAPS. Symptom experiences and behavioral responses the result of complex, bidirectional interaction between psychosocial factors (e.g., stessors, social support) and gut physiology (i.e., inflammation, visceral sensory afferent function). Abnormal modulation and interpretation of afferent signals from the intestine within the gut-brain axis lead to the experience of chronic abdominal pain, and consequently increased use of health-care resources and reduced quality of life.[47,118] *CNS*, Central nervous system; *HPA*, hypothalamic-pituitary-adrenal. (From Van Oudenhove L, Crowell MD, Drossman DA, et al. Biopsychosocial aspects of functional gastrointestinal disorders. *Gastroenterology*. 2016. https://doi.org/10.1053/j.gastro.2016.02.027. Adapted from Drossman DA, Camilleri M, Mayer EA, Whitehead WE. AGA technical review on irritable bowel syndrome. *Gastroenterology*. 2002;123(6):2108–2131.)

The Gut-Brain Axis (GBA)

The GBA is a bidirectional network of communication between the somatosensory and effector nerve networks of the gastrointestinal tract (enteric nervous network, ENS) and the CNS (brain and spinal cord). The ENS and CNS are "hardwired" allowing for nerve communication in both a "bottom-up" (ENS to CNS) and a "top-down" (CNS to ENS) direction. As a result, descending signaling within the GBA allows for central modulation of bowel function and sensorimotor signaling, and moreover mediates gut responses to thoughts and emotions. Inversely, gut to brain communication inputs are not only found in sensory brain regions, but also the emotional-arousal and cognitive regions of the brain, resulting in patient's perceptive, affective and interpretive experiences of abdominal pain. The CNS responses to pain also elicit the patient's behavioral responses to chronic abdominal pain. GBA signaling is further regulated by autonomic nervous system (sympathetic and parasympathetic) inputs as well as neuroimmune and neuroendocrine system influences via biochemical and electrophysiologic interactions with the viscerosensory network. The gut microbiome (trillions of resident commensal organisms in the gut lumen) more recently has gained recognition as important in its interaction with the GBA and the regulation of gut homeostasis. Perturbations in this broader "microbiota-GBA" (MGBA) may lead to pathologic derangements in intestinal sensorimotor function (Fig. 13.3).[48,49] Conceptually, enhanced perception of visceral pain signals, or "visceral hypersensitivity," can result from imbalances in MGBA function within any component of this complex network.[50] Alterations in MGBA function have particular importance to the development of chronic abdominal pain and related DGBI (formerly functional GI disorders), including IBS and FD.[51]

The Autonomic and Enteric Nervous Systems

The main function of the ANS is to maintain physiologic balance "homeostasis" in an unconscious, involuntary fashion throughout the body. This homeostasis is maintained through neuronal interconnections involving the parasympathetic, sympathetic, and enteric nervous systems with central input from higher cortical centers.

The ENS complex of the ANS comprises an estimated 500 million individual intrinsic enteric neurons and glia embedded between the mucosa and circular and longitudinal muscle layers of

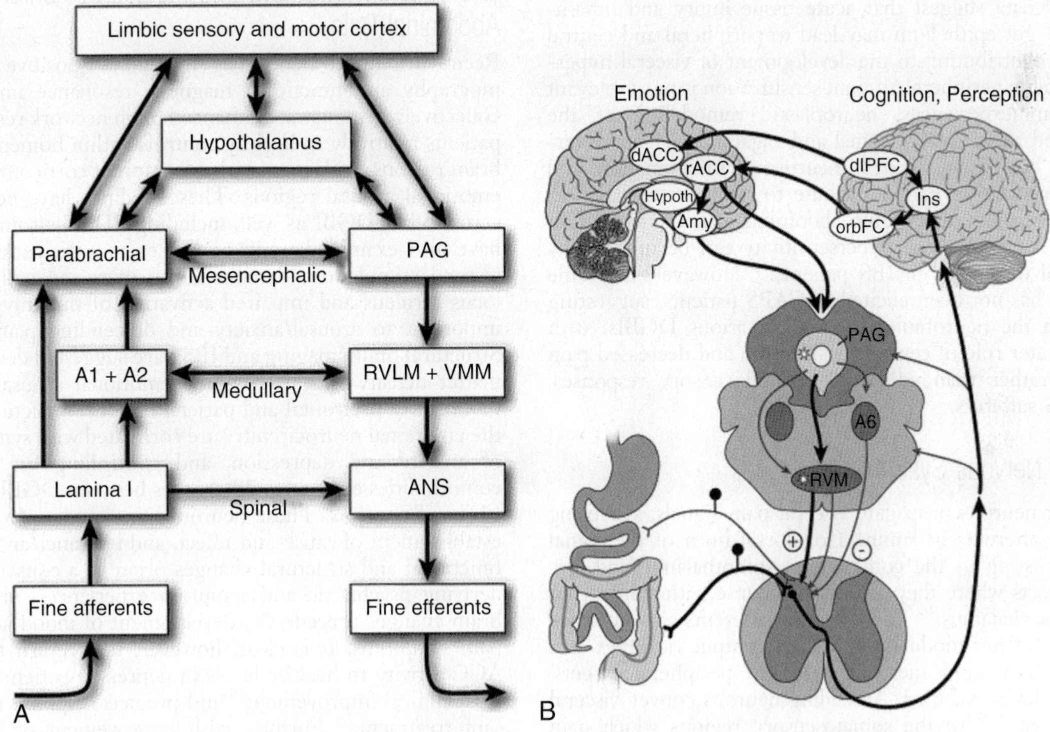

Fig. 13.3 Pain sensation pathways and signals. (A) Visceral pain sensation homeostatic reflex pathways. First-order neurons "homeostatic afferents" convey visceral sensory signals from the bowel, and synapse in the dorsal horn of the spinal cord. These neuronal projections form reflex arcs at the spinal, medullary and mesencephalic levels. Limbic, paralimbic, and prefrontal centers modulate the gain of these reflexes. Second-order neurons from the dorsal horn ascend via the spinothalamic, spinoreticular and reticulothalamic tracts to converge in the thalamus with third-order neurons. These neurons then network with the limbic system (Ins) and anterior cingulate cortex (ACC) and primary somatosensory cortex.[119] *MCC,* Midcingulate cortex. (B) Cortical modulation of homeostatic afferent visceral signals. Prefrontal cortical (PFC) regions [dorsolateral PFC (dlPFC), orbitofrontal cortex (orbFC)] modulate limbic and paralimbic networks [amygdala (amy), (dorsal ACC [dACC], rostral ACC [rACC]), and hypothalamus (Hypoth)], which in turn provide input to descending inhibitory and facilitatory descending pathways via periaqueductal gray (PAG) and pontomedullary nuclei. Corticolimbic pontine networks mediate emotional and cognitive interpretation of homeostatic feelings (e.g., abdominal symptoms and pain).[46] ((A) Adapted from Craig AD. How do you feel? Interoception: the sense of the physiological condition of the body. *Nat Rev Neurosci*. 2002;3(8):655–666. (B) From Mayer EA, Naliboff BD, Craig AD. Neuroimaging of the brain-gut axis: from basic understanding to treatment of functional GI disorders. *Gastroenterology*. 2006;131(6):1925–1942.)

the bowel. Most neurotransmitter and modulator classes represented within the CNS also participate in this "connectome," or system of neurons in close proximity and functional connectivity.[52] The ENS can function independently of CNS input and hence is often referred to as the "second brain of the body."[53] These diverse neurons (e.g., motor neurons, interneurons, and intrinsic primary sensory afferent) organize to form to large plexuses. The myenteric (Auerbach's) plexus is organized structurally similar to the CNS and includes sensory receptors (i.e., chemoreceptors and mechanoreceptors) that communicate sensory signals to the ENS interneurons. The myenteric plexus also controls longitudinal and circular muscular contraction. As the parasympathetic nucleus of origin for the vagus nerve, the myenteric plexus interacts with the medulla oblongata via the anterior and posterior vagal nerves. The submucosal (Meissner's) plexus effectors control secretory function.

Ascending transmission of visceral pain signals occurs via first-order extrinsic afferent neurons housed in the dorsal root ganglia and conveys visceral sensory signals via the thoracolumbar sympathetic system to synapse in the dorsal horn of the spinal cord.[46] Repeated peripheral stimulation may evoke upregulation of afferent pain signaling, increasing gut sensitization and resulting in visceral hyperalgesia (enhanced pain response to noxious stimuli) and susceptibility to chronic pain.

Preclinical data suggest that acute tissue injury and inflammation in the gut epithelium may lead to peripheral and central sensitization, contributing to the development of visceral hyperalgesia.[54] Though peripheral afferent sensitization is most relevant to acute pain experiences, neuroplastic remodeling of the epithelium and alterations to spinal and vagal afferent nerve terminals in the bowel may result in neurogenic inflammation, and peripheral sensitization may contribute to intermittent pain experiences in a subset of chronic abdominal pain patients.[55] In experimental settings, rectal hypersensitivity can be induced by noxious rectal distention in IBS patients.[56] However, the same phenomenon has not been elicited in CAPS patients, suggesting differences in the neurobiologic basis of various DGBIs, with perhaps a greater role of central sensitization and decreased pain modulation, rather than enhanced visceral sensory responses, among CAPS sufferers.

The Central Nervous System

Second-order neurons propagate visceral pain signals, synapsing with primary afferents in lamina I of dorsal horn of the spinal cord, then crossing to the contralateral spinothalamic and spinoreticular tracts where they ascend to synapse with third order neurons in the thalamus.[46] These visceral afferents also interface with ANS to further modulate autonomic output via reflex arcs (spinal, medullary, and mesencephalic) to peripheral targets, including the intestinal tract. Ascending neurons convey visceral afferent pain signals to the somatosensory regions which pain localization and intensity is perceived, as well as the limbic, paralimbic, and prefrontal centers that modulate the "gain" of the afferent signals and conduct noxious stimulus appraisal (salience) and measured cognitive and emotional responses. The insular cortex integrates input received from the sensory thalamus and nucleus tractus solitarius, functioning as a "limbic sensory cortex" that processes visceral sensory and emotional information.[57] Prefrontal cortical (PFC) regions, including the orbitofrontal cortex and dorsolateral PFC, are involved in visceral pain perception and related cognitive interpretation of those signals. Further cortical modulation of homeostatic visceral afferent activity occurs in key limbic and paralimbic regions, including anterior cingulate cortex (ACC) subregions, the hypothalamus, and amygdala, where emotional interpretation and arousal responses to noxious stimuli are generated (Fig. 13.3; see also Chapter 4).[46] Collectively, the processing of visceral afferent signals by these corticolimbic pontine networks yields the cognitive and emotional perception of homeostatic sensory input. This complex central processing of pain signals partially accounts for the variability of pain experiences, even in the same individual, and likely is enhanced in chronic abdominal pain patients.

Limbic regions further regulate pain experiences through descending inhibitory and faciliatory pathways, providing "gate control" of visceral sensory input from the spinal cord via endorphin-, enkephalin-, and serotonin-based neural networks that converge in the midbrain (periaqueductal gray) and rostral ventral medulla.[58] This regulation of ascending nociceptive impulses tracking among the dorsal horn of the spinal cord thus allows for further modulation (upregulation or downregulation) of pain signals from the intestinal tract. It has been observed that DGBI patients with chronic abdominal pain have diminished diffuse noxious inhibitory control of visceral stimuli.[58] The recognition that descending modulation of homeostatic input originates in brain networks responsible for emotion generation and attention to pain provides a physiologic basis for the potential benefit of psychological therapies, such as cognitive behavioral therapy (CBT), in the management of centrally-mediated abdominal pain.

Altered Brain Structure and Function in Chronic Abdominal Pain

Rectal distention neuroimaging studies [positive emission tomography and functional magnetic resonance imaging (MRI)] collectively demonstrate enhanced brain network responses in IBS patients relatively to healthy controls within homeostatic afferent brain regions, with increased activation of corticomodulatory and emotional arousal regions. These findings have been consistent across other DGBI as well, including FD. Neuroimaging studies have also examined brain responses to anticipation of noxious visceral stimulation, demonstrating increased activation in the locus ceruleus and impaired activation of the amygdala, regions important to arousal/anxiety and descending pain modulation. Structural brain imaging and IBS have suggested decreases in gray matter density within the same emotional arousal and cortical modulatory prefrontal and parietal regions. Structural changes in the emotional neurocircuitry are correlated with symptom reports of anxiety and depression, and controlling for psychological comorbidities eliminates differences between DGBI (i.e., IBS and FD) and controls. These neuroimaging studies do not allow for establishment of cause-and-effect, and it is unclear whether these functional and structural changes occur as a consequence of underlying psychiatric and symptom experiences, or whether the brain changes precede the development of mood and abdominal pain symptoms. It is clear, however, that return to baseline of ACC activity to healthy levels in depressed patients is associated with clinical improvement[59] and predicts response to antidepressant treatment.[60] Further, with improvement of IBS pain and emotional distress, activity within the ACC correspondingly normalizes.[59]

Gut Microbiota Role in Gut-Brain Signaling

Host–microbial interactions in susceptible individuals may trigger the development of abdominal pain syndromes following infectious gastroenteritis. The potential for development of postinfectious IBS (PI–IBS) is now well-established and demonstrated to occur in approximately 10% of patients experiencing bacterial enteritis. Risk factors for the development of PI-IBS include psychosocial stressors and psychiatric comorbidities present at the time of infection (see *Psychiatric and Functional Somatic Syndrome Comorbidities* below).

Residual alterations in neuroimmune and sensory responses may lead to persistence of abdominal pain symptoms beyond the resolution of the inciting infection. Gut microorganisms (microbiota), present throughout the intestinal tract, but most prevalent in the colon, are an important contributor to gut-brain communications.[48,59,60] Changes to the intestinal bacterial milieu may precipitate a number of physiologic effects salient to the development of chronic abdominal pain symptoms, including intestinal microinflammation, alterations in gut permeability, visceral nociception and autonomic tone (Fig. 13.4).[61] Alterations in intestinal microbiota composition (decreased *Bifidobacterium* levels) have been associated with more severe abdominal pain symptoms in healthy individuals.[62] Animal studies have demonstrated that exaggerated HPA axis stress responses can be abolished by gut colonization with *Bifidobacterium* species, and conversely that transplantation of IBS patient microbiota into germ free rats may precipitate visceral hypersensitivity in those animals.[63] Finally, a double-blind study of *Bifidobacterium* probiotic administration in IBS patient population resulted in decreased emotional arousal network responses to negative stimuli on functional MRI.[64] In a top-down fashion, stress exposures have been shown to precipitate alterations in gut microbiota composition.[65] Together, there is an emerging recognition of the neurobiochemical influences of intestinal microbiota on gut-brain function and visceral nociception, leading to the concept of a bidirectional "microbiota-gut-brain" axis pertinent to chronic abdominal pain experiences.[49,66]

Psychiatric and Functional Somatic Syndrome Comorbidities

Psychiatric Comorbidity

Psychological distress is very common in DGBI and can exist in multiple forms. including comorbid mood disorders (e.g., major depression and anxiety), life stressors, poor social support, and experiences of abuse (physical, sexual, emotional).[67] As emphasized by the biopsychosocial model, psychiatric burden is an important risk factor for the development of DGBI and furthermore can exacerbate abdominal pain experiences. Inversely, chronic abdominal pain may perpetuate or worsen the severity of psychological comorbidity.[47]

The prevalence of psychiatric comorbidity in DGBI varies by the patient population. In the case of IBS as a prototypical DGBI, approximately 18% of patients in the community satisfy criteria for at least one primary psychiatric disorder, whereas upwards of 90% of patients meet *Diagnostic and Statistical Manual of Mental Disorders (DSM)* Axis I psychiatric diagnostic criteria in tertiary

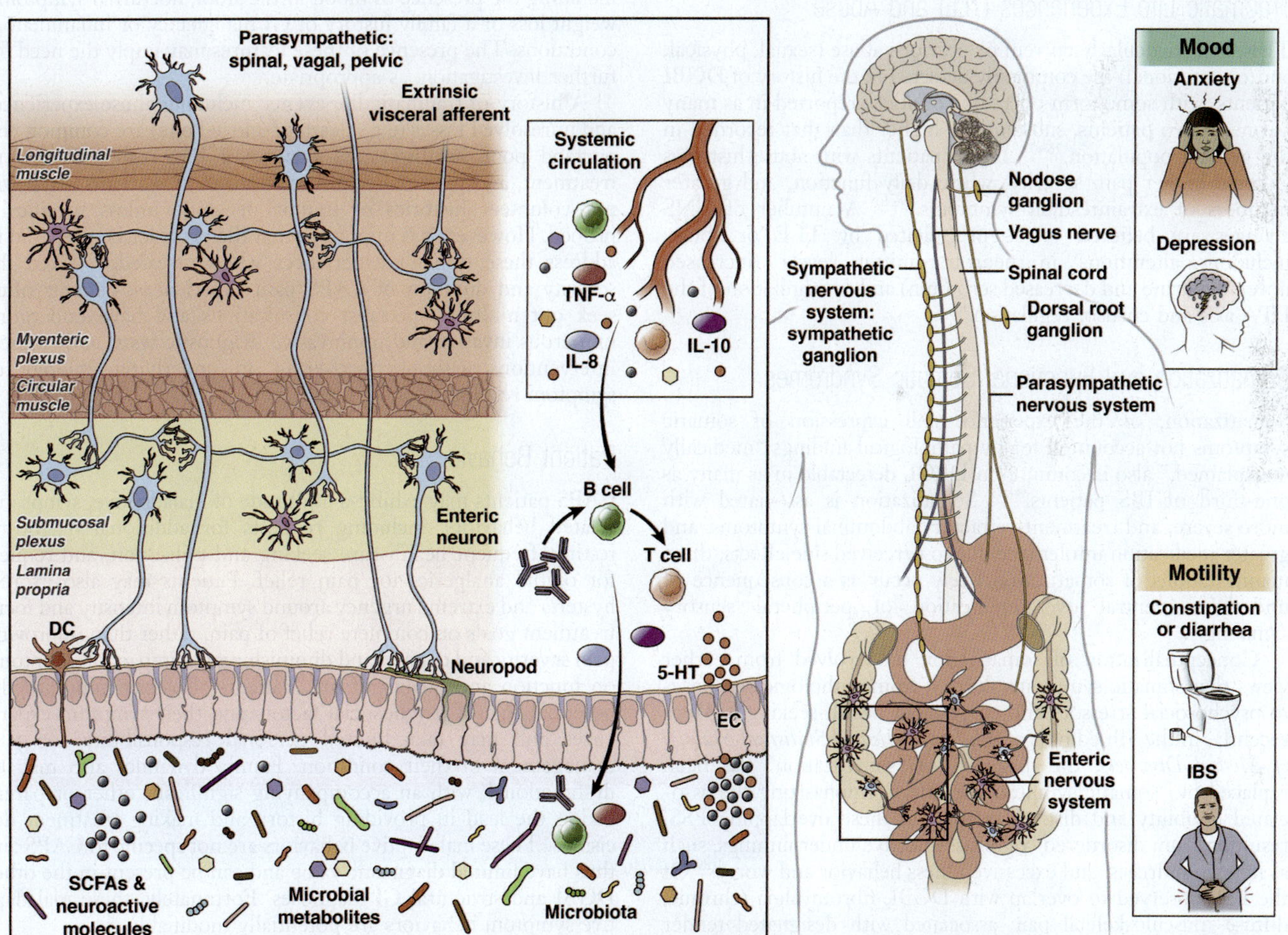

Fig. 13.4 The local and central influences of the microbiota-gut-brain axis. Gut microbiota hold the potential to modulate gut-brain interactions via direct, local effects [e.g., neurotransmitter production (γ-amino butyric acid (GABA), dopamine, norepinephrine)], intestinal permeability, and microinflammation. Indirect modulation of gut-brain function can occur via production of neuroactive microbial metabolites, induction of enteroendocrine cell (EEC) release of GI hormones, and neuropod transduction of intestinal sensory signals centrally via the vagus nerve through synapse-like connections. Collectively, these microbiota-gut-brain interactions can influence abdominal symptoms (i.e., centrally mediated abdominal pain) and the emotional responses to noxious symptom experiences.[120] (From Margolis KG, Cryan JF, Mayer EA. The microbiota-gut-brain axis: from motility to mood. *Gastroenterology*. 2021;160(5):1486–1501.)

referral populations.[68–70] Psychiatric diagnoses and current mood symptoms are more common among patients with multiple GI and non-GI functional diagnoses.[71] Anxiety disorders are most commonly encountered in DGBI, accounting for perhaps as much as half of the detected psychiatric comorbidity in this patient population.[47] The enhanced autonomic arousal and CNS responses to stress in patients with overlapping anxiety disorders may increase vulnerability to abdominal pain experiences via enhanced sensitivity to noxious stimuli and diminished tolerance of abdominal symptoms. Epidemiologic evidence supports a relationship of psychosocial stressors and the onset or exacerbation of IBS abdominal pain symptoms. Acute, experimental stress exposure also has been demonstrated to lead to the development of stress-induced visceral hyperalgesia.[72,73] Evidence from preclinical and clinical studies supports the importance of central corticotropin releasing factor (CRF) and CRF1 receptor systems in the development of acute and chronic stress-related visceral hyperalgesia.[74] The influence of psychiatric comorbidity on pain symptom experiences is not unique to abdominal pain; for instance, depression and anxiety have been observed to mediate pain effects on patient function in chronic low back pain sufferers.[75]

Traumatic Life Experiences (TLE) and Abuse

TLE, and particularly current or previous abuse (sexual, physical, and/or emotional) are commonly detected in the history of DGBI patients, with some form of trauma or abuse reported in as many as one in two patients, substantially higher than that recorded in the general population.[76–78] DGBI patients with abuse histories endorse higher pain severity, worse daily function, and greater numbers of extraintestinal symptoms.[79–82] A number of CNS changes are believed to be precipitated by TLE or abuse, including alterations in neurotransmitter levels (increased norepinephrine and decreased serotonin) and dysregulation of the HPA axis and cortisol regulation.[83]

Somatization and Functional Somatic Syndromes

Somatization, or the experience and expression of somatic symptoms not accounted for by pathological findings "medically unexplained," also is common in DBGI, detectable in as many as one-third of IBS patients.[84,85] Somatization is associated with more severe, and treatment-refractory abdominal symptoms, and greater medication intolerance due to perceived side effects; these manifestations of somatization likely occur as a consequence of underlying central overamplification of peripheral sensory signaling.[86–88]

Conceptualization of somatization has evolved from earlier views that somatic symptoms derived from pathologic responses to psychosocial stressors and consequent health-seeking.[47] More recently, in the 5th edition of the *Diagnostic and Statistical Manual of Mental Disorders*, the diagnosis of "somatization" has been replaced by "somatic symptom disorder," emphasizing the associated disability and distress relating to these overlapping FSS, resulting from disordered cognitive-affective underpinnings, such as hypochondriasis, and excessive illness behavior and worry.[89] Of the FSS observed to overlap with DGBI, fibromyalgia (chronic, diffuse musculoskeletal pain associated with designated tender points on exam) is the most common somatic comorbidity. While only affecting an estimated 2% of the general population, fibromyalgia is detected in nearly one-third of IBS patients; conversely, IBS diagnoses are present in one out of two fibromyalgia patients. Other commonly codiagnosed FSS include headaches, chronic pelvic pain, interstitial cystitis, and chronic fatigue syndrome. Overall, two-thirds of DGBI patients have overlapping FFS conditions.[47,85]

Clinical Features

History

CAPS can affect both sexes and patients across a spectrum of ages but is most commonly encountered in middle-aged females. The clinical history is that of chronic abdominal pain, present for at least 6 months but often reported to be experienced for years or even decades. Some CAPS patients can relate the onset of symptoms back to childhood.[41] Pain is often very severe in intensity, constantly present or frequently recurrent, and widespread in anatomical location. Qualitatively, patients may describe the pain as colicky, though burning pain may also be reported particularly with postsurgical onset.[38] Patients will often report experiencing pain on a daily basis. An important distinction between CAPS and other DGBI is the lack of pain association with eating, bowel movements, or other GI symptoms. Though CAPS patients may endorse other GI symptoms such as abnormal bowel habits, these other symptoms are neither temporally nor qualitatively associated with CAPS pain experiences. CAPS may coexist with other DGBI or non-GI functional somatic symptoms (e.g. musculoskeletal pain, headaches, pelvic pain) and often overlaps with psychiatric diagnoses, including depression, anxiety, and somatization. History of alarm features or "red flag" symptoms should be elicited, including the presence of blood in the stool, nocturnal symptoms, weight loss or a family history of GI malignancy or inflammatory conditions. The presence of these features may imply the need for further investigation, as appropriate.

A history of traumatic life events, including abuse experiences and unresolved losses (e.g., death of a loved one) are common and portend poor health-related quality of life, responsiveness to treatment, and greater health-care utilization. Patients often will not volunteer histories of trauma or abuse unless specifically probed. However, it is important that the provider be prepared to address these difficult experiences when revealed.[90] Given the severity and duration of CAPS pain experiences, patients often seek out multiple specialist consultations and have undergone numerous invasive and noninvasive diagnostic tests, and surgical interventions without uncovering an underlying etiology or symptom resolution.

Patient Behavior

CAPS patients may exhibit a multitude of maladaptive, symptom-related behaviors, including requests for additional diagnostic testing, frequent health-care seeking and utilization, and request for opioid analgesics for pain relief. Patients may also express hysteria and extreme urgency around symptom intensity and focus treatment goals on complete relief of pain, rather than improving pain severity and coping, and diminishing the impact of symptoms on function and quality of life. Patients also may minimize the potential role of psychosocial factors and their symptom experiences and may take limited personal responsibility for self-management of their condition. Family dynamics also may be dysfunctional, with an accompanying significant other or parent taking the lead in providing history and making treatment decisions. These maladaptive behaviors are not specific to CAPS and thus have limited diagnostic value and can be present in the other DGBI and structural GI diagnoses. Fortunately, these maladaptive symptom behaviors are potentially modifiable.[38]

Physical Examination

The physical exam is not itself diagnostic and rarely reveals alternative diagnoses or structural etiologies to explain the chronic pain of a CAPS patient. Exam should begin with inspection of the abdomen for the presence of surgical scars suggestive of previous procedures related to be chronic abdominal pain. The palpation of the abdomen is initiated away from the reported area of maximal intensity and should begin with superficial pressure to elicit potential abdominal wall sources. Observation during palpation for changes in the patient's behavior and response to palpation, particularly with distraction maneuvers, can be useful. The "stethoscope sign," a distracting gentle compression of the abdomen using the diaphragm of the stethoscope, may elicit a diminished behavioral and nonverbal response despite pressing in a previously identified painful location. The "closed eyes sign" has also been described with CAPS patients, wherein abdominal palpation results in patient wincing with closed eyes. Conversely, abdominal palpation in the setting of acute pain of structural etiology is more likely to produce a wide-eyed, anxious patient response in anticipation of an uncomfortable physical exam.[91]

Diagnosis and Differential Diagnosis

Following the completion of a patient history and physical examination, the clinician will have a strong inclination toward a CAPS diagnosis. Further evaluation and support of a CAPS diagnosis includes routine laboratory testing and abdominal imaging. Often, these tests have been completed in the recent past and generally should not be repeated without a change in symptoms or new alarm features. Incidental findings may be encountered (e.g., gastritis on upper endoscopy, liver cysts, gallstones) and should not distract the clinician from a diagnosis of CAPS without good cause. Ultimately, the CAPS diagnosis relies on established symptom criteria (see Box 13.2) and the absence of any other plausible etiology to explain the patient's chronic abdominal pain (see Box 13.2). The evaluation of a suspected CAPS diagnosis can be facilitated through the implementation of an expert proposed algorithm (Fig. 13.5).

Treatment

Patient-Physician Relationship

An important initial step in the effective management of CAPS symptoms is the establishment of an effective rapport between the provider and patient. This patient-physician relationship is an essential foundation upon which a CAPS management strategy is built (see Fig. 13.6). A key aspect of this therapeutic relationship is listening intently as the patient describes their symptoms and the burden they impose, then offering validation of illness to the patient and his/her family. This can come through the provision of a specific, legitimate diagnosis (CAPS) and an explanation of our current understanding of the pathophysiology and mechanisms underlying the disorder. Education of the patient and family will enhance knowledge with regard to the syndrome, address concerns, and provide reassurance and the alleviation of fears relating to a potentially ominous, unrecognized etiology of pain symptoms. Where appropriate, this includes a discussion of the important influence of psychological

BOX 13.2 Rome IV Diagnostic Criteria* for Centrally Mediated Abdominal Pain Syndrome[‡,†]

Must include all the following:

1. Continuous or nearly continuous abdominal pain.
2. No or only occasional relationship of pain with physiological events (e.g., eating, defecation, menses).‡
3. Pain limits some aspect of daily functioning.[§]
4. Pain is not feigned.
5. Pain is not explained by another structural or functional GI disorder or other medical condition.

*Criteria fulfilled for the past 3 months, with symptom onset at least 6 months prior to diagnosis.

‡Some degree of GI dysfunction may be present.

†Centrally mediated abdominal pain syndrome is typically associated with psychosocial comorbidity, but there is no specific profile that can be used for diagnosis.

§Daily function could include impairments in work, intimacy, social/leisure, family life, and caregiving for self or others.

From Whorwell PJ, Keefer L, Drossman DA, et al. Centrally mediated disorders of gastrointestinal pain. In: Drossman DA, Chang L, Chey WD, Kellow J, Tack J, Whitehead WE, eds. *Rome IV: Functional Gastrointestinal Disorders: Disorders of Gut-Brain Interaction. I.* Raleigh, NC: The Rome Foundation; 2016:1059–1116.

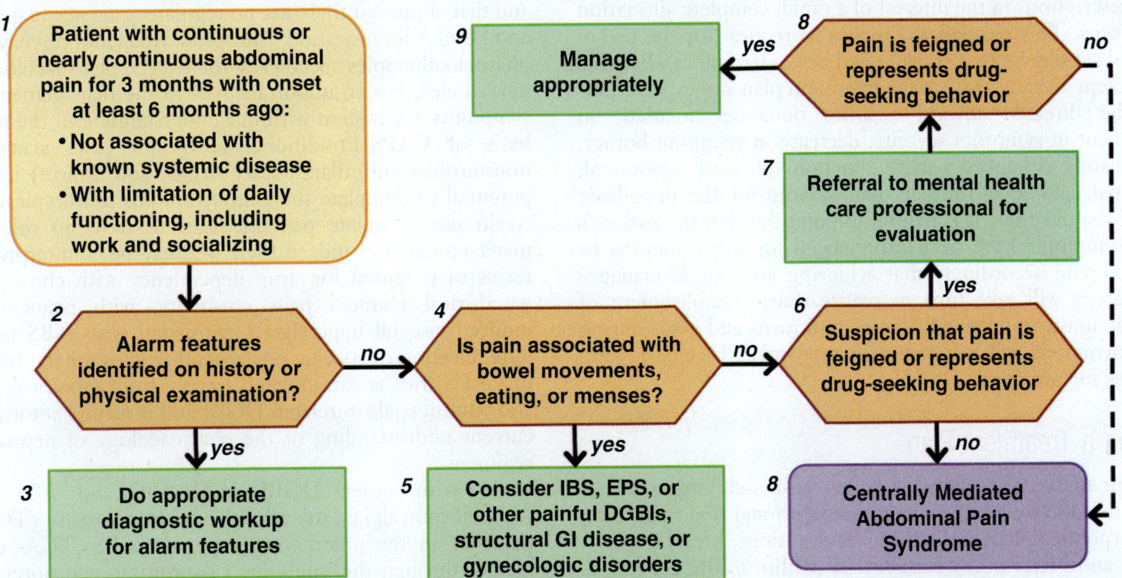

Fig. 13.5 Algorithm for the diagnosis of centrally mediated abdominal pain syndrome (CAPS). *EPS,* Epigastric pain syndrome; *DGBIs,* disorders of gut-brain interaction.[38] (Reprinted from Sperber AD, Drossman DA. Functional abdominal pain syndrome: constant or frequently recurring abdominal pain. *Am J Gastroenterol* 2010;105:770–774)

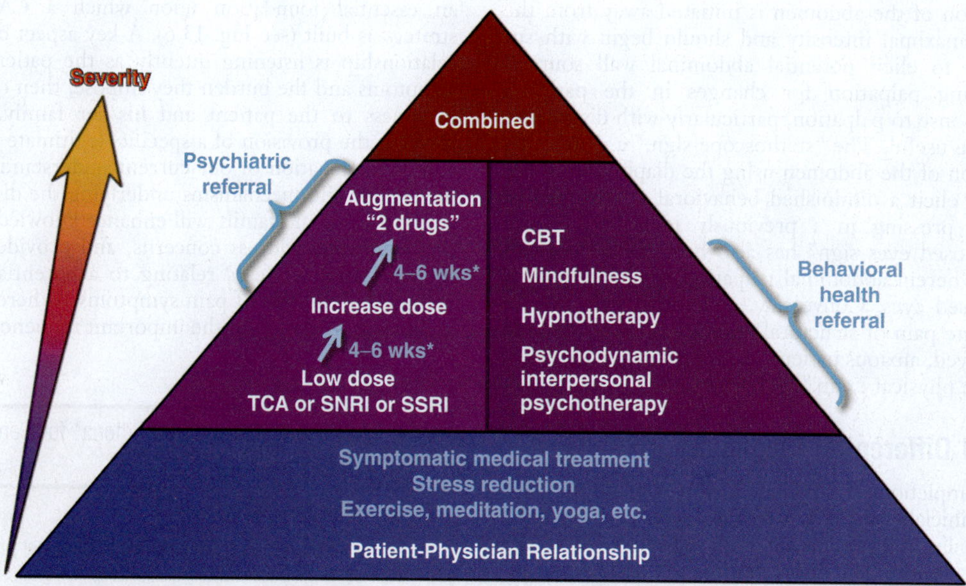

Fig. 13.6 Management strategy for centrally mediated abdominal pain syndrome (CAPS). Strong physician-patient relationships serve as a foundation for CAPS. Symptom-directed therapy, lifestyle changes (e.g., exercise, sleep, stress reduction), and education are key additions. Tricyclic antidepressants (*TCAs*) or serotonin and norepinephrine reuptake inhibitor (*SNRIs*) are often useful as neuromodulators in CAPS management. Augmentation therapy (multiple pharmacotherapeutic agents) and mental health intervention [e.g., cognitive behavioral treatment (*CBT*) or hypnotherapy] can address pain symptoms and psychological distress in refractory cases. Combination therapy with both a medication and a mental health intervention may be required in severe cases.[38] (From Keefer L, Drossman DA, Guthrie E, et al. Centrally mediated disorders of gastrointestinal pain. *Gastroenterology*. 2016. https://doi.org/10.1053/j.gastro.2016.02.034)

factors on pain experiences. An empathetic approach with an acknowledgment of the impact of symptoms on patient physical well-being and psychosocial function will facilitate rapport and enhance satisfaction, adherence to treatment plans, and, ultimately, clinical outcomes.[92]

Empathy and support cannot, however, extend to an over accommodation of the patient's desires for further unnecessary diagnostic testing, or inappropriate or potentially unsafe medication prescriptions in the interest of a rapid, complete alleviation of symptoms. This particularly applies to request for the use of controlled substances (e.g., opiates and benzodiazepines). Patients should accept an active role in the treatment plan and expectations should be directed toward realistic outcomes focused on improvement in symptom severity, decrease in symptom bother, and ultimately enhanced patient function (physical, emotional, professional, and social) rather than striving for the unrealistic "cure" of the disorder. It is helpful to point out that the patient's chronic symptoms have been experienced for many months or even years, and accordingly that achieving an optimal management strategy will take time to realize. Early establishment of reasonable limits in terms of time commitment and goals during patient encounters will help maintain appropriate boundaries and milestones for progress.

Instituting a Treatment Plan

Treatment of CAPS is never a "one-size-fits-all" approach; it requires the development of a multidimensional treatment plan that incorporates pharmacological interventions, lifestyle modifications, and behavioral treatments all within in the context of regular interactions and frequent contacts with the patient to gauge progress and adjust strategy based on responses. It should be expected that augmentative approaches and combinations of different therapeutic options context of a biopsychosocial treatment plan will lead to the best potential for patient improvement.

Pharmacotherapy

Recognizing that there are limited prospective, controlled data to support the benefit of medication treatment specifically in CAPS, and that at present there are no regulatory agency (e.g., U.S. Food and Drug Administration, European Medicines Agency) approved pharmacotherapies specifically for CAPS, pharmacologic therapy nevertheless has an important role in the management of CAPS symptoms. Consistent with our understanding of the mechanistic basis of CAPS, traditional analgesics (e.g., acetaminophen, nonsteroidal antiinflammatory drugs, and aspirin) have limited potential to modulate the pain symptoms prototypical to CAPS. Again use of opiate pain medications have no role in CAPS management, and indeed their use may be counterproductive in terms of potential for drug dependency with chronic use, and paradoxical elevated pain sensitivity, with resultant narcotic induced visceral hyperalgesia consistent with NBS (see below). The selection of specific pharmacotherapies for the management of CAPS thus is extrapolated largely from empirical experience and clinical trials in related DGBI and is further informed by our current understanding of the pharmacology of neuromodulator regimens.[93]

As with other DGBI (e.g., IBS and FD) and FSS (e.g., fibromyalgia), the tricyclic antidepressants (TCAs) are a mainstay in the pharmacotherapy of CAPS. TCAs exert their benefit through the inhibition of serotonin and norepinephrone reuptake, as well as direct receptor effects. Antidepressants improve not only abdominal pain symptoms, but also symptom bother via modulation of brain responses (emotional and

13

cognitive) to peripheral bowel signals. The pain benefit of TCAs is expected to be unrelated to their antidepressant effects, as these agents typically are used to treat chronic pain at low dosages from a psychiatric perspective (i.e., "subpsychiatric" regimens).[94,95] Indeed, in the largest TCA trial to date in IBS, patient response to desipramine was the independent of dosage or blood levels.[96] It is important that the patient understand the rationale for use of these "neuromodulator" agents, making it clear that the intent of TCA treatment is not to treat psychiatric symptoms or a mood disorder as the etiology of pain experiences.

Anticholinergic side effects, such as xerostomia, sedation, constipation, and urinary retention can be limiting with TCA agents. Selection of secondary amine TCAs (e.g., nortriptyline, desipramine), with their lesser affinity for cholinergic muscarinic, histaminergic, and alpha-adrenergic receptors relative to the tertiary amines (e.g., amitriptyline, imipramine, doxepin) may help to mitigate some of these undesirable TCA adverse effects. It is also recommended that the patient initiate TCA treatment at low doses (10–25 mg) and slowly titrate based on response and tolerance (maximal dose 100–150 mg in 25 mg increments every 2–4 weeks). Patients who exceed this dose range or who are on other antidepressants or medications that may prolong the cardiac QT interval should have an electrocardiogram following dose adjustments. Meta-analysis of TCAs in the treatment of IBS has shown them to be quite effective at improving global symptoms [number needed to treat (NNT) around 4].[97] While some patients respond rapidly to the initiation of a TCA, it should be expected that maximal benefit may not be achieved for several months, possibly relating to gradual effects on remodeling of CNS networks.

The selective serotonin reuptake inhibitors (SSRIs; e.g., citalopram) have also been studied in the treatment of global symptoms and IBS, with a similar NNT. However, the available SSRI studies are fewer in number and enrolled smaller patient cohorts. Anecdotally, SSRIs are less effective at addressing pain symptoms in DGBI; this diminished visceral analgesic benefit of SSRIs may relate to their lack of norepinephrine transporter inhibition. SSRIs are used at conventional depression and anxiety dosages, and accordingly may convey some psychiatric benefit. SSRIs generally are better tolerated than TCAs, though nausea, diarrhea, sexual dysfunction, and paradoxical worsening of mood symptoms may be experienced.

The serotonin norepinephrine reuptake inhibitors (SNRIs; e.g., duloxetine, venlafaxine, milnacipran), with their effects on synaptic norepinephrine levels, may be preferable over SSRIs in terms of their potential to modulate central pain experiences. SNRIs are used at typical depression doses, and thus may have a dual benefit of improving both mood and visceral hyperalgesia.[98] Though not specifically studied in CAPS, SNRI such as duloxetine have demonstrated efficacy in IBS.[99]

Atypical (second-generation) antipsychotics (e.g., quetiapine[100]), other contemporary antidepressant or antianxiety agents (e.g., buspirone, mirtazapine) and the alpha-2 delta ligands (e.g., gabapentin, pregabalin) also can be used to treat chronic abdominal pain symptoms, either in combination with other antidepressant agents (augmentation therapy) in the case of suboptimal response to an initial neuromodulator regimen, or alone as monotherapy.[99–101] Potential exists for drug–drug interactions when implementing multiple psychotropic agents, and as a result the provider must be familiar with the pharmacology and neurotransmitter effects of these agents. It is important that these complex regimens be selected in collaboration with the patient's psychiatrist and medical doctor. Detailed descriptions of these neuromodulator medications and considerations for use in DGBI have been reviewed elsewhere. Future directions include profiling of gene expression to inform the selection of a psychotropic agent (i.e., pharmacogenetics) as an individualized approach to the treatment of DGBI-related symptoms.[99,102,103]

Psychological and Gut-Brain Behavioral Treatments (GBBT)

Psychological therapies and gut-brain behavioral treatment have established efficacy in the management of DGBI, and are a mainstay in the treatment of related visceral pain symptoms.[104] Psychological therapies may benefit patients through modulation of higher brain function (enhanced coping strategies and cognitive adaptation), as compared to the targeting of subcortical regions with antidepressant medications. These differential effects enhance the theoretical appeal of implementing combined treatment strategies with both pharmacotherapy and psychological intervention. Combined therapeutic strategies may achieve overall symptom responses that exceed the potential effect of the individual treatments as monotherapy.[105]

Several different psychological treatment options may be considered in the CAPS patient. CBT seeks to identify and reframe the patient's maladaptive thoughts, behaviors, and perceptions. CBT has proven benefit in multiple studies and IBS and is becoming increasingly accessible to patients without access to a health psychologist through minimal contact/self-help workbooks and web/smartphone based applications.[106,107] CBT also has demonstrated efficacy in pediatric CAPS patients.[108,109] Mindfulness-based stress reduction focuses on the theoretical framework of being grounded in the moment and the recognition that pain experiences may be inevitable yet suffering can be diminished, leading to a reduction in physical vulnerability to stress. Several randomized control trials have demonstrated efficacy of mindfulness therapy in IBS and other chronic pain syndromes. Gut-directed hypnotherapy emphasizes a heightened state of focus and awareness, leading to an increase receptiveness to suggestions for change. Hypnotherapy has proven useful in several different DGBI, including IBS and FD, and also has demonstrated benefit in children with CAPS.[110] Follow-up studies have shown hypnotherapy to have durable effects over time.[111] Gut-directed hypnotherapy is a useful option for patients with severe and refractory symptoms, and high levels somatization. Online and digital options for hypnotherapy are available. Psychodynamic interpersonal psychotherapy (PIP) establishes a trusting collaborative relationship that helps to facilitate change for the patient. Through psychoeducation, it is helpful in targeting negative emotions, abuse, and traumatic early life experiences. PIP requires an experienced mental health professional for delivery and can be effective in severe and refractory symptoms, patients with somatizations, and interpersonal challenges. It has been shown to be effective in meta-analysis for FSS and IBS. Regardless of the psychological therapy recommended by the provider, it is important that the patient understand that psychological interventions will be implemented in parallel with continued medical care, minimizing the potential perception of physician rejection or stigmatization of symptoms being "all in the patient's head."

NARCOTIC BOWEL SYNDROME (NBS) OPIOID-INDUCED GASTROINTESTINAL HYPERALGESIA

Introduction

Opioid pain medications are well known to decrease gastrointestinal motility, leading to potential for delayed gastric emptying, ileus, and constipation. In cases of continued to use, patients may develop "opioid-induced constipation," or in the setting of preexistent constipation, "opioid-exacerbated constipation" due to the peripheral effects of opioids on GI motility.[112] NBS is a distinct condition of opioid-induced centrally-mediated hyperalgesia, characterized by paradoxical increases in abdominal pain symptoms in the setting of chronic opiate use (Box 13.3).[113] Though NBS has only recently been described over the last

BOX 13.3 Rome IV Diagnostic Criteria for Narcotic Bowel Syndrome/Opioid-Induced Gastrointestinal Hyperalgesia

Must include all the following:

1. Chronic or frequently recurring abdominal pain* that is treated with acute high-dose or chronic narcotics.
2. The nature and intensity of the pain is not explained by a current or previous GI diagnosis.†
3. Two or more of the following:
   a. The pain worsens or incompletely resolves with continued or escalating doses of narcotics.
   b. There is marked worsening of pain when the narcotic dose wanes and improvement when narcotics are reinstituted "soar and crash."
   c. There is a progression of the frequency, duration, and intensity of pain episodes.

*Pain must occur on most days.

†A patient may have a structural diagnosis (e.g., IBD, chronic pancreatitis), but the character or activity of the disease process is not sufficient to explain the pain. From Whorwell PJ, Keefer L, Drossman DA, et al. Centrally mediated disorders of gastrointestinal pain. In: Drossman DA, Chang L, Chey WD, Kellow J, Tack J, Whitehead WE, eds. *Rome IV: Functional Gastrointestinal Disorders: Disorders of Gut-Brain Interaction. I.* Raleigh, NC: The Rome Foundation; 2016:1059–1116.

couple of decades, opioid-induced hyperalgesia (OIH) is a well-recognized condition in the neurophysiological and anesthesia literature. OIH manifests as either allodynia (pain resulting from a stimulus that normally would not evoke pain) or hyperalgesia (increased sensitivity to noxious stimuli). NBS thus represents a subgroup of OIH, or "opioid-induced gastrointestinal hyperalgesia."

Epidemiology

Though less common than opioid-induced constipation, NBS has become more prevalent in parallel with the opioid epidemic in the United States, driven by the more liberal use of opioid prescriptions for the management of noncancer pain etiologies.[114,115] NBS prevalence from large epidemiologic studies is estimated to be approximately 4%, and even more prevalent in pain management clinics. NBS initially may go unrecognized by the pain specialist, and often is detected upon referral to GI specialist for a possible DGBI diagnosis. The pain indication for opiate prescriptions may be predominantly gastrointestinal but can also be musculoskeletal. In some cases, NBS may develop postoperatively. From a demographic perspective, NBS tends to affect well-educated, younger to middle-aged women. Patients often have symptoms for years prior to receiving a formal diagnosis. Risk factors for NBS include a background of other DGBI or psychological comorbidities, as well as histories of past physical or sexual abuse.[114] Substantial levels of disability are encountered (over 80% NBS patients are out of work) and NBS sufferers are high health-care utilizers.[116]

Pathophysiology

Several mechanisms have been suggested to be relevant to the development of NBS, with insights gained from work conducted in the study of OIH. A notable theory is the opioid-induced inflammatory activation of spinal glial cells (microglia and astrocytes), leading to diminished analgesic effects of opiates, opioid tolerance, and neuropathic pain. Other posited mechanisms include: augmentation of pain signaling in the dorsal horn of the spinal cord via G-protein coupled excitatory opioid receptors, spinal cord *N*-methyl-D-aspartate receptor activation of pain facilitatory pathways, dynorphin-mediated ascending facilitation of nociceptive signals at the level of the rostral ventral medulla, and central abnormalities and pain processing, similar to that seen in CAPS.[117]

Clinical Presentation

Patients develop NBS following opioid prescriptions for either gastrointestinal disease (e.g., chronic pancreatitis, inflammatory bowel disease, or DGBI) or extraintestinal conditions (e.g., musculoskeletal pain, migraines, fibromyalgia). Abdominal pain subsequently develops, and eventually progresses over time, despite escalating doses of opiate medications. NBS is a positive diagnosis, rather than a diagnosis of exclusion, that can be made in the setting of the appropriate clinical scenario. Cross-sectional imaging may identify fecal loading, and also can help exclude other diagnoses including bowel obstruction, inflammation, or ischemia. When GI diagnoses are the primary indication for opiate prescription, NBS symptoms often can be misattributed to the underlying structural or functional bowel disorder. NBS can exist alongside opioid-induced constipation (OIC) and other peripheral-mu-opioid receptor-mediated effects on GI motility, including delayed gastric emptying, nausea, biliary pain, ileus, and pseudo-obstruction. The vicious cycle of increasing pain and demand for escalating doses of opiates to achieve relief often results in patient frustration and maladaptive patient-physician relationships. Concerns about potential dependence, abuse, opioid diversion, and overdose all are additional challenges that face the provider and patient.

Treatment

Establishing a strong patient physician relationship based on solid communication skills is requisite to the successful management of NBS. A multicomponent detoxification program that follows a described protocol systematic opioid reduction in conjunction with TCAs to manage pain, anxiolytics (e.g., lorazepam or quetiapine), and treatment of withdrawal symptoms (e.g., clonidine), and psychological support is the only effective way of managing NBS.[116,117] This detoxification is best conducted in an inpatient setting. In one series, nearly 90% of patients completed detoxification, resulting in substantial improvements in abdominal pain symptoms. Unfortunately, over 40% of this same NBS cohort had restarted opiate pain medications within 3 months, often with a recurrence of abdominal symptoms.

Full references for this chapter can be found at https://ebooks.health.elsevier.com.

14 Symptoms of Esophageal Disease

Kenneth R. DeVault

IN THIS CHAPTER

Common symptoms that affect the esophagus include dysphagia, odynophagia, globus sensation, hiccups, chest pain, heartburn, regurgitation, and a number of "supraesophageal" complaints that have been attributed to gastroesophageal reflux. A carefully taken history can clarify many of these symptoms and is followed by selected testing, therapeutic trials, or both. Dysphagia is either proximal or distal and can be to solids only or to liquids and solids. Barium testing, manometry, and endoscopy are appropriate tests in a patient with dysphagia. Odynophagia usually indicates mucosal disease and should lead to endoscopy in most situations. The evaluation of globus sensation and hiccups usually does not yield a specific disorder, and the management is thus challenging. Chest pain can originate from the esophagus and frequently responds to gastric acid suppression. If reflux is not present, the evaluation and treatment of chest pain become challenging. Typical (heartburn and regurgitation) and extraesophageal symptoms potentially caused by gastroesophageal reflux disease (GERD) may respond to a diagnostic and therapeutic trial of acid suppression. Ambulatory pH testing is the best method to confirm reflux in these patients. Many of these esophageal symptoms may also occur in a patient with no objective evidence of pathology and are then considered and treated as functional disorders.

Symptoms related to the esophagus are among the most common in general medical as well as gastroenterologic practice. For example, dysphagia becomes more common with aging and affects up to 15% of persons age 65 or older.[1] Heartburn, regurgitation, and other symptoms of GERD are also common. A survey of healthy subjects in Olmsted County, Minnesota, found that 20% of persons, regardless of gender or age, experienced heartburn at least weekly.[2] Mild symptoms of GERD rarely indicate severe underlying disease but must be addressed, especially if they have occurred for many years. Frequent or persistent dysphagia or odynophagia suggests an esophageal problem that necessitates investigation and treatment. Other less specific symptoms of possible esophageal origin include globus sensation, chest pain, belching, hiccups, rumination, and extraesophageal complaints like wheezing, coughing, sore throat, and hoarseness, especially if other causes have been excluded. A major challenge in evaluating esophageal symptoms is that the degree of esophageal damage often does not correlate well with the patient's or physician's impression of symptom severity.[3] This is a particular problem in older patients, in whom the severity of gastroesophageal reflux-induced injury to the esophageal mucosa is increased despite an overall decrease in the severity of symptoms.[4]

DYSPHAGIA

Dysphagia, from the Greek *dys* (difficulty, disordered) and *phagia* (to eat), refers to the sensation that food is hindered in its passage from the mouth to the stomach. Most patients complain that food sticks, hangs up, or stops, or they feel that the food "just won't go down right." Occasionally they complain of associated pain. If asked, "Do you have trouble swallowing?", some patients with dysphagia in the lower esophagus will actually say no because they may only think of swallowing as the transfer of food from the mouth to the esophagus. Patients with a dilated esophagus, particularly due to achalasia, may incorrectly interpret dysphagia as regurgitation or even vomiting. Dysphagia usually indicates malfunction of some type in the oropharynx or esophagus, although associated psychiatric disorders can amplify this symptom, and a functional basis for dysphagia is possible in some patients. It is also now clear that chronic narcotic use can result in esophageal symptoms and motility disturbances that may resolve after discontinuation of those medications.

Pathophysiology

Inability to swallow is caused by a problem with the strength or coordination of the muscles required to move material from the mouth to the stomach or by a fixed obstruction somewhere between the mouth and stomach. Occasionally patients may have a combination of the two processes. The oropharyngeal swallowing mechanism and the primary and secondary peristaltic contractions of the esophageal body that follow usually transport solid and liquid boluses from the mouth to the stomach within 10 seconds. If these orderly contractions fail to develop or progress, the accumulated bolus of food distends the esophageal lumen and causes the discomfort associated with dysphagia. In some patients, particularly older adults, dysphagia is the result of low-amplitude primary or secondary peristaltic activity that is insufficient to clear the esophagus. High-resolution manometry has identified areas of weak or absent peristalsis of varying lengths (peristaltic gaps) that may explain dysphagia in some patients who have a normal conventional manometry result.[5] Other patients have a primary or secondary motility disorder that grossly disturbs the orderly contractions of the esophageal body. Because these motor abnormalities may not be present with every swallow, dysphagia may wax and wane (see also Chapter 46).

Mechanical narrowing of the esophageal lumen may interrupt the orderly passage of a food bolus despite adequate peristaltic contractions. Symptoms vary with the degree of luminal obstruction, associated esophagitis, and type of food ingested. The normal esophagus distends in advance of a bolus's arrival. Patients with a poorly distensible esophagus (e.g., due to eosinophilic esophagitis or radiation esophagitis) may experience dysphagia even though the esophagus does not appear to be narrowed during esophagogastroduodenoscopy (EGD) or barium swallow (see later).[6] Although minimally obstructing lesions cause dysphagia only with large, poorly chewed boluses of foods like meat and dry bread, lesions that obstruct the esophageal lumen completely lead to symptoms with solids and liquids. GERD may produce dysphagia related to an esophageal stricture, but some patients with GERD clearly have dysphagia in the absence of a demonstrable stricture and perhaps even without esophagitis.[7] Abnormal sensory perception in the esophagus may lead to the feeling of dysphagia even when the bolus has cleared the esophagus. Because some normal test subjects experience the sensation of dysphagia when the distal esophagus is distended by a balloon, as well as by other intraluminal stimuli, an aberration in visceral perception could explain dysphagia in patients who have no definable cause.[8] This mechanism may also apply to amplification of symptoms in patients with spastic motility disorders, in whom the frequency of psychiatric disorders is increased.[9] The concept of "functional dysphagia" has been refined by the Rome Foundation and is a reasonable diagnosis when testing does not identify a cause for dysphagia and therapeutic trials do not lead to symptom improvement.

BOX 14.1 Causes of Oropharyngeal Dysphagia

NEUROMUSCULAR*

Amyotrophic lateral sclerosis (ALS, Lou Gehrig disease)
CNS tumors (benign or malignant)
Idiopathic UES dysfunction
Manometric dysfunction of the UES or pharynx†
Multiple sclerosis
Muscular dystrophy
Myasthenia gravis
Parkinson disease
Polymyositis or dermatomyositis
Postpolio syndrome
Stroke
Thyroid dysfunction

STRUCTURAL

Carcinoma
Infections of pharynx or neck
Osteophytes and other spinal disorders
Prior surgery or radiation therapy
Proximal esophageal web
Thyromegaly
Zenker diverticulum

*Any disease that affects striated muscle or its innervation may result in dysphagia.
†Many manometric disorders (hypertensive and hypotensive UES, abnormal coordination, and incomplete UES relaxation) have been described, although their true relationship to dysphagia is often unclear.
UES, Upper esophageal sphincter.

Differential Diagnosis and Approach

When faced with a patient who complains of dysphagia, the health care provider should approach the problem in a systematic way. Most patients can localize dysphagia to the upper or lower portion of the esophagus, although occasional patients with a distal esophageal cause of dysphagia will present with symptoms referred only to the suprasternal notch or higher. The approach to dysphagia can be divided into oropharyngeal and esophageal dysphagia, although considerable overlap may occur in certain groups of patients. An attempt should be made to determine whether the patient has difficulty only with solid boluses or with both liquids and solids.

Oropharyngeal Dysphagia

With processes that affect the mouth, hypopharynx, and upper esophagus, the patient is often unable to initiate a swallow and must repeatedly attempt to swallow. Patients frequently describe coughing or choking when they attempt to eat. The inability to propel a food bolus successfully from the hypopharyngeal area through the upper esophageal sphincter (UES) into the esophageal body is called *oropharyngeal* or *transfer dysphagia*. The patient is aware that the bolus has not left the oropharynx and locates the site of symptoms specifically to the region of the cervical esophagus. Dysphagia that occurs immediately or within 1 second of swallowing suggests an oropharyngeal abnormality. At times, a liquid bolus may enter the trachea or nose rather than the esophagus. Some patients describe recurrent bolus impactions that require manual dislodgement. In severe cases, saliva cannot be swallowed, and the patient drools. Families are tempted to perform the Heimlich maneuver in such instances, but this is not appropriate unless the bolus is producing airway compromise. They should be informed that if the patient can speak, the airway is functional, and forcing an esophageal bolus proximally may cause rather than prevent aspiration. Abnormalities of speech like dysarthria or nasal speech may be associated with oropharyngeal dysphagia. Systemic neurologic and neuromuscular conditions, such as Parkinson disease, amyotrophic lateral sclerosis, and polymyositis, can present with dysphagia as a predominant and occasionally only symptom. Oral pathology should be considered well; poor teeth or poorly fitting dentures may disrupt mastication and result in an attempt to swallow an overly large or poorly chewed bolus. Loss of salivation—caused by medications, radiation, or primary salivary dysfunction—may result in a bolus that is difficult to swallow.

Recurrent bouts of pulmonary infection may reflect spillover of food into the trachea because of inadequate laryngeal protection. Hoarseness may result from recurrent laryngeal nerve dysfunction or intrinsic muscular disease, both of which cause ineffective vocal cord movement. Weakness of the soft palate or pharyngeal constrictors causes dysarthria and nasal speech as well as pharyngonasal regurgitation. Swallowing associated with a gurgling noise may be described by patients with Zenker diverticulum. Finally, unexplained weight loss may be the only clue to a swallowing disorder; patients avoid eating because of the difficulties encountered. Potential causes of oropharyngeal dysphagia are shown in Box 14.1.

After an adequate history is obtained, the initial test is a carefully conducted barium radiographic examination, which is optimally performed with the assistance of a swallowing therapist (modified barium swallow). If the study is normal with liquid barium, the examination is repeated after the patient is fed a solid bolus to bring out the patient's symptoms and thereby aid in localizing any pathology. If the oropharyngeal portion of the study is normal, the remainder of the esophagus should be examined. The modified barium swallow usually identifies the problem and directs initial therapy.

Esophageal Dysphagia

Most patients with esophageal dysphagia localize their symptoms to the lower sternum or, at times, the epigastric region. A smaller

14

BOX 14.2 Common Causes of Esophageal Dysphagia

NEUROMUSCULAR (MOTILITY) DISORDERS*

Primary

Achalasia
Distal esophageal spasm
Hypercontractile (jackhammer) esophagus
Hypertensive LES
Nutcracker (high-pressure) esophagus
Other peristaltic abnormalities

Secondary

Chagas disease
Reflux-related dysmotility
Scleroderma and other rheumatologic disorders

STRUCTURAL (MECHANICAL) DISORDERS

Intrinsic

Carcinoma and benign tumors
Diverticula
Eosinophilic esophagitis
Esophageal rings and webs (other than Schatzki ring)
Foreign body
Lower esophageal (Schatzki) ring
Medication-induced stricture
Peptic stricture

Extrinsic

Mediastinal mass
Spinal osteophytes
Vascular compression

*Peristaltic abnormalities include absent peristalsis and weak peristalsis, as well as hypertensive peristalsis (nutcracker esophagus).
LES, Lower esophageal sphincter.

number of patients describe a sensation in the suprasternal notch or higher even though the bolus stops in the lower esophagus. Esophageal dysphagia can frequently be relieved by various maneuvers like repeated swallowing, raising the arms over the head, throwing the shoulders back, and using the Valsalva maneuver. Motility disorders or mechanical obstructing lesions can cause esophageal dysphagia. To clarify the origin of symptoms of esophageal dysphagia, the answers to three questions are crucial:

1. What type of food or liquid causes symptoms?
2. Is the dysphagia intermittent or progressive?
3. Does the patient have heartburn?

On the basis of these answers, distinguishing the several causes of esophageal dysphagia (Box 14.2) as a structural (mechanical) or a neuromuscular (motility) defect and postulating the specific cause are often possible (Fig. 14.1).

Patients who report dysphagia with solids and liquids are more likely to have an esophageal motility disorder than mechanical obstruction. Achalasia is the prototypical esophageal motility disorder; in addition to dysphagia, many patients with achalasia complain of bland regurgitation of undigested food, especially at night, and weight loss. By contrast, patients with a spastic motility disorder like distal esophageal spasm may complain of chest pain and sensitivity to hot or cold liquids. Patients with scleroderma (systemic sclerosis) involving the esophagus usually have Raynaud phenomenon and may have heartburn and regurgitation. In these patients, complaints of mild dysphagia can be due to a motility disturbance or esophageal inflammation, but severe dysphagia almost always signals the presence of a peptic stricture or (less commonly) malignancy (see Chapters 39, 46, 48, and 50).

In patients who report dysphagia only after swallowing solid foods and never with liquids alone, mechanical obstruction should be suspected. A luminal obstruction of sufficiently high grade, however, may be associated with dysphagia for solids and liquids. If food impaction develops, the patient frequently must regurgitate for relief. If a patient continues to drink liquid after the bolus impaction, large amounts of that liquid may be regurgitated. When asking about liquid dysphagia, it is important to distinguish the patient who has true liquid dysphagia only when drinking from the patient who has liquid dysphagia only after a solid bolus has become impacted. Hypersalivation is common during an episode of dysphagia and provides even more liquid to regurgitate.

Episodic and nonprogressive dysphagia without weight loss is characteristic of an esophageal web or a distal esophageal (Schatzki) ring. The first episode typically occurs during a hurried meal, often with alcohol. The patient notes that the bolus of food sticks in the lower esophagus; it can often be passed by drinking large quantities of liquids. Many patients finish the meal without difficulty after the obstruction is relieved. Initially, an episode may not recur for weeks or months, but subsequent episodes may occur frequently (see Chapter 46). Daily dysphagia, however, is likely not caused by a lower esophageal ring unless it is very tight.

If solid food dysphagia is clearly progressive, the differential diagnosis includes peptic esophageal stricture and carcinoma. Benign esophageal strictures develop in some patients with GERD (see Chapter 48). Most of these patients have a long history of associated heartburn. Weight loss seldom occurs in patients with a benign lesion, because these patients have a good appetite and convert their diet to high-calorie soft and liquid foods to maintain weight. Patients with carcinoma differ from those with peptic stricture in several ways. As a group, patients with carcinoma are older and present with a history of rapidly progressive dysphagia. They may or may not have a history of heartburn, and heartburn may have occurred in the past but not the present. Most have anorexia and weight loss (see Chapter 50). True dysphagia may be seen in patients with pill, caustic, or viral esophagitis, but the predominant complaint of patients with these acute esophageal injuries is usually odynophagia (see Chapter 47).

Patients may present with a food bolus impaction, and eosinophilic esophagitis should be considered in the differential diagnosis of all patients who present with dysphagia (see Chapter 30).[10] Eosinophilic esophagitis was initially described in young adult men, but subsequent series have found this disorder in both sexes and all age groups.[11]

Surgical causes of dysphagia include prior fundoplication or other surgery at the esophagogastric junction, and bariatric surgery can also present with dysphagia (see Chapter 9). Such dysphagia can be due to mechanical obstruction, but there have also been reports of motility disturbances after surgery up to and including a manometric appearance consistent with achalasia.[12] Motility dysfunction is most common with gastric banding but can occur with any of the bariatric surgeries.

After a focused history of the patient's symptoms is obtained, a barium study, including a solid bolus challenge, is often advocated as the first test. Alternatively, many experts have advocated endoscopy as the first test, especially in patients with intermittent dysphagia for solid food suggestive of a lower esophageal ring or with pronounced reflux symptoms. Choice of the initial test should be based on local expertise and the preference of the individual health care provider. If the barium examination demonstrates an obstructive lesion, endoscopy is usually done for confirmation and biopsy. Endoscopy also permits dilation of strictures, rings, and neoplasms. Empirical dilation of the esophagus is often performed in patients with a history suggestive of obstructive dysphagia and a normal endoscopic examination,[13] but the safety and efficacy of this approach have been questioned.[14] If the barium examination is normal, esophageal manometry is often performed to look for a motility disorder. Some patients with

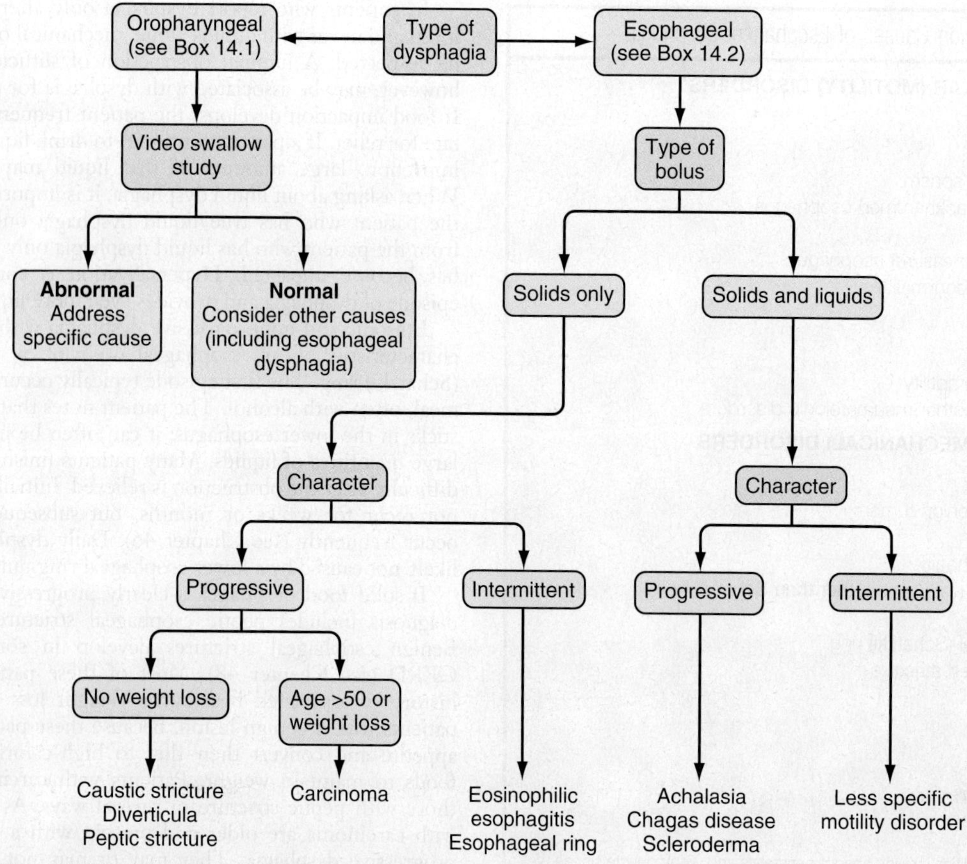

Fig. 14.1 Diagnostic algorithm for patients with dysphagia. For details of the approach to each type of dysphagia, see text and boxes. Less specific motility disorders include nutcracker esophagus, distal esophageal spasm, and other disorders of ineffective esophageal motility. (Modified from Castell DO, Donner MW. Evaluation of dysphagia: a careful history is crucial. *Dysphagia*. 1987;2:65-71.)

reflux symptoms and dysphagia, a normal barium study or endoscopy, or both, will respond to a trial of gastric acid suppressive therapy.

ODYNOPHAGIA

Like dysphagia, odynophagia, or painful swallowing, is specific for esophageal involvement. Chest pain that is spontaneous and not usually related to swallowing is not odynophagia and will be discussed below. Odynophagia may range from a dull retrosternal ache on swallowing to a stabbing pain with radiation to the back so severe the patient cannot eat or even swallow his or her own saliva. Odynophagia usually reflects an inflammatory process that involves the esophageal mucosa or, in rare instances, the esophageal muscle. The most common causes of odynophagia include caustic ingestion, pill-induced esophagitis, radiation injury, and infectious esophagitis (*Candida*, herpesvirus, cytomegalovirus (CMV) [Box 14.3]) (see Chapters 39 and 47). In these diseases, dysphagia may also be present, but pain is the dominant complaint. Odynophagia is an infrequent complaint of patients with GERD and, when present, is usually associated with severe ulcerative esophagitis. In rare cases, a nonobstructive esophageal carcinoma can produce odynophagia. Because many of the diseases that cause odynophagia have associated symptoms and signs, a carefully taken history can often suggest a diagnosis. For example, a teenager who takes tetracycline for acne and in whom odynophagia develops most likely has pill-related dysphagia; an immunocompromised patient with odynophagia is likely to have an infectious cause (see Chapters 34, 35, and 47); and a patient with GERD is likely to have severe peptic esophagitis. EGD to visualize and obtain biopsy specimens of the esophageal mucosa is required to confirm a specific diagnosis in most patients with odynophagia.

GLOBUS SENSATION

Globus sensation is a feeling of a lump or tightness in the throat, unrelated to swallowing. Up to 46% of the general population experience globus sensation at one time or another.[15] The sensation can be described as a lump, tightness, choking, or strangling feeling, as if something is caught in the throat. Globus sensation is present between meals, and swallowing solids or large liquid boluses may give temporary relief. Frequent dry swallowing and emotional stress may worsen this symptom. Globus sensation may occur after a traumatic event like swallowing a rough bolus (fish bone) or even after endoscopy—despite the lack of identifiable mucosal injury—if intubation with the endoscope was psychologically traumatic.[16] Globus sensation should not be diagnosed in the presence of dysphagia or odynophagia.

Pathophysiology

Detection of physiologic and psychological abnormalities in patients with globus sensation has been inconsistent and controversial. Although frequently suggested, manometrically detectable UES dysfunction has not been identified directly as the cause of globus sensation, nor does the UES appear to be hyperresponsive

BOX 14.3 Causes of Odynophagia

CAUSTIC INGESTION

Acid
Alkali

PILL-INDUCED INJURY

Alendronate and other bisphosphonates
Aspirin and other NSAIDs
Emepronium bromide
Iron preparations
Potassium chloride (especially slow-release form)
Quinidine
Tetracycline and its derivatives
Zidovudine

INFECTIOUS ESOPHAGITIS

Viral

CMV
EBV
HIV
HSV

Bacterial

Mycobacteria (tuberculosis or *Mycobacterium avium* complex)

Fungal

Candida albicans
Histoplasmosis

Protozoan

Cryptosporidiosis
Pneumocystis jirovecii

SEVERE REFLUX ESOPHAGITIS

ESOPHAGEAL CARCINOMA

to esophageal distention, acidification, or mental stress.[17] Furthermore, esophageal distention can cause globus sensation unrelated to a rise in UES pressure, and stress can induce an increase in UES pressure that is not associated with globus sensation in normal subjects and in patients who complain of globus sensation. Heartburn has been reported in up to 90% of patients with globus sensation,[18] yet documentation of esophagitis or abnormal gastroesophageal reflux by esophageal pH monitoring is found in fewer than 25% (see later). Balloon distention of the esophagus produces globus sensation at lower balloon volumes in globus sufferers than in controls; this finding suggests the perception of esophageal stretch may be heightened in some patients with globus sensation.

Psychological factors may be important in the genesis of globus sensation. The most common associated psychiatric diagnoses include anxiety, panic disorder, depression, hypochondriasis, somatic symptom disorder, and introversion.[19] Indeed, globus sensation is the fourth most common symptom in patients with somatic symptom disorder (see Chapter 23).[20] A combination of biological factors, hypochondriacal traits, and learned fear after a choking episode provides a framework for misinterpretation of the symptoms and intensifies the symptoms of globus or the patient's anxiety.[21]

Approach

The approach to globus sensation involves excluding a more sinister underlying disorder and then offering symptom-driven therapy. A nasal endoscopy to rule out pharyngeal pathology and a barium swallow to rule out a fixed pharyngeal lesion are often helpful.[22] Patients with globus sensation often have erythema and other changes in the larynx that may be interpreted as consistent with laryngopharyngeal reflux. Most reflux experts consider these changes to be nonspecific and not diagnostic of pathologic reflux.[23] If a patient has heartburn, gastric acid suppressive therapy is the first step, but reflux may be the cause of globus sensation even in the absence of heartburn. A trial of a proton pump inhibitor (PPI) (usually given twice daily before meals) is diagnostic and therapeutic in some patients. Ambulatory reflux monitoring may show acid or nonacid reflux in some patients (see Chapter 48).[24] Alternatively, if the patient has obvious anxiety and has already failed a trial of acid suppression, therapy directed toward the psychological component of the problem should be considered.

HICCUPS

The symptom of hiccups (hiccoughs and singultus) is caused by a combination of diaphragmatic contraction and glottic closure. Therefore it is not classically an esophageal symptom but is a common complaint in primary care and gastroenterology. Most cases of hiccups are idiopathic, but the symptom has been associated with many conditions (trauma, masses, infections, and uremia) that affect the central nervous system, thorax, or abdomen. Hiccups associated with uremia may be particularly difficult to control. GI causes include GERD, achalasia, gastropathies, and peptic ulcer. Hiccups often occur after a large meal. Because most cases are self-limited, intervention is not usually required. The evaluation of chronic or difficult cases should include select tests to exclude esophageal, thoracic, or systemic diseases. Because GERD has been associated with hiccups, a trial of gastric acid suppressive therapy may be reasonable in some patients.[25] Many agents have been used to suppress hiccups, with varying success: chlorpromazine, nifedipine, haloperidol, phenytoin, metoclopramide, baclofen, and gabapentin.[26] Alternative modalities, including acupuncture, have also been tried in refractory cases.[27] Ablation and stimulation of the phrenic nerve have been reported but should only be considered in truly refractory cases in which the patient's quality of life is severely reduced by the condition and only after all other less invasive approaches have been attempted.[28]

CHEST PAIN OF ESOPHAGEAL ORIGIN

Chest pain of esophageal origin may be indistinguishable from angina pectoris to patients and their health care providers. The esophagus and heart are anatomically adjacent and share innervation. In fact, once cardiac disease is excluded, esophageal disorders are probably the most common causes of chest pain. Of the approximately 1,000,000 patients in the United States who undergo coronary angiography yearly for presumed cardiac pain, almost 40% have normal epicardial coronary arteries; in many of these persons, esophageal disease is implicated as a cause of pain.[29,30]

Esophageal chest pain is usually described as a squeezing or burning substernal sensation that radiates to the back, neck, jaw, or arms. Although not always related to swallowing, the pain can be triggered by ingestion of hot or cold liquids. It may awaken the patient from sleep and can worsen during periods of emotional stress. The duration of pain ranges from minutes to hours and may occur intermittently over several days. Although pain can be severe, causing the patient to become ashen and perspire, it often abates spontaneously and may be eased with antacids. Occasionally the pain is so severe that narcotics or nitroglycerin are required for relief.

The clinical history is important but does not always enable the physician to reliably distinguish a cardiac from an esophageal cause of chest pain.[31] In fact, gastroesophageal reflux may be triggered by exercise[32] and cause exertional chest pain that mimics angina pectoris, even during treadmill testing. Features suggestive of an esophageal origin include pain that continues for hours, is retrosternal without lateral radiation, interrupts sleep or is related to meals, and is relieved with antacids. The presence of other esophageal symptoms helps establish an esophageal cause of pain. However, as many as 50% of patients with cardiac pain also have one or more symptoms of esophageal disease.[33] Furthermore, relief of pain with sublingual nitroglycerin has been shown not to be specific for a coronary origin of pain.[34] Cardiac and esophageal disease increase in frequency as people grow older, and both problems may not only coexist but also interact to produce chest pain. The esophagus can be blamed for musculoskeletal pain, so the examination should include careful palpation of the chest wall.

Pathophysiology

The specific mechanisms that produce esophageal chest pain are not well understood. Chest pain that arises from the esophagus has commonly been attributed to stimulation of chemoreceptors (by acid, pepsin, or bile) or mechanoreceptors (by distention or spasm); thermoreceptors (stimulated by cold) may also be involved. Gastroesophageal reflux causes chest pain primarily through acid-sensitive esophageal chemoreceptors. Acid-induced dysmotility may be a cause of esophageal pain. Early studies showed that perfusion of acid into the esophagus in patients with gastroesophageal reflux increases the amplitude and duration of esophageal contractions and induces simultaneous and spontaneous contractions, with the occurrence of pain.[35] Distal esophageal spasm has also been demonstrated during spontaneous acid reflux. Subsequent studies with modern equipment, however, have shown that such changes in motility are rare.[36] In addition, studies using 24-hour ambulatory esophageal pH and motility monitoring have shown that the association between abnormal motility and pain is uncommon, and that spontaneous acid-induced chest pain is rarely associated with abnormalities in esophageal motility.[37,38]

Patients with chest pain suspected to be esophageal in origin have an increased frequency of esophageal contractions of high amplitude and a slightly increased frequency of simultaneous contractions when compared with a normal control population.[39] In addition, intraluminal US has been able to identify abnormal sustained contractions of the longitudinal smooth muscle in a subset of patients with chest pain.[40] How these contractions cause pain is unknown. One possible explanation is that pain occurs when high intramural esophageal tension resulting from altered motility inhibits blood flow to the esophagus for a critical period (i.e., myoischemia). MacKenzie and colleagues found that rates of esophageal rewarming are decreased after infusions of cold water into the esophagus of patients with symptomatic esophageal motility disorders as compared with age-matched controls.[41] Because the rate of rewarming after cold water infusion in patients with Raynaud phenomenon correlates directly with blood flow, the authors theorized that esophageal ischemia is the cause of the reduced rate of rewarming. None of the patients with a symptomatic esophageal motility disorder, however, experienced chest pain during the study. Furthermore, the extensive arterial and venous blood supply to the esophagus makes it unlikely that blood flow is compromised after even the most abnormal esophageal contractions. Complicating the relationship between esophageal chest pain and abnormal esophageal contractions is the consistent observation that most of these patients are asymptomatic when the contraction abnormalities are identified. In addition, the amelioration of chest pain does not correlate predictably with a reduction in the amplitude of esophageal contractions.[42] The possibility exists that chest pain-associated motility changes represent an epiphenomenon of a chronic pain syndrome rather than the direct cause of the pain. In fact, experimentally induced stress can produce manometric changes and lower the tolerance to balloon or acid provocation in both normal subjects and patients with gastroesophageal reflux.[43]

Other potential causes of esophageal chest pain include excitation of temperature receptors and luminal distention. Ingestion of hot or cold liquids can produce severe chest pain. This association was previously thought to be related to esophageal spasm, but subsequent studies have shown that cold-induced pain produces esophageal aperistalsis and dilatation, not spasm.[44] This observation suggests that the cause of esophageal chest pain may be activation of stretch receptors by acute distention. Esophageal distention and pain are experienced during an acute food impaction, drinking carbonated beverages (in some patients), and dysfunction of the belch reflex.[45] In susceptible persons, esophageal chest pain can be reproduced by distention of an esophageal balloon to volumes lower than those that produce pain in asymptomatic persons.[46] Therefore altered pain perception may contribute to the patient's reaction to a painful stimulus. Panic disorder is a commonly overlooked coexisting condition in patients with chest pain[47] and should be sought specifically during history taking. The observation that anxiolytics and antidepressants can raise pain thresholds as well as improve mood states may explain why these medications may improve esophageal chest pain in the absence of manometric changes.[48,49]

Approach

The approach to patients with esophageal chest pain has evolved over the years.[50] Before the esophagus is considered the cause of chest pain, a cardiac cause must be excluded. Appropriate testing may include an exercise stress test, noninvasive cardiac imaging, and coronary angiography.

Insufficiency of coronary blood flow with normal-appearing epicoronary arteries (microvascular angina) has been suggested as a cause of chest pain in some patients.[51] Diagnosing microvascular angina on the basis of a therapeutic trial is difficult because the medications reported to improve this condition also have effects on the esophagus; however, the prognosis of most patients with microvascular angina is thought to be good.[52]

The recognition that chest pain is often associated with GERD has been a major advance in our understanding of esophageal chest pain. Ambulatory pH testing can document pathologic amounts of acid reflux or a correlation between acid reflux and chest pain in up to 50% of patients in whom a cardiac cause has been excluded.[53] In addition, a trial of therapy with a PPI produces symptomatic improvement in many such patients.[54] The association between chest pain and GERD is easy to recognize when the patient has coexisting reflux symptoms but not so clear when typical reflux symptoms are absent. A 10- to 14-day trial of an oral PPI taken twice daily has been shown to be sensitive and specific for the diagnosis of esophageal chest pain when compared with ambulatory intraesophageal pH testing.[55] The results of a randomized placebo-controlled trial in 2013 support a trial of a PPI in primary care patients with chest pain (after cardiac disease has been excluded).[56] Chest pain may respond to gastric acid inhibition even if a coexisting motility disturbance is present.[57] If a patient fails this trial, the next practical approach may be a trial of agents such as citalopram, imipramine, or trazodone that raise the pain threshold.[58]

Some authorities recommend esophageal testing with stationary manometry at this point to exclude a motility disorder and ambulatory pH testing to exclude gastroesophageal reflux unresponsive to the initial trial of the PPI therapy. Rarely, patients with chest pain will have a specific manometric disorder such as achalasia or distal spasm, but more frequently, abnormalities are nonspecific and difficult to attribute to an individual patient's symptoms. The advent of a tube-free wireless system for gastroesophageal reflux monitoring has allowed a longer and more comfortable monitoring period, which increases the likelihood of observing a correlation between pain and an acid event.[59] If gastroesophageal reflux is confirmed by ambulatory pH testing, an additional trial of acid suppressive therapy is warranted. If a spastic or hypercontractile motility disorder is discovered on manometry, an attempt at lowering esophageal pressure with nitrates or a calcium channel blocker is appropriate, although some patients with chest pain and a motility disorder will respond better to agents directed at lowering visceral sensitivity. Surgery (myotomy) for patients with esophageal spasm and with chest-pain-predominant type-III achalasia or esophagogastric outflow obstruction should be avoided in the absence of significant dysphagia (see Chapter 46).

HEARTBURN AND REGURGITATION

Heartburn (pyrosis) is one of the most common GI complaints in Western populations.[2] In fact, it is so common that many people assume it to be a normal part of life and fail to report the symptom to their health care providers. They seek relief with over the-counter antacids; indeed, heartburn accounts for most of the $1 billion/year sales of these nonprescription drugs. Despite its high prevalence, the term *heartburn* is frequently misunderstood. It has many synonyms, including *indigestion*, *acid regurgitation*, *sour stomach*, and *bitter belching*. The physician should listen for these descriptors if the patient does not volunteer a complaint of heartburn. A study from Europe has suggested that using a word-picture description of "a burning feeling rising from the stomach or lower chest up toward the neck" increases the ability to identify patients with gastroesophageal reflux.[60] The burning sensation often begins inferiorly and radiates up the entire retrosternal area to the neck, occasionally to the back, and rarely into the arms. Heartburn due to gastroesophageal reflux of acid may be relieved, albeit only transiently, by ingestion of antacids, baking soda, or milk. Interestingly, the severity of esophageal damage (esophagitis or Barrett esophagus) does not correlate with the severity of heartburn (e.g., patients with severe heartburn may have a normal-appearing esophagus on endoscopy, and those with severe esophagitis or Barrett esophagus may at times have mild or even no symptoms [see Chapters 48 and 49]).[61]

Heartburn is most frequently noted within 1 hour after eating, particularly after the largest meal of the day. Sugars, chocolate, onions, carminatives, and foods high in fat may aggravate heartburn by decreasing lower esophageal sphincter (LES) pressure. Other foods commonly associated with heartburn (e.g., citrus products, tomato-based foods, and spicy foods) irritate the inflamed esophageal mucosa because of their acidity or high osmolarity.[62] Beverages, including citrus juices, soft drinks, coffee, and alcohol, may also cause heartburn. The relationship between alcohol and heartburn is complicated. It appears that most heartburn associated with alcohol is related to increased sensitivity to acid by "loosening" of tight junctions between esophageal epithelial cells, thereby allowing normal amounts of acid to reach deeper into the mucosa and produce symptoms.[63] Many patients have exacerbation of heartburn if they go to sleep shortly after a late meal or snack, and others note that their heartburn is more pronounced, while they lie on their right side.[64] Weight gain frequently results in development of new symptoms of GERD and worsening of symptoms in patients with preexisting GERD.[65]

Activities that increase intra-abdominal pressure (e.g., bending over, straining at stool, lifting heavy objects, and performing isometric exercises) may aggravate heartburn. Running may also aggravate heartburn, and stationary bike riding may be a better exercise for those with GERD.[32] Because nicotine and air swallowing reduce LES pressure, cigarette smoking exacerbates the symptoms of reflux.[66] Emotions (anxiety, fear, and worry) may exacerbate heartburn by lowering visceral sensitivity thresholds rather than increasing the amount of gastroesophageal acid reflux.[67] Some patients with heartburn complain that certain drugs initiate or exacerbate their symptoms by reducing LES pressure and peristaltic contractions (e.g., theophylline and calcium-channel blockers) or by irritating the inflamed esophagus (e.g., aspirin, other NSAIDs, and bisphosphonates).

Heartburn may be accompanied by the appearance of fluid in the mouth, either a bitter acidic material or a salty fluid. *Regurgitation* describes the return of bitter, acidic fluid into the mouth and, at times, the effortless return of food, acid, or bilious material from the stomach. Regurgitation is more common at night or when the patient bends over. The absence of nausea, retching, and abdominal contractions suggests regurgitation rather than vomiting (see Chapter 16). "Water brash" is an uncommon and frequently misunderstood symptom that should be used to describe the sudden filling of the mouth with clear, slightly salty fluid. This fluid is not regurgitated material but is secreted from the salivary glands as part of a protective, vagally mediated reflex from the distal esophagus.[68] Regurgitation and symptoms similar to water brash can occur in patients with achalasia, who may be misdiagnosed as having GERD.

Regurgitation must be distinguished from the syndrome of rumination (see Chapter 16). *Rumination* is a clinical diagnosis and is best described by the Rome IV Consensus Committee diagnostic criteria. Patients must have persistent or recurrent regurgitation (not preceded by retching) of recently ingested food into the mouth, with subsequent remastication and swallowing. Supportive criteria include the absence of nausea, cessation of the process when the regurgitated material becomes acidic, and content consisting of recognizable food with a pleasant taste in the regurgitant.[69] Rumination is essentially a diagnosis of exclusion when there is clinical suspicion. There have been reports of a fairly specific pattern often seen during prolonged manometry, although an episode must occur during the study for the manometric pattern to be helpful.[70] Patients with bulimia sometimes report regurgitation and may be mistakenly diagnosed as having GERD (see Chapter 10). Both rumination and bulimia may produce esophagitis, a positive ambulatory pH test, or both, thereby making the clinical differentiation even more challenging.

Nocturnal reflux symptoms have special significance. In a survey of patients with frequent reflux symptoms, 74% reported nocturnal symptoms.[71] These nighttime symptoms interrupt sleep and health-related quality of life to a greater degree than daytime reflux symptoms alone. Patients who have prolonged reflux episodes at night are also at increased risk of complications of GERD, including severe reflux esophagitis and Barrett esophagus (see Chapters 48 and 49).

Pathophysiology

The physiologic mechanisms that produce heartburn remain poorly understood. Although reflux of gastric acid is most commonly associated with heartburn, the same symptom may be elicited by esophageal balloon distention,[72] reflux of bile salts,[73] and acid-induced motility disturbances. The best evidence that the pain mechanism is probably related to stimulation of mucosal chemoreceptors is the sensitivity of the esophagus to acid perfused into the esophagus and acid reflux demonstrated by monitoring pH. The location of these chemoreceptors is unknown. One suggestion is that the esophagus is sensitized by repeated acid exposure, resulting in the production of symptoms from smaller boluses after repeated exposure to acid. This hypersensitivity has been reported to resolve with gastric acid suppressive therapy.[74]

The correlation between discrete episodes of acid reflux and symptoms, however, is poor. For example, postprandial gastroesophageal reflux is common in healthy people, but symptoms are uncommon. Intraesophageal pH monitoring of patients with endoscopic evidence of esophagitis typically shows excessive periods of acid reflux, but fewer than 20% of these reflux episodes are accompanied by symptoms.[75] Moreover, one-third of patients with Barrett esophagus, the most advanced form of GERD, are insensitive to acid.[76] As patients age, their sensitivity to acid in the esophagus seems to decline; this finding may explain the common observation that mucosal damage is fairly severe, but symptoms are minimal in older patients with GERD.[77] Therefore the development of symptoms must require more than esophageal contact with acid. Mucosal disruption and inflammation may be contributing factors, but on endoscopy the esophagus appears normal in most symptomatic patients. Other factors that possibly influence the occurrence of heartburn include the acid clearance mechanism, salivary bicarbonate concentration, volume of acid refluxed (as measured by the duration and proximal extent of reflux episodes), frequency of heartburn, and interaction of pepsin with acid (see Chapter 48). Studies in which acid reflux is monitored for more than 24 hours have demonstrated considerable daily variability in esophageal acid exposure.[78,79]

As noted earlier, heartburn strongly suggests gastroesophageal acid reflux, but peptic ulcer disease (PUD), delayed gastric emptying, and even gallbladder disease can produce symptoms similar to those caused by reflux (see Chapters 52, 55, and 67). Regurgitation is not quite as specific for acid reflux as heartburn, and the differential diagnosis of regurgitation should include an esophageal obstruction (e.g., ring, stricture, and achalasia) or a gastric abnormality such as gastroparesis or outlet obstruction. Heartburn can also be a functional symptom as discussed in the Rome IV guidelines.[80] Functional heartburn is defined as retrosternal burning discomfort or pain refractory to optimal antisecretory therapy in the absence of GERD, histopathologic mucosal abnormalities, major motor disorders, or structural explanations. Reflux hypersensitivity is the designation applied to patients with esophageal symptoms (heartburn or chest pain) who lack evidence of reflux on endoscopy (e.g., esophagitis) or an abnormal acid burden on reflux monitoring but experience symptoms with physiologic reflux.

Approach

The approach to patients with heartburn and regurgitation is discussed extensively in Chapter 48. In brief, published guidelines support an initial trial of gastric acid suppressive therapy, generally with a PPI, as a diagnostic and therapeutic maneuver, although diagnosing erosive esophagitis on an early endoscopy is gaining traction as a way to firm up the diagnosis prior to long-term PPI therapy.[81] This concept is cost-effective but plagued by limitations in sensitivity and specificity.[82] If the cause of symptoms remains uncertain after a therapeutic trial, ambulatory intraesophageal pH testing is the best test to document pathologic esophageal acid exposure. Endoscopy of the esophagus is reserved for patients with symptoms suggestive of a complication (e.g., dysphagia, weight loss, and signs of bleeding), but the predictive value of using a symptom profile to predict esophageal damage is questionable at best. Although not without controversy, most guidelines also suggest endoscopy to screen for Barrett esophagus in patients with chronic reflux symptoms[83]; the risk is particularly increased in white male, older, and obese persons.[84,85] Guidelines as recent as 2012 have continued to challenge the utility of screening for Barrett esophagus, particularly in women.[86]

EXTRAESOPHAGEAL SYMPTOMS OF GASTROESOPHAGEAL REFLUX DISEASE

Extraesophageal symptoms of GERD are listed in Box 14.4. Although these symptoms may be caused by esophageal motility disorders, they are most frequently associated with GERD. In patients with extraesophageal symptoms, the classic reflux symptoms of heartburn and regurgitation often are mild or absent (see Chapter 48).

BOX 14.4 Extraesophageal Manifestations of GERD

- Asthma
- Chronic cough
- Excess mucus or phlegm
- Globus sensation
- Hoarseness
- Laryngitis
- Pulmonary fibrosis
- Sore throat

Gastroesophageal reflux is thought to cause chronic cough and other extraesophageal symptoms as a result of recurrent microaspiration of gastric contents, a vagally mediated neural reflex, or, in many patients, a combination of both.[87] Although bronchodilators reduce LES pressure, most persons with asthma have gastroesophageal reflux with or without bronchodilator therapy. In animal studies, instillation of small amounts of acid in the trachea or on the vocal cords[88] can produce marked changes in airway resistance, as well as vocal cord ulcers. Direct evidence for aspiration is more difficult to identify in adults and rests primarily on the presence of fat-filled macrophages in sputum,[89] radioactivity in the lungs after a tracer is placed in the stomach overnight,[90] increased pepsin levels in lung secretions,[91] and a high degree of esophageal or hypopharyngeal acid reflux recorded by 24-hour pH monitoring with dual probes.[92] Data from animal and human studies suggest that a neural reflex is another pathophysiologic basis for these symptoms. Acid perfusion into the distal esophagus increases airway resistance in all subjects, but the changes are most marked in patients with both asthma and heartburn.[93]

Abnormal amounts of gastroesophageal acid reflux recorded by prolonged intraesophageal pH monitoring have been identified in 35%–80% of asthmatic adults.[94] Symptoms that suggest reflux-induced asthma include the onset of wheezing in adulthood in the absence of a history of allergies or asthma, nocturnal cough or wheezing, worsening of asthma after meals, by exercise, or in the supine position, and asthma that is exacerbated by bronchodilators or is glucocorticoid dependent. In patients with reflux, symptoms strongly suggestive of aspiration include nocturnal cough and heartburn, recurrent pneumonia, unexplained fever, and an associated esophageal motility disorder. Silent aspiration after lung transplantation has been implicated as an important cause of declining graft function and even rejection.[95] In addition to reflux, significant esophageal dysmotility can occur in patients with more advanced pulmonary disease, including those recovering from lung transplantation.[96]

Ear, nose, and throat complaints associated with gastroesophageal reflux include postnasal drip, voice changes, hoarseness, sore throat, persistent cough, otalgia, halitosis, dental erosion, and excessive salivation. Many patients with GERD complain of only head and neck symptoms. Examination of the vocal cords may help in evaluating patients with suspected acid reflux-related extraesophageal problems. Some patients have redness, hyperemia, and edema of the vocal cords and arytenoids. In more severe cases, vocal cord ulcers, granulomas, and even laryngeal cancer, all secondary to GERD, have been reported. Normal results of a laryngeal examination, however, are not incompatible with acid reflux-related extraesophageal symptoms, nor are the aforementioned laryngeal signs specific for a GERD-related pathogenesis.

The options in a patient with suspected extraesophageal GERD are to study them with an ambulatory intraesophageal pH test or initiate a trial of therapy to confirm the diagnosis and treat the symptom (Fig. 14.2). Either approach is reasonable, but many experts favor an initial trial of acid suppressive therapy with a PPI twice

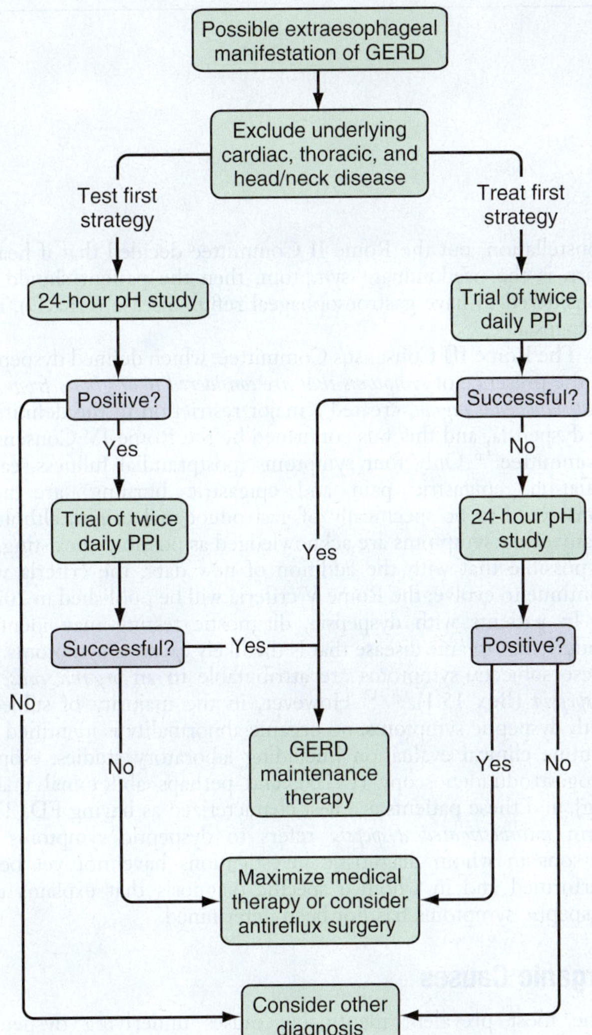

Fig. 14.2 Algorithm for the approach to patients with extraesophageal manifestations of GERD, including noncardiac chest pain. The approach to exclusion of an underlying disease varies, depending on the symptom underevaluation (see text). A PPI is given before breakfast and before the evening meal. The duration of the trial depends on the symptom. For example, a 10–14-day trial may be sufficient for noncardiac chest pain, whereas a 3-month trial may be needed for chronic cough.

daily.[97] Ambulatory pH testing is then reserved for those who fail the initial trial, although it is not clear whether pH testing should be done while the patient continues or after the patient discontinues acid suppressive therapy (see Chapter 48). Interpreting pH data in patients with extraesophageal symptoms and normal amounts of acid exposure is particularly challenging. Many studies have shown a poor correlation between reflux events and cough when cough is recorded by the patient, but a better correlation when acoustic cough monitoring (an experimental yet-to-be-approved technology) is used to quantify and time the cough episodes.[98]

The association between gastroesophageal reflux and extra-esophageal symptoms, particularly laryngeal symptoms, has been challenged. In one study, pH monitoring of the hypopharynx and proximal and distal esophagus was performed in patients with presumed gastroesophageal acid reflux-related endoscopic laryngeal findings.[99] An abnormal result was noted in only 15% of hypopharyngeal probes, 9% of proximal esophageal probes, and 29% of distal esophageal probes, indicating that most patients (70%) with symptoms and signs of laryngeal reflux do not have

BOX 14.5 Diagnostic Criteria for Functional Disorders of the Esophagus as defined by the Rome Foundation (version x)

FUNCTIONAL CHEST PAIN

1. Retrosternal chest pain or discomfort
2. Absence of associated esophageal symptoms, such as heartburn and dysphagia
3. Absence of evidence that gastroesophageal reflux or eosinophilic esophagitis is the cause of the symptom
4. Absence of major esophageal motor disorders

FUNCTIONAL HEARTBURN

1. Burning retrosternal discomfort or pain
2. No symptom relief despite optimal antisecretory therapy
3. Absence of evidence that gastroesophageal reflux or eosinophilic esophagitis is the cause of the symptom
4. Absence of major esophageal motor disorders

REFLUX HYPERSENSITIVITY

1. Retrosternal symptoms, including heartburn and chest pain
2. Normal endoscopy and absence of evidence that eosinophilic esophagitis is the cause of the symptoms
3. Absence of major esophageal motor disorders
4. Evidence of triggering of symptoms by reflux events despite normal acid exposure on pH- or pH-impedance monitoring

GLOBUS

1. Persistent or intermittent, nonpainful sensation of a lump or foreign body in the throat with no structural lesion identified on physical examination, laryngoscopy, or endoscopy
2. Occurrence of the sensation between meals
3. Absence of dysphagia or odynophagia
4. Absence of a gastric inlet patch in the proximal esophagus
5. Absence of evidence that gastroesophageal reflux or eosinophilic esophagitis is the cause of the symptom
6. Absence of major esophageal motor disorders

FUNCTIONAL DYSPHAGIA

1. Sense of solid and/or liquid foods sticking, lodging, or passing abnormally through the esophagus
2. Absence of evidence that esophageal mucosal or structural abnormality is the cause of the symptom
3. Absence of evidence that gastroesophageal reflux or eosinophilic esophagitis is the cause of the symptom
4. Absence of major esophageal motor disorders

documentable abnormal acid exposure. That preliminary study was followed by a randomized placebo-controlled trial of esomeprazole (40 mg twice daily) in the same patients, with response rates of 42% in those treated with esomeprazole and 46% in those treated with placebo.[100] A randomized controlled trial of therapy with a PPI in asthmatics produced similar results.[101] Despite the contradictory data, a trial of PPI therapy in patients with symptoms suggestive of extraesophageal GERD is reasonable, but the patient and physician should not be surprised if this therapy fails.

Function Esophageal Symptoms

While functional symptoms have been discussed throughout this chapter, the most recent ROME criteria are presented in Box 14.5. Unfortunately, a great deal of testing is needed to confirm these functional syndromes, including combinations of endoscopy (with esophageal biopsy), esophageal manometry, ambulatory reflux testing, and therapeutic trials of acid blockers (Box 14.5).

Full references for this chapter can be found at https://ebooks.health.elsevier.com.

15 Dyspepsia

Brian E. Lacy, David J. Cangemi

IN THIS CHAPTER

DEFINITION

Dyspepsia is not a new condition. Described by the ancient Greeks [the Greek words "δυς-" (dys-) and "πέψη" (pepse) literally mean "difficult digestion"], it was the subject of a London medical journal in 1789 (A treatise upon indigestion and the hypochondriac disease). At present, *dyspepsia* refers to a heterogeneous group of symptoms in the upper abdomen. Broadly defined as pain or discomfort centered in the upper abdomen,[1,2] patients with dyspepsia often report a variety of other symptoms, including postprandial fullness, early satiation, anorexia, belching, nausea, vomiting, upper abdominal bloating, and even heartburn and regurgitation.[1–4]

Earlier definitions considered dyspepsia to comprise all upper abdominal and retrosternal sensations—in effect, all symptoms referable to the proximal alimentary tract.[5] Definitions of dyspepsia have evolved over time to become more restrictive and now focus on symptoms thought to arise from the gastroduodenal region, not the esophagus.[4–6] Several consensus definitions for dyspepsia and functional dyspepsia (FD) have been proposed, with the Rome Consensus Committees providing the most influential classification system.

The Rome I and II Consensus Committees both defined dyspepsia as *pain or discomfort centered in the upper abdomen*.[2,7] Discomfort includes postprandial fullness, upper abdominal bloating, early satiation, epigastric burning, belching, nausea, and vomiting. Heartburn may occur as part of the symptom constellation, but the Rome II Committee decided that if heartburn is the predominant symptom, then the patient should be considered to have gastroesophageal reflux disease (GERD), not dyspepsia.

The Rome III Consensus Committee, which defined dyspepsia as the presence of *symptoms that are considered to originate from the gastroduodenal region*, created a major restriction in the definition of dyspepsia, and this was confirmed by the Rome IV Consensus Committee.[4,6] Only four symptoms (postprandial fullness, early satiation, epigastric pain and epigastric burning) are now considered to be specifically of gastroduodenal origin, although many other symptoms are acknowledged as possibly coexisting. It is possible that with the addition of new data, the criteria will continue to evolve; the Rome V criteria will be published in 2026.

In patients with dyspepsia, diagnostic testing may identify underlying organic disease that is the likely cause of symptoms. In these subjects, symptoms are attributable to an *organic cause of dyspepsia* (Box 15.1).[1,8–12] However, in the majority of subjects with dyspeptic symptoms, no organic abnormality is identified by routine clinical evaluation [including laboratory studies, esophagogastroduodenoscopy (EGD), and perhaps abdominal imaging], and these patients are best characterized as having FD. The term *uninvestigated dyspepsia* refers to dyspeptic symptoms in persons in whom diagnostic investigations have not yet been performed and in whom a specific diagnosis that explains the dyspeptic symptoms has not been determined.

Organic Causes

The most prevalent identifiable causes underlying dyspeptic symptoms are peptic ulcer disease (PUD) and GERD. Malignancies of the upper gastrointestinal (UGI) tract and celiac disease are less common but clinically important organic causes of dyspeptic symptoms[8–12] (see Box 15.1). Initial testing in a patient with uninvestigated dyspepsia should include laboratory tests (e.g., complete blood count, basic metabolic profile, and liver chemistries). Some providers routinely order a marker of inflammation, such as CRP or ESR, although the clinical utility of this strategy is unknown, as is the value of routinely ordering TSH and lipase. The diagnostic test of choice in a patient with uninvestigated dyspepsia is EGD, which allows identification of erosive esophagitis, Barrett's esophagus, PUD, gastric or duodenal infections, and gastric or esophageal cancer. Imaging of the abdomen, such as with x-ray, computed tomography (CT) or magnetic resonance imaging, may be considered depending on the severity and nature of symptoms (i.e., pain-predominant symptoms), particularly in older patients who have not been investigated with abdominal imaging previously. In addition, a gastric emptying study (GES), such as 4-hour gastric emptying scintigraphy, may warrant consideration in a patient with predominant symptoms of early satiety and/or postprandial nausea and vomiting.

Systematic studies indicate that 20%–25% of patients with dyspeptic symptoms in Western societies have erosive esophagitis, 20% are estimated to have endoscopy-negative reflux disease, 10% have PUD, 2% have Barrett's esophagus, and 1% or less have malignancy.[9,12] Minor endoscopic or histopathologic findings like duodenitis or gastritis do not seem to correlate with the presence or absence of dyspeptic symptoms.

BOX 15.1 Organic Causes of Dyspepsia

LUMINAL GI TRACT

Gastroesophageal reflux and chronic/recurrent esophagitis
Peptic ulcer disease (gastric or duodenal)
Chronic gastritis (secondary to alcohol, medications, infections, inflammation)
Food intolerance (carbohydrates, foods high in FODMAPs)
Gastric infections—viral, bacterial, fungal or parasitic (e.g., CMV, HIV, tuberculosis, syphilis, *Helicobacter pylori*, candidiasis, *Giardia lamblia, Strongyloides stercoralis)*
Celiac disease
Gastric or esophageal neoplasms
Infiltrative gastric disorders (Ménétrier disease, Crohn disease, eosinophilic gastroenteritis, sarcoidosis, amyloidosis)
Mast cell disorders
Recurrent or chronic gastric volvulus
Recurrent or chronic gastric or intestinal ischemia

MEDICATIONS

Acarbose
Aspirin or other NSAIDs (including COX-2 selective agents)
Cholesterol lowering agents (gemfibrozil)
Colchicine
Digitalis preparations
Estrogens
Glucocorticoids
Iron
Levodopa
Opioids
Niacin
Nitrates
Orlistat
Potassium chloride
Quinidine
Sildenafil
Theophylline

PANCREATICOBILIARY DISORDERS

Cholelithiasis and choledocholithiasis
Sphincter of Oddi dysfunction
Chronic pancreatitis
Pancreatic neoplasms

SYSTEMIC CONDITIONS

Adrenal insufficiency
Diabetes mellitus
Heart failure
Hyperparathyroidism
Intraabdominal malignancy
Median arcuate ligament syndrome
Mesenteric ischemia
Myocardial ischemia
Pregnancy
Renal insufficiency
Superior mesenteric artery syndrome
Thyroid disease

Intolerance to Food and Medications

Contrary to popular beliefs, ingestion of specific foods (e.g., spices, coffee, alcohol, or red meat) has not been convincingly established as a cause of dyspepsia. Gluten, dietary fat and foods high in fermentable oligo-, di- and monosaccharides and polyols (FODMAPs) may play a role in symptom generation in some patients.[13,14] Although ingestion of food often aggravates dyspeptic symptoms, the effect is most likely related to the sensorimotor response to food rather than specific food intolerances or allergies. However, acute ingestion of capsaicin has been shown to induce dyspeptic symptoms in healthy persons and those with FD, with greater intensity in the latter group.[15]

Dyspepsia is a common side effect of many drugs, including iron, antibiotics, opioids, digitalis, estrogens and oral contraceptives, theophylline, and levodopa (see Box 15.1). Medications may cause symptoms through direct gastric mucosal injury, changes in GI sensorimotor function, facilitation of gastroesophageal reflux (GER), or idiosyncratic mechanisms. Nonsteroidal anti-inflammatory drugs (NSAIDs) have received the most attention because of their potential to induce ulceration in the GI tract. Chronic use of aspirin and other NSAIDs may provoke dyspeptic symptoms in up to 20% of subjects, but the occurrence of dyspepsia correlates poorly with the presence of an ulcer. In controlled trials, dyspepsia developed in 4%–8% of persons treated with NSAIDs, with an odds ratio ranging from 1.1 to 3.1 compared with placebo. The magnitude of this effect depends on the dose and type of NSAID.[16] Compared with NSAIDs, COX-2 selective inhibitors are associated with a lower frequency of dyspepsia and peptic ulceration (see Chapter 55).[17]

Peptic Ulcer Disease

PUD is a well-established cause of dyspeptic symptoms and is an important consideration for clinicians in the management of these patients. However, the frequency of peptic ulcer in persons with dyspepsia is only 5%–10%.[8,9,12] Increasing age, NSAID use, and *Helicobacter pylori* (*Hp*) infection are the main risk factors for PUD (see Chapter 55).

Gastroesophageal Reflux

Erosive esophagitis is a diagnostic marker for GER, but most patients with symptoms attributable to reflux of stomach contents into the esophagus have no endoscopic signs of esophageal injury; these patients are most accurately diagnosed as having nonerosive GER. Erosive esophagitis is found in approximately 20% of dyspeptic patients, and a similar number of patients may have nonerosive GERD.[8,9,12,18] Empiric therapy with an acid suppressant decreases the likelihood of finding erosive esophagitis in persons with dyspepsia (see Chapter 48).

Gastric and Esophageal Cancer

The risk of gastric or esophageal malignancy in patients with dyspeptic symptoms is estimated to be less than 1%.[11,12] The risk of gastric cancer is increased among persons with *Hp* infection, a family history of gastric malignancy, or a history of gastric surgery or those who emigrated from areas endemic for gastric malignancy. The risk of esophageal cancer is increased in men, smokers, persons with high alcohol consumption, and those with long-standing heartburn (see Chapter 50).

Biliary and Pancreatic Tract Disorders

Despite the high prevalence of both dyspepsia and gallstones in adults, epidemiologic studies have confirmed that cholelithiasis is not associated with dyspepsia. Therefore persons with dyspepsia should not be investigated routinely for cholelithiasis, and cholecystectomy in persons with cholelithiasis is not indicated for dyspepsia alone. The clinical presentation of biliary pain is easily distinguishable from that of dyspepsia (see Chapter 67).

Pancreatic disease is less prevalent than cholelithiasis, but symptoms of acute or chronic pancreatitis or pancreatic cancer may initially be mistaken for dyspepsia. Pancreatic disorders are usually associated with more severe pain and are often

BOX 15.2 Rome IV Criteria for Functional Dyspepsia, Postprandial Distress Syndrome, and Epigastric Pain Syndrome

Diagnostic criteria* for functional dyspepsia†	1. *One or more* of the following: Bothersome postprandial fullness Bothersome early satiation Bothersome epigastric pain Bothersome epigastric burning AND 2. No evidence of structural disease (including at EGD) that is likely to explain the symptoms
Diagnostic criteria* for postprandial distress syndrome (PDS)	Must include *one or both* of the following at least 3 days a week: 1. Bothersome postprandial fullness (i.e., severe enough to impact usual activities) 2. Bothersome early satiation (i.e., severe enough to prevent finishing a regular-sized meal) 3. No evidence of organic, systemic, or metabolic disease that is likely to explain the symptoms on routine investigations (including at EGD) *Supportive Criteria* 1. Postprandial epigastric pain or burning, epigastric bloating, excessive belching, and nausea can also be present 2. Vomiting warrants consideration of another disorder 3. Heartburn is not a symptom of dyspepsia but often may coexist with PDS 4. Symptoms that are relieved by evacuation of feces or gas should generally not be considered part of the dyspepsia symptom complex 5. Other individual digestive symptoms or groups of symptoms (e.g., from GERD or IBS) may coexist with PDS
Diagnostic criteria* for epigastric pain syndrome (EPS)	Must include *one or both* of the following symptoms at least 1 day a week: 1. Bothersome epigastric pain (i.e., severe enough to impact on usual activities) 2. Bothersome epigastric burning (i.e., severe enough to impact usual activities) 3. No evidence of organic, systemic, or metabolic disease that is likely to explain the symptoms on routine investigations (including at EGD) *Supportive Criteria* 1. Pain may be induced by ingestion of a meal, relieved by ingestion of a meal, or may occur while fasting 2. Postprandial epigastric bloating, belching, and nausea can also be present 3. Persistent vomiting likely suggests another disorder 4. Heartburn is not a symptom of dyspepsia but may often coexist with EPS 5. The pain does not fulfill criteria for biliary pain 6. Symptoms that are relieved by evacuation of feces or gas generally should not be considered part of the dyspepsia symptom complex 7. Other digestive symptoms (such as GERD and IBS) may coexist with EPS

*Criteria fulfilled for the previous 3 months with symptom onset at least 6 months prior to diagnosis
†Must fulfill criteria for PDS and/or EPS.

accompanied by anorexia, rapid weight loss, or jaundice (see Chapters 60 to 62).

Other GI or Systemic Disorders

Several GI disorders may cause dyspepsia-like symptoms: infectious (e.g., *Giardia lamblia* and *Strongyloides stercoralis* infections, tuberculosis, fungal infections, syphilis); inflammatory (celiac disease, Crohn disease, sarcoidosis, lymphocytic gastritis, eosinophilic gastroenteritis); or infiltrative (lymphoma, amyloid, Ménétrier disease) disorders of the UGI tract. Most of these disorders will be identifiable at EGD with mucosal biopsies. Persons with recurrent gastric volvulus and chronic mesenteric or gastric ischemia may also present with dyspeptic symptoms, though these are uncommon conditions (see Chapter 120).

The symptom pattern associated with gastroparesis (idiopathic, drug-induced, or secondary to a metabolic, systemic, or neurologic disorder) is similar to dyspepsia, as specified by older definitions.[1–7] The distinction between idiopathic gastroparesis and FD with delayed gastric emptying is a matter of ongoing debate (see later and Chapter 52).[19] Nausea and vomiting are cardinal symptoms in persons with gastroparesis and were not considered symptoms of dyspepsia by the Rome III and Rome IV Consensus Committees, thereby allowing the potential for symptom-based differentiation between dyspepsia and gastroparesis.[3,6,19] Dyspepsia may be the presenting or accompanying symptom of acute myocardial ischemia, pregnancy, acute or chronic renal failure, thyroid dysfunction, adrenal insufficiency, and hyperparathyroidism (see Box 15.1).

FUNCTIONAL DYSPEPSIA

According to the Rome IV criteria, FD is defined as the presence of early satiation, postprandial fullness, epigastric pain, or epigastric burning in the absence of organic, systemic, or metabolic disease that is likely to explain the symptoms (Box 15.2).[6]

Dyspepsia Symptom Complex

Pattern and Heterogeneity

The dyspepsia symptom complex is broader than the four cardinal symptoms that constitute the Rome IV definition and includes other frequently reported symptoms, such as epigastric fullness or discomfort, upper abdominal bloating, belching, loss of appetite, nausea, and vomiting. Although some patients have daily persistent symptoms, most patients have symptoms that are more intermittent in nature, even during highly symptomatic episodes.[1,8,19] The most frequent symptoms reported by patients with FD at a tertiary care center are postprandial fullness and bloating,

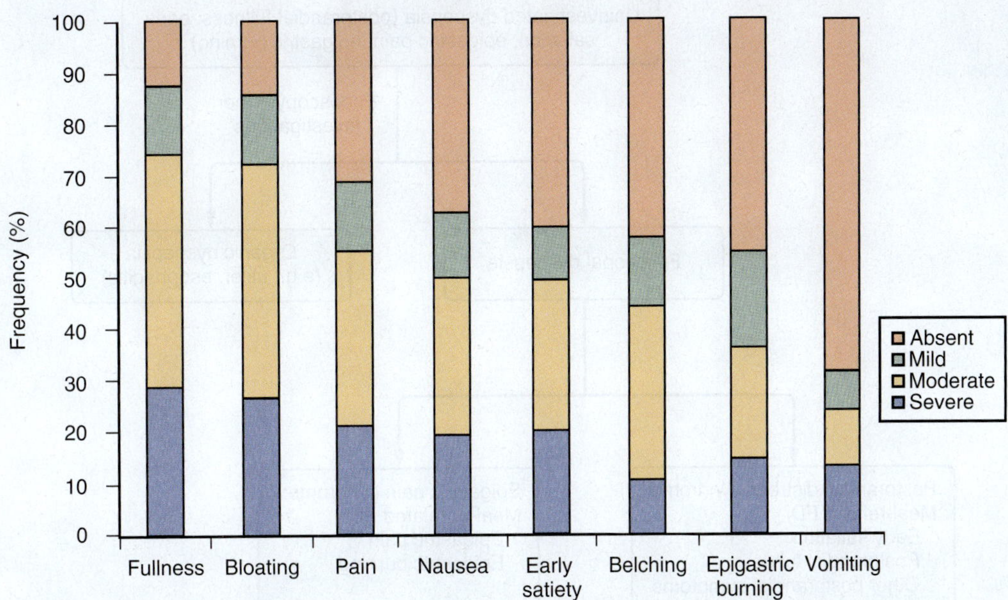

Fig. 15.1 Frequency of symptoms (percent of patients) and their severity ratings in 674 patients with functional dyspepsia seen at a tertiary referral center. (Unpublished, University of Gasthuisberg, Leuven, Belgium.)

followed by epigastric pain, early satiation, nausea, and belching.[3,20–23] There is considerable heterogeneity, however, as demonstrated, for example, in the number of symptoms that patients report (Fig. 15.1). In the general population, the most frequent dyspeptic symptoms are postprandial fullness, early satiation, upper abdominal pain, and nausea.[24–26]

Weight loss is traditionally considered an "alarm" symptom, pointing towards potentially serious organic disease. However, studies in tertiary care patients with FD have shown a high frequency of unexplained weight loss,[20,21] while population-based studies in Australia and Europe have shown an association between uninvestigated dyspepsia and unexplained weight loss.[25,26] Thus unintentional weight loss in the patient with dyspepsia may not be the serious warning sign once thought, although a careful history (e.g., diet, caloric intake, exercise, medications), physical examination, and appropriate laboratory studies should be performed.

Another consideration in patients presenting with unexplained weight loss is the possibility of an underlying eating disorder. In particular, avoidant/restrictive food intake disorder (ARFID), an eating disorder classification newly recognized by the *Diagnostic and Statistical Manual of Mental Disorders* (DSM-5) and characterized by avoiding or restricting food intake resulting in a failure to meet nutritional needs, has gained increased attention as an underrecognized condition in patients with gastrointestinal disorders—particularly disorders of gut-brain interaction (DGBI), such as FD. The prevalence of ARFID symptoms in patients presenting to a tertiary neurogastroenterology clinic was estimated to be nearly 25% in a recent retrospective study, and dyspepsia was identified as an independent risk factor for ARFID.[27]

Subgroups

Dyspepsia and FD are heterogeneous disorders. This is critical to understand, as it explains the array of reported symptoms and why no single diet or medication will resolve FD symptoms in all patients. Factor analysis of dyspepsia symptoms in the general population, and in tertiary care patients with FD, have demonstrated that FD is not a homogeneous (i.e., unidimensional) condition.[25,26,28] Unfortunately, although these studies have confirmed the heterogeneity of the dyspepsia symptom complex, they have not provided a clinically meaningful classification system.

Several attempts have been made to identify clinically meaningful subgroups of persons with dyspepsia to simplify the intricate heterogeneity of the dyspepsia symptom complex and to guide management. The Rome II Consensus Committee proposed a subdivision based on a predominant symptom of pain or discomfort.[2] Although correlations were found between this classification and the presence or absence of *Hp* infection, absence or presence of delayed gastric emptying, and response or lack of response to acid suppressive therapy,[29,30] the classification has been criticized because of the difficulty in distinguishing pain from discomfort, lack of a widely accepted definition of "predominant," uncertainty about overlap between the symptom subgroups, absence of an association with putative pathophysiologic mechanisms, and, especially, lack of stability of the predominant symptom over short time periods.[4,31–34]

The Rome III Consensus Committee proposed a different classification (Fig. 15.2).[4] Studies in patients with FD seen at a tertiary care center and persons with uninvestigated dyspepsia in the general population have revealed that between 40% and 75% of dyspeptic persons report aggravation of symptoms after ingestion of a meal.[26,35,36] Assuming that a distinction between meal-related and meal-unrelated symptoms might be pathophysiologically and clinically relevant, the Rome III Consensus Committee proposed that FD be considered an umbrella term and that the *postprandial distress syndrome* (PDS)—characterized by meal-related dyspeptic symptoms, postprandial fullness, and early satiation be distinguished from the *epigastric pain syndrome* (EPS)—characterized by meal-unrelated dyspeptic symptoms, epigastric pain, and epigastric burning.[4] In population-based studies, the Rome III-based classification of FD into EPS and PDS showed the existence of both entities, with little overlap between them.[37–39] In contrast, studies of persons with FD who sought consultation with a physician demonstrated significant overlap in Rome III-defined PDS and EPS.[1,40,41] The Rome IV

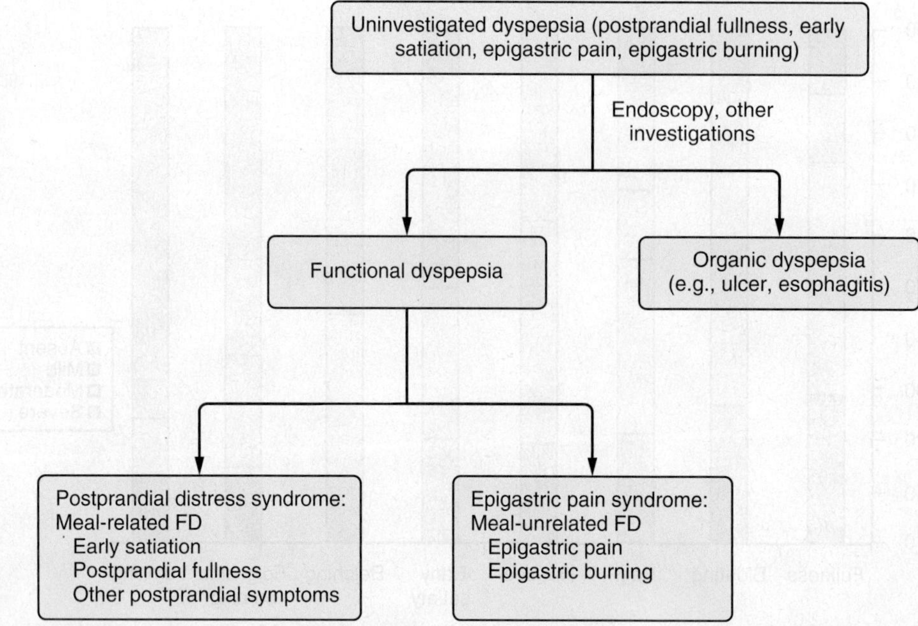

Fig. 15.2 Schematic representation of the classification of uninvestigated dyspepsia, functional dyspepsia (FD), and subtypes of functional dyspepsia according to the Rome IV criteria.

Consensus Committee aimed to reduce this overlap by considering all postprandially occurring symptoms to be part of PDS.[6] Therefore, when epigastric pain occurs postprandially in patients with early satiation or postprandial fullness, the patient is still categorized as having PDS (see Fig. 15.2). Epidemiologic studies and studies in patient cohorts have shown that PDS is the dominant subgroup and that overlap with EPS is small using Rome IV classification.[5,42,43]

Overlap With Heartburn and IBS

The issue of overlap between dyspepsia and GERD has been a challenging one. Although earlier investigators considered a group of patients with reflux-like dyspepsia,[5] the Rome Consensus Committees did not consider heartburn to arise primarily from the gastroduodenal region, and this symptom was excluded from the definition of dyspepsia.[2,4,6,7] Heartburn commonly coexists with dyspepsia, however, in both the general population and patients with FD.[18,26,30,44] Moreover, distinguishing GERD from dyspepsia is hampered by a number of confounding factors, such as the presence of dyspepsia-type symptoms in many patients with GERD[18,26,45] and difficulties in recognizing heartburn by patients and physicians.[18,46,47]

The Rome II Consensus Committee stated that patients with typical heartburn as a dominant complaint almost invariably have GERD and should be distinguished from patients with dyspepsia.[2] Although this distinction is valid,[33,48,49] the Rome III Consensus Committee proposed identifying patients with frequent heartburn and using a word-picture questionnaire to identify patients with FD who will respond to acid-suppressive therapy or in whom pathologic esophageal acid exposure can be demonstrated.[48,49] The Rome III and IV Consensus Committees state that heartburn is not a gastroduodenal symptom, although it often occurs in association with symptoms of FD and its presence does not exclude a diagnosis of FD.[4,6]

Similarly, the frequent cooccurrence of FD and IBS[50] is explicitly recognized in the Rome III and IV consensus guidelines and does not exclude a diagnosis of FD.[4,6]

Epidemiology

Dyspeptic symptoms are common in the general population, with frequencies ranging from 10% to 45%.[1,8,26,35,37–39,51–53] The frequency of dyspepsia is slightly higher in women than men and in smokers and NSAID users; the influence of age varies across studies. Results of prevalence studies are strongly influenced by the criteria used to define dyspepsia, and several studies have either included patients with typical symptoms of GERD or not incorporated the presence of dyspepsia-type symptoms in many patients with GERD. When heartburn is excluded, the frequency of uninvestigated dyspepsia in the general population ranges from 5% to 15%.[26,35,37–39,51,52] An internet, cross-sectional survey study of 6300 adults in Canada, the United Kingdom, and the United States identified a 10% prevalence of FD using Rome IV criteria.[53] The annual incidence of dyspepsia has been estimated to range from 1% to 6%.[19] Long-term follow-up studies have suggested that symptoms improve or resolve in more than half of patients.[19,54]

Quality of life is significantly affected by dyspepsia, especially FD.[52] Although the majority of patients do not seek medical care, a significant proportion will eventually seek consultation, which results in substantial costs.[19,26,55–58] Factors that influence healthcare seeking are symptom severity, fear of underlying serious disease, psychological distress, and lack of adequate psychosocial support.[57,58]

Pathophysiology

Several pathophysiologic mechanisms have been suggested to underlie dyspeptic symptoms: delayed or rapid gastric emptying; impaired gastric accommodation to a meal; hypersensitivity to gastric distention; low-grade mucosal inflammation; elevated levels of duodenal eosinophils or mast cells; altered duodenal sensitivity to lipids or acid; abnormal intestinal motility; and CNS dysfunction[1,3,8] (Fig. 15.3). The heterogeneity of FD seems to be confirmed by the contribution of one or more of these disturbances in subgroups of patients. Many studies that investigated the pathophysiologic mechanisms of FD predated the Rome IV

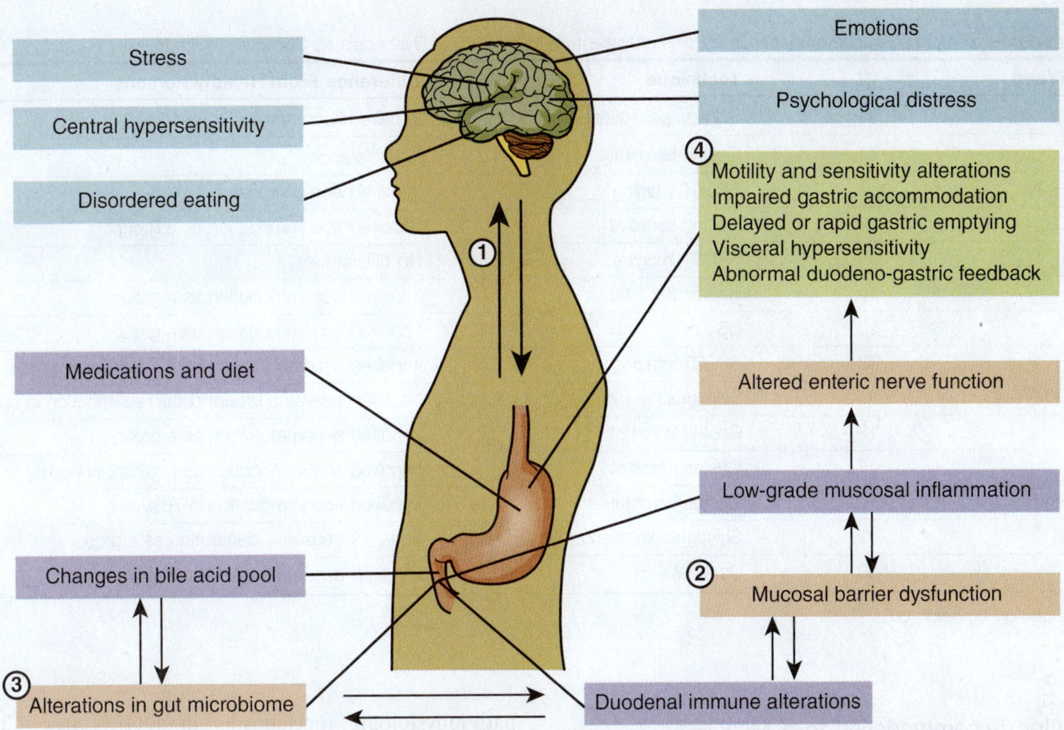

Fig. 15.3 Pathophysiology of functional dyspepsia. FD symptoms may develop due to changes in the brain-gut axis (1). Contributing factors include changes in duodenal barrier function (2), alterations in the gut microbiome (3), and abnormalities in gastric sensorimotor function (4).

guidelines and classification, and thus defined FD according to the Rome I and II consensus definitions.

Delayed or Rapid Gastric Emptying

Several studies have investigated gastric emptying and its relationship to the pattern and severity of symptoms in patients with FD. The frequency of delayed gastric emptying ranges from 20% to 50% (Table 15.1).[1,3,8] In a meta-analysis of 17 studies involving 868 dyspeptic patients and 397 controls, a significant delay in solid gastric emptying was present in almost 40% of patients with FD.[59] Most of the studies, however, were performed in small groups of patients. In the largest studies, gastric emptying of solids was delayed in about 30% of the patients with FD.[3,23,60] In the NIH sponsored FD Treatment Trial (Rome II criteria), 21% of patients had delayed gastric emptying.[61] Delayed gastric emptying was found in 23% of FD patients (Rome III criteria) in a large study involving breath testing; there was no preferential association with PDS.[62] Most studies failed to find a convincing relationship between delayed gastric emptying and the pattern of symptoms. Large-scale single-center studies from Europe showed that patients with delayed gastric emptying of solids are more likely to report postprandial fullness, nausea, and vomiting,[23,60,62] although two large multicenter studies in the United States found no or a weak association.[63,64] In general, the relationship between delays in gastric emptying and the presence of dyspeptic symptoms is weak, an important point to consider when considering treatment options.

Rapid gastric emptying is present in 5%–7% of patients with FD.[1,8,61] Symptoms cannot reliably distinguish between rapid, delayed or normal emptying in these patients. Gastric emptying scans play an important role in identifying these patients as empiric treatment with a prokinetic agent could worsen symptoms in a patient with FD and rapid emptying.

However, in discussing the relevance of gastric emptying with regard to FD, it is important to recognize that gastric emptying may change over time. A recent study conducted by the Gastroparesis Clinical Research Consortium involving 944 patients (24% of which had FD) found that 37% of patients with FD were reclassified as having gastroparesis based on GES results at 48 weeks, compared to baseline. Further, 42% of patients initially diagnosed with gastroparesis were reclassified as having FD at study conclusion.[65] These findings speak to the lability of gastric emptying over time for some patients, as well as to the significant overlap which exists between FD and gastroparesis. Thus in the evaluation of dyspeptic symptoms, it is important to interpret the results of an individual GES with the understanding that the results may not necessarily predict symptoms and may change over time.

TABLE 15.1 Frequency of Delayed Gastric Emptying in Studies of Patients With Functional Dyspepsia

Investigator (Year)	*N*	Frequency (%)
Asano (2017)	94	11
Jian (1989)	28	59
Klauser (1993)	69	35
Maes (1997)	344	30
Perri (1998)	304	33
Sarnelli (2003)	392	23
Scott (1993)	75	28
Stanghellini (1996)	343	34
Talley (1989)	32	30
Talley (2001)	551	24
Talley (2006)	864	34
Vanheel (2017)	560	23
Waldron (1991)	50	42
Wegener (1989)	43	30

TABLE 15.2 Evidence of Impaired Accommodation in Studies of Patients With Functional Dyspepsia as Compared With Healthy Persons

Investigator (Year)	N	Technique	Difference From Healthy Persons
Asano (2017)	94	Scintigraphic distribution	Impaired accommodation in 15%
Boeckxstaens (2001)	44	Gastric barostat	No difference
Bredenoord (2003)	151	SPECT imaging	Impaired accommodation in 43%
Caldarella (2003)	30	Gastric barostat	Impaired accommodation as a group
Castillo (2004)	35	SPECT imaging	No difference
Coffin (1994)	10	Gastric barostat	Impaired accommodation as a group
Gilja (1996)	20	US	Impaired accommodation as a group
Kim (2001)	33	SPECT imaging	Impaired accommodation as a group; abnormal in 41%
Piessevaux (2004)	40	Scintigraphic distribution	No difference as a group; distal redistribution in up to 50%
Salet (1998)	12	Gastric barostat	Impaired accommodation as a group
Tack (1998)	40	Gastric barostat	Impaired accommodation as a group; abnormal in 40%
Thumshirn (1999)	17	Gastric barostat	Impaired accommodation in 70%
Troncon (1994)	11	Scintigraphic distribution	Altered intragastric distribution as a group
Vanheel (2017)	560	Barostat	Impaired accommodation in 37%

SPECT, Single photon emission CT.

Impaired Gastric Accommodation to a Meal

The motor functions of the proximal and distal stomach differ remarkably. Whereas the distal stomach regulates gastric emptying of solids by grinding and sieving the content until the particles are small enough to pass the pylorus, the proximal stomach serves mainly as a reservoir during and after ingestion of the meal. Accommodation of the stomach to a meal is a vagally mediated reflex relaxation of the proximal stomach and provides the meal with a reservoir, thereby enabling the stomach to handle large intragastric volumes without a rise of intragastric pressure.[66] Studies using intragastric manometry have shown that ingestion of a meal is associated with a drop in intragastric pressure followed by a gradual recovery of the pressure during continued ingestion of nutrients, with increasing meal-induced satiation.[67]

Studies using a gastric barostat, scintigraphy, US, single-photon emission CT, or noninvasive surrogate markers (e.g., satiation drinking test) have all identified impaired accommodation in approximately 40% of patients with FD (Table 15.2).[3,20,22,62,66] A barostat study of gastric accommodation in patients with Rome III-defined subtypes of FD found impaired accommodation in 37% but showed no preferential association with PDS.[62] Lack of accommodation of the proximal stomach during and after the ingestion of a meal may be accompanied by increased intragastric pressure and activation of mechanoreceptors in the gastric wall, thus inducing symptoms. Although a number of studies have found an association between impaired accommodation and early satiation and weight loss, others have failed to find such an association.[3,20,22,62] The mechanism(s) by which impaired accommodation can cause symptoms is still unclear. Meal ingestion in the absence of proper relaxation of the proximal stomach may be accompanied by activation of tension-sensitive mechanoreceptors in the proximal stomach. Alternatively, insufficient accommodation of the proximal stomach may rapidly propel the meal into the distal stomach, thereby activating tension-sensitive mechanoreceptors in a distended antrum.[66]

Hypersensitivity to Gastric Distension

Visceral hypersensitivity, defined as abnormally enhanced perception of visceral stimuli, is considered one of the major pathophysiologic mechanisms in DGBIs (see Chapter xx).[68] Several studies have established that, as a group, patients with FD are hypersensitive to isobaric gastric distention.[3,21,62] A study in patients with Rome III-defined FD subgroups identified hypersensitivity in 37%, but there was no preferential association with any of the subtypes.[62] The level at which visceral hypersensitivity is generated is unclear, and there is evidence for involvement of tension-sensitive mechanoreceptors as well as changes at the level of visceral afferent nerves or of the central nervous system.[69–71]

Mucosal Inflammation and Duodenal Eosinophilia and Mast Cells

Low-grade mucosal inflammation in the duodenum, substantiated by increased duodenal mucosal mast cells and eosinophils, may contribute to FD symptom generation in some patients.[72–75] The investigation of immune dysfunction in FD was initially triggered by observations in patients with postinfection FD, but it is now clear that increased eosinophil and mast cell numbers are present in a large subset of patients with FD, many of whom likely had a preceding infection.[75] The inflammatory cell infiltrate (eosinophils and mast cells) in the duodenum has been correlated with increased mucosal permeability and altered expression of tight junction proteins with impaired activity and integrity of neurons in the submucous plexus.[73,75] To what extent low-grade duodenal inflammation is associated with the changes in gastric sensorimotor function described earlier, or with increased sensitivity to duodenal luminal contents discussed later, remains to be evaluated.

Intestinal Barrier Dysfunction

More recently, attention has been directed to the potential role of impaired intestinal barrier function, and resulting increased intestinal permeability, as a relevant pathophysiologic mechanism in patients with FD. In the first study of its kind, patients with FD with PDS (with or without concomitant EPS, $n = 16$) and healthy controls ($n = 18$) underwent upper endoscopy with confocal laser endomicroscopy (CLE), a technique which allows high power magnification of the intestinal lining and identification of epithelial gaps, biopsies of the duodenum for identification of inflammatory/immune cells and cell pyroptosis, as well as measurement of transepithelial electrical resistance of ex vivo tissue samples. Patients with FD were found to have significantly higher epithelial gap density in the third portion of the duodenum as detected by CLE, compared to controls, and significant changes in duodenal biopsy specimens were identified, including reduced transepithelial resistance (indicative of impaired musical integrity), and an increase in the number of cells undergoing pyroptosis.[76] Though the study was small and data is limited, such findings have added increased focus on the microenvironment of the duodenum as it relates to the pathophysiology of FD, not only with respect to increased inflammatory cells but also impaired barrier function and increased intestinal permeability. However, further research is needed to better understand the relevance of these findings and to determine if intestinal barrier inflammation and dysfunction represent novel therapeutic targets.

Altered Duodenal Sensitivity to Lipids or Acid

In healthy persons and in patients with FD, perfusion of the duodenum with nutrient lipids, but not glucose, enhances the perception of gastric distention through a mechanism that requires lipid digestion and subsequent release of CCK.[77–79] Duodenal infusion of hydrochloric acid induces nausea in patients with FD but not in healthy subjects, suggesting duodenal hypersensitivity to acid.[80] Duodenal aspirates revealed higher fasting luminal pH in FD patients off PPI therapy compared to healthy volunteers. Interestingly, symptoms, duodenal permeability, and duodenal eosinophil and mast cell numbers all improved with PPI therapy.[81] On the basis of these observations, increased duodenal sensitivity to lipids and acid may contribute to symptom generation in some patients with FD, although more research is needed in this area.

Other Mechanisms

Rapid gastric emptying, present in a small subset of patients with FD, may be responsible for symptoms, especially in the postprandial period.[82,83] Abnormalities in gastric myoelectrical activity, as measured by cutaneous electrogastrography, may be present in some patients with FD, although whether this is the cause or simply an epiphenomenon is unclear.[84] Small bowel motor alterations, most commonly hypermotility with burst activity or clusters and an increased proportion of duodenal retrograde contractions, have been reported in patients with FD, but no clear correlation with symptoms has been found.[85] Alterations in the duodenal microbiome could potentially trigger symptoms in some FD patients, although this area remains largely unexplored. A recent meta-analysis found that small intestine bacterial overgrowth (SIBO) was more common in patients with FD than healthy controls.[86]

Pathogenic Factors

The cause of symptoms in patients with FD has not been established, but evidence exists for genetic susceptibility, infective agents, and psychological factors. The relationship between potential pathogenic factors and putative pathophysiologic mechanisms has not been addressed in depth.

Genetic Predisposition

Population studies have suggested that genetic factors contribute to FD. The frequency of dyspepsia is increased in first-degree relatives of affected patients compared with the frequency in their spouses.[87] Polymorphisms of the G-protein beta-polypeptide 3 gene (*GNB3*) and TGFB1 have been associated with the risk of FD,[88,89] although larger confirmatory studies are required to determine whether these polymorphisms truly predispose a patient to develop FD or are simply associated.

Infection

Hp Infection

Depending on the region and population studied, a variable proportion of patients with FD are infected with *Hp*.[1,3,8] Although *Hp* is associated with a number of organic causes of dyspepsia, there is only limited evidence to support a causal relationship between *Hp* and FD.[90] No consistent differences in the pattern of symptoms or putative pathophysiologic mechanisms have been found between *Hp*-positive and *Hp*-negative subjects.[3,8,91] The best evidence in support of a role for *Hp* in the pathogenesis of FD is the small, but statistically significant, beneficial effect of eradication therapy on symptoms in patients with FD.[90,92] These considerations have led to the Kyoto consensus, which defines *Hp*-associated dyspepsia as dyspepsia in an *Hp*-infected person with the absence of an alternative cause of dyspepsia on endoscopy and sustained control of symptoms after eradication of *Hp*.[93] Determination of the size of this group, both in Western and non-Western clinical practices, and the long-term outcome require further studies.

Postinfection Functional Dyspepsia

Postinfection FD was first proposed as a clinical entity on the basis of a large retrospective study from a tertiary referral center.[22] Compared with patients who had FD of unspecified-onset, patients with a history suggestive of postinfection FD were more likely to report symptoms of early satiation, weight loss, nausea, and vomiting and had a significantly higher frequency of impaired accommodation of the proximal stomach, which was attributed to dysfunction at the level of gastric nitrergic neurons.[22] The frequency of *Hp* infection is not increased in postinfection FD, indicating that *Hp* is not the causal infectious agent. Patients with postinfection FD have more prominent mucosal inflammation in the duodenum.[75] In a prospective cohort study, development of FD was increased fivefold 1 year after acute salmonella gastroenteritis, compared with subjects who had not had gastroenteritis.[94] Acute gastroenteritis was a risk factor (12-fold) for the development of FD (Rome III criteria) in a prospective study of 345 consecutive adults (age and gender matched to healthy controls).[95] Additional studies are required to identify the underlying pathophysiology and risk factors and to assess the long-term prognosis.

Psychosocial Factors

A review of the literature reveals a clear association between psychosocial factors and FD.[1,3,8,96] The most common psychiatric comorbidities in patients with FD are anxiety, depressive or somatoform disorders, and a recent or remote history of physical or sexual abuse. Psychological distress has long been a recognized feature of healthcare-seeking behavior in patients with DGBI, including FD. Studies have confirmed an association between dyspeptic symptoms in the general population and psychosocial factors, such as somatization, anxiety, and stressful life events; this association argues against a mere healthcare–seeking effect.[27,36,96,97] Symptom severity in patients seen at a tertiary care center is more strongly related to psychosocial factors (especially depression, abuse history, and somatization) than to abnormalities of gastric sensorimotor function.[97]

Although these observations show a close interaction between different psychosocial variables and the presence and severity of symptoms of FD, they do not establish whether psychosocial factors and FD are separate manifestations of a common predisposition or whether psychosocial factors play a direct causal role in the pathophysiology of dyspeptic symptoms. Longitudinal studies support the idea of a common predisposition, as FD has been reported to both precede and follow the development of a mood disorder in population-based studies and each component increases the risk for the other.[98,99]

The presence of psychosocial comorbidities is also associated with greater symptom severity in patients with FD, and this association may be mediated in part by visceral hypersensitivity.[28,100] Acutely induced anxiety in healthy volunteers, however, is not associated with increased visceral sensitivity but with decreased gastric compliance and inhibition of meal-induced accommodation.[101] In patients with FD, a correlation between anxiety and gastric sensitivity was found in a subgroup of "hypersensitive" patients with FD but not in the overall group of patients with FD.[100] A history of abuse was associated with visceral hypersensitivity in patients with FD.[102]

APPROACH TO UNINVESTIGATED DYSPEPSIA

The high prevalence of dyspepsia and the large number of patients referred to a healthcare provider for symptom evaluation underscores the importance of effective patient management. A key first step is to determine which patients can be managed empirically and which patients should be referred for additional diagnostic evaluation.

History and Physical Examination

A complete clinical history should be obtained and a physical examination performed in all patients with dyspepsia. The nature, frequency, and chronicity of the symptoms, as well as the relationship to ingestion of meals and the possible influence of specific dietary factors, should be assessed. The onset of symptoms (acute after an infectious gastroenteritis or more gradual in nature) and the identification of consistent aggravating and alleviating factors are of interest. The amount of weight loss, if present, should be determined, as should other alarm symptoms, such as anemia, blood loss, dysphagia, and intractable vomiting. Distinguishing the EPS from PDS symptom subgroup according to the Rome IV classification may influence the choice of treatment (see later).[5] In patients with long-standing symptoms, the reason for seeking health care at this time should be elicited, so that specific fears and concerns can be addressed. Further assessment of symptoms or signs of a systemic disorder (e.g., diabetes mellitus, cardiac disease, thyroid disease) and of the patient's family and personal history (i.e., history of UGI malignancy) will indicate whether the patient is at risk for a particular organic disease that may present as dyspepsia. Physical findings, such as an abdominal mass, abdominal bruit, organomegaly, ascites, lymphadenopathy, or a positive fecal occult blood test result, warrant further evaluation. Chronic abdominal wall pain should be considered in the differential diagnosis and patients should be evaluated for Carnett's sign.

Attention should be paid to elicit a history of heartburn, and a word-picture questionnaire may help the patient recognize the typical symptom pattern.[46] Burning pain confined to the epigastrium is a cardinal symptom of dyspepsia and is not considered heartburn unless it radiates retrosternally. The presence of frequent and typical reflux symptoms should lead to a provisional diagnosis of GERD rather than dyspepsia, and the patient should be treated initially for GERD (see Chapter 48). Overlap of GERD with dyspepsia is frequent and should be considered if the patient's symptoms do not respond to appropriate management of GERD.[18] The possible presence of overlapping IBS should also be assessed,[50] and symptoms that improve with bowel movements or are associated with changes in stool frequency or consistency should lead to a presumptive diagnosis of IBS. A structured questionnaire with pictograms that incorporates the heartburn word-picture may help identify the nature of symptoms as distinct from nausea, GERD, and IBS.[103]

The use of prescription and nonprescription medications should be reviewed, and medications commonly associated with dyspepsia (especially NSAIDs; see Box 15.1) should be discontinued if possible.

Laboratory Testing

The cost-effectiveness of routine laboratory testing, especially in younger patients with uncomplicated dyspepsia, has not been established. Nevertheless, most clinicians will consider routine tests (CBC, serum electrolytes, serum calcium, and liver chemistries) after the age of 45. Other studies, such as a serum lipase, antibodies for celiac disease, thyroid stimulating hormone and thyroid hormone levels, stool testing for ova and parasites or Giardia antigen, and a pregnancy test, may be considered in selected cases.[1,3,5,8,10]

Initial Management Strategies

In many cases, the patient's history and physical examination will allow dyspepsia to be distinguished from symptoms suggestive of esophageal, pancreatic, or biliary disease, but both primary care physicians and gastroenterologists should be aware that the patient's history and physical findings, and even the presence of alarm symptoms, are unreliable in distinguishing functional from organic causes of dyspepsia.[5,8,9,11,103–105] Therefore most guidelines and recommendations advocate prompt endoscopy when risk factors for dyspepsia (e.g., NSAID use, age above 40–60, alarm symptoms) are present.[106–108] The optimal management strategy for the majority of patients who do not have a risk factor for an organic cause of dyspepsia remains a matter of debate and controversy, and several approaches have been proposed. Available options include: (1) prompt diagnostic endoscopy, followed by targeted medical therapy; (2) noninvasive testing for *Hp* infection, followed by treatment based on the result ("test-and-treat" strategy); and (3) empirical antisecretory therapy. In the two latter strategies, endoscopy is performed in patients who do not respond to treatment or experience recurrent symptoms. In theory, empirical prokinetic therapy could also be considered as an initial option but is generally not recommended because of the lack of widely available prokinetic drugs with established efficacy.[107]

Prompt Endoscopy and Directed Treatment

Diagnostic EGD allows direct detection of organic causes of dyspepsia, such as PUD, erosive esophagitis, severe gastritis, or a malignancy. Endoscopy before any therapy has been instituted is still considered the gold standard for the diagnosis of UGI disorders.[109] The procedure may also have a reassuring effect on patients and physicians.[110–112] Gastric mucosal biopsies facilitate diagnosis of *Hp* infection, which should be followed by eradication therapy if the results are positive. Endoscopy has been claimed to detect early gastric cancer at a curable stage but evidence for this claim is weak at best.[113,114] Similar to colonoscopy withdrawal time, longer endoscopy time increases the likelihood of detecting malignant lesions.[115] Endoscopy is both expensive and invasive and may not have such a major impact on initial treatment. Patients found to have a peptic ulcer or erosive esophagitis or gastritis will receive antisecretory therapy, while those with a normal upper endoscopy may still be treated empirically with antisecretory therapy with the working diagnoses of FD and/or nonerosive GERD. Some experts argue that initial empirical antisecretory therapy will only delay endoscopy, because both FD and GERD are likely to recur after discontinuation of empirical therapy, at which time the patient will be referred for endoscopy. As well, empiric therapy prior to EGD may obscure the underlying cause (i.e., severe esophagitis or gastritis) if symptoms persist and upper endoscopy is performed later.

15

A number of randomized controlled trials have compared prompt endoscopy with empirical noninvasive management strategies. A meta-analysis of five trials that compared initial endoscopy with a test-and-treat strategy concluded that initial endoscopy may be associated with a small reduction in the risk of recurrent dyspeptic symptoms but that this gain was not cost-effective (Table 15.3).[116] Most relevant studies found that the direct and indirect costs associated with prompt endoscopy are higher than those associated with empirical therapy and are not completely offset by reduced medication use or subsequent physician visits.[107–119] Available data, therefore, do not support early endoscopy as a cost-effective initial management strategy for all patients with uncomplicated dyspepsia.

Nevertheless, most relevant practice guidelines advocate initial endoscopy in all patients above a certain age threshold (usually 45–60 years old) to detect potentially curable UGI malignancy.[106–108] The rationale for this approach is that the vast majority of gastric malignancies occur in persons over 45 years of age and that the rate of cancer detection rises in persons with dyspepsia who are 45 years of age or older.[113–115] Risk factors for gastric cancer should be assessed at the initial evaluation (e.g., *Hp* status, family history of gastric cancer, male sex, older age, cigarette smoking, alcohol use, prior gastric surgery, pernicious anemia, diet). Most patients with newly diagnosed gastric cancer are already incurable at the time of diagnosis, however, and many will have an alarm feature that would have warranted immediate endoscopy.[114] In patients younger than age 45 who have a family history of gastric cancer, who emigrated from a country with a high rate of gastric cancer, or who have undergone partial gastrectomy, early endoscopy is also recommended.

Test and Treat for *Hp* Infection

Hp is causally associated with the majority of peptic ulcers and is the most important risk factor for gastric cancer (see Chapters 54 to 56).[120] Because of the involvement of *Hp* in PUD, several consensus panels and guidelines have advocated noninvasive testing for *Hp* in young patients (<45–60 years of age) with uncomplicated dyspepsia.[5,8,106–108] Persons with a positive test result should receive eradication therapy (a PPI and see Chapter 55), whereas patients with a negative test result should be treated empirically, usually with a PPI.[121] The benefits of this test-and-treat strategy are the cure of PUD or prevention of future peptic ulcers and symptom resolution (≈7% above the rate with placebo) in a small subset of patients with dyspepsia who are infected with *Hp*.[92,93,107,116,117,121] Eradication of *Hp* eliminates chronic gastritis and may thereby contribute to a reduction in the risk of *Hp*-associated gastric cancer.[122]

In Western countries, the prevalence of *Hp* infection in patients with uninvestigated dyspepsia is declining rapidly, and infection rates are especially low (10%–30%) in persons younger than 30 years of age. Widespread use of antibiotics has the disadvantage of inducing resistance and occasionally causing drug allergies. Whether eradication of *Hp* causes or worsens GERD has long been debated,[123] but a randomized controlled trial in *Hp*-positive patients with GERD failed to demonstrate any worsening of GERD.[124] Furthermore, the accuracy of noninvasive testing depends on both the prevalence of *Hp* in the population and the sensitivity and specificity of the test. Serologic tests for *Hp* are the least expensive but also the least accurate. If the prevalence of *Hp* in a population is less than 60%, the urea breath test and the fecal antigen test are preferred, because their higher accuracy reduces inappropriate treatment for patients without *Hp* infection (see Chapter 55).[125]

Randomized placebo-controlled trials have shown only a modest reduction in symptoms of dyspepsia after a test-and-treat approach in primary care.[126–128] A meta-analysis of studies comparing a test-and-treat strategy with empirical antisecretory therapy in patients with dyspepsia found little difference in the frequency of symptom resolution or costs between the two strategies.[129] Although earlier models that assumed higher prevalence rates of *Hp* infection suggested a greater benefit to a test-and-treat strategy,[130–132] economic models have suggested that the test-and-treat approach may be equally or less cost-effective than empirical antisecretory therapy.[133,134] The test-and-treat strategy as an initial approach to uninvestigated dyspepsia is most likely to be beneficial in areas where the *Hp* infection rate is high.

Empirical Antisecretory Drug Therapy

Initial empirical antisecretory therapy is widely used in primary care for patients with uninvestigated dyspepsia. The approach is attractive because it controls symptoms and heals lesions in most patients with underlying GERD or PUD and may be beneficial for up to one-third of patients with FD.[135,136] PPIs provide superior symptom relief compared with H2RAs, and the response usually occurs within 2 weeks of therapy.[106–108] Disadvantages of empirical PPI therapy are rapid symptomatic relapse after therapy is discontinued and the potential for rebound gastric hypersecretion,[137] so many patients require long-term PPI therapy. As noted earlier, a meta-analysis of studies that compared a test-and-treat approach with empirical antisecretory therapy in patients with dyspepsia found little difference in symptom resolution or costs between the two strategies[129]; however, economic analyses indicate that empirical antisecretory therapy may be equally or more cost-effective.[133,134]

Recommendations

The optimal cost-effective approach to the initial management of uncomplicated dyspepsia remains unclear. Clinical decision-making should consider specific aspects of a patient's case and weigh risk-benefit factors. In a young dyspeptic patient (age <45) without alarm features, initial endoscopy cannot be recommended because the yield is low and the test is unlikely to lead to improved outcomes. This position can be reconsidered if the patient is worried about an underlying disease, has alarm symptoms, a family history of cancer, or has emigrated from an area with a high incidence of gastric or esophageal cancer. In a population with a high prevalence (>20%) of *Hp* infection, the test-and-treat approach remains attractive because patients with PUD will be

TABLE 15.3 Two Meta-analyses of Initial Management Strategies in Patients With Uninvestigated Dyspepsia

Investigator (Year)	Relative Risk (95% CI)
Prompt Endoscopy vs. Empirical Acid Suppression	
Bytzer (1994)	0.99 (0.61–1.63)
Delaney (2001)	0.93 (0.78–1.10)
Duggan (1999)	0.86 (0.63–1.18)
Lewin (1999)	0.75 (0.54–1.05)
Overall	**0.89 (0.77–1.02)**
An *Helicobacter pylori* Test-and-Treat Strategy vs. Endoscopy	
Arents (2003)	1.05 (0.90–1.21)
Duggan (1999)	1.38 (1.03–1.84)
Heany (1999)	0.82 (0.60–1.11)
Lassen (2001)	0.84 (0.59–1.19)
McColl (2002)	0.78 (0.51–1.19)
Overall	**0.98 (0.81–1.18)**

Neither analysis demonstrated a difference between strategies. *CI*, Confidence interval.

cured. The tests of choice are the urea breath test or the fecal antigen test. *Hp*-positive patients should be given a course of *Hp* eradication therapy (see Chapter 55). In those who are negative for *Hp*, a PPI can be prescribed for 1–2 months. In populations in which the prevalence of *Hp* infection is low, empirical antisecretory therapy (once daily PPI for 1–2 months) appears to be the preferred option. Patients who fail to respond to these initial approaches, and possibly those in whom symptoms recur after cessation of antisecretory therapy, should undergo endoscopy, although the yield is likely to be low.

In patients older than age 45–60 without alarm features, most guidelines recommend initial diagnostic endoscopy, although the benefit in terms of detection of early-stage malignancies remains unproved. In these cases, management will depend on endoscopic findings and detection of *Hp*, but PPI therapy is likely the first agent to be prescribed to most patients.

Additional Investigations

Additional investigations may be pursued in patients with progressive or refractory symptoms who do not respond to initial management approaches. Testing for celiac disease and *Giardia* infection is useful for patients with refractory symptoms, especially when accompanied by weight loss. In patients with severe pain or weight loss, In patients with severe pain or weight loss, a mesenteric duplex US can screen for stenosis of large abdominal arteries and assess for pancreaticobiliary disease.

In case of severe postprandial fullness, and especially in case of refractory nausea and vomiting, a GES using scintigraphy or a breath test can be considered. When gastric emptying is severely delayed, a small bowel x-ray can rule out mechanical obstruction as a contributing factor. In cases of refractory intermittent epigastric pain or burning, esophageal pH with impedance monitoring is useful for diagnosing atypical manifestations of GERD not responding sufficiently to empirical antisecretory drug therapy. Psychological or psychiatric assessment is recommended for patients with long-standing refractory or debilitating symptoms. Electrogastrography, barostat studies, or simple nutrient challenge tests have been used in pathophysiologic studies but have no established role in the clinical management of dyspeptic patients.

TREATMENT OF FUNCTIONAL DYSPEPSIA

General Measures

Reassurance and education are of primary importance in patients with FD. Despite normal findings at endoscopy, the patient should be given a confident diagnosis. In IBS, a positive physician-patient interaction has been shown to reduce healthcare-seeking behavior, and this approach is applicable to patients with FD as well.[138]

Lifestyle and dietary measures are usually prescribed to patients with FD, but the impact of dietary interventions has not been studied systematically.[14] Advising patients to eat more frequent, smaller meals seems logical. Because the presence of lipids in the duodenum enhances gastric sensitivity, avoiding meals with a high fat content may be advisable.[77,78] Similarly, physicians tend to discourage consumption of spicy foods containing capsaicin and other irritants.[15] One prospective study of 184 patients with FD randomized to a low FODMAP diet or traditional dietary advice found that both groups reported symptom improvement at the end of the 4-week study, although there was no significant difference between the two different diets.[139] However, symptoms of bloating and patients with PDS seemed to respond better to the low FODMAP diet. Coffee, smoking, and alcohol consumption may induce or aggravate symptoms in some patients, and thus limiting intake may help the occasional patient, although data from large RCTs is not available to guide therapy. Avoidance of aspirin and other NSAIDs is commonly recommended and seems sensible, although not of established value.[8,16] If the patient has an apparent coexisting anxiety disorder, depression, posttraumatic stress disorder, or displays behaviors suspicious for an eating disorder, psychiatry and/or psychology referral should be strongly considered.

Pharmacologic Treatment

Many patients with FD will not improve with dietary modifications and medication cessation and thus pharmacotherapy is warranted. The efficacy of pharmacologic treatments for FD is limited, however.

Acid-Suppressive Drugs

In patients with GERD, a trial of antisecretory therapy often has both therapeutic and diagnostic value. Based on meta-analyses of therapeutic outcomes in FD, the efficacy of antacids, sucralfate, and misoprostol has not been demonstrated.[140] A meta-analysis of 12 randomized placebo-controlled trials that evaluated the efficacy of H2RAs in patients with FD reported a significant benefit over placebo, with a relative risk reduction of 23% and a number needed to treat of 7.[140] However, many of these trials included patients with GERD under a broad interpretation of FD, thereby limiting the value of the data. In clinical practice, H2RAs infrequently improve global FD symptoms.

A meta-analysis of 15 placebo-controlled, randomized trials of PPIs for FD confirmed that this class of agents is superior to placebo, with a number needed to treat of 10 (Table 15.4).[107,141] The relative risk reduction was lower (13%) than for H2RAs, probably reflecting more stringent entry criteria and better exclusion of patients with GERD. No difference in efficacy was found between standard and low-dose PPI therapy, and double-dose PPI therapy was not superior to single-dose PPI therapy.[107,141] The patient's *Hp* status did not affect the response to PPI therapy. Subgrouping of FD using previous Rome classifications showed a trend for PPI therapy to be most effective in the group with overlapping reflux and less effective in the group with epigastric pain (likely corresponding to EPS), and those classified as having dysmotility (likely corresponding to PDS).[140,141] Prospective studies of PPI therapy for FD in patients subgrouped according to the Rome IV classification are lacking.

Eradication of *Hp* Infection

A meta-analysis has reported a 9% reduction in the frequency of dyspepsia after *Hp* eradication compared with placebo at 12 months of follow-up, with a number needed to treat of 12.5 (Table 15.5).[107] Arguments against eradication therapy are the low number of responders and the delayed occurrence of demonstrable symptomatic benefit. It has been argued, however, that *Hp* eradication can induce sustained remission in dyspepsia, albeit in a minority of patients.[142] These patients are referred to as having "*Hp*-associated dyspepsia" according to the Kyoto Global Consensus Conference report.[93] Other arguments in favor of the use of eradication therapy are protection against PUD, presumed protection against gastric cancer, and the short-term nature and relatively low cost of treatment.

Prokinetic Agents

Gastric prokinetic agents are a heterogeneous class of compounds that exert a stimulatory effect on gastric motility through a variety of mechanisms. The efficacy of available prokinetic agents in patients with FD has been controversial.[107,140,143–145] A meta-analysis has suggested that therapy with a prokinetic agent is superior to placebo in patients with FD, with a number needed to

TABLE 15.4 Meta-analysis of Randomized, Controlled Trials of PPI Therapy in Patients With Functional Dyspepsia

	PPI		Placebo		Risk Ratio	Relative Risk
Investigator (Year)	**Events**	**Total**	**Events**	**Total**	**Relative Risk (95% CI)**	**95% CI**
Blum (2000)	272	395	170	203	0.82 (0.75, 0.90)	
Bolling-Sternevald (2002)	71	100	80	97	0.86 (0.74, 1.01)	
Farup (1999)	6	14	8	10	0.54 (0.27, 1.06)	
Fletcher (2011)	45	70	33	35	0.68 (0.56, 0.83)	
Gerson (2005)	16	21	9	19	1.61 (0.95, 2.74)	
Hengels (1998)	50	131	77	138	0.68 (0.53, 0.89)	
Iwakiri (2013)	194	253	71	85	0.92 (0.82, 1.03)	
Peura (2004)	474	613	271	308	0.88 (0.83, 0.93)	
Suzuki (2013) (ELF)	16	23	28	30	0.75 (0.56, 0.99)	
Talley (1998) (BOND)	242	423	162	219	0.77 (0.69, 0.87)	
Talley (1998) (OPERA)	277	403	141	203	0.99 (0.88, 1.11)	
Talley (2007)	653	853	84	111	1.01 (0.90, 1.13)	
Van Rensburg (2008)	93	207	116	212	0.82 (0.68, 1.00)	
Van Zanten (2006)	84	109	100	115	0.89 (0.78, 1.00)	
Wong (2002)	231	301	107	152	1.09 (0.97, 1.23)	
Total	–	**3916**	–	**1937**	**0.87 (0.82, 0.94)**	
Total events	**2724**	–	**1457**	–		

0.5 0.7 1 1.5 2

Favors PPI **Favors Placebo**

Events signify the number of patients with symptomatic improvement. Total signifies the total number of patients treated. *CI*, Confidence interval.
From Moayyedi PM, Lacy BE, Andrews CN, et al. ACG and CAG clinical guideline: management of dyspepsia. *Am J Gastroenterol*. 2017;112:988–1013.

TABLE 15.5 Meta-analysis of Randomized, Controlled Trials of *Helicobacter pylori* Eradication in Patients With Functional Dyspepsia

	Treatment		Control		Risk Ratio	Relative Risk
Investigator (Year)	**Events**	**Total**	**Events**	**Total**	**Relative Risk (95% CI)**	**95% CI**
Ang (2006)	49	71	45	59	0.90 (0.73, 1.12)	
Blum (OCAY) (1998)	119	164	130	164	0.92 (0.81, 1.03)	
Froehlich (2001)	31	74	34	70	0.86 (0.60, 1.24)	
Gilbert (2004)	13	34	8	16	0.76 (0.40, 1.46)	
Gonzalez Carro (2004)	22	47	31	46	0.69 (0.48, 1.00)	
Gwee (2009)	31	41	38	41	0.82 (0.67, 0.991	
HSU (2001)	34	81	36	80	0.93 (0.66, 1.33)	
Koelz (2003)	67	89	73	92	0.95 (0.81, 1.111)	
Koskenpato (2001)	61	77	63	74	0.93 (0.80, 1.081)	
Lan (2011)	86	98	94	97	0.91 (0.83, 0.981)	
Matfertheiner (2003)	338	534	177	266	0.95 (0.85, 1.061)	
Martinek (2005)	5	20	12	20	0.42 (0.18, 0.961)	
Mazzoleni (2006)	39	46	40	43	0.91 (0.79, 1.061)	
Mazzoleni (2011)	166	201	175	203	0.96 (0.88, 1.041)	
McColl (1998)	121	154	143	154	0.85 (0.77, 0.931)	
Mlwa (2000)	33	48	28	37	0.91 (0.70, 1.18)	
Ruiz (2005)	46	79	64	79	0.72 (0.58, 0.89)	
Sodhi (2013)	164	259	188	260	0.88 (0.78, 0.99)	
Talley (ORCHID) (1999)	101	133	111	142	0.97 (0.85, 1.11)	
Talley (United States) (1999)	122	150	120	143	0.97 (0.87, 1.08)	
van Zanten (2003)	45	75	55	82	0.89 (0.70, 1.14)	
Varannes (2001)	74	129	86	124	0.83 (0.68, 1.00)	
Total	–	**2604**	–	**2292**	**0.91 (0.88, 0.94)**	
Total events	**1767**	–	**1751**	–		

0.5 0.7 1 1.5 2

Favors Treatment **Favors Control**

Events signify the number of patients with symptomatic improvement. Total signifies the total number of patients treated. *CI*, Confidence interval.
From Moayyedi PM, Lacy BE, Andrews CN, et al. ACG and CAG clinical guideline: management of dyspepsia. *Am J Gastroenterol*. 2017;112:988–1013.

treat of 7, but this effect was largely driven by cisapride and removal of data for cisapride increased the number needed to treat to 12 (Table 15.6).[145] Metoclopramide and domperidone are dopamine receptor antagonists with a stimulatory effect on UGI motility. Unlike metoclopramide, which may cause serious neurologic adverse effects, domperidone does not cross the blood-brain barrier but has been associated with QT interval prolongation on electrocardiography and may precipitate cardiac arrhythmias. Moreover, placebo-controlled studies of domperidone in patients with FD are lacking.[107,145] Cisapride facilitates the release of acetylcholine in the myenteric plexus via 5-hydroxytryptamine 4 (5-HT_4) receptor agonism and accelerates gastric emptying. The available trials with these drugs, however, were of poor quality, concerns were raised about publication bias, and cisapride was withdrawn from the market in the United States for safety concerns.[144,145] Other agents with evidence of efficacy are tegaserod and acotiamide (see later).[145–147] Tegaserod showed only a small benefit over placebo[146] and is currently not available in most countries because of concerns about potentially associated cardiovascular risk although an adjudicated analysis of a large data bank of IBS patients disproved these safety concerns.[148]

Unfortunately, studies of other types of prokinetic agents have generally been unsuccessful in providing convincing evidence of symptomatic relief in patients with FD.[149] On the basis of a systematic analysis, the efficacy of prokinetic agents is not thought to be driven by their stimulatory effect on gastric emptying but rather by effects on accommodation and visceral hypersensitivity.[144,147] Although some prokinetic agents impair gastric accommodation and increase gastric sensitivity, others may enhance gastric accommodation (see later).[144]

Agents that Enhance Gastric Accommodation

Impaired gastric accommodation is the most commonly found motor abnormality in FD, occurring in approximately 30% of patients (see earlier). In a mechanistic proof-of-concept study, the anxiolytic 5-HT_{1A} agonist buspirone improved both symptoms of early satiation and gastric accommodation, without effects on anxiety to explain the symptomatic benefit.[150] A multicenter 4-week study of tandospirone, another 5-HT_{1A} agonist, also demonstrated alleviation of epigastric pain and discomfort independent of changes in anxiety and depression levels.[151] The first-in-class agent acotiamide is both a presynaptic muscarinic autoreceptor inhibitor and a cholinesterase inhibitor and enhances both gastric emptying and accommodation.[152] A single 4-week phase 3 study was conducted in Japan and showed favorable effects of acotiamide on early satiation, postprandial fullness, and upper abdominal bloating in patients with PDS.[147] The drug was well tolerated, and the findings were confirmed in a one-year open-label study in Europe.[153] Acotiamide is available in Japan, India, and several countries in Latin America.

Centrally Acting Neuromodulators

Psychotropic agents, such as antidepressants, anxiolytics, and antipsychotics, are often used for the treatment of functional GI disorders that do not respond to initial conventional approaches. Rationale for their treatment includes their potential to alter pain-processing pathways in the brain. Based on this concept, they are now referred to as centrally acting neuromodulators (see Chapters 52 and 124).[154] A meta-analysis has confirmed that centrally acting neuromodulators may be effective for treating FD, but convincing evidence is available only for atypical antipsychotics and tricyclic antidepressants; trials of other agents are limited in size and numbers.[154,155]

In a multicenter trial of patients with FD randomized to treatment with placebo, amitriptyline, or escitalopram for 8 weeks, only amitriptyline resulted in symptomatic improvement, which was confined to the subgroup characterized by epigastric pain (EPS-like subgroup).[156] Antidepressant therapy did not significantly alter the gastric emptying rate or nutrient volume tolerance, but amitriptyline increased gastric accommodation as assessed by single-photon emission CT imaging (see earlier).[157] Treatment with amitriptyline and escitalopram did not significantly improve anxiety, depression, or somatization scores, but sleep was improved modestly by amitriptyline.[158]

A large controlled trial with the selective serotonin and norepinephrine reuptake inhibitor venlafaxine in patients with FD failed to show any symptomatic benefit, and tolerance was poor.[159] Mirtazapine, an antidepressant with activity on diverse neurotransmitter receptors, was efficacious in nondepressed and non-anxious patients with FD and major weight loss.[159,160] In addition to increased body weight, mirtazapine improved overall symptoms, early satiation nausea, and nutrient volume tolerance.

Other Pharmacotherapeutic Approaches

On the basis of a meta-analysis of four trials, bismuth salts seemed efficacious but this analysis had marginal statistical significance.[140] Simethicone was superior to placebo in one controlled trial.[161] Peppermint oil has also been evaluated in the treatment of FD. In a controlled trial, specially formulated capsules of caraway oil and L-menthol were superior to placebo in alleviating symptoms of both EPS and PDS within 24 hours, with good tolerance, though no statistically significant benefit was demonstrated at 2 and 4 weeks, respectively.[162] The mode of action remains to be established, but previous mechanistic studies showed that peppermint oil relaxes the proximal stomach.[163] In a study from Hong Kong, rifaximin, 400 mg three times daily for 2 weeks, was well tolerated and superior to placebo in providing adequate relief of belching and postprandial fullness and bloating in patients with FD (Rome III criteria) without SIBO.[164] This result requires confirmation before the use of nonabsorbable antibiotics can be recommended for the treatment of FD.

Various studies have reported improvement in symptoms during treatment with mixed herbal preparations, Japanese Kampo medicine, Chinese herbals, or artichoke leaf extract.[165–170] The basis for improvement remains to be determined. One study reported that long-term administration of red pepper was more effective than placebo in decreasing the intensity of dyspeptic symptoms in patients with FD.[171] Probiotic-containing products have become popular as self-management or prescribed treatment for bowel symptoms; upper abdominal symptoms including PDS have been less well studied. Limited data suggest potential efficacy, but more studies are needed.[172,173] Finally, a recent randomized, placebo-controlled trial involving 72 patients with FD (Rome IV criteria) with refractory symptoms despite PPI therapy, demonstrated that treatment with pregabalin resulted in significant improvement in global dyspeptic symptoms, though improvement was limited to epigastric pain and burning and sensation of reflux in the analysis of individual symptom scores.[174] Pregabalin is a second-generation gabapentinoid agent acting on the $\alpha 2$-δ subunit of calcium channels.

Psychological Interventions

Although patients with FD have a higher prevalence of psychosocial comorbidities, the role of psychosocial factors in the generation of symptoms remains unclear. In part because of these comorbidities, psychological interventions, such as group support with relaxation training, cognitive behavioral therapy, psychotherapy, and hypnotherapy, have been used in patients with FD. A systematic review of clinical trials of psychological interventions for FD found that all trials claimed benefit from psychological interventions, with effects persisting for over 1 year, but all studies were limited by inadequate statistical analysis.[175] The authors concluded that evidence to confirm the efficacy of psychological

TABLE 15.6 Meta-analysis of Randomized, Controlled Trials of Selected Prokinetic Agents in Patients With Functional Dyspepsia

	Prokinetic		Placebo		Risk Ratio	Relative Risk
Investigator (Year)	**Events**	**Total**	**Events**	**95% CI**	**Relative Risk (95% CI)**	**95% CI**
CISAPRIDE VS PLACEBO						
AJ-Quorain (1995)	22	48	47	50	0.49 (0.36, 0.67)	
Champion (1997)	43	83	26	40	0.80 (0.59, 1.08)	
De Groot (1997)	26	61	35	60	0.73 (0.51, 1.05)	
De Nutte (1989)	6	17	11	15	0.48 (0.24, 0.98)	
Francois (1987)	8	17	14	17	0.57 (0.33, 0.99)	
Hanson (1998)	101	109	99	110	1.03 (0.95, 1.12)	
Holtmann (2002)	51	59	52	61	1.01 (0.88, 1.17)	
Kellow (1995)	26	30	25	31	1.07 (0.86, 1.34)	
Rosch (1987)	27	57	45	57	0.60 (0.44, 0.81)	
Teixeira (2000)	9	22	11	16	0.60 (0.33, 1.09)	
Wang (1995)	137	414	145	169	0.39 (0.33, 0.45)	
Yeoh (1997)	46	52	47	52	0.98 (0.86, 1.12)	
Subtotal	–	**969**	–	**678**	**0.71 (0.54, 0.93)**	
Total events	**502**	–	**557**	–		
ACOTIAMIDE VS PLACEBO						
Kusunoki (2012)	15	21	18	21	0.83 (0.60, 1.15)	
Matsueda (2010-1)	187	216	94	107	0.99 (0.90, 1.08)	
Matsueda (2010-2)	290	346	99	116	0.98 (0.90, 1.07)	
Matsuoda (2012)	383	452	405	445	0.93 (0.89, 0.98)	
Tack (2011)	87	193	53	96	0.82 (0.64, 1.04)	
Talley (2008)	195	312	71	104	0.92 (0.78, 1.07)	
Subtotal	**1540**	–	**889**	–	**0.94 (0.91, 0.98)**	
Total events	**1157**	–	**740**	–		
ITOPRIDE VS. PLACEBO						
Holtmann (2006)	174	406	86	142	0.71 (0.59, 0.84)	
Ma (2012)	53	119	79	120	0.68 (0.53, 0.86)	
Shen (2014)	14	40	22	40	0.64 (0.38, 1.06)	
Talley (2008-1)	124	264	226	260	0.54 (0.47, 0.62)	
Talley (2008-2)	288	315	309	830	0.98 (0.93, 1.02)	
Wong (2014)	3	16	4	14	0.66 (0.18, 2.44)	
Subtotal	**1160**	–	**906**	–	**0.70 (0.47, 1.03)**	
Total events	**656**	–	**726**	–		
TEGASEROD 6 MG BID VS PLACEBO						
Vakil (2008-1)	423	685	452	675	0.92 (0.85, 1.00)	
Vakil (2008-2)	356	652	420	655	0.85 (0.78, 0.93)	
Subtotal	1337	–	1330	–	0.89 (0.82, 0.96)	
Total events	779	–	872	–		
Mosapride vs. Placebo						
Hallerback (2002)	171	425	57	141	1.00 (0.79, 1.25)	
Lin (2009)	21	30	26	30	0.81 (0.61, 1.06)	
Subtotal	**455**	–	**171**	–	**0.91 (0.73, 1.13)**	
Total events	**192**	–	**83**	–		
ABT-229 VS. PLACEBO						
Talley (2000)	253	488	47	121	1.33 (1.05, 1.70)	
Subtotal	**488**	–	**121**	–	**1.33 (1.05, 1.70)**	
Total events	**253**	–	**47**	–		
Total	–	**5949**	–	**4095**	**0.81 (0.74, 0.89)**	
Total events	**3539**	–	**3025**	–		

0.2 0.5 1 2

Favors Prokinetic **Favors Placebo**

Events signify the number of patients with symptomatic improvement. Total signifies the total number of patients treated. *CI*, Confidence interval.
From Moayyedi PM, Lacy BE, Andrews CN, et al. ACG and CAG clinical guideline: management of dyspepsia. *Am J Gastroenterol*. 2017;112:988–1013.

interventions in FD is insufficient. A recent meta-analysis of 14 RCTs reported that psychological interventions may be effective in alleviating the symptoms and psychology of FD, although benefits may be limited to psychotherapy.[176]

RECOMMENDATIONS

In patients with FD with mild or intermittent symptoms, reassurance, education, and dietary changes may be sufficient. Drug therapy can be considered in patients with more severe symptoms or those who do not respond to reassurance and lifestyle changes. Testing for *Hp* infection is recommended, and, if positive, eradication therapy should be prescribed. An immediate impact on symptoms is unlikely, however, and any potential benefit is observed mainly over a longer period of follow-up (Fig. 15.4). PPIs and, if available, prokinetic agents may also be used as initial pharmacotherapy. The symptom pattern may help determine the most appropriate initial choice of treatment, and a change in drug class is advisable in case the therapeutic response is insufficient.

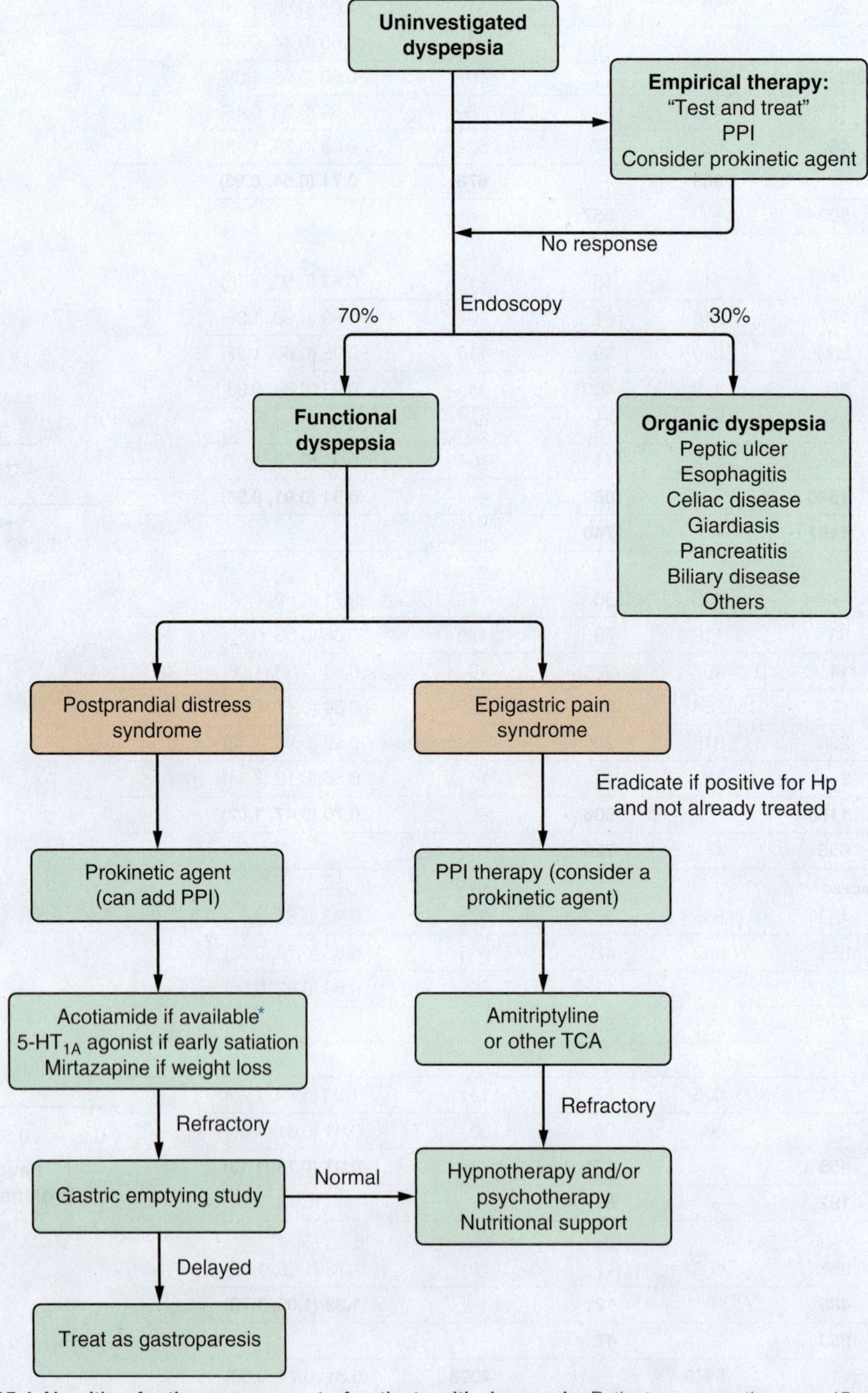

Fig. 15.4 Algorithm for the management of patients with dyspepsia. Patients younger than age 45–55 who do not have alarm features may be treated empirically, whereas all others should be evaluated initially by esophagogastroduodenoscopy. *5-HT*, 5-hydroxytryptamine; *TCA*, tricyclic antidepressant. *Not available in the United States.

A 4–8-week trial of once daily PPI therapy should be given to all patients with coexisting heartburn and to those with EPS. In case of symptomatic relief, treatment should be interrupted and intermittent or chronic therapy with a PPI tried for patients with repeated relapses. In those with PDS, a motility modifying drug with an attractive safety profile (e.g., acotiamide, where available) can be considered. Metoclopramide and cisapride should not be used because of the risk of serious adverse events, and clinicians should be aware that domperidone has also been associated with QT prolongation. Theoretically, combinations of PPIs and prokinetic agents may have additive symptomatic effects, although single-drug therapy is always preferable to reduce costs and minimize the potential for adverse effects.

In patients with bothersome symptoms of EPS that persist despite initial treatment, a trial of a low-dose neuromodulator, such as a tricyclic antidepressant, may be considered, even in the absence of apparent anxiety or depression. Higher doses can be considered in patients with significant anxiety or depression. The SNRI venlafaxine was not shown to be beneficial and should, thus, not be prescribed for the treatment of FD. There is limited data supporting the use of pregabalin in patients with pain-predominant dyspeptic symptoms, such as EPS.

In patients with bothersome symptoms of PDS, treatment with a 5-HT_{1A} agonist or mirtazapine can be used for refractory early satiation. In patients with persisting symptoms, gastric emptying should be measured; in cases with severely delayed gastric emptying, the patient should be diagnosed as having idiopathic gastroparesis, and prokinetic agents can be considered (see Chapter 52).

A trial of simethicone, peppermint oil, or a medically prescribed herbal preparation with apparent benefit in controlled trials may also be considered in refractory patients. Opioids should not be prescribed for the treatment of FD-related pain.

Referral to a psychiatrist or psychotherapist can be considered in patients with obvious coexisting psychiatric disease, a history of abuse, or a debilitating impact of severe symptoms on daily life activities. Motivated patients may benefit from psychological approaches, such as psychotherapy, hypnotherapy, cognitive behavioral therapy, or relaxation therapy.

Full references for this chapter can be found at https://ebooks.health.elsevier.com.

16 Nausea and Vomiting

Parth Patel, C. Prakash Gyawali

IN THIS CHAPTER

Nausea is an unpleasant subjective sensation of impending vomiting and can be associated with salivation, anorexia, perspiration, disinterest in ongoing activities, and anxiety.[1] In many instances, the sensation cannot be localized, although it can sometimes be felt in the epigastrium or throat. Nausea typically occurs prior to or during vomiting but can happen in isolation.

Retching or *dry heaving* consists of spasmodic respiratory movements with the glottis closed. When part of the emetic sequence, retching is associated with intense nausea and usually, but not invariably, culminates in the act of vomiting.

Vomiting or *emesis* is a partially voluntary act of forcefully expelling gastric or intestinal content through the mouth. This can occur in isolation, but is often part of the emetic sequence that includes nausea and retching and requires central neurogenic coordination.

Vomiting must be differentiated from *regurgitation*, the effortless reflux of gastric contents into the esophagus that sometimes reaches the mouth but without the forceful ejection typical of vomiting (see Chapter 14). Regurgitation can be esophageal, whereby the regurgitate tastes exactly like recently eaten food, or gastric, whereby the regurgitate tastes sour and may be associated with retrosternal or throat burning. Esophageal regurgitation can occur in disorders associated with esophageal outflow obstruction, such as achalasia.[2] By contrast, gastric regurgitation can occur with GERD[3] or rumination syndrome (a behavioral disorder) (see Chapter 14).[4] The differential diagnosis of vomiting needs to be kept in mind because patients often report vomiting without distinction, and a detailed clinical history is needed to distinguish regurgitation from vomiting.

PATHOPHYSIOLOGY

The mechanism of vomiting requires synchronized contraction and/or relaxation of several muscles, including the diaphragm, abdominal wall muscles, pharyngeal muscles, and muscles responsible for breathing, in conjunction with postural changes to accommodate oral emptying of gastric contents (Fig. 16.1).[1,5–7] Although a network of neurons in the brainstem controls the motor elements of the emetic response, important neural circuits in the medulla initiate vomiting.[8] Afferent neural signals for initiating emesis arise from many locations in the body, including the pharynx, stomach, and small intestine, as well as from extra-intestinal organs such as the heart and the testicle. Abdominal pain by itself can be a trigger for initiation of nausea and vomiting.[7] Pathways from the chemoreceptor trigger zone (CTZ) located in the area postrema on the floor of the fourth ventricle also activate vomiting. Despite its central location, the CTZ is outside (at least in part) the blood-brain barrier and serves primarily as a sensitive detection apparatus for circulating endogenous and exogenous molecules that may activate emesis. Finally, pathways arising from other CNS structures, including the cortex, brainstem, and vestibular system via the cerebellum, can also initiate symptoms.

The perception of nausea requires intact neural circuits in the supratentorial regions.[9,10] Afferent signals that mediate vomiting are carried by vagal fibers to the nucleus tractus solitarius, but nausea may occur even following bilateral abdominal vagotomy,[11] indicating the existence of alternative pathways for the development of nausea such as input from vestibular apparatus, cerebellum, and splanchnic nerves. Nausea and vomiting, therefore, only share part of the neural circuitry used to generate these symptoms, which explains why nausea and vomiting are clinically and pharmacologically separable.[11] In some patients, nausea may be present continuously and become quite troublesome.

The circuitry of the emetic reflex involves multiple receptors.[7] The following elements are the most relevant to clinical issues:

Stimulation of brain 5-hydroxytryptamine$_3$ (5-HT$_3$) serotonin receptors through release of 5-HT from enterochromaffin cells provokes release of several pro-emetic peptides and neurotransmitters, including dopamine, acetylcholine, and substance P, which in turn stimulate dopamine D2 receptors in the brainstem, thereby activating the emetic sequence. This sequence is the basis for the pharmacodynamic action of antiemetic agents like ondansetron, a 5-HT$_3$ receptor inhibitor (effective in treating acute chemotherapy-induced vomiting within 0–24 hours), and metoclopramide, a dopamine D2-receptor antagonist.[12] Toxins and drugs (including chemotherapeutic agents) that act on the GI

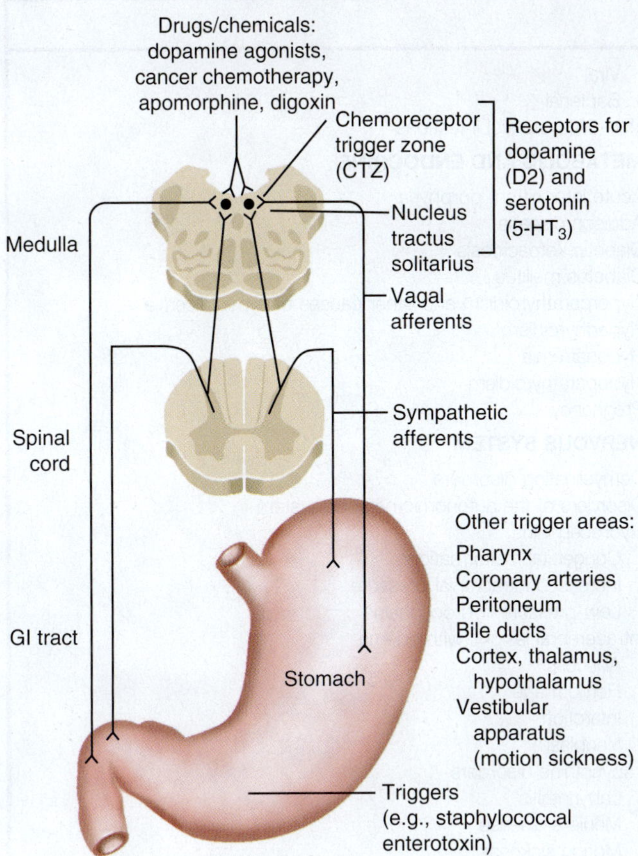

Fig. 16.1 Schematic representation of the proposed neural pathways that mediate vomiting. *5-HT3*, 5-hydroxytryptamine.

tract are detected by enteroendocrine cells that release 5-HT, which in turn activates 5-HT_3 receptors on vagal afferents.[11]

Histamine H_1 and muscarinic M1 receptors, which are abundant in the vestibular center and solitary nucleus, constitute the preferred pharmacologic targets for inhibiting motion sickness, vestibular nausea, and pregnancy-related emesis.[13] Other mediators of emesis being studied include prostaglandins that have a role in pregnancy and chemotherapy-related emesis, and corticosteroids that have therapeutic role in inhibiting synthesis of prostaglandins in managing these disorders.[14]

Cannabinoid CB1 receptors in the dorsal vagal complex inhibit the emetic reflex.[15] Cannabinoid agonists also modulate 5-HT_3 ion channels. The CB and 5-HT_3 receptor systems colocalize and interact in the brainstem.[16] Activation of somatodendritic 5-HT_{1A} autoreceptors in the dorsal raphe nucleus by cannabinoids reduces nausea and emesis provoked by emetogenic drugs.[17]

Neurokinin-1 (NK-1) receptors located in the area postrema and the solitary nucleus bind to substance P and are part of the terminal emetic pathways. Activation of NK-1 receptors by substance P constitutes the basis of chemotherapy-induced emesis (i.e., emesis 24–72 hours after administration of chemotherapeutic drugs).[12] NK-1 antagonists reduce emesis induced by both peripherally and centrally acting emetogens. 5-HT_3 receptors appear to be involved to a greater extent in centrally induced emesis compared to peripherally induced emesis. Therefore NK-1 receptor antagonists are more efficacious than $5HT_3$-receptor inhibitors and other known antiemetic drugs in reducing vomiting induced by a variety of causes, and are useful in preventing delayed emesis induced by chemotherapeutic agents.[7] Conversely, they may have less potent antinausea effects.

When activated, the brainstem sets into motion, through neural efferents, the various components of the emetic sequence (see Fig 16.1).[7] First, nausea develops as a result of activation of the cerebral cortex, the stomach relaxes concomitantly, and antral and intestinal peristalsis is inhibited. Second, retching occurs as a result of activation of spasmodic contractions of the diaphragm and intercostal muscles combined with closure of the glottis. Third, the act of vomiting occurs when somatic and visceral components are activated simultaneously. The components include brisk contraction of the diaphragm and abdominal muscles, relaxation of the lower esophageal sphincter, and a forceful retrograde peristaltic contraction in the jejunum that pushes enteric content in the oral direction.[18] Simultaneously, protective reflexes are activated. The soft palate is raised to prevent gastric content from entering the nasopharynx, respiration is momentarily inhibited, and the glottis is closed to prevent pulmonary aspiration, a potentially serious complication of vomiting. Other reflex phenomena that may accompany nausea include hypersalivation, cardiac dysrhythmias, and passage of gas and stool rectally. Emesis may alleviate nausea.[7]

CLINICAL CHARACTERISTICS

Certain clinical features may be characteristic of specific causes of nausea and vomiting. Symptoms in the morning or on an empty stomach, with swallowed saliva or gastric secretions in the emesis, suggest direct activation of the brainstem or CTZ, most typical of pregnancy, drugs, toxins (e.g., alcohol), and metabolic disorders (e.g., diabetes mellitus, uremia); functional vomiting may also exhibit these characteristics. Although excessive nocturnal postnasal drip is thought to demonstrate a similar pattern, direct evidence for this association is lacking. Vomiting of retained and partially digested food beyond the immediate postprandial period is typical of gastroparesis or slowly developing gastric outlet obstruction.[19] Bilious vomiting is commonly seen after multiple and repetitive vomiting episodes because of retrograde entry of intestinal content into the stomach or in the presence of a surgical gastroenteric anastomosis. Acute vomiting associated with a specific location or pattern of abdominal pain may indicate intra-abdominal organ inflammation such as pancreatitis, appendicitis, enteritis, pyelonephritis, or gallbladder disease. Vomitus with a feculent odor or taste suggests intestinal obstruction, ileus, longstanding gastric outlet obstruction, or a gastrocolic fistula. Vomiting that develops abruptly without preceding nausea or retching (projectile vomiting) is characteristic of, but not specific for, direct stimulation of the brainstem from an intracerebral lesion (tumor, abscess) or increased intracranial pressure.[20]

CAUSES

Establishing the etiology of nausea and vomiting allows specific management targeting the underlying mechanism. The urgency of diagnostic investigation is determined by the clinical presentation. Aggressive investigation is warranted when vomiting is bilious, when neurologic deficits are present, or if vomiting is acutely worsening. Short-term symptoms (<1 week) should be evaluated urgently, whereas chronic symptoms may be investigated electively in the outpatient setting. Causes of nausea and vomiting are listed in Box 16.1.

Acute Vomiting

In the patient with acute vomiting, the following two questions must be answered first (Fig. 16.2):

Is emergent evaluation or management needed? The patient is assessed for shock, dehydration, hypotension, and serious

BOX 16.1 Principal Causes of Nausea and Vomiting

ABDOMINAL

- Mechanical obstruction
  - Gastric outlet obstruction
  - SBO
- Motility disorders
  - Chronic intestinal pseudo-obstruction
  - Functional dyspepsia
  - Gastroparesis
- Other intra-abdominal causes
  - Acute appendicitis
  - Acute cholecystitis
  - Acute hepatitis
  - Acute mesenteric ischemia
  - Crohn disease
  - Gastric and duodenal ulcer disease
  - Pancreatitis and pancreatic neoplasms
  - Peritonitis and peritoneal carcinomatosis
  - Retroperitoneal and mesenteric pathology

DRUG*

- Aspirin and other NSAIDs
- Antidiabetic agents
- Antigout drugs
- Oral contraceptives (estrogen/progestrone)
- Antimicrobial agents
  - Acyclovir
  - Antituberculosis drugs
  - Erythromycin
  - Sulfonamides
  - Tetracycline
- Cancer chemotherapy
  - Cisplatin
  - Cytarabine
  - Dacarbazine
  - Etoposide
  - 5-Fluorouracil
  - Methotrexate
  - Nitrogen mustard
  - Tamoxifen
  - Vinblastine
- Cardiovascular drugs
  - Antidysrhythmics
  - Antihypertensives
  - Calcium channel blockers
  - Digoxin
  - Diuretics
  - β-Receptor blocking agents
- CNS drugs
  - Antiparkinsonian drugs (levodopa and other dopamine agonists)
  - Anticonvulsants
  - Acetylcholine esterase inhibitors
- GI medications
  - Azathioprine
  - Sulfasalazine
- Narcotics
  - Oral contraceptives
  - Theophylline

INFECTIOUS

- Acute gastroenteritis
  - Viral
  - Bacterial
- Non-GI (systemic) infections

METABOLIC AND ENDOCRINE

- Acute intermittent porphyria
- Addison disease
- Diabetic ketoacidosis
- Diabetes mellitus
- Hyperparathyroidism and other causes of hypercalcemia
- Hyperthyroidism
- Hyponatremia
- Hypoparathyroidism
- Pregnancy

NERVOUS SYSTEM

- Demyelinating disorders
- Disorders of the autonomic nervous system
- Hydrocephalus
  - Congenital malformations
  - Increased intracranial pressure
  - Low-pressure hydrocephalus
- Intracerebral lesions with edema
  - Abscess
  - Hemorrhage
  - Infarction
  - Neoplasm
- Labyrinthine disorders
  - Labyrinthitis
  - Ménière disease
  - Motion sickness
- Meningitis
  - Migraine headaches
  - Otitis media
  - Seizure disorders
  - Visceral neuropathy

OTHERS

- Anxiety and depression
- Cannabinoid hyperemesis syndrome
- Cardiac disease
  - Heart failure
  - Myocardial infarction, ischemia
  - Radiofrequency ablation for dysrhythmias
- Collagen vascular disorders
  - Scleroderma
  - SLE
- Cyclic vomiting syndrome
- Eating disorders
- Ethanol abuse
- Functional disorders
- Hypervitaminosis A
- Intense pain
- Paraneoplastic syndrome
- Postoperative state
- Postvagotomy
- Radiation therapy
- Starvation

*Partial list.

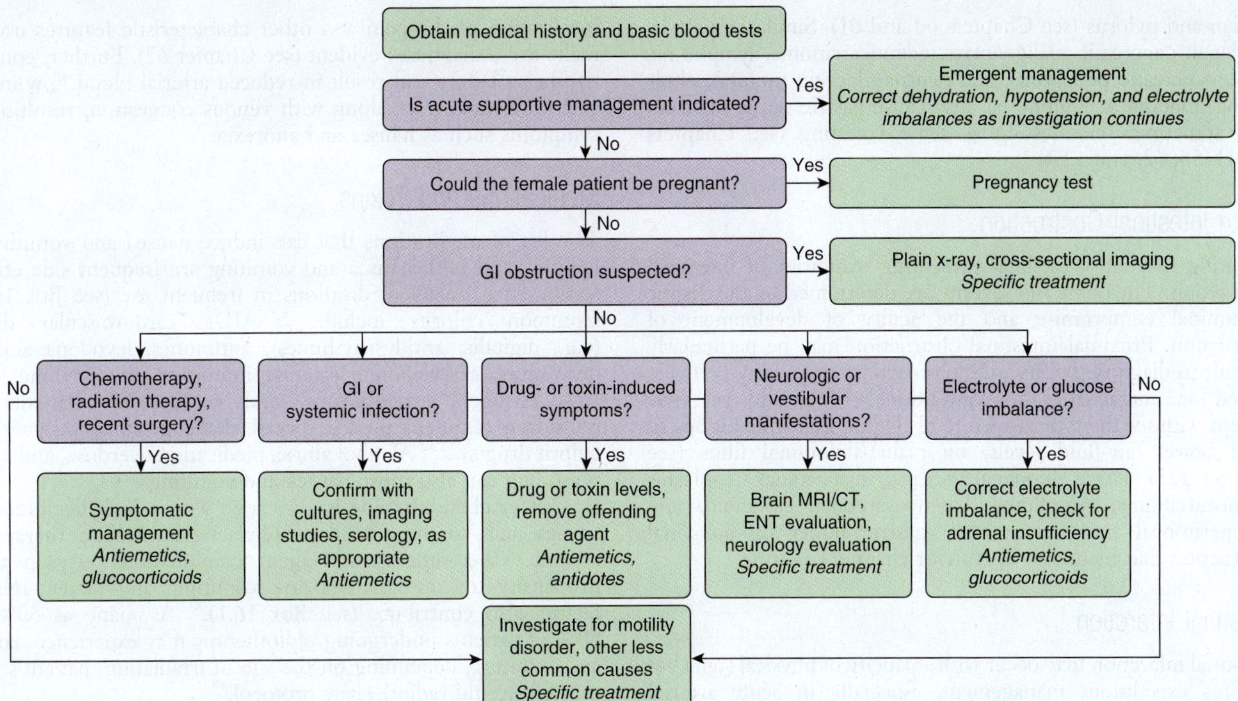

Fig. 16.2 Algorithm for the management of a patient with acute vomiting. Potential treatments are shown in italics. *ENT*, ear, nose, and throat.

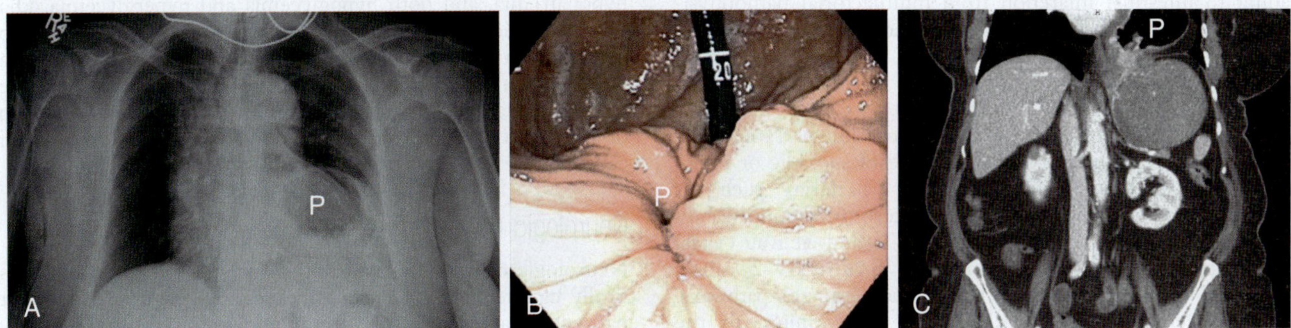

Fig. 16.3 Abdominal film (A), endoscopic image (B), and CT scan (C) in a patient with an obstructing paraesophageal hernia (P) presenting with nausea and vomiting. Note the presence of the air-containing viscus in the left thoracic cavity on the imaging studies. On retroflexion in the stomach during EGD, the opening into the paraesophageal hernia is visualized. Emergent surgery was performed to repair the paraesophageal hernia.

electrolyte disturbances with a carefully taken history and basic laboratory testing (CBC, comprehensive metabolic panel, and serum amylase and lipase levels). Intestinal obstruction, hollow viscus perforation, infectious processes, acute pancreatitis, organ infarction, cerebral edema, acute adrenocortical (Addisonian) crisis, and poisoning are some of the emergent etiologies to be considered.

Is the female patient pregnant? In women of reproductive age, pregnancy must be considered and excluded before alternative etiologies are considered.

Once these two issues are addressed, a number of potentially emergent diagnostic possibilities should be considered.

Gastric Outlet Obstruction

In the past, PUD was a major cause of gastric outlet obstruction (see Chapter 55), resulting from edema due to an active pyloric channel ulcer or stenotic narrowing of the pylorus from prior PUD. Vomiting can develop acutely but can also be chronic and slowly progressive due to gastric emptying delay mimicking gastroparesis (see Chapter 52). Although the incidence of gastric outlet obstruction is not well established in the literature, it has likely decreased with early and effective treatment of PUD, since complicated peptic ulcers are now relatively infrequent.[21] Gastric volvulus, paraesophageal hernias, and posttraumatic diaphragmatic hernias are other relatively uncommon but important causes of acute vomiting; symptoms may be relapsing because of intermittent obstruction and spontaneous resolution (Fig. 16.3) (see Chapter 27).[22] Excessive splenic mobility (i.e., wandering spleen) and outlet obstruction from a pseudopolypoid antral mass (e.g., heterotopic pancreas) are other uncommon but well-described causes of acute vomiting.[23,24]

Both acute and chronic pancreatitis, with associated inflammatory masses, necrosis, pseudocysts, or secondary infection, may lead to gastric outlet obstruction at the duodenum (from external compression or luminal stricture), and less commonly, at the antrum and pylorus (see Chapters 60 and 61). Similarly, gastric, duodenal, pancreatic malignancies (adenocarcinoma, lymphoma, cystic pancreatic neoplasms, and neuroendocrine tumors), cholangiocarcinoma or lymphoma, may cause gastric outlet obstruction, sometimes manifesting as acute vomiting (see Chapters 41–43, 56, 62, and 127).[25]

Acute Intestinal Obstruction

Vomiting may be a cardinal presenting symptom of intestinal obstruction. The onset and severity are determined by the degree of luminal compromise and the acuity of development of obstruction. Proximal intestinal obstruction may be particularly difficult to diagnose because the obstructing lesion may be overlooked or unreachable by conventional EGD and yet may present without the typical picture of dilated fluid-filled loops of small bowel (air-fluid levels) on plain abdominal films (see Chapter 125). Distal duodenal and proximal jejunal neoplasms (adenocarcinoma, lymphoma, leiomyosarcoma, carcinoid, and retroperitoneal mass) may cause gastric outlet or intestinal obstruction that manifests as acute or chronic vomiting.

Intestinal Infarction

Intestinal infarction may occur with a paucity of physical signs but requires expeditious management, especially in acute arterial mesenteric infarction, because the in-hospital mortality rate is greater than 60%.[24] This diagnosis should be considered in the appropriate clinical setting,[26] especially in patients with vascular disorders, thrombotic diatheses and in older adults (see Chapter 120). SARS-CoV-2 can result in mesenteric vascular events leading to intestinal infarction from multifactorial pathophysiology, including the inflammatory state and hypercoagulability.[27]

Infectious and Inflammatory Causes

Vomiting is common in acute infectious illness. Norovirus-induced gastroenteritis is a common cause of sporadic or infectious viral illness.[28] Toxin-producing bacteria, such as *Staphylococcus aureus* and others result in enterotoxin stimulation of enterochromaffin cells that release 5-HT and activate vagal afferent pathways to cause vomiting.[29] SARS-CoV-2 causes nausea and vomiting via both the central and peripheral pathways. Similar to enteroviruses, SARS-CoV-2 causes injury to the mucosal barrier, thereby activating afferent vagal receptors to release cytokines, prostaglandins, and neuroactive agents from enteroendocrine cells targeting the area postrema in the dorsal medulla, resulting in nausea and emesis, among other gastrointestinal symptoms.[30] During the early stages of illness, nausea and vomiting may be the predominant or even exclusive clinical manifestation (see Chapters 112 and 113). Systemic infections (septicemia, urosepsis, pneumonia, and meningitis) can also result in nausea and vomiting.

Intraperitoneal or retroperitoneal inflammatory conditions (e.g., acute appendicitis, acute cholecystitis, peritonitis, acute pancreatitis—in general, any cause of acute abdominal pain) may be associated with vomiting. Vomiting is occasionally so intense (and rarely, the only symptom) that it causes diagnostic confusion (see Chapters 12, 60, and 122).

Extraintestinal Causes

A primary extraintestinal condition may cause nausea and vomiting. Myocardial infarction may manifest initially as acute vomiting because of afferent connections between the heart and brainstem. Similarly, renal colic, biliary pain, and ovarian or testicular torsion may manifest with intense vomiting, although localization of the pain and other characteristic features usually make these diagnoses evident (see Chapter 67). Further, congestive heart failure can result in reduced arterial blood flow in the gastrointestinal tract along with venous congestion, resulting in symptoms such as nausea and anorexia.

Medications and Toxins

The list of medications that can induce nausea and vomiting is lengthy, and both nausea and vomiting are frequent side effects attributed to many medications in frequent use (see Box 16.1). Common culprits include NSAIDs, cardiovascular drugs (e.g., digitalis, antidysrhythmics), antibiotics, levodopa and its derivatives, acetylcholine esterase inhibitors, theophylline, opiates, estrogen, progesterone, and azathioprine. Patients on multidrug regimens pose a special challenge in identifying the culprit drug(s).[31,32] Alcohol abuse, medication overdose, and acute poisoning can also cause nausea and vomiting.

Cancer chemotherapy is associated with a high likelihood of nausea and vomiting, and prophylactic antiemetic therapy is routine. Chemotherapeutic agent combinations vary in their propensity to cause nausea and vomiting, and patient-related factors also contribute (see Box 16.1).[33] As many as 50% to 80% of patients undergoing radiotherapy may experience nausea and vomiting, depending on the site of irradiation, patient's susceptibility, and radiotherapy protocol.[34]

Metabolic Causes

Practically any electrolyte disturbance can cause nausea and vomiting, including but not limited to uremia, hypercalcemia, hyponatremia, and both hypoglycemia and hyperglycemia. Diabetic ketoacidosis, hypoaldosteronism (Addison's disease), hyponatremia, hypercalcemia, and porphyria have a particular propensity to be associated with nausea and vomiting. Diabetes mellitus can also cause nausea and vomiting through development of gastroparesis. Correction of the underlying process will typically lead to resolution of nausea and vomiting.

Neurologic Causes

Neurologic disorders are an important and sometimes diagnostically elusive cause of chronic nausea and vomiting. Migraine, particularly atypical forms without an aura or family history and with delayed or no headache, is an important neurologic cause of chronic or relapsing vomiting. Cyclic vomiting syndrome (CVS) and abdominal migraine are thought to represent migrainoid disorders (see later). Hydrocephalus and lesions that compress or irritate the base of the brain may also account for chronic vomiting.

Nausea and vomiting associated with motion sickness involves stimulation of 5-HT_{1B} and 5-HT_{1D} receptors expressed in the vestibular apparatus.[35] Meningeal inflammation or meningitis can manifest as nausea and vomiting as the sole or predominant manifestation. Nausea and vomiting may be associated with vertigo in patients with vestibular or cerebellar disorders. Intracerebral lesions associated with increased intracranial pressure, interference with intracerebral fluid flow, or direct compression of the brainstem may manifest with nausea and vomiting, sometimes projectile. Migraine headaches may be accompanied by nausea and vomiting with little or no headache, making the diagnosis difficult. Ictal vomiting is an uncommon manifestation, most often associated with right temporal lobe epilepsy.[36] A rare autoimmune condition associated with antibodies against a brain water channel may cause severe nausea and vomiting.[37] Exercise-induced nausea and vomiting may provide a clue to the diagnosis of pheochromocytoma or paraganglioma.

Postoperative Nausea and Vomiting

Up to 43% of patients undergoing surgery who do not receive prophylactic antiemetic therapy will experience nausea and vomiting after surgery, one of the more common morbidities associated with surgical procedures. Numerous factors play a causative role, including age, gender, time, since the last meal, type of anesthesia, and type of surgery. The risk is highest with abdominal, gynecologic, eye, and middle ear surgery and is three times as common in women as in men.[38] General and epidural anesthesia carry the highest risk, whereas the risk is much lower for IV anesthesia.[39,40] Administration of volatile anesthetics, nitrous oxide, and opioids are also associated with postoperative nausea and vomiting.[41] The differential diagnosis of postoperative nausea and vomiting includes complications of surgery (intestinal perforation, peritonitis), electrolyte disturbances, and cardiac disease ("silent" myocardial infarction, heart failure).

Chronic or Relapsing Vomiting

The same causes of acute vomiting discussed earlier must also be considered in patients with chronic vomiting, but with specific features as discussed later. Other etiologies for relapsing vomiting include pregnancy, functional vomiting, CVS, cannabinoid hyperemesis syndrome, intermittent partial bowel obstruction, and hereditary angioedema.

Partial Intestinal Obstruction

Although complete intestinal obstruction manifests with the acute onset of abdominal symptoms that prompt urgent evaluation, partial intestinal obstruction may present with relapsing vomiting that waxes and wanes as intestinal transit is intermittently interrupted and spontaneously restored. Stricturing Crohn disease, neoplasms of the intestine, radiation enteritis, and ischemic strictures are the main identifiable causes of partial mechanical intestinal obstruction (see Chapters 39, 117, 120, and 125). Intermittent or chronic gastric outlet obstruction from PUD was an additional potential cause in the past, but this diagnosis is relatively infrequent in modern times. Adhesions from surgery or pelvic inflammatory disease can cause intermittent bowel obstruction, but establishing their pathogenic role is sometimes difficult. Advanced intra-abdominal cancer is another cause of intestinal obstruction. Angioedema of the gastrointestinal tract and enterolithiasis are other rare causes of partial bowel obstruction.[42,43] Long-standing partial intestinal obstruction can mimic chronic intestinal pseudo-obstruction, and indeed, occult partial intestinal obstruction needs to be excluded before a diagnosis of pseudo-obstruction can be made (see Chapters 125 and 126). In older, debilitated individuals, particularly with psychiatric comorbidities, constipation, and obstipation may lead to a presentation similar to intestinal obstruction when the colon becomes impacted with stool and ileal outflow is partially impeded (see Chapter 20).[44]

GI Motility Disorders

Gastroparesis and chronic intestinal pseudo-obstruction may produce chronic vomiting (see Chapter 52).[45,46] Recurrent or chronic vomiting is the presenting manifestation of gastroparesis, but a similar presentation can be seen with functional dyspepsia, chronic functional nausea and vomiting, and CVS (where clear symptom-free periods are interspersed between stereotypical symptom episodes, see later).[45,47,48] Vomiting in gastroparesis and functional disorders may lead to food aversion, poor oral intake, trace nutrient and vitamin deficiencies, and malnutrition.[49] The stomach may become dilated, and the vomitus may contain partially digested food, but these findings are not constant. Marked gastric stasis tends to be associated with more severe vomiting and early satiety.[50] Although delayed gastric emptying is the hallmark of gastroparesis, gastric emptying can also be delayed in functional dyspepsia, and the degree of emptying delay may not necessarily predict negative health outcomes or refractoriness to therapy.[51–53] Recent research suggests a significant overlap between gastroparesis and functional dyspepsia, and gastric emptying study findings can change from normal to prolonged or vice versa in over a third of patients when repeated after a year.[54] Diminished accommodation of the proximal stomach can explain some of the symptomatology in gastroparesis,[55] and decreasing gastric stasis may improve symptoms.[56] Diabetes mellitus is a major cause of gastroparesis,[57] in which cellular abnormalities such as loss of growth factors for the interstitial cells of Cajal (which generate pacemaker activity), enteric nerve abnormalities, and increased immune cells have been reported.[50,58–60] Patients with prior stroke, Parkinson disease, and spinal cord injury have delayed gastrointestinal motility resulting in several symptoms including nausea. In multiple sclerosis, there is dysregulation of sacral parasympathetic outflow resulting in anorectal dyssynergia and delayed colonic transit which can rarely present as chronic nausea and vomiting.[32] Iatrogenic gastroparesis may occur in patients with diabetes mellitus treated with incretins (pramlintide or exenatide).[57] Idiopathic gastroparesis can develop after an acute viral (e.g., CMV, EBV) illness, in which abdominal pain may be a prominent feature.[50,61–63] There are reports of delayed gastric emptying after SARS-CoV-2 infection.[64] Demyelination, similar to that found in Guillain-Barré syndrome, has been observed.[65] Postviral gastroparesis is often self-limited.[62]

Chronic gastroparesis with recurrent nausea and vomiting can be observed transiently or chronically after fundoplication for GERD or after bariatric surgery and arises mainly from altered gastric accommodation, although vagal injury may contribute (see Chapters 9 and 48).[66] Gastroparesis may also develop after pulmonary or combined heart-lung transplantation.[67,68]

Chronic nausea and vomiting, clinically indistinguishable from idiopathic gastroparesis but with normal gastric emptying, has been described.[60,69] Intestinal pseudo-obstruction can manifest with nausea and vomiting in addition to abdominal pain and distention and is characterized by partial or complete intestinal obstruction in the absence of a restricting or occlusive luminal lesion (see Chapter 126).[70] The distinction between gastroparesis and chronic intestinal pseudo-obstruction often requires specific diagnostic tests (Chapters 52 and 126).

Nausea and Vomiting During Pregnancy

Both nausea and vomiting are commonly experienced during pregnancy, with a frequency between 50% and 80%.[71] These symptoms tend to develop early in pregnancy, peak around 6–12 weeks' gestation, and rarely continue beyond 22 weeks' gestation. Although nausea and vomiting tend to occur more often in the morning (hence the designation "morning sickness"), symptoms can occur at any time of day. Symptoms may start before a woman realizes she is pregnant; therefore a pregnancy test should be administered in any fertile woman with a new complaint of nausea and vomiting. Although morning nausea and vomiting may be regarded as a normal manifestation of pregnancy, excessive or severe symptoms may warrant pharmacotherapy.

The pathogenesis of nausea and vomiting during pregnancy remains unclear, although hormonal and psychological influences are thought to contribute. Specific risk factors have been identified for hyperemesis gravidarum, described below. Whereas estrogen and progesterone have been thought to slow gastric emptying, increased HCG levels during the first trimester may stimulate gastric CCK receptors and trigger symptoms. Higher HCG levels (as seen in molar pregnancies and multiparity) have been associated with more frequent nausea and vomiting.[72,73]

Hyperemesis Gravidarum

Hyperemesis gravidarum refers to severe and persistent vomiting that leads to complications and occurs in 0.3%–3% of pregnant women. Risk factors for vomiting in pregnancy include multiple gestation, underlying GERD, migraines, younger age, first pregnancy, and family history of hyperemesis gravidarum. Maternal complications include weight loss of more than 5% of prepregnancy weight, electrolyte imbalance, dehydration, ketosis, Mallory-Weiss tears, pneumothorax, splenic avulsion, and rarely, Wernicke's encephalopathy. Hyperemesis gravidarum is more common among young, primiparous mothers, especially of Asian and Middle Eastern ethnicities, especially in the presence of risk factors described above.[74] A genome-wide association study found that the genetic variant of GDF15 (missense mutation) was associated with hyperemesis gravidum. GDF15 is secreted from placenta during pregnancy and is also released in response to cellular stress and certain nutritional deficiencies. GDF15 binds to receptor (GFRAL) located in area postrema, which can result in altered taste, reduced appetite, nausea, and vomiting.[75,76] A variety of nutritional deficiencies have been reported as consequences of severe emesis, including deficiencies of fat-soluble vitamins and of B vitamins, rarely resulting in Wernicke's encephalopathy.[77] Disturbances in serum electrolytes can result in profound hypokalemia. The psychosocial burden of hyperemesis includes fear of subsequent pregnancy.[78] Fetal outcomes have been less well described, with higher rates of low birth weight and preterm delivery in infants born to women with hyperemesis gravidarum.[79]

Hyperemesis gravidarum is the most common cause of hospitalization during the first half of pregnancy in the United States, second only to preterm labor.[80] Exclusion of alternative pathologic causes of nausea and vomiting (such as PUD, cholecystitis, appendicitis, and pyelonephritis) is essential before a diagnosis of hyperemesis gravidarum is made. Initial laboratory testing includes CBC, comprehensive metabolic panel, thyroid function studies, serum lipase levels, urinalysis for ketones, and a serum β-HCG level for evaluation of possible molar and multiple gestations. Hyperemesis gravidarum is often associated with failure to respond to outpatient management and often requires hospitalization for fluid and electrolyte replacement therapy and parenteral antiemetics.

Simple lifestyle changes, including eating frequent, small meals, avoiding known dietary triggers and strong odors, and utilizing over-the-counter remedies such as ginger, pyridoxine (vitamin B6), and acupressure wristbands or acupuncture, are first-line therapies. Randomized trials show benefit with use of ginger extract compared with placebo, regardless of ginger dose or preparation.[81–84] Pyridoxine and acupressure (P6 pressure point) can provide symptomatic benefit.[85–87] Second-line treatments include antiemetic medications, IV fluids, and repletion of electrolytes. Dopamine antagonists improve symptoms as well as serotonin antagonists, but with a higher likelihood of adverse effects, particularly for metoclopramide.[88,89] Antihistamines can be used but should not be combined with serotonin 5-HT_3 inhibitors if possible.[90] Advanced management of refractory cases may include, glucocorticoids and enteral feeding when symptoms are severe and life-threatening.[91,92] There is some evidence to support the use of mindfulness-based cognitive behavioral therapy in conjunction with the options described above.[93]

Functional Vomiting

Population-based data indicate that vomiting that occurs at least once a month is seen in 2%–3% of the general population.[48,94] The prevalence of chronic nausea and vomiting syndrome is reported to be 0.8%–1.2%.[95] Rome IV criteria for functional vomiting include one or more episodes of vomiting per week for 3 months, with the onset of symptoms at least 6 months prior to diagnosis and with symptoms that are not cyclical in nature.[48] Eating disorders, rumination, self-induced vomiting, major psychiatric disorders, chronic cannabinoid use, and other structural or organic causes of vomiting should be excluded first. Psychosocial stressors and underlying depression or anxiety often play important roles and should be addressed.[48,96]

Prevailing hypotheses regarding the pathophysiology of functional vomiting involve visceral hypersensitivity, altered gut-brain interactions, motility disturbances, altered gut microbiota or mucosal immune function, and psychosocial stressors. The lack of biochemical markers or anatomic abnormalities poses a diagnostic challenge.

Evaluation includes a comprehensive history, and diagnostic testing to exclude organic causes of vomiting. EGD, contrast radiography (UGIS and small bowel follow-through), and cross-sectional imaging (e.g., CT, MRI) should be performed when indicated to rule out structural or obstructive processes. Tests assessing motor function (e.g., radionuclide gastric emptying study, antroduodenal manometry) may reveal findings suggestive of gastroparesis or intestinal pseudo-obstruction, although delayed gastric emptying can be seen in conjunction with functional dyspepsia (which can also be associated with nausea and vomiting), as well as other causes of nausea and vomiting (e.g., CVS, medication-induced nausea and vomiting). Antroduodenal manometry can differentiate mechanical from functional obstructive processes, although this has a low diagnostic specificity. If manometry is performed in a patient with vomiting, the diagnosis of intestinal pseudo-obstruction is essentially ruled out with the detection of strong antral phasic waves and a normal intestinal pressure pattern during fasting and postprandial periods.[97,98] Cutaneous electrogastrography (EGG) measures the pacemaking ability of the stomach and can identify gastric dysrhythmias[97] but does not establish whether gastric dysrhythmias are the cause or consequence of nausea and vomiting.[98]

Beyond avoiding triggering foods that worsen symptoms, specific dietary therapy adds little to management. Coexisting nutritional deficiencies and metabolic disturbances also need correction. Psychotherapy, behavioral therapy, and psychotropic agents are all used in practice, even in the absence of formal studies demonstrating their efficacy. Reassurance and a supportive physician-patient relationship are crucial in the management of functional vomiting.[99]

Cyclic Vomiting Syndrome and Cannabinoid Hyperemesis Syndrome

Cyclic Vomiting Syndrome

CVS is characterized by clustered, recurrent episodes of vomiting in the absence of an alternative etiology. Although initially described in children, CVS is now known to occur in adults, with an estimated frequency of 1.9%–2.3%; it is most common in white males.[95] Rome IV criteria define CVS as the presence of stereotypical episodes of vomiting (acute in onset and a duration of less than 1 week), 3 or more discrete episodes in the prior year and 2 or more episodes in the past 6 months (each occurring at least 1 week apart), and the absence of vomiting between episodes.[48,95,100] A personal or family history of migraine is supportive of the diagnosis of CVS, particularly in children.[95,101] Regular use of cannabinoids can be associated with a syndrome indistinguishable from CVS, termed cannabinoid hyperemesis syndrome, which resolves with cessation of cannabinoid use (see later).

The characteristic clinical presentation consists of the acute onset of nausea and/or vomiting with associated abdominal pain, anorexia, and fatigue. Episodes can last for hours to days, with symptom-free intervals between episodes. Physical examination findings are usually nonspecific but may reflect dehydration.

Patients often consult multiple health care providers over time and undergo an extensive laboratory and diagnostic workup, including blood tests, endoscopy, cross-sectional imaging, and even exploratory surgery.[102] The differential diagnosis includes gastroenteritis, PUD, gallbladder disease, pancreatitis, pregnancy in a female patient, or an underlying metabolic or psychiatric disorder. In the pediatric age group, various mitochondrial, ion channel, and autonomic disorders have also been associated with intermittent episodes of vomiting and may have to be ruled out. Similarly, food allergy (sensitivity to cow's milk, soy, or egg white protein) or food intolerances (to chocolate, cheese, nuts, or monosodium glutamate) may manifest with vomiting spells and should be excluded (see Chapter 11).[102,103]

Abortive treatment is typically initiated during the prodrome, if present. Antimigraine drugs, especially serotonin 5-HT_1 agonists (e.g., sumatriptan) administered subcutaneously, transnasally, or orally, have been utilized. Conventional antiemetics and benzodiazepines (e.g., lorazepam) administered intravenously can be of value during the acute phase. Neurokinin-1 receptor antagonists such as aprepitant can be used as abortive therapy.[104] Anecdotal reports demonstrate benefits of intravenous haloperidol in an acute management of CVS.[105] Dehydration and metabolic complications may require admission to the hospital and IV corrective measures.[102]

Tricyclic antidepressants (e.g., amitriptyline, nortriptyline, imipramine, desipramine) are effective as prophylaxis in about two-thirds of both adults and children.[100,106] β-adrenergic receptor antagonists (e.g., propranolol) have also been used for prophylaxis. There is limited evidence to support use of aprepitant and mitochondrial supplements such as coenzyme Q10 in prophylaxis,[107] while more robust evidence exists for the use of antiepileptic drugs such as zonisamide and levetiracetam.[108] Olanzapine is reported to be effective in preventing episodes of CVS in pediatric patients.[109] Other agents reported anecdotally to help improve symptoms include serotonin reuptake inhibitors, cyproheptadine, naloxone, carnitine, valproic acid, and erythromycin. The psychological aspects of CVS require special consideration. Although 20% of adult patients with CVS have an overt anxiety disorder or other psychiatric disease, anticipatory anxiety prior to an episode is common and may precipitate episodes. Consequently, management of concurrent anxiety or depression can be of therapeutic value.[100,110]

Cannabinoid Hyperemesis Syndrome

In a subset of patients with CVS, symptoms can be precipitated and exacerbated by chronic cannabis use, a variant termed *cannabinoid hyperemesis syndrome*, with symptom relief if there is sustained cessation of cannabis use.[111,112] Cannabinoid CB_1 receptors are distributed in the brain as well as the GI system, whereas CB_2 receptors are found in lymphoid tissue where they regulate immune function.[113,114] Stimulation of CB_1 receptors by endogenous cannabinoids results in inhibition of the hypothalamo-pituitary-adrenal axis and sympathetic response to stressful stimuli and modulates gastric motility and sensation, among other roles.[113] Fatty acid amide hydrolase and monoacylglycerol lipase are responsible for degradation of endocannabinoids. One of the proposed hypotheses is that regular cannabis use leads to downregulation and desensitization of CB_1 receptors, leading in turn to abdominal pain and intractable vomiting that resolves when the receptors regain their original sensitivity following abstinence from cannabinoids.[115] Genetic polymorphisms in endocannabinoid receptors may also play a role, although further research is needed.[116]

The manifestations of cannabinoid hyperemesis syndrome are indistinguishable from those of CVS, with a similar onset, duration, and frequency of episodes. A history of regular cannabis use and relief of symptoms with abstinence from cannabinoids are hallmarks of the syndrome.[48] Ritualistic hot baths are reported by up to 67% of affected persons although this feature is not specific for cannabinoid hyperemesis syndrome and can be reported by patients with CVS in general. Symptoms consistently improve or resolve with total abstinence from cannabis use.[115,117] The liberalization of marijuana policies in the U.S. has led to an increase in emergency department visits for cannabis-related syndromes, including cannabinoid hyperemesis syndrome, particularly in states like Colorado, where the increase is higher in out-of-state visitors than residents of Colorado.[118] The maximum duration for detection of cannabinoids in urine following the most recent reported use varies from a few days to 4 weeks, with prolonged duration of urine excretion reported in patients with chronic heavy cannabinoid use.[119] Urine cannabinoid testing can provide objective information regarding cannabinoid usage, as significant discordance is common between patient reports and objective test findings in as many as a third of patients,[120] despite the urine test having high accuracy when the detection threshold is 50 µg/L.[121]

In conjunction with abstinence, abortive and prophylactic approaches similar to those for CVS are effective.[122] In addition, topical application of capsaicin cream to the abdominal wall results in activation of TRPV1 receptors, which further depletes neurokinin and substance P, resulting in symptom improvement. Parenteral haloperidol and olanzapine oral disintegrating tablet administration have been reported to abort episodes in a small randomized controlled trial and case series, respectively.[122–126]

Superior Mesenteric Artery Syndrome

Although some objective basis exists for superior mesenteric artery (SMA) syndrome, the diagnosis tends to be applied inappropriately to patients with functional vomiting or CVS, who then are unfortunately subjected to unnecessary surgery.[127] The SMA branches off the aorta at an acute angle, travels in the root of the mesentery, and crosses over the duodenum, usually just to the right of the midline (see Chapter 120). The angle between the aorta and the SMA can become more acute under certain circumstances (increased lordosis with a body cast, loss of muscle tone or weight, prolonged bed rest), leading to partial obstruction of the distal duodenum.[128] Symptoms include epigastric fullness and pressure after meals, nausea and vomiting (often bilious), and mid-abdominal pain that may improve in the prone or knee-chest position. The diagnosis is supported by imaging tests (UGIS or CT) that show dilatation and stasis proximal to the location of the SMA in the third portion of the duodenum. The appearance may be misleading, however, because duodenal dilatation may be caused by atony rather than mechanical obstruction.[127] Stasis proximal to the site of duodenal obstruction should be demonstrated on contrast studies and/or scintigraphic tests prior to corrective surgery to avoid overdiagnosis. Antroduodenal and small bowel manometry may demonstrate characteristic patterns that distinguish mechanical obstruction from a motility disorder. Relief of vomiting with feeding through an enteric catheter placed across the obstruction into the proximal jejunum supports the diagnosis.

Precipitating factors should be corrected first whenever possible. Acute symptoms may resolve with gastric decompression and IV fluid replacement. Nutritional optimization has been shown to improve the aorta-SMA angle with improvement in adipose tissue fat pad and lymphatic tissue around the SMA which can subsequently resolve symptoms attributed to the SMA syndrome.[129] Therefore surgical correction should only be undertaken in well-investigated patients with chronic relapsing episodes of SMA syndrome despite conservative management. The surgical technique performed most commonly is a laparoscopic proximal duodenojejunostomy; a gastrojejunostomy may not be effective because the proximal duodenum is not decompressed by this approach.[130]

Rumination Syndrome

Rumination is a distinct and unique functional gastroduodenal disorder characterized by repetitive effortless regurgitation of small amounts of recently ingested food into the mouth, followed by re-chewing and re-swallowing or expulsion (see also Chapter 14).[131] Although rumination resembles vomiting, it does not involve an integrated somatovisceral response coordinated by the emetic center. Characteristically, nausea and autonomic manifestations (e.g., hypersalivation, cutaneous vasoconstriction, and sweating) that usually accompany vomiting are absent. Rumination typically begins during or immediately following a meal and may stop when the regurgitated material becomes noticeably acidic. Rumination is relatively common in infants, typically developing between 3 and 6 months of age. There is no apparent distress, and rumination may cease with distraction or sleep. Rumination occurs in adults of any age with equal gender distribution.[94]

The clinical significance of rumination varies. Some otherwise healthy individuals ruminate frequently without considering the practice abnormal. Others, under pressure from family or friends, consult a health care provider, who may mistakenly interpret rumination as habitual vomiting, GERD, or gastroparesis, which delays diagnosis and definitive management. Some ruminators seek medical attention because of the concern that they are unable to control the process. Alternatively, rumination may be associated with heartburn, epigastric discomfort, and changes in bowel habits in patients who have concomitant GERD, functional dyspepsia, or IBS, respectively. Weight loss may occur and suggests a possible eating disorder.

Rumination may be diagnosed clinically in most patients with careful history taking. Achalasia, other esophageal motility disorders, gastric outlet obstruction, and gastroparesis should be excluded. Detection of esophagitis on EGD does not exclude rumination. Combined UGI manometry with pH-impedance testing may show sharp phasic pressure spikes (r waves) recorded in the antrum and duodenum on manometry, which correspond to abrupt increments in intra-abdominal pressure as the patient involuntarily or voluntarily forces subdiaphragmatic intragastric content toward the esophagus through a relaxed lower esophageal sphincter. High-resolution esophageal manometry and impedance testing after a meal may help distinguish rumination from other belching and regurgitation disorders.[132,133] Evidence of postprandial reflux events extending to the proximal esophagus, typically with prompt symptom reporting, and with concomitant gastric pressure of greater than 30 mm Hg, supports the diagnosis of rumination syndrome.[134,135] Because rumination is a behavioral disorder, the coexistence of rumination with another functional disorder should be considered (see Chapter 46).

The pathophysiology of rumination syndrome has only partially been elucidated. Rumination may reflect adaptation of the belch reflex (see Chapter 18). During the abrupt retrograde movement of gastric content, the gastroesophageal junction appears to move into the thorax, thereby creating a "pseudohernia" that facilitates opening of the lower esophageal sphincter.[136] A distinct subgroup of ruminators has "reflux-related" rumination with abdominogastric strain that is synchronized with transient lower esophageal sphincter relaxation occurring as part of a reflux episode.[137]

Treatment of rumination involves several steps. Reassurance and careful explanation of the phenomenon may allow some patients to control rumination on their own. Behavior modification is the most effective therapy and may be accomplished by teaching the patient special diaphragmatic breathing techniques or with the help of biofeedback training, because rumination and diaphragmatic contraction cannot be performed simultaneously.[138] Patients trained to control their abdominothoracic muscles by viewing EMG recordings displayed on a monitor experienced a reduction in the frequency of rumination episodes after just three sessions. Patients with heartburn and endoscopic evidence of esophagitis should be treated with a PPI. Further pharmacologic treatment includes baclofen (up to 10 mg orally three times daily), a γ-aminobutyric acid agonist that increases lower esophageal sphincter pressure, reduces frequency of transient lower esophageal sphincter relaxation and decreases the swallowing rate.[139,140]

EVALUATION

Acute Vomiting

Evaluation of a patient with acute vomiting begins with a carefully taken history and physical examination that focuses on the patient's volume status and important causes of acute vomiting. An algorithm for management of the patient with acute vomiting is shown in Fig. 16.2. A pregnancy test should be performed in all women of childbearing age. Routine blood studies should include a CBC, tests of kidney function, thyroid function tests, liver biochemical tests, electrolyte, glucose, serum amylase and lipase levels, and in some cases, arterial blood gases to assess the patient's acid-base status. Medication and toxin levels are ordered when indicated.

Imaging

Plain abdominal films, supine and upright, should be obtained. If the films suggest SBO, further testing to ascertain the cause of obstruction (including cross-sectional imaging and urgent surgical exploration when appropriate) should be undertaken (see Chapter 125).

If plain abdominal films are negative, additional tests can be considered. EGD can evaluate for mucosal lesions, ulcers, neoplasia, and gastric outlet or duodenal obstruction. CT or MRI of the abdomen may demonstrate intra-abdominal inflammatory or infectious processes (e.g., appendicitis, diverticulitis), acute intestinal ischemia, obstruction, or pseudo-obstruction. US of the abdomen tends to be less revealing in this setting. MRI of the brain can be performed to look for a mass lesion or other neurologic mechanisms of vomiting.

Additional Tests

Further testing can include blood levels of drugs and toxins (specifically digoxin, opioids, theophylline, ethanol, and carbamazepine), cultures of blood or body fluids when an infection is suspected, analysis of cerebrospinal fluid following lumbar puncture, and serologic tests for viral hepatitis, if indicated. If appropriate, blood levels of cortisol, corticotropin-releasing factor, and catecholamines can be determined.

Chronic Vomiting

A detailed clinical history and careful physical examination are central to diagnosing functional dyspepsia, functional vomiting, CVS, and rumination syndrome. EGD and/or a UGIS are the tests of choice for partial gastric outlet obstruction and partial duodenal obstruction. Barium contrast radiography may suggest a diagnosis of achalasia, gastroparesis, or neoplasm. CT of the abdomen is particularly useful for identifying intestinal obstruction, intra-abdominal masses, and retroperitoneal pathology and also provides information on the degree of bowel dilatation, bowel wall thickness, and a transition point in bowel lumen diameter that helps localize the obstruction.[141] By contrast, plain films of the abdomen are often unreliable, particularly in the presence of fluid-filled loops of bowel. Magnetic resonance enterography is an alternative to CT enterography and has the advantage of not exposing patients to radiation.[142] MRI of the brain is useful for diagnosis of CNS lesions that may cause vomiting, including slow-growing tumors, hydrocephalus, and inflammatory, vascular, and ischemic lesions. Motility studies are useful for evaluating motor disorders including gastroparesis and chronic intestinal pseudo-obstruction, which are relatively uncommon but important causes of nausea and vomiting (see Chapters 52, 101, and 126).

Esophageal Manometry

Esophageal manometry, preferably high-resolution manometry, is used to assess esophageal motor activity. Patients with esophageal motility disorders such as achalasia and other spastic disorders may present with vomiting or, more frequently, regurgitation that is misinterpreted as vomiting (see Chapter 46).

Measurement of Gastric Emptying

Radioscintigraphy is the preferred and most accurate method of assessing gastric emptying and should be performed over a 4-hour period for accurate assessment of gastric emptying after ensuring patients have been off opioid medication and cannabinoid agonists. Ideally, dual markers (separating solids from liquids) should be used and the test performed with a dual-headed gamma camera. Symptoms of gastroparesis are primarily associated with delayed solid phase gastric emptying.[143] Alternative, but less precise, methods of assessing gastric emptying include three-dimensional gastric US to assess emptying of a liquid meal and the ^{13}C breath test with octanoate acid, a fatty acid that is labeled with a stable isotope and incorporated into a test meal.[144] The rate at which $^{13}CO_2$ is exhaled reflects the rate of gastric emptying and subsequent duodenal absorption of the lipid marker, but the diagnostic reliability of this breath test is not firmly established (see Chapter 52).[145] Other potential diagnostic modalities, include the wireless motility capsule, MRI, and single-photon emission CT.[144,146] If the result of the gastric emptying study does not fit the overall clinical impression, an alternate diagnosis should be considered, and there is role for repeating the gastric emptying test as studies have shown variable gastric emptying rates on repeat testing.[147]

Cutaneous Electrogastrography

EGG with cutaneously placed electrodes identifies dysrhythmia (e.g., bradygastria or tachygastria) of the gastric pacemaker and changes in the frequency of pacemaker activity in response to feeding. There has been advancement in EGG techniques using 25 sequential cutaneous electrodes placed 2 cm apart on the abdominal wall, providing high-resolution-EGG topographic maps of gastric electrical activity. High-resolution-EGG has been validated in healthy volunteers to quantify gastric slow wave propagation.[148] A case-control study demonstrated abnormal slow wave propagation in functional dyspepsia with abdominal pain, but the sample size was small.[149] Although noninvasive and rather simple, EGG and high-resolution-EGG findings require further large studies to establish parameters in healthy individuals and to demonstrate correlation of findings with clinical symptoms.[63,97] It is likely that some EGG findings may be secondary to rather than the cause of nausea (see Chapter 52).

Antroduodenal Manometry

Antroduodenal manometry is the most specific physiologic test for assessing foregut motor disturbances distal to the esophagus. Intraluminal pressure changes are recorded in the antrum and proximal small bowel using a pressure-sensitive catheter. The test is cumbersome, expensive, technically challenging to perform, and available at only a few centers that specialize in GI motility disorders. Manometry may distinguish myogenic from neurogenic forms of pseudo-obstruction and may help detect partial SBO on the basis of wave pattern analysis (see Chapters 52, 125, and 126). If antroduodenal manometry is abnormal, a laparoscopic full-thickness biopsy of the small bowel can be considered to diagnose genetic and acquired myogenic or neurologic causes of chronic intestinal pseudo-obstruction.

Autonomic Function Tests

Tests of autonomic function can assess sympathetic function and include the tilt table test (an orthostatic challenge to blood pressure and cardiac rate regulation) and the cold hand test (a pain reflex test in which the hand is immersed in cold water to produce vasoconstriction and a significant increase in systolic arterial pressure). Parasympathetic function can be assessed by measuring variations in the RR interval on the electrocardiogram in response to bradycardia induced by deep respiration (via a vasovagal reflex) and by a voluntary Valsalva maneuver. Results of such tests can help distinguish visceral autonomic neuropathies (e.g., due to amyloidosis or diabetes mellitus) from a central autonomic disorder (e.g., Shy-Drager syndrome, pandysautonomia).

Histopathologic Studies

In some patients, a further diagnostic step may involve histopathologic examination of mucosal biopsies for quantification of nerve density and morphology as evidence of autonomic neuropathy.[150] Intravenous immunoglobulin was effective in reducing symptoms of nausea, vomiting, early satiety, and abdominal pain in an open-label study of 14 patients with medically refractory delayed gastric emptying in the context of immune abnormalities. In these patients, evidence of immune pathophysiology included gastric biopsies showing significantly fewer interstitial cells of Cajal or positive serum antibodies against AchR, striated muscle, anti-RNP, voltage-gated potassium channel, or calcium channel antibodies.[151]

COMPLICATIONS

Vomiting, particularly when protracted or recurrent, can lead to a number of potentially life-threatening complications.

Emetic Injuries to the Esophagus and Stomach

Chronic protracted vomiting often produces esophagitis, ranging from mild erythema to erosions and ulcerations on endoscopy. Characteristically, esophagitis from vomiting extends uniformly throughout the esophageal body, in contrast to the distal esophagitis associated with GERD. Patients can experience heartburn or retrosternal pain after an acute bout of vomiting. By contrast, patients with chronic vomiting rarely complain of chest symptoms, and esophagitis associated with long-standing vomiting is often asymptomatic.

Abrupt retching or vomiting episodes may also induce longitudinal mucosal and, rarely, transmural lacerations at the level of the gastroesophageal junction. Acute bleeding and hematemesis associated with mucosal lacerations at the gastroesophageal junction constitute the *Mallory-Weiss syndrome* (see Chapters 21 and 47). *Boerhaave syndrome* refers to spontaneous rupture of the esophageal wall, with free perforation and secondary mediastinitis and carries a high mortality rate.[152] It is more common in persons with alcohol use disorder, although esophageal rupture may develop in any person during vomiting (see Chapter 47).

Multiple purpuric lesions may appear on the face and upper neck after prolonged episodes of vomiting, probably because of repetitive increases in intrathoracic pressure and rupture of blood vessels. Dental caries and erosions may result from chronic vomiting.

Spasm of the Glottis and Aspiration Pneumonia

Spasm of the glottis and transient asphyxia may develop during vomiting as a result of irritation of the pharynx by acidic or bilious material. Similarly, vomiting during insertion of an NG tube, during sedated endoscopy, in an older person, or when the cough reflex is depressed may result in aspiration of gastric contents into the bronchi, with resulting acute asphyxia and a subsequent risk of aspiration pneumonia. Aspiration is more likely to occur when the stomach contains food, fluid, or enteric secretions, which should be suctioned from the stomach during endoscopy.

Fluid, Electrolyte, and Metabolic Alterations

Fluid, electrolyte, and metabolic abnormalities may develop rapidly after protracted vomiting. Dehydration, hypotension, hemoconcentration, oliguria, muscle weakness, and cardiac dysrhythmias can result. Hypochloremic alkalosis is usually the first metabolic abnormality to develop and is due to loss of fluid, as well as of hydrogen and chloride ions. Hypokalemia results from loss of potassium ions in the vomitus and renal potassium wasting due to alkalosis. Hyponatremia may occur in severe cases because of loss of sodium and release of antidiuretic hormone in an attempt to conserve intravascular volume. Metabolic derangements, especially metabolic alkalosis with low urinary sodium excretion, may be a sign of chronic functional or self-induced vomiting.

Nutritional Deficiencies

Nutritional deficiencies may result from reduced caloric intake or loss of nutrients in the vomitus. Regardless of cause, chronic nausea and vomiting can result in malnutrition, weight loss, and deficiency states that require supplementation (see Chapters 6 and 7).

TREATMENT

Effective management of the patient with nausea and vomiting requires correction of clinically relevant metabolic complications, pharmacologic therapy, and treatment of the underlying cause.

Correction of Metabolic Complications

Patients with acute, severe, or repeated vomiting may become dehydrated rapidly and develop metabolic imbalances, secondary circulatory collapse, and kidney failure. If oral hydration is not adequate, IV fluids and electrolytes should be administered promptly. Adequate replacement generally consists of a normal saline solution in volumes sufficient to correct deficits (and in addition to maintenance fluids) with potassium supplementation (60–80 mEq/24 hours). The normal saline can be administered with glucose (e.g., 5% dextrose in normal saline); in some cases a 10% glucose solution may be required. When oral intake can be resumed, glucose-containing fluids are preferred because they are easily absorbed from the intestine. A split-meal, low-fat, and low-fiber solid diet can be gradually introduced.

Patients with long-standing chronic vomiting are at risk of developing malnutrition, so enteral or parenteral feeding should be considered when the patient is unable to resume adequate oral nutrition after 5–8 days. Although enteral nutrition is a good option, even orogastrojejunal catheters placed with guidewires may be dislodged during episodes of vomiting. When resuming enteral or parenteral nutrition, refeeding syndrome is a consideration and can be evaluated through close monitoring of electrolyte derangements, such as hypophosphatemia, hypokalemia, and hypomagnesemia. Preventing refeeding syndrome can occur through optimal nutritional supplementation (such as thiamine) and starting refeeding at lower caloric values with gradual increase to goal calorie requirements.[153] For long-term treatment, percutaneous enteral feeding tubes or home parenteral nutrition may be required (see Chapter 7).

Pharmacologic Treatment

Drugs used to treat nausea and vomiting belong to one of two main categories: centrally acting antiemetic agents and peripherally acting prokinetic agents. Some drugs share both mechanisms of action, with variable predominance of one or the other. [Doses indicated are for adult patients (Table 16.1)].

Central Antiemetic Agents

Central antiemetic agents are classified according to the predominant receptor on which the drug acts. These can be administered orally, parenterally (single bolus, repeat boluses, or continuous IV infusion), or transdermally when available.[154]

Dopamine D2 Receptor Antagonists

Benzamides

The main antiemetic effect of benzamides (e.g., metoclopramide, clebopride) is through antagonism of the dopamine D2 receptor in the brainstem. These agents also stimulate peripheral 5-HT_4 receptors, thereby facilitating acetylcholine release for antroduodenal prokinetic activity.

Side effects limit the use of these drugs. When administered rapidly by the IV route, metoclopramide may cause acute restlessness and anxiety. Repeated oral administration may induce somnolence in some patients. In about 1% of treated patients, distressing extrapyramidal effects, including dystonic reactions and tremor, may appear and limit their use, particularly at high doses. Older patients are at particular risk of tardive dyskinesia.[155] Metoclopramide may prolong the QT interval and thus has a dysrhythmogenic potential. This agent is subject to tachyphylaxis and may lose efficacy with continued use.

The most common indications for these drugs are nausea and vomiting of pregnancy, postoperative nausea and vomiting, and chemotherapy- and radiotherapy-induced nausea and vomiting. Because of their associated gastric prokinetic action, the drugs can be used for gastroparesis related to diabetes mellitus, prior vagotomy, and prior partial gastrectomy. The standard dose of metoclopramide is 10–20 mg three or four times daily orally or intravenously.

Benzimidazole Derivatives

Domperidone is the main benzimidazole derivative but is not available in the United States.[156] The drug crosses the blood-brain barrier poorly and acts primarily as a peripheral dopamine D2 receptor antagonist. It blocks the receptors centrally in the area postrema (which is partly outside the blood-brain barrier) and in the stomach, where D2 receptor inhibition decreases proximal gastric relaxation and facilitates gastric emptying. Although domperidone is a weaker antiemetic than metoclopramide, it may be particularly useful for the management of nausea and vomiting associated with treatment with levodopa in patients with Parkinson's disease, because it antagonizes the proemetic side effects of levodopa without interfering with antiparkinsonian action in brain centers protected by the blood-brain barrier. The standard dose is 10–20 mg three or four times daily orally. A review of domperidone use in the treatment of diabetic gastroparesis has concluded that the drug is probably useful but has not been properly evaluated by well-designed controlled trials. Responses may be

TABLE 16.1 Centrally and Peripherally Acting Agents Useful in the Management of Nausea and Vomiting[a]

	Drug	Category	Indications	Dose[b]	Side Effects
Centrally acting antiemetic agents	Metoclopramide Clebopride	Benzamides (Dopamine D2 antagonist) Peripheral 5-HT_4 agonist	Nausea and vomiting of pregnancy Postoperative nausea and vomiting Chemotherapy- and radiotherapy-induced nausea and vomiting Nausea and vomiting related to gastroparesis	10 mg PO four times daily 25 mg PO three times daily	Restlessness, anxiety Dystonic reactions and tremor Tardive dyskinesia QT prolongation
	Chlorpromazine Perphenazine Prochlorperazine Promethazine Thiethylperazine	Phenothiazines (Dopamine D2 antagonist) Muscarinic M1 antagonist Histamine H1 antagonist	Vertigo, migraines, motion sickness Chemotherapy or postoperative nausea and vomiting	10–25 mg PO every 4–6 h 8–16 mg PO daily 2.5–10 mg IV every 4 h 12.5–25 mg IV every 4–6 h 10 mg IV every 8 h	Extrapyramidal effects
	Droperidol Haloperidol	Butyrophenones (Dopamine D2 antagonist) Muscarinic M1 antagonist		2.5 mg IV once 1 mg IV every 6 h	
	Diphenhydramine Cinnarizine Meclizine Hydroxyzine	Histamine H1 antagonist	Motion sickness and/or vestibular disease Additional antipruritic effect	25–50 mg PO every 6–8 h 25–75 mg PO every 8 h 25–50 mg PO every 24 h 25–100 mg IM every 24 h	Drowsiness Anticholinergic effects
	Ondansetron Granisetron Dolasetron Tropisetron	5-HT_3 antagonist	Postoperative, chemotherapy- and radiotherapy-induced nausea and vomiting	0.15 mg/kg IV every 8 h 12–24 mg PO every 8 h 100 mg PO 1 h before chemotherapy or 12.5 mg IV ~15 min before cessation of anesthesia 5 mg IV before chemotherapy, then 5 mg PO daily for 5 days	Headache
	Dexamethasone	Glucocorticoid	Postoperative, chemotherapy- and radiotherapy-induced nausea and vomiting	8–20 mg IV every 6 h 4 mg PO every 6 h	Hyperglycemia Worsening of PUD and gastritis
	Nabilone Dronabinol	Cannabinoid	Refractory chemotherapy-induced nausea and vomiting	1–2 mg PO every 12 h 2.5–10 mg PO every 6–8 h	Hypotension Psychotropic reactions
	Aprepitant Fosaprepitant	Neurokinin-1 antagonist	Chemotherapy-induced nausea and vomiting Postoperative nausea and vomiting	40 mg PO within 3 h of anesthesia130 mg IV ~30 min before chemotherapy	Fatigue Neutropenia
Peripherally-acting prokinetic agents	Prucalopride Cinitapride	Peripheral 5-HT_4 agonist	Nausea and vomiting related to gastroparesis	2 mg PO every 24 h 1 mg PO every 8 h	Cardiac dysrhythmias
	Erythromycin	Motilin agonist	Nausea and vomiting related to gastroparesis	3 mg/kg IV every 8 h	QT prolongation

[a]Agents used commonly in practice; additional drugs are discussed in the text.
[b]Adult doses.
HT, Hydroxytryptamine.

influenced by genetic characteristics.[157] Domperidone (as well as benzamides) may increase the release of prolactin and is occasionally associated with breast tenderness and galactorrhea. Domperidone has also been noted to prolong the QT interval and therefore has dysrhythmogenic potential.

Phenothiazines and Butyrophenones

The phenothiazines (chlorpromazine, perphenazine, prochlorperazine, promethazine, and thiethylperazine) and butyrophenones (droperidol and haloperidol) also block D2 dopaminergic receptors in addition to muscarinic M1 receptors; phenothiazines also block histamine H_1 receptors. These drugs tend to induce relaxation and somnolence and are generally used parenterally or as suppositories in patients with acute intense vomiting of central origin, as in vertigo, migraine headaches, and motion sickness. They are also useful for patients with vomiting from toxic agents, from chemotherapy and after surgery.[158,159] Safety concerns, especially extrapyramidal effects, have limited the use of all these agents to some degree.[160] For this reason, the dose of droperidol should not exceed 1 mg.

Olanzapine, a second-generation neuroleptic agent, is an attractive alternative because of its strong antinausea and antiemetic action and lack of extrapyramidal side effects.[161,162] Side effects of the use of olanzapine, include mild sedation, weight gain, and increased risk of diabetes mellitus. A double-blind trial that compared olanzapine, 10 mg, with placebo, both in combination with dexamethasone, oral aprepitant, or IV fosaprepitant and a 5-HT_3 receptor antagonist demonstrated a clinically significant reduction in chemotherapy-induced nausea and vomiting, with benefits extending up to 120 hours after administration. Patients who received olanzapine had significantly increased sedation, which was severe in 5% of cases, particularly at Day 2 as compared with baseline. These symptoms improved by Days 3–5 despite continued use of oral olanzapine. Olanzapine therefore may also be used in combination with other agents such as dexamethasone or an NK-1 antagonist.

Antihistamines and Antimuscarinic Agents

Antihistamines and antimuscarinic agents act primarily by blocking histamine H_1 receptors (cyclizine, diphenhydramine, cinnarizine, meclizine, and hydroxyzine) and muscarinic M1 receptors (scopolamine, which may be applied transdermally) at a central level.[163] Scopolamine may induce annoying visual accommodation disturbances.[164] Although promethazines belong to the phenothiazine class, they also act as antihistaminic H_1 and antimuscarinic agents with strong sedative properties. Cyclizine and diphenhydramine are commonly used to treat motion sickness and have been shown to decrease gastric dysrhythmia, so their antiemetic effect may be mediated in part by their peripheral action. A standard antiemetic dose of cyclizine is 50 mg given three times daily orally or 100 mg as a suppository. The main indication is nausea and vomiting associated with motion sickness and vestibular disease. Cyclizine is useful for postoperative and other forms of acute vomiting. Some of these drugs are also used as antipruritic agents. Drowsiness is the major limiting side effect, particularly with older agents, but this effect may be advantageous in the treatment of acute vomiting. Anticholinergic effects are potentially troublesome in patients with glaucoma, prostatic hyperplasia, and asthma.

Serotonin Antagonists

Serotonin 5-HT_3 receptor antagonists (ondansetron, granisetron, dolasetron, and tropisetron) are potent antiemetics that selectively block 5-HT_3 receptors in the brainstem and in gastric wall receptors that relay afferent emetic impulses through the vagus nerve. In addition to their antiemetic effect, they have a modest gastric prokinetic action. The main indication for this class of drugs is nausea and vomiting associated with chemotherapy and radiation therapy or following surgery. They are often prescribed in combination therapy with haloperidol and dexamethasone, with or without an NK-1 antagonist.[165] Headache is a common side effect. Ondansetron appears to be safe in pregnancy. It may be given as a single dose of 8–32 mg, intravenously in a dose of 0.15 mg/kg every 8 hours, or orally in a dose of 12–24 mg every 24 hours in three divided doses. There is a risk of QT prolongation with high doses of ondansetron.[166] Granisetron is available in a transdermal patch form.[167]

Palonosetron, a second-generation agent, exhibits unique interactions with the 5-HT_3 receptor and appears to be more effective than first-generation 5-HT_3 receptor antagonists. It has better efficacy when used in combination with netupitant (NK-1 receptor antagonist).[168] It is the only effective agent for preventing delayed nausea and vomiting.[169–173]

Glucocorticoids

The antiemetic mechanism of glucocorticoids is not well understood and may relate to inhibition of central prostaglandin synthesis, release of endorphins, or altered synthesis or release of serotonin. The principal indication is treatment of nausea and vomiting in the postoperative period or as a result of chemotherapy or radiation. Glucocorticoids may also be used to reduce cerebral edema and alleviate vomiting due to increased intracranial pressure. Dexamethasone is the formulation used acutely, in doses ranging from 8 to 20 mg intravenously and 4 mg every 6 hours orally. Side effects are uncommon because treatment is usually administered for short periods. In diabetic patients, however, careful monitoring of blood glucose levels is required. In patients with a history of peptic ulcer or with a gastroenteric anastomosis, concurrent administration of a gastric antisecretory agent is advisable. In practice, dexamethasone is often used in combination with another antiemetic agent, such as haloperidol, olanzapine, metoclopramide, 5-HT_3 antagonist, or aprepitant.[174,175]

Cannabinoids

Although cannabinoids cause or exacerbate nausea and vomiting (e.g., CVS, cannabinoid hyperemesis syndrome), cannabinoid agents have demonstrated utility in managing some forms of chronic nausea and vomiting. The benefits of cannabinoids are limited to patients with chronic nausea and vomiting; by contrast, intermittent stereotypical nausea and vomiting may develop from cannabinoid use and has a high likelihood of being part of a migrainoid disorder that may worsen with continued cannabinoid use. Two oral synthetic cannabinoids are part of the standard therapeutic armamentarium: nabilone and dronabinol. Both agents are approved by the FDA for use in chemotherapy-induced nausea and vomiting refractory to conventional antiemetic therapy. The combination of a dopamine antagonist and a cannabinoid may be particularly effective in preventing nausea that has a major negative impact on a patient's quality of life.[176,177] Mood-enhancing properties make cannabinoids attractive to patients, but these drugs are potentially more toxic than conventional antiemetic agents. Hypotension and psychotropic reactions are relatively common side effects. These drugs should be used with caution in older adults and in patients with a history of mental illness. Cannabinoids are no longer first-line agents in the management of chemotherapy-induced emesis because of their side effects and the availability of more attractive alternatives including combination regimens, although they remain useful for breakthrough nausea and vomiting.[175,178]

Neurokinin-1 Receptor Antagonists

NK-1 receptor antagonists, which inhibit substance P and NK-1, are potent antiemetic agents. Two formulations are available, aprepitant (oral) and fosaprepitant (parenteral); other preparations (e.g., rolapitant) are undergoing evaluation.[179,180] These drugs provide better protection against postoperative vomiting but not nausea when compared with 5-HT_3 antagonists. NK-1 receptor antagonists may be particularly useful when combined with other drugs like 5-HT_3 antagonists and dexamethasone and are approved by the FDA for use in preventing vomiting in patients undergoing cancer chemotherapy.[165]

Adjuvant Agents and Therapies

Patients with acute nausea and vomiting associated with chemotherapy, radiotherapy, and surgery often have anxiety that may exacerbate their symptoms. The anxiolytic effects of benzodiazepines (e.g., lorazepam, alprazolam) may potentiate the antiemetic action of agents like 5-HT_3 receptor antagonists and glucocorticoids that are devoid of psychotropic effects. Gabapentin may help prevent delayed nausea and vomiting after chemotherapy.[181] Ginger has shown some useful antinausea effects.[182] Acupuncture, acustimulation, aromatherapy, and acupressure have also been shown to decrease the nausea associated with motion sickness induced by illusory self-motion and nausea associated with cancer radiotherapy and chemotherapy, but the evidence is somewhat controversial.[183,184] Alternative therapies including gut directed hypnotherapy alone or in combination with medical therapy has been shown to be an effective option in managing nausea symptoms in pediatric population.[185]

Gastric Prokinetic Agents

Serotonin 5-HT_4 Receptor Agonists

Drugs in the benzamide class share the peripheral 5-HT_4 agonist effect of metoclopramide (also a benzamide) without the dopamine D2 antagonist action that is primarily responsible for the potentially troublesome central side effects of metoclopramide. Prucalopride, an agent primarily intended for treatment of constipation but with some prokinetic effects in the UGI tract as well, can be used in this regard (see Chapter 20).[186] Cinitapride is another agent with pharmacodynamic properties similar to those of cisapride, an older drug that was associated with cardiac dysrhythmias and withdrawn from the market. At a dose of 1 mg orally three times daily, cinitapride appears to be free of cardiac side effects but is not yet available in the United States. Other new generation 5-HT_4 antagonists, such as velusetrag, have shown good efficacy in phase 2 clinical trial as a prokinetic agent without significant cardiac side effects.[187] The main indication for 5-HT_4 agonist drugs is the management of nausea and vomiting associated with gastroparesis, intestinal pseudo-obstruction, and functional dyspepsia.

Motilin Receptor Agonists

Motilin receptor agonists include the antibiotic erythromycin and other agents—none of which is commonly available—that act as motilin receptor ligands on smooth muscle cells and enteric nerves. The pharmacodynamic effects in humans are dose dependent. In low doses (0.5–1 mg/kg as an IV bolus), erythromycin induces sweeping gastric and intestinal peristaltic motor activity that resembles phase III of the interdigestive migrating motor complex but may empty the stomach inefficiently (see Chapters 52 and 101). In higher doses (3 mg/kg every 8 hours given as a slow IV infusion), antral activity becomes intense and empties the stomach rapidly, although the burst of motility does not always migrate down the small intestine. A simultaneous increase in small bowel contractions may induce abdominal cramps and diarrhea. When used clinically as an antibiotic, generally at higher doses, erythromycin may cause nausea and vomiting.

In clinical practice, erythromycin may be used to treat acute nausea and vomiting associated with gastroparesis (diabetic, postsurgical, or idiopathic) and to clear the stomach of retained food, secretions, and blood prior to EGD (see Chapter 21). Although the prokinetic effect is well established, its symptom-relieving effects have been questioned; there is evidence that erythromycin modulates vagal nerve traffic, a potential antinausea mechanism.[188,189] Erythromycin may be administered intravenously in boluses of 200–400 mg every 4–5 hours. The lower doses are more appropriate for patients with pseudo-obstruction, which is associated with reduced interdigestive sweeping motor activity in the small bowel.

Erythromycin is not suitable for prolonged treatment, first because of relatively prompt tachyphylaxis and second because its efficacy by the oral route is uncertain and its inherent antibiotic properties carry the potential risk of complications, including pseudomembranous colitis and QT prolongation. Azithromycin, a structurally similar drug, has been proposed for the treatment of gastroparesis in slowly administered IV boluses of 250 or 500 mg, but an FDA warning has alerted the public of the potential danger of azithromycin use in patients with heart disease.[190] New synthetic motilin agonists devoid of antibiotic activity are in development.

Ghrelin is a peptide structurally and functionally related to motilin that acts to accelerate postprandial gastric emptying. Ghrelin receptor agonists (e.g., ulimorelin, atilmolin, mitemcinal, and relamorelin) have prokinetic action and may have a future therapeutic role as prokinetic agents to treat nausea and vomiting in patients with gastroparesis.[191,192]

Surgery and Endoscopic Interventions for Gastric Outlet Obstruction

Refractory nausea and vomiting from gastric outlet obstruction can be managed with surgical or endoscopic interventions. Endoscopic interventions for gastric outlet strictures include the dilation of luminal stricture or enteric metal stent placement. For malignant obstruction, an endoscopic gastrojejunostomy technique has been successfully used to bypass the obstructed lumen.[193,194] Surgical management includes open and laparoscopic gastrojejunostomy to bypass the obstruction, surgical tumor resection (if deemed to be surgical candidate). The choice of the intervention is a personalized decision and requires multidisciplinary discussions and patient counseling to select an appropriate intervention.[195]

Gastric Electrical Stimulation

There are two main technical approaches to gastric electrical stimulation. The first is low-frequency/high-energy stimulation "gastric pacing" that involves application of high-energy currents to entrain the gastric slow waves and generate phasic contractions. This technique may achieve correction of gastroparesis and amelioration of nausea and vomiting but requires external energy sources that limit the autonomy of the patient. A technical variation, 2-channel gastric pacing, has achieved some success in normalizing gastric dysrhythmia and delayed emptying.[196] A second approach, gastric neurostimulation, delivers high-frequency/low-energy impulses to the stomach with the use of an implantable neurostimulator (Enterra system), similar to devices used to control chronic pain. The gastric neurostimulator does not entrain slow-wave activity and does not consistently accelerate emptying, but it appears to relax proximal gastric tone, reduce discomfort associated with gastric distension, and produce significant improvement in nausea and vomiting, as well as the patient's nutritional status and quality of life, even in patients with normal gastric emptying.[197–199] In responders, symptoms may be ameliorated for at least 5 years, on average.[200] Addition of a pyloroplasty has been proposed to boost the effectiveness of neurostimulation in patients with nausea and vomiting associated with gastroparesis.[201]

Gastric neurostimulation is not without risk; commonly reported complications include electrode dislodgement, infection, and bowel obstruction.[198] The device is also expensive and may be recommended with caution only for long-standing (at least 1 year's duration) refractory gastroparesis. A trial of temporary neurostimulation via endoscopically placed electrodes is feasible.[202]

Acknowledgment

The authors acknowledge the contributions of Drs. Juan-R. Malagelada, Carolina Malagelada, and Arvind Rengarajan to this chapter in previous editions of the book.

Full references for this chapter can be found at https://ebooks.health.elsevier.com.

17 Diarrhea

Dejan Micic

IN THIS CHAPTER

INTRODUCTION

Diarrhea is a universal human experience. In the United States, the 30-day prevalence of diarrhea is 7.6% leading to an annualized rate of 0.92 cases/person/year.[1] In essence, diarrhea is an expected symptom. While the majority of cases of acute diarrhea are self-limited and less than 20% of cases of diarrhea will result in a health care encounter,[1] over 2.5 million ambulatory visits still occur for diarrhea in the United States[2] with expenditures of over $13.5 billion annually for combined causes of intestinal infection, noninfectious gastroenteritis, and inflammatory bowel disease (IBD).[2] Globally, an estimated 2.39 billion cases of acute diarrheal disease occur annually, trailing only upper respiratory infections[3] as the leading cause of an acute medical condition. Diarrhea is, therefore, the eighth leading cause of death and fifth leading cause of death in children under the age of 5 years.[4] Separate from acute causes of diarrhea, over the course of a year, the prevalence of chronic diarrhea based on stool consistency in the United States was an estimated 6.6%[5] with higher rates reported when, including stool frequency, in the definition[6] and with stable rates when measured over time.[7]

DEFINITION

Diarrhea can be defined as an excess of gastrointestinal losses that is accompanied by an increase in stool frequency or liquidity. Any process that stimulates intestinal epithelial chloride secretion and/or inhibits sodium/chloride absorption, decreases intestinal epithelial surface area for absorption, or alters motility, intraluminal digestion, or the autonomic nervous system can cause diarrhea.

It is important to recognize that diarrhea is a clinical symptom and not a disease process in itself. Therefore individual clinical conditions, alterations in diet, medical therapies, and surgical treatments can all result in the clinical symptom of diarrhea with or without additional clinical findings.

Using a strict quantitative definition, diarrhea is defined as having more than three bowel movements per day.[8,9] In a sampling of the United States population, normal bowel movement frequency ranged from three bowel movements per week to three bowel movements per day.[9]

Stool liquidity holds up as a criterion most often used by patients.[10] Most patients with self-reported diarrhea will describe their stool patterns in a qualitative sense, with loose or watery stools and urgency.[11] To standardize assessments of stool consistency, measures of stool form using pictorial images and written descriptors have been developed to aid in describing stool consistency, showing correlation with intestinal transit time[12] and stool frequency.[13]

Stool weight is often used when assessing the composition and contents of stool. In healthy adults, stool weight ranges from 100 to 200 g with a composition of 60%–85% water[14,10] with diarrhea defined as a fecal weight of over 200 g.[14,15] However, stool weight can exceed 200 g when a fiber is added to a controlled diet[16,17] or 300 g when high-fiber diets are consumed as they are in developing countries.[18]

Roughly 20% of individuals presenting with diarrhea are found to have a normal stool weight of less than 200 g.[19] This can result from frequent small volume bowel movements or impaired mechanisms of stool continence.[15] While alterations in stool composition can be identified in individuals with a fecal weight of less than 200 g,[19] the primary disorder is often not one of impaired absorption; therefore, individuals reporting diarrhea should be asked about the presence of fecal incontinence.

Normal Intestinal Physiology

To appreciate the basic mechanisms of acute diarrhea or the subclassifications of chronic diarrhea (watery, fatty, and inflammatory), it is important to understand normal intestinal absorption and regulation of fluids and solutes.

Flow through the intestines should be considered, starting with oral intake. Whether a hypotonic meal, such as steak and iced tea, is consumed or a hypertonic meal consisting of doughnuts and juice, gastric and small intestinal secretions render the contents isotonic to plasma within the small intestinal lumen.[20]

Fluid passing the mid-small bowel is mainly an isotonic salt solution. By the time chyme reaches the ileum, most of the dietary sugars, amino acids, and fats have been absorbed. If one considers the fact that glucose and other actively absorbed nonelectrolytes stimulate small bowel fluid absorption, the fluid absorptive capacity of the normal small bowel is enormous and far surpasses the volume of absorption of the colon. In contrast to the small bowel, the colon can absorb ions against steep electrochemical gradients,[21–23] allowing for extraction of the remaining sodium and water. To illustrate the above points, if one were to perfuse an isotonic solution with half of the osmolarity accounted for by mannitol and half by sodium chloride, the colon would absorb fluid, whereas there would be a net fluid secretion by the jejunum.[363] Together, the small intestine and colon absorb 99% of the fluid load passing beyond the ligament of Treitz—a total volume of roughly 9–10 L daily (Fig. 17.1).

At the cellular level, sodium and chloride are absorbed by nutrient-dependent and nutrient-independent transporters on the apical surface of the intestinal epithelium. The sodium-potassium (Na^+-K^+) ATPase pumps on the basolateral surface of the epithelial cells generate a low intracellular sodium concentration and negative intracellular electrical potential gradient that favors

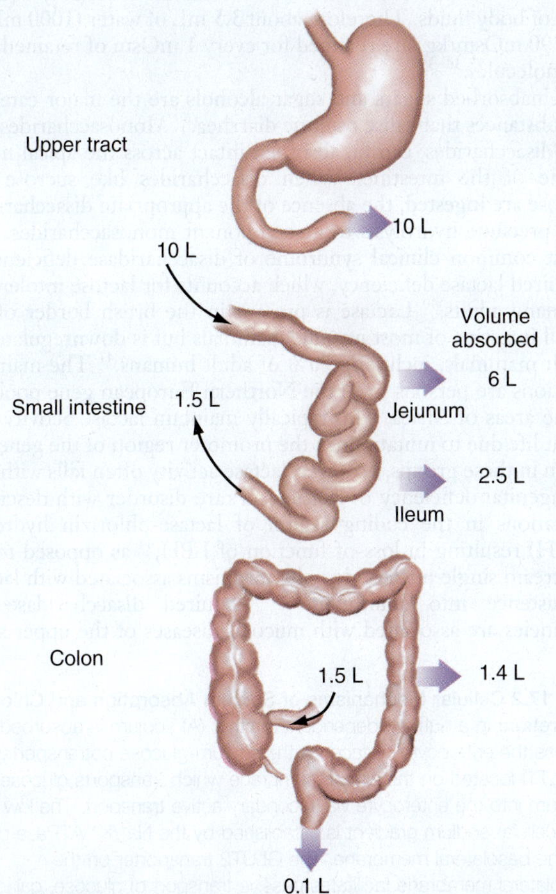

Fig. 17.1 Fluid loads along the GI tract. Each day, close to 10 L of fluid composed of ingested food and drink and secretions from the salivary glands, esophagus, stomach, pancreas, bile duct, and duodenum pass the ligament of Treitz. The jejunum absorbs approximately 6 L and the ileum 2.5 L, leaving about 1.5 L to pass into the colon each day. The colon absorbs more than 90% of this load, leaving about 0.1 L in feces. The overall efficiency of water absorption is 99%, and a reduction of this efficiency by as little as 1% may lead to diarrhea. (From Schiller LR. Chronic diarrhea. In: McNally P, ed. *GI/Liver Secrets*. 2nd ed. Philadelphia: Hanley & Belfus; 2001:411.)

movement of sodium into the cell (Fig. 17.2). In a nutrient-independent paired exchanger model, sodium absorption occurs via the Na^+/H^+ antiporter [e.g., Na^+/H^+ exchange isoform 3 (NHE3)], with hydrogen efflux driving chloride absorption via Cl^-/HCO_3^- exchange [chloride anion exchanger, also known as the down regulated in adenoma (DRA) anion transporter]. The alkalinization of the cytoplasm further facilitates electroneutral NaCl absorption. The sodium gradient across the cell and electrical potential gradient also acts as the driving force for glucose, amino acid, vitamin, and bile acid absorption via specific sodium coupled cotransport proteins on the apical surface of the enterocyte. The absorbed nutrients are then carried out of the cell into the bloodstream by diffusion carriers in the basolateral membrane, such as GLUT2 for passive glucose, fructose, and galactose absorption.[24] The generated transcellular osmotic gradient in turn facilitates water absorption via paracellular and intracellular pathways.

While the intestinal surface epithelium facilitates a net absorption of nutrients, water and electrolytes, secretory mechanisms exist to maintain the hydration and passage of luminal contents (Fig. 17.2). In the intestinal crypt cells, the low intracellular sodium concentrations generated by the Na^+-K^+ ATPase aid in the uptake of chloride across the basolateral membrane via a sodium-potassium-2 chloride cotransporter, NKCC1.[25,26] Chloride channels along the apical cell surface then allow for chloride release into the intestinal lumen, principally via the cystic fibrosis transmembrane conductance regulator (CFTR) and the calcium-activated chloride channel (TMEM16A).[364] The chloride secretory mechanisms are under tight regulatory control, principally through the extrinsic sympathetic nervous system and intrinsic neurohormonal agents that act through intracellular cyclic adenosine monophosphate (cAMP), cyclic guanosine monophosphate (cGMP), or calcium[25] and downstream signaling protein kinases and phosphatases.[26] Cyclic nucleotide-stimulated secretion is strong and sustained, whereas calcium dependent secretion is weaker and transient. Combined stimulation, however, results in a synergistic enhancement of chloride secretion.[25]

The normal colon absorbs 90% of the fluid entering it per day and has substantial reserve capacity, being able to compensate for an additional 2 L/day.[27] The colonic electrogenic sodium transport mechanisms extract sodium from the stool, and as a result, the sodium content of stool decreases to 30–40 mEq/L.[363] Potassium is secreted and increases from 5 to 10 mEq/L in the small bowel to 75–90 mEq/L in the colon, and poorly absorbed divalent cations, such as magnesium and calcium, are concentrated in stool to values of 5–100 mEq/L.[364]

Any perturbations to the finely tuned mechanisms that control intestinal absorption, including inhibition of the low intracellular sodium concentrations,[28] impairment of sodium cotransport mechanisms,[29] or activation of chloride[30] or potassium secretion,[31] can contribute to both acute and chronic diarrhea pathogenesis.

Diarrhea Mechanisms

Diarrhea results from an excess of stool water in relation to the water-holding capacity of fecal solids.[10] Alterations in absorption or secretion by as little as 1% in the small bowel or colon can result in diarrhea. This may occur when the *rate* of mucosal water and electrolyte transport is altered. Reduced net water absorption may also result from rapid transit, which reduces the *time* available for water absorption, especially when fluid is hurried through the colon. A third mechanism that may contribute to the degree of stool looseness is the presence of water insoluble solids (fiber, fat, or bacterial components) and their ability to hold and bind water.[10,32] Whereas psyllium fiber has a high water-holding capacity (and improved stool consistency), reductions in water binding (as seen with stool fats) may produce looser stools and the complaint of diarrhea.

Acute (and often self-limited) infectious diarrhea can result from impaired electrolyte absorption or toxin-mediated activation of secretory mechanisms [e.g., cholera toxin (CT)]. Likewise, for the purposes of clinical classification, chronic diarrhea is often subcategorized as chronic watery (secretory or osmotic), fatty, or inflammatory. Diarrhea due to disordered electrolyte transport is termed *secretory diarrhea*, even though it is more commonly caused by reduced electrolyte absorption rather than by net secretion.[32] Reduced paracellular and transcellular water absorption due to retention of osmotically active substances (e.g., magnesium ion, lactulose, and lactose) causing retention of water in the gastrointestinal lumen is known as *osmotic diarrhea*. Fat malabsorption (*steatorrhea*) results from impaired digestion (decreased bile salts or pancreatic dysfunction) or impaired absorption (loss of villous surface area or lymphatic obstruction) of dietary fats. In addition to loss of mucosal surface area, inflammatory causes of diarrhea often include complex underlying and overlapping mechanisms, such as impaired sodium absorption (e.g., loss of barrier epithelial function resulting in paracellular water efflux), in IBD.[33–35]

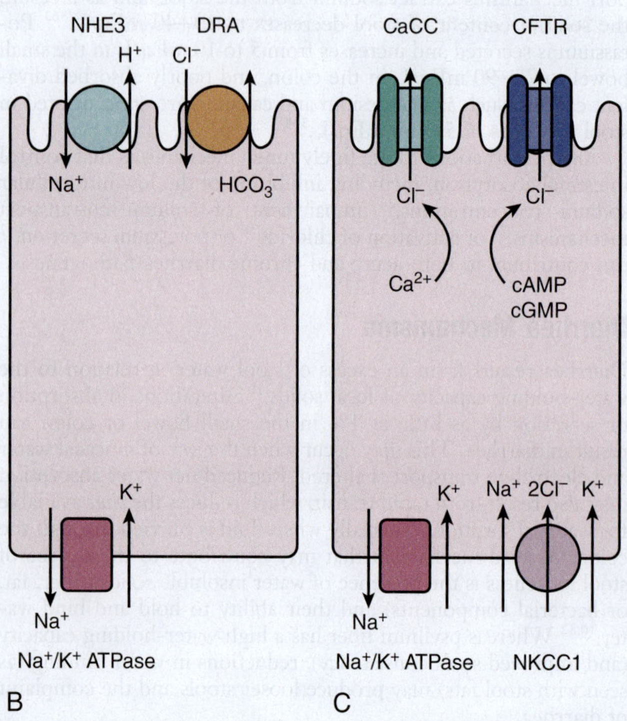

Osmotic Diarrhea

Osmotic diarrhea specifically refers to the presence of an *osmotically active*, poorly absorbable solute. Prototypically this is a carbohydrate, sugar alcohol, or divalent/trivalent cation (Mg^{2+}) or anion ($SO_4^=$, $PO_4^=$)[36] that retains water in the intestinal lumen.

The causative ions are transported actively by mechanisms that are saturated at low intraluminal ion concentrations and passively by mechanisms that are limited in capacity. Because neither the small intestine nor the colon can maintain an osmotic gradient relative to plasma, poorly absorbed divalent/trivalent ions (and their counter ions) remain in the intestinal lumen and obligate retention of water to maintain an intraluminal osmolality equal to that of body fluids. Therefore about 3.5 mL of water (1000 mL/kg ÷ 290 mOsm/kg) are retained for every 1 mOsm of retained ions or molecules.[36–39]

Unabsorbed sugars and sugar alcohols are the major category of substances that cause osmotic diarrhea.[39] Monosaccharides, but not disaccharides, can be absorbed intact across the apical membrane of the intestine. When disaccharides like sucrose and lactose are ingested, the absence of the appropriate disaccharidase will preclude hydrolysis to its component monosaccharides. The most common clinical syndrome of disaccharidase deficiency is acquired lactase deficiency, which accounts for lactose intolerance in many adults.[40] Lactase is present in the brush border of the small intestine of most juvenile mammals but is downregulated in adult mammals, including 70% of adult humans.[41] The main exceptions are persons from the Northern European gene pool and some areas of Africa, who typically maintain lactase activity into adult life due to mutations in the promoter region of the gene.[42,43] Even in these groups, however, lactase activity often falls with age. Congenital deficiency of lactase is a rare disorder with described mutations in the coding region of lactase-phlorizin hydrolase (LPH) resulting in loss-of-function of LPH,[44] as opposed to the upstream single nucleotide polymorphisms associated with lactase persistence into adulthood.[45,46] Acquired disaccharidase deficiencies are associated with mucosal diseases of the upper small

Fig. 17.2 Cellular Mechanisms of Sodium Absorption and Chloride Secretion: In a nutrient-dependent manner (A) sodium is absorbed across the enterocyte surface via the sodium-glucose cotransporter (SGLT1) located on the apical membrane which transports glucose and sodium into the enterocyte via secondary active transport. The low intracellular sodium gradient is established by the Na^+/K^+ ATPase pump on the basolateral membrane. The GLUT2 transporter on the basolateral membrane facilitates passive transport of glucose, galactose and fructose into the bloodstream. Via paracellular route, sodium and water move across tight junctions into the bloodstream, contributing to absorption. In a nutrient-independent manner (B), sodium is absorbed in exchange for hydrogen export via the sodium-hydrogen exchanger (NHE3). The hydrogen efflux drives chloride absorption via Cl-/HCO3-exchange via the down regulated in adenoma [DRA] anion transporter. Chloride secretion (C) occurs along the apical cell surface via the cystic fibrosis transmembrane conductance regulator (CFTR) and the calcium-activated chloride channel (CaCC; TMEM16A) in response to intracellular cyclic adenosine monophosphate (cAMP), cyclic guanosine monophosphate (cGMP) or calcium signaling.

intestine, such as celiac disease. Congenital sucrase and trehalase deficiencies are rare and prevent adequate digestion of sucrose (table sugar) and trehalose (a disaccharide found in mushrooms and lobsters and used as an additive in processed foods), respectively. Lactulose is a synthetic disaccharide that cannot be hydrolyzed by human disaccharidases; it causes an osmotic diarrhea when given in sufficient quantity.[47]

Knowledge of impaired absorption of concentrated sugars, disaccharides, and sugar alcohols has led to the low *f*ermentable *o*ligosaccharides, *d*isaccharides, *m*onosaccharides, *a*nd *p*olyols (FODMAPs) diet that has been shown to improve stool consistency and fecal frequency among individuals with irritable bowel syndrome (IBS), particularly the diarrhea subtype.[48,49]

Secretory Diarrhea

Secretory diarrhea has many underlying causes. Although the term *secretory* implies net secretion of monovalent anions (Cl^- or HCO^{3-}) or cations (K^+), any disorder altering the *handling* of the monovalent electrolytes (sodium, potassium, bicarbonate, or chloride) and water can result in secretory diarrhea. Therefore both increased secretory mechanisms *and* impaired absorption of electrolytes can result in the net secretion (fecal loss) of sodium, potassium, chloride or bicarbonate, and water.

The stimuli for altered electrolyte transport (both absorption and secretion) arise from toxins, drugs, hormones, and inflammatory mediators that alter the messenger systems that regulate ion transport pathways. In rare cases, congenital absence of specific transport molecules limits sodium or chloride absorption, resulting in diarrhea. In other cases, loss of villous surface area, intestinal length, or impaired barrier function critically limits electrolyte, particularly sodium, absorption.

The most common cause of secretory diarrhea is infection.[29] Enterotoxins from various infectious agents (primarily bacteria, but also parasites and viruses) interact with receptors that modulate intestinal electrolyte transport and can lead to increased anion secretion and/or impaired sodium absorption. For example, *Escherichia coli* heat-stable enterotoxin interacts with the guanylate cyclase C receptors on the enterocyte luminal surface resulting in elevated levels of cellular cGMP. This elicits a signaling cascade involving protein kinases that stimulates chloride secretion via CFTR.[50] In addition to stimulating secretion, the heat-stable enterotoxin can inhibit NHE3 activity by dysregulating trafficking of the transporter.[29] In the prototypical secretory diarrhea, *Vibrio cholerae* causes diarrhea via its major virulence factor, CT. The exotoxin, once internalized, locks adenylate cyclase in a GTP-bound activated state, resulting in enhanced cAMP production, thus driving chloride and bicarbonate export primarily via the stimulation of CFTR.[29,51] CT also inhibits sodium absorption by downregulating both sodium-hydrogen exchanger 2 (NHE2) and NHE3, although via different mechanisms (posttranslational vs. posttranscriptional).[29]

Genetic mutations may result in the absence or disruption of specific transport pathways. For example, rare congenital syndromes (e.g., congenital chloride diarrhea and congenital sodium diarrhea) are caused by the absence of specific transport molecules resulting in intrauterine diarrhea and clinically manifesting often in the first weeks of life with severe watery diarrhea and failure to thrive.[50–55] In congenital chloride diarrhea, mutations in the SLC26A3 gene (DRA anion transporter) impair chloride/bicarbonate exchange activity in the ileum and colon (chloride absorption and bicarbonate secretion), resulting in secondary disruption of sodium/hydrogen transport and intestinal losses of both NaCl and water.[56] Diarrhea resulting from congenital chloride diarrhea can be reduced by inhibiting gastric chloride secretion[57] or by stimulating chloride absorption with short-chain fatty acids.[53] Reduced activity of NHE3 is responsible for congenital sodium diarrhea.[55] Another familial diarrhea syndrome results from a mutation in the guanylate cyclase C receptor that markedly increases production of intracellular cGMP resulting in a similar signaling cascade and stimulation of chloride secretion via CFTR, as with *E. coli* heat-stable enterotoxin.[50]

Chronic secretory diarrhea can also result from peptides produced by endocrine tumors.[58] The prototypical diarrhea resulting from a circulating agent is due to tumor-related secretion of vasoactive intestinal peptide (VIP) (also described as Verner-Morrison syndrome, VIPoma, pancreatic cholera, and watery diarrhea hypokalemia hypochlorhydria syndrome). VIP results in active chloride and bicarbonate secretion via intracellular cAMP production[30] leading to large intestinal fluid losses (averaging 1.8–4.5 L/day), metabolic acidosis, and hypokalemia.[58,59] While tumor-induced diarrhea is usually large in volume and associated with dehydration, this occurs most often with VIPomas but is not true for most other neuroendocrine tumor-induced diarrheas.[60] In Zollinger-Ellison syndrome (ZES), gastrin-producing tumors cause acid hypersecretion with large gastric fluid volumes that overwhelm the absorptive capacity of the intestines. The acidic environment of the duodenum further inactivates pancreatic digestive enzymes and disrupts the emulsification of fat by bile acids.[365] In medullary carcinoma of the thyroid, circulating calcitonin reduces sodium absorption and activates chloride secretion via calcium-dependent signaling pathways involving CFTR.[58,61,62]

Other neurotransmitters, such as acetylcholine, histamine, or serotonin [5-hydroxytryptamine (5-HT)], can act as potent secretory stimuli. Most of these endogenous regulators of intestinal transport elicit diarrhea by altering intracellular messengers, such as cAMP, cGMP, and calcium, that control specific transport pathways.[25] In carcinoid syndrome, in addition to alterations in gut motor function,[63] 5-HT-induced, calcium-mediated chloride secretion contributes to the development of diarrhea.[64,65] Similarly, postprandial plasma 5-HT levels are increased in patients with IBS with diarrhea[144,366] or postinfectious IBS.[66,25] Systemic mastocytosis is a rare myeloproliferative disorder characterized by excessive numbers of mast cells with release of serine proteases (e.g., tryptase) and histamine, resulting in impaired intestinal absorption similar to ZES with gastric acid hypersecretion.[67,25] Other exogenous agents, such as drugs and some poisons, lead to secretory diarrhea, presumably by interacting with intracellular regulators or messengers of the enterocytes.

Bile acids are amphipathic end products of cholesterol metabolism with multiple physiological functions.[68] Bile acids that are synthesized in the hepatocyte, conjugated, and released in bile to aid in digestion are absorbed via the apical sodium bile acid transporter in the distal ileum, facilitating their enterohepatic circulation. Roughly 5%–10% of the conjugated primary bile acids [cholic acid (CA) and chenodeoxy CA (CDCA)] that are unabsorbed by the ileum reach the colon and are deconjugated by bacterial bile salt hydrolases and dehydroxylated by bacterial 7α-dehydroxylase to form secondary bile acids, predominantly deoxy CA (DCA), litho CA, and ursodeoxy CA.[69] Dihydroxy bile acids, such as CDCA and DCA, cause colonic secretion of fluid and electrolytes if they reach the colon in sufficient concentrations (3–5 mmol/L).[70] Additionally, primary bile acids stimulate colonic motor activity,[71] alter rectal sensory thresholds,[72] and alter mucosal permeability.[73] As such, ileal dysfunction, either secondary to surgical resection or due to inflammatory disease of the ileum (e.g., Crohn disease) interrupts the normal enterohepatic circulation, thereby resulting in an increase in synthesis of bile acids by the liver and more bile acids entering the colon, contributing to diarrhea.[74] In the absence of apparent ileal disease, inappropriate downregulation of the ileal bile acid transporter,[75] genetic variation in bile acid receptors,[76] or insufficient generation of fibroblast growth factor-19 (FGF-19)[77] alters the enterohepatic circulation, resulting in excessive bile acid production and an expanded bile acid pool that can overwhelm the absorptive capacity of the ileum contributing to a secretory bile acid diarrhea (BAD).[78]

While mucosal inflammation is implicated in the diarrhea of microscopic colitis, stool outputs are consistent with a secretory diarrhea. Colonic perfusion studies have shown that absorption of water and salt is impaired in lymphocytic colitis and collagenous colitis with colonic water absorption correlating inversely with the cellularity of the lamina propria.[79] Sodium malabsorption results from inhibited upregulation of epithelial sodium channels in response to aldosterone,[80] and impaired water absorption results from reduced expression of colonocyte aquaporins.[81] Bile acid malabsorption has also been identified in microscopic colitis, further resulting in a secretory diarrhea.[82]

Fatty Diarrhea (Steatorrhea)

Due to the range of physiologic intraluminal and cellular processes required, dietary fats are the most difficult nutrients to absorb. Dietary fat absorption requires appropriate intraluminal digestive components (e.g., pancreatic enzymes, bile salts, and adequate pH), surface area for intestinal absorption, and appropriate transit time in the small intestine to allow for absorption. Steatorrhea, therefore, encompasses a wide range of clinical disorders ranging from lipase deficiency, obstructed flow or loss of bile acids, mucosal disorders, and lymphatic obstruction.

Mechanistically, in maldigestion, nonpolar triglyceride emulsions have little osmotic load leading to smaller volume loose stools due to the altered water holding capacity of the fecal fats. In contrast, in malabsorption, digested free intraluminal fatty acids can impair water and electrolyte absorption[83,84] leading to a more voluminous diarrhea. In intestinal malabsorption due to disorders of mucosal surface area, concurrent malabsorption of water, electrolytes, fat, and often other macronutrients occurs.

For intestinal fluid, fat, and electrolyte absorption to be complete, the intestine must have an adequate surface area and adequate contact time with luminal contents. Redundancy in the small intestine and colon surface area allows for handling of the large volumes of gastrointestinal fluid passage. The average length of small intestine ranges from 300 to 800 cm with variations based on measurement technique to include radiologic, surgical, or postmortem techniques.[85] In addition, in comparison to its luminal volume, the small intestine has an increased surface area due to the presence of folds (plicae circulares), villi, and enterocyte microvilli, which increase the surface area to greater than 30 m^2.[86] Similarly, the adult colon, responsible for water and electrolyte handling, measures roughly 150 cm in length,[87] with variations in intestinal transit time leading to differences in stool form, consistency, and frequency.[88]

Substantial loss of surface area as in short bowel syndrome (<200 cm of small intestine) or mucosal disease processes, such as celiac disease or Crohn disease, can compromise water and nutrient absorption. Even though the reserve absorptive capacity in the small intestine and colon is large, sufficiently large surgical resections inevitably cause diarrhea. In some cases, the problem is temporary because, over time, the intestine may improve its capacity for absorption by the process of adaptation.[85,89] However, such compensation is impossible following resection of certain segments of the intestine with highly specific absorptive functions. For example, ileocecal resection is followed by permanent inability to absorb sodium chloride against a concentration gradient that cannot be overcome by more distal parts of the colon.[90] Ileal resection also may lead to excessive bile acid malabsorption that can impair colonic water and electrolyte absorption[91] and when greater than 100 cm of ileum is resected, depletions in the bile acid pool can further impair fat digestion.[92]

Inflammatory Diarrhea

Inflammatory diarrhea is suggested by the presence of blood, pus, or inflammatory markers in the stool. Disruption of the integrity of the intestinal mucosa due to inflammation and ulceration results in loss of plasma proteins and blood. Infectious examples resulting in mucosal invasion include protozoa or bacteria, such as *Entamoeba histolytica*, *Shigella*, *Salmonella*, *Campylobacter jejuni*, *Yersinia enterocolitica*, and Enteropathogenic *E. coli*.

While destructive loss of the mucosal surface area is typically considered to be the underlying cause of diarrhea, a variety of overlapping mechanisms contribute to the pathogenesis of diarrhea. In IBD, altered expression and/or loss of function of ion transport mechanisms and channels, increased paracellular permeability and increased intestinal transit lead to inadequate water and solute absorption.[93] Altered expression of the NHE3 antiporter has been demonstrated in IBD,[94,95] as has reduced expression of DRA, resulting in impaired chloride absorption.[96] Disease complexity is only further enhanced when considering the potential immunomodulatory effects of altered transporter expression as reflected in enhanced inflammation in NHE3 knockout mice (KO)[93] and impaired mucus barrier expression in DRA KO mice.[97,93] Cytokines also stimulate fluid secretion and may directly influence tight junction barrier function,[98–100,34] while epithelial cells can secrete cytokines that enhance polymorphonuclear leukocyte (neutrophil) function (e.g., IL-6).[101]

Reduced intestinal blood flow has an important but yet poorly defined role in diarrhea. Colonic ischemia can produce findings that range from subepithelial hemorrhage and edema to a transient colitis, chronic colitis, stricture formation, or fulminant universal colitis requiring surgical resection.[102] Whether mesenteric ischemia has a direct effect on absorption or whether low blood flow prompts secondary responses (e.g., via cytokines or neurotransmitters) that affect fluid transport and produce a secretory diarrhea is not clear.

Radiation-induced injury to the small bowel or colon can exist in both an acute and chronic form with chronic disease occurring often between 18 months and 6 years after the completion of therapy.[103] Disease location and extent can vary widely, resulting in several clinical presentations. Ionizing radiation can result in acute inflammation in the lamina propria, crypt abscess formation, and mucosal ulceration. The resultant epithelial dysfunction leads to nutrient and fluid loss, whereas the associated increase in intestinal permeability to gut pathogens can exacerbate mucosal inflammation.[104] Obliterative endarteritis can lead to local tissue ischemia and submucosal fibrosis, which can progress to stricture or fistula formation[104] requiring surgical resection or diversion in a subset of individuals.[105] In less severe cases, given typical injury of the distal small intestine, loss of the sodium-dependent bile acid transporter[106] and bile acid malabsorption have been implicated in radiation enteritis.[107]

Complex Diarrhea

Multiple overlapping pathophysiologic mechanisms can participate in producing diarrhea in specific clinical entities. Most clinically important diarrhea is therefore complex in nature. As observed in IBD, altered sodium handling and bile acid malabsorption can occur as a result of inflammation or post-surgical resection. Similarly, altered motility can result in altered sodium absorption, potassium secretion, and nutrient absorption.

Abnormal motility can disturb the typical digestive and absorptive patterns in the small intestine and alter the composition of chyme entering the colon. For fluid and electrolyte absorption to be complete, the contact time between luminal contents and the epithelium must be sufficient to permit absorption. Rapid intestinal transit, often a result of autonomic dysfunction, can lead to glucose malabsorption[108,109] due to inadequate time for absorption.[32] Unabsorbed carbohydrates are rapidly fermented to short-chain fatty acids but can also overwhelm the colonic absorptive capacity due to an increased osmotic load.[27,110] In some patients with intestinal hurry, and in those with short bowel syndrome, the oral-cecal transit time may be as short as 10 minutes. Under such circumstances, the diarrhea is exacerbated by malabsorption of nutrients. While failure to absorb carbohydrates leads to an osmotic diarrhea, bile acids, once deconjugated in the colon, can stimulate secretion and inhibit absorption,[70] and long-chain fatty acids have an irritant effect on the colon.[111] Many endocrine diarrheas, such as those caused by peptide-secreting tumors (i.e., carcinoid syndrome) or hyperthyroidism, may lead to diarrhea not only by affecting intestinal electrolyte transport but also by accelerating intestinal motility.[112]

Slow intestinal transit can also lead to diarrhea by promoting small intestinal bacterial overgrowth (SIBO)[113–115] or through the decreased mixing of intraluminal contents leading to impaired micelle formation and fat absorption.[116] Excess bacteria in the small intestine can disrupt intraluminal digestion and may alter electrolyte transport. The best documented example of diarrhea related to this mechanism is scleroderma (systemic sclerosis). In a classical sense, excess small intestinal bacteria lead to deconjugation of bile acids, rapid absorption of deconjugated bile acids by the small bowel, and impaired micelle formation.[117] Enterocyte injury and villous blunting leads to a loss of absorptive surface area, reduced activity of brush-border disaccharidases and altered permeability of the intestine,[118] resulting in osmotic and in severe cases fatty diarrhea. Disruption of the intrinsic factor-cobalamin complex by intestinal bacteria can furthermore result in vitamin B_{12} deficiency.[119] While motionless dilated loops of bowel are most often associated with impaired digestion and absorption, secretory diarrhea can develop in patients with colonic pseudo-obstruction due to active potassium secretion in the colon.[31]

Although diabetes mellitus is often suspected of causing diarrhea by slow transit and stasis, such a pathophysiologic mechanism is not always established.[120,121] Slow motility can lead to a stasis syndrome predisposing individuals to impaired digestive processes and SIBO. However, hypermotility in diabetes mellitus can also result from sympathetic inhibition and lead to intestinal hurry.[122] Medications (metformin and α-glucosidase inhibitors) result in diarrhea due to alterations in the bile acid pool and carbohydrate malabsorption, respectively.[123] Celiac disease occurs in approximately 6% of individuals with type 1 diabetes mellitus with the highest rates in children.[124] Type 1 diabetes is more commonly encountered among individuals with microscopic colitis, although this association may be confounded by medication use among diabetic patients.[125] Lastly, diabetic neuropathy can contribute to anorectal dysfunction and fecal incontinence with demonstrated associations with disease duration.[126]

Alterations in transit due to foregut surgeries are common. For many years, peptic ulcer disease was treated surgically by vagotomy with pyloroplasty or antrectomy. The introduction of highly selective vagotomy in the 1980s led to a decrease in the frequency of postoperative diarrhea. Postvagotomy diarrhea is thought to result from alterations in gastric emptying, impaired pancreatic function, or alterations in the excretion of bile salts[127] that respond to bile acid binding agents.[128,129]

The most common syndrome after gastric surgery is now dumping syndrome, which refers to the gastrointestinal and vasomotor symptoms following the ingestion of a meal. Dumping syndrome symptoms and severity are proportional to the rate of gastric emptying.[130] As the pylorus meters gastric emptying, any operation in which the pylorus is removed, altered, or bypassed can result in dumping. While typically described after a truncal vagotomy and pyloroplasty for peptic ulcer disease,[27] dumping can also occur in 15%–20% of individuals with a partial gastrectomy[131] and in 50%–70% of individuals after a Roux-en-Y gastric bypass in the early postoperative period.[132] When bypassed with a gastrojejunostomy, the duodenal feedback inhibition is lost,[129] resulting in rapid emptying of gastric contents. Symptoms of sweating, lethargy, and lightheadedness result from accelerated gastric emptying of a hyperosmolar load into the small bowel, leading to fluid shifts from the intravascular compartment into the intestinal lumen and increased small bowel distention and contractility.[131] This correlates with a precipitous rise and then fall in blood glucose levels. Late symptoms (1–3 hours after a meal) are characterized by the systemic vascular symptoms of flushing, dizziness, and a desire to lie down.[131] Low blood sugar, a contraction of blood volume due to profuse intestinal secretions or altered release of vasoactive gastrointestinal hormones all contribute to symptoms that are made worse after a meal containing a high simple sugar content.[27,131]

IBS is another example of a disorder with a complex pathophysiology and is the most common diagnosis made in individuals with chronic diarrhea. In the current Rome IV criteria, abdominal pain is the central feature of the disorder, and the temporal connection between pain and bowel habits gives the criteria their specificity,[133] in contrast to *functional diarrhea.*[134] While, historically, IBS was considered not to have an underlying pathologic or biochemical basis, recent studies have uncovered several mechanisms leading to IBS.[135] Initial studies have centered on alterations in gastrointestinal motility[136] or visceral sensory function.[137] However, more recent evidence has revealed genetic factors,[138,139] disturbances in intestinal microbiota,[140] low-grade mucosal inflammation with immune activation,[141] altered permeability,[142] disordered bile salt metabolism,[143] and abnormalities in serotonin metabolism[66,144] as causative factors. Additionally, dietary factors, including intake of osmotically active and poorly absorbed sugars (FODMAPs), may exacerbate symptoms in a subgroup of patients due to their fermentation and osmotic effects.[135] As fructose is absorbed by limited capacity facilitated diffusion,[145] consumption of processed foods containing high fructose corn syrup makes it easier to overwhelm the absorptive capacity of the gut.[146,147] When administered to healthy adults undergoing magnetic resonance imaging (MRI) studies, fructose results in small bowel distention.[148] The myriad of underlying pathophysiologic factors contributing to IBS is demonstrated in the complexity of management of the disease process.

Clinical Presentation

The basic clinical classifications allow for insight into the etiology of diarrhea and its management. The initial classification of the time course, volume, and composition of the stool breaks down the broad differential of causes of diarrhea into manageable subsets and offers insight into the underlying pathology. For the clinician, classification is useful when it delineates a diagnostic and management approach in a given patient. In this regard, no single scheme is perfect; the experienced physician uses all these classifications to facilitate patient care. Common clinical scenarios and the diagnoses that should be considered are shown in Box 17.1.

Acute Versus Chronic

Acute diarrhea is defined as less than 2 weeks in duration[149] and is most commonly due to an infectious agent or drug exposure that is self-limited in nature.[150] Clinical history, including age, exposure history, immunocompromised status, and travel history, are important to understand as risk factors for an infectious diarrhea. Diagnostic testing is typically reserved for individuals with a clinical history of invasive infection (fever or bloody diarrhea), immune compromise, or those at increased risk for involvement in an outbreak setting.[151–153] When identified, viral agents (norovirus) are the most common cause of foodborne illness in the United States, followed by bacterial infections (nontyphoidal *Salmonella* spp., *Clostridium perfringens,* and *Campylobacter* spp.).[154] Persistent diarrhea (>7–14 days)[155,156] increases the possibility of a protozoal cause of diarrhea, such as giardiasis or cryptosporidiosis. Chronic diarrhea is then somewhat arbitrarily defined as lasting greater than 4 weeks.[157,15] Although some infectious agents, such as *Aeromonas*

BOX 17.1 Likely Causes of Diarrhea in Well-Defined Patient Groups or Settings

TRAVELERS

Bacterial infection (mostly acute)
Protozoal infections (e.g., amebiasis, giardiasis)
Tropical sprue

EPIDEMICS AND OUTBREAKS

Bacterial infection
Epidemic idiopathic secretory diarrhea (e.g., Brainerd diarrhea)
Protozoal infection (e.g., cryptosporidiosis)
Viral infection (e.g., rotavirus, COVID-19*)

PATIENTS WITH DIABETES MELLITUS

Altered motility (increased or decreased)
Associated diseases
 Celiac disease
 Pancreatic exocrine insufficiency
 SIBO
Drug side effects (especially acarbose, metformin)

PATIENTS WITH PRIOR INTESTINAL SURGERY

Bile acid malabsorption
Dumping syndrome
Impaired pancreatic secretion
Postvagotomy diarrhea
Short bowel syndrome
SIBO

INSTITUTIONALIZED AND HOSPITALIZED PATIENTS

Clostridioides difficile toxin–mediated colitis
Drug side effects
Fecal impaction with overflow diarrhea
Ischemic colitis
Tube feeding

BOX 17.2 Historical Features to Consider in Patients Presenting With Diarrhea

Duration: acute (<2 weeks) vs. chronic (≥4 weeks)
Onset: congenital, abrupt, gradual
Pattern: continuous, intermittent
Epidemiology (see Box 17.1)
Iatrogenic factors: drugs (see Box 17.3), radiation, surgery
Factitious diarrhea
Systemic diseases: endocrine, collagen vascular, neoplastic, immunologic
Stool appearance: bloody, fatty, watery
Fecal incontinence: present, absent
Abdominal pain: location, relation to meals or bowel movements, aggravating and relieving factors
Weight loss
Aggravating factors: diet, stress
Alleviating factors: diet, over-the-counter drugs, prescription drugs
Previous evaluation

spp., *Yersinia* spp., or *Clostridioides difficile*, can result in diarrhea lasting greater than 4 weeks, chronic diarrhea is usually not caused by an infectious agent, requiring the clinician to consider noninfectious causes first.

Large Versus Small Volume

Although patients often have difficulty in quantifying the volume of stool passage, the distinction between small- and large-volume stools may guide further diagnostic studies. Passage of small volume, frequent stools suggests a disorder of the colon reservoir capacity—the left colon or rectum. Inflammatory, luminal obstructing lesions or impaired motility/compliance of the rectum or left colon are often accompanied by the clinical symptoms of tenesmus or painful passage of stool and the stool can contain mucus, pus, or blood.[157] Large volume, infrequent, and painless stools suggest normal compliance of the left colon, and rectum and the pathology instead can lie in the small bowel or right colon. Since volume can be difficult for patients to quantify, measured stool volumes can assist in the identification of an underlying pathology. IBS typically produces normal or slightly elevated 24-hour fecal weights[157,158] while those with fecal weights in a 24-hour period of over 1000 g are more likely to have pancreatic cholera syndrome resulting in dehydration and electrolyte disturbances.[157]

Watery Versus Fatty Versus Inflammatory

By characterizing stools as watery, fatty, or inflammatory with simple stool tests, evaluation of the patient with chronic diarrhea can be expedited by limiting the number of conditions that must be considered in the differential diagnosis.[15] Watery diarrhea implies either secretory or osmotic diarrhea. Fatty diarrhea implies defective intraluminal digestion or absorption of fats and often other nutrients in the small intestine and inflammatory diarrhea implies the presence of one of a number of destructive inflammatory, infectious, or neoplastic diseases. Complex overlap of the three primary subgroups of chronic diarrhea can commonly coexist.

EVALUATION

History

A careful medical history is crucial to the evaluation of a patient with diarrhea. Categorizing patients based on historical clues allows for a directed work-up. A checklist for findings in the clinical history is provided in Box 17.2.

An essential clinical feature is the duration of symptoms and volume. Patients with acute diarrhea (<2–4 weeks in duration) should be distinguished from those with chronic diarrhea, in whom the differential diagnosis is much broader. For all cases of diarrhea, the characteristics of the diarrhea should be ascertained. Stool frequency is the easiest characteristic of diarrhea for patients to define but does not necessarily correlate with stool weight. Patients often have a poor notion of stool volume; some persons pass small amounts of stool frequently, but others have less frequent and more voluminous evacuations. Qualitative measures of stool consistency correlate to intestinal transit time[12] and stool frequency.[13] Among patients with self-reported diarrhea, loose, watery stools and urgency are the most common symptoms as compared to a feeling of incomplete evacuation among individuals with alternating diarrhea and constipation.[11]

The pattern of stool passage allows for an anatomical localization of the underlying clinical condition. The presence of small frequent stools with urgency and tenesmus is commonly seen in colitis and distal colonic irritability.[159] Pain, when present, is likely to be in the hypogastrium, in the left or right lower quadrants, or in the sacral region, reflecting the established zones of pain reference from the colon and rectum. The discomfort is usually relieved to some extent by a bowel movement or even the passage of flatus. Conversely, large volume, soupy, pale, or malodorous stool often arises from disorders of the small bowel or proximal colon. When pain accompanies this large volume diarrhea, it is likely to be in the periumbilical region or localized to the right lower quadrant, reference regions of pain from the small intestine and cecum. The pain in such instances is often intermittent, cramp-like and accompanied by borborygmi.

The physician should also ask about the relationship of defecation to meals or fasting, passage of stool during the day versus the night, and the presence of fecal urgency or incontinence. The essential characteristic of osmotic diarrhea is that it resolves with fasting or cessation of ingestion of the offending substance. This characteristic can be used clinically to differentiate osmotic diarrhea from secretory diarrhea, which typically continues with fasting. Nocturnal diarrhea that awakens the patient from sleep strongly suggests an organic rather than a functional disorder, such as IBS. Individuals reporting diarrhea should be asked about the presence of fecal incontinence. If present, especially in the absence of rectal urgency or loose stools, the patient should be evaluated for incontinence and not diarrhea. Impaction of the distal colon and rectum can also lead to incontinence (overflow diarrhea) when the internal anal sphincter relaxes in response to the rectal distention. Impaired anorectal sensation, decreased anal squeeze pressures, reduced integrity of the sphincter and/or pelvic muscles, and neurogenic abnormalities can promote incontinence in the presence of fecal impaction.[160]

Severity of diarrhea can be characterized by the frequency of stool passage or by symptoms of volume depletion, such as dry mouth, increased thirst, headaches, and dizziness upon standing, suggesting dehydration resulting from high intestinal losses. Acute anorexia suggests a serious inflammatory disorder or malignancy as does the presence of fever. Chronic weight loss is a concerning finding associated with the development of malnutrition and requires assessment for IBD, malignancy, chronic infections, and endocrine disorders, such as hyperthyroidism. Other coexisting symptoms, such as abdominal pain, flatulence, bloating or gaseous distention, and cramping, should be noted. Excessive flatus or bloating suggests increased fermentation of carbohydrates by colonic bacteria as a result of the ingestion of poorly absorbable carbohydrates or maldigestion of carbohydrates in the small intestine.

Stool characteristics are important. Blood in the stool signals the possibility of malignancy or IBD, although it is often caused by hemorrhoids in patients with frequent evacuations. In patients with acute infectious diarrhea, visible blood in the stool is highly specific for infection with an invasive organism.[161] Watery stools suggest an osmotic or secretory process, and the presence of oil or food particles is suggestive of malabsorption, maldigestion, or intestinal hurry. The phenomenon of floating stools generally represents an increase in the gas content (carbohydrate malabsorption) rather than the fat content of stools.

Recent foreign travel, particularly to underdeveloped countries, makes the diagnosis of travelers' diarrhea likely. The globalization of commerce has increased the frequency of once exotic infections in those without grossly obvious exposures.[162] The physician should also consider whether the patient lives in a rural or urban environment, the source of the patient's drinking water, and the patient's occupation, sexual history, and use of alcohol or illicit drugs. Potential secondary gains from illness or a history of attempted weight loss and fixation on body image should raise the possibility of laxative abuse.

The past medical history may be important, particularly, in patients with chronic diarrhea. Seronegative spondyloarthropathy may precede the recognition of IBD by many years. A history of diabetes, thyroid disorders, or other autoimmune conditions has a particular pertinence. Because iatrogenic causes of diarrhea (e.g., drugs, previous surgery, and radiation therapy) are common, the health care provider should explore the history for prior abdominal surgeries and ingestion of prescription drugs and over-the-counter remedies, including nutritional and herbal therapies.

The most common syndrome seen after gastric surgery is *dumping syndrome*, characterized by postprandial flushing, hypotension, diarrhea, and hypoglycemia resulting from unregulated gastric emptying, osmotic shifts, and the rapid release of peptide hormones from the intestine.[163] Gastrointestinal surgery may also predispose patients to SIBO, bile acid malabsorption, and pancreatic exocrine insufficiency as a result of poor stimulation of pancreatic secretion and/or inadequate mixing of pancreatic enzymes with intestinal contents.

Pelvic radiation therapy can result in chronic inflammation to the distal small bowel or colon, leading to stricturing disease or impaired compliance resulting in both diarrhea and impaired intestinal transit. In patients with prior surgical resections, the location of surgery, length of resections, and remaining small bowel length/anatomy should be documented. Loss of the ileocecal valve and extensive resections of the ileum (>75–100 cm) result in impaired sodium absorption,[90] electrolyte deficiencies,[164] and fat malabsorption due to depletions in the bile acid pool.[92] Due to the enhanced ability of the ileum to adapt to intestinal resections, extensive resections of the jejunum are better tolerated than loss of ileum and the ileocecal valve with respect to fluid and electrolyte losses.[89]

Drug-induced gastrointestinal injury can affect any part of the gastrointestinal tract, including the mouth,[165] esophagus,[165,166] stomach,[165,167] small intestine,[168] and colon[169] (Box 17.3). Immunosuppressive agents, such as mycophenolate mofetil, calcineurin inhibitors, and chemotherapeutics (cytotoxic, targeted, and biologic), are commonly associated with the occurrence of diarrhea. Diarrhea occurs in over 40% of individuals exposed to combination checkpoint inhibitor therapies for cancer[168] requiring both drug discontinuation and immune suppression to control symptoms. Sprue-like enteropathy has been associated with olmesartan use that was first described in 2012.[170] Drug discontinuation often leads to symptomatic improvement, although parenteral nutrition support may be required in cases of severe malnutrition.

Known therapies that inhibit gastrointestinal digestion are associated with malabsorption and gastrointestinal side effects. By inhibiting α-glucosidase, acarbose reduces carbohydrate absorption and therefore results in abdominal bloating, flatulence, and diarrhea.[168] Microscopic colitis has been associated with prior proton-pump inhibitor use, nonsteroidal anti-inflammatory use, and selective serotonin reuptake inhibitors.[168] Increasingly, therapies are being identified to derive their metabolic benefits and toxicities through alterations in the gut microbiota and bile acid profiles as with the antihyperglycemic agent metformin.[171] Prior antibiotic

BOX 17.3 Medications Associated With Diarrhea

- Acid-reducing agents (e.g., H_2RAs, PPIs)
- Antacids (e.g., those that contain magnesium)
- Antiarrhythmics (e.g., quinidine)
- Antibiotics (most)
- Anti-inflammatory agents (e.g., 5-aminosalicylates, gold salts, ixekizumab, NSAIDs)
- Antihypertensives (e.g., β-adrenergic receptor blocking drugs, olmesartan)
- Antineoplastic agents (many)
- Immune checkpoint inhibitors (e.g., nivolumab, pembrolizumab)
- Antiretroviral agents
- Cholinergic agents
- Colchicine
- Heavy metals
- Herbal products
- Immunosuppresive therapies (e.g. calcineurin inhibitors, mycophenolate)
- Prostaglandin analogs (e.g., misoprostol)
- Theophylline
- Vitamin and mineral supplements

exposures are associated with the development of antibiotic-associated diarrhea, *C. difficile* infection,[172,173] and antibiotic-associated hemorrhagic colitis as a result of *Klebsiella oxytoca* infection.[174]

Family history of any diarrheal disease may be helpful. Hereditary pancreatitis and multiple endocrine neoplasia with medullary carcinoma of the thyroid are autosomal dominantly inherited diseases associated with steatorrhea or diarrhea. The pooled prevalence of celiac disease in first degree family members is 7.5% (95% CI, 6.3%–8.8%).[175] Studies of family history in IBD show a greater proportion of Crohn disease patients have a family history than ulcerative colitis[176] with the most pronounced effect seen in twin studies, where participants have shared genes and similar early life environments. Among monozygotic twins, concordance for IBD is 30%–50% in Crohn disease compared with 15%–18% in ulcerative colitis; concordance rates for dizygotic twins are 2%–6% in Crohn disease and 1%–4% in ulcerative colitis.[177,178] In twin studies, concordance of a diagnosis of IBS is more common in monozygotic twins than in dizygotic twins; however, having a parent with IBS is a strong predictor, suggesting that environmental developmental factors are more important than genetic factors.[179,180]

Specific foods and diets are often incriminated as causes of diarrhea, some with good evidence and others less so.[181,182] A careful dietary history, therefore, is important, particularly in patients with chronic diarrhea. Patients frequently are concerned about how diet may be precipitating or exacerbating symptoms leading to restrictions in diet, placing the patient at risk for malnutrition.[183,184] In assessing these associations with foods, one must consider the following: (1) substances that in excess quantities cause diarrhea in an otherwise normal gut (e.g., fructose); (2) foods or additives that are poorly or not absorbed (e.g., dairy products in lactase deficiency and sugar alcohols); (3) gastrointestinal disorders that limit digestion or absorption of nutrients (e.g., short bowel syndrome and exocrine pancreatic insufficiency); (4) idiosyncratic food intolerances; and (5) true food allergies. Food diaries that record the time and amount of food ingestion and the onset of symptoms may aid in the identification of a dietary cause of diarrhea.

TABLE 17.1 Potential Implications of Physical Findings in Patients With Chronic Diarrhea

Finding	Potential Implication
Orthostasis, hypotension	Dehydration, neuropathy
Muscle wasting, edema	Malnutrition
Urticaria pigmentosa, dermatographism	Mast cell disease (mastocytosis)
Pinch purpura, macroglossia	Amyloidosis
Hyperpigmentation	Addison disease
Migratory necrotizing erythema	Glucagonoma
Flushing	Carcinoid syndrome
Malignant atrophic papulosis	Kohlmeier-Degos disease
Dermatitis herpetiformis	Celiac disease
Thyroid nodule, lymphadenopathy	Medullary carcinoma of the thyroid
Tremor, lid lag	Hyperthyroidism
Oculomasticatory myorhythmia	Whipple disease
Right-sided heart murmur, wheezing	Carcinoid syndrome
Hepatomegaly	Endocrine tumor, amyloidosis
Abdominal bruit	Chronic mesenteric ischemia
Arthritis	IBD, yersiniosis, Whipple disease
Lymphadenopathy	HIV infection, lymphoma, cancer
Anal sphincter weakness	Fecal incontinence

HIV, Human immunodeficiency virus.
From Schiller LR, Pardi DS, Spiller R, et al. Gastro 2013 APDW/WCOG Shanghai Working Party Report. Chronic diarrhea: definition, classification, diagnosis. *J Gastroenterol Hepatol*. 2014;29:6–25.

PHYSICAL EXAMINATION

Physical exam findings are usually more useful in determining the severity of diarrhea than in determining its cause. Characteristic physical findings that should be sought are listed in Table 17.1. The patient's volume status can be assessed by looking for orthostatic changes in blood pressure and pulse. Fever and other signs of toxicity should be noted. A careful abdominal examination is important, with particular attention to the presence or absence of bowel sounds, abdominal bruit, abdominal distention, localized or generalized tenderness, masses, and an enlarged liver. Hyperpigmentation (Whipple disease) and characteristic skin lesions can be identified in IBD (e.g., erythema nodosum or pyoderma gangrenosum) and celiac disease (e.g., blistering and pruritic rash of dermatitis herpetiformis). Clubbing of the fingers can be seen in small intestinal malabsorptive disorders, and detailed examination for the presence of malnutrition includes an assessment of fat loss and muscle mass depletion of the temporalis muscle, deltoids, interosseous muscles, and quadriceps. Presence of a perianal fistula or enlarged "elephant ear" skin tag suggests an underlying IBD, in particular Crohn disease. Rectal examination can assess for rectal masses, impaction, and sphincter tone.[185]

DIFFERENTIAL DIAGNOSIS

As diarrhea is a clinical symptom as opposed to a disease process, the list of conditions manifesting with diarrhea as part of the clinical presentation is broad. From a system-based approach, the underlying causes of diarrhea are numerous: endocrine, allergic, autoinflammatory, medication side effects, neoplastic, vascular, genetic, and postsurgical, and infectious. In considering a differential list of conditions, the time course and presentation should be considered. Early on, diarrhea can be divided into manageable subgroupings—acute, chronic watery, inflammatory, and fatty (Box 17.4). The time course, clinical presentation, and basic studies on the composition of the stool allow for a directed workup aimed at determining the underlying etiology of the clinical symptom.

Acute Diarrhea

Acute diarrhea is defined as lasting less than 2 weeks in duration, although many cases last fewer than 4 days.[186,187] The usual infectious causes of acute diarrhea include viruses, bacteria, protozoa, and multicellular parasites with increased risk for protozoa and helminths in those with an increased duration of symptoms (Box 17.5).[188] Food poisoning as a result of preformed toxins results in a rapid onset of symptoms (between 30 minutes and 16 hours) with symptoms ranging from vomiting to diarrhea.[189] Acute diarrhea as a result of medications often correlates to the onset of medication initiation, although for immunotherapy-related colitis, the onset of symptoms can occur 1–3 months after therapy initiation.[190] Abdominal pain, an urgent need to defecate, and bloody diarrhea are common features of ischemic colitis often occurring within 3 days of clinical presentation and associated with clinical risk factors, such as hypovolemia, cardiac

BOX 17.4 Differential Diagnosis of Diarrhea

ACUTE DIARRHEA

- Infection (see Box 17.5)
  - Bacteria
  - Parasites
  - Protozoa
  - Viruses
- Food allergies
- Food poisoning
- Medications
- Initial presentation of chronic diarrhea

CHRONIC DIARRHEA

Watery

- Osmotic diarrhea
  - Carbohydrate malabsorption
  - Osmotic laxatives (e.g., Mg^{2+}, PO_4^{3-}, SO_4^{2-})
- Secretory diarrhea
  - Bacterial toxins
  - Congenital syndromes (e.g., congenital chloridorrhea)
  - Disordered motility, regulation
    - Diabetic autonomic neuropathy
    - IBS
    - Postsympathectomy diarrhea
    - Postvagotomy diarrhea
  - Diverticulitis
  - Endocrinopathies
    - Addison disease
    - Carcinoid syndrome
    - Gastrinoma
    - Hyperthyroidism
    - Mastocytosis
    - Medullary carcinoma of the thyroid
    - Pheochromocytoma
    - Somatostatinoma
    - VIPoma
  - Idiopathic secretory diarrhea
    - Epidemic secretory (Brainerd) diarrhea
    - Sporadic idiopathic secretory diarrhea
  - Ileal bile acid malabsorption
  - IBD
    - Crohn disease
    - UC
  - Laxative abuse (stimulant laxatives)
  - Medications and toxins
    - Microscopic colitis
    - Collagenous colitis
    - Lymphocytic colitis
  - Neoplasia
    - Colon carcinoma
    - Lymphoma
    - Villous adenoma in rectum
  - Vasculitis

Fatty

- Malabsorption syndromes
  - Mesenteric ischemia
  - Mucosal diseases (e.g., celiac disease and Whipple disease)
  - Short bowel syndrome
  - SIBO
- Maldigestion
  - Inadequate luminal bile acid concentration
  - Pancreatic exocrine insufficiency

Inflammatory

- Diverticulitis
- Infectious diseases
  - Invasive bacterial infections (e.g., tuberculosis and yersiniosis)
  - Invasive parasitic infections (e.g., amebiasis and strongyloidiasis)
  - Pseudomembranous colitis (*Clostridioides difficile* infection)
  - Ulcerating viral infections (e.g., CMV, HSV)
- IBD
  - Crohn disease
  - UC
  - Ulcerative jejunoileitis
- Ischemic colitis
- Neoplasia
  - Colon cancer
  - Lymphoma
- Radiation colitis

arrhythmias, atherosclerosis, or specific associated medications/drug use.[191] Chronic diarrhea initially starts as an acute diarrhea; therefore, basic risk factors specific for acute diarrhea—travel, sexual history, antibiotic exposures, and medication initiation—should be evaluated for all patients presenting with diarrhea before considering etiologies of chronic diarrhea.

Chronic Watery Diarrhea

Chronic watery diarrhea can be subdivided into osmotic and secretory. As osmotic diarrhea results from ingestion of poorly absorbed osmotically active substances, the primary causes include carbohydrate malabsorption (lactose, fructose, and sugar alcohols) and surreptitious magnesium or phosphate containing laxative use. By contrast, chronic secretory diarrhea results from the impaired absorption and/or secretion of fluid and electrolytes. Drugs that enhance intracellular cGMP or cAMP levels (e.g., caffeine, theophylline, and phosphodiesterase 4 inhibitors) or drugs that impair the low intracellular sodium concentrations and electrochemical gradient (e.g., digoxin) can result in diarrhea due to excess secretion or impaired absorption, respectively.[28] Alternatively, cholinergic stimulation for therapeutic purposes (e.g., acetylcholine esterase inhibitors) or in environmental exposures (e.g., organophosphate poisoning) results in acetylcholine-induced intestinal secretion[192] and enhanced gastrointestinal motility[193] resulting in diarrhea.

In addition to medications causing secretory diarrhea, endocrine disorders and neuroendocrine secreting tumors can result in net intestinal secretion. Rare endocrine tumors produce diarrhea, typically by altering electrolyte absorption or speeding intestinal transit. Eight different neoplastic disorders can cause chronic diarrhea attributable to a peptide-mediated diarrhea. These include pancreatic endocrine tumor syndromes (gastrinomas, VIPomas, glucagonomas, somatostatinomas, and pancreatic endocrine tumors secreting calcitonin), carcinoid syndrome, medullary thyroid cancer, and systemic mastocytosis.[60] The rarity of these tumors makes the pretest probability of finding these conditions low, especially in the absence of liver metastases, so screening tests are often falsely positive. Hypercalcemia is a common finding in multiple endocrine neoplasia type 1 (MEN-1), which is one of the four inherited syndromes associated with pancreatic endocrine syndromes (duodenal somatostatinoma in neurofibromatosis-1 and pancreatic endocrine tumors in von Hippel-Lindau, and tuberous sclerosis).[60]

BOX 17.5 Infections that Cause Diarrhea

BACTERIA

Aeromonas spp.
Campylobacter spp.
Clostridioides difficile
Escherichia coli (enterotoxigenic, enteroinvasive, and enterohemorrhagic)
Mycobacterium tuberculosis
Plesiomonas spp.
Salmonella spp.
Shigella spp.
Yersinia spp.

VIRUSES

Adenovirus
Coronavirus
Cytomegalovirus
Norovirus
Rotavirus

PARASITES, PROTOZOA, AND FUNGI

Cryptosporidium spp.
Cyclospora spp.
Entamoeba histolytica
Giardia lamblia
Microsporidia spp.

Relatively common endocrine disturbances like hyperthyroidism can be complicated by chronic secretory diarrhea[194] due to enhanced gastrointestinal transit. Among individuals with longstanding diabetes mellitus, 7%–22% will develop diarrhea attributable to altered motility or impaired fluid absorption[195–197] often associated with fecal incontinence and autonomic neuropathy. Alternative causes of diarrhea to consider in diabetes include the use of sugar-free substitutes in foods or snacks, bacterial overgrowth, celiac disease, and pancreatic insufficiency.[198] Adrenal insufficiency, and in particular aldosterone deficiency, can impair sodium absorption.[199] Other causes of dysmotility contributing to diarrhea include postsympathectomy (e.g., celiac plexus block) diarrhea,[200] amyloidosis, and diarrhea-predominant IBS/functional diarrhea.[201]

The di-hydroxy bile acids (CDCA and DCA) cause colonic secretion of fluid and electrolytes and may stimulate colonic transit if they reach the colon in sufficient concentrations resulting in BAD.[70] Mechanistically, BAD has been divided into four categories related to the underlying pathophysiology. Type 1 BAD results from ileal dysfunction, either secondary to surgical resection or to inflammatory disease of the ileum (e.g., Crohn disease) interrupting the normal enterohepatic circulation of bile acids.[74] Type 2 or "idiopathic" BAD occurs in the setting of a morphologically normal terminal ileum[202] and encompasses the roughly 30% of patients with diarrhea-predominant IBS and/or functional diarrhea with evidence of bile acid malabsorption.[78] Type 3 BAD is a collection of diarrheal diseases that have been attributed to bile acid malabsorption from other gastrointestinal conditions (e.g., celiac disease and enteropathy) or biliopancreatic disease, including cholecystectomy.[202,69] Postcholecystectomy diarrhea may occur in as many as 20% of patients after gallbladder surgery[203,204] and has been attributed to changes in the enterohepatic cycling of bile acids, but evidence in support of this mechanism is limited.[205] A separate category of type 3 (sometimes called type 4) BAD results from excessive bile acid synthesis without a clear source of impaired reabsorption (e.g., metformin use).[69,206] Lastly, a congenital defect of the apical bile salt transporter in the ileum is an extremely rare cause of neonatal diarrhea.[207]

Other tumors cause watery diarrhea by obstructing bowel, blocking lymphatic drainage, interfering with absorption, or causing electrolyte secretion. Examples of such conditions include colon carcinoma (bowel obstruction), retroperitoneal lymphoma (lymphatic obstruction in the small bowel and mesentery), and villous adenomas of the rectum (secretion of a large amount of potassium-rich gelatinous fluid into the lumen). Villous adenomas found more proximally in the colon rarely cause this type of diarrhea.

The last category of chronic watery diarrhea is idiopathic secretory diarrhea, including epidemic secretory diarrhea (also known as *Brainerd diarrhea*) and sporadic idiopathic secretory diarrhea. Both disorders are protracted but self-limited conditions.[208,209]

Fatty Diarrhea

Chronic fatty diarrhea results from maldigestion or malabsorption. Malabsorption syndromes are caused by mucosal diseases, most commonly celiac disease. Rare entities, such as Whipple disease and niacin deficiency,[210] can also produce fatty diarrhea. Short bowel syndrome or postresection diarrhea can also present with this pattern, although if the resection is relatively limited, the diarrhea may be watery secondary to bile acid malabsorption. SIBO causes steatorrhea by deconjugation of bile acids and at times modest villous blunting. Mesenteric ischemia affecting the small intestine may impair intestinal absorption of fat, but weight loss is more often due to postprandial pain resulting in sitophobia (fear of eating). Maldigestion due to pancreatic exocrine insufficiency or inadequate duodenal bile acid concentrations produces steatorrhea. Although fatty, the stools may not be very loose in maldigestive conditions, because in the absence of fat digestion, triglycerides remain intact and have little effect on colonic electrolyte absorption. By contrast, malabsorption in the presence of normal digestion may produce voluminous diarrhea because of the cathartic action of free fatty acids in the colon.

Inflammatory Diarrhea

Chronic inflammatory diarrhea includes infectious, autoimmune, inflammatory, and neoplastic processes. Idiopathic IBD, including ulcerative colitis and Crohn disease, often occurs in a bimodal age distribution with peaks in the ages of 20–29 and 70–79 years.[211] Infections that cause chronic inflammatory diarrhea include bacterial infections (e.g., tuberculosis, yersiniosis, *C. difficile*), viral infections that ulcerate [e.g., cytomegalovirus (CMV) and herpes simplex virus (HSV)], and invasive parasitic infections (e.g., strongyloidiasis, and amebiasis). In immunocompromised persons, a broader range of infectious agents should be considered.[212] Noninfectious diseases that cause chronic inflammatory diarrhea include ischemic colitis and neoplasms (e.g., colon cancer and lymphoma). Although IBD typically produces diarrhea characterized by the presence of blood and pus, other inflammatory diseases without ulceration (e.g., microscopic colitis) may cause diarrhea with the characteristics of chronic secretory diarrhea.

DIAGNOSTIC APPROACH

Acute Diarrhea

Most cases of acute diarrhea result from an infectious disease with a limited time course and often do not come to the attention of a physician. In most cases of acute diarrhea, no testing is needed unless the patient is immunosuppressed or experiences a complication of volume depletion or systemic toxicity. The initial

17

TABLE 17.2 Management of Acute Diarrhea Based on the Patient's Appearance

Appearance of Patient	Treatment and Evaluation
Nontoxic	Symptomatic therapy, rehydration
Toxic	Fluid and electrolyte repletion Complete blood count Abdominal radiograph Serum electrolytes, blood urea nitrogen, serum creatinine Stool tests: culture (if fecal leukocytes are present), ova and parasite examination, *Giardia* and *Cryptosporidium* antigens, *Clostridioides difficile* testing; and/or PCR multiplex panel Sigmoidoscopy or colonoscopy

workup should assess for fever and include an evaluation of volume status and cardiovascular function. A checklist for evaluating patients with acute diarrhea is shown in Table 17.2. A complete blood count can assess for hemoconcentration. Leukocytosis can be present with bacterial infections, particularly those with invasion of the intestinal mucosa.[213,214] Leukopenia can result from an underlying immunodeficiency or be observed in systemic infections with *Salmonella*.[215,216] Lymphopenia can be observed in severe viral infections (e.g., coronavirus and CMV)[217,218] in severe sepsis[219] or acquired immunodeficiency syndrome (AIDS). Measurements of serum electrolyte concentrations and blood urea nitrogen and serum creatinine levels can be used to assess the extent of fluid and electrolyte depletion and its effect on kidney function.

Stool samples should be obtained for an assessment of inflammatory markers. Recent developments have improved on the traditional methods of stool examinations for white blood cells (WBCs) for inflammation and culture for bacterial infections. Microscopic examination for fecal leukocytes aids in the diagnosis of invasive bacterial infections but can be negative in viral causes of diarrhea, cholera, and noninvasive toxigenic *E. coli*.[220] Occult blood testing by guaiac card testing offers similar sensitivity to fecal leukocyte testing[221,161] and has a high negative predictive value in excluding invasive infections.[222] Detection of fecal lactoferrin, an iron-binding protein found in neutrophils, improves the ability to recognize inflammatory diarrhea with higher sensitivity compared to guaiac-based examinations for occult blood.[223–225] Fecal calprotectin, a soluble protein residing in neutrophils, offers the greatest sensitivity for the detection of intestinal inflammation[225,226] and can differentiate bacterial from viral causes of infectious diarrhea.[227] As with any marker of inflammation, no stool test is specific for infection compared to alternative causes of inflammation (e.g., IBD).

Testing for microbial causes of diarrhea traditionally has included conventional bacterial cultures, microscopic examination of stool for ova and parasites, and (rarely) viral cultures. These have been supplemented by enzyme-linked immunosorbent assays for giardiasis and cryptosporidiosis that are more accurate than microscopy.[228] Increasingly, detection of viral, bacterial, and parasitic DNA by multiplex polymerase chain reaction techniques offers the greatest sensitivity for detection of infectious pathogens with improved diagnostic yield and time to diagnosis.[229] Enhanced detection and sensitivity, however, must be balanced with the potential for overdiagnosis resulting from asymptomatic pathogen colonization or persistence of DNA in successfully treated and already cleared infections.[230] Clinical context, presentation, and decision-making are therefore required in the interpretation of the sensitive DNA-based assays. This can be best exemplified by the varying assays for detection of *C. difficile*. Treatment of toxin-negative *C. difficile* infection (detected by nucleic acid amplification techniques) alters the intestinal microbiome and potentially increases the risk of drug-resistant bacterial isolates[231,232] without altering clinical patient outcomes.[233] Therefore specificity of infection by *C. difficile* has been advocated for by the added direct detection of expressed toxin in the stool.[234]

Abdominal x-rays should be performed in toxic-appearing patients to assess for bowel distention, presence of ileus, perforation, or megacolon. Endoscopic examination of the colon by flexible sigmoidoscopy or colonoscopy offers little value in the diagnosis of acute infectious colitis but can be of value in the evaluation of patients that are clearly toxic with infection, those with persistent acute diarrhea, or in the evaluation of an infectious proctitis where the presence of ulcerations may suggest lymphogranuloma venereum, HSV, or syphilis infection. Rectal swab testing for nucleic-acid amplification testing for *Chlamydia trachomatis*, *Neisseria gonorrhoeae*, and HSV can aid in the diagnosis of infectious proctitis. In patients with AIDS-related diarrhea, colonoscopy is preferable because a substantial proportion of infections, and lymphomas may be present only in the right colon,[235] although this approach has been questioned.[236] If sigmoidoscopy or colonoscopy is done, mucosal biopsy specimens should be obtained even if the mucosa does not appear to be grossly inflamed; pathologic examination can identify important clues to facilitate a specific diagnosis.[237] By contrast, biopsy of a normal-appearing terminal ileum is generally unhelpful.

Chronic Diarrhea

Given the broad differential diagnosis of chronic diarrhea, when compared to acute diarrhea, the evaluation is more complex[15,25,238,133,239] and can become costly and cumbersome if not evaluated systematically. The clinician first should reevaluate the history and any prior evaluations and then consider five possibilities: (1) fecal incontinence masquerading as chronic diarrhea; (2) iatrogenic diarrhea due to drugs, surgery, or radiation therapy; (3) chronic infection; (4) IBS with diarrhea; and (5) functional diarrhea (loose stools without pain and in the absence of demonstrated structural or biochemical abnormalities). The first possibility can be excluded with careful history taking and a digital rectal examination. The second possibility can be evaluated by reviewing the patient's medication list and history. The third possibility requires looking for stool pathogens with traditional testing techniques or a multiplex PCR assay to assess for chronic infectious processes, in particular, in individuals with a history of travel, sick contacts, immune suppression, or antibiotic use. The fourth and fifth possibilities are defined by published criteria, normal physical, and rectal examination, the absence of alarm features (age >45 years, nocturnal diarrhea, weight loss >10% over 3 months, rectal bleeding, or family history of colon cancer), and absence of serologic evidence of celiac disease, inflammation (C-reactive protein), and fecal inflammatory markers (e.g., fecal calprotectin)[240,134] (Box 17.6).

The consequences of missing a diagnosis of celiac disease can be serious with the potential for nutritional deficiencies, neurologic sequalae, and an increased risk of gastrointestinal malignancies.[241] Among patients with suspected IBS, the odds of biopsy-proven celiac disease are over four times higher compared to healthy controls.[242] Serologic evaluation includes a quantitative assessment of serum immunoglobulin A (IgA) to identify individuals with concomitant IgA deficiency and serum IgA anti–tissue transglutaminase (TTG) antibodies due to their high sensitivity (94%) and specificity (97%). Among individuals with IgA deficiency, IgG anti-TTG antibodies or deamidated gliadin peptide antibodies of the IgG class can be measured due to their slightly better sensitivity and specificity. Antiendomysial IgA antibodies have nearly 100% specificity and are used as a confirmatory test in individuals with borderline positive or potentially false-positive anti-TTG antibodies. Testing for HLA-DQ2 and HLA-DQ8 risk alleles has a high negative predictive value and is useful in at risk-persons, such as those with a family history of celiac disease.[243]

Additional factors that suggest a diagnosis of IBS include a long history of symptoms, passage of mucus, and exacerbation of symptoms by stress. If patients meet criteria and have no alarm features, they are unlikely to have structural disease but may have one of the following three treatable conditions often overlapping with IBS and functional diarrhea: food intolerances, BAD, or SIBO[133] (Table 17.3). Emerging diagnostic tests or therapeutic trials with elimination diets, bile acid-binding agents, or antibiotics can identify these problems.

In the absence of alarm features but severe, complicated, persistent, or refractory diarrhea, the next level of evaluation often includes an endoscopic assessment. Most patients with chronic diarrhea who reach this point in their evaluation without a diagnosis will need colonoscopy with examination of the ileum and cross-sectional abdominal imaging with CT or MRI (with preferred enterography techniques). These tests can identify or exclude IBD, microscopic colitis, ischemic colitis, cancer, and pancreatic disorders. Colonoscopy has the highest diagnostic yield, leading to a diagnosis in up to 30% of patients referred for chronic diarrhea.[244] In the setting of endoscopically normal tissue, random biopsies should be obtained from several locations in the colon to give the pathologist the best chance of making a diagnosis.[245] Diseases in which the colonic mucosa appears normal endoscopically, but which can be diagnosed histologically, include microscopic colitis (lymphocytic and collagenous colitis), amyloidosis, granulomatous infections, and schistosomiasis.

Although esophagogastroduodenoscopy (EGD) often is done as part of the evaluation of chronic diarrhea, no studies have documented its diagnostic yield in the absence of markers of celiac disease or steatorrhea. Visualization and biopsy of the mucosa of the small bowel by EGD or enteroscopy can be valuable, but whether push enteroscopy adds much to standard EGD for evaluating for small bowel diseases is uncertain.[246] Diseases that can be detected by small intestinal biopsy include celiac disease, Crohn disease, giardiasis, intestinal lymphoma, eosinophilic gastroenteritis, tropical sprue, Whipple disease, lymphangiectasia, abetalipoproteinemia, amyloidosis, mastocytosis, and several infectious processes. The role of wireless capsule endoscopy in the diagnosis of diarrhea caused by small bowel disease is limited. One retrospective review demonstrated a positive diagnostic yield of 42.9%, but most findings were of uncertain importance.[247] Guidelines for the use of video capsule endoscopy recommend against employing this technique in the evaluation of chronic diarrhea unless Crohn disease is suspected.[248]

If no diagnosis is apparent at this point in the evaluation, further chemical analysis of stool can be used to categorize the diarrhea as watery, inflammatory, or fatty. In the setting of severe diarrhea, malnutrition, dehydration/volume depletion, or electrolyte abnormalities, inpatient evaluation may be necessary allowing for adequate parenteral volume replacement and electrolyte monitoring. Absent these features, outpatient stool collections can be performed.

Stool analyses can be obtained on a random or timed (24-, 48-, or 72-hour) stool collection, although the necessary duration of the timed collection has not been defined for clinical purposes.[157] The benefits of a timed collection include the ability to analyze diet over the course of the timed study as well as obtain a stool weight allowing for accurate measures of total output and stool components, such as fat and bile acids. Stool volume may clarify the degree of the patient's diarrhea and can help localize the potential cause of the diarrhea. Stool volumes over 500 mL/day are rarely seen in individuals with IBS[249,158] and stool volumes over 1000 mL/day are suggestive of pancreatic cholera syndrome. In microscopic colitis, the typical stool weights of 500–1000 g/24 hours are consistent with little or no fluid absorption by the colon. Additionally, the presence of very large volumes will alert the physician for the potential need for intravenous hydration support.

BOX 17.6 Basic Laboratory Tests to Consider in Patients With Chronic Diarrhea

BLOOD TESTS

CBC
Comprehensive metabolic profile
IgA tissue transglutaminase antibody, IgA level
C-reactive protein

STOOL TESTS

Fecal occult blood test
Fecal leukocytes (Wright stain) or fecal calprotectin or lactoferrin
Bacterial culture, ova and parasite examination, and giardia and *Cryptosporidium* antigens or multiplex PCR testing
Qualitative or quantitative stool fat

TABLE 17.3 Differential Diagnosis of IBS With Diarrhea (IBS-D)

Diagnosis	Estimated Prevalence in IBS-D (%)	Diagnostic Strategy
Food intolerances	20–67	Diet and symptom diary → exclusion diet
Postinfection IBS	28–58	Anticytolethal distending toxin B and antivinculin antibody assays
SIBO	23–45	Quantitative culture of small intestinal aspirate, breath hydrogen testing; trial of antibiotic therapy
Bile acid malabsorption	10–40	^{75}SeHCAT retention, C4 or FGF19 assay; trial of bile acid sequestrant
Microscopic colitis	5–10	Colon biopsies (from above rectum)
Celiac disease	0.4–4	IgA tissue transglutaminase antibody and total IgA assays; duodenal biopsy
Pancreatic exocrine insufficiency	Unknown	Fecal elastase-1 concentration; trial of pancreatic enzyme replacement
Rapid or slow intestinal transit	Unknown	Scintigraphic or capsule-based transit study

C4, 7α-hydroxy-4-cholesten-3-one; *FGF19*, fibroblast growth factor 19; *IgA*, immunoglobulin A; ^{75}*SeHCAT*, ^{75}selenium-labeled homotaurocholic acid.
From Schiller LR. Evaluation of chronic diarrhea and irritable bowel syndrome with diarrhea in adults in the era of precision medicine. *Am J Gastroenterol.* 2018;113:660–669.

For quantitative stool collections, necessary equipment includes preweighed collection containers with airtight lids (often holding 1–2 L per container), disposable collection units that allow separation of stool, and urine and a receptacle to keep the collection containers cold during the collection period with ice packs. Prior to and during the collection period, it is helpful to have the patient record their oral food and liquid intake to allow for an estimation of calories and grams of fat, carbohydrate, and/or fiber. It is encouraged, but not required, to have an estimation of fat intake during the course of the collection study. Patients should be encouraged to eat three regular meals of moderately high fat content per day (80–100 g of fat per day) for 2 days prior to the stool collection and continue the high fat diet throughout the collection period. Diet examples and sample menus are helpful if provided to the patient. Fecal fat output can be adjusted for intake by calculating output as a percentage of intake (coefficient of fat absorption). During the course of the collection, other diagnostic tests that would alter the normal course of eating (e.g., breath tests or enteral contrast media) should be avoided as should the use of antidiarrheal medications. For most patients with diarrhea, a 48-hour collection is sufficient. If stool output is not representative during that time, the collection can be extended. In special instances, stool collections can be continued during a 48-hour fast; if the diarrhea is caused by an ingested substance, fasting should abolish the diarrhea. Persistence of diarrhea during fasting is a criterion for secretory diarrhea.[250,157]

Full analysis of a stool collection includes the measurement of stool weight, fat content, osmolality, electrolytes, pH, occult blood/inflammatory markers and when appropriate studies of pancreatic function and laxative screens. If these tests cannot be performed locally, representative aliquots of the homogenized stool collection can be taken, frozen, and sent to reference clinical laboratories. Fecal electrolytes, osmolality, and pH are obtained after homogenization of the stool collection and centrifugation, allowing for the collection of the supernatant (stool water) for analysis.

In the absence of a timed collection, the assessment of stool characteristics on a random, or "spot" collection still provides many clues to the correct diagnosis. These assessments include stool electrolyte concentrations, pH, a fecal occult blood test, and an examination of stool for WBCs or a test for the presence of a surrogate inflammatory marker, such as fecal calprotectin or lactoferrin.[251–253] In appropriate circumstances, stool samples can also be analyzed for fat content and laxatives.

Electrolytes and Calculation of an Osmotic Gap

Measurement of stool sodium and potassium concentrations allows calculation of an osmotic gap in stool water. The *fecal osmotic gap* is calculated by subtracting twice the sum of the sodium and potassium concentrations from 290 mOsm/kg, the osmolality of stool in the body.[37] A small osmotic gap (<50 mOsm/kg) signifies that the osmolality of stool water is due mostly to incompletely absorbed, or excessively secreted electrolytes, which is characteristic of secretory diarrhea (Fig. 17.3). A large gap (>100 mOsm/kg) is characteristic of an osmotic diarrhea, usually resulting from ingestion of some poorly absorbed substance like magnesium salts or nonelectrolytes that retain water in the stool. When the sum of sodium and potassium concentrations doubled is higher than 290 mOsm/kg, ingestion of a poorly absorbed multivalent anion (e.g., phosphate and sulfate) is likely.[37] The negative osmotic gap is the result of an excess of cations obligated by the multivalent anions. The osmolality of the stool in the distal intestine (estimated as 290 mOsm/kg because it equilibrates with plasma osmolality) should be used for the calculation as opposed to the measured osmolality as the stool osmolality increases in the collection container when carbohydrates are converted to active organic acids by bacterial fermentation.[39,157] In mixed cases of secretory and osmotic diarrhea and in cases of modest carbohydrate malabsorption (in which case the converted organic acids obligate the fecal excretion of sodium and potassium), the osmotic gap may lie between 50 and 125 mOsm/kg.[157]

Measured Osmolality

Measured fecal osmolality should not be used for calculation of the osmotic gap as values >290 mOsm/kg are commonly seen as a result of bacterial fermentation (up to 600 mOsm/kg).[157] A low measured osmolality, however, can be useful in patients with unexplained diarrhea as it can indicate the contamination of stool with water or dilute urine,[254] a fistula to a bladder urine reservoir, or the presence of a gastrocolic fistula with ingestion of hypotonic fluids. Excessively high osmolality can be observed with ingestion of poorly absorbable carbohydrates or dietary fiber, fecal contamination with concentrated urine, or a gastrocolic fistula with intake of hypertonic fluids.[157]

Fecal pH

The pH of stool water provides useful information about the possibility of carbohydrate malabsorption.[37,39] Carbohydrate that reaches the colon is promptly fermented by the bacterial flora, with the release of CO_2 and H_2 gases and short-chain fatty acids. As a result of fermentation, the pH is acidic, usually dropping to less than 6, a finding that indirectly indicates excess carbohydrate fermentation in the colon. In experimentally induced diarrhea (with lactulose or sorbitol), the fecal fluid pH was always <5.6 and usually <5.3.[37] In generalized malabsorption, including

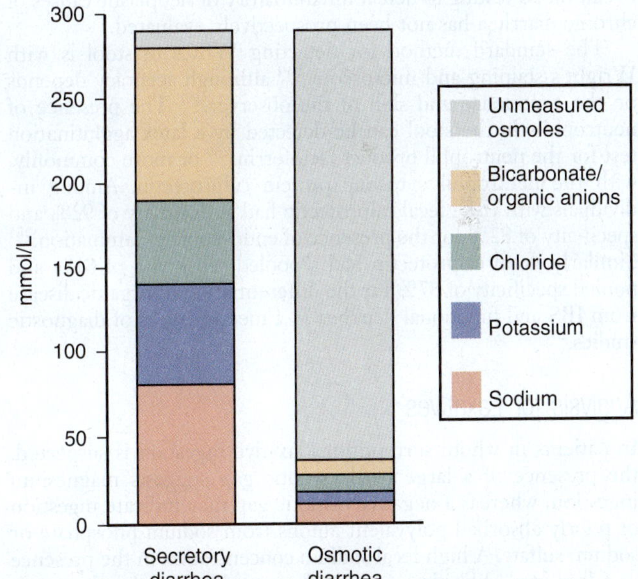

Fig. 17.3 Fecal electrolytes and the fecal osmotic gap. The osmolality of colonic fluid and body fluids is in equilibrium and is approximately 290 mOsm/kg. Total concentration of electrolytes, therefore, cannot exceed 290 mmol/L. In secretory diarrhea, almost all the osmotic activity of colonic contents is caused by electrolytes, so the estimate of electrolyte content by the formula 2 × ($[Na^+] + [K^+]$) is approximately 290 mmol/L. In osmotic diarrhea, electrolytes account for only a small part of the osmotic activity; unmeasured osmoles resulting from ingestion of a poorly absorbed substance account for most of the osmotic activity, and the calculated osmotic gap will be high. (From Schiller LR. Chronic diarrhea. In: McNally P, ed. *GI/Liver Secrets*. 2nd ed. Philadelphia: Hanley & Belfus; 2001:411.)

carbohydrates, amino acids, and fatty acids, the fecal pH is usually higher (e.g., 6.0–7.5).[157]

Fecal Fat Concentration and Output

Stool fat output can be measured quantitatively by nuclear MR spectroscopy on a timed (48- to 72-hour) collection[255] or estimated by use of a Sudan stain on a random specimen. Sudan staining can be performed on a sample of homogenized stool using a dedicated approach of counting the size and number of fat globules. This approach can detect steatorrheas with 94% sensitivity and 95% specificity with a good correlation with quantitative fat excretion.[256] However, a high level of observer skill and experience is critical to the accuracy of the microscopic interpretation.[157]

Steatorrhea is formally defined as excessive loss of fat in the stool in a timed collection (>7 g or >9% of intake for 24 hours), but this definition may not be valid for the diagnosis of fat malabsorption or maldigestion in all patients with chronic diarrhea. In a study of subjects with experimentally induced diarrhea, 35% of normal subjects had fecal fat excretion above the upper limit of normal, with values as high as 13.6 g/day.[157,257] Therefore, in patients with diarrhea, an abnormal fecal fat value of 7–14 g/24 hours has a low specificity for the diagnosis of defective fat absorption. However, fat excretion over 14 g/24 hours strongly indicates a disorder of fat digestion or absorption.[257]

Occult Blood/White Blood Cells

Fecal occult blood testing and examination of stool for leukocytes allow for identification of an inflammatory diarrhea. Diarrheal conditions that cause occult bleeding include lymphoma of the small intestine and celiac disease.[258] However, the role of fecal occult blood testing to detect inflammatory or neoplastic causes of chronic diarrhea has not been prospectively evaluated.

The standard method for detecting WBCs in stool is with Wright's staining and microscopy,[259] although accuracy depends on the experience and skill of the observer.[157] The presence of neutrophils in the stool can be detected by a latex agglutination test for the neutrophil product lactoferrin,[260] or more commonly, with the neutrophil cytosolic protein calprotectin. Among individuals with IBD, fecal calprotectin had a sensitivity of 92% and specificity of 82% for the presence of endoscopic inflammation.[261] Similarly, fecal calprotectin had a pooled sensitivity of 81% and pooled specificity of 87% for the differentiation of organic disease from IBS and functional diarrhea in a meta-analysis of diagnostic studies.[262]

Analysis for Laxatives

In patients in whom surreptitious laxative ingestion is suspected, the presence of a large fecal osmotic gap suggests magnesium ingestion, whereas a negative osmotic gap may indicate ingestion of poorly absorbed polyvalent anions from sodium phosphate or sodium sulfate. A high fecal sodium concentration in the presence of a low fecal chloride concentration should also raise the suspicion of ingestion of sodium sulfate or sodium phosphate.[157] Stool water can also be analyzed for laxatives by chemical or chromatographic methods, although reference centers performing such studies for bisacodyl and its metabolites and anthraquinone derivatives are increasingly limited.

Because some patients exaggerate stool volume by adding urine or water, stool osmolality should be measured as well; a value lower than 290 mOsm/kg suggests dilution of the stool with water or hypotonic urine. Admixture of stool with hypertonic urine often leads to an impossibly high fecal osmolality (typically >600 mOsm/kg) and to a negative fecal osmotic gap because of high concentrations of sodium and potassium in the urine ($Na^+ + K^+ > 165$). Stool water measurements for creatinine and urea can aide in the detection of urine contaminating the stool collection.[157]

Analysis for Protein-Losing Enteropathy

Protein-losing enteropathy should be considered when a patient has hypoalbuminemia without a diagnosis of nephrotic syndrome or hepatic dysfunction[157] and should not be considered part of a routine evaluation in a patient with chronic diarrhea. Enteric protein losses can be detected by the measurement of the fecal clearance of α_1-antitrypsin. A radioimmunoassay is used to measure α_1-antitrypsin concentrations in the stool and plasma, and total fecal output is determined from a timed stool collection and the reported α_1-antitrypsin concentration. This is divided by the plasma concentration establishing a clearance in mL per day of protein.[263] On average, the serum albumin falls to <3.0 g/dL when the α_1-antitrypsin clearance exceeds 180 mL/day.[263]

Once stool analysis is completed, chronic diarrhea can be categorized as watery (with subtypes of secretory or osmotic diarrhea), inflammatory, or fatty to help further differentiate its cause. A retrospective review of a series of stool analyses done at a tertiary referral center showed findings clustered into 10 groups that have diagnostic significance (Table 17.4).[19]

Chronic Secretory Diarrhea

Secretory diarrhea has a broad differential diagnosis, and a wide investigative net must be cast to identify a specific cause (Box 17.7). At this point of the investigation, gastrointestinal infection and risk factors for chronic infections, such as immunosuppression or human immunodeficiency virus, should be elucidated. Although most bacteria that cause diarrhea are cleared spontaneously within 4 weeks, some organisms (e.g., *Aeromonas* spp., *Plesiomonas*) may produce a chronic diarrhea,[264] although it should be noted that these agents can also be isolated from the stools of healthy individuals. Special microbiological techniques are required to find pathogens like coccidia and microsporidia.[265] Increasingly, multiplex PCR techniques have the ability to simultaneously detect bacterial, viral, and parasitic causes of diarrhea,[266] although concerns exist over the potential for false positive testing based on the highly sensitive nature of the DNA-based test. Examination of a mucosal biopsy allows for detection of *Tropheryma whippelii* (by PCR), the agent of Whipple disease, or CMV (based on special stains or PCR).

Few secretory causes of chronic watery diarrhea require colonoscopy for diagnosis that would not otherwise be evident from the clinical history. SIBO may result in secretory diarrhea, presumably caused by bacterial toxins, as well as a fatty diarrhea caused by bile salt deconjugation or villous blunting.

Microscopic colitis, including lymphocytic colitis and collagenous colitis, is a common cause of watery secretory diarrhea, particularly among middle-aged females with associations with autoimmune conditions, smoking, and nonsteroidal anti-inflammatory medication use.[267,268] While mucosal inflammation is present, traditional markers of inflammation, such as lactoferrin, are often absent,[269] although emerging data suggests mild increases in fecal calprotectin may be present.[270] Mechanistically, colonic perfusion studies have shown that absorption of water and salt is impaired in lymphocytic colitis and collagenous colitis,[79] leading to a secretory diarrhea.[271] While net secretion of water and salt by the colon is not noted frequently, in vitro studies using human colon specimens have demonstrated decreases in sodium chloride absorption accompanied by changes in diffusion and the function of tight junctions.[272]

The clinical diagnosis of BAD is problematic. The gold-standard diagnosis assesses for the retention of a radiolabeled orally administered conjugated bile acid analog (^{75}selenium-labeled

TABLE 17.4 Implications of Stool Characteristics in Patients With Chronic Diarrhea

Characteristic	Implications
Stool weight ≤200 g/24 hours	
No objective evidence of diarrhea	Change in stool frequency, intermittent diarrhea, fecal incontinence, treatment with antidiarrheal drugs during collection
Hyperdefecation (increased frequency without excess volume)	Possible IBS, proctitis, abnormal rectal reservoir function
Abnormal consistency (unformed to runny stools)	Possible IBS
Elevated fecal osmotic gap	Presumed mild carbohydrate malabsorption or excess Mg intake from supplements
Steatorrhea	Malabsorption or maldigestion
Stool weight >200 g/24 hours	
Secretory diarrhea without steatorrhea	Microscopic colitis or other cause of secretory diarrhea
Carbohydrate malabsorption without steatorrhea	Ingestion of poorly absorbed carbohydrates, malabsorption
Steatorrhea with or without carbohydrate malabsorption	Small bowel mucosal disease, SIBO, bile acid deficiency, pancreatic insufficiency
Osmotic diarrhea	Ingestion of poorly absorbed ions (e.g., magnesium, phosphate, sulfate) or osmotically active polymers (e.g., polyethylene glycol)
Unclassified	Blood or pus suggests an inflammatory cause of diarrhea

From Steffer KJ, Santa Ana CA, Cole JA, et al. The practical value of comprehensive stool analysis in detecting the cause of idiopathic chronic diarrhea. *Gastroenterol Clin North Am*. 2012;41:539–560.

homotauro CA) after 7 days. A retention value of <10%–15% is usually considered diagnostic with lower values signifying less bile acid retention.[273,274] When strict diagnostic criteria are used (<5%–10% retention at 1 week), the test can predict responsiveness to bile acid–binding drugs.[15,275] The test is limited by the fact that diarrhea itself can make the test abnormal[276] and its availability only outside of the United States.

Outside of the ^{75}selenium-labeled homotauro CA test (^{75}SeHCAT), a bile acid profile can be performed on a quantitative 48-hour stool collection on a high fat diet (100 g/day). Interestingly, there appears to be an increase in primary bile acids in BAD, which suggests that there is less bacterial deconjugation of endogenous bile acids, perhaps related to rapid transit in the colon.[277] Total and primary fecal bile acid levels have significant associations with ^{75}SeHCAT retention[278,279] as well as associations with stool weight, frequency, and consistency.[280–282] Three criteria can be used for a diagnosis of BAD: total fecal bile acids >2337 μmol/48 hours, primary bile acids >10%, or total fecal bile acids >1000 μmol/48 hours with a primary bile acid profile >4%.[91,277,283,69]

Alternatively, in place of quantitative stool collections, serum fasting levels of 7α-hydroxy-4-cholesten-3-one (7αC4) can be measured as an indirect measure of bile acid synthesis. Morning serum samples have been validated against the ^{75}SeHCAT (cut-off value >48.4 ng/mL; sensitivity 90% and specificity 79%)[284] and against a 48-hour fecal collection for total bile acids (cut-off value >52.5 ng/mL; sensitivity 25% and specificity 90%).[285,69] Similarly, a serum fasting level of FGF-19 is inversely related to 7αC4[283] and a level <145 pg/mL had a sensitivity of 58% and specificity of 84% against a ^{75}SeHCAT (<10% retention).[286] Given the low sensitivities, serum tests have an inability to act as stand-alone tests for the diagnosis of BAD, and responsiveness to bile acid binders remains to be fully determined.[275]

In most clinical situations, an empirical trial of a bile acid sequestering resin may be the best way of establishing the diagnosis of BAD. The dose and timing of administration may be critical but need to be assessed scientifically. Unlike the use of bile acid sequestrants in hypercholesterolemia, where the sequestration of bile acid needs to occur in the proximal small intestine when bile acids are present postprandially, in BAD, bile acids need to be bound in the colon, so it makes sense to give the bile acid binders at bedtime and away from meals. A clinical response suggests that BAD may be playing a role.

Diarrhea caused by a peptide-secreting tumor is an intellectually interesting form of chronic watery diarrhea that is quite rare. The pretest probability of having a peptide-secreting tumor in a patient with chronic diarrhea is so low that screening these patients with a panel of serum peptide levels is far more likely to produce a false-positive than a true-positive result.[287] Testing should be limited to those patients with chronic diarrhea with symptoms and signs consistent with a tumor syndrome (e.g., flushing or a large, hard liver in carcinoid syndrome, or CT demonstrating tumor).[58,288] In carcinoid syndrome, elevated serotonin is detected by measuring plasma or urine 5-hydroxyindoleacetic acid (5-HIAA), the major metabolite of serotonin. Measurement of 5-HIAA is preferred over serotonin, as the interpretation of serotonin levels may be challenging owing to fluctuation.[289] ZES is supported by a serum gastrin >1000 pg/mL in the setting of a gastric pH < 3.[289] Cross-sectional imaging using somatostatin receptor radioligands with positron emission

BOX 17.7 Diagnostic Approach to the Patient With Chronic Secretory Diarrhea

EXCLUSION OF INFECTION

Bacterial cultures ("standard" enteric pathogens, *Aeromonas*, *Plesiomonas*)

Tests for other pathogens (microscopy for ova and parasites, *Giardia* and *Cryptosporidium* antigens, special techniques for *Cyclospora*, coccidia, microsporidia), and/or multiplex PCR assay

EXCLUSION OF STRUCTURAL DISEASE

CT or MRI of abdomen and pelvis

Sigmoidoscopy or colonoscopy with mucosal biopsies

Small bowel mucosal biopsy and aspirate for quantitative culture

Capsule enteroscopy

SELECTIVE TESTING

Plasma peptides: calcitonin, chromogranin A, gastrin, somatostatin, vasoactive intestinal polypeptide

Urine autacoids and metabolites: histamine, 5-hydroxyindoleacetic acid, metanephrines

Other tests: ACTH stimulation, immunoglobulins, serum protein electrophoresis, TSH

EMPIRICAL TRIALS

Food exclusion diets (e.g., low-FODMAP diet)

Bile acid–binding agent

Antibiotic for SIBO

tomography can also be used to identify a peptide-secreting tumor.[290] Plasma chromogranin, a secretory protein from neuroendocrine cells, is an ineffective diagnostic test for neuroendocrine tumors given lack of specificity and elevations in cardiac, renal, and inflammatory conditions, as well as with acid-suppressive therapy.[291] The clonal accumulation of mast cells in systemic mastocytosis is supported by elevations in serum tryptase, urine histamine, or endoscopic biopsy showing mast cell infiltrates.[289]

More common endocrinologic diseases that cause diarrhea are diabetes mellitus, hyperthyroidism, and Addison disease. In many cases, other symptoms and signs, such as an enlarged thyroid or skin pigmentation characteristic of Addison disease, suggest the presence of these conditions.[112] Blood glucose, thyroid-stimulating hormone, and serum cortisol levels before and after injection of an ACTH analog should be measured selectively in these patients.

Other blood tests that may be relevant in evaluating secretory diarrhea include serum protein electrophoresis and immunoglobulin electrophoresis. Selective IgA deficiency may present with recurrent intestinal infections, such as giardiasis, whereas combined variable immune deficiency can be associated with both colonic inflammation and small bowel enteropathy, mimicking celiac disease.[292]

Chronic Osmotic Diarrhea

Osmotic diarrhea has a more limited differential diagnosis compared to secretory diarrhea, and therefore its evaluation is more straightforward (Box 17.8). For practical purposes, osmotic diarrhea is a result of: (1) ingestion of osmotic laxatives (e.g., magnesium salts, phosphate salts, sulfate salts, or polyethylene glycol) or (2) consumption of poorly absorbed carbohydrates. Ingestion of other osmotically active substances is unusual.

Osmotic laxatives can be measured directly in stool water by chemical tests.[38] Excretion of more than 15 mmol (30 mEq) of magnesium daily or concentrations in stool water of more than 44 mmol/L (90 mEq/L) strongly suggests magnesium-induced diarrhea. Phosphate excretion of more than 15 mmol/day or concentrations of more than 33 mmol/L is suspicious for phosphate-induced diarrhea.[293] The laxative ingestion may be intentional, as in a patient with surreptitious laxative ingestion, or accidental, as in a patient who uses magnesium-containing antacids or mineral supplements.

Ingestion of poorly absorbed carbohydrates or carbohydrate malabsorption typically leads to a low fecal pH because of bacterial fermentation in the colon. A fecal pH lower than 6 is highly suggestive of carbohydrate malabsorption.[37,39] Isolated carbohydrate malabsorption is usually due to ingestion of a poorly absorbable carbohydrate, such as lactose in a person with lactase deficiency. Other common causes include ingestion of poorly absorbed sugar alcohols that are used as artificial sweeteners (e.g., sorbitol and mannitol) or excessive ingestion of sugars with a limited absorption capacity (e.g., fructose).[294]

Breath hydrogen tests can be used to implicate specific carbohydrates, including lactose and fructose.[295,296] In these tests, a previously fasting patient ingests a fixed dose of carbohydrate dissolved in water, and exhaled breath is assayed for hydrogen content at baseline and at intervals for several hours. Because hydrogen is not a normal product of human metabolism, any increase in breath hydrogen concentration is the result of bacterial fermentation and indicates that unabsorbed carbohydrate has reached an area with high concentrations of intraluminal bacteria, typically the colon.

Once the clinical picture or stool analysis suggests carbohydrate malabsorption, a careful review of the patient's diet may indicate the likely source. Once a specific cause of osmotic diarrhea has been postulated, a therapeutic trial of an elimination diet can often confirm the diagnosis.

BOX 17.8 Diagnostic Approach to the Patient With Osmotic Diarrhea

- Measurement of fecal osmotic gap; if elevated (>50 mosm/kg):
  - Stool magnesium output
  - Stool polyethylene glycol output
- Measurement of fecal osmotic gap; if negative (<0 mosm/kg):
  - Stool phosphorus, sulfate output
- Determination of stool pH; if <6 (consistent with carbohydrate malabsorption):
  - Diet review
  - Breath hydrogen test with lactose; mucosal lactase assay if available
  - Measurement of stool-reducing substances; anthrone reaction

BOX 17.9 Diagnostic Approach to the Patient With Chronic Fatty Diarrhea

EXCLUSION OF STRUCTURAL DISEASE

- CT or MRI of abdomen and pelvis
- Small bowel biopsy and aspirate for quantitative culture

EXCLUSION OF PANCREATIC EXOCRINE INSUFFICIENCY

- Empirical trial of pancreatic enzyme replacement therapy
- Stool elastase or chymotrypsin concentration
- Secretin test

EXCLUSION OF DUODENAL BILE ACID DEFICIENCY

- Empirical trial of bile acid replacement therapy
- Postprandial duodenal aspirate for bile acid concentration

Chronic Fatty Diarrhea

Steatorrhea implies the disruption of fat solubilization, digestion, or absorption in the small intestine. Evaluation of chronic fatty diarrhea is designed to distinguish maldigestion (inadequate luminal breakdown of triglycerides) from malabsorption (inadequate mucosal transport of the products of digestion) (Box 17.9).

The major causes of maldigestion are pancreatic exocrine insufficiency (e.g., chronic pancreatitis) and lack of intraluminal bile acids (e.g., advanced primary biliary cholangitis, extensive ileal resections). Mucosal diseases (e.g., celiac disease) and reduced mucosal surface area (e.g., short bowel syndrome) are common causes of fat malabsorption.

The absolute amount of steatorrhea and the fecal fat concentration (grams of fat/100 g of stool) provide clues to the cause of steatorrhea.[297] The degree of steatorrhea tends to be higher (often >30 g fat/day) with maldigestion than with mucosal diseases (other than extensive small bowel resections) because of the greater disruption of fat assimilation. Fecal fat concentration tends to be higher with maldigestion when compared to mucosal disorders because fluid and electrolyte absorption may also be defective with mucosal disorders, and stool fat content is then diluted by unabsorbed water. Fat digestion is also usually intact in mucosal disorders, so triglycerides are hydrolyzed to free fatty acids that can inhibit colonic electrolyte and water absorption, further diluting the fat content of stool.[84] By contrast, triglyceride hydrolysis, which is reduced in maldigestion, does not result in fatty acid–mediated inhibition of fluid and electrolyte transport in the colon, so in maldigestion, unabsorbed fat is dispersed in a smaller stool volume and is thus more concentrated. A fecal fat concentration over 9.5 g/100 g strongly suggests a pancreatic or biliary cause of steatorrhea.

Further evaluation of patients with chronic fatty diarrhea is relatively straightforward. The first step is to assess for a structural problem involving the small bowel or pancreas. Structural disorders of the small bowel, including diverticula (predisposing to SIBO), can be best seen using small bowel radiography or cross-sectional imaging of the small bowel. Small bowel imaging can further suggest a mucosal disorder of the small bowel as in jejunoileal fold pattern reversal in celiac disease[298] or abnormal small bowel folds showing a "hide-bound" appearance in scleroderma.[299] Unaugmented small bowel follow-through can also aide in the determination of the small bowel transit time that can be helpful in the evaluation of extensive small bowel resections.[300]

Small intestinal biopsies are required for the detection of villous blunting that can be seen in celiac disease, SIBO, malnutrition, common variable immune deficiency, tropical sprue, and drug-induced enteropathy. Adequate biopsies from the duodenal bulb and postbulbar duodenum are recommended for evaluation of mucosal disorders.[301] Because celiac disease is the most common cause of mucosal disease that leads to malabsorption, TTG antibodies should be determined with an appropriate immunoglobulin level assessment.[302,303]

When a small bowel biopsy is performed, luminal contents can also be aspirated and a sample sent for quantitative culture to exclude SIBO in select clinical centers. Given the lack of availability of quantitative culture, breath hydrogen testing has been adapted to detect SIBO with the use of glucose, a substrate that ordinarily should be absorbed completely before reaching the colon.[295,296] Lactulose, a nonabsorbable but easily fermented disaccharide, has also been used to detect SIBO, but because of the wide variability of intestinal transit time, use of lactulose for this purpose is problematic.[296,367] Lactulose can be used as a substrate for determining the oral-cecal transit time. For most purposes, breath hydrogen testing provides only supportive evidence when the pretest likelihood of a particular diagnosis is high.

Initial cross-sectional imaging with an abdominal computed tomography scan is widely accepted as the first-line imaging modality of choice when investigating an individual with clinical suspicion of chronic pancreatitis.[304] If suggested by history, MR cholangiopancreatography with or without secretin stimulation allows for more subtle detection of pancreatic ductal irregularities[304] and more advanced imaging techniques by endoscopic ultrasound may further play a future role in the assessment of early chronic pancreatitis.[305]

If no intestinal abnormalities are discovered or if imaging evidence of chronic pancreatitis is detected, pancreatic exocrine insufficiency should be considered.[306] Available tests of pancreatic function in general all have limitations. The secretin stimulation test, in which exogenous secretin is used to stimulate the pancreas and bicarbonate output is measured by aspiration of duodenal contents, is the most time-honored of these tests but is rarely performed because of its complexity.[307] Determination of pancreatic enzyme concentrations in stool has been advocated as a simpler screening test for pancreatic exocrine insufficiency. Direct measurement of stool chymotrypsin activity has poor sensitivity and specificity in patients with chronic diarrhea.[308] Evaluation of pancreatic elastase had a clinical sensitivity of 0.96 in patients with a high pretest probability of exocrine pancreatic insufficiency, although the sensitivity drops when considering all patients with diarrhea.[309] Therefore pancreatic elastase testing can only safely rule out exocrine pancreatic insufficiency in patients with a low pretest probability of the disorder (those with IBS-D). A high false-positive rate exists in individuals with a low level of fecal elastase (<200 μg/g),[309] often related to abnormal reporting in watery stools.[310]

In reality, the best way to determine pancreatic exocrine insufficiency may be a therapeutic trial of pancreatic enzyme supplementation. If such a trial is conducted, adequate enzyme doses should be prescribed[311] with some objective measurement, such as change in fecal fat excretion, weight gain, or stool characteristics, to assess response to treatment.[306,312]

Inadequate bile salt solubilization of dietary fat can usually be inferred from the patient's history or physical examination (e.g., cholestatic jaundice, ileal resection, and known enterocolic fistula). If proof of the mechanism is required, analysis of a postprandial duodenal aspirate can demonstrate reduced conjugated bile acid concentrations.[205] As this test may not be available at most centers, a therapeutic trial of exogenous conjugated bile acids (ox bile) may be the best way of establishing the diagnosis. Supplementation with bile acids reduces steatorrhea and can improve the patient's nutritional status without aggravating diarrhea in cases of short bowel syndrome.[313]

Chronic Inflammatory Diarrhea

In addition to the detection of inflammation in the setting of infectious colitis, fecal markers of inflammation, including the presence of WBCs, fecal lactoferrin, and calprotectin, are central to the evaluation of chronic inflammatory diarrhea. Among patients presenting with GI symptoms, a combination of a low level of C-reactive protein and fecal calprotectin <40 μg/g effectively rules out the diagnosis of IBD.[226]

In contrast to chronic secretory diarrhea, endoscopic examination by colonoscopy is the hallmark diagnostic in the evaluation of chronic inflammatory diarrhea. Colonoscopy should be undertaken initially to look for structural and histologic changes (Box 17.10). Biopsy specimens must be obtained from the colon to aid in making the correct diagnosis.[314] In the setting of acute exacerbations of an underlying inflammatory diarrhea, such as IBD, colonoscopy or flexible sigmoidoscopy, also aids in the diagnosis of superimposed infection from CMV.[315] The pathogens most likely to cause chronic inflammatory diarrhea are *C. difficile*, CMV, *E. histolytica*, *Yersinia* spp., and *Mycobacterium tuberculosis*. In addition to biopsies, appropriate cultures or culture-independent tests should be obtained to exclude these infections. Although colonoscopy is best utilized to exclude IBD, as isolated disease of the ileum or right colon can occur in Crohn disease, flexible sigmoidoscopy is likely sufficient for a diagnosis of microscopic colitis[316,317] and immunotherapy-related colitis.[318]

When the clinical suspicion for a chronic inflammatory diarrhea is high, but endoscopic examination is unrevealing, alternative imaging modalities, including cross-sectional enterography protocols, capsule endoscopy, and deep enteroscopy, can aide in the detection of small bowel inflammation. When compared to cross-sectional imaging, capsule endoscopy has the highest sensitivity for detection of proximal and mid-small bowel inflammation in Crohn disease[319,320] and can aid in the detection of complications of refractory celiac disease, such as ulcerative jejunoileitis or enteropathy-associated T-cell lymphoma.[321,322] The primary risk of capsule endoscopy includes capsule retention with the highest rates in individuals with suspected Crohn disease

BOX 17.10 Diagnostic Approach to the Patient With Chronic Inflammatory Diarrhea

- Exclusion of structural disease
  - CT or MRI of abdomen and pelvis
  - Sigmoidoscopy or colonoscopy with mucosal biopsies
  - Enteroscopy with mucosal biopsies
- Exclusion of tuberculosis, parasites, and viruses

(1.6%) or known Crohn disease (13%).[323] A dissolvable patency capsule test performed prior to capsule endoscopy allows for safe evaluation of the small bowel in individuals with risk factors for luminal strictures or obstructive symptoms.[324]

MANAGEMENT

The most important factor in the management of diarrhea (either acute or chronic) is the recognition of volume depletion and appropriate replenishment of intravascular volume with intravenous fluids or oral rehydration therapy. Oral rehydration therapy takes advantage of the basic principles of nutrient-dependent sodium absorption in the small bowel allowing for a convenient oral and inexpensive therapeutic option. Its major impact has been in decreasing morbidity and mortality from cholera and other infectious diarrheas in less developed countries.[325] Because nutrient absorption enhances sodium and fluid absorption in the jejunum even when other forms of sodium absorption are impaired, or in the presence of activated secretory mechanisms, orally ingested saline solutions that contain glucose, amino acids, or more complex nutrients that can be hydrolyzed will be readily absorbed. Although the earliest oral rehydration solutions used glucose to accelerate sodium absorption in the jejunum, hypoosmolar high-amylose maize starch oral rehydration solutions that also enhance production of short-chain fatty acids and absorption of fluid in the colon are now thought to be superior.[325]

Although oral rehydration solutions increase fluid and electrolyte absorption, they do not reduce stool output, and stool weight may actually increase with the use of these solutions. Use of oral rehydration solutions is also precluded in patients who are vomiting frequently. Most sports drinks (e.g., Gatorade) are designed to replenish modest electrolyte losses from sweat and do not contain enough sodium to adequately replace diarrheal losses. These solutions can be used if additional sources of sodium and absorbable nutrients (e.g., pretzels or crackers) are ingested concomitantly. Care should be taken to avoid products with artificial sweeteners or no sugar calories as these can impair sodium absorption and worsen diarrhea. Solutions that more closely approximate the World Health Organization oral rehydration solution or cereal-based rehydration solutions are available commercially (e.g., Ceralyte 90).

Acute Diarrhea

Because infection is a frequent cause of acute diarrhea, empirical trials of antibiotic therapy are often considered by care providers.[326] If the prevalence of bacterial or protozoal infection is high in a community or a specific situation, empirical use of an antibiotic is logical, as in the treatment of travelers' diarrhea with a fluoroquinolone or rifaximin, even without bacteriologic proof of infection.[162]

Traditionally, empiric antibiotic therapy is used for more severely ill patients, while bacterial culture results are pending, but this approach has been called into question. Patients in whom hemolytic-uremic syndrome develops in response to infection with *E. coli* are more likely to have received empirical antibiotic therapy.[327] Experts also often advise against empirical antibiotic treatment of salmonellosis unless enteric fever is present or unless patients are at high risk for extraintestinal spread of the infection.[328] For patients with persistent diarrhea (lasting >1 week), an empirical trial of metronidazole or nitazoxanide for a potential protozoal infection is sometimes considered. However, multiplex PCR assays, given their demonstrated superior diagnostic yield and time to diagnosis when compared to standard culture techniques in infectious diarrhea, may result in improved antibiotic use patterns and subsequent healthcare utilization.[329–331]

TABLE 17.5 Nonspecific Drug Therapy for Chronic Diarrhea

Drug Class	Agent	Dose[a]
Opiates (mu opiate receptor selective)	Codeine	15–60 mg four times daily
	Diphenoxylate	2.5–5 mg four times daily
	Loperamide	2–4 mg four times daily
	Morphine	2–20 mg four times daily
	Tincture of opium	2–20 drops four times daily
Enkephalinase inhibitor (delta opiate receptor effects)	Racecadotril[b] (acetorphan)	1.5 mg/kg three times daily
α_2-Adrenergic agonist	Clonidine	0.1–0.3 mg three times daily
Somatostatin analog	Octreotide	50–250 µg three times daily (subcutaneously)
Bile acid–binding resin	Cholestyramine	4 g one to four times daily
	Colesevelam	1.875 g twice daily
	Colestipol	4 g one to four times daily
Fiber supplement	Calcium polycarbophil	5–10 g daily
	Psyllium	10–20 g daily

[a]Oral unless otherwise indicated.
[b]Not approved in the United States.

Nonspecific antidiarrheal agents can reduce stool frequency, stool weight, and coexisting symptoms of abdominal cramps (Table 17.5). Opiates, such as loperamide or diphenoxylate with atropine, are frequently prescribed.[332] The concern that these antiperistaltic agents slow the clearance of pathogens from the intestines largely has not been substantiated. Opiate antidiarrheals have been abused by some individuals, and only a small supply should be needed to mitigate acute diarrhea. Intraluminal agents, such as bismuth subsalicylate (Pepto-Bismol) and adsorbents (e.g., kaolin), may also help reduce the fluidity of bowel movements. Racecadotril, a drug that inhibits enkephalinase and thereby increases the effects of endogenous opiates on the mu opiate receptor, is available for the treatment of acute diarrhea in some countries.[333]

Chronic Diarrhea

Empirical therapy is used in patients with chronic diarrhea in the following three situations: (1) as temporizing or initial treatment before diagnostic testing; (2) after diagnostic testing has failed to confirm a diagnosis; and (3) when a diagnosis has been made but no specific treatment is available or specific treatment has failed to produce an improvement in symptoms. Generally, empirical antibiotic therapy is less useful for chronic diarrhea than for acute diarrhea, because infection is a much less likely cause. Although some clinicians try an empirical course of metronidazole or a fluoroquinolone before committing a patient to extensive diagnostic testing, this approach is not supported by data and is not recommended.

In the appropriate clinical setting, therapeutic trials of pancreatic enzyme replacement and conjugated bile acid supplementation in patients with unexplained steatorrhea may be diagnostic and therapeutic. In such clinical scenarios, objective improvement in steatorrhea should be pursued. By contrast, when pancreatic enzyme supplements are tried empirically for so-called idiopathic chronic diarrhea, they rarely yield satisfactory results.

In contrast to supplementation with bile acids in steatorrhea, bile acid sequestrants are empirically used in the management of IBS/functional diarrhea and in the workup of BAD. Cholestyramine, colestipol, and colesevelam are available, vary in effectiveness and tolerance, and may need to be tried sequentially.[334–336] A clinical response suggests that BAD may be playing a role. Nevertheless, because such agents may also bind toxins or have other actions, the possibility of a nonspecific effect must be considered.

Symptomatic treatment with an opiate is often necessary in patients with chronic diarrhea, because specific treatment may not be available.[332] Loperamide (4 mg, four times daily) is often tried but may not be potent enough for some patients. More potent opiates, such as codeine or opium, are often underused in the management of these patients, largely because of fear of abuse. In fact, these agents are rarely abused by patients with chronic diarrhea, especially if a few simple measures are taken. First, the patient needs to be informed about the abuse potential of the medication and should be warned not to increase the dose without consulting the physician. Second, the dose should be low initially and titrated up until efficacy is achieved. Third, use of the opiate should be monitored closely, and the prescription should not be refilled until an interval appropriate with the anticipated usage has passed. Because tolerance to the GI effects of opiates does not develop, the dose needed to control diarrhea should be stable over time; frequent requests to increase the dose may indicate abuse.

Other agents used as antidiarrheal therapies include octreotide and clonidine. Octreotide, a somatostatin analog, has been shown to improve diarrhea in patients with the carcinoid syndrome and other endocrinopathies, dumping syndrome, chemotherapy-induced diarrhea, and AIDS.[337] Clonidine, an α2-adrenergic agent that has effects on intestinal motility and transport, may have a special role in diabetic diarrhea[338] and short bowel syndrome,[339] but its hypotensive effect limits its usefulness in many patients with diarrhea. Telotristat ethyl is an approved inhibitor of tryptophan hydroxylase, the enzymatic rate-limiting step in the conversion of tryptophan to serotonin, leading to improvements in diarrhea in individuals with carcinoid syndrome.[340] Crofelemer, an agent approved by the FDA for noninfectious diarrhea in AIDS patients on antiretroviral therapy, inhibits both CFTR and the calcium-activated chloride channel, TMEM16A, thereby reducing chloride secretion.[341] Whether crofelemer will be useful in other forms of secretory diarrhea remains to be seen.

The glucagon-like peptides (GLP)-(1 and 2) are peptide hormones released by the enteroendocrine L-cells of the ileum and colon in response to oral intake and digested nutrients. GLP-1 reduces gastric acid secretion, gastric motility and small bowel motility in addition to its incretin effects.[342] GLP-2 reduces gastric emptying in addition to its effects on small intestinal blood flow and increases in villous length and small bowel absorptive surface area.[343,344] Given reductions in gastrointestinal transit and improved absorptive function,[345–347] there is considerable interest in the use of these agents for control of diarrhea. However, current approved use is limited to diabetes mellitus and obesity for GLP-1 analogs and short bowel syndrome with intestinal failure for GLP-2 therapies.

Interest in the use of probiotics as nonspecific therapy for diarrhea has been increasing, but evidence of effectiveness remains limited.[348] When applied in special situations, such as infectious diarrhea, these agents may alter intestinal microbiota, and speed resolution of diarrhea.[349,350] Despite conflicting reports, a large randomized controlled study in inpatient older adults demonstrated no benefit of a probiotic combination for the prevention of antibiotic associated diarrhea.[351] Herbal remedies for diarrhea include those containing berberine (goldenseal and barberry), which appears to stimulate fluid and electrolyte absorption, and arrowroot, the mechanism of which is unknown.[352,353]

Stool-modifying agents such as bulk forming fermentable fibers (e.g., psyllium/ispaghula) alter stool consistency but do not reduce stool weight.[354–358] The bulk forming fibers can therefore be helpful in patients with coexisting fecal incontinence[359,360] and in some patients with low stool weights. The change from watery to semiformed stools may be sufficient to alleviate symptoms. In addition, pectin may delay transit through the proximal intestine and increase luminal viscosity, thereby serving as an adjunctive empirical treatment.[361] Calcium supplementation with 1–2 g elemental calcium daily may be simple and effective therapy in some patients; the mechanism of this effect is not well established.[362]

Full references for this chapter can be found at https://ebooks.health.elsevier.com.

18 Intestinal Gas

Fernando Azpiroz

IN THIS CHAPTER

Although many patients encountered in clinical practice complain about intestinal gas, systematic investigation of this subject did not begin until the 1960s, when a series of brilliant studies by Levitt et al. began to shed light on the pathophysiology of intestinal gas.[1]

COMPOSITION AND VOLUME OF GASTROINTESTINAL GAS

The GI tract normally contains a relatively small amount of gas. The volume of gas within the intestinal lumen is determined by the balance between gas input and output, a highly dynamic process. Gas input may result from swallowing, chemical reactions, bacterial fermentation, and diffusion from the blood, whereas output involves belching, bacterial consumption, absorption into the blood, and anal evacuation. Despite this variety of factors, the volume of gas within the GI tract is remarkably constant and similar among healthy persons,[2,3] suggesting that it is under tight homeostatic control. Measurements of intestinal gas volume have been performed using a specifically designed CT technique.[2] Data acquisition is relatively simple, but analysis is fairly elaborate and has been carefully validated. This technique has confirmed previous measurements by other techniques showing about 100–200 mL of gas in the fasting state and somewhat larger volumes (65% increase) after ingestion of a meal (Figs. 18.1 and 18.2). Techniques using magnetic resonance imaging have been developed to measure intestinal gas.[4–7] Since this method does not involve radiation, it is suitable for repeat testing either for research purposes or in clinical practice, but the analysis of the images is less precise.

Analysis of gas composition is technically challenging, and still only few and relatively old data are available. In a study of 11 healthy fasting subjects, the overall composition of gas within the GI tract was assessed using a washout technique in which a rapid infusion of argon into the jejunum via an intraluminal tube was used to flush out the intestinal gases.[8] Gas effluent was collected via a rectal tube and analyzed. Five gases—N_2, O_2, CO_2, H_2, and methane (CH_4)—were found to account for more than 99% of intestinal gas; many additional gases were present in trace concentrations. During fasting, N_2 was usually predominant, O_2 was present in low concentrations, and the concentrations of CO_2, H_2, and CH_4 were highly variable. The latter three gases are related to fermentation of meal residues and may predominate in the postprandial period (see later).

GAS METABOLISM AND EXCRETION

GI gas is distributed in three compartments: stomach, small intestine, and colon. In each compartment the volume and composition of gas depend on gas metabolism and diffusion of gas between the lumen and blood. Part of the gas in one compartment is propelled to the next, and the end product is evacuated per anus. Fig. 18.3 schematically depicts gas homeostasis in various segments of the GI tract.

Diffusion of Gas Between the Intestinal Lumen and Blood

The rate and direction of diffusion of each gas are a function of the three factors: diffusivity, difference in partial pressure between lumen and blood, and exposure of the gas to the mucosal surface. The diffusivity of a gas across the mucosa of the GI tract depends on its solubility in water. For a given partial pressure difference, CO_2 diffuses much more rapidly than H_2, CH_4, N_2, and O_2. Luminal gases with a partial pressure (concentration) higher than that in venous blood pass into the circulation and vice versa. Gas absorption also depends on the extent of the mucosal area and the time of exposure. H_2 and CH_4 absorbed from the bowel are not metabolized by the host and are excreted in expired air. Breath analysis provides a simple means of estimating the production of these gases in the GI tract. Breath excretion of these gases is the product of the alveolar ventilation rate and their alveolar concentrations. Because alveolar ventilation is relatively constant in sedentary conditions, the end-alveolar breath concentration of H_2 and CH_4 can be used as a simple indicator of their total breath excretion and intestinal production.

Mouth to Stomach

The stomach normally contains a relatively small amount of gas ($\approx$10–20 mL).[2,3] Its location within the stomach is determined by flotation and gravitational forces. In the upright position, gas forms a bubble in the fundus of the stomach. By contrast, in the supine position, gas forms a thin film lining the anterior wall of the gastric corpus and antrum close to the abdominal wall (see Fig. 18.1). Air swallowing (rather than intraluminal production) is believed to be the major source of stomach gas, as suggested by the absence of the gastric bubble in patients with advanced

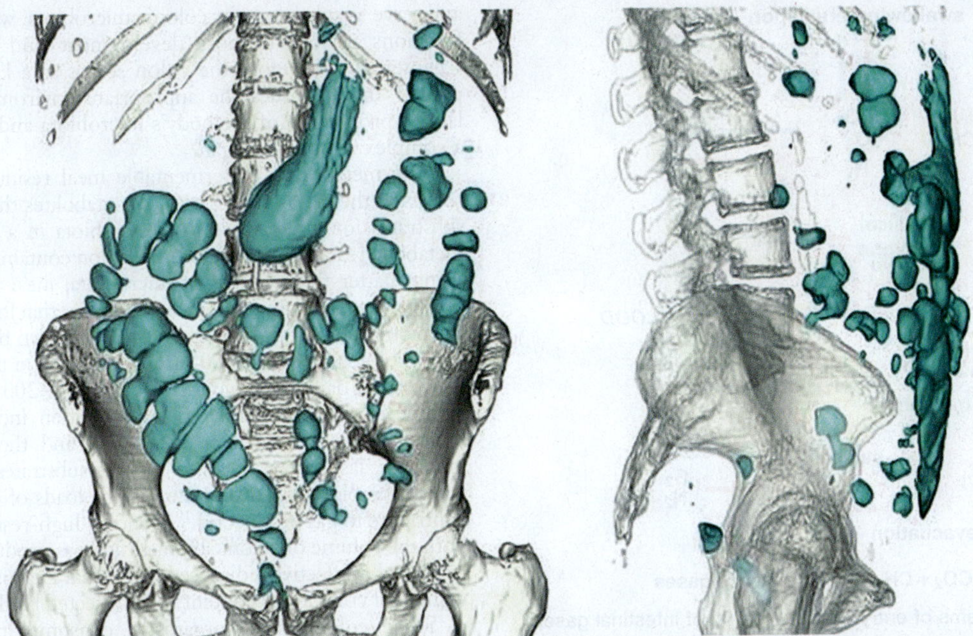

Fig. 18.1 CT image analysis of abdominal gas content (*green*) in a healthy subject in a supine position. An anterior view is shown on the left. Note in the lateral view (*right*) that in the supine position, most luminal gas is located close to the anterior abdominal wall. (From Accarino A, Perez F, Azpiroz F, et al. Intestinal gas and bloating: effect of prokinetic stimulation. *Am J Gastroenterol.* 2008;103:2036–2042.)

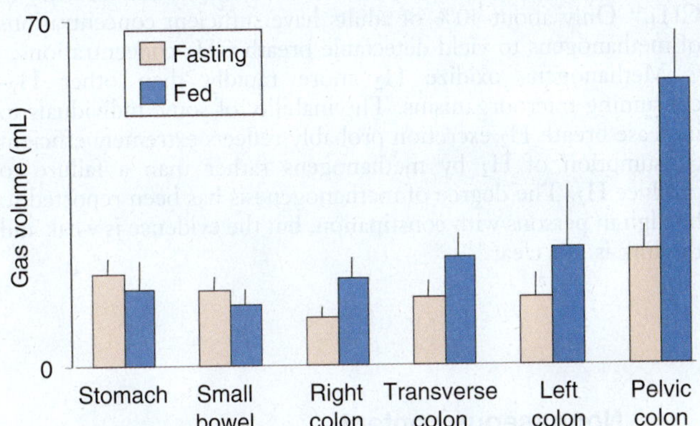

Fig. 18.2 Abdominal gas volume in various segments of the GI tract in fasting and fed states as determined by CT volumetric analysis. The postprandial increment in intestinal gas is located predominantly in the pelvic portion of the colon. (From Perez F, Accarino A, Azpiroz F, et al. Gas distribution within the human gut: effect of meals. *Am J Gastroenterol.* 2007;102:842–849.)

achalasia (see Chapter 46), but the normal amount of air swallowing is not clear. Gas leaves the stomach via belching, absorption, or emptying into the duodenum. The belching process has been well documented, but there is hardly any information related to the passage of gases across the gastric mucosa or the emptying of gas into the duodenum. Given the lower proportion of CO_2 and a higher proportion of O_2 in swallowed air compared with that in blood, in theory, CO_2 should diffuse from blood into the stomach bubble and O_2 from the lumen to blood. Because N_2 diffuses poorly across the mucosa, luminal N_2 throughout the GI tract presumably derives from swallowed air.

Small Intestine

From 10 to 20 mL of gas is normally present in the small intestine, usually in the form of small bubbles scattered along the intestinal lumen.[2,3] Theoretically, in the upper small intestine, a large amount of CO_2 is liberated from the interaction of bicarbonate and acid; however, studies using CT-based volumetric analysis did not detect changes in gas volume within the small bowel in the postprandial period.[2] The gas produced should diffuse into the blood (which is plausible for CO_2) or be transported to the colon. An increase in colonic gas, although relatively small, is observed after a meal (see later). Gas production by small bowel microbiota is considered negligible in normal conditions, but direct evidence of this conclusion is lacking.

Colon

The colon normally contains around 50–100 mL of gas (see Fig. 18.2).[2,3,9] A study comparing gas content based on CT images taken during fasting and 99 ± 22 minutes after a meal showed an increase in gas in the pelvic colon (see Fig. 18.2), earlier than would be expected for gas derived from colonic fermentation of food substrates.[2] Therefore gas of proximal GI tract origin is presumably propelled into the colon after ingestion of a meal, possibly by a gastroileal reflex. However, colonic gas originates primarily by the metabolic activity of the microbiota and is eliminated by mucosal absorption, microbiota gas consumption, and anal evacuation. With the growing interest in intestinal microbiota, the study of intestinal gas production and evacuation has become particularly important, because it reflects the metabolic activity of intestinal microbiota, and monitoring intestinal gas evacuation may serve as an on-line indicator of microbiota gas metabolism.

Colonic Endoluminal Microenvironment and Gas Metabolism

The upper part of the digestive tract primarily has a nutritional function: Useful components, such as nutrients, water, and minerals, are extracted from ingested material by a process of digestion and absorption. Nonabsorbed residues pass into the colon

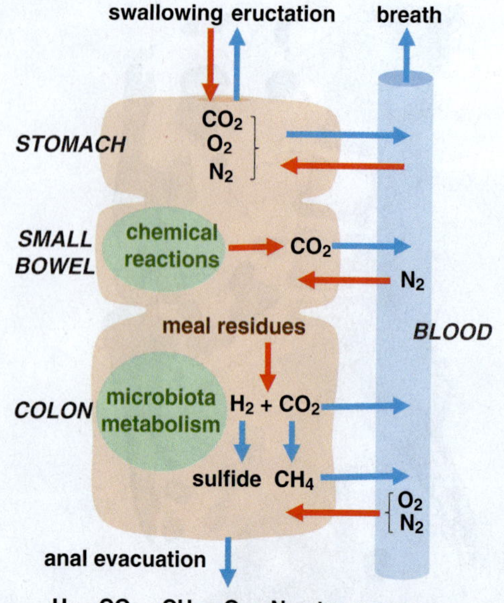

Fig. 18.3 Mechanisms of entry and elimination of intestinal gases. Air and CO_2 (in carbonated drinks) are swallowed, and a sizable fraction is eructated. CO_2 and some O_2 in swallowed air diffuse into the gastric mucosa. The reaction of acid and bicarbonate in the duodenum yields CO_2, which diffuses into the blood, while N_2 diffuses into the lumen down the gradient established by CO_2 production. In the colon, gas-producing microorganisms ferment unabsorbed residues, thereby releasing CO_2, H_2, and CH_4, as well as a variety of trace gases. A large proportion of H_2 is consumed by other microorganisms to reduce sulfate to sulfide, CO_2 to acetate, and CO_2 to CH_4, thereby reducing the net volume of gas derived from bacterial metabolism. N_2 and O_2 diffuse from the blood into the colonic lumen down a gradient created by gas production by bacteria. Gas is ordinarily propelled down the GI tract and evacuated per anus. The net result of all of these processes determines the volume and composition of gas in the different GI tract compartments.

and serve as substrates for colonic microbiota, which carry out key functions related to host development and homeostasis (see Chapter 3). Therefore the colon serves as a kind of "marsupial pouch" that provides the appropriate environment to host the largest proportion of the body's microbiota and thereby serves as a complex metabolic organ.

The metabolism of fermentable meal residues by microbiota results in the release of a series of metabolites that in turn serve as substrates for other subsets of microbiota in a dynamic chain of metabolic reactions. Therefore the colon contains an active mass of living matter that consists of microbiota, meal residues, and secondary metabolic products, including gases, that form bubbles within the biomass (see Fig. 18.4). Studies have shown that the colon contains a biomass of 500–800 mL, depending on the residues of the diet, with a daily dynamic turnover of 100–200 mL, which is the volume of fecal output.[4,5,9] Gas production increases as soon as fermentable residues enter the colon, and the activity declines gradually, lasting for hours as long as substrates remain available within the biomass, so that the residue loads of consecutive meals contribute to gas production.[10] Hence, a high-residue diet increases both the volume of colonic biomass and gas production, but the gas produced is effectively disposed (see "Anal Evacuation") so that the volume of colonic gas content is not affected by the diet.[5]

Some colonic microorganisms consume intraluminal gases (H_2, CO_2, and O_2), and this catabolism accounts for a proportion of intraluminal gas disposal. Three types of microorganisms consume H_2: acetogens, sulfate-reducing organisms, and methanogens.[11] Acetogens consume H_2 and CO_2 to synthesize short-chain fatty acids. Sulfate-reducing microorganisms use H_2 to reduce sulfate to sulfide. Methanogens use H_2 to reduce CO_2 to CH_4.[12] Only about 40% of adults have sufficient concentrations of methanogens to yield detectable breath CH_4 concentrations.

Methanogens oxidize H_2 more rapidly than other H_2-consuming microorganisms. The inability of some individuals to increase breath H_2 excretion probably reflects extremely efficient consumption of H_2 by methanogens rather than a failure to produce H_2. The degree of methanogenesis has been reported to be high in persons with constipation, but the evidence is weak and the link is not clear.[11]

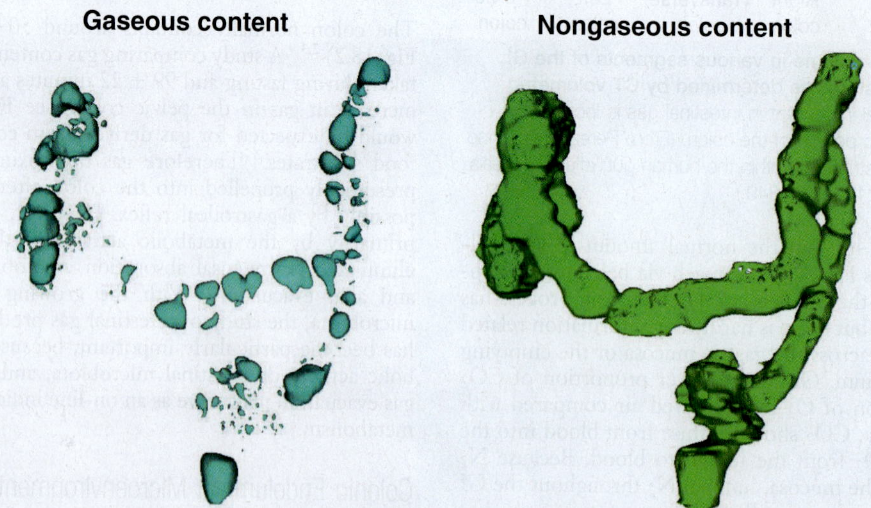

Fig. 18.4 Independent representation of gaseous and nongaseous components of colonic content on CT in a healthy subject. (From Bendezu RA, Barba E, Burri E, et al. Colonic content in health and its relation to functional gut symptoms. *Neurogastroenterol Motil*. 2016;28:849–854.)

Plasticity of Microbiota and Gas Metabolism

The composition of the colonic microbiota (and therefore the amount of gas produced on a given diet) varies considerably among individuals, depending on early environmental conditions as well as factors encountered later in life, such as diet and antibiotic exposures.[13] Even in the same individuals, dietary habits influence microbiota composition: whereas fiber-rich diets increase its diversity, diets low in fermentable residues induce the opposite effect.[14,15,5,16] One study showed that a 3-day diet rich in flatulogenic residues increased the relative abundance of methanogens in healthy subjects.[14] Chronic ingestion of high doses of an intestinally malabsorbed disaccharide (e.g., lactulose by patients with constipation or lactose by persons with intestinal lactase deficiency) results in diminished breath H_2 excretion following a challenge dose of the same disaccharide.[17] This phenomenon may result from colonic proliferation of organisms such as *Bifidobacterium* spp. that ferment lactose or lactulose via nonH_2 releasing pathways or of gas-consuming microorganisms. Similarly, oral administration of some prebiotics, such as a galacto-oligosaccharide or resistant dextrin, has been shown to increase the volume of gas produced within the intestine; the volume then declines to baseline by 7–10 days of administration.[18,19] Conceivably, the initial increase in gas production is due to the fermentation of the prebiotic, and the subsequent decline is due to adaptation by the microbiota. Indeed, changes in the microbiota composition are detected by the end of the administration period.[18,19] Another study indicated that adaptation of microbiota to regular prebiotic consumption involves a shift in microbiota metabolism toward low-gas–producing pathways, with a nonsignificant upregulation of gas-consuming activity.[20]

Odoriferous Gases

None of the quantitatively important gases has an odor; the unpleasant odor of feces is due to gases present in trace quantities. The intensity of the noxious odor of flatus samples correlates with concentrations of hydrogen sulfide and methanethiol.[21] Odoriferous gases are difficult to study, among other reasons, because they pass across rubber or plastic membranes that are impermeable to other gases. For example, these gases diffuse from the intracolonic milieu into an intrarectal latex balloon inflated with air, and the air recovered by deflating the balloon has the characteristic odor of these gases.

Anal Evacuation

Intestinal gas that is not absorbed or metabolized is eliminated via anal evacuation. Therefore anal gas evacuation is the net result of gas dynamics along the entire GI tract, but in fact, anal evacuation is by and large determined by colonic gas homeostasis. Anal gas evacuation can be monitored in two different settings: in laboratory conditions, measuring the volume of gas collected via a rectal tube or an anal cannula, or in daily life conditions, measuring the number of anal gas evacuations by an event marker (see Fig. 18.5). A study in 20 healthy subjects showed that on their normal diets, the rate of gas evacuation 6 hours after breakfast was about 40 mL/h; on a highly flatulogenic diet, the rate increased to around 120 mL/h after a high-residue meal (see Fig. 18.5).[14] The average number of anal gas evacuations by healthy subjects on their normal diets is roughly 10 during the day, with an upper limit of normal of about 20 a day.[14,5,18,19,22,23] The number of evacuations is two to three times higher on a highly flatulogenic diet (see Fig. 18.5).[5,14] Neither age nor gender correlates significantly with the frequency of flatus.

About 200 mL of N_2 are evacuated per anus daily independently of the diet. The volume of O_2 evacuated is much smaller and not influenced by diet.[24,25] It is not clear to what extent N_2

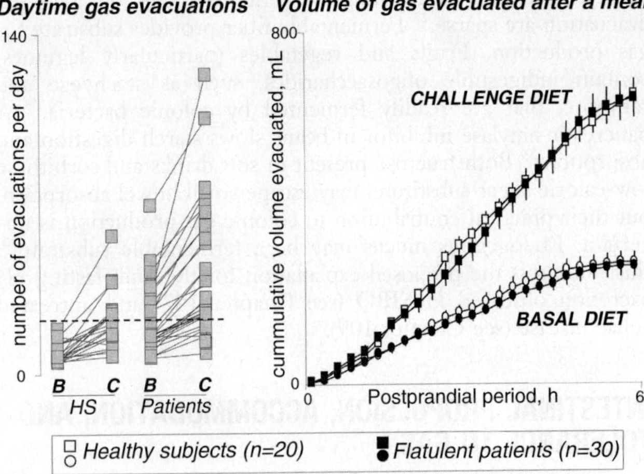

Fig. 18.5 Anal gas evacuation. The number of daytime anal gas evacuations (left panel; individual data) and the volume of gas evacuated after a meal (right panel; mean ± SE) increased with a high flatulogenic challenge diet (C), as compared to a basal diet (B). The number of gas evacuations was higher in patients complaining of flatulence than in healthy subjects (HS), but the volume evacuated was similar in both groups. (From Manichanh C, Eck A, Varela E, et al. Anal gas evacuation and colonic microbiota in patients with flatulence: effect of diet. *Gut*. 2014;63:401–408.)

and O_2 in flatus are derived from swallowed air or diffuses from blood. The volumes of H_2, CO_2, and CH_4 excreted in flatus are highly variable and depend on fermentative activity in the colon. In the presence of fermentable residues in the colon, their volumes increase. Conversely, after a 48-hour liquid fiber-free diet, anal evacuation of H_2, CO_2, and CH_4 is almost abolished.[25]

Studies have measured the volume of endogenous gas produced within the intestine using a washout technique. High-rate infusion of labeled exogenous gas directly into the jejunum washes endogenous gas from the intestine and thereby prevents its absorption and consumption.[10,20] To determine the proportion of endogenous gas eliminated from the lumen, volumes of endogenous gas collected per anus in paired studies with and without gaseous washout have been compared; the volume of endogenous gas measured in the washout experiments approximates the total volume of gas produced, whereas gas evacuated through the anus in basal experiments (without washout) represents the volume produced minus the fraction absorbed or consumed. These studies have consistently shown that a large proportion of the gas produced after a meal is rapidly eliminated from the intestinal lumen either by absorption into the blood and excretion by breath or by gas-consuming microorganisms, and only a modest proportion, about 20%–25%, is eliminated per anus; however, the proportion of gas clearance by absorption versus consumption was not discriminated in these experiments.[10,20]

In a classic study, long-term simultaneous measurements of rectal and breath H_2 excretion were performed in adult subjects maintained in an airtight environment,[26] and the proportion of gas particularly H_2, CO_2, and CH_4 removed from the colon via intestinal absorption and anal evacuation was found to depend on the rate of gas production. When H_2 production was low, breath accounted for 65% of total H_2 excretion, with 35% of H_2 eliminated per anus; however, when H_2 production was high, only 20% was eliminated via the breath, and the major part (80%) was eliminated per anus. Because the intestinal absorption process for H_2 is not saturatable, the decreasing proportion of H_2 excreted in the breath is presumably a result of more rapid propulsion of the gas to the anus. Likewise, the concentration of CO_2 in flatus tends to be highest during periods of high gas production and rapid anal evacuation.

Scientific data concerning the effect of diet on anal gas evacuation are sparse.[27] Fermentable fiber provides substrate for gas production. Fruits and vegetables (particularly legumes) contain indigestible oligosaccharides, such as stachyose and raffinose, that are readily fermented by colonic bacteria.[28] A pancreatic amylase inhibitor in beans slows starch digestion and absorption.[29] Both fructose present in soft drinks and sorbitol, a low-calorie sugar substitute, may escape small bowel absorption, but their practical contribution to colonic gas production is uncertain. Endogenous mucus may be a fermentable substrate[30]; this finding is the proposed explanation for the high fasting H_2 excretion observed in SIBO (see Chapter 107) and untreated celiac disease (see Chapter 109).

INTESTINAL PROPULSION, ACCOMMODATION, AND TOLERANCE TO GAS

The aboral propulsion of gas in the gastrointestinal tract determines the residence time of gas in the intestinal lumen; absorption and bacterial consumption of gas are influenced by transit time, as is the composition of gas evacuated from the anus. Therefore the increase in anal gas evacuation may be related in some conditions to increased intestinal gas propulsion, rather than to increased production. Gas movement along the intestine has been studied using experimental models of intestinal gas infusion, but it is not known how much gas moves from one compartment to the next in normal conditions. In contrast to the gastric cardia, which allows belching, the normal ileocecal valve is highly competent and does not allow ileal gas reflux even during experimental inflation of the colon.[31]

Visceral Responses to Intestinal Gas

Intestinal gas transit and tolerance have been measured using a gas challenge test in which a mixture of gases is continually infused into the jejunum and anal gas output is quantified. A dose-response study using infusion rates of up to 30 mL/min (1.8 L/h) showed that most healthy subjects evacuate gas as rapidly as it is infused, with little or no discomfort.[32] Transit of gas, like that of solids and liquids, is modulated by a series of reflex mechanisms. Intraluminal nutrients, particularly lipids, delay gas transit,[33] whereas mechanical stimulation of the intestine (e.g., mild rectal distention) has a strong prokinetic effect.[34] Gas is moved along the GI tract far more rapidly than solids and liquids, but the type of motor activity that determines gas transit is not known. Conceivably, movement and displacement of large masses of low-resistance gas is produced by subtle changes in tonic activity and capacitance of the intestine that do not affect the movement of solids and liquids.[35] This activity can be detected by a barostat[34,35] but not by conventional manometry.

Gas boluses infused into the left colon have been shown to elicit forceful peristaltic contractions that precede anal gas expulsions,[36] but this type of phasic event has not been recorded during continuous gas infusion with a barostat located inside the rectum. Therefore these phasic events could be a response to focal distention produced by abrupt delivery of intraluminal gas.

Gas transit is normally effective, but when an appreciable amount of gas is retained within the GI tract, subjects may develop abdominal distention and symptoms. Different experimental models of gas retention have been used to show that, although abdominal distention is related to the volume of gas within the GI tract, perception of abdominal symptoms depends on both intestinal motor activity and the intraluminal distribution of gas.[37,38] The intestine normally relaxes to accommodate gas, and pooling of gas is better tolerated in a relaxed segment with high capacitance than in a noncompliant intestine.

Somatic Response to Intestinal Gas Retention

The abdominal wall actively adapts to its contents. Retention of gas in the intestine (as any change in intra-abdominal volume) stimulates an abdominal accommodation reflex, that adapts the muscular activity of the anterior abdominal wall and the diaphragm to the volume load.[39] This reflex has been studied in healthy subjects using experimental models of intestinal gas retention. Considerable colonic gas retention produces relatively small increments in girth in healthy persons, because the anterior abdominal wall contracts and the diaphragm relaxes, thereby expanding the abdominal cavity in a cephalad direction.[39] The thorax participates in the accommodation reflex: cephalad displacement of the diaphragm is associated with intercostal contraction and compensatory expansion of the costal wall, to limit the impact on lung volume and function.[40] Therefore this abdomino-phreno-thoracic coordination limits the increase in abdominal girth that results from an increase in intestinal contents.

CLINICAL GAS PROBLEMS

Symptoms commonly attributed to excess gas are among the most frequently encountered GI complaints.[41] The understanding of the clinical problems related (or presumably related) to intestinal gas has substantially evolved over the past few years. Patients frequently complain of a generic problem with gas, and the initial step for the clinician is to determine whether the patient is referring to chronic eructation, visible, that is, objective, abdominal distention, sensation of increased abdominal pressure or fullness, that is, abdominal bloating, passage of excessive gas per anus, that is, flatulence, rumbling, that is, borborygmi, or impaired anal gas evacuation. A specific questionnaire for the evaluation of gas-related symptoms has been developed.[42,43] Recent studies indicate that abdominal bloating, sensation of flatulence, impaired anal gas evacuation, and borborygmi are nonspecific sensations of visceral origin, part of the spectrum of functional digestive disorders. By contrast, visible abdominal distention and chronic eructation are somatic manifestations of functional digestive disorders that have a behavioral origin. Somatic manifestations are frequently, but not always, associated with visceral sensations; particularly, most patients with visible distention refer to an abdominal bloating sensation, and a fraction of patients with a bloating sensation complain of visible distention.[44–46] Pneumatosis cystoides intestinalis, a condition characterized by the presence of gas-filled cysts in the intestinal wall, will also be discussed in this section.

Sensations Attributed to Intestinal Gas

In clinical practice, subjective gas-related symptoms, for example, abdominal bloating, borborygmi, impaired gas evacuation, and flatulence, tend to lump together and occur largely in the context of functional gastrointestinal disorders, particularly IBS and functional dyspepsia; hence, they may be associated with other symptoms, such as early satiety, abdominal pain, constipation, and diarrhea. Studies using structured questionnaires showed that regardless of the specific primary inclusion criterium, patients reported the whole spectrum of gas-related symptoms, including abdominal bloating, distention, borborygmi, flatulence, and abdominal pain.[14,47–51]

Pathophysiology

Gas-related sensations are produced by the same pathophysiological mechanisms as other functional gut symptoms, primarily through increased visceral sensation. Data on the specific roles of intestinal sensitivity and gas content, production, handling, and evacuation are discussed below.

Intestinal Sensitivity

It has been consistently shown that patients with functional GI symptoms have visceral hypersensitivity and hypervigilance[52] (see Chapter 124). Specifically, patients with IBS whose predominant complaint was abdominal bloating exhibited reduced tolerance to colonic gas infusion and reported significantly more severe symptoms than healthy subjects.[31,53] A prospective controlled study reported that patients with bloating were more likely to have experienced recent weight gain than healthy controls,[54] suggesting that fat accumulation in the abdomen may be perceived as bloating sensation.

Intestinal Gas Content

Abdominal CT studies, using validated analysis techniques, systematically showed that the volume of intestinal gas in patients with functional digestive disorders complaining of gas-related symptoms is within the normal range[14,55–58]; likewise, no abnormalities in nongaseous content were detected.[9] Thorough analysis of intestinal gas distribution in a large cohort of patients failed to detect abnormalities, such as localized gas accumulations, in most patients with symptoms.[3] Of note, the same findings were observed in patients in whom a bloating sensation was associated with visible abdominal distention (see "Visible Abdominal Distention").

Intestinal Gas Production

Intestinal gas production may be increased in some conditions that result in true carbohydrate malabsorption (e.g., celiac disease). Patients with IBS who complain of frequent bloating have been reported to have increased gas production caused by SIBO, intestinal dysbiosis or intestinal malabsorption (see Chapters 107 and 124). However, this finding has not been supported by other well-designed studies.[59,60] It has been shown that in patients complaining of flatulence, bloating and abdominal distention, the net production of intestinal gas (and the content of abdominal gas) is similar to that of healthy subjects.[14,61] Hence, the indication to investigate sugar malabsorption or small intestinal bacterial overgrowth in this context, primarily by breath testing, is debatable. Like most mammals, a large population of humans lose the capability to synthetize lactase after weaning, and undigested lactose is fermented in the colon, releasing gas. The gas released by moderate lactose ingestion is effectively disposed of via the lung and anal evacuation, without changes in intestinal gas content; only in persons with associated intestinal hypersensitivity or hypervigilance does the amount of gas released by lactose fermentation induce symptoms. Cognitive factors and beliefs may play also a role: a double-blind crossover study in people who regarded themselves as severely lactose intolerant did not find differences in symptoms when comparing daily ingestion of 250 mL of milk or lactose-hydrolyzed milk.[62]

Intestinal Gas Handling

Multiple studies using intestinal gas infusion have shown consistently that patients with bloating have impaired handling of the infused gas. In response to large exogenous gas loads, these patients exhibit gas retention, abdominal symptoms, or both.[61,63–66] These abnormalities apparently reflect impaired reflex control of gas transit and increased sensation.[33,67–69,3,70] Therefore these gas challenge tests provide a sensitive method for identifying subtle intestinal motor disturbances that are not detectable by conventional diagnostic tests; however, the normal volume and distribution of intestinal gas in these patients indicates that the disturbances in gas propulsion do not affect handling of endogenous gas under everyday conditions.[3,9,71]

Anal Gas Evacuation

A study of 30 consecutive patients, whose predominant complaint was flatulence, showed that in 18, the number of daytime gas evacuations measured with an event marker was within the normal range.[14] Interestingly, the volume of gas collected after a test meal in flatulent patients, in those with either a normal or excessive number of measured passages was similar to that in healthy subjects (see Fig. 18.5); furthermore, intestinal gas volume measured by CT was also within the normal range. These data indicate that the distorted appreciation in the subgroup of patients with a normal number of gas evacuations was related to hypervigilance. The other subgroup, with increased number of evacuations but normal volume of gas evacuated, conceivably had lower tolerance for and more efficient evacuation of gas arriving into the rectum.[72] More frequent passages of smaller volumes could be a behavioral response to rectal gas sensation. Increased rectal sensitivity may also result in a false impression of impaired anal gas evacuation.

Conclusion

The data discussed above suggest that gas-related symptoms mainly result from a poor tolerance of normal gas (and nongaseous) intestinal content; in the case of a hypersensitive gut, even normal intraluminal contents may induce abdominal bloating and gas-related sensations.

Treatment

Treatment of the Underlying Condition

In patients with an identifiable condition that results in intestinal carbohydrate malabsorption (e.g., celiac disease), treatment of the underlying condition reduces gas production.

In patients with gas-related symptoms in the context of a functional digestive disorder (e.g., IBS or functional dyspepsia), the basic approach to treatment should be similar to that for these conditions because they share a common pathophysiology (see Chapters 15 and 124). Although intestinal gas production and intraluminal volumes appear to be normal in patients with functional digestive disorders and gas-related complaints, the sensitivity of their intestines to normal volumes of bowel contents suggests that reducing gas production and intestinal content may be beneficial.

General Measures

Intestinal clearance of perfused gas is increased by mild exercise and the erect posture, which may explain anecdotal observations that activity (as opposed to resting in the supine posture) improves bloating in some patients.[73–75] Weight loss may improve bloating sensation in overweight patients.

Pharmacological Treatment

The effectiveness of rifaximin in the treatment of gas symptoms remains controversial; although studies have suggested that antibiotics, particularly rifaximin, can reduce symptoms of IBS,[76] IBS may first appear after antibiotic therapy.[77] Neostigmine, a potent prokinetic agent, has been reported to reduce abdominal symptoms resulting from an intestinal infusion of gas.[64] Chronic administration of pyridostigmine improves symptoms in patients complaining of bloating but has only marginal effects on intestinal gas content.[55] Other prokinetic agents may also be effective. Inhibition of intestinal motor activity enhances gas tolerance.[38] A meta-analysis of the efficacy of smooth muscle relaxants in the treatment of IBS has concluded that these drugs are superior to placebo in the management of symptoms, specifically abdominal pain and distention.[78] Peppermint oil has an antispasmodic effect on the GI tract because of the calcium channel blocker activity of its active constituent, menthol, but its benefit in IBS is questionable.[79] Drugs with antinociceptive action may also be useful (see Chapter 124).

Commercial preparations of β-galactosidase (e.g., Beano) are touted to enhance digestion of the indigestible oligosaccharides present in legumes and other vegetables,[80] but efficacy has only been demonstrated for the liquid preparation; tablets containing this enzyme may not be effective. Simethicone has defoaming properties that eliminate bubbles that might trap gas,[81] but it does not reduce the volume of gas. Activated charcoal has been reported to reduce breath H_2 excretion,[82] but another study showed that charcoal does not bind H_2 (or any other quantitatively important intestinal gas) and does not reduce breath H_2 excretion.[83] These products are well tolerated and, in some patients, exert a welcome placebo effect. Bismuth subsalicylate in high doses may reduce odoriferous flatus, but its use may not be justifiable because of its potential toxicity.[84]

Correction of Constipation

Abdominal bloating (or postprandial fullness) and other gas-related symptoms in patients with constipation-predominant IBS or with functional dyspepsia are frequently associated with constipation. In these patients, correction of constipation by biofeedback in the case of dyssynergic defecation improves abdominal bloating and associated symptoms[47,85]; conceivably, this effect is related to improved bulking and gas evacuation. Hence, patients with abdominal bloating, distention, and other gas-related symptoms should be systematically questioned about bowel habits and defecation, even if constipation is not spontaneously reported.

Dietary Interventions

Gas production can be effectively reduced by a low-flatulogenic diet. Foods thought to increase gas include legumes, cauliflower, Brussels sprouts, eggplant, onion, celery, carrots, raisins, bananas, and whole wheat bread.[27] Selective restriction of specific foodstuffs, such as onion and garlic, may reduce odoriferous gases, but experimental evidence is lacking. Foods that provide minimal substrate to colonic bacteria include proteins (e.g., meat, fowl, fish, and eggs), lipids (e.g., animal fat, and oil), and certain carbohydrates (e.g., rice, rice bread, and gluten-free bread). In general, after a 1-week low-flatulogenic diet, patients usually experience relief of symptoms,[86] even though their basal gas production is within the normal range; a bulking effect of the low-flatulogenic diet may also be involved. Restriction of fiber supplements, either fermentable or nonfermentable (due to the bulking effect) is particularly important. By an orderly reintroduction of eliminated foodstuffs, patients may learn to identify the offending meal components. The low-flatulogenic diet is particularly effective in patients complaining of flatulence.[14]

Diets low in fermentable oligosaccharides, disaccharides, monosaccharides, and polyols (FODMAPs) have become popular[87]; these diets are complex to design and cumbersome to follow and do not seem to offer documentable advantages over simpler low-residue alternatives.[88,89] Some data indicate that FODMAP restriction has deleterious effects on "good" intestinal microbiota,[90] and it is not known whether the same is true for other low-residue diets (see Chapter 124). Similarly, little experimental support is available to recommend a gluten-free diet in the absence of celiac disease or wheat intolerance (see Chapter 109).

Pre- and probiotics may influence the composition of colonic microbiota and thereby reduce anal gas evacuation. As discussed earlier, a galacto-oligosaccharide prebiotic induces the adaptation of colonic microbiota so that gas-producing metabolism is reduced.[18,20] A study has shown that the benefit of this prebiotic administered for 4 weeks is similar to that of a low-FODMAP diet; however, whereas the improvement persisted 2 weeks after termination of administration of the prebiotic, a rebound effect was observed after the discontinuation of the low-FODMAP diet.[49] Whether the benefit is specific to this galacto-oligosaccharide prebiotic is unknown. Some data indicate that the use of probiotics may reduce symptoms of IBS, particularly abdominal bloating and distention.[91,23,92] Results with probiotic agents are variable and depend on the bacterial species used, dose, duration of treatment, and endpoints used for evaluation.[93]

Visible Abdominal Distention

Pathophysiology

Visible abdominal distention may be related to an increase in abdominal contents, particularly intestinal gas, or to an incoordination of the abdominal wall. In addition, some patients with a normal or just a fatty abdomen are convinced of having abdominal distention.

Excessive gas has been observed in patients with intestinal obstruction or with severe motility disorders, such as chronic intestinal pseudo-obstruction (see Chapter 126)[94] (Fig. 18.6). Radiologic images of intestinal air-fluid levels in the erect position indicate that liquid is present below the gas bubble and is seen only with abnormal fluid retention (see Chapters 125 and 126). The origin and mechanisms of gas accumulation remain unclear; intestinal neuropathy is associated with impaired transit of gas,[63] but a mucosal barrier dysfunction leaking gas (and possibly also liquid) from the blood to the lumen could also play a role.[95] Nevertheless, patients with intestinal neuropathy or myopathy are rare and usually seen in referral centers.

In patients with functional digestive disorders, that is, without underlying organic cause, visible abdominal distention usually develops following meals or at the end of the day and resolves after an overnight rest. Measurements using inductance plethysmography and CT have objectively demonstrated a clear-cut increase in abdominal girth with episodes of distention (Fig. 18.7).[57,96,97] This observation was corroborated by a series of studies of patients with functional digestive disorders, in which abdominal CT images were compared under basal conditions and during an episode of visible distention, showing that the sensation of distention is associated with a real increase in girth and in the anteroposterior diameter of the abdomen.[56,58] These studies further showed that distention is associated with a significant diaphragmatic descent but only a modest increment in intestinal gas content (see Fig. 18.7). A recent analysis of a large series of

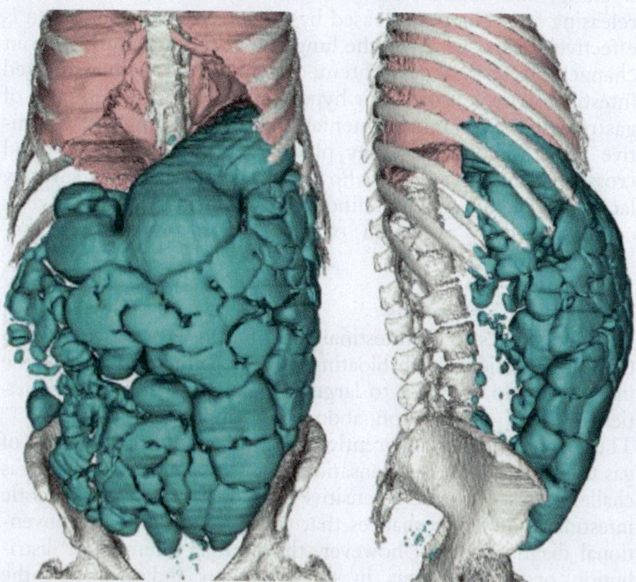

Fig. 18.6 Tridimensional reconstruction of CT images in a patient with intestinal dysmotility. Note large pooling of gas (in *blue*).

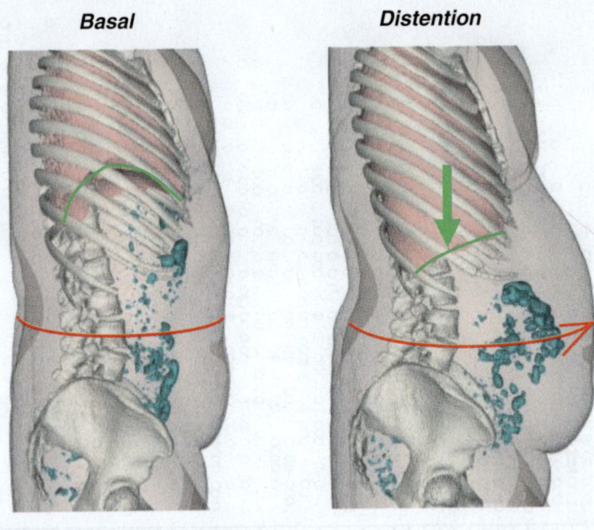

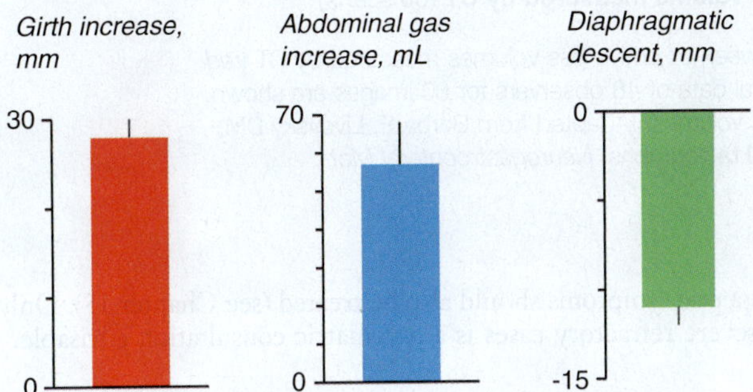

Fig. 18.7 Mechanisms of functional abdominal distention. (*Upper panel*) CT images in the same patient during basal conditions (no distention) and during an episode of abdominal distention. (Lower panel) Differences during distention versus basal conditions (n = 104). Note the increase in *girth* (*red*), modest increase in abdominal gas (*blue*), and diaphragmatic descent (*green*). (Adapted from Barba E, Burri E, Accarino A, et al. Abdominothoracic mechanisms of functional abdominal distention and correction by biofeedback. *Gastroenterology*. 2015;148:732–739; distentionand Barba E, Burri E, Quiroga S, et al. Visible abdominal distention in functional gut disorders: objective evaluation. *Neurogastroenterol Motil*. 2023;35:e14466.)

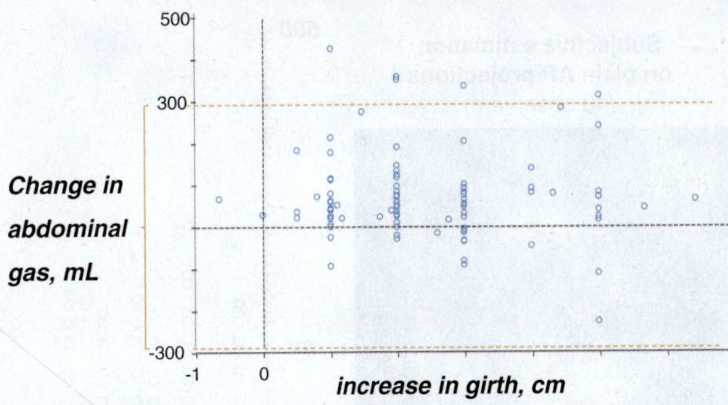

Fig. 18.8 Changes in abdominal gas and girth from basal to distention (n = 104). Girth was larger during the distention episodes than on basal conditions all but 1 patient. In CT scans obtained during distention episodes, intestinal gas volume was within ±300 mL from basal scans in all but 5 patients with a larger increment, who nevertheless exhibited a marked diaphragmatic descent (abdominophrenic dyssynergia). (Adapted from Barba E, Burri E, Quiroga S, et al. Visible abdominal distention in functional gut disorders: objective evaluation. *Neurogastroenterol Motil*. 2023;35:e14466.)

patients convincingly shows that, in contrast to pseudo-obstruction functional distention is not explained by intestinal gas (Fig. 18.8).[56] Electromyographic studies have shown that the abdomen normally adapts to an increase in contents via a coordinated abdomino-phrenic response (abdominal accommodation).[39] Patients with functional digestive disorders and visible abdominal distention have an uncoordinated response, with paradoxical diaphragmatic contraction and anterior wall relaxation, a phenomenon termed abdomino-phrenic dyssynergia.[53,98] Whereas normal accommodation of abdominal contents seems to be a reflex response, some data suggest that abnormal accommodation in patients with distention is a behavioral response, because it can be reversed by biofeedback techniques.[58,50] The conditioning mechanism and the trigger for this somatic response is not known, but it could be speculated that a sensation of bloating in hypersensitive patients triggers the episode of visible abdominal distention. In some patients, distention develops suddenly after a precipitating event, and cognitive or emotive factors may play a role.[99,100]

In contrast to the common episodic presentation, some patients complain of steady, unremitting abdominal distention, which may be related to a fatty abdomen or a delusory appreciation.

Management

Patients complaining of self-limited episodes of visible distention deserve credibility, and if the report is clear, comparative exams during distention versus basal conditions are not required. In patients fulfilling criteria for a functional gut disorder, abdomino-phrenic dyssynergia is the rule, and the possibility of excess gas, a common belief, is very unlikely. Evidence by CT or MR imaging may be required very rarely; gas volumes over 300 mL raise the suspicion of intestinal neuro-myopathy.[56] Gas estimations by plain abdominal radiographs have proven completely unreliable (Fig. 18.9).[101]

Since perception of symptoms, particularly bloating, may facilitate or trigger distention,[8] treatment of abdominal symptoms by conventional therapy for functional gut disorders, including dietary interventions and correction of constipation, is a reasonable first step. If identifiable, other triggers involving cognitive or emotive factors, could also be targeted.[99] Hypnosis has been reported to reduce symptoms of IBS, including bloating and visible abdominal distention.[102]

Patients complaining of episodes of visible abdominal distention can be trained to correct the activity of the diaphragm and the anterior abdominal wall using biofeedback techniques.[50,58] The original technique is complex, but new simpler modalities are under development, and may have widespread application.[102a,102b]

Repetitive Eructation

Pathophysiology

The occasional belch expels air from the stomach that has been swallowed with ingested solids or liquids. Repetitive eructation results from inadvertent and compulsive aspiration of air into the hypopharynx and esophagus, most of which is immediately expelled before reaching the stomach[103]; aspiration of air into the esophagus may be produced by pharyngeal injection, thoracic suction, or both.[103,104] Bredenoord and Smout have proposed the terms *aerophagia* (air swallowing) and *gastric belching* (venting air from the stomach), in contrast to *supragastric*

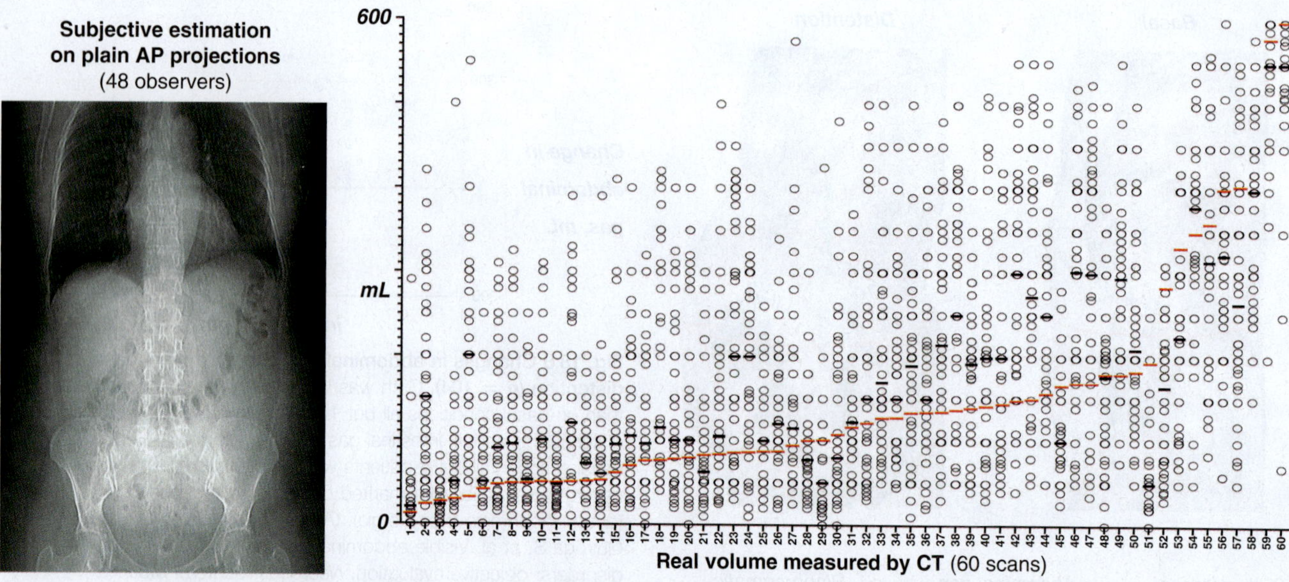

Fig. 18.9 Evaluation of intestinal gas content. Relation between objective gas volumes measured by CT (*red lines*) and estimated volumes on plain AP projections. Individual data of 48 observers for 60 images are shown. Note, great overlap of estimated values, even with largest gas volumes. (Adapted from Barba E, Livovsky DM, Relea L, et al. Evaluation of abdominal gas by plain abdominal radiographs. *Neurogastroenterol Motil.* 2023;35:e14485.)

belching (repetitive eructation of air aspirated into the esophagus).[103,104]

Repetitive eructation is frequently triggered by emotional stress. Episodes of continuous belching often occur after meals; in a proportion of cases, careful interrogation reveals underlying dyspeptic-type postprandial symptoms that patients misinterpret as excessive gas in the stomach. Attempting to evacuate the air presumably retained in the stomach, patients inadvertently aspirate air, which increases their discomfort, and eructation produces partial relief. This reinforces the false impression of the patient, and a vicious cycle develops. Therefore chronic eructation is almost always a behavioral disorder, but it is not known why and how these patients learn this maneuver and acquire the habit. Prior work has described patients with aerophagia, in whom swallowed air passed into the intestine, leading to massive distention and/or severe flatulence without excessive eructation.[27] However, laboratory studies showed that most healthy subjects evacuate gas as rapidly as it is infused in the intestine, with little or no discomfort; only patients with intestinal hypersensitivity, for example, IBS, or dysmotility, for example, intestinal neuropathy, develop symptoms and/or retention.[32,63] Difficulty with eructation after fundoplication for GERD results in the gas-bloat syndrome (see Chapter 48).

Treatment

Treatment of repetitive eructation begins with providing a clear pathophysiologic explanation for the patient's repetitive belching: that air swallowing rather than gas production in the GI tract is the problem. Distress is diminished by an understanding of the benign nature of chronic eructation. Esophageal impedance monitoring may be performed to reassure reluctant patients, and radiologic and endoscopic evaluation should be reserved for patients who have associated symptoms or signs suggestive of thoracic or abdominal pathology.[105] Patients should be instructed to refrain from belching; holding a pencil between the teeth during episodes of repetitive belching may help a patient become aware of swallowing and stop the cycle. If present, underlying dyspeptic symptoms should also be treated (see Chapter 15). Only in severe refractory cases is a psychiatric consultation advisable.

Pneumatosis Cystoides Intestinalis

Pneumatosis cystoides intestinalis and coli is a condition characterized by the presence of gas-filled cysts in the wall of the small bowel, colon, or both (see Chapter 130). The clinical presentation ranges from completely asymptomatic to life-threatening intraabdominal complications.[106] Pneumatosis cystoides may be idiopathic (15%) or secondary (85%); the etiology appears to be multifactorial, but the precise pathophysiology is poorly understood.[107] Many patients with pneumatosis have extremely high breath H_2 concentrations, a finding indicative of high luminal concentrations of H_2.[108,109] The feces of three patients with pneumatosis of the colon were found to have unusually low concentrations of H_2-consuming organisms. Therefore the high luminal H_2 of these subjects appears to reflect H_2 production that is relatively unopposed by H_2 consumption.

How a high luminal H_2 tension results in pneumatosis is controversial. One proposal is that small intramural gas collections normally occur with some frequency but are quickly absorbed into the circulation. In the presence of high H_2 production, rapid diffusion of luminal H_2 into the cyst dilutes other cyst gases (e.g., N_2). Therefore the cyst N_2 tension remains lower than or equal to that in the blood. As a result, N_2 in the cyst cannot be absorbed and the cyst persists. The most effective treatment to eliminate the cysts is administration of high concentrations of O_2 via inhalation.[110] This maneuver reduces the blood N_2 tension to a value below that of the cyst, allowing N_2 to diffuse from the cyst into the blood, with resolution of the cyst. Other forms of therapy that may be effective are antibiotics that inhibit H_2 production and dietary manipulations that reduce the delivery of fermentable substrate to colonic bacteria.

Full references for this chapter can be found at https://ebooks.health.elsevier.com.

19 Fecal Incontinence

Satish S.C. Rao

IN THIS CHAPTER

Fecal incontinence is defined as the involuntary leakage of fecal matter through the anus or inability to control the discharge of bowel contents. Its severity can range from occasional unintentional loss of flatus to seepage of liquid fecal matter or complete evacuation of bowel contents. Consequently, the problem has been difficult to characterize from an epidemiologic and pathophysiologic standpoint, but it causes considerable embarrassment, loss of self-esteem, social isolation, and diminished quality of life (QOL).[1]

EPIDEMIOLOGY

Fecal incontinence affects people of all ages, but its prevalence is disproportionately higher in middle-aged women, older adults, and nursing home residents. Estimates of its prevalence vary greatly and depend on the clinical setting, definition of incontinence, frequency of occurrence, and influence of social stigma and other factors.[2] The embarrassment and social stigma attached to fecal incontinence make it difficult for patients to seek health care; treatment is often delayed for several years. Fecal incontinence not only causes significant morbidity but also consumes substantial health care resources.

A systematic review of 80 population-based studies reported that the polled global prevalence of FI was 8.0%.[3] In the United Kingdom, two or more episodes of fecal incontinence per month were reported by 0.8% of patients who presented to a primary care clinic.[4] In an older (age >65) self-caring population, fecal incontinence occurred at least once a week in 3.7% of patients and in more men than women (ratio of 1.5:1).[5] The frequency of fecal incontinence increases with age, from 7% in women younger than 30%–22% in women in their seventh decade.[6,7] By contrast, 25%–35% of institutionalized patients and 10%–25% of hospitalized geriatric patients have fecal incontinence.[1] In the United States, fecal incontinence is the second leading reason for placement in a nursing home.

A National Institute of Diabetes and Digestive and Kidney Diseases workshop of experts concluded that the frequency of fecal incontinence in community-dwelling women and men averages from 7% to 15%.[8] In another prospective survey of patients who attended either a gastroenterology or primary care clinic, over 18% reported fecal incontinence at least once a week.[9] Only one-third had ever discussed the problem with a physician, thereby suggesting that fecal incontinence is underreported. When stratified for the frequency of episodes, 2.7% of patients reported incontinence daily, 4.5% weekly, and 7.1% monthly.[9] In another survey, fecal incontinence was associated with urinary incontinence in 26% of women who attended a urology-gynecology clinic.[10] A high frequency of mixed fecal and urinary incontinence was also reported in nursing home residents.

Fecal incontinence has a significant impact on the QOL, including loss of self-respect, confidence, and modesty.[8,11] It also has an impact on psychological domains, including coping strategies, anxiety, fear, embarrassment, personal hygiene/odor issues, and unpredictability of stool habit.[8] Furthermore, there is a significant correlation between symptom severity and QOL.[12] Moreover, persons with incontinence were 6.8 times as likely to miss work or school and missed an average of 50 work or school days per year compared with those without incontinence or other functional GI symptoms.[13]

The cost of health care related to fecal incontinence includes measurable components such as evaluation, diagnostic testing, and treatment of incontinence, as well as use of disposable pads and other ancillary devices, skin care, and nursing care. Roughly $1.8 billion per year was spent on adult diapers in the United States alone and globally $10.7 billion,[14] and between $1.5 and $7 billion/year is spent on care for incontinence among institutionalized older patients.[1,2,15] When adjusted for 2012 dollars, the total per patient annual cost was slightly higher in the United States ($84,111) than in the Netherlands ($83,521).[16] The potential economic impact of nonsurgical therapy for fecal incontinence, such as sacral nerve stimulation (SNS), was estimated in the United Kingdom to be more than $35,000 per year,[17] but there are no prospective cost-effectiveness comparative trials. In a long-term facility, the annual cost for a patient with mixed fecal and urinary incontinence was $9711.[18] In the outpatient setting, the average estimated cost per patient (including evaluation) is $17,166.[19] These persons also incur costs that cannot be easily measured and result from their impaired QOL and social dysfunction.[7] Fecal incontinence causes a significant economic burden, including increased use of health care resources and has a major impact on QOL.

PATHOPHYSIOLOGY

Functional Anatomy and Physiology of the Anorectum

A structurally and functionally intact anorectal unit is essential for maintaining normal continence of bowel contents.[20] The rectum is a hollow muscular tube composed of a continuous layer of longitudinal muscle that interlaces with the underlying circular muscle. This unique muscle arrangement enables the rectum to serve as both a reservoir for stool and a pump for emptying stool. The anus is a muscular tube 2–4 cm in length that at rest forms an angle with the axis of the rectum (Fig. 19.1). At rest, the anorectal angle is approximately 90 degrees; with voluntary squeeze, the angle becomes more acute, about 70 degrees; and during defecation the angle becomes obtuse, about 110–130 degrees (see Chapter 20).

The anal sphincter consists of two muscular components: the internal anal sphincter (IAS), a 0.3–0.5-cm thick expansion of the circular smooth muscle layer of the rectum, and the external anal sphincter (EAS), a 0.6–1.0-cm thick expansion of the levator ani muscles. Morphologically, both sphincters are separate and heterogeneous.[21] The IAS is composed predominantly of slow-twitch, fatigue-resistant smooth muscle and generates mechanical activity with a frequency of 15–35 cycles/min as well as ultraslow waves at 1.5–3 cycles/min.[20] The IAS contributes 70%–85% of the resting anal sphincter pressure, but only 40% of the pressure after sudden distention of the rectum and 65% during constant rectal distention; the remainder of the pressure is provided by the EAS or puborectalis, or both.[22] Therefore the IAS is chiefly responsible for maintaining anal continence at rest.

The anus is normally closed by the tonic activity of the IAS. This barrier is reinforced during voluntary squeeze by the EAS. The EAS, although circumferential in its inner layers, may also have a purse string configuration in some of its outer layers anteriorly with fibers inserting into the contralateral transverse perineal and bulbospongiosus muscles and pubic rami.[23] This unique configuration may have implications for episiotomy and anal sphincter reconstruction. The anal mucosal folds, together with the expansive anal vascular cushions (see later), provide a tight seal.[24] These barriers are augmented by the puborectalis muscle, which forms a flap-like valve that creates a forward pull and reinforces the anorectal angle.[20] Studies using high-definition three-dimensional (3D) manometry have revealed that the puborectalis muscle contributes significantly to the pressure profiles and plays an integral role in maintaining continence, sensory motor response, and the rectoanal inhibitory reflex (see later).[25]

The anorectum is richly innervated by sensory, motor, and autonomic nerves and by the enteric nervous system. Traditionally it has been believed that the principal nerve to the anorectum is the pudendal nerve, which arises from the second, third, and fourth sacral nerves (S2, S3, and S4), innervates the EAS, and subserves sensory and motor function.[26] However, more recent work suggests that the anorectal nerve innervation is more

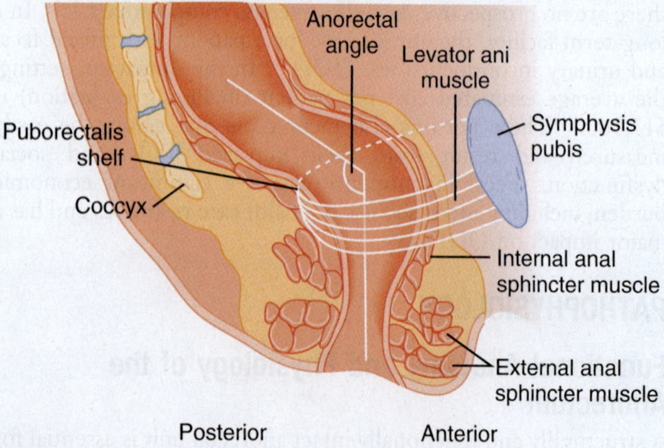

Fig. 19.1 Sagittal diagrammatic view of the anorectum. (*Source*: From Rao SSC. Pathophysiology of adult fecal incontinence. *Gastroenterology*. 2004;126:S14–22.)

complex and involves the lumbar and sacral sympathetic and parasympathetic pathways as well as a complex network of nerves.[26] A pudendal nerve block creates a loss of sensation in the perianal and genital skin and weakness of the anal sphincter muscle but does not affect rectal sensation.[22] A pudendal nerve block also abolishes the rectoanal contractile reflexes (see later), an observation that suggests that pudendal neuropathy may affect the rectoanal contractile reflex response. The sensation of rectal distention is most likely transmitted along the S2, S3, and S4 parasympathetic nerves. These nerve fibers travel along the pelvic splanchnic nerves and are independent of the pudendal nerve.[20]

How humans perceive stool contents in the anorectum is not completely understood. Earlier studies failed to demonstrate rectal sensory awareness.[20] Subsequent studies have confirmed that balloon distention is perceived in the rectum and that such perception plays a role in maintaining continence.[24,27] Furthermore, sensory conditioning can improve hyposensitivity[28,29] and hypersensitivity[30] of the rectum. Mechanical stimulation of the rectum can produce cerebral-evoked responses,[31] confirming that the rectum is a sensory organ. Likewise, electrical stimulation of the anus and rectum also triggers cortical-evoked potentials, both in health[32] and in patients with fecal incontinence.[33]

Although organized nerve endings are not present in the rectal mucosa or myenteric plexus, myelinated and unmyelinated nerve fibers are present.[20] These nerves most likely mediate the distention or stretch-induced sensory responses as well as the viscerovisceral,[31] rectoanal inhibitory, and rectoanal contractile reflexes. The sensation of rectal distention is most likely transmitted via the parasympathetic nervi erigentes along the S2, S3, and S4 splanchnic nerves. Rectal sensation and the ability to defecate can be abolished completely by resection of the nervi erigentes.[34] If parasympathetic innervation is absent, rectal filling is perceived only as a vague sensation of discomfort. Even persons with paraplegia or sacral neuronal lesions may retain some degree of sensory function, but almost no sensation is felt if lesions occur in the higher spine.[17,21,35] Studies using novel noninvasive magnetic stimulation of lumbosacral plexus and recordings of anal and rectal motor-evoked potentials (MEPs) have shown that patients with spinal cord injury and fecal incontinence exhibit significant lumbosacral neuropathy.[36,37] Therefore the sacral nerves are intimately involved in the maintenance of continence.

The suggestion has been made that bowel contents are sensed periodically by anorectal sampling,[38] the process whereby transient relaxation of the IAS allows the stool contents from the rectum to come into contact with specialized sensory organs in the upper anal canal. Specialized afferent nerves may exist that subserve sensations of touch, temperature, tension, and friction, but the mechanisms are incompletely understood.[20] Incontinent persons appear to sample rectal contents less frequently than continent persons. The likely role of anal sensation is to facilitate discrimination between flatus and feces and the fine-tuning of the continence barrier, but its precise role has not been well characterized.

Rectal distention is associated with a reflex decrease in anal resting pressure known as the *rectoanal inhibitory reflex*. The amplitude and duration of this relaxation increases with the volume of rectal distention up to a maximum of 100–150 cm^3 and then plateaus.[39] This reflex is mediated by the myenteric plexus and caused by the release of nitric oxide and vasoactive intestinal peptide[40] and is present in patients in whom the hypogastric nerves have been transected and in those with a spinal cord lesion. The reflex is absent after transection of the rectum, but it may recover.[27] The rectoanal inhibitory reflex may facilitate discharge of flatus and stool. Rectal distention is also associated with a rectoanal contractile response, a subconscious reflex effort to prevent release of rectal contents such as flatus.[41,42] This response involves contraction of the EAS and is mediated by the pelvic splanchnic and pudendal nerves. The amplitude and duration of the rectoanal contractile reflex also increases with rectal distention, up to a maximum volume of 30 mL. Abrupt increases in intra-abdominal pressure, as caused by coughing or laughing, are associated with an increase in anal sphincter pressure. A number of mechanisms, including reflex contraction of the puborectalis, may be involved. More recently, a rectoanal sensorimotor reflex response has been described, whereby the conscious perception of a desire to defecate (induced by balloon distention) evokes a contractile response in the anal canal.[43] This response is primarily mediated by contraction of the puborectalis[39] and is significantly impaired in patients with rectal hyposensitivity.[44]

The blood-filled vascular tissue of the anal mucosa also plays an important role in producing optimal closure of the anus. An in vitro study has shown that even during maximal involuntary contraction, the internal sphincter ring is unable to completely close the anal orifice; a gap of some 7 mm remains. This gap is filled by the anal cushions, which may exert pressures of up to 9 mm Hg and thereby contribute 10%–20% to the resting anal pressure.[41]

Pathogenic Mechanisms

Fecal incontinence occurs when one or more mechanisms that maintain continence are disrupted to the extent that other mechanisms cannot compensate. Therefore fecal incontinence is often multifactorial.[2,42] In a prospective study, 80% of patients with fecal incontinence had more than one pathogenic abnormality (Fig. 19.2).[20] Although pathophysiologic mechanisms often overlap, they can be categorized under four broad groups (Table 19.1).

Abnormal Anorectal and Pelvic Floor Structures

Anal Sphincter Muscles

Disruption or weakness of the EAS muscle causes urge-related or diarrhea-associated fecal incontinence. By contrast, damage to the IAS muscle or anal endovascular cushions may lead to a poor seal and an impaired sampling reflex. These changes may cause passive incontinence or fecal seepage (see later), often under resting conditions. Both sphincters may be defective in many patients. The extent of muscle loss can influence the severity of incontinence.[20]

The most common cause of anal sphincter disruption is obstetric trauma, which may involve the EAS, IAS, or pudendal nerves. However, why most women who have sustained an obstetric injury in their 20s or 30s typically do not present with fecal incontinence until their 50s is unclear. In a prospective study,

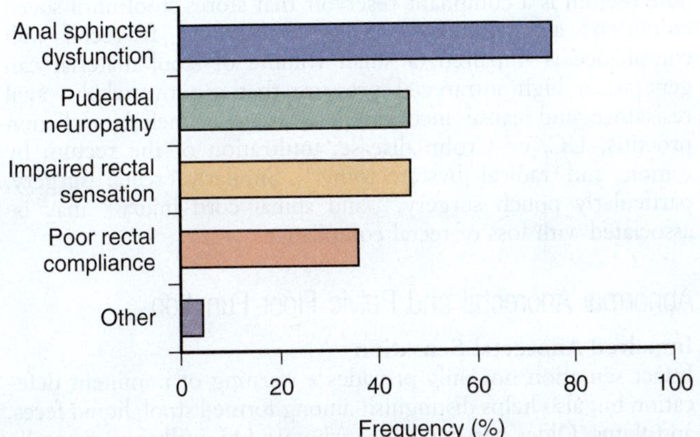

Fig. 19.2 Relative frequencies of common mechanisms that lead to fecal incontinence. In many patients, more than one mechanism is involved.

35% of primiparous (normal antepartum) women showed evidence of anal sphincter disruption after vaginal delivery.[45,46] Other important risk factors include a forceps-assisted delivery, prolonged second stage of labor, large birth weight, and occipitoposterior presentation.[20] A prospective study of 921 primiparous women has shown that the frequencies of fecal incontinence at 6 weeks and 6 months postpartum are 27% and 17%, respectively, in women with vaginal delivery and a sphincter tear; 11% and 8%, respectively, in women with vaginal delivery but without a tear; and 10% and 7.6%, respectively, in women who underwent cesarean section.[47] This study showed clearly that the occurrence and severity of fecal incontinence were due to an anal sphincter tear that occurred at the time of vaginal delivery.

Episiotomy is believed to be a risk factor for anal sphincter disruption. In one study, medial episiotomy was associated with a ninefold higher risk of anal sphincter dysfunction.[48] Regardless of the type of delivery, however, incontinence of feces or flatus occurred in a surprisingly large percentage of middle-aged women, thereby suggesting that age-related changes in the pelvic floor may predispose to fecal incontinence.

Aging affects anal sphincter function.[49] In men and women older than age 70, sphincter pressures decrease by 30%–40%, compared with younger persons.[50] In all age groups, anal squeeze pressure is lower in women than men,[50] with a rapid fall after menopause.[51] Estrogen receptors have been identified in the human striated anal sphincter, and ovariectomy in rats leads to atrophy of the striated anal sphincter muscle.[20,52] These observations suggest that the strength and vigor of the pelvic floor muscles are influenced by hormones. Pudendal nerve terminal motor latency (PNTML) is prolonged in older women, and pelvic floor descent is excessive on straining (see later).[50] These mechanisms may contribute to progressive damage to the striated anal sphincter muscle. Aging is also associated with increased thickness and echogenicity of the IAS.[53]

Other causes of anatomic disruption include anorectal surgery for hemorrhoids, fistulas, and fissures. Anal dilation or lateral sphincterotomy may result in incontinence secondary to fragmentation of the anal sphincters.[54] Hemorrhoidectomy can cause incontinence by inadvertent damage to the IAS[55] or loss of endovascular cushions. Accidental perineal trauma or a pelvic fracture may also cause direct sphincter trauma that leads to fecal incontinence,[56] but anoreceptive intercourse is not associated with anal sphincter dysfunction.[57] Finally, IAS dysfunction may also occur because of myopathy, degeneration, or radiotherapy.[20]

Puborectalis Muscle

The puborectalis muscle is important for maintaining continence by forming a flap valve mechanism.[58] Studies using 3D US have shown that 40% of women with fecal incontinence have major abnormalities, and another 32% have minor abnormalities, of the puborectalis muscle, compared with 21% and 32%, respectively, of asymptomatic parous controls.[59] Assessment of puborectalis function by a perineal dynamometer revealed impaired puborectalis (levator ani) contraction in patients with fecal incontinence, and this finding was an independent risk factor for and correlated with the severity of fecal incontinence.[60] Furthermore, improvement in puborectalis strength following biofeedback therapy was associated with clinical improvement, in part because the upper portion of the puborectalis muscle receives its innervations from branches of the S3 and S4 sacral nerves rather than the pudendal nerve. Because the puborectalis muscle and EAS have separate neurologic innervations, pudendal blockage does not abolish voluntary contraction of the pelvic floor[61] but completely abolishes EAS function.[22]

Nervous System

Intact innervation of the pelvic floor is essential for maintaining continence. Sphincter degeneration due to pudendal neuropathy

TABLE 19.1 Mechanisms, Causes, and Pathophysiology of Fecal Incontinence

Mechanism	Causes	Pathophysiology
Abnormal Anorectal or Pelvic Floor Structures		
Anal sphincter muscles	Hemorrhoidectomy, neuropathy, obstetric injury	Sphincter weakness, loss of sampling reflex
Puborectalis muscle	Aging, excessive perineal descent, trauma	Obtuse anorectal angle, sphincter weakness
Pudendal nerve	Excessive straining, obstetric or surgical injury, perineal descent	Impaired reflexes, sensory loss, sphincter weakness
Nervous system, spinal cord, autonomic nervous system	Avulsion injury, diabetes mellitus, head injury, multiple sclerosis, spinal cord injury, spine surgery, stroke	Impaired reflexes, loss of accommodation, loss of sensation, secondary myopathy
Rectum	Aging, IBD, IBS, prolapse, radiation	Hypersensitivity, loss of accommodation, loss of sensation
Abnormal Anorectal or Pelvic Floor Function		
Impaired anorectal sensation	Autonomic nervous system disorders, CNS disorders, obstetric injury	Loss of stool awareness, rectoanal agnosia
Fecal impaction	Dyssynergic defecation	Fecal retention with overflow, impaired sensation
Altered Stool Characteristics		
Increased volume and loose consistency	Bile salt malabsorption, drugs, infection, IBD, IBS, laxatives, metabolic disorders	Diarrhea and urgency, impaired accommodation, rapid stool transport
Hard stools, retention	Drugs, dyssynergia	Fecal retention with overflow
Miscellaneous		
Physical mobility, cognitive function	Aging, dementia, disability	Multifactorial changes
Psychosis	Willful soiling	Multifactorial changes
Drugs[a]	Anticholinergics Antidepressants Caffeine Laxatives Muscle relaxants	Constipation Altered sensation, constipation Relaxation of sphincter tone Diarrhea Relaxation of sphincter tone
Food intolerance	Fructose, lactose, or sorbitol malabsorption	Diarrhea, flatus

[a]Pathophysiology is noted for each class of drugs.

and obstetric trauma may cause fecal incontinence in women.[45] Neuropathic injury is often sustained during childbirth, probably as a result of stretching of the nerves during elongation of the birth canal or direct trauma during passage of the fetal head. Nerve damage is more likely to occur when the fetal head is large, the second stage of labor is prolonged, or forceps are applied, especially with a high forceps delivery or prolonged labor.

The role of extrinsic autonomic innervation is controversial. Animal studies have shown that the pelvic nerves convey fibers that relax the rectum[62]; these nerves may play a role in accommodating and storing feces and gas. Damage to the pelvic nerves may lead to impaired accommodation and rapid transit through the rectosigmoid region, thereby overwhelming the continence barrier mechanisms. Sympathetic efferent activity, as studied by stimulating the presacral sympathetic nerves, tends to relax the IAS, whereas parasympathetic stimulation may cause contraction of the anal sphincter. The upper motor neurons for voluntary sphincter muscle lie close to those that innervate the lower limb muscles in the parasagittal motor cortex and adjacent to the representation of the genitalia and perineum in the sensory cortex.[20] Damage to the motor cortex from a CNS lesion may lead to incontinence. In some patients with neurogenic incontinence, the sensory and motor nerve fibers may be damaged, resulting in sensory impairment.[63] This damage can impair conscious awareness of rectal filling as well as the associated reflex responses in the striated pelvic floor sphincter muscles.

Approximately 10% of patients with fecal incontinence may have a lesion more proximal than the intrapelvic or perianal nerves. The primary abnormality in these patients is cauda equina nerve injury,[64] which may be occult and not evident through clinical evaluation. These patients have a prolongation of nerve conduction along the cauda equina nerve roots without an abnormality in PNTML.[65] In a minority of patients, however, a combination of peripheral and central lesions is present. Other disorders such as multiple sclerosis, diabetes mellitus, and demyelination injury (or toxic neuropathy from alcohol or traumatic neuropathy) may also lead to incontinence.[20]

Rectum

The rectum is a compliant reservoir that stores stool until social conditions are conducive to its evacuation.[2] If rectal wall compliance is impaired, a small volume of stool material can generate a high intrarectal pressure that can overwhelm anal resistance and cause incontinence.[66] Causes include radiation proctitis, UC, or Crohn disease, infiltration of the rectum by tumor, and radical hysterectomy.[67] Similarly, rectal surgery, particularly pouch surgery,[68] and spinal cord injury[69] may be associated with loss of rectal compliance.

Abnormal Anorectal and Pelvic Floor Function

Impaired Anorectal Sensation

Intact sensation not only provides a warning of imminent defecation but also helps distinguish among formed stool, liquid feces, and flatus. Older persons, those who are physically and mentally challenged, and children with fecal incontinence[70] often show blunted rectal sensation. Impaired rectal sensation may lead to excessive accumulation of stool, thereby causing fecal impaction, megarectum (extreme dilatation of the rectum), and fecal overflow. Causes of impaired sensation include neurologic damage due to multiple sclerosis, diabetes mellitus, and spinal cord injury.[69] Less well known is that analgesics (particularly opiates) and antidepressants may also impair rectal sensation and produce fecal incontinence. The importance of the rectum in preserving continence has been demonstrated conclusively through surgical studies in which preservation of the distal 6–8 cm of the rectum, along with its parasympathetic nerve supply, helped patients avoid incontinence.[71] By contrast, rectal sensation and the ability to defecate can be abolished completely by resection of the nervi erigentes (see earlier).[34]

An intact sampling reflex allows an individual to choose whether to discharge or retain rectal contents. Conversely, an impaired sampling reflex may predispose a subject to incontinence.[38] The role of the sampling reflex in maintaining continence, however, remains unclear. In children who have undergone colonic pull-through surgery, some degree of sensory discrimination is preserved.[72] Because the anal mucosal sensory zone is absent in these children, the suggestion has been made that sensory receptors, possibly located in the puborectalis muscle, may play a role in facilitating sensory discrimination; traction on the muscle is a potent stimulus for triggering defecation and a sensation of rectal distention. Because abolition of anal sensation by the topical application of 5% lidocaine does not reduce resting sphincter pressure (it affects voluntary squeeze pressure but does not affect the ability to retain saline infused into the rectum), the role of anal sensation in maintaining fecal continence has been questioned.[20]

Dyssynergic Defecation and Incomplete Stool Evacuation

In some patients, particularly older adults, prolonged retention of stool in the rectum or incomplete evacuation may lead to seepage of stool or staining of undergarments.[73] Most of these patients show obstructive or dyssynergic defecation,[74] and many of them also exhibit impaired rectal sensation, whereby anal sphincter and pudendal nerve function is intact but the ability to evacuate a simulated stool is impaired. Similarly, in older adults and in children with functional incontinence, prolonged retention of stool in the rectum can lead to fecal impaction, which may also cause prolonged relaxation of the IAS, thereby allowing liquid stool to flow around impacted stool and escape through the anal canal.[70]

Descending Perineum Syndrome

In women with long-standing constipation and a history of excessive straining for many years (perhaps even without prior childbirth), excessive straining may lead to progressive denervation of the pelvic floor muscles.[75] Most of these patients demonstrate excessive perineal descent and sphincter weakness that may lead to rectal prolapse, but fecal incontinence is not an inevitable consequence. Whether or not incontinence develops will depend on the state of the pelvic floor and the strength of the sphincter muscles.

Altered Stool Characteristics

The consistency, volume, and frequency of stool and the presence or absence of irritants in stool may also contribute to the pathogenesis of fecal incontinence.[2] In the presence of large-volume liquid stools, which often transit the hindgut rapidly, continence can only be maintained through intact sensation and a strong sphincteric barrier. In patients with bile salt malabsorption, lactose or fructose intolerance, or rapid dumping of osmotic material into the colon, colonic transit of gaseous and stool contents is too rapid and can overwhelm the continence mechanisms.[2]

Miscellaneous Mechanisms

Various medical conditions and disabilities may predispose to fecal incontinence, particularly in older adults. Immobility and lack of access to toileting facilities are primary causes of fecal incontinence in this population.[76] Several drugs may inhibit sphincter tone; some are used to treat urinary incontinence and detrusor instability, including anticholinergics like tolterodine tartrate (Detrol) and oxybutynin (e.g., Ditropan), and muscle relaxants like baclofen (e.g., Lioresal) and cyclobenzaprine (e.g., Flexeril). Stimulants (e.g., caffeinated products, fiber supplements, laxatives) produce fecal incontinence by causing diarrhea.[20]

EVALUATION

History

The first step in evaluating a patient with fecal incontinence is to establish a trusting relationship and assess the duration and nature of the symptoms, with specific attention to (1) whether the leakage consists of flatus, liquid stool, or solid stool; and (2) the impact of the symptoms on QOL (Box 19.1). Because many people misinterpret fecal incontinence as diarrhea or urgency,[77] a detailed characterization of the complaint is important. The clinician should ask about the use of pads or other devices and the patient's ability to discriminate between formed or unformed stool and gas (lack of such discrimination is termed *rectal agnosia*).[2] An obstetric history, dietary history, and history of coexisting urinary incontinence and conditions like diabetes mellitus, pelvic radiation, neurologic problems, or spinal cord injury are important. A prospective stool diary, specifically the FI stool smartphone application, can be useful.

The circumstances under which incontinence occurs should also be determined. Such a detailed inquiry may facilitate recognition of the following types of fecal incontinence:

1. *Passive incontinence*, the involuntary discharge of fecal matter or flatus without any awareness. This pattern suggests a loss of perception or impaired rectoanal reflexes, with or without sphincter dysfunction.
2. *Urge incontinence*, the discharge of fecal matter or flatus despite active attempts to retain these contents. Predominant causes of this pattern are disruption of sphincter function and a decrease in rectal capacity to retain stool.
3. *Fecal seepage*, the undesired leakage of stool, often after a bowel movement, with otherwise normal continence and evacuation. This condition results primarily from incomplete evacuation of stool or impaired rectal sensation.[73,74] Sphincter function and pudendal nerve function are mostly intact.

BOX 19.1 Features of the History that Should be Elicited from a Patient with Fecal Incontinence

- Onset and precipitating event(s)
- Duration and timing
- Severity
- Stool consistency and rectal urgency
- History of fecal impaction
- Coexisting problems (e.g., diarrhea, IBD)
- Drugs, caffeine, diet
- Past history: spine surgery, urinary incontinence, back injury, diabetes mellitus, neurologic disorders
- Clinical subtypes: passive or urge incontinence or fecal seepage
- Obstetric history: use of forceps, tears, presentation of the infant, repairs

Although overlap exists among the three types, useful insights can be gained regarding the underlying mechanism(s) and preferred management by determining the predominant pattern.

Symptom assessment may not correlate well with manometric findings (see later). In one study, leakage had a sensitivity of 98.9%, specificity of 11%, and positive predictive value of 51% for detecting a low resting anal sphincter pressure on manometry.[78] The positive predictive value for detecting a low anal squeeze pressure was 80%. Therefore for an individual patient with fecal incontinence, the history and clinical features alone are insufficient to define the pathophysiology, and objective testing is essential (see later).[79,80]

A number of self-reporting QOL and fecal incontinence severity scales are available that have been validated, including FI-QOL (Fecal Incontinence-QOL), St. Mark's/Vaizey score,[81] Fecal Incontinence Severity Index,[82] Fecal Incontinence Severity Score,[12,83] and International Consultation on Incontinence Questionnaire-Bowels.[84] On the basis of the clinical features, several grading systems have been proposed. A modification of the Cleveland Clinic grading system[85] has been validated by investigators at St. Mark's Hospital[81] and provides an objective method of quantifying the degree of incontinence. It can also be useful for assessing the efficacy of therapy. This grading system is based on seven parameters: the character of the anal discharge as (1) solid, (2) liquid, or (3) flatus; (4) the degree of alterations in lifestyle; the need to (5) wear a pad or (6) take antidiarrheal medication; and (7) the ability to defer defecation. The total score ranges from 0 (continent) to 24 (severe incontinence). As noted earlier, however, clinical features alone are insufficient to define the pathophysiology. The use of validated questionnaires such as the symptom checklist 90-R and short form 36 and FI-QOL surveys may provide additional information regarding psychosocial issues and the impact of fecal incontinence on the patient's QOL. However, a stool diary that prospectively records key symptoms associated with fecal incontinence can provide useful perspectives on the problem and can also be used for the assessment of the percentage of bowel movements that are associated with fecal incontinence, a key parameter for the evaluation of treatment success.[86] An electronic stool diary using a smartphone application (FI stool app) is available for recording bowel symptoms and could prove extremely useful.

Physical Examination

A detailed physical examination, including a neurologic examination, should be performed in any patient with fecal incontinence because incontinence may be secondary to a systemic or neurologic disorder. A stepwise approach for performing a digital rectal examination in a patient with suspected fecal incontinence and documentation and scoring of the abnormal examination findings has been described.[87] The focus of the examination is on the perineum and anorectum. Perineal inspection and digital rectal examination are best performed with the patient lying in the left lateral position and with good illumination. On inspection, the presence of fecal matter, prolapsed hemorrhoids, dermatitis, scars, skin excoriations, or a gaping anus and the absence of perianal creases may be noted. These features suggest sphincter weakness or chronic skin irritation and provide clues regarding the underlying cause.[2] Excessive perineal descent or rectal prolapse can be demonstrated by asking the patient to attempt defecation. An outward bulge that exceeds 3 cm is usually defined as excessive perineal descent.[88]

First, perianal sensation should be checked. The anocutaneous reflex examines the integrity of the connections between the sensory nerves and skin; the intermediate neurons in spinal cord segments S2, S3, and S4; and the motor innervation of the EAS. This reflex can be assessed by gently stroking the perianal skin in each perianal quadrant with a cotton bud. A normal response consists of a brisk contraction of the EAS "anal wink". An impaired or absent anocutaneous reflex suggests either afferent or efferent neuronal injury.[2]

After inserting a lubricated, gloved index finger into the anus and rectum, the clinician should assess the resting sphincter tone, length of the anal canal, strength of the puborectalis sling, acuteness of the anorectal angle, strength of anal sphincter squeeze, and elevation of the perineum during voluntary squeeze. The presence of a rectocele or impacted stool may be noted.

The accuracy of the digital rectal examination has been assessed in several studies. In one study of 66 patients, digital rectal examination by an experienced surgeon correlated somewhat with resting sphincter pressure ($r = 0.56$; $P < .001$) or maximum squeeze pressure ($r = 0.72$; $P < .001$).[89] In a study of 280 patients with various anorectal disorders, a reasonable correlation was reported between digital examination and manometric findings, but the sensitivity, specificity, and positive predictive values of digital examination were low.[90] In another study of 64 patients, correlations between digital rectal examination with resting and squeeze pressure were 0.41 and 0.52, respectively.[91] These data suggest that digital rectal examination provides only an approximation of sphincter strength. The findings are influenced by many factors, including the size of the examiner's finger, technique used, and cooperation of the patient. Moreover, trainees lack adequate skills for recognizing the features of fecal incontinence on digital rectal examination.[92] Although digital rectal examination can identify patients with fecal impaction and overflow, it is not accurate for diagnosing sphincter dysfunction and should not be used as the basis for decisions regarding treatment.[2]

Diagnostic Testing

An important step in assessing a patient with fecal incontinence is to determine whether the incontinence is secondary to diarrhea or independent of stool consistency. If diarrhea coexists with incontinence, appropriate tests should be performed to identify the cause of the diarrhea (see Chapter 17). Such testing may include flexible sigmoidoscopy or colonoscopy to exclude colonic mucosal inflammation, a rectal mass, or stricture and stool studies for infection, volume, osmolality, electrolytes, fat content, and pancreatic dysfunction. Biochemical tests should be performed to look for thyroid dysfunction, diabetes mellitus, and other metabolic disorders. Breath tests may be considered for lactose or fructose intolerance or small intestinal bacterial overgrowth (SIBO).[2] A history of cholecystectomy may suggest bile salt malabsorption and prompt a therapeutic trial of a bile salt–binding agent.

Specific tests are available for defining the underlying mechanisms of fecal incontinence and are often used in a complementary fashion. The most useful tests are anorectal manometry, anal endosonography, the balloon expulsion test (BET), special neurophysiologic tests including translumbosacral anorectal magnetic stimulation (TAMS), and PNTML,[2,93–96] as well as newer tests such as fecobionics for defining the anal sphincteric region.[97]

Anorectal Manometry

Anorectal manometry is a useful method for assessing IAS and EAS pressures (Fig. 19.3) as well as rectal sensation, rectoanal reflexes, and rectal compliance. Several types of probes and pressure recording devices are available. Each system has distinct advantages and drawbacks; however, an international survey of experts showed significant variability in methodology, performance characteristics, and interpretation of the tests.[98] Although traditionally a water-perfused probe with closely spaced sensors has been used,[2] increasingly, solid-state probes with

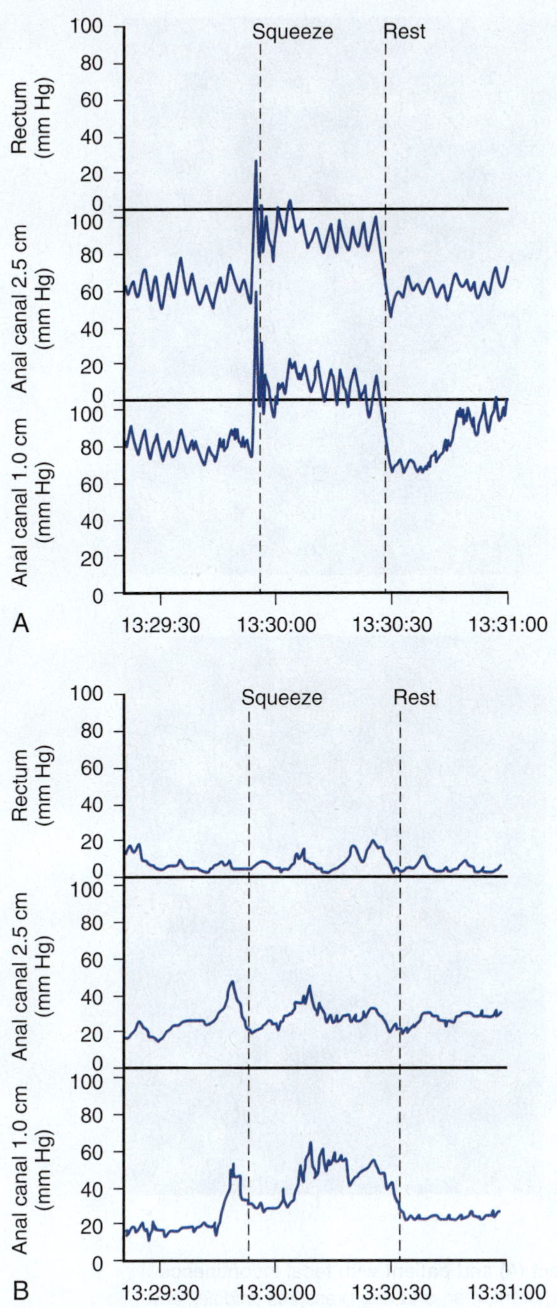

Fig. 19.3 Anorectal manometry profiles in (A) a healthy normal subject in whom squeeze (external anal sphincter) and resting (internal anal sphincter) pressures are normal and (B) a patient with fecal incontinence in whom squeeze and resting pressures are weak. *Upper tracings,* rectal pressure activity; *middle tracings,* anal pressure activity at 2.5 cm; *lower tracings,* anal pressure activity at 1.0 cm from the anal margin.

microtransducers or air-filled miniaturized balloons are being adopted globally. A solid-state probe with 12 circumferential sensors spaced at 1-cm intervals with a 4.2-mm outer diameter and
4-cm-long balloon (Given Imaging) provides high resolution.[99] This device uses a novel pressure transduction technology (TactArray) that allows each of the pressure-sensing elements to detect pressure over a length of 2.5 mm and in each of 12 radially

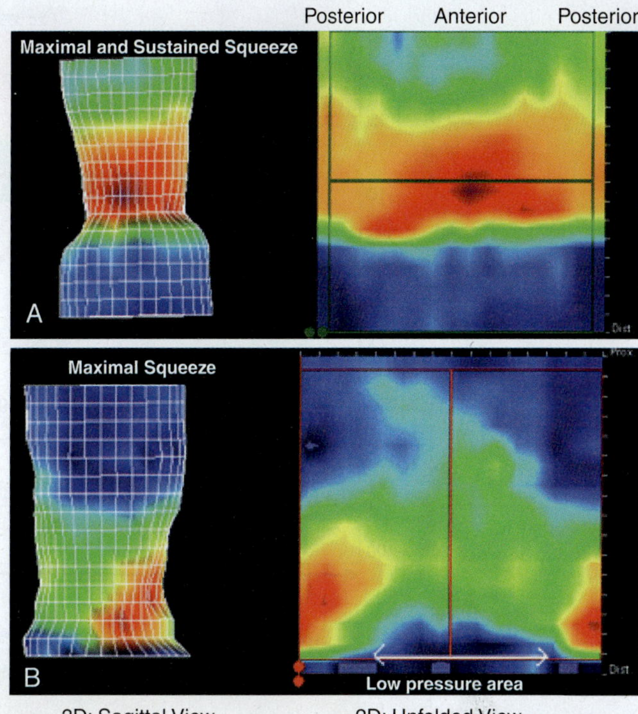

Fig. 19.4 High-definition anal sphincter vector topography showing pressure changes during maximal squeeze in a three-dimensional sagittal view (*left*) and a two-dimensional unfolded view (*right*). (A) Changes in a healthy control subject. (B) Changes in a subject with fecal incontinence. The subject with incontinence has significant anal sphincter weakness, with an asymmetrical squeeze and a change in some vectors (*predominantly yellow and green*), whereas the healthy subject shows a robust squeeze (*orange and red*) and symmetrical decrease in sphincter diameter.

dispersed sectors. The data can be displayed in isobaric contour plots that can provide a continuous dynamic representation of pressure changes, although anal sphincter pressures are higher than those recorded with water-perfused manometry. A high-definition 3D manometry system with 256 circumferentially arrayed sensors in a 5-cm probe is also being used in many laboratories and provides anal sphincter pressure profiles and topography (Fig. 19.4). The fecobionics is a newer system that is composed of a simulated stool with a balloon housing multiple impedance sensors, rear and front pressure sensors, gyroscopes, and provides a comprehensive profile of the anal high-pressure zone, quantification of the anal sphincter distensibility, and an assessment of anal resistance, opening forces, and compliance (Fig. 19.5). Preliminary study in FI subjects shows that distensibility indices and defecatory resistances are significantly different compared to controls.[97]

Anal sphincter pressures can be measured by stationary or station pull-through techniques.[85,94] Resting anal sphincter pressure predominantly represents IAS function, and voluntary anal squeeze pressure represents EAS and puborectalis function. Patients with fecal incontinence have low resting and low squeeze pressures (see Figs. 19.3 and 19.4), indicating IAS and EAS weakness, respectively.[2,90] The duration of sustained squeeze pressure provides an index of sphincter muscle fatigue. The ability of the EAS to contract reflexively can be assessed during abrupt increases in intra-abdominal pressure, as when the patient coughs. This reflex response causes the anal sphincter pressure to rise above that of the rectal pressure to preserve continence. The response may be triggered by receptors in the pelvic floor and mediated through a spinal reflex arc. In patients with a spinal cord

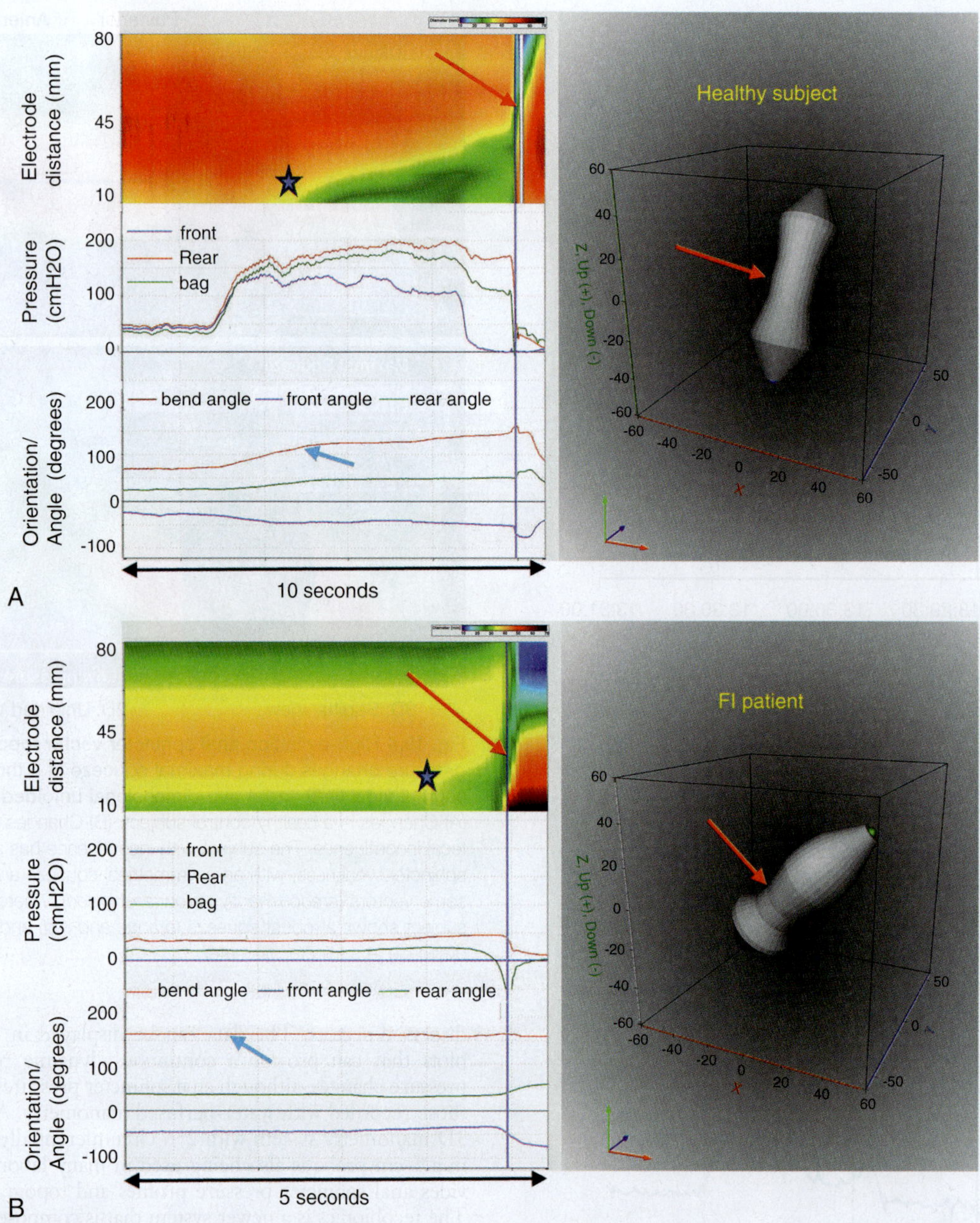

Fig. 19.5 Images from Fecobionics study in a healthy subject (A) and patient with fecal incontinence (FI) (B). The left panels show diameter color topography (*upper*), front, rear, and bag pressures (*middle*), and the orientations at the front and rear and bend angle of the device (*lower*). The right panel shows the 3D shape of device during evacuation. The *red arrows* point to the minimum anal diameter in color topography and 3D diagram, and *blue arrows* point to the bend angle (anorectal angle). The *stars* indicate when the device starts to move during evacuation. During evacuation, in the healthy subject, the abdominal/rectal pressure increases, the angle straightens, the anal sphincter relaxes, and the device moves through the anal canal. In the FI patient, the front pressure was 0 cm H_2O (atmospheric pressure) even before the evacuation attempt, indicating weak anal sphincter, and the bend angle was more obtuse and the smallest anal diameter was larger than the healthy subject, suggesting low anal resistance and faster evacuation.

lesion above the conus medullaris, this reflex response is preserved even though voluntary squeeze may be absent, whereas in patients with a lesion of the cauda equina or sacral plexus, both the reflex and voluntary squeeze responses are absent.[2,100,101]

Anorectal manometry can provide useful information regarding anorectal function.[93,95,102] The American Motility Society has recommended guidelines and minimal standards for manometry testing.[95] Although data regarding normal values are insufficient, and results between healthy subjects and patients with fecal incontinence overlap,[90] with large confidence intervals for test reproducibility,[103] manometry testing can be useful in an individual patient with fecal incontinence.[95] Manometric tests of anorectal function may also be useful for assessing objective improvement following drug therapy, biofeedback therapy, or surgery (see later).[28,104,105] International efforts to develop consensus among experts regarding testing methodology and interpretation of tests could pave the way for standardizing the test and improving clinical diagnosis and patient management.[106]

Rectal Sensory Testing

Rectal balloon distention with air or water can be used to assess sensory responses and compliance of the rectal wall. By distending a balloon with incremental volumes in the rectum, the thresholds for first perception, first desire to defecate, and urgent desire to defecate can be assessed. A higher threshold for sensory perception indicates rectal hyposensitivity.[2,100,107] The balloon volume required for partial or complete inhibition of anal sphincter tone can also be assessed. The volume required to induce reflex anal relaxation is lower in incontinent patients than in controls.[108]

Because sampling of rectal contents by the anal mucosa may play an important role in maintaining continence,[38] quantitative assessment of anal perception using electrical or thermal stimulation has been advocated but is not used clinically.[2] Rectal compliance can be calculated by assessing the changes in rectal pressure during balloon distention with air or fluid.[94,109] Rectal compliance is reduced in patients with colitis,[66] patients with a low spinal cord lesion, and diabetic patients with incontinence but is increased in those with a high spinal cord lesion. Recent studies show that patients with FI have both rectal hyposensitivity and rectal hypersensitivity.[110]

Imaging the Anal Canal

Anal Endosonography

Anal endosonography is performed by using a 7–15-mHz rotating transducer with a focal length of 1–4 cm.[111] The test provides an assessment of EAS and IAS thickness and structural integrity and can detect scarring, loss of muscle tissue, and other local pathology (Fig. 19.6).[112] Higher-frequency (10–15-mHz) probes and 3D reconstruction of the anal sphincter that provide improved delineation of the sphincter complex have become available.[112]

After vaginal delivery, anal endosonography has revealed occult sphincter injury in 35% of primiparous women; most of these lesions were not detected clinically. In another study, sphincter defects were detected in 85% of women with a third-degree perineal tear, compared with 33% of patients without a tear.[113] In studies that compared EMG (see later) mapping with anal endosonography, the concordance rate for identifying a sphincter defect was high,[114,115] but the technique is operator dependent and requires training and experience.[94] Although endosonography can distinguish internal from external sphincter injury, it has a low specificity for demonstrating the cause of fecal incontinence.[2] Because anal endosonography is more widely available, less expensive, and certainly less painful than EMG, which requires needle insertion, it is the preferred technique for examining the morphology of the anal sphincter muscles and detecting anal sphincter defects.[98]

MRI

Endoanal MRI can provide superior imaging with excellent spatial resolution, particularly for defining the anatomy of the EAS.[116,117] One study,[118] but not another,[116] has shown that MRI is less accurate than anal endosonography. A major contribution of anal MRI has been the recognition of EAS atrophy, which may adversely affect sphincter repair (see later)[119]; atrophy may be present without pudendal neuropathy.[120] The addition of dynamic pelvic MRI using fast imaging sequences or MRI colpocystography, which involves filling the rectum with ultrasound gel as a contact agent and having the patient evacuate while lying inside the magnet, may define the anorectal anatomy more precisely.[121] Use of an endoanal coil enhances resolution and allows more precise definition of the sphincter muscles. Comparative studies of costs, availability, technical factors, clinical utility, and role in treatment decision making are warranted.

Defecography

Defecography uses fluoroscopic techniques to provide morphologic information about the rectum and anal canal.[122] It is used to assess the anorectal angle, measure pelvic floor descent and the length of the anal canal, and detect the presence of a rectocele, rectal prolapse, or mucosal intussusception. About 150 mL of contrast material is placed into the rectum, and the subject is asked to squeeze or cough and expel the contrast. Although defecography can detect a number of abnormalities, these findings can also be seen in otherwise asymptomatic persons,[94,123] and their presence correlates poorly with impaired rectal evacuation. Agreement between observers in the measurement of the anorectal angle is also poor. Whether one should use the central axis of the rectum or the posterior wall of the rectum when measuring the angle is unclear. The functional significance of identifying morphologic defects has been questioned. Although defecography can confirm the occurrence of incontinence at rest or during coughing, it is most useful for demonstrating rectal prolapse[2,124] or poor rectal evacuation (see Chapter 20). In selected patients, magnetic resonance

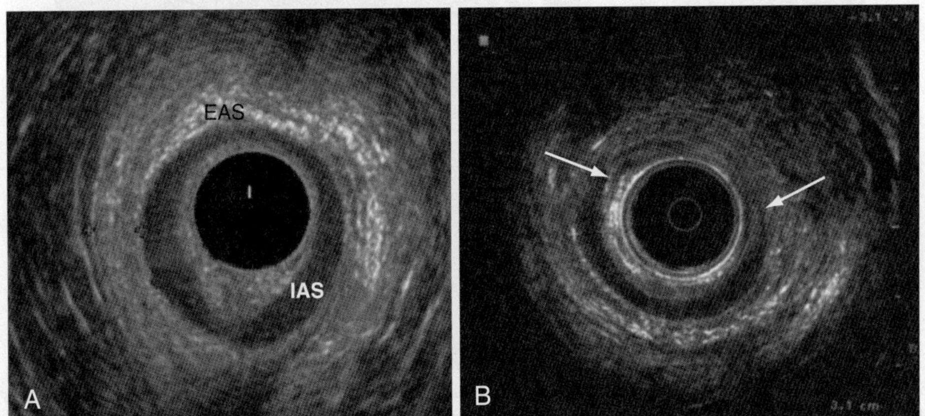

Fig. 19.6 Anal endosonograms. (A) Normal, healthy subject with an intact hypoechoic internal anal sphincter (*IAS*) and an intact thicker and hyperechoic external anal sphincter (*EAS*). (B) Subject with fecal incontinence secondary to an obstetric injury, causing a large anterior sphincter defect that involves the IAS and EAS and spans the circumference between the 10 and 2 o'clock positions (*arrows*).

defecography can be used to evaluate evacuation and identify coexisting problems (e.g., rectocele, enterocele, cystocele, and mucosal intussusception).[112]

Balloon Expulsion Test (BET)

Normal patients can expel a 50-mL water-filled balloon[125] or a silicone-filled artificial stool from the rectum in less than 1 minute.[2] Some studies have used a Foley balloon for performing this test[126]; however, one study has shown that use of a Foley balloon is an inappropriate method, and up to 50% of normal subjects may experience difficulty expelling this device.[127] Most patients with fecal incontinence have little or no difficulty with evacuation, but patients with fecal seepage[74] and many older persons with fecal incontinence secondary to fecal impaction[73] demonstrate impaired evacuation. In these patients, a BET may help identify coexisting dyssynergia or a lack of coordination between the abdominal, pelvic floor, and anal sphincter muscles during defecation. One study has shown a high frequency of dyssynergia in residents of nursing homes (see Chapter 20).[128]

Neurophysiologic Testing

EMG of the muscle activity from the anal sphincter is a useful technique for identifying sphincter injury as well as denervation-reinnervation potentials that can indicate neuropathy.[31] EMG can be performed using a fine-wire needle electrode or a surface electrode, such as an anal plug. Abnormal EMG activity like fibrillation potentials and high-frequency spontaneous discharges provides evidence of chronic denervation, which is commonly seen in patients with fecal incontinence secondary to pudendal nerve injury or cauda equina syndrome.[129] However, EMG is rarely used clinically.

The PNTML measures neuromuscular integrity between the terminal portion of the pudendal nerve and the anal sphincter. Injury to the pudendal nerve leads to denervation of the anal sphincter muscle and muscle weakness. Therefore measurement of the nerve latency time can help distinguish muscle injury from nerve injury as the cause of a weak sphincter muscle. A disposable electrode [St. Mark's electrode (Dantec, Denmark)] is used to measure the latency time.[130] Prolonged nerve latency time suggests pudendal neuropathy. Women who have delivered vaginally with a prolonged second stage of labor or have had forceps-assisted delivery have been found to have a prolonged PNTML compared with women who delivered by cesarean section or spontaneously.[131,132] An American Gastroenterological Association (AGA) technical review did not recommend PNTML,[94] although an expert review has noted that patients with pudendal neuropathy generally have a poor surgical outcome.[133] A normal PNTML does not exclude pudendal neuropathy, because the presence of a few intact nerve fibers can lead to a normal result, whereas an abnormal latency time is significant. PNTML may be useful for the assessment of patients prior to anal sphincter repair and is particularly helpful in predicting surgical outcome.

A better test of the neuromuscular integrity of the efferent motor pathways that control anorectal function is by recording the MEPs of the rectum and anal sphincter in response to magnetic stimulation of the lumbar and sacral nerve roots, using a novel noninvasive modality—TAMS—bilaterally.[26,36,37,134] The technique is based on Faraday's principle, which states that in the presence of a changing electrical field, a magnetic field is generated. Consequently, when a current is discharged rapidly through a conducting coil, a magnetic flux is produced around the coil. The magnetic flux causes stimulation of neural tissue. TAMS allows more precise localization of the nerve pathways between the spinal cord and the anal sphincter, as well as subcomponent analysis of the efferent peripheral nervous system, rectum, and anal sphincter. Electrical or magnetic stimulation of the lumbosacral nerve roots facilitates measurement of the conduction time within the cauda equina and can diagnose sacral motor radiculopathy as a possible cause of fecal incontinence.[135,136] One study has shown that recording of translumbar MEPs and transsacral MEPs of the rectum and anus provides delineation of peripheral neuromuscular injury in patients with fecal incontinence

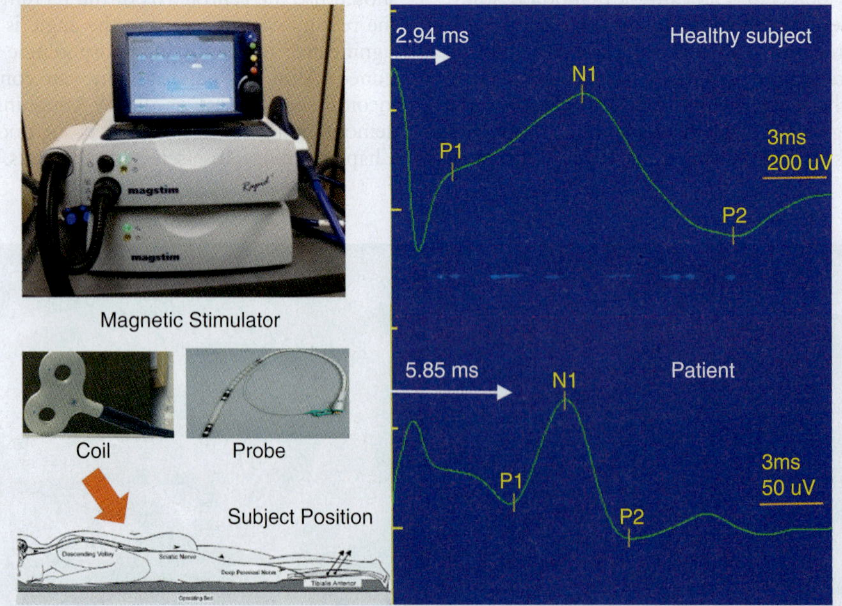

Fig. 19.7 Equipment for the translumbosacral anorectal magnetic stimulation (TAMS) test (*left*) and anal motor evoked potential (MEP) responses following translumbar magnetic stimulation (*right*). The equipment consists of a magnetic stimulation device, a magnetic coil, and an anorectal MEP probe. The subject's position is illustrated at the bottom left. The MEP response from a healthy subject (*top right*) shows a normal MEP latency of 2.94 ms. The lower right profile from a patient with fecal incontinence shows a prolonged latency and a smaller amplitude of the MEP response, indicating anorectal neuropathy.

(Fig. 19.7)[26,37] and can reveal hitherto undetected changes in patients with back injury. Another study assessed the locus of efferent in patients with fecal incontinence and showed that although the transcranial-anorectal MEPs were prolonged in patients with fecal incontinence when compared with healthy controls, the primary locus for nerve dysfunction in patients with fecal incontinence was between the spinal nerve roots and the anorectum; the segment between the brain and spinal cord was mostly intact.[33]

Clinical Utility of Tests for Fecal Incontinence

In one prospective study, history taking alone could detect an underlying cause in only 9 of 80 patients (11%) with fecal incontinence, whereas physiologic tests revealed an abnormality in 44 patients (55%).[137] In a large retrospective study of 302 patients with fecal incontinence, an underlying pathophysiologic abnormality was identified, but only after manometry, EMG, and rectal sensory testing were performed.[138] Most patients had more than one pathophysiologic abnormality. In another large study of 350 patients, incontinent patients had lower resting and squeeze sphincter pressures, a smaller rectal capacity, and earlier leakage following saline infusion in the rectum.[102] Nevertheless, results of a single test or a combination of three different tests (anal manometry, rectal capacity, and saline continence test) provided a low discriminatory value between continent and incontinent patients. This finding emphasizes the wide range of normal values and the ability of the body to compensate for the loss of any one mechanism involved in fecal incontinence.

In a prospective study, anorectal manometry with sensory testing not only confirmed a clinical impression but also provided new information that was not detected clinically.[93] Diagnostic information obtained from these studies can influence both management and outcomes of patients with incontinence. A single abnormality was found in 20% of patients, whereas more than one abnormality was found in 80% of patients. In another study, abnormal sphincter pressure was found in 40 patients (71%), and altered rectal sensation or poor rectal compliance was present in 42 patients (75%).[137] These findings were confirmed by another study, which showed that physiologic tests provided a definitive diagnosis in 66% of patients with fecal incontinence.[138] Still, on the basis of the test results alone, it is not possible to predict whether an individual patient is continent or incontinent. An abnormal test result must be interpreted in the context of the patient's symptoms and the results of other complementary tests. Tests of anorectal function provide objective data and define the underlying pathophysiology. Table 19.2 summarizes the key tests, information gained from them, and evidence to support their clinical use.

TREATMENT

Treatment goals for patients with fecal incontinence are to restore continence and improve QOL. Strategies that include supportive and specific measures may be used. An algorithmic approach to the evaluation and management of patients with fecal incontinence is presented in Fig. 19.8

Supportive Measures

Supportive measures like avoiding offending foods, ritualizing bowel habits, improving skin hygiene, and instituting lifestyle changes may serve as useful adjuncts to managing fecal incontinence. For older or institutionalized patients with fecal incontinence, the availability of personnel experienced in the treatment of fecal incontinence, timely recognition of soiling, and immediate cleansing of the perianal skin are of paramount importance.[76] Hygienic measures such as changing undergarments, cleaning the perianal skin immediately following a soiling episode, using moist wipes rather than dry toilet paper, and using barrier creams like zinc oxide and calamine lotion [Calmoseptine (Calmoseptine, Huntington Beach, CA)] may help prevent or heal skin excoriation. Perianal fungal infections should be treated with topical antifungal agents. More importantly, scheduled toileting with a commode at the bedside (or bedpan) and supportive measures to improve the patient's general well-being and nutritional status may prove effective. Stool deodorants [e.g., Bedside-Care Perineal Wash (Coloplast Manufacturing, North Mankato, MN); Derifil (Integra, Plainsboro, NJ); Devrom (Parthenon, Salt Lake City, UT)] can help disguise the smell of feces. In an institutionalized patient, ritualizing the bowel habit and instituting cognitive training may prove beneficial. Using these measures, short-term (3–6 months) success rates of up to 60% have been reported in case series.[139] Patients in whom these measures fail have been shown to have a higher mortality rate than those without incontinence and those with incontinence who respond to these measures.[140]

Other supportive measures include dietary modifications like reducing caffeine or fiber intake. Caffeinated coffee enhances the gastrocolic (or gastroileal) reflex, increases colonic motility,[141] and induces fluid secretion in the small intestine.[142] Reducing caffeine consumption, particularly after meals, may help lessen postprandial urgency and diarrhea. Brisk physical activity, particularly after meals or immediately after waking, may precipitate fecal incontinence, because these physiologic events are associated with increased colonic motility[143] and enhanced colonic transit.[144] In a study of 2565 adults that monitored exercise activity and fecal incontinence, after adjustments, fecal incontinence was positively associated with moderate-to-vigorous exercise but not with light-intensity physical activity.[145] A food and symptom diary may identify dietary factors that cause diarrheal stools and incontinence. Frequent culprits are lactose and fructose, which may be malabsorbed[146]; eliminating food items containing these constituents may prove beneficial.[2] Fiber supplements such as psyllium are often advocated in an attempt to increase stool bulk and reduce watery stools. In a single case-controlled study, psyllium led to modest improvement,[147] but fiber supplements can potentially worsen diarrhea by increasing colonic fermentation of unabsorbable fiber.

Specific Therapies

Pharmacologic Therapy

The antidiarrheal agents loperamide hydrochloride (Imodium) and diphenoxylate and atropine sulfate (Lomotil) remain the mainstays of drug treatment for fecal incontinence, although other drug treatments have been proposed.[2,148] In placebo-controlled studies, loperamide, 4 mg three times daily, has been shown to reduce the frequency of incontinence, improve stool urgency, and increase colonic transit time,[104] as well as increase anal resting sphincter pressure[149] and reduce stool weight. An 8-week randomized crossover study of 80 patients with fecal incontinence showed an approximate 40% reduction in fecal incontinence episodes with both loperamide and psyllium, but there was no difference between the two treatments.[150] Clinical improvement was also reported with diphenoxylate and atropine,[151] but objective testing showed no improvement in the patient's ability to retain saline or spheres in the rectum. Although most patients temporarily benefit from antidiarrheal agents, many report cramping, lower abdominal pain, or difficulty with evacuation after a few days. Careful dose titration is required to produce the desired result. Another randomized controlled study tested clonidine, an α2-adrenergic agonist, 0.1 mg twice daily, in patients with incontinence and found that, although diarrhea decreased, the number of episodes of fecal incontinence did not change.[152]

TABLE 19.2 Diagnostic Tests for Fecal Incontinence[a]

Test	Clinical Use: Advantages	Clinical Use: Disadvantages	Quality of Evidence	Comments
Physiology				
Anorectal manometry (high resolution and 3D-high definition)	Quantifies normal or weak EAS and IAS and puborectalis pressures; identifies rectal hyposensitivity, rectal hypersensitivity, impaired rectal compliance, dyssynergic defecation	Lack of standardization	Good	Useful for detecting anal sphincter weakness, altered rectal sensation and accommodation, and dyssynergia
Anorectal EndoFLIP	Measures the cross-sectional area of the anal sphincter, distensibility index, and sphincter compliance	Lack of normative data and availability	Fair	Mostly used in research labs; clinical utility not fully known
Needle EMG	Quantifies spike potentials and reinnervation pattern indicating neuropathy or myopathy	Invasive, painful; not widely available	Fair	Useful but used largely in research laboratories
Surface EMG	Displays EMG activity; can provide information on normal or weak muscle tone	Inaccurate, frequent artefacts	Fair	Used largely for neuromuscular training
Pudendal nerve terminal motor latency (PNTML)	Measures latency of the terminal portion of the pudendal nerve, simple to perform	Minimally invasive, low sensitivity, interobserver differences	Fair	Conflicting data; correlation with other tests and surgical outcome unclear
Translumbosacral anorectal magnetic stimulation (TAMS) test	Quantifies the nerve conduction time of the entire spinoanal and spinorectal pathways; minimally invasive	Lack of training and availability	Good	Noninvasive test; objective and higher yield than PNTML; quantifies anal and rectal neuropathy
Colonic transit study with radiopaque markers	Evaluates the presence of fecal retention; inexpensive and widely available	Inconsistent methodology; validity has been questioned	Good	Useful for identifying patients with fecal seepage and older persons with impaction
Balloon expulsion test (BET)	Simple, inexpensive, bedside assessment of ability to expel a simulated stool; identifies dyssynergic defecation	Lack of standardization	Good	Normal BET does not exclude dyssynergia; should be interpreted in the context of other anorectal test results
Imaging				
Anorectal US	Visualizes IAS and EAS defects, thickness, and atrophy and puborectalis muscles	Interobserver bias; scars difficult to identify	Good	Most widely available test
Defecography	Detects prolapse, intussusception, obtuse anorectal angle, and pelvic floor weakness, as well as rectoceles and megarectum	Radiation exposure, embarrassment, availability, interobserver bias, inconsistent methodology	Fair	Useful and complementary with other tests
MRI	Simultaneously evaluates global pelvic floor anatomy and dynamic motion; reveals sphincter morphology and pathology outside the anorectum	Expensive, lack of standardization and availability	Fair	Used as an adjunct to other tests
Plain abdominal film	Identifies excessive amount of stool in the colon; simple, inexpensive, widely available	Lack of standardization of interpretation, lack of controlled studies	Poor	Not recommended for routine evaluation but useful in older adults and children with incontinence and fecal impaction
Barium enema	Identifies megacolon, megarectum, stenosis, diverticulosis, extrinsic compression, and intraluminal masses	Lack of standardization, embarrassment, radiation exposure, lack of controlled studies	Poor	Not recommended as part of routine evaluation
Endoscopy				
Flexible sigmoidoscopy and colonoscopy	Directly visualizes the colon to exclude mucosal lesions (e.g., solitary rectal ulcer syndrome, inflammation, malignancy)	Invasive, risks related to procedure (perforation, bleeding) and sedation	Poor	Indicated in patients with unexplained diarrhea and seepage and patients > age 50

[a]Evidence-based summary.

3D, 3-Dimensional; *EAS*, external anal sphincter; *EndoFLIP*, endoluminal functional lumen imaging probe; *IAS*, internal anal sphincter.

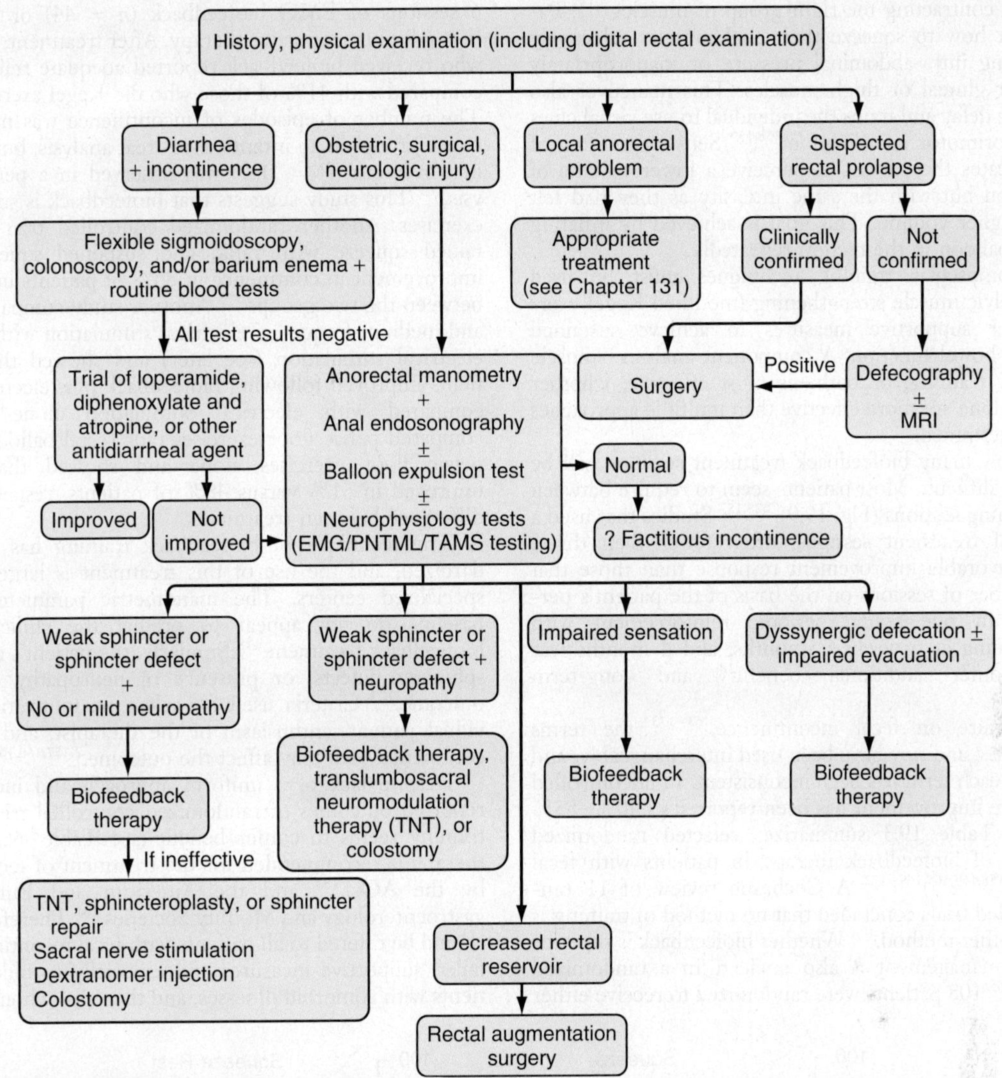

Fig. 19.8 Algorithm for the evaluation and management of patients with fecal incontinence. *PNTML*, Pudendal nerve terminal motor latency; *TAMS*, translumbosacral anorectal magnetic stimulation.

Idiopathic bile salt malabsorption may be an important underlying cause of diarrhea and fecal incontinence (see Chapters 17 and 66).[153] Patients with this problem may benefit from titrated doses of ion exchange resins like cholestyramine (Questran) (2–6 g daily), colestipol (Colestid), or colesevelam (Welchol). Alosetron (Lotronex), a 5-hydroxytryptamine-3 receptor antagonist approved for treatment of IBS and diarrhea, may serve as an adjunctive therapy for fecal incontinence, but the drug's side effects restrict its use (see Chapter 124).[154]

Postmenopausal women with fecal incontinence may benefit from estrogen replacement therapy.[155] An open-label study has shown that oral amitriptyline, 20 mg, is useful in treating patients who have urinary or fecal incontinence without evidence of a structural defect or neuropathy.[156] Suppositories or enemas may also have a role in the treatment of incontinent patients with incomplete rectal evacuation or in those with postdefecation seepage. In some patients, constipating medications alternating with periodic enemas may provide more controlled evacuation of bowel contents, but these interventions have not been tested prospectively.

Biofeedback

Neuromuscular and sensory training, usually referred to as *biofeedback therapy* (or simply biofeedback), improves symptoms of fecal incontinence, restores QOL, and improves objective parameters of anorectal function. Biofeedback training is useful in patients with a weak sphincter or impaired rectal sensation. The method is based on operant conditioning techniques whereby an individual acquires a new behavior through a learning process of repeated reinforcement and instant feedback.[2,157] The goals of biofeedback therapy in a patient with fecal incontinence are to (1) improve anal sphincter muscle strength; (2) improve coordination between the abdominal, gluteal, and anal sphincter muscles during voluntary squeeze and following rectal perception; and (3) enhance anorectal sensory perception.

Because each goal requires a specific method of training, the treatment protocol should be customized for each patient on the basis of the underlying pathophysiologic mechanism(s). Biofeedback training is often performed using visual, auditory, or verbal feedback techniques, and the feedback is provided via a manometry or EMG probe placed in the anorectum.[2,157] When a patient is asked to squeeze, the anal sphincter contraction is displayed as an increase in anal pressure or EMG activity. This visual cue provides instant feedback to the patient.

The aim of rectoanal coordination training is to achieve a maximum voluntary squeeze in less than 2 seconds after a balloon is inflated in the rectum. In reality, this maneuver mimics the arrival of stool in the rectum and prepares the patient to react appropriately by contracting the right group of muscles.[2,157] Patients are taught how to squeeze their anal muscles selectively without increasing intra-abdominal pressure or inappropriately contracting their gluteal or thigh muscles. This maneuver also identifies sensory delay and trains the individual to use visual clues to improve sensorimotor coordination.[158,159] Sensory training of the rectum educates the patient to perceive a lower volume of balloon distention but with the same intensity as they had felt earlier with a higher volume. This goal is achieved by inflating and deflating a balloon in the rectum repeatedly.

These neuromuscular training techniques must be used together with pelvic muscle strengthening (modified Kegel exercises) and other supportive measures to achieve sustained improvement in bowel function. A component analysis—muscle training, sensory training, or both—is most effective; whether Kegel exercises alone are more effective than multiple approaches has not been determined.

Predicting how many biofeedback treatment sessions will be required is often difficult. Most patients seem to require between four and six training sessions (Fig. 19.9).[2,28,157] Studies that used a fixed number of treatment sessions, often fewer than three, showed a less favorable improvement response than those that titrated the number of sessions on the basis of the patient's performance.[160,161] In one study, periodic reinforcement with biofeedback training at 6 weeks, 3 months, and 6 months was thought to confer additional benefit[28] and long-term improvement.[162]

In the literature on fecal incontinence,[163–173] the terms *improvement*, *success*, and *cure* have been used interchangeably, and the definition of each term has been inconsistent. In uncontrolled studies, subjective improvement has been reported in 40%–85% of patients.[2,160] Table 19.3 summarizes selected randomized controlled trials of biofeedback therapy in patients with fecal incontinence.[157,158,164,165,169–172] A Cochrane review of 11 randomized controlled trials concluded that no method of training is better than any other method.[174] Whether biofeedback is superior to conservative management is also unclear. In a randomized controlled trial,[165] 108 patients were randomized to receive either 6 sessions of EMG biofeedback ($n = 44$) or Kegel exercises ($n = 64$) plus supportive therapy. After treatment, 77% of patients who received biofeedback reported adequate relief of symptoms compared with 41% of those who did Kegel exercises ($P < .001$). The number of episodes of incontinence was not different between groups in an intention-to-treat analysis, but a trend toward improvement ($P = .042$) was observed in a per-protocol analysis.[165] This study suggests that biofeedback is superior to Kegel exercises. Another randomized controlled trial compared sustained squeeze with rapid and sustained squeeze and found improvement in continence in 86% of patients but no difference between the two groups.[175] Another study compared biofeedback and medium-frequency electrical stimulation with low-frequency electrical stimulation (see later) and showed that 54% of patients improved following biofeedback plus electrical stimulation compared with electrical stimulation alone.[176] One study compared pelvic floor exercises plus rectal balloon training with pelvic floor exercises alone and showed that incontinence improved in 51% versus 48% of patients, respectively, with no difference between treatments.[177]

The technique of biofeedback training has not been standardized, and the use of this treatment is largely restricted to specialized centers. The manometric parameters obtained at baseline do not appear to predict the clinical response to biofeedback treatment.[178] Similarly, the patient's age, presence of sphincter defects, or presence of neuropathy do not predict outcome.[179] Criteria used for selection, motivation of the individual patient, enthusiasm of the therapist, and severity of incontinence each may affect the outcome.[2,157,160,161,171]

Despite lack of a uniform approach and inconsistencies in reported outcomes of randomized controlled trials, biofeedback training seems to confer benefit (see Table 19.3). Biofeedback therapy is recommended for the treatment of fecal incontinence by the ACG,[180] and the American and European Neurogastroenterology and Motility Societies.[181] Therefore biofeedback should be offered to all patients with fecal incontinence who have failed supportive measures and especially to older patients, patients with comorbid illnesses, and those for whom reconstructive

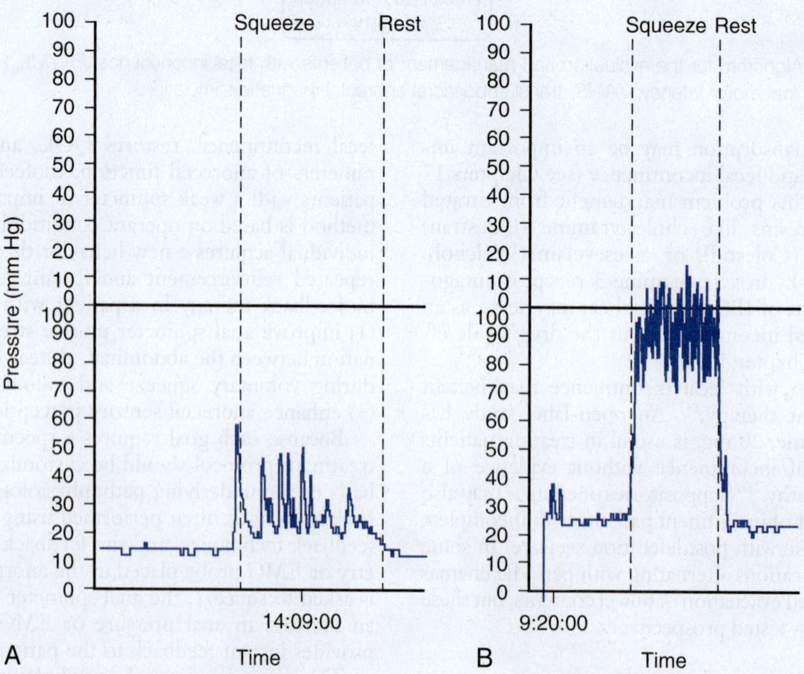

Fig. 19.9 Anal manometric pressure tracings in a patient with fecal incontinence before (A) and after (B) neuromuscular training (biofeedback) while squeezing and at rest. Before neuromuscular training, the patient has a weak and poorly sustained squeeze and makes multiple ineffective attempts to squeeze. After 6 sessions of training, the patient's ability to generate and sustain the squeeze has improved significantly.

TABLE 19.3 Outcome of Biofeedback Therapy and/or Exercises for Fecal Incontinence in Adults[a]

Reference(s)	Subjects (F/M)	Treatment	Control	Outcome
156	17/8	Manometric BFB + rectal sensory training + coordination training (weekly, 4 weeks)	Sham training (crossover design)	Treatment improved symptoms
162	40/0	BFB + electrical stimulation (augmented) (weekly, 12 weeks)	Vaginal manometric biofeedback	Greater symptom improvement in treatment group than control group ($P < .001$)
163	83/25	BFB + PFMT + sensory training (biweekly, 12 weeks)	PFMT	Treatment improved symptoms more than PFMT alone (77% vs. 41%; $P = .001$)
167	60/0	BFB (weekly, 12 weeks) + electrical stimulation	BFB	NSD between groups
168	49/0	BFB + home exercises	Electrical stimulation	Both groups improved NSD between groups in symptoms and QOL
169	159/12	4 groups: 1. Education + advice 2. As per group 1 + PFMT 3. As per group 2 + manometric BFB 4. As per group 3 + home BFB (biweekly, 6 sessions, 3 months)	N/A	≈54% improved in all groups NSD between groups in symptoms and QOL
170	107/13	3 groups: 1. PFMT 2. PFMT + anal ultrasound BFB 3. PFMT + manometric BFB (monthly, 5 sessions)	N/A	NSD between groups in symptoms, QOL, and manometry changes
173	53/19	Sustained squeeze (5 sessions, 8 weeks)	Rapid and sustained squeeze (5 sessions, 8 weeks)	Continence improved in 86% NSD between groups
174	65/15	Biofeedback and medium-frequency electrical stimulation (twice daily, 6 months)	Low-frequency electrical stimulation (twice daily, 6 months)	Anal continence improved 54% in treatment group but 0% in control group
175	72/8	PFMT and RBT (twice weekly for 3 weeks, then once a week; 12 sessions)	PFMT (twice a week for 3 weeks, then once a week; 12 sessions)	Incontinence improved in both groups; 51% in treatment group and 48% in control group NSD between groups
249, 250	26/4	Home biofeedback with novel electrical stimulation and anal resistance training (once a day, 6 weeks)	Office biofeedback with ARM probe (once a week, 6 weeks)	Incontinence improved in both groups; rates of response (≥50% reduction in incontinence events) were 65% in home group and 60% in office group

[a]Selected randomized controlled trials.
ARM, Anorectal manometry; *BFB*, biofeedback (using EMG probe unless otherwise specified); *F*, females; *M*, males; *N/A*, not applicable; *NSD*, no significant difference; *PFMT*, pelvic floor muscle training; *QOL*, quality of life; *RBT*, rectal balloon training.
Adapted from Norton C. Fecal incontinence and biofeedback therapy. *Gastroenterol Clin North Am*. 2008;37:587–604.

surgery is being considered. Severe fecal incontinence, pudendal neuropathy, and an underlying neurologic disorder are associated with a poor response to biofeedback therapy.[182–184] One study has suggested that biofeedback training may be most beneficial in patients with urge incontinence.[185] Biofeedback also seems to be useful for patients who have undergone anal sphincteroplasty,[186] postanal repair (see later),[187] or low-anterior resection[188] and children who have undergone correction of a congenital anorectal anomaly.[189]

Plugs, Sphincter Bulking Agents, and Electrical Stimulation

Disposable anal plugs have been used to help temporarily occlude the anal canal and prevent stool leakage.[190] Unfortunately, many patients are unable to tolerate prolonged insertion of the device.[191,192] A plug may be useful for patients with impaired anal canal sensation, those with neurologic disease,[193] and those who are institutionalized or immobilized. In some patients with fecal seepage, insertion of an anal plug made of surgical cotton may prove beneficial.[194] A multicenter, prospective, single-arm, nonrandomized controlled study assessed a silicone insert (Renew Medical Inc., Foster City, CA) in 91 patients with fecal incontinence. A greater than or equal to 50% reduction in fecal incontinence episodes was seen in 62% of the treated patients, who also had a reduction in incontinence severity scores. About 78% of patients who completed 12 weeks of treatment reported extreme satisfaction with the device in preventing stool leakage.[195] A vaginal bowel control system [Eclipse System (Pevalon, Sunnyvale, CA)] using an inflatable, self-retaining balloon, akin to a pessary, operates by providing extrinsic compression of the anorectum.[196] In an open labeled 4-week trial, 61 of 110 patients were successfully fitted with the device, and 79% of this group reported a greater than or equal to 50% reduction in the number of incontinence episodes,[196] with improvement in QOL. Pelvic discomfort or pain, vaginal spotting, and erythema and urinary leakage were the main adverse events. A long-term controlled trial is awaited.

Many people with fecal incontinence choose not to wear a pad. Small anal dressings may be useful for minor soiling contained between the buttocks but can become costly if several dressings are needed each day. Diapers are generally thought to be unsatisfactory for providing security or comfort, for skin protection, or for disguising odor. However, the rising global sales and improvement in diaper technology suggest that diapers may be more acceptable than previously appreciated.

Bulking the anal sphincter to augment its surface area and thereby provide a better seal for the anal canal has been attempted with a variety of agents, including autologous fat,[197] glutaraldehyde-treated collagen,[198] and synthetic macromolecules.[199] These materials are usually injected submucosally at the site where the sphincter is deficient or circumferentially if the whole muscle is degenerated or fragmented. Studies have shown definite improvement in the short term in patients with passive fecal incontinence. Injection of dextranomer beads above the dentate line has been shown to be superior to placebo injection in a randomized controlled trial of 206 patients. Response was defined as a 50% or more decrease in the number of incontinence episodes compared with baseline, with response rates of 52% with injection of the beads and 31% with placebo.[200] A 36-month long-term efficacy assessment showed that 52.2% of patients reported sustained benefit (≥50% reduction in the number of episodes) and 13.25% reported complete continence.[201] Another injectable bulking agent, polyacrylate-polyalcohol, has also been assessed in a prospective uncontrolled trial of 58 patients. The injections were given subcutaneously through the perianal skin into the submucosa of the anorectum, above the dentate line. About 60% of patients were adjudicated as having treatment success, based on 50% improvement in the Cleveland Clinic score for fecal incontinence.[202] Lack of a control group and selection bias are significant limitations of this study.

Electrical stimulation of striated muscle at a frequency sufficient to produce a tonic involuntary contraction (usually 30–50 Hz) can increase muscle strength, the conduction rate of the pudendal nerve, and the size of motor units, as well as encourage neuronal sprouting and promote local blood flow.[203,204] Stimulation at lower frequencies (5–10 Hz) can modulate autonomic function, including sensation and overactivity. Studies of electrical stimulation for fecal incontinence have been small, uncontrolled, and confounded by the effects of exercise, biofeedback, or other interventions. A Cochrane review of 4 randomized controlled trials with 260 participants concluded that electrical stimulation may have some effect.[205] One study found that anal electrical stimulation with anal biofeedback produces short-term benefits greater than those with biofeedback alone,[164] whereas another study found no additional benefit to electrical stimulation over exercises and biofeedback alone.[169] Patients have been shown to improve equally with stimulation at 1 and 35 Hz.[157] Two randomized controlled trials have reported that biofeedback and electrical stimulation are equally effective[170,206]; therefore, whether electrical stimulation by itself is helpful remains unclear.

A critical barrier in our understanding of the treatments for fecal incontinence has been a lack of comparative effectiveness trials that involve two or more therapies. Consequently, it is not known which treatment is most effective for which type of patient and who is likely to benefit the most.

Surgery

Surgery should be considered for selected patients who have failed conservative measures or biofeedback therapy.[207] The choice of surgical procedure must be tailored to the need of the individual patient and can be described under four broad clinical categories: (1) simple structural defects of the anal sphincters, (2) weak but intact anal sphincters, (3) complex disruption of the anal sphincter complex, and (4) extrasphincteric abnormalities. Table 19.4 summarizes success rates for various surgical procedures.[208]

In most patients, particularly those with obstetric trauma, overlapping sphincter repair is often sufficient. The torn ends of the sphincter muscle are plicated together and to the puborectalis muscle. Overlapping sphincter repair, as described by Parks and McPartlin,[209] involves a curved incision anterior to the anal canal with mobilization of the external sphincter, which is divided at the site of the scar; the scar tissue is preserved to anchor the sutures, and overlap repair is carried out using two rows of sutures. If an IAS defect is identified, a separate imbrication (overlapping

TABLE 19.4 Success Rates of Minimally Invasive Surgical Interventions for Fecal Incontinence

Procedure	Outcome Measures	Success Rate (%)	Quality of Evidence
Currently Available			
Injection of dextranomer beads	>50% improvement in incontinence episodes compared with baseline	52 vs. 31 (dextranomer vs. placebo)	Fair
Anal sphincter repair	Clinical, physiologic	50–66[a]	Fair[b]
Sacral nerve stimulation	Complete continence Improvement in continence by ≥50%	40–75 75–100	Good
Dynamic gracilis neosphincter	Restoration of continence	42–85	Poor[c]
Artificial bowel sphincter	Full continence	50–100[d]	Poor
Under Study			
Radiofrequency therapy (Secca procedure)	Improvement in continence by ≥50%	84	Poor
Rectal augmentation	Avoidance of stoma	64	Poor

[a]5-year success rates fall to 50%.
[b]Derived from a Cochrane review, but in some cases data were extrapolated from only one study.
[c]Based on a systematic review of case series; no comparative studies available.
[d]Explantation rates in case series of approximately 50%.
Adapted from Gladman MA. Surgical treatment of patients with constipation and fecal incontinence. *Gastroenterol Clin North Am*. 2008;37:605–25, With permission.

repair) of the IAS may be undertaken. Symptom improvement rates of 70%–80% have been reported, although one study reported an improvement rate of only about 50%.[209–213] Some patients may experience problems with evacuation after surgery. Long-term outcomes of sphincteroplasty (over 5–10 years) have been disappointing, with only 30% of patients showing a good outcome.[214]

In patients with incontinence caused by a weak but intact anal sphincter, postanal repair has been tried.[215] The anorectal angle is made more acute via an intersphincteric approach, thereby improving continence. Long-term success of this approach ranges from 20% to 58%.[216]

In patients with severe structural damage of the anal sphincter and significant incontinence, construction of a neosphincter has been attempted using two approaches: (1) use of autologous skeletal muscle, often the gracilis and rarely the gluteus,[133,217] and (2) use of an artificial bowel sphincter (ABS).[218] The technique of stimulated gracilis muscle transposition (dynamic graciloplasty) has been tested in many centers, but results have been disappointing.[219,220] Implantation of an ABS consists of an inflatable cuffed device filled with fluid from an implanted balloon reservoir, which is controlled by a subcutaneous pump. The cuff is deflated to allow defecation.[221,222] A randomized controlled trial has demonstrated that an ABS is better than conservative treatment in improving continence.[223] Long-term outcome studies with median follow-up periods of approximately 7 years, however, have documented success rates of less than 50%, explantation rates as high as 49%, and infection rates of up to 33%.[158,224] Evacuation problems occur in 50% of patients.

Rectal augmentation is a novel approach to correcting physiologic abnormalities in a subgroup of patients with intractable fecal incontinence secondary to reservoir or rectal sensorimotor dysfunction.[225]

No controlled studies have compared surgical management with pharmacologic or biofeedback therapy, and no controlled studies of the different surgical approaches have been published. Because the outcome of most procedures ranges from significant improvement initially to a less satisfactory result in the long term, no single procedure is universally accepted. In the future, a better understanding of the underlying pathophysiology and development of safer and better techniques, followed by prospective controlled trials, may allow selection of younger patients with well-defined sphincter defects for appropriate surgery.

Other Procedures

Radiofrequency energy can be delivered deep to the mucosa of the anal canal via multiple needle electrodes with use of a specially designed probe [Secca System (Rayfield Technology, Houston, TX)] inserted into the anal canal of patients with fecal incontinence.[226] The proposed mechanism of action is heat-induced tissue contraction and remodeling of the anal canal and distal rectum. In one study, symptomatic improvement was sustained at 2 and 5 years after treatment.[227] A multicenter trial has confirmed the improvements in continence and QOL, at least in the short term (6 months). Complications include ulceration of the mucosa and delayed bleeding.[228] Interestingly, no changes were seen in the results of anorectal manometry, PNTML measurement, or anal endosonography. A 6-month European controlled study showed that radiofrequency was better than sham treatment, but the clinical impact was negligible and QOL was unchanged.[229] Results of a randomized controlled trial of this method completed in the United States are pending.

The Malone, or antegrade continent, enema procedure[230] consists of fashioning a cecostomy button or appendicostomy[231] to allow periodic antegrade washout of the colon. This approach may be suitable for children and patients with neurologic disorders.[231–233]

Colostomy

If none of the aforementioned techniques is suitable or all have failed, a colostomy remains a safe, although aesthetically less preferable, option for many patients.[133,234–236] It is particularly suitable for patients with spinal cord injury, immobilized patients, and those with severe skin problems or other complications. A colostomy should not be regarded as a failure of medical or surgical treatment.[208] For many patients with fecal incontinence, restoration of a normal QOL and amelioration of symptoms can be rewarding. Use of a laparoscopic-assisted approach, a trephine colostomy, may help to fashion a stoma with minimal morbidity for the patient.[237] In one study, the total direct costs were estimated to be $31,733 for a dynamic graciloplasty, $71,576 for a colostomy including stoma care, and $12,180 for conventional treatment of fecal incontinence.[238]

Sacral Nerve Stimulation (SNS)

SNS has emerged as a useful treatment option in selected patients, although how SNS improves fecal incontinence remains unclear.[239] The benefit may relate to direct peripheral effects on colorectal sensory or motor function or to central effects at the level of the spinal cord or brain.[240] Earlier studies were performed in patients with a morphologically intact anal sphincter, but subsequent reports have described the treatment in patients with EAS defects,[241] IAS defects,[242] cauda equina syndrome,[243] and spinal injuries.[244]

The SNS technique consists of two phases. The first is a temporary trial phase of 2 weeks during which electrodes are implanted in the second or third sacral nerve roots and the nerves are stimulated with a neurostimulator device. If the patient reports satisfactory improvement of symptoms, a permanent neurostimulator device is placed in the second phase (Fig. 19.10). Initial reports of SNS have described marked improvements in clinical symptoms and QOL and marginal effects on physiologic parameters.[213,245] Results of multicenter studies of SNS have reported marked and sustained improvement in fecal incontinence and

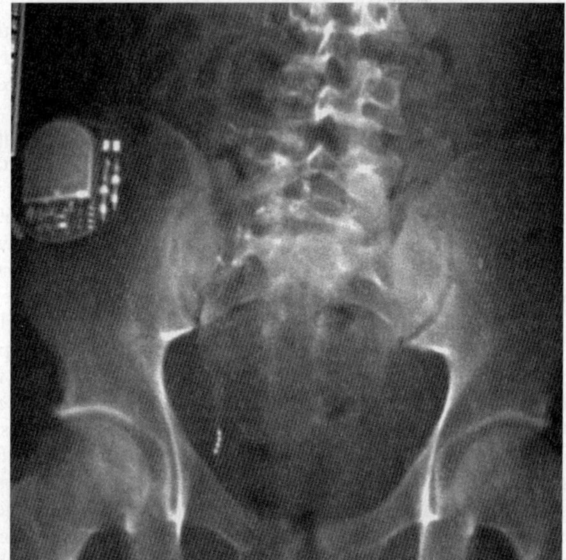

Fig. 19.10 Plain abdominal film showing a nerve stimulator device (RLQ) along with electrodes (radiopaque) permanently implanted into the sacral nerves. This patient presented with fecal incontinence and underwent a colonic transit study that revealed significant retention of radiopaque markers, which were located mostly in the distal colon, suggesting anorectal outlet dysfunction.

QOL.[246–248] A randomized controlled trial found SNS to be superior to supportive therapy (pelvic floor exercises, bulking agents, and dietary manipulation),[249] but long-term outcomes are not yet available. A morphologically intact anal sphincter may not be a prerequisite for success with SNS, and patients with EAS defects of less than 33% can be treated effectively with this method.[241] A systematic review of the published outcomes of trials of SNS revealed that 40%–75% of patients achieve complete continence, and 75%–100% experience improvement, with a low (10%) frequency of adverse events.[239]

Percutaneous Tibial Nerve Stimulation

Percutaneous tibial nerve stimulation (PTNS) uses a 34-gauge needle to stimulate the posterior tibial nerve, and through this the L4-S3 nerve roots, to improve fecal incontinence.[250] In a large multicenter randomized controlled trial of 227 patients, there was no difference in efficacy ($\geq$50% reduction in FI) between the PTNS and sham groups (38% vs. 31%), suggesting a lack of benefit in all comers with fecal incontinence.[250] Another approach for PTNS is to use cutaneous pads, but data are limited.

Novel Therapies

Several new innovative approaches are being explored to remedy fecal incontinence. A new home biofeedback system that combines mechanical resistance training of the anal sphincter with a self-titrating inflation balloon and gradual escalation of the electrical stimulation of anal sphincter with a voice-guided program has been tested in a randomized controlled trial.[251,252] Home biofeedback appeared to be as effective as office biofeedback, with a clinical response rate of 65% in the home group compared with 60% in the office group in a 6-week randomized controlled trial.[251,252] Another approach has been to augment the anal sphincter by encircling it with magnetic leads. An uncontrolled prospective study of 35 patients reported 5-year follow-up data in 23 patients (65%) with a therapeutic success in 63% at 1 year, 66% at 3 years, and 53% at 5 years. Adverse events included seven device explantations, defecatory dysfunction (20%), pain (14%), and infection (11%).[253] Another novel approach has been to use adult stem cells, especially myoblasts, obtained from muscle biopsies that have the potential for repairing and regenerating damaged anal sphincter tissue.[254] In a randomized controlled trial, intrasphincteric injections of autologous myoblasts or placebo showed similar degrees of improvement in Cleveland Clinic incontinence score at 6 months (primary outcome measure), but at 12 months improvement continued in the myoblast group whereas the placebo group reverted to baseline. Subsequently, the placebo group received open-labeled myoblasts and showed 60% improvement in fecal incontinence symptoms.[255] However, another study that used stem cells derived from adipose tissue showed no improvement in fecal incontinence.[256] A phase II RCT, compared autologous skeletal muscle derived cells at a low cell count plus electrical stimulation versus a high cell count plus electrical stimulation versus controls.[257] The responder rate was similar among three groups, but fecal incontinence episodes and QOL were significantly better in the two cell therapy groups. A pilot randomized controlled trial evaluated the efficacy and safety of translumbosacral neuromodulation therapy using repetitive magnetic stimulation of the lumbar and sacral nerves.[33] Magnetic stimulation at a frequency of 1 Hz showed significant superiority in improving fecal incontinence, with an 88% response rate when compared with the 5 Hz group (25% response rate) and 15 Hz group (42% response rate). Such noninvasive neuromodulatory therapies may prove beneficial in the future.

In summary, conservative therapies and biofeedback are the first-line treatments.[258] If unsuccessful, sphincter bulking with dextranomer followed by SNS may be considered. PTNS is not recommended, but sphincteroplasty should be considered in postoperative incontinence. An evidence-based summary of current therapies for fecal incontinence is shown in Table 19.5.

Specific Subgroups of Patients

Patients with Spinal Cord Injury

Patients with a spinal cord injury demonstrate delayed colonic motility or anorectal dysfunction that may manifest as incontinence, seepage, difficulty with defecation, or rectal hyposensitivity.[259] Anal sphincter pressures and rectal compliance are low in these patients, but the correlation between manometric findings and bowel dysfunction is poor. Studies of translumbar and transsacral MEPs have shown profound neuromuscular dysfunction affecting the entire spinoanal and spinorectal pathways.[36] Patients with a spinal cord injury may have fecal incontinence due to a supraspinal lesion or lesion of the cauda equina.[100,101] In the former group, the sacral neuronal reflex arc is intact, and the cough reflex is preserved. Therefore reflex defecation is possible through digital stimulation or with suppositories. In patients with a low spinal cord or cauda equina lesion, digital stimulation may not be effective because the defecation reflex is often impaired. In these cases, management consists of antidiarrheal agents to prevent continuous soiling with stool, followed by periodic administration of enemas or use of laxatives or lavage solutions at convenient intervals.[2] A cecostomy procedure may also be appropriate.[260] In some patients, colostomy may be the best option.[234]

Patients with Fecal Seepage

Because patients with fecal seepage show dyssynergic defecation with impaired rectal sensation, neuromuscular conditioning with biofeedback techniques to improve dyssynergia can be useful (see Chapter 20).[74,261] Therapy that consists of sensory conditioning

TABLE 19.5 Treatment Options for Fecal Incontinence[a]

Treatment	Quality of Evidence
Medications	
Diphenoxylate and atropine	Fair
Loperamide	Fair
Amitriptyline	Poor
Cholestyramine	Poor
Biofeedback	Good
Anal Plug Devices	Poor
Surgery	
Sacral nerve stimulation	Good
Sphincter bulking	Good
Artificial bowel sphincter	Fair
Dynamic graciloplasty	Fair
Sphincteroplasty	Fair
Colostomy	Poor
Radiofrequency therapy (Secca procedure)	Poor
Novel Treatments	
Autologous myoblast/stem cell therapy	Fair
Electrical/mechanical resistance training	Fair
Translumbosacral neuromodulation therapy	Fair

[a]Evidence-based summary.

and rectoanal coordination of the pelvic floor muscles to evacuate stools more completely has been shown to substantially reduce the number of fecal seepage events and improve bowel function and anorectal function by objective measures.[74]

Older Persons

Fecal incontinence is a common problem in older adults and may be a marker of declining health and increased mortality in patients in nursing homes.[76] In one study, fecal incontinence developed in 20% of nursing home residents during a 10-month period after admission, and long-lasting incontinence was associated with reduced survival.[140] In one report, immobility, dementia, and the use of restraints that precluded a patient from reaching the toilet in time were the most important risk factors for development of fecal incontinence.[18] Usual mechanisms of incontinence include impaired anorectal sensation, weak anal sphincter, and weak pelvic floor muscles. Decreased mobility and lowered sensory perception are also common causes of incontinence.[262] Many of these patients have fecal impaction and overflow.[73,263] Fecal impaction, a leading cause of fecal incontinence in institutionalized older adults, results largely from a person's inability to sense and respond to the presence of stool in the rectum. A retrospective screening of 245 permanently hospitalized geriatric patients[264] revealed that fecal impaction (55%) and laxatives (20%) are the most common causes of diarrhea and that immobility and fecal incontinence are strongly associated with fecal impaction and diarrhea. One study showed that impaired anal sphincter function (a risk factor for fecal incontinence), decreased rectal sensation, and dyssynergia are seen in up to 75% of nursing home residents with fecal incontinence.[50,265]

Stool softeners, saline laxatives, and stimulant laxatives are frequently administered as prophylactic treatments to prevent constipation and impaction.[266] In a study of institutionalized older patients, use of a single osmotic agent with a rectal stimulant and weekly enemas to achieve complete rectal emptying reduced the frequency of fecal incontinence by 35% and the frequency of soiling by 42%.[139] If fecal impaction is not relieved by laxatives and better toileting, a regimen of manual disimpaction, tap water enemas two or three times weekly, and rectal suppositories should be considered.[267] In the presence of impaired sphincter function and decreased rectal sensation, however, liquid stools may be counterproductive. Similarly, neuromuscular training to improve dyssynergia in older adults, ritualizing the patient's bowel habits, improving mobility, and cognitive training may be useful.[76]

Children

Incontinence is seen in 1%–2% of otherwise healthy 7-year-old children.[268] It is due to functional fecal retention (previously described as *encopresis*), functional nonretentive fecal incontinence,[269] congenital anomalies, developmental disability, or mental retardation.

In children with functional fecal retention, bowel movements are irregular, often large and bulky, and painful. Consequently, when the child experiences an urge to defecate, he or she assumes an erect posture, holds the legs close together, and forcefully contracts the pelvic and gluteal muscles. Over time, this conscious suppression of defecation leads to excessive rectal accommodation, loss of rectal sensitivity, and loss of the normal urge to defecate. The retained stools become progressively more difficult to evacuate, thereby leading to a vicious cycle. The ultimate result is overflow incontinence, with seepage of mucus or liquid stool around an impacted fecal mass. This aberrant behavior may lead to unconscious contraction of the external sphincter during defecation and cause dyssynergic defecation.[263,270]

By contrast, functional nonretentive fecal incontinence represents repeated and inappropriate passage of stool at a place other than the toilet by a child older than 4 years of age with no evidence of fecal retention. According to criteria established by the Rome III Consensus Committee,[269] children with functional nonretentive fecal incontinence often pass stools daily in the toilet but in addition have almost complete stool evacuations in their underwear more than once a week. They have no palpable abdominal or rectal fecal mass nor evidence of fecal retention on a plain abdominal film, and colonic radiopaque marker studies are normal.[271] The frequency of daytime and nighttime enuresis is higher (40%–45%) in children with functional nonretentive fecal incontinence than in those with fecal retention. Children with functional nonretentive fecal incontinence have significantly more behavioral problems and more externalizing or internalizing of psychosocial problems than control subjects.

Treatment goals are to remove any fecal impaction, restore normal bowel habits (including passage of soft stools without discomfort), and ensure self-toileting and passage of stools at appropriate places.[271] Disimpaction is best accomplished with oral medication or enemas. High doses of polyethylene glycol 3350 (1–1.5 g/kg/day for 3 days) have been shown to be effective.[272] Once disimpaction has been achieved, the treatment should focus on preventing a recurrence through dietary interventions, behavioral modification, and laxatives. Treatment of functional nonretentive fecal incontinence is based on education, a nonaccusatory approach, regular toilet use with rewards, and referral to a psychologist. Successful resolution of symptoms may require prolonged treatment and follow up.[273,274] Resolving parental conflicts and psychosocial stressors and alleviating the fear of painful bowel movements may be critical to a successful outcome.[261,275]

The most common congenital anomalies are neural tube defects (e.g., meningomyelocele, spina bifida) and anal atresia [imperforate anus (see Chapter 100)]. Children with a neural defect or malformation may benefit from behavioral therapy, including a stimulated defecation program (see earlier).[276] Anal atresia is best treated by surgery, but about 20% may have unsatisfactory results.[271] Surprisingly, children with anorectal malformations seem to cope well with their illness.[277] Children with mental retardation or those with a developmental delay may be slow to (or never) achieve full bowel control and require lifelong supportive therapy.

Acknowledgment

The author is most grateful for the excellent assistance of Ms. Helen Smith and Dr. Yun Yan. This work was supported in part by Grants U01DK115572-05 and 5R01DK121003-05 and R01DK131488-02 from the National Institutes of Health.

Full references for this chapter can be found at https://ebooks.health.elsevier.com.

20 Constipation

Johanna C. Iturrino, Anthony J. Lembo

IN THIS CHAPTER

Constipation is a term used to describe a person's perception of altered bowel movements that includes hard stools, difficulty with defecation, and a sensation of incomplete evacuation, among others. Chronic constipation is diagnosed when a person describes symptoms of constipation for at least 3 consecutive months. Chronic constipation is usually due to a disorder of colonic propulsion and/or rectal evacuation[1] and can be divided into three categories: slow-transit constipation, normal-transit constipation, and rectal evacuation disorder. Significant overlap can exist among these entities.[1,2] Secondary causes of chronic constipation are less common and include mechanical, neurologic, hormonal, and metabolic conditions, as well as the effects of pharmacotherapy.

Chronic constipation affects a substantial portion of the population and is particularly prevalent in women, children, and older adults. Most people do not seek medical attention for their constipation, and nearly two-thirds do not discuss their constipation with their doctor,[3] but because constipation affects between 3% and 31% of the population, it still resulted in approximately 2.5 million office and over 320,000 emergency department visits in the United States in 2010.[4] For most affected people, minimal or no intervention is required, whereas for others, constipation can be challenging to treat and have a negative impact on quality of life. In these cases, secondary causes of constipation must be excluded.

DEFINITION AND PRESENTING SYMPTOMS

It is important to ask patients what they mean when they say, "I am constipated." Most patients describe constipation as the perception of difficulty with bowel movements or a discomfort related to bowel movements. The most common terms used by young, healthy adults to define constipation are *straining* (52%), *hard stools* (44%), and *inability to have a bowel movement* (34%).[5] Constipation among Asian adults was characterized by *straining* (83%), *hard stool* (74%), and *sensation of incomplete evacuation* (68%).[6] Similarly, analysis of the National Health Interview Survey (NHIS) data found that in 10,875 subjects older than age 60, straining and hard bowel movements were most strongly associated with self-reported constipation.[7]

The definition of constipation also varies among health care providers.[8] The traditional medical definition of constipation, based on the 95% lower confidence limit for healthy adults in the United States, has been 3 or fewer bowel movements per week.[9] Reports of stool frequency, however, are often inaccurate and correlate poorly with complaints of constipation,[10] and people who complain of constipation frequently have a broader set of symptoms, including hard stools, a feeling of incomplete evacuation, abdominal discomfort, bloating, excessive straining, a sensation of blockage during defecation, and abdominal distention.[2]

In an attempt to standardize the definition of constipation, a consensus definition was initially developed by international experts in 1992 (Rome I Consensus Committee criteria)[11] and has since been updated in 1999,[12] 2006,[13] and 2016[14] (Rome II, III, and IV criteria, respectively [Box 20.1]).

BOX 20.1 Rome IV Criteria for Functional Constipation

1. Must include 2 or more of the following:*
   a. Straining during more than 25% of defecations
   b. Lumpy or hard stools† during more than 25% of defecations
   c. Sensation of incomplete evacuation during more than 25% of defecations
   d. Sensation of anorectal obstruction/blockage during more than 25% of defecations
   e. Manual maneuvers (e.g., digital evacuation, support of the pelvic floor) to facilitate more than 25% of defecations
   f. Fewer than 3 spontaneous bowel movements per week
2. Loose stools are rarely present without the use of laxatives
3. Insufficient criteria for IBS

*Criteria fulfilled for the past 3 months with symptom onset at least 6 months prior to diagnosis.
†Bristol stool form scale Types 1 or 2 (see Fig. 20.2)
From Lacy BE, Mearin F, Chang L, et al. Bowel disorders. *Gastroenterology*. 2016; 150:1393–1407.e5.

The Rome criteria incorporate the multiple symptoms of constipation, of which stool frequency is only one of several, and require that a minimum of two symptoms be present in at least 25% of bowel movements. The Rome criteria include symptoms suggestive of pelvic floor dyssynergia or outlet obstruction (e.g., a sensation of anorectal blockage or obstruction and use of maneuvers to facilitate defecation) and allow patients to have rare episodes of loose stools without the use of laxatives. The Rome criteria require symptoms to be present for the previous 3 months, with the onset of symptoms 6 months prior to diagnosis. The Rome IV criteria recognize that functional bowel disorders, such as IBS with constipation and chronic constipation, exist on a spectrum and that there may be overlapping symptoms.[14]

The American College of Gastroenterology (ACG) defined constipation as unsatisfactory defecation characterized by infrequent stools, difficult stool passage, or both.[15] Difficult stool passage includes straining, a sense of difficulty passing stool, incomplete evacuation, hard/lumpy stools, prolonged time to stool, or need for manual maneuvers to pass stool.

EPIDEMIOLOGY

Prevalence

A worldwide study using the Rome IV Criteria for constipation that included an internet survey sample of 54,127 individuals in 26 countries and a household survey sample of 18,949 individuals in 9 countries found the prevalence of chronic constipation to be 11.7%.[16] A meta-analysis of 41 population-based studies with over 261,000 subjects throughout the world using a variety of definitions estimated the prevalence of constipation to be 14.[17] In individual studies, the prevalence of constipation has varied from 3% to 31%[18–38] depending on the demographics of the population, definition of constipation (e.g., self-report, questionnaire, or specific symptom-based criteria), and method of questioning (e.g., postal questionnaire and interview). In general, the prevalence is highest when constipation is self-reported[18] and lowest when criteria are applied. The frequency is higher among women, older adults, and those with a lower socioeconomic status. Using the National Health and Nutrition Examination Survey (NHANES), the prevalence of constipation in the general US population was found to be higher when defined by stool consistency (i.e., Type 1 or 2 on the Bristol stool form scale,[39] see Fig. 20.2) rather than by stool frequency (i.e., fewer than 3 bowel movements per week) (7.2%, 95% CI 7–8, vs. 3.1%, 95% CI 3–4, respectively).[40]

BOX 20.2 Risk Factors for Constipation

Advanced age
Female gender
Low level of education
Low level of physical activity
Low socioeconomic status
Multiracial ethnicity
Use of certain medications (see Box 20.3)

Incidence

A survey of 690 nonelderly residents of Olmsted County, Minnesota, at baseline and after 12–20 months found constipation present in 17% at the baseline survey and 15% on the follow-up survey.[41] The rate of new constipation in this study was 50/1000 person-years, whereas the disappearance rate was 31/1000 person-years. In a similar study, residents of Olmsted County, Minnesota, were surveyed at baseline and about 12 years later. The cumulative incidence of constipation over a 12-year period was 17.4%, and, in subjects younger than age 50, it was higher in women (18.3%) than men (9.2%).[42,43]

Public Health Perspective

Constipation is a common reason for health care visits, and the frequency of these visits and associated costs appears to be on the rise. In 2014 there were 1.7 million ambulatory and nearly 800,000 emergency department visits for constipation as well as a similar number of visits in 2014 for hemorrhoids, which is associated with constipation.[44] According to data from the National Emergency Department Sample (NEDS), the frequency of ED visits for constipation in the United States increased by 41.5% between 2006 and 2011, and the associated costs increased by 121.4%.[45] Some 85% of physician visits for constipation lead to a prescription for laxatives or cathartics.[46] The mean annual costs for patients with commercial insurance in the United States with chronic constipation were $8700 (2010 US dollars) more than matched controls.[47] Over a 15-year period, constipated women incur direct medical costs that were more than double that of nonconstipated women.[48] In 2004 the direct costs for constipation were nearly $1.6 billion, with indirect costs of $140 million, making constipation among the top 10 digestive disorders in attributable direct costs.[49] Constipation is treated by a variety of physicians; in an analysis of physician visits for constipation in the United States between 2001 and 2004, 33% of patients who required medical attention were seen by internists and family practitioners, followed in frequency by pediatricians (21%) and gastroenterologists (14.1%).[50] However, not all patients seek medical attention for their constipation. As shown in a National Canadian Survey, only 34% of people who reported constipation had seen a physician for their symptoms.[18]

RISK FACTORS

Although risk factors for constipation have not been systematically evaluated, female gender, advanced age, multiracial ethnicity, lower levels of income and education, and a low level of physical activity have been associated with chronic constipation.[10,17,32,51,52] Other risk factors include use of certain medications (e.g., acetaminophen [>3.5 g tablets/week], aspirin, and other NSAIDs)[22] and certain underlying medical disorders (discussed later). Diet and lifestyle may also play a role in the development of constipation (Box 20.2).

Gender

The prevalence of self-reported constipation is two to three times higher in women,[20,28,32,53] particularly women of reproductive age, than men, and infrequent bowel movements (e.g., once a week) are reported almost exclusively by women.[39] In a meta-analysis of 26 studies, the pooled prevalence of constipation in women was 17.4% (95% CI 13.4–21.8), almost double the 9.2% in men (odds ratio 2.2, 95% CI 1.87–2.62).[17] The reason for the female predominance is unknown. Colonic transit is significantly delayed in women during the luteal phase of the menstrual cycle, compared with the follicular phase, when estrogen levels are relatively low.[54] A reduction in levels of steroid hormones has been observed in women with severe idiopathic constipation, although the clinical significance of this finding is unclear.[55] Overexpression of progesterone receptors on colonic smooth muscle cells has been reported to downregulate contractile G proteins and upregulate inhibitory G proteins.[56] Overexpression of progesterone receptors in colonic epithelial cells is also associated with reduced serotonin transporter, high 5-hydroxytryptamine (5-HT), and normal tryptophan hydroxylase levels.[57] In addition, overexpression of progesterone receptor B on colonic muscle cells, which makes them more sensitive to physiologic concentrations of progesterone, has been proposed as an explanation for severe slow-transit constipation in some women.[58]

Age

The prevalence of self-reported constipation among older adults ranges from 15% to 30%, with many,[20,51,59,60] but not all,[17,18,20,22,32,61] studies showing an increase in prevalence with age. Constipation in older adults is most commonly characterized by excessive straining and hard stools[7,62] rather than a decrease in stool frequency. In a community sample of 209 people aged 65–93 years, the main symptom used to describe constipation was the need to strain at defecation; only 3% of men and 2% of women reported that their average bowel frequencies were less than 3 per week.[63] Possible causes for the increased frequency of straining in older adults include decreased food intake, reduced mobility, weakening of abdominal and pelvic wall muscles (descending perineum syndrome), chronic illness, psychological factors, and medications, particularly pain-relieving drugs.[64] Older adults also tend to seek medical assistance for constipation more commonly than their younger counterparts. In an analysis of physician visits for constipation in the United States between 1958 and 1986, the frequency was about 1% in people younger than 60 years of age, 1%–2% in those 60–65 years, and 3%–5% in those older than 65 years.[46]

Constipation is particularly problematic in nursing home residents, among whom constipation is reported in almost half, and 50%–74% of residents use laxatives on a daily basis.[64] Similarly, hospitalized older patients appear to be at high risk of developing constipation. A study of patients on a geriatrics ward in the United Kingdom showed that up to 42% had a fecal impaction while hospitalized.[65] A study of 34 nursing homes in the United States found the frequency of chronic constipation to be 71%, with a frequency of self-reported fecal impaction of 47%.[66] A study from Finland revealed that 79% of women and 81% of men in a nursing home reported chronic constipation or a rectal evacuation disorder.[67–70]

Constipation is also common in children younger than age 4.[71] In Great Britain, the frequency of a consultation for constipation in general practice was 2%–3% in children aged 0–4 years, about 1% in women aged 15–64 years, 2%–3% in both genders aged 65–74 years, and 5%–6% in persons aged 75 years or older. Fecal retention with fecal soiling is a common cause of impaired quality of life and the need for medical attention in childhood.

Ethnicity and Nationality

In North America, constipation is reported more commonly by non-Whites than Whites. In a survey of 15,014 persons, the frequency of constipation was 17.3% in non-Whites and 12.2% in Whites.[10,32,72] Age-specific increases in prevalence were found in both groups.[10] Data regarding constipation in developing countries are limited. A meta-analysis that included studies mostly from North America and Northern Europe with a few studies from South America and the Middle East found that the prevalence of chronic constipation was similar in all countries, between 14% and 16%.[17] A study comparing the prevalence in South America and Asia found comparable frequencies of constipation, with rates of 21.7% in Colombia and 16.7% in South Korea.[60] In Asian countries, including China, Korea, Hong Kong, and India, the prevalence of constipation ranges from 8.2% to 16.8%.[34–36] In Sri Lanka, constipation (as defined by the Rome III criteria using a self-administered survey) was reported by 15.4% of children between 10 and 16 years of age. The worldwide Rome IV internet global survey found the lowest prevalence of chronic constipation to be in Japan (7.7%) and highest in Australia (16.6%).[16] The frequency of constipation was significantly higher in children with a family history of constipation (49% vs. 14.8%), those living in a war-affected area (18.1% vs. 13.7%), and those attending an urban school (16.7% vs. 13.3%).[73]

Socioeconomic Status and Education Level

Lower socioeconomic status and education levels have been found to be risk factors for chronic constipation. In population-based surveys, people with a lower income status have higher rates of constipation than those who have a higher income status.[10,13,30,32] Similarly, persons who have a lower education level tend to have a higher prevalence of constipation than those who have a higher education level.[10,18,32,72] Pooled data from a meta-analysis showed a modest increase in the prevalence of chronic constipation in persons of lower socioeconomic status compared with those of higher socioeconomic status.[17] These results have been reproduced in other countries, such as Brazil, Germany, and Croatia.[74–76]

Diet and Physical Activity

Cross-sectional studies have not linked a low intake of fiber with constipation.[40,77] Yet data suggest that increased consumption of fiber decreases colonic transit and increases stool weight and frequency.[78] An analysis from the Nurses' Health Study, which assessed the self-reported bowel habits of 62,036 women between 36 and 61 years of age, demonstrated that women who were in the highest quintile of fiber intake (median intake, 20 g/day) and who exercised daily were 68% less likely to report constipation, defined as fewer than 3 bowel movements per week, than women who were in the lowest quintile of fiber intake (median intake, 7 g/day) and exercised less than once a week.[51] Although other observational studies have supported a protective effect of physical activity on constipation, results from trials designed to test this hypothesis have been conflicting. In one trial, symptoms of constipation did not improve after a 4-week exercise program.[79] Likewise, among Department of Veterans Affairs employees, physical activity levels did not differ between those with or without constipation.[80]

Dehydration has been identified as a potential risk factor for constipation. Some, but not all, observational studies have found an association between slow colonic transit and dehydration.[81,82] Among female Japanese dietetic students, however, total water intake was not associated with constipation.[77] Although patients with constipation are routinely advised to increase their fluid intake, the benefits have not been thoroughly investigated.

Medication Use

In a review of 7251 patients with chronic constipation (and non-constipated controls) from a general practice database, medications that were significantly associated with constipation were opioids, diuretics, antidepressants, antihistamines, antispasmodics, anticonvulsants, and aluminum antacids (Box 20.3).[61] The use of acetaminophen (>3.5 g tablets weekly), aspirin, and other NSAIDs has also found to be associated with an increased risk of constipation.[22]

COLONIC FUNCTION

Microbiome and Luminal Contents

The main contents of the colonic lumen are food residue, water and electrolytes, bacteria, and gas. Unabsorbed carbohydrates, such as starches and nonstarch polysaccharides, that enter the cecum serve as substrates for bacterial proliferation and fermentation, yielding short-chain fatty acids and gas (see Chapter 18). On average, bacteria represent about 50% of stool weight.[83] In an analysis of feces from nine healthy subjects on a metabolically controlled British diet, bacteria constituted 55% of the total solids, and fiber represented approximately 17% of the stool weight.[84] While several studies have demonstrated dysbiosis of the gut microbiota in patients with chronic constipation compared to healthy controls,[85–89] no clear microbial signature for constipation has been identified. A study using 16S rRNA metagenomics analysis (V3–V5) found the microbiota profile in the colonic mucosa discriminated patients with constipation from healthy individuals even after adjusting for diet and colon transit time. Specifically, patients with constipation had increased levels of genera from *Bacteroidetes* in their colonic mucosa.[89] The role of intestinal microbiota in constipation is just beginning to be explored (see Chapter 3).[90,91]

A meta-analysis has suggested that wheat bran increases stool weight and reduces mean colonic transit in healthy volunteers.[84] The effect of bran may primarily be the result of increased bulk within the colonic lumen with consequent stimulation of propulsive motor activity. The particulate nature of some fibers may also stimulate the colon. Ingestion of coarse bran (10 g twice daily) was shown to reduce colonic transit by about one-third, whereas ingestion of the same quantity of fine bran led to no significant decrease.[83] Similarly, ingestion of inert plastic particles comparable in size to coarse bran increased fecal output by almost three times their own weight and reduced colonic transit.[92]

BOX 20.3 Secondary Causes of Constipation

MECHANICAL OBSTRUCTION
- Anal stenosis
- Colorectal cancer
- Extrinsic compression
- Rectocele or sigmoidocele
- Stricture

MEDICATIONS
- Acetaminophen (>3.5 g tablets weekly)
- Antacids (aluminum containing)
- Anticholinergic agents (e.g., antiparkinsonian drugs, antipsychotics, antispasmodics, and tricyclic antidepressants)
- Anticonvulsants (e.g., carbamazepine, phenobarbital, and phenytoin)
- Antineoplastic agents (e.g., vinca derivatives)
- Calcium channel blockers (e.g., verapamil)
- Calcium supplements
- Diuretics (e.g., furosemide)
- 5-Hydroxytryptamine$_3$ antagonists (e.g., alosetron)
- Iron supplements
- NSAIDs (e.g., ibuprofen)
- μ-opioid agonists (e.g., fentanyl, loperamide, morphine)

METABOLIC AND ENDOCRINOLOGIC DISORDERS
- Diabetes mellitus
- Heavy metal poisoning (e.g., arsenic, lead, and mercury)
- Hypercalcemia
- Hyperthyroidism
- Hypokalemia
- Hypothyroidism
- Panhypopituitarism
- Pheochromocytoma
- Porphyria
- Pregnancy

NEUROLOGIC AND MYOPATHIC DISORDERS
- Amyloidosis
- Autonomic neuropathy
- Chagas disease
- Dermatomyositis
- Intestinal pseudo-obstruction
- Multiple sclerosis
- Parkinsonism
- Shy-Drager syndrome
- Spinal cord injury
- Stroke
- Systemic sclerosis

Absorption of Water and Sodium

The colon avidly absorbs water and sodium (see Chapter 103). The colon extracts most of the 1000–1500 mL of fluid that crosses the ileocecal valve and leaves only 100–200 mL of fecal water daily. Sodium-chloride exchange and short-chain fatty acid transport are the principal mechanisms for stimulating water absorption in the colon. The absorption of water in the colon also depends on an intact epithelial barrier function to prevent the back diffusion of electrolytes and other solutes once they have been absorbed across the epithelium.[1] One proposed pathophysiologic mechanism of constipation is that delayed transit allows more time for bacterial degradation of stool solids and increased sodium and water absorption, thereby decreasing stool weight and frequency and increasing its firmness.[93,94]

Diameter and Length

A wide or long colon may lead to a slow colonic transit rate (see Chapter 102). Although only a small fraction of patients with constipation have megacolon or megarectum, most patients with dilatation of the colon or rectum report constipation. A colonic width of more than 6.5 cm at the pelvic brim on a barium enema film is abnormal and has been associated with chronic constipation.[95]

Motor Function

Colonic muscle has four main functions (see Chapter 102): (1) delay passage of the luminal contents to allow time for water absorption; (2) mix the contents and allow contact with the mucosa; (3) allow the colon to store feces between defecations; and (4) propel the contents toward the anus. Muscle activity is affected by sleep and wakefulness, eating, emotion, colon contents, and drugs. Neural control is partly intrinsic and partly extrinsic by the sympathetic nerves and the parasympathetic sacral outflow.

The mean colonic transit in healthy volunteers is 34–35 hours, with an upper limit of normal of 72 hours.[96,97] In some patients, slow colonic transit is driven by delay in the passage of material in the ascending and transverse colon (proximal colon) rather than in the left colon.[98–100] Other patients show slow transit in both the right and left sides of the colon.[101]

Peristalsis is intrinsic to the gut and consists of segmental contraction combined with distal relaxation. Excitatory motor neurons activated by acetylcholine cause intestinal smooth muscle contractions, whereas inhibitory neurons activated by ATP and nitric oxide cause intestinal smooth muscle relaxation.[1] Peristalsis can be activated by chemical or mechanical stimuli that are sensed by the enterochromaffin cells and mechanoreceptors in the enteric ganglia. Once initiated, peristalsis can be propagated for long distances, thereby moving material through the gut.[1] Enterochromaffin cells synthesize serotonin (5-HT) in response to nutrients, short-chain fatty acids, bile salts, and mechanical stimuli. 5-HT activates upstream excitatory motor neurons and downstream inhibitory motor neurons, thereby resulting in peristalsis.

Colonic propulsions are of two basic types: low-amplitude propagated contractions and high-amplitude propagated contractions (HAPCs).[102] The frequency and duration of HAPCs are reduced in some patients with constipation. In one study that included 14 patients with slow-transit constipation, during a 24-hour period, 4 patients had no peristaltic movement, whereas in the remaining 10 patients peristaltic, movements were fewer in number and shorter in duration compared with healthy controls.[103] In contrast to propulsive contractions, there are also repetitive retrograde contractions predominantly in the rectosigmoid, which appear to serve as a "braking" mechanism ("rectosigmoid brake") to limit rectal filling.[104]

Innervation and the Interstitial Cells of Cajal

Constipation, particularly slow-transit constipation, may be related to autonomic dysfunction.[105,106] Histologic studies have shown abnormal numbers of myenteric plexus neurons involved in excitatory or inhibitory control of colonic motility, thereby resulting in decreased amounts of the excitatory transmitter substance P[107] and increased amounts of the inhibitory transmitters vasoactive intestinal polypeptide or nitric oxide (see Chapter 4).[108]

The interstitial cells of Cajal (ICCs) are intestinal pacemaker cells and play a part in mediating the excitatory and inhibitory signals between the enteric nervous system and the smooth muscle cells (see Chapters 101 and 102).[1] ICCs initiate slow waves throughout the GI tract. Confocal images of ICCs in patients with slow-transit constipation show not only reduced numbers but also abnormal morphology of ICCs, with irregular surface markings and a decreased number of dendrites. In patients with slow-transit constipation, the number of ICCs has been shown to be decreased in the sigmoid colon[109] or the entire colon.[110,111] Pathologic examination of colectomy specimens of 14 patients with severe intractable constipation revealed decreased numbers of ICCs and myenteric ganglion cells throughout the colon.[112]

Defecatory Function

The process of defecation in healthy persons begins with a predefecatory period during which the frequency and amplitude of propagating sequences (three or more successive pressure waves) are increased. Stimuli, such as waking and meals (*gastroileal reflex*, also referred to as *gastrocolic reflex or response*), can stimulate this process. In patients with slow-transit constipation, this predefecatory period is blunted and may be absent.[102] The gastroileal reflex is also diminished in persons with slow-transit constipation. Stool is often present in the rectum before the urge to defecate arises. The urge to defecate is usually experienced when stool comes into contact with receptors in the upper anal canal. When the urge to defecate is resisted, retrograde movement of stool may occur, and transit time increases throughout the colon (see Chapter 102).[113]

Although the sitting or squatting position seems to facilitate defecation, the benefit of squatting has not been well studied in patients with constipation.[114] Full flexion of the hips stretches the anal canal in an anteroposterior direction and straightens the anorectal angle, thereby promoting emptying of the rectum.[115] Contraction of the diaphragm and abdominal muscles raises intrapelvic pressure, and the pelvic floor relaxes simultaneously. Striated muscular activity expels rectal contents, with little contribution from colonic or rectal propulsive waves. Coordinated relaxation of the puborectalis muscle (which maintains the anorectal angle) and the external anal sphincter at a time when pressure is increasing in the rectum results in expulsion of stool (Fig. 20.1).

The length of the colon emptied during spontaneous defecation most commonly extends from the descending colon to the rectum.[116] When the propulsive action of smooth muscle is normal, defecation usually requires minimal voluntary effort. If colonic and rectal waves are infrequent or absent, however, the normal urge to defecate may not occur.[117]

Size and Consistency of Stool

In a study of healthy persons who were asked to expel single hard spheres of different sizes from the rectal ampulla, the intrarectal pressure and time needed to pass the objects varied inversely with their diameters. Small, hard stools are more difficult to pass than large, soft stools. When larger stimulated stools were tested, a hard stool took longer to expel than a soft silicone rubber object of roughly the same shape and volume. Similarly, more subjects were able to expel a 50-mL water-filled compressible balloon than a hard 1.8-cm sphere.[118]

Human stools may vary in consistency from small hard lumps to liquid. The water content of stool determines consistency. Rapid colonic transit of fecal residue leads to diminished water absorption and (perhaps counterintuitively) an increase in the bacterial content of the stool. The Bristol stool form scale[39] is used in the assessment of constipation and is regarded as the best descriptor of stool form and consistency (Fig. 20.2). Stool consistency appears to be a better predictor of whole-gut transit time than of defecation frequency or stool volume.[119,120]

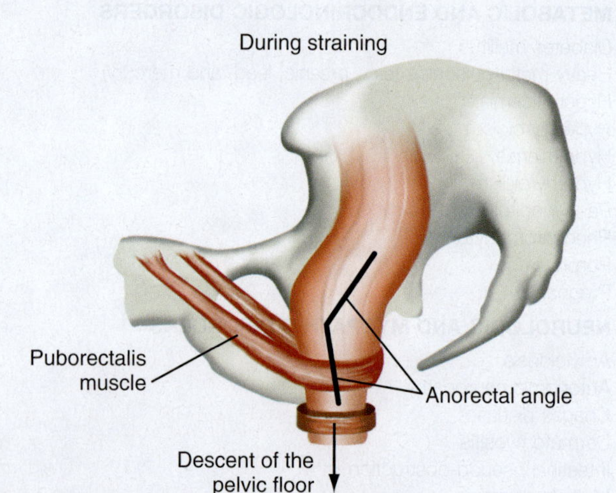

Fig. 20.1 Physiology of defecation. Defecation requires relaxation of the puborectalis muscle with descent of the pelvic floor and straightening of the anorectal angle during straining, as well as relaxation of the internal anal sphincter. (From Lembo A, Camilleri M. Chronic constipation. *N Engl J Med*. 2003;349:1360–1368.)

Whole-gut transit time	Type of stool	Description	Pictorial representation
Long transit (e.g., 100 hours)			
	Type 1	Separate hard lumps, like nuts, hard to pass	
	Type 2	Sausage shaped but lumpy	
	Type 3	Like sausage but with cracks on its surface	
	Type 4	Like sausage or snake, smooth and soft	
	Type 5	Soft blobs with clear-cut edges (passed easily)	
	Type 6	Fluffy pieces with ragged edges, a mushy stool	
	Type 7	Watery, no solid pieces	Entirely liquid
Short transit (e.g., 10 hours)			

Fig. 20.2 The Bristol stool form scale. Common stool forms and their consistency in relation to whole-gut transit time are shown. (From Heaton KW, Radvan J, Cripps H, et al. Defecation frequency and timing, and stool form in the general population: a prospective study. *Gut*. 1992;33:818–824.)

TABLE 20.1 Clinical Classification of Functional Constipation

Category	Features	Physiologic Test Results
Normal-transit constipation	Incomplete evacuation; abdominal pain may be present but not a predominant feature	Normal
Slow-transit constipation	Infrequent stools (e.g., ≤1/week), lack of urge to defecate, poor response to fiber and laxatives, generalized symptoms (e.g., malaise, fatigue); more prevalent in young women	Delay in colonic transit (e.g., retention in colon of >20% of radiopaque markers 5 days after ingestion)
Defecatory disorder*	Frequent straining, incomplete evacuation, need for manual maneuvers to facilitate defecation	Abnormal balloon expulsion test and/or anorectal manometry

*Pelvic floor dysfunction, anismus, descending perineum syndrome, and rectal prolapse.

CLASSIFICATION

Secondary causes of constipation (e.g., small or large bowel obstruction, medications, and systemic illnesses) must be excluded, especially in patients presenting with new-onset constipation (see Box 20.3). Most often, chronic constipation is due to disordered function of the colon or rectum (sometimes referred to as functional constipation). Chronic constipation can be divided into three broad categories—normal-transit constipation, slow-transit constipation, and defecatory or rectal evacuation disorders (Table 20.1). In a study of more than 1000 patients with chronic constipation who were evaluated at the Mayo Clinic, 59% were found to have normal-transit constipation, 25% had defecatory disorders, 13% had slow-transit constipation, and 3% had a combination of a defecatory disorder and slow-transit constipation.[121]

PATHOPHYSIOLOGY

Normal-Transit Constipation

In normal-transit constipation, stool travels along the colon at a normal rate.[122] Patients with normal-transit constipation may have misperceptions about their bowel frequencies and often exhibit psychosocial distress.[123] Some patients have abnormalities of anorectal sensory and motor function indistinguishable from those in patients with slow-transit constipation.[124] Whether increased rectal compliance and reduced rectal sensation are effects of chronic constipation or contribute to these patients' failure to experience an urge to defecate is unclear, but most patients have normal results of physiologic testing (see later).

Slow-Transit Constipation

Slow-transit constipation is most common in young women and characterized by infrequent bowel movements (<1 bowel movement/week). Associated symptoms include abdominal pain, bloating, and malaise. Symptoms are often intractable, and conservative measures, such as fiber supplements and osmotic laxatives, are usually ineffective.[125,126] The onset of symptoms is gradual and usually occurs around the time of puberty. Slow-transit constipation arises from disordered colonic motor function. Patients who have mild delays in colonic transit have symptoms similar to those seen in persons with IBS (see Chapter 124).[127] In patients with more severe symptoms, the pathophysiology includes delayed emptying of the proximal colon and fewer HAPCs after meals as well as altered bile acid metabolism.[128] *Colonic inertia* is a term used to describe the disorder in patients with symptoms at the most severe end of the spectrum. In this condition, colonic motor activity fails to increase after a meal,[129] ingestion of bisacodyl,[130] or administration of a cholinesterase inhibitor such as neostigmine.[131]

Defecatory Disorders

Rectal evacuation disorders arise from failure to empty the rectum effectively due to an inability to coordinate the abdominal, rectoanal, and pelvic floor muscles. Many patients with defecatory disorders also have slow-transit constipation.[132] Defecatory disorders are also known as *anismus*, *dyssynergia*, *pelvic floor dyssynergia*, *spastic pelvic floor syndrome*, *obstructive defecation*, or *outlet obstruction*. These disorders appear to be acquired and may start in childhood. They may be a learned behavior to avoid discomfort associated with the passage of large, hard stools or pain associated with attempted defecation in the setting of an active anal fissure or inflamed hemorrhoids. Individuals with defecatory disorders commonly have inappropriate contraction of the anal sphincter when they bear down (Fig. 20.3). This phenomenon can occur in asymptomatic persons but is more common among those who complain of difficult defecation.[133] Some patients with a defecatory disorder are unable to raise intrarectal pressure to a level sufficient to expel stool, a disturbance that manifests clinically as failure of the pelvic floor to descend on straining.[134]

Rectal evacuation disorders are particularly common in older adults with chronic constipation and excessive straining, many of whom do not respond to standard medical treatment.[135] Occasionally, rectal evacuation disorders are associated with structural abnormalities (e.g., rectal intussusception, obstructing rectocele, megarectum, and excessive perineal descent).[136]

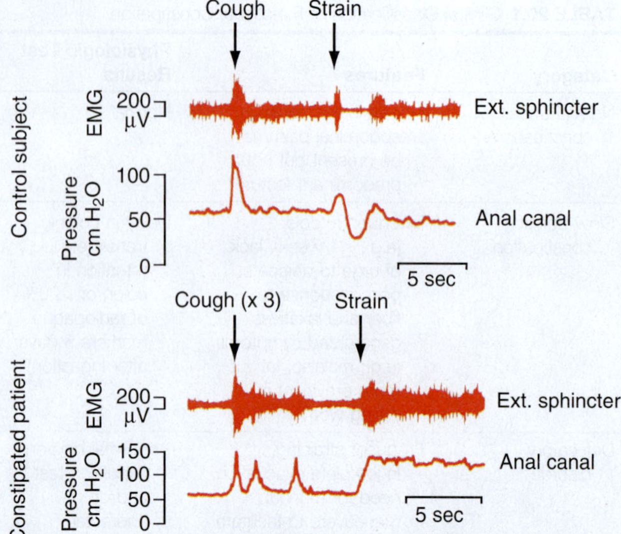

Fig. 20.3 EMG and pressure tracings during defecation in a normal (control) subject and a constipated patient with a defecatory disorder. In both the control subject and constipated patient, a cough produces a rise in pressure. When a normal subject strains *(upper tracing)*, EMG activity of the external anal sphincter is inhibited, and pressure in the anal canal falls. In a constipated patient with a defecatory disorder, EMG activity of the anal sphincter is not inhibited on straining, and pressure within the anal canal increases *(lower tracing)*. This paradoxical contraction has been termed *anismus*, *anal dyssynergia*, and *spastic perineum*. (From Preston DM, Lennard-Jones JE. Anismus in chronic constipation. *Dig Dis Sci*. 1985;30:413–418.)

BOX 20.4 Rome IV Criteria for Functional Defecation Disorders*

1. The patient must satisfy diagnostic criteria for functional constipation and/or IBS with constipation
2. During repeated attempts to defecate, there must be features of impaired evacuation, as demonstrated by two of the following three test results:
   a. Abnormal balloon expulsion test
   b. Abnormal anorectal evacuation pattern with manometry or anal surface EMG
   c. Impaired rectal evacuation by imaging

*Criteria fulfilled for the previous 3 months, with symptom onset at least 6 months prior to diagnosis.

From Rao SSC, Bharucha AE, Chiarioni G, et al. Anorectal disorders. *Gastroenterology*. 2016; 150(6):1430–42.

Patients with rectal evacuation disorders may report infrequent bowel movements, ineffective and excessive straining, and the need for manual disimpaction, but symptoms—particularly in the case of pelvic floor dysfunction—do not reliably correlate with physiologic findings.[137] For a diagnosis of a rectal evacuation disorder, a Rome working group has specified the criteria listed in Box 20.4.[138] To meet the Rome criteria for a defecatory disorder, patients must meet the Rome criteria for constipation and have evidence of dysfunction of the pelvic floor muscles as determined by physiologic tests (see later). Pelvic floor dyssynergia affects a subset of these patients in whom the anal sphincter fails to relax more than 20% of its basal resting pressure during attempted defecation, despite the presence of adequate propulsive forces in the rectum. Patients with rectal evacuation disorders have a greater rectal gas volume compared with that found in other subtypes of constipation, thereby suggesting that imaging of the rectum (i.e., by CT) may provide a sensitive (>70%) and reasonably specific (>60%) method of distinguishing a rectal evacuation disorder from other subtypes of constipation.[139]

Functional fecal retention is the most common defecatory disorder in children. It is a learned behavior that results from withholding defecation, often because of fear of a painful bowel movement or for social reasons.[140] The symptoms are common and may result in secondary encopresis (fecal incontinence) due to leakage of liquid stool around a fecal impaction. Functional fecal retention is the most common cause of encopresis in childhood (see Chapter 19).[141]

CAUSES

Disorders of the Anorectum and Pelvic Floor

Rectocele

A rectocele is the bulging or displacement of the rectum through a defect in the anterior rectal wall. In women, the perineal body supports the anterior rectal (posterior vaginal) wall above the anorectal junction, and a layer of fascia runs from the rectovaginal pouch of Douglas to the perineal body and adheres to the posterior vaginal wall. The anterior rectal wall is unsupported above the level of the perineal body, and the rectovaginal septum can bulge anteriorly to form a rectocele (Fig. 20.4). Rectoceles can arise from damage to the rectovaginal septum or its supporting structures during vaginal childbirth. These injuries are exacerbated by repetitive increases in intra-abdominal pressure and the long-term effects of gravity. Prolapse of other pelvic organs may be present. Urinary incontinence and previous hysterectomy are more common in patients with a rectocele than in patients with difficult defecation and no demonstrable rectocele.[142]

Studies using defecating proctography (see later) have shown that rectoceles are common in symptomless healthy women and may protrude as much as 4 cm from the line of the anterior rectal wall without causing bowel symptoms, although 2 cm is the generally accepted lower limit of a rectocele that may be regarded as clinically significant.[143] Symptomatic patients report the inability to complete fecal evacuation, perineal pain, sensation of local pressure, and appearance of a bulge at the vaginal opening on straining. Women may report the need to use their thumb or fingers to support the posterior vaginal wall to complete defecation.[142] Women may also report the need to use a finger to digitally evacuate the rectum.

Defecography can be used to demonstrate a rectocele, measure its size, and determine whether barium becomes trapped within the rectocele. In one study, trapping of barium in rectoceles changed with the degree of rectal emptying and was related to the size of the rectocele.[144] However, rectocele size or degree of emptying on defecation have not been shown to correlate with the outcomes of surgical repair.[145,146]

Asymptomatic women with rectoceles do not require surgical treatment. Kegel exercises (designed to strengthen pelvic floor muscles that support the urethra, bladder, uterus, and rectum) and instructions to avoid repetitive increases in intra-abdominal pressure may help prevent progression of the rectocele.[147] Surgery should be considered only for patients in whom contrast is retained during defecography and patients in whom constipation is relieved with digital vaginal pressure to facilitate defecation.[148] Surgical repair can be performed by an endorectal, transvaginal, or transperineal approach. Other types of genital prolapse may also be present, and collaboration between the surgeon and gynecologist may be appropriate. In carefully selected patients, surgical repair benefits 75% of patients. In a review of 89 women who underwent a combined transvaginal and transanal rectocele repair for symptoms of obstructive defecation, the repair was successful in 71% of patients, as assessed by the absence of

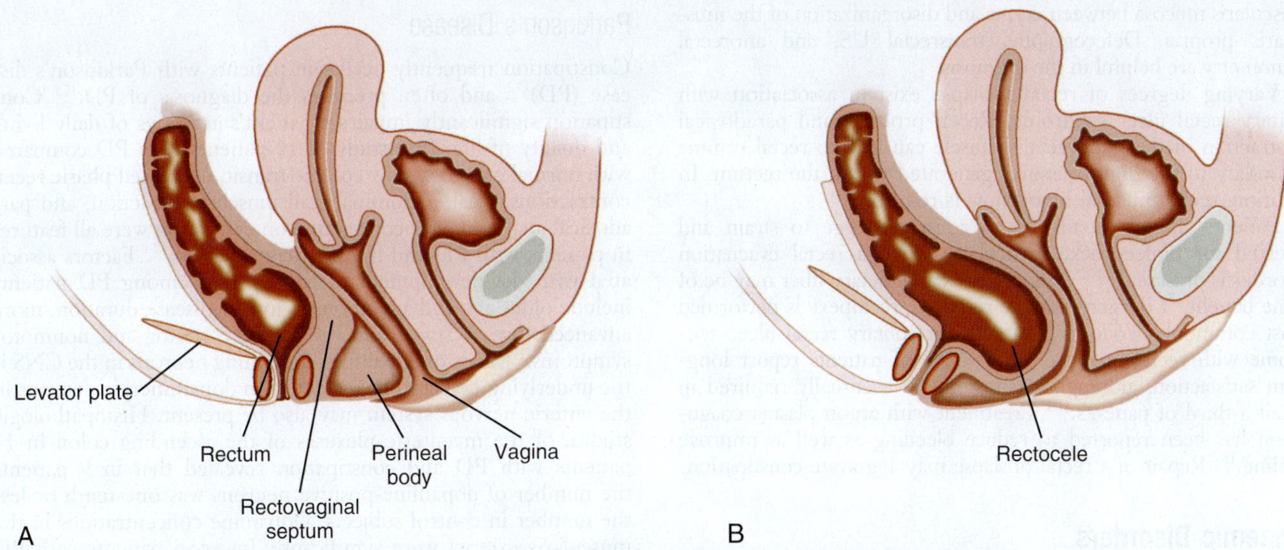

Fig. 20.4 Development of a rectocele. (A) Normal anatomy of the female pelvis. The levator plate is almost horizontal, supporting the rectum and vagina. The perineal body provides support for the lower posterior vaginal wall; above it lies the rectovaginal septum. (B) Pelvic floor weakness leads to a more vertical levator plate. The perineal body is attenuated, which favors formation of a rectocele. Pelvic floor laxity also favors rectal mucosal prolapse. (From Loder PB, Phillips RKS. Rectocele and pelvic floor weakness. In: Kamm MA, Lennard-Jones JE, eds. Constipation. Petersfield: Wrightson Biomedical; 1994:281.)

symptoms after 1 year.[149] A subsequent study[150] found that bowel symptoms improved in 50% of patients and that a longer history of splinting was a risk factor for persistent postoperative symptoms. Reduction in rectocele size, as judged by defecography, does not appear to correlate clearly with symptomatic improvement.[146]

Descending Perineum Syndrome

In descending perineum syndrome, the pelvic floor descends to a greater extent than normal (1–4 cm) when the patient strains during defecation, and rectal expulsion is difficult. The anorectal angle is widened as a result of pelvic floor weakness, and the rectum is more vertical than normal. The perineal body is weak (facilitating rectocele formation), and lax muscular support favors intrarectal mucosal intussusception or rectal prolapse. The pelvic floor may not provide the resistance necessary for extrusion of solid stool through the anal canal. A common reason for pelvic floor weakness is trauma or stretching during parturition. In some cases, repeated and prolonged defecation appears to be a damaging factor. Symptoms include constipation, incomplete rectal evacuation, excessive straining, and the need for digital rectal evacuation.[151] Electrophysiologic studies show partial denervation of the striated muscle and evidence of pudendal nerve damage (see later). Histologic examination of operative specimens of the pelvic floor muscles confirms loss of muscle fibers.

Diminished Rectal Sensation

The urge to defecate depends in part on tension within the rectal wall (determined by the tone of the circular muscle of the rectal wall), rate and volume of rectal distention, and size of the rectum. Some patients with constipation appear to feel pain normally as the rectum is distended to the maximal tolerable volume, but with intermediate volumes they fail to experience an urge to defecate.[152] In a study of women with severe idiopathic constipation, a higher than normal electrical stimulation current applied to the rectal mucosa was required to elicit pain, suggesting a possible rectal sensory neuropathy.[153]

Rectal hyposensitivity (RH) is defined as insensitivity of the rectum to balloon distention on anorectal physiologic investigation, although the pathophysiology of RH is not entirely clear. Constipation is the most common presenting symptom of RH. In an investigation of 261 patients with RH, 38% had a history of pelvic surgery, 22% had a history of anal surgery, and 13% had a history of spinal trauma.[154]

Rectal Prolapse and Solitary Rectal Ulcer Syndrome

Full-thickness rectal prolapse and solitary rectal ulcer syndrome are part of a spectrum of defects that arise from pelvic floor weakening. Some patients complain of many fruitless visits to the bathroom, with prolonged straining in response to a constant desire to defecate. The patient has a sense of incomplete evacuation and may spend an hour or more daily on the toilet. Infrequent passage of small hard stools is common, as are other features of a functional bowel disorder, such as abdominal pain and distention.

Rectal prolapse refers to complete protrusion of the rectum through the anus (see Chapter 131). Occult (asymptomatic) rectal prolapse has been found in 33% of patients with clinically recognized rectoceles and defecatory dysfunction[155] and can easily be detected on physical examination by asking the patient to strain as if to defecate. A laparoscopic rectopexy—in which the prolapsed rectum is raised and secured with sutures to the adjacent fascia—is the recommended treatment.[156]

Solitary rectal ulcer syndrome is a rare disorder characterized by erythema or ulceration, generally of the anterior rectal wall, as a result of chronic straining (see Chapter 121). Mucus and blood may be passed when the patient strains during defecation.[157,158] Endoscopic findings may include erythema, hyperemia, mucosal ulceration, and a polypoid lesion. The syndrome's heterogeneous findings and misleading name (an ulcer need not be present) can lead to misdiagnosis. In a study of 98 patients with solitary rectal ulcer syndrome, 26% were initially diagnosed incorrectly. In patients with a rectal ulcer or mucosal hyperemia, the most common misdiagnoses were Crohn's disease and UC. In those with a polypoid lesion, the most common misdiagnosis was a neoplastic polyp.[159] Histology of full-thickness specimens of the lesion reveals extension of the muscularis mucosa between crypts and disorganization of the muscularis propria. Defecography, transrectal US, and anorectal manometry are helpful in the diagnosis.

Varying degrees of rectal prolapse exist in association with solitary rectal ulcer syndrome. Rectal prolapse and paradoxical contraction of the puborectalis muscle can lead to rectal trauma secondary to the high pressures generated within the rectum. In addition, rectal mucosal blood flow is reduced.[160]

Patients should be advised to resist the urge to strain and referred for biofeedback, particularly when a rectal evacuation disorder is present.[161,162] Bulk laxatives and dietary fiber may be of some benefit.[163] Surgery may be required; rectopexy is performed most commonly. Following surgery for solitary rectal ulcer syndrome with rectal prolapse, 55%–60% of patients report long-term satisfaction, although a colostomy is eventually required in about a third of patients.[164] Treatment with argon plasma coagulation has been reported to reduce bleeding as well as improve healing.[165] Repair of a rectal prolapse may aggravate constipation.

Systemic Disorders

Hypothyroidism

Constipation is the most common GI complaint in patients with hypothyroidism. The pathologic effects are due to alteration of intestinal motor function and possible infiltration of the intestine by myxedematous tissue. The basic electrical rhythm that generates peristaltic waves in the duodenum decreases in hypothyroidism, and small bowel transit time is increased.[166] Myxedema megacolon is rare but can result from myxedematous infiltration of the muscle layers of the colon. Symptoms include abdominal pain, flatulence, and constipation (see Chapter 35).[167]

Diabetes Mellitus

The mean colonic transit time is longer in diabetics than in healthy controls. In one study, mean total colonic transit time in 28 diabetic patients (34.9 ± 29.6 hours; mean ± SD) was significantly longer than that in 28 healthy subjects (20.4 ± 15.6 hours; $P < .05$).[168] Among the 28 diabetic patients, 9 of 28 (32%) met the Rome II criteria for constipation, and 14 of 28 (50%) had cardiovascular autonomic neuropathy. Mean colonic transit times in diabetic patients with and without cardiovascular autonomic neuropathy were similar. By contrast, a previous study reported that asymptomatic diabetic patients with cardiovascular autonomic neuropathy had significantly longer whole-gut transit times (although still within the range of normal) than a control group without neuropathy.[169] In another study, diabetic patients with mild constipation demonstrated delayed colonic myoelectrical and motor responses after ingestion of a standard meal, whereas diabetics with severe constipation had no increases in these responses after food. Neostigmine increased colonic motor activity in all diabetic patients, suggesting the defect was neural rather than muscular (see Chapter 35).[170]

Hypercalcemia

Constipation is a common symptom of hypercalcemia resulting from hyperparathyroidism.[171] It may also be a manifestation of hypercalcemia due to other conditions (e.g., sarcoidosis, malignancy involving bone [see Chapter 35]).

Nervous System Disease

Loss of Conscious Control

Cerebral disability or dementia with a decrease in or complete loss of bodily perception can lead to defecatory failure, possibly because of inattention.

Parkinson's Disease

Constipation frequently occurs in patients with Parkinson's disease (PD)[172] and often precedes the diagnosis of PD.[173] Constipation significantly impairs a patient's activities of daily living and quality of life. In a study of 12 patients with PD compared with normal controls, slow colonic transit, decreased phasic rectal contractions, weak abdominal wall muscle contraction, and paradoxical anal sphincter contraction on defecation were all features in patients with PD and frequent constipation.[174] Factors associated with the development of constipation among PD patients include older age and age of onset, longer disease duration, more advanced disease stage, and more severe motor and nonmotor symptoms.[172] Loss of dopamine-containing neurons in the CNS is the underlying defect in PD; a defect in dopaminergic neurons in the enteric nervous system may also be present. Histopathologic studies of the myenteric plexuses of the ascending colon in 11 patients with PD and constipation revealed that in 9 patients the number of dopamine-positive neurons was one-tenth or less the number in control subjects. Dopamine concentrations in the muscularis externa were significantly lower in patients with PD than in controls.[175]

Another possible contributor to constipation is the inability of some patients with PD to relax the striated muscles of the pelvic floor on defecation. This finding is a local manifestation of the extrapyramidal motor disorder that affects skeletal muscle. Preliminary observations suggest that injection of botulinum toxin into the puborectalis muscle is a potential therapy for this type of outlet dysfunction (see Chapter 35).[176,177]

Multiple Sclerosis

Constipation is common among patients with multiple sclerosis (MS).[178] In an unselected group of 280 patients with MS, the frequency of constipation (defined as diminished bowel frequency, digitation to facilitate defecation, or use of laxatives) was 43%. Almost 25% of the subjects passed fewer than 3 stools/week, and 18% used a laxative more than once a week. Constipation correlated with the duration of MS but did not correlate with immobility or use of medications.[179] Similar to Parkinson's disease, constipation may predate the diagnosis of MS in approximately a third of patients based on a 14-year cohort study.[180] In another questionnaire study of 221 patients with MS, the frequency of constipation was as high as 54%.[181] The cause of constipation in patients with MS can be multifactorial and related to a reduction in postprandial colonic motor activity, limited physical activity, and medications.

Patients with advanced MS and constipation have evidence of a visceral neuropathy. In a group of patients with advanced MS and severe constipation, all had evidence of disease in the lumbosacral spinal cord and decreased compliance of the colon. The usual increase in colonic motor activity after meals is absent. Among less severely affected patients, slow colonic transit and manometric evidence of pelvic floor muscular and anal sphincter dysfunction have been demonstrated. Patients may have fecal incontinence.[182,183] Therapy with biofeedback has been reported to relieve constipation and fecal incontinence, although in a study of 13 patients with MS with either constipation or incontinence, only 38% improved with biofeedback (see Chapters 19 and 35).[184]

Spinal Cord Lesions

Lesions Above the Sacral Segments. Spinal cord lesions or injury above the sacral segments lead to an upper motor neuron disorder with severe constipation. The resulting delay in colonic transit primarily affects the rectosigmoid colon.[185,186] In a study of patients with severe thoracic spinal cord injury, colonic compliance was abnormal, with a rapid rise in colonic pressure on instillation of relatively small volumes of fluid. Motor activity after meals did not increase, but the colonic response to neostigmine was normal, thereby excluding myopathy.

Studies of anorectal function in patients with severe traumatic spinal cord injury have shown that rectal sensation to distention is abolished, although a dull pelvic sensation is experienced by some patients at maximum levels of rectal balloon distention. Anal relaxation on rectal distention is exaggerated and occurs at a lower balloon volume than in normal subjects. Distention of the rectum leads to a linear increase in rectal pressure, without the plateau at intermediate values seen in normal subjects, and ends in high-pressure rectal contractions after a relatively small volume (100 mL) has been instilled. As expected, the rectal pressure generated by straining is lower in patients than in control subjects and is less with higher than lower spinal cord lesions. Patients demonstrate a loss of conscious external anal sphincter control, and the sphincter does not relax on straining, suggesting that in normal subjects, descending inhibitory pathways are present.[187] These findings explain why some patients with spinal cord lesions experience not only constipation but also sudden, uncontrollable rectal expulsion with incontinence. Other patients cannot empty the rectum in response to laxatives or enemas, possibly because of failure of the external anal sphincter to relax, and may require manual evacuation.

Electrical stimulation of anterior sacral nerve roots S2, S3, and S4 via electrodes implanted for urinary control in paraplegic patients leads to a rise in pressure within the sigmoid colon and rectum and contraction of the external anal sphincter. Contraction of the rectum and relaxation of the internal anal sphincter persist for a short time after the stimulus ceases. By appropriate adjustment of the stimulus, it was possible for 5 of 12 paraplegic patients to evacuate feces completely and for most of the others to increase the frequency of defecation and reduce the time spent emptying the rectum.[188] In another series, left-sided colonic transit time decreased with regular sacral nerve stimulation.[189]

Lesions of the Sacral Cord, Conus Medullaris, Cauda Equina, and Nervi Erigentes (S2–S4). Neural integration of anal sphincter control and rectosigmoid propulsion occurs in the sacral segments of the spinal cord. The motor neurons that supply the striated sphincter muscles are grouped in the Onuf's nucleus at the level of S2. There is evidence that efferent parasympathetic nerves that arise in the sacral segments enter the colon at the region of the rectosigmoid junction and extend distally in the intermuscular plane to reach the level of the internal anal sphincter and proximally to the midcolon via the ascending colonic nerves, which retain the structure of peripheral nerves (see Chapter 102).[190]

Damage to sacral segments of the spinal cord or to efferent nerves leads to severe constipation. Fluoroscopic studies show a loss of progression of contractions in the left colon. When the colon is filled with fluid, the intraluminal pressure generated is lower than normal, in contrast to the situation after higher lesions of the spinal cord. The distal colon and rectum may dilate, and feces may accumulate in the distal colon. Spasticity of the anal canal can occur. Loss of sensation of the perineal skin may extend to the anal canal, and rectal sensation may be diminished. Rectal wall tone depends on the level of the spinal lesion. In a study of 25 patients with spinal cord injury, rectal tone was significantly higher than normal in patients with acute and chronic supraconal lesions, but significantly lower than normal in patients with acute and chronic conal or cauda equina lesions.[191]

Structural Disorders of the Colon, Rectum, and Anus

Obstruction

Anal atresia in infancy, anal stenosis later in life, or obstruction of the colon may manifest as constipation. Obstruction of the small intestine generally manifests as abdominal pain and distention, but constipation and inability to pass flatus may also be features (see Chapters 100 and 125).

Disorders of Smooth Muscle

Myopathy Affecting Colonic Muscle. Congenital or acquired myopathy of the colon usually manifests as pseudo-obstruction. The colon is hypotonic and inert (see Chapter 126).

Hereditary Internal Anal Sphincter Myopathy. Hereditary internal anal sphincter myopathy is a rare condition characterized by constipation with difficulty in rectal expulsion and episodes of severe *proctalgia fugax*, defined as the sudden onset of brief episodes of pain in the anorectal region.[192–194] Three affected families have been reported. The mode of inheritance appears to be autosomal dominant with incomplete penetrance. In symptomatic persons, the internal anal sphincter muscle is thickened, and resting anal pressure is greatly increased. In two patients, treatment with a calcium channel blocker improved pain but had no effect on constipation. In another family, two patients were treated by internal anal sphincter strip myectomy; one showed marked improvement, and one had improvement in constipation but only slight improvement in pain. Examination of the muscle strips showed myopathic changes with polyglucosan bodies (glucose polymers) in the smooth muscle fibers and increased endomysial fibrosis.

Systemic Sclerosis. Systemic sclerosis (scleroderma) may lead to constipation.[195] In patients with systemic sclerosis and constipation, 9 of 10 had no increase in colonic motor activity after ingestion of a 1000-kcal meal. Histologic examination of colonic specimens from these subjects revealed smooth muscle atrophy of the colonic wall (see Chapter 35).[196]

Muscular Dystrophies. Muscular dystrophies are usually regarded as disorders of striated muscle, but visceral smooth muscle may also be abnormal. In myotonic muscular dystrophy, a condition in which skeletal muscle fails to relax normally, megacolon may be found, and abnormal function of the anal sphincter is demonstrable.[197] Cases associated with intestinal pseudoobstruction have been reported (see Chapter 126).[198]

Disorders of Enteric Nerves

Congenital Aganglionosis or Hypoganglionosis. Congenital absence or reduction in the number of ganglia in the colon leads to functional colonic obstruction with proximal dilatation, as seen in Hirschsprung disease and related conditions (see Chapter 100). In Hirschsprung disease, ganglion cells in the distal colon are absent because of an arrest in caudal migration of neural crest cells in the intestine during embryonic development. Although most patients present during early childhood, often with delayed passage of meconium, some patients with a relatively short segment of involved colon present later in life.[199] Typically, the colon narrows at the area that lacks ganglion cells, and the bowel proximal to the narrowing is usually dilated. Two genetic defects have been identified in patients with Hirschsprung disease—a mutation in the rearranged during transfection (RET) proto-oncogene, which is involved in the development of neural crest cells, and a mutation in the gene that encodes the endothelin B receptor, which affects intracellular calcium levels.[200,201]

Hypoganglionosis is reported when small, sparse myenteric ganglia are seen. Neuronal counts can be made on full-thickness tissue specimens and compared with published reference values obtained from autopsy material. Because of variations in the normal density of neurons, establishing the diagnosis of hypoganglionosis is not easy.[202] Quantitative declines in the number of neurons in the enteric nervous system are also seen in patients with severe slow-transit constipation and characterized morphologically as oligoneuronal hypoganglionosis.[203]

Congenital Hyperganglionosis (Intestinal Neuronal Dysplasia). Congenital hyperganglionosis, or intestinal neuronal dysplasia, is a developmental defect characterized by hyperplasia of the submucosal nerve plexus. Clinical manifestations of the disease are similar to those seen in Hirschsprung disease and include young age of onset and symptoms of intestinal obstruction (see Chapter 100). In contrast to functional constipation, affected children do not have symptoms of soiling or evidence of a fecaloma.[204] A multicenter study of interobserver variation in histologic interpretation of findings in children with constipation caused by abnormalities of the enteric nervous system showed complete agreement in the diagnosis of Hirschsprung disease but accord in only 14% of children with colonic motility disorders other than aganglionosis. Some of the clinical features and histologic changes previously associated with congenital hyperganglionosis may evolve to normal as children age.[202] A diagnosis of congenital hyperganglionosis can be made on the basis of hyperganglionosis of the submucous plexus with giant ganglia and at least one of the following features in rectal biopsy specimens: (1) ectopic ganglia, (2) increased acetylcholinesterase activity in the lamina propria, and (3) increased acetylcholinesterase nerve fibers around the submucosal blood vessels. Most patients with congenital hyperganglionosis respond to conservative treatment, including laxatives. Internal anal sphincter myectomy may be performed if conservative management fails.[205]

Acquired Neuropathies. Chagas disease, which results from infection with *Trypanosoma cruzi*, is the only known infectious neuropathy. The reason for neuronal degeneration in this disorder is unclear but may have an immune basis.[206] Patients with Chagas disease present with progressively worsening symptoms of constipation and abdominal distention resulting from a segmental megacolon that may be complicated by sigmoid volvulus (see Chapter 115).

Paraneoplastic visceral neuropathy may be associated with malignant tumors outside the GI tract, particularly small cell carcinoma of the lung and carcinoid tumors. Pathologic examination of the affected intestine reveals neuronal degeneration or myenteric plexus inflammation.[207] An antibody against a component of myenteric neurons has been identified in some patients with this disorder (see Chapter 126).[208] Disruption of the ICCs has been associated with a case of small cell lung carcinoma–related paraneoplastic colonic motility disorder.[209]

Neuropathies of Unknown Cause. Severe acute neuropathies that present mainly with obstructive symptoms and not principally with constipation have been described. As noted earlier, neuropathic features affecting the colon may occur in some patients with severe idiopathic constipation.

Medications

Constipation may be a side effect of a drug or preparation taken long term. Drugs commonly implicated are listed in Box 20.3 (see earlier). Common offenders include opioids used for chronic pain, anticholinergic agents (including antispasmodics), calcium supplements, some tricyclic antidepressants, NSAIDs, phenothiazines used as long-term neuroleptics, and antimuscarinic drugs used for PD.

Psychological Disorders

Constipation may be a symptom of a psychiatric disorder or a side effect of its treatment (see Chapter 23). Healthy men who are socially outgoing, energetic, and optimistic—and not anxious—and who described themselves in more favorable terms than others have heavier stools than men without these personality characteristics.[210] Psychological factors associated with a prolonged colonic transit time in constipated patients include a highly depressed mood state and frequent control of anger.[211] In one study, women with constipation had higher somatization and anxiety scores than healthy controls, and the psychological scores correlated inversely with rectal mucosal blood flow (used as an index of innervation of the distal colon).[212] In a study that assessed psychological characteristics of older persons with constipation, a delayed colonic transit time was related significantly to symptoms of somatization, obsessive-compulsiveness, depression, and anxiety.[81] In a study of 28 consecutive female patients who underwent psychological assessment for intractable constipation, 60% had evidence of a current affective disorder. One-third reported distorted attitudes toward food. Patients with slow-transit constipation reported more psychosocial distress on rating scales than those with normal-transit constipation.[213]

Depression

For some patients, constipation can be a somatic manifestation of an affective disorder. In a study of patients with depression, 27% said that constipation developed or became worse at the onset of the depression.[214] Constipation can occur in the absence of other typical features of severe depression, such as anorexia or psychomotor retardation with physical inactivity. Psychological factors are likely to influence intestinal function via autonomic efferent neural pathways.[212] In an analysis of 4 million discharge records of US military veterans, major depression was associated with constipation, and schizophrenia was associated with both constipation and megacolon.[215] A study using the NHANES from 2009 to 2010 found depressed individuals were more likely than nondepressed individuals to report constipation (9.1% vs. 6.7%) as well as diarrhea (15.6% vs. 6.1%).[216]

Eating Disorders

Patients with anorexia nervosa or bulimia often complain of constipation, and a prolonged whole-gut transit time has been demonstrated in patients with these disorders.[217] Colonic transit time returns to normal in most patients with anorexia nervosa once they are consuming a balanced diet and gaining weight for at least 3 weeks.[218] Pelvic floor dysfunction is found in some patients with an eating disorder and does not improve with weight gain and a balanced diet.[219]

Anorexia nervosa should be considered a possible diagnosis in young underweight women who present with constipation. Patients with an eating disorder often resort to regular use of laxatives to treat constipation or to facilitate weight loss or relieve the presumed consequences of binge eating. Treatment of such patients is directed at the underlying eating disorder (see Chapter 10).

Denied Bowel Movements

Patients may deny or fail to report defecation when solid inert markers have been demonstrated to disappear from the abdomen by radiologic examination, proving that elimination has occurred (see later). Such patients need skilled psychiatric help.

Fecal Impaction

Fecal impaction is defined by a large mass of stool in the rectum or colon that cannot be evacuated[220] and usually presents as a complication (rather than a cause) of chronic or severe constipation. Fecal impaction is seen more commonly in older adults[221] but can also be present in children and in patients with spinal cord injury or neuromuscular disease.[65,222] Institutionalized older adults are at particularly high risk of developing fecal impaction.[66,223,224]

A variety of factors can contribute to the development of fecal impaction. These often include chronic constipation, inadequate fiber and water intake, obstructing lesions of the colon, or lack of mobility resulting from old age, spinal cord injury, or neuromuscular disease. Medications that slow gastrointestinal motility (e.g., opioids, anticholinergics, calcium channel blockers, antacids, antipsychotics, antihypertensives, iron, and laxative abuse) may also contribute in some patients.[221,222,225]

Fecal impaction often presents with symptoms similar to those associated with intestinal obstruction, including nausea, vomiting, abdominal pain and distension, and anorexia.[225] Other symptoms of fecal impaction include rectal discomfort, paradoxical diarrhea, fecal incontinence, urinary frequency, and urinary overflow incontinence.[221] Fecal impaction may be accompanied by serious morbidity and a high mortality rate. Morbidities include intestinal perforation, intestinal obstruction, stercoral colitis or ulceration, rectovaginal fistulation, and megarectum or megacolon.[221,226–228] A study of 32 patients with fecal impaction seen at a tertiary care hospital found 41% experience serious morbidities related to fecal impaction, and 22% died while in the hospital.[229] Emergency department visits for fecal impaction are common in the late elderly (i.e., >85 years of age).[230] In up to 30% of hospital cases, mortality can occur secondary to complications of fecal impaction.[227]Common methods for relieving fecal impaction include digital disimpaction, use of enemas, and oral laxative administration. Subsequent to successful disimpaction of the stool burden, colonic workup, including colonoscopy or barium enema, should be performed to evaluate the patient for a stricture or malignancy.[225] Endocrine and metabolic screening should also be performed to rule out extraintestinal causes of constipation and fecal impaction.[221] If no anatomic abnormalities are found, measures should be employed to reduce the likelihood of recurrence. As in the prevention of constipation, increased fiber intake, hydration, and appropriate laxative use (but not overuse) may help reduce risk of reimpaction.[225] If applicable, other risk factors, including constipating medication regimens and lack of mobility, should be addressed.

CLINICAL ASSESSMENT

History

It is important to determine exactly what a patient considers constipation. A detailed history that includes duration of symptoms, frequency of bowel movements, and associated symptoms, such as abdominal discomfort and distention, should be obtained. The history should include an assessment of stool consistency, stool size, and degree of straining during defecation. The presence of warning symptoms or signs—unintentional weight loss, rectal bleeding, change in the caliber of stool, severe abdominal pain, or family history of colon cancer—should be elicited. A long duration of symptoms that have been refractory to conservative measures is suggestive of a functional colorectal disorder. By contrast, the new onset of constipation may indicate a structural disease.

A dietary history should be obtained. The amount of daily fiber and fluid consumed should be assessed. Many patients tend to skip breakfast,[231] and this practice may exacerbate constipation, because the postprandial increase in colonic motility is greatest after breakfast.[232,233] Although caffeinated coffee (150 mg of caffeine) stimulates colonic motility, ingestion of a meal has a greater effect.[234]

A patient's past medical history must be reviewed. Obstetric and surgical histories are particularly important. Neurologic disorders may also explain some cases of constipation. A carefully taken drug history, including use of over-the-counter laxatives and herbal medications and their frequencies of intake, is important.

A detailed social history may provide useful information as to why the patient has sought help for constipation at this time; potentially relevant behavioral background information may also be obtained. In patients with IBS, the frequency of a history of sexual abuse is increased as compared with healthy controls.[235] In a survey of 120 patients with dyssynergia, 22% reported a history of sexual abuse, and 32% reported a history of physical abuse. Bowel dysfunction adversely affected sexual life in 56% and social life in 76% of patients.[236] The physician should be alert to manifestations of depression, such as insomnia, lack of energy, loss of interest in life, loss of confidence, and a sense of hopelessness. A history of physical or sexual abuse may not emerge during the initial visit. However, if the physician indicates that a history of abuse is common in patients with intestinal symptoms, while maintaining a sensitive, encouraging attitude, a complete history more often emerges gradually during subsequent visits, provided that there is privacy, confidentiality, and adequate time (see Chapter 23).

Physical Examination

The patient's general appearance or voice may point to a clinical diagnosis of hypothyroidism, PD, or depression. The physical examination should exclude major CNS disorders, especially spinal lesions. If spinal disease is suspected, the sacral dermatomes should be examined for loss of sensation. The abdomen should be examined for distention, hard feces in a palpable colon, or an inflammatory or neoplastic mass. If the abdomen appears distended, a hand should be passed under the lumbar spine while the patient is lying supine to exclude anterior arching of the lumbar spine as a cause of postural bloating (see Chapter 18).

The rectal examination is paramount in evaluating a patient with constipation.[237] Placing the patient in the left lateral position is most convenient for performing a thorough rectal examination. Painful perianal conditions and rectal mucosal disease should be excluded, and defecatory function should be evaluated. The perineum should be observed both at rest and after the patient strains as if to have a bowel movement. Normally, the perineum descends between 1 and 4 cm during straining. With the patient in the left lateral position, descent of the perineum below the plane of the ischial tuberosities (i.e., >4 cm) usually suggests excessive perineal descent. A lack of descent may indicate the inability to relax the pelvic floor muscles during defecation, whereas excessive perineal descent may indicate descending perineum syndrome. Patients with descending perineum syndrome strain excessively and achieve only incomplete evacuation because of a lack of straightening of the anorectal angle. Eventually, excessive descent of the perineum may result in injury to the sacral nerves from stretching, a reduction in rectal sensation, and ultimately incontinence due to denervation.[151] Rectal prolapse may be detected when the patient is asked to strain.

The perianal area should be examined for scars, fistulas, fissures, and external hemorrhoids. A digital rectal examination should be performed to evaluate the patient for the presence of a fecal impaction, anal stricture, or rectal mass. A patulous anal sphincter may suggest prior trauma to the anal sphincter or a neurologic disorder that impairs sphincter function. Other important functions that should be assessed during the digital examination are summarized in Box 20.5. Specifically, inability to

BOX 20.5 Clinical Clues to an Evacuation Disorder

HISTORY

Prolonged straining is required to expel stool

Assumption of unusual postures on the toilet to facilitate stool expulsion

Support of the perineum, digitation of rectum, or application of pressure to the posterior vaginal wall are required to facilitate rectal emptying

Inability to expel enema fluid

Constipation after subtotal colectomy for constipation

RECTAL EXAMINATION (WITH PATIENT IN THE LEFT LATERAL POSITION)

Inspection

The anus is "pulled" forward during attempts to simulate strain during defecation

The anal verge descends <1 cm or >4 cm (or beyond ischial tuberosities) during attempts to simulate straining at defecation

The perineum balloons down during straining; rectal mucosa partially prolapses through anal canal

Palpation

High anal sphincter tone at rest precludes easy entry of the examining finger (in the absence of a painful perianal condition [e.g., anal fissure])

Anal sphincter pressure during voluntary squeeze is only minimally higher than anal pressure at rest

The perineum and examining finger descend <1 cm or >4 cm during simulated straining at defecation

The puborectalis muscle is tender to palpation through the rectal wall posteriorly, or palpation reproduces pain

Palpable mucosal prolapse occurs during straining

"Defect" in anterior wall of the rectum, suggestive of rectocele

ANORECTAL MANOMETRY AND BALLOON EXPULSION TEST (WITH PATIENT IN LEFT LATERAL POSITION)

Elevated resting anal sphincter pressure

Delay in balloon expulsion (normal values for women <50 years: 4–75 sec; normal values for women ≥50 years of age: 3–15 sec)[246]

insert the examining finger into the anal canal may suggest an elevated anal sphincter pressure, and tenderness on palpation of the pelvic floor as it traverses the posterior aspect of the rectum may suggest pelvic floor spasm. The degree of descent of the perineum during attempts to strain and expel the examining finger provides another way of assessing the degree of perineal descent. Compared with high-resolution manometry and balloon expulsion (see later), the sensitivity, specificity, and positive predictive value of a digital rectal examination in the diagnosis of dyssynergia were 93.2%, 58.7%, and 91.0%, respectively, with moderate agreement seen between the two diagnostic modalities (κ-coefficient = 0.542, $P < .001$).[238] A thorough history and physical examination can exclude most secondary causes of constipation (see Box 20.3).

DIAGNOSTIC TESTS

Further diagnostic testing is unnecessary for most patients who complain of mild symptoms, especially adolescents, young adults, and those without alarm features. Investigations may be indicated for 1 of 2 reasons: (1) to exclude a systemic illness or structural disorder of the GI tract as a cause of constipation or (2) to elucidate the underlying pathophysiologic process when symptoms are unresponsive to simple treatment.

Tests for Systemic Disease

Determination of the hemoglobin level, ESR, and biochemical screening test levels (e.g., thyroid function, serum calcium, glucose, and other appropriate investigations) are indicated if the clinical picture suggests that symptoms may be due to an inflammatory, neoplastic, metabolic, or other systemic disorder.

Tests for Structural Disease

Imaging of the colon by a CT, MRI, or barium enema study reveals the width and length of the colon and may be indicated to exclude an obstructing lesion severe enough to cause constipation. When fecal impaction is present, a limited enema study with a water-soluble contrast agent outlines the colon and fecal mass without aggravating the condition. Imaging of the small bowel is indicated only if obstruction or pseudo-obstruction involving the small bowel is suspected (see Chapters 125 and 126). Endoscopy allows direct visualization of the colonic mucosa. The yield of colonoscopy in the absence of "alarm" symptoms in patients with chronic constipation is low and comparable to that for asymptomatic patients who undergo colonoscopy for colon cancer screening.[239] Among 786 patients who underwent colonoscopy for constipation, only 5.5% had a polyp, and no cancers were found.[240] A colonoscopy is recommended only when there has been a recent change in bowel habits, blood in the stool, or other alarm symptoms (e.g., weight loss and fever).[241] All adults 45 years of age and older should undergo screening for colorectal cancer, as widely recommended (see Chapter 128).[242]

Physiologic Measurements

Physiologic testing is reserved for patients with refractory symptoms. Testing can be performed to measure colonic transit time, evaluate pelvic floor functioning during defecation, and exclude anatomic abnormalities that could cause constipation.

Colonic Transit Time

Studies that measure colonic transit time are important for confirming and quantifying a patient's complaint of constipation and identifying slow transit and regional delay. The American and European Neurogastroenterology and Motility Societies recommend three methods for assessing colonic transit time: radiopaque markers, wireless motility capsule, and scintigraphy.[243]

Radiopaque Markers. Radiopaque marker testing is used to distinguish normal from slow colonic transit, assess segmental transit times, and evaluate the response to new treatments.[243] Colonic transit time is measured by performing abdominal radiography at predetermined times after the patient ingests plastic beads or rings and counting the number of retained markers (Fig. 20.5). Before the study, patients should be maintained on a high-fiber diet and should avoid laxatives, enemas, or medications that may affect bowel function. Because the markers are eliminated only with defecation, the process of measuring colonic transit is discontinuous, and the result of a transit measurement should be regarded with caution, taking recent defecation into account. If the markers are retained exclusively in the sigmoid colon and rectum, the patient may have a defecatory disorder. The presence of markers throughout the colon, however, does not exclude the possibility of a defecatory disorder. Therefore anorectal physiologic testing should be considered in appropriate patients prior to performing radiopaque marker testing (see later).[243] Measurements of transit through different segments of the colon are of doubtful value in planning treatment, except for megarectum, in which all the markers move rapidly to the rectum and are retained there. Assessment of stool burden by plain film

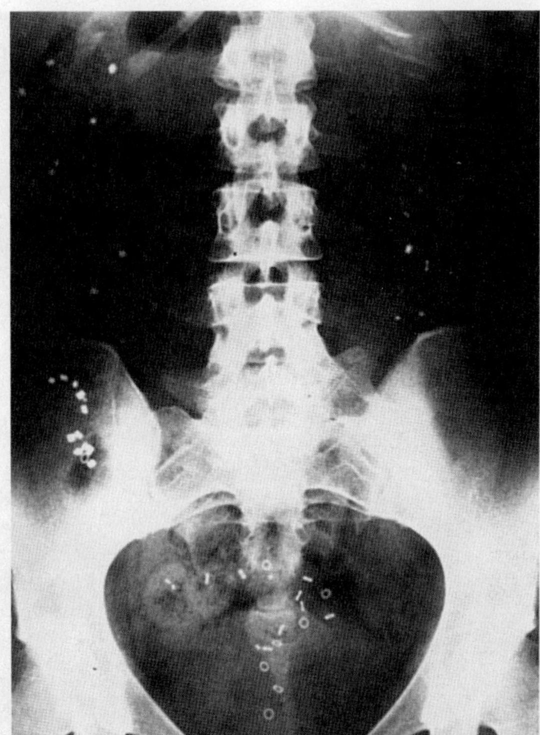

Fig. 20.5 Abdominal film from a colonic transit study. This constipated patient had ingested 20 inert ring markers 120 h previously and 20 cube-shaped markers 72 h previously. Most markers are still present, indicating slow whole-gut transit.

abdominal x-ray has been proposed as a reliable alternative to radiopaque marker study.[244]

In nonconstipated subjects, the mean colonic transit time using radiopaque marker testing is 30–40 hours, with an upper limit of normal of 72 hours (see earlier).[245] Women often have longer maximal colonic transit times than men (70–106 hours vs. 50 hours).

Wireless Motility Capsule.[120] The wireless recording capsule is a single-use capsule that assesses colonic transit without radiation exposure. It is used to distinguish normal from slow colonic transit and can also be used in patients with a suspected motility disorder of the upper GI tract because it measures gastric emptying, small bowel transit, and colonic transit times (Fig. 20.6). The wireless motility capsule is ingested following a standardized meal and 50 mL of water. The capsule continuously sends temperature, pH, and pressure measurements to a data receiver as it moves along the GI tract. Patients wear a data receiver on their waists for 5 days, or until the capsule is passed, and keep a log of daily activities such as meals, sleep, and bowel movements.

Most studies that have compared the wireless motility capsule with conventional radiopaque marker testing have found concordance between the two methods (a wireless motility capsule specificity of 0.95 and sensitivity of 0.46 for identifying an abnormal transit time, compared with a radiopaque marker testing specificity of 0.95 and sensitivity of 0.40).[246–248] In one retrospective study, however, the wireless motility capsule showed only 86% positive test agreement and 43% negative test agreement with radiopaque marker testing.[249] The wireless motility capsule has also been found to be comparable to both gastric emptying scintigraphy and whole-gut scintigraphy.[250,251]

The normal colonic transit time using the wireless motility capsule is 10–59 hours, with delayed colonic transit considered greater than 44 hours in men and 59 hours in women.[247] The difference in colonic transit times between radiopaque marker testing and a wireless motility capsule is not unexpected, given the different methods of quantifying colonic transit time and the larger size of the wireless motility capsule compared with the smaller plastic beads used in radiopaque marker testing.[247,248] Wireless motility capsule testing is particularly useful in patients being considered for colectomy as treatment for severe constipation when assessment of upper GI transit is recommended (see later).[252] Although the wireless motility capsule is well tolerated and permits ambulatory testing, device failure is reported in about 3% of cases,[243] and its use is not recommended in patients with pacemakers or defibrillators, swallowing disorders, suspected strictures or fistulas, or a high risk for strictures.

Colonic Transit Scintigraphy. Colonic transit scintigraphy is used to measure whole-gut and regional colonic transit in patients with diffuse disorders involving the stomach or small intestine or with a suspected colonic motility disorder.[253] Transit time is measured by capturing serial abdominal images using a gamma camera at specified times after ingestion of a labeled meal (^{111}In-diethylenetriamine pentaacetate-labeled water with a standard ^{99m}Tc egg sandwich[235] or ^{111}In-labeled activated charcoal particles contained in a capsule).[254,255] Anterior and posterior images of the colon are obtained at specified times over 2–3 days following ingestion of the meal. Using ^{111}In-diethylenetriamine pentaacetate-labeled water with the standard ^{99m}Tc egg sandwich allows gastric, small bowel, and colonic transit times to be measured in the same study.[256] The capsule containing ^{111}In-labeled activated charcoal particles, however, does not dissolve until it reaches the distal ileum, where it releases the labeled particles into the colon, thereby permitting measurement of only colonic transit.[254] Results are reported as ascending colon emptying (indicating the time for 50% emptying) or overall colonic transit expressed as the geometric center (weighted average of the radioactivity distribution within the colon and stool).[243]

Using scintigraphy, the mean colonic transit, expressed as the geometric center, is 2.7 ± 1.05 at 24 hours. A 24-hour colonic transit time less than 1.7 is considered slow transit.[254] A low geometric center is considered slow transit because the majority of the radioactivity is in the proximal colon, whereas a high geometric center is considered accelerated transit because the majority of the radioactivity has moved to the left side of the colon or into the expelled stool. Colonic transit scintigraphy has been shown to be comparable with radiopaque marker testing, except in the descending colon,[257] but is available in only a limited number of specialized centers.

Tests to Assess the Physiology of Defecation

Clinical tests to assess a patient for a defecatory disorder include defecography, balloon expulsion test, anorectal manometry, and EMG. To diagnose dyssynergic defecation, the Rome criteria require a combination of 2 of the following 3 abnormal tests of the pelvic floor on attempted defecation: (1) impaired evacuation on balloon expulsion or defecography; (2) inappropriate contraction of the pelvic floor muscles on manometry, imaging, or EMG; and (3) inadequate propulsive forces as assessed by manometry or imaging.[138]

A meta-analysis of 79 studies in patients with chronic constipation found that dyssynergic defecation is common in patients with chronic constipation. The pooled frequencies of abnormal findings differed depending on the test: anorectal manometry, 48%; balloon expulsion, 43% (by any criteria); defecography, 15% (absent opening of the anorectal angle) and 37% (excessive perineal descent); and EMG, 44% (increased activity of the puborectalis muscles).[258]

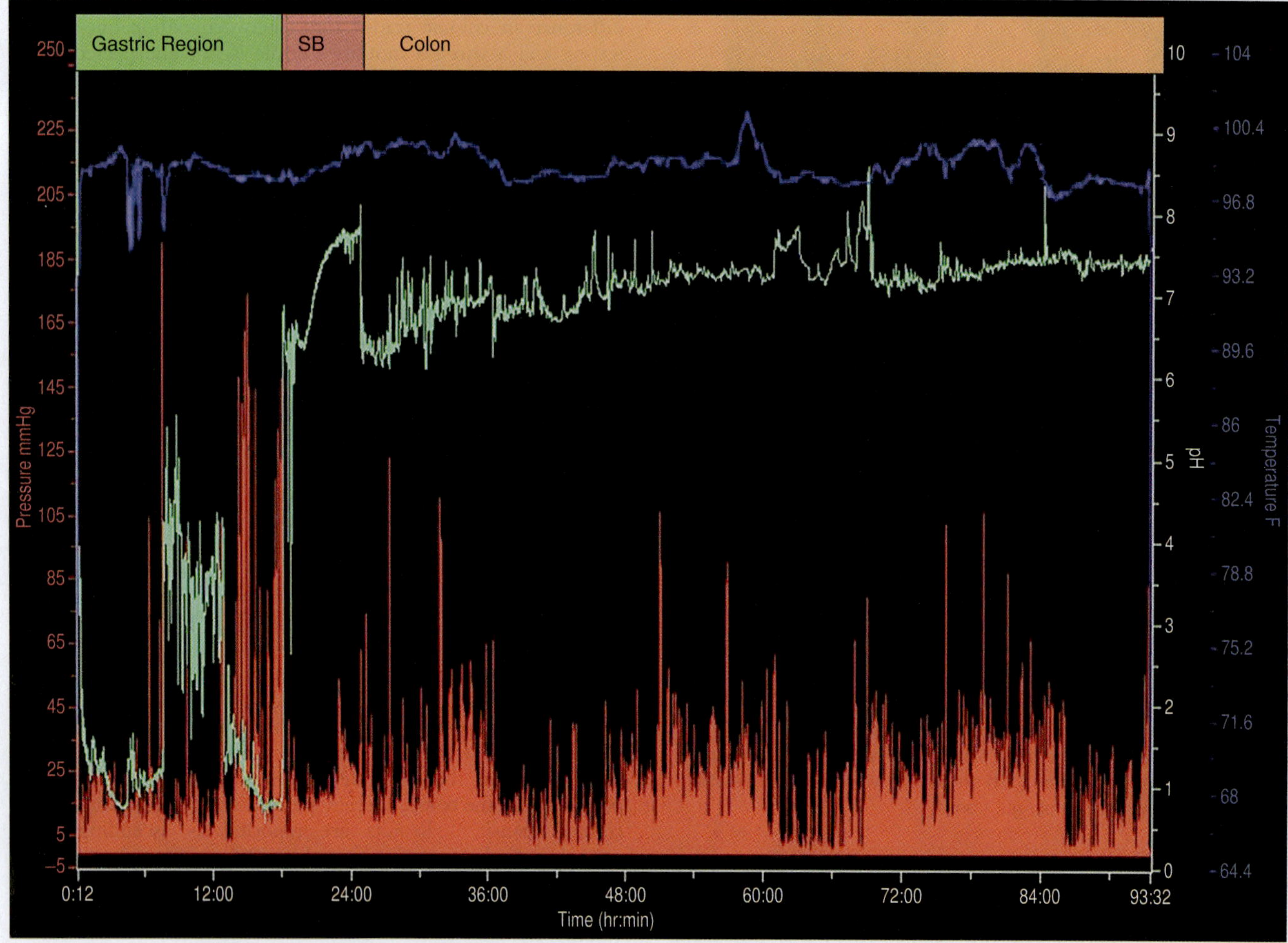

Fig. 20.6 Tracing from a wireless motility capsule study in a constipated patient. After the wireless motility capsule is swallowed, temperature *(blue line)*, pressure *(red line)*, and pH *(green line)* are recorded. Gastric emptying time is determined by a rise in pH, signifying that the capsule has passed into the duodenum. A drop in pH (at ≈ 24 h) occurs when the capsule passes into the colon. The time when the capsule is passed through the rectum and into the toilet is determined by a drop in temperature. In this patient, colonic transit is prolonged. *SB*, Small bowel.

DEFECOGRAPHY

Defecography evaluates the rate and completeness of rectal emptying, anorectal angle, and amount of perineal descent and identifies structural abnormalities (e.g., large rectocele, internal mucosal prolapse, and intussusception). Thickened barium is instilled into the rectum, and films or videos are taken during fluoroscopy with the patient sitting on a radiolucent commode while resting, deferring defecation, and straining to defecate. Importantly, identified anatomic abnormalities are not always functionally relevant. For example, a rectocele is only relevant if it fills preferentially (i.e., instead of the rectal ampulla) and fails to empty after simulated defecation. The limitations of defecography include variability among radiologists in interpreting studies, inhibition of normal rectal emptying because of patient embarrassment, and differences in texture between barium paste and stool. Magnetic resonance defecography may offer advantages over standard barium defecography, such as lack of radiation exposure and increased detection of abnormalities during the defecation phase.[259,260] Additionally, magnetic resonance defecography may also be more sensitive for detecting pelvic organ abnormalities in a dynamic fashion, including cystoceles and colpoceles,[261,262] but is not yet widely available and rarely can be performed with the patient in a sitting position.

Balloon Expulsion Test

The balloon expulsion test can suggest a defecatory disorder in a patient with no or delayed evacuation of a 50-mL water-filled balloon from the rectum; the test is generally performed, while the patient is sitting on a commode.[263,264] In a study of 359 patients with constipation, the balloon expulsion test was abnormal in 21 of 24 patients with pelvic floor dyssynergia (as determined by manometry and defecography). By contrast, an abnormal balloon expulsion test was also found in 12 of 106 patients who did not have pelvic floor dyssynergia.[265] Therefore the balloon expulsion test is often used in conjunction with anorectal manometry. In healthy women, balloon expulsion time decreases with age; normal values range from 4 to 75 seconds in those younger than 50 years of age and from 3 to 15 seconds in those 50 years or older.[266] The sensitivity and specificity for diagnosing a rectal evacuation disorder using a 60 second cut for balloon expulsion time were reported to be 39% and 93%, respectively, while the sensitivity and specificity of a cutoff of 22 seconds were 78% and 70%, respectively.[267]

Anorectal Manometry

Anorectal manometry can assess the resting and maximum squeeze pressures of the anal sphincters, the presence or absence of relaxation of the anal sphincter during balloon distention of the rectum (rectoanal inhibitory reflex), rectal sensation, and ability of the anal sphincter to relax during straining.[239,268] A high resting anal pressure suggests the presence of an anal fissure or anismus (paradoxical contraction of the external anal sphincter in response to straining or pressure within the anal canal). RH suggests a neurologic disorder, but the volume of rectal content necessary to induce rectal urgency may also be increased in patients with fecal retention, so the results of rectal sensitivity testing must be interpreted with caution. The absence of a rectoanal inhibitory reflex raises the possibility of Hirschsprung disease.

Patients with a defecatory disorder commonly have inappropriate contraction of the anal sphincter when they bear down. A positive rectoanal gradient (i.e., higher rectal than anal pressure) is generally thought to be necessary for normal defecation, whereas a negative rectoanal gradient (i.e., lower rectal than anal pressure) is associated with a defecatory disorder; however, asymptomatic persons often have abnormal anal sphincter contraction during anorectal manometry. In a study of healthy subjects, 36% had dyssynergia in the left lateral position, but the presence or the absence of dyssynergia did not predict the ability to expel a balloon.[269] In a subsequent study using high-resolution anorectal manometry, the rectoanal gradient was negative in a majority of asymptomatic women.[266] A retrospective clinical database study of 475 constipated individuals who underwent high resolution manometry, balloon expulsion test, and defecography showed that a reduced rectoanal gradient was the best predictor of prolonged balloon expulsion test or reduced rectal evacuation. A combination of prolonged balloon expulsion test and reduced rectoanal gradient has a 75% probability of having a defecatory disorder, while either one alone has a probability of 45%.[270] Although a negative rectoanal gradient can be supportive of a diagnosis of a defecatory disorder, it is not conclusive by itself and should be used in conjunction with other physiologic testing.

With the purpose to standardize and classify disorders of anorectal function, an international anorectal physiology working group (IAPWA) was created in the first attempt to standardized maneuvers to test rectoanal reflexes, anal tone, anal contractibility, rectoanal coordination, and rectal sensation.[271] Based on these measurements, a London classification system was created. However, this classification system has not been clinically tested, and therefore clinical meaningfulness is still to be determined.[272–274] Also, it is important to mention that the anorectal function tests should be interpreted with reference to age- and sex-matched normal values. The reproducibility of high-resolution manometry and the intra-subject variability are still under investigation.[275]

EMG of Striated Muscle Activity. In general, EMG studies of the external anal sphincter and puborectalis muscles using concentric needle or surface electrode recordings are not essential and rarely indicated. An exception is the use of EMG in patients with a suspected spinal cord or cauda equina lesion, in whom bilateral or unilateral dysfunction of the external anal sphincter can be demonstrated.

Rectal Sensitivity and Sensation Testing. Rectal sensitivity to distention can be measured by introducing successive volumes of air into a rectal balloon and recording the volume at which the stimulus is first perceived, the volume that produces an urge to defecate, and the volume above which further addition of air can no longer be tolerated owing to discomfort.

TREATMENT

Initial treatment of constipation is based on nonpharmacologic interventions. If these measures fail, pharmacologic agents may be used. If a defecatory disorder is present, initial treatment should include biofeedback. Whereas many patients with disordered evacuation do not respond well to fiber supplementation or oral laxatives, up to 75% respond to biofeedback. Otherwise, treatment should include increased physical activity and increased fluid and fiber intake through changes in diet or use of commercial fiber supplements. Patients who do not improve with fiber supplementation should be given an osmotic laxative such as milk of magnesia or polyethylene glycol (PEG). The dose should be adjusted until soft stools are attained. Stimulant agents (e.g., bisacodyl and senna derivatives) should be reserved for patients who do not respond to fiber or osmotic laxatives. Prescription pharmacologic agents, such as lubiprostone, linaclotide, plecanatide, and prucalopride, should be considered for patients who have not responded to initial therapy. Fig. 20.7 provides an algorithm for the evaluation and treatment of patients with moderate-to-severe constipation.

General Measures

Reassurance

Some patients can be helped by being told that an irregular bowel habit and other mild defecatory symptoms are common in the healthy general population and that their symptoms are not harmful. Patients who are concerned that their symptoms may indicate disease may be reassured by appropriate investigation.

Lifestyle Changes

Lifestyle modifications and dietary changes are often used as the first line of management for patients with chronic constipation. The need to set aside an unhurried and, if possible, regular time for defecation and always to respond to a defecatory urge should be emphasized. If patients experience difficulty in expelling stool, they should be advised to place a support approximately 6 inches in height under their feet when sitting on a toilet so that the hips are flexed toward a squatting posture. For persons with an inactive lifestyle, physical activity should be encouraged. Use of constipating drugs, including over-the-counter medications (see Box 20.3), should be avoided.

Psychological Support

Constipation may be aggravated by stress or may be a manifestation of emotional disturbance (e.g., previous sexual abuse [see Chapter 23]). For such patients, an assessment of the person's circumstances, personality, and background and supportive advice may help more than any pharmacologic or physical measures of treatment. Behavioral treatment (see later) offers a physical approach with a psychological component and is often acceptable and beneficial.

Fluid Intake

Dehydration or salt depletion is likely to lead to increased salt and water absorption by the colon, leading in turn to the passage of small hard stools. Low fluid intake has been found to be an independent predictor of constipation.[40] In the absence of clinical dehydration, however, no data support the notion that increasing fluid intake relieves constipation.[276,277] Increasing water intake to 1.5–2 L daily may enhance the effects of fiber intake in patients with constipation.[278]

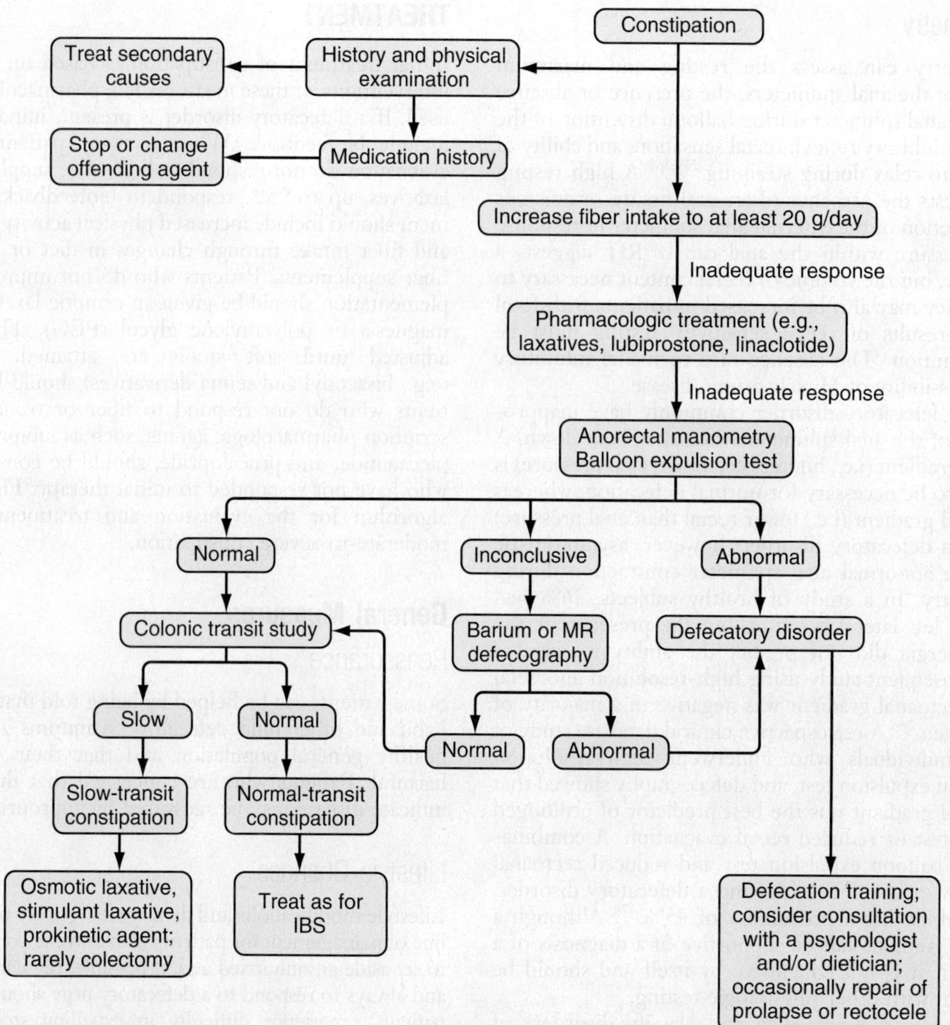

Fig. 20.7 Algorithm for the evaluation and treatment of moderate-to-severe constipation.

Dietary Changes and Fiber Supplementation

Based on the dietary and stool patterns of rural Africans in the early 1970s, Dr. Denis Burkitt speculated that a deficiency in dietary fiber was contributing to constipation and other colonic diseases in Western societies.[279] Since then, studies have shown that when nonconstipated persons increase their intake of dietary fiber, stool weight increases in proportion to the baseline stool weight and frequency of defecation and correlates with a decrease in colonic transit time.[280] Every gram of wheat fiber ingested yields approximately 2.7 g of stool expelled. It follows that when an increased intake of dietary fiber leads to an increase in stool weight in constipated subjects who pass small stools, the resulting stool weight may still be lower than normal. For this reason, the therapeutic results of a high-fiber diet are often disappointing as a treatment for constipation. In a study of 10 constipated women who supplemented their diets with wheat bran (20 g/day), average daily stool weight increased from roughly 30–60 g/day, with only half of patients achieving a normal average stool weight. Bowel frequency increased from a mean of 2–3 bowel movements weekly.[281] In a controlled crossover trial, 24 patients received either 20 g of bran or placebo daily for 4 weeks. Although bran was more effective than placebo in improving bowel frequency and oroanal transit rate, the occurrence and severity of constipation experienced by the patients did not differ between the two treatment periods,[282] possibly due to difficulty in defecation rather than decreased frequency of bowel movements.

Dietary fiber appears to be effective in relieving mild to moderate[92] but not severe constipation,[125] especially if severe constipation is associated with slow colonic transit, an evacuation disorder, or medications. Although dietary modification may not succeed, most constipated subjects should be advised initially to increase their dietary fiber intake as the simplest, most physiologic, and cheapest form of treatment. Guidelines for the treatment of constipation recommend a fiber intake of at least 25–30 g/day[15,283,284] of soluble fiber, as there are conflicting data on the role of insoluble fiber. A systematic review of six randomized controlled trials (four with soluble fiber and two with insoluble fiber) found that soluble fiber improved symptoms of constipation, and evidence in support of insoluble fiber was conflicting.[285] Soluble fiber seems to be better tolerated in patients with chronic constipation and IBS with constipation.[286] Therefore increased intake of soluble fiber, such as oat bran, nuts, barley, seeds, beans, lentils, peas, some fruits and vegetables, and psyllium fiber supplements, should be considered. Insoluble fiber, such as wheat bran, whole grains, and some vegetables, seems to be less tolerated and can aggravate symptoms, especially in patients with IBS with constipation.[15,285–287] Insoluble fiber particles can be coarse and large (such as bran) and can cause mechanical irritation to the colon and mucus secretion. By contrast, soluble fiber (e.g., psyllium) has a high water-holding capacity that helps pull water into the colon and avoids dehydration, thereby improving stool consistency.[1,288] Patients should be encouraged to consume approximately 25 g of nonstarch polysaccharides (NSPs) daily by eating whole-wheat bread, unrefined cereals, plenty of fruits and vegetables, and, if necessary, a supplement of raw bran, either in breakfast cereals or with cooked foods. Specific dietary counseling is often needed.

Side effects of fiber supplementation include abdominal distention, bloating, and flatulence, and, along with its poor taste, can lead to poor patient adherence, especially for the first several weeks. Most controlled studies of the effects of fiber have shown that the minimum amount needed to consistently and significantly alter bowel function or colonic transit time is 12 g/day. To improve adherence, patients should be instructed to increase their dietary fiber intake gradually over several weeks to about 20–25 g/day. If results of therapy are inadequate, commercially packaged fiber supplements should be tried (Table 20.2). Fiber and bulking agents are concentrated forms of NSPs based on wheat, plant seed mucilage (ispaghula), plant gums (sterculia), or synthetic methylcellulose derivatives (methylcellulose, carboxymethylcellulose [see later]).

Some patients, particularly women with markedly delayed colonic transit, find that fiber aggravates abdominal distention. If patients fail to respond to a dietary fiber trial, slow-transit constipation and/or a defecatory disorder could be suspected.[125] Bran may also be unhelpful in young people with megacolon and in older adults, in whom it may lead to fecal incontinence. For these patients, a reduction in fiber intake may relieve symptoms.

Low-FODMAP Diet

Restricting poorly absorbed fermentable carbohydrates (fermentable oligosaccharides, disaccharides, monosaccharides, and polyols; FODMAPs) has been shown to be favorable in some patients with IBS with constipation, although evidence is poor and further trials are necessary (see Chapter 124).[286] No clinical trials of a low-FODMAP diet have been conducted in patients with chronic constipation unassociated with IBS.

Specific Therapeutic Agents

Commercial Fiber Products

Methylcellulose. Methylcellulose is a semisynthetic NSP of varying chain length and degree of methylation. Methylation reduces bacterial degradation in the colon. One study of constipated patients with an average daily fecal weight of only 35 g showed an increase in fecal solids with 1, 2, and 4 g of methylcellulose/day, but fecal water increased only with the 4 g dose. Bowel frequency in this group of patients increased from an average of two to four stools a week, but the patients did not report marked improvement in consistency or ease of passage of stools (see Table 20.2).[289]

Ispaghula (Psyllium). Ispaghula is derived from the husks of the *Plantago ovata* plant, which has high water-binding capacity, is fermented in the colon to a moderate extent, and increases bacterial cell mass. It is available as effervescent suspensions, granules, and a powder. The suspensions, which are popular, have to be consumed quickly before the husk absorbs water. The granules may be stirred briskly in a half-glass of water and swallowed at once; carbonated water may be preferred. Some people prefer to swallow the solid granules and then drink a glass of water.

Ispaghula has been shown to increase fecal bulk to the same extent as methylcellulose 1–4 g daily in constipated subjects. Although both stool dry and wet weights increase, the total weekly weights remain less than those of a healthy control group without treatment. In an observational study, 149 patients were treated with psyllium in the form of *P. ovata* seeds (15–30 g daily) for a period of at least 6 weeks. The response to treatment was poor among patients with slow colonic transit or a disorder of defecation, whereas 85% of patients without abnormal physiologic testing results improved or became symptom free. Nevertheless, the authors recommend a trial of dietary fiber before diagnostic testing is undertaken.[125]

Ispaghula can cause an acute allergic immunoglobulin E–mediated response, with facial swelling, urticaria, tightness in the throat, cough, and asthma.[290] Workers who inhale the compound during manufacture or preparation can have a similar reaction (see Table 20.2).[291]

Calcium Polycarbophil. Calcium polycarbophil is a hydrophilic polyacrylic resin that is resistant to bacterial degradation and thus may be less likely to cause gas and bloating. In patients with IBS, calcium polycarbophil appears to improve global symptoms and ease of stool passage but not abdominal pain (see Table 20.2).[292]

Guar Gum. Guar gum is a natural high molecular weight polysaccharide extracted from the seed of the leguminous shrub *Cyamopsis tetragonoloba*. It hydrates rapidly to form a highly viscous solution. Guar gum is approved for use in a number of foods and cosmetics and as a supplement. When used in high doses, guar gum has been reported to cause intestinal obstruction.

Flaxseed. Flaxseed, also known as *linseed*, has not been well studied in patients with constipation, and conflicting results have been reported in small studies of patients with IBS.[293,294]

Mixed Soluble and Insoluble Fiber. The combination of soluble and insoluble fiber has been proposed to be as effective as soluble fiber alone and perhaps slightly better tolerated and, therefore, is a reasonable option for patients looking to increase fiber in their diet.[295] In a 4-week trial, 10 g/day of a plum-derived mixed fiber supplement was equally efficacious as 10 g/day of psyllium in improving constipation and quality of life but more effective in relieving flatulence and bloating and dissolved better.

TABLE 20.2 Commercial Fiber Products

Agent	Starting Daily Dose (g)	Comments
Methylcellulose	4–6	Semisynthetic cellulose fiber that is relatively resistant to colonic bacterial degradation and tends to cause less bloating and flatus than psyllium
Psyllium	4–6	Made from ground seed husk of the ispaghula plant; forms a gel when mixed with water, so an ample amount of water should be taken with psyllium to avoid intestinal obstruction; undergoes bacterial degradation, which may contribute to side effects of bloating and flatus; allergic reactions (e.g., anaphylaxis, asthma) have been reported but are rare
Polycarbophil	4–6	Synthetic fiber made of polymer of acrylic acid, which is resistant to bacterial degradation
Guar gum	3–6	Soluble fiber extracted from seeds of the leguminous shrub *Cyamopsis tetragonoloba*

Other Laxatives

The main groups of laxatives other than fiber are osmotic agents and stimulatory laxatives. Stool softeners and emollients are additional therapeutic agents (see later) (Tables 20.3 and 20.4).

Osmotic Laxatives. Osmotic laxatives increase fecal volume and reduce stool consistency by creating an intraluminal osmotic gradient that drives the secretion of water and electrolytes into the intestinal lumen.

Poorly Absorbed Ions

Magnesium, sulfate, and phosphate ions are poorly absorbed by the intestine and thereby create a hyperosmolar intraluminal environment. Their primary mode of action appears to be osmotic, but they may have other possible effects with unclear consequences, such as increasing prostaglandin concentrations in the stool.[296] Stool weight increases by 7.3 g for each additional millimole of soluble magnesium excreted.[297] Standard doses of magnesium hydroxide (see Table 20.3) typically produce a bowel movement within 6 hours. Magnesium sulfate is a more potent laxative that tends to produce a large volume of liquid stool and often leads to abdominal distention and sudden passage of a foul-smelling liquid stool.

A small randomized, double-blind placebo-controlled study that included 34 female Japanese patients with constipation who were randomized to magnesium oxide (0.5 g 3 times a day) or placebo for 28 days. The primary endpoint, "overall improvement," was defined as "significantly improved" or "improved" for at least 2 out of 4 weeks and was met by 70.6% of patients receiving magnesium and 25.0% of patients receiving placebo.[298] In this study magnesium also improved stool form and colon transit time but not complete spontaneous bowel movements (CSBM). A second study, also in 90 constipated Japanese patients, compared magnesium oxide (0.5 g 3 times a day), senna (0.5 mg twice a day), or placebo.[299] In this study, overall improvement was met by 68.3% of patients receiving magnesium, 69.2% receiving senna, and 11.7% receiving placebo. Improvement was also seen for patients receiving magnesium and senna in bowel frequency and quality of life. No serious adverse events were reported. Use of magnesium, particularly in older adults, can be limited by adverse effects such as flatulence, abdominal cramps, and intravascular volume shifts. A small percentage of magnesium is actively absorbed in the small intestine; the remainder draws water into the intestine along an osmotic gradient.[300] Hypermagnesemia can occur particularly in patients with renal failure and in children. Hypermagnesemia-induced paralytic ileus is a rare complication,[301] and hypermagnesemia with coma requiring hemodialysis has occurred in a child given 18 g/day of magnesium hydroxide for 7 days.[302] Patients with renal insufficiency or cardiac dysfunction can experience electrolyte and volume overload from the absorption of magnesium. With excessive use, even patients who are otherwise healthy can experience these complications, in addition to dehydration.

Because phosphate is absorbed by the small intestine, a substantial dose must be ingested to produce an osmotic laxative effect, which is not ideal for daily use. A rare but serious form of acute kidney injury has been associated with sodium phosphate solution used before colonoscopy, even in patients with normal baseline renal function (see Chapter 40). Risk factors for kidney injury from phosphate include hypertension, advanced age, volume depletion, and use of angiotensin-converting enzyme inhibitors or NSAIDs.[303,304]

Poorly Absorbed Sugars

Lactulose

Lactulose is a nonabsorbable synthetic disaccharide that consists of galactose and fructose linked by a bond resistant to lactase. Lactulose is not absorbed by the small intestine but undergoes fermentation in the colon to yield short-chain fatty acids, hydrogen, and carbon dioxide, with consequent lowering of the fecal pH. When healthy volunteers receive lactulose 20 g (30 mL) daily, the sugar is not detectable in the stool. In larger doses, some passes through the colon unchanged.

The recommended dose of lactulose in adults is 15–30 mL once or twice daily. The time to onset of action is longer than that of other osmotic laxatives, and 2 or 3 days are required for lactulose to achieve an effect. Some patients report that lactulose is effective initially but then loses its effect, possibly due to alteration in the intestinal flora in response to the medication.[305] Adverse effects related to lactulose include abdominal distention or discomfort, presumably as a result of colonic gas production. Cases of lactulose-induced megacolon have been reported.[305]

In a group of young, chronically constipated volunteers who reported fewer than 3 stools/week, lactulose increased bowel frequency and percentage of stool moisture and softened stools when compared with a control syrup that contained only sucrose. The effectiveness of lactulose was dose dependent.[306] The effect of lactulose in older patients has been studied in two double-blind, placebo-controlled trials. In one trial, only about half of patients were found to be truly constipated; among these patients, lactulose was effective in 80%, as compared with 33% of those who received placebo (glucose) ($P < .01$).[307] The second trial was conducted in a nursing home over 8–12 weeks in 42 older patients with constipation.[308] The initial dose of lactulose was 30 mL/day, and the dose was reduced temporarily or permanently to 15 mL, depending on bowel frequency. Lactulose showed an advantage over placebo (a 50% glucose syrup) by increasing the mean number of bowel movements each day and markedly reducing episodes of fecal impaction ($P < .015$) and the need for enemas.

Sorbitol and Mannitol

Sorbitol is widely used in the food industry as an artificial sweetener but is rarely used in clinical practice. Ingestion of as little as 5 g causes a rise in breath hydrogen, and 20 g produces diarrhea in about half of normal subjects.[309] Sorbitol is as effective as lactulose and less expensive. A randomized double-blind cross-over trial of lactulose (20 g/day) and sorbitol (21 g/day) in ambulatory older men with chronic constipation showed no difference between the two compounds with regard to frequency or normality of bowel movements or patient preference.[310] The frequency of side effects was similar except for nausea, which was more common with lactulose. Mannitol is another sugar alcohol that can be used as a laxative. Like sorbitol, it is rarely used clinically for constipation.

Polyethylene Glycol

PEG is an isosmotic laxative that is metabolically inert and able to bind water molecules, thereby increasing intraluminal water retention.[311] PEG is not metabolized by colonic bacteria. Ingestion of PEG leads to an increase in stool volume and softer stools, which may become liquid depending on the volume of PEG consumed. PEG is excreted mostly unchanged in the feces. Electrolytes are added to PEG solutions used for colonic lavage before colonoscopy to avoid the potential adverse effects associated with diarrhea, such as dehydration and electrolyte imbalance. PEG-3350 without electrolytes is available in the United States as an over-the-counter powder that is mixed in smaller doses with water for regular use to treat constipation.

Several high-quality studies have demonstrated the efficacy of PEG in the treatment of chronic constipation.[312] A randomized control trial of 304 patients with chronic constipation showed symptom improvement for 6 months in 52.0% of the patients treated with the PEG solution compared with 11% in the placebo group. Similar efficacy was seen in a subgroup of 75 elderly subjects. No electrolyte abnormalities or intestinal malabsorption were noted.[312]

TABLE 20.3 Laxatives Commonly Used for Constipation

Type of Laxative	Generic Name(s)	Dose	Comments
Osmotic laxatives			
Poorly Absorbed Ions			
Magnesium	Magnesium hydroxide	15–30 mL once or twice daily	Hypermagnesemia can occur particularly in patients with renal failure and in children.
	Magnesium citrate	75–150 mL or 2–4 tablets once daily	Often used as part of a bowel preparation. Prolonged use of more than 1650 g of magnesium has been associated with hypermagnesemia.
	Magnesium sulfate	5–10 g once daily	
Sulfate	Sodium sulfate (Glauber salt)	5–10 g once daily	Sodium sulfate is generally not used by itself as a laxative agent.
Phosphate	Sodium phosphate	0.5–10 mL with 12 oz of water	Hyperphosphatemia can occur, especially in patients with renal failure.
Poorly Absorbed Sugars			
Disaccharides	Lactulose	15–30 mL once or twice daily	Gas and bloating are common side effect.
Sugar alcohols	Sorbitol	15–30 mL once or twice daily	Sorbitol is commonly used as a sweetener in sugar-free products. In older adults, sorbitol has an effect similar to lactulose but costs less.
	Mannitol	15–30 mL once or twice daily	Rarely used as a laxative.
Polyethylene glycol	Polyethylene glycol electrolyte	17–34 g once or twice daily	Tends to cause less bloating and cramps than other agents; tasteless and odorless, it can be mixed with noncarbonated beverages. Typically used to prepare the colon for diagnostic examinations and surgery; also available as a powder without electrolytes for regular use.
Stimulant Laxatives			
Anthraquinones	Cascara sagrada Senna	325 mg (or 5 mL) at bedtime One to two 7.5-mg tablets daily	Cause apoptosis of colonic epithelial cells that are phagocytosed by macrophages; result in a lipofuscin-like pigmented condition known as *pseudomelanosis coli*; no definitive association has been established between anthraquinones and colon cancer or myenteric nerve damage (cathartic colon).
Ricinoleic acid	Castor oil	15–30 mL at bedtime	Cramping is common.
Diphenylmethane derivatives	Bisacodyl Phenolphthalein	5–10 mg at bedtime 30–200 mg at bedtime	Has effects in the small intestine and colon. Removed from the United States and other markets because of teratogenicity in animals.
	Sodium picosulfate	5–15 mg at bedtime	Likely has effects only on the colon. Although widely used in Europe, it is only available in the United States as part of a colonoscopy preparation.
Stool Softener	Docusate sodium	100 mg twice daily	Efficacy in constipation is not well established.
Emollient	Mineral oil	5–15 mL at bedtime	Long-term use can cause malabsorption of fat-soluble vitamins, anal seepage, and lipoid pneumonia in patients predisposed to aspiration of liquids.
Enemas, Suppositories	Phosphate enema Mineral oil retention enema Tap water enema Soapsuds enema Glycerin suppository Bisacodyl suppository	120 mL 100 mL 500 mL 1500 mL 60 g 10 mg	Serious damage to rectal mucosa can result from extravasation of the enema solution into the submucosa. Hypertonic phosphate enemas and large-volume water or soapsuds enemas can lead to hyperphosphatemia and other electrolyte abnormalities if the enema is retained. Soapsuds enemas can cause colitis. Prescribed on an as-needed basis.
Chloride Channel Activator	Lubiprostone	8–24 μg twice daily	Increases secretion in the intestine. Its mechanism of action is presumed to be via the chloride 2 channel.
Guanylate Cyclase C (GC-C) Agonists	Linaclotide	72–145 μg once daily	Increase secretion in the intestine through cyclic guanosine monophosphate. Also approved at a dose of 290 ug for IBS with constipation.
	Plecanatide	3 mg once daily	pH-dependent GC-C agonist. May cause less diarrhea requiring discontinuation.
5-HT_4 Agonist	Prucalopride	1–2 mg once daily	Increases propulsion through the bowel by stimulation of 5-hydroxytryptamine$_4$ receptors.
Sodium-Hydrogen	Tenapanor	50 μg twice daily	Inhibitor of sodium absorption in the small intestine.
Exchanger 3 Inhibitor	Colon resulting in increased fluid secretion and accelerated		Intestinal transit, approved for IBS with constipation.

TABLE 20.4 Summary of the Results of the ACG Monograph on Interventions for Chronic Idiopathic Constipation

Statement	No. of Trials	No. of Patients	RR of Symptoms (95% CI)	NNT (95% CI)	Recommendation	Quality of Evidence
Some fiber supplements increase stool frequency in patients with chronic idiopathic constipation (CIC)	3	293	0.25 (0.16–0.37)	2 (1.6–3)	Strong	Low
PEG is effective in increasing stool frequency and improving stool consistency in CIC	4	573	0.52 (0.41–0.65)	3 (2–4)	Strong	High
Lactulose is effective in increasing stool frequency and improving stool consistency in CIC	2	148	0.48 (0.27–0.86)	4 (2–7)	Strong	Low
Sodium picosulfate and bisacodyl are effective in CIC	2	735	0.54 (0.42–0.69)	3 (2–3.5)	Strong	Moderate
Prucalopride is more effective than placebo at improving symptoms of CIC	8	3140	0.81 (0.75–0.86)	5 (4–8)	Strong	Moderate
Linaclotide is effective in CIC	3	1582	0.84 (0.80–0.87)	6 (5–8)	Strong	High
Lubiprostone is effective in the treatment of CIC	4	651	0.67 (0.58–0.77)	4 (3–6)	Strong	High
Biofeedback is effective in patients with CIC and demonstrated evidence of pelvic floor dyssynergia	3	216	0.33 (0.22–0.50)	2 (1.6–4)	Weak	Low

CI, Confidence interval; *NNT*, number needed to treat; *PEG*, polyethylene glycol; *RR*, relative risk.
From Ford AC, Moayyedi P, Lacy BE, et al. American College of Gastroenterology monograph on the management of irritable bowel syndrome and chronic idiopathic constipation. *Am J Gastroenterol*. 2014;109(S1):S2–26.

In post hoc analyses using the US Food and Drug Administration (FDA) endpoint for chronic idiopathic constipation (i.e., ≥3 CSBM/week and an increase of ≥1 CSBM/week from baseline for ≥9/12 weeks, including 3 of the last 4 weeks), a greater percentage of patients receiving PEG-3350 compared with those receiving placebo met this endpoint (42% vs. 13%). In another trial in which 70 ambulatory outpatients were treated for 4 weeks with a 14.6 g PEG-electrolyte solution twice daily, patients who responded to PEG (less than 3 bowel movements per week) at the end of the 4 weeks were then randomized to continue PEG or a placebo for 20 weeks at a dose of 17 g or 34 g daily. Compared with placebo, PEG resulted in improvement in bowel frequency and consistency. At the end of follow-up, the complete remission of constipation was reported by 77% of patients randomized to PEG compared with only 20% of those randomized to placebo. The dropout rate in the placebo group, mostly secondary to treatment failure, was 46%.[313]

Another randomized multicenter trial compared standard and maximum doses of 2 PEG formulations of different molecular weights (PEG-3350 and PEG-4000) in 266 outpatients; most patients had their first stool within 1 day of initiating PEG treatment, and stool consistency improved in both treatment groups. The lowest dose of PEG produced the most normal stool consistency, whereas higher doses produced more liquid stools.[314] Low-dose PEG appears to be more effective than lactulose in the treatment of chronic constipation[315] and seems to be noninferior to prucalopride (a 5-HT_4 receptor agonist, see later) with better tolerability.[316]

PEG solutions may be useful for short-term treatment of fecal impaction. In one study,[317] 16 severely ill patients aged 26–87 years who, despite treatment with various laxatives, had not had a bowel movement in the hospital for 5–23 days; all had a fecal impaction on clinical examination and were treated with a PEG solution, 1 L taken as 2 portions of 500 mL, each over 4–6 hours. The regimen was repeated on a second and third day if necessary. The full dose was taken by 12 patients on the first day, and the remainder took at least half the recommended dose; only 8 patients needed treatment on the second day and 2 patients on the third day. The treatment was highly effective; after the last dose, most patients were passing moderate or large volumes of soft stool, with resolution of impaction. No adverse side effects apart from abdominal rumbling occurred, and only one patient, who was paraplegic, experienced fecal incontinence. Successful treatment with PEG has been described in outpatients with refractory constipation and older adults (with administration of PEG by mouth or by a nasogastric tube).[318]

The most common adverse events of PEG include abdominal bloating and cramps.[311] The most commonly reported adverse effects of PEG used for colonoscopy preparation include electrolyte imbalances, allergic reactions, and Mallory-Weiss tears.[319] Cases of fulminant pulmonary edema have been reported after administration of PEG solution by nasogastric tube, with one fatality.[320,321] In each case, the patient had emesis, suggesting aspiration of PEG. PEG also may delay gastric emptying.[322]

Stimulant Laxatives. Stimulant laxatives are often used when patients have no response to osmotic laxatives. Stimulant laxatives increase intestinal motility, water and electrolyte secretion into the lumen, prostaglandin secretion,[323] and accelerate colon transit.[1,324] They begin working within hours and are often associated with abdominal cramps. Stimulant laxatives include anthraquinones (e.g., cascara, aloe, and senna) and diphenylmethanes (e.g., bisacodyl, sodium picosulfate, and phenolphthalein). Castor oil is used less commonly because of its side effect profile. The effect of stimulant laxatives is dose dependent. Low doses prevent absorption of water and sodium, whereas high doses stimulate secretion of sodium, followed by water, into the colonic lumen.

Stimulant laxatives are sometimes abused, especially in patients with an eating disorder (see Chapter 10),[325] even though at high doses they have only a modest effect on calorie absorption. Although a cathartic colon (i.e., a colon with reduced motility) has been attributed to prolonged use of stimulant laxatives, no animal or human data support this effect. Rather, cathartic colon, as seen on a barium enema examination, is probably a primary motility disorder.

Stimulant laxatives can produce normal, soft, formed stools in some patients but are often associated with abdominal cramps and diarrhea even in standard doses. They act rapidly and are particularly suitable for use in a single dose for temporary constipation. Most clinicians are cautious about recommending daily dosing of stimulant laxatives indefinitely for chronic constipation. Stimulant laxatives vary widely in clinical effectiveness, and some patients with severe constipation are not helped by them.

Anthraquinones

Anthraquinones (e.g., cascara, senna, aloe, and frangula) are produced by a variety of plants. The compounds are inactive glycosides. When ingested, they pass unabsorbed and unchanged through the small intestine and are hydrolyzed by colonic bacterial glycosidases to yield active metabolites that increase the transport of electrolytes into the colonic lumen and stimulate myenteric plexuses to increase intestinal motility. The anthraquinones typically induce defecation 6–8 hours after oral dosing.

Anthraquinones cause apoptosis of colonic epithelial cells, which are then phagocytosed by macrophages and appear as a lipofuscin-like pigment that darkens the colonic mucosa, a condition termed *pseudomelanosis coli* (see Chapter 130).[326] Anthraquinone laxatives do not appear to cause significant adverse functional or structural changes in the intestine. Animal studies have shown neither damage to the myenteric plexus after long-term administration of sennosides[327] nor a functional defect in motility.[328] A case-control study in which multiple colonic mucosal biopsy specimens were examined by electron microscopy showed no differences in the submucosal plexuses between patients taking an anthraquinone laxative regularly for 1 year and those not taking one.[329] An association between use of anthraquinones and colon cancer or myenteric nerve damage and the development of so-called cathartic colon has not been established.[330]

Senna has been shown in controlled trials to soften stools[331] and increase the frequency and weight, both wet and dry, of stool. The formulations available for clinical use vary from crude vegetable preparations to purified and standardized extracts to a synthetic compound. As discussed above, senna (0.5 g twice a day) has been shown to improve constipation-related symptoms though the dose used in this study is higher than typically used in clinical practice.

Castor Oil

Castor oil is obtained from the castor bean. After oral ingestion, it is hydrolyzed by lipase in the small intestine to ricinoleic acid, which inhibits intestinal water absorption and stimulates intestinal motor function by damaging mucosal cells and releasing neurotransmitters.[332] Cramping is frequent, and consequently castor oil is not commonly used in clinical practice.

Diphenylmethane Derivatives

Diphenylmethane compounds include bisacodyl, sodium picosulfate, and phenolphthalein. After oral ingestion, bisacodyl and sodium picosulfate are hydrolyzed to the same active metabolite, but the mode of hydrolysis differs. Bisacodyl is hydrolyzed by intestinal enzymes and thus can act in the small and large intestines. Sodium picosulfate is hydrolyzed by colonic bacteria. Like anthraquinones, the action of sodium picosulfate is confined to the colon, and its activity can be unpredictable because its activation depends on the bacterial flora.

The effects of bisacodyl, and presumably sodium picosulfate, on the colon are similar to those of the anthraquinone laxatives. When applied to the colonic mucosa, bisacodyl induces an almost immediate, powerful, propulsive motor activity in healthy and constipated subjects, although the effect is sometimes reduced in the latter.[333] These laxatives also stimulate colonic secretion.

Like the anthraquinone laxatives, bisacodyl leads to apoptosis of colonic epithelial cells, the remnants of which accumulate in phagocytic macrophages, but these cellular remnants are not pigmented.[334] Aside from these changes, bisacodyl does not appear to cause adverse effects with long-term use.[335]

Bisacodyl is a useful and predictable laxative, especially suitable for single-dose use in patients with temporary constipation. Its possible effect on the small bowel is a disadvantage, in contrast to anthraquinones and sodium picosulfate. Long-term use of bisacodyl or related agents is sometimes necessary for patients with chronic severe constipation. In the doses used, liquid stools and cramps tend to result, which is difficult to adjust the dose to produce soft, formed stools. In a multicenter randomized double-blind, placebo-controlled study, 247 patients with chronic constipation were randomized to bisacodyl 10 mg once daily for 4 weeks. Patients in the bisacodyl group reported a greater number of CSBM per week during the treatment period compared with those in the placebo group (1.1 ± 0.1 at baseline in both groups increased to 5.2 ±0.1 in the bisacodyl group and 1.9 ± X.Y in the placebo group). Those who received bisacodyl reported improvements in straining, feeling of anal obstruction, and stool form and had increased quality-of-life scores compared with those who received placebo. However, 72% of patients in the bisacodyl group reported at least one adverse event (diarrhea and abdominal pain most commonly), with a decrease in frequency after the first week of treatment. In addition, despite being able to reduce the dose of bisacodyl from 10 to 5 mg a day, adverse events caused 18% of patients in the bisacodyl group to withdraw from the study, compared with 5% of those in the placebo group.[336]

Sodium picosulfate is commonly used outside the United States. It is available in the United States as part of a colonoscopy preparation. In a randomized, double-blind, placebo-controlled study conducted in Germany, 233 patients with chronic constipation were randomized to sodium picosulfate (10-mg drops) or placebo once daily for 4 weeks. Patients in the sodium picosulfate group reported a greater number of CSBM per week during the treatment period compared with those in the placebo group (0.9 ± 0.1 at baseline increased to 3.4 ± 0.2 in the sodium picosulfate group and 1.1 ± 0.1 at baseline increased to 1.7 ± 0.1 in the placebo group). Patients who received sodium picosulfate reported improvement in straining, incomplete evacuation, a feeling of anal obstruction, and improvement in stool form and had increased quality-of-life scores compared with those who received placebo. Diarrhea was reported by 32% of patients who received the sodium picosulfate.[337]

A systematic review and meta-analysis of pharmacotherapies for chronic constipation showed that bisacodyl and sodium picosulfate met the primary endpoints of responder analysis with greater than or equal to 3 CSBM per week and an increase over baseline of greater than or equal to 1 CSBM per week.[338] However, bisacodyl may be superior to other prescription drugs in secondary endpoints, including an increase from baseline in the number of spontaneous bowel movements (SBM) per week and in the number of CSBM per week. Although a network meta-analysis found bisacodyl and sodium picosulfate to rank first at 4 weeks to achieve >3 CSBM/week, bisacodyl ranked last for adverse events (abdominal pain and diarrhea).[339]

Phenolphthalein inhibits water absorption in the small intestine and colon by effects on eicosanoids and the Na^+/K^+-ATPase pump present on the surface of enterocytes (see Chapter 103). The drug undergoes enterohepatic circulation (see Chapter 66), which may prolong its effects. Although effective, a 2-year feeding study in rodents found increased incidences of ovarian, adrenal gland, renal, and hematopoietic neoplasms in treated animals,[340] and in 1997 the FDA proposed that phenolphthalein be reclassified as "not generally recognized as safe and effective." Since then, most phenolphthalein-containing laxatives have been voluntarily withdrawn from the US and other markets. Subsequent studies have failed to show an association between phenolphthalein laxatives and cancers.[341]

Stool Softeners and Emollients

Docusate Sodium. Although the detergent dioctyl sodium sulfosuccinate (docusate sodium) is available as a stool softener, further studies of its efficacy are needed. The compound stimulates fluid secretion by the small and large intestines but does not increase the volume of ileostomy output or the weight of stools in normal subjects.[342,343] A double-blind cross-over trial showed benefit in 5 of 15 older constipated subjects, as judged by patients and their caregivers, and a significant increase in bowel frequency.[344] In a multicenter, double-blind randomized trial in adults, however, docusate sodium was less effective than psyllium for treating chronic idiopathic constipation.[345]

Mineral Oils. Mineral oils alter the stool by undergoing emulsification into the stool mass and providing lubrication for stool passage. Because long-term use can cause intestinal malabsorption of fat-soluble vitamins, anal seepage, and lipoid pneumonia in patients predisposed to aspiration of liquids, they are rarely used.

Enemas and Suppositories

Compounds may be introduced into the rectum to stimulate contraction by distention or chemical action, soften hard stools, or both. Serious damage to the rectal mucosa can result from extravasation of the enema solution into the submucosal plane. The anterior rectal mucosa is the site most vulnerable to trauma from the tip of a catheter introduced through the backward-angulated anal canal (see Chapter 131). The enema nozzle should be directed posteriorly after the anal canal has been passed.

Phosphate Enemas. Hypertonic sodium phosphate enemas cause distention and stimulation of the rectum. A histologic study in normal subjects showed that a single hypertonic phosphate enema caused disruption of the surface epithelium in 17 of 21 biopsy specimens. Scanning electron microscopy showed patchy denudation of the surface epithelium, with exposure of the lamina propria and the absence of goblet cells. The proctoscopic appearance of the mucosa was abnormal in every case but returned to normal within 1 week.[346] Therefore superficially damaged mucosa appears to heal rapidly. Phosphate enemas are used widely, although studies documenting their efficacy are lacking.

A phosphate enema, if given to a patient who cannot evacuate it promptly, can lead to dangerous hyperphosphatemia and hypocalcemic tetany; one patient (age 91 years) died after a single phosphate enema,[347] and coma developed in an adult who was given six phosphate enemas at hourly intervals without evacuation.[348] Severe hyperphosphatemia, hypocalcemia, and seizure have been reported in a 4-year-old child with normal renal function after retention of two phosphate enemas.[349] Phosphate enemas are *not* recommended in children age 3 and younger.[350,351]

Saline, Tap Water, and Soapsuds Enemas. Saline, tap water, or soapsuds enemas can be effective mainly by distending the rectum and softening feces. Stool evacuation typically occurs 2–5 minutes following administration. A saline enema does no damage to the rectal mucosa and may be effective.[346] Water enemas and soapsuds enemas also may be used, but with large volumes, dangerous water intoxication can occur if the enema is retained. Large-volume water or soapsuds enemas can also lead to hyperphosphatemia and other electrolyte disturbances if the enema is retained. Soapsuds enemas can cause rectal mucosal damage and necrosis.

Stimulant Suppositories and Enemas. Glycerin can be administered as a suppository and is often clinically effective. The rectum is stimulated by an osmotic effect. The effect of glycerin, if any, on the rectal mucosa is unknown. Bisacodyl 10 mg is available as a suppository that appears to act topically by stimulating enteric neurons.[335] In normal subjects, a single-bisacodyl suppository or an enema containing 19 mg of bisacodyl in 100 or 200 mL of water produced marked changes in 23 of 25 rectal mucosal biopsy specimens. The epithelium of the surface and within the crypts was altered; with the use of the enema, the surface epithelium was absent.[346] Regular use of bisacodyl suppositories, therefore, appears unwise. Oxyphenisatin (Veripaque), which is no longer available in the United States, is a stimulant enema that was used in the past mainly before diagnostic procedures. When given by mouth, this compound led to cases of chronic hepatitis.

Prosecretory Laxatives

Chloride Type-2 Channel Activator

Lubiprostone is a bicyclic fatty acid derived from prostaglandin E_1 that is reported to work predominantly by activating the intestinal chloride two channels at the level of the intestinal epithelial cell, thereby increasing chloride secretion in the lumen, followed by sodium and water, thereby causing intestinal fluid secretion and acceleration of transit[352] without altering serum electrolyte levels. Lubiprostone was approved for the treatment of chronic idiopathic constipation for men and women in the United States in 2006. In 24-week phase 3 randomized placebo-controlled trials, lubiprostone (24 μg twice daily) increased the number of SBM (i.e., bowel movements that occur without laxative use in the previous 24 hours) in patients with chronic constipation as defined by the Rome II criteria (5.89 at week 1 in lubiprostone-treated patients vs. 3.99 at week 1 in placebo-treated patients).[353] Lubiprostone also significantly decreased straining, improved stool consistency, and reduced the overall severity of symptoms while increasing the frequency of SBM in both men and women, as well as older patients. A rebound effect after withdrawal was not evident.[354] Nausea was the most common adverse event reported, occurring in up to 31.7% of patients and leading to discontinuation in 5%.[348] Lubiprostone is also approved in the United States for the treatment of opioid-induced constipation as well as for women with IBS with constipation at a dose of 8 μg twice daily.

Guanylate Cyclase C Agonists

Linaclotide

Linaclotide is a minimally absorbed 14-amino acid peptide that activates the guanylate cyclase C receptor on the luminal surface of the intestinal epithelium, resulting in increased levels of cyclic guanosine monophosphate and increased secretion of chloride and bicarbonate into the intestinal lumen. In animal models, cyclic guanosine monophosphate also appears to reduce firing of afferent nerves in the bowel.[355] In 2 phase 3 studies involving 1276 patients with chronic constipation, linaclotide significantly increased the percentage of people who reported 3 or more CSBM (i.e., associated with the sensation of complete emptying) per week and an increase of one or more from baseline during at least 9 of the 12 weeks (20% of patients who received linaclotide 145 or 290 μg, compared with 5% of patients who received placebo). Linaclotide also increased stool frequency, improved stool consistency, and reduced straining, abdominal bloating, and discomfort as compared with placebo. Diarrhea was the most common adverse event, leading to discontinuation of treatment in about 4% of patients.[356] Linaclotide also has been shown to improve bowel and abdominal symptoms in patients with chronic constipation with moderate-to-severe abdominal bloating.[357] Linaclotide, 145 μg once daily and subsequently 72 mg daily, was approved by the FDA in 2012 for the treatment of men and women with chronic constipation and in a dose of 290 μg once daily for those with IBS with constipation. Linaclotide is contraindicated in children younger than 2 years of age due to the risk of serious dehydration. The safety and efficacy of linaclotide in children less than 18 years has not been established; however, there does not appear to be age-dependent trend in GC-C intestinal expression in children 2–18 years of age.

Plecanatide

Plecanatide is a guanylate cyclase C agonist mechanistically similar to linaclotide. In contrast to linaclotide, plecanatide is pH-sensitive with a higher affinity to the GC-C in the acidic environment of the proximal duodenum. Two phase 3 trials with plecanatide once daily for 12 weeks showed an increase in the overall percentage of CSBM responders (>3 CSBM/week and >1 CSBM over baseline for 9 out of 12 weeks and 3 of the last 4 weeks of the trial) in patients with chronic constipation.[358] At a dose of 3 and 6 mg, 19.5%–20.1% and 20.0%–21.0% of patients were responders compared with 10.2%–12.8% in patients who received placebo. Plecanatide also significantly improved stool consistency and stool frequency. Diarrhea was reported in 5.1% of patients and led to discontinuation in 2.7%.[359] Plecanatide, 3 mg once daily, was approved by the FDA in 2017 for the treatment of chronic constipation and IBS with constipation.

Tenapanor

Tenapanor, the first sodium-hydrogen exchanger three inhibitor, was approved by the FDA in 2019 for the treatment of IBS with constipation in a dose of 50 mg twice daily. It inhibits sodium absorption in the small intestine and colon and thereby results in an increase of intestinal fluid secretion and accelerates intestinal transit. In a phase 3 trial in patients with IBS with constipation, a greater percentage of patients receiving tenapanor were CSBM responders, defined as an increase of ≥1 CSBM/week from baseline for ≥9 of 12 treatment weeks, including ≥3 of the final 4 weeks, compared to patients receiving placebo (16.0% vs. 4.7%, respectively).[360] Tenapanor has not been studied in patients specifically with chronic constipation.

Serotonergic Laxatives. Stimulation of the 5-HT_4 receptor on afferent nerves in the wall of the GI tract induces peristaltic contraction of the intestine. Several 5-HT_4 agonists have been tested for treating constipation. Cisapride, a benzodiazepine, has had variable results in treating constipation.[361] Potentially lethal cardiac dysrhythmias led to its withdrawal from the commercial US market in July 2000. Tegaserod was removed from the US market in 2007 due to cardiovascular concerns; however, it was recently reapproved by the FDA for women with IBS-C under the age of 65 without a history of myocardial infarction, stroke, transient ischemic attack, or angina. Tegaserod is discussed because of the extensive previous experience in the treatment of constipation. Prucalopride is a newer full 5-HT_4 agonist without cardiac effects that was FDA approved for chronic constipation in 2018.

Tegaserod

Tegaserod, a partial 5-HT_4 agonist, is an aminoguanidine indole derivative of serotonin that is structurally different from cisapride. Because of cardiovascular safety concerns, tegaserod was withdrawn from the market in April 2007 due to cardiovascular concerns. Specifically, the frequency of cardiovascular events in previous clinical trials was 13 in 13,614 (0.11%) in patients receiving tegaserod compared with 1 in 7031 (0.01%) in patients receiving placebo. The cardiovascular events reported were myocardial infarction ($n = 3$), sudden cardiac death ($n = 1$), unstable angina ($n = 6$), and stroke ($n = 3$). The FDA's decision to withdraw the drug has been the subject of debate.[362] Prior to its withdrawal, tegaserod was approved for use in chronic constipation and IBS-C. In a 12-week randomized double-blind, placebo-controlled trial of 1348 subjects with chronic constipation, response rates were 41.4%, 43.2%, and 25.1% for tegaserod 2 mg twice daily, tegaserod 6 mg twice daily, and placebo, respectively.[363] Diarrhea was more common with tegaserod 2 and 6 mg twice daily (4.5% and 7.3%, respectively) than with placebo (3.8%).[363] Tegaserod was reapproved in 2019 only for women with IBS-C (see Chapter 124) under the age of 65 without cardiovascular risk factors at a dose of 6 mg twice daily.[364(p5)]

Prucalopride

Prucalopride, a full 5-HT_4 agonist, is a benzofuran derivative that accelerates colonic transit in healthy humans and patients with chronic constipation.[365] Three large 12-week randomized placebo-controlled phase 3 trials of similar design that evaluated the efficacy and safety of prucalopride 2 or 4 mg once daily versus placebo in patients with chronic constipation have been published.[366–368] In one of these studies, the percentage of patients achieving more than 3 CSBM/week was 30.9% for those receiving prucalopride 2 mg and 28.4% for those receiving prucalopride 4 mg, compared with 12.0% in those receiving placebo ($P < .001$ for both comparisons). All other secondary efficacy endpoints, including patients' satisfaction with their bowel function and treatment and their perception of the severity of their symptoms of constipation, were improved significantly at week 12 with the use of 2 or 4 mg of prucalopride as compared with placebo. A meta-analysis of 7 randomized controlled trials of 2639 constipated patients found the number needed to treat to be 6; the percentage of patients who responded to prucalopride was 28.3%, compared with 13.3% for placebo.[369] The most frequent adverse effects were headaches, nausea, and diarrhea. Although cardiac side effects had been reported in patients who received tegaserod and cisapride, which are both partial 5-HT_4 agonists, no cardiovascular side effects have been observed to date with prucalopride, nor have any electrocardiographic abnormalities been reported. In addition, in a study of elderly constipated patients in nursing homes, no differences in vital signs, electrocardiograph parameters, or Holter-monitoring results were found in patients receiving prucalopride and placebo. Approximately 88% of the patients had a history of cardiovascular disease.[370] Prucalopride was approved by the FDA for chronic constipation in 2018 and is also available in the European Union, Canada, and elsewhere.

Ileal Bile Acid Transporter Inhibitor

Elobixibat is a novel, minimally absorbed ileal bile acid–transporter inhibitor that increases the flow of bile into the colon (see Chapter 66) that was approved in Japan in 2018 for the treatment of chronic constipation. In a phase 2 study, 190 patients with chronic constipation (defined using modified Rome III criteria) were randomized to elobixibat (5, 10, or 15 mg) or placebo once daily for 8 weeks. Elobixibat increased stool frequency for week 1 by 2.5, 4.0, and 5.4 SBM in patients who received 5, 10, and 15 mg of elobixibat, respectively, compared with 1.7 for those who received placebo; the improvement was maintained over 8 weeks. Abdominal bloating and straining were also improved with elobixibat compared with placebo. The most commonly reported adverse events were abdominal pain and diarrhea.[371]

In a phase 3 trial involving 132 Japanese patients with chronic constipation, they were randomized to elobixibat 10 mg once a day or placebo for 2 weeks. Patients receiving elobixibat had a greater increase in the number of SBMs/week compared with those receiving placebo (week 1: 6.4 vs. 1.7, respectively; week 2: 5.0 vs. 1.8, respectively). The most common adverse events reported with elobixibat and placebo were diarrhea (13% vs. 0%, respectively) and mild abdominal pain (19% vs. 2%, respectively).[372]

Other Agents

Colchicine, a drug used for gout, and misoprostol, a prostaglandin analog, have been used to treat patients with severe chronic constipation. In a randomized placebo-controlled, double-blind cross-over trial, colchicine increased the frequency of bowel movements as compared with placebo (3/week at baseline compared with 10/week while on colchicine 0.6 mg three times a day); however, abdominal pain was greater during administration of colchicine than placebo.[373] Data for misoprostol are limited, and side effects of the drug are common.[374]

Cholinergic Agents. Cholinergic agents have also been used to treat constipation. Bethanechol, a cholinergic agonist, appears to benefit patients in whom constipation results from therapy with tricyclic antidepressants; data to support its use in patients with other causes of constipation are limited. A single intravenous dose of neostigmine, a cholinesterase inhibitor, has been shown to be remarkably effective in decompressing the colon in patients with acute colonic pseudoobstruction[375] (see Chapter 126), but controlled studies of this class of drugs have not been completed in patients with normal-transit or slow-transit constipation. A study of neostigmine administered subcutaneously to patients with postoperative ileus, acute colonic pseudoobstruction, or refractory constipation showed that the median time for a bowel movement in patients with refractory constipation (n = 10) was 39.23 hours (interquartile range, 19.95–57.56). The majority of patients (>75%) needed a repeat dosing, with nearly half of the cohort requiring 5 or more doses before a bowel movement was produced.[376] Side effects, such as bradycardia, increased salivation, vomiting, and abdominal cramping, are common.

Oral cholinergic agents, such as pyridostigmine, have been shown to accelerate colonic transit in diabetic patients with chronic constipation in a dose of 360 mg daily in the majority of the patients or 180 mg daily in a subset of patients. Compared with placebo, pyridostigmine accelerated overall colonic transit at 24 hours (1.96 ± 0.18 (baseline), 2.45 ± 0.2 units (treatment), P < .01), but not gastric emptying or small-intestinal transit. Stool frequency, consistency, and ease of passage also improved. Cholinergic side effects were somewhat more common with pyridostigmine than with placebo.[377]

In a study of 31 patients with systemic sclerosis treated with pyridostigmine for at least 4 weeks, 51.6% reported improvement in constipation. Fifteen of 31 patients reported adverse effects, most commonly diarrhea. Pyridostigmine was continued by 81.3% of patients who reported symptomatic benefit and 58.1% of patients overall.[378]

Botulinum Toxin. *Clostridium botulinum* toxin type A (Botox), a potent neurotoxin that inhibits presynaptic release of acetylcholine, has been injected intramuscularly into the puborectalis muscle to treat defecatory disorders. Preliminary data suggest that botulinum toxin may be effective for patients in whom spastic pelvic floor dysfunction causes outlet delay,[379] including those who also have PD.[176,177] In one study, 19 of 24 patients experienced improvement in symptoms and physiologic measurements of pelvic floor function at 2 months.[380] Controlled trials have not been performed, however, and this approach is not recommended in lieu of biofeedback, for which clinical experience is greater (see later).

Vibrating Capsule

An orally ingested, nonpharmacological, vibrating capsule that mechanically stimulates the bowel wall, increasing circadian rhythm of colon activity, received FDA clearance as a medical device in 2022.[381] An 8-week, phase 3 trial, including 312 patients with chronic constipation, was randomized to the vibrating capsule (2 separate vibration cycles over 1 day period; each cycle lasted 2 hours, and vibration comprised 3 seconds of stimulation followed by 16 seconds rest [3 seconds/minute]). A greater percentage of patients receiving the vibrating capsule compared with placebo achieved an increase of ≥1 or 2 CSBM/week for ≥6 of the 8 weeks (≥1 CSBM/week: 39.3% vs. 22.1%, respectively; ≥2 CSBM: 22.7% vs. 11.4%, respectively). In addition, straining, stool consistency, and quality-of-life measures also improved with the vibrating capsule compared to placebo. Adverse events were mild; a mild vibrating sensation was reported by 11% of patients in the vibrating capsule group, but none withdrew from the trial. Another vibrating capsule using different stimulation paradigms is being studied and has reported improvement in constipation in a smaller number of Chinese patients.[382]

Future Agents

Chenodeoxycholate

Chenodeoxycholic acid is a bile acid previously used to treat patients with gallstones (see Chapter 68). Diarrhea was reported in 40% of patients receiving 750–1000 mg/day.[383] A double-blind placebo-controlled study of 36 female patients with IBS with constipation was randomized to delayed-release sodium chenodeoxycholate (500 or 1000 mg) or placebo for 4 days. Colonic transit time, stool consistency, and stool frequency were improved in both chenodeoxycholate groups, compared with placebo. The most common side effect was abdominal cramping or pain.[384] Studies in patients with chronic constipation have not been performed.

Relamorelin

Relamorelin is a pentapeptide selective agonist of ghrelin receptor 1a that is known to have gastric effects. In a randomized, double-blind clinical trial of 48 female patients with chronic constipation, relamorelin accelerated colonic transit at 32 hours (P = .040) and 48 hours (P = .017), increased SBM, and accelerated the time to first bowel movement after the first dose compared with placebo. Relamorelin did not affect stool form. The most common side effects reported were increased appetite, fatigue, and headache.[385]

Velusetrag

Velusetrag is a full 5-HT_4 agonist. In a 4-week phase 2 trial, 401 patients with chronic constipation were randomized to receive velusetrag 15, 30, or 50 mg or placebo once daily. SBM increased by 3.6 (15 mg), 3.3 (30 mg), and 3.5 (50 mg)/week in the patients who received velusetrag compared with an increase of 1.4 per week for placebo.[386] Improvement with velusetrag had a relative risk of 4.86, with a wide 95% CI of 2.02–11.71, which suggests that the drug might be less efficacious when compared with prucalopride.[338]

Transabdominal Electrical Stimulation

Similar to sacral nerve stimulation, which involves neuromodulation of the sacral nerves (S2–S4), transcutaneous interferential therapy has recently been proposed as an alternative for neuromodulation, which uses two medium frequency currents that bisect intra-abdominally to produce the therapeutic low frequency current within the bowel. In a single-blind randomized sham-controlled pilot study involving 33 women who received the active treatment (6 weeks × 1 hour per day), they were more likely to report improvement in bowel function and reduced their use of laxatives compared to patients who received sham treatment 3 months after treatment.[387]

Other Forms of Therapy

Defecation Training

Defecation training typically involves three to five treatment sessions, each lasting at least 30 minutes. During these sessions, the normal defecation process is taught, and misconceptions are dispelled. Patients are encouraged to give a detailed description of their bowel symptoms, prompted by a sympathetic listener who is familiar with the full range of problems experienced by those with defecatory dysfunction. This process is in itself therapeutic because it enables patients to discuss symptoms that otherwise might be regarded as a private burden. Recommendations regarding the proper amount of fiber intake are often given. For patients with infrequent defecation, the importance of developing a regular bowel habit and not ignoring the urge to defecate is emphasized. For those who spend excessive time in the bathroom due to ineffective straining, a regimen of less frequent visits to the bathroom and more effective defecation is recommended. The optimal posture for defecation, including the benefit of raising the feet above floor level when using a Western-type toilet, is described. Following each visit, patients are encouraged to practice the techniques they are taught. At each visit, patients are encouraged to reduce any dependence on laxatives, enemas, and suppositories. Progress is praised.

Anorectal Biofeedback

During anorectal biofeedback, which typically follows defecation training, a patient receives visual or auditory feedback, or both, on the functioning of his or her anal sphincter and pelvic floor muscles. Biofeedback can be used to train patients to relax their pelvic floor muscles during straining and to coordinate this relaxation with abdominal maneuvers to enhance entry of stool into the rectum. Biofeedback can be performed with an EMG or anorectal manometry catheter. Simulated evacuation with a balloon or silicone-filled artificial stool is commonly taught to patients to emphasize normal coordination of successful defecation.[388] Patient education and rapport between the therapist and patient are integral components of successful biofeedback.[389] Patients typically complete from 6 sessions in 6 weeks to 3 sessions/day for 10 successive days.

A systematic review of biofeedback studies performed up to 1993 revealed an overall success rate of 67%, although controlled studies were lacking.[390] Biofeedback may be less effective for patients with descending perineum syndrome than for those with spastic pelvic floor disorders.[151] In a review of 38 biofeedback studies, psychological factors were found to influence the response to biofeedback.[391] Successful biofeedback training, as defined by an improvement in global bowel satisfaction, was also found to correlate with harder stool consistency, greater willingness to participate, higher resting anal pressure, and prolonged balloon expulsion time, but not with age, duration of symptoms, stool frequency, compliance with therapy, straining rectal pressure, or relaxation of the anal sphincter on straining.[392]

More recently, several controlled trials have found biofeedback to be more effective than sham feedback or standard therapy,[393,394] diazepam,[395] or laxatives.[396,397] Patients with pelvic floor dyssynergia who failed fiber (20 g/day) plus enemas or suppositories were randomized to 5 weekly biofeedback sessions (n = 54) or PEG (14.6–29.2 g/day) plus 5 weekly counseling sessions (n = 55). At 6 months, major improvement was reported by 80% of patients who underwent biofeedback compared with 22% of the laxative-treated patients ($P < .001$). The benefits of biofeedback were sustained at 12 and 24 months and produced greater reductions in straining, sensations of incomplete evacuation and anorectal blockage, use of enemas and suppositories, and abdominal pain (all $P < .01$). Stool frequency increased in both groups. All biofeedback-treated patients reporting major improvement were able to relax the pelvic floor and defecate a 50-mL balloon at 6 and 12 months.[396] In another controlled trial, 77 patients with dyssynergic defecation were randomized to biofeedback, sham therapy, or standard therapy for 3 months. Patients who received biofeedback were significantly more likely to correct dyssynergia, improve the defecation index, decrease balloon expulsion time, increase the number of CSBM per week, and decrease the use of digital maneuvers; global bowel satisfaction was also higher.[393] Thirteen patients from each group elected to participate in a long-term follow-up trial. The number of CSBM per week increased significantly in the biofeedback group after 1 year (1.91 at baseline compared with 4.85 after 1 year) but not in a standard-treatment control group (1.66 at baseline compared with 1.43 after 1 year). The 3-month improvement in dyssynergia, defecation index, and decreased balloon expulsion time in the biofeedback group was also maintained after 1 year, and colonic transit time normalized.[394(p)]

Originally, biofeedback training was intensive and initiated during an admission to the hospital,[398] but subsequent experience has shown that training as an outpatient is satisfactory. A small comparative trial has shown no difference in outcome with or without use of an intrarectal balloon or home training.[399] Results are similar when training is conducted with or without access to a visual display of muscular activity. In the absence of a visual display, the instructor gives continuous information and encouragement to the patient and assesses the effect of instruction by observing how the patient strains and by sensing the effectiveness of straining through gentle tension on a rectal balloon.

Most patients who complete defecation training continue to report improvement in symptoms up to 2 years later.[398,399] Symptoms reported to improve include bowel frequency, straining, abdominal pain, bloating, and the need for laxatives.[400] Physiologic measurements before and after treatment have shown that training results in appropriate relaxation of the puborectalis and external anal sphincter muscles,[401–403] an increase in intrarectal pressure,[132] a widened rectoanal angle on straining during defecation, an increased rate of rectal emptying, an increased rate of colonic transit, and increased rectal mucosal blood flow.

Most published series have restricted defecation training and anorectal biofeedback to patients with a defecatory disorder (i.e., paradoxical contraction of pelvic floor muscles). At one center, however, such training appeared to benefit a high proportion of unselected patients with chronic constipation, regardless of the results of investigation of colonic transit or pelvic floor dysfunction, including patients with slow colonic transit.[402,404] In another series, treatment results did not depend on the presence or absence of a rectocele, intussusception, or perineal descent.[400] Other investigators, however, have shown that patients who fail to respond to defecation training and biofeedback have a greater degree of perineal descent than those who respond.[151] Defecation training has benefited some patients in whom constipation developed after hysterectomy[405] and some patients with solitary rectal ulcer syndrome.[406]

Complementary and Alternative Medical Therapies

Many complementary and alternative therapies are used by patients with constipation,[407] but clinical studies are limited and generally of poor quality (see Chapter 132), and no definitive recommendations regarding their use in constipation can be made.

Acupuncture. A multicenter Chinese trial assessed the efficacy of electroacupuncture (28 sessions of EA over 8 weeks) compared with sham electroacupuncture (i.e., shallow needling at non-acupoints without electrical activity) in 1075 patients with severe chronic constipation. Patients receiving electroacupuncture had a mean weekly CSBM increase during week 1 that was significantly greater compared to patients receiving sham electroacupuncture (1.8 vs. 0.9, respectively).[408] Similar results were seen during the subsequent 11 weeks after completion of acupuncture. There were few acupuncture-related adverse events, and all were mild or transient.

Probiotics. The popularity of probiotics continues to grow, yet few studies have been conducted to date. One prospective study showed that in women with chronic constipation, *Bifidobacterium animalis* and fructooligosaccharide improved bowel frequency and consistency, straining, and pain with defecation ($P < .010$).[409]

Traditional Chinese Medicine. The role of traditional Chinese medicine in constipation remains unclear. Traditional Chinese medicine is a significant part of what is known as complementary and alternative medicine (CAM), which has been practiced for treating diseases and promoting the health of humans for thousands of years. A systematic review and meta-analysis of the herbal formula MaZiRenWan (Hemp Seed Pill) that included 17 trials, including 2 high-quality studies from East Asia, found evidence to support its improvement in CSBM and overall response in patients with chronic constipation.[410] However, in general, there is insufficient evidence to support any specific traditional Chinese medicines for chronic constipation.[411]

Sacral Nerve Stimulation

Data suggest that sacral nerve stimulation may be helpful for patients with severe constipation.[412] Sixty-two patients with chronic constipation who failed treatment with laxatives, suppositories, enemas, and biofeedback underwent a 21-day test period with a temporary stimulation wire connected to an external pulse generator. Successful treatment was defined as improvement in any of the following: (1) increase in bowel frequency from 2 or less to 3 or more bowel movements per week, (2) 50% or greater reduction in the proportion of defecation episodes associated with straining, or (3) 50% or greater reduction in the proportion of defecation episodes associated with a sense of incomplete evacuation. Forty-five patients met a criterion for successful treatment and had a permanent neurostimulator implanted. Of the patients who received a permanent neurostimulator, 87% met the criteria for successful treatment. During the follow-up period, which ranged from 1 to 55 months with a median of 28 months, the number of bowel movements per week increased from 2.3 to 6.6.[413] Although promising, the magnitude of the benefit and which patients are most likely to benefit from sacral nerve stimulation remain unclear.[414]

Surgery

The goal of surgical treatment for patients with severe constipation is to increase bowel frequency and ease of defecation; a possible additional benefit is relief of abdominal pain and distention. Surgery should only be considered a last resort and after medical treatments have failed. Physiological testing is critical for planning the appropriate surgical treatment.[415]

Surgical procedures may be divided into three groups: partial or total colectomy, construction of a stoma, and anorectal operations undertaken to improve defecatory function.[416]

Colectomy. Colectomy for constipation produces variable results. A review of 32 published studies of surgery for chronic constipation found considerable variability in the rates of patient satisfaction (39%–100%).[417] The most common complications following surgery are small bowel obstruction, diarrhea, and incontinence, but diarrhea and incontinence tend to improve after the first year following surgery.

Selection of Patients

Preoperative psychological assessment is essential because poor results are common among patients who are psychologically disturbed.[418] Because the aim of surgery is to increase bowel frequency, slow colonic transit must be demonstrated by an objective method. Also, defecatory function must be assessed. Finally, a generalized intestinal dysmotility or pseudoobstruction syndrome should be excluded (as much as possible) by radiologic study of the small intestine and, when available, studies of gastric emptying and small bowel transit.

Series in which these steps have been taken to select a homogeneous group of patients have shown the best results, although longer follow-up is awaited. At one center, only 74 of 1009 patients referred for possible surgical treatment of chronic constipation underwent surgery. Measurement of intestinal transit and tests of pelvic floor function revealed that 597 patients had no quantifiable abnormality and that 249 patients had pelvic floor dysfunction without slow colonic transit. Colectomy with an ileorectal anastomosis was performed in 52 patients with demonstrable slow colonic transit and normal defecatory function. The operation was also performed in 22 patients with slow colonic transit and pelvic floor dysfunction after the latter had been treated by a training program. Of the 74 patients treated surgically, 97% were satisfied with the result, and 90% had a good or improved quality of life after a mean follow-up of 56 months. There was no operative mortality, but seven patients had a subsequent episode of small bowel obstruction.[121]

Type of Operation

The results of colectomy with cecorectal or ileosigmoid anastomosis are inferior to those for a subtotal colectomy with an ileorectal anastomosis.[419] Occasional reports have described proctocolectomy with ileoanal anastomosis and construction of an ileal pouch, usually following failure of colectomy and ileorectal anastomosis.[420] In one patient, ileorectal anastomosis failed because the rectal capacity was larger than normal.[421] Laparoscopic subtotal colectomy appears to be as effective as an open approach.[422,423]

Construction of a Stoma. A colostomy is occasionally performed for slow-transit constipation, because it is reversible and the results of colectomy are uncertain. Most patients report subjective improvement after a colostomy performed as a primary procedure for slow-transit constipation or for neurologic disease.[417] Many patients, however, continue to require laxatives or regular colonic irrigation.

An ileostomy is occasionally performed after failure of colectomy and ileorectal anastomosis for slow-transit constipation, either because constipation persists or because severe diarrhea and incontinence occur. Patients who do not benefit from colectomy with ileorectal anastomosis are likely to be those with a generalized disorder of intestinal motility or those with a psychological disturbance.

Creation of a continent catheterizable appendicostomy or cecostomy through which antegrade enemas can be administered can sometimes benefit patients with paraplegia or those unable or unwilling to undergo colectomy. A retrospective study of 32 patients who underwent this procedure and were followed for a median of 36 months (range, 13–140 months) reported satisfactory long-term results in about half of the patients. Revisions were frequently required.[424] Such a procedure can decrease the time and medication needed for bowel care; most of the experience is in children.[425]

Operations for Defecatory Disorders. The stapled transanal rectal resection (STARR) procedure has been used with some success, particularly for patients who also have a rectocele and intussusception.[426–428] Puborectalis or internal anal sphincter muscle division is unsuccessful in patients with slow-transit constipation.[429] In a single center, retrospective review of 215 patients with symptomatic obstructive defecation (97%), feeling of vaginal prolapse/bulge (81%), and a rectocele of >4 cm, who underwent tissue transvaginal rectocele repair, it was found that in-hospital complication rate was 11.2%, with the most common complication being urinary retention (8.4%). The mean length of follow-up was 12.7 months (SD 13.9, range 1.4–71.5), with 87.9% of the cases reporting global improvement of symptoms, 80% reporting improvement in feeling of vaginal bulge, and 58% reporting improvement of obstructive defecation-related symptoms.[430] Procedures to correct a rectocele should be considered when conservative management has failed in patients with symptomatic rectocele >4 cm[430] and in those who have evidence of retained contrast during defecography or women in whom constipation is relieved with digital vaginal pressure.[148]

Full references for this chapter can be found at https://ebooks.health.elsevier.com.

21 Gastrointestinal Bleeding

Thomas J. Savides, Dennis M. Jensen

IN THIS CHAPTER

The annual rate of hospitalization for any type of GI hemorrhage in the United States is estimated to be 350 hospital admissions/100,000 population, with more than 1000,000 hospitalizations each year.[1] Approximately 50% of admissions for GI bleeding are for UGI bleeding (from the esophagus, stomach, and duodenum), 40% are for LGI bleeding (from the colon and anorectum), and 10% are for obscure bleeding (from the small intestine).

Severe GI bleeding is defined as documented GI bleeding (hematemesis, melena, hematochezia, or positive NG lavage) accompanied by shock or orthostatic hypotension, a decrease in the hematocrit value by at least 6% (or a decrease in the hemoglobin level of at least 2 g/dL), or transfusion of at least two units of packed red blood cells (RBCs). Most patients with severe GI bleeding are admitted to the hospital for resuscitation and treatment. Overt bleeding implies visible signs of blood loss from the GI tract. *Hematemesis* is defined as vomiting of blood, which is indicative of bleeding from the nasopharynx, esophagus, stomach, or duodenum. Hematemesis includes vomiting of bright red blood, which suggests recent or ongoing bleeding, and dark material (coffee-ground emesis), which suggests bleeding that stopped some time ago. *Melena* is defined as black tarry stool and results from the degradation of blood to hematin or other hemochromes by intestinal bacteria. Melena can signify bleeding that originates from a UGI, small bowel, or proximal colonic source and generally occurs when 50–100 mL or more of blood is delivered into the GI tract (usually the upper tract), with passage of characteristic stool occurring several hours after the bleeding event.[2,3] *Hematochezia* refers to bright red blood per rectum and suggests colonic or anorectal bleeding or active UGI or small bowel bleeding. *Occult GI bleeding* refers to subacute bleeding that is not clinically visible. *Obscure GI bleeding* is bleeding from a site that is not apparent after routine endoscopic evaluation with EGD (upper endoscopy), and colonoscopy, and possibly push enteroscopy. An algorithm for the initial management of severe acute UGI bleeding is shown in Fig. 21.1.

INITIAL ASSESSMENT AND MANAGEMENT OF ACUTE GASTROINTESTINAL BLEEDING

History

Initial assessment of the patient with acute GI bleeding includes taking a medical history, obtaining vital signs, performing a physical examination, including a rectal examination, and NG lavage. Patients should be questioned about risk factors such as medication that may cause ulcers or bleeding, prior GI surgeries, and historical features that help identify diagnostic possibilities for the bleeding source (Table 21.1).

Physical Examination

On initial evaluation, physical examination should focus on the patient's vital signs, with attention to signs of hypovolemia, such as hypotension, tachycardia, and orthostasis. The abdomen should be examined for surgical scars, tenderness, and masses. Signs of chronic liver disease include spider telangiectasias, palmar erythema, gynecomastia, ascites, splenomegaly, caput medusae, and Dupuytren contracture. The skin, lips, and buccal mucosa should be examined for telangiectasias, which are suggestive of HHT, or Osler-Weber-Rendu disease. Subungual telangiectasias and characteristic changes of the skin of the fingers may indicate scleroderma (systemic sclerosis), which is associated with GAVE or UGI telangiectasias. Pigmented lip lesions may suggest Peutz-Jeghers syndrome. Purpuric skin lesions may suggest Henoch-Schönlein purpura. Acanthosis nigricans may suggest underlying malignancy, especially gastric cancer. The patient's feces should be observed to identify melena or maroon and red stool; however, the subjective description of stool color varies greatly among patients and physicians.[4]

NG or orogastric tube placement to aspirate and visually characterize gastric contents can be useful for determining the presence or absence of large amounts of red blood, coffee-ground material, or nonbloody fluid; it is particularly useful in patients with melena in the absence of hematemesis. Occult blood testing of an NG tube aspirate is not useful, however, because trauma from the NG tube may induce sufficient, although scant, bleeding to cause a false-positive result. Patients who have coffee-ground emesis or fresh bloody emesis that is witnessed do not require

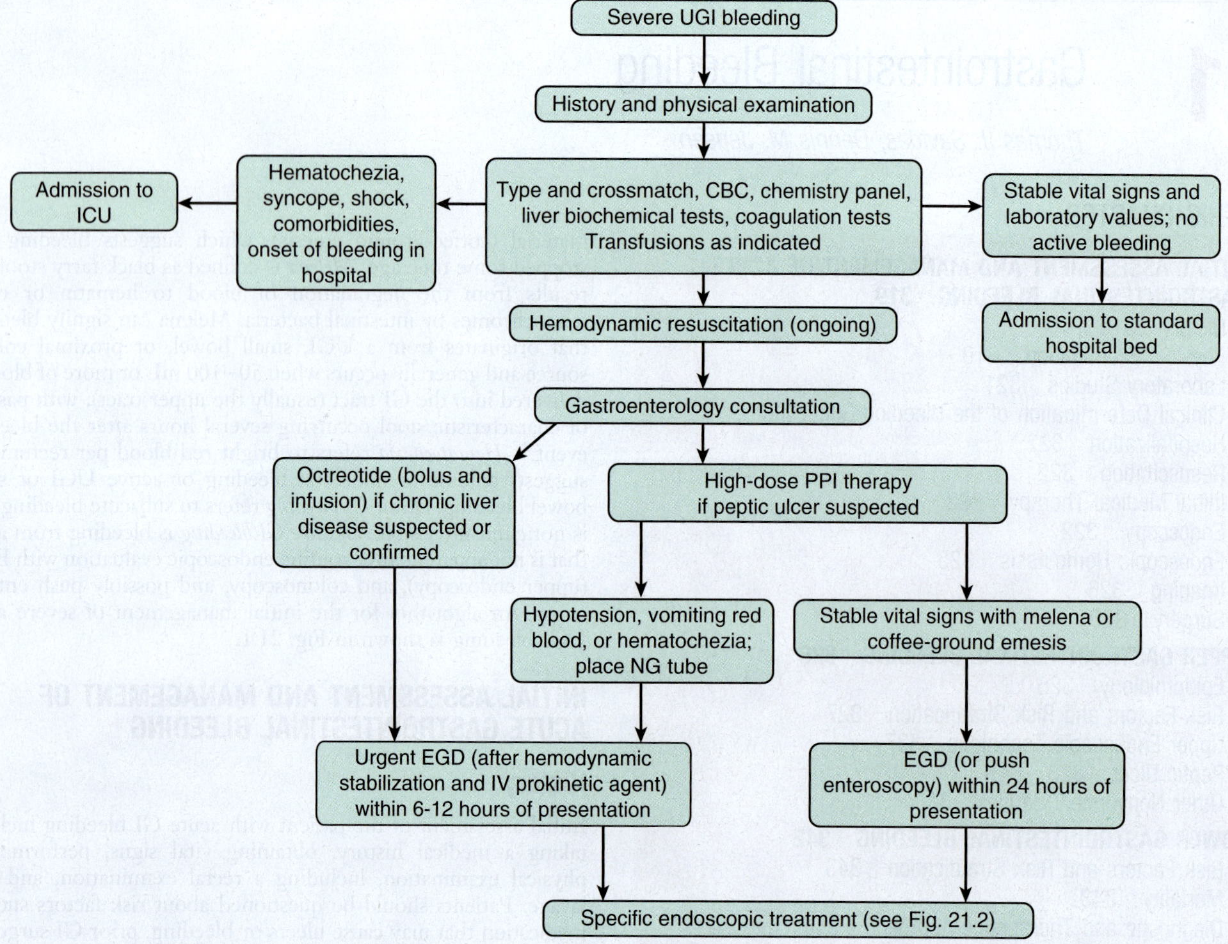

Fig. 21.1 Algorithm for the initial management of severe UGI bleeding. Some steps may take place simultaneously or in varying order and in the emergency department, depending on the clinical situation.

TABLE 21.1 Suspected Source of GI Bleeding as Suggested by a Patient's History

Suspected Source of Bleeding	History
Nasopharynx	History of nasopharyngeal radiation Prior nasopharyngeal malignancy Recurrent epistaxis
Lungs	Hemoptysis
Esophageal ulceration	GERD Heartburn Heavy alcohol use Odynophagia Pill ingestion Traumatic NG tube placement
Esophageal cancer	Dysphagia History of Barrett esophagus Weight loss
Mallory-Weiss tear	Alcohol binge Vomiting
Cameron lesions	Large hiatal hernia
Esophageal or gastric varices or portal hypertensive gastropathy	Chronic liver disease Cirrhosis Morbid obesity
Gastric angiodysplasia	Aortic stenosis Chronic kidney disease Systemic sclerosis

TABLE 21.1 Suspected Source of GI Bleeding as Suggested by a Patient's History—cont'd

Suspected Source of Bleeding	History
Peptic ulcer	Hp infection Epigastric discomfort Frequent aspirin or other NSAID use History of PUD
Gastric cancer	Early satiety Weight loss
Primary aortoenteric fistula	Prior severe acute unexplained bleeding and abdominal aortic aneurysm without surgery
Secondary aortoenteric fistula	Prior surgical repair of an abdominal aortic aneurysm with synthetic graft
Ampulla of Vater	Recent endoscopic sphincterotomy
Bile ducts	Recent liver biopsy, cholangiography, or TIPS
Pancreatic ducts	Pancreatitis Pseudocyst Recent pancreatography
Small intestinal malignancy	Hereditary nonpolyposis colorectal cancer History of intra-abdominal metastatic cancer Intermittent SBO Recurrent unexplained GI bleeding Weight loss
Meckel diverticulum	Unexplained GI bleeding in patient ≤40 years of age
Small intestinal or colonic ulcerations	IBD Use of aspirin or other NSAID
Small intestinal telangiectasias	Frequent nosebleeds HHT (Osler-Weber-Rendu disease)
Small intestinal angiodysplasia	Age >60 years Chronic GI blood loss Iron deficiency anemia
Colonic diverticulosis	Hematochezia without abdominal pain History of diverticulosis
Colonic neoplasia	Change in bowel habits Chronic bleeding Personal or family history of colon neoplasia Weight loss
Ischemic colitis	Cardiovascular disease Hematochezia with or without abdominal pain
UC	Bloody diarrhea Family history of IBD History of UC
Crohn disease	Chronic abdominal discomfort Family history of IBD History of Crohn disease
Anal fissure	Hematochezia with anal pain Severe constipation
Hemorrhoids	Dripping blood with bowel movements Hematochezia with otherwise normal bowel movements
Postpolypectomy ulcer	Recent colonoscopy with polypectomy Use of anticoagulants or antiplatelet drugs
Colonic or small intestinal angioectasias	Age >70 years Cardiovascular disease Chronic LGI bleeding/iron deficiency anemia Recurrent bleeding of variable severity
Anastomotic ulceration	Prior intestinal surgical anastomosis
Radiation enteritis or proctitis	History of abdominal radiation therapy

placement of an NG tube for diagnostic purposes but may need an NG tube to help clear the gastric blood for better endoscopic visualization and to minimize the risk of aspiration.

Laboratory Studies

Blood from the patient with acute GI bleeding should be sent for standard hematology, chemistry, liver biochemical, and coagulation studies and for typing and crossmatching for packed RBCs. The hematocrit or hemoglobin values immediately after the onset of bleeding may not reflect blood loss accurately because it takes more than 24–72 hours for the vascular space to equilibrate with extravascular fluid and hemodilution results from IV administration of saline.[5] A mean corpuscular volume (MCV) lower than 80 fL suggests chronic GI blood loss and iron deficiency, which can be confirmed by the finding of low blood iron, high total iron-binding capacity (TIBC), and low ferritin levels. A low MCV and negative fecal occult blood test (FOBT) result raise the possibility of celiac disease. A high MCV (>100 fL) suggests chronic liver disease or folate or vitamin B_{12} deficiency. An elevated WBC count may occur in more than half of patients with UGI bleeding and has been associated with greater severity of bleeding.[6] A low platelet count can contribute to the severity of bleeding and suggests chronic liver disease or a hematologic disorder. In patients with UGI bleeding, the blood urea nitrogen level typically increases to a greater extent than the serum creatinine level because of increased intestinal absorption of urea after the breakdown of blood proteins by intestinal bacteria.[7] The prothrombin time (PT) and INR assess whether a patient has impairment of the extrinsic coagulation pathway. Values can be elevated in chronic liver disease or with warfarin.

Clinical Determination of the Bleeding Site

Presentation with hematemesis, coffee-ground emesis, or NG lavage with return of a large amount of blood or coffee-ground emesis indicates a UGI source of bleeding. A small amount of coffee-ground material or pink-tinged fluid that clears easily may represent mucosal trauma from the NG tube rather than active bleeding from a UGI source. A clear (nonbloody) NG aspirate does not necessarily indicate a more distal GI source bleeding, because at least 16% of patients with actively bleeding UGI lesions have a clear NG aspirate.[8] The presence of bile in the NG aspirate makes acute UGI bleeding unlikely but can be seen with an intermittently bleeding UGI source.

Melena generally indicates a UGI source but can be seen with small intestinal or proximal colonic bleeding. Hematochezia generally implies a colonic or anorectal source of bleeding unless the patient is hypotensive, which could indicate a severe, brisk UGI bleed with rapid transit of blood through the GI tract.[4,9] Maroon-colored stool can be seen with an actively bleeding UGI source or a small intestinal or proximal colonic source.

Hospitalization

Patients with severe GI bleeding require hospitalization, whereas those who present with only mild acute bleeding (self-limited hematochezia or infrequent melena) and who are hemodynamically stable (not suspected to be volume depleted), have normal blood test results, and can be relied on to return to the hospital if symptoms recur may be candidates for semiurgent outpatient endoscopy rather than direct admission to the hospital.[10,11] Patients should be hospitalized in an ICU if they have large amounts of red blood in the NG tube or per rectum, have unstable vital signs, or have had severe acute blood loss that may exacerbate other underlying medical conditions. Patients who have had an acute GI bleed but are hemodynamically stable can be admitted to a monitored bed (step-down unit) or standard hospital bed, depending on their clinical condition. Urgent endoscopy performed in the emergency department in patients with a suspected UGI bleed can help determine optimal hospital placement.[12,13]

Resuscitation

Resuscitation efforts should be initiated at the same time as initial assessment in the emergency department and continue during the patient's hospitalization. At least 1 large-bore (14- or 16-ga) catheter should be placed intravenously, and 2 should be placed when the patient has ongoing bleeding. Normal saline is infused as fast as needed to keep the patient's systolic blood pressure higher than 100 mm Hg and pulse lower than 100/min. Patients should be transfused with packed RBCs, platelets, and fresh frozen plasma as necessary to keep the hemoglobin level greater than 7 g/dL, platelet count higher than 50,000/mm^3, and PT less than 15 seconds, respectively. In a large study from Barcelona, patients with severe UGI bleeding were randomized to receive transfusions either when the hemoglobin level was less than 7 g/dL or when the hemoglobin level was less than 9 g/dL.[14] The former "restrictive" transfusion strategy was associated with a higher survival rate and lower rebleeding rate in patients with bleeding owing to peptic ulcer and in those with Child-Pugh class A or B cirrhosis but a lower survival rate and higher rebleeding rate in those with Child-Pugh class C cirrhosis (see Chapter 96). Decisions about the timing of transfusion need to be individualized based on a patient's clinical status and comorbidities and the rapidity of blood loss.

An endoscopist should be consulted as soon as possible to expedite the patient's assessment and determine the optimal timing of endoscopy. In hospitals with an LT program, the transplantation hepatology service should also be notified if the patient is known to have cirrhosis and is a potential transplant candidate (see Chapter 99).

The patient's vital signs should be monitored frequently, as appropriate to the level of hospitalization. Laboratory-determined hematocrit and hemoglobin values (not fingerstick hematocrit values, which are less reliable) should be obtained every 4–8 hours until the hematocrit and hemoglobin values are stable. In patients with active bleeding, an indwelling urinary catheter should be placed to monitor the patient's urine output.

Endotracheal intubation should be considered in patients with active ongoing hematemesis or with altered mental status to prevent aspiration pneumonia. Patients who are older than 60 years of age, have chest pain, or have a history of cardiac disease should be evaluated for myocardial infarction with electrocardiography and serial troponin measurements. A chest x-ray should also be considered.

Initial Medical Therapy

Administration of a PPI is useful for reducing rebleeding rates in patients with PUD (see later). Starting a PPI in the emergency department or ICU before endoscopy is performed in patients with severe UGI bleeding has become a common practice but is still controversial.[15] Several clinical studies and meta-analyses have shown that infusion of a PPI in a high dose before endoscopy accelerates the resolution of endoscopic stigmata of recent hemorrhage (SRH) in ulcers (see later) and reduces the need for endoscopic therapy but does not result in improvement in clinical major outcomes.[16–19] Patients with a strong suspicion of portal hypertension and variceal bleeding should be started empirically on IV octreotide [bolus followed by infusion (see later and Chapter 96)], which can reduce the risk of rebleeding to a rate similar to that following endoscopic therapy (Fig. 21.2; also see Fig. 21.1).[20,21]

Endoscopy

GI endoscopy will identify the bleeding site and permit therapeutic hemostasis in most patients with GI bleeding.[22] There is a controversy about the timing of endoscopy for patients with severe UGI bleeding. The consensus is that for patients with severe comorbidities (such as American Society of Anesthesiologists Physical Status class 3–4) (see Chapter 40), the optimal period for performing EGD associated with the least mortality is after the patient has been hemodynamically resuscitated but within 12–20 hours of presentation. Emergency endoscopy before or after this interval is associated with higher mortality rates. For hemodynamically stable patients with less severe comorbidity (American Society of Anesthesiologists class 1–2), EGD within 24 hours is associated with lower mortality. Endoscopy should be done only when it is safe to do so and when the information obtained from the procedure will influence patient care. Ideally, the patient should be hemodynamically stable, with a heart rate of less than

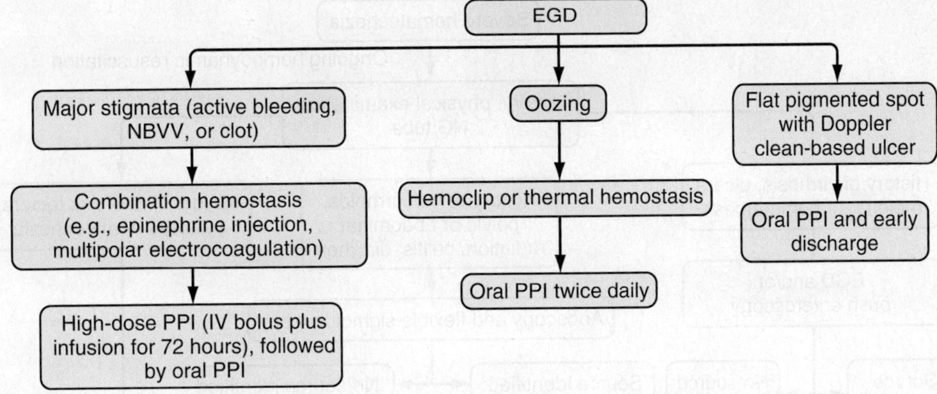

Fig. 21.2 Algorithm for the endoscopic and medical management of severe peptic ulcer hemorrhage following hemodynamic stabilization. *NBVV*, Nonbleeding visible vessel.

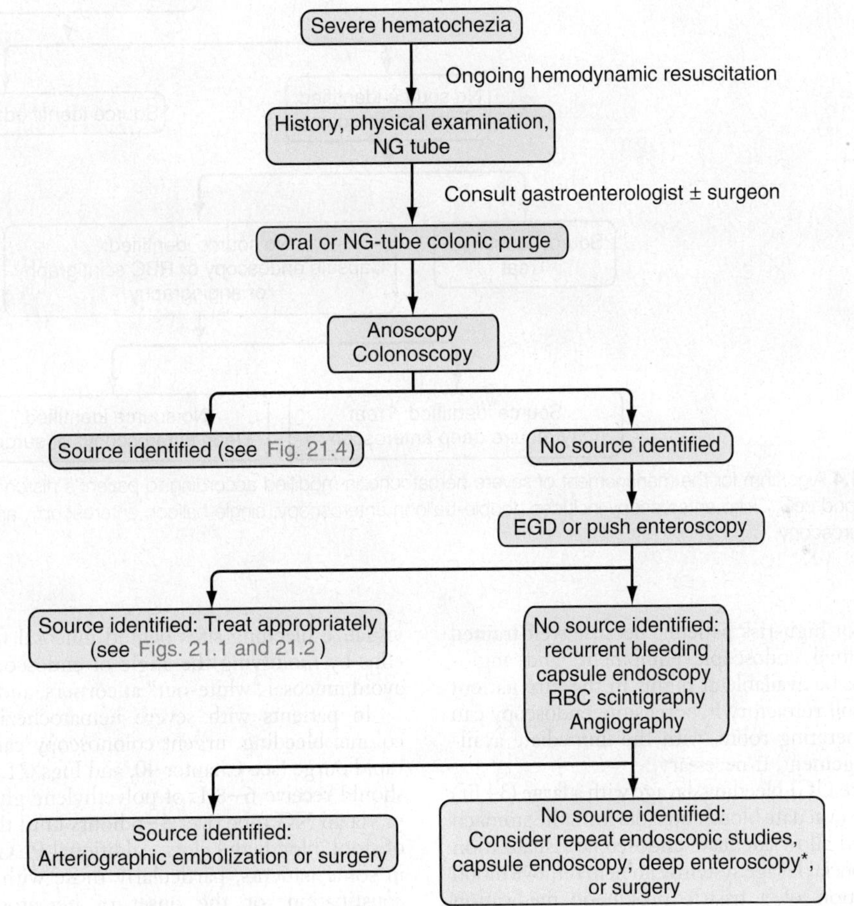

Fig. 21.3 Algorithm for the management of severe hematochezia. *RBC*, Red blood cell. *Deep enteroscopy includes double-balloon enteroscopy, single-balloon enteroscopy, and spiral enteroscopy.

100/min and a systolic blood pressure higher than 100 mm Hg. Respiratory insufficiency, altered mental status, or ongoing hematemesis indicates the need for endotracheal intubation before emergency EGD to stabilize the patient and protect the airway. Proper medical resuscitation will not only allow safer endoscopy but also ensure a better diagnostic examination for lesions, such as varices, that are volume dependent, and it will allow more effective hemostasis because of the correction of coagulopathy (Figs. 21.3 and 21.4; also see Figs. 21.1 and 21.2).

Patients with active hemorrhage (i.e., a high-volume bloody NG lavage or ongoing hematochezia) should undergo emergency EGD soon after medical resuscitation. In general, emergency endoscopy is best performed once the patient has reached an ICU bed, rather than in the emergency department, because resources (personnel, medications, and space) are more readily available in the ICU. Patients suspected of having cirrhosis or an aortoenteric fistula, or who rebleed in the hospital, should undergo emergent endoscopy as soon as they are hemodynamically resuscitated. Patients who are hemodynamically stable without evidence of ongoing bleeding can undergo urgent endoscopy (within 24 hours), often in the GI endoscopy unit rather than the ICU. Middle-of-the-night endoscopy should be avoided, except for the

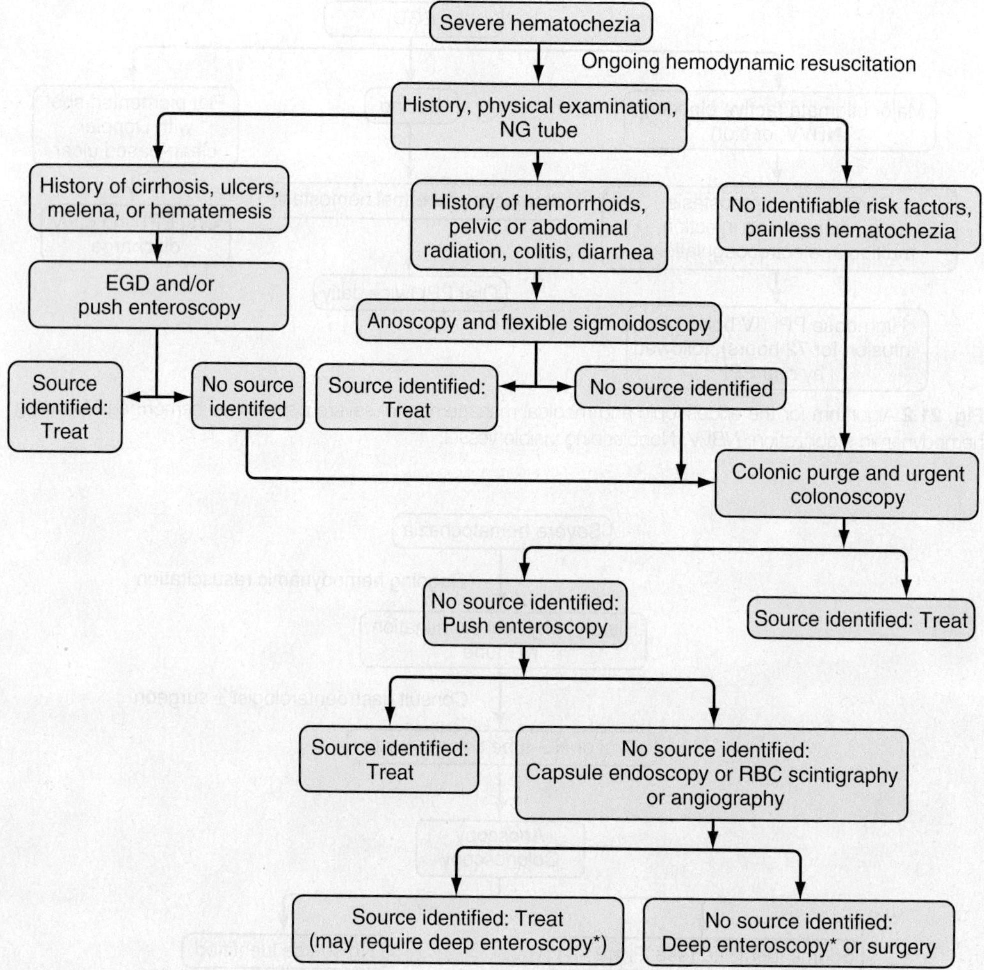

Fig. 21.4 Algorithm for the management of severe hematochezia modified according to patient's history. *RBC*, Red blood cell. *Deep enteroscopy includes double-balloon enteroscopy, single-balloon enteroscopy, and spiral enteroscopy.

most severely bleeding or high-risk patients, because well-trained endoscopy nurses, optimal endoscopic equipment, and angiographic backup may not be available at night. In the rare patient with massive bleeding and refractory hypotension, endoscopy can be performed in the operating room, with the immediate availability of surgical management, if necessary.

In patients with severe UGI bleeding, lavage with a large (34 Fr) orogastric tube may help evacuate blood and clots from the stomach to prevent aspiration and allow adequate endoscopic visualization (see also Chapter 40). Special lavage systems can help remove blood rapidly. IV administration of a gastric prokinetic medication (e.g., erythromycin and metoclopramide) 30–90 minutes before EGD to induce gastric contraction and propel blood from the stomach into the small intestine helps endoscopic visualization and decreases the need for repeat endoscopy but does not reduce the transfusion requirement, length of hospitalization, or need for surgery.[23–25] Therapeutic single- or double-channel endoscopes with large-diameter suction channels should be used to allow rapid removal of fresh blood from the GI tract during endoscopy. Additionally, a water pump is useful for irrigating target lesions through an accessory channel and for diluting blood to allow suctioning, thereby facilitating visualization. Iced saline lavage is of no value in the management of UGI bleeding and may impair coagulation and cause hypothermia. NG lavage with lukewarm tap water is as safe as lavage with sterile saline and much less expensive. A clear plastic cap placed on the tip of the endoscope can help to visualize bleeding sites behind mucosal folds, deploy endoscopic clips by modifying the angle of endoscopic approach (see later), avoid mucosal "white-out" at corners, and remove blood clots.[26]

In patients with severe hematochezia and suspected active colonic bleeding, urgent colonoscopy can be undertaken after a rapid purge (see Chapter 40, and Figs. 21.3 and 21.4).[27,28] Patients should receive 6–8 L of polyethylene glycol (PEG) purge orally or via an NG tube over 4–6 hours until the rectal effluent is clear of stool, blood, and clots. Additional PEG purge may be required in some patients, particularly those with active bleeding, severe constipation, or the onset of hematochezia in the hospital. Metoclopramide, 10 mg given intravenously before the purge and repeated every 4–6 hours, may facilitate gastric emptying and reduce nausea. In patients with severe or ongoing active hematochezia, urgent colonoscopy should be performed within 12–14 hours, but only after thorough cleansing of the colon. Patients with mild or moderate self-limited hematochezia should undergo colonoscopy within 24 hours of admission after a colonic purge. Patients with maroon stool in whom there is pretest uncertainty about the bleeding source should be considered for an urgent PEG preparation as well. Colonoscopy immediately after push enteroscopy (see later) while the patient is still sedated will expedite a patient's care if push enteroscopy does not provide a diagnosis (Fig. 21.5).

Wireless video capsule endoscopy (see later) is useful in patients with overt GI bleeding who have normal push enteroscopy

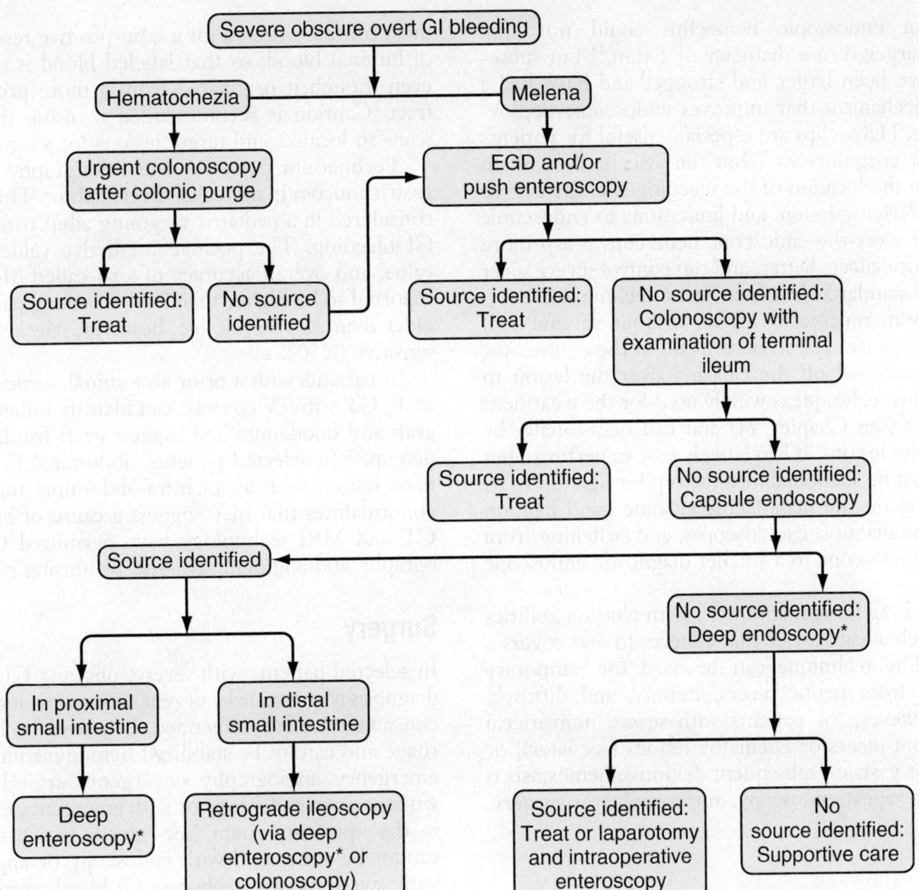

Fig. 21.5 Algorithm for the management of severe obscure overt GI bleeding. *Deep enteroscopy includes double-balloon enteroscopy, single-balloon enteroscopy, and spiral enteroscopy.

and colonoscopy results and in whom a small bowel source of bleeding is suspected.[29] Capsule endoscopy has the advantage of directly visualizing the small intestine to identify potential sources or active bleeding. Disadvantages are that the procedure takes 8 hours to complete and additional time to download and review the images, does not permit therapeutic hemostasis, and may be difficult to perform in inpatients because of limited availability of staff trained to place the capsule during off-hours. A follow-up endoscopic procedure, such as single- or double-balloon enteroscopy or retrograde ileoscopy, may be indicated for definitive diagnosis and treatment if a focal bleeding site is found on capsule endoscopy.

Complications related to emergency endoscopy and endoscopic hemostasis may occur in up to 1% of patients, depending on the type of endoscopy and treatment performed.[30,31] The most common complications include aspiration pneumonia, induced hemorrhage, an adverse medication reaction, hypotension, hypoxia, and GI tract perforation (see Chapter 40).

Endoscopic Hemostasis

Thermal contact probes have been the mainstay of endoscopic hemostasis since the 1970s. These probes come in diameters of 7 and 10 Fr and in lengths that can fit through panendoscopes, enteroscopes, or colonoscopes. Contact probes can physically tamponade a blood vessel to stop bleeding and interrupt underlying blood flow; thermal energy is then applied to seal the underlying vessel (coaptive coagulation). The most commonly used probe is a multipolar electrocoagulation (MPEC) probe, also referred to as a bipolar electrocoagulation probe, with which heat is created by current flowing between intertwined electrodes on the tip of the probe. In animal studies, optimal coagulation has been shown to occur with low-power settings (12–16 W) applied for a moderate amount of time (8–10 seconds) with moderate pressure on the bleeding site.[32] Heater probes provide a predetermined amount of joules of energy, which does not vary with tissue resistance and can effectively coagulate arteries up to 2 mm in diameter, a diameter considerably larger than most secondary or tertiary branches of arteries (usually 1 mm) found in resected bleeding human peptic ulcers.[33,34] The main risk of using a thermal probe is perforation with excessive application of coagulation or pressure, especially in acute or nonfibrotic lesions. Thermal probes can also cause a coagulation injury that can make lesions larger and deeper and may induce delayed bleeding in patients with a coagulopathy. Argon plasma coagulation is a noncontact thermal therapy (see later).

Injection therapy is most commonly performed with a sclerotherapy needle and submucosal injection of epinephrine, diluted to a concentration of 1:10,000 or 1:20,000, into or around the bleeding site or stigma of hemorrhage (see later). The advantages of this technique are its wide availability, relatively low cost, and safety in patients with a coagulopathy and lower risk of perforation (and absence of thermal burn damage) than thermal techniques. Epinephrine injection is not as effective, however, for definitive hemostasis as thermal coagulation, hemostatic clip placement [hemoclipping (see later)], or combination therapy.[35,36] Injection therapy can also be performed with a sclerosant, such as ethanolamine or alcohol, but these agents are associated with increased tissue damage and other risks.

Endoscopic hemoclips (or clips) have been available since 1974 and have become popular following technical improvements.[37] Hemoclips serve to apply mechanical pressure to a bleeding site.

The first-generation endoscopic hemoclips could not stop bleeding in vessels larger than a diameter of 1 mm,[38] but subsequent hemoclips have been larger and stronger and have had a grasp-and-release mechanism that improves endoscopic deployment and hemostasis. Hemoclips are especially useful for patients with malnutrition or coagulopathy[39] but can also be difficult to deploy depending on the location of the bleeding site, the degree of fibrosis of the underlying lesion, and limitations to endoscopic access. Newer, large, over-the-endoscope hemoclips grasp more tissue, adhere to fibrotic ulcers better, and can control severe ulcer bleeding better than standard ulcer hemostatic techniques.[40]

With band ligation, mucosal (with or without submucosal) tissue is suctioned into a cap placed on the end of the endoscope, and a rubber band is rolled off the cap and over the lesion to compress its base. This technique is widely used for the treatment of esophageal varices (see Chapter 94) and can occasionally be used for other bleeding lesions. It is relatively easy to perform, but sufficient mucosa must be suctioned into the cap for ligation to be successful. Depending on the manufacturer, some band ligation devices can only fit on diagnostic endoscopes, and switching from a larger therapeutic endoscope to a smaller diagnostic endoscope is necessary.

Hemostatic spray is an inorganic powder with clotting abilities that can create a mechanical barrier that adheres to and covers a bleeding site.[41–44] The technique can be used for temporary control of bleeding from peptic ulcers, tumors, and diffusely bleeding lesions; however, for patients with severe nonvariceal bleeding [such as from ulcers or Dieulafoy lesions (see later)] or varices (esophageal or gastric), subsequent definitive hemostasis is usually required with repeat endoscopy, angiography, or surgery.

Imaging

Angiography may be used to diagnose and treat severe bleeding, especially when the cause cannot be determined by upper and lower endoscopy. Angiography is generally diagnostic of extravasation into the intestinal lumen only when the arterial bleeding rate is at least 0.5 mL/min.[45] The sensitivity of mesenteric angiography is 30%–50% (with higher sensitivity rates for active GI bleeding than for recurrent acute or chronic occult bleeding), and the specificity is 100%.[46] Angiography permits therapeutic intra-arterial infusion of vasopressin or transcatheter embolization for hemostasis if active bleeding is detected, without the need for bowel cleansing. The rate of major complications, including hematoma formation, femoral artery thrombosis, contrast dye reactions, acute kidney injury, intestinal ischemia, and transient ischemic attacks, is 3%.[47] Moreover, angiography does not usually identify the specific cause of bleeding, only its location.

Radionuclide imaging is occasionally helpful for patients with unexplained GI bleeding, although it is used less frequently now than in the past because of the widespread use of endoscopy and lack of availability of nuclear medicine services for emergencies, particularly at night and on weekends. Radionuclide imaging can be performed relatively quickly and may help localize the general area of bleeding and thereby guide subsequent endoscopy, angiography, or surgery. The technique involves IV injection of a radiolabeled substance into the patient's bloodstream, followed by serial scintigraphy to detect focal collections of radiolabeled material. Radionuclide imaging has been reported to detect bleeding at a rate of 0.04 mL/min.[48] RBCs are generally labeled with technetium pertechnetate because they remain in the circulation for up to 24 hours so that scanning can be repeated in patients with either active or intermittent GI bleeding.[49]

The overall rate of a tagged RBC scan for the diagnosis of hematochezia is low (<30%), and up to 25% of scans suggest a site of bleeding that proves to be incorrect.[50–52] The rate of true-positive scans is higher when bleeding is active and associated with hemodynamic instability than when bleeding is less severe.[53] The most common reason for a false-positive result is the rapid transit of luminal blood, so that labeled blood is detected in the colon even though it originated from a more proximal site in the GI tract. Caution is recommended in using the results of delayed scans to localize and target lesions for surgical resection.[54]

Technetium pertechnetate scintigraphy can identify ectopic gastric mucosa in a Meckel diverticulum. This diagnosis should be considered in a pediatric or young adult patient with unexplained GI bleeding. The positive predictive value, negative predictive value, and overall accuracy of a so-called Meckel scan have been reported to be higher than 90% in young patients.[55,56] In patients older than 25 years of age, however, Meckel scans are much less sensitive (<50%).[57]

In patients with a prior abdominal aortic aneurysm repair and graft, CT with IV contrast can identify inflammation between the graft and duodenum and suggest graft fistulization into the duodenum.[58] In selected patients, abdominal CT can also identify a mass lesion, such as an intra-abdominal tumor, or small bowel abnormalities that may suggest a cause of bleeding. Advances in CT and MRI technology have permitted CT and MRI enterography and angiography, with promising results.[59,60]

Surgery

In selected patients with severe, ongoing GI bleeding in whom a diagnosis is not made by urgent endoscopy or colonoscopy, surgical consultation is recommended. Patients who have massive hemorrhage and cannot be stabilized hemodynamically should undergo emergency angiography or urgent surgical exploration [either without prior endoscopy or with emergency endoscopy performed in the operating room (see later)]. Patients with bleeding that cannot be controlled with endoscopy or angiography and those with severe recurrent obscure GI bleeding may also benefit from surgery with intraoperative enteroscopy (see later).

UPPER GASTROINTESTINAL BLEEDING

Epidemiology

Of the potential causes of severe UGI bleeding, peptic ulcer is the most common, accounting for approximately 40% of cases (Table 21.2).[61,62] Despite advances in medical therapy, ICU care,

TABLE 21.2 Causes of Severe UGI Bleeding in the UCLA CURE Database (n = 968)

Cause	Frequency (%)
Peptic ulcer	35.2
Esophageal or gastric varix	21.9
Portal hypertension-related lesion[a]	4.6
Esophagitis	4.6
Angioectasia[b]	4.0
Mallory-Weiss tear	4.0
Dieulafoy lesion	3.2
UGI tract neoplasm	3.1
Epistaxis	2.2
Erosions	1.2
Other	8.8
No cause found	7.3

[a]Other than an esophageal or gastric varix.
[b]Angioectasia and telangiectasia.
CURE, Center for Ulcer Research and Education; *UCLA*, University of California, Los Angeles.

endoscopy, and surgery, the mortality rate of 5%–10% for severe UGI bleeding has not changed since the 1970s[1,61–65] in part because of an increase in the proportion of older patients with GI bleeding who die of severe comorbid conditions rather than exsanguination, and an increase in the number of patients with cirrhosis and variceal bleeding.

Bleeding is self-limited in 80% of patients with UGI hemorrhage, even without specific therapy.[63,66] Of the remaining 20% who continue to bleed or rebleed, the mortality rate is 30% –40%.[8] Patients at high risk for continuous bleeding or for rebleeding potentially benefit the most from acute medical, endoscopic, angiographic, or surgical therapy.

Risk Factors and Risk Stratification

Scoring tools have been developed to try to identify patients with nonvariceal UGI bleeding at greatest risk for mortality and rebleeding and to triage patients to a higher level of hospital care or more urgent endoscopy. Preendoscopy scoring systems for nonvariceal bleeding include the Blatchford Score, the Clinical Rockall Score, an artificial neural network score, and the AIMS65 score. The Blatchford Score uses preendoscopy variables, including blood pressure, blood urea nitrogen level, hemoglobin level, heart rate, syncope, melena, liver disease, and heart failure, to assess a patient's risk for needing clinical interventions to control bleeding (e.g., blood transfusions, endoscopic therapy, and surgery).[67] The Clinical Rockall Score is based on the patient's age, shock, and coexisting illnesses.[68] The artificial neural network instrument uses 21 clinical variables to help predict the presence of SRH at endoscopy (see later) and the need for endoscopic therapy.[69] AIMS65 is an aggregate score of 5 preendoscopy variables (serum albumin <3.0 g/dL, INR >1.5, altered mental status, systolic blood pressure ≤90 mm Hg and age >65); an AIMS65 score less than two is associated with a lower risk of mortality, length of stay, and cost of hospitalization than a score of two or more.[70]

The most commonly used postendoscopy scoring system is the Complete Rockall Score (Table 21.3).[68] The Complete Rockall Score includes the Clinical Rockall Score (preendoscopy variables—patient age, shock, and coexisting illnesses) and endoscopic findings, including endoscopic SRH (see later). The Rockall Score after endoscopic therapy correlates well with mortality but not as well with the risk of rebleeding.[71–73] The Rockall risk stratification schemes can also be used to identify patients at low risk for poor outcomes (i.e., Rockall Scores of 0–2) who should be considered for early discharge from the hospital.[74]

Other scoring systems to predict outcomes from UGI bleeding after endoscopy include the Baylor Scoring System and the Cedars-Sinai Bleeding Index.[75–78] In general, all of these scoring systems are better at determining mortality than rebleeding.[79]

Upper Endoscopic Technique

A therapeutic endoscope facilitates aspiration of blood and the use of large accessories. Target jet water irrigation with a foot pump through a separate small channel should be available. Patients should be hemodynamically resuscitated medically prior to EGD (see earlier), and, if active bleeding is severe, consideration should be given to prophylactic endotracheal intubation to minimize the risk of airway aspiration.

Once the endoscope is inserted, the first thing to look for is blood in the GI tract lumen. Examining all the nonbloody mucosa quickly is often best to document that these areas are free of any lesions. Then, any liquid blood that can be aspirated should be removed. Aspiration of blood can be aided by water irrigation to dilute the blood. Other options to remove blood and clots are to

TABLE 21.3 Rockall Scoring System for UGI Bleeding

	Points			
Variable	**0**	**1**	**2**	**3**
Age (year)	<60	60–79	≥80	–
Pulse rate (beats/min)	<100	≥100	–	–
Systolic blood pressure (mm Hg)	Normal	≥100	<100	–
Comorbidity	None	–	Ischemic heart disease, cardiac failure, other major illness	Renal failure, hepatic failure, metastatic cancer
Diagnosis	Mallory-Weiss tear or no lesion observed	All other benign diagnoses	Malignant lesion	–
Endoscopic stigmata of recent hemorrhage	No stigmata or dark spot in ulcer base	–	Blood in UGI tract, adherent clot, visible vessel, active bleeding	–
Total Score	**Frequency (% of Total)**	**Rebleeding Rate (%)**	**Mortality Rate (%)**	
0	4.9	4.9	0	
1	9.5	3.4	0	
2	11.4	5.3	0.2	
3	15.0	11.2	2.9	
4	17.9	14.1	5.3	
5	15.3	24.1	10.8	
6	10.6	32.9	17.3	
7	9.0	43.8	27.0	
≥8	6.4	41.8	41.1	

Modified from Rockall TA, Logan RF, Devlin HB, Northfield TC. Selection of patients for early discharge or outpatient care after acute upper gastrointestinal haemorrhage. National Audit of Acute Upper Gastrointestinal Haemorrhage. *Lancet*. 1996;347:1138–1140.

use an endoscope with a very large (6 mm) suction channel or to use an accessory on a therapeutic endoscope that suctions directly through the suction port, bypassing the umbilical cord of the instrument. If large clots cannot be removed with suction, the patient can be turned onto his or her back or right side, provided that the patient is intubated to protect against aspiration. Raising the head of the bed can also help move a clot distally from the gastric fundus. Any visualized adherent fresh blood or clot should be followed to find its origin. If too much blood is present in the stomach to allow detection of a bleeding lesion, another dose (or an initial dose) of a prokinetic agent (e.g., erythromycin and metoclopramide) should be considered, lavage should be repeated with a large orogastric tube, or the examination should be repeated in the next 24 hours if the patient has stabilized. If bleeding from the duodenum is suspected but not identified with a forward-viewing endoscope, a side-viewing duodenoscope should be used to examine the duodenal wall and ampulla.

Peptic Ulcer

In the past, peptic ulcer, most commonly gastric or duodenal ulcer, accounted for 50% of UGI bleeds and approximately 100,000 hospitalizations/year in the United States.[80,81] Some data have suggested that the incidence of bleeding peptic ulcer decreased between 1993 and 2002, whereas the proportion of ulcers caused by NSAIDs increased.[82] Other data, however, found no change in overall rates of bleeding ulcers between 1990 and 2000, but an increase in the rate in the subgroup of older patients taking NSAIDs (Fig. 21.6).[83] The mortality rate associated with peptic ulcer bleeding is 5%–10%.[61,62] The costs of hospitalization for peptic ulcer bleeding are estimated to be more than $2 billion per year in the United States (see Chapter 55).[84] Clinical and endoscopic factors in patients with peptic ulcer bleeding associated with increased morbidity and mortality are shown in Box 21.1.

Pathogenesis

Peptic ulcers are most commonly caused by a decrease in mucosal defense mechanisms attributable to aspirin or other NSAIDs, Hp infection, or both (see Chapters 54 and 55).[85,86] In one large multicenter study of patients with severe peptic ulcer bleeding, 57% of those with bleeding from a gastric ulcer ($n = 2057$) took aspirin or another NSAID, and 45% were infected with Hp, whereas 53% of those with a bleeding duodenal ulcer ($n = 2033$) took aspirin or another NSAID, or both, and 50% were infected with Hp.[87] Of the patients with a bleeding peptic ulcer in this study, 10% had no obvious cause for the ulcer (Hp-negative, no aspirin or other NSAID use, no cancer, no gastrinoma).

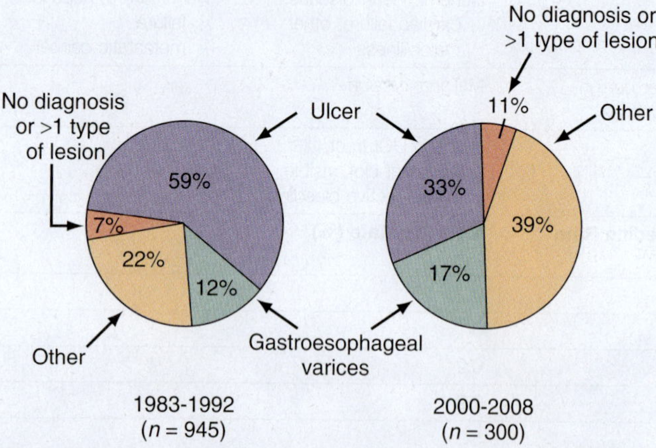

Fig. 21.6 Frequencies of major causes of severe UGI bleeding during two time periods in patients seen at UCLA CURE. (All differences between the two time periods are statistically significant; $P < .05$.) Note that in the more recent period, the overall number of cases of severe UGI bleeding and the percentage of cases caused by peptic ulcer have declined. *CURE*, Center for Ulcer Research and Education; *UCLA*, University of California, Los Angeles

BOX 21.1 Factors Predictive of a Poor Prognosis After Hemorrhage From Peptic Ulcer

- Age >60 years
- Bleeding onset in hospital
- Severe comorbid medical illness
- Shock or orthostatic hypotension
- Fresh blood in NG tube
- Coagulopathy
- Multiple transfusions required
- Higher lesser curve gastric ulcer (adjacent to left gastric artery)
- Posterior duodenal bulb ulcer (adjacent to gastroduodenal artery)
- Endoscopic finding of arterial bleeding or visible vessel
- Residual arterial blood flow after endoscopic treatment

The prevalence of Hp infection is more than 80% of the population in many developing countries and 20%–50% in industrialized countries.[88] Hp gastritis most commonly involves the antrum and predisposes patients to duodenal ulcers, whereas gastric body-predominant gastritis is associated with gastric ulcers. The lifetime risk of peptic ulcer disease from Hp infection ranges from 3% in the United States to 25% in Japan (see Chapter 52).

NSAIDs are the most widely used medication in the United States, with 11% of the adult population using NSAIDs on a daily basis.[89] Many are bought over the counter and without a doctor's prescription.[87] NSAIDs, including aspirin, predominantly cause ulceration by inhibiting COX-mediated prostaglandin synthesis and thereby impairing mucosal protection, rather than by causing direct topical injury.[86] Gastroduodenal ulcers are found at endoscopy in 15%–45% of patients who take NSAIDs regularly.[90,91] Gastric ulcers are approximately four times as common as duodenal ulcers in patients who take NSAIDs.[92] In a large study of patients with UGI hemorrhage and NSAID-associated ulcers, however, gastric and duodenal ulcers occurred with equal frequencies (see Chapter 53).[87]

Histopathology

In a landmark study by Swain et al., the pathologic examination of 27 surgically resected bleeding gastric ulcers with endoscopically visible vessels revealed an underlying artery in 96% of specimens.[33] Approximately 50% of the vessels protruded above the surface of the ulcer, whereas the other 50% had an adherent clot in continuity with a breach in the artery wall. The bleeding arteries had a mean diameter of 0.7 mm, with a range of 0.1–1.18 mm.

Endoscopic Risk Stratification

In the United Kingdom, Asia, and some other countries, the Forrest classification is used to categorize findings during endoscopic evaluation of bleeding peptic ulcers as follows: active spurting bleeding (Forrest IA), oozing of blood (Forrest IB), pigmented protuberance or nonbleeding visible vessel [NBVV (Forrest IIA)], adherent clot (Forrest IIB), flat pigmented spot (Forrest IIC), and clean-based ulcer (Forrest III).[93] Descriptive terms are used in the United States and other countries. Overall interobserver agreement among experts for classifying these SRH to the Forrest classification is only fair to moderate, with poor agreement for NBVVs.[94,95]

Endoscopic SRH from an ulcer is shown in Fig. 21.7, and the risk of rebleeding associated with each stigma is shown in Fig. 21.8. Patients at high risk of rebleeding without treatment are those with active arterial bleeding (90%), an NBVV (50%), or an adherent clot (33%).[96,97] These patients benefit from endoscopic hemostasis (see later). An endoscopically identified NBVV that has a translucent (pearl or whitish) color has a higher risk of rebleeding than a darkly colored pigmented protuberance (clot), because the translucent stigma likely represents the arterial wall.[98,99] A multivariate analysis of predictors of persistent or recurrent bleeding in patients with nonvariceal UGI bleeding is shown in Table 21.4. Patients with major SRH (spurting, NBVV, or adherent clot) benefit most from endoscopic hemostasis, whereas those with a clean ulcer base do not. Patients with oozing bleeding or flat spots and no other stigma (e.g., a clot or NBVV) may benefit from endoscopic hemostasis but not from infusion of high-dose PPI (see later).

The risk of rebleeding from a peptic ulcer decreases significantly 72 hours after the initial episode of bleeding. This conclusion is based on studies in which only active bleeding was treated endoscopically, all other stigmata were observed, and all patients were treated with an IV H2RA and cessation of aspirin and other NSAIDs.[98–102] Natural history studies of untreated NBVVs have found that these lesions resolve over 4 days, and adherent clots tend to resolve over 2 days.[103]

Doppler Endoscopic Probe

Portable Doppler endoscopic probes (DEPs) can be passed through the working channel of an endoscope and applied to an ulcer to determine if blood flow is present beneath a stigma in the ulcer base (Fig. 21.9).[104] DEP has been utilized to risk stratify patients with SRH into high risk for rebleeding [active arterial bleeding (Forrest

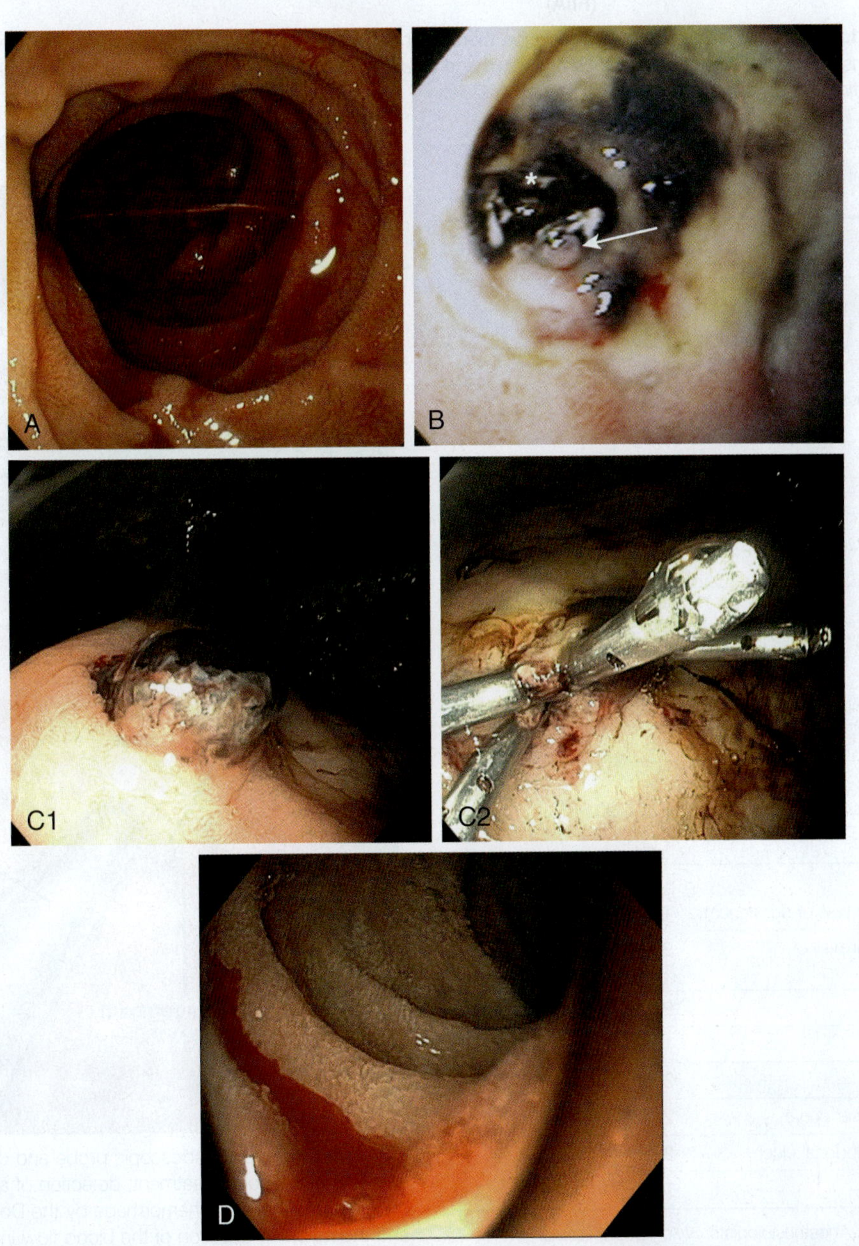

Fig. 21.7 Endoscopic stigmata of recent peptic ulcer bleeding. (A) Active bleeding with spurting. (B) Visible vessel (*arrow*) with adjacent clot. (C1) Adherent clot. (C2) Clips applied to lesion. (D) Slight oozing of blood after washing in the center of the ulcer, without clot or a visible vessel. (E) Small clot with pigmented spots. (F) Clean based.

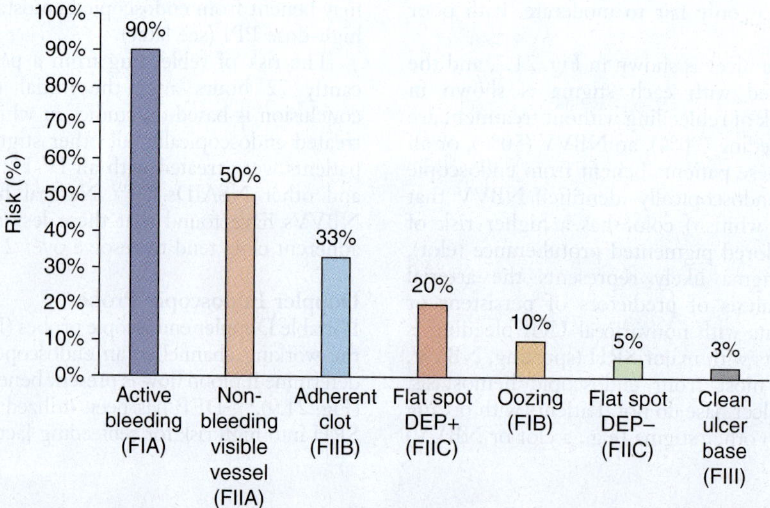

Fig. 21.8 Rebleeding rates without endoscopic therapy or administration of a PPI in patients with ulcers demonstrating various stigmata of recent hemorrhage at UCLA CURE. *CURE*, Center for Ulcer Research and Education; *UCLA*, University of California, Los Angeles.

TABLE 21.4 Independent Risk Factors for Persistent or Recurrent GI Tract Bleeding

Risk Factor	Range of Odds Ratios for Increased Risk
CLINICAL FACTORS	
Health status (ASA class 1 vs. 2–5)	1.94–7.63
Comorbid illness	1.6–7.63
Shock (systolic blood pressure <100 mm Hg)	1.2–3.65
Erratic mental status	3.21
Ongoing bleeding	3.14
Age ≥70 years	2.23
Age >65 years	1.3
Transfusion requirement	N/A
PRESENTATION OF BLEEDING	
Hematemesis	1.2–5.7
Red blood on rectal examination	3.76
Melena	1.6
LABORATORY FACTORS	
Initial hemoglobin ≤10 g/dL	0.8–2.99
Coagulopathy	1.96
ENDOSCOPIC FACTORS	
Ulcer location on superior wall of duodenum	13.9
Ulcer location on posterior wall of duodenum	9.2
Active bleeding	2.5–6.48
High-risk stigmata	1.91–4.81
Ulcer size ≥2 cm	2.29–3.54
Ulcer location high on lesser curve	2.79
Diagnosis of gastric or duodenal ulcer	2.7
Clot over ulcer	1.72–1.9

ASA, American Society of Anesthesiologists; *N/A*, not applicable.
Data from Barkun A, Bardou M, Marshall JK. Consensus recommendations for managing patients with nonvariceal upper gastrointestinal bleeding. *Ann Intern Med*. 2003;139:843–857.

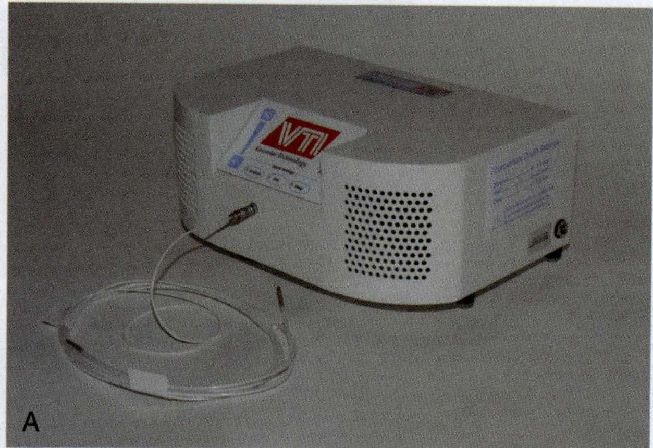

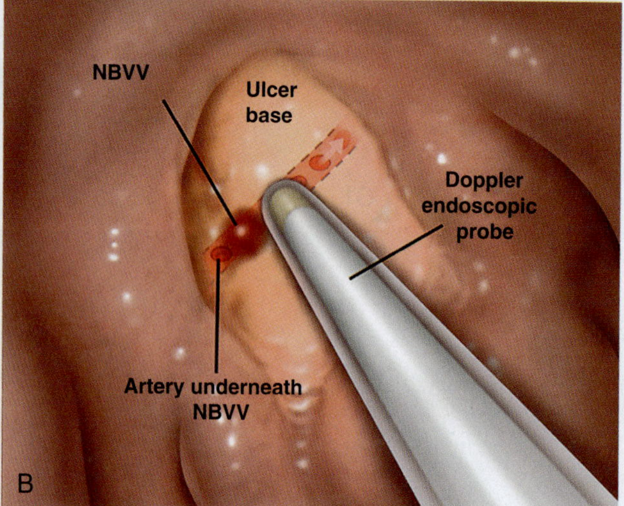

Fig. 21.9 (A) Doppler endoscopic probe and control unit. (B) Prior to and after endoscopic treatment, detection of arterial blood flow underneath stigmata of hemorrhage by the Doppler endoscopic probe and the mapping direction of the blood flow in the artery facilitate risk stratification, endoscopic hemostasis, and reduction in the rate of rebleeding (if arterial blood flow is obliterated). *NBVV*, Nonbleeding visible vessel.

FIA), NBVV (Forrest FIIA), and adherent clot (Forrest FIIB)]; intermediate risk [oozing bleeding (Forrest FIA) and flat spots (Forrest FIIC)]; and low risk [clean ulcer base (Forrest FIII)].[105,106] The presence of a blood flow signal correlates with the risk of rebleeding before and after endoscopic therapy. The DEP has also been used to map the direction of the artery underneath stigmata, stratify the risk of rebleeding, and confirm completion of nonvariceal hemostasis and obliteration of the underlying arterial blood flow. Prior conflicting results have been reported, however, as to whether use of the DEP improves the outcome of endoscopic hemostasis in patients with acute peptic ulcer bleeding.[107,108] A decision-analysis study found that the DEP is the preferred cost-minimizing strategy over conventional endoscopic therapy alone in patients with acute peptic ulcer bleeding.[109] The University of California, Los Angeles (UCLA) Center for Ulcer Research and Education (CURE) Hemostasis Group reported in a randomized controlled trial that rebleeding rates were significantly reduced in the group randomized to DEP compared with the group randomized to standard visually guided hemostasis, and the treatment was safe and effective.[110] Rebleeding rates correlated highly with residual arterial blood flow after endoscopic hemostasis. In another study, patients with severe nonvariceal UGI bleeding treated with the DEP by the UCLA CURE group were compared with matched historical controls; rates of rebleeding and surgery were also significantly reduced in the patients treated with the DEP but not in those treated with standard visually guided endoscopic hemostasis (see Fig. 21.7A).[111]

Endoscopic Hemostasis

Active Bleeding and Nonbleeding Visible Vessels

Many well-conducted randomized controlled trials, meta-analyses, and consensus recommendations have concluded that endoscopic hemostasis with epinephrine injection or coaptive thermal probe therapy significantly decreases the rates of ulcer rebleeding, urgent surgery, and mortality in patients with high-risk stigmata, such as active arterial bleeding and NBVVs.[22,112–115] The rebleeding rates for peptic ulcers with various endoscopic stigmata are shown in Fig. 21.8. These rebleeding rates are based on studies that were performed before the widespread use of high-dose PPI infusions and that predominantly used injection therapy, MPEC therapy, or a combination of injection and thermal probe therapy. In general, for the lesions with the highest risk of ongoing bleeding or rebleeding, including active bleeding (90% risk of ongoing bleeding) or NBVVs (50% risk of ongoing bleeding), endoscopic hemostasis alone decreases the rebleeding rate to approximately 15%–30% (Table 21.5). The adjunctive IV administration of a high-dose PPI (e.g., pantoprazole, 80-mg bolus and 8 mg/h for 72 hours) decreases this rate even further, as discussed in the next section. IV formulations of pantoprazole, lansoprazole, and esomeprazole are available in the United States.

The most commonly used treatment for ulcer bleeding worldwide is epinephrine injection therapy; it is widely available, easy to perform, safe, and inexpensive. Therapy with epinephrine alone seems to be more effective when used in high doses (13–20 mL) than in low doses (5–10 mL).[116] Injection of epinephrine results in a fivefold increase in circulating plasma epinephrine levels but is rarely thought to cause clinically significant cardiovascular events.[117] Numerous studies and meta-analyses have shown that the addition of a thermal or mechanical hemostatic modality further decreases the rates of rebleeding, surgery, and mortality.[35,118,119] Several studies have suggested that the only benefit to adding epinephrine injection to thermal probe therapy is in patients with active bleeding and that no benefit is seen in patients with NBVVs.[120,121]

Endoscopic hemostatic clips have not been studied as well as injection and thermal probe techniques but are more effective than epinephrine injection alone and have shown mixed results when compared with thermal probe therapy.[122–125] In a meta-analysis of outcomes of ulcer hemorrhage, the outcome with the application of hemoclips was shown to be superior to that for epinephrine injection alone but comparable to that for thermocoagulation.[36]

TABLE 21.5 Endoscopic Stigmata of Recent Ulcer Hemorrhage and Risk of Rebleeding

Endoscopic Stigma (Forrest Class)	Frequency (%)	Risk of Rebleeding (%)	Risk of Rebleeding After Endoscopic Hemostasis (%)[a]
Active arterial bleeding (IA)	12	90	15–30
Nonbleeding visible vessel (IIA)	22	50	15–30
Adherent clot (IIB)	10	33	0–5
Oozing without stigmata (IB)	14	10–14[b]	0–5
Flat spot (IIC)	10	10–25[b]	0
Clean base (III)	32	3	N/A

[a]Reduction in bleeding risk is without the administration of a PPI.
[b]The risk depends on whether arterial blood flow is detected before endoscopic hemostasis.[111,112]
N/A, Not applicable.

Adherent Clots

An *adherent clot* is generally defined as a blood clot over an ulcer that is resistant to several minutes of vigorous target jet water irrigation. The rebleeding rate for ulcers with an adherent clot treated with medical therapy alone is 8%–35%, with most large studies reporting rebleeding rates of 30%–35%.[126–129] Randomized controlled studies have shown that endoscopic treatment of an adherent clot can decrease the rebleeding rate to less than 5% (see Table 21.5). In DEP studies (see earlier), adherent clot has been reported to have underlying arterial blood flow in 69% of ulcer patients, indicating an increased risk of rebleeding if not treated endoscopically.[105,110] A meta-analysis has found that endoscopic therapy is superior to medical therapy for preventing recurrent bleeding from peptic ulcers with an adherent clot, but with no differences in the need for surgery, duration of hospitalization, number of transfusions, or mortality rate.[130] These studies were performed prior to the widespread use of PPIs, which also decrease rates of rebleeding (see earlier).

Clean-Based Ulcers

Patients with a clean-based ulcer at endoscopy after target irrigation have a rebleeding rate of less than 5%. Laine et al. found no difference in outcomes between patients who immediately resumed eating and those who waited several days before they resumed eating after a UGIB.[131] Longstreth and Feitelberg showed that selected low-risk patients with clinically mild UGIBs and clean-based ulcers can be discharged safely to home, with a significant saving in cost.[10,11]

Techniques for Endoscopic Hemostasis

The goals of endoscopic hemostasis are control of active bleeding and prevention of rebleeding. Since the 1980s the standard approach has been based on treating SRH; however, with the DEP, some investigators have reported an additional goal of

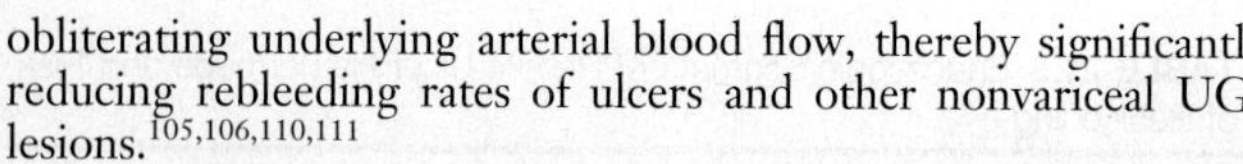

obliterating underlying arterial blood flow, thereby significantly reducing rebleeding rates of ulcers and other nonvariceal UGI lesions.[105,106,110,111]

Active Arterial Bleeding

The standard visually guided technique used at UCLA CURE for actively spurting ulcer bleeding (Forrest IA) is to inject 0.5–1-mL aliquots of epinephrine (1:20,000) via a sclerotherapy needle into 4 quadrants of the ulcer within 1–2 mm of the bleeding site (Table 21.6). When combination therapy is performed, coagulation is performed with a large 10 Fr multipolar probe. After epinephrine injection, the thermal probe is placed directly on the bleeding site to tamponade the site and stop the bleeding, and coagulation is applied with long (10-second) pulses and firm pressure at a low (12–15 W) power setting (Fig. 21.10). The probe is then removed slowly from the ulcer (sometimes with gentle irrigation to prevent pulling coagulated tissue), and thermal coagulation is repeated as required to stop bleeding and flatten any underlying visible vessel. Epinephrine injection can be repeated if bleeding persists. With successful endoscopic hemostasis, the rebleeding rate can be decreased to 30% with monotherapy and 15% with combination therapy (see Table 21.5). Alternatively, injection of epinephrine followed by hemoclip placement directly across the actively bleeding site can also be effective. Some investigators recommend that clips be placed prior to injection of epinephrine to allow placement of the clip directly on the vessel rather than on a submucosal epinephrine-filled cushion. The initial goal with DEP guidance is to trace the direction of the artery. The CURE Hemostasis Group now first interrogates the ulcer base to determine the direction and location of the underlying artery, injects epinephrine to reduce arterial flow, and then coagulates or places hemoclips on top of the bleeding point to stop the bleeding and on either side along the artery to seal it and prevent rebleeding (see Fig. 21.7B). Rebleeding rates are further reduced by DEP guidance and obliteration of underlying arterial blood flow.[105,106]

Nonbleeding Visible Vessel

In contrast to active arterial bleeding, no significant difference in results between thermal therapy alone and combination thermal and epinephrine injection therapy is seen with NBVVs (Forrest IIA). We use the same technique as that used to stop active bleeding: flattening of visible vessels using a large probe, firm pressure, and a low-power setting (Fig. 21.11). Hemoclipping can also be effective for preventing rebleeding from an NBVV if the clip is placed across the NBVV and a high-dose PPI is administered intravenously for 72 hours (Fig. 21.12).[87,132] With successful endoscopic hemostasis, the rebleeding rate can be reduced to 30% with injection alone and 10%–15% with thermal coagulation, hemoclipping, or combination therapy (see Table 21.5).

Adherent Clot

For standard, visually guided hemostasis, our recommendations for treating an adherent clot on an ulcer (Forrest IIB) are to inject epinephrine (1:20,000) in 1-mL increments in 4 quadrants around the pedicle of the clot and then use a rotatable cold snare to guillotine the clot piecemeal, without pulling it off the base, until an underlying stigma of hemorrhage is identified in the ulcer base or a 3 mm or smaller clot pedicle is left. Coagulation or hemoclipping is performed if active bleeding, a visible vessel, or residual pedicle is seen (Fig. 21.13). The combination technique decreases the rebleeding rate from up to 35% (with medical therapy alone) to 5%. Adherent clots are considered a high-risk stigma, and administration of a high-dose PPI is recommended after endoscopic hemostasis.[129,130] More recently, we recommend DEP interrogation of the clot near the pedicle before injection of epinephrine—69% have underlying arterial flow.[105,110] DEP is

TABLE 21.6 Endoscopic Technical Parameters for Using Multipolar Electrocoagulation in the Treatment of Bleeding Lesions

	Peptic Ulcer							
	Active Bleeding	**Nonbleeding Visible Vessel**	**Adherent Clot**	**Mallory-Weiss Tear**	**Dieulafoy Lesion**	**Gastric Angioectasia**	**Colon Diverticulum with Visible Vessel**	**Colon Angioectasia**
Epinephrine injection	Yes[a]	No	Yes[b]	May be	Yes	No	May be[c]	No
Probe size[d]	Large	Large	Large	Large or small	Large	Large	Large or small	Large or small
Pressure[e]	Firm	Firm	Firm	Moderate	Firm	Light	Light	Light
Power setting (W)[f]	12–15	12–15	12–15	10–15	10–15	10–15	10–15	10–15
Pulse duration (second)	8–10	8–10	8–10	4	8–10	2	2	2
End point	Bleeding stops	Flat vessel	Flat spot	Bleeding stops	Flat vessel	White	Flat vessel	White

[a]Epinephrine (1:20,000) injected in 1-mL aliquots into each of 4 quadrants should be used to control bleeding initially, followed by coagulation.
[b]Epinephrine (1:20,000) injected in 1-mL aliquots into each of 4 quadrants should be injected around clot initially, followed by piecemeal snare resection of the clot and treatment of underlying stigmata.
[c]Colonic diverticulum with active bleeding can be treated with epinephrine (1:20,000) injected into the neck or base. If a visible vessel is seen at the neck, it can be treated with multipolar electrocoagulation.
[d]Large probe is 10 Fr (3.2 mm diameter) and fits through a 3.8-mm endoscope channel. Small probe is 7 Fr (2.4 mm) and fits through a 2.8-mm endoscope channel.
[e]Pressure is the tamponade pressure exerted en face or tangentially via the contact probe directly on the lesion.
[f]Power setting using BICAP II generator. Power settings are general guidelines and may vary based on the generator used.
These guidelines from UCLA CURE have been derived from experimental and randomized endoscopic studies. Power, pressure, and duration settings must be reduced for small, acute, or deep bleeding lesions. *CURE*, Center for Ulcer Research and Education; *UCLA*, University of California, Los Angeles; *W*, watts.

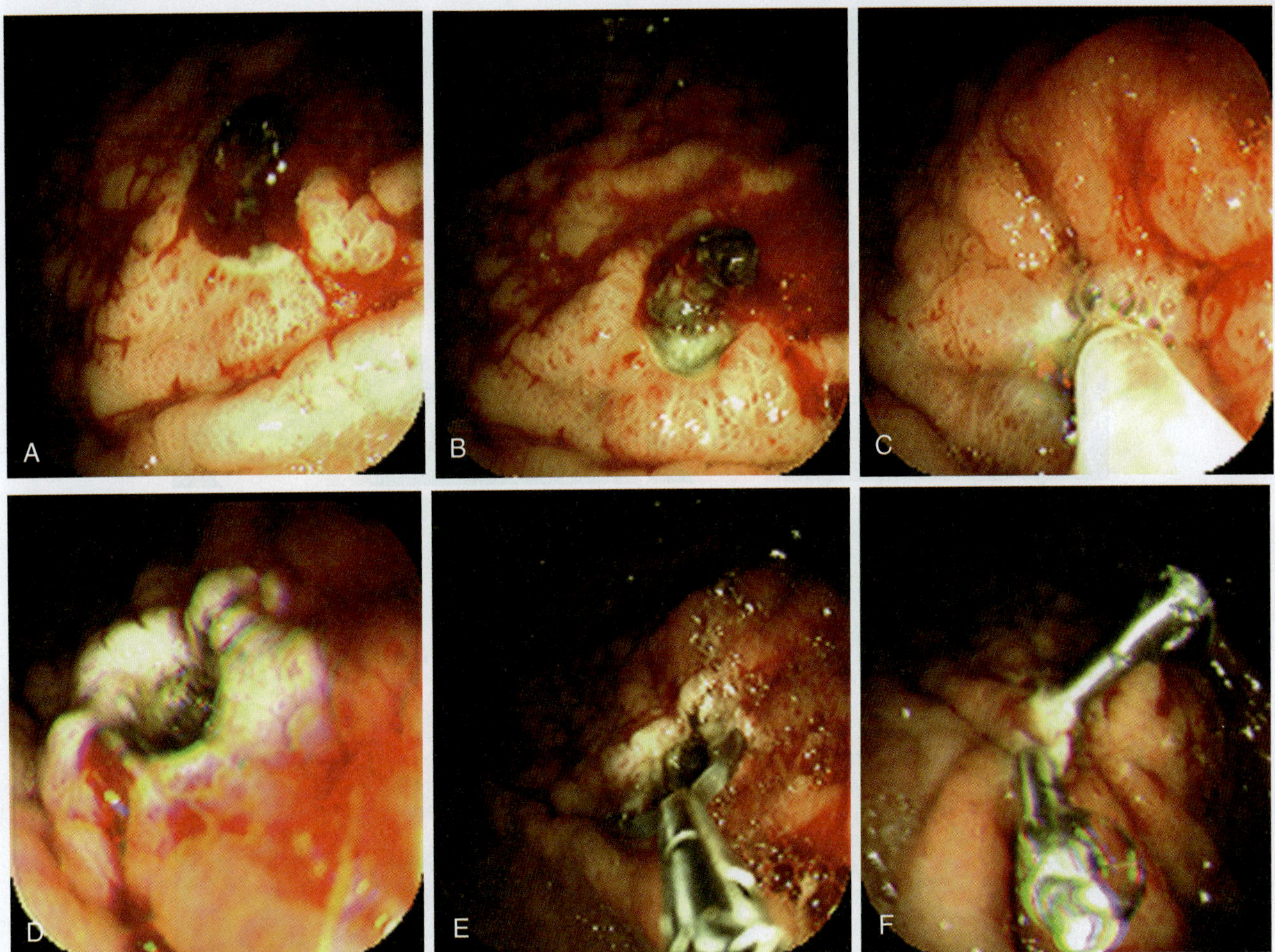

Fig. 21.10 An actively bleeding gastric ulcer treated with a combination of epinephrine injection, multipolar electrocoagulation, and hemoclip placement. (A) Clot with oozing of blood is seen. (B) After injection of epinephrine, oozing has subsided; the edge of the ulcer is seen inferior to clot. (C) Multipolar electrocoagulation is applied with a probe. (D) Appearance of the ulcer after electrocoagulation; some oozing is noted at the 7 o'clock position at the crater's edge. (E) A single hemoclip has been applied; bleeding has ceased entirely. (F) A second hemoclip has been applied.

repeated after hemostasis to ensure the absence of arterial flow and a low risk of rebleeding.

Oozing of Blood From an Ulcer Without Other Stigmata

Minor bleeding from the edge or base of an ulcer (without other stigmata) that continues despite water irrigation and observation (Forrest IB) suggests the need for endoscopic treatment. The rebleeding rate for ulcers with persistent oozing treated medically varies from 10% (UCLA CURE) to 27% (Hong Kong). Monotherapy with a thermal probe or epinephrine injection reduces the rebleeding rate to less than 5%. In patients with oozing, the bleeding arteries may be small, and the outcomes are better than those in patients with active arterial bleeding.[105,133] Patients with oozing and no other stigma of hemorrhage (e.g., a clot or NBVV) can be treated effectively with epinephrine injection alone because there is no added benefit to combination therapy.[133] After successful endoscopic hemostasis, patients with oozing and no other stigma do not benefit from administration of a high-dose PPI.[133] With DEP guidance, underlying arterial flow was detected in 46% of oozing ulcers, and hemostasis was achieved with an MPEC probe or hemoclips; none had residual blood flow, and after treatment with oral PPIs twice daily, none rebled.[105] Oozing ulcers should be considered to have an intermediate risk of rebleeding.[105,106,110,111,134]

Flat Spots

In the past, patients with flat spots in ulcers (Forrest IIC) were considered at low risk for rebleeding, and endoscopic hemostasis was not recommended; however, in studies with DEP, 40%–49% of ulcers with flat spots had underlying arterial blood flow. When those with a positive DEP for blood flow were not treated endoscopically and managed medically, half rebled.[110] Similar to oozing bleeding (Forrest 1A), we now classify patients with flat spots (Forrest IIC) as having an intermediate risk of rebleeding.[105,110,134] Epinephrine injection alone only transiently reduced arterial blood flow. When DEP is positive, either MPEC or hemoclips are recommended to obliterate underlying arterial blood flow and to prevent rebleeding.[110]

Clean-Based Ulcers

Patients with a clean-based ulcer (Forrest III) at endoscopy have a rebleeding rate of less than 5% and do not require endoscopic therapy. If the patient has a clean-based gastric ulcer, biopsies of the ulcer edge and gastric muscosa should be considered to exclude underlying malignancy (see Chapter 56). These patients can be fed after the endoscopy and treated with oral acid suppression medication; they do not require continued hospitalization unless indicated for other medical problems.

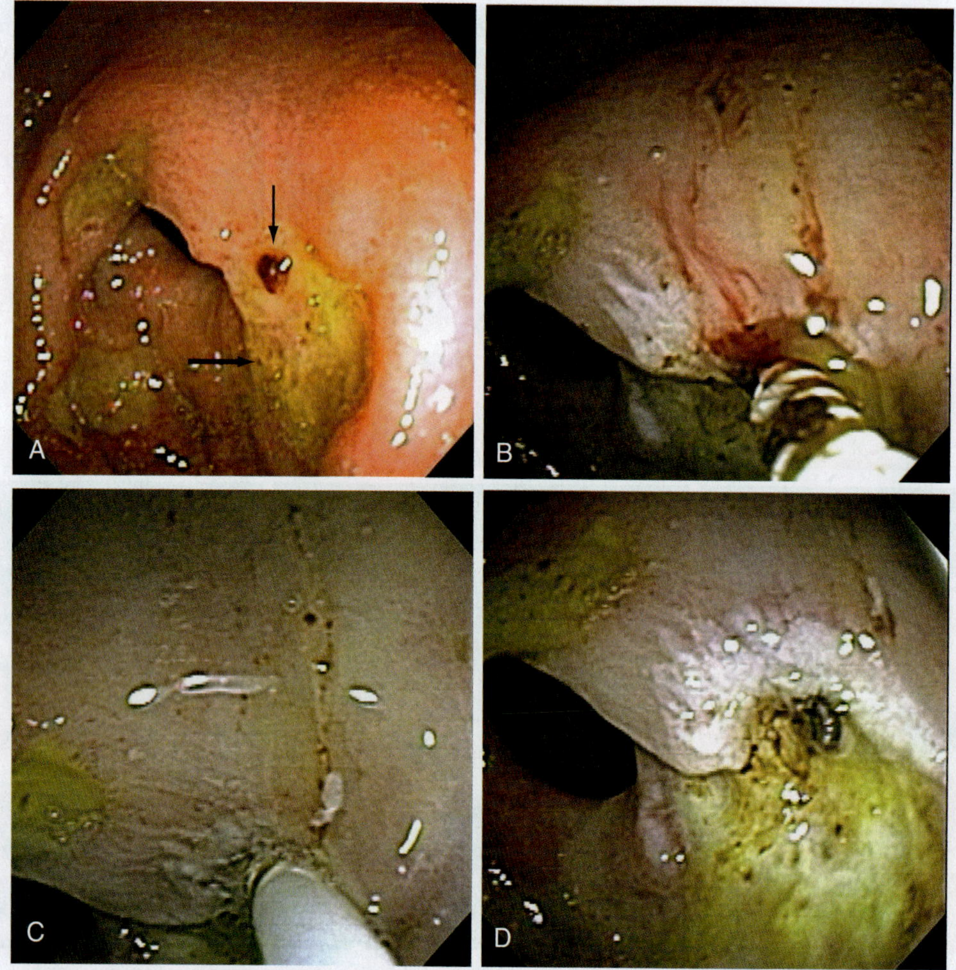

Fig. 21.11 (A) Epinephrine injection and multipolar electrocoagulation for hemostasis of a chronic gastric ulcer (*thick arrow*) with a nonbleeding visible vessel (*thin arrow*). (B) The nonbleeding visible vessel is injected with epinephrine, after which blanching and swelling of surrounding mucosa occur. (Note that epinephrine injection for a nonbleeding visible vessel is not recommended in Table 21.6.) (C) A multipolar electrocoagulation probe is applied with firm pressure and coagulation. (D) After completion of treatment, the visible vessel has been coagulated and flattened.

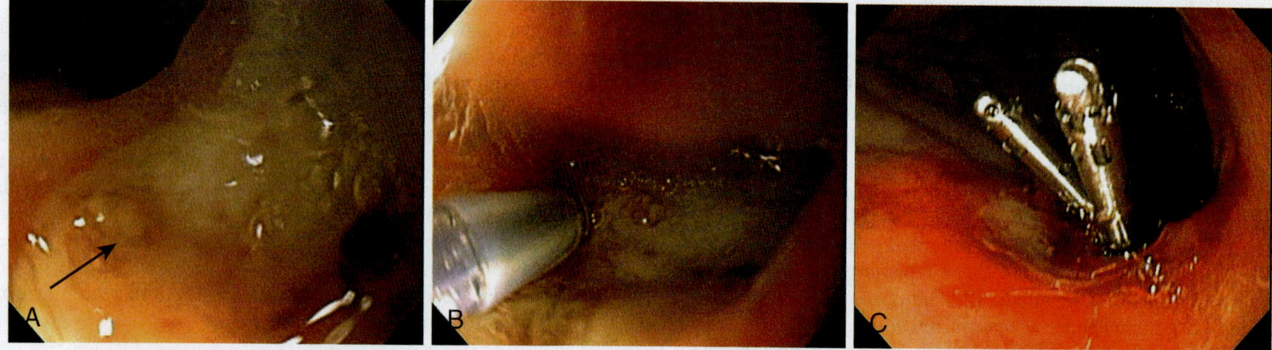

Fig. 21.12 (A) Gastric ulcer with a nonbleeding visible vessel (*arrow*) treated by endoscopy with epinephrine injection (B) and hemoclip placement (C). Note that epinephrine injection of a nonbleeding visible vessel is not recommended in Table 21.6.

Newer Endoscopic Techniques

Hemospray

Hemospray has been reported to stop active bleeding both from nonvariceal UGI lesions, varices, and tumors, but hemospray does not treat underlying arterial or variceal blood flow. Therefore the risk of rebleeding is high, and definitive hemostasis with standard techniques is usually required in patients with varices or ulcers with major stigmata. Current guidelines recommend utilization of hemospray as a stopgap or adjunct technique.[115] Further studies,

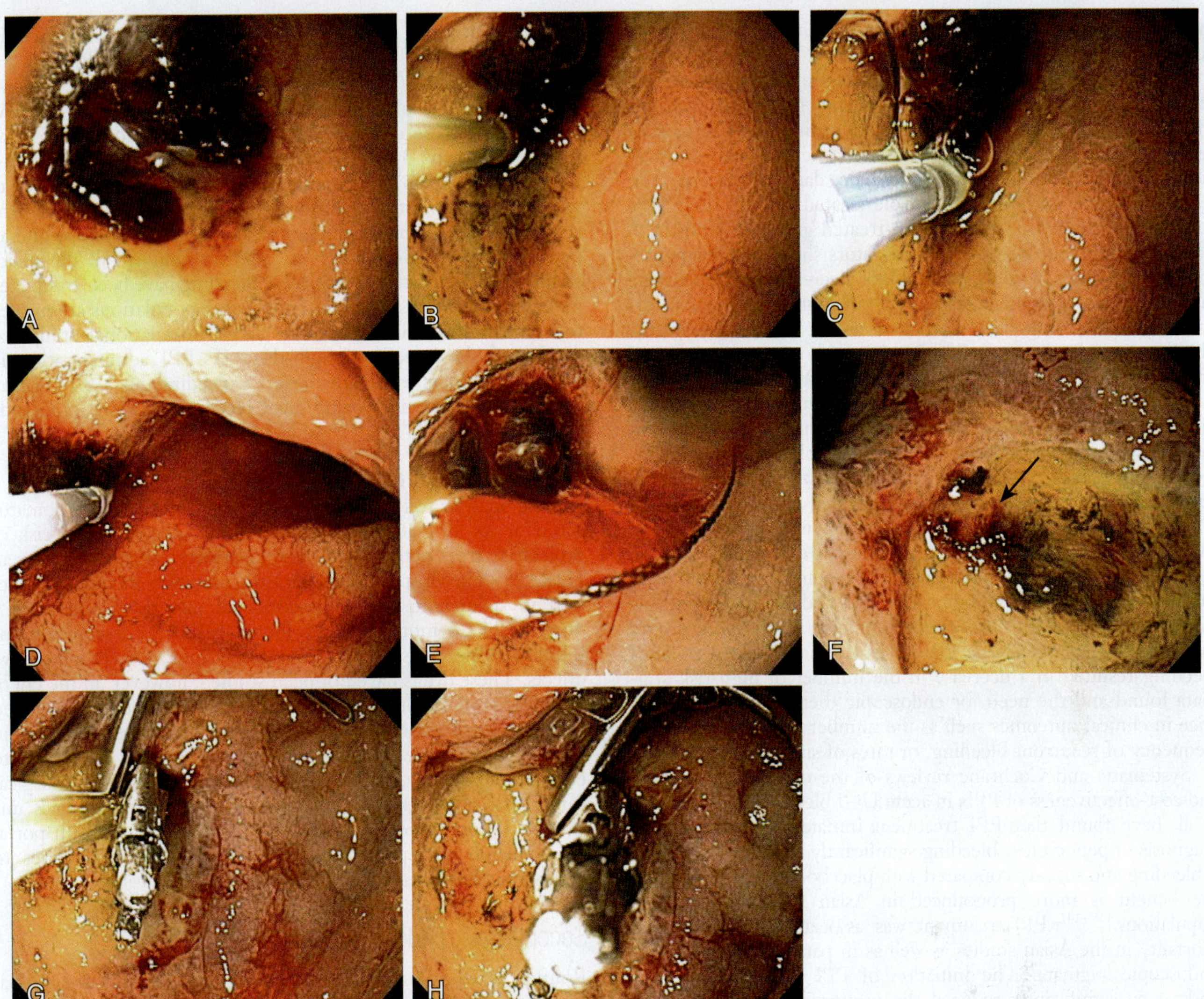

Fig. 21.13 (A) Endoscopic treatment of a duodenal ulcer with an adherent clot. (B) The clot was injected with epinephrine, followed by piecemeal snare polypectomy to trim away the clot (C–E), after which an underlying vessel was revealed [F (*arrow*)]. (G and H) Two endoscopic hemoclips were placed across the visible vessel.

including randomized controlled trials, are required to determine the efficacy and role of hemospray in the clinical management of GI bleeding.

Over-the-Scope Hemoclip

A large over-the-scope (OTSC) hemoclip (OVESCO Endoscopy AG, Tübingen, Germany) has been reported in a randomized controlled trial to significantly reduce rebleeding rates compared with standard hemostasis in patients with recurrent ulcer bleeding. Case series have also reported good results using the OTSC hemoclip as primary treatment, but no randomized controlled trials of ulcer bleeding have been reported to demonstrate whether OTSC hemoclipping is superior to standard hemostasis as initial therapy. We have documented that, when successfully applied, OTSC hemoclipping more effectively obliterates underlying arterial blood flow in the peptic ulcer base with high-risk SRH than standard hemostasis with through-the-scope hemoclips or MPEC.

Testing for Hp Infection

In a patient with a bleeding gastric or duodenal ulcer, endoscopic mucosal biopsy specimens of the normal-appearing antrum and mid-body greater curvature should be obtained to assess for the presence of Hp infection. Biopsy specimens can be obtained safely after successful endoscopic hemostasis, but bleeding reduces the sensitivity of rapid urease testing. Therefore stool antigen and other tests for Hp infection are recommended (see Chapter 52).

Pharmacologic Therapy

Acid Suppression Medication

In vitro studies have shown that a luminal gastric pH higher than 6.8 is required for normal clotting function (platelet aggregation and fibrin formation) and that a pH less than 5.4 almost abolishes platelet aggregation and plasma coagulation.[135] Platelet aggregates lyse at an acidic pH, an effect that is enhanced by the presence of pepsin; thus, reducing the risk of acute bleeding and rebleeding from a peptic ulcer is theoretically possible by maintaining a gastric pH higher than 6. IV H2RAs can raise the intragastric pH acutely, but tolerance to these agents develops rapidly, and the pH usually returns to 3–5 within 24 hours. Several studies have shown that in normal subjects, IV administration of a PPI can consistently keep the gastric pH higher than four (and often higher than 6) over a 72-hour infusion.[136,137] Trials of IV H2RAs for the prevention of recurrent ulcer bleeding have shown no definite benefit.[138,139]

Several studies have shown that PPIs are effective in reducing rebleeding rates from peptic ulcer. In a study from India, patients with endoscopic high-risk SRH (active bleeding, NBVV, clot, or oozing) who did not undergo endoscopic hemostasis were randomized to omeprazole, 40 mg orally twice daily, or placebo. The rebleeding rate in the omeprazole-treated group was 11% compared with 36% in the placebo-treated group ($P < .001$).[140] Another study from the same investigators showed that omeprazole, 40 mg orally twice daily for 5 days, decreased the rebleeding rate after endoscopic hemostasis with injection therapy for ulcers with active bleeding, an NBVV, or a clot from 21% in the placebo-treated group to 7% in the oral omeprazole-treated group ($P = .02$).[141] In a study from Hong Kong, patients who had undergone successful endoscopic hemostasis for active bleeding or an NBVV were randomized to high-dose IV omeprazole, 80-mg bolus followed by 8 mg/h or placebo. The 30-day rebleeding rate was 6.7% in the omeprazole-treated group, compared with 22.5% in the placebo-treated group ($P < .05$).[142] The same investigators from Hong Kong found that the 30-day rebleeding rate in patients with an adherent clot or NBVV who received IV omeprazole alone was 12%, compared with 1% in those who received IV omeprazole and underwent endoscopic hemostasis ($P < .05$).[143] Another study from Hong Kong found that starting IV omeprazole before EGD in patients with UGI bleeding resulted in a decrease in the number of high-risk stigmata found and the need for endoscopic therapy, but no difference in clinical outcomes such as the number of units transfused, frequency of recurrent bleeding, or rates of surgery and death.[144]

Systematic and Cochrane reviews of the clinical effectiveness and cost-effectiveness of PPIs in acute UGI bleeding by Leontiadis et al. have found that PPI treatment initiated after endoscopic diagnosis of peptic ulcer bleeding significantly reduces the rates of rebleeding and surgery compared with placebo or H2RAs and that the benefit is more pronounced in Asian than in non-Asian populations.[145–147] PPI treatment was associated with decreased mortality in the Asian studies as well as in patients with high-risk endoscopic stigmata. The initiation of PPI treatment prior to endoscopy significantly reduced the proportion of patients with SRH at index endoscopy compared with placebo or H2RAs but did not reduce the rate of mortality, rebleeding, or surgery.

Caution is advised in generalizing the results of PPI trials in Asian patients with peptic ulcer hemorrhage to heterogeneous non-Asian populations. Asian patients are generally more responsive than heterogeneous populations or whites to PPIs.[148] Asian patients have a smaller average parietal cell mass, are slower metabolizers of PPIs, and often have Hp infection, all of which increase the effectiveness of PPIs. These factors may explain the lower mortality rates in Asians compared with non-Asians in meta-analyses of trials of PPI therapy for peptic ulcer hemorrhage.

Whether a PPI should be given before or after EGD is uncertain. Although some small randomized studies have not shown that preendoscopy administration of a PPI improves clinical outcomes (although the number of high-risk stigmata that require treatment is reduced), most modeling studies have suggested that preendoscopy administration of a PPI is cost-effective.[16,18,19,144,147] The optimal effective PPI dose after endoscopic hemostasis is uncertain, with a meta-analysis finding no difference between high-dose IV continuous infusion of a PPI (80 mg bolus followed by 8 mg/h for 3 days) and nonhigh-dose intermittent or oral administration (for 3 days).[149] Whether oral administration is as effective as IV administration of a PPI is unclear, although studies have shown that high-dose oral administration (e.g., omeprazole, 40 mg twice daily) reduces rebleeding to rates that would be expected from endoscopic hemostasis. In fact, the increase in intragastric pH with high-dose oral PPI administration is almost identical (although delayed by 1 hour) to that with IV PPI administration.[139,150] Whether IV administration of a PPI alone is sufficient therapy (without endoscopic hemostasis) in patients with recent UGI bleeding and some SRH, such as an NBVV, oozing, or clot, is controversial. In an Asian study, Sung et al. reported that the 30-day rebleeding rate with IV PPI administration alone (12%) was similar to that in previous studies of endoscopic hemostasis, although they also found that the rebleeding rate with a combination of endoscopic therapy and an IV PPI was even lower (1%).[151] Because almost all the major studies of PPIs in acute peptic ulcer bleeding have been conducted in Asian populations, studies in non-Asian populations are needed to confirm the Asian data. One large international study has confirmed the benefit of high-dose IV PPI administration in high-risk patients with active arterial bleeding, an NBVV, or an adherent clot, but not oozing ulcer bleeding, in a predominantly white population.[134,152]

Somatostatin and Octreotide

A meta-analysis has suggested that IV administration of somatostatin or its long-acting form, octreotide, decreases the risk of rebleeding from peptic ulcers when compared with placebo or an H2RA.[153] The proposed mechanisms of action include a reduction in splanchnic and gastroduodenal mucosal blood flow, a decrease in GI motility, inhibition of gastric acid secretion, inhibition of pepsin secretion, and gastric mucosal cytoprotective effects. These drugs have not been studied, however, in the era of endoscopic or PPI therapy and, therefore, cannot be considered for routine use.[154] Somatostatin or octreotide can be considered in patients with severe ongoing bleeding who are not responsive to endoscopic therapy, an IV PPI, or both, and are not surgical candidates, although their effectiveness in these patients is uncertain. IV octreotide may also be useful in patients with portal hypertension and peptic ulcer hemorrhage as an adjunct to endoscopic hemostasis and a PPI (see Chapter 94).

Second-Look Endoscopy

Routine repeat, or second-look, endoscopy 24 hours after initial endoscopic hemostasis, with additional endoscopic hemostasis if persistent high-risk endoscopic stigmata are found, has been proposed to improve patient outcomes. A meta-analysis of four prospective randomized trials of patients with PUD and high-risk endoscopic stigmata revealed that second-look endoscopy reduced the rates of rebleeding and surgery but not mortality; however, the only trial in which high-dose PPI therapy was administered to patients showed no benefit to second-look endoscopy, and most trials did not use what has become standard-of-care endoscopic hemostasis techniques.[155] Therefore routine second-look endoscopy is not recommended for most patients with peptic ulcer bleeding,[113] except in those in whom the initial endoscopic examination was suboptimal because excessive blood obscured the view, technical problems with hemostasis occurred, clinically significant bleeding recurred, or less effective endoscopic techniques, such as epinephrine injection alone, were used.

Rebleeding After Endoscopic Treatment

The risk of rebleeding from peptic ulcers, which started bleeding in the outpatient setting and required endoscopic hemostasis, is greatest in the first 72 hours after diagnosis and treatment. Patients should be kept on a PPI in high doses for at least 72 hours following endoscopic hemostasis, after which they can be switched to a standard dose. Before the widespread use of IV PPIs, the rebleeding rate after endoscopic hemostasis of actively bleeding ulcers or those with an NBVV was as high as 30%; with the use of PPIs and improved endoscopic techniques, the rate is less than 10% in most studies.

TABLE 21.7 Comparison of the Onset of Peptic Ulcer Bleeding in Outpatients Versus Inpatients

	Onset	
Parameter	**Outpatient**	**Inpatient**
Frequency (%)	80–90	10–20
American Society of Anesthesiologists Physical Status score[a]	≤3	>3
Time to rebleeding (%)		
≤72 hours	70–80	40–50
4–7 days	10–15	15–20
8–30 days	1–5	15–20
>30 days	0	5–10

[a]One point signifies a healthy person; 5 points signifies high likelihood of mortality within 24 hours.
CURE, Center for Ulcer Research and Education; *UCLA*, University of California, Los Angeles.
Data from the UCLA CURE database.

The difference between ulcer hemorrhage that starts in the outpatient setting and hemorrhage that starts in the inpatient setting is substantial (Table 21.7). Owing to the fact that the time to rebleeding can be much longer for inpatient (than outpatient) ulcer hemorrhage and the risk of rebleeding is high, combination endoscopic hemostasis and high-dose IV PPI administration for more than 72 hours should be considered. Further studies are warranted in this high-risk group to define optimal management.

If rebleeding from a peptic ulcer is severe, an urgent repeat EGD (rather than immediate surgery) should be performed. A large, well-designed, randomized trial from Hong Kong found that when endoscopic hemostasis is repeated in patients with hemodynamically significant rebleeding after initial endoscopic hemostasis, 73% of patients achieve sustained hemostasis and do not require surgery.[156] The overall mortality rate was the same in those who achieved and those who did not achieve hemostasis, but the rate of serious complications was significantly higher in the latter group (who required surgery). Factors that predicted failure of endoscopic retreatment included an ulcer size of at least 2 cm and hypotension on initial presentation.

Angiography, Surgery, and Over-the-Scope Hemoclips

Patients with recurrent bleeding despite two sessions of endoscopic hemostasis can be considered for angiographic embolization or surgical therapy. Several retrospective series have reported no significant differences between angiography with embolization and surgery in rates of rebleeding and mortality, despite the older age and more serious medical problems of patients treated by angiography.[157,158] These studies suggest that angiography can be considered after failure of endoscopic therapy. If embolization therapy does not control the bleeding, surgery remains an option.

A randomized controlled trial has suggested that OTSC hemoclipping for recurrent peptic ulcer bleeding was more effective than standard endoscopic hemostasis (mostly by hemoclipping). This new treatment has the potential to reduce the need for surgery or angiography for recurrent ulcer bleeding. OTSC hemoclipping is also more effective than standard hemostasis in eradicating underlying arterial blood flow, which, when present, correlates with a risk of rebleeding.[105,110] Immediate surgical intervention is indicated for patients who have exsanguinating bleeding and those who cannot be medically resuscitated. Surgery should also be considered if the endoscopist does not feel comfortable treating a large or pulsating visible vessel (e.g., one in a deep, posterior duodenal ulcer that may represent the gastroduodenal artery) or if a bleeding malignant ulcerated mass is found on endoscopy.

Immediate Postendoscopic Management

High-Risk Endoscopic Stigmata

Patients who have undergone endoscopic hemostasis for active arterial bleeding, an NBVV, or an adherent clot should be observed in the hospital for 72 hours while they receive high-dose IV infusions of a PPI. After successful endoscopic treatment and recovery from sedation, the patient can be started on a liquid diet, with subsequent advancement of the diet. For patients who have been on and need to continue antiplatelet agents or an anticoagulant, a cardiologist or vascular physician should be consulted to help determine whether, and for how long, these agents can be held.[115,159] For patients with severe atherosclerotic cardiovascular disease who require aspirin, however, a dose of 81 mg/day should be started within 7 days.

Intermediate-Risk Stigmata

Patients with flat spots and arterial blood flow detected underneath, those with oozing bleeding from an ulcer and no other stigmata (e.g., spurting, NBVV, and clot), and those with severe comorbidity or shock on presentation should undergo endoscopic hemostasis. Initiation of a twice daily oral PPI and observation in the hospital for 24–48 hours after successful endoscopic hemostasis are recommended. Such patients do not benefit from high-dose IV PPIs after successful endoscopic hemostasis.[105,134]

Low-Risk Endoscopic Stigmata

Patients with a clean-based ulcer or flat spot with no arterial blood flow detected in the ulcer base can generally resume a normal diet immediately, begin an oral PPI once daily, and be discharged early after endoscopy when stable.[131] These patients can often avoid hospitalization entirely or be discharged early.[10,11,74,160] Generally, they are young and hemodynamically stable with no severe coexisting medical illnesses, a hemoglobin level higher than 10 mg/dL, normal coagulation parameters, and good social support systems at home in case bleeding recurs.

Prevention of Recurrent Ulcer Bleeding

Hp Infection

All patients with peptic ulcer bleeding should be tested for Hp infection (see earlier) and, if the result is positive, should receive standard therapy for Hp infection (see Chapter 54).[88] One caveat is that bleeding can lead to a false-negative rapid urease test result, and the patient may need to undergo an alternative method of testing for Hp in this setting. Antibiotic therapy does not have to be started immediately and can be initiated on an outpatient basis when the patient has resumed a normal diet. In patients who are found to have an Hp-induced ulcer, the confirmation of the eradication of Hp after treatment is strongly recommended (see Chapter 54).

Aspirin, Other NSAIDs, and Antiplatelet Drugs

Ideally, patients with ulcer bleeding caused by aspirin or another nonselective NSAID should stop the drug. If the patient is also positive for Hp, the organism should be eradicated with standard therapy (see Chapter 52).[161] In patients with a history of ulcer bleeding who are positive for Hp and need to continue taking low-dose aspirin (81 mg daily), eradication of Hp alone results in ulcer rebleeding rates similar to those associated with daily PPI therapy (if Hp is not eradicated).[162] By contrast, in patients with a history of ulcer bleeding who are positive for Hp and need to continue full-dose NSAID therapy, eradication of Hp alone without a PPI leads to a significantly higher rebleeding rate than use of a daily PPI in conjunction with the NSAID. In patients with ulcer bleeding who do not have Hp infection but who need to continue daily aspirin, cotherapy with a daily PPI significantly reduces the rebleeding rate compared with placebo.[163] Patients who require an antiplatelet medication, such as clopidogrel, and have a history of ulcer bleeding will have less chance of recurrent bleeding if they take aspirin (81 mg) and a PPI daily compared with taking clopidogrel alone.[164]

Patients who require an NSAID after an ulcer bleed may be considered for a selective COX-2 inhibitor. Selective COX-2 inhibitors cause fewer ulcers than nonselective NSAIDs but are associated with a greater rate of cardiovascular complications. Because selective COX-2 inhibitors result in rebleeding rates similar to those associated with a nonselective NSAID and PPI cotherapy, their use may not be worth the increased cardiovascular risk.[165]

Repeat Endoscopy to Confirm Gastric Ulcer Healing

Repeat EGD should be considered in patients with a gastric ulcer after 6–10 weeks of acid suppressive therapy to confirm healing of the ulcer and absence of malignancy (see Chapters 54 and 55). In areas of the world where the population is at intermediate risk for gastric cancer, 2%–4% of repeat upper endoscopies to confirm ulcer healing have been reported to disclose gastric cancer.[166–168] Some experts have suggested that when the index endoscopy with biopsies is negative for malignancy and the ulcer appears benign endoscopically, a follow-up endoscopy is unnecessary.[169] A small retrospective study has found that when gastric cancer is detected on repeat endoscopy to evaluate gastric ulcer healing, survival is no better than that for patients who did not undergo the recommended follow-up endoscopy.[170]

Other Nonvariceal Causes

Esophagitis

Patients with severe erosive esophagitis can present with hematemesis or melena. A multivariate analysis from a center in France, in which 8% of all UGI bleeding was caused by erosive esophagitis, found that independent risk factors for bleeding esophagitis were grade 3 or 4 (moderate to severe) esophagitis by the Savary-Miller grading system (see Chapter 48), cirrhosis, a poor performance status, and anticoagulant therapy.[170] A history of heartburn was obtained in only 38% of patients. Severe bleeding from gastroesophageal reflux-induced esophagitis is treated medically with a PPI (see Chapter 48). EGD is essential for diagnosing severe erosive esophagitis, but endoscopic therapy generally has no role unless a focal ulcer with an SRH is found. These patients should be treated with a daily PPI for 8–12 weeks and undergo repeat endoscopy to exclude underlying Barrett's esophagus (see Chapter 49).

Patients can sometimes present with mild UGI bleeding from esophagitis not related to GERD but to infections (e.g., *Candida*, HSV, and CMV) or pill-induced esophagitis. Endoscopy with biopsies and brushings is critical for making these diagnoses and determining the appropriate pharmacologic therapy (see Chapter 47).

Ulcer Hemorrhage in Hospitalized Patients

Hemorrhage from an ulcer or erosions in hospitalized patients typically falls into two categories. The classic cause is stress-related mucosal injury (SRMI or stress ulcers), characterized by diffuse bleeding from erosions and superficial ulcers. The second category is inpatient ulcers, which are large, focal, chronic-appearing ulcers that are painless and present with severe UGI hemorrhage manifested by hematochezia, melena, or bloody emesis. On emergency endoscopy, focal inpatient ulcers are often actively bleeding or demonstrate a visible vessel or adherent clot and are marked by high rebleeding rates, despite combination endoscopic therapy, and delayed healing on a high-dose PPI.

SRMI occurs in the UGI tract of severely ill inpatients in an ICU and is likely caused by a combination of decreased mucosal protection and mucosal ischemia. SRMI usually occurs in the stomach but can also be seen in the duodenum, esophagus, and even rectum. Diffuse oozing is common, and patients have a poor prognosis and high rebleeding rate, often related to impaired wound healing and multiple organ failure.

Bleeding from SRMI is now uncommon, with a frequency of approximately 1.5% of patients in an ICU. The two main risk factors are severe coagulopathy and mechanical ventilation for longer than 48 hours.[171] The frequency of clinically significant GI bleeding with either or both of these risk factors is 3.7%, compared with 0.1% when neither risk factor is present. Other proposed risk factors include a history of UGI bleeding, sepsis, an ICU admission longer than 7 days, occult GI bleeding for more than 5 days, and treatment with high-dose glucocorticoids.

ICU patients with risk factors for bleeding are the main target groups for pharmacologic prevention of bleeding SRMI. Therapy with an H2RA has been shown to decrease the rate of clinically significant bleeding in ICU patients at high risk of SRMI.[172] One large multicenter study found that prophylactic treatment with oral omeprazole or IV cimetidine results in similar bleeding rates, but that omeprazole is more effective than cimetidine in maintaining the luminal gastric pH above 4.[173] A potential harmful effect of gastric acid suppression to prevent stress ulcers is proliferation of bacteria in the stomach secondary to the increased gastric pH and the associated risk of aspiration and ventilator-associated pneumonia; however, randomized trials in which acid suppression (with an H2RA or antacids) and sucralfate (which does not lower gastric pH) were compared have not shown convincingly that raising gastric pH increases the risk of pneumonia.[174,175]

Generally, if a patient with SRMI or an inpatient ulcer is supported hemodynamically and medically, the lesion will heal as the patient's overall medical status improves. Because SRMI is diffuse, endoscopic therapy is generally not feasible. By contrast, focal inpatient ulcer hemorrhage often requires endoscopic hemostasis for severe hemorrhage (see Fig. 21.9); however, rebleeding rates are higher and healing is slower than in patients in whom bleeding starts before hospitalization (see Table 21.7).[176,177] A study in which epinephrine injection plus hemoclip placement was compared with epinephrine injection plus MPEC in a cohort of patients who had a high frequency of in-hospital ulcers found a significantly lower rebleeding rate in the group that underwent injection and hemoclip placement.[132]

Dieulafoy Lesion

A Dieulafoy lesion is a large (1–3 mm) submucosal artery that protrudes through the mucosa, is not associated with a peptic ulcer, and can cause massive bleeding. It is usually located in the gastric fundus, within 6 cm of the gastroesophageal junction, although lesions in the duodenum, small intestine, and colon have been reported. The cause is unknown, and congenital and acquired (related to mucosal atrophy or an arteriolar aneurysm) causes are thought to occur (see Chapter 36).

Dieulafoy lesion can be difficult to identify at endoscopy because of the intermittent nature of the bleeding; the overlying mucosa may appear normal if the lesion is not bleeding. An NBVV or adherent clot without an ulcer may be seen on endoscopy. If a massive UGIB seems to be emanating from the stomach, careful inspection of the proximal stomach should be carried out to look for a protuberance that might be a Dieulafoy lesion. DEP has been used to help identify a Dieulafoy lesion not visualized on endoscopy.[178] Owing to the difficulty of identifying the bleeding site and because rebleeding is not uncommon, we recommend that if a Dieulafoy lesion is found and treated, the site should be marked with submucosal injection of ink to tattoo the area in case of rebleeding and the need for retreatment.

Endoscopic hemostasis of a Dieulafoy lesion can be performed with injection therapy, a thermal probe, hemoclipping, OTSC hemoclipping, or rubber band ligation.[110,178–183] Large case series have reported an initial hemostasis rate of approximately 90%, with the need for surgery in 4%–16% of cases.[181] Rebleeding rates may be lower with combination therapy or OTSC hemoclipping because underlying arterial blood flow is eradicated more effectively than by injection or monotherapy.[110] Although all the endoscopic hemostasis techniques seem to be effective, perforation and delayed rebleeding have been reported after band ligation (see Chapter 40).

Mallory-Weiss Tears

Mallory-Weiss tears are mucosal or submucosal lacerations that occur at the gastroesophageal junction and usually extend distally into a hiatal hernia (Fig. 21.14). Patients generally present with hematemesis or coffee-ground emesis and a history of nonbloody vomiting followed by hematemesis, although some patients do not recall vomiting. The tear is thought to result from increased intra-abdominal pressure in combination with a shearing effect caused by negative intrathoracic pressure above the diaphragm, which is often related to vomiting. Mallory-Weiss tears have been reported in patients who vomit while taking a bowel purge before colonoscopy.[184] Endoscopy usually reveals a single tear that begins at the gastroesophageal junction and extends several millimeters distally into a hiatal hernia sac. Occasionally, more than one tear is seen. A retroflexed view in the stomach may provide better visualization than a forward view. The bleeding stigmata of Mallory-Weiss tears can include a clean base, adherent clot, NBVV, oozing, or, rarely, active spurting. Usually, the bleeding is self-limited and mild, but occasionally it can be severe, especially in patients with esophageal varices or coagulopathies. Mucosal (superficial) Mallory-Weiss tears can start healing within hours and can heal completely within 48 hours.

Although approximately 50% of patients hospitalized with UGI bleeding from a Mallory-Weiss tear receive blood transfusions, the tear manifests as mild, self-limited hematemesis in most patients, who do not seek medical care.[185] The rebleeding rate among patients hospitalized for a Mallory-Weiss tear is approximately 10%; risk factors for rebleeding include shock at presentation and active bleeding at endoscopy.[186] Owing to the risk of continued and recurrent bleeding, patients with active bleeding from a Mallory-Weiss tear should undergo endoscopic therapy, which can be performed successfully with epinephrine injection, MPEC, hemoclip placement, or band ligation. Randomized trials that compared MPEC and medical therapy with an H2RA have found that endoscopic therapy reduces the rates of rebleeding, blood transfusions, and emergency surgery.[187]

Our current endoscopic technique for treating actively bleeding Mallory-Weiss tears in patients without portal hypertension or esophageal varices is to apply endoscopic hemoclips to stop the bleeding and close the tear. If hemoclips are unavailable, epinephrine injection to slow bleeding and focal hemostasis of the bleeding site with MPEC at a low-power setting (12–14 W) and with light pressure applied for 1–2 seconds are recommended. The management of patients with esophageal varices caused by portal hypertension who have also a Mallory-Weiss tear should be targeted toward the esophageal varices, with esophageal band ligation or variceal sclerotherapy (see later and Chapter 94).

Patients with a Mallory-Weiss tear are also treated with antiemetics if they have nausea or vomiting and a PPI to accelerate mucosal healing. Long-term treatment with a PPI is not required.

Cameron Lesions

Cameron lesions are linear erosions or ulcerations in the proximal stomach at the end of a large hiatal hernia, near the diaphragmatic pinch (Fig. 21.15).[188] Cameron lesions are thought to be caused by mechanical trauma and local ischemia as the hernia moves against the diaphragm and only secondarily by acid and pepsin. They can be a source of acute UGI bleeding but more commonly may present as chronic GI bleeding and iron deficiency anemia. Cameron lesions are a common cause of obscure GI bleeding (see later) and, not uncommonly, are missed by an unsuspecting endoscopist. Endoscopic management has been reported.[189] Long-term medical management is usually with iron supplements and an oral PPI.[190,191] Surgical repair of the hiatal hernia may be

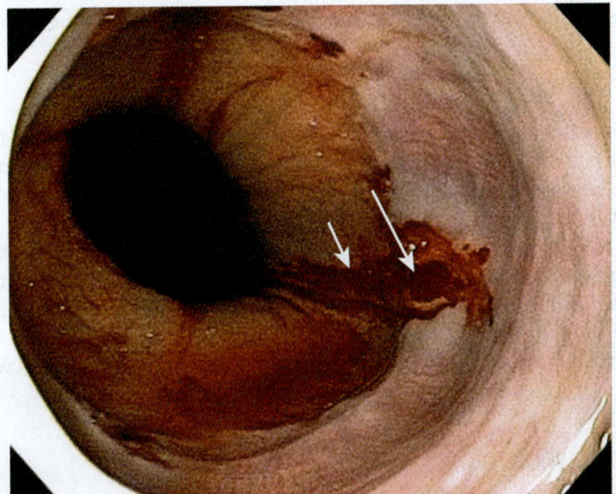

Fig. 21.14 Endoscopic appearance of a Mallory-Weiss tear with mild oozing. Note that the tear starts at the gastroesophageal junction (*long arrow*) and extends distally into the hiatal hernia (*short arrow*).

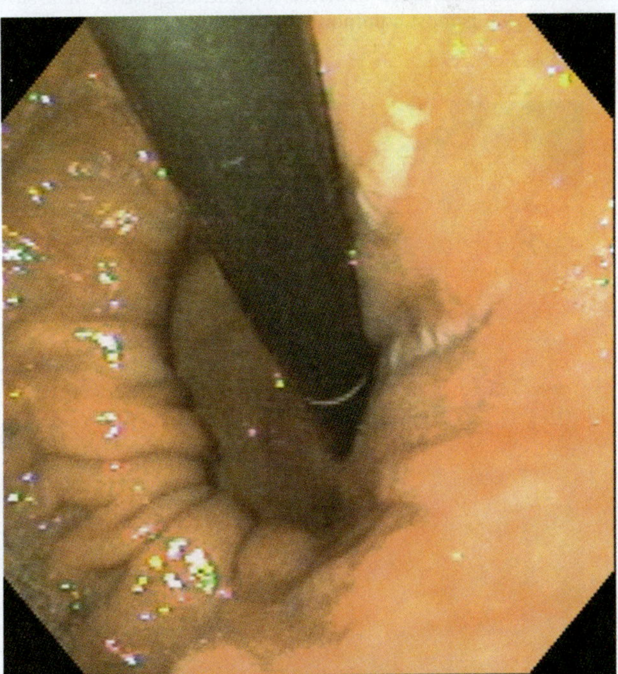

Fig. 21.15 Endoscopic appearance of Cameron lesions. Note that these linear ulcerations (*arrows*) are located at the distal end of a hiatal hernia.

needed for patients with severe acute or chronic GI bleeding and failure of medical management (see Chapter 27).[190]

UGI Malignancy

Malignancy accounts for 1% of severe UGIBs. The tumors are usually large, ulcerated masses in the esophagus, stomach, or duodenum. Endoscopic hemostasis with MPEC, laser, injection therapy, or hemoclips can temporarily control acute bleeding in most patients and allow time to determine the appropriate long-term management.[192,193] Patients with an ulcerated subepithelial mass (usually a GIST or leiomyoma) should undergo surgical resection of the mass to prevent rebleeding and, in the case of a GIST, the risk of metastasis. Angiography with embolization should be considered for patients with severe UGI bleeding caused by malignancy who do not respond to endoscopic therapy. External beam radiation can provide palliative hemostasis for patients with bleeding from advanced gastric or duodenal cancer (see Chapter 54). Hemospray has been used to manage oozing bleeding from UGI tumors in a small case series (see earlier).[42]

GAVE

GAVE, also described as "watermelon stomach," is a variant of gastric vascular ectasia (see Chapter 94) characterized by rows or stripes of ectatic mucosal blood vessels that emanate from the pylorus and extend proximally into the antrum (Fig. 21.16). The cause is uncertain, and the lesion may represent a response to mucosal trauma from contraction waves in the antrum. GAVE has been associated with cirrhosis and systemic sclerosis (scleroderma) (see Chapters 39, 40, and 76). Patients with GAVE who do not have portal hypertension demonstrate linear arrays of angiomas (classic GAVE), whereas those with portal hypertension have more diffuse antral angiomas.[194] The diffuse types of antral angiomas and, occasionally, classic GAVE are sometimes mistaken for gastritis by an unsuspecting endoscopist. Such cases are a common cause of obscure GI bleeding in referral centers (see later).[57]

Patients usually present with iron deficiency anemia or melena, with a mildly decreased hematocrit value suggestive of a slow UGIB. GAVE is most commonly reported in older women[194] and also seems to be more common in patients with end-stage renal disease.

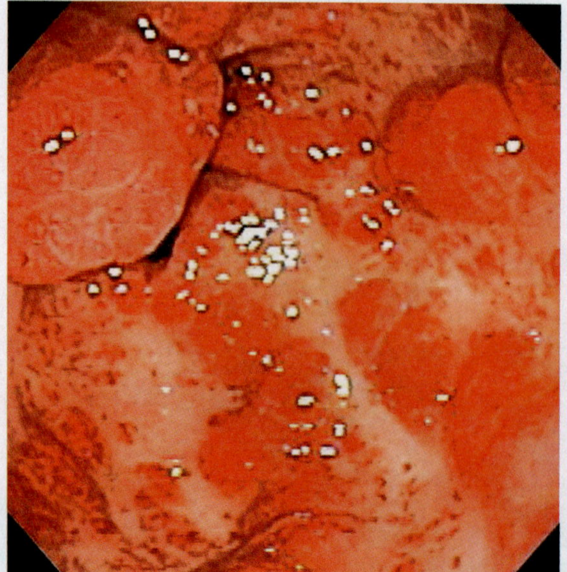

Fig. 21.16 Endoscopic appearance of GAVE, or watermelon stomach. The pattern seen in this view is considered classic, with rows of ectatic mucosal blood vessels emanating from the pylorus.

Endoscopic hemostasis with thermal heat modalities, such as laser, MPEC, or argon plasma coagulation, has been used successfully. Endoscopic hemostasis and ablation with thermal modalities can result in good palliation with an increase in the hematocrit value and a decrease in the need for blood transfusions and hospitalization.[194,195] Usually, several sessions approximately 4–8 weeks apart are required to achieve eradication of the lesions and a reduction in bleeding from the antral ectasias. Endoscopic therapy with argon plasma coagulation has been shown to be equally (80%) effective in cirrhotic and noncirrhotic patients with GAVE.[196] Pilot studies have demonstrated that mucosal band ligation, radiofrequency ablation, and cryotherapy can also lead to eradication of GAVE in selected patients.[197–199]

Placement of a TIPS in patients with portal hypertension and cirrhosis does not decrease bleeding from GAVE or diffuse antral angiomas. Patients who have ongoing severe chronic bleeding from GAVE rarely require surgical antrectomy to control symptoms (see Chapters 36 and 94).[200]

Portal Hypertensive Gastropathy

Portal hypertensive gastropathy (PHG) is caused by increased portal venous pressure and severe mucosal hyperemia that results in ectatic blood vessels in the proximal gastric body and cardia and oozing of blood. Less severe grades of PHG appear as a mosaic or snakeskin pattern and are not associated with bleeding.[201] Usually, patients with severe PHG present with chronic blood loss, but they can occasionally present with acute bleeding.

Severe PHG with diffuse bleeding is treated by measures that decrease portal pressure, usually with β-adrenergic receptor blocking agents or possibly with placement of a TIPS or surgical portacaval shunt. Endoscopic management has no role unless an obvious focal bleeding site is identified. The best treatment is LT (see Chapter 99).

Hemobilia

Hemobilia may occur in patients who have experienced liver trauma, undergone a liver biopsy or manipulation of the hepatobiliary system (as occurs with ERCP, percutaneous transhepatic cholangiography, or TIPS), or have HCC or a biliary parasitic infection.[202] Patients may present with a combination of GI bleeding and elevated liver biochemical tests with the blood clot acting similarly to a bile duct stone. The diagnosis can be confirmed by using a side-viewing duodenoscope to identify bleeding from the ampulla (Fig. 21.17). Ongoing or recurrent bleeding is treated with arterial embolization via arteriography.

Hemosuccus Pancreaticus

Hemosuccus pancreaticus is a rare form of UGI bleeding that occurs most commonly in patients with acute pancreatitis, chronic pancreatitis, pancreatic pseudocyst, or pancreatic cancer or after ERCP with pancreatic duct manipulation (see Chapters 60, 61, 62, and 63). It can also result from rupture of a splenic artery aneurysm into the pancreatic duct.[203] CT can demonstrate pancreatic pathology if previously unsuspected. Endoscopy with a side-viewing duodenoscope reveals blood coming out of the ampulla. Management of severe hemorrhage is usually with angiographic embolization or surgery.

Postsphincterotomy Bleeding

Bleeding following endoscopic sphincterotomy occurs in approximately 2% of patients (see Chapter 40).[204] Potential risk factors include coagulopathy, use of anticoagulants, portal

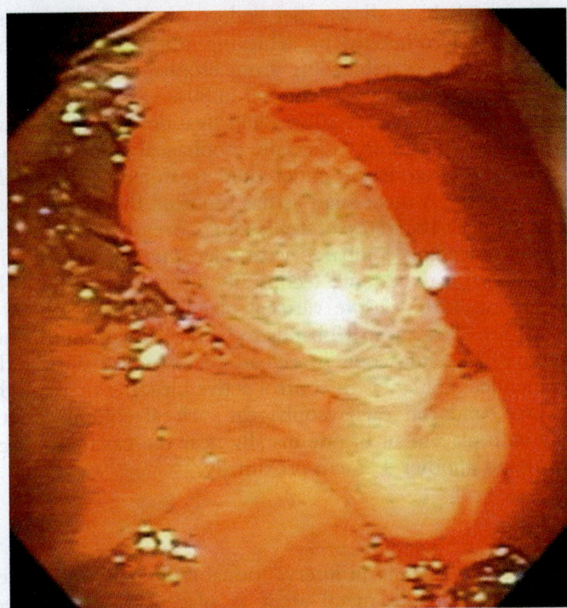

Fig. 21.17 Endoscopic appearance of the ampulla of Vater and hemobilia. Note fresh red blood on the right side exuding from the ampulla of a patient who earlier that day had undergone a percutaneous liver biopsy.

hypertension, renal failure, and the type and length of sphincterotomy. Successful hemostasis of postsphincterotomy bleeding is usually achieved with endoscopic methods such as injection of epinephrine, hemoclips, or MPEC (see Chapter 40).

Aortoenteric Fistula

Bleeding from an aortoenteric fistula is usually acute and massive, with a high mortality rate.[205] A primary aortoenteric fistula is a communication between the native abdominal aorta (usually an atherosclerotic abdominal aortic aneurysm) and, most commonly, the third portion of the duodenum.[206] Often, a self-limited herald bleed occurs hours to months before a more severe exsanguinating bleed. Occasionally, the diagnosis of an aortoenteric fistula is suspected by a history of an abdominal aortic aneurysm or by palpation of a pulsatile abdominal mass. The diagnosis can be difficult to make on endoscopy in the absence of active bleeding. Demonstration of an aortic aneurysm on abdominal CT or MRI (with IV contrast) suggests the diagnosis of a fistula.[58] Secondary aortoenteric fistulas are more common and usually occur between the small intestine and an infected abdominal aortic surgical graft. The fistula typically occurs between the third portion of the duodenum and the proximal end of the graft but may occur elsewhere in the GI tract. The fistula usually forms between 3 and 5 years after graft placement. Patients often experience a herald bleed that is mild and self-limited, and occasionally intermittent, before massive bleeding occurs.[207] A secondary fistula can also occur between the third part of the duodenum and an endovascular stent, in which case the fistula may be caused by pressure from the stent against the duodenum, infection of the stent, or possibly expansion of the native aneurysm.[208]

Patients with an acute UGIB and a history of an aortic aneurysm repair should undergo urgent CT with IV contrast or MR angiography first. CT or MRI may show inflammation around the graft and may demonstrate the fistula. If these are not diagnostic, push enteroscopy should be considered to evaluate the third portion of the duodenum for compression, blood, or graft material, as well as to exclude other bleeding sources. A vascular surgery consultation should also be obtained. Surgical treatment is required to remove the infected graft. Therapeutic endoscopy plays no role in the management of bleeding from an aortoenteric fistula (see Chapter 40).

Varices

Variceal hemorrhage is an important cause of UGI bleeding and is discussed in more detail in Chapter 94. Esophageal variceal bleeding related to portal hypertension is the second most common cause of severe UGI bleeding (after PUD). The acute mortality rate with each bleed is approximately 30%, and the long-term survival rate is less than 40% after 1 year with medical management alone.[209] Despite advances in medical therapy, endoscopic hemostasis, and angiographic procedures and TIPS, overall long-term survival rates have not improved for patients with variceal bleeding. Survival in nontransplanted patients with variceal bleeding is heavily influenced by the severity of underlying liver disease, with poorer survival rates for patients with higher MELD scores or Child-Pugh class C cirrhosis than for those with Child-Pugh class A or B cirrhosis (see Chapters 76, 94, and 99). LT can improve survival in selected patients.

Bleeding gastric varices are a difficult therapeutic problem because in contrast to bleeding esophageal varices, most available nonsurgical treatments are ineffective, except when isolated gastric varices are found without accompanying esophageal varices, as occurs with splenic vein thrombosis and often in association with pancreatitis or pancreatic cancer. The diagnosis of splenic vein thrombosis can be made with Doppler US, MRI, or routine angiography. Bleeding from gastric varices caused by splenic vein thrombosis is treated by splenectomy. Focal gastric varices with bleeding can be treated with injection of cyanoacrylate glue or radiologic procedures such as balloon-occluded retrograde transvenous obliteration (see Chapter 92).

Medical Management of Acute Variceal Bleeding

Somatostatin and its long-acting analog, octreotide, cause selective splanchnic vasoconstriction and lower portal pressure without causing the cardiac complications seen with vasopressin (even in combination with nitroglycerin). Studies have shown mixed results as to whether somatostatin is more effective than placebo in managing variceal bleeding, but it seems to be at least as effective as vasopressin and is much safer. A meta-analysis has shown that vasoactive drugs [e.g., octreotide, somatostatin, and terlipressin (a long-acting vasopressin analog)] are as effective as sclerotherapy for controlling variceal bleeding and cause fewer adverse events.[21] No studies have shown a survival benefit to vasopressin or somatostatin in patients with variceal bleeding. Given the potential ability of octreotide to control acute variceal hemorrhage, its low toxicity, and its availability in the United States, octreotide has been the pharmacologic drug of choice as an adjunct to endoscopic therapy for the treatment of variceal hemorrhage. The dose of octreotide for acute variceal hemorrhage is a 50 µg bolus followed by a continuous IV infusion of 50 µg/h for up to 5 days.

Patients with a prolonged PT that does not correct with fresh frozen plasma may benefit from infusion of human recombinant factor VIIa, although prolongation of the PT does not correlate with bleeding risk (see Chapters 76 and 94). In one uncontrolled trial, a single 80 µg/kg dose of recombinant factor VIIa normalized the PT in all 10 patients within 30 minutes, with immediate control of bleeding in all patients.[210] In a large randomized, placebo-controlled study, the administration of recombinant factor VIIa in addition to endoscopic hemostasis decreased rebleeding rates in patients with Child-Pugh class B and C cirrhosis who had bled from varices.[211] Because recombinant factor VIIa is expensive and associated with a risk of thrombosis, its use should be reserved for patients with severe ongoing bleeding and irreversible coagulopathy, pending the results of additional clinical and cost-effectiveness studies.

Up to 20% of cirrhotic patients who are hospitalized with GI bleeding have a bacterial infection at the time of admission to the hospital, and infection develops during the hospitalization in up to 50% (see Chapter 93). Meta-analyses suggest that the administration of an antibiotic to cirrhotic patients with variceal bleeding is associated with a decrease in the rates of mortality and bacterial infections.[212,213] Commonly prescribed antibiotics are fluoroquinolones, such as oral norfloxacin (400 mg twice daily) (not available in the United States), IV ciprofloxacin (400 mg every 12 hours), IV levofloxacin (500 mg every 24 hours), and, most commonly, IV ceftriaxone, 1 g every 24 hours, administered for 7 days.

Balloon Tamponade

Although balloon tamponade of varices is seldom used now to control gastroesophageal variceal bleeding, it may be used to stabilize a patient with massive bleeding prior to definitive therapy (see Chapter 94). Three types of tamponade balloons are available. The Sengstaken-Blakemore tube has gastric and esophageal balloons, with a single aspirating port in the stomach. The Minnesota tube has also gastric and esophageal balloons and has aspiration ports in the esophagus and stomach. The Linton-Nachlas tube has a single large gastric balloon and aspiration ports in the stomach and esophagus. Most reports suggest that balloon tamponade provides initial control of bleeding in 85%–98% of cases, but variceal rebleeding recurs soon after the balloon is deflated in 21%–60% of patients.[214] The major problem with tamponade balloons is a 30% rate of serious complications, such as aspiration pneumonia, esophageal rupture, and airway obstruction. Patients should be intubated before placement of a tamponade balloon to minimize the risk of pulmonary complications. Clinical studies have not shown a significant difference in efficacy between vasopressin administration and balloon tamponade.

Endoscopic Sclerotherapy

Endoscopic variceal sclerotherapy involves injecting a sclerosant into or adjacent to esophageal varices. The most used sclerosants are ethanolamine oleate, sodium tetradecyl sulfate, sodium morrhuate, and ethanol. Cyanoacrylate, a glue that effectively stops bleeding when injected into esophageal or gastric varices, is difficult to use and not approved by the FDA. Various techniques are used; their common goals are to achieve initial hemostasis and reduce the risk of rebleeding by performing sclerotherapy on a scheduled basis until the varices are obliterated. Esophageal varices are much more amenable than gastric varices to eradication with endoscopic therapy.

Prospective randomized trials have suggested that immediate hemostasis is improved and the risk of acute rebleeding is reduced with sclerotherapy compared with medical therapy alone for bleeding esophageal varices.[215–218] Hemostasis can be achieved in 85%–95% of cases, with a rebleeding rate of 25%–30%.[219] Complications of endoscopic variceal sclerotherapy include esophageal ulcers that can bleed or perforate, esophageal strictures, mediastinitis, pleural effusions, aspiration pneumonia, acute respiratory distress syndrome, chest pain, fever, and bacteremia and account, in part, for the use of esophageal variceal band ligation as the preferred endoscopic therapy for variceal bleeding.

Endoscopic Band Ligation

The technique of endoscopic band ligation is similar to that used for band ligation of internal hemorrhoids (see Chapter 131). A rubber band is placed over a varix, which subsequently undergoes thrombosis, sloughing, and fibrosis. Prospective randomized controlled trials have shown that endoscopic band ligation is as effective as sclerotherapy in achieving initial hemostasis and reducing the rate of rebleeding from esophageal varices. Acute hemostasis can generally be achieved in 80%–85% of cases, with a rebleeding rate of 25%–30%. Band ligation is associated with fewer local complications, especially esophageal strictures, and in one study required fewer endoscopic treatment sessions than sclerotherapy.[220] A meta-analysis has reported that variceal band ligation reduces the rates of rebleeding, overall mortality, and death from bleeding compared with sclerotherapy.[221] Band ligation, however, may be more technically difficult to perform than sclerotherapy during active variceal bleeding. Devices used for band ligation allow up to 10 bands to be placed without the need to remove the endoscope to reload the banding device. The recommended strategy is to control active bleeding first and then place two bands on each esophageal variceal column, starting distally with placement of one distally near the gastroesophageal junction and another 4–6 cm proximally.[222,223]

TIPS

Placement of a TIPS is an interventional radiologic procedure in which an expandable metal stent is placed via percutaneous insertion between the hepatic and portal veins, thereby creating an intrahepatic portosystemic shunt. TIPS is effective for short-term control of bleeding gastroesophageal varices, especially those that fail endoscopic therapy.[223,224] Initially envisioned as a bridge to LT, it has been used with increased frequency in non-transplantation situations. Randomized trials that have compared TIPS with endoscopic sclerotherapy suggest that TIPS is more effective for the long-term prevention of rebleeding.[225] The main problems with TIPS are a rate of shunt occlusion of up to 80% (less with use of polytetrafluoroethylene-coated stents) within 1 year and the development of new or worsening hepatic encephalopathy in approximately 20% of patients.[226] Most relevant studies have shown that TIPS does not prolong survival of patients with variceal bleeding compared with endoscopic treatment. In the management of acute variceal bleeding, TIPS is generally reserved for patients who fail endoscopic treatment. In one study of patients with predominantly alcoholic cirrhosis and active drinking, those with Child-Pugh class B cirrhosis who were stabilized with vasoactive and endoscopic therapy were randomized to either urgent TIPS within 72 hours after initial stabilization or therapy with a β-adrenergic receptor blocking agent and endoscopic band ligation as maintenance therapy, and those who underwent a TIPS had a lower rate of rebleeding and improved 1-year survival.[227] The findings may not be as applicable to patients with nonalcoholic cirrhosis (see also Chapter 94).

Portosystemic Shunt Surgery

A variety of portosystemic shunt operations have been performed to reduce portal venous pressure. When compared with sclerotherapy, surgical shunts decrease the rebleeding rate significantly but do not improve survival.[219,228–231] Surgical shunts may be associated with hepatic encephalopathy and can make future LT technically more difficult, but they have an advantage over endoscopic variceal therapy in reducing portal hypertension and treating gastric variceal bleeding. Surgical shunts are performed infrequently now but are considered for selected patients who have failed endoscopic therapy and are not expected to become candidates for LT (see Chapters 94 and 99).

LOWER GASTROINTESTINAL BLEEDING

LGI bleeding generally signifies bleeding from the colon or anorectum. The annual incidence of LGI bleeding is

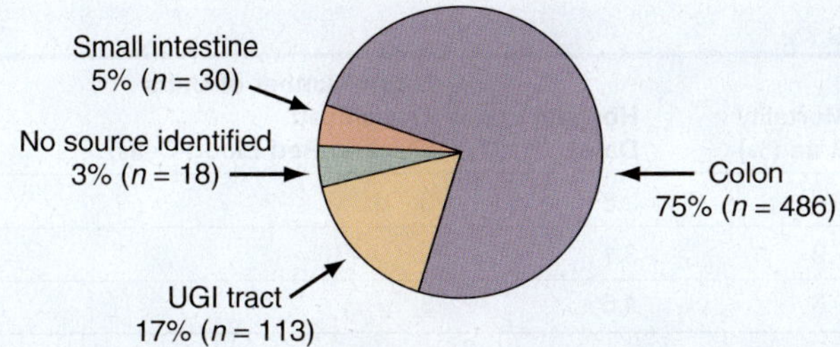

Fig. 21.18 Frequencies of sources of severe hematochezia in patients seen at UCLA CURE. Note that in most cases (75%), severe hematochezia is from the colon, 17% is from a UGI (esophagus, stomach, or duodenum) source, and 5% is from a small intestinal source. *CURE*, Center for Ulcer Research and Education; *UCLA*, University of California, Los Angeles.

approximately 20 cases/100,000 population, with an increased risk in older adults.[232] The rate of hospitalization for LGI bleeding is lower than that for UGI bleeding. Most patients are older than 70 years of age. Patients usually present with painless hematochezia and a decrease in the hematocrit value but without orthostasis. If orthostasis is associated with hematochezia, a briskly bleeding UGI source should be excluded (see earlier); severe painless hematochezia results from a foregut source in approximately 15% of noncirrhotic patients.[233] The sites of origin within the GI tract of severe hematochezia at UCLA CURE are shown in Fig. 21.18.

Patients with LGI bleeding should initially be resuscitated medically. After they have been stabilized, they should generally undergo urgent colonoscopy after a PEG purge.[27] For patients with cirrhosis, a recent history of melena or hematemesis, or a history of PUD, "panendoscopy" (upper and lower endoscopy) is recommended first.[233,234] In early reports, urgent colonoscopy resulted in a diagnosis in approximately 70% of cases;[235,236] however, in subsequent reports, the combination of urgent colonoscopy and, if necessary, push enteroscopy, anoscopy, and capsule endoscopy has resulted in a diagnosis in 95% of cases (see Fig. 21.4).[233,234]

The most common causes of LGI bleeding are shown in Table 21.8. Diverticulosis is the most common cause of acute LGI bleeding and occurs in approximately 30% of cases.[2] Colonic polyps or cancer, colitis, and anorectal disorders each account for approximately 20% of cases.[237]

In most cases, acute LGI bleeding will stop spontaneously, thereby allowing nonurgent diagnosis and treatment. For patients with ongoing or recurrent hematochezia, urgent diagnosis and treatment are required to control the bleeding. In a large series of patients at the UCLA Medical Center and Wadsworth Veterans Administration Hospital, 64% of patients with severe hematochezia required a therapeutic intervention to control continued bleeding or rebleeding[27]: 39% underwent endoscopic hemostasis, 1% underwent angiographic embolization, and 24% underwent surgery.

TABLE 21.8 Colonic Causes of Severe Hematochezia (%)

	Study		
Lesion	**Reference 239**	**Reference 240**	**UCLA CURE[a] (2018)**
Diverticulosis	30	33	33
Colon cancer or polyps	18	21	5.2
Colitis	17	17	N/A
Ischemic colitis	N/A	7	11.9
IBD	N/A	4	3.6
Noninfectious colitis	N/A	5	2.7
Infectious colitis	N/A	1	1.2
Angioectasia	7	6	5.0
Postpolypectomy ulcer	6	N/A	7.8
Rectal ulcer	N/A	1	8.4
Hemorrhoids	N/A	20	10.3
Anorectal source (other)	4	3	1.8[b]
Radiation colitis	0	0.5	2.2
Colon anastomotic ulcer	N/A	N/A	2.1
Other	8	3	4.1
Unknown	16	0	0

[a]*N* = 823.
[b]Anal fissure following rubber band ligation, ulcer, rectal cancer, or other anorectal lesion.
CURE, Center for Ulcer Research and Education; *UCLA*, University of California, Los Angeles; *N/A*, not available.

Risk Factors and Risk Stratification

Nonselective NSAIDs increase the risk of LGI bleeding compared with placebo.[238,239] The main risk factors for NSAID-associated LGI bleeding appear to be an age of 65 years or older and a prior history of LGI bleeding.[240] Whether use of long-term selective COX-2 inhibitors is associated with a lower risk of LGI bleeding than nonselective NSAIDs is uncertain.

Table 21.9 shows clinical factors that are predictive of severe LGI bleeding (defined as continued bleeding within the first 24 hours of hospitalization, with a transfusion requirement of at least 2 units of packed RBCs or a decrease in the hematocrit value of 20% or more) or recurrent bleeding after 24 hours of stability (defined as the need for additional transfusions, a further decrease in the hematocrit value of at least 20%, or readmission for LGI bleeding within 1 week of discharge). Predictive factors include tachycardia, hypotension, syncope, a nontender abdomen, witnessed rectal bleeding on presentation, aspirin use, and more than two comorbid illnesses.[241,242] These risk factors are used in a prognostic scoring system that identifies patients at the highest risk for severe LGI bleeding, who account for 19% of patients with LGI bleeding and may benefit most from urgent colonoscopy.

A single-institution case series of 94 patients admitted for LGI bleeding[243] found that 39% of all cases of LGI bleeding requiring hospitalization were severe, as defined by the passage of red blood after the patient had left the emergency department and associated hypotension or tachycardia or the need for a transfusion of more than 2 units of packed RBCs during hospitalization. Independent risk factors for severe LGI bleeding were an initial hematocrit value of 35% or lower, abnormal vital signs (a systolic blood pressure <100 mm Hg or a heart rate >100/min) on admission, and gross blood on initial rectal examination.

Artificial neural networks have also been used to develop prediction models for severe LGI bleeding,[244,245] but from a clinical point of view, the large number of variables that have to be entered into a computer program for analysis limit their widespread use.

Mortality

A large U.S. database study of 227,000 patients with a discharge diagnosis of LGI bleeding reported an overall mortality rate of

TABLE 21.9 Clinical Prediction Score and Outcomes of Severe Acute LGI Bleeding

Total Risk Points[a]	Frequency (%)	Risk of Severe Bleeding (%)	Need for Surgery (%)	Mortality Rate (%)	Hospital Days	Mean Number of Units Transfused (Packed Red Blood Cells)
0	6	6	0	0	2.8	0
1–3	75	43	1.5	2.9	3.1	1
≥4	19	79	7.7	9.6	4.6	3

[a]Risk factors (1 point each): aspirin use; more than two comorbid illnesses; heart rate ≥100/min; nontender abdominal examination; rectal bleeding within the first 4 hours of evaluation; syncope; systolic blood pressure ≤115 mm Hg.

Severe LGI bleeding is defined as continued bleeding within the first 24 hours of hospitalization (transfusion of two or more units of packed red blood cells and/or hematocrit value drop of 20% or more) and/or recurrent bleeding after 24 hours of stability (need for additional transfusions, further hematocrit value decrease of 20% or more, or readmission to the hospital for LGI bleeding within 1 week of discharge).

Data from Strate LL, Saltzman JR, Ookubo R, et al. Validation of a clinical prediction rule for severe acute lower intestinal bleeding. *Am J Gastroenterol.* 2005;100:1821–1827.

3.9% in 2008.[237] Multivariate analysis found that independent predictors of in-hospital mortality are age older than 70 years, intestinal ischemia, at least two comorbid illnesses, onset of bleeding after hospitalization for an unrelated condition, coagulopathy, hypovolemia, transfusion of packed RBCs, and male gender. Colorectal polyps and hemorrhoids were associated with a lower mortality risk. The low risk of death from LGI bleeding identified in this study is consistent with data from smaller series, such as those from Kaiser San Diego (2.4%) and the University of California, San Francisco (3.2%).[232,243] The Kaiser study also found an increased risk of death with in-hospital LGI bleeding.

Diagnostic and Therapeutic Approach

Patients with hematochezia should undergo the same careful history taking, physical examination, and laboratory testing described earlier for the general approach to the patient with acute GI bleeding (see Table 21.1). The history should focus specifically on identifying sources of LGI bleeding. Diverticular bleeding should be suspected in patients with painless, severe, acute hematochezia and a history of diverticulosis, although ischemic colitis may also be painless.[245]

Patients should be medically resuscitated. Because LGI bleeding is generally less severe than UGI bleeding, blood transfusions may not be required. Most patients should undergo initial evaluation with colonoscopy after bowel preparation, although in selected cases anoscopy or flexible sigmoidoscopy without any bowel cleansing or after an enema may be performed. Other diagnostic tests, including radionuclide bleeding scans or angiography, may be used in selected cases or when colonoscopy fails to detect a source of bleeding.

Anoscopy

Anoscopy can be useful for patients in whom bleeding internal hemorrhoids or other anorectal disorders (e.g., fissures, fistulas, and proctitis) are suspected from the medical history. For internal hemorrhoids, immediate treatment with rubber band ligation is recommended (see Chapter 131). Most patients, however, especially if older than 50 years of age, will also require colonoscopy, at least electively, to evaluate the remainder of the colon.

Flexible Sigmoidoscopy

Flexible sigmoidoscopy can evaluate the rectum and left side of the colon for a bleeding site and can be performed without a standard colonoscopy bowel preparation. Although not adequate for evaluation of the anal canal, flexible sigmoidoscopy alone will result in a diagnosis in approximately 9% of cases.[247] If the distal colon can be adequately cleansed with enemas, an urgent flexible sigmoidoscopy can be useful for patients suspected of having a solitary rectal ulcer, UC, radiation proctitis, postpolypectomy bleeding (in the rectosigmoid), or internal hemorrhoids (see Chapters 40, 117, 130, and 131). Therapeutic hemostasis can be provided with injection therapy, hemoclip placement, band ligation, or MPEC. Monopolar electrocautery (e.g., argon plasma coagulation, snare polypectomy, and hot biopsy forceps) should not be used if a bowel preparation has not been administered to avoid the risk of ignited flammable colonic gas (see Chapter 18).

Radionuclide Imaging

Radionuclide imaging involves injecting a radiolabeled substance into the patient's bloodstream and performing serial scintigraphy to detect focal collections of radiolabeled material (see earlier). This technique has been reported to detect bleeding at a rate as low as 0.04 mL/min,[48] with an overall positive diagnostic rate of approximately 45% and an accuracy rate of 78% for localizing the true bleeding site.[235] The disadvantages of radionuclide imaging are that delayed scans may be misleading, and determining the specific cause of bleeding often depends on endoscopy or surgery. False-positive results are most likely to occur when transit of luminal blood is rapid, so that radiolabeled blood is detected in the colon even though it originated in the UGI tract. Radionuclide imaging may be helpful in cases of obscure GI bleeding (see later) or prior to angiography to help localize a lesion, particularly if an early scan (e.g., 30 minutes to 4 hours after injection of the radiolabeled material) is positive for RBC extravasation.

Angiography

Angiography is most likely to detect a site of bleeding when the rate of arterial bleeding is at least 0.5 mL/min.[45] The diagnostic yield depends on patient selection, the timing of the procedure, and the skill of the angiographer, with positive results in 12%–69% of cases. An advantage of angiography is that embolization can be performed to control some bleeding lesions. Major complications, however, occur in 3% of cases and include bowel ischemia, hematoma formation, femoral artery thrombosis, contrast dye reactions, acute kidney injury, and transient ischemic attacks.[47] Other disadvantages of angiography are the absence of active bleeding in most patients at the time of angiography, inability to detect nonbleeding SRH (NBVV, clot, or spot), expense of the test, and inability to determine the specific lesion responsible for bleeding in many cases.[233,234] A small retrospective case series of 11 patients with colonic bleeding who underwent angiographic embolization reported that the bleeding ceased in 10, mesenteric ischemia developed in 7, and 6 died.[248] Another study of 65 patients with acute LGI bleeding who did not undergo colonoscopy as a first diagnostic step found that diagnostic angiography provided little additional clinical information because the bleeding stopped spontaneously in most patients. Moreover, angiography did not help guide subsequent surgery and was associated with a complication rate of 11%.[249]

CT and CT Colonography

Multidetector CT can identify abnormalities in the colon that could be a source of bleeding, such as diverticulosis, colitis, masses, and varices. CT is often performed if the patient is having hematochezia with abdominal pain. One study from France reported that CT accurately identified 17 of 19 LGI bleeding sites, including diverticula, tumors, angiomas, and varices.[250] Multidetector CT has been shown to be more accurate than technetium-tagged RBC scanning in patients with LGI bleeding.[251]

CT colonography is being used increasingly to screen persons for colonic polyps and cancer and may be of some benefit in patients with LGI bleeding (see Chapter 128). CT colonography detects large polyps (>1 cm) or cancers with a sensitivity rate of 90%.[252] Faster multidetector scanners also allow CT angiography to be performed, as well as evaluation of the small bowel. This capability could allow detection of masses and vascular lesions and is a potential advantage of CT angiography over other radiologic imaging techniques.

Multidetector CT has been proposed as an early diagnostic step in patients with suspected colonic bleeding to help direct colonoscopic evaluation.[253] Because this approach may expose the patient to unnecessary radiation, and because nearly all patients will undergo either urgent or elective colonoscopy anyway, CT colonography is unlikely to play an important role in the acute evaluation of patients with LGI bleeding. Moreover, CT angiographic IV contrast can cause acute kidney injury in patients with renal insufficiency.

Colonoscopy

Urgent colonoscopy following a rapid bowel purge has been shown to be safe, provide important diagnostic information, and allow therapeutic intervention.[233,234] Patients usually ingest 6–8 L of PEG solution orally or via an NG tube over 4–6 hours until the rectal effluent is clear of stool, blood, and clots. Metoclopramide, in a dose of 10 mg, may be given intravenously before the purge and repeated every 3–4 hours to facilitate gastric emptying and reduce nausea. Owing to the potential risks of high sodium and phosphate loads, sodium phosphate bowel preparations should probably be avoided in patients with suspected LGI bleeding.

Urgent colonoscopy for LGI bleeding is generally performed 6–24 hours after the patient is admitted to the hospital. Most bleeding stops spontaneously, and thus colonoscopy is often performed semielectively on the day after initial hospitalization to allow the patient to receive blood transfusions and the bowel preparation on the first day of hospitalization.

The overall rate of detecting a presumed or definite cause of LGI bleeding by colonoscopy ranges from 48%–90%, with an average of 68%, based on a review of 13 studies.[235] The problem with interpreting these data, however, is that making a definite diagnosis of the cause of the bleeding is often not possible unless a bleeding stigma such as active bleeding, a visible vessel, an adherent clot, a flat spot, mucosal friability or ulceration, or the presence of fresh blood limited to a specific segment of the colon is seen.

The optimal time for performing urgent bowel preparation and colonoscopy is unknown. Theoretically, the sooner an endoscopy is performed, the higher the likelihood of finding a lesion (e.g., bleeding diverticulum and polyp stalk) with stigmata that might be amenable to endoscopic hemostasis. A retrospective study from the Mayo Clinic, however, suggested that in patients with diverticular bleeding, the timing of endoscopy (0–12 hours, 12–24 hours, or more than 24 hours after admission) is not significantly associated with the finding of active bleeding or other stigmata that would prompt colonoscopic hemostasis.[254] A prospective study revealed no difference between urgent (≤12 hours after presentation) and elective (36–60 hours after presentation) colonoscopy in terms of further bleeding, blood transfusions, hospital days, or hospital charges.[9] Early colonoscopy (soon after admission) has been associated with a shorter length of hospitalization, principally because of improved diagnostic yield rather than therapeutic intervention.[255]

A consensus on a single approach to patients with severe hematochezia has not been reached, and the approach used depends on local resources and expertise. In large centers, the approach detailed in Fig. 21.4 is recommended. With the use of an urgent endoscopic approach for diagnosis and treatment, the diagnostic yield of definitive and presumptive bleeding sites is more than 90%, and the estimated direct costs are significantly less than the costs associated with an elective evaluation.[28]

Barium Enema

Emergency barium enema has no role in patients with LGI bleeding. This test is rarely diagnostic because it cannot demonstrate vascular lesions and may be misleading if only diverticula are seen. It fails to detect 50% of polyps larger than 10 mm.[256] In addition, the barium contrast liquid can make urgent colonoscopy more difficult by impairing visualization and delaying other studies such as angiography. Subsequent colonoscopy is required for any suspicious lesions seen on barium enema or for lesions that require therapy.

Role of Surgery

Surgical management is rarely needed in patients with LGI bleeding because most bleeding is self-limited or easily managed with medical or endoscopic therapy. The main indications for surgery are malignancy, diffuse bleeding that fails to cease with medical therapy (as in ischemic colitis or UC), and recurrent bleeding from a diverticulum. At present, most patients are managed on a medical service rather than on a surgical service.

Causes and Management

Visualizing active bleeding during colonoscopy is not always possible, but colonoscopy permits identification of SRH (visible vessels, adherent clot, or spots) and provides information on the location of the lesion and on risk stratification. The earlier a colonoscopy is carried out, the higher the chance of detecting an actively bleeding lesion or SRH. A definite diagnosis of a bleeding lesion can usually be made if active bleeding, a visible vessel, or a clot is seen. A presumptive diagnosis of the cause of bleeding can be made if a lesion that is a potential cause of bleeding is seen and no other possible sources are identified by anoscopy, full colonoscopy with intubation of the terminal ileum, and, in some cases, push enteroscopy.[28]

Diverticulosis

Colonic diverticula are herniations of colonic mucosa and submucosa through the muscular layers of the colon (see Chapter 123). Histopathologically, diverticula in the colon are actually pseudodiverticula because they do not contain all layers of the colonic wall. Diverticula form when colonic tissue is pushed out by intraluminal pressure at points of entry of the small arteries (vasa recta), where they penetrate the circular muscle layer of the colonic wall. The entry points of the vasa recta are areas of relative weakness through which the mucosa and submucosa can herniate when intraluminal pressure is increased.[257] Diverticula vary in diameter from a few millimeters to several centimeters and are located most commonly in the left colon. Most colonic diverticula are asymptomatic and remain uncomplicated. Bleeding may occur from vessels at the neck or base of a diverticulum.[257] In our experience with definitive diverticular hemorrhage (see later), bleeding was from the base in 52% and from the neck in 48% of diverticula.[258]

Diverticula are common in Western countries, with a frequency of 50% in older adults.[259] By contrast, diverticula are found in fewer than 1% of continental African and Asian populations.[260] It has been hypothesized that the regional differences in prevalence rates can be explained by the low amount of dietary fiber in Western diets (see Chapter 123). Diverticular bleeding develops in an estimated 3%–5% of patients with diverticulosis.[261] Although most diverticula are in the left colon, several series have suggested that diverticula in the right colon are more likely to bleed.[261–263] Two-thirds of definitive diverticular bleeds (with SRH) emanate from the region of the splenic flexure of the colon or proximally.[258]

Diverticular hemorrhage should be classified carefully based on findings at colonoscopy, angiography, or surgery,[28] particularly in the case of older patients with severe hematochezia who are likely to have colonic diverticulosis. *Definitive diverticular hemorrhage* is diagnosed, when SRH (e.g., active bleeding, visible vessel, and adherent clot) are seen on colonoscopy or active bleeding is demonstrated on angiography or radionuclide imaging, with later confirmation of a diverticulum in that location as the source of bleeding by colonoscopy or surgery. *Presumptive diverticular hemorrhage* is diagnosed when colonoscopy reveals diverticulosis without stigmata, and no other significant lesions are seen in the colon and by anoscopy, terminal ileum examination, and push enteroscopy. The term *incidental diverticulosis* is used when another lesion is identified as the cause of hematochezia, and colonic diverticulosis is evident. In a large prospective cohort study in which the management algorithm shown in Fig. 21.4 was used in our institutions to classify patients with hematochezia, colonic diverticulosis was incidental in 52%, presumptive diverticular hemorrhage occurred in 31%, and definitive diverticular hemorrhage was established in 17% of cases.[234]

Patients with diverticular bleeding are typically older, have been taking aspirin or other NSAIDs, and present with painless hematochezia.[264,265] In at least 75% of patients with diverticular bleeding, the bleeding stops spontaneously, and these patients require transfusion of fewer than 4 units of packed RBCs. In one surgical series, surgical segmental colonic resection was performed in 60% of patients, most of whom had had continued bleeding despite transfusion of four units of blood.[262] Patients who underwent resection for a bleeding diverticulum had a rebleeding rate of 4%. Among patients who stopped bleeding spontaneously, the rebleeding rate from colonic diverticulosis has been reported to range from 25%–38% over the next 4 years, with most patients having mild rebleeding.[232,262] These data, however, are not based on colonoscopic documentation of diverticular bleeding, and the actual rate of rebleeding appears to be lower. In a large prospective cohort study of patients with documented colonic diverticular hemorrhage (definitive or presumptive) by our group, the overall rate of rebleeding was 18% in 4 years—9% from recurrent diverticular hemorrhage and 9% from other GI sources.[258]

Endoscopic Stigmata

About one-third of patients with true diverticular hemorrhage (presumptive or definitive) during urgent colonoscopy following adequate cleansing have a stigma of recent bleeding, such as active bleeding, a visible vessel, an adherent clot, or a flat spot in a single diverticulum.[234,258] As noted earlier, colonoscopy for LGI bleeding is likely to result in a greater frequency of finding SRH, although a small case series study from the Mayo Clinic did not find any difference in the rate of detection of these stigmata whether colonoscopy was performed between 0 and 12, 12 and 24, or more than 24 hours from the time of hospital admission.[254]

Stratifying the risk of diverticular rebleeding by applying the same endoscopic stigmata used in high-risk peptic ulcer bleeding (active bleeding, NBVV, and clot) has been advocated. For example, as in histopathologic examination of resection specimens of bleeding ulcers with visible vessels, the pigmented protuberance found on the edge of some diverticula is an organized clot over an underlying ruptured blood vessel on histopathology (Fig. 21.19).[266] The short-term natural history associated with each of these stigmata has been reported to be similar to that for stigmata associated with peptic ulcer hemorrhage.[267] Of medically treated patients with active bleeding from a diverticulum, 83% (15 of 18) rebled and 56% required intervention (surgery or angiographic embolization) for hemostasis. In patients with an NBVV in a single diverticulum, the rate of rebleeding was 60%, and the rate of intervention for hemostasis was 40%. In patients with an adherent clot treated medically, the rebleeding rate was 43%, and the rate of intervention was 29%. For the entire group of 37 patients with these high-risk stigmata, the rebleeding rate on medical therapy was 65%, and the rate of intervention was 43%. These rebleeding and intervention rates are worse than those for peptic ulcer hemorrhage because there are no drugs similar to PPIs that can be used to reduce the rebleeding risk in patients with high-risk SRH.

UCLA CURE hemostasis studies using a DEP have detected underlying blood flow in 91% of patients with major SRH (active bleeding, NBVV, or adherent clot) but in no patient without these stigmata. The DEP has also been used for risk stratification of patients with flat spots in diverticula during urgent colonoscopy for hemorrhage and as a guide to the completeness of hemostasis in patients with SRH.[268] With DEP guidance to obliterate blood flow, the rebleeding rates have been less than 5% in 30 days.[267,268]

Endoscopic Hemostasis

Colonoscopic hemostasis of actively bleeding diverticula has been reported using MPEC, epinephrine injection, hemoclips, fibrin glue, rubber band ligation, endoloops, or combinations of epinephrine and MPEC or hemoclips.[28,266,269–273] If fresh red blood is seen in a focal segment of the colon that segment should be irrigated vigorously with water to remove the blood and identify the underlying bleeding site. If bleeding is coming from the edge of a diverticulum or a pigmented protuberance is seen on the edge, a sclerotherapy needle can be used for submucosal injection of epinephrine (diluted 1:20,000 in saline) in 1 mL aliquots into 4 quadrants around the bleeding site. Subsequently, MPEC at a low-power setting (10–15 W) and light pressure can be carried out for a 1-second pulse duration to cauterize the diverticular edge and stop bleeding or flatten the visible vessel, or hemoclips can be applied. A nonbleeding adherent clot can be injected with 1:20,000 epinephrine into 4 quadrants, 1 mL/quadrant, after which the clot can be removed piecemeal by guillotining it with a cold polyp snare until it extends 3 mm above the diverticulum. The underlying stigma is treated with MPEC or hemoclips (see earlier).

After endoscopic hemostasis of a bleeding diverticulum is completed, a permanent submucosal tattoo should be placed around the lesion to allow identification of the site in case colonoscopy is repeated or surgery is performed for recurrent bleeding. After colonoscopic hemostasis, patients should be told to avoid aspirin and other NSAIDs and take a daily fiber supplement on a long-term basis.

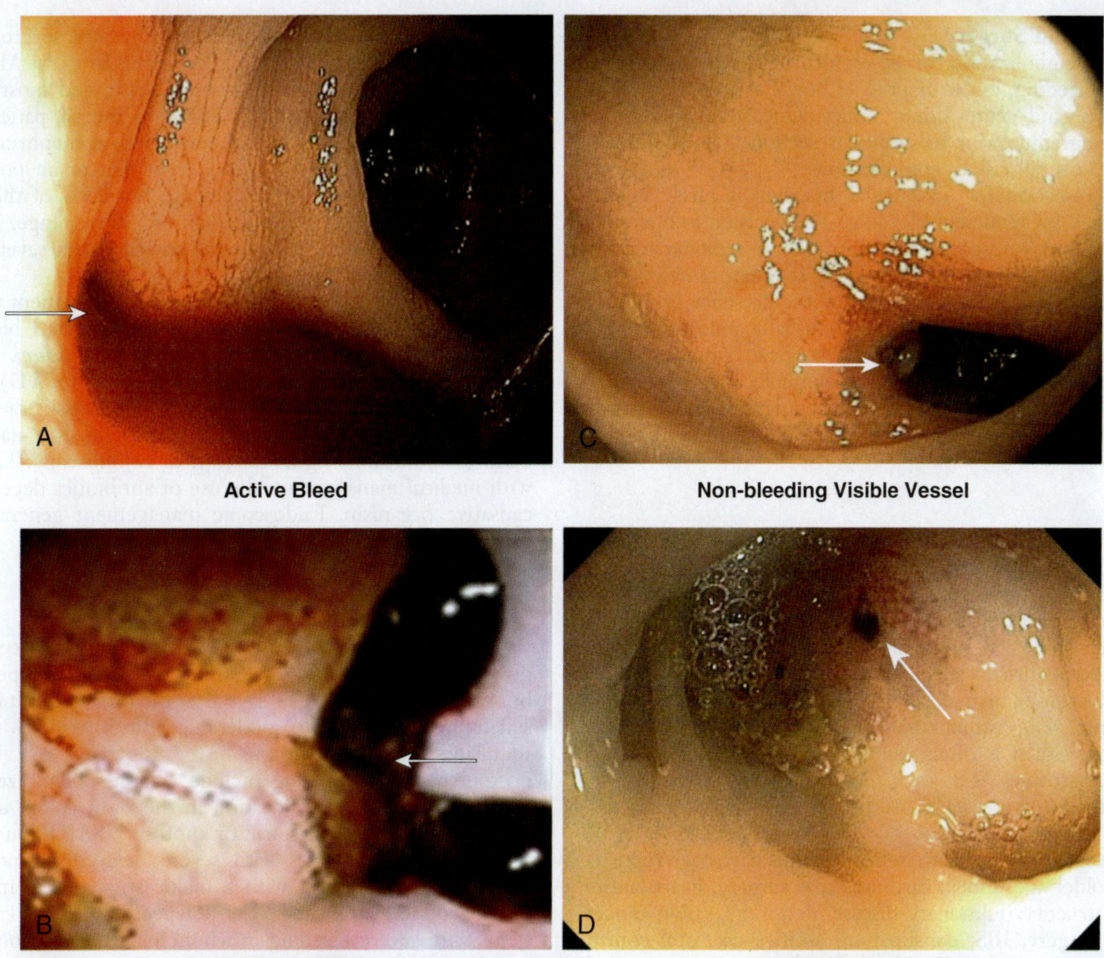

Fig. 21.19 Endoscopic stigmata of recent colonic diverticular bleeding. (A) Active bleeding (*arrow*). (B) Adherent clot (*arrow*). (C) Nonbleeding visible vessel (*arrow*). (D) Flat spot (*arrow*).

In 2000 Jensen and the UCLA CURE group published their results on urgent colonoscopy for the diagnosis and treatment of severe diverticular hemorrhage[28] and reported that 20% of patients with severe hematochezia had endoscopic stigmata, suggesting a definitive diverticular bleed. This group of patients, who underwent colonoscopic hemostasis, had a rebleeding rate of 0% and an emergency hemicolectomy rate of 0%, compared with 53% and 35%, respectively, in a historical control group of patients who had high-risk stigmata but did not undergo colonoscopic hemostasis. No rebleeding had occurred after 3 years of follow-up in the patients who underwent colonoscopic hemostasis.

In another report from the UCLA CURE group of 63 patients with definitive diverticular hemorrhage who were treated with endoscopic hemostasis, the rebleeding rate was 4.8%, and the rate of surgery or angiographic embolization for rebleeding was only 3.2%.[268] The investigators carried out treatment with injection of epinephrine and hemoclipping of the SRH in the base of the diverticulum (and on either side of a stigma to obliterate the underlying arterial blood flow) and injection of epinephrine and MPEC of SRH at the neck. Approximately 50% of the diverticular SRH were located at the neck and 50% at the base; more than 55% of the diverticula with SRH were found at or proximal to the splenic flexure. Complete hemostasis was documented with a DEP by the absence of blood flow after treatment, and the absence of blood flow correlated with a lack of rebleeding.

A 2012 study from Japan of 87 patients who underwent endoscopic clip placement at the mouth of a diverticulum for acute bleeding revealed a 34% early rebleeding rate, with the majority of rebleeding episodes occurring from diverticula located in the ascending colon.[274] The high rebleeding rate in this study[274] can be explained by the vascular anatomy of colonic diverticula and the placement of hemoclips away from SRH that lie in the base of a diverticulum. Because there is bidirectional arterial flow in diverticula and an arcade of two different arteries, treating with hemoclips at the neck of the diverticulum when the SRH is in the base will not seal the artery under the stigma; therefore, rebleeding rates would be expected to be high. The acute rebleeding rate in this study[274] is similar to that for the medically treated patients in a report from UCLA CURE of the natural history of diverticular bleeding, in which 65% of patients rebled and 43% required surgery or interventional radiology.[267]

Endoscopic band ligation has also been reported as a treatment of colonic diverticular hemorrhage. A 2012 study from Japan of 29 patients showed that band ligation was successful and safe, with an 11% rate of early rebleeding and the need for surgical resection in only one patient with bleeding from an ascending colon diverticulum.[275] Owing to the potential risk of full-thickness wall entrapment in the right colon, however, band ligation may increase the risk of perforation.[276] Diverticulitis has also been reported after band ligation. In a Japanese study, banding was reported to yield lower rebleeding rates than hemoclipping[277]; however, many of the patients were treated by remote hemoclipping treatment, that is, placement of the clips at the neck for diverticular closure when the bleeding point was in the base of the diverticulum.

Angiography and Surgery

Angiographic embolization can be performed in selected cases of diverticular bleeding, but with a risk of bowel infarction, contrast dye reactions, and acute kidney injury. One study found that routine angiography prior to surgical resection is not helpful in reducing the overall risk of complications.[249]

Surgical resection for diverticular bleeding is rarely needed and is reserved for recurrent bleeding. The decision to operate is best guided by colonoscopic, angiographic, or radionuclide imaging studies that demonstrate the likely segment of colon from which the bleeding is emanating and by the presence of medical comorbidities. Diverticular bleeding is usually mild in patients without major SRH, and the risk of surgical complications is increased in older patients. Blind subtotal colectomy, often performed in the past when a definite bleeding site could not be identified, should be avoided if possible.

Colitis

The term *colitis* refers to any form of inflammation of the colon. Severe LGI bleeding may be caused by ischemic colitis, IBD, or infectious colitis.

Ischemic colitis can present as painless or painful hematochezia with mild left-sided abdominal discomfort (see Chapter 120). The painless subtype usually results from mucosal hypoxia and is thought to be caused by hypoperfusion of the intramural vessels of the intestinal wall, rather than by large-vessel occlusion or embolization, which is often painful and clinically more severe with worse outcomes. The incidence of ischemic colitis is estimated to be 4.5–44 cases/100,000 person-years.[278] Most cases do not have a recognizable cause.

Risk factors associated with ischemic colitis have been reported to include older age, shock, cardiovascular surgery, heart failure, chronic obstructive pulmonary disease, ileostomy, colon cancer, abdominal surgery, IBS, constipation, laxative use, oral contraceptive use, and use of an H2RA.[278–281] The superior mesenteric artery supplies blood to the right colon (cecum, ascending colon, hepatic flexure, proximal transverse colon, and midtransverse colon), whereas the inferior mesenteric artery supplies blood to the left colon (distal transverse colon, splenic flexure, descending colon, sigmoid colon, and rectum). The colon has an abundant blood supply, but the watershed area between the superior and inferior mesenteric arteries has the fewest collateral vessels and is at most risk for ischemia. The colon normally receives 10%–35% of cardiac output, and ischemia can occur if blood flow decreases by more than 50%. Although ischemia is most likely to occur in the watershed area of the splenic flexure, it can occur anywhere in the colon.[282]

The diagnosis of ischemia is usually made by colonoscopy, but in severe cases of large-vessel ischemia, "thumbprinting" may be noted on plain films or colonic wall thickening on CT. The colonoscopic appearance of the mucosa includes erythema, friability, exudate, and superficial ulceration. Mucosal biopsy specimens may suggest ischemic changes but are generally used to exclude infectious or Crohn's colitis. Ischemic colitis usually resolves in a few days and generally does not require colonoscopic hemostasis or antibiotic therapy. In the UCLA CURE experience, approximately 10% of patients with ischemic colitis and severe hematochezia had a focal ulcer with a major stigma of hemorrhage on urgent colonoscopy.[283] After detection of arterial blood flow with DEP, the recommended treatment in these cases is epinephrine injection and hemoclipping, similar to that for other ulcers. In a large retrospective series from Kaiser, no episodes of rebleeding from ischemic colitis occurred over a 4-year follow-up period.[232] On the other hand, patients with large-vessel mesenteric ischemia usually have worse outcomes, including higher rates of rebleeding, perforation, surgery, and death.

IBD that involves the colon can rarely cause severe acute LGI bleeding (see Chapter 117). In a case series from the Mayo Clinic, most of these patients had Crohn disease, and most were successfully treated medically.[284] Three of the 31 patients in this series underwent endoscopic therapy with epinephrine injection alone or with MPEC for an adherent clot or an oozing ulcer. These 3 patients had no rebleeding, but 23% of the other 28 patients had rebleeding at a median of 3 days (range, 1–75 days) after the initial bleed; 39% of the patients with severe bleeding eventually required surgery.

Infectious colitis should be excluded in any patient with severe LGI bleeding and colitis (see Chapter 112). LGI bleeding can occur with infection caused by *Campylobacter jejuni*, *Salmonella*, *Shigella*, enterohemorrhagic *Escherichia coli* (O157:H7), CMV, or rarely *Clostridioides difficile*. Significant blood loss is rare except in patients with severe coagulopathy. The diagnosis is made by stool cultures and flexible sigmoidoscopy or colonoscopy. Treatment is with medical management; the use of antibiotics depends on the causative organism. Endoscopic management generally has no role in infectious colitis.

Postpolypectomy Bleeding

Painless bleeding occurs after approximately 1% of colonoscopic polypectomies. It is most common 5–7 days after polypectomy but can occur from 1 to 14 days after the procedure. It is generally self-limited and mild to moderate, with 50%–75% of patients requiring blood transfusions.[285–288] Reported risk factors for postpolypectomy bleeding include a large polyp size (>2 cm), thick stalk, sessile type, location in the right colon, use of anticoagulants, and use of aspirin or another NSAID. During urgent colonoscopy of patients with severe delayed postpolypectomy bleeding, an ulceration with a major stigma of hemorrhage is usually found at the site of the polypectomy (Fig. 21.20). In patients with severe bleeding in whom an SRH is found in the ulceration,[289,290] a DEP can be used to detect underlying arterial blood flow and the need for endoscopic hemostasis. Endoscopic management techniques for delayed postpolypectomy bleeding depend on the stigma found and are similar to those used for peptic ulcer hemorrhage, including epinephrine injection, thermal coagulation, hemoclip placement, and combination therapy. Most major SRH in postpolypectomy ulcers are treated with

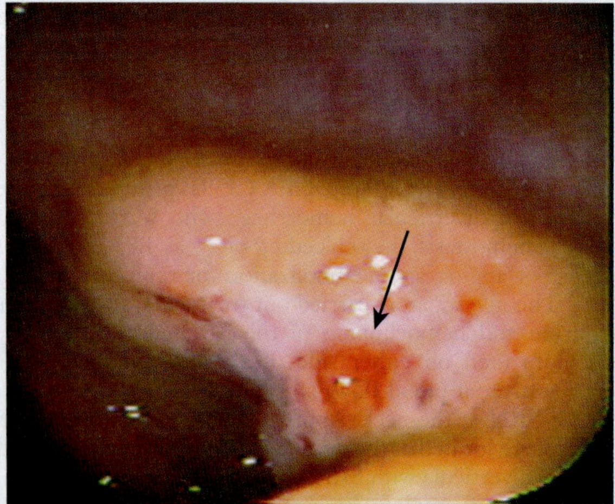

Fig. 21.20 Endoscopic appearance of postpolypectomy bleeding in the colon. Bleeding occurred 7 days after snare polypectomy of a large pedunculated polyp. Note the nonbleeding visible vessel (*arrow*) in the ulcerated polypectomy site.

hemoclipping (with or without epinephrine injection) because hemoclips do not cause tissue damage, as is seen with thermal coagulation.

Colon Neoplasia

Patients with colon polyps and cancer can present with acute hematochezia. Often, these patients have a microcytic iron deficiency anemia consistent with slow GI blood loss (see later) before more overt bleeding occurs. Colonic neoplasia was the eighth most common cause of severe hematochezia in a large CURE series.[291] At colonoscopy, epinephrine can be injected into the lesion to slow active bleeding, and hemoclips can be applied to treat SRH on ulcerated lesions that cannot be resected endoscopically. Hemostatic powder may have a palliative role in reducing acute bleeding prior to definitive treatment (see earlier).[43] When possible, colon polyps can be removed to stop bleeding. Surgical resection is usually required to prevent rebleeding from a large, ulcerated sessile lesion (see Chapters 128 and 129); however, most patients with colon polyps or cancer and severe hematochezia have advanced stage disease and high early mortality and should be considered for nonsurgical therapies.[291]

Radiation Proctitis

Radiation proctitis usually causes mild chronic hematochezia but occasionally can cause acute severe LGI bleeding. Ionizing radiation can cause acute and chronic damage to the normal colon and rectum when used to treat pelvic tumors—gynecologic, prostatic, bladder, or rectal (see Chapter 39). Acute self-limited diarrhea, tenesmus, abdominal cramping, and, rarely, bleeding develop for a few weeks in approximately 75% of patients who have received a radiation dose of 4000 cGy. Chronic radiation effects occur 6–18 months after completion of treatment and manifest as bright red blood with bowel movements. Bowel injury resulting from chronic radiation is related to vascular damage, with subsequent mucosal ischemia, thickening, and ulceration. Much of this damage is thought to result from chronic hypoxic ischemia and oxidative stress.

Flexible sigmoidoscopy or colonoscopy reveals telangiectasias, friability, and sometimes ulceration in the rectum (Fig. 21.21). Oozing bleeding is common, and often other nonbleeding rectal telangiectasias are seen. Internal hemorrhoids are often seen as well and are frequently misdiagnosed as the cause of the rectal bleeding by those unfamiliar with radiation telangiectasias.

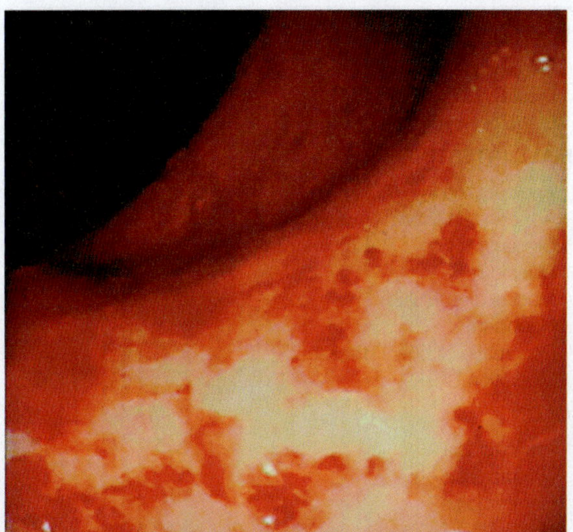

Fig. 21.21 Endoscopic appearance of radiation proctitis. Note diffuse oozing and telangiectasias.

Treatment initially focuses on avoidance of aspirin and other NSAIDs, consumption of a high-fiber diet, and iron supplementation if the patient is anemic. Medical therapy with topical or oral 5-aminosalicylic acid (mesalamine), sucralfate, or glucocorticoids may be prescribed but is not generally effective.[292] Thermal therapy is usually successful, but repeated treatments with MPEC or argon plasma coagulation are necessary to achieve good outcomes.[284] Topical formalin applied directly to the rectal mucosa can reduce bleeding,[294] as can the use of hyperbaric oxygen.[295] Antioxidant vitamins, such as vitamins E and C, have also been reported to decrease bleeding from chronic radiation proctitis (see Chapter 41).[296]

Colonic Angioectasia

Colonic bleeding from angioectasia, an important cause of LGI bleeding in the older adults, is discussed in the section on small bowel and obscure bleeding (see later). When angioectasia is the cause of bleeding in the colon, the lesions are often multiple, making endoscopic hemostasis a challenge (see also Chapter 36).

Internal Hemorrhoids

Hemorrhoidal bleeding is painless and characterized by bright red blood per rectum that can coat the outside of the stool, drip into the toilet bowl, be seen on tissue after wiping, and often appear as a large amount of fresh blood in the toilet. Usually, bleeding is mild, intermittent, and self-limited, but occasionally, severe transfusion-requiring bleeding may occur from hemorrhoids.[297] In a large study of patients with hematochezia discharged from the hospital, 20% were thought to have had bleeding from hemorrhoids.[237] In the UCLA CURE series of patients hospitalized for severe hematochezia (see earlier), internal hemorrhoids were the second most common cause (see Table 21.8).[234] Hemorrhoids were documented by urgent anoscopy and colonoscopy after a colonic cleansing preparation. The diagnosis can be made with anoscopy, sigmoidoscopy, or colonoscopy, especially if performed while bleeding is ongoing.

The treatment of internal hemorrhoids usually starts with medical therapy consisting of fiber supplementation, stool softeners, lubricant rectal suppositories (with or without glucocorticoids), and warm sitz baths. Anoscopic therapy can also be used and includes injection sclerotherapy, rubber band ligation, cryosurgery, infrared photocoagulation, MPEC, and direct current electrocoagulation. Although most patients with mild hemorrhoidal bleeding respond to medical therapy, those with severe or recurrent bleeding are likely to require rubber band ligation, some other endoscopic treatment, or, if these measures fail, surgery (see Chapter 131).

Anal Fissures

Patients with an anal fissure usually present with constipation followed by painful bowel movements with or without hematochezia. The hematochezia is usually mild and is noticed with wiping; rarely, hematochezia is moderate to severe. Treatment focuses on healing the anal fissure rather than using specific hemostasis techniques. A topical calcium channel blocker (e.g., 2% topical diltiazem cream) and control of constipation with fiber supplementation and stool softeners plus sitz baths will heal most anal fissures (see Chapter 131).

Rectal Varices

Ectopic varices may develop in the rectal mucosa between the superior hemorrhoidal veins (portal circulation) and middle and inferior hemorrhoidal veins (systemic circulation) in patients with portal hypertension. On sigmoidoscopy, rectal varices are seen during retroflexion as venous structures located several centimeters above the dentate line and extending into the rectum. They are distinct from internal hemorrhoids. The frequency of rectal varices increases with the degree of portal hypertension. Approximately 60% of patients with a history of bleeding esophageal varices have rectal varices, but they are a rare cause of severe hematochezia.[27,227,289] The treatment of bleeding rectal varices is similar to that for esophageal varices, with sclerotherapy, band ligation, or a portosystemic shunt (see Chapter 94).[298–300]

Rectal Dieulafoy Lesions

Dieulafoy lesions are large submucosal arteries without overlying mucosal ulceration that can cause massive bleeding. They can occur anywhere in the GI tract, although usually in the foregut (see earlier). Bleeding Dieulafoy lesions in the rectum, which have been treated successfully with endoscopic hemostasis, have been described in several reports.[178,301]

Rectal Ulcers

Several case series have described seriously ill hospitalized patients with the sudden onset of painless severe hematochezia from a solitary or multiple rectal ulcer(s) located 3–10 cm above the dentate line. In one series of 19 cases from Taiwan, 2.7% of patients evaluated for severe hematochezia were diagnosed with acute hemorrhagic rectal ulcer syndrome.[302] The patients had a mean age of 71 years and had been hospitalized for other medical problems from 3 to 14 days (average 7.5 days) prior to the onset of bleeding. All developed hypotension and required transfer to an ICU and blood transfusions. Colonoscopy revealed an equal number of cases of multiple and solitary ulcers located 1–7 cm from the dentate line; most of the ulcers were large (more than 1 cm) and circumferential or geographic in appearance. The patients were treated with combinations of thermal coagulation, injection therapy, and suture ligation and had a mortality rate of 26% because of multiorgan failure. The pathology of the lesions revealed necrosis suggestive of mucosal ischemia, as seen with gastric stress ulcers (see earlier). This entity appears to be a different disease from solitary rectal ulcer syndrome, colitis cystica profunda, infectious ulcers, radiation ulcers, NSAID ulcers, or constipation-induced stercoral ulcers and can be considered a type of stress ulcer of the rectum, similar to that seen in the duodenum, in extremely ill, hospitalized patients (see Chapter 130).

Solitary or multiple painless rectal ulcers were the third most common cause of severe hematochezia developing in inpatients in the UCLA CURE study (see Table 21.8). In contrast to solitary rectal ulcer syndrome, they occur in older patients with severe constipation, ICU patients, and persons who are bedridden. On colonoscopy, ulcers are chronic-appearing, large, and single or multiple. They often have SRH and can be treated endoscopically (Fig. 21.22).[303] Patients with inpatient hematochezia from a rectal ulcer have a higher rate of rebleeding than those who present from home. For acute hemostasis of large, firm ulcers with stigmata, treatment with OTSC hemoclips is recommended.

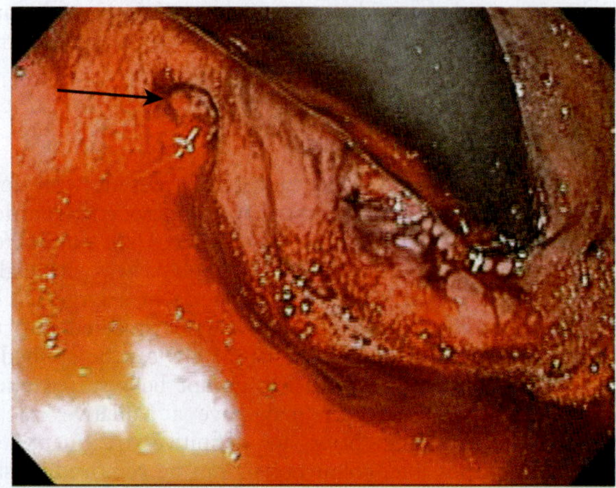

Fig. 21.22 Endoscopic appearance of bleeding from a solitary rectal ulcer with a visible vessel (*arrow*) seen on a retroflexed view.

OBSCURE OVERT GASTROINTESTINAL BLEEDING

Obscure GI bleeding is traditionally defined as GI bleeding of uncertain cause after a nondiagnostic EGD, colonoscopy, and barium small bowel follow-through.[304] Obscure GI bleeding may have an overt or occult presentation. *Obscure overt GI bleeding* refers to visible acute GI bleeding (e.g., melena, maroon stool, and hematochezia) in patients with a nondiagnostic EGD, colonoscopy, and small bowel series. *Obscure occult GI bleeding* refers to a positive FOBT result, usually in association with unexplained iron deficiency anemia. In most large series, the cause of bleeding is not found on EGD and colonoscopy in 5% of hospitalized patients with overt GI bleeding. In 75% of these patients, a bleeding site is located in the small intestine.

In patients with obscure GI bleeding, the following possibilities exist: (1) the lesion was within reach of a standard endoscope and colonoscope but not recognized as the bleeding site (e.g., Cameron lesions, angioectasias, and internal hemorrhoids); (2) the lesion was within reach of the endoscope and colonoscope but was difficult to visualize (e.g., a blood clot obscured visualization of the lesion; varices became inapparent in a hypovolemic patient; and a lesion was hidden behind a mucosal fold) or presented with intermittent bleeding (e.g., Dieulafoy lesion and angioectasias); or (3) the lesion was in the small intestine beyond the reach of standard endoscopes (e.g., neoplasm, angioectasias, and Meckel diverticula). In several series, 50% or more patients referred to a tertiary medical center for evaluation of obscure bleeding were found to have a lesion within reach of standard endoscopes (i.e., a missed lesion or difficult-to-see lesion that accounted for the bleeding) (Box 21.2).[305]

BOX 21.2 Causes of Obscure GI Bleeding

UPPER GI TRACT

- Cameron lesions
- Dieulafoy lesions
- GAVE

SMALL INTESTINE

- Angioectasia
- Aortoenteric fistula
- Dieulafoy lesion
- Diverticulosis
- Meckel diverticulum
- Neoplasm
- Pancreatic or biliary disease
- Ulceration

COLON

- Angioectasia
- Diverticulosis
- Hemorrhoids

*After exclusion of common causes of UGI bleeding.

In a patient with recurrent severe unexplained hematochezia without hypotension, a colonic source should be suspected, and a repeat colonoscopy with a good colon preparation by an experienced endoscopist is warranted. Colonic lesions that can bleed profusely and then stop, such as diverticulosis or hemorrhoids, should be considered. In patients with recurrent severe melena, push enteroscopy to reexamine the esophagus, stomach, and duodenum, as well as the proximal jejunum, for a missed or unrecognized lesion should be considered. Duodenoscopy may be useful for blood or lesions in the second to fourth portions of the duodenum.[57]

Once it is certain that a bleeding lesion in the UGI or LGI tract was not missed, the evaluation should focus on the small intestine. In the past, the principal imaging modality of the small intestine was barium radiography, but this technique was limited by the length, mobility, and motility of the small bowel and by overlying loops of bowel. Because small bowel bleeding is often intermittent, radionuclide imaging or angiography has limited value in the diagnostic evaluation. Since the late 1990s, diagnostic options for evaluating the small intestine have expanded greatly and have been revolutionized by the development of new small bowel imaging techniques, including wireless video capsule endoscopy, deep enteroscopy, and CT enterography, which now allow greater visualization and more therapeutic options than in the past (see later).[306]

Causes

A number of lesions can cause obscure GI bleeding (see Box 21.2). In persons younger than age 40, bleeding is more likely to be caused by a tumor, Meckel diverticulum, or Crohn disease. Angioectasias or an NSAID-induced ulcer are common causes in persons 40 years of age and older.

Angioectasia

A variety of vascular lesions may cause bleeding from the GI tract (see Chapter 36). *Angioectasia*, also referred to as *angiodysplasia*, is the formation of aberrant blood vessels found throughout the GI tract that develop with advancing age. The lesions are distinct from arteriovenous malformations (AVMs), which are congenital, and angiomas, which are neoplastic. *Telangiectasia* is the lesion that results from dilatation of the terminal aspect of a blood vessel. Any of the vascular lesions may cause overt or obscure GI bleeding in adults, particularly in older adults and those who take antiplatelet and anticoagulant drugs. Acquired vascular lesions (angioectasia and telangiectasia) occur in association with various disorders, such as chronic kidney disease, cirrhosis, rheumatologic disorders, and severe heart disease.[57] Although angioectasia may present as overt bleeding, they often manifest as occult bleeding or iron deficiency anemia. The most common locations are the colon and small intestine.

The histopathology of angioectasias in the colon is characterized by ectatic, dilated submucosal veins.[307,308] A proposed mechanism for their formation in the colon is that partial, intermittent, low-grade obstruction of submucosal veins during muscular contraction and distention of the cecum results in dilatation and tortuosity of the submucosal veins. Over time, the increased pressure also results in dilatation of the venules, capillaries, and arteries of the mucosal vasculature. Finally, precapillary sphincters can become incompetent, thereby causing arteriovenous communications to develop and possibly result in local mucosal ischemia. Because angioectasia can occur elsewhere in the GI tract, other mechanisms are postulated, including a response to mucosal irritation or local ischemia, as occurs after radiation.

Most angioectasias occur in patients older than 60 years of age and can involve any segment of the GI tract. Usually, the lesions are multiple in a given segment of intestine. Approximately 20% (and probably more) of patients have angioectasias in at least two sections of the GI tract.[309,310]

In studies of asymptomatic persons who underwent colonoscopy, angioectasias were found in 1%–3%.[311,312] In these persons, the angioectasias were mostly in the right colon, with the following distribution: cecum, 37%; ascending colon, 17%; transverse colon, 7%; descending colon, 7%; sigmoid colon, 18%; and rectum, 14%. Among asymptomatic persons found incidentally to have colonic angioectasia, no bleeding occurred during a 3-year follow up.

Several conditions appear to be associated with an increased frequency of angioectasia. Patients with chronic kidney disease and uremia have an increased rate of intestinal angioectasias. A study of patients with and without chronic kidney disease who had obscure GI bleeding found angioectasia as the presumptive source in 47%, compared with 18% of those without kidney disease.[313] The increased risk of bleeding from angioectasia in patients with chronic kidney disease may be associated with uremia-induced platelet dysfunction.

von Willebrand disease (congenital or acquired) has also been associated with bleeding angioectasia.[314] von Willebrand's factor is needed for effective platelet aggregation. A well-controlled prospective study found that almost all patients with bleeding UGI and colonic angioectasias, as opposed to nonbleeding angioectasias or bleeding diverticulosis, had acquired von Willebrand disease associated with selective loss of the largest multimeric forms of von Willebrand factor, as well as with aortic stenosis.[315] Because the large von Willebrand multimers promote primary hemostasis in a microcirculation characterized by high shear forces, as occurs in angioectasia, the loss of the large multimers may explain why bleeding occurs in some patients with angioectasias.

Aortic stenosis has been associated with GI bleeding from angioectasia (Heyde syndrome).[316] This association is controversial because both conditions are common, and an association may not imply cause and effect.[317] Nevertheless, aortic stenosis has been shown to be associated with an acquired form of von Willebrand disease in 67%–92% of patients because of mechanical disruption of von Willebrand proteins during passage through the stenotic aortic valve; the acquired von Willebrand disease, in turn, increases the risk of bleeding from angioectasia.[318,319] Several series have reported cessation of bleeding from angioectasia after aortic valve replacement, even though the angioectasias persisted, an observation consistent with the hypothesis that bleeding was the result of the damaged von Willebrand factors that normalized after aortic valve replacement.[320]

Overt or obscure GI bleeding occurs in approximately 20% of patients with a left ventricular assist device, especially in older patients, with angioectasia as one of the most frequent causes of bleeding.[321–323] Possible pathophysiologic mechanisms for angioectasia formation and bleeding include loss of von Willebrand factor related to shear stress, which results in impaired platelet aggregation, and intestinal hypoperfusion related to increased vascular luminal pressure and lowered pulse pressure.[323] Because many older persons with bleeding from intestinal angioectasia have cardiovascular disease but not severe aortic stenosis, other cardiovascular disorders such as mild to moderate aortic stenosis, aortic sclerosis, hypertrophic cardiomyopathy, and peripheral vascular disease may result in sufficiently high shear stress to disrupt von Willebrand factors and contribute to bleeding angioectasias.[320]

On endoscopy, an angioectasia appears as a 2–10 mm red lesion, with arborizing ectatic blood vessels that emanate from a central vessel (Fig. 21.23). Application of pressure on an angioectasia with an endoscopic probe may cause the lesion to blanch. One study has suggested that sedation of a patient with a narcotic during endoscopy can make visualization of angioectasia difficult because of transient mucosal or submucosal hypoperfusion, which leads to decreased filling or causes

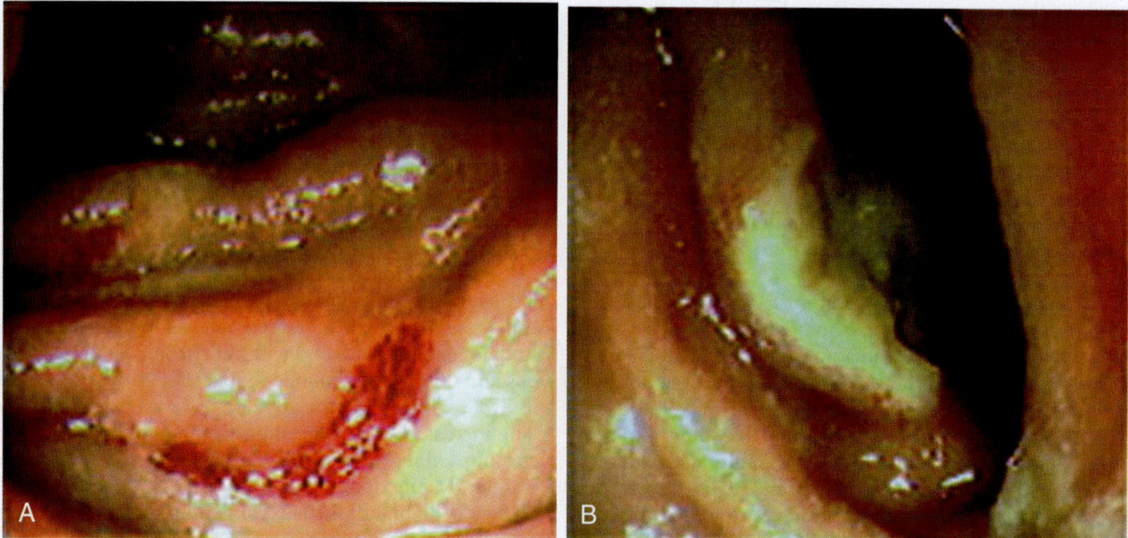

Fig. 21.23 Endoscopic appearance of jejunal angioectasia before (A) and after (B) multipolar probe electrocoagulation.

vasoconstriction, and that reversal with naloxone, an opioid antagonist, can make the angioectasia more prominent.[324] In practice, however, this maneuver is unlikely to be useful clinically and might make the patient more uncomfortable.

Angioectasias can be treated endoscopically with various modalities, including epinephrine injection, thermal probe coagulation, argon plasma coagulation, hemoclips, and band ligation. Assessing efficacy can be difficult, given the heterogeneity of affected patients and intermittent nature of the blood loss. One series of 16 patients with transfusion-requiring bleeding from angioectasia found no difference in the frequency of continued bleeding (50%) whether treatment was with surgery, endoscopic therapy, or blood transfusions alone, presumably because of the diffuse locations of the angioectasias.[325] In another study of 33 patients with iron deficiency anemia and small bowel angioectasias seen on push enteroscopy, no changes in clinical or endoscopic findings were found in most patients 1 year after endoscopic therapy.[326] By contrast, in another study of patients with GI bleeding suspected from small bowel angioectasia, treatment with electrocoagulation led to a significant decrease in (but not elimination of) the need for blood transfusions compared with observation alone.[327] In a pilot study of double-balloon enteroscopy, endoscopic treatment was performed in approximately one-half of patients with angioectasia, and rebleeding rates during follow up were similar in the treated and nontreated patients.[328]

In a small case series, hormonal therapy with estrogen was suggested to have a benefit in controlling bleeding from telangiectasia in patients with chronic kidney disease.[329] Case reports have suggested that estrogen also decreases bleeding in patients with HHT [Osler-Weber-Rendu disease (see later)] and von Willebrand disease. A multicenter randomized controlled trial involving 72 patients, however, found no difference between an estrogen-progesterone combination and placebo in the rates of rebleeding, which were 39% and 46%, respectively.[330] Therefore routine use of hormones for managing bleeding from angioectasia cannot be recommended.

Thalidomide is an angiogenesis inhibitor that may be effective in selected patients with vascular malformations. A randomized trial that compared thalidomide with oral iron in patients with angiodysplasia or GAVE revealed that thalidomide-treated patients experienced a significant decrease in the number of bleeding episodes, transfusions, and hospitalizations and in vascular endothelial growth factor levels.[331] Until these data are confirmed, however, caution is required in the use of thalidomide, given its potential for serious side effects including profound and distinctive birth defects.

Most patients with intermittently bleeding GI angioectasia require medical treatment in addition to endoscopic hemostasis. Medications that can exacerbate chronic low-level bleeding (in particular, aspirin, other NSAIDs, warfarin, other antiplatelet agents such as clopidogrel, and direct-acting oral anticoagulants) should be avoided or at least minimized. Many patients can be managed with chronic administration of iron (orally or intravenously), and, occasionally, those with renal insufficiency may need erythropoietin injections as well to maintain adequate blood counts, despite ongoing bleeding.

HHT

HHT, also known as *Osler-Weber-Rendu disease*, is a hereditary condition characterized by diffuse telangiectasias and large AVMs (see also Chapters 36 and 87). The most striking clinical feature is telangiectasias on the lips, oral mucosa, and fingertips. Additionally, up to one-third of patients have pulmonary, hepatic, or cerebral AVMs (see Chapter 87). Patients generally present with recurrent severe nosebleeds, GI bleeding, and iron deficiency anemia. Usually the epistaxis, rather than GI bleeding, causes the more profound blood loss and anemia. HHT can be life-threatening because of embolic strokes or brain abscesses related to the pulmonary and cerebral AVMs. Symptoms of HHT generally develop in childhood or early adulthood.

HHT is inherited as an autosomal dominant trait, with varying phenotypic expression. Mutations occur in at least four genes [*ENG* (encodes endoglin, type 1 HHT or HHT1), *ALK-1* (encodes activin receptor-like kinase 1, type 2 HHT or HHT2), *SMAD4*, and *HHT3*] that encode proteins needed to maintain the integrity of the vascular endothelium; defects in these proteins allow the formation of AVMs.

The diagnosis of HHT is based on four criteria: (1) spontaneous and recurrent epistaxis, (2) multiple mucocutaneous telangiectasias, (3) visceral AVMs (GI, pulmonary, brain, liver), and (4) a first-degree relative with HHT.[332] Genetic testing to detect mutations in the *ENG*, *ALK-1*, or *SMAD4* genes may be helpful in selected cases. Patients suspected of having HHT should be screened for cerebral and pulmonary AVMs, and family members of the patient should consider genetic testing.

Telangiectasias can occur anywhere in the small intestine in patients with HHT. In a case series in which capsule endoscopy was performed in 32 patients with and 48 patients without HHT who were being evaluated for small bowel bleeding, small bowel telangiectasias were found in 81% of patients with HHT compared with 29% of those without HHT.[333] The telangiectasias were evenly distributed throughout the small bowel, but all actively bleeding lesions were found in the duodenum or proximal jejunum and within reach of a standard push enteroscope. The detection of five or more telangiectasias had a sensitivity of 75% and a positive predictive value of 86% for a diagnosis of HHT.

The treatment of HHT is generally focused on the control of acute bleeding (epistaxis and GI bleeding), prevention of rebleeding, and treatment of anemia (with iron supplements). Patients with GI bleeding should undergo endoscopy (or push enteroscopy) and colonoscopy to look for any GI tract lesions that may be bleeding. Focal GI tract bleeding can be treated with endoscopic coagulation. Hormonal therapy has also been reported as a treatment for small bowel bleeding in HHT.[334] Patients who have symptomatic or large cerebral or pulmonary AVMs should be considered for radiologic embolization of these lesions (see Chapter 38).

Blue Rubber Bleb Nevus Syndrome

Blue rubber bleb nevus syndrome is rare and characterized by venous malformations in the skin, soft tissues, and GI tract.[335,336] Bleeding usually occurs in childhood and continues into adulthood and results in chronic iron deficiency requiring iron replacement and transfusions. On endoscopy, lesions appear as large, protuberant, polypoid, blue venous blebs; they can occur anywhere in the GI tract, but especially in the small bowel and colon, and can be treated by endoscopic band ligation or surgical resection (see Chapter 36).

Meckel Diverticulum

A Meckel diverticulum is a congenital, blind, intestinal pouch that results from incomplete obliteration of the vitelline duct during gestation (see Chapter 100).[337] Characteristic features of Meckel diverticula have been described by the "rule of 2s": they occur in 2% of the population, are found within 2 feet of the ileocecal valve, are 2 inches long, result in a complication in 2% of cases, have two types of ectopic tissue (gastric and pancreatic) within the diverticulum, present clinically most commonly at age 2 (with intestinal obstruction), and have a male-to-female ratio of more than 2:1. The most common complications of Meckel diverticula are bleeding, obstruction, and diverticulitis, which can occur in children or adults. Histopathologic evaluation of bleeding diverticula reveals ectopic gastric mucosa, which can lead to acid secretion and ulceration in up to 75% of patients. The diagnostic test for a Meckel diverticulum is a ^{99m}Tc-pertechnetate scan (Meckel scan) because technetium pertechnetate has an affinity for gastric mucosa. Meckel scans have a high specificity (almost 100%) and positive predictive value but can be negative in the 25%–50% of patients in whom the diverticulum does not contain ectopic gastric mucosa.[338] The accuracy of the Meckel scan can be improved with the administration of an H2RA for 24–48 hours before the test. Meckel diverticula have also been diagnosed by CT enterography, capsule endoscopy, or double-balloon enteroscopy (via an oral or rectal approach).

NSAID–Induced Small Intestinal Erosions and Ulcers

Mucosal erosions or ulcers that can be seen on capsule endoscopy develop in 25%–55% of patients who take full-dose nonselective NSAIDs.[339–343] Patients who take selective COX-2 inhibitors have lower rates of mucosal ulcers on capsule endoscopy (see Chapter 121).

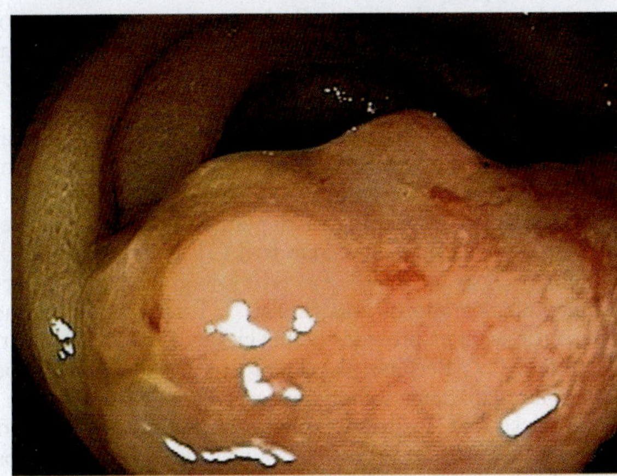

Fig. 21.24 Ileal adenocarcinoma detected on deep enteroscopy in a patient with a history of hereditary nonpolyposis colorectal cancer who had obscure overt GI bleeding. The lesion was initially visualized on a capsule endoscopy study.

Small Intestinal Neoplasms

Tumors of the small intestine comprise only 5%–7% of all GI tract neoplasms but are the most common cause of obscure GI bleeding in patients younger than age 50.[344] The most common small intestine neoplasms are adenomas (usually duodenal), adenocarcinomas (Fig. 21.24), carcinoid tumors (usually ileal), GISTs, lymphomas, hamartomatosis polyps (Peutz-Jeghers syndrome), and juvenile polyps (see Chapters 127 and 128).

Small Intestinal Diverticula

The duodenum is the most common site of small intestinal diverticula. In one large series,[345] 79% of small intestinal diverticula occurred in the duodenum, 18% were in the jejunum or ileum, and only 3% were in all three segments—duodenum, jejunum, and ileum. Duodenal diverticula are noted in up to 20% of the population, with an increasing frequency with age.[345–348] They are usually located along the medial wall of the second part of the duodenum within 1–2 cm of the ampulla of Vater. Bleeding from a duodenal diverticulum is rare. Several reports have described bleeding from a duodenal diverticulum that was managed endoscopically.[348,349] Jejunal and ileal diverticula occur in 1%–2% of the population, are most associated with scleroderma, another motility disorder, or SIBO, and only rarely have been associated with bleeding (see Chapters 26 and 107).

Dieulafoy Lesion of the Small Intestine

Several reports have described Dieulafoy lesions of the duodenum, jejunum, and ileum (see Chapter 36).[350] Most affected persons are younger than age 40, in contrast to those with gastric Dieulafoy lesions, who tend to be older (see earlier). The lesions are often challenging to find and in the past were detected by angiography and intraoperative endoscopy. Capsule endoscopy can also localize and diagnose these lesions, which can be treated via a single- or double-balloon enteroscope.

Diagnostic Tests

Imaging

Barium small bowel follow-through is no longer utilized because it has a low yield for determining the cause of obscure GI bleeding (with limited ability to distend the bowel and visualize mucosal lesions such as angiodysplasia). Barium studies are not recommended for patients with acute bleeding; residual barium contrast in the GI tract can make urgent endoscopy, colonoscopy, or angiography more difficult to perform.

CT of the abdomen has the advantage of imaging extraluminal structures as well as mucosal and intramural lesions in the small bowel. High-quality abdominal CT (with and without oral contrast) can show thickening of the small bowel, suggestive of Crohn disease or malignancy. Standard CT is less accurate than barium enteroclysis for the diagnosis of low-grade bowel obstruction, mucosal ulcerations, and fistulas. CT enteroclysis using a multidetector scanner provides better views of the small intestine than standard CT. Because placement of a nasoduodenal tube is usually required, patients sometimes receive moderate sedation for CT enteroclysis.[351] CT enterography with a high volume of an oral contrast agent to distend the small bowel may have a diagnostic yield similar to that for CT enteroclysis, without the need for a nasoduodenal tube. MRI enteroclysis and enterography have also been described, but preliminary studies suggest that results to date are inferior to those with a multidetector CT. MRI techniques have the advantage of not exposing the patient to radiation.

Nuclear medicine studies and angiography can be used to evaluate obscure GI bleeding. A Meckel (^{99m}Tc-pertechnetate) scan can be useful for the diagnostic evaluation of a Meckel diverticulum, particularly in younger patients, as discussed earlier. Radionuclide scanning with technetium-labeled RBCs has limited utility because of its poor ability to localize the bleeding site in the small bowel. Angiography can be useful for patients with active, acute small bowel bleeding because of the possibility of therapeutic embolization. Small case series have described provocative angiography, in which heparin or another anticoagulant is administered to provoke GI bleeding that has been intermittent. The technique increases the yield of detecting a bleeding lesion but at the risk of causing a life-threatening complication.[352]

Endoscopy

Push Enteroscopy

Push enteroscopy can be performed with a colonoscope (160–180 cm in length) or dedicated push enteroscope (220–250 cm in length).[353] These endoscopes can be used to evaluate the esophagus, stomach, duodenum, and proximal jejunum approximately 50–150 cm beyond the ligament of Treitz. Insertion is often limited by looping of the endoscope in the stomach. Push enteroscopy identifies a potential bleeding site in 50% or more patients, and roughly 50% of lesions found are within reach of a standard upper endoscope, suggesting that the lesion was missed or unrecognized on the initial examination.[304,305,353] The overall diagnostic yield of push enteroscopy is approximately 40%, with a range of 3%–80% in various studies; the most commonly detected lesions are angioectasias.[304] In the UCLA CURE hemostasis experience in patients with recurrent, severe, obscure, overt GI bleeding manifesting as melena, the diagnostic yield has been 80%.[57] The lesions were categorized as those missed by EGD, those in the duodenum (first to fourth portion), and those in the jejunum; most lesions were within reach of a push enteroscope. Focal lesions were treated endoscopically, biopsied, or tattooed. Patients in whom a diagnosis was not made by push enteroscopy underwent further studies (see Fig. 21.5).

Intraoperative Endoscopy and Surgical Exploration

Surgical exploration of the small intestine can be performed when other studies are nondiagnostic. At surgery, the small bowel should be palpated "running the bowel" to detect mass lesions. In general, a standard exploratory laparotomy or laparoscopy is performed first to lyse any adhesions and look for obvious tumors, a Meckel diverticulum, or large vascular lesions. The small bowel is usually extracted through the abdominal incision to allow the surgeon to assist with advancement of an endoscope within the lumen of the GI tract, which allows mucosal visualization as well as transillumination. Various endoscopes can be used (standard upper endoscope and colonoscope, pediatric colonoscope, or push enteroscope), depending on the route of access. The endoscope can be passed transorally for a natural orifice luminal examination or via an enterotomy with the use of a sterile endoscope.[354] Because air insufflation will distend the entire small intestine and thereby make laparoscopic or open visualization difficult, the surgeon should pinch the intestine, manually or with an atraumatic clamp, distal to the tip of the endoscope, to trap enough air to permit visualization. Additionally, the insufflation of the bowel with carbon dioxide, rather than room air, allows faster diffusion of gas out of the bowel. The surgeon helps advance the endoscope by pleating the small bowel over the endoscope. Any lesion identified can be addressed surgically or endoscopically, depending on the nature of the lesion. Most series report complete enteroscopy of the entire small bowel in 50%–75% of cases.[355,356] The diagnostic yield of intraoperative enteroscopy ranges from 58% to 88%, but rebleeding after intraoperative enteroscopy has also been reported in 13%–60% of patients.[304] The moderate performance characteristics, as well as risks of surgical exploration, limit this procedure as a diagnostic tool, but in selected patients, combined endoscopic and surgical evaluation can be useful and definitive.

The role of intraoperative endoscopy in the management of severe obscure GI bleeding before versus after the introduction of capsule endoscopy and deep enteroscopy has been reported.[356] Before an operation in the precapsule endoscopy era, a presumptive diagnosis or localization of bleeding site was achieved in 36% of patients compared with 63% in the postcapsule endoscopy era. In the precapsule endoscopy era, a definitive diagnosis was made intraoperatively in 100% of patients compared with 76% in the postcapsule endoscopy era. For lesions that were surgically resectable—small bowel tumors, Meckel diverticula, aortoenteric fistula, and focal ischemic ulcers—no patient experienced postoperative bleeding during long-term follow-up; however, rebleeding rates were high in other patients—67% with vascular lesions, 44% with small bowel ulcers, 50% with Crohn disease, and 63% with no definitive diagnosis.[356] Preoperative diagnosis with capsule endoscopy or deep enteroscopy has become more important, particularly in older patients who may have significant complications or death from surgery. Careful selection of patients is required (see Fig. 21.5).[357]

Capsule Endoscopy

With capsule endoscopy, the patient ingests a pill camera that transmits images of the small intestine for 8 hours or more. In patients with severe recurrent GI bleeding, this technique can identify a transition point at which fresh blood appears in the small bowel and thereby localize the bleeding site and sometimes identify a specific source lesion.[357] Capsule endoscopy does not permit the application of therapy and can only localize a lesion in the small bowel on the basis of the time of passage down the small intestine, as determined by sensors on the abdomen and telemetry. The information can be useful, however, in directing subsequent therapeutic procedures such as deep enteroscopy, angiography, or surgery. Although capsule endoscopy may occasionally detect gastric, duodenal, or colonic lesions, it is not a substitute for EGD and colonoscopy.

Compared with small bowel barium studies, capsule endoscopy has significantly improved detection rates for small bowel lesions (67% vs. 8%) and findings that influence clinical management (42% vs. 6%).[357,358] A small series found capsule endoscopy to be superior to CT enteroclysis for the diagnosis of obscure GI bleeding because of its ability to identify angioectasias.[359]

An evaluation of published studies that have compared push enteroscopy with capsule endoscopy in patients with obscure bleeding (79% overt, 21% occult) found that the average rate of positive findings was 23% for push enteroscopy and 63% for capsule endoscopy.[304] A similar result was found in a meta-analysis of published trials and abstracts; the diagnostic yield for push enteroscopy was 28% and 63% for capsule endoscopy.[358] A randomized trial that compared push enteroscopy with capsule endoscopy as a first-line approach to obscure GI bleeding reported identification of a bleeding source in 24% of the push enteroscopy examinations and 50% of the capsule studies ($P = .02$).[360] In this study, capsule endoscopy missed lesions in 8% of patients, and all the missed lesions were within reach of a standard upper endoscope.

A study of patients with acute, overt, unexplained GI bleeding (melena or hematochezia with nondiagnostic EGD and colonoscopy) who were randomized to capsule endoscopy or angiography reported a significantly higher diagnostic rate for capsule endoscopy than for angiography (53% vs. 20%) but no difference in the long-term outcomes, including transfusions, hospitalizations, and mortality.[361] Capsule endoscopy was compared with intraoperative endoscopy in one study of 47 patients who underwent both procedures, primarily for obscure overt GI bleeding.[362] Using intraoperative endoscopy as the gold standard, capsule endoscopy had a sensitivity of 95%, specificity of 75%, positive predictive value of 95%, and negative predictive value of 85%. Most of the bleeding lesions were angioectasias.

Several studies have found that the diagnostic yield of capsule endoscopy increases in the setting of ongoing or recent (<2 weeks) overt GI bleeding or severe chronic GI bleeding (hemoglobin <10 g/dL, iron deficiency anemia, or more than one overt bleeding episode).[362–364] In a study from Greece of 34 patients who had active mild to moderate overt GI bleeding and negative EGD and colonoscopy results and who underwent an urgent capsule endoscopy study while still in the hospital, the diagnostic yield was 92%, as defined by the identification of a bleeding lesion (18 angioectasias, 3 ulcers, 2 tumors) or the segment of intestine with bleeding (11 patients).[29] By contrast, the same group from Greece found that the diagnostic yield of capsule endoscopy in patients with obscure occult bleeding and iron deficiency anemia was 57% (angioectasias in 24%, multiple jejunal or ileal ulcers in 12%, multiple erosions in 8%, solitary ulcers in 6%, polyps in 4%, and other tumors in 4%).[365]

Deep Enteroscopy of the Jejunum and Ileum

Specially designed, ultraflexible, 200-cm-long enteroscopes are used in conjunction with an overtube to advance the endoscope by pleating the small intestine over it. The available systems include a double-balloon endoscope (with a balloon on the tip of the endoscope and another balloon on the overtube), a single-balloon system (a balloon on the overtube only), and a spiral overtube (no balloon used). All enteroscopes work by pleating the small intestine over the endoscope. These enteroscopes can be inserted orally (antegrade) and advanced into the proximal to midileum or inserted rectally (retrograde) and advanced to the distal to midileum. Rarely, a complete enteroscopy of the small intestine to the cecum can be performed via the antegrade approach using the double-balloon enteroscope, whereas total enteroscopy (complete visualization of entire small bowel) using a combined antegrade and retrograde occurred in 44% of cases in a large review of published studies.[366] Deep enteroscopy allows not only visualization but also interventions such as biopsy, hemostasis, and tattooing of lesions. The endoscopes used for deep enteroscopy have standard working channels that allow passage of accessories such as biopsy forceps, MPEC probes, hemoclips, and injection needles that fit through a standard colonoscope. The risk of major complications with double-balloon enteroscopy is approximately 1%; complications include perforation, pancreatitis, bleeding, and aspiration pneumonia (see Chapter 40).[367]

A compilation of 12 case series of double-balloon enteroscopy for obscure bleeding in 723 patients found an overall diagnostic yield of 65% (Table 21.10).[304] Comparative studies of capsule endoscopy and double-balloon enteroscopy have revealed a slightly higher diagnostic yield for capsule endoscopy. The agreement between these approaches in one large multicenter study of 115 patients was 74% for angioectasias, 96% for ulcers, 94% for polyps, and 96% for other large tumors.[368] Another comparative study found that for patients with obscure bleeding, the agreement was 92%, but the yield in a given segment of intestine in patients with polyposis was only 33% for capsule endoscopy compared with 67% for double-balloon enteroscopy; however, capsule endoscopy may detect polyps beyond the reach of the double-balloon enteroscope.[368]

TABLE 21.10 Small Intestinal Lesions Found in 488 Patients During Double-Balloon Enteroscopy for Obscure GI Bleeding

Lesion	Frequency, % (Range)
None	40 (0–57)
Angioectasias	31 (6–55)
Ulcerations	13 (2–35)
Malignancy	8 (3–26)
Other	6 (2–22)

Data from Raju GS, Gerson L, Das A, Lewis B. American Gastroenterological Association (AGA) Institute technical review on obscure gastrointestinal bleeding. *Gastroenterology*. 2007;133:1697–1717.

Overall Approach

For patients with unexplained overt GI bleeding and negative upper endoscopy and colonoscopy results, capsule endoscopy is generally recommended as the next step. If capsule endoscopy reveals a lesion in the proximal jejunum, push enteroscopy can be performed. If a lesion is found in the mid-small intestine, deep enteroscopy or surgery may be considered, depending on the nature of the lesion. A lesion in the terminal ileum may prompt deep enteroscopy via the colonic route. If no lesion is detected on capsule endoscopy, but a high suspicion for a lesion remains, capsule endoscopy should be repeated or deep enteroscopy performed. With the increased availability of deep enteroscopes and accessories, deep enteroscopy could become the preferred initial diagnostic step (before capsule endoscopy). Modeling studies have suggested that this approach may be a cost-effective strategy,[369,370] but the question ideally should be addressed in a randomized study.

The UCLA CURE group's algorithm for the management of patients who have had unexplained severe overt GI bleeding with a history of melena and the need for blood transfusions is shown in Fig. 21.5. For such patients, the diagnostic yield is more than 80%.[57]

OBSCURE OCCULT GASTROINTESTINAL BLEEDING AND IRON DEFICIENCY ANEMIA

Fecal Occult Blood

Occult GI bleeding is usually detected with a routine guaiac-based FOBT or fecal immunochemical test (FIT) and occurs (by definition) with no visible blood in the stool, with or without iron deficiency. Normal fecal blood loss is 0.5–1.5 mL/day.[371] Many FOBTs are available for detecting increased amounts of blood in the stool and are described in detail in Chapter 129.

The approach to the patient with a positive FOBT result depends on why the test was obtained. If the FOBT or FIT was obtained for colon cancer screening in a patient 50 years of age or older, the patient should undergo colonoscopy and possibly EGD, even in the absence of iron deficiency anemia. This recommendation is based on results of a study of 248 patients with fecal occult blood in whom more lesions were found in the UGI tract by EGD (mostly esophagitis, gastropathy, and ulcers) than in the colon by colonoscopy (mostly large adenomas and cancer).[372] Whether patients with a positive FIT result (which detects only human hemoglobin from the LGI tract) and normal colonoscopy result require EGD is uncertain (and unlikely).[373] If an FOBT was performed for iron deficiency anemia, the patient should be evaluated with EGD and colonoscopy. If the results of both examinations are negative, the small bowel should be imaged, as described earlier, with capsule endoscopy, possibly followed by deep enteroscopy if a lesion is detected on capsule endoscopy.

Although colon cancer screening with FOBTs is generally based on six samples of spontaneously passed stool, a positive FOBT result (not uncommonly) may be found when stool is obtained during digital examination of the rectum. Although a digital rectal examination could potentially cause trauma to the anal canal, several studies have found no increase in the false-positive rate of FOBTs when stool is obtained by a digital examination.[374,375] Therefore a positive FOBT result should be approached in the same manner regardless of the method by which the stool sample is obtained. Additionally, a single negative FOBT result on digital rectal examination is not considered adequate colon cancer screening and does not reduce a patient's chances of having advanced neoplasia.[376]

Iron Deficiency Anemia

Iron deficiency anemia is common, with a frequency of 2%–5% in adult men and postmenopausal women.[377] Iron deficiency anemia represents 4%–13% of all referrals for outpatient gastroenterology consultation.[378]

The approach to iron deficiency anemia depends on the patient's gender and the presence or absence of clinically significant overt non-GI blood loss.[379] Young women with iron deficiency anemia should be considered to have menstrual blood loss as the cause of anemia and, depending on clinical circumstances, may not need a GI evaluation. By contrast, men and postmenopausal women with iron deficiency anemia should always be evaluated for a GI cause of iron deficiency. Iron deficiency anemia should be considered in patients with a low MCV and anemia.

In iron deficiency anemia, the serum iron concentration is decreased and the level of transferrin (TIBC) is increased. A transferrin saturation index (serum iron divided by TIBC) lower than 15% is a sensitive indicator of iron deficiency anemia. A serum ferritin level lower than 15 ng/mL has a sensitivity of 59% and specificity of 99% for iron deficiency, whereas a cutoff ferritin level of 41 ng/mL has a sensitivity and specificity of 98%.[380] A bone marrow aspirate can provide information about body stores of iron but is rarely necessary.

Iron deficiency can result from overt or occult blood loss (from GI tract luminal lesions, menses, epistaxis, pulmonary lesions, or urinary tract lesions), intestinal iron malabsorption (as in celiac disease or gastric atrophy, or after gastric bypass surgery), treatment with erythropoietin (because of excess iron requirements), and RBC destruction (hemolysis). The GI evaluation of a patient with iron deficiency should focus on endoscopy (upper and lower) to detect treatable lesions, especially malignancies. Recognizing iron malabsorption from the GI tract as a cause of iron deficiency is especially important. The duodenum is the site of iron absorption in the small intestine. Most dietary iron is in the ferric form, but only the ferrous form of iron can be absorbed by the duodenum. Ascorbic acid at a low pH is required to release nonheme iron and convert it to the ferrous form for absorption in the small intestine.[381] Several studies have shown that 20%–30% of patients with iron deficiency anemia have gastric atrophy and therefore do not produce an acid milieu that facilitates iron absorption.[377,382,383] Iron deficiency anemia has also been associated with Hp infection.[384] Therefore gastric biopsies should be obtained during upper endoscopy in patients with unexplained iron deficiency anemia (see Chapters 52, 53, and 54).

Celiac disease commonly manifests as iron deficiency anemia, primarily because of iron malabsorption resulting from blunted duodenal villi. Patients with celiac disease have been reported to have higher rates of positive FOBT results than healthy controls, but subsequent studies in which radiolabeled RBCs were used did not find a true increase in blood loss.[385,386] The cause of iron deficiency anemia in patients with celiac disease may, in fact, be multifactorial. Any patient who is evaluated for iron deficiency anemia and undergoes EGD should have duodenal biopsy samples obtained to look for celiac disease (see Chapter 109).

Patients who have undergone Roux-en-Y gastric bypass surgery are at high risk of iron malabsorption because of bypass of the duodenum, where most iron is absorbed. These patients can present with severe unexplained iron deficiency without occult blood in the stool. They often have extremely low body stores of iron and require IV iron supplementation (see Chapter 7).

The differential diagnosis of iron deficiency anemia includes anemia of chronic disease and thalassemia. In anemia of chronic disease, both the serum iron level and TIBC are low, with a normal serum ferritin level. Patients with thalassemia have a family history of anemia, splenomegaly, target cells on peripheral blood smear, and normal serum ferritin levels.

Patients with unexplained iron deficiency anemia should undergo EGD and colonoscopy to rule out a GI tract lesion that may cause chronic blood loss. In a prospective study of 100 patients with iron deficiency anemia, GI tract lesions were found in 62 patients, with 36 having lesions in the UGI tract (mostly ulcers), 25 in the colon (mostly cancer), and 1 in both the UGI tract and colon.[387] In patients with unexplained iron deficiency anemia who undergo EGD, duodenal biopsy specimens should be obtained to exclude celiac disease as a cause of iron malabsorption. Gastric biopsy samples also should be obtained to rule out gastropathy and Hp infection. Depending on the severity of iron deficiency anemia, even without a positive FOBT result, the evaluation of the small intestine for a bleeding lesion, as discussed earlier, should be considered. If a specific cause of anemia is not identified, patients should be advised to avoid antiplatelet and anticoagulant drugs and take supplemental iron.

Full references for this chapter can be found at https://ebooks.health.elsevier.com.

22 Jaundice

Steven D. Lidofsky

IN THIS CHAPTER

Jaundice, a condition manifested by a distinctive yellowing of the sclera, skin, and mucous membranes, takes its name from the Old French word for yellow (*jaundice*). It is also known as *icterus* (derived from the Greek *ikteros*, a golden bird believed to possess the power to cure icteric individuals). Jaundice results from tissue deposition of the compound bilirubin. Although jaundice is commonly thought to be a sign of liver and biliary tract disease, the differential diagnosis is broad. Consequently, identification of the cause of jaundice and selection of an appropriate treatment plan may not always be straightforward.

The quest to elucidate the origins of jaundice has a rich history (the interested reader is encouraged to delve into a recently published monograph on the subject).[1] Clinical descriptions of disorders associated with jaundice can be found as early as the classical Greek texts that comprise the Hippocratic Corpus. By the late 19th century (e.g., see *Osler's Principles and Practice of Medicine*), important distinctions had been made between jaundice as a result of biliary tract obstruction and nonobstructive causes of jaundice. By the end of the 20th century, parallel revolutions in molecular biology and clinical imaging had led, respectively, to elucidation of fundamental mechanisms of bilirubin metabolism and membrane transport, and to technical approaches that made it possible to pinpoint the cause of jaundice in most cases. Despite these advances, the final chapter concerning the pathophysiology of jaundice has yet to be written, and optimization of diagnostic and therapeutic strategies remains in evolution.

BILIRUBIN METABOLISM AND MEASUREMENT

Metabolism

Bilirubin is an end-product of heme degradation. Its internally hydrogen-bonded tetrapyrrole structure renders it hydrophobic, and its elimination requires conversion to water-soluble conjugates. At physiological concentrations, the antioxidant properties of bilirubin and its interactions with selected circulating and cell membrane proteins have revealed important antiinflammatory and immunomodulatory roles for this molecule,[2] and it can influence metabolic programming, for example, by binding to the transcription factor peroxisome proliferator-activated receptor alpha, with resultant regulation of target gene expression.[3] By contrast, at high concentrations, bilirubin can cross the blood-brain barrier and induce neuronal death. Efficient metabolism of this compound is critical to prevent this complication.

Bilirubin metabolism is summarized briefly in Fig. 22.1. Much of the literature concerning the metabolism of this substance was published over 35 years ago, and the interested reader is encouraged to seek more recently published reviews for in-depth detail.[4,5] Each day, a healthy adult produces an average of 4 mg/kg of bilirubin (i.e., almost 0.5 mmol in a 70-kg person). Most bilirubin (70%–80%) results from breakdown of hemoglobin released from senescent erythrocytes. The remainder derives primarily from catabolism of other heme-containing proteins (e.g., catalase, cytochrome oxidases) in hepatocytes. Although other hemoproteins (e.g., myoglobin) are present in extrahepatic tissues, their turnover rate is low. Consequently, in healthy individuals, their overall contribution to bilirubin production is minimal.

The conversion of heme to bilirubin involves the sequential actions of two enzymes: (1) *heme oxygenase (HO)* and (2) *biliverdin reductase (BVR)*. HO has two isoforms: (1) HO-1, an inducible ubiquitously expressed protein, and (2) HO-2, which is expressed constitutively in selected tissues (including hepatocytes).[6,7] These proteins catalyze the opening of the heme ring to produce biliverdin (BV), a water-soluble compound. Isomer-selective BVR,[8] a ubiquitously expressed cell surface membrane protein, converts BV IXα to bilirubin IXα, the predominant adult form of this molecule. The major sites of bilirubin production depend upon the tissue sources of the hemoprotein precursors. Conversion of erythrocyte-derived hemoglobin to bilirubin occurs primarily in macrophages in the spleen, bone marrow, and liver (where they are known as Kupffer cells). By contrast, free hemoglobin, haptoglobin-bound hemoglobin, and methemalbumin are predominantly processed to bilirubin in hepatocytes.

Bilirubin (in its native hydrophobic form, also known as unconjugated bilirubin) circulates in plasma tightly and noncovalently bound to albumin. Excretion of bilirubin requires uptake by hepatocytes, where it is converted into water-soluble conjugates, which are subsequently exported primarily into bile for delivery to the gut. Bilirubin metabolism and elimination is a multistep process for which several inherited disorders have been identified (see later).

Unconjugated bilirubin is taken up across the sinusoidal (basolateral) membrane of hepatocytes. How this occurs remains unresolved. Considerable debate has revolved around the relative roles of passive diffusion versus carrier-mediated transport,[9] and the mechanisms responsible for hepatocyte bilirubin uptake have not been clarified. Because the uptake of unconjugated bilirubin is competitively inhibited by certain organic anions [e.g., bromosulfophthalein (BSP), indocyanine], it has been speculated, based upon studies in transfected cells, that a member

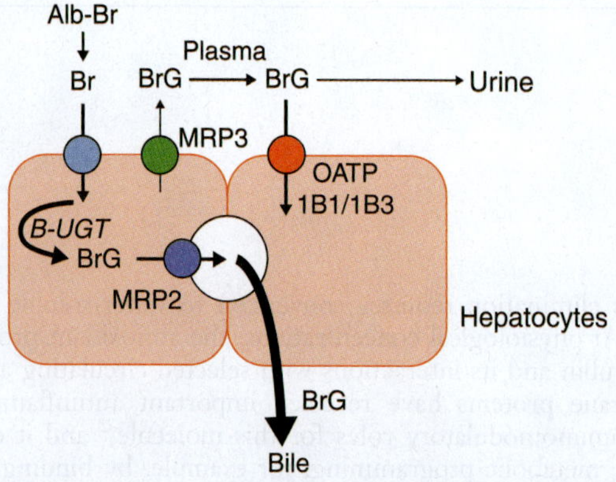

Fig. 22.1 Schematic overview of bilirubin formation, metabolism, and transport. Heme from hemoglobin and other hemoproteins is converted to biliverdin and then to bilirubin (*Br*), predominantly in macrophages in bone marrow and spleen. Br is released into plasma (in its unconjugated form), where it is tightly but reversibly bound to albumin (*Alb*). Br is then taken up at the sinusoidal membrane of hepatocytes, possibly via a member of the organic anion transporter (*OATP*) family. Br is conjugated via the activity of bilirubin uridine diphosphate-glucuronyl transferase (*B-UGT*) to form bilirubin mono- and diglucuronides (*BrG*). Biliary secretion of BrG occurs at the canalicular membrane by the multispecific organic anion transporter MRP2. Under physiologic conditions, the vast majority of BrG is eliminated in bile. Small amounts of BrG are transported at the sinusoidal membrane back into plasma via the multispecific organic anion transporter MRP3 and are recaptured primarily via uptake by OATP (OATP1B1 and OATP1B3). Remaining plasma BrG enters the renal circulation, where it undergoes glomerular filtration and elimination into urine. Therefore under normal conditions, at least 95% of bilirubin in plasma is present in the unconjugated form. If abnormally high concentrations of BrG are retained over a prolonged period, BrG-Alb complexes, which do not dissociate and cannot undergo glomerular filtration, are formed. *MRP*, Multidrug resistance-associated protein.

of the organic anion transport protein (OATP) family is involved (see Chapter 66). Although OATPB1 clearly plays a role in the sinusoidal membrane uptake of conjugated bilirubin (see later), its importance in unconjugated bilirubin uptake by hepatocytes has been disputed.[4,9,10] The subsequent steps of bilirubin metabolism are better understood.

After uptake by hepatocytes, unconjugated bilirubin binds to selected cytosolic proteins (e.g., glutathione *S*-transferase B, and fatty acid binding protein), which transport bilirubin to the endoplasmic reticulum by diffusion. There, bilirubin is converted to hydrophilic products by conjugation with uridine diphosphate (UDP)-glucuronic acid, and this is mediated by the enzyme bilirubin UDP–glucuronyl transferase (B-UGT). The bilirubin glucuronides that are formed (also known as conjugated bilirubin) then diffuse to the plasma membrane. At the canalicular (apical) domain, conjugated bilirubin is transported into bile by multidrug resistance–associated protein-2 (MRP2, gene symbol *ABCC2*), an adenosine triphosphate (ATP)-dependent export pump. MRP2 can also transport a variety of other anionic organic compounds, including BSP, glutathione, and conjugated bile salts.[4,10,11] The canalicular membrane is not the only locus of conjugated bilirubin export from the hepatocyte. Conjugated bilirubin is also transported into plasma across the sinusoidal (basolateral) domain, and this is mediated by the protein MRP3 (gene symbol *ABCC3*), a distinct multispecific organic ion export pump.[4,11] Once secreted across the sinusoidal membrane, conjugated bilirubin has two potential fates: (1) reuptake into hepatocytes by the sinusoidal transporters OATP1B1 and OATP1B3 (gene symbol *SLCO1B3*),[4,10] and (2) release into the circulation, uptake by renal tubular epithelial cells (which express OATP family members and MRP2), and export into urine (see Fig. 22.1). In disorders characterized by cholestasis (attenuated bile flow), MRP3-mediated export of conjugated bilirubin from hepatocytes can be upregulated,[11] and this leads to a disproportionate elevation in the serum concentration of conjugated bilirubin under these conditions (see later). With prolonged cholestasis [or selected isolated metabolic disorders associated with reduced delivery of conjugated bilirubin to the bile canaliculus (see later)], excess amounts of conjugated bilirubin in plasma become covalently bound to albumin, and these complexes cannot be excreted into urine.

Under physiological conditions, virtually all bilirubin in bile is conjugated, and only trace amounts are unconjugated. In humans, approximately 80% of bilirubin in bile is in the diglucuronide form, and almost all the rest is in the form of monoglucuronides. Resorption of conjugated bilirubin by the gallbladder and intestine is negligible; the bulk of bilirubin released from the biliary tract is eliminated in feces. It should be noted, however, that bilirubin can be deconjugated by bacteria in the terminal ileum and colon and converted to nonpigmented tetrapyrroles known as *urobilinogens*.[12] Up to 20% of urobilinogens undergo resorption within the gut, and these are ultimately excreted in bile and urine.

Measurement

Measurement of serum bilirubin is essential in diverse clinical situations, which range from managing neonatal jaundice[13] to determining priority for liver transplantation.[14] In adults, normal serum bilirubin concentration is 1.0 mg/dL (17.1 μmol/L) or less. In general, jaundice is not evident until the serum bilirubin concentration exceeds 3 mg/dL, and intermediate concentrations are not typically associated with recognizable icterus. In healthy individuals, most bilirubin circulates in blood in its unconjugated form; less than 5% of bilirubin in plasma is present in its conjugated form. In cholestatic conditions, however, the proportion of conjugated bilirubin in plasma may increase as a consequence of impaired canalicular export and increased sinusoidal export driven by compensatory upregulation of MRP3 expression. Therefore the concentration and composition of bilirubin in plasma can vary widely between health and disease.

Techniques that are commonly used by clinical laboratories for determination of serum bilirubin concentration are based upon the diazo reaction (sometimes given the eponymous label van den Bergh reaction, after its developer), which was pioneered in the early part of the 20th century. For these assays, bilirubin is cleaved by compounds (diazo reagents) such as diazotized sulfanilic acid, to form an azodipyrrole that can be quantified by spectrophotometry. Conjugated bilirubin is cleaved rapidly (directly) by diazo reagents. By contrast, formation of azodipyrroles from unconjugated bilirubin occurs more slowly, because internal hydrogen bonding reduces the accessibility of the diazo reagent to the site of chemical cleavage. Therefore reliable measurement of total bilirubin concentration (i.e., the sum of the conjugated and unconjugated bilirubin fractions) requires addition of another (accelerator) compound (e.g., ethanol, urea) that disrupts this hydrogen bonding and facilitates cleavage of unconjugated bilirubin by the diazo reagent. Using this technique, the "directly" reacting bilirubin, determined in the absence of accelerator compound, is reported as the direct bilirubin concentration, whereas the total bilirubin concentration is measured in the presence of the accelerator compound. The numerical difference between the total and direct bilirubin concentrations is then reported as the indirect bilirubin concentration.

Some confusion has arisen about the clinical significance of direct and indirect bilirubin concentrations. Although the direct serum bilirubin concentration is influenced by changes in conjugated bilirubin levels, direct and conjugated bilirubin are not equivalent to each other. Similarly, the indirect serum bilirubin concentration is not equivalent to the concentration of unconjugated bilirubin. In particular, reliance on direct and indirect bilirubin measurements can lead to errors in the diagnosis of isolated disorders of bilirubin metabolism [e.g., suspected Gilbert syndrome (see later)]. Consequently, a number of clinical laboratories instead use automated reflectance spectroscopic assays that more accurately estimate serum conjugated and unconjugated bilirubin concentrations. These assays can provide useful information for the management of neonatal jaundice, in which the therapy of unconjugated hyperbilirubinemia is distinct from that for other conditions (see later discussion). In disorders characterized by prolonged cholestasis, however, such assays may underestimate the conjugated bilirubin concentration, because they do not accurately detect albumin-bound conjugated bilirubin (so-called delta bilirubin, the numerical difference between the total bilirubin concentration and the sum of the measured conjugated and unconjugated bilirubin concentration). This may not be a high impact issue in the adult, where in general, accurate measurement of conjugated bilirubin concentration is not critical. A potential exception is when the diagnosis of a specific disorder of bilirubin metabolism is suspected. In the past, resolution of this issue required the use of sophisticated (and not widely available) chromatographic techniques, which specifically measured the concentrations of unconjugated, monoglucuronidated, and diglucuronidated bilirubin, as well as conjugated bilirubin-albumin complexes. This need may no longer be pressing, given the availability of advanced molecular methodology, which can identify mutations in genes that encode proteins involved in bilirubin metabolism (see the following section). It should be emphasized that determination of conjugated and unconjugated bilirubin concentrations cannot distinguish hyperbilirubinemia that results from hepatic disease from hyperbilirubinemia that results from biliary obstruction. Therefore in most adult cases, precise measurements of conjugated and unconjugated bilirubin concentrations in serum are of limited use.

DIFFERENTIAL DIAGNOSIS OF HYPERBILIRUBINEMIA

Serum bilirubin levels reflect the balance between production of bilirubin and its hepatobiliary clearance. Inability of bilirubin clearance to meet the demands of its production can thus lead to jaundice. From a practical standpoint, conditions associated with hyperbilirubinemia (and jaundice) can be classified under the broad categories of disorders of bilirubin metabolism, liver disease, and bile duct obstruction (Table 22.1).

Disorders of Bilirubin Metabolism

Isolated Unconjugated Hyperbilirubinemia

Isolated unconjugated hyperbilirubinemia (i.e., in the absence of hepatobiliary disease) can be subdivided conceptually into three

TABLE 22.1 Differential Diagnosis of Jaundice and Hyperbilirubinemia

Disorder	Examples
ISOLATED DISORDERS OF BILIRUBIN METABOLISM	
Unconjugated Hyperbilirubinemia	
Increased bilirubin production	Hemolysis, ineffective erythropoiesis, blood transfusion, resorption of hematomas
Decreased hepatocellular uptake	Possibly drugs (e.g., rifampin, cyclosporine A)
Decreased conjugation	Gilbert syndrome, Crigler-Najjar syndrome, physiologic jaundice of the newborn, drugs (e.g., indinavir, atazanavir)
Conjugated or Mixed Hyperbilirubinemia	
Dubin-Johnson syndrome	–
Rotor syndrome	–
LIVER DISEASE	
Hepatocellular Dysfunction	
Acute or subacute hepatocellular injury	Viral hepatitis, hepatotoxins (e.g., ethanol, acetaminophen, *Amanita phalloides*); drugs (e.g., isoniazid, phenytoin); ischemia (e.g., caused by hypotension), vascular outflow obstruction; metabolic disorders (e.g., Wilson disease); pregnancy-related as in acute fatty liver of pregnancy, preeclampsia
Chronic hepatocellular disease	Viral hepatitis; hepatotoxins (e.g., ethanol, vinyl chloride, vitamin A); autoimmune hepatitis; metabolic disorders (e.g., nonalcoholic fatty liver disease, hemochromatosis, Wilson disease, α_1-antitrypsin ZZ disease)
Hepatic Disorders with Prominent Cholestasis	
Infiltrative diseases	Granulomatous diseases such as mycobacterial infections, sarcoidosis, lymphoma, granulomatosis with polyangiitis; malignancy; amyloidosis
Cholangiocyte injury	PBC; graft-versus-host disease; drugs (e.g., amoxicillin–clavulanic acid); cystic fibrosis
Miscellaneous conditions	Benign recurrent intrahepatic cholestasis; drugs (e.g., estrogens, anabolic steroids); TPN; bacterial infections; paraneoplastic syndromes; intrahepatic cholestasis of pregnancy
BILE DUCT OBSTRUCTION	
Choledocholithiasis	
Bile Duct Diseases	
Inflammation, infection	PSC, AIDS cholangiopathy, injury caused by hepatic arterial chemotherapy/chemoembolization, postsurgical strictures
Neoplasms	Cholangiocarcinoma
Extrinsic Compression	–
Neoplasms	Pancreatic carcinoma, metastatic lymphadenopathy, hepatocellular carcinoma, ampullary adenoma/carcinoma, lymphoma
Pancreatitis	–
Vascular enlargement	Aneurysm, cavernous transformation of the portal vein (portal cavernoma)

AIDS, Acquired immunodeficiency syndrome; *PBC*, primary biliary cholangitis; *PSC*, primary sclerosing cholangitis.

basic mechanisms: (1) increased bilirubin production, (2) decreased hepatocellular uptake of unconjugated bilirubin, and (3) decreased bilirubin conjugation by hepatocytes. In each of these conditions, serum bilirubin is increased in isolation, and global liver function and biochemical markers of hepatocellular injury and cholestasis are normal (see Chapter 75).

Increased Bilirubin Production

A variety of extrahepatic processes can generate excessive bilirubin production. These include hemolysis, ineffective erythropoiesis, and resorption of a hematoma.[15] With these disorders, bilirubin concentration generally does not exceed 4–5 mg/dL. Jaundice can also follow massive blood transfusion, as a consequence of the increased fragility of stored erythrocytes, hemoglobin release, and amplification of the bilirubin load. This can be a major contributor to hyperbilirubinemia in patients with major trauma.[16]

Decreased Bilirubin Uptake by Hepatocytes

Selected drugs can interfere with hepatocellular uptake of bilirubin. For example, the antibiotic rifampin and the immunosuppressive agent cyclosporine A competitively inhibit the sinusoidal transport protein OATP1B1, and this has been proposed to be a contributing mechanism for these agents.[17] However, whether drug-induced inhibition of bilirubin uptake is a clinically important cause of unconjugated hyperbilirubinemia has been a source of debate.[4,9,10]

Decreased Hepatocellular Bilirubin Conjugation

Three autosomally inherited disorders of unconjugated hyperbilirubinemia, Gilbert syndrome, and Crigler-Najjar syndromes type I and II, arise from defects in bilirubin conjugation (Table 22.2). They are distinguished from each other by the extent of reduction of B-UGT activity. In Gilbert syndrome, the most common of these, enzymatic activity is reduced the least. Gilbert syndrome has a prevalence of approximately 3%–7% in the United States, which varies across ethnic groups (highest in the Middle East, lowest in East Asia). Patients with Gilbert syndrome typically present when isolated hyperbilirubinemia is detected as an incidental finding on routine biochemical screening for unrelated health conditions, and clinically evident jaundice is uncommon.[18] Serum bilirubin levels may rise two- to three-fold with fasting or dehydration but are generally below 4 mg/dL. The molecular basis of Gilbert syndrome has been linked to a reduction in transcription of the *UGT1A1* gene that encodes B-UGT1A, as a result of mutations in the promoter region (most commonly found in Caucasian populations) as well as in the coding region.[4,5,18] Although Gilbert syndrome has generally been thought to be an entirely benign condition, individuals with this disorder may be at increased risk for gallstones and for toxicity of selected drugs, like irinotecan, which undergo glucuronidation for metabolic clearance.[18] On the other hand, based upon the physiological properties of bilirubin as an anti-inflammatory, immunomodulatory, and metabolic regulatory compound, it has been speculated that mild hyperbilirubinemia with Gilbert syndrome confers an evolutionary advantage. Indeed, individuals with Gilbert syndrome appear to be at decreased risk for atherosclerotic heart disease, selected cancers, and complications of type II diabetes.[18]

Mutations in the coding region of *UGT1A1* underlie the Crigler-Najjar syndromes.[4,19] In type I Crigler-Najjar syndrome, B-UGT activity is absent, and markedly increased serum levels of unconjugated bilirubin are evident shortly after birth. The major morbidity associated with type I Crigler-Najjar syndrome is accumulation of bilirubin in the brain (kernicterus), and the resulting neurotoxic effects can lead to neonatal death (see Table 22.2). Phototherapy (see later) is required to prevent kernicterus, and liver transplantation can be lifesaving. At the time of this writing, gene therapy for the management of this disorder

TABLE 22.2 Hereditary Disorders of Bilirubin Metabolism and Transport

	Syndrome				
Parameter	**Gilbert**	**Type I Crigler-Najjar**	**Type II Crigler-Najjar**	**Dubin-Johnson**	**Rotor**
Incidence	6%–12%	Very rare	Uncommon	Uncommon	Rare
Gene affected	*UGT1A1*	*UGT1A1*	*UGT1A1*	*MRP2*	*OATP1B1* and *OATP1B3*
Metabolic defect	↓Bilirubin conjugation	No bilirubin conjugation	↓↓Bilirubin conjugation	Impaired canalicular export of conjugated bilirubin	Impaired sinsusoidal extraction of conjugated bilirubin
Plasma bilirubin (mg/dL)	≤3 in absence of fasting or hemolysis, almost all unconjugated	Usually >20 (range, 17–50), all unconjugated	Usually <20 (range, 6–45), almost all unconjugated	Usually <7, about half conjugated	Usually <7, about half conjugated
Liver histology	Usually normal, occasional ↑lipofuscin	Normal	Normal	Coarse pigment in centrilobular hepatocytes	Normal
Other distinguishing features	↓Bilirubin concentration with phenobarbital	No response to phenobarbital	↓Bilirubin concentration with phenobarbital	↑Bilirubin concentration with estrogens; ↑↑urinary coproporphyrin I/III ratio	Mild ↑urinary coproporphyrin I/III ratio
Prognosis	Normal (theoretical risk of selected drug toxicity)	Death in infancy if untreated	Usually normal	Normal (theoretical risk of selected drug toxicity)	Normal (theoretical risk of selected drug toxicity)
Treatment	None	Phototherapy as a bridge to liver transplantation	Phenobarbital for ↑↑bilirubin concentration	Avoid estrogens	None available

MRP2, Multidrug resistance–associated protein-2 gene; *OATP*, organic anion transporter; *UGTIA1*, bilirubin uridine diphosphate-glucuronyl transferase gene.

remains experimental, but findings from a small clinical trial appear promising.[20]

In contrast to persons with type I Crigler-Najjar syndrome, those with type II Crigler-Najjar syndrome have limited B-UGT activity, and serum bilirubin levels are lower (see Table 22.2). Patients with type II Crigler-Najjar syndrome are not ill during the neonatal period and may not be diagnosed until early childhood. Most patients with type II Crigler-Najjar syndrome can be treated successfully with phenobarbital, an agonist for the constitutive androstane receptor CAR, which increases UGT1A1 expression.[21] Following phenobarbital treatment, serum bilirubin levels generally decrease to within the range of 2–5 mg/dL.

A related disorder of bilirubin metabolism is physiologic jaundice of the newborn, which results from delayed developmental expression of B-UGT and generally resolves rapidly in the neonatal period.[22] A brief course of phototherapy (see later) may be required to prevent kernicterus.

B-UGT is inhibited competitively by the HIV protease inhibitors atazanavir and indinavir, which produce hyperbilirubinemia in more than 25% of patients who receive these agents; patients with Gilbert syndrome appear to be at higher risk for this complication.[18]

Isolated Conjugated or Mixed Hyperbilirubinemia

Two autosomally inherited disorders, Dubin-Johnson syndrome and Rotor syndrome, are associated with isolated conjugated or mixed hyperbilirubinemia (i.e., increase in serum concentrations of both conjugated and unconjugated bilirubin). In each, the serum concentration of bilirubin is selectively increased, and global liver function and biochemical markers of hepatocellular injury and cholestasis are normal (see Chapter 75). The underlying mechanisms of Dubin-Johnson syndrome and Rotor syndrome are distinct. In Dubin-Johnson syndrome, an absence of expression or defective canalicular targeting of MRP2 impairs secretion of conjugated bilirubin into the bile canaliculus.[4] Compensatory upregulation of MRP3 permits sinusoidal export of potentially toxic organic anions that are normally secreted by MRP2 (and serves to prevent overload of these compounds in hepatocytes), and in addition, drives sinusoidal conjugated bilirubin export, with resultant hyperbilirubinemia. The molecular basis of Rotor syndrome is more complex. Studies in transgenic mice have demonstrated that conjugated bilirubin, which is secreted into plasma by MRP3, is taken up by the sinusoidal transport proteins OATP1B1 and OATP1B3.[23] Combined deficiency of OATP1B1 and OATP1B3 results in Rotor syndrome and impaired hepatocyte reuptake of conjugated bilirubin.

Dubin-Johnson and Rotor syndromes can be distinguished biochemically and histologically (see Table 22.2). In Dubin-Johnson syndrome, hepatocyte lysosomes contain a characteristic black pigment, which is thought to be formed by aromatic amino acid metabolites that are putative MRP2 substrates.[4] The advent of next generation DNA sequencing panels (now commercially available), which can identify mutations in multiple genes implicated in hyperbilirubinemia and cholestatic liver disease, is anticipated to simplify the diagnostic process.[24] The availability of these tests, as well as the fact that neither Dubin-Johnson nor Rotor syndrome is associated with progressive hepatic damage, should serve to negate the need for liver biopsy in distinguishing these disorders from each other. As an aside, patients with Rotor syndrome may be at increased risk for toxicity from selected drugs (e.g., statin-induced myopathy) that undergo metabolic disposal via OATP1B-mediated hepatic uptake.[4]

Liver Disease

Jaundice is a common feature of a broad spectrum of liver diseases; in which hyperbilirubinemia is generally associated with other biochemical liver test abnormalities (see Chapter 75). In this section, disorders in which hyperbilirubinemia and jaundice are manifestations of global hepatocellular dysfunction are distinguished from those in which cholestasis is the predominant problem.

Acute Hepatocellular Dysfunction

Jaundice can develop in the setting of extensive hepatocyte injury produced by a variety of causes, which include viral hepatitis, exposure to hepatotoxins, ischemic processes, and certain metabolic derangements. Serum aminotransferase levels are characteristically elevated (see later). Acute viral hepatitis is often heralded by anorexia, malaise, and myalgias before jaundice develops (see Chapters 80–85). Five hepatotropic viruses have been isolated: hepatitis A and E viruses, which are transmitted enterally and are generally self-limited, and hepatitis B, C, and D, which are transmitted parenterally and may lead to chronic disease. The diagnosis of each of these disorders is aided by serologic testing (see later).

One of the most common causes of toxic liver injury is ingestion of large quantities of the analgesic acetaminophen (see Chapter 90), which can lead to jaundice and overt liver failure within several days after exposure. In patients who survive (and do not have preexisting liver disease) jaundice resolves and hepatic function recovers completely. Drugs and other chemical agents that produce idiosyncratic (i.e., dose-independent) hepatocellular injury and jaundice are discussed elsewhere in this text (see Chapters 90 and 91). Alcohol-associated hepatitis should be a diagnostic consideration in the jaundiced patient with a history of ongoing immoderate alcohol intake (see Chapter 88).

Jaundice can be a manifestation of hepatic ischemia. This may result from hypotension, hypoxia, hyperthermia, obstruction to hepatic venous outflow (Budd-Chiari syndrome), or sinusoidal obstruction syndrome (see Chapter 87).

Wilson disease, an inherited disorder of hepatobiliary copper secretion, may manifest de novo with clinical features indistinguishable from those of acute viral hepatitis (see Chapter 78). The diagnosis should be considered particularly in younger individuals with jaundice (but cases in middle-aged patients have been reported). Hemolytic anemia is a part of the spectrum of Wilson disease and contributes to disproportionate hyperbilirubinemia in these patients. The diagnosis of Wilson disease is confirmed by specialized slit-lamp examination of the eyes for corneal copper deposits (Kaiser-Fleischer rings) and/or liver copper analysis.

Chronic Hepatocellular Dysfunction

In contrast to acute hepatocellular injury, jaundice does not typically develop in chronic liver disease unless cirrhosis is present. Chronic viral hepatitis should be a diagnostic consideration in patients with suspected cirrhosis, especially in the presence of historical risk factors for parenteral exposure to causative agents (see Chapters 81–83). Diagnosis is aided by molecular testing (see later). Cirrhosis is part of the spectrum of steatotic liver disease, either in the context of chronic immoderate alcohol use [alcohol-associated liver disease (ALD)], as a component of metabolic syndrome (metabolic dysfunction associated steatotic liver disease), or both (MetALD). Details about each of these can be found in Chapters 88 and 89. Certain inherited metabolic diseases may progress to cirrhosis. Hemochromatosis, a disorder of hepatocellular injury due to excessive iron absorption, is the most common of these (see Chapter 77). Decades of hepatic iron overload are generally required to produce symptoms, and hemochromatosis often is not diagnosed until middle age. The diagnosis of hemochromatosis is confirmed by detection of characteristic mutations in the *HFE* gene or by hepatic iron analysis. Copper-induced hepatic injury in Wilson disease may also progress to cirrhosis (see Chapter 78). In a jaundiced patient with chronic lung disease, α_1-antitrypsin ZZ disease should be suspected (see Chapter 79). In this disorder, misfolded mutant α_1-antitrypsin (ZZ phenotype) accumulates in the endoplasmic reticulum of hepatocytes, which can trigger liver injury and progressive fibrosis. Serological proteotyping facilitates screening, and liver biopsy is required for diagnosis. Autoimmune hepatitis may be associated with systemic symptoms such as fatigue, arthralgias, and rash, but jaundice may be the only presenting manifestation of cirrhosis in this disorder (see Chapter 92). The diagnosis is aided by serologic testing and liver biopsy (see later).

Hepatic Disorders with Prominent Cholestasis

Intrahepatic cholestatic disorders are characterized by impaired bile formation in the absence of widespread hepatocellular injury or biliary obstruction. Because the presentation of these disorders and associated biochemical abnormalities may be difficult to distinguish from biliary obstruction, hepatobiliary imaging studies may be needed to clarify the diagnosis. Intrahepatic cholestatic disorders can be categorized histologically as infiltrative, those associated with injury to cholangiocytes within intrahepatic bile ductules, and those in which major histologic changes are not evident.

Infiltrative Diseases

Infiltrative diseases of the liver disrupt the network of intrahepatic bile ductules and are often associated with striking cholestasis, and ultimately jaundice. Predominant causes are granulomatous diseases, malignancy, and amyloidosis. A diverse number of disorders, including infectious, toxins, lymphoma, and other systemic diseases (e.g., sarcoidosis) can produce granulomatous disease that involves the liver.[25] The most common of these disorders that produce jaundice are tuberculosis and sarcoidosis.[26,27] Although malignant hepatic infiltration can often be suspected by the clinical history and hepatic imaging studies (see later), it can rarely present with acute liver failure in the absence of overt radiological findings.[28] Granulomatous diseases should be suspected, in particular, when jaundice accompanies fever of undetermined origin. Physical examination often reveals hepatosplenomegaly, and lymphadenopathy may be present. Radiographic chest abnormalities often provide a clue to the diagnosis of sarcoidosis or mycobacterial infection. Ultimately, diagnosis may require liver biopsy if other tissue is unavailable. Jaundice is an unusual manifestation of amyloidosis, but when present, it is invariably accompanied by marked hepatomegaly.[29] The diagnosis of amyloidosis should also be suspected in the jaundiced patient if there are signs of involvement of other organs (e.g., macroglossia, malabsorption, heart failure, peripheral neuropathy, and proteinuria). In the absence of other clues, liver biopsy may be necessary.

Disorders Involving Cholangiocyte Injury

A broad spectrum of disorders can lead to cholangiocyte damage. In many of these, the cholangiocyte is a target of an immune-mediated inflammatory response, as exemplified by primary biliary cholangitis (PBC, see Chapter 93). PBC occurs primarily in women. By the time jaundice develops, cirrhosis is invariably present, and the prognosis is guarded. Biochemical and serologic testing (mitochondrial antibodies) is generally sufficient to make a diagnosis of PBC, but liver biopsy may be necessary if there is uncertainty. The cholangiocyte is a target of graft-versus-host disease (see Chapter 34), a complication of transplantation of solid organs and hematopoietic stem cells; the implementation of preventative management strategies in the latter has been associated with a reduction in posttransplant jaundice.[30] Certain drugs also produce cholestasis as a result of cholangiocyte injury (see Chapter 90). The most common of these is amoxicillin–clavulanic acid, and more can be found on the National Library of Medicine LiverTox website: available at https://www.ncbi.nlm.nih.gov/books/NBK547852. In general, cholestasis resolves within several months following discontinuation of the causative drug. Cholestasis from cholangiocyte injury occurs in about 30% of adults with cystic fibrosis (see Chapters 59 and 64), a genetic disorder of the cystic fibrosis transmembrane conductance regulator ion channel protein that is expressed in secretory epithelia, including cholangiocytes.

Cholestasis with Minimal Histologic Abnormalities

Jaundice may accompany intrahepatic cholestasis in the absence of hepatic infiltration, or injury to hepatocytes or cholangiocytes. Several mechanisms may be responsible, including mutations in the genes that encode canalicular membrane transport proteins involved in bile formation, and conditions that interfere with the functional expression of such proteins.

Benign recurrent cholestasis (BRIC) is an autosomally inherited disorder associated with mutations in the genes that encode: (1) the familial intrahepatic cholestasis 1 protein (FIC1, gene symbol *ATP8B1*) and (2) the bile salt export pump [BSEP, gene symbol *ABCB11* (see Chapter 79)].[31] FIC1 is a P-type ATPase believed to function in hepatocytes as a canalicular membrane "flippase" for aminophospholipids, and FIC1 dysfunction appears to cause cholestasis by increasing the susceptibility to canalicular membrane damage by hydrophobic bile acids and/or interfering with the localization of proteins that regulate BSEP expression or function. BSEP is an ATP-dependent BSEP, and impaired BSEP activity leads to cholestasis by reduction in bile salt secretion. BRIC represents one end of a spectrum of disorders associated with FIC1 and BSEP mutations; the other end is progressive familial intrahepatic cholestasis (PFIC) types 1 and 2, diseases that can lead to liver failure in childhood and necessitate liver transplantation.[32]

Patients with BRIC typically present before the second decade of life with recurrent episodes of malaise and pruritus in association with jaundice; fever and abdominal pain are uncommon. The findings on liver biopsy, if performed during an icteric episode, are generally confined to centrilobular cholestasis; portal-based inflammatory cell infiltrates are uncommon. As mentioned in an earlier section, the need for histological diagnosis in suspected cases has been largely supplanted the availability of cholestasis gene panels. Symptomatic episodes in BRIC may last up to several months and are separated by periods of clinical remission. Although quality of life may be adversely affected, the disease does not lead to progressive liver damage, and (unlike PFIC) liver failure does not occur.

A number of drugs produce histologically bland intrahepatic cholestasis (see Chapter 90). Estrogens reduce bile formation principally by inhibiting bile salt secretion.[33] There are several mechanisms by which this occurs, including downregulation of the sinusoidal bile salt uptake protein Na^+-taurocholate cotransporting peptide (NTCP, gene symbol *SLC10A1*), competitive inhibition of BSEP, and interference with MRP2 function. Jaundice related to the use of oral contraceptives usually develops within 2 months of initiation of therapy and is generally accompanied by pruritus; these symptoms resolve promptly with discontinuation of the drug. Anabolic steroids can produce a syndrome that is clinically indistinguishable from estrogen-induced cholestasis (see the related LiverTox website: available at https://www.ncbi.nlm.nih.gov/books/NBK548931). The clinical features of cholestasis associated with total parenteral nutrition (possibly related to altered enterohepatic circulation and diminished neuroendocrine stimulation of bile flow) may also resemble those related to estrogen and anabolic steroids, but progressive hepatic fibrosis has also been described.[34]

Cholestasis and jaundice also may develop during bacterial infections, likely because of cytokine-dependent downregulation of the transporters NTCP, MRP2, and BSEP.[35] As in other cholestatic disorders, the clinical features may be difficult to distinguish from biliary obstruction, and imaging studies may be required to resolve this issue.

Jaundice due to intrahepatic cholestasis has been reported as a paraneoplastic phenomenon (i.e., in the absence of malignant infiltration of the liver) in patients with lymphoma, and in selected nonhematological malignancies, known as *Stauffer syndrome*.[36] In the latter, originally described in renal cell carcinoma, successful treatment of the primary tumor leads to resolution of cholestasis. The pathogenesis remains unclear but may relate to tumor-derived secretion of cytokines that interfere with NTCP, MRP2, and BSEP function.

Atypical Presentations of Cholestasis

Acute viral hepatitis rarely may cause profound cholestasis, with pruritus and jaundice.[37] Unless the patient has risk factors for viral hepatitis, no features reliably distinguish this disorder from other cholestatic syndromes or biliary tract obstruction. A high level of suspicion and appropriate laboratory testing will help establish the diagnosis. Alcohol-associated hepatitis manifesting as fever, jaundice, abdominal pain, and leukocytosis may also be difficult to distinguish from bile duct obstruction.[38] Liver biopsy may be required to confirm the diagnosis.

Jaundice in Pregnancy

Several cholestatic disorders are uniquely encountered in pregnancy (see Chapter 38).[39] Jaundice uncommonly may accompany hyperemesis gravidarum, a generally self-limited disorder of the first trimester, but liver failure is not a feature of this illness. Intrahepatic cholestasis of pregnancy typically occurs in the third trimester and presents with pruritus and occasionally with jaundice. Cholestasis generally resolves within 2 weeks of delivery and often recurs with subsequent pregnancies. Polymorphisms in the genes encoding the canalicular transporters BSEP, FIC1, MRP2, and MDR3 (gene symbol *ABCB4*), and the canalicular membrane tight junction protein TJP2 have been associated with this disorder.[40] Functional alterations in these transporters may enhance their sensitivity to the inhibitory effects of estrogens with respect to bile formation. A far more serious syndrome is acute fatty liver of pregnancy, which typically occurs in the third trimester and is associated with hepatocellular injury. Jaundice, when present, is usually accompanied by nausea, abdominal pain, and evidence of liver failure. Liver biopsy (if performed) demonstrates microvesicular steatosis. The disorder may be fatal unless obstetrical delivery is performed promptly. Preeclampsia, a microvascular disorder of the third trimester, is heralded by hypertension and proteinuria and affects the liver in about 10% of cases. A particularly severe form, the HELLP (*h*emolysis, *el*evated *l*iver enzyme levels, and a *l*ow *p*latelet count) syndrome, is treated by prompt obstetric delivery.

Jaundice in the Critically Ill Patient

Establishing the cause of jaundice in the critically ill patient can present a challenge to intensivists and their consultants. Simple explanations are the exception rather than the rule, as multiple predisposing factors are often present. Among these are hepatic ischemia, medications associated with liver injury, infection, blood transfusions, and parenteral nutrition.[41,42] Furthermore, the presence of kidney injury may exacerbate the situation by impairment of extrahepatic elimination of conjugated bilirubin. The persistence of icterus can be a source of dismay and frustration to concerned relatives and other advocates for the patient, who may view jaundice as the cause rather than a manifestation of critical illness. The health care team may issue requests for urgent biliary drainage, even in the absence of evidence of bile duct obstruction on noninvasive imaging studies (see later), and this can amplify the tension. Additional confusion can arise when despite evidence of clinical recovery; there is lag in the resolution of jaundice. With these issues in mind, management of jaundice in intensive care settings requires not only a careful search for reversible causes but also a great deal of patience.

Bile Duct Obstruction

Obstructive disorders of the biliary tract include occlusion of the bile duct lumen, intrinsic disorders of the bile ducts, and extrinsic biliary compression.

Choledocholithiasis

The most common cause of biliary obstruction is occlusion of the bile duct lumen by a stone (choledocholithiasis). Three types of stones have been implicated in this process, with cholesterol gallstones, which typically form in the gallbladder, responsible for the majority of cases. In patients with unconjugated hyperbilirubinemia, calcium bilirubinate stones (so-called black pigment gallstones) can also form in the gallbladder but may also form in situ at any level of the biliary tract. Brown pigment gallstones, a distinct type of bilirubinate stone, can lead to repeated bouts of cholangitis (recurrent pyogenic cholangitis), particularly in patients from certain regions of eastern Asia and in patients with prior biliary tract surgery or endoscopic intervention (see Chapter 67).

Bile Duct Diseases

Intrinsic narrowing of the bile ducts occurs in inflammatory, infectious, or neoplastic biliary disease. Congenital disorders of the bile ducts, including cysts and biliary atresia, are discussed in Chapter 64. Primary sclerosing cholangitis, a progressive inflammatory disorder of the bile ducts, is characterized by focal and segmental biliary strictures (see Chapter 70). A similar appearing syndrome of discrete narrowing and localized obstruction of the bile ducts is an unusual complication of acquired immunodeficiency syndrome [so-called AIDS cholangiopathy (see Chapter 33)]. Biliary strictures may also follow hepatic arterial infusion or embolization of certain chemotherapeutic compounds,[43] or they can result from surgical injury to the common bile duct or hepatic artery.[44] Neoplasms of the biliary tract are discussed in Chapter 71.

Extrinsic Compression

Extrinsic compression of the biliary tract may occur with neoplastic involvement or inflammation of surrounding viscera. Rarely, marked enlargement of the surrounding vasculature [e.g., arterial aneurysms, cavernous transformation of the portal vein (portal cavernoma)] can compress the bile ducts (see Chapter 87).

Painless jaundice is a classic feature of carcinoma of the head of the pancreas (see Chapter 62). Occasionally, hepatocellular carcinoma or periportal lymph nodes enlarged by metastatic tumor or lymphoma obstructs the extrahepatic bile ducts. Pancreatitis may lead to biliary compression from edema or pseudocyst formation (see Chapter 60). Rarely, gallstones in the cystic duct or infundibulum of the gallbladder compress the common hepatic duct (Mirizzi syndrome) and produce jaundice.[45]

DIAGNOSTIC APPROACH TO JAUNDICE

A general algorithm for evaluating the patient with jaundice is depicted in Fig. 22.2. A logical approach involves four basic steps:

(1) a carefully taken patient history, thorough physical examination, and screening laboratory studies; (2) formulation of a working differential diagnosis; (3) selection of specialized tests to narrow the diagnostic possibilities; and (4) development of a strategy for treatment or further testing if unexpected diagnostic possibilities arise.

History and Physical Examination

The history and physical examination provide important clues regarding the cause of jaundice (Table 22.3). A history of biliary tract surgery, fever, and abdominal pain, particularly in the right upper quadrant, is suggestive of biliary obstruction with

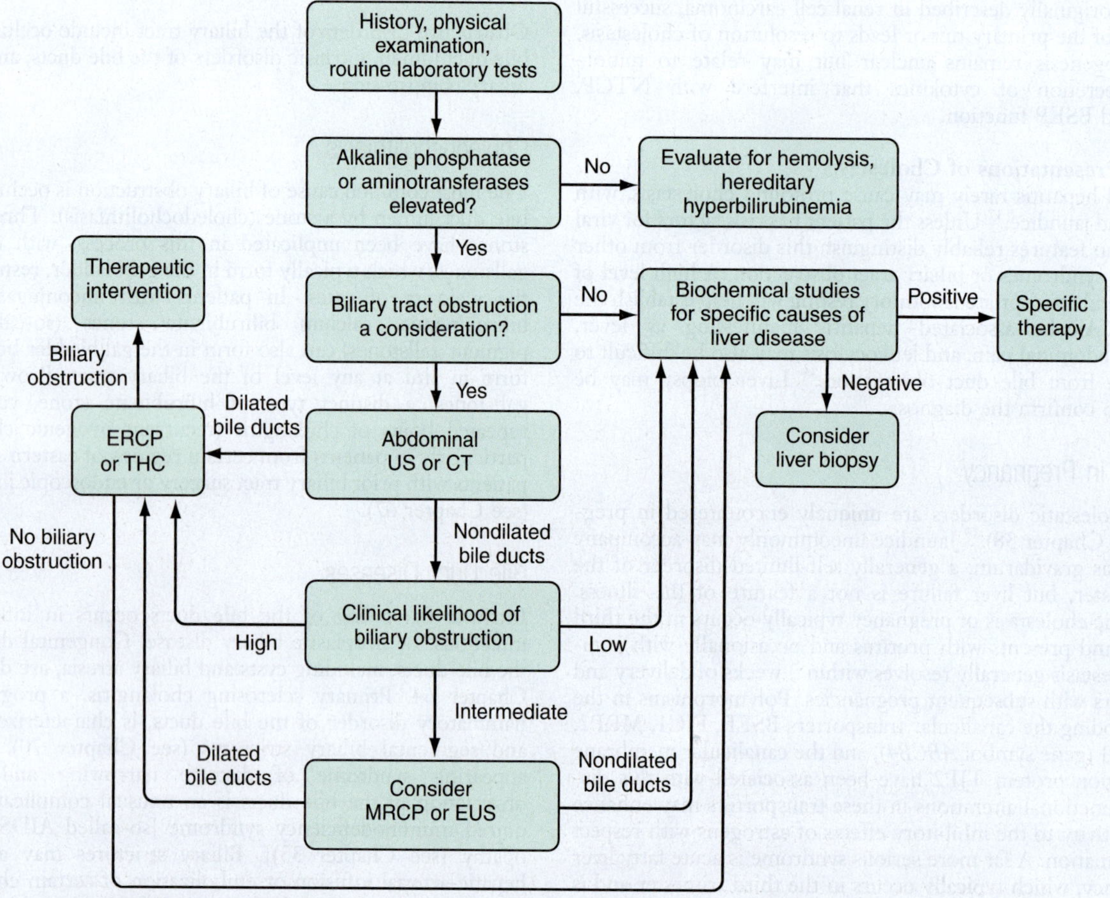

Fig. 22.2 Algorithm for evaluation and management of jaundice and hyperbilirubinemia. *THC*, Transhepatic cholangiography.

TABLE 22.3 Clues to the Differential Diagnosis of Jaundice: Biliary Obstruction versus Liver Disease

Parameter	Biliary Obstruction	Liver Disease
History	Abdominal pain Fever, rigors Prior biliary surgery Older age	Anorexia, malaise, myalgias (viral prodrome) Known viral exposure History of blood product receipt or injection drug use Exposure to known hepatotoxin Family history of liver disease
Physical examination	Fever Abdominal tenderness Palpable abdominal mass Abdominal surgical scar	Spider telangiectasias Stigmata of portal hypertension (e.g., prominent abdominal veins, splenomegaly, ascites) Asterixis
Laboratory studies	Predominant elevation of serum alkaline phosphatase relative to aminotransferases[a] Prothrombin time (INR) normal or normalizes with vitamin K administration Leukocytosis Elevated serum amylase or lipase level	Predominant elevation of serum aminotransferase levels relative to alkaline phosphatase Prolonged prothrombin time that does not normalize with vitamin K administration Thrombocytopenia Serologies indicative of specific liver disease

[a]Except early after acute obstruction when the opposite pattern may be seen transiently.

cholangitis. On the other hand, symptoms compatible with a viral prodrome (e.g., anorexia, malaise, myalgias) make acute viral hepatitis a strong diagnostic possibility, especially if there are risk factors for potential infectious exposure. A carefully taken history may suggest that contact with environmental hepatotoxins, or use of ethanol, or medications (including over-the-counter agents or herbal supplements) are responsible for liver injury. A family history of jaundice raises the possibility of an inherited disorder of bilirubin metabolism or genetic liver disease. All clues must be interpreted with caution; for example, fever and abdominal pain accompany diseases other than biliary obstruction, and viral hepatitis may occur coincidentally in patients with a history of prior biliary surgery. Moreover, anorexia and malaise are not specific for viral hepatitis, and gallstones can develop in patients with chronic liver disease. Nevertheless, when details from the patient's history are evaluated in the context of the physical findings and results of routine laboratory tests, jaundice can be characterized correctly as obstructive or nonobstructive in about 75% of cases, and this rate has not yet been surpassed by computer-based modeling.[46]

Clues offered by the physical examination are also important in the patient with jaundice. Fever or abdominal tenderness (particularly in the right upper quadrant) suggests cholangitis, and a palpable abdominal mass suggests a neoplastic cause of obstructive jaundice. The presence of cirrhosis may be suggested by signs of portal hypertension (e.g., ascites, splenomegaly, prominent abdominal veins), spider telangiectasias, gynecomastia, and asterixis.

Initial Laboratory Studies

Essential laboratory tests in the patient with jaundice include serum total bilirubin, alkaline phosphatase, aminotransferases, complete blood count, and prothrombin time (see Chapter 75). Serum alkaline phosphatase activity derives from related isoenzymes expressed on the membranes of multiple cell types; the hepatobiliary "liver" alkaline phosphatase isoform is a membrane linked protein predominantly localized on the apical poles of hepatocytes and cholangiocytes. In hepatocytes and cholangiocytes, enzymatic cleavage under physiologic conditions releases alkaline phosphatase from the apical membranes into bile; small amounts are released from the basolateral membrane into plasma as well. Biliary obstruction and intrahepatic cholestasis increase the basolateral release of alkaline phosphatase, and serum alkaline phosphatase activity increases under these conditions. Consequently, in a jaundiced patient, a predominant increase in serum alkaline phosphatase (relative to aminotransferase) activity suggests the presence of biliary tract obstruction or intrahepatic cholestasis. An increase in serum alkaline phosphatase activity (especially if aminotransferase activity is normal), however, may reflect release of alkaline phosphatase isoenzymes from extrahepatic tissues. If there is diagnostic uncertainty, elevated serum activities of other proteins (e.g., gamma glutamyl transpeptidase, 5′-nucleotidase, alkaline phosphatase isoenzymes) confirm the presence of hepatobiliary disease (see Chapter 75).

The aminotransferases—alanine aminotransferase, a cytosolic enzyme found predominantly in hepatocytes, and aspartate aminotransferase, isoforms of which are found within hepatocytes and cells from several other tissues—are ordinarily detected in serum in low concentrations. Conditions that produce hepatocellular injury [e.g., viral hepatitis, toxic liver injury, hepatic ischemia (see earlier)] increase plasma membrane permeability and release of aminotransferases into plasma. A predominant elevation of serum aminotransferase levels (relative to alkaline phosphatase) suggests that jaundice is due to hepatocellular injury. There are exceptions to this generalization, however. For example, transient biliary obstruction from choledocholithiasis may cause a brief but dramatic elevation (>10–20 times normal) of serum aminotransferase activity.[47]

A complete blood count provides information that complements findings from biochemical testing described above. Leukocytosis may be a clue to the presence of biliary tract obstruction or another inflammatory disorder associated with cholestasis. The presence of anemia raises the possibility that a hemolytic disorder is responsible for jaundice, especially if isolated hyperbilirubinemia (without other abnormalities in biochemical liver tests) is detected. Thrombocytopenia is a characteristic finding in cirrhosis and appears to result from reduced hepatic synthesis of the platelet production regulator thrombopoietin or from increased splenic sequestration associated with portal hypertension.

The prothrombin time reflects the activities of coagulation factors I, II, V, VII, and X. With impaired hepatocellular synthesis of these proteins, prothrombin time is prolonged (often reported as an increase in the international normalized ratio), but this finding is not specific for conditions associated with hepatocellular injury. Prolongation of prothrombin time can also be seen with intrahepatic cholestasis or prolonged biliary obstruction, as a result of impaired absorption of vitamin K, a fat-soluble cofactor required for synthesis of factors II, VII, IX, and X. Exogenously administered vitamin K will generally normalize the prothrombin time in intrahepatic cholestasis or prolonged biliary obstruction but not in conditions associated with hepatocellular injury.

Overall Approach

Integration of the patient's history, physical examination, and laboratory study results will refine a determination of the likelihood that jaundice is due to a disorder of bilirubin production or metabolism, intrinsic liver disease, or biliary obstruction. At one extreme is the asymptomatic patient with no abnormalities (other than jaundice) on physical examination. Under these conditions, if the serum alkaline phosphatase and aminotransferase activities, platelet count, and prothrombin time are normal, liver disease or biliary obstruction is highly unlikely. In this situation, further testing for specific disorders, such as an isolated defect in bilirubin metabolism or hemolysis, is warranted (see Fig. 22.2). On the other hand, if the history, physical examination, and laboratory test results raise the possibility of biliary obstruction, hepatobiliary imaging is appropriate. Selection of the appropriate imaging study depends on the likelihood of bile duct obstruction and the diagnostic accuracy, complication rate, cost, and availability of each test (see later), especially if there is clinical urgency, and therapeutic intervention at the time of the study is anticipated. The following section provides an overview. Because much of the literature concerning the performance of imaging studies in the context of jaundice is over 35 years old, the interested reader is encouraged to delve into more recently published reviews that have been cited in the references.

Imaging Studies

Abdominal Ultrasound (US)

Abdominal ultrasound (US) is usually the initial imaging test in jaundiced patients with suspected hepatobiliary disease.[48,49] US can demonstrate cholelithiasis (although bile duct stones may not be well seen) and intrahepatic lesions more than 1 cm in diameter. US has the advantages of being noninvasive, portable, and less expensive than other imaging studies (Table 22.4). Disadvantages include issues related to operator-related variability, as well as potential technical difficulty in patients with significantly increased abdominal adiposity or in situations in which portions of the biliary tree are obscured by bowel gas.

TABLE 22.4 Imaging Studies for Evaluation of Jaundice

Test	Sensitivity (%)	Specificity (%)	Morbidity (%)	Mortality (%)	Advantages and Disadvantages
Abdominal US	55–91	82–95	0	0	*Advantages:* noninvasive, portable *Disadvantages:* bowel gas may obscure bile duct; difficult in obese persons, operator dependent
Abdominal CT	63–96	93–100	See disadvantages	0	*Advantages:* noninvasive, higher resolution than US, not operator dependent *Disadvantages:* ionizing radiation, potential for contrast-induced anaphylaxis
MRCP	82–100	94–98	See disadvantages		*Advantages:* noninvasive, imaging of bile ducts superior to US and CT *Disadvantages:* requires breath holding, may miss small-caliber bile duct disease
ERCP	89–98	89–100	5	0.2	*Advantages:* provides direct imaging of bile ducts; permits direct visualization of periampullary region and acquisition of tissue distal to bifurcation of hepatic ducts; permits simultaneous therapeutic intervention, especially useful for lesions distal to the bifurcation of the hepatic ducts *Disadvantages:* requires sedation, cannot be performed if altered anatomy precludes endoscopic access to the ampulla (e.g., Roux-en-Y loop); may cause complications (e.g., pancreatitis)
Percutaneous THC	98–100	89–100	3.5	0.2	*Advantages:* provides direct imaging of the bile ducts, permits simultaneous therapeutic intervention, especially useful for lesions proximal to the common hepatic duct *Disadvantages:* more difficult with nondilated intrahepatic bile ducts; may cause complications
EUS	89–97	67–98	See disadvantages	0	*Advantages:* imaging of the bile ducts is superior to US and CT; permits needle aspiration of suspected neoplasms *Disadvantages:* requires sedation

CT, Computed tomography; *ERCP,* endoscopic retrograde cholangiopancreatography; *EUS,* endoscopic ultrasound; *MRCP,* magnetic resonance cholangiopancreatography; *THC,* transhepatic cholangiography; *US,* ultrasound.

Abdominal Computed Tomography (CT)

Computed tomography (CT) of the abdomen with intravenous contrast is an alternative noninvasive means of evaluating hepatobiliary disease.[50] Abdominal CT permits accurate measurement of bile duct caliber, with sensitivity and specificity rates comparable to those for US.[48] Abdominal CT detects intrahepatic space-occupying lesions as small as 5 mm, is not operator-dependent, and does not have the limitations of US with respect to body habitus or increased bowel gas. However, it lacks portability, exposes the patient to ionizing radiation, and is more expensive than US (Table 22.4).

Magnetic Resonance Cholangiopancreatography

Magnetic resonance cholangiopancreatography (MRCP) is a technical refinement of standard magnetic resonance imaging (MRI) that permits rapid clear-cut delineation of the biliary tract. MRCP is superior to conventional US or CT for the detection of biliary tract obstruction[51] and plays an important role as a diagnostic test in this setting (Table 22.4). Moreover, standard MRI can be performed during the same examination if there is a question of a hepatobiliary mass or if a contrast allergy precludes CT. It is more expensive than US or CT.

Endoscopic Retrograde Cholangiopancreatography

Endoscopic retrograde cholangiopancreatography (ERCP) permits direct visualization of the biliary tract.[52] ERCP is more invasive than US, CT, and MRCP (see Table 22.4) and comparable in cost to MRCP. After endoscopic identification of the ampulla of Vater, insertion of a catheter permits contrast injection into the biliary tract; sedation and analgesia are necessary. ERCP is highly accurate in the diagnosis of biliary obstruction. If a focal cause (e.g., choledocholithiasis, biliary stricture) is identified, maneuvers to relieve obstruction (e.g., sphincterotomy, stone extraction, stricture dilation, and stent placement) can be performed during the same session (see Chapter 72). Similarly, if there is concern about a neoplasm, biopsy and brushings for cytology can be obtained. In this setting, acquisition of biopsy specimens and therapeutic interventions via ERCP are limited largely to lesions distal to the bifurcation of the right and left hepatic bile ducts.[53] However, advances in catheter design (cholangioscopy) have permitted improved optical visualization of lesions incompletely characterized by conventional ERCP, and which have expanded its diagnostic and therapeutic reach.[54] The technical success rate of diagnostic ERCP is higher than 90%; the technique fails when the ampulla of Vater cannot be cannulated, as may be the case in patients with prior abdominal surgery and altered anatomy (e.g., gastric bypass, choledochojejunostomy). The major complication of ERCP is pancreatitis, which occurs in at least 5% of cases, and the mortality rate is approximately 0.2%. These rates are influenced in part by the patient's baseline characteristics and need for therapeutic instrumentation during the procedure.[55]

Percutaneous Transhepatic Cholangiography

Percutaneous transhepatic cholangiography (THC) (also known as PTC) is a procedure that complements ERCP. Percutaneous THC requires passage of a needle through the skin and subcutaneous tissues into the liver and advancement into a peripheral bile duct. When bile is aspirated, a catheter is introduced through the needle, and radiopaque contrast medium is injected. The sensitivity and specificity of percutaneous THC for the diagnosis of biliary tract disease are comparable with those for ERCP.[56] Like ERCP, interventional procedures like balloon dilation and stent placement can be performed at the time of percutaneous THC to relieve focal obstructions of the biliary tract, and cholangioscopy is also feasible by this route (see Chapter 72). Percutaneous THC is particularly technically advantageous when the level of biliary obstruction is proximal to the common hepatic duct or altered anatomy precludes ERCP (see earlier). Percutaneous THC may be challenging in the absence of dilatation of the intrahepatic bile ducts; in this situation, multiple passes may be required, and visualization of the biliary tract may be unsuccessful in approximately 10% of attempts.[57] With percutaneous THC, about 2% of patients experience complications as a result of bleeding, perforation, and infection; death is rare. Percutaneous THC is more expensive than abdominal US and CT (see Table 22.4).

Endoscopic US

Endoscopic US (EUS) can also detect obstruction of the bile duct and major intrahepatic bile ducts, with sensitivity and specificity comparable to those for MRCP.[58,59] EUS has the potential advantage of permitting biopsy of suspected malignant lesions, and under appropriate circumstances, the operator can proceed directly to ERCP for definitive biliary decompression (see Table 22.4). The risk of diagnostic EUS is comparable with that of diagnostic upper endoscopy; when needle biopsy is used, the mortality rate is roughly 0.1%. EUS may be most useful in circumstances in which the patient is thought to be at high risk for complications of ERCP or percutaneous THC, and there is uncertainty about the presence of biliary obstruction.

Nuclear Imaging Studies

Nuclear scintigraphy of the biliary tract, although helpful in the diagnosis of cholecystitis,[60,61] is not routinely used in the diagnostic evaluation of adults with jaundice, given the availability of techniques described above, which permit hepatobiliary imaging with higher spatial resolution. There are two potential exceptions. In the very early phases of biliary obstruction, dilation of the bile ducts may not be observable, and this may be a setting in which nuclear medicine imaging could be advantageous.[60] Nuclear scintigraphy also has an important role in the diagnosis of a potential bile leak, an uncommon cause of jaundice following hepatobiliary surgery or blunt abdominal trauma.[62,63]

Suggested Strategies for Imaging

The order of imaging studies depends largely on the clinical likelihood of obstructive jaundice (see Fig. 22.2). Several diagnostic strategies have been compared by clinical decision analysis in the era that predated MRCP and EUS[64]; no subsequent refinements to this comparison have been published. Based upon the analysis, if the probability of biliary obstruction is approximately 20%, the positive and negative predictive values of a strategy that uses US as the initial test are estimated to be 96% and 98%, respectively. If the probability of biliary obstruction is 60%, a strategy that uses US as the first test would yield a positive predictive value of 99%, whereas the negative predictive value would fall to 89%. The implication is that if the level of suspicion for biliary tract obstruction is high and US does not show dilated bile ducts, further studies to visualize the biliary tract should be pursued. A similar logic has been used in more recently published radiology guidelines.[65]

Based upon previous information, in jaundiced patients in whom biliary obstruction is a possibility, abdominal US (or CT) is an appropriate initial approach. If the bile ducts are dilated, the biliary tract should be imaged directly with ERCP (or percutaneous THC) and appropriate therapy undertaken if biliary obstruction is found. If the bile ducts are not dilated on abdominal US (or CT), the next step depends on the clinical likelihood of biliary obstruction. If the likelihood of biliary obstruction is thought to be low, the patient should be evaluated for intrinsic liver disease (see later). If the likelihood of biliary obstruction is thought to be intermediate, EUS or MRCP is a reasonable next step prior to biliary intervention or evaluation for a hepatic disorder. Among patients in whom biliary obstruction is thought to be likely, ERCP (or percutaneous THC) should be considered the next step. If ERCP or percutaneous THC does not show biliary obstruction, the patient should be evaluated for cholestatic liver disease. The choice between ERCP and percutaneous THC will be influenced by various factors (see Table 22.4), including the availability of each procedure at a particular institution, presence or absence of dilated bile ducts on initial imaging (which would hamper percutaneous THC), history of prior gastrointestinal surgery that would hamper endoscopic access (e.g., gastric bypass, choledochojejunostomy), and suspected level of biliary obstruction. Under most circumstances, ERCP should be the procedure of choice because it is comparable to percutaneous THC in accuracy, technical success rate, and frequency of major complications; tends to be more widely available; and may offer better postprocedure tolerability (e.g., no need for an external biliary drainage tube). It is tempting to speculate that in the future, advances in artificial intelligence will simplify the selection of imaging studies and therapeutic interventions in complex cases.

Other Studies

Serologic Testing

Jaundiced patients with biochemical evidence of hepatocellular dysfunction or cholestasis, in whom imaging studies do not suggest biliary obstruction, should be evaluated for underlying liver disease. Depending on the disorder suspected, screening laboratory studies may include viral serologies; serum levels of iron, transferrin, and ferritin (for hemochromatosis); ceruloplasmin (for Wilson disease); mitochondrial antibodies (for PBC); and antinuclear antibodies, smooth muscle antibodies, and serum immunoglobulins (for autoimmune hepatitis). Confirmation of these diagnoses, as well as elucidation of diagnoses not revealed by serologic analysis, may be made by liver biopsy.

Liver Biopsy

Liver biopsy provides precise information regarding lobular architecture and the extent and pattern of hepatic inflammation and fibrosis, and it is most helpful for patients with persistent and undiagnosed jaundice. With histological analysis (and if appropriate, quantification of iron or copper content), liver biopsy permits the diagnosis of steatotic liver disease (alcohol-associated, metabolic dysfunction-associated, or both, as guided by patient history), hemochromatosis, Wilson disease, autoimmune hepatitis, PBC, granulomatous hepatitis, and neoplasms. Occasionally, liver biopsy findings provide clues to otherwise unsuspected biliary tract obstruction, classical histologic features of which are shown in Fig. 22.3. However, liver histology may be entirely normal in acute biliary obstruction. Liver biopsy is associated with a low but definite complication rate, predominantly from bleeding and perforation, and the need for hospitalization in 1% of cases; the mortality rate is about 0.01%.[66]

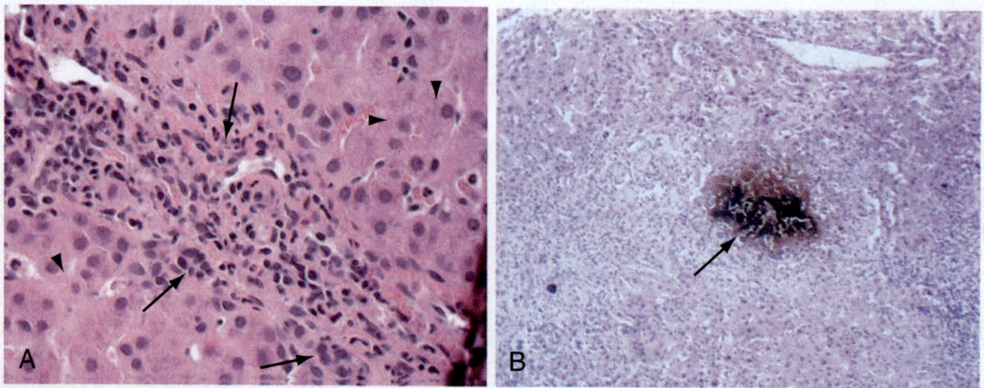

Fig. 22.3 Liver histology in biliary tract obstruction. (A) Prominent bile duct proliferation (*arrows*) and a mixed portal-based inflammatory infiltrate are evident. Periportal hepatocytes show feathery degeneration (*arrowheads*) indicative of cholate stasis, cytologic changes caused by prolonged cholestasis (H&E, ×200). (B) The periportal bilirubin-stained region (*arrow*) surrounded by necrotic cells represents a bile infarct (H&E, ×40).

THERAPEUTIC APPROACHES

Obstructive Jaundice

In the patient with bile duct obstruction, therapy is typically directed at relieving the obstruction. Interventional endoscopic or radiologic approaches include sphincterotomy, balloon dilation of focal strictures, and placement of drains or stents (see Chapter 72); the alternative approach is surgery. The therapeutic strategy chosen depends in part on the location and likely cause of the obstructing lesion. Focal intrahepatic strictures may be amenable to an interventional radiologic approach, whereas lesions distal to the bifurcation of the hepatic ducts may be more suitably managed endoscopically (e.g., sphincterotomy for choledocholithiasis); surgery should be considered for neoplasms if feasible.

Nonobstructive Jaundice

When jaundice is due to liver disease, optimal treatment is directed toward the underlying cause (e.g., cessation of ethanol, discontinuation of the offending drug, administration of antiviral therapy for hepatitis B or hepatitis C, immunosuppressive agents for autoimmune hepatitis), and in some cases, liver transplantation may be the only viable option (see Chapter 99). Therapy for hyperbilirubinemia *per se* is generally unnecessary in adults, because the neurotoxicity of bilirubin is limited to disorders characterized by extreme elevations of unconjugated bilirubin in neonates and infants (e.g., physiologic jaundice of the newborn, type I Crigler-Najjar syndrome). In these disorders, the risk of neurotoxicity can be reduced with phototherapy, in which exposure to blue-green light (wavelength range 460–490 nm) produces photoisomerization of bilirubin to more water-soluble enantiomers that do not require conjugation for excretion in bile.[67]

Ursodiol (ursodeoxycholic acid), an orally administered bile acid that potently stimulates bile flow, has been used successfully as a treatment for several cholestatic disorders. In PBC, ursodiol improves biochemical indices and slows disease progression in the majority of patients (see Chapter 93).[68] Ursodiol has also been shown to improve biochemical markers and symptoms in patients with intrahepatic cholestasis of pregnancy,[69] and it appears to prevent hyperbilirubinemia following hematopoietic stem cell transplantation.[70] Additional treatments for cholestatic disorders are directed toward complications that are independent of hyperbilirubinemia, such as malabsorption of fat-soluble vitamins (A, D, E, and K), and pruritus. These are discussed in Chapters 70 and 93.

Full references for this chapter can be found at https://ebooks.health.elsevier.com.

23 Factitious Gastrointestinal Diseases

Christopher Vélez, Braden Kuo

IN THIS CHAPTER

INTRODUCTION

An accepted principle of the patient-physician relationship is that the patient should make every attempt to regain health, including faithfully and unreservedly communicating to his or her physician the supposed cause of illness.[1–3] In factitious disorders (FD), this assumption fails. Patients may deviate from this covenant by self-inducing disease, feigning illness, withholding information regarding the cause of illness, exaggerating the severity of symptoms, or presenting a false medical history or medical records. When a gastroenterologist is concerned about FD, it is incumbent on her to ensure that: (1) similarly presenting disorders—such as somatic symptom disorder (SSD)—are not misdiagnosed as FD; (2) behaviors that may appear as FD but are related to other diseases (such as eating disorders) are not falsely attributed to FD; and (3), nondisease related actions (such as malingering) are not attributed to an incorrect FD diagnosis.

The purposes of this chapter are to discuss the possible etiologies of these abnormal illness behaviors, provide suggestions on how to recognize them, and point out ethical conflicts that confront physicians taking care of such patients. We will emphasize the types of deceptive behaviors most likely to be encountered in the practice of gastroenterology and the iatrogenic diseases that are most likely to develop because of them. FD are stigmatizing and have been reported in women in manners that historically have reinforced implicit bias toward people of female sex (who still in the 21st century are more likely to receive care that dismisses disease as having an emotional basis compared to patients of male sex).[4] Care must be taken to understand historical descriptions of these disorders when applying them to modern patient care, particularly when one considers that all too often women's illnesses are minimized compared to men's complaints. FD should be diagnoses of exclusion, and even once recognized, empathy must be shown for people with such serious illnesses. Note is made a priori of cases being described in this chapter mostly in women; this should be balanced against the cases of male patients.

FACTITIOUS DISORDER IMPOSED ON SELF

The subtle form of FD was first described in 1864 by Hector Gavin.[5] He observed it mainly in those who "mimicked or counterfeited illness to gain compliance with their wishes, or to excite interest, or for the pleasure of deceiving." While in the 21st century physicians should be loathed to describe patients in such a negative manner, this description does capture vividly a physician's sense of betrayal. It is extremely difficult to determine prevalence in the population, but prior reports have suggested a predominance of younger women. Patients may lead an outwardly normal life, be employed and medically insured, and be highly cooperative with their caregivers. FD is considered a psychiatric illness,[6] but the patients seek medical care from nonpsychiatric physicians. Case Study 23.1 illustrates subtle FD, which is also referred to as the "socially conformist" type of FD.[7–9]

Etiology and Motives

Generally, patients with FD present themselves with disabilities and disturbances that fall within the purview of physicians.[10] There are several possible explanations for FD behaviors, and one can draw on various theoretical frameworks. While exploring these theoretical frameworks is interesting from a historical perspective, there are two important limitations to this approach: (1) gastroenterologists are not equipped in training to explore whether or not these theories can be applied in routine clinical care; and (2) many of these constructs reinforce the paternalistic, hierarchical view of the physician in the patient-doctor relationship in ways that are uncomfortable in the 21st century. Unfortunately, given the near impossibility of research being performed to address FD constructs, it is important to understand these constructs' role in our profession and to move beyond the biases that are inherent in them.

It has been posited that excessive or deceptive illness behavior learned earlier in life is the best response the person knows. Psychodynamic theories draw on a number of possible conflicts—particularly in the child-parent relationship—resulting in the need to be cared for, the need to deceive, the need for revenge, the need to feel in control, the need for mastery over abusive parents, and the need to be punished or hurt.[11] By focusing on a physical illness, the patient can avoid the underlying painful feelings prompting these needs. The longing for nurturance and the need for distraction from authentic life problems[12] are also possible motivations. Behavioral theories point to

CASE STUDY 23.1 A 37-YEAR-OLD WOMAN WITH DIARRHEA

The patient began to have diarrhea a few days after undergoing reconstructive jaw surgery. Extensive evaluations failed to reveal a cause of diarrhea, and the patient was referred for gastrointestinal consultation. By quantitative stool collection, her average stool weight was 1008 g/day (normal stool weight for women is 87 ± 8 g/day.) The diarrhea was secretory in nature according to electrolyte analysis. Fecal fat output was within normal limits. Serum gastrin and vasoactive intestinal polypeptide concentrations were normal, and stool culture revealed no pathogens.

Due to inability to find a cause of the patient's chronic secretory diarrhea, and because of multiple other medical and surgical illnesses prior to the onset of diarrhea (see later), surreptitious laxative ingestion with bisacodyl or senna was suspected. However, the patient denied ingestion of laxatives, a urine and stool laxative screen (Toxi-Lab) was negative, and the patient did not have pseudomelanosis coli on colonic biopsy specimens (see Chapter 128). Her personal belongings were not searched, and she was not confronted with the clinicans' suspicion. She was discharged with advice on fluid and electrolyte replacement and symptom management, and with an offer to return at any time.

Approximately 1 year after her evaluation, the patient went to another medical center, where endoscopies were repeated, but no diagnosis was forthcoming. A colonoscopy with biopsy was complicated by severe bleeding, and she required transfusion of multiple units of blood. Owing to continuing weight loss, parenteral nutrition was begun. After the diarrhea had been present for about 4 years, she returned to the original institution. At this time, bisacodyl testing was positive.

The patient was confronted in a supportive manner (see later) and in the presence of her husband, who was with her continuously during her outpatient evaluation. With a few tears, she calmly said that she had "absolutely not" been taking laxatives and added, "I don't know what bisacodyl is." After discharge, her husband searched her closet at home and found an empty box of correctol for Women, which contains bisacodyl. The husband and her local physician agreed to obtain psychiatric help for the patient.

According to her family, there was no evidence of an eating disorder or sexual abuse. For the previous 6 years, she had worked in a doctor's office, where her knowledge of medicine had increased. "She's always been a great believer in medicine, and she doesn't see the risks." She had undergone multiple orthopedic surgeries without any clear need, and the jaw surgery was done for a questionable indication. These surgeries made her the center of attention. She was married to a loving and caring husband. The diarrheal illness started about 3 months after her diagnosis of infertility. (Others have observed that the onset of FD often begins shortly after a stressful event).[7,8]

About 3 years after the diagnosis of FD, the patient's family and some of her local physicians were contacted again for an update. Generally, things were much better. Although the decision to confront the patient was probably wise, the patient had felt betrayed. She never accepted the diagnosis and refused to see a psychiatrist. She still had various medical problems with frequent appointments with specialists. Two weeks before these conversations, the patient had had hip surgery, and several months before she had had a cholecystectomy. Earlier in the year she had had surgery to correct damage caused by teeth grinding. "She's probably not taking laxatives anymore, but several times a year her potassium level is low, and on one occasion a diuretic was found in her urine." These could be compatible with factitious disorder, with involvement of different organ systems.

TABLE 23.1 Manifestations of Factitious Diseases by Mechanism[a]

Mechanism	Manifestations
Self-induced infection	Abscesses, bacteremia, fever, sepsis, wound infection
Surreptitious ingestion of medicines, vitamins, minerals	Bartter syndrome, bleeding or purpura from coagulation disorder (warfarin, heparin), bone marrow depression, diarrhea, hyperthyroidism, hypoglycemia, hypokalemia (laxatives and/or diuretics), hypomagnesemia, liver disease, pheochromocytoma (epinephrine injection), renal failure, salt poisoning, vomiting
Self-induced injury	Bruises, complex regional pain syndrome (reflex sympathetic dystrophy), deformities, dermatoses (may also be induced by ingestion of certain drugs), unhealed wounds
Phlebotomy (self or animal)	Anemia, hematemesis, hematochezia, hematuria, melena
Thermometer manipulation or substitution of thermometer	Fever
Simulation of the clinical manifestations of specific diseases or syndromes (sometimes using falsified medical records or contamination of body fluids)	AIDS, cancer, CF, depression, multiple sclerosis, pain syndromes, pancreatitis, proteinuria, seizures, psychosis, renal stones

[a]Organization was modified from Ref. [15].

exposure to and reinforcement of sick-role activity. The self-enhancement model[11,13] suggests that individuals covet the specialness of their ailments and their relationships with high-status professionals (especially doctors).

There is usually no apparent symbolic significance to the selection of the illness that is induced or feigned.[14] Patients with FD can simulate authentic disease in almost all organ systems (Table 23.1). Indeed, a given patient may use different manufactured symptoms and diseases at different times. It is generally believed that patients with FD are aware of what they are doing, as evidenced by careful planning in most cases. They know right from wrong. Their intelligent quotients are usually normal or high (even if their educational attainment is relatively limited), and only very few are psychotic. Some are depressed and may have thoughts of suicide. As a group, they are sometimes described as being immature and lacking interpersonal skills.[15]

Risk of Iatrogenic Disease

Patients with FD are usually willing and sometimes appear eager to accept dangerous diagnostic procedures to sustain the sick role. As a result of their deception, unneeded invasive and potentially dangerous diagnostic tests, procedures, and treatments are prescribed, and these may, in turn, result in iatrogenic disease. In most cases, the greatest damage to these patients is due to doctors' actions, rather than from any direct action by the patient.[16] FD patients presenting with GI symptoms or signs may receive needless laparotomies, gastric, or intestinal resections, pancreatectomy, renal biopsy, adrenalectomy, or prolonged treatment with glucocorticoids. Case Study 23.2 illustrates some of these points.

Diagnosis and Detection

Early recognition of patients with FD is the best way to prevent iatrogenic disease, but most internists and gastroenterologists never consider FD in the differential diagnosis of patients with idiopathic physical symptoms. A factitious etiology of symptoms destroys the reasoned ordering of potential disease conditions when generating differential diagnoses in ways that can trouble a physician. The tests are repeated, new doctors are consulted, tests with low specificity for extremely rare authentic diseases may be performed and false-positive results lead to more tests.

Even if FD is considered in the differential diagnosis, several factors make it difficult for physicians to recognize the subtle form of FD. First, these patients do not appear to be different from other patients with similar symptoms caused by authentic disease.[17,18] Second, the psychiatric illnesses they have are not easily recognized,[19] and there is usually no obvious excessive secondary gain that these patients are receiving. Third, the patients convincingly deny self-induced illness if they are asked.[18,20] Fourth, there is a lack of communication between current and previous doctors, as well as a failure to study old medical records (previously due to their being in paper form, currently due to vast amount of information available electronically and lack of electronic medical record system interoperability). Fifth, physicians can be afraid to discuss the possibility of FD with their patients.

Several clues, if present, increase the likelihood of FD in a particular patient (Box 23.1); however, the diagnosis of FD cannot be made solely on the basis of clues, so some form of confirmation must be obtained. Box 23.2 provides a list of some of the methods that have been used to bolster or confirm a suspicion of self-induced illness.

If the attending physician considers FD and obtains a psychiatric consultation, it is important to recognize that even an

CASE STUDY 23.2 IATROGENIC DISEASE IN A 33-YEAR-OLD WOMAN

The patient felt well until 8 years earlier when she developed constipation requiring laxatives; later that year she developed diarrhea. Colonoscopy revealed mild colitis, and x-rays suggested ileitis. Over the next 2 years, the diarrhea persisted despite many different diets and medications, including prednisone. Salt depletion occurred frequently, requiring multiple hospitalizations. The patient developed aseptic necrosis of both hips, presumably the result of prednisone therapy, and had a total left hip replacement. Severe diarrhea continued, and she underwent several surgical procedures: exploratory laparotomy, loop ileostomy without bowel resection, and subsequently a total colectomy with standard ileostomy. The pathology report showed nonspecific chronic inflammation. Postoperatively, the patient had severe ileostomy diarrhea. A neuroendocrine tumor syndrome was suspected, and she was referred for further studies.

A balance study revealed that the ileostomy volume was 2561 mL/day (normal 600), the diarrhea was secretory in type, and intestinal absorption of dietary fat was normal. Intestinal perfusion studies showed normal small bowel absorption of water and electrolytes. The patient denied use of laxatives since the onset of her diarrhea. However, her room was secretly searched, and a box of Carter's Little Pills was discovered, which contained several anthraquinones including podophyllum and aloin (see Chapter 20). A review of her medical records near the time of her colectomy revealed a pathology report on a rectal biopsy specimen that described pseudomelanosis coli.

BOX 23.1 Clues That Increase the Likelihood of Subtle Forms of Factitious Disorder

- Predominantly women (prevalence is difficult to estimate; as women's medical complaints are taken less seriously than men's, it is critical to minimize implicit bias and misdiagnose female patients with factitious disorders)
- Previous experience in the medical field, which provides an unusual grasp of terminology and access to medical supplies
- Multiple surgeries, multiple procedures
- Inexplicable laboratory test results
- Inconsistency and implausibility of certain aspects of the history
- Visits to 3 or more medical centers previously for the same symptoms or to a nationally known referral center, despite residing far away
- History of substance abuse or prior psychiatric disorder
- Reluctance to allow release of previous medical records

BOX 23.2 Methods That Have Been Used to Bolster or Confirm a Suspicion of a Factitious Disorder Imposed on Self

- Review old medical records and discuss the case with previous doctors and family members, if appropriate. Identify discrepancies and inconsistencies and estimate the influence of gain derived from the sick role; be aware of implicit bias and arriving inappropriately at an FD diagnosis. Inquire about psychiatric illness, previous psychiatric treatment, suicide attempts, stress in the patient's life, childhood abuse, marital/sexual problems, eating disorders, etc.
- Review previous biopsy slides to look for foreign body material in wounds,[71] pseudomelanosis coli,[72] and other clues, as appropriate for the patient's symptoms.
- Obtain a psychiatric evaluation to help determine if criteria are met for psychiatric illness which may argue against factitious disease.
- If symptoms and signs may be explained by surreptitious ingestion of medications and poisons, obtain appropriate medication and toxicology screens. Consider obtaining a urine test for diuretics even in the absence of renal or electrolyte abnormalities. Evaluate the results of such screens in light of the sensitivity and specificity of the tests used.
- When possible, compare patient-submitted specimens with those obtained directly under clinical supervision. For example, compare fecal material obtained at an "unprepped" sigmoidoscopy with fecal material submitted by the patient.
- If appropriate, review with risk management at your institution prior to initiating a search of a patient's personal belongings (see text).

experienced psychiatrist cannot reliably make or rule out a diagnosis of FD by taking a psychiatric history from a patient who is suspected of having FD but denies it.

Management

Two main assumptions form the basis for the proposed management recommendations. The first is that FD represents the patient's attempt to cope with emotional distress. The second is that a supportive attitude by the healthcare team will make it possible for the patient to process an FD diagnosis. Unfortunately, almost all management recommendations that have been reported were based on experience with patients who were hospitalized. We know of no suggested recommendations for outpatients, despite most people with FD being ambulatory. Additionally, data are limited to case series. When gastrointestinal symptoms predominate, close collaboration with internists and psychiatrists are key to reduce aforementioned harms.

Techniques that have been used for the management of FD include the confrontation of the patient, psychotherapy, pharmacotherapy, behavioral therapy, and multidisciplinary approaches. Eastwood and Bisson[21] attempted to evaluate the effectiveness of these management methods by reviewing 32 case reports and 13 case series. Based on their review, these authors concluded that the evidence in the literature is insufficient to evaluate the effectiveness of any management technique. Little progress has been made since then.

Nevertheless, there appears to be a general consensus in the literature on several aspects of the treatment of FD, as listed in Box 23.3. Although these recommendations are probably accepted by most experts, differences of opinion exist on the value and wisdom of confronting a patient with a diagnosis of FD. Combining the recommendations from the authors of three studies,[15,22,23] there seems to be a consensus that confrontation of patients with "confirmed FD" should be done when there is a danger of significant iatrogenic disease. All agree that the confrontation should be supportive, as enumerated in Box 23.4. There is no consensus on whether confrontation should be done when FD is suspected but "unproved" or when the danger of iatrogenic disease is judged to be small.

Management without confrontation is sometimes referred to as a "face-saving technique."[24,25] Here the patient is gently given the message that the doctors suspect that disease is not present and the patient is offered a chance to abandon factitious disease before it is exposed. The patient may be told that "if the next treatment fails to work, we will need to question whether or not an illness exists." The next treatment (almost any treatment) is then applied, and a surprising number of patients will undergo miraculous improvement rather than risk being exposed as a fraud. One report concluded that after such nonconfrontational approaches, about one-third of the patients' complaints remitted. They may have vigorously denied what they were doing, but if the doctors somehow allowed them to save face, the behavior stopped for some time. Therefore the embarrassment of discovery is avoided in a substantial minority of patients. Even if patients admit to some or all the deceptions, however, most will continue to induce or feign disease. This trade-off is acceptable, provided the danger of iatrogenic disease is judged to be small, with the recognition that no therapeutic technique is consistently effective.[24] Although this face-saving technique is favored by several experts, the authors are not aware of results of this method in a case series of patients with the subtle form of FD. With growing emphasis on patient autonomy and shared decision-making in the 21st century, this technique may be challenging to apply.

In general, the treatment of FD seldom leads to "cure." Some patients temporarily discontinue their illness-seeking behavior, but most are unwilling to accept psychiatric referral and probably will continue to complain of illness. Whenever possible, a psychiatrist should assess the patient for comorbid psychiatric/personality disorders that may predispose the patient toward, or contribute to expressions of, factitious illness behavior. If the underlying mental condition can be recognized and treated, the psychological forces driving the FD may be lessened. The patient should also be assessed for suicidality and, when appropriate, should be transferred to a more secure setting. Psychiatric hospitalization is indicated when a patient has suicidal ideation or attempts suicide, has a deteriorating social situation, or manifests potentially dangerous behavior.[22,26] When recovery occurs, it most often results from changes in the patient's life situation rather than from medical intervention.[27]

BOX 23.3 Consensus Opinions on the Treatment of Factitious Disorder*

- Achievement of insight should not be the principal early goal of treatment, because it can weaken the patient's defenses.
- One person should have primary responsibility for patient management.
- There should be a comprehensive the psychiatric evaluation of the patient, including assessment for suicide risk.
- All members of a multidisciplinary team should be aware of the assessment and treatment plan.
- The treatment plan should be individualized.
- Comorbid illness should be treated appropriately.
- If confrontational techniques are used, they should be nonpunitive and supportive.

*Derived from the literature.

BOX 23.4 Features of Supportive Confrontation

- Tell the patient what you suspect without outright accusation.
- Provide empathetic and face-saving comments*.
- Avoid probing to uncover the patient's underlying feelings and motivations†‡.
- Assure the patient that the physician will not release the diagnosis to others without the patient's permission, unless required to do so by law‡.
- Make sure the staff demonstrate continued acceptance of the patient.
- Engage in shared decision-making regarding mental health.

*"Maybe you didn't know what you were taking; this medication could cause you to be sick"; "Maybe you took it in your sleep"; "We realize you must be in great distress"; "We want to continue to take care of you."

†This is done to minimize the disruption of essential emotional defenses.

‡Later it may be decided to break this promise in patients with potentially fatal factitious disease, such as patients who are creating sepsis by injecting contaminated material into their bodies. This promise should only be broken after consultation and consensus opinion has been obtained by an ethics committee, legal personnel, and others, as described in the text.

Ethical and Legal Issues

The management of FD may potentially place physicians in precarious situations related to potential breaches in protection of sensitive patient health information. There may be potential litigation targeting clinicians (including for failing to diagnose FD in the setting of invasive diagnostic/management interventions). The best approach to such dilemmas is to consult with risk management and other physicians, such as the hospital's chief medical officer, and with the ethical and legal committees of the institution. The issues are best discussed thoroughly in a team setting so that a consensus can be reached.

RELATED ABNORMAL ILLNESSES AND BEHAVIORS

Somatic Symptom Disorder

SSD can be defined as idiopathic physical symptoms that over time are located in different parts of the body, and that cause disproportionally severe disability and impaired function. The main symptom is pain, which may be described as gastrointestinal in nature. There is no evidence that pain in patients with SSD is intentionally feigned or exaggerated, but there is no way to prove that it is not (see also Chapters 5 and 13).

The onset of physical symptoms often closely follows a traumatic event, and the physical symptoms may coexist with other psychiatric disorders such as depression. A female predominance has been reported. The patients seek medical care for their symptoms, but no authentic medical explanation can be found. Secondary gain from assumption of the "sick role" is often apparent. In some patients, symptoms and illness become a means of communication,[28] and a way of controlling their environment. The dysfunction and disability attributed to the symptoms often appear to be out of proportion to the severity of the symptoms. The course of SSD is usually chronic. Once established at a young age, it can continue into advanced age.[29] An example of SSD is presented in Case Study 23.3.

The underlying etiology of SSD is unknown, but several mechanisms have been proposed. They include the hypothesis that patients with SSD experience psychologic distress in the form of physical symptoms.[30] Another theory is that the patient learns the behavior that manifests his or her belief in the supposed affliction and that the resulting "illness" helps the patient to cope.[31] The boundaries of SSD are obviously not sharp, merging imperceptibly with illness anxiety disorder on one side and with FD on the other side.[31]

Diagnosis of SSD depends on recognizing two features of the patient's illness. First, there has been illness-seeking behavior for multiple idiopathic symptoms related to different organ systems; and second, the disability and dysfunction attributed to the symptoms are disproportionally high. In one report, patients with SSD spent 7 days in bed each month, compared with 0.48 days for a general population.[32] Patients with SSD potentially do not prize as highly the relationship with their doctors as patients with FD.

Unfortunately, even highly skilled physicians repeatedly fail to recognize SSD,[29] and they, therefore obtain diagnostic tests for rare and then very rare conditions. These patients are highly vulnerable to such practice because repeated diagnostic tests often reveal questionable abnormalities that can lead to complications from medical treatments (e.g., glucocorticoids or narcotics), invasive procedures, or surgeries.

For the management of patients with the SSD, a "caring" rather than "curing" approach is recommended.[33] An empathetic, long-term relationship should be established, preferably by one physician. Regular appointments should be scheduled, and brief physical examinations are preferred over extensive diagnostic tests and procedures.[34] Prescribed medication should be kept to a minimum, and opioids should be avoided.[33] Because depression is common, and these patients should be evaluated for suicide risk.[6] Confrontation should be avoided because motivation in SSD is unconscious, but some awareness of emotional components can be achieved.[33] In a randomized controlled clinical trial, it was found that cognitive behavioral therapy was associated with significant improvement in self-reported functioning, and somatic symptoms and decreased health care costs.[35] These improvements, however, could have been due to the increased attention and extra time that was invested in the experimental cognitive behavioral therapy treatment.[33]

CASE STUDY 23.3 A 20-YEAR-OLD WOMAN WITH ABDOMINAL PAIN

A college student developed left-sided periumbilical pain associated with nausea. She was so disabled by the pain that she had to drop out of school. She was placed on opioids, but the pain persisted. CT showed a jejunal intussusception. The patient was scheduled for abdominal surgery, but her family decided to obtain a second opinion.

During the evaluation with the gastroenterologist, she described her pain as constant, aching, and burning (10 of 10 in severity), and located in the left mid-abdomen. The pain was not related to meals, bowel movements, or her menstrual cycle. She did not have constipation or diarrhea. Her past medical history revealed an inguinal hernia, right knee arthroscopies, chronic back pain, chronic pelvic pain, depression, fatigue, and a menstrual disorder. During physical examination she demonstrated a depressed affect and did not appear to be in severe pain. There was minimal tenderness to palpation.

Review of CT images with a radiologist confirmed intermittent jejunal intussusception without obstruction. Because it is known that most small bowel intussusceptions discovered incidentally by CT scans are asymptomatic, transient, and do not warrant surgical management,[70] we doubted that the jejunal intussusception was the cause of her abdominal pain. Endoscopy to the mid-ileum revealed no abnormalities. A surgical consultant agreed that the patient's pain was not caused by the jejunal intussusception seen on CT scan. The gastroenterologist and the surgeon made a diagnosis of SSD. The patient was referred to a psychiatrist to evaluate her for depression and suicidal risk.

Several years later, her condition was more or less unchanged. She still had pain, but it was located in the chest rather than the abdomen. There was continued biopsychosocial distress.

Malingering

As with the subtle form of FD, Gavin was the first to describe malingering.[5] Malingering is defined as conscious and intentional production or exaggeration of symptoms and signs of disease for material gain, such as money, lodging, food, narcotics, avoidance of military duty, and escape from criminal prosecution. Malingering is not always a reflection of greed. It might instead be the result of financial desperation or an attempt to escape physical or emotional abuse.[36] For example, a patient may malinger through surreptitious laxative ingestion to induce illness due to a fear of spousal abandonment. A careful medical and social history is obviously required to put this medical deception into proper context.[36]

As with FD, people who malinger seek medical care for the symptoms and signs they feign or produce, and they hide the true etiology of their symptoms from their physicians. They typically are not as willing as patients with FD to accept dangerous diagnostic or therapeutic procedures, and they may attempt to minimize contact with health care professionals to avoid detection.[36]

The distinction between malingering and FD is based on the perception of motive: material gain for malingering and emotional gain from the sick role for FD. Perception of motive, however, is not always correct and is subject to bias.[36] Clinicians should also be aware that an individual's goals, whether internal or external, conscious or unconscious, can vary over time or coexist.[37] Unlike FD and SSD, malingering is not considered to be a mental disorder as per the *Diagnostic and Statistical Manual of Mental Disorders*, fifth edition.[6]

SPECIAL ISSUES RELATED TO GASTROENTEROLOGY

Gastrointestinal Distress Associated With Eating Disorders

Patients with eating disorders often develop GI symptoms, many of which are caused by excessive laxative usage or self-induced vomiting (see Chapter 10).[38] When seeking medical care for these symptoms, it can be challenging to identify that the patient is suffering from an eating disorder (particularly since the inducing factors can be multifactorial).[73] Others have reported that they sought medical care only once their families insisted and can state that they have no desire to engage in the sick role as a relief of emotional stress. Empathy is critical in such patients—there can be intense shame from symptoms themselves or for concealing behaviors from doctors (particularly when evaluations have progressed so far as to result in abdominal surgery).

Surreptitious Laxative Ingestion

Diarrhea caused by surreptitious ingestion of laxatives is often associated with abdominal pain, weight loss, electrolyte derangements, and/or postural hypotension. Depending on which of these manifestations are revealed to the physician and which are hidden, the clinical presentation can be highly variable. Diarrhea in association with hypokalemia, abdominal pain, weight loss, or postural hypotension have different well-known connotations that provoke specific diagnostic studies that may further complicate management by involving other specialists, including nephrologists and endocrinologists.[39,40] In any case, the usual tools of gastroenterology will not reveal the correct diagnosis and will often be misleading. Only gastroenterologists who know the information in Boxes 23.1 and 23.2 will be likely to make the correct diagnosis. If laxative use disorders are suspected, empathy must be practiced to enhance the likelihood of a positive therapeutic alliance that can help the patient achieve improvement.

Factitious Diarrhea

When gastroenterologists refer patients with chronic idiopathic diarrhea to a medical center that has a special interest in diarrheal disease, once organ-based disorders such as steatorrhea or disordered gut-brain interaction such as functional diarrhea or irritable bowel syndrome with diarrhea have been excluded, the most common specific diagnosis that can be made is the ingestion of laxatives (see Chapter 17).[41] To a significant degree, the diagnosis of laxative ingestion in patients who deny laxative intake depends on the ability to detect laxatives or their metabolic products in stool or urine by analytical methods. It is important to recognize, however, that any mistakes in the determination of laxative intake could have serious deleterious consequences. False-negative results delay the diagnosis of factitious disease for years and contribute to complications from unnecessary or inappropriate medical or surgical therapy. Conversely, false-positive results prematurely stop the diagnostic evaluation for an authentic disease and may result in a patient's being incorrectly accused of self-induction of disease, which can be catastrophic for the physician-patient relationship (as well as offering substandard care).

Bisacodyl and senna are the most common laxatives ingested surreptitiously to produce factitious diarrhea.[42] While research laboratories have reported 100% sensitivity and specificity for identification of these drugs by thin layer chromatography (TLC) of urine, there are conflicting reports of such claims (Fig. 23.1).[18,19] Additionally, the reported frequency of bisacodyl-induced diarrhea among patients with cryptogenic diarrhea under the care of a general practitioner is about 2.4%.[42] At this frequency, the vast majority of positive urine tests for bisacodyl would show false-positive results. Aside from analytical mistakes in the testing procedure, part of the problem with TLC may be that the results are reported as "none detected" or "positive," rather than quantitatively in terms of weight per liter or weight per day. Theoretically, miniscule quantities of contamination (too small to induce diarrhea) from ingested substances or from endogenous metabolism might produce false-positive results. Any positive result obtained on a patient with osmotic diarrhea would almost surely be falsely positive because bisacodyl and senna do not cause osmotic diarrhea. Based on all information available to us in the 2020s, we believe that these tests should not be ordered unless there is judged to be a high likelihood of factitious disease (see Boxes 23.1 and 23.2) and unless stool analysis has revealed secretory diarrhea.

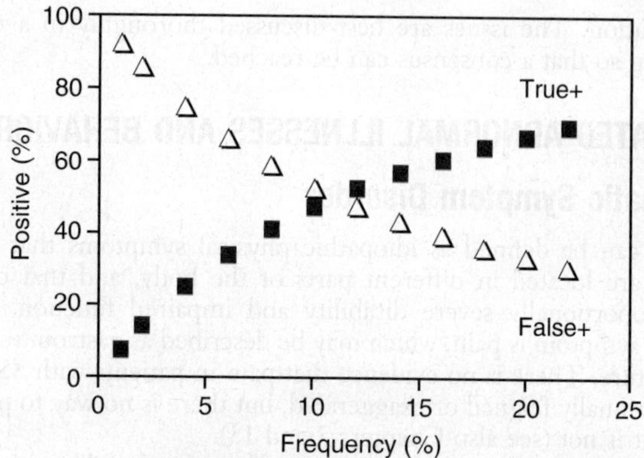

Fig. 23.1 Correlation between the likelihood that a positive urine test for bisacodyl by thin-layer chromatography is a true- or a false-positive result and the frequency of bisacodyl-induced diarrhea in tested populations.

In patients with chronic idiopathic diarrhea, analysis of fecal fluid for monovalent electrolytes (Na, K, and Cl), pH, and osmolality can identify the presence of osmotic or secretory diarrhea (see Chapter 17). When osmotic diarrhea is induced by an ingestion of poorly absorbed solutes such as magnesium, sulfate, phosphate, or polyethylene glycol, chemical methods can quantitatively determine their percent content in fecal fluid.[43] The effects of these osmotic laxatives have been studied in normal subjects, and the fecal fluid concentrations from normal people and from normal people with laxative-induced diarrhea have been established for each solute. When this method of testing was evaluated in 158 patients with chronic idiopathic diarrhea, 8% (12 of 158) were found to have diarrheagenic concentrations of one of these osmotic laxatives in their fecal fluids.[43] (Lactulose also causes osmotic diarrhea, but by fecal analysis it would be indistinguishable from dietary causes of carbohydrate malabsorption.) These results indicate that early use of simple chemical tests in patients with idiopathic chronic osmotic diarrhea would markedly reduce the utilization of expensive and sometimes dangerous diagnostic procedures that have no ability to detect laxative ingestion.

Finding a true positive test for laxative ingestion in a patient with idiopathic chronic diarrhea is not conclusive evidence for surreptitious laxative ingestion or factitious diarrhea, because the patient may have been unknowingly ingesting the laxative in a medication (magnesium in an antacid, for example) or in a health supplement (which may contain anthraquinones). An empathetic gathering of patient history and medication administration must occur prior to diagnosis of FD.[44]

A patient with factitious disorder can mimic diarrheal consistency and volume of stool by diluting stool with water. This dilution can be carried out in vitro after a stool specimen is collected or in vivo by giving oneself a tap water enema and then collecting the rectal effluent. This type of factitious diarrhea can be identified by measuring osmolality of the fecal fluid supernatant and finding values far below the average physiological level of 290 mOsm/kg. This dilutional form of factitious diarrhea would not be detectable by measurement of fecal fluid osmolality if stools were diluted with normal saline.

As discussed in Chapter 130, pseudomelanosis coli develops in more than 70% of patients who use anthraquinones laxatives (e.g., cascara, aloe, and senna), on average within 9 months of regular intake of these products. However, this finding may also be seen in patients with chronic constipation and inflammatory bowel disease, so care should be taken prior to settling on a diagnosis of factitious diarrhea.[45] The effect is said to be reversible within 1 year of discontinuing the intake of an anthraquinone. Finding this pigment (lipofuscin) at colonoscopy or in biopsy specimens is suggestive, but not diagnostic, of recent anthraquinone ingestion. Other apparent causes for this condition include ingestion of an NSAID.[46]

Concealed Vomiting

In the early part of the 20th century, gastroenterologists and surgeons recognized that persistent vomiting due to gastric outlet obstruction could lead to severe toxemia, with volume depletion, hypochloremic metabolic alkalosis, hypokalemia, uremia, and tetany.[47] Based on subsequent clinical research, it was discovered that the pathogenesis of vomiting-induced electrolyte abnormalities is as follows: vomiting → loss of HCl and volume contraction → metabolic alkalosis → increased renal excretion of bicarbonate → increased renal excretion of potassium and sodium → hypokalemia, and more volume contraction. The alkalosis also causes potassium to move from extracellular fluid into the intracellular spaces, further reducing the serum potassium concentration.

When patients surreptitiously self-induce vomiting and then present to physicians seeking a cause for their vomiting, identifying the factitious nature of the vomiting can be difficult. When patients conceal episodes of induced vomiting and present with hypochloremic alkalosis and hypokalemia, they will be subjected to diagnostic studies that suggest rare diseases with similar features (such as Bartter syndrome). A useful clue to concealed vomiting as the cause of hypokalemia and alkalosis is an extremely low rate of urine chloride excretion, even when a patient is ingesting a diet containing a normal amount of chloride; this is not present in Bartter syndrome or surreptitious thiazide ingestion.[48] Due to the highly stigmatizing nature of disordered gut-brain interactions such as chronic nausea vomiting syndrome or cyclic vomiting syndrome, it is critical to consider these conditions prior to believing a patient has factitious vomiting.

Factitious Anemia and Factitious GI Blood Loss

Factitious anemia should be considered when there are repeated instances of unexplained sharp drops in the hemoglobin concentration, with appropriate but unsustainable responses to blood transfusions.[49] Care must be taken to distinguish factitious anemia from vascular conditions that can present similarly (such as periodic assessments of complete blood count in people with intermittently bleeding angioectasias, arteriovenous malformations, or Dieulafoy lesions). Patients with FD usually use phlebotomy and/or placed IV lines for self-bloodletting to create factitious anemia. They may also ingest collected blood by mouth to mimic hematemesis and melena or add the blood to urine or stool samples to create hematuria and hematochezia, respectively. There have been reports in the literature of bleeding intentionally caused through use of knitting needles, razors, peripherally inserted central catheters, and ingested blood during intentional venesection.[50–53] If a patient withdraws blood after being injected with isotope-labeled red blood cells and then drinks the blood or injects it into the abdominal cavity, bleeding scans can be abnormal and may lead to inappropriate treatment.[54,55]

Factitious Cancer

People with factitious disorder can enter a new institution seeking to continue treatment for their "cancer" and claim that they were referred to by doctors in another city or state. They provide a convincing history, have scars compatible with previous surgical treatment for cancer, and often provide a (false) pathology report. They claim that their other medical records will be sent shortly. Alternatively, or in addition, some patients will gain entrance into cancer support groups. One such patient participated in classes on death and dying. The class was so moved by her courage that it raised money for her to ride in a hot air balloon—one of her "final wishes."[56]

Several motivations apparently cause people to feign cancer. One is secondary material gain (malingering, perhaps to obtain opiate analgesia). Another is an unconscious need to deceive the medical system and be subjected to diagnostic tests and therapeutic procedures. Some may seek the social status associated with the diagnosis of cancer (e.g., being lauded as a "survivor") and take advantage of displays of sympathy and gifts from friends, co-workers, and others.[56] Some apparently feign cancer because someone they loved had cancer. One woman later stated that she was hoping to die as a result of immunosuppression.[57] Several of these motives may be present simultaneously and can make such factitious behaviors distinct from malingering ones. Whatever the motivation, the onset of factitious cancer seems to commonly occur after rejection by a loved one or after some other type of loss. Loneliness and isolation seem to be the precipitating factors in many people who begin to behave in this manner.

Medical records would almost always be required before a patient is given chemotherapy for cancer or is subjected to cancer surgery. Patients may steal and alter authentic records from other patients' medical charts and pass them off as their own. In one case, a patient scanned and modified records, making it even more difficult to recognize their fraudulence.[57] Gaining access to medical terminology, symptomatology, pathology reports, and diagnostic and treatment plans would be easiest for a hospital employee, probably explaining why the best and most complete forgeries are from people who work in hospitals. Despite oncologists' efforts to review medical records carefully, fabrications have been good enough in some cases to allow people with FD to obtain chemotherapy.[57]

The diagnosis of factitious cancer is usually made by the detection of inconsistencies in the medical history, evidence of fabrication of medical record, health insurance documentation, or fortuitous doubts about the patient's story raised by doctors. Claims of prolonged survival with a usually lethal cancer have helped reveal factitious cancer in some cases.

Lessons From Case Reports

Table 23.2 lists brief summaries of selected case reports to further illustrate the wide variety of factitious diseases that can occur in the practice of gastroenterology. They also demonstrate the potential pitfalls, including simply deferring to psychiatry colleagues (Case Study 23.4). They also emphasize the importance of being an astute gastroenterologist who generates a comprehensive differential diagnosis that includes factitious disorder as a potential explanation for an elusive diagnosis (provided that thoughtful evaluations have been performed and that implicit bias that may result in premature narrowing of the differential diagnoses has been recognized).

TABLE 23.2 Cases of Factitious Disorder (FD) in Gastroenterology

Presentation	Comments
Fistulizing Crohn's disease with stomal bleeding[60]	Histology revealed only nonspecific abnormalities, and inflammation was more severe in the serosa than in the mucosa, suggesting extrinsic trauma. The disease was caused by self-inflected wounds using a needle inserted through the vagina, rectum, and stoma
Refractory celiac disease[61]	The patient had celiac disease that initially responded to a gluten-free diet. She later developed severe diarrhea, believed to be due to refractory celiac disease. The diagnosis was established by fecal analysis, which revealed that the diarrhea was caused by ingestion of milk of magnesia. Had the correct diagnosis of FD not been established, the patient would have received immunosuppressive therapy
Porphyria[62,63]	A patient with abdominal pain and red urine. Freshly passed urine was red, but in porphyria, freshly passed urine is normal in color and turns red or brown when exposed to daylight. A room search revealed a drug containing rubazonic acid, a red-in-acid solution A patient with a complaint of various neuromuscular symptoms who self-reported porphyria. Discovered to have presented to multiple hospitals with different ailments
Death from liver failure[64]	Nosebleeds, anemia, alopecia, hepatomegaly, and elevated liver biochemical test levels in a 29-year-old woman. A liver biopsy done about 18 months before her death revealed changes suggestive of hypervitaminosis A (including fat-laden stellate cells). Although her serum vitamin A level was high, she denied excess intake of vitamin A. Just before death, she admitted that she had surreptitiously ingested grossly excessive amounts of cod liver oil
Intestinal pseudo-obstruction[65]	An 18-year-old man had GI and urinary findings that led to a diagnosis of intestinal pseudo-obstruction. He became bedridden and required TPN and repeated daily bladder catheterizations, but physiologic testing revealed no evidence of a GI or bladder motility disorder. The patient's mother was suspected of factitous disorder imposed on another (previously called Munchausen syndrome by proxy). The patient's stool and urine tested positive for emetine, a component of ipecac. The patient was completely well after 1 week of court-ordered separation from his mother
Bartter syndrome[39,40]	This patient developed episodic paralysis associated with hypokalemia and metabolic alkalosis. Plasma concentrations of renin and aldosterone were high, and a renal biopsy specimen revealed hyperplasia of the juxtaglomerular apparatus, yielding a diagnosis of Bartter syndrome.[39] Subsequently, it was discovered that the patient was surreptitiously ingesting phenolphthalein but had been hiding the fact that she had diarrhea[40]
Recurrent wound infection in a woman who had recently donated part of her liver for transplantation[66]	Five weeks after liver donation, a postsurgical wound infection with septic shock developed. The donor's hospital bill was huge and was sent to the recipient's insurance, thereby threatening the recipient's lifetime benefits. FD was suspected because antibiotic-sensitive polymicrobial bacteria were cultured. Past medical records revealed evidence of previous FD
Induced vomiting to create treatment-resistant hypertension[67]	A 25-year-old woman with hypertension used self-induced vomiting to increase her blood pressure by eliminating the effect of her antihypertensive medication. Her motive was to achieve a prolonged hospitalization to avoid a stressful home environment
Fatal nonthrombotic pulmonary embolization[68]	A 32-year-old woman was on TPN following complications of a Roux-en-Y gastric bypass and pancreatic auto-islet cell transplantation. She presented with recurrent episodes of bacteremia with atypical pathogens. Sudden cardiac arrest with right-sided heart failure resulted in her death. The cause of death at autopsy was attributed to complications from pulmonary microcrystalline cellulose emboli, which likely resulted from self-injection of oral medication through a central line
Recurrent pancytopenia in a woman with Crohn's disease[69]	A 50-year-old woman with a history of fistulizing Crohn's disease was previously treated with 6-mercaptopurine (6-MP) but was told to stop the medication due to drug-induced pancreatitis. 2 Months later she presented with recurrent pancytopenia. Results of a repeat bone marrow biopsy were nondiagnostic. Thiopurine metabolite testing showed that 6-MP was present with levels that predispose to toxicity even though 6-MP had been discontinued several months earlier. The patient denied refilling the old prescription and taking the 6-MP, but her community pharmacist confirmed that a refill of 6-MP had been dispensed recently. Pancytopenia was attributed to surreptitious ingestion of 6-MP

CASE STUDY 23.4 A 31-YEAR-OLD MAN WITH ABDOMINAL PAIN

This patient was admitted to our hospital because of severe abdominal pain during the previous 6 weeks.[73] The pain was mid-abdominal in location and was present mainly after meals. He had lost about 12 pounds in weight. Physical examination revealed no signs of peritonitis. The results of EGD, colonoscopy, CT, US, and ERCP were normal except for a small benign gastric ulcer. His pain did not respond to potent antiulcer medications, so the ulcer was not believed to be the cause of his pain.

A psychiatrist examined the patient and noted major depression, with somatization, and an amphetamine was prescribed. The medication seemed to help initially, and the patient was feeling better the next day; however, on the following day, he was again having severe abdominal pain after meals. His abdomen was soft and without tenderness, and bowel sounds were normal. Demerol was given. Progress notes stated, "Pattern of complaints and his response to antidepressant are indicative of psychogenic pain problem coupled with dependent/oppositional personality disorder," and "Patient continues to be quite regressed. He makes the most secondary gain of each and every somatic concern."

On the 10th day of hospitalization, the patient was lying in the fetal position with constant severe abdominal pain. Periumbilical tenderness was present, but there was no rebound tenderness. A progress note said, "His mom and friends hovering over him. He does seem depressed, but the pain syndrome seems psychogenic in origin (not a depressive equivalent) and secondary to his dependent narcissistic personality structure." Two days later a feeding tube was placed, and the patient was transferred to a psychiatry unit, where later he was found unresponsive. An abdominal film showed air under the diagram. The patient died a short time later. An autopsy revealed that patient's superior mesenteric artery was completely occluded by atherosclerosis, which led to necrosis and perforation of his small intestine.[73]

23

PITFALLS IN THE DIAGNOSIS AND MANAGEMENT OF ABNORMAL ILLNESS BEHAVIOR

In Case Study 23.4, no organic cause was found to explain his severe abdominal pain and weight loss. This led a gastroenterologist to suspect a psychiatric explanation for the patient's symptoms, and a psychiatrist was consulted. After taking a psychiatric history and observing the patient, the psychiatrist made a diagnosis of "psychogenic pain," a term that implies that pain is caused primarily and maintained by emotional distress. This diagnosis was fully accepted by the gastroenterologist, and the patient was transferred to a psychiatric unit of the hospital.

The thought processes were erroneous for two reasons. First, physical (or organic) disease cannot be excluded with certainty, and failure to discover an organic disease to explain severe abdominal pain did not constitute evidence for a psychiatric etiology in this case. Moreover, there were no clues suggesting positive evidence for abnormal illness behavior. Although consulting a psychiatrist to help manage any associated depression may have been wise, the gastroenterologist should have known that a psychiatrist cannot accurately diagnose emotional distress as the primary cause of severe abdominal pain by performing a psychiatric evaluation. Second, the psychiatrist should have known that secondary gain is part of normal illness behavior, and he should have recognized that there was no supporting evidence for abnormal illness behavior. He should not have made a diagnosis of "psychogenic pain," which closed the door to a further search for a medical cause of this patient's severe abdominal pain, which was classic abdominal angina.[58]

In this regard, the advice of Nadelson rings true: "The psychiatrist must encourage the referring physician to confront the patient on the basis of clinical evidence, recognizing that the psychiatrist's own diagnostic acumen may fall short of divining the hidden truth."[59] According to our interpretation of this advice, a diagnosis of abnormal illness behavior as the primary cause of physical symptoms should be based on clinical evidence (such as that discussed in Boxes 23.1 and 23.2), rather than on information gained from a psychiatric evaluation. In this case, the negative clinical evidence could have been compiled by either the gastroenterologist or the psychiatrist. Unfortunately, no one did it.

CONCLUSION

Gastroenterologists may be called on to care for patients with FD. The desire to make the correct diagnosis (as to spare the patient unnecessary diagnostic testing and treatment) of FD must be balanced with the role that physicians have played in ignoring the complaints of patients due to implicit bias (particularly female patients). Multidisciplinary efforts and careful review of the patient history are key to making these diagnoses when gastrointestinal complaints are reported.

Acknowledgment

The authors thank Marc D. Feldman, MD, John S. Fordtran, and Anahit A. Zeynalyan for their contributions to prior chapters.

Full references for this chapter can be found at https://ebooks.health.elsevier.com.

PART IV Processes Involving Multiple Organs

24 Oral Diseases and Oral Manifestations of Gastrointestinal and Liver Diseases

Ginat W. Mirowski, Callie B. Burgin

IN THIS CHAPTER

LIP DISORDERS

The lips are paired structures that are highly visible in the mid face and function to facilitate mastication, speech, and numerous habits. The lips are symmetric from left to right and extend from the base of the nose to the upper chin. The philtrum extends from columella to slightly keratinized vermilion. The commissure (angle) is the junction of upper and lower lip. Separating the cutaneous aspect of the lip from the vermilion aspect is a slightly raised border called the vermilion border.

Cheilitis

Cheilitis, inflammation of the lips, may include the vermilion, the mucosa, and the perioral skin, including the oral commissures. Angular cheilitis (angular cheilosis and angular stomatitis) presents as painful edema and fissures due to inflammation and irritation at the oral commissures. Treatment involves targeting or discontinuing the underlying cause of the inflammation. Etiologies include trauma; primary dermatologic disorders, including contact mucositis, lichen planus, psoriasis, lupus erythematosus, and erythema multiforme; disorders of the minor salivary glands; and drug reactions. Vitamin B_2 (riboflavin) or iron deficiency may cause cheilitis. Infections may cause irritation to the lips. Oral habits, like lip licking and lip biting, may also predispose patients to angular cheilitis.[1]

Exfoliative cheilitis (chronic chapped lips) is a chronic inflammation of the vermilion. Patients complain of dryness or itching in the setting of a wide variety of disorders (e.g., atopic dermatitis, psoriasis, chronic irritation, and allergies). Topical glucocorticoids or calcineurin inhibitors may be effective for symptomatic treatment.

Contact cheilitis, precipitated by an irritant or allergic reaction, presents with lip and perioral edema, erythema, and scale. Fragrances, lanolin, dodecyl gallate, and benzoyl peroxide in personal hygiene products and cosmetics, foods, personal habits, and topical medications (e.g., gentamicin) have been indicted as etiologies of allergic contact cheilitis. The most common allergens include fragrance mix and balsam of Peru.[2]

Granulomatous cheilitis is a rare condition that presents with recurrent lip swelling associated with chronic enlargement and firmness of the lips.[3] Lip biopsy shows noncaseating granulomas.

Granulomatous cheilitis is associated with Crohn disease and tuberculosis and is a component of Melkersson-Rosenthal syndrome (a rare condition characterized by fissured tongue and granulomatous cheilitis, with or without facial palsy and migraine).[3–5]

Lip Neoplasms

Actinic cheilitis (solar cheilosis) is a premalignant epithelial dysplasia linked to chronic solar or ultraviolet radiation. Fair-skinned individuals, especially those with occupational exposure, older age individuals, and those with a history of solid organ transplant (with subsequent immunosuppression), have a higher risk of developing actinic cheilitis.[6,7] While the presentation is variable, loss of the vermilion border, with diffuse erythema, patchy whiteness, dryness, and vermilion scaling, are the most typical symptoms. Lip biopsies from multiple sites should be taken, as location and degree of lip dysplasia cannot be predicted by clinical presentation alone. While there are currently no Food and Drug Administration (FDA)-approved therapies for this disorder, treatment of the entire lip is indicated, as actinic cheilitis may progress to squamous cell carcinoma (SCC).

Proliferative Verrucous Leukoplakia

Proliferative verrucous leukoplakia (PVL) is a rare variant of oral leukoplakia with high malignant potential that typically occurs on the oral mucosa that has been reported on the lip.[8]

SCC is the most common oral neoplasm and most commonly affects the lower lip.[9] Fair-skinned Caucasian men, and HPV 16 or 18 infection may predispose patients to malignant transformation of lip epithelial cells. Because SCC is a high-risk source of metastases, the diagnosis should include staging at initial evaluation. Treatment includes surgical excision and radiation therapy.

SALIVARY DISORDERS

Oral health is predicated on adequate saliva. Saliva helps remove food debris from tooth and mucosal surfaces, thus cleansing the mouth and clearing the esophagus. Saliva functions to lubricate the mucosa that helps with speech, chewing, taste, and swallowing. In addition, it provides the essential chemical milieu for function and protection of the oral mucosa and teeth, including antimicrobial and immunologic roles (specifically IgA), and neutralizes acids in the mouth and helps with remineralization.[10–12]

Xerostomia

Xerostomia (dry mouth) and burning sensation that occur concurrently are common complaints that result from atrophy or destruction of the salivary glands. Polypharmacy (>5 medication) is the etiology in 40% cases (Tables 24.1 and 24.2).

Xerostomia can predispose to oral candidiasis.[13] It is not surprising that as patients age, the increasing number of medications and associated predisposing conditions may further contribute to the development of xerostomia.[14]

Beyond physical exam, sialometric tests measuring salivary flow rate or stimulated salivary production and salivary gland scintigraphy may be helpful in the diagnosis and therapeutic management of xerostomia.[15] Sucking and chewing gum or sugarless mints helps stimulate increased salivary flow, which, in turn, assists in debris removal without increasing the risk of developing caries. Patients with xerostomia should avoid sweets and acidic foods or beverages to limit caries induction. Patients should be encouraged to sip water and suck ice chips frequently.

TABLE 24.1 Etiologies of Xerostomia[13,14]

Neuropathic	Diabetes I polyuria, dehydration, autonomic dehydration) Parkinson's disease
Autoimmune	Thyroid disease Sjögren syndrome Rheumatoid arthritis Systemic lupus erythematosus Primary biliary cirrhosis Celiac disease Scleroderma
Inflammatory/infectious illnesses	HIV EBV CMV HTLV-1 Periodontal disease (linear gingival erythema, acute necrotizing ulcerative gingivostomatitis) Actinomyces Herpes viruses (EBV, CMV) Hepatitis C Tuberculosis
Lifestyle factors	Mouth breathing, heavy snoring Alcohol use Smoking (tobacco, marijuana) Caffeinated beverages
Genetic disorders	Ectodermal dysplasia
Granulomatous or infiltrative reactions	Sarcoidosis Hemochromatosis Amyloidosis
Dehydration	
ESRD	

TABLE 24.2 Medication Associated with Xerostomia (partial list)

Anticholinergics	Atropine Ipratropium	Omeprazole Scopolamine
Antidepressants	Amitriptyline Bupropion Citalopram	Fluoxetine Paroxetine Sertraline
Antihistamines	Chlorpheniramine Diphenhydramine Fexofenadine	Hydroxyzine Loratadine
Antihypertensives	Chlorothiazide Clonidine Furosemide Methyldopa	Metoprolol Nifedipine Reserpine Terazosin
Antipsychotics	Haloperidol	Phenothiazine
Decongestants	Phenylephrine	
Sedatives and anxiolytics	Benzodiazepines Gabapentin	Opioids

Preparations containing 1% sodium carboxymethylcellulose may be used to moisten the oral cavity. Salivary stimulants, such as cevimeline (Evoxac), 30 mg three times daily, or pilocarpine (Salagen), 5 mg three to four times daily, are effective sialogogues.[16] Preventative pilocarpine use during radiation therapy may lessen the grade of radiation-induced xerostomia.[17] Acupuncture, intraoral electrostimulation, and hyperbaric oxygen or amifostine for radiation therapy patients are emerging as further management tools.[15]

Sjögren Syndrome

Sjögren syndrome is a chronic autoimmune disease classified by the triad of xerostomia, keratoconjunctivitis sicca (dry eyes), and arthritis, but other systemic effects (extraglandular) are recognized (see Chapter 35).[16] Over 4 million Americans are affected, with women outnumbering men by 9:1. Sjögren syndrome is characterized as *primary* in the absence of other disorders or *secondary* when other systemic diseases are present. Oral manifestations of Sjögren syndrome are due to destruction of the salivary glands by a lymphocytic infiltrate that results in diminished or absent saliva, resulting in difficulty chewing, odynophagia, diminished taste and smell, mucosal erythema, increased incidence of dental caries, oral candidiasis, and salivary gland calculi. Marginal zone lymphoma, a non-Hodgkin lymphoma, is the most serious complication of Sjögren syndrome. Diagnosis is usually made based on clinical presentation, though laboratory demonstration of associated anti-SSA, anti-SSB antibodies, and/or rheumatoid factor, the Schirmer test for oral and ocular dryness, or sialometry may be useful.[16] Salivary gland scintigraphy is used to objectively assess the severity and extent of salivary gland involvement and may be helpful in the diagnosis and therapeutic management of Sjögren.[18] Treatment strategies for general xerostomia are also helpful in the management of Sjögren-induced xerostomia.

TONGUE DISORDERS

The tongue, a muscular organ in the mouth, is critical for gustation, mastication, swallowing, and speech. The dorsal surface of the tongue is characterized by extensive 1- to 2-mm filiform or keratotic papillae and far fewer erythematous 1-mm smooth, domed papules. In individuals of color, benign pigmentation of individual fungiform papillae may be present.

Glossitis, Glossodynia, and Oral Dysesthesia

Glossitis, inflammation, and irritation of the tongue occur in a heterogeneous group of disorders (Box 24.1). Patients may complain of lingual pain (glossodynia) or a burning sensation (glossopyrosis). Loss of filiform papillae results in a spectrum of changes, from patchy erythema with or without erosive changes to a completely smooth, atrophic, erythematous surface (Fig. 24.1). Median rhomboid glossitis manifests as an asymptomatic, well-defined erythematous patch in the mid-posterior dorsum of the tongue. *Candida* infection, predominantly with *Candida albicans*,[19] may present with a loss of the filiform papillae in such a pattern.

Glossodynia is defined as pain in the absence of clinical or histologic evidence of inflammation or irritation and may be associated with anxiety or depression. Glossodynia occurs commonly in postmenopausal women, but hormonal replacement therapy is of little value.[19] Serologic evaluation for hypomagnesemia, vitamin B_2, vitamin B_9 (folic acid), or vitamin B_{12} (cobalamin) deficiency, as well as a complete medication history, may occasionally yield a correctable cause.[21] Box 24.2 may be used as a guide to considerations in the treatment of both primary and secondary causes of glossodynia. Olanzapine may be a treatment option.[22]

Oral dysesthesia, also known as burning mouth, is characterized by a burning sensation in the tongue and oral cavity and most commonly affects postmenopausal women.[23] Burning mouth syndrome (BMS) is also characterized by oral dysesthesia and is a diagnosis of exclusion. The pathophysiology of this condition is incompletely understood. Reports have suggested peripheral small fiber neuropathy, sleep disturbances, circadian rhythm abnormalities, mood disorders, or hormone-mediated changes in salivary composition may contribute to symptoms.[24,25] Vitamin B_3 (niacin), vitamin B_{12} (cobalamin), or zinc deficiency, diabetes mellitus, hyperthyroidism, and Sjögren syndrome have also been linked to oral dysesthesia.[21,26] Oral dysesthesia is not specifically associated with higher rate of *Candida* infection,[27] but burning symptoms have been correlated to the presence of *Helicobacter pylori* in the oral cavity.[25] Treatment is difficult, and response is

BOX 24.1 Primary and Secondary Glossodynia and Associated Etiologies

Primary (idiopathic)	Normal-appearing tongue with no other etiology found by taking history or physical examination
Secondary oral disorders	Infection (candidiasis, fusospirochetal, and viral) Allergic/contact hypersensitivity (dentures, amalgams, additives) Mechanical trauma (abnormal tongue habit, dentures) Xerostomia Geographic tongue Fissured tongue Vesiculobullous disease Temporomandibular dysfunction Referred pain from teeth or tonsils
Systemic disorders	Anemia (iron deficiency, pernicious) Nutritional deficiency (folate, zinc, vitamin B_{12}, B-complex vitamins) Diabetes mellitus GERD Sjögren syndrome Hypothyroidism AIDS Menopause (controversial)
Drug related	Antibiotics, psychiatric medications, chemotherapy agents, others Any medication that can cause xerostomia
Neurologic	Peripheral neuropathy Diabetic neuropathy Trigeminal neuralgia Acoustic neuroma
Psychiatric	Depression Anxiety Cancerophobia Somatoform disorder Obsessive-compulsive disorder

Modified from Gick CL, Mirowski GW, Kennedy JS, et al. Treatment of glossodynia with olanzapine. *J Am Acad Dermatol*. 2004;51:463–465.

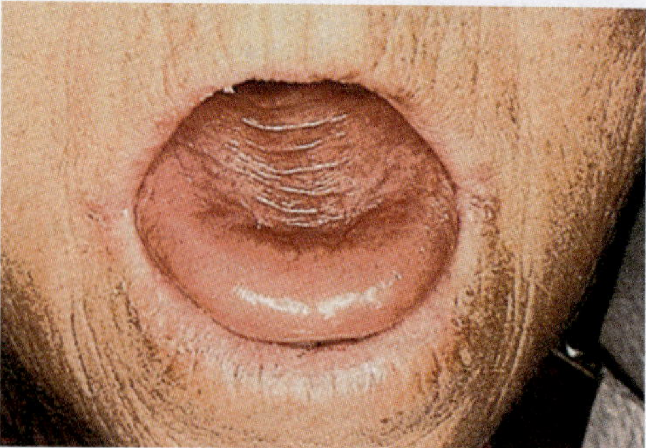

Fig. 24.1 Glossitis in a patient with diabetes mellitus and malabsorption. The tongue is smooth (depilated) and red. Angular cheilitis is also present.

BOX 24.2 Treatments Employed in Glossodynia and Glossopyrosis

Eliminate identifiable etiologies of glossodynia (see Box 24.1)
Avoid irritants, including foods and dental appliances
Nutritional and vitamin replacement
Topical antifungals
Topical glucocorticoids
Viscous lidocaine (provides temporary relief)
Sialogogues (e.g., cevimeline, pilocarpine)
Benzodiazepines (e.g., clonazepam, chlordiazepoxide)
Tricyclic antidepressants (e.g., amitriptyline, doxepin)
Antipsychotics (e.g., olanzapine)

Modified from Gick CL, Mirowski GW, Kennedy JS, et al. Treatment of glossodynia with olanzapine. *J Am Acad Dermatol*. 2004;51:463–465.

often incomplete or temporary. Any underlying nutritional deficiency should be corrected, and systemic disease management should be optimized. Treatment options may include topical or systemic clonazepam, tricyclic antidepressants, gabapentin, capsaicin, alpha-lipoic acid, or cognitive-behavioral therapy.[23,28,29] Large, randomized clinical trials are lacking, and treatment should be individualized to the patient.

Hypogeusia and Dysgeusia

Hypogeusia (diminished sense of taste) and dysgeusia (distortion of normal taste) are other oral complaints and are sometimes associated with glossitis. Hypogeusia and dysgeusia have been attributed to various neurologic, nutritional, and metabolic disorders, including eosinophilic granulomatosis with polyangiitis, several medications, and aging.[30–32] Hypogeusia has even been noted in otherwise healthy children.[33] Tobacco smokers, denture wearers, and patients with anxiety or other psychiatric disorders commonly complain of hypogeusia and dysgeusia. Radiation therapy to the head and neck may result in altered taste. Infection with severe acute respiratory SARS-CoV-2 has been associated with ageusia.[34] The mechanisms whereby taste buds and their receptors are affected by aging, medications, or disease states are not well understood; taste bud changes could be associated with changes in the expression of taste-associated genes (see Chapter 4).[35] Therapy is empirical and includes identifying and correcting any associated condition. Patients may be treated with zinc supplementation, a low-dose anxiolytic, or an antidepressant medication such as SSRIs. Paradoxically, tricyclic antidepressant medications block responses to a wide range of taste stimuli and may contribute to clinical reports of hypogeusia and dysgeusia.[20,36]

Geographic Tongue

Geographic tongue (benign migratory glossitis, erythema migrans, and glossitis areata migrans) is benign and has no known associations with malignancy. Geographic tongue is characterized by loss of filiform papillae, forming irregular patchy configurations that resemble geographic landmarks on a map. The role of Th17 is highly suggestive.[37] Geographic tongue has been linked to changes in lingual microbiota ecology[38] or as an oral symptom in patients with psoriasis associated with fissured tongue.[39] Patients may complain of pain or difficulty in eating acidic, spicy, or salty foods. Recurrent episodes are common. Histologically, spongiosus and neutrophilic microabscesses are found in the epithelium, with no evidence of candidiasis. Treatment consists of tacrolimus swish and spit bid,[40] topical anesthetics, magnesium and aluminum hydroxide (Maalox) protective coatings, and topical glucocorticoids, along with control of the underlying cutaneous psoriasis if present. Benzocaine (Orabase) has been associated with a rare risk of methemoglobinemia and is no longer recommended by the US FDA for treatment of this disorder.

Fissured Tongue

Fissured tongue (lingua plicata, furrowed tongue, and scrotal tongue) presents as a benign central groove on the dorsal tongue. It is commonly seen with aging but is also associated with geographic tongue, Sjögren syndrome, and Melkersson-Rosenthal syndrome (characterized by fissured tongue, granulomatous cheilitis, and migraines, with or without facial palsy). Food and bacteria may get trapped in the fissures and lead to halitosis and inflammation. Symptomatic relief may be obtained by gently brushing the tongue after meals and before sleeping.[41]

Black Hairy Tongue

In black hairy tongue, the dorsal surface of the tongue appears yellow, green, brown, or black due to exogenous pigment trapped within the elongated keratin strands of filiform papillae. This benign condition is seen most commonly in chronic smokers and often follows a course of systemic antibiotics, the use of hydrogen peroxide, or drinking coffee or tea.[42] Elderly individuals are more prone to hairy tongue.[43] Off-label treatment consists of 25% podophyllum or topical tretinoin (Retin-A) gel.[42] Chronic debridement with a tongue scraper may also be helpful.

Strawberry Tongue

Strawberry tongue is a form of glossitis characterized by swollen, enlarged fungiform papillae on the surface of the tongue. These enlarged fungiform papillae are most commonly associated with scarlet fever and Kawasaki disease. Scarlet fever, caused by an infection with *Streptococcus pyogenes* (Group A *Streptococcus*), often presents with strawberry tongue in addition to pharyngitis, a sandpaper-like rash, and circumoral pallor. Treatment is with penicillin.

Kawasaki disease, or mucocutaneous lymph node syndrome, is a medium- to large-vessel vasculitis (see Chapter 35). It generally affects children younger than 5 years and has replaced rheumatic fever as the primary cause of childhood heart disease in the United States. It is more common in East Asia and in children of East Asian descent. Diagnostic criteria include at least five of the following: (1) acute cervical adenopathy; (2) peripheral extremity edema, erythema, or desquamation; (3) bilateral painless conjunctival injection; (4) a polymorphous exanthem; and (5) oral mucosal erythema or strawberry tongue. Kawasaki disease also can cause colonic edema. IVIG and oral aspirin are the usual treatment.

Atrophic Tongue

Atrophic tongue (atrophic glossitis) is characterized by the absence of filiform papillae and glossodynia. It is implicated in many nutritional deficiencies, such as filiform papillae atrophy as a result of protein-calorie malnutrition: long-standing iron-deficiency anemia, vitamin B_2 (often with a magenta hue), vitamin B_6 (pyridoxine), vitamin B_9 (with erythema and swelling of the tongue), and vitamin B_{12}.[21] Atrophic glossitis is also seen in Plummer-Vinson syndrome (characterized by a triad of iron-deficiency anemia, upper esophageal webbing, and atrophic glossitis) and is linked to conditions that cause xerostomia.[44] It is also an oral manifestation of *Candida* infections, primarily from *C. albicans*, though *Candida glabrata*, *Candida tropicalis*, *Candida krusei*, and *Candida parapsilosis* have been cultured from *Candida* atrophic glossitis patients.[19,45] Advanced age and malnutrition, associated with decreased tongue thickness, can also predispose patients to the development of atrophic glossitis.[44] Treatment involves targeting the underlying nutritional deficiency or condition, and a soft, bland diet may be recommended for symptomatic relief.

Hypertrophic Tongue

Hypertrophic tongue (macroglossia) is an enlargement of the tongue beyond the mouth and jaws that can impair mastication, swallowing, and speech. It is associated with a number of disorders, including congenital hypothyroidism, acromegaly, Down syndrome, Beckwith-Wiedemann syndrome, and primary amyloidosis.[46]

Congenital hypothyroidism can manifest with a hypertrophic tongue and jaundice and progresses to intellectual disability if left untreated. Acromegaly results from the excess production of growth hormone, such as from a pituitary adenoma, and may present with a hypertrophic, fissured tongue in addition to oral soft tissue hypertrophy and metabolic changes that progress to bone enlargement and diabetes mellitus.[47] Beckwith-Wiedemann syndrome is a congenital overgrowth syndrome characterized by a hypertrophic tongue and is associated with omphalocele and organomegaly.

While treatment for macroglossia depends on treating the underlying disorder, surgical management of severe macroglossia includes anterior wedge or keyhole resection of the tongue.[48]

Leukoplakia

Hairy leukoplakia (oral hairy leukoplakia, HL) is an asymptomatic infection with Epstein-Barr virus and appears as corrugated white plaques on the lateral borders and dorsal surface of the tongue (Fig. 24.2). Although HL occurs predominantly in patients with HIV infection, renal and other organ transplant recipients are susceptible as well (see Chapter 34). The presence of HL in an HIV-infected person has a poor prognostic implication. Of 198 cases of HL, the median time to onset of AIDS was 24 months, and the median time to death (in the absence of ART) was 41 months.[49] Candidiasis, which coexists in about half of cases of HL, must be treated as well. A prudent first step in management is the administration of anticandidal therapy. Because HL is usually asymptomatic, off-label use of oral acyclovir, topical retinoic acid, and podophyllum is optional.[41] When such treatment is discontinued, however, HL usually returns. Introduction of ART has decreased the incidence of HL.

Other white mucosal lesions, such as oral leukoplakia (Fig. 24.3), can resemble HL lesions; biopsy confirmation and serologic testing for HIV are indicated if the diagnosis of HL is considered.

Oral leukoplakia is a clinical white plaque in the oral cavity that is not associated with an identifiable cause. A diagnosis is made by excluding other causes of a white oral lesion, including *Candida* infection and HL. These conditions should be ruled out and eliminated before diagnosing a patient with oral leukoplakia. Oral leukoplakia is most commonly seen in older individuals, with 73%–81% of affected patients having a history of tobacco use.[50] While oral leukoplakia itself is usually asymptomatic, this lesion is clinically relevant because of its association with oral SCC.[50] If the elimination of other possible causes (e.g., candidiasis) does not result in the resolution of the lesion, biopsy of the lesion is warranted to examine the oral epithelium for dysplastic changes or carcinoma. While there is not yet randomized controlled trial data to support the treatment, retrospective data suggest that excised higher risk oral leukoplakia lesions are less likely to undergo malignant transformation, although it does not completely eliminate the risk of recurrence or malignant transformation.[50]

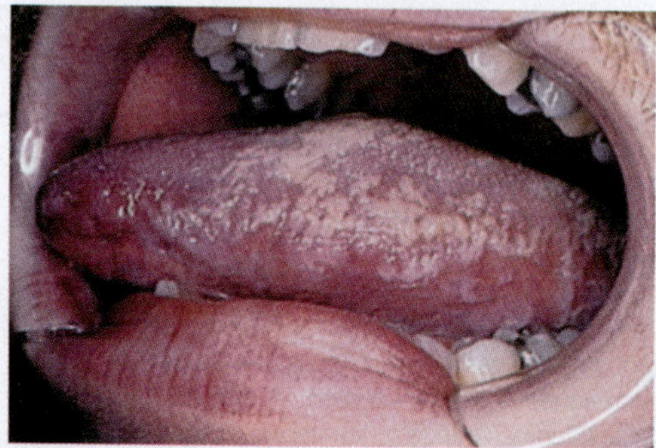

Fig. 24.2 Hairy leukoplakia involving the tongue in a patient with AIDS. (Courtesy Dr. Sol Silverman, Jr., DDS, and Dr. Victor Newcomer.)

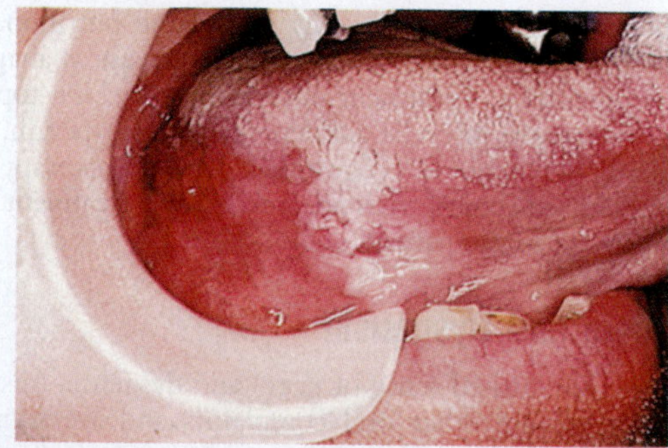

Fig. 24.3 Oral leukoplakia and associated squamous cell carcinoma.

PVL is a rare variant of oral leukoplakia characterized by a high risk for malignant transformation.[8] The etiology of this multifocal process is unknown. Women outnumber men four to one, and smoking is documented in only a third of cases. Early lesions appear as white patches, but over time these benign hyperkeratotic plaques thicken and develop a verrucous exophytic appearance and develop severe dysplasia. More than 70% of patients develop invasive SCC.[51]

Herpetic Geometric Glossitis

Herpetic geometric glossitis (HGG) is characterized as painful, geometric, linear fissures on the dorsal surface of the tongue, making it difficult for patients to eat. HGG tends to present in immunosuppressed patients as a reactivation of chronic oral herpes simplex infection but can present in immunocompetent individuals.[52] It is responsive to oral antiviral therapy, such as acyclovir.

GINGIVAL DISORDERS

Gingival Enlargement

Gingival enlargement (gingival hyperplasia, strawberry gingivitis, and gingival hypertrophy) is characterized by either an increased number or size of gingival cells. Gingival enlargement is a frequent manifestation of granulomatosis with polyangiitis (see Chapter 35).[53] It has also been noted in the rare lysosomal storage disorder, I-cell disease, and is linked to a number of medications, including cyclosporine, phenytoin, and nondihydropyridine calcium channel blockers such as verapamil.

Gingivostomatitis

Gingivostomatitis presents as painful inflammation of both the gingiva and oral mucosa and is a common presentation of primary herpesvirus infection (discussed below).

Acute Necrotizing Ulcerative Gingivitis

Acute necrotizing ulcerative gingivitis (ANUG) is an acute inflammatory and necrotic infection affecting the interdental papillae. Treatment consists of surgical debridement, oral rinses, and systemic antibiotics.[54]

Lead Poisoning

Chronic lead poisoning may be evident as asymptomatic *gingival lead lines* (Burton lines), a thin blue-black line of deposited lead sulfide along the gingival margin. Affected patients may also have abdominal pain and sideroblastic anemia.

ORAL MANIFESTATIONS OF INFECTIONS, NEOPLASMS, AND OTHER SELECTED DISORDERS

Candidiasis

Candida spp. (chiefly *C. albicans*) are normal oral commensal organisms in almost half of the population.[19] A diagnosis of oral candidiasis (thrush, candidosis, and moniliasis) requires clinical and cytologic evidence of an infection or clinical overgrowth. Symptoms include pain, dry mouth, lip swelling, and altered taste. When dysphagia and/or upper GI bleeding accompany oral thrush, concurrent candidal esophagitis is likely (see Chapter 47). Oral candidiasis appears as white curd-like patches (pseudomembranous) or as red (atrophic) or white and red friable lesions on any mucosal surface (Fig. 24.4). All newborns experience initial overgrowth of *Candida* associated with colonization of the GI tract. Oral candidiasis, especially of *C. albicans*,[13] can occur in 11% −15% of children during their first year of life, especially with environmental exposure to pets and siblings.[55] The presence of pseudohyphae and budding yeast on a smear using a potassium hydroxide (KOH) preparation is evidence of infection with *C. albicans;* however, a negative KOH preparation does not exclude active infection. Candidiasis can occur during or after initiation of antibiotic or oral glucocorticoid therapy, in denture wearers, during pregnancy, and in patients with xerostomia, atrophic glossitis, diabetes mellitus, Hashimoto thyroiditis, Cushing disease, or familial hypoparathyroidism.[13,19,56] Systemic and environmental risk factors include smoking, diet, age extremes, or nutritional deficiency.[13] Immunosuppression caused by AIDS, other debilitating illnesses, or cancer chemotherapy may lead to candidiasis. Systemic candidiasis may result when normal barriers to infection are lost. *C. albicans* is the predominant species cultured. However, *C. glabrata*, *C. krusei*, *C. tropicalis*, *C. parapsilosis*, and other azole-resistant species must be considered in resistant cases.[57] The incidence of *C. glabrata* and *C. parapsilosis* varies depending on region, patient's predisposing conditions, and local hospital epidemiology.[57] Cultures are necessary to speciate and to determine resistance.

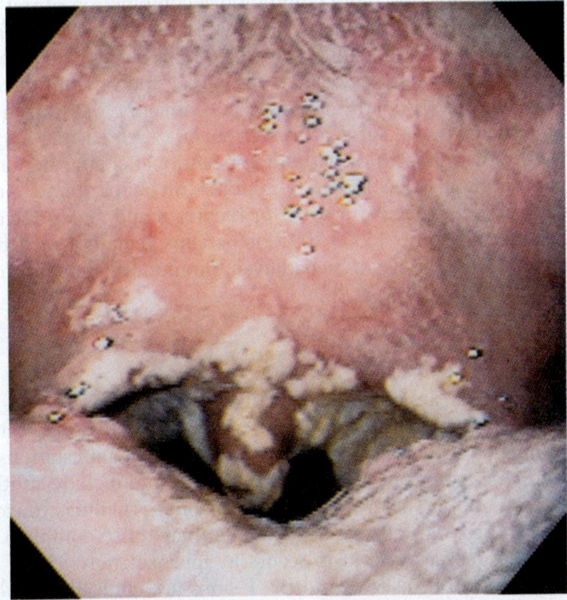

Fig. 24.4 Oral candidiasis; multiple white and yellow plaques are seen on the soft and hard palate, uvula, and tongue.

Early treatment of oral candidiasis relieves the symptoms and prevents any potential, albeit rare systemic spread of localized disease as discussed in Chapters 33, 34, and 35. While *C. albicans* is the most common cause of candidemia, treatment options for candidiasis include topical suspensions, creams, ointments, lozenges, and oral capsules and tablets. Topical treatments are effective in healthy patients when inciting risks have been removed. In denture wearers, regular cleaning of dentures by soaking them in a dilute bleach solution and taking the dentures out overnight is important for clearing infection. However, dosing schedules, unpalatable taste, and the concomitant use of oral appliances may lead to noncompliance and treatment failure. A variety of systemic therapies are reserved to treat refractory disease, immunocompromised hosts, or when topical treatment is precluded by appliances or other factors (see Chapters 33, 34, 35, and 47).[13] Systemic antifungals such as ketoconazole and itraconazole are associated with increased potential for adverse drug-drug interactions owing to their strong inhibition of the cytochrome P450 3A4 hepatic metabolic pathway, in addition to increasing in vitro resistance,[58] and are therefore less frequently utilized in patients requiring chronic prophylactic therapy. The most common HIV-associated infection of the mouth is candidiasis (see Chapters 37 and 47).

Herpesvirus Infections

Primary herpetic gingivostomatitis is caused by herpes simplex virus (HSV) type 1 (occasionally, type 2). Primary infection occurs in up to 90% of the population before puberty. The illness is often mild and mistaken for a routine upper respiratory tract infection; it may include varying degrees of fever, malaise, and adenopathy, together with oral and gingival ulcers. Lesions may appear on the lips. They generally heal in 1 to 2 weeks. Management is palliative, but acyclovir, 400 mg three times a day, may shorten the course and reduce severity. Secondary bacterial infection is common and can be treated topically.

Recurrent orolabial HSV is caused by reactivation of virus that had been dormant in regional ganglia, with no associated increase in HSV antibody titers. Episodes may be precipitated by febrile illnesses, sunlight, and physical or emotional stress. Recurrences vary in frequency and severity. Typically, the lesions involve the lips (cold sores) and are preceded by several hours of prodromal symptoms such as a burning sensation, tingling, or pruritus. Vesicles then appear but soon rupture, leaving small, irregular, painful ulcers. Coalescence of ulcers, crusting, and weeping of lesions are common. Intraoral recurrent herpetic ulcers occur on keratinized mucosa (i.e., hard palate or gingiva; see Table 24.3). They appear as shallow, irregular, small ulcerations and may coalesce. Labial and oral herpetic ulcers normally heal in less than 2 weeks. Recurrent HSV is the most common cause of recurrent erythema multiforme. HGG (discussed earlier) is an additional manifestation of this HSV reactivation.

TABLE 24.3 Distinctions Between Aphthous and Herpetic Oral Ulcers

Condition	Mucosa	Location
Aphthous ulcers	Unkeratinized	Lateral tongue, floor of the mouth, labial and buccal mucosa, soft palate, pharynx
Herpetic ulcers	Keratinized	Gingiva, hard palate, dorsal tongue

In immunocompromised patients, HSV may affect any mucocutaneous surface and can appear as large, irregular, pseudomembrane-covered ulcers. This is especially true in HIV-infected persons, in whom all perineal and orolabial ulcerations should be considered manifestations of HSV until proved otherwise (see Chapter 33). Care should be taken to avoid ocular autoinoculation.

HSV infection or reactivation is usually diagnosed from the history and clinical findings. A history of a prodrome or of vesicles, the site of lesions, and reappearance of lesions in the same location help differentiate HSV from other ulcerative disorders. A cytologic smear (Tzanck) showing multinucleate giant cells is suggestive, although viral cultures and monoclonal antibody staining of smears are more sensitive and specific tests for diagnosing HSV infection. Topical acyclovir is of little benefit in recurrent labial herpes and is of limited benefit in recurrent genital HSV. Systemic acyclovir is regularly used for treatment of primary or recurrent attacks in immunosuppressed patients (2 g orally in divided doses or 5 mg/kg intravenously three times daily until lesions heal). Famciclovir, 125 mg twice daily, or valacyclovir, 500 mg twice daily, are also effective. Oral treatment should optimally begin within the first few hours of the prodrome. For patients with more than four recurrent episodes per year, longer term suppressive therapy may be accomplished with acyclovir, 200 mg orally three times daily or 400 mg twice daily. Acyclovir is used for the prevention of recurrent oral and genital HSV associated with bone marrow transplantation (see Chapter 36). Antivirals are also used to prevent recurrent herpes infections in other immunocompromised patients, such as those with leukemia or HIV infection or after solid organ transplantation.

Herpes zoster (shingles) is caused by a reactivation of the varicella-zoster virus (VZV, HHV-3). Oral lesions can occur and resemble aphthous ulcers, except for the following features: the ulcers are unilateral; lip and/or skin lesions may coexist; and the onset is sudden and acutely painful, usually tracking along a dermatome, and is often associated with fever. High dosages of acyclovir (4 g/d orally), famciclovir (500 mg every 8 hours), or valacyclovir (1 g every 8 hours), within 72 hours of the onset of the illness may be helpful in accelerating healing and reducing postherpetic neuralgia. Vaccination is available to reduce the risk of shingles in elderly individuals, even those who have recovered from an attack.

Human Papillomavirus Infection

Oral manifestations of HPV infection include verrucous papules on the lips.[1] In infants and children, HPV 6 and 11 most commonly present with oral papillomas or, rarely, laryngeal papillomatosis.[59] Malignant transformation to verrucous carcinoma has been reported in 3%–5% of cases, but nearly all cases are associated with the previous radiation of the papillomas. While current evidence supports the view that HPV can be transmitted vertically from mother to child, cesarean section is not indicated to prevent HPV transmission. HPV vaccination reduces the incidence of HPV infection.

Kaposi Sarcoma

Kaposi sarcoma (KS) is a common consequence of HIV infection and is caused by infection with human herpesvirus 8. A significant decline in the incidence of KS occurred during 1996 and 1997, which corresponded to the introduction of ART. Although KS is usually found on the skin, more than half of patients also have intraoral lesions (Fig. 24.5). The first manifestation of KS occurred in the mouth in 22% of patients; in another 45%, KS occurred in the mouth and skin simultaneously.[49] Oral lesions may vary in appearance from minimal asymptomatic, flat, purple, or red macules to large nodules. The hard palate is the most frequent location, followed by the gingiva and tongue (see Fig. 24.5).

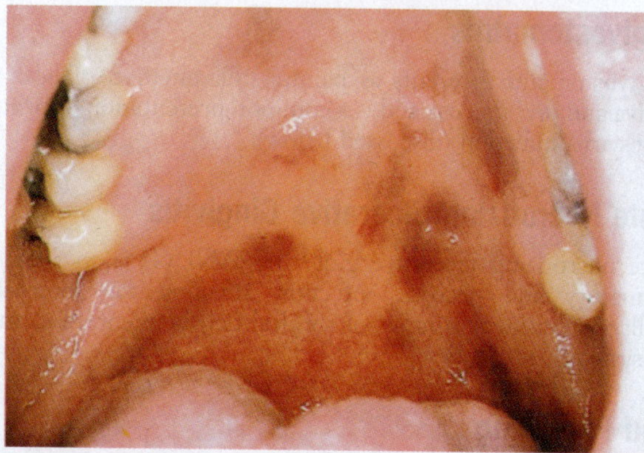

Fig. 24.5 Kaposi sarcoma involving the palate. (Courtesy Dr. Sol Silverman, Jr., DDS, and Dr. Victor Newcomer.)

Other HIV-Related Conditions

Other oral conditions associated with HIV infection include lymphoma; extensive oral, genital, or cutaneous warts; recurrent aphthae; chronic mucocutaneous HSV infections; lymphocytic infiltrates of major salivary glands leading to secondary Sjögren syndrome; and drug reactions, including drug-induced Stevens-Johnson syndrome and ANUG.

Squamous Cell Carcinoma

Leukoplakia as a precursor lesion accounts for 15% of oral SCC cases, but the clinical presentation of oral SCC is quite variable, ranging from an asymptomatic erythematous patch to a white verrucous plaque and, more commonly, a combination of red and white changes (erythroleukoplakia) that may be asymptomatic or rarely associated with pain.[50] Staging of SCC through clinical documentation of any associated ipsilateral and/or contralateral cervical lymphadenopathy, biopsy, and imaging is warranted. Treatment involves surgical resection of affected tissue and adjuvant radiation with or without conventional chemotherapy.[50] Immunotherapy checkpoint inhibitors (nivolumab and pembrolizumab) have been approved for recurrent and metastatic oral SCC, although only 15%–20% of patients benefit from these treatments.[60,61] Trials of neoadjuvant immunotherapy for oral SCC are ongoing.

Inflammatory Bowel Disease

Crohn disease is an inflammatory disorder that can involve the entire GI tract with transmural inflammation and noncaseating granulomas (see Chapters 117 and 118). Oral manifestations of Crohn disease occur in 4%–14% of patients and include aphthae (Fig. 24.6), lip fissures, cobblestone plaques, cheilitis, mucosal tags, and perioral erythema. Patients may also complain of metallic dysgeusia. Aphthosis occurs in approximately 5% of patients with Crohn disease, and the lesions are clinically and histologically indistinguishable from typical aphthae. In comparison, aphthosis and perianal-perifistular ulcerations are not seen in

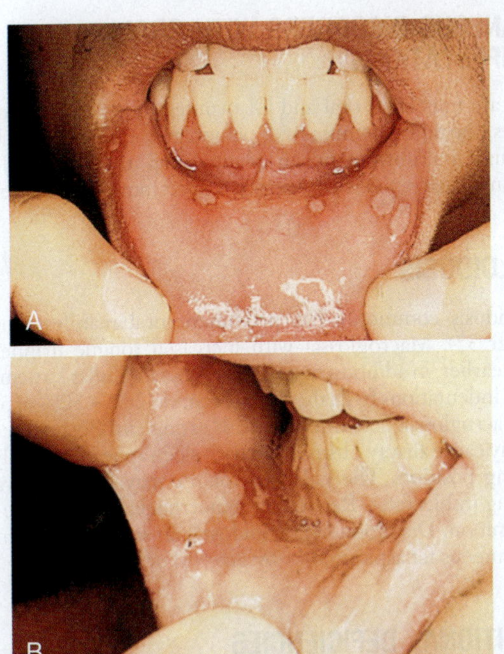

Fig. 24.6 (A) Multiple minor aphthous ulcers. (B) A major aphthous ulcer.

ulcerative colitis. In rare cases, Crohn disease may be associated with granulomatous cheilitis (discussed earlier). *Pyostomatitis vegetans* (see Fig. 25.4) is a specific marker of IBD, both of Crohn and ulcerative colitis, and may precede the GI symptoms by months to years.[62] Pyostomatitis vegetans is characterized by pustules, erosions, and vegetations involving the labial mucosa of the upper and lower lips, buccal mucosa, and gingival mucosa, as well as the skin of the axillae, genitalia, trunk, and scalp. Histologically, intraepithelial and subepithelial eosinophilic miliary abscesses are characteristic. Superficial pustules coat the friable, erythematous, and eroded mucosa of the oral cavity, least commonly the floor of the mouth and tongue. Symptoms may be severe or minimal. Eosinophilia and anemia are common. Diagnosis is made from biopsy findings, and treatment is with topical or systemic glucocorticoids, dapsone, or sulfasalazine.[63]

GASTROESOPHAGEAL REFLUX

Chronic exposure to acidic fluids in the oral cavity results in dissolution of the tooth surfaces (enamel erosion), most commonly seen on the palatal surfaces of the maxillary teeth with exposed underlying dentin, a softer and more opaque yellow substance. The teeth become sensitive to temperature changes as a result of the enamel erosion. The prevalence of caries is not increased in persons with gastroesophageal reflux, possibly because the acidic environment interferes with the formation of dental bacterial biofilms. Erosion of enamel is irreversible. The most effective medical therapy in adults is proton pump inhibitors, though H_2-receptor antagonists may be beneficial. Patients may also benefit from decreased consumption of acidic foods and beverages.

LIVER DISEASE

Jaundice may be seen orally in patients with chronic liver disease, where the oral mucosa may appear yellow due to deposition of bilirubin into the submucosa. The sublingual and soft palate mucosae are very thin, and they are often first to develop this yellow hue. Examination of these regions may provide useful diagnostic clues in patients with darker skin or physiological conjunctival pigmentation.

RECURRENT APHTHOUS ULCERS

Recurrent aphthous ulcers (RAUs, recurrent aphthous stomatitis, canker sores) are painful shallow ulcers, often covered with a grayish-white or yellow exudate and surrounded by an erythematous margin. In immunocompetent individuals, they appear almost exclusively on unkeratinized oral mucosal surfaces (see Table 24.3). Rarely, RAUs may occur in the esophagus, upper and lower GI tracts, and anorectal epithelium. RAUs are the most common cause of oral ulcers and develop at some time in 25% of individuals in the general population and recur at irregular intervals.

Three clinical forms of aphthous ulcers are recognized: minor aphthae (most common), major aphthae (less common), and herpetiform aphthae (least common). Minor aphthae typically are smaller than 5 mm and heal in 1–3 weeks (see Fig. 24.6A). Major aphthae may exceed 6 mm (see Fig. 24.6B) and require months to heal, often leaving scars. Herpetiform aphthae are 1–3 mm in diameter, occur in clusters of 10 to hundreds of ulcers, and resolve quickly.[64]

The mechanism for development of RAU is thought to be multifactorial, with precipitating factors including: (1) immunologic abnormalities, such as celiac disease and increased allergen presentation caused by impaired constitutive oral barriers (putatively from sodium lauryl sulfate use in dental products); (2) chronic trauma, such as from ill-fitting dentures[65]; (3) deficiencies of iron, folate, and/or cobalamin[21]; (4) genetic predisposition; (5) stress and anxiety; (6) allergies to foods or medications, such as to cyclooxygenase 2 inhibitors or sertraline; and (7) xerostomia.[21,64] *H. pylori* infection may be associated with RAUs, as eradication of *H. pylori* from the stomach appears to be associated with a reduction of recurrences of canker sores, as well as a decrease in the number of ulcers and days of symptoms.[64]

Morphologically identical aphthous lesions (aphthae; aphthosis) may be observed in patients with IBD and in Behçet syndrome (discussed below). The workup for RAUs may include, as directed by history and review of systems, a complete blood cell count, erythrocyte sedimentation rate, serum iron and ferritin, serum folate and B_{12} levels, KOH stain, Tzanck smear, viral culture, biopsy of coexisting skin lesions to exclude infection with HSV, and colonoscopy to address the possibility of IBD. Histologically, lesional tissue shows an ulcerated mucosa with chronic mixed inflammatory cells.

Management of RAU includes palliative and curative measures. First, deficient vitamins, if found, should be replaced. Otherwise, patients should be advised to use multivitamins with iron and avoid crusty, salty, or spicy foods to minimize irritation of oral lesions. Using soft toothbrushes, repairing dentition, and other measures to avoid unnecessary oral trauma should be instituted. Analgesics and topical anesthetics, such as 2% viscous lidocaine, may be helpful, along with topical bismuth subsalicylate (Kaopectate) and sucralfate to protect lesions and accelerate healing. Aphthous ulcers can be treated effectively with a topical glucocorticoid, such as fluocinonide (Lidex) or clobetasol (Temovate) gel or ointment. Second-line therapy includes colchicine, 0.6 mg three times daily; tetracycline, 250 mg four times daily; cimetidine, 400–800 mg/d; azathioprine, 50 mg/d; or thalidomide, 200 mg/d. Short courses of systemic prednisone (20–60 mg/d) are reproducibly effective when more conservative approaches are not satisfactory. An elimination diet may be helpful for patients with allergic reactions to certain foods or medications, including a trial of sodium lauryl sulfate-free dental products.[66] A gluten-free diet is required for patients with gluten-sensitive enteropathy (see Chapter 109). Dexamethasone elixir, 0.5 mg/5 mL; doxycycline rinse, 100 mg/100 mL; or chlorhexidine gluconate oral rinse, 0.12&/15mL, may also be helpful.

BEHÇET DISEASE

Behçet disease is a small-vessel vasculitis characterized by RAUs, genital ulcerations, uveitis, and erythema nodosum (see Chapter 35). Recurrent oral aphthous ulcers are the most common symptom of this disorder and are usually accompanied with genital aphthous ulcers. These genital aphthous ulcers tend to be larger, more painful, and carry a higher risk of scarring than oral ulcers.[67] Rare GI manifestations include mucosal inflammation and ulcers, usually localized to the ileocecal region, and hepatic involvement secondary to Budd-Chiari syndrome.[67] Because Behçet disease may be mistaken for complex RAUs, especially in nonendemic areas, a detailed history must be taken. Diagnosis is made clinically by noting oral aphthae and the concurrent presence of at least two of the following: genital ulcers, skin lesions, ocular involvement, and pathergy test positivity.[67] Apremilast 30 mg BID is now approved for treatment of Behçet disease.[61] Treatment is discussed in Chapter 35.

CUTANEOUS DISORDERS WITH ORAL MANIFESTATIONS

There are important oral and GI manifestations of numerous skin diseases, including pemphigoid, pemphigus, epidermolysis bullosa, erythema multiforme, lichen planus, and the Stevens-Johnson syndrome/toxic epidermal necrolysis spectrum (see Chapter 25).

AMYLOIDOSIS

Amyloidosis commonly has prominent oral manifestations (see Chapter 37). Macroglossia with increased tongue firmness, discussed earlier, in addition to enlarged submandibular structures and lingual indentations from the teeth, occurs in 20%–50% of patients. The macroglossia may interfere with eating and closing the mouth and may cause airway obstruction with sleep apnea, especially in the reclining position. The enlarged tongue may be highly vascular, resulting in bleeding. Recurrent hemorrhagic bullae in the mouth are common. Diagnosis of amyloidosis can sometimes be made by subcutaneous fat aspiration or by gingival or tongue biopsy.

NUTRITIONAL DEFICIENCIES

See Table 24.4 (also see Chapters 6, 25, and 106).[21]

TABLE 24.4 Selected Nutritional Abnormalities and Associated Oral Findings

Nutritional Abnormality	Causes	Clinical Features
Riboflavin deficiency (vitamin B_2)	Alcohol abuse GI disease Chlorpromazine	Erythema of pharyngeal and oral mucous membranes Atrophic glossitis with a magenta color Glossodynia Cheilosis Angular cheilitis
Niacin deficiency (vitamin B_3)	Inadequate diet Medication (e.g., isoniazid) Congenital defects of tryptophan transport in intestine and/or kidneys Carcinoid syndrome	Mucosal edema Cheilosis Angular cheilitis Bright red glossitis Burning mouth Gingival erythema Dental caries 4 Ds: dermatitis, diarrhea, dementia, death
Pyridoxine deficiency (vitamin B_6)	Advanced age Alcohol abuse Chronic renal failure Liver disease Malnutrition	Atrophic glossitis Cheilosis Angular stomatitis Gingival erythema
Folate deficiency (vitamin B_9)	Malnutrition Malabsorption diseases (e.g., Celiac, IBD) Medications (e.g., methotrexate, valproic acid)	Atrophic glossitis with erythema and swelling of the tongue Angular cheilitis Tongue soreness or burning Dysphagia
Cobalamin deficiency (vitamin B_{12})	Pernicious anemia Insufficient diet	Generalized stomatitis Taste disturbance Red, atrophic, beefy, burning tongue with loss of filiform papillae
Retinol deficiency (vitamin A)	Malnutrition Malabsorption Alcohol abuse	Xerostomia Periodontal disease Increased intraoral infection Impaired tooth development (in children)
Vitamin K deficiency	Exclusively breast-fed infants Malabsorption Medications (e.g., warfarin)	Submucosal hemorrhage Gingival bleeding
Iron deficiency		Angular cheilitis Atrophic glossitis Glossodynia Recurrent aphthous stomatitis

TABLE 24.4 Selected Nutritional Abnormalities and Associated Oral Findings—cont'd

Nutritional Abnormality	Causes	Clinical Features
Zinc deficiency (acrodermatitis enteropathica if genetic) Deficiency of essential fatty acids Biotin deficiency	Congenital metabolic abnormalities Alcoholics with cirrhosis Hyperalimentation Crohn disease	Burning mouth syndrome Recurrent aphthous stomatitis Perioral or intraoral erosions Dysgeusia (taste alteration)
Vitamin C deficiency (scurvy)	Alcohol abuse Crohn disease Whipple disease	Mucosal petechiae Hemorrhagic gingivitis Gingival bleeding Gingival hypertrophy Interdental infarcts

TABLE 24.5 Drug-Induced Oral Findings

Condition	Drug Class/ Medications	Notes
Gingival Hyperplasia	Anticonvulsants—**phenytoin**, sodium valproate, phenobarbital, vigabatrin, primidone, mephenytoin, ethosuximide Immunosuppressants—**cyclosporine**, sirolimus, tacrolimus Calcium-channel blockers—**nifedipine**, nitrendipine, felodipine, amlodipine, nisoldipine, verapamil, diltiazem. Antibiotics—erythromycin, trimethoprim-sulfamethoxazole Sertraline Lithium Oral contraceptives Estrogens Amphetamines	Stop offending medication Can use azithromycin for cyclosporine-induced gingival hyperplasia
Tooth Discoloration	Extrinsic: mouth rinses with fluoride, chlorhexidine gluconate Antimicrobials—amoxicillin-clavulanic acid, linezolid, ciprofloxacin Intrinsic: tetracyclines, tigecycline	
Fixed Drug Eruption	Trimethoprim-sulfamethoxazole NSAIDS Tetracyclines Pseudoephedrine	
Stevens-Johnson Syndrome	Sulfonamides Aromatic anticonvulsants Lamotrigine Allopurinol NSAIDS NNRTIs—nevirapine	
Pemphigus Vulgaris	Thiols: penicillamine, captopril, tiopronin Phenols: aspirin, heroin, rifampin, levodopa Other: NSAIDS, calcium-channel blockers	
Pemphigoid	Gliptins PD-1/PD-L1 inhibitors Loop diuretics Penicillins NSAIDS Thiazides PUVA	

TABLE 24.6 Teeth Findings

Anhidrotic Ectodermal Dysplasia	Peg Teeth
Nevoid basal cell carcinoma syndrome (Gorlin syndrome)	Pits
Congenital syphilis	Mulberry molars Hutchinson incisors
Tuberous sclerosis	Enamel pits
Incontinentia pigmenti	Hypodontia, conical teeth
Familial colorectal polyposis (Gardner syndrome)	Multiple nonerupted teeth, polydontia/supernumerary teeth
Congenital erythropoietic porphyria (Günther syndrome)	Maroon discoloration of dentin
Tetracyclines	Tetracycline and doxycycline—irreversible Minocycline—reversible
Fluorosis	White discoloration, large pits
Bulimia nervosa, chronic gastroesophageal reflux disease	Dissolution of enamel
Acromegaly	Diastema
Radiation-induced changes	Severe xerostomia Caries Complete loss of enamel Mummification of dentin
Drug-induced changes	See Table 24.5

DRUG-INDUCED ORAL FINDINGS

See Table 24.5.

CONDITIONS WITH CHARACTERISTIC TEETH FINDINGS

See Table 24.6.

Full references for this chapter can be found at https://ebooks.health.elsevier.com.

25 Cutaneous Manifestations of Gastrointestinal and Liver Diseases

Lawrence A. Mark, Valeriya Skorobogatko

IN THIS CHAPTER

VESICULOBULLOUS SKIN DISEASES

The vesiculobullous skin diseases include pemphigoid, pemphigus, epidermolysis bullosa (EB), erythema multiforme (EM), and the Stevens-Johnson/toxic epidermolysis spectrum. They may have oral and GI manifestations, as discussed later.

Pemphigoid

Pemphigoid is a general term for heterogeneous blistering disorders characterized by serum immunoglobulin (Ig)G or IgA autoimmune antibodies directed against 230- and 180-kd hemidesmosomal proteins (among other keratinocyte antigens) located at the squamous epithelial basement membrane. This antigen-antibody reaction leads to loss of adhesion between the epithelium and its supportive basement membrane substrate. Pemphigoid clinically presents with tense bullae and ulcers affecting the mucosa of the oral cavity, pharynx, esophagus, anus, conjunctiva, and skin. Oral findings appear as highly inflamed (erythematous) mucosa on the buccal and gingival mucosa.

Two types of pemphigoid have been identified: bullous pemphigoid (autoimmune and drug-induced variants) and cicatricial (mucous membrane) pemphigoid. Patients with bullous pemphigoid typically have skin lesions, and about one-third also have mucous membrane lesions. The autoimmune subtype most often presents in the older population and may be preceded by a nonbullous, intensely pruritic, "urticarial" phase of disease. Drug-induced bullous pemphigoid has been associated with dipeptidyl peptidase-4 (DPP-4) inhibitors (e.g., vildagliptin and linagliptin),[1] programmed cell death protein-1 (PD-1) and programmed cell death ligand-1 inhibitors (e.g., nivolumab and pembrolizumab),[2] diuretics (loop, thiazide, and aldosterone antagonist), NSAIDs, aspirin, sulfasalazine, antibiotics (e.g., penicillins, vancomycin, and levofloxacin), angiotensin-converting enzyme inhibitors (e.g., captopril), and possibly angiotensin receptor blockers (e.g., valsartan), among many others with less literature support for their causative nature.[3] Discontinuation of a suspected offending agent is primary therapy. In contrast to bullous pemphigoid, all patients with cicatricial pemphigoid have mucosal lesions, and about one-third also have skin lesions. Ocular symblepharon (i.e., adhesion between the tarsal and bulbar conjunctiva) commonly occurs with cicatricial pemphigoid. Potentially fatal upper GI bleeding from esophageal involvement by pemphigoid has been reported.[4]

For all types of pemphigoid, immunofluorescence staining of involved mucosa and skin is diagnostic, showing linear deposition of antibody and complement in the basement membrane zone. Patients with elevated serum IgG and IgA autoantibodies are more likely to respond to systemic medications. Treatment ranges from low-dose to high-dose prednisone. Alternative therapies for patients with contraindications to glucocorticoid use or with systemic toxicities from glucocorticoids include dapsone, tetracycline and nicotinamide in combination, azathioprine, chlorambucil, plasma exchange, IVIG, cyclosporine, cyclophosphamide, methotrexate, rituximab, and infliximab. Topical tacrolimus has shown efficacy for localized oral disease.[5]

Pemphigus

Pemphigus vulgaris differs from pemphigoid in that the serum autoantibodies are directed against intercellular keratinocyte proteins, causing loss of cell-to-cell adhesion. This antigen-antibody reaction leads to bullous skin lesions, often flaccid, that can be life-threatening if untreated. Oral involvement can be extensive. Mucosal involvement can cause poor nutrition and severe pain. Half of patients with *pemphigus vulgaris* present with oral lesions, and oral lesions occur in almost 100% of patients during the illness. Direct immunofluorescence of biopsy material is diagnostic, showing IgG antibodies and complement on the surface of squamous epithelial cells. Indirect immunofluorescence detects circulating IgG antibodies in most patients with *pemphigus vulgaris*. Treatment consists of various regimens of topical or systemic prednisone, sometimes supplemented with cytotoxic or immunosuppressive drugs. Rituximab has been demonstrated to be highly effective and well tolerated in moderate-to-severe *pemphigus vulgaris*.[6]

Paraneoplastic pemphigus shares features of pemphigus vulgaris and EM. It is associated with GI malignancies, lymphomas, leukemias, thymomas, and soft tissue sarcomas. Features that characterize paraneoplastic pemphigus include the following: (1) painful mucosal erosions and a polymorphous skin eruption; (2) intraepidermal acantholysis, keratinocyte necrosis, and vacuolar interface reaction; (3) deposition of IgG and C3 intercellularly and along the epidermal basement membrane zone; (4) serum autoantibodies that bind to skin and mucosa epithelium in a pattern characteristic of pemphigus, as well as binding to simple, columnar, and transitional epithelia; and (5) immunoprecipitation of a complex of four proteins (250, 230, 210, and 190 kd) from keratinocytes by the autoantibodies.[7] The prognosis of paraneoplastic pemphigus is generally poor because symptomatic improvement depends on successful treatment of the underlying malignancy.

Epidermolysis Bullosa

EB is a heterogeneous group of rare inherited disorders of skin fragility (Fig. 25.1). They are characterized by the formation of blisters with minimal trauma and are divided into dystrophic (scarring), junctional, simplex, and Kindler forms.[8] Oral erosions, premature caries, and gingival involvement, as well as GI disease, are not only common in the dystrophic form but also occur in some patients with the junctional form. In addition to oral erosions, esophageal strictures are the most common GI complication in dystrophic EB.[9] They most commonly occur in the upper third of the esophagus but may also be found in the lower third. The esophageal strictures are probably induced by repeated trauma from food and/or refluxed gastric contents; therefore, strict adherence to a soft food diet remains a cornerstone of management. Although dilations with bougienage historically have been shunned because of an unacceptable risk of increasing esophageal stenosis over the long term, evidence supports the use of balloon dilation as a safe and efficacious method of palliating esophageal strictures without this risk. Esophageal resection, feeding gastrostomy, and colonic interpositioning have been effectively used in dystrophic EB patients with severe esophageal strictures. Esophageal webs in the postcricoid area have also been described. Anal stenosis and constipation (with or without stenosis) are frequent in patients with dystrophic EB. Junctional EB has been uniquely associated with pyloric atresia. Anemia and growth retardation frequently develop in patients with severe dystrophic and junctional EB, partly because of GI and oral complications.

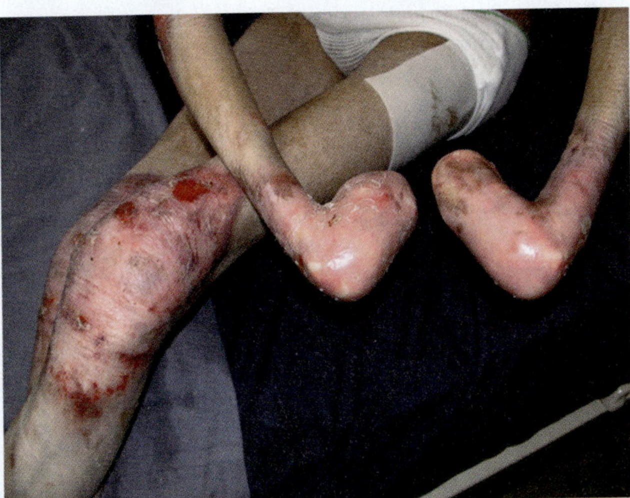

Fig. 25.1 Characteristic lesions resulting from skin fragility caused by severe recessive dystrophic epidermolysis bullosa. (Courtesy Dr. Benjamin Lockshin, Silver Spring, MD.)

Patients with clinical lesions identical to the dystrophic forms of EB but with no family history and an adult onset have been identified; their condition is called *acquired EB* or *EB acquisita* (EBA). EBA, like pemphigus and pemphigoid, is an autoimmune disease. The autoantibodies in EBA are directed against type VII collagen. The diagnosis of EBA is established by routine histology and direct immunofluorescence examination of skin biopsy specimens. Like patients with cicatricial pemphigoid, EBA patients may have significant mucosal involvement, especially oral and esophageal disease. Coexistent Crohn's disease has been reported in a number of patients with EBA. Hepatitis C infection and diabetes mellitus have also been associated. Treatment is with high-dose colchicine, dapsone, and immunosuppressive agents.[10]

Erythema Multiforme

EM is an acute mucocutaneous eruption associated with underlying infections (especially HSV and *Mycoplasma pneumoniae*) and, less commonly, medications (e.g., NSAIDs and sulfonamides). It is often preceded or accompanied by low-grade fever, malaise, and symptoms suggesting an upper respiratory tract infection. The eruption consists of alternating pink and red target lesions on the elbows, knees, palms, and soles, and of shallow, broad oral erosions. Patients with EM may only have oral involvement. Variable degrees of nonspecific erythema are found, with or without ulcers. Crusting, hemorrhagic, and moist lip ulcers may be present. Severe oral and pharyngeal pain, secondary bacterial and fungal infections, and bleeding are common complications. Involvement of the esophagus leading to esophagitis is rare but has been reported.[11] The diagnosis is made by clinical characteristics, excluding other specifically diagnosable diseases, and by response to treatment. The biopsy reveals a nonspecific interface reaction. Oral EM can be self-limited or chronic, and often the inciting process goes unidentified. Management includes palliative measures and the elimination of any offending agent. Often, glucocorticoids and/or other immunosuppressive drugs are needed. Recurrences and flares have variable patterns. Herpes-associated EM lesions are treated with episodic or suppressive antiviral therapy with acyclovir, valacyclovir, famciclovir, or foscarnet.[12]

Stevens-Johnson Syndrome/Toxic Epidermal Necrolysis Spectrum

Stevens-Johnson syndrome (SJS, with between 10% and 30% skin sloughing) and toxic epidermal necrolysis (TEN, with more than 30% skin sloughing) are diagnosed when severe, acute, painful targetoid lesions and skin sloughing occur in association with eye, skin, and mucous membrane involvement. In contrast to EM, which is usually infection related, SJS and TEN are almost always caused by a reaction to a medication, such as an antibiotic (especially a sulfonamide), an anticonvulsant (e.g., lamotrigine and phenytoin), or a checkpoint inhibitor (e.g., nivolumab and pembrolizumab).[13] Diffuse oral and pharyngeal ulceration may prevent oral intake. At endoscopy, the esophagus may show diffuse erythema, friability, and whitish plaques that can be mistaken for candidiasis. Diffuse gastric and duodenal erythema and friability may be present without esophageal involvement. The colonoscopic appearance may resemble severe ulcerative or pseudomembranous colitis. However, colonic biopsies show extensive necrosis and lymphocytic infiltration, without crypt abscesses or neutrophils.[14] This pattern is reminiscent of graft-versus-host disease (see Chapter 34). The mucosa of large portions of bowel may slough in SJS, accounting for reports of hematemesis, melena, and intestinal perforation. Treatment largely consists of discontinuation of offending pharmaceutical agents (often anticonvulsants or antibiotics), hospital admission to a burn unit, if possible, and supportive care by a multiteam approach. No reliable evidence exists for the use of systemic glucocorticoids, intravenous immune globulin, TNF-alpha inhibitors, *N*-acetylcysteine, or plasmapheresis in the treatment of SJS/TEN, but weak evidence suggests that cyclosporine may reduce disease progression and mortality when used early in the disease course.[15]

LICHEN PLANUS

Lichen planus (LP) is a common chronic inflammatory disorder involving the mucosa and skin. The disease usually begins in adulthood, and two-thirds of patients are women. Oral lesions are variable in their presentation and may appear as white, lace-like, and/or punctate patterns on any mucosal surface (Fig. 25.2). Mucosal erythema or ulceration is common. Oral lesions may appear as asymptomatic lace-like plaques on the buccal mucosal or as painful erythematous or erosive plaques involving the tongue, buccal mucosa, or gingiva. Topical and/or systemic glucocorticoids are effective in decreasing the signs and symptoms in almost all cases of oral and cutaneous LP. Topical tacrolimus is an effective steroid-sparing treatment alternative. Esophageal LP may present with progressive dysphagia and odynophagia, upper GI bleeding, strictures, and squamous cell carcinoma.[16] The endoscopic findings include erythema, ulcers, proximal esophageal webs, and erosions throughout the esophagus. An increased prevalence of chronic liver disease, including chronic hepatitis C and PBC, has been reported in patients with LP. Oral LP may be associated with an increased risk of squamous cell carcinoma arising in areas of atrophy or erosion, regardless of treatment.[17] Bullous LP may occur with cancer immunotherapy agents that inhibit programmed death-1 (anti-PD).[18]

CUTANEOUS MANIFESTATIONS OF INFLAMMATORY BOWEL DISEASE

Both Crohn's disease and UC may be accompanied by cutaneous manifestations (see Chapters 117 and 118). Skin lesions are more common (up to 44%) and often more specific in Crohn's disease than in UC. It is rare for cutaneous involvement by Crohn's disease to appear before symptomatic bowel disease. The most common cutaneous complication of Crohn's disease is granulomatous inflammation of the perianal or perifistular skin, which occurs by direct extension from underlying diseased bowel. *Metastatic Crohn's disease* refers to rare ulcerative lesions, plaques, or nodules that occur at sites distant from the bowel. Such lesions favor intertriginous areas such as the retroauricular and inframammary regions. On histologic study, local cutaneous extension and metastatic Crohn's disease show sarcoid-like granulomatous inflammation, and both occur with greater frequency in patients with colonic involvement by Crohn's disease.[19]

Oral manifestations of Crohn's disease occur in 4%–14% of patients and include aphthae, lip fissures, cobblestone plaques, cheilitis, mucosal tags, and perioral erythema. Patients may also complain of metallic dysgeusia. Aphthosis occurs in approximately 5% of patients with Crohn's disease, and the lesions are clinically and histologically indistinguishable from typical aphthae. Aphthosis and perianal-perifistular ulcerations are not seen in ulcerative colitis. Granulomatous cheilitis is a rare condition with recurrent lip swelling that leads to enlargement and firmness of the lips. A lip biopsy shows noncaseating granulomas. In rare cases associated with Crohn's disease,[20] this condition may be a component of Melkersson-Rosenthal syndrome (scrotal tongue, lip swelling, with or without facial palsy, and migraine) or may be idiopathic.

Pyostomatitis vegetans (Fig. 25.3) and its cutaneous counterpart, *pyoderma vegetans*, are characterized by pustules, erosions, and vegetations involving the labial mucosa of the upper and lower lips, buccal mucosa, and gingival mucosa, as well as the skin of the axillae, genitalia, trunk, and scalp. Both pyostomatitis vegetans and pyoderma vegetans are specific markers of IBD (Crohn's and ulcerative colitis) and may precede the GI symptoms by months to years. Histologically, intraepithelial and subepithelial eosinophilic miliary abscesses are characteristic. Superficial pustules coat the friable, erythematous, and eroded mucosa of the oral cavity, least commonly the floor of the mouth and tongue. Symptoms may be severe or minimal. Eosinophilia and anemia are common. Diagnosis is made from biopsy findings, and treatment is with topical or systemic glucocorticoids, dapsone, or sulfasalazine.

Erythema nodosum is a common inflammatory disorder of the subcutaneous fat, with a marked predilection for women. Lesions characteristically appear as 1 cm or larger, shiny, tender, deep red nodules on the anterior shins. The pathogenesis is unknown. The causes of erythema nodosum are infections (especially streptococcal, systemic fungal, and tuberculous), medications (especially oral contraceptives), and leukemias. Erythema nodosum develops in 4%–15% of patients with Crohn's disease and 3%–10% of patients with ulcerative colitis.[21] In addition, GI infections with *Yersinia enterocolitica*, *Shigella flexneri*, and *Campylobacter jejuni* have been associated with erythema nodosum. Treatment of the underlying disease, strict bed rest, and elevation of the legs, as well as the use of anti-inflammatory drugs or potassium iodide, are effective.

Pyoderma gangrenosum is a noninfectious ulcerative cutaneous disorder of unknown pathogenesis (Fig. 25.4). The classic lesion is

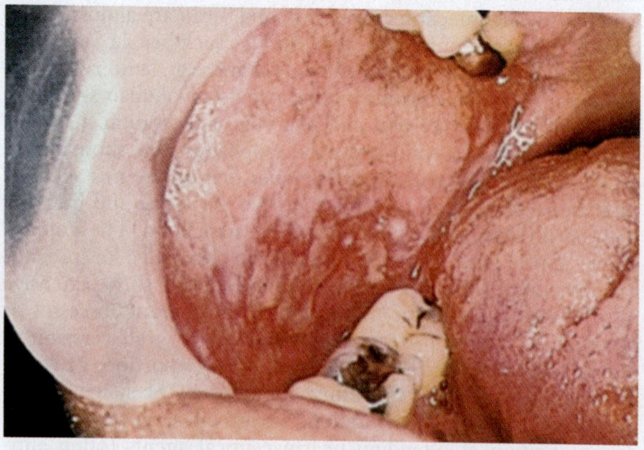

Fig. 25.2 The erosive form of oral lichen planus involving the buccal mucosa. Note the lace-like keratoses, erythema, and ulceration.

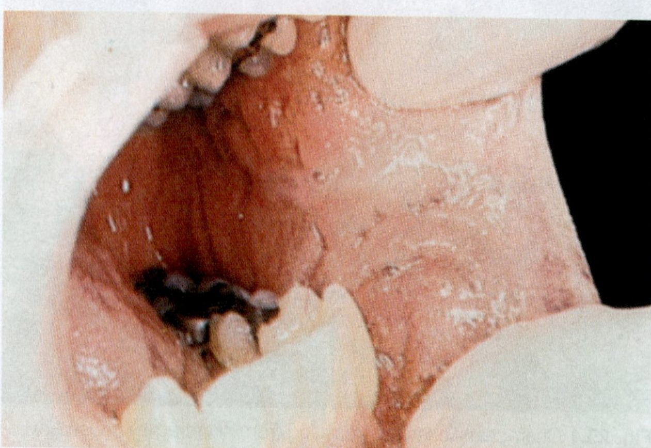

Fig. 25.3 Pyostomatitis vegetans in a patient with UC. A biopsy specimen revealed microabscesses.

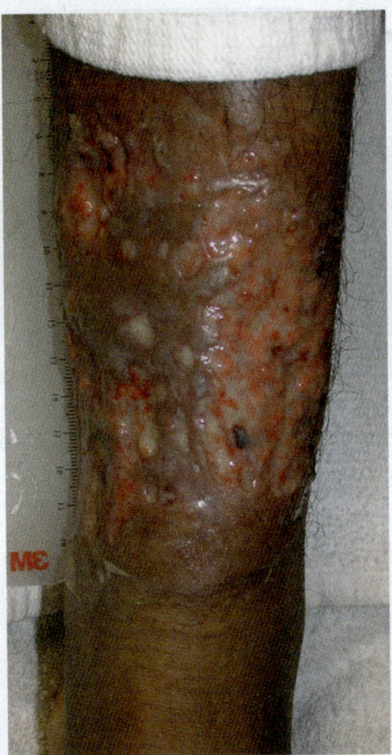

Fig. 25.4 Pyoderma gangrenosum in a patient with UC. (Courtesy Dr. Benjamin Lockshin, Silver Spring, MD.)

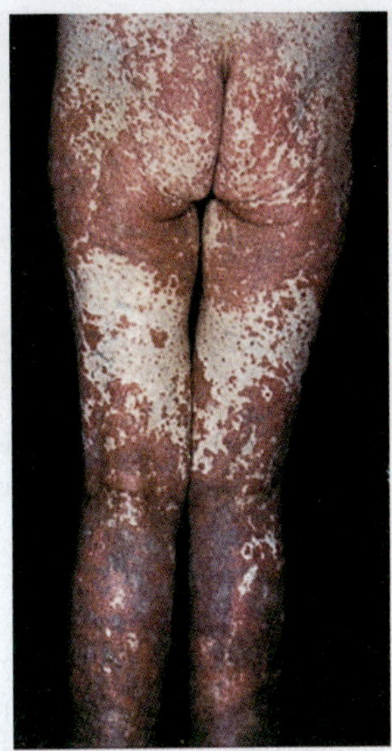

Fig. 25.5 Cryoglobulinemic vasculitis caused by a drug. This type of vasculitis may also be seen in patients with chronic hepatitis C, although generally not as severe as shown here.

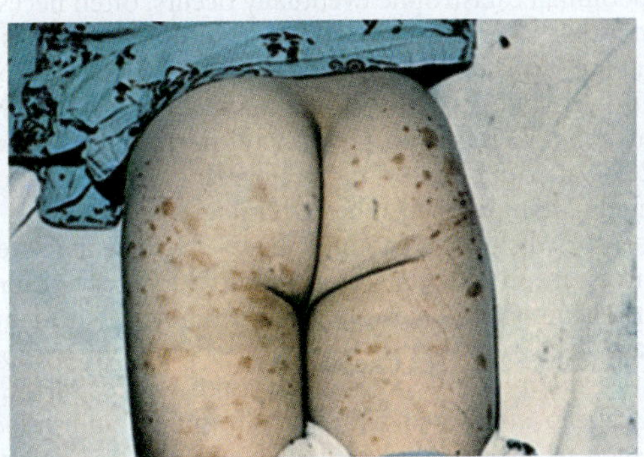

Fig. 25.6 Skin lesions of Henoch-Schönlein purpura.

a tender or painful ulcer with an elevated, dusky purple border that is widely undermined. One or multiple lesions may occur. Lesions begin as small papulopustules that break down very rapidly. *Pathergy*, the appearance of new ulcers at sites of minor trauma or surgery, is often present. The diagnosis is one of exclusion, in that infectious and other causes of ulceration, including factitious dermatitis, must be ruled out. Most cases of pyoderma gangrenosum occur in patients with no underlying disease. Pyoderma gangrenosum develops in approximately 0.4% –2.6% of patients with IBD, more commonly affecting patients with UC.[22] It may recur following successful treatment in 25% of cases, often presenting in the same place as the initial lesion.[23] The bowel disease may be subclinical when the skin lesions appear, and therefore bowel evaluation, especially of the rectum and distal colon, is essential in cases of pyoderma gangrenosum. If the disorder is associated with underlying bowel disease, therapy of the bowel disease may lead to improvement of the skin lesions. The usual management of pyoderma gangrenosum includes local wound care, high-dose systemic glucocorticoids, or steroid-sparing immunosuppressive agents, such as azathioprine, mycophenolate mofetil, methotrexate, tacrolimus, and cyclosporine.[22]

VASCULAR AND CONNECTIVE TISSUE DISORDERS

Connective tissue diseases, like SLE, dermatomyositis (DM, discussed later), and progressive systemic sclerosis (PSS), all have characteristic skin and GI manifestations (see Chapter 35). SLE patients prototypically have malar erythema with photosensitivity and often erythematous raised patches with follicular plugging (discoid lupus). SLE patients can have oral ulcers. Patients with PSS often demonstrate generalized sclerotic skin or, less commonly, morphea (sclerotic plaques with ivory-colored centers), matted telangiectasia, and Raynaud phenomenon.

Immune complex vasculitis of small vessels (leukocytoclastic vasculitis) appears on the skin of dependent sites as crops of palpable purpura and is mediated by deposition of immune complexes in postcapillary venules (Fig. 25.5; see Chapter 36). Although GI involvement can occur in any case of small vessel vasculitis, it occurs in up to 72% of patients with Henoch-Schönlein purpura (Fig. 25.6).[24] Vasculitic hemorrhage, bowel wall edema, and intussusception affect the jejunum and ileum most commonly. Intussusception is the most common life-threatening gastrointestinal complication and occurs in 3%–4% of patients.[25] Direct immunofluorescence of early skin lesions reveals deposits of IgG in most cases of small vessel vasculitis and deposits of IgA in Henoch-Schönlein purpura.

Polyarteritis nodosa, sometimes associated with hepatitis B, is a vasculitis of the medium-sized and small arteries. Arterial lesions of the abdominal viscera can lead to infarction of the gut, liver, and gallbladder and to ischemic pancreatic necrosis, as well as to GI infarcts or perforation. Involvement of the appendix, gallbladder, or pancreas can simulate acute appendicitis, cholecystitis, or pancreatitis. Cutaneous involvement occurs in 25% of cases, most typically manifesting as 5–10-mm nodules distributed along the course of the superficial arteries. A mottled livedo vascular pattern is also frequently seen.

Malignant atrophic papulosis (Degos disease, Köhlmeier-Degos syndrome, progressive arterial mesenteric vascular occlusive disease, or disseminated intestinal and cutaneous thromboangiitis) is a vasculopathic disorder that may occasionally be familial; approximately 200 cases have been described. There is a purely cutaneous form, but the multisystem subtype is important because of its implications for a nearly uniformly fatal outcome due to GI perforation (see Chapter 37). Cutaneous lesions are the initial

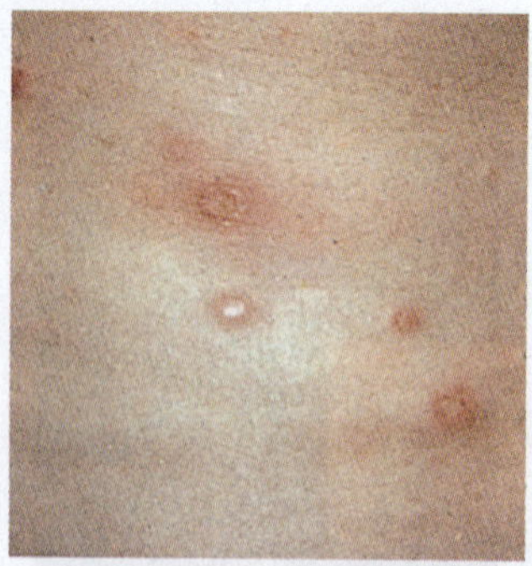

Fig. 25.7 Malignant atrophic papulosis (Degos disease) with cutaneous lesions of different stages.

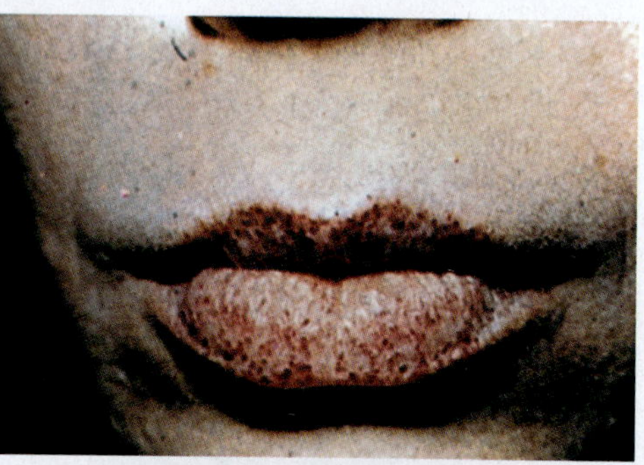

Fig. 25.8 Flat telangiectasias of the lips and vermillion border in a patient with hereditary hemorrhagic telangiectasia (Osler-Weber-Rendu disease).

manifestations, appearing most commonly in early adulthood. They appear as crops of asymptomatic, pink, 2–15-mm papules that rapidly become umbilicated and develop a characteristic atrophic, depressed, porcelain white center (Fig. 25.7). These lesions represent cutaneous infarcts. Similar infarcts may occur in the GI tract in up to 60% of cases but may also involve the nervous system, heart, lung, liver, and kidney. Although GI involvement may initially be asymptomatic or nonspecific, an acute abdominal catastrophe eventually occurs, often necessitating laparoscopy or laparotomy. Perforation of the intestine is usually found, along with multiple white, yellowish, or rose-colored flat or slightly depressed patches below an intact serosa, usually in the small intestine. Cerebral and peripheral nerve infarcts develop in about 20% of patients, leading to neurologic complications that can include hemiparesis, aphasia, cranial neuropathies, monoplegia, sensory disturbances, and seizures. Microscopy reveals that the infarcts are consequences of noninflammatory thromboses. The pathogenesis of Degos disease is unknown, but identical lesions have been reported in SLE and in a patient without SLE with anticardiolipin antibodies and a lupus anticoagulant. Treatment has been attempted with antithrombotic and vasodilatory agents such as aspirin, ticlopidine, pentoxifylline, heparin, and dipyridamole, with limited success.[26] Eculizumab, which prevents the generation of the terminal complement complex C5b-9, has shown improvement in both cutaneous and intestinal lesions but does not impede the development or advancement of systemic involvement. The combination of eculizumab and treprostinil, a prostacyclin analog, has been employed with success to treat GI involvement.[27] Annual follow-up is mandatory due to the potential for life-threatening complications and includes skin examinations, gastroscopy, colonoscopy, and various other imaging modalities.[28]

Hereditary hemorrhagic telangiectasia (HHT), or Osler-Weber-Rendu disease, is a group of autosomal dominant disorders characterized by vascular lesions, including telangiectasias, arteriovenous malformations, and aneurysmal vessels involving the skin and internal organs (lung, brain, and GI tract). Epistaxis (80%–90%) and GI hemorrhage are the most common complications (see Chapter 36). The skin lesions are 1–3-mm macular telangiectasias of the face, lips, tongue, conjunctiva, fingers, chest, and feet (Fig. 25.8). Skin lesions appear later than the epistaxis, usually in the second or third decade of life. In the fifth to sixth decades, recurrent upper and lower GI hemorrhage may occur. Vascular malformations have been reported in the GI tract, liver, lungs, central nervous system, genitourinary tract, and almost every other organ system in the body. Management of the GI bleeding may be difficult, but the use of bipolar electrocoagulation or laser techniques has been beneficial (see Chapter 21). Associated von Willebrand factor deficiency may be present, and therapy with desmopressin has been successful in treating massive GI bleeding. Chronic therapy with estrogen and progesterone may reduce bleeding from GI telangiectases. Although there is presently no FDA-approved treatment to prevent the development of telangiectatic lesions in patients with HHT, current research is focused on the proposed genetic pathway involved. Mutations in the transforming growth factor β signaling pathway, including *ENG*, *ACVRL1*, and *SMAD4*, might be targets for antiangiogenesis drugs such as bevacizumab and thalidomide.[29] Numerous case reports demonstrating improvement of HHT bleeds after bevacizumab have been published without any severe adverse effects reported. Preclinical studies have isolated novel molecular targets involved in the signaling pathway of HHT, including FKBP12, PI3-kinase, and angiopoietin-2, further expanding the potential for additional therapies.[30]

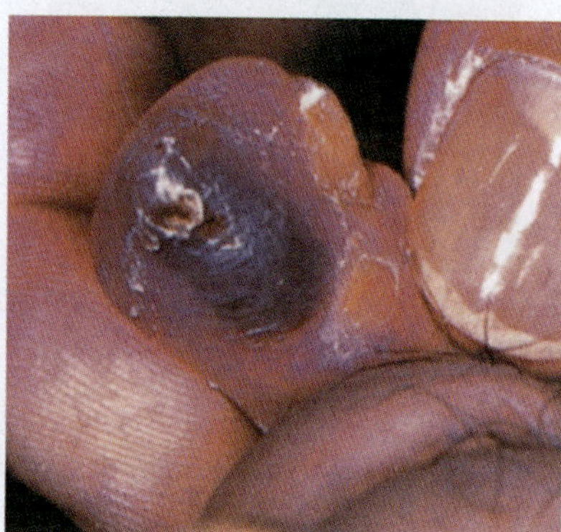

Fig. 25.9 Fingertip lesion in a patient with the blue rubber bleb nevus syndrome.

Blue rubber bleb nevus syndrome is a rare disorder of the skin and GI tract comprising a constellation of multiple cutaneous and GI venous malformations. Most cases are sporadic. In affected patients, blue, subcutaneous, and compressible nodules develop on the skin (Fig. 25.9). GI vascular malformations are common, especially in the small intestine or colon, and bleeding is an almost universal feature. Acute GI hemorrhage, intussusception, volvulus, bowel infarction, and rectal prolapse have been described. Treatment is primarily surgical or with photocoagulation.

Amyloidosis commonly has prominent cutaneous and oral manifestations (see Chapter 35). Waxy papules around the eyes, nose, and central face, as well as purpura involving the face, neck, and upper eyelids, are frequently noted. If a waxy papule is pinched, hemorrhage will ensue (pinch purpura). Orbital purpura after endoscopy, vomiting, or coughing is almost diagnostic. Macroglossia, increased tongue firmness, enlarged submandibular structures, and lingual indentations from the teeth occur in 20%–50% of patients. The macroglossia may interfere with eating and closing the mouth and may cause airway obstruction with apnea, especially in the reclining position. The enlarged tongue may be highly vascular, resulting in bleeding. Recurrent hemorrhagic bullae in the mouth are common. Patients may have carpal tunnel syndrome, edema, the shoulder pad sign (amyloid deposits in soft tissues around shoulders), GI bleeding, peripheral neuropathies, rheumatoid arthritis–like deposits in small joints, and cardiac involvement. Congestive heart failure or arrhythmias account for death in 40% of patients with systemic amyloidosis. Diagnosis of amyloidosis can be made by subcutaneous fat aspiration or by bone marrow, rectal, skin, or tongue biopsy.

Pseudoxanthoma elasticum is a rare autosomal recessive disorder of the *ABCC6* gene characterized by aberrant calcification of mature elastic tissue. Skin lesions are usually the initial manifestation, appearing in the second decade as yellow to orange papules (plucked chicken skin) on the lateral neck (Fig. 25.10). Skin lesions may progress caudally, involving other flexural areas (e.g., axilla, groin, antecubital, and popliteal fossae). Calcification of the elastic tissue of arteries leads to the major complications of retinal bleeding, intermittent claudication, premature coronary artery disease, and GI bleeding. Up to 10% of patients experience GI bleeding,[31] which is usually from the stomach, and often no specific bleeding point is found. As opposed to the other complications of pseudoxanthoma elasticum just noted, GI bleeding tends to occur in younger patients (average age, 26 years), often occurs during pregnancy, and may be recurrent. Skin lesions may not be visible at the time of bleeding. Because apparently normal flexural or scar skin may yield diagnostic findings, a blind skin biopsy may be indicated in a young person with GI bleeding with no other explanation. Lesions identical to those seen on the skin may also be present on the lower lip and the rectal mucosa.[32]

Neurofibromatosis type 1 (NF1, von Recklinghausen disease) is defined by its cutaneous manifestations of six or more café au lait spots (each with a diameter >5 mm in prepubertal persons and >15 mm in postpubertal persons), multiple soft papules [neurofibromas (Fig. 25.11)], or a single plexiform neurofibroma, and freckling of the axillae or inguinal areas. GI involvement occurs in 10%–15% of patients with NF1. Intestinal neurofibromas may arise at any level of the GI tract, although small intestinal involvement is most common. These tumors are generally submucosal but may extend to the serosa. Dense growths known as *plexiform neurofibromatosis* of the mesentery or retroperitoneal space may lead to arterial compression or nerve injury. Other tumors may occur in neurofibromatosis. There is an increased incidence of pheochromocytoma, with or without the multiple endocrine neoplasia type IIB syndrome.[33] Duodenal and ampullary carcinoid tumors (sometimes producing obstructive jaundice; see Chapter 43), gastrointestinal stromal tumors, malignant schwannomas, sarcomas, and pancreatic adenocarcinomas are seen with increased frequency. GI manifestations of NF1 include abdominal pain, constipation, anemia, melena, and an abdominal mass. Serious complications that have been reported include intestinal or biliary obstruction, ischemic bowel, perforation, and intussusception. Involvement of the myenteric plexus has resulted in megacolon.

Mastocytosis is characterized by mast cell infiltration of the bone marrow, skin, liver, spleen, lymph nodes, and GI tract. It occurs in adult and pediatric patients (see Chapter 37). In children, the most common lesions consist of a large red to brown plaque (solitary mastocytoma), multiple red to brown papules or plaques (urticaria pigmentosa), or diffuse cutaneous involvement, with or without flushing or blistering. In adult patients, most have urticaria pigmentosa–type lesions (Fig. 25.12), sometimes with prominent telangiectasia. Lesions are often on the trunk. The spectrum of clinical symptoms is due to either organ infiltration by mast cells or the release of mast cell mediators (e.g., histamine and prostaglandins), leading to headache, syncope, flushing, sweating, shortness of breath, wheezing, or even anaphylaxis. The most common GI complaint is dyspepsia, and often peptic ulcer disease is caused by histamine-induced gastric acid hypersecretion (see Chapter 53). Diarrhea and abdominal pain are also common problems and can be accompanied by malabsorption.[34] In children, the lesions usually involute spontaneously, and systemic disease is uncommon. In adults, cutaneous lesions may resolve as well, but without improvement in systemic symptoms. In the rare pediatric case with a solitary mastocytoma and significant systemic

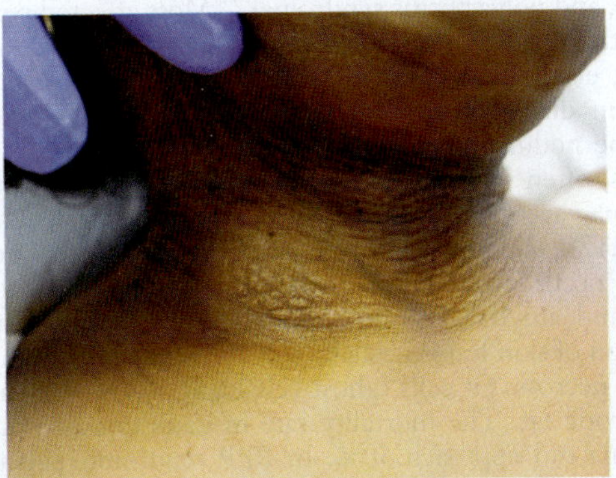

Fig. 25.10 Characteristic "plucked chicken skin" appearance in a patient with pseudoxanthoma elasticum. (Courtesy Dr. Benjamin Lockshin, Silver Spring, MD.)

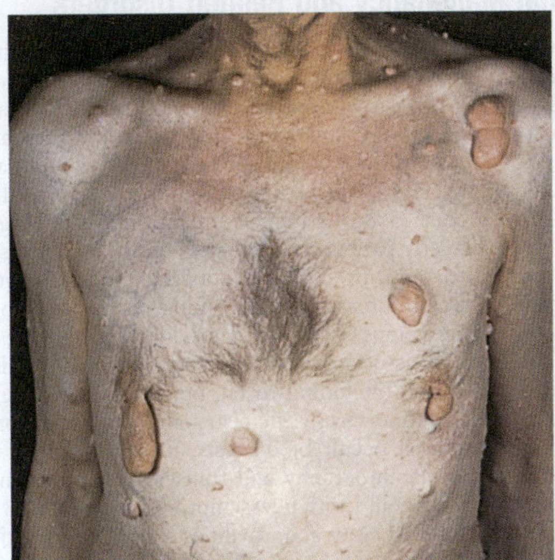

Fig. 25.11 Neurofibromatosis.

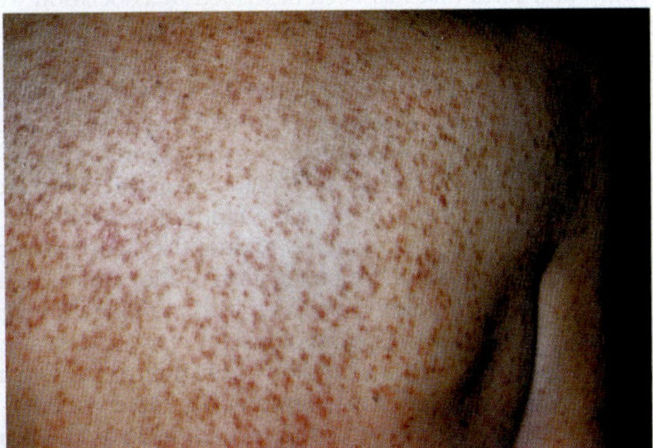

Fig. 25.12 An adult with urticaria pigmentosa. Reddish-brown freckle-like lesions are characteristic of the adult form of this disease. The term *urticarial* is a misnomer, as these lesions do not resemble hives.

symptoms, excision of the skin lesion may resolve the systemic complications. Extracutaneous involvement should be considered for adult patients with cutaneous mastocytosis because management of symptoms can easily be achieved.

CUTANEOUS MANIFESTATIONS OF GASTROINTESTINAL MALIGNANCIES

Cutaneous manifestations may be of importance in recognizing individuals with cancer or from a kindred with a high risk for the development of cancer. These cutaneous markers are discussed in three sections: syndromes with GI polyposis and skin findings, cutaneous markers of internal malignancy, and cutaneous manifestations of metastatic GI carcinoma.

Polyposis Syndromes

The polyposis syndromes, discussed in Chapter 126, have a number of cutaneous findings that are key to clinical identification and unique discrimination. Table 25.1 reviews the pertinent mucocutaneous and clinical findings, as well as the genetics associated with polyposis syndromes, hereditary nonpolyposis colorectal cancer (HNPCC, Lynch syndrome), Muir-Torre syndrome, and Peutz-Jeghers syndrome (Fig. 25.13). A thorough review of this topic is available.[35]

Internal Malignancy and Related Disorders

DM manifested by a violaceous color of the eyelids, often with edema (heliotrope); keratotic papules over the knuckles [Gottron papules (Fig. 25.14)]; a widespread erythema, often with accentuation over the elbows and knees (Gottron sign), resembling psoriasis; photosensitivity; and nail cuticle abnormalities, including telangiectases, thickening, roughness, overgrowth, and irregularity. About 25% of patients with DM have internal malignancy, particularly patients older than 40 years.[36] Cancers most commonly associated with DM are esophageal, gastric, colorectal, pancreatic, ovarian, breast, cervical, lung, and non-Hodgkin lymphoma. There appears to be a predilection for the male sex.[37] To detect an associated cancer, a complete medical history, physical examination (including rectal, pelvic, and breast examinations), CBC, routine serum chemistry analysis, serum protein electrophoresis, fecal occult blood tests, urinalysis, chest x-ray, and (in women) mammography and transvaginal ultrasound are recommended yearly, and with new symptoms, for the first 3 years after the onset of DM. Any abnormalities should be investigated further.[38,39]

Keratosis palmaris et plantaris (Howel-Evans syndrome, tylosis, and esophageal cancer) is an adult-onset diffuse hyperkeratosis of the palms and soles that has been described in association with a very high incidence of esophageal carcinoma in several kindred in Liverpool, England. It is an autosomal dominant phenotype caused by loss of heterozygosity of the TOC (tylosis esophageal cancer) gene, *RHBDF2*, located on chromosome 17q.[40] The skin lesions appear during adolescence or early adulthood, and the carcinomas appear on average at 45 years. Esophageal carcinoma develops in almost all patients in these kindred with tylosis.

Acanthosis nigricans is a cutaneous finding that manifests with a velvety hyperplasia and hyperpigmentation of the skin of the neck and axillae (Fig. 25.15), often associated with multiple skin tags. It is most commonly a manifestation of insulin resistance. However, some patients with acanthosis nigricans have internal malignancy, so-called malignant acanthosis nigricans. In these patients, the extent of involvement may be severe and include the hands, genitalia, and oral mucosa. When acanthosis nigricans affects the hands, it is known as *tripe palms* (acanthosis palmaris, pachydermatoglyphy, palmar hyperkeratosis, and palmar keratoderma). Tripe palms present as a moss-like or velvety texture with pronounced dermatoglyphics or by a cobbled or honeycombed surface of the palms and fingers. The associated carcinoma is usually present simultaneously with the acanthosis nigricans but may not yet be clinically evident. Intra-abdominal adenocarcinomas constitute more than 85% of associated malignancies, with gastric carcinomas representing more than 60%. Survival is short, and more than 50% of patients die in less than 1 year.[41]

Paraneoplastic acrokeratosis of Bazex is a rare but distinctive syndrome associated with a primary malignant neoplasm of the upper aerodigestive tract or metastatic carcinoma to the lymph nodes of the neck. All of the more than 50 patients reported to date have had malignancy, including esophageal carcinoma and one gastric carcinoma with cervical nodal metastases. The skin eruption begins as thickening of the periungual skin and marked nail dystrophy. The rash progresses proximally and also involves the tip of the nose and ears. Thickening of the palms and soles ensues initially, with central sparing, which can make walking very painful. Eventually the face and scalp become involved. Treatment of the underlying carcinoma is usually associated with improvement or resolution of the skin lesions.

Hypertrichosis lanuginosa, another rare paraneoplastic syndrome consisting of fine, thin, down-like, unpigmented lanugo-type hair, is typically noted on the face, forehead, ears, nose, axillae, limbs, and trunk. Associated manifestations include glossodynia, papillary hypertrophy of the tongue, disturbances of taste and smell, diarrhea, scleroderma, acanthosis nigricans, seborrheic keratoses, adenopathy, and weight loss. Colorectal carcinomas are second only to lung carcinoma in the frequency of associated malignancies. Rarely, it may be associated with autoimmune hepatitis.[42]

Carcinoid tumors produce a number of vasoactive substances that can induce cutaneous flushing (see Chapter 43). The most common carcinoid tumors (appendix and small bowel) do not produce flushing until the vasoactive substances reach the systemic circulation. Flushing, therefore, generally denotes metastasis to the liver or a different primary tumor site (e.g., lung or ovary). Glucagonoma is a very rare neuroendocrine tumor of the alpha cells of the pancreas that may cause a *necrolytic migratory erythema* of the skin. The rash is common around orifices, flexural regions, and the fingers. Lesions are typically papulovesicular, with secondary erosions, crusting, and fissures appearing in a geographic circinate pattern (Fig. 25.16). Patients can also often have weight loss, diarrhea, anemia, psychiatric disturbances, hypoaminoacidemia, and diabetes. The rash typically clears with successful removal of the tumor (discussed in more detail in Chapter 43).

Subcutaneous fat necrosis and polyarthralgia are associated with pancreatic acinar cell carcinoma and pancreatitis. It is less commonly associated with pancreatic pseudocysts, pancreatic divisum, and vascular pancreatic fistulas. This constellation is now increasingly referred to as the *PPP syndrome* (pancreatitis, panniculitis, and polyarthritis syndrome).[43] Most affected persons are men with a history of prior or current alcohol use. Deep subcutaneous, erythematous nodules ranging from 1 to several centimeters in diameter usually appear on the legs. In uncommon cases, the nodules may break down, exuding a creamy material. Arthritis, often involving several joints, especially the ankles and knees, may accompany the nodules or occur without skin lesions (Fig. 25.17). Abdominal pain may be absent when skin lesions or arthritis occur. In addition to the expected elevations of serum lipase (and amylase), eosinophilia is common. Histopathologic evaluation of skin lesions usually reveals diagnostic findings—pale staining necrotic fat cells (ghost cells) and deposits of calcium in the necrotic fat. The mortality rate in cases not associated with carcinoma can approach 50%. In PPP syndrome, subcutaneous nodules usually manifest on the anterior shins.

A bluish discoloration of the skin (ecchymosis) around the umbilicus, sometimes associated with hemorrhagic pancreatitis, is

TABLE 25.1 Pertinent Cutaneous Findings and Genetics of the Polyposis Syndromes

Syndrome (Inheritance)	Cutaneous/Mucosal Presentation	Other Findings	Gene Defect (OMIM#)
Gardner syndrome Familial adenomatous polyposis variant (autosomal dominant)	Prepubertal epidermoid (inclusion) cysts Lipomas Desmoid tumors Dental abnormalities: Osteomas Odontomas Supernumerary teeth Multiple unerupted teeth Long, pointed posterior tooth roots	100–1000 adenomatous colon polyps Congenital hypertrophy of the retinal pigment epithelium (CHRPE) Malignancies: Colon/rectum Duodenum Ampulla of Vater Thyroid Medulloblastoma Adrenal gland Hepatoblastoma	APC (tumor suppressor gene defect) OMIM #175100
Muir-Torre syndrome Lynch syndrome variant (autosomal dominant)	Sebaceous adenomas and carcinomas Epitheliomas Keratoacanthomas	Malignancies: Colorectal mucinous adenocarcinoma (proximal colon usually) Stomach Small bowel Ampulla of Vater Endometrium Urologic tract Ovary Live/biliary	Mismatch repair gene defects in *MLH1*, *MSH2*, *MSH6*, and *PMS2* OMIM #158320
Peutz-Jeghers syndrome (autosomal dominant)	Early onset mucocutaneous melanocytic macules: Perioral area Lips/vermillion border Buccal mucosa Lingual mucosa Digits Periocular area Perianal area	Hamartomatous GI polyps (any part of GI tract) Malignancies: Small and large intestine Pancreas Breast Uterus Cervix Testes	*STK11* (serine/threonine kinase germline mutation) OMIM #175200
Cowden syndrome Multiple hamartoma syndrome (autosomal dominant)	Trichilemmomas Facial papules Lipomas Acral keratosis Penile lentigines Oral findings: Papillomatosis Scrotal tongue/lingual fissuring Buccal/lingual cobblestoning	Polyposis: Esophagus Stomach Colon/rectum Hamartomas: Bone CNS Eyes GU tract Pectus excavatum Scoliosis Macrocephaly Malignancies: Colon/rectum Breast Thyroid Endometrium	*PTEN* tumor suppressor gene defect OMIM #158350
Cronkhite-Canada syndrome (sporadic)	Alopecia (patchy) Hyperpigmentation (diffuse) Nail dystrophy: Thinning Splitting Onycholysis Onychomadesis (periodic shedding of nails)	Diffuse polyposis throughout the GI tract, sparing the esophagus, leading to diarrhea, weight loss, anorexia, GI bleeding, intussusception, and a protein-losing enteropathy	OMIM #175500

CNS, Central nervous system; *GU*, genitourinary; *OMIM*, Online Mendelian Inheritance in Man.

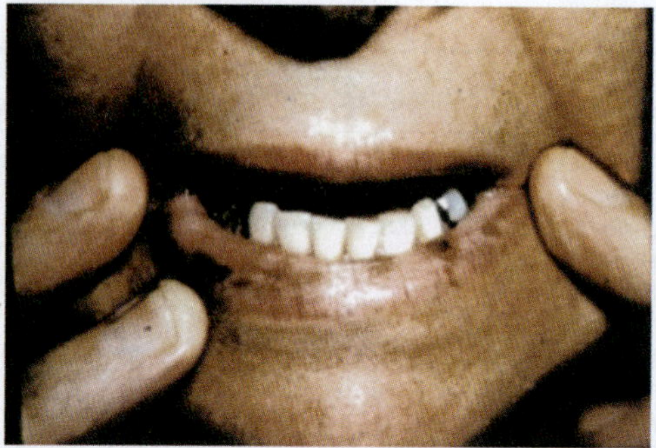

Fig. 25.13 Mucocutaneous pigmentation in a patient with Peutz-Jeghers syndrome.

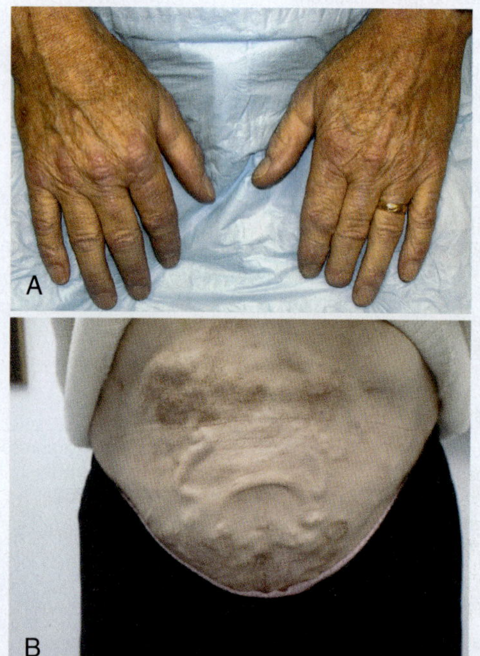

Fig. 25.14 (A) Dermatomyositis with erythematous plaques, especially over the knuckles (Gottron papules). (B) Calcinosis cutis from dermatomyositis with caput medusae. (Courtesy Dr. Benjamin Lockshin, Silver Spring, MD.)

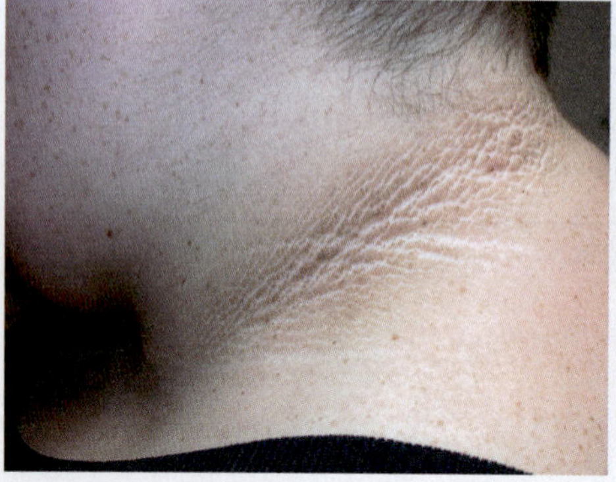

Fig. 25.15 Acanthosis nigricans on the neck. (Courtesy Dr. Benjamin Lockshin, Silver Spring, MD.)

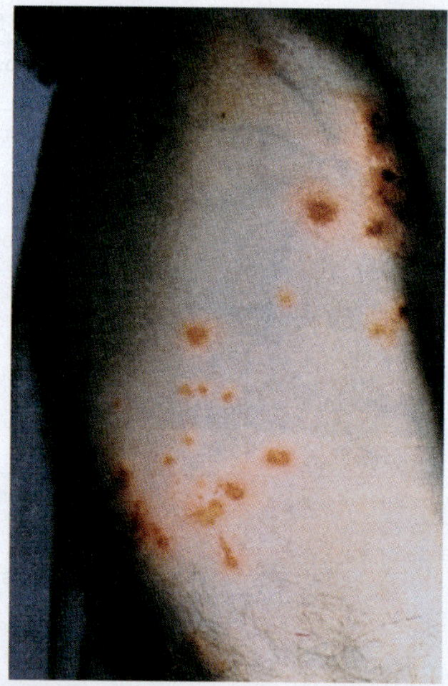

Fig. 25.16 Necrolytic migratory erythema in a patient with glucagonoma, characterized by rapidly eroding, superficial blisters. Lesions are usually localized to the buttocks, groin, perineum, elbows, hands, feet, and perioral area. (Courtesy Dr. Carl Grunfeld, San Francisco, CA.)

called the *Cullen sign*; when a similar process occurs in the flank, it is called the *Grey Turner sign* (see Chapter 58).

Some cutaneous markers historically thought to be associated with internal malignancies have more recently been dismissed as having no direct relationship. These include Bowen disease (cutaneous squamous cell carcinoma in situ) and skin tags. Leser-Trélat sign (sudden appearance of multiple seborrheic keratoses) remains controversial but may be more specific for a GI or lung adenocarcinoma when associated with another paraneoplastic finding, such as malignant acanthosis nigricans.[44] Sweet syndrome (acute febrile neutrophilic dermatoses) might be associated with a lymphoproliferative neoplasm.

Cutaneous Metastases

Cutaneous metastases occur rarely with GI adenocarcinomas. They may appear anywhere on the skin and are often nonspecific, very firm, dermal, or subcutaneous nodules. When metastasis to the umbilicus occurs, intra-abdominal GI carcinoma is found in more than half of cases and gastric carcinoma in 20%. This lesion is called the *Sister Mary Joseph nodule*. Immunoperoxidase markers have assisted pathologists in predicting the primary site of origin from biopsy specimens of metastatic nodules.

CUTANEOUS MANIFESTATIONS OF LIVER DISEASE

Liver disease can result in a variety of cutaneous manifestations, especially in relation to hepatitis B and C (Boxes 25.1 and 25.2).

Pruritus is a distressing complication of cholestatic, inflammatory, and malignant liver diseases. The itching of liver disease is not relieved by scratching or topical glucocorticoids, may be especially prominent in the palms and soles, and can be difficult to manage. Amelioration of pruritus with ultraviolet B light treatment, cholestyramine, or rifampin does not help in elucidating the pathogenesis of this distressing condition. Opiate antagonists may relieve pruritus of liver disease, and the pruritus associated with

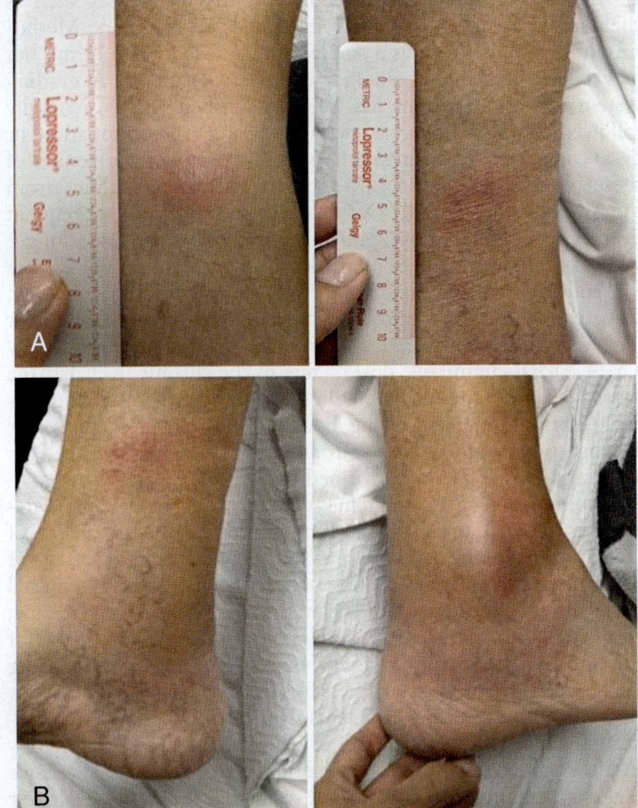

Fig. 25.17 (A and B) Pancreatitis, panniculitis, and polyarthritis syndrome. A 69-year-old alcoholic man with chronic calcific pancreatitis, a pseudocyst, and marked hyperlipasemia (>6000 U/L) developed acute bilateral ankle pain with redness and swelling. Three days later he noticed painful red bumps in his right posterior forearm and right ankle area, with later spread to the right ankle. He had pain and swelling in several metacarpophalangeal and interphalangeal joints and bilateral swelling of the Achilles tendon. Biopsy of one of the subcutaneous nodules showed fat necrosis. The lesions and arthritis gradually resolved without scarring over several weeks. (Courtesy Ann Malbas, MD.)

BOX 25.1 Cutaneous Manifestations of Selected Liver Diseases

LIVER DISEASE IN GENERAL

Jaundice
Vascular spider angiomata
Corkscrew scleral vessels
Palmar erythema
Telangiectasia
Striae
Caput medusa

HEMOCHROMATOSIS

Generalized bronze-brown skin color with accentuation over sun-exposed sites

PRIMARY BILIARY CHOLANGITIS

Xanthomas of trunk, face, or extremities, including striking plane xanthomas on palmar creases

HEPATITIS B AND C

See Box 25.2

BOX 25.2 Cutaneous Manifestations of Hepatitis B and C

HEPATITIS B MORE THAN IN HEPATITIS C

Polyarteritis nodosa
Urticaria
Serum sickness
Infantile papular acrodermatitis (Gianotti-Crosti syndrome)
Erythema nodosum

BOTH HEPATITIS B AND C

Small vessel vasculitis
Urticarial vasculitis
Pruritus
Erythema multiforme

HEPATITIS C MORE THAN IN HEPATITIS B

Leukocytoclastic vasculitis with cryoglobulinemia
Porphyria cutanea tarda

HEPATITIS C

Lichen planus
Livedo reticularis
Necrolytic acral erythema

metastatic disease to the liver has been successfully treated with ondansetron, a 5-HT$_3$ receptor antagonist. Intense ongoing research is being applied to the field of itch, and multiple potential itch pathways have been proposed, including receptor activations of TRPV1, opioid receptors, 5-HT, histamine receptors, GABA receptors, neurokinin-1, TRPA1, and others.[45]

Frequently administered to patients with liver disease and hypoprothrombinemia, *vitamin K cutaneous reactions*, although rare, may occur after subcutaneous, intramuscular, or intravenous administration. Large, erythematous, indurated, and pruritic plaques occur within a few days to a few weeks. These reactions may be a delayed hypersensitivity reaction, in that dermal testing can reproduce the reactions. When tested, patients have been found to be allergic to the vitamin K not the benzyl alcohol vehicle. However, vitamin K$_3$ (Synkayvite), which is water-soluble, has not been reported to cause similar reactions. If reactions occur after buttock injections of vitamin K, there is an almost diagnostic tendency of these plaques to spread around the waist and down the thigh, reproducing what has been called a "cowboy gun belt and holster" pattern. These reaction sites resolve over days to weeks but may persist for months to years. After an erythematous reaction, or without prior reaction, expanding sclerotic plaques with violaceous borders similar to those of morphea have occurred months to years after injections. The latter pattern usually occurs after large parenteral doses of vitamin K. In addition to these local reactions, anaphylaxis after intravenous administration that may be fatal may occur.

The association between *polyarteritis nodosa* and hepatitis B is well documented. Urticaria and serum sickness classically occur in patients with hepatitis B, although both have been reported in association with hepatitis C (see Chapters 79 and 80). Chronic hepatitis C virus is associated with leukocytoclastic vasculitis with cryoglobulinemia. Petechiae and palpable purpura are noted on the skin.

Porphyria cutanea tarda (PCT) is a disorder of porphyrin metabolism characterized by skin fragility, blisters, hypertrichosis, and hyperpigmentation in sun-exposed skin (Fig. 25.18). PCT is the most common form of porphyria and is characterized by a deficiency of uroporphyrinogen decarboxylase. Diagnosis is typically made with a 24-hour urine collection demonstrating elevated uroporphyrin levels. Alcohol consumption, estrogens,

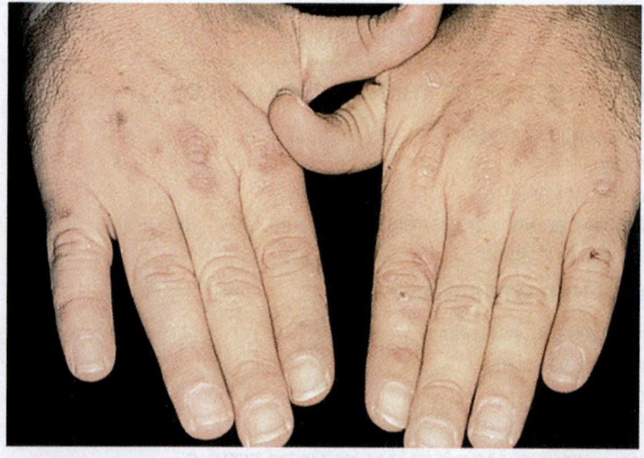

Fig. 25.18 Porphyria cutanea tarda characterized by noninflammatory blisters and erosions of the dorsa of the hands. Affected patients are frequently infected with HCV. (Courtesy Dr. Timothy Berger, San Francisco, CA.)

iron, and sunlight all are known to exacerbate PCT. There is a clear and substantial link between PCT and hepatitis C.[46] The prevalence of hepatitis C in patients with PCT demonstrates regional variation, ranging from 65% in Southern Europe and North America to 20% in Northern Europe and Australia.[47] Treatment involves phlebotomy and antimalarial agents. Antiviral treatment has demonstrated that HCV clearance promotes the resolution of PCT lesions and decreases urinary porphyrins.[48]

LP is a common idiopathic inflammatory disorder that can affect skin, hair, mucous membranes, and nails (see earlier). The prototypical presentation of LP is violaceous, polygonal, and flat-topped papules of flexural areas of the wrists, arms, and legs. The papules often have an overlying reticulated white scale known as *Wickham striae*. An association between LP and hepatitis C exists but is not as prominent as the link between PCT and hepatitis C.[49]

DRUG-INDUCED LIVER DISEASE IN PATIENTS WITH SKIN DISEASE

Dermatologists frequently consult gastroenterologists for evaluation of patients who are being treated with methotrexate or retinoids, because these medications can cause acute and chronic liver disease (see Chapter 88). Methotrexate is commonly used for severe psoriasis and psoriatic arthritis but is also used for cutaneous T-cell lymphoma, connective tissue diseases such as rheumatoid arthritis, and other inflammatory disorders. Methotrexate is usually given as a single weekly dose of 10–25 mg but may be used in higher dosages in selected patients. A grading system for liver biopsies has been established and is generally followed by dermatologists, with decisions on continuation or discontinuation of treatment frequently based on the results of these biopsies (Table 25.2).[50] Latest consensus guidelines from the American Academy of Dermatology recommend less frequent liver biopsies than those previously prescribed and no longer suggest pretreatment liver biopsies in patients without risk factors for additive hepatotoxicity (e.g., chronic alcohol use, obesity, diabetes mellitus, and active or chronic hepatitis). Notably, liver biopsy is still recommended for monitoring in psoriasis (every 3.5–4 g total cumulative dose)[51] due to the chronic liver damage caused by the inherent metabolic disorder that accompanies severe psoriasis, but a growing body of work suggests that liver elastography or other noninvasive tests may supplant the need for as many biopsies as are performed today.[52]

Retinoids (e.g., isotretinoin, acitretin, and bexarotene), derivatives of vitamin A, are currently used for the treatment of certain forms of severe psoriasis, cystic acne, and other disorders of keratinization. Regular evaluation of liver chemistry tests is required during this treatment. Mild elevations of serum triglyceride, cholesterol, ALT, and AST levels are common (20%–30% of patients treated), usually transient, or easily managed by reducing the dose. Severe or even fatal hepatitis has been reported, however. Retinoids may be used for patients with psoriasis who were previously treated with methotrexate or who have preexisting liver disease contraindicating the use of methotrexate. Limited experience suggests that these patients do not suffer the progression of their liver disease with such retinoid therapy. As with methotrexate, there is a poor correlation between liver chemistry test results and liver histology during retinoid therapy. Therefore, pretreatment and intermittent liver biopsies may be required for certain high-risk patients being chronically treated with oral retinoids.

PARASITIC DISEASES OF THE SKIN AND GASTROINTESTINAL TRACT

The larval forms of human and animal nematodes may cause migratory erythematous skin lesions called *creeping eruptions* (see Chapter 116). The most common pattern is cutaneous larva migrans, caused by dog and cat hookworms (Fig. 25.19). Pruritic linear papules migrate at a rate of 1–2 cm daily on skin sites that

TABLE 25.2 Grading System for Liver Biopsy Findings in Patients Taking Methotrexate and Guidelines for Continuation/Discontinuation of Methotrexate

Grade	Criteria	Guidelines
I	Normal, mild fatty infiltration, nuclear variability, and portal inflammation	May continue to receive methotrexate
II	Moderate-to-severe fatty infiltration; nuclear variability; portal tract expansion, portal tract inflammation, and necrosis	May continue to receive methotrexate
IIIA	Mild fibrosis (formation of fibrotic septa extending into the lobules)	May continue to receive methotrexate but should have a repeat liver biopsy after approximately 6 more months of methotrexate. Alternative therapy should be considered.
IIIB	Moderate-to-severe fibrosis	Should not administer further methotrexate. Exceptional circumstances, however, may require continued methotrexate, with follow-up liver biopsies.
IV	Cirrhosis (regenerative nodules as well as bridging of portal tracts)	Should not administer further methotrexate. Exceptional circumstances, however, may require continued methotrexate, with follow-up liver biopsies.

Modified from Roenigk HH Jr, Auerbach R, Maibach H, Weinstein GD. Methotrexate in psoriasis: revised guidelines. *J Am Acad Dermatol*. 1988;19:145–156.

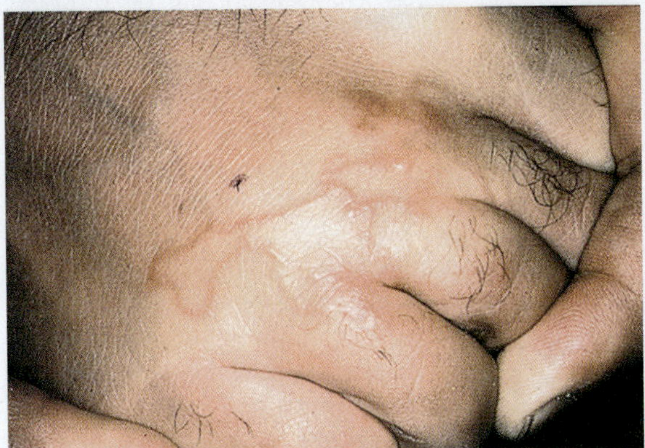

Fig. 25.19 Cutaneous larva migrans characterized by a serpiginous erythematous migratory lesion caused by an infection with dog hookworm. (Courtesy Dr. Timothy Berger, San Francisco, CA.)

have come in contact with fecally contaminated soil, usually the feet, buttocks, or back. Lesions resolve spontaneously over weeks to months. Larva currens is due to *Strongyloides stercoralis* larvae migrating in the skin. It occurs in two forms: one localized to the perirectal skin in immunocompetent hosts and another disseminated form occurring in immunosuppressed hosts. *S. stercoralis* has the unique capacity among nematodes to develop into infective larvae within the intestine. These infective larvae may invade the perirectal skin in infected immunocompetent individuals, causing urticarial, erythematous, and linear lesions that migrate up to 10 cm a day, usually within 30 cm of the anus. Skin lesions may occur intermittently, making diagnosis difficult. In immunosuppressed hosts, repeated autoinfection through the intestine leads to a tremendous parasite burden (hyperinfection), manifested most commonly by pulmonary disease. In association with hyperinfection, disseminated larva currens–type lesions may appear over the whole body, especially the trunk. Petechial or purpuric serpiginous lesions may also occur periumbilically.

Parasitic infections are classically considered in the differential diagnosis of urticaria. Except for fascioliasis and hydatid disease, however, a direct relationship with urticaria has rarely been proved. If blood eosinophilia and GI symptoms are absent, stool examination for parasites is rarely beneficial.

DERMATITIS HERPETIFORMIS AND CELIAC DISEASE

Dermatitis herpetiformis (DH) is an extremely pruritic skin disorder most commonly appearing during early adulthood (see Chapter 109). The cutaneous eruption consists of urticarial, vesicular, or bullous lesions characteristically localized to the scalp, shoulders, elbows, knees, and buttocks.[53] The disorder is so pruritic that often all the skin lesions have been excoriated, and the diagnosis must be suspected on the basis of this and the distribution (Fig. 25.20).

The diagnosis of DH is established by skin biopsy and direct immunofluorescence examination of the skin. Deposits of IgA are found in the dermal papillae at sites of itching and where vesicles are forming. Patients with DH commonly have an enteropathy indistinguishable from celiac disease (CD). Their HLA patterns, including haplotypes B8, DR3, and DQw2, intestinal malabsorption, presence of antibodies to endomysium (EMA), gliadin (AGA), and tissue transglutaminase (TG), and small bowel biopsy findings are similar to those of patients with CD. Approximately 75% of DH patients have villous atrophy in the small intestine.[53] Despite these striking similarities, fewer than 5% of patients with DH have symptomatic GI disease.

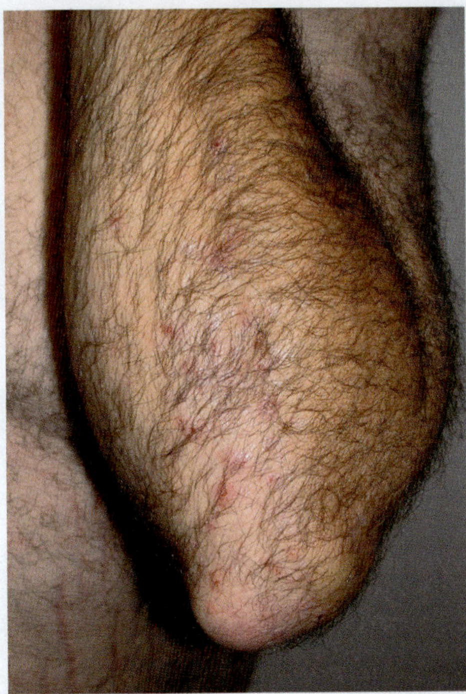

Fig. 25.20 Dermatitis herpetiformis characterized by pruritic, urticarial papules, and small blisters concentrated over the elbows, knees, and buttocks. (Courtesy Dr. Benjamin Lockshin, Silver Spring, MD.)

Gluten has been shown to be the dietary trigger of DH. Even patients with such minimal bowel disease that bowel biopsy findings are normal improve on a gluten-free diet. Reintroduction of gluten in a symptom-free patient on a gluten-free diet leads to the reappearance of pruritus and skin lesions.

A pathogenic mechanism has been proposed to explain the relationship between DH and CD. In patients with CD, IgA antibodies are produced in response to tissue TG2 that is cross-linked to deamidated gliadin peptides (derived from dietary wheat, barley, or rye and presented by HLA-DQ2 or -DQ8 molecules on antigen-presenting cells). IgA antibodies to the epidermal form of TG, TG3, are then thought to form as a result of epitope spreading, and these antibodies eventually form antigen-antibody complexes with TG3 in the papillary dermis, resulting in the clinical and pathologic findings of DH. This model would explain why DH more commonly presents at a later age than symptomatic CD, and with less severe intestinal disease, in that epitope spreading likely requires time and continued exposure to gluten.[54]

Because it is occasionally difficult to distinguish DH from other blistering skin diseases, a patient with an extremely pruritic eruption may be referred for endoscopy. The finding of an abnormal small intestine consistent with CD in a patient with a pruritic eruption would highly be suggestive of DH (see Chapter 109). The skin lesions of DH respond dramatically to sulfa drugs (dapsone or sulfapyridine), but the gut pathology and skin immunofluorescence are unchanged by sulfa drugs. Treatment with a gluten-free diet leads to gradual clearing of skin lesions, improvement of the intestinal abnormality, disappearance of the IgA from the skin, and decreased dependence on dapsone for control of the cutaneous eruption.[53]

VITAMIN AND MINERAL DEFICIENCIES

Though many vitamin deficiencies result in various skin findings (Figs. 25.21 and 25.22), those of most relevance to GI and liver

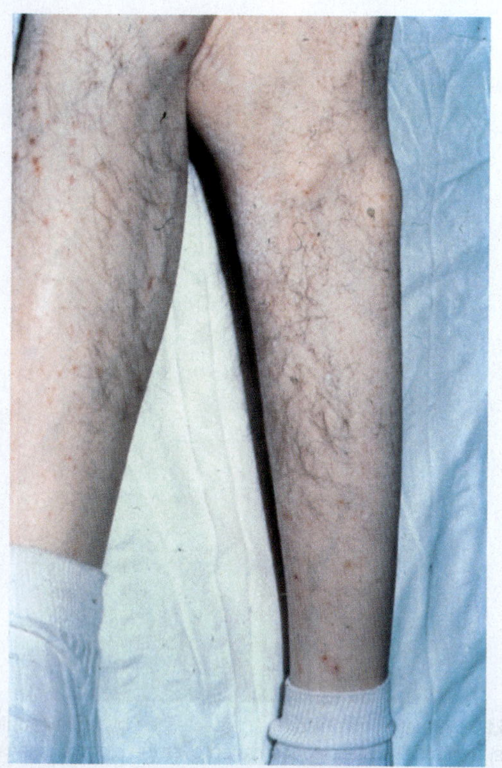

Fig. 25.21 Lower extremities of an older man with Whipple disease. Perifollicular hemorrhage is apparent. Plasma vitamin C levels were decreased. The skin lesions rapidly disappeared after vitamin C supplementation. (Courtesy Dr. Mark Feldman, Dallas, TX.)

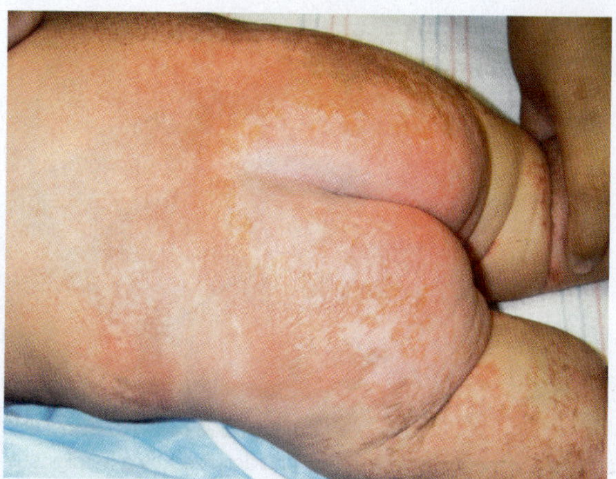

Fig. 25.22 Infant girl with acrodermatitis enteropathica secondary to nutritional zinc deficiency. She was subsisting on a diet of rice cereal and water. (Courtesy Dr. Genevieve Wallace, Dallas, TX.)

disease are summarized in Table 25.3, along with treatment algorithms[55] (also see Chapters 7 and 106).

Full references for this chapter can be found at https://ebooks.health.elsevier.com.

TABLE 25.3 Nutritional Abnormalities and Associated Skin Findings

Nutritional Abnormality	Causes	Clinical Features	Treatment
Niacin deficiency (pellagra)	Inadequate diet Medication (isoniazid) Carcinoid syndrome	Symmetrical brown-red, blistering, or scaling plaques in sun-exposed areas Glossodynia, atrophic glossitis 4 Ds: dermatitis, diarrhea, dementia, death	Nicotinic acid: *Mild:* 50 mg orally 3 times daily *Symptomatic:* 25 mg intravenously or intramuscularly 3 times daily *Advanced:* 50–100 mg intravenously or intramuscularly 3 times daily × 3–4 days, followed by oral therapy
Zinc deficiency (acrodermatitis enteropathica if genetic) Deficiency of essential fatty acids Biotin deficiency	Congenital metabolic abnormalities Alcoholics with cirrhosis Hyperalimentation without adequate supplementation Crohn's disease	Superficial scaling eruption, accentuated in groin and around the mouth Alopecia	Zinc: 1–2 mg/kg/day orally for acquired form; 3 mg/kg/day for congenital form, acrodermatitis enteropathica Biotin: 10–40 mg/day orally, intramuscularly
Vitamin C deficiency (scurvy)	Alcohol abuse Crohn's disease Whipple disease	Follicular hyperkeratosis and perifollicular hemorrhage Ecchymoses Xerosis Poor wound healing Corkscrew body hairs Gingivitis with gum hemorrhage	Ascorbic acid, 800 mg/day orally
Glucagonoma syndrome (necrolytic migratory erythema)	Glucagon-secreting neuroendocrine tumors of the pancreas Also in the setting of cirrhosis and subtotal villus atrophy of the jejunal mucosa	Intense erythema progressing to flaccid bullae and crusting with rupture Most commonly on the central face, intertriginous sites, thighs, buttocks, and distal limbs Often painful or pruritic	Surgical removal of the tumor Somatostatin analog or zinc supplementation sometimes beneficial while awaiting surgery

Modified from Nieves D, Goldsmith L. Cutaneous changes in nutritional disease. In: Freedberg I, Eisen A, Wolff F, eds. *Fitzpatrick's Dermatology in General Medicine*. New York: McGraw-Hill; 2003:1399–1412.

26 Diverticula of the Pharynx, Esophagus, Stomach, and Small Intestine

Divya B. Bhatt, D. Rohan Jeyarajah

IN THIS CHAPTER

Diverticula are outpouchings from tubular structures. True diverticula involve all layers of the intestinal wall, whereas false diverticula occur due to herniation of mucosa and submucosa through the muscular wall. Many diverticula contain attenuated portions of the muscular wall of the intestine and hence may be difficult to define as true or false. True diverticula are often assumed to be congenital lesions, whereas false diverticula are assumed to be acquired, but this is not always the case. Some authors reserve the terms *false diverticula* or *pseudodiverticula* for diverticula caused by an inflammatory process. This chapter addresses diverticula of all parts of the GI tract, except for Meckel diverticulum and colonic diverticula, which are covered in Chapters 98 and 121.

ZENKER DIVERTICULUM

A Zenker diverticulum is defined as a posterior false pulsion diverticulum that occurs superior to the cricopharyngeus muscle Ludlow first described a patient with a hypopharyngeal diverticulum in 1767, and in 1877 Zenker and Von Ziemssen reported 23 such patients.[1,2]

Epidemiology, Etiology, and Pathophysiology

The prevalence of Zenker diverticulum has been estimated to be between 0.1% and 0.01%. Patients generally present in the seventh or eighth decade of life. Twice as many men as women develop Zenker diverticula.[3,4]

Zenker diverticula are acquired. They develop when abnormally high pressures occur during swallowing, leading to mucosa that protrudes through an area of anatomic weakness in the pharynx known as *Killian triangle* (see Chapter 43). Killian triangle is located posteriorly where the transverse fibers of the cricopharyngeus muscle of the upper esophageal sphincter (UES) intersect with the oblique fibers of the inferior pharyngeal constrictor muscle. The size of this area of weakness varies among individuals. Relatively large defects may predispose to the development of Zenker diverticula.[4]

A Zenker diverticulum can form when the opening of the UES is impaired, generating high pressures with swallowing. In addition, several pathophysiologic changes, such as inflammation and fibrosis of the cricopharyngeus, can cause abnormal relaxation.[5,6] These changes lead to a reduction in compliance and decreased opening of the UES.[3] The main pathophysiology is the pulsion of the mucosa above a relative high-pressure zone, similar to epiphrenic diverticula that occur with LES hypertension (see below). Other types of similar diverticula, in appearance to Zenker diverticulum, have been reported as a complication of anterior cervical spine surgery.[7,8] Killian-Jamieson diverticula have a similar presentation to Zenker diverticulum but occur just inferior to the cricopharyngeus muscle.[9]

Clinical Features and Diagnosis

Common presenting symptoms are listed in Box 26.1, with dysphagia and regurgitation as the most frequent complaints. Patients with small diverticula may be asymptomatic. In some patients, *Boyce sign*, a palpable nodule or swelling on the left anterior neck that may gurgle on palpation, can be found.[10]

Zenker diverticulum should be suspected after obtaining a careful history. Barium swallow is the most useful diagnostic study. The radiologist should be alerted in advance so that proper views are taken (Fig. 26.1A; see also Chapter 43). Small diverticula may be seen only transiently. Barium swallow in the lateral view, using video fluoroscopy, is helpful for detecting small diverticula. The opening of a large Zenker diverticulum often becomes aligned with the axis of the esophagus and therefore may be obscured unless an oblique film is obtained. Oral contrast will preferentially fill the diverticulum and empty slowly from it. Large diverticula are therefore often obvious, even on delayed images. Zenker diverticulum occurs more often on the left side of the neck.

Zenker diverticulum may be discovered incidentally during barium swallow or upper endoscopy (see Fig. 26.1B), performed

BOX 26.1 Presenting Symptoms in Patients with a Zenker Diverticulum

Aspiration
Choking
Dysphagia
Halitosis
Regurgitation
Voice changes
Weight loss

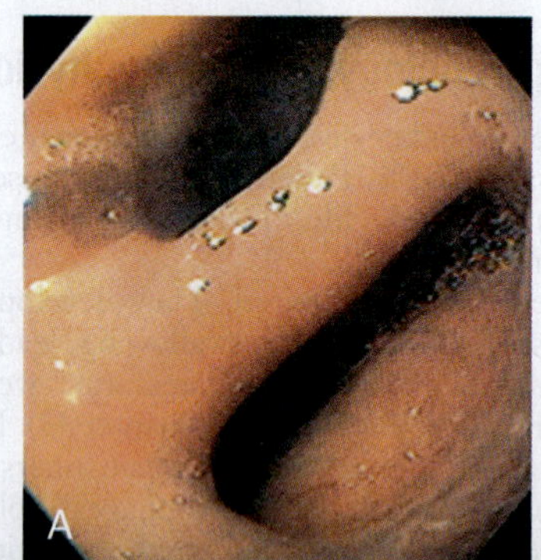

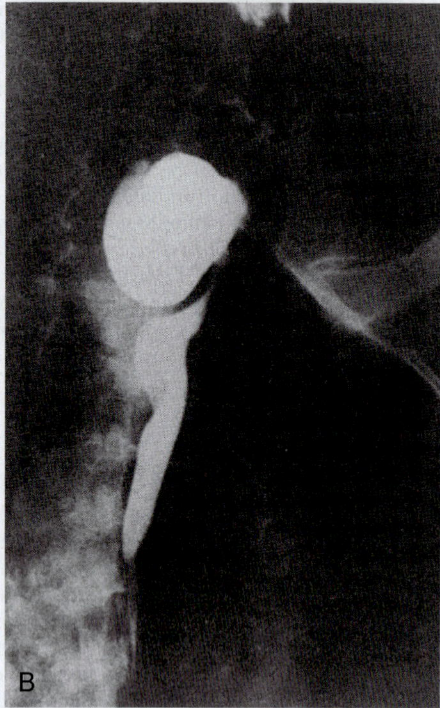

Fig. 26.1 Zenker diverticulum. (A) Barium esophagogram showing a diverticulum large enough to cause esophageal obstruction when it fills. (B) Endoscopic view. It is often difficult to distinguish the lumen of the esophagus from the lumen of the diverticulum. ((A) Courtesy of the late Dr. David Langdon; (B) Courtesy Dr. Charles E. Pope, Seattle, WA.)

to investigate unrelated problems. When evaluating patients with symptoms suspicious for the presence of a Zenker diverticulum, consider obtaining a barium swallow prior to endoscopic evaluation. During endoscopy, upon entering the pharynx, a Zenker diverticulum should be suspected if the UES cannot be easily located. In such cases, the endoscopy should be stopped, and a barium swallow performed.

Complications

Squamous cell cancer may develop in a Zenker diverticulum; the estimated incidence is 0.4%–1.5%.[3,11] If myotomy without diverticulectomy is planned, it is prudent to carefully inspect the lining of the diverticulum for any evidence of cancer.

Bleeding may occur from ulcerated Zenker diverticulum.[12] Aspiration of retained food contents may lead to aspiration pneumonia.[13,14] Medications may become lodged in Zenker diverticulum and can cause ulceration and pain, as well as decreased medication effectiveness.[15,16] Because a Zenker diverticulum is occasionally palpable on physical exam, it can be difficult to distinguish from a large thyroid nodule, and accumulation of radioactive iodine tracer in a Zenker diverticulum has been reported to lead to erroneous diagnosis of metastatic thyroid cancer.[17] The video capsules used for capsule endoscopy may also become lodged in Zenker diverticulum and should be delivered into the stomach with an endoscope when such studies are required.[18]

Intubation of the trachea or the esophagus may be complicated by the presence of a Zenker diverticulum. A large diverticulum displaces the lumen of the esophagus. The tip of the intubation instrument is often directed preferentially into the diverticulum. During endoscopy, it may be difficult to distinguish the lumen of the diverticulum from the true lumen of the esophagus (see Fig. 26.1B). Endotracheal intubation, placement of a nasogastric tube, and intubation of the esophagus for upper endoscopy, endoscopic retrograde cholangiopancreatography, or transesophageal echocardiography may be difficult. Perforation can occur. Intubation of the esophagus in patients with Zenker diverticulum should be performed under direct vision. However, when a large Zenker diverticulum causes marked anatomic distortion or when intubation with a side-viewing endoscope is required, direct intubation is not prudent. In such cases, a forward-viewing endoscope can be used to pass a soft-tipped guidewire into the esophageal lumen.[19] The guidewire is then back-loaded into the endoscope, and the endoscope is advanced into the esophagus over the guidewire. An alternative technique consists of passing a forward-viewing endoscope loaded with an overtube. Once the endoscope has been passed into the esophagus, the overtube is advanced into the esophageal lumen, the forward-viewing endoscope can be withdrawn, and the side-viewing endoscope can be advanced through the overtube.[20]

Treatment and Prognosis

Patients with small asymptomatic or minimally symptomatic diverticula can be followed, because progressive enlargement is uncommon.[21,22] Patients with large and symptomatic Zenker diverticulum should be offered treatment.[22,23]

Zenker diverticulum may be treated by open surgical procedures or by transoral endoscopic techniques using rigid or flexible endoscopes. Open surgery for Zenker diverticulum is typically performed through the left neck in patients with large (>5 cm) diverticula that extend into the thorax.[24] Young patients and patients with small diverticula (<3 cm) may also be candidates for open surgery.[25] Large diverticulum can be resected (diverticulectomy), inverted, or suspended (diverticulopexy). Cricopharyngeal myotomy is the key aspect to treating this disorder; the hypertonic cricopharyngeus muscle must be divided to relieve distal obstruction. Cricopharyngeal myotomy is the key element of any intervention as this is the main impetus for the diverticulum. If diverticula are resected without myotomy, there is an increased risk of postoperative leaks and an increased frequency of recurrence.[25,26] This is due to the fact that the high-pressure zone is still present distal to the staple line of the diverticulectomy. Complications of open surgery include anastomotic leaks, mediastinitis, esophagocutaneous fistula, and vocal cord paralysis from injury to the recurrent laryngeal nerve, which runs in the tracheoesophageal groove. One review of 22 research studies, including 1793 patients who underwent open surgery for Zenker diverticulum, found an initial success rate of 96%, a morbidity rate of 11%, a 5% perforation or leak rate, and a 3.5% symptom recurrence rate over a median of 36 months of follow-up.[23]

Endoscopic treatment of Zenker diverticulum can be performed using a rigid endoscope or flexible endoscope, with a division of the fibrotic septum between the esophagus and the diverticulum.[25,27] Compared with open surgical approaches, endoscopic approaches are associated with shorter anesthesia times, reportedly lower complication rates, and shorter hospital stays. Endoscopic techniques are suitable for patients with medium-sized diverticula (2–5 cm). Rigid diverticuloscopes and flexible endoscopes have been used. The diverticuloscope provides a visualization of the lumen of the esophagus and diverticulum and the septum between them (Fig. 26.2). This septum is composed of the posterior wall of the esophagus and the anterior wall of the diverticulum and includes the UES. The muscular layers of this septum (and UES) are incised, restoring a single lumen.

The incision can be performed by several techniques. With a rigid diverticuloscope, the incision can be made using a CO_2 laser, surgical stapling, argon plasma coagulation, electrocautery, or harmonic scalpel.[22,25] Stapling is performed by placing one leg of the stapler in the esophagus and the other into the diverticulum. The septum is then divided and stapled with two rows of staples on each side of the division line. The Zenker diverticulum must be at least 3 cm in length to be able to seat the stapler. However, modified staplers and other techniques may improve results in short diverticulum.[28] Complications of rigid endoscopic procedures include bleeding, perforation, mediastinitis, vocal cord injury, and leaks; however, these are less common if a stapler-assisted technique is used. In a review of rigid endoscopic treatment of Zenker diverticulum, combining 11 studies of 494 patients, the median initial success rate was 95%, with a 4% rate of conversion to open surgery, a 3% rate of major morbidity, with a recurrence of symptoms in 5% over a median follow-up of 16 months.[23]

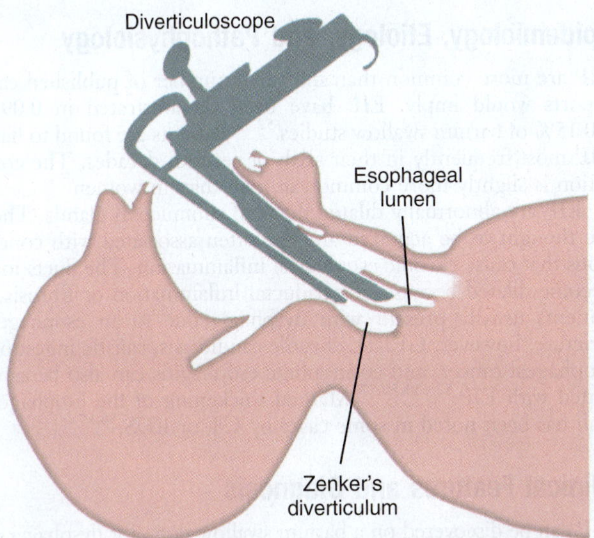

Fig. 26.2 Diverticuloscope. The instrument is positioned to expose the common wall between the lumen of the esophagus and the Zenker diverticulum.

Flexible endoscopic techniques are increasingly used to treat Zenker diverticulum, especially for patients with limited neck extension or mouth opening.[26] Transparent caps or a soft diverticuloscope may be attached to the endoscope to improve visualization.[29–31] A variety of techniques can be used to perform the endoscopic myotomy, including needle knife, argon plasma coagulation, monopolar forceps, or harmonic scalpel.[22,29] Endoscopic through-the-scope clips can be used to close defects and prevent delayed perforations.[30] Complications of flexible endoscopic techniques are similar to those of rigid endoscopic procedures; however, recurrence is more likely after flexible endoscopic techniques.[31] In a review of 20 studies of flexible endoscopic treatment of 813 patients with Zenker diverticulum, the initial success rate was 91%, with an 11% adverse event rate, and an 11% recurrence rate after a median of 23 months of follow-up.[32] Flexible endoscopic treatment of Zenker diverticulum can be performed by highly trained surgeons and endoscopists (Video 26.1).[4]

DIVERTICULA OF THE ESOPHAGEAL BODY

Diverticula of the esophageal body are most commonly located in the middle or lower third of the esophagus (Fig. 26.3).

Epidemiology, Etiology, and Pathophysiology

Estimates of the frequency of esophageal body diverticula vary from a prevalence of 0.015% seen on autopsy to 2% in patients referred to for a radiologic evaluation of swallowing disorders.[33,34] These diverticula can be divided into two types: *traction* and *pulsion diverticula*. Traction diverticula are related to an inflammatory, fibrotic, or neoplastic process outside of the esophagus. Traction diverticula are often related to mediastinal inflammation associated with tuberculosis or histoplasmosis.[35] Enlarged mediastinal lymph nodes from lung malignancies or inflammatory conditions, such as sarcoidosis, can also lead to traction diverticula. Pulsion diverticula are typically caused by motility disorders.

The most common type of pulsion diverticulum is an *epiphrenic diverticulum*, which is located near the diaphragmatic hiatus (Fig. 26.4). About 80% of epiphrenic diverticula are associated with esophageal motility disorders, such as achalasia or distal esophageal spasm, which are discussed in Chapter 45.[36,37] Epiphrenic diverticula have been reported as a complication of band-based obesity surgery, due to an obstruction of the esophagus and upper stomach by the band (see Chapter 8).[38,39] Congenital bronchopulmonary-foregut malformations can also present with esophageal diverticula.[40]

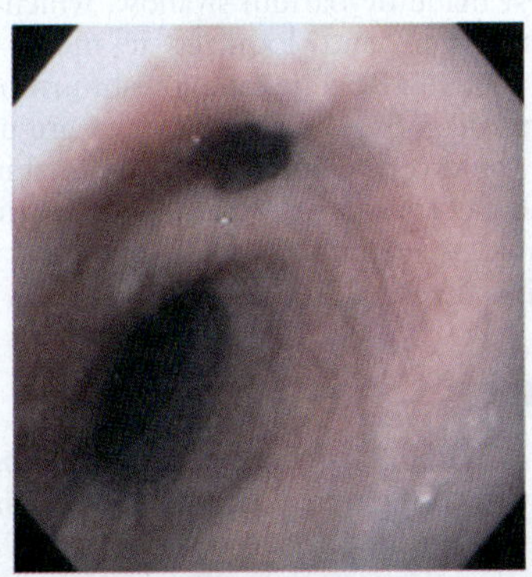

Fig. 26.3 Endoscopic view of a midesophageal diverticulum. These diverticula are most apparent when the esophagus is well-insufflated.

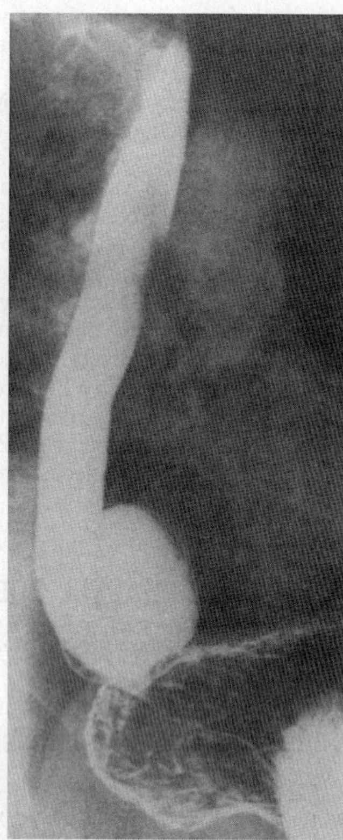

Fig. 26.4 Barium esophagogram showing an epiphrenic diverticulum immediately above the stomach. In this projection, the diverticulum may be confused with a hiatal hernia. (Courtesy Dr. Charles A. Rohrmann and Dr. Charles E. Pope, Seattle, WA.)

Clinical Features and Diagnosis

Congenital and traction diverticula of the esophagus are usually asymptomatic, particularly when located in the mid and lower esophagus. If symptoms are not present at diagnosis, they rarely occur during follow-up. When symptoms occur, the most common are dysphagia, food regurgitation, reflux, weight loss, and chest discomfort.[41] Dysphagia is typically caused by an underlying motility disorder. Less commonly, preferential filling of the diverticulum leads to an extrinsic compression of the esophagus, causing dysphagia.[36,37,42] Bronchopulmonary-foregut fistulas can develop, leading to cough, pneumonia, and recurrent bronchopulmonary infections.[43] Diagnosis of epiphrenic diverticula can be made during endoscopy or barium radiography. An epiphrenic diverticulum may be mistaken for a diaphragmatic hernia or duplication cyst on chest radiography. Endoscopy may show an empty diverticulum or the presence of food debris (Fig. 26.5A). Diagnosis is best made by barium swallow, which serves to visualize the diverticulum and localizes it more precisely than endoscopy (see Fig. 26.5B). The radiologist must be alerted to the possibility of this diagnosis, as oblique views are usually required to demonstrate the diverticulum. Cross-sectional imaging such as CT should also be considered to evaluate for mass lesions or associated pathologic adenopathy that might be the underlying cause of a pulsion diverticulum.

Complications

Squamous cell carcinoma has been reported in epiphrenic diverticula.[44,45] As with Zenker diverticulum, accumulation of radioactive iodine tracer in esophageal diverticula has been mistaken for metastatic thyroid cancer.[46] Bleeding from an ulcerated esophageal diverticulum has been reported.[47] Regurgitation and aspiration of the contents of the diverticulum may complicate induction of anesthesia. Perforation is possible during nasogastric intubation or UGI endoscopy. As mentioned above, fistulization can rarely occur.

Treatment and Prognosis

Asymptomatic diverticula of the esophagus require no treatment. Only patients with symptoms clearly related to their diverticula should be treated. If surgical treatment is planned, preoperative endoscopy and manometry are advisable. A diagnosis of achalasia or distal esophageal spasm is helpful for guiding treatment, even though passing a manometry catheter beyond the diverticulum may be challenging.[48] Surgical treatment of esophageal diverticula can be performed by laparoscopic, combined laparoscopic-thoracoscopic, or robotic techniques.[49,50] Rarely, open surgery is needed in cases when a minimally invasive approach is not technically feasible. It must be understood that the symptoms are usually related to the underlying motility disorder and not the diverticulum itself. Therefore, treating the underlying condition, usually with myotomy, is the key component of surgery. Epiphrenic diverticula are often amenable to a laparoscopic approach, which has the advantages of a shorter hospital stay and a quicker return to normal activities (see Fig. 26.5C). Large diverticula may be inverted or resected. Given the high prevalence of associated motility disorders such as achalasia or a hypertonic LES, esophageal myotomy is performed in most cases.[41,49] Small diverticula can be treated by myotomy without resection. The advantage to forgoing the diverticulectomy is that there is no staple line to heal, decreasing the risk of a leak. To prevent gastroesophageal reflux after myotomy, a partial posterior (Toupet) or anterior (Dor) fundoplication may be performed.[41,49] More recently, per-oral endoscopic myotomy has also been used to treat esophageal diverticula (see Chapter 43). The prognosis for patients who undergo intervention for esophageal diverticula is good, with rates of symptom improvement of 88.5%, and even better response rates when diverticulectomy is performed.[49]

ESOPHAGEAL INTRAMURAL PSEUDODIVERTICULA

Esophageal intramural pseudodiverticula (EIP) were first described in 1960.[51] The pseudodiverticula are flask-shaped outpouchings from the lumen of the esophagus, ranging in size from 1 to 4 mm.

Epidemiology, Etiology, and Pathophysiology

EIP are more common than the small number of published case reports would imply. EIP have been demonstrated in 0.09%–0.15% of barium swallow studies.[52,53] Patients are found to have EIP most frequently in their sixth or seventh decades. The condition is slightly more common in men than in women.[54]

EIP are abnormally dilated ducts of submucosal glands. They are thought to be acquired and are often associated with conditions that cause chronic esophageal inflammation. The ducts may become dilated because of periductal inflammation or fibrosis.[55] Patients usually present with dysphagia due to an esophageal stricture; however, GERD, chronic candidiasis, caustic ingestion, esophageal cancer, and eosinophilic esophagitis can also be associated with EIP.[52–54,56,57] Marked thickening of the esophageal wall has been noted in some cases by CT or EUS.[58,59]

Clinical Features and Diagnosis

EIP can be discovered on a barium swallow done for dysphagia or heartburn (Fig. 26.6A). EIP may also be an incidental finding in patients without related symptoms. The esophageal pseudodiverticula are localized in 60% of cases but can be diffusely scattered

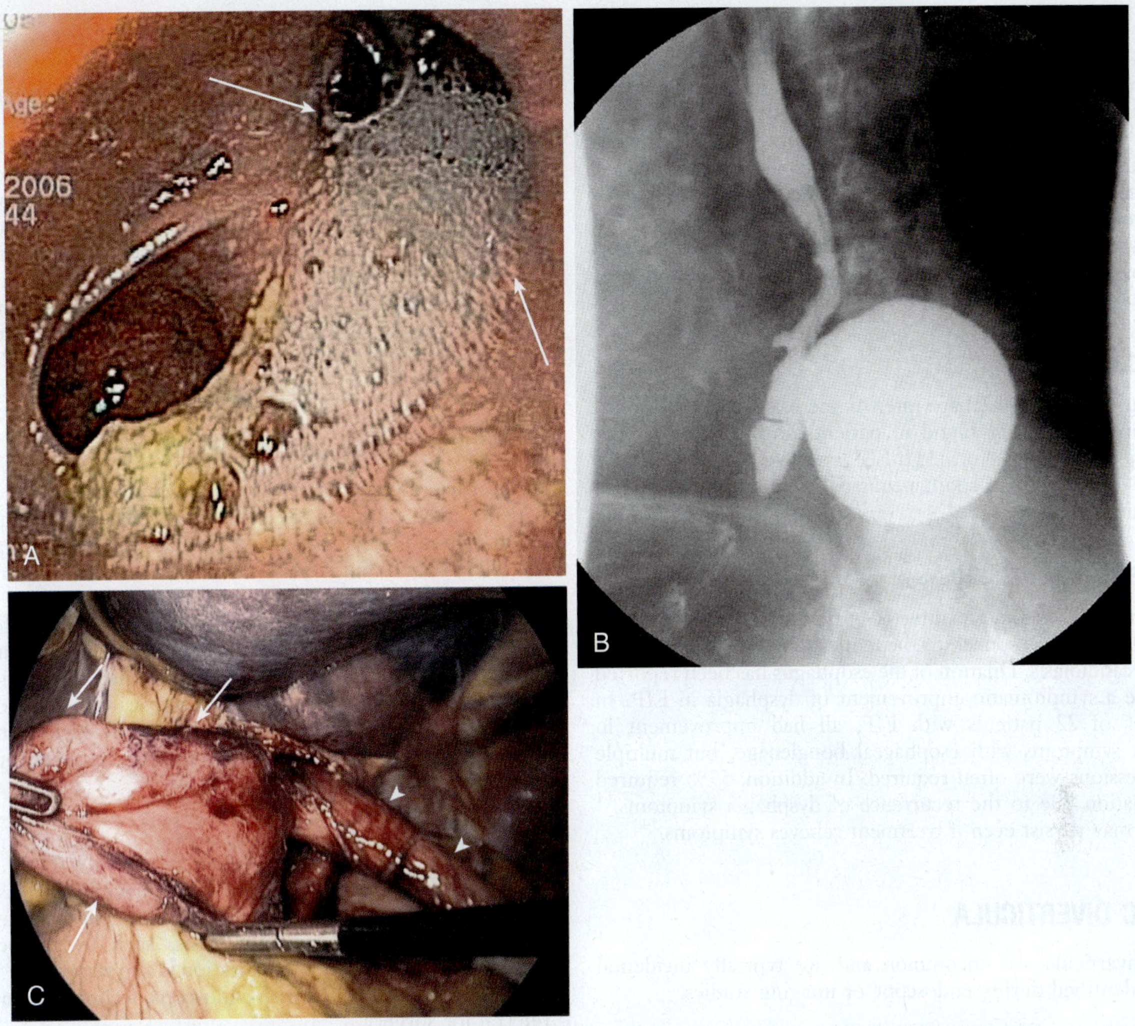

Fig. 26.5 Giant esophageal diverticulum. (A) Endoscopic view of a large esophageal diverticulum with food and liquid (*arrows*). (B) Barium esophagogram showing a large esophageal diverticulum. (C) Laparoscopic resection of a large diverticulum (*arrows*) of the esophagus (*arrowheads*). ((B and C) Courtesy Dr. Thai Pham, Dallas, TX.)

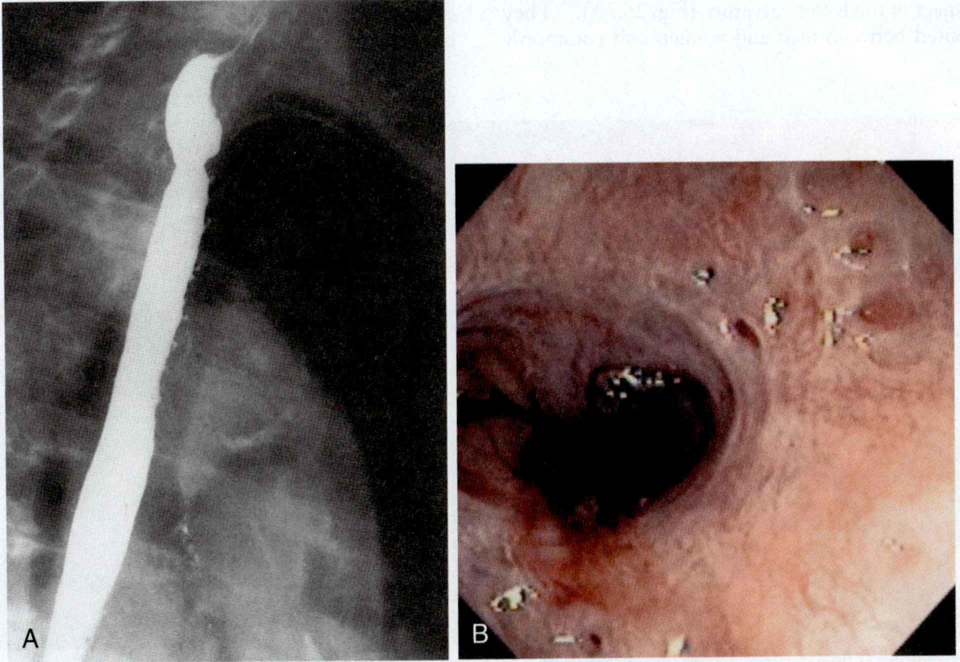

Fig. 26.6 Esophageal intramural pseudodiverticula. (A) Barium esophagogram showing numerous small outpouchings. (B) Endoscopic view. Tiny openings of the pseudodiverticula are seen in this patient, who also has a distal esophageal peptic stricture.

throughout the esophagus.[54] Strictures are common, and tracking or communication between adjacent pseudodiverticula can also occur.[60,61] The differential diagnosis on barium swallow examination includes esophageal ulceration. Although the endoscopic appearance of EIP is characteristic (see Fig. 26.6B), the openings of EIP are small and are often missed. EIP located within an area of stricture are particularly difficult to appreciate during endoscopy. Symptoms are generally related to the associated condition, such as stricture or candidiasis, rather than to the EIP.

Complications

Complications due to EIP are rare. As increased rates of esophageal cancer have been found in patients with EIP, an upper endoscopy should be performed if EIP is suspected.[52] There have been rare case reports of spontaneous EIP perforation leading to mediastinitis.[62,63]

Treatment and Prognosis

Treatment of EIP should be directed at the underlying condition, such as eosinophilic esophagitis, benign esophageal stricture, acid reflux, or candidiasis. Dilation of the esophagus has been reported to provide a symptomatic improvement of dysphagia in EIP. In one series of 22 patients with EIP, all had improvement in dysphagia symptoms with esophageal bougienage, but multiple dilation sessions were often required. In addition, 57% required repeat dilation due to the recurrence of dysphagia symptoms.[61] The EIP may persist even if treatment relieves symptoms.[54]

GASTRIC DIVERTICULA

Gastric diverticula are uncommon and are typically incidental findings identified during endoscopy or imaging studies.

Epidemiology, Etiology, and Pathophysiology

Gastric diverticula are found in only 0.04% of UGI x-rays and 0.02% of autopsies.[64]

Juxtacardiac diverticula make up 75% of all gastric diverticula. These are most often located near the gastroesophageal junction on the posterior aspect of the lesser curvature (Fig. 26.7A).[65] They are equally distributed between men and women and commonly occur in middle-aged patients, although cases have been reported in children and adolescents.[66] They typically range in size from 1 to 3 cm in diameter but are occasionally larger. Intramural or partial gastric diverticula are formed by projection of the stomach mucosa through the muscularis. These diverticula are found most commonly on the greater curvature.[67,68] Deformities caused by peptic ulcers or other inflammatory processes can resemble prepyloric diverticula on barium studies or at endoscopy (see Fig. 26.7B). Gastric diverticula have been reported as a complication of obesity surgery, particularly from vertical banded gastroplasty, although they have also been seen after Roux-en-Y gastric bypass.[69,70]

Clinical Features and Diagnosis

Juxtacardiac diverticula are almost always asymptomatic. Rarely, patients may complain of pain or dyspepsia attributable to a diverticulum. During endoscopy, juxtacardiac diverticula are best seen on a retroflexed view. They may be missed on barium study unless lateral views are taken. On CT, they may appear as air- or contrast-filled suprarenal masses and can be mistaken for an adrenal mass or cyst.[71] If fluid-filled, a gastric diverticulum can be mistaken for a pancreatic cystic lesion. The combination of air and fluid within a gastric diverticulum leads the radiologist to consider a pancreatic abscess in the differential. Intramural diverticula do not usually cause symptoms, however, but can be mistaken for ulcers on barium studies.

Complications

Complications of gastric diverticula are uncommon. Cancer has rarely been reported.[72,73] Bleeding is infrequent and may require combination therapy for hemostasis, such as hemoclips and epinephrine injection.[74,75] Perforation is also very rare.[75] Bleeding that cannot be controlled with endoscopic techniques may require referral for surgery.

Treatment and Prognosis

Intramural diverticula generally do not require intervention. Juxtacardiac diverticula almost never require treatment. A clear association with a specific symptom complex should be firmly established before considering resection, as UGI symptoms can be caused by more common diagnoses (e.g., dyspepsia and reflux)

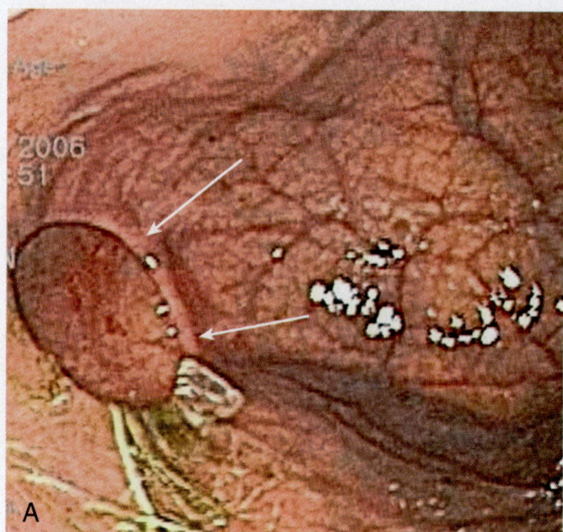

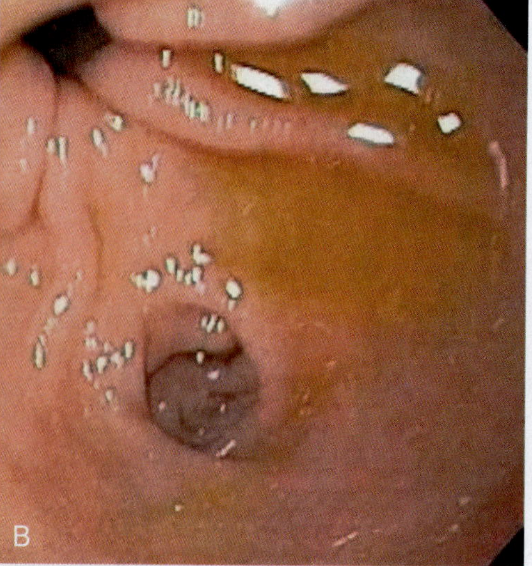

Fig. 26.7 (A) Juxtacardiac gastric diverticulum. This wide-mouthed diverticulum (*arrows*) was seen on a retroflexed view of the cardia. The mucosa within the diverticulum was normal. (B) Prepyloric gastric diverticulum.

and can be treated with acid suppression. If a patient with a juxtacardiac diverticulum is referred to for surgery, it may be prudent to place an endoscopic tattoo near the diverticulum, to assist with localization during surgery. For symptomatic management or in the case of perforation, simple resection can be performed via laparoscopic diverticulectomy.[76] During diverticulectomy, the stomach is mobilized laparoscopically and the diverticulum is stapled, leaving the majority of the stomach intact. In cases where there is a broad-based diverticulum, the surgeon will generally try to perform a sleeve-type resection rather than a gastrojejunostomy. Proximal diverticula near the esophagogastric junction are handled with care; the placement of a bougie while stapling can help avoid narrowing of the gastroesophageal junction. Laparoscopic diverticulectomy is considered a safe and feasible option for symptomatic gastric diverticula.[76]

DUODENAL DIVERTICULA

Duodenal diverticula can be extraluminal or intraluminal.

Extraluminal Diverticula

Epidemiology, Etiology, and Pathophysiology

Extraluminal duodenal diverticula are noted in about 5% of UGI x-rays and seen in roughly 20%–30% of ERCP studies.[77,78] They are thought to be acquired and are typically seen in patients older than age 50.[78] They arise in an area of the duodenal wall where a vessel penetrates the muscularis or where the dorsal and ventral pancreas fuse in embryologic development. About 75% are located within 2 cm of the ampulla, on the medial wall of the duodenum, and are termed *juxtapapillary diverticula* (JPD) (Fig. 26.8A).

Clinical Features and Diagnosis

Duodenal diverticula are sometimes diagnosed on UGI x-rays. They can be missed on endoscopy unless a side-viewing endoscope is used. A duodenal diverticulum may be mistaken for a pancreatic pseudocyst, peripancreatic fluid collection, pancreatic abscess, cystic pancreatic neoplasm, hypermetabolic mass, or distal bile duct stone on various imaging modalities (ultrasonography, CT, MRI, or PET-CT).[79–83]

Especially on cross-sectional imaging, a duodenal diverticulum can appear similar to a pancreatic cystic neoplasm. If a diverticulum is suspected on CT or MRI, the diagnosis can be clarified by having the patient drink water and repeating the scan, or by using negative contrast agents during MRI.[84,85]

Complications

Although extraluminal duodenal diverticula are relatively common, complications are rare. Complications associated with extraluminal duodenal diverticula include perforation, diverticulitis, bleeding, acute pancreatitis, and bile duct stones.[77,86–88] Rarely, a periampullary duodenal diverticulum filled with debris can obstruct the bile duct in the absence of bile duct stones or tumor, leading to cholangitis (Lemmel syndrome).[88] Duodenal diverticulitis may also present as a free or contained perforation. Patients present with pain in the upper abdomen, often radiating to the back, and may have signs and symptoms of sepsis. An abdominal CT scan may reveal thickening of the duodenum, retroperitoneal air, phlegmon, or abscess.

Bleeding has been reported from Dieulafoy-like lesions or ulcers within duodenal diverticula.[89,90] Bleeding from duodenal diverticula may be very difficult to diagnose, requiring examination with a side-viewing endoscope or angiography. In some patients, the site of bleeding is discovered only at the time of surgery.

Patients with multiple duodenal diverticula may develop bacterial overgrowth and malabsorption (see Fig. 26.8B) (see Chapters 104 and 105).[91] JPD have been associated with bile duct stones, cholangitis, sphincter of Oddi dysfunction (see Chapter 63), and recurrent pancreatitis, thought to be caused by an abnormal entrance of the pancreatic duct into the diverticulum.[77,92–95] Delayed emptying of the bile duct may occur, even after sphincterotomy. Stasis within diverticula can result in bacterial overgrowth, leading to bile salt deconjugation and increasing the risk of primary bile duct stones.[77,96]

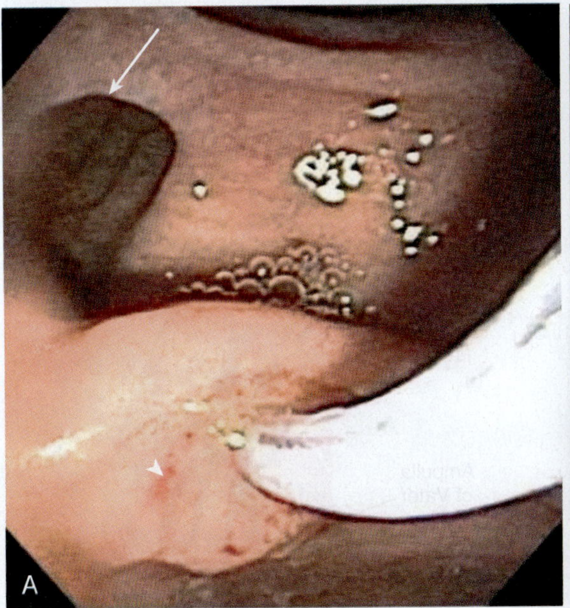

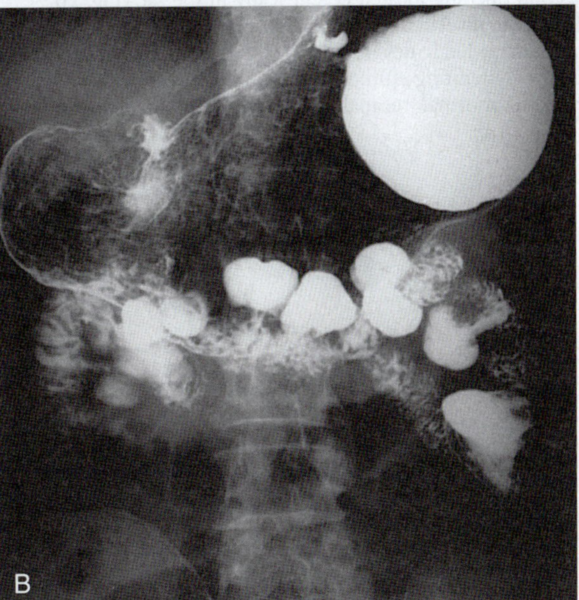

Fig. 26.8 (A) Juxtapapillary diverticulum identified during ERCP (*arrow*). A sphincterotome is inserted into the nearby ampulla (*arrowhead*). (B) Upper GI radiograph showing multiple large duodenal diverticula. ((A) Courtesy Dr. Zeeshan Ramzan, Dallas, TX.)

JPD can increase the difficulty of cannulation or the risk of complications during ERCP, even when performed by experienced therapeutic endoscopists.[78,97] However, several techniques have been described to overcome difficulties associated with an ampulla situated deep within a diverticulum.[78,97]

Treatment and Prognosis

Extraluminal duodenal diverticula rarely require therapeutic intervention. Resection of duodenal diverticula should never be performed for vague abdominal complaints.

Bleeding, diverticulitis, and perforation are the most common problems associated with duodenal diverticula. Endoscopic control of bleeding from diverticula has been accomplished using various techniques, including bipolar cautery, epinephrine injection, and hemoclips.[89,90,98] If the diagnosis is not made preoperatively, arterial embolization can be performed in select cases. Definitive surgical control of bleeding can be accomplished through a duodenotomy.

Some patients with duodenal perforation or diverticulitis may require surgery for diagnosis and treatment including drainage and resection of the involved diverticulum. However, stapling of a medially perforated duodenal diverticulum can result in occlusion of both the bile duct and the pancreatic duct and can result in pancreatic duct leaks, complications from pancreatitis, and even death. If the diagnosis of duodenal diverticulitis is made preoperatively, conservative therapy with percutaneous drainage and antibiotics is preferred.[87] Whipple procedure is a last resort and may be required in a patient with inadvertent transection of the bile duct and pancreatic duct at time of diverticulectomy.

Intraluminal Diverticula

Epidemiology, Etiology, and Pathogenesis

Intraluminal duodenal diverticula are very rare. Most patients present between the ages of 30 and 60, with men and women equally affected.[99] Intraluminal duodenal diverticula (windsock diverticula) are single saccular structures that originate in the second portion of the duodenum. They are connected to the entire circumference or only to part of the wall of the duodenum and may project as far distally as the fourth part of the duodenum. There is often a second opening located eccentrically in the sac (Fig. 26.9). Both sides of the diverticulum are lined by duodenal mucosa.

During early fetal development, the duodenal lumen is occluded by proliferating epithelial cells and later recanalized (see Chapter 49). Abnormal recanalization may lead to a duodenal diaphragm or web. Over time, peristaltic stretching may transform the diaphragm into an intraluminal diverticulum.

Clinical Features and Diagnosis

Intraluminal diverticula are often asymptomatic but may become symptomatic at any age. The most common symptoms are those of incomplete duodenal obstruction, including nausea, vomiting, and abdominal pain.[99] The typical radiographic appearance is that of a barium-filled globular structure of variable length, originating in the second portion of the duodenum, with its fundus extending into the third portion and outlined by a thin radiolucent line. The CT appearance has been reported as a ring-like soft tissue density in the lumen of the second portion of the duodenum, outlined with oral contrast and containing oral contrast and a small amount of air (halo sign).[100]

At endoscopy, an intraluminal diverticulum is a sac-like structure with an eccentric aperture or a large, soft, polypoid mass if the diverticulum is inverted orad.[101,102] Endoscopic diagnosis may be difficult. A long sac may be mistaken for the duodenal lumen, whereas an inverted diverticulum may be mistaken for a large polyp.

Complications

Obstruction may be precipitated by the retention of vegetable material or foreign bodies within the diverticulum, which commonly include food and less commonly coins or marbles.[103–105] Pancreatitis and bleeding have also been reported.[92,101] Gastric retention or dilation of the duodenal bulb may result from chronic partial obstruction caused by the diverticulum.

Treatment and Prognosis

Treatment may include resection in patients with symptoms of obstruction or bleeding, which can be performed laparoscopically.[99] Successful endoscopic resection of intraluminal duodenal diverticula has also been reported.[106]

JEJUNAL DIVERTICULA

In 1881, Sir William Osler wrote about a patient with jejunal diverticula who, for years, "had suffered much from loud rumbling noises in his belly, particularly after each meal. So loud were they that it was his habit, shortly after eating, to go out and

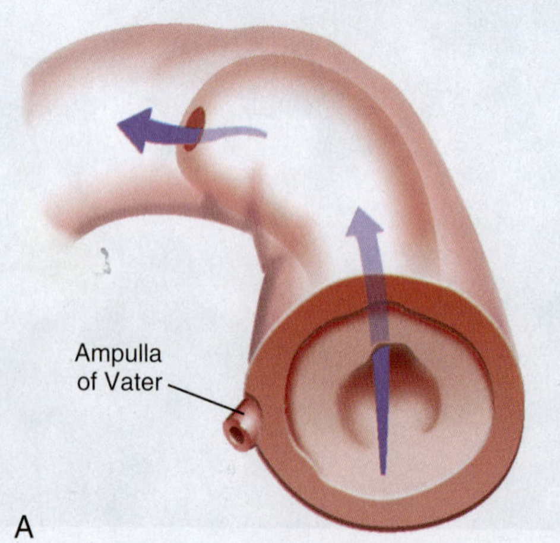

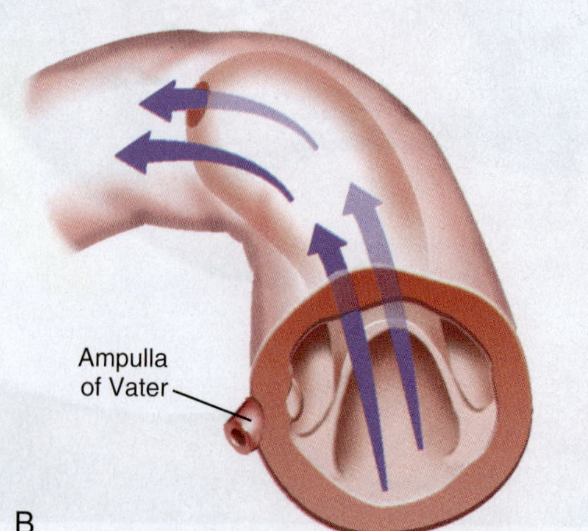

Fig. 26.9 Intramural duodenal diverticulum (windsock diverticulum). (A) Diverticulum attached to entire duodenal circumference. (B) Diverticulum attached to only part of the duodenal circumference.

take a walk to keep away from people, as the noises could be heard at some distance."[107]

Epidemiology, Etiology, and Pathophysiology

Diverticula of the small bowel (apart from duodenal and Meckel diverticula) are most commonly found in the proximal jejunum and are seen in approximately 1% of the population.[108] About 80% of jejunoileal diverticula arise in the jejunum, 15% in the ileum, and 5% in both; small bowel diverticula have been found in about 0.5%–5% of small bowel x-rays and autopsies.[109,110] They are commonly multiple and can vary from a few millimeters to several centimeters in size. They are usually located on the mesenteric border of the small bowel. Small bowel diverticula generally lack a true muscular wall and are considered acquired rather than congenital.

The cause of jejunoileal diverticula is largely unknown. Many patients have an underlying intestinal motility disorder. Periodically, elevated intraluminal pressures can lead to herniation through areas of weakness at the mesenteric border where blood vessels penetrate the muscularis. Visceral neuropathies and myopathies, including progressive systemic sclerosis, can lead to chronic atrophy and fibrosis of the intestinal wall, with resultant herniation and diverticula formation (see Chapter 37).[111]

Clinical Features and Diagnosis

Jejunal diverticula are best diagnosed by UGI radiography with small bowel follow-through or CT with oral contrast and can also be identified via small bowel enteroscopy and video capsule endoscopy.[112–115] Jejunal diverticula most commonly occur on the mesenteric border of the bowel, in contrast to Meckel diverticulum, which occur on the antimesenteric border.

Many cases of jejunoileal diverticulosis are asymptomatic or associated with nonspecific symptoms for which patients may not seek medical attention. About 40% of cases are discovered incidentally.[110] Various symptoms and clinical problems may occur with jejunal diverticula. The most common clinical features are recurrent abdominal pain, early satiety, and bloating. Loud borborygmi and intermittent diarrhea may occur; these symptoms may be caused by an underlying motility disorder.[116] Patients can present with pain related to diverticulitis, which can be difficult to diagnose. The finding of inflammation surrounding a small bowel diverticulum on cross-sectional imaging should raise the suspicion of jejunal diverticulitis.

Complications

Similar to diverticula of the colon, complications of jejunal diverticula include bleeding, diverticulitis, and perforation. Bleeding jejunal diverticula have been treated during double-balloon enteroscopy, although there is a small risk of perforation.[117–119] Malabsorption may result from associated small bowel bacterial overgrowth (see Chapters 106 and 107).[110,120] Patients with jejunal diverticulosis and severe dysmotility can develop intestinal pseudo-obstruction (see Chapter 124). Patients with intestinal pseudo-obstruction may periodically have small amounts of free intraperitoneal air (pneumoperitoneum) without overt perforation.[121] If such patients are otherwise well, they should be carefully observed. Surgical intervention is often not necessary.

Bleeding from small bowel diverticula may be difficult to localize.[117,122] If a source of bleeding is discovered in the small bowel at angiography, it may be useful to leave a small catheter within the feeding vessel if the patient requires surgical intervention. When the patient is explored, a small amount of dye can be injected through the catheter, staining the involved bowel. This may help the surgeon localize an otherwise obscure lesion. Diverticulitis may result in free perforation or an abscess contained within the mesentery.[123] The finding of an inflammatory mass in the mesentery should raise the possibility of a perforated small bowel diverticulum.[124] Because jejunal diverticula usually project into the mesentery, they can be difficult to detect, even during surgery.

Large enteroliths can form in jejunal diverticula and lead to mucosal erosion, with bleeding, diverticulitis, perforation, or intestinal obstruction.[123,125,126] Jejunal diverticulosis has also been associated with small bowel volvulus.[127]

Treatment and Prognosis

In patients with small bowel diverticulosis and suspected dysmotility, the use of oral antibiotics to treat associated bacterial overgrowth may lead to improvement in bloating and diarrhea, as well as malabsorption (see Chapters 106 and 107).[128]

Patients with bleeding, perforation, or diverticulitis who have not responded to less invasive therapies should undergo a limited surgical resection of the affected section of the bowel, However, this may be difficult to localize with precision.[123,129] In patients with symptoms of chronic intestinal pseudo-obstruction, surgery should generally be avoided, although carefully selected patients may benefit.[130] If a long segment of bowel is resected in an attempt to remove all the diverticula, the patient may be left with short bowel syndrome, which can lead to severe disability (see Chapter 106).

Full references for this chapter can be found at https://ebooks.health.elsevier.com.

27 Abdominal Hernias and Gastric Volvulus

D. Rohan Jeyarajah, Kerry B. Dunbar

IN THIS CHAPTER

A *hernia* is a protrusion of an organ or structure into an opening or pouch, usually through a structure that is meant to contain the contents of that cavity. Abdominal wall hernias protrude through the muscular and fascial walls of the abdomen and have two parts: (1) the orifice or defect in the aponeurotic wall of the abdomen, and (2) the hernia sac, which consists of peritoneum and contains abdominal contents. Abdominal wall hernias are *external* if the sac protrudes through the abdominal wall or *interparietal* if the sac is contained within the abdominal wall. *Internal hernias* are contained within the abdominal cavity and do not always have a hernia sac.

Hernias are *reducible* when the protruding contents can be returned to the abdomen and *irreducible* or *incarcerated* when they cannot. A hernia is *strangulated* when the vascular supply of the protruding organ is compromised, and, as a consequence, the organ becomes ischemic or necrotic. An incarcerated hernia is often associated with a bowel obstruction and is generally repaired because there is danger of strangulation, which can result in necrosis of the bowel. Because it can be difficult to determine whether a hernia is incarcerated or strangulated, incarcerated hernias are presumed strangulated, and treated with urgent surgical intervention. Another type of hernia is a *Richter hernia*, where only one side of the bowel (most often the antimesenteric side) protrudes through the hernia orifice. In contrast to other hernias, strangulation may occur in a Richter hernia *without* intestinal obstruction, making this type of hernia a diagnostic challenge.

DIAPHRAGMATIC HERNIAS

There are three main types of diaphragmatic hernias: hiatal and paraesophageal hernias (both involve the hiatus), congenital hernias, and traumatic hernias.

Hiatal and Paraesophageal Hernias

The most common diaphragmatic hernias are sliding hernias of the stomach through the esophageal hiatus, which include hiatal and paraesophageal hernias. Technically, all these hernias are hiatal hernias because they pass through the esophageal hiatus of the diaphragm. These are *centrally* located hernias.

Etiology and Pathophysiology

Sliding hiatal hernias (type I) occur when the gastroesophageal junction and some portion of the stomach are displaced above the diaphragm, but the orientation of the stomach axis is unchanged. The frequency of sliding hiatal hernias increases with age. The phrenoesophageal membrane normally anchors the gastroesophageal junction to the diaphragm (see Chapters 43 and 46). Hiatal hernias may be caused by age-related deterioration of this membrane, combined with normal positive intra-abdominal pressure and traction of the esophagus on the stomach as the esophagus shortens during swallowing.[1]

Paraesophageal hernias (type II) occur when the stomach protrudes through the esophageal hiatus alongside the esophagus (Fig. 27.1A). The gastroesophageal junction remains in a normal position at the level of the diaphragm, because there is preservation of the posterior phrenoesophageal ligament and normal anchoring of the gastroesophageal junction, and only the stomach moves proximally.[2] The entire stomach can pass into the chest (see Fig. 27.1B). Most paraesophageal hernias contain a sliding hiatal component, in addition to the paraesophageal component, and are thus mixed diaphragmatic hernias [type III (see Fig. 27.1C)].[3] With a paraesophageal hernia, other intra-abdominal structures (e.g., omentum, colon, spleen) may also herniate (type IV). A barium study may be obtained to evaluate for the presence of hiatal and paraesophageal hernias. However,

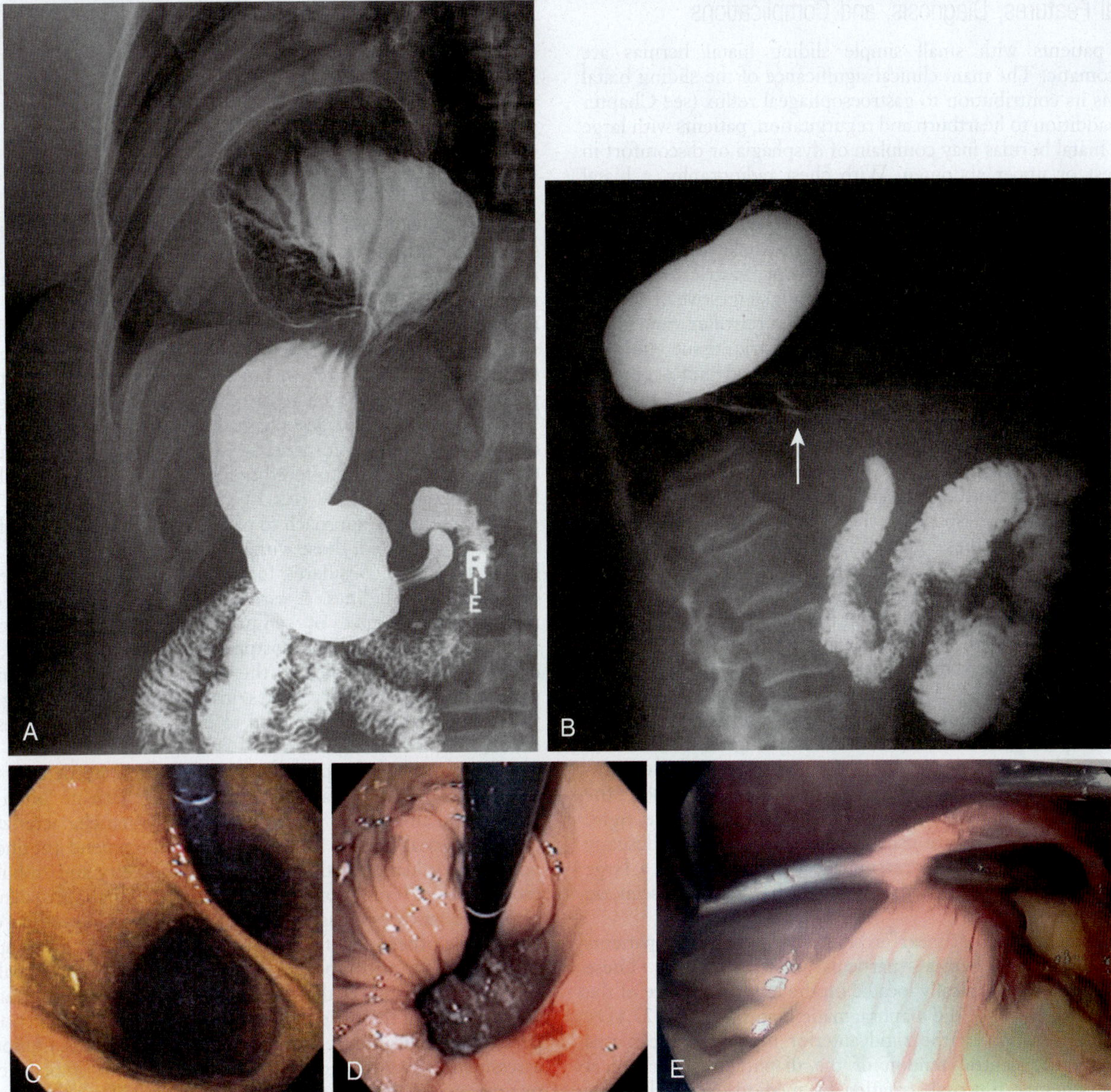

Fig. 27.1 (A) Paraesophageal (type II) hernia. Barium study showing a paraesophageal hernia with a portion of the stomach above the diaphragm. (B) This barium study showing a paraesophageal hernia complicated by an organoaxial volvulus of the stomach (see Fig. 27.5). The gastroesophageal junction remains in a relatively normal position below the diaphragm (*arrow*). (C) The retroflexed endoscopic view of the proximal stomach demonstrates the endoscope traversing a sliding hiatal hernia adjacent to a large paraesophageal hernia. (D) Cameron lesion. A large hiatal hernia is seen on endoscopic retroflexed view, with a Cameron lesion at the level of the diaphragmatic hiatus at the 5-o'clock position. (E) Laparoscopic view of a paraesophageal hernia. (B, Courtesy Dr. Herbert J. Smith, Dallas, TX.)

cross-sectional imaging with CT scan is the test of choice to document a type IV defect, as the barium study will not identify organs prolapsing through the hiatus. When diagnosing a hiatal or paraesophageal hernia, important questions for the radiologist to address include: (1) Does the gastroesophageal junction lie at or above the hiatus? (2) Does the stomach or any other visceral structure lie above the gastroesophageal junction? For example, if the gastroesophageal junction is above the hiatus and there is stomach above it, the patient has a type III (mixed) hernia. These two landmarks can help the surgeon and radiologist to be aligned in their definitions.[255]

Epidemiology

Estimates of the prevalence of hiatal hernia vary widely, ranging from 14% to 84% of patients examined, depending on the patient population, method of diagnosis, and presence of symptoms.[4–8] In general, hiatal hernias are more frequent in patients with GERD.[8] About 90%–95% of hiatal hernias found by imaging are sliding (type I) hernias; the remainder are paraesophageal hernias.[3,7] Most sliding hiatal hernias are small and of little clinical significance. Patients with symptomatic paraesophageal hernias are most often middle-aged to older adults.

Clinical Features, Diagnosis, and Complications

Many patients with small simple sliding hiatal hernias are asymptomatic. The main clinical significance of the sliding hiatal hernia is its contribution to gastroesophageal reflux (see Chapter 48). In addition to heartburn and regurgitation, patients with large sliding hiatal hernias may complain of dysphagia or discomfort in the chest or upper abdomen. With chest radiography, a hiatal hernia may appear as a soft tissue density or an air-fluid level in the retrocardiac area. Hiatal hernias can also be identified on UGI barium studies. CT can demonstrate the proximal stomach above the diaphragmatic hiatus. During endoscopy, gastric folds identified proximal to the diaphragmatic pinch is suggestive of a hiatal hernia. Hiatal hernias are often identified on retroflex view in the stomach, showing a gap between the gastric tissue and the endoscope. Hiatal hernia size can be described endoscopically using the Hill grade.[256]

Patients with paraesophageal or mixed hiatal hernias are rarely completely asymptomatic if closely questioned. Many patients with paraesophageal hernias have gastroesophageal reflux, particularly those with larger paraesophageal hernias.[3,9] Other symptoms include dysphagia, chest pain, vague postprandial discomfort, and shortness of breath, and some patients will have iron deficiency anemia due to chronic GI blood loss.[9,10]

A paraesophageal or mixed hiatal hernia may be seen on a chest radiograph as an abnormal soft tissue density (often with an air bubble) in the mediastinum or left chest (see Fig. 27.1A). CT scanning can demonstrate that part of the stomach is above the diaphragm in the chest. Differences between UGI radiography and CT scan can sometimes be seen, as the latter is performed in the supine position where the stomach may migrate further into the chest. The former is usually performed with the patient upright and the stomach may reduce into the abdomen. Of note, the stomach usually migrates into the *left* chest and not the right. Paraesophageal hernias are usually obvious on upper endoscopy (see Fig. 27.1B), but the paraesophageal component of a large mixed hernia may be missed. These hernias are best seen on retroflexion.

Cameron lesions or linear erosions may develop in patients with sliding hiatal hernias, particularly large hernias. These mucosal lesions are typically located on the lesser curvature of the stomach at the level of the diaphragmatic hiatus (see Fig. 27.1D). This is the location of the rigid anterior margin of the hiatus formed by the central tendon of the diaphragm. Mechanical trauma, ischemia, mucosal irritation by medications, and peptic injury have been proposed as the cause of Cameron lesions. As the size of the hiatal hernia increases, so does the prevalence of Cameron lesions. They are identified in about 5% of patients with hiatal hernia undergoing endoscopy and approximately 30% of patients with paraesophageal hernias referred for surgical repair.[11–13] Cameron lesions may cause acute or chronic UGI bleeding with a reduced response to acid suppression therapy.[14] Iron deficiency anemia due to chronic bleeding is seen in 30%–40% of patients with paraesophageal hernia.[9,13] Paraesophageal hernia repair can be considered for treatment of occult GI bleeding and persistent iron deficiency anemia secondary to Cameron lesions or a trial of proton pump inhibitor therapy.[14] Prior to surgical repair of hiatal hernia for treatment of occult GI bleeding and iron deficiency anemia, it is important to rule out other causes for occult bleeding with a thorough gastrointestinal evaluation including colonoscopy and small bowel evaluation.

Gastric volvulus is a life-threatening complication of paraesophageal hernia. Symptoms include acute abdominal pain and retching, and it can progress rapidly to a surgical emergency (see "Gastric Volvulus"). With UGI radiography or CT, lack of filling the gastric lumen with contrast or gastric wall thickening with pneumatosis should increase suspicion for a volvulus and associated gastric necrosis.[15] Usually, a CT scan has been performed when they are evaluated in the emergency department with acute inability to swallow and vomiting. The CT will show the stomach in the chest and no further evaluation needs to be undertaken. Endoscopy may be difficult if the hernia is associated with gastric volvulus, and reaching the pylorus may be a challenge due to positioning of the stomach.[16]

Treatment and Prognosis

Simple sliding hiatal hernias do not require treatment, unless symptomatic from reflux (see Chapter 46). Patients with symptomatic large sliding hiatal hernias, paraesophageal hernias, and mixed hernias should be offered surgery. When closely questioned, most patients with type II, III, or IV hernias will have symptoms.[9,10] In the past, all paraesophageal hernias were thought to be a surgical emergency, but it is now clear that the risk of progression to gastric necrosis is lower than initially believed.[17] Elective repair of paraesophageal hernias is more frequently offered to symptomatic patients, although some experts suggest that surgery should be offered to all patients with paraesophageal hernias because of the risk of future complications.[3,9,18,19] In general, a selective approach to patients with large paraesophageal hernias is warranted; those with symptoms that may be due to the hernia should be considered for surgical intervention, depending on other comorbidities. A careful history is essential for determining the presence of symptoms. One should pay careful attention to chest pain and postprandial shortness of breath; these may be symptoms related to the paraesophageal hernia. Indeed, patients with pulmonary issues may benefit from having their paraesophageal hernias repaired to create room in the chest and decrease aspiration events.

The extent of the preoperative evaluation needed for paraesophageal hernia repair is controversial. Patients often have already had an imaging study or endoscopy that characterizes the paraesophageal hernia. Many surgeons recommend routine preoperative evaluation with esophageal manometry and ambulatory esophageal pH monitoring because of the high prevalence of associated gastroesophageal reflux and esophageal motility disorders, while others may forgo pH testing and use reflux symptoms as a guide for the type of repair chosen.[20] The rationale for omitting pH testing is that the result will not change the surgical management of the patient, who will receive hernia reduction and partial fundoplication regardless of pH testing results. Options for assessment of esophageal pH include 24-hour impedance/pH testing and 48- or 96-hour wireless capsule pH monitoring. The object of manometric evaluation is to determine whether the patient has a significant motility disorder, such as achalasia or aperistalsis, which may affect fundoplication type or whether myotomy is needed. Manometric evaluation is particularly important if the patient has dysphagia. Performing esophageal manometry can be challenging when a paraesophageal hernia is present due to anatomic distortion from the hernia.[257]

The principles of surgery for repair of hiatal or paraesophageal hernias include four main elements: (1) reduction of the hernia from the mediastinum or chest, with excision of the hernia sac; (2) reconstruction of the diaphragmatic hiatus, with simple posterior closure with or without bolstering with prosthetic mesh; (3) providing bulk at the hiatus to prevent prolapse into the chest with consideration of a fundoplication, which may lessen postoperative reflux; and (4) addition of a gastropexy or gastrostomy tube to provide an additional tacking mechanism for the stomach intra-abdominally. Minimally invasive surgical techniques (i.e., laparosocopy, robotic-assisted) are most common, although open operations performed through the abdomen or chest are occasionally performed.[3,18,21–23] Minimally invasive surgery through the abdomen leads to a shorter hospital stay, less postoperative pain, and an equivalent risk of hernia recurrence (see Fig. 27.1E).[22,23] Reduction of chronic paraesophageal hernias via the chest can be difficult and can be approached through a combined thoracoscopic and abdominal procedure. Injury to the lung can occur with vigorous traction. As the diaphragmatic defect is central (medial) rather than peripheral (lateral), lung adhesions are uncommon, as the hernia sac lines the visceral structures. Reconstruction of the diaphragm can be performed by placing nonabsorbable sutures posterior to the esophagus.[24,25] Use of prosthetic mesh has resulted in fewer recurrences in some studies.[26–28] The use of mesh is still controversial as there has been no clear long-term results demonstrating a decreased risk of hernia recurrence. However, most surgeons are wary of using synthetic mesh close to the esophagus, and therefore "biological" products are favored. The shape of the mesh is also an area of controversy. Keyhole mesh can be used, in which the esophagus is completely encircled with mesh, with the concern being dysphagia in this situation.[27,29] Alternatively, U-shaped mesh can be used, where the anterior portion is left open, therefore, reinforcing only posteriorly (the major area of recurrence). Fixation of the stomach in the abdomen is usually achieved by using a fundoplication, which provides some bolstering effect at the hiatus to keep the stomach in the abdomen and can reduce postoperative gastroesophageal reflux. Additional use of gastropexy, with suturing of the stomach to the abdominal wall, left diaphragm, or gastrostomy tube placement for 2 weeks to allow the stomach to mature to the abdominal wall, may result in fewer recurrences.[30] Newer developments in surgical management of hiatal and paraesophageal hernias include the use of impedance planimetry, which measures esophageal distensibility. Intraoperative use of impedance planimetry is being studied to guide surgical management of the LES.[258] Addition of gastropexy may reduce the recurrence rate after hernia repair.[21,30] In a recent study, crural closer with intraoperative impedance planimetry-guided fundoplication and gastropexy to the left diaphragm showed good results (manuscript in review). It is important to discuss expectations with the patient prior to surgical repair, as some symptoms may be present after surgery. For example, mild reflux symptoms may be present, which can be managed with PPIs, and this may be preferred over the presurgery symptom of dysphagia.

Patients with sliding hiatal or paraesophageal hernias may have shortening of the esophagus. This makes it difficult to restore the gastroesophageal junction below the diaphragm without tension, a key factor in decreasing recurrence. In such cases, an extra length of neoesophagus can be constructed from the proximal stomach (Collis-Nissen procedure).[31] In this situation, a stapler is fired parallel to the axis of the esophagus along a bougie that is passed into the stomach, creating a lengthened esophagus. Alternatively, transmediastinal dissection of the esophagus for more than 5 cm into the chest will usually result in adequate intra-abdominal length of esophagus without the need for additional stapling.[32] Potential surgical complications include esophageal and gastric perforation, pneumothorax, and liver laceration. Resection of the hernia sac can lead to a capnothorax, with carbon dioxide from laparoscopy present in the pleural space. This can require chest tube placement. More often, the resultant capnothorax resorbs very quickly and even a significant capnothorax can be observed for resolution. Potential long-term complications may include dysphagia if the fundoplication is too tight or gastroesophageal reflux if the fundoplication breaks down or migrates into the chest. When examined closely, radiographic recurrence after paraesophageal hernia repair is 15%–25%.[23] However, the clinical impact of a recurrence may be minimal because most of these patients remain symptom-free and do not require further treatment. The patient who develops both reflux and dysphagia after paraesophageal hernia repair should be evaluated for a symptomatic recurrence. Upper endoscopy, barium studies, and CT can be helpful in evaluation of symptom recurrence.

Recurrence of hiatal and paraesophageal hernia is higher in patients with obesity. Roux-en-Y gastric bypass (RYGB) can be considered for patients with a BMI greater than 35 kg/m^2.[33,34] Simple hernia reduction and crural closure and fundoplication patients with obesity is less successful for symptom management and hernia recurrence is more common. Referral to a surgeon with expertise in all aspects of foregut surgery, including Roux-en-Y gastrojejunostomy, is important for ideal patient outcomes. RYGB may also be needed for repair of recurrent paraesophageal hernias associated with a vagal injury and gastroparesis. Interestingly, nonobese patients with vagal injury who undergo repeat hiatal hernia repair with RYGB do not have the dramatic weight loss seen in patients with obesity who undergo RYGB.[259]

Congenital Diaphragmatic Hernias

Congenital diaphragmatic hernias (CDHs) are rare but can have significant complications. Many are diagnosed at birth.

Etiology and Pathophysiology

CDHs result from failure of fusion of the multiple developmental components of the diaphragm (Fig. 27.2). Embryologically, the diaphragm is derived from the septum transversum, which separates the peritoneal and pericardial spaces, the mesentery of the esophagus, the pleuroperitoneal membranes, and muscle of the chest wall. *Morgagni hernias* form anteriorly at the sternocostal junctions of the diaphragm, and *Bochdalek hernias* form posterolaterally at the lumbocostal junctions of the diaphragm.[35] Bochdalek hernias most commonly manifest immediately after birth and are commonly associated with pulmonary hypoplasia.

Epidemiology

CDHs occur in about 1/2000 to 1/10,000 births, with some types seen more frequently in males.[36–40] Hernias manifesting in neonates are most often Bochdalek hernias. With the routine use of prenatal ultrasound, CDHs can be discovered in the prenatal period. The presence of intra-abdominal contents in the chest during fetal development results in significant hypoplasia of the lung. It is the degree of pulmonary dysfunction, not the presence of the hernia, which determines the child's prognosis. Prenatal measures are then taken to prepare for the pulmonary hypoplasia that invariably accompanies a large CDH. Only a few Bochdalek hernias are first discovered in adulthood.[41] Bochdalek hernias occur on the left side in about 80% of cases (Fig. 27.3).[42–44] Right-

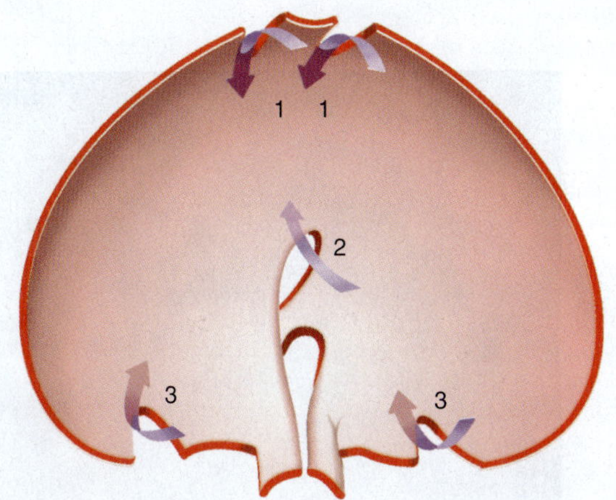

Fig. 27.2 Congenital diaphragmatic hernias. Diagram of the diaphragm viewed from below with areas of potential herniation shown. *1*, Sternocostal foramina of Morgagni anteriorly. *2*, Esophageal hiatus. *3*, Lumbocostal foramina of Bochdalek posteriorly. *Arrows* indicate the direction of herniation.

sided Bochdalek hernias usually contain liver in the right chest. Morgagni hernias make up about 2%–3% of surgically treated diaphragmatic hernias (Fig. 27.4).[45] Although thought to be congenital, they usually manifest in adults and occur on the right side in 80%–90% of cases.[46]

Clinical Features, Diagnosis, and Complications

The clinical presentation of CDHs varies greatly, from death in the neonatal period to an asymptomatic serendipitous finding in adults. Newborns with Bochdalek hernia have respiratory distress, absent breath sounds on one side of the chest, and a scaphoid abdomen.[47] Serious chromosomal anomalies are found in 30% of cases, but in many cases the exact mutation (or mutations) cannot be identified.[48] Pulmonary hypoplasia occurs on the side of the hernia, but some degree of hypoplasia may also occur in the contralateral lung. Pulmonary hypertension is common. The major causes of mortality in infants with Bochdalek hernias are respiratory failure and associated anomalies, which can include cardiac abnormalities and musculoskeletal defects.[47] Most of these neonates are diagnosed in utero with routine use of prenatal ultrasound, which visualizes stomach or loops of bowel in the chest. The pregnancy is considered high risk when CDH is diagnosed in the prenatal period. These babies are delivered electively and preparations are made for immediate extracorporeal membrane oxygenation (ECMO).

In older children and adults, a Bochdalek hernia may manifest as an asymptomatic chest mass. The differential diagnosis includes mediastinal or pulmonary cyst or tumor, pleural effusion, or empyema. Symptoms, when present, can include pain, pulmonary symptoms, and obstructive symptoms and are due to herniation of the stomach, omentum, colon, or small bowel.[44] About 30% of adult patients present with acute emergencies caused by strangulation, and gastric volvulus can occur.[44] Other patients may have chronic intermittent symptoms, including chest discomfort, shortness of breath, dysphagia, nausea, vomiting, and constipation. The diagnosis may be suspected on a chest radiograph, particularly a lateral view. The key finding is a posterior chest mass, as the defect of Bochdalek is posterior. The diagnosis may be confirmed by barium UGI radiography (useful if only the stomach is involved), CT, or MRI.[36,44]

Morgagni hernias are most likely to manifest in adult life. They may contain omentum, stomach, colon, or liver. Bowel sounds may be heard in the chest if bowel has herniated through the defect. As with Bochdalek hernias, the diagnosis is often made by chest radiography, particularly the lateral view, because Morgagni hernias are anterior, differentiating this hernia from a Bochdalek defect (see Fig. 27.4). The contents of the hernia can be confirmed with barium radiography or CT (see Figs. 27.3A and B and 27.4C and D). The differential diagnosis is similar to that of Bochdalek hernias. Many patients have no symptoms or nonspecific symptoms, such as chest discomfort, cough, dyspnea, and upper abdominal distress. Gastric, omental, or intestinal incarceration with obstruction and ischemia may cause acute symptoms.[45,46]

Treatment and Prognosis

For infants with Bochdalek hernias, intubation and mechanical ventilation are often needed at the time of delivery. ECMO is useful in some cases with cardiac dysfunction and pulmonary hypertension.[47] Once the infant's pulmonary issues have stabilized, surgical repair is performed, either open or laparoscopically, using a mesh prosthesis. Despite advances in critical care and surgical techniques, the mortality rate is still around 60%, although higher survival rates have been reported by some centers.[47] The abdomen may not be able to tolerate the increased pressure when the intestinal contents are reduced, and therefore a gradual abdominal closure can also be used.[49]

Laparoscopic and thoracoscopic repair of Bochdalek hernias have been reported.[44,50] Morgagni hernias have been repaired through the chest or abdomen, using open, thoracoscopic, and/or laparoscopic techniques.[45,46] An abdominal laparoscopic approach is favored in small diaphragmatic hernias. One must be careful to note the inferior epigastric vessels that are present in the location of the Morgagni hernia. This anterior defect can be bridged with synthetic mesh. Larger Bochdalek defects require open approach with use of prosthetic mesh.

Traumatic and Posttraumatic Diaphragmatic Hernias

Etiology and Pathogenesis

Traumatic diaphragmatic hernias are caused by blunt trauma, such as motor vehicle accidents, in about 75% of cases, and by penetrating trauma, such as stab or gunshot wounds, in the remainder.[51] During blunt trauma, abrupt changes in intra-abdominal pressure may lead to large rents in the diaphragm. A huge impact is needed to cause a diaphragmatic injury. As such,

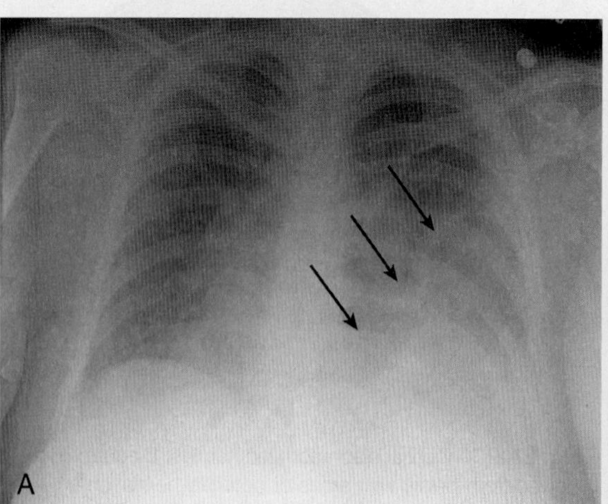

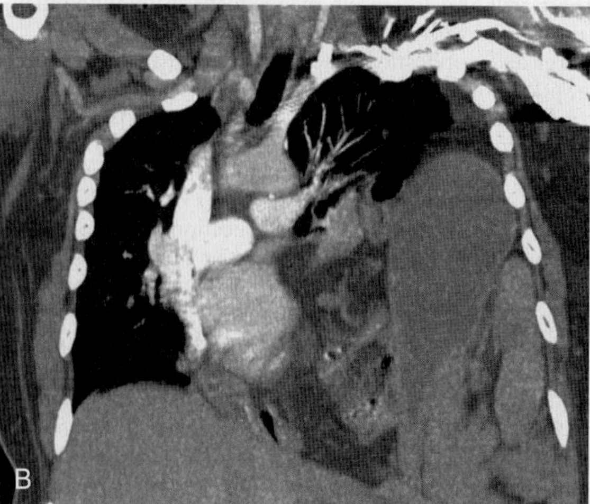

Fig. 27.3 Bochdalek hernia. (A) This plain chest film shows a Bochdalek hernia as a small opacity in the posterior chest at the level of the diaphragm, with bowel in the left chest (*arrows*). (B) CT of the same patient showing bowel above the diaphragm and causing a mediastinal shift.

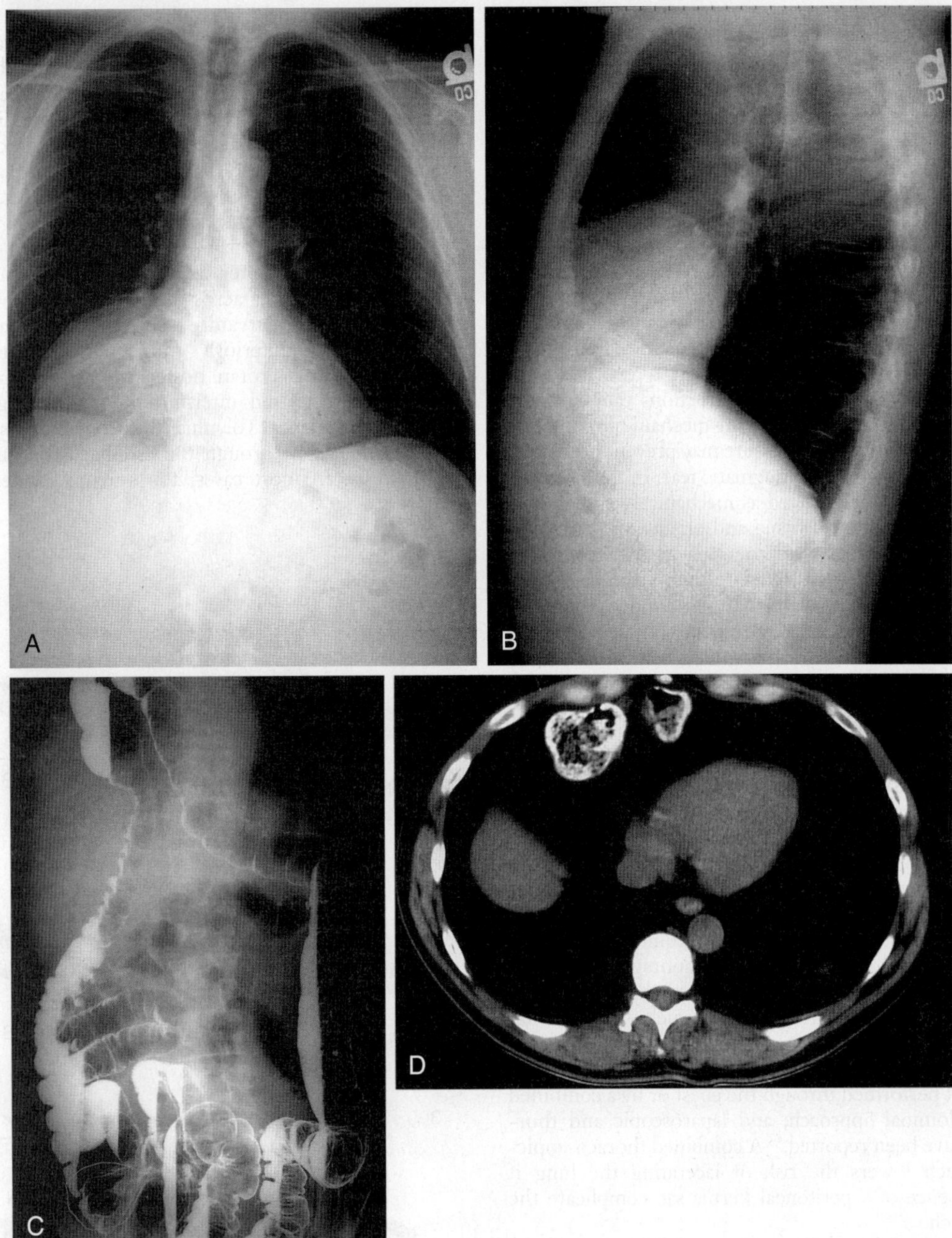

Fig. 27.4 Morgagni hernia. (A) A mass is noted in the right chest on a chest film (posteroanterior view). (B) Lateral chest film shows that the mass is in the anterior chest. (C) Barium enema shows that a portion of the transverse colon is the hernia (*top left*). (D) CT shows a contrast-filled colon in the right anterior chest (11-o'clock position).

associated injuries are commonly life threatening in the circumstance of a blunt diaphragmatic injury. Penetrating injuries often cause only small lacerations. Blunt trauma is more likely than penetrating trauma to eventually lead to a herniation of abdominal contents into the chest, because the defect is usually larger. The right hemidiaphragm is somewhat protected by the liver during blunt trauma. Thus, in one series, 68% of diaphragmatic injuries from blunt trauma occurred on the left side, 24% on the right side, 1.5% were bilateral, 1% pericardial, and 5% unclassified.[51] Diaphragmatic injury may not result in immediate herniation, but with time, normal relative negative intrathoracic pressure may lead to gradual enlargement of a small diaphragmatic defect and protrusion of abdominal contents through the defect, leading to a delayed diagnosis in about 15% of cases.[52] Stomach, omentum, colon, small bowel, spleen, and even kidney may be found in a posttraumatic diaphragmatic hernia. Left-sided traumatic hernia defects often have more clinical consequences as the right diaphgragm is protected by the liver.

Epidemiology

The incidence of posttraumatic diaphragmatic hernia is uncertain. Diaphragmatic injury occurs in about 5% of patients with multiple traumatic injuries who undergo laparotomy and was found in approximately 1% of patients in a large trauma database.[53,54]

Clinical Features, Diagnosis, and Complications

Posttraumatic diaphragmatic hernias may cause respiratory or abdominal symptoms. After serious trauma, rupture of the diaphragm is often masked by other injuries.[55] Penetrating injuries between the fourth intercostal space and the umbilicus should raise the level of suspicion of a diaphragmatic injury. Respiratory or abdominal symptoms manifesting several days to weeks after injury should suggest the possibility of a missed diaphragmatic injury. The diaphragm must be closely inspected to detect injury at the time of exploratory laparotomy or laparoscopy, as these injuries can easily be missed. In particular, the posterior aspect of the left diaphragm should be carefully examined, as a missed defect in this area can become clinically significant. Chest radiograph and CT are diagnostic in 40%–80% of cases, depending on the type of CT performed.[56] The coronal and sagittal reconstructions can show the defect in the diaphragm. In patients receiving mechanical ventilation after trauma, positive intrathoracic pressure may prevent herniation or organs and tissue through a diaphragmatic tear. In this case, the diaphragmatic defect may be detected as mechanical ventilation is discontinued, with, herniation of tissue and organs into the chest causing respiratory compromise. Symptoms may also manifest long after diaphragmatic injury. Delays of more than years have been reported.[52] In such cases, the patient may not connect the acute symptoms with remote trauma. The treating physician should consider a traumatic cause when a diaphragmatic defect is not hiatal and is not located in the usual locations of congenital defects.

Treatment and Prognosis

Acute diaphragmatic rupture is most commonly approached from the abdomen during exploratory laparotomy or laparoscopy. However, a chest approach can be considered in some cases. Diagnostic laparoscopy has been used in patients thought to have a high risk of diaphragmatic injury but appear to have no other visceral injury (e.g., after a stab wound to the lower chest).[57] Use of thoracoscopy in the stable patient, as this requires single-lung ventilation, can aid in the diagnosis of a diaphragmatic injury. Chronic posttraumatic diaphragmatic hernias are characterized by a lack of a peritoneal lining or hernia sac. As such, these hernias are commonly associated with extensive adhesions to adjacent lung, reduction of which can cause significant bleeding. In such cases, repair is best performed through the chest or by a combined thoracoscopic-abdominal approach, and laparoscopic and thoracoscopic repair have been reported.[57] A combined thoracoscopic-abdominal approach lowers the risk of lacerating the lung if adhesions and absence of a peritoneal hernia sac complicate the abdominal approach.

GASTRIC VOLVULUS

Gastric volvulus results when the stomach twists on itself but rarely occurs unless there is an associated diaphragmatic hernia. Paré described the first case of gastric volvulus in 1579 in a patient who had a diaphragmatic injury from a sword wound. Gastric volvulus may be transient and produce few symptoms, or it may lead to obstruction and ischemia.

Etiology and Pathophysiology

The stomach is normally fixed in position by ligamentous attachments to the spleen, liver, and diaphragm. When there is normal intestinal rotation, the duodenum is fixed to the retroperitoneum, which results in pexy of the distal stomach. Laxity of these ligamentous attachments, elevation of the left hemidiaphragm, or fixation of an otherwise mobile stomach to a specific point can result in volvulus. Focal adhesions, gastric tumor, or masses in adjacent organs may predispose to gastric volvulus. In two-thirds of cases, the volvulus occurs above the diaphragm in association with a paraesophageal or mixed diaphragmatic hernia. In the other third of cases, volvulus occurs below the diaphragm.

Gastric volvulus may be mesenteroaxial or organoaxial (Fig. 27.5).[58] In mesenteroaxial volvulus, the stomach folds on its short axis, which runs across the stomach from the lesser curvature to the greater curvature (see Fig. 27.5, 1A and 1B), with the antrum twisting anteriorly and superiorly. In rare cases, the antrum and pylorus rotate posteriorly. Mesenteroaxial volvulus is often incomplete and intermittent, manifesting chronic symptoms. In organoaxial volvulus, the stomach twists along its long axis, which passes through the esophagastric junction region to the pylorus. In most cases, the antrum rotates anteriorly and

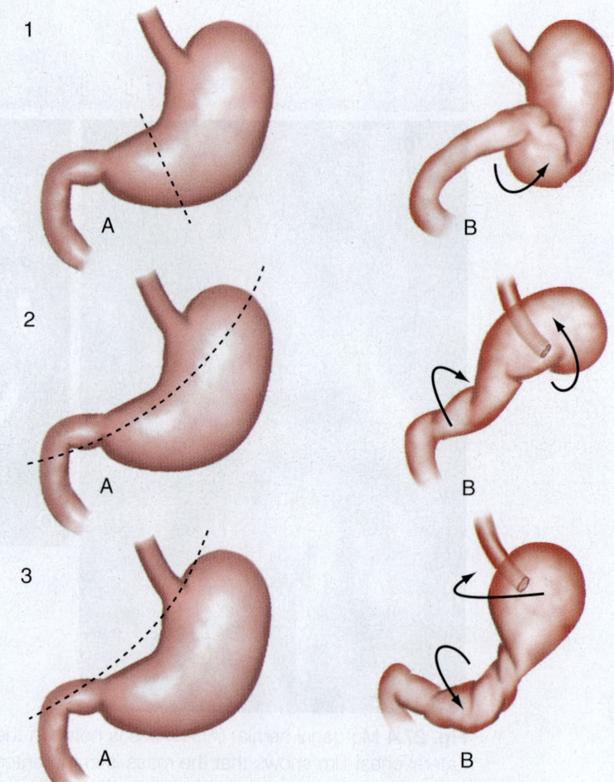

Fig. 27.5 Pathogenesis of gastric volvulus. (1A) Axis for potential mesenteroaxial volvulus bisecting the lesser and greater curvatures. (1B) Mesenteroaxial volvulus resulting from anterior rotation of the antrum along this axis. (2A) Axis for potential organoaxial volvulus passing through the body of the stomach. (2B) Organoaxial volvulus resulting from anterior-superior rotation of the antrum along this axis. (3A) Axis for potential organoaxial volvulus passing through the gastroesophageal junction and the pylorus. (3B) Organoaxial volvulus resulting from anterior-superior rotation of the antrum and posterior-inferior rotation of the fundus along this axis. (Adapted from Carter R, Brewer 3rd LA, Hinshaw DB. Acute gastric volvulus. A study of 25 cases. *Am J Surg*. 1980;140:101–106.)

superiorly and the fundus posteriorly and inferiorly, twisting the greater curvature at some point along its length (see Fig. 27.5, 3A and 3B). Less commonly, the long axis passes through the body of the stomach itself, in which case the greater curvature of the antrum and fundus rotate anteriorly and superiorly (see Fig. 27.5, 2A and 2B). This type of volvulus is commonly associated with a diaphragmatic hernia. Organoaxial volvulus is usually an acute event. Mixed mesenteroaxial and organoaxial volvulus has also been reported.[59]

Epidemiology

The incidence and prevalence of gastric volvulus are unknown. It is difficult to estimate how many cases are intermittent and undiagnosed. About 15%–20% of cases occur in children younger than 1 year of age, most often in association with a congenital diaphragmatic defect. The peak incidence in adults is in the fifth decade. Men and women are equally affected.[60,61]

Clinical Features, Diagnosis, and Complications

Acute gastric volvulus causes sudden severe pain in the upper abdomen or lower chest, associated with the inability to swallow, nausea, vomiting, and persistent retching. In cases of complete volvulus, it is impossible to pass a nasogastric tube into the stomach. Hematemesis is rare but may be due to an esophageal tear or gastric mucosal ischemia.[61] Vascular compromise and gastric infarction may occur. The combination of pain, unproductive retching, and inability to pass a nasogastric tube is called *Borchardt triad*.[62] If the volvulus is associated with a diaphragmatic hernia, plain chest or abdominal films will show a large gas-filled structure in the chest.[61] CT is often obtained in the emergency department and will show the stomach in the chest. While a barium UGI can also identify gastric volvulus, this may result in aspiration and should be avoided. Upper endoscopy may show twisting of the gastric folds (Fig. 27.6C). Acute gastric volvulus is a surgical emergency. Delay in surgery can result in gastric necrosis, which has a high mortality.

Chronic gastric volvulus is associated with mild and nonspecific symptoms like dysphagia, epigastric discomfort or fullness, bloating, and heartburn, particularly after meals. Symptoms may be intermittent and present for months to years.[61] A substantial number of cases likely go unrecognized. The diagnosis should be suspected in the proper clinical setting if a UGI radiograph or CT shows a large diaphragmatic hernia, even if the stomach is not twisted at the time of the radiograph. During imaging exams, the stomach may twist and untwist, securing the diagnosis.

Treatment and Prognosis

Acute gastric volvulus is an emergency, with a mortality rate of approximately 30%.[58] Placement of a nasogastric tube can allow for reduction of the stomach and conversion of an emergency surgery to an urgent, but not emergent, surgery. If signs of gastric infarction are not present, acute endoscopic detorsion may be considered. Using fluoroscopy, the endoscope is advanced to form an alpha loop in the proximal stomach.[63] The tip is passed through the area of torsion into the antrum or duodenum if possible, avoiding excess pressure. Torque may then reduce the gastric volvulus. This technique is most often used in chronic gastric volvulus without signs of ischemia.[63,64] Definitive surgical intervention should not be delayed for endoscopy. Surgery for gastric volvulus is usually performed using minimally invasive techniques. Insufflation of the abdomen may not be hemodynamically tolerated in a critically ill patient, as this results in decreased venous return and an acute drop in preload leading to

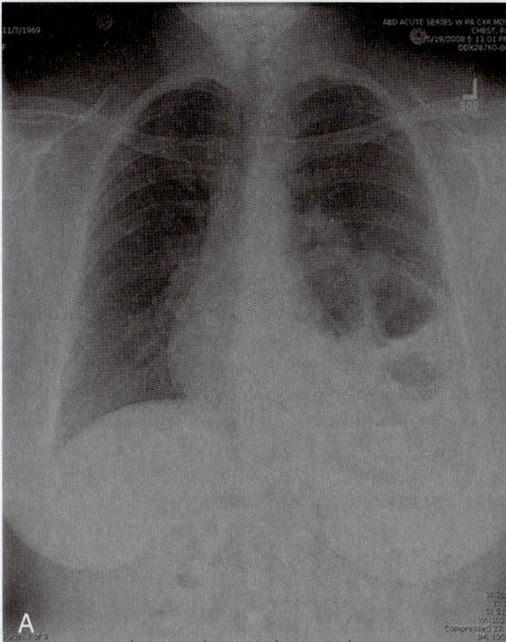

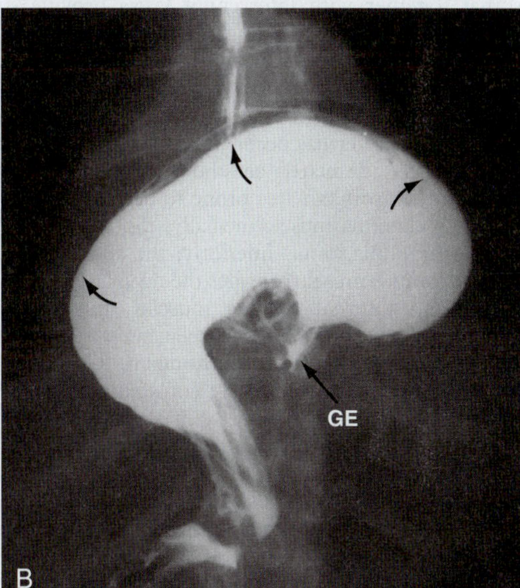

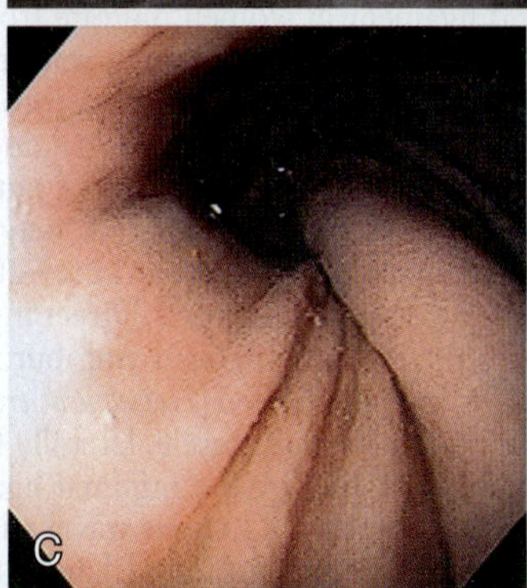

Fig. 27.6 Gastric volvulus with paraesophageal hernia. (A) Chest film showing a gas-filled mediastinal mass. (B) Barium examination showing that the greater curvature and lesser curvature of the stomach are reversed in position (upside-down stomach). (C) Twisting of the gastric folds at the point of torsion is noted in this endoscopic view of a gastric volvulus. (A, Courtesy Dr. Mark Feldman, Dallas, TX.)

hypotension. In this circumstance, an acute gastric volvulus should be repaired by open techniques.[60,61] After the torsion is reduced, the stomach is fixed by gastropexy or tube gastrostomy and the associated diaphragmatic hernia is repaired.[61,65] However, in the circumstance of a critically ill patient, the surgeon may elect to place a gastrostomy tube and return at a later date to complete the other components of the repair. Combined endoscopic and laparoscopic repair or simple endoscopic gastropexy by placement of a percutaneous gastrostomy tube has been reported.[65–68]

Chronic gastric volvulus is treated in the same manner as acute volvulus. If the patient is clinically stable, the surgeon may elect to treat the underlying cause of the volvulus (e.g., associated paraesophageal hernia) in the usual manner. Occasionally, gastric volvulus is caused by an elevated left hemidiaphragm, which may challenging to repair. In these cases, plication of the diaphragm in the position of inhalation with gastropexy can be considered.

INGUINAL AND FEMORAL HERNIAS

Etiology and Pathophysiology

The abdominal wall is protected from hernia formation by several mechanisms. In the lateral abdominal wall, there are layers of muscles that together with intervening fascia provide support. These muscles travel at oblique angles to each other and, therefore, handle forces in various planes, affording greater support than if they were parallel to each other. In the central abdomen, the bulky rectus abdominis muscles provide a barrier to herniation. Abdominal wall hernias occur in areas where these muscles and fascial layers are attenuated, and the hernias can be congenital or acquired. In the groin, an area prone to herniation is bounded by the rectus abdominis muscle medially, the inguinal ligament laterally, and the pubic ramus inferiorly; the aponeurosis of the transversus abdominis muscle provides the deep layer. In this area, the external and internal oblique muscles thin to a fascial aponeurosis only, so there is no muscular support of the transverse abdominal fascia and the peritoneum. Upright posture causes intra-abdominal pressure to be constantly directed to this area. During transient increases in abdominal pressure (e.g., coughing, straining, heavy lifting), reflex abdominal muscle wall contraction narrows the myopectineal orifice and tenses the overlying fascia (shutter mechanism).[69] Chronic cough, smoking, increasing age, and male gender are associated with an increased risk of hernia.[70,71]

During embryologic development, the spermatic cord and testis in men and the round ligament in women migrate from the retroperitoneum through the anterior abdominal wall to the inguinal canal, along with a projection of peritoneum (processus vaginalis). The defect in the abdominal wall (internal inguinal ring) associated with this process represents an area of potential weakness through which an indirect inguinal hernia may form (Fig. 27.7). The processus vaginalis may persist in 12%–20% of adults, further predisposing to hernia formation.[72] Direct inguinal hernias do not pass through the internal inguinal ring but rather protrude through defects in an area called *Hesselbach triangle*, bounded medially by the rectus abdominis muscle, laterally by the inferior epigastric artery, and inferiorly by the inguinal ligament (see Fig. 27.7). Therefore indirect inguinal hernias travel with the spermatic cord (or round ligament) and are found lateral to the inferior epigastric vessels, whereas direct hernias are found in the floor of the inguinal canal—an area supported only by the weak transversalis fascia—and are medial to the inferior epigastric vessels.

Femoral hernias pass through the opening associated with the femoral artery and vein. They manifest inferior to the inguinal ligament and medial to the femoral artery (see Fig. 27.7).[69] Clinical examination cannot easily differentiate indirect from direct inguinal hernias. The importance of distinguishing these two entities preoperatively is not critical, because the operative approach and repair are identical. However, it is important to accurately diagnose femoral hernias because they can be mistaken for lymph nodes in the groin. Misinterpreting an incarcerated loop of bowel in a femoral defect as a lymph node can lead to fine-needle aspiration of the mass and bowel injury. *Any mass that is medial to the femoral arterial pulsation and inferior to the inguinal ligament should be evaluated for a femoral hernia.*

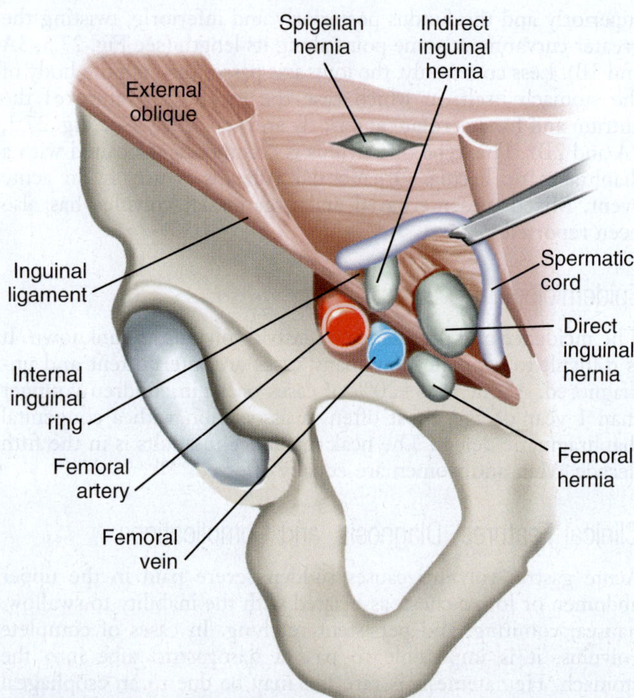

Fig. 27.7 Anatomic diagram of Spigelian hernia, indirect and direct inguinal hernias, and femoral hernia. The external oblique muscle has been omitted, and the spermatic cord (the round ligament in women) is retracted. Spigelian hernia occurs through defects in the fused aponeurosis of the internal oblique and transverse abdominal muscles. Indirect inguinal hernia occurs through the internal inguinal ring. Direct inguinal hernia occurs through defects in the transversalis fascia in Hesselbach triangle. Femoral hernia occurs inferior to the inguinal ligament and medial to the femoral vein and femoral artery.

The omentum, colon, small bowel, and bladder are the most common contents of groin hernias, although the appendix, Meckel diverticulum, fallopian tube, and ovary have been reported to herniate.[73–78] In a *Richter hernia*, only the antimesenteric side of the bowel protrudes. In this situation, the patient can have strangulation of the bowel without evidence of bowel obstruction, which is typically present when bowel is incarcerated in a hernia. The surgeon must be wary of the Richter hernia, as this can result in intestinal necrosis, despite the lack of the typical association with a bowel obstruction.

Epidemiology

The lifetime risk of groin hernia requiring repair is 27% for men and 3% for women, with repair seen most often in children under age 5 and adults older than 70.[79,80] The incidence increases with age, from 1% in men younger than age 45 to 3%–5% in those older than 45. About 800,000 groin hernia repairs are performed annually in the United States.[81] Of these, 80%–90% are performed in men.[79] Indirect inguinal hernias account for about 65%–70% of groin hernias in men and women. In men, direct inguinal hernias account for about 30% and femoral hernias for about 1%. In women, about 25% of groin hernias requiring repair are femoral, and the occurrence increases with age.[79,82] Groin hernias are somewhat more common on the right than on the left side.

Congenital hernias are more common in males because they represent a patent processus vaginalis. These pediatric hernias are commonly bilateral, and pediatric surgeons are taught to always evaluate the contralateral side.

Clinical Features, Diagnosis, and Complications

Many groin hernias are asymptomatic. The most common symptom is a mass in the inguinal or femoral area that enlarges when the patient stands or strains. An incarcerated hernia may produce constant discomfort. Strangulation causes increasing pain. Symptoms of bowel obstruction or ischemia may occur. In a Richter-type hernia, pain from bowel strangulation may occur without symptoms of obstruction, as only one wall of the intestine is involved in the hernia. The patient should be questioned about risk factors for hernia formation (e.g., patients who smoke, have a chronic cough, constipation). These factors, if not corrected prior to herniorrhaphy, can lead to recurrence.[83,84]

On physical examination, inguinal hernias present as a soft mass in the groin. The mass may be larger on standing or straining. It may be slightly tender. It may be possible to palpate the fascial defect associated with the hernia. The patient should be examined upright, the examiner's finger should be inserted into the inguinal canal, and a prolonged Valsalva maneuver should be initiated; it is normal to feel a small impulse against the examining finger with coughing. However, when a hernia is present, a prolonged Valsalva maneuver will result in protrusion of the sac, which is tender against the examiner's finger. Direct and indirect hernias may be difficult to distinguish. Groin hernias may also be noted on a plain abdominal radiograph (Fig. 27.8), barium radiograph, sonogram, or CT, and MRI may be helpful for identifying other causes of groin pain.[85]

Femoral hernias are more difficult to diagnose than other groin hernias, and 30%–40% manifest as surgical emergencies due to strangulation.[70,82] The correct diagnosis is often not made before surgery. The neck of femoral hernias is usually small. Even a small femoral hernia that is difficult to palpate may cause obstruction or strangulation. Richter hernias are most common in the femoral area, further complicating the diagnosis. Femoral hernias are most common in women, in whom clinicians may have a lower level of suspicion for hernia than in men. Femoral hernias also occur in children.[86] Delay in diagnosis, strangulation, and need for emergency surgery are common.[82,87] Any mass below the inguinal ligament and medial to the femoral artery should raise the suspicion of femoral hernia. Femoral hernias are commonly mistaken for femoral adenopathy or groin abscess.[87] Obviously, bedside incision and drainage of an incarcerated femoral hernia must be avoided, and, therefore, liberal use of sonography or CT is useful for distinguishing a hernia from adenopathy, abscess, or other masses.[85] The radiologist should perform these examinations with and without a prolonged Valsalva maneuver to demonstrate small defects. Of course, clinical acumen with a high suspicion for a missed hernia is of utmost importance.

Treatment and Prognosis

Some surgeons recommend repair of direct and indirect inguinal hernias even if they are asymptomatic, but this is controversial. A study by the American College of Surgeons has shown that males with minimally symptomatic groin hernias can be safely watched.[88] This study randomized 720 male patients to elective hernia repair or watchful waiting. Only 2 of the 364 patients in the watchful waiting arm of the study developed complications related

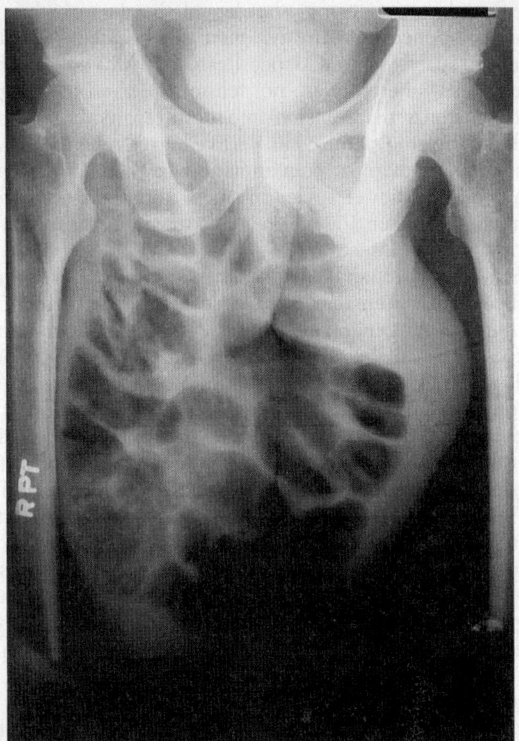

Fig. 27.8 Plain film in a 28-year-old man with a giant incarcerated inguinal hernia. (Courtesy Dr. Michael J. Smerud, Dallas, TX.)

to their hernia in 4.5 years. This suggests that minimally symptomatic patients can be watched safely and have their hernia repaired when symptoms increase.[89] Femoral hernias must be repaired promptly because the risk of strangulation is higher.[75,80]

When a patient presents with an incarcerated hernia and does not have clear signs and symptoms of ischemic bowel, it is reasonable to try to reduce the hernia manually. This will convert an emergent surgery into a semielective one. The patient can be sedated and placed in Trendelenburg position. Two hands must be used to coax the hernia back through the hernia defect. The patient must be watched closely to ensure dead bowel has not been reduced into the peritoneal cavity, a situation that can cause peritonitis and death. Often, ischemic bowel is so edematous that manual reduction is not possible. Repair of the hernia should occur within that same hospitalization, unless there are medical issues that justify a delay (e.g., recent acute myocardial infarction).

Groin hernias can be repaired using various techniques, including open or minimally invasive techniques, and is the source of ongoing debate for surgeons. Historically, tissue repairs have been performed. However, in the modern era, synthetic mesh repair is the standard of care.[90–93] The type of mesh used is of great debate also, as there are many choices available at this time.

The traditional tissue-based repairs were performed exclusively until the 1990s. There are two key components to successful hernia repair: (1) high ligation of the hernia sac, which treats the direct defect, and (2) repair of the floor of the canal, which treats the indirect defect. Even if there is no direct component, a repair of the floor is routinely undertaken. Open repairs involve approach to the inguinal canal through a small incision parallel to the inguinal ligament and centered over the internal inguinal ring. Dissection is continued through the external oblique muscle, exposing the internal inguinal ring. The cord structures are then isolated and explored thoroughly to identify an indirect hernia sac, which is ligated and transected. The floor of Hesselbach triangle is then reinforced and strengthened by apposing the lateral border of the rectus abdominis aponeurosis to the inguinal ligament (Bassini or Shouldice repair) or to Cooper ligament (McVay repair).[94–96] Tissue repairs inherently are not tension-free and pose a greater risk of recurrence than tension-free mesh repairs. Use of mesh is considered the gold standard in elective hernia repair.[81] However, in cases where there is contamination (e.g., in a strangulated hernia requiring bowel resection), it is important to perform a primary tissue repair and not a mesh repair, because there is a high risk of mesh infection.

Open mesh repairs are most commonly performed as described by Lichtenstein.[93,97] These can be performed under local, regional, or general anesthetic.[98,99] The major components of successful repair begin with high ligation of the sac, but the floor is repaired using synthetic mesh to bridge the gap between the conjoint tendon (edge of the rectus aponeurosis) and inguinal ligament, thus reconstructing the floor of the canal. The mesh can be sutured or stapled in place. Mesh plug repairs have also been developed and appear to have outcomes similar to other repairs.[100] In these cases, minimal dissection is undertaken, and the mesh plug, which looks like a badminton shuttlecock, is laid into the defect and tacked in place with a few sutures. The mesh causes fibroblast ingrowth and scarring that leads to strengthening of the floor of the inguinal canal. Mesh repairs have the advantage of being somewhat simpler to perform than tissue repairs and have less tension, less acute pain, and a decreased rate of recurrence.[90–92] Bilateral, very large, or complex abdominal hernias can be repaired with a large mesh that reinforces the entire ventral abdominal wall. This is called giant prosthetic reinforcement of the visceral sac, or the Stoppa procedure.[101]

Several series have compared open hernia repair with laparoscopic repair. One large study was performed by the Veterans Cooperative group.[102] Almost 1700 patients were followed for 2 years after being randomized to open versus laparoscopic repair of inguinal hernias. Patients who had their hernias repaired laparoscopically had less pain initially and returned to work 1 day sooner than those who had open repair. However, the recurrence rate was higher in the laparoscopic group (10% vs. 4% in the open group), and complication rates were higher and more serious in the laparoscopic group than in the open repair group. Meta-analyses of open versus laparoscopic repair have suggested that laparoscopic repair causes less pain, but recurrence rate is higher, as is the risk of complications.[103–105] This study in veterans changed the face of hernia repair in the 1990s and early 2000s. However, newer robotic transabdominal approaches have led to a resurgence of this technique for groin hernia repair that appears to be very safe.[260]

Minimally invasive hernia repair can be performed via a totally extraperitoneal approach or transabdominal preperitoneal approach (TAPP).[106–108] In the former case, the dissection is performed just above the peritoneum using a balloon for dissection. The mesh is then placed in this plane. In the TAPP procedure, the abdomen is entered and a peritoneal flap is raised. The mesh is placed and the flap is reattached to prevent the mesh from being in contact with bowel. The TAPP approach can cause intra-abdominal adhesions and future risk for adhesive bowel obstruction, a down side to this approach. The robotic TAPP approach has become the procedure of choice for many surgeons for repair of groin hernias.

Postsurgery Complications and Recurrence

Elective groin hernia repair is safe, and serious complications are unusual.[102–104] Lacerations of the bowel, bladder, or blood vessels may occur, particularly during a TAPP repair, and may cause serious consequences if not detected early. Damage to the bowel may also occur during reduction of an incarcerated hernia.

Minor acute complications include acute urinary retention, seroma, hematoma, and infection.[88,100,109] Serious infection occurs in less than 1% of cases. Damage to the spermatic cord may lead to ischemic orchitis.[88] Tissue dissection predisposes to thrombosis of the venous drainage of the testis. Symptoms are swelling and pain of the cord and testis. The condition persists for 6–12 weeks and may result in testicular atrophy. Fortunately, this is a rare complication, occurring after about 0.04% of tissue repairs.[110,111] Hydrocele or vas deferens injury occurs in less than 1% of cases.[111] Damage to sensory nerves is not uncommon during inguinal hernia surgery, and can be related to the division or preservation of the ilioinguinal nerve as it traverses the inguinal canal.[112–114] Chronic paresthesias and pain of the medial aspect of the scrotum are reported by about 10% of patients, either caused by damage to the sensory nerves or neuroma. This can be treated by local nerve block, desensitization therapy, and neurectomy.[114–116]

Some recurrent hernias are indirect hernias missed during the first hernia repair. The risk of recurrence is related to conditions that lead to tissue deterioration, such as malnutrition, liver or renal failure, glucocorticoid therapy, and malignancies.[117] Patients with scrotal hernias and recurrent hernias are at higher risk for recurrence or re-recurrence, respectively.[84] Recurrent hernias are also more common among smokers than nonsmokers.[71] In patients with cirrhosis, portal hypertension, and no ascites or moderate ascites, inguinal hernia repair is reported to be safe, although the recurrence rate is increased in some series.[118,119] Ideally, the ascites is aggressively controlled prior to elective herniorrhaphy, and a TIPS or liver transplantation should be considered for control of ascites. Post-operative leakage of ascites can lead to infection and death and can be challenging to manage. Preoperative consultation with a hepatologist is essential to assess for portal hypertension and evaluate surgical risk. Despite initial data that suggested that minimally invasive TAPP repair resulted in higher recurrence rates, more recent data suggests that this is not true in the current era.[260] Routine use of mesh has become standard and has contributed towards a tension free repair and lower recurrence rates. Overall, recurrence rates are higher after tissue repairs than after tension-free mesh repairs.[91,104] Recurrence rates for groin hernia repair using mesh are now reported to be in the 0%–4% range.[90,94,96,102,104]

Inguinal Hernias and Colorectal Cancer Screening

Some practitioners recommend that patients aged 50 years or older with inguinal hernias be screened for colorectal neoplasms before hernia repair. One older prospective study using flexible sigmoidoscopy to screen primarily middle-aged or elderly men with inguinal hernias reported the prevalence of colorectal polyps to be 26% and the prevalence of colorectal cancers to be 3.6%.[120] However, more recent data have clearly shown that there is no increased risk of colorectal cancer in patients who have groin hernias. In a prospective study of colonoscopy for screening of asymptomatic U.S. veterans, the prevalence of polyps was 37.5% and of colorectal cancer 1%.[121] Thus the prevalence of colorectal neoplasms is substantial in middle-aged or older men with or without inguinal hernias. In several more recent studies, the risk of colorectal cancer was found to be similar in patients with hernias (5%) compared with a control group that did not have hernias (4%).[122] Large inguinal hernias, particularly incarcerated hernias, may cause difficulty during sigmoidoscopy or colonoscopy. In such patients, it may be advisable to defer the examination until after hernia repair. Incarceration of colonoscopes within hernias has been reported.[123]

Inguinal Hernias and Benign Prostatic Hyperplasia

Inguinal hernia and symptomatic benign prostatic hyperplasia commonly occur in older men.[124] Straining to void may cause worsening of inguinal hernia. Conversely, the risk of postoperative urinary retention after hernia repair is increased by prostatic hyperplasia, and older male patients with any symptoms of prostate disease should be counseled on the risk of urinary retention after hernia repair. It is important that prostate symptoms are addressed prior to elective hernia repair. This will avoid urinary retention postoperatively that can be painful and extend length of stay. If elective inguinal hernia repair and transurethral prostatic therapy are required, some surgeons would consider performing these procedures concurrently,[125,126] but more frequently, concerns about infection of mesh lead to sequential surgery.

OTHER VENTRAL HERNIAS

True ventral hernias include incisional, epigastric, umbilical, and Spigelian hernias. Patients often mistake diastasis recti for ventral hernia. *Diastasis recti* is a separation of the rectus abdominis muscles without a defect in the abdominal fascia and can be demonstrated as a midline defect exaggerated by a Valsalva maneuver. No fascial ring can be palpated, and the defect is often very wide and long. This condition does not require repair and is cosmetic only. There is no fascial defect and visceral contents cannot become incarcerated in this defect.

INCISIONAL HERNIAS

Incisional hernias, as the name implies, are hernias that occur after a prior operation. Incisional hernias include postlaparotomy hernias, parastomal hernias, and trocar-site hernias.

Etiology and Pathophysiology

Several factors contribute to incisional hernias. Patient-specific risk factors include obesity, collagen vascular diseases, a history of surgically repaired aorta, nutritional deficiencies, and ascites.[119,127–129] Conditions that impair healing, such as smoking or glucocorticoid therapy, can also increase postoperative hernia formation.[130] Surgery-related risk factors include the type and location of the prior surgical incision and postoperative wound infection. It is more common for hernias to develop after a vertical midline incision than after a transverse incision, although this has been brought into question by some recent data. This has led some surgeons to use transverse incisions in patients who are predisposed to hernias due to glucocorticoids or other immunosuppressants. Development of a postoperative wound infection can lead to a higher incidence of hernia formation.[131]

Placement of a stoma (ileostomy or colostomy) results in an intentional creation of a hernia through which the intestine runs. The risk of a parastomal hernia can be reduced by placing these intentional hernias within the rectus muscle rather than lateral to the rectus, and by using mesh to reinforce the area.[132]

Trocar-site hernias have become more common with the widespread adoption of minimally invasive surgery. The rate of hernia formation is related to the size of the trocar used (trocars >10 mm in diameter are more commonly associated with hernia formation), length of surgery, obesity, and advancing age.[133] Lateral trocar placement has a lower chance of hernia formation than midline placement.

Epidemiology

Incisional hernias are common after laparotomy. When followed carefully over a long period, up to 20% of patients can be found to develop a hernia. This incidence increases to 35%–50% of cases when there is wound infection or dehiscence.[134,135] Up to 50% of such hernias manifest more than 1 year after surgery.[134] Vertical incisions, obesity, advanced age, diabetes, sepsis, postoperative pulmonary complications, immunosuppression, and glucocorticoid use increase the risk.[131]

Parastomal hernias are reported to occur in as many as 50% of cases after stoma placement.[132] Specific measures are taken at the time of surgery to decrease the incidence of hernia formation. For example, the smallest fascial defect is created within the rectus sheath, rather than lateral to it. The use of biological mesh in primary stoma placement may reduce the incidence of subsequent hernia formation, but this routine use of mesh is controversial. A multicenter randomized controlled trial showed no impact in parastomal hernia occurrence with mesh placement.[132,136,269] Conditions that lead to bowel dilation prior to stoma placement (e.g., obstruction) can result in subsequent bowel shrinkage after stoma placement. This shrinkage can increase the space between the bowel wall and fascia, facilitating hernia formation.

Trocar-site hernias are estimated to occur after 0.5% of laparoscopic cholecystectomies.[133] They usually occur at the site of the largest trocar, which is typically larger than 10 mm in diameter and is at the umbilical location.

Clinical Features, Diagnosis, and Complications

Incisional hernias can cause chronic abdominal discomfort. Because the fascial defect of incisional hernias is usually large, strangulation is unusual even with incarceration. Reduced ability to voluntarily increase intra-abdominal pressure interferes with defecation and urination. Lordosis and back pain may occur, due to weakness and imbalance in core muscles.[135] Large incisional hernias may lead to "eventration disease." With the loss of integrity of the abdominal wall, the diaphragm cannot contract against the abdominal viscera during inspiration, but rather forces the viscera into the hernia. The diaphragm thus becomes inefficient, and the hernia tends to enlarge. The viscera may lose the "right of domain" in the abdominal cavity. Surgeons should use caution repairing these large hernias, as the acute increase in abdominal pressure can lead to pulmonary failure and reduced venous return, resulting in an effective abdominal compartment syndrome.[137]

Parastomal hernias often interfere with ostomy function and the fit of appliances. This can lead to leakage of stool that can be incapacitating. Prolapse of the bowel through the stoma can occur. This results in the stoma appearing as a long protrusion. The patient may bring in pictures of an engorged and protruding stoma that is intussusscepted bowel. Incarceration and strangulation of bowel may occur within the parastomal defect, presenting as a bowel obstruction.[132]

Trocar site hernias usually cause pain and a bulge at the trocar site. Because of the small opening, it is more likely intra-abdominal contents could become strangulated in the defect. Richter hernia has been reported, and other organs (e.g., stomach) can herniate into trocar hernias.[138,139]

Diagnosis of an incisional hernia can be difficult if the defect is small, tender, or of obesity is present. Ultrasound and CT can be used for evaluation of incisional hernias, and the radiologist should be alerted to this indication, as specific maneuvers can be performed during imaging to demonstrate the hernia defect. For example, ultrasound can be performed with the patient in an upright position or CT in the prone position.[140] Parastomal hernias can also be identified with intrastomal ultrasound,[141] although CT is the diagnostic modality of choice. Trocar site hernias are especially challenging to diagnose, as the site of fascial entry can be tangential to the skin incision site, hence the defect and the symptomatic area may not be over the visible trocar incision. This is because the abdomen is insufflated with carbon dioxide at the time of trocar placement, leading to different fascial entry point than when the abdomen is desufflated. The finding of localized pain at a site that is close to a trocar site should trigger evaluation with CT scan.

Treatment and Prognosis

Incisional hernias are best repaired with prosthetic mesh; the recurrence rate is substantially lower than after traditional tissue repair.[131] Synthetic mesh and biologic mesh (which provides a tissue matrix into which ingrowth occurs with remolding) are available for use.[262] The key element in hernia repair is to achieve a tension-free repair. In general, every attempt should be made to bring the fascia together with placement of mesh in one of several spaces to reinforce the repair. In fact, the term "abdominal wall reconstruction" or "abdominal core health" is used to describe this type of surgery.[263] These terms emphasize the attempt to restore anatomy, with medialization of the components of the abdominal wall. Every attempt is made to place a layer of peritoneum or hernia sac between the abdominal contents and synthetic mesh. However, if this cannot be done, special double-sided mesh is available with a barrier of some kind on one side, to prevent adhesions to viscera. This material does not stick to bowel and is therefore unlikely to erode into the intestine.[137] There has been a trend toward using biological mesh in patients who are high risk for poor wound healing, such as patients with obesity, diabetes, or a smoking history. If diaphragmatic dysfunction (eventration disease) is suspected, the abdominal wall may have to be stretched by repeated progressive pneumoperitoneum before repair.[142] Recurrences of incisional hernia are reported in 2%−60% of cases, depending on the method used for repair and the duration of follow-up.[143] Minimally invasive repair of ventral defects can be performed. There is some suggestion that minimally invasive repair results in fewer recurrences and lower morbidity.[131,144]

Minimally invasive hernia repair is performed by insufflating the abdomen and gradually creating a working space by carefully lysing adhesions. Double-sided mesh is then placed in the preperitoneal position and fixed by tacks and sutures. More recently, suturing of the fascial edges prior to placement of mesh has been performed more readily with the robotic platform. Prior iterations of the minimally invasive technique bridged the gap between the fascial edges and left the patient with the sensation that the hernia was still present. Some surgeons perform a minimally invasive components separation, where the lateral components are incised and slide to meet at the midline. This results in medializing the fascial defect under no tension. Mesh is always used in these repairs and can be placed in many spaces, including intra-abdominal, retro-rectus, transverse abdominus, or onlay.[264] Chronic pain at suture or tack sites appears to be a greater issue with laparoscopic hernia repair than with open repair.[145,146]

Small and minimally symptomatic parastomal hernias may be treated with a modified ostomy belt. If surgery is necessary, there are several modes of treatment. The best treatment is to eliminate the stoma completely. This requires the ability to reconstruct the patient, an option not possible in the patient who has undergone abdominoperineal resection. The stoma can be relocated another quadrant of the abdomen. Primary repair of the parastomal defect is no longer considered adequate treatment and mesh placement is advocated. A piece of mesh shaped with a keyhole defect through which the stoma can be exteriorized can be used.[132] Alternatively, the "Sugarbaker technique" can be performed, where a flat piece of mesh is placed over the piece of bowel as it exits the abdominal cavity to the stoma. This changes the angle of the bowel to parallel to the abdominal wall and creates a physiologic effect preventing future hernia formation. In this case, it is important for the gastroenterologist to know that the scope will travel parallel to the abdominal wall before diving into the abdomen. These parastomal repairs can all be performed through minimally invasive techniques.[147,148]

To decrease the incidence of trocar site hernias, it is recommended that trocar ports be removed under direct vision and the defects for ports greater than 10 mm in size be sutured closed.

Biological mesh can be used in place of synthetic mesh in patients in whom there has been contamination, such as when bowel resection is needed or there is an associated fistula. Biological mesh substrates are thought to be degradable over time, with tissue ingrowth and remodeling, and development of a scar that can provide strength similar to mesh. However, hernia recurrence is still a significant issue with biological mesh and can occur in up to 21% of patients.[149] Because of the significant recurrence rate, bridging of defects should be avoided when using biological mesh.

Epigastric and Umbilical Hernias

Etiology and Pathophysiology

Epigastric hernias occur through midline defects in the aponeurosis of the rectus sheath (linea alba) between the xiphoid and umbilicus. These defects are usually small and frequently multiple. Because of the location in the upper part of the abdominal wall, it is unusual for bowel to become incarcerated in epigastric hernias. The falciform ligament lies in this location, providing protection from bowel incarceration. More commonly, preperitoneal fat or omentum protrude through these hernias.[150]

Umbilical hernias in infants are congenital (see Chapter 98). They often close spontaneously. In general, these defects will close spontaneously by 4 years of age.[168] If they are still evident after this age, surgical repair is indicated. In adults, umbilical hernias may develop consequent to increased intra-abdominal pressure due to ascites, pregnancy, or obesity.

Epidemiology

Epigastric hernias are found in 0.5%−10% of autopsies.[150] Many are asymptomatic or undiagnosed during life. They generally occur in the third through fifth decades. Risk factors for epigastric hernia include obesity, smoking, and heavy lifting.[150] Epigastric hernia has also been reported after deep inferior epigastric perforator flap breast reconstruction.[151]

Umbilical hernias occur in about 30% of African American infants and 4% of white infants at birth, and are present in 13% and 2%, respectively, by 1 year of age.[152] Umbilical hernias are more common in low-birth-weight infants than in those of normal weight. Other risk factors include obesity and pregnancy. Umbilical hernias occur in roughly 20% of patients with cirrhosis and ascites.[153]

Clinical Features, Diagnosis, and Complications

The main symptom of epigastric hernia is upper abdominal pain, usually localized to the abdominal wall, rather than the deep visceral pain that accompanies intestinal pathology. A specific tender nodule or point of tenderness can be palpated in the nonobese patient. Diagnosis may be difficult, particularly in obese patients. However, symptoms are sometimes mistaken for those of a peptic ulcer or biliary disease. Determining that the discomfort is in the abdominal wall, rather than deep within the peritoneum, can help distinguish incarcerated bowel from fat in the hernia. Sonography and CT may be helpful in the diagnosis.[154,155] Complications of epigastric hernia are very rare, with reports of acute pancreatitis from incarceration of the head of the pancreas, perforation of a gastroduodenal ulcer incarcerated in the hernia, and strangulation of bowel in the hernia.[156−158]

Umbilical hernias in children are usually asymptomatic. Adults may be asymptomatic or report some discomfort with palpation of the hernia. Incarceration and strangulation may occur in children and adults. Spontaneous rupture of umbilical hernias may occur in patients with ascites and, rarely, in pregnant women.[159,160] Skin changes with maceration and ulceration generally occur prior to frank rupture. Therefore the findings of skin changes in a patient with an umbilical hernia should warrant urgent repair. Care must be taken when performing a therapeutic paracentesis in patients with umbilical hernias; the hernia must be reduced and kept reduced during the paracentesis, because strangulation of umbilical hernias may occasionally be precipitated by rapid removal of ascites.[153,161]

Treatment and Prognosis

If surgery is performed for epigastric hernia, the linea alba should be widely exposed because multiple defects called *Swiss cheese defects* may be found. A minimally invasive approach is preferred in this circumstance, where excellent visualization of the midline can be achieved with just a few 5-mm ports. A single defect can be fixed easily, and a Swiss cheese–type scenario can also be fixed minimally invasively without opening the whole midline of the abdomen. Mesh is laid within the abdomen to cover all of these defects. Surgical repair is typically successful, with a low recurrence rate.

Umbilical hernias are most often left untreated in children; complications are unusual, and they usually close spontaneously if smaller than 1.5 cm in diameter. Repair should be considered if they are larger than 2 cm or if they are still present after 4 years of age.[152] Repair of umbilical hernias should be recommended for adults if they are difficult to reduce or symptomatic. Techniques for repair of all abdominal wall defects rely on a tension-free repair to decrease the risk of recurrence. Open or minimally invasive techniques can be used to achieve this end.[162] Data support routine use of mesh in repair of these defects, because this results in a decrease in recurrences.[163] Mesh is always used in minimally invasive repair.

When complications develop in patients with umbilical hernias, the prognosis worsens significantly. Those patients requiring bowel resection at the time of umbilical herniorrhaphy or who have ascites and cirrhosis have increased mortality.[161,164] Repair of umbilical hernias in patients with cirrhosis and ascites can be challenging, and consultation with a hepatologist is needed for appropriate presurgical risk assessment and management. In general, ascites should be aggressively controlled and TIPS or liver transplantation can be considered (see Chapters 94 and 99). Repair of an umbilical hernia in a patient with ascites should be triggered by skin changes, indicating imminent rupture, or incarceration of bowel has occurred. Spontaneous rupture of umbilical defects in patients with ascites portends a poor prognosis, with reported mortality of up to 60%.[153,159,165] Minimally invasive techniques and earlier repair of hernias in patients with cirrhosis can be considered, although leakage of ascites from incisions can lead to infection and death. The morbidity of elective umbilical hernia repair in patients with ascites appears not to be as high as once thought, with one trial reporting a mortality rate of 3.7% for elective repair, with even lower rates (1.3%) for patients with a MELD score less than 15.[166] Outcome after surgical repair is directly dependent on nutritional status and control of ascites. Control of ascites may require frequent paracentesis to keep the abdomen flat to allow healing. Topical fibrin sealant has been used to successfully treat a leaking umbilical hernia in a patient with ascites.[167] In general, one should undertake umbilical hernia repair with caution in cirrhotic patients with ascites with consultation with a hepatologist.

Spigelian Hernias

Etiology and Pathophysiology

Spigelian hernias occur through defects in the fused aponeurosis of the transversus abdominis muscle and internal oblique muscle, lateral to the rectus sheath; they most commonly occur just below the level of the umbilicus (see Fig. 27.7). This area is called the *spigelian fascia*, named after the Belgian anatomist Adriaan van den Spiegel. This fascia is where the linea semilunaris, the level at which the transversus abdominis muscle becomes aponeurosis rather than muscle, meets the semicircular line of Douglas. The epigastric vessels penetrate the rectus sheath in this area. The combination of all these anatomic features can lead to a potential defect and a spigelian hernia. The spigelian fascia is covered by the external oblique muscle, and therefore, Spigelian hernias do not penetrate through all layers of the abdominal wall, making the diagnosis of a hernia challenging.[168]

Epidemiology

Spigelian hernias are very rare. Only about 1000 cases have been reported.[169] The largest series of patients included 81 patients.[170] They are twice as common in females as in males and are somewhat more common on the left side of the abdomen.[171,172] They generally occur in patients around age 60 years.[170–172]

Clinical Features, Diagnosis, and Complications

Spigelian hernias can be difficult to diagnose because the external oblique muscle overlies the defect in the deeper fascia. Therefore this defect only involves the inner two layers of the abdominal wall. Only 75%–80% of patients with a Spigelian hernia are correctly diagnosed before surgery.[170,172] The examiner must have a high degree of suspicion when a patient complains of pain at the lateral edge of the rectus, inferior to the umbilicus. Careful examination will suggest that the pain originates in the abdominal wall and not in the peritoneal cavity. This determination is critical because a Spigelian hernia can be mistaken for conditions like acute appendicitis and diverticulitis.[173–175] Frequently, only omentum is present in the hernia, but large or small bowel, ovary, appendix, or fallopian tube may herniate.[170,174,176] A Richter hernia or a bowel obstruction caused by incarcerated small intestine may occur.[177] The differential diagnosis includes rectus sheath hematoma, lipoma, or sarcoma. Sonography and CT are useful for diagnosing a Spigelian hernia.[170,172,178] An astute radiologist will perform these studies using various techniques (e.g., Valsalva maneuver) to increase detection of even a small Spigelian hernia. The finding of a visceral structure penetrating through the two inner layers of the abdominal wall at the correct location will lead to the diagnosis of a Spigelian hernia.

Treatment and Prognosis

Spigelian hernias may be approached by open or minimally invasive techniques.[179] Laparoscopy can be helpful as a diagnostic tool in patients suspected of having a Spigelian hernia, even if open repair is anticipated.[180] The hernia can be best identified from within the peritoneal cavity. Preperitoneal laparoscopic techniques can be used, with the advantage of staying outside the peritoneal cavity, thereby avoiding adhesions.[181] Intraperitoneal laparoscopic repair can be performed using mesh that is coated on one side to avoid adhesion to the underlying bowel.[181,182] Minimally invasive approaches result in decreased pain and decreased length of hospital stay compared with open techniques.[183] However, these hernias are so rare, the surgeon's choice of technique should be based on personal experience. It is the authors' preference to at least start with a laparoscopic approach, as this can confirm the diagnosis and help locate the hernia itself. As with other hernias, most Spigelian hernias are closed using mesh repairs, a technique that appears to have a lower recurrence rate than primary repair.[170,181]

PELVIC AND PERINEAL HERNIAS

The three main types of pelvic and perineal hernias are obturator, sciatic, and perineal hernias.

Etiology and Pathogenesis

Obturator hernias are rare and occur in older women.[184] Obturator hernias occur through the greater and lesser obturator foramina. The obturator foramen is larger in women than in men and is ordinarily filled with fat. Marked weight loss predisposes to herniation.[185]

Sciatic hernias occur through the foramina formed by the sciatic notch and the sacrospinous or sacrotuberous ligaments. Abnormal development or atrophy of the piriform muscle may predispose to sciatic hernia. Sciatic hernias may contain ovary, ureter, bladder, or large or small bowel.[186]

Perineal hernias occur in the soft tissues of the perineum and are very rare. They may be primary or postoperative. Primary perineal hernias occur anteriorly through the urogenital diaphragm or posteriorly through the levator ani muscle or between the levator ani and coccygeus muscles. Secondary perineal hernias occur most often after surgery, such as abdominal-perineal resection, pelvic exenteration, or hysterectomy.[187–189] Radiation therapy, wound infection, and obesity predispose to the development of secondary perineal hernias.[190,191]

Epidemiology

Obturator hernias typically occur in older, cachectic, multiparous women. About 800 cases have been reported.[192] In Asia, obturator hernias account for about 1% of all hernia repairs, but in the West, they account for 0.07% of all hernias.[193,194]

Sciatic hernias are even less common than obturator hernias, with fewer than 100 cases reported.[186] They are most common in older women, although are occasionally seen in children.[195]

Perineal hernias are also rare. Primary perineal hernias are most common in middle-aged women. Secondary perineal hernias occur after less than 3% of pelvic exenterations and less than 1% of abdominal-perineal resections for anorectal cancer.[191,196]

Clinical Features, Diagnosis, and Complications

Obturator hernias occur almost exclusively in older women and are more common on the right side.[192,197] They commonly cause cramping lower abdominal pain, nausea, and vomiting. Almost all patients present with symptoms of small bowel obstruction.[197] Because the hernia orifice is small, Richter hernia and strangulation are common, and bowel necrosis is not uncommon.[197,198] There are three signs specific for an incarcerated obturator hernia.[197] The first is obturator neuralgia, manifesting as paresthesia that extends along the medial aspect of the thigh. Second is the Howship-Romberg sign, caused by pressure on the obturator nerve and resulting in paresthesias and pain in the hip and inner thigh. The pain is diminished by hip flexion and increased by hip extension, adduction, or medial rotation. This sign is seen in 25% −50% of patients with obturator hernia and is considered pathognomonic. Third is the Hannington-Kiff sign, elicited by percussing the adductor muscle above the knee. Absence of the normal adductor reflex contraction is a strong indicator of obturator nerve impingement caused by an obturator hernia. Occasionally, a mass may be palpable in the upper medial thigh or in the pelvis on pelvic or rectal examination. The diagnosis is difficult, often delayed, and usually not made preoperatively. The treating physician must have a low threshold for entertaining this diagnosis in an elderly female patient with a bowel obstruction in the pelvis. Preoperative diagnosis is sometimes evident on ultrasound or CT.[197,199,200] Most patients with signs of a bowel obstruction will have a CT scan in the emergency department. The point of obstruction in the pelvis maybe difficult to ascertain, and the surgeon will need to be prepared to repair an obturator defect.

Sciatic foramen hernias may manifest as a mass or swelling in the gluteal or infragluteal area, but are generally difficult to palpate because they occur deep to the gluteal muscles. Chronic pelvic pain caused by incarceration of a fallopian tube and/or ovary may occur.[201] Impingement on the sciatic nerve may also produce pain deep in the buttock or radiating to the thigh.[202] Intestinal or ureteral obstruction may occur. The differential diagnosis includes lipoma or other soft-tissue tumor, cyst, abscess, and aneurysm.[203] The diagnosis is often difficult, with only 37% of patients diagnosed by physical exam findings.[186] CT and MRI may be helpful, but many patients are diagnosed at laparotomy or laparoscopy.

In women, primary perineal hernias manifest anteriorly in the labia majora (pudendal hernia) or posteriorly in the vagina.[190] In men, they manifest in the ischiorectal fossa. Primary and postoperative perineal hernias are usually soft and reducible. Most patients complain of a mass that produces discomfort on sitting. Because the orifice of the hernia is usually wide, incarceration is rare. If the bladder is involved, urinary symptoms may occur.[204] Postoperative perineal hernias may be complicated by cutaneous ulceration. The differential diagnosis includes sciatic hernia, tumor, hematoma, cyst, abscess, and rectal or bladder prolapse.[205]

Treatment and Prognosis

The treatment of pelvic hernias is surgical. Laparoscopic repair of obturator, sciatic, and perineal hernias has been reported.[187,206,207] However, most patients with pelvic hernias present with an acute surgical condition, often bowel obstruction, and it is often necessary to perform an open procedure to manage the problem. Repair of perineal hernias can be complex. When bowel resection is required, mesh placement is usually not used because of the high risk of infection. The advent of biologic mesh has allowed these materials to be used in contaminated fields.[186] Peritoneal flaps or muscle advancement flaps can be used to perform tissue repairs of these defects.[208] The prognosis is poor when patients present with an acute illness, and is more related to the underlying medical conditions rather than the hernia itself. Nutritional depletion, advanced age, and poor medical health are all confounding variables.

LUMBAR HERNIAS

Etiology and Pathophysiology

Lumbar hernias can occur in two separate triangular areas of the flank. The superior triangle (Grynfeltt lumbar triangle) is bounded by the 12th rib superiorly, the internal oblique muscle inferiorly, and the sacrospinous muscles medially. The inferior triangle (Petit lumbar triangle) is bounded by the latissimus dorsi muscle posteriorly, the external oblique muscle anteriorly, and the iliac crest inferiorly (Fig. 27.9).[209] Grynfeltt hernias are more common than Petit hernias. Lumbar hernias are more common on the left than on the right side. This may be because the liver pushes the right kidney inferiorly in development, leading to protection of the lumbar triangles. Pseudohernia may occur in the lumbar area as the result of paresis of the thoracodorsal nerves.[209–211] This is caused by loss of muscle control and tone,

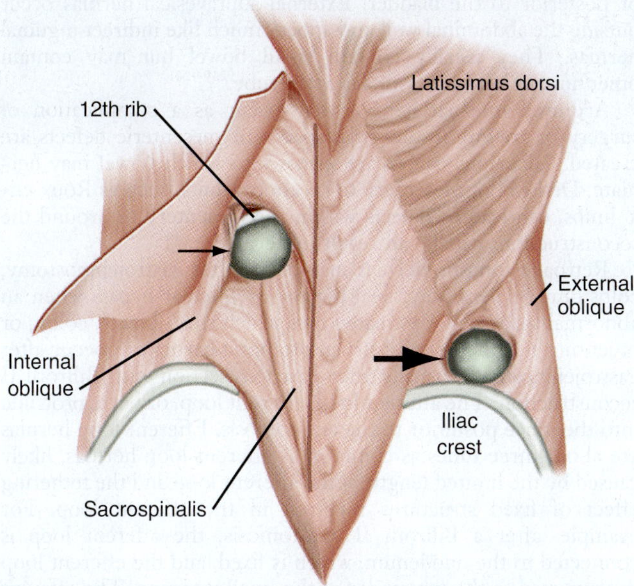

Fig. 27.9 Anatomic diagram of lumbar hernias. The inferior triangle hernia, Petit hernia (*thick arrow*), is bounded by the latissimus dorsi muscle, the external oblique muscle, and the iliac crest. The superior triangle hernia, Grynfeltt hernia (*thin arrow*), is bounded by the 12th rib, the internal oblique muscle, and the sacrospinalis muscle.

but there is no associated fascial defect. Causes of pseudohernia include diabetic neuropathy, herpes zoster infection, nerve injury, and syringomyelia.[212]

Of the acquired lumbar hernias, about half are spontaneous and the rest are incisional or posttraumatic hernias. Flank incisions are used to access the retroperitoneum for procedures such as nephrectomy, and hernias can result, which may be true hernias or pseudohernias caused by postoperative muscle paralysis.[213,214] Lumbar hernias have also been reported after harvest of bone from the iliac crest.[215] Motor vehicle accidents are the most common cause of posttraumatic lumbar hernias. If a lumbar hernia is found after a motor vehicle accident, it is critical to assume that the patient has other intra-abdominal injuries. Most of these patients will undergo urgent laparotomy; more than 60% of them will have major intra-abdominal injuries.[216,217]

Epidemiology

Lumbar hernias are rare, with about 300 cases reported.[210] Some 20% are congenital, and they are rarely bilateral.[218,219]

Clinical Features, Diagnosis, and Complications

Lumbar incisional hernias generally present as a large bulge that may produce discomfort. These are especially evident when the patient strains or is in the upright position. Because of the large size of the defect, incarceration is not common. Moreover, the location, in the retroperitoneum, makes incarceration of intraabdominal structures rare. Superior and inferior lumbar triangle hernias may occur through small defects and can manifest with incarceration (24%) and strangulation (18%).[220] The differential diagnosis includes lipoma, renal tumor, abscess, and hematoma. Bowel, mesentery, spleen, ovary, and kidney have been reported to herniate.[218] Occasionally, a small lumbar hernia may impinge on a cutaneous branch of a lumbosacral nerve, causing pain referred to the groin or thigh. Most patients have had a CT scan prior to seeing the surgeon for this disorder.[221]

Treatment and Prognosis

Closure of large lumbar hernias, as well as superior and inferior lumbar triangle hernias, often requires the use of prosthetic mesh or an aponeurotic flap. Identifying fascia with good tensile strength and repairing the defect with mesh in a tension-free manner is critical to preventing recurrence.[218,222] Fixation of mesh to bony structures (e.g., rib, iliac crest) may be required. Preperitoneal as well as transperitoneal laparoscopic repair has been reported and can result in less pain and quicker return to activity.[210,214,223,224] The open surgical approach is a reliable way to get good fixation to stable structures. Large and symptomatic lumbar pseudohernias should be treated by managing the underlying condition. Resolution of lumbar pseudohernia symptoms has been reported following treatment of herpes zoster.[212]

INTERNAL HERNIAS

Internal hernias are protrusions into pouches or openings within the abdominal cavity, rather than through the abdominal wall. Internal hernias may be the result of developmental anomalies or may be acquired, most commonly after an RYGB procedure.[225]

Etiology and Pathophysiology

Internal hernias caused by developmental anomalies include paraduodenal, foramen of Winslow, mesenteric, and supravesical hernias. During gestation, the intestines are extra-abdominal. During fetal development, the mesentery of the duodenum, ascending colon, and descending colon becomes fixed to the posterior peritoneum. These segments of the bowel become reperitonealized and attach to the retroperitoneum. Anomalies of mesenteric fixation may lead to abnormal openings through which internal hernias may occur. The extreme example of this is a complete intestinal malrotation, in which the ligament of Treitz does not assume its appropriate location to the left of the spine. This condition predisposes to midgut volvulus and can lead to extensive mesenteric ischemia (see Chapter 98).[226,227] Lesser anomalies of fixation lead to defects such as paraduodenal and supravesical hernias. Abnormal mesenteric fixation may lead to abnormal mobility of the small bowel and right colon, which facilitates herniation. During fetal development, abnormal openings may occur in the pericecal, small bowel, transverse colon, or sigmoid mesentery, as well as the omentum, leading to mesenteric hernias.[225] Unusual hernias can occur on structures like the broad ligament.[228]

Abnormal fixation of the mesentery of the descending or ascending colon may lead to paraduodenal hernias. Paraduodenal hernias occur on the left side in 75% of cases and have a 3:1 male predominance.[229–232] Patients most commonly present in the fourth decade. In cases of left paraduodenal hernia, an abnormal foramen (the fossa of Landzert), develops through the mesentery close to the ligament of Treitz, tracking under the distal transverse and descending colon and posterior to the superior mesenteric artery. Small bowel may protrude through this fossa and become fixed in the left upper quadrant of the abdomen. The mesentery of the colon thus forms the anterior wall of a sac that encloses a portion of the small intestine. Right paraduodenal hernia occurs in the same fashion through another abnormal foramen, the fossa of Waldeyer, leading under the ascending colon.[225,233]

Foramen of Winslow hernias may occur when this foramen is abnormally large, particularly if there is abnormal mesenteric fixation of the small bowel and right colon. Most commonly, the right colon is abnormally fixed to the retroperitoneum, resulting in a patulous foramen of Winslow. Abnormally mobile small bowel and colon may herniate through the foramen of Winslow into the lesser sac. Symptoms of small bowel or colonic obstruction may occur, and these may be intermittent as the hernia reduces spontaneously. Impingement on the portal structures can occur but rarely results in biliary obstruction or compression of the portal vein.[234,235] Gastric symptoms may also occur if the herniated bowel becomes distended, because the herniated bowel loops are located in the lesser sac, behind the stomach.

Mesenteric hernias occur when a loop of intestine protrudes through an abnormal opening in the mesentery of the small bowel or colon. These mesenteric defects can be congenital, although they may also be acquired as a result of surgery, trauma, or infection. The most common area for such an opening is in the mesentery of the small intestine, most often near the ileocolic junction. Defects have been reported in the mesentery of the appendix, sigmoid colon, and a Meckel diverticulum.[236–238] The intestine finds its way through the defects through normal peristaltic activity. Various lengths of intestine may herniate posteriorly to the right colon into the right paracolic gutter (Fig. 27.10). Compression of the loops may lead to obstruction of the herniated intestine. Strangulation may occur by compression or by torsion of the herniated segment. Obstruction may be acute, chronic, or intermittent. The herniated bowel may also compress arteries in the margins of the mesenteric defect, causing ischemia of nonherniated intestine. Similar defects may occur in the mesentery of the small bowel, transverse mesocolon, omentum, and sigmoid mesocolon.

There are three types of mesenteric hernias involving the sigmoid colon. Transmesosigmoid hernias have no true hernia sac and occur through both layers of the mesocolon. Generally, the bowel becomes trapped in the left paracolic gutter, lateral to the sigmoid colon. Intermesosigmoid hernias are hernias that occur within the leaves of the sigmoid colon. This results in the hernia contents being contained within the mesentery of the sigmoid colon, generally posterior to the sigmoid colon. Intersigmoid hernias occur between the retroperitoneal fusion plane, between the sigmoid colon mesentery and the retroperitoneum. These hernias are contained in the retroperitoneum and generally lift and dissect the sigmoid colon on its mesentery out of the left paracolic gutter.[231]

Supravesical hernias protrude into abnormal fossae around the bladder. They are classified as internal or external supravesical hernias. Internal supravesical hernias occur within the abdomen and thus are internal hernias. They may extend anterior, lateral,

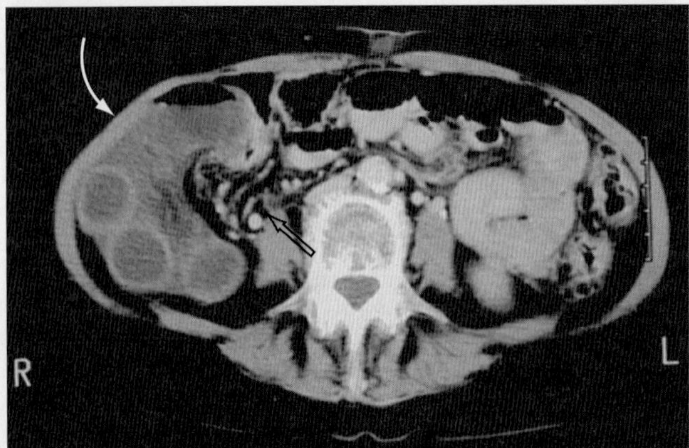

Fig. 27.10 CT of an internal (pericecal) hernia with strangulation. A mass of infarcted small intestine is seen in the right side of the abdomen (*white arrow*). The area of herniation (*open arrow to right of spine*) shows twisting of the small bowel as it passes through the mesentery. (Courtesy Dr. Michael J. Smerud, Dallas, TX.)

or posterior to the bladder. External supravesical hernias occur outside the abdominal wall and appear much like indirect inguinal hernias. They usually contain small bowel but may contain omentum, colon, ovary, or fallopian tube.[239–241]

Acquired internal hernias may occur as a complication of surgery or trauma if abnormal spaces or mesenteric defects are created. Adhesions can create spaces into which bowel may herniate. Division of mesentery to create conduits, such as Roux-en-Y limbs, can lead to defects within the mesentery or around the reconstruction, which can result in herniation.[242–244]

Retroanastomotic hernias may occur after gastrojejunostomy, colostomy or ileostomy, ileal bypass, or vascular bypass when an abnormal space may be created into which small bowel, colon, or omentum may herniate. Retroanastomotic hernia can occur after gastrojejunostomy, usually after gastric resection with Billroth II reconstruction. The afferent loop, efferent loop, or both, protrude into the space posterior to the anastomosis. Efferent loop hernias are about three times as common as afferent loop hernias, likely caused by the limited length of the afferent loop and the tethering effect of fixed structures involved in the afferent loop. For example, after a Billroth II anastomosis, the afferent loop is connected to the duodenum, which is fixed, and the efferent loop is connected to the remainder of the small intestine. The efferent loop is therefore more mobile and can herniate into potential spaces.[231,245] Colostomy, ileostomy, ileal bypass, and vascular bypass procedures may also lead to the creation of a space into which organs can protrude. Obstruction secondary to retroanastomotic hernia has been reported after liver transplantation.[246] Renal transplant procedures are extraperitoneal, but an unrecognized inadvertent rent in the peritoneum can lead to pararenal intestinal herniation.[247]

Hernias after RYGB procedures have become more common with the increasing demand for this operation. These can be internal or external hernias through the incision or port sites. Small bowel obstruction related to internal hernias after RYGB occurs in 2%–3% of patients.[242,243,248] There are three potential spaces created during the RYGB that can result in internal herniation. The *Peterson defect* occurs to the right of the jejunum as it traverses the mesentery of the transverse colon to reach the pouch of the stapled stomach. By definition, the Roux limb has to travel in the retrocolic location for this to occur. The endoscopist encounters this as a narrowing that occurs in the Roux limb at around 40–60 cm distal to the pouch-jejunum anastomosis. The *jejunojejunostomy mesenteric defect* occurs between the divided leaves of the small intestinal mesentery. The mesentery is divided to create the Roux limb, which is brought up to the gastric pouch. The two edges of the transected mesentery are then sewn together to prevent this defect. However, despite these measures, a defect can develop resulting in herniation of intra-abdominal contents. The *transverse mesocolic defect* occurs through the defect in the transverse mesocolon through which the jejunal limb is brought to reach the stomach pouch. The Peterson and transverse mesocolic defects can be avoided by placing the jejunal limb in an antecolic position, the position that is favored by most bariatric surgeons in the modern era. In this case, the jejunum is not placed through a rent in the transverse mesocolon, but rather is brought anterior to the transverse colon. With the majority of RYGB being performed minimally invasively, there are fewer adhesions being formed after surgery; this in fact allows for greater mobility of the small intestine and a greater ability to prolapse through hernia defects. Adhesions that occur with open surgery can actually reduce the risk for this type of internal hernia. However, adhesive causes for bowel obstruction occur more frequently in the open gastric bypass cases. The Duodenal Switch surgery carries similar risk of internal hernias. In this surgery, the Roux limb is typically brought anterior to the transverse colon, avoiding the Peterson's defect and the transmesocolic defect.

Hernias can occur in the mesentery of the colon very rarely after colonoscopy.[249,250] This likely occurs as a rent develops in the sigmoid mesocolon with insufflation of the colon.

Hernias may occur through the broad ligament of the uterus, most commonly through tears occurring during pregnancy, because the majority of these hernias occur in parous women. Other cases may be developmental or caused by surgery.[228,251]

Epidemiology

Internal hernias are rare and occur most often in adults. They are found in 0.2%–0.9% of autopsies, but a substantial proportion of these remain asymptomatic.[231] About 5% of bowel obstructions are caused by internal hernias.

Although half of developmental internal hernias are paraduodenal hernias, 1% or fewer of all cases of intestinal obstruction are caused by paraduodenal hernias.[225,232,252] They are more common in males than in females. They may occur in children or adults but typically manifest between the third and sixth decades of life; most (75%) paraduodenal hernias occur on the left side.[229–232]

Foramen of Winslow hernias are very rare, accounting for 8% of internal hernias.[225,252] Mesenteric hernias are rare and can occur at any age.[231,245] Supravesical hernias are extremely rare, with limited case reports. They are more common in men than in women. Almost all reported cases have occurred in adults, most commonly in the sixth or seventh decade.[241] Similarly, broad ligament hernias are exceedingly rare.[228] Postgastroenterostomy internal hernias have become less common because the frequency of surgery for peptic ulcer disease has declined. Other post-anastomotic internal hernias are also rare.[231] Internal hernias related to RYGB procedures have become more common because surgeries for morbid obesity have become more widely performed. Small bowel obstruction related to internal hernias in most patients occurs with an incidence of 2%–3% after RYGB.[242,243,248]

Clinical Features and Diagnosis

Any of the various forms of internal hernias may manifest with symptoms of acute or chronic intermittent intestinal obstruction. The diagnosis is difficult in patients with chronic symptoms and is rarely made preoperatively in patients who present with acute obstruction and strangulation.[225,231,245]

Intestinal obstruction, which may be low-grade, chronic, and recurrent or high-grade and acute, develops in about half of patients with paraduodenal hernias.[231,232] UGI tract contrast radiography has been shown to have excellent accuracy. Barium radiographs may show the small bowel to be bunched up or agglomerated as if it were contained in a bag, and displaced to the left or right side of the colon. Small bowel is often absent from the pelvis, and appears to be present in the lesser sac, posterior to the stomach. The colon may be deviated by the internal hernia sac. Bowel proximal to the hernia may be dilated.[231,253] However, barium radiographs may be normal if the hernia has reduced at the time of the study. Endoscopy is not reliable for the diagnosis of paraduodenal hernias. Displacement of the mesenteric vessels can be noted if CT with intravenous contrast or arteriography is performed.[229,231] However, CT may miss a paraduodenal hernia unless specific attention is paid to the relationship of the small intestine to the colon and mesenteric vessels.

In hernias of the foramen of Winslow, small bowel herniates behind the portal structures in about two-thirds of cases; in the remaining cases, the right colon herniates into the lesser sac. Herniation of the gallbladder has been reported.[234] Patients may have symptoms of gastric or proximal intestinal obstruction, even in the case of colon herniation, because of pressure of the herniated bowel on the stomach. Occasionally, an epigastric mass is palpable. Plain abdominal radiographs may show the stomach displaced anteriorly and to the left. Bowel, most commonly right colon, will be seen posterior to the stomach in the lesser sac. Contrast enema may show displacement of the cecum into the epigastrium. CT is accurate for the diagnosis of foramen of Winslow hernias. The herniated bowel is posterior to the stomach within the lesser sac. There may be associated dilation of the biliary tree or portal vein narrowing caused by compression of the portal structures.[231,235]

Mesenteric hernias are difficult to diagnose preoperatively. Symptoms and signs are those of acute or chronic intermittent bowel obstruction or acute strangulation.[245] Plain abdominal radiographs may show evidence of bowel obstruction or displacement of the normal gas pattern. For example, with hernias through the sigmoid mesentery, the small intestine gas pattern lies laterally to the sigmoid gas pattern.[231] This finding, in association with bowel obstruction, may increase the suspicion for an internal hernia.

Internal supravesical hernias produce symptoms of bowel obstruction. Associated symptoms of bladder compression occur in about 30% of cases. Anterior supravesical hernias may result in a suprapubic mass or tenderness. Patients with supravesical hernia may also have an inguinal hernia. Barium radiography or abdominal CT with oral contrast may be helpful in the diagnosis.[239,241]

Hernias of the broad ligament of the uterus cause symptoms of bowel obstruction in about half of cases and can cause chronic pelvic pain.[251] Other cases are discovered incidentally at surgery. Small bowel, sigmoid colon, appendix, omentum, and ureter have been reported to herniate. CT scanning may show dilation of small bowel and deviation of the uterus.

Retroanastomotic hernias cause symptoms and signs similar to those of other internal hernias. Postgastrojejunostomy hernias cause symptoms of gastric outlet obstruction. The efferent loop herniates most often. Afferent loop hernias are a cause of the afferent loop syndrome (see Chapter 55). About 50% of postgastrojejunostomy hernias occur within the first month after surgery, 25% occur during the first year, and the rest occur later.[252] The physical examination is not specific. The serum amylase and lipase level is often elevated with afferent limb obstruction. Plain abdominal radiographs may show gastric distention and a fluid-filled loop. Barium UGI radiographs are most useful for documenting efferent limb obstruction versus afferent limb obstruction. Sonography or CT may show dilation of the afferent limb, or the "whirl sign," where the mesenteric vessels and small bowel appear to twist around a point[253] (Fig. 27.11). Biliary scintigraphy will show excretion of radionuclide into the biliary tree but retention of the tracer in an obstructed afferent limb.[231]

The clinical presentation of post-RYGB hernias is similar to that of other internal hernias. Most commonly, bowel obstruction is present. Herniation of the afferent limb of the jejunojejunostomy (the limb that carries pancreaticobiliary secretions) can present an interesting diagnostic dilemma because this loop does not carry food material. Therefore vomiting may not occur. As a consequence, herniation of the afferent limb may present with biliary obstruction and pancreatitis rather than classic bowel obstruction. CT and plain films will show evidence of duodenal distention, and on biliary scintigraphy there is lack of progression of radionuclide from the dilated duodenum into the distal small intestine. Herniation of the distal small intestine manifests with signs and symptoms of a bowel obstruction. The finding of a "whirl sign" after RYGB in a patient with symptoms should lead to *immediate* surgical evaluation. Delay in treatment can result in bowel loss and death. Strictures at the base of the Roux limb can present with a similar obstructive syndrome. However, findings of a more distal bowel obstruction should increase suspicion for an internal hernia.

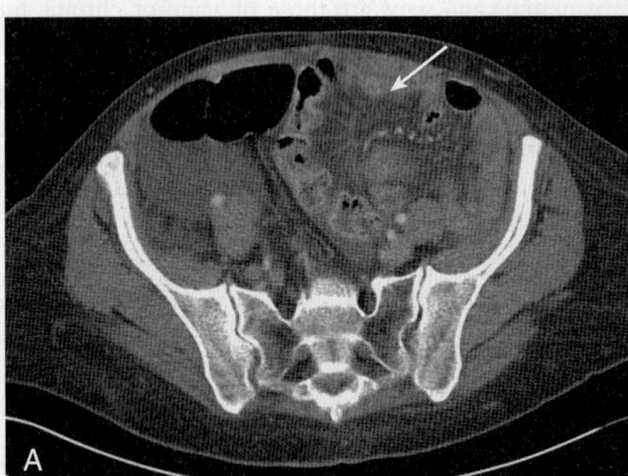

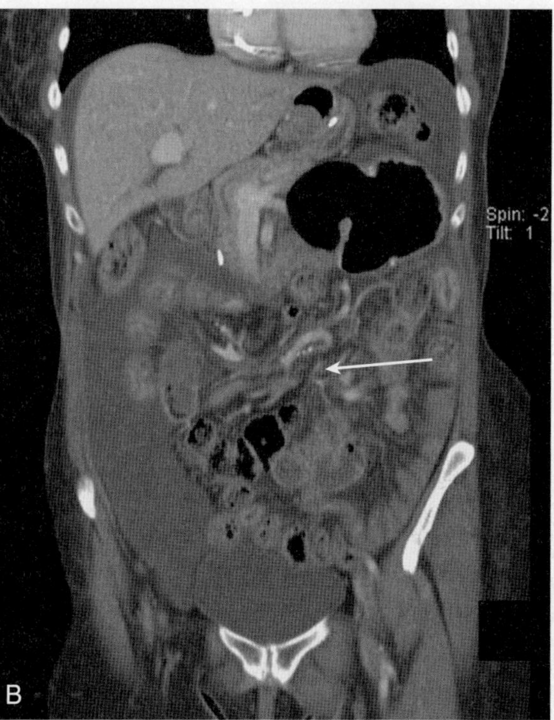

Fig. 27.11 CT on an internal hernia showing the "whirl sign." (A) Whirl sign is seen in a patient with an internal hernia after Roux-en-Y gastric bypass (*arrow*). (B) Upright view of same patient shows the point of twisting of the bowel and mesentery (*arrow*).

Treatment and Prognosis

Symptomatic internal hernias require surgery.[225,231,245,252] Laparoscopic repair is preferred if the hernia is detected prior to complications.[235,241,251] Once the patient has developed signs and symptoms of bowel obstruction, it is reasonable to explore the patient, reduce the hernia, ensure the bowel is viable, and repair the defect. Acute obstruction leads to strangulation, bowel ischemia, and death if not promptly treated.[238]

Paraduodenal hernias are usually corrected by incising the enclosing mesentery. Care must be taken to avoid injuring the superior or inferior mesenteric arteries, because they follow an abnormal course within the border of the hernia. Sometimes the small bowel can be reduced through the opening of the hernia without incising the mesentery.[229,232] Thereafter, the paraduodenal defect must be closed. This may involve performing a formal Ladd procedure if the hernia is associated with a true malrotation (see Chapter 100).[226,227] If there is a patulous paraduodenal space, a simple resection of the hernia sac and plication of the defect can afford adequate repair. Once incarceration has occurred, mortality can be higher than 20%,[232] so it is recommended that all paraduodenal hernias be repaired electively if possible.

Broad ligament hernias and supravesical hernias can all be successfully repaired laparoscopically.[228,241,251]

Post-RYGB hernias are a common event in the current era, and the gastroenterologist must have a working knowledge of the anatomy and the possible defects that can occur. The post-RYGB patient who is unable to eat may have an internal hernia if there is no obstruction of the pouch-jejunal anastomosis. CT will usually show the "whirl sign" that should alert the treating physician to a possible internal hernia.[254] The surgeon should have a low threshold to operate on these patients, as missing an internal hernia can lead to bowel necrosis and short gut syndrome.

Full references for this chapter can be found at https://ebooks.health.elsevier.com

28 Foreign Bodies, Bezoars, and Caustic Ingestions

Patrick R. Pfau, Mark Benson

IN THIS CHAPTER

GI foreign bodies (GIFBs) are composed of food bolus impactions and intentionally and unintentionally ingested or inserted foreign objects. *Bezoars* are ingested materials (food or other materials) that accumulate in a normal or abnormal stomach. *Caustic ingestions* present following ingestion of acid or alkaline materials, which may result in acute and/or chronic injury to the esophagus and stomach. These topics are discussed in detail in this chapter.

GASTROINTESTINAL FOREIGN BODIES

GIFBs are a common problem encountered by gastroenterologists. Most resolve without serious clinical sequelae.[1] Annual incidence in the United States is estimated to be 120,000 cases per year.[2] Older studies have suggested that between 1500 and 2750 deaths occurred in the U.S. secondary to GIFBs.[3–5] More recent studies have shown mortality related to foreign bodies as high as 0.85% of cases to extremely rare with no deaths reported in over 850 adults and only one death in 2200 children with reported GIFBs.[6–13] Regardless of imprecise morbidity and mortality rates, serious complications and deaths can result from foreign body ingestions.[14–16] Because of their frequent occurrence and potential for negative consequences, it is important to understand which patients are at risk and know how to diagnose and treat GIFBs and deal with their complications.

Epidemiology

GIFBs may result from unintentional or intentional ingestion. The most common patient group that unintentionally ingests foreign bodies is children, particularly those between ages 6 months and 3 years. Children account for 80% of foreign body ingestions.[17] Children's natural oral curiosity leads to placing objects in their mouths and occasionally swallowing them. Coins are the most common objects swallowed by children, but other frequently swallowed objects include marbles, magnets, batteries, toys, crayons, and safety pins.[8,12,18,19]

Accidental ingestion due to loss of tactile sensation during swallowing may also occur in adults with dental covers or dentures[20]; mistakenly ingesting one's own dentures is not uncommon.[21] Patients with altered mental status or sensorium, including the elderly, demented, or intoxicated, are at risk for accidental foreign body ingestions (Fig. 28.1). Accidental coin ingestion has been noted in college-aged adults during a tavern beer drinking game called "Quarters," in which the coin may become lodged in the esophagus.[22] Finally, those in certain occupations (e.g., roofers, carpenters, seamstresses, and tailors) are at risk of accidental ingestion when nails or pins are held in the mouth during work.

The most common groups that intentionally ingest foreign bodies are psychiatric patients and prisoners,[23] in whom ingestion is often done for secondary gain; they often ingest objects multiple times and often the most complex foreign bodies.

Iatrogenic foreign bodies are increasing in prevalence because of complications from capsule endoscopy, migrated stents (esophageal, enteral, and biliary), and migrated enteral access tubes and bolsters.[24,25]

Esophageal food impaction is the most common GIFB requiring medical attention in the United States, with an incidence of 16/100,000.[26] The vast majority (75%–100%) of patients with an esophageal food impaction have an underlying predisposing esophageal pathology,[27,28] most often peptic strictures, Schatzki rings, and increasingly eosinophilic esophagitis (EoE).[29] Patients with recurrent food impactions almost universally have preexisting esophageal disease, particularly EoE.[30] Esophageal cancer rarely presents with acute food bolus impaction.[31] Other causes that contribute to esophageal food impactions include altered surgical anatomy following esophagectomy, fundoplication, or bariatric

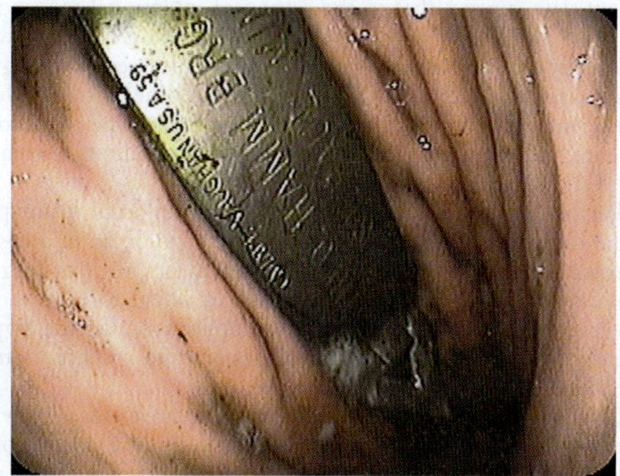

Fig. 28.1 Endoscopic image of a bottle opener (in the stomach) ingested by an intoxicated patient.

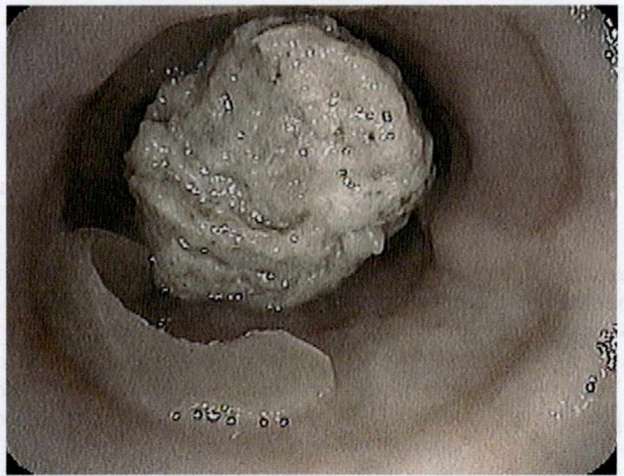

Fig. 28.2 Endoscopic image of bratwurst with sauerkraut impacted in the esophagus while the patient was tailgating at a football game.

surgery and motility disorders such as achalasia and distal esophageal spasm.[32]

Food impactions most commonly occur in adults in their fourth or fifth decade of life but are becoming more prevalent in young adults because of the rising incidence of EoE. Cultural and regional dietary habits influence GIFBs. Fishbone injury is common in Asian countries and the Pacific Rim, whereas impactions due to meats (e.g., hot dogs, pork, beef, chicken) are common in the United States (Fig. 28.2).[33,34]

Symptomatic rectal foreign bodies are more often the result of insertion through the anus rather than oral ingestion and transit. This is reported most commonly in young adult males with a male-to-female ratio of 6:1 with increasing incidence over the last decade.[35,36] Rectal foreign bodies that come to medical attention are most commonly inserted with the intention of autoeroticism but may present following consensual sexual acts or sexual assault.[37] Less common but still prevalent causes of rectal foreign bodies include concealment of illegal drugs during smuggling efforts, loss of objects during attempts by the patient to relieve constipation, and even reports of falling on objects.[38]

Pathophysiology

The majority (≈80%–90%) of GIFBs pass through the GI tract without any clinical sequelae and cause no harm to the patient.[1,39] The remaining 10%–20% of GIFBs will require endoscopic intervention, and 1% of GIFBs may require operative therapy.[7,40] Recent data suggest that in the setting of intentional ingestions, the need for endoscopic and surgical intervention is higher with endoscopy being performed in two-thirds of cases and surgery needed in greater than 10% of patients.[41] To help stratify therapeutic interventions, it is important to understand the conditions, patients, and anatomic locations in which complications associated with GIFBs are apt to occur.

Perforation and obstruction from GIFBs can occur in any part of the digestive tract, but they are more apt to occur in areas of narrowing, angulation, anatomic sphincters, or previous surgery (Fig. 28.3).[42] The pharynx is the first area where foreign bodies may become entrapped and cause complications. In the hypopharynx, short sharp objects like fishbones and toothpicks may lacerate the mucosa or become lodged.[43,44]

Once in the esophagus, there are four areas of narrowing where food boluses and foreign bodies become lodged: upper esophageal sphincter, level of the aortic arch, level of the mainstem bronchus, and esophagogastric junction. These areas all have luminal narrowing to 23 mm or less.[45] However, food and foreign bodies more commonly lodge in the esophagus at areas of

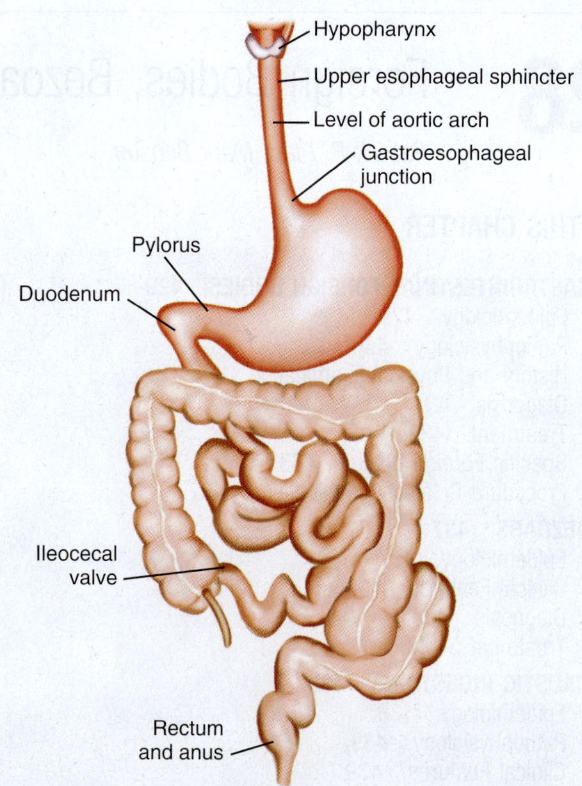

Fig. 28.3 Gastrointestinal areas of luminal narrowing and angulation that predispose to foreign body impaction and obstruction.

pathology, including rings, webs, or strictures. Multiple esophageal rings associated with EoE contribute to esophageal food impaction at an increasing prevalence in young adults and have become the most common cause of esophageal food impaction overall.[29,46,47] Similarly, esophageal motor abnormalities (such as distal esophageal spasm or achalasia) may lead to food or foreign body impaction in the esophagus.[48–51] Foreign body and food impaction in the esophagus have the highest incidence of overall adverse events, with the complication rate proportional to the duration it is lodged in the esophagus. Esophageal foreign bodies in children have a significantly lower spontaneous passage rate, as low as 12% compared with other GIFBs.[52] Serious complications of esophageal foreign bodies include perforation, abscess, mediastinitis, pneumothorax, fistula formation, and cardiac tamponade.[53,54]

If a GIFB passes through the esophagus, the vast majority will pass through the entire GI tract without further difficulty or complication. Exceptions are sharp, long, and large objects. Sharp or pointed objects may have a perforation rate as high as 35%. Large objects (>2.5 cm in diameter) may not be able to pass through the pylorus. Long objects (>5 cm) such as pens, pencils, and eating utensils may not negotiate around the duodenal sweep or through the pylorus.

Objects may become impacted in the small intestine at the ligament of Treitz or ileocecal valve. Adhesions, inflammatory strictures, and surgical anastomoses within the small intestine may also be sites where foreign bodies lodge and obstruct. However, most objects, even sharp ones, rarely cause damage once in the small intestine and colon, because the bowel naturally protects itself through peristalsis and axial flow. These factors tend to keep the foreign body concentrated in the center of fecal residue, with the blunt end leading and the sharp end trailing.[55,56]

Inserted rectal objects are often tenaciously retained because of anal sphincter spasm and edema, making spontaneous passage of the object difficult. The angulation and valves of Houston may also impede the passage of objects through the rectum.

History and Physical Examination

The history of children or noncommunicative adults with altered sensorium or a psychiatric history is often unreliable. Most gastric and up to 20%–30% of esophageal foreign bodies in children are asymptomatic.[57] Most present after having been witnessed or suspected by a parent or caregiver but in up to 40% of cases, there is no history of a witnessed ingestion.[58] Thus symptoms are often subtle in children, presenting as drooling, not wanting to eat, and failure to thrive.

For communicative adults, history of the timing and type of ingestion is usually reliable. Patients are able to relate exactly what they ingested, when they ingested it, and symptoms of pain and/or obstruction. Patients with esophageal food bolus impactions are symptomatic with complete or intermittent obstruction. They are unable to drink liquids or retain their own oral secretions. Sialorrhea is common. Ingestion of an unappreciated small, sharp object, including obscured fish or animal bones, may cause odynophagia or a persistent foreign body sensation because of mucosal laceration. If the patient presents with dysphagia, odynophagia, or dysphonia, there is an 80% likelihood a foreign body is present, causing at least partial obstruction. Symptoms of drooling and inability to handle secretions are indicative of a near-total esophageal obstruction. If symptoms are restricted to retrosternal chest pain or pharyngeal discomfort, less than 50% of patients will still have a foreign body present.[59] Patient localization of where an ingested foreign object is lodged is not accurate, with only a 30%–40% correct localization in the esophagus and essentially a 0% accuracy for foreign bodies in the stomach.[57,60] Once the object reaches the stomach, small intestine, or colon, the patient will not report symptoms unless a complication occurs (e.g., obstruction, perforation, bleeding).

Patients with rectal foreign bodies are frequently asymptomatic,[37] but embarrassment may interfere with obtaining an accurate history. Presentation is often after the patient or another person has made multiple attempts to remove the object.[43] Symptoms may include anorectal pain, bleeding, and pruritus, with a small number of patients presenting with more serious complications, including obstruction, perforation, and peritonitis.

Past medical history is useful to identify previous foreign body ingestion; repeat offenders are likely to ingest multiple and more complex foreign objects. A history of dysphagia in a person with a food impaction or esophageal foreign body suggests a high likelihood of underlying esophageal pathology. Previous food impaction or need for esophageal dilation makes recurrent episodes more likely. A history of allergies (e.g., asthma, allergic rhinitis, and food allergy) may be a clue that a patient may have EoE.[61]

Physical examination does little to secure the diagnosis or location of a retained foreign body, but it is crucial to identify complications related to foreign body ingestion. Assessment of the patient's airway, ventilatory status, and risk for aspiration are crucial prior to initiating therapy to remove a GIFB. A neck and chest examination looking for crepitus, erythema, and swelling can suggest a proximal perforation. A lung examination should be performed to detect the presence of aspiration or wheezing. An abdominal examination should be performed to evaluate for signs of perforation or obstruction.

Diagnosis

Imaging

Plain films of the chest and abdomen are recommended for patients presenting with suspected foreign body ingestion to determine the presence, type, number, and location of foreign objects present. Radiologic evaluation is not routinely needed for patients with nonbony food impactions who have no complications.[62] Both anteroposterior and lateral chest films are needed because lateral films will aid in determining if a foreign body is in the esophagus or the trachea[63] and may detail foreign bodies obscured by the overlying spine in an anteroposterior film. Biplanar neck films are recommended if there is a suspected object or complication in the hypopharynx or cervical esophagus. Plain films are also useful in identifying complications like free air, aspiration, or subcutaneous emphysema (Fig. 28.4).[64]

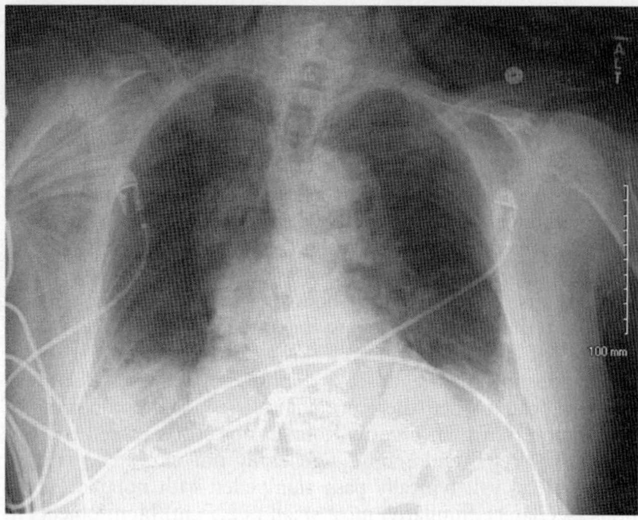

Fig. 28.4 Chest film demonstrating pneumomediastinum and bilateral pneumothoraces in a patient who developed esophageal perforation secondary to a food impaction left untreated for longer than 24 hours.

Unfortunately, radiography cannot image nonradiopaque objects (e.g., plastic, glass, and wood) and may miss small bones, particularly fishbones in the proximal esophagus. The false-negative rate for plain film investigation of foreign bodies is as high as 47%, with false-positive rates up to 20%. False-negative rates for food impactions have been reported as high as 87%.[65] If continued clinical suspicion or symptoms warrant, the individual should undergo further clinical investigation.[66]

Use of plain films in children is more controversial because of the inability of the child to give a history and the associated radiation exposure. Some have suggested mouth-to-anus screening films to detect the presence of foreign bodies in children. Bedside ultrasound has been effective in identifying esophageal foreign bodies in children without the need of radiation.[67,68] Also to limit radiation, handheld metal detectors have been used, with a sensitivity ranging from 89% to 95% for detection and localization of metallic foreign bodies.[69,70]

Barium studies are generally not recommended for evaluating GIFBs. Aspiration of hypertonic contrast agents in patients with complete or near-complete esophageal obstruction may lead to aspiration pneumonitis.[71] Barium may also delay or impair the performance of a therapeutic endoscopic intervention by interfering with endoscopic visualization.[72] Even if a barium study is considered normal, an endoscopy is still recommended if symptoms persist or suspicion of a foreign body is high.[43]

CT or MRI are not routinely needed for the diagnosis of GIFBs. However, CT has been found to detect foreign bodies missed by other modalities[73] and has been found to be superior to radiography in the detection of fishbones (90% sensitivity vs. 32%).[74] CT should be performed in any patient with suspected complications such as perforation or abscess, prior to the use of endoscopy[74] CT of the cervical esophagus or hypopharynx prior to the endoscopic investigation may benefit diagnosis.[75]

Endoscopy

Endoscopy provides the most precise means to diagnose suspected foreign bodies or food impactions. This ensures an almost 100% diagnostic accuracy for objects within the reach of the endoscope, including nonradiopaque objects that are not visualized by radiography.

Endoscopy allows the most accurate diagnosis of the underlying pathology, such as esophageal strictures, which may have led to an impacted esophageal foreign body. Endoscopy also allows visualization of mucosal defects, abrasions, or ulcerations that may have resulted from the foreign body. Diagnostic endoscopy is also linked to the most efficacious therapy for GIFBs, the use of therapeutic endoscopy to remove or treat the object.

Diagnostic upper endoscopy for foreign bodies is relatively contraindicated when there are clinical or radiographic signs of perforation. Once an ingested foreign object has passed the ligament of Treitz, endoscopy is generally not indicated, because these objects will typically pass unimpeded with notable exceptions (see later). Similarly, most small (<2.5 cm) blunt objects in an adult patient's stomach do not require endoscopic retrieval; most will pass without complication.

Treatment

Nonendoscopic Methods

Treatment of GIFBs should always be planned with the knowledge that 80%–90% of GIFBs will spontaneously pass through the GI tract without complication.[7,10] This has led some investigators to suggest that all foreign bodies can be managed with conservative observation.[76,77] Although conservative management is effective in most cases of GIFB, it is more appropriate to perform selective endoscopy for treatment based on the location, size, and type of foreign body ingested.[23,78]

Several medical therapies have been considered primary treatment of esophageal foreign bodies and food impactions. The smooth muscle relaxant glucagon is the most widely used and studied drug for the treatment of esophageal food and foreign object impactions. Glucagon, given in intravenous doses of 0.5–2 mg, can produce relaxation of the lower esophageal sphincter by as much as 60%, with the potential to permit passage of the impacted food or foreign body.[79,80] Success with glucagon has been reported to be from 12% to 58% in treating food impactions.[81–83] However, a multicenter study showed glucagon to be effective in only 14% of cases and a meta-analysis of >1100 patients showed no increase in treatment success with glucagon.[84,85] Glucagon may cause nausea, vomiting, and abdominal distention and has little effect when a fixed obstruction is present. Nifedipine and nitroglycerin are not recommended because of hypotension-related side effects and no proven efficacy. Similarly, anticholinergic agents and benzodiazepines have been used but without proven efficacy.

Gas-forming agents like carbonated beverages or preparations consisting of sodium bicarbonate and citric acid have been described for treating esophageal impactions. They are purported to release carbon dioxide gas to distend the lumen and act as a piston to push the object from the esophagus into the stomach.[86] A retrospective study did show a success rate in treating food impaction of 55% with effervescent agents, superior to glucagon or no therapy.[87] However, perforations and aspiration have been reported with the use of gas-forming objects and should be used with caution.[88] The meat tenderizer papain is not recommended for the treatment of esophageal meat impactions; its lack of efficacy and risk of complications (e.g., perforation and mediastinitis) have been described.[89,90]

Under fluoroscopic guidance, Foley catheters, suction catheters, wire baskets, and magnets attached to tubes have been used to retract objects.[64] The most described extraction device is the Foley catheter; its tip is passed beyond the object, the balloon is inflated, and then the object is withdrawn into the oropharynx. Success with this method under fluoroscopy has been described as better than 90%. However, all radiographic methods suffer from lack of control of the object, particularly at the level of the upper esophageal sphincter and hypopharynx. Complications include nosebleeds, laryngospasm, aspiration, perforation, and even death.[91] Radiographic methods are recommended only if flexible endoscopy is unavailable.

Endoscopic Methods

Flexible endoscopy has become the treatment of choice for GIFBs because it is safe and highly efficacious. Multiple large series have reported the success rate for endoscopic treatment of GIFBs to be more than 95%, with complication rates of less than 5%.[7,40,70,78,92–94] The risk for complications is increased when sharp or multiple objects are ingested and when ingestion is intentional as opposed to accidental.

Because most GIFBs pass spontaneously without causing symptoms, it is important to understand the indications and timing for endoscopic intervention. Generally, all foreign bodies lodged in the esophagus require urgent intervention. Patients with complete esophageal obstruction should undergo a more emergent endoscopy within 2–6 hours. The risk for an adverse outcome from an esophageal foreign body or food impaction is directly related to how long the object or food dwells in the esophagus.[95] Ideally, no object should be left in the esophagus longer than 24 hours with a risk of complications increasing by greater than 14-fold for impacted objects left in longer.

Once in the stomach, most ingested objects will pass spontaneously, and the risk of complications is lower, making observation acceptable. There are notable exceptions. Sharp and pointed objects are associated with perforation rates as high as 15%–35% and should undergo endoscopy within 24 hours or less.[95] Magnets, batteries, and objects longer than 5 cm and round objects wider than 2.5 cm that may not pass should undergo endoscopy within 24 hours as well. If a more complex or sharp object has progressed beyond the stomach and cannot be retrieved, periodic radiographs should be obtained every 3–5 days to document progression through the GI tract.[96] The patient should be followed for any symptoms suggestive of obstruction or perforation (e.g., fever, tachycardia, abdominal pain, and distention).

With the increasing use of double and single balloon enteroscopy, case series have detailed the use of these scopes to safely and effectively retrieve various foreign bodies from the small bowel, in particular lodged video capsules.[97,98] Given that most foreign bodies pass without sequelae upon reaching the small intestine, use of balloon-assisted enteroscopy should take into consideration the type of object and the patient who ingested it. Accessories including baskets, hoods, and forceps have been designed for balloon enteroscopes to enable foreign body retrieval.

Sedation to facilitate endoscopy for the management of food impactions and ingested foreign objects should be individualized. Conscious sedation is adequate for treating most food impactions and simple foreign bodies in the adult population, but anesthesia assistance may be required for uncooperative patients or patients who have swallowed multiple complex objects, or patients who need protection of the airway. As trends shift for all endoscopic procedures being performed with anesthesia assistance, more patients with food impactions and foreign bodies are sedated with the aid of anesthesiology. Endoscopy for the treatment of foreign bodies in the pediatric population is usually performed with the aid of anesthesia and endotracheal intubation.[99]

For the management of impactions and ingestions below the level of the laryngopharynx, flexible endoscopy is preferred.[100] Rigid esophagoscopy and flexible nasoendoscopes can be used but

BOX 28.1 Equipment for Treatment and Removal of Gastrointestinal Foreign Bodies and Food Impactions

ENDOSCOPES

Flexible endoscope
Rigid endoscope
Laryngoscope

OVERTUBES

Standard esophageal overtube
45- to 60-cm foreign body overtube

ACCESSORY EQUIPMENT

Retrieval net
Grasping forceps
Dormia basket
Polypectomy snare
Transparent cap
Latex protector hood
Kelly or McGill forceps

provide no additional benefit and are often available to only a few endoscopists.[9,101] A meta-analysis of rigid versus flexible endoscopes to treat esophageal foreign bodies found no difference in success rate but greater than 2.5-fold more perforations with rigid endoscopes.[102] Laryngoscopes with the aid of a Kelly or McGill forceps can be useful for proximal foreign bodies and small sharp objects in the hypopharynx.

Availability of and familiarity with multiple endoscopic retrieval devices for the removal of foreign bodies and food impactions is critical (Box 28.1). An endoscopy suite and/or travel cart should be equipped with at least rat-tooth or alligator grasping forceps, polypectomy snare, Dormia basket, multiprong graspers, transparent caps, and retrieval net.[103] Overtubes of 45 and 60 cm in length should be available to the endoscopist. An overtube allows protection of the airway, multiple exchanges of the endoscope, and mucosal protection from sharp objects.[104] The longer 60-cm overtube enables retrieval of sharp and complex objects from the stomach and encompasses the lower esophageal sphincter. An alternative adjunct for the extraction of sharp objects is a latex protection hood that fits onto the tip of the endoscope (discussed later).[105,106]

When planning for extraction of complex, sharp, or pointed objects that were ingested, and when opportunity permits, it may be valuable to go through an ex vivo dry run on a similar object when considering retrieval devices and extraction technique.[7] Success and speed of retrieval of the foreign body have been shown to be directly related to endoscopist experience.[107] When personnel or facilities are not available to accomplish relief endoscopically, consideration should be given to transferring the patient to another center.

Specific Foreign Bodies

Food Impaction

Food impaction is the most common ingested foreign body in the United States.[32] The most common foods to cause impactions in the United States are meat products, including beef, hot dogs, and chicken. Fishbone impactions are more common in coastal areas and Asian countries. Imbibing alcohol while eating large cuts of meat may increase the risk for food impactions and has led to the terms *backyard barbecue syndrome* and *steakhouse syndrome*.

Given that food boluses may pass spontaneously, the need for endoscopic intervention is based on the persistence of symptoms.

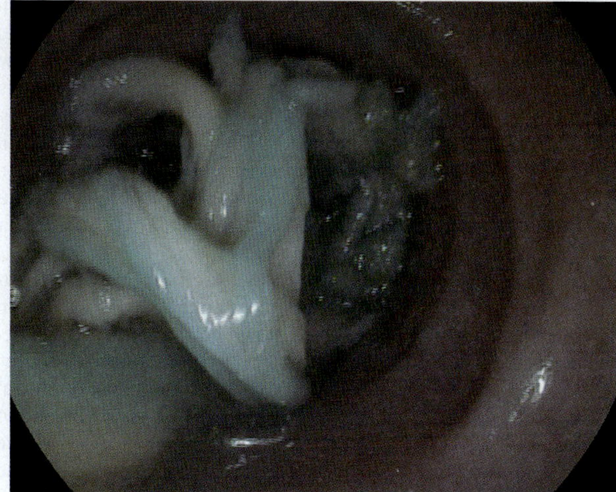

Fig. 28.5 Food impaction in a patient with multiple concentric rings and known diagnosis of eosinophilic esophagitis.

Patients with signs of complete or near-complete obstruction with drooling or excessive salivation should undergo emergent upper GI endoscopy within 2–6 hours of presentation. Endoscopic intervention in noncomplete obstruction should be achieved within 24 hours of onset of symptoms. Longer duration of the food impaction may decrease the endoscopy success rate[108] and increase risk for complications.[1,20,109]

The primary method to treat food impaction is the push method, with success rates well over 90% and minimal complications.[27] Before the food impaction is pushed into the stomach, an attempt to steer the endoscope around the food into the stomach should be made. Generally, if the endoscope can be passed around the food impaction into the stomach, the impaction can be safely pushed into the stomach without difficulty. This also allows the assessment of any obstructive esophageal pathology beyond the impaction. Even if the endoscope cannot steer around the food impaction, *gentle* pushing pressure can be safely attempted. Larger boluses of impacted meat can be broken apart with the endoscope or an accessory prior to safely pushing the smaller pieces into the stomach. Balloon dilation of an obstructing stricture distal to the food bolus to facilitate the push method has been shown to be safe and effective.[110]

EoE has increasingly been associated with esophageal food impactions resulting in an overall increase in food impactions with EoE as an etiology increasing at the highest rate[111] (Fig. 28.5). Food impactions tend to occur more frequently in EoE patients with visible endoscopic rings and higher eosinophil density on biopsy.[112] Reports indicate that food impaction in patients with EoE can be treated effectively and safely with the push method,[46] but care should be taken to minimize inducing mucosal tears.[113] While perforation is overall low with EoE, the majority of these perforations occur with a prolonged food bolus impaction.[114] Particular care should be taken when using rigid endoscopes if EoE is suspected; perforation rates with rigid scopes in this patient population have been reported as high as 20%.[115] If EoE is suspected, mucosal biopsies should be obtained after the food impaction is treated. However, only 34% of endoscopists take esophageal biopsies at the time of food impaction significantly decreasing the chance for diagnosis and proper treatment.[116] Treatment of EoE with proton pump inhibitors or topical glucocorticoids reduces the risk of subsequent food bolus impactions and should be started immediately after the initial endoscopy.[117]

Food impactions that cannot be gently pushed into the stomach must be dislodged and withdrawn. Retrograde removal can be achieved with various retrieval devices, including snares, baskets, nets, and forceps. Initial manual disruption of the food bolus into smaller pieces typically makes removal easier. An esophageal overtube may be useful because it protects the airway and allows multiple exchanges of the endoscope during retrieval. A retrieval net can be useful for removing large pieces of food without the use of an overtube, because the food can be satisfactorily secured within the net, reducing the risk of aspiration of the ingestate.[118] All pull methods can also be used effectively and safely in EoE patients, but care should be taken when placing overtubes, particularly in patients with a narrow caliber esophagus.

Transparent plastic hoods or caps, such as those used to perform variceal band ligation and endoscopic mucosal resection, have been successfully used to remove large, tightly impacted meat boluses (Fig. 28.6). Use of the cap may be a more effective method with less complications than using other devices to pull out the food impaction. A randomized controlled study has shown cap-assisted treatment of food impactions to be more effective, less costly, and have a shorter procedure time than conventional endoscopic removal.[119] With the cap secured to the tip of the endoscope, the device can be used to suction the food into the vacuum chamber and withdraw the bolus per os.[120,121]

More than 75% of patients with food impactions have associated esophageal pathology,[7,28] and about half of patients with food bolus impactions have abnormal 24-hour esophageal pH studies and/or esophageal manometry. If an esophageal stricture or Schatzki ring is present after the food bolus is cleared, it can be safely and effectively dilated with no increase in complications. Dilation is performed in less than 20% of food impaction cases leading to a loss of patients for interval dilation and recurrent impactions.[122] Empiric proton pump inhibitor therapy should be prescribed until follow-up. Lack of appropriate follow-up for patients has been described as high at 50%−79% of food impaction patients, particularly those with strictures or rings, and this lack of follow-up has been shown to be a predictor for recurrent food impactions, continued esophageal symptoms, and need for further dilations.[123]

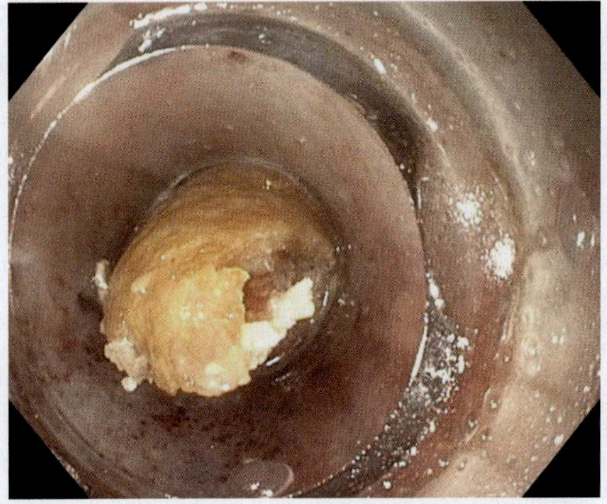

Fig. 28.6 Use of a transparent plastic cap to remove a large meat bolus food impaction.

Sharp and Pointed Objects

Sharp and pointed objects may cause a perforation in up to 15% −35% of patients and account for one-third of all perforations from GI foreign bodies, with a 2.5-fold greater risk of complications compared to other GIFB.[124,125] Sharp and pointed objects, particularly toothpicks and animal bones, are the most likely ingested foreign objects to cause a perforation that necessitates surgical management.[126] Patients with psychiatric illness and incarcerated patients are more likely to ingest more complex and multiple sharp and pointed objects, such as razor blades (Fig. 28.7), pins, needles, and writing and eating utensils (Fig. 28.8). If a patient with a history of a sharp ingested foreign body has negative radiographs, a CT scan and endoscopy should still be strongly considered.

Sharp objects above the cricopharyngeus should be seen by otolaryngology for removal with a laryngoscope. Sharp and pointed objects retained in the esophagus are considered a medical emergency and should be removed in less than 6 hours. Time of impaction and delayed time to endoscopy have been shown to significantly increase the perforation rate in sharp esophageal foreign bodies.[127] Any sharp and pointed object within the reach of the endoscope should be removed if this can be safely done. When removing sharp and pointed objects, the foreign body should be grasped and oriented so that the pointed end trails on withdrawal to reduce the risk of perforation and mucosal laceration.[128]

For sharp and pointed objects, retrieval is best achieved with grasping forceps, polypectomy snare, or biliary stone retrieval basket.[107] All these devices can secure the object; orient the device with the sharp end pointing distally as described earlier. Retrieval nets tend to shear in the removal of sharp objects and may compromise visualization.

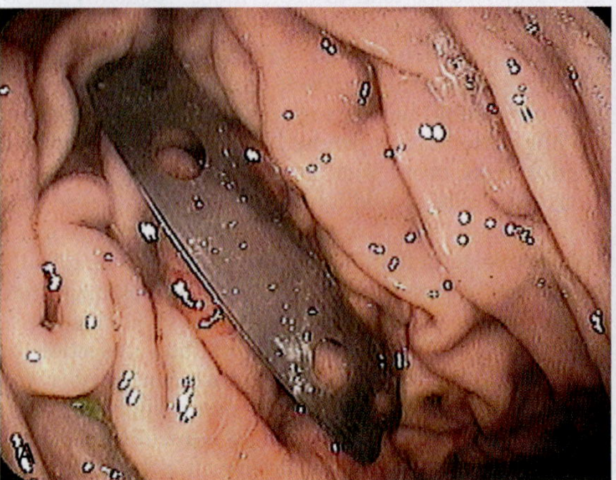

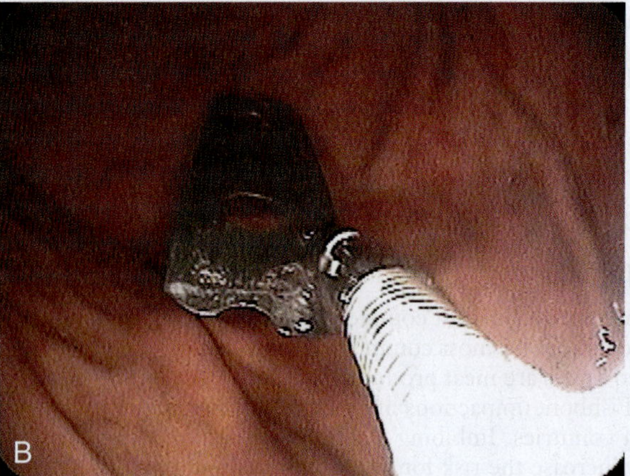

Fig. 28.7 (A) A razor blade (in the stomach) ingested by a prisoner. (B) Removal of the razor blade with a grasping forceps and overtube.

Use of an overtube should be considered to protect the esophagus and pharynx. Long, pointed objects can be grasped and directed into the overtube; the entire assembly, including the sharp and pointed object, endoscope, and overtube, are then removed in unison (Fig. 28.9).

An alternative to an overtube for the extraction of sharp and pointed objects is a retractable latex hood that can be affixed to the tip of the endoscope (Fig. 28.10). When the endoscope is pulled back through the lower esophageal sphincter, the hood flips over the grasped object and protects the mucosa during withdrawal.[105,129]

Although associated with an increased risk of perforation, most sharp or pointed objects beyond the reach of the endoscope will pass unimpeded and be eliminated through the GI tract without complication. Because of the increased risk of perforation, sharp and pointed objects should be followed by serial daily radiographs to ensure progression. If a sharp or pointed object fails to progress over 3 days, operative intervention should be considered.

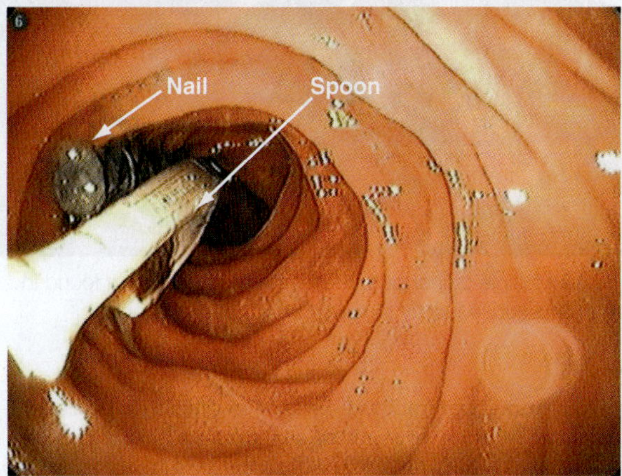

Fig. 28.8 Endoscopic image of a nail and a long spoon that became impacted in the duodenal sweep after being swallowed by a psychiatric patient.

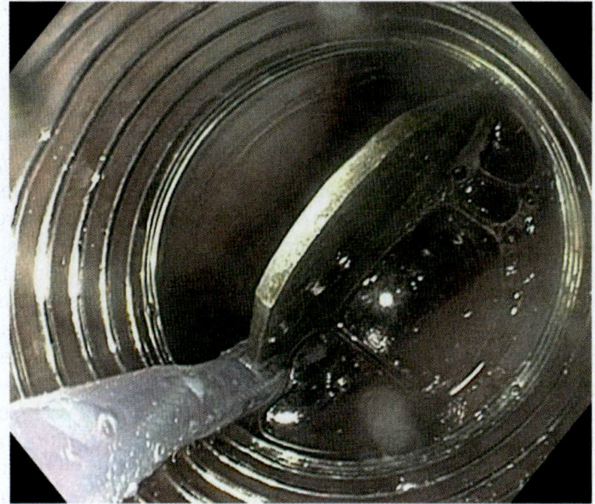

Fig. 28.9 Removal of a sharp foreign body with the pointed end of the object downwards pulled through an overtube by a rat-tooth forceps.

Long Objects

Ingested objects longer than 5 cm, especially those longer than 10 cm, have difficulty passing through the pylorus and duodenal sweep and can get hung up, causing obstruction or perforation at these locations (Fig. 28.11). The most commonly ingested long objects are pens, pencils, toothbrushes, and eating utensils as well as migrated luminal and biliary stents. Grasping forceps and polypectomy snares are the most commonly used devices to secure and remove long objects. Long objects should be grasped at one end and oriented longitudinally to permit removal. For extraction of long objects, use of the 60-cm overtube endoscope assembly, as described earlier, should be considered.

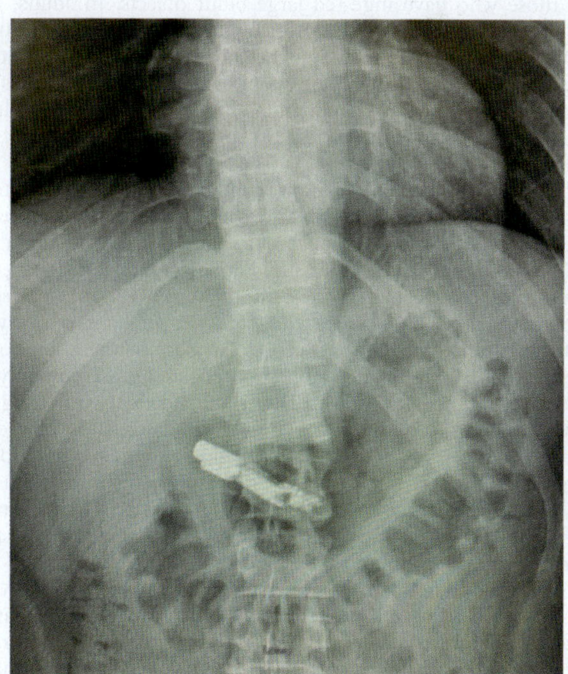

Fig. 28.11 Abdominal film of a long object, a swallowed vibrator, unable to pass through the pylorus necessitating endoscopic removal.

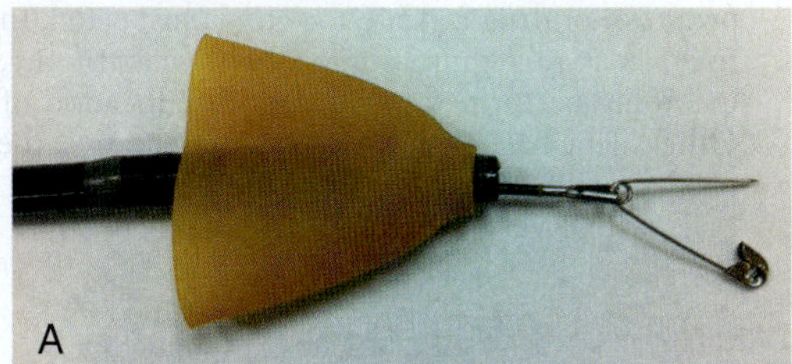

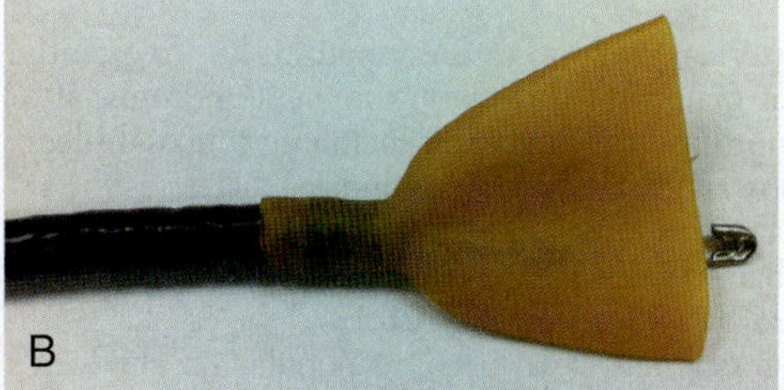

Fig. 28.10 (A) A latex protector hood with the hood pulled back. This position enables full visualization and allows the endoscopist to grasp a sharp object easily. (B) As the protector hood is pulled back through the lower esophageal sphincter, the hood flips forward, protecting the GI mucosa from the sharp object.

Blunt Objects: Coins, Batteries, and Magnets

Small blunt objects, such as pieces of toys and coins, are the most commonly ingested objects by children. Disc (button) battery and magnet ingestions are uncommon but pose unique potential dangers. Blunt objects in the esophagus should be removed within 24 hours. Impacted coins can result in pressure necrosis of the esophageal wall, resulting in perforation and fistula. CT scan should be considered if a coin has been in the esophagus for 3–4 days or greater to evaluate for complications prior to endoscopy. A coin of any size can become lodged in the esophagus of children, but ingested coins—in particular, dimes and pennies measuring 17 and 18 mm—will usually pass through the adult esophagus. Coins located in the distal esophagus on imaging are twice as likely as coins in the proximal esophagus to pass spontaneously.[130]

Retrieval nets allow the capture and secure removal of coins and most small blunt objects.[107] Grasping forceps and biliary stone retrieval baskets are also effective. Standard biopsy forceps and snares are not recommended because they fail to secure coins reliably during extraction. If it is difficult to capture a blunt object in the esophagus, it is safe to push the object into the stomach, where there is more room to negotiate.

Once a small blunt object enters the stomach, conservative outpatient management is appropriate.[131] Exceptions to this include patients with surgically altered digestive tract anatomy and those who have ingested large blunt objects. In adults, the pylorus will allow passage of most blunt objects up to 25 mm in diameter. Otherwise, once in the stomach, a regular diet is appropriate, with radiographic monitoring every 1–2 weeks to confirm progression or elimination. If after 3–4 weeks a blunt object has not passed, endoscopic removal should be performed.[132]

Disc and lithium batteries are contained in many small toys and electronic devices accessible to young children. Disc battery ingestion is of particular concern because batteries contain an alkaline solution that can cause rapid liquefaction necrosis and the creation of an electric current in the esophagus. Data from emergency rooms have suggested the use of sucralfate or honey to coat the battery and reduce mucosal exposure before endoscopic intervention.[133] Disc battery ingestion occurs most commonly in younger children and is increasing in incidence, with roughly 10% becoming symptomatic.[134] Any clinical suspicion of a disc battery in the esophagus should prompt emergent endoscopy. Most button batteries will be identified on plain films prior to endoscopy with larger batteries (>2 cm) more likely to remain in the esophagus and cause complications.[135] Grasping forceps and snares are generally ineffective for disc battery removal, but the use of a retrieval net permits successful removal in almost 100% of cases.[136] Protection of the airway with an overtube or, in pediatric patients, endotracheal intubation is crucial in the retrieval of disc batteries. Half of patients with disc batteries in the stomach have mucosal damage and thus gastric batteries should also be removed via the endoscope within 24 hours.[137] Once in the small intestine, disc batteries rarely cause clinical problems and can be observed radiographically, with 85% passing through the GI tract within 72 hours.[138]

Cylindrical batteries appear to cause symptoms less frequently, with no reports of major life-threatening injuries and only 20% having minor symptoms after ingestion including mucosal ulceration and rarely bowel obstruction.[138] Cylindrical batteries should be removed from the esophagus and, if in the stomach, ones larger than 20 mm or batteries that have not progressed in 48 hours should be removed by endoscopy (Fig. 28.12).

Small coupling magnets have become popular as children's toys with numbers of ingestions and associated morbidity increasing. Ingested magnets within the reach of the endoscope should be removed on an emergent basis. Pretreatment imaging with chest and abdominal radiographs is crucial to determine the number and location of ingested magnets and other metallic objects. Although a single magnet will rarely be a cause of symptoms, concern exists if multiple magnets are ingested or if magnets are ingested with other metal objects. This can result in magnetic attraction and coupling between interposed loops of the bowel, with subsequent pressure necrosis, fistula formation, and bowel perforation.[139,140] Removal can be achieved with grasping forceps, retrieval net, or basket. Magnetic attraction to metallic retrieval devices may ease the task of removal.

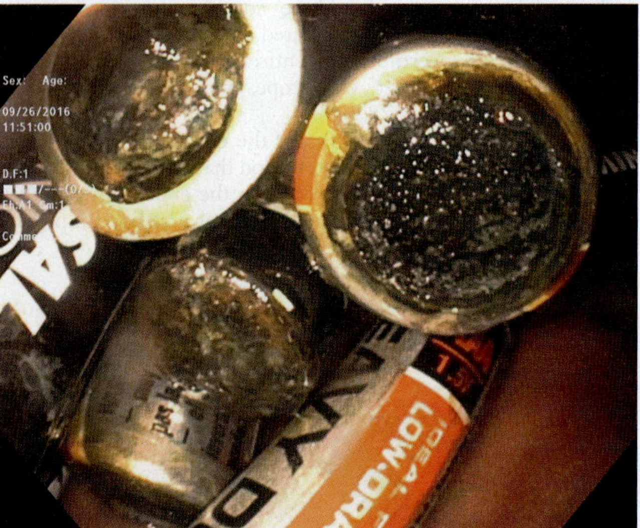

Fig. 28.12 Multiple cylindrical batteries greater than 2 cm found in stomach and subsequently removed with the endoscope.

Narcotic Packets

Ingested packets of illicit narcotics in the GI tract are present in two general groups: body stuffers and body packers. *Body stuffers* are drug users or traffickers who quickly ingest small amounts of drugs, but in poorly wrapped or contained packages that are prone to leakage. *Body packers* are "mules" used by drug smugglers for drug transport; they ingest large quantities of carefully prepared packages intended to withstand GI transit.[141,142] These patients may present with intestinal obstruction due to the packages or with symptoms related to the drug ingested. The latter may result in serious toxicity and death in 5% of individuals.[143]

Diagnosis is initiated with plain film radiology or CT scan, with multiple round or tube-shaped packets seen. Endoscopic removal has been traditionally contraindicated because of the high risk of package perforation, with resultant drug overdose though a small study suggested endoscopic retrieval was possible with fewer complications and shorter hospital stay.[1,144] Observation on a clear liquid diet is recommended with serial radiographs. Operative intervention is indicated when bowel obstruction, failure to progress, or drug leakage/toxicity is suspected. In a large study, up to 45% may require surgery with gastrotomy, enterotomy, or colotomy performed based upon the location of the packages.[145] Other data has suggested that conservative therapy of narcotic packers with just observation led to surgery in less than 3% of cases with a very low complication rate.[146,147]

Colorectal Foreign Bodies

Ingested objects uncommonly become lodged in the colorectum. More commonly, colorectal foreign bodies were inserted into the rectum intentionally or unintentionally. Radiographs should be obtained prior to attempting the removal of colorectal foreign bodies for better visualization of the location, orientation, and configuration of the object (Fig. 28.13). To avoid health care provider injury, attempts at manual removal or digital rectal examination should be deferred until the presence of a sharp or pointed object has been excluded.

Manual digital extraction may be successful for the removal of small, blunt, palpable objects in the distal rectum. Conscious sedation may be adequate for manual removal in some patients, but examination and extraction under general anesthesia may be required in others to allow greater anal sphincter relaxation and successful object extraction.

Nonpalpable and sharp or pointed objects should be removed under direct visualization with the use of a rigid proctoscope or flexible sigmoidoscope.[148] Standard retrieval devices can be used as described earlier for the upper digestive tract. Proximal objects can be repositioned with an endoscope to the distal rectum where the object may more easily be removed manually. A latex hood or overtube can be particularly useful in removing long, sharp, pointed objects to protect the rectal mucosa from laceration and to overcome the tendency of the anal sphincter to contract on an attempted removal of objects. General anesthesia can allow maximum dilation of the anal sphincter to help remove larger and more complex objects. Greater than 90% of rectal foreign bodies can be removed via a transanal approach either manually, via an endoscope, or in combination.[149]

Operative intervention is indicated for any suspected complications secondary to a rectal or colon foreign body, including perforation, abscess, and obstruction or failure of transanal removal. Complications are more common when the object is proximal to the rectum.[150]

Procedure-Related Complications

Although the reported complication rate associated with endoscopic removal of GIFBs and food impactions is low (0%–1.8%), it is thought to be much higher in practice.[7,11,26,27,40,72] Perforation is the most feared complication, although aspiration and sedation-related cardiopulmonary complications may also occur. Factors that increase the risk for complications include objects in the esophagus, removal of sharp objects, an uncooperative patient, multiple and/or deliberate ingestion, and extended duration of time from ingestion to endoscopy.[14,151]

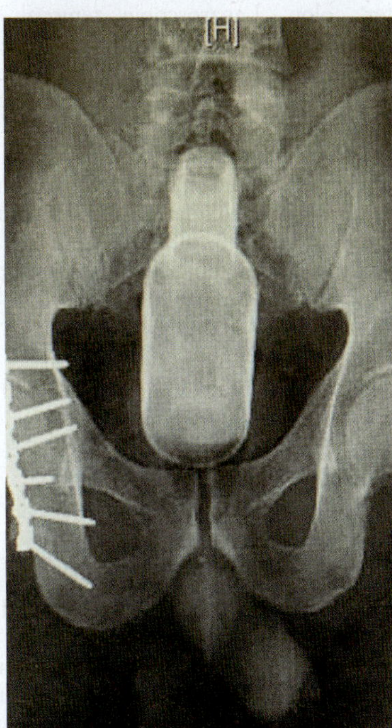

Fig. 28.13 Plain film showing a self-introduced rectal foreign body.

BEZOARS

Bezoars are collections of indigestible material that accumulate in the GI tract, most frequently in the stomach. The three most common types of bezoars encountered are phytobezoars, composed of vegetable or fruit matter; trichobezoars, made up of hair or hair-like fibers; and medication bezoars (pharmacobezoars) (Fig. 28.14 and Box 28.2).

Epidemiology

Phytobezoars are the most common type of bezoar. Offending fruits and vegetables include celery, pumpkin, prunes, raisins, leeks, beets, and persimmon.[7] All these foods contain large

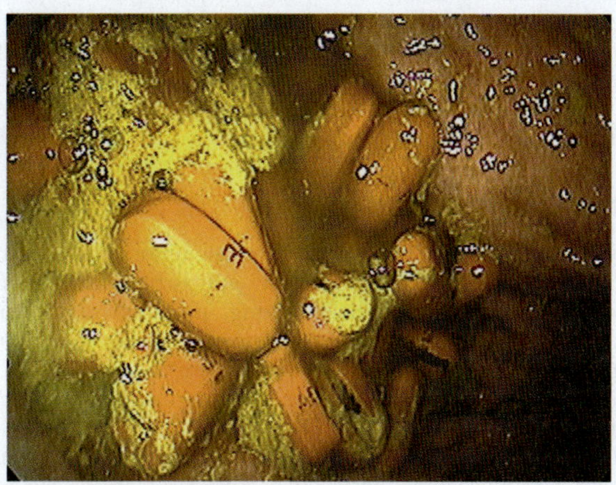

Fig. 28.14 Endoscopic image of a pharmacobezoar in a patient with a history of a pancreaticoduodenectomy who had obstructive symptoms. The pills were removed with an endoscopic net, with subsequent relief of the patient's symptoms.

BOX 28.2 Oral Pharmacologic Agents Associated with Medication Bezoar Formation

- Nonabsorbable antacids
- Bulk laxatives
- Cardiovascular medications
  - Nifedipine
  - Verapamil
  - Procainamide
- Vitamins and minerals
  - Vitamin C
  - Vitamin B_{12}
  - Ferrous sulfate
- Miscellaneous agents
  - Sucralfate
  - Guar gum
  - Cholestyramine
  - Enteral feeding formulations
  - Theophylline
  - Sodium polystyrene sulfonate (Kayexalate) resin

amounts of insoluble and indigestible fibers such as cellulose, hemicellulose, lignin, and fruit tannin.[152] A phytobezoar develops when large quantities are ingested and accumulate.

Trichobezoars occur most commonly in young women, less than 30 years old, and children from ingestion of large amounts of hair (tricophagia), carpet fiber, or clothing fiber. Trichobezoars are more often associated with psychiatric disorders such as trichotillomania, mental disabilities, or pica.[153]

Medication bezoars occur with fiber-containing medications, resin-water products, medication gels, or extended-release medications designed to resist digestion.[154] Medication bezoars can result in decreased pharmacologic efficacy when the active agent is trapped in the bezoar and cannot be absorbed or, alternatively, toxicity and overdose when the contents of a large gastric medication bezoar are released all at once into the small intestine.[155] The clear majority of patients with bezoars (other than trichobezoars) have a predisposing factor that decreases the emptying of gastric contents. Prior gastric surgery is evident in as many as 70%–94% of patients with bezoars. Retained gastric contents may be observed in up to 65%–80% of patients who have undergone a vagotomy with or without pyloroplasty.[60] Bezoar formation after gastric surgery results from delayed gastric emptying, decreased gastric accommodation and reduced acid-peptic activity.[156] Gastroparesis is commonly seen in patients with gastric bezoars. Patients with poor mastication, very high-fiber intake, histamine two receptor agonists use, diabetes or end-stage renal disease, and patients on mechanical ventilation are at greater risk for bezoar formation.[157]

Clinical Features

Patients with gastric bezoars may be asymptomatic, but most (80%) have vague symptoms of epigastric discomfort.[157] Associated anorexia, nausea, vomiting, palpable mass, weight loss, and early satiety may also be present. Bezoars can cause gastric ulceration secondary to pressure necrosis. Bezoar-induced gastric ulcers can cause bleeding and gastric outlet obstruction.[158]

Bezoars may also accumulate in the small bowel and usually present with mechanical obstruction. *Rapunzel syndrome* is a term used to describe trichobezoars located primarily in the stomach that extend past the pylorus and into the duodenum and jejunum, causing bowel obstruction or even jaundice or pancreatitis because of obstruction at the level of the ampulla of Vater.[159,160]

Diagnosis

A careful history is helpful in the diagnosis of bezoar, with a focus on the amount and types of food or medications consumed. A history of psychiatric illness, previous bezoar, gastric surgery, or gastric dysmotility, and dysautonomia should be considered. Physical examination usually assists little in the diagnosis, although occasionally a palpable abdominal mass may be appreciated. Halitosis due to the putrefying materials of the bezoar residing in the stomach may be present. Baldness and a patchy hair pattern may be present in patients who suffer from trichotillomania.

A plain abdominal radiograph may demonstrate the outline of the bezoar. On contrast radiography, a gastric bezoar classically presents as filling defects within the stomach.[152] Plain films and contrast studies will detect only 25% of bezoars detected at upper endoscopy. A CT scan may aid in identifying small bowel bezoars and predict, based on size and degree of vegetable matter the bezoar is made of, whether an obstruction will occur.[161] Gastric bezoars are more definitively diagnosed with upper endoscopy; phytobezoars are seen as a dark brown, green, or black mass of amorphous vegetable material in the stomach. Trichobezoars tend to have a hard, blackened, and almost concrete appearance. Medication bezoars will be seen as whole pills or pill fragments in the midst of the material (Fig. 28.14).

Treatment

Smaller bezoars may be treated with conservative medical management, usually this consists of a liquid diet for a short period of time and a prokinetic agent to promote gastric emptying.[152] Chemical dissolution, most commonly with cellulase, has been reported successful in up to 85% of patients with small bezoars.[158] Cellulase can be taken as a tablet or instilled into the stomach as a liquid via an endoscope or nasogastric tube. Nasogastric lavage may aid in the physical dissolution of small bezoars. Carbonated soda (e.g., Coca-Cola) may be effective in the dissolution of over 50% of cases of phytobezoars and over 90% when combined with endoscopic methods.[161] Additional medications that have been shown to effectively treat gastric bezoars include pancreatin and ursodeoxycholic acid, alone or in combination with cellulase and carbonated beverages.[162]

For larger bezoars and bezoars resistant to medical therapy, endoscopic therapy may be effective. The endoscope is used to fragment the bezoar into smaller pieces. Fragmentation can be performed with the endoscope itself, with accessory devices like forceps or snares, endoscopic scissors, or with the instillation of saline or water flushes through the endoscope. The fragments of the bezoar can be pushed into the small bowel or removed by mouth. If most of the bezoar is to be removed, an overtube is recommended to facilitate frequent passes of the endoscope and to protect the airway. Mechanical disruption and endoscopic removal will be successful in 85%–90% of gastric bezoars. Resistant gastric bezoars may be treated with mechanical lithotripsy, electrohydraulic lithotripsy, laser, or a needle-knife sphincterotome.[163–165]

Operative intervention may be needed if endoscopic therapy fails or if there is a complication related to the bezoar (e.g., perforation, obstruction, bleeding). Trichobezoars more often require surgery than phytobezoars. Gastric bezoars are usually removed via a small gastrostomy.[158,160] Small bowel bezoars are removed via an enterotomy or can be transmurally milked to the cecum, where they rarely cause a problem in the larger diameter colon. Laparoscopic removal can first be attempted in bezoar removal but conversion to an open surgery may occur in just over half of patients.[166] When operative intervention is contemplated, care must be made to exclude multiple bezoars in more than one location.

Preventing bezoar recurrence is as important as active treatment. If the underlying causes of bezoar formation are not corrected, recurrence is likely. Avoidance of high-fiber and other nondigestible foods should be followed. Cellulase can be taken prophylactically by patients who have recurring bezoars. Prokinetic drugs may be useful for patients with underlying motility disorders. In particularly refractory patients with recurring gastric bezoars, repeated periodic endoscopy with physical disruption of food material may prevent larger and clinically significant bezoar formation.

CAUSTIC INGESTIONS

Epidemiology

Some 5000 caustic ingestions are reported annually in the United States.[167] Most occur as accidental ingestions by children younger than 6 years.[168] Caustic ingestions in adults occur as suicide attempts, in patients with mental health problems, and in intoxicated persons as a result of alcohol or recreational drug ingestion. Adults can ingest larger amounts of caustic substances, so they tend to have more serious injuries than children, who will typically spit out or throw up the caustic agent they swallowed. In addition, adults or adolescents will ingest larger volumes of caustic substances, in intentional ingestions, in attempts at self-harm.[169]

Broadly, two types of caustic agents are most commonly ingested: alkali agents or acidic agents. Alkali agents are most commonly in household cleaners like drain, toilet bowl, and oven cleaners as well as bleach products. Lye is an alkali ingestion that contains sodium or potassium hydroxide. Alkali solutions are often odorless and tasteless, which can result in large amounts being swallowed accidentally. There has been a more recent increase in the ingestion of laundry pods leading to serious health consequences.[170] Finally, as noted, disc batteries may also cause alkali-induced damage.

Acid ingestion usually comes from swallowing toilet bowl cleaner, swimming pool cleaner, rust remover, mold or mildew remover, or battery acid. Acid ingestion often causes immediate pain, which results in the agent being rapidly expelled. Household bleach may contain both acid and alkali products but rarely causes severe injury because of their diluted concentration.

Pathophysiology

Alkali

Alkaline ingestion causes liquefactive necrosis by fat saponification that very rapidly extends through the mucosa, submucosa, muscularis of the esophagus, and stomach.[171] Vascular thrombosis occurs following the necrosis. The initial alkali injury can be transmural and result in perforation, mediastinitis, and peritonitis.[172] External sloughing and ulceration occur a few days after ingestion. Finally, extensive granulation tissue, fibroblastic activity, and collagen deposition occur over weeks, leading to chronic stricture formation. With alkali ingestion, the esophagus is most affected; neutralization by gastric acid limits damage in the stomach. A minority of patients have damage in the small intestine as well.[173] The degree of injury is also dependent on the agent ingested, its quantity, and duration of exposure.[174]

Acid

Acidic agents cause coagulative necrosis by denaturing proteins, with thromboses of mucosal blood vessels and a more limited superficial necrosis. Despite the superficial mucosal damage, caustic acidic agent ingestion can lead to severe systemic complications.[169] Acidic agents are more apt to damage the stomach, particularly the antrum, more than the esophagus (Fig. 28.15). Acidic agents tend to be ingested in smaller quantities because of their offensive taste and immediate pain, so they are associated with less overall damage than alkali agents.

Clinical Features

Initially, patients may present with oropharyngeal pain, epigastric pain, chest pain, dysphagia, or odynophagia. Oropharyngeal involvement can cause sialorrhea and drooling. Hoarseness, stridor, and dyspnea suggest injury to the epiglottis, larynx, and upper airway. Persistent chest or back pain may suggest esophageal perforation and mediastinitis, whereas severe abdominal pain can be related to gastric perforation and peritonitis. Of importance is that early signs and symptoms do not always correlate with the amount of caustic injury and likelihood for late complications.[175] On physical examination, patients may have evidence of burns to the oral cavity, with edema, ulceration, and exudate, but as many as 20%–45% of patients will have a normal physical examination. Delayed complications of caustic ingestions include esophageal stricture formation leading to significant dysphagia and malnutrition.[176]

Diagnosis

Radiologic images such as chest x-ray and abdominal films will not aid in the direct diagnosis or grading of severity of injury but will indicate the presence of perforation by showing a pneumomediastinum, pneumothorax, or pneumoperitoneum. CT of the neck, chest, and/or abdomen should be considered when a high degree of suspicion remains for perforation, despite negative plain films. If perforation is present, surgery rather than endoscopy should be performed emergently (Fig. 28.16).

Symptoms and the physical examination may not match the degree of injury after caustic ingestion, so an upper endoscopy examination should be performed in the first 24–48 hours after ingestion in patients without perforation.[177] An upper endoscopy allows diagnosis of injury to the GI tract, permits grading of the

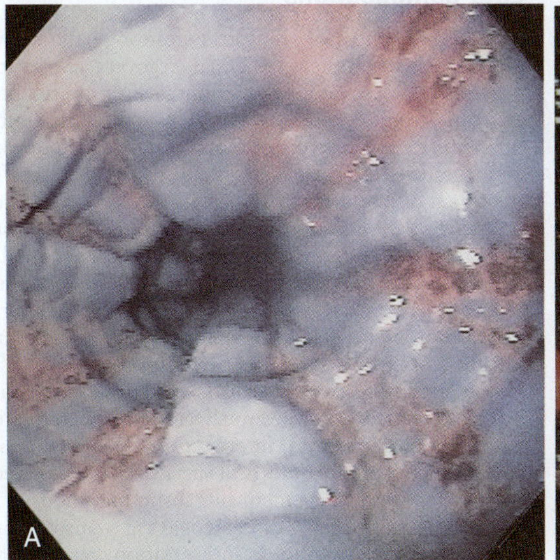

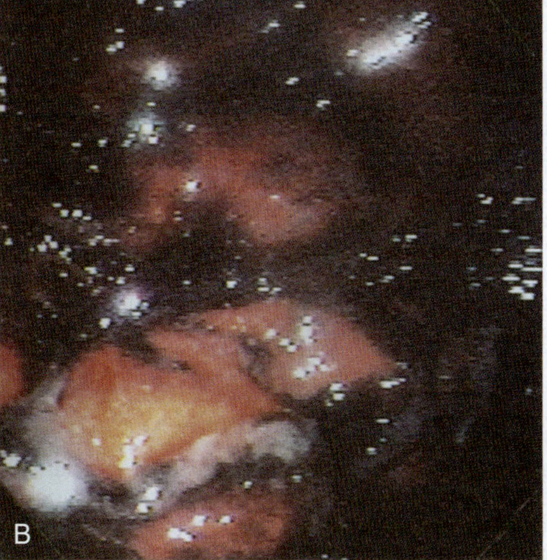

Fig. 28.15 Caustic injury to the esophagus and stomach by acid. (A) After the ingestion of acid, the squamous mucosa of the esophagus has sloughed in a linear pattern. The esophageal mucosa is edematous and has a bluish discoloration. (B) The gastric mucosa in this patient is hemorrhagic and edematous. (From Wilcox MC. *Atlas of Clinical Gastrointestinal Endoscopy*. Philadelphia, PA: WB Saunders; 1995:85.)

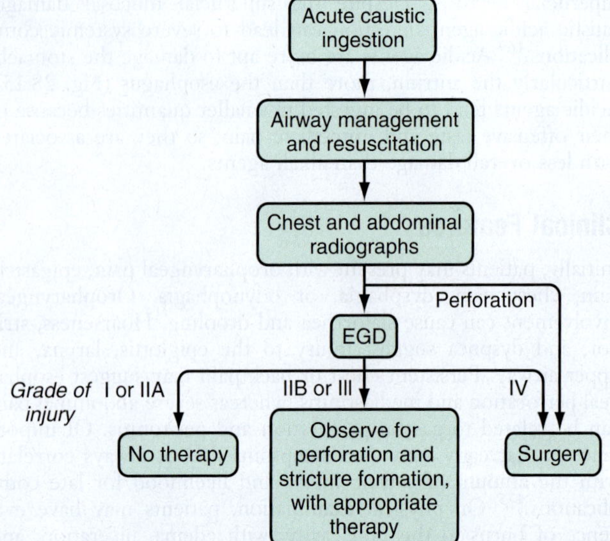

Fig. 28.16 Algorithm for the approach to acute caustic injury. For the definitions of endoscopic grades of injury, see Table 28.1.

TABLE 28.1 Endoscopic Grades of Caustic Injury

Grade	Endoscopic Findings
I	Edema and erythema
IIA	Hemorrhage, erosions, blisters, ulcers with exudate
IIB	Circumferential ulceration
III	Multiple deep ulcers with brown, black, or gray discoloration
IV	Perforation

degree of injury, establishes prognosis, and guides therapy (see Fig. 28.16). A relook endoscopy at 5 days postingestion may be performed as well, as it can better predict esophageal and gastric complications than an endoscopy performed in the first 24 hours.[178] It is important to note that 40%–80% of patients with reported caustic ingestion will have no evidence of injury on endoscopic examination.[179] Emergency CT imaging scan can also be used to grade mucosal injury at the time of caustic ingestion and accurately predict the depth of transmural necrosis and overall clinical outcomes.[180,181]

The degree of injury seen on endoscopic examination can be graded and provides prognostic information (Table 28.1). Initial endoscopic grading can predict overall survival. Grades I and IIA burns, which correspond to first- and second-degree burns, will usually heal without sequelae.[173] However, strictures will develop in 70%–100% of patients with grade IIB injury, which causes circumferential ulceration, and grade III injury with associated necrosis.[182] Grade IV injury with perforation carries a mortality rate of up to 65% and requires urgent surgery.

Treatment

Initial management should address the ABCs of resuscitative management: *a*irway, *b*reathing, and *c*irculation. Attempts should be made to identify the volume, type, and timing of the caustic agent ingested as well as whether the ingestion was intentional or not. Once initially stabilized, management is based on the clinical status of the patient and the grade of injury seen on endoscopy. Asymptomatic patients who have a normal endoscopic examination or only grade I or IIA injury can be started on oral intake in the first 24–48 hours and usually discharged within that same time frame.

Clinically ill patients with hypotension, respiratory distress, and grade IIB (circumferential ulceration) or III necrosis on endoscopy should be admitted to an intensive care unit and managed with intravenous fluid resuscitation and close monitoring for evidence of perforation. Leukocytosis, elevated CRP, acidosis, renal failure, and elevated liver function tests have been associated with poor clinical outcomes.[183] Laryngoscopy should be performed in patients with respiratory distress. A patient with an edematous, necrotic laryngopharynx should not undergo endotracheal intubation and will need a tracheotomy to maintain an airway.

Perforations are uncommon for most caustic ingestions. Emergency surgery with esophagectomy or gastrectomy is required for perforation. Colonic interposition is sometimes required. Operator and institutional experience affect mortality and morbidity of emergent esophagogastrectomy and is best undertaken at referral centers when circumstances allow.[184]

The need for and timing of operative intervention in patients with severe ulceration or necrosis without clear evidence of perforation remains controversial. Comparative analyses are difficult in this patient population. Some authorities have suggested that early operative exploration decreases mortality,[185,186] but others cite lower mortality rates and complete healing in patients with nonoperative supportive care.[174] Advanced age, tracheobronchial injuries, extended resections, and emergent esophagectomy are negative predictors for survival in those undergoing early surgical management.[186] As such, management must be considered on an individualized basis.

Inducing emesis or placing a nasogastric tube to clear or dilute the GI tract of the caustic agent is contraindicated because it may reexpose the esophagus, oropharynx, and airway to the caustic agent. Induced retching and vomiting may increase the risk of perforation. The use of neutralizing agents is not recommended because they have not been shown to be efficacious, may lead to increased thermal injury, and may also promote retching and emesis.[187] The routine use of glucocorticoids[171] and systemic antibiotics[167] is not recommended, but the use of a PPI may reduce complications.[188]

Late Complications

Up to one-third of caustic ingestion patients will develop esophageal stricture after initial recovery. Stricture formation presents most commonly at 2 months after injury but can occur at any time from 2 weeks to many years after the initial injury.[173] Stricture formation occurs more commonly following more severe (grade IIB or III) injuries (see Table 28.1). The primary treatment of esophageal strictures secondary to caustic ingestion is frequent dilation. Endoscopic management of caustic strictures must be deliberate, with gradual and incremental progressive dilation to 15 mm or until symptom relief is obtained.[189] Endoscopic injection of triamcinolone into the stricture or use of topical mitomycin has been reported to be beneficial in treating caustic strictures.[190,191] The perforation rate is 0.5% for endoscopic dilation of chronic caustic strictures, and as many as 10%–50% of patients will eventually require operative intervention. Those requiring surgical intervention for late complications have better functional outcomes and survival than those requiring early surgery for the management of caustic ingestions.[184] Esophageal resection with an esophagogastric anastomosis, esophagojejunostomy, or colonic interposition may be considered.[192] Case reports have described successful treatment with the use of temporary esophageal stents soon after caustic ingestion, but there is insufficient evidence to support recommendations for

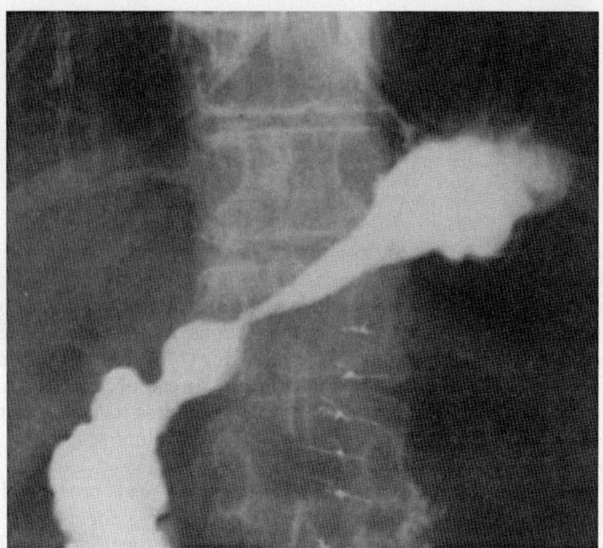

Fig. 28.17 Barium study of a chronic antral stricture caused by a caustic ingestion. (Courtesy Dr. Robert N. Berk, San Diego, CA.)

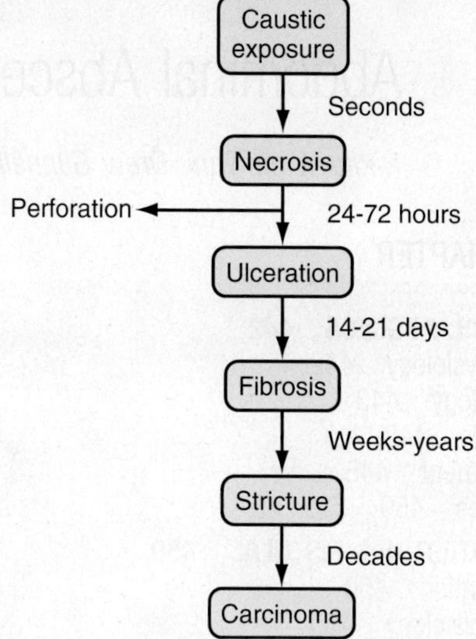

Fig. 28.18 Sequence of the consequences of caustic injury to the gastrointestinal tract as a function of time after ingestion.

routine prophylactic stenting or for prophylactic early endoscopic dilation to prevent caustic-related strictures.[187]

Antral and pyloric strictures may also occur after caustic injury (Fig. 28.17). Antral and pyloric stenoses will usually develop 1–6 weeks after caustic ingestion but can also occur years later.[166] The risk of antral stenosis is also related to the degree of injury. Endoscopic dilation with the addition of acid suppression is successful in many patients, but many others will require antrectomy.

Alkaline caustic ingestion is associated with an increased risk for squamous cell cancer of the esophagus. Patients with a history of lye ingestion have a 1000-fold increased risk of developing esophageal cancer, with a lag time from injury of approximately 40 years.[193] Periodic endoscopic surveillance is advocated every 1–3 years, beginning 20 years after the caustic ingestion.

Fig. 28.18 summarizes the time course of complications from caustic ingestions reviewed in this section.

Full references for this chapter can be found at https://ebooks.health.elsevier.com.

29 Abdominal Abscesses and Gastrointestinal Fistulas

Nikita Wadhwani, Drew Gunnells, Jr.

IN THIS CHAPTER

ABDOMINAL ABSCESS

An *abdominal abscess* (AA) is a localized abdominal infection arising in the background of infectious peritonitis. *Primary peritonitis* (spontaneous bacterial peritonitis, discussed in Chapter 93) is not usually associated with the development of abscesses, whereas *secondary peritonitis*, peritoneal infection due to an inflammatory process in the GI tract, is commonly associated with abscess formation (see Chapter 37). Most cases of AA arise in the setting of secondary peritonitis due to bowel perforation (Box 29.1). *Tertiary peritonitis*, a persistent or recurrent infection arising 48 hours after treatment of secondary peritonitis, often arises in the setting of preexisting comorbidities and may be associated with AA (see Chapter 37).[1,2] Abscesses in solid organs are discussed in Chapters 58, 61, and 84.

Pathophysiology

Sterility in the peritoneal cavity is maintained as the host defense mechanisms designed to clear bacterial contamination and protect against the bacterial factors fostering microbial primacy. Bacteria commonly gain access to the peritoneal cavity through perforation of the intestinal wall or bacterial translocation due to an impaired mucosal barrier.[3] The bulk of these bacteria are delivered to the reticuloendothelial system for clearance via the continuous lymphatic drainage caused by the function of the diaphragm.[2] Lymphatic clearance is usually efficient enough to prevent abscess formation, except when adjuvant substances such as hemoglobin, barium, or necrotic tissue are present.[4] These adjuvant substances may block lymphatic vessels (barium, fecal particulate matter), provide bacterial nutrients (iron from hemoglobin), or impair bacterial killing, all fostering bacterial infection. Shortly after bacterial contamination, the predominant phagocytic cell types are peritoneal macrophages, which are also cleared by the lymphatic system. As bacteria proliferate, polymorphonuclear leukocytes invade the contaminated area and become abundant. The resultant peritoneal inflammation leads to an increase in splanchnic blood flow, with exudative fluid loss into the peritoneal cavity. The delivery of fibrinogen combined with the procoagulatory effects of the inflammatory process and reduced levels of plasminogen activator activity enhance fibrin deposition, leading to entrapment of bacteria and localization of infection.[5] The peritoneal cavity contains numerous recesses, pouches, and potential spaces that allow for compartmentalization of abdominal infection to prevent further spread of infection and the dreaded occurrence of sepsis.[6,7] Thus abscess formation ultimately may be regarded as a means of controlling severe intra-abdominal infection.

Although peritoneal defense mechanisms can prevent the spread of bacterial infection, they can have adverse effects as well. Lymphatic clearance of bacteria may be so effective that it results in sepsis. Exudation of fluid into the peritoneal cavity can lead to hypovolemia and shock; it can also dilute the opsonins that target bacteria for phagocytosis. Furthermore, fibrin entrapment of bacteria can impair antimicrobial drug penetration and phagocytic migration.[1]

A number of host factors interact with bacterial contamination to increase the risk of AA (Box 29.2). Diabetes, malnutrition, advancing age, preexisting organ dysfunction, underlying malignancy, and transfusion are all factors that predispose to abscess formation.[8–10] In all these conditions, the immune system's ability to combat bacterial contamination is weakened, whether it is in the setting of secondary or tertiary peritonitis.

Clinical manifestations of IBD, specifically Crohn's, offer insights into the pathogenesis of AA. The transmural inflammation, characteristic of Crohn's, leads to wall weakening and subsequent translocation and/or micro perforation leading to AA formation. As the disease stems from a complex interaction between host immunological processes and environmental triggers, current medical management comprises immunomodulators, in addition to standard antibiotics and drainage.[11] In addition, pharmacological agents used for the treatment of IBD have been associated with the development of AA, especially in postsurgical patients.

BOX 29.1 Causes of Intra-Abdominal Abscesses

- Abdominal trauma
- Appendicitis
- Cholecystectomy and other operations or invasive procedures
- Crohn's disease
- Diverticulitis
- Neoplastic disease
- Pancreatitis
- Perforated hollow viscus (e.g., duodenal or gastric ulcer)

BOX 29.2 Clinical Risk Factors for Intra-Abdominal Abscess

- Chronic glucocorticoid use
- Increasing age
- Malnutrition
- Preexisting organ dysfunction
- Transfusion
- Underlying malignancy

Chronic glucocorticoid administration is associated with an increased risk of AA.[12] Similarly, preoperative use of azathioprine for IBD increases the risk of intra-abdominal septic complications.[13] In contrast, two recent large studies showed that anti-TNF-α therapy for IBD within the 12 weeks before surgery did not increase the incidence of AA.[14–16]

Bacteriology

Classic studies have shown that the polymicrobial nature of the abdominal infection may in fact be from synergy between the various bacterial subspecies. Facultative anaerobic organisms such as *Escherichia coli* can provide the ideal anaerobic environment for *Bacteroides fragilis* to multiply.[17] Consequently, the increased number of anaerobic organisms such as *B. fragilis* will make it more difficult for host defenses to engage against the *E. coli*, because local effects will reduce the efficacy of phagocytosis.

The bacteria associated with abdominal infections and abscesses in ICU patients are subjected to broad-spectrum antimicrobial selection pressure and as such are different from those in non-ICU patients with abscesses due to secondary bacterial peritonitis.[18] The organisms that cause tertiary peritonitis are no longer dominated by *E. coli* and *B. fragilis*. Rather, nosocomial infections with resistant Gram-negative organisms, *Enterococcus* species, and/or yeast are more common.[19,20] A microbiological analysis of abscesses in severely ill patients (Acute Physiology and Chronic Health Evaluation II score >15) revealed that 38% had monomicrobial infections. The most common organisms were *Candida* (41%), *Enterococcus* (31%), and *Enterobacter* (21%) species and *Staphylococcus epidermidis* (21%); *E. coli* and *Bacteroides* species accounted for only 17% and 7%, respectively.[21]

Diagnosis

The classic presentation of AA is abdominal pain, fever, shaking chills, and palpable abdominal mass, but this tetrad of symptoms is rarely observed in practice. The presence of additional symptoms and signs may be observed, depending on the location of the abscess. Subphrenic abscesses may cause pleurisy; lesser sac or perigastric abscesses may result in nausea and early satiety. Interloop abscesses may present with ileus or obstructive symptoms. Pelvic abscesses may cause tenesmus or urgency. In older adults and patients with underlying comorbidities, the signs and symptoms of AA may be more varied and subtle, mandating a high clinical suspicion.[22] While routine laboratory tests provide nonspecific clues for ongoing systemic infection/inflammation, imaging is at the forefront of AA diagnosis, be it in the patient presenting to the emergency department or in the hospitalized patient experiencing a clinical downturn.

CT

CT is the gold standard for the diagnosis of AA. Detection of abscess is optimized following oral and intravenous contrast. The classic CT appearance of AA is a rim-enhancing complex fluid collection containing gas.[23] Multidetector CT with helical acquisition allows for rapid scanning and affords the creation of coronal and sagittal images that optimally characterize complex-appearing and insinuating collections (Fig. 29.1).[24] CT exams following proper protocols afford diagnosis of associated bowel obstruction, pylephlebitis, and may suggest or confirm the presence of a fistula.[25] Despite the sensitivity of CT for detecting intraperitoneal collections, the a priori correct diagnosis of infection in an intra-abdominal collection has been reported recently to be 83%, with a specificity of only 39%.[26] Detection of extraluminal gas remains the most specific indicator of infection using CT but is observed in fewer than 40% of patients.[27] Presence of a fluid collection with attenuation greater than 20 Hounsfield units is also predictive of an abscess.[26] Hematomas, seromas, pseudocysts, and necrotic tumors may all confound the diagnostic accuracy of CT for AA, though it is important to note that the walls of these collections are usually not enhanced by intravenous contrast.[28] Thus fluid aspiration followed by Gram stain and culture of the aspirate remains requisite for definitive diagnosis of abscess.

An important pitfall in the detection of AA is confusing fluid-filled bowel loops for an abscess. This diagnostic dilemma is best prevented by administration of oral contrast 90 minutes (or more) before the CT. Occasionally, despite oral contrast administration, slow bowel transit time will leave some bowel nonopacified. These cases require a longer delay and repeat scanning to allow more time for oral contrast migration distally (Fig. 29.2). Importantly, there is a growing trend in emergency departments to perform abdominal CT without oral contrast to increase patient throughput.[29,30] As a result, some patients presenting to the emergency department may require repeat scanning with oral contrast administration and repeat scanning to confirm the diagnosis of abscess.

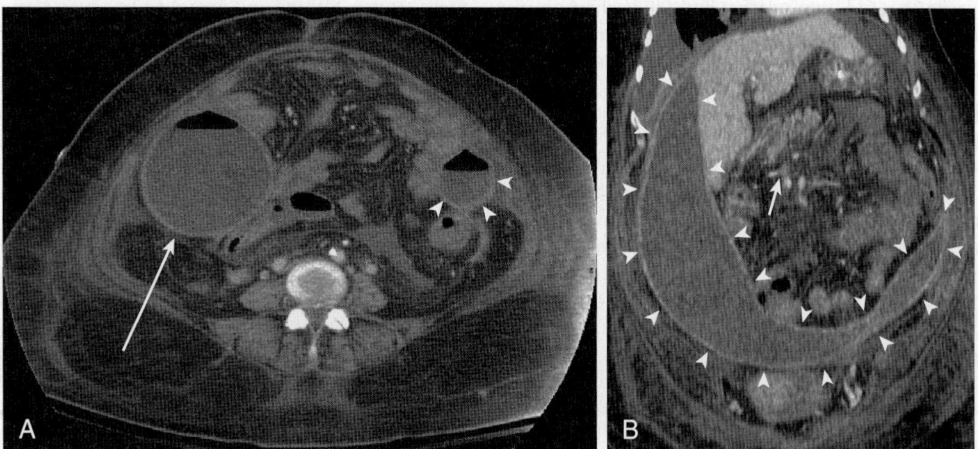

Fig. 29.1 (A) Axial CT image shows a large rim-enhancing structure containing an air–fluid level in the right lower quadrant (*arrow*) and a smaller similar structure in the left lower quadrant (*arrowheads*). (B) Coronal image in the same patient shows that the two collections constitute a single large C-shaped collection that crosses the midline in the low pelvis (*arrowheads*) and demonstrates thrombosis of the superior mesenteric vein (*arrow*), one of the potential complications of the abscess.

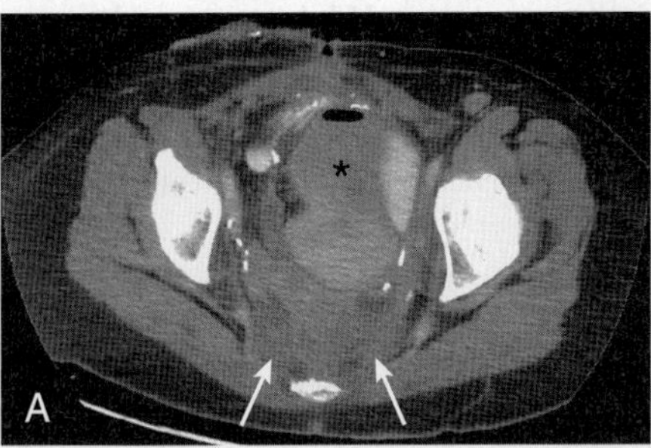

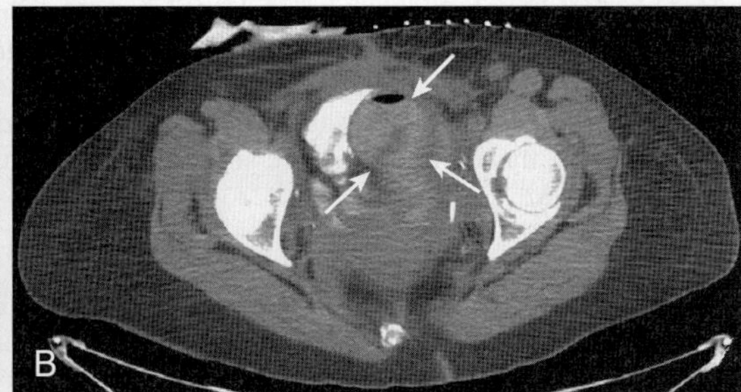

Fig. 29.2 (A) Axial CT image shows an apparently rim-enhancing structure containing gas (*asterisk*) in the deep pelvis adjacent to tethered bowel loops in a patient with prior pelvic irradiation. The structure could represent an abscess or a dilated loop of small bowel. The presacral inflammation (*arrows*) is related to radiation change. (B) CT image obtained 2 hours later shows ingested oral contrast in this structure (*arrows*), confirming that this is a bowel loop rather than an abscess.

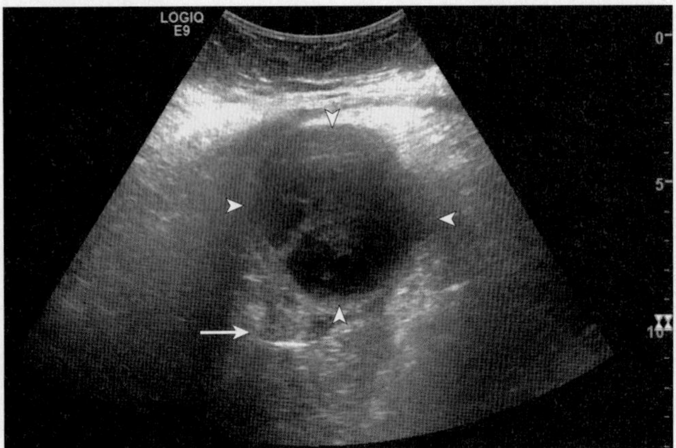

Fig. 29.3 Abdominal US of a typical abscess (*arrowheads*) demonstrating central decreased echogenicity, thickened wall, and debris arising anterior to the descending colon (*arrow*) in a patient with diverticulosis, compatible with a diverticular abscess. *US*, Ultrasound.

Ultrasound

Ultrasound (US) is a commonly used screening exam that is readily available, rapid, and does not expose the patient to radiation, making it especially useful in pediatric and pregnant patients. It can also serve as rapid, noninvasive bedside evaluation in critically ill patients for whom transport to the radiology department is unsafe.[28] The appearance of an abscess may vary from a relatively simple anechoic fluid collection to a more complex fluid with heterogeneous echogenicity, a reflection of the amount of debris and gas present (Fig. 29.3).[31] US is an excellent modality for the evaluation of suspected solid abdominal visceral AA and for pelvic collections. Fluid in the urinary bladder serves as an ultrasonographic window for the localization of AA. Transvaginal imaging affords US detection of most pelvic abscesses. Gas prevents US beam penetration, and gas-containing bowel in the midabdomen hampers abscess detection, with detection rates of 43% in a recent report.[32] Furthermore, surgical wounds, ostomies, dressings, and drains may preclude or limit the use of US in the postoperative period. Lastly, technical challenges may occur with obese individuals and differences in operator.

MRI

Improvements in MRI protocols and scanners in conjunction with increasing awareness of the radiation dose associated with CT have resulted in increased utilization of MRI for acute and subacute indications. The use of MRI initially was spawned by advances in MRI that allow for the accurate diagnosis of appendicitis in pregnancy.[33] Now, MRI is more commonly being performed in patients presenting to the emergency department with acute intra-abdominal pain.[34,35] Moreover, a recent multicenter study demonstrated that in experienced hands, MRI compares favorably with CT in the diagnosis of appendicitis, which will likely increase the role of MRI use in these patients.[36] One advance that has become standard in the evaluation of Crohn's disease is magnetic resonance enterography.[37] This technique combines intravenous administration of a gadolinium-based contrast agent with high-resolution coronal MRI to detect abnormalities in the bowel wall, a common finding in Crohn's disease. On contrast-enhanced MRI enterography, abscesses are extraluminal, rim-enhancing collections with heterogeneous signal elevation on fluid-sensitive sequences (Fig. 29.4).[37,38] Diffusion-weighted imaging may increase the ability to discriminate abscesses from cysts.[39] MRI is also extremely useful for pelvic abscesses/inflammatory disorders due to its superior soft tissue contrast and high sensitivity for inflammation.[40] Barriers to mainstream use of MRI in the diagnosis of AA are limited to the availability of MRI in the acute setting, radiologist/clinician comfort with CT, and time and cost of the exam compared with CT.[34]

Radiographic Studies

Radiographs may demonstrate large abscesses that have significant mass effects. Supine and upright films may reveal an air-fluid level in a large abscess cavity, or associated ileus or bowel obstruction that may help clue in on the diagnosis. Overall, however, radiographs are insensitive for the detection of the majority of AA, and sizeable abscesses may be overlooked. CT is far superior to radiography in sensitivity, specificity, and accuracy of diagnosing acute nontraumatic abdominal pathology, with rates of 96%, 95%, and 96% for CT versus 30%, 88%, and 56% for radiography, respectively.[41]

Nuclear Medicine Studies

Nuclear medicine studies that can be used to diagnose AA include the gallium scan, labeled leukocyte scan, and PET/CT scan, among others.[42] Historically, the gallium scan has been used most frequently for diagnosis of AA, but normal uptake in bowel and tumors may give rise to false-positive results. Radiolabeled leukocyte scans afford whole-body imaging with high sensitivity and specificity. Still, these scans have drawbacks; they are not readily available owing to the time required for synthesis of the radiolabel, and they typically require 18 and possibly up to 72 hours to perform.[43] Furthermore, upper quadrant abscess

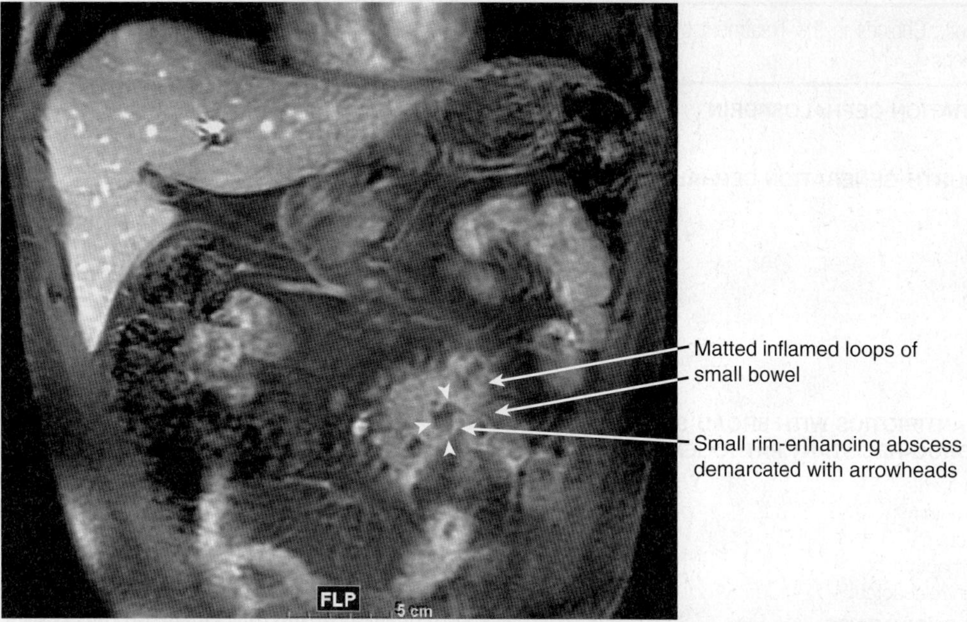

Fig. 29.4 Coronal MRI with gadolinium contrast of a patient with Crohn's disease showing a small rim-enhancing collection (*arrowheads*) interposed between several loops of inflamed bowel (*arrows*), compatible with an interloop abscess. Interloop abscesses are not amenable to percutaneous drain placement.

detection may be confounded by tracer uptake, both in the liver and spleen, which may require the addition of a sulfur colloid scan to distinguish physiologic uptake from infection.[44] PET/CT scans have great potential for an important role in the diagnosis of AA. Cells involved in the inflammatory process take up great quantities of glucose, making the use of[45] F-FDG PET scans extremely useful.[45] F-FDG uptake, combined with the CT component of the scan, allows for accurate anatomic localization of abnormalities, a problem that has long plagued nuclear medicine studies. In the persistently bacteremic patient, whole-body images obtained using PET/CT may uncover unsuspected AA.[46] PET/CT is the test of choice in the setting of fever of unknown origin; it can detect infectious, inflammatory, and neoplastic sources for fever.[47] The greatest disadvantage of PET/CT and gallium scanning is their inability to differentiate between sterile inflammation and infection.[42] Although CT will remain the first-line test of choice for AA in the foreseeable future, PET/CT scans and other nuclear medicine studies can be of utility in diagnosing challenging cases.

Management

Stabilization

Initial management entails fluid and electrolyte resuscitation and support of vital organ function, especially if there is a presentation with sepsis or septic shock. Fluid resuscitation in septic shock entails aggressive crystalloid infusion, at least 30 cm^3/kg of IV crystalloids within the first 3 hours of presentation, per the Surviving Sepsis Campaign.[25,48]

Antibiotic Therapy

Empirical therapy should be started once the presumptive diagnosis of AA is made, optimally after obtaining blood cultures. The antibiotics should be administered within the first 3 hours of recognition, ideally within first hour.[49] Although an important component of early management, antibiotics may not be fully effective prior to drainage of an abscess, owing to the inability to penetrate the area of infection. This is due to both host factors (e.g., tissue necrosis, an acidic environment, and lack of adequate perfusion) and pathogenic factors (e.g., high colony count, slow growth rate of bacteria and their byproducts). Such factors can present specific obstacles for certain antibiotics: for example, β-lactams are less effective in dense bacterial populations, and aminoglycosides have reduced activity at a lower pH.

An initial choice of antibiotics should be based on the clinical scenario of each individual patient. In AA associated with secondary peritonitis, antibiotics should target usual bowel flora such as *E. coli* and other coliforms, including *B. fragilis*. These cases are usually less complicated and do not have extraintestinal manifestations like bacteremia. Unfortunately, there are no randomized controlled trials showing that one agent is superior to another. Multiple noninferiority trials have been published, however, providing a variety of options (Box 29.3). Antibiotic selection will follow patient factors such as renal function and prior allergies. Hospital antibiograms are also helpful; for example, some institutions have high rates of *E. coli* resistance to fluoroquinolones.

Guidelines issued by the Infectious Diseases Society of America and Surgical Infection Society recommend that single agents (e.g., β-lactams with β-lactamase inhibitors, carbapenems, the second-generation cephalosporin cefoxitin, the fluoroquinolone moxifloxacin, and the glycylcycline tigecycline) are considered appropriate for mild to moderate disease (see Box 29.3).[18] For patients with a high risk for methicillin-resistant *Staphylococcus aureus* (MRSA) infection, appropriate antibiotics with MRSA coverage should be started early in the course. Gram stain and cultures can be useful, but the updated guidelines point out that there have been no studies to validate this practice. Combination choices can also be selected by the clinician. Most experts recommend reserving antipseudomonal coverage for those cases with a more severe illness or with high-risk comorbid conditions.

Important points to consider in the selection of empirical antibiotics come from more recent published reports. Certain pathogens are less likely to play a role in those patients who present with community-associated AAs. MRSA is unusual in these cases, so vancomycin or other anti-MRSA antibiotics are not usually recommended at the time of initial presentation.

BOX 29.3 Antibiotic Choices in the Treatment of Intra-Abdominal Infections

SECOND-GENERATION CEPHALOSPORIN

Cefoxitin[a]

THIRD- AND FOURTH-GENERATION CEPHALOSPORINS

Ceftriaxone[a,b]
Ceftazidime[b]
Cefepime[b]

CARBAPENEMS

Imipenem-cilastatin
Meropenem
Ertapenem[a]

COMBINATION ANTIBIOTICS WITH BROAD-SPECTRUM ACTIVITY FOR DRUG-RESISTANT PATHOGENS

Piperacillin/tazobactam
Ceftolazone/tazobactam[b]
Ceftazidime/avibactam[b]
Meropenem/vaborbactam
Imipenem-cilastatin/relebactam

TETRACYCLINE DERIVATIVES

Tigecycline[a]
Eravacycline[a]
Omadacycline[a]

FLUOROQUINOLONES

Ciprofloxacin[b]
Levofloxacin[b]
Moxifloxacin[a]

[a]Provides no coverage for *Pseudomonas* spp.
[b]Add metronidazole IV or PO for anaerobic activity.

Enterococci are not usually pathogenic at this stage of infection, so antibiotic choices do not typically require adequate enterococcal coverage.[18]

The traditional practice of adding an aminoglycoside or clindamycin can no longer be routinely recommended; more recent studies have shown that aminoglycosides are associated with higher rates of nephrotoxicity without additional benefit[50] and that rates of resistance to clindamycin, especially with *B. fragilis*, have been on the increase in the past decade. Cefotetan has been shown to have diminished efficacy against anaerobes such as *B. fragilis*, and ampicillin/sulbactam is no longer routinely recommended owing to increasing rates of *E. coli* resistance to ampicillin.

AA associated with tertiary peritonitis includes those cases at later or more aggressive stages of abdominal infection as well as "health care–associated infections" with more resistant nosocomial pathogens (see Chapter 37). Empirical choices in these patients will have to provide broader coverage, considering the possibility of *Pseudomonas aeruginosa*, enterococci, MRSA, drug-resistant Gram-negative bacilli, and even *Candida* species. Antipseudomonal β-lactams, carbapenems, or combination therapy with an antipseudomonal cephalosporin or antipseudomonal quinolone added to metronidazole are considered equally good choices. Of the β-lactams, piperacillin/tazobactam is the most widely used. Carbapenems can be imipenem-cilastin, doripenem, or meropenem; however, ertapenem has no antipseudomonal activity. Cefepime and ceftazidime are both active against *Pseudomonas* species, but anaerobic coverage should be added with metronidazole. Ciprofloxacin or levofloxacin can be used with metronidazole in patient populations where quinolone resistance is uncommon (defined as <10% of hospital isolates on an antibiogram). As selection pressure from prior antibiotics alters the flora of AA in tertiary peritonitis, microbiology from the abscess may be helpful to guide antibiotic choice.[18]

For enterococci, older surgical literature indicated coverage of these organisms was unnecessary, but it is now known that these species can develop a pathogenic role.[18] Piperacillin/tazobactam and vancomycin both have activity against *Enterococcus faecalis* and *Enterococcus faecium* in community-associated cases. Penicillin resistance has been on the increase, however, and at times only vancomycin will be effective. Vancomycin-resistant enterococci are typically not found in routine intra-abdominal infections, except for hospitalized/vulnerable patient cohorts such as liver transplant cases where vancomycin-resistant enterococci have been a pernicious problem.[51]

MRSA has not commonly been described in AA. Vancomycin remains the antibiotic of choice for MRSA. The FDA has granted approval to linezolid and tigecycline against MRSA infections of the abdomen, but there are few published clinical trials, so most experts do not routinely recommend their use at the onset.

Nosocomial drug-resistant, Gram-negative bacilli are becoming an obstacle in the management of complicated abdominal infections. In patients with prior infections and extensive antibiotic exposure, multidrug-resistant organisms can be found in their abscess cultures. Most notable have been the extended-spectrum β-lactamase producers seen with *E. coli*, as well as other Enterobacteriaceae that are usually only sensitive to carbapenems (hence, no oral agents are available) and more recently, the *Klebsiella*-producing carbapenemase, which are even resistant to the carbapenems and present few antimicrobial options to the clinician except perhaps for the use of tigecycline, aminoglycosides, or novel carbapenemase inhibitor–based antibiotics such as ceftazidime/avibactam. Additional newer combination antibiotic formulations are coming to the market, but clinical data are presently lacking.

Lastly, *Candida* species can play a role in these most advanced cases of AA. Traditionally fluconazole had been the drug of choice, but in some centers, non-*albicans Candida* species resistant to fluconazole are on the rise, making echinocandins such as micafungin or caspofungin the preferred agents. Amphotericin is no longer recommended in fungal AA except for the most unusual circumstances.

Once culture results are available, the empirical antibiotic(s) chosen should be adjusted to tailor therapy. This is common practice, but, curiously, little evidence supports this from the perspective of patient outcome. Antimicrobial stewardship is experiencing a renaissance at most medical centers, so this will likely continue to be a practice in evolution. Importantly, several studies have shown that inadequate antibiotic choices have been associated with worse patient outcomes.[52]

In some cases, the patient may develop further signs of infection with fever, abdominal complaints, or leukocytosis. These patients should undergo repeat abdominal imaging to confirm adequate source control (discussed next). It is, however, important to note that superinfection may occur and could mandate additional cultures to guide changes in antimicrobial therapy.

Antibiotics should be given at the time of diagnosis of the AA and are often continued until the patient is clinically better, usually for 5–7 days. In the STOP-IT trial, patients with complicated abdominal infection were treated with source control plus antibiotics for either 2 days after resolution of the pathophysiologic abnormalities related to abdominal infection (maximum, 10 days of therapy) or for 4 ± 1 days, with no significant differences in outcomes.[53]

Risk of relapse after therapy is higher in patients with persistent leukocytosis following therapy (37%) and higher still in patients with leukocytosis and fever (57%).[54] In patients who have poor intestinal absorption, persistent ileus, large draining abscess, and poor immunologic/nutritional status, there are less data to guide clinical choices. With the greater variety of microbiological resistance and unusual pathogens now encountered, some centers have relied more on outpatient intravenous antibiotics to achieve cures in those patients with multiple risk factors.

Source Control and Drainage

Percutaneous Drainage of Abscesses. Percutaneous drainage (PD) of abscesses has become the standard of care for abscesses amenable to this technique,[55,56] because the efficacy compared with surgical drainage has been well-established.[57] The majority of cases of AA (85%–90%) are amenable to PD.[55,58] Contraindications to PD include lack of a safe drainage route, irreversible coagulopathy, generalized peritonitis, and/or bowel perforations associated with free air or ascites.[58,59] For patients with peritonitis in whom surgery is not possible, PD placement may be performed selectively. Ill-defined or phlegmonous collections are not appropriate for PD. Small collections, usually less than 3 cm in diameter, are typically treated with percutaneous aspiration without drain placement, although no trial has validated this practice.[57,60]

Advances in interventional techniques have expanded the role of PD to include AA in locations previously considered unreachable percutaneously[58,61] (e.g., instillation of sterile saline into the retroperitoneal space may allow drainage of AA adjacent to the stomach, duodenum, colon[61]). If the clinical scenario mandates, the liver, or stomach may be traversed with a small-bore PD catheter, but the large and small intestine should not be violated with a catheter. Thus intramesenteric or interloop abscesses that may arise from Crohn's disease or other conditions may prohibit the use of PD (see Fig. 29.4). Studies indicate that patients who have AA from complicated Crohn's disease have fewer postoperative intra-abdominal septic complications and a lower rate of stoma creation if PD is performed prior to surgery.[62,63] In patients with Crohn's disease and interloop abscess, it may be technically feasible to traverse the small bowel with a small-gauge needle to aspirate the interloop abscess without percutaneous abscess drainage (PAD) placement, but no studies have validated this practice.[58,60] Patients with numerous separate AAs are better served with surgery than PD (Fig. 29.5). Even though it is technically feasible to place any number of PDs in patients with numerous contemporaneous AAs, patient discomfort and complexity of drain management prohibit this practice. Lastly, symptomatic collections associated with vascular grafts or surgical mesh, among other causes, should only have PD after establishing the presence of infection as placing a drain in a sterile collection can lead to infection.[58] Technical factors to consider for PD use include the size, location, and perhaps the viscosity of the collection to be drained. Physicians may use US, CT, or fluoroscopy for guidance, depending upon abscess location and their preference. CT usually offers the most comprehensive evaluation of viscera, blood vessels, and nerves in relation to the abscess being drained, but US is faster and well suited to draining superficial abdominal collections. The primary limitation of US is the possibility of traversing intervening bowel; however, transrectal and transvaginal US may be utilized for deep pelvic collections. If multiloculated AA is encountered at diagnosis or if a post-PD imaging check reveals evidence of undrained septated components, thrombolytics may be instilled to achieve drainage, with success rates as high as 96%.[64]

After a safe percutaneous route is identified, the cavity is accessed using a trocar method or a needle and guidewire method

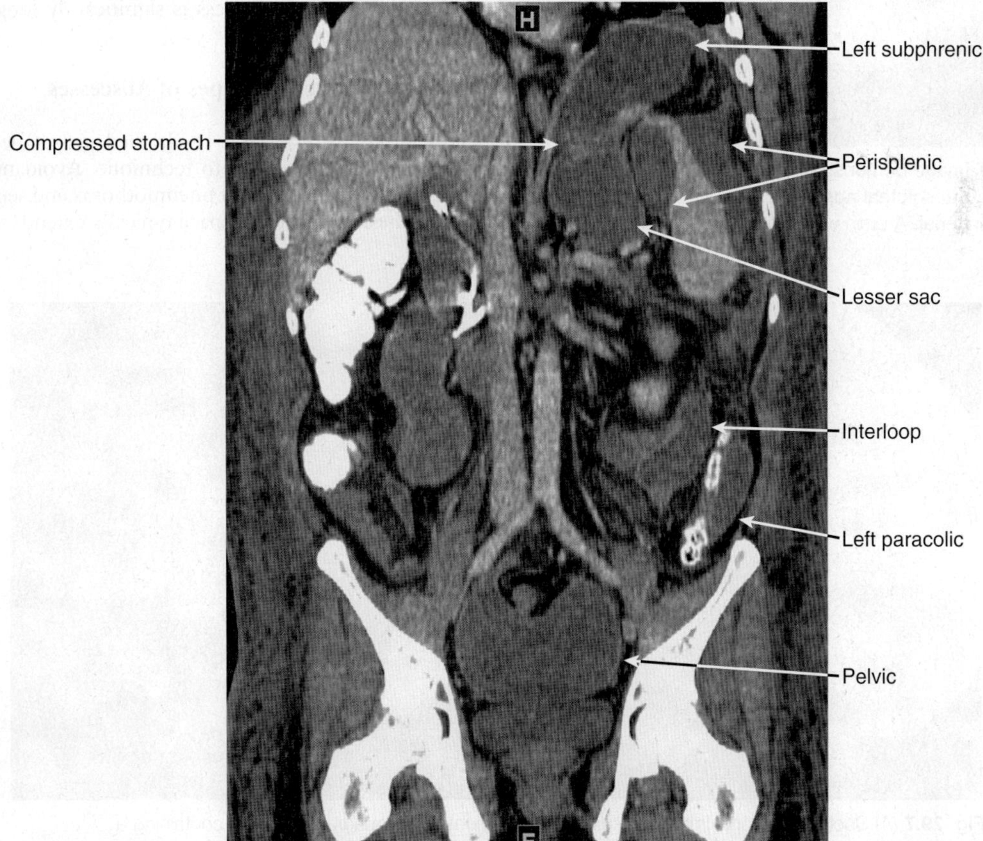

Fig. 29.5 Coronal CT image showing numerous rim-enhancing collections (*arrows*) in the abdomen and pelvis in a liver transplant recipient. Left subphrenic, perisplenic, lesser sac, interloop, left paracolic, and pelvic abscesses are seen. Cases such as this are best managed surgically.

(Fig. 29.6). The tract is dilated to a diameter approximating that of the planned catheter, and the catheter is advanced into the cavity. An initial 8- or 10-Fr catheter size is likely adequate, although upsizing and exchanges are frequently needed.[65] Once the catheter is placed, its position should be confirmed by repeat imaging to ensure that all catheter side holes are within the abscess. The cavity is typically aspirated dry, followed by flushing with sterile saline solution to clear any residual debris. The catheter is then placed to suction or gravity drainage and secured to the skin. A sample of the fluid is generally sent to the laboratory for Gram stain and culture. Following placement, the catheter is flushed daily with sterile saline solution to maintain patency. Catheter output and character of the output should be documented daily. Clinical status should be monitored for adequate response by assessing body temperature and blood leukocyte counts.

PD endpoints and decisions to obtain follow-up imaging studies depend on the clinical response, amount and nature of catheter drainage, and presence of suspected enteric communications. If the clinical response has been satisfactory and the catheter drainage has diminished to less than 20 mL/day, the catheter can be safely removed. If clinical response is inadequate, repeat imaging is warranted. Persistently high catheter output raises suspicion of a fistula. A catheter imaging study, performed by instilling water-soluble contrast medium through the catheter under fluoroscopy, is the best method to assess for the presence of a fistula (Fig. 29.7). If a fistula is located, the catheter can be repositioned adjacent to the opening into the bowel for better control of bowel effluent. Poor clinical responses to PD can also be caused by catheter dislodgment from the major abscess cavity, undrained loculations, multiple abscesses, or the formation of new abscesses. Repeat CT can evaluate these possible causes and guide additional percutaneous interventions when appropriate. Thick debris may occlude the catheter and inhibit daily flushing. In this case, a larger catheter can be exchanged for the catheter currently in use.[65]

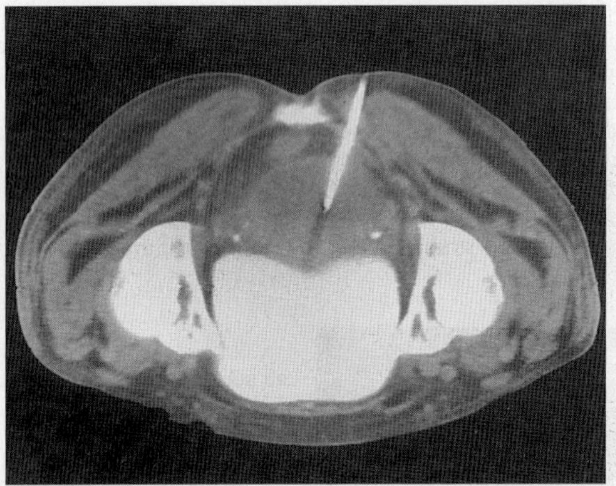

Fig. 29.6 Prone CT image demonstrating a pelvic abscess accessed with a needle via a transgluteal approach through the sciatic notch, yielding purulent material. A drain was subsequently placed.

The success rate for PD varies depending on the underlying etiology of the AA and patient comorbidities. Success rates of 64%–90% or better may be seen in the setting of perforated appendicitis and postoperative AA, challenging prior assertions that postoperative AA drainage is more often successful than nonpostoperative AA drainage.[66–70] Factors associated with a high rate of successful PD drainage in postoperative AA are the presence of a single abscess, lack of residual collection, and development of the abscess within 8 days after surgery.[67,69,70] In the setting of Crohn's disease, success rates of about 80% have been described for AA.[67]

The complication rate of PD ranges from 4% to 15%.[57,71–73] Complications include sepsis, organ injury, hemorrhage, pneumothorax, peritonitis, empyema, and pain. AA recurrence rates range from 1% to 9%.[57,72,74,75] Even when an abscess recurs, repeat secondary PD should be considered and can be curative. Success rates up to 91% for secondary PD have been achieved in recurrent abscesses, although the mean duration of drainage necessary to achieve success is significantly longer with the secondary procedure.[74]

Drainage of Specific Types of Abscesses

Subphrenic Abscesses

Subphrenic abscesses can be drained percutaneously so long as there is careful attention to technique. Avoidance of the pleural space is optimal to prevent pneumothorax and seeding of infection to the chest. The pleural space typically extends to the level of the

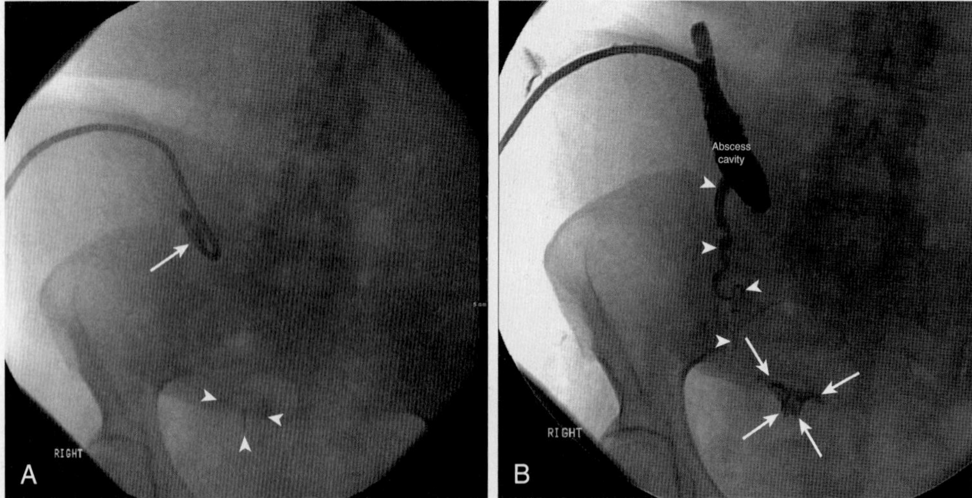

Fig. 29.7 (A) Spot fluoroscopic image in a patient with a right lower quadrant abscess containing a percutaneous drain (*arrow*). Note an IUD in the pelvis (*arrowheads*). (B) Same patient after instilling contrast into the drainage catheter showing contrast filling the abscess cavity, which communicates with the fallopian tube (*arrowheads*), indicating a fistula, with contrast filling the uterine cavity around the IUD (*arrows*). *IUD*, Intrauterine contraceptive device.

eighth thoracic vertebra (T8) anteriorly, T10 laterally, and T12 posteriorly. These landmarks can be used to prevent penetration of the pleural space. Some subphrenic fluid collections may not allow an extrapleural approach, in which case risks of surgical drainage should be weighed against the increased risk of pneumothorax and empyema posed by a transpleural PD procedure.[76] Endoscopic drainage of subphrenic abscesses has also been reported, which can mitigate the risk of pneumothorax and empyema.[77]

Pelvic Abscesses

If anterior access to pelvic abscesses is limited by intervening bowel, bladder, uterus, and/or vascular structures, a posterior transgluteal approach through the sciatic notch with the patient in prone position may be used to drain deep pelvic fluid collections (see Fig. 29.6).[78] Care must be taken to avoid the gluteal vasculature and sciatic nerve. US-guided transvaginal and transrectal drainage techniques have been increasingly used for drainage of deep pelvic abscesses that are inaccessible through other routes. A comparison of transrectal and transvaginal techniques demonstrated better patient tolerance of the transrectal drainage route; pain is more severe with transvaginal drainage.[79] Endoscopic transrectal US is another viable approach.

Appendiceal Abscesses

Periappendiceal abscesses can often be diagnosed on initial CT (see Chapter 120). PD has been increasingly accepted as the initial management of sepsis associated with a periappendiceal abscess, allowing the surgeon to perform a subsequent appendectomy, often laparoscopically, on an elective basis.[80,81] Thus avoiding an extended resection in the acute period. Studies show that the presence of a poorly defined collection or collections associated with an extraluminal appendicolith is predictive of clinical failure with PD (Fig. 29.8).[66] For a low-grade abscess, defined as periappendiceal phlegmon or abscess smaller than 3 cm, CT guidance and a transgluteal approach have been shown to be associated with a successful resolution.[69]

Diverticulutis-Associated Abscesses

PD of diverticulitis-associated abscesses has been an increasingly accepted procedure (see Chapter 121). In patients with diverticular abscess who ultimately require colon surgery, drainage can allow initial control of symptoms and obviate a diverting colostomy by allowing a one-stage rather than a two-stage procedure (see Fig. 29.3).[82]

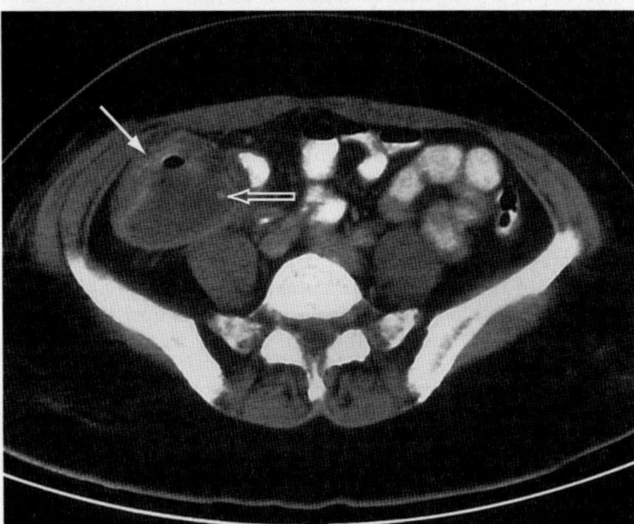

Fig. 29.8 Axial CT demonstrating a right lower quadrant abscess (*closed arrow*) with an appendicolith (*open arrow*). Such extraluminal appendicoliths may predict clinical failure with percutaneous drainage.

Pancreatitis-Related Abscesses

The Revised Atlanta classification describes various fluid collections associated with acute pancreatitis.[83] While the details of these pancreatitis-associated fluid collections are beyond the scope of this chapter, it is important to understand the management of pancreatic abscess (infected pancreatic necrosis), which results most commonly because of secondary infection of pancreatic necrosis and devitalized retroperitoneal tissues seen in necrotizing pancreatitis.[84] These are classically diagnosed on CT scans with the presence of gas within pancreatic necrosis. Historically these were treated with open surgical debridement which carried significant risks and high mortality rates for this patient population. However, with the advances in nonsurgical interventions such as endoscopic and PD modalities, surgical debridement is often the last resort in today's practice. The use of a minimally invasive step-up approach has been shown to reduce overall complications and mortality in these patients.[85]

Endoscopic Management

Spawned by success with managing pancreatic pseudocysts and walled-off pancreatic necrosis (see Chapters 58, 59, and 61) and paralleling technical improvements in EUS, endoscopic-guided drainage of AA is an emerging paradigm.[77,86,87] Although no large randomized controlled trials have validated this approach, case series have shown favorable results with transgastric and transcolonic drainage of IAA, allowing access to subphrenic, perihepatic, lesser sac, pericolonic, and pelvic collections.[77,87,88] Drainage of AA is precluded by this method if the abscess cavity is more than 20 mm from the transducer if there are intervening vessels or intervening ascites.[88]

If a review of cross-sectional imaging (CT, MRI, and US) reveals a collection amenable to drainage, the cavity is localized with EUS and cannulated with a 19-ga EUS FNA needle. A stiff guidewire is placed into the collection. The wall of the abscess is punctured with an over-the-wire-needle knife catheter or via cannulation with an ERCP cannula. The tract is then dilated, and double pigtail plastic stents (7–10 Fr) are placed. A sample of the AA is sent for Gram stain and culture. Follow-up CT is performed 2–3 days after the procedure. If the abscess has decreased significantly in size and the patient has clinically improved, the stents may be removed prior to patient discharge. If a sizable collection persists, the stents are left in place and a repeat CT is performed in 6–8 weeks. If the abscess remains, additional stent deployment, PD, or surgical management may be undertaken.[87] Stent migration has been reported in a minority of available case reports.[88] Case series suggest that endoscopic drainage of postoperative fluid collections is comparable to PD in success rate and complications.[89]

Surgical Management

Surgical management of AA is indicated in the setting of generalized peritonitis, uncontained GI perforation, in patients without a safe PD or endoscopic drainage option, or in patients who have failed PD or endoscopic drainage. Prime examples of the need for surgical management still include intramesenteric or interloop abscesses and numerous separate abscesses (see Fig. 29.5). Patients who have failed PD management owing to the presence of a continued source of infection require surgery for removal of the contaminant (e.g., extraluminal appendicoliths, dropped gallstones, and large debris).[66,90]

Patients with complex abdominal trauma, abdominal septic shock, abdominal hemorrhagic shock, or abdominal compartment syndrome are increasingly managed with damage control laparotomy (DCL), giving rise to laparostomy or "open abdomen"

(OA),[91] a technique whereby the fascia and skin are intentionally left open at the initial surgery, with a plan for definitive closure at a later time. DCL affords brief therapy for acute abdominal issues, with the aim of precluding complications associated with coagulopathy, acidosis, and hypothermia that arise in these patients. Treatment failure or overwhelming infection at the time of the initial DCL can cause patients with abdominal septic shock and secondary peritonitis to progress to tertiary peritonitis, with the need for multiple debridements and washouts. AA in this subset of patients presents special challenges, chief among them antibiotic selection to cover nosocomial infection, as detailed earlier. Development of AA and enteric fistula in these patients is associated with failure to achieve fascia closure and contributes to the high mortality rate associated with OA, usually over 20%.[91] Negative-pressure devices like the vacuum-assisted closure (VAC) device remain a cornerstone in OA management, but techniques to increase closure rates of the OA are under continual investigation and include such novel solutions as injection of botulinum toxin into abdominal wall musculature to permit closure.

Outcomes

Outcomes after treatment of AA are dependent on many factors. Mortality rates range from less than 5% for simple secondary bacterial peritonitis to 65% or higher for complicated tertiary peritonitis.[19,20,92–94] Simple abscesses associated with perforated appendicitis that respond to surgical drainage and antibiotics have a low mortality rate. Higher mortality rates occur in older patients, those who have complex abscesses, high Acute Physiology and Chronic Health Evaluation II and multiple organ dysfunction scores, or in patients who experience a therapeutic delay or who receive glucocorticoids or are otherwise immunosuppressed.[1,95] Other risk factors for high mortality include multiple reoperations to control intra-abdominal sepsis, malnutrition, poor physiologic reserve, high New York Heart Association class, and multiple organ dysfunction syndrome. It has been suggested that continued intra-abdominal infection is another manifestation of organ failure and not a cause[96]—that is, patients die *with* infection, not *of* infection. Aggressive surgical, antibiotic, and supportive care is needed in this group of patients, and they may benefit from defined clinical pathways that minimize variability in practice.[97]

GASTROINTESTINAL FISTULAS

A *fistula* is any abnormal anatomic connection between two epithelialized surfaces, a definition that includes many clinical entities. Fistulas arising in the abdomen can originate from any epithelialized surface of a hollow viscus or drainage duct in the GI or genitourinary tract, liver, or pancreas.

Classification

In general, fistulas are classified by their anatomy and physiology. Anatomic classifications are based on the fistula's origin and drainage point. Inherent in this anatomic classification system is whether the fistula is internal or external; *internal fistulas* drain between two epithelial surfaces, whereas *external fistulas* drain to the outside surface of the body. Physiologic or volume classifications are based on the output of a fistula in a 24-hour period, and they are generally divided into high (>500 cm^3) or low output (<500 cm^3) (Box 29.4). Both fistula classifications are often used clinically when describing a fistulous tract (e.g., a high-output gastrocutaneous fistula). A special case is the *enteroatmospheric fistula*, defined as a fistula between a hollow viscous and the atmosphere (discussed later). This chapter largely focuses on enterocutaneous fistulas; for specific discussions of biliary and pancreatic fistulas, see Chapters 58, 59, and 61.

BOX 29.4 Classification of Fistulas

ANATOMIC

Internal (e.g., ileocolic, colovesical)
External (e.g., enterocutaneous)

PHYSIOLOGIC

High output (>500 mL/day)
Low output (<200 mL/day)

Pathophysiology

GI fistulas can occur spontaneously or following medical procedures. Spontaneous fistulas account for 15%–25% of fistulas and arise in association with inflammatory/infectious processes, cancer, and radiation treatment.[98–106] Inflammatory processes contributing to spontaneous fistula formation include colonic diverticulitis, IBD, AA, peptic ulcer disease, appendicitis, radiation enteritis, and distal obstruction/neoplasms. These fistulas can be internal or external, and depending on the special circumstances, they can have different rates of spontaneous closure. The remaining 75%–85% of fistulas are due to surgical or other procedures [107–112]; most of these are postoperative and represent anastomotic disruptions or missed injuries to the bowel. Risk factors for postoperative fistula formation include malnutrition, sepsis, shock, hypotension or need for vasopressor therapy, glucocorticoid therapy, associated comorbidities, foreign body such as suture/mesh, and technical difficulties with surgical anastomosis.[113]

Determining the cause of fistula formation is important because it often influences therapy. Fistulas that arise in the setting of IBD may respond to anti-inflammatory therapy, whereas those due to direct involvement from malignancy are unlikely to close spontaneously and often require surgical intervention. Postoperative low-output fistulas arising from a partial anastomotic dehiscence frequently close with conservative management. Conditions associated with the failure of spontaneous fistula closure are listed in Box 29.5.

Diagnosis

Accurately diagnosing fistulas largely depends on anatomic considerations. An external enterocutaneous fistula is often diagnosed based on visual confirmation of external enteric drainage. Suspicious wound drainage can be tested for elevated levels of bilirubin and amylase to confirm that the fluid is enteric in origin. Fistulas with external drainage are often more obvious than internal fistulas, which may be more difficult to diagnose. This would be the case, for example, in a cholecystoduodenal fistula, which may not manifest unless a gallstone ileus develops (see Chapter 65). In a colovesical fistula, the presenting signs are often urinary tract infection, fecaluria, and pneumaturia.

Occasionally, especially in the setting of associated infection, it may be more difficult to confirm the presence of a fistula on a physical exam. In cases where there is suspicion of a fistula, stabilization of the patient is paramount, after which radiographic studies are often helpful in establishing the diagnosis of a fistula, determining the cause and source of the fistula, confirming

BOX 29.5 Conditions Associated with Nonhealing Spontaneous GI Fistulas

Foreign body within the fistula tract (see Chapter 28)
Radiation enteritis involving the affected bowel (see Chapter 41)
Infection or inflammation at the fistula origin
Epithelialization of the fistula tract
Neoplasm at the fistula origin
Distal obstruction of intestine

adequate drainage, and defining the tract. This information is then used in formulating an appropriate treatment plan. These studies can include fluoroscopy after administration of oral or rectal contrast medium, depending on the site of suspicion. Internal fistulas can be diagnosed when injecting contrast medium into one hollow viscus (e.g., urinary bladder) results in the opacification of another viscus [e.g., rectosigmoid (Fig. 29.9)]. Alternatively, contrast can be injected retrograde into the drainage site (fistulography) and followed to its site of origin (Fig. 29.10; also see Fig. 29.7). CT with contrast or MRI, especially when performed with an enterography protocol, may reveal a fistula tract (Fig. 29.11). Such cross-sectional imaging protocols have the added advantage of determining whether any undrained collections are present. Lastly, endoscopy may be useful to visualize the luminal origin of the fistula.

Management

Stabilization

Initial management of GI fistulas is directed at stabilizing the patient, controlling sepsis, and management of fluid and electrolyte derangements. This can be a daunting task if the patient presents with severe sepsis or if the fistula has a high output (>500 mL/day; see Box 29.4). Output greater than 1000 mL/day is not uncommon if the fistula originates in the proximal small bowel. To prevent intravascular volume depletion and electrolyte imbalance, fluid and electrolyte replacement must be a priority and should be addressed before more detailed diagnostic studies of the fistula are undertaken. Administration of replacement fluids should account for the volume and electrolyte content lost through the fistula. In general, fistula output is isosmotic and rich in potassium. Initially, fistula

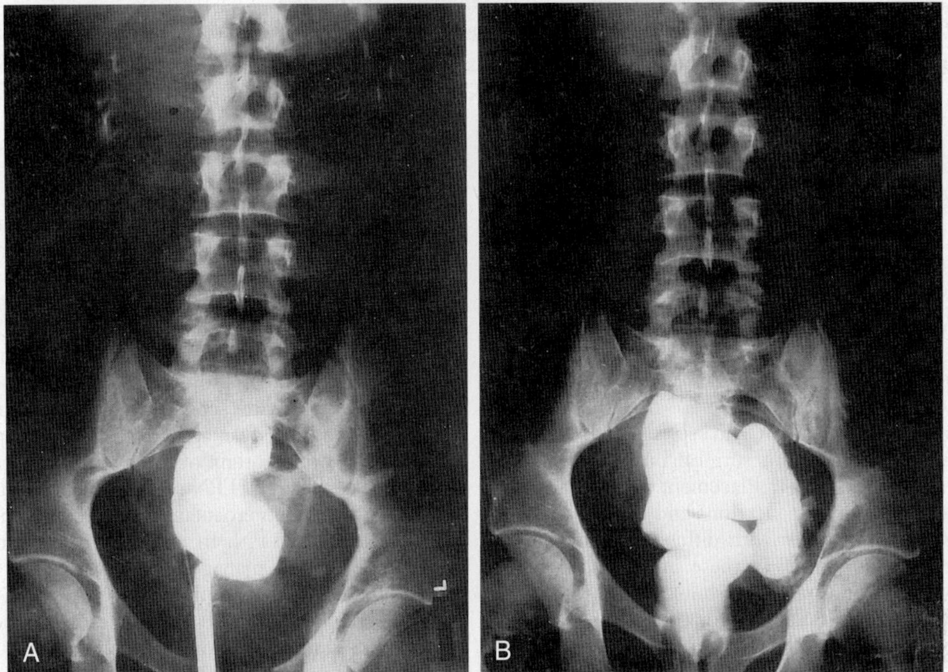

Fig. 29.9 Abdominal films showing a rectovesical fistula in a patient with Crohn's disease, pneumaturia, and urinary tract infection. (A) Catheter in the bladder, with contrast beginning to fill the bowel. (B) Contrast has filled the sigmoid colon and rectum through the fistulous tract. (Courtesy Dr. Mark Feldman, Dallas, TX.)

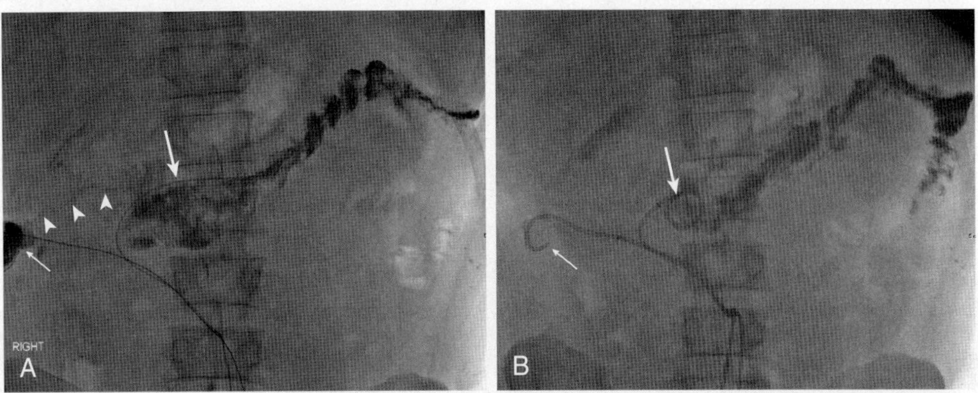

Fig. 29.10 (A) Fluoroscopic image of a patient with Crohn's disease with two draining abdominal wounds in whom guidewires have been placed within each tract, one within the transverse colon (*large arrow*) and the other within a loop of jejunum (*small arrow*). Note an additional thin enterocolonic fistula connecting the jejunum and transverse colon (*arrowheads*). (B) Same patient after placement of drainage catheters into the transverse colonic (*large arrow*) and jejunal (*small arrow*) components of this complex fistula.

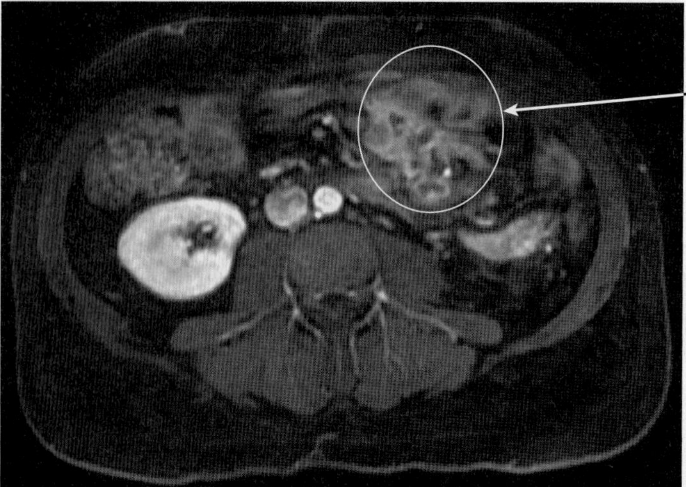

Fig. 29.11 Axial MRI after gadolinium contrast of a patient with Crohn's disease, showing matted loops of small bowel (*circle*) in a tethered stellate configuration typical of enteroenteric fistulas (*arrow*).

output should be replaced milliliter for milliliter with a balanced crystalloid solution that contains added potassium.

Establishment of Adequate Drainage

A cornerstone of the early management strategy in the treatment of enterocutaneous fistulas is establishing adequate drainage. This issue requires immediate attention because if drainage is not facilitated, pooling of fistula contents within the abdominal cavity can lead to infection, abscess formation, and sepsis. Minor surgical maneuvers, such as opening a recent surgical incision to allow adequate drainage, are often required. Placement of percutaneous catheters may be needed to drain collections and control the fistula effluent. Some patients present with diffuse peritonitis that cannot be managed with PD alone. In these situations, patients may require abdominal exploration and washout. Definitive repair of such fistulas at the time of operation for peritonitis is rarely successful. In these circumstances, the goal of surgery is to remove contamination and establish drainage, often with a placement of drains during surgery.

Diverting enterostomies and surgical feeding tubes are placed when appropriate.[114] Once ongoing peritoneal contamination is resolved and external drainage is established, the effluent from the fistula must be controlled. Because most enterocutaneous fistulas occur postoperatively, some ingenuity may be required when trying to protect the skin from the caustic effects of the fistula output. Most acute postoperative enterocutaneous fistulas decompress through the surgical incision. Because the incision shows signs of infection and drainage, it must be opened. A reopened incision that is draining intestinal contents is not amenable to a simple placement of an ostomy bag to collect the drainage. There are multiple options for containment, but an experienced enterostomal therapist should be consulted when dealing with this difficult problem.[115] A recent adjunct in the management of enterocutaneous fistulas has been local wound care with the VAC system described earlier. The VAC device has simplified the management of these difficult wounds because control of the effluent and the open wound can be managed simultaneously.[107,116–118]

With the increasing popularity of DCL and OA, enteroatmospheric fistulas have become more common.[119–121] These "exposed fistulas" are often very difficult to manage and give rise to drainage challenges. Many inventive strategies have been used to care for these complex fistulas.[122–125]

Nutritional Support

Well-nourished patients without infectious complications are more likely to experience spontaneous fistula closure and are at lower risk for operative complications if surgical repair is required.[102,126–129] Thus nutritional evaluation and support must be aggressively pursued (see Chapters 5 and 6). The causes of malnutrition in the patient with a GI fistula are multifactorial, including underlying disease states, lack of protein intake, protein losses through the fistula, and underlying sepsis with hypercatabolism.[113] Soon after diagnosis of a GI fistula, aggressive caloric support must be given. Once the anatomic origin of the fistula is determined, the route of feeding is considered. TPN seems to be the natural first choice for a patient with an enterocutaneous fistula, but not all patients need to be placed on TPN. In a study of 335 patients with external fistulas, 85% were managed solely with enteral feedings.[130] In a subgroup of patients with uncomplicated fistulas in this study, 50% healed spontaneously with this mode of nutritional therapy alone. In another study, initiation of enteral feeding within 2 weeks of admission in patients with GI fistulas complicated with severe sepsis resulted in more rapid abdominal wound closure and decreased mortality compared with later initiation.[131] Enteral feeding enhances mucosal proliferation and villous growth through direct and indirect mechanisms. Nutrients in contact with the bowel mucosa provide direct stimulation to the enterocyte, and feedings high in glutamine may be particularly beneficial because glutamine is the main source of energy for the enterocyte.[132] Furthermore, nutrients within the gut lumen cause the release of gut-derived hormones that have an indirect trophic effect on the intestinal mucosa (see Chapter 4). TPN, in contrast, has been shown to lead to gut mucosal atrophy. This may in part be because standard TPN solutions do not contain glutamine, which crystallizes out of solution. In a small study of patients on TPN, spontaneous resolution of fistula drainage was more likely in patients supplemented with oral glutamine.[133] Despite recent advances in enteral feeding of patients with GI fistulas, TPN remains the mainstay of nutritional support for most patients because they are unable to absorb sufficient calories enterally.[134] Consequently, aggressive nutritional support is vital to improving outcomes in patients with GI fistulas.[135]

The decision to support the patient with a GI fistula with enteral nutrition or TPN is based on anatomic and physiologic considerations. In most patients, a trial of enteral feeding should be initiated after stabilization. Often, fistula output is not increased significantly despite feeding. If the output does increase significantly, decreasing or stopping enteral feeding should be considered. If the fistula is in the proximal intestine and distal access to the intestine has been established, as in many post-operative fistulas in which a feeding jejunostomy has been placed at the time of surgery, enteral feeding into the distal bowel should be started. Along with the commencement of enteral feeding, infusion of the proximal fistula drainage into the distal bowel has been shown to make fluid and electrolyte management easier, as well as decrease the output of the proximal fistula.[105,136] In addition, fistuloclysis or tube feeding directly into the efferent limb of a fistula has been shown to be effective in selected patients.[137] It is not mandatory to provide full nutritional support via the enteral route to obtain the benefits of enteral feeding; protein and caloric requirements can be supplemented by TPN.

Medical Therapy

Somatostatin Analogs. Somatostatin analogs such as octreotide or lanreotide may be adjunctive to TPN in the management of a patient with a GI fistula. Octreotide has been shown to decrease fistula output by several mechanisms. First, it inhibits the release of gastrin, cholecystokinin, secretin, and many other GI hormones. This inhibition decreases the secretion of electrolytes, water, and pancreatic enzymes into the intestine, subsequently decreasing intestinal volume. Second, octreotide relaxes intestinal smooth muscle, thereby allowing for a greater intestinal capacity. Third, octreotide increases intestinal water and electrolyte absorption.[138]

Meta-analyses of the randomized studies evaluating somatostain analogs in the treatment of enterocutaneous fistulas show an increased closure rate, with decreased fistula output, time to closure, and hospital stay, without an effect on mortality.[139,140] Octreotide results in an increased fistula closure rate by converting a high-output fistula to a low-output fistula.[141] We advocate a time-limited trial to evaluate whether an addition of octreotide reduces fistula output. If the output does not decrease within 72 hours of initiation of treatment, octreotide should be discontinued.

Other pharmacologic agents, such as proton pump inhibitors and loperamide, have also been used, similar to their application in controlling the output from "high output" ostomy, with variable success. Teduglutide, a recombinant GLP-2 analog, has been shown to stimulate mucosal hypertrophy and is being used in patients with short bowel syndrome to increase absorptive capacity and potentially help wean off TPN. However, the data for its use in enterocutaneous fistulas is currently lacking.[142]

Management of Crohn's Disease

Historically, conservative management of fistulas associated with Crohn's disease had been uniformly unrewarding because most abdominal and perianal fistulas required surgical correction. The observation that TNF-α production in the intestinal mucosa is increased in patients with Crohn's disease[143] has led to the development of chimeric monoclonal antibodies against TNF-α (infliximab), as well as other anti-inflammatory monoclonal antibodies (ustekinumab and vedolizumab) for the treatment of Crohn's disease (see Chapter 116). For the initial management of fistulas in Crohn's disease, a trial of an anti-TNF-α antibody regimen should be considered and has been supported by a Cochrane database review.[144] A number of small series advocate for the use of aggressive immunosuppression of fistulizing Crohn's patients with methotrexate or tacrolimus or other biologics when other nonoperative therapy has failed.[145,146]

The data for medical treatment of fistulizing Crohn's disease are heavily weighted toward the treatment of perianal disease, with little data specifically for enterocutaneous fistulas. Meta-analysis suggests variable quality evidence for the role of TNF antagonists, mesenchymal stem cell therapy, immunosuppressive agents, and therapy with TNF antagonists in combination with antibiotics in the treatment of fistulizing Crohn's disease.[147,148] In the setting of failed medical management, surgical intervention should be pursued.

Nonsurgical Intervention

Nonsurgical interventions in the management of refractory fistulas include the use of covered stents, clips, endoluminal vacuum (E-vac) therapy, endoscopic suturing, occlusive plugs, and fibrin glue placed endoscopically or percutaneously. Although reports are limited to case series at this time, a variety of nonsurgical techniques, including fistuloscopy, fluoroscopy, and endoscopy, have been reported.[149–152] Success with endoscopic clipping of the internal fistula opening has also been seen, and over-the-scope clips now available may allow for endoscopic closure of larger defects.[153–158]

E-vac therapy is very promising in the management of upper and lower GI fistulas and leaks. It has theoretical advantages over other techniques, with improved drainage of infection and enteric effluents through the negative pressure suction applied. Additionally, this can improve blood flow to the healing defect. This technique involves endoscopic evaluation of the luminal defect, irrigation, and aspiration of any associated abscess cavity or fistulous track, followed by insertion of an open pore polyurethane sponge cut to the appropriate size and attached to the end of a nasogastric tube (there is currently no available commercial E-vac product in the United States). Once the sponge is in place, it is placed to continuous negative pressure of 100–125 mm Hg. Sponge changes are performed every 3–5 days until the closure of the cavity and defect. Data from the case series are quite encouraging.[159–162]

Endoscopic and nonoperative techniques may serve as a useful adjunct for fistulas refractory to conservative management or increasingly as front-line treatment options. Initial attempts of nonsurgical interventions do not preclude surgery and may spare some patients having to undergo highly morbid procedures.

Surgical Intervention

Surgical therapy remains the mainstay of management of enterocutaneous fistula in which conservative and/or endoscopic interventions have failed.[102,105] Indications for early surgery include inability to control the fistula without surgical drainage, uncontrolled sepsis, abscess formation, intestinal obstruction distal to the fistula, and bleeding. Early surgical intervention often involves temporizing measures to eliminate the source of sepsis and establish fistula control, such as washout and drainage and/or stoma formation. More complex fistulas may require surgery to remove mesh or other foreign bodies before spontaneous closure can occur or definitive surgery is undertaken. The goal of surgical therapy is to resolve infection and restore intestinal continuity, usually requiring resection.[163] Attempts at direct fistula closure are rarely successful and generally should be avoided. Minimally invasive surgery is an option in selected patients.[149,164]

There are no firm data to dictate the timing of a definitive operation, but timing of surgery should take into account the clinical scenario for the case at hand. In the case of the post-operative enterocutaneous fistula, further surgery should occur either in the favorable "window period," 7–12 days after laparotomy, or deferred at least 6–8 weeks thereafter to allow improvement of intra-abdominal inflammation and adhesions.[165] The rationale for waiting is to avoid an operation until the severe inflammatory response in the abdomen has resolved and the associated dense vascular adhesions have diminished. If operative intervention is performed beyond the window period, it is often doomed to fail. Moreover, these patients have an increased likelihood of developing additional enterotomies and subsequent complications. In the setting of sepsis, the general consensus in the literature is to wait at least 6 weeks after stabilization and resolution of sepsis, with many advocating for longer waiting periods.[165,166]

TABLE 29.1 Prognostic Indicators of Spontaneous Fistula Closure with Nonoperative Management

Favorable	Unfavorable
Surgical etiology	Ileal, jejunal, nonsurgical etiology
Appendicitis, diverticulitis	IBD, cancer, radiation
Transferrin >200 mg/dL	Transferrin <200 mg/dL
No obstruction, bowel in continuity, no infection, no inflamed intestine	Distal obstruction, bowel discontinuity, adjacent infection, adjacent active inflammation
Length >2 cm, end fistula	Length <2 cm, lateral fistula, multiple fistulas
Output <200 mL/24 h	Output >200 mL/24 h
No sepsis, balanced serum electrolytes	Sepsis, electrolyte disturbances
Initial referral to tertiary care center and subspecialty care	Delay getting referral to tertiary care center and subspecialty care

IBD, Inflammatory bowel disease.
Adapted from Gribovskaja-Rupp I, Melton GB. Enterocutaneous fistula: proven strategies and updates. *Clin Colon Rectal Surg.* 2016;29:130–137.

The mainstay of surgical treatment is resection of the involved segment of the bowel, with anastomosis. Different techniques have been used in the surgical treatment of fistulas, and some success has been seen with innovative techniques such as pedicled flaps.[167]

Outcomes

Early morbidity and mortality in the management of external fistulas result from initial fluid and electrolyte derangements that go unchecked. However, the major cause of mortality in patients with GI fistulas is sepsis with multiple organ failure. The typical setting for septic complications is provided by complex fistulas for which there is inadequate or uncontrolled drainage. In this setting, pooling of enteric contents occurs within the abdominal cavity and acts as a nidus of infection. Therefore, as noted, aggressive attempts must be made to ensure that fistulous drainage is well controlled. The mortality rate from all causes in patients with fistulas ranges from 10% to 30%.[99–103,105–108,127–129,165,168] Higher mortality rates are seen in those with comorbidities, age older than 55, who are septic, are malnourished, have had previous radiation therapy, or have complex fistulas associated with postoperative abdominal wall dehiscence.[108,128,165] Another major risk of mortality in patients with GI fistulas is severe underlying disease, most frequently cancer. Often, patients who are terminally ill secondary to malignancy forgo further operative procedures.[169]

Fistula recurrence after surgery has been noted in 5%–38% of postoperative patients. Factors associated with fistula recurrence after surgery include IBD, poor nutritional status, complex fistula, delayed fascial closure, mesh implantation, infection, advanced underlying disease states, and oversewing the fistula instead of resection and reanastomosis.[99–101,107,127,163,165] It has been reported that patients with high-output fistulas had a four-time greater chance of recurrence than patients with low-output fistulas.[167] In a univariate analysis, factors associated with the greatest chance of recurrence after surgery for fistula closure included high output, enteroatmospheric fistula, and/or a history of OA. The authors' recommendation was to treat any recurrence as a "new" fistula and to follow standard treatments.[167]

Beyond the prevention of morbidity and mortality, the ultimate goal in fistula management is closure. Often this is accomplished spontaneously with supportive measures. The rate of spontaneous closure of fistulas varies in the literature from 15% to

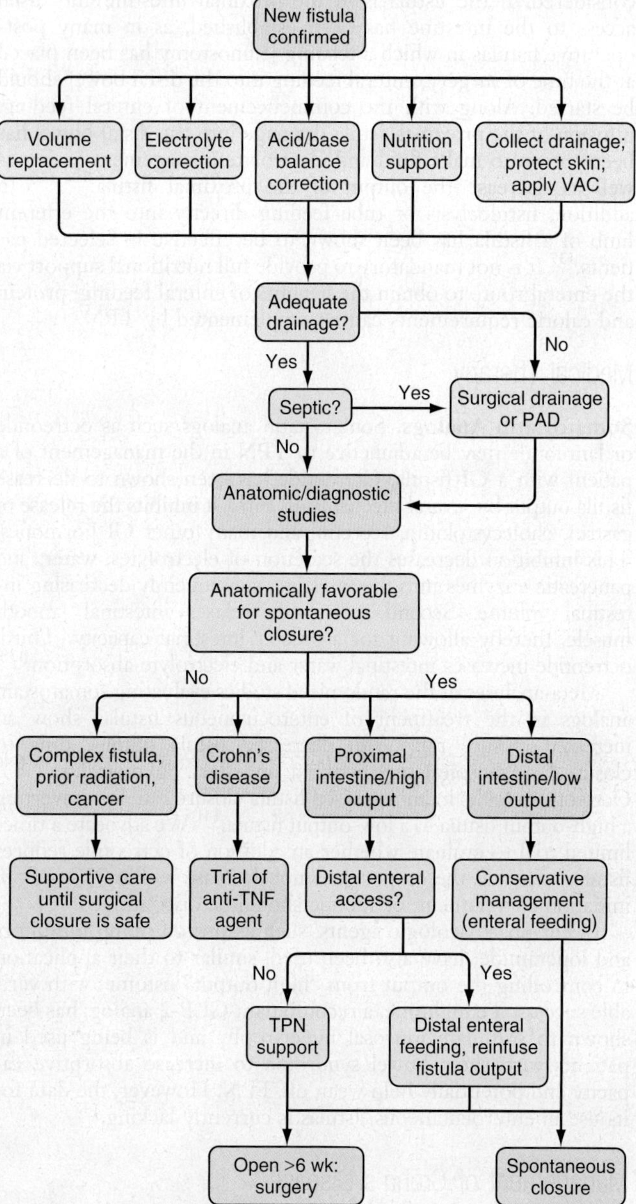

Fig. 29.12 Algorithm for the management of GI fistulas. See text for details. *PAD*, Percutaneous abscess drainage; *VAC*, vacuum-assisted closure.

71%. Of those fistulas that close spontaneously, about 90% will do so within 30 days of stabilization and control of sepsis. Important factors for resolution are control of sepsis, control of fistula output, and nutritional support. Table 29.1 lists some prognostic factors important in determining the rate of spontaneous fistula closure.[170] Fistulas that ultimately require surgical closure are more often associated with high output, short tract, and ongoing sepsis.

Although innovative therapy and supportive care have resulted in improving spontaneous closure rates, management of these difficult problems requires a multidisciplinary approach that includes a nutritional support service, an enterostomal therapist, a surgeon, an interventional radiologist, and a gastroenterologist.[171] An algorithm to manage GI fistulas is presented in Fig. 29.12.

Full references for this chapter can be found on https://ebooks.health.elsevier.com.

30 Eosinophilic Disorders of the Gastrointestinal Tract

Marc E. Rothenberg, Simin Zhang

IN THIS CHAPTER

INTRODUCTION

Eosinophilic GI disorders (EGIDs) are a group of disorders characterized by eosinophil infiltration into various segments of the GI tract. These include eosinophilic esophagitis (EoE), eosinophilic gastritis (EoG), eosinophilic enteritis (EoN), and eosinophilic colitis (EoC). EoE is the most well studied and understood. Genetic factors[1–3] and environmental factors[4–6] have been shown to contribute to EGIDs. Allergens,[4–6] cytokines, including IL-13, chemokines,[7] and skewing toward type 2 immunity, contribute to disease pathophysiology.[7] There have been significant advances of our understanding of EGIDs in the last decade, including dupilumab, the first FDA-approved drug for EoE, and the approval of orodispersible budesonide tablets for EoE in Europe and some other locations outside the United States.

EOSINOPHIL BIOLOGY AND POTENTIAL DIAGNOSTIC AND THERAPEUTIC TARGETS

Eosinophils originate from pluripotent stem cells in the bone marrow and develop under the globin transcription factor (GATA-1), cytokines IL-3, IL-5, and granulocyte-macrophage colony-stimulating factor.[8] Eosinophils are characterized by primary and secondary granules containing major basic protein (MBP)-1 and MBP-2, eosinophil peroxidase, and eosinophil cationic protein that are toxic to tissues, including the intestinal epithelium,[9] and expression of Charcot-Leyden Crystal Protein (CLC), also known as galectin-10, which is a potent immune-stimulating adjuvant.[10]

IL-5 is responsible for eosinophil differentiation,[11] release from bone marrow,[12] and survival.[13] Murine studies show positive correlation of *IL-5* with blood eosinophilia, with decreased IL-5 levels causing reduced eosinophils after allergen challenge in blood, lungs, and GI tract.[14–17] These results contributed to development of anti-IL-5 therapies, such as reslizumab and mepolizumab,[18,19] as well as the eosinophil-depleting antibody benralizumab that binds to the IL-5 receptor and mediates antibody-dependent cytotoxicity.[20] Clinical trials of these and other biologics have shown mixed results in EGIDs, with clinical trial data of lirentelimab (anti-siglec-8) for EoG and eosinophilic duodenitis (EoD) (ENIGMA)[21] and benralizumab (anti-IL-5) for EoE (MESSINA),[22] suggesting that therapies that eosinophils do not improve clinical symptoms of EGIDs; however, it remains to be determined whether subgroups of patients may benefit.

RNA sequencing of EoE has shown a robust IL-13 signature,[23] and eosinophils are known to respond to and express Th2 cytokines.[24,25] IL-4 and IL-13 induce intercellular adhesion molecule-1 and vascular cell adhesion molecule-1 expression on endothelium, which bind β1 and β2 integrins on eosinophils.[25] IL-4 and IL-13 signal through the common receptor subunit IL-4Rα that results in downstream activation of the STAT6 pathway,[26] which is required for IL-13's potent ability to activate gene transcriptions at hundreds of sites across the human genome, most notably induction of the eosinophil chemokine eotaxin-3 as well as the product of a chief EoE genetic risk loci, calpain-14. *Stat6* knockout in mice has impaired GI Th2-associated response development.[27] STAT6 gain-of-function mutations cause severe atopy, including EGID.[28] Dupilumab is a monoclonal antibody directed against IL-4Rα, which blocks the action of IL-4 and IL-13, and in clinical trials showed clinical, endoscopic, and histologic improvement for patients with EoE, which led to its approval as the first FDA-approved treatment of EoE.

Eotaxins are chemokines that are constitutively expressed throughout the GI tract and regulate eosinophil localization to the GI lamina propria.[29] Overexpression of eotaxin-3 mRNA in the esophagus has 89% sensitivity for identifying those with EoE from those without.[23] There are currently CCR3 inhibitors and an eotaxin-1 antibody that have been developed and are in clinical trials for various indications.[25,30,31]

EOSINOPHILIC GASTROINTESTINAL DISORDERS

Multiple GI disorders have eosinophil infiltration, including gastroesophageal reflux disease (GERD),[32,33] drug reactions, parasitic infections, fungal infections, inflammatory bowel disorders (IBD), celiac disease, food-protein induced enterocolitis syndrome (FPIES), hypereosinophilic syndromes (HESs), classic IgE-mediated food allergy,[34–36] allergic colitis,[37,38] esophageal leiomyomatosis, myeloproliferative disorders, carcinomatosis, polyarteritis, allergic vasculitis, collagen vascular disease, pemphigus vegetans, drug injury, and EGIDs[29,39] (Box 30.1). EGIDs are chronic immune-mediated disorders that present

BOX 30.1 Causes of Gastrointestinal Eosinophilia

Gastroesophageal reflux disease
Eosinophilic gastrointestinal disorders
Eosinophilic esophagitis
Connective tissue disease-associated eosinophilic esophagitis
Familial eosinophilic esophagitis
Eosinophilic gastritis
Eosinophilic enteritis
Eosinophilic colitis
Infections
Schistosomiasis
Anisakiasis
Gastrointestinal basidiobolomycosis (*Basidiobolus ranarum*)
Toxacariasis (*Toxocara canis*)
Celiac disease
Hypereosinophilic syndrome
Drug hypersensitivity response
Inflammatory bowel disease
Transplant-associated eosinophilic enteritis
Churg-Strauss syndrome/vasculitis
Toxic injury
Graft-versus-Host disease

BOX 30.2 Diagnostic Work-Up for Eosinophilic Gastrointestinal Disorders

General
Complete blood count and differential
Total IgE level
Erythrocyte sedimentation rate
Skin prick testing
Infection work-up (stool or colonic aspirate analysis)
Upper and lower gastrointestinal endoscopy with biopsies
(pH probe impedance study, skin patch testing, tests for specific IgE)
Consideration of exome sequencing
In the presence of hypereosinophilia
Bone marrow analysis
Serum tryptase
Serum vitamin B_{12}
Echocardiogram
Genetic analysis for *FIP1L1-PDGFRA* fusion gene
(Evaluation and biopsy of any other potentially involved tissue)

Reproduced from Rothenberg ME. Eosinophilic gastrointestinal disorders (EGID). *J Allergy Clin Immunol.* 2004;113:11–28, with permission from the American Academy of Allergy, Asthma, and Immunology.

histologically with eosinophilic infiltration of the GI tract after exclusion of secondary causes of intestinal eosinophilia.[40] EGIDs are classified by location of eosinophilia in the GI tract, including EoE, EoG, EoN, and EoC.[41] EoN can be further classified into EoD, eosinophilic jejunitis, and eosinophilic ileitis. Clinical symptoms are nonspecific, and different EGIDs can have similar symptoms, such as abdominal pain. Non-EoE EGIDs (EoG, EoN, and EoC) can present with iron deficiency anemia and protein-losing enteropathy and interestingly do not have the male predominance seen in EoE.[42] Endoscopy and histologic assessment for eosinophils are necessary for EGID diagnosis. Due to nonspecific symptoms and lack of endoscopic/histologic evaluation, there can be a long delay of years before diagnosis. There is also a genetic component to EGIDs, as evidenced by ~10% of patients with EGIDs having an immediate family member with EGID[1,2] (Box 30.2).

EOSINOPHILIC ESOPHAGITIS

Etiology

The etiology of EoE involves a complex interplay between environmental and genetic factors and is evidenced by the improvement of EoE with food elimination diets and elemental formula.[43,44] EoE is associated with atopy[45] and frequently occurs in patients with asthma, eczema, and food anaphylaxis.[46] Patients report seasonal variations in their symptoms. Patients with allergic rhinitis to pollen have also been noted to have esophageal eosinophil infiltration during the allergic pollen season.[47] Epicutaneous antigen exposure has also been shown to prime the esophagus for eosinophilia following airway antigen challenge.[48] Additionally, the majority of patients with EoE have food and aeroallergen sensitization on skin prick testing and/or allergen-specific IgE testing.[49] However, only a few have food anaphylaxis,[50] and food elimination based on skin prick/IgE testing has not yielded promising results.[51] While EoE is the most common EGID in the United States and Europe, Japan has reported a lower prevalence compared with non-EoE EGID.[52]

EoE is also associated with a type 2 immune mechanism, with increases in T cells and mast cells in addition to eosinophils.[53,54] Pathogenic effector memory $CD4^+$ T cells accumulate in the esophagus and express high levels of IL-5 and IL-13 locally.[55] In addition, mast cells also accumulate in the esophagus, but unlike eosinophils, they locally proliferate and remain abnormal, poised for activation, even in patients with remission (defined by eosinophil levels).[56] Esophageal inflammation is also linked with pulmonary inflammation, as shown by studies in which repeated lung allergen challenge and IL-13 challenge, or the transgenic overexpression of IL-13 in the lung, induce experimental EoE.[57–59]

The analysis of EoE tissue by genome-wide RNA expression analysis was a landmark study that established the importance of eotaxin-3 for disease pathogenesis, and mice deficient in the eotaxin receptor have attenuated eosinophil recruitment to the esophagus.[60] Eotaxin-3 overexpression has an 89% predictive value of diagnosing EoE from an esophageal biopsy.[23] Multiple genome-wide association studies have implicated several atopic risk loci (*TSLP*, *LRRC32*, *IL33*, *LPP*) and *CAPN14*, an EoE disease-associated, esophagus-specific element.[61,62]

EoE has a prevalence of about 1 in 2000 people in the general population in most countries, about 5%–15% in patients who underwent endoscopy for dysphagia, and >50% in patients with food impaction.[63] EoE has a familial component in terms of atopic disease, EoE, and esophageal dilations, and a sibling recurrence risk ratio of approximately 80, which means an increased risk of disease compared to the general population.[2] Twin studies have revealed a high concordance rate in monozygotic twins (40%), indicating a genetic element in disease susceptibility.[64] Interesting, dizygotic twins have a 10-fold increased risk for EoE compared with nontwin siblings, suggesting a key role for early life exposures.[64] Indeed, multiple studies have substantiated prenatal and perinatal exposures (such as antibiotic usage and cesarean section delivery) as risk factors.[65–68] These findings support the role an interaction between early life microbiome established commensal flora and genetic variants. Interestingly, the esophagus expresses a unique microbiome, which includes anti-inflammatory species such as *Lactobacillus* underhealth homeostatic conditions, and a dysbiosis occurs in patients with EoE.[69] *Streptococcus* and *Gemella* were found to be associated with active EoE compared to controls.[70] Experiments with germ-free mice and mice treated with antibiotics demonstrate elevated IgE and esophageal eosinophil responses under these conditions.[69]

Clinical Features and Diagnosis

Predominant clinical features depend on the age of the patient. Infants present with feeding difficulties and failure to thrive; school-age children present with difficulty eating, vomiting, and chest and/or abdominal pain; and adolescents present with dysphagia and food impaction.[71,72] Adults present with dysphagia as the most common symptom, chest pain/abdominal pain, and food impaction, the latter requiring endoscopic bolus removal in about 40% of adults.[73,74] These complaints are different than GERD (Table 30.1).

The normal esophagus is devoid of eosinophils (Table 30.1).[40,50] Diagnosis of EoE requires (1) exclusion of secondary causes of esophageal eosinophilia as previously mentioned and (2) consideration of clinical and pathologic information. New consensus criteria published in 2018 define EoE as symptoms of esophageal dysfunction and at least 15 eosinophils per high-power field (HPF) on esophageal biopsy after exclusion of non-EoE disorders that may account for esophageal eosinophilia.[75] Previously, a proton pump inhibitor (PPI) trial showing persistent eosinophilia was required before diagnosis, but due to substantial evidence showing eosinophil reduction with PPIs[76] and several potential underlying anti-inflammatory mechanisms of PPIs, including activation of the aryl hydrocarbon receptor,[77–80] PPI responsiveness is now no longer a requirement in EoE diagnosis.

Endoscopic features of the disease include trachealization, transient esophageal rings, exudates, furrows, edema, esophageal narrowing, and mucosal fragility, which gives the esophagus a crepe paper appearance (Fig. 30.1). The endoscopic reference score is a validated scoring system for endoscopy in EoE.[81]

EoE histology shows ≥15 esophageal eosinophils/HPF, basal zone hyperplasia, dilated intracellular spaces, lamina propria fibrosis, eosinophil abscesses, surface epithelial alterations, and dyskeratotic epithelial cells; these are quantified and validated in the EoE histology scoring system[82] (Fig. 30.2).

Treatment

Dietary Therapy

Food elimination reduces esophageal eosinophilia in patients with EoE.[4,83] Elemental diet, which consists of an amino acid–based formula without any potential allergens, has the best response rate around 88%,[43] but a solely liquid formula is hard to tolerate, especially for adult patients. Patients on elemental diet may

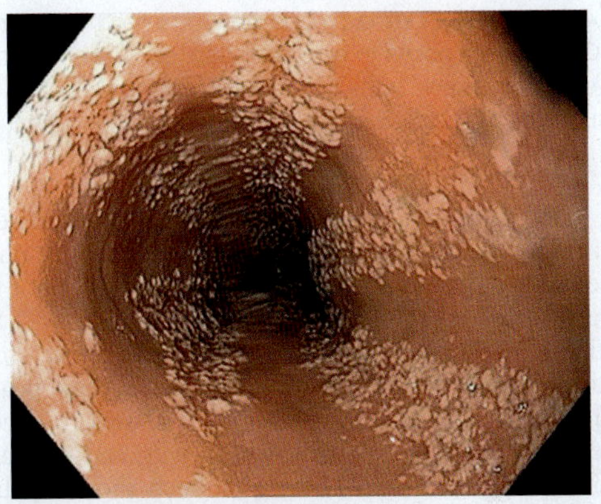

Fig. 30.1 Endoscopic view of eosinophilic esophagitis, with furrowing and exudates.

TABLE 30.1 Comparison of Eosinophilic Esophagitis (EoE) and Gastroesophageal Reflux Disease (GERD)

Characteristic Features	EoE	GERD
Clinical		
Prevalence	~1:1000	~1:10
Prevalence of atopy	Very high	Normal
Prevalence of food sensitization	Very high	Normal
Gender preference	Male	None
Abdominal pain and vomiting	Common	Common
Food impaction	Common	Uncommon
Investigative findings		
pH probe/impedance study	Normal	Abnormal
Endoscopic furrowing	Very common	Occasional
Histopathology/pathogenesis		
Involvement of proximal esophagus	Yes	No
Involvement of distal esophagus	Yes	Yes
Epithelial hyperplasia	Severely increased	Increased
Eosinophil levels in mucosa	>15/HPF	0–7/HPF
Elevated eotaxin-3 level	Yes	No
Treatment		
H_2 antihistamines	Not helpful	Helpful
Proton pump inhibitors	Sometimes helpful (but eosinophil levels remain >15/HPF)	Helpful
Glucocorticoids	Helpful	Not helpful
Specific food antigen elimination	Sometimes helpful	Not helpful
Elemental diet	Helpful	Not helpful

Modified from Rothenberg ME. Eosinophilic gastrointestinal disorders (EGID). *J Allergy Clin Immunol* 2004;113:11–18, with permission from the American Academy of Allergy, Asthma, and Immunology.

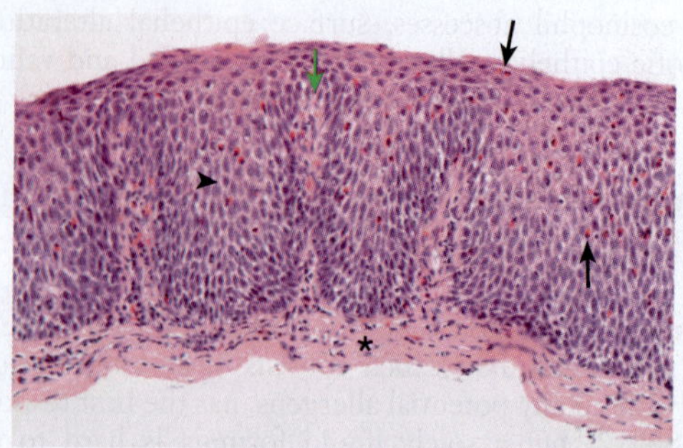

Fig. 30.2 Hematoxylin and eosin staining of the esophagus from a patient with eosinophilic esophagitis. *Arrows* point to eosinophils, including at the surface. *Arrowhead* points to dilated intercellular spaces. *Asterisk* marks lamina propria showing inflammation and fibrosis. *Green arrow* points to elongated papillae. There is also marked basal layer hyperplasia with the basal layer reaching almost to the luminal surface.

require placement of a gastrostomy tube for adequate caloric support. Allergy testing has also been used to identify potentially causative foods to be eliminated, but this method was not found to be more effective than empiric food elimination.[84,85] Six-food elimination diet consists of avoidance of the most commonly allergenic foods, including cow milk, soy, wheat, egg, peanut/tree nut, and seafood/shellfish, which has been shown to have a high response rate.[43] Four-food (milk, wheat, egg, and soy) and one-food elimination diets (milk) have also been shown to be effective. A recently conducted randomized multisite study comparing one-food elimination (milk) to six-food elimination diets in adults revealed that both were equally effective, yet only about 35% of patients responded.[44] Based on these findings, it is reasonable to start EoE patients on a milk-elimination diet as an initial approach.

Proton Pump Inhibitors

The diagnostic criteria of EoE used to require a trial of adequate treatment with PPI therapy prior to finding ≥15 eosinophils/high power field (HPF) for diagnosis to rule out PPI-responsive esophageal eosinophilia (PPI-REE).[86] However, several papers have shown that there is no clinical, histologic, or endoscopic difference between EoE and PPI-REE.[87–89] There is also significant overlap in the transcriptome signatures of EoE and PPI-REE.[90,91] So, more recent consensus guidelines have classified PPIs as a treatment option for EoE instead of part of the diagnostic criteria.[75] There are several mechanisms by which PPIs reduce esophageal eosinophilia in EoE, one of which is partially through the aryl hydrocarbon receptor signaling pathway[77] and through inhibition of eotaxin production.[79,80]

Swallowed Glucocorticoids

Swallowed topical glucocorticoids are another mainstay of treatment to provide long-term control. Off-label use of asthma inhalers containing fluticasone or budesonide using a puff and swallow technique or a budesonide slurry made from a mixture of budesonide and sucralose is commonly used.[92,93] Swallowed topical fluticasone has been shown to induce disease remission, including a reduction in inflammatory cells (eosinophils, mast cells, CD8 T cells) and degree of epithelial hyperplasia in children.[94] Budesonide oral suspension improves symptomatic, endoscopic, and histologic parameters.[95] In Europe, an orodispersable budesonide tablet[96,97] is available for treatment of EoE. Swallowed steroids have much fewer side effects compared to systemic steroids because they undergo first-pass metabolism in the liver after GI absorption.[98] However, patients can develop esophageal candidiasis as a side effect.

Biologics

Early murine work showed that IL-13 could induce EoE-like changes in the esophagus,[58] and an anti-human IL-13 mAb (QAX576) reversed EoE-like changes.[99] In a proof of principal clinical trial, adults treated with QAX576 had decreased esophageal eosinophilia and a trend for improved symptoms.[100] In subsequent clinical trials, dupilumab, an anti-IL-4Rα blocker that acts on the IL-4 and IL-13 receptors, resulted in decreased esophageal eosinophils, symptom improvement, endoscopic improvement, and biomarker improvement.[101–103] In 2022 dupilumab became the first FDA-approved medication for EoE. Another biologic targeting IL-13 (cendakimab) is in an advanced stage of development.[104]

Other biologics that have undergone clinical trials include omalizumab, an anti-IgE antibody, and those that deplete eosinophils, including mepolizumab, reslizumab, and benralizumab. Unfortunately, early clinical trials for these were unsuccessful.[19,105,106] There are ongoing clinical trials for etrasimod, an S1P receptor modulator, lirentelimab, an anti-Siglec-8 biologic that targets eosinophils and mast cells, and CALY-002, which targets IL-15.[104]

Surgical Intervention

In patients with dysphagia and/or food impaction from esophageal strictures or narrow-caliber esophagus, esophageal dilation can provide relief of dysphagia.[107] This can be achieved by through-the-scope and bougie dilators. Although risk of perforation is low, a more conservative approach in dilation technique is advised for patients with EoE,[108] especially if the dilation is performed gradually in multiple sessions for a lumen of 16–18 mm.[107]

Esophageal intramural tears are identified endoscopically as deep lacerations into esophageal submucosa or radiographically by contrast within the esophageal wall but outside the esophageal lumen. A partial rupture consists of air or contrast extravasation into the mediastinum and is managed conservatively. A full-thickness tear permits esophageal and/or gastric contents to enter the chest cavity and requires surgical intervention.

Prognosis

Similar to other allergic diseases, EoE requires prolonged treatment, with the vast majority of patients having ongoing symptoms.[109] Complications of EoE include narrow-caliber esophagus, food impaction, esophageal strictures/rings, and perforation. Food impaction prevalence ranges from 30% to 55%.[110,111] The prevalence of strictures ranges from 11% to 31%.[108,112–114] Untreated EoE has been associated with progressive fibrostenosis in several studies, substantiating the need for therapy.[115]

EOSINOPHILIC GASTRITIS/EOSINOPHILIC ENTERITIS

Due to considerable variability in the nomenclature of EGIDs, international consensus recommendations were published in 2022 to standardize the terms. EoG is the standardized term for EoG, and EoN is used to refer to small bowel involvement. Most of the data for EoN comes from EoD.

In contrast to the esophagus, the rest of the GI tract contains baseline levels of eosinophils in healthy people, which makes diagnosis of EoG, EoN, and EoC more complex (Table 30.2). Primary subtypes include atopic, nonatopic, and familial variants. Secondary subtypes are divided into systemic eosinophilic disorders, like HES, and noneosinophilic disorders.

TABLE 30.2 Gastrointestinal Eosinophils (Cells Per High Power Field) in Normal Pediatric Endoscopy Biopsies

	Lamina Propria		Villous Lamina Propria		Surface Epithelium		Crypt/Glandular Epithelium	
Gastrointestinal Segment	**Mean ± SD**	**Max**	**Mean ± SD**	**Max**	**Mean ± SD**	**Max**	**Mean ± SD**	**Max**
Esophagus	N/A	N/A	N/A	N/A	0.03 ± 0.10	1	N/A	N/A
Stomach (antrum)	1.9 ± 1.3	8	N/A	N/A	0	0	0.02 ± 0.04	1
Stomach (fundus)	2.1 ± 2.4	11	N/A	N/A	0	0	0.008 ± 0.03	1
Duodenum	9.6 ± 5.3	26	2.1 ± 1.4	9	0.06 ± 0.09	2	0.26 ± 0.36	6
Ileum	12.4 ± 5.4	28	4.8 ± 2.8	15	0.47 ± 0.25	4	0.80 ± 0.51	4
Ascending colon	20.3 ± 8.2	50	N/A	N/A	0.29 ± 0.25	3	1.4 ± 1.2	11
Transverse colon	16.3 ± 5.6	42	N/A	N/A	0.22 ± 0.39	4	0.77 ± 0.61	4
Rectum	8.3 ± 5.9	32	N/A	N/A	0.15 ± 0.13	2	1.2 ± 1.1	9

Max, Maximum; *N/A*, not applicable; *SD*, standard deviation of the mean.
From Straumann A, Bauer M, Fischer B, Blaser K, Simon HU. Idiopathic eosinophilic esophagitis is associated with a TH2-type allergic inflammatory response. *J Allergy Clin Immunol*. 2001;108(6):954–961.

The primary subtypes include the atopic, nonatopic, and familial variants, and the secondary subtype is divided into two groups, one composed of systemic eosinophilic disorders (HES) and the other of noneosinophilic disorders (see Box 30.1). Primary EoG and EoN have also been called idiopathic or allergic gastroenteropathy or previously primary eosinophilic gastroenteritis, which has been redefined and only be used to indicate gastric and small bowel involvement.[41] The familial forms of EoG and EoN have not been well characterized but are seen in about 10% of the authors' own patients (unpublished findings).[1] Of note, any layer of the GI tract can be involved in EoG and EoN; thus endoscopic biopsy can be normal in patients with the muscularis and/or serosal subtypes rather than the mucosal subtype.

Etiology

Eosinophilic Gastritis

EoG is characterized by stomach eosinophilia. Early transcriptome analysis of EoG showed that proliferating cells, mast cells, and T cells were increased.[116] Transcripts of Th2 cytokines, including IL-4, IL-5, IL-13, IL-17, and CCL-26, and mast cell transcripts were also increased, and IL-33 transcripts were decreased.[116] Recent transcriptome analysis of EoG shows 18 differentially expressed genes in patients with EoG versus control subjects, especially genes involved in type 2 immune pathways, including increased TSLP in blood.[117] Eight of the differentially expressed genes in EoG were upregulated, comprising *CCL26*, *CCL18*, *IL13RA2*, *IL5*, *CLC*, *CDH26*, *KLK7*, and *MUC4*. The other 10 differentially expressed genes in EoG were downregulated, comprising *DEFB1*, *BMP3*, *COL2A1*, *SLC26A7*, *GABRA1*, *GLDN*, *NPY*, *TACI*, *ATP4A*, and *SST*.

In a murine model, enteric-coated allergen beads induced EGID of the esophagus, stomach, and intestine[118] and caused gastromegaly, delayed food transit, and weight loss, which were eotaxin 1 dependent.[119] Mast cells are increased in EGIDs, and a murine model of oral allergen–induced diarrhea showed a critical role of IL-9.[120,121] T cells are also involved, as patients with EGID with gastric and/or enteric involvement have T cells with increased secretion of IL-4 and IL-5.[122] When stimulated with milk proteins, lamina propria T cells from the duodenum of patients with EGID preferentially secrete Th2 cytokines, including IL-13.[123] Furthermore, there are increased $CD3^+CD4^+FOXP3^+$ T regulatory cells and $CD3^+CD4^+GATA3^+$ Th2 cells in EoG that correlate with eosinophil levels, endoscopic, and histologic features.[124] The Th2 cells were also found to produce increased levels of IL-4, IL-5, and IL-13.[124]

Eosinophilic Enteritis

Recent transcriptome and histologic analysis found 382 differentially expressed genes between the EoD transcriptome and control patients, including those with celiac disease.[125] Transcripts for eosinophils, mast cells, and myeloid and granulocyte progenitors were increased. Upregulated functional processes include IL-4 and 13 signaling and extracellular matrix organization. Downregulated functional processes include metabolic process and transporter activity. The genes with the largest fold change in EoD compared to controls include upregulated ones (*DUOX2*, *CCL26*, *CLC*, *CCL18*, *DUOXA2*, *ANKRD30B*, *POSTN*, *ITLN1*, *TNXB*, *ADGRG3*, *LCN2*, *CTSG*, and *F13A1*) and downregulated ones (*SLC1A7*, *MS4A18*, *PLA2G4C*, *BEST4*, and *BTNL8*).

EGIDs and dietary protein–induced enterocolitis/enteropathy/colitis may represent a continuum of EGID with similar mechanisms. Additionally, EGIDs can be associated with protein-losing enteropathy.[126]

Clinical Features and Diagnosis

Eosinophilic Gastritis

Current estimates of EoG are approximately 6 cases per 100,000 people,[42,127] although higher prevalence may exist in Japan.[52] Patients with EoG have a higher prevalence of asthma, food allergy, and food anaphylaxis.[116] Blood eosinophilia is also significantly higher in patients with EoG.[116] Differential diagnosis for gastric eosinophilia includes parasitic infections, bacterial infections like *Helicobacter pylori*, inflammatory bowel syndrome, HES, myeloproliferative disorders, vasculitis, and drug injury/hypersensitivity.

Symptoms can include nausea, vomiting, early satiety, abdominal bloating, abdominal pain, and diarrhea.

There are eosinophils in the stomach and small intestine at baseline in healthy individuals. Unlike EoE, EoG diagnosis criteria lack consensus and include ≥30 gastric eosinophils/HPF in ≥5 HPF and ≥70 gastric eosinophils/HPF in ≥3 HPF.[128,129] In a transcriptomic analysis of EoG, where a cutoff of ≥30 eosinophils in ≥5 HPF was used, the 10 genes that correlated most highly with tissue eosinophils were *CCL26*, *CLC*, *IL13RA2*, *BMP3*, *IL5*, *CDH26*, *CCL18*, *NPY*, *HPGDS*, and *SST*.

Endoscopic features include gastric mucosal nodularity.[116] Endoscopic severity in EoD was associated with *CCL26*, *GLDN*, *IL13RA2*, *SST*, *DEFB1*, *GABRA1*, *IL5*, *TAC1*, *CLC*, and *IL13*, and most associated with gastric granularity and nodularity.[117]

Common histologic features include eosinophil sheets in expanded lamina propria, eosinophilia in epithelium, eosinophil abscesses, and eosinophils in submucosa and muscularis mucosa.[130] Genes that tracked most closely with histologic severity include *CCL26*, *IL13RA2*, *CLC*, *SST*, *BMP3*, *IL5*, *CDH26*, *GLDN*, *ANXA1*, and *DEFB1* and were most strongly associated with periglandular circumferential collars.[117]

Eosinophilic Enteritis

Estimates of EoN are approximately 5 cases per 100,000 people,[131] although higher prevalence may exist in Japan.[52] For EoD, proposed thresholds include ≥30 eosinophils/HPF in 3 HPF[21] and ≥52 eosinophils in 1 HPF,[132] which is twice the upper limit of normal duodenal eosinophils.[133] A transcriptomic analysis of duodenal eosinophilia showed that the criteria of ≥52 eosinophils in 1 HPF (vs. 30 eosinophils in 1 HPF) provides a better separation of EoD from controls by principal component analysis.[125]

Generally, EoG and EoN present with symptoms related to the degree of inflammation and area(s) affected. However, even those with a single area affected can have a range of symptoms. Symptoms can include nausea, vomiting, early satiety, abdominal bloating, abdominal pain, and diarrhea.

Six histologic features significantly associated with EoD compared to controls are as follows, including the 10 most significantly associated genes with each: lamina propria eosinophil sheets (*UTS2*, *ANKRD30B*, *VSTM1*, *CCL26*, *ITLN1*, *TNC*, *CPA3*, *ADGRG3*, *ACTC1*, and *MUC12*), pericryptal circumferential eosinophil collars (*VSTM1*, *NME8*, *AC011511.4*, *DDIAS*, *TNC*, *FAM189A1*, *ADGRG3*, *WARS2*, *CLC*, and *ELN*), eosinophilic cryptitis (*TMEM229A*, *UTS2*, *CCL26*, *TREML2*, *EFNA1*, *PCK1*, *CYP3A4*, *MS4A8*, *HTR4*, and *SLC2A2*), eosinophils in surface epithelium (*CLEC1A*, *BMX*, *SLC6A16*, *GPR42*, *NBPF10*, *DDIAS*, *WDR72*, *FCGR2B*, *LGR6*, and *GAPT*), reactive epithelial changes (*KCNK10*, *HACL1*, *TNC*, *BEST4*, *WDR72*, *TMEM229A*, *ITLN1*, *SCN3B*, *TMEM132E*, and *CPA3*), and eosinophils in muscularis (*ITLN1*, *C1QTNF1*, *MS4A18*, *C11orf53*, *C15orf48*, *THRB*, *DUOX2*, *ANKRD30B*, *PMP22*, and *TMEM52*).[125]

Endoscopic findings of EoD include normal appearance, erythema, erosion, and granularity.[125]

Treatment

Dietary Therapy

Similar to EoE, empiric food elimination diet or an elemental diet can be trialed for 4–6 weeks for EoG and/or EoN. After disease remission is obtained, specific food groups are slowly reintroduced at ~3-week intervals for each food group, and endoscopy can be performed every 3 months for disease remission or relapse. Cromoglycate, montelukast, ketotifen, mycophenolate mofetil, and alternative medicines have been studied[1,134] without widespread success in the authors' experience.

Glucocorticoids

In addition to dietary modification, systemic and topical glucocorticoids are mainstays of therapy. For systemic glucocorticoids, 2–6 weeks of therapy with relatively low dosing seem to work better than a 1-week burst of high-dose glucocorticoids. In terms of topical glucocorticoids, there are formulations made to deliver to specific segments of the GI tract, such as Entocort EC, which is designed to deliver the drug to the ileum and proximal colon. In severe refractory cases, total parenteral nutrition and immunosuppressive/antimetabolite therapy with azathioprine or 6-mercaptopurine have been used. PPIs may also improve symptoms, even if GERD is not present.

Biologics

A single center open label clinical trial of omalizumab (anti-IgE mAb) in patients with EoG and/or EoD resulted in significantly decreased blood eosinophil counts, a trend toward decreased tissue eosinophil counts, and improvement in symptom scores.[135] A Phase 2 trial of lirentelimab (anti-Siglec 8 mAb, which depletes eosinophils and inactivates mast cells) in EoG and EoN significantly depleted eosinophils and reduced symptoms.[21] Unfortunately, although the Phase 3 trial of lirentelimab met the primary endpoint of decreased eosinophils, it did not meet the coprimary endpoint on symptom improvement (unpublished).

Prognosis

The natural history of these diseases is not well documented but appears to wax and wane chronically. Patients with EoG in particular have abnormally high levels of circulating eosinophils. Given that eosinophilia may be a systemic manifestation, routine surveillance of the cardiopulmonary system for eosinophils is recommended. If the disease presents in infancy, there is a high likelihood of remission by late childhood.

EOSINOPHILIC COLITIS

Etiology

The immunologic mechanisms underlying EoC are not well understood. There are some suggestions that it is a T cell–mediated process,[136] with a murine model of oral antigen–induced diarrhea showing disease transfer by STAT6-dependent mechanisms.[27] Compared with the transcriptomes of other EGIDs, the EoC transcriptome contains a lower type 2 signature with evidence of increased apoptosis and decreased cell proliferation.[137] The EoC transcriptome also shows minimal overlap with Crohn's disease, substantiating a unique disease mechanism.[137] Additionally, eotaxin-1 was more highly regulated compared to eotaxin 2 and 3.[137]

Clinical Features and Diagnosis

EoC affects approximately 2 per 100,000 people.[127,138,139] However, the diagnosis is often confounded by other causes of colonic eosinophilia. The differential diagnoses for colonic eosinophils include parasitic infection, drug reaction, vasculitis, IBD, dietary protein–induced proctocolitis of infancy, and EoC.[140–143] In fact, one retrospective study found that definitive EoC only accounted for 2% of patients who had an ICD code for EoC, and that the colonic eosinophilia was actually due to other causes, including inflammatory bowel disease, unknown causes, dysmotility, and other EGIDs.[139] In another, only 7% of pediatric cases and 55% of adult cases that had an ICD code for EoC met clinical and histopathologic criteria for EoC; the top final diagnoses at two pediatric hospitals include FPIES and allergic colitis of infancy.[144]

There is a bimodal age distribution at around 60 days[145] and at adolescence/early adulthood.[1] In infancy, symptoms can include bloody diarrhea and anemia from blood loss in an otherwise healthy infant. In older patients, symptoms can include diarrhea, abdominal pain, weight loss, fatigue, and anorexia.

Eosinophils are present in normal colon at different ranges in distinct segments so various cutoff values may be used, but there is presently no consensus criteria of eosinophils for diagnosis of EoC.[130] Cutoffs in one study were ≥100 eosinophils/HPF in

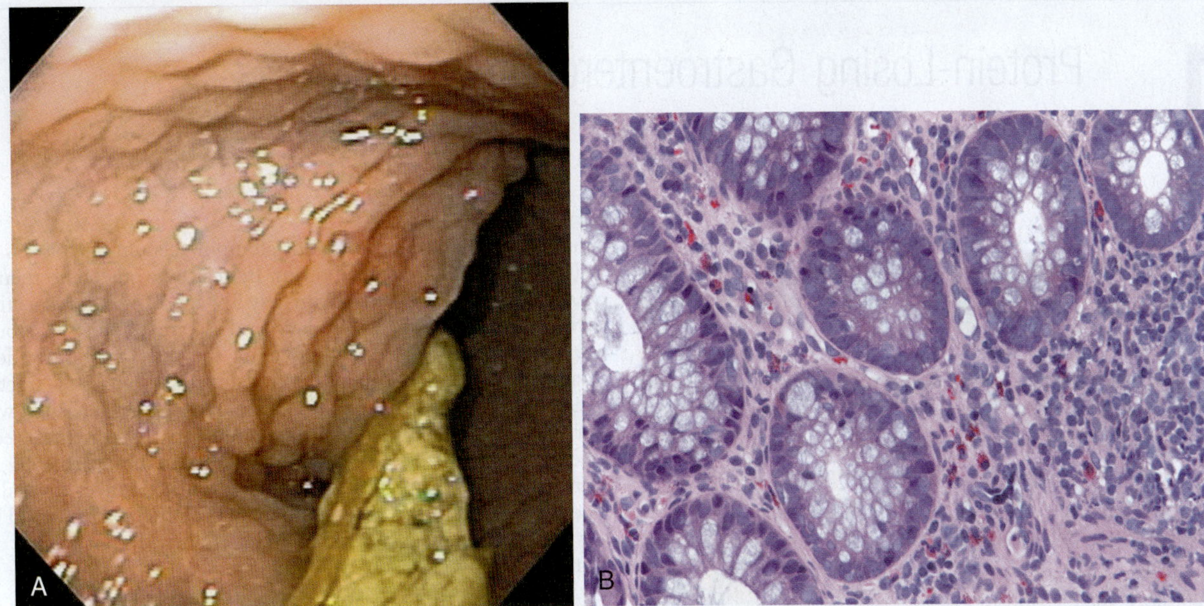

Fig. 30.3 *(A)* Eosinophilic proctitis. This is an endoscopic image of the rectum in an infant presenting with guaiac positive stools and anemia. Mucosal nodularity with central umbilication characteristic of nodular lymphoid hyperplasia is evident, findings often associated with food allergies. (B) Photomicrograph of a rectal mucosal biopsy shows increased numbers of eosinophils in the lamina propria that are forming aggregates and, occasionally, encroaching on the epithelium and crypts (hematoxylin and eosin, ×40). (Courtesy Dr. Robert Garola, Department of Pathology, Wilmington, Delaware.)

ascending colon, ≥85 eosinophils/HPF in descending colon, and/or ≥65 eosinophils/HPF in sigmoid colon.[137]

Endoscopy shows patchy edema, erythema, loss of vascularity, patchy granularity,[146] and lymphonodular hyperplasia[136] (Fig. 30.3).

Histologic abnormalities include increased eosinophils in the epithelium, eosinophil cryptitis, crypt architectural abnormalities, and eosinophilia in submucosa and muscularis mucosa.[130] The EoC transcriptome closely correlates with histologic features, including eosinophilic inflammation, pericryptal circumferential eosinophil collars, and lamina propria eosinophil sheets.[137]

Treatment

EoC in infancy is thought to be generally a benign disease, with improvement of bloody diarrhea within days of withdrawal of the offending dietary trigger.[38,147] In older patients, although there are no clinical trials, anti-inflammatory drugs and systemic and topical glucocorticoids have been used. In steroid-refractory cases, total parenteral nutrition and/or oral immunosuppressives, including azathioprine or 6-mercaptopurine, have been used.

Prognosis

EoC in infancy has a good prognosis, and the majority of patients are able to tolerate culprit foods by 1–3 years of age. The prognosis for older patients is not well documented and is considered a chronic waxing and waning disorder. Routine surveillance for additional eosinophilic involvement in the body for HESs or other EGIDs is recommended.

FUTURE DIRECTIONS

There has been significant progress made in the field of EGIDs in the past three decades, including the FDA approval of dupilumab for EoE, but much work remains to be done. The natural history of non-EoE EGIDs still needs to be further characterized. It is crucial that clinically meaningful endpoints are used through development of consensus clinical trial endpoint assessment criteria. Furthermore, a curriculum for understanding EGIDs targeted toward clinicians and other health professionals needs to be developed so that patients can be promptly recognized and treated. The efforts of the Consortium of Eosinophilic Gastrointestinal Diseases will undoubtedly continue to help with disease elucidation, treatment, as well as advocacy and education.[148,149]

As shown by variable molecular signatures in different EGIDs, different mechanisms are likely driving pathology in different segments of the GI tract. Elucidating these mechanisms will allow more opportunities for biologics to be investigated as potential treatments. Additionally, there may be different phenotypes/endotypes of these diseases that may respond better to certain biologics. Collaborations among patients, advocates, researchers, clinicians, regulatory agencies, and industry are necessary for additional FDA-approved medications for EGIDs through clinical trials of potential drug targets.[150]

Full references for this chapter can be found at https://ebooks.health.elsevier.com.

31 Protein-Losing Gastroenteropathy

Amanda K. Cartee

IN THIS CHAPTER

DEFINITION AND NORMAL PHYSIOLOGY

Protein-losing gastroenteropathy describes a diverse group of disorders associated with excessive loss of serum proteins into the GI tract.[1–16] This excess serum protein loss can result in hypoproteinemia and may present as edema, ascites, and malnutrition. Box 31.1 lists disorders associated with protein-losing gastroenteropathy.[17–76]

In 1947 Maimon et al. postulated that fluid emanating from the large gastric folds in patients with Ménétrier disease was rich in protein. In 1949 Albright and Forbes discovered, using IV infusions of albumin, that hypoproteinemia resulted from excessive catabolism of albumin rather than decreased albumin synthesis.[1] By 1956, Kimbel et al. demonstrated an increase in gastric albumin production in patients with chronic gastritis. A year later, Citrin et al. were able to show that the GI tract was the actual site of excess protein loss in patients with Ménétrier disease.[2] They demonstrated that the excess loss of IV-administered radioiodinated albumin could be explained by the appearance of labeled protein in the gastric secretions of such patients.

Subsequent research using radiolabeled polyvinylpyrrolidone, albumin, and other proteins, as well as immunologic methods measuring enteric loss of α_1-antitrypsin (α_1-AT), has further characterized the role of the GI tract in the metabolism of serum proteins. In fact, GI tract loss of albumin normally accounts for only 2%–5% of the total body degradation of albumin, but in patients with severe protein-losing GI disorders, this enteric protein loss may extend to up to 60% of the total albumin pool.[3–6]

Under physiologic conditions, most endogenous proteins found in the lumen of the GI tract are derived from sloughed enterocytes and pancreatic and biliary secretions.[7,8] Studies of serum protein loss into the GI tract measured by various methods (e.g., ^{67}Cu-ceruloplasmin, ^{51}Cr-albumin, and α_1-AT clearance) have shown that daily enteric loss of serum proteins accounts for less than 1%–2% of the serum protein pool in healthy individuals, with enteric loss of albumin accounting for less than 10% of total albumin catabolism. In healthy women and men, the total albumin pool is approximately 3.9 and 4.7 g/kg, respectively, with a half-life of 15–33 days and a rate of hepatic albumin synthesis of 0.15 g/kg/day, equaling the rate of albumin degradation.[9,10] Excess proteins that enter the upper GI tract are metabolized by existing proteases similar to other peptides, which are broken down into constituent amino acids and reabsorbed. In healthy individuals, GI losses play only a minor role in total protein metabolism, and serum protein levels reflect the balance between protein synthesis and total protein metabolism. However, this balance can be markedly altered in patients with protein-losing gastroenteropathy.[5,11]

PATHOPHYSIOLOGY

Excessive plasma protein loss across the GI epithelium can result from several pathologic mucosal processes. First, mucosal injury can result in increased permeability to plasma proteins. Mucosal erosions and ulcerations can result in weeping of an inflammatory, protein-rich exudate. Second, lymphatic obstruction or increased lymphatic hydrostatic pressure can result in direct leakage of lymph, which contains plasma proteins. Lastly, changes in vascular permeability can affect the concentration of serum proteins in the interstitial fluid, which influences the amount of enteric mucosal protein loss.[12,16]

Bode et al. have suggested that protein-losing gastroenteropathy may be related to loss of heparan sulfate proteins found on the surface of intestinal epithelial cells.[11,13,14] Heparan sulfate proteoglycans affect the integrity of the intestinal barrier through their large extracellular domains that bind to the plasma membrane, known as *syndecans*, or are attached to a membrane glycolipid called a *glypican*.[15] Syndecans help maintain tight intercellular junctions.

Mice that were genetically altered to lack syndecans or other heparan sulfate proteins have alterations to the normal tight intercellular barrier and leak protein via paracellular pathways into the intestinal lumen (Fig. 31.1). Moreover, the treatment of such mice with proinflammatory cytokines, such as TNF-α or interferon-γ, leads to significant intercellular junction defects and greater protein loss into the intestine.[13] The combination of a syndecan-deficient state and exposure to proinflammatory cytokines leads to even greater albumin flux and protein loss. Finally, the reintroduction of heparan sulfate or other syndecans abolishes the protein loss into the lumen of the bowel.[13]

The loss of serum proteins in patients with protein-losing gastroenteropathy is independent of their molecular weight, and therefore the fraction of the intravascular pool degraded daily remains the same for various proteins, including albumin, immunoglobulin (IgG, IgA, and IgM), and ceruloplasmin.[5,11,16] In contrast, patients with nephrotic syndrome selectively lose lower molecular weight proteins such as albumin. As proteins enter the GI tract, the synthesis of new proteins occurs in a compensatory fashion. Proteins that enter the GI tract are metabolized into constituent amino acids by gastric, pancreatic, and small intestinal enzymes, reabsorbed by specific transporters, and recirculated. When the rate of gastric or enteric protein loss, or both, exceeds

BOX 31.1 Disorders Associated With Protein-Losing Gastroenteropathy

DISEASES WITHOUT MUCOSAL EROSIONS OR ULCERATIONS

AIDS-associated gastroenteropathy[17]
Acute viral gastroenteritis[18]
Allergic gastroenteropathy[19]
Celiac disease[20]
Cobalamin deficiency[21]
Collagenous colitis[22]
Cytomegalovirus infection[23]
Eosinophilic gastroenteritis[24]
Giant hypertrophic gastropathy (Ménétrier disease)[25,26]
Giardiasis, schistosomiasis, nematodiasis (capillariasis), strongyloidiasis
Graft-versus-host disease
Helicobacter pylori gastritis
Henoch–Schönlein purpura[27]
Hypertrophic hypersecretory gastropathy
Intestinal parasitosis[28–30]
Lymphocytic colitis[22]
Lymphocytic gastritis
Mixed connective tissue disease[31]
Paracoccidiomycosis
Postmeasles diarrhea
SIBO[32]
Sjögren syndrome[33]
Systemic lupus erythematosus (SLE)[34–40]
Tropical sprue[41]
Vascular ectasia (gastric, colonic)[42]
Whipple disease[43]

DISEASES WITH MUCOSAL EROSIONS OR ULCERATIONS

α-Chain disease[44]
Amyloidosis[45]
Behçet disease[46]
Carcinoid syndrome
Crohn's disease[47,48]
Duodenitis[49]
Erosive gastritis[49]
GI carcinomas
Graft-versus-host disease[50]
H. pylori gastritis[51–53]
Idiopathic ulcerative jejunoileitis[54]
Infectious diarrhea (e.g., *Clostridium difficile*[55] and *Shigella* spp.[56])
Ischemic colitis
Kaposi sarcoma[57]
Leukemia/lymphoma
Melanoma
Multiple myeloma
Neurofibromatosis[58]
NSAID enteropathy[59]
Sarcoidosis[60]
Toxic shock syndrome (*Streptococcus pyogenes*)
Waldenström macroglobulinemia[62]

DISEASES WITH LYMPHATIC OBSTRUCTION OR ELEVATED LYMPHATIC PRESSURE

Budd–Chiari syndrome[68]
Cardiac disease[63,64]
CD55 deficiency[69]
Constrictive pericarditis, heart failure, tricuspid regurgitation, Fontan procedure[70,71]
Crohn disease[47,48]
Intestinal endometriosis[65]
Intestinal lymphangiectasia (congenital, acquired)[66,67]
Lymphatic-enteric fistula[28]
Lymphoma, including mycosis fungoides
Mesenteric TB and sarcoidosis[60]
Mesenteric venous thrombosis[73]
Neoplastic disease involving mesenteric lymphatics
Portal hypertensive gastroenteropathy[74]
Posttransplant lymphoproliferative disease[75]
Retroperitoneal fibrosis
Sclerosing mesenteritis[76]
Superior vena cava thrombosis
SLE[35–40]
TB peritonitis
Whipple disease[43]

the body's capacity to synthesize new protein, hypoproteinemia develops.[7,8] Hypoalbuminemia is common in protein-losing gastroenteropathy and results when there is an imbalance between hepatic albumin synthesis and albumin loss. Hepatic albumin synthesis is limited and can increase only by 25%. Reductions in the total body albumin pool and albumin half-life contribute to albumin loss.[12]

Adaptive changes in endogenous protein catabolism may compensate for excessive enteric protein loss, resulting in unequal loss of specific proteins. For example, proteins, like insulin, some clotting factors, and IgE, have rapid catabolic turnover rates (short half-lives). Since rapid synthesis of these proteins ensues, these proteins are relatively unaffected by GI losses. In contrast, enhanced synthesis of albumin and most immunoglobulins (IgG, IgA, and IgM) is limited, and gastrointestinal protein loss will be manifested by hypoproteinemia (hypoalbuminemia and hypoglobulinemia).[11] Impaired hepatic protein synthesis and increased endogenous degradation of plasma proteins can also contribute to the excessive enteric protein loss seen in various diseases.

In addition to causing hypoproteinemia, protein-losing gastroenteropathy can be associated with reduced concentrations of other serum components such as lipids, iron, and trace metals.[11] Lymphatic obstruction can result in lymphopenia, which subsequently alters cellular immunity.

CLINICAL FEATURES

Hypoproteinemia and edema are the principal clinical manifestations of protein-losing gastroenteropathy. Pleural and pericardial effusions and malnutrition are also common. Most other clinical features reflect the underlying disease process, accounting for the varied clinical presentations of patients with protein-losing gastroenteropathy (Box 31.2).[17–76] Protein-losing gastroenteropathy is seen in both pediatric and adult populations.[77] Hypoproteinemia, the most common clinical sequela, is manifested by a decrease in serum levels of albumin, most immunoglobulins (IgG, IgA, and IgM, but not IgE), fibrinogen, lipoproteins, α_1-AT, transferrin, and ceruloplasmin.[11] Levels of rapid-turnover proteins, such as retinal binding protein and prealbumin, are typically preserved, despite hypoproteinemia.[78] Dependent edema results from diminished plasma oncotic pressure and is frequently a clinically significant issue. Anasarca is rare in protein-losing gastroenteropathy. Unilateral edema, upper

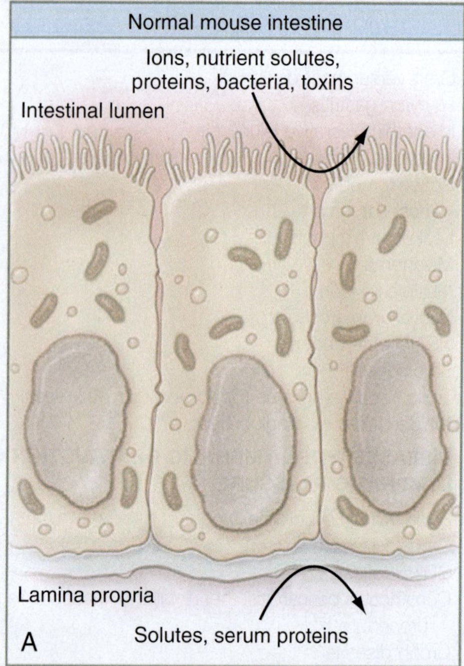

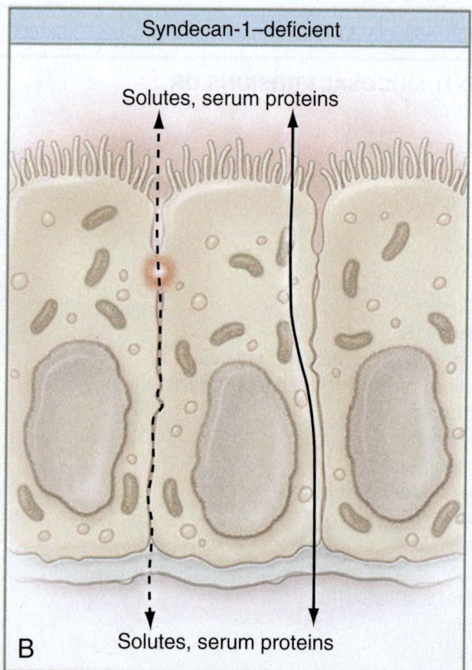

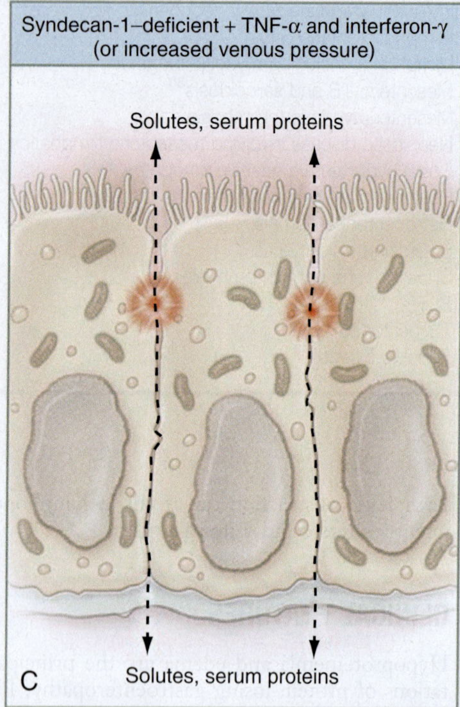

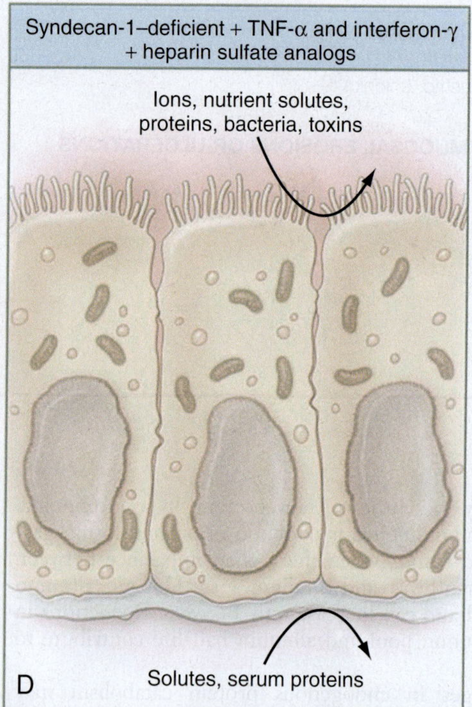

Fig. 31.1 Diagrams illustrating the factors that contribute to intestinal integrity in the mouse. (A) The normal mouse intestine is an effective barrier against the free diffusion of certain ions, nutrient solutes, proteins, bacteria, and toxins to separate the intestinal lumen (outside) from the lamina propria (inside) effectively. (B) Syndecan-1–deficient mice have decreased intestinal barrier function as a result of defective intercellular junctions and increased paracellular leaks (*dashed line*) or increased transcellular protein transport (*solid line*).[13] (C) Syndecan-1–deficient mice that were given inflammatory cytokines (TNF-α and interferon-γ) or operated on to increase their portal venous pressure have massively defective intercellular junctions and large intercellular protein leaks (*dashed lines*), consistent with protein-losing enteropathy. (D) Infusions of heparin sulfate analogs completely reverse the intestinal barrier dysfunction seen in syndecan-1–deficient mice given inflammatory cytokines. See text for more details. (From Lencer WI. Patching a leaky intestine. *N Engl J Med*. 2008;359:526–528, with permission.)

BOX 31.2 Clinical Manifestations of Protein-Losing Gastroenteropathy

SYMPTOMS AND SIGNS

Edema (dependent, upper extremity, facial, macular; unilateral in lymphangiectasia)
Diarrhea
Retinal detachment (in lymphangiectasia)[79]

LABORATORY ABNORMALITIES

Hypoproteinemia
Hypoalbuminemia
Decreased serum gamma globulins (IgG, IgA, and IgM)
Decreased serum proteins—ceruloplasmin, α_1-antitrypsin, fibrinogen, transferrin, hormone-binding proteins
Decreased serum lipoproteins
Evidence of fat malabsorption
Evidence of carbohydrate malabsorption
Evidence of fat-soluble vitamin malabsorption or deficiency
Altered cellular immunity[80]
Lymphopenia

Ig, Immunoglobulin.

extremity edema, facial edema, macular edema (with reversible blindness), and bilateral retinal detachments have been seen as a consequence of intestinal lymphangiectasia.[79] Despite the decrease in serum gamma globulin levels, increased susceptibility to infections is uncommon. Although clotting factors may be lost into the GI tract, resynthesis is rapid, and, in general, coagulation status typically remains unaffected. On the other hand, angiopathic thrombosis has been noted in certain situations, discussed below.[69] Circulating levels of proteins that bind hormones, such as cortisol-binding globulin and thyroid-binding globulin, may be substantially decreased, but levels of circulating free hormones are not significantly altered.

Most of the clinical findings in patients with protein-losing diseases are the result of the underlying disease state and are not caused by the protein loss itself. For example, small bowel disorders with protein loss as a feature (e.g., celiac disease and tropical sprue) may be associated with malabsorption and resultant diarrhea, vitamin deficiencies, and anemia. Lymphatic obstruction from lymphangiectasia may result in lymphopenia or abnormal cellular immunity.[80]

DISEASES ASSOCIATED WITH PROTEIN-LOSING GASTROENTEROPATHY

Diseases associated with protein-losing gastroenteropathy can be divided into three broad categories: (1) diseases without GI mucosal erosions or ulcerations; (2) diseases with GI mucosal erosions or ulcerations; and (3) diseases leading to elevated lymphatic and interstitial pressure (see Box 31.1). More than one of these mechanisms may contribute, as in some infectious diseases.

Diseases Without Mucosal Erosions or Ulcerations

Diseases that damage the GI epithelium without causing erosions or ulcers may lead to surface epithelial cell shedding, resulting in excess protein loss. Lesions of the small intestine that cause malabsorption are often associated with enteric leakage of plasma proteins. In addition, vascular injury can increase permeability and subsequent protein loss, which occurs in lupus vasculitis, allergic IgE-mediated type 1 hypersensitivity reactions, parasitic and viral infections, bacterial overgrowth, increased intercellular permeability, or increased capillary permeability.[28–38]

Ménétrier Disease

Giant hypertrophic gastropathy (Ménétrier disease; see Chapter 54) is the most common gastric lesion causing severe protein loss.[25,26] Patients usually have dyspepsia, nausea, emesis, edema, weight loss, and hypoproteinemia. Prominent, thick gastric folds with substantial mucus and protein-rich exudates are seen endoscopically. Mucus-secreting cells replace normal gastric glands and reduce the number of parietal cells, resulting in hypochlorhydria or achlorhydria. An increase in intercellular permeability results in protein loss. In this disorder, tight junctions between cells are wider than those found in healthy people, which is believed that proteins traverse the gastric mucosa through these widened spaces. H_2RAs, anticholinergic agents, and octreotide may be used to improve symptoms, but patients with persistent abdominal pain or severe unrelenting protein loss require subtotal or total gastrectomy.[26] As discussed in Chapter 54, there is a possible causal relationship between *Helicobacter pylori* infection and Ménétrier disease with protein-losing gastroenteropathy. *Helicobacter pylori* eradication can lead to normalization of gastric fold configuration and resolution of the hypoproteinemia.[51–53]

H. pylori Gastritis

Helicobacter pylori gastritis in the absence of Ménétrier disease (see Chapter 54) has been associated with protein-losing gastropathy and responds with *H. pylori* eradication.[51–53] Some of these patients may have gastric erosions, which also contributes to protein loss.

Allergic Gastroenteropathy

Although allergic gastroenteropathy (see Chapters 11, 30, and 54) is often considered a disease of childhood, it may be seen in adults as well. Patients with this syndrome experience abdominal pain, vomiting, and sporadic diarrhea. Findings include hypoproteinemia, iron deficiency anemia, and peripheral eosinophilia. Serum levels of total protein and albumin, as well as IgA and IgG, are markedly reduced, whereas levels of IgM and transferrin are only moderately diminished. Characteristic histology of the small bowel in patients with this disorder includes a marked increase in the number of eosinophils in the lamina propria, and Charcot–Leyden crystals may be found on stool examination.[19]

SLE

SLE is a systemic autoimmune disease not infrequently associated with protein-losing gastroenteropathy. The entity has been termed *lupus protein-losing enteropathy*, and several mechanisms contribute to the gastrointestinal protein loss (Fig. 31.2).[34–39] First, mesenteric vasculitis results in intestinal ischemia, edema, and altered intestinal vascular permeability. Second, patients with SLE can have gastritis and mucosal ulcerations that contribute to excess protein loss. Protein-losing gastroenteropathy may be the initial clinical presentation of SLE. Therapy with systemic glucocorticoids, as well as other immunomodulatory agents such as azathioprine, cyclophosphamide, and tacrolimus, can lead to remission with resolution of clinical symptoms, including protein-losing gastroenteropathy.[38–40]

Diseases With Mucosal Erosions or Ulcerations

Mucosal erosions or ulcerations resulting in protein-losing gastroenteropathy can be localized or diffuse and can be caused by

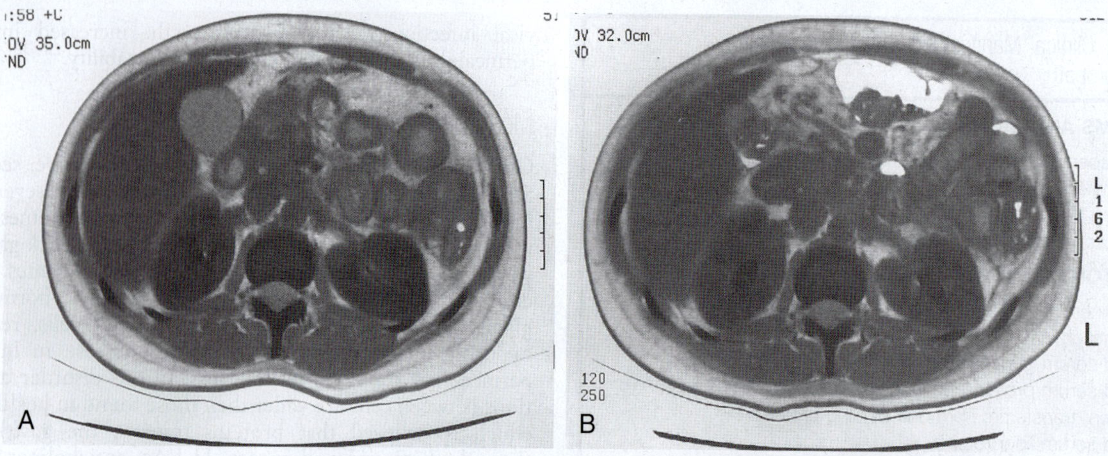

Fig. 31.2 (A) CT of the abdomen in a 29-year-old woman with severe watery diarrhea and diffuse nonradiating abdominal pain. The serum albumin level was 2.9 g/dL, and the creatinine level was 0.6 mg/dL. Stool studies were negative for pathogens. The CT shows diffuse small bowel wall thickening. The titer of antinuclear antibodies was 1:1280, and she was started on methylprednisolone. Her symptoms improved rapidly, with much less diarrhea and resolution of abdominal pain. (B) Repeat CT 5 days later showed marked improvement of the bowel wall thickening, at which time the serum albumin level was 3.4 g/dL. Renal biopsy confirmed changes consistent with lupus nephritis.

benign or malignant disease (see Box 31.1). The severity of protein loss depends on the degree of cellular loss and the associated inflammation and lymphatic obstruction. Diffuse ulcerations of the small intestine or colon, as seen with Crohn's disease, ulcerative colitis, and pseudomembranous colitides, can result in severe protein loss.[47,48,61] The hypoalbuminemia commonly seen in patients with GI tract malignancies is typically due to a decrease in albumin synthesis, but excessive enteric protein loss has also been reported. In addition, protein-losing gastroenteropathy can result from therapy for malignant disease, including chemotherapy, radiation-related injury, and bone marrow transplantation.

Diseases With Lymphatic Obstruction or Elevated Lymphatic Pressure

Lymphatic obstruction results in dilatation of intestinal lymphatic channels and can result in rupture of lacteals rich in plasma proteins, chylomicrons, and lymphocytes. When central venous pressure is elevated as in heart failure or constrictive pericarditis, bowel wall lymphatic vessels become congested, resulting in a loss of protein-rich lymph into the GI tract.[8,63,64] Tortuous, dilated mucosal and submucosal lymphatic vessels are also seen in patients with primary intestinal lymphangiectasias (Fig. 31.3). These patients often present by 30 years of age with edema, hypoproteinemia, diarrhea, and lymphopenia from both lymphatic leakage and rupture.[66,67] Patients with an autosomal dominant homozygous loss-of-function mutation in the gene encoding CD55 (decay accelerating factor) have been identified; these patients have abdominal pain, diarrhea, and protein-losing gastroenteropathy with intestinal lymphangiectasia, edema, malabsorption, recurrent infections, and angiopathic thromboembolic disease.[69] Retroperitoneal processes, such as adenopathy, fibrosis, and pancreatitis, can also impair lymphatic drainage. Budd–Chiari syndrome after liver transplantation has also been associated with protein-losing gastroenteropathy.[68]

An association between protein-losing gastroenteropathy and heart disease is seen after the Fontan procedure, a surgical correction for a congenital univentricular heart or severely hypoplastic left ventricle. The surgery creates a wide anastomosis between the right atrium and pulmonary artery, with venous blood bypassing the right ventricle. Hemodynamic studies in patients after the Fontan procedure reveal increased central venous pressures. Protein-losing gastroenteropathy occurs in up to 15% of patients in the ensuing 10 years.[8,70–72]

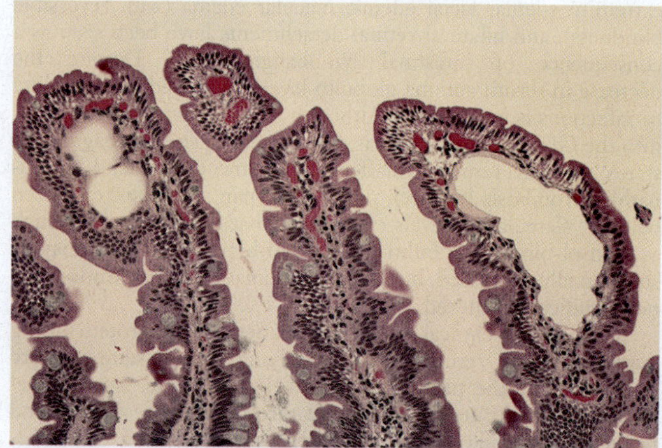

Fig. 31.3 Intestinal lymphangiectasia. This small intestinal biopsy specimen was obtained from a patient with protein-losing enteropathy. It shows focal lymphangiectasia (i.e., two villi are involved and two are spared), consistent with an acquired (secondary) lymphangiectasia. A more diffuse lymphangiectasia would favor a congenital type of lymphangiectasia. (Courtesy Dr. Edward Lee, Washington, DC.)

DIAGNOSIS

Laboratory Tests

Because hypoproteinemia and edema are seen in many other disorders, the documentation of excessive protein loss from the GI tract is important. Patients with unexplained hypoproteinemia in the absence of proteinuria, liver disease, and malnutrition should be investigated for evidence of protein-losing gastroenteropathy. The previous gold standard for diagnosing protein-losing gastroenteropathy, measurement of the fecal loss of radiolabeled IV-administered macromolecules (e.g., ^{51}Cr-albumin), has significant limitations, such as exposure to radioactive material and a 6–10-day collection period. Therefore this test is not clinically practical or widely used.[81]

α_1-AT is a useful marker of intestinal protein loss. α_1-AT is a 50-kd glycoprotein similar in size to albumin (67 kd). Like albumin, α_1-AT is synthesized in the liver and is neither actively absorbed nor secreted in the intestine; it is also resistant to luminal proteolysis. α_1-AT is normally present in the stool in low concentrations.[6,81,82] Enteric protein loss can be demonstrated by quantifying the concentration of α_1-AT in the stool or by measuring its clearance from plasma; the latter is the more reliable indicator. Therefore the optimal test is to measure the clearance of α_1-AT from the plasma during a 72-hour stool collection, with α_1-AT plasma clearance expressed in milliliters/day using this formula:

$$\alpha_1 - \text{AT plasma clearance} = ([\text{Daily stool volume}] \times [\text{Stool } \alpha 1 - \text{AT}])/\text{Serum } \alpha 1 - \text{AT}$$

Plasma clearance of α_1-AT can also be used to monitor response to therapy.

An α_1-AT clearance in excess of 24 mL/day in patients without diarrhea is abnormal. Since diarrhea alone can increase α_1-AT clearance, an α_1-AT clearance exceeding 56 mL/day in patients with diarrhea is abnormal. In addition, there is an inverse correlation between α_1-AT plasma clearance and serum albumin concentration; as serum albumin levels fall below 3 g/dL, the clearance of α_1-AT exceeds 180 mL/day. In infants, meconium can interfere with α_1-AT results and result in false positives because of the higher concentration of α_1-AT in meconium. Therefore this test should not be performed on infants suspected of having protein-losing enteropathy.[6,81–83] Intestinal bleeding also leads to false elevations of α_1-AT clearance. In patients who test positive for fecal occult blood, interpretation of α_1-AT clearance can be difficult because of increased clearance rates.[6,81–83] Finally, α_1-AT is degraded by pepsin at a gastric pH below 3 and, thus, may be falsely negative in patients with gastric protein loss. Use of a PPI to prevent peptic degradation of α_1-AT in the stomach may improve detection of protein-losing gastropathy.[83]

Nuclear medicine studies are available to aid in the diagnosis of protein-losing gastroenteropathy. These tests include technetium-99m (^{99m}Tc)-labeled human serum albumin (^{99m}Tc-HSA), ^{99m}Tc-labeled methylene diphosphonate (^{99m}Tc-MDP), ^{99m}Tc-labeled dextran scintigraphy, ^{99m}Tc-labeled human immunoglobulin, and indium-111 (^{111}In)-labeled transferrin.[84–88] Nuclear imaging may be useful to quantify protein loss, localize a site-specific area of protein loss, and diagnosis when the α_1-AT clearance results are equivocal. Of these tests, ^{99m}Tc-labeled dextran scintigraphy may be more sensitive than ^{99m}Tc-HSA.[89] However, neither test is widely available. Studies in children and adults have used ^{99m}Tc-HSA for detecting the specific site of gastric or enteric protein loss and to monitor the response to therapy. ^{99m}Tc-labeled human immunoglobulin and ^{111}In-labeled transferrin also may help quantify and localize protein loss into the GI tract.[84–88] MRI has been described as a useful tool for the diagnosis of primary protein-losing gastroenteropathy because it can characterize lesions associated with gastrointestinal protein loss, such as dilated mesenteric lymphatics in the abdomen and prominent subcutaneous lymphatics in the extremities.[90] MR enterocolonography has been reported as a useful diagnostic tool in confirming suspected protein-losing gastroenteropathy detected on scintigraphy, identifying inflamed areas of the small bowel and colon where protein loss occurs.[91] Video capsule endoscopy can identify characteristic changes suggestive of protein-losing gastroenteropathy, and biopsy samples may be obtained through deep enteroscopy.[92]

Approach to the Patient With Suspected Protein-Losing Gastroenteropathy

The diagnosis of protein-losing gastroenteropathy is based on an increase in α_1-AT clearance in the absence of confounding variables and nuclear testing such as ^{99m}Tc-HSA to confirm, localize to a specific organ, and quantitate the extent in certain patients (Fig. 31.4).[84,85] Testing to confirm protein loss from the GI tract is critical to establishing the diagnosis of protein-losing gastroenteropathy because many other diseases can present with edema and hypoproteinemia without enteric protein loss. Examples include nephrotic syndrome, cirrhosis, malignancy, eating disorders including bulimia and anorexia, malnutrition, and diuretic or laxative abuse.

Following confirmation of enteric protein loss, further evaluation is necessary to identify the underlying disease process. Initial evaluation should include a thorough history and physical examination. Blood testing typically would include a complete blood count with differential (specifically looking for eosinophilia) and red cell indices, electrolytes, calcium, magnesium, serum protein electrophoresis and immunoelectrophoresis, C-reactive protein, erythrocyte sedimentation rate, antinuclear antibody (ANA) and rheumatoid factor, coagulation studies, HIV testing, iron and iron-binding capacity, and thyroid studies. In those patients with diarrhea, a 72-hour fecal fat may be useful if not previously performed, as well as collection of stool specimens for ova and parasites, *Giardia* antigen, *Clostridium difficile* toxin, and Charcot–Leyden crystals if peripheral eosinophilia is present. A chest radiograph may reveal granulomatous disease or evidence of cardiomegaly. Electrocardiography or echocardiography may be indicated if increased venous pressure is suspected. In the presence of steatorrhea, diagnostic studies should concentrate on the upper GI tract, and radiologic and endoscopic evaluation of the small intestine, including capsule endoscopy, deep enteroscopy, and MR enterography, might be performed.[91,92]

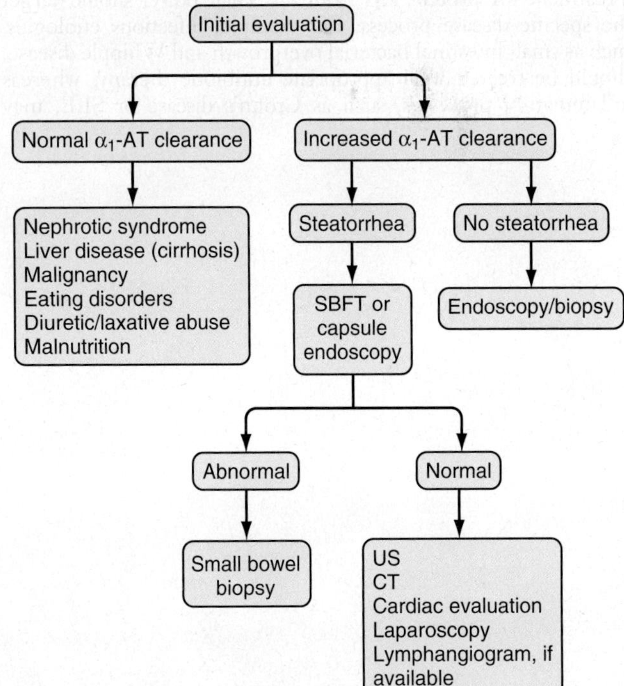

Fig. 31.4 Approach to the patient with protein-losing gastroenteropathy. Initial evaluation includes a complete history and physical examination, laboratory evaluation (see text), and determination of α_1-antitrypsin (α_1-AT) plasma clearance. *SBFT*, Small bowel follow-through.

EGD and colonoscopy may help detect mucosal inflammation, ulceration, neoplastic disease, or other luminal abnormalities. Biopsies should be obtained from any abnormal-appearing areas; random biopsies may have a role since certain conditions, such as collagenous or lymphocytic colitis, can appear endoscopically normal. Contrast studies of the small and large bowel may demonstrate ulcers and mucosal abnormalities. Disorders that might lead to lymphatic obstruction (e.g., retroperitoneal fibrosis, pancreatic diseases, and malignancies) can be evaluated by CT or MRI of the abdomen and pelvis. Video capsule endoscopy is useful in evaluating for protein-losing gastroenteropathy to identify the presence of intestinal lymphangietases.[93] Lymphangiography may be useful for select patients, but this test is rarely performed at most centers. When the diagnosis remains unclear, exploratory laparotomy or laparoscopy to exclude the possibility of occult malignancy is sometimes appropriate.

TREATMENT AND PROGNOSIS

Because protein-losing gastroenteropathy is a syndrome and not a specific disease, treatment is directed not only at correction of the underlying disease but also includes supportive care and dietary modifications. Protein loss may be offset in part by a high-protein diet, and a diet lower in fat appears to have a beneficial effect on albumin metabolism.[94] Moreover, octreotide may be useful for some patients with protein-losing gastroenteropathy to decrease fluid secretion and protein exudation from the bowel.[95] There is some suggestion in experimental mouse models that infusion of heparan analogs may restore intestinal mucosal tight junctions and prevent protein loss across the surface of the bowel; further clinical work is needed to define efficacy.[15]

For diseases affecting the stomach, such as giant hypertrophic gastropathy (Ménétrier disease), gastrectomy reverses protein loss. However, *H. pylori* infection should be excluded and treated, if present, before surgical consideration (see Chapter 54).[51,52] Treatment for protein loss from the small bowel should target the specific disease process. For example, infectious etiologies, such as small intestinal bacterial overgrowth and Whipple disease, should be treated with appropriate antibiotic therapy, whereas inflammatory processes, such as Crohn's disease or SLE, may require immunosuppressive therapy.[38,40,96,97] In the colon, protein loss from ulcerative colitis and collagenous colitis may require long-term immunomodulators or surgery, and infectious colitides require antibiotic treatment. Malignancy-induced enteric protein loss requires cancer-specific therapy. Enteric protein loss and lymphocytopenia seen in cardiac diseases (e.g., heart failure and constrictive pericarditis) can be ameliorated with medical and surgical management of the underlying cardiac condition.[8,64,97] Budesonide and high-dose spironolactone have been advocated for some patients with protein-losing gastroenteropathy after the Fontan procedure.[98,99]

Acquired intestinal lymphangiectasia should be treated by correction of the primary disease, whereas congenital intestinal lymphangiectasia can be partially controlled with dietary modifications. Enteric protein loss in patients with the latter condition can be reduced by a low-fat diet enriched with medium-chain triglycerides, which do not require lymphatic transport and, therefore, do not stimulate lymph flow.[100,101]

Supportive care can reduce the incidence of secondary symptoms. Diuretics typically are not indicated because the edema is caused by a decrease in plasma oncotic pressure. However, diuretics may reduce dependent edema from hypoalbuminemia, thereby improving comfort. Support stockings, if used appropriately, can reduce lower extremity edema in patients with lymphedema and hypoalbuminemia. Exercise and adequate ambulation should be encouraged to reduce the risk of venous thrombosis. Meticulous skin care is critical to prevent skin breakdown and cellulitis. Although these measures do not affect enteric protein loss, they can minimize secondary complications.

Most causes of the protein-losing disorders of the GI tract are easily detectable and treatable, and many can be cured. As such, the goal of therapy in protein-losing gastroenteropathy is to identify the cause and direct dietary, medical, or surgical intervention, or a combination, at the underlying disease.[5,11] With reversal or control of the primary disease, a significant proportion of patients will have a partial or complete remission of enteric protein loss, edema, and other associated conditions.

Full references for this chapter can be found at https://ebooks.health.elsevier.com.

32

32 Gastrointestinal and Hepatic Manifestations of Coronavirus Infection

Shahnaz Sultan, Jose Debes

IN THIS CHAPTER

CORONAVIRUSES

Coronaviruses are enveloped, positive-sense RNA viruses that belong to the Coronaviridae family and infect various mammalian and avian species.[1] They derive their name because of the crown-like appearance of their spike protein on the exterior surface as seen when viewed under an electronic microscope. In the past two decades, coronaviruses have been responsible for the three epidemics, namely, Severe Acute Respiratory Syndrome in 2003 (SARS-CoV), Middle Eastern Respiratory Syndrome in 2012 (MERS-CoV), and Coronavirus disease 2019, or COVID-19 (SARS-CoV-2).[2,3] The SARS-CoV-2 virus had the distinction of being the leading a cause of death by a single infectious agent, with an estimated 6 million deaths worldwide during the pandemic, replacing tuberculosis.[4]

SARS-COV

The earliest record of coronavirus infections was among animals in the late 1920s, where acute respiratory infections occurred in domesticated chickens in North America.[5] Human coronaviruses were discovered in the 1960s with several identified strains known to cause human disease.[6–9] Outbreaks of SARS-CoV-1 and MERS-CoV infections occurred in 2002 and 2012, respectively. The first case of SARS-CoV-1 was discovered in Foshan, China, in November 2002, but by July 2003, SARS-CoV had spread to over 30 countries, causing 8096 reported cases and 774 deaths with transmission of infection occurring through either direct or indirect contact.[10,11] After that, no additional infections were detected, and the SARS pandemic was declared over. The virus, SARS-CoV, was isolated from civets from a live-animal market in Guangdong, China, but bats were recognized as an important reservoir for several coronaviruses.[11–13]

MERS

MERS, transmitted through the virus MERS-CoV, was first found in 2012 in a lung sample from a 60-year-old patient who died of respiratory failure in Jeddah, Saudi Arabia.[14] This virus also belongs to the coronavirus family and is believed to be originally from bats.[15] However, the virus is typically transferred to humans from infected camels either during direct contact or indirectly through respiratory droplets. MERS has a 35% mortality rate, and since it emerged in the human population in June 2012, it has caused substantial morbidity and mortality.[15] Risk to the global population is limited since spread between humans typically requires close contact with an infected person.

SARS-COV-2

SARS-CoV-2 has many genetic similarities to these coronaviruses sharing approximately 79% of its genome sequence with SARS-CoV-1 and about 50% with MERS-CoV.[2] SARS-CoV-2 was identified as a novel coronavirus in December 2019. Like other coronaviruses, SARS-CoV-2 is an enveloped single-stranded positive-sense RNA. It has a relatively large genome composition of 26–32 kbs and contains four main structural proteins—spike (S), envelope (E), and membrane (M) proteins in the viral membrane, with genomic RNA complexed with nucleocapsid (N) protein.[16] The SARS-CoV-2 virus particles are formed from an envelope and membrane, with the spike protein forming the viral envelope and the nucleocapsid protein holding the virus's RNA genome.[17] The spike (S) plays a pivotal role in viral attachment, fusion, and entry to the host cell (Fig. 32.1).

INFECTION

SARS-CoV-2 relies on its obligate receptor, angiotensin-converting enzyme 2 (ACE2), to enter cells, and the expression and distribution of ACE2 receptor in humans serve as potential routes of infection.[18–22] ACE2 is highly expressed in the ciliated, goblet, and epithelial cells.[23] SARS-CoV-2 primarily attacks the respiratory tract of the host. In the respiratory tract, ACE2 expression is much higher in the nasal epithelium, especially in the ciliated cells, followed by the upper bronchial epithelia, and

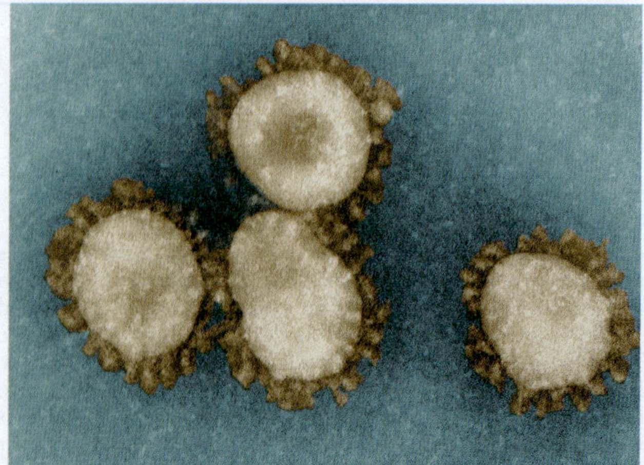

Fig. 32.1 Electron microscope view of coronavirus depicting its characteristic halo or crown-like (corona) appearance. Content provi-ders(s): CDC/Dr. Fred Murphy This media comes from the Centers for Disease Control and Prevention's Public Health Image Library. This image is in the public domain and thus free of any copyright restrictions. As a matter of courtesy we request that the content provider be credi-ted and notified in any public or private usage of this image.

relatively limited in the lower lungs (type II alveolar cells).[23–27] The nasal ciliated cells are primary targets for SARS-CoV-2 replication in the early stage of infection.

Infection with SARS-CoV-2 starts with binding of the spike protein to the cell surface ACE2 receptor, which induces a conformational change that results in endocytosis or fusion of the viral envelope with the host cell plasma membrane.[18] The transmembrane serine protease (TMPRSS2) is the main host cell protease, which cleaves the spike protein and facilitates entry of the virus into the cytoplasm of the host cell. Coexpression of ACE2 and TMPRSS2 is considered critical for entry of SARS-CoV-2 into the cells. After entry, the viral RNA is released into the cytoplasm, and gene expression is triggered ultimately resulting in mature virus particles being exocytosed from the host cell.[28] The SARS-CoV-2 infection then triggers an inflammatory immune response, during which helper T cells and cytotoxic T cells infiltrate the site of infection to eliminate virus-infected cells (Fig. 32.2).

COVID-19

COVID-19, the illness caused by SARS-CoV-2, was first detected in Wuhan, China, in December 2019.[29–31] As the virus spread worldwide, the World Health Organization (WHO) declared COVID a global pandemic on March 11, 2020.[32] A year after the

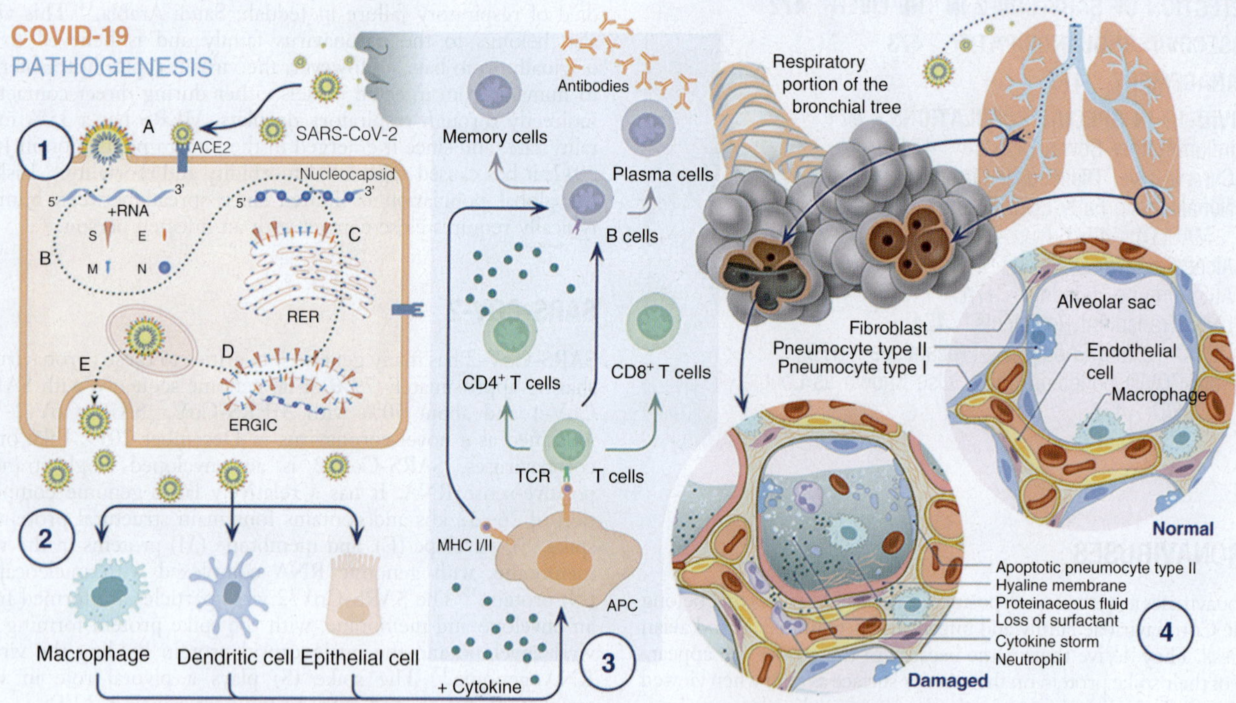

Fig. 32.2 Illustration of COVID-19 pathogenesis: (1) SARS-CoV-2 enters the epithelial cell through binding (A) to ACE2 receptor and releasing its RNA into the cytoplasm. Viral RNA uses the cell's machinery to translate (B) its viral proteins and replicate its RNA. Viral structural proteins S, E, and M assemble (C) in the rough endoplasmic reticulum (RER). Viral structures and nucleocapsid subsequently assemble (D) in the endoplasmic reticulum golgi intermediate (ERGIC). New virion packed in golgi vesicles fuse with the plasma membrane and get released (D) via exocytosis. (2) SARS-CoV-2 infection induces inflammatory factors that lead to activation of macrophages and dendritic cells. (3) Antigen presentation of SARS-CoV-2 via major histocompatibility complexes I and II (MHC I and II) stimulates humoral and cellular immunity resulting in cytokine and antibody production. (4) In severe COVID-19 cases, the virus reaches the lower respiratory tract and infects type II pneumocytes leading to apoptosis and loss of surfactant. The influx of macrophages and neutrophils induces a cytokine storm. Leaky capillaries lead to alveolar edema. Hyaline membrane is formed. All of these pathological changes result in alveolar damage and collapse, impairing gas exchange. (*From* Chams N, Chams S, Badran R, et al. COVID-19: a multidisciplinary review. *Front Public Health*. 2020;8:383. https://doi.org/10.3389/fpubh.2020.00383. Date 29 July 2020. https://commons.wikimedia.org/wiki/File:Fpubh-08-00383-g003.jpg;)

initial cases (December 12, 2019), the disease was present in all populated continents, with around 76.2 million people infected (0.97% of the world's population), causing 1.8 million deaths (2.3%) of those infected, according to the WHO coronavirus (COVID-19) dashboard.[33]

From late 2019 and early 2020, data from multiple sources highlighted the distinct waves of infection associated with the emergence of variants.[34] These variants reflected the natural mutation rate in viruses. As they appeared, the international consensus named variants by Greek letters of the alphabet and a code of the letter B followed by a numerical designation based on molecular genetics (using the Phylogenetic Assessment of Named Global Outbreak).[35] The most important mutations were those that lead to changes in the tertiary structure of the spike protein, often labeled as "variants of concern" or "variants under investigation" resulting in changes in the behavior of the variant with regard to transmissibility, infectivity, immune escape, and pathogenicity. Notable variants of SARS-CoV-2 have been reported, such as alpha (B.1.1.7), beta (B.1.351), gamma (P.1), delta (B.1.617.2), and omicron (B.1.1.529), the latter identified in late 2021 led to significant cases worldwide. The exact number of waves varied by country and region due to differences in factors such as public health responses, population density, and population immunity, as well as variability in how cases and deaths were reported, frequency of testing, with some countries releasing limited data.

COVID-19-ASSOCIATED GASTROINTESTINAL (GI) MANIFESTATIONS

Pyrexia, cough, dyspnea, pharyngitis, rhinorrhea, and malaise were the most common presenting symptoms of COVID-19. Respiratory symptoms resulting from pneumonia and subsequent acute respiratory distress syndrome accounted for most of the morbidity and mortality from COVID-19. However, COVID-19 was considered a multisystem disease associated with hemostatic abnormalities and thrombotic complications, cardiac dysfunction and arrhythmias, liver dysfunction and hepatitis, central nervous system/peripheral nervous system complications, acute kidney injury, and various skin rashes and eruptions.[36] Much of our understanding of the GI manifestations of COVID is based on clinical presentations of earlier variants of SARS-CoV-2 infection.

GI symptoms were an important part of the clinical spectrum of this multisystemic disease with varying reports of GI symptoms based on population and geographic setting. Commonly reported GI symptoms included anorexia, nausea/emesis, heartburn, abdominal pain, and diarrhea.[37] Early in the pandemic, the incidence of any GI symptoms in patients with COVID-19 varied between different studies, ranging from 3% in the initial reports from Wuhan, up to 61.3% in a multicenter cohort from the United States.[38] Based on a systematic review and meta-analysis of 47 studies and more than 10,000 patients, GI symptoms were observed in around 10% of patients with acute COVID-19.[38] Higher incidences of gastrointestinal manifestations were reported in the later periods of the pandemic than in the early period.[39] Additionally, a subset of patients with COVID-19 developed isolated GI symptoms that preceded the development of respiratory symptoms, or they presented only with digestive symptoms throughout the disease. Most GI symptoms associated with COVID-19 were perceived to be mild.[40]

In patients with COVID-19, the following prevalence of gastrointestinal symptoms was reported in systematic reviews and meta-analysis: diarrhea (8%–20%), nausea or vomiting (4% –20%), loss of appetite or anorexia (2%–27%), and abdominal pain (2%–20%).[38,41–54] Anorexia was frequently associated with the other GI symptoms and was thought to be due to acute viral prodrome and inflammation and cytokine modulation as well as be exacerbated by change in taste (dysgeusia). Diarrhea caused by SARS-CoV-2 was sometimes the first, and occasionally the only, symptom of COVID-19. As described above, wide ranges of prevalence rates of diarrhea were reported across studies.[55–58] COVID-19 diarrhea was usually mild and self-limited, with less than six loose or watery bowel movements daily (low or modest volume). In patients with COVID-19 who had diarrhea as their only symptom, diagnosis was often delayed compared with those presenting with respiratory symptoms. Abdominal pain was also reported in some patients with COVID-19, but there was no consensus regarding the severity, duration, or location of the pain, and the precise underlying mechanism was unclear. One hypothesis was that SARS-CoV-2 exerted cytopathic/inflammatory changes resulting in visceral pain.[59]

Early in the pandemic, GI symptoms were commonly seen in severe and critically ill patients and were associated with longer illness duration.[48,60–62] The presence of GI symptoms of COVID-19 was variably associated with clinical outcomes; while some studies suggested that GI symptoms portended a worse outcome, other studies showed no correlation between GI symptoms, such as abdominal pain, and severity of disease.[48–50,52,63] Several case reports described more severe GI complications ranging from ileus to hemorrhagic colitis or life-threatening mesenteric ischemia were reported in critically ill patients with COVID-19 during their frequently lengthy hospitalization[39] (Fig. 32.3).

COVID-19 ASSOCIATED LIVER MANIFESTATIONS

Abnormal liver biochemistry tests were present with high frequency in individuals with COVID-19, and multiple studies showed elevation of liver enzymes associated with overall severity of infection.[64–66] Liver abnormalities were most commonly characterized as mild elevations of alanine transaminase (ALT) and aspartate transaminase (AST) <5 times the upper limit of normal (ULN) occurring with a frequency of 40%–70% depending on the studied population, and whether individuals were hospitalized versus ambulatory, and on the geographic location. There was a slight tendency for higher transaminase

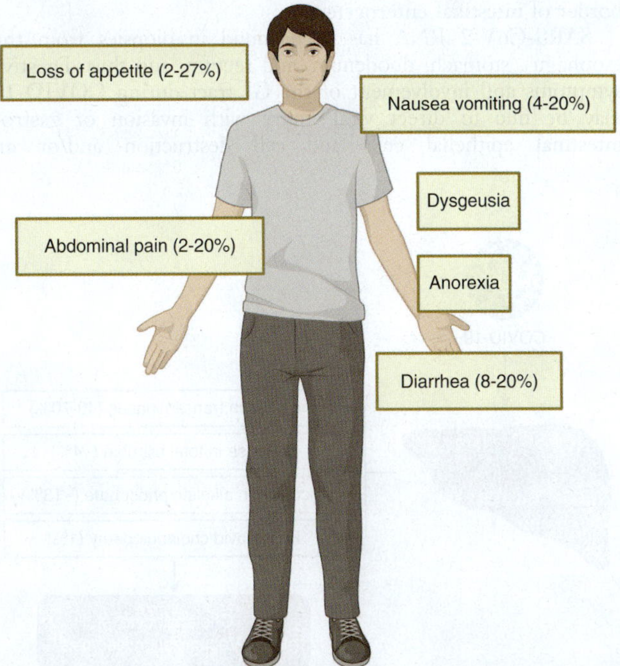

Fig. 32.3 Common gastrointestinal manifestations of COVID-19.

elevation in reports from North America compared to initial reports from China.[64–66] The majority of these abnormal levels of transaminases were limited to five ULN (>60%), with a small proportion of patients expressing severe liver injury (SLI): <6% (when SLI was defined as >5ULN) and <1% (when SLI was defined as >20ULN). Higher transaminase levels, in particular SLI, were associated with worse clinical outcomes, including ICU admission and mechanical ventilation.[65] The transaminase pattern also favored a higher frequency of abnormal AST (~60%) compared to abnormal ALT (~40%) levels.[64,65] Interestingly, this pattern of liver injury with AST-predominant elevations was also reported during the influenza H1N1 outbreak and believed to be related to systemic or liver-related hypoxia.[67,68] Other liver enzyme elevations were relatively uncommon with alkaline phosphatase being abnormal in 13.5% and total bilirubin in 4.3% of hospitalized individuals with COVID-19 in one of the largest series in the United States.[69] Because of the direct correlation of elevated liver enzymes and worse clinical outcomes, it was recommended that hospitalized patients with COVID-19 undergo frequent measurement of liver biochemistries during the course of the disease.

The etiology of elevated liver enzymes in individuals with SARS-COV-2 infection was mainly based on four hypothesis: (1) An extrahepatic components is considered with muscle inflammation leading to elevated transaminases; (2) direct hepatocyte infection related to the presence of ACE2 receptor and DPP4 in liver cells; (3) immune-mediated as general inflammatory markers (including C-reactive protein and specific cytokines) are elevated in these patients; and (4) vascular mechanisms, particularly related to micro-thrombi and ischemia of the liver[68,70] (Fig. 32.4).

DETECTION OF SARS-COV-2 IN THE GI SYSTEM

The presence of ACE2 in the GI tract has been suggested as an explanation for gastrointestinal complications of SARS-CoV-2 infection. ACE2 receptors are highly expressed in the stomach and small intestine.[57,71,72] In gut epithelial cells, ACE2 is needed for maintaining amino acid homeostasis, antimicrobial peptide expression, and the ecology of the gut microbiome, and there is high ACE2 on the brush border of the proximal and distal small intestinal epithelium with the highest expression seen at the brush border of intestinal enterocytes.

SARS-CoV-2 RNA has been found in biopsies from the esophagus, stomach, duodenum, and rectum, and thus digestive symptoms and involvement of the GI tract during COVID-19 may be due to direct viral injury with invasion of gastrointestinal epithelial cells and cell destruction and/or an inflammatory immune response.[73] This may lead to disruption of the tight and adherent junctions of the endothelium and intestinal epithelium, which in turn may lead to leaky gut syndrome, local and systemic invasion of normal microbiota, immune activation and inflammation, activation of the enteric nervous system causing nausea, vomiting, and diarrhea.[59 57] In addition, this disruption of the normal gastrointestinal function may cause nausea and vomiting.[74]

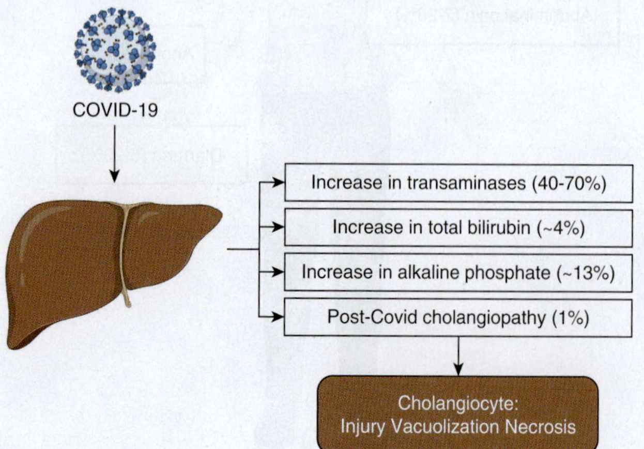

Fig. 32.4 Common hepatic manifestations of COVID-19.

DETECTION OF SARS-COV-2 IN SALIVA AND STOOL

In individuals with COVID, viral SARS-CoV-2 particles were isolated from various bodily fluids, including saliva, stool (feces), urine, semen, and tears, raising concern about transmission through these routes[75,76] Indeed, the presence of SARS-CoV-2 RNA in saliva was used for diagnostic testing during the acute phase and had some advantages over nasopharyngeal swabs, such as ease of sampling, with less risk to health care workers and lower cost.[77,78]

The detection of viral particles in stool was of particular importance, as it raised concerns about transmission of SARS-CoV-2 through the fecal-oral route. In several reports, a large proportion (29.0%–53.4%) of patients with COVID-19 tested positive for SARS-CoV-2 RNA in stool with persistent fecal shedding even after respiratory samples turned negative.[42,55,74,79,80] Patients with GI symptoms had a higher proportion of detectable fecal SARS-CoV-2 RNA as compared with those without GI symptoms, especially in patients who developed diarrhea. Despite these data, no cases of direct fecal-oral transmission were reported, thereby questioning the viability and infectivity of SARS-CoV-2 virus found in fecal matter. Importantly, wastewater evaluation was used as surveillance strategy for tracking and predicting rates of prevalent COVID-19[81] (Fig. 32.5).

DETECTION OF SARS-COV-2 IN THE LIVER

SARS-CoV-2 infection related molecules, such as TMPRSS2 and dipeptidyl peptidase-4 (DPP-4), are expressed in the liver, but no connection between these molecules and viral infection or liver damage has been established.[82,83] Multiple studies have also

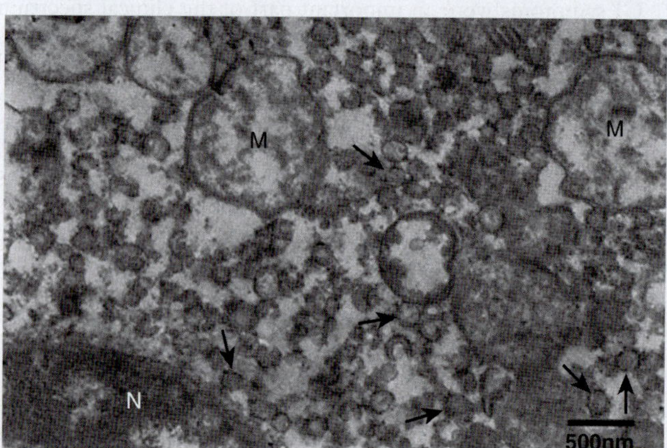

Fig. 32.5 Ultrastructural examination identifying amounts of typical coronavirus particles (*arrow*) with size of 60–120 nm in cytoplasm of hepatocytes. Ultrastructural impairment manifesting conspicuous mitochondria (marked as M) swelling and glycogen granule decrease (original magnification Å ~ 15,000). (From Wang Y, Liu S, Liu H, et al. SARS-CoV-2 infection of the liver directly contributes to hepatic impairment in patients with COVID-19. *J Hepatol*. 2020;73(4):807–816. doi: 10.1016/j.jhep.2020.05.002.)

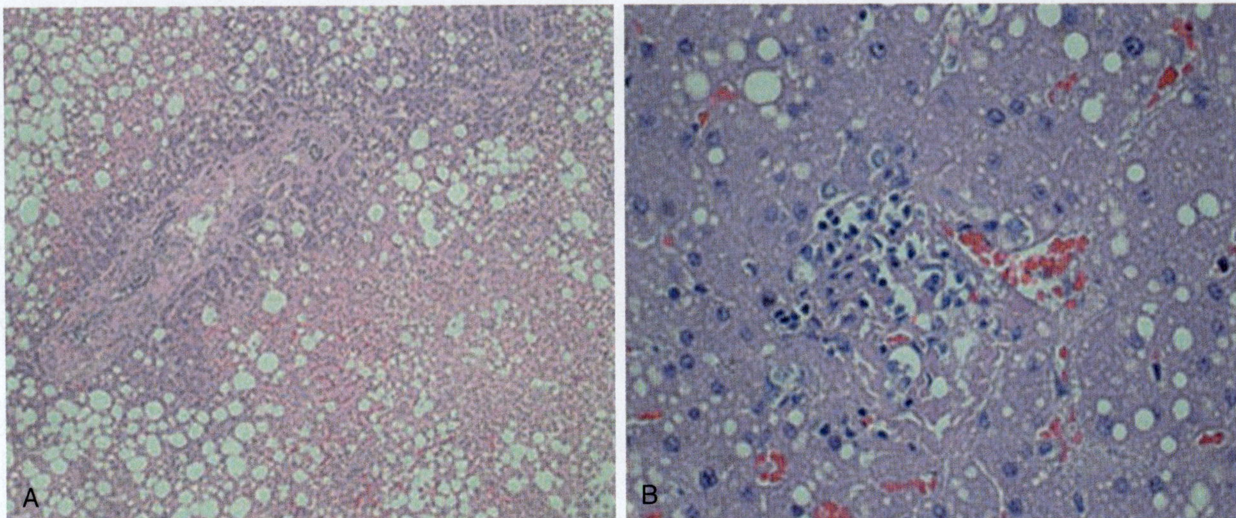

Fig. 32.6 Hematoxylin and eosin stained slides of liver showing (A) marked steatosis involving all three zones (×100) and (B) lobular necroinflammation, comprised predominantly of lymphocytes admixed apoptotic debris (×600). (From Lagana SM, Kudose S, Iuga AC, et al. Hepatic pathology in patients dying of COVID-19: a series of 40 cases including clinical, histologic, and virologic data. *Mod Pathol.* 2020;33(11):2147–2155. doi: 10.1038/s41379-020-00649-x.)

confirmed expression of SARS-CoV-2 in the liver and cholangiocytes, suggesting that the virus could infect these cells.[84–86] In 1 study of 60 COVID-19 patients, 22% of them expressed SARS-CoV-2 RNA or nucleocapsid protein in the liver.[84,85,87] Nonetheless, no study directly established a pathophysiologic connection between the presence of the virus and liver damage or dysfunction. Interestingly, one study showed viral presence via immunohistochemistry in the liver up to 6 months after clinical recovery of viral infection. However, this study was performed in less than five patients, and much of the expression was in immune cells in the liver, highlighting the complexities of understanding hepatic infection by the virus.[88] Not all studies assessing liver histology found detectable virus particles in the liver with 1 study of 24 autopsies finding evidence of severe hepatic necrosis and steatosis but no viral particles, and 1 study using single-cell sequencing only found RNA reads in nonnuclear locations in the liver.[89,90]

Furthermore, histologically defined acute hepatitis cases did not correlate with higher serum transaminases levels, and laboratory values were essentially identical in those with histologic acute hepatitis as compared with no hepatitis, suggesting a disparity of histological and clinical findings pertaining to liver disease.[91] Reported histological findings included necrosis and mild periportal lymphocytic inflammation, mild-to-moderate lobular inflammation, mild portal inflammation, parenchymal confluent necrosis, steatosis, vascular thrombosis, and vascular alterations, including portal vein parietal fibrosis and lobular necroinflammation and portal inflammation.[70,89] Steatosis had also been a consistent finding in multiple studies. However, the populations included individuals with diabetes mellitus, hypertension, and obesity, or those that had received steatosis-inducing medications, including steroids.[70] Some authors, however, postulated that the steatosis findings were not characteristic of diabetes and, therefore, warranted further study.[91] Signs of vascular thrombosis, including VOD-like phlebosclerosis and sinusoidal thrombosis, were initially reported in a great number of reports (with a limited number of samples).[92] A meta-analysis of early cases found that ~30% of evaluated liver tissue showed evidence of vascular thrombosis.[70] However, further reports found minimal to no evidence of vascular events related to the liver.[84,91] The ACE2 receptor is also expressed in cholangiocytes leading to a heightened search for findings related to cholangiopathy in individuals with COVID-19 infection. Nonetheless, most studies assessing histological damage did not find any cholestatic pattern of injury or affection of cholangiocytes[91,93] (Figs. 32.5 and 32.6).

POSTCOVID CHOLANGIOPATHY

A rare but worth mentioning liver-related complication of SARS-CoV-2 infection is post COVID cholangiopathy.[94] This entity occurred in less than 1% of hospitalized patients with COVID-19 and developed in average 5–6 months after initial infection with an overwhelming predilection for males (>90%). Patients presented with jaundice and elevation of alkaline phosphatase (median of 1855 IU in the largest series) and frequently elevated erythrocyte sedimentation rate.[95] Magnetic resonance cholangiopancreatography findings included beading of intrahepatic bile ducts and bile duct wall thickening with enhancement. Liver biopsy showed extensive degenerative cholangiocyte injury, with prominent cholangiocyte vacuolization, and necrosis of the cholangiocyte epithelial layer of terminal bile ducts and marginal ductules.[95,96] The great majority of patients that developed cholangiopathy had a severe course of COVID-19, frequently needing mechanical ventilation. Indeed, the clinical and histological findings resembled sclerosing cholangitis seen in critical ill patients, only at a much later stage. Some of these patients showed progressive biliary tract damage requiring liver transplantation.[95] A more recent European study reported a strong association between chronic liver disease (CLD) and postcovid cholestasis and sclerosis cholangitis with approximately 20% of patients with CLD developing progressive cholestasis after SARS-CoV-2 infection.[97]

MANAGEMENT

As most virus-induced GI manifestations were mild and self-limiting, supportive care and symptomatic treatment were usually sufficient. In such patients, no further investigations specific to the GI system were needed. Routine endoscopy was not recommended, as there was limited value with respect to diagnosis or evaluation and potential risk for health care workers. In reports of endoscopic evaluation of the GI tract in COVID-19 patients (in the acute or immediate postacute stage of COVID-19) findings were usually unremarkable with "normal" histological appearance of intestinal tissues, often with a scant neutrophilic infiltrate or mild increase in intraepithelial lymphocytes.[98]

In published case series of endoscopies performed in hospitalized subjects with substantial burden of critical or prolonged illness, there were reports of mucosal injury ranging from erosions or ulcers (multiple round herpetic-like erosions) inflammation (with moderate lymphocytic infiltration on histology) to ischemic enteritis or acute necrosis.[39,55,73,99] Despite the high prevalence of GI symptoms, the indications and findings (mucosal damage) on endoscopy were judged more likely to reflect overall systemic illness or prolonged hospitalization rather than direct viral injury from COVID-19.[100]

COVID-19 IN SPECIAL POPULATIONS

Inflammatory Bowel Disease

Early in the pandemic, there was heightened concern that inflammatory bowel disease (IBD) patients may be at increased risk of COVID-19 given their underlying immune dysregulation and high utilization of immunosuppressive or immunomodulatory agents; however, studies demonstrated that the overall incidence of COVID-19 in this cohort was comparable to the rate in the general population.[101] A multinational study of 23,879 patients from 12 centers demonstrated that the incidence of COVID-19 in the IBD cohort matched the incidence observed in the general population, further supporting the conclusion that IBD patients were not at increased risk of acquiring SARS-CoV-2 infection.[102] Furthermore, among individuals with IBD who acquired COVID-19, there was no evidence to suggest that these individuals had more severe disease or worse outcomes. Data from the comprehensive longitudinal database, Surveillance Epidemiology of Coronavirus Under Research Exclusion for IBD demonstrated that the overall mortality did not differ significantly from mortality reported in patients without IBD. Furthermore, the database demonstrated no increased risk of adverse outcomes with the use of biologics; however, systemic corticosteroid use was associated with worse outcomes from SARS-CoV-2 infection.[103]

Chronic Liver Disease or Cirrhosis

Multiple studies showed an association between CLD and an increased likelihood of being diagnosed with COVID-19, which may have been attributed to a higher likelihood of testing for SARS-CoV-2.[64,104] One large U.S. study showed a higher overall mortality in those with alcohol-related liver disease (ALD), decompensated cirrhosis, and hepatocellular carcinoma.[105,106] Multiple international studies in different geographic regions of the world demonstrated that individuals with decompensated cirrhosis who contracted COVID had an increased risk of complications and death: mortality in patients with cirrhosis following COVID-19 infection was found to be 32% in a large registry cohort of across 29 countries with increasing mortality related to Child-Pugh (CP) scores: 8% no cirrhosis, 19% with CP-A, 35% with CP-B, and 51% with CP-C. This trend remained the same even after matching for age and other comorbidities.[107]

A large retrospective French cohort (>259,000 hospitalized patients with COVID-19 and >15,000 with CLD) highlighted that patients with decompensated cirrhosis were at an increased adjusted risk for COVID-19 mortality.[108] A study from Northern Italy during the early phase of the pandemic reported a 30-day mortality of 30% in those with cirrhosis.[109] A multicountry Asian study showed increasing complications with increasing degree of liver disease decompensation, and a South American study reported increased mortality in those with cirrhosis.[110,111]

Nonalcoholic Fatty Liver Disease (NAFLD, Now MASLD)

An association between nonalcoholic fatty liver disease (NAFLD, now MASLD) and COVID-19 has been heavily studied, as NAFLD-associated variables, such as obesity, T2DM and cardiovascular disease, are well-established risk factors for SARS-CoV-2 infection and worst prognosis.[104] Moreover, as mentioned above, multiple studies find that liver steatosis as a common histopathological finding in patients infected with SARS-CoV-2.[70] Nonetheless, beyond that of epidemiological association, studies looking a direct causality, once controlling for multiple variables, showed inconsistent results.[107,112–116] Moreover, as the NAFLD impact on morbidity and mortality seemed somewhat related to geographic location and specific subtype (i.e., lean NAFLD and T2DM-associated NAFLD).[117] In view of the significant comorbidities associated with NAFLD, it was advised that these patients be managed with greater care.

Alcoholic Liver Disease

ALD has shown to have an independent deleterious effect enhancing COVID-19 mortality, even within different causes of CLD. A large U.S. multicenter study found a 2.4 hazard ratio of mortality for ALD, which was similar to that of cirrhosis of any cause.[105] Other studies have confirmed this association after controlling for multiple cofactors and coexisting liver disease etiologies.[107,110] The underlying factors related to a higher impact of ALD on COVID-19 are likely related to functional immunosuppression, poor nutritional status, and late presentation to a health care facility. Equally important has been the impact that the COVID-19 pandemic has had on alcohol consumption and increase in ALD. The rise of unhealthy alcohol consumption accelerated dramatically during the pandemic, likely related to stay-at-home orders, social isolation, loss of support systems, and disruptions to work and recreational routines.[68] This has reflected, among other issues, in ALD becoming the most common indication for listing and the fastest increasing cause for liver transplant in the United States since the COVID-19 pandemic.[118]

Autoimmune Hepatitis

Patients with autoimmune hepatitis (AIH) represented a group of concern initially as it was assumed that their ongoing immunosuppression (in those treated for AIH) would predispose them to worse outcomes. Multiple studies, including 1 study involving 34 centers from 10 countries in Europe and the Americas, showed no worse outcomes than patients with CLD and no association of AIH and COVID-19 severity.[119,120] Another study, retrospective in nature and involving several authors from the previous cohort, found an association with the use of steroids and thiopurines and COVID-19 severity in patients with AIH when compared to those with AIH not using immunosuppressive medications before acquiring COVID-19.[121] This effect was more evident with a higher dose of steroids (i.e., prednisolone equivalent >5 mg/day compared to 5 mg a day). This is not entirely surprising as previous studies in individuals with inflammatory bowel disease have shown worse outcomes related to COVID-19 on those taking glucocorticoids.[122]

Liver Transplant Recipients

The COVID-19 pandemic affected the liver transplant world in a dynamic and comprehensive manner. Initially during the pandemic, multiple centers around the world temporarily stopped performing solid organ transplants as there were too many uncertainties on the new pandemic.[123] Later on, as centers started performing transplants, there was hesitancy to use SARS-CoV-2 infected organs. Following important studies on the safety profile of such organs, they then became accepted for transplantation. Indeed, a worldwide survey conducted in 2020 showed that ~15% of centers transplanted organs from previously SARS-CoV-2-infected donors, and more recent data suggests that SOT from such donors is feasible and safe.[123,124] It should be noted though that active COVID-19 still remains a clinical contraindication to both donation and allocation of liver (and other solid organs) transplantation.

LT recipients were diagnosed with COVID-19 more frequently than nontransplant recipients.[125] However, this seemed related to closer monitoring and a lower threshold for testing in this patient population as opposed to an increased risk of SARS-CoV-2 infection.[68] When infected with SARS-CoV-2, liver transplant recipients reported more frequent GI symptoms, particularly diarrhea occurring approximately in 30%–40% of patients.[126] Interestingly, the frequency of elevated liver enzymes seems similar between LT recipients and nontransplant patients, and a study from the U.S. found that when age- and sex-matched with nontransplant patients with CLD, the incidence of acute liver injury was lower in LT recipients.[126,127] Multiple studies showed high mortality rates in SOT recipients with COVID-19, particularly LT.[127,128] However, LT recipients frequently had higher rates of chronic kidney disease, overweight-obesity, and T2DM, all of which are risk factors for worse outcomes in COVID-19. Some studies suggested that after controlling for multiple comorbidities, LT recipients may not be at an increased risk of severe COVID-19 or death compared with non-LT recipients.[125,129] In terms of management, decreasing or altering immunosuppression medications did not seem to affect liver biochemistries.[125,127,130]

COVID-19 and Endoscopy Precautions

Due to the high risk of human-to-human transmission and the potential for transmission of infection with SARS-CoV-2 during routine performance of endoscopy, there was a lack of clarity regarding the necessity of PPE.[131] Since the initial SARS infection in the early 2000s, there was ongoing recognition that certain medical interventions, labeled aerosol generating procedures, increased the risk of potential infection due to aerosol generation.[132] According to the WHO, an AGP is any medical or patient care procedure that results in the production of airborne particles, or aerosols, which are "associated with an increased risk of pathogen transmission" and therefore require enhanced precautions.[133]

There was significant controversy as to whether upper or lower endoscopy qualified as AGPs.[134] AGF classification was critical in informing infection prevention and control policies, specifically the requirements for respiratory protective devices, such as N95 or N99 masks/respirators or filtering facepiece respirators (such as FFP2 or FFP3) or masks at endoscopy.[135] In the context of COVID-19, a classification of a procedure as an AGP necessitated a higher grade of PPE to protect against aerosolized virus and potential airborne transmission risk. Possible sources of aerosolization during endoscopy include intubation and removal of the endoscope, coughing, belching during endoscopy, heavy breathing from sedation, patient expulsion of gas and liquid, and dispersion of contaminated fluid during insertion and removal of tools through the working channel of the endoscope, adjustment of the air/water button, retrieval of tissue from a biopsy channel, and during precleaning of the endoscope.[136] During the course of the pandemic, our knowledge of the role of aerosol generation during endoscopy expanded with increasing consensus that upper gastrointestinal endoscopy should be classified as an AGP, and periprocedural management, including PPE recommendations, should follow the AGP protocols to minimize transmission.

In March 2020 when the COVID-19 outbreak was declared a global pandemic, all endoscopy services came to a virtual halt.[137] Considering the escalating rates of hospitalizations and deaths, limited PPE availability, limited COVID-19 test availability, and the burden on the health care system, routine elective endoscopy services were temporarily discontinued. HCWs, physicians, and nursing staff were redeployed, and protocols were developed for triaging of endoscopies to identify and perform only endoscopic procedures for urgent or emergent indications. After the initial phase, many centers resumed limited endoscopy services with the implementation of stringent infection prevention and control policies. Moreover, the use of preprocedure testing in asymptomatic individuals became a common path to triage for risk stratification. A critical aspect of resuming endoscopy services included providing reassurance to patients and importantly to reassure HCWs, including endoscopists, nurses, and staff.

The rapid development and widespread implementation of vaccination programs and the availability of relatively effective treatments helped decrease morbidity and mortality from COVID-19. Within the GI community, as universal screening and testing for SARS-CoV-2 and PPE became widely available, many endoscopy centers again revised their testing policies. In contrast to early reports of high rates of HCW infections early in the pandemic (in the setting of limited PPE) accumulating evidence demonstrated low rates of COVID-19 infections among HCWs performing endoscopy.[138] This evidence, along with data demonstrating the relative effectiveness of vaccines in decreasing rates of transmission of infection, prompted a recommendation against routine preprocedure testing and a ramp up of endoscopic services across endoscopy centers. However, the impact of the pandemic on cancer-related care due to disruptions in screening, follow-up, diagnosis, and receipt of timely care has been well documented, with declines in incidence rates for all GI cancers in 2020 compared with prior years and lower rates for early-stage disease and concurrent increased mortality rates for specific GI cancers, for example, colorectal cancer and esophageal adenocarcinoma.[139,140]

Post-COVID Condition (PCC), also Known as Long COVID

According to the WHO, post-COVID condition (PCC) is defined as a syndrome that occurs in individuals with a history of probable or confirmed SARS-CoV-2 infection that develops usually 3 months after the onset of COVID-19 and includes symptoms that last at least 2 months and cannot be explained by another diagnosis. Symptoms can be new in onset after initial recovery or persist from the acute phase and may fluctuate or relapse over time. PCC is considered a multiorgan disorder involving the cardiopulmonary, neurologic, GI, nephrological, and other systems.[141–143] The prevalence of PCC varies across different studies and populations. According to a meta-analysis and systematic review, the global estimated pooled prevalence of PCC is approximately 43% (39%–46%) at 28+ days from infection.[144]

While GI manifestations of acute COVID-19 have been well described, some individuals experience persistent GI complaints even after recovery from COVID infection.[145–147] However, accurate reporting of the GI manifestations of PCC is confounded by evolutions in definitions of disease and inaccuracy in the diagnosis and reporting of symptoms, as well as differences in populations and health systems.[148]

Based on 1 systematic review and meta-analysis of 12 studies, including 158,731 individuals with PCC, the frequency of GI symptoms was reported in 22% of individuals (95% CI,

10%–41%).[149] The pooled frequency for abdominal pain and nausea/vomiting was 14% and 6%, respectively. Additionally, the frequency for loss of appetite and loss of taste was 20% and 17%, respectively, and the pooled frequency for diarrhea was 10% in PCC individuals. Persistent GI symptoms were commonly reported in individuals who had acute COVID but did not met criteria for PCC with similar rates for abdominal pain (7%), nausea/vomiting (6%), loss of appetite/taste (9%–10%), and diarrhea (5%). The GI manifestations of long COVID were not related to severity of underlying COVID-19 and occurred even in those with mild initial disease. While the mechanism underlying GI symptoms of PCC is poorly understood, it is hypothesized that persistence of the virus in the GI tract, ensuing inflammation, and alteration of the microbiome, intestinal permeability, and changes in the absorption and metabolism of neurotransmitters are all likely mediators of the effects of SARS-CoV-2 virus on the gut.[150] Notably, a significant number of patients developed dyspepsia (17%), irritable bowel syndrome (20%), or new-onset constipation (19%) as a sequelae of COVID-19 infection.[149,151] Long-term GI impact of SARS-CoV-2 infection is increasingly recognized as a disorder of the gut-brain axis or functional GI disorders. The development of functional GI disorders after episodes of viral gastroenteritis is well recognized. The management of GI sequelae of COVID-19 includes supportive care and symptom management on an individual basis.[141]

Full references for this chapter can be found at https://ebooks.health.elsevier.com.

33 Gastrointestinal Consequences of Infection With Human Immunodeficiency Virus

C. Mel Wilcox

IN THIS CHAPTER

In 1981 the first cases of what we now recognize as acquired immunodeficiency syndrome (AIDS) were described. Subsequently, the world witnessed an explosion of cases typically manifested by opportunistic infections (OIs) such as *Pneumocystis jirovecii* pneumonia and neoplasms such as Kaposi sarcoma, which is caused by human herpesvirus 8. Over 35 million people have died from AIDS; it is estimated that over 36 million people worldwide are currently living with human immunodeficiency virus (HIV) infection, and there are about 5000 infections per day.[1] Early in the epidemic, the focus of attention was on identifying the etiology of the disease (HIV-1 and HIV-2), characterizing these disorders, and when effective, using prophylactic antimicrobial therapy. In 1995 the concept of highly active antiretroviral therapy (HAART) was born, and the face of the epidemic changed rapidly. Now, simply referred to as antiretroviral therapy (ART), fully active treatment blocks viral replication and, consequently, circulating HIV. In most patients, HIV RNA (also known as "viral load") becomes undetectable in the blood. Associated with a reduction in viral load, there is substantive improvement in immune function that can be assessed by objective measures such as an increase in the CD4 lymphocyte count, clinically by a decrease in OIs, and a marked improved survival.[2,3] In developed countries, the current focus centers around viral control, whereas in resource-poor nations, OIs such as TB abound, mimicking what was first witnessed in the early stages of the epidemic in the developed world.[4,5] Despite the scale of the epidemic, there is much to be optimistic about, including data showing a reduced risk of transmission with preexposure prophylaxis; use of ART in HIV-discordant couples, which virtually eliminates the risk of transmission to the seronegative partner when the seropositive partner is on effective ART (PARTNER Study), often referred to as "treatment is prevention"; reduction in mother-to-child transmission with ART; male circumcision, which effectively reduces transmission by over 60% (Gray et al.); earlier use of ART, which may improve the rates of full immunologic recovery; and increasing use of ART worldwide.[6]

With the immune reconstitution associated with effective ART, there also has been a shift to the management of chronic diseases, as well as drug side effects. Mortality among HIV-infected patients on ART is most often due to non-AIDS events such as chronic liver disease secondary to infection with HCV.[7,8] Similarly, HIV-infected patients responding to ART who have GI complaints are more likely to have drug-induced side effects or nonopportunistic GI infections, shifting management strategies back to disorders prevalent in immunocompetent hosts.[9]

Because patients are generally approached based on clinical presentation, accordingly, this chapter is organized primarily around symptom diagnosis. Specific HIV-related disorders (limited to HIV-1, which is the most common and virulent form of the disease) and their treatments are presented within the context of their most common associated symptoms and signs. In addition, the effect of ART in relation to these symptom complexes and diseases is discussed. Throughout this chapter, when referring to patients with AIDS, we specify those patients with a CD4 count of less than 200/mm^3 who are at risk for or have developed opportunistic disorders. Generally, these patients with AIDS are not yet receiving, are unable to receive, or have failed ART.

Although ART has dramatically altered the occurrence of GI complications, many of the same principles of management established before ART remain applicable. In general, the approach to investigating GI symptoms in the patient with AIDS parallels that of non-HIV-infected patients. Several general points must be considered when evaluating GI symptoms in AIDS:

1. Clinical signs and symptoms infrequently suggest a specific diagnosis.
2. GI symptoms in a patient on ART are most often drug-induced or nonopportunistic in etiology.
3. Risk stratification for an opportunistic disorder, in the absence of ART, may be predicted on the basis of the extent of immunocompromise [i.e., CD4 count >200/mm^3 favors common bacteria and other nonopportunistic diseases (e.g., Kaposi sarcoma); CD4 count <100/mm^3 favors CMV, fungi, *Mycobacterium avium* complex (MAC), and unusual protozoa] (Fig. 33.1).
4. In patients with AIDS, the GI tract is commonly involved in opportunistic processes, oftentimes multiple ones (Fig. 33.2). GI pathogens are usually part of a systemic infection (e.g., CMV and MAC). Thus identification of a pathogen outside the gut in the appropriate clinical setting may negate the need for GI evaluation.
5. Evaluation should proceed from less invasive to more invasive and should be dictated by the severity and acuity of symptoms and signs.
6. Evidence of tissue invasion should be sought as a hallmark of pathogenicity.
7. Without improvement of immune function (by ART), recurrence of OIs is almost uniform, necessitating maintenance of antimicrobial therapy.
8. Treatment of all opportunistic disorders should include ART; the timing of initiation of ART is typically coincident with the initiation of antimicrobial therapy with the exception of tuberculosis (within 2 weeks, depending on CD4 count) and *Cryptococcus* (within 2 weeks).

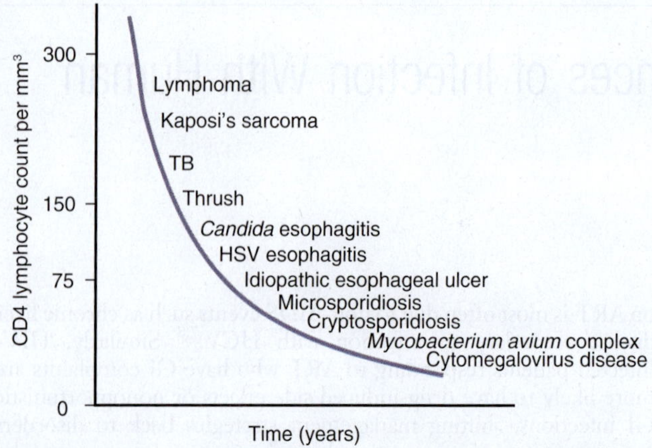

Fig. 33.1 Timeline of *opportunistic* disorders based on CD4 lymphocyte count. (From Wilcox CM, Saag MS. Gastrointestinal complications of HIV infection: changing priorities in the HAART era. *Gut*. 2008;57:861–870.)

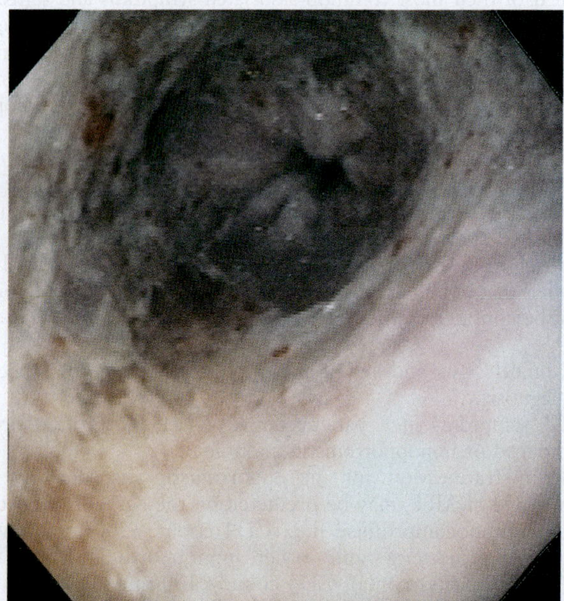

Fig. 33.2 Cytomegalovirus and HSV esophagitis. Diffuse circumferential ulceration is seen on this endoscopic view, and the esophagogastric junction is seen in the distance. In patients with AIDS, multiple pathogens are frequently found. (From Wilcox CM. *Atlas of Clinical Gastrointestinal Endoscopy*. Philadelphia, PA: Saunders; 1995:28.)

ODYNOPHAGIA AND DYSPHAGIA

Before HAART was available, these esophageal complaints (dysphagia and odynophagia) occurred in at least one-third of patients during the course of HIV disease. Because of effective ART, the incidence of esophageal disease has markedly fallen, and the number of patients with diseases not unique to AIDS (e.g., GERD) has risen.[10]

Candida albicans, the most frequent esophageal infection in AIDS, often coexists with other disorders in this setting. Although most cases occur in the setting of AIDS, *Candida* esophagitis may occur during primary HIV infection as a result of transient immunosuppression.[11] Oral thrush often predicts concurrent esophagitis in patients with esophageal complaints, though thrush

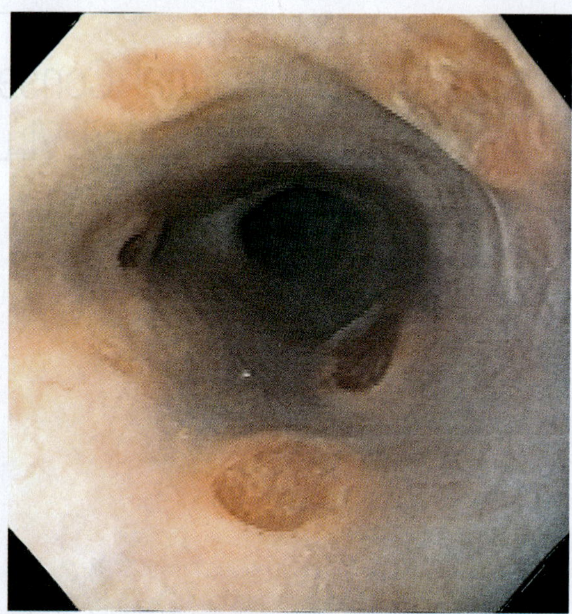

Fig. 33.3 HIV-associated idiopathic ulcers. Multiple well-circumscribed ulcerations throughout the esophagus are evident in this endoscopic view. The ulcers have a punched-out appearance, with normal-appearing intervening mucosa, and seem to be raised, resulting in a heaped-up appearance. (From Wilcox CM. *Atlas of Clinical Gastrointestinal Endoscopy*. Philadelphia, PA: Saunders; 1995:75.)

is not invariably present (see Fig. 33.2); the absence of thrush does not exclude the possibility of esophageal candidiasis.[12]

Patients with esophageal candidiasis generally complain of substernal dysphagia.[13] Odynophagia, when present, is usually not severe. Definitive diagnosis is established by upper endoscopy, which reveals either focal or diffuse plaques in association with mucosal hyperemia and friability. A well-circumscribed ulcer or ulcers suggest(s) other or additional process. Biopsies show desquamated epithelial cells with typical-appearing yeast forms; fungal invasion is usually present only in the superficial epithelium.[14]

Although CMV is the most commonly identified pathogen in advanced untreated AIDS, its association with esophageal disease is less frequent than *Candida*. CMV characteristically causes mucosal ulceration. Thus patients with CMV esophagitis complain of odynophagia or substernal chest pain, characteristically severe.[15] Dysphagia is much less common than in patients with *Candida* esophagitis and is rarely the primary complaint. Fever is rare. Generally, upper endoscopy reveals extensive ulcerations that are large and deep, although the endoscopic pattern is variable (see Fig. 33.2).[16] *Candida* coinfection is common. Mucosal biopsies should demonstrate viral cytopathic effect in mesenchymal and/or endothelial cells in the granulation tissue. Characteristic inclusions may be absent, necessitating confirmation by immunohistochemical stains. Biopsy of granulation tissue in the ulcer base provides the highest yield for viral cytopathic effect, whereas viral culture is less sensitive, and cytologic brushings are unhelpful.[17]

A syndrome of nonspecific (idiopathic and aphthous) esophageal ulceration is common (Fig. 33.3).[15] The clinical presentation and endoscopic appearance are indistinguishable from esophageal CMV infection. Criteria for diagnosis of idiopathic ulcers include the following: (1) endoscopic ulcer confirmed by histopathology, (2) no evidence of viral cytopathic effect (CMV and HSV) by both routine histology and immunohistochemical studies, and (3) no clinical or endoscopic evidence of GERD or pill-induced

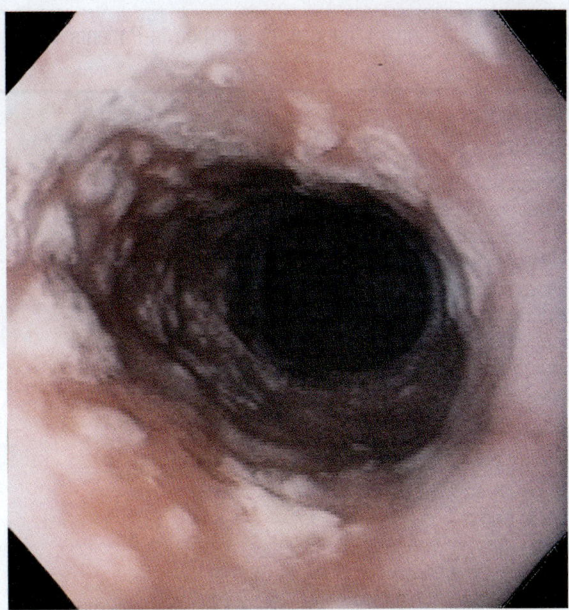

Fig. 33.4 HSV esophagitis. This endoscopic view demonstrates diffuse erythema that surrounds multiple whitish plaques, which represent shallow ulceration. Islands of normal-appearing esophageal mucosa are still present.

esophagitis. As with CMV ulcers, nonspecific ulcers occur in late-stage disease, with most patients having a CD4 count less than 50/mm^3. However, they have also been described in acute HIV infection.[11] The pathogenesis of these ulcers remains unknown.

In contrast with other immunocompromised hosts, HSV esophagitis is infrequent in AIDS.[15] In immunocompetent patients, herpetic esophagitis is usually due to HSV type 1. However, AIDS patients may have esophagitis due to either type 1 or type 2 HSV. The disease is similar to herpetic infections of other mucous membranes in that the pathogenetic features follow a predictable sequence. Discrete vesicles form, then shallow ulcers occur, and finally coalesce into regions of diffuse shallow ulceration. In contrast to CMV esophagitis and nonspecific ulcer, the ulcers tend to be shallow; large, deep ulcers are rare (Fig. 33.4). Biopsies and cytologic brushings taken from the margin of the ulcers (the sites of active viral replication) are most likely to show epithelial cell invasion and nuclear changes typical of herpes infections. Viral cultures of biopsy specimens are usually positive.[17]

Isolated cases of esophagitis/ulcerations have been reported from a variety of other infections as well as pills.

AIDS patients may also be at increased risk for esophageal neoplasms. Reported neoplasms include Hodgkin and various non-Hodgkin lymphomas, Kaposi sarcoma, squamous cell carcinoma, and adenocarcinoma.

A specific cause of esophageal complaints in the AIDS patient cannot be made based on symptoms or physical examination alone (Box 33.1). Nevertheless, a few generalizations may be made. The presence of oral thrush associated with mild-to-moderate dysphagia without odynophagia is likely caused by *Candida* esophagitis. In contrast, the patient with severe odynophagia without dysphagia or thrush is more likely to have ulcerative esophagitis (viral and idiopathic). The patient complaining of substernal burning and regurgitation is most likely to have GERD, especially if on ART.

Endoscopy with biopsy is the only means of establishing a specific etiology for the cause of dysphagia and odynophagia. Multiple mucosal biopsies are preferred over brush cytology for ulcerated lesions.[17] Barium swallow radiography may play a diagnostic role in the HIV-infected patient with preserved immune function when a motility disorder is suspected.

BOX 33.1 Differential Diagnosis of Dysphagia and Odynophagia in Patients With AIDS

INFECTIONS

*Candida albicans**
CMV*
HSV
Histoplasma capsulatum
Mycobacterium avium complex
Cryptosporidium spp.
Toxoplasma gondii
Idiopathic ulcerations*
GERD*
Neoplasms
Kaposi sarcoma
Lymphoma
Squamous cell carcinoma
Adenocarcinoma
Pill-induced esophagitis

*More frequent cause.

Given the preponderance of *Candida* infection, an empirical approach to the management of esophageal symptoms is reasonable in most patients with AIDS. Patients with dysphagia and/or odynophagia who also have oral thrush should be treated empirically with fluconazole 100 mg/day after a 200-mg loading dose.[18] Itraconazole or fluconazole suspensions are effective alternatives. If symptoms persist despite a 1-week empirical trial, endoscopy with biopsy should be performed rather than initiation of other empirical trials or escalation of the dose of fluconazole. Relapse of *Candida* esophagitis is invariable unless immune function is improved with ART. Furthermore, despite chronic prophylaxis, relapse of esophagitis due to antifungal resistance frequently occurs.

CMV and HSV infections should be treated similarly to other gut involvement with these viruses (see following). Idiopathic ulcers respond in more than 90% of patients to oral glucocorticoids (e.g., 40 mg prednisone per day initially and tapered over 4 weeks). The basis for glucocorticoid efficacy is unknown; infectious causes should be assiduously excluded before administering glucocorticoids in this setting. Thalidomide is also highly effective and may be curative when prednisone fails.[19] The devastating teratogenic effects mandate its use be limited to men or women of nonchildbearing potential. ART itself has been shown to result in ulcer healing.

DIARRHEA

Before ART, diarrhea occurred in up to 90% of patients during the course of HIV disease, especially those from resource-poor countries.[20] In the era of effective ART, diarrhea is a less frequent complaint and etiologically is now most often medication-induced (e.g., ART) or caused by disorders unrelated to HIV infection.[21,22]

HIV infection results in a rapid CD4 T cell depletion throughout the GI tract, as well as an enteropathy characterized by increased inflammation of the lamina propria and damage to the GI epithelial cell layer, which is associated with microbial translocation and immune activation.[23] Alterations in the mucosal immune system in AIDS predispose to intestinal infections, may lead to untreatable chronic infection by organisms that typically cause self-limited infection in immunocompetent hosts (e.g., *Cryptosporidium parvum*), and may contribute to a more virulent clinical course of common enteric infections (e.g., *Salmonella*, *Shigella*, and *Campylobacter* species). Clinical and socioenvironmental factors are associated with intestinal OIs, including low CD4 lymphocyte count and nonuse of ART, low socioeconomic status, lack of availability of safe drinking water, and exposure to farm animals.[20] Despite the vast spectrum of protozoal, viral, bacterial, and fungal organisms that can cause diarrhea in the patient with AIDS, a differential diagnosis can be developed on the basis of the clinical presentation and degree of immunodeficiency (Box 33.2).

Protozoa are the most prevalent diarrheal pathogens in most series,[24–26] largely because many of these infections can lead to chronic diarrhea and are refractory to treatment. *Cryptosporidia* species such as *C. parvum*, a cause of self-limited diarrhea in healthy hosts, remain the most frequent protozoa identified in HIV-infected patients worldwide. Clinical presentation and outcome are related to the degree of immunocompromise and the subtype of organism.[26] The small bowel is the most common site of infection, although the organisms can be recovered in all regions of the gut as well as in biliary and respiratory epithelium. Diarrhea is typically severe, with stool volumes of several liters per day not uncommon. Borborygmi, nausea, and weight loss are frequently associated symptoms; right upper quadrant pain suggests biliary tract involvement (see later). The pathogenesis of this infection is uncertain. The diagnosis of intestinal cryptosporidiosis is most often made by acid-fast stain of the stool, where the organisms appear as bright-red spherules similar in size to red blood cells. The sensitivity of stool testing varies and depends on the burden of organisms, character of the stool (formed vs. liquid), and primary site of infection. Stool antigen detection and PCR markedly increase sensitivity of stool testing. *Cryptosporidia* may be identified in small bowel or rectal biopsies even when the stool examination is negative.[27]

Specific antimicrobial treatment of cryptosporidial infection remains disappointing. Numerous antimicrobial agents have been tested, most without significant effect (Table 33.1).[28] Currently, the most effective therapy for cryptosporidia is ART, in which the improvement of immune function results in a clinical remission of diarrhea and clearance of cryptosporidia from the stool and on small bowel biopsy.[29] For patients failing ART and/or in whom antimicrobial therapy is ineffective, symptomatic treatment should include fluid support and antidiarrheal agents, occasionally including opiates to control the diarrhea.

Cystoisospora belli is a sporozoan and, like *C. parvum*, is a cause of both acute and chronic diarrhea in patients with AIDS. The disease is rare in the United States, but it is more frequent and endemic in resource-poor countries. The organism may be identified by acid-fast stain of the stool or duodenal secretions or on mucosal biopsy. Unlike cryptosporidiosis, infection with *C. belli* can be effectively treated with antibiotics, specifically trimethoprim/sulfamethoxazole or ciprofloxacin.[30]

Cyclospora species are coccidian parasites and infrequently cause acute or chronic diarrhea in both immunocompetent and immunodeficient individuals. Its prevalence in AIDS is low. The organism is detectable by stool studies and is treatable with trimethoprim/sulfamethoxazole or ciprofloxacin.

Microsporidia emerged as common intestinal infections in AIDS, but their prevalence has markedly fallen in the HAART era.[31] Intestinal and hepatobiliary disease may be caused by two species of microsporidia: *Enterocytozoon bieneusi* (most common species) and *Encephalitozoon intestinalis*. The reported prevalence of microsporidia without ART varies from 15% to 39%.[32] Typical symptoms include watery, nonbloody diarrhea of mild-to-moderate severity, usually without associated crampy abdominal pain. Infection is associated with severe immunodeficiency, with median CD4 counts of infected individuals of less than 100/mm^3.[27]

BOX 33.2 Differential Diagnosis of Diarrhea in Patients With AIDS

INFECTIONS

Protozoa

*Microsporidium**
Cryptosporidia spp.*
Cystoisospora belli
Cyclospora spp.
Giardia lamblia
Entamoeba histolytica
Leishmania donovani
Pneumocystis jirovecii
Toxoplasma spp.

Bacteria

Clostridium difficile
Salmonella spp.*
Shigella spp.*
*Campylobacter jejuni**
Mycobacterium avium complex
Mycobacterium tuberculosis
SIBO

Viruses

CMV*
HSV
Adenoviruses
Rotavirus spp.
Norovirus
HIV?

Fungi

Histoplasmosis
Coccidioidomycosis
Cryptococcosis
Candidiasis
Talaromyces marneffei

Neoplasms

Lymphoma
Kaposi sarcoma

Idiopathic

"AIDS enteropathy"

Drug-Induced

HIV protease inhibitors

Pancreatic Disease

Pancreatic insufficiency
Chronic pancreatitis
Infectious pancreatitis (CMV and MAC)
Drug-induced pancreatitis (e.g., pentamidine)

*More frequent cause.

As with infection from cryptosporidia, the pathogenesis of disease remains poorly defined. Microsporidia can be discerned by light microscopy when tissue is embedded in plastic or paraffin (Fig. 33.5). Staining of embedded mucosal biopsies with Brown-Brenn, Gram stain, or modified Masson trichrome stain is superior to routine H&E staining. *E. intestinalis* can usually be differentiated from *E. bieneusi* by its larger size and infection of lamina propria macrophages; electron microscopy is definitive. Stool staining techniques are only moderately sensitive, whereas small bowel biopsies are generally positive. Although albendazole has shown effective for *E. intestinalis*,[33] no widely available therapy

TABLE 33.1 Treatment of Infectious Causes of Diarrhea in Patients With AIDS

Pathogen	Treatment	Duration (Days)
PROTOZOA		
Cryptosporidia spp.	Paromomycin, azithromycin, and nitazoxanide	14–28
Cyclospora spp.	Trimethoprim/sulfamethoxazole or ciprofloxacin	14–28
Cystoisospora belli	Trimethoprim/sulfamethoxazole or ciprofloxacin	14–28
Microsporidia	Albendazole (*Encephalitozoon intestinalis*)	14–28
	Metronidazole, atovaquone, and fumagillin (not available in the United States)	
VIRUSES		
Cytomegalovirus	Ganciclovir or valganciclovir	14–28[a]
	Foscarnet	14–28[a]
	Cidofovir	14–28[a]
HSV	Acyclovir or valacyclovir	5–10[a]
BACTERIA		
Salmonella, Shigella, and *Campylobacter* spp.	Fluoroquinolone (e.g., ciprofloxacin) or azithromycin	10–14[a]
Clostridium difficile	Metronidazole and vancomycin	10–14
SIBO	Metronidazole and ciprofloxacin	10–14
Mycobacterium tuberculosis	Rifampin, isoniazid, pyrazinamide, and ethambutol (RIPE)	270–365 (9–12 months)
Mycobacterium avium complex	Multidrug regimens for symptomatic infection	270–365 (9–12 months)
FUNGI		
Histoplasmosis	Amphotericin B and then itraconazole	28
Coccidioidomycosis	Amphotericin B and then fluconazole	28
Cryptococcosis	Amphotericin B and then fluconazole	28

[a]Duration of therapy dictated by immune reconstitution with HAART.

is effective for *E. bieneusi*. As with cryptosporidiosis, ART is the best therapy, resulting in the resolution of diarrhea with clearance of this pathogen.[29]

For unclear reasons, infections by the protozoa *Giardia lamblia* and *Entamoeba histolytica* are not consistently seen with increased frequency or virulence in AIDS. However, in East Asia, where *E. histolytica* is endemic, amebic colitis was identified as a common cause of diarrhea.[34] The nonpathogenic *Entamoeba dispar* is morphologically similar to *E. histolytica* and can only be distinguished by more specific stool or enzyme-linked immunosorbent assay tests.[35] *Blastocystis hominis*, *Endolimax nana*, and *Entamoeba coli* are nonpathogenic protozoa that are seen more commonly in men who have sex with men (MSM) and are often found in association with other protozoal parasites. Rare cases of enteric leishmaniasis (endemic), *P. jirovecii* infection, and toxoplasmosis have been reported.

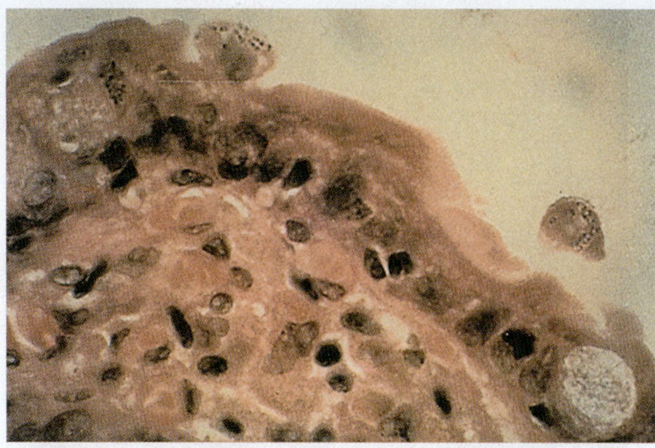

Fig. 33.5 Endoscopic biopsy specimen of small bowel microsporidiosis. This thin plastic section demonstrates shedding of an epithelial cell containing microsporidial oocysts. (From Gazzard BG. Diarrhea in human immunodeficiency virus antibody-positive patients. *Semin Gastroenterol.* 1991;2:3.)

Helminths, particularly *Strongyloides stercoralis* and *Ascaris lumbricoides*, are uncommon pathogens in AIDS patients.[36] Infected patients may present with abdominal pain, diarrhea, and eosinophilia. The clinical syndrome and recurrence rate associated with these parasites do not appear to be altered in the setting of HIV infection.

Viral infection of the large bowel, and rarely the small bowel, is an important cause of diarrhea in HIV infection. CMV is the most common viral cause of diarrhea and the most frequent cause of chronic diarrhea in patients with advanced AIDS and multiple negative stool tests.[37] This infection characteristically occurs late in the course of HIV infection when the CD4 lymphocyte count is below 50/L (see Fig. 33.1). Infection is most common in the colon, but concomitant disease in the esophagus, stomach, or small bowel may be observed (see Fig. 33.2). Isolated gastric or small bowel disease often presents as abdominal pain, typically in the cecum, rather than a diarrheal illness.

The clinical manifestations of enteric CMV infection vary greatly and include asymptomatic carriage, nonspecific symptoms of weight loss and fevers, and focal enteritis/colitis, including appendicitis or diffuse ulcerating hemorrhagic involvement with bleeding or perforation. As a result, patients can present with any of several constellations of symptoms, including abdominal pain, peritonitis, watery nonbloody diarrhea, or hematochezia.[38] The most common presentation, however, is abdominal pain associated with chronic diarrhea. Although the endoscopic spectrum is variable, the hallmark of CMV enteritis/colitis is subepithelial hemorrhage and mucosal ulceration (Fig. 33.6).[38] Whenever CMV is present in the GI track, it is imperative to look for the pathogen elsewhere, especially in the retina.

As noted previously, the diagnosis of GI CMV infection is best established by demonstrating viral cytopathic effect, including confirmation by immunostaining in tissue specimens. If inclusions are few and demonstrable in tissue that appears macroscopically normal, the patient should be considered to have CMV colonization rather than true CMV infection.

Several effective therapies are available for the treatment of CMV (see Table 33.1). Ganciclovir, an acyclovir derivative typically given intravenously, is effective in approximately 75% of

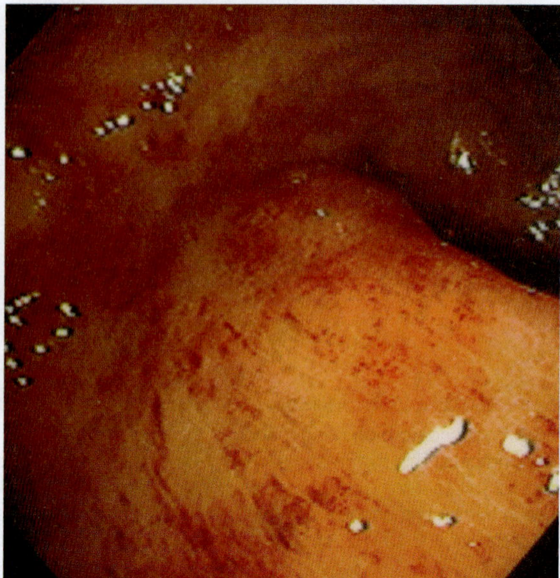

Fig. 33.6 CMV colitis. Endoscopic photograph of the sigmoid colon showing edema and diffuse subepithelial hemorrhage typical for CMV. This endoscopic appearance is similar to that of idiopathic ulcerative colitis.

cases.[39] Valganciclovir, an oral prodrug of ganciclovir, has excellent GI absorption and efficacy for CMV retinitis but has not been well studied for induction therapy in GI disease. Immune reconstitution with ART will negate the need for long-term suppressive therapy. At the time of diagnosis of GI CMV infection, all patients should have an ophthalmologic examination to exclude CMV retinitis, because this site of infection requires close follow-up to ensure remission, thereby preventing blindness. Although widely used in the transplant setting, the role of CMV antigenemia or DNA concentrations by PCR to predict subsequent disease and guide the use of preemptive therapy remains less well defined.[40]

A number of other viruses (e.g., Norwalk, adenovirus, and rotavirus), as well as novel noroviruses, have been identified in symptomatic and asymptomatic patients, but their overall contribution to diarrheal disease in AIDS is small.

The evidence for a role of HIV itself as a diarrheal pathogen is limited. An idiopathic AIDS enteropathy has been proposed to account for the diarrhea in AIDS patients who lack an identifiable pathogen and may reflect indirect effects of HIV on enteric homeostasis. With improvements in diagnostic techniques, greater awareness of the spectrum of diarrheal pathogens in AIDS, recognition of the importance of adverse drug effects as additional causes of diarrhea, and use of panendoscopy with biopsy for patients with negative stool tests, a diminishing fraction of AIDS patients have truly "idiopathic diarrhea." Institution of HAART has been shown to improve chronic unexplained diarrhea.[41]

Infections by enteric bacteria are more frequent and more virulent in HIV-infected individuals compared with healthy hosts. *Salmonella*, *Shigella*, and *Campylobacter* have higher rates of bacteremia and antibiotic resistance. Diagnosis is straightforward because the organisms usually can be grown from stool samples (see Chapter 110). These enteric infections typically present with high fever, abdominal pain, and diarrhea that may be bloody. Abdominal pain can be severe, mimicking an acute abdomen. As noted, bacteremia is common, and parenteral antibiotics should be administered empirically in severely ill patients when these infections are suspected until results of stool and blood cultures and sensitivities are available, after which antibiotics can be tailored to the pathogen isolated.

Diarrhea due to *Clostridium difficile* has emerged as a common bacterial pathogen, not because it is an OI but rather because antibiotic use is far greater and hospitalization is more frequent in this population than in healthy hosts.[42] The clinical presentation, response to therapy, and relapse rate are no different than in immunocompetent patients.[43] Diagnosis rests on standard assays of stool for *C. difficile* enterotoxin (see Chapter 112).

Small bowel bacterial overgrowth (see Chapter 105) is uncommon in AIDS patients,[44] and its role in causing diarrhea appears limited.

Mycobacterial involvement of the bowel with *M. avium intracellulare* (MAC) or TB may lead to diarrhea, abdominal pain, and, rarely, obstruction or bleeding in patients with late-stage AIDS. A large number of patients with MAC have an asymptomatic GI infection, whereas *Mycobacterium tuberculosis* appears to be symptomatic in all cases. Duodenal involvement by MAC is most common and may be suspected at endoscopy by the presence of yellow mucosal nodules, often in association with malabsorption, bacteremia, and systemic infection. Diagnosis of GI MAC infection is best made by endoscopic biopsy; fecal acid-fast smear is much less sensitive than culture. The organism is readily seen on biopsy specimens with acid-fast staining, and the number of organisms is often striking (Fig. 33.7). Blood culture positivity may suggest the diagnosis. Affected patients have severe malabsorption and weight loss in association with blunting of villi and suffusion of macrophages with mycobacteria. A pseudo–Whipple syndrome with periodic acid–Schiff (PAS)-positive macrophages has been noted, although in contrast to MAC, acid-fast bacilli (AFB) positivity rather than PAS-positive macrophages are identified; electron microscopy will distinguish Whipple versus this pseudo–Whipple disease. As is typical of MAC infection, in AIDS there is a poorly formed inflammatory response, and granulomas are rarely present. Response to multidrug antibiotic therapy is variable and depends in part on the extent of immunocompromise. However, eradication is rarely achieved without ART. As with other OIs, the institution of ART improves immune function, hastens clinical resolution of the infection, prevents relapse (such that long-term antimicrobial therapy will become unnecessary), and enhances survival.

Although extrapulmonary TB is characteristic of AIDS, luminal GI tract involvement remains infrequent but, when present, usually involves the ileocecal region or colon.[42] Fistula formation, intussusception, and perforation, as well as peritoneal and rectal involvement, have been reported. Tuberculous involvement of the gut in HIV infection is most commonly found in resource-poor countries. In contrast with MAC, TB infections in AIDS generally respond to multidrug antituberculous therapy [e.g., rifampin, isoniazid, pyrazinamide, and ethambutol (see Table 33.1)].[39]

Infections caused by mycobacteria (e.g., MAC lymphadenitis) and viruses (e.g., CMV uveitis) have been described following institution of ART. This immune reconstitution inflammatory syndrome (IRIS) results in an exuberant inflammatory response directed toward previously quiescent or incubating pathogens.[45] In addition, following the diagnosis of the OI and institution of ART, paradoxical exacerbations of these infections may lead to a worse outcome.

Among fungal infections of the gut in AIDS, histoplasmosis is most commonly described and occurs in the setting of disseminated infection, often in association with pulmonary and hepatic histoplasmosis. Histoplasmosis may manifest as a diffuse colitis with large ulcerations and diarrhea, as a mass, or as serosal disease in association with peritonitis.[46] The diagnosis of disseminated histoplasmosis may be suspected in a patient with high fever and markedly elevated serum LDH levels.[46] The diagnosis is established by fungal smear and culture of urine, infected tissue, or blood; urinary histoplasmosis antigen assay often is strongly positive and is diagnostic in the setting of typical symptoms. Rare

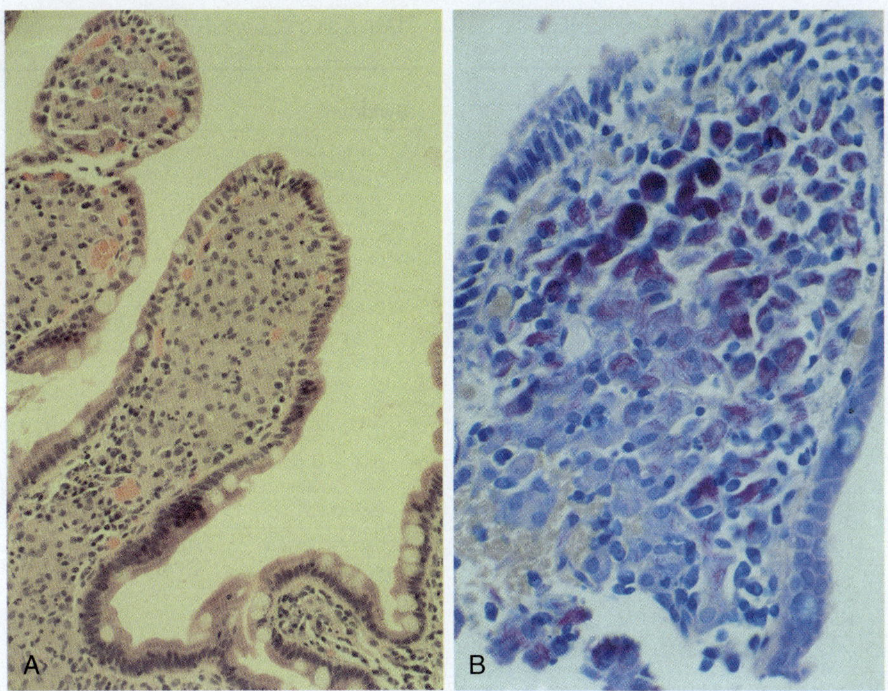

Fig. 33.7 Intestinal *Mycobacterium avium* complex. (A) H&E staining of a small bowel biopsy specimen shows marked thickening of the villi, with a cellular infiltrate. (B) High-power view with acid-fast staining shows numerous macrophages filled with mycobacteria.

cases of systemic cryptococcosis, coccidioidomycosis, and *Talaromyces marneffei* infection (principally in Southeast Asia) with gut involvement have also been described.

With the advent of effective ART, drug-induced diarrhea became increasingly important. Although almost any therapeutic regimen is associated with diarrhea, the most common agents associated with diarrhea are the protease inhibitors, with nelfinavir (not used currently) having the highest rate, with the boosting agent, ritonavir, having a high rate of loose stools.[47] Generally, the diarrhea is mild to moderate in severity and is not associated with weight loss. The mechanism(s) for diarrhea due to these agents is poorly understood. Symptomatic therapies are generally effective. A botanical agent, crofelemer, may be useful for diarrhea in this setting.[48] A suggested approach to the evaluation of diarrhea is outlined in Box 33.3.

BOX 33.3 Evaluation of Diarrhea in Patients With AIDS

ALL PATIENTS

Stool specimen for bacterial culture; *Clostridium difficile* toxin

Stool smear for fecal leukocytes, ova and parasite testing, and acid-fast stain

PATIENTS WITH RECTAL BLEEDING, TENESMUS, OR FECAL LEUKOCYTES

Flexible sigmoidoscopy or colonoscopy with biopsy of the mucosa for histopathology, viruses, and protozoa

Cultures of rectal tissue for bacteria (especially *Campylobacter* spp.) and for viruses in some cases

PATIENTS WITH PERSISTENT DIARRHEA AND WEIGHT LOSS AND OTHERWISE NEGATIVE ABOVE EVALUATION

Upper endoscopy with small bowel mucosal biopsies

ABDOMINAL PAIN

The frequency of abdominal pain in patients with AIDS is unknown, but like other GI complications of AIDS, the prevalence and etiology have been altered by ART. In most patients with AIDS, abdominal pain, when severe, is directly related to HIV and its consequences. However, clinicians must consider not only the manifestations of OIs and neoplasms but also the more common causes of abdominal pain in the general population.

The differential diagnosis of abdominal pain in AIDS is presented in Table 33.2. This table does not include AIDS-unrelated diagnoses that have assumed more importance in the ART era. Table 33.3 describes abdominal pain in terms of the four most common pain syndromes, their suspected diagnoses, most likely causes, and the diagnostic approaches indicated. Generally, the duration and severity of symptoms dictate the urgency of evaluation.

The history is helpful in localizing the origin of abdominal pain. Associated symptoms and signs should suggest the particular organ involved, and the quality and duration of the abdominal pain may implicate specific diseases. Generally, the same work-up as for a patient without AIDS should be initiated. Abdominal CT scanning is especially useful early in the assessment of abdominal pain. In patients with acute pancreatitis, drug-induced causes must be considered.[49] Management of abdominal pain falls broadly into surgical versus nonsurgical options. Indications for surgical intervention in AIDS patients are the same as for patients without AIDS. All tissue specimens must be submitted for viral and fungal culture and for pathologic examination, and enlarged mesenteric nodes should undergo biopsy.

TABLE 33.2 Differential Diagnosis of Abdominal Pain in Patients With AIDS

Organ	Causes
Stomach	
Gastritis	CMV,[b] cryptosporidia (see Chapter 52)
Gastric ulcer	CMV,[b] PUD
Gastric outlet obstruction	Cryptosporidia, CMV, lymphoma, and PUD
Mass	Lymphoma, KS, and CMV
Small bowel	
Enteritis	Cryptosporidia,[b] CMV, and MAC
Obstruction	Lymphoma[b] and KS
Perforation	CMV[b] and lymphoma
Colon	
Colitis	Enteric bacteria,[b] CMV, and HSV
Obstruction	Lymphoma,[b] KS, and intussusceptions
Perforation	CMV,[b] lymphoma, and HSV
Appendicitis	KS,[b] cryptosporidia, and CMV
Liver and spleen	
Infiltration	Lymphoma,[b] CMV, and MAC
Biliary tract	
Cholecystitis	CMV,[b] cryptosporidia,[b] and microsporidia
Papillary stenosis	CMV,[b] cryptosporidia,[b] and KS
Cholangitis	CMV[b]
Pancreas	
Pancreatitis	CMV,[b] KS, and medication-induced
Tumor	Lymphoma and KS
Mesentery and peritoneum	
Infiltration	MAC,[b] *Cryptococcus* spp., KS, lymphoma, histoplasmosis, TB, coccidioidomycosis, and toxoplasmosis

[a]The differential diagnosis does not include many non–AIDS-specific conditions.
[b]More frequent diagnosis.
KS, Kaposi sarcoma; *MAC*, *Mycobacterium avium* complex.

TABLE 33.3 Evaluation of Abdominal Pain Syndromes in Patients With AIDS

Syndrome	Suspected diagnosis	Diagnostic approach
Dull pain, diarrhea, mild nausea, and vomiting	Infectious enteritis	Stool culture, stool for ova and parasite testing, and sigmoidoscopy
Acute severe pain with peritoneal irritation	Perforation and infectious peritonitis	Abdominal and upright chest plain films, surgical consultation, CT or US, paracentesis if ascites is present, and laparoscopy
Right upper quadrant pain and elevated liver biochemical test levels	Cholecystitis, cholangitis, hepatic infiltration, and cholangiopathy	US or CT, MRCP, ERCP, and liver biopsy
Subacute pain, severe nausea, and vomiting	Intestinal obstruction	Abdominal plain films, CT, small bowel series, endoscopy, and barium enema

BOX 33.4 Differential Diagnosis of Anorectal Disease in Patients With AIDS

INFECTIONS

Bacteria

*Chlamydia trachomatis**
Lymphogranuloma venereum
*Neisseria gonorrhoeae**
Shigella flexneri
Mycobacterium tuberculosis

Protozoa

Entamoeba histolytica
Leishmania donovani

Viruses

HSV*
CMV*
HPV

Fungi

Candida albicans
Histoplasma capsulatum

Neoplasms

Lymphoma*
Kaposi sarcoma
Squamous cell carcinoma
Cloacogenic carcinoma
Condyloma acuminatum

Other

Idiopathic ulcers*
Perirectal abscess, fistula*

*More frequent diagnosis.

ANORECTAL DISEASE

The frequency of anorectal disease among AIDS-infected MSM is higher than in other AIDS patients primarily related to sexually transmitted infections. Common findings in HIV-infected patients include perirectal abscesses, anal fistulas, perianal HSV infection, idiopathic ulcerations, and infectious proctitis, but lymphoma, ulcerations due to CMV, TB, and histoplasmosis may also be seen (Box 33.4). The frequency of anorectal squamous cell carcinomas is strikingly higher in MSM than in other groups, and this risk increases as HIV disease progresses. Despite the use of ART, however, the incidence of anorectal tumors continues to rise.[49] These neoplasms result from HPV infections acquired through sexual contact, particularly HPV types 16 and 18. Morphologic studies have documented histologic progression, often in the same lesion, from a benign lesion, condyloma acuminatum, to high-grade intraepithelial neoplasia or squamous cell carcinoma; however, the rate and risk factors for progression are poorly understood. High-grade intraepithelial neoplasia is associated with oncogenic HPV16 or HPV18 and low nadir $CD4^+$ cell count and may progress rapidly to cancer.[50] Cytologic specimens of the anal canal, similar to Papanicolaou smears, are used for screening and have high predictive value for dysplasia.[51]

Risk factors for liver injury associated with medication use have most consistently been associated with chronic viral hepatitis, most notably HBV or HCV, increasing the rate threefold or greater. Other reported risk factors include preexisting liver fibrosis, pretreatment elevation in liver chemistry tests, older age, alcohol abuse, and concomitant treatment with antituberculous agents.[56,57]

Mechanisms by which ART results in liver injury include drug-induced toxicity and/or metabolism, direct hypersensitivity reactions, mitochondrial toxicity, IRIS, and steatosis.[58] Hypersensitivity reactions are idiosyncratic, immune related, and typically occur within the first 4–6 weeks of starting the offending agent.

The lactic acidosis syndrome, typically caused by the nucleoside reverse transcriptase inhibitors, namely, zidovudine, didanosine, or stavudine, is characterized by marked hepatomegaly, microvesicular steatosis, and metabolic lactic acidosis, leading to liver failure. Given that these drugs are not used much in current ART regimens, this syndrome is rarely seen.[59]

IRIS-related liver injury occurs after initiating ART, coincident with subsequent CD4 cell recovery, especially in those coinfected with chronic HBV. The syndrome generally manifests within the first 2 months of ARV drug initiation and is accompanied by a precipitous decline in HIV RNA and a rise in CD4 count. Elevated serum aminotransferase levels and high levels of HBV DNA are predisposing factors.[60] The degree of liver injury ranges from mild with minimally abnormal liver chemistry test results to fatal with acute hepatic failure.

A high prevalence and incidence of viral hepatitis B and C is common in this population, given the shared risk factors for viral hepatitis acquisition, including IV drug use and sexual transmission. Clinical manifestations and histologic features of infection from HBV (+/−HDV), HCV, and HAV are altered in the presence of HIV coinfection, but in remarkably different ways for each virus.

Prior exposure to HBV has been reported in up to 90% of AIDS patients, with active infection in 5%–20% of patients, but with marked worldwide differences.[61] In Africa and Asia, vertical transmission is the most common route of HBV acquisition, whereas in the Western world, drug use and sexual transmission predominate. More recent studies suggest lower infection rates, perhaps due to use of HBV vaccines.[62] Concurrent HIV and HBV infections lead to alterations of HBV antigen-antibody display, viral replication, and clinical consequences. Patients with HIV have a lower rate of spontaneous clearance of hepatitis B e antigen (HBeAg), increased HBV replication, a higher rate of loss of anti-HBs, and reactivation of HBV, and are much more likely to develop chronic HBV infection after an acute exposure to this virus. Like HCV, HBV/HIV-coinfected patients have an increased and more rapid rate of progression to cirrhosis and mortality compared to HBV-infected individuals without HIV. Recurrence of HBsAg may arise from either reinfection or reactivation with advanced immunodeficiency. With loss or reduction in immunity to HBV, there is an increased prevalence of HBeAg expression, elevated mean levels of DNA polymerase, and increased titers of antibody to hepatitis B core antigen. Increased serum HBV DNA viral load also translates into an increased risk of hepatocellular carcinoma (HCC). Acquisition of the chronic carrier state is also much more likely in the HIV-infected patient, especially if infection occurs when immunodeficiency is more advanced. Thus a larger proportion of patients with HIV/HBV coinfections have a chronic HBV carrier state, with highly infectious serum and body fluids, compared with those who are HIV negative.

Although HIV infection leads to more prevalent chronic HBV carriage, it appears to attenuate the severity of biochemical and histologic liver disease. The mechanism for reduced HBV-related liver injury following HIV infection is not certain but has been attributed to a diminution in lymphocyte-mediated hepatocellular injury as a result of HIV's effects on immune system activity. In those PWH without serologic evidence of past or present HBV infection, the efficacy of HBV vaccination is related to the stage of immunocompromise and degree of HIV viremia.[63] Immune response to HBV vaccination can be improved by vaccinating after initiation of ART and improvement in immune function, using high-dose vaccination, and repeating vaccination.[64]

Conversely, the institution of ART in a chronic carrier of HBV can have catastrophic consequences following immune reconstitution (IRIS). Patients may develop an acute flare of viral hepatitis that can be severe, leading to fulminant hepatic failure. However, the proportion of HIV/HBV coinfected patients who develop an acute hepatitis B flare following use of ART is low.[65] It is believed that reconstitution of immune function with HAART leads to production of antibody that is directed to infected hepatocytes as in the normal host. Seroconversion to anti-HBe and/or anti–hepatitis B surface antigen (anti-HBs) may also be observed. Inclusion of lamivudine, which has potent antiviral effects on HBV, in the HAART regimen may reduce the likelihood of an acute flare of hepatitis B. Long-term lamivudine monotherapy often results in resistance mutations and precipitates acute hepatitis. Treatment of either HIV or HBV must take into account each infection because many antiretroviral agents have dual activity against both viruses. If treatment is indicated for either infection, treatment should be initiated with a combination of tenofovir (TDF or TAF) and emtricitabine or lamivudine plus a third agent against HIV. Current recommendations are to include two drugs that are active against HBV to prevent the emergence of resistant variants. In patients with advanced immunosuppression, cure of HBV is unlikely; thus the goal should be to reduce HBV DNA as low as possible. Such treatment may reduce disease progression and perhaps reduce the risk for HCC. These observations mandate that all patients who are to receive ART should be screened for active or past HBV infection. Vaccination should be considered in all eligible patients. Treatment options for HBV infection in the setting of HIV have been summarized.[66] Triple infection with HIV, HBV, and HDV is rare. The consequences of HIV infection on HDV appear similar to those of HBV, although some data suggest that liver disease may be more aggressive.[67]

The primary risk factors for HAV acquisition germane to this population include travel and high-risk sexual behavior. Outbreaks of HAV have been described in MSM.[68] Although HAV infection occurring in HIV-infected patients may result in higher serum titers of HAV RNA and prolonged viremia, there is no evidence to suggest a more severe course. As with hepatitis B, the immune response to HAV vaccine is less in those immunocompromised, but when immune function is preserved, the response rate is high and the durability prolonged, especially when three rather than two doses of vaccine are administered.[69] Given the fecal-oral route of transmission, vaccination should be considered in all nonimmune MSM.

The prevalence of HCV infection in HIV is variable, being highest in IV drug users and hemophiliacs (≈50%–90%) as compared to heterosexual individuals and MSM (1%–10%).[70] HIV infection profoundly alters the natural history of HCV coinfection. Liver disease is now an important cause of mortality in HIV-infected patients, and much of this is related to coinfection with HCV. Unlike HBV, the clinical course of HCV worsens as HIV-related immunocompromise advances. HIV-infected patients acutely infected with HCV are less likely to clear HCV viremia, have much higher HCV RNA levels, and have an accelerated progression to fibrosis, with decompensated cirrhosis and fatal liver disease occurring a decade or more sooner than in HIV-negative patients.[71] Fibrosis progresses more rapidly in coinfected individuals, first observed in the hemophiliac population. There is a twofold higher risk of developing cirrhosis, a sixfold higher relative risk of developing decompensated liver disease, and a higher risk for developing liver cancer. Factors that predict fibrosis and progression to cirrhosis in coinfected patients include older age at infection, higher serum ALT levels, higher inflammatory activity, alcohol consumption of more than 50 g/day, and CD4 count less than 500 cells/mm^3.[72] Steatohepatitis also may play a role.[73] Mechanisms underlying this rapid progression to fibrosis are multifactorial but similarly recognized in other immunocompromised patients. Survival is poor in patients with decompensated cirrhosis who are coinfected, with a median survival of approximately 1 year. Sustained virologic responders are less likely to experience liver-related events and mortality, supporting the urgent need for implementation of effective therapy, which is now widely available.[74,75] Indeed, all PWH coinfected with HCV should be treated for HCV, assuming their HCV RNA levels are detectable (indicating chronic infection). Although much of the mortality related to liver disease in these patients is due to HCV infection, HCC is rising in incidence, with AIDS patients having a four times higher rate than the general population.[76] Like hepatitis B, HCV does not cause progression of HIV disease. Triple infection (HCV, HBV, and HIV) or even quadruple infections (HCV, HBV, HDV, and HIV) are rare, associated with injection drug use, and may be associated with a worse outcome, including higher rate of cirrhosis.

With the advent of new simplified oral agents for HCV (Chapter 80), the treatment of, response to, and natural history of coinfected patients is transformed. For many patients, cure of HCV is now a reality with these new DAAs. Prior interferon-based therapies were associated with side effects and poor efficacy. The use of DAA typically with ART results in equivalent sustained viral response (SVR) as in HCV+/HCV− patients (>95%).[77,78] In addition, earlier treatment may reduce fibrosis and the incidence of HCC. Reinfection has been observed.

Hepatitis E coinfection appears to be rare and endemic, and any additional impact on pregnant women is uncertain.[79]

NAFLD is increasingly recognized worldwide, associated with the obesity epidemic. Increasingly in HIV-infected patients, this disease is playing a role in the development of abnormal liver tests, liver fibrosis, and cirrhosis, especially in the setting of the metabolic syndrome.[80] Moreover, the cause may be multifactorial, including HCV infection, alcohol use, and HAART itself or its effect on lipogenesis.

Nodular regenerative hyperplasia and noncirrhotic portal hypertension, while rare, have been increasingly reported in the HIV population. Associated risk factors are didanosine use (not used any longer) and thrombophilia.[81]

MAC infection is consistently the most frequent specific hepatic finding in AIDS in late-stage HIV disease.[82] The pathologic hallmark of this infection is the presence of poorly formed granulomas containing AFB within foamy histiocytes. In developing countries, TB is the most common OI involving the liver in HIV-infected individuals. TB, in contrast to MAC, may occur before HIV-infected patients are profoundly immunocompromised. TB is commonly extrapulmonary (≈80%) in HIV-infected patients.[83] Hepatic disease as part of miliary tuberculosis has been noted. Rarer manifestations include tuberculous abscesses and bile duct tuberculomas.[84] The diagnosis of hepatic TB is made by culture of the organism from liver tissue obtained by percutaneous or laparoscopic biopsy. PCR may allow earlier diagnosis. As with MAC, appropriate staining of biopsy specimens can demonstrate typical-appearing mycobacteria.

CMV is an uncommon liver pathogen, most often found at autopsy in HIV patients. However, it rarely is a cause of clinical hepatitis or cause of other hepatic symptoms. Typical viral inclusions are usually identified in Kupffer cells but can sometimes be seen in hepatocytes or sinusoidal endothelial cells or in association with granulomas.

Fungal infections of the liver are not unusual in HIV infection when immunocompromise is advanced. Hepatic histoplasmosis, cryptococcosis, and coccidioidomycosis may be observed in patients with disseminated fungal disease, predominantly but not exclusively in regions of high prevalence of the organism.[84] *Candida* infection of the liver is rare, in contrast to its high prevalence in mucosal sites.

Kaposi sarcoma is most often found at postmortem or incidentally at liver biopsy but may occasionally cause elevated serum aminotransferase levels or even jaundice.

Hepatic involvement by non-Hodgkin lymphoma may be the index manifestation of AIDS and the primary site of the neoplasm. This tumor in the AIDS patient tends to be more aggressive, spreading rapidly to extranodal sites, making liver involvement more likely.[85] The lesions are typically focal and may be large. The prognosis is determined largely by the extent of underlying immunocompromise and performance score rather than the lymphoma itself. Improvements in survival have been demonstrated in those receiving ART.[86]

A number of other isolated cases of hepatic involvement by a variety of pathogens have been reported, including *P. jirovecii*, cryptosporidia, microsporidia, *Dicrocoelium dendriticum*, and *Leishmania* species.[87]

Bacillary peliosis hepatis, caused by either *Bartonella henselae* or *Bartonella quintana*, is a systemic infection that may be associated with fever, skin lesions, abdominal pain, and lytic bone lesions.[88] Liver chemistry tests usually show a disproportionate elevation of serum alkaline phosphatase. Liver biopsies demonstrate regions of a myxoid stroma in association with granular purple material, which with Warthin-Starry stain or electron microscopy reveal clumps of organisms.

Biliary tract disease is currently most likely related to cholelithiasis, choledocholithiasis, or chronic pancreatitis. A syndrome resembling sclerosing cholangitis with papillary stenosis is well recognized and has been termed *AIDS cholangiopathy*.[89] Patients characteristically develop significant upper abdominal pain in association with marked elevation of serum alkaline phosphatase, as well as minimal elevations of bilirubin, AST, and ALT.

Ductular changes consist of papillary stenosis alone, sclerosing cholangitis-like lesions alone, a combination of both, or long extrahepatic strictures. Most series have found papillary stenosis with intrahepatic disease as the most common findings (Fig. 33.8). US or CT detects ductular abnormalities, usually dilation, in most of those with cholangiographically proved disease, implying that a negative imaging study does not definitively exclude the diagnosis. The etiology in most cases is due to infection of the duodenal and biliary epithelium with cryptosporidia, CMV, microsporidia, or *Cystoisospora*. For patients with predominantly papillary stenosis, biliary sphincterotomy results in a symptomatic improvement in most patients.[89] However, the serum alkaline phosphatase may continue to rise, probably reflecting progression of associated intrahepatic disease. ART may lead to improvement of the radiographic abnormalities in some patients.[89] Survival in AIDS cholangiopathy is linked to severity of immunodeficiency.[90]

Other less common causes of biliary tract disease in AIDS include primary bile duct lymphoma, obstruction of the biliary tree by lymphomatous lymph nodes in the porta hepatis, Kaposi sarcoma, and extrahepatic collections of bile (biloma).

Acalculous cholecystitis has also been described in AIDS patients, presenting as severe abdominal pain and occasionally peritonitis. This syndrome is usually caused not only by a specific infection, most frequently CMV, but also from microsporidia, cryptosporidia, and *C. belli*.[91] Cholelithiasis may occur. Laparoscopic cholecystectomy is the treatment of choice.

The clinical history and the finding of symptomatic hepatomegaly or abnormal liver chemistry tests are nonspecific, and further evaluation is always necessary. Nevertheless, some generalizations can be made. Significant elevation of the serum aminotransferase levels favors a drug-induced or viral cause. In contrast, marked elevation of the serum alkaline phosphatase level

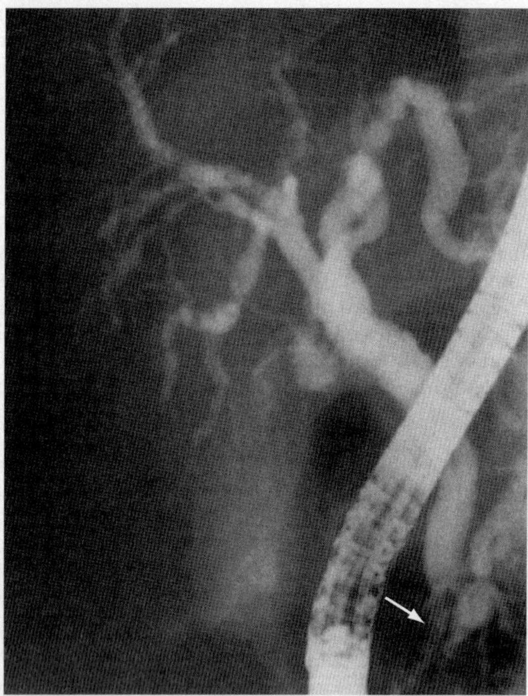

Fig. 33.8 ERCP in a patient with AIDS cholangiopathy. Papillary stenosis is present (*arrow*).

correlates statistically with the presence of hepatic MAC infection in AIDS when extrahepatic obstruction is absent. US, CT, and MR cholangiography should be used early because they are especially useful in identifying ductal dilation, gallbladder pathology, and focal hepatic lesions.

The indications for liver biopsy for the patient with suspected intrahepatic disease are limited. Although a specific diagnosis is likely in most patients, liver biopsy rarely identifies a previously undiagnosed OI, suggesting that the liver is rarely the site of disease not manifest elsewhere. This observation underscores the importance of reserving liver biopsy for those circumstances in which less invasive diagnostic methods such as blood cultures and bone marrow examination have not yielded a diagnosis.[92] Liver biopsy or elastography may play a role in the treatment decision for HCV therapy, as in the normal host. Focal hepatic lesions identified by abdominal imaging can be sampled under US or CT guidance. Use of transjugular liver biopsy may be favored over percutaneous biopsy in selected settings such as hemophilia. Specific infections or neoplasms are usually evident on tissue sections of appropriately stained biopsy material.

An extrahepatic cause for jaundice is suggested on CT or US by the presence of dilated bile ducts or other biliary and/or pancreatic abnormalities. Once extrahepatic obstruction is recognized, the possibility of papillary stenosis associated with AIDS cholangiopathy must be considered, as well as the possibility of choledocholithiasis or other disorders, depending on the imaging studies and clinical setting. Additional testing with CT, MRCP, or endoscopic US may better delineate the underlying cause, reserving ERCP for those in whom endoscopic therapy is planned. Bile duct, ampullary, and duodenal biopsy specimens or bile and/or biliary cytology (with appropriate staining) collected during ERCP can be examined for the presence of viruses, protozoa, or neoplastic cells.

Full references for this chapter can be found at https://ebooks.health.elsevier.com.

34 Gastrointestinal and Hepatic Complications of Solid Organ and Hematopoietic Cell Transplantation

David M. Hockenbery, Anne M. Larson

IN THIS CHAPTER

Transplantation of a solid organ is an immunologic mirror of the transplantation of allogeneic hematopoietic cells. Thus solid organs can be rejected by the patient in whom they are placed, whereas allogeneic hematopoietic cells can damage or "reject" the organs of their recipient. There are similarities in the intestinal and hepatic complications of these transplant procedures, particularly regarding infections and the side effects of immunosuppressive drugs. However, there are extreme differences in the patient populations being transplanted, in the preparation for transplant, and in the degree and length of immune suppression. For this reason, this chapter presents separate problem-oriented approaches to the complications of solid organ and hematopoietic cell transplantation (HCT).

COMPLICATIONS OF SOLID ORGAN TRANSPLANTATION

GI complaints after solid organ transplant (SOT) are reported in up to 40% of recipients, with a frequency as high as 60% reported in India. Most of the problems relate to opportunistic infections, graft dysfunction, adverse effects of medications, or malignancy[1–4] (Table 34.1). Infections in the setting of SOT are categorized into those occurring within the first 6 months after SOT and those after 6 months.[4] Infectious complications remain a major source of morbidity and mortality, particularly within the first 6 months after SOT.[5] Infection following the first 6 months, however, occurs in up to 16% of SOT recipients.[6] During the first month following SOT, infections include those present prior to transplant (e.g., urinary tract infection), those related to technical complications of the procedure itself (e.g., biliary sepsis), or those transmitted with the allograft. Opportunistic viral, fungal, and parasitic infections are more likely to develop after the first month, with herpesvirus infections being the most common (Fig. 34.1).[5] Universal prophylaxis—prophylactic antimicrobials, antivirals, and antifungals—may reduce the occurrence of these infections.[7,8] There are several noninfectious complications that can mimic infection (see Table 34.1).

Cytomegalovirus (CMV) is a ubiquitous viral infection, with rates of infection ranging from about half of the adults in the United States to over 95% across the globe.[9,10] CMV infection is the predominant viral pathogen occurring within the first year after SOT. Without antiviral prophylaxis, 40%–60% of seropositive recipients will develop viremia.[11] It can lead to significant morbidity, including allograft rejection and reduced graft survival and mortality.[12–15] Several factors predispose to the development of CMV infection[12,13]: (1) Increased immunosuppression, such as antilymphocyte antibody in addition to conventional immunosuppression or high-dose maintenance mycophenolate mofetil (MMF) therapy[5]; (2) CMV donor and recipient mismatch[12,13,16]; and (3) allograft rejection or coinfection with immunomodulating viruses (i.e., human herpesvirus [HHV]-6, HHV-7), bacteria, or fungi.[5,17] The peak incidence of CMV infection is generally 4–6 months after transplantation, once antiviral prophylaxis has been discontinued. Presentations include asymptomatic viremia, CMV syndrome (fevers, malaise, leukopenia, neutropenia, atypical lymphocytosis, elevated liver aminotransferases), and tissue-invasive disease (e.g., GI and hepatobiliary infection, pneumonitis, retinitis) (see Fig. 34.1).[9,18] Between 70% and 80% of cases of organ-invasive disease in SOT recipients are secondary to GI CMV.[19,20] Active disease can be identified in several ways, including quantitative CMV DNA testing, antigenemia, culture, histopathology, and immunologic assays, which reflect cellular immune response to CMV.[18,21] Quantitative CMV DNA testing is the preferred diagnostic testing method, due to its high sensitivity.[22] However, in the setting of GI disease, virus may not be detectable in the bloodstream in up to 50% of patients, and CMV must be recovered from intestinal or liver biopsy tissue.[23,24] The use of prevention strategies is standard of care in patients at risk.[22] The two main prevention strategies are posttransplant universal antiviral prophylaxis or preemptive therapy (treating if CMV viremia develops).[25,26] Both strategies are effective in minimizing the incidence of CMV-associated disease.[27,28] Clinical guidelines tend to favor prophylaxis over preemptive therapy in high risk recipients (D+/R−)[29]; however, preemptive therapy has been recently shown to decrease incidence of late-onset CMV in liver transplant recipients.[30] Ganciclovir, valacyclovir, or valganciclovir

TABLE 34.1 Causes of Intestinal and Hepatobiliary Disorders in Solid Organ Transplantation Recipients

	Esophageal Symptoms	Nausea, Vomiting, Anorexia	Abdominal Pain	GI Bleeding	Diarrhea	Malignancy	Hepatobiliary Disorders
Infections	*Candida albicans* Other fungal species CMV HSV (VZV) (*Mycobacterium tuberculosis*) (Parasites)	CMV HSV Hp-related ulcers (VZV) (*Giardia lamblia*) (Cryptosporidiosis) (Norovirus) (Rotavirus) (EBV-PTLD)	CMV *Clostridium difficile* Hp-related ulcers Perforation with abscess, peritonitis Acute cholecystitis (Viral pancreatitis) (VZV) (Fungal infection)	CMV Fungal infection (*Candida*, molds) Hp-related ulcers (EBV-PTLD) *C. difficile* (HSV esophagitis)	CMV Other viruses *C. difficile* (Parasites) (EBV-PTLD) (Enteric bacterial pathogens)	EBV-PTLD MALT lymphoma (Hp-related) (Kaposi sarcoma)	Sepsis-related cholestasis (cholangitis lenta) Herpesviruses (CMV, HSV, VZV, EBV) HBV HCV Abscess (fungal, bacterial)
Noninfectious causes	Acid reflux ± peptic stricture Pill esophagitis Thoracostomy tube	Medications Obstruction Uremia Dialysis Pancreatitis Hepatitis Cholecystitis Gastroparesis GVHD	Intestinal obstruction Pseudo-obstruction Narcotic bowel syndrome Immunosuppressive drugs Diverticulitis Ischemic colitis Appendicitis Acute pancreatitis (acute GVHD) Intestinal motility disorder (intestinal transplant) Biliary leak (LT)	NSAID gastroduodenal ulcers Peptic esophagitis Diverticulosis (especially KT) Ischemic colitis (especially KT) Biliary or Roux-en-Y anastomotic bleeding (LT) Liver biopsy (hemobilia caused by liver biopsy) Variceal bleeding (Acute GVHD)	Promotility drugs Immunosuppressive drugs (Sorbitol colitis) Ischemic colitis Mg^{++} salts Antibiotic-associated diarrhea	Lymphoma Skin cancer Colon cancer Recurrent HCC Lung cancer	Drug toxicity Vascular injury (LT) Nodular regenerative hyperplasia Biliary tract disease Recurrent hepatocellular carcinoma

*Conditions that are described in the literature but rarely seen are in parentheses.
GVHD, Graft-versus-host disease; *KT*, kidney transplant; *MALT*, mucosa-associated lymphoid tissue; *MMF*, mycophenolate mofetil; *PTLD*, posttransplant lymphoproliferative disorder; *VZV*, varicella-zoster virus.

In symptomatic HIV-infected patients and patients with AIDS, physical examination should include careful inspection of the skin and mucous membranes, as well as palpation of the lymph nodes. Visual inspection of the anus for ulcers, fissures, and masses should precede digital rectal examination. Palpation of the perianal area and buttocks for abscess should be performed. The presence of severe pain on rectal examination strongly suggests ulcerative disease, thrombosed hemorrhoids, or neoplasms. Palpation of the anal canal may reveal masses or fissures not otherwise evident. All patients with anorectal symptoms should have anoscopy and sigmoidoscopy (rigid or flexible) with mucosal biopsy. High-resolution anoscopy plays a vital role in follow-up to abnormal screening anal cytology. Evaluation under general anesthesia may be necessary when pain is severe. Specimens should be evaluated for evidence of neoplasm or infection; when appropriate, they should be examined with bacterial (including gonococcal and chlamydial), viral, and fungal cultures or nucleic acid amplification tests. CT scan may define the extent of disease if a neoplasm is identified. Healing of anorectal disease following surgical or medical therapy will largely be determined by the stage of HIV infection. The survival of patients with squamous cell cancer has improved in the ART era.[52]

GASTROINTESTINAL BLEEDING

OIs and neoplasms seen with AIDS can rarely cause GI bleeding (Box 33.5). However, the causes of upper GI bleeding in patients with HIV are most frequently due to disorders not linked to AIDS, including peptic ulcer disease; in contrast, the most common cause of lower GI bleeding in patients with AIDS is an OI, namely, CMV colitis.[53] Infections causing mucosal ulceration (e.g., CMV, HSV, and invasive enteric bacteria) are the most common etiologies of bleeding. Enteric lymphoma (e.g., Burkitt), Kaposi sarcoma lesions, or adenocarcinoma may ulcerate and bleed spontaneously, although most enteric Kaposi sarcoma lesions are asymptomatic.

The initial evaluation of GI bleeding in a patient with AIDS parallels the approach taken in patients without HIV infection (see Chapter 20). Endoscopy is preferred in all patients, especially those with severe immunodeficiency, given the likelihood of opportunistic diseases that require mucosal biopsy for diagnosis and because endoscopic therapy for hemostasis can be performed.

BOX 33.5 Differential Diagnosis of GI Bleeding in Patients With AIDS (Excluding Non-AIDS-Specific Diagnoses)

ESOPHAGUS

Candida spp.*
CMV*
HSV
Idiopathic ulcer

STOMACH

CMV*
Kaposi sarcoma*
Cryptosporidiosis
Lymphoma

SMALL INTESTINE

Kaposi sarcoma*
Lymphoma*
CMV
Salmonella spp.
Cryptosporidia spp.

COLON

CMV*
Kaposi sarcoma*
Entamoeba histolytica
Campylobacter jejuni
Clostridioides difficile
Shigella spp.
Idiopathic ulcerations
Lymphoma

*More frequent diagnosis.

HEPATOBILIARY DISEASE

Effective ART has markedly changed the causes, approach, and outcome of liver disease and abnormal liver biochemical tests in patients with HIV infection (Box 33.6). Hepatobiliary disease can broadly be classified into either hepatic parenchymal abnormalities, biliary abnormalities, or a combination of both. As noted earlier, liver disease has emerged as common non-AIDS-related causes of death; a third or more patients on HAART die from complications of liver disease.[54,55] In the modern ART era, the most common causes of parenchymal liver disease relate to viral hepatitis, most importantly chronic HCV, medication-related hepatotoxicity, fatty liver disease, and alcohol-related liver disease.

Drug-induced liver injury is the most prevalent cause of liver test abnormalities and is often related to the increasing array of antiretroviral medications. Before ART, drug hepatotoxicity was most commonly due to sulfonamides, and the increased frequency of adverse reactions to these medications is well recognized in AIDS. Use of additional prescription (or nonprescription) drugs, as well as herbal remedies, must always be considered, either individually or as potential drug-drug interactions, as a cause of abnormal liver chemistry tests.

BOX 33.6 Differential Diagnosis of Hepatomegaly and Elevated Biochemical Liver Test Levels in Patients With AIDS

HEPATIC PARENCHYMAL DISEASE

Infection

Hepatitis C*
Mycobacterium avium complex*
*Mycobacterium tuberculosis**
CMV
Bacillary peliosis hepatis (*Bartonella* sp.)
Cryptococcus spp.
Hepatitis B, D
Pneumocystis jirovecii
Microsporidia

Drugs[†]

Neoplasms

Lymphoma
Kaposi sarcoma

BILIARY TRACT DISEASE

Cholangitis

CMV*
Cryptosporidia*
Microsporidia
Neoplasm
Lymphoma*
Kaposi sarcoma

*More frequent diagnosis.
[†]Especially sulfonamides and protease inhibitors.

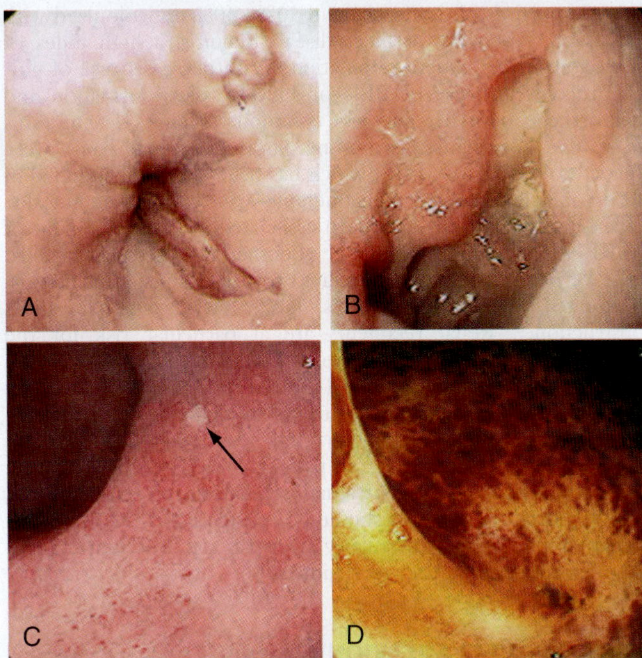

Fig. 34.1 Endoscopic photographs of intestinal infections following a solid organ transplant. (A) Distal esophageal ulcerations caused by cytomegalovirus (CMV). (B) Duodenal ulceration caused by HSV, with a deep, irregular ulcer surrounded by edematous mucosa. (C) Colon mucosa in CMV infection, showing focal ulceration (*arrow*) and pale ulceration and intramucosal hemorrhage in the surrounding mucosa. (D) Colonic mucosa in CMV infection with diffuse mucosal friability and ulceration.

significantly reduces the incidence of CMV disease in transplant recipients; the drug used depends on the organ transplanted. Valganciclovir is generally preferred, although it is not FDA approved in the United States for use in the setting of liver transplantation due to a higher rate of tissue-invasive disease seen in clinical trials. Ganciclovir-resistant CMV has been reported and is an emerging problem in management of CMV disease.[31] Letermovir has been approved for CMV prophylaxis in hematopoietic stem cell transplantation and is associated with less toxicity. Data in SOT look promising; however, the emergence of resistance has been reported.[32–34]

The herpes simplex viruses (HSV1/HHV-1 and SV2/HHV-2) and varicella-zoster virus (VZV/HHV-3) are the next most commonly seen viral infections and characteristically represent reactivation of latent virus within the recipient.[31,35–37] If antiviral prophylaxis is not used, manifestations of HSV or VZV infection can develop in up to 70% of transplant recipients.[36] HSV has tropism for squamous epithelium (nose, mouth, esophagus, and genital) but can involve the intestine, lungs, and liver if patients are not receiving prophylactic antiviral therapy (see Fig. 34.1B). Primary HSV infection is uncommon but is generally more severe and prolonged in the SOT recipient. HSV reactivation is common and often asymptomatic. Symptomatic lesions are similar to those seen in primary infection. Rarely, disseminated HSV can occur, presenting with fever, leukopenia, and hepatitis.[36] Primary VZV infection may also lead to end-organ damage. Fortunately, few adult SOT recipients are susceptible because only 2%–4% of adults are seronegative for VZV.[38] Reactivated disease most often presents as localized shingles, although severe disseminated disease is possible.[38] Up to 20% of SOT recipients will develop symptomatic infection.[31,39] Lung and heart recipients have the greatest risk, followed by liver and kidney recipients.[38–42] Prophylaxis with acyclovir, valacyclovir, valganciclovir, or famciclovir reduces recurrence of HSV and VZV following SOT.[43,44] There are reports of development of HSV antiviral drug resistance in up to 11% of immunocompromised hosts, but little data in the SOT setting.[31]

Infections caused by EBV and other human herpesviruses (HHV-6, -7, and -8) are less common. As with the other herpesviruses, EBV infection can be either primary or secondary. Clinical disease ranges from asymptomatic viremia to symptomatic disease, including infectious mononucleosis and posttransplant lymphoproliferative disorder (PTLD).[45] Primary infection is often symptomatic and associated with more significant disease .[46] The incidence of EBV-associated PTLD varies (0.6%–18%), depending on the organ transplanted and whether the recipient is an adult or a child.[47,48] PTLD continues to be a problem for SOT recipients who require continued high-level immune suppression; both B- and T-cell lymphomas can be seen (Fig. 34.2). HHV-6 causes clinical disease in fewer than 1%–2% of SOT recipients.[31,49–51] Primary infections are rare, and reactivation leads predominantly to subclinical, short-lived infection. It has been reported to cause GI disease.[52,53] Conclusive evidence of HHV-7 as a pathogen is lacking.[31,54] Both HHV-6 and -7 predispose the SOT recipient to other opportunistic infections. The role of antiviral prophylaxis in this setting has not been proven, and prophylaxis is currently not recommended.[31] HHV-8 is oncogenic and can lead to Kaposi sarcoma, Castleman disease, and primary effusion lymphomas (a form of non-Hodgkin lymphoma). HHV-8 may also cause a syndrome of fever, bone marrow suppression, and multiorgan failure.[31] Screening for these viruses has not been standardized.[55]

Fungal infections usually develop after the first month posttransplant, particularly among those who have discontinued antifungal prophylaxis. The incidence of fungal infection in SOT recipients is estimated to be less than 5%.[56,57] The most common fungi are candidal species (*Candida albicans*, *Candida tropicalis*), but molds, such as *Aspergillus* and Zygomycetes, are increasing in incidence.[37,58,59] Beyond the first 6 months following SOT, opportunistic fungal infections occur less frequently, but recipients remain at risk for community-acquired infections. Less common infections (*Histoplasmosis* [<1%], *Coccidioides* [1.5%–8.7%], *Nocardia*, *Pneumocystis*, *Toxoplasma*, and *Strongyloides*) also may occur after the first month.[52,60–62]

KIDNEY AND KIDNEY/PANCREAS TRANSPLANTATION

GI complications are among the most prevalent complications of kidney transplant (KT), seen in up to 50% of patients, and correlate with patient long-term survival.[63–65] It has been reported that KT patients who experience GERD or dyspepsia have an increased risk of graft loss and death, the mechanism of which is unclear.[66] Graft pancreatitis and graft duodenitis generally occur early after kidney/pancreas transplant (KPT) and may lead to intra-abdominal infection.[67,68] The frequency of HCV or HBV infection ranges from 5% to 66% of KT and KPT recipients, depending on country of origin.[69,70] The effect of HCV on patient and graft outcomes has been controversial.[71] Many have shown outcomes to be inferior in patients who are chronically infected with either HCV or HBV.[72–75] Cirrhotic patients who undergo KT have traditionally shown a significantly worse 10-year survival compared to noncirrhotics, with HCV cirrhotics faring worse than HBV cirrhotics. The appropriate use of combined kidney-liver transplantation in this setting remains debated. Both HBV and HCV antiviral therapies have significantly improved the clinical outcome of the KT and KPT recipients.[76]

Many serious infections reported in KT recipients are now less common because of more intense surveillance, anti-infective

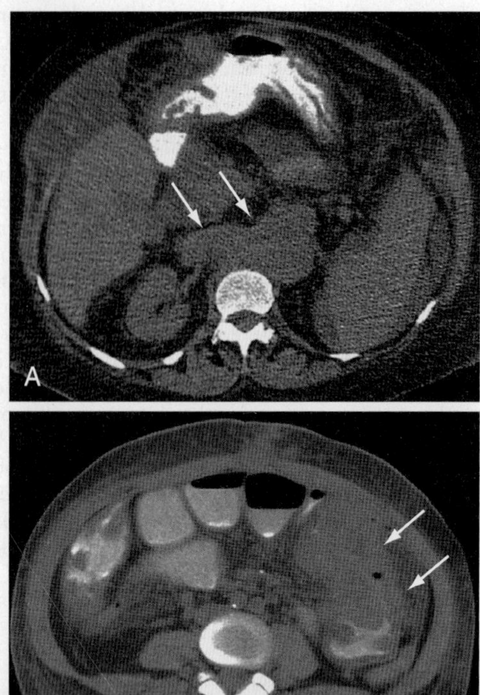

Fig. 34.2 Computed tomographic findings in lymphoproliferative disease following a solid organ transplant. (A) A retroperitoneal mass (*arrows*) following a liver transplant, caused by an EBV-positive B-cell lymphoma. (B) Distal small intestinal mass (*arrows*) following a renal transplant, caused by a T-cell lymphoma. The mass was causing intestinal obstruction, with dilated loops of small intestine seen proximal to the mass.

prophylaxis, and preemptive treatment of viral and fungal infections. However, if untreatable life-threatening infection should develop, immunosuppressive drugs can be discontinued, and the patient must be maintained on dialysis, if necessary. This option is unavailable to recipients of other organs. CMV infection is reported in up to 100% of patients after KT or KPT transplant, with a significant portion developing symptomatic disease.[77–79] Age and CMV serostatus (D+/R−) are significant risk factors for CMV disease. GI CMV infection is seen in up to about 50% of KT and KPT recipients, with pancreas recipients at greater risk owing to higher levels of immunosuppression.[20,69,80,81] EBV-associated PTLD has been reported in up to 10% following KT.[48] *Clostridium difficile* infection is reported in about 3.5% of adults following KT and 15.5% in KPT .[82] About 4% develop intestinal fungal infections, most often with candidal species, and parasitic infections must also be considered (*Enterocytozoon bieneusi, Strongyloides stercoralis, Cryptosporidium, Microsporidia*).[83,84] HSV infection post KT is generally asymptomatic and self-limited but may present as stomatitis, mononucleosis, hepatitis, or pneumonia.[85] Cholecystitis is seen in KT recipients, and the incidence is higher among diabetic patients.[86]

Historically, peptic ulcer disease and GI hemorrhage occurred in up to 20% of KT recipients. Although the incidence has decreased to about 5%, GI bleeding remains a significant cause of morbidity and mortality.[87,88] Surgical outcomes have improved from those seen in the past.[89,90] Many KT recipients with gastroduodenal ulcers will have no past history of gastroduodenal disease. Up to 40% will be asymptomatic, approximately 50% will have complaints of dyspepsia, and 30%−40% are colonized with *Hp*.[83,91,92] Discovery of ulcer disease requires a high index of suspicion in this patient population. With decreased use of glucocorticoids and use of PPIs or H2RAs, ulcer formation and hemorrhage have become less common.[3] Many GI symptoms (e.g., diarrhea, nausea, vomiting, and abdominal pain) were related to the use of MMF, which has been largely abandoned in favor of enteric-coated mycophenolic acid, with fewer gut side effects.[93,94] MMF has also been associated with development of MMF-related colitis.[95] An acute abdomen may be seen in up to 10% of patients and can be related to pancreatitis, cholecystitis, perforated ulcer, diverticulitis, appendicitis, and intestinal obstruction.[96] Renal recipients are at particular risk for the development of intestinal ischemia compared with other SOT recipients. The incidence is low (<5%), however, and the etiology is multifactorial.[97] Recipients with polycystic kidney disease more often develop intestinal ischemia and obstruction.[98] This group also has a higher percentage of patients with diverticular disease and complications.[83,98,99] Intestinal ischemia in this setting carries a high mortality. Ischemia should be considered in KT recipients with abdominal pain, particularly older patients (>40 years of age) who have received a cadaveric kidney.[97]

LIVER TRANSPLANTATION

As also discussed in Chapter 97, GI complications unique to orthotopic liver transplantation (OLT) are generally related to the surgery itself and include intra-abdominal hemorrhage, hepatic arterial stenosis or thrombosis, biliary tract dysfunction, bowel perforation, bowel obstruction, and GI bleeding.[100] Hepatic artery thrombosis develops in 1%−9% of adult recipients and presents with a spectrum of consequences, ranging from mildly elevated liver enzymes with or without fever to acute hepatic failure necessitating urgent retransplantation.[101–103] Moreover, the biliary tree receives its entire blood supply from the hepatic artery following OLT, and loss of this arterial flow results in bile duct necrosis and leakage, with development of intrahepatic bilomas and abscesses (Fig. 34.3A and B).[104,105] Gradual loss of hepatic arterial flow can also result in hepatic ductopenia, which is indistinguishable from ductopenic rejection. Hepatic artery stenosis is less common. Pseudoaneurysms of the hepatic artery are rare (1%−2%).[106]

Portal vein thrombosis has been reported in up to 12% of transplants and can lead to hepatic ischemia and severe hepatic dysfunction if it occurs early in the posttransplant course; later, signs of portal hypertension develop. Portal vein thrombosis and stenosis are now less common, with an incidence of 1%−3%. Rarely, hepatic vein thrombosis and inferior vena cava thrombosis or stenosis can create a Budd-Chiari-like syndrome.

Biliary complications are the most common cause of morbidity after OLT, ranging from 5% to 30%.[107–109] Bile leakage (7.1% −11.8%), with bilomas, and stricture formation, generally at the anastomotic site, are the most common of the biliary abnormalities (see (Fig. 34.3A and B).[107–110] Anastomotic strictures account for up to 80% of stricturing disease. They generally present within 2−6 months post OLT but can occur in the newly transplanted patient as well. Strictures and leaks in patients with duct-to-duct anastomoses are often amenable to endoscopic therapy, whereas those with choledochojejunostomies may require percutaneous or surgical correction. Endoscopic stenting of anastomotic strictures carries a resolution rate of 94%−100%.[111] Nonanastomotic strictures raise the concern of hepatic artery insufficiency and are associated with graft loss up to 46%.[112,113] Biliary casts may develop in up to 6% of recipients and generally occur within the first year post OLT.[54,114] Clinical factors associated with development of biliary casts include hepatic ischemia and biliary strictures. Endoscopic and percutaneous therapy are

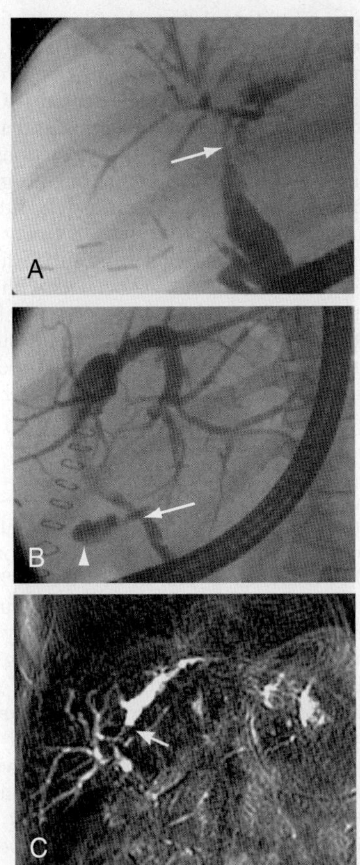

Fig. 34.3 Hepatobiliary imaging following a liver transplant. (A) Endoscopic retrograde cholangiogram showing an ischemic stricture (*arrow*) of the bile duct following the transplant. (B) Endoscopic retrograde cholangiogram showing a bile leak (*arrowhead*) at the biliary anastomosis (*arrow*) following transplant. (C) Magnetic resonance cholangiogram of the intrahepatic biliary system showing recurrent sclerosing cholangitis in the liver graft. The *arrow* points to a stricture, with upstream biliary dilatation.

successful in up to 70%, but surgical intervention may be required, and mortality has been reported at 10%–30%.[54,115]

Infection is the most common cause of morbidity and mortality post OLT, seen in up to 75% of recipients.[116] Immediately following transplant, hospital-acquired infections and wound infections can be seen (accounting for approximately 70% of tissue-invasive CMV in this population). GI CMV infection is reported in up to 40% of liver recipients.[20] CMV hepatitis is the most common manifestation of CMV post OLT and is more severe in OLT recipients than in recipients of other organs.[117,118] Patients often have elevations in serum aminotransferases, which can be confused with rejection; therefore liver biopsy is essential for diagnosis. The diagnosis can usually be confirmed by the detection of CMV DNA in the bloodstream.[119] Asymptomatic low-level CMV viremia usually does not require antiviral therapy but must be followed closely.[120] The incidence of EBV-associated PTLD is 1% in adult recipient, with EBV seronegative recipients at 3.5-fold higher risk.[121] Cohort studies have reported a 1-year rate of invasive fungal disease of 4%–8% in SOT recipients.[122] OLT recipients more often develop invasive fungal infections than other SOT recipients, with a high mortality. In the absence of antifungal prophylaxis, invasive infections occur in up to 42% of recipients, and *Candida* and *Aspergillus* species account for the majority.[123,124] Nonalbicans *Candida* species are becoming more common. A serum galactomannan assay is useful for detecting mold infections, particularly invasive aspergillosis.[125,126] Invasive fungi are becoming increasingly resistant to antifungal therapy. Acute pancreatitis is rare but has been reported in up to 5.7% of OLT recipients and carries a high mortality (up to 64%).[54,127]

There is a risk for recurrence of the underlying liver disease following OLT, including HCV, HBV, autoimmune hepatitis, NASH, PBC, and PSC (see Fig. 34.3C).[128–131] Recurrence of HCV in the liver allograft is nearly universal (see Chapters 80 and 97). Historically, this led to significant increased graft loss.[132–135] With the development of multiple highly effective direct-acting antiviral (DAA) drugs, however, this is no longer an issue. In fact, the use of HCV-infected donor organs in noninfected recipients is becoming more common with cure of the infection following transplant.[121] HBV recurrence may be prevented with the use of a low dose, short course of hepatitis B immune globulin (HBIG) and antiviral medications. Life-long antiviral therapy is undertaken to reduce HBV viral relapse. PBC and PSC recur in about one-third of patients post OLT (see Chapter 99).[129] OLT recipients are susceptible to SARS-CoV-2 infection with an incidence of COVID-19 of 0.1%–1.25% with mortality reported up to 23%.

HEART, LUNG, AND HEART-LUNG TRANSPLANTATION

Up to half of heart (HT), lung (LT), and heart-lung transplantation (HLT) recipients experience GI complications, with up to 50% requiring surgery.[136–140] The most common complications include diarrhea, GERD, dyspepsia, nausea and vomiting, abdominal pain, acute abdomen, pancreatitis, herpesvirus infections (especially CMV), cholelithiasis, ulcers, and hepatobiliary disease.[136,137,141] Biliary disorders have been reported in up to 40% of patients, and they carry a high mortality with surgical intervention.[140,142,143] GERD and gastroparesis are particularly problematic after LT or HLT and may be related to medications and vagal nerve injury during the operation.[136,144–149] Symptomatic gastroparesis has been described in 25% of LT recipients and up to 80% of HLT recipients.[150–152] The course is often waxing and waning, suggesting a neuropathic, infectious (CMV), or medication-induced etiology.[152,153] Recipients with GERD and/or gastroparesis are at particular risk for the development of bronchiolitis obliterans syndrome, which significantly threatens the longevity of LT recipients.[144,151,152] PPIs can be used to help control reflux; however, if reflux disease is unremitting, laparoscopic fundoplication may be successful.[154–156]

LT recipients may develop giant gastric ulcers (>3 cm in diameter), which occur despite routine use of acid suppression. These ulcers carry significant morbidity and mortality and are more often associated with bilateral LT, use of high-dose NSAIDs after transplant, acute rejection requiring high-dose glucocorticoids, and cyclosporine immunosuppression.[138] For this reason, some authors believe NSAIDs should not be used in the posttransplant setting. Recipients of LT and HT more often develop CMV infection (15%–25%) than other SOT recipients. Generally, CMV infection presents as pneumonitis, but GI CMV infection remains a major cause of morbidity (see Fig. 34.1).[16] LT and HLT recipients have the highest incidence of fungal infection in the SOT setting, and noncandidal species predominate.[157–159]

Patients undergoing LT for CF experience a unique set of GI complications.[160] Pancreatic insufficiency, a marker for severe CF, is common. CF-induced secondary biliary cirrhosis can complicate absorption of immunosuppressive medications such as cyclosporine. If severe liver disease is detected prior to LT, lung-liver transplant can be considered. Distal intestinal obstruction syndrome occurs in up to 10% and is similar to the incidence in CF in the nontransplant setting.[161] CF patients may also experience cholecystitis, PUD, and GERD.[162]

Primary HCV infection following HT previously led to significantly increased 1- and 3-year mortality. With newer antiviral medications now available for hepatitis C virus infection, this will become less of an issue. Acquisition of HBV following HT does not appear to affect survival, at least up to 5 years.[163,164]

INTESTINAL TRANSPLANTATION

Most complications are related to underlying diseases, graft rejection, intestinal ischemia, and anastomotic leaks. Bacterial and fungal infections are common, often associated with mucosal disruption following surgery, but a source may not be identifiable. Two types of malignancy related to intense immune suppression have been reported: EBV-lymphoproliferative disease (LPD) and de novo cancers of nonlymphomatous origin.[165,166] Surveillance for EBV DNA and preemptive treatment by reducing immunosuppression or using rituximab reduces the frequency of LPD. Altered intestinal motility and anorexia have been reported. SOT graft-versus-host disease (GVHD) is seen in up to 9%–10% of intestinal transplant recipients.[167]

PROBLEM-ORIENTED APPROACH TO DIAGNOSIS IN SOLID ORGAN TRANSPLANTATION RECIPIENTS

Upper Intestinal Symptoms and Signs

The approach to SOT patients with esophageal or gastric symptoms is influenced by a high frequency of nonspecific symptoms as harbingers of serious infection (e.g., CMV infection presenting as nausea and vomiting) and by the rapidity with which disease can progress. GERD is the most common cause of heartburn and mid-chest pain, particularly following LT, but viral and fungal esophagitis may underlie these symptoms, particularly after antimicrobial prophylaxis has been discontinued. Candidal esophagitis is seen with high frequency in those with diabetes; other risk factors include use of broad-spectrum antibiotics, high-dose immunosuppression, and the presence of a Roux-en-Y anastomosis in OLT recipients. Severe necrotizing fungal esophagitis can lead to perforation, which can have a fatal outcome in up to one-third of cases. Odynophagia, dysphagia, or hematemesis should lead to consideration of an esophageal infection; herpesviruses (CMV, HSV) and fungal species (*Candida*) are responsible for the largest proportion, but unusual organisms can be seen.[168] Dysphagia secondary to pill esophagitis may develop in SOT recipients who are ingesting antibiotics, antivirals, potassium chloride, bisphosphonates, NSAIDs, and iron pills. Esophageal strictures following severe esophageal infection have been reported and may present long after eradication of the organism.

Anorexia, nausea, and/or vomiting are common following SOT, particularly early in the posttransplant course.[65,136,137] These symptoms are often related to herpesvirus infections or medications (including immunosuppressive drugs); thus endoscopic evaluation is necessary for diagnosis in most patients. Tacrolimus is a macrolide lactone that can cause nausea, abdominal pain, and diarrhea, often leading to anorexia, food aversion, and weight loss. These side effects are dose-dependent and can be managed with dose reduction or, more rarely, drug discontinuation. Sirolimus (Rapamune), also a macrolide immunosuppressant, has a GI side-effect profile similar to tacrolimus. MMF is an inhibitor of nucleic acid synthesis with well-described GI side effects of nausea, vomiting, and diarrhea, often requiring dosing modifications. The formulation of mycophenolic acid delayed-release tablets has significantly fewer GI side effects, with similar therapeutic efficacy.[93,94,169] Less common causes of anorexia and nausea include pancreatitis, cholecystitis, or cystitis.

Rarely following SOT (~1%) and within the first 2–6 weeks after transplantation, GVHD presents with fever, rash, and GI symptoms, particularly nausea, vomiting, and diarrhea.[170,171] Endoscopic evaluation with biopsy is essential if GVHD is suspected and skin lesions are absent, recognizing that other conditions, such as viral infections and drug reactions, can have a GVHD-like histologic pattern.[172] Symptomatic gastroparesis is frequently seen in the setting of LT but is less often reported in the setting of other SOT.[152] CMV and VZV may rarely involve intestinal neural plexuses, leading to intestinal dilation or gastroparesis. *Hp* infection may be associated with symptomatic dyspepsia, gastritis, and gastroduodenal ulceration, but there is no relationship between the use or degree of immunosuppression and *Hp* colonization; its incidence is similar to that seen in the nontransplant setting.[2] *Hp* infection is common in dialysis and KT patients.[83]

Diarrhea and Constipation

Colonic and small bowel complications (diverticulitis, ischemic colitis, malignancy, and infections) have been reported following all types of SOT. Diarrhea is seen in between 20% and 50% of patients.[173] Early in the posttransplant setting, infections predominate, and diarrhea may be accompanied by fever (37%), abdominal pain (46%), nausea (32%), and vomiting (22%).[174–176] The microbes predominantly responsible are CMV and *C. difficile*, but the literature describes a wide range of organisms in SOT recipients, particularly when they are cared for in infection-endemic areas [e.g., adenovirus, norovirus, rotavirus, coxsackievirus, bacterial enteric pathogens, enterohemorrhagic *Escherichia coli*, *Yersinia enterocolitica*, *Giardia lamblia*, *Candida* species, cryptosporidia, microsporidia (*E. bieneusi*), *Isospora belli*, *S. stercoralis*].[175–177] Bacterial intestinal tract infections occur more often if the patient also has concomitant systemic CMV.[82] Diagnosis can be made by examination of stool specimens in nearly all cases; the exceptions are CMV, certain parasites, and EBV-associated lymphoproliferative disorders (EBV-LPD). Small intestinal involvement with CMV often causes profuse watery diarrhea with protein-losing enteropathy, particularly if the diagnosis is delayed. Colonic involvement may appear as an inflammatory colitis resulting in bloody diarrhea and is often associated with fever, abdominal distention, and pain.[178,179] Diagnosis of colonic CMV requires mucosal biopsy, particularly if blood specimens are negative for CMV DNA or antigen. *C. difficile* occurs in 2%–30% of hospitalized SOT recipients, a greater incidence than in the general hospitalized population (1%–3%).[173,180] The most important risk factor in development of *C. difficile* is the use of antimicrobials. Additional risk factors include age over 55 years, use of antithymocyte globulin (ATG), retransplantation, and type of organ (greatest in OLT).[177,181] *C. difficile* infection may present with a more severe course post SOT; patients with fulminant colitis, intestinal obstruction, abscess, and toxic megacolon require prompt surgical intervention to prevent perforation and peritonitis.[175,177] Signs of colitis may be subtle and are because of concomitant immune suppression. Treatment is discussed in Chapter 114. Recurrence may develop in up to 20% of cases, and mortality rates range between 2.3% and 8.5%.[173,177,182]

The use of certain probiotics (e.g., *Saccharomyces boulardii*) in SOT recipients remains controversial because there have been reports of yeast dissemination and infection in the immunocompromised host.[183,184] However, it appears that the use of bacterial probiotics may help prevent infection,[185] and transplantation of normal colonic bacterial flora can be useful in treating recurrent *C. difficile* colitis (see Chapter 114). Intestinal fungal infections can be seen in up to 25% of SOT recipients. In the absence of prophylaxis, intestinal fungal overgrowth and diarrhea can result from antibiotic use or intestinal dysmotility. Common parasitic infections must also be considered in an immunocompromised host, particularly in areas of high endemicity. The protozoa and metazoan parasites are a much less frequent cause of acute diarrhea post SOT but must be considered. Microsporidia (*E. bieneusi*) is a more rarely reported cause of chronic diarrhea, perhaps reflecting the fact that it is often not sought out in the post-SOT setting.[186] Clinically, patients with this infection experience fatigue, intermittent diarrhea, and weight loss. There are no clearly effective therapies for *E. bieneusi*. Symptoms of colitis or toxic megacolon are most often associated with infection, but in up to 20% of cases, no clear etiology can be found.[175,187] Early recognition, diagnosis, and treatment of colitis can decrease disease-associated mortality. There are reports of donor-transmitted infections with *S. stercoralis*, which carries a high mortality rate. This pathogen should be considered when donors hail from endemic regions. Eosinophilic colitis with diarrhea has been reported with the use of both tacrolimus and cyclosporine. Histologically, this is characterized by eosinophilic colonic infiltrates and peripheral eosinophilia; elevated serum immunoglobulin (Ig) E may be present in some patients. Colonoscopy is generally only needed if noninvasive testing for infectious causes is unrevealing. Intestinal GVHD and PTLD must be considered in those patients in whom an infectious etiology cannot be found.

Drug-related diarrhea is seen in up to two-thirds of SOT patients, most commonly with tacrolimus or sirolimus.[175,176,188,189] MMF causes watery diarrhea in up to 30% of patients and may require dose reduction or discontinuation. The mechanism of MMF-induced diarrhea is unclear. It is dose dependent and may be related inhibition of de novo purine synthesis within the enterocyte. Histology shows focal inflammatory lesions similar to GVHD with loss of villous architecture of the duodenum.[190] The use of enteric-coated mycophenolic acid has decreased this side effect. ATG and anti-T-cell antibody (OKT3) therapies are both associated with diarrhea, which predictably lasts for 3–4 days and resolves spontaneously. Most cases of immunosuppressant-induced diarrhea can be managed with dose manipulation, but some are so severe that the discontinuation of the immunosuppressant is required. Diarrhea can also be caused by magnesium-containing preparations prescribed to correct renal magnesium wasting and by antibiotics prescribed either prophylactically or therapeutically. Noninfectious diarrhea has been reported to increase the risk of graft loss and mortality.[188]

Constipation is seen in less mobile SOT recipients who are receiving certain medications (e.g., narcotics, calcium- and aluminum-containing antacids, and anticholinergics). The constipation is generally responsive to increased patient mobility, decreased use of narcotics, use of methylnaltrexone in those receiving narcotics,[191] and therapy with polyethylene glycol laxatives and senna.

Abdominal Pain

Abdominal complications are common following SOT, affecting up to 30% of patients.[191] Symptoms may be mild despite the presence of life-threatening complications. All patients with abdominal pain should be aggressively evaluated, with attention as to whether the patient requires urgent surgery or a specific medical treatment. Most recipients with abdominal pain will not need surgery.

The intra-abdominal conditions presenting with pain that require urgent surgery are abscess, perforation, severe colitis, appendicitis, intestinal obstruction, intestinal ischemia, and acute cholecystitis. These disorders may appear in the early posttransplant period. Immunosuppression may mask symptoms and suppress the host response, leading to a delay in diagnosis and an increase in mortality. Most transplant patients with acute appendicitis will have typical right lower quadrant pain, although complications are more frequent.[192] Overall, intestinal perforation occurs in fewer than 5% of SOT recipients, although the incidence may be slightly higher in the setting of lung transplant.[63,193] Perforation may occur spontaneously without clear etiology, but it is associated with colon diverticula in up to two-thirds of cases (particularly kidney recipients) and ischemia in 15%. Perforation, especially diverticular, carries a high mortality.[97,178] Risk factors for the development of colonic perforation include diverticular disease, immunosuppression (particularly glucocorticoids), CMV infection, fungal infections (e.g., mucormycosis), unrecognized lymphoma (EBV-LPD), colon cancer, and ischemia.[2,178] Abdominal x-rays and CT can confirm the presence of perforation but may not reveal its source before surgery. Diverticular perforation is especially common after renal transplant, often leading to abscess formation and fistulization, sometimes without causing severe pain or findings of peritonitis. Pretransplant colonic screening in patients younger than 50 years does not predict posttransplant colonic perforations. SOT recipients are also at increased risk for the development of cholelithiasis.[194] Factors related to gallstones include cyclosporine, obesity, and CF as an underlying disorder. Abdominal pain is frequently associated with tissue-invasive CMV disease. CMV may also cause focal ulceration, perforation, high-grade stricture, and intestinal obstruction (see Fig. 34.1) while generally producing a diffuse pattern of mucosal edema. The first manifestation of disseminated VZV infection is often severe abdominal pain related to pseudo-obstruction and visceral neuropathy. Early treatment of both CMV and VZV infections results in improved survival.

Abdominal pain may also be a manifestation of transplant-related complications that do not usually have a dire outcome. Generalized abdominal pain has been reported with oral tacrolimus, sirolimus, and MMF. Abdominal pain secondary to MMF is seen in up to 19% of those receiving it and can significantly limit its use.[195,196] The etiology of MMF-induced pain has been postulated to involve inflammatory ulcers (seen at endoscopy), as well as interference with rapidly dividing intestinal cells, a hypothesis supported by studies showing fewer GI complications with delayed-release mycophenolic acid compared to MMF.[93,94,169] Narcotic- or anticholinergic-induced pseudo-obstruction is common after surgery. Care must be taken to rule out an infectious etiology such as CMV or VZV, both of which can involve the intestinal nerve plexuses.[2] Noninfectious pseudo-obstruction often can be managed conservatively, with nasogastric decompression, vigorous correction of electrolyte imbalance, and withdrawal of opiates. Mu-agonist opioid-related gut symptoms can also be blocked with the use of methylnaltrexone without interfering with central pain relief.[191] Neostigmine can be safely used for treatment of pseudo-obstruction in the transplant setting.[178] Surgical intervention may be required in the setting of massive colon dilation. Acute pancreatitis has been reported in 1%–2% of renal transplant recipients, up to 6% of LT recipients, and up to 18% of HT recipients; it may have a fatal outcome.[197] Acute pancreatitis is associated with CMV infection, hypercalcemia, cholelithiasis, biliary manipulation, malignancy, recent alcohol ingestion, and medications such as azathioprine, cyclosporine, tacrolimus, and glucocorticoids. Treatment of pancreatitis in the posttransplant setting is identical to that in the nontransplant setting, except for the need to exclude CMV infection and some immunosuppressive medications (see Chapter 58).

Pneumatosis intestinalis may be discovered during abdominal imaging after SOT as an incidental finding but can also be a manifestation of life-threatening intestinal ischemia or infection with a gas-forming organism.[198] Pneumatosis intestinalis can be associated with CMV infection, *C. difficile* colitis, and sepsis and can be seen in patients receiving glucocorticoid therapy. Most patients require no specific intervention, and the gas collections resolve spontaneously unless caused by ischemia or an infection with a clostridial organism.[198]

Gastrointestinal Bleeding

When GI bleeding occurs, it is often secondary to infectious ulcers. Noninfectious causes of hemorrhage include NSAID-induced gastroduodenal ulcers, diverticular bleeding, anastomotic bleeding, and ischemic colitis. The current incidence of gastroduodenal ulcer disease in the transplant population is now about 5%, with perforation rates of less than 1%.[3] Prophylaxis with H2RAs or PPIs decreases the occurrence of ulcer disease in this population; these two therapies are equally effective in KT recipients.[3] Patients infected with *Hp* prior to transplantation are more likely to develop PUD following transplant.[199] In the absence of effective antiviral prophylaxis, viral ulcerations are the most common cause of GI bleeding. HSV-associated esophageal ulcers may present with severe bleeding even in the absence of esophageal symptoms. CMV can lead to ulceration throughout the entire intestinal tract. Whereas CMV esophageal ulcers are usually shallow (see Fig. 34.1A), ulcers in the stomach or intestine can be deep, erode into vessels, and lead to severe bleeding. CMV can also cause diffuse colonic inflammation resembling that seen in IBD (see Fig. 34.1C and D). VZV and EBV are much less often associated with GI bleeding. Although EBV itself does not cause mucosal ulceration, EBV-associated LPD can form mucosal tumors that can ulcerate and bleed (see Fig. 34.2). Massive bleeding has been reported in the setting of invasive fungal infection.[200]

Gastrointestinal Malignancy

PTLD, lymphoid proliferations, or lymphomas associated with EBV infection occur in up to 20% of transplant recipients.[45,201] Although most PTLD is of B-cell origin, T-cell lymphoma has been reported.[202] The incidence of PTLD is organ specific with small ranging from up to 32% (small intestinal recipients), 3%−12% (pancreas, heart, lung, and liver recipients), to 1%–2% (renal recipients).[203] EBV reactivation generally presents in the early posttransplant setting as a mononucleosis-like syndrome with diffuse adenopathy and fever; detection of EBV DNA in the bloodstream may allow preemptive therapy, with lower doses of immune suppression or treatment with rituximab.[204] PTLD manifesting later than a year after transplant is more insidious, often presenting with extranodal disease or visceral involvement. GI PTLD can present with diarrhea, intestinal obstruction (see Fig. 34.2B), bleeding, or perforation. Mucosa-associated lymphoid tissue–type lymphomas have also been reported in the posttransplant setting.[205] Fortunately, they often respond to reduction in immunosuppression, antibiotics (if associated with *Hp*), surgery, or chemotherapy (see Chapter 41).

The risk of cancer in long-lived transplant recipients is higher than in the general population, particularly for lymphomas, skin cancers, colon and anal cancers, head and neck cancers, and Kaposi sarcoma.[206,207] Patients who underwent OLT for cirrhosis secondary to PSC are at high risk for the development of colonic dysplasia and diffuse colon cancer related to underlying ulcerative colitis.[208] If severe dysplasia is discovered, colectomy can be performed safely as early as 10–12 weeks following transplant.

Hepatobiliary Complications

Drug-induced hepatotoxicity can be problematic after SOT because this diagnosis is often one of exclusion. Azathioprine hepatotoxicity presents as an elevation in serum aminotransferase enzyme levels in up to 10% of recipients; injury is generally cholestatic with centrilobular hepatocyte damage. A less common presentation is the slow, insidious development of sinusoidal obstruction syndrome (SOS; formerly veno-occlusive disease), which often manifests as portal hypertension, usually regressing following withdrawal of the drug. Azathioprine is used less often now following organ transplant, having been largely replaced by mycophenolic acid. Cyclosporine- or tacrolimus-induced cholestasis can occur when their blood levels are high. Sirolimus has been reported to cause dose-dependent elevations in serum aminotransferase levels. Transplant recipients are exposed to numerous other pharmacologic agents that, alone or in combination, can produce cholestasis, fatty liver, hepatitis, or a mixed histologic picture.

Bacterial sepsis can have profound effects on liver function (see Chapter 75), with severe cholestasis the most common finding (a syndrome sometimes called *cholangitis lenta* or *hyperbilirubinemia of sepsis*).[209] CMV infection may lead to elevations in hepatic enzymes, with either a cholestatic or hepatocellular picture. CMV hepatitis is more frequent and severe in LT recipients compared to recipients of other organs.[117] VZV and HSV infections can lead to hepatitis and fulminant liver failure.[36,85] EBV hepatitis is seen in 2%–3% after SOT but is generally mild. Primary or recurrent disease with either HCV or HBV can lead to liver disease in the posttransplant setting. These viruses may also be passaged by any solid organ. Fortunately, antiviral therapy for both has improved outcomes significantly.[135] The treatment of HCV in the posttransplant setting has improved greatly with development of DAAs, curing up to 98%–99% of recipients.[210] In fact, at the time of this writing, the success of these medications has led to the consideration of the use of HCV viremic donors for HCV-negative recipients.[121,211,212] Chronic HBV carriers (hepatitis B surface antigen–positive recipients) may develop a flare following transplant if not treated with serum HBIG and antiviral agents (see Chapter 81).

Vascular injury associated with OLT may lead to liver dysfunction. Nodular regenerative hyperplasia with subsequent portal hypertension and peliosis hepatis has both been reported following renal transplantation.

Organ transplant recipients, particularly those with LT, are at high risk for biliary tract disease. Presentation includes acalculous cholecystitis, gallbladder sludge, thickened gallbladder wall, dilated bile ducts, or cholelithiasis.[143] Diseases of gallbladder and biliary necessitating cholecystectomy have a posttransplant incidence of 1%–6%. Emergent cholecystectomy in the posttransplant setting carries a high mortality (29%).[143] However, pretransplant biliary screening and prophylactic cholecystectomy remain controversial. The etiology of biliary tract disease is multifactorial, including obesity, use of TPN, fasting, biliary strictures, and medications. Cyclosporine, excreted in the bile where it may precipitate, has been implicated in an increased incidence of cholelithiasis and cholangitis.[86,213] Some centers recommend that biliary calculi be removed prior to transplantation or immediately upon discovery after transplantation.

Patients who have undergone OLT for hepatocellular carcinoma are at risk for recurrence in the graft, particularly if the lesions were multiple or large prior to transplant. PTLD may also involve the liver.

COMPLICATIONS OF HEMATOPOIETIC CELL TRANSPLANTATION

HCT uses one of three sources of hematopoietic and immune cells: bone marrow, peripheral blood hematopoietic cells, or cord blood.[214] Transplanted cells can be one's own (autologous HCT), from an identical twin (syngeneic HCT), or from another person (allogeneic HCT). Allogeneic cells can come from a sibling who is HLA matched with the recipient, from a family member who is half-matched with the recipient (haploidentical HCT), from an HLA-matched unrelated donor, or from an HLA-mismatched unrelated donor (as with cord blood donors).[215] HCT differs from SOT in three important ways: (1) The indication for HCT often involves a potentially fatal malignancy, bone marrow failure (aplastic anemia), a congenital immune deficiency, or a genetic hematologic disorder such as thalassemia or sickle cell disease; (2) preparation for HCT requires either high-dose myeloablative therapy or intense immune suppression, resulting in extreme susceptibility to infection and, with some preparative regimens, damage to the liver, kidneys, lungs, and heart; and (3) recipients of allogeneic donor cells commonly develop acute and chronic GVHD (cGVHD). HCT patients face combined morbidity from the toxicity of chemotherapy drugs, infections, acute and cGVHD, and recurrent malignancy.[214] GI and hepatic complications of HCT have now become far less frequent, and some past problems have disappeared.[214,216,217] Guides to the sometimes arcane HCT terminology and abbreviations can be useful to those unfamiliar with HCT.[218]

Evaluation of Intestinal and Liver Disorders Before Hematopoietic Cell Transplantation

Ulcers and Tumors in the Intestinal Tract

In immunocompromised patients who are candidates for HCT, mucosal ulcers may have an infectious etiology that requires specific antimicrobial treatment.[219] CMV, *Entamoeba histolytica*, and *C. difficile* are infectious causes of colonic ulceration that may mimic IBD. Intestinal ulcerations should be healed before the start of conditioning therapy to avoid major bleeding during post-HCT thrombocytopenia. Patients with ulcerative colitis and Crohn disease have undergone both allogeneic and autologous HCT without complications of bleeding, perforation, or dissemination of unusual microorganisms .[220] Long-term resolution of Crohn's disease has been observed following myeloablative allogeneic HCT, and autologous HCT has resulted in improvement as well.[221] Monogenic autoimmune syndromes, including many patients with very early onset IBD, can be cured after allogeneic HCT.[222] Any recent history of GI bleeding should prompt both colonoscopy and upper endoscopy before HCT. Endoscopic biopsy may be required for staging some malignant disorders with a predilection for gut involvement (e.g., mantle cell lymphoma; see Chapter 41).

Diarrhea

Patients with diarrhea should be investigated for organisms that may cause morbidity after HCT (*E. histolytica*, *S. stercoralis*, *G. lamblia*, cryptosporidia, microsporidia, clostridia, CMV, rotavirus, norovirus, adenovirus).[223,224] Many, but not all, of these pathogens are included in multiplex molecular panels now available, and specific therapy is available for clostridia, CMV, adenovirus, amebiasis, giardiasis, strongyloidiasis, and other helminths, and microsporidia.[225] Cryptosporidiosis is resistant to therapy in an immunosuppressed patient, but restoration of normal immunity after allogeneic HCT can result in clearance of cryptosporidia.[226] Typhlitis is a syndrome of cecal edema, mucosal barrier injury, and ulceration in neutropenic patients, often associated with polymicrobial sepsis; its cause is usually an intestinal clostridial infection, particularly with *Clostridium septicum*.[227] After treatment and recovery, the risk of post-HCT typhlitis is similar to other patients.

Perianal Pain

Pain near the anal canal in a granulocytopenic patient is due to bacterial infection until proved otherwise. Administration of broad-spectrum antibiotics with anaerobic coverage is adequate treatment in most cases, with surgical incision and drainage reserved for progressive infections.[228] Extensive supralevator and intersphincteric abscesses may be present without being apparent on external examination but can be diagnosed by CT, MRI, or transperineal sonography.[229] Proctitis and genital ulcers due to HSV and CMV infections may also lead to perianal pain.[230]

Fungal Liver Infections

Diagnosis depends on liver imaging (high-resolution CT or MRI) in conjunction with fungal biomarkers (galactomannan and glucan assays), PCR, or culture of liver biopsy material.[231] Fungal liver infection should be treated with echinocandins that offer reduced toxicity, fewer drug-drug interactions, and a broader range of coverage than older drugs.[232] A fully engrafted patient can then clear intractable fungal liver abscesses after HCT.

Viral Hepatitis in Allogeneic Hematopoietic Cell Transplant Donors

Donors who are viremic with HBV or HCV will likely transmit virus to their recipients. When two equally HLA-matched donors are available, the uninfected donor is preferred. If the most suitable donor has chronic hepatitis B, treating that donor and recipient with entecavir or tenofovir and passive or active immunization of the recipient may prevent passage of virus.[233] HBsAg-negative, anti-HBc-positive donors can be used if their serum and harvested cell product are HBV DNA–negative, with monthly monitoring of serum HBV DNA in recipient after transplant, or alternatively, administering antiviral prophylaxis starting 1–2 days before stem cell infusion and continuing for at least 4 weeks. A donor who is naturally anti-HBc positive may be the preferred donor if the recipient is HBsAg positive or anti-HBc positive, because adoptive transfer of natural immunity can effect clearance of virus.[234]

If a donor is infected by HCV and if time permits, treatment of the donor prior to harvest of donor cells can render them nonviremic and much less likely to transmit infection.[235] New DAA drug combinations are the treatment of choice for this indication (see Chapter 82 and www.HCVguidelines.org).[236] If HCV is transmitted, the acute phase of HCV infection may cause elevated liver enzymes by 2–3 months post-HCT after recovery of T-cell function. Increased 1- to 2-year nonrelapse-related mortality has been observed in HCV-infected patients than HCV-negative controls, including excess deaths related to bacterial infections.[237] Fibrosing cholestatic hepatitis C has rarely been described after HCT, possibly related to use of MMF for immune suppression.[238] Antiviral treatment of hepatitis C-infected recipients with DAAs can reduce nonrelapse mortality, relapse of HCV-associated non-Hodgkin lymphomas, and the longer term risk for development of cirrhosis and hepatocellular carcinoma.[239]

Liver Disease in Candidates for Hematopoietic Cell Transplantation

The risks faced by patients with fibroinflammatory liver disease include fatal SOS following some myeloablative regimens with liver toxicity.[218] Child-Pugh B or C cirrhosis is a contraindication to most high-dose conditioning regimens because of the risk of developing fatal sinusoidal injury; these patients may also develop fatal sepsis or hepatic decompensation after HCT even if given a reduced-intensity conditioning regimen.[240,241] Liver biopsy or transient elastography should be considered if there is a clinical suspicion of cirrhosis or extensive fibrosis resulting from chronic viral infection, alcohol, or NASH. Myeloproliferative neoplasms can present with noncirrhotic portal hypertension and an increased incidence of early posttransplant hepatotoxicity.[242,243] Patients with Gilbert syndrome exhibit increased nonrelapse mortality after conditioning with busulfan (BU)-containing regimens.[244] More recent liver injury caused by chemotherapy or radiation in the months before transplant can also pose risk. Many chemotherapy drugs cause liver dysfunction either directly (cholestatic injury, hepatocyte necrosis, or sinusoidal damage) or indirectly (cholestasis caused by sepsis or endotoxemia; i.e., cholangitis lenta).[245] Although exposure to standard chemotherapy per se has not been associated with an increased risk of fatal SOS, patients presenting for HCT with persistent jaundice and elevations of aminotransferase enzymes are at risk.[246] Liver injury has been associated with prolonged exposure to antimetabolites such as 6-thioguanine, as well as agents such as imatinib (Gleevec) and newer tyrosine kinase inhibitors.[247] Gemtuzumab ozogamicin (Mylotarg) predisposes patients to SOS after hepatotoxic myeloablative regimens, particularly if the patient is transplanted within 3 months of high-dose gemtuzumab exposure.[248] Similar findings have been reported with inotuzumab ozogamicin (Besponza), possibly related to IgG Fc receptor expressed on sinusoidal endothelial cells.[249]

Gallbladder and Bile Duct Stones

HCT candidates with asymptomatic gallstones [incidentally discovered during CT or ultrasound (US)] do not require operative intervention. Patients with symptomatic cholelithiasis or stones in the common duct should be considered for pretransplant cholecystectomy or an endoscopic biliary procedure with stone removal.

Iron Overload

HCT candidates with diseases, such as thalassemia, aplastic anemia, myelodysplastic syndrome, and chronic leukemia or lymphoma, may come to HCT with marked hepatic iron overload. Moderate elevations in liver iron content (best assessed by T2-weighted MRI) have been inconsistently associated with increased nonrelapse mortality post-HCT.[250] In patients with thalassemia major, effective pre-HCT chelation therapy improves post-HCT survival. In most other patients, however, the quantitation of tissue iron stores and consideration of iron removal can be deferred until after recovery from HCT.

Problems From the Time of the Transplant Through the First Year

Nausea, Vomiting, and Anorexia

Mucositis caused by high-dose conditioning therapy leads to oral mucosal swelling, pain, and, in severe cases, sloughing of pharyngeal and esophageal epithelium, intense gagging, an inability to swallow, vomiting, retrosternal pain, and airway obstruction. Some regimens, notably those that contain 5-fluorouracil, cytarabine, etoposide, high-dose melphalan (MEL), or multiple alkylating agents, may cause unusually severe intestinal mucosal necrosis and further delay the return of eating. Oral cryotherapy has been shown to decrease severity and duration of oral mucositis after 5-fluorouracil and high-dose MEL.[251] Myeloablative conditioning therapy makes most patients nauseated and anorexic, with delayed gastric emptying and poor oral intake, with the worst problems at Day 10–12 posttransplant but often extending to Day 20.[252] 5-hydroxytryptamine receptor antagonist (5-HT_3RA) drugs are very effective in relieving acute symptoms during conditioning therapy.[253] Addition of a neurokinin receptor-1 antagonist (NK1RA) such as aprepitant and fosaprepitant to block substance P action at the vomiting center in the brainstem increases the efficacy of (5-HT_3RAs).[254] Dexamethasone also potentiates the efficacy of 5-HT_3RAs. Olanzapine, a multiacting, receptor-targeted antipsychotic, has demonstrated activity in breakthrough nausea and vomiting.[255] Protracted anorexia may be related to circulating interleukin (IL)-1, IL-6, and TNF-α, cytokines known to affect appetite centers.[252]

Upper gut acute GVHD is the most common cause of these symptoms in allograft recipients. Early signs include loss of appetite, absence in pleasure from eating, and satiety, often followed by nausea and vomiting. When the onset of GVHD is before Day 15 following a peripheral blood allograft, for example, the histologic features of GVHD may be indistinguishable from those resulting from conditioning therapy. After Day 20, over 80% of allografted patients with intractable anorexia, nausea, or vomiting will have gastric and duodenal GVHD as the sole explanation.[256] Endoscopy shows edema of the gastric antral and duodenal mucosa, patchy erythema, and bilious gastric fluid (Fig. 34.4), with severe cases showing partial or complete denudation of the duodenal mucosa.[257] Histology may show epithelial cell apoptosis and drop-out, often with localized lymphocytic infiltrates.[257–259] The gamut of clinical presentation, endoscopic appearance, absence of infection, and histology needs to be integrated to arrive at a diagnosis when histology is equivocal. Immunosuppressive therapy using a 10-day induction course of prednisone 0.5 mg/kg/day plus oral beclomethasone dipropionate 8 mg/day is an effective therapy for upper gut–predominant GVHD that avoids prolonged prednisone exposure.[260,261] Recipients of autologous grafts may also develop a syndrome of anorexia, nausea, and vomiting that is associated with diffuse gastric edema and erythema.[262]

Endoscopy also serves to rule out GI infection with herpesviruses, bacteria, and fungi as causes of upper gut symptoms. CMV infection of the esophagus, stomach, and upper intestine accounted for a third of patients with unexplained nausea and vomiting during the preganciclovir era, but CMV infection is now an uncommon cause of these symptoms.[256] CMV infections in the GI tract are usually diagnosed between 50 and 150 days after HCT but can appear earlier if patients have CMV infection before HCT or receive cord blood transplants.[219,263] CMV infections can be detected in the GI tract in the absence of CMV antigen or DNA in peripheral blood. Nausea and vomiting may be prominent symptoms of some parasitic infections (if missed during pre-HCT screening) and infections caused by enteric viruses (norovirus, rotavirus, and astrovirus).[223,225,226] Anorexia and vomiting may also be manifestations of increased intracranial pressure related to central nervous system infection, posterior reversible encephalopathy syndrome, or subdural hematomas.

Oral nonabsorbable antimicrobial drugs (particularly nystatin), cyclosporine, MMF, trimethoprim/sulfamethoxazole, voriconazole, posaconazole, itraconazole, amphotericin, and high-dose opioids also cause nausea and occasionally vomiting. Deterioration in nutritional status during the early posttransplant period is associated with acute GVHD and early mortality.[264] If feasible, enteral nutrition is preferred to parenteral nutrition, as it reduces bloodstream infections, intestinal mucosal atrophy, and incidence of severe acute GVHD.[265] Even after parenteral nutrition has been stopped, appetite suppression may linger for 1–2 weeks.[266]

Jaundice, Hepatomegaly, and Abnormal Liver Tests

Development of jaundice following HCT is a poor prognostic sign, whether caused by SOS, cholangitis lenta, GVHD, or infection (Table 34.2 and Fig. 34.5).[267,268] Preventive approaches have lessened the incidence of several liver complications of transplant.[218,269]

Sinusoidal Obstruction Syndrome

SOS (see Fig. 34.5A and B) is a syndrome of tender hepatomegaly, fluid retention with weight gain, and an elevated serum bilirubin

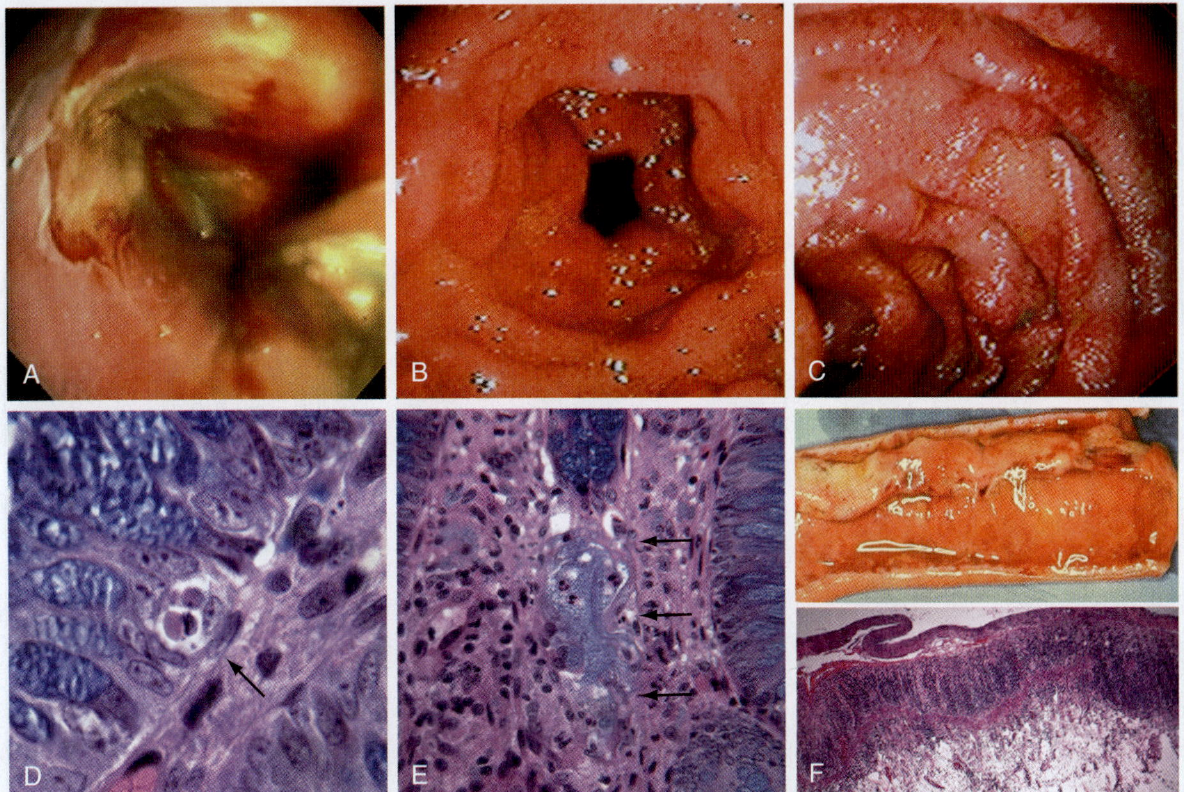

Fig. 34.4 Endoscopic and histopathologic manifestations of acute graft-versus-host disease (GVHD) of the GI tract. (A) Esophagus: Desquamation of squamous epithelium of the distal esophagus in severe GVHD. (B) Stomach: Diffuse mucosal edema and erythema in the gastric antrum in moderately severe GVHD. (C) Small intestine: Mucosal edema, focal bleeding, and ulceration in severe GVHD. (D) Histopathology: Focal apoptosis (*arrow*) caused by GVHD in crypt epithelium from a rectal biopsy (H&E, Alcian blue). (E) Histopathology: Bottom of a colon crypt (*arrows*) is missing epithelial cells; apoptotic debris is admixed with mucus at the base of the crypt (H&E, Alcian blue.). (F) Gross and histopathologic findings in fatal GVHD: Autopsy photograph of a small intestinal segment opened to reveal sloughing of the mucosa (*top*); histopathology shows complete absence of epithelial cells, lymphoid infiltrate, and submucosal edema (*bottom*) (H&E).

concentration associated predominantly with certain conditioning regimens.[270] Because this form of liver injury is initiated by damage to hepatic sinusoid endothelial cells, the older term "veno-occlusive disease" is inaccurate. SOS is caused by toxins in certain conditioning regimens; important contributors to variability in the incidence of SOS are (1) variations in the metabolism of CY from patient to patient in CY/TBI regimens; (2) underlying fibroinflammatory liver diseases; (3) the order of delivery of drugs in multidrug conditioning regimens[271]; and (4) concomitant use of drugs during and after conditioning therapy that either affect the metabolism of myeloablative drugs (e.g., itraconazole) or that cause concomitant liver injury (e.g., methotrexate, sirolimus, and norethisterone).

The onset of SOS is heralded by an increase in liver size, right upper quadrant tenderness, renal sodium retention, and weight gain, occurring 10–20 days after the start of CY and later after other conditioning regimens.[218] Hyperbilirubinemia follows in 4–10 days, although anicteric SOS has been increasingly reported in pediatric patients.[272] Concomitant ascites and refractory thrombocytopenia strongly suggest SOS.[246,270] Severe but transient elevations of serum AST/ALT may herald the clinical onset of SOS.[273] Doppler US is useful for demonstrating hepatomegaly, ascites, periportal edema, attenuated hepatic venous flow, and gallbladder wall edema consistent with SOS, as well as for excluding other causes of hepatomegaly and jaundice.[274] Abnormal findings later in the course of SOS may include an enlarged portal vein diameter, slow or reversed flow in the portal vein or its segmental branches, high congestion index, portal vein thrombosis, and increased resistive index to hepatic artery flow. Shear-wave US elastography is an emerging technology that may help detect SOS earlier than traditional Doppler US.[275] Liver biopsy, via a transvenous approach that allows hepatic venous pressure measurements, is the most accurate diagnostic test.[276] A hepatic venous pressure gradient above 10 mm Hg in this clinical setting is highly specific for SOS.[277] Initial histologic changes are dilation of sinusoids, extravasation of red cells through the space of Disse, necrosis of perivenular hepatocytes, and widening of the subendothelial zone in central veins.[278] The later stages of SOS are characterized by activation and proliferation of stellate cells, extensive collagenization of sinusoids, and a variable degree of obstruction of venular lumens, leading to obliteration of sinusoidal blood flow.[278] Intensity of collagenization of sinusoids and central veins and the degree of hepatocyte necrosis correlate with outcome.[278] Complete recovery from SOS occurs in over 70% of patients with treatment of fluid retention. Patients with severe SOS seldom die of liver failure, but rather from renal and cardiopulmonary failure.[270] Adverse prognostic findings include the rapidity with which weight is gained and serum bilirubin rises, serum ALT levels over 1500 U/L, renal insufficiency, and hypoxemia.

The key to prevention of SOS is understanding its pathogenesis.[270,278,279] Toxic damage to hepatic sinusoidal endothelial

TABLE 34.2 Liver Diseases After Hematopoietic Cell Transplantation

Disease	Frequency	Timing	Diagnosis	Treatment	Prevention
Sinusoidal obstruction syndrome	<10% (regimen-dependent)	Onset before Day +20	Typical clinical features Imaging WHVPG, histology (see Fig. 34.5A and B) Note atypical presentations (acute hepatitis, anasarca)	None proved Defibrotide successful in ≈40% of patients with severe SOS	Assess patient risk Choose "liver-friendly" conditioning regimen
Cholestasis of sepsis (cholangitis lenta)	Common in neutropenic patients	Follows sepsis or neutropenic fever (usually before Day +30)	Exclude other causes of cholestasis Clinical diagnosis	Treat underlying infection	Infection prophylaxis or expectant treatment Ursodiol
Acute GVHD	≈20% of allograft recipients Rare after autograft	Day +15–50	Confirm GVHD in skin, gut Exclude other causes of cholestasis Histology (see Fig. 34.5C and D)	Glucocorticoids (2 mg/kg/day) Ursodeoxycholic acid	Optimal donor selection Complete GVHD prophylaxis T-cell-depletion protocols Ursodiol
Acute viral hepatitis	Uncommon when prophylaxis is used against herpesviruses, hepatitis B	HSV, Day +20–50 Adenovirus, Day +30–80 VZV, Day +80–250 HBV and HCV, during immune reconstitution	Pretransplant serology and PCR results Isolation of virus from other sites (stool and urine for adenovirus) PCR of serum for specific viruses Liver histology/PCR/immunostains (see Fig. 34.5E and F)	HSV, VZV: acyclovir Adenovirus: cidofovir HBV: entecavir or tenofovir HCV: consider direct-acting antiviral drugs if liver injury is severe	HSV and VZV infection: acyclovir prophylaxis for all patients If the patient is at risk for an HBV infection: lamivudine or entecavir, choose an HBV immune donor
Fungal abscess	Rare when prophylaxis is used	Day 10–60	Hepatic pain, fever Liver imaging Serum fungal antigen	Antifungal drugs	Pretransplant screening Oral antifungal prophylaxis for all patients
Drug-induced liver injury	Common	Day 0–100	Clinical diagnosis	Discontinue drug	None
Ischemic liver disease	Confined to patients with septic or hemorrhagic shock or respiratory failure	Day 0–50	Clinical diagnosis	Restore cardiac output, blood oxygenation	Early treatment of sepsis, bleeding
Biliary obstruction	Transient biliary sludge is common Stones, chloromas rarely	Day 15–60	History, examination Biliary US study	Papillotomy ± stent if obstruction persists	None
Idiopathic hyperammonemia	Rare	Day 10–50	Venous blood ammonia	None proved	Unknown, probably genetic defect
Chronic hepatitis C	Declining	After Day 80	HCV RNA in serum Elevations of serum AST, ALT after immune reconstitution	Anti-HCV therapy after full immune reconstitution (www.HCVguidelines.org)	Screen hematopoietic cell donors
Iron overload	Very common	Pretransplant Long-term follow-up after transplant	MRI specific for iron quantitation Transferrin saturation Marrow iron quantitation Liver iron quantitation	May not be necessary Phlebotomy, chelation therapy if iron burden is very high (see text)	Avoid medicinal iron supplements
Chronic GVHD	Common	After Day 80	Prior acute GVHD Chronic GVHD in other organs Characteristic ALT, alkaline phosphatase levels Histology (see Fig. 34.5D)	Immunosuppressive drug therapy Ursodeoxycholic acid	Screening for chronic GVHD at Day 80

GVHD, Graft-versus-host disease; *SOS*, sinusoidal obstruction syndrome (veno-occlusive disease); *VZV*, varicella-zoster virus; *WHVPG*, wedged hepatic venous pressure gradient.

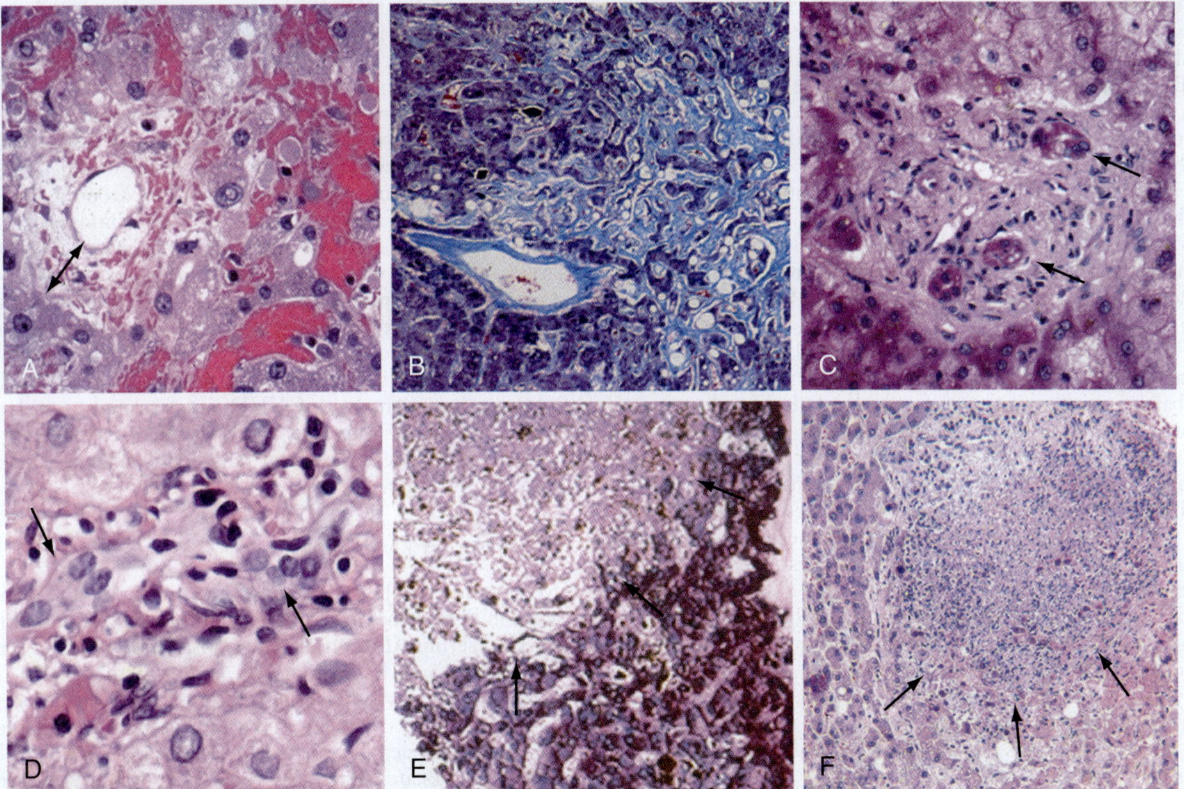

Fig. 34.5 Histopathology of liver diseases following hematopoietic cell transplantation. (A) Sinusoidal obstruction syndrome (also known as *veno-occlusive disease of the liver*) at 23 days post transplant; high-power view of hemorrhage into the space of Disse, hepatocyte necrosis, disrupted sinusoids, and subendothelial edema of the central vein (*arrow*). The lumen of the vein is patent (H&E). (B) Sinusoidal obstruction syndrome caused by gemtuzumab ozogamicin; high-power view of Zone 3 of the acinus, showing extensive sinusoidal fibrosis, hepatocyte dropout, and a patent central vein (Masson trichrome). (C) Acute graft-versus-host disease (GVHD) at Day 82 post transplant; portal area containing abnormal small bile ducts (*arrows*) with epithelial cell dropout, cytoplasmic eosinophilia, and vacuolization (H&E). (D) Chronic GVHD at Day 184 post transplant; high-power view of a portal area with damaged small bile ducts (*arrows*) infiltrated by lymphocytes (H&E). (E) Varicella-zoster virus hepatitis; low-power view of confluent necrosis of hepatocytes (*arrows, pointing to pale area*) adjacent to hepatocytes that are normal (Periodic acid-Schiff). (F) Adenovirus hepatitis; low-power view of a focal area of confluent hepatocyte necrosis (*arrows, pointing to basophilic area*) with remnants of hepatocytes that contain intranuclear inclusions typical of adenovirus ("smudge cells"), best seen at higher power (H&E).

cells, not venular damage and not thrombosis within the liver vasculature, is the proximate cause of SOS. SOS is associated with elevated plasma proteins, including endothelial markers (suppression of tumorigenicity-2, angiopoietin-2, hyaluronic acid, and vascular cell adhesion molecule-1).[280] The linkage between regimens that contain CY/TBI and SOS has been rigorously investigated. Patients who generate a greater quantity of toxic CY metabolites are more likely to develop fatal SOS.[281] A total CY dose of 100–110 mg/kg, instead of 120 mg/kg, will lower the frequency of organ toxicity in the CY/TBI regimen.[281] When combined with CY 120 mg/kg, the total dose of TBI is related to the frequency of severe SOS—approximately 1% after CY/TBI 10 Gy, 4%–7% after CY/TBI 12–4 Gy, and 20% after CY/TBI over 14 Gy. BU is another component of regimens with a high frequency of SOS, although BU itself does not appear to be hepatotoxic.[282] BU may contribute to liver injury by inducing oxidative stress, reducing glutathione levels in hepatocytes and sinusoidal endothelial cells, and altering CY metabolism.[271] Giving CY before IV targeted BU leads to less liver toxicity than with targeted BU/CY.[271] MEL pharmacokinetics, also widely variable from patient to patient, can be normalized using therapeutic drug monitoring.[283] Genetically determined differences in drug metabolism or susceptibility to toxic injury might explain some of the variability in the frequency of SOS, but there is no current method of altering drug dosing or determining susceptibility of individual patients to sinusoidal injury based on genomic data.

One way to prevent fatal SOS is to avoid damage to hepatic sinusoidal endothelial cells, especially in patients at risk. Prevention of severe sinusoidal liver injury begins with an assessment of the risk in patients with underlying liver disease for a given myeloablative conditioning regimen. Patients at increased risk for fatal SOS have several options: (1) a reduced-intensity conditioning regimen; (2) a myeloablative regimen that does not contain CY—for example, targeted BU-fludarabine for allogeneic[284] or BEAM for autologous[285] HCT; (3) modification of CY-based regimens with either a change in the order (e.g., CY/targeted BU[271]) or reduction in CY dose to 100–110 mg/kg; and (4) use of pharmacologic approaches to prevent sinusoidal liver injury. If a CY/TBI regimen must be used for a patient at risk for fatal SOS, modifications should be considered for both CY (100–110 mg/kg) and TBI (≤12 Gy) dosing. If a BU/CY regimen must be used for a patient at risk for fatal SOS, liver toxicity is less frequent if CY is given before targeted BU or if dosing of CY is delayed for 1 or 2 days after completion of BU. The metabolism of IV BU is variable, with a several-fold range in the area under the curve (AUC_{BU}), a problem that can be addressed by therapeutic drug monitoring.[286] Use of therapeutic drug monitoring to normalize exposure to MEL is also feasible.[283] Another approach to decreasing the toxicity of regimens that contain BU and MEL is to give them in reverse order (MEL/BU). Treosulfan, a prodrug of an alkylating agent related to BU with highly predictable pharmacokinetics and reduced hepatotoxicity due to lack of conjugation to glutathione, has supplanted BU in some conditioning regimens.

For the more than 70% of patients with SOS who will recover spontaneously, treatment involves management of sodium and water balance, preservation of renal blood flow, and repeated paracenteses for ascites that is associated with discomfort and/or pulmonary compromise. Patients with a poor prognosis can be recognized soon after disease onset by steep rises in total serum bilirubin and body weight, serum ALT values over 1500 U/L, portal pressures above 20 mm Hg, splenomegaly, ascites, and especially by multiorgan failure requiring dialysis, hemofiltration, or mechanical ventilation.[270,273,287,288]

Defibrotide, a mixture of single-stranded DNA oligonucleotides purified from pig intestine, is approved in the United States and Europe for treatment of severe SOS.[289,290] A phase 3, historically controlled, multicenter trial in patient with SOS and multiorgan failure demonstrated day +100 survival following HCT of 38.2% versus control survival of 25.0% using a propensity-adjusted analysis.[290] Intravenous administration of defibrotide is proposed to preserve sinusoidal endothelial cell function and structure.[291] In the event of severe SOS unresponsive to pharmacologic and supportive therapies, successful OLTs for severe SOS have been reported.[292] However, in most centers, patients at risk for recurrent malignancy are low-priority candidates for a liver transplant.

Defibrotide infusion also has been shown to reduce incidence of SOS in pediatric patients with one or more risk factors for SOS.[293] Prospective studies have shown no benefit from use of prophylactic heparin, antithrombin III, or *N*-acetyl cysteine in preventing fatal SOS. A meta-analysis suggests that ursodiol may prevent SOS,[269] although a large randomized trial showed no effect of ursodiol on the frequency of SOS but a large effect on the frequency of cholestatic jaundice.[294]

Cholestatic Disorders

Prophylactic ursodeoxycholic acid reduces the frequency of cholestasis in general and GVHD-related cholestasis specifically and improves outcomes compared to placebo.[216,294] Now that the frequency of SOS has declined, the leading cause of post-HCT jaundice is cholestatic liver injury.[218,268]

Cholangitis Lenta

Hyperbilirubinemia is common when patients are neutropenic, febrile and have gut mucosal injury from the conditioning regimen. Hepatocyte retention of conjugated bilirubin is mediated by endotoxins, IL-6, and TNF-α.[209] Although this disorder is often referred to as "cholestasis of sepsis," it occurs in patients with fever alone and in the presence of localized infection in the lungs and soft tissues (see Chapter 35).

Acute Graft-Versus-Host Disease

Acute GVHD (see Fig. 34.5C) develops in up to 70% of allograft recipients. Prophylaxis with ursodiol has greatly decreased the frequency of jaundice after transplant and has altered the clinical phenotype of GVHD.[216] In retrospect, what had been called "hepatic GVHD" is a mélange of three processes. The first process is jaundice occurring early in GVHD, where cholestasis is caused by cytokines such as IL-6.[295] The second process is characterized by increases in serum bilirubin, alkaline phosphatase, and GGTP, usually in patients with GI GVHD in whom liver biopsies show lymphocytic infiltration of small bile ducts with nuclear pleomorphism, epithelial cell dropout, and cholestasis in Zone 1 of the liver acinus.[296,297] Inflammatory infiltrates may be minimal because of immune suppression. Persistent hepatic GVHD and worsening jaundice are associated with ductopenia. The third process in hepatic GVHD is most commonly seen in allograft recipients on minimal immunosuppression or after donor lymphocyte infusion, in whom GVHD presents as an acute hepatitis with marked elevation of serum ALT.[298,299] Prognosis in patients with GVHD is not related to peak severity of signs and symptoms, but rather to the area under a disease activity curve, where persistent jaundice is an independent predictor of mortality.[300]

Drug-Induced Liver Injury

Cyclosporine inhibits canalicular bile transport and commonly causes mild increases in serum bilirubin concentrations without an effect on serum ALT or alkaline phosphatase levels. Tacrolimus causes cholestasis less commonly, except in the setting of toxic blood levels. Many other drugs used after HCT have been associated with liver dysfunction (e.g., trimethoprim/sulfamethoxazole, voriconazole, fluconazole, posaconazole, and ruxolitinib), although drugs are usually not responsible for severe liver injury in this setting.

Acute Hepatocellular Injury

The incidence of severe hepatocellular injury after HCT has declined remarkably since the 1990s.[216] A sudden rise in serum aminotransferase enzymes (AST and ALT) following HCT is usually due to a noninfective cause, such as Zone 3 hepatocyte necrosis in SOS (peaking around Day 20), hypoxic liver injury (as in septic or cardiogenic shock or respiratory failure), acute biliary obstruction (choledocholithiasis), drug-induced liver injury, or the acute hepatitic presentation of GVHD discussed earlier.[218] If a likely cause is not apparent, acute viral hepatitis should be suspected; early diagnosis and treatment may prevent a fatal outcome.

Acute hepatitis caused by HSV, VZV, adenovirus, and HBV can lead to fatal fulminant hepatic failure after HCT, whereas hepatic infections caused by CMV and HCV are seldom severe (see Fig. 34.5E and F). With routine use of prophylactic acyclovir or valacyclovir, acute hepatitis due to HSV and VZV is now rare; however, HHV-6 and HHV-8 reactivation and HEV as causes of hepatitis have been reported after HCT.[301,302] When there is uncertainty about the cause of rising serum ALT and AST levels, serum PCR tests for herpesviruses, adenovirus, HCV, HBV, and HEV should be performed. Blood tests for viruses have largely replaced the need to obtain liver tissue for viral diagnosis, but transvenous measurement of the wedged hepatic venous pressure gradient with liver biopsy can be useful in diagnosis of unsuspected SOS. If acyclovir is not being given, it should be started empirically, particularly if the patient presents with abdominal complaints typical of VZV infection.[303] Adenovirus hepatitis should be suspected if the patient has concomitant pulmonary, renal, bladder, or intestinal symptoms but may present only with fevers, raised liver enzymes, and hypodense regions in the liver on abdominal CT, along with features of bone marrow suppression[304]; the most effective treatment is cidofovir when given early in the course of adenovirus infection, but many cases are fatal.[305] New agents are in development.[306]

Fulminant hepatitis B may develop during immune reconstitution in patients at risk but can be prevented with prophylactic antiviral agents.[307] If severe hepatitis B reactivation does occur, usually because a diagnosis of HBV was not made prior to HCT, antiviral therapy with the most potent anti-HBV drug available (entecavir or tenofovir) should be initiated immediately; however, progression to fatal liver failure is not uncommon.[308] Fulminant hepatitis B has also been reported following discontinuation of prophylactic antiviral therapy, and all patients, particularly those with high pretransplant HBV DNA levels, should be monitored following antiviral drug withdrawal.[309,310]

Chronic hepatitis C in HCT recipients usually results in asymptomatic elevation of serum ALT from Days 60–120, coinciding with the tapering of immunosuppressive drugs.[237] However, in recent years, the treatment of chronic HCV infection in patients with hematologic malignancies with DAAs has become the standard of care. HCT recipients without contraindications to DAAs and who do not receive treatment prior to transplantation should be treated for HCV once the patient has ceased all immunosuppressive drugs and has no evidence of active GVHD.[239,311] DAAs might also offer an effective treatment in the rare case of severe hepatitis and fibrosing cholestatic hepatitis due to HCV after HCT.[238]

Fungal and Bacterial Infections

Antifungal prophylaxis has significantly reduced the incidence of hepatic fungal disease in HCT recipients.[312] Presenting features include fever, tender hepatomegaly, and increased serum alkaline phosphatase levels; resistant *Candida* species or molds should be suspected.[312] High-resolution CT or MRI may demonstrate multiple fungal abscesses, and serologic tests for fungal antigens may be useful for diagnosis.[231,232] Return of neutrophil function after HCT can affect resolution of a previously treatment-refractory *Aspergillus* infection.[313] Bacterial liver abscesses are rare in HCT recipients, probably because systemic antibiotics are so widely used; however, latent mycobacterial infection (including *Bacille Calmette-Guérin*) may reactivate within the liver with prolonged immunosuppressive therapy. Disseminated clostridial infection and gallbladder infection with gas-producing organisms may lead to air in the liver and biliary system.

Gallbladder and Biliary Disease

Biliary sludge (calcium bilirubinate) is very common in HCT recipients.[314] Sludge obstructing the distal common bile duct may cause epigastric pain, nausea, and abnormal serum liver enzymes. Biliary sludge may be a cause of acute "acalculous" cholecystitis, acute pancreatitis, and bacterial cholangitis.[315,316] Acute cholecystitis is uncommonly seen in HCT recipients and is more commonly acalculous.[317] Cholecystitis in this setting may also be due to leukemic relapse with gallbladder involvement or infection by CMV, fungi, or rarely by other organisms such as *Haemophilus influenzae*. Diagnosis of cholecystitis after HCT is difficult because of the high frequency of gallbladder abnormalities on US or CT in asymptomatic patients.[318] Pericholecystic fluid, gallbladder wall necrosis, or localized tenderness suggest cholecystitis. Nonvisualization of the gallbladder after a radionuclide bile excretion study with morphine infusion suggests cholecystitis. Biliary obstruction is a rare event caused by a variety of disorders: common bile duct calculi or inspissated biliary sludge; GVHD of the ampullary mucosa; lymphoblastic infiltration of the common bile duct, gallbladder, and ampulla of Vater in EBV-LPD; CMV-related biliary disease; dissecting duodenal hematoma complicating endoscopic biopsy; and leukemic relapse (chloroma) in the head of the pancreas.[316,319] In patients undergoing autologous HCT, biliary strictures are commonly due to recurrent malignancy.[320] The use of ursodiol to stimulate bile flow in patients with biliary sludge after HCT is ineffective, likely due to the absence of cholesterol crystals[314] ERCP is indicated in patients with clinical evidence of cholangitis and radiologic evidence of biliary obstruction and allows for biliary stenting or dilation with acceptable risk.[320]

Malignant Hepatic Disorders

EBV-LPD is now an infrequent complication of HCT, largely because of EBV DNA surveillance and preemptive treatment with rituximab. The highest incidence was in recipients of HLA-mismatched, T-cell-depleted grafts and those receiving potent anti-T-cell therapies for GVHD. Symptoms include fever, sweats, generalized malaise, enlarged tonsils, and cervical lymphadenopathy, often with involvement of the liver and spleen (abnormal serum alkaline phosphatase and hepatosplenomegaly) and GI invasion. Malignancies that were the indication for transplant can appear in the liver as part of relapse.

Idiopathic Hyperammonemia and Coma

A syndrome of hyperammonemia and coma has been described in patients who received high-dose chemotherapy, including conditioning for HCT.[321] Patients present with progressive lethargy, confusion, weakness, incoordination, vomiting, and hyperventilation with respiratory alkalosis. The diagnosis is confirmed when the plasma ammonia exceeds 200 μmol/L and there is no evidence of liver failure. Rare cases associated with *Ureaplasma urealyticum* and *Ureaplasma parvum* have been reported with subsequent improvements in ammonia levels and symptoms after treatment.[322,274]

GI Bleeding

Minor bleeding is very common, particularly when platelet counts are below 50 × 10^9/L (Fig. 34.6). Causes include retching-induced trauma to the esophageal or gastric mucosa, mucosal injury from conditioning therapy, reflux esophagitis, *C. difficile* colitis, anal fissures, internal hemorrhoids, and acute GVHD. The incidence of severe GI bleeding after HCT is 1%–2%, lower than in the past because of effective prophylaxis against viruses, fungi, and acute GVHD.[323] Mortality from severe GI bleeding, however, remains at 40%.[323,324] A common cause of severe bleeding is refractory acute GVHD with bleeding from extensive ulceration in the small intestine and cecum.[325] Bleeding is an independent predictor of mortality in patients with severe gut GVHD.

Transplant-associated thrombotic microangiopathy (TA-TMA) can affect the small vasculature of the intestine, accompanied by abdominal pain and bleeding caused by ischemic changes.[326] Histologic signs of microangiopathy are endothelial swelling of small vessels, withering crypts with cytoplasmic depletion, and platelet microthrombi.[327,328] Intestinal TMA (iTMA) can coexist with acute GVHD or mimic steroid-refractory GVHD and may occur independently of renal or other systemic manifestations of TMA.[329] Recognition of iTMA in patients with suspected acute GI GVHD is crucial, as continued treatment with calcineurin inhibitors can worsen microangiopathy.[327] One prospective study in children and young adults identified iTMA as the most common cause of severe GI bleeding.[330] Based on severity of symptoms and plasma levels of the soluble membrane attack complex (sC5b-9), complement inhibitors such as eculizumab.[331] Current models of TA-TMA pathogenesis involve aberrant activation of complement pathways in patients sustaining endothelial damage from immunosuppressive drugs (calcineurin and mammalian target of rapamycin inhibitors or GVHD, with underlying genetic predisposition or preexisting endothelial injury.[332]

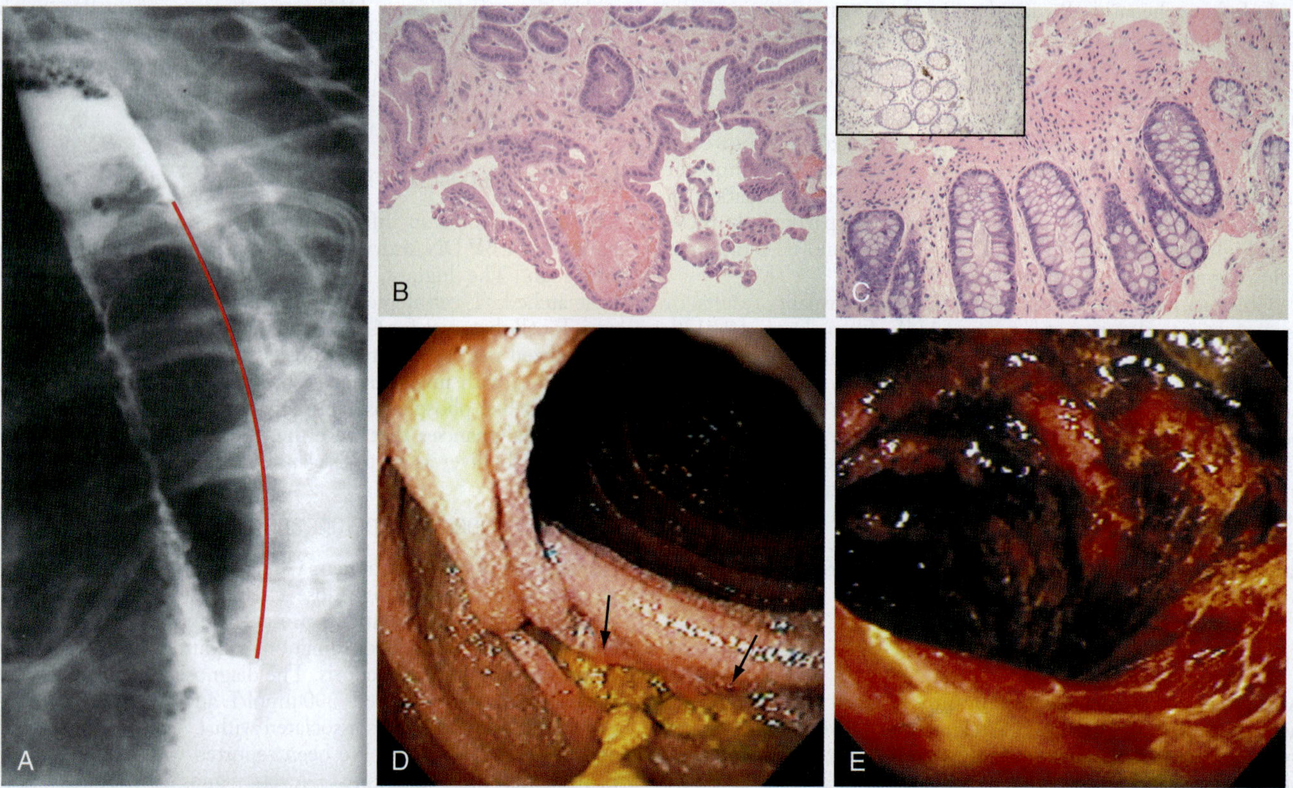

Fig. 34.6 Other GI problems in hematopoietic cell transplant recipients. (A) Esophagus: Barium contrast demonstration of an intramural hematoma that occupies one wall of the esophagus from the aortic arch to the lower esophagus. The *red line* approximates the normal esophageal contour. This hematoma was caused by retching in a thrombocytopenic patient. (B) Thrombotic microangiopathy: Photomicrograph of gastric tissue taken with 20× objective with swollen endothelial cells, double-tracked vessel walls, and extravasated red blood cells. Note loss of mucin and atrophy of the surface epithelial cells. (C) Thrombotic microangiopathy: Photomicrograph of colonic tissue taken with 20× objective with small vessels that have platelet thrombi. Inset: anti-CD61 immunohistochemistry showing platelet thrombi. (D) Duodenum: Linear duodenal ulceration with yellow exudates (*arrows*) caused by *Rhizopus* infection in a transplant patient receiving immunosuppressive therapy for graft-versus-host disease (GVHD). The surrounding mucosa is abnormal because of GVHD. (E) Colon: Sigmoid colon in adenovirus colitis, showing diffuse mucosal edema, ulceration, and hemorrhage.

With ganciclovir prophylaxis and preemptive therapy, bleeding CMV ulcers have become rare. Gastric ulcerations may also be caused by infection by VZV, invasive bacteria (phlegmonous gastritis), or EBV (LPD) (see Chapter 55). Although now rare after HCT, EBV-LPD involves the GI tract in 20%–25% of cases and can present as GI bleeding. GAVE can be a cause of severe upper intestinal bleeding in HCT recipients, particularly those who have received oral BU.[333] Diffuse areas of hemorrhage are seen in the gastric antrum and occasionally small and large intestine, but the underlying mucosa is intact.[333–335] Histology is diagnostic, revealing abnormal dilated capillaries, thromboses, and fibromuscular hyperplasia in the lamina propria. Patients who are transplanted for advanced systemic sclerosis may bleed from similar vascular lesions. Endoscopic laser therapy or argon plasma coagulation are treatments of choice to control bleeding from vascular ectasia, but multiple treatments may be required to obliterate ectatic lesions.[333] Other rare causes of bleeding post HCT include ulcers caused by molds, Dieulafoy lesions, Curling (stress) ulcers, duodenal biopsy sites, mycophenolate-induced enteritis, adenovirus enterocolitis, and *C. septicum* infection (typhlitis). Patients with severe amyloidosis who undergo autologous HCT may bleed from multiple ischemic ulcers throughout the intestine.[336]

There is no effective therapy for mucosa that is diffusely oozing blood, other than platelet transfusions to raise the platelet count to greater than 50 × 10^9/L and treating the underlying condition, if possible. In GVHD, reepithelialization of ulcerated intestinal mucosa is very slow. Focal lesions, especially mucosal infections, can be treated with endoscopic cautery, heater probe, hemostatic clips, or epinephrine injection, but these therapies are futile in mucosa that is oozing blood diffusely. Topical hemostatic agents applied via the endoscope can have temporizing effects for 24–72 hours.[337] Unless the underlying disease process is eliminated, endoscopic methods will not cure the bleeding problem. Attempts to resect large segments of diffusely bleeding intestine involved with GVHD have not been successful.[325]

Dysphagia, Painful Swallowing, and Esophageal Pain

Oral and hypopharyngeal mucositis from conditioning therapy, reflux esophagitis, and pill esophagitis are currently the leading causes of dysphagia and esophageal pain. Infections of the esophagus (fungal, viral, and bacterial) have largely disappeared because of antimicrobial prophylaxis; when fungal esophagitis is discovered, the organism is likely to be a resistant candidal species or a mold.[338] Rarely, fungal esophagitis can lead to perforation.[339] Nonhealing esophageal ulcerations, strictures, and dysphagia may uncommonly result from conditioning therapy.[340] In patients with gastric stasis related to acute GVHD or recurrent vomiting, painful esophagitis is common, caused by reflux of both gastric acid and bilious fluid. In patients with severe acute GVHD, esophageal edema, erythema, and a peeling epithelium lead to ulcerations.[341]

Pill esophagitis occurs after ingestion of some medications in use after HCT—for example, phenytoin, foscarnet, oral bisphosphonates, ciprofloxacin, clindamycin, trimethoprim-sulfamethoxazole, and oral potassium chloride.

The abrupt onset of severe retrosternal pain, hematemesis, and painful swallowing suggests a hematoma in the wall of the esophagus, a result of retching when platelet counts are very low (see Chapter 47).[342] CT is the diagnostic test of choice. The course of intramural hematomas is one of slow resolution over 1 or 2 weeks.

Diarrhea Conditioning Therapy

Diarrhea caused by mucosal damage from high-dose conditioning therapy is seldom severe, usually resolving by Day 12–15, with some exceptions. Cytarabine-containing regimens, high-dose MEL ($\geq$200 mg/m^2), and regimens containing multiple alkylating agents may cause more severe and protracted diarrhea. IV infusion of octreotide and oral loperamide may be effective for severe diarrhea associated with conditioning therapy.[343]

Graft-Versus-Host Disease

Acute GVHD (Table 34.3; also see Fig. 34.4) is the most common cause of diarrhea after Day 15.[344] However, GVHD may not be the sole cause of diarrhea in an individual patient, especially in patients receiving prolonged immune suppression, in whom reassessing the cause of diarrhea may detect infections or iTMA not present at baseline.[345,346] GVHD may also be exacerbated by emerging off-label therapies (i.e., immune checkpoint inhibitors) for the treatment of relapsed hematologic malignancies after HCT.[347] The onset of GVHD diarrhea can be sudden, with stool volumes in excess of 2 L daily in severe cases. GVHD in patients who were grafted after reduced-intensity conditioning regimens may have its presentation delayed, occurring after Day 100 in many patients.[348] The diarrheal fluid of GVHD is watery with ropy strands of mucoid material that reflect transmucosal protein loss. This presentation is almost diagnostic of intestinal GVHD, particularly when accompanied by decreasing serum albumin levels and negative stool studies for infection.[349] In atypical cases where GVHD is suspected, abdominal imaging by CT, MRI, or US may reveal intestinal edema and mucosal enhancement, particularly in the ileum and right colon, although the appearances of acute GVHD and CMV infection can overlap.[350–353] Pneumatosis intestinalis, which may be associated with GVHD or CMV enteritis, may be seen by plain x-ray, CT, or MRI, and in the absence of ancillary evidence of clinical severity, managed conservatively.[354] A definitive diagnosis of GVHD requires endoscopic views of mucosa, histology of GI mucosal tissue, and exclusion of infection. What the endoscopist sees should carry equal diagnostic weight to what the pathologist sees through the microscope.[257] Moderately severe GVHD causes diffusely edematous and erythematous mucosa throughout the GI tract. Severe GVHD may lead to ulcerations and large areas of mucosal sloughing in the stomach, small intestine, and colon.[355] Even when the appearance is normal, mucosal biopsies may reveal intestinal crypt necrosis and apoptotic bodies diagnostic of acute GVHD. The diagnostic yield of mucosal biopsy is best when biopsies are obtained either from the distal colon and stomach or from the colon and ileum.[345,355,356] Ileal biopsies may reveal higher histologic grading of GVHD than other sites.[357] The use of capsule endoscopy for diagnosis of GVHD can provide visual inspection of the jejunum and ileum that cannot usually be seen with routine endoscopy.[358] Other histologic findings that support the diagnosis of GVHD include pericapillary hemorrhage, infiltrating neutrophils or eosinophils, and evidence of endothelial damage.

In severe cases of GVHD, individual crypts are destroyed, then adjacent crypts, and finally whole segments of intestinal mucosa. Successful treatment of severe acute GVHD with glucocorticoid (2 mg/kg prednisone equivalent) therapy results in a dramatic reduction in stool volume, with resolution of accompanying symptoms of abdominal pain, nausea, and vomiting. Lesser grades of acute GVHD (upper GI symptoms, <1 L/day of diarrhea, rash involving <50% of body surface area, and no hepatic GVHD) can be treated with lower doses of glucocorticoids (0.5 mg/kg/day prednisone equivalent) or nonsteroid alternatives.[261,359] Other methods of predicting outcomes in patients with GVHD include calculation of the Acute GVHD Activity Index, measurement in decline of serum albumin level from baseline, and panels of serum biomarkers.[300,349,360]

Ruxolitinib, a JAK1/2 kinase inhibitor, is the first (and only) drug approved by the FDA for steroid-refractory GVHD in adult and pediatric patients 12 years and older, defined as disease progression after at least 3 days of high-dose system glucocorticoid therapy, lack of response after 7 days, treatment failure during glucocorticoid taper, or an inability to taper glucocorticoids to <0.6 mg/kg/day of prednisone for a minimum of 7 days.[361,362] Extracorporeal photopheresis (ECP), a cell-based immunotherapy with reinfusion of autologous mononuclear cells after exposure to 8-methoxypsoralen and ultraviolet A light irradiation, increases levels of regulatory T cells and may improve responses in ruxolitinib-refractory aGvHD cases.[363]

In allograft recipients, infectious causes of diarrhea are far less common than GVHD, accounting for only 10%–15% of diarrheal episodes.[324,344,364] Common bacterial pathogens are extremely rare after HCT,[364] except in geographic areas where such infections are prevalent.[365] *C. difficile* colitis is usually a relatively mild, treatable disease when diagnosed at the onset of diarrhea.[344,366,367] A significant fraction of these patients may be *C. difficile* carriers, as identified by screening for toxin A/toxin B by PCR at admission.[368] Among HCT recipients with recurrent or refractory *C. difficile* colitis, fecal microbiota transplantation appears to be safe and effective with careful donor and recipient selection.[369] Commercial sources of fecal microbiota are on the horizon, with the first product approved by the FDA for recurrent *C. difficile* in 2022. One often overlooked factor is the inappropriate use of PPIs for marginal indications, which increases the risk of *C. difficile* colitis twofold.[370] Norovirus may spread within hospitals as a nosocomial infection in HCT patients, with devastating consequences.[371] Susceptibility to norovirus infection is determined by human histo-blood group antigen secretor status, even among immunocompromised patients.[372] Some serotypes of adenovirus cause necrotizing enteritis and rapidly fatal multiorgan failure involving the gut, liver, lungs, and kidneys.[338,373] There should be a sense of urgency in identifying adenovirus as a cause of enteritis; delayed treatment is often ineffective, and reduction of immunosuppression is usually required.[374–377] However, not all patients in whom adenovirus is found in diarrheal stools have adenovirus enteritis or develop disseminated infection.[378]

CMV is the only common infectious cause of enteritis after HCT that requires an intestinal biopsy for diagnosis .[344] As with adenovirus, CMV DNA can be detected in diarrheal stool specimens from patients who do not have demonstrable mucosal CMV disease. CMV can be found in mucosal biopsies in patients whose blood is negative for CMV antigen or DNA.[219,379] Otherwise, the predictive value of a negative stool examination for other viruses, bacteria, fungi, and parasites is high, particularly if molecular methods are used.[380] After HCT, watery diarrhea secondary to intestinal parasite infection (*Cryptosporidium parvum*, *G. lamblia*, *E. histolytica*, and helminths) is rare, but sporadic cases are seen that can be confused with GVHD.[226,381] *Strongyloides* infection and hyperinfection syndrome have been described after HCT; patients from endemic areas should be screened before HCT.[223] Nontuberculous mycobacterial infection of the small intestine has been described post HCT.[382]

TABLE 34.3 Causes of Diarrhea After Hematopoietic Cell Transplantation

Cause	Frequency	Diagnosis	Severity	Treatment
Myeloablative conditioning therapy	Common	Exclude infection, hyperacute GVHD	Usually mild, can be severe after some regimens	Self-limited; octreotide useful in severe cases
Acute GVHD	Common after allografts; occurs in ≈10% of autografts	Association with skin and liver GVHD; exclude infection Abrupt decline in serum albumin is a marker of more severe GVHD Mucosal histology in problematic cases	Ranges from mild to intractable high-volume diarrhea	Immunosuppressive drugs, usually prednisone initially
Viral Infection				
CMV	Now uncommon	CMV antigen or DNA in blood; viral culture, immunohistology of mucosal biopsy	Potentially fatal if not detected early	Ganciclovir or foscarnet
Adenovirus	Sporadic	Adenovirus DNA in blood or stool; viral culture, immunohistology of mucosal biopsy	Serotype dependent; may be rapidly fatal	Cidofovir
Norovirus	Uncommon; can be acquired by nosocomial spread in hospitals	PCR on stool specimen	Can be severe and protracted if immunodeficiency persists	None
Astrovirus	Uncommon	ELISA, PCR of stool	Self-limited	None
Rotavirus	Rare	ELISA, PCR of stool	Serotype dependent; can be severe	None
EBV (lymphoproliferative disease)	Now rare	EBV DNA in blood; mucosal biopsy	Usually fatal when lymphomatous gut involvement develops	Rituximab when detected early; withdrawal of immunosuppressive drugs
Bacterial Infection				
Clostridioides difficile	Common	PCR, toxin and antigen in stool	Usually mild to moderate	Oral vancomycin > fidaxomicin > metronidazole
Clostridioides septicum	Sporadic	Clinical syndrome of typhlitis	Potentially fatal	Imipenem, oral vancomycin
Enteric pathogens	Rare except in endemic areas	Stool, blood culture	Potentially fatal	Based on organism's sensitivities
Parasitic Infection				
Giardia lamblia	Rare	Stool ELISA	Can be protracted	Metronidazole
Cryptosporidium hominis	Rare	Stool microscopy, PCR	Often protracted	Recovery of immunity
Entamoeba histolytica	Rare	Stool microscopy, antigen, PCR; serum EIA	Potentially fatal	Metronidazole or tinidazole, followed by paromomycin
Strongyloides stercoralis	Rare	Stool microscopy	Potentially fatal	Ivermectin
Osmotic Diarrhea				
Oral magnesium salts	Common	Clinical diagnosis	Dose dependent	Reduce dose; IV Mg^{++}
Carbohydrate malabsorption	Common with gut GVHD, infection	Clinical diagnosis	Diet dependent	Disaccharide dietary restriction
Antibiotic use	Common	Clinical diagnosis	Medication dependent	Discontinue antibiotic
Medication				
Tacrolimus	Unusual	Clinical diagnosis	Dose dependent	Reduce dose; loperamide
Mycophenolate mofetil	Common	Clinical diagnosis, endoscopic findings	Dose dependent	Reduce dose; substitute enteric-coated mycophenolic acid formulation; loperamide
Metoclopramide	Unusual	Clinical diagnosis	Medication dependent	Discontinue

EIA, Enzyme immunoassay; *ELISA*, enzyme-linked immunosorbent assay; *GVHD*, graft-versus-host disease.

Other Causes of Diarrhea

In addition to infection, several other conditions may occur after HCT, including brush border disaccharidase deficiency, bile salt malabsorption, pancreatic insufficiency, mucosal toxicity from MMF, and iTMA. Intestinal inflammation often results in reduced expression of lactase and sucrase/isomaltase, leading to diarrhea if lactose or sucrose is ingested. Failure of bile salt absorption in the small intestine as a cause of diarrhea can be treated with bile acid sequestrants.[383] Steatorrhea and pancreatic insufficiency have been associated with calcineurin-inhibitor therapy, and transient pancreatic insufficiency has been described as a consequence of mucosal edema at the ampulla of Vater.[384,385] MMF causes intestinal ulcerations and apoptotic crypt cells similar to the histology of acute GVHD.[386] Fewer GI side effects have been reported after conversion to enteric-coated mycophenolic acid in SOT recipients.[93] A cord colitis/diarrheal syndrome has been reported in cord blood recipients. Pathology of endoscopic biopsies shows chronic active colitis with granulomas, and DNA sequencing of endoscopic biopsies identified a novel bacterium, *Bradyrhizobium enterica*, associated with cord colitis.[387,388] However, other centers have not identified cord colitis as a cause of post-HCT diarrhea.[389]

Abdominal Pain

Abdominal pain may be an indicator of a rapidly progressive, fatal illness, or an illness with a benign natural history that requires only conservative management (Table 34.4). The illnesses that may be rapidly fatal include intestinal perforation, some infections (e.g., typhlitis caused by *C. septicum*, adenovirus enteritis, visceral VZV infection, and angio-invasive *Aspergillus*), cholecystitis, and pyogenic liver abscess. More common causes of abdominal pain are intestinal pseudo-obstruction, narcotic bowel syndrome, acute GVHD, liver pain related to SOS, and hemorrhagic cystitis. The first question to answer is whether a patient with abdominal pain needs urgent surgery. Surgical intervention for abdominal pain after HCT is a rare event but is indicated for intestinal perforation, acute cholecystitis, drainage of abscesses, appendicitis, and in some patients with intestinal or biliary obstruction, typhlitis, and dissecting hematomas.[390] Surgical decision-making depends on the clinical situation, abdominal examination, and imaging findings. Current imaging tests and careful examination should allow the surgeon to be highly selective in choosing candidates for operation, but clinical judgment may lead to surgical exploration or laparoscopy in difficult cases when one cannot exclude the possibility of a surgical disease, such as in pneumoperitoneum of unknown cause or possible gallbladder necrosis. Intestinal perforation may develop in the setting of therapy-induced necrosis of a transmural lymphoma shortly after conditioning therapy or later from CMV ulcers or a diverticular perforation. Perforation may present with only mild to moderate abdominal pain and pneumoperitoneum on abdominal CT, especially in granulocytopenic patients. Pneumoperitoneum can also be a manifestation of pneumatosis intestinalis, a much more benign process without peritonitis, usually caused by CMV or GVHD.[391] Recognition of acute cholecystitis can be difficult because right upper quadrant pain and fever are common in the early post-HCT period, and imaging studies show gallbladder wall thickening and luminal sludge in asymptomatic patients. A radionuclide study with morphine that shows filling of the gallbladder suggests that surgical cholecystitis is not present.[392] When pain is localized to the right lower quadrant, typhlitis (*C. septicum* infection) and appendicitis are diagnoses that can be made by imaging. Symptoms of typhlitis include fever, right lower quadrant pain, nausea and vomiting, diarrhea, occult blood in the stool, and shock; the diagnosis of typhlitis is usually made by imaging studies showing cecal edema, although ileal and ascending colon extension are commonly seen.[393,394] Surgical resection for typhlitis is rarely necessary, provided that antibiotic therapy (e.g., piperacillin-tazobactam and clindamycin) for *C. septicum* is started along with systemic coverage for luminal bacteria and fungi in febrile patients.[395]

The most common cause of moderate to severe abdominal pain is intestinal pseudo-obstruction with bowel distention; the clinical findings of distention and tympany on percussion in the setting of opioid, anticholinergic, or prior vinca alkaloid drug exposure are virtually diagnostic. In visceral VZV infection, abdominal distention, severe pain, fever, and rising serum ALT levels may precede cutaneous manifestations by up to 10 days, a presentation that occurs only among patients not receiving acyclovir prophylaxis.[303,396] Acyclovir should be started on clinical suspicion, while serum is analyzed by PCR for VZV DNA. Clinical pancreatitis is an uncommon cause of abdominal pain in HCT patients; subclinical pancreatitis does occur, with symptoms masked by immunosuppressive drugs.[315] Patients with thrombocytopenia or coagulopathy may rarely bleed into the retroperitoneum, abdominal wall, or intra-abdominal viscera, particularly after duodenal biopsy, causing significant pain. In patients with intestinal pseudo-obstruction, medical management is almost always effective, and perforation is rare. Although some infections of gut neurons (VZV and CMV) lead to pseudo-obstruction, mu-agonist opioid and anticholinergic medications are the usual causes, particularly in patients with gut inflammation. There are three approaches to opioid-related pseudo-obstruction: (1) decreasing the opioid dose; (2) peripherally acting mu-opioid receptor antagonist such as methylnaltrexone or naloxegol[191]; or (3) switching to a κ-opioid agonist (e.g., butorphanol). Anticholinergic medications are contraindicated in pseudo-obstruction, and drugs with anticholinergic side effects should be discontinued. Neostigmine (2 mg IV) has been successfully used in patients with acute colonic pseudo-obstruction after HCT.[397] Octreotide is useful for treating gut distention with fluid related to pseudo-obstruction.[398]

Acute GI GVHD can present with abdominal pain as a sole manifestation, but more commonly, rash, nausea, vomiting, anorexia, or diarrhea accompany pain. The presentation can include a rigid abdomen with rebound tenderness, but more commonly crampy and periumbilical pain are present. Empiric treatment may be considered without definitive evidence of GVHD, and biopsy confirmation of acute GVHD can be obtained within several days after starting glucocorticoid therapy.

Perianal Pain

Perianal pain after HCT can be caused by an anal fissure, a thrombosed external hemorrhoid, cellulitis related to tissue maceration, and infections. In patients with granulocytopenia, infections in the perineum or perianal spaces are usually polymicrobial, arising either from anal glands or from tears in the anal canal. Extensive supralevator and intersphincteric abscesses may be present without being apparent on external examination.[399] CT, MRI, endoscopy, or transperineal US can give a clear view of the anatomy involved, particularly if there is pus present.[400] When antibiotics covering both anaerobic and aerobic bacteria are given to patients with "cryptitis" (incipient perianal infection), far fewer patients require surgical drainage than in the past. Unusual causes of perianal pain include giant condyloma acuminata (genital warts) caused by HPV, HSV infection, fungal infection, and CMV-induced cutaneous vasculopathy with perianal ulcers.[401,402]

Problems in Long-Term Transplant Survivors

GI and hepatobiliary problems that occur in the years after allogeneic HCT are usually a continuation of symptoms of protracted acute GVHD, cGVHD, medication side effects, and infection related to immune suppression.[403,404]

TABLE 34.4 Causes of Acute Abdominal Pain After Hematopoietic Cell Transplantation

Cause	Frequency	Diagnosis	Severity	Treatment
Sinusoidal obstruction syndrome (SOS)	Now less common	Tender hepatomegaly, weight gain, jaundice	Potentially fatal	See text
Intestinal damage from conditioning therapy	Unusual	Examination, imaging	Can be protracted after some regimens	None
Colonic pseudo-obstruction	Common, particularly in patients taking mu-opioid or anticholinergic medications May also occur with GVHD and VZV or CMV infection Prior vincristine exposure increases risk	Distention, tympany, abdominal plain film	When medication related, usually resolves; when a sign of GVHD or viral infection, may be severe	Reduce opioid, anticholinergic drug exposure; rule out treatable underlying causes; consider methylnaltrexone; neostigmine if persistent and severe
Hemorrhagic cystitis	Common after cyclophosphamide and with viral bladder infection	Suprapubic pain, hematuria, viral cultures (JC/BK virus or adenovirus)	Can be protracted with viral infection	Urologic therapy, antiviral drugs if appropriate
Acute GVHD	Common, particularly with more severe GVHD	Evaluate skin, gut symptoms, serum bilirubin Intestinal imaging (CT, US, MRE, PET) Mucosal biopsy	Potentially severe but not immediately fatal	Immunosuppressive drug therapy
Biliary pain	Unusual	RUQ/epigastric localization; gallbladder sludge, gallbladder edema, gas; biliary dilatation on US	Passage of sludge is usually self-limited; necrotic gallbladder requires surgery	Persistent biliary obstruction requires stent placement; surgery for gallbladder necrosis
Pancreatitis	Unusual	Serum lipase	Usually self-limited, but hemorrhagic pancreatitis occurs	Treat biliary, infectious, and medication causes
Hematomas	Rare can be seen after duodenal biopsy	Examination, abdominal imaging, endoscopy	Can be protracted	Restoration of platelet counts; intestinal obstruction may require surgery
Intestinal infection	Unusual	Diagnostic and imaging tests for clostridial infection, VZV, CMV, adenovirus, norovirus, molds	Potentially fatal if not treated (especially *Clostridium septicum*, viral, or mold infection)	Treat the organism discovered
Intestinal perforation (CMV ulcer, intestinal tumor necrosis, diverticula)	Now rare	Abdominal plain film, CT scan	Potentially fatal	Surgery
Liver abscess/bacterial infection	Rare (usually fungal)	Liver imaging (MRI preferred), examination, serum fungal antigen detection	Potentially fatal if not treated	Antifungal therapy, antibacterial therapy
Intestinal infarction (usually due to disseminated *Aspergillus* infection)	Rare	Intestinal imaging, examination, chest x-ray, galactomannan ELISA	Uniformly fatal	Antifungal drugs
EBV-lymphoproliferative disease	Rare with surveillance for EBV DNA in serum	Abdominal imaging, endoscopic biopsy	Usually fatal once tumor masses form	Rituximab when detected early; withdrawal of immunosuppressive drugs

EIA, Enzyme immunoassay; *GVHD*, graft-versus-host disease; *JC/BK*, polyomaviruses; *MRC*, magnetic resonance cholangiography; *MRE*, magnetic resonance enterography; *VZV*, varicella-zoster virus.

Esophageal Symptoms

Heartburn may be worse if cGVHD is present because salivary gland destruction reduces bicarbonate production. cGVHD may involve the esophagus, leading to dysmotility and failure to clear refluxed acid.[405] Protracted acute GVHD involving the stomach leads to gastric stasis and reflux of both acid and bile. Less common causes of esophagitis in survivors include fungal and viral infections and inflammation caused by retained pills (pill esophagitis). Common causes of dysphagia include esophageal and oral cGVHD, infection, xerostomia, and poor dentition.[404] Patients with extensive cGVHD often complain of dysphagia for solid food and pills; children also present with insidious weight loss, retrosternal pain, and aspiration of gastric contents, leading to pulmonary disease that can be mistaken for GVHD-related bronchiolitis obliterans syndromes.[406] The diagnosis of esophageal cGVHD is made by barium contrast x-ray or endoscopy, the latter of which should be done with caution because perforations have been reported. Radiologic findings include bullae, webs, concentric rings, tapering strictures, and aperistalsis.[407] Characteristic endoscopic findings include desquamation of the upper esophagus and distinctive upper esophageal webs. Histologic findings include submucosal infiltration of the esophageal mucosa with lymphocytes, vacuolization of basal layer epithelium, and submucosal fibrosis. Patients with esophageal cGVHD may need endoscopic dilation to avoid progressive luminal narrowing, but dilations must be done with extreme care because the perforation risk is higher than with peptic strictures. Topical glucocorticoid therapy can be effective. The risk of squamous cell carcinoma of the esophagus is 8.5-fold higher after HCT than among controls; cGVHD is the major risk factor.[408]

Upper Gut Symptoms: Anorexia, Nausea, Vomiting, Satiety

Gastroduodenal GVHD in long-term survivors is called persistent, recurrent, or late acute GVHD because symptoms, endoscopic appearance, and histology are identical whether they occur before Day 100 or years after transplant.[409] Herpesviruses (HSV, CMV, and VZV) may cause nausea, vomiting, and satiety in survivors if prophylactic antiviral medications and viral surveillance have been discontinued. When upper gut symptoms appear along with abdominal distention and elevated serum ALT levels, visceral VZV infection should be suspected and confirmed with PCR for VZV DNA in blood. Gastroparesis may develop after HCT and typically responds to prokinetic agents.[410]

Mid-Gut and Colonic Symptoms: Diarrhea and Abdominal Pain

Late acute GVHD or overlap disease with both acute and cGVHD can cause GI symptoms for many years after transplant.[411] Some patients who have had more severe GVHD in the past may develop intestinal strictures.[411,412] Sporadic cases of gut infection may occur with *C. difficile*, norovirus, CMV, and rarely *G. lamblia* and *C. parvum*.[226,338,413] Narcotic bowel syndrome may present with increasing abdominal pain and constipation in patients requiring opiates.[414] Bile acid malabsorption in the ileum may contribute to persistent low-volume diarrhea in patients receiving lenalidomide; bile acid sequestering agents may be helpful.[415] Rare cases of "transmission" of intestinal diseases such as celiac sprue via donor T cells have been reported.[416]

Graft-Versus-Host Disease of the Liver

There are three presentations of liver GVHD in long-term survivors of HCT[218,403,404]: (1) Asymptomatic elevation of serum ALT, alkaline phosphatase, and GGTP in the absence of jaundice; (2) slowly progressive cholestatic jaundice with elevated serum alkaline phosphatase, a result of damage to small bile ducts (see Fig. 34.5D); and (3) acute hepatocellular injury (hepatitic GVHD), with abrupt elevations of serum ALT to over 500 U/L without preceding hepatic dysfunction. In long-term survivors, the differential diagnosis of jaundice is narrower than it is before Day 100. The differential diagnosis of cholestatic jaundice includes GVHD, biliary obstruction, DILI, and fibrosing cholestatic hepatitis B or C.[218] If a cause of elevated liver enzymes is not apparent, a biopsy may be indicated to identify GVHD as a cause. The addition of ursodiol (12–15 mg/kg/day) to the immunosuppressive regimen results in significant biochemical improvement in liver GVHD.[417,418] Severe hepatic GVHD can progress to ductopenia and deep jaundice and may require a course of several months of therapy with prednisone, a calcineurin inhibitor, and ursodiol therapy to resolve.[296] Several case series, but no randomized trials, have touted the following as effective steroid-sparing treatments: pulse CY,[419] ECP,[420] switching calcineurin inhibitors, or adding sirolimus. Oral beclomethasone dipropionate or budesonide could be used for hepatic GVHD, because 40% and 90% of these "topical" glucocorticoids, respectively, reach the portal circulation[421] and the liver; this approach to other inflammatory liver diseases, such as autoimmune hepatitis, has been effective.[422] OLT, including living-donor transplantation from the original hematopoietic cell donor, has been performed in patients with refractory cholestasis or end-stage liver disease due to GVHD.[292,423,424] Hepatitic GVHD can occur after discontinuation or tapering of immunosuppressive therapy or after donor lymphocyte infusion.[298,299] Patients who present with steeply rising serum ALT levels, with or without jaundice, present a differential diagnosis of viral infection, DILI, and hepatitic GVHD. These patients require urgent diagnosis and treatment. Hepatic histologic findings include hepatocellular injury, lobular inflammation, lymphocytic infiltration in and around small bile ducts, extensive damage to (and loss of) small bile duct epithelial cells, cholestasis, portal fibrosis, and piecemeal necrosis.[298] Blood tests for viral antigen or viral DNA/RNA will exclude acute hepatitis due to a herpesvirus (HSV or VZV), hepatitis viruses A–E, or adenovirus. Acyclovir should be started pending results of tests for herpesviruses; if viral studies are negative, a calcineurin inhibitor and prednisone (1–2 mg/kg/day) should be begun, while histology is pending to prevent extensive ductular damage from GVHD.[298]

Chronic Viral Hepatitis and Cirrhosis

In long-term HCT survivors with chronic hepatitis C, cirrhosis develops with a median time of 10–18 years, compared to 40 years in controls.[425,426] Confirmation of cirrhosis using either liver biopsy or noninvasive methods, such as transient elastography,[427] is crucial so that patients can be monitored for complications, including esophageal varices and hepatocellular carcinoma. Chronic hepatitis C may also be a risk factor for development of lymphoma and other lymphoproliferative disorders after transplant.[428,429] All survivors with chronic HCV, including those with cirrhosis, should be offered antiviral therapy unless contraindications exist.[239] DAA drug combinations are highly effective and well tolerated. This website provides continuously updated recommendations for treatment of patients with HCV infection: www.HCVguidelines.org. Interferon-free treatment regimens are particularly attractive in post-HCT patients where the potential for interferon-induced activation of cGVHD is a concern.

The serologic pattern of HBV infection may be atypical in HCT survivors because of immunosuppression. Clearance of surface antigenemia may be observed and is particularly likely if the donor was anti-HBs positive from prior HBV infection or a robust response to vaccination.[234,430] Patients who remain HBsAg positive after HCT are at risk of flares of hepatitis B activity, particularly at times of reduction of immunosuppression, such as during tapering or cessation of treatment for cGVHD; these patients should be taking antiviral agents such as tenofovir or entecavir for 12 months after discontinuation of immunosuppressive treatment.[431] All long-term survivors with chronic hepatitis B should be regularly monitored to assess virologic and disease status and the need for antiviral therapy.[432] Pegylated interferon cannot be recommended in allogeneic HCT survivors because of the concern for flares of cGVHD. HBV viral status should be reassessed prior to reintroduction of chemotherapy.[431] B-cell-depleting agents, such as rituximab used in the treatment of B-cell malignancies, have a particularly high risk of reactivation of occult hepatitis B (HBsAg negative and anti-HBc positive), and prophylactic antiviral therapy is recommended .[433] As in the peritransplant period, patients with HBsAg should receive an antiviral agent whenever they receive immunosuppressive or cytotoxic therapy.

Ascites

The most common causes of new ascites in HCT survivors are cirrhosis (e.g., accelerated development of cirrhosis in patients with chronic hepatitis C[425,426] and rarely in patients with hepatic GVHD) and, in noncirrhotic patients, nodular regenerative hyperplasia of the liver (within the spectrum of idiopathic noncirrhotic portal hypertension).[434,435] The diagnosis of nodular regenerative hyperplasia can be challenging because both liver imaging and wedged hepatic venous pressure measurements can be misleadingly normal.[436] The prognosis of nodular regenerative hyperplasia after HCT is mixed, and frequent large volume paracenteses or a TIPS may be required for management of ascites.[437] Other causes of enigmatic ascites after HCT include constrictive pericarditis, pancreatic ascites, peritoneal carcinomatosis, and a serositis syndrome related to cGVHD.[438]

Other Liver Disorders

DILI in patients receiving HCT is associated with statins, NSAIDs, amoxicillin-clavulanate, sulfamethoxazole/trimethoprim, azoles, or herbal preparations.[245] Although most DILI responds to drug withdrawal, some drug reactions can result in chronic liver disease. Compared with the general population, patients develop new solid organ malignancies at twice the expected rate.[439] Because of the increased rate of chronic hepatitis C infection, the risk of hepatocellular carcinoma is particularly elevated.[439] Transplant survivors with risk factors for hepatocellular carcinoma (HCV cirrhosis, chronic HBV infection, or cirrhosis of any cause) should undergo surveillance every 6 months with liver US, according to international guidelines.[440] In one series of pediatric survivors of HCT undergoing liver MRI, incidental focal nodular hyperplasia lesions were present in 5.2%.[441] These lesions have characteristic central scars that differentiate them from hepatocellular carcinomas and fungal lesions. Because their appearance is so characteristic on MRI,[442] liver biopsy is often not necessary. In this age group without background cirrhosis, fibrolamellar hepatocellular carcinoma may also present with a central scar and can be distinguished by contrast-enhanced US.[443] Liver infections caused by fungi and bacteria are now rare late complications. Nonsterile herbal remedies contaminated by molds may lead to liver abscesses in survivors.[444]

Gallbladder and Biliary Diseases

Long-term HCT survivors have an increased incidence of gallstones and gallstone complications related to the formation of calcium bilirubinate microliths (biliary sludge) following myeloablative conditioning therapy.[314,445] Cyclosporine, and possibly tacrolimus, can predispose to cholesterol gallstones.[446,447] Biliary sludge and gallstones may cause cystic duct obstruction, bile duct obstruction, and acute pancreatitis.[316]

Pancreatic Disease

Acute pancreatitis is very uncommon in long-term HCT survivors, with most cases related either to biliary stone passage or (rarely) to tacrolimus-related pancreatic damage.[448] Pancreatic insufficiency caused by pancreatic atrophy, detected by CT or MRI, after HCT has been described.[449,450]

Iron Overload

Secondary iron overload is caused by both repeated transfusions and increased GI iron absorption in the setting of ineffective erythropoiesis. Morbidity from severe iron overload comes mostly from cardiac iron accumulation, which is only marginally correlated with liver iron content.[451] Iron-specific MRI methods can accurately measure not only liver iron but also iron accumulation in the heart, pituitary, pancreas, and thyroid.[452] The effects of persistent iron overload on long-term HCT outcomes have not been fully investigated except in patients transplanted for thalassemia, in whom very high iron burdens translate to increased mortality from cardiac causes. Iron overload could be a risk factor for morbidity and nonrelapse mortality among HCT survivors with less extreme iron burdens than in thalassemia patients, although the best measure of iron status remains to be determined.[218,453] Multiply transfused patients who died before Day 100 after allogeneic HCT had levels of liver iron in the hemochromatosis range (1832–13,120 mg/g dry weight).[454]

Full references for this chapter can be found at https://ebooks.health.elsevier.com.

35 Gastrointestinal and Hepatic Manifestations of Systemic Diseases

Adam Edwards, Frederick Weber

IN THIS CHAPTER

Numerous systemic diseases have GI and hepatic manifestations, but only the more common diseases and those with recent developments will be discussed in this chapter. Involvement can occur via changes in GI/hepatic structure, function, or both and may relate directly to the systemic disorder, associated disorders, or via effects of therapy. It should be noted that rarer conditions such as systemic sclerosis (PSS) (scleroderma) and amyloidosis are likely to be studied in tertiary care centers, which may be biased toward the sicker patient. The reader is also referred to other chapters where the GI and hepatic manifestations of specific systemic disorders are discussed in greater detail.

COLLAGEN VASCULAR AND INFLAMMATORY DISEASES

Rheumatoid Arthritis

Rheumatoid arthritis (RA) has a prevalence of 0.5%–1% in North America and Europe (Table 35.1).[1,2] Increasing evidence suggests that dysbiosis plays a role in systemic autoimmunity development with microbiome changes preceding clinical RA onset by years and RA therapy partly restoring the microbiome.[3] GI symptoms are common and are largely due to medications, particularly NSAIDs. Oropharyngeal symptoms occur as a result of xerostomia [associated Sjögren syndrome (SS)] and involvement of the temporomandibular joint, cervical spine, and larynx (particularly the cricoarytenoid joint).[4,5] Atlantoaxial subluxation may result in dysphagia associated with other signs of spinal cord compression; endoscopy is a high-risk procedure in these patients. Esophageal dysmotility, characterized by low peristaltic pressure in the lower two-thirds of the esophagus and reduced lower esophageal sphincter (LES) pressure, is associated with heartburn, dysphagia, and esophagitis. Associated rheumatoid vasculitis (RV), SS, or amyloidosis (all discussed later) may also cause esophageal symptoms and dysmotility, and vasculitis may induce esophageal strictures from ischemia.

PUD may occur in relation to anti-inflammatory medications or RV. Chronic superficial and chronic atrophic gastritis is

TABLE 35.1 Gastrointestinal Manifestations of Collagen Vascular and Inflammatory Diseases

Disease	Abnormality/Disorder	Clinical Manifestations
RA	Temporomandibular arthritis	Impaired mastication
	Esophageal dysmotility	Dysphagia, heartburn
	Vasculitis	Intestinal ulceration and infarction, perforation, bleeding
	Amyloidosis	Pseudo-obstruction, malabsorption, PLGE, intestinal ulceration and infarction, gastric outlet obstruction
	Felty syndrome	Hepatosplenomegaly, abnormal liver biochemical tests
Adult-onset Still disease	Liver disease	Hepatosplenomegaly, abnormal liver chemistry tests, hyperferritinemia
Systemic sclerosis	Esophageal dysmotility	Dysphagia, heartburn, Barrett esophagus, esophageal candidiasis
	Gastroparesis	Nausea, dyspepsia
	Intestinal dysmotility	Constipation, pseudo-obstruction, malabsorption, PLGE, SIBO, pneumatosis cystoides intestinalis, true diverticula
	Pancreatic disease	Pancreatic exocrine dysfunction, calcific pancreatitis
	Anal dysfunction	Incontinence, rectal prolapse
	GI bleeding	Gastric antral vascular ectasia, telangiectasias
SLE	Mesenteric vasculitis	Bowel ischemia, ulceration
	Esophageal dysmotility	Dysphagia, heartburn
	Pancreatic disease	Pancreatitis
	Serositis	Ascites, peritonitis
	Liver disease	Abnormal liver chemistry tests, hepatitis
Polymyositis/ dermatomyositis	Skeletal muscle dysfunction	Impaired glutition, tongue weakness, aspiration, dysphagia
	Dysmotility	Heartburn, dysphagia, gastroparesis, pseudo-obstruction, pneumatosis cystoides intestinalis
Sjögren syndrome	Xerostomia	Angular cheilitis, tooth decay, oral candidiasis, hoarseness
	Esophageal dysmotility	Dysphagia
	Pancreatic disease	Pancreatitis
	Liver disease	Abnormal liver biochemistry chemistry tests, PBC, AIH, HCV infection
Mixed connective tissue disease	Esophageal dysmotility	Heartburn, dysphagia
	Sclerodermatous changes	Malabsorption, PLGE, pseudo-obstruction, pneumatosis cystoides intestinalis
	Vasculitis	Bowel ischemia, ulceration, perforation
Polyarteritis nodosa	Vasculitis	Bowel ischemia, ulceration, perforation, arterial aneurysms, acalculous cholecystitis, sclerosing cholangitis, pancreatic diseases, association with HBV infection
Henoch-Schönlein purpura	Vasculitis	Abdominal pain, GI bleeding, intussusception
Eosinophilic granulomatosis with polyangiitis	Eosinophilic phase	Eosinophilic gastroenteritis, eosinophilic ascites
	Vasculitic phase	Abdominal pain, bleeding, intestinal ulceration, perforation
Granulomatosis with polyangiitis	Oral disease	Oral ulcers, gingival hyperplasia (strawberry gums), lingual infarction
	Vasculitis	Esophageal and gastric ulcers, bowel ischemia with ulceration and perforation, pancreatitis, gangrenous cholecystitis
Behçet disease	Vasculitis	Oral ulcers, ileocecal ulcers and perforation, amyloidosis
	Large-vessel disease	Portal or hepatic vein thrombosis, aneurysms
Spondyloarthropathies	Associated intestinal inflammation	Acute disease resembles bacterial enteritis
		Chronic disease resembles Crohn disease
Familial Mediterranean fever	Serositis/amyloidosis	Peritonitis, symptoms resembling an acute abdomen
Cogan syndrome	Crohn disease	Bloody diarrhea, abdominal pain, fistulas, fissures
	Mesenteric vasculitis (rare)	Hemorrhage, ulceration, intestinal infarction, intussusception
Marfan/Ehlers–Danlos syndrome/Joint hypermobility syndrome	Defective collagen	Megaesophagus, hypomotility, diverticula, megacolon, malabsorption, perforation, arterial rupture
IgG4-related disease	Infiltration/fibrosis	Autoimmune pancreatitis, sclerosing cholangitis, hepatitis, retroperitoneal fibrosis, inflammatory pseudotumor, aortitis, sclerosing mesenteritis, enteritis, colitis, pouchitis

AIH, Autoimmune hepatitis; *PLGE*, protein-losing gastroenteropathy.

seen in 30% and 65%, respectively, of biopsy specimens from patients with RA. About one-third of patients with RA have hypochlorhydria or achlorhydria, predisposing them to small bowel bacterial overgrowth (SBBO). Hypergastrinemia may be associated with achlorhydria, antiparietal cell antibodies, intrinsic factor antibodies, vitamin B_{12} deficiency, or pernicious anemia.[4,6,7]

RA is sometimes associated with ulcerative colitis and celiac disease, and RV may mimic IBD.[8–10] Unlike RA, IBD-related peripheral arthropathy is usually rheumatoid factor (RF)-negative, nondeforming, and nonerosive. RA may rarely be associated with pneumatosis cystoides intestinalis (Fig. 35.1).

RV, an inflammatory condition of the small- and medium-sized vessels, affects about 1%–5% of patients with RA,

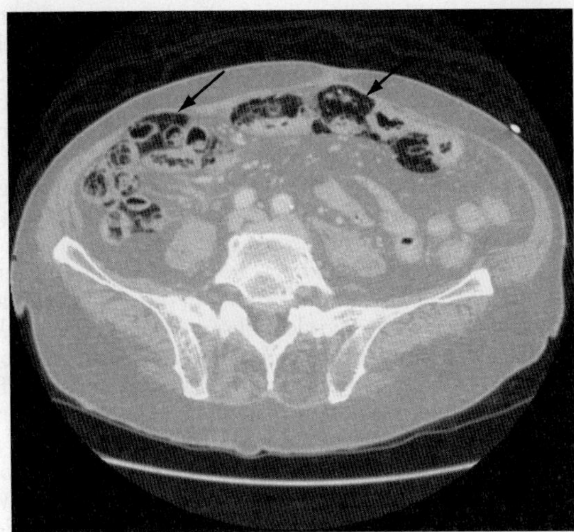

Fig. 35.1 CT showing pneumatosis cystoides intestinalis (*arrows*) in a patient with RA. (From Ebert EC, Hagspiel KD. Gastrointestinal and hepatic manifestations of rheumatoid arthritis. *Dig Dis Sci.* 2011;56:295–302, with permission from Springer.)

typically those with severe disease and high RF titers.[11,12] About 10%–38% of these cases have intestinal involvement, often associated with cutaneous manifestations (digital gangrene, cutaneous ulcers) and peripheral nervous system (neuropathy, mononeuritis multiplex). Involvement of small vessels in the gut results in ischemia with ulcers, pain, and hemorrhage. Involvement of large vessels may lead to bowel infarction, stricture formation, bowel perforation, pancreatic necrosis, appendicitis, aortic aneurysmal rupture, or hemoperitoneum. Therapy may include glucocorticoids and/or cyclophosphamide based on small uncontrolled studies. Notably, an increased rate of lower GI tract perforations has also been found in RA patients managed with corticosteroids, tofacitinib, or tocilizumab but not TNF inhibitors.

Hepatic Involvement

Clinical evidence of liver disease is generally absent in RA. Serum aminotransferase and bilirubin levels are usually normal, whereas serum alkaline phosphatase (both liver and bone isoenzymes) may be elevated.[13–15] Liver histology is nonspecific, including portal tract inflammation, congestion, fatty change, sinusoidal dilatation, amyloid, periportal fibrosis, and nodular regenerative hyperplasia.[16] RA is rarely associated with PBC, autoimmune cholangiopathy, and autoimmune hepatitis (AIH).[15,17,18]

Felty syndrome, a triad of neutropenia, splenomegaly, and severe RA, may be associated with hepatomegaly and abnormal liver chemistry tests. Portal hypertension may occur due to distorted liver microarchitecture (from nodular regenerative hyperplasia) or increased splenic blood flow from splenomegaly. In the latter case, splenectomy may decompress varices.[19] Because HCV infection and RA are common diseases, they may be found concurrently in the same patient. Patients with HCV often have arthralgias, sicca syndrome, and myalgias and express RF and ANAs.[20] A subset of HCV patients develop mixed cryoglobulinemia with arthritis that may be confused with RA. It is usually a nondestructive mono or oligoarthritis affecting large- and medium-sized joints. Anticyclic citrullinated peptide antibodies are rarely found in such subjects and are thus reliable markers of RA when present.[21] Treatment of RA patients with TNF-α antagonists may not reactivate underlying HCV although long-term effects are unknown.[22] A review of 216 HCV-infected patients exposed to one or more TNF antagonists over 260 cumulative patient years revealed only 3 cases of drug withdrawal due to hepatic issues.[23] In contrast, anti-TNF-α therapy and other immunosuppressive agents may exacerbate HBV, and antiviral therapy may be needed in selected HBV-infected individuals.[24] About 2% of patients who are either HB surface antigen-positive or HB core antibody-positive receiving conventional immunosuppressive therapy for RA will experience HBV reactivation.[25]

Drug-Induced Side Effects

Salicylate-induced hepatotoxicity is often asymptomatic, most commonly occurring with high doses of the drugs.[4,26] Elevated serum ALT levels correlate with salicylate levels, are dose-related, and normalize within a few days after aspirin is discontinued or the dose reduced. Biopsies show mononuclear cell infiltrates in portal triads with little hepatocellular necrosis, although rare cases of severe hepatic necrosis occur. NSAIDs may rarely be hepatotoxic, especially when used with other potentially hepatotoxic medications.[27] Ibuprofen has been associated with a hepatocellular or cholestatic picture, including the vanishing bile duct syndrome.

Sulfasalazine may cause a delayed hypersensitivity reaction, occasionally leading to liver failure.[28] Patients may develop a rash, lymphadenopathy, nausea, vomiting, eosinophilia, and either a hepatocellular or mixed liver pattern generally within 6 weeks of starting the medication.

Methotrexate (MTX) has been associated with hepatic fibrosis and cirrhosis, particularly in patients with psoriatic rather than RA. Single nucleotide polymorphisms related to MTX transport and metabolism are associated with this hepatotoxicity.[29] Up to 25% of RA patients may have modest serum aminotransferase elevations, but it is not clear these correlate with fibrosis or cirrhosis. Although cofactors, such as diabetes, obesity, alcohol use, and NAFLD, may play a role, chronic hepatitis B and C do not.[30] Azathioprine and mercaptopurine have been associated with transient asymptomatic rises in serum aminotransferases, cholestatic injury, and chronic hepatic injury marked by peliosis hepatitis, nodular regenerative hyperplasia, and sinusoidal obstruction syndrome, usually occurring in the first 5 years of therapy. There also appears to be an increased risk for lymphoma and possibly hepatocellular carcinoma. Hepatosplenic T-cell lymphoma has been reported rarely in mostly young males on combination azathioprine and TNF inhibitor therapy and presents with fever, fatigue, pancytopenia, and hepatosplenomegaly. The diagnosis is established by bone marrow or liver biopsy, and prognosis is poor. Leflunomide can cause diarrhea, lymphocytic or collagenous colitis, colitis with surface erosion and histologic crypt abscesses, and hepatotoxicity usually within the first 6 months of treatment and is associated with abnormal liver stiffness, especially in the presence of MTX.[31]

Adult-Onset Still Disease

Adult-onset still disease (the adult form of juvenile RA) is an inflammatory disorder presenting with spiking fevers, pharyngitis, evanescent maculopapular rash, arthralgias/arthritis, and neutrophilic leukocytosis.[32–34] Abdominal pain is usually mild and transient but may be severe. Occasionally, small bowel distention and air-fluid levels are found. Hepatosplenomegaly and lymphadenopathy are common. Ferritin is often extremely elevated;[35] C-reactive protein and ESR are high, whereas ANA and RF are negative or low titer.[36] Abnormal liver chemistry tests occur in 50%–75% of patients and are usually mild and transient, correlating with disease activity. Severe hepatitis and even fulminant hepatic failure occasionally occur, leading to death or liver transplantation. Liver histology may be normal, show portal mononuclear cell infiltration, or interface hepatitis with lymphoplasmacytic inflammation similar to AIH. Portal vein thrombosis has been described.[37] Treatment may include NSAID(s), glucocorticoids, MTX, cyclosporine, tocilizumab, canakinumab, and anakinra, with rare hepatotoxicity being reported with anakinra.[38]

Systemic Sclerosis

PSS has a female and African-American predominance with increased severity also noted in African-Americans. Symptoms may be reported in 90% of patients and can effect any region of the GI tract, although esophageal symptoms typically predominate.[37] Patients most commonly complain of anorexia, reflux, dysphagia, early satiety, nausea, distension, diarrhea, constipation, fecal incontinence, and a decline in social and emotional well-being.[39,40] Malnutrition is common, occasionally requiring parenteral nutrition.[40] Among its causes are microstomia, dental caries, anorexia, delayed gastric emptying, malabsorption, SBBO, and slow small bowel transit.

The long-standing theory is that a neuropathic process occurs first, followed by a myopathic process as the muscles atrophy and fibrosis develops. Only in the first stage would prokinetic agents be effective.[41,42] Serum antimuscarinic-3 acetylcholine autoantibodies that may block neurotransmission may then lead to secondary tissue/muscle atrophy.[43] Myositis-related antibodies may also be found in a subset of PSS patients.[44]

Esophageal Involvement

Esophageal symptoms in PSS include heartburn, regurgitation, and dysphagia. Reflux is due to (1) low/absent esophageal peristalsis, (2) reduced LES pressure, (3) hiatal hernia (from a foreshortened esophagus), (4) gastroparesis, (5) autonomic nerve dysfunction, (6) sicca syndrome with loss of salivary bicarbonate, and (7) increased abdominal pressure from coughing and straining.[45]

Patients with PSS develop Barrett esophagus with an increased risk of esophageal adenocarcinoma, although the most common malignancy is probably lung cancer.[46,47] Delayed esophageal transit, treatment with immunosuppressive drugs, and gastric acid suppression predispose to candidal esophagitis. Pill-induced esophagitis may occur secondary to increased mucosal contact. PSS mainly affects the smooth muscle in the lower two-thirds of the esophagus. The upper esophagus, composed mainly of striated muscle, is usually spared unless affected by proximal reflux.[48] The dysmotility documented by esophageal manometry can diagnose PSS. It classically shows low-amplitude contractions or aperistalsis in the lower two-thirds of the esophagus, and low or absent LES pressure (Fig. 35.2). These findings, however, are not universally seen nor specific to PSS and can be seen in other diseases such as amyloidosis, diabetes, chronic alcoholism, esophageal candidiasis, severe reflux, hypothyroidism, and other connective tissue diseases.[45] In 200 patients with scleroderma (117 limited, 83 diffuse) who underwent high-resolution manometry and had their findings classified according to the Chicago classification, the most common findings were absent contractility (56%), normal motility (26%), and ineffective motility (10%), irrespective of whether they had limited or diffuse disease. Classic scleroderma esophagus was observed in only 33%. Severe dysmotility was associated with disease duration, interstitial lung disease, and GI symptom scores.[49] Moreover, in 111 patients with PSS (89 women) who underwent high-resolution manometry that involved multiple rapid swallows, peristaltic amplification during multiple rapid swallows was much less frequent (18%) than in young healthy controls (100%). Abnormal peristaltic reserve was the most common manometric abnormality in patients with PSS.[50] Impedance studies show incomplete bolus clearance.[46,51,52] Like achalasia, the esophagus may be dilated on imaging studies but in PSS there is no mechanical obstruction and, therefore, air-fluid levels are usually not seen unless a stricture is present. Endoscopy often shows abnormalities even without symptoms.[53] Endoluminal ultrasonography shows hyperechoic abnormalities in the muscularis propria thought to represent fibrosis.[45] Reflux may contribute to pulmonary disease by aspiration of gastric contents and/or vagal stimulation from gastric contents in the esophagus. Conversely, pulmonary disease may contribute to

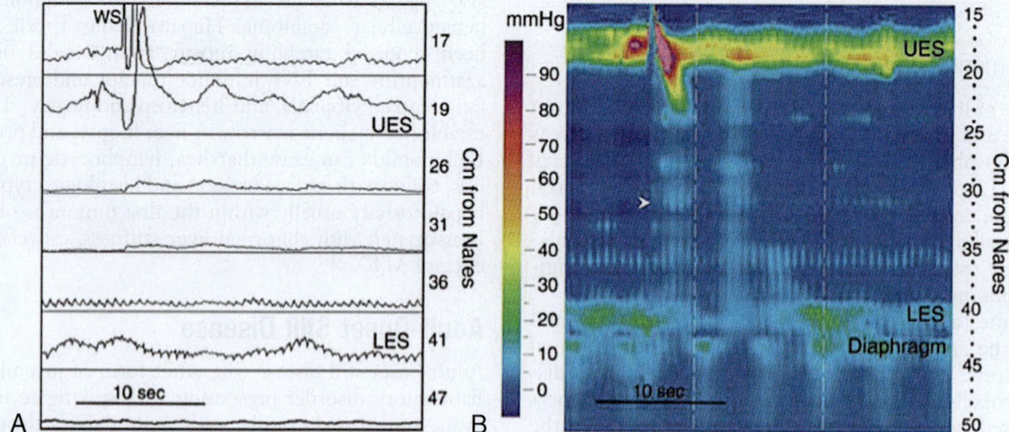

Fig. 35.2 (A) High-resolution manometry (HRM) in line mode from a patient with PSS. A wet swallow (WS) generates normal relaxation of the upper esophageal sphincter (UES) but no esophageal peristalsis. It is difficult to determine whether the lower esophageal sphincter (LES) relaxes. (B) In the HRM color contour, the UES and peristalsis in the striated muscle esophagus are normal. There is aperistalsis of the smooth muscle esophagus. At the gastroesophageal junction, there is a small hiatal hernia, and the LES relaxes appropriately. The WS generates a bolus pressure (seen as a simultaneous shift to the lighter blue or higher pressure) (*arrowhead*) coinciding with the opening of the UES. Without a peristaltic pressure wave, the lighter blue color only slowly returns toward the darker blue seen in the empty esophagus, indicating that the bolus was not cleared from the esophagus. (From Conklin J, Pimentel M, Soffer E. Color atlas of high resolution manometry. New York: Springer Science and Business Media; 2009. Fig. 2.23, p 38, with permission.)

reflux by greater negative intrathoracic pressure required for ventilation and by the effect of bronchodilators lowering LES pressure.

Esophageal reflux is associated with interstitial lung disease in PSS;[45,54,55] these manifestations may evolve together. Although a cause-effect relationship has not been definitively proved, centrilobular fibrosis with a bronchocentric distribution is found in 21% of PSS patients with intraluminal basophilic content consistent with peptic necrosis, suggesting a pulmonary reaction to aspiration of gastric contents.[56] Pulmonary disease is a major cause of death in PSS and responds poorly to treatment. Aspiration precautions and lifestyle modifications for reflux are essential.

PPIs may heal esophagitis and may even reverse esophageal fibrosis.[57] Higher than standard doses of PPIs may be needed but likely do not prevent progression of dysmotility.[58] Whether PPIs help pulmonary disease is not known. Prokinetic agents may help in the early stage of disease. Buspirone (a 5-HT_1 receptor agonist) may have a favorable effect on esophageal peristalsis and LES function. An open-label trial of buspirone 20 mg daily in PPI—refractory patients with PSS showed a significant increase in resting LES pressure and significant reductions in heartburn and regurgitation scores at 4 weeks.[59] Limited data have suggested benefit from alginic acid, domperidone, or vonoprazan 20 mg daily. Surgical therapy with fundoplication has a limited role due to concern that dysphagia could worsen in an aperistaltic esophagus.[45] A Roux-en-Y gastric bypass is an alternative.[60]

Gastric Involvement

Gastric emptying, particularly for solids, is often delayed in PSS and may result in early satiety, bloating, nausea, and vomiting or may be asymptomatic.[61,62] Gastric outlet obstruction and PUD, especially in the presence of NSAIDs, should be ruled out. EUS may show thickening of the gastric wall, particularly the submucosa and muscularis.[63] Treatment of delayed gastric emptying has not been extensively studied in PSS.[64] In other gastroparetic disorders, benefit from metoclopramide, erythromycin, domperidone, prucalopride, and mirtazepine has been described in some patients. When refractory, venting gastrostomy and jejunal tube feedings may be necessary. Gastric antral vascular ectasia may be found.

Small Bowel Involvement

The true prevalence of small bowel dysfunction is unknown. The absorptive capacity is normal except with SBBO or the rare association with celiac sprue.[65] Small bowel permeability may be increased in PSS, resulting in protein-losing gastroenteropathy (PLGE) or generalized malabsorption.[66] In severe cases, intestinal failure requires intravenous nutrition and has a poor outcome.

Delayed orocecal transit time is common.[67] Manometric abnormalities of the small bowel are frequent.[68,69] Absent, abnormal, or uncoordinated migrating motor complexes suggest a neuropathic process, whereas reduced amplitudes of contraction may suggest a myopathic process.

The small bowel may be dilated with flocculation and pooling of barium. A "hide-bound" bowel pattern consists of diffuse dilatation with closely packed valvulae conniventes from atrophy of the longitudinal fibers of the muscularis propria that foreshortens the bowel.[70] The jejunum and colon may have true diverticula containing all of the layers of the bowel wall, with wide necks that do not predispose to diverticulitis.[62] They may be asymptomatic or associated with abdominal pain, vomiting, bleeding, perforation, or SBBO. Rarely, pneumatosis cystoides intestinalis (see Fig. 35.1), intestinal pseudo-obstruction, or pneumoperitoneum may develop.[71,72]

SBBO is common[73] and due to delayed orocecal transit time, loss of normal migrating motor complexes, the presence of diverticula, and raised gastric pH with PPIs. Symptoms may improve with antibiotics, sometimes in combination with daily low-dose octreotide, which may improve phase III of the migrating motor complex in PSS patients. An open-label pilot trial of a combination of the probiotic *Saccharomyces boulardii* (SB) and metronidazole treatment was 22% more effective in eradicating SIBO than SB treatment alone and 30% more effective than metronidazole treatment alone.[74] Refractory symptoms may require enteral feedings or total parenteral nutrition.

Colonic Involvement

Colonic involvement in PSS occurs in 50% but is frequently asymptomatic. Symptoms may include abnormal stool consistency, bloating, incomplete evacuation, fecal incontinence, and rectal bleeding.[75] Typical findings on barium enema include an increase in luminal fluid, post-evacuation residuals, and lack of haustrations with bowel dilation.[62]

Complications of colonic involvement include pseudo-obstruction, stercoral rectosigmoid ulcers from chronic impaction, volvulus, perforation, colonic strictures, rectal prolapse, pneumatosis cystoides intestinalis, and benign pneumoperitoneum.[61,62]

Oral mineral oil should be avoided in those with impaired esophageal function and at risk for aspiration. Osmotically active agents may worsen pseudo-obstruction. Data on prokinetics are limited. A report describes successful use of prucalopride, a 5-HT_4 receptor agonist, in two PSS patients, but further studies are needed.[76] Pyridostigmine has been shown to be beneficial as a prokinetic in PSS, especially with regard to constipation improvement.[77] Octreotide may be useful in refractory cases and can be tried in combination with erythromycin.[78,79]

Anal Involvement

The anal sphincter is the second most common part of the GI tract affected by PSS. Incontinence of feces is due to diarrhea, anal dysfunction, rectal prolapse, and chronic straining. The internal anal sphincter (IAS), composed of smooth muscle, is atrophic and thin as shown by endoanal ultrasonography and functional lumen imaging probe.[80,81] Resting anal sphincter tone may be reduced, the anal sensory threshold attenuated, rectal compliance reduced, and the rectoanal inhibitory reflex impaired.[82,83] Treatment includes biofeedback (often unsuccessful) and sacral nerve stimulation, although data are limited.[84] Similar to gastric antral vascular ectasia, patients may develop watermelon-like vascular stripes in the rectum, with dilated and thrombosed capillaries in the lamina propria.[85] In addition, telangiectasias have been described throughout the GI tract and may be sources of bleeding.

Miscellaneous Problems

Case reports document idiopathic calcific pancreatitis and arteritis resulting in ischemic pancreatic necrosis.[62,86] Anticentromere antibody, a hallmark antibody of PSS, is reported in 9%–30% of patients with PBC, and 25% of PSS patients are positive for AMA. Patients with PBC associated with PSS have slower liver disease progression compared to those with PBC alone.[13,14,87]

Systemic Lupus Erythematosus

Systemic lupus erythematosus (SLE) is a multisystemic female-predominant autoimmune disorder.[88,89] GI symptoms (e.g., nausea/vomiting, anorexia, and abdominal pain) are common, usually mild, but can be fulminant and life-threatening. In adults, they are caused by diverse etiologies, sometimes unrelated to lupus, with wide ranges of severity. In children, abdominal pain is usually related to the SLE, most commonly from vasculitis, pancreatitis, and/or peritonitis/ascites.[90,91]

Vasculitis

Vasculitis, also termed *lupus enteritis* when pathology is unavailable, affects up to 9.7% of patients with SLE and up to 65% of those presenting with an acute abdomen.[92] This typically small vessel disease should be distinguished from mesenteric artery atherosclerotic disease, to which SLE patients are predisposed via proinflammatory cytokines and corticosteroid use. The inflammatory form is characterized by leukocytoclastic vasculitis due to immune complex deposition in vessel walls, whereas the thrombotic form is caused by thrombosis of vessels associated with antiphospholipid antibodies. These processes may activate one another. Its presentation, ranging from mild symptoms to an acute abdomen, is almost always accompanied by systemically active disease.[92–94] There is usually pain, nausea and vomiting, tenderness, hypocomplementemia, and leucopenia. Complications include symptomatic ischemia, infarction, stricture formation, bleeding, and perforation. Lower levels of CH50 at presentation are a predictor of inadequate treatment response.[95]

CT findings typically include bowel wall thickening, target or double halo sign, dilatation of intestinal segments, comb sign (prominent mesenteric vessels with palisade pattern), ascites, or in more advanced cases, pneumatosis intestinalis or mesenteric venous gas.[96] The jejunum and ileum are most commonly affected, with involvement being segmental or multifocal rather than restricted to a vascular territory as in thromboembolic ischemia.[93] Mesenteric angiography, although useful in excluding polyarteritis nodosa (PAN), may be negative in SLE, which generally involves medium to small arteries. Endoscopic exams may show ischemia and punched-out ulcers with intervening normal mucosa, although colonoscopy has been documented to rarely precipitate ischemic colitis and/or perforation.[97]

Endoscopic biopsies are often unrevealing unless submucosal vessels are sampled. Pathology shows small vessel arteritis and venulitis, leading to diffuse concentric fibrosis, fibrinoid necrosis with thrombosis of affected vessels, leukocytoclasis, and inflammatory infiltrates.[92]

Patients usually respond well to high dose glucocoricoids,[88,89,92,93] although cyclophosphamide can be used acutely in difficult cases and to prevent recurrences. Surgical intervention should be considered when a rapid response to immunosuppressive agents is lacking to prevent potential complications like intestinal perforation or significant bowel ischemia. In 1 series, all 33 mesenteric vasculitis patients who received surgery between 24 and 48 hours of presentation survived, while 10 of 11 patients who underwent surgery after 48 hours died.[98] The differential diagnosis includes antiphospholipid antibody syndrome and opportunistic infections, which may mimic GI vasculitis in these immunocompromised patients.[99]

Oral, Esophageal, Gastric, and Intestinal Involvement

Oral ulcers are the most common area of mucosal involvement in SLE and are part of the diagnostic criteria. SLE esophageal involvement manifests as heartburn and sometimes dysphagia exacerbated by esophageal dysmotility and decreased saliva production from associated SS. Dysmotility has been found in different parts of the esophagus, although it is less frequent than in PSS or mixed connective tissue disease (MCTD).[100] The upper esophagus and pharynx may be involved; whether this is due to SLE or to an overlap with polymyositis is controversial. Aperistalsis in the lower esophagus with a hypotonic LES can be due to SLE itself or PSS/MCTD overlap. Immunosuppressive therapy may be required when esophageal involvement is histologically vasculitic.

Gastric involvement manifests as dyspepsia. It is unclear whether lupus confers an additional or synergistic ulcerogenic effect above that seen with NSAIDs and/or glucocorticoids. Patients with SLE may have low serum B_{12} levels, intrinsic factor antibodies, or (rarely) pernicious anemia.[88,89]

Although hypoalbuminemia in SLE is usually ascribed to nephrotic syndrome, disease exacerbation, liver disease and excess intestinal losses should be considered. PLGE, sometimes an initial manifestation of SLE and often found in young women, is characterized by marked hypoalbuminemia, ascites, pleural or pericardial effusions, peripheral edema, and low serum complement levels[101–103]; GI symptoms, such as abdominal pain or diarrhea, may be infrequent. The source of protein loss is usually the small bowel and, less commonly the colon.[102] Possible mechanisms include increased microvascular/endothelial permeability, complement-mediated vascular injury, and vasculitis. Other causes of PLGE in SLE include pericardial effusion/constriction and SBBO (see Chapter 31).

A relationship between SLE and celiac disease has been suggested in the past. Although a threefold increased risk of SLE has been reported in patients with celiac disease, this translates into a low absolute risk of at most 2 individuals in 1000 developing SLE in 10 years.[104] SLE has been described with IBD, eosinophilic enteritis, and collagenous colitis; these may represent chance associations.[88,89,105]

Immunocompromised SLE patients may acquire CMV that could mimic a lupus flare with enteritis and/or pancreatitis.[106,107] Salmonellosis is also a common infection in SLE.[108,109] Bacteremia with fever and abdominal pain is seen more frequently than diarrhea, and the organism is more commonly isolated from blood than stool. Risk factors include immunosuppression, low complement levels, impaired clearance of the organism, and hyposplenism. SLE and salmonellosis share certain clinical features such as pleurisy, synovitis, cytopenias, and rashes. An increased incidence of giardiasis in SLE patients compared with healthy controls has been suggested.[110]

Pneumatosis cystoides intestinalis (see Fig. 35.1) and pneumoperitoneum are rare, generally benign lesions associated with SLE.[111] Intestinal pseudo-obstruction (see Chapter 126) usually occurs in the setting of active lupus, sometimes as an initial manifestation of disease and has many proposed etiologies. It is associated with ureterohydronephrosis and interstitial cystitis.[88,112,113] Patients often respond to glucocorticoids but may require immunosuppressives or cyclophosphamide for maintenance therapy.

Pancreatic and Gallbladder Involvement

The annual incidence of SLE-associated pancreatitis is said to be 0.4–1 per 1000 in SLE patients,[114] but subclinical cases may be missed, and other causes of pancreatitis are common in SLE.[115] In about 22% of cases, pancreatitis is the initial presentation. Patients usually have active lupus.[116] Only an occasional patient will have vascular lesions associated with antiphospholipid antibodies.[114] Glucocorticoids reduce mortality;[114] addition of azathioprine may be needed. Chronic pancreatitis is extremely rare, is usually preceded by episodes of acute pancreatitis, and is not associated with exocrine or endocrine pancreatic insufficiency.[117]

Primary sclerosing cholangitis and autoimmune cholangiopathy have been found in patients with SLE.[88,118] Pronounced irregularity of the common bile duct may be due to previous subclinical vasculitic episodes affecting the delicate intramural capillary network. Acute acalculous cholecystitis may be due to vasculitis or thrombosis.[119] Although usually treated surgically, it may respond to glucocorticoids if the gallbladder is not distended and if there is no evidence of septicemia.

Ascites and Peritonitis

SLE predisposes to ascites from many causes, such as infection, heart failure, bowel infarction, nephrotic syndrome, PLGE, constrictive pericarditis, pancreatitis, mesenteric vasculitis, Budd-Chiari, or serositis.[120] Serositis more commonly presents as pleuritis or pericarditis rather than peritonitis.[121] In acute lupus peritonitis, the ascites tends to develop rapidly and is associated with pain and a lupus flare. In chronic peritonitis, the ascites develops slowly and is painless. The sterile ascitic fluid may show a low complement level, positive ANA, elevated anti-DNA antibody, and typically a low (<1.1 g/dL) serum ascites albumin gradient. Peritonitis may respond to glucocorticoids or may require additional immunosuppressive therapy.

Hepatic Involvement

Abnormal liver chemistry tests are common, while end-stage liver disease is rare.[14,122] Multiple etiologies of liver disease are found [e.g., fatty liver, hepatic arteritis, PBC, AIH, nodular regenerative hyperplasia, viral hepatitis, drug reaction (discussed previously under RA)]. Hepatitis from SLE, considered a variant of AIH by some investigators, is associated with antiribosomal-P antibodies and deposits of complement 1q on liver immunohistochemistry can differentiate lupus hepatitis from other hepatic disorders.[13,14,88,122] HCV can mimic SLE clinically and serologically,[123] and interferon treatment can induce SLE.[124] Infliximab induces ANA and anti–double stranded DNA in 53% and 35% of patients with IBD, but drug-induced lupus is rare.[125] Vascular disorders of the liver include Budd-Chiari syndrome and hepatic infarction, often due to antiphospholipid syndrome.[13,14,126] Focal disturbances of the hepatic blood supply may account for an increased frequency of focal nodular hyperplasia and hepatic hemangiomas in SLE patients.

Myopathies

The inflammatory myopathies—polymyositis, dermatomyositis, and inclusion body myositis—are diagnosed by a combination of muscle weakness, elevated muscle enzyme levels, electromyographic evidence of a myopathy, and typical muscle histology.[127] Serum AST and ALT levels are roughly equal, because the greater release of AST is counteracted by its greater clearance.[128] Often, an ALT of 100 U/L is accompanied by creatine phosphokinase levels of about 1000 U/L,[129] although many exceptions occur. Of the drugs used in GI diseases, myositis can be caused by anti-TNF agents, interferon, and occasionally PPIs.[130] Myositis can also be associated with IBD, celiac disease, infection with HBV or HCV, and PBC.[127,131] Dermatomyositis may also be associated with a GI vasculopathy, a grave but rare manifestation resulting in vascular ectasias, ulcers, and bowel perforation.[132] Dermatomyositis and, less commonly, polymyositis may be paraneoplastic associated with malignancy involving the stomach, colon, pancreas, and other organs.

Involvement of the pharynx and upper esophageal sphincter (UES), both composed of skeletal muscle, results in nasal regurgitation, tracheal aspiration, tongue weakness, and dysphagia for both solids and liquids.[133,134] This occurs in one-third of such patients and is one of the more treatment refractory manifestations. Low-amplitude pharyngeal contractions and decreased UES pressure are found on esophageal motility studies. Smooth muscle may also be involved, with delayed esophageal and gastric emptying.[127] Reduced LES pressure and nonperistaltic low-amplitude simultaneous esophageal contractions are associated with heartburn. Treatment of pharyngoesophageal involvement includes immunosuppressive therapy (e.g., glucocorticoids), intravenous immunoglobulin, mycophenolate, rituximab, calcineurin inhibitors, cricopharyngeal myotomy, and pharyngeal dilatation, resulting in variable success rates.[133,134]

Sjögren Syndrome

SS occurs alone (primary) or associated with an autoimmune disease (secondary). SS is characterized by lymphocytic infiltration of lacrimal and salivary glands with keratoconjunctivitis sicca and xerostomia. The mouth (discussed in Chapter 24) and esophagus are most commonly involved.[135] Reduced salivary neutralization may increase esophageal acid exposure time and predispose to reflux symptoms and/or mucosal damage. Although salivary flow rates are reduced and a variety of motility disturbances may be found in the esophagus, neither of these abnormalities generally correlates with dysphagia.[135,136] Although chronic atrophic gastritis is common, low vitamin B_{12} levels and/or pernicious anemia are rare.[135] Whether the prevalence of *Helicobacter pylori* (Hp) gastritis is increased in SS is controversial; treatment of Hp does not reduce gastric lymphocytic infiltration, atrophy, or dyspepsia.[137,138] There is a well-known association with mucosa-associated lymphoid tissue lymphoma. Gastric lymphoma is the most common extraglandular site for lymphoma in SS. A risk for gastric adenocarcinoma has been suggested, which may parallel the disease severity association with inflammatory markers, IgA level, and SS-B antibody. The role for gastric cancer screening or surveillance in SS is unclear. Associated celiac disease is found in up to 15% of SS patients.[139] Vasculitis is a rare manifestation of SS and is usually associated with cryoglobulins.

Pancreatitis has been documented in up to 7% of patients with SS,[135] often presenting as autoimmune pancreatitis[140] or chronic pancreatitis. Chronic pancreatitis, with morphologic changes and/or an abnormal secretin test may occur in about 25% of patients with SS[141] but is usually clinically silent.

Abnormal liver chemistry tests, found in 10%–49% of SS patients, are usually mild and have no definite pattern and little clinical significance.[142,143] Hepatomegaly occurs in 11%–21% of patients.[135] The most common causes of liver disease are nonalcoholic fatty liver disease, PBC, AIH, and HCV. Sicca syndrome, abnormal salivary histology, and abnormal sialograms are common in PBC, whereas anti–SS-A/B antibodies are not. Although xerostomia, decreased salivary flow rates, and sialadenitis are seen in HCV, anti–Ro/SS-A/B antibodies are rare.[144] The pathogenesis of HCV-related SS may be due to HCV infection of salivary glands, molecular mimicry, and/or the formation of immune complexes containing HCV.[135]

Mixed Connective Tissue Disease

MCTD is an overlap syndrome, including characteristics of SLE, PSS, and polymyositis associated with antibodies to ribonucleoprotein. Patients can present with heartburn and dysphagia.[145] Delayed esophageal transit, pathologic gastroesophageal reflux on 24-hour pH study, and reduced amplitude and coordination of esophageal peristalsis are found in the majority of patients.[145–147] The diagnosis of MCTD is suggested if there is dysmotility of the entire esophagus, both upper and lower, similar to that seen in polymyositis and PSS, respectively. Upper and LES hypotonia may also be observed. Like in PSS, esophageal abnormalities usually correlate with pulmonary abnormalities in MCTD.[145,146] The role of glucocorticoid therapy in esophageal disease is uncertain.

Changes similar to those of PSS may be seen in the intestine.[148] Occasionally, patients may have a vasculitis, amyloidosis, or pancreatitis.[149] There may be hepatomegaly, splenomegaly, AIH, idiopathic portal hypertension,[150] or Budd-Chiari syndrome.

Polyarteritis Nodosa

PAN is a vasculitis affecting mainly medium-sized arteries; it causes necrotizing inflammation, fibrinoid necrosis, neutrophilic infiltration, and fibroblast proliferation of the vessel wall.[151,152] In addition to GI involvement, skin, joint, kidney, peripheral nerve, and testicular involvement may occur. Mesenteric arterial aneurysms, stenosis, thrombosis, occlusion, and arterial rupture may occur. The result is impaired intestinal perfusion, ulcerations, bleeding, and ischemia if damage is limited to the mucosa or submucosa, and perforation if there is transmural involvement. In 65% of patients the GI tract may be involved, small bowel involvement is most common.[153] Liver involvement, usually subclinical, includes necrotizing vasculitis leading to atrophy of a liver lobe, liver infarction, or nodular regenerative hyperplasia.[154] Rarely, aneurysmal rupture occurs in the liver resulting in hemobilia, subcapsular hemorrhage, or intrahepatic hemorrhage. HBV-associated PAN, which generally occurs early in HBV infection, has a higher association with GI disease, more severe vasculitis, and a higher mortality rate than PAN without HBV.[151,152] HBV-PAN is characterized by circulating immune complexes containing hepatitis B surface antigen and antihepatitis B surface antibodies, supporting the concept that it is mediated by deposition of viral Ag/Ab complexes. Hepatitis B is silent in most cases, with only mild increases in serum aminotransferases.[155] HCV can occasionally be associated with PAN but unlike the early onset after HBV exposure, PAN usually occurs several years after viral exposure; like HBV-PAN, it usually manifests with severe vasculitis.[156]

Pancreatic involvement occurs in 35%–37% of autopsy cases, with acute pancreatitis, pancreatic infarcts, pseudocysts, pancreatic masses, or pancreatic insufficiency.[151] Vasculitis of arteries supplying small bile ducts leads to intrahepatic sclerosing cholangitis, whereas cystic arteritis leads to acalculous gangrenous cholecystitis.[153,157] Ascites due to vasculitis is rare.[158]

Angiography, which is abnormal in more than 60% of patients,[159,160] shows arterial aneurysms, irregularities, and thrombosis, all of which may progress to stenosis and occlusion of the vessels. Aneurysms are focal and segmental, in different stages of development, with a predilection for branch points of vessels. They tend to be multiple, intraparenchymal, and measure up to 1 cm in diameter. Rupture, especially in the presence of hypertension, occurs occasionally. Microaneurysms are sometimes seen as in other conditions [e.g., RA, SLE, and granulomatosis with polyangiitis (GPA)]. A normal visceral angiogram does not exclude PAN; aneurysms may be thrombosed or healing. CT may show bowel wall thickening and the target sign.[161] 3D CT angiography detects aneurysms with diameters as small as 3 mm, as well as early vasculitic changes such as increased wall thickness and calcification, not seen on routine angiography.

Biopsy sites include skin lesions, sural nerve, and muscle. Endoscopic biopsies are usually too superficial to make the diagnosis; deeper biopsies risk perforation.[153]

Glucocorticoids, along with a potent immunosuppressive agent, particularly cyclophosphamide, dramatically decrease mortality. HBV-PAN or HCV-PAN is usually treated with immunosuppressive agents and an antiviral agent, sometimes with plasma exchanges (to remove immune complexes).[151,152,155]

IgA Vasculitis

IgA vasculitis, formerly known as Henoch-Schönlein purpura (HSP), is the most common systemic vasculitis in childhood and occasionally affects young adults. HSP is clinically characterized by palpable purpura, arthritis, and renal and GI involvement. It is associated with the HLA-DRB1*01 allele. Triggers may include drugs, allergens, immunizations, and infections and there is an association with inflammatory bowel disease. Adults typically have a more severe clinical syndrome with higher frequency of renal involvement. HSP is mediated by immune deposits (typically IgA), resulting in leukocytoclastic vasculitis that causes necrosis of small blood vessel walls.[162–164] GI involvement occurs in the majority of patients and sometimes precedes the rash. The abdominal pain is usually colicky, periumbilical or epigastric, and sometimes worsens with eating. There is occult or, less commonly, overt, usually melenic bleeding. The small intestine is most frequently involved with the second portion of the duodenum involved more than the bulb.[162,164] The main differential diagnosis is Crohn disease. Intussusception is usually ileoileal or ileocolic and due to an ileal lead-point (intramural hemorrhage or edema). It often resolves spontaneously or may be reduced with air or contrast enemas performed gently to minimize perforation risk.[165] If intussusception is still present after 24 hours, surgery should be considered. Rarely, the patient may develop acute acalculous cholecystitis, ascites with serositis, or pancreatitis.[162] Recurrences are usually stereotypic, milder, and shorter in duration than the first episode.

Endoscopic findings include petechiae, erosions and ulcers, hyperemia, and ecchymoses (Fig. 35.3). Mucosal biopsies usually show IgA deposition and inflammation. Sampling of the submucosa may reveal vasculitis. Capsule endoscopy may determine the extent of disease and location of bleeding.[166] CT shows thickened bowel walls with skip lesions, ileus, and bowel dilation. To avoid irradiation in children, abdominal ultrasonography is considered the study of choice by some and may help determine prognosis.[167]

Glucocorticoids should be considered in those at high risk for renal involvement; their effects on GI disease are unknown, as more than 80% of cases resolve spontaneously.[162,168] Other modalities (plasma exchange, dapsone, rituximab, and intravenous immunoglobulins) have been tried.

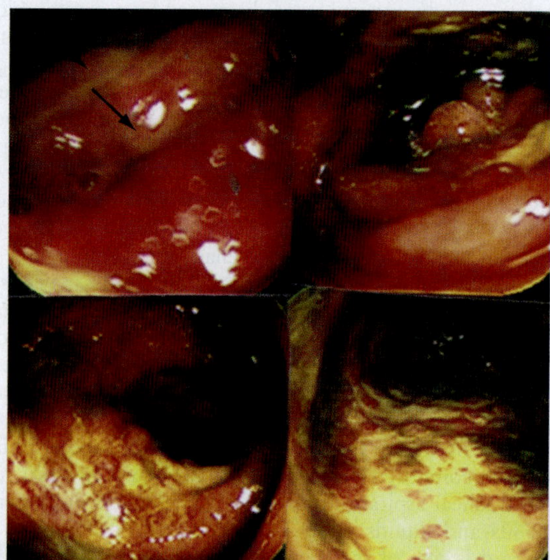

Fig. 35.3 Endoscopic views in a patient with Henoch-Schönlein purpura. The upper views show jejunal mucosa that is diffusely thickened and nodular with superficial linear ulcers (*black arrow*). The lower views show ileal mucosa with a cobblestone appearance. (From Ebert EC. Gastrointestinal manifestations of Henoch-Schönlein purpura. *Dig Dis Sci*. 2008;53:2011–19, with permission from Springer.)

Eosinophilic Granulomatosis With Polyangiitis

Eosinophilic GPA (EGPA) (formerly Churg-Strauss syndrome) is a small- and medium-vessel vasculitis with GI involvement in up to 59% of cases.[169] Of the three phases of this disease (prodromal, eosinophilic, and vasculitic), the GI tract can be involved in the last two. An eosinophilic gastroenteritis can occur with peripheral eosinophilia and an eosinophilic infiltrate in the GI mucosa.[169,170] Abdominal pain, diarrhea, nausea/vomiting, and bleeding are the most common symptoms. Vasculitis may cause ulcerations, perforation, and rarely stenosis.[171] The ulcers characteristically have an erythematous rim.[172] Unusual complications include acalculous cholecystitis, pancreatitis, or eosinophilic ascites from involvement of the peritoneum.[170] Intestinal resection specimens and submucosal biopsies reveal vasculitis with fibrinoid necrosis, eosinophilic infiltrates, and/or granulomas. Glucocorticoids achieve remission in 90%, but close monitoring for intestinal perforation is needed. Involvement of the GI tract, kidneys, CNS, or heart and glucocorticoid–refractory disease may be treated with cyclophosphamide, intravenous immunoglobulin, or plasma exchange.[173] Severe GI tract involvement is associated with a poor outcome.

Granulomatosis With Polyangiitis

GPA (formerly Wegener granulomatosis) along with EGPA and microscopic polyangiitis make up the ANCA-associated vasculitides. Most of the GI tract can be involved in GPA, which is a necrotizing vasculitis affecting small- and medium-sized vessels. The incidence of GI involvement is difficult to determine as it is often asymptomatic. Oral involvement includes ulcers, lingual infarction, and the pathognomonic "strawberry gums," representing gingival hyperplasia studded with petechiae mimicking a ripe strawberry.[174] Esophageal and gastric ulcers occur, with pathology showing necrotizing granulomatous inflammation.[175] Vasculitis leads to intestinal ulcerations, ischemia, infarction, strictures, and perforation. It may resemble or be associated with IBD.[176] Arteritis may lead to pancreatitis or a gangrenous gallbladder.[177] Liver involvement is usually nonspecific, although unusual findings such as incomplete septal fibrosis from ischemia have been described.[178] Superficial intestinal biopsies may reveal only nonspecific findings, and angiography may be normal. Perinuclear-staining antibody ANCA (*p*-ANCA) specific for myeloperoxidase may be positive but the cytoplasmic-staining antibody ANCA (*c*-ANCA) directed at the proteinase 3 antigen of myeloid lysosomes (PR3) is more specific. Most lesions respond to induction with pulse corticosteroids, or cyclophosphamide. Plasma exchange or rituximab may also be effective.

Cryoglobulinemia

Cryoglobulins are immunoglobulins that precipitate in vitro at temperatures below 37°C.[179] Cryoglobulinemia may produce organ damage through hyperviscosity or vasculitis, the latter being the main mechanism for GI involvement. Although cryoglobulinemia is associated with infections, autoimmune diseases, and cancer, the most common cause is HCV. Up to 7% of patients with cryoglobulinemia have GI involvement, usually manifesting as mesenteric vasculitis (see RA, SLE, and PAN).[180] Severe GI involvement is an independent factor associated with poor outcome in non–HCV-related vasculitis. Treatment is aimed at the underlying disease and may include corticosteroids, colchicine, or dapsone for mild disease but more severe disease will require immunosuppressive drugs, plasma exchange, and/or rituximab.

Behçet Disease

This multisystemic vasculitis typically includes recurrent oral and genital ulcers, arthritis, uveitis, and characteristic skin lesions. CNS symptoms, GI lesions, hypercoagulability, and visceral artery aneurysms may also be seen. Although Behçet disease (BD) is most common in the ancient "Silk Road" countries, GI involvement in this disease is most common in certain other countries (e.g., Japan and United Kingdom).[181,182] Small vessel vasculitis primarily affecting veins and venules presents with mucosal inflammation causing ulcers; large vessel disease results in ischemia and infarction. This vasculitis mainly affects the ileocecal region resembling Crohn disease. Extraintestinal manifestations of oral aphthae, uveitis, arthritis, and erythema nodosum may mimic IBD. Pathergy testing (skin papules or pustules after needle prick) can be helpful diagnostically. Several other features distinguish BD from Crohn disease.[183–185] Unlike Crohn disease, BD rarely causes strictures, perianal disease, or rectal ulcers and multisegmental or diffuse GI involvement is rare. BD frequently causes oral ulcers, mucosal edema, intestinal perforation, and venulitis (without bowel inflammation, fibrosis, or granulomas), and it often resolves spontaneously. Infectious processes may mimic or complicate BD.[186] Endoscopic studies should be done with caution due to a risk of perforation, because the intestinal ulcers are often quite deep. There may be amyloidosis (discussed later), aneurysm formation, or hepatic or portal vein thrombosis.[187] Thrombophlebitis, thought to be due to venulitis, may not benefit from anticoagulation. Acute pancreatitis, Budd-Chiari syndrome, multiple aseptic hepatic and splenic abscesses,[188] and sclerosing cholangitis are reported in BD. Therapy of GI involvement includes mesalamine, immunomodulators, and TNF inhibitors. Whether glucocorticoids prolong the healing process and provoke perforation is unclear.[189] A phase 2 study found that the oral phosphodiesterase inhibitor apremilast significantly reduced oral ulcer formation in patients with BD. However, the treatment was brief (12–24 weeks) and associated with diarrhea, nausea, and vomiting. Furthermore, effects of apremilast on other aspects of the disease, including the GI manifestations, remain to be elucidated.[190] Recurrences after surgery, often at the anastomotic site, occur in 50%.[191]

Spondyloarthropathies

Subclinical gut inflammation has been described in up to two-thirds of patients with various spondyloarthopathies.[192–194] The presence of ileitis may be associated with chronicity of the articular disease. The acute form of spondyloarthropathy (typically reactive arthritis) has gut inflammation that mimics bacterial enteritis with neutrophil infiltration but preserved gut architecture. The chronic form (typically ankylosing spondylitis) mimics Crohn disease, with a mononuclear cell infiltrate and disturbed architecture. Although it may be histologically indistinguishable from Crohn's ileitis, spondyloarthropathy-associated ileitis is usually asymptomatic, radiologically inapparent, and patients are usually HLA-B27 positive. Ankylosing spondylitis is found in up to 15% of IBD patients in general and in 50% of IBD patients with HLA-B27. For axial involvement, NSAIDs reduce joint pain and stiffness but may worsen underlying IBD. Glucocorticoids are rarely effective in spondyloarthropathies and decrease bone mineral density. Sulfasalazine and possibly MTX may have some efficacy in spondyloarthropathies, particularly in patients with appendicular involvement. TNF-α blocking agents, including etanercept, which is not used in IBD, as well as JAK inhibitors are also quite effective.

Familial Mediterranean Fever

Familial Mediterranean fever (FMF), an autosomal recessive disease, is characterized by recurrent self-limited attacks of fever, joint pain, and abdominal pain, most commonly in people of Mediterranean origin.[195,196] The gene responsible for FMF, *MEFV* on chromosome 16, encodes the protein pyrin. *MEFV* gene analysis assists in diagnosis.

Patients develop what appears to be an acute abdomen due to peritonitis. Their severe abdominal pain is reduced by lying motionless with hips flexed. The abdomen is rigid with rebound tenderness, reduced bowel sounds, and abdominal distension. There may be multiple air-fluid levels, a leukocytosis with a left shift, an increased ESR, and elevated acute-phase reactants. The attack begins to subside after 24 hours. Peritonitis results in protein-rich sterile exudates with fibrin and neutrophils that, when organized, may lead to adhesions and small bowel obstruction, sometimes with strangulation and necrosis. Patients are asymptomatic between episodes, although acute-phase reactants may be elevated, indicating subclinical inflammation.

Serum amyloid concentration increases dramatically during febrile attacks [see the "amyloidosis" section (under infiltrative diseases)]. AA amyloidosis may develop independent of the frequency, duration, and intensity of flare-ups. Kidney impairment is the most clinically significant result, but amyloid can deposit in the GI tract and cause symptoms after many years. FMF is associated with other diseases such as IBD[197] some vasculitides, and irritable bowel syndrome. GI mucosal involvement may suggest IBD but mucosal healing can be achieved with colchicine alone.

Abnormal esophageal motility may occur regardless of amyloid status.[198] Liver disease is usually from amyloid, and splenomegaly is from ongoing inflammation.[195,196] Although there is no specific treatment for acute attacks, colchicine at daily doses up to 2 mg/day reduces the attack frequency, severity, and duration in most FMF patients. Because it can prevent, arrest, and even reverse renal amyloidosis and treats subclinical inflammation, colchicine should be continued for life. Refractory cases may respond to the anti-IL-1 beta 1 monoclonal antibody canakinumab, TNF-α inhibitors, or tocilizumab.

Disorders of Connective Tissue

GI manifestations have been reported in a variety of connective tissue disorders. These may be classified as structural or functional abnormalities.

GI manifestations of *Marfan syndrome* are typically overshadowed by cardiac, ophthalmic, and musculoskeletal manifestations. Fibrillin-1 gene mutations lead to qualitative and/or quantitative alterations to the glycoprotein fibrillin-1, with subsequent myofibril deficiency and connective tissue instability. In the GI tract, this may lead to visceral herniation, abdominal wall hernias, diverticula/pseudodiverticula, and clinical events such as acute appendicitis or acute diverticulitis at unusually young ages. There also appears to be an increased frequency of hepatic cysts, renal cysts, and cholelithiasis. Functional GI disorders, such as IBS, may also be more common than in control groups.[199]

In *Ehlers–Danlos syndrome* (EDS), functional GI disorders predominate but epiphrenic diverticula, diaphragmatic eventration, megaesophagus, spontaneous GI perforations, and acute GI bleeding may occur. One large retrospective study found that 378 of 687 patients with EDS (56%) had associated GI manifestations in the classic, hypermobility, and vascular subtypes. The vascular subtypes all had frequent GI symptoms, but such symptoms were somewhat less common than in the hypermobility variant. Typical symptoms included abdominal pain (56%), nausea (42%), constipation (39%), heartburn (38%), and IBS symptoms (28%). Gastric and colonic transits were delayed in 12% and 28%, respectively. All abdominal aneurysms occurred in the Villefranche EDS type IV vascular subtype, which accounts for 5%–10% of EDS.[200] This results from mutations in the gene for type III procollagen (COL3Ar). This mutation results in quantitative and qualitative abnormalities of mature type III collagen. Systemic arteries that are rich in type III collagen may undergo dissection, aneurysms or rupture. In addition to vascular complications, spontaneous rupture of hollow viscera that is also rich in type III collagen, such as the uterus or intestine, may occur.

The *benign joint hypermobility syndrome* may be found with increased frequency in unselected tertiary functional GI disorder patients when compared with a 10%–20% frequency in normal individuals. Joint hypermobility incidence was evaluated in 129 unselected new tertiary referrals (97 female) to a neurogastrointestinal clinic and 63 (49%) had evidence of joint hypermobility; an unknown etiology of GI symptoms was more frequent in those with joint hypermobility than in those without it. A clinical impression of joint hypermobility was confirmed by a rheumatologist in 23 of 25 patients evaluated.[201]

IgG4-Related Disease

This rare multisystem inflammatory and fibrotic disorder typically affects the pancreas (type I or II autoimmune pancreatitis; see Chapter 61) or bile ducts and can mimic pancreatic cancer, cholangiocarcinoma, or PSC. Reports of other intra-abdominal involvement include retroperitoneal fibrosis, aortitis, sclerosing mesenteritis, inflammatory pseudotumor, hepatitis, enteritis, colitis, and pouchitis. Serum IgG4 is elevated in only 60%–70% of patients; frequently, diagnostic biopsies of the affected organ are necessary and typically reveal a dense lymphoplasmacytic IgG4 staining infiltrate, storiform fibrosis, and obliterative phlebitis. Initial therapy with glucocorticoids is usually effective therapeutically but relapses are common and maintenance immunomodulators, mycophenolate, abatacept, or rituximab are sometimes required.

ONCOLOGIC AND HEMATOLOGIC DISEASES

Metastases to the Gastrointestinal Tract

Metastases to the gut occur by hematogenous or lymphatic spread or by intraperitoneal seeding, most commonly from breast cancer.[202] Metastases are distinguished from primary tumors by the absence of a transition between normal and cancer cells and by histologic and immunohistochemical similarities between the primary and the secondary deposits.

GI metastases are more commonly seen at autopsy than clinically because many are asymptomatic. The most common presentations are abdominal pain, anemia, GI bleeding, obstruction, weight loss, and (rarely) PLGE.[202,203] Some metastases, particularly melanoma (Fig. 35.4), breast cancer, and renal cell carcinoma, may present decades after the primary tumor is found.[204,205]

Polypoid metastatic lesions in the intestinal mucosa may initiate intussusception[207] or result in bleeding from ulceration or cavitation as the growth of the metastasis exceeds its blood supply. Deposition in the submucosa causes a submucosal mass or diffuse infiltration with wall thickening and rigidity. With central ulceration, a "bull's eye" lesion may appear.[204,208] Carcinomatosis with malignant ascites may occur with rupture of tumor into the peritoneal cavity.[204] Perforation may occur, sometimes from tumor necrosis caused by chemotherapy.

Gastric metastases are most commonly from lung, breast, esophagus, and melanoma.[208] Small bowel involvement is most commonly due to lobular breast cancer or malignant melanoma. Pancreatic metastases are rare and due to renal cancer in 60% of

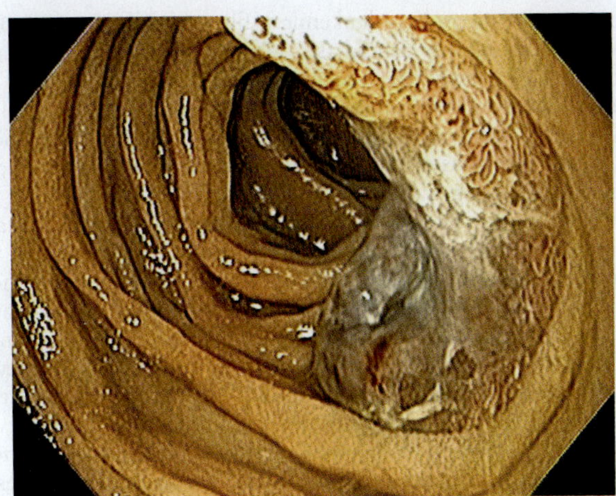

Fig. 35.4 Endoscopic view of an ulcerated metastatic melanoma lesion involving the second portion of the duodenum in a young man who presented with upper GI bleeding.

cases.[209] Renal cancer appears as an enhancing mass on CT and is hypervascular on angiography.[210] Resection of a pancreatic metastasis may increase survival.[209,210]

Melanoma metastases, pigmented or amelanotic, are most often found in the small bowel[204,205] followed by the colon and stomach.[206] Surgical resection of the metastasis, usually for anemia or obstruction, improves symptoms with minimal morbidity or mortality although disease recurrence is common postoperatively. Melanoma has been reported to metastasize to the gallbladder.[211] Primary mucosal melanoma of the GI tract is rare, most commonly affecting the anorectum.[206]

The most common type of breast cancer to metastasize to the GI tract is lobular carcinoma, even though most breast cancers are ductular carcinomas.[212] Patients occasionally present with oropharyngeal dysphagia, pseudoachalasia, or an esophageal stricture. Gastric metastases may mimic linitis plastica with an infiltrative picture, involvement of the terminal ileum may resemble Crohn disease, and rectal infiltration may mimic primary rectal cancer (Schnitzler metastasis). Metastatic breast cancer may consist of signet ring cells without gland formation, mimicking a primary GI malignancy. Estrogen receptors are commonly expressed in the tumor, helping in the diagnosis. GI metastases from lung cancer, although rare, are usually due to large cell carcinoma.[213]

Paraneoplastic Syndromes

Paraneoplastic GI dysmotility presents with pseudoachalasia, gastroparesis, constipation, or pseudo-obstruction.[214,215] It is most commonly due to small cell lung cancer, with GI symptoms usually preceding the tumor diagnosis by weeks or months. Other primary neoplasms associated with paraneoplastic GI dysmotility include breast, bladder, prostate, kidney, testicular, ovary, neuroblastoma, and primary GI malignancies such as pancreatic carcinoma. The most commonly described autoantibodies are type 1 antineuronal nuclear antibodies reactive against tumor cells and neuronal nuclei, including those in the myenteric plexus. Anti-HuD antibodies induce neuronal apoptosis.[216] The presence of this and similar antineuronal antibodies should prompt a search for malignancy. Neuropathy is the most common manifestation of type 1 antineuronal antibodies, but GI dysmotility is found in about 30% of patients.

Patients present with acute and rapidly progressive weight loss, dysphagia, nausea and vomiting, early satiety, constipation, and/or abdominal pain, usually with normal chest x-rays despite the presence of small cell lung cancer.[215] Esophageal dysmotility, delayed gastric emptying, slow intestinal transit, and abnormal autonomic reflex tests are common.[217] Antroduodenal manometry shows a neuropathic type of GI dysmotility. The differential diagnosis of altered GI motility includes viral infections, medications (especially opioids), chemotherapy (e.g., vincristine), and radiation damage.

Conventional therapeutic measures, such as prokinetics, antiemetics, and laxatives, have limited benefit.[215] Even chemotherapy that shrinks the tumor may not palliate the GI symptoms.

Paraneoplastic hepatopathy describes the rare phenomenon of intrahepatic cholestasis as a paraneoplastic phenomenon, most commonly associated with renal cell carcinoma (Stauffer syndrome) and lymphoma. Alkaline phosphatase abnormalities are most characteristic, and hyperbilirubinemia or jaundice is more unusual. Paraneoplastic hepatopathy has also been associated with pheochromocytoma, prostate carcinoma, medullary thyroid carcinoma, ovarian dysgerminoma, and neuroendocrine tumors. Such cholestasis has been associated with nonspecific hepatic inflammation or sinusoidal dilation histologically, typically resolves after tumor resection, and may recur with tumor recurrence. Paraneoplastic biliary ductal damage (secondary sclerosing cholangitis) and the vanishing bile duct syndrome have been associated with lymphoma.[218]

POEMS syndrome (polyneuropathy, organomegaly, endocrinopathy, M-protein, and skin changes) is a rare multisystem neoplastic disorder of plasma cells. It frequently has an insidious onset manifesting in the fifth to sixth decade of life. Mandatory criteria include polyneuropathy and a monoclonal plasma cell dyscrasia (usually lambda light chain); major criteria may also include Castleman disease, sclerotic bone lesions, and vascular endothelial growth factor (VEGF) elevation; minor criteria include organomegaly, extravascular fluid accumulation [edema, low SAAG (75%) ascites, pleural effusions], skin changes, endocrinopathy, papilledema, and polycythemia/thrombocytosis. The clinical manifestations are likely caused by elevated VEGF, which markedly increases microvascular permeability. Most patients have solitary or multiple plasmacytomas. Bone marrow evaluation often shows plasma cell clonality, and therapy is directed at the underlying plasma cell dyscrasia. Hepatomegaly and ascites may falsely suggest underlying chronic liver disease.[219]

Hematologic Malignancies

The liver, as part of the reticuloendothelial system, is frequently involved in disseminated lymphoproliferative disease and usually signifies an advanced stage.[220] Hematologic malignancies are frequently associated with elevated liver chemistry tests but typically do not cause clinically significant hepatic dysfunction. The frequency of liver involvement varies widely depending upon the type of malignancy. Alternatively, some hepatic abnormalities may be due to drug toxicity, infections, amyloidosis, or extrahepatic obstruction from porta hepatis lymphadenopathy.

Liver Involvement in Systemic Lymphomas

The liver may be the site for a rare primary lymphoma or, more commonly, for spread from systemic lymphomas. There is an association of lymphoma with HIV, HCV, or EBV (post-transplant) infection, common variable immunodeficiency (CVID), rheumatologic disorders, celiac disease, IBD, thiopurine therapy, and possibly TNF inhibitor therapy. HBV-infected patients also have a two- to threefold increased risk of developing non-Hodgkin lymphoma (NHL), although a cause-effect relationship has not been proven.[221]

Almost 90% of hepatic lymphomas are NHL, with most being of B cell origin.[220,222] NHL more commonly has malignant involvement of the liver than does Hodgkin lymphoma (HL).

Imaging is often normal or shows multiple or diffusely infiltrating lesions. The less common focal liver lesions are usually hypoechoic on ultrasonography and hypoattenuating on CT scan.[223,224] Splenic involvement and lymphadenopathy support the diagnosis of lymphoma. Nonspecific histologic findings in both NHL and HL are portal lymphocytic infiltrates, hemosiderosis, steatosis, and granulomas (usually noncaseating), the last more common in HL than in NHL.[220,222,225] Immunotyping can characterize the phenotype of these cells.

Many patients have no clinical or biochemical suggestion of hepatic involvement. Hepatomegaly or abnormal liver chemistry tests, such as a moderately elevated serum alkaline phosphatase level, do not correlate well with lymphomatous involvement.[226] Rarely, massive hepatic infiltration by tumor can result in acute liver failure, with an average survival of 10 days.[227]

In NHL, diffuse large B-cell lymphoma is the most common subtype. This presents predominantly with tumor nodules distributed diffusely throughout the liver with a dense lymphomatous infiltrate.[220,222] T-cell–rich B-cell lymphoma, in contrast, is characterized by a scattered portal tract infiltrate with few neoplastic cells, often misdiagnosed as a reactive inflammatory condition or as T-cell lymphoma infiltration of the liver. The less common T-cell lymphoma lacks a typical infiltration pattern and may be confused with a drug-induced or viral hepatitis when biopsies just show increased numbers of T cells. A distinction between these possibilities would necessitate clonality analysis by T-cell receptor or immunoglobulin heavy locus PCR.

In HL, hepatic involvement is virtually always associated with splenic involvement, but the converse is not always true. Liver disease is usually diffuse with miliary lesions more often than masses. A predominantly portal infiltration is the most common histologic feature, with Reed-Sternberg cells detected only occasionally.[220,222]

Cholestasis is most commonly due to intrahepatic tumor infiltration, but extrahepatic bile duct obstruction by enlarged lymph nodes should be kept in mind. Rare conditions include idiopathic cholestasis and vanishing bile duct syndrome.[228] The degree of cholestasis is often disproportionate to the apparent tumor load and may respond to chemotherapy or lead to fatal liver damage.

GI Involvement in Primary Cutaneous T-cell and B-cell Lymphomas

Mycosis fungoides, nasal-type extranodal natural killer cell/T-cell lymphoma, primary cutaneous gamma-delta T-cell lymphoma, and Sézary syndrome have all been documented to involve the GI tract, most often the stomach, small bowel, and pancreas. Autopsy studies have shown GI involvement in 50 of 146 patients with mycosis fungoides. The severity of skin burden, typically the nodular-tumorous stage with inguinal lymph node involvement, appears to be correlated with visceral involvement. Mycosis fungoides affecting the GI tract may present with malabsorption, diarrhea, perforation, bleeding, dysphagia, and obstruction.[206]

GI and Liver Involvement in Leukemia

Leukemias can involve any part of the GI tract, with about 10% of patients being symptomatic.[229] GI involvement usually occurs during relapse due to leukemic infiltration of the bowel wall, immunodeficiency, coagulation disorders, or chemotherapy. Treatment reduces proliferation of normal cells, causes myelosuppression, and weakens areas of the bowel wall as it destroys the underlying malignancy. Although most patients are asymptomatic, others may complain of abdominal pain, bleeding, or diarrhea.

Common oral problems include xerostomia, gingival bleeding, mucositis, infections (particularly candidal), and dental disease.[230] The esophagus may have leukemic infiltrates, infectious esophagitis (most commonly candidiasis, HSV, or CMV), hemorrhagic lesions (e.g., petechiae, ecchymoses, erosions, ulcers), or chemotherapy-induced mucositis.[229,231]

Leukemic infiltration of the bowel may present as ulcerations or as nodular lesions resulting in intussusception, obstruction, or a picture resembling cancer.[229,232,233] It can extend through the bowel wall, resulting in perforation. Less common are PLGE and malabsorption. Leukemic infiltrates are found particularly in the terminal ileum and appendix, owing to the abundant lymphoid tissue in these areas. The picture may mimic IBD or be associated with pneumatosis cystoides intestinalis or pneumoperitoneum.[229,234] Immunodeficiency may lead to agranulocytic ulcers with bacterial invasion and bleeding. Coagulation defects can produce intramural hematomas and hemorrhagic necrosis of the bowel. Painful anorectal lesions include thrombosed hemorrhoids, stercoral and neutropenic ulcers, fistulas, and abscesses.

Neutropenic enterocolitis or typhlitis (from the Greek word *typhlon*, meaning "cecum") is a necrotizing process involving the terminal ileum, cecum, and ascending colon.[229,234–237] It usually occurs during the onset or relapse of acute myelogenous leukemia, often following chemotherapy, and is a common source of fever. Other conditions associated with neutropenia may also be complicated by neutropenic enterocolitis. Distension of the cecum, sometimes associated with hypotension, impairs perfusion, leading to mucosal breaches and entry of organisms that proliferate profusely given the neutropenia.[229,238]

Patients present with fever, right lower quadrant abdominal pain, diarrhea, bleeding, nausea and vomiting, dehydration and sepsis, and occasionally an acute abdomen. With sepsis, Gram-negative bacteria are the most frequently identified pathogens. Bowel wall thickness of greater than 10 mm is seen on CT and ultrasonography and is associated with 60% mortality.[236,239] Most patients can be managed with intravenous fluids, transfusion of blood and platelets, granulocyte colony-stimulating factor, and broad-spectrum antibiotics, with surgery reserved for complications.

Infiltration of liver, spleen, and lymph nodes is common in leukemia, but the possible hemorrhagic complications resulting from liver biopsy make it difficult to discern the relative contributions of leukemic infiltrates, extramedullary hematopoiesis (EMH), and other infectious and toxic complications of these diseases. Although often asymptomatic, acute liver failure may develop.[240] Rarely, the pancreas, gallbladder, or bile ducts (cholangiopathy) may be involved.[241–243] Splenic rupture in acute leukemia, mainly with splenomegaly, may be due to leukemic infiltration, splenic infarction, or defects in coagulation, particularly thrombocytopenia.[244]

A diffuse nondestructive infiltration of the liver is usually asymptomatic and without significant laboratory abnormalities. In chronic lymphocytic leukemia, the leukemic infiltrate involves the portal areas, usually leaving the limiting plate intact, although in some cases it may cause hepatocellular necrosis, bridging necrosis, and occasionally pseudo-lobule formation.[222] In other leukemias, sinusoidal involvement may be seen with or without portal infiltrates.

Systemic Mastocytosis

Systemic mastocytosis is characterized by multiple dense infiltrates of mast cells (MCs) in bone marrow or extracutaneous organs, mutations in the *c-kit* gene (*CD117*), and elevated serum tryptase concentrations.[245,246] The classical skin finding of urticaria pigmentosa is seen with or without systemic involvement. The frequency of GI involvement is highly variable but probably second only to pruritus as a cause of morbidity.[247] Symptoms are thought to be due mainly to mediator release (e.g., histamine, leukotrienes, heparin, and proteases), and less commonly to MC

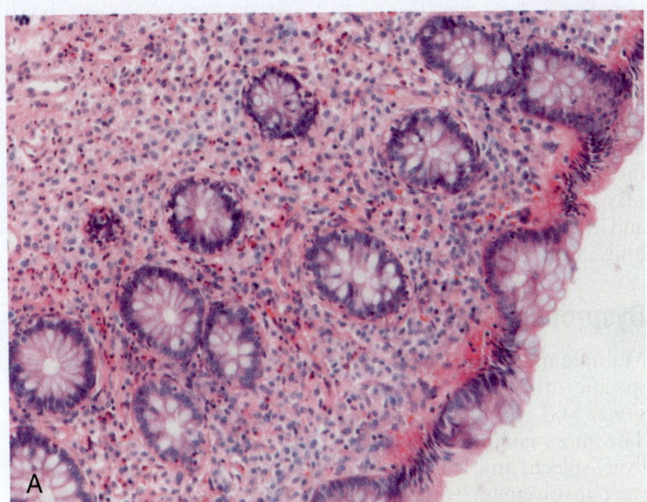

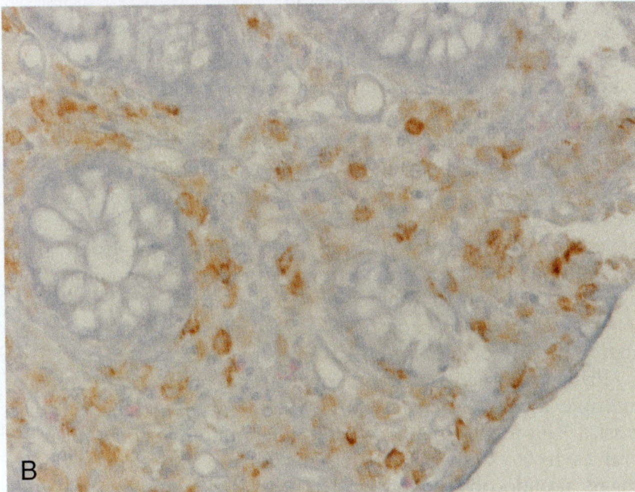

Fig. 35.5 Systemic mastocytosis involving the colon. (A) An interstitial infiltrate of mast cells with pale cytoplasm is present (H&E, ×100). (B) A mast cell tryptase immunohistochemical stain highlights the interstitial infiltrate (×400). The patient also had bone marrow involvement. (Courtesy Shahab I, MD, Dallas, TX.)

infiltration of the gut. Inflammatory and vasoactive mediator release leads to symptoms, most commonly diarrhea and bloating, but also abdominal pain and nausea/vomiting, often exacerbated by precipitants such as drugs, stress, and certain foods. Pain may be either dyspeptic or lower abdominal cramping. Direct infiltration of the gut mucosa by MCs may lead to malabsorption and weight loss symptoms.[248] Occasionally the esophagus is affected leading to heartburn/esophagitis or motor disorders.[249] PUD may be underdiagnosed and can be caused by histamine-mediated gastric acid hypersecretion. Diarrhea also may be related to gastric hypersecretion, as well as to intestinal malabsorption, overproduction of prostaglandin D_2, or occasionally to altered intestinal transit.[245–247,250]

Endoscopic features are nonspecific (nodularity, erythema, ulcerations, urticaria-like lesions, thickened folds, and purple pigmented lesions).[247] Histology may be diagnostic or nonspecific, with a mixed infiltrate that may include MCs, although MCs are commonly seen in other disorders (Fig. 35.5). However, unlike other inflammatory diseases, the histology in systemic mastocytosis may include high numbers of MCs, MCs in aggregates or confluent sheets, abnormal MC morphology, and positive staining for CD25.[251,252] Often, infiltrates contain plasma cells and eosinophils, but the presence of numerous MCs would be atypical for eosinophilic gastroenteritis. There may be expansion and distortion of crypt architecture as in IBD.[253] Crypt abscesses, however, are unusual. Also, although villous atrophy is found, the crypt hyperplasia typical of celiac sprue is usually not seen.

Hepatomegaly and abnormal liver chemistry tests are common. The liver chemistry tests may be either a mixed pattern or an isolated alkaline phosphatase elevation, often from bone.[246] Liver biopsies may show portal MC infiltrates, eosinophilic infiltrates, EMH, portal fibrosis, and sometimes cirrhosis. Portal hypertension may develop, although splenomegaly may also be due to MC infiltration. Liver stiffness by transient elastography may be seen.[254]

Treatment is aimed at limiting MC degranulation and controlling pathologic MC tissue infiltration.[245] GI symptoms may improve with H_1- and/or and H_2-receptor antagonists, oral disodium cromoglycate, or glucocorticoids. For aggressive disease with organ dysfunction, cytoreductive therapy with interferon or cladribine has shown limited response rates and duration. The KIT D816V (Asp-→Val) mutation is present in 90% of patients with systemic mastocytosis, and an uncontrolled, observational multinational study of 116 such patients reported that a multiple kinase inhibitor (midostaurin) is effective both in advanced mastocytosis and its highly lethal variant, MC leukemia. Imatinib (Gleevec) is currently FDA-approved for patients with this D816V mutation.[255] Patients should also be informed of the potential triggers of MC activation, including emotional distress, infections, allergies, alcohol, and some medications, including NSAIDs and opiates.[248]

The prognosis is good for the indolent or smoldering type (the latter with organ infiltration without organ dysfunction) but poor for the aggressive type (organ infiltration with dysfunction) or transformation to MC leukemia.

Unlike systemic mastocytosis, the MC activation syndrome does not occur due to an increased MC number but rather a hyperresponsiveness of MCs that leads to an inflammatory mediator-driven multisystemic disorder. MC activation syndrome may be associated with CVID, postural orthostatic tachycardia syndrome, Lyme disease, and EDS but may also be idiopathic. Symptoms typically are dermatologic (hives, flushing, and burning), cardiovascular (dizziness and presyncope/syncope), GI (diarrhea, abdominal cramping, nausea/vomiting, and dysphagia), neurologic (brain fog, altered memory, and headache), respiratory (dyspnea, wheezing, and nasal congestion), and constitutional (fatigue/malaise). Laboratory clues may include baseline elevation of serum tryptase, elevated 24-hour urinary histamine, elevation of 24-hour urine prostaglandin D2 or its metabolite prostaglandin F2, or documentation of these markers being significantly elevated above baseline when symptomatic. Treatment includes H1 and H2 receptor antagonists, antileukotrienes, MC stabilizers, and the IgE-binding monoclonal antibody omalizumab.[248,256,257]

Myelophthisic and Myeloproliferative Disorders

EMH is a reactive process from bone marrow failure and/or infiltration or from chronic hemolytic anemias.[258,259] The most common extramedullary sites for blood formation include the liver and spleen. As a result, EMH commonly presents as hepatosplenomegaly from diffuse infiltration associated with vague abdominal symptoms. Liver chemistry tests may be abnormal, but clinically significant liver dysfunction rarely occurs. Histology shows clumps of erythroid and myeloid precursors along with megakaryocytes in the sinusoids, space of Disse, and portal tracts. The pleomorphism differentiates this from leukemic infiltration. The most common form is diffuse infiltration, but well-defined nodules or masses, usually multiple, may be seen. They are hypoechoic or inhomogeneous on ultrasonography and hypodense on unenhanced CT scan. MRI appearance varies depending upon the activity of the EMH and the degree of iron deposition.[260,261] EMH may rarely be found in the GI tract, causing bowel obstruction, abdominal pain, bleeding, or ascites.[262,263] Ascites could be due to implants of EMH in peritoneum, omentum, mesentery, or bowel wall.

Myelofibrosis is characterized by clonal myeloproliferation with bone marrow fibrosis and EMH. Portal hypertension may be due to increased portal blood flow related to massive splenomegaly, increased intrahepatic resistance and sinusoidal narrowing from EMH, and/or a hypercoagulable state resulting in Budd-Chiari syndrome or portal vein thrombosis.[264,265] Splenectomy can improve the hyperdynamic circulation due to EMH but cannot reduce the increased portal pressure due to obstruction of the intrahepatic portal veins. Complications of splenectomy include thrombocytosis with thrombotic events, as well as hepatomegaly, sometimes massive, due to transfer of the EMH to the liver. Thrombotic complications have been associated with myelofibrosis, polycythemia vera, and essential thrombocytosis.[266] Splenic infarction can cause left upper quadrant abdominal pain. Up to 50% of patients with Budd-Chiari syndrome have an overt myeloproliferative syndrome.

Langerhans cell histiocytosis (also called *histiocytosis X*, *eosinophilic granuloma*, *Letterer–Siwe disease*, and *Hand–Schüller–Christian disease*) is an uncommon disorder involving mainly infants and children.[267,268] Infiltration of the GI tract is rare (1.6%–2.6%) and usually associated with severe systemic disease, the characteristic rash, and a poor prognosis, with more than 50% dying within 18 months of diagnosis. Affected patients complain of vomiting, bleeding, diarrhea, constipation, and/or perianal disease. Malabsorption, PLGE, and even bowel perforation may occur. The diverse endoscopic findings include nodules, ulcers, polyps, luminal narrowing, and colitis. Liver disease may be found in 18%–20%; the incidence of hepatomegaly is variable. Pathologic evidence of Langerhans cell histiocytosis may be found in the skin, liver, and GI tract. Hepatobiliary abnormalities include portal triaditis, bile duct proliferation, fibrosis with histiocytic changes, cholestasis, sclerosing cholangitis, and cirrhosis.[269,270]

Hemophagocytic lymphohistiocytosis (HLH), also known as hemophagocytic syndrome, is an uncommon hematologic disorder categorized as one of the cytokine storm syndromes. It is life-threatening with severe inflammation caused by uncontrolled natural killer cell activity of the innate immune system, leading to lymphocyte and macrophage hyperreactivity and resulting in massive overproduction of cytokines. Primary HLH is a heterogeneous autosomal recessive disorder with an increased frequency of parental consanguinity. Secondary HLH occurs after strong immunologic activation as may occur with rheumatic diseases such as adult-onset Still disease (discussed earlier), with systemic infection, or in patients with immunodeficiency syndromes or underlying malignancy. Secondary HLH is also known as the macrophage activation syndrome. Resultant overwhelming T lymphocyte and macrophage activation leads to clinical and hematologic disturbances, which culminate in death if untreated. Clinical manifestations include fever, lymphadenopathy, hepatosplenomegaly, and rash (60%). Laboratory studies typically show pancytopenia, low fibrinogen, hypoalbuminemia, elevated liver chemistry tests sometimes with jaundice, and marked elevations of C-reactive protein, ESR, serum triglycerides, and ferritin. Hemophagocytosis can be identified in the bone marrow, lymph nodes, and spleen. An elevated CD25 is often noted. Therapy involves treating the underlying cause when possible. Often concomitant therapy using high-dose glucocorticoids, etoposide, cyclosporine, MTX, or intravenous immunoglobulin may be required.[271]

Erdheim-Chester disease or polyostotic sclerosing histiocytosis is a rare disease characterized by abnormal proliferation of non-Langerhans histiocytes due to a disturbance of the RAS/MARK intracellular signaling pathway. Onset is typically in middle age, manifesting as bone marrow infiltration and nearly universal long bone sclerosis by inflammatory infiltrates of lymphocytes and histiocytes. Extraskeletal involvement is infiltrative, and GI manifestations are uncommon, but liver biopsy may include xanthogranulomatous infiltration. Retroperitoneal fibrosis may lead to chylous ascites[272] and PLGE. Mortality rates are high and therapy may include high-dose glucocorticoids, vinca alkaloids, anthracyclines, cyclosporine, or interferon-alpha.[273]

Dysproteinemias

Multiple myeloma may affect the GI tract by direct invasion of a specific organ, mass effect, or production of a malignant effusion.[274] GI involvement from AL amyloidosis is described later. The most common sites of myelomatous involvement are the liver, spleen, and lymph nodes. Clinically significant liver or GI tract involvement is rare, usually occurs late in disease, and is associated with a poor prognosis. Hepatomegaly occurs in up to 58% of patients, often with splenomegaly. Diffuse involvement of the liver is most common, although nodular patterns have been found.[275] An elevated serum alkaline phosphatase level is seen with tumor infiltration.

The stomach, intestine, pancreas, and peritoneum are sites of spread. Symptoms are due to direct invasion resulting in perforation or hemorrhage in the stomach or intestine; mass-like effects with gastric, intestinal, or biliary obstruction; and production of ascites. Ascites may be due to portal hypertension from amyloidosis, malignant infiltration of the liver, heart failure, malignant seeding of the peritoneal cavity, or infectious (e.g., tuberculous) peritonitis. Multiple myeloma may be associated with IBD or present an IBD-like picture.[276]

Primary extramedullary plasmacytomas without evidence of multiple myeloma account for 3%–5% of all plasma cell dyscrasias. Gut involvement, although uncommon, is noted from the oral cavity to anus. Manifestations include dysphagia, hemorrhage, pseudo-obstruction, and polyposis.[277] Some gastric plasmacytomas improve with Hp treatment, although these may in fact be mucosa-associated lymphoid tissue lymphomas with extreme plasmacytic differentiation.[278] Although usually treated surgically or by radiation, endoscopic resection should be kept in mind.[279]

Waldenström macroglobulinemia is characterized by malignant proliferation of B lymphocytes producing IgM. Although hepatosplenomegaly and lymphadenopathy are common, lumenal GI tract involvement is rare. GI disease may be due to (1) deposition of immunoglobulin light chain fragments as amyloid protein, (2) infiltration of the gut wall with lymphoplasmacytic cells producing monoclonal IgM (negative Congo red staining), or (3) lymphatic dilatation and obstruction from high viscosity of the interstitial fluid.[280,281] IgM deposits, which may stain with periodic acid–Schiff, may lead to blunted and distended villi and lymphangiectasia. Its interference with function may result in malabsorption, PLGE, or pseudo-obstruction. Portal hypertension may develop from infiltration of portal tracts with lymphoplasmacytoid cells and/or an increased splenic vein inflow secondary to splenomegaly.[282] Ascites is rare.

Red Blood Cell Dyscrasias

Sickle Cell Disease

Sickle cell disease (SCD) is an autosomal recessive abnormality of the β-globin chain of hemoglobin (Hb).[283,284] The resulting HbS polymerizes when deoxygenated to form a gelatinous network that stiffens the erythrocyte membrane and increases viscosity.

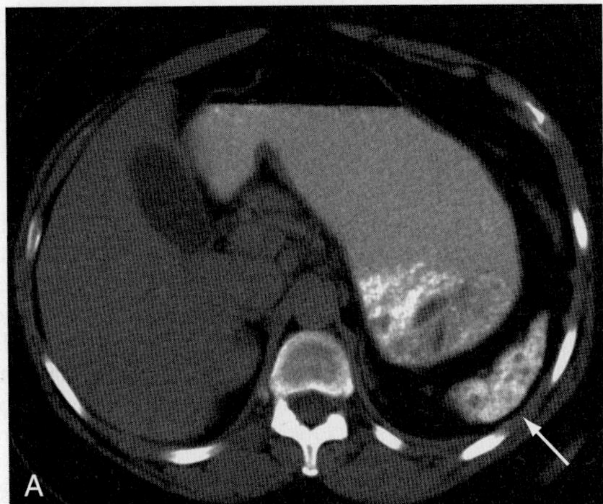

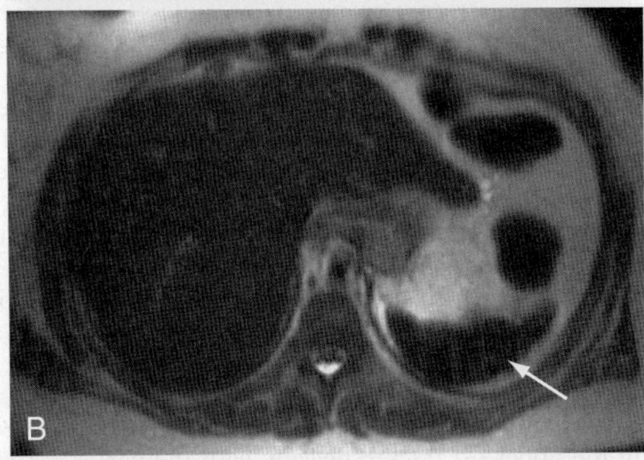

Fig. 35.6 Imaging studies in a patient with sickle cell disease and autosplenectomy. Unenhanced CT of the abdomen (A) shows increased density of the small spleen (*arrow*). On MRI (B), the spleen is also small and diffusely hypointense in all sequences (*arrow*), consistent with the finding of dense calcification on CT. The calcifications and small size make detection of the spleen difficult on US. (From Ebert EC, Nagar M, Hagspiel KD. Gastrointestinal and hepatic complications of sickle cell disease. *Clin Gastroenterol Hepatol*. 2010;8:483–489.)

This results in microvascular occlusion, with ischemia and infarction of the organs and red blood cell destruction. Some 8% of African-Americans are heterozygous for HbS trait, and 0.2% are homozygotes.

Splenic Involvement. In the first 6 months of life, splenic congestion and sickling lead to functional asplenia.[285] As hemorrhages and infarctions occur, the spleen becomes smaller and is eventually replaced by fibrous tissue, termed *autosplenectomy* (Fig. 35.6). It is usually infarcted within the first 18–36 months of life, paralleling the disappearance of protective HbF. Splenic atrophy results in increased susceptibility to infection with encapsulated bacteria and the appearance of Howell-Jolly bodies in red blood cells. Radiologically, the spleen is small and often calcified.[285]

Acute splenic infarction is more common in SC-HbC or SC-thalassemia than in homozygous SCD, owing to the combination of splenomegaly with near-normal Hb levels and relatively high blood viscosity.[283] It may even occasionally occur with SC trait in nonhypoxic conditions. Splenic infarction presents with left upper quadrant pain, nausea and vomiting, a friction rub over the splenic area, and leukocytosis; it may result in abscesses or pseudocysts. The spleen may occasionally rupture or be involved with EMH or hemosiderosis.

Acute splenic sequestration, or the sudden pooling of blood in the spleen, may cause rapid splenic enlargement and a drop in Hb.[286] Rarely, hypovolemic shock and death may occur within hours if not prevented by transfusions. In homozygous SCD, it occurs only in infants and children; subsequent progressive fibrosis of the spleen impairs sequestration. In SC-thalassemia, acute splenic sequestration can occur at any age, and there is a high recurrence rate that can be prevented by splenectomy or chronic transfusions.

Biliary Tract Involvement. Cholelithiasis, occurring in about 70% of patients during their lifetime, consists of pigmented stones resulting from elevated bilirubin excretion due to chronic hemolysis.[287–289] Calcium bilirubinate gallstones are often radiopaque and thus seen on plain films. The incidence of choledocholithiasis in SCD with cholelithiasis ranges from 18% to 30%, greater than that found in patients with cholesterol gallstones.

Laparoscopic cholecystectomy in asymptomatic SCD patients is controversial.[290,291] Perioperative management includes monitoring changes in arterial oxygen tension and pH, hydration, possible perioperative blood transfusion, early ambulation, and sometimes continuous positive airway pressure postoperatively to avoid atelectasis and SCD-related postoperative complications. A search for choledocholithiasis should be considered preoperatively or postoperatively, using MRCP or EUS.[292]

Sickle cell cholangiopathy presents as cholestatic jaundice without choledocholithiasis and may be due to ischemic bile duct injury.[293] Such patients need to be followed for the possibility of developing bile duct stones.

Hepatic Involvement. *Acute sickle hepatic crisis*, which affects about 10% of patients admitted for painful crisis, is due to stagnation of sickled cells in the hepatic sinusoids with decreased hepatic blood flow.[283,287] Patients present with right upper quadrant pain, nausea, tender hepatomegaly, low-grade fever, leukocytosis, and elevated serum aminotransferase and conjugated bilirubin levels. The aminotransferases are usually one to three times normal but may reach levels greater than 1000 IU/L. Treatment is supportive; in some cases, exchange transfusions are used.

Sequestration of blood, although seen most commonly in the lungs and spleen, can occasionally affect the liver. Obstruction of blood flow through the sinusoids by sickled erythrocytes leads to compression of the bile ducts. The pooling of blood leads to acute hepatic enlargement, a rapid drop in hematocrit, increase in reticulocyte count, and mild increase in liver enzymes and bilirubin. Reverse sequestration results in a decrease in hepatic size and increase in hematocrit, suggesting that not all sequestered cells are destroyed. Occasionally, this results in hypervolemia, heart failure, and intracerebral hemorrhage.

Acute sickle intrahepatic cholestasis is a rare, potentially fatal complication caused by widespread sickling in the sinusoids and results in hypoxia and intracanalicular cholestasis.[294] It is thought to represent a severe form of hepatic crisis with severe hyperbilirubinemia, coagulopathy, and renal insufficiency/failure, ultimately resulting in liver failure. Early treatment, including exchange transfusion, is essential.

Acute hepatic failure rarely occurs, usually in the presence of underlying chronic liver disease.[295] It is characterized by jaundice, variable serum aminotransferase elevations, progressive coagulopathy, and encephalopathy. Liver transplantation is an option in these patients.

Of patients admitted to a hospital with homozygous SCD or sickle-thalassemia, there was a 39% prevalence of acute veno-occlusive involvement of the liver. It was not associated with the severity of the crisis, was either mixed cholestatic-hepatocellular or cholestatic, and generally had a benign course.[296,297] Hepatic infarction, appearing as a peripheral hypodense wedge-shaped lesion on CT, is a relatively rare clinical event. Liver abscesses, with fever and pain, perhaps due to a secondarily infected hepatic infarct, may occur as a result of diminished removal of bacteria from the bloodstream from functional asplenism and reduced IgG antibodies to polysaccharide antigens. Focal nodular hyperplasia, perhaps due to obstructive portal venopathy, may also be seen. Cocaine, if being consumed, hepatotoxicity may markedly worsen liver function and its arterial vasoconstriction likely contributes to tissue hypoxia, vaso-occlusion, and further sickling.[298] Occasionally, hepatic or portal vein obstruction may occur in SCD.

Miscellaneous GI Problems. *Abdominal pain* frequently accompanies vaso-occlusive crisis and may be difficult to distinguish from acute abdominal disease. It tends to be diffuse and associated with pain elsewhere, such as in the limbs and chest. The pain of vaso-occlusive crises is typically relieved with hydration and oxygen within 48 hours. The abdominal crisis is thought to be due to small infarcts of the mesentery and abdominal viscera causing severe pain, peritoneal irritation, and a generalized ileus.[283] *Acute pancreatitis* is not common despite the frequency of gallstones. It may be due to gallstones or to microvascular occlusion with ischemic injury.[299] *Duodenal ulcers* in SCD may not be associated with high gastric acid outputs, suggesting that they are instead due to reduced mucosal resistance, possibly from ischemia. *Ischemic bowel* due to intravascular sickling and the resulting microvascular occlusion occasionally occurs.[300]

Diagnosis of GI Involvement. The elevated serum bilirubin, mostly unconjugated, is from the increased load of red cell heme on an acutely damaged liver. There is some enhancement of bilirubin conjugation by bilirubin induction of uridine diphosphate glucuronyltransferase, which is elevated in these patients.[301] The serum bilirubin correlates with LDH levels, suggesting that chronic hemolysis and ineffective erythropoiesis, rather than liver disease, are the sources of hyperbilirubinemia. Elevated serum AST may be partly due to erythrocyte AST and to muscle breakdown, so hepatocyte injury is better reflected by an increase in serum ALT levels. The serum alkaline phosphatase level is often elevated during pain crises, mainly due to bone rather than liver isoenzymes.

Liver biopsy, although not usually performed during an acute sickle crisis, may show intrasinusoidal sickling, Kupffer cell enlargement and erythrophagocytosis, and hemosiderosis, with variable fibrosis. Shrunken hepatocytes or perivenular necrosis, features characteristically seen in ischemic livers, are generally not seen in SCD.[283,287] The safety of liver biopsies has been questioned, especially during acute sickling crisis.[302] Patients with complications from biopsies have chronic venous outflow obstruction, marked hepatic sequestration of erythrocytes, and sinusoidal dilatation.

Hemosiderosis. With multiple transfusions and hemolysis in SCD, hemosiderosis develops, with iron first found in the sinusoids where erythrocytes are taken up by the Kupffer cells.[303] As iron accumulation increases, it is then found in the hepatocytes, increasing the risk of liver damage. In thalassemia, iron is found in both the sinusoids and hepatocytes. Patients with thalassemia tend to require more transfusions than patients with SCD and have increased intestinal uptake of iron from ineffective erythropoiesis and, therefore, more iron visceral loading.[304] On CT, the density of the liver and spleen increases with hemosiderosis. On MRI, the magnetic signal diminishes in the liver as the iron concentration increases.[305,306] MRI T2 techniques correlate with hepatic iron content and can be used to guide therapy. There is a lack of correlation, however, between liver and cardiac iron content, so both organs should be evaluated. Ferritin is a poor measure of iron overload, because it is an acute-phase reactant. The available iron chelators are deferoxamine (given parenterally) and the oral agents, namely deferiprone and deferasirox.

Coagulation Disorders

Intramural hematomas due to trauma or bleeding diatheses most commonly involve the duodenum or jejunum, respectively.[307,308] The second and third portions of the duodenum are vulnerable to damage from trauma. They are fixed between the anterior abdominal wall and the vertebral column, so they may be either compressed or torn away from the more mobile areas. Spontaneous hematomas are most commonly due to overanticoagulation or bleeding diatheses. Patients present with a range of symptoms; complications include bowel obstruction and intussusception. Unenhanced CT findings include homogeneous and symmetric intramural thickening that is hyperdense in the first 10 days, evolving into a hypodense area. Rapid clinical remission usually occurs with conservative management unless involvement is extensive. A lesion persisting for more than 2 months suggests another etiology.

In *von Willebrand disease*, which is the most common inherited bleeding disorder, GI bleeding commonly occurs associated with GI angioectasias or without visible lesions. Heyde syndrome, the association of calcific aortic valve stenosis and GI bleeding, may be due to an acquired deficiency of von Willebrand factor as the multimers are reduced in size from the shear stress.[309,310] This abnormality is corrected or improved with aortic valve replacement. A similar phenomenon occurs after left ventricular assist device (LVAD) placement and accounts for angioectasia-related GI bleeding in 30%–40% of such patients.

Hemophilia is commonly associated with mucosal GI bleeding, often in the upper GI tract, especially with the use of traditional NSAIDs.[311,312] Concomitant chronic liver disease related to factor-acquired HCV is commonly present and can exacerbate GI bleeding potential.

Hemolytic-uremic syndrome (HUS) consists of a triad of renal impairment, microangiopathic hemolytic anemia, and thrombocytopenia (see Chapter 112). Triggers of HUS include nonenteric infections (especially *Streptococcus pneumoniae*), malignancies, pregnancy, transplantation, anticancer molecules, immunosuppressive agents, and antiplatelet agents.[313] Shiga toxin-producing *Escherichia coli* 0157:H7 accounts for the majority of cases of HUS. Undercooked hamburger is the most common vector, with other foods (e.g., apple juice, lettuce) also implicated.[314] Other modes of transmission include the fecal-oral route (particularly child daycare centers), water consumption (including swimming pools), and animal contact. Children are predominantly involved, mainly during summer and autumn. After an average incubation period of 3 days, patients develop abdominal cramps, vomiting, fever, and diarrhea that becomes hemorrhagic in 70% of cases. HUS develops in 3%–7% of patients in sporadic cases and up to 30% in some outbreaks. Stool cultures may be negative because excretion of *E. coli* is intermittent and bacterial counts are low. CT shows colonic wall thickening, often with a target sign and pericolonic stranding.[315] Rarely, pancreatitis, hemoperitoneum, colonic perforation, or stricture may occur.[316,317] The suggestion that antibiotic therapy of *E. coli* 0157:H7 increases the risk of developing HUS has been challenged in a meta-analysis.[318] Antimotility agents are contraindicated because they may delay clearance of the pathogen and may even increase the risk of developing HUS.

Thrombotic thrombocytopenic purpura consists of a microangiopathic hemolytic anemia and thrombocytopenia, with or without neurologic dysfunction and renal insufficiency.[319–321] Most patients have low activity of the protease ADAMTS13, which degrades large von Willebrand factor multimers, predisposing to a thrombotic microangiopathy and platelet consumption. With profound thrombocytopenia, bleeding may also occur.

Unlike HUS, the peak age is in the fourth decade. About 70% of patients have GI symptoms, which may include lumenal ischemia and GI bleeding. Plasma exchange allows 80% of patients with thrombotic thrombocytopenic purpura to survive an episode without permanent organ damage.

ENDOCRINE DISEASES

Diabetes Mellitus

Whether GI symptoms are increased in patients with diabetes mellitus (DM) is controversial.[322] The populations studied are quite variable, confounding by population obesity of control groups is increasingly problematic, and publication bias is likely present. Symptoms suggestive of autonomic dysfunction (e.g., postural dizziness, lack of sweating, impaired erection or ejaculation, difficulty with bladder emptying, xerostomia, gustatory sweating) should be identified. Acute variations in blood glucose can influence GI motor function and the perception of sensations.[323–325] Poor glycemic control delays gastric emptying, which, in turn, affects glycemic control. Metformin is a common cause of diarrhea and fecal incontinence;[326] GLP-1 agonists may exacerbate preexisting gastric emptying delay.

Loss of interstitial Cajal cells,[327] imbalances in the numbers of excitatory and inhibitory enteric neurons,[328] autonomic neuropathy, and impaired vagal and sympathetic innervations can alter GI motor function. Central processing may perceive GI events in an abnormal way,[329] and there may be a reduction in sensory neuropeptides (e.g., substance P), impaired smooth muscle contractility, or ischemia from microvascular disease.[324]

Diabetes and Cancer

DM is probably associated with an increased risk of certain GI malignancies (e.g., cancers of the pancreas, liver, and colon), although the data are conflicting.[322,330–332] The association may be due in part to shared risk factors such as aging, obesity, diet, and physical inactivity. Metformin may reduce the risk of cancer, whereas insulin may increase it.[332,333]

DM occurring with cancer increases mortality in general and in cancer-associated surgery.[334] Insulin resistance with secondary hyperinsulinemia lowers the concentration of insulin-like growth factor (IGF)-binding proteins, leading to an increase in bioavailable IGF-1 concentrations,[331,332,335] which may stimulate cancer growth.

There is a modest increase in pancreatic cancer among patients who have DM for more than 5 years.[336,337] Conversely, pancreatic cancer causes DM, as evidenced by the development of new-onset DM followed by the diagnosis of pancreatic adenocarcinoma and its improvement in some individuals with tumor resection. Chronic pancreatitis with pancreatic insufficiency increases the risk of both DM and pancreatic cancer (see later). Pancreatic ductal adenocarcinoma (PDAC) should be considered in an older patient with new-onset poorly controlled DM, especially with weight loss. In a retrospective Israeli study, 23% (1245/5408) of new-onset diabetes patients were classified as high-risk of which 32 (2.6%) developed PDAC. The median follow-up time from initial DM detection to PDAC diagnosis was 609 days (interquartile range, 367–997). The hazard ratio for PDAC diagnosis among individuals in the high-risk group compared with the low-risk group was 5.7.[338] A glucagonoma is much rarer but may present similarly with new-onset DM perhaps also with cheilitis, glossitis, and the characteristic annular, crusted, and bullous rash *necrolytic migratory erythema* (see Chapter 31).

DM is a risk factor for HCC.[339,340] Confounding factors are that patients with cirrhosis (who are at increased risk of HCC) may be glucose intolerant, and 30% may develop overt DM, and that comorbid HBV, HCV, obesity, fatty liver disease, or alcohol may increase HCC risk.

DM is also associated with an increased risk of colorectal cancer.[335,341] High circulating levels of insulin, C-peptide, or IGF-1 and chronic insulin use increase this risk. Poor glycemic control (as evidenced by an HbA_{1c} >7.5%) is associated with a younger age at presentation, more advanced tumors, and poorer survival than diabetics with a low HbA_{1c} or nondiabetics.[342]

Esophageal Involvement

Although esophageal dysmotility may occur in up to 50% of diabetic patients, the prevalence of symptoms is only 25%.[322] Defects include decreased LES pressure, delayed transit, multipeaked or spontaneous contractions, and reduced amplitude of contractions.[343] Esophageal dysmotility has been correlated with peripheral motor neuropathy measured by nerve conduction velocity.

The frequency of gastroesophageal reflux in DM varies considerably, with endoscopic esophagitis in up to 40% of patients,[344] aggravated by obesity, reduced parotid gland secretion of bicarbonate, and hyperglycemia. Delayed esophageal transit does not necessarily correlate with gastric emptying, suggesting that the GI tract is not uniformly affected by DM and that reflux is not mainly a consequence of delayed gastric emptying. With odynophagia and/or dysphagia, oral and esophageal candidiasis should be considered; diabetic predisposing factors include impaired immunity, esophageal stasis from dysmotility, and hyperglycemic impairment of neutrophil function and opsonization.

Gastric Involvement

Gastric emptying in DM is extremely variable and does not closely correlate with symptoms. Patients with type 1 DM have a 15%–20% incidence of parietal cell antibodies, autoimmune atrophic gastritis (5%–10%), and pernicious anemia (2.6%–4%).[345] Autoimmune atrophic gastritis can lead to iron deficiency anemia (due to hypochlorhydric iron malabsorption); there is an increased risk for type I gastric carcinoids and probably gastric cancer. Type 1 diabetics should be tested for parietal cell antibodies periodically. Those with such antibodies should have a complete blood count, fasting serum gastrin, serum iron, and vitamin B_{12} levels periodically.

Although the association between DM and PUD is controversial, there is some evidence that DM increases the risk of ulcer bleeding, perhaps secondary to diabetes-related microcirculatory changes that may impair mucosal integrity.[346] There appears to be no clear association between Hp and DM when looking at prevalence of the infection, relationship to symptoms, gastric emptying, or eradication rate.[347]

Small Bowel Involvement

Celiac disease is found in an average of 4% of patients with type 1 DM from the United States and Western Europe, compared to a prevalence of about 0.5% in that population without DM.[348,349] Shared HLA class II genes and non-HLA loci suggest common autoimmune origins.[350] GI symptoms may be absent in celiac disease; patients may present with non-GI disorders such as short stature, pubertal delay, fat-soluble vitamin deficiencies, anemia, osteoporosis, and/or reproductive disorders. Type 1 diabetics with celiac disease may have poor glycemic control, hypoglycemic episodes, and microvascular complications.[351] These patients have a propensity to develop other autoimmune disorders such as pernicious anemia, Addison disease, and autoimmune thyroid diseases. Screening all type I diabetics for celiac disease is controversial.

The small bowel transit time in DM is quite variable and does not necessarily correlate with transit times in the stomach or colon. Diarrhea is found in up to 22% of diabetic patients, but constipation is even more common.[322] Diarrhea is often episodic, painless, and sometimes nocturnal and must be differentiated from fecal incontinence (see later). Steatorrhea may occur in as many as 75% of diabetics with diarrhea. Metformin is the most common diabetic medication to cause diarrhea, even after years of treatment.[326,352] Etiologies of diarrhea related to DM include drugs, fast transit, autonomic and/or enteric neuropathy, celiac disease, SBBO, excess use of sugar-free sweeteners, pancreatic insufficiency, and hormones. Neuropathy may cause diarrhea by altering fluid and electrolyte transport and by altering motility. Rare hormone-producing tumors induce both DM and diarrhea, such as those secreting glucagon or somatostatin. Treatment of diarrhea should be geared toward the specific etiology or otherwise be symptomatic with loperamide, diphenoxalate, or bile acid sequestrants. Clonidine stimulates α_2-adrenergic receptors but may worsen orthostatic hypotension. A patch form may be tried if the oral form is not tolerated.[322] Octreotide, or the long-acting octreotide analog lanreotide, may help.[353,354] Also reported is the use of selective serotonin 5-HT_3 receptor antagonists.[355]

Diabetic radiculopathy of thoracic nerve roots may cause otherwise unexplained upper abdominal pain in patients with diabetic neuropathy. Pain may be associated with anorexia and weight loss, mimicking an intra-abdominal malignancy. Affected dermatomal sensory loss and muscle atrophy/weakness may be physical examination clues. Electromyography of the abdominal muscles may show denervation.[356]

Colonic and Anal Involvement

Constipation occurs in over half of patients with long-standing DM and is partly due to an impaired gastrocolic reflex and delayed colonic transit. Occasionally, megacolon and (rarely) intestinal pseudo-obstruction may result. DM can lead to ischemic colitis with capillary basement membrane thickening and luminal narrowing of submucosal arterioles in the colon.[357] Fecal incontinence may be associated with dysfunction of the IAS and/or reduced sensitivity of the rectum to distension.[322] Control of hyperglycemia and perhaps biofeedback may improve fecal incontinence.

Pancreatic Involvement

Exocrine pancreatic insufficiency is common in DM and associated with reduced pancreatic size and changes of chronic pancreatitis by MRI and MRCP.[358–360] Possible mechanisms by which DM causes pancreatic insufficiency include diabetic vascular changes in the pancreas and autonomic neuropathy with impaired enteropancreatic reflexes. In type 1 DM, the autoimmune process may damage both endocrine β cells and adjacent exocrine cells; low insulin levels also reduce its trophic effects on acinar cells. Half of type I diabetics have demonstrable changes in the exocrine pancreas.

Alternatively, pancreatic disease may result in DM (*type 3 DM*), a condition that is probably underdiagnosed.[361,362] Etiologies include chronic pancreatitis, hemochromatosis, pancreatic cancer (discussed earlier), autoimmune pancreatitis, and a partial pancreatectomy. In hemochromatosis, iron usually accumulates in pancreatic acinar cells but may also affect islet cells. DM usually occurs before or concurrently with the diagnosis of autoimmune pancreatitis, and glucocorticoids have variable effects.[363] The effects of pancreatic resection depend upon the portion of pancreas removed because glucagon-producing cells are mainly in the tail, pancreatic polypeptide-secreting cells are located in the head, and insulin-secreting cells are more evenly distributed. Unlike types 1 and 2 DM, pancreatic DM is characterized by a deficiency in nutrient-stimulated pancreatic polypeptide and glucagon release with consequent predisposition to hypoglycemia and a reduced incidence of diabetic ketoacidosis (DKA). Hypoglycemia will be accentuated by alcohol use and/or loss of glycogen stores in the liver. The role of pancreatic enzyme replacement in glucose control is controversial. These patients can develop many of the same complications as other diabetics over the long term, but their low incidence of obesity and hyperlipidemia, presumably from maldigestion, reduces the risk of vascular complications.

DM occurs in 50% of patients with cystic fibrosis by the age of 30 years. It increases mortality and worsens lung function.[364,365] Abnormal chloride channel function results in thick, viscous secretions causing obstructive damage to the pancreas, resulting in fibrosis, fatty infiltration, and severe pancreatic atrophy. There is loss of alpha, beta, and pancreatic polypeptide cells and development of insulin resistance. Hypoglycemia is a problem due to a blunted glucagon increase with stimuli, liver disease, and malnourishment, but patients are rarely ketosis prone. Insulin, rather than oral diabetic agents, is recommended when the patient displays poor growth, low weight, or unexpected decline in pulmonary function. A high-calorie, high-fat diet should be used to maintain nutrition.

DM is associated with an increased incidence of acute pancreatitis, a risk that is reduced by taking antidiabetic drugs.[366] Acute pancreatitis can complicate DKA in 11% of cases; transient hypertriglyceridemia is thought to be a contributing factor.[367] Abdominal pain may be mild or absent. Acute pancreatitis may worsen volume depletion and hyperglycemia associated with DKA. DKA itself can be associated with abdominal pain and mild elevations of amylase and lipase without pancreatic inflammatory changes being identified.

Gallbladder Involvement

Fasting gallbladder volume by ultrasonography can be normal or increased in diabetics.[368] Possible causes of gallbladder dysfunction in DM include a defect in the cholinergic pathway, reduced α-adrenergic tone, deficiency of cholecystokinin receptors,[369] arteriolar disease impairing muscle contraction, hyperglycemia, and hyperinsulinemia.

Proving that DM is a risk factor for gallstones has been difficult because of associated clearly established risk factors for gallstones, particularly obesity, hypertriglyceridemia, advancing age, and hyperinsulinemia.[322] The natural history of cholelithiasis in DM and surgical risks is probably similar to that in nondiabetics when controlling for the associated cardiovascular and renal diseases.[370] Hyperglycemia, vascular disease, and impaired host defenses increase diabetics' susceptibility to infection; emphysematous cholecystitis is an uncommon condition usually associated with DM. It is probably due to ischemia of the gallbladder from vascular compromise, with proliferation of gas-forming organisms.

Hepatic Involvement

Abnormal liver chemistry tests are common in type 2 DM, especially serum ALT.[371] If within three times the upper limit of normal and no cause can be found, oral antidiabetic or lipid-modifying therapy can be started; these regimens often decrease serum ALT levels as tighter blood glucose levels are achieved. Hepatotoxicity is rare with currently available antidiabetic medications. Hepatitis or acute liver failure has been described with thiazolidinediones, and cholestasis with sulfonylureas.[372] Metformin has not been associated with hepatotoxicity. Fatty liver, common in DM, is a manifestation of insulin resistance, often found in conjunction with the metabolic syndrome. DM has been shown to increase the risk of acute hepatic failure independent of underlying liver disease.[373]

Cross-sectional and longitudinal studies have shown that HCV-positive patients have an increased risk of type 2 DM (odds ratio of 1.6–2.1) compared to uninfected controls, those with HBV, or those with other liver diseases.[372,374,375] Similarly, HCV is a strong predictor of new-onset DM after liver transplantation.[376] Insulin resistance accelerates fibrogenesis, and upregulation of TNF-α in HCV promotes insulin resistance.[377] HCV eradication improves insulin sensitivity and reduces the incidence of DM.

Rarely, in poorly controlled diabetics, acute liver injury manifesting as RUQ pain, hepatomegaly, and marked elevations of serum aminotransferases can occur related to glycogenic hepatopathy. Differentiating this condition from hepatic steatosis can require liver biopsy to show extensive PAS-positive glycogenation of hepatocytes; there is reversibility with glycemic control.

Hepatogenous diabetes affects 30%–60% of cirrhotic patients.[378,379] It is characterized by insulin resistance in muscular, hepatic, and adipose tissues, as well as hyperinsulinemia and an impaired response of pancreatic islet cells. There is a reduced frequency of micro- and macroangiopathic complications, perhaps due to lower body mass index, lipids, and blood pressure compared to type 2 DM. Also, they may die of liver disease before diabetic complications have time to develop. They are at risk for hypoglycemia due to minimal glycogen storage in the liver, impaired hepatic insulin extraction, high catabolic rate, and sometimes superimposed alcoholism. These patients should generally have no dietary restrictions, because they are often malnourished. Oral hypoglycemic drugs are metabolized by the liver, so they may lead to hypoglycemia. Although biguanides may be helpful because they reduce insulin resistance, metformin is associated with a risk of lactic acidosis and is relatively contraindicated in cirrhotic patients who drink alcohol.[380] Acarbose may reduce ammonia levels in patients with hepatic encephalopathy.[381] Liver transplantation cures DM in 67% of cirrhotic-diabetic patients.[382,383]

Thyroid Disease

Hyperthyroidism

Clinical manifestations of hyperthyroidism range from apathetic thyrotoxicosis to thyroid storm (with fever, tachycardia, agitation, and delirium). GI symptoms include abdominal pain, vomiting, weight loss, and change in bowel habits.[384] Hyperthyroidism may be associated with other autoimmune diseases such as pernicious anemia, celiac disease, and ulcerative colitis.[384–387]

Dysphagia is a rare manifestation that may be related to direct compression from a goiter or nodule, excess thyroid hormone causing a myopathy affecting the striated muscles of the pharynx and upper third of the esophagus, or increased esophageal contraction velocity. Gastric emptying has been shown to be normal, rapid, or delayed.[384] Low acid secretion and hypergastrinemia are found in some studies. Autoimmune thyroid disease is linked to atrophic gastritis.[388]

Up to 25% of patients have diarrhea.[389] Accelerated transit time and excess fecal fat excretion are common. Mechanisms of steatorrhea include dietary fat hyperphagia and accelerated transit. The diarrhea in hyperthyroidism may be due to associated ulcerative colitis or celiac disease.[384,387] Diarrhea may decrease with propranolol, suggesting improvement of a relative adrenergic stimulatory state.

Although mild abnormalities in serum aminotransferases or alkaline phosphatase commonly occur in hyperthyroidism due to the thyroid dysfunction itself, drug therapy (propylthiouracil) or concomitant overlapping autoimmune liver disease (AIH and PBC) clinically significant abnormalities in thyroid function are rare. Severe cholestatic hepatitis, jaundice, and/or acute hepatic failure are rare but may occur due to a mismatch between increased hepatic oxygen consumption and hepatic blood flow. Predominant zone 3 hepatic necrosis with or without concomitant right-sided heart failure is typical. Responses to pharmacologic therapy of thyrotoxicosis may occur, but emergent thyroidectomy and/or hepatic transplantation may be required.

Hypothyroidism

Hypothyroidism is most commonly due to Hashimoto thyroiditis or to thyroid ablation for hyperthyroidism. The former is an autoimmune disease that is sometimes associated with other autoimmune processes such as ulcerative colitis, pernicious anemia, DM, celiac disease, and PBC.[384,387] The most common GI complaints in hypothyroidism are constipation, anorexia, nausea/vomiting, and abdominal pain.

Esophageal manifestations of dysphagia and reflux may be due to a motility disorder with low LES pressure and reduced amplitude of contractions.[384] Patients may have reduced acid secretion or delayed gastric emptying, the etiology of which is unclear. Phytobezoars may be found in the stomach or intestine, occasionally resulting in obstruction.

Hypothyroidism is associated with SBBO, causing abdominal discomfort, flatulence, and bloating; these symptoms often respond to antibiotics.[390] Small bowel transit time may be normal or delayed.[386] Colonic hypomotility may result in obstipation, ileus, megacolon, or volvulus. Megacolon and pseudovolvulus are rare, usually associated with severe hypothyroidism or myxedema coma, and may respond to intravenous thyroid hormone.[391] There may be transverse thickening of colonic haustrations or distended loops of bowel with air-fluid levels that must be differentiated from intestinal obstruction. Surgery in these patients may be complicated by prolonged ileus.[392] Pathology may suggest a neuropathy or, alternatively, accumulation of glycosaminoglycans in the interstitial tissues.[384] Ascites in myxedema is characterized by high protein concentration (>2.5 g/dL) with a variable serum ascites albumin gradient and a low white blood cell count with a predominance of lymphocytes.[393] Resolution occurs with thyroid replacement, not with diuretics.

Medullary Carcinoma of the Thyroid

Medullary carcinoma of the thyroid is a calcitonin-producing tumor of the C cells of the thyroid gland. It may be associated with MEN syndrome type 2. Diarrhea is seen in one-third of patients, particularly in those with extensive metastatic disease.[384] Its mechanism varies, being attributed to calcitonin, prostaglandins, 6-hydroxyindoleacetic acid, or nonhormonal causes.

Papillary and Follicular Carcinoma of the Thyroid

Papillary carcinoma of the thyroid occurs in up to 15% of patients with familial polyposis coli and has a distinct female preponderance and indolent behavior despite typical multicentricity. Both papillary and follicular cancer have been described in Cowden syndrome and the Bannayan–Riley–Ruvalcaba syndrome (PTEN hamartomatous syndromes).

Parathyroid Disease

Hyperparathyroidism

With the advent of multichannel biochemical screening that includes serum calcium measurements, severe hyperparathyroidism is now unusual and milder cases predominate. GI complaints include abdominal pain, constipation from large bowel atony, nausea/vomiting from gastric atony, anorexia, and weight loss.[394,395] Measurement of serum calcium is therefore an important part of the evaluation of abdominal pain. Abdominal pain could be due to PUD, pancreatitis, or related to smooth muscle atony. Whether the incidence of PUD increases in hyperparathyroidism is controversial. Gastric acid hypersecretion and/or hypergastrinemia have been found in some but not all studies, and hyperparathyroidism potentiates mucosal damage in MEN-1-associated gastrinomas. Constipation may be due to a reduction in neuromuscular excitability by high calcium levels.

Hyperparathyroidism accounts for <1% of acute pancreatitis. The incidence of acute pancreatitis in hyperparathyroidism ranges from 1% to 12%. Pancreatic calculi, mainly intraductal, have been noted in 80% of patients with pancreatitis and hyperparathyroidism.[394] In addition, calcium can promote conversion of trypsinogen to trypsin, resulting in damage to acinar cells. In converse, acute (often severe) pancreatitis can lead to hypocalcemia from a relative deficiency of parathyroid hormone secretion, as shown by correction of the calcium level with administration of parathyroid hormone. In addition, the hypocalcemia may be due to resistance to parathyroid hormone action in bones and kidneys resulting from fluid sequestration and reduction in effective arterial blood volume. Rarely, there are genetic factors such as mutations in serine protease inhibitor Kazal type 1 and CFTR in hyperparathyroidism and pancreatitis.[396] Once a diagnosis of hyperparathyroid-induced acute pancreatitis is established, a parathyroidectomy should be performed. Acute pancreatitis may follow parathyroid surgery, perhaps because of acute rises in calcium with manipulation of the parathyroid glands or to a blunted response of calcitonin-producing cells from cellular fatigue.[394] Hyperparathyroidism may also be associated with chronic pancreatitis and colon cancer.[397]

Hypoparathyroidism

The main GI manifestation of hypoparathyroidism is steatorrhea. It may be due to insufficient endogenous cholecystokinin release by duodenal mucosa following a meal, thereby reducing gallbladder contraction and pancreatic enzyme secretion.[398] Replacement of dietary long-chain triglycerides with medium-chain triglycerides reduces fecal fat losses, thus reducing fecal calcium losses from saponification. Calcium and vitamin D supplementation are important therapeutically as well.

Hypoparathyroidism may occasionally be associated with celiac disease, with the malabsorption responding to a gluten-free diet.[399] Underlying celiac disease should be suspected even in the absence of diarrhea in a hypoparathyroid patient whose serum calcium levels do not respond to treatment.

Hypoparathyroidism may cause a low serum alkaline phosphatase, but zinc deficiency, magnesium deficiency, malnutrition, Wilson disease, and hypophosphatasia deserve consideration in the evaluation.

Adrenal Gland Disease

Over half the patients with adrenal insufficiency (Addison disease) have GI symptoms, such as nausea, vomiting, diarrhea, and abdominal pain.[400] Cutaneous hyperpigmentation, electrolyte abnormalities, and hypotension may be absent, making the diagnosis elusive. Associated celiac disease is described in 8%–12% of patients, with both diseases having similar HLA associations.[401] Poor absorption of glucocorticoids due to associated celiac disease may complicate the therapy of Addison disease, whereas glucocorticoid treatment may mitigate celiac sprue. Atrophic gastritis and pernicious anemia may also be present.[402] Elevated serum aminotransferases may occur in Addison disease and resolve on glucocorticoid replacement therapy.[403]

Pheochromocytoma, a rare catecholamine-secreting tumor, presents with hypertension, palpitations, headaches, and diaphoresis. GI manifestations include nausea, vomiting, abdominal pain, and, less commonly, constipation, ileus, megacolon, ischemic colitis, and perforation.[404,405] Catecholamines decrease intestinal motility and tone by relaxation of intestinal smooth muscle and cause ischemia from vasoconstriction of splanchnic arterioles. The effects can be relieved by α-adrenergic blockers such as phentolamine. Hypertensive emergencies can occur with the use of opioids and other medications (as during endoscopic procedures).

Pituitary Disease

The hypothalamic-pituitary-adrenal axis provides an important link between the brain and the gut.[406,407] Pituitary disorders infrequently affect the GI tract, except in association with MEN-1 syndrome. Hypercortisolism, caused by the inappropriate secretion of corticotropin in Cushing disease, may be associated with an increased incidence of gastric ulceration when concomitant NSAIDs are used. Paraneoplastic Cushing syndrome may arise from lung cancers or neuroendocrine tumors when tumor secretion of ACTH or CRF results in production and release of cortisol from the adrenal glands. Acromegaly, a rare disorder characterized by hypersecretion of growth hormone, is associated with increased length and circumference of the colon and slow colon transit time, so that the standard bowel preparation is often inadequate.[408] Upper and lower functional GI tract disorders (defined by Rome IV diagnostic criteria) are significantly more prevalent in patients with acromegaly compared with healthy age- and sex-matched controls.[409] Acromegalic patients may have an increased risk of colorectal cancer, colonic polyps, and other GI tract cancers.[410] Increased growth hormone and IGF-1, which promote epithelial cell proliferation and reduce apoptosis, are thought to play a role. Whether colonoscopic colorectal cancer screening should begin before age 50 in acromegaly is controversial. A total of 3–5-year surveillance intervals may be appropriate in acromegalics with adenomas or elevated IGF-1 levels. Octreotide treatment in acromegalics increases gallstone formation, probably owing to suppression of cholecystokinin release and gallbladder emptying.[411] Symptomatic gallstone disease may occur following withdrawal of octreotide.[412]

DISORDERS OF LIPID METABOLISM

Hypertriglyceridemia to levels above 1000 mg/dL can cause acute and recurrent pancreatitis but rarely also chronic pancreatitis.[413] Usually the patient has a familial hyperlipoproteinemia along with a secondary factor such as poorly controlled DM, alcohol intake, or use of certain medications such as estrogen. The serum amylase level may be normal or minimally elevated as hypertriglyceridemia interferes with the amylase measurement. Familial hyperlipoproteinemia, particularly type IV, has a high incidence of gallstones.[414]

Hypobetalipoproteinemia can be acquired secondary to malnutrition or severe liver disease.[415] Primary causes include abetalipoproteinemia, chylomicron retention disease, and familial hypobetalipoproteinemia.[416] Abetalipoproteinemia is a rare autosomal recessive disorder with fat malabsorption, low or absent serum cholesterol, LDL, and VLDL levels, and acanthocytosis. Spinocerebellar degeneration and retinitis pigmentosa may also be seen. Elevated serum aminotransferases are commonly associated with hepatomegaly due to lipid-laden hepatocytes, occasionally progressing to cirrhosis. Lipid droplets are found in enterocytes, seen particularly with electron microscopy, owing to their lack of transport to the Golgi apparatus.[417] Patients with familial hypobetalipoproteinemia are usually heterozygotes who are asymptomatic with or without fatty liver disease.

Wolman disease, an autosomal recessive disorder involving absence of lysosomal acid lipase (LAL), is a rare but important cause of hepatosplenomegaly, progressive liver disease, premature atherosclerotic disease, and adrenal calcification. It is caused by a mutation in the LAL gene and may present in infancy or adulthood. A milder form of LAL deficiency where some enzyme activity is present is known as cholesteryl ester storage disease. Laboratory studies may reveal moderate anemia, abnormal liver chemistries, and markedly elevated total cholesterol (high LDL, low HDL). Liver biopsy usually reveals a bright yellow-orange color, lipid accumulation in hepatocytes and Kupffer cells, and a mixed microvesicular and macrovesicular steatosis. The diagnosis can be established by measuring enzyme activity from a dried blood smear or by genetic testing. Enzyme replacement therapy with sebalipase alpha is available.

Fabry disease, an X-linked deficiency of α-galactosidase A, is associated with GI symptoms, mainly abdominal pain and diarrhea, in 50%–60% of patients.[418–420] It is the most common lysosomal storage disorder and may be confused with diarrhea-predominant irritable bowel syndrome. Acroparesthesias precipitated by stress, extremes of heat or cold, or physical exertion, or the presence of characteristic cutaneous angiokeratomas, occur in more than 70% of Fabry patients and may serve as important clinical clues. Deposition of globotriasosylceramide in autonomic ganglia of the bowel and mesenteric vasculature may lead to gastroparesis, vomiting, autonomic neuropathy, bowel dilatation, formation of diverticula, reduced peristalsis, and SBBO. Symptoms may improve with enzyme replacement therapy using agalsidase alfa or beta.

Gaucher disease, a disorder of the recycling of cellular glycolipids with deficiency of glucocerebrosidase, results in the accumulation of glucosylceramide within cells of monocyte/macrophage origin.[421,422] Involvement of visceral organs, bone marrow, and bones is typically present in affected patients. The characteristic Gaucher cells are macrophages engorged with lipid with a crumpled tissue paper appearance and displaced nuclei. Hepatosplenomegaly due to glycolipid-laden reticuloendothelial cells in the hepatic sinusoids is common. Hepatocytes are spared, so liver failure is uncommon. Portal hypertension, also uncommon, may be due to increased forward portal blood flow secondary to splenic enlargement and/or to intrahepatic obstruction from extensive deposits of Gaucher cells. The former abnormality is managed by splenectomy, and both are managed by enzyme replacement therapy. Splenectomy, however, may increase hepatic glycolipid deposition with loss of the spleen as a storage site. The incidence of gallstones, mainly composed of cholesterol, is increased, particularly after splenectomy.[422]

Niemann–Pick disease type B, with deficiency of acid sphingomyelinase, is characterized by accumulation of sphingomyelin within lysosomes, mainly in monocytes/macrophages.[423] Early on, hepatic accumulation is isolated to Kupffer cells, but other cell types, particularly hepatocytes, are affected as the disease progresses. Portal hypertension, liver failure, and cirrhosis are uncommon.

Tangier disease is an autosomal recessive disorder characterized by accumulation of cholesterol esters in macrophages in tonsils, thymus, lymph nodes, bone marrow, liver, and the gut. Tangier disease is caused by a mutation in the adenosine triphosphate-binding cassette protein, ABCA1, which mediates the efflux of excess cellular sterol to apolipoprotein A–I, a step leading to the formation of HDL. These patients have very low levels of plasma cholesterol and HDL, owing to a lack of apolipoprotein A–I. The striking clinical findings include yellow-orange "streaked" tonsils in 80% of cases, hepatosplenomegaly, premature coronary artery disease, and peripheral neuropathy. Patients may have diarrhea without steatorrhea. Colonoscopy reveals orange-brown mucosal spots throughout the colon and rectum, and laparoscopy reveals similar yellow patches on the surface of the liver due to cholesterol esters in hepatic reticuloendothelial cells.

RENAL DISEASES

Anorexia, nausea, vomiting, abdominal pain, and constipation are common in renal failure.[424–426] Nausea has many causes, including the dialysis disequilibrium syndrome, uremic toxins, hypotension, and rapid changes in osmolality. Gastroesophageal reflux also occurs, particularly in those undergoing peritoneal dialysis; minimizing exchange volumes, especially at night, may help.[427] Gastric emptying studies have yielded conflicting results and do not correlate with symptoms. Gastric dysfunction may be associated with impaired gastric myoelectric activity,[428] increased levels of GI hormones (e.g., cholecystokinin, gastrin) that modulate GI motility,[425] uremic toxins, DM, autonomic nerve dysfunction, and the physical restriction caused by PD.

Gastroduodenal lesions—usually inflammation, erythema, and erosions—are common in patients with renal failure but do not correlate with symptoms.[429] Whether gastric acid or serum gastrin is altered is controversial. The prevalence of Hp infection is usually normal or reduced in patients with renal failure.[430]

Occult and overt GI bleeding are common in renal failure. For those admitted for upper GI bleeding, the mortality and rebleeding rates are greater than for those bleeding patients without renal failure.[431,432] GI bleeding is probably aggravated by the effects of uremia on the GI mucosa, platelet dysfunction, and antiplatelet agents, NSAIDs, and/or heparinization during hemodialysis. The prevalence of angioectasias in the upper or lower GI tract may be increased in patients with renal failure and may be discovered by investigation of GI bleeding.[433] These vascular lesions tend to bleed more often in patients with renal failure than in the general population.

Acute mesenteric ischemia is generally nonocclusive and may be due to episodes of hemodynamic instability during hemodialysis.[434–436] It tends to involve the right side of the colon or multiple areas and has a poor prognosis. Risk factors include NSAID use and aggressive erythropoietin administration.

Constipation and fecal impaction are significant problems for patients on hemodialysis and, to a lesser extent, those on peritoneal dialysis. Causes include inactivity, dehydration, reduced fiber intake (due to potassium-restricted diets), metabolic abnormalities, phosphate binders, aluminum antacids, ion exchange resins, comorbidities, and prolonged colonic transit time.[424–426,437,438] Diarrhea due to SBBO from small bowel dysmotility,[439] abnormal bile acid metabolism, exocrine pancreatic insufficiency, or amyloidosis (the last two discussed later) may also occur.

Oral sodium phosphate used as a bowel preparation may result in phosphate nephropathy, hyperphosphatemia, hypocalcemia, hypokalemia, and/or hyper- or hyponatremia, although heterogeneity of the studies makes the risk unclear.[440–443] Magnesium-containing laxatives could result in hypermagnesemia. GI necrosis may occur with sodium polystyrene sulfonate (Kayexalate), commonly used to treat hyperkalemia, in combination with sorbitol to prevent constipation. Cleansing enemas may decrease the risk. Aluminum-containing antacids or sucralfate could lead to aluminum toxicity or fecal concretions, causing obstruction and/or perforation.

Patients on hemodialysis may have an increased risk of perforation during colonoscopy. This is partly due to deposition of β_2-microglobulin, suggesting that GI amyloidosis is involved (see later).[444] The mortality after emergency abdominal surgery is high for patients on hemodialysis.[445]

Peritonitis related to the dialysis catheter in patients on peritoneal dialysis is most commonly caused by a single organism and usually resolves with appropriate antibiotics. However, a nonresolving peritonitis, polymicrobial pathogens, and an increase in effluent amylase concentration suggest bowel perforation.[446] Diagnosis of perforation may be delayed, and hence mortality increased, because patients are given antibiotics for presumed peritonitis from peritoneal dialysis, partially treating the infection. Abdominal pain is diffuse with reduced intensity, owing to lack of contact of parietal and visceral peritoneum. In addition, continuous peritoneal lavage dilutes the bacterial load, reducing abscess formation, so that CT may be unrevealing. To complicate the picture, pneumoperitoneum is seen in patients on peritoneal dialysis, especially with catheter-induced peritonitis, although the incidence is improving with better technique.[447]

Encapsulating peritoneal sclerosis (EPS, also known as abdominal cocoon or sclerosing encapsulating peritonitis), a rare and lethal condition in peritoneal dialysis, is characterized by an acquired, inflammatory fibrocollagenous peritoneal thickening that encapsulates the bowel, causing obstruction.[448–450] Given how rare the condition is, the incidence and prevalence are unknown, though available data from peritoneal dialysis patients suggest an annual incidence of 0.14%–2.5%. Duration of peritoneal dialysis appears to be the most important risk factor. Mortality in a peritoneal dialysis patient approaches 50% 1 year after a diagnosis of EPS. The most common presenting symptoms are abdominal pain, abdominal distention, and nausea with vomiting. CT shows peritoneal thickening and calcification, loculated fluid collections, and tethered, dilated small bowel loops. Treatment includes cessation of peritoneal dialysis with transition to hemodialysis, withdrawal of any potential contributing medications (e.g., MTX, antiepileptic drugs), and treatment of any associated intra-abdominal infection. Despite these measures, EPS is frequently chronic with resolution unlikely. Thus nutritional support, often with total parenteral nutrition, is usually required. Observational studies support a potential role for corticosteroid therapy aimed at the inflammatory component of EPS, and tamoxifen, a selective estrogen receptor modulator with antifibrotic properties, has been used with some improvement in mortality. If symptoms remain severe despite medical therapy, then surgical intervention such as enterolysis or limited lysis of adhesions may be considered.[450]

Hernias are common in patients on peritoneal dialysis, especially at the catheter insertion site, inguinal canal, umbilicus, and sites of previous surgeries. Peritoneal dialysis fluid, under increased intra-abdominal pressure, can dissect through the peritoneal membrane into the soft tissues of the anterior abdominal wall, causing edema.

Pancreatic parenchymal changes and exocrine insufficiency have been found in patients on peritoneal dialysis.[451,452] High serum parathyroid hormone levels, hypertriglyceridemia, elevated pancreatic-stimulating hormones (e.g., cholecystokinin), irritation of the pancreas, increased intra-abdominal pressure by the dialysate, and amyloidosis have been implicated. Whether the incidence of pancreatitis is increased in patients with renal failure or on hemodialysis is controversial. Although serum amylase levels are elevated from reduced clearance, a serum amylase (or lipase) above threefold normal and/or positive CT findings suggests pancreatitis.

NEUROLOGIC DISEASES

Because of the importance of nerves and neurotransmitters on GI function (see Chapter 4), it is not surprising that a wide variety of neurologic diseases are frequently associated with GI symptoms.

Diseases of the Central Nervous System

Abdominal migraine affects 1%–4% of children, particularly girls, with an onset between ages 7 and 12 years; it is also occasionally seen in adults.[453,454] It is characterized by recurrent attacks of noncolicky, intense, acute periumbilical pain. The attacks last from 1 to 72 hours and are associated with anorexia, nausea, vomiting, and/or pallor. Headache is not a necessary feature. The intervening periods are pain free. A family history of migraine is common. Nonpharmacologic therapy involves the removal of triggers (e.g., certain foods, stress, prolonged fasting, altered sleep patterns, travel). Antimigraine therapies (e.g., propranolol, cyproheptadine, triptans, tricyclic antidepressants, pizotifen) may be successful.

Abdominal epilepsy is a rare condition, found more commonly in children than adults. It is characterized by (1) paroxysmal GI complaints, usually abdominal pain, nausea, and vomiting of unclear etiology; (2) symptoms of a CNS disturbance, usually lethargy and confusion; (3) an abnormal encephalogram indicating a seizure disorder; and (4) sustained improvement with anticonvulsant medication.[455,456] The abdominal pain usually lasts for minutes and is sharp or colicky. The abdominal and CNS complaints in adults may be more diverse than in children. There is probably a spectrum, with GI symptoms associated with seizures (abdominal auras) or more subtle neurologic symptoms. The primary problem is often in the brain, usually in the temporal lobe, although it may arise from visceral stimuli with connections to the brain. Response to anticonvulsant therapy is not by itself a diagnostic criteria, because antiepileptic drugs may improve abdominal pain via a sedating or placebo effect, and some cases of abdominal epilepsy are refractory to medication.

Head trauma is associated with stress gastropathy and delayed gastric emptying.[457] Such patients often do not tolerate enteral feedings and develop vomiting, abdominal distension, increased gastric residual volumes, reflux, aspiration, and pneumonia. Gastric emptying delay is due to suppressed vagal nerve activity from increased intracranial pressure, elevated corticotropin-releasing factor, hyperglycemia, medications (sedatives, opioids, and catecholamines), inflammation, electrolyte disturbances, and altered enteric flora. Enteral nutrition can be started even with a mild ileus, because it promotes gut integrity and motility. Treatment includes prokinetic therapies and perhaps an opioid receptor antagonist.[457,458]

Cerebrovascular accidents may cause pharyngeal dysphagia, especially a brainstem lesion that involves the swallowing center.[459,460] According to a recent stroke registry study, up to 75% of patients report dysphagia following stroke,[461] and up to half of these patients will continue to experience dysphagia after hospital discharge.[462] Cerebrovascular accidents also result in stress gastropathy with ulcers and GI bleeding. GI bleeding occurs in up to 8% of stroke patients, with risk increased by the use of calcium channel blockers, steroids, and nonsteroidal anti-inflammatory drugs.[463] Constipation is due to a prolonged colonic transit time, immobility, and altered diets. Paralytic ileus is the second most common GI symptom in patients with brainstem infarcts, occurring in up to 45%.[463]

Multiple sclerosis (MS) is the most frequent chronic neurologic disease in young persons in developed countries. GI disturbance is present in around 40% of MS patients, particularly constipation and fecal incontinence.[464,465] Also seen are early satiety, nausea and vomiting, and postprandial discomfort associated with delayed gastric emptying. There is an increased prevalence of celiac disease (and in their first-degree relatives), but not of DQ2 and DQ8 genetic markers.[466] Constipation may be associated with prolonged colonic transit time, pelvic floor dysfunction, reduced colonic compliance, immobility, paradoxical anal contractions, and an absence of postprandial colonic motor and myoelectric responses. Defecography may demonstrate pelvic outlet obstruction with failure of the puborectalis and anal sphincter muscles to relax.[467] Occasional patients develop intrarectal intussusception, reduced by perineal pressure. Medications commonly used in MS (e.g., muscle relaxants, anticholinergics, antidepressants, opiates) can also contribute to constipation, as will generalized muscle weakness, which impairs generation of intra-abdominal pressure. Fecal incontinence in MS may be due to reduced external anal sphincter tone, reduced anorectal sensation, and spontaneous rectal contractions. It should not be confused with overflow incontinence secondary to fecal overloading. Typical pharmacologic therapy is usually effective, but mechanical evacuation is sometimes required. Biofeedback may help, especially in mild disease.[468]

Spinal Cord Injury

Patients with spinal cord injury (SCI) most commonly have constipation, distension, abdominal pain, bowel accidents, and autonomic hyperreflexia.[469,470]

Spinal shock occurs for several weeks after the injury when all autonomic and reflex activities are lost below the level of cord transection. The abdomen is distended and flaccid, with no sensation below the level of injury and with absent or hypoactive bowel sounds due to gastric dilatation and a paralytic ileus. The incidence of ulcer disease and hemorrhage is increased. Acute abdominal pathology is difficult to diagnose during this period. When spinal shock ends, there is a return and then exaggeration of autonomic reflex activity below the level of injury.

Autonomic hyperreflexia is a potentially dangerous, intense reflex vasoconstriction in patients whose SCI lies above T6 or the greater splanchnic outflow. The result is hypertension, diaphoresis, bladder spasms, and diarrhea. It can be precipitated by rectosigmoid distension and anal manipulation and can be reduced by anesthetic suppositories.[471]

The diagnosis of an acute abdomen may be delayed in a high-level SCI, raising the mortality rate, because rigidity and rebound tenderness may be absent.[472] Those with appendicitis have a perforated appendix in over 90% of cases.[469] Early clues include autonomic hyperreflexia, referred shoulder pain, dull and poorly localized abdominal pain, distension, increased spasticity, nausea, and vomiting.

Abdominal operations are challenged by deformities or spasticity, making the procedures technically difficult. Retention sutures may be needed to close wounds due to tension from abdominal spasticity. Patients may have hyperreflexic hypertension, decreased pulmonary excursion, prolonged ileus, and chronic septic foci, increasing the risk of wound infections.

Patients with SCI are predisposed to gastroesophageal reflux from their supine position, increased intra-abdominal pressure due to constipation, and use of intra-abdominal muscles for transfers.[473] Because the posterior wall of the pharynx lies adjacent to the cervical vertebrae, cervical trauma may impinge upon or even perforate the pharynx. Defective UES relaxation in those with cervical SCI reduces clearance of oral secretions and impairs swallowing.[474] This may be due to injury of the UES and/or its innervations and to interventions such as tracheostomy and anterior spinal surgery.

Gastric emptying is either delayed or normal in SCI patients.[469] Promotility agents can be effective because the enteric nervous system and smooth muscle layers are intact. Superior mesenteric artery syndrome (Wilkie's syndrome, cast syndrome), where the third portion of the duodenum is intermittently compressed by the overlying superior mesenteric artery, may occur following rapid weight loss, prolonged supine positioning, and the use of spinal orthoses.

Constipation and fecal incontinence are common in patients with SCI. Fecal impaction, megacolon, stercoral ulcers, and hemorrhoids may also result.[475,476] Delay in colon transit time is frequently found. The ability to increase intra-abdominal pressure is lost in lesions above T7, promoting constipation. The external anal sphincter is tight, such that stool is retained. When spinal reflexes are lost, there is more incontinence and less constipation. The external anal sphincter does not contract with increased intra-abdominal pressure or with rectal distension.

Colon evacuation should be done after a meal to take advantage of the gastrocolic reflex.[477] A laxative may be introduced, followed by digital stimulation of the anus and rectum to dilate the anal canal and relax the puborectalis muscle. Other techniques used are abdominal massage, manual evacuation, transanal irrigation, and neostigmine with glycopyrrolate (an anticholinergic agent that reduces the side effects of neostigmine).[478,479] More aggressive modalities are anterior sacral root stimulators, sometimes combined with an S2–S4 posterior sacral rhizotomy, antegrade continence enemas, and placement of a colostomy.[469,480]

In the first 6 months after SCI, biliary sludge rather than gallstones is found. Afterward, the prevalence of gallstones or cholecystectomy is high (17%–31% of SCI patients) for unclear reasons, although some patients have other risk factors for gallstones.[481] These patients are usually accurately diagnosed with acute cholecystitis, and morbidity and mortality from the cholecystectomy are acceptable.[482]

Extrapyramidal (Movement) Disorders

Movement disorders arising from basal ganglia are classified as hypokinetic (Parkinson disease) and hyperkinetic (Huntington disease). Lewy bodies, the pathognomonic feature of Parkinson disease, are found in the enteric nervous system of the esophagus, stomach, and colon.[483] Dopaminergic deficiency in the enteric nervous system and involvement of the dorsal motor nucleus of the vagus, reducing parasympathetic innervation to much of the GI tract, may be pathogenic features.

In Parkinson disease, saliva is excessive, not because of increased production but rather from reduced effectiveness of swallowing,[484] sometimes resulting in drooling from a stooped posture and a tendency for the mouth to remain open. Local delivery of anticholinergic agents may be useful.

All stages of swallowing—oral, pharyngeal, or esophageal—may be affected by Parkinson disease. There is a delay in triggering the swallowing reflex associated with impaired tongue movement and a prolonged pharyngeal stage.[485] The result is vallecular pooling, leading to aspiration (often asymptomatic), worsened by a decreased cough reflex, and contributing to pneumonia, a leading cause of death in Parkinson disease. Various esophageal abnormalities have been found in Parkinson disease, including aperistalsis and multiple simultaneous contractions.[486]

Delayed gastric emptying, particularly of solids, with impaired gastric myoelectric activity,[487–489] is found in the majority of Parkinson disease patients, does not necessarily correlate with symptoms, and may be present early in disease. Nausea may be a medication side effect rather than due to delayed gastric emptying. Gastroparesis may interfere with levodopa absorption, whereby increased gastric dwell time allows for breakdown by gastric DOPA decarboxylase to dopamine, which cannot be absorbed by the intestine. This effect may be ameliorated by giving levodopa between meals, using soluble levodopa, or using alternative routes of administration (parenteral, nasal, sublingual, rectal, or jejunal).[490] Metoclopramide is contraindicated; it aggravates Parkinson disease by blocking central dopamine receptors. The dopaminergic D_2 receptor antagonist domperidone can be used safely because it does not cross the blood-brain barrier, and 5-HT_4 receptor agonists [e.g., mosapride (not available in the United States) and tegaserod (limited United States. availability)] may improve gastric emptying, presumably by increasing acetylcholine release.

Gastritis caused by Hp may interfere with levodopa absorption; an improved response to levodopa occurs after its eradication.[491] SBBO is more prevalent in patients with Parkinson disease than in controls, presumably from gut dysmotility, and is associated with bloating and flatulence.[492]

Constipation is frequent and even found in patients who have not yet developed clinical Parkinson disease.[493,494] It is aggravated by certain medications, reduced mobility, and weak abdominal straining pressure (from muscle rigidity and failure of coordinated glottis closure). Rarely, megacolon, pseudo-obstruction, volvulus, or even perforation may occur. Prolonged orocecal transit time is the main cause of constipation.[494] Muscles involved in defecation may not act in a coordinated fashion. Dystonia may prevent the anal sphincter from relaxing, resulting in an abnormally large postdefecation residual. Botulinum toxin injection of the puborectalis muscle and/or external anal sphincter may help,[495] but fecal incontinence could result. Apomorphine injections (an opiate/dopamine agonist) may ameliorate paradoxical anal sphincter contraction.

Huntington disease is an autosomal dominant neurodegenerative disease characterized by involuntary movements, psychiatric disturbance, and cognitive decline. The dysphagia in Huntington disease occurs in the preparatory oral phase (postural instability, tachyphagia, poor lingual control), the oral phase, the pharyngeal phase,[496] or esophageal phase.[497] Gastritis or esophagitis are commonly found endoscopically in asymptomatic patients,[498] but gastric emptying is normal.[499]

Diseases of the Autonomic Nervous System

Autonomic nervous system dysfunction is usually measured by cardiovascular abnormalities (heart rate variability to breathing or Valsalva maneuver or measurement of orthostatic blood pressure) but can also be assessed by quantitating sweat production or function of postganglionic sympathetic axons. Associated features may be orthostatic hypotension, dry eyes and mouth, cold hands and feet with color or trophic changes, changes in sweating, and dysfunction of the urinary bladder and sexual performance.[500,501] Autonomic dysfunction is often preceded by a viral syndrome. The spectrum ranges from panautonomic to selective adrenergic or cholinergic failure. GI symptoms (e.g., abdominal pain, bloating, nausea, vomiting, constipation, and diarrhea) occur in up to 85% of patients. There may be associated hypomotility or uncoordinated contractile activity of the GI tract. The etiology may be immune mediated, as suggested by a perivascular mononuclear cell infiltrate in the epineurium and the association with ganglionic acetylcholine receptor antibodies in some patients.

Secondary causes of autonomic neuropathy include the porphyrias, infections with herpesviruses, rubella, DM, paraneoplastic autonomic neuropathy, amyloidosis, myasthenia gravis, Chagas disease, and botulism.

Disease of the Neuromuscular Junction

Myasthenia gravis is a disorder of neuromuscular transmission causing fatigable muscle weakness. Dysphagia and aspiration are common and occasionally may be the sole manifestation of the disease.[502,503] The pharynx is usually involved, and esophageal abnormalities may occur. Classically, contractions weaken with repetitive swallows and may improve with edrophonium (Tensilon test). Myasthenia gravis occasionally develops during interferon therapy and may be associated with other autoimmune diseases such as pernicious anemia, AIH, or PBC.[504,505]

Muscular Dystrophy

Duchenne muscular dystrophy (MD) is caused by a mutation of the dystrophin gene, which results in abnormal dystrophin, critical for muscle structure and function.[506] Dystrophin is found not only in skeletal muscle but also in smooth muscle cells and myenteric neurons, and thus GI symptoms may occur. *Myotonic MD* is characterized by progressive muscular weakness. Most of the GI tract can be involved, although the severity generally does not correlate with degree of skeletal muscle involvement.[507]

The elevated serum aminotransferases in patients with MD may be confused with liver disease. Although the amount of AST in muscle is much greater than that of ALT, the values are about equal in the serum in MD (generally no more than about 600 IU/L) owing to greater clearance of AST.[508] Creatine phosphokinase is usually at least 20-fold higher than serum AST and ALT, indicating muscle rather than liver disease. Another distinction is the normal serum γ-glutamyl transferase level in patients with MD.[509]

Oropharyngeal symptoms are typical and may lead to aspiration. Pharyngeal contractions may be asymmetric or low amplitude, and UES pressure is low.[507] The esophagus may be dilated, and the amplitude of esophageal contractions may be low with poor coordination; some patients may have complete atony of the esophageal body. LES pressure may be normal or reduced. Patients often have few to no symptoms despite esophageal dysmotility.

Patients often have early satiety, nausea and vomiting, epigastric pain, and/or bezoars related to delayed gastric emptying and a reduced postprandial increase in motilin levels.[510] Response to metoclopramide suggests some preserved smooth muscle function and implies an underlying neuropathy in some patients.

Episodic severe diarrhea, malabsorption, nonspecific abdominal pain, and fecal incontinence are common complaints.[507] Delayed small bowel transit may lead to SBBO, with 70% of patients responding to antibiotics.[511] Jejunal manometry is more sensitive than barium studies to detect motor abnormalities of the small bowel. Megacolon with risk of volvulus or perforation may be seen.

Anorectal manometry shows low anal resting and squeeze pressures in some studies. Electromyography may show myopathic potentials with myotonia or decreased duration and amplitude of the motor units of the external anal sphincter. Pathology may show an atrophic, fibrotic EAS with skeletal muscle replaced by smooth muscle from the IAS.

PULMONARY DISEASE

Chronic obstructive pulmonary disease and its therapy are associated with gastroesophageal reflux. Chronic obstructive pulmonary disease predisposes to PUD and increases mortality associated with perforated or bleeding ulcers, especially with use of glucocorticoids. The contribution of smoking per se to ulcer disease is discussed in Chapter 55. The GI manifestations of cystic fibrosis and α_1-antitrypsin deficiency are discussed in Chapters 57 and 79, respectively.

CRITICAL ILLNESS

ICU patients are difficult to study because they are a heterogeneous and complex group. Frequent upper GI dysmotility[512] manifests as high gastric residual volumes, abdominal distension, vomiting, regurgitation, and aspiration.[513,514] The resulting intolerance of enteral nutrition, along with a predominance of catabolism over anabolism, leads to malnutrition, which is associated with increased morbidity and mortality. Bacterial colonization of the upper airways may originate from flora in stagnant gastric contents and lead to pneumonia.[515] Whether acid-reducing therapy worsens this is unclear. Intolerance to feeding is associated with changes in gut flora and organic acids; such patients have a higher incidence of bacteremia and mortality than those without feeding intolerance.[516]

LES pressure is low to absent, and esophageal body contractions are infrequent and of low amplitude in ventilated and sedated patients.[513] Salivary secretion is diminished and when combined with frequent straining (usually coughing from endotracheal tube suctioning), these factors all contribute to reflux and aspiration. Acute stress-induced gastropathy is common, with hemorrhage increased in patients on mechanical ventilation and those with significant coagulopathies. Ileus[517] is discussed in more detail in Chapter 126. Constipation, with no bowel movement in the first 96 hours in the ICU, occurs in 50% of patients.[518] The main risk factors are opioid intake and disease severity. Routine administration of stimulant or osmotic laxatives should be considered. Fiber laxatives should be used with caution because they may result in fecal impaction if fluid intake is inadequate. Ischemic colitis may be seen following hypotensive episodes.

Acalculous cholecystitis is also commonly seen in severely ill ICU patients and manifests as acute abdominal pain, unexplained leukocytosis, or abdominal sepsis.

SEPSIS

Hepatic involvement in sepsis is the most common cause of jaundice in ICU patients. The liver can be involved in sepsis in two phases. In the first, hepatic hypoperfusion occurs initially with septic shock, leading to poor synthetic function of the liver and elevated serum aminotransferases. In phase 2, hepatic dysfunction is caused by the liver's response to sepsis as the major protective organ. Hepatic Kupffer cells detoxify bacterial endotoxin and remove bacteria from the circulation.[519–521] Their activation causes recruitment of neutrophils, which, in turn, injure hepatocytes. Hepatic endothelial cells acquire procoagulant and proinflammatory activities.[522] Endothelial damage, decreased blood flow through the sinusoids, and formation of fibrin microthrombi are the result of endotoxin-mediated compromise of the hepatic microvasculature, causing pronounced hepatocellular necrosis. The importance of the liver's role in defense against systemic infections is illustrated by the fact that when compared to patients with normal livers, patients with cirrhosis more commonly have hospitalizations associated with sepsis and an increased likelihood of death from sepsis.[523]

Hepatic involvement in sepsis is much more common in neonates than in adults and is usually from Gram-negative bacteria such as *E. coli*.[522] Hepatic involvement most often occurs in critically ill septic patients, and contributions by such factors as hemolysis, disseminated intravascular coagulation, heart failure, ischemic hepatitis, total parenteral nutrition, drug toxicity, renal insufficiency, or biliary obstruction may also be contributory. Hepatic involvement in sepsis associated with lobar pneumonia, in contrast, mainly affects men, perhaps exacerbated by alcoholism.[522] Most cases of pneumonia are due to *S. pneumoniae*, although *Klebsiella pneumoniae* and other organisms have been described. Hepatic involvement in sepsis occurs within a few days after the onset of bacteremia, with mild hepatomegaly in 50% of patients but without pruritus or abdominal pain.[519,520,522] Manifestations of the underlying infection dominate the presentation. It resolves slowly with treatment of the infection. Peak serum bilirubin levels, mostly direct, are usually between 5 and 10 mg/dL but can be much higher. Serum alkaline phosphatase is elevated in almost 50% of patients; it is rarely more than two to three times normal, although marked elevations can occur. Serum aminotransferases are usually normal but can be slightly elevated. Serum LDH is usually normal, as opposed to hypoxic/ischemic hepatitis, where it is markedly elevated. Serum albumin may be low but probably no lower than in nonjaundiced sepsis. Prothrombin time is normal or correctable with vitamin K.

Contributions to jaundice include increased bilirubin load from associated red blood cell transfusion and hemolysis.[519] In addition, hepatocyte dysfunction resulting in reduced bilirubin uptake, intrahepatic conjugation, and canalicular excretion promotes hyperbilirubinemia. Bile ducts and cholangiocytes may be involved. Bile duct injury from sepsis and trauma can lead to progressive sclerosing cholangitis, usually small duct disease. This should be in the differential diagnosis when there is persistent hyperbilirubinemia and elevated serum alkaline phosphatase levels after resolution of the sepsis.[519]

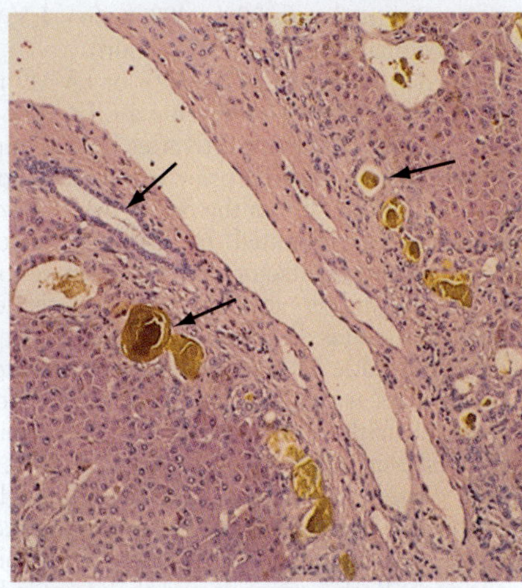

Fig. 35.7 Liver biopsy specimen obtained from a septic patient with marked hyperbilirubinemia and normal serum alkaline phosphatase levels showing "cholangitis lenta." Bile is inspissated in proliferated periportal bile ductules (*arrows*). The interlobular bile ducts in the portal tract are normal in appearance, without bile stasis or injury (H&E, ×25).

Liver histology in sepsis, although usually not obtained, reveals portal inflammation, centrilobular necrosis, lobular inflammation, hepatocellular apoptosis, cholangitis/cholangiolitis, steatosis (both macrovesicular and microvesicular), and cholestasis without damage to bile duct epithelium.[522,524,525] Ductular cholestasis, a sepsis-specific hepatic lesion related to "cholangitis lenta," is associated with increased mortality (Fig. 35.7).[526]

No specific treatment for hepatic involvement in sepsis is indicated. Antibiotics excreted by the liver into bile (e.g., ceftriaxone), if indicated, should be used at reduced doses. Prognosis is unrelated to hepatic involvement or to the height of the hyperbilirubinemia in patients with sepsis, but rather to the underlying process.

CARDIOVASCULAR DISEASES

The association of cardiac and liver disease can occur in several settings.[527] Heart diseases may secondarily cause congestive hepatopathy, ischemic hepatopathy, or even cardiac cirrhosis with ascites. Liver diseases may secondarily affect the heart and lungs and include hepatopulmonary syndrome, portopulmonary hypertension, pericardial effusions in cirrhosis, cirrhotic cardiomyopathy,[528] and high-output heart failure caused by intrahepatic arteriovenous fistulae in the noncirrhotic liver (as in Osler–Weber–Rendu). Nonalcoholic fatty liver disease patients have an increased risk of developing cardiovascular disease, and hepatic steatosis is an independent cardiovascular risk factor.[529] Other diseases affecting both the liver and the heart/circulation include sepsis and infiltrative disorders such as hemochromatosis, amyloidosis, and sarcoidosis. Finally, cardiovascular disease is the leading cause of non-graft-related death in liver transplant recipients.[530]

Heart disease (heart failure, constrictive pericarditis, cor pulmonale) can also affect the GI tract through intestinal malabsorption or PLGE. Ischemic heart disease is a risk factor for ischemic colitis.[531] Fibromuscular dysplasia, a nonatherosclerotic, noninflammatory vasculopathy, usually affects the renal and carotid arteries but may affect the mesenteric arteries, causing abdominal angina and acute intestinal ischemia.[532] Symptomatic GI angioectasias may occur in patients with aortic stenosis (Heyde syndrome) and many patients (30%–40%) after LVAD placement (see the "Coagulation Disorders" section).

GI bleeding (GIB) occurs in 15%–30% of LVAD recipients, and among LVAD recipients who develop a GIB, 40% will have recurrent bleeding. Risk factors for GIB after LVAD implantation include older age, history of GIB prior to LVAD implantation, and lower device pulsatility. Given the risk of device thrombus, all LVAD recipients are committed to lifelong anticoagulation therapy. However, additional factors likely contribute to the post-LVAD GIB risk, including aberrant angiogenesis leading to angiodysplasia formation (as described above) and an acquired von Willebrand syndrome due to increased clearance of von Willebrand factor multimers as they traverse the LVAD. Endoscopy is typically performed in the evaluation of LVAD recipients with GIB, including esophagogastroduodenoscopy (EGD), colonoscopy, and video capsule endoscopy. EGD has the highest diagnostic yield, though a bleeding source is not identified in 19%–22% of patients. Anticoagulation dose reduction is commonly a part of management. Both octreotide and thalidomide have been used in cases of recurrent GIB after LVAD implantation despite endoscopic intervention.[533]

INFILTRATIVE DISEASES

Amyloidosis

Amyloidosis is a group of infiltrative disorders that result from the extracellular deposition of amyloid fibrils composed of a variety of serum protein precursors, along with the nonfibrillar glycoprotein serum amyloid P and glycosaminoglycans.[534–536] Over 20 different proteins have been identified as causative agents. The letter *A* is used to designate amyloid fibril protein and is modified by a second letter or letters to indicate the specific fibrillar protein. Thus with primary amyloidosis, the most common form is called *AL*, with the *L* representing the fragment of immunoglobulin light chains found in the majority of patients, whether "primary" or associated with multiple myeloma.

Secondary (AA) amyloidosis is due to deposition of serum amyloid A (SAA) associated with a variety of infectious, inflammatory, or (less commonly) neoplastic disorders. The number of patients with AA amyloidosis has declined in frequency in the last 40 years, partly because of fewer chronic infections (e.g., tuberculosis), better control of chronic inflammatory diseases (e.g., RA, IBD, FMF), and increased recognition of AL amyloidosis. Although overproduction of SAA is necessary for the development of AA amyloidosis, it is not sufficient; SAA is an acute-phase reactant that increases with many inflammatory diseases.

Dialysis-related amyloidosis (Aβ_2M) is due to deposition of β_2-microglobulin, a protein found in all nucleated cells that is normally metabolized in the kidney.[537] There are several types of hereditary amyloidosis, the most common caused by a mutant transthyretin (TTR) produced by the liver. The resulting amyloidosis (ATTR) is called *familial amyloidotic polyneuropathy*, an autosomal dominant disorder mainly affecting nerves and cured by liver transplantation.[538] Senile systemic amyloidosis involves the heart, lung, and GI tract with deposition of wild-type (nonmutated) TTR in subserosal veins.[539]

Systemic manifestations include nephrotic syndrome, peripheral neuropathy, restrictive cardiomyopathy with heart failure and cardiac conduction disturbances, purpura (raccoon eyes), macroglossia, joint involvement, carpal tunnel syndrome, and weight loss. Autonomic dysfunction manifests as orthostatic hypotension, diarrhea, and impotence. In the GI tract, amyloid is often deposited in submucosal vessel walls, narrowing and eventually occluding the lumen and resulting in ischemia, infarction, and/or ulceration of the area served by the vessel. Amyloid deposited between smooth muscle fibers causes pressure atrophy of adjacent fibers, resulting in gut dysmotility. Amyloid deposited in the nerves of the GI tract can also cause dysmotility, particularly in ATTR amyloidosis. Mucosal architecture usually remains normal until massive deposits of amyloid destroy it, resulting in malabsorption.

Oral, Esophageal, and Gastric Involvement

Macroglossia, found most frequently in AL amyloidosis, is virtually pathognomonic, with a tongue that may be dry, fissured, ulcerated, and indented by teeth.[540,541] It may cause airway obstruction, speech difficulties, oral dysphagia, and malocclusion of teeth. Involvement of the submandibular glands may result in xerostomia. Gingival biopsy is of questionable value.

The esophagus was involved in 13% of patients in a radiologic study and 22% in an autopsy series.[534,535] The main symptoms are dysphagia, chest pain, heartburn, and hematemesis. There may be an atonic esophagus, ulcerations, or masses suggestive of carcinoma. Basal LES pressure is normal or low, and the amplitudes of esophageal contractions are decreased. Occasionally secondary achalasia may develop, with rapid onset of symptoms and significant weight loss.

Gastric involvement occurs in 12% by autopsy and 8% on biopsy during endoscopy; only 1% are symptomatic, with early satiety, nausea, abdominal pain, vomiting, or hematemesis. Gastric outlet obstruction may occur. There may be gastroparesis, especially with familial amyloidotic polyneuropathy, which affects the autonomic nervous system. Thickened irregular folds may have hypoechoic thickening of the mucosa and submucosa with loss of sonographic wall layer structure.[542] Loss of rugal folds and decreased motility occur when smooth muscle is replaced by amyloid. The most common endoscopic findings are granularity, friability, polyps, erosions/ulcers, and enlarged folds.[543]

Small and Large Bowel Involvement

The greatest amount of GI amyloid is deposited in the small bowel (Fig. 35.8), presenting as diarrhea, steatorrhea, PLGE, hemorrhage, obstruction, ischemia and infarction, pneumatosis

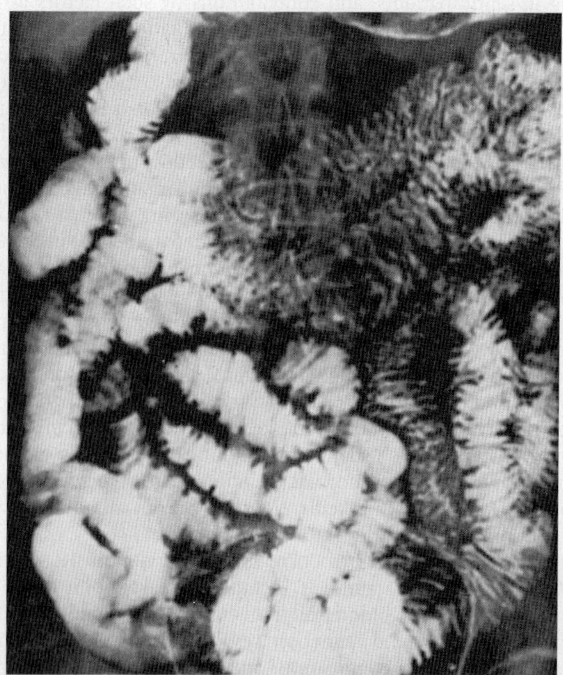

Fig. 35.8 Film from a small bowel series in a patient with amyloidosis; small bowel shows symmetric, sharply demarcated thickening of the valvulae conniventes throughout the small intestine. (Courtesy Marshak RH, MD, New York.)

cystoides intestinalis, intussusception, constipation, pseudo-obstruction, mesenteric infiltration, and perforation (sometimes due to diverticula).[543,544] Many types of duodenal lesions have been described: scalloped edges, duodenitis, ulcers, masses, hypotonia, and dilation.[534,535] Thickened folds may be due to amyloid in the vasculature causing ischemic enteritis, amyloid in the wall, or edema from hypoalbuminemia. Hypoalbuminemia results from malabsorption, PLGE, and/or nephrotic syndrome.[545–547] Polypoid protrusions and thickening of the valvular conniventes can be seen in patients with AL amyloidosis, with diffuse deposition of amyloid associated with mechanical obstruction and chronic intestinal pseudo-obstruction.[534,535] In contrast, AA amyloidosis is associated with a fine granular appearance, with deposits in the mucosa associated with diarrhea, malabsorption, and occult blood in the stool. $A\beta_2M$ amyloidosis is associated with delayed intestinal transit and bowel dilatation due to amyloid deposition in the muscularis propria.

Amyloid in the large intestine may be less readily discernible than in the small bowel, with luminal narrowing or dilation, loss of haustrations, thickened folds, nodularity, polypoid lesions, and ulcerations. It may mimic IBD, malignancy,[548] or ischemic colitis. Acute pseudo-obstruction, found particularly in AA amyloidosis with deposits in the myenteric plexus, may be reversible. Patients with AL amyloidosis and obstructive symptoms due to amyloid infiltrating smooth muscle have a poor prognosis.[534]

Diarrhea may be due to rapid transit from autonomic dysfunction,[549] delayed transit resulting in SBBO, bile acid malabsorption from fast transit or SBBO, or pancreatic insufficiency from ischemia of acinar tissue by amyloid deposition in vessels. Although often resistant to conventional therapies, somatostatin analogs and enterostomy have provided relief of diarrhea in case studies.[534,535,546] Steatorrhea is common in familial amyloidotic polyneuropathy but not AL amyloidosis. Weight loss (often severe) and malnutrition adversely influence survival.

Hemorrhage may be due to direct vascular and tissue infiltration, with increased friability or ischemia, specific amyloid lesions, or fragility of blood vessels and impaired vasoconstriction.[550] Acquired coagulation abnormalities, such as factor X deficiency, are found, particularly in AL amyloidosis. A prolonged prothrombin time may be due to liver dysfunction, malabsorption, decreased vitamin K intake, or reduced factor X.

Amyloidosis occurs clinically in 0.9% of patients with Crohn disease and in 0.07% of patients with ulcerative colitis, although the prevalence is higher in autopsy data. It is associated with suppurative complications, found particularly in Crohn disease, usually taking about 15 years to develop.[551]

Hepatic Involvement

Hepatic amyloidosis has no clinical significance in the majority of patients, except in familial amyloidotic polyneuropathy, where the liver is the main organ involved. Symptoms, when present, include weight loss, fatigue, abdominal discomfort, and anorexia.[552] In patients with primary amyloidosis and biopsy-proved liver involvement, hepatomegaly (sometimes massive) and an elevated serum alkaline phosphatase level are the most frequent findings, although the degree of liver chemistry test abnormality does not correlate with the extent of hepatic amyloid deposition. Ascites is more often due to cardiac failure than to liver disease. Stigmata of chronic liver disease (e.g., portal hypertension, jaundice) are uncommon. Splenomegaly is usually associated with hepatomegaly; occasionally the spleen or liver may rupture.[553] Amyloid may be a cause of increased liver stiffness.[554] Amyloid deposits can be sinusoidal or vascular. They usually begin periportally in the space of Disse, followed by hepatocyte atrophy due to compression by amyloid fibrils.[534] When amyloid blocks the sinusoids, portal hypertension develops. Sometimes amyloid infiltrates the portal blood vessel walls. In those with suspected hepatic amyloidosis, a subcutaneous fat aspirate or a bone marrow biopsy is usually positive (80% and 82%, respectively), providing a diagnostic alternative to liver biopsy, which may carry an increased bleeding risk from hepatic amyloid infiltration.[552] Hyperbilirubinemia is associated with a poor prognosis.

Diagnosis

In AL amyloidosis, serum and urine should be tested for monoclonal light chains, which are found in 89% of patients by immunoelectrophoresis with immunofixation. The latter is used so as not to miss a small monoclonal (M) spike. A bone marrow aspirate and biopsy should be performed to quantify the number and monoclonality of plasma cells.

Common biopsy sites include the kidneys, liver, subcutaneous fat, bone marrow, and the GI tract; gastroduodenal biopsies correlate well with renal biopsies and are much less risky.[555] The positivity of GI tract biopsies increases if submucosal vessels are sampled. Amyloid in oral biopsies is demonstrated in 88% in the subepithelial connective tissue from diseased areas,[556] whereas blind biopsies of the mouth are of little diagnostic use. The risk of bleeding with percutaneous liver biopsies is controversial, with some investigators reporting an increased risk of hemorrhage.[534] Bleeding may be due to coagulopathies from reduced hepatic synthesis or malabsorption of vitamin K dependent clotting factors, factor X deficiency, and amyloid infiltration of vessels, which, once lacerated, may not vasoconstrict normally. According to one study, those with bleeding from a procedure had normal clotting studies but a history of bleeding problems.[534]

Amyloid stains pink with H&E (Fig. 35.9A). With Congo red staining, it has a red appearance in normal light and an apple-green birefringence in polarized light (see Fig. 35.9B). Pretreatment with potassium permanganate does not affect staining affinity for Congo red in AL amyloid but often eliminates this affinity in AA amyloid. Immunohistochemistry performed on biopsy samples is important because it impacts treatment.[557,558]

Treatment and Prognosis

AL amyloidosis is treated with myeloma-type chemotherapy or high-dose chemotherapy plus hematopoietic autologous stem cell transplantation to eliminate the B or plasma cell clones.[559,560] Morbidity is high, but the median survival is greatly increased, and amyloid deposition may regress. For AA amyloidosis, control of the underlying inflammatory disorder leads to reduction of SAA and disease progression. Anti-TNF agents result in clinical improvement in patients with AA amyloidosis associated with Crohn disease.[561] Colchicine decreases symptoms and prevents amyloid deposition in patients with familial amyloidotic polyneuropathy and FMF and appears to benefit patients who have already developed amyloidosis.[534] For dialysis-related amyloidosis, renal transplantation results in a fall in serum β_2M levels and a slower decrease in amyloid deposition. For hereditary amyloidosis, where the precursor protein (mutant TTR) is produced solely by the liver, such as in familial amyloidotic polyneuropathy, liver transplantation is curative, with improvement in GI symptoms and nutritional status in a substantial proportion of patients.[562] The explanted liver is normal, other than its production of amyloidogenic proteins, and is not a site of amyloid deposition.

Octreotide has been used to treat refractory diarrhea in patients with AA amyloidosis.[534] Dysmotility may respond to prokinetic agents, according to anecdotal reports. Surgery is difficult and carries a number of risks: bleeding, impaired wound healing, anastomotic dehiscence (perhaps related to amyloid deposits in the resection margins), malnutrition, and multiorgan failure, particularly heart and renal failure.

Patients with AL hepatic amyloidosis have a median survival of less than 1 year, particularly those with heart failure and/or

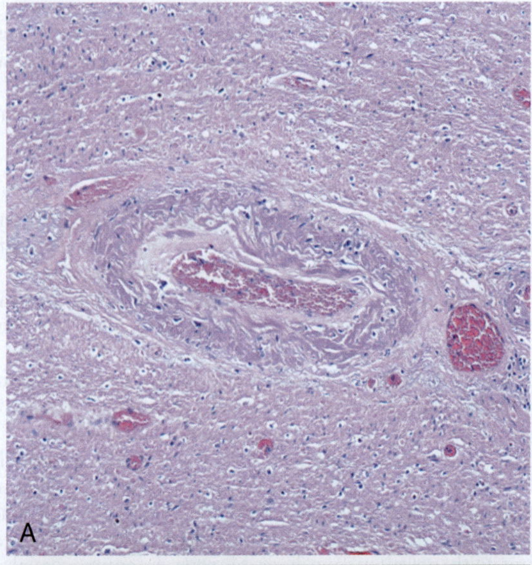

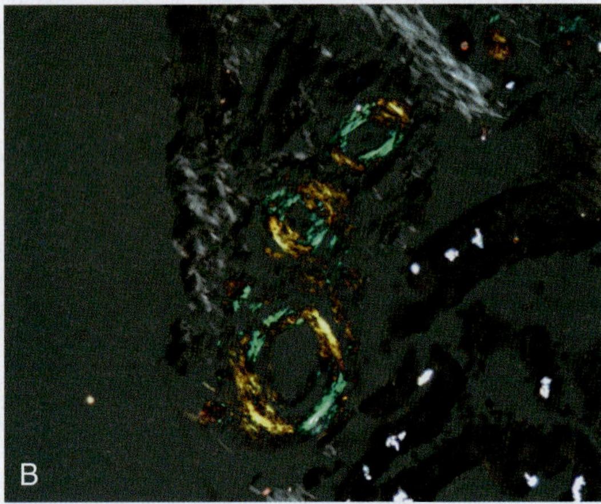

Fig. 35.9 (A) Histopathology specimen showing submucosal vessels with amorphous eosinophilic material (amyloid) within the tunica media of a mesenteric artery. (B) Submucosal vessel showing apple-green birefringence by Congo red stain. (From Ebert EC, Nagar M. Gastrointestinal manifestations of amyloidosis. *Am J Gastroenterol*. 2008;103:776–787, with permission from Nature Publishing Group.)

hyperbilirubinemia. The majority of deaths are related to cardiac or renal complications or, in the case of multiple myeloma, to progression of the underlying malignancy.[552] Morbidity and mortality are rarely determined by extent of hepatic involvement.

Granulomatous Liver Disease

Granulomas, an organized collection of immune cells that attempt to wall off what the body sees as foreign, are often found in the liver as a primary process or a manifestation of a systemic disease.[563–566] They are found in 2%–15% of liver biopsies, most often near portal tracts. Many etiologies must be considered (Table 35.2), with 10%–30% being idiopathic. Probably the most common cause in the developed world is PBC, whereas the most common etiologies in the developing world (and in older studies) are infectious diseases, especially tuberculosis. Although usually asymptomatic, patients with hepatic granulomas may present with hepatomegaly, right upper quadrant pain, fever, and/or weight loss. Granulomas associated with infections that require a macrophage-based pathway for clearance commonly comprise a mixed infiltrate and tend to be caseating with central necrosis. Those in immunologically mediated diseases are usually associated with dense lymphocytic infiltrates. Foreign-body granulomas from indigestible particulate matter such as starch, silicone, or mineral oil, and lipogranulomas have minimal inflammatory infiltrates. Epithelioid granulomas, as in sarcoidosis, certain infections, toxins, and drugs, contain activated macrophages resembling epithelial cells. Fibrin ring granulomas consist of an epithelioid granuloma with a central lipid vacuole surrounded by a fibrin ring, classically described in association with Q fever but seen in a variety of other diseases.[566] Granulomatous inflammation is characterized by poorly formed granulomas with indistinct edges, often associated with hepatocellular and/or duct damage. The pathologist reading the liver biopsy should attempt to determine the location of the granulomas, the presence/absence of necrosis, the type of accompanying infiltrate, any organisms or foreign material in the granuloma, and associated findings.

Rare complications are usually due to compression of adjacent structures by the granulomas, resulting in portal hypertension, intrahepatic cholestasis, biliary stricture, hepatic vein thrombosis, and cirrhosis.[564] Work-up, where appropriate, includes a chest x-ray; cultures for bacteria (including *Brucella* species), mycobacteria, and fungi; serum AMA; serologies for Q fever, brucellosis, syphilis, HBV, and HCV; PCR for infectious pathogens; and TB testing.

Sarcoidosis

Sarcoidosis is a multisystem granulomatandous disorder of unknown cause.[567] This disease generally occurs in those ages 20–40, with an increased incidence and mortality in African-Americans compared to Caucasians. Patients may have constitutional symptoms, lung disease, adenopathy, granulomatous uveitis, proximal myopathy, lupus pernio, cranial nerve palsies, erythema nodosum, hypercalcemia, and granulomas in many organs. Increased levels of angiotensin-converting enzyme, produced by the epithelioid cells in the granulomas, are a weak diagnostic test. The Kveim–Siltzbach test is the intradermal injection of sarcoid tissue extract, followed 4 weeks later by a biopsy of the papule that develops in the area; availability and ethical constraints limit its use.

Gastrointestinal Involvement

GI involvement in sarcoidosis is rare.[568–570] Mucosal granulomas may be an incidental finding, and other diagnoses, such as tuberculosis or Crohn disease, must be thoroughly ruled out, particularly before embarking on immunosuppressive therapy. The esophagus is rarely involved, resulting in dysphagia or reflux. Mucosal involvement can cause aphthous lesions, plaques, or nodules.[571–574] Muscular or neuropathic involvement causes a dysmotility in the cricopharynx or produces an achalasia-like picture responding to glucocorticoids. Mechanical obstruction of the esophagus may occur from compression by hilar or mediastinal lymph nodes, and infiltrative esophagogastric junction outflow obstruction may be seen on high-resolution esophageal manometry.

The most common GI site involved is the stomach, and, although usually asymptomatic, such involvement may cause pain, early satiety, nausea, and vomiting (see Chapter 54). A variety of lesions, particularly affecting the antrum, have been reported: ulcers, thickened folds, a linitis plastica-type picture, and extrinsic compression by retroperitoneal adenopathy.[572,575] Whether the granulomas are incidental findings or causing symptoms is often unclear. Isolated granulomas of the stomach are more commonly due to Crohn disease than to sarcoidosis. Duodenal involvement from sarcoidosis is rare.[576]

TABLE 35.2 Some Causes of Hepatic Granulomas*

Infections	Neoplasms	Medications	Miscellaneous Causes
Bacteria			
	Hodgkin lymphoma	Allopurinol	Autoimmune hepatitis
Bartonella henselae (cat scratch disease)	Non-Hodgkin lymphoma	Carbamazepine	Bacille Calmette-Guérin
Borrelia species (Lyme disease)		Cephalexin	Biliary obstruction
Brucella species	Renal cell carcinoma	Chlorpropamide	Common variable, immunodeficiency
Francisella tularensis (tularemia)		Chlorpromazine	
Listeria monocytogenes (listeriosis)		Dapsone	Crohn disease
Mycobacterium avium intracellulare		Diazepam	Foreign body (talc, starch)
Mycobacterium leprae (leprosy)		Diclofenac	Green juice
Mycobacterium tuberculosis		Dicloxacillin	Idiopathic
Nocardia species		Diltiazem	Metal toxicity (beryllium, copper)
Salmonella typhi (typhoid fever)		Etanercept	PBC
Treponema pallidum (syphilis)		Glyburide	PSC
Tropheryma whipplei (Whipple disease)		Gold	Sarcoidosis
Yersinia enterocolitica		Hydralazine	Silicone injections
Rickettsia species		Infliximab	SLE
Coxiella burnetii (Q fever)		Interferon	Granulomatosis with polyangiitis
Viruses			
		Isoniazid	
CMV		Mesalamine	
EBV		Methyldopa	
HCV		Nitrofurantoin	
Fungal Diseases			
		Oral contraceptives	
Actinomycosis		Oxacillin	
Coccidioides immitis (coccidioidomycosis)		Penicillin	
Cryptococcosis neoformans (cryptococcosis)		Phenytoin	
Histoplasma capsulatum (histoplasmosis)		Procainamide	
Parasitic Diseases			
		Procarbazine	
Fasciola hepatica (fascioliasis)		Quinidine	
Leishmaniasis		Quinine	
Schistosomiasis		Rosiglitazone	
Toxocara canis and *cati* (visceral larva migrans)		Saridon (excedrin)	
Toxoplasma gondii (toxoplasmosis)		Sulfonamides	

*Also see Chapters 35, 84, 88, and 91.

There may be an association between celiac disease and sarcoidosis, perhaps because both disorders are linked to HLA-DQ2 and HLA-DR3, result from defective antigen processing, and involve an increased expression of class II HLA molecules.[577]

Bowel involvement is rare in sarcoidosis, the main differential diagnosis being Crohn disease. Distinguishing features suggesting sarcoidosis are the rare Schaumann bodies (concentrically laminated intracellular inclusion bodies), granulomas outside the GI tract, and a dramatic response to glucocorticoids. Fistulas, architectural distortion, and acute inflammation are uncommon. Patients may present with intestinal obstruction (from masses, strictures, or external compression from lymphadenopathy), pain, chronic diarrhea, PLGE,[578] or bleeding from ulcers or colitis.[576,579]

Pancreatic sarcoidosis is quite rare, presenting as an enlarged pancreas, biliary obstruction, abdominal pain, acute pancreatitis, or pancreatic insufficiency.[580] Serum amylase and rarely lipase may be mildly elevated.[581] Acute cholecystitis may occur secondary to extrinsic compression of the cystic duct by lymph nodes or by granulomatous inflammation of the gallbladder.[582] Obstructive jaundice may develop from granulomatous involvement of the bile ducts or surrounding lymph nodes. Granulomas in the gallbladder wall may be discovered after cholecystectomy for cholecystitis.

Unlike lymphoma, abdominal adenopathy in sarcoidosis is characterized by lymph nodes that are generally less than 2 cm in diameter, discrete (rather than confluent), and spare the retrocrural area.[583] Sarcoidosis must be differentiated from "sarcoid-like reactions" found in lymph nodes of patients with cancer. EUS with fine-needle aspiration can identify granulomas in most patients.[584]

Ascites is rare and usually due to right heart failure or portal hypertension. However, peritoneal studding with small nodules may cause a lymphocytic ascites.[585] CT may show infiltration of peritoneal ligaments and mesenteries.[586] Peritoneal biopsy is needed to confirm the diagnosis and rule out tuberculosis, fungal infections, and malignancies. Ascites usually resolves spontaneously or with a short course of glucocorticoids.

Sarcoidosis may uncommonly be triggered by interferon therapy (generally within the first 6 months), usually involving the lungs and skin. Most patients improve after stopping interferon, although a few require glucocorticoids.[587,588] Occasionally, treatment-naïve patients with HCV may develop sarcoidosis. Sarcoidosis has been described in patients receiving natalizumab for Crohn disease; it is unclear if this may occur with vedolizumab.[589]

Hepatic and Splenic Involvement

Hepatic involvement is usually asymptomatic, with normal liver chemistry tests.[568,570,590,591] The most common symptom is abdominal pain. Jaundice is rare and may be due to intrahepatic cholestasis, hemolysis, hepatocellular dysfunction, or obstruction of the extrahepatic bile ducts by enlarged lymph nodes. Hepatomegaly is found clinically in about 21% of patients and in more than half of patients on abdominal CT. About 20%–40% have abnormal liver chemistry tests, usually with high serum alkaline phosphatase levels and less prominent elevations in serum aminotransferases.[568,592] Hyperglobulinemia is quite common. One-fourth of patients in a report had liver without lung involvement.[593]

Finding granulomas on liver biopsy can aid in the diagnosis of sarcoidosis. Granulomas are mainly in the portal and periportal zones with a cluster of large epithelioid cells, often with multinucleated giant cells (Fig. 35.10A). There is a high turnover rate of granulomas, and large confluent granulomas lead to hyalinized scar formation. Only rarely do hepatic granulomas contain Schaumann bodies or asteroid bodies (stellate-shaped inclusion bodies). Although frank caseation is not seen, central necrosis of granulomas may occur.

A wide array of histologic features may occur, categorized as cholestatic, necroinflammatory, and vascular. Cholestasis may be due to sarcoidosis of extrahepatic bile ducts, bile duct compression by enlarged perihilar lymph nodes, involvement of the pancreas, or associated PBC and PSC.[590] Patients with intrahepatic cholestasis may have progressive destruction of bile ducts by granulomas, leading to depletion of interlobular bile ducts, periportal fibrosis, and biliary cirrhosis similar to PBC.[568,590] Others may have a pattern of periductular fibrosis reminiscent of PSC. Unlike PBC and PSC, patients with sarcoidosis usually have normal serum IgM levels, negative AMA, and negative ANCA. In addition, they may have rapid improvement with glucocorticoids not seen with PBC or PSC. Both PBC and PSC may be associated with hepatic granulomas (see Table 35.2), but the typical bile duct findings of these diseases are less conspicuous or absent in sarcoidosis. Rarely, PBC or PSC coexists with sarcoidosis. Some patients have acute cholangitis suggestive of mechanical obstruction without true ductal obstruction. Necroinflammatory disease or hepatitis-like changes may be found, as well as vascular changes such as nodular regenerative hyperplasia or sinusoidal dilatation, mainly affecting the pericentral zone. Rarely, hepatic vein thrombosis results from veins narrowed by extrinsic compression or granulomas in the vessel walls. Fibrosis may be limited to the portal-periportal area or progress to portal-portal bridging fibrosis or even cirrhosis. A small proportion of patients develop portal hypertension due to a presinusoidal block or pre- and

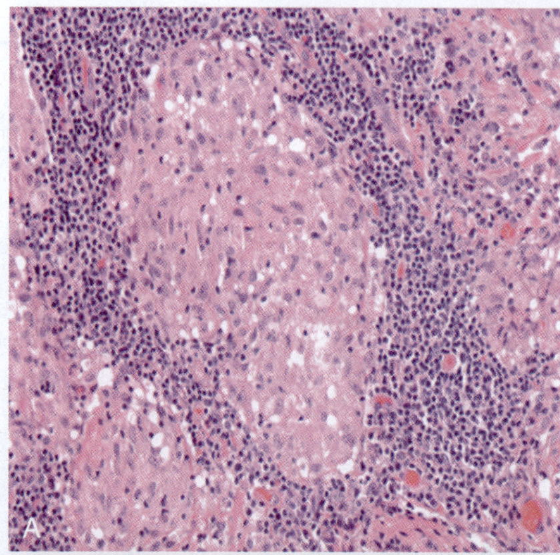

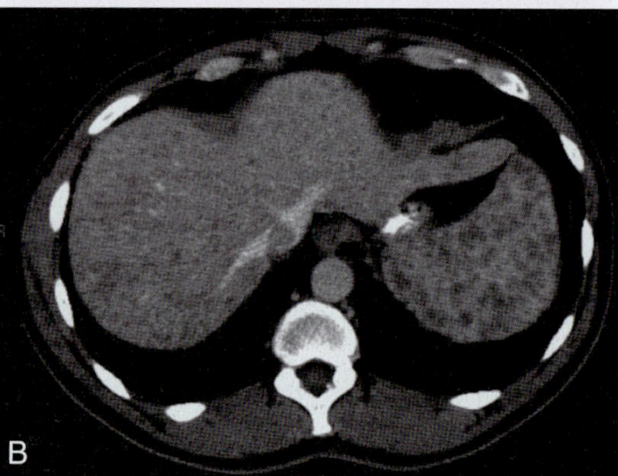

Fig. 35.10 Sarcoidosis. (A) Histopathology showing noncaseating granuloma within a lymph node. There are aggregates of epithelioid histiocytes and Langhans-type giant cells surrounded by lymphocytes, with no central necrosis. (B) CT of the abdomen shows multiple hypodense lesions in the liver and spleen, proved to be granulomas in a patient with sarcoidosis. (From Ebert EC, Kierson M, Hagspiel KD. Gastrointestinal and hepatic manifestations of sarcoidosis. *Am J Gastroenterol.* 2008;103:3184–3192, with permission from Nature Publishing Group.)

postsinusoidal resistance from hepatic ischemia secondary to granulomatous phlebitis of portal and hepatic veins.[591] Because cirrhosis is rare and liver function is usually preserved, encephalopathy and liver failure are unusual. In a retrospective study of 350 patients with sarcoidosis, hepatic involvement occurred in 19 (6%). Sixteen underwent liver biopsy, and noncaseating granulomas were found in 88% of them. Four patients developed cirrhosis over a mean follow-up of 10 years after diagnosis of hepatic sarcoid.[594]

Sarcoid granulomas are typically small and not detectable by radiographic studies. However, if they cluster to form large aggregates, perhaps surrounded by fibrosis and/or inflammation, they may appear as innumerable small nodules on imaging studies (see Fig. 35.10B). On CT, they are low-attenuating and nonenhancing after contrast injection.[590] On T1- and T2-weighted MRI, they present as hypodense lesions without enhancement after gadolinium injection. Lesions take up fludeoxyglucose on positron emission tomography and can be used to monitor disease progression or remission.

Sarcoidosis has a high rate of spontaneous remission, and because there are no large controlled trials evaluating treatment, it is unclear if and when to treat hepatic sarcoidosis.[595] Liver chemistry tests, but not necessarily liver histology, may improve on glucocorticoids, and progression to cirrhosis may still occur. Only case reports support the use of other agents, such as ursodeoxycholic acid, chlorambucil, azathioprine, or MTX. Disease recurrence after liver transplantation can be a rare cause of graft loss or patient death.[596]

Splenic involvement in sarcoidosis is usually asymptomatic but may present with left upper quadrant abdominal pain, constitutional symptoms, hypersplenism, and rarely rupture. Splenic nodules tend to be small, discrete, and multiple, but coalesce with increasing size (see Fig. 35.10B).[597] Up to 50% have associated hepatic lesions. The differential diagnosis includes infections (tuberculosis and histoplasmosis), benign lesions such as hamartomas and hemangiomas, and malignant lesions such as lymphoma. MRI is useful in characterizing these lesions. Glucocorticoids may be helpful for severe splenomegaly.

Others

Eosinophilic infiltration of the GI mucosa occurs in eosinophilic gastroenteritis (see Chapter 30), the hypereosinophilic syndrome, EGPA, PAN, parasitic disorders, and gold toxicity. Langerhans cell granulomatosis (histiocytosis X, eosinophilic granuloma) also may infiltrate the GI tract.

Small vessel hyalinosis is a rare familial syndrome consisting of diarrhea, rectal bleeding, malabsorption, and PLGE, combined with poikiloderma, hair graying, and cerebrovascular calcifications.[598] Pathologically, basement membrane–like deposits can be seen in the subepithelial space of intestinal capillaries, arterioles, and small veins.

PRIMARY IMMUNODEFICIENCY DISEASES

Selective IgA Deficiency

Selective IgA deficiency (sIgAD) represents the most common immunodeficiency disorder and may predispose to respiratory, urogenital, and GI infections as well as autoimmune disorders, allergic disorders, and anaphylactic transfusion reactions. Immunologic redundancy, however, allows many affected individuals to remain asymptomatic. It has a prevalence of between 0.1% and 1% of the population with significantly increased risk conferred by a family history of sIgAD or CVID. It is characterized by low or absent GI mucosal and serum IgA levels and predisposes particularly to infections with giardia lamblia, celiac disease, nodular lymphoid hyperplasia, and inflammatory bowel disease.[599] Rare patients may have a celiac-like malabsorptive enteropathy that is unresponsive to a gluten-free diet and may require immunosuppressive therapy.

Common Variable Immunodeficiency

CVID is a genetically and clinically variable disorder characterized by low serum IgG, variably low other serum immunoglobulin levels, and variable T-cell defects. Most cases are sporadic and manifest in adulthood as recurrent respiratory and GI infections. This disorder predisposes not only to infectious complications (Hp, giardia lamblia, cytomegalovirus, norovirus, and bacterial enteric pathogens) but also to nodular lymphoid hyperplasia, autoimmune disorders, and neoplastic disorders such as lymphomas and gastric adenocarcinoma (complicating the increased frequency of seronegative atrophic gastritis). Enteropathy that is inflammatory/autoimmune and noninfectious occurs in 15%–20% of CVID patients. Intestinal involvement can lead to the clinical and endoscopic picture of Crohn disease, ulcerative colitis, celiac disease, or a nongluten-dependent enteropathy, which rarely can be severe with high-volume diarrhea, malabsorption, and weight loss. In these latter patients, endoscopic findings rarely show extensive ulceration, and histologic findings may include increased intraepithelial lymphocytes, villous atrophy, paucity of plasma cells, lamina propria T-cell infiltrates, nodular lymphoid hyperplasia, granulomas, or a graft-versus-host-like histologic picture.[600]

Patients with mild enteropathy can be treated symptomatically. Notably, IV immunoglobulin is not helpful, consistent with the understood pathophysiology involving abnormal T-cell rather than B-cell function. In a large cohort of 473 individuals with CVID, autoimmune or autoinflammatory conditions occurred in 68%, and noninfectious GI manifestations in 15.4%. Individuals with CVID enteropathy primarily complain of bloating, pain, and diarrhea.[601] Enteropathy associated with CVID can be resistant to a gluten-free diet and is histologically distinct from celiac disease. Guidelines regarding treatment for CVID enteropathy are lacking. Budesonide has been reported to be successful in case reports. Prednisone and IV corticosteroids have considerable risks of infectious complications in this population. Immunomodulators such as azathioprine have shown some benefit in autoimmune enteropathy unassociated with CVID, but there is limited experience in CVID, and the thiopurine-related lymphoma risk is problematic in a patient population already at increased risk for lymphoma.TNF inhibitors such as infliximab have shown efficacy in limited case series, although infectious complications have been noted and are of particular concern in the setting of CVID.[602] Vedolizumab, a humanized monoclonal antibody against the leukocyte $\alpha 4\beta 7$ integrin receptor that interacts with the gut mucosal addressin cell adhesion molecule-1 (MAdCAM-1), is a mechanistically attractive approach in CVID enteropathy in that it affects lymphocyte trafficking to the intestinal mucosa and has a limited risk of opportunistic infections outside the GI tract. Reports of vedolizumab therapy in severe CVID-associated enteropathy are quite limited and have shown variable results. Sifers et al. described one of seven patients with sustained success after vedolizumab therapy; however, the group was clinically heterogeneous, and several were later found to have infections.[603] Another case series showed sustained improvement in two of three anti-TNF naïve patients with vedolizumab and noninfectious enteropathy; one of the two responders had a Crohn-like phenotype, however.[604] High-quality trials are needed to further assess safety and efficacy of vedolizumab in this setting.

Hepatic manifestations of CVID occur in 10%–50% and include asymptomatic elevations of alkaline phosphatase, hepatic infections, AIH (usually seronegative), nodular regenerative hyperplasia, sinusoidal obstruction syndrome, PBC, PSC, lymphoproliferative disorders, and cirrhosis with portal hypertension. Patients with CVID-related enteropathy are more likely to have concomitant CVID-related liver disease.[605]

Allergic Diseases

Drug Reaction With Eosinophilia and Systemic Symptoms

This is also known as drug-induced hypersensitivity syndrome. Rarely, a severe drug-induced T-cell–mediated hypersensitivity reaction may occur, leading to exanthema, fever, eosinophilia, lymphadenopathy, and hepatitis. Other organs such as the heart, lungs, kidneys, CNS, and pancreas may also be affected. The diagnosis can be challenging, especially in the prodromal stage with initial nonspecific symptoms consistent with an infectious or autoimmune disorder and long latency from drug exposure of up to 8 weeks. Quite significantly, aggravation of signs and symptoms of drug reaction with eosinophilia and systemic symptoms (DRESS) by adding drugs distinctly different from the offending agent is common, possibly due to generalized immune system activation. DRESS has a 5%–10% overall mortality. There is increasing recognition that DRESS shares features with secondary

HLH, including hemophagocytosis in some cases, suggesting overlap and a possible shared immunopathogenesis.

Hepatic involvement in DRESS is quite common, occurring in up to 85%. Liver involvement can demonstrate a wide range of biochemical abnormalities ranging from mild hepatitis to fulminant hepatic failure. Most patients respond to corticosteroid therapy, but some may require intravenous immunoglobulin, cyclosporine, mycophenolate mofetil, or rituximab. Severe hepatic disease suggests a mortality of 75%. Fulminant hepatic failure requiring liver transplantation has been reported, with fatal recurrences post-transplantation in some cases.[606]

Lesser known GI manifestations include esophagitis, gastritis, enteritis, colitis, and pancreatitis, including beta cell injury causing new DM. Of these nonhepatic manifestations, acute or chronic pancreatitis and colitis are the most common.[607]

Alpha-Gal Allergy

First documented in 2006, alpha-gal (galactose-a-1,3-galactose) is an allergy to mammalian meat manifesting as isolated GI symptoms. Remnant alpha-gal from a previous tick bite is transmitted to humans via the saliva of *Amblyomma americanum* (lone star tick), which is endemic to the southern United States, Australia, Europe, Africa, Central and South America, and Asia. Ingested alpha-gal is packaged into chylomicrons and carried to the thoracic duct where IgE is deployed. This sugar causes an allergic reaction to mammalian meat such as beef or pork with a delayed onset (3–8 hours after ingestion) of abdominal pain, nausea, vomiting, and diarrhea, is characteristic and may not be accompanied by urticaria. Elevated alpha-gal IgE titers are highly sensitive and specific. Symptoms are caused by IgE-mediated degranulation of MCs acting on histamine receptors in the GI tract. In one observational series of 16 patients, symptoms were episodic in 68.8% and chronic in 31.25%. Nine patients met Rome IV criteria for diarrhea-predominant irritable bowel syndrome.[608] GI symptoms may occur without more traditional allergic symptoms such as urticaria, angioedema, or anaphylaxis. Treatment involves mammalian meat avoidance and epinephrine pen prescription due to the risk of anaphylaxis.

Full references for this chapter can be found at https://ebooks.health.elsevier.com.

36 Vascular Lesions of the Gastrointestinal Tract

Daniel Behin, Lawrence J. Brandt

IN THIS CHAPTER

Vascular lesions and disorders of the GI tract are being more accurately documented as our diagnostic modalities become more sophisticated. Among the diagnostic techniques commonly used today are upper- and lower-tract endoscopy, single- and double-balloon enteroscopy (SBE and DBE), video capsule endoscopy (VCE), and advanced radiologic imaging techniques, such as CTA and MRA. Vascular lesions are a common cause of GI hemorrhage and may be solitary or multiple; benign or malignant; isolated, grouped, or diffuse; part of a syndrome or systemic disorder; or due to an anatomic abnormality of the vasculature; or develop as a result of treatment. It is important at the outset to understand the nomenclature of vascular lesions. *Vas* and its derivative *vascular* are Latin words meaning "vessel"; the Greek equivalent is *angeion*. *Ectasia* is a word of Greek derivation that refers to the process whereby a blood vessel becomes dilated or lengthened; the resulting lesion also can be referred to as an ectasia. Telangiectasia is the lesion that results from dilatation of the terminal aspect *(tele)* of a vessel. Angiodysplasia is used as a general term to describe the lesion or process whereby an abnormally formed (*dys*, "bad"; *plasis*, "molded") vessel develops. An arteriovenous (AV) malformation (AVM) is a congenital lesion, whereas an angioma is a neoplasm. This chapter discusses the clinically important vascular lesions of the GI tract, most of which cause GI bleeding.

PRIMARY VASCULAR LESIONS

Colonic Angioectasia

AE of the colon is a distinct clinical and pathologic entity.[1–3] It is the most common vascular abnormality of the GI tract and probably the most frequent cause of recurrent or chronic lower intestinal bleeding in persons older than 60 years of age.[4] AEs are acquired with aging, and there does not appear to be a gender predominance. In contrast to congenital or neoplastic vascular lesions of the GI tract, acquired AEs are not associated with lesions of the skin or other viscera, although some 10% of patients with colonic AE have similar lesions in the small intestine when evaluated by angiography or enteroscopy.[3,5,6] AEs almost always are confined to the cecum or ascending colon, often are multiple rather than single, and usually are smaller than 10 mm in diameter. They are seldom identified by the surgeon at operation or by the pathologist using standard histologic techniques, but usually they can be diagnosed by angiography (discussed later), colonoscopy (Figs. 36.1 and 36.2), or helical CTA.[7]

The roles of CT and MRI for vascular lesions of all types are evolving but are certain to increase as these sophisticated modes of diagnosis become more widely available; it is also clear that conventional angiography now is more important for therapy than for diagnosis. To determine the precise nature of a vascular lesion, histologic examination, with or without injection studies of the vasculature, is necessary. For example, in one publication in which histologic confirmation of vascular lesions was not performed, AEs reportedly occurred distal to the hepatic flexure in 46% of patients[8]; Subsequent review of tissue sections from the supposed AEs in the small bowel or left colon revealed histologic changes different from those of AEs in the right colon (personal review by S.J. Boley and L.J. Brandt).

Pathology

Histologic identification of AEs is difficult unless special techniques are used.[1] Although usually less than one-third of lesions are found by routine pathologic examination, almost all can be identified by injecting the colonic vasculature with silicone rubber, dehydrating the cells with increasing concentrations of ethyl alcohol, clearing the specimen by immersing it for 24 hours in a bath of methylsalicylate, and then viewing the specimen by dissecting stereomicroscopy (Fig. 36.3).[1] In a study using these methods, surgically resected colons were found to have 1 or more mucosal AEs that measured 1–10 mm in diameter. AEs were usually multiple, and all were located in the cecum and ascending colon.[1]

Microscopically, mucosal AEs consist of ectatic, distorted, thin-walled venules, capillaries, and arterioles. The earliest abnormality is the presence of dilated, tortuous, submucosal veins (Fig. 36.4A), often in areas where overlying mucosal vessels appear normal. More advanced lesions show increasing numbers of dilated and deformed vessels traversing the muscularis mucosa and involving the mucosa (see Fig. 36.4B and C) until, in the most severe lesions, the mucosa is replaced by a maze of distorted, dilated vascular channels (see Fig. 36.4D). Enlarged arteries and thick-walled veins occasionally are seen in advanced lesions, in which the dilated arteriolar-capillary-venular unit has become a

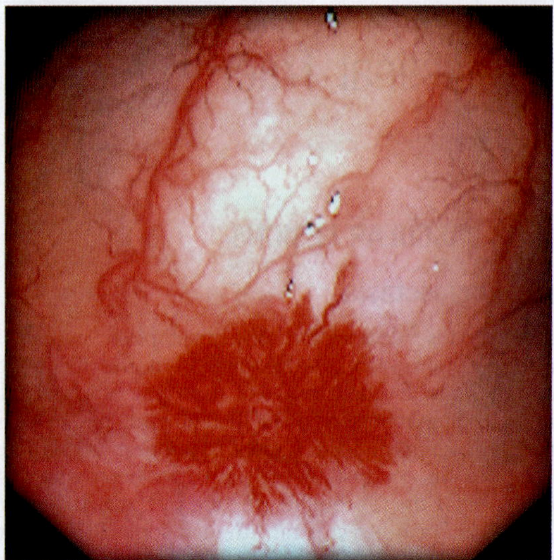

Fig. 36.1 Endoscopic image of an AE in the ascending colon. This AE has a typical coral reef-like pattern of small vessels distorting the mucosa and submucosa. A tortuous submucosal vein, which is the earliest stage in the development of an AE, probably is present among the linear vessels intersecting the ectasia but cannot be distinguished.

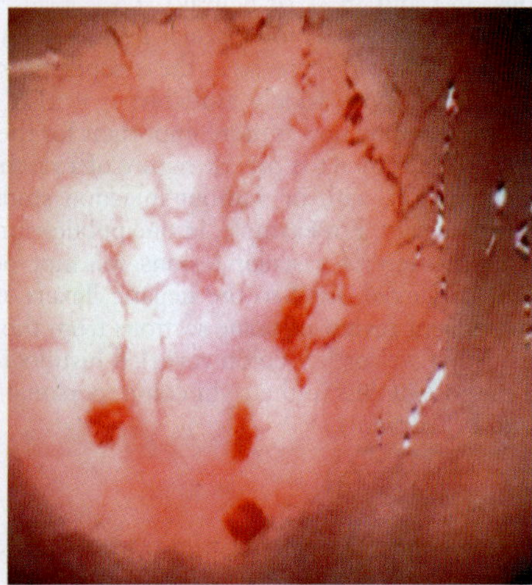

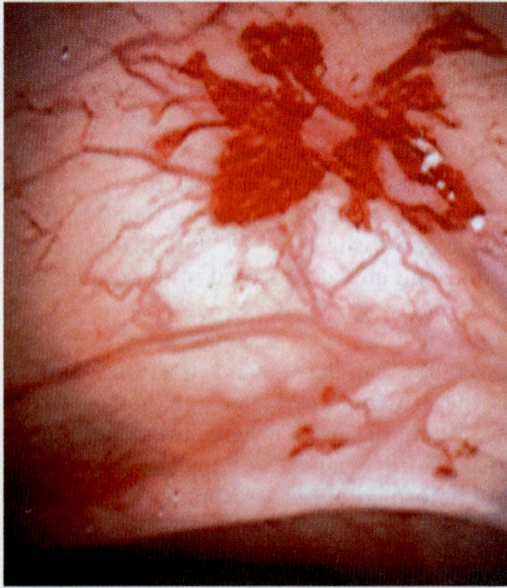

Fig. 36.2 Endoscopic images of multiple AEs in the ascending colon of an older adult patient who presented with the recurrent bouts of LGIB. AEs can be single or, as shown here, multiple and of various shapes and sizes. Draining veins are seen adjacent to the AEs.

small AV fistula because of loss of prearteriolar sphincter function. Large thick-walled arteries, however, are more typical of congenital AVMs.

Pathogenesis

The previously described studies using injection and clearing techniques indicated that AEs are acquired with aging and that they represent a unique clinical and pathologic entity.[1] Clinically, AEs are frequently identified at colonoscopy in older adults and in injected colons resected from older patients with no history of bleeding.[1,9] Boley postulated that the likely cause of AEs is partial, intermittent, low-grade obstruction of submucosal veins at the site where these vessels pierce the muscular layers of the colon (Figs. 36.5 and 36.6).[1] He then went on to propose a schema for their development, suggesting that repeated episodes of transiently elevated pressure during muscular contraction and distention of the cecum over many years result in dilatation and tortuosity of the submucosal vein and, later, of the venules and capillaries of the mucosal units that drain into it. He further suggested that, ultimately, the capillary rings dilate, the precapillary sphincters lose their competency, and a small AV fistula is produced; the latter is responsible for the "early-filling vein," which was the original angiographic hallmark of this lesion (Fig. 36.7). Prolonged increased flow through the AV fistula can then produce alterations in the arteries supplying the area and in the extramural veins that drain it. This developmental concept of the cause of AEs was based on the finding of (1) a prominent submucosal vein, either in the absence of any mucosal lesion, or underlying only a minute mucosal AE supplied by a normal artery; (2) dilatation of the veins, starting where they traverse the muscularis propria (see Fig. 36.5); and (3) previous studies showing that venous flow in the bowel may be diminished by increases in colon motility, intramural tension, and intraluminal pressure.[10] Following this logic, the prevalence of AEs in the right colon can be attributed to the greater tension in the cecal wall compared with that in other parts of the colon, according to Laplace's principle: $T \propto PR$ (where T is tension, P is intraluminal pressure, and R is radius).

An alternative concept for the development of AEs is based on the demonstration that AEs have been shown to express vascular endothelial growth factor (VEGF) and its receptors along their endothelial lining in surgical specimens from patients who have undergone colectomy for recurrent bleeding[11]; this indicates a proliferative phase of angiogenesis. VEGF and VEGF receptor 1 have been shown to be upregulated by hypoxia,[12] and therefore a role also has been suggested for hypoxia in the pathogenesis of AEs. It further has been proposed that von Willebrand factor (vWf) regulates angiogenesis through multiple "cross-talking" pathways that involve VEGF receptor 2 signaling, angiopoietins, and integrin $\alpha v\beta 3$. In a mouse model, inhibition of vWf in endothelial cells results in increased in vitro angiogenesis and increased VEGF receptor proliferation and migration, coupled to decreased integrin $\alpha v\beta 3$ levels and increased angiopoietin release.[13] Further research still is needed to clarify the pathophysiology of AEs.

Clinical Features and Associated Conditions

In 1961 Baum et al. used intraoperative angiography to show that cecal AEs may bleed.[8] Today such an observation is well documented in daily practice by colonoscopy. Recent publications have cited AEs and diverticulosis to be responsible for 3%–15% and 20%–65%, respectively, of acute LGIB episodes (see Chapters 21 and 123).[14] The problem of attributing bleeding to one or the other cause, when bleeding from the lesion is not demonstrated by colonoscopy or by extravasation of contrast material on vascular imaging studies, is compounded by the frequency and

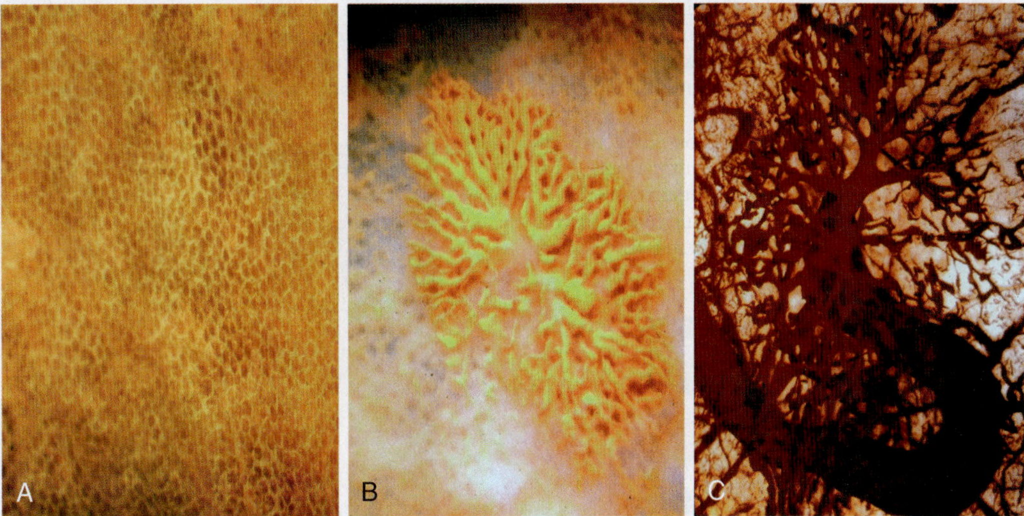

Fig. 36.3 (A) A specimen of resected colon that has been injected with silicone rubber but not cleared (see text for details). Stereomicroscopy reveals the honeycomb-like pattern of normal colon crypts. (B) Coral reef appearance of an AE in an injected, but not cleared, colon. The normal crypts are seen surrounding the AE. (C) Injected, cleared, and transilluminated colon showing a mucosal ectasia surrounded by normal crypts with ectatic venules leading to a large, distended, tortuous underlying submucosal vein. ([A and B] From Mitsudo S, Boley SJ, Brandt LJ, et al. Vascular ectasias of the right colon in the elderly: a distinct clinical entity. *Hum Pathol*. 1979;10:589; [C] from Boley SJ, Sammartano RJ, Adams A, et al. On the nature and etiology of vascular ectasias of the colon: degenerative lesions of aging. *Gastroenterology*. 1977;72:650–660, with permission.)

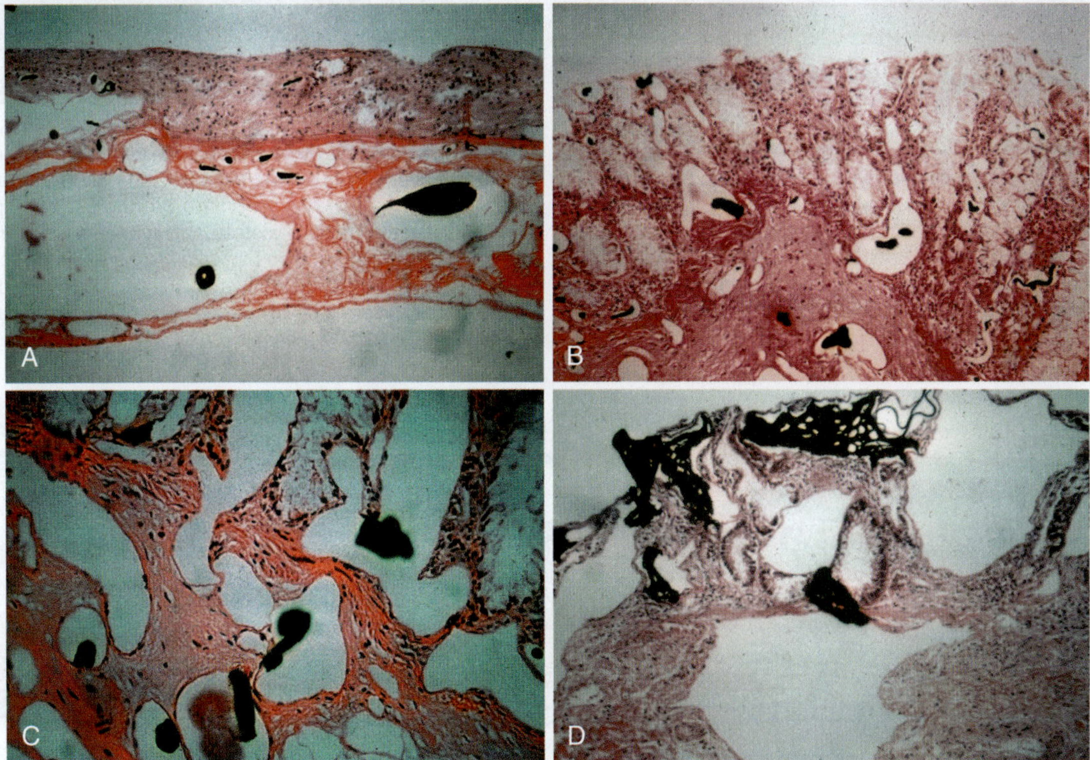

Fig. 36.4 Histopathology of AE. (A) Large distended veins filling the submucosa with a few dilated venules in the overlying mucosa. This appearance is the hallmark of an early AE. The black material in the lumen of the vessels is Microfil^{R}. (B) A more advanced AE lesion in which dilated tortuous veins in the submucosa extend into the mucosa. (C) A further stage in the development of an AE lesion in which the ectatic vessels are disrupting and replacing the mucosa. (D) A late stage of AE shows total disruption of the mucosa with replacement by ectatic vessels. Only one layer of endothelium separates the lumen of the cecum from those of the dilated vessels (H & E, ×50). (From Boley SJ, Sammartano RJ, Adams A, et al. On the nature and etiology of vascular ectasias of the colon: degenerative lesions of aging. *Gastroenterology*. 1977;72:650–660, with permission.)

coexistence of these disorders without bleeding in people older than 60 years of age. The prevalence of diverticulosis is estimated to be as high as 50% in the population older than age 60. Mucosal and submucosal AEs of the right colon can be found by injection studies of colons removed at surgery in more than 25% and 50%, respectively, of patients in this age range without evidence of bleeding.[1,15] In large series of colonoscopic examinations, AEs have been seen in 0.2%–2.9% of nonbleeding persons and 2.6% –6.2% of patients evaluated specifically for occult blood in the stool, anemia, or hemorrhage.[3,9,16] In a patient being studied for GI bleeding, in whom the site of active bleeding is unproven, the only basis for determining that an identified AE or diverticulum is responsible is the indirect evidence provided by the patient's course after ablation or resection of the suspected lesion. It is

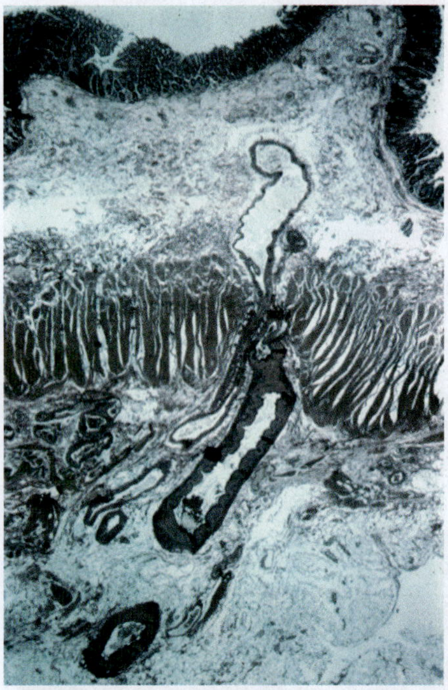

Fig. 36.5 Vasa rectum and accompanying vein traversing the cecal muscularis propria. Compression of the vein is the functional anatomic explanation for its intermittent, partial low-grade venous obstruction (Elastin-van Gieson, ×50). (From Boley SJ, Sammartano RJ, Adams A, et al. On the nature and etiology of vascular ectasias of the colon: degenerative lesions of aging. *Gastroenterology*. 1977;72:650–660, with permission.)

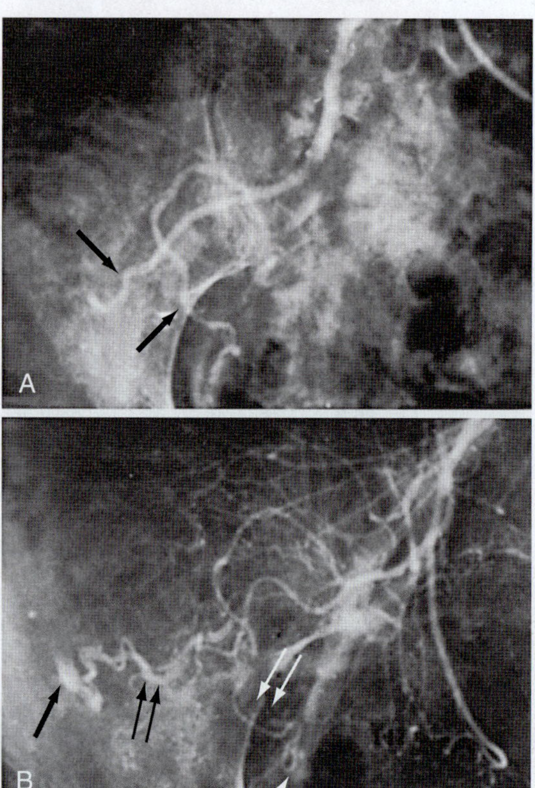

Fig. 36.7 Angiography of AE. (A) Superior mesenteric artery arteriogram from a patient with AEs shows 2 densely opacified, slowly emptying, dilated tortuous cecal veins (*arrows*). Note the late visualization of the ileocolic vein after the other veins have cleared. (B) Arterial phase of the same arteriogram shows 2 vascular tufts (*thick arrows*) and 2 early-filling veins (each shown by a pair of *thin arrows*). (From Boley SJ, Sprayregen S, Sammartano RJ, et al. The pathophysiologic basis for the angiographic signs of vascular ectasias of the colon. *Radiology*. 1977;125:615–621, with permission.)

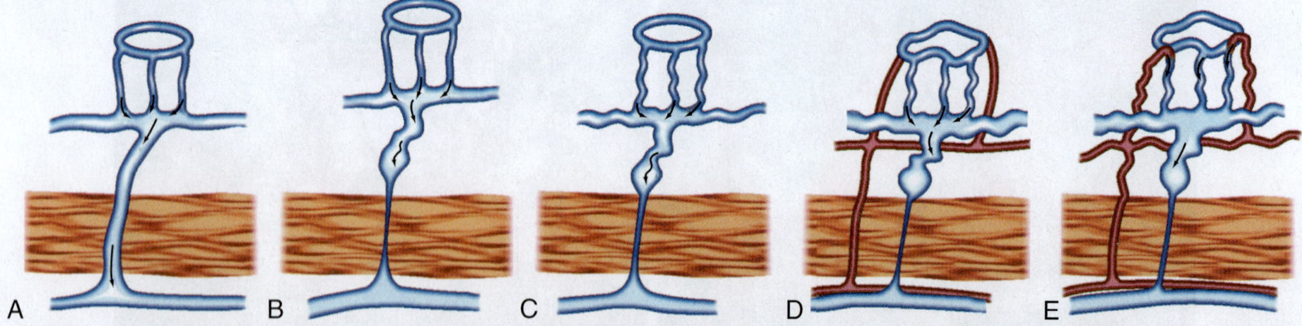

Fig. 36.6 Proposed concept of the development of cecal AE. (A) Normal state of the vein perforating the muscular layers. (B) With muscular contraction or increased intraluminal pressure, the vein is partially obstructed. (C) After repeated episodes over many years, the submucosal vein becomes dilated and tortuous; this is the stage that accounts for the slowly emptying vein on mesenteric angiography. (D) Later, the veins and venules draining into the abnormal submucosal vein become similarly involved. (E) Ultimately, the capillary ring becomes dilated, the precapillary sphincter becomes incompetent, and a small arteriovenous communication is present through the AE; this stage accounts for the early-filling vein seen on mesenteric angiography. (From Boley SJ, Sammartano RJ, Adams A, et al. On the nature and etiology of vascular ectasias of the colon: degenerative lesions of aging. *Gastroenterology*. 1977;72:650–660, with permission.)

unusual for incidentally found AEs to bleed, and an AE, even in a patient with a history of bleeding, cannot be assumed to be the cause.[17]

Bleeding from AEs typically is recurrent and low-grade, although patients can present with massive hemorrhage. The nature and degree of bleeding frequently vary in the same patient with different episodes: Patients may have bright red blood, maroon stools, or melena on separate occasions. This spectrum reflects the varied rates of bleeding from the ectatic capillaries, venules, and AV communications, which depends on the developmental stage of the lesions. In one study, bleeding from AEs was characterized by tarry stools in 20%–25% of cases, whereas the minority (10%–15%) of patients exhibited solely iron deficiency anemia, with stools that were intermittently positive for occult blood.[4] Another study reported that AEs resulted in hemodynamically significant LGIB in 21% of cases, although 42% exhibited chronic LGIB or anemia without evidence of acute hemorrhage.[17] Today, AEs are thought to be asymptomatic or to result in occult obscure GI bleeding in most patients. Bleeding from AEs stop spontaneously in more than 90% of cases.

In 1958 Heyde described what is still a controversial association: AE, GI bleeding, and aortic stenosis (AS); aortic valve replacement (AVR) had even been recommended for "Heyde syndrome" when bleeding could not be managed by medical means. Numerous reports of Heyde syndrome appear in the literature, although some analyses[18] and studies[19] have failed to support the association. The existence of Heyde syndrome has been suggested again[20] in a retrospective study in which the frequency of AS was 31.7% in patients with "AVMs" compared with 14% in the general population. It has been postulated that deficiencies of the largest forms of vWf multimers [von Willebrand disease (vWD), type 2A] result in hemostatic abnormalities that may predispose preexisting AEs to bleed.[21] It is now believed that increased shear stress results in unfolding of the globular von Willebrand polymer into an elongated highly asymmetric protein, which exposes the A2 domain.[22] ADAMTS13 then binds to the A2 domain, which results in cleavage of this high molecular weight multimer into smaller polymers, which are less hemostatic than their parent molecules.[22] Preoperative deficiency of these multimers reverses after AVR,[23] with a resolution of bleeding in most patients with Heyde syndrome who underwent AVR. In a study by Goltsein et al. in 2022, 70 patients with Heyde syndrome underwent transcatheter aortic valve implantation (TAVI). Within the first postoperative year, GI bleeding ceased in 62% of patients, bleeding episodes decreased from 3.2 to 1.6, and 83% of patients had no GI bleeding during a 5-year follow-up.[166] Currently, it is our opinion that AVR or TAVI should be considered to control GI bleeding from AS-associated AEs, only if blood loss cannot be controlled by available endoscopic or angiographic methods.

GI bleeding is a major occurrence in those with a left ventricular assist device (LVAD) and now recognized to result most commonly from UGI tract angiodysplasia (discussed later). A meta-analysis of 17 case-control and cohort studies showed a pooled prevalence of GI bleeding in continuous-flow LVAD patients to be 23% with potential risk factors of older age and elevated creatinine.[24] A subsequent meta-analysis in 2019 that reviewed 24 studies found the mean time to the first episode of bleeding was 54 days; 59% of patients had a single episode of bleeding and 40% experienced multiple episodes.[167] The mechanism of LVAD-associated GI bleeding is still not well understood but has been attributed to impaired vWf-dependent primary hemostasis.[25] Such impairment may be a result of decreased specific activity of vWf, shear stress that results in release of preformed vWf from endothelial cells, and decreased high molecular weight multimers in nonpulsatile flow regimens leading to acquired von Willebrand syndrome.[24] It has been noted that wide pulse pressures are associated with increased von Willebrand multimers,[25] but that patients with LVADs and AS have narrow or zero pulse pressures. Studies are underway to determine whether decreasing the speed of these devices and hence inducing more "pulsatile" flow will result in a reduction in GI bleeding, although preliminary results do not show improvement in acquired von Willebrand syndrome with these maneuvers. Patel et al. published a novel approach using nasal endoscopy to determine the risk of GI bleeding for patients with LVADs. The presence of nasal hypervascularity as a potential surrogate for GI vascular lesions helped determine the risk of GI bleeding in patients who were to undergo LVAD. They found that nasal hypervascularity was equally common in patients with heart failure regardless of whether or not they received an LVAD (63% in the LVAD group and 57% in the heart failure group vs. 20% in the control group), but there was a statistically significant association between GI bleeding in patients with LVAD and nasal hypervascularity with an incidence of 32%. There was no statistically significant association between GI bleeding and heart failure patients with hypervascularity but without an LVAD. Thus nasal endoscopy may be a potential surrogate marker for GI mucosal vascular alterations. Further studies are being done to compare nasal endoscopy findings in LVAD patients with and without small bowel vascular lesions diagnosed by VCE to confirm this hypothesis.[26]

Diagnosis and Management

Management of colonic AEs begins with suspecting the lesion in an older person who has acute or chronic LGIB (see Chapter 21). Colonoscopy is the primary means of both diagnosis and treatment. If the suspected lesion cannot be found, or if bleeding is massive and colonoscopy cannot be performed, the radionuclide scintigraphy followed by CTA should be performed. One retrospective study compared CTA to ^{99}mTc-labeled red blood cell scintigraphy (RBCS) for the overall evaluation and management of acute LGIB and found that both CTA and RBCS could be used to identify active bleeding (38% of cases), but the site of bleeding was localized with CTA in a significantly higher proportion of studies. Of 24 patients in whom the site of LGIB was accurately localized by CTA, 2 patients were diagnosed with "AVMs." RBCS did not establish the causation of bleeding in any patient.[7] A novel telemetric capsule recently has been developed with an optical sensor for a real-time detection of bleeding from lesions within the GI tract. Capsule use for detection of upper- and mid-small-bowel bleeding is currently in phase 3 trials and its use in the large bowel is currently reported only in one case.[168]

The endoscopist's ability to diagnose the specific nature of a vascular lesion is limited by the similar appearance of different types of lesions. AEs, spider angiomas, telangiectasias, angiomas, the focal hypervascularity of radiation colitis, UC, Crohn disease, ischemic colitis, certain infections, hyperplastic and adenomatous polyps, and malignancies, including lymphoma and leukemic infiltrations, can all, on occasion, resemble each other (Box 36.1). Because traumatic and endoscopic suction artifacts may resemble vascular lesions, all lesions must be evaluated on the insertion of the colonoscope, rather than during withdrawal. Pinch biopsy samples obtained from small, flat vascular lesions during endoscopy usually are nonspecific; therefore the risk of performing biopsies of these abnormalities is not justified. Sometimes the prominent feeding vessel of an AE might be appreciated at the time of endoscopy, and the mucosa at the AE margin may be paler than distant mucosa, although such a "pale halo" also may be seen in other vascular lesions.[27]

Because the appearance of vascular lesions is influenced by a patient's blood pressure and blood volume, such lesions may not be evident in those with significant anemia or hypotension; thus accurate evaluation may not be possible until red cell and volume

BOX 36.1 Lesions That May Be Confused With AE on Endoscopy

COLITIDES

IBD
Infectious
Ischemic
Radiation

NEOPLASMS

Adenomatous polyps
Leukemic infiltration
Lymphoma

NONNEOPLASTIC POLYPS

Hyperplastic
Lymphoid

NONVASCULAR LESIONS

Trauma

VASCULAR LESIONS

Angiomas
Arteriovenous malformations
Phlebectasias
Spider telangiectasias
Telangiectasias
Varices
Venous stars

deficits are corrected. Meperidine also may diminish the prominence of finer vascular abnormalities (e.g., AEs, the telangiectasias of HHT); use of meperidine, therefore, should be avoided and, if used, its effects reversed by naloxone so that vascular lesions can be detected accurately; such a masking effect does not occur with fentanyl.[28] In patients who have received meperidine, naloxone has been shown to enhance the appearance of normal colonic vasculature in approximately 10% of patients and to cause existing AEs to appear (2.7%) or increase in size (5.4%) (Fig. 36.8).[29] For these reasons, naloxone is an important adjunctive medication for patients undergoing endoscopic evaluation for lower intestinal bleeding and who have received meperidine. Cool water lavage, to cleanse the mucosal surface during colonoscopy, also may cause underlying AEs to vasoconstrict and disappear transiently.[30]

Angiography is used to determine the site and nature of vascular lesions during active bleeding and can identify some vascular lesions even after bleeding has ceased. The three reliable angiographic signs of AEs are a densely opacified, slowly emptying, dilated, tortuous vein; a vascular tuft; and an early-filling vein (see Fig. 36.7).[31] A fourth sign, extravasation of contrast material, identifies the site of bleeding when the rate of bleeding is at least 0.5 mL/min but is not specific for AE. The slowly emptying vein (see Fig. 36.7A) persists late into the venous phase, after the other mesenteric veins have emptied. Vascular tufts (see Fig. 36.7B) are created by the ectatic venules that join the mucosal component of the AE and its submucosal vein. They are seen best in the arterial phase; are usually located at the termination of a branch of the ileocolic artery; appear as small candelabra-like or oval clusters of vessels; and still are seen in the

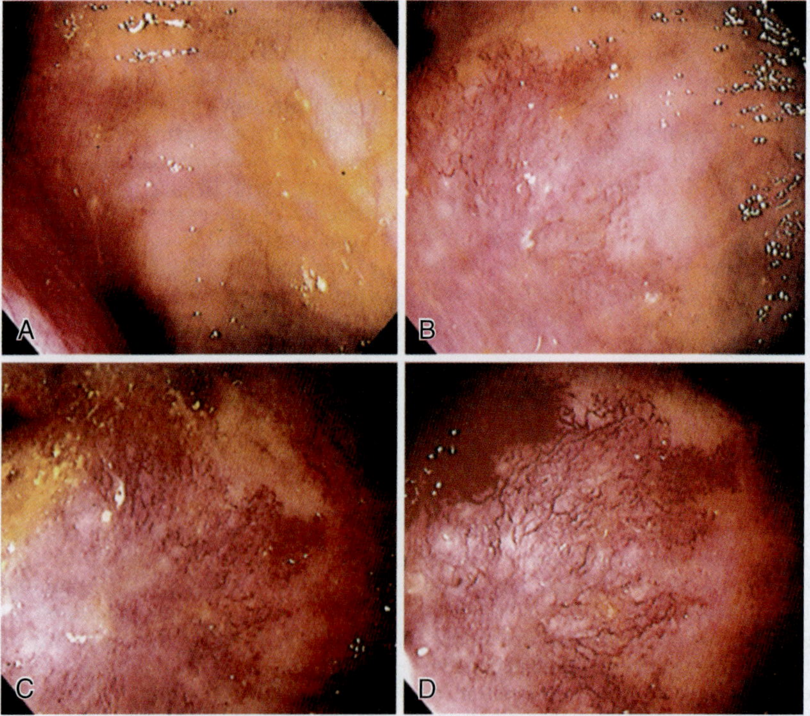

Fig. 36.8 Endoscopic images showing progressive changes in the appearance of a cecal AE (A) after the administration of naloxone in a patient who had received meperidine sedation. Subtle at first, the AE becomes a pale (B) and then deep red, fan-shaped obvious vascular lesion (C,D). (From Brandt LJ, Spinnell M. Ability of naloxone to enhance the colonoscopic appearance of normal color vasculature and colon vascular ectasias. *Gastrointest Endosc*. 1999;49:79–83.)

venous phase communicating with a dilated, tortuous, intramural vein. The early-filling vein is seen in the arterial phase within 4 or 5 seconds of injection (see Fig. 36.7B) but is not a valid sign of AE if vasodilators such as papaverine or tolazoline (Priscoline) have been used to enhance the study. When the lesion is bleeding, intraluminal extravasation of contrast material usually appears during the arterial phase and persists throughout the study. Extravasation identifies a site of active bleeding, but in the absence of other signs of AEs, it suggests another cause for the bleeding.

Management of nonbleeding AEs incidentally found at colonoscopy is expectant. In such cases, endoscopic therapy is not indicated[32] because the risk of bleeding in asymptomatic patients with AEs has been shown in a prospective study to be low (0% in 3 years),[30] which clearly does not warrant the potential risks of bleeding and perforation with colonoscopic ablation.[17,33,34]

Bleeding from AEs can be controlled endoscopically or angiographically in most patients, thereby avoiding the morbidity and mortality of emergency operation. Today, superselective microcoil embolization has replaced intra-arterial vasopressin infusion for the treatment of LGIB. Such embolization is highly effective and safe although complications occur in 5%–9% of cases; serious complications (e.g., gangrene, hematoma formation, arterial dissection, thrombosis, and pseudoaneurysm formation) are reported in less than 2% of cases. Vasopressin still is recommended, however, when intestinal vascular lesions are diffuse throughout the bowel or when superselective catheterization is not possible.[27]

Hormonal therapy, using estrogens in combination with progestins, had been used to treat patients with a variety of bleeding vascular lesions of the GI tract. The mechanisms by which such agents work are not known, although procoagulant effects and enhanced endothelial integrity are popular theories. A long-term observational study[35] showed that combination hormonal therapy stopped bleeding in patients with occult GI bleeding of obscure origin (likely to have resulted from angiodysplasias in the small intestine), although a recent meta-analysis detailed two case-control studies in which hormonal therapy was ineffective for bleeding cessation.[36] It is conceivable that vascular lesions in the small intestine may respond differently to such treatment than similar appearing lesions in the colon; no study of hormonal therapy has been done for proven colonic AEs.

Somatostatin analogs are another option for the treatment of bleeding from GI vascular lesions. These agents work by inhibiting angiogenesis, decreasing splanchnic blood flow, increasing vascular resistance, and improving platelet aggregation. In the meta-analysis mentioned previously, four cohort studies were found assessing the efficacy of either daily or monthly octreotide. The pooled odds ratio for bleeding cessation was 14.5 [95% confidence interval (CI): 5.9–36], and there was a decrease in transfusion requirements seen after 1 year of therapy with an odds ratio of 0.55 (95% CI: 0.29–0.82).[36] In 2021 Goltstein et al completed a systemic review and individual patient data meta-analysis looking at 212 patients with gastrointestinal "angiodysplasia." During a median treatment duration of 12 months and follow-up period of 12 months, they found that patients who received somatostatin analogs had at least a 50% reduction in the number of red blood cell transfusions.[169]

A novel therapy for AEs, and perhaps other vascular lesions in the GI tract, is the use of antiangiogenic factors, including thalidomide, bevacizumab, and lenalidomide. Thalidomide was developed in the 1950s as a sedative, sleeping pill, and antiemetic for pregnant women, but it soon became notorious for causing phocomelia and other malformations in the newborn.[36] In 1994 D'Amato et al. reported that thalidomide inhibited VEGF and basic fibroblast growth factor-mediated angiogenesis.[37,38] Data suggest the mechanism for its antiangiogenic effect is related to reduced expression of integrin genes with resultant decreased cell-cell surface interactions and response to angiogenic cytokines.[39] Several case reports and case series have described the successful use of thalidomide to treat life-threatening or refractory bleeding from intestinal AEs and Crohn disease with refractory bleeding.[40–43] After treatment with thalidomide for 3 months, substantial reductions in the number, size, and color intensity of AEs were documented by VCE.[41] A controlled trial of patients with GI angiodysplasias and GAVE (see later) randomized patients to thalidomide or iron supplementation and reported a 50% or greater decrease in bleeding episodes at the 1-year follow-up in 71.4% patients in the thalidomide group compared with 3.7% in the iron supplementation group; these patients had lesions that were predominantly confined to the stomach and small intestine and there still is no experience with these treatments for colonic AEs.[44]

Bevacizumab (Avastatin) is a humanized monoclonal antibody against VEGF that is effective against colon and renal cancers and also has strong antiangiogenic activity.[45] Curiously, dose-dependent nasal and GI bleeding is observed in up to 59% of patients during treatment, possibly caused by a loss of vascular integrity as a result of bevacizumab-induced endothelial-cell shedding in highly regenerative mucosal tissues with active angiogenesis. It is unclear why some antiangiogenic substances like bevacizumab cause mucosal bleeding and others like thalidomide do not; this disparity effect may be related to the phase of angiogenesis that is antagonized or might reflect a particularly strong antiangiogenic activity. A retrospective study in 2020 by Albitar et al looked at 21 patients with at least a 6-month follow-up after receiving IV bevacizumab for refractory bleeding from gastric antral vascular ectasias or small bowel angioectasia. They found a significant reduction in the need for endoscopic procedures and a 10-fold reduction in RBC transfusion requirements 1 year after treatment; 25.4% of patients remained transfusion-free at 6 months.[170]

Lenalidomide is a newer angiogenesis inhibitor that is an analog of thalidomide but with fewer adverse effects. Lenolidamide potentially is a new therapeutic asset for AEs, although its role remains to be evaluated in controlled studies.[27] VEGF-based antiangiogenic therapy is a promising therapy, but a more detailed understanding of the angiogenic cascade and how antiangiogenic substances act within it will be needed to resolve this issue. A small retrospective chart review by Khatri et al. in 2018 looked at patients who had confirmed vWD with angiodysplasias throughout the GI tract and who were receiving lenalidomide; the authors found a significant reduction in the number of endoscopic interventions needed for GI bleeding compared to pretherapy (0.25 vs. 5.50).[171]

In the past, neodymium-yttrium-aluminum garnet laser,[3,6,46] endoscopic sclerosis,[9] monopolar[47] and bipolar[48] electrocoagulation, and heater probe[48] had been used to ablate a variety of vascular lesions throughout the GI tract and to control active bleeding. More recently, however, hemoclips in combination with cautery,[49] endoscopic band ligation,[50] APC,[51] and radiofrequency ablation (RFA)[172] have been used for this purpose (Fig. 36.9). For AEs, electrocoagulation (heater probe or gold probe), and APC are most commonly used. Control of bleeding has been obtained with a variety of endoscopic thermal means in 47%–88% of cases,[3] and no technique has been established as superior.[9] Severe delayed bleeding occurs in 5% of patients with colonic AEs after thermal therapy.[47] Recurrent bleeding from colonic AEs appears to be reduced after endoscopic therapies, but more than 1 treatment session may be necessary.[48] Rebleeding can be expected to increase with time and has been seen in 28%–52% of patients over a follow-up period ranging from 15 to 36 months.[3] The "elevate, snare, resect, and coagulate" method was introduced by Sriram, in a study of 6 patients with a total of 14 colonic angioectasias. Submucosal lifting injections with saline or

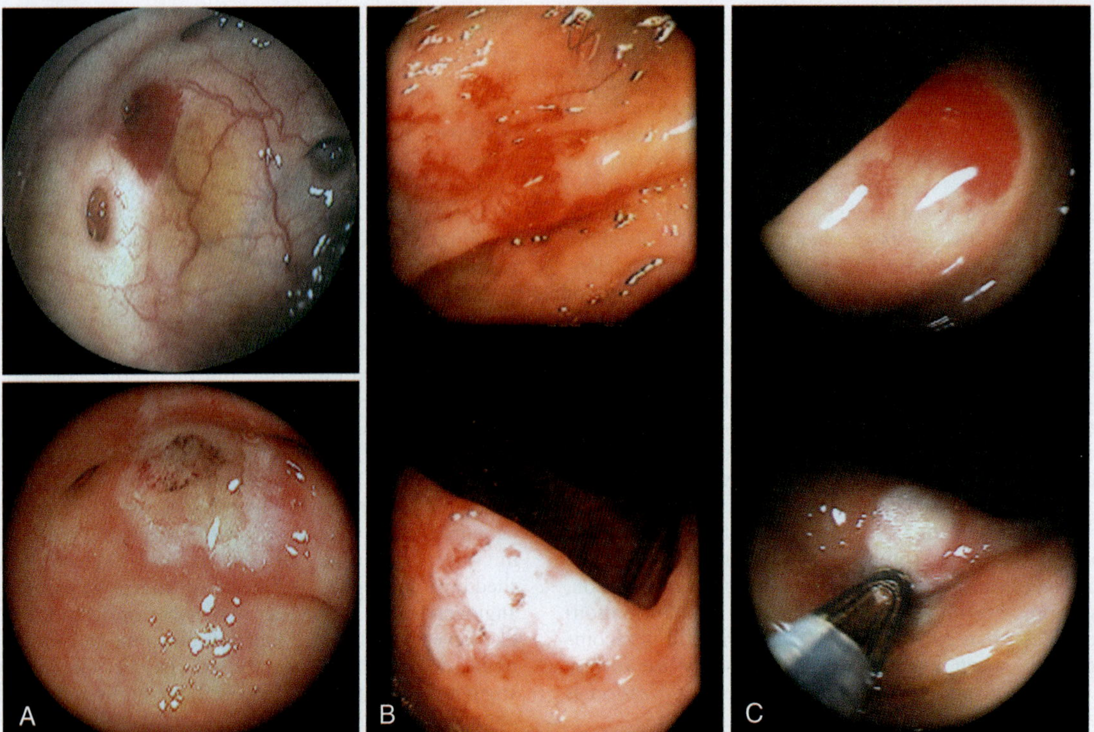

Fig. 36.9 Endoscopic images showing AE and diverticulosis of the colon. (A, upper) A single AE nestled among diverticula in the ascending colon of an older adult man with LGIB. AEs and diverticula are the 2 most common causes of major recurrent LGIB in older adults; therefore finding them together in the same patient is not unusual. (A, lower) The AE after treatment with APC (B, upper) Multiple AEs in the ascending colon. (B, lower) AEs after treatment with a heater probe. (C, upper) A solitary AE. (C, lower) A heater probe is being used to ablate the AE.

succinylate gelatin are made, the mucosal lesion is resected via EMR, and the underlying feeding vessel is identified and cauterized using a soft-coagulation forceps. The defect is then closed with endoscopic clips. In this small study, no patient required blood transfusion, iron replacement therapy or repeat endoscopic procedures, although the follow-up period was not addressed.[173]

In preparation for endoscopic ablation of vascular lesions, aspirin and aspirin-containing drugs, other NSAIDs, anticoagulants, and antiplatelet agents should be withdrawn, if possible, at least several days before the procedure and depending on the agent. Aspiration of some intraluminal gas just before thermal therapy is applied adds a measure of safety as the colon wall is not so thinned with a smaller diameter lumen. Right hemicolectomy is indicated when AE has been identified by either colonoscopy or angiography and when therapy by either or both of these modalities is unsuccessful, cannot be performed, or is unavailable and the patient has continuous or recurrent LGI bleeding. The presence or absence of diverticulosis in the left colon does not alter the extent of colonic resection in this circumstance; only the right half of the colon is removed, but it is important that the entire right half of the colon be removed to ensure that no AEs are left behind. If the site of bleeding (and its cause) is not identified, and bleeding recurs or is continuous, a subtotal colectomy (STC) is appropriate. Morbidity and mortality rates of an STC are not statistically different from those accompanying a "blind" hemicolectomy, that is, when the bleeding site is not identified.[52,53] In one surgical review, mortality and rebleeding rates for STC, directed limited colectomy, and blind limited colectomy were 0%–40% and 0%–8%; 2%–22% and 0%–15%; and 20%–57% and 35%–75%, respectively.[52]

Angiodysplasia

Angiodysplasias are most commonly found in the stomach and small intestine of patients with chronic kidney disease (see Chapter 35) but are also found in approximately 10% of patients with colonic AEs. Other vascular lesions that occur in the small intestine include the blue rubber bleb, hemangioma, angioma, Dieulafoy lesion, and portal hypertensive enteropathy (discussed later). Although SBE and DBE (Fig. 36.10) are used for diagnosis and treatment of many of these lesions, VCE (Fig. 36.11) is currently the mainstay for their diagnosis and for evaluating patients with obscure and occult GI bleeding because it is noninvasive, easily performed, and enables inspection of the entire small intestine. In a prospective multicenter study, VCE had an overall diagnostic yield of 67% for overt small bowel bleeding, with AE as the most commonly identified source.[54] VCE also has been shown to be superior to push enteroscopy and small bowel series in a meta-analysis comparing these three techniques: VCE showed an incremental yield of 30% over push enteroscopy and 36% over small bowel series.[55] The diagnostic yield of VCE also has been demonstrated to exceed that of angiography (53% vs. 20%) in patients with acute overt obscure GI bleeding.[56]

Vascular lesions are the most frequently identified culprit lesion in patients who undergo VCE for occult obscure GI bleeding, particularly those older than 65 years of age.[57] Younger patients tend to exhibit more sinister pathology (e.g., small intestinal tumors) as the cause of their anemia.[57]

SBE and DBE can be used to examine the small intestine by either an anterograde or retrograde approach and allow for implementation of endoscopic therapy at the time of diagnosis (Video 36.1). The rate of complete enteroscopy has been reported

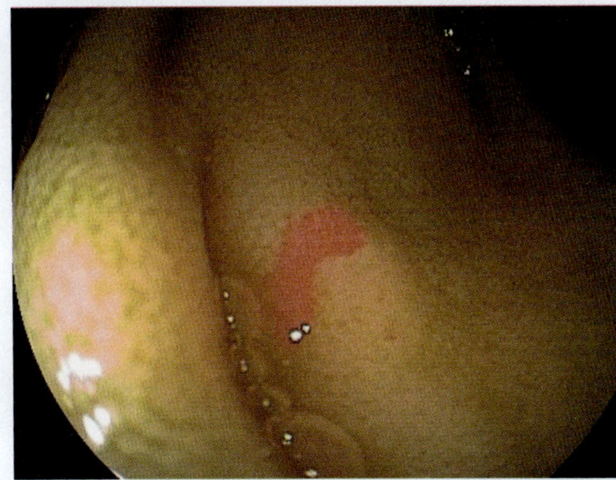

Fig. 36.10 Angiodysplasia demonstrated by double-balloon enteroscopy. (Courtesy Dr. Daniel Mishkin, Boston, MA.)

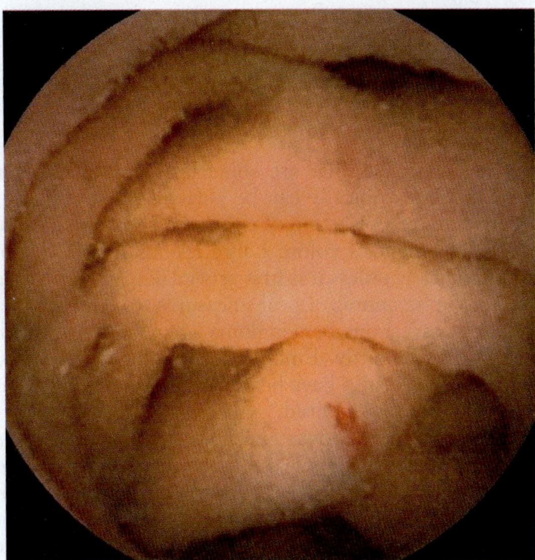

Fig. 36.11 Angiodysplasia demonstrated by video capsule endoscopy. (Courtesy Dr. Daniel Mishkin, Boston, MA.)

as 57% for DBE compared with 0% for SBE, justifying a preferred use for DBE.[58] A meta-analysis of 10 studies comparing VCE and DBE in patients with obscure GI bleeding showed comparable diagnostic yields of 60%–57%, respectively, although the diagnostic yield of DBE was significantly higher when performed after a positive VCE compared with a negative VCE (75% vs. 27.5%; $P = .02$).[59] A study from 2012 that investigated long-term outcomes in patients undergoing DBE for obscure GI bleeding identified small intestinal vascular lesions (i.e., angiodysplasias, telangiectasias, blue rubber blebs, and Dieulafoy's) as suspected causes in 51% of patients; these lesions were successfully treated by APC in 97% of patients with a cumulative rebleeding rate of 46% at 36 months.[60] In a systematic review and meta-analysis, it was shown that approximately 34% of patients with angiodysplastic lesions and approximately 45% of patients with isolated small bowel angiodysplastic lesions rebled after endoscopic therapy.[24] The meta-analysis also included four studies that looked at the impact of octreotide analogs on rebleeding rates for patients who were refractory to endoscopic therapy and showed a significant decrease in both rebleeding rates and transfusion requirements. The standard mean reduction in number of transfusions after 1 year of therapy was 0.55 (95% CI: 0.29–0.82). Two studies analyzed the use of thalidomide for refractory bleeding, and both showed a decrease in rebleeding rates and transfusion requirements.[40,41]

Dieulafoy Lesion

This vascular lesion is an unusual cause of massive GI hemorrhage and may occur anywhere in the GI tract from esophagus to rectum (Fig. 36.12).[61] It is twice as common in men as in women and presents at a mean age of 52 years. The abnormality is the presence of an artery of persistently large caliber in the submucosa and, in some instances the mucosa, typically with a small, overlying mucosal defect. Dieulafoy called the lesion *exulceratio simplex* because he thought it was the initial stage of a gastric ulcer. This lesion also has been called an atherosclerotic aneurysm, an inaccurate term because the caliber of the artery's walls is uniform throughout and shows no unusual degree of arteriosclerosis. It is believed that focal pressure from these large "caliber-persistent" vessels thins the overlying mucosa, leading to erosion of the exposed vascular wall with resultant hemorrhage. Massive hematemesis or melena typically is not preceded by any GI symptoms and usually is followed by intermittent and severe bleeding over several days. The most common site of bleeding is 6 cm distal to the cardioesophageal junction, where the arteries that supply the stomach are largest, but, as mentioned previously, Dieulafoy lesions have been reported in extragastric locations, including the esophagus, small bowel, rectum,[61] and even outside the GI tract in the bronchus. Endoscopically, a Dieulafoy lesion appears as an isolated protruding vessel surrounded by normal mucosa that may be difficult to find in a patient with UGI bleeding because the overlying mucosal defect may be small and hidden between the gastric rugae, and the caliber-persistent vessel may constrict and retract after the bleeding episode. If found, tattooing of the lesion is advocated by some authorities to allow for rapid identification of the lesion should rebleeding occur. EUS also has been used to enhance detection of these aberrant submucosa vessels and can help determine whether endoscopic therapy was successful. Mesenteric angiography is used when endoscopy fails to localize a site of hemorrhage and may be of particular benefit in patients with lesions in the colon or rectum where the view could be obscured by active bleeding and poor bowel preparation.[62]

Endoscopic techniques to localize and treat Dieulafoy lesions have decreased the need for surgical intervention and dramatically reduced the mortality of bleeding from 80% to 8%. Endoscopic treatments are considered safe and effective at achieving hemostasis with success rates reaching 75%–100%. Therapeutic approaches to bleeding Dieulafoy lesions include injection therapy, heater probe, APC, band ligation, hemoclips, and the use of over-the-scope clips. Combination endoscopic therapy with injection followed by thermal or mechanical therapy is superior to monotherapy and has achieved hemostasis in 95% of cases.[63] Rebleeding from these lesions is reported between 9% and 40%[62] and is higher after endoscopic monotherapy compared with combination therapy.[64]

Hemangioma

Considered by some to be true neoplasms, hemangiomas generally are thought to be hamartomas. Hemangiomas are the second most common vascular lesion of the colon and may occur as solitary or multiple lesions limited to the colon or as part of diffuse GI or multisystem angiomatoses. Hemangiomas are structurally complicated lesions characterized by an excess of blood vessels, usually veins and capillaries, in a focal area of submucosal connective tissue.[65] Hemangiomas may be classified as cavernous, capillary, or mixed types; however, the most common hemangioma found in the GI tract is of the capillary variety.[65]

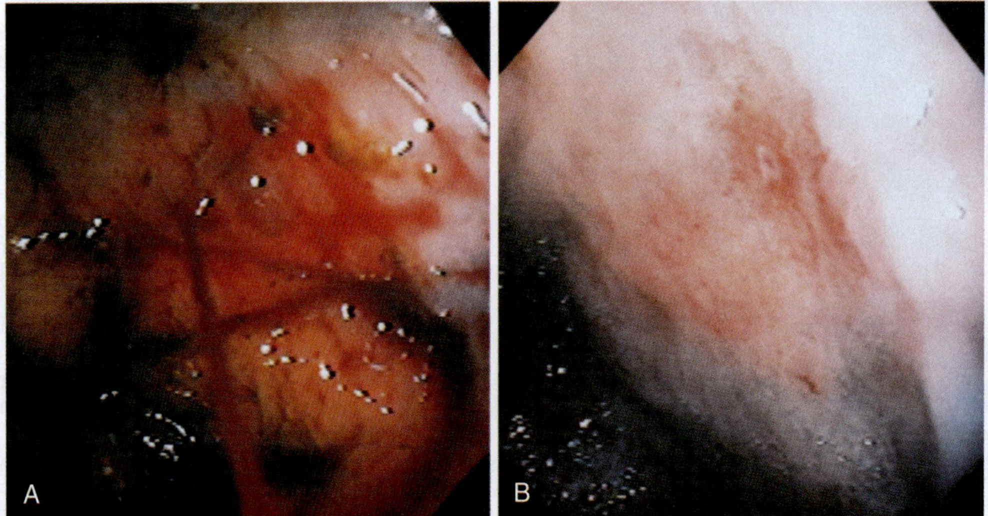

Fig. 36.12 Endoscopic images of a Dieulafoy lesion. (A) Arterial bleeding (spurting) just distal to the gastroesophageal junction. (B) The bleeding point was a small defect without the endoscopic evidence of ulceration. (From Wilcox CM. *Atlas of Clinical Gastrointestinal Endoscopy*. Philadelphia: WB Saunders; 1995:122.)

Most hemangiomas are small, ranging from a few millimeters to 2 cm, but larger lesions occur, especially in the rectum. Bleeding from colonic hemangiomas usually is slow, producing occult blood loss with anemia or melena. Hematochezia is less common, except with large cavernous hemangiomas of the rectum, which may cause massive hemorrhage. The diagnosis is best established by endoscopy, including enteroscopy because radiologic studies, even including angiography, frequently are normal. The diagnosis of *cavernous hemangioma of the rectum* often can be suggested on plain films of the abdomen by the presence of phleboliths and displacement or distortion of the rectal air column (Fig. 36.13). On barium enema, the affected rectal lumen typically shows narrowing and rigidity, scalloping of the rectal wall, and widening of the presacral space (see Fig. 36.13). Endoscopically, one sees elevated plum-red nodules or vascular congestion; ulcers and proctitis also may be present. Imaging with CT and MRI are highly accurate in delineating cavernous hemangiomas and EUS also can help identify the extent of invasion into the anal canal and adjacent structures.[66] Angiography can demonstrate these lesions but seldom is necessary to establish the diagnosis.

Grossly, cavernous hemangiomas appear as polypoid or mound-like reddish purple mucosal lesions. Histologically, numerous dilated, irregular blood-filled spaces are seen within the mucosa and submucosa and sometimes extend through the muscular wall to the serosal surface. The vascular channels are lined by flat endothelial cells with flat or plump nuclei depending on their age. Younger hemangiomas have plump endothelial nuclei and often demonstrate mitotic activity, a feature not present in older lesions; vascular lumina remain small and irregular.[65] As the lesion matures, the endothelial cells flatten and decrease in number. During involution, the fibrous septa thicken, the endothelial cells are replaced by adipocytes, and the vascular structures atrophy.[65] Although lacking a capsule, the capillary hemangioma is often well circumscribed and there typically is a central feeding vessel with radiating, lobular extensions.[65] Capillary hemangiomas are plaque-like or mound-like reddish purple lesions composed of a proliferation of fine, closely packed, newly formed capillaries separated by little stroma. The endothelial cells are large, usually hypertrophic, and in some areas may form solid cords or nodules with ill-defined capillary spaces.

Small hemangiomas that are solitary or few in number and approachable endoscopically can be ablated. Most large or multiple lesions require a resection of either the hemangioma alone or the involved segment of colon. Large lesions should not be ablated endoscopically unless it is first proved (e.g., by EUS) that the lesion is not transmural. Local measures to control massive bleeding from cavernous hemangioma of the rectum usually are effective only temporarily. Embolization and surgical ligation of major feeding vessels also have been used, but ultimately, excision of the rectum often is required.[67]

In a particular entity known as *diffuse intestinal hemangiomatosis*, numerous lesions, usually of the cavernous type, involve the stomach, small bowel, and colon; hemangiomas of the skin or soft tissues of the head and neck frequently are present. The occurrence of bleeding or anemia in childhood typically leads to the diagnosis, and surgical intervention may be required for continuous, slow bleeding or for intussusception.[68] Intraoperative endoscopy had been helpful in finding small lesions, but today SBE and DBE probably would be tried first. Inhibitors of the VEGF receptor (bevacizumab) and multitargeted tyrosine kinases, including sunitinib [inhibits VEGF, platelet-derived growth factor (PDGF)], vatalanib (inhibits VEGF, PDGF, c-kit), and semaxanib (inhibits VEGF and PDGF), have been used for treatment of hemangioblastoma, another highly vascularized lesion of uncertain histogenesis that occurs most frequently in patients with von Hippel-Lindau disease (vHLD).[69] In vHLD, a loss of von Hippel-Lindau protein results in an accumulation of hypoxia-inducible factor and, subsequently, excessive production of VEGF.[70] Bevacizumab, a humanized monoclonal antibody against VEGF may, in patients with vHLD, result in stabilization or regression of CNS hemangioblastomas with resultant improvement in visual acuity in the setting of macular and optic nerve hemangioblastomas[69]; these results suggest there may be a role for the use of VEGF inhibitors in the management of other types of hemangiomas. Definitive treatment can be provided with surgery.

Congenital Arteriovenous Malformation

AVMs are embryonic growth defects and are considered to be developmental anomalies. Although AVMs are found mainly in the extremities, they may occur anywhere in the vascular system.

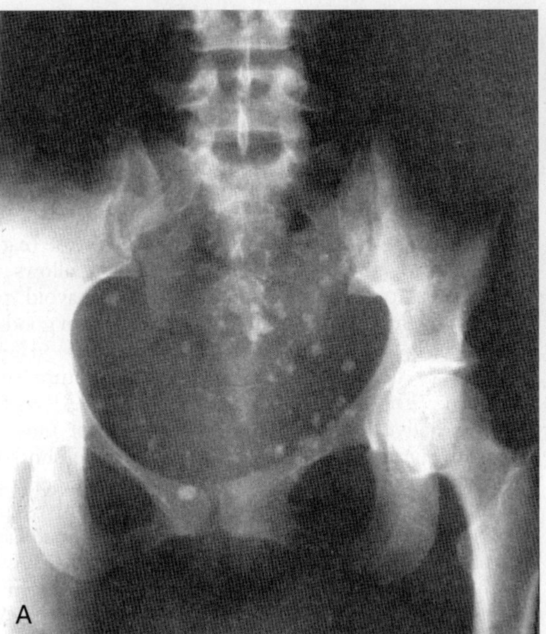

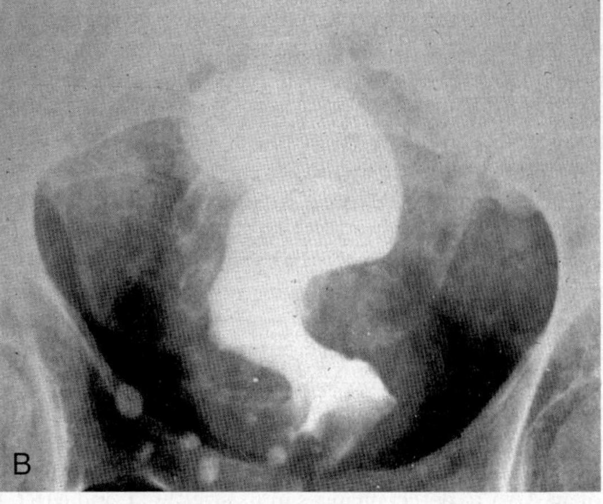

Fig. 36.13 Two imaging examples of cavernous hemangioma of the rectum. (A) Plain film of the pelvis reveals a soft tissue mass with foci of calcification in abnormal vascular channels. This appearance of pelvic phleboliths in a child is pathognomonic for a cavernous hemangioma. (B) A barium enema film shows the characteristic phlebolith pattern outside the colon, with scalloping of the bowel lumen caused by pressure from the vascular lesion.

In the colon, they may be small and resemble AEs or they may involve a long segment of bowel. The most extensive AVMs typically are in the rectum and sigmoid. Histologically, AVMs are persistent congenital communications between arteries and veins located primarily in the submucosa. Characteristically, there is "arterialization" of the veins (i.e., tortuosity, dilatation, and thick walls with smooth muscle hypertrophy and intimal thickening or sclerosis). In long-standing AVMs, the arteries are dilated and exhibit atrophic and sclerotic degeneration. Angiography is the primary means of diagnosis (Fig. 36.14). Early-filling veins in small lesions and extensive dilatation of arteries or veins in large lesions are typical. Patients with significant bleeding from large AVMs should undergo a resection of the involved segment; transendoscopic therapy may be beneficial for smaller lesions.

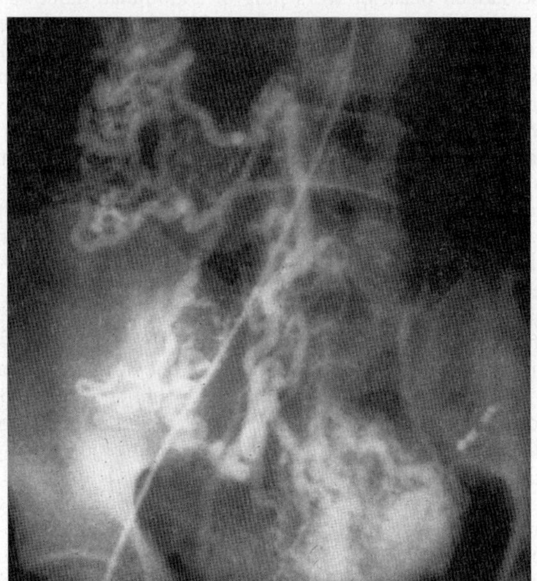

Fig. 36.14 Mesenteric angiogram in a patient who presented with recurrent LGIB. The angiogram shows a complex, racemose configuration of vessels in a large congenital arteriovenous malformation involving the superior and inferior mesenteric arterial circulations.

ANEURYSMS

Abdominal Aortic Aneurysm

Approximately 95% of abdominal aortic aneurysms (AAA) are atherosclerotic in origin, although genetic predisposition is also an important factor; less common causes include trauma, vasculitis, infection, and congenital abnormalities. Risk factors associated with the development of an AAA include age older than 60 years, male gender, white race, smoking, and hypertension. Population-based studies in adults older than 50 years have found that the prevalence of AAA is 3.9%−7.2% in men and 1.0%−1.3% in women.[71] Familial clustering of AAA has been noted in 15%−20% of cases, and, in some families, an abnormality has been identified in chromosome 16[72]; defects in procollagen III in patients with Ehlers-Danlos syndrome type IV and altered gene expression causing abnormalities of the elastin and collagen content of AAA have been shown in other families.[72] The two genes with the strongest supporting evidence to date of contribution to the genetic risk for AAA are the *CDKN2BAS* gene, also known as *ANRIL*, which encodes an antisense RNA that regulates expression of the cyclin-dependent kinase inhibitors CDKN2A and CDKN2B; and *DAB2IP*, which encodes an inhibitor of cell growth and survival.[73]

Most AAAs are asymptomatic until rupture and are incidentally detected on abdominal US, CT, or MRI performed for other indications; as a result, current guidelines support screening with "one-time" abdominal US in men between the ages of 65 and 74 years who have a history of smoking.[71] The most common symptom of AAA is epigastric pain, often radiating through to the back; severe pain may presage rupture. On physical examination, a pulsatile epigastric mass may be palpable. Distinguishing an aneurysm from an overlying abdominal mass with transmitted pulsations may be difficult on physical examination and is best done by imaging studies. A bruit may be present, but unless recent in onset, is usually of no diagnostic help.[71]

Abdominal plain films may show a soft tissue mass with peripheral calcification in the region of the abdominal aorta. With large aneurysms, the erosion of the lumbar vertebrae or displacement of surrounding viscera, including bowel, kidneys, and ureters, may be seen. Because plain film studies are not sufficiently sensitive to establish the presence or size of an aneurysm, US, CT, and MRI have become the standard means of evaluation. US is the imaging screening modality of choice for AAA because it is highly sensitive (95%–100%) and specific (100%) and relatively inexpensive. Additionally, US is the preferred test for serial monitoring of an AAA to detect changes in its size.[71] CT and MRI are used preoperatively to demonstrate aortic and vascular anatomy and to help tailor stent grafts. Preoperative angiography is not used as frequently as in the past and is most appropriate in patients with evidence of peripheral vascular disease, severe hypertension, symptoms of chronic mesenteric ischemia (see Chapter 120), if thoracic or iliac artery involvement is suspected, and in cases of horseshoe or pelvic kidneys to demonstrate renal artery anatomy. Angiography is not used to estimate the size of the aneurysm because intraluminal laminated thrombus limits the delineation of the entire lumen and, more importantly, simpler, less invasive, and less expensive imaging modalities are now readily available.

The major complication of AAA is rupture, which is heralded by the sudden onset or worsening of abdominal, flank, or back pain; an insidious presentation characterized by several weeks of pain can occur when "leakage" precedes overt rupture. Pain may be exacerbated by lying recumbent and relieved by sitting or leaning forward. Severe abdominal pain also may be seen with aortic dissection as the splanchnic vessels become compromised and acute intestinal ischemia develops. The consensus among vascular surgeons is that the most important predictor of AAA rupture is the size of the aneurysm. The annual risk for rupture is nearly 0% for AAAs between 3.0 and 3.9 cm in diameter, 1% for those between 4.0 and 4.9 cm in diameter, and 11% for those between 5.00 and 5.99 cm in diameter.[71] Risk factors associated with rupture include hypertension and the presence of chronic obstructive pulmonary disease. AAA most commonly ruptures into the retroperitoneal tissues that surround the aorta. Less commonly, the aneurysm may communicate with the peritoneal cavity, in which case hemorrhagic shock develops rapidly. Aneurysmal rupture into the small intestine usually occurs in the third or fourth portion of the duodenum and typically presents as massive GI bleeding; intermittent bleeding can occur with clot formation and subsequent dislodgement from the eroded bowel or fistulous opening. Indeed, many of these patients will have a "herald bleed" followed by massive hemorrhage several hours or days later.[74] Endoscopy is the most sensitive method for diagnosing this complication. Rarely, AAA ruptures into the inferior vena cava; if so, a loud bruit can be heard.

Asymptomatic patients with an AAA larger than 5.5 cm or symptomatic patients with aneurysms of any size should undergo surgical repair to prevent rupture. Surveillance ultrasound examination is recommended to assess for interval change of AAAs every 3 years for aneurysms of 3.0–3.9 cm, annually for those of 4.0–4.9 cm, and every 6 months for aneurysms larger than 5 cm.[174] The growth rate of AAAs is variable and has been less in recent studies than in older ones. In a large population of patients with small aneurysms (average initial size of 4 cm) studied over an average of 3.3 years, 58.4% of patients had no change or a decrease in aneurysm size, 25.3% had an expansion between 0.1 and 0.25 cm, 12.6% had an increase of greater than 0.25 cm, and only 3.7% had an enlargement of greater than 0.5 cm.[72] On average, the growth rate of an AAA is 0.35 cm per year.

Operative repair of an AAA includes an open approach either retroperitoneally or transabdominally, or an endovascular repair, which involves insertion of an endograft into the vascular lumen to exclude the aneurysm from blood flow, thus minimizing the risk of rupture. In elective cases, preoperative angiography is useful to demonstrate additional vascular disease (e.g., stenosis or occlusion of the splanchnic arteries) and allows for planned vascular reconstruction, which may help avoid postoperative bowel ischemia. The mortality of AAA repair in good-risk patients is 1%–4%[74]; mortality increases sharply to 34%–85% when surgery is done as an emergency for rupture or impending rupture.[75] Endovascular aneurysm repair (EVAR) is being used as an alternative to open repair of an AAA for most cases in the United States. EVAR may provide selective short-term advantages over open surgery, such as avoidance of general anesthesia, reduced operative time, reduced blood loss, and less postoperative pain. A meta-analysis of four major trials published in 2018 revealed an early survival advantage in the EVAR group compared with the open repair group, but this was lost within 3 years, and aneurysm-related mortality was higher in the EVAR group, mostly because of secondary rupture or reinterventions; there was no difference in total morality between groups.[175] Current recommendations support open repair of an AAA in patients who are at low- or average-risk for operative complications and EVAR in those who at high risk for complications.[76–78] EVAR also should be considered in patients who are not at high surgical risk, although evidence supporting benefit in this group is not well established.[76]

Splanchnic Artery Aneurysms

The prevalence of splanchnic artery aneurysms (SAAs) has been estimated to be up to 10% based on autopsy reports, although the natural history of SAAs is not well understood.[79,80] SAAs are usually asymptomatic and detected incidentally on imaging studies. In a retrospective review from Yale New Haven Medical Center, 138 SAAs in 122 patients were documented on imaging studies and their annual growth rate and risk of rupture assessed. The growth rate of SAAs was slow (0.064 ± 0.18 cm/year), and the smallest aneurysm rupture was seen at 2.3 cm; hence the recommendation to observe asymptomatic patients with SAAs less than 2.5 cm.[80,176] When symptomatic, SAAs can present with abdominal pain or GI bleeding. On physical exam, a bruit may be heard on auscultation, but an abdominal mass is rarely palpable because the aneurysms are small. Up to 25% of SAAs may be complicated by rupture that has an estimated mortality rate of 25%–70%.[81] Like aneurysms of the aorta, if a SAA erodes into the GI lumen, this can present with sporadic GI bleeding, the so-called herald bleed. Rupture into a mesenteric vein can result in an AV fistula and can lead to portal hypertension with variceal bleeding. If an SAA is sufficiently calcified, it may be seen on plain films of the abdomen, but the diagnosis is usually made with CT, MRI, or splanchnic angiography, which has the added benefit of a potential therapeutic intervention. Treatment depends on the presentation, location, and size of the aneurysm. In general, treatment is considered if the diameter of the aneurysm is greater than 2 cm even if asymptomatic. Treatment options include embolization, surgical repair, or endovascular stenting.[80] Embolization may be preferred for aneurysms difficult to manage surgically and for high-risk patients.

Splenic Artery Aneurysms

Splenic artery aneurysms are usually saccular, and 20% of patients have multiple aneurysms. Symptoms if present are left upper quadrant or epigastric pain that may radiate to the left shoulder. The common causes are atherosclerosis and portal hypertension, whereas less common causes include splenic arterial dissection, septic emboli, hypertension, polyarteritis nodosa, SLE, Ehlers-Danlos syndrome, fibromuscular dysplasia, and neurofibromatosis. There is a female to male predominance of 3–4:1, and it is associated with pregnancy.[79–82] The increased prevalence in pregnant women may be related to an increase in splenic blood flow and the effects of estrogen on the elastic tissue of the tunica media, which can result in dilatation of the splenic artery and predispose to aneurysm formation. Similarly, increased splenic blood flow is considered the cause of splenic artery aneurysms in portal hypertension. Aneurysmal rupture occurs in less than 2% of patients except for in pregnant women in whom the risk of rupture is much higher. More than 95% of aneurysms in pregnant woman are diagnosed after rupture and are associated with a 75% maternal and 95% fetal mortality rate.[79] If the aneurysm ruptures into the lesser sac, the patient can remain hemodynamically stable, but once the blood overflows into the greater intraperitoneal sac through the foramen of Winslow, diffuse abdominal pain and hypovolemic shock will develop; this is the "double-rupture" phenomenon. It is said that the period in which the bleeding is localized in the lesser sac allows time for surgical intervention in about 25% of patients.[79] Treatment options for splenic artery aneurysms depend on the location as well as its presentation. Ruptured aneurysms are usually treated with splenectomy. Mortality after emergency surgery is as high as 40%, compared with a very low mortality rate after elective repair. A symptomatic aneurysm or an aneurysm of any size in a pregnant woman or a woman planning to get pregnant should undergo repair before pregnancy. If the location of the aneurysm is proximal and it is larger than 2 cm, surgical management should be considered and would include resection and an end to end vascular repair; if the location is distal or involves the hilum, splenectomy is recommended. Aneurysms between 1 and 2 cm should be monitored with imaging. If surgery is not an option, embolization may be performed. For patients with portal hypertension, embolization is preferred because the extensive collateral circulation makes surgery more difficult. Complications of embolization include splenic infarction and reperfusion of the aneurysm which can occur in 5%–20% of patients. Yearly follow-up imaging with CT or MRI is recommended to evaluate for leak and subsequent growth.[79,81]

Celiac Artery Aneurysms

Historically, the most frequent cause of celiac artery aneurysms was infection due to either syphilis or tuberculosis, and most cases were diagnosed at autopsy after an aneurysm ruptured. Now that syphilis and tuberculosis are more readily identified and treated, the more common causes of CA aneurysm are atherosclerosis, trauma, dissection, and Takayasu arteritis.[79,81] Association with other aneurysms is common and in one series occurred in 66% of patients.[82] CA aneurysms are usually asymptomatic. Symptoms, when present, can mimic pancreatitis due to location. The lifetime risk of rupture is about 6%. CA aneurysms greater than 2.5 cm should be considered for repair, whereas asymptomatic lesions less than that size can be followed with imaging.[81] Traditional open repair can be performed through a transabdominal route or thoracolumbar approach. Ligation can be performed followed by aortohepatic bypass or direct aortic reimplantation. In patients undergoing revascularization, prosthetic grafts have a lower risk of occlusion than saphenous vein grafts but are difficult to place due to its location. If the aneurysm ruptures, intervention may include ligation or percutaneous transcatheter embolization.[79]

Superior Mesenteric Artery Aneurysms

Superior mesenteric artery (SMA) aneurysms are rare. They usually involve the proximal 5 cm of the SMA. Aneurysm-related thrombus or dissection can occur, which can cause symptoms of intestinal ischemia. Historically, the most common etiology was infectious, with septic emboli accounting for a third of all SMA aneurysms. In recent series, the common causes include atherosclerosis, polyarteritis nodosa, pancreatitis, biliary tract disease, neurofibromatosis, and trauma.[82] More than 90% of SMA aneurysms are symptomatic with associated abdominal pain and GI bleeding. Up to 50% of the patients present with rupture and a mortality rate of 30%. β-Adrenergic blockers can have a protective effect against rupture.[79] Intervention is recommended for all symptomatic patients and for all patients at low surgical risk because of the high rate of complications. Although earlier recommendations were to follow asymptomatic SMA aneurysms smaller than 2.5 cm with CT imaging, the Society for Vascular Surgery Clinic Practice Guidelines currently recommends repair of all true SMA aneurysms regardless of size[81,177] The surgical approach includes aneurysmectomy and either interposition vein grafting or ligation of a branch of a mesenteric artery to treat the aneurysm. In addition, resection of any ischemic segment of bowel is performed. Transcatheter embolization and endovascular stenting can be used as well but the latter may increase the risk of mesenteric ischemia if the branches of the SMA are blocked by the stent. β-Adrenergic blockers should be used for individuals who are reluctant to undergo interventional procedures.[79,81]

Mycotic Aneurysm

Mycotic aneurysms of the aorta and splanchnic vessels are rare. They were so named by Sir William Osler because their appearance reminded him of fungi (*mykes*, fungus). In the past, mycotic aneurysms were most commonly caused by septic emboli from bacterial endocarditis. Today, the main risk factor is IV drug use. Other important risk factors include contiguous spread from adjacent infectious processes, arterial manipulation, and immunocompromise (e.g., alcoholism, diabetes mellitus, chemotherapy, treatment with glucocorticoids). *Salmonella* (especially *Salmonella choleraesuis*) and *Staphylococcus* are the most common infecting organisms. The CA is most often affected, followed by the SMA and IMA. Early in the course, symptoms of mycotic aneurysms are nonspecific; fever, chills, and abdominal pain typically occur later. Diagnosis is by imaging the vasculature: mycotic aneurysms typically are lobulated and saccular (Fig. 36.15). The destructive process can develop quickly, leading to rapid expansion and rupture. Treatment is typically surgical, usually with the resection of the aneurysm and vascular reconstruction followed by IV antibiotics for 6 weeks. A multicenter European study showed that endovascular treatment is a feasible option, and for most patients a durable treatment option, but carries a higher risk of late secondary infections.[178] Life-long suppressive oral antibiotic therapy also has been used to prevent prosthetic graft infection.[83,84]

PARAPROSTHETIC-ENTERIC AND AORTOENTERIC FISTULAS

An uncommon but potentially catastrophic complication of aortic aneurysmectomy and other procedures in which vascular prostheses are placed in the retroperitoneum or abdomen is the formation of a fistula between the graft and the adjacent bowel, usually the third or fourth portion of the duodenum because of its proximity to the infrarenal abdominal aorta (Fig. 36.16).[85] This complication is known as a secondary aortoenteric fistula, and its frequency ranges between 0.36% and 2%.[86] The reported mean

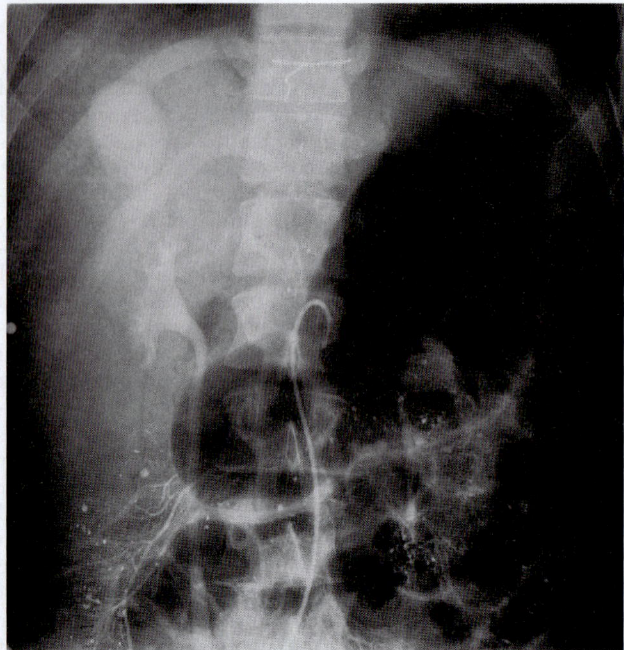

Fig. 36.15 Splanchnic angiogram of a patient with a large mycotic aneurysm of the hepatic artery. (Courtesy Dr. Lawrence J. Brandt, Bronx, NY.)

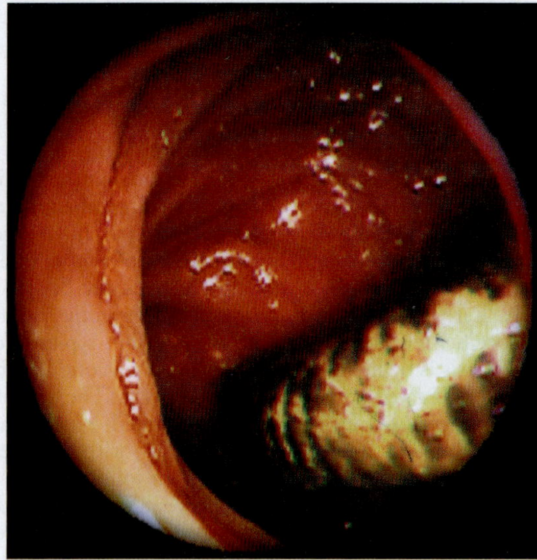

Fig. 36.16 The endoscopic view of the third portion of the duodenum, where part of an aortic graft is seen. Patients with aortoenteric fistulas typically present with GI bleeding, abdominal pain, and fever because the graft usually has become infected by the time it erodes into the GI tract. (Courtesy, Dr. Lawrence J. Brandt, Bronx, NY.)

interval between aortic surgery and the development of a secondary aortoenteric fistula is 44 months, but such fistulas have been reported as early as 21 days and as late as 14 years postoperatively; fistulas develop sooner, at a mean interval of 22 months, when concomitant intra-abdominal infections are present.[86] Secondary aortoenteric fistulas are thought to result from local conditions at the time of, or subsequent to, graft placement, including infection, damage to the duodenum or its blood supply during the dissection, and subsequent erosion of the duodenal wall by the graft. Newer surgical techniques, including the use of endovascular grafts, nonabsorbable sutures, antibiotics, strict hemostasis, and coverage of suture lines with retroperitoneal tissue and peritoneum, may reduce the frequency of fistula formation. Primary aortoenteric fistulas develop in the absence of prior aneurysm repair and are associated with atherosclerosis, infection (most commonly *Salmonella* spp. and *Klebsiella* spp.; other organisms that are less common include *Staphylococcus* spp., *Streptococcus* spp., *Escherichia coli*, *Enterococcus faecalis*, *Clostridium septicum*, and *Lactobacillus*), malignancy, radiotherapy, trauma, and foreign body. Primary aortoenteric fistulas are less common than secondary aortoenteric fistulas, with an incidence of 0.04% –0.07%.[87]

Patients with aortoenteric fistulas present with upper or LGIB that if untreated may be massive and rapidly fatal. EGD combined with CT imaging is used to exclude other diagnoses and plan management.[88] To make the diagnosis, a high index of suspicion is required—typically in a patient who has had aortoiliac graft surgery and presents with GI bleeding, and prompt diagnosis and expedient surgical repair are essential for survival. CT angiography is useful to diagnose secondary aortoenteric fistula. Findings suggesting infection include periaortic gas, effacement of the periaortic or perigraft fat plane and the fat plane between the aorta and bowel, perigraft soft tissue thickening and/or fluid, perigraft hematoma, and pseudoaneurysm or aneurysm bulge. These findings, however, also can be seen in graft infection or inflammation without AEF.[179]

VASCULAR LESIONS ASSOCIATED WITH SYSTEMIC DISORDERS OR MANIFESTATIONS

Hereditary Hemorrhagic Telangiectasia

This autosomal dominant familial disorder, also known as Osler-Weber-Rendu disease, is characterized by telangiectasia of the skin and mucous membranes, as well as recurrent GI bleeding.[89–91] In some patients, the pathogenesis follows mutations of the endoglin (*ENG*) and activin receptor-like kinase-1 (*ALK-1*) genes, which have an important role in determining the properties of endothelial cells during angiogenesis.[92] Lesions typically are noticed in the first few years of life, and recurrent epistaxis in childhood is characteristic. By age 10, about half of patients have had some GI bleeding. Severe hemorrhage is unusual before the fourth decade and has a peak incidence in the sixth decade. In most patients, bleeding presents as melena; BRBPR and hematemesis are less frequent. Hematochezia in a patient with HHT suggests bleeding from a source other than telangiectasia. Bleeding is intermittent and chronic and may be severe; patients may receive more than 60 transfusions in a lifetime. A family history of the disease has been reported in 80% of patients with HHT but is less common in those who bleed later in life. Telangiectasias usually are present on the lips, oral and nasopharyngeal membranes, tongue, and periungual areas; lack of involvement of these sites casts suspicion on the diagnosis (Fig. 36.17).

The diagnosis of HHT currently requires the presence of at least three of four relevant clinical criteria. These so-called Curaçao criteria include epistaxis (spontaneous and recurrent nosebleeds); telangiectasias (multiple lesions at characteristic sites, e.g., lips, oral cavity, fingers, nose); visceral lesions (e.g., pulmonary, hepatic, cerebral, spinal, GI); and a positive family history (a first-degree relative with HHT)[93]; clinical diagnosis can be confirmed by molecular genetic analysis. In most cases, HHT is caused by mutations in one of the two known HHT genes. Mutations of the *ENG* gene lead to type 1 HHT.[94] The *ENG* gene is located on chromosome 9 and encodes for endoglin, a type III transforming growth factor-β (TGF-β) receptor. Mutations of the *activin* gene lead to type 2 HHT. People

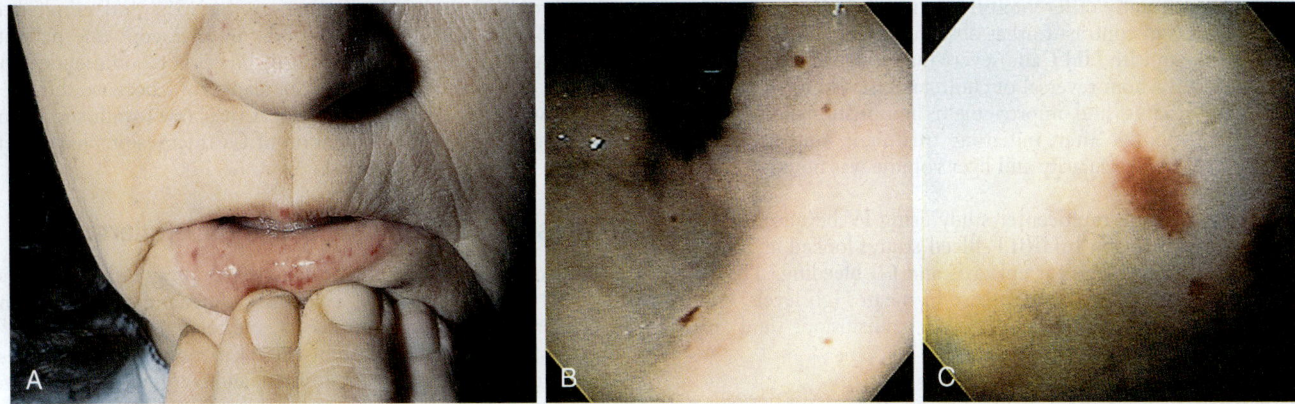

Fig. 36.17 Telangiectasias of HHT. (A) Multiple telangiectasias on the nose and lips. Telangiectasias of varying size and shape in the proximal gastric body (B), antrum (C). (From Wilcox CM. *Atlas of Clinical Gastrointestinal Endoscopy*. Philadelphia: WB Saunders; 1995:123.)

with type 1 HHT tend to develop symptoms earlier than those with type 2 HHT and are more likely to have blood vessel malformations in the lungs and brain; liver involvement with portal hypertension is more common in patients with type 2 HHT. The *activin* gene is located on chromosome 12 and encodes for the ACVRL1 protein, a type I TGF-β receptor.[91] Both receptors are expressed predominantly on vascular endothelium and play essential roles in maintaining vascular integrity. Evidence for the existence of two other as yet unidentified HHT genes has been reported.[95,96] Mutation of the *SMAD4* gene (involved in the TGF-β signaling cascade), which is known to cause juvenile polyposis, also has been reported in a few patients with HHT[97,98]; these patients have an overlap syndrome of juvenile polyposis and HHT and, therefore, are at significant risk for colorectal cancer (CRC), which necessitates aggressive CRC screening.[97] Despite genotypic heterogeneity in HHT, clinical expression of the different HHT genotypes appears similar. HHT and nonhereditary intestinal AE are both characterized by increased production of VEGF. High serum levels of VEGF, which also correlate with a severity of bleeding, are found in patients with HHT.[99,100] Vascular involvement of the liver is common in HHT, especially type 2, and frequently is asymptomatic. Hepatic manifestations during the course of the disease are seen in 8%–31% of patients and include high-output heart failure resulting from AV shunting, portal hypertension, and biliary tract disease.[101,102] Expert panelists from the Second International Guidelines for the Diagnosis and Management of HHT recommend offering screening by ultrasonography to patients with definite or suspected HHT for liver vascular malformations.[180] Liver involvement is associated with complications, including liver failure necessitating liver transplantation, and significant morbidity and mortality.[103] In one study that followed patients with HHT and known hepatic vascular malformations for a median of 44 months, 5.2% of patients died and 25.3% experienced complications, including high-output heart failure, atrial fibrillation, portal hypertension, and GI bleeding. Complete response was achieved in 63% with the implementation of multidisciplinary therapy that included supportive care, medical treatment of high-output heart failure and portal hypertension, and RFA in those who developed atrial fibrillation, transarterial embolization of hepatic vascular malformations, and orthotopic liver transplantation.[103]

Telangiectasias in patients with HHT also occur in the colon but are more common in the stomach and small intestine, where they are more apt to cause major bleeding. Telangiectasias are seen easily on endoscopy, although in the presence of severe anemia, blood loss, or hypotension, they transiently may become less obvious or even invisible; after correction of blood volume and blood pressure, they once again become more prominent. Evaluation by conventional angiography or newer techniques, such as helical CTA[104,105] and MRA, may be unrevealing or demonstrate heterogeneous enhancement of hepatic parenchyma, dilated and tortuous intrahepatic arterial branches, conglomerate masses of abnormal vessels, aneurysms, AV communications, phlebectasia, and hepatic artery and portal vein enlargement.[105,106] Angiography may be misleading when it demonstrates multiple vascular abnormalities because some of these lesions may be in the mesentery rather than in the intestine and are not potential sites of GI blood loss.

Grossly, the telangiectasias of HHT are the size of millet seeds and typically appear as cherry red, smooth hillocks. Pathologically, the major changes involve the capillaries and venules, but arterioles also may be affected. Lesions consist of irregular, ectatic, tortuous blood spaces lined by a delicate single layer of endothelial cells and supported by a fine layer of fibrous connective tissue. No elastic lamina or muscular tissue is present in these vessels, so they cannot contract; this property may explain why telangiectasias tend to bleed. Arterioles show intimal proliferation and commonly have thrombi in them, suggesting vascular stasis. In contrast to the thinned venules of AEs, venules are abnormally thick in HHT; have prominent, well-developed longitudinal muscles; and are thought to play a major role regulating blood flow within the telangiectasia.[104]

Many forms of treatment have been recommended for telangiectasias, including estrogens,[107] aminocaproic acid,[108] tranexamic acid,[181] endoscopic thermal ablation,[6,46] and resection of involved bowel. Success of endoscopic ablation, including APC and thermal contact devices, is most promising when lesions are within reach of the endoscope and not diffusely distributed along the length of the small intestine. The availability of SBE and DBE, however, extends the range of endoscopic therapy to the entire GI tract. Endoscopic therapy may be performed during active bleeding or between bleeding episodes and has reduced the need for emergency bowel resection. Long-term follow-up studies are necessary to evaluate the ultimate efficacy of the various forms of therapy. Repeated sessions are not recommended unless necessary to maintain an acceptable Hgb level.

In suspected or proven SMAD4-HHT, screening colonoscopy is recommended starting at age 15 with repeat examinations every 3 years if no colon polyps are found or every year along with EGD if colon polyps are found.[180]

Bevacizumab was used in a study of 25 patients with HHT and associated severe hepatic vascular malformations with high cardiac output; it resulted in decreased cardiac output and a reduction in epistaxis; however, liver vascularity, liver volume, and liver tests were not significantly different at the 6-month follow-up.[109] This experience was in contrast to that observed in one report of a 47-year-old woman with HHT and severe liver involvement treated 4 years earlier in whom reversal of cholestasis, resolution of cardiac failure, and ascites, and improvement in nutritional status was observed 3 months after initiating treatment, and a marked reduction in liver vascularity and liver volume was noted over a 6-month interval.[110–113]

An international, multicenter study using IV bevacizumab for bleeding in HHT (the InHIBIT-Bleed study) looked at 238 patients receiving the drug for epistaxis and GI bleeding. The majority of patients showed an increase in mean Hgb levels, and a decreased need for red blood cell transfusion, and iron infusions.[182]

Blue Rubber Bleb Nevus Syndrome

In 1860 an association of cutaneous vascular nevi, intestinal lesions, and GI bleeding was described, and almost a century later this constellation of findings was named *blue rubber bleb nevus syndrome* (BRBNS) by Bean to distinguish it from other cutaneous vascular lesions (Fig. 36.18). Other sites in addition to the GI tract may be affected, including the eyes, nasopharynx, parotid glands, lungs, liver, spleen, heart, brain, skeletal muscles, urinary bladder, and penis. Orthopedic abnormalities may be present, and calcification, thrombosis, and consumptive coagulopathy (with thrombocytopenia) may occur within the lesions.[114] A familial history is infrequent, although a few cases of autosomal dominant transmission have been reported,[115] and one analysis has identified a responsible locus on chromosome 9. A recent study hypothesized that BRBNS may be due to somatic mutations in *TEK*, the gene encoding TIE2, which is the endothelial cell tyrosine kinase receptor for the angiopoietins. This study found that *TEK* mutations were present in 15 of 17 individuals with BRBNS, supporting the hypothesis that these genetic mutations was the cause of the cutaneous and mucosal venous malformations.[116]

The lesions are distinctive: they are blue and raised and vary from 0.1 to 5 cm in diameter. Characteristically, the contained blood can be emptied by direct pressure, leaving a "wrinkled sac" remaining until it fills again. Lesions may be single or numerous and are usually found on the trunk, extremities, and face. They may involve any portion of the GI tract but are most common in the small bowel. In the colon they are more common distally. They are detected infrequently by barium or angiographic studies and are seen better with CT and MRI. Endoscopy is the most important diagnostic test for this syndrome but VCE has also been used.[117] Originally the lesions were thought to be hemangiomas, but they are now considered to be venous malformations. A prospective study in 2021 looked at the use of sirolimus in 11 pediatric and adult patients with BRBNS.[183] Sirolimus reduced the size of the venous malformations by 13% and eliminated transfusion dependence at 12 months in all except one patient. Resection of the involved segment of bowel is recommended for recurrent hemorrhage. APC may be dangerous because these lesions may involve the full thickness of the bowel wall; successful sclerotherapy and the band ligation of GI tract lesions have been reported.

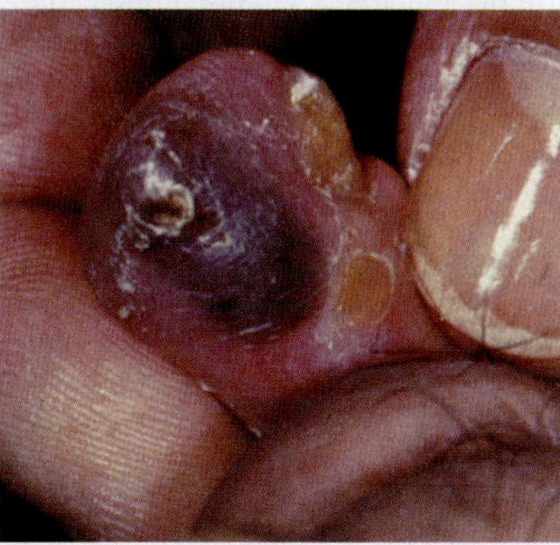

Fig. 36.18 Fingertip lesion in a patient with the blue rubber bleb nevus syndrome.

Progressive Systemic Sclerosis (Scleroderma)

Telangiectasia is a prominent feature of progressive systemic sclerosis, especially in the calcinosis, Raynaud phenomenon, esophageal dysmotility, scleroderma, and telangiectasia variant.[118] Sites most frequently involved by these lesions are the hands, lips, tongue, and face, but gastric, intestinal, and colorectal lesions have been reported. These tiny lesions may be the source of occult or clinically significant bleeding and are best treated, if possible, by endoscopic thermal ablation.[119]

PIK3CA-related Overgrowth Spectrum

In its initial description, the Klippel-Trénaunay syndrome (KTS) consisted of (1) a vascular nevus that involved the lower limb; (2) varicose veins that were limited to the affected side and appeared at birth or in childhood; and (3) hypertrophy of all tissues of the involved limb, especially the bones.[120] In 2018, KTS was grouped under PIK3CA-related Overgrowth Spectrum (PROS) by the International Society for the Study of Vascular Anomalies. KTS is now believed to harbor somatic heterozygous gain-of-function mutations in the phosphatidylinositol-4,5-bisphospate 3-kinase (PIK3CA) gene in a mosaic pattern, which may or may not include vascular anomalies.[184] This overgrowth spectrum includes KTS; Fibroadipose Hyperplasia or Overgrowth; Hemi-Hyperplasia Multiple Lipomatosis; Congenital Lipomatous Overgrowth, Vascular malformations, Epidermal nevi, Scoliosis/skeletal and spinal syndrome (CLOVES); macrodactyly; fibroadipose-infiltrating lipomatosis/facial-infiltrative lipomatosis; Megalencephaly-CAPillary malformation and Dysplastic MEGalencephaly. For the purposes of this chapter, we will focus on KTS as well as Parkes-Weber syndrome, which is not considered a PROS.

Klippel-Trénaunay and Parkes Weber; the former is a pure low-flow condition, whereas the latter is characterized by higher flow AV fistulas. Several genetic defects in the regulation of the angiogenic factor VG5Q have been shown in patients with KTS.[121] The cause of bony elongation is controversial, but one theory invokes in utero venous hypertension and stasis.[120] Edema of the involved leg is common, and if the thigh is involved (Fig. 36.19A), a variety of lymphatic abnormalities are usually present (e.g., chylous mesenteric cysts, chyloperitoneum, protein-losing enteropathy; see Chapter 31).

Visceral lesions have been described involving the GI tract, liver, spleen, bladder, kidney, lung, heart, and genital organs (see Fig. 36.19B). Involvement of the GI tract is more common than previously thought and may occur in as many as 20% of patients, some of whom may not be recognized to have visceral involvement because they are asymptomatic. GI bleeding is the major symptom of visceral GI involvement and initially is intermittent, beginning in the first decade of life; subsequently GI bleeding from KTS may vary from occult to massive.[122] In the largest series, the most common GI symptom was hematochezia, although reported by only 6 of 588 patients.[120] The most common bleeding sites in the GI tract are the distal colon and rectum, and involvement of the whole GI tract is uncommon.[122] GI bleeding usually is caused by a rectal vascular lesion, localized rectovaginal varices resulting from the obstruction of the internal iliac system, or portal hypertension with varices (see Fig. 36.19C). Bleeding may be intensified by consumption coagulopathy, which may

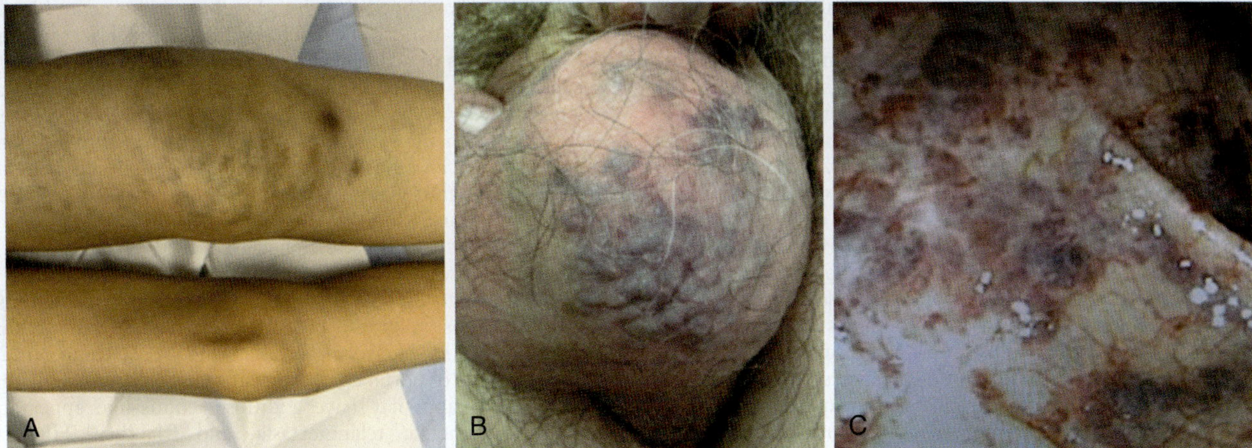

Fig. 36.19 Images of Klippel-Trénaunay syndrome. (A) Edema of the involved leg and associated vascular lesions are seen. (B) Involvement of the scrotum in another patient. (C) Endoscopic image of the same patient in part (B) showing an example of extensive rectal vascular lesions that can be a cause of GI bleeding. (Courtesy, Dr. Lawrence J. Brandt, Bronx, NY.)

occur within the smaller sinusoids of the vascular lesion. Physical examination is diagnostic, but various imaging techniques are used to define the anatomy and plan surgical repair.[123] MRA is used for diagnosis and to detect AV shunting[124]; angiography remains the gold standard and may allow for therapeutic intervention.[122] Endoscopic thermal ablation therapy is useful in controlling hemorrhage and preventing or minimizing recurrent GI bleeding, especially when the lesions are relatively well localized (L. Brandt, personal experience); however, patients with clinically significant hemorrhage often require surgical resection.[122]

In 2016 Adams et al. published the first prospective trial of children and young adults using sirolimus for complicated vascular anomalies such as Generalized Lymphatic Anomaly and Kaposiform-lymphangiomatosis. Although GI bleeding was not an end point of the study, they showed an improvement in the quality of life and function.[185]

Radiation-Induced Mucosal Injury

Radiation injury can induce a progressive obliterative endarteritis and endothelial proliferation leading to neovascularization and telangiectasia formation that may bleed.[125] As discussed in Chapter 39, radiation injury can occur anywhere in the GI tract but is most commonly described in the rectosigmoid as a result of pelvic radiation for prostate and cervical cancers.[126,127]

GAVE (Watermelon Stomach) and Portal Hypertensive Gastropathy, Enteropathy, and Colopathy

GAVE

GAVE (watermelon stomach) describes a vascular lesion of the gastric antrum that consists of tortuous, dilated vessels radiating outward from the pylorus like the spokes of a wheel and resembling the dark stripes on the surface of a watermelon.[128] This lesion may cause acute hemorrhage, chronic occult bleeding, or both. Its cause is unknown, although it has been proposed that gastric peristalsis causes prolapse of the loose antral mucosa with consequent elongation of the mucosal vessels (Fig. 36.20).[128,129] GAVE also has been postulated to result from delayed gastric emptying, as well as from hypergastrinemia, prostaglandin E_2, 5-hydroxytryptamine (serotonin), and vasoactive intestinal polypeptide.

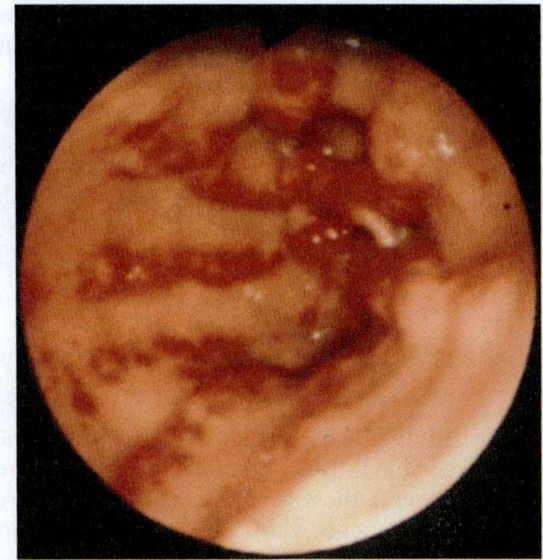

Fig. 36.20 Endoscopic appearance of GAVE, also referred to as "watermelon stomach."

GAVE is seen particularly in middle-aged or older women and in association with achlorhydria/atrophic gastritis, cirrhosis and portal hypertension, chronic kidney disease, cardiac diseases, autoimmune and connective tissue disorders, as well as after bone marrow transplantation.[118,130,131] The association with cirrhosis and portal hypertension is seen in approximately 40% of reported cases of GAVE; thus GAVE may be caused by portal hypertension or hepatic veno-occlusive disease,[132] although GAVE may not respond to therapies directed at reducing portal pressure. Given case reports of GAVE resolution after liver transplantation, however, it is possible that hepatic insufficiency may play a role in its pathophysiology.[133] Although not pathognomonic, microscopic features of GAVE include mucosal capillary ectasia and congestion, focal thrombosis, spindle cell proliferation (smooth muscle cell and myofibroblast hyperplasia), and fibrohyalinosis that surrounds the ectatic capillaries of the lamina propria.[131] Some researchers believe that GAVE and portal hypertensive gastropathy (PHG) are different manifestations of the same pathogenetic process, but the literature suggests that these are distinct entities[134] and distinguishing them is important to implement appropriate therapeutic intervention.[131]

Limited pharmacotherapy options are available for treating GAVE. Estrogen-progesterone has been tried[135] and appears to have some efficacy. Successful use of tranexamic acid, an antifibrinolytic agent,[136,137] and thalidomide[138] also have been reported. In a randomized controlled trial, thalidomide was found to markedly reduce recurrent bleeding in patients with GAVE and other GI angiodysplasia.[139] In a small study of 21 patients, which included subjects with GAVE and small bowel AE, IV bevacizumab was shown to reduce the need for endoscopic intervention and RBC transfusions 1 year after treatment.[170] TIPS does not appear to be effective for GAVE in the absence of portal hypertension.[140] Antrectomy has been a last resort for patients in whom pharmacologic and endoscopic therapies have failed.[141]

Transendoscopic therapy is the current mainstay of management for GAVE. Multiple studies have shown that APC improves anemia and decreases transfusion requirement, particularly in cirrhotic patients; side effects are minimal, although multiple treatments are usually needed. An analysis of 10 studies by Mohan et al., in 2021, looked at endoscopic band ligation for GAVE. The pooled rate of treatment responders was 81%. Recurrence was 15.4% with a mean number of endoscopic banding treatment sessions of 2.4.[186] Other therapies that can be considered if APC is not available include RFA, cryotherapy, and the use of cyanoacrylate spray.[142] Portal hypertension in a patient with GAVE and GI bleeding makes the bleeding more difficult to manage because bleeding is usually greater and more resistant to treatment in this situation.[143] Several case reports have a detailed reversal of GAVE after liver transplantation.[144] However, the data are insufficient to recommend this therapy unless the patient is otherwise a liver transplant candidate. TIPS offers another modality when GAVE is associated with portal hypertension or when bleeding resulting from GAVE associated with PHG cannot controlled endoscopically (see also Chapters 21 and 94).

Portal Hypertensive Gastropathy (PHG), Enteropathy, and Colopathy

The prevalence of PHG in patients with cirrhosis varies from 20% to 98%, likely due to lack of uniform diagnostic criteria and classification; in general, there is an association with more severe portal hypertension. Patients with PHG can be asymptomatic or exhibit symptoms related to chronic GI bleeding, which has been reported to occur in 3%−60% of patients. Acute GI bleeding is less common, with a prevalence reported between 2% and 12%.[145] PHG manifests three endoscopic patterns: (1) the fine red speckling of the mucosa; (2) superficial reddening, especially at the tips of the gastric rugae; and, most commonly, (3) the presence of a mosaic pattern with red spots (snakeskin appearance) in the gastric fundus or body (Fig. 36.21). Histologically, PHG occurs in oxyntic mucosa and manifests with dilated, tortuous, irregular veins without fibrin thrombi, sometimes with intimal thickening, and usually in the absence of significant inflammation.[133]

Management of PHG is focused on the reduction of portal pressures mostly with pharmacotherapy. Nonselective β-adrenergic blockers are first-line therapy. Propranolol is a nonselective beta blocker that was investigated in the classic randomized controlled trial evaluating the role of beta blockade in preventing recurrent bleeding in severe PHG.[145] In this study, patients who received propranolol had a significantly lower rebleeding rate at 12 months (35% vs. 62%) and at 30 months (48% vs. 93%) compared with patients taking placebo. If a patient is refractory to beta blocker therapy, TIPS is indicated and has been effective in most cases.[141,146–148] Somatostatin analogs such as octreotide, which are established as effective treatment for acute variceal bleeding, also have been shown to be effective for acute bleeding from PHG. In two studies that evaluated the effect of these vasoactive drugs in acute hemorrhage from PHG,[149,150] bleeding was successfully treated in all patients who received somatostatin or octreotide. Vasopressin and its analog, terlipressin, also have been tried, with mixed results.[149,151] In patients with refractory bleeding, APC can be used as a limited, but potentially beneficial therapy, although it is not practical for those with a large portion of involved stomach.[187]

Varices and spider-like telangiectasias also may be seen in the small intestine, warranting the term *portal enteropathy*. *Portal colopathy* is the term used to describe the vascular manifestations of portal hypertension in the colon, which include hemorrhoids, varices, and spider-like telangiectasias (Fig. 36.22A and 36.22B). Mucosal lesions of portal colopathy endoscopically resemble those seen in PHG and may have a diffuse, colitis-like appearance, including erythema, telangiectasia, and friability. Histologic changes of portal colopathy and enteropathy are similar to those of portal gastropathy.[152] The lesions of portal enteropathy and colopathy are amenable to the same thermal therapies used for GAVE and PHG, so long as they are within reach of the endoscope.[153]

ANATOMIC ABNORMALITIES OF THE VASCULATURE

Superior Mesenteric Artery (SMA) Syndrome

The third portion of the duodenum is cradled in an angle of approximately 45 degrees formed by the root of the SMA and the wall of the aorta. When this angle is narrowed to less than 25 degrees, the SMA impinges on the duodenum, thereby leading to gastric and intestinal obstruction, a condition referred to as Wilkie's syndrome or the SMA syndrome (Fig. 36.23).[154,155] The latter term may be confusing and does not imply vascular insufficiency. Symptoms may be acute or chronic and typically include epigastric pain, vomiting, and early satiety. The syndrome has been associated with immobilization in a body cast; rapid growth in children; and marked, rapid weight loss in adults, particularly young women with eating disorders (see Chapter 10). Rarely, anatomic anomalies predispose to the condition, including a high ligament of Treitz or low origin of the SMA.

Barium studies may show an abrupt cutoff in the third portion of the duodenum with dilatation proximally, particularly when the patient is supine. CTA and MRA can provide noninvasive and detailed anatomic information that can be used to diagnose the condition and plan a surgical approach.[156,157] When CTA or MRA are not available, Doppler ultrasonography can be used for diagnosis.[188] Symptoms typically improve after the restoration of lost weight or removal of a body cast. Surgery is necessary only rarely. Duodenojejunostomy may relieve the symptoms and has been performed for this condition laparoscopically.[158]

Celiac Axis Compression (Median Arcuate Ligament) Syndrome

Whether celiac axis compression syndrome (CACS) is a cause of GI ischemia has been a subject of controversy ever since postprandial pain and an epigastric bruit were described in a patient in whom angiography showed narrowing of the CA caused by compression from a fibrotic celiac ganglion.[159] After release of the artery, the murmur and postprandial pain disappeared. Since that description in 1963 by Harjola, compression of the CA by the median arcuate ligament of the diaphragm and the celiac ganglion has been increasingly identified but still is not well understood.

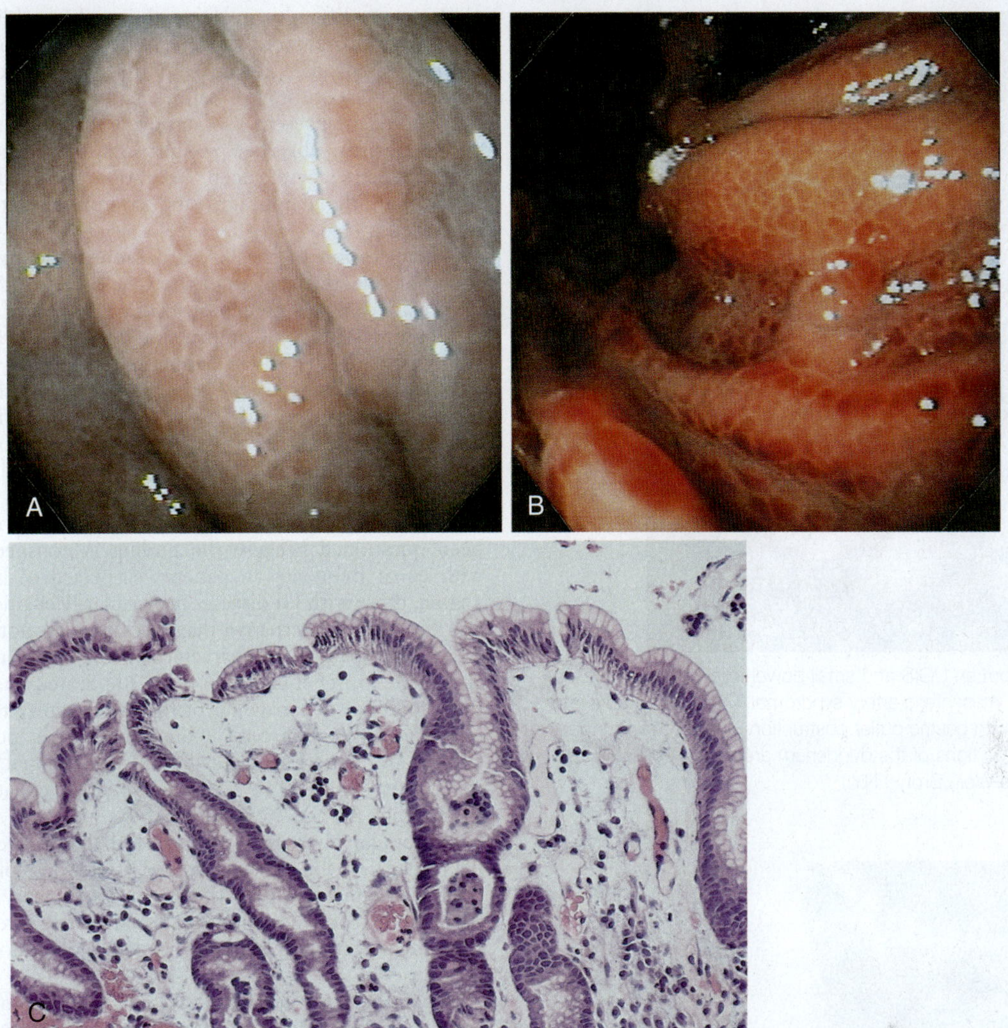

Fig. 36.21 Portal hypertensive gastropathy. (A) Mild gastropathy is manifested by prominence of the areae gastricae, with areas of erythema and subepithelial hemorrhage. This appearance is not pathognomonic and may be noted with other disorders that induce mucosal edema, such as *Helicobacter pylori* gastritis. (B) Severe gastropathy with diffuse subepithelial hemorrhage in a snakeskin pattern. (C) Low-power photomicrograph showing prominent edema of the mucosa involving the lamina propria with multiple congested blood vessels. No histologic evidence of gastritis is seen. (From Wilcox CM. *Atlas of Clinical Gastrointestinal Endoscopy*. Philadelphia: WB Saunders; 1995:109.)

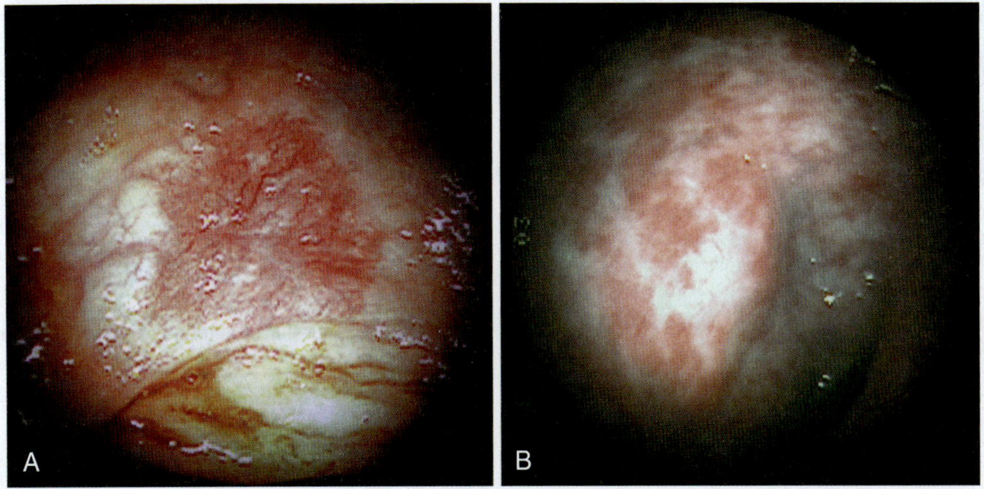

Fig. 36.22 Endoscopic images showing 2 examples of portal colopathy. (A) A solitary lesion that resembles a spider-like telangiectasia or AE is seen in the rectosigmoid. (B) Patchy foci of erythema in the descending colon of a patient with cirrhosis and portal hypertension. (Courtesy Dr. Lawrence J. Brandt, Bronx, NY.)

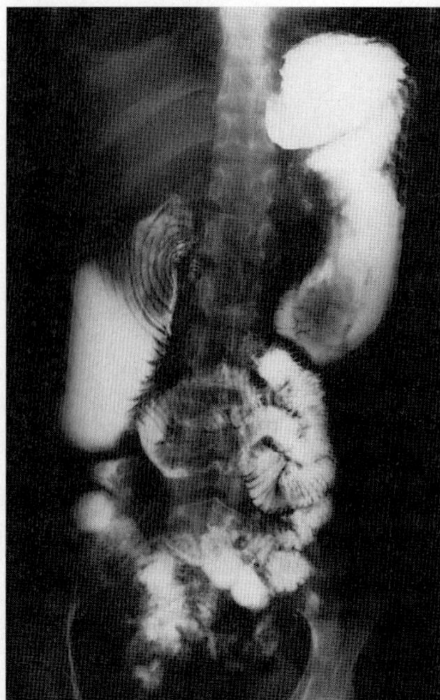

Fig. 36.23 Film from an UGIS and small bowel follow-through in a patient with superior mesenteric artery syndrome. The patient had symptoms compatible with gastric outlet obstruction, and on this film the second and third portions of the duodenum are markedly dilated. (Courtesy Dr. Ellen Wolf, Bronx, NY.)

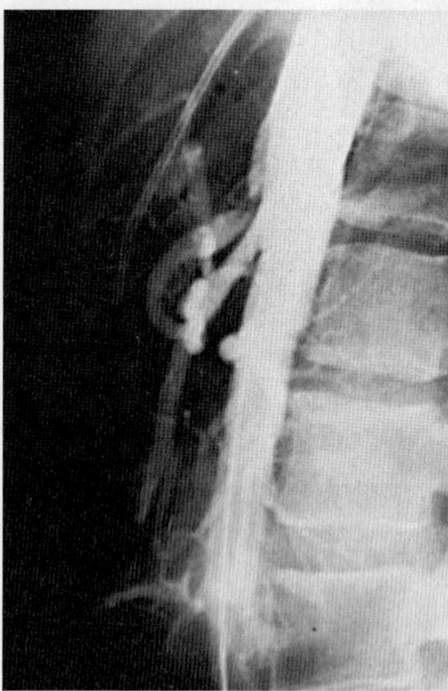

Fig. 36.24 Film from a lateral flush aortogram revealing the findings of celiac axis compression syndrome: a typical hook-like compression of the origin of the celiac axis with some poststenotic dilatation. The angiogram was performed on a patient with no GI complaints related to these findings. (From Boley SJ, Brandt LJ, Veith FJ. Ischemic disorders of the intestines. *Curr Probl Surg*. 1978;15:1.)

A major difficulty in determining the validity of CACS as an entity, also sometimes referred to as Harjola syndrome or Dunbar syndrome, arises from the different criteria used by various investigators to define it.[160,161] The clinical features that should be present to diagnose CACS include postprandial epigastric pain, diarrhea, weight loss, and an abdominal bruit that intensifies with deep expiration when the CA ascends more than the diaphragm and compression of the artery is increased.

Compression of the CA is demonstrated by lateral aortography or selective studies of the CA. EUS, CTA, and MRA are noninvasive means of demonstrating the vascular anatomy and CA compression.[162] Compression by the crural fibers of the diaphragm or the celiac ganglion produces a smooth, asymmetrical narrowing of the superior aspect of the CA and displaces it toward the SMA (Fig. 36.24). These findings are best shown at end-expiration and not end-inspiration, which is the phase in which respiration is typically halted during angiographic studies.

The clinical significance of a narrowed CA on angiography has been questioned because the finding is nonspecific and occurs with equal frequency in patients suspected of having intestinal angina, those with GI diseases not primarily characterized by pain, and those with alternative diagnoses that do not involve the GI tract. The pain that characterizes CACS is most frequently attributed to ischemia because the implicated anatomic lesion in this syndrome is narrowing of the major artery that perfuses the upper abdominal viscera. This concept has persisted, despite clinical and experimental evidence that isolated compromise of the CA is almost always compensated by collateral circulation from either the SMA or the IMA.

A popular alternative theory to that of ischemia is that the pain arises in the celiac ganglion itself, possibly secondary to pressure or throbbing by the compressed artery. The increased splanchnic blood flow and dilatation of the artery that accompany the ingestion of food may explain the relationship of pain to meals.

Operative approaches to CACS include division of the median arcuate ligament, with or without ganglionectomy, arterial reconstruction, or bypass; a laparoscopic approach has been successful in releasing the compression.[162] Results of operations for CACS have varied as much as have the criteria used to diagnose them. In a long-term follow-up study of patients treated for CACS, Evans found that 83% of patients were asymptomatic 6 months after a decompression procedure, but only 41% remained asymptomatic 3–11 years later.[163] In another study of 400 patients who underwent either open or laparoscopic division of the median arcuate ligament for the treatment of CACS, immediate postoperative symptom relief was reported in 85% and 96%, respectively. Symptom recurrence was reported in 6.8% and 5.7% of patients in the open and laparoscopic groups, respectively, when these patients were followed for 6–229 months after surgery.[164]

The controversy concerning CACS continues. A small number of patients who have otherwise unexplained abdominal pain not helped by standard regimens have exhibited relief by some aspect of the operations performed for CACS.[165] To keep unnecessary procedures to a minimum, surgery should be performed only in patients who manifest the clinical features described earlier.

Full references for this chapter can be found at https://ebooks.health.elsevier.com.

37 Surgical Peritonitis and Other Diseases of the Peritoneum, Mesentery, Omentum, and Diaphragm

Jeffrey B. Matthews, Kiran Turaga

IN THIS CHAPTER

Secondary inflammation of the peritoneum frequently presents with the patient *in extremis* requiring a procedural intervention and is commonly referred to as "surgical peritonitis." Primary peritonitis or spontaneous bacterial peritonitis (SBP), has a distinct pathophysiology, is discussed in Chapter 93.

This chapter discusses the disease processes that affect the peritoneum, mesentery, omentum, and diaphragm.

ANATOMY AND PHYSIOLOGY

Gross Anatomy

The peritoneum is the largest serous membrane of the human body, with an estimated surface area of 1.8 m^2, which is almost the same area as the skin (or total body surface area). The embryological development of the peritoneum occurs in the gastrulation phase, where the three layers of the embryo: ectoderm, mesoderm, and endoderm, further differentiate into the visceral plate mesoderm and the parietal plate mesoderm. The parietal peritoneum secretes serous fluid, while the visceral peritoneum invests organs and the mesentery that suspends the gut tube from the abdominal wall, thus providing a pathway for vessels, nerves, and lymphatics. The peritoneal sac, as it is often referred to, is sealed in men and open to the exterior via the ostia of the fallopian tubes in women.[1]

The parietal peritoneum in a completely developed fetus covers the internal surfaces of the abdominal wall, including the diaphragms and the pelvis, while the visceral peritoneum invests all intraperitoneal organs (such as small intestine, gallbladder, and stomach) and the anterior surface of retroperitoneal organs (pancreas, kidneys, ascending and descending colon). Remarkably, the understanding of the anatomy of the peritoneum, omentum, and mesentery is evolving. Meyers identified numerous ligaments and two mesenteries including the coronary, gastrohepatic, hepatic, duodenal, falciform, gastrocolic, duodenocolic, gastrosplenic, splenorenal, and phrenicocolic ligaments and the transverse mesocolon and the small bowel mesentery. While important in understanding and predicting spread of disease and inflammation that manifests in clinically relevant situations, this is an oversimplification of the anatomy. For instance, patients with perforated peptic ulcer disease may present with right lower quadrant pain due to dependent drainage along the right paracolic gutter. Prior to imaging techniques, patients would be placed in semi-recumbent positions (Fowler's position) to encourage the dependent accumulation of infected fluid with the goal that the eventually encapsulated pelvic abscess could be drained transrectally.

Current understanding of the mesentery and the parietal peritoneum suggest that the mesentery distal to the duodenojejunal flexure is a contiguous and extra-retroperitoneal organ.[2] The right and left mesocolic regions and the mesosigmoid are flattened against the abdominal wall, held in place by Toldt's fascia. It has been suggested that the intestine and mesentery are contiguous from diaphragm to pelvic floor and that the mesogastrium and mesoduodenum are indeed contiguous with the mesentery. This description of the mesentery is broken into six flexures: duodenojejunal, ileocecal, hepatic, splenic, between descending and sigmoid, and sigmoid and rectum. The peritoneal reflections, while contiguous, are variably named Jackson's membrane, anterior reflection, pouch of Douglas, and the lateral peritoneal reflection (Fig. 37.1). This understanding is translating into "total mesocolic or mesorectal" excisions for oncological purposes.

The greater omentum is an intraperitoneal organ derived from the greater curvature of the stomach and spleen, draping across the transverse colon, which separates the abdomen into the greater and lesser sacs. The lesser omentum attaches the lesser curvature of the stomach to the liver and is also referred to as the gastrohepatic omentum. The right edge of the lesser omentum is also known as the hepatoduodenal ligament, and the opening posterior to this (the epiploic foramen of Winslow) is the only connection between the lesser and greater sacs.

Microscopic Anatomy

The word peritoneum is derived from the Greek *peri*, meaning "around" and *tonos*, meaning "a stretching around." The visceral and parietal peritoneum have a similar structure and consist of three layers: mesothelium, basal lamina, and submesothelial stroma. The mesothelium is formed by a monolayer of cuboidal mesothelial cells approximately 25 μm in diameter. Mesothelial cells possess both epithelial and mesenchymal characteristics, and peritoneal pathology can lead to epithelial–mesenchymal transitions. The peritoneum contains *stomata*, which are direct portals to the lymphatic system. These are abundantly present on the diaphragm. At the apical surface of the peritoneum are numerous microvilli and occasional cilia in which lamellar bodies are embedded. These release surfactant that allows a friction-free state. On top of the microvilli and lamellar bodies, a glycocalyx is present consisting of proteoglycans and glycosaminoglycans.[3] These are responsible for intercellular contact, inflammatory regulation, tissue remodeling, and possibly transport. Mesothelial cells are joined by well-defined intercellular junctional complexes, including tight junctions, adherens junctions, gap junctions, and desmosomes that establish and maintain the semipermeable barrier for fluid, solutes, and particles.

Blood Supply and Innervation

The visceral peritoneum is supplied by the splanchnic blood vessels, and the parietal peritoneum by intercostal, subcostal, lumbar, and iliac vessels. The venous blood from the visceral peritoneum returns via the portal vein while the parietal peritoneum drains via the inferior vena cava. The visceral peritoneum is supplied by nonsomatic nerves, whereas the parietal peritoneum is supplied by somatic nerves. Therefore visceral pain is poorly localized, diffuse, and vague (see Chapter 13). Visceral pain is caused by stretching, distention, torsion, and twisting. The visceral peritoneum does not produce pain when it is cut or burned. When visceral pain fibers of midgut structures are stimulated, a vague periumbilical discomfort results because the visceral pain fibers enter the spinal cord at the same level as the T10 dermatome somatic fibers (see Chapters 12 and 13). This sensation is, therefore, experienced as discomfort in a dermatomal distribution. Likewise, visceral stimulation from foregut structures produces epigastric (T8 distribution) discomfort, whereas visceral stimulation in the hindgut produces suprapubic (T12) discomfort. Parietal (somatic) pain fibers are activated by such stimuli as cutting, burning, and inflammation. This type of pain is sharply localized. A good example of this process is acute appendicitis. Early in the disease process, the patient experiences periumbilical discomfort secondary to distention of the appendiceal lumen, and this progresses to localized right lower quadrant pain and tenderness as the inflammation becomes transmural and involves the parietal peritoneum.

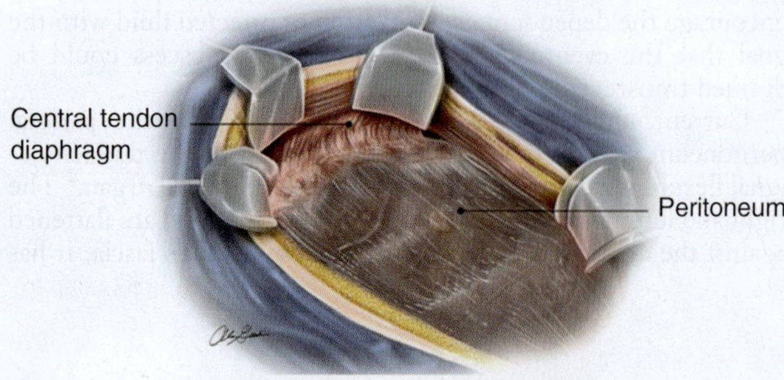

Fig. 37.1 The anterior parietal peritoneum is shown after having been stripped from the anterior abdominal wall.

Physiology

The mesothelial cell maintains the homeostasis of the peritoneal cavity and synthesizes the matrix proteins on the basal surface that maintain the architecture of the peritoneal membrane[4] (Fig. 37.2). The peritoneum can regenerate after injury or surgery. The

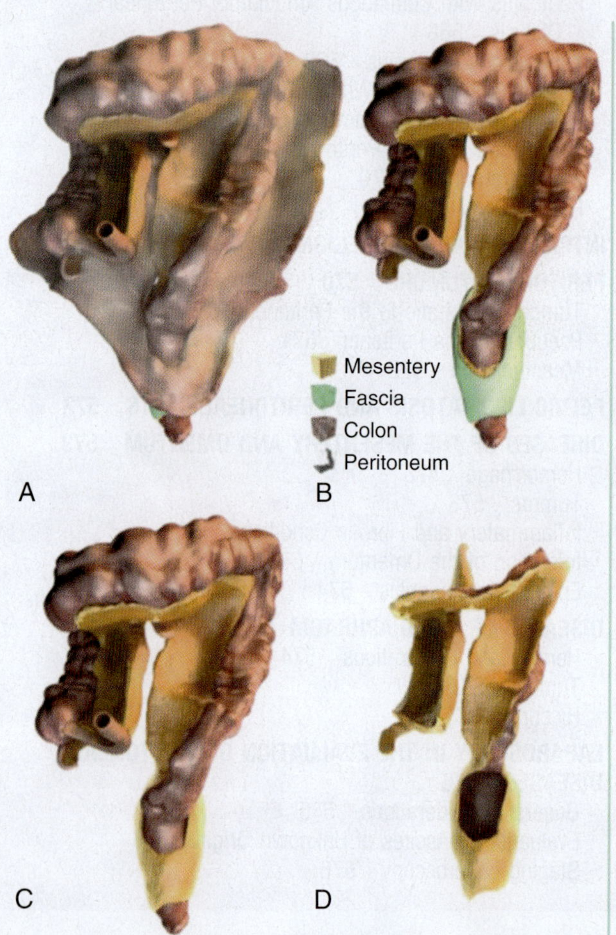

Fig. 37.2 Digital representations of peritoneum, mesentery, fascia, and intestine. (A) Peritoneum, mesentery, fascia, and intestine. (B) Mesentery, fascia, and intestine. (C) Mesentery and intestine. (D) Mesentery.

peritoneum can also cause fibrosis by exerting epithelial–mesenchymal transitions. In addition, these cells can also promote the degradation of fibrin by converting plasminogen to plasmin, thus activating tissue plasminogen activator. In animal models of abdominal wall hernias repaired with composite mesh grafts, a functional neoperitoneum covers the graft in 7–14 days.[5,6]

Under conditions of inflammation, the mesothelial cell initiates and regulates the inflammatory response by the synthesis of cytokines, chemokines, and growth factors. The peritoneal mesothelial cell is capable of phagocytosis and can serve as an antigen-presenting cell.[7]

Finally, in health and in inflammatory conditions, the mesothelial cell facilitates transport of fluids, solutes, and particulate matter across the peritoneal membrane. Fluid and solute movement are governed by convection and diffusion.[8] Particles are absorbed from the peritoneal cavity by two different anatomic routes. Particles smaller than 2 kd may be absorbed through peritoneal venous pores and are directed to the portal circulation. Particles larger than 3 kd are absorbed through peritoneal lymphatics, entering the lymphatic thoracic duct and from there the systemic circulation. This last route of absorption plays an important role in controlling abdominal infections because it has a huge capacity for absorption. The anatomic structure of these large channels between the peritoneal cavity and the diaphragmatic vessels and the negative pressure of the thorax during inspiration make this mechanism extremely effective in the removal of bacteria and cells. The large surface area and semipermeability of the peritoneal membrane can be exploited therapeutically in peritoneal dialysis (Fig. 37.3).

SECONDARY (SURGICAL) PERITONITIS

Secondary (surgical) peritonitis is a result of an inflammatory process in the peritoneal cavity secondary to inflammation, perforation, or gangrene of an intra-abdominal or retroperitoneal structure. Surgical intervention is usually required to treat these processes. However, in certain situations such as perforated peptic ulcer, nonoperative treatment may also be successful (see Chapter 55). Antibiotics play only an adjunctive role in severe intra-abdominal infection. If untreated, secondary peritonitis will, in most cases, lead to septic shock and death. It is common medical parlance to equate nonoperative management and "conservative" therapy; however, the reverse is more often the case for secondary peritonitis (i.e., operative intervention is in fact the "conservative" approach).

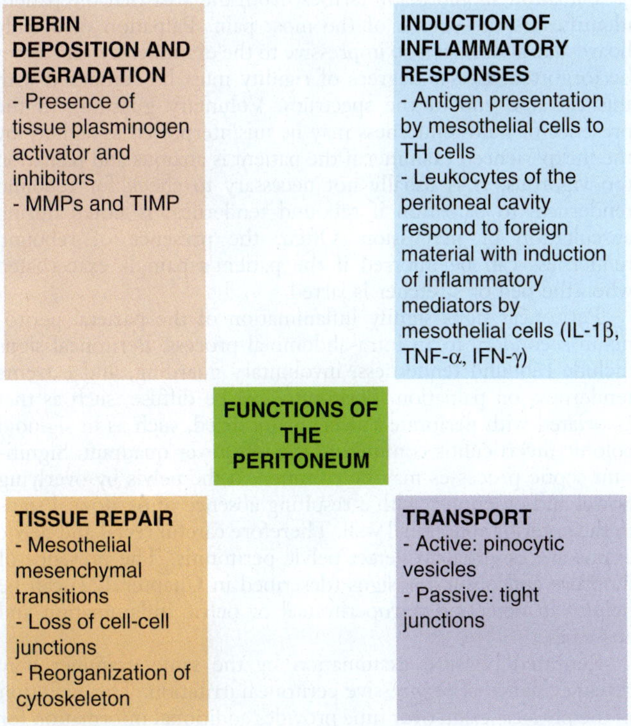

FIBRIN DEPOSITION AND DEGRADATION
- Presence of tissue plasminogen activator and inhibitors
- MMPs and TIMP

INDUCTION OF INFLAMMATORY RESPONSES
- Antigen presentation by mesothelial cells to TH cells
- Leukocytes of the peritoneal cavity respond to foreign material with induction of inflammatory mediators by mesothelial cells (IL-1β, TNF-α, IFN-γ)

FUNCTIONS OF THE PERITONEUM

TISSUE REPAIR
- Mesothelial mesenchymal transitions
- Loss of cell-cell junctions
- Reorganization of cytoskeleton

TRANSPORT
- Active: pinocytic vesicles
- Passive: tight junctions

Fig. 37.3 Functions of the peritoneum. *IFN-γ*, Interferon gamma; *IL-1β*, interleukin 1 beta; *MMP*, metalloproteinase; *TIMP*, tissue inhibitor of metalloproteinase; *TH*, T helper; *TNF-α*, tumor necrosis factor-alpha.

Causes and Pathogenesis

The diagnosis of secondary peritonitis is based on history, physical examination, imaging studies, and operative exploration. History and physical examination are very important in secondary peritonitis, and a good history and physical examination can often reduce or eliminate the need for further studies. Secondary peritonitis has numerous causes. Some of the more common causes of secondary peritonitis include perforated peptic ulcer disease, appendicitis, diverticulitis, acute cholecystitis, pancreatitis, and postsurgical complications. Other sources of inflammation such as autoimmune serositis (e.g., SLE), endometriosis, and malignancies cause peritoneal inflammation but rarely cause clinical peritonitis.

Other nonbacterial causes of peritonitis include leakage of blood into the peritoneal cavity due to rupture of a tubal pregnancy, ovarian cyst, or aneurysmal vessel. Blood is highly irritating to the peritoneum and may cause abdominal pain (hemorrhagic peritonitis) similar to that found in septic peritonitis. Bile leakage into the peritoneal cavity also can cause signs and symptoms of peritonitis, especially when there is also bacterial contamination of the bilious contents. However, sterile bile in the abdomen can be surprisingly asymptomatic. Large bilomas may have minimal symptoms.

Bacteria can reach the peritoneal cavity by a variety of pathologic processes: transmural inflammation with luminal obstruction (see Chapter 125), perforation of the GI tract, bacterial translocation (see Chapter 60), and intestinal ischemia (see Chapter 120). The initial inoculum of bacteria is determined by the normal flora in the involved portion of the GI tract (see Chapter 3).

Flora

Although the flora of the gut, especially of the large bowel, is diverse and extensive, the numbers of types of organisms rapidly decrease after leakage of gut contents into the peritoneal cavity.[9] Aerobes such as *Escherichia coli* and enterococci and anaerobes such as *Bacteroides fragilis* and *Clostridium* organisms predominate. A study of infections associated with ruptured colonic diverticulitis reported anaerobes only in 15% of cases, aerobic bacteria only in 11%, and mixed aerobic and anaerobic flora in 74%; cultures from peritoneal abscesses detected anaerobic bacteria alone in 18%, aerobes alone in 5%, and mixed aerobic and anaerobic flora in 77%.[10] In addition to bacteria, fungi in intra-abdominal infection are more frequently recognized and may have clinical significance. For example, a positive fungal culture is quite common in perforated peptic ulcer disease (PUD) and may adversely affect outcome.[11]

On the basis of an animal model of monomicrobial and polymicrobial peritonitis with various combinations of bacteria, it is apparent that *E. coli* is the organism most often responsible for death from this form of iatrogenic peritonitis, at least in part because of its ability to cause bacteremia, and that combinations of anaerobes and facultative organisms lead to abscess formation.[12] Other adjuvant substances, such as devitalized tissue, mucus, bile, hemoglobin, and barium, can act synergistically with microorganisms to increase mortality in surgical peritonitis through their ability to interfere with phagocytosis and killing of bacteria. These considerations form the basis for the treatment of surgical peritonitis, which is described later.

The peritoneal cavity possesses several lines of defense against bacterial infection[13–15] (Box 37.1). Peritonitis results when these defenses are overwhelmed.

Peritoneal Clearance of Bacteria

Once bacteria enter the peritoneal cavity, clearance of the offending microorganisms begins immediately. Within 6 minutes of intraperitoneal inoculation of bacteria in dogs, bacteria can be cultured in thoracic lymph, indicating passage of organisms through the diaphragm. Twelve minutes later, bacteremia may be evident. This clearance mechanism is probably important in survival because blockade of the thoracic duct in an animal model of peritonitis decreases bacteremic episodes but increases mortality and induces liver necrosis. This appears to be directly related to the amount of endotoxin to which the liver is exposed.[16] Decades before it was known that the diaphragm was the predominant site of clearance of bacteria, Fowler, in 1900, proposed his head-up, pelvis-down position for the prevention of absorption of toxins from infected peritoneal cavities. In the preantibiotic era, the documentation of the delayed clearance of bacteria from experiments in infected dogs in the head-down position confirmed the wisdom of this positioning for patients with peritonitis.

History and Physical Examination

Clinical history and careful physical examination are the key factors in making a timely diagnosis of surgical peritonitis. In general, the sooner the diagnosis is made, the better the prognosis. Abdominal pain is the hallmark of peritonitis. The exact details of the onset of pain can be helpful in drawing attention to the affected organ (see Chapter 12). The pain's character, location, area of radiation, change over time, and provocative and palliative factors are key pieces of information in assisting with the diagnosis. Peritoneal inflammation is typically associated with ileus, and therefore nausea and vomiting are common symptoms.

BOX 37.1 Peritoneal Defense Mechanisms Against Bacteria

REMOVAL MECHANISMS

Peritoneal clearance of bacteria through the diaphragm via the thoracic duct

LEUKOCYTE-ATTRACTING MECHANISMS

Microvilli of the mesothelial cell
ICAM-1 (CD 54) and VCAM-1 (CD 106)
Neutrophil recruitment through omental high endothelial venules (HEV)

KILLING MECHANISMS

Macrophages (with glutamate metabolic bursts)
Neutrophils
Opsonins
- Complement C3b
- Immunoglobulin G
- Fibronectin
- Mast cell–derived leukotrienes

SEQUESTRATION MECHANISMS

Fibrin trapping of bacteria
Formation of fibrinous adhesions
Omental loculation of foci of inflammation

ICAM, Intercellular adhesion molecule; *VCAM*, vascular cell adhesion molecule.

The ability of the clinician to elicit an accurate history of abdominal pain and peritoneal signs is limited in patients with neurologic and immunologic compromise. The pain of peritonitis can be reduced or even absent in older adult patients. Infants and children may be incapable of furnishing any history or cooperating with the physical examination. Patients notoriously difficult to assess for secondary peritonitis include emergency room patients under the influence of alcohol or illicit drugs, trauma patients with central nervous system or spinal cord injuries, and sedated and ventilated ICU patients. Analgesics typically will not relieve the findings of peritonitis on physical examination but may relieve some discomfort. Diabetic patients may have deficits in both neurologic and immune function. Patients receiving immunosuppressive and anti-inflammatory drugs, such as glucocorticoids and chemotherapeutic drugs, may have blunted perception of pain and minimal signs of peritoneal irritation. Patients with cirrhosis and ascites may show no pain during episodes of SBP unless the parietal peritoneum becomes involved with the inflammatory process.

On examination, the patient with surgical peritonitis usually prefers to remain immobile because any movement acutely worsens the pain. Fever of 100°F or higher is typical, as is tachycardia, which may be in part secondary to pain. Hypotension is usually a late finding in sepsis. Fever is a fundamental endogenous mechanism to help fight infection. In fact, the increase in body temperature that is usually found during bacterial infections, including peritonitis, seems to be essential for optimal host defense against bacteria.[17] The absence of hepatic dullness to percussion suggests the presence of free air in the peritoneal cavity. Exquisite tenderness to percussion should lead to very gentle palpation. Overly vigorous palpation of a very tender abdomen may cause patients such pain that they are subsequently unable to cooperate for the remainder of the examination.

Palpation should begin farthest from the area that the patient identifies as the source of the most pain. Palpation of a truly board-like abdomen is so impressive to the examiner that it cannot be forgotten. Lesser degrees of rigidity must be compared with this extreme end of the spectrum. Voluntary guarding in the presence of mild tenderness may be misinterpreted as rigidity by the inexperienced examiner if the patient is anxious and palpation too vigorous. It is usually not necessary to check for rebound tenderness to palpation if rebound tenderness is noted during auscultation or percussion. Often, the presence of rebound tenderness can be inferred if the patient's pain is exacerbated when the bed or stretcher is jarred.

Peritoneal signs signify inflammation of the parietal peritoneum secondary to an intra-abdominal process. Peritoneal signs include rebound tenderness, involuntary guarding, and extreme tenderness on palpation. Peritonitis can be diffuse, such as that associated with perforated ulcer, or localized, such as in sigmoid colonic diverticulitis confined to the left lower quadrant. Significant septic processes may be confined to the pelvis by overlying bowel and omentum, with a resulting absence of peritoneal signs in the anterior abdominal wall. Therefore careful rectal and pelvic exams are essential to detect pelvic peritonitis. The presence of iliopsoas and obturator signs (described in Chapter 122) can be helpful in detecting retroperitoneal or pelvic inflammation and abscesses.

Repeated physical examination by the same examiner may reveal evidence of progressive peritoneal irritation. The evolution of the physical exam over time provides additional information for diagnosis and evaluation of response to initial nonoperative therapy. This, together with laboratory tests and imaging procedures described below, may indicate the need for surgical intervention.

Laboratory Tests and Imaging

The most common and widely available laboratory test that is abnormal in otherwise immunocompetent patients with peritonitis is an increased WBC count with left shift. The presence of circulating juvenile forms (i.e., bands) reflects an increasing demand of new white cells from the bone marrow. A low WBC count during a bacterial infection, associated at times with Gram-negative septicemia, may indicate the presence of an exhausted bone marrow and carries a poorer prognosis. In addition, metabolic acidosis, hemoconcentration, and prerenal azotemia may be present.

Free air may be evident on upright chest radiograph or on upright or decubitus abdominal films, but the finding of pneumoperitoneum by radiography has limited sensitivity in gut perforation.[18] The absence of free air should not delay surgical intervention in an otherwise appropriate clinical setting. US can be helpful in demonstrating abscesses, bile duct dilation, and large fluid collections but is usually not the best first-line choice for diagnostic imaging. CT of the abdomen and pelvis, generally with both oral (and occasionally rectal) and IV contrast, is increasingly preferred as the most sensitive and specific imaging modality for acute abdominal pain. Multidetector CT scanners are capable of imaging the entire abdomen and pelvis in a single breath-hold. The axial images are of extremely high resolution and can be reconstructed in coronal, sagittal, and 3D sets of images.[19] CT is much more sensitive than plain films for the detection of free air, and with multidetector CT it is possible to visualize the actual site of perforation. Although CT images are increasingly accurate and the images compelling, they should not delay surgical consultation, resuscitation, and operation in a patient with suspected peritonitis.

Diagnosis

The diagnosis of surgical peritonitis is suspected on the basis of history, physical examination, and laboratory and imaging tests and is confirmed at laparotomy or laparoscopy when purulent fibrinous peritonitis is found. In those patients whose history and physical examinations are unreliable, CT and peritoneal lavage are valuable in confirming the diagnosis of surgical peritonitis. CT is less invasive, but if not available, or if a patient is too hemodynamically unstable to undergo scanning, peritoneal lavage is an effective alternative that can be rapidly performed. Peritoneal lavage involves insertion under sterile conditions of a catheter into the peritoneal cavity and infusing 1 L of normal saline. If the effluent contains more than 500 WBCs/mm^3, effluent amylase or bilirubin levels greater than the corresponding serum value, or bacteria are visible on Gram stain, there is approximately a 90% likelihood of surgical peritonitis. Surgery is usually indicated in this setting. Finally, diagnostic laparoscopy is highly accurate in the diagnosis of surgical peritonitis, and many of the underlying diseases can be dealt with laparoscopically, avoiding the need for laparotomy.[20]

Treatment

Two principles in the management of secondary peritonitis cannot be overemphasized. First, not all patients with peritonitis require surgery. For example, a patient with localized left lower quadrant peritonitis secondary to sigmoid colonic diverticulitis can be managed with bowel rest and IV antibiotics alone. Another patient with the same clinical presentation and findings of a diverticular abscess on CT scan can be successfully treated with antibiotics and percutaneous drainage (see Chapter 29). The second principle is that the *absence* of peritonitis does not exclude the possibility of surgical emergency. The classic example of this clinical situation is early acute mesenteric ischemia with abdominal pain out of proportion to findings on physical examination findings (see Chapter 120). Likewise, a complete mechanical small bowel obstruction generally requires emergency operation *before* the development of peritoneal signs that indicate progression to perforation or vascular compromise (see Chapter 125).

For most cases of secondary peritonitis, fluid resuscitation, and antibiotic therapy followed by urgent laparotomy or laparoscopy are the mainstays of treatment. The patient should be aggressively fluid resuscitated to treat intravascular volume depletion secondary to movement of fluid out of the vascular space. Fluid resuscitation (bolus of 30 mL/kg) is guided by frequent monitoring of physiologic parameters in an intensive care setting, including blood pressure (by arterial line if shock is present), heart rate, central venous pressure, mixed venous oxygen saturation, and urine output. Hematocrit, WBC, electrolytes, glucose, creatinine, and blood gases should also be monitored. Hypovolemia, hypotension, metabolic acidosis, hypoxia, and hemoconcentration from loss of plasma into the peritoneal cavity are expected. Vasopressor therapy should be initiated only after adequate volume resuscitation has failed to correct hypotension and hypoperfusion. Measurement of serum lactate levels to guide resuscitative efforts has been included in the new update for surviving sepsis guidelines.[21] Glucocorticoids that were previously empirically administered, are restricted to patients who fail to respond to fluid and vasopressor therapy. Surgical intervention for source control should be pursued as soon as the patient is hemodynamically stable for operation.

Antibiotics

Antibiotic therapy is required before, during, and after surgical intervention. The type of bacteria causing secondary peritonitis depends in part on the normal flora of the part of the GI tract that is the source of sepsis and in part on the clinical setting. Two recent sets of guidelines for the management of complicated intra-abdominal infections recommend broader antimicrobial therapy for hospital-acquired infections than in community-acquired infections.[22,23] In community-acquired peritonitis, susceptible Gram-negative bacilli, strict anaerobic bacteria, and enterococci are typically found. In health care–associated infections, the flora may have been altered by previous antibiotic exposure and previous disease, with more antibiotic-resistant organisms present. In general, antibiotics directed against the most likely pathogens should be chosen. For example, colonic processes require coverage for Gram-negative aerobes and anaerobes. In animal models, antibiotics directed against Gram-negative enteric aerobic organisms minimize mortality, and drugs effective against anaerobes prevent abscess formation. It has been shown that there is synergy between aerobic and anaerobic bacteria in experimental models of peritonitis. The coverage of all potential organisms is not necessary. The flora of surgical peritonitis simplifies with time, even before initiation of antibiotics. Killing certain key species may change the microenvironment sufficiently to prevent growth and allow killing of other flora. If a *Candida* species is cultured from the peritoneal cavity, this organism should be treated if the patient is in septic shock, in an immunocompromised state, or in a hospital-acquired setting.[24] On the other hand, hemodynamically stable immunocompetent patients with secondary peritonitis in a community setting do not need treatment for *Candida.* Examination of short-course antibiotics (4 ± 1) days versus antibiotics until a resolution of fever/leukocytosis (approximately 8 days) after source control suggested equivalence in the STOP-IT trial.[25]

A variety of antibiotic regimens have been proposed using the following classes of antibiotics alone or in combination: second-generation cephalosporins, third-generation cephalosporins, broad-spectrum beta-lactams, fluoroquinolones and metronidazole, and aminoglycosides with clindamycin or metronidazole.

Many controlled trials of antibiotic regimens show equivalency. For example, it has been shown that monotherapy with a broad-spectrum beta-lactam is as effective as combination therapy with a beta-lactam and an aminoglycoside.[26] Data-supported guidelines regarding optimal treatment have been hampered by suboptimal study design and nonuniform efficacy criteria in the controlled trials that have been performed. A Cochrane review of 40 randomized trials involving 16 different regimens showed no difference in mortality.[27] The specific antibiotics chosen should take into account other considerations such as the avoidance of toxicities, the sensitivity profile of cultured organisms, the ease and route of administration, the risk of emergence of antibiotic resistance, and cost.[22] The availability of broad-spectrum antibiotics, including beta-lactams, fluoroquinolones, and third- and fourth-generation cephalosporins, makes it unnecessary to use aminoglycosides with their potential nephrotoxicity in patients with compromised renal function.

The failure to clear secondary peritonitis after an appropriate course of antibiotic therapy or the recurrence of peritonitis is termed *tertiary peritonitis*. Nosocomial infections occurring in patients after long periods of hospitalization may include infections with multiresistant *Pseudomonas*, *Enterobacter*, *Enterococcus*, *Staphylococcus*, and *Candida* species. The development of multiple organ dysfunction syndrome after an initial operation should prompt an aggressive search for inadequate source control and for abscesses, involving repeat CT, percutaneous or operative drainage of abscesses, and culture of persistent fluid collections, in addition to antimicrobial therapy.[28]

Surgical Intervention

Antibiotics help treat or prevent fatal bacteremia but do not cure most patients with surgical peritonitis unless operative intervention is also undertaken. Neither free leakage of gut contents nor large abscesses can be sterilized by antibiotics alone in the absence of drainage. Surgical intervention should occur as soon as possible after the patient has been stabilized and resuscitated and antibiotics have been given. Laparotomy remains the gold standard for definitive diagnosis and mainstay of therapy in surgical peritonitis. However, a recent review confirms the success of an increasing number of laparoscopic procedures for some forms of peritonitis.[20] With either laparoscopic or conventional open operations, the aims of surgical treatment are source control, peritoneal decontamination, and prevention of recurrent infection.

Repeat laparotomy after temporary abdominal closure may be useful when control of the source of infection is not possible at the initial operation. Surgical reexploration may be undertaken for the following reasons: (1) tenuous control of the source of infection; (2) reassessment of bowel viability; (3) inadequate or poor drainage; (4) hemodynamic instability; (5) infected pancreatic necrosis or diffuse fecal peritonitis at the initial operation; (6) reassessment of a tenuous anastomosis; and (7) the development of intra-abdominal hypertension (abdominal compartment syndrome). Abdominal compartment syndrome, which is described in more detail in Chapter 12, develops when the closure of the abdomen at either the level of the fascia or skin causes intra-abdominal pressure to rise to a degree that impairs respiratory, hepatic, and/or renal function.[29]

Preoperative and postoperative fluid and nutritional support are crucial to prompt wound healing and survival. Peritonitis has been compared with a 50% total body surface area burn, and even a calorie intake of 3000–4000 kcal/day may not achieve positive nitrogen balance. Inability to achieve positive nitrogen balance may, however, be secondary to accelerated proteolysis, and negative nitrogen balance associated with pathologic proteolysis cannot be reversed by any amount of caloric intake. This proteolysis may only be thwarted with treatment of the septic process and recovery of the patient. The enteral route of nutrition is preferred over parenteral (see Chapter 6). Placement of a feeding jejunostomy tube at the initial operation is therefore prudent in these critically ill patients.

Prognosis

Despite the modern approach to the diagnosis and treatment of secondary (surgical) peritonitis, mortality remains high in certain subgroups of patients, especially older adult patients and patients who suffer multiple organ failure before the development of peritonitis. In general, peritonitis-related mortality may be as high as 30%,[30] with appendicitis and perforated duodenal ulcer at the low end of the spectrum ($\approx$10%) and postoperative (tertiary) peritonitis at the high end (up to 50%).

PERITONITIS OF OTHER CAUSES

Primary Peritonitis

SBP, or peritonitis without a known surgical source, is the most common cause of primary peritonitis (Box 37.2). This occurs predominantly in patients with cirrhosis and ascites and is discussed in Chapter 95. Primary peritonitis may also occur in patients with ascites due to nephrotic syndrome. Primary peritonitis in the absence of cirrhosis or nephrosis is much less common and usually occurs in children. Primary peritonitis is treated without surgical intervention, using antibiotics directed against the offending organism.

Peritonitis With Continuous Ambulatory Peritoneal Dialysis

Continuous ambulatory peritoneal dialysis (CAPD) is a common treatment of end-stage kidney disease, particularly outside of the United States.[31] Rates of bacterial peritonitis vary widely by dialysis program, with a reported range of 0.06–1.66 episodes per patient-year of treatment.[32] The most common isolates are *Staphylococcus epidermidis* and other skin flora. Other pathogens, such as Gram-negative bacilli including *Pseudomonas* species, fungi, or *Mycobacterium tuberculosis*, are less frequent. The most probable explanation for this high incidence of infection is inadvertent contamination of the indwelling catheter, but gastrointestinal, gynecologic, and bacteremic sources have been implicated. Because of this, a variety of recommendations for the prevention of peritonitis have been proposed.[32] Peritonitis in this group of patients is a major source of morbidity and the largest single cause of patient failure on CAPD.

Abdominal pain and tenderness are found in about 80% of patients, but fever is found in only about one-third. A consistent feature is cloudy effluent, noted in 84%.[33] The diagnosis is suspected on the basis of signs and symptoms and is confirmed by a

BOX 37.2 Causes of Nonsurgical Peritonitis

SBP (see Chapter 95)
Chronic ambulatory peritoneal dialysis
Mycobacterium tuberculosis
AIDS associated
Chlamydia trachomatis
Neisseria gonorrhoeae (Fitz-Hugh-Curtis syndrome)
Rare causes

1. Polyarteritis nodosa
2. SLE
3. PSS
4. Familial Mediterranean fever

fluid WBC count greater than 100 neutrophils/mm^3 or the presence of organisms on Gram stain. Treatment should be started immediately without waiting for the culture results, similar to the empirical treatment of patients with cirrhosis and neutrocytic ascites. Initial treatment of suspected CAPD peritonitis should cover the most frequently isolated bacteria. Vancomycin or a cephalosporins are good options if monotherapy is considered. The intraperitoneal route of administration is now preferred to the IV route.[33] The sensitivity of the organism isolated determines the subsequent antibiotic choice. Most of these patients are successfully treated on an outpatient basis without stopping dialysis. Prompt treatment ensures survival; however, recurrent infection is common and may lead to catheter removal or scarring of the peritoneum. Addition of heparin to the dialysis bag in cases of peritonitis may decrease the formation of fibrin and thereby the incidence of postinfection adhesions, but there was no beneficial role for urokinase administration. Fungal infections and recurring bacterial infections require removal of the catheter. Repeated infections lead to sclerosing encapsulating peritonitis (abdominal cocoon syndrome) and loss of surface area for effective dialysis.[34]

Tuberculous Peritonitis

Tuberculous peritonitis is an uncommon site of extrapulmonary infection caused by *M. tuberculosis*. Patients with HIV infection, cirrhosis, diabetes mellitus, and underlying malignancy are at increased risk.[35] Noncirrhotic patients with tuberculous peritonitis usually have ascites with a high protein content, low glucose concentration, and a low serum-to-ascites albumin gradient (<1.1 g/dL).[36] Patients almost always have an elevated ascitic fluid WBC count with a lymphocytic predominance. The algorithm in evaluation of patients with ascitic fluid that has a high lymphocyte count includes cytologic evaluation of the fluid and consideration of laparoscopy. Patients with lymphocytic ascites and fever usually have tuberculous (TB), whereas afebrile patients usually have malignancy-related ascites. Cancer is the cause of lymphocytic ascites about 10 times more frequently than TB (see Chapter 95). If peritoneal metastases are present, the cytologic findings are positive more than 90% of the time, and the laparoscopy can be avoided. If the cytology is negative, laparoscopy is performed and is nearly 100% sensitive in detecting TB peritonitis. However, a number of noninvasive diagnostic tests are available to diagnoses extrapulmonary disease. Adenosine deaminase levels are typically elevated in the ascitic fluid in tuberculous ascites, and this finding can help differentiate tuberculous peritonitis from peritoneal carcinomatosis.[37] An enzyme-linked immunospot assay (ELISPOT) and PCR assay (Xpert MTB/RIF) are novel, rapid, noninvasive tests for *M. tuberculosis*.[38,39] Tuberculous peritonitis may also appear as a pelvic mass on CT, with high serum levels of CA125, making the diagnosis difficult to distinguish from metastatic ovarian cancer.

Serum tests such as quantiferon gold have poor test characteristics in diagnosing active tuberculous peritonitis, especially in TB-endemic countries where Bacillus Calmette-Guérin (BCG) vaccine is still administered. A 6-month treatment course consisting of isoniazid, rifampin, pyrazinamide, and ethambutol for the first 8 weeks, followed by isoniazid and rifampin for the next 4 months, is considered adequate. More antituberculous drugs may be necessary, depending on local susceptibility testing and the emergence of resistant strains. The hepatotoxicity of the first-line drugs in cirrhotic patients may necessitate a change in drug therapy. Antituberculous therapy must be supervised carefully by public health personnel as well as physicians. Erratic treatment leads to emergence of resistant strains.

Peritonitis Associated With AIDS

With advances in antiretroviral therapy, there has been a several-fold reduction in the mortality rate from AIDS, a decline in the prevalence of opportunistic GI disease, and a major decrease in the number of operations for AIDS-related surgical illness (see Chapter 35).

Patients with AIDS may develop peritonitis from many different pathogens: bacteria (monomicrobial or polymicrobial); viruses (cytomegalovirus, herpes, and others) and fungal organisms (*Histoplasma*, cryptococci, and *Coccidioides*); parasites (*Pneumocystis jirovecii*, *Trypanosoma cruzi*); and mycobacteria (*M. tuberculosis* and *Mycobacterium avium-intracellulare*). Also, neoplastic lesions, such as Kaposi sarcoma and non-Hodgkin's lymphoma, may involve the peritoneum. Like other forms of peritonitis, the common features of presentation are abdominal pain, anorexia, fever, and ascites, which typically has a high protein content, occurring in an AIDS patient. The treatment of these opportunistic infections involving the peritoneum is generally pharmacologic (e.g., antibiotics, amphotericin B, and ganciclovir) unless bowel involvement has led to gut perforation, which may occur with cytomegalovirus, for example. Also, laparotomy may be indicated for obstructive symptoms, as with lymphoma. Bowel resection is required in this instance. HIV-infected patients with preserved immune function should be managed as with another patient with peritoneal disease.

Fitz-Hugh-Curtis Syndrome

Fitz-Hugh-Curtis syndrome, or perihepatitis (Fig. 37.4), was formerly most commonly associated with *Neisseria gonorrhoeae* infection. However, in recent years *Chlamydia trachomatis* is increasingly implicated in perihepatitis.[40] Chlamydia perihepatitis occurs only in women, owing to seeding of bacteria into the peritoneal cavity from the fallopian tubes. Symptoms in these patients include inflammatory ascites, pain in the right upper abdominal quadrant, fever, and a hepatic friction rub. If there is enough ascitic fluid to be clinically detectable, it has an elevated white cell count with a predominance of neutrophils and a high protein content, even in excess of 9 g/dL. Laparoscopy is very helpful in confirming the diagnosis, revealing "violin strings" and "bridal veil" adhesions from the abdominal wall to the liver (see Fig. 37.4). Doxycycline is usually curative. When these adhesions are an incidental finding during laparoscopy or laparotomy performed for another reason, no treatment is required.

Fungal and Parasitic Peritonitis

Fungal peritonitis can be due to gut perforation, especially perforation of the upper GI tract. It can also be a complication of

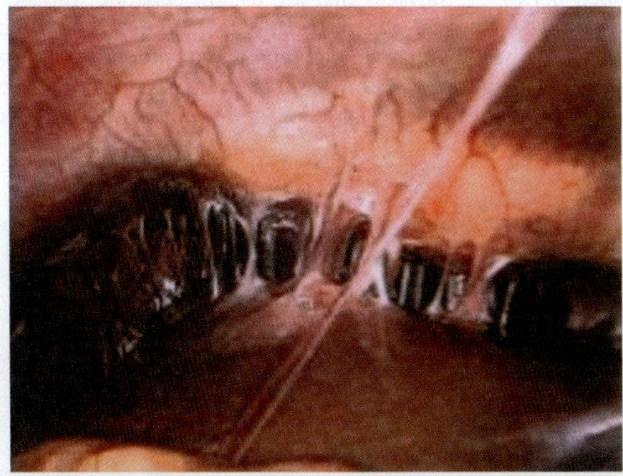

Fig. 37.4 Laparoscopic photograph of perihepatitis (Fitz-Hugh-Curtis syndrome) showing adhesions on the surface of the liver. (From Frumovitz MM. eMedicine.com, Inc.; 2004.)

acquired immunodeficiency (see Chapter 33). Fungal peritonitis may be limited to the pelvis in cases of a gynecologic source; this may be treated with fluconazole.[41] The most common isolates are *Candida* species, probably because routine blood culture media can detect *Candida*. As mentioned earlier, fungal peritonitis has occurred in patients undergoing CAPD.

Although rare, peritoneal histoplasmosis, coccidioidomycosis, and cryptococcal infection can be seen in the setting of AIDS. Schistosomiasis, pinworms, ascariasis, strongyloidiasis, and amebiasis also may involve the peritoneal cavity (see Chapters 115 and 116).

Starch Peritonitis

Years ago, approximately 1 of 1000 patients who underwent laparotomy developed fever and migratory abdominal pain 2–3 weeks postoperatively due to contamination of the peritoneum by glove powder starch. After 1980 manufacturers replaced cornstarch with more inert substances. Glove cornstarch potentiates wound infection, forms peritoneal adhesions, induces granulomatous peritonitis, and serves as a carrier of the latex allergen.[42] Glove powder granulomas also may mimic peritoneal carcinomatosis. These lesions should be biopsied and sent for frozen section if the etiology is in question and if the results could change the operative procedure. Starch peritonitis is a difficult diagnosis to make, and a high index of suspicion is required. Treatment is nonoperative, and glucocorticoids may be of benefit.

Rare Causes

Connective tissue diseases lead to peritonitis as a manifestation of serositis in approximately 5% of patients with lupus[43] and approximately 10% of patients with polyarteritis and scleroderma. Treatment of the underlying disease usually controls the serositis (see Chapter 35).

Familial Mediterranean fever is an autosomal recessive hereditary disease that affects the peritoneum, as well as other serous membranes. It is more frequently found in patients of Ashkenazi Jewish, Armenian, and Arabic ancestry. It is an aseptic form of recurrent peritonitis. Patients usually present with sporadic episodes of abdominal pain and fever; synovitis and pleuritis may also be present. Treatment with colchicine prevents attacks and renal amyloidosis (see Chapter 35).

INTRA-ABDOMINAL ADHESIONS

Formation of intra-abdominal adhesions, abnormal fibrous bands between peritoneal surfaces that are usually separate, can be the aftermath of secondary peritonitis and the surgery performed to correct it. Adhesions may be congenital, but the vast majority is acquired as result of peritoneal injury. Intraperitoneal foreign bodies such as suture material, clips, and mesh also contribute to adhesion formation. Intra-abdominal adhesions can be a considerable source of morbidity and mortality. They are the most common cause of small bowel obstruction (see Chapter 125). Adhesions are a leading cause of secondary infertility in women, accounting for 15%–20% of cases. Pelvic adhesions may be a source of chronic lower abdominal and pelvic pain. Adhesions may preclude peritoneal dialysis or intraperitoneal chemotherapy should they be necessary. Extensive adhesions may preclude laparoscopic procedures and have been shown to increase blood loss, operative time, and risk of enterotomy in reoperative surgery. These patients are then at increased risk for postoperative complications and prolonged hospital stay. The socioeconomic cost of adhesive disease is considerable.[44]

Formidable effort has been devoted to the prevention of adhesion formation. Tissue damage, hemorrhage, and inflammation in the peritoneal cavity lead to fibrin deposition on the peritoneal surfaces, allowing adjacent surfaces to adhere in this sticky matrix. Various strategies for prevention of adhesion formation include reduction of peritoneal injury, inhibition of the inflammatory response, prevention of fibrin formation, promotion of fibrinolysis, prevention of collagen deposition, and barrier separation of the peritoneal surfaces. Although various experimental strategies in animal experiments have reduced the number and severity of adhesions, few of these have translated into clinical practice. The preponderance of evidence in human as well as animal studies shows decreased adhesions at the incision sites and at the operative site in laparoscopic surgery compared with open surgery.[45] Seprafilm, a hyaluronic–carboxymethylcellulose membrane, has been shown in human trials to reduce intra-abdominal adhesions after general surgical procedures, but there has been no demonstrable reduction in subsequent bowel obstruction.[46] In patients undergoing gynecological surgery, low-quality evidence suggests that oxidized regenerated cellulose (Interceed), expanded PTFE (Gore-Tex) and Seprafilm may reduce adhesions, although the evidence is rather low quality.

PERITONEAL TUMORS

Tumors Metastatic to the Peritoneum

Metastatic cancer is by far the most common peritoneal tumor (Fig. 37.5). Tumors that preferentially metastasize to the peritoneum include adenocarcinomas of the ovary, stomach, colon and rectum, appendix, pancreas, and lobular carcinoma of the breast. Primary tumors of the peritoneum include mesothelioma and desmoplastic round-cell tumors.

Clinical Features

Patients with peritoneal metastases are often diagnosed late due to inadequate imaging. The pathognomonic manifestations of peritoneal metastases are ascites and malignant bowel and ureteral obstructions, which may occur independent of each other. Some

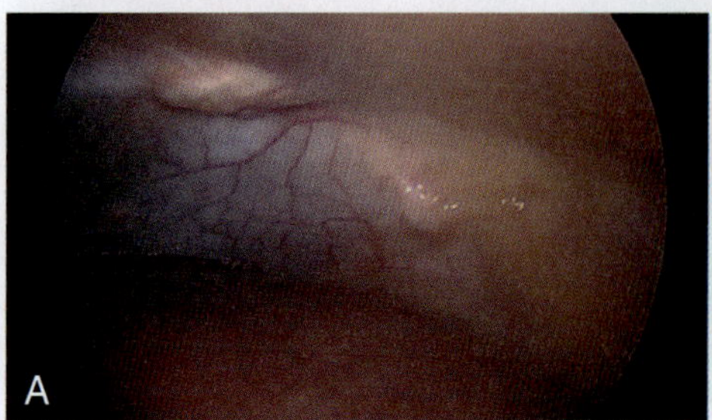

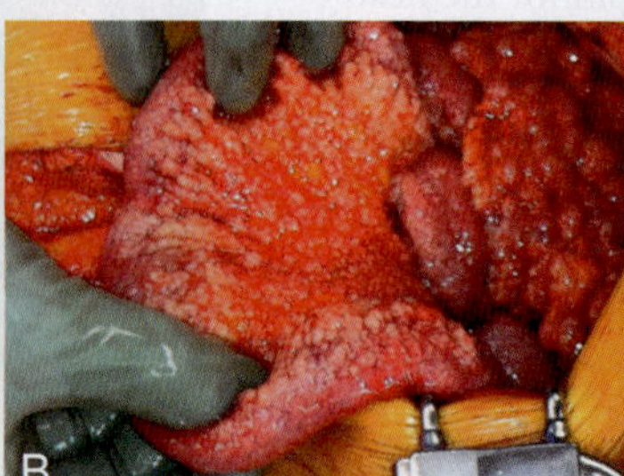

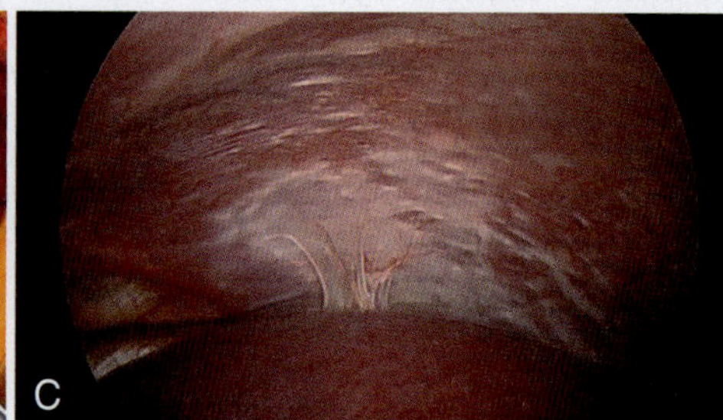

Fig. 37.5 Appearance of peritoneal metastases. (A) Nodular type metastases, (B) diffuse nodular metastases with mesenteric involvement, (C) scirrhous or scar-like metastases (commonest).

patients present with abdominal wall metastases (including umbilical nodules known by the eponym "Sister Mary Joseph" nodules) that are easy to detect. In patients with high risk of peritoneal metastases, such findings should promptly trigger a laparoscopy to examine the peritoneum.

Presence of such symptoms generally portend a worse prognosis, and interventions at this stage are generally limited in their therapeutic benefit with curative intent. This has led many investigators to attempt diagnosis of peritoneal metastases with proactive laparoscopies. The recent PROPHYLOCHIP trial is one such study, in which patients with high-risk colon cancers (perforated tumors, T4 lesions, and small burden peritoneal disease/tumor deposits) that underwent complete resection were randomized to second-look laparotomy after completing their chemotherapy if there was no peritoneal disease visible on imaging. Peritoneal metastases were diagnosed in 52% of patients.[47] Similar trials are underway for gastric and other solid tumor malignancies. The incidence of visualizing otherwise undetectable peritoneal metastases in resectable (and borderline resectable) pancreas cancer ranges from 8% to 20%.

Peritoneal fluid is generally not seen on conventional imaging studies. Thus the presence of peritoneal fluid in the absence of inflammatory processes is suspicious for metastases. Exudative ascites appears in patients as evidence of an advanced manifestation of a known tumor with a large tumor burden, rather than as a primary manifestation of cancer. Weight loss, abdominal pain, and early satiety are common. In the absence of peritoneal metastases, massive liver metastases, hepatocellular carcinoma with or without cirrhosis, malignant lymph node obstruction as in lymphoma, and Budd–Chiari syndrome with or without inferior vena cava obstruction are also associated with ascites. Ascitic fluid characteristics often allow their distinction, which is important because each may require different treatment (see Chapter 93 for details of pathogenesis and ascitic fluid analysis). Cytology can often detect peritoneal metastases (except in certain histologies such as mesothelioma) and the ascites is more often serous and mucinous than sanguineous (see Chapter 93).

Patients with ureteral obstruction are generally incidentally found to have hydronephrosis on imaging. Progression of hydronephrosis can lead to uremia, with nausea and vomiting mimicking bowel obstruction. Prompt relief of the obstruction with ureteral stents or percutaneous nephrostomy tubes can alleviate worsening renal dysfunction.

Malignant bowel obstruction is a common terminal event for patients presenting with peritoneal metastases. Commonly, there are multifocal areas of obstruction, although a dominant obstruction may be suggested. Patients often present with abdominal pain, cramping from closed-loop obstruction, and emesis. The sigmoid colon and proximal jejunum are common sites of obstruction from metastatic disease.

General Treatment

Management of patients with peritoneal metastases requires expertise and such patients are best managed in a multidisciplinary approach. Symptomatic management and early goal-setting are important and can facilitate decision making.

Surgery and Intraperitoneal Chemotherapy. Not all peritoneal metastases portend a poor prognosis. Some patients can be treated with curative intent depending on the burden of disease and histology.

Patients with low-grade appendiceal epithelial neoplasms, peritoneal mesothelioma (discussed later), low burden colorectal metastases, and ovarian cancers will often live at least 5 years, with a significant percentage of patients living 10 years or more.[48]

Techniques of cytoreductive surgery have been employed in the management of such patients and can include peritonectomy procedures in which the parietal peritoneum is systematically removed from the lining of the abdominal wall. Peritonectomy was previously considered a high-risk procedure, but advances in techniques and high volume centers have now yielded morbidity and mortality rates in line with other major oncological resections. Morbidity is directly related to the burden of disease, and hence early detection with proactive approaches might render these operations amenable to minimally invasive approaches. The achievement of complete cytoreduction is of significant therapeutic benefit.

The use of intraperitoneal chemotherapy in a single setting, such as *h*yperthermic *i*ntra*pe*ritoneal *c*hemotherapy, or HIPEC) or subsequent catheter-based intraperitoneal therapy has been widely used in patients with peritoneal metastases.[49] The use of HIPEC is well studied in patients with ovarian cancer, appendiceal epithelial neoplasms, mesothelioma, gastric and colorectal malignancies. The added use of intraperitoneal therapy increases 30 and 90 day morbidity and requires management by an experienced team. Management strategies in patients with peritoneally metastatic malignancies are outlined in Table 37.1.

Malignant Bowel Obstruction. The management of malignant bowel obstruction often requires placement of a nasogastric tube. Soft sialistic nasogastric tubes can provide more comfort than conventional Salem sump tubes. Supplemental management options include the use of octreotide, proton pump inhibitors (to reduce acid secretion), anticholinergics such as hyoscyamine to reduce spasms, and analgesia. Glucocorticoids have been suggested to reduce edema and nausea, providing an adjunct in nonoperative treatment. Surgical consultation is appropriate to determine whether intervention can be of therapeutic or palliative benefit. Early placement of gastrostomy tubes must be considered, especially since episodes of malignant obstruction frequently recur. Patients are generally counseled that 40%–80% of obstructions resolve spontaneously and that adherence to low-fiber diets may reduce future occurrences. Placement of endoluminal stents are generally futile in this setting due to the extent of extrinsic compression caused by tumor but may be considered in selected instances in consultation with a multidisciplinary team. Early attention to palliative care helps patients with symptom relief.

Therapeutic

Paracentesis. Therapeutic paracentesis for symptom palliation is performed for the majority of patients with peritoneal carcinomatosis. Repeated paracentesis often leads to protein calorie malnutrition, failure to thrive, and inanition. Patients who are considering hospice or end-of-life measures, benefit greatly from indwelling catheters that can be drained at home. The recommendation to use diuretics for treatment was based largely on supposition rather than hard data and should be restricted.

Pseudomyxoma Peritonei

Pseudomyxoma peritonei is not truly a diagnosis in and of itself but represents a syndrome of mucinous ascites that, while primarily associated with appendiceal epithelial neoplasms, can also occur with ovarian, pancreatic, colorectal, and gastric mucinous tumors. The histological origin of the mucinous ascites predicts the outcome. Presenting symptoms and signs are usually painless abdominal distention. Definitive diagnosis is made when characteristic jelly-like material is encountered at laparotomy or laparoscopy. When arising from appendiceal neoplasms, it is important to distinguish between low-grade appendiceal mucinous neoplasms (previously referred to as mucinous cystadenoma, mucocele) or

TABLE 37.1 Management Strategies in Peritoneal Surface Malignancies

Histological Subtype	Systemic Therapy	Cytoreductive Surgery	Regional Therapy
PRIMARY			
Primary peritoneal	Taxane/carboplatin (neoadjuvant/adjuvant)	Optimal cytoreduction	Intraperitoneal chemotherapy (cisplatin/paclitaxel) for optimally debulked patient ±HIPEC (cisplatin/carboplatin)
Malignant mesothelioma	Cisplatin/pemetrexed	Optimal cytoreduction	HIPEC (cisplatin /adriamycin/mitomycin-C)
DSRCT	Cyclophosphamide, doxorubicin, vincristine alternating with ifosfamide and etoposide Autologous stem cell rescue Whole abdominal radiation	Optimal cytoreduction	HIPEC (cisplatin)
SECONDARY			
Low-grade appendiceal neoplasms		Optimal cytoreduction	HIPEC (mitomycin-C)
High-grade appendiceal neoplasms (including goblet cell carcinoid, signet ring cell histology)	Fluoropyrimidine, oxaliplatin, irinotecan, anti-EGFR antibodies (cetuximab/panitumumab), anti-VEGF antibodies (bevacizumab)	Optimal cytoreduction	HIPEC (mitomycin-C)
Colorectal carcinoma	Fluoropyrimidine, oxaliplatin, irinotecan, anti-EGFR antibodies (cetuximab/panitumumab), anti-VEGF antibodies (bevacizumab)	Optimal cytoreduction	HIPEC (mitomycin-C/oxaliplatin)
Ovarian carcinoma	Taxane/carboplatin (neoadjuvant/adjuvant)	Optimal cytoreduction	Intraperitoneal chemotherapy (cisplatin/paclitaxel) for optimally debulked patient HIPEC (cisplatin)
Gastric carcinoma	Cisplatin/fluoropyrimidine Docetaxel/epirubicin Trastuzumab for HER2/neu+ tumors Checkpoint inhibitors	Optimal cytoreduction being investigated	±HIPEC (cisplatin/mitomycin-C) ±IP docetaxel/paclitaxel
Esophageal/pancreatic/hepatobiliary	Fluoropyrimidine/oxaliplatin/irinotecan Gemcitabine/cisplatin Nab-palitaxel Gastric regimens Checkpoint inhibitors		
Sarcomas (non-GIST)	Adriamycin/ifosfamide Eribulin Pazaponib	Optimal cytoreduction	±HIPEC (cisplatin/Adriamycin)
Sarcomas (GIST)	Tyrosine kinase inhibitors imatinib/sunitinib/pazopanib/regorafenib		

HIPEC, Hyperthermic intraperitoneal chemotherapy; *IP*, intraperitoneal.
From the American Cancer Society Oncology in Practice, Turaga KK (Feb 2018).

high-grade tumors including adenocarcinoma. This condition is effectively treated by cytoreductive surgery and HIPEC. Visceral resection including right hemicolectomy can be avoided in patients in whom complete cytoreductive surgery is possible without removing the colon because nodal metastases are rare.

Mesothelioma

Most (65%–70%) of mesotheliomas arise in the pleura, and 25% in the peritoneum. Most peritoneal mesotheliomas are malignant, associated with asbestos exposure, and detected 35–40 years after initial asbestos exposure. The families of asbestos workers are also at risk. Mesothelioma can have a rather indolent course in patients with well-differentiated papillary mesothelioma and multicystic mesotheliomas. Diagnosis is usually made at laparotomy or laparoscopy, but occasionally malignant mesothelial cells are found on ascitic fluid analysis. Patients with malignant peritoneal mesothelioma often harbor sporadic and occasionally germline BRCA-associated protein-1 mutations. Patients are best treated in a multidisciplinary setting. Cytoreductive surgery and HIPEC have been shown to improve survival with a 5 year survival ranging from 29% to 70%.[50]

PELVIC LIPOMATOSIS AND PERITONEAL CYSTS

Fat deposits normally found in the perirectal and perivesical spaces may develop nonmalignant overgrowth and are recognized as a distinct clinicopathologic entity, pelvic lipomatosis. It occurs predominantly in African-American men (male-to-female ratio 18:1) between 20 and 60 years of age and may cause or be associated with hypertension, cystitis, urinary tract obstruction, and occasionally GI symptoms.[51] The abnormal proliferation of fat is accompanied by varying degrees of fibrous reaction. Transrectal US and CT are important in diagnosis, particularly in differentiating pelvic lipomatosis from liposarcoma. The disease does not progress in most patients, although urinary tract obstruction may require diversion.

Peritoneal cysts are rare. Benign cystic lymphangiomas affect young men, present as mass lesions, and seldom recur after resection.

DISEASES OF THE MESENTERY AND OMENTUM

Diseases of the mesentery and omentum include, in decreasing order of frequency, hemorrhage, tumors and cysts, inflammatory and fibrotic conditions, and infarction. Mesenteric abscesses are covered in Chapter 29.

Hemorrhage

Mesenteric, intraperitoneal, and retroperitoneal bleeding and their complications can be classified as traumatic or spontaneous. Both types are aggravated by anticoagulation. Traumatic hematomas may or may not require surgical intervention, depending on the site of the lesion and whether the trauma was blunt or penetrating. The etiology of spontaneous hemorrhage can be due to gynecologic (e.g., ruptured ovarian cyst), hepatic (e.g., rupture of a hepatocellular carcinoma), splenic (e.g., rupture due to infection with Epstein–Barr virus), vascular (e.g., rupture of a splanchnic arterial aneurysm), and coagulopathic causes.[52]

Symptoms usually are pain and those from mass effects of the hematoma such as intestinal obstruction. Diagnosis depends on a high index of suspicion and US or CT, which demonstrates the collection of blood. A US-guided fine-needle aspiration (FNA) may help in confirming the diagnosis. Treatment consists of discontinuation of anticoagulants (in those being so treated) and reversal of anticoagulation. In others treatment is dictated by the local or systemic symptoms of hemorrhage. In certain cases, angiographic embolization may help treat intraperitoneal hemorrhage.[53]

Tumors

Tumors originating in the mesentery and omentum are rare and include soft tissue tumors (e.g., cysts, fibromas, sarcomas, and desmoids) and tumors specific to this site, such as leiomyomatosis peritonealis disseminata, and Castleman disease. Most tumors are large when detected in this site because of the large potential space in which they can grow. They may also be detected incidentally when an imaging study is performed for an unrelated reason. These typically present with nonspecific symptoms such as abdominal discomfort or low-grade obstructive symptoms.

Mesenteric Cysts

Mesenteric cysts are rare tumors that can arise in a variety of intra-abdominal locations and have a variable presentation. They occur in children and adults. These are typically large (averaging ~13 cm), fluid-filled (~2000 mL) and, despite their size, are malignant in only 3% of cases. The most common presenting symptom is pain (58%), and the most common physical finding is abdominal distention (68%).[54] Some cases may present with fever and chills, and others are asymptomatic, discovered incidentally, and misdiagnosed before laparotomy. If a small mesenteric cyst is found incidentally at laparotomy, it does not require resection. Excision is the treatment of choice for a cyst complication such as rupture or hemorrhage, and this may be performed laparoscopically. Mesenteric cysts are usually cured by complete excision (Fig. 37.6).

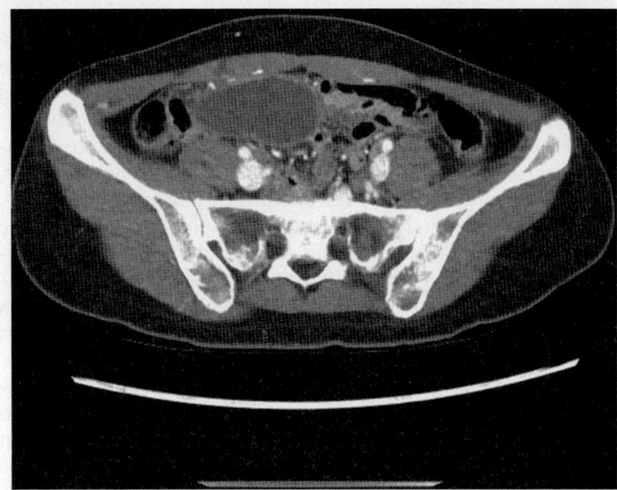

Fig. 37.6 Mesenteric cyst characterized by anatomical location and homogeneous appearance with fluid-filled density.

Solid Tumors

Solid tumors of the mesentery are less common than mesenteric cysts. Most (67%) are benign, including fibromas, xanthogranulomas, lipomas, leiomyomas, capillary and cavernous hemangiomas, neurofibromas, and mesenchymomas. Malignant tumors include hemangiopericytomas, fibrosarcomas, liposarcomas, leiomyosarcomas, and malignant mesenchymomas. Solid tumors of the omentum are remarkably similar in histologic type and prevalence of malignancy. Typical symptoms and signs of mesenteric and omental tumors include pain and distention with large lesions. Treatment is surgical resection. While about 18% of patients die of the tumor, the overall 5-year survival rate for patients with malignant tumors is only 21%.[55] Needle biopsy may be attempted with these tumors, although laparoscopy or laparotomy may be required for diagnosis as well as treatment.

Multifocal Leiomyomas (Leiomyomatosis Peritonealis Disseminata)

Multifocal leiomyomatous tumors are even less common than other tumors, can be malignant, and can mimic peritoneal carcinomatosis. They may appear together with other leiomyomatous lesions or endometriosis. These lesions consist of small, rubbery nodules and appear to be hormone sensitive, developing sometimes during pregnancy or on estrogen therapy and regressing with hormone withdrawal. These tumors can cause abdominal pain or GI bleeding. This condition must be differentiated from multifocal leiomyosarcoma that has been described to occur after uterine morcellation of endometrial sarcomas.

Castleman Disease

Castleman disease (giant or follicular lymph node hyperplasia) is rare. There is considerable heterogeneity in the disease, but it is classified in unicentric and multicentric forms. Castleman disease is caused in some cases by infection with human herpesvirus 8 (HHV-8). The central lymph nodes of the mesentery or mediastinum are more frequently involved in the unicentric form of the disease. In this form, the surgical removal of the mass is successful and prognosis is good. The multicentric form is treated with systemic therapies with variable success. The prognosis is considerably worse, with patients at risk for conversion to frank lymphoma.[56]

Inflammatory and Fibrotic Conditions

Inflammatory conditions of the retroperitoneum are heterogeneous and their understanding is evolving. Recent advances in the understanding of this field has suggested that these are manifestations of IgG4-related disease, characterized by a lymphoplasmacytic infiltrate, obliterative phlebitis, and moderate eosinophilia (Chapter 37). Other IgG4-related diseases include autoimmune cholangitis, autoimmune pancreatitis, and Riedel thyroiditis among others.[57]

Inflammatory conditions of the retroperitoneum are histologically classified into three basic diseases: retractile mesenteritis, mesenteric panniculitis, and retroperitoneal fibrosis.

Retractile mesenteritis represents the fibrotic end of the spectrum and has been known as sclerosing mesenteritis, multifocal subperitoneal sclerosis, fibromatosis, and mesenteric desmoid tumor (Fig. 37.7). The inflammatory end of the spectrum has been called mesenteric panniculitis, mesenteric lipodystrophy, lipogranuloma of the mesentery, liposclerotic mesenteritis, mesenteric Weber-Christian disease, and systemic nodular panniculitis. There have been attempts to subclassify this disease into diffuse, single, and multiple forms and to suggest an association with lymphoma.[58]

Overlapping names such as sclerosing lipogranuloma, the well-documented progression and conversion of mesenteric panniculitis to retractile mesenteritis over a 12-year period, and the concurrence of sclerosing mesenteritis and retroperitoneal fibrosis indicate that these are simply stages of one common underlying process.

Although mesenteric panniculitis and retractile mesenteritis are usually manifested by abdominal pain, symptoms of gut obstruction, and a mass lesion, cases associated with prolonged high-grade fever and autoimmune hemolytic anemia without abdominal symptoms have been described. Retractile mesenteritis and mesenteric panniculitis are always idiopathic, but retroperitoneal fibrosis has a cause approximately 30% of the time, including drugs, malignancy, trauma, or inflammation. Most of the reported cases have been drug induced (methysergide and ergotamine). The process of fibrosis may lead to ureteral or vascular obstruction.

Histologically, retractile mesenteritis and mesenteric panniculitis can have inflammation with lymphocytes and neutrophils, fat necrosis, fibrosis, and calcification. In contrast, only mesenteric panniculitis has multinucleate giant cells, cholesterol clefts, lipid-laden macrophages, and lymphangiectasia. Retroperitoneal fibrosis consists of dense connective tissue, with or without inflammation. The presence of IgG4 plasma cells, storiform fibrosis, and obliterative phlebitis should prompt evaluation for an IgG4-related fibrosis.

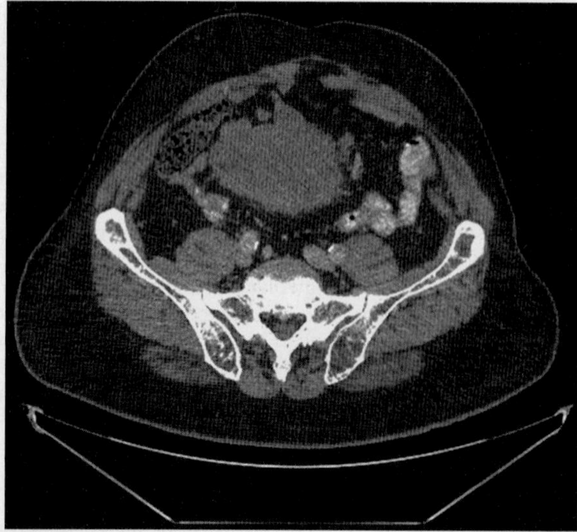

Fig. 37.7 Axial CT section of a patient with a mesenteric desmoid tumor.

Diagnosis and Treatment

These diseases were previously only recognized at laparotomy or autopsy; however, noninvasive techniques such as CT (Fig. 37.8) or MRI may assist in preoperative diagnosis. Radiologic findings suggestive of mesenteric panniculitis have been found in 0.6% of patients in a large series of abdominal CT scans.[59] There was a female predominance and an association with malignancy in 34 of 49 patients with radiologic features of mesenteric panniculitis. Patients with retroperitoneal fibrosis often present with hydronephrosis.

Retroperitoneal fibrosis is more common in men and typically causes the ureters to deviate medially on radiographic evaluation. Treatment usually consists of removal of the offending agent and a trial course of glucocorticoids (see Fig. 37.8). The use of rituximab has shown promising results in early phase II trials. Often surgical intervention can be avoided except when encased ureters cannot be managed by endoluminal stents. Treatment may be necessary in patients with retractile mesenteritis if it obstructs the intestine. Administration of progesterone has been reported to downregulate fibrogenesis. The prognosis of patients with retroperitoneal fibrosis seems to be better than in the past.

Infarction of the Omentum

Infarction of the omentum occurs when a portion of the omentum twists around a narrow vascular pedicle. If a diagnosis by imaging techniques (e.g., CT and US) is achieved preoperatively, conservative management can be pursued. However, the diagnosis is difficult, often delayed, and sometimes made only at surgery. Laparoscopic resection of the necrotic mass is curative.

Epiploic Appendagitis

Epiploic appendagitis (primary inflammation of the colonic epiploic appendices) is an entity that is occasionally seen and is often confused with the diagnosis of appendicitis. The diagnosis of epiploic appendagitis requires a high index of suspicion. It typically presents with right lower quadrant abdominal pain. However, constitutional symptoms, such as nausea, vomiting, and anorexia, are less frequent, and the pain tends to have a more sudden onset. The patient can typically locate the exact location of the pain with one finger, and the point of tenderness and pain tends to be more localized and slightly more cephalad than in appendicitis. Epiploic appendagitis can be diagnosed by CT, and the treatment is nonoperative if the diagnosis can be made.

DISEASES OF THE DIAPHRAGM

Hernias and Eventrations

Diaphragmatic hernias consist of herniation of an abdominal organ through the diaphragm into the thorax and are discussed in detail in Chapter 27. Eventration is not a true hernia but consists of a localized weakness in the dome of the diaphragm that can lead to bulging of abdominal viscera into the thorax. This is usually an incidental finding on chest films, but large eventrations can cause shortness of breath by loss of lung volume on the affected side and mediastinal shift to the unaffected side. Symptomatic patients can be surgically corrected with thoracoscopic plication of the diaphragm.

Tumors

Diaphragmatic tumors are usually of connective tissue origin and may be benign or malignant or may consist of simple cysts. They are often detected by screening chest films or in evaluation of pleuritic chest pain. Surgical resection involves a consideration of

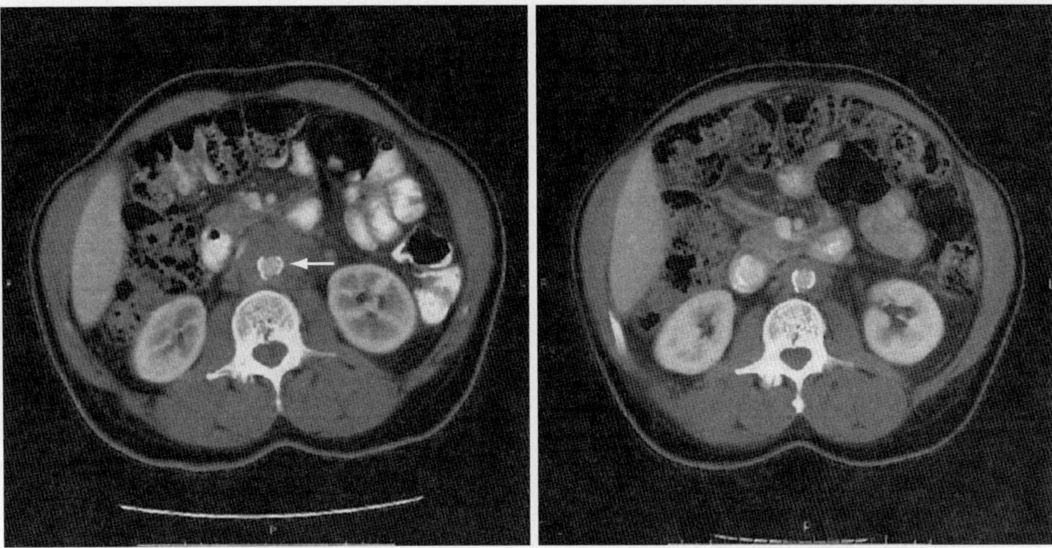

Fig. 37.8 CT of the abdomen in a 63-year-old man with nausea, periumbilical pain, and a 10-pound weight loss. The scan on the *left* shows a soft tissue mass in the retroperitoneum encasing the aorta *(arrow)*. Open biopsy of the mass showed inflammation and fibrosis with no evidence of tumor, which is compatible with retroperitoneal fibrosis. Symptoms resolved, and the mass regressed on glucocorticoid therapy. The scan on the *right* was taken 9 months after diagnosis and therapy. (Courtesy Jeffrey H. Phillips, MD, Dallas, TX.)

a thoracic or an abdominal approach with preservation of the phrenic nerve.

Hiccups

Hiccups are quick inhalations that follow abrupt rhythmic involuntary contractions of the diaphragm and closure of the glottis. When they last only a few minutes, they are considered a form of physiologic myoclonus. For persistent hiccups (defined as >48 hours duration), home remedies include breath-holding, sudden fright, rebreathing from a paper bag, eating dry granulated sugar, and drinking cold liquids. Intractable hiccups (defined as >1 month duration) can be familial and are usually due to diaphragmatic irritation, gastric distention, thoracic or central nervous system irritation or tumors, hyponatremia, or other metabolic derangements.

There is a paucity of evidence to guide therapy among attempted treatments, including acupuncture, pharmacologic agents, noninvasive phrenic nerve stimulation, phrenic nerve crush, or implantable diaphragmatic pacemakers. Drugs that have been reported to be successful include chlorpromazine, metoclopramide, quinidine, phenytoin, valproic acid, baclofen, sertraline, gabapentin, and nifedipine. Postoperative hiccups after abdominal surgery may be due to subphrenic abscess or other sources of diaphragmatic irritation such as acute gastric dilatation, and this should be considered before assuming a more benign cause.

LAPAROSCOPY IN THE EVALUATION OF PERITONEAL DISEASES

General Considerations

Diagnostic laparoscopy, as first described by Kelling in 1901, is a safe and effective means of evaluating the abdominal cavity. It allows direct visualization of the liver surface, peritoneal lining, and mesentery for directed biopsies. Ascitic fluid can be collected easily. Although less invasive imaging techniques such as CT have reduced its necessity, laparoscopy continues to have a role in the evaluation of liver and peritoneal diseases. In a large retrospective review of diagnostic laparoscopy, the procedure had a mortality rate of 0% and an overall morbidity rate of 1.2%. Possible complications include prolonged abdominal pain, vasovagal reaction, viscus perforation, bleeding (either from biopsy sites or within abdominal wall), splenic laceration, ascites fluid leakage, and fever. It has been shown in animal models of peritonitis that abdominal insufflation during laparoscopy could increase bacterial translocation,[60] raising the concern that laparoscopy is dangerous in the clinical setting of septic peritonitis. Despite these concerns, laparoscopy is becoming a common technique in patients requiring operation for diseases causing peritonitis. The adverse hemodynamic consequences of abdominal insufflation can be overcome in the vast majority of patients with aggressive resuscitation and careful anesthetic management. A laparoscopic approach has been effective in treating perforated gastroduodenal ulcer. Laparoscopic appendectomy is advocated as the treatment of choice for patients with acute appendicitis and complicated appendicitis. Laparoscopic cholecystectomy is safe and effective treatment of acute cholecystitis. Laparoscopic colectomy can be performed for complicated diverticulitis.[60] Evidence-based guidelines for the application of laparoscopic operation in surgical peritonitis have been developed.

Evaluation of Ascites of Unknown Origin

Clinical presentation, conventional laboratory examinations, and ascitic fluid analysis identify the cause of ascites in the majority of patients (see Chapter 93). However, conventional paracentesis occasionally fails to make a diagnosis. In these instances, diagnostic laparoscopy affords direct and sensitive technique for obtaining specimens for histology and culture. In the United States, occult cirrhosis and peritoneal malignancy account for the majority of cases. In studies from Asian countries, peritoneal malignancy is also the most common cause of unexplained ascites, but tuberculous peritonitis accounts for an increasing number of cases. In patients with AIDS, peritoneal involvement may result from a variety of opportunistic infections and neoplasms (see the earlier section and Chapter 33). Non-Hodgkin's lymphoma accounts for the majority of these peritoneal lesions revealed by laparoscopy, but *M. tuberculosis*, *M. avium-intracellulare*, and *P. jirovecii* may be revealed.

Staging Laparoscopy

Laparoscopy has found increasing utility in the staging of malignant solid tumors of the GI tract (Fig. 37.9). Diagnostic laparoscopy coupled with laparoscopic US, peritoneal fluid cytology, and biopsy allow for an improved selection of patients that will benefit from larger, definitive operations for curative intent. In GI malignancies, the use of diagnostic laparoscopy finds that some patients with potentially resectable disease have metastatic or locally advanced disease and can be spared unnecessary laparotomy with both reduction of costs and preservation of quality of life.[62] In laparoscopic staging for pancreatic cancer, 11%–48% of patients will be shown to have metastatic disease after an initial negative CT. Laparoscopic staging has been recommended for gastric cancer and changes management for 12%–60% of patients.[63] The finding of metastatic disease on staging laparoscopy in esophageal and gastric cancers may obviate the need for palliative operations.

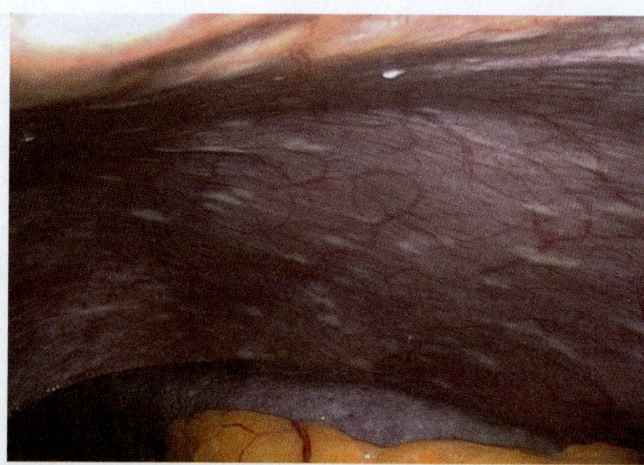

Fig. 37.9 Laparoscopy revealing left hemidiaphgramatic disease not visualized on preoperative imaging.

Full references for this chapter can be found at https://ebooks.health.elsevier.com.

38 Gastrointestinal and Hepatic Disorders in the Pregnant Patient

Clara Y. Tow, John F. Reinus

IN THIS CHAPTER

GASTROINTESTINAL AND HEPATIC FUNCTION IN NORMAL PREGNANCY

The GI tract undergoes dramatic modifications during pregnancy. Intra-abdominal organs move to accommodate uterine growth, hormonal factors alter motility, and the immunologic adaptation to pregnancy affects response to disease. Heartburn, nausea, abdominal cramps, and altered bowel habits, the most common GI symptoms of pregnant women, are caused by normal physiologic changes in gut motility. These symptoms are usually transitory and easily treated with conservative measures. It may be a challenge, however, to distinguish between symptoms of pregnancy-induced altered motility and those that signal the onset or worsening of problems that require immediate medical attention.

Esophageal Function

The amplitude and duration of esophageal muscle contractions in pregnant and nonpregnant women are similar.[1] In the distal esophagus, the velocity of peristaltic waves decreases by approximately one-third during pregnancy but remains within the normal range.[2] In contrast, resting lower esophageal sphincter tone progressively declines during gestation, most likely a consequence of inhibition of smooth muscle contraction by progesterone.[2–4] This effect coupled with increased abdominal pressure during gestation is responsible for the gastroesophageal reflux symptoms that occur in 70% of pregnant women.[5]

GI Function

The effects of pregnancy on gastric motility are unclear. Delayed gastric emptying has been demonstrated by some authors, especially during delivery,[6] whereas no effect on gastric emptying has been found by others.[7] Estrogen inhibits acetylcholine-induced contraction of gastric smooth muscle cells.[8] Pregnant women have normal gastric secretion.[9] The absorptive capacity of the small intestine increases during pregnancy to meet the metabolic demands of the fetus. Animal experiments have revealed pregnancy-induced increases in small intestinal weight and villous height in conjunction with mucosal hypertrophy.[10,11] The activity of some brush border enzymes increases during lactation and then decreases after weaning.[12,13] Increased absorption of calcium, amino acids, and vitamins has been demonstrated.[14–17] Furthermore, intestinal transit time is prolonged during gestation, particularly during the third trimester, and is associated with slowing of the migrating motor complex.[18,19] Colonic transit time is prolonged in pregnant animals as well. Progesterone is thought to have a direct inhibitory effect on gut smooth muscle cells that slows motility.[20] A role for endogenous opioids has also been suggested.[21] Together, these changes often result in mild physiologic constipation.

Immune Function and the Intestinal Microbiota

During pregnancy, the maternal immune system must adapt to the presence of the fetus. Adaptive changes can influence the response to infection and modulate the course of underlying autoimmune disease. There is a shift from cellular to humoral responses, with downregulation of Th1 and upregulation of Th2 cytokines. Pregnancy modulates natural killer cell cytotoxicity and induces T-regulatory cells that affect the maternal immune response.[22,23] Unfortunately, we still do not understand the effects of pregnancy on the mechanisms responsible for autoimmune diseases such as autoimmune hepatitis and Crohn's disease well enough to allow us to predict clinical outcomes during pregnancy. The maternal intestinal flora changes during pregnancy, potentially altering the host-microbial interaction in a beneficial fashion.[24] Bacteria from the mother colonize the neonate's gut, establishing the microbiota with potential long-lasting health consequences.[25] Although the establishment of the human GI microbiota previously was thought to begin at birth, the finding of bacterial products in meconium, placenta, and amniotic fluid suggests that seeding occurs in utero.[26,27]

Gallbladder Function

Pregnancy causes an alteration in bile composition, including cholesterol supersaturation, decreased chenodeoxycholic acid, increased cholic acid concentrations, and increased size of the bile acid pool.[28] These changes are associated with greater residual gallbladder volumes in the fasting as well as fed states. Sex-steroid hormones may inhibit gallbladder contraction in pregnant women, promoting precipitation of cholesterol crystals and stone formation.[29,30]

Hepatic Function

During pregnancy, maternal blood volume increases progressively until week 30 of gestation when it is 50% greater than normal and remains so until confinement.[31] This volume expansion, attributed to the effects of steroid hormones and elevated plasma levels of aldosterone and renin, is responsible for dilution of some blood constituents such as red blood cells (physiologic anemia). As a result, total serum protein concentrations diminish 20% by mid-pregnancy, largely as a result of a reduced serum albumin level. Maternal proteins passively diffuse across the placenta to the fetal circulation.[32] Similarly, alpha fetal fetoprotein (AFP) moves across the placenta from the fetal to the maternal circulation and raises maternal serum levels. Active transport may be involved in the transplacental movement of some macromolecules.

Despite increases in maternal blood volume, the levels of many serum proteins measured to assess hepatic injury are unchanged or even increased during gestation. Progesterone causes a proliferation of smooth endoplasmic reticulum, whereas estrogens promote the formation of rough endoplasmic reticulum and associated protein synthesis. Pregnant women synthesize the products of the cytochrome P450 gene superfamily and other proteins at an accelerated rate, including coagulation factors, binding globulins, and ceruloplasmin.[33] Maternal serum alkaline phosphatase levels are normally elevated during the third trimester of pregnancy, largely due to placental production; for this reason, measurement of alkaline phosphatase in pregnant women is only of clinical use early in gestation. Alterations in maternal concentrations of plasma proteins may persist for several months postpartum. Mild leukocytosis and increased erythrocyte sedimentation rates are also common in normal pregnancy.

DRUG SAFETY IN PREGNANT PATIENTS

Patients and physicians tend to avoid treatment with medications during pregnancy because they fear harming the fetus.[34,35] No medication or other therapeutic intervention can be considered definitely safe during pregnancy. Withholding medical intervention, however, may adversely affect the mother's health and the pregnancy outcome. The placenta is not a reliable barrier to the passage of most drugs. The distribution of a drug within the fetal compartment cannot be accurately predicted. Data on long-term effects of in utero fetal drug exposure are practically impossible to collect. The necessity of any proposed drug therapy should be discussed with the patient, and known and unknown risks of treatments must be carefully evaluated. For this reason, the FDA in 2014 required a change in the content and format of prescription-drug labels required by the Physician Labeling Rule.[36] Letter categories (A, B, C, D, X) are no longer used. Instead, the FDA now requires labels to contain a narrative explanation of risk and supporting data.

ENDOSCOPY DURING PREGNANCY

It is estimated that 20,000 pregnant women undergo endoscopy each year.[37] Recommendations concerning endoscopy in this setting are largely based on expert opinion and case reports.[38] Although the safety of endoscopy during pregnancy has not been completely established, it is performed routinely if there is a clear indication.[39] Pregnant women have safely undergone EGD, colonoscopy, sigmoidoscopy, ERCP, and percutaneous gastroscopy.[40] Although a recent large Swedish cohort study found endoscopy during pregnancy to be associated with an increased risk of preterm birth or small-for-gestational-age neonates, the authors concluded that the risks were small and likely due to intrafamilial factors or disease activity and not because of endoscopy alone.[41] In addition to general contraindications to endoscopic procedures, specific contraindications during pregnancy include imminent or threatened delivery, ruptured membranes, placental abruption, and pregnancy-induced hypertension.[42]

Several precautions should be observed to avoid complications when performing endoscopy in a pregnant patient.[42] Given the extreme sensitivity of the fetus to maternal hypoxia, pregnant women should receive supplemental oxygen with continuous saturation monitoring. When the fetus is capable of surviving outside the uterus, usually around 24 weeks of gestation, maternal monitoring for contractions before, during, and after invasive procedures is advisable to enable prompt delivery if fetal distress occurs. In the second and third trimesters, the supine position and external abdominal pressure should be avoided because resulting compression of the vena cava and aorta may cause hypotension and placental hypoperfusion. ERCP should be performed only with therapeutic intent and by expert endoscopists. Every effort should be made to avoid fetal radiation (see later).[40] Opioid (narcotic) analgesics cross the placenta, and benefits during endoscopy must be weighed against risks for the mother (see Chapter 40) and the fetus. Sedation with benzodiazepines should be avoided, especially during the first trimester, because diazepam has been reported to cause fetal malformations.[43,44] Extensive experience with propofol is lacking, and its high lipid solubility is a reason for concern.[45] Lactating patients are advised to avoid breastfeeding and to discard breast milk for 4 hours after a procedure requiring sedation.[42]

IMAGING AND RADIATION EXPOSURE DURING PREGNANCY

The National Commission on Radiation Protection recommends limiting exposure to ionizing radiation during pregnancy to less than 5 cGy.[46] Well-referenced guidelines for imaging of pregnant women with ionizing radiation have been published by the American College of Radiology Guidelines and Standards Committee[47] and by the American College of Obstetricians and Gynecologists Committee on Obstetric Practice.[48] The potential for radiation damage to the fetus is determined by dose and gestational age at the time of exposure (Table 38.1).

CT should be performed only when its potential benefits clearly outweigh its risks and should be done, if possible, after completion of organogenesis.[49] Helical CT may be associated with less fetal radiation exposure than conventional CT. MRI is often a superior alternative to CT; MRI without contrast has not been associated with adverse pregnancy outcomes, and magnetic fields are not considered harmful to living organisms.[50] There is a

TABLE 38.1 Fetal Effects of Radiation During Gestation

Gestational Age (Days)	Effects of Radiation
0–9	Death
13–50	Teratogenesis
	Growth restriction
51–280	Growth restriction
	CNS abnormalities
	Possible cancer risk

*Effects listed are related to dose of radiation also.

theoretical risk of thermal injury to the fetus from MRI in early pregnancy, though clinical studies have shown that MRI without contrast is safe in the first trimester.[51] Contrast agents may cross the placenta, and their safety in pregnant women has not been formally assessed. Neonatal hypothyroidism has been associated with use of some iodinated agents. Paramagnetic contrast agents used during MRI (e.g., gadolinium) have not been studied in pregnant women. While chelated gadolinium is generally considered safe, free gadolinium is toxic. Prolonged, high doses of gadolinium-based products in the amniotic fluid increase the potential for gadolinium to dissociate from the chelate.[48] Animal studies have shown teratogenicity at high doses; however, a large retrospective clinical study found no increased risk of fetal or neonatal death or neonatal intensive care admission with gadolinium exposure.[52] Given controversial and limited data, the American College of Obstetricians and Gynecologists Committee on Obstetric Practice suggests only using gadolinium in limited situations where benefits clearly outweigh the possible risks.[48] Less than 0.04% of a dose of gadolinium-labeled contrast is excreted in breast milk during the first 24 hours after administration, and a negligible amount of this is absorbed from the infant GI tract.[53] Therefore breastfeeding should not be interrupted after imaging with gadolinium. US is widely used and safe during pregnancy.

GI DISORDERS AND PREGNANCY

Nausea, Vomiting, and Hyperemesis Gravidarum

In the first trimester, 60%–70% of pregnant women report having some nausea, and more than 40% report vomiting (see Chapter 16).[54,55] Onset of these symptoms is typically in the 4th to 6th week of gestation, with a peak occurrence in the 8th to 12th week and resolution by week 20. Although nausea and vomiting may vary from mild to severe, most affected individuals are still able to obtain adequate oral nutrition and hydration, in some cases by eating frequent small meals of dry starchy foods. Hp infection in pregnant women may contribute to the development of vomiting.[56]

Severe persistent vomiting demanding medical intervention, or *hyperemesis gravidarum*, is less common, occurring in 2% or less of pregnancies.[57,58] Hyperemesis is accompanied by fluid, electrolyte, and acid-base imbalances, nutritional deficiency, and weight loss and is defined by the presence of ketonuria and a 5% decrease from prepregnancy weight. It may be associated with pyrosis, hematemesis, and hypersalivation (ptyalism).[59] Although the prognosis of hyperemesis gravidarum is generally favorable, severe untreated disease may lead to significant maternal and fetal morbidity.[60] Symptoms usually begin at weeks 4–5 and improve by weeks 14–16 of gestation. In up to 20% of affected patients, however, vomiting persists until delivery.[61] Hyperemesis frequently recurs in subsequent pregnancies. Reported risk factors for hyperemesis include a personal or family history of the disorder, a female fetus, multiple gestation, gestational trophoblastic disease, fetal trisomy 21, hydrops fetalis, and maternal infection.[62,63]

The etiology of hyperemesis gravidarum is likely multifactorial, including contributions by hormonal changes, GI dysmotility, Hp infection, and psychosocial factors. A genetic predisposition is suggested by familial clusters of the disease. Pregnancy-related hormones, specifically HCG and estrogen, have been implicated as important causes of hyperemesis.[64] Symptoms worsen during periods of peak HCG concentrations, and conditions associated with higher serum HCG levels, such as multiple gestation, trophoblastic disease, and trisomy 21, are associated with an increased incidence of hyperemesis.[65] Elevated serum estrogen concentrations, as seen in obese patients, have also been associated with this disorder.[66] Estrogen and progesterone are thought to cause nausea and vomiting by altering gastric motility and slowing GI transit time.[67] Other hormones implicated in the pathogenesis of hyperemesis include thyroid hormones and gut-derived hormones, ghrelin, and leptin.[68,69] Abnormal thyroid function test results are found in two-thirds of patients with hyperemesis gravidarum.[70] The alpha subunit of HCG has thyroid-stimulating hormone-like activity that suppresses endogenous thyroid-stimulating hormone release and causes a slight rise in free thyroxine (T_4) levels.[71] Despite these findings, this transient gestational thyrotoxicosis is not associated with unfavorable pregnancy outcomes and does not usually require treatment. An increased risk of hyperemesis has been found in two meta-analyses of *Helicobacter pylori* infection during pregnancy.[72,73] Some authors have documented symptomatic improvement in pregnant patients with vomiting after *H. pylori* eradication.[74,75]

Vomiting in patients with hyperemesis gravidarum is often triggered by olfactory and even auditory and visual stimuli. A pregnancy-unique quantification of nausea and emesis (PUQE score) can be used to evaluate the number of hours of nausea and the number of episodes of emesis and retching per day in affected women and is helpful in tailoring therapy.[76] Hospital admission for IV fluid and electrolyte replacement and, sometimes, nutritional support is indicated when affected individuals develop hypotension, tachycardia, ketosis, weight loss, or muscle wasting. Abnormal laboratory test results in such patients include hypokalemia, hyponatremia, and ketonuria. Hyperemesis is associated with slight increases in serum aminotransferase and bilirubin levels in 25%–40% of cases. Hyperamylasemia, seen in a quarter of affected patients, is caused by excessive salivary gland production stimulated by prolonged vomiting.[77]

Severe hyperemesis gravidarum is associated with poor maternal and fetal outcomes. In a study of more than 150,000 singleton pregnancies, infants born to women with hyperemesis who had gained less than 7 kg of weight during pregnancy were more likely to have low birth weights, be premature and small for gestational age, and to have low Apgar scores.[57] These findings were confirmed by meta-analysis.[78] Severe, albeit rare, maternal complications of hyperemesis include Mallory-Weiss tears with upper GI bleeding, Boerhaave syndrome, Wernicke encephalopathy with or without Korsakoff psychosis, central pontine myelinolysis, retinal hemorrhage, and spontaneous pneumomediastinum.[79] Patients with hyperemesis may have depression and post-traumatic stress disorder during pregnancy and postpartum.[80] Lastly, severe depression after elective termination of pregnancy has been reported.[81] Fortunately, mortality from severe hyperemesis gravidarum has declined in the last decade and is likely attributable to early intervention with modern therapies.[60]

Given the potential for morbidity and mortality in hyperemesis gravidarum, affected individuals should be treated aggressively. Obstetric management should be overseen, if possible, by physicians qualified in maternal-fetal medicine. The goals of therapy are maintenance of adequate maternal fluid intake and nutrition as well as symptom control. Patients should be advised to eat multiple small meals as tolerated and to avoid an empty stomach, which may trigger nausea. Also, avoidance of offensive odors, separation of ingestion of solid and liquid foods, and consumption of a high-carbohydrate diet may be helpful.[82] Antiemetic and antireflux medications are first-line pharmacologic therapy for outpatients who have failed dietary modifications. Ginger, phenothiazines (chlorpromazine and prochlorperazine), the dopamine antagonist metoclopramide, and pyridoxine (vitamin B_6) have proved beneficial in this setting.[83,84] Extensive data show lack of teratogenesis and good fetal safety for many of these drugs.[85–87] Treatment with ondansetron, a 5-hydroxytryptamine-3 (5-HT_3) receptor antagonist, or metoclopramide should be considered in patients who do not respond to the above measures.[88] The safety of ondansetron therapy during pregnancy is supported by a controlled trial,[89] case reports, and widespread clinical experience. Glucocorticoids may benefit individuals with severe symptoms. Failure of oral medical therapy can be managed in the home setting with IV fluid replacement, medications, and multivitamins. It should be noted, however, that as many as 50% of pregnant patients treated through central venous catheters, including those peripherally inserted, have catheter-related complications,[90] most likely as a result of the relative hypercoagulable state and increased susceptibility to infections seen in pregnant women. Enteral feeding through a nasoenteric tube or surgically placed feeding tube is sometimes required to maintain maternal nutrition.[91]

GERD

GERD, also referred to as pyrosis, commonly occurs in pregnancy (see Chapter 48). By the end of the third trimester, 50%–80% of pregnant patients have had new, or an exacerbation of preexisting, heartburn.[92,93] Pyrosis, however, is rarely accompanied by overt esophagitis or its complications.[94] Pregnant women with heartburn may also have nausea and vomiting as well as atypical reflux symptoms, such as persistent cough and wheezing. Symptoms may develop at any time during pregnancy, with a peak incidence in the third trimester.[95] Symptoms may persist until delivery and may be predictive of recurrent GERD later in life.[92] Risk factors for reflux include multiparity, older maternal age, and reflux complicating a prior pregnancy.[5,92,96] The contributions of pre-pregnancy BMI and excessive weight gain are controversial.[97]

The pathogenesis of GERD in pregnant women is related to the effects of gestational hormones on esophageal motility, lower esophageal sphincter tone, and gastric emptying. Compression of the stomach and increased intra-abdominal pressure caused by the enlarging uterus also contribute to the development of this disorder.

EGD is rarely required for the assessment of pregnant women with symptoms of GERD.[98] There are no data assessing the use of 24-hour ambulatory pH monitoring in this setting, and use of a barium esophagogram is undesirable because it entails fetal radiation exposure. Thus evaluation of suspected GERD in a pregnant woman depends on the clinical experience and judgment of the physician and requires due consideration of the patient's history and all potential, reasonable causes for the patient's present symptoms.

Mild reflux symptoms can often be controlled by modifications of diet and lifestyle. Liquid antacids and sucralfate are prescribed as first-line pharmacologic therapy.[99] Magnesium-containing antacids should be avoided during the late third trimester because they theoretically may impair labor. Ranitidine remains the treatment of choice for patients who have persistent heartburn despite liquid antacid therapy.[100] PPIs should be reserved for refractory cases. A large population study and two meta-analyses have found no significant risk of fetal malformations in babies exposed to PPIs during the first trimester of pregnancy.[101,102] Omeprazole, however, has dose-related neonatal fetal toxicity in rats and rabbits and is avoided in clinical use.[103] An association between use of PPIs or H2RAs by pregnant women and development of childhood asthma in their offspring has been noted in a survey of Danish medical registries,[104] but the significance of this observation is unclear. The pro-motility agent metoclopramide has not been used extensively to treat GERD during gestation, although it is used during obstetric anesthesia and to treat hyperemesis gravidarum.

PUD

Case studies and retrospective series suggest that the incidence of peptic ulcer disease (PUD) is lower in pregnant women than in nonpregnant individuals (see Chapter 55).[105,106] This finding may be related to decreased use of NSAIDs by cautious patients or possibly to increased use of antacid medications to treat nausea or heartburn. It is conceivable, though equally unproven, that gestational steroids promote GI mucosal cytoprotection. PUD is likely underdiagnosed during pregnancy, given the reluctance of physicians to perform diagnostic tests on pregnant women. Gastric acid secretion and the natural history of Hp infection, as far as we know, are not altered by gestation.

The dyspeptic symptoms that often accompany pregnancy, especially nausea, vomiting, and heartburn, may make diagnosis of PUD difficult. Because PUD is exceedingly common in the population as a whole, physicians who care for pregnant women should be vigilant for its occurrence. A trial of empirical acid suppression may be useful in women with suspected PUD and is thought to be safe.[107–110] In confusing cases, diagnostic EGD may be indicated (see earlier). First-line therapies of PUD in pregnancy include ranitidine and sucralfate, although most PPIs are also effective. Patients with Hp infection may be given antibiotics during pregnancy or after delivery.

IBD

Physicians who treat patients with IBD are likely to encounter the disorder in pregnant women (see Chapters 117 and 118).[111] The majority of cases of IBD in women first present before age 30, the years of peak fertility.[112] Some authors report women to have an approximately 30% greater risk than men of developing UC or Crohn's disease.

There is controversy regarding the effects of IBD on fertility. Pregnancy rates in IBD patients may be spuriously low because of sexual avoidance and voluntary childlessness.[113] Fear of IBD in offspring and fear of fetal malformation from maternal drug therapy are often cited as major causes of childlessness by affected women.[114] Female fertility in IBD patients is variable and dependent upon disease activity and medical therapies. Fertility does not appear to be impaired in those with quiescent IBD and without prior pelvic surgery.[115,116] A notable exception is fertility in UC patients with prior total colectomy and ileoanal J-pouch anastomosis.[117,112] A meta-analysis found a threefold increase in the risk of infertility in IBD patients who had undergone this procedure.[118] Infertility in these individuals is most likely caused by pelvic adhesions and fallopian tube scarring. Potential infertility should be discussed with patients of childbearing age who are considering this operation. Fertility in men with IBD is impaired by sulfasalazine treatment, which causes decreased sperm counts, which usually return to normal within 6 months of discontinuing the drug.[119] Methotrexate can impact sperm morphology, though findings can be reversed after 3–6 months of drug cessation.[120]

If the initial presentation of IBD is during pregnancy, the disease is often diagnosed during the first trimester.[121,122] Cases of this type are no more severe than those in nonpregnant individuals. Likewise, pregnancy does not appear to increase the severity of or morbidity due to preexisting IBD. Evidence suggests that active disease around the time of conception increases the risk of disease relapse during pregnancy; UC patients relapse more often during pregnancy than Crohn's disease patients.[123]

The goals of the treating physician are to minimize IBD symptoms and morbidity prior to conception. Most experts agree that during gestation, affected patients should continue optimized prepregnancy therapy to avoid possible flares resulting from medication withdrawal. Exacerbations of IBD that occur during pregnancy should be managed aggressively to avoid complications, including hemorrhage, perforation, sepsis, fetal demise, and premature labor. Treatment of fulminant colitis is the same as in nonpregnant individuals, namely, high-dose glucocorticoids, IV antibiotics, cyclosporine, and salvage biological therapies. The indications for bowel surgery likewise are the same as in nonpregnant IBD patients, although bowel surgery is associated with premature labor as well as maternal and fetal mortality.[124,125] A colostomy to achieve colonic decompression and fecal diversion may be safer than total colectomy.[126] Synchronous cesarean section and subtotal colectomy have been advocated for patients with fulminant colitis after 28 weeks of gestation.[127] IBD patients are at increased risk for poor pregnancy outcomes, even if they have mild or inactive disease.[128] Major complications include premature birth, low-birth-weight and small-for-gestational-age infants, and increased cesarean section rates.[129] The risk of fetal malformations in this setting is unclear.[130] Pregnant women with UC may be at increased risk for thromboembolic events.[131]

The majority of IBD patients require several medications to remain symptom-free. Some safety data are available regarding the teratogenicity of the most commonly used IBD drugs, but there are no long-term studies of their potential adverse effects on the offspring of affected patients. It is important to carefully review the possible risks and known benefits of therapy with patients before conception. Potentially teratogenic drugs should be discontinued before conception, if at all possible. Methotrexate and thalidomide are known teratogens and abortifacients and should be used with caution in patients of childbearing age. If these medications are necessary for disease control, two forms of birth control are required. The optimum period of abstinence from these medications before conception is unknown; however, a minimum of 6 months is recommended. 5-Aminosalicylates are widely used during pregnancy to treat mild IBD. A prospective study of pregnant patients treated with mesalamine, as well as a large case series, did not show any increased risk of teratogenicity from this therapy.[132,133]

Azathioprine and its metabolite, 6-mercaptopurine, are among the most studied and widely used immunosuppressant medications in pregnant patients. Their metabolites are found in cord blood and excreted in small quantities in breast milk. Data concerning human use of these agents have failed to confirm the teratogenicity seen in animal studies.[134] Many studies of pregnant IBD patients treated with 6-mercaptopurine have not shown an increase in preterm delivery, spontaneous abortion, congenital abnormalities, or childhood neoplasia.[135–137] Based on these data and extensive experience with this drug and its metabolites in pregnant women, experts concur that their discontinuation before or during pregnancy is not advisable. Instead, careful monitoring of metabolite levels in the mother is recommended.[138]

Glucocorticoids have been used for decades to treat pregnant patients with moderate to severe IBD, as well as other more common glucocorticoid-responsive diseases such as asthma. Early reports suggested an increased risk of congenital malformations in the infants of treated mothers.[133] Subsequent prospective studies and substantial experience with drugs in this class confirm that the risk of malformations secondary to their use is extremely low. Glucocorticoid treatment during pregnancy is, however, associated with other complications, including maternal glucose intolerance and hypertension (risks factor for preeclampsia), macrosomia, and fetal adrenal suppression.[139] Prednisolone is more efficiently metabolized by the placenta than other glucocorticoids and may pose less risk of adrenal suppression.[140] Adverse outcomes have not been reported after use of oral budesonide in a small number of pregnant patients.[141]

Many pregnant organ transplant recipients have been treated with cyclosporine as immunosuppressive therapy, without reports of significant teratogenicity. TNF-α antagonists have been used extensively to treat IBD and other inflammatory diseases. Serum infliximab levels increase, whereas serum adalimumab levels are stable, during pregnancy.[142] These immunoglobulins reach the fetal compartment, especially during the third trimester. An exception may be certolizumab, which lacks the Fc fragment required for active transport. The drugs are concentrated in the fetus and are detectable in the infant's blood for months after birth.[121,143] Postmarketing registries of safety data and case series have not identified an increased incidence of fetal malformations or miscarriage in women treated during pregnancy with infliximab or adalimumab.[144] Recently published guidelines recommend that TNF-α antagonists be continued throughout pregnancy, unless otherwise indicated.[145] Some experts have expressed concerns about potential detrimental effects of fetal exposure to TNF-α antagonists on the development of the neonatal immune system. For this reason, babies exposed in utero to drugs in this class should not receive live vaccines during the first 6 months of life; however, other vaccines are recommended.[146] There has been no increase in the short- or long-term incidence of infections in children who have been exposed in utero to TNF-α antagonists.[147]

There is still limited data on the effects of treatment with anti-integrin and anti-IL-12/23 antibodies (vedolizumab or natalizumab and ustekinumab, respectively) during pregnancy. Although no problems were identified in one small study of pregnancy outcomes in women exposed to vedolizumab, use of these drugs in pregnant women should be judicious.[148]

Vaginal delivery is not contraindicated in IBD patients, but cesarean section is recommended for patients with active perineal disease. Patients with ileoanal pouches are often advised to avoid vaginal delivery in order to avoid anal sphincter injury.

Appendicitis

Suspected acute appendicitis is the most common nonobstetric indication for exploratory laparotomy in pregnant women (see Chapter 122).[149] Appendicitis complicates approximately 1 in 1500 pregnancies and may develop at any time during the course of gestation.[150] Diagnosis may be difficult because the enlarging uterus displaces the cecum and appendix cephalad, altering the location of pain caused by appendiceal inflammation and resulting in increasingly delayed detection as pregnancy progresses.[151] Late diagnosis of an inflamed appendix is responsible for complications that are associated with excess maternal and fetal morbidity and mortality.[152] During all three trimesters of pregnancy, right lower quadrant (RLQ) pain is the most common presenting symptom of appendicitis.[153] In addition to pain, affected individuals frequently complain of nausea, but this symptom is often difficult to interpret during gestation. Graded-compression US of the appendix is the diagnostic test of choice for pregnant patients suspected of having appendicitis. Helical CT has also been reported to be helpful in this setting.[150] Pregnant patients with appendicitis during any trimester may be treated with laparoscopic appendectomy,[154] although potential interference by the gravid uterus may be a relative contraindication to this procedure during the third trimester.[155] Appropriate supportive care can prevent fetal loss associated with appendiceal perforation.[156]

GALLBLADDER AND PANCREATIC DISORDERS AND PREGNANCY

Gallstone Disease

Pregnant women tend to form gallstones because of changes in gallbladder contractility and bile acid composition (see earlier) (see Chapter 67). Gallstones are frequently noted during gestation when US examination is performed to evaluate the fetus[157]; the prevalence of gallstones in asymptomatic pregnant women is reported to be between 2.5% and 12%. Despite this high prevalence, the incidence of acute cholecystitis is not increased by pregnancy. When necessary, surgical intervention for gallstone-related disease does not increase the risk of preterm labor or of fetal or maternal mortality.[77,158] Endoscopic extraction of bile duct stones with minimal use of fluoroscopy and appropriate maternal shielding is acceptable when necessary to treat choledocholithiasis during pregnancy.[159] Endoscopic intervention was found to be associated with fewer hospital admissions and a lower cesarean section rate than conservative treatment in one study.[160]

Acute Pancreatitis

Acute pancreatitis is uncommon during gestation, occurring once in every 1066–3300 pregnancies (see Chapter 60).[161,162] Most cases are caused by gallstones and present during the third trimester or the puerperium. The mild hypertriglyceridemia normally seen in pregnant women may be more severe in persons with familial hyperlipidemia, predisposing them to develop pancreatitis on this basis.[163] The clinical characteristics of acute pancreatitis during gestation are similar to those in nonpregnant women, although complications of pancreatitis do not develop in the majority of pregnant women with this disorder.[164]

HEPATIC DISORDERS UNIQUE TO PREGNANCY

Pregnant women may develop liver diseases that are etiologically related to gestation or its complications.[165] As a rule, these disorders become clinically evident during the third trimester or just after delivery. They may be severe, even life-threatening, but affected individuals are expected to survive with prompt diagnosis and appropriate management. Liver diseases unique to pregnancy are also associated with increased fetal morbidity and mortality.

Cholestasis of Pregnancy

Cholestasis of pregnancy is a form of intrahepatic cholestasis associated with pruritus, elevated serum bile acid levels, and the finding of bland cholestasis on liver biopsy.[166,167] This disorder may have a variable course, making it difficult to diagnose; nevertheless, it has serious implications for fetal well-being, and cases must be identified as promptly as possible.[168]

Cholestasis of pregnancy usually presents in the third trimester but may be seen earlier in gestation, even in the first trimester. Its first and most characteristic symptom is pruritus, and as a result, patients may be referred to a dermatologist for initial evaluation. As in other forms of cholestasis, the pruritus of cholestasis of pregnancy is most severe in the skin of the palms and soles and experienced most intensely at night. Only 10%–25% of affected individuals later develop jaundice. Elevated serum bile acid levels (>10 μmol/L) confirm the presence of cholestasis; some patients with the disorder also have bilirubinuria and even mild hyperbilirubinemia.[169] Serum alkaline phosphatase concentrations are modestly increased, but GGTP levels are normal or only marginally elevated. The latter pattern of test results is typical of adult cholestasis but is seen in pediatric patients with progressive familial intrahepatic cholestasis, as in Byler syndrome.[170] Serum aminotransferase levels are elevated in affected women, sometimes to values of 1000 U/L or higher, making it difficult, on occasion, to distinguish cholestasis of pregnancy from viral hepatitis. An increased serum autotaxin level has been shown to be a sensitive and specific diagnostic test that can distinguish cholestasis of pregnancy from other pregnancy-related liver diseases.[171] Symptoms and laboratory test abnormalities of affected patients may wax and wane. Intense cholestasis is associated with steatorrhea that is usually subclinical but can cause fat-soluble vitamin deficiencies, most notably deficiency of vitamin K.

Improvement of symptoms and laboratory test results begins with delivery of the infant, and usually, although not invariably, is prompt and complete. Rare patients experience prolonged cholestasis that may be indicative of underlying biliary tract disease, such as PBC or sclerosing cholangitis.[172,173] Women with ordinary cholestasis of pregnancy have no residual hepatic defect after resolution of the disorder, but they are at increased risk for development of gallstones, cholecystitis, and pancreatitis in the future.[174] In addition, 60%–70% of affected individuals develop cholestasis during subsequent pregnancies (although recurrent episodes may be less severe than the initial one) or with use of oral contraceptives. The risk of recurrence with subsequent pregnancies is increased by interval cholecystectomy.[175]

Cholestasis of pregnancy has serious implications for fetal well-being. There are many reports of increased frequencies of fetal distress, unexplained stillbirth, and the need for premature delivery of the babies of women with this disorder.[176] Fetal hypoxia and meconium staining have been reported at delivery in 19% of Swedish women with cholestasis of pregnancy.[177] These complications were shown to correlate with maternal bile acid levels higher than 40 μmol/L.[178] Although the risk to the fetus may be reduced by close monitoring of affected mothers, it cannot be eliminated completely.[179–182] Planned early elective delivery as soon as the fetal lungs have matured has been recommended for this reason.

As discussed in Chapter 66, a number of the molecular mechanisms of bile formation have been elucidated in recent years, resulting in a more sophisticated understanding of many cholestatic disorders.[183,184] Mutations of the *MDR3 (ABCB4)* gene are likely responsible for approximately 15% of cases of cholestasis of pregnancy.[185–188] The *MDR3* gene product is a phospholipid flippase that translocates phosphatidylcholine from the inner to the outer leaflet of the canalicular hepatocyte membrane where it is solubilized by bile acids to form mixed micelles. There is, however, no relationship of cholestasis of pregnancy to HLA type.[189]

Environmental, hormonal, and other factors also likely contribute to the development of cholestasis in pregnant women. In Chile and Scandinavia, where cholestasis of pregnancy is common, the disorder occurs most often during colder months. The incidence of cholestasis of pregnancy in Chile has declined, possibly owing to a fall in mean plasma selenium levels.[190] An increased sensitivity to the cholestatic effects of exogenous estrogen has been demonstrated in family members, including male relatives, of patients who develop cholestasis while pregnant.[191] Therapeutic or experimental administration of estrogen compounds to susceptible women can precipitate the disorder.[192,193] Similarly, progesterone therapy during gestation is associated with development of cholestasis.[194,195] The finding that ursodeoxycholic acid alters the metabolism of progesterone may explain its therapeutic effect in this setting.[196,197] It is possible that some women with cholestasis of pregnancy have inherited an enhanced sensitivity to estrogen or a variation in the metabolism of progesterone that causes cholestasis in response to a variety of stimuli, including some medications and dietary factors.[198] The incidence of cholestasis of pregnancy is significantly higher in women with hepatitis C than in other pregnant women.[199]

The differential diagnosis of cholestasis of pregnancy includes other cholestatic disorders such as PBC, PSC, benign recurrent intrahepatic cholestasis, cholestatic viral hepatitis, toxic liver injury, and bile duct obstruction. Liver biopsy specimens of affected individuals reveal bland changes typical of cholestasis due to a variety of etiologies, but biopsy is not usually necessary to make the diagnosis. It is important to remember that pregnancy may exacerbate a preexisting subclinical cholestatic disorder.[165]

Management of cholestasis of pregnancy is primarily palliative.[200,201] Ursodeoxycholic acid is helpful in relieving symptoms,[197] may reduce fetal complication rates,[185] and is well tolerated by mother and fetus.[202,203] Studies of treated individuals have demonstrated a change in the bile acid content of maternal serum and amniotic fluid, as well as increased placental bile acid transport.[204–206] Most investigators have prescribed a conventional dose (15 mg/kg/day), although one report suggests that a higher dose (20–25 mg/kg/day) is more effective.[186] In clinical practice, patients are often given the conventional dose and only given the higher dose if symptoms persist. Treatment with bile-acid binders such as cholestyramine[203] and guar gum may also relieve symptoms,[207] but it is important to keep in mind that therapy with these agents worsens steatorrhea and resultant fat-soluble vitamin deficiencies.[208] Administration of *S*-adenosyl-L-methionine to patients with cholestasis of pregnancy has had mixed therapeutic results[209–211]; its use in combination with ursodeoxycholic acid may increase its benefit.[212] A short course of a glucocorticoid (e.g., oral dexamethasone 12 mg/day for 7 days) has been reported to reduce itching and serum bile acid levels in persons with this disorder[213] but was also associated with clinical deterioration in one case.[214] Sedatives, such as phenobarbital, may relieve itching in cholestasis patients but may adversely affect the fetus. Exposure to ultraviolet B light has been suggested as therapy in this setting. As in other cholestatic syndromes, no treatment is uniformly effective in women with cholestasis of pregnancy, with the usual exception of delivery.

Preeclampsia

Preeclampsia is a multisystem disorder characterized by de novo hypertension associated with endothelial damage and maternal organ dysfunction, possibly including the liver, that may produce severe, even life-threatening, complications and affect pregnancy outcome.[215] The placenta is essential to the development of this disorder, and severe cases are associated with pathologic evidence of placental ischemia.[216] Preeclampsia complicates 3%–10% of pregnancies, occurring in the second half of pregnancy or the puerperium and more commonly in primiparous women or women with multiple gestations.[217] Usual criteria for making the diagnosis include a sustained systolic blood pressure of ≥140mmHg or diastolic blood pressure ≥90 mmHg after the 20th week of pregnancy in a previously normotensive woman, accompanied by either proteinuria (≥0.3 g in 24 hours), platelet count <100,000/µL, serum creatinine >1.1 mg/dL, liver transaminases at least twice the upper limit of normal, pulmonary edema, new-onset persistent headache, and/or visual symptoms.[218] Many patients may develop hyperreflexia and edema.

Liver disease is recognized as a common and potentially ominous complication of severe preeclampsia. The HELLP syndrome, first described by Weinstein in 1982,[219] is the most usual form of preeclamptic liver disease and may underlie development of hepatic hematoma, rupture, and infarction.[220–222] Evidence suggests that there are different preeclampsia phenotypes and that HELLP syndrome may be a distinct genetic and clinical entity.[223,224] Although preeclampsia is common in patients with acute fatty liver of pregnancy (AFLP) and may play a role in the pathogenesis of this disorder, AFLP is not usually classified as a preeclamptic liver disease.[225]

HELLP Syndrome

HELLP is seen in up to 12% of women with severe preeclampsia, occurring in 0.2%–0.8% of all pregnancies.[226–228] In the past, clinicians have relied on two major HELLP diagnostic classification systems: the Tennessee classification and the Mississippi Triple-Class classification, which further categorizes affected individuals on the basis of the nadir of the maternal platelet count (Box 38.1). The diagnostic criteria for HELLP syndrome have been standardized by the American College of Obstetricians and Gynecologists Task Force in Hypertension in Pregnancy (Box 38.2).[218] In addition to the diagnostic abnormalities of hemolysis, elevated serum aminotransferase levels, and thrombocytopenia in conjunction with hypertension and proteinuria, patients with typical HELLP syndrome frequently have complaints of chest, epigastric, and RUQ abdominal pain (Table 38.2). These symptoms are often accompanied by nausea, vomiting, headache, and blurred vision in varying combinations. Some pregnant patients may present with an asymptomatic fall in the platelet count during observation for preeclampsia or initially have no hypertension or proteinuria.[229] Other women may complain of malaise, suggesting the diagnosis of a viral syndrome.[230] Most affected individuals seek treatment after week 27 of gestation, but up to 11% may do so earlier. It is important to note that a delayed presentation of HELLP syndrome after delivery, despite absence of signs of preeclampsia at delivery, occurs in up to 30% of cases.[218]

The diagnosis of HELLP syndrome is based on an assessment of the clinical circumstances and features of the illness at the time of presentation because there is no single diagnostic test that is specific for the disorder.[228,231] Hemolysis in patients with HELLP is mild. Fragmented red blood cells (schistocytes) are seen on smears, and the serum LDH level is elevated, while serum haptoglobin level is low. Serum aminotransferase levels are also elevated, sometimes minimally and other times to greater than

BOX 38.1 The Tennessee and Mississippi Triple-Class Diagnostic Classification Systems of the HELLP Syndrome

TENNESSEE CLASSIFICATION

1. Microangiopathic hemolytic anemia with abnormal blood smear, low serum haptoglobin, and elevated serum LDH levels
2. Serum LDH level >600 IU/L or twice the laboratory upper limit of normal and serum AST level >70IU/L or twice the laboratory upper limit of normal, or serum bilirubin level >1.2 mg/dL
3. Platelet count <100,000/µL
4. Incomplete HELLP syndrome is defined as the presence of only 1 or 2 of these abnormalities and may be less severe

MISSISSIPPI TRIPLE-CLASS CLASSIFICATION

Class I: platelet count nadir ≤50,000/mm^3
Class II: platelet count nadir >50,000 and ≤100,000/mm^3
Class III: platelet count nadir >100,000 and ≤150,000/mm^3

BOX 38.2 Recommended Criteria for Diagnosis of HELLP Syndrome (ACOG Task Force in Hypertension in Pregnancy)

1. LDH ≥ 600 IU/L
2. AST and ALT elevated more than twice the upper limit of normal
3. Platelet count <100,000 cells/µL

TABLE 38.2 Clinical Characteristics and Maternal Complications of Patients with HELLP Syndrome

Presenting Symptom	Percent Affected
Abdominal pain (RUQ, epigastric)	65
Nausea or vomiting	36
Headache	31
Bleeding	9
Jaundice	5
Laboratory Test Level (Normal Value)	**Median (Range)**
Serum AST (<40 U/L)	249 (70–633)
Serum bilirubin (<1 mg/dL)	1.5 (0.5–25)
Platelet count (>125 × 10^3/mm^3)	57 (7–99)
Maternal Complications	**Percent Affected**
DIC	21
Abruption placentae	16
Acute kidney injury	8
Hepatic subcapsular hematoma	1
Death	1

From Sibai BH, Ramadan MK, Usta I, et al. Maternal morbidity and mortality in 442 pregnancies with hemolysis, elevated liver enzymes and low platelets (HELLP) syndrome. *Am J Obstet Gynecol*. 1993;169:100–106.

1000 U/L in association with laboratory signs of cholestasis.[226,232] Serum bilirubin levels can often be mildly elevated, compatible with the finding of hemolysis. Elevated serum levels of glutathione *S*-transferase alpha,[233] D-dimer,[234] tissue polypeptide antigen,[235] and fibronectin[236] have been described in persons with HELLP syndrome, and these tests may have some use in predicting the presence or severity of liver disease.

Abdominal imaging, especially CT and MRI, may be useful in making the diagnosis of HELLP syndrome and detecting cases of intrahepatic hemorrhage and infarction (discussed later). Imaging should be performed in patients with complaints of severe abdominal pain, neck or shoulder pain, or a sudden drop in blood pressure. One report documented abnormal imaging findings in 45% of such patients.[220]

Liver biopsy specimens in patients with HELLP syndrome demonstrate periportal hemorrhage, intrasinusoidal fibrin deposition, and irregular areas of liver cell necrosis with mild reactive hepatitis, findings characteristic of preeclampsia (Fig. 38.1). If hepatic steatosis is present, it is modest and does not have the appearance of the extensive pericentral microvesicular fat accumulation that occurs in patients with AFLP (discussed later). There is little if any correlation between the severity of liver biopsy lesions and laboratory test abnormalities in patients with HELLP syndrome; thus mild thrombocytopenia and mild increases in serum aminotransferase levels do not necessarily connote insignificant liver damage.[237] Liver biopsy, however, is rarely necessary to make a diagnosis in these patients and may possibly precipitate the development of intraparenchymal hepatic hematoma or contained hepatic rupture.

Although most pregnant women with low platelet counts and preeclampsia have HELLP syndrome, the differential diagnosis includes other causes of thrombocytopenia, including immune thrombocytopenic purpura, thrombotic thrombocytopenic purpura,[238] and antiphospholipid antibody syndrome, which itself may be associated with early onset of HELLP.[239,240] Elevated serum aminotransferase levels in patients with preeclampsia are most frequently misdiagnosed as being caused by viral hepatitis.[241] A diagnosis of AFLP should also be considered

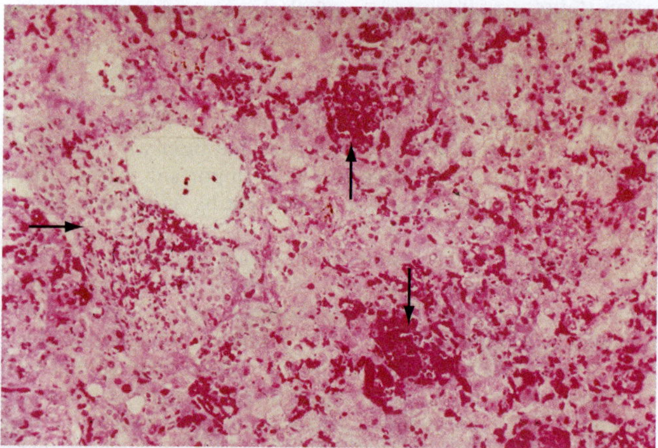

Fig. 38.1 Histopathology of HELLP syndrome. The portal triad on the *left* of the figure (the *horizontal arrow* points to an interlobular bile duct in the portal triad) is surrounded by pockets of hemorrhage (*vertical arrows*) and by an area of fibrin deposition (to the left of the portal triad).

in patients with clinical findings of HELLP syndrome, but AFLP is usually associated with signs of more significant liver dysfunction and possibly liver failure, albeit with lower serum aminotransferase levels, and is not necessarily associated with thrombocytopenia.

Preeclampsia and HELLP syndrome are now thought to be consequences of abnormal placental formation. Failures of trophoblast invasion of the uterine lining and dilation of the spiral arteries result in the physiologic inability to increase uteroplacental perfusion appropriately as gestation progresses, with the secondary release of placental products that initiate clinical disease.[242,243]

Female relatives, including the mothers of patients with preeclampsia, often have a history of the disorder. Evidence exists in some populations for its inheritance as either an autosomal recessive trait or an autosomal dominant trait with variable penetrance.[223,244,245] A number of maternal genetic variants have been associated with an increased risk of developing HELLP syndrome.[246–249] Early onset of HELLP or preeclampsia may be predicted by detection of specific serum factors, many of which have effects on angiogenesis.[250–254] Furthermore, women with a hypercoagulable condition (e.g., with factor V Leiden or anticardiolipin antibodies) are at risk for developing early and severe preeclampsia.[255,256] There is convincing evidence that development of this disorder is mediated by excessive release of soluble fms-like tyrosine kinase 1 (sFlt1) into the circulation; sFlt1 is a potent antagonist of vascular endothelial growth factor, placental growth factor, and soluble endoglin (sEng), an inhibitor of capillary formation.[257,258] Pregnant rats that overexpress both sFlt1 and sEng develop proteinuria, severe hypertension, laboratory findings of HELLP syndrome, and intrauterine growth restriction.[259] Women with preeclampsia similarly produce excessive amounts of sFlt1 and sEng.[258]

The clinical abnormalities that characterize HELLP syndrome usually resolve rapidly after childbirth.[260,261] Rarely, HELLP syndrome becomes gradually worse prior to delivery, with subsequent development of postpartum liver failure, sepsis, consumptive coagulopathy, and, rarely, even death.[262] In the absence of appropriate supportive therapy and expedited delivery, affected patients may progress to renal failure, hepatic hematoma, and hepatic rupture. Neither serum aminotransferase levels nor platelet counts are predictive of outcome in women with HELLP syndrome.[263] The disorder can recur during subsequent pregnancies but usually does not.[264,265]

Management of HELLP syndrome is primarily supportive[254]; patients should be treated in an intensive care setting prior to delivery, preferably by an obstetrician qualified in the practice of maternal-fetal medicine. Some affected patients may have a decline in serum aminotransferase levels and a rise in platelet counts with supportive care.[266] Under such circumstances, a delay in delivery may be appropriate in cases of fetal immaturity, but the fetus usually fails to grow in the setting of preeclampsia. Patients with severe preeclampsia and HELLP syndrome may require antepartum platelet transfusions and hemodialysis. Plasmapheresis after delivery has been advocated for some patients to prevent postpartum thrombotic microangiopathy.[267,268] Many affected women receive glucocorticoids before delivery, not as disease treatment but to promote fetal lung maturity; however, glucocorticoid therapy has also been used as therapy in this setting.[269] Glucocorticoid therapy of HELLP syndrome may improve platelet counts and serum ALT levels and reduce hospital and ICU stays but has not been associated with a significant improvement in maternal morbidity and mortality.[270] Orthotopic liver transplantation may be appropriate treatment for some HELLP syndrome patients,[271–273] but early diagnosis and prompt delivery almost always make this and other extreme therapeutic measures unnecessary in these individuals. Full recovery without sequelae is anticipated for the vast majority of affected patients. Those supportive measures just discussed are also employed in the nearly one-third of patients who develop HELLP syndrome postpartum, usually within the first 2 weeks after delivery.

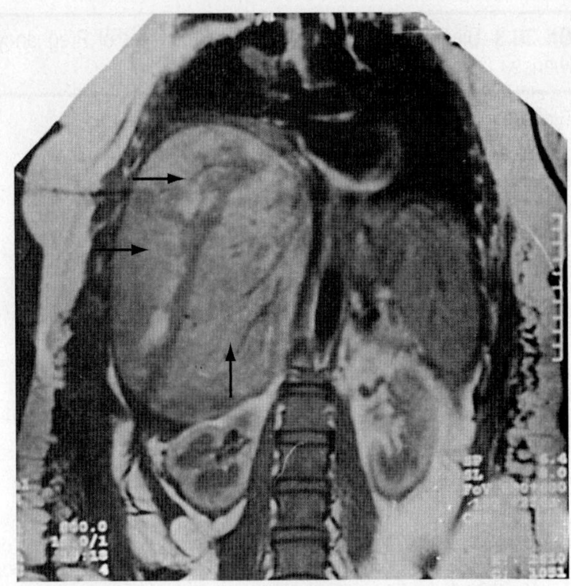

Fig. 38.2 Subcapsular hepatic hematoma in a patient with preeclampsia. This coronal section of a T1-weighted MRI scan demonstrates the subcapsular clot or hemorrhage (*horizontal arrows*) adjacent to the liver (*vertical arrow*). (From Barton JR, Sibai BM. Hepatic imaging in HELLP syndrome. *Am J Obstet Gynecol*. 1996; 174:1820–1825.)

Hepatic Rupture, Hematoma, and Infarct

Spontaneous rupture of the liver may complicate preeclampsia and HELLP syndrome, usually in the third trimester of pregnancy close to term or in the early postpartum period. Patients with this potentially fatal disorder present with abdominal distention and pain, with cardiovascular collapse.[274,275] In contrast to other patients with preeclampsia, women with spontaneous hepatic rupture tend to be older and to have had multiple previous pregnancies. Diagnosis is made by signs of liver rupture on US, CT, or MRI in conjunction with aspiration of blood on paracentesis.[220,276] Imaging studies often show that affected patients have a partially contained subcapsular hematoma (Fig. 38.2).[277] In this situation, hepatic artery embolization may be effective in controlling bleeding and limiting morbidity and mortality.[278] Management must be aggressive, with rapid delivery of the fetus by the obstetrician and, if embolization is inadequate to control bleeding, repair of the liver by an experienced liver surgeon.[279] Postoperatively, patients have a protracted course that may include DIC and hepatic failure. Patients with hepatic rupture have undergone orthotopic liver transplantation after emergent hepatectomy and interval portosystemic shunt as a temporizing measure, while a donor graft is sought.[272,273,280,281] Survivors of hepatic rupture may have uneventful subsequent pregnancies,[282] but recurrences of hematoma and rupture have also been reported.[283]

Some pregnant women with preeclampsia, HELLP syndrome, and abdominal pain have contained subcapsular hematoma.[284] In this circumstance, patients can be observed with serial CT and managed without surgery.[220,283] Angiographic embolization of hepatic artery branches supplying blood to the affected portion of the liver may be helpful.[278]

Hepatic hematoma and rupture complicating preeclampsia presumably result from extravasation of blood from one or several microscopic areas of periportal hemorrhage under Glisson capsule. Periportal hemorrhage is a typical pathologic finding in the livers of patients with preeclampsia and HELLP syndrome.[285] The capsule is believed to be stretched and torn away from the surface of the liver by the enlarging hematoma. Ultimately, the capsule may rupture, allowing the liver surface to bleed freely into the peritoneal cavity.

Hepatic infarcts may also complicate preeclampsia. Affected individuals present with fever, leukocytosis, anemia, and marked elevation of serum aminotransferase levels[220,222,286] and in the most severe cases develop multiorgan failure, including liver failure. Cross-sectional imaging demonstrates confluent hepatic infarcts. Needle aspiration of these areas yields blood and necrotic tissue; immediately adjacent liver parenchyma contains periportal hemorrhage and fibrin deposition typical of preeclampsia and HELLP syndrome. Hepatic infarction is sometimes associated with the presence of a hypercoagulable condition, such as factor V Leiden or antiphospholipid antibody.[287]

Acute Fatty Liver of Pregnancy

AFLP, a form of microvesicular fatty liver disease unique to human gestation, presents late in pregnancy, sometimes as fulminant hepatic failure with sudden onset of coagulopathy and encephalopathy in a woman without a prior history of liver disease.[288,289] AFLP is diagnosed on the basis of typical clinical and pathologic manifestations in approximately 1 of 6700 third-trimester pregnancies,[290] but it is also recognized that subclinical cases exist.[225] A prospective study of more than 1 million pregnant women using the United Kingdom Obstetric Surveillance System and standard diagnostic criteria [Swansea criteria (Box 38.3)][291] identified only 57 cases of AFLP.[292] The pathophysiologic mechanisms underlying development of this disorder are unknown, although at least some patients with AFLP have an inherited fatty-acid oxidation defect that also affects the fetus.[293–297] The disorder is most common in primiparous women and in women with multiple gestations.[298] Affected individuals have a much greater than expected number of male fetuses.[299] Of note, preeclampsia, an accompanying diagnosis in 21%–64% of cases of AFLP, is also associated with first pregnancies, twin pregnancies, and male fetuses.[290,291,300]

AFLP presents late in pregnancy, usually between 34 and 37 weeks of gestation, although cases beginning as early as weeks

BOX 38.3 Diagnostic Criteria for Acute Fatty Liver of Pregnancy (Swansea Criteria)

≥6 of the following, in absence of another explanation:

Abdominal pain
Ascites or bright liver on hepatic US
Coagulopathy (PT > 14 sec or aPTT > 34 sec)
Elevated serum ammonia levels (>47 μmol/L)
Elevated serum AST or ALT levels (>42 IU/L)
Elevated serum bilirubin levels (>14 μmol/L or 0.8 mg/dL)
Elevated serum urate levels (>340 μmol/L or 5.7 mg/dL)
Encephalopathy
Hypoglycemia (<4 mmol/L or 72 mg/dL)
Leukocytosis (>11,000/mm^3)
Microvesicular steatosis on liver biopsy
Polydipsia/polyuria
Renal impairment (creatinine >150 μmol/L or 1.7 mg/dL)
Vomiting

Adapted from Ch'ng CL, Morgan M, Hainsworth I, et al. Prospective study of liver dysfunction in pregnancy in Southwest Wales. *Gut*. 2002;51:876–880; and Knight M, Nelson-Piercy C, Kurinczuk JJ, et al. A prospective national study of acute fatty liver of pregnancy in the UK. *Gut*. 2008; 57:951–956.

19–20 of gestation have been reported. Rarely, the onset of AFLP is after delivery. Initial symptoms usually include nausea and vomiting and are often associated with abdominal pain. Pruritus may be an early complaint; overlap with cholestasis of pregnancy has occurred but is rare.[301] Patients with AFLP are frequently confused and have pregnancy-related complications, such as premature labor, vaginal bleeding, and decreased fetal movement.

On laboratory evaluation, women with AFLP often have prolonged prothrombin times and decreased serum fibrinogen levels, as well as leukocytosis. Their serum aminotransferase levels are usually moderately elevated (≈750 U/L) but, rarely, may be very high or even normal. Jaundice is common but not invariable. Renal dysfunction with elevations of serum creatinine, blood urea nitrogen, and uric acid levels is often present.

The course of AFLP is quite variable. Hypoglycemia and hyperammonemia occur and should be suspected when at-risk patients exhibit signs of altered central nervous system function. Other complications of liver failure, including ascites, pleural effusion, acute pancreatitis, respiratory failure, renal failure, and infection, may develop in patients with AFLP. Vaginal bleeding or post-cesarean section bleeding is also common in these individuals. Transient diabetes insipidus is sometimes seen.[302] More rarely, affected patients have myocardial infarction[303] or pulmonary fat emboli.[304]

Diagnosis of AFLP is almost always based on the appearance of typical clinical features of the disorder, including laboratory test results, during the later stages of pregnancy. Hepatic imaging may confirm the presence of hepatic steatosis in patients with suspected AFLP[305] and plays a crucial role in identifying hepatic hematoma, rupture, and infarction.

Liver biopsy is usually unnecessary to make the diagnosis, but histologic results may be pathognomonic and, therefore, useful if the obstetrician has reservations about delivery. Transvenous sampling of liver tissue, however, may be necessitated due to coagulopathy. The histologic hallmark of AFLP is small-droplet fatty infiltration of the liver that is most prominent in hepatocytes surrounding central veins (zone 3) and spares hepatocytes surrounding portal areas (Fig. 38.3). Steatosis of this type has a relatively homogeneous appearance on light microscopy and may be difficult to discern on examination of ordinary H&E-stained specimens. To confirm the diagnosis, special techniques must be used; frozen tissue may be stained for fat with oil-red O, or

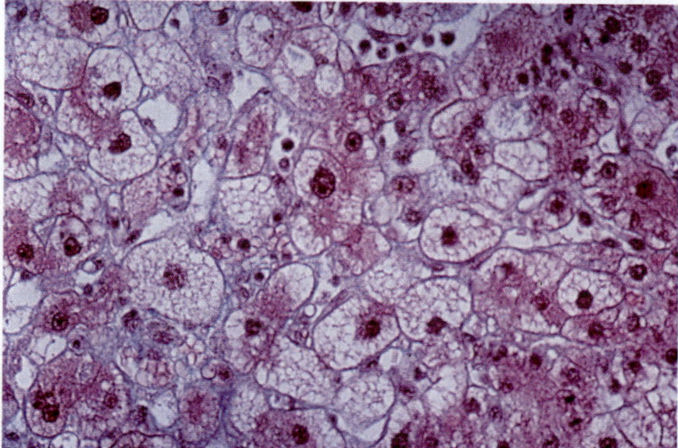

Fig. 38.3 Histopathology of acute fatty liver of pregnancy. The perivenular hepatocytes are pleomorphic and vacuolated, and there is lobular disarray. Large fat droplets are not seen.

electron microscopy can be used to examine a glutaraldehyde-fixed specimen. Plans must be made prior to the biopsy for appropriate handling of the liver tissue. Other histologic findings in affected patients can be misleading, including lobular disarray suggestive of viral hepatitis and biliary ductular proliferation and inflammation suggestive of cholangitis.[225,306] Patients with AFLP do not have the periportal hemorrhage and sinusoidal fibrin deposition seen in the livers of individuals with preeclampsia and HELLP syndrome.

The differential diagnosis in suspected cases of AFLP includes those causes of acute hepatic failure not associated with pregnancy, as discussed later, especially viral hepatitis and toxic liver injury. Uncommon types of viral hepatitis, such as hepatitis E and herpes simplex hepatitis, may be more severe in pregnant than in nonpregnant individuals.[307,308] These viral agents can be identified by appropriate serologic tests. A more difficult problem is distinguishing AFLP from other liver diseases that complicate pregnancy, particularly HELLP syndrome and hemorrhagic or ischemic liver injury. For example, patients with AFLP may develop preeclampsia and DIC with attendant thrombocytopenia, thereby meeting the diagnostic criteria for HELLP syndrome (see Box 38.1). Fortunately, it is not usually necessary to distinguish among these various diagnoses because AFLP, HELLP syndrome, and preeclampsia are treated by expedited delivery of the infant. It is, however, of crucial importance to recognize hepatic hematoma and rupture rapidly (see earlier discussion).

The pathogenesis of AFLP has not been elucidated. Initially, AFLP was thought to be caused by exposure to a toxin. For example, microvesicular steatosis of the liver can be caused by treatment with sodium valproate or IV tetracycline. Despite an intensive search, however, no toxin that might be responsible for development of AFLP has been identified. Because of the coincidental occurrence of preeclampsia and AFLP in many patients, the disorder has been considered by some experts to be a severe form of preeclamptic liver disease.[225,309,310] Placental oxidative stress, thought to be responsible for development of preeclampsia, is accompanied by the release of toxic mediators that may play a role in the pathogenesis of AFLP.[311] Arguing against this conclusion is the absence of the usual histologic features of preeclampsia in liver biopsy specimens from patients with AFLP and the absence of the usual clinical features of preeclampsia in many patients with AFLP.

There is a well-established association between AFLP and inherited defects in beta oxidation of fatty acids.[294,295,312,313] This connection is empirically supported by similar clinical and histologic findings in patients with AFLP and those with Jamaican vomiting sickness, a liver disease caused by a toxin in unripe akee fruit that disables intramitochondrial beta oxidation of fatty acids. Maternal liver disease (HELLP or AFLP) has been reported in 62% of the mothers of infants with defects of fatty-acid oxidation.[294] AFLP may develop regardless of maternal genotype if the fetus is deficient in long-chain 3-hydroxyacyl-coenzyme A dehydrogenase (LCHAD) and carries at least 1 allele for the G1528C *LCHAD* mutation.[293,314] Other mitochondrial oxidation defects, including carnitine palmitoyltransferase-1 deficiency, short- and medium-chain acyl-CoA dehydrogenase deficiency, and mitochondrial trifunctional protein deficiency, have also been associated with AFLP.[315–318] Prenatal genetic diagnosis based on chorionic villus sampling has proved to be feasible and accurate in pregnant members of affected families.[319,320] Not every investigator, however, has been able to confirm the association between AFLP and mitochondrial oxidation defects,[321] and other as yet unknown mechanisms may play a role in the pathogenesis of this disorder.

Patients with AFLP should be managed in an intensive care setting, preferably by obstetricians qualified in the practice of maternal-fetal medicine, in cooperation with other appropriate specialists. Early diagnosis and prompt delivery of the infant are imperative to minimize maternal and fetal morbidity and mortality. Affected individuals may be very ill postpartum until the physiologic defects responsible for their clinical abnormalities resolve and the livers recover. Supportive care may include infusion of blood products, mechanical ventilation, hemodialysis, and antibiotic therapy. Hepatic encephalopathy is treated as indicated by measures intended to evacuate feces and bacteria from the colon and eliminate ammonia via hemodialysis. Infusion of concentrated glucose solution may be required to treat or prevent hypoglycemia. Although many patients with AFLP have DIC and depressed antithrombin III levels, treatment with heparin or antithrombin III is not recommended.[322] Patients with diabetes insipidus may be managed with 1-deamino-8-D-arginine-vasopressin.[302] Some individuals with liver failure secondary to AFLP have been successfully treated with plasmapheresis.[323] Others may require emergency orthotopic liver transplantation as a potentially life-saving measure.[273,324,325] Most affected women, however, recover completely with appropriate supportive care. Persistent or even increasing hyperbilirubinemia and multiple complications after delivery do not necessarily indicate the need for liver transplantation.

Survival of patients with AFLP has been reported to be nearly 100% with prompt diagnosis, delivery of the infant, and intensive care.[290,290,326,327] Infants of affected women have perinatal mortality rates of less than 7%. Surviving babies may have LCHAD deficiency and develop nonketotic hypoglycemia and obtundation. Recurrence of AFLP has been documented, particularly in women with LCHAD deficiency.[328,329] In all cases of AFLP, the mother, father, and child should be tested for the *G1528C LCHAD* mutation.[293]

OTHER HEPATIC DISORDERS AND PREGNANCY

Viral Hepatitis

Viral hepatitis is the most common form of liver disease worldwide and frequently affects women of childbearing age, either as an acute infection or as a chronic disease.[330,331] Hepatitis A, unless unusually severe, does not appear to alter the normal course of pregnancy, nor does pregnancy appear to influence the natural history of hepatitis A. Acute and chronic viral hepatitis of other types, however, may have implications for maternal and fetal well-being.

HEV

HEV is an enterically transmitted RNA virus with four genotypes and one serotype (see Chapter 84).[308,332] Genotypes 1 and 2 only infect humans and usually cause epidemic disease during the monsoon season in Central and South Asia and India. Genotypes 3 and 4 infect humans and numerous animal species, particularly swine and chickens and possibly cattle and sheep, as well as rats. These HEV genotypes are responsible for sporadic cases of hepatitis in farmers and may spread to others by consumption of undercooked meat.[333] The prevalence of HEV antibody has declined in blood samples collected in the U.S. from 2009 to 2010, as compared to those collected from 1998 to 1994.[331] Most recently, the HEV antibody prevalence was 6% for individuals aged 6 years or above. Two recombinant-protein anti-HEV vaccines have been tested in clinical trials,[334] and one of them was approved for use in China by the State Food and Drug Administration in December 2011.

Acute hepatitis E during the third trimester of pregnancy is a cause of fulminant hepatic failure and has a mortality rate of up to 20%.[308] Maternal HEV infection has also been associated with intrauterine fetal death.[335,336] The risks of intrauterine death and abortion in any trimester are greater in pregnant women with hepatitis E than they are in their uninfected counterparts. Maternal-fetal transmission of HEV resulting in symptomatic neonatal hepatitis has occurred,[337] and no known therapy prevents vertical transmission of this virus. Pregnant women should avoid traveling to endemic areas during monsoon season and outbreaks of the disease.

HSV

Subclinical hepatitis associated with primary HSV infection is common (see Chapter 85). In pregnant or immunosuppressed individuals, this virus may cause severe liver disease.[338] Infection during pregnancy, particularly the third trimester, can result in fulminant hepatic failure. Affected individuals are obtunded and usually anicteric with elevated serum aminotransferase levels and coagulopathy. They may have subtle oropharyngeal or genital herpetic lesions. Encephalopathy may result from herpes encephalitis. The diagnosis of HSV infection can be confirmed by serologic testing and PCR assay for viral DNA. Liver biopsy specimens from affected patients usually demonstrate characteristic intracytoplasmic inclusion bodies and areas of focal hemorrhage. Treatment with oral acyclovir or valacyclovir is effective and appears to prevent viral transmission to the fetus.[339,340]

HBV and HDV

HBV infection in pregnant women is the most important factor perpetuating the worldwide epidemic of chronic hepatitis B (see Chapter 81).[341–343] Universal HBV screening in pregnant women is recommended.[344] Although HBV can be passed from infected mothers to their infants during gestation, at the time of delivery, or after birth, most mother-to-infant transmission occurs during delivery, a time when the neonate's immune system is incapable of clearing the virus. Vertical transmission of HBV is responsible for most cases of chronic hepatitis B in endemic areas, especially Southeast Asia and Africa.[345]

Maternal infectivity is proportional to viral load.[346] Mothers with a reactive serum test for hepatitis B e antigen have more circulating virus and higher rates of perinatal transmission[347] than mothers who have undetectable serum hepatitis B e antigen with a reactive serum test for hepatitis B e antibody,[348] although the latter individuals can still be a source of neonatal infection.[349] Without treatment, 90% of infants born to hepatitis B e antigen–positive mothers and 10% of infants born to hepatitis B e antigen–negative mothers develop chronic HBV infection. Antiviral therapy beginning in the third trimester is recommended for pregnant women with inactive hepatitis B and serum HBV DNA levels greater than 200,000 IU/mL.[350] For pregnant women with active hepatitis B, management should be the same as that recommended for nonpregnant women.[351] Appropriate therapy during pregnancy significantly reduces the risk of mother-to-infant viral transmission.[352] If, however, the risk of transmission is low, antiviral therapy in addition to recommended prophylaxis of the infant offers no advantage.[353] Invasive procedures during pregnancy, such as amniocentesis, may pose a risk of HBV transmission from mother to child, especially when the maternal HBV-DNA level is greater than or equal to 7 log copies/mL.[354]

The infants of mothers with a reactive serum test for hepatitis B surface antigen should receive hepatitis B immunoglobulin and hepatitis B vaccine within 12 hours of delivery.[355] This treatment is highly effective, but despite appropriate passive-active immunoprophylaxis immediately after birth, 1%–2% of treated infants will become chronically infected with HBV.[346,356] Breastfeeding by mothers with chronic hepatitis B poses no additional risk of viral transmission as long as the baby has received appropriate immunoprophylaxis.[357]

Most women of childbearing age with chronic HBV infection are healthy virus carriers with a very low risk of developing disease complications. A flare of hepatitis, however, and in some cases even acute liver failure, may occur in previously asymptomatic individuals during the peripartum period.[358,359] One study found that approximately 25% of women with chronic hepatitis B had disease flares in the first few months after delivery.[360] Investigators have also found an increased incidence of spontaneous preterm birth in association with the presence of HBV DNA in umbilical cord blood.[361] For these reasons, pregnant and postpartum patients with hepatitis B should be monitored closely for up to 6 months after delivery.[362]

The only hepatitis B treatments that have been studied in pregnant women are lamivudine, telbivudine, and tenofovir disoproxil fumarate (TDF). Of these, TDF is preferred because of its reliable efficacy and high barrier to the emergence of viral resistance. TDF therapy during the third trimester in pregnant women with high serum levels of HBV DNA has been shown to significantly reduce the incidence of mother-to-child viral transmission.[352,363] There was no difference between treated and untreated women in the rates of prematurity, congenital malformations, and Apgar scores. Other studies have shown no difference in the incidence of adverse effects between TDF-exposed and -unexposed infants.[364–366] Women with chronic hepatitis B are not treated with interferon during pregnancy.[367] Vaccination of nonimmune pregnant women against HBV infection is safe and effective.[368] An accelerated vaccination schedule may be used in women at high risk for exposure to HBV.[369] When the indication for hepatitis B therapy is a third-trimester serum HBV DNA level greater than 200,000 IU/mL, stopping treatment at, or within 4 weeks of, delivery is recommended.[370] Continued treatment for up to 12 weeks postpartum does not protect the mother from disease flares.[371]

HDV infection requires simultaneous acute or chronic hepatitis B virus infection. Pregnant patients with hepatitis B who are most likely to have HDV coinfection include those with HIV and immigrants from areas of high HDV endemicity. These individuals should be tested for the presence of anti-HDV antibody, which indicates infection.[359]

There is no evidence that pregnancy changes the natural course of hepatitis D. Prevention of vertical transmission of HDV is best accomplished by vaccination of the mother against infection with hepatitis B virus, or appropriate therapy of existing maternal hepatitis B prior to pregnancy in conjunction with vaccination and administration of hepatitis B immunoglobulin to the infant. A case report has documented prevention of vertical transmission of hepatitis B and D viruses by this management.[372]

HCV

Recommendations for the diagnosis and management of hepatitis C in pregnant women (and others) are continually updated by the hepatitis C guidance panel of the AASLD and the Infectious Diseases Society of North America (see Chapter 82)[373] and are available on the internet at https://www.hcvguidelines.org. Since 2020 the CDC has recommended universal HCV screening of pregnant women. Patients with reactive antibody tests should have confirmatory HCV nucleic-acid testing.[374,375]

Mother-to-infant transmission is the principal cause of hepatitis C in children. Between 1% and 2.5% of pregnant women in the US have HCV infection.[376] The incidence of HCV vertical transmission is reported to be 5.8% in the children of HCV RNA-positive, HIV-negative women and 10.8% in the children of HCV RNA-positive, HIV-positive women.[377,378] Greater serum levels of HCV RNA, as seen in HIV and HCV coinfection, increase the risk of vertical transmission: serum HCV-RNA levels of 10^6 or greater copies/mL have been associated with vertical transmission in as many as 36% of cases.[379] Intrapartum exposure to infected maternal blood, prolonged rupture of membranes, and internal fetal monitoring have also been identified as possible risk factors for neonatal HCV infection.[380,381] The incidence of perinatal HCV infection does not seem to be related to whether the baby is delivered vaginally or by cesarean section.[379] Although HCV RNA can be detected in breast milk,[382] breastfeeding is not considered to be a risk factor for neonatal HCV infection,[383] nor are there data that amniocentesis significantly increases the risk of fetal infection.

Population-based and case-control studies of the effects of maternal HCV infection on pregnancy outcomes have had inconsistent results. Chronic hepatitis C may be independently associated with development of gestational diabetes, preterm delivery, low birth weight, retarded fetal development, and cholestasis of pregnancy.[384–387] Cirrhosis, in particular, is associated with increased maternal and fetal morbidity.[388,389] There are no convincing data to suggest that pregnancy alters the natural history of hepatitis C infection, although pregnant women with hepatitis C have a higher incidence of cholestasis of pregnancy than uninfected controls.[192]

When possible, women of reproductive age with hepatitis C should receive antiviral therapy before becoming pregnant; direct-acting antiviral agents are not approved for use during pregnancy. No intra- or postpartum intervention has been shown to reduce the risk of vertical HCV transmission, including treatment of the infant with immunoglobulin.[390] Patients with hepatitis C are not treated with interferon/ribavirin during pregnancy; ribavirin is a well-established teratogen. Previously infected individuals may have spontaneous HCV-RNA clearance after delivery.[391]

Chronic Liver Disease and Portal Hypertension

Women with significant chronic liver disease and cirrhosis often have anovulatory menstrual cycles or are amenorrheic and therefore are unlikely to become pregnant (see Chapters 94 and 96). Only 37 cases of cirrhosis were identified using ICD-9 codes in more than 2 million pregnant women recorded in the California Birth Registry Database between 2005 and 2009.[378]

Portal hypertension, ascites, and compensatory dilation of submucosal esophageal veins connecting the portal circulation to the azygos vein can occur in pregnant women with noncirrhotic portal hypertension aggravated by physiologic increases in circulating blood volume. Even in the absence of pathologic causes of portal hypertension, these esophageal venous collaterals may become engorged during gestation owing to normal circulatory changes, including increased blood flow and compression of the inferior vena cava by the enlarging uterus, and may be seen on endoscopy. Enlarged veins of the latter type do not bleed spontaneously.

Normal pregnancy-associated increases in maternal blood volume appear to aggravate the risk of variceal bleeding in individuals with underlying portal hypertension.[392,393] Esophageal variceal bleeding has been reported in 18%–32% of pregnant women with cirrhosis and as many as 50% of those with known portal hypertension and 78% of those with preexisting varices. In addition to variceal bleeding, women with chronic liver disease and portal hypertension who become pregnant may be at increased risk of death, hepatic decompensation, splenic artery rupture, and uterine hemorrhage, according to reports published between 1950 and 1980.[377,381] Cirrhosis appears to significantly increase the risk of preeclampsia, preterm delivery, low birthweight, and neonatal death.[378,394]

Endoscopic band ligation is accepted as the preferred initial therapy of variceal bleeding in pregnant women, although no studies of its safety and efficacy have been done in this setting. Infusion of the somatostatin analog octreotide is also used on the basis of its effectiveness in nonpregnant patients. Vasopressin and octreotide infusions may theoretically cause uterine ischemia and induce premature labor. Despite the risks of associated radiation exposure, placement of a transjugular intrahepatic portosystemic shunt may be indicated when variceal bleeding cannot be controlled by any other means.[395–397] The American College of Gastroenterology recommends endoscopic screening for esophageal varices in women during the second trimester.[398] If large varices are present, nonselective beta blockers or endoscopic band ligations are recommended to prevent variceal bleeding.

Ascites and hepatic encephalopathy in pregnant women with chronic liver disease are managed in the customary manner. The only therapy available for severe hepatic decompensation during pregnancy is liver transplantation. Orthotopic liver transplantation has been performed successfully during pregnancy.[399,400] The MELD score can help predict clinical decompensation in a cirrhotic woman during pregnancy. For example, a MELD score of 10 or greater at the time of conception had an 83% sensitivity and an 83% specificity in predicting development of ascites, encephalopathy, or variceal hemorrhage prior to delivery in one study.[401]

Wilson Disease

Wilson disease in women of childbearing age is associated with amenorrhea and infertility (see Chapter 78). Treatment of affected individuals to remove excess copper may result in resumption of ovulatory cycles and a subsequent pregnancy. Pregnant patients must remain on medication to treat Wilson disease because discontinuation of therapy can cause sudden copper release, hemolysis, acute liver failure, and death.[402] D-Penicillamine is potentially teratogenic in humans[403] but has been used safely during pregnancy at doses necessary for copper chelation.[404] Similarly, trientine is teratogenic in animals but appears to be safe in humans as treatment for copper overload. Zinc salts such as zinc acetate do not appear to be teratogenic, and some experts favor use of zinc during pregnancy as therapy for Wilson disease for this reason.[405]

Autoimmune Liver Diseases

Autoimmune diseases of most types, including autoimmune hepatitis, are more common in women than in men (see Chapter 92). Autoimmune liver disease has a variety of clinical phenotypes. In women, classic (type 1) autoimmune hepatitis typically presents around the expected time of menarche but is associated with amenorrhea. When women with autoimmune hepatitis become pregnant, they have a greater-than-expected incidence of spontaneous abortion and preterm delivery.[406] Affected patients may also have disease flares during pregnancy and postpartum.[407,408] For this reason, treated individuals with autoimmune hepatitis who conceive a child should continue taking immunosuppressive medications during pregnancy. The doses of azathioprine prescribed as part of standard treatment regimens are not thought to be teratogenic. Autoimmune hepatitis patients should be carefully monitored during pregnancy and in the postpartum period.

PBC is much more common in postmenopausal women than it is in their fertile counterparts. Women with PBC may experience an exacerbation of pruritus during pregnancy.[409] Pruritus can be ameliorated by treatment with ursodeoxycholic acid,[410] although the safety of this therapy during pregnancy has not been formally proved.

Hepatic Tumors and Mass Lesions

Mass-like defects of the hepatic parenchyma may be discovered during pregnancy, usually as an incidental finding on US (see Chapter 98). Benign liver lesions found commonly in women of childbearing age include adenomas, focal nodular hyperplasia, and hemangiomas. Hepatic adenomas are associated with oral contraceptive use and may enlarge during pregnancy. Enlarging lesions can bleed and rupture into the abdominal cavity. Focal nodular hyperplasia and hemangiomas in pregnant patients have also been reported to hemorrhage. Women known to have a benign hepatic nodular defect should be evaluated with serial US to measure mass size and look for evidence of intralesional bleeding.

Hepatocellular carcinoma occurs almost exclusively in persons with chronic liver disease and may present in the absence of cirrhosis in young people with chronic HBV infection. At-risk patients should have standard screening for liver cancer during pregnancy. It must be borne in mind that maternal serum alpha-fetoprotein (AFP) levels are always modestly elevated during normal pregnancy[411] and can increase further in cases of fetal Down syndrome, neural-tube defects, and hydatidiform mole, thereby limiting the positive predictive value for diagnosing hepatocellular carcinoma during pregnancy.

Hepatic fibrolamellar carcinoma has been reported to occur in pregnant women.[412] Fibrolamellar carcinoma is a slow-growing liver cancer usually found in young adults (median age, 25 years).[413] Unlike typical primary liver cancer, this neoplasm has no known association with cirrhosis or chronic liver disease and is not a cause of increased serum AFP levels. It is an aggressive neoplasm with a 5-year survival rate below 50%.

Hepatic metastases from other cancers are rare in women of childbearing age.

Hepatic Vein Thrombosis (Budd–Chiari Syndrome)

Pregnancy is a predisposing factor for the development of venous thrombosis (see Chapter 87). Hepatic vein thrombosis may occur in association with HELLP syndrome[414] and with preeclampsia in women who have an antiphospholipid antibody.[415] Pregnant women who develop hepatic vein thrombosis should be evaluated for the presence of antiphospholipid antibody and other circulating procoagulants (e.g., factor V Leiden), and also for JAK-2, and possibly other gene mutations.[416]

Pregnancy After Liver Transplantation

Women of childbearing age may become pregnant after successful orthotopic liver transplantation and deliver normal infants (see Chapter 99).[134,417,418] Delaying pregnancy until the second post-transplant year may be associated with a lower risk of prematurity. Transplant patients must continue immunosuppressive therapy during gestation but may need to have their treatment modified. Mycophenolate mofetil, a part of many post-transplant immunosuppressive regimens, is highly teratogenic[419] and must be avoided in women of childbearing age who may become pregnant. Adverse effects of other immunosuppressive medications, including hypertension and hyperglycemia, may increase the incidence of fetal distress and preeclampsia in pregnant liver transplant recipients. In rare instances, pregnancy has been complicated by organ rejection.

Full references for this chapter can be found at https://ebooks.health.elsevier.com.

39 Acute and Chronic Gastrointestinal Side Effects of Radiation Therapy

Alex J. Gooding, Christopher G. Willett, Brian G. Czito

IN THIS CHAPTER

Early and late GI organ injury may occur following irradiation of thoracic, abdominal, and pelvic malignancies of GI and non-GI origin. As with all toxicities associated with radiation therapy (RT), GI side effects are categorized broadly into two types: early or late reactions. Early reactions, such as diarrhea and nausea, occur during and soon after completion of a treatment course, and late or chronic effects, such as ulceration, stricture formation, and bowel obstruction, can develop months to years later. Severe acute reactions can lead to treatment breaks and, in turn, a suboptimal treatment course, whereas the concern for chronic toxicity, particularly to the small bowel, is commonly a dose-limiting consideration in the creation of a treatment plan. The incidence and severity of radiation-induced GI morbidity depend on both total dose and fraction size, treatment volumes and techniques, the presence or absence of other treatment modalities such as systemic therapy and surgery, and underlying patient comorbidities. This chapter discusses the early and late toxicities of RT and combined chemoradiation therapy (CRT) regimens to the esophagus, stomach, small intestines, colon, rectum, anus, pancreas, and liver.

The sections to follow will focus on the various radiation toxicities that can occur in each of the individual organs of the GI tract, as well as the steps radiation oncologists take to reduce the likelihood and severity of said toxicities. Prior to that, we present a brief general discussion of the cellular mechanisms of radiation damage and introduce the concept of an organ that functions in series versus one that functions in parallel, which informs radiation dose constraints.

MOLECULAR MECHANISMS OF RADIATION-INDUCED GI DAMAGE

At the cellular level, both the therapeutic and injurious acute effects of RT are consequences of its ability to induce DNA double-strand breaks through the creation of free radicals. In some cell types, this damage will lead to programmed cell death (apoptosis), which proceeds through a well-defined signaling cascade that is commonly disrupted during the process of oncogenesis. In rapidly dividing cancer cells, which generally lack important components of the normal DNA-damage response system and the apoptotic cascade, RT-induced DNA double-strand breaks can result in lethal chromosomal aberrations that cause cell death when division is attempted, a phenomenon known as mitotic catastrophe.

The acute effects of radiation exposure to the normal GI tract have been studied in animal models, where a rapid increase in the rate of apoptosis of intestinal crypt/stem cells can be observed after exposure to low-dose irradiation (1−5 cGy). The rate of apoptosis is dose-dependent and reaches a plateau at 1 Gy. Radiation exposure increases expression of the *TP53* gene product, p53, in GI epithelium, which induces expression of PUMA (p53 upregulated modulator of apoptosis, also known as BBC3 or Bcl-2-binding component 3), a proapoptotic protein that causes cell death via the intrinsic apoptotic pathway. Conversely, the rate of radiation-induced apoptosis in endothelial cells is significantly reduced in animals lacking the proapoptotic bcl-2 multidomain proteins, bax and bak.[1,2] It is therefore postulated that p53 promotes apoptosis after irradiation, whereas antiapoptotic members of the bcl-2 family protect the normal mucosa.

Beyond the acute loss of cells through apoptosis and mitotic catastrophe, radiation injury is the consequence of a complex set of interactions between cells involving multiple cytokines and molecular pathways that can acutely lead to mucosal edema and chronically to fibrosis and organ dysfunction through excess deposition of extracellular matrix coincident with a reduction in the expression of remodeling enzymes such as matrix metalloproteinases. Radiation-induced fibrosis is, essentially, improper wound healing and, when combined with mucosal stem cell loss, underlies the chronic toxicities associated with RT such as dysmotility, stenosis, and fistula formation.[3,4] This process typically begins several months to a year after the conclusion of a course of RT and can progress over the following years.

The initial step in this process is the recruitment of immune cells to the site of RT-induced injury, which, in turn, results in the increased local expression of a number of cytokines, including platelet-derived growth factor and transforming growth factor (TGF)-β. Platelet-derived growth factor promotes the migration of fibroblasts to the injured area, whereas TGF-β promotes both the proliferation of fibroblasts and their transdifferentiation into profibrotic myofibroblasts.[5,6] Ongoing local expression of active TGF-β is thought to be the primary mediator of radiation-induced fibrosis. In addition to promoting the creation of myofibroblasts, TGF-β promotes the production of extracellular matrix proteins and reduces the expression of matrix metalloproteinases.[7,8] Pathologic examination of bowel specimens from patients who underwent surgery for radiation enteropathy showed increased TGF-β in areas with vascular sclerosis and fibrotic areas of the serosa and muscularis propria as compared with patients who had surgery for other causes.[9] In rat liver, TGF-β expression was found to be upregulated in a dose-dependent manner in hepatocytes up to 9 months after irradiation.[10] Neutralizing antibodies to TGF-β and small molecule inhibitors have been shown to suppress or reverse fibrosis in preclinical models, but this has not been used in clinical practice to date.[11–13]

The acute to subacute formation of fibrotic tissue and loss of epithelium can in turn lead to chronic and permanent fibrosis, although the ultimate risk of developing a pathologic outcome is influenced by patient-specific factors such as comorbidities, including smoking status, nutrition, diabetes, and certain inflammatory diseases.[14] A further emerging mechanistic determinant of acute and chronic GI toxicities is the composition and function of the gut microbiome preceding, during, and following radiation, as several studies have revealed that the local inflammatory response to radiation is impacted by the immunomodulatory and metabolic effects of specific microbial species populating the gut.[15,16] Regardless of the underlying molecular mediators, the overall picture is thought to be a product of the initial insult and damage response that leads to vascular changes with an end result of tissue ischemia and progressive fibrosis.[17]

SERIAL VERSUS PARALLEL ORGAN FUNCTION

Through the loss of epithelial stem cells and the formation of scar tissue, RT can cause segments of organs of the GI tract to become less functional. Whether this manifests clinically is partly related to the functional arrangement of the organ, of which there are two types: serial and parallel.

Organs arranged in series are composed of segments that are reliant on the functionality of the preceding segment such that the loss of any individual segment will make the organ dysfunctional or even nonfunctional downstream and possibly upstream from the insult. The prototypical organ with this arrangement is the spinal cord, where significant damage at a single spinal level can cause loss-of-function at every level downstream of the injury. With respect to the GI system, much of the luminal GI tract has this type of organization.

Organs with parallel architecture, on the other hand, have some functional redundancy built in such that the loss of segments up to a point may not manifest clinically. The liver has this type of arrangement, although debate continues on exactly how much liver need be preserved to remain fully functional, particularly in patients with underlying liver disease.

When creating RT plans, the consideration of these arrangements informs the types of dose constraints that are used. Organs that function in series are subject to maximum dose constraints, because an ablative dose to a small area can manifest as dysfunction of the entire organ, such as small bowel obstruction (SBO). Organs with a parallel functional architecture are subject to constraints that allow for the protection of an adequate relative volume of functional tissue. As will be discussed in the case of the liver, it is important to constrain an absolute volume to receive less than a certain dose of radiation.

SMALL INTESTINE

The first case of radiation injury of the small bowel, or radiation enteropathy, was described in 1897 in the context of irradiating the skin of the abdomen.[18] RT can damage the small bowel during the treatment of virtually all GI and gynecologic cancers, while rarely being used as part of the primary treatment of cancers of the small bowel. Mitigating the risk and severity of radiation enteritis and chronic small bowel injury is commonly the dose-limiting factor in the radiotherapeutic management of most abdominal and pelvic malignancies.

Incidence and Clinical Features

The epithelium of the GI tract has a high proliferative rate, with turnover every 3–5 days, making it susceptible to radiation- and chemotherapy-induced mucositis. Irradiation of intestinal mucosa primarily affects the clonogenic intestinal stem cells within the crypts of Lieberkühn (cells that provide, via self-replication and eventual maturation, replacement cells in the intestinal villi). Stem cell damage, as a result of direct radiation damage or radiation-induced microvascular damage, leads to a decrease in cellular reserves for the intestinal villi. This results in mucosal denudement, shortened villi, a decreased absorptive surface area, and associated intestinal inflammation and edema. Histologic changes are seen within hours of irradiation.

Within 2–4 weeks, an infiltration of leukocytes with crypt abscess (microabscess) formation can be observed, leading to ulcer formation (Fig. 39.1). This acute injury can result in impaired absorption of fats, carbohydrates, proteins, bile salts, and vitamin B_{12}, with loss of water, electrolytes, and proteins. Impaired ileal bile-salt absorption increases loads of conjugated bile salts entering the colon, which are deconjugated by colonic bacteria, causing intraluminal salt and water accumulation and subsequent diarrhea. Furthermore, impaired digestion of lactose may occur following radiation, leading to increased bacterial fermentation with associated flatulence, distention, and diarrhea. There is also evidence of acutely altered gut motility following RT.[19]

Patients with acute radiation enteritis experience diarrhea, abdominal cramping or pain, nausea and vomiting, anorexia, and malaise. Radiation-induced diarrhea often appears during the third week of a fractionated radiation course, with reported rates of 20%–70%.[20] Acute radiation enteropathy with diarrhea may be seen in some patients after delivery of doses of 18–22 Gy using conventional fractionation, which coincides with the start of the third week of therapy and is seen in most patients by 40 Gy. The symptoms and pathologic findings typically subside 2–6 weeks following completion of RT, although evidence suggests that

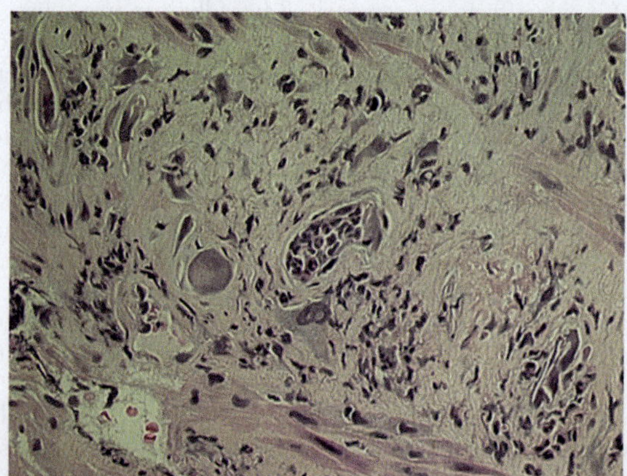

Fig. 39.1 Histopathology showing microabscesses and radiation-related fibroblasts. Submucosal reaction shows large, bizarre radiation fibroblasts that have both cytomegaly and nucleomegaly. Smooth muscle cells also have reactive changes. Microabscesses composed of excess neutrophils infiltrate the stroma. (Courtesy Dr. Robin Amirkahn, Dallas, TX.)

patients who develop acute small intestinal toxicity may be at higher risk for chronic effects.[21]

Histologic changes of chronic toxicity to the small intestine include progressive occlusive vasculopathy with foam cell invasion of the intima and hyaline thickening of the arteriolar walls, with collagen deposition and fibrosis. The small bowel becomes thickened, with development of telangiectasias, whereas the vessel walls of small arterioles are obliterated, causing ischemia (Fig. 39.2).[22] As the vasculopathy progresses, mucosal ulceration, necrosis, and occasionally perforation of the intestinal wall can be seen, leading to fistula and abscess formation. Lymphatic damage contributes to mucosal edema and inflammation. Histologically, the mucosa atrophies, with atypical hyperplastic glands and intestinal wall fibrosis (Fig. 39.3).[23] As the ulcers heal, there can be fibrosis and narrowing of the intestinal lumen, with subsequent stricture formation and even obstruction with dilatation of the proximal bowel. Bacterial overgrowth may be an indirect complication arising from stasis in a dilated loop of bowel proximal to the stricture,[24] and the untoward effects of this bacterial proliferation are amplified by radiation-induced disruption of intestinal epithelium tight junctions, which allows for increased bacterial translocation capable of inducing a local and systemic inflammatory response.[15] Although the affected segments of intestine and serosa appear thickened with areas of telangiectasias,[25] it should be noted that even if the gut appears normal, patients can still be at risk of spontaneous perforation.[26]

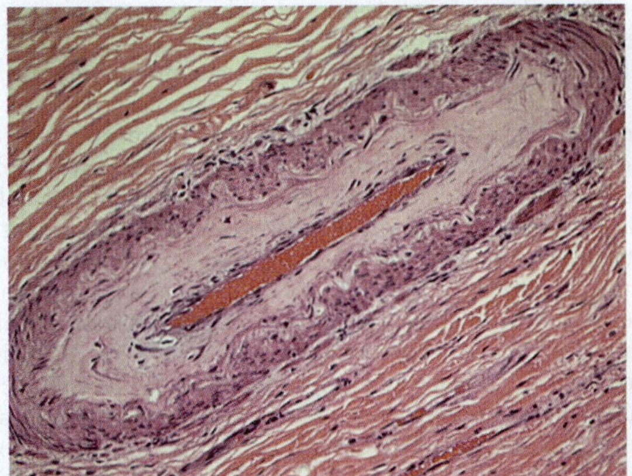

Fig. 39.2 Histopathology showing a submucosal arteriole in chronic radiation enteropathy. Radiation-induced changes include thickening of the blood vessel walls, subintimal hydropic change, and fibrosis, which results in luminal narrowing and occlusion and subsequent tissue ischemia. (Courtesy Dr. Robin Amirkahn, Dallas, TX.)

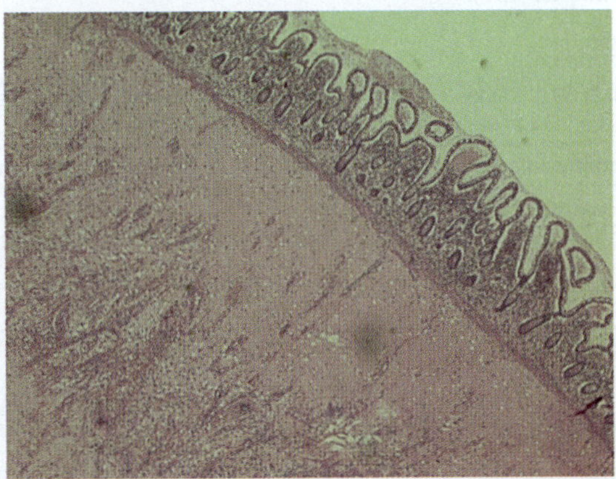

Fig. 39.3 Histopathology showing small intestinal submucosal fibrosis following radiation therapy. The patient presented with small intestinal obstruction due to this stricture. (Courtesy Dr. Robin Amirkahn, Dallas, TX.)

Chronic radiation enteritis can cause significant morbidity. This complication tends to be progressive, with an onset at least 6 months after radiotherapy. Late radiation injury to the small intestine occurs at a median of 8–12 months following RT, although it can appear years later.[27] There are many clinical manifestations of the chronic phase of radiation enteritis (Table 39.1). Fibrosis and vasculitis of the bowel may lead to dysmotility, stricture formation, and malabsorption.[28,29] More rapid transit times can occur in the affected bowel, which can cause chronic malnutrition and resultant anemia and hypoalbuminemia. Malabsorption and other complications may require surgical intervention and parenteral alimentation. Patients with severe chronic radiation enteritis have a poor long-term prognosis and a mortality rate of approximately 10%.[30–35]

The overall incidence of chronic radiation enteritis has not been precisely defined. Retrospective series suggest an incidence of 20%,[36] but questionnaire-based cohort studies suggest perceptible chronic alterations in bowel habits occur much more frequently than anticipated following pelvic radiation (e.g., 50% –80%).[37,38] However, these studies often use imprecise definitions of enteritis and included a large number of patients who were lost to follow-up or died between the end of RT and the completion of the study.[36] A review of randomized trials of neoadjuvant and adjuvant RT for rectal cancer shows severe long-term complications as low as 1.2% and as high as 15%, which is greatly improved in comparison with older trials, suggesting that technical advances have reduced chronic small bowel toxicity rates.[39–41]

Certain factors have been found to predispose patients to radiation toxicity to the small intestine. Women, older patients, and thin patients may have a larger amount of small bowel in the pelvic cul-de-sac, which can increase the likelihood of radiation injury in the treatment of pelvic malignancies.[42] Patients with a history of pelvic inflammatory disease or endometriosis also appear to be at higher risk of radiation complications.[43,44] Patients who have had previous abdominal surgery can develop adhesions that decrease the mobility of the small bowel, allowing it to be consistently exposed to fractionated RT.[45,46] In addition, patients with prior pelvic surgery may have an increase in the amount of small bowel within the pelvis. In one study, the risk of small bowel complications was significantly higher in women who had undergone a previous laparotomy.[47]

Smokers, and patients with diabetes, hypertension, and cardiovascular disease, also have an increased risk of preexisting vascular damage or occlusion.[48–50] These comorbid conditions are

TABLE 39.1 Clinical Complications of Chronic Radiation Enteritis or Proctitis

Complication	Lesion(s)	Clinical Features
Obstruction	Stricture	Constipation, nausea, vomiting, postprandial abdominal pain
Infection	Abscess	Abdominal pain, fever, chills, sepsis, peritonitis
Fistulization	Fistula	Fecal, vaginal, or bladder discharge; pneumaturia
Bleeding	Ulceration	Rectal pain, tenesmus, rectal bleeding, anemia
Malabsorption	Small bowel damage	Diarrhea, steatorrhea, weight loss, malnutrition, cachexia

From Girvent M, Carlson GL, Anderson I, et al. Intestinal failure after surgery for complicated radiation enteritis. *Ann R Coll Surg Engl.* 2000;82:198–201.

compounded by the pathologic changes of chronic radiation injury, which include vasculopathy and ischemia, predisposing the patients to radiation-related small bowel toxicity. Interestingly, however, retrospective studies indicate that the use of statins and/or ACE inhibitors during the course of pelvic radiotherapy may in fact reduce the incidence of acute and chronic bowel toxicity,[51] perhaps stemming from the anti-inflammatory effect exerted by these drugs on endothelial cells.[52] Additionally, patients with collagen vascular and inflammatory bowel diseases have a higher risk of acute as well as chronic radiation-induced injury. Patients with these diseases may have pathologic changes that include transmural fibrosis, collagen deposition, and inflammatory infiltration of the mucosa. The late effects induced by RT to the small bowel are likely additive to these preexisting changes, and studies have shown that these patients have a lower GI tolerance to RT.[53,54] Patients whose IBD or nonmalignant systemic disease is quiescent or well controlled appear to fare better than patients with active disease.

Studies have also addressed the effect of radiation dose on occurrence of small bowel toxicity. Volume of the treatment field, volume of irradiated small bowel, total dose, fraction size, treatment time, and treatment technique all influence small bowel tolerance. The TD5/5 (dose at which there is a 5% risk of toxicity at 5 years) for small volumes of small bowel has been estimated to be 50 Gy. Patients can generally receive 45–50 Gy in 1.8- to 2-Gy daily fractions to a pelvic field without a significant rate of toxicity.[55] Retrospective analysis of patients with locally advanced pancreatic cancer treated with CRT found a maximum dose of 55 Gy to 1 mL of the duodenum to be an important metric for preventing long-term toxicity.[56]

For postoperative patients, radiation to 45–50 Gy in 5 weeks is associated with an approximately 5% incidence of SBO requiring surgery, whereas at doses greater than 50 Gy the incidence rises to as high as 25%–50%.[42] Doses greater than 2 Gy per fraction in the postoperative setting also increase the risk of toxicity.[57] At radiation doses of 70 Gy or greater, the incidence of toxicity rises precipitously.[58]

Studies that have analyzed dose-volume parameters associated with acute small bowel toxicity in patients undergoing treatment with 5-fluorouracil (5-FU)–based CRT therapy for rectal cancer found strong correlations between acute toxicity and the amount of small bowel irradiated at each dose level analyzed.[59,60] A study of different treatment techniques to minimize the effect of pelvic radiation on the small bowel showed that irradiating smaller volumes of bowel yielded less toxicity.[61] In addition, treating patients in the prone position with external compression and bladder distention decreased side effects, likely from exclusion of portions of the small bowel from the radiation field (Fig. 39.4).[62]

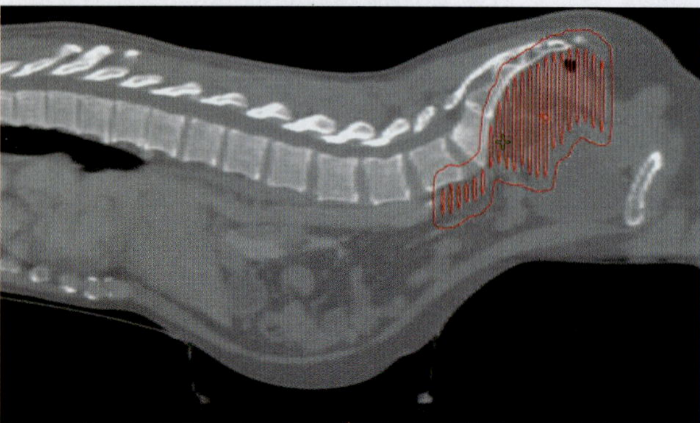

Fig. 39.4 Image from a planning scan performed on a patient with rectal cancer. The patient was positioned prone on a belly board, which allows the small bowel to fall out of the anatomic area to which the prescription dose is planned (illustrated in *red*).

Chemoradiation therapy, commonly with concurrent 5-FU or capecitabine, is used in the treatment of GI malignancies and is known to increase the risk of small bowel toxicity. In the Fédération Francophone de Cancérologie Digestive trial, which randomized patients to RT or CRT with 5-FU and leucovorin, the rate of acute toxicity was 2.7% with RT and 14.6% with the addition of chemotherapy to RT.[63] A second trial conducted by the European Organization for Research and Treatment of Cancer randomized patients with advanced rectal cancer to preoperative RT or CRT, with or without adjuvant chemotherapy. The addition of chemotherapy resulted in higher grade 3 acute toxicity rates: 13.9% versus 7.4%. Rates of grade 2 diarrhea occurred more frequently in patients receiving concurrent chemotherapy: 37.6% versus 17.3%, with no differences in late toxicity.[64]

There is ongoing investigation into the integration of novel chemotherapeutic and "targeted" agents with RT in neoadjuvant therapy for GI cancers. Promising results from early phase II studies incorporating concurrent oxaliplatin into the neoadjuvant regimen were shown later to be more toxic and to offer no disease benefit in subsequent randomized trials.[65] Data from phases I and II trials using novel agents such as irinotecan, EGF receptor inhibitors, and the VEGF inhibitor bevacizumab suggest that the addition of these agents may significantly increase grades 3 and 4 GI toxicity rates relative to standard 5-FU-based chemoradiotherapy (CRT) regimens,[66,67] further emphasizing the importance of careful radiation planning to maximize normal tissue sparing in these patients.

Diagnosis of chronic (late) radiation enteropathy is made clinically (Table 39.2). The cause of symptoms can vary from patient to patient, and individualization of diagnostic and therapeutic approaches is indicated. Therapeutic options are displayed in Table 39.3. Consultation with the treating radiation oncologist should be requested if the clinical presentation is consistent with radiation enteritis. Review of the patient's previous radiation treatment record will reveal the total dose, fractionation, volume of treatment, and other radiation parameters. Analysis of the treatment plan may show areas of high dose, especially if the patient had an intracavitary implant or brachytherapy. Lesions encountered at endoscopy or imaging studies are usually localized in the area of high dose. Ulceration of the mucosa, thickening of jejunal folds, and thickening of the intestinal loops are radiologic signs that suggest radiation damage to the small bowel (Fig. 39.5). Faster intestinal transit and reduced bile acid and lactose absorption can be observed in patients with chronic radiation enteritis.[68] These effects may be improved after the administration of antimotility agents such as loperamide. Antibiotics are indicated if there is small intestinal bacterial overgrowth syndrome (see Chapter 107).[69,70]

TABLE 39.2 Pathophysiologic Features of Patients With Chronic (Late) Radiation Enteropathy and Their Clinical Manifestations

Pathophysiologic Feature	Clinical Manifestations
Mucosal dysfunction	Lactose intolerance Vitamin B_{12} deficiency Steatorrhea
Stricture or blind loop syndrome with SIBO	Diarrhea
Intestinal dysmotility	Bloating Constipation Diarrhea
Abnormal bile acid recirculation	Cholerheic diarrhea

SIBO, Small intestinal bacterial overgrowth.

From Hauer-Jensen M, Wang J, Denham J. Bowel injury: current and evolving management strategies. *Semin Radiat Oncol.* 2003;13:357–371.

TABLE 39.3 Therapeutic Options for Patients With Chronic (Late) Radiation Enteropathy

Pathophysiologic Feature	Therapeutic Options
Nutritional deficits	Correction of specific deficits Low-fat diet Lactose-free diet Elemental diet TPN
Intestinal dysmotility (increased or decreased)	Loperamide Octreotide Prokinetic agent
Bile acid malabsorption	Bile-salt binding agent
SIBO	Antibiotics

SIBO, Small intestinal bacterial overgrowth.
From Hauer-Jensen M, Wang J, Denham J. Bowel injury: current and evolving management strategies. *Semin Radiat Oncol*. 2003;13:357–371.

Treatment and Prevention

The management of acute radiation small bowel toxicity should be based on the severity of symptoms. Most cases of acute radiation enteritis are self-limited, requiring only supportive treatment. Diarrhea, nausea, vomiting, and abdominal cramping are treated symptomatically. Antidiarrheal medications such as loperamide, diphenoxylate atropine, or opiates can be used. Antiemetic agents may also be effective. A low-fat, lactose-free diet with incorporation of long-chain omega-3 and probiotics may improve symptoms.[71] A study of oral sucralfate in patients receiving pelvic irradiation showed a decrease in frequency and an improvement in consistency of bowel movements at both early and late time points.[72] Cholestyramine to treat diarrhea from bile acid malabsorption has also shown some benefit,[73] and treatment with aspirin has been effective.[74] Intractable diarrhea during combined-modality treatment (CRT) may require hospital admission for administration of parenteral fluids and electrolyte repletion. Patients who are refractory to conventional antidiarrheal medications may benefit from administration of a synthetic somatostatin analog such as octreotide.[75]

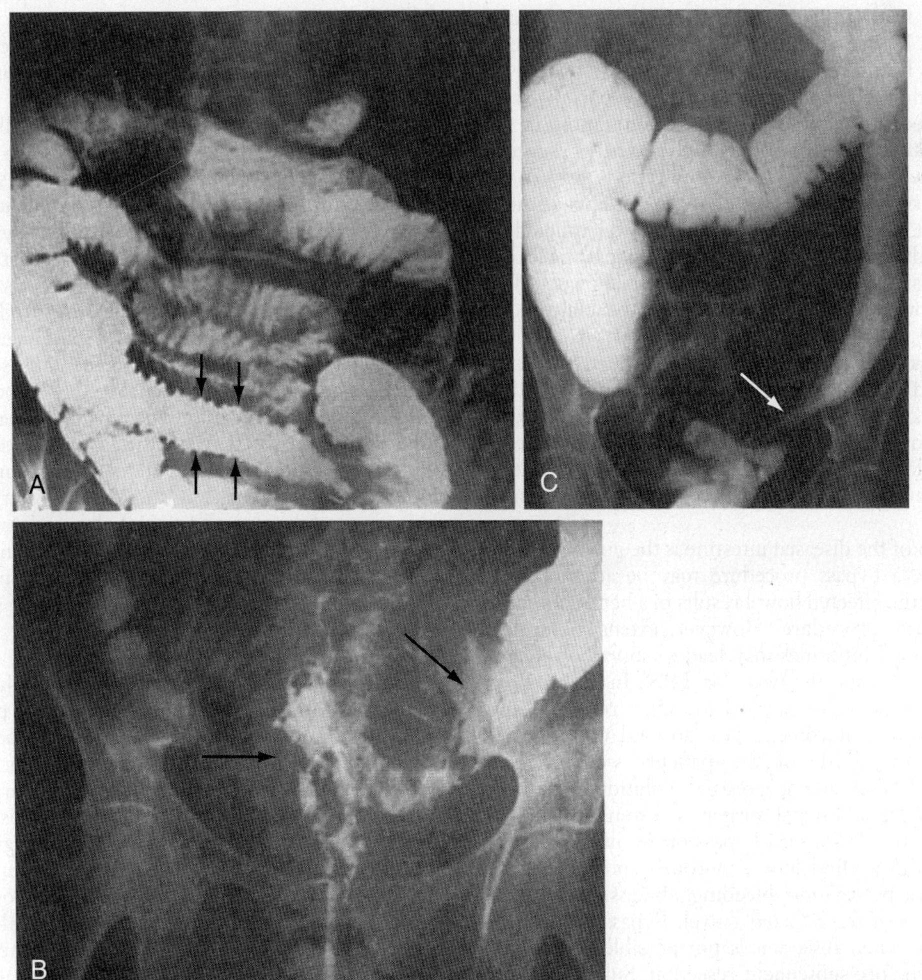

Fig. 39.5 Radiologic evidence of radiation injury of the intestine. (A) In early injury, bowel and mesenteric edema may cause separation of intestinal loops, lead to thickening and straightening of mucosal folds, and impart a spiked appearance (*arrows*) to the small bowel mucosa. (B) Severe abnormalities of the rectosigmoid colon are evident on this film from a barium enema performed 2 months after the patient underwent radiation therapy for cervical carcinoma. Subacute radiation injury of the colon may present as edematous, occasionally ulcerated mucosa with asymmetrical areas of narrowing suggestive of Crohn colitis or recurrent tumor (*arrows*). (C) Late radiation change in the colon, with stricture formation (*arrow*) after a cumulative dose of approximately 55 Gy.

The management of chronic radiation enteritis remains a major challenge, given the progressive evolution of the pathophysiology, including obstructive endarteritis and fibrosis. The treatment should be conservative, given the diffuse nature of the process and the high morbidity associated with surgery; however, surgical intervention is indicated in intestinal obstruction, perforation, fistulas, and severe bleeding.

Chronic effects of diarrhea are managed symptomatically with a low-residue diet. Fiber supplementation (e.g., Metamucil, Citrucel) has shown benefit in some cases. In the rare setting of malnutrition related to chronic radiation injury, TPN can improve clinical outcome, and methylprednisolone may add to the effects of TPN.[43] Despite these interventions, the 5-year survival rate for patients undergoing TPN ranges from 36% to 54%.[35,76] It has been estimated that overall mortality rate associated with chronic radiation enteropathy is approximately 10%.[77]

Endoscopic techniques are sometimes required for diagnosis of bleeding intestinal ulcers. Double-balloon enteroscopy and capsule endoscopy may help facilitate this diagnosis.[78] The double-balloon enteroscope method may allow therapeutic intervention in certain situations, including coagulation of small bowel telangiectasias. Significant bleeding refractory to endoscopic intervention may be managed surgically or via arterial embolization.

SBO is generally managed conservatively with bowel rest and tube decompression. In rare situations, the obstruction is severe or chronic enough that bowel resection or lysis of adhesions may be required. It can be difficult to perform surgery for chronic radiation enteritis because of the diffuse fibrosis and alterations in the intestine and mesentery, resulting in high rates of surgical morbidity and reoperation.[79,80] These complications lead to an estimated 5-year survival rate of only 69% in patients without recurrent disease but who undergo resection of bowel afflicted by chronic radiation-induced injury.[81] The risk of anastomotic leak is high if the anastomosis is performed using irradiated bowel.[77] The risk of leak can be lowered if at least one limb of the anastomosis involves previously unirradiated bowel. However, it may be difficult to distinguish between normal and irradiated tissues at time of surgery and even on pathologic evaluation.[82] Another method the surgeon can use to circumvent this technical difficulty is to create the anastomosis with unirradiated colon. The accuracy in localizing injured bowel may be improved by intraoperative endoscopic examination, which can detect radiation-induced mucosal injury.[83]

Limited resection of the diseased intestine is the goal, but if the lesion is too diffuse, a bypass procedure may be attempted. If feasible, resection of the affected bowel results in a better outcome than an enteric bypass procedure. However, extensive surgical resection of the diseased intestines may lead to short bowel syndrome (see Chapter 108) and the need for TPN. In selected patients who underwent extensive surgical intestinal resection and experienced short bowel syndrome, 5-year survival was approximately 65%, with two-thirds of the patients weaned from parenteral nutrition.[84] Given the progressive evolution of fibrosis, the patient may require additional surgery if extensive surgical resection is not performed. Surgical bypass of the injured bowel may be associated with a blind loop syndrome, and the patient may still be at risk for perforation, bleeding, abscess, and fistulas due to the persistence of the affected bowel. Bypass procedures should be performed when resection is not possible or as temporary management before subsequent resection. Surgery should be performed by an experienced team familiar with the management of radiation enteritis. Perforations and fistulae are best managed surgically. It should be noted that many patients with chronic small bowel radiation toxicity are nutritionally depleted and more susceptible to anastomotic leakage and dehiscence after surgery. The postoperative mortality of these patients may be significant and must be taken into consideration before a decision to proceed with surgery is made.

Hyperbaric oxygen has been used in the treatment of chronic radiation enteritis, the rationale being that the creation of an oxygen gradient in hypoxic tissue will stimulate neoangiogensis.[85,86] In a retrospective study of 36 patients with severe radiation enteritis refractory to medical management, improvement of clinical symptoms was reported in two-thirds of the patients treated with hyperbaric oxygen.[87] Hyperbaric oxygen may be helpful in management of bleeding due to chronic radiation enteritis in patients who are not controlled with conservative measures such as formalin and laser therapy (discussed later).[87–89] A clinical series of 65 consecutive patients with chronic radiation enteritis (small bowel and rectum), primarily manifested as chronic bleeding, were treated with hyperbaric oxygen. Response rates for rectal and more proximal sites were 65% and 73%, respectively. The response rate for bleeding was 70%, and for other symptoms (pain, diarrhea, weight loss, fistula, obstruction), it was 58%. The authors concluded that hyperbaric oxygen therapy resulted in clinically significant improvement in two-thirds of patients with chronic radiation enteritis.[90] Moreover, a comprehensive meta-analysis, including 330 patients with radiation-induced enteritis, suggests the benefit of hyperbaric oxygen may be even more notable, with 81% of patients having partial or complete resolution of GI bleeding and 75% with improvement in diarrhea following hyperbaric oxygen treatment.[91]

Other agents to reduce the incidence of chronic enteritis have been investigated. There is some suggestion that pentoxifylline may abrogate radiation-associated fibrosis through antioxidant effects and inhibition of TGF-β1. In a small study, patients with radiation enteropathy were treated with pentoxifylline and vitamin E, with response assessment by subjective, objective, management, and analytic scales. Regression of symptoms by subjective, objective, management, and analytic scales was seen in 40% of patients by 6 months and 80% of patients at 18 months.[92]

Given that chronic radiation enteritis is complex and rarely curable, prevention is key, and measures to decrease its incidence are imperative. Pancreatic enzymes can exacerbate acute intestinal radiation toxicity, and reducing pancreatic secretion with a synthetic somatostatin receptor analog such as octreotide may reduce early and delayed radiation enteritis in animal studies; however, a randomized phase III trial showed that octreotide was unable to diminish the incidence of acute diarrhea in anorectal patients.[93,94] Further recent preclinical studies suggest that the HMG-CoA reductase inhibitor pravastatin helps maintain intestinal epithelial integrity and delay chronic fibrotic changes following radiation,[95,96] indicating that clinical investigations may be warranted to determine the potential utility of this safe and commonly prescribed medication in mitigating the onset of radiation enteritis.

One of the major risk factors for injury is the previous abdominopelvic surgery, which leads to the prolapse of the small intestines into the pelvis and exposure to radiation. Anticipation for the need of radiation and chemotherapy before or after surgery requires close collaboration among surgical, radiation, and medical oncologists. If gross residual tumor is found unexpectedly at surgery, outlining the tumor bed with surgical clips to facilitate postoperative treatment planning and surgical techniques to keep the small intestine outside the pelvis (e.g., omentoplasty or polyglycolic mesh) may significantly decrease the rate of complications. Postoperative bowel adhesions may increase the volume of bowel irradiated compared with normal small intestine, which is usually mobile. If RT is anticipated after surgery, attempts should be made at the time of surgery to displace the bowel outside the radiation field.[97] One simple technique is the surgical placement of a polyglycolic, biodegradable mesh that moves the intestines out of the pelvis.[98,99] This procedure has minimal morbidity and does not significantly increase operating time. It also does not require a second operation to remove the mesh, because it is absorbed 3 to 4 months after surgery. MRI can be used after surgery to verify the position of the mesh, the small bowel, and eventual disappearance of the mesh. A reduction of 50% of the volume of the small bowel exposed to the radiation has been demonstrated with placement of a mesh during surgery, allowing a higher dose of radiation to be given postoperatively where indicated.[100,101] Other techniques such as pelvic reconstruction, omentoplasty, and transposition of the colon may also significantly decrease the volume of bowel exposed to RT.[101–103]

RT technique is critical in reducing the rate of complications. The use of only anterior and posterior fields for pelvic radiation should be avoided, if possible, because of the high dose and large volume of bowel irradiated. The toxicity of RT correlates with the volume of small bowel irradiated.[104] In many patients, treatment in the prone position with a "belly board" allows the displacement of the small intestines out of the radiation field.[105,106] Patients should be instructed to maintain a full bladder during the radiation session, which further displaces the intestines out of the pelvis.[45] Three-dimensional (3D) treatment planning optimizes the treatment technique by facilitating more accurate dose distributions. A 3D treatment algorithm ensures the sparing of excessive radiation dose to normal tissues by the judicious use of multiple fields to the target volume from multiple geometries.[107] Moreover, utilization of modern techniques such as intensity-modulated radiotherapy (IMRT), which uses sophisticated planning techniques to deliver conformal radiation dose that allows avoidance of critical structures, is becoming standard of care for pelvic and abdominal radiation. In patients undergoing abdominopelvic radiation, IMRT has been shown to reduce the unintended dose to small bowel by ~60% compared to 3D treatment, a dosimetric advantage that leads to significantly reduced gastrointestinal toxicity (including grade 3 chronic GI toxicity) in patients treated with IMRT.[108,109] Finally, technological advances have allowed for the incorporation of adaptive planning techniques that allow for patient-specific assessments of day-to-day anatomical variation to ensure that organs at risk (e.g., bowel bordering a target) do not inadvertently enter a high-dose treatment volume. Such adaptive planning techniques can take many forms, including on-board cone beam CT images obtained prior to administering treatment and even the use of magnetic resonance-guided linear accelerators (MR-linacs), which allow for the acquisition of real-time MR cine images used to administer gated RT that helps ensure bowel does not receive untoward radiation doses.

Treatment of radiation enteritis is often only partially successful. Management is patient specific and should be as conservative as possible because of the relentless progression of the disease, which can be exacerbated by further injury to the area. A better understanding of the mechanism of fibrosis and the interaction of the molecular events controlling apoptosis and fibrosis may assist in the identification of the patient at risk for radiation complications and in the development of new therapeutic approaches.

ESOPHAGUS

Incidence and Clinical Features

Early and late effects on the esophagus following RT of thoracic and upper abdominal malignancies (e.g., esophageal/esophagogastric junctional carcinomas, lung carcinomas) are common. Normal esophageal mucosa undergoes continuous renewal. Acute esophageal injury is believed to be primarily related to radiation damage to the basal epithelial layer, manifested histologically by vacuolization, resulting in epithelial thinning followed by denudation (Fig. 39.6). These changes manifest clinically as dysphagia, odynophagia, and substernal discomfort, usually occurring within 2–3 weeks following initiation of RT. Patients may describe a sudden, sharp, severe chest pain radiating to the back. As treatment progresses, pain may become constant and may not necessarily be related to swallowing. The symptoms may be confused with *Candida* esophagitis, which may occur in conjunction with radiation esophagitis. Concurrent chemotherapy exacerbates these toxic effects. Endoscopically, mucositis and ulceration may be observed. Perforation and bleeding are rare in the acute phase.[110] Shortly after treatment completion, basal proliferation returns and regeneration occurs.[111] CRT, common for the therapy of both lung and esophageal cancer, escalates the rates of grade 3 or greater acute esophagitis approximately fivefold.[112]

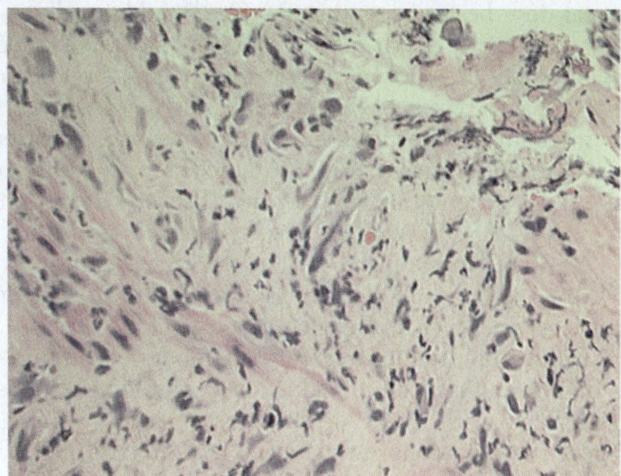

Fig. 39.6 Histopathology of acute radiation-induced esophageal injury showing esophageal ulceration with abundant fibroblasts.

Following recovery from acute injury, late effects such as benign stricture leading to persistent dysphagia, ulceration, and fistula formation may occur months to years following treatment. These effects are believed primarily due to inflammation and scar formation within the esophageal muscle. The connective tissues surrounding the esophagus may also exhibit severe fibrosis over time, and small vessel telangiectasias may be seen endoscopically. Histologic studies of the esophagus in previously irradiated patients have demonstrated epithelial thickening, chronic inflammation, and fibrosis of the submucosa and muscularis propria but rarely chronic ulceration. Complete epithelial recovery from radiation effects may take 3–24 months.[23] Late effects often manifest as dysphagia due to stricture, as well as altered motility due to fibrosis or muscular damage, possibly with accompanying nerve injury. Fistula formation is unusual and radiation dose dependent. Barium swallow examination may show strictures and disruption of peristalsis at the level of the irradiated esophagus, with repetitive and nonperistaltic waves above and below the irradiated region. Abnormal peristalsis has been reported at 1–3 months following treatment completion, whereas most strictures occur 4–8 months following treatment completion. Late effects are usually not seen until 3 months following completion of RT, with a median time to onset of 6 months in some series.[27,113,114]

Development of radiation-related late complications is dose related. Much of the randomized data regarding the dependence of acute radiation esophagitis on different dose-fractionation schemes are from lung cancer trials. The Intergroup 0096 trial of patients with limited stage small cell lung cancer compared CRT regimens of 1.5-Gy fractions delivered twice daily over 3 weeks against 1.8-Gy fractions delivered daily over 5 weeks to the same total dose of 45 Gy. Grade 3 esophagitis was nearly three times as likely in the group receiving treatment twice daily.[115] In the RT Oncology Group (RTOG) 0617 trial, comparing total doses of 60 Gy versus 74 Gy in the treatment of locally advanced non–small cell lung cancer, a threefold increase in grade 3 or greater esophagitis was also noted.[116] Historically the TD5/5 (i.e., dose at which 5% of patients will develop complications at 5 years) has been estimated to be 60 Gy when one-third of the length of the esophagus is irradiated.[117] Cumulatively, it is recommended that the mean esophageal dose be kept less than 34 Gy.[118] Additionally, a dosimetric analysis of the patients in RTOG 0617 demonstrated that the risk of grade ≥2 esophagitis increases precipitously if the volume of esophagus receiving 60 Gy exceeds 17%.[119]

Few randomized trials in esophageal cancer have reported late esophageal toxicities. In the RTOG study 0113, which used doses of 50.4 Gy with chemotherapy, the rate of severe late esophageal toxicity was 12% (3% grade 5 toxicity, which is death).[120] In RTOG 85-01, a randomized trial comparing definitive radiotherapy to 64 Gy and CRT to 50 Gy, nearly 20% of patients in each arm experienced severe late esophageal toxicity.[121] More recent analyses of patients treated with modern planning techniques have found significant reduction in the long-term esophageal sequelae, with rates of long-term grade 3 or higher esophageal complications estimated at ~7% (10.1007/s13566-012-0048-5).[122,123] However, even contemporary studies using sophisticated radiation techniques (e.g., IMRT with a simultaneous integrated boost) to definitively treat esophageal cancer patients to a high dose of 61.6 Gy report high grade 5 toxicity rates of 8%, the majority from esophageal bleeds and fistulas.[124]

Brachytherapy (the temporary insertion of a radioactive source into or adjacent to a tumor) has also been used as a technique for radiation dose escalation in esophageal cancer. Although some institutions have reported low rates of fistula associated with brachytherapy, Gaspar and colleagues reported the results of a phase I/II study examining the role of brachytherapy in addition to external beam RT in the treatment of esophageal cancer. The 1-year actuarial fistula formation rate was 18%, and the authors recommended caution in the use of this approach, particularly in conjunction with concurrent chemotherapy.[125,126] A more contemporary series of 115 patients treated with external beam and brachytherapy resulted in a 38% rate of stricture formation, 9% rate of fistula formation, and 7% rate of acute esophageal bleeding.[127]

The intensity of cancer treatment, such as use of concurrent chemotherapy with RT, increases the rate of acute esophagitis.[128] Maguire and colleagues evaluated 91 patients treated with RT for non–small cell lung cancer and found that the percentage esophageal volume and surface area treated to greater than 50 Gy predicted late esophageal toxicity. Patients who had preexisting GERD and esophageal erosions secondary to tumor were at increased risk for late toxicity. Hyperfractionation (multiple daily radiation treatments) was also associated with increased acute toxicity.[129] Singh and associates studied patients with non–small cell lung cancer who received conformal daily RT with or without concurrent chemotherapy. They found that a maximal esophageal "point" dose of 69 Gy (RT alone) and 58 Gy (with concurrent chemotherapy) predicted significant toxicity. Overall, 26% of patients receiving concurrent CRT developed grade 3 or higher esophageal toxicity, whereas only 1.3% of patients who received RT alone experienced this degree of toxicity.[130] The precise chemotherapeutic agents utilized during concurrent therapy can also influence the risk of toxicity, as the risk of grades 3-4 esophagitis is increased when taxanes are combined with 5-FU-based regimens, as opposed to their combination with platinum agents.[131]

Ahn and colleagues found that the most powerful predictor of late esophageal toxicity in 254 patients treated for non–small cell lung cancer was the severity of acute esophageal toxicity. Severe acute toxicity was predicted using twice-daily radiation, older age, increasing nodal stage, and a variety of dosimetric parameters. The overall incidence of late toxicity was 7%, with a median and maximal time to onset of 5 and 40 months, respectively.[113] Wei and coworkers, evaluating 215 patients who received concurrent chemotherapy, found that the relative esophageal volume receiving greater than 20 Gy predicted for grade 3 or greater acute toxicity, and a second series found that when greater than 30% of the esophageal volume received greater than 50 Gy (V50), this resulted in grade 1 or higher acute toxicity.[132,133] Similarly, patients undergoing chemoradiation in the aforementioned RTOG 0617 had a 25% greater risk of grade ≥3 esophagitis for every 10% increase in esophageal V50.[119] Multivariate analysis in this same study showed that grade ≥3 esophagitis portended worse overall survival for patients compared to those who did not develop substantial esophageal toxicity.[134] Based on these and other data, it is clear that the addition of concurrent chemotherapy to RT increases the incidence of both acute and chronic esophageal toxicity.

Treatment and Prevention

The treatment and prevention of radiation-induced esophagitis have come under increased attention with the use of aggressive combination chemotherapy and RT regimens. Treatment interruptions may ease the symptoms of acute esophagitis but may also compromise treatment efficacy and are generally reserved for severe cases. The management of acute esophagitis usually includes symptomatic management such as topical anesthetics (including viscous lidocaine-based regimens), oral analgesics (including anti-inflammatory agents and narcotics), gastric antisecretory drugs (histamine blockers, proton pump inhibitors [PPIs]), promotility agents (e.g., metoclopramide), and treatment of superimposed infection (candidiasis). Dietary modification, including bland foods, pureed or soft foods, and soups, can help patients maintain oral intake. Other modifications include avoidance of smoking, alcohol, coffee, spicy or acidic foods, chips, crackers, and fatty foods. A study of dietary modifications and pharmacologic prophylaxis for radiation-induced esophagitis reported decreased toxicity and fewer treatment interruptions. It was recommended to drink between meals and to eat six smaller meals per day, consisting of semisolid food, soup, high-calorie supplements, purees, puddings, milk, and soft breads.[135] In addition, ingestion of hot or cold foods should be avoided if possible; instead, foods and liquids should be at room temperature. In severe cases, feeding tube placement may be required.

Radioprotective chemical agents have been investigated as a means of mitigating radiation-induced normal tissue toxicity. The best studied radioprotector, amifostine, is an organic thiophosphate. This agent is a scavenger of free radicals and serves as an alternative target to nucleic acids for alkylating or platinum agents.[136] Trials have had conflicting results and are limited by small patient numbers.[137–141] In the largest randomized trial, patients treated with chemotherapy and RT for non–small cell lung cancer were randomized to receive amifostine or no drug. Although amifostine did not significantly reduce grade 3 or higher esophagitis, patient self-assessments suggested a significantly lower incidence of acute esophagitis in those who received amifostine. Patients receiving amifostine, however, experienced significantly higher rates of nausea, vomiting, infection, febrile neutropenia, and cardiac events.[142] Given these side effects, amifostine is not routinely recommended in the prevention of radiation esophagitis.[143]

A second radioprotector, glutamine, has generated clinical interest. In hypercatabolic states, such as cancer, glutamine deficiency can develop. A retrospective study in 41 patients with lung cancer demonstrated that glutamine was well tolerated, with supplemented patients experiencing a lower incidence of grades 2–3 esophagitis, typically resulting in weight gain during treatment.[144] A second analysis from the same institution evaluated 104 patients, 56 of whom received glutamine. Glutamine was associated with less grade 3 esophagitis, treatment breaks, and weight loss, and administration was not associated with differences in time to event endpoints.[145] A pilot study of 75 patients corroborated retrospective data demonstrating no glutamine intolerance or toxicity. Most patients (73%) were treated with sequential chemoradiation, and 49% of those treated with concomitant chemoradiation did not develop esophagitis.[146] A recent retrospective analysis of 122 patients with advanced lung cancer noted that patients treated prophylactically with glutamine had significantly less acute esophagitis and, consequently, significantly less weight loss.[147] In contrast, preliminary results of a randomized trial investigating whether glutamine decreases the incidence or severity of acute esophagitis in patients undergoing radiotherapy for advanced thoracic malignancies indicate that glutamine does not provide any protective effects against esophagitis, as compared to placebo.[148] In contrast, a prospective randomized phase II trial indicated that the alternative radioprotector epigallocatechin gallate, a naturally occurring polyphenol known to act as a scavenger of reactive oxygen species, is capable of both preventing onset and mitigating the severity of acute esophagitis during RT when randomized against conventional therapy.[149,150] Epigallocatechin gallate did not appear to negatively impact disease-specific outcomes; however, its effect on local control and overall survival has only been reported in patients with small cell lung cancer, necessitating further studies.[151]

The most efficacious means to reduce esophageal toxicity during RT is to minimize the radiation dose to esophageal mucosa that is not part of the treatment target itself. Technological advances have allowed for substantial sparing of the esophagus in nonesophageal primary disease (e.g. locoregionally advanced lung cancer patients). IMRT allows for decreased dose delivered to the esophagus when compared to 3D-conformal radiation techniques, despite IMRT requiring larger treatment volumes in this patient cohort.[152] Furthermore, IMRT can allow sparing of dose to the esophagus on a smaller level, as techniques have emerged that allow radiation oncologists to avoid administering high dose to the full circumferential volume of esophageal mucosa. This so-called contralateral esophagus-sparing technique has been shown to decrease the rates of esophagitis in advanced lung cancer patients, including in a cohort of 27 patients receiving high-dose chemoradiation, with no grade 3 esophagitis nor local failures reported, despite gross tumors frequently situated within 1 cm of the esophagus.[153,154]

The management of late esophageal radiation-induced stricture consists of serial endoscopic dilatation for symptomatic improvement. Dilations in advanced stricture can result in esophageal rupture and therefore should be approached cautiously. Long-term use of gastric antisecretory drugs, as well as prokinetic agents such as metoclopramide, has been recommended to decrease gastroesophageal (GE) reflux effects. Uncommonly, tube feedings may be required for patients with significant weight loss who are unable to maintain weight or for those only able to take in liquids. Surgical intervention may be required for patients who develop perforation or fistula. Finally, it is important to note that the clinical symptoms associated with late radiation injury are often difficult to distinguish from those caused by recurrent or new primary malignancies. Patients with strictures or ulcerations should also be evaluated to differentiate chronic radiation changes from cancer recurrence.

STOMACH

Incidence and Clinical Features

The stomach may be damaged following irradiation of the upper abdomen for cancer, including esophageal-GE junctional, gastric, hepatobiliary, and pancreatic carcinomas. Radiation to the stomach in animals using a very high single dose results in erosive and ulcerative gastritis. A slightly lower single dose results in gastric dilatation and gastroparesis, with replacement of the normal gastric mucosa by hyperkeratinized squamous epithelium. With even lower doses, gastric obstruction occurring months after irradiation was observed, with an atrophic gastric mucosa and intestinal metaplasia seen in surviving animals.[155]

Studies in which serial gastric biopsies were obtained following irradiation of patients for PUD noted necrosis of chief and parietal cells, with mucosal thinning, edema, and chronic inflammatory infiltration.[27,156] In addition, gastric acid production decreased after relatively low doses of gastric irradiation. In the past, RT had been used to decrease acid production in patients with PUD. Even with a relatively low dose of 18 Gy delivered in 10 fractions, approximately 40% of ulcer patients had a 50% reduction in gastric acid secretion that lasted for a year or more.[157]

Clinically, radiation-induced gastritis may occur within a week of starting radiotherapy, with microscopic changes including edema, hemorrhage, and exudation. Histologic changes include disappearance of cytoplasmic details and granules in parietal and chief cells as early as 1 week into therapy. Cell damage and subsequent cell death are often seen first in the depths of glands, followed by thinning of the gastric mucosa. Additional mucosal changes include deepening of the glandular pits and proliferation of cells in the glandular neck. Loss of glandular architecture and thickening of the mucosa can be seen by the third week of radiotherapy. Histologic recovery begins approximately 3 weeks after completing radiotherapy. Signs of recovery of early radiation injury to the stomach include re-epithelialization and fibrosis.

Symptoms of acute radiation injury of the stomach consist primarily of nausea and vomiting, dyspepsia, anorexia, abdominal pain, and malaise. These are more common with the concurrent administration of chemotherapy. Radiation-induced nausea and vomiting may occur within the first 24 hours following treatment. It is estimated that approximately half of patients receiving upper abdominal radiation will experience emesis within 2–3 weeks following radiation initiation.[158]

Late effects of gastric irradiation have been classified into four categories: (1) acute ulceration (occurring shortly after completion of RT); (2) gastritis with smoothened mucosal folds and mucosal atrophy on endoscopy, accompanied by radiographic evidence of antral stenosis (1–12 months following irradiation) (see Chapter 54); (3) dyspepsia, consisting of vague gastric symptoms without obvious clinical correlate (6 months to 4 years following irradiation); and (4) late ulceration (averaging 5 months after irradiation).[27,159] The TD5/5 for treatment of the entire stomach has been estimated to be 50 Gy.[117] Large studies of upper abdominal irradiation have suggested that prior abdominal surgery, as well as using a higher radiation dose per fraction, may increase the risk of late effects.[160]

Studies from Walter Reed Army Medical Center, delivering abdominal radiation using now-antiquated techniques in testicular cancer patients, have suggested that higher radiation doses lead to an increasing risk of late gastric ulceration and perforation, with ulceration occurring in approximately 6% of patients treated to 45–50 Gy, 10% of patients treated to 50–60 Gy, and 38% of patients treated to greater than 60 Gy. Perforation rates were 2% and 14% after doses less than 50 Gy and 50 Gy or greater, respectively. Symptomatic gastritis occurred approximately 2 months following radiation completion, with ulcer formation occurring at a median of 5 months. Six of 233 patients (3%) required surgery for ulcer hemorrhage or pain related to ulcer disease, almost all of whom had received doses of greater than 50 Gy.[27,161] Other studies of patients treated with RT for Hodgkin lymphoma or testicular, gastric, or cervical cancer have established tolerance limits for gastric irradiation.[160–163] These studies delivered doses of 40–60 Gy. Patients who received doses greater than 50 Gy experienced gastric ulceration and gastric ulcer–associated perforation at rates of 15% and 10%, respectively. If indicated, the dose to the entire stomach with conformal RT is limited to 45–50 Gy, with an estimated 5%–7% risk of severe radiation toxicity, primarily ulceration.[164]

As in the esophagus, combining chemotherapy with RT decreases the tolerance of the gastric mucosa to RT. 5-FU-based chemotherapy is the most common agent delivered concurrently with RT in the management of GI tumors. This agent can be delivered in the adjuvant or neoadjuvant setting or as "definitive" therapy for GE junction, gastric, peripancreatic, and biliary cancers. 5-FU is a radiation sensitizer but has historically been given safely with RT at doses of 45−50 Gy without substantial increases in toxicity. Contemporary studies reiterate the safety of 5-FU-based chemoradiation strategies, with, for example, interim results from the TOPGEAR study, investigating the role of neoadjuvant 5-FU + 45 Gy gastro-abdominal RT in addition to neoadjuvant chemotherapy, showing that rates of gastric toxicities and surgical complications following chemoradiation are modest and equivalent to those undergoing systemic therapy alone.[165]

Newer systemic agents have been shown to increase acute gastric toxicity when delivered with radiotherapy, including taxanes, gemcitabine, and EGF receptor inhibitors. A phase I study evaluated 5-FU, gemcitabine, and radiotherapy in locally advanced pancreatic cancer. Of the seven patients enrolled, three experienced gastric or duodenal ulcers with severe bleeding, requiring transfusion.[166] However, several recent studies have demonstrated good disease control and excellent tolerability of RT combined with gemcitabine alone in the setting of neoadjuvant treatment of pancreatic cancer, with no reports of ulceration or severe bleeding.[167,168] Similarly, a large, randomized phase 3 trial investigating postoperative chemotherapy versus postoperative chemoradiation in resected gastric cancer (~50% subtotal gastrectomy) demonstrated that combining cisplatin with 5-FU during a 45 Gy course of radiation to the abdomen was well tolerated, with GI toxicities similar to adjuvant chemotherapy alone and only a ~1% risk of fistula, perforation, or GI bleed.[169] These studies demonstrate that careful selection of concurrent chemotherapeutic regimens can effectively mitigate gastric toxicity when modern treatment regimens are employed.

Treatment and Prevention

Acute symptoms of gastric radiation toxicity are treated with antiemetics (5-hydroxytryptamine-3 [5-HT_3] antagonists, phenothiazines, metoclopramide, glucocorticoids, benzodiazepines, antihistamines, or anticholinergics), as well as consumption of a light meal prior to delivery of RT. Randomized trials of prophylactic 5-HT_3 inhibitors have shown efficacy compared with placebo in preventing radiation-induced nausea and vomiting.[170] A randomized trial of 211 patients receiving upper abdominal radiation compared the 5-HT_3 inhibitor ondansetron given twice daily with or without dexamethasone delivered daily for the first 5 fractions of treatment. Patients receiving dexamethasone showed a trend toward improved complete control of nausea (50% vs. 38%) and significant improvement in complete control over emesis. The authors concluded that the addition of dexamethasone resulted in modest improvement in protection against radiation-induced emesis.[171] Narcotic and nonnarcotic agents are often used for pain. In addition, it is recommended that patients be placed on acid antisecretory medications, including PPIs. Careful nutritional support along with antiemetic therapy is essential for patients undergoing radiotherapy to the abdomen. Acute symptoms generally resolve within 1−2 weeks following completion of RT. Similar to that observed during pelvic radiation or thoracic radiation, modern radiation techniques in the form of intensity-modulated RT (IMRT) have been shown to prevent gastric toxicity, with one large institutional study indicating that patients undergoing preoperative chemoradiation for gastric cancer have significantly lower rates of grades 3 and 4 acute toxicities compared to their counterparts undergoing 3D conformal radiation, including decreased rates of nausea and malnutrition with less requirement for IV hydration, feeding tube use, and hospitalization.[172]

Late gastritis-related symptoms are often treated with acid antisecretory drugs, including histamine antagonists and PPIs, and/or sucralfate. These may be used on a long-term basis to avoid late ulceration. With more severe complications of bleeding, ulceration, gastric outlet obstruction, fistula formation, or perforation, patients may require endoscopic therapeutic approaches or rarely surgical intervention with partial gastrectomy.

COLON AND RECTUM

Incidence and Clinical Features

The large bowel is less radiosensitive than the small bowel. Nevertheless, the mechanisms underlying acute and chronic injuries of the large intestine are similar to those of the small intestine. There is a decrease in the stem cell mitotic rate, resulting in a depletion of precursor cells required to replenish the epithelium as it normally sheds. Acute injury can be accompanied by superficial mucosal erosions and lamina propria hemorrhage. There is also a thickening of the mucosa, with proliferation of fibroblasts (Fig. 39.7).[173] Late changes include vascular fibrosis with associated ischemia and formation of telangiectasias, which can be a source of bleeding (Fig. 39.8). Late radiation large bowel changes can lead to fluid and electrolyte malabsorption, obstruction, chronic proctitis, and fistula formation. Ischemic changes also include ulceration (Fig. 39.9), perforation, and fistulae.[25] Bowel wall fibrosis may occur, causing decreased motility and compliance, and stricture.[174] A decrease in rectal compliance can reduce the ability of the rectum to act as a reservoir, leading to frequent low volume stools, urgency, and incontinence.

Acute colitis from RT manifests clinically as diarrhea, cramping, tenesmus, urgency, incontinence, and, less commonly, mucoid or bloody rectal discharge. These symptoms can result from rectal inflammation, edema, and spasm. Symptoms often begin 2−3 weeks into treatment and usually resolve within several weeks to 3 months following radiation completion. The relationship between the incidence of acute and chronic radiation injury is uncertain.[175,176] Chronic changes appear within 6 months to 2 years and beyond following completion of RT, with symptoms similar to acute injury. Patients may present with tenesmus, bleeding, low-volume diarrhea, rectal pain, and occasionally low-grade obstruction or fistulae (see Table 39.1).[177] Possible risk factors for the development of chronic colitis or proctitis include tobacco use, history of pelvic or abdominal surgeries, and the development of a specific "cluster" of symptoms to include pain, fecal urgency, rectal bleeding, and rectal mucus production (as opposed to nausea, diarrhea, or incontinence).[178] Patients can also develop a pancolitis that mimics IBD. In addition, pelvic

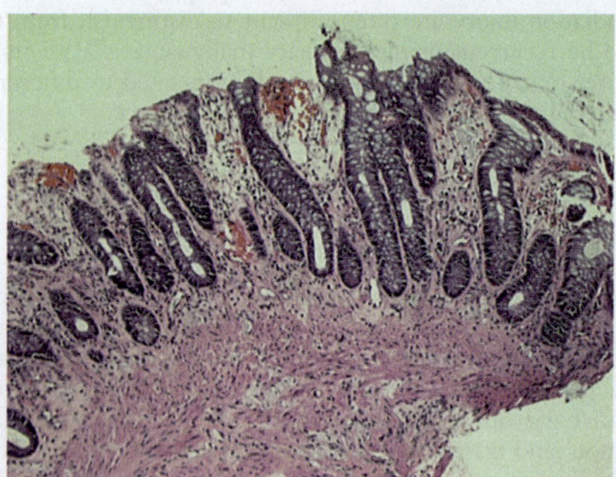

Fig. 39.7 Histopathology of acute radiation injury to the rectum with superficial rectal mucosal erosion and focal lamina propria hemorrhage. (Courtesy Dr. Robin Amirkahn, Dallas, TX.)

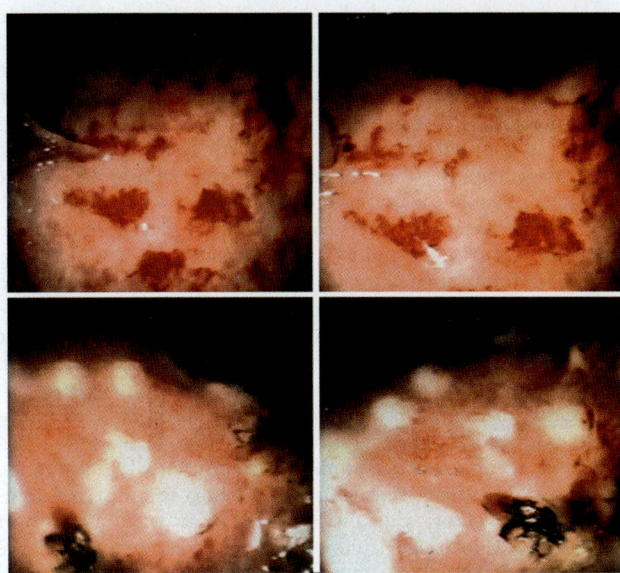

Fig. 39.8 Typical colonoscopic findings of radiation proctitis in a patient treated for prostate cancer. *Top panels*: Endoscopic view of the rectum reveals the characteristic fine tortuosity and curling of the new vessels. *Lower panels*: These demonstrate superficial burns from argon plasma coagulation, which was used to stop this patient's bleeding. It is not necessary to ablate the lesions completely but merely to cause mucosal and submucosal fibrosis, thereby entrapping the vessels in the scarring process. (Courtesy Lawrence J. Brandt, MD, Bronx, New York.)

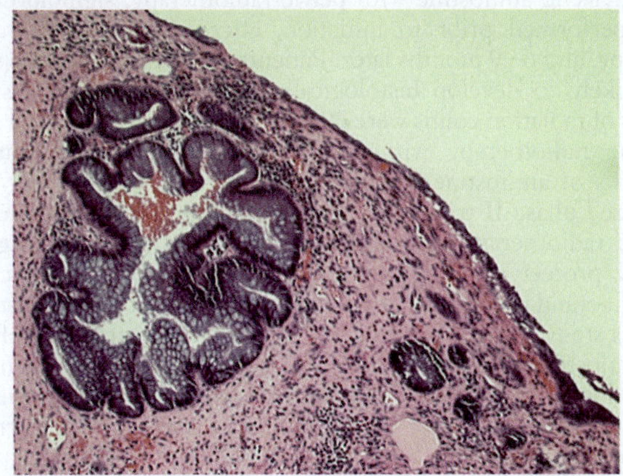

Fig. 39.9 Histopathology of the rectal mucosa after radiotherapy with residual malformed rectal crypts and flat, regenerating surface mucosa in the region of a radiation-induced rectal ulcer. Note the fibrosis and inflammation of the lamina propria. (Courtesy Dr. Robin Amirkahn, Dallas, TX.)

irradiation is a risk factor for development of rectal cancer, and there is evidence that those patients who have received prostate-directed RT have a risk for rectal cancer similar to that of having a first-degree relative with rectal cancer.[179]

The lower radiosensitivity of the colon and rectum than the small intestine may be partially explained by the fact that higher doses of radiation are often delivered to smaller volumes of the rectum compared with small intestine (i.e., focal "collateral" rectal irradiation in prostate and gynecological cancer therapy). The rectum is also a readily accessible organ by endoscopy, allowing early diagnosis and intervention, possibly preventing symptomatic progression. Data suggest that although rectal mucosal changes are present for up to 5 years posttreatment, there is often recovery after complications and resolution of mucosal changes.[180]

Series have reported the risk of serious late rectal complications is 5% or less when less than 80 Gy is delivered.[27] Radiation injury of the large intestine occurs most frequently in the rectum, owing to its location adjacent to the prostate, bladder, cervix, uterus, and ovaries, exposing it to a collateral radiation dose with treatment of these organs.[23] There have been recent improvements in this derived from procedural techniques aimed at displacing the rectal interface from its radiation target, namely by introducing an absorbable hydrogel between the rectal-prostate space preceding treatment for prostate cancer, which has led to sustained benefits in reducing late rectal toxicity following 79.2 Gy RT to the prostate.[181] Acute rectal injury is often self-limited, but the incidence of chronic radiation proctitis is increasing with increased use of pelvic RT and radiation dose escalation.[182,183]

As is true with other sites, the incidence of large bowel toxicity is associated with radiation dose, volumes treated, and the use of CRT. The treatment of rectal cancer commonly uses doses of 45–54 Gy, whereas treatment of prostate and cervical cancer uses higher doses ranging from 60 to 80 Gy. The incidence of severe rectosigmoid toxicity in cervical cancer patients was 4% or less for patients receiving doses less than 80 Gy and 13% for doses greater than 95 Gy; modern brachytherapy-based treatment techniques for cervical cancer show that the incidence of grades 2–4 rectal toxicity is below 10% even when the rectum receives a maximum point dose up to 107 Gy.[184,185] The treatment of prostate cancer with doses of 60–70 Gy has been associated with an incidence of severe proctitis less than 8%.[186] Radiation doses of 60–70 Gy for anal cancer yield an incidence of severe rectal toxicity of 5% or less.[187–189]

Collectively, it is recommended that less than 20% of the rectum should receive doses greater than 70 Gy. This is associated with grade 2 or higher rectal toxicity in the range of 6%–23%.[190] Treatment using conformal radiation, 3-field, and 4-field techniques further decreases the risk of rectal toxicity.[184,191] A trial of conformal versus conventional radiation for prostate cancer reported less radiation proctitis (5% vs. 15%, respectively).[192] The use of IMRT may further improve this rate, as demonstrated by an updated analysis of nearly 1000 prostate cancer patients treated to doses greater than 80 Gy. The actuarial rate of grade 2 or higher rectal toxicity at 7 years was 4.4%, and the incidence of late grade 3 toxicity was 0.7%; no patients experienced grade 4 toxicity.[193] The safety of IMRT remained durable well after these patients were treated, with only 1.0%, 1.0%, and 0% of these prostate cancer patients experiencing late grade 2, grade 3, or grade 4 GI toxicities, respectively, at 15 years posttreatment.[194] Even as moderate to severe hypofractionation, including stereotactic body radiotherapy (SBRT), has become more commonly used in the treatment of prostate cancer, late GI toxicities have remained acceptably low with modern planning techniques and image guidance.[195–198]

Combining chemotherapy with RT increases toxicity rates. A combination of 5-FU and mitomycin C with radiation doses of 40–55 Gy in the treatment of anal cancer was associated with a less than 5% risk of severe rectal complications.[199] Multiple trials have combined 5-FU–based chemotherapy and RT as neoadjuvant and adjuvant treatment for rectal cancer.[200–203] The toxic effect of combined chemotherapy and radiation has varied from no significant increase in toxicity to a 24% incidence of severe diarrhea and a 25% incidence of chronic bowel injury.[204] Given the increase in toxicity observed with single or opposed-only radiation fields, the use of conformal and multifield techniques is necessary when using combination therapy. The increasing use of neoadjuvant CRT has also raised the concern of increased postoperative complications in these patients, although a large, randomized trial showed a significant reduction in the rates of acute and chronic GI toxicity, as well as improved local control in patients treated neoadjuvantly, which now represents the standard of care.[203,205]

In contrast to small bowel injury, previous abdominopelvic surgery does not appear to predispose the rectum to radiation injury, likely due to the fact it is not otherwise mobile. Given the similarity of vascular changes seen with small bowel radiation injury, a history of diabetes, hypertension, cardiovascular disease, or peripheral vascular disease may predispose the large bowel to radiation toxicity.[48,53,54,206] Patients with collagen vascular disease and IBD also have an increased propensity for large bowel radiation toxicity.

Treatment and Prevention

Management of large bowel radiation toxicity is based on symptom control. Acute toxicity is treated with antimotility agents such as loperamide or diphenoxylate with atropine and a low-residue diet. Opiates and anticholinergics may also be of benefit. Glucocorticoid-containing suppositories may be helpful in the management of patients with anorectal inflammation. Colonoscopy should be avoided if possible because of the potential risk of perforation associated with friable rectal mucosa during radiation.[207] It is recommended that screening colonoscopies be done prior to prostate brachytherapy to reduce rectal complications.[208] This is also a reasonable approach prior to the initiation of external beam RT.

For chronic diarrhea due to decreased rectal compliance, stool softeners or fiber supplements may alleviate symptoms. As in acute proctitis, glucocorticoid suppositories may be beneficial. The benefit of glucocorticoid retention enemas is unclear.[209] Short-chain fatty acids and amino acid derivatives, which nourish and protect the colonic mucosa, have been studied in acute radiation proctitis.[210] Initial relief of symptoms can be seen, but symptoms recur shortly after stopping treatment.[211] Additionally, randomized data suggest that oral probiotics taken during the course of pelvic radiotherapy decrease the incidence of proctitis and associated radiation-induced diarrhea.[212,213] Hyperbaric oxygen has been used to stabilize bleeding related to telangiectasias, but this treatment is not widely available and requires many sessions before any effect is seen.[214] Nonetheless, a randomized trial in patients with refractory chronic radiation proctitis reported that hyperbaric oxygen therapy significantly improved healing, with a more recent study showing response rates as high as 95% in patients with chronic proctitis undergoing HBO.[215,216]

Treatment of colorectal ulcerations associated with bleeding is initially endoscopic, with the use of coagulation techniques, such as argon plasma coagulation. Bleeding due to radiation proctopathy is usually minor and often controlled endoscopically with conservative measures such as cauterization of the telangiectasias with laser treatment (see Fig. 39.8).[217] Application of formalin or colonic irrigation with oral antibiotics may result in long-lasting therapeutic effect.[218–222] Sucralfate enemas may alleviate radiation proctopathy by forming a protective complex with the rectal mucosa. It also increases the local levels of fibroblast growth factors and prostaglandins. Sucralfate enemas appear to be helpful in chronic proctopathy, but their benefit is unclear during the acute period.[223–225] Short-chain fatty acid enemas may also be helpful for management of chronic hemorrhagic radiation proctopathy by inhibiting the inflammatory response, including the nuclear factor κB pathway.[226,227]

Strictures can also be endoscopically dilated. For patients who have refractory bleeding, stricture, perforation, or fistulae, surgical management may rarely be necessary. Management of a pelvic fistula (e.g., vaginal or bladder fistula) is complex and generally requires fecal diversion before corrective surgery. A thorough radiographic investigation with barium enema, small bowel follow-through, or enterography to delineate the extent of the fistula should be performed before surgery. Patients with fistulas may present with additional challenges such as electrolyte imbalance, malnutrition, and infections. Many surgical techniques have been described to repair fistulas, but corrective surgery is best done when the patient is medically stable, and enough time has elapsed after surgical diversion. This allows healing and decreased inflammation of the affected tissues.[228,229]

Prevention of large bowel toxicity from radiation has been studied. Prostaglandins have been investigated as a potential radioprotector. Prostaglandin E_2 and prostaglandin analogs display radiation protection in animal studies.[230–233] Clinically, misoprostol suppositories have also been shown to reduce symptoms of acute radiation enteritis in patients undergoing RT for prostate cancer. However, a randomized placebo-controlled trial from Germany in patients with prostate cancer undergoing irradiation found that significantly more patients experienced rectal bleeding in the misoprostol group.[234,235]

Amifostine has been investigated for the prevention of chronic radiation enteritis and has demonstrated protection of the small and large intestines in preclinical studies.[236] The drug has also been shown to reduce the incidence of early and delayed radiotherapeutic injuries at several anatomic sites. In a randomized study, the late effects of radiation were significantly reduced in the rectal cancer patients receiving parenterally administered amifostine.[237] However, the median follow-up was quite short (24 months), and longer follow-up is necessary to confirm the benefits of the medication, given the incidence of late bowel complications increases with time. Another randomized trial evaluated 205 patients with pelvic malignancies who received RT alone or with IV amifostine. Patients receiving amifostine experienced a significantly lower incidence of grades 2 and 3 bladder and lower GI tract toxicity, with no significant difference between the two groups in tumor response to treatment.[238] There is also evidence to suggest that intrarectal application of amifostine may reduce the risk of proctitis in patients undergoing radiotherapy for prostate cancer.[239] In a phase II study of patients receiving prophylactic amifostine with pelvic radiotherapy, sigmoidoscopy was performed prior to initiation, after completion of radiotherapy, and 6–9 months later. Patients receiving amifostine were less likely to develop histologically detectable mucosal lesions. Rates of radiation colitis were 29% in the amifostine arm and 52% in the radiotherapy without amifostine arm.[240] The durable benefits of amifostine are less clear, however, as a further randomized phase II trial assessing the benefit of amifostine during pelvic radiotherapy demonstrated that it was unable to significantly protect against chronic radiation colitis.[240] The lack of benefit could potentially be related to the lower dose administered in this study (e.g., 500 mg daily), given that the protective effects of amifostine appear to be dose dependent and most notable at daily doses of 1000 mg, which are well tolerated.[241] Nevertheless, such uncertainties make clinical utility of amifostine in current-day practice unclear.

A preclinical study showed a possible role for anti-TGF-β1 interventions to reduce delayed radiation fibrosis and enteropathy.[242] Many special diets and nutrients such as fiber, elemental diets, short-chain fatty acids, and amino acids, such as glutamine, may reduce radiation toxicity to the intestine. However, consistent clinical results were not observed.[243–247] Preventive therapy must have high efficacy, low toxicity, and low cost and not protect the tumor from RT. Unfortunately, no currently available therapy fulfills all of these objectives. As described previously, careful radiation planning and delivery are of paramount importance.

ANUS

Incidence and Clinical Features

The anal canal is typically spared from significant radiation exposure except in treatment of anal, low rectal, and gynecologic cancers. The primary acute toxicity from anal cancer irradiation is diarrhea from large bowel exposure. Damage to the anus itself can occur in the form of acute desquamation or ulceration, with later development of ulcers, strictures, anorectal fistulae, and incontinence.[248] The primary data on anal toxicity from RT come from studies using RT or CRT for the treatment of anal cancer. Anal toxicity manifests as mucosal edema and friability.[249] These changes are often exacerbated by diarrhea that occurs from rectal toxicity. Chronically, anal fibrotic changes may evolve.

Anal toxicity presents initially as a perianal skin reaction that ranges from minimal skin changes and erythema to moist desquamation and diarrhea. These changes are self-limited and usually resolve within a few weeks of treatment completion. Acute toxicity can lead to an interruption of therapy, although this may be less common with modern radiation treatment techniques.[249–251] The incidence of acute toxicity is high and is increased with concurrent chemotherapy delivery or use of a large dose per fraction.[188,199,252,253] Phase III studies and series of patients treated with combined chemotherapy and RT have noted an incidence of skin toxicity of grade 3 or greater in 26%–78% of patients using doses of 45–60 Gy in 1.8–2.25-Gy fractions.[199,248,250,254–257] In a multi-institutional experience of anal cancer patients treated with IMRT-based CRT, grade 3 skin toxicity was seen in 38% of patients, with no grade 4 toxicity observed, comparing favorably to the results of previous randomized trials.[251] A study comparing IMRT with conventional RT found that patients treated with conventional RT had longer elapsed treatment days with significantly more breaks from treatment with higher rates of grade 2 or greater toxicity.[258] A more recent study similarly revealed that anal cancer patients treated with IMRT have reduced rates of grade 3 GI and dermatologic toxicities compared to historic controls treated with non-conformal RT.[259]

Late anal toxicity occurs within months to years following completion of therapy. The most common late complication is anorectal ulceration. Patients also may develop anal stricture or stenosis, incontinence, anal pain, or anorectal fistulae.[199,248,256,260] There does not appear to be an increase in the occurrence of chronic anal toxicity with the addition of chemotherapy to RT.[250,260,261] Doses of 45–60 Gy in fractions of 1.8–2 Gy are considered safe, resulting in chronic grade 3 or higher toxicity rates of zero to 22%.[187,189,199,253,262–264] Doses greater than 65 Gy or fraction size greater than 2 Gy result in a high incidence of anal toxicity.[252] Patients with HIV and anal cancer treated with CRT have an increased risk of both acute and late anal toxicity, although updated analyses indicate that modern antiretroviral therapy likely alleviates these chronic toxicities.[265,266]

Treatment

Treatment of acute toxicity is primarily supportive, including skin care, dietary modifications, pain medications, and topical glucocorticoid medications, with treatment breaks if severe. The effects are self-limited and usually resolve within weeks of therapy completion. Treatment for chronic toxicity, such as anal stricture and stenosis, includes sphincter dilatation. Rarely, patients can require colostomy for severe symptoms. Small studies of hyperbaric oxygen therapy have shown efficacy in treating chronic anorectal ulcers.[267] There is also a report of oral vitamin A therapy for treatment of anorectal ulceration, but confirmatory studies are lacking.[249] Other limited investigations have shown some benefit to sacral nerve stimulation or topical phenylephrine for radiation-induced fecal incontinence.[268,269]

PANCREAS AND LIVER

Incidence and Clinical Features

Pancreas

A Japanese study that randomized patients with resectable pancreatic adenocarcinoma to surgery versus CRT noted respective 3-year survival rates of 20% and 0%, suggesting that surgery is requisite for long-term survival even in the most favorable patients.[270] In turn, the long-term sequelae of irradiation of the pancreas remain poorly defined. Irradiation of the pancreas has a greater impact on exocrine than on endocrine function in animal studies.[271] A study that evaluated the early and late effects of intraoperative RT following resection of pancreatic head lesions noted a larger, transient decrement in exocrine function in the immediate postoperative period in the patients who received RT versus those who did not, with this difference resolving on longer follow-up.[272] The risk of exocrine dysfunction was nevertheless confirmed in a cohort of gastric cancer patients requiring postoperative RT, wherein 60%–70% of patients had evidence of exocrine pancreatic insufficiency up to 5 years following abdominal RT.[273] More recent studies have investigated pancreatic function in a cohort of 53 gastric cancer patients who either required postoperative RT or were simply observed without adjuvant therapy. The 37 patients requiring adjuvant radiotherapy, all with a substantial dose to the pancreas, were significantly more likely to develop pancreatic endocrine dysfunction and sustain a substantial decrease in pancreatic volume, as compared to patients avoiding abdominal irradiation.[274,275] These studies provide evidence for the need to exercise greater vigilance in reducing radiation dose to the pancreas.

Liver

Radiation-induced liver disease (RILD) is seen in approximately 5% of patients when the whole-liver radiation dose reaches 30–35 Gy at 2 Gy per fraction.[276] The pathologic lesion in RILD is central vein thrombosis at the lobular level (veno-occlusive disease), which results in marked sinusoidal congestion, leading to lobular hemorrhage and secondary injury to surrounding hepatocytes.[277] Fibrin deposition in the central veins is thought to be the cause of the veno-occlusive injury. It is unknown what stimulates the fibrin deposition, but hypotheses suggest that TGF-β is increased in the setting of exposure to radiation, which, in turn, stimulates fibroblast migration to the site of injury, causing fibrin and collagen deposition. Foci of necrosis are found in the affected portion of the lobules.[278] Severe acute hepatic toxicity may progress to fibrosis, cirrhosis, and liver failure.

Classic RILD is a clinical syndrome consisting of anicteric hepatomegaly, ascites, and elevated liver enzymes. RILD occurs typically between 2 weeks and 4 months after completion of RT. Patients note fatigue, weight gain, increased abdominal girth, and occasionally RUQ pain. Serum alkaline phosphatase levels are elevated out of proportion to other liver enzymes, and initially the total serum bilirubin level is normal. A nonclassic form of RILD consists of markedly abnormal liver enzyme and bilirubin levels and is more likely in patients with underlying liver disease like viral hepatitis or cirrhosis. Abdominal imaging with CT scan or MRI can be used in diagnosis. RILD can progress to a chronic phase in which patients can develop increasing fibrosis and liver failure.[279]

Given the parallel architecture of the liver, the volume of liver spared from a certain dose of RT, underlying liver function notwithstanding, is an important factor in predicting the likelihood of RILD. Although radiation hepatopathy can occur after doses of 35–40 Gy to the entire liver, significantly higher doses can be given with few clinical complications if sufficient normal liver is spared. Studies by Lawrence and colleagues report that if less than 25% of the normal liver is treated with RT, there may be no upper limit on the dose associated with radiation hepatopathy.[277] Estimates of the hepatic irradiation doses associated with a 5% risk of RILD for uniform irradiation of one-third, two-thirds, and the whole liver are 90, 47, and 31 Gy, respectively. Combining chemotherapy and radiation can increase liver damage, particularly if the chemotherapeutic agents are hepatotoxic. Chlorambucil, busulfan, and platinum drugs are used with RT in bone marrow transplantation patients and are potentially hepatotoxic agents. In contrast, fluoropyrimidines do not seem to increase radiation-related hepatotoxicity.[276,280]

When evaluating the appropriateness of liver-directed therapy, consideration of baseline liver function is important. Patients are presently stratified based upon their Child-Pugh score. Other grading systems exist (e.g., MELD score and ALBI score), but they have not been fully evaluated in patients receiving RT. Most trials investigating the use of RT in the treatment of HCC have excluded patients with the poorest liver function.

Because baseline liver function is typically worse in patients with HCC versus those with cancer that originated outside of the liver, guidelines have suggested adhering to a lower mean liver dose in patients with primary liver cancers.[281] Findings extrapolated from trials using SBRT in the treatment of liver metastases have suggested that a volume of 700 mL of normal liver be spared.[282] In three-fraction SBRT regimens, this constraint requires that at least 700 mL receive less than 15 Gy over the course of treatment, although it is important to keep in mind that this was in patients without underlying liver disease, in whom the volume to spare may be 800 mL and additionally impacted by mean liver doses exceeding ~18 Gy.[283,284] Even more stringent dose constraints are required in patients with Child-Pugh class B cirrhosis undergoing SBRT, with suggested mean liver doses to remain below 8–10 Gy and at least 500–700 mL of normal liver receiving less than 10 Gy, therefore requiring extreme care when considering SBRT for advanced cirrhotic patients.[285,286]

Treatment

Pancreas

Exocrine pancreatic insufficiency is a consequence of both pancreatic volume loss and anatomic alteration in patients who have successfully undergone a Whipple procedure, although it is also commonly seen in patients who underwent a distal pancreatectomy. Fat malabsorption is the predominant cause of symptoms, and dietary modification is often the first recommendation. Pancreatic enzyme replacement has shown success in increasing fat absorption and in turn reducing the severity of steatorrhea, but there is no trial evaluating enzyme replacement in postoperative patients.[287] Nonetheless, pancreatic enzyme replacement is FDA-approved for this indication and should be used in this population with close attention paid to dosing recommendations, including total dose, timing relative to meals, and whether a PPI or antacid is necessary to optimize efficacy. Endocrine pancreatic insufficiency is amenable to insulin replacement similar to that seen in type 1 diabetes mellitus, although underlying insulin resistance must be ruled out or addressed to allow for proper management.

Liver

Supportive care is the mainstay of RILD management. A randomized trial comparing a course of pentoxifylline, ursodeoxycholic acid, and low-molecular-weight heparin versus no treatment in patients receiving interstitial brachytherapy for the treatment of liver metastases noted a significant reduction in radiation-induced liver injury 6 weeks after treatment.[288] This group also prophylactically treated a cohort of 93 patients undergoing radioembolization with this same regimen, noting low rates of RILD and excellent tolerability, albeit in a relatively healthy cohort of breast cancer metastasis patients.[289] Unfortunately, RILD may be fatal given the lack of proven effective treatments and, commonly, the patient's lack of reserve hepatic function.

THERAPEUTIC TECHNIQUES TO REDUCE TOXICITY

GI toxicity is a significant obstacle in the management of many malignancies, resulting in patient morbidity and impeding tumor control by limiting the timely delivery of radiation dose. Maximal avoidance of RT to normal tissue with delivery of adequate therapeutic doses to targets is the primary goal of the radiation oncologist. As discussed, different techniques may be implemented to decrease the volume of nontarget GI tissues treated, including the use of multiple treatment fields to avoid hotspots, treating in the prone position, use of a belly board or false tabletop, as well as treating the patient with a full bladder to displace bowel out of the radiation field.

In the past, RT plans were based on two-dimensional planning in which treatment fields were defined using plain films and known anatomic landmarks. With improvements in imaging and computing capabilities, 3D treatment planning became available in the 1980s. An advanced form of 3D planning, IMRT, has now been implemented in clinical practice.[290,291] As opposed to conventional "static" fields, IMRT uses the principle of multiple "fields-within-fields" that more accurately conform radiation dose to target tissues while sparing normal structures. IMRT requires target tissues and normal organs to be accurately defined. Dose constraints are assigned to these organs, along with a desired prescription dose to the target volume(s). "Inverse planning," whereby computer-searched algorithms establish multiple (and sometimes unconventional) beam or field designs, is then performed, attempting to meet the prescribed target dose and normal tissue dose constraints. Individual fields are treated with multiple, small "beamlets" rather than one uniform beam, and each beam delivers a different dose intensity to the different parts of the target. This allows close conformation of radiation dose to the shape of the target and preferential sparing of nearby normal tissues.

Collectively, early clinical results in varying cancers using IMRT-based CRT have shown significant reductions in treatment-related toxicities, with cancer-related outcomes similar to conventional radiotherapy approaches. For example, Mundt and associates showed a marked improvement in small bowel dosimetry for patients with gynecologic malignancies treated with IMRT compared with conventional 3D planning. An experience of 36 patients with gynecologic malignancies treated with intensity-modulated whole-pelvic radiotherapy was compared with outcomes of 30 patients treated at the same institution with 3D conformal radiotherapy. Patients were well matched with respect to demographic and treatment factors. Significantly lower rates of chronic GI toxicity were seen in the IMRT group, with only 11% of women treated with IMRT experiencing grades 1–3 toxicity (0% grade 3) versus 50% in the non-IMRT group.[292] In a different series, Salama and colleagues reported on 53 patients with anal carcinoma treated with IMRT-based CRT. The median radiation doses to the pelvis and the primary disease were 45 and 52 Gy, respectively. Fifteen percent of patients experienced acute grade 3 GI toxicity, with no grade 4 toxicity observed, comparing favorably with observed rates of severe GI toxicity in contemporary trials using conventional radiation planning.[251] IMRT is now the primary modality used in the treatment of anal canal cancer and is very commonly used in the treatment of esophageal, hepatobiliary, and pancreatic cancer.

Full references for this chapter can be found at https://ebooks.health.elsevier.com.

40 Preparation for and Complications of GI Endoscopy

Adam Slivka, Stephanie Romutis

IN THIS CHAPTER

PREPARATION OF THE PATIENT FOR ENDOSCOPY

Many complications can be prevented before the patient even arrives in the endoscopy suite. Proper patient preparation is crucial for procedural safety and success.

History and Physical Examination

A thorough and pertinent medical history should be obtained prior to endoscopy. A careful review of previous endoscopic procedures should also be performed. This should include the recognition of any adverse events, the targeted level of sedation, and the patient's satisfaction with the sedation. A list of current medication usage along with relevant allergies should also be obtained. Use of sedatives, analgesics, and alcohol by the patient can predict the need for larger doses of sedatives and analgesics or the use of monitored anesthesia care. A focused physical examination, including the airway, heart, lungs, and abdomen, should be performed prior to each endoscopy. Assignment of an American Society of Anesthesiology (ASA) Physical Status (PS) category (Table 40.1) is strongly encouraged because it has been shown to predict adverse cardiopulmonary events.[1]

Informed Consent

Written informed consent should be obtained by the endoscopist before performance of any endoscopic procedure. The components of the informed consent should include a discussion of the procedure itself, including the risks, benefits, and alternatives. The frequency and severity of complications should also be reviewed.[2] The process of obtaining informed consent is a legal requirement as well as a basic ethical obligation. It allows the patient to gain a thorough understanding of the proposed procedure, including the potential risks involved, possible alternatives, and to have all questions answered.

Management of Anticoagulant and Antiplatelet Drugs

The management of antithrombotic and antiplatelet medication should be based on the urgency of the endoscopic procedure and the bleeding risk associated with the procedure if the agent is not discontinued.[3] A good framework is required to classify endoscopic procedures as low versus high risk for bleeding and the underlying disease condition as high versus low risk for a thrombotic complication. With the advent of newer antiplatelet and anticoagulant medications, it is important for the practicing gastroenterologist to be familiar with the pharmacokinetics of these agents to decrease bleeding and thrombotic complications.

Several societies, including the ASGE and ESGE, provide position statements on the management of antithrombotic agents for patients undergoing GI endoscopy.[4–7] For procedures with low perceived bleeding risk, including diagnostic EGD/colonoscopy with biopsy, diagnostic EUS without FNA, and ERCP with stent placement only, medications, including aspirin, warfarin, and clopidogrel, can be continued without interruption. Procedures with high perceived bleeding risk include polypectomy, ERCP with sphincterotomy or sphincteroplasty, stricture dilation,

TABLE 40.1 ASA PS* Classification System Used to Assess Risk of GI Endoscopic Procedures

ASA PS Category	Preprocedure Health Status
1	Healthy (normal)
2	Mild systemic disease
3	Severe systemic disease
4	Severe systemic disease that is a constant threat to life
5	Moribund (not expected to survive without the procedure)
6	Brain death (for organ harvest)

**ASA PS*, American Society of Anesthesiologists Physical Status.

injection or banding of varices, percutaneous gastrostomy, EUS with FNA, and ampullectomy. In this setting, it is recommended that warfarin be held for a minimum of 5 days and direct oral anticoagulants (DOACs) for a minimum of 48–72 hours depending on their pharmacokinetics.[4,6,7]

While thienopyridines (e.g., clopidogrel and prasugrel) and direct P2Y12 antagonists (e.g., ticagrelor) can be continued during low-risk procedures, general consensus is to hold these agents for 5–7 days prior to endoscopic procedures. In the setting of recent percutaneous coronary intervention (PCI), it is recommended to delay elective endoscopic procedures until at least 6 months post-PCI in an effort to minimize potential antiplatelet agent disruption.[4,6,7] When antithrombotic therapy is temporary, such as in the treatment of acute venous thromboembolism, elective GI procedures should be delayed if possible until the anticoagulation is no longer indicated.[3,4] The decision to "bridge" patients with low-molecular-weight heparin should depend on whether there is a high risk of venous thromboembolism, including prosthetic mitral/aortic valves, a prosthetic valve with concurrent atrial fibrillation, history of atrial fibrillation and recent cerebral vascular accident (within ≤3 months), and recent VTE (≤3 months).[6]

The resumption of antiplatelet and anticoagulant agents following endoscopy is based on the perceived continued bleeding risk. Generally, warfarin can be resumed on the evening following the procedure with DOACs and antiplatelet agents resumed 48–72 hours postprocedure.[4,6]

Antibiotic Prophylaxis

There are several GI endoscopic procedures in which antibiotic prophylaxis is warranted (Table 40.2).[8] The strongest level of evidence for prophylactic administration of antibiotics is prior to percutaneous endoscopic gastrostomy (PEG) placement to reduce the risk of peristomal cellulitis.[8–10] Intended or unintended manipulation of sterile pancreatic necrosis or a pancreatic pseudocyst during ERCP or EUS, as well as EUS-guided FNA of cystic structures within and surrounding the GI tract, should receive antibiotic prophylaxis.[8,10] Patients undergoing ERCP with anticipated incomplete drainage of the biliary tree (such as in cases of extensive primary sclerosing cholangitis or hilar tumors) should also receive antibiotic prophylaxis.[8,10] Antibiotic prophylaxis has also been recommended in all liver transplant patients undergoing ERCP[8,10]; however, data are inconclusive on the necessity of antibiotics in such patients.[11]

TABLE 40.2 Conditions and Procedures Requiring Antibiotic Prophylaxis for Endoscopic Procedures

Patient Condition	Procedure	Goal of Prophylaxis
Bile duct obstruction without cholangitis	ERCP with anticipated incomplete biliary drainage	Prevention of cholangitis
Sterile pancreatic fluid collections that communicate with the pancreatic duct	ERCP	Prevention of cyst infection
Sterile pancreatic fluid collection	Transmural drainage	Prevention of cyst infection
Cystic lesions along the GI tract, including the mediastinum	EUS-FNA	Prevention of cyst infection
Cirrhosis with acute GI bleeding	All endoscopic procedures	Prevention of infectious complications including SBP
Any condition	Percutaneous endoscopic feeding tube placement	Prevention of peristomal infection (cellulitis)

Transient bacteremia is not uncommon during endoscopic procedures, but the infectious sequelae from bacteremia, such as endocarditis or seeding of other sites, are so rare that current recommendations from the American Heart Association and the ASGE recommends antibiotic prophylaxis for only very specific situations.[12,13] Contrary to previous supposition, not all patients with cardiac valvular conditions, synthetic vascular grafts, and prosthetic joints should receive antibiotic prophylaxis. Data have not demonstrated a clear link between GI procedures and infectious complications or demonstrated that antibiotic prophylaxis prevents infectious complications after endoscopic procedures.[8,12] However, it is recommended that patients with high-risk cardiac conditions and concurrent established GI tract infections receive prophylaxis prior to endoscopy.[8] When prophylactic antibiotics are given, the choice of antibiotic(s) depends upon the specific GI procedure, clinical scenario, and allergy history of the patient (e.g., cephalosporins or quinolones in suspected variceal bleeding).[14,15]

Endoscopy in Pregnancy

Generally, endoscopic procedures should be deferred until after pregnancy; however, there are instances where nonelective procedures may be warranted. Pregnant patients may require endoscopic evaluation in the setting of uncontrolled gastrointestinal bleeding, uncontrolled diarrhea, severe/refractory nausea, dysphagia, and biliary complications, including cholangitis, biliary pancreatitis, and symptomatic choledocholithiasis.[16] While endoscopic procedures can be performed safely during pregnancy, cohort studies have demonstrated that pregnant women undergoing endoscopic evaluation have an increased risk for preterm birth and delivering infants that are small for their gestational age.[16] Although cohort studies have not demonstrated a difference in adverse outcomes based on trimester, general consensus is that if an endoscopic procedure is needed, it should be performed in the second trimester in an effort to avoid the period of organogenesis and limit the potential maneuver restrictions from a gravid uterus.[17] Generally, the greatest risk to mother and fetus during endoscopy is related to procedural sedation, and it is recommended that procedures include both anesthesia and obstetrics involvement.[16–18] ERCP can be performed safely with a mindful use of fluoroscopy using ALARA principles as the radiation dose is typically far less than the exposure limit for a developing fetus.[17]

PREPARATION OF THE ENDOSCOPY SPACE

In addition to proper preparation of the patient, a proper setup of the endoscopy space enables procedural efficiency while ensuring both patient and staff safety. Special consideration should be given toward creating a workspace that incorporates ergonomics in an effort to decrease potential work-place injuries by endoscopists and support staff.

Staffing

The number of personnel required for endoscopic procedures in part depends on the type of sedation planned, in instances where sedation is provided by the endoscopist and additional RN should be present to help monitor the patient. While it is felt that this RN can participate in brief endoscopic tasks (e.g., taking a biopsy), if the endoscopic task is more time intensive, then a separate RN or technician should be available to assist.[19,20] Certain jurisdictions have limitations on what tasks can be performed by technicians versus RNs; however, in certain areas, properly trained technicians can perform snare polypectomy, biopsy, injection for lift or tattoo placement, submucosal injection, and contrast injection during ERCP.[20]

Ergonomics

Proper placement of endoscopic equipment can help mitigate the risk of musculoskeletal injuries amongst staff. Endoscopy monitors should ideally be placed at or within 15–25 degrees below eye level to help reduce the risk of neck strain. Adjustable beds enable endoscopists to position patients at a recommended bed height that falls at the level of the elbow to 10 cm below the elbow.[20–23] Ideally, endoscopy suites should have an absolute minimum of 180 ft^2 of space to allow for adequate equipment positioning and staff mobility. However, if additional equipment and procedural complexity is expected, larger rooms akin to standard operating rooms may be required. Cushioned mats can help reduce back strain and consideration of endoscopic monitors with rounded or cushioned edges can help reduce potential head-strike injuries.[24] While many interventions are geared toward reducing endoscopist injury, endoscopic support staff are also at risk of musculoskeletal injuries. Patient handling, including transfers and providing abdominal compression, place staff at risk for possible injury.[21,22,24] For staff involved in fluoroscopic procedures, consideration of two piece lead aprons may help to reduce the associated musculoskeletal strain that can come with prolonged lead use while minimizing radiation exposure.[24]

Infection Control

All staff involved in endoscopic procedures or endoscopic equipment reprocessing should have ready access to appropriate personal protective equipment (PPE). It is recommended that staff directly involved in endoscopic procedures wear gloves, eyewear, a face mask, and gown. When possible, equipment should be single-use, and proper hand hygiene should be observed both before and after the use of PPE.[20,24,25]

Endoscope Cleaning and Maintenance

It has been estimated that the rate of transmission of infection via GI endoscopy is 1 per 1.8 million in the United States.[8,26,27] Infectious adverse events are a consequence of a failure to follow established reprocessing guidelines for endoscopic devices and accessories, failure to follow sterile technique using sedatives such as propofol, or from the procedure itself.[8,25,28–30] Per Spaulding classification, most endoscopic equipment is considered semi-critical and can undergo high-level disinfection (HLD) that removes most potential infectious agents, including hepatitis B and C as well as HIV.[25,30,31] Although prions, such as the Jakob-Creutzfeldt agent, are not inactivated by HLD, prions are not found in saliva, intestinal tissue, feces, and blood and hence are judged by the WHO as being noninfectious for the purposes of infection control.[26] It is recommended that equipment used for EUS and ERCP undergo sterilization.

The process of HLD includes mechanical cleaning of channels and the exterior of the endoscope, followed by soaking in disinfectant solutions such as glutaraldehyde or peracetic acid followed by thorough rinsing and drying of the instruments. Ideally, HLD should be performed in an automated endoscope reprocessor.[30] If possible, it is recommended that single-use accessories be used to minimize infections risk.[25]

Single-Use Duodenoscopes

Despite adherence to regimented cleaning recommendations, infectious complications have occurred. An outbreak of carbapenem-resistant enterococci infection from duodenoscopes highlighted how endoscope design limitations can enable potential pathogen reservoirs.[30,32] The recessed area of the elevator mechanism and the accessory channel are thought to create a rich environment for biofilm formation.[33] Studies have shown that even after proper reprocessing, up to 5% of duodenoscopes can continue to culture pathogenic organisms.[33] Use of disposable duodenoscope endcaps may help to reduce this infectious risk, but do nothing for channel contamination and are associated with a surge in adverse events, including dislodgement of the removable caps.[33] The advent of single-use endoscopes and duodenoscopes aims to further reduce endoscopic infectious risk; however, questions still remain regarding the cost-effectiveness, comparable maneuverability, and environmental ramifications of these new devices.[34] Several studies have demonstrated that while single-use duodenoscopes perform similarly in terms of ERCP maneuvers, the increased stiffness of the scopes can lead to increased difficulty with positioning and consequently potential for increased luminal injury.[33,35,36]

Electrosurgery

It is of extreme importance to understand the operational capabilities of the electrosurgical unit used. This should include understanding the various settings on the device and their correlation with the desired tissue effect. Additionally, the endoscopist should be able to troubleshoot the device, should an error message or a disruption in the circuit be noted.[37,38]

The presence of a cardiac pacemaker or implantable cardiac defibrillator (ICD) requires special consideration because electrocautery performed during an endoscopic procedure can inhibit cardiac pacemaker function and can lead to an inappropriate discharge of a defibrillator. It is therefore prudent to place the grounding pad away from the pacemaker on the patient's thigh or buttock and to use brief bursts of electrosurgical output. Temporary deactivation of the ICD with an external magnet, coupled with continuous cardiac monitoring of the patient's cardiac rhythm and a readily available defibrillator, should be used. Additionally, utilizing a bipolar platform or, in the case of endoscopic hemostasis, a mechanical or thermal device can minimize risk.[39]

SEDATION

Sedation is used for most endoscopic procedures to provide a comfortable and safe setting for the conduct of the procedure. The majority of ambulatory cases, including EGD and colonoscopy are performed by targeting a moderate level of sedation. Deep sedation or general anesthesia is usually targeted for advanced endoscopic procedures such as ERCP, EUS, ESD, peroral endoscopic myotomy (POEM), and in those patients in whom medications used to target moderate sedation could be problematic. This may potentially include patients using narcotic and/or sedative agents as well as those with significant comorbidities who would be at risk for untoward cardiopulmonary events, including decompensated heart failure, critical aortic stenosis, and patients with known or suspected gastric outlet obstruction. Patients with hemodynamic instability or respiratory compromise may also benefit from anesthesia-assisted sedation. All patients undergoing endoscopic procedures should undergo a presedative assessment, including ASA status and whether or not there is a history of obstructive sleep apnea or class III obesity. Proper preprocedure evaluation can help determine the need for anesthesia assistance in achieving optimal patient sedation.[19,40,41]

In cases of moderate sedation, typically, a combination of a benzodiazepine and opiate is used. Outside of the United States, there is also potential for nonanesthesiologist administration of propofol. Regardless of the medications administered, if anesthesia is not present, it is recommended that sedation be provided by staff who have sufficient training in advanced life support and thorough understanding of the medications to be used and their potential reversal-agents if available (e.g., flumazenil for benzodiazepines and naloxone for narcotics). Furthermore, the nurse administering sedation should have no other tasks that would distract from patient monitoring. Having a posted placard in the endoscopy suite with this information readily accessible is prudent. At a minimum, vitals should be checked preprocedure, after any medication administration, every 5 minutes, postprocedure, and prior to patient discharge. At a minimum, vitals should include heart rate, blood pressure, and pulse oximetry with limited data available regarding the utility of capnography during endoscopic procedures.[19,40–42]

In the recovery area, there is a risk of re-sedation once the stimulus of the procedure has been removed. Recovery to baseline vital signs is an important discharge criterion. It should be emphasized that psychomotor recovery can be delayed even in patients receiving fast-acting agents such as propofol.[43] It is therefore advisable to have the patient accompanied by another individual on discharge and to recommend that the patient not drive or operate machinery until the day following the procedure.

Topical Anesthesia

There are limited data on the efficacy of topical anesthetic agents prior to endoscopic procedures.[44] Although occasional applied in an effort to minimize the amount of systemic sedation required or suppress patient reflexes such as coughing, topical anesthetics are not without risk. Topical anesthetic agents such as benzocaine and lidocaine have been associated with serious adverse events, including methemoglobinemia and severe anaphylactoid reactions. Methemoglobinemia is manifested by clinical evidence of cyanosis coupled with a low-O_2 saturation on pulse oximetry despite a normal arterial pO_2. Methemoglobinemia can be reversed with the administration of IV methylene blue.[45,46] There may also be an increased risk for aspiration with use of topical anesthetics. Currently, there is insufficient data regarding topical anesthesia in endoscopy and their use is not promoted in current guidelines.

Cardiopulmonary Events

Unplanned cardiopulmonary events such as hypotension and hypoxemia occur in 0.9% of procedures.[1,47] Cardiopulmonary adverse events related to sedation and analgesia account for 30% −60% of all adverse events with EGD.[1,48,49] Adverse events can include hypoxia, apnea, hypotension/shock, aspiration, respiratory arrest, pneumonia, myocardial infarction, and cerebral vascular accidents. The risk of cardiopulmonary events is related to increasing complexity of the procedure and severity of comorbid conditions.[1,47] Risk factors for these events include age, ascending ASA PS category (see Table 40.1), inpatient procedures, as well as procedures that are targeted for prolonged deep sedation or general anesthesia, such as ERCP.[1]

Risk factors for hypoxemia include increased BMI, advancing age, and higher doses of narcotic analgesics during the procedure.[50,51] Alveolar hypoventilation can be due either to central nervous system depression or to relaxation of the hypopharyngeal muscles. Use of pulse oximetry allows for an early identification of hypoxemia, and the routine use of supplemental O_2 can prevent hypoxemia in most cases. The use of capnography to measure effective CO_2 elimination significantly decreases the occurrence of apnea in patients undergoing colonoscopy, ERCP, and EUS in which deep sedation is used.[52,53] However, there are currently no data supporting routine use of capnography in subjects undergoing EGD or colonoscopy when targeting moderate sedation.

Hypotension during endoscopy is usually due to medication-induced venous dilation in patients who are volume depleted and is usually responsive to IV fluid boluses. Vasovagal reactions are the most common cause of arrhythmias seen during endoscopy. These reactions are usually due to a painful stimulus and can usually be remedied by improving endoscope positioning and reducing bowel distention. Occasionally, intravenous atropine or glycopyrrolate and fluid boluses are required.[40,42,44]

TIMING AND SEVERITY OF COMPLICATIONS

Endoscopic complications can occur during a procedure or may be delayed. Knowledge of the potential complication(s) is a critical element of the informed consent process (see earlier). Just as important, patients should be educated on signs and symptoms that may indicate a delayed complication and have access to a streamlined process for contacting the endoscopist about a potential complication for appropriate management. From a quality-improvement and treatment perspective, it is important to use this standard set of definitions for adverse outcomes, which would include elements of timing, attribution, severity, and ultimate outcome.[54]

EGD

Perforation

Perforation of the upper GI tract during diagnostic EGD has been estimated to occur in 1 in 2500 to 1 in 11,000 cases.[55,56] The mortality from esophageal perforation can range from 2% to 36%.[57] The most common site of perforation is the oropharynx or cervical esophagus. As such, patients with proximal esophageal strictures and cancers, as well as those with Zenker diverticula or large anterior cervical osteophytes, are at particular risk for perforation. Development of crepitus with associated neck or chest pain should prompt an urgent evaluation. Typically, either an esophagogram with water-soluble contrast or a CT scan of the neck and chest using an oral contrast agent should be considered. When recognized early, most perforations in the neck can be managed conservatively, in concert with the appropriate surgical services, using broad-spectrum antibiotics and nasogastric suctioning. Intrathoracic perforations can also be managed in this manner. In the appropriate setting, an array of endoscopic devices can be used to treat perforations, including metallic clips, over-the-scope (OTS) tissue apposition devices, stents, and suturing platforms.[58–63]

Endoscopic Hemostasis

Rare complications of endoscopic hemostasis include aspiration pneumonia, perforation, and peritonitis. The risk of perforation or exacerbation of bleeding is felt to be $<0.5\%$ with an increased risk of perforation to 2% if a heater probe is used. Dual therapy of injection plus thermal therapy is felt to be as effective as either thermal therapy alone or hemostatic clip placement.[57,64,65]

In terms of variceal bleeding management, complications vary on the modality of treatment used. Following band-ligation, ulceration development can occur in 5%−15% of cases with rare incidences of postbanding perforation and stricture formation.[57] In contrast, ulceration following variceal sclerotherapy can occur in up to 78% of patients.[66] Significant immediate bleeding with sclerotherapy can occur in up to 6% of patients with significant delayed bleeding in 109%–124% of patients.[57,67] Stricture formation following sclerotherapy can occur in up to 20% of cases, and the rate of perforation is estimated to be 0.5%–5%.[57] Other sclerotherapy complications include aspiration, perforation, pericardial and pleural effusions, as well as mediastinitis.[68,69] Injection hemostasis with agents such as polidocanol and ethanol have been infrequently reported to cause perforation or exacerbation of bleeding.[70,71]

Enteral Access Procedures

Endoscopy is often used to provide enteral access routes. Endoscopic placement of nasoenteric feeding tubes ensures delivery of the feeding tube into the small intestine and is associated with minor, self-limited complications. Epistaxis is the most common, occurring in up to 5% of patients. Proximal migration as well as tube dislodgement may also occur.[72,73]

Adverse events with PEG placement range from 1.5% to 9.4% with peristomal wound infection being the most common.[57,74,75] Other adverse events include aspiration, bleeding, perforation, necrotizing fasciitis, intestinal obstruction (Fig. 40.1), and injury to other organs.[76,77] A single, preprocedure dose of a cephalosporin or beta lactam significantly reduces the rate of peristomal wound infections.[77] Bleeding during or following PEG placement is usually minor and self-limited but occasionally can require endoscopic hemostasis. Anticoagulants should be held, and

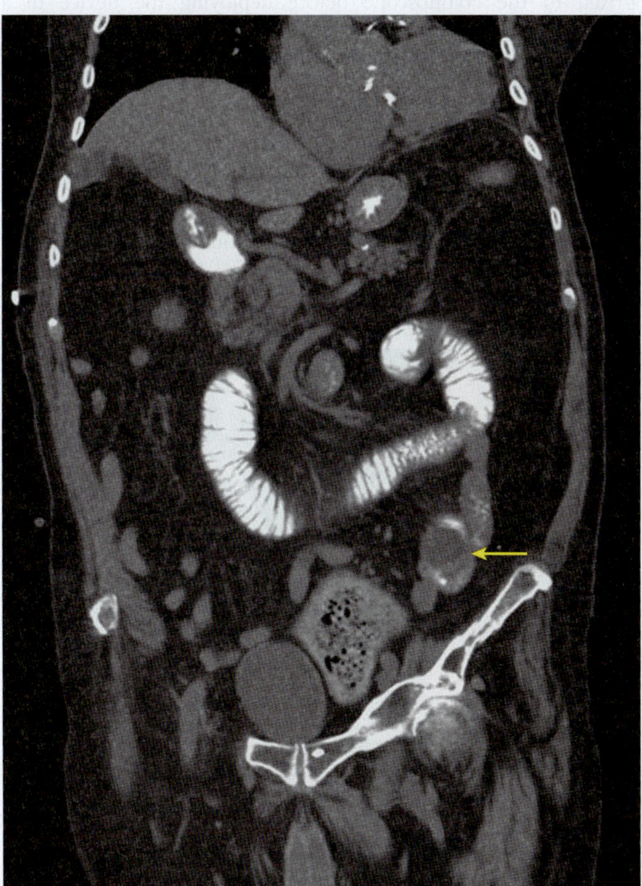

Fig 40.1 Magnetic resonance enterography showing a migrated, water-filled PEG bumper in the proximal ileum (*yellow arrow*). The patient presented with a 7-day history of small bowel obstruction. Single-balloon enteroscopy was performed; the balloon was deflated with an injection needle, and the bumper was captured with a snare and removed per os, with full recovery.

documentation of normalization of coagulation parameters should be documented prior to PEG placement.[3] The "buried bumper syndrome" occurs when the external bumper of the PEG remains too tight and causes the migration of the internal bumper into the gastric wall.[78] Treatment involves removal of the tube and placement of another tube at a different site. Metastasis developing at the PEG insertion site has been described in patients with oropharyngeal and esophageal malignancy. It is unknown whether the metastasis is[72,73] a result of local or hematogenous spread. In patients with these cancers, an alternative route for enteral nutrition, such as a radiologically assisted tube placement, may be considered.[79] Accidental dislodgement of the PEG tube within 1 month of placement can result in peritonitis if a mature fistulous tract has not developed. In the setting of a mature tract and tube dislodgement, a replacement tube should be inserted as soon as possible.[80] Contrast injection can be used with fluoroscopy to determine appropriate positioning. Adverse events with percutaneous endoscopic jejunostomy are like those of PEG placement, although the rates of clogging, migration, and unintentional removal may be higher.[81] Aspiration pneumonia may develop either due to aspiration of oropharyngeal contents or the tube feedings themselves. Risk factors for aspiration may include neuromuscular or structural problems of the oropharynx, prolonged supine positioning, history of documented aspiration, reduced level of consciousness, or vomiting/regurgitation.[82]

Mucosal Ablation and Resection

Esophageal ablative therapy for Barrett's esophagus (with or without dysplasia) and mucosal carcinoma (see Chapters 49 and 50), with thermal electrocoagulation, radiofrequency ablation, cryotherapy, and photodynamic therapy have been associated with postprocedure dysphagia, odynophagia, chest pain, dyspepsia, ulceration with bleeding, and perforation.[83–86] The rate of stricture formation following treatment therapy approaches 11%–42% for photodynamic therapy, 2%–8% for RFA, and 4%–10% for cryotherapy.[57]

Endoscopic mucosal resection in the upper GI tract has an incidence of serious advents such as perforation and bleeding between 0.5% and 5%.[57,87] When EMR involves greater than 50% of the luminal circumference, the incidence of esophageal stricture formation is 12%–50%. Most of these strictures can be adequately treated with esophageal dilation.[88] Gastric EMR has an intraprocedure bleeding risk of 0%–11.5% and an incidence of perforation of 1%. In comparison, duodenal EMR carries an intraprocedure bleeding risk of 11.5%–19.3% and an incidence of perforation of 2%.[89]

Endoscopic submucosal dissection allows for an en bloc resection using a variety of specialized tools and using the submucosal layer as the dissection plane. Adverse events with ESD of the upper GI tract are similar to EMR, although the incidence of bleeding (11%) and perforation (6%) are higher.[57,87,90] Immediate bleeding during ESD has an incidence approaching 10%; however, it is often manageable with the use of a coagulation knife/graspers.[91] The incidence of delayed bleeding following ESD ranges from 4.5% to 10%, while the incidence of post-ESD esophageal structure ranges from 12% to 17% with greater incidence when more luminal circumference is involved.[91,92]

Other Therapeutic Procedures

Complications from endoscopic removal of foreign bodies from the upper GI tract include aspiration, perforation, and GI hemorrhage (see Chapter 28). The risk of foreign body aspiration can be reduced using an overtube or endotracheal intubation. Risk factors for perforation include a more than 24-hour delay in endoscopic intervention or the presence of an irregular or sharp object.[93–95]

Colonoscopy

The overall risk of complications during colonoscopy is 0.28%.[96] Risk factors include patient age, comorbid conditions (e.g., history of stroke, atrial fibrillation, or heart failure), and undergoing a polypectomy.[96,97] The main complications of colonoscopy are cardiovascular and pulmonary events (Fig. 40.2), perforation, bleeding, and a postpolypectomy electrocoagulation syndrome.[98]

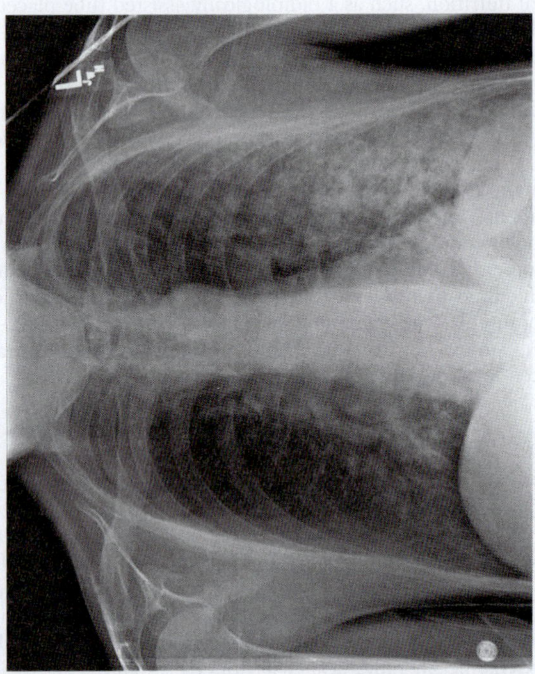

Fig 40.2 Chest film showing bilateral aspiration pneumonia in a patient who had undergone a colonoscopy with monitored anesthesia care. There was no history of gastroparesis.

Perforation

The rate of perforation with colonoscopy varies from 0.05% to 0.3%.[54,99,100] Perforations can be caused by tearing of the antimesenteric border of the colon from excessive pressure on colonic loops, by excessive air/gas pressure (barotrauma), following polypectomy or from injury at the site of electrosurgical application. Colonic tears occur mainly in the sigmoid colon, where looping of the colonoscope is most frequently encountered. Barotrauma is most often encountered in the cecum, where the colonic diameter is the greatest and, therefore, the tension on the colonic wall is the highest. Ablative treatment of angioectasias, particularly in the right colon, is associated with a perforation rate of up to 2.5%.[101] There is a 2% risk of perforation with the placement of a colonic decompression tube in patients with pseudo-obstruction.[102–104] Balloon dilation of colonic Crohn's disease is associated with nearly a 2% risk of perforation.[105] Perforation should be considered in patients with abdominal or shoulder pain who have abdominal distention that does not improve. Frequently a perforation can be recognized at the time of colonoscopy (Fig. 40.3A). Defect closure using endoscopic clips in concert with antibiotics and close observation can be effective in many cases and avoid the need for surgical intervention (see Fig. 40.3B).[106,107] Careful observation by the gastroenterologist in conjunction with a surgeon is advisable in this situation. In cases with larger tears or frank peritonitis, operative intervention should be considered. OTS full thickness closure devices are very effective at treating acute perforations. They require suction of the defect and surrounding tissue in and endcap affixed to the colonoscope before deploying the device in a mechanism akin to band ligation. Entrapment of omental fat, adjacent organs, or nearby blood vessels can be reduced by using tissue grasping devices to the pull the injured wall into the device cap rather than relying entirely on suction.[108]

Bleeding

The most common cause of immediate or delayed bleeding with colonoscopy is performing a polypectomy. Immediate postpolypectomy bleeding occurs at a rate of 0.4%–10.2%, while

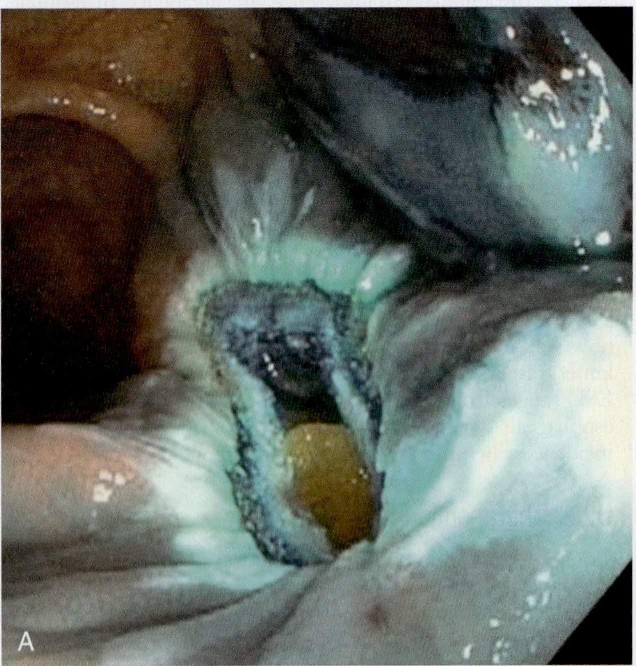

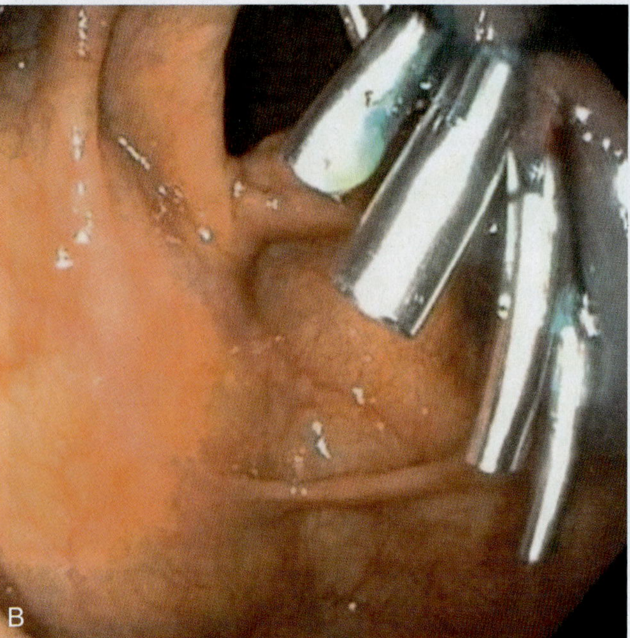

Fig 40.3 (A) Colonoscopic view of an ascending colon perforation following polypectomy of a 2-cm sessile polyp. (B) Endoscopic closure of the perforation site using metallic clips. The patient was observed for 48 hours on antibiotics, remained asymptomatic, and was discharged.

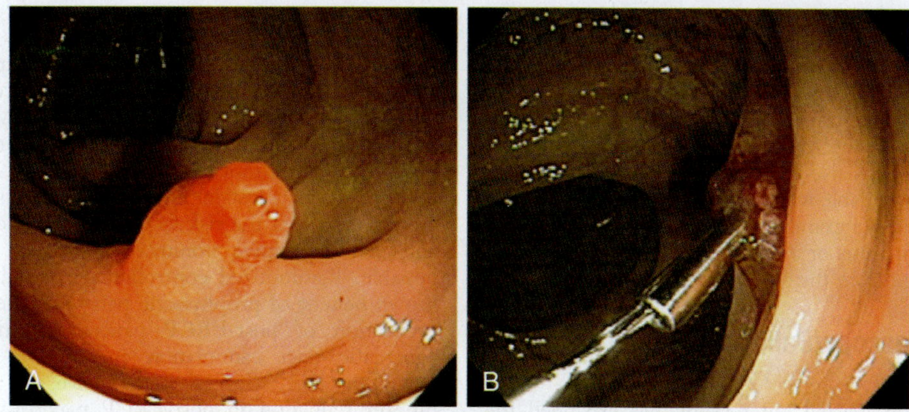

Fig 40.4 (A) Colonoscopic view of a polypectomy site in a patient presenting with hematochezia 5 days after colon polypectomy. This polyp stalk was thought to be the cause of the bleeding. (B) Although no bleeding was encountered during the second colonoscopy, a hemostatic clip was placed in an effort to reduce the risk of further bleeding.

delayed postpolypectomy bleeding is felt to occur at a rate of 0.6%–1.9%.[109,110] Risk factors for both immediate and delayed bleeding include polyp size >10 mm, pedunculated lesions, polyps located in the right colon, and degree of endoscopist experience.[109]

Patient age, cardiovascular comorbidities, and use of antithrombotic and/or antiplatelet agents are associated with increased risk for polypectomy-associated bleeding.[97,111–113] Polyp size may be an additional risk factor for postpolypectomy bleeding.[111,113,114] While prophylactic clipping of resection sites has not been shown to uniformly prevent bleeding, studies have shown that prophylactic clipping following a removal of sessile lesions ≥20 mm or pedunculated lesions with a stalk ≥10 mm may reduce the risk of delayed postpolypectomy hemorrhage especially in the right colon.[109,110,115,116] Acute postpolypectomy hemorrhage is usually amenable to a variety of endoscopic therapeutic measures (Fig. 40.4).[117,118]

Postpolypectomy Electrocoagulation Syndrome

Postpolypectomy electrocoagulation syndrome is defined by the constellation of fever, localized abdominal pain with rebound tenderness, and leukocytosis. Caused by electrocoagulation-induced transmural thermal injury with localized peritonitis, this syndrome typically occurs 1–5 days after colonoscopy with polypectomy. The reported incidence of this complication varies from 0.003% to 0.1%.[99] Typically, patients are managed with IV hydration, broad-spectrum parenteral antibiotics, and NPO status until symptoms improve.[119] Abdominal CT should also be obtained to rule out the possibility of a localized perforation. CT should also be undertaken if worrisome findings are noted on serial, frequent abdominal examinations. Milder cases of postpolypectomy electrocoagulation syndrome have been treated with oral antibiotics in an outpatient setting.[120]

Complications Related to Colon Preparation

Polyethylene glycol is generally safer than sodium phosphate preparations in patients with fluid/electrolyte imbalances or with chronic kidney disease, heart failure, and/or liver failure. Medications such as angiotensin-converting enzyme inhibitors, NSAIDs, and diuretics can contribute to fluid/electrolyte problems in such patients about to undergo colonoscopy. In general, patients with predisposing conditions for fluid and electrolyte disorders who are taking the aforementioned medications should have a more gradual bowel preparation and be monitored closely, with a baseline serum creatinine level determined.[121–124]

Others

Rarer complications of colonoscopy include splenic rupture, appendicitis, and chemical colitis after accidental contamination with disinfectant solutions.[125–128] Colonoscopy-specific mortality is rare, occurring in 7 per 100,000 procedures. Gas explosion has been rarely reported and is thought to be due to combustible levels of methane or hydrogen present in the colonic lumen when electrocautery or argon plasma coagulation is used. Risk factors may include incomplete colonic cleansing and the use of nonabsorbable or (incompletely absorbable) preparations such as sorbitol, lactulose, and mannitol.[129–131]

Capsule Endoscopy

Contraindications to wireless capsule endoscopy include known or suspected intestinal obstruction, stricture, fistula or extensive Crohn's disease, swallowing disorders, and ileus or intestinal pseudo-obstruction (see Chapter 125).[132] More relative contraindications include pregnancy, long-standing use of NSAIDs, Zenker diverticulum, gastroparesis, previous pelvic or abdominal surgery or radiation therapy, and the presence of cardiac pacemakers or ICDs and left ventricular assist devices. There is a theoretical risk of electromagnetic interference between these cardiac devices and capsule endoscopes; however, studies of this issue have not demonstrated this to be a clinically significant problem.[133–136]

Perhaps the most dreaded complication is the retained capsule within the small bowel. Patients at risk for this condition include those with a history of IBD, prior radiation therapy, previous surgery, and use of NSAIDs.[132] A capsule retention rate of 1.4% was seen in a large case series. In almost all instances, significant small bowel pathology was identified that necessitated surgical intervention.[132] In those individuals with capsule retention, no obstructive symptoms, no indication for immediate surgery, and whose underlying disease is potentially treatable medically or endoscopically, the use of double-balloon enteroscopy can be successful in retrieving the capsule and treating lesions such as diaphragmatic strictures from NSAIDs.[137] In patients in whom luminal patency needs to be assessed prior to performing capsule endoscopy, use of a patency capsule system is a useful tool in determining whether sufficient luminal narrowing is present to result in capsule retention and subsequent complications.[138–140]

In patients with dysphagia, appropriate structural and motility evaluation should be performed prior to capsule endoscopy such as a barium swallow coupled with a 13-mm barium pill. Capsule retention at the cricopharyngeus as well as inside a Zenker diverticulum has been described, with successful endoscopic removal.[141] Aspiration of the capsule endoscope with successful bronchoscopic retrieval has also been reported.[142,143] Endoscopic placement devices are available which can bypass the stomach and lead to a successful capsule examination of the small intestine in the presence of gastroparesis or a postsurgical anatomy that may lead to delayed passage from the stomach.[144]

Small Bowel Endoscopy/Balloon-Assisted Enteroscopy

The advent of balloon-assisted enteroscopy has expanded the horizon of diagnostic and therapeutic vistas into the small bowel. Complication rates for diagnostic double-balloon enteroscopy are 0.8% and 4.3% for therapeutic procedures.[145] A multicenter survey of double-balloon procedures found bleeding (0.8%), perforation (0.3%), and pancreatitis (0.3%) as the most common complications.[145] Virtually all the bleeding complications occurred in therapeutic procedures in which polypectomy was performed. A perforation rate following the balloon dilation of 2.9% was also reported. Although the data on single-balloon enteroscopy are not as voluminous, they appear to have a similar complication profile.[146,147]

ERCP

With the continued advances in EUS and MRCP, ERCP has become almost exclusively a therapeutic technique. Severe complications of therapeutic ERCP are fortunately rare (Fig 40.5; also see Chapters 63 and 72), and it is imperative that endoscopists minimize complications by using less invasive tests whenever possible. The incidence of adverse events following ERCP include pancreatitis at 3.5%–9.7%, cholangitis/cholecystitis at 1.4% (combined incidence), bleeding at 1.3%, and perforation at 0.6%.[148]

Pancreatitis

Post-ERCP pancreatitis is discussed in Chapter 60. Both patient and procedural factors have been identified as risk factors for post-ERCP pancreatitis (Box 40.1) and may amplify this risk to over 20%. While the majority of cases are mild, post-ERCP pancreatitis has a mortality rate of 0.1%–0.7%.[148]

Perhaps the most important components of ERCP planning are ensuring that the risk factors listed in Box 40.1 are respected and that alternative noninvasive imaging studies are used if possible. Randomized controlled trials and meta-analyses have shown benefit of prophylactic pancreatic stent placement in the prevention of post-ERCP pancreatitis following inadvertent pancreatic duct cannulation and/or use of the double-wire technique.[148–150] Several studies have also demonstrated a significant reduction in post-ERCP pancreatitis following use of intraprocedure rectal indomethacin.[148,151] A recent large multicentered random controlled trial exploring whether pancreatic duct stents added to rectal indomethacin have added protection against post-ERCP pancreatitis has been completed and we await results. Treatment of post-ERCP pancreatitis remains supportive

BOX 40.1 Risk Factors for Post-ERCP Pancreatitis (see also Chapter 60)

- Balloon dilation of an intact sphincter
- Failed or difficult cannulation
- History of post-ERCP pancreatitis
- Normal serum bilirubin level
- Pancreatic duct injection
- Pancreatic guidewire placement
- Pancreatic sphincterotomy
- Pancreatic tissue sampling
- Precut sphincterotomy
- Suspected Sphincter of Oddi (SOD)
- Young age

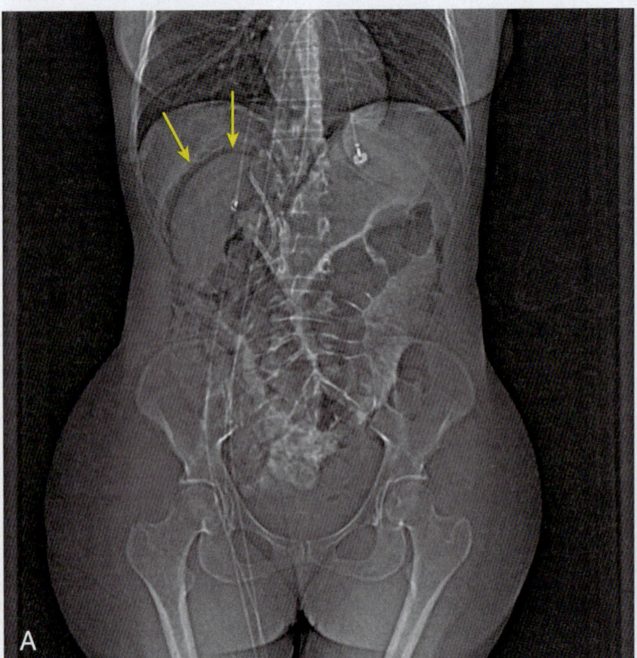

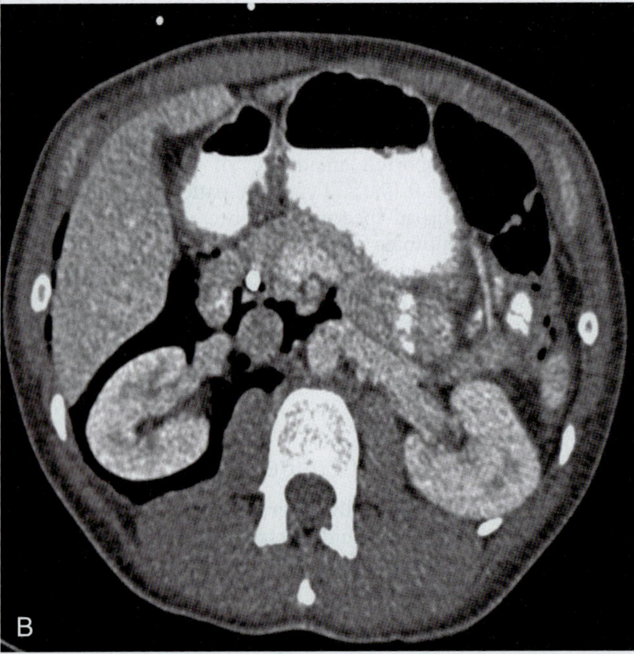

Fig 40.5 (A) Radiologic image showing right perinephric air following a biliary sphincterotomy (*arrow*). The perforation was identified, and a biliary stent was placed. (B) CT showing the retroperitoneal air. The patient was observed for 48 hours on antibiotics and was discharged after an uneventful course.

(see Chapter 60), and there is no role for repeat ERCP in this setting. Whether particular electrocautery cutting currents influence the risk of pancreatitis remains controversial.[152,153]

Infection

Cholangitis and cholecystitis occur in 1% and less than 0.5% of patients undergoing ERCP, respectively.[154] Risk factors for ascending cholangitis include combined percutaneous/endoscopic procedures, stenting of malignancy, and failed biliary access or drainage.[154] Use of additional imaging modalities, such as MRCP to further define complex biliary anatomy prior to the ERCP, may be useful. Management of these conditions may include a reattempt at endoscopic therapy, a percutaneous approach, or a surgical intervention. Prophylactic antibiotics have not been shown to reduce the risk of cholangitis following uncomplicated ERCP; however, current guidelines recommend prophylactic antibiotics in those patients undergoing ERCP with anticipated incomplete drainage.[8,10,155] Infection of a pseudocyst, if present, is always a possibility with ERCP. Plans for drainage of the cyst should be considered in concert with the ERCP. In most cases, this can be rendered via an endoscopic cyst gastrostomy or cyst duodenostomy.[156] The use of single operator cholangioscopy to visualize the bile duct has a similar complication profile to ERCP except for an increased risk of cholangitis. A prospective study of the risk of bacteremia in directed cholangioscopic examination of the common bile duct when indicated appears to be as safe as ERCP, even in older patients.[157]

Bleeding

Most bleeding complications following ERCP are related to sphincterotomy, which occur in 1% to 2% of cases.[154,158] Risk factors for sphincterotomy bleeding include thrombocytopenia, coagulopathy, cholangitis, and initiation of anticoagulant therapy within 3 days after the procedure. Additionally, endoscopists who had performed less than one biliary sphincterotomy per week were noted to have a higher bleeding rate following sphincterotomy.[154] Treatment of sphincterotomy bleeding can include the injection of dilute epinephrine, thermal methods such as using a BiCAP probe, use of metallic clips, or mechanical methods such as balloon tamponade within the sphincterotomy or placement of covered expandable metallic stents. In instances where the bleeding is not controlled, therapeutic angiography or surgery may be necessary.

Perforation

Perforation occurs in less than 1% of ERCP cases.[148,154,158,159] Lateral wall duodenal perforations tend to be large and usually require surgical intervention. With the advent of OTS clipping devices, endoscopic closure is sometimes feasible.[160] Periampullary perforation following biliary sphincterotomy or stone extraction is less likely to require surgical intervention if recognized early (see Fig. 40.5). Endoscopic management can include the placement of plastic or fully covered metal stents.[161,162] Perforation of the biliary tree usually occurs as a result of instrumentation with a guidewire or basket near an obstruction. Most of these can be managed conservatively with the placement of a plastic or fully coated metallic stent. In patients with failed closure, delayed access, or clear evidence of retroperitoneal extravasation, surgical intervention should be considered.

EUS

Diagnostic EUS carries a risk profile that is similar to standard endoscopy. Esophageal perforation stemming from the passage of an echoendoscope is rare (0.06%).[163,164] Risk factors for esophageal perforation include older patient age, lack of operator experience, and a difficult esophageal intubation.[163] In up to one-third of patients with esophageal malignancy, there is difficulty or an inability in passing the echoendoscope. Sequential esophageal dilation can often be achieved in these patients, allowing the completion of the EUS.[165,166]

FNA of cystic lesions carries an increased risk of infection of the targeted cyst and subsequent sepsis. Current guidelines recommend prophylactic antibiotics periprocedurally with consideration of continuing antibiotics for up to 48 hours post-procedure.[8,164,167,168] Current data do not support the use of prophylactic antibiotics during FNA of lymph nodes or solid masses. Studies have also shown that the incidence of infection following EUS fiducial placement for pancreaticobiliary malignancy is low.[169]

Mild intraluminal GI bleeding may be encountered in up to 4% of FNA cases,[170] and extraluminal hemorrhage may occur in 1.3%.[171] Pancreatitis, reported in up to 2% of patients, is most likely secondary to passage of the FNA needle through pancreatic tissue.[164,172] Celiac plexus block can result in transient diarrhea (4%–15%), orthostasis (1%), and transient increased pain (9%).[164] It is recommended that patients receive adequate fluid hydration both in pre- and postprocedure to help mitigate these risks.

Endoscopic Stent Placement

Insertion of self-expanding metallic stents (SEMS) can be used to treat both malignant and benign refractory strictures. Immediate complications for esophageal stent placement occur at a rate of 2%–12% and include aspiration, tracheal compression, and perforation.[57,173–175] Worsening reflux can result when the esophagogastric junction is bridged by the stent, making high-dose acid suppressive therapy with a PPI necessary. Late adverse events of esophageal SEMS placement occur at a rate of 20%–40% and include pyrosis, regurgitation, recurrent occlusion in up to 30% (from food impaction, tissue ingrowth, or tumor progression), and stent migration, especially following malignancy treatment with radiation therapy.[57,174,176,177]

Gastric SEMS placement has been associated with risk of bleeding and perforation in 1%–5% of cases with stents placed for malignant obstruction often requiring repeat intervention (20%–30%).[57] In addition to perforation, duodenal SEMS placement carries the risk of development of pancreatitis and obstructive jaundice from ampullary obstruction.[174,175] Enteric SEMS is often associated with better short-term outcomes (return to feeding, resolution of obstructive symptoms), but worse long-term durability compared to surgical options.[175]

Complications from colonic SEMS placement include perforation (3.8%–10%), migration (10%–11.8%%), and stent occlusion (7.3%–10%).[175] Stricture dilation of malignant colonic strictures before or after stent placement is not recommended owing to the high risk of perforation.[178–180]

Lumen Apposing Metal Stents

The advent of lumen apposing metal stents has expanded the repertoire of endoscopic therapeutic interventions, including improved pancreatic fluid collection drainage, endoscopic gallbladder drainage in poor surgical candidates, and creation of gastroenteric anastomosis to circumvent obstructive lesions. Endoscopic drainage has become the therapy of choice for the management of complex pancreatic fluid collection and walled off pancreatic necrosis (see Chapter 60). Lumen-opposing metallic stents have an excellent safety profile, with complications requiring intervention that include stent migration (4.2%), infection (3.8%), bleeding (2.4%), and stent occlusion (1.9%).[181–183]

COMPLICATIONS OF NEWER ENDOSCOPIC TECHNIQUES

The "scope" of GI endoscopy continues to expand with novel therapeutic interventions such as POEM, endoscopic bariatric procedures, and novel third space endoscopic procedures offering new avenues to treat various conditions. With such expansion, understanding the risks associated with these techniques and balancing them against the potential benefits is imperative. The importance of this process cannot be minimized. Complications are inevitable, but proper recognition of optimal technical and cognitive abilities is crucial to minimizing their occurrence.

Esophageal POEM

Esophageal POEM (E-POEM) performs comparatively to Heller myotomy in terms of effectiveness and durability for the treatment of achalasia (see Chapter 46). Although an increase in post-procedure reflux can be seen in E-POEM versus Heller myotomy, E-POEM is otherwise associated with lower rates of adverse events and lower postoperative pain compared to standard myotomy. Current panel recommendations recommend E-POEM or myotomy for achalasia subtypes I and II with a preference for E-POEM in treatment subtype III.[184] Potential complications arising during E-POEM include bleeding, mucosal injury from thermal therapy, capnomediastinum, and mediastinitis.[185,186] It is recommended that patients receive prophylactic antibiotics and continue on PPI therapy for at least 4 weeks postprocedure in an effort to minimize complications. It is also recommended that CO_2 be used for insufflation to minimize the risk of developing pneumomediastinum, pneumoperitoneum, and abdominal compartment syndrome.[185,186]

Endobariatrics

Endoscopic bariatric procedures span the gamut of minimally invasive procedures such as intragastric balloons to endoscopic sleeve gastroplasty (see Chapter 8). The appropriate indications for such procedures continue to evolve. Adverse events following intragastric balloon placement include development of post-procedural nausea, dyspepsia, and reflux with a small risk of migration of the balloon into the small bowel (<1%).[187] Gastric aspiration devices carry a similar risk profile as standard PEG placement with an overall estimated complication rate of 3.6%.[187] Endoscopic sleeve gastrectomy has an overall associated complication rate of 0.82% with complications, including postprocedure hematemesis, abdominal pain, nausea and more rarely, intra-abdominal abscess formation, splenic laceration, and pneumoperitoneum.[187,188] Several novel devices are currently undergoing investigation, including duodenal bypass liners and duodenal resurfacing techniques that carry potential risk for ampullary occlusion/disruption leading to hepatic abscess or pancreatitis development, as well as concern for bleeding and perforation at the site of device attachment.[188] Regardless of the modality chosen, patient's undergoing endobariatric procedures should still receive adequate preprocedure dietary, exercise, and behavioral modifications that can be continued in the postprocedure period.[189]

Emerging Third Space Endoscopic Procedures

Advances in submucosal tunneling continue to broaden the scope of endoscopic interventions. Gastric POEM has emerged as a potential intervention for gastroparesis, and Z-POEM has been described as a method of treating Zenker's diverticulum. Additional advances in endoscopic equipment are reigniting the potential for natural orifice transluminal endoscopy surgery. There is currently limited data regarding potential negative outcomes in these newer procedures such as rates of bleeding, perforation, and mediastinitis/intra-abdominal infection.[190,191] As these techniques become more commonplace, it is imperative that performing endoscopists are adequately trained not only in the techniques but also in recognizing potential complications so that patients can be appropriately counseled and monitored.

Full references for this chapter can be found at https://ebooks.health.elsevier.com.

PART V Neoplasia Involving Multiple Organs

41 Gastrointestinal Lymphomas*

Mayur Narkhede

IN THIS CHAPTER

Lymphomas are solid malignancies of the lymphoid system and are subdivided into Hodgkin and non-Hodgkin lymphomas (NHLs). It was estimated that in 2017 there would be 8260 and 72,240 new diagnoses of Hodgkin and NHL, respectively, in the United States.[1] The GI tract is very rarely involved with Hodgkin lymphoma and will not be discussed in this chapter.

This chapter deals with primary GI lymphoma (PGIL), where the main bulk of disease is in the GI tract, with or without an involvement of adjacent lymph nodes. PGILs constitute 1%–4% of all GI malignancies, 10%–15% of all NHLs, and 30%–40% of all extranodal NHLs,[2] making the GI tract the most common site of extranodal NHL. The incidence of PGIL among nations varies from 0.58 to 1.31 per 100,000 people, and the usual age of diagnosis is between 50 and 70 years. Lymphomas that involve the GI tract but have the bulk of the disease in nodal areas are managed in a similar fashion to those that do not involve the GI tract.

In broad terms, the immune system can be thought of as a highly structured and tightly regulated interaction between lymphoid and nonlymphoid tissues aimed at protecting the host from harmful agents (see Chapter 2).[3] Lymphoid cells are produced in the bone marrow and thymus and then arrayed in the lymphoid tissues, which include the lymph nodes, spleen, Waldeyer ring, and mucosa-associated lymphoid tissue (MALT). The GI tract lymphoid tissue is MALT, typified by the Peyer patches of the terminal ileum. MALT contains B cells at various stages of differentiation, organized into different zones (Fig. 41.1A). B cells that have encountered antigen diffusing across the mucosa enter the germinal center of MALT and undergo repeated immunoglobulin gene mutations (somatic mutations).[4] The resultant B-cell subclones whose immunoglobulins are highly specific for antigen have a survival advantage over B cells whose immunoglobulins are less specific. These more specific B cells then leave the germinal center, enter the circulation, differentiate into memory B cells or antibody-producing plasma cells, and return to the intestinal mucosa. Memory B cells reside in the marginal zone of MALT. Some marginal zone B cells occupy the epithelial tissue that covers the Peyer patches; these cells are called intraepithelial marginal zone B cells. B cells that have not encountered any antigen make up the mantle zone of MALT. T cells play a role in the coordination and delivery of the immune system and thus are also found in MALT (see Fig. 41.1A). Therefore MALT is composed of B and T cells at various stages of differentiation; immune cells at a given stage of differentiation have characteristic histologic, immunophenotypic, and genetic features. Malignant transformation may occur in a cell at any one of these stages of differentiation, leading to a malignancy with distinct clinical pathologic features (see Fig. 41.1B). This way of understanding lymphomas has led to the WHO lymphoma system, which recognizes over 60 different clinical pathologic subtypes of NHL.[5,6]

Most lymphomas of the GI tract are B-cell lymphomas, with most of these resulting from transformation of marginal zone B cells, classified by the WHO system as extranodal marginal zone B-cell lymphomas. However, B-cell lymphomas can also arise from other cells of MALT, such as centrocytes of the germinal center [follicular lymphomas (FLs)] or cells of the mantle zone [mantle cell lymphoma (MCL)]. The precise histogenesis of large B-cell lymphomas likely varies from case to case. T-cell lymphomas of the GI tract are less common and usually involve a malignant transformation of intraepithelial T cells in patients with celiac disease (see Chapter 109).

PGILs most commonly involve the stomach or small intestine; the oral pharynx, esophagus, colon, or rectum may be involved uncommonly. In developed countries, the stomach is the most common site of involvement (approximately 60% of cases), but in the Middle East, the small intestine is the most common site of GI involvement. The first definition of PGIL was proposed by

*Hsiao C. Li and Robert H. Collins, Jr. contributed to an earlier version of this chapter.

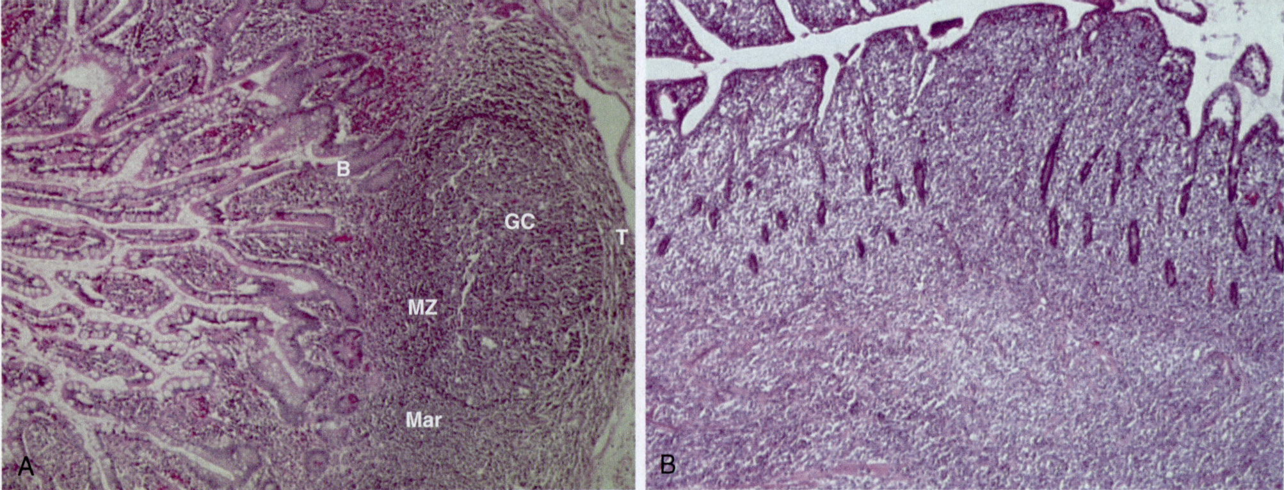

Fig. 41.1 (A) Normal mucosa-associated lymphoid tissue of small intestine. The T zone is situated toward the serosal aspect (*T*). Intraepithelial B cells are also present (B). (B) Large B-cell lymphoma of the small intestine. Note the infiltration and expansion of the mucosa by the neoplastic cells, with atrophy of the native epithelial structures. *GC*, Germinal center; *Mar,* pale external marginal zone; *MZ,* dark surrounding mantle zone. (Courtesy Dr. Pamela Jensen, Dallas, TX.)

Dawson et al.[7] using restricted criteria, namely, the presence of a predominant GI lesion with or without expansion to regional lymph nodes but without an involvement of distant lymph nodes and the exclusion of patients with a leukemic presentation and those with bone marrow, spleen, or liver involvement.[7] This definition was later expanded to include cases involving the adjacent liver and spleen, and allowing for distant nodal disease, provided the extranodal GI lesion was the presenting site and the site of predominant bulk (>75% of total tumor volume), to which primary treatment should be directed.[8–10]

Clinicians dealing with GI lymphoma are faced with a specific pathologic diagnosis of lymphoma occurring in a specific site and, in some cases, modified by important patient's characteristics, such as HIV infection. This chapter discusses the main clinicopathologic entities that a clinician may encounter.

GENERAL PRINCIPLES OF LYMPHOMA MANAGEMENT

Diagnosis

Because of the many subtypes of NHL, lymphoma should be diagnosed and categorized accurately by an expert. Sufficient tissue is required for an accurate diagnosis. In the GI tract, this often means multiple endoscopic biopsies. Fine-needle aspiration biopsy is not considered sufficient for diagnosis because it only permits analysis of the morphology of individual cells and not an in-depth examination of the background milieu in which those cells reside. The minimal pathologic workup should include light microscopy and immunophenotypic analysis, either by flow cytometry or immunohistochemistry (IHC). Staining for immunoglobulin light chains assists in the documentation of monoclonality when there is a clear-cut light chain restriction (κ/λ ratio or λ/κ ratio $\geq$10:1), strongly suggesting B-cell lymphoma. Occasionally, molecular genetic analysis by Southern blot testing or PCR assay is indicated to document monoclonal immunoglobulin B-cell receptor or T-cell receptor gene rearrangements, or to assess characteristic oncogene rearrangements. One must keep in mind though that clonality markers might be positive in various inflammatory conditions and are not necessarily pathognomonic of a malignancy. Therefore an evaluation of a biopsy sample by an expert hematopathologist is extremely important to render an accurate diagnosis.

Staging and Prognostic Assessment

The extent of involvement by NHL is assessed by careful history and physical examination; CT of the neck, chest, abdomen, and pelvis; PET in cases of high-grade NHL; bone marrow examination in certain cases; and EUS for PGILs.[11] A Waldeyer ring is often involved in GI lymphomas, and examination of the pharynx is therefore indicated. Prior to the initiation of treatment, serologies for HIV, hepatitis B, and hepatitis C and screening for *Helicobacter pylori* (*Hp*) in gastric lymphomas should also be obtained. The Ann Arbor staging system[12] was originally developed for Hodgkin lymphoma and is also used for NHL but is deemed by many to be inadequate for staging of PGILs. Alternative systems have been proposed (Table 41.1).[13]

Prognosis is assessed by defining the distinct lymphoma subtype and evaluating clinical features, including tumor stage, age of the patient, performance status, and serum LDH level. The International Prognostic Index (IPI) is a model used to predict outcome in patients with aggressive NHL.[14] This model has been revised as R-IPI to reflect the use of the monoclonal antibody, rituximab, directed against CD20[15] and has been prospectively validated; retaining its predictive value in the rituximab era.

Treatment

Treatment varies according to lymphoma subtype and stage, but it should be noted that the best treatment for many GI lymphomas remains controversial. Whereas many large controlled trials have defined the best treatment for many nodal lymphomas, this is not the case for GI lymphomas. Thus many treatment recommendations are based on small case series and extrapolation from results with nodal lymphomas. Prior to the initiation of treatment with systemic chemotherapy, interested patients should receive counseling regarding fertility preservation in addition to the side effect profile of drugs being used.[16] We also routinely screen patients for chronic infections such as HIV, HBV, HCV, and *Hp* in lymphomas involving the MALT. We consider this important

TABLE 41.1 Staging Systems for Primary Gastrointestinal Lymphomas

Stage	Modified Paris Staging System[a]	TNM Staging System (Modified for Gastric Lymphoma)	Ann Arbor Staging System	Tumor Involvement
I	TI N0 T2 N0	T1 N0 M0 T2 N0 M0 T3 N0 M0	I_E I_E I_E	Mucosa, submucosa Muscularis propria Serosa
II	Extending into abdomen II_1 = local nodal involvement II_2 = distant nodal involvement	 T1-3 N1 M0 T1-3 N2 M0	 II_E II_E	 Perigastric or peri-intestinal lymph nodes More distant regional lymph nodes
II_E	Penetration of serosa to involve adjacent organs or tissues	T4 N0 M0	II_E	Invasion of adjacent structures
IV	Disseminated extranodal involvement or concomitant supradiaphragmatic nodal involvement	T1-4 N3 M0 T1-4 N0-3 M1	III_E IV_E	Lymph nodes on both sides of the diaphragm Distant metastases (e.g., bone marrow or additional extranodal sites)

[a]Modified from Ruskoné-Fourmestraux A, Dragosics B, Morgner A, et al. Paris staging system for primary gastrointestinal lymphomas. *Gut*. 2003;52:912–913.
GI, Gastrointestinal; *TNM*, tumor node metastasis.

because a sizeable percentage of low-grade lymphomas will undergo spontaneous regression, after the chronic infection driving them is adequately treated.

GASTRIC LYMPHOMAS

Primary gastric lymphomas account for 5% of gastric neoplasms, with an increasing trend worldwide.[17] The stomach is the most common extranodal site of lymphoma and accounts for 68%–75% of PGILs.[18] Most of these gastric lymphomas are classified as marginal zone B-cell lymphoma of the MALT type or as diffuse large B-cell lymphoma (DLBCL).[2]

Gastric Extranodal Marginal Zone B-Cell Lymphoma of Mucosa-Associated Lymphoid Tissue (Lymphomas)

Extranodal marginal zone B-cell lymphoma of MALT, also known as MALT lymphoma, was first described by Isaacson and Spencer in 1983[19] and comprises about 8% of all NHLs.[20] These lymphomas arise from malignant transformation of B cells from the marginal zone of MALT.[21] They may arise from MALT that exists under normal physiologic circumstances (e.g., in Peyer patches of the gut) or from MALT associated with infection or an autoimmune process. For example, gastric tissue normally does not contain MALT but may acquire it in response to chronic *Hp* infection (see Chapter 54).[22] The phenomenon of *lymphocytic homing*, which involves interaction between circulating lymphocytes and endothelial venules mediated by lymphocyte integrins and tissue-specific addressins, is key to extranodal lymphomagenesis.[23]

Malignant transformation occurs in a small percentage of patients with acquired gastric MALT and results in a lymphoma with generally indolent behavior. The malignant process appears to be driven to a large degree by chronic *Hp* infection because eradication of this infection leads to a regression of the lymphoma in 50%–80% of cases.[24,25]

Epidemiology

Gastric marginal zone B-cell lymphoma of MALT represents 38%–48% of gastric lymphomas.[26] The incidence varies according to the incidence of *Hp* in the population being assessed. Thus the incidence in northeastern Italy, where the rate of *Hp* infection is very high, is roughly 13 times the incidence in the United Kingdom.[27] The median age at diagnosis of gastric MALT lymphoma is approximately 60 years, with a wide age range, with men and women affected equally. The male-to-female ratio is equal.[28]

Cause and Pathogenesis

_Hp_ Infection

Several lines of evidence support the key role of *Hp* in the development of gastric MALT lymphoma (see Chapter 54). Infection by *Hp* is present in the vast majority of cases of gastric MALT lymphoma.[29] The epidemiologic studies cited earlier have shown a close correlation between the prevalence of *Hp* infection and gastric lymphoma in a given population,[30,31] and case-control studies have shown an association between previous *Hp* infection and subsequent development of gastric lymphoma.[32] In vitro studies have shown that gastric MALT lymphoma tissue contains T cells that are specifically reactive to *Hp*. These *Hp*-reactive T cells support the proliferation of neoplastic B cells.[33] Gastric MALT lymphoma can be induced in murine models by chronic *Helicobacter* infection.[34] Many groups have documented the regression of gastric MALT lymphoma after eradication of *Hp*.[24,25,35] Of interest, responses of small intestinal and rectal lymphoma to *Hp* eradication have been reported,[36,37] although a consistent role of the organism at these nongastric sites is not clear. Lymphomas have also been reported in patients with *Helicobacter heilmannii* infections, with resolution after eradication of the infection.[38]

Evidence for Antigen-Driven B-Cell Proliferation

As noted previously, the B-cell immunoglobulin variable region (V) genes undergo somatic hypermutation during the T-cell-dependent B-cell response to antigen,[4] which leads to the production of new antigen receptors with altered antigen-binding affinity. Resultant B-cell clones that express higher affinity antigen receptors have a survival advantage over B-cell clones containing receptors with lower affinity. Thus somatic mutation is a marker for an antigen-driven selection of B-cell clones. Sequence analysis of malignant B cells from gastric MALT lymphoma shows that the immunoglobulin genes have undergone somatic mutation.[39]

Genetic Studies

There are four main chromosomal translocations in extranodal marginal zone lymphomas: t(11;18)(q21;q21) BIRC3::MALT1, t(14;18)(q32;q21) IGH::MALT1, t(1;14)(p22;q32) IGH::BCL10, and t(3;14)(p14.1;q32) IGH::FOXP1. The most common translocation, t(11;18)(q21;q21), is found in 30% of cases, but its incidence varies with disease site: It is more common in cases involving the stomach (and lung), but rare in other sites.[40,41] The t(11;18)(q21;q21) translocation results in the reciprocal fusion of the *API-2* and *MALT-1* genes. *API-2* is an apoptosis inhibitor, and *MALT-1* is involved in nuclear factor κB (NF-κB) activation. MALT lymphomas with this translocation do not respond as well to antibiotic therapy aimed at eradicating *Hp* infection similar to lymphomas without this infection.[24] However, these lymphomas are also less likely to have other chromosomal translocations or transform to more aggressive large cell lymphomas.[40,42]

The t(14;18)(q32;q21) variant results in the translocation of the *MALT-1* gene on chromosome 18q21 to the immunoglobulin gene heavy-chain enhancer region, leading to its overexpression, thus differing from the t(14;18) translocation of FL, which involves the *bcl-2* gene. The t(14;18)(q32:q21) translocation occurs in about 20% of MALT lymphomas overall, although the incidence varies according to the disease site; it is rare in the GI tract but more common in lymphomas occurring in the salivary glands and ocular adnexa.[40]

Approximately 5% of gastric MALT lymphomas have a t(1;14)(p22;q32) translocation.[43] In this translocation, the *bcl-10* gene is brought under the control of the immunoglobulin heavy-chain gene enhancer, deregulating its expression. This translocation has been detected only in patients with MALT lymphomas, but those with it often have concurrent trisomies of chromosomes 3, 12, and 18. It is more commonly found in advanced-stage cases, which are less likely to respond to *Hp* eradication.

Finally, the t(3;14)(p14.1;q32) translocation results in a juxtaposition of the gene for the transcription factor *FOXP1* on 3p14.1, next to the immunoglobulin gene heavy-chain enhancer region, leading to a deregulation of *FOXP1*,[44] that is necessary for B cell development.[45]

Common Molecular Pathways From Mucosa-Associated Lymphoid Tissue Lymphoma Chromosomal Translocations

The first three translocations listed earlier all activate NF-κB, a transcription factor that increases cell activation, proliferation, and survival (see Chapters 1 and 2).[46,47] In unstimulated B and T lymphocytes, NF-κB is sequestered in the cytoplasm because it is bound to IκB, an inhibitory protein. Phosphorylation of IκB targets it for ubiquitination and degradation, thus releasing NF-κB, which then translocates to the nucleus to function as a transcription factor. The pathways through which IκB is phosphorylated are tightly regulated and involve *BCL-10* and *MALT-1*. Excessive *BCL-10* or *MALT-1* activity occurring as a consequence of t(11;18), t(14;18), or t(1;14) leads to constitutive NF-κB activation.[40]

Model for the Pathogenesis of Gastric Mucosa-Associated Lymphoid Tissue Lymphoma

A model for the pathogenesis of gastric MALT lymphoma suggests that the evolution of the disease is a multistage process, comprising the sequential development of *Hp* gastritis, low-grade B-cell lymphoma, and then high-grade B-cell lymphoma.[43] This model is supported by gastric biopsies obtained from patients with chronic gastritis taken years before the onset of lymphoma showing B-lymphocytic clones that later gave rise to a clinically evident lymphoma. In this model, *Hp* infection elicits an immune response in which T and B cells are recruited to the gastric mucosa, where MALT is then formed. *Hp*-specific T cells provide growth help to abnormal B-cell clones. The abnormal B cells may not be *Hp*-specific and may even be autoreactive. However, their continued proliferation, initially, depends on T-cell help. The pivotal role of *Hp*-reactive T cells in driving B-cell proliferation may explain why tumor cells tend to remain localized and why the tumor regresses after the eradication of *Hp*. However, continued B-cell proliferation eventually leads to an accumulation of additional genetic abnormalities, resulting in autonomous growth and more aggressive clinical behavior.

Because only a small percentage of *Hp*-infected individuals develop lymphoma, additional currently unknown environmental, microbial, or genetic factors must play a contributory role. Genetic polymorphisms affecting genes, such as *IL1RN* and *GSTT1* involved in inflammatory responses and antioxidative capacity, may be partly responsible for the genetic background for MALT lymphomagenesis.[48] *Hp* strains expressing certain proteins, such as CagA and oxidative damage, have been suggested to play a role in the development of gastric lymphoma.[49]

Pathology

Gross Appearance and Location

Low-grade gastric MALT lymphomas may present as a single lesion or as multiple lesions. Unifocal disease usually presents as ulcerated, protruding, or infiltrating masses, but may also manifest as erosions or simply erythema. They are most commonly located in the antrum.

Histology

The key histologic feature of low-grade MALT lymphoma is the presence of "lymphoepithelial lesions" (Fig. 41.2).[19,50] These lesions are defined as the unequivocal invasion and partial destruction of gastric glands or crypts by tumor cell aggregates. It should be noted, however, that these lesions can sometimes be seen in cases of florid chronic gastritis. Tumor cells are small- to medium-sized lymphocytes, with irregularly shaped nuclei and moderately abundant cytoplasm. The morphology of these cells can vary from small lymphoplasmacytoid cells to monocytoid cells that have abundant pale cytoplasm and well-defined borders.[51] Scattered larger cells or transformed lymphoblasts may also be seen. The lymphoma cells infiltrate the lamina propria diffusely and grow around reactive follicles; the germinal centers may be invaded, a phenomenon termed *follicular colonization*. Because there is a continuous spectrum from the transition of gastritis to

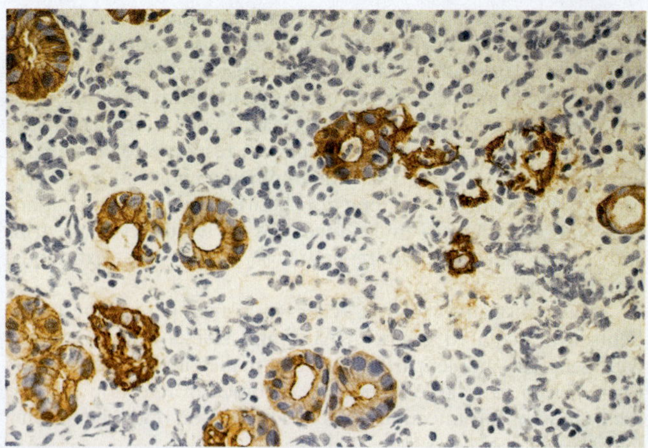

Fig. 41.2 Photomicrograph showing a "lymphoepithelial lesion" characteristic of gastric mucosa–associated lymphoid tissue lymphoma. Cytokeratin stain demonstrates invasion and destruction of some gastric glands by a monomorphic population of lymphocytes. Note for comparison the uninvolved normal glands in the *bottom center* of the photograph. Special stains (not shown) demonstrated *Hp*. (Courtesy Dr. Edward Lee, Washington, DC.)

lymphoma, diagnosis of borderline cases can be difficult. Various parameters may assist in the distinction, such as the prominence of lymphoepithelial lesions, degree of cytologic atypia, and presence of plasma cells with Dutcher bodies (periodic acid–Schiff-positive intranuclear pseudoinclusions).

The presence of large cells can add further complexity to the diagnosis.[17] The low-grade MALT lymphoma may have scattered large cells, but the tumor is composed predominantly of small cells. At the other end of the spectrum, gastric lymphomas that contain only large cells or only small areas of small cell MALT-like lymphoma should be classified as DLBCLs (see later).[5] In between the ends of this spectrum are low-grade lymphomas in the process of evolving into more aggressive lymphoma, with increasing numbers of large cells being observed with transformation.

Immunophenotype

Gastric MALT lymphoma cells have the typical immunophenotype of marginal zone B cells. They express pan-B antigens (CD19, CD20, and CD79a) and they lack expression of CD5, CD10, CD23, and cyclin D1.[2] Further immunostaining by experienced pathologists can aid in identifying lymphoepithelial lesions (see Fig. 41.2) and in distinguishing follicular colonization from FL (a rare occurrence in the stomach; see later).

Molecular Tests of Monoclonality

Southern blotting or PCR assay of immunoglobulin heavy-chain rearrangement can assist in the documentation of monoclonality. It should be noted that B-cell monoclonality may be detected in *Hp*-associated gastritis (see Chapter 54). Although monoclonality may predict for later development of lymphoma, monoclonality alone does not allow a diagnosis of lymphoma; thus molecular tests should always be considered in the context of histologic findings.

Clinical Features

Symptoms, Signs, and Laboratory Tests

The most common symptoms are dyspepsia and epigastric pain. Other less common symptoms include anorexia, weight loss, nausea and/or vomiting, and early satiety.[43] Gastric bleeding and B symptoms (fevers, night sweats, and weight loss) are rare. Serum levels of LDH and β_2-microglobulin are usually normal.[52]

Diagnosis and Staging

Patients are evaluated by EGD. PPI therapy should ideally be withheld for at least 2 weeks prior to endoscopy to avoid a false-negative result for *Hp*. Endoscopic findings include erythema, erosions, and/or ulcers. Diffuse superficial infiltration is typical for MALT lymphoma, whereas masses are more commonly seen in DLBCL (Fig. 41.3), an aggressive NHL. The most common site of involvement in the stomach is the antrum, but biopsies should be taken from all abnormal areas and randomly from each area of the stomach, as well as the duodenum and gastroesophageal junction, because disease is often multifocal. Because some lymphomas infiltrate the submucosa without involving the mucosal membrane, biopsies need to be sufficiently deep and large for histopathologic and immunohistochemical analyses. *Hp* infection should be established by histologic studies, breath test, or fecal antigen testing (see Chapter 54).[53] EUS can determine the depth of infiltration and assess for the presence of enlarged perigastric lymph nodes.[11] Additional staging consists of upper airway examination, CT of the chest, abdomen, and pelvis, bone marrow aspiration and biopsy, and measurement of the serum LDH level. PET is not usually helpful in gastric MALT lymphoma because of low uptake of fluorodeoxyglucose (FDG) but can assist if there is a concern of transformation of gastric MALT lymphoma to aggressive lymphomas.[54,55]

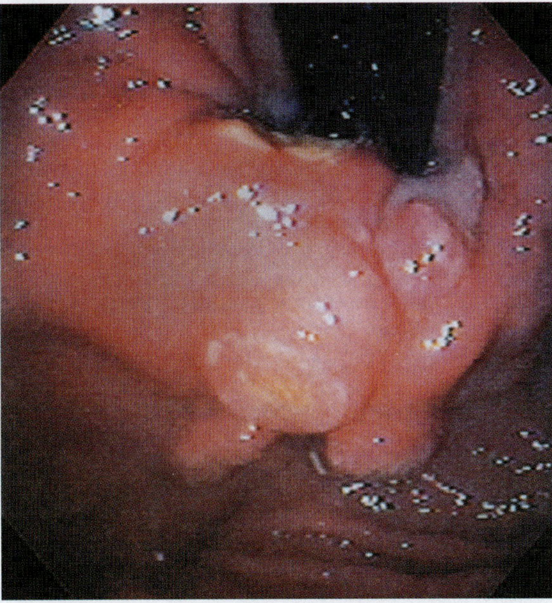

Fig. 41.3 Endoscopic appearance of diffuse large B-cell lymphoma of the stomach with multiple umbilicated lesions adjacent to the gastroesophageal junction. One large ulceration is seen just beyond the squamocolumnar junction.

Staging System and Prognostic Assessment

In 1994 an international workshop on the staging of GI tract lymphomas proposed the Lugano staging system,[56] a modification of the Blackledge system. The Paris staging system (see Table 41.1) is a modification of the TNM system and incorporates the depth of infiltration as well as lymph node involvement based on EUS.[57] Approximately 75% of gastric MALT lymphomas are confined to the stomach (stage I) at diagnosis[43] and behave in a clinically indolent fashion; thus prognosis is good for most patients, with overall survival rates of 80%–95% at 5 years. Prognosis is poor in the rare patient with more advanced disease. Additional features associated with a worse prognosis are deep infiltration of the stomach wall, which is associated with a higher likelihood of regional lymph node involvement,[58] and a high percentage of large cells on histologic evaluation.

A MALT lymphoma–specific prognostic index (MALT-IPI) has been developed and validated with these three key parameters: age ≥70 years, stage III or IV disease and an elevated LDH serum level. The 5-year event–free survival rates in the low-, intermediate-, and high-risk groups per the MALT-IPI in the studied patient cohort were 70%, 56%, and 29%, respectively. This easily reproducible tool retained utility in both gastric and nongastric MALT-lymphomas and in different treatment strategies used in the study group.[59]

Treatment

Large, randomized clinical trials have not been performed in MALT lymphoma because of the rarity of the disorder. Therefore treatment recommendations are based on case series and expert opinion. Wotherspoon and colleagues[25] first reported that gastric MALT lymphoma could completely regress by endoscopic, histologic, and molecular criteria after eradication of *Hp*. Numerous studies have confirmed these observations,[60–63] and antibiotics aimed at eradicating *Hp* (see Chapter 54) have become the mainstay of therapy for low-grade gastric MALT lymphoma. Even patients with advanced stages of disease can regress with eradication of *Hp*. However, it is important to recognize that the current literature in this field is less than optimal in several respects. Older studies are limited by insufficient staging procedures and outdated classification systems. Moreover, none of the reports is a controlled or randomized trial, and long-term follow-up is lacking. Nevertheless, the current literature is sufficient to suggest that early-stage disease is best managed with a trial of *Hp*-directed antibiotics (Chapter 54), reserving more toxic therapies such as radiation, chemotherapy, or surgery for cases without concomitant *Hp* infection or for those that do not respond to antibiotics, keeping in mind that it may take several months before remission is achieved.

Table 41.2 indicates treatment options by stage using the Lugano staging system.

Stage I Disease

Most patients fall into this category and can be treated with antibiotic therapy aimed at eradication of *Hp*. Any of the treatment regimens discussed in Chapter 54 may be used. Follow-up endoscopy with multiple biopsies should be done 3–6 months after the completion of therapy to document clearance of infection and to assess lymphoma regression.[58] Regression of lymphoma, but not necessarily complete regression, is usually evident at this initial posttreatment examination. Patients with persistence of infection should be treated with a second-line antibiotic regimen (see Chapter 54).[64] Histopathology at this initial posttreatment examination can predict ultimate response, with biopsies showing only small foci of lymphoma being predictive of subsequent complete regression and biopsies showing diffuse persistent disease, thus predicting a low likelihood of subsequent complete regression. The Wotherspoon index was initially proposed (1993) as a histologic tool to evaluate therapy response, but its utility has been more for initial diagnosis. The Groupe d'Etude des Lymphomes de l'Adulte posttreatment histologic evaluation system (2003)[65] is an effective, reproducible criterion to monitor therapeutic courses of gastric lymphomas (Table 41.3). Patients are then followed with endoscopy approximately every 6 months for 2 years and then yearly. Overall, approximately 75% of patients with stage I disease confined to the mucosa and submucosa achieve complete remission.[31] The median time to remission is 5 months, with remission usually occurring within 12 months. However, time to remission has been reported to be as long as 45 months.[24,66] Of patients in clinical remission, a majority will still have tumor clones detected by PCR.[60] With a continued follow-up of these patients, the malignant clone decreases; current studies have suggested that a positive PCR at histologic remission does not predict subsequent relapse, but a longer follow-up of this issue is necessary. Approximately 90% of patients who had a complete clinical remission to *Hp* eradication remain in remission,[31] but late relapses can occur. Relapse may occur in association with *Hp* reinfection and can be cured by eradicating the organism again. In the absence of *Hp* reinfection, relapse is frequently transient.[67] A randomized trial of patients who responded to *Hp* treatment did not show a benefit with chlorambucil when compared to observation.[68]

TABLE 41.2 Treatment of Gastric Marginal Zone B-cell Lymphoma of MALT Type[a]

Lugano Stage	Treatment[b,c]
I, with disease limited to mucosa and submucosa	Antibiotics alone
II, with involvement of muscularis propria or serosa	Best treatment unknown currently. Radiation or chemotherapy is probably a better option than surgery (see text)
IV, with involvement beyond stomach wall	Chemotherapy for symptomatic disease. Local management with radiation or surgery may be indicated in selected cases

[a]According to Lugano staging system.
[b]Patients with *Hp* infection should be treated with antibiotics to clear the infection, regardless of stage (see Chapter 54).
[c]Patients with a high percentage of large cells and disease limited to the mucosa may respond to antibiotics alone, although further study of this issue is necessary.
Patients with a high percentage of large cells and more advanced-stage disease should be treated as in Table 41.4 for diffuse large B-cell lymphoma. *MALT*, Mucosa-associated lymphoid tissue.

Approximately 25% of patients do not respond to *Hp* eradication.[69] Lack of response is more common in patients with the t(11;18)(q21;q21) BIRC3::MALT1 translocation; in one study, 67% of nonresponders harbored this abnormality, whereas only 4% of responders did.[70,71] Lack of response to antibiotic therapy used in *Hp* infection is also seen in *Hp*-negative gastric MALT lymphomas[72] and in patients with lymph node involvement at diagnosis.[58]

The optimal management of disease unresponsive to *Hp* eradication is not certain. Options include surgical resection, chemotherapy, and radiation. These options are discussed in the section on treatment of stage II_E disease (see later).

The management of patients with localized disease, but a significant percentage of large cells, is also uncertain. More recent studies have documented remission after *Hp* eradication, in contrast to earlier studies. For example, in one study of 34 patients with high-grade histology, 18 had disease regression with *Hp* eradication and were free of lymphoma after a median follow-up of 7.7 years.[73] If this approach is taken, the patient should be followed closely and, if the response is suboptimal, treated with one of the approaches discussed in the following section.

As mentioned, occasional cases of gastric MALT lymphoma are *Hp*-negative and these patients are much less likely to respond

TABLE 41.3 Histological Evaluation System Proposed to Evaluate MALT Gastric Lymphomas Following Antibiotic Therapy

Treatment Outcome	Definition	Histological Characteristics
CR	Complete histological remission	Normal or empty lamina propria and/or fibrosis with absent or sparse plasmacytes and lymphoid cells in the lamina propria without lymphoepithelial lesions
pMRD	Probable minimal residual disease	Empty lamina propria and/or fibrosis with disease aggregates or lymphocyte nodules in the lamina propria, in the muscularis mucosae, and/or in the submucosa
rRD	Residual disease in regression	Lamina propria focally empty and/or fibrosis; dense, diffuse, or nodular-infiltrated lymphoid, which extends around the glands in the lamina propria. Focal or absent lymphoepithelial lesions
NC	No change	Lymphocytic infiltration dense, diffuse, or nodular, +/− lymphoepithelial lesions

As Proposed by the Groupe d'Etude des Lymphomes de l'Adulte.

to antibiotic treatment. However, anti-*Hp* treatment should still be attempted because of possible false-negative results for *Hp* or in the event that another helicobacter, *H. heilmannii*, caused the lymphoma.[58]

Locally Advanced Disease: Stage I with Involvement of Muscularis or Serosa or Poor Response to Hp Eradication (stage II_E). Patients with more advanced-stage disease who are *Hp*-positive should also receive antibiotic therapy, but antibiotic therapy alone is usually not sufficient to eradicate the lymphoma. There is currently no consensus regarding the optimal management of this group of patients. Total gastrectomy can cure more than 80% of patients with stage II_E disease but diminishes patients' quality of life and has not been shown to achieve superior results when compared with more conservative approaches.[74] Involved field radiation therapy (30–40 Gy delivered in 15–20 fractions to the stomach and perigastric nodes) produces excellent results with a complete remission rate of 90%–100% and a 5-year disease-free survival of approximately 80%.[75,76] Radiation therapy is usually well tolerated and preserves gastric function. Thus it has become the preferred therapy for patients with advanced-stage disease, those who are negative for *Hp*, and those with persistent disease despite *Hp* treatment.[77] Other treatment options in this group include chemotherapy, immunotherapy, combined chemo-immunotherapy or newer novel, target-specific chemotherapeutics such as bruton tyrosine kinase inhibitors. Older data suggest that single-agent oral chemotherapy drugs such as cyclophosphamide[24] or chlorambucil have activity, as does treatment with purine analogs such as cladribine (2 CdA), and monoclonal antibodies against CD20 such as rituximab that may be more effective in patients with t(11;18)(q21;q21) BIRC3::MALT1.[78] Chemoimmunotherapy with rituximab, a monoclonal antibody against CD20, in combination with chlorambucil,[79,80] fludarabine,[81] cladribine,[82] and bendamustine,[43] an approach similar to treatment of other low-grade B-NHL, has shown response rates of 80%–100% with acceptable toxicity.

Stage II or IV Disease

Low-grade gastric MALT lymphoma that has spread to distant lymph nodes or extranodal sites should be treated as advanced low-grade B-cell NHL. Various regimens are used, most incorporating rituximab.[83,84] Such disease is usually not considered curable but is generally indolent, with transient responses to chemotherapy.[85] Asymptomatic patients may be followed expectantly.

Diffuse Large B-Cell Lymphoma of the Stomach

Epidemiology

Approximately, 50% of gastric lymphomas are DLBCLs. The incidence may be higher in developing than in developed nations, but clinical features are to be similar. The median age is approximately 60 years, with a slight male predominance.[18]

Cause and Pathogenesis

The pathogenesis of gastric DLBCL is poorly understood. Many large cell tumors have components of low-grade MALT tissue and are assumed to have evolved through transformation of low-grade lesions. Frequently, these bear identical rearranged immunoglobulin genes. According to the WHO classification, this is now referred to as "Transformations of indolent B-cell lymphomas."[6] However, other DLBCLs have no evidence of associated low-grade MALT tissue. It is unclear whether de novo gastric DLBCL has a worse prognosis than transformations of indolent B-cell lymphomas.[86]

If the large-cell lesions commonly arise from progression of low-grade lesions, then conceivably *Hp* may have a role in the initial pathogenesis. One study suggested that *Hp* infection is more common in patients whose large-cell lesions had a low-grade component.[87] Moreover, the observation of a response of early-stage large-cell lymphomas to *Hp* eradication has suggested a role for the organism, at least in some cases.[73,88] As outlined earlier in the discussion of tentative models for *Hp*-induced lymphoma, large-cell transformation resulting from genetic events, including loss of p53 and p16, may lead to tumor cells losing their dependence on *Hp* for growth.[2] A high incidence of somatic mutations in rearranged immunoglobulin heavy-chain variable genes in one study of DLBCLs of the stomach has implicated antigen selection in the genesis of the lymphoma.

Pathology

DLBCL may appear grossly as large ulcers, protruded tumors (see Fig. 41.3), or multiple shallow ulcers.[89,90] The most common sites of involvement are the body and antrum of the stomach. Tumors with a low-grade component are more likely to be multifocal than tumors with no low-grade component. Large-cell lymphomas typically invade the muscularis propria layer or even more deeply.

Microscopic examination reveals compact clusters, confluent aggregates, or sheets of large cells that resemble immunoblasts or centroblasts, most often with a mixture of the two (Fig. 41.4).[2] From 25% to 40% of cases show evidence of derivation from MALT, including dense infiltration of centrocyte-like cells in the lamina propria and typical lymphoepithelial lesions.[87]

Immunophenotypic analysis shows an expression of one or more B-cell antigens (CD19, CD20, CD22, and CD79a) and CD45. Lesions with evidence of low-grade MALT tissue do not express CD10, consistent with their having evolved from the CD10-negative marginal zone low-grade lesions. Lesions, without evidence of MALT, may or may not express CD10. Genetic analysis reveals monoclonal immunoglobulin gene rearrangements. *BCL6* is frequently mutated or rearranged[91]; if this is seen along with translocation involving *myc and bcl-2*, the lymphoma is referred to as a "double hit" DLBCL, or based on WHO 2022 classification, diffuse large B-cell lymphoma/high-grade B-cell lymphoma, with *MYC* and *BCL2* rearrangements.[6]

MYC translocation along with rearrangements in either *BCL2* are increasingly being recognized as adverse prognostic features and most experts modify treatments based on it, using more

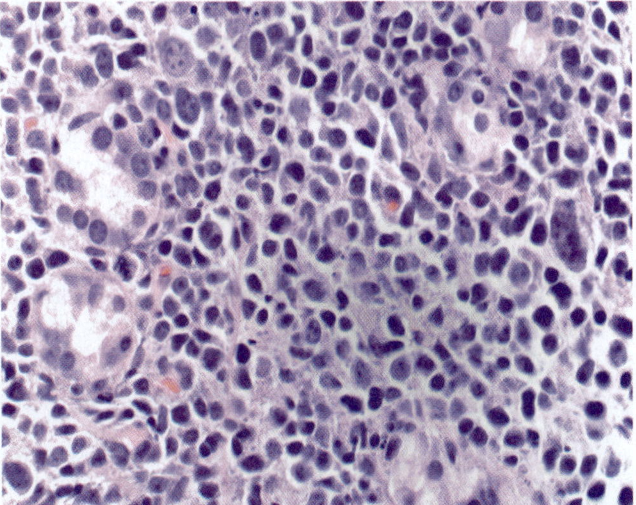

Fig. 41.4 Photomicrograph showing diffuse large B-cell lymphoma in stomach. There is a dense infiltrate of medium-sized to large B-lymphoid cells within gastric mucosa. (Courtesy Dr. Weina Chen, UT Southwestern Medical Center, Dallas, TX.)

intense chemo-immunotherapy regimens. Similarly, an increased expression of *myc* and *bcl2* by IHC staining is associated with relatively poor outcomes; although colloquially referred to as *double expressor*, this category is not formally recognized by WHO yet and outside of the setting of a clinical trial; most experts continue to use standard R-CHOP for it.

It is worth discussing the evolution in terminology regarding DLBCLs of the stomach. Many pathologists have referred to lymphomas arising in MALT with high-grade features (with or without a component of low-grade disease) as high-grade gastric MALT lymphomas. However, those involved in the development of the WHO classification were concerned that many clinicians had come to regard the term *gastric MALT lymphoma* as synonymous with a lesion that responds to antibiotics. This is usually not the case with high-grade lesions arising in MALT. Therefore those involved in formulating the WHO classification[5] agreed to use the term *extranodal marginal zone B-cell lymphoma of MALT type* for low-grade lesions, and the term *diffuse large B-cell lymphoma* for high-grade lesions, leaving out the term *MALT*. Low-grade lesions involving MALT often contain varying proportions of large cells, with a worse prognosis in relation to increased percentage of large cells. However, at this point, a precise grading system for this situation has not been devised and remains a goal of ongoing research.

Clinical Features

Patients present with epigastric pain (70%) or dyspepsia (30%), symptoms similar to those patients with gastric adenocarcinoma.[89,92] Large tumors may cause obstruction. Ulcerating lesions may be associated with GI bleeding. B symptoms (fevers, night sweats, and weight loss) and elevated serum LDH levels are uncommon.

Staging consists of EGD (see Fig. 41.3), upper airway examination, CT of the chest, abdomen, and pelvis or PET-CT scan, bone marrow aspiration and biopsy, and measurement of the serum LDH level. In addition, EUS plays an important role in assessing the depth of stomach wall involvement. *Hp* infection should be assessed; it is detected in 35% of patients with DLBCL of the stomach and is more common in those with concomitant gastric MALT.[89] Most patients have stage I or II disease by the Ann Arbor staging system.[93] However, as other staging systems have been developed, the use of various systems has made it difficult to compare results of different series.

Treatment

The optimal management of gastric DLBCL is controversial, but the current consensus recommends chemoimmunotherapy with or without radiotherapy as a replacement for surgery (Table 41.4).[89] Traditionally, localized disease was approached with surgery alone or followed by radiation and/or chemotherapy for patients with poor prognostic features.[94] This approach had the advantage of providing diagnostic and staging information and avoided the risk of gastric perforation or bleeding that was believed to result from treatment with chemotherapy or radiation. Approximately 70% of patients with stage I disease are disease-free 5 years after surgery.[95] However, several investigators have questioned the role of surgery in the management of localized gastric DLBCL. They noted that with the availability of endoscopy, surgery was no longer necessary for diagnosis and, with the availability of CT and EUS, surgery was no longer necessary for staging. In addition, the risk of gastric bleeding or perforation during chemotherapy is lower than 5% and only a few of those who bleed require urgent gastrectomy.[96] Surgery, however, carries a 5%–10% risk of mortality and is associated with significant morbidity.

TABLE 41.4 Treatment of Diffuse Large B-cell Lymphoma of the Stomach[a]

Lugano Stage	Treatment
I	CHOP[b] × 3–4 cycles + RT[c] + rituximab[d]
II, II_E	CHOP × 3–4 cycles + RT + rituximab
IV	CHOP × 6–8 cycles + RT + rituximab

[a]According to the Lugano staging system, optimal management of this entity is controversial. However, a developing consensus seems to favor combined chemotherapy and radiation and avoidance of surgery (see text).

[b]Cyclophosphamide, doxorubicin (hydroxydaunorubicin), vincristine (Oncovin), prednisone.

[c]RT (radiotherapy); usually, 30–40 Gy in 20–30 fractions.

[d]The suggestion for the addition of rituximab in this setting involves extrapolation of randomized data from nodal diffuse large B-cell lymphoma.

Thus chemotherapy and radiation were investigated as alternatives to surgery. Retrospective studies have shown similar outcomes in patients treated with surgery alone versus chemotherapy alone.[18] A prospective study of patients with DLBCL of the stomach who were randomized to surgery, surgery plus radiotherapy, surgery plus chemotherapy, or chemotherapy alone showed improved complete response rates and overall survival for patients who received surgery plus chemotherapy and chemotherapy alone when compared with those who received surgery alone or surgery plus radiotherapy.[97] The German Multicenter Study GIT NHL 01/92 was a prospective nonrandomized study of surgery in conjunction with chemotherapy and radiation versus chemotherapy and radiation alone for primary gastric lymphoma in localized stages. Whether the treatment included surgery was left to the discretion of each participating center. There was no difference in survival rate between those who received surgery followed by chemoradiotherapy and those who received chemoradiotherapy alone.[98] These results were confirmed in a subsequent, larger, prospective nonrandomized trial, GIT NHL 02/96.[99]

For patients with advanced-stage nodal DLBCL, the addition of rituximab, a monoclonal antibody against CD20, to CHOP (*c*yclophosphamide, doxorubicin [*h*ydroxydaunorubicin], vincristine [*O*ncovin], *p*rednisone) chemotherapy improves overall survival when compared with CHOP alone.[100–103] This combination has also been administered to patients with gastric DLBCL and found to be safe and effective.[104,105]

The necessity of radiation therapy in the management of gastric DLBCL is controversial. A small retrospective study of patients with stage I or II primary gastric high-grade DLBCL treated with chemotherapy with or without radiotherapy has shown decreased relapse rates in patients who received consolidative radiotherapy.[96] However, this study included only 21 patients, of whom 3 relapsed, and it is thought that a prospective randomized trial is needed.

Thus standard management of gastric large B-cell lymphoma follows standard management of nodal large B-cell lymphomas. The treatment of localized (stage I or II) nodal large B-cell lymphoma consists of three to six cycles of combination chemotherapy (typically the CHOP regimen) given with rituximab, with radiation generally given if using abbreviated chemotherapy (three cycles instead of six).[106,107] Experts are increasingly using a more intense regimen, DA-R-EPOCH (dose-adjusted rituximab, etoposide, prednisone, and vincristine [*O*ncovin], *c*yclophosphamide, doxorubicin [*h*ydroxydaunorubicin]) for patients with

DLBCL/high-grade B-cell lymphoma with *myc* and *bcl2* rearrangement. This regimen is primarily based on retrospective data, which show increasing numbers of complete remissions achieved with this regimen and patients achieving complete remission having the best chance of long-term disease-free survival. No prospective data comparing the two regimens for DLBCL/high-grade B-cell lymphoma with *myc* and *bcl2* rearrangement are available. DA-R-EPOCH, however, for routine DLBCL does not lead to better outcomes and carries a risk of more prominent side effects based on data from a prospective trial (CALGB/Alliance 50303) presented at American Society of Hematology Annual Meeting in 2016.[108] Similarly, the increased expression of *myc* and *bcl2* by IHC staining is associated with relatively poor outcomes. Although colloquially referred to as "double expressor," this category is not formally recognized by WHO as yet and, outside of the setting of a clinical trial, most experts continue to use the standard R-CHOP regimen for it. DLBCL patients with evidence of *Hp* infection should be treated, as response of large-cell lymphoma has been reported after the eradication of *Hp*.[109,110] However, these studies must be considered preliminary, and most patients treated with antibiotics alone have had disease limited to the mucosa; most patients with DLBCL of the stomach have more advanced disease, and antibiotics alone are considered inadequate treatment.

For patients with relapsed/refractory DLBCL after failing two lines of therapy (including anthracycline-based regimen) or refractory to frontline therapy, anti-CD19 directed chimeric-antigen receptor T-cell therapy is an emerging treatment option recently approved by the FDA. Although durable remissions are being observed with this treatment, long-term data on treatment outcomes are being discerned.[111,112]

Uncommon Gastric Lymphomas

B-cell lymphomas other than marginal zone or diffuse large B cell may involve the stomach uncommonly [e.g., MCL (1%) and FL (0.5%–2%)]. Gastric lymphomas of T-cell origin have rarely (1.5%–4%) been reported.[113–115]

SMALL INTESTINAL LYMPHOMAS

Small intestinal lymphomas may be divided into B- and T-cell tumors and account for 20%–30% of PGILs.[116] The B-cell tumors include immunoproliferative small intestinal disease (IPSID) and various non-IPSID subtypes, including marginal zone B-cell lymphoma of MALT type, DLBCL, MCL, FL, and Burkitt lymphoma. Relatively few reports have described the various non-IPSID small intestinal lymphomas, and large series have tended to group together all the lymphoma subtypes when cataloguing manifestations and treatment outcomes.[117–119] Given the lack of information about these diseases with regard to their behavior in the intestine, it is probably best to consider them in light of the well-described features of their nodal counterparts. Thus marginal zone and FLs are regarded as indolent processes, incurable but controllable by chemotherapy, and often associated with a relatively long survival. DLBCLs, MCLs, and Burkitt lymphomas are more aggressive processes, which generally require chemotherapy as part of their management. T-cell lymphomas of the small intestine are usually enteropathy-type intestinal T-cell lymphomas; other forms of T-cell lymphoma have been rarely reported. Recent reports have suggested the existence of a rare natural killer (NK) cell or NK-type T-cell intestinal lymphoma.[120–123]

Marginal Zone B-Cell Lymphoma of MALT Type

Lymphoma arising in the small intestine may have the characteristics of marginal zone B-cell lymphoma, with the same histologic and immunophenotypic features described earlier for gastric marginal zone B-cell lymphoma.[122,124] However, an association with *Hp* infection has not been documented, although rare responses to antibiotics have been reported. Most cases occur in older patients who present with melena. The disease usually presents as a single annular or exophytic tumor,[125] which may be present anywhere in the small intestine; disease is usually confined to the intestine or to local nodes. Treatment is generally surgical. Some patients have received chemotherapy, but few data are available regarding regimens and outcome. It should be noted that in nodal marginal zone lymphoma, chemotherapy is usually reserved for patients with symptoms, because the disease is slow-growing and sensitive to chemotherapy, but not curable by it. The 5-year survival rate is approximately 75%. As in gastric marginal zone B-cell lymphoma, the small intestinal variety may have varying components of large-cell transformation. This feature probably confers a worse prognosis, but data are scanty.

Diffuse Large B-Cell Lymphoma

DLBCL of the small intestine is similar to its gastric counterpart in histology and clinical behavior. Patients may present with abdominal pain, weight loss, obstruction, abdominal mass, bleeding, and/or perforation. The tumor is usually an exophytic or annular lesion. Histologic findings are similar to those described earlier for gastric DLBCL, with some patients having a low-grade component and others having only a large-cell component. Approximately half of patients have localized disease, and the other half have disease spread to regional or distant nodes. Surgery is usually required because of obstruction or perforation,[126] and additional therapy includes anthracycline-containing chemotherapy and the anti-CD20 monoclonal antibody, rituximab.[127] In addition, radiotherapy is sometimes indicated. Prognosis depends on disease stage and patient factors, such as age and performance status.

Mantle Cell Lymphoma

MCL is a subtype of B-cell NHL.[128] It is a heterogeneous lymphoma in terms of its clinical behavior, with disease in some patients having an indolent course like a low-grade B-NHL and in others an extremely aggressive course similar to high-grade B-cell malignancies. Patients typically present with widespread adenopathy and frequently have bone marrow and extranodal involvement. The GI tract is involved in more than 80% of patients (Fig. 41.5), although not all patients with GI involvement are symptomatic.[129] The most common manifestation of GI disease is multiple "lymphomatous polyposis," in which multiple lymphoid polyps are present in the GI tract.[130,131] The most common site of involvement is the ileocecal region, but any other area may be involved from the stomach to the rectum; occasionally patients have the involvement of all these regions (Fig. 41.6; see also Fig. 41.5). Involvement of the GI tract may also occur without the appearance of multiple polyps, and the isolated GI tract involvement has been reported. When patients have symptoms related to GI involvement, they usually include pain, obstruction, diarrhea, or hematochezia. It should be noted that multiple lymphomatous polyposis can also be seen with other lymphomas, especially marginal zone B-cell lymphomas of MALT and FLs. Microscopically, MCL involves the mucosa and submucosa and the malignant cells have the appearance of small atypical lymphocytes, which may surround benign-appearing germinal centers or may efface the lymphoid tissue. The tumor cells express pan-B markers and the T-cell marker CD5. The disease is characterized by t(11;14)(q13;q32) IGH::CCND1, a translocation that results in rearrangement and overexpression of the *bcl-1* gene encoding the protooncogene cyclin D1.[132] Patients with obstructive tumor masses require surgical therapy, but the

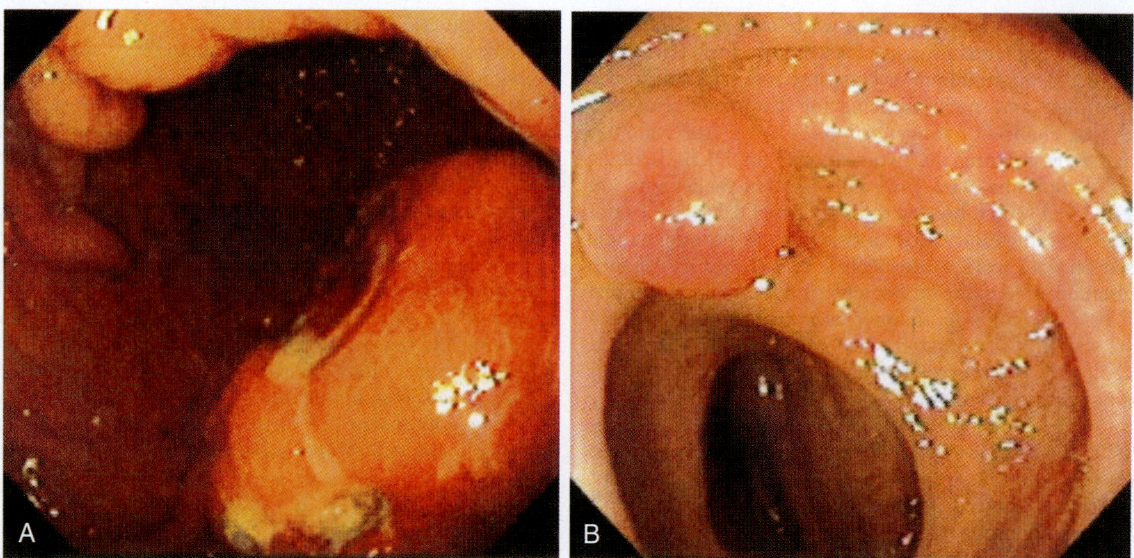

Fig. 41.5 Endoscopic appearance of mantle cell lymphoma presenting as multiple lymphomatous polyposis in the stomach (A) and in the colon (B).

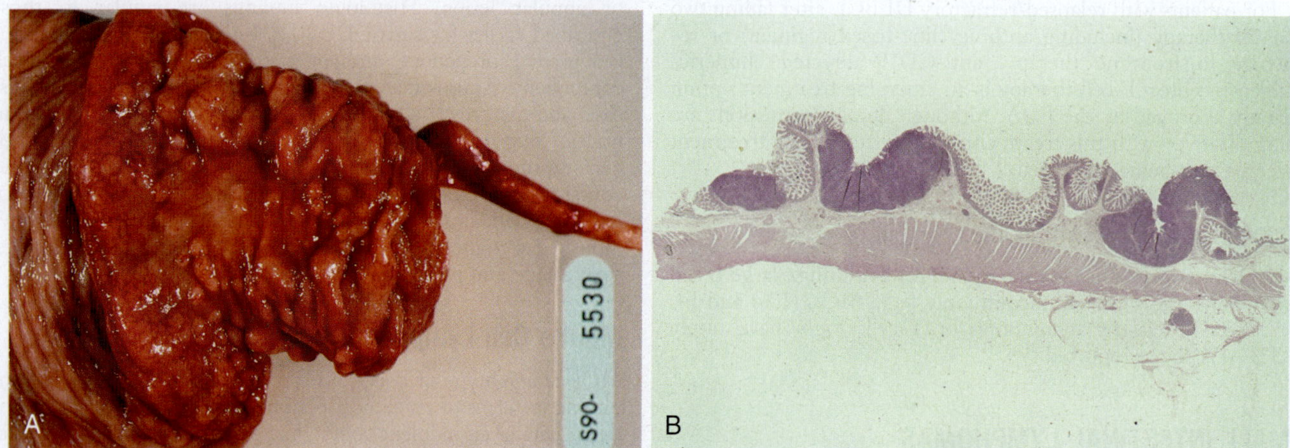

Fig. 41.6 Multiple lymphomatous polyposis (mantle cell lymphoma). (A) Gross specimen showing numerous small polypoid lesions in the cecum. Additional synchronous and metachronous lesions were present or later developed in the ileum and the duodenum, as well as the rectum and sigmoid colon. (B) Low-power photomicrograph of ileum shows multiple discrete sites of mucosal and submucosal involvement by lymphomatous polyposis. (Courtesy Dr. Edward Lee, Washington, DC, United States.)

mainstay of treatment is chemo-immunotherapy. Aggressive presentations of MCL are also usually consolidated with an autologous stem cell transplant in first remission after induction chemotherapy followed by maintenance rituximab.[133] Although MCL is initially responsive to chemotherapy, it eventually becomes refractory; median survival is 3– 5 years. Bruton tyrosine kinase inhibitors (ibrutinib, acalabrutinib, zanubrutinib, and pirtobrutinib) have been approved for use in refractory or relapsed MCL.[134,135]

Follicular Lymphoma

Follicular B-cell lymphomas of the GI tract are rare.[136] The most common presentation is as an obstructing lesion in the terminal ileum. As noted, patients with this diagnosis may also present with the gross appearance of multiple lymphomatous polyposis. Microscopically, most FLs are composed of small cleaved lymphocytes, or centrocytes (Fig. 41.7), with a varying admixture of large cells. The disease is characterized by t(14;18)(q24;q32), a translocation that results in overexpression of the *bcl-2* gene.[137]

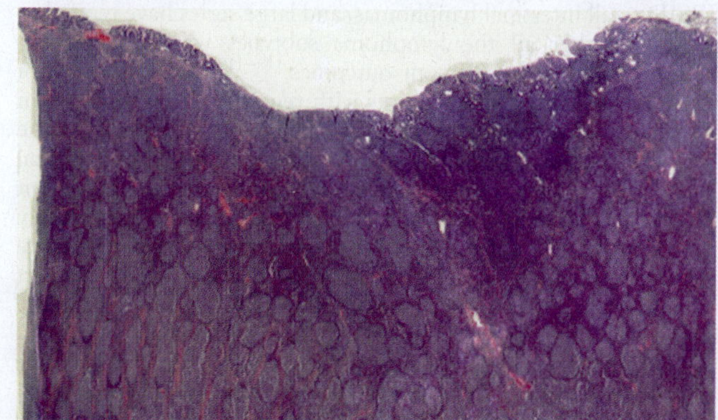

Fig. 41.7 Photomicrograph showing follicular lymphoma, World Health Organization grade II. Neoplastic lymphoid follicles are evident, involving the wall of the small intestine and effacing the normal architecture (H&E, low power). (Courtesy Dr. Imran Shahab and Dr. Pamela Jensen, Dallas, TX.)

Obstructing lesions require surgical management. Chemotherapy and radiation are sometimes indicated for the management of this indolent but incurable disorder.

Duodenal-type FL (D-FL) is a newly recognized entity in the 2016 WHO classification and maintained in the 2022 update. Unlike other FLs, D-FL is almost always incidentally detected on endoscopy (solitary or multiple nodules, or polypoid lesions, between 1 and 5 mm), diagnosed at a low grade and stage, and stays localized to most commonly the second portion of the duodenum. By gene expression profile and pathogenesis, it appears more closely related to MALT lymphoma than FL. Due to the excellent prognosis (median survival >12 years) associated with this disorder, most experts recommend a "wait and watch" strategy to management.[138,139]

Burkitt Lymphoma

Burkitt lymphoma is a highly aggressive malignancy that presents either as an endemic form, observed in Africa, or a sporadic form.[140] In the sporadic form, patients usually present with disease in the abdomen, with involvement of the distal ileum, cecum, and/or mesentery. Burkitt tumor cells are monomorphic, medium-sized cells with round nuclei, multiple nucleoli, and basophilic cytoplasm (Fig. 41.8). The involved lymphoid tissue microscopically has a starry sky appearance caused by numerous benign macrophages that have ingested apoptotic tumor cells.[141] The tumor cells express B-cell-associated antigens and surface immunoglobulin. Most cases have a translocation of the *c-myc* gene on chromosome 8, either to the immunoglobulin heavy-chain region on chromosome 14 or to one of the immunoglobulin light-chain regions on chromosome 2 or 22, resulting in a t(8;14), t(2;8), or t(8;22) translocation.[142] Burkitt lymphoma is rapidly fatal without treatment but responds rapidly to the institution of aggressive chemotherapy. Treatment carries a high risk of tumor lysis syndrome. Cure rates are 50%–90%, depending on the extent of the disease.[143,144]

Immunoproliferative Small Intestinal Disease

Epidemiology

IPSID (also known as α heavy-chain disease and as Mediterranean lymphoma) is confined to certain regions of the world, especially North Africa, Israel, and the surrounding Middle Eastern and Mediterranean countries.[145] IPSID is seen less often in other areas, including Central and South Africa, India and East Asia, and South and Central America. A diagnosis in North America or Europe should be questioned, unless the patient has previously lived in an endemic area. The disease occurs in individuals with lower socioeconomic status who live in conditions of poor hygiene and sanitation.[146] The disease generally occurs in the second or third decade of life, although it has been observed in older individuals. The incidence in males and females is equal.

Cause and Pathogenesis

Several observations suggest that IPSID may be initiated by an infectious agent or agents[147]: (1) an association of the disease with lower socioeconomic status and poor sanitation; (2) a high prevalence of intestinal bacterial overgrowth and parasitosis; (3) a decrease in incidence when living conditions have improved in endemic areas; and (4) a response of early lesions to antibiotic therapy. In addition, it is known that enteric microbiota stimulate IgA-producing cells, and intestinal biopsies from apparently normal individuals from endemic regions have shown an increase in lamina propria lymphocytes and plasma cells, reminiscent of findings in patients with IPSID. An association with *Campylobacter jejuni* infection has been demonstrated.[148,149]

As discussed later, IPSID is associated with the production of an unusual IgA heavy-chain protein, called α heavy chain, which is secreted by plasma cells and is detectable in various body fluids.[150,151] The plasma cells, which are the predominant histologic feature in the superficial mucosa, possess surface and cytoplasmic α chain protein. Centrocyte-like cells proliferating deeper in the mucosa have mainly cytoplasmic α-chain protein. It is likely that these centrocyte-like cells, stimulated by microbial antigens, differentiate into the plasma cells that secrete the α-chain protein characteristic of the disease. Genetic analyses have revealed that cellular proliferations are monoclonal, even in early lesions.[152,153]

Thus it can be proposed that, in a way somewhat analogous to *Hp*-associated gastric MALT, lymphocytes in intestinal MALT may be stimulated by infectious agents, in particular *C. jejuni*,[149] and proliferate in response. The lymphocytic response becomes monoclonal and initially depends on the presence of antigen. However, with time, the malignant cells acquire additional genetic changes, causing them to lose their dependence on antigen persistence. This loss of antigen dependence is associated with the development of more aggressive clinical features.

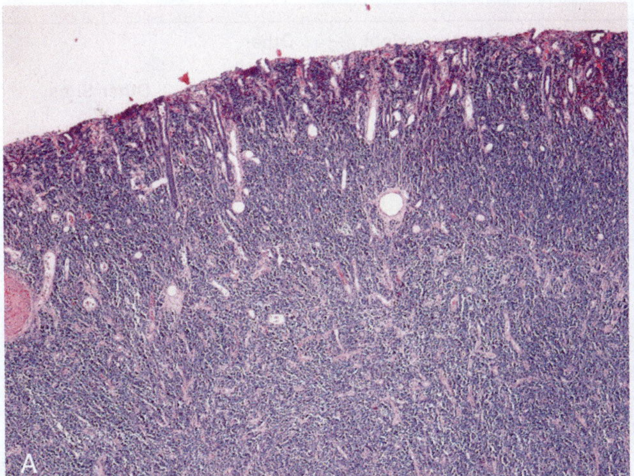

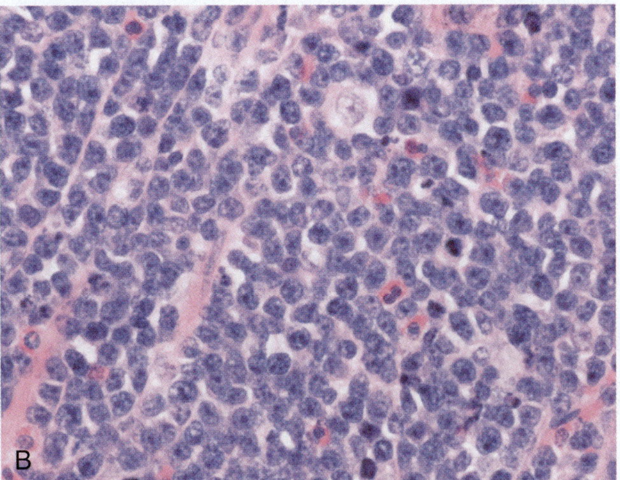

Fig. 41.8 Burkitt lymphoma. (A) Diffuse involvement of the small bowel by Burkitt lymphoma. Note infiltration around native glandular structures. (B) High-power view showing brisk mitotic activity and background macrophages. CD20 immunostaining (not shown) was strongly positive within the tumor population [(A) H&E, ×20; (B) H&E, ×600]. (Courtesy Dr. Pamela Jensen, Dallas, TX.)

Pathology

Gross lesions are generally confined to the proximal small intestine, with adenopathy of adjacent mesenteric nodes.[154] Although some patients have thickening of mucosal folds only, others have a generalized thickening of the bowel wall, discrete masses, nodules, or polypoid lesions. Although grossly only the proximal bowel wall is involved, histologically the disease is characterized by a dense mucosal and submucosal cellular infiltrate that extends continuously throughout the length of the small intestine. Various pathologic staging systems have been proposed (Table 41.5).[154,155] In early-stage disease, the cellular infiltrate is composed of benign-appearing plasma cells or lymphoplasmacytic cells. However, as already noted, various studies assessing immunoglobulin gene rearrangements or light-chain restriction have suggested that even the earliest infiltrate is monoclonal. This early infiltrate broadens villi and shortens and separates crypts, but epithelial cells remain intact. A histologic variant, the follicular lymphoid type, has been described in some patients (see Fig. 41.7). This variant features a diffuse involvement of the mucosa, with lymphoid follicle-like structures. As the disease progresses to intermediate and late stages, the villi are further broadened and may become completely effaced, crypts are fewer, and the immunoproliferation extends more deeply. Atypical lymphoid cells infiltrate the benign-appearing plasma cells and lymphoplasmacytic cells. With time, the process evolves into overt lymphoma. Mesenteric lymph nodes are enlarged in early lesions, with preserved architecture, although follicles may be encroached on by a histologically benign-appearing lymphocytic or plasmacytic infiltrate. As the disease progresses, the lymph node may acquire a more dysplastic appearance.

Clinical Features

Patients usually present with diarrhea, colicky abdominal pain, anorexia, and significant weight loss, with a duration of symptoms from months to years. The diarrhea initially may be intermittent but becomes voluminous and foul-smelling as malabsorption develops. About half of the patients have fever. Physical examination reveals evidence of malnutrition, digital clubbing, and peripheral edema. Late physical manifestations are ascites, hepatosplenomegaly, an abdominal mass, and peripheral lymphadenopathy. Endoscopy may reveal thickened mucosal folds, nodules, ulcers, or evidence of submucosal infiltration, rendering the intestine immobile, tender, and indistensible. Small bowel barium radiographs show diffuse dilation of the duodenum, jejunum, and proximal ileum, with thickened mucosal folds. Patients are frequently anemic because of vitamin deficiencies, and the erythrocyte sedimentation rate is elevated in one-third of cases. The circulating lymphocyte count is low, and measures of humoral and cellular immunity are impaired. Stool examination frequently reveals *Giardia lamblia* infestation. As noted, *C. jejuni* has been implicated in a high percentage of patients by PCR assay, DNA sequencing, fluorescence in situ hybridization, and immunohistochemical studies on intestinal biopsy specimens.[149] Serum IgG and IgM levels may be high or low; IgA levels are usually low or undetectable.

The characteristic and unique laboratory abnormality is the presence of the α-chain protein.[156] This 32–34-kD protein is a free

TABLE 41.5 Pathologic Staging Systems for Immunoproliferative Small Intestinal Disease

World Health Organization

1. Diffuse, dense, compact, and apparently benign lymphoproliferative mucosal infiltration
   a. pure plasmacytic
   b. mixed lymphoplasmacytic
2. As in (1), plus circumscribed "immunoblastic" lymphoma, in either the intestine and/or mesenteric lymph nodes
3. Diffuse "immunoblastic" lymphoma with or without demonstrable, apparently benign, lymphoplasmacytic infiltration

Salem et al.[145]

Stage 0: Benign-appearing LPI, no evidence of malignancy
Stage I: LPI and malignant lymphoma in either intestine (Ii) or mesenteric lymph nodes (In), but not both
Stage II: LPI and malignant lymphoma in both intestine and mesenteric lymph nodes
Stage III: Involvement of retroperitoneal and/or extra-abdominal lymph nodes
Stage IV: Involvement of noncontiguous nonlymphatic tissues
Unknown or inadequate staging

Al-Saleem et al.[148]

Stage	Small Intestine: Site I	Mesenteric Lymph Nodes: Site IIA	Other Abdominal and Retroperitoneal Lymph Nodes: Site IIB	Other Lymph Nodes: Site III	Other Sites: Site IV
A	Mature[a] plasmacytic infiltration of lamina propria[b], with no or limited disorganization of general lymph node architecture; inconstant and variable villus atrophy	Infiltrate in these sites cytologically like that in site I			
B	Atypical plasmacytic or lymphoplasmacytic infiltrate, with presence of more or less atypical immunoblast-like cells, extending at least to the submucosa; subtotal or total villus atrophy	Atypical plasmacytic or lymphoplasmacytic infiltrate, with the presence of more or less atypical immunoblast-like cells; total or subtotal obliteration of nodal architecture			Infiltrate cytologically similar to that in site I
C	Lymphomatous proliferation invading the whole depth of intestinal wall	Lymphomatous proliferation with total obliteration of nodal architecture[b]			Lymphomatous proliferation similar to that in site I

[a]Rare cells may show an immature pattern.
[b]Limited and superficial extensions to submucosa may be observed.
LPI, Lymphoplasmacytic mucosal infiltrate.
Modified from Fine KD, Stone MJ. Alpha-heavy-chain disease, Mediterranean lymphoma, and immunoproliferative small intestinal disease: a review of clinicopathological features, pathogenesis, and differential diagnosis. *Am J Gastroenterol.* 1999;94:1139–1152

α_1 heavy chain with an internal deletion of the variable (V_H) and C_H1 regions. It is devoid of light chains and thus corresponds to the Fc portion of the α_1 subunit of IgA. The α-chain protein amino terminal contains sequences that are not homologous to any known immunoglobulin sequence. These changes are often the result of insertions or deletions, usually involving the V_H–J_H and C_H2 regions,[148] but the source of inserted genetic material is unknown.

The α-chain production migrates as a broad band within the α_2 and β regions on serum protein electrophoresis. In addition to electrophoresis, the protein can be detected by immunoelectrophoresis or immunoselection (the most sensitive and specific methods)[148] in serum, urine, saliva, or intestinal secretions. Detection of α-chain protein from these sources is more likely in patients with early disease than in patients with more advanced disease, but, regardless of stage, α-chain protein can be detected in tissue sections in most cases of IPSID by immunofluorescence or immunoperoxidase staining of plasma or lymphoma cells.[156]

It has been postulated that chronic antigenic stimulation of the intestinal IgA secretory apparatus results in the expansion of several plasma cell clones. Eventually, a structural mutation occurs in a particular clone, resulting in an internal deletion of part of the α heavy chain. This leads to an inability to make light chains and results in secretion of α-chain protein rather than intact IgA.[145,148]

Diagnosis and Staging

Because the more malignant-appearing histology may be present only in deeper layers of the intestine, endoscopic biopsy alone is often considered an inadequate evaluation; staging laparotomy is therefore strongly recommended by some authors to allow full-thickness intestinal biopsy and biopsy of mesenteric lymph nodes.[157] However, some investigators do not routinely perform laparoscopy or laparotomy; instead, upper and lower GI endoscopy, small bowel series, bone marrow biopsies, and fine-needle aspiration of enlarged lymph nodes are performed.[158] One of the staging systems may then be applied (see Table 41.5). More advanced disease, poor performance status, and comorbid illnesses portend a worse prognosis.

Treatment

Because of the relative rarity of this lymphoma, no large trials investigating therapy have been carried out.[158,159] Patients often require intensive nutritional support.[160] Patients with early disease (e.g., Salem stage 0 disease; see Table 41.5) are generally treated with antibiotics for 6 months or more. The two most commonly used regimens are tetracycline alone and a combination of metronidazole and ampicillin. Response rates have ranged from 33% to 71%[161]; in one study, the complete response rate was 71%, with a disease-free survival of 43% at 5 years.[158] In patients who do not significantly improve by 6 months or who do not achieve complete remission by 12 months, or who have advanced disease at presentation, chemotherapy should be given. Most investigators recommend anthracycline-containing regimens such as CHOP.[162,163] For example, one investigator has reported a complete response rate of 67% and a survival rate of 58% at 3.5 years in patients treated with antibiotics, total parenteral nutrition, and anthracycline-based combination chemotherapy.[163] However, good results have been reported with nonanthracycline-containing regimens as well; in one report, 56% of patients with advanced disease were free of disease at 5 years.[158] Finally, because total abdominal radiotherapy has been used in only a small number of patients, it is difficult to assess its proper role.[164]

Enteropathy-Associated T-Cell Lymphoma

Enteropathy-associated T-cell lymphoma (EATL) occurs as a complication of celiac disease (see Chapter 109).[165] Malignant transformation of intraepithelial T cells leads to an aggressive malignancy, causing most patients to die within a few months of diagnosis.[166,167] Treatment of celiac disease with a gluten-free diet may decrease the risk of this malignancy.[168]

Epidemiology

EATL is a rare malignancy with an incidence of only 0.016 per 100,000 population, though the overall age-adjusted incidence is increasing.[169] Celiac disease has a prevalence of 0.5%–1% in the United States and Europe[170,171] and is more common in whites compared with African-Americans and Asians. In patients with symptomatic celiac disease, the most common cause of death was NHL.[172] The diagnosis of lymphoma is usually made concomitantly with or shortly after the diagnosis of celiac disease, although the two conditions are commonly diagnosed simultaneously, especially in patients who have a long history of malabsorption. Adherence to a strict gluten-free diet appears to reduce mortality.[173] The median age at diagnosis of EATL is 60 years and the incidence in men and women is equal.[174]

Cause and Pathogenesis

EATL occurs in patients with adult celiac disease.[175] As discussed in Chapter 109, celiac disease is characterized by a hereditary sensitivity to gluten.[176] Gluten peptides are presented by celiac disease–specific HLA-DQ2 and HLA-DQ8 positive antigen-presenting cells and thus elicit an immune response in which gluten-specific intraepithelial lymphocytes damage intestinal epithelium. Intraepithelial T cells in celiac disease have a normal immunophenotype ($CD3^+/CD8^+$) and are polyclonal.[177,178] Malignant transformation of these T cells results in a monoclonal population of intraepithelial T cells that have an abnormal phenotype.[179–182] Monoclonal populations of intraepithelial T cells in celiac mucosa may result in any one of several interrelated processes.[182,183] The first condition is refractory celiac disease, a condition in which patients lose responsiveness to a gluten-free diet.[184] The second condition, ulcerative jejunitis, is characterized by inflammatory jejunal ulcers and unresponsiveness to a gluten-free diet.[185] The third condition is EATL, an aggressive malignancy of the small intestine.[180,181] In patients with any of these three conditions, uninvolved mucosa adjacent to the lesions can contain monoclonal T cells containing the same rearranged T-cell receptor genes.[186] In addition, patients with ulcerative jejunitis can subsequently develop EATL, in which the same clone is isolated in the jejunitis and the subsequent lymphoma. Thus these three conditions have come to be considered to represent a spectrum of disorders mediated by monoclonal intraepithelial T cells.

Comparative genomic hybridization studies have shown recurrent chromosomal gains in EATL at chromosomes 9q, 7q, 5q, and 1q and recurrent losses at 8p, 13q, and 9p. A gain at 9q is the most common, seen in 58% of cases examined.[187] Another study has shown that loss of heterozygosity at 9q21 is a frequent finding.[188] In addition, one study has suggested that gain of chromosome 1q may be an early event in lymphomagenesis.[189]

Pathology

Tumors typically occur in the jejunum but may be seen in other sites of the small intestine. Lymphoma may occur in single or multiple sites. Grossly, the lymphomas commonly appear as ulcerating lesions, with circumferential involvement of the small bowel. Lesions may also appear as nodules, plaques, or strictures, but large masses are uncommon. Mesenteric lymph nodes are often enlarged, either because of tumor involvement or of edema and reactive changes. Distant sites, especially the bone marrow or the liver, are sometimes involved.

Histologically, the lymphoma is generally characterized by large, highly pleomorphic cells with numerous, bizarre, multinucleated forms, with an inflammatory background. A minority of patients (10%–20%) may have monomorphic medium-sized cells (Fig. 41.9). This was previously termed type II EATL and is currently called monomorphic epitheliotropic intestinal T-cell lymphoma (MEITL)[6] and may occur in the absence of celiac disease. MEITL has an increased incidence in Asian and Hispanic populations. Uninvolved mucosa usually has the typical appearance of celiac disease, with villous atrophy, crypt hyperplasia, plasmacytosis in the lamina propria, and an increase in intraepithelial lymphocytes (see Chapter 109). However, the enteropathy may be subtle in some cases, with only an increase in the intraepithelial lymphocytes.

According to 62 patients identified to have EATL in the International Peripheral T-cell Lymphoma Project, immunophenotyping typically shows that the malignant cells are $CD3^+$, $CD2^+$, $CD5^-$, $CD4^-$, $CD8^+$, $CD30^+$, $CD103^+$, and contain cytotoxic granules recognized by the antibody TIA-1.[190] Monoclonal T-cell populations can also be detected in mucosa not involved by lymphoma. Whole-genome analysis and HLA genotyping has identified two subtypes of EATL.[191] Type I is CD56 negative, pathogenically linked to celiac disease, and shares an HLA-DQB1 genotype pattern with refractory celiac disease. MEITL (previously type II EATL) is $CD56^+$, MYC^+, and shows an HLA-DQB1 genotype pattern like that of the normal Caucasian population.

Clinical Features

Patients may have a history of documented celiac disease, with the time to development of lymphoma varying widely. However, at least half of patients have celiac sprue diagnosed at the same time as the lymphoma. The most common symptoms at presentation are abdominal pain, weight loss, diarrhea, or vomiting. Less common symptoms may include fever, night sweats, and small bowel obstruction or perforation. It is rare for patients to have palpable abdominal masses or peripheral lymphadenopathy, but extraintestinal sites of involvement may include the liver, spleen, thyroid, skin, nasal sinus, and brain.[165] In one series, β_2-microglobulin and serum LDH were elevated in 85.7% and 62% of patients, respectively, and anemia and low serum albumin levels were seen in 91% and 88% of patients, respectively.[192]

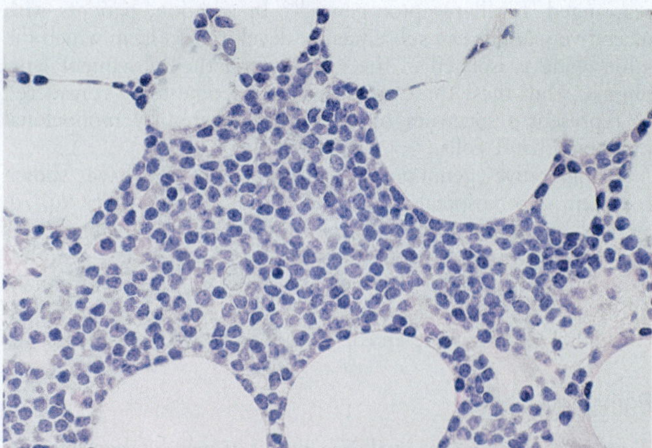

Fig. 41.9 Photomicrograph of enteropathy-type intestinal T-cell lymphoma in a patient with celiac disease. Mesenteric fat of the small bowel wall is involved with a monomorphic population of small-to-intermediate-sized irregular T lymphocytes. Cells were positive for CD2, CD3, and CD7, and negative for CD5. T-cell gene rearrangement studies were positive (i.e., showed a clonal band indicating a clonal T-cell process). (Courtesy Dr. Edward Lee, Washington, DC.)

Diagnosis is usually made by endoscopic biopsies or full-thickness, laparoscopic small bowel biopsies. Traditionally, patients were staged with CT and bone marrow biopsies, but ^{18}F-FDG PET-CT appears to be more sensitive and specific than CT in differentiating EATL from refractory celiac disease.[193] The Lugano system has been proposed as a staging system, but its utility in assessing prognosis is unclear.[56]

Treatment

No large controlled trials of therapy for EATL have been reported. Thus standard treatment is not well defined. Typically, patients are treated with a combination of surgery and chemotherapy.[192] Surgery involves the removal of as much tumor as is feasible. Intensive chemotherapy is then administered postoperatively, with the most common regimens being the ones that contain anthracyclines such as CHOP in older adults and CHOEP (CHOP with etoposide) in younger adults.[174] The 5-year overall survival rate with anthracycline-based chemotherapy alone is approximately 10%–20%. For this reason and based on retrospective data, most experts recommend an autologous stem cell transplant in first remission for the more robust patients with no or minimal medical comorbidities. Nutritional status is commonly poor, requiring parenteral nutrition. Because of poor nutritional and performance status, less than 50% of patients are candidates for systemic chemotherapy and of those, less than 50% can complete the prescribed treatment regimen. Relapse occurs at a median of 6 months from the time of diagnosis in approximately 80% of patients, usually in small bowel sites. Various salvage regimens have been tried for patients with relapsed disease, but few relapsed patients have survived.[194] Poor results with conventional chemotherapy have led to the investigation of high-dose chemotherapy followed by autologous stem cell transplantation in the minority of patients with an adequate performance status. A retrospective study of autologous stem cell transplantation by the European Group for Blood and Marrow Transplantation, including 44 patients, transplanted between 2000 and 2010 showed a 4-year relapse incidence, progression-free survival, and an overall survival rate of 39%, 54%, and 59%, respectively.[195] Therapy with novel agents has also been attempted. Alemtuzumab (Campath), an anti-CD52 monoclonal antibody, has been used to treat refractory celiac disease,[196] as well as brentuximab vedotin, an anti-CD30 monoclonal antibody conjugated to monomethyl auristatin E, an antimitotic agent.[197] Conceivably, earlier diagnosis may improve the outcome. The diagnosis should be considered for patients who present in midlife with celiac disease and for those who have clinical deterioration after having been stable on a gluten-free diet.

Uncommon Small Intestinal Lymphomas

Natural Killer Type T-Cell Intestinal Lymphoma

Extranodal NK T-cell lymphoma, nasal type, is a distinct pathologic entity in the WHO classification of hematolymphoid malignancies.[6] Very rare cases of intestinal NK cell lymphomas have been described.[198] Most of the cases reported have not involved patients with celiac sprue or sensitivity to gluten.[121,122] Optimal management of this very rare disorder has not been determined. Most data come from East Asian countries, and traditional regimens, such as CHOP and CHOEP, have high treatment failure rates. Aggressive regimens such as DeVIC (dexamethasone, etoposide, ifosfamide, and carboplatin), DDGP (cisplatin, dexamethasone, gemcitabine, and pegaspargase), and SMILE (dexamethasone, methotrexate, ifosfamide, L-asparaginase, and etoposide), with and without radiation, have been used with some degree of success. Immunotherapy with anti-PD1 checkpoint inhibitors such as pembrolizumab is showing promising responses in the relapsed/refractory subset of patients with this disease entity.[199]

OTHER GASTROINTESTINAL SITES

NHL less commonly occurs in other sites of the GI tract, including the oropharynx, esophagus, liver, pancreas, biliary tree, appendix, colon, and rectum. Signs and symptoms reflect the site of presentation. Because of the relative rarity of these disorders, the literature is fairly limited. Therefore definitive conclusions cannot be reached about the optimal management of these more unusual GI lymphomas. Standard principles of lymphoma management dictate diagnostic procedures, staging, prognostic assessment, and treatment. As is the case for all lymphomas, histology, and stage guide treatment.

Waldeyer ring lymphomas are usually diffuse large cell lymphomas, but other histologies may be present instead.[200,201] Endoscopy and imaging of the remainder of the GI tract should be included in the staging workup, because lymphomatous involvement in other sites may accompany Waldeyer ring involvement. Ann Arbor stage I or II diffuse large-cell lymphoma is managed with combined anthracycline-based chemotherapy and/or local radiotherapy.[107]

Primary hepatic lymphoma is more common in men and has a median age of onset of approximately 50 years.[202,203] Primary hepatic lymphoma can present as a single, large, multilobulated mass or as single or multiple nodules. The histology is usually diffuse large B cell, but MALT lymphoma (extranodal marginal B-cell lymphoma) has been reported as well. Rare cases of T-cell hepatic lymphoma have been reported. Diagnosis is usually made by needle biopsy. Because of the rarity of the disease, optimal therapy is uncertain. Long-term disease-free survival has been reported after resection, but multiagent chemo-immunotherapy is probably most appropriate for DLBCL. Less aggressive chemo-immunotherapy or single-agent rituximab may be appropriate for lymphomas with marginal zone histology. An association of HCV with hepatic and splenic marginal zone lymphoma has been established, and response of the lymphoma to hepatitis C treatment has been documented[204,205]; whether there may be an association with other hepatitis viruses and hepatic lymphomas is unknown.

Pancreatic lymphomas are rare (<0.5% of all pancreatic tumors).[206] Patients have a clinical presentation similar to that of pancreatic adenocarcinoma, with abdominal pain and obstructive jaundice; chylous ascites have also been reported. Histology is diffuse large B cell in over 80% of the cases and published literature supports use of combined modality therapy with anthracycline-containing chemotherapy (e.g., CHOP) with rituximab along with radiation. Patients with biliary obstruction may require a biliary drainage procedure before being treated with chemotherapy to avoid excessive chemotherapy-related toxicity.

Primary colorectal lymphomas most commonly involve the cecum,[207,208] with high- or intermediate-grade histology. Most colorectal lymphomas are Ann Arbor stage I_E or II_E. Therapy is dictated by histology and stage. Resection is the standard therapy, with adjuvant chemotherapy given for patients with aggressive histology.

IMMUNODEFICIENCY-RELATED LYMPHOMAS

Post-Transplantation Lymphoproliferative Disorders

The post-transplantation lymphoproliferative disorders (PTLDs)[209–211] complicate 0.8%–20% of cases of those with solid organ transplants (see Chapter 34), with the incidence being highest in heart-lung transplant recipients. PTLDs are also seen in bone marrow transplant recipients, particularly in patients receiving T-cell-depleted allografts. PTLD results from proliferation of Epstein-Barr virus (EBV)-transformed B-cell clones that have developed in part because of immunosuppression.[212] The histologic appearance of PTLD is highly variable, with lesions being polymorphic or monomorphic (resembling a lymphoma); the histology may reflect infectious mononucleosis, aggressive NHL, or plasmacytoma. Lesions may be polyclonal, oligoclonal, or monoclonal. Monoclonal lesions, similar in appearance to low-grade lymphomas such as FL, marginal zone lymphoma, small lymphocytic lymphomas, by convention, are not considered PTLD. The clinical presentation also varies greatly, with some patients having a syndrome resembling infectious mononucleosis and some having a more lymphoma-like presentation, with nodal or extranodal disease. Involvement of extranodal areas is common, with the GI tract being a common site. The literature regarding the treatment of PTLD suffers from a lack of prospective trials and lack of standardized histologic classification.

The treatment approach varies but usually consists initially of a withdrawal/modulation of immunosuppression for polymorphic PTLD.[213] For monomorphic PTLD that is $CD20^+$, in addition to minimizing immunosuppression, the preferred treatment is immunotherapy with the anti-CD20 antibody rituximab or subsequently, combining it with an anthracycline-based chemotherapy for patients who fail to respond to this first maneuver. This sequential approach to treatment is based predominantly on European data which supports long-term disease-free survival in early responders to rituximab therapy, thereby avoiding the need for toxic chemotherapeutics altogether in patients with CD20 positive PTLD.[214]

Surgical or radiation therapy may cure patients with localized disease in highly selected cases. Other treatments have included acyclovir or ganciclovir directed at EBV, allogeneic cytotoxic EBV specific T cells or EBV-CTL and interferon-α. Donor leukocyte infusions are frequently used for patients with PTLD that develops after allogeneic bone marrow transplantation.[215]

IATROGENIC LYMPHOPROLIFERATIVE DISORDERS

Increasingly, a spectrum of lymphoproliferative conditions is being recognized and described in the setting of use of immunosuppressive drugs outside the setting of transplant (other iatrogenic immunodeficiency-associated lymphoproliferative disorders).[216] Methotrexate-driven lymphomas have been well recognized and described. We are increasingly seeing patients with IBD, on or with a history of immune suppression, including biologics such as TNF inhibitors, present with these conditions. EBV is a central driving force behind many of these conditions, and management is extrapolated from the PTLD literature (see the section on "Post-transplantation Lymphoproliferative Disorders").

Polymorphic lymphoproliferation is thought to be reactive and is predominantly treated with withdrawing immunosuppression. Monomorphic lymphoproliferation can resemble any NHL or Hodgkin lymphoma and treatment is based predominantly on grade, type, and extent of lymphoma at the time of presentation.

Close observation after stopping immunosuppression for patients with low-grade disease and a low tumor burden is favored if possible. Spontaneous regression can be seen in as many as 40% of these patients. Upfront chemotherapy is generally offered to patients with a high-grade lymphoma in the setting of extensive organ involvement or visceral crisis.

The WHO 2022 classification has a unique disorder, generally affecting older adults, called EBV-positive muco-cutaneous ulcer that has some pathologic features of Hodgkin lymphoma (Fig. 41.10). This disease is often seen in the setting of immune suppression, and predominantly presents as well-circumscribed oropharyngeal lesions but can involve skin and any site along

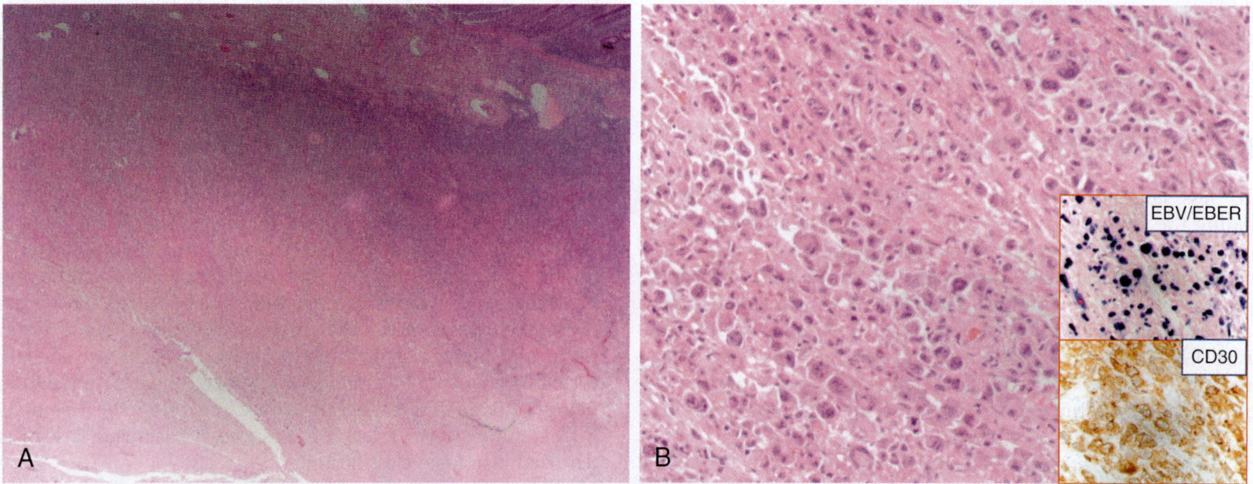

Fig. 41.10 Photomicrograph showing Epstein-Barr virus (EBV) positive mucocutaneous ulcer in the small bowel. (A) A polymorphous infiltrate, including small lymphocytes, histiocytes, and large atypical lymphoid cells in small bowel mucosa with ulceration. (B) Large lymphoid cells with irregular nucleus, prominent nucleolus, and abundant cytoplasm, variably resembling Hodgkin cells that express EBV/EBER and CD30 (insets). (Courtesy Dr. Weina Chen, UT Southwestern Medical Center, Dallas, TX.)

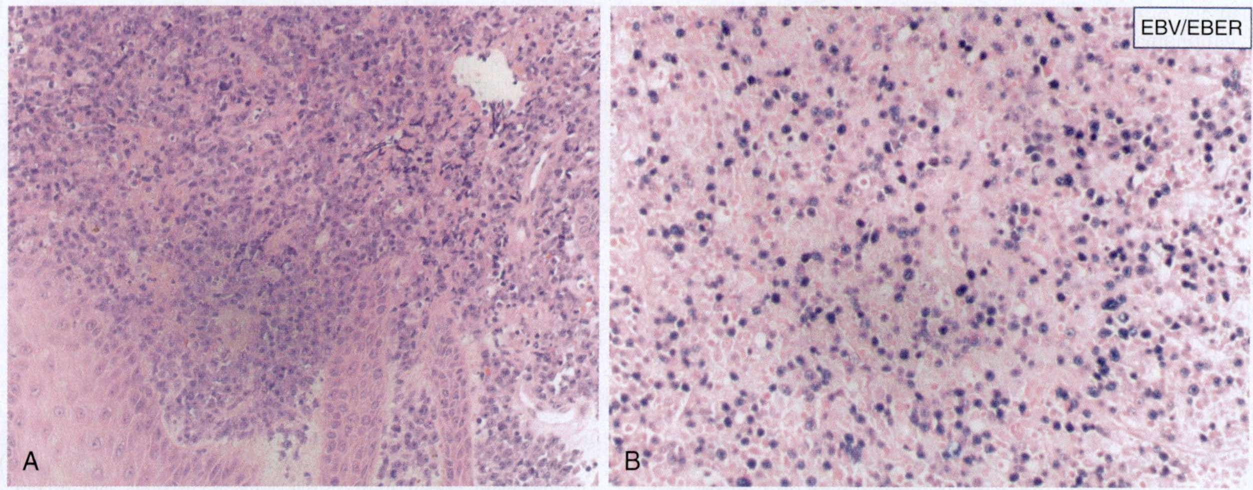

Fig. 41.11 Photomicrograph showing plasmablastic lymphoma involving the rectum. (A) Large lymphoma cells infiltrating rectum mucosa (underneath squamous epithelium). (B) Lymphoma cells with Epstein-Barr virus/EBER expression. (Courtesy Dr. Weina Chen, UT Southwestern Medical Center, Dallas, TX.)

the length of the GI tract. These lesions predominantly have an indolent course (45% spontaneous remission, 15% relapsing/remitting course), and clinicopathologic correlation is important to distinguish this from Hodgkin lymphoma, which seldom presents with extranodal involvement.[217]

HIV-ASSOCIATED NON-HODGKIN LYMPHOMA

The risk of developing NHL is markedly increased in patients with HIV (see Chapter 33), and the development of lymphoma is considered an AIDS-defining condition. These malignancies are B-cell neoplasms,[218] with most cases having small noncleaved cell or diffuse large cell histology. EBV is implicated in about half of non–central nervous system HIV-related lymphomas. HIV-associated NHL typically has an aggressive presentation, with rapidly growing disease and prominent B symptoms. The GI tract is a common site, including unusual sites such as the anus and rectum. Historically, chemotherapy has been poorly tolerated, and lower-dose chemotherapy regimens have been used. However, patients with higher $CD4^+$ T-cell counts (as is more commonly seen in view of the standard current usage of HAART) may be better able to tolerate full-dose chemotherapy regimens and may have a better prognosis than has been seen in previous studies.[219]

Plasmablastic lymphoma (PBL), an aggressive variant of DLBCL, was initially described in the oral cavity in HIV patients. Most GI PBL cases involve the anal canal in HIV-infected patients. PBL is essentially negative for CD20, CD45, and PAX5 and expresses plasma cell–associated proteins, including CD38, CD138, and VS38c. The majority of cases are EBV-positive and HHV8-negative. *MYC* rearrangements are detected frequently (Fig. 41.11). Aggressive chemo-immunotherapy strategies such as V-EPOCH [bortezomib (Velcade) with EPOCH] are showing promising responses in this difficult to treat disorder.[220]

Primary effusion lymphoma is a clinicopathologic entity associated with the herpesvirus HHV-8 (Kaposi sarcoma–associated virus).[221,222] Histology shows a distinctive morphology that bridges large-cell immunoblastic lymphoma and anaplastic large-cell lymphoma.[223] Tumor cells show monoclonal immunoglobulin gene rearrangements but typically lack B-cell-associated antigens. HHV-8 is detectable by PCR assay. Patients are usually HIV-positive, but the syndrome has been reported in HIV-negative patients. Patients present with malignant effusions in the pleural or peritoneal cavity, which remain localized to the body cavity of origin. Disease progression is rapid, with survival of only a few weeks to months. Optimal therapy has not been defined.

Full references for this chapter can be found at https://ebooks.health.elsevier.com/.

42 Gastrointestinal Stromal Tumors

Tamas Ordog, Thanh P. Ho

IN THIS CHAPTER

GI stromal tumors (GISTs) comprise 1%–3% of all malignant GI tumors and are considered a rare disease by the National Institutes of Heath (https://rarediseases.info.nih.gov/diseases/8598/gastrointestinal-stromal-tumors). However, they are the most common mesenchymal tumor of the GI tract. The groundbreaking discoveries of the type III receptor tyrosine kinase (RTK) KIT as a marker for GISTs and the role of activating *KIT* mutations in GIST oncogenesis in 1998[1,2] set the stage for investigations into the molecular pathogenesis of GISTs, and have been translated into highly effective, molecularly targeted therapies, such as imatinib mesylate and related drugs, for the majority of patients with GISTs.[3,4]

PATHOLOGY

The term *gastrointestinal stromal tumor* was initially coined as a purely descriptive term by Mazur and Clark in 1983 to define intra-abdominal tumors that were not carcinomas (i.e., nonepithelial tumors) but exhibited histologic features of smooth muscle and neural elements.[5] At that time, the morphology of the tumor cells was the dominant feature driving the diagnosis. Expression of differentiation antigens used as markers for muscle cells (e.g., smooth muscle actin) and for neural crest-derived cells (e.g., S100) was noted to vary widely in GI mesenchymal lesions, leading to interesting hypotheses about whether GIST lesions from different patients were attempting to recapitulate distinct myogenic or neural programs of differentiation. To accommodate these empirical observations, it was proposed that approximately one-third of GIST lesions differentiated along smooth muscle lineages, another third were neurogenic in origin, and the final third lacked any detectable lineage-specific markers (null phenotype) by immunohistochemical analysis.[6–8]

Before 1999, there was no objective, reproducible, and clearly defined criteria for the diagnosis and classification of GISTs. They were often misdiagnosed as *leiomyomas* or *leiomyosarcomas* because of the histologic resemblance to these smooth muscle neoplasms. Other terms that were often applied to GISTs included *benign leiomyoblastomas*[9] and, recognizing some of the neural characteristics, *plexosarcoma*[10] or *GI autonomic nerve tumors*.[11] Insightful studies by several pathology groups noted that the panoply of tumors lumped together as smooth muscle tumors of the GI tract were likely not simply leiomyosarcomas nor benign leiomyomas; a subset of these tumors originating in the bowel wall had several unique histologic features, probably representing a totally different diagnostic group altogether.[12,13] The interpretation of published GIST series accumulated before 2000 is difficult given the heterogeneity reflected by the diagnostic term *gastrointestinal stromal tumors* as well as the underdiagnosis of the entity before widespread use of specific kinase-directed diagnostic and molecular markers.

Immunohistochemical analyses of GISTs in the early 1990s attempted to find specific markers that might distinguish GISTs from other spindle cell tumors of the GI tract, such as schwannomas and sarcomatoid carcinomas. There was some initial enthusiasm for the CD34 antigen as such a marker; however, this antigen is also expressed by hematopoietic stem cells and by vascular and myofibroblastic cells. Moreover, the sensitivity and specificity of CD34 are low because only about half of GIST cases express CD34, and other smooth muscle, myofibroblastic (e.g., desmoid), or Schwann cell tumors can also express CD34.[14,15]

A critical advance in the understanding of GISTs at the molecular level occurred in the late 1990s with the recognition that the cells of these tumors exhibited some histopathologic similarities with *interstitial cells of Cajal* (ICCs),[2] mesodermally derived mesenchymal cells that regulate GI motility by modulating smooth muscle excitability, facilitating efferent and afferent neural control, and generating electrical slow waves underlying peristalsis and segmentation[16–18] (see Chapters 100 and 101). GIST cells and ICCs have certain common ultrastructural features, with GIST cells showing more undifferentiated and sometimes more myoid phenotypes.[19]

By immunohistochemical staining, GISTs characteristically (>95%) exhibit the expression of KIT [KIT proto-oncogene, RTK; aliases: CD117, mast/stem cell factor (SCF) receptor].[3] KIT expression is generally diffuse and strong in the spindle cell GIST subtype (Fig. 42.1). In contrast, in the epithelioid GIST subtype, KIT expression is often focal and weakly positive in a dot-like pattern (Fig. 42.2). As discussed later, there are rare KIT-negative GISTs.

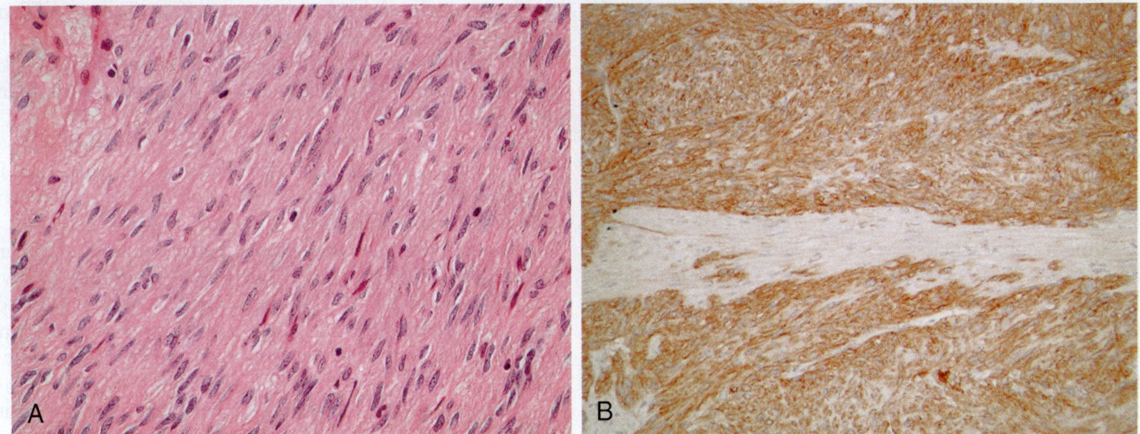

Fig. 42.1 (A) Photomicrograph of a typical spindle cell GIST. The cells are monomorphic, have abundant pale, eosinophilic, fibrillary cytoplasm, and lack mitotic activity. (H&E, ×100.) (B) KIT (CD117) immunostaining. This medium-power photomicrograph of a spindle cell GIST shows diffuse and strong cytoplasmic immunoreactivity for KIT. The entrapped muscle fibers from the bowel wall are negative by CD117 immunostaining for KIT. (CD117 immunostain, ×100.) (Courtesy Dr. Brian P. Rubin, Cleveland, OH.)

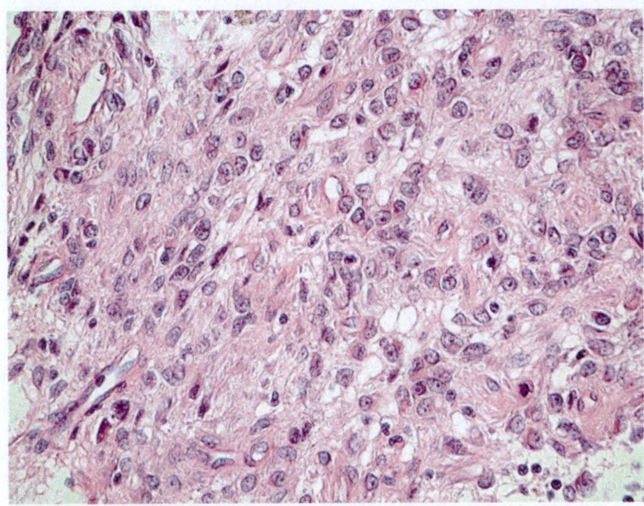

Fig. 42.2 Photomicrograph of a gastrointestinal stromal tumor showing epithelioid cytomorphology, fibrillary cytoplasm, and lack of mitotic activity. (H&E, ×200.) (Courtesy Dr. Brian P. Rubin, Cleveland, OH.)

True leiomyosarcomas express two smooth muscle markers, smooth muscle actin and desmin, but fail to express KIT. Schwannomas are usually positive for S100 but are also negative for KIT. Normal mast cells and ICCs within the surrounding stromal tissues serve as ideal positive internal controls because these normal cells strongly express KIT.

GIST lesions can be heterogeneous in the expression of KIT, even within a single tumor. It is, therefore, possible that a needle biopsy may yield cells histologically consistent with a GIST yet be KIT-negative simply due to sampling bias. There are rare subsets of GISTs (<5% of cases overall) that have no KIT expression; these are most likely dependent on an alternative kinase, such as mutated platelet-derived growth factor receptor-alpha (PDGFRA), another type III RTK (see the "Molecular Pathogenesis" section).[20] The definitive diagnostic criteria of uncommon KIT-negative GISTs has been aided by the identification of anoctamin 1 (ANO1)[21] (aliases: DOG-1 for "discovered on GIST," TMEM16A) a Ca^{2+}-activated chloride channel universally expressed in ICCs[22] and important for ICC functions.[18] Since ANO1 has been found to be positive in 98% of GISTs, including in those that have *PDGFRA* mutations and may not express KIT, it has become a standard for GIST diagnosis in many pathology departments. An additional marker reported to aid in the diagnosis of KIT-negative GIST is PKC-θ (PRKCQ),[23] a gene expressed in some ICC classes[24] and 96% of KIT-negative GISTs. Therefore the diagnosis of a GIST should be made on the grounds of morphologic, clinical-pathologic, and immunohistochemical data, as well as molecular analysis if there is any ambiguity from the other pathologic assessments (see the "Molecular Pathogenesis" section). It is also possible for a KIT-positive GIST to dedifferentiate as it becomes anaplastic and loses its ability to express KIT.[25]

Criteria for estimating the risk of malignant behavior of GIST were initially based on a consensus published by pathologists with expertise in GISTs who met at the National Cancer Institute.[26] This consensus conference defined the two most reliable prognostic factors for behavior of a primary GIST as (1) the size of the primary tumor and (2) the number of mitoses, reflecting the proliferative activity of the cells.[26] Additional factors are now recognized as important in terms of prognosis. Tumor location is also relevant, with primary tumors of the stomach having a better prognosis compared to those arising at other sites. In addition, primary tumors that undergo perforation prior to or during resection have a particularly poor prognosis.[27,28] Other factors besides size and mitoses, such as the specific histologic subtype [epithelioid vs spindle cell (see Figs. 42.1 and 42.2)], degree of cellular pleomorphism, and patient age, may have some contribution to prognosis but are most likely to play a minor role in determining the clinical outcome.

Nomograms and staging systems have also been published to assess the risk of recurrence after primary resection.[29,30] The GIST Nomogram, developed by investigators at Memorial Sloan Kettering Cancer Center,[29] is available online (https://www.mskcc.org/nomograms/gastrointestinal/stromal_tumor). Although simple, there is concern that the risk assigned to tumors arising in the stomach is too high compared to other risk criteria. The population-based topographical maps of disease recurrence by Joensuu and colleagues provides the greatest clarity, as size and mitotic count are measured as continuous variables; this tool also takes into account evidence of rupture.[30] A simplified "rule of 5s" has been advocated in which size larger than 5 cm *and* more than 5 mitoses per 50 high-power fields (HPFs) define an intermediate-high risk gastric GIST and in which size larger than 5 cm *or* more than 5 mitoses per 50 HPFs defines an intermediate-high risk nongastric GIST.[31]

MOLECULAR PATHOGENESIS

Driver mutations have been identified in nearly 99% of GISTs,[32] making this tumor a paradigm for the development of precision medicine treatment approaches.[33] Nearly 95% of all GISTs carry mutations in *KIT* (~70%) or *PDGFRA* (~15%), or deficient in the tricarboxylic acid cycle and mitochondrial electron transfer chain protein complex succinate dehydrogenase (SDH; complex II) (~9%).[4] NF1 (neurofibromin 1)-deficient,[34] *BRAF* (B-Raf proto-oncogene, serine/threonine kinase),[35] *KRAS* (KRAS proto-oncogene, GTPase),[36] or *PIK3CA* [phosphatidylinositol-4,5-bisphosphate 3-kinase (PI3K) catalytic subunit alpha]-mutant tumors,[37] as well as GISTs harboring neurotrophic RTK 3 (NTRK3) or fibroblast growth factor receptor 1 (FGFR1) fusion proteins[38] account for a minority of the cases with known driver mutations.

The first breakthrough toward understanding the molecular pathogenesis of GISTs was the discovery of the role of gain-of-function *KIT* mutations by Hirota et al.[1] This same team also expanded these observations to patients with familial GISTs harboring germline activating mutations in *KIT*.[39] KIT and its ligand, SCF (*NCBI* gene: KITLG, KIT ligand; alias: mast cell growth factor), play essential roles in development and maintenance of normal ICCs, as well as other cells, including melanocytes, erythrocytes, germ cells, and mast cells. In wild-type cells, KIT is kept in an auto-inhibited conformation until SCF binds[40] and induces the homodimerization of the receptor and cross-phosphorylation of critical tyrosine residues in the intracellular domains of KIT, which then activates downstream signal transduction pathways.[32] These include the PI3K-PDPK1 (3-phosphoinositide-dependent protein kinase 1)-AKT (AKT serine/threonine kinase) pathway, the mitogen-activated protein kinase (MAPK) cascade consisting of RAF (Raf-1 proto-oncogene serine/threonine-protein kinase), MEK (including the MAP2K1 and MAP2K2 mitogen-activated protein kinase kinases), ERK (MAPK1 and MAPK3), and the JAK (Janus kinase)-STAT3 (signal transducer and activator of transcription 3) pathway. These mechanisms prevent apoptosis, promote cell survival, and drive proliferation in part by stimulating gene transcription.[32] An important aspect of KIT-induced ERK MAPK signaling, discovered by Chi and colleagues,[41] is the stabilization of ETS variant transcription factor 1 (ETV1), which is required for the development of most ICC classes via the stimulation of *KIT* transcription through binding to a cell type-specific superenhancer,[42–44] completing a self-reinforcing loop. The net physiologic effect of normal ligand-induced KIT activation is the *controlled* stimulation of cell proliferation and enhanced cell survival. For example, PI3K signaling is required for the postnatal development of mouse jejunal ICC and slow wave activity, with dependence on this mechanism waning in fully developed adults[45] when ICC turnover is reduced.[46] In contrast, ERK MAPK activation remains robust in adults and contributes to the regulation of KIT and ICC populations in response to hyperglycemia and in aging.[46,47] Activating mutations in *KIT* were identified in five of six cases of human GISTs originally analyzed by Hirota et al.,[1] with evidence that the mutations resulted in *uncontrolled ligand-independent* or *constitutive* activation of KIT manifesting in phosphorylation of the receptor in the absence of ligand. Genetically engineered cells harboring the mutant overactive KIT proteins were tumorigenic in nude mice, serving as proof of concept that the malignant phenotype was directly induced by the aberrant signaling pathways associated with uncontrolled ligand-independent KIT activation. Additional lines of evidence supporting the oncogenic nature of activating *KIT* mutations include the consistent detectability of phosphorylated KIT in GIST tumor extracts[48] and the development of GIST-like tumors in mice engineered to express KIT with mutations found in human GISTs.[49–52]

The oncogenic potential of mutant, constitutively activated KIT in the pathogenesis of GISTs in humans, has also been supported by the identification of familial syndromes (see the "Familial Gastrointestinal Stromal Tumors" section) with an autosomal dominant inheritance pattern and an abnormally high incidence of GISTs, usually occurring as multiple foci within any affected individual.[39,53,54] Genetic analysis of such kindreds reveals that they harbor activating *KIT* mutations in the germline similar to the mutations that were first described in sporadic cases of GISTs.

Gain-of-function mutations have been most commonly identified in exon 11 of *KIT*, an exon that encodes the intracellular juxtamembrane domain of KIT.[48,55–59] Certain mutations in exon 11 that result in stop codons or deletions convey a poorer prognosis.[59] Exon 11 mutations disrupt the secondary structure that normally prevents kinase activation in the absence of the ligand, leading to constitutive signaling.[40,60] As will be discussed, imatinib mesylate [and some other tyrosine kinase inhibitors (TKIs)] can block this aberrant activation and kinase activity in these mutated tumors. Mutations have also been identified in *KIT* exon 9,[56] the extracellular domain of the kinase, which mimic the conformational change that the extracellular KIT receptor undergoes when SCF is bound,[61] and, less commonly, in exons 13 (ATP-binding region) and 17 (kinase activation loop),[48,55–57,62] with rare occurrences of mutations in exon 8 (extracellular domain).[58] The frequency of particular mutations varies between primary tumors and metastatic GISTs (Table 42.1).[63,64]

It is noteworthy that some aspects of the signaling cascades activated in GISTs appear to differ from KIT signaling in hematologic cancers. For example, the STAT5 pathway of leukemic cells is not typically activated in GISTs, whereas STAT1 and STAT3 are activated at a high level.[55] Other differences may in part reflect the cell type-specific expression, function, and KIT signaling-mediated regulation of transcription factors.[41,43,44,65]

The recognition of histopathological similarities between GISTs and ICCs,[1,2,66] together with the dependence of ICCs on KIT signaling for development and maintenance,[67–69] have led

TABLE 42.1 Frequency of Particular *KIT* and *PDGFRA* Mutations in Newly Diagnosed Gastrointestinal Stromal Tumors as Compared With Metastatic Gastrointestinal Stromal Tumors

	Newly Diagnosed[63]	Metastatic Disease[64]
GISTs (*N*)	106	414
KIT Mutations	67%	81%
Exon 8	Not reported	<1%
Exon 11	53%	71%
Exon 9	9%	8%
Exon 13	4%	1%
Exon 17	1%	1%
PDGFRA Mutations	16%	2%
Exon 12	2%	<1%
Exon 14	0%	0%
Exon 18	15%	2%
Wild-type *KIT* and *PDGFRA*	17%	17%

PDGFRA, Platelet-derived growth factor receptor-alpha.

several investigators to propose that the cells of GISTs and normal ICCs may share a common precursor, likely a stem cell residing within the wall of the gut, which can then differentiate incompletely toward the ICC phenotype.[1,2,66] The discovery of $KIT^{low}CD34^{+}$ adult stem cells for ICC in mice[46,47,70–72] gave support to this notion as these immune-evading, antiinflammatory precursors[73] were hyperplastic in mice with germline *Kit* K641E mutation and formed GIST-like tumors following spontaneous transformation.[71,74] Recently, stem-like cells with the same $KIT^{low}CD34^{+}$ phenotype and ability to self-renew and differentiate into KIT^{+} progeny have also been described in human GIST cell lines and imatinib-treated tumors, extending the concept of an ICC/GIST stem cell to humans.[75]

Another key advance in the understanding of GISTs was the recognition that signaling through other uncontrolled kinases besides KIT could drive the neoplastic phenotype of GIST cells. Specifically, it is now recognized that approximately 15% of GIST cells have mutational activation of the structurally related kinase known as the *PDGFRA*, most often in exon 18 (kinase domain activation loop), but also in exon 12 (juxtamembrane domain) and exon 14 (ATP-binding pocket) (see Table 42.1).[4,20,32,64,76] *PDGFRA* and *KIT* mutations activate the same signaling pathways and, due to their functional overlap, are mutually exclusive.[76] Familial cases of GIST have also been identified with germline *PDGFRA* mutations and are discussed later.[77–79]

Although *PDGFRA*-mutant GIST have variable or sometimes no expression of KIT, they are typically positive for the ICC marker ANO1.[32] While ICCs only very rarely express PDGFRA, both fetal and adult ICC precursors, as well as most *KIT*-mutant GISTs coexpress KIT and PDGFRA.[71,72,80,81] Therefore most *PDGFRA*-mutant GISTs likely share precursors with *KIT*-mutant GISTs. However, in a kindred with a rare inherited *P653L* mutation in exon 14 of *PDGFRA*, GISTs with a $PDGFRA+CD34+KIT^{-}ANO1^{-}$ phenotype have been reported.[79] These tumors may have originated from PDGFRA-expressing interstitial cells, which are distinct from ICCs and perform specific functions in the regulation of GI motility.[18] While some authors refer to these cells as *telocytes*,[82] this term is not used in this review because it has been variably applied to cells with or without KIT expression in several GI and extra-GI locations and also to the transcriptionally distinct tunica muscularis and subepithelial PDGFRA+ cells.[79,82–85]

KIT and *PDGFRA* mutations have been documented even in small GISTs (<1 cm in greatest dimension often called *micro-GISTs*).[86,87] Such morphologically benign lesions have been found in approximately one-third of the general population[88] and are most often detected incidentally (e.g., gastric or esophageal GISTs during upper endoscopy for reflux symptoms). These findings support the hypothesis that activating mutations in the *KIT* or *PDGFRA* proto-oncogenes represent an early event in the transformation from a normal precursor cell into a GIST lesion and may only rarely progress to malignancy. Because lesions in familial GISTs with germline *KIT* or *PDGFRA* mutations (see the "Familial Gastrointestinal Stromal Tumors" section) may not present clinically until the second or third decade of life, or even much later, it is likely that second hits are necessary to attain a more aggressive malignant phenotype.

There is now consensus that the *KIT* genotype alone cannot account for differences between GISTs that may behave in an indolent manner (and which, when small, are likely to be curable by resection alone) versus those that are clearly aggressive and malignant by all functional definitions. Well-differentiated benign cell morphology alone should not provide any reassurance that an individual GIST lesion will pursue a benign clinical course. However, gastric GIST lesions smaller than 2 cm are considered benign and if removed do not require follow-up.[89]

Importantly, most GIST cells at initial presentation demonstrate a single site of mutation in *KIT*. However, additional genetic events play important roles in aggressive malignant behavior associated with clinical progression.[32] These include secondary *KIT* mutations in most cases of *KIT*-mutant GIST with acquired resistance to TKIs.[88] Monosomy of chromosome 14 or partial loss of chromosome 14q and 22q deletion are early and common events and involve tumor suppressor genes important for GIST formation.[32] Mutational dysregulation of the cell cycle, for example, via genomic inactivation, copy number variation, or loss of heterozygosity of cell cycle control genes such as RB transcriptional corepressor 1 (*RB1*), cyclin-dependent kinase inhibitors 2A/B (*CDKN2A/B*), and tumor protein 53 (*TP53*), is key to progression from low-risk to malignant GIST and may sensitize cells to cyclin-dependent kinase 4 or MDM2 (transformed 3T3 cell double minute 2, P53-binding protein) inhibitors.[88] Mutations in spliceosome-related genes have been found in a minority of metastatic GISTs. In contrast, the inactivation of the tumor suppressor dystrophin (*DMD*) is a common late event in GIST progression.[90]

Up to 15% of GISTs are wild-type for *KIT* and *PDGFRA* (i.e., have no mutations in these genes).[4] The majority (approximately 9% of all GISTs) have a loss of expression and function of SDH proteins SDH A, B, C, and D, which are subunits of a mitochondrial tricarboxylic acid cycle and electron transfer chain complex (complex II) that oxidizes succinate to fumarate and supplies electrons to the respiratory chain. SDH loss leads to succinate accumulation and the inhibition of α-ketoglutarate-dependent dioxygenases, including procollagen prolyl hydroxylases, enzymes that degrade hypoxia-inducible transcription factors HIF1A and EPAS1 (alias: HIF2A), the HIF1A inhibitor HIF1AN, ribosomal oxygenases, Jumonji C domain-containing histone lysine demethylases (KDMs), *N*-methyl DNA/RNA demethylases, tRNA oxidases, and 10–11 translocation (TET) DNA demethylases.[91] Reflecting impaired TET function, promoter hypermethylation and consequent silencing of the DNA damage repair enzyme 6-*O*-methylguanine-DNA methyltransferase (*MGMT*) makes SDH-deficient GISTs vulnerable to the alkylating agent temozolomide, which is currently being tested in a phase II clinical trial (NCT03556384). In contrast, a phase II trial of the hypomethylating agent guadecitabine in children and adults with SDH-deficient tumors, including in seven GIST patients, did not result in objective responses despite global demethylation in peripheral blood mononuclear cells.[92]

In some cases, SDH genes are mutated, but in others there is hypermethylation of the gene promoters, leading to loss of expression and activity. These tumors can be identified by loss of SDHB staining in tumor cells; they have also been found to express high levels of insulin-like growth factor-1 receptor.[93–98] These tumors are now called SDH-deficient GISTs; Carney triad and the Carney-Stratakis dyad (discussed in the "Familial Gastrointestinal Stromal Tumors" section) are syndromes whose GISTs have this oncologic mechanism. SDH-deficient GIST arises in the stomach, may be multifocal and metastasize to lymph nodes, but most behave in an indolent fashion.[4] Tumors are more common in females and tend to be diagnosed at an earlier age than typical mutant GIST; most GISTs in the pediatric age group are SDH-deficient GIST. Pediatric GISTs do not carry karyotypic changes.[99]

PIK3CA mutations[37] lead to GISTs through the stimulation of the AKT pathway, whereas NF1-deficient,[34] *BRAF*-mutant,[35] and *KRAS*-mutant[36] GISTs arise via excessive stimulation of ERK MAPK signaling.[4] Some *PIK3CA*- and *KRAS*-mutant GISTs also have an activating *KIT* mutation.[36] Interestingly, GISTs that develop from activating *BRAF* V600E mutations may originate from either the ICC lineage or smooth muscle cells.[100,101]

In addition to the genes and proteins already discussed, other genes, transcription factors, microRNAs, and pathways have been reported to play a role in the pathogenesis, behavior, diagnosis, and prognosis of GISTs.[102–119] Some of these will be undoubtedly important predictors of outcome or provide therapeutic targets in the future. A detailed discussion of these many factors is beyond the scope of this chapter.

MOLECULAR PHARMACOLOGY

Identification of *KIT* mutations provided critical understanding of the pathobiology of GIST and provided an appealing therapeutic target. It was serendipitous that a medication being developed for an entirely different purpose showed a dramatic inhibition of KIT activity. The initial concept for this molecularly targeted approach came from efforts to develop small molecules against BCR-ABL, the fusion oncoprotein between the breakpoint cluster region protein activator of RhoGEF and GTPase (BCR) and the Abelson murine leukemia viral oncogene homolog (ABL), which is critical to the pathogenesis of chronic myelogenous leukemia (CML). A small molecule in the 2-phenylaminopyrimidine class was identified by Druker et al. at Novartis that demonstrated potent inhibitory in vitro activity for ABL and the dysregulated BCR-ABL.[120,121] Additional screening studies from the laboratories of Druker and Buchdunger and associates demonstrated that this agent, signal transduction inhibitor-571, subsequently called *imatinib mesylate* (Gleevec in the United States, Glivec elsewhere), could also potently inhibit the tyrosine kinase activity of both KIT and PDGFRA.[122] Subsequent studies performed in a human mast cell leukemia cell line that harbored a *KIT* mutation similar to the mutations noted in GISTs documented that imatinib could inhibit both wild-type and mutant KIT protein.[123] Laboratory experiments testing imatinib in human GIST cell lines with defined activating mutations of *KIT* revealed dramatic evidence of anti-GIST activity. Addition of imatinib to cultured human GIST cells rapidly inhibited KIT activation, arrested cell proliferation, and induced apoptosis in the tumor cells.[124] By all criteria, therefore, the clinical development of imatinib was promising as a treatment of GIST to target the fundamental molecular pathogenesis of this disease. Treatment of GISTs with imatinib mesylate and other tyrosine receptor kinase inhibitors are discussed later.

EPIDEMIOLOGY

It has been difficult to obtain accurate data regarding the true incidence of GISTs. This is because of referral bias, which concentrates GIST cases with a worse prognosis and a more malignant behavior into academic cancer centers, and the lack of definitive diagnostic techniques before the molecular definitions of GISTs in 1998 and beyond. Before 2000, the number of new GIST cases was both underestimated and underreported. With the understanding of the molecular underpinnings of GISTs and the availability of molecularly targeted drugs, there has been an increase in the diagnostic accuracy of the disease.[125] A study using the Surveillance, Epidemiology, and End Results database of cases diagnosed between 2001 and 2011 found an increase in the age-adjusted incidence from 0.55/100,000 in 2001 to 0.78/100,000 in 2011. The incidence increased with age and was highest in the 70–79-age group, at 3.06/100,000.[126] Another study based on the United States Cancer Statistics reported an overall incidence of 0.70 per 100,000 people per year between 2001 and 2015.[127] Overall incidence rates were greatest for males, blacks, localized disease, primary location in the stomach, and the Northeast. Studies of gastrectomy specimens resected for nonneoplastic diseases and autopsy studies have documented a remarkably high incidence of occult microscopic GIST lesions, in the range of 20%–35%.[128,129]

CLINICAL FEATURES

Most GISTs (60%–70%) arise in the stomach; 20%–30% originate in the small intestine, and less than 10% in the esophagus, colon, and rectum. GISTs can also occur in extra-GI abdominal or pelvic sites such as the omentum, mesentery, or retroperitoneum,[130–143] including the pancreas; extra-GI tumors are termed E-GISTs.[84]

The clinical presentation of patients with GISTs depends on the anatomic location of the primary lesion, as well as other factors like tumor size and presence or absence of symptomatic metastases. For many patients, an initial detection of GISTs may be an incidental finding or result from evaluation of nonspecific symptoms. Symptoms from GISTs per se are usually noted only after tumors are larger than 5 cm in size or have impinged on a specific anatomic region (e.g., a gastric GIST causing gastric outlet obstruction). Symptoms at presentation may include a palpable abdominal mass or abdominal swelling, abdominal pain, nausea, vomiting, anorexia, and early satiety. It has been reported that up to 40% of patients with GISTs present with acute hemorrhage into the GI tract or into the peritoneal cavity from tumor rupture; however, such reports are likely dependent on referral bias of patients with large GIST lesions or multifocal disease. Some will present with anemia due to chronic blood loss. Because a GIST may not be identified by routine endoscopy, abdominopelvic imaging should be considered part of an iron deficiency anemia workup with negative GI endoscopy studies for a source of bleeding (see Chapter 21).

The vast majority of metastases from GISTs, at presentation or with disease recurrence, are intra-abdominal, with metastases to the liver, omentum, or peritoneal cavity.[131] Metastatic spread to lymph nodes and other regions is rare; most lesions thought to be nodal metastases by imaging studies simply represent metastatic deposits of tumor nodules in the omentum or peritoneum rather than true lymphatic spread of the disease. Sites of metastases seen in advanced disease can also include the lung and bone. GISTs can express a thyroid hormone-inactivating enzyme (type 3 iodothyronine deiodinase) that can result in a consumptive type of hypothyroidism, requiring supranormal doses of thyroid hormone therapy.[144]

Esophageal Tumors

GISTs may arise within the esophagus, although this is a rare presentation for larger lesions.[135–137] Most esophageal GIST lesions are noted incidentally during upper endoscopy performed for some other unrelated symptom or disorder, such as reflux esophagitis. Esophageal GISTs may be small (only a few millimeters in size) and may be resected using endoscopic techniques.[138] Margins may be involved if a lesion, unsuspected as a GIST and thought to be benign, is simply enucleated endoscopically. It remains unclear whether watchful waiting with serial endoscopic follow-up is appropriate for any patient with small GIST lesions (<1 cm in maximal dimension). Larger esophageal GISTs may perforate.[139] On imaging, they appear like GISTs elsewhere in the GI tract[135]; they tend to be well-circumscribed, ^{18}F-fluorodeoxyglucose (^{18}F-FDG) avid, hypoattenuating, and spread locally (e.g., to the pleura) or hematogenously (e.g., to the liver).[137]

As noted, histopathology showing putatively benign GIST cells cannot be viewed reassuringly because histology does not perfectly predict the malignant behavior of GISTs. Retrospective studies, including a review of over 100 patients, show that large tumor size and high mitotic rate are associated with poor survival;

KIT exon 11 mutation has also been associated with metastasis.[145–147] A careful risk-based assessment includes accounting for such aspects of the tumor, as well as patient-specific factors (e.g., age, comorbidities, and patient preferences) are pertinent given preoperative imatinib may be a consideration for large tumors or enucleation may be an option for small tumors.

Gastric Tumors

The most common primary site for GISTs is the stomach (Figs. 42.3 and 42.4). They can be asymptomatic or present with bleeding, pain, or obstruction. Most GIST lesions as seen endoscopically are submucosal rather than mucosal, without overlying ulceration. This explains why many GIST masses may only be visualized on endoscopy as a subtle, smooth protrusion with overtly normal mucosa.[140] However, ulceration is common with large lesions. Moreover, this submucosal localization can make diagnostic biopsy through an endoscope difficult. It is not uncommon for superficial biopsies to reveal only normal mucosa, whereas deeper biopsies or histopathology from a definitive resection would show the true underlying GIST cells. The use of EUS often allows for appropriate sampling and adequate diagnostic biopsies.

Duodenal and Jejunoileal Tumors

The second most common site for GISTs is the small intestine.[141,142] In one report, approximately half of all small bowel tumors identified on small bowel capsule endoscopy were GISTs.[143,148] GISTs in the small intestine tend to occur in the jejunum, followed by the ileum and then the duodenum. More investigators are now separating duodenal GISTs from other small intestinal GISTs because of differences in presentation and behavior. Duodenal GISTs seem to have a more favorable prognosis than jejunoileal GISTs, even with resections that are more conservative and limited (i.e., without performing a pancreaticoduodenectomy).[149–153] Small intestinal GISTs often present with significantly larger lesions than other primary sites. The large lesions may be highly vascularized and present significant risks of bleeding, even with only a biopsy. Because complete surgical resection is the treatment of choice for GISTs, there is some controversy over whether any preoperative biopsy is necessary, or whether biopsy represents an extra risk for the patient (discussed further below). This is a challenging subject because other disease entities enter the differential diagnosis of a large abdominal mass involving the small intestine and mesentery. In general, clinical practice guidelines have suggested that resection may be performed without antecedent biopsy if a GIST is strongly suspected and if surgery can be accomplished without significant risk of morbidity to the patient. If only radical surgery, leading to significant functional impairment, could remove the lesion, it may be in the patient's best interest to consider a preoperative biopsy to establish the diagnosis of a GIST and allow for neoadjuvant therapy (see below).

Colonic and Anorectal Tumors

GISTs in the rectum and colon are rare, accounting for roughly 5% of GIST cases, and they present unique management challenges.[154–159] As in other sites, small GIST lesions in the rectum may present as small, hard nodules less than 1 cm in diameter found incidentally during a rectal examination or proctoscopy. However, much larger tumors can ulcerate and bleed

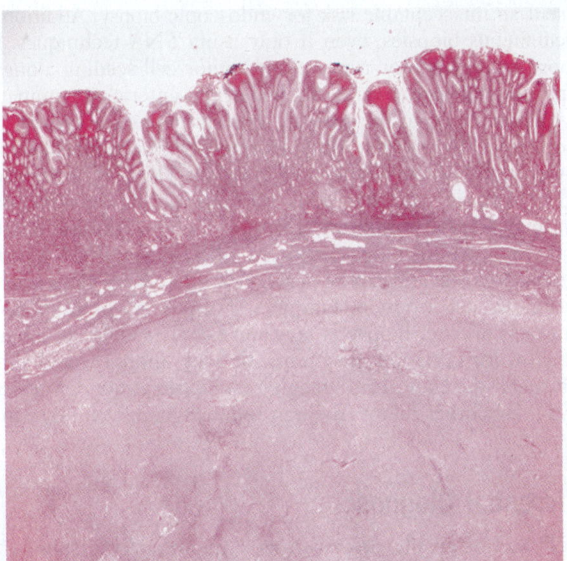

Fig. 42.3 Photomicrograph of a spindle cell submucosal gastrointestinal stromal tumor in the stomach. The lesion is well circumscribed and does not invade the overlying muscularis mucosa. Invasion of the muscularis mucosa is considered an adverse prognostic factor. (H&E, ×50.) (Courtesy Dr. Brian P. Rubin, Cleveland, OH.)

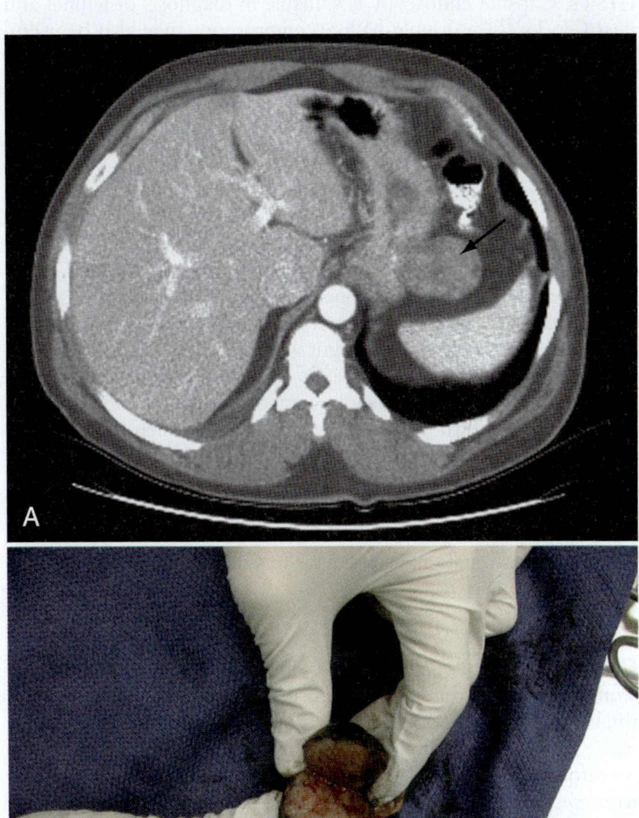

Fig. 42.4 Gastric GIST. (A) CT showing a 4–5-cm exophytic gastric GIST arising from the greater curvature of the stomach *(arrow)*. (B) Gross photograph of the 3.5 × 4.5 × 4–cm³ tumor after it was resected and cut open. Histology showed a spindle cell gastric GIST that was positive for KIT (CD117) immunoreactivity. (Courtesy Dr. Jay N. Yepuri and Dr. Christopher Bell, Dallas, TX.)

acutely or chronically, mimicking a rectal adenocarcinoma. Diagnosis can be challenging because the epithelioid or mixed cell variants of GISTs can also be misclassified as adenocarcinomas, especially if small biopsies are confounded by severe inflammatory changes or associated abscess formation.

DIAGNOSIS

Several professional organizations have developed consensus-based (and, whenever possible, evidence-based) clinical practice guidelines. The National Comprehensive Cancer Network has developed extensive publicly accessible guidelines to assist clinicians in the diagnosis and treatment of GIST patients.[160] The European Society of Medical Oncology also has published expert-driven clinical practice guidelines.[161]

The diagnostic evaluation of a suspected or proven GIST resembles that of other GI neoplasms. The most important element is to keep GISTs in the differential diagnosis of any mass lesion noted throughout the length of the GI tract, as well as in extra-intestinal sites of the abdomen and pelvis. As for any GI evaluation, the site of lesion determines which diagnostic tools are most appropriate for the patient. Endoscopy plays a major role in the diagnosis of gastric, duodenal, esophageal, colonic, and anorectal GISTs. Capsule endoscopy is valuable in diagnosis of jejunal and ileal GISTs[143,148]; double-balloon enteroscopy may also be useful in diagnosis of these small intestinal GISTs, especially those that bleed.[162]

Imaging

EUS

EUS is a useful technology for evaluating possible GISTs because of the submucosal localization of these tumors (see Video 42.1). GISTs visualized by EUS appear as hypoechoic masses contiguous with the fourth (muscularis propria) or second (muscularis mucosae) layers of the normal gut wall. In one study,[163] the seven EUS features, most predictive of so-called benign GI GISTs, were regular margins, tumor size 3 cm or less, and a homogeneous echogenicity pattern. Multivariate analysis identified the presence of cystic spaces and irregular margins as independent predictors of malignant potential. A second study identified tumor size larger than 4 cm, irregular extraluminal borders, echogenic foci larger than 3 mm, and cystic spaces larger than 4 mm as factors that correlated with malignant behavior in GIST.[164]

CT and MRI

CT is the most effective way to image primary lesions in the stomach, because the oral contrast will outline masses and gastric thickening (see Fig. 42.4). The differential diagnosis with inadequate gastric distention can be a challenge, especially when monitoring for recurrence following surgery. CT is also essential to stage the extent of disease. For measurable GISTs, it is particularly useful to perform CT with noncontrast image acquisition as well as assess early and late images following the administration of IV contrast. Routine MRI is inferior to CT for visualizing a gastric GIST because of uncontrollable movement of the gastric wall and surrounding tissues. However, diffusion weighted imaging with MRI may be comparable to PET/CT.[165] MRI can be useful for the assessment of liver metastases because some GIST lesions can be fully isodense to normal tissues and thus invisible against surrounding hepatic parenchyma on CT.

Baseline CT imaging is critical for patients with GISTs, because endoscopic imaging alone may only reveal a small fraction of the underlying tumor. Additionally, imaging patterns can be interpreted qualitatively to assess the impact of targeted therapy using metrics other than tumor size.[166,167] Response to kinase inhibitors will lead to a decrease in tumor density on CT, even in the absence of a change in size of the lesion (CHOI criteria); hypodense lesions on CT have been correlated with loss of metabolic activity on FDG PET imaging.[167]

PET/CT

^{18}F-FDG PET scans can provide functional information on GISTs to complement conventional anatomic imaging such as CT or MRI's size assessment (Fig. 42.5). The actual mechanisms responsible for the high-level avidity of GISTs for the ^{18}F-FDG tracer is likely due to signaling through the overactive KIT, RTK, and glucose transport proteins, such as GLUT4.[168] With TKI therapy, there is decreased cell viability and glucose uptake associated with decreased GLUT4 expression, thus explaining the rapid changes in PET imaging associated with inhibition of KIT signaling by pharmacologic means.[169,170] Large GISTs can demonstrate centers with predominantly cystic or low-attenuation characteristics noted on CT or MRI. It is clear by ^{18}F-FDG PET scans that the internal mass of large GIST lesions can often be viewed as metabolically quiescent, likely because of tumor necrosis of these large lesions in their central portions. Even though GIST lesions can be vascular, the internal portion can nonetheless represent a confluent mass of necrotic material, with the more viable portions of the GIST pushing out toward the edges of the lesion. Much of the added value of ^{18}F-FDG PET imaging in serial imaging can also be obtained by a qualitative assessment of tumor density obtained via CT.[167] However, occasionally, metastatic GIST lesions in the omentum can be subtle and easy to overlook on CT because small lesions could blend into the folds of the bowel walls and be difficult for even the most experienced radiologist to detect. ^{18}F-FDG PET imaging can detect lesions about 1 cm or larger in size without difficulty because neither the normal bowel nor omentum will take up the ^{18}F-FDG tracer with excess avidity. National guidelines, however, do not encourage the routine use of ^{18}F-FDG PET imaging and it is not a substitute for CT.

Biopsy

As discussed earlier, GISTs can be highly vascular, which may present an unacceptable risk for endoscopic biopsy. Additionally, percutaneous biopsies, even if only using FNA techniques, may impose risks of tumor rupture and tumor cell seeding along the biopsy tract or spread via peritoneal or mesenteric contamination. To minimize risk to the patient, some surgeons recommend that preoperative biopsy not be performed if resection is planned. However, biopsy must be performed in cases of unresectable GIST to make the diagnosis and justify preoperative (neoadjuvant) administration of imatinib therapy (discussed later). Furthermore, FNA biopsy of gastric GISTs using EUS guidance can be diagnostic and can be performed safely,[171] as can a mucosal incision-assisted biopsy technique.[172] For patients presenting with metastatic disease, biopsy is appropriate to establish a diagnosis and allow for initiation of systemic therapy. Biopsy would also be indicated if the clinical and imaging evaluation is not definitive for GIST, since other tumors (benign and malignant) can occur in the GI tract.

Differential Diagnosis

GIST was originally described as a monomorphic spindle cell neoplasm. However, it is now clear that GIST can exhibit a wide variety of histologic appearances, ranging from an epithelioid form with large round cells (see Fig. 42.2) to the spindle cell form (see Fig. 42.1), and lesions with mixed histology. The spindle cell GIST variant is far more common, representing some 70% of

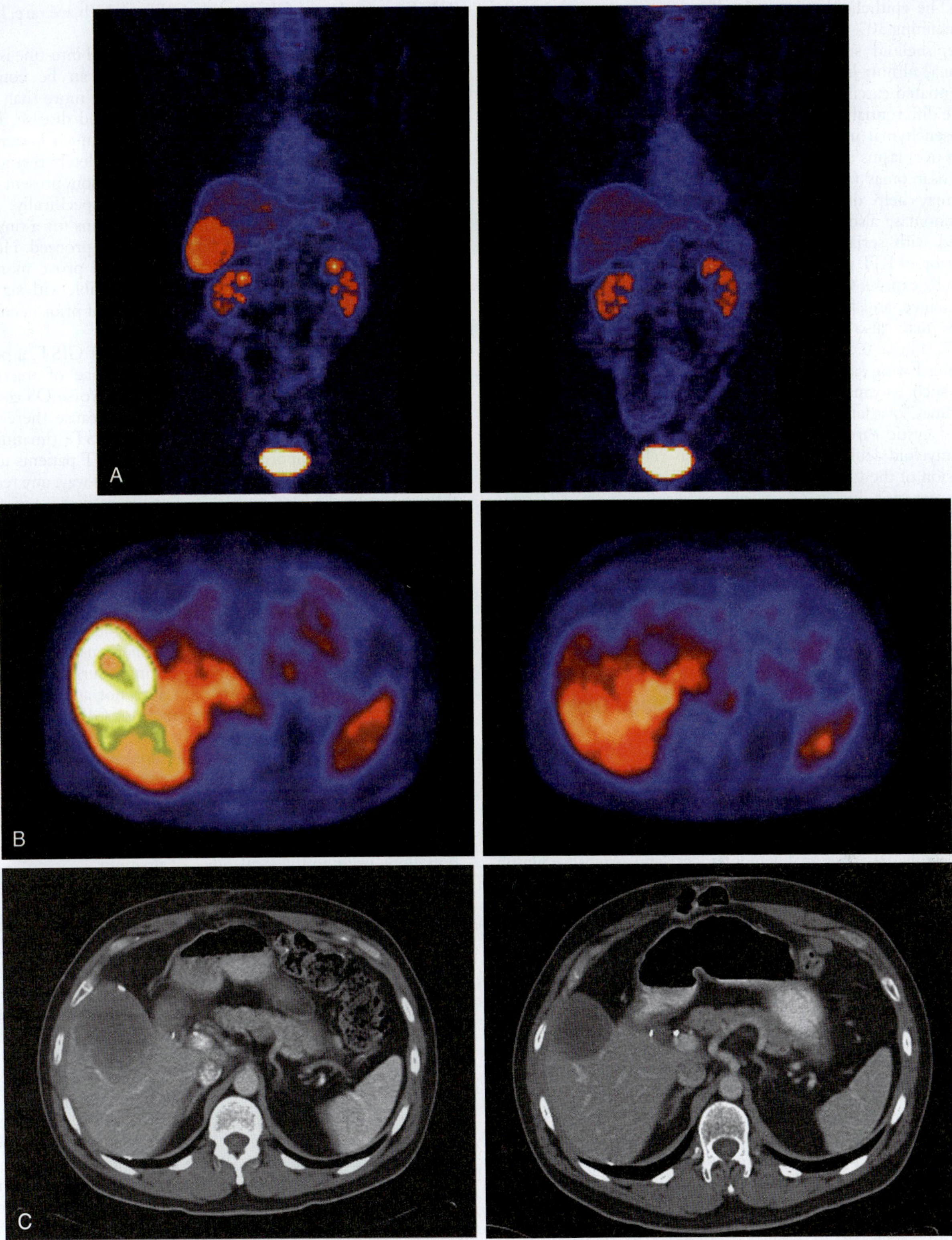

Fig. 42.5 Metastatic GIST. PET (A and B) and CT (C) in a patient with a GIST metastatic to the liver, before (*left*) and after (*right*) treatment with imatinib mesylate. Partial tumor regression with reduced ^{18}F-FDG uptake is seen after treatment. (Courtesy Dr. A. Van den Abbeele, Boston, MA; and modified from Demetri GD, Benjamin RS, Blanke CD, et al. NCCN Task Force report: management of patients with gastrointestinal stromal tumor [GIST]—update of the NCCN clinical practice guidelines. *J Natl Compr Canc Netw*. 2007;5(suppl 2):S1–S29.)

cases. The epithelioid, or round cell, pattern represents most of the remaining 30% and may contain an admixture of spindle cells. The epithelioid subset was previously diagnosed as leiomyoblastoma, although some may have been mistaken for poorly differentiated carcinomas.

The differential diagnosis of GI tract neoplasms that appear to be mesenchymal in origin includes GISTs (80%), true smooth muscle neoplasms of the GI tract, including true leiomyomas and leiomyosarcomas (≈15%), and schwannomas (≈5%). CT features may help distinguish small gastric GISTs from gastric schwannomas; also, gastric GISTs tend to grow faster when assessed with serial CTs than schwannomas.[173] As noted, the expression of KIT is not limited to GIST cells. Normal ICCs and mast cells express CD117 and depend on KIT for development, maintenance, and function. A relatively limited number of other tumors may also express immunohistochemically detectable CD117. These include certain subsets of soft tissue sarcomas, including Ewing sarcoma and angiosarcoma, as well as other tumors, such as small cell lung cancers, melanomas, desmoids, seminomas, ovarian carcinomas, mastocytomas, neuroblastomas, adenoid cystic carcinomas, and rare subsets of lymphoma and acute myeloid leukemia.[174–177] It is also relevant to note that expression of the CD117 antigen does not imply activation of the KIT target, nor does it necessarily correlate with any *KIT* gene mutation. The same CD117 antigen is expressed by cells harboring normal (wild-type) *KIT* as those that have activating *KIT* mutations. Moreover, the expression of KIT protein does not necessarily mean that the protein is involved in the pathogenesis of that specific cancer.

TREATMENT

Primary Localized Disease (Early-Stage Disease)

Surgery

Definitive surgery remains the mainstay of treatment for patients with primary localized GISTs (early-stage GISTs). The surgical approach to resection of primary disease must account for the specific growth and behavior characteristics of this disease. GISTs rarely involve the regional lymph nodes, and extensive lymph node exploration or resection is rarely indicated. GIST lesions are highly vascularized and often exhibit a fragile pseudocapsule; therefore surgeons should be careful to minimize the risk of tumor rupture, which subsequently increases the risk of peritoneal dissemination. The margins of resection from the tumor specimen should be carefully oriented and examined, and biopsy samples from several different areas of the tumor should be evaluated by the surgical pathologist. Increasingly, laparoscopic[178–182] and endoscopic[183,184] resections are being used with good outcomes.

The natural history of early-stage primary GIST has been examined in studies from single-institution referral centers. These studies are certainly prone to selection bias, and it is clear in this evolving field that many early-stage GIST patients have likely been managed by physicians from multiple specialties, including gastroenterology and general surgery. The Memorial Sloan Kettering Cancer Center's series evaluated 200 patients that were followed prospectively[131]; 80 of these patients (40%) had primary disease managed with complete surgical resection. This subgroup with primary resected GISTs demonstrated 5-year disease-specific survival rates of only 54%, supporting the fact that GISTs, as seen at such an academic referral center, can exhibit a high risk for recurrence and ultimately prove to be life-threatening. On multivariate analysis, large tumor size (>10 cm) was the only factor that reduced disease-specific survival. Anatomic location of the primary tumor also appears to be an important prognostic factor for primary localized GIST.[133] Small intestinal GISTs have a less favorable prognosis than gastric GISTs; colon/rectal GIST and E-GISTs, which are rare, have the poorest outcome.

The prognosis of GISTs involving the small intestine is related to the adequacy of resection.[131,185] Most can be completely resected, with median overall survival (OS) of more than 5 years for patients with localized or locally advanced disease. Patients who underwent complete resections exhibit much better 5-year OS than those whose lesions cannot be completely resected.

GISTs in the rectal and perirectal location present similar challenges to those in the small intestine; specifically, if non-mutilating surgery can achieve negative margins for a tiny GIST (<1 cm), that is probably a reasonable way to proceed. However, many GIST lesions in the rectal region will prove more challenging to resect, and surgery may only be feasible with significant functional morbidity, especially if done without prior neoadjuvant therapy.

For patients with intermediate to high-risk GIST, a post hoc observational study showed that the presence of microscopic positive margin (R1) was not associated with worse OS compared to R0 unless tumor rupture occurred.[186] Because there is now effective medical treatment for advanced GISTs (imatinib, discussed later), it is important that resected GIST patients undergo regular surveillance following resection. In this way, any recurrent disease can be detected and treated at the earliest stage, thereby avoiding complications (e.g., tumor hemorrhages) that might stem from treatment of recurrent large, bulky disease.

Adjuvant Radiation Therapy

Only a limited number of case reports and small series have investigated the role of adjuvant treatment using conventional modalities, such as radiotherapy following a surgical resection of an early-stage GIST. Radiotherapy does not appear to have an important role in the adjuvant treatment of GIST; this in part is due to the inability to administer effective doses given the toxicity to small bowel and other intra-abdominal structures. There also have only been small series of patients who have received adjuvant systemic or intraperitoneal chemotherapy, and these data have not identified any clear benefits. The standard of care after complete surgical resection of primary GISTs has therefore been observation alone prior to the availability of imatinib.

Adjuvant Therapy With Imatinib

It is now clear that administration of imatinib in the postresection (adjuvant) setting delays tumor recurrence, especially for patients who present with large tumors and who are at high risk of disease recurrence and metastatic spread.[187–191] Risk stratification for adjuvant therapy is based on tumors estimated to be at intermediate to high risk of recurrence, using the GIST nomogram, population topographical charts, or the rule of 5s discussed earlier.[29–31]

The activity of adjuvant imatinib in GIST patients has been investigated in several large multicenter trials.[187–191] In the first randomized adjuvant trial Z9001, conducted by the American College of Surgical Oncology Group (ACOSOG), imatinib (or placebo) was administered for 1 year. Administration of imatinib following resection of primary limited GIST significantly prolonged recurrence-free survival compared with placebo (98% vs. 83% free of recurrence at 1 year; hazard ratio 0.35), although no OS benefit has been noted.[187] The ACOSOG trial enrolled patients with any size GIST. Analysis of the benefit from therapy based upon size (i.e., 3–6, 6–10, and 10 cm or larger) identified that although there was a numerical benefit in all groups, it was only statistically significant in the tumors larger than 10 cm. The European Organization for the Research and Treatment of Cancer (EORTC) tested 2 years of adjuvant therapy versus none, and originally had OS as the primary endpoint.[189] It became clear

TABLE 42.2 Antitumor Responses to Imatinib in Patients With Metastatic or Unresectable Gastrointestinal Stromal Tumors

References	GISTs (*N*)	Imatinib Dose (mg/day)	CR (%)	PR (%)	DSD (%)
211	36	400-1000	0	53	17
169	147	400 or 600	0	54	28
214	946	400 vs. 800	5	47	32
213	746	400 vs. 800	4	41	23

There were no significant differences in antitumor responses among doses in these studies. *CR*, Complete remission; *DSD*, durable stable disease; *GISTs*, gastrointestinal stromal tumors; *PR*, partial remission.

that the results of this trial would potentially require more than a decade and so the endpoint was switched to the time to imatinib-resistant disease. Patients who were on imatinib for 2 years and progressed were allowed to restart imatinib, and those on the placebo arm who progressed initiated therapy. There was no statistically significant difference in the time to imatinib resistance in the two groups. In the Scandinavian trial,[191] patients with KIT-positive GISTs by immunostaining who had a high likelihood of recurring postoperatively due to their size, mitotic rate, and/or tumor rupture were randomized to receive adjuvant imatinib mesylate (400 mg daily) for either 1 or 3 years beginning 1–12 weeks postoperatively. Imatinib therapy for 3 years resulted in significantly better OS than when taken for 1 year (91.9% vs. 85.3%, HR, 0.60, $P = 0.036$), although there was a higher imatinib discontinuation rate in the 3-year group, usually for adverse effects or patient preferences. In addition, this trial demonstrated a survival advantage for those receiving adjuvant therapy and the 10-year update showed 53% recurrence-free survival and 79% OS with 3 years of adjuvant imatinib.[191] The PERSIST-5 study was a single-arm phase II study that enrolled patients with high-risk GIST, defined as a primary GIST (any site) ≥2 cm with a mitotic count ≥5/50 HPF or nongastric primary GIST ≥5 cm. This study showed estimated 5-year recurrence-free survival of 90% although approximately half of patients stopped treatment early because of patient choice (21%), adverse events (16%), or other reasons (12%).[192] The benefit of adjuvant activity of imatinib is clear and merits a thoughtful discussion of possible risks and benefits in all patients with resected GISTs who are at moderate to high risk of disease recurrence by current risk classification systems.[26,29,30] Guidelines recommend treatment for at least 3 years. Studies are now ongoing to assess the benefit of longer-term therapy (check clinicaltrials.gov).

Neoadjuvant Therapy

With the advent of highly effective drug therapy, current guidelines recommend that surgical resection of GISTs be undertaken as the first intervention only if there is an acceptably low risk of functional deficit or morbidity from the surgery. If a large GIST is detected, and there is a risk for perioperative morbidity, neoadjuvant (preoperative) imatinib should be considered. In this scenario, a tissue biopsy is required prior to starting therapy. The tissue from such a diagnostic biopsy is too small to provide detailed risk stratification but should be sufficient to obtain molecular testing. Trials have shown that such neoadjuvant drug administration can be effective at downsizing tumors and, hence, facilitating effective surgical intervention.[193–195] Following the maximal response to imatinib (median time to maximal response being 6 months or longer), definitive surgery can be performed. In such patients, postoperative imatinib adjuvant therapy is also recommended for a total of at least 3 years of therapy.

Advanced-Stage Disease

Systemic and Locoregional Chemotherapy, Radiotherapy, and Debulking Surgery

Historically, leiomyosarcomas of the GI tract were noted to be resistant to standard chemotherapy regimens; these leiomyosarcomas proved largely to represent GISTs. Studies in patients with advanced GISTs receiving conventional cytotoxic chemotherapy demonstrated little benefit with objective antitumor response to various chemotherapy agents routinely reported to be 0%–4%.[3,196] Some investigators attempted to improve on these dismal results with chemotherapy by administering the drugs via an intraperitoneal route.[197] However, because GISTs rarely remain confined to the peritoneal surfaces, with hematogenous spread to the liver and other intra-abdominal locations, and because most of the life-threatening complications of GISTs arise from hepatic involvement or from bulk disease affecting the omentum, this intraperitoneal approach was not particularly promising. Based on these disappointing results, conventional cytotoxic chemotherapy is regarded as ineffective for the treatment of patients with GIST.

The high levels of resistance to chemotherapy exhibited by GISTs may result, in part, from the expression of increased levels of *P*-glycoprotein (the product of *MDR1*). GISTs have been shown to have increased expression of *P*-glycoprotein compared with leiomyosarcomas.[198] These cellular efflux pumps prevent some types of chemotherapy from reaching effective intracellular concentrations in the target GIST cells.

There are single-institution data demonstrating control of metastatic GIST for a limited time by locoregional, surgical or interventional radiology techniques, such as hepatic resection,[199] hepatic artery embolization/chemoembolization,[200] or radiofrequency ablation.[201] Although a subset of patients with metastatic GISTs involving the liver have demonstrated antitumor responses and a somewhat limited progression-free survival (PFS) following chemoembolization, the benefits are generally measured in months rather than years. Similarly, radiation therapy has a limited role in advanced/metastatic GIST, with infrequent response but potential durable stability for over 1 year at the radiated site.[202] Generally, these local therapy modalities are reserved for palliation, such as to treat painful metastasis or bleeding tumor, or in conjunction with other therapies such as TKI and surgery.[203]

Debulking surgery has a limited role in selected patients with metastatic GIST. If a patient presents with metastatic disease involving the liver and peritoneal surfaces, the first line of therapy is systemic treatment with a TKI. Once the disease has responded to the TKI, the role of debulking surgery has been hypothesized to be of benefit by eliminating tumor that contains resistant clones and may prolong disease control, supported by PFS on imatinib being correlated with bulk of disease.[204] The EORTC developed a trial to test this hypothesis in which patients were to be randomized to continued imatinib therapy versus resection of disease with continued imatinib, with a primary endpoint of PFS. The study accrued poorly and was closed before answering the question.

Large series from several institutions have also reported on the benefit of limited resection in patients with progressive disease on TKI therapy.[205–209] The majority have reported on outcomes for patients on imatinib therapy. Although surgery is feasible with sunitinib, it is complicated by the vascular endothelial growth factor receptor targeting of sunitinib, requiring the drug to be stopped for 2 weeks or longer prior to surgery due to increased risk of bleeding and wound complications.[206] In the setting of progressive disease on imatinib, patients with isolated progressive disease that is resected achieve approximately an extra year on imatinib therapy. There is limited benefit of surgery for diffuse progression and patients are better served by changing their systemic therapy.

For patients with metastatic or unresectable GISTs, prognosis was dismal before the advent of molecularly targeted therapy. For patients with metastatic or recurrent GISTs or GI sarcomas (most of which were likely to have been a true GIST), most studies prior to the introduction of targeted therapy with kinase inhibition documented poor survival rates, with fatal outcomes from disease progression generally occurring within 1–2 years from the date of first recurrence or metastasis.[131]

Imatinib Mesylate

The collaborative worldwide clinical development of imatinib as a molecularly targeted therapy of GIST proceeded at a dramatic pace. In 2000 a single-patient pilot study in a patient with advanced, heavily pretreated, and widely metastatic GIST was undertaken. The patient had a rapid response with sustained clinical benefit from imatinib for nearly 3 years.[210] Based on the dramatic and durable benefits in this patient, as well as striking scientific rationale and strong preclinical data, other studies testing imatinib for GISTs were started. A dose-finding study, begun by the EORTC Sarcoma Group, enrolled primarily patients with GISTs.[211] The maximal tolerated dose of imatinib was judged to be 800 mg/day (given as 400 mg twice daily); at the higher dose level of 1000 mg daily (given as 500 mg twice daily), unacceptably severe, dose-limiting toxicities such as nausea, vomiting, and severe edema were reported. A multicenter United States-Finland collaborative study randomized 147 patients with metastatic GISTs between two dose levels of the drug (400 mg daily or 300 mg twice daily).[169] There did not appear to be differences in response rates or duration of disease control between the two dose levels, but the study was not powered to detect differences. The EORTC group went on to expand its exploration of imatinib in GISTs and other forms of sarcomas. In this trial, the high levels of antitumor activity against GISTs were again confirmed, whereas there was no demonstrable benefit for patients with other forms of soft tissue sarcomas.[212] The results from these wholly independent trials were remarkably concordant (Table 42.2). These data supported the hypothesis that targeting the mutations in KIT and PDGFRA believed to be the molecular drivers critical to GIST cell growth and survival leads to meaningful therapeutic benefit. Without such a target to inhibit (as in sarcomas other than GISTs), imatinib treatment does not have major anticancer activity.

Further assessment of the optimal dose of imatinib for advanced unresectable GIST was obtained in two large trials designed and run concurrently by the Southwest Oncology Group (SWOG) and the EORTC.[213,214] These studies enrolled 1700 patients and were powered to determine whether 400 mg twice daily (compared to 400 mg daily) would translate into significant clinical benefits as measured by improved response rates, PFS (SWOG trial), or survival (EORTC trial). In addition, progressing patients on the lower-dose arm were allowed to cross over to the higher-dose arm. There was no survival difference documented in either trial between these dose levels. Although the SWOG study demonstrated only a favorable trend in the duration of disease control associated with the higher-dose of imatinib, the European study noted a modest, but statistically significant, benefit in favor of the higher-dose arm for PFS. In a combined meta-analysis, benefit of the higher dose of imatinib was limited solely to the relatively small subset of GIST patients whose tumors harbored mutations in *KIT* exon 9, encoding a mutation in the extracellular KIT domain that promotes dimerization of kinase molecules.[213] This has led to the recommendation by some experts to use the higher dose of imatinib as first-line therapy for advanced GIST in patients whose tumors have documented exon 9 *KIT* mutations. The benefit, however, should be weighed against the additional toxicities, because the higher dose of imatinib was associated with a greater incidence of adverse effects and led to a greater number of dose reductions for toxicity. This increase in toxicity can be mitigated, however, by initiating therapy at 400 mg/day and then escalating to 400 mg twice a day after 1–2 months; a lower incidence of toxicity was noted in the patients who crossed over to the higher dose of 400 mg twice daily.[214]

The results from these trials in the United States and Europe confirmed the exceptional activity of imatinib in controlling metastatic GIST, with objective responses in 45%–53%, as well as control of symptoms and prolonged survival in comparison with historical controls. The median time to objective response was more than 3 months, although some patients experienced dramatic disease regressions within a week after starting imatinib oral dosing. Imatinib was well tolerated overall in both studies. Based on these trials, the FDA approved the use of imatinib for treatment of metastatic or unresectable GIST in 2002 in the United States. Approval in Europe and the rest of the world followed quickly thereafter.

Correlative molecular studies were performed in conjunction with the United States-Finland trial as well as the phase III trials run by SWOG and EORTC.[64,215] These studies documented differences in the activity of imatinib based on the genotype of the GIST lesions treated. Specifically, patients whose GISTs harbored *KIT* mutations in exon 11 (the most common molecular subtype) had higher rates of objective response and more durable disease control than patients whose disease had exon 9 *KIT* mutations or no detectable *KIT* mutations. The meta-analysis of the phase III SWOG and EORTC studies demonstrated a benefit in PFS in those with *KIT* exon 9 mutations who initiated therapy at 400 mg twice daily, although OS was not different, and may have reflected the ability to increase from 400 mg/day to 400 mg twice daily in the setting of disease progression.[216] Patients with *PDGFRA* mutations also benefited, with the exception of those with the *D842V* mutation.[20,64,215]

The studies of imatinib in advanced GIST have consistently documented the tolerability of imatinib overall.[169,211,213,214] It is fortunate that normal physiologic processes (e.g., hematopoiesis and GI motility) that depend on the normal receptor-ligand signaling through the KIT receptor do not fail with fatal consequences when KIT function is blocked by imatinib therapy. The adverse effects of imatinib are generally mild (grade 1 or 2) and include edema, especially notable in the loose subcutaneous tissues of the facial periorbital region, diarrhea, myalgia or musculoskeletal pain, rashes, and headache. Myelotoxicity has been much less common in GIST patients than in patients with CML treated with imatinib. Nonetheless, GIST patients treated with imatinib can occasionally exhibit severe cytopenias; because of this risk, patients should be monitored carefully. The most worrisome adverse events observed in imatinib treatment of patients with advanced GIST have included hemorrhages from abdominal or GI sites in approximately 5% of GIST patients, largely related to bleeding from bulky tumor masses; bleeding is thought to be induced by the potent and rapid antitumor effects of imatinib. In patients with toxicity from imatinib, dose reductions may reduce toxicity and allow for continued therapy.

Most side effects of imatinib therapy become milder over time, suggesting that some sort of tachyphylaxis mechanism may be present.[217] For example, the edema associated with imatinib therapy of GIST often improves with continued dosing over time, although diuretics may be used judiciously and are often effective at managing this side effect. Counseling GIST patients on the use of a low-salt diet may also aid in controlling this side effect. Nausea with imatinib administration is usually mild and self-limited. Patients should be counseled to take the daily dose with a low-fat meal and a large glass of water; antiemetics can be used if symptoms are more severe. Diarrhea is typically managed with antidiarrheal drugs as needed. Muscle cramps, frequently in the calves, are usually transient and self-limited, often mitigated by increased fluid and electrolyte intake.

Imatinib rapidly and dramatically leads to decrease in the tumors' ^{18}F-FDG tracer uptake on functional PET imaging (see Fig. 42.5).[168] The decreased ^{18}F-FDG in tumors can be detected as early as 24 hours following a single dose of imatinib. The PET findings were also highly reliable, correlating both with beneficial response to imatinib and documenting progressive disease in the small subset of patients with primary resistance to imatinib. These data indicate that functional imaging of GIST with ^{18}F-FDG PET scanning represents a useful diagnostic modality for early response assessment with imatinib therapy. PET, however, should not be considered the standard imaging modality for ongoing treatment assessment given the increased exposure to radiation as well as greater cost associated with its use.

The optimal duration of imatinib for patients with metastatic GIST has been defined as lifelong therapy based on current evidence.[218,219] A randomized study by the French Sarcoma Group tested the impact of discontinuing imatinib therapy in GIST patients whose disease was stable or had responded following 1, 3, or 5 years of therapy. Discontinuation of imatinib was associated with rapidly recurring disease. This is due to the persistence of some tumor cells, which in response to imatinib become metabolically quiescent and do not proliferate but can reenter the cell cycle upon treatment discontinuation.[4,220] Imatinib-persistent cells may also provide a source of TKI-resistant clones. Mechanisms of persistence include escape from apoptosis by upregulating macroautophagy[221] and withdrawal from the cell cycle due to the proteasomal degradation of the cyclin-dependent kinase inhibitor 1B (CDKN1B; p27^{Kip1})-regulator S-phase kinase-associated protein 2[222], and the formation of the DREAM complex (DP, p130/RBL2, E2F4, and MuvB).[223] Imatinib-treated GISTs may also lose KIT expression due to tumor cell dedifferentiation[25] or selection for KIT^{low}CD34^{+} ICC/GIST stem cells.[71,75,220]

Resistance to imatinib can be primary and manifest as rapid progression of disease despite initial imatinib dosing. However, primary imatinib resistance is relatively uncommon and has been found to be primarily associated with *PDGFRA* D842V and other nonimatinib sensitive oncologic drivers (see Table 42.2).[64] Alternatively, imatinib-resistant disease may emerge after more than 1 or 2 years of durable response due to the clonal evolution of the GIST.[224] This secondary resistance to imatinib in GIST is overall similar to the resistance mechanisms that have been described in imatinib-resistant CML.[225]

Sunitinib Malate

Sunitinib (Sutent) inhibits multiple RTKs, including KIT; PDGFRA and platelet-derived growth factor receptor-beta; VEGF receptors 1, 2, and 3; FMS-like tyrosine kinase-3 receptor (FLT3); macrophage colony-stimulating factor receptor (CSF1R); and glial cell-line derived neurotropic factor receptor (RET, rearranged during transfection).[226] Sunitinib demonstrated antineoplastic activity in GISTs in the first phase I clinical trial.[226] The study tested several doses and schedules and picked 50 mg orally for 28 days, with 14 days of rest as the schedule to be developed. The patients included in the phase 1 and subsequent phase 2 trials of sunitinib were for the most part refractory to imatinib and had extensive metastatic disease. PET scans demonstrated metabolic response during the 4 weeks of sunitinib treatment, but with reactivation of metabolic activity during the 2-week rest period (washout). Similar to imatinib, CT scan responses evolved more slowly. Response data in the early trials as well as the pivotal placebo-controlled, phase 3 trial were markedly similar, with no complete responses and partial responses ranging from 7% to 13%.[226–228] Median time to tumor progression was 7.8 months and median survival was 19.8 months in the early-phase studies.

In the phase III trial that led to the regulatory approval of sunitinib, 312 patients with metastatic or surgically unresectable GIST following failure of imatinib therapy due to resistance or intolerance were randomized to receive sunitinib 50 mg/day (n = 207) or to placebo (n = 105) using the dosing schedule of 4 weeks of drug dosing followed by a 2-week period off drug.[227,228] The primary endpoint of the study was disease control as assessed by time to progression (TTP). The trial was unblinded early when a planned interim efficacy analysis showed that sunitinib was associated with a significant improvement in median TTP of more than fourfold compared with placebo. The PFS for patients receiving sunitinib was significantly greater than for those receiving placebo (sunitinib, 24.1 weeks vs. placebo, 6.0 weeks with a hazard ratio of 0.335, P = 0.0001). In the initial analysis, sunitinib also significantly improved OS (hazard ratio, 0.49). In the final analysis, TTP was similar to the findings of the interim analysis (6.7 months vs. 1.6 months). The OS was also improved in the patients who initiated therapy on sunitinib, despite the cross-over design of the study (18.2 months vs. 16.2 months); 87% of patients assigned to the placebo arm received therapy with open label sunitinib.

Molecular analysis of GIST samples from the initial phase I and II trials indicated that primary and secondary mutations in *KIT* affected treatment outcomes with sunitinib in patients with imatinib-resistant GISTs; insufficient numbers of patients with *PDGFRA* mutations limited assessment of this group.[229] Responses and clinical benefit were observed more frequently in patients with mutations that are less sensitive to imatinib such as *KIT* exon 9 and wild-type *KIT*, compared to those with exon 11 mutations. TTP was longest for patients whose tumors contained a *KIT* exon 9 mutation, followed by wild-type *KIT*, exon 11 mutated, and worst for a tumor with both an exon 11 mutation and a new mutation. Patients with *KIT* exon 9 and wild-type mutations had the best OS. This does not suggest that sunitinib is inactive in exon 11 tumors; rather, it represents the fact that patients with exon 11 mutations who have progressed on imatinib have developed resistance, and typically have clones with additional mutations. Further study has shown that secondary mutations involving KIT exons 13 or 14 are sensitive to sunitinib, whereas those with exon 17 and 18 secondary mutations tend to be resistant to sunitinib.[229,230] Structural biology analyses of these mutated kinases have provided insight as to how sunitinib can inhibit kinase function when mutations encode certain amino acid changes that induce steric hindrance to the binding and inhibition of imatinib.[231]

For some patients, the treatment schedule with a 2-week treatment break was accompanied by resumption of disease-related symptoms. However, they clearly needed a dose interruption to manage side effects. The most common grades 3 and 4 sunitinib toxicities in GIST patients included fatigue, asymptomatic serum lipase and amylase increases, and hypertension.[226–228] Other side effects included nausea, diarrhea, stomatitis, hand-foot syndrome, anemia, and skin discoloration. Bleeding has also been described at sites of tumor biopsies when patients were on the drug. Patients on sunitinib also experienced a greater incidence of skin abnormalities, including palmar-plantar erythrodysesthesia (hand-foot syndrome) and oral cavity mucosal irritation. In addition, some patients with a history of coronary artery disease were found to have asymptomatic cardiac enzyme elevations. Certain patients may also have cardiac dysfunction, which in general reverses with discontinuation of sunitinib dosing.[232] Hypothyroidism has also been observed and mandates monitoring for emergence during therapy.[233]

A phase 2 trial of continuous daily but lower sunitinib dosing was tested in patients with GISTs.[234] This dosing schedule sought to mitigate drug-related side effects, but also to control disease-related symptoms seen during the 2-week break. The study demonstrated safety and tolerability using a starting sunitinib dose of 37.5 mg daily. Types of toxicities are similar with either schedule, but of less intensity with the lower dose, allowing for continuous dosing. There was a suggestion of longer disease control with the daily dosing schedule. This regimen is preferred by most practitioners.

Thus sunitinib appears to have unique activity for the management of imatinib-resistant GIST as second-line therapy, but the powerful inhibition of a number of other kinase signaling pathways is associated with more unpleasant or medically relevant adverse effects that require close monitoring and possibly adjustment of dosing.

Regorafenib

Regorafenib (Stivarga) has multiple targets, including KIT, PDGFRB, vascular endothelial growth factor receptors FLT1, KDR, and FLT4, TEK RTK (TEK or TIE2), RET, FGFR1, RAF, and p38 mitogen-activated protein kinase.[235,236] The initial phase II trial in GIST demonstrated a response rate of 17.6% and a clinical benefit rate of 76%, defined as those with objective responses or stable disease for ≥16 weeks. In addition, the median PFS was 13.2 months.[235,236]

These compelling phase II data led to the GRID study, an international double-blind phase III trial of regorafenib compared with placebo using the same criteria for study entry regarding prior treatment as in the phase II study.[237] The trial randomized 199 patients in a 2:1 fashion to regorafenib versus placebo, allowing for open-label therapy with regorafenib at the time of progression for both patients on either arm. The overall response rates (ORRs) were very low at 4.5% for regorafenib and 1.5% for placebo (one partial response). The median PFS was 4.8 months with regorafenib versus 0.9 months on placebo. OS was not statistically significant and anticipated, given that 85% of the patients on placebo crossed over to active therapy.

Toxicities for this agent were more like sunitinib than imatinib. The most common toxicities noted in the phase II trial were hand-foot syndrome, fatigue, diarrhea, and hypertension, affecting 91%, 85%, 79%, and 76%, respectively, of patients, most commonly during the first cycle of therapy.[235] Overall, 67% of patients experienced at least one or more grade 3 or 4 toxicity while on the study. In the phase III study, drug-related adverse events were more common in the regorafenib arm than in the placebo arm (98.5% vs. 68.2%, respectively), with grade 3 or higher events noted in 61.4% versus 13.6%, respectively. The most common grade 3 or higher events in the regorafenib arm were hypertension (23.5%), hand-foot skin reaction (19.7%), and diarrhea (5.3%).[235]

Analysis of factors associated with improved PFS with regorafenib from the phase III study determined a benefit for tumors with both primary mutations in *KIT* exon 11 and 9, irrespective of what line of therapy third or beyond.[237] The only factor that trended toward favoring placebo was prior imatinib therapy of less than 6 months' duration. An analysis of clinical benefit from the phase II study documented 76% of patients benefited, with the greatest benefit being in SDH deficient tumors (100%), exon 11 mutated tumors (79%), and exon 9 mutated tumors (67%).[237] There was one patient with a BRAF exon 15 mutation who did not benefit. There were three patients with unknown genotype, two of whom derived clinical benefit.

Avapritinib

Avapritinib, also known as BLU-285, was optimized to inhibit kinase mutations involving the distal kinase domain, where secondary mutations commonly occur.[238] This region is also the location of the *PDGFRA* D842V mutation that is refractory to standard therapies and is the single most common *PDGFRA* mutation in GIST.[239,240] With the D842V mutation, which is in *PDGFRA* exon 18 (activation loop), the protein is a persistent active state, causing resistance to tyrosine kinase inhibitors such as imatinib that only bind the inactive conformation. Avapritinib selectively inhibits the active conformation of KIT and PDGFRA, including PDGFRA with the D842V substitution. It was initially evaluated in the phase I NAVIGATOR study, which showed that in 56 patients with *PDGFRA* exon 18 D842V mutation, 88% had an overall response with 9% complete response and 79% partial response.[241] In the long-term follow-up (with a median follow-up of 27.5 months), the median PFS was 34.0 months and median OS was not reached; the duration of response was 27.6 months.[242] This subsequently led to the phase III VOYAGER study, comparing avapritinib 300 mg once daily to regorafenib as third or later-line therapy in GIST.[243] In this study, which included patients with and without D842V mutation, the median PFS was similar (4.2 months for avapritinib compared to 5.6 months for regorafenib). For patients on avapritinib, the objective response rate was 17.1% and disease control rate was 41.7%, with 7.6 months response duration.

Based on the NAVIGATOR data specifically in patients with PDGFRA exon 18 mutated GIST (including D842V), the FDA and European Union approved avapritinib (Ayvakit) for these individuals with unresectable or metastatic disease in 2020. However, the phase III study did not lead to changes in the sequence of tyrosine kinase inhibitor therapy for patients without the mutation.[243] The most common treatment-related adverse events were anemia (40.2%), nausea (39.3%), fatigue (35.1%), increased blood bilirubin (27.6%), periorbital edema (27.6%), with 8.3% rate of discontinuation due to treatment-related adverse events. Treatment-related serious adverse events occurred in 19.7% of patients on avapritinib, and the most common was anemia (5.9% had grade 3 or higher anemia). Cognitive effects (which included cognitive disorder, memory impairment, confusional state, and encephalopathy) occurred in 25.9% of patients on avapritinib, most of whom reported memory impairment (11.7%) or cognitive disorder (11.7%). Three patients (1.3%) had grade 3 or higher cognitive disorder. Intracranial bleeding occurred in three patients (1.3%) on avapritinib, two with grade 3 or higher (intracranial hemorrhage and subdural hematoma), leading to treatment discontinuation.

Ripretinib

Ripretinib (DCC-2618) uses a novel approach to treatment for GIST.[244,245] KIT has an interior switch pocket, with two portions of the kinase serving as an inhibitory switch (exon 11 juxtamembrane domain) or an activation switch (exon 17 activation loop). Mutations in exon 11 render the kinase constitutively active, which can fortunately be inhibited by approved kinase inhibitors that function as ATP-competitive inhibitors. However, mutations in exon 17 are not inhibited. Ripretinib is a switch-control tyrosine kinase inhibitor of KIT and PDGFRA, designed to block access to the switch pocket by the activation loop, rendering the kinase inactive and halting downstream activation. Ripretinib also inhibits PDGFRB, TEK, KDR, and BRAF kinases.[246] The first-in-human phase I study of ripretinib in 184 patients with GIST established the tolerated dose at 150 mg once daily.[247] Although no patients had complete response, 11.3% had partial response, and 61.3% had stable disease with ORR of 11.3%. The median duration of response was 18.4 months in the phase I study.

This subsequently led to the phase III INVICTUS double-blinded, randomized study that compared the efficacy of fourth-line ripretinib versus placebo in 154 patients with advanced GIST. This included patients who developed disease progression or had intolerance to imatinib, sunitinib and regorafenib; patients on placebo were permitted to cross over to the ripretinib arm at the time of disease progression. INVICTUS demonstrated significant improvement in PFS (6.3 months with ripretinib compared to 1.0 month with placebo).[248] The median OS in ripretinib arm was 15.1 months (compared to 6.6 months in placebo arm). In the ripretinib arm, 9.4% of patients had confirmed objective response (all partial responses) and 66% had stable disease. The most common treatment-related, treatment-emergent adverse events in patients receiving ripretinib were alopecia (49%), myalgia (27%), nausea (25%), fatigue (24%), palmar-plantar erythrodysesthesia (hand-foot syndrome, 21%), and diarrhea (20%). The most common grade 3 or 4 treatment-related treatment-emergent adverse events for ripretinib were lipase elevation (5%), hypertension (4%), fatigue (2%), and hypophosphatemia (2%). There was one treatment-related death in the ripretinib arm, with unknown cause of death (the patient died in sleep). Treatment-related serious adverse events were reported in 9% of patients on ripretinib. Treatment-related adverse events leading to dose reduction was reported in 6% and discontinuation in 5% of patients on ripretinib. The findings of INVICTUS study led to FDA approval in 2020 for ripretinib (Qinlock) in patients with advanced GIST who have received three or more kinase inhibitors including imatinib. Ripretinib was endorsed by the European Medicines Agency in 2021. For patients who develop disease progression on ripretinib 150 mg once daily, the phase I study of intrapatient dose escalation demonstrated benefit at higher dose of 150 mg twice daily, with median PFS (from date of dose increase to disease progression or death) ranging from 3.3 to 5.6 months depending on the line of therapy.[249]

INTRIGUE was a phase III randomized study comparing ripretinib to sunitinib as second line for patients with advanced GIST who previously received imatinib. It did not achieve the primary endpoint of superior PFS; rather, PFS was similar for ripretinib (8.0 months) and sunitinib (8.3 months).[250] Specifically, no difference in PFS was observed in *KIT* exon 11 mutant GIST, although ripretinib did have higher objective response rate (23.9%) compared to sunitinib (14.6%) for this cohort. Patients on ripretinib reported fewer grade 3 or 4 treatment-emergent adverse events compared to sunitinib (41.3% compared to 65.6%, respectively).

Alternative Agents

Several other agents have been evaluated in GIST, with a certain level of clinical efficacy demonstrated largely in limited phase II trials, which have not led to FDA approval. The review of all these agents is beyond the scope of this chapter. Some agents approved for alternative indications can have a role in patients with advanced disease who are physically well enough to continue therapy and for whom there is not an appropriate clinical trial option. Table 42.3 lists the agents and studies supporting their use.

Nilotinib is the best studied agent. Initial phase I data testing nilotinib alone or with imatinib demonstrated safety and tolerability, with some suggestion of activity.[251] Subsequent studies, including two phase III studies, were conducted that did not support its indication in GIST.[252,253] In first-line therapy in patients with metastatic GIST, compared to imatinib, nilotinib was found to be not as effective as imatinib, particularly for tumors with exon 9 mutations.[252] There has been much discussion of the phase III trial in patients with advanced disease who failed both imatinib and sunitinib that allowed ongoing kinase therapy in the control arm; had the study been placebo controlled, some have speculated the trial would have been positive for an improvement in PFS.[253]

Other single agent kinase inhibitors available (FDA approved for other indications) have some evidence of limited benefit in GISTs, including sorafenib, pazopanib, and dasatinib (primarily for *PDGFRA* D842V-mutant GIST) (see Table 42.3).[254–264]

TABLE 42.3 Non-FDA Approved Agents in the Management of Gastrointestinal Stromal Tumors

Agent	Disease Setting	Study Phase	References
Nilotinib		I/Ib	251
	Metastatic first line compared to imatinib	III	252
	Metastatic third line following progression on imatinib and sunitinib, compared to best supportive care and ongoing kinase therapy	III	253
Sorafenib	Second-line setting or beyond	II	255–257
Pazopanib	Third- and fourth-line setting	II	258, 259
Dasatinib	Third- and fourth-line setting	II	260
Everolimus	Second- and third-line setting	I/II	261
Cabozantinib	Metastatic following progression on imatinib and sunitinib	II	266
Dabrafenib	FDA approved for unresectable/metastatic tumors with *BRAF* V600E mutation in combination with trametinib (MEK inhibitor)	Case report	254
Larotrectinib	Approved for tumors with NTRK positive fusion	I	267
Entrectinib	Approved for tumors with NTRK positive fusion	I/II	268

Combination therapies have been assessed with the rationale of inhibiting the KIT pathway as well as another molecule in the same pathway or alternate pathway. Imatinib plus everolimus, an inhibitor of the serine-threonine kinase mTOR, was evaluated in patients who progressed following imatinib and at least one other TKI.[261] Investigators found that 37% of patients were free of progression when receiving imatinib 600 mg with everolimus 2.5 mg daily. The addition of the MEK inhibitor binimetinib to imatinib has been shown to be safe; a phase II study showed objective response rate of 69% with median PFS 29.9 months in patients with advanced GIST who were treatment-naïve.[265] The European Organization for Research and Treatment of Cancer phase II trial 1317 (CaboGIST) assessed the safety and activity of cabozantinib, a multitargeted TKI inhibitor that can overcome compensatory MET signaling occurring on TKI treatment, in patients with GIST who had progressed on imatinib and sunitinib.[266] This trial met its primary endpoint of progression free at week 12 of treatment in 24 of 41 patients, demonstrating partial response (14%) or stable disease (68%).

For rare patients with *BRAF* mutations, dabrafenib has demonstrated activity.[254] More recently, NTRK fusion positive tumors including GIST have been reported to respond to larotrectinib and entrectinib, leading to FDA approval in 2018 and 2019, respectively, for these agents.[267,268] The use of targeted agents highlights the importance of next-generation sequencing to identify actionable mutations. In addition, immune checkpoint inhibitors have been investigated in the use of GIST. A randomized phase II study of nivolumab or nivolumab + ipilimumab in patients with advanced/metastatic GIST refractory to at least imatinib showed stable disease in 52.6% of nivolumab-treated patients and complete response and stable disease in 6.7% and 25.0%, respectively, of patients treated with nivolumab + ipilimumab, but the primary endpoint of response rate >15% was not observed.[269] This suggests that a combination regimen of immunotherapy with a targeted agent may be needed to elicit response in metastatic GIST. Additional novel treatment strategies under investigation such as antibody-drug conjugates and radioligand therapies have been recently reviewed.[4]

SPECIAL CONSIDERATIONS

Imaging of Clonal Progression

When monitoring malignancies for disease response to therapy, progression is associated with an increase in size of disease. In clinical research this has been standardized with the use of RECIST criteria that defines progression as an increase of measurable lesions by 20% or more, as well as the appearance of new disease.[270] As discussed above (see the "CT and MRI" section), with the use of TKI therapy in GIST, benefit from therapy can also be assessed by a decrease in tumor density using CHOI criteria. Within metastatic lesions that are responding, progression can be identified with the development of a new nodule that has increased density or enhancement.[271] Genomic studies of these new lesions have identified new mutations accounting for resistance to therapy and thus progression.[272] Review of CT and MRI imaging must be done with care to identify these lesions.

Carney Triad and the Carney-Stratakis Dyad

The Carney triad was first described in the 1970s.[273] Young patients, often females, were reported to present with gastric leiomyosarcomas, paragangliomas, and pulmonary chondromas.[274] We now appreciate that the gastric tumors were GISTs, often multifocal with lymph node involvement.[274] The description of the triad has evolved and may now include adrenal adenomas and esophageal leiomyomas.[275] The Carney-Stratakis dyad (Carney-Stratakis syndrome) was described and included patients with a family history of paragangliomas and GIST.[276,277] Both of these syndromes have GIST that lack mutations in *KIT* or *PDGFRA*; they are characterized by lack of expression of SDHB by immunohistochemistry staining. Evaluation of these tumors and genetic testing has identified that tumors that are part of the dyad carry mutations in the SDH family of genes, whereas those associated with the triad do not have such mutations.[98] For clinicians and patients, the importance of the distinction is imperative. Patients who present with gastric GISTs that are found to lack SDHB expression by immunohistochemistry staining require a referral for genetic counseling to determine if the patient has the dyad with a germline mutation; those with the dyad need ongoing screening for paragangliomas that can occur in the neck, chest, and abdomen, as well as consideration of genetic counseling and screening of other family members.

Management of patients with SDH-deficient GIST has unique features. These tumors are often multifocal and can present with bleeding. At presentation, it is not unusual to find lymph node metastases and they can metastasize to the liver. However, their clinical course can be quite indolent, so care of these patients must balance the control of symptoms with the potential morbidity of symptoms. Aggressive gastric resections to eradicate disease are not recommended; rather, these patients are best managed with selective surgical procedures to manage lesions that are causing symptoms.[278]

For patients who do have disease that is metastatic and progressing, the benefit of kinase inhibitors is not entirely clear. This is in part because of the evolution of tumor mutation testing. Earlier studies used assays that missed mutations in *KIT* or *PDGFRA* or did not even require testing. Although there are reports of imatinib being of benefit,[60,215,216] it is now believed that for most patients it is ineffective. There are reports of benefit for sunitinib and regorafenib in patients with SDH-deficient GIST, including a phase II study evaluating first-line regorafenib in wild-type GIST (NCT02638766).[236,279] The potential utility of temozolomide is discussed in the section on molecular pathogenesis.

Familial Gastrointestinal Stromal Tumors

In addition to the Carney-Stratakis dyad, GIST can rarely be associated with familial inheritance patterns.[39,53,54,77–79,277] In several of these families, *KIT* mutations have been reported. These familial cases tend to have autosomal-dominant germline mutations, and the GISTs seen in affected members tend to be multifocal. Additional clinical characteristics of affected family members include cutaneous lesions such as hyperpigmentation or skin lesions that resemble the clinical appearance of urticaria pigmentosa. These skin pigmentation abnormalities may be due to the effect of the mutationally activated KIT kinase function on melanocyte growth and development. The mechanisms whereby such pigmentation disorders remain focal rather than disseminated may provide clues as to why GIST lesions may take decades to appear in these rare familial cases.

It should be noted that there also are reports of familial PDGFRA-associated mutations. Familial cases of GIST have also been identified with germline *PDGFRA* mutations[77–79]; members of the family with the mutation were noted to have large hands as well as GIST in contrast to nonaffected family members. Another case of a germline *PDGFRA* mutation described an association with multiple fibrous polyps and lipomas of the intestine.[78] More recently, a PDGFRA Mutant syndrome has been described that includes GIST, inflammatory fibroid polyps and fibrous tumors.[79] This syndrome is associated with mutations in *PDGFRA* exon 14, which is an uncommon mutation in GIST.

Other Genetic Tumor Syndromes Associated With Gastrointestinal Stromal Tumors

Patients with neurofibromatosis type I (NF1) have an increased risk of GIST, as well as other malignancies.[280–283] Molecular analysis of GIST lesions arising in patients with NF1 has documented that these GISTs often do not harbor detectable mutations in the *KIT* or *PDGFRA* gene, but molecular testing should still be performed.[280,281] Tumors with the classic mutations respond to standard therapies as would be expected. For those that do not have the typical genetic alterations, systemic therapy with standard agents appears to have limited benefit, although the literature on outcomes in this small subset of tumors is very limited. One would not anticipate response based on targeting KIT and PDGFRA, but the antiangiogenic effects may have some utility. In NF1-driven tumors, the disease may present with multifocal lesions in the abdominal cavity, with an indolent course over time. Surgery is performed if feasible; otherwise, watchful waiting is a very reasonable option in this group of patients.

Gastrointestinal Stromal Tumors in Children

GISTs rarely can affect children.[99,284,285] Pediatric GISTs typically are what was formerly called wild-type GISTs and now are understood to be SDH-deficient GISTs. Initial evaluation of these tumors identified few molecular alterations.[99,285] Guidelines for GISTs in children and young adults have been published.[286]

Full references for this chapter can be found at https://ebooks.health.elsevier.com/.

43 Neuroendocrine Tumors

Jonathan R. Strosberg, Taymeyah Al-Toubah

IN THIS CHAPTER

Neuroendocrine tumors (NETs) originate from the diffuse neuroendocrine system discussed in Chapter 4.[1,2] Gastroenteropancreatic NETs (GEP-NETs) can originate in the GI tract (GI-NETs, also known as carcinoid tumors) and pancreas (pNETs). GEP-NETs are characterized by a propensity to produce hormones and other vasoactive substances. Tumors that secrete hormones resulting in a clinical syndrome are also known as "functional tumors" (Table 43.1),[3–18] whereas tumors that are nonsecretory or secrete inactive proteins are termed "nonfunctional." GI-NETs and pNETs have many similarities, and in these similar areas, they are discussed together. Where there are important differences, they are discussed separately.

HISTORICAL ASPECTS

Langerhans described the histology of a carcinoid tumor in 1869. Lubarsch in 1888 described ileal carcinoid tumors at autopsy. The term *carcinoid* (karzinoide) was coined by Oberndorfer to describe a tumor that was less aggressive than an adenocarcinoma.[19] Scholte in 1931 described the carcinoid syndrome in a patient experiencing edema, sweating, flushing, and diarrhea, with a 1-cm ileal carcinoid and a thickened tricuspid valve. Lembeck in 1952 showed that the enterochromaffin (EC) cell, described by Kulchitsky in 1897, was the putative carcinoid cell of origin and synthesized and secreted serotonin.[19] The first pancreatic hormone-producing tumor syndrome was described in 1927 (5 years after the discovery of insulin) in a hypoglycemic patient with a metastatic islet cell tumor; extracts from the tumor had hypoglycemic effects.[20] Many other hormone-producing pNETs have since been described or proposed (see Table 43.1).

EPIDEMIOLOGY

The annual incidence of clinically significant GEP-NETs is rising significantly (Fig. 43.1). Data from the Surveillance, Epidemiology and End Results (SEER) 18 database (2000–2012) demonstrated an annual incidence of 3.56 per 100,000 for GEP-NETs and 0.84 per 100,000 for NETs of unknown primary site.[21] The incidence of GI-NET on autopsy is even higher at 8.4 per 10,000, demonstrating that many are clinically silent.[22–24] The principal cause of the rising incidence of NETs is not clear, as there are no known environmental risk factors. It is likely that this

TABLE 43.1 Syndromes Associated with Pancreatic Neuroendocrine Tumors[a]

Syndrome	Incidence/10^6/Year	Symptoms/Signs	Malignancy (%)	Hormone
Insulinoma	1-2	See Table 43.5	<10	Insulin
Gastrinoma (ZES)	0.5-1.5	See Table 43.6	60-90	Gastrin
VIPoma (Verner-Morrison syndrome, WDHA, pancreatic cholera)	0.05-0.2	See Table 43.7	>60	VIP
Glucagonoma	0.01-0.1	See Table 43.7	50-80	Glucagon
GRFoma	Unknown	Acromegaly	>30	GH-RF
ACTHoma	Uncommon	Ectopic Cushing syndrome	>95	ACTH
pNET secreting PTH-rP	Rare	Symptoms from hypercalcemia	84	PTH-rP
Pancreatic carcinoid tumor	Rare (<1% of all carcinoids)	Carcinoid syndrome (see Table 43.11)	77	Serotonin, tachykinins
pNET secreting renin	Rare	Hypertension	Unknown	Renin
pNET secreting erythropoietin	Rare	Polycythemia	Unknown	Erythropoietin
pNET secreting luteinizing hormone	Rare	Masculinization (female) Loss of libido (male)	Unknown	Luteinizing hormone
pNET secreting cholecystokinin (CCKoma)	Rare	Diarrhea, gallstones, peptic ulcer, weight loss	Unknown	CCK

[a]These syndromes may also be caused by a GI-NET (carcinoid).
GH-RF, Growth hormone–releasing factor; *PP*, pancreatic polypeptide; *PTH-rP*, parathyroid hormone–related protein; *VIP*, vasoactive intestinal polypeptide; *WDHA*, watery diarrhea, hypokalemia, achlorhydria.

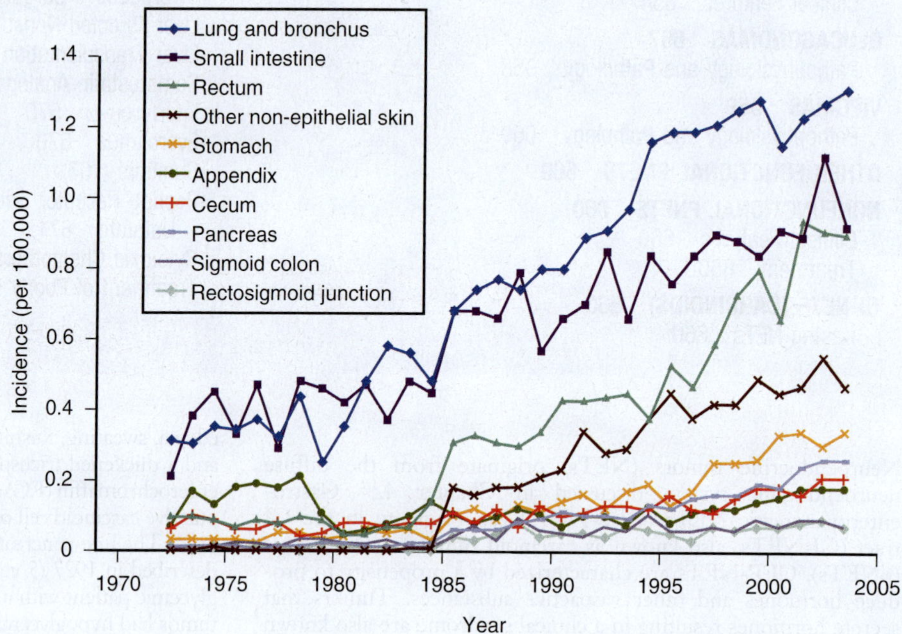

FIG. 43.1 Incidence of different subtypes of neuroendocrine tumors, 1970–2005. (From Modlin IM, Oberg K, Chung DC, et al. Gastroenteropancreatic neuroendocrine tumours. *Lancet Oncol.* 2008;9:61–72.)

increase is related to greater use of endoscopic procedures, increased imaging, and improved recognition of NETs by pathologists.[22–24]

pNETs account for 1%–10% of tumors arising in the pancreas.[25–27] The overall prevalence of functional pNETs is low, reported to be approximately 1 in 100,000.[5] In contrast, the prevalence of pNETs in autopsy studies is 0.5%–1.5%.[28] The annual incidence of pNETs is approximately 0.8 per 100,000.[24] The overall incidence of pNETs increases with age and peaks in the sixth and seventh decades. Nonfunctional pNETs account for 60%–80% of all pNETs in recent studies.[12,29,30] The incidence of functional pNETs varies, with insulinomas and gastrinomas representing the most common subtypes, with annual incidences of 0.5–3 in 1,000,000 (see Table 43.1).[12,31–34]

ORIGIN AND HISTOCHEMICAL FEATURES

GI-NETs arise from EC cells which form part of the diffuse neuroendocrine cell system scattered throughout the GI tract, respiratory tract, and other tissues[22,35]; pNETs may originate from the islets of Langerhans which are also a component of the diffuse neuroendocrine system.[12,36,37] Cells of this system share certain cytochemical properties and were originally proposed to have a common embryonic origin from neural crest cells, although more current studies support both a neural crest and endodermal origin.[35] Ultrastructurally, the neuroendocrine cells often have electron-dense granules that contain multiple regulatory hormones and amines, neuron-specific enolase, synaptophysin, and chromogranin.

GI-NETs and pNETs have marked histologic similarities.[38] Well-differentiated tumors consist of relatively homogeneous small round cells with uniform nuclei and cytoplasm, often arrayed in islets or trabeculae (Fig. 43.2). Mitotic figures are characteristically infrequent (<2 mitoses/high-power field), and necrosis is uncommon.[39] Malignancy can be determined only by metastases or tissue invasion and cannot be predicted by light microscopic or ultrastructural studies.[40] Controversy surrounds the exact cell of origin for pNETs.[36,41] pNETs are often called "islet cell tumors," but it is uncertain that they originate from the pancreatic islets.[11,34,36] These tumors frequently contain ductular structures, and they often produce hormones not normally present in the adult pancreas, such as gastrin and vasoactive intestinal polypeptide (VIP).[42] Finding of ductular structures in many pNETs and the budding off of endocrine cells from ductules during ontogenesis of the pancreas (see Chapter 57), has led to the speculation that these tumors are ductular in origin.[41] GI-NETs and pNETs can produce multiple GI hormones, which can be localized by immunocytochemical methods.[38,39] In many studies, most functional and nonfunctional GI-NETs (carcinoid) and pNETs have cells containing peptides that were not causing clinical symptoms.[39,42] It is unclear why usually only one syndrome or no clinical syndrome is seen, despite the presence of multiple hormones in the tumor.[40,42] As discussed later, a functional pNET syndrome or the carcinoid syndrome should, therefore, be diagnosed only if the appropriate clinical symptoms are present and not only based on immunocytochemistry alone.

Well-differentiated GI-NETs, pNETs, and respiratory tract NETs appear similar histologically. Thus predicting the site of the primary NET in a patient with a metastasis is difficult. Recent studies report that NETs from varying sites can differentially express transcription factors, including CDX-2, pancreatic and duodenal homeobox factor-1, TTF, PAX-1, and ISL-1. A panel of these factors can be used to localize the source of the primary NET from a metastatic focus.[43,44]

CLASSIFICATION

Tumors are classified by their grade and differentiation, which are vitally important prognostic markers. Grade refers to the proliferative activity of the tumor, measured using both mitotic rate and Ki-67 index. Differentiation refers to the extent to which tumor morphology resembles endocrine cells of origin. The term "carcinoma" is used to describe poorly differentiated histology. Poorly differentiated neuroendocrine carcinomas (NECs) are often characterized as sheets of pleomorphic cells with regions of necrosis.[45] NECs tend to be highly aggressive malignancies with high proliferative activity: Virtually all poorly differentiated carcinomas are high grade.

Well-differentiated GEP-NETs are classified as low grade defined as having 0–1 mitoses per 10 high-powered fields (HPF) and Ki-67 index of <3%, intermediate-grade tumors having a mitotic rate of 2–20 per 10 HPF or Ki-67 3%–20%, and high-grade tumors as having mitotic rate >20 per 10 HPF or Ki-67 index >20% (Table 43.2a).[46,47]

Formal TNM staging classifications have been introduced for GEP-NETs in the last decade by the American Joint Committee

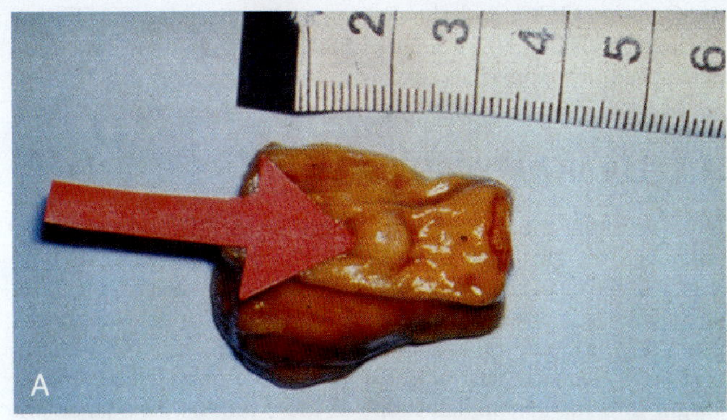

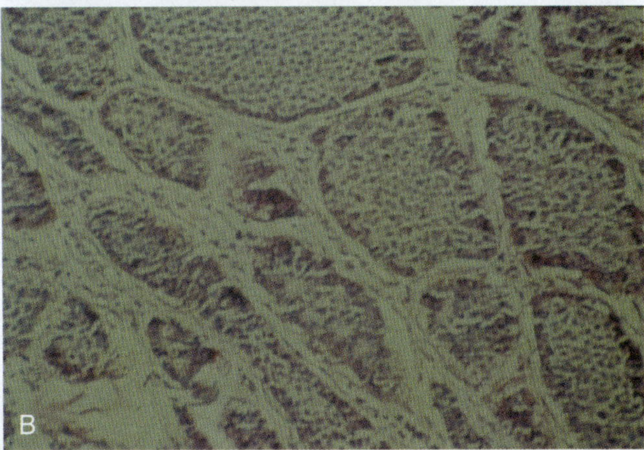

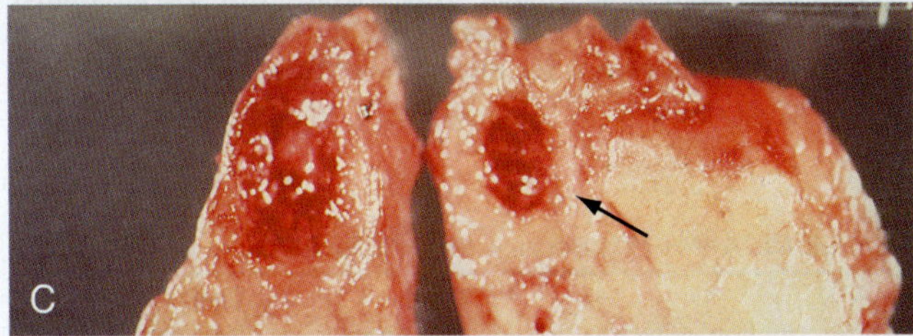

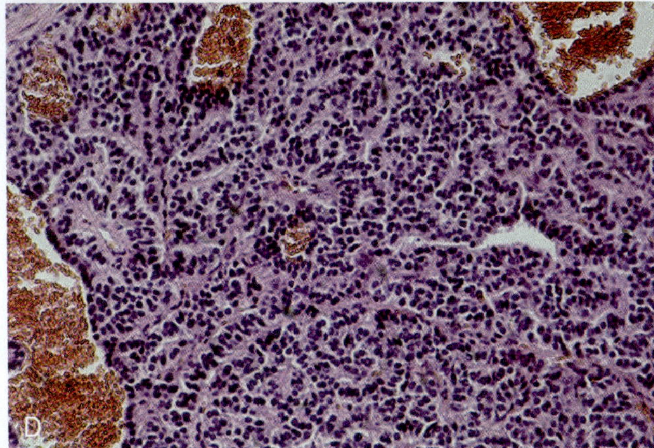

Fig. 43.2 Gross and histologic sections of a GI-NET (carcinoid) and a pNET. (A) Gross section of a carcinoid in the small intestine. The size is typical for primary small intestinal carcinoids, and the tumor is subepithelial in location. (B) Histopathology of a small intestinal carcinoid with its characteristic insular growth pattern. (H&E, ´80.) (C) Hemorrhagic and cystic 2-cm pNET (gastrinoma) in the tail of the pancreas (*arrow*). (D) Histopathology of gastrinoma, similar to that of other pNETs. This highly vascular tumor is composed of tubules of bland endocrine cells.

on Cancer (AJCC) and the European Neuroendocrine Tumor Society (ENETS). Validations of both staging systems have been performed on population and institutional databases.

MOLECULAR PATHOGENESIS

Until recently, the molecular pathogenesis of NETs was largely unknown.[48–51] In contrast to many nonendocrine GI tumors (e.g., colonic or pancreatic adenocarcinoma), mutations in common oncogenes (e.g., *ras*, *fos*, *myc*, *src*, and *jun*) and tumor suppressor genes (e.g., *p53* and *rb*) are rare in well-differentiated NETs.[12,28]

Recent genomic analyses of pNETs have provided significant insight into the genetic landscape of these tumors. In a landmark whole-exome study of 68 sporadic pNETs, somatic mutations of *MEN1* were observed in 44% of cases, whereas mutations in DAXX (death-domain-associated protein) or ATRX (α-thalassemia/mental retardation syndrome X-linked) were seen in 43%.[50]

All three genes are associated with chromatin remodeling. Also, 14% of samples had mutations in mammalian target of rapamycin (mTOR) pathway genes, including *PTEN*, *TSC2*, and *PIK3CA*. Similar findings were reported in a whole-genome sequencing study of 102 primary pNETs. Four dysregulated signaling pathways were described: (1) DNA damage repair; (2) chromatin remodeling; (3) telomere maintenance; and (4) mTOR activation. A higher-than-expected proportion of germline mutations was found in clinically sporadic pNETs, with mutations of *MUTYH*, *CHEK2*, and *BRCA2* occurring in 11% of patients.[52]

The precise sequence of gene mutations driving the development and progression of pNETs is currently unknown. Loss of DAXX/ATRX expression is associated with activation of the alternative lengthening of telomeres pathway and chromosomal instability. Additional mutations can accumulate over time and are associated with clinical progression. The genetic landscape of poorly differentiated pNECs is markedly distinct from well-differentiated pNETs. Mutations of *KRAS* and loss of Rb have been reported in 55% and 49% of patients with pNECs. Overall, frequency of mutations is substantially higher in NEC versus NET.[53]

The molecular landscape of GI-NETs is much less well understood than pNETs. Loss of chromosome 18 has been reported in over 60% of small intestinal (SI) NETs, but the biological significance of this alteration is uncertain.[54] Overall, a low mutational rate (0.1 somatic single nucleotide variants/10^5 nucleotides) has been observed in SI NETs, with mutations or deletions of the cyclin-dependent kinase inhibitor gene *CDKN1B* observed in 8% of patients.[55] Epigenetic changes appear to play a fundamental role in progression of SI NETs. Global DNA hypomethylation is a characteristic feature of SI NETs, whereas tumors with high methylation index tend to be clinically aggressive. Progressive changes in DNA methylation have been detected between primary tumors and their metastases.[56,57]

The mTOR pathway appears to be significantly dysregulated in many GEP-NETs, even in the absence of identifiable mutations in pathway components. mTOR is a serine/threonine kinase that modulates cell survival and proliferation, angiogenesis, and metabolism. Overexpression of mTOR and/or its downstream targets is frequently detected in NETs and is associated with poorer prognosis.[58] Expression of tuberous sclerosis-2 (TSC-2) and phosphatase and tensin homolog (PTEN), inhibitors of the mTOR pathway, is decreased in the majority of pNETs. Furthermore, decreased expression of TSC-2 and PTEN correlates with reduced survival.[59]

NETs are highly vascular tumors, and angiogenesis has been identified as a key event in NET progression. Overexpression of proangiogenic factors, including fibroblast growth factor (FGF), platelet-derived growth factor (PDGF), and vascular endothelial growth factor (VEGF), as well as of their receptors, has been reported.[60]

TABLE 43.2A WHO Classification for GI NETs: 2010

Differentiation	Grade	WHO Grading	WHO Nomenclature
Well differentiated	Low (G1)	<2 mitoses/10 HPF and <3% Ki-67 index	NET grade 1
	Intermediate (G2)	2–20 mitoses/10 HPF or 3%-20% Ki-67 index	NET grade 2
Poorly differentiated	High	>20 mitoses/10 HPF or >20% Ki-67 index	Neuroendocrine carcinoma, grade 3 (large-cell or small-cell type)

HPF, High-powered fields; *NET*, neuroendocrine tumors; WHO, World Health Organization.

MULTIPLE ENDOCRINE NEOPLASIA AND OTHER INHERITED SYNDROMES

MEN-1

MEN-1 (Wermer syndrome) is characterized principally by hyperparathyroidism, multifocal pancreaticoduodenal NETs, and pituitary adenomas. The genetic defect in MEN-1 is located on chromosome 11q13 and is caused by germline mutations in a 10-exon gene encoding for a 610–amino acid protein, menin (Table 43.3).[61,62] Menin is a nuclear protein that interacts with many proteins, including the AP-1 transcription factor, nuclear factor (NF)-κβ, RPA2 (a DNA processing factor), FAN CD2 (a DNA repair factor), and various cytoskeleton-associated proteins and histone-modifying enzymes.[61–63] Menin has important roles in transcriptional regulation, genomic stability, cell division, and cell cycle control.[61,63,64] The exact mechanism of carcinogenesis is unclear.[65,66]

Development of endocrine tumors in patients with MEN-1 conforms to Knudsen's[11,61] two-hit model theory of neoplasm,

TABLE 43.2B WHO Classification for GEP-NETs

Differentiation	Grade	WHO Grading	WHO Nomenclature
Well differentiated	Low (G1)	<2 mitoses/10 HPF and <3% Ki-67 index	NET grade 1
	Intermediate (G2)	2–20 mitoses/10 HPF or 3%-20% Ki-67 index	NET grade 2
	High (G3)	>20 mitoses/10 HPF or >20% Ki-67 index	NET grade 3
Poorly differentiated	High	>20 mitoses/10 HPF or >20% Ki-67 index	Neuroendocrine carcinoma, grade 3 (large-cell or small-cell type)

HPF, High-powered fields; *NET*, neuroendocrine tumors.

TABLE 43.3 Inherited GI Neuroendocrine Tumor Syndromes

Syndrome	Prevalence/10^5	Genetic Defect(s): Altered Protein(s)	NET Frequency	Types of pNET
Multiple endocrine neoplasia type 1 (MEN-1)	1-10	11q13: Menin, a 610–amino acid nuclear protein that interacts with pathways involved in cell growth, cell cycle regulation, genomic stability, and apoptosis	pNETs 80%-100% (microscopic), 20%-80% (clinical) Carcinoids: gastric (15%-35%), pulmonary (0%-8%), thymic (0%-8%)	NF-pNETs: 80%-100% microscopic; 0%-20% large) Functional pNETs: Gastrinoma (54%) Insulinoma (18%) Glucagonoma (3%) VIPoma (3%) GRFoma (<1%) SSoma (<1%)
von Hippel–Lindau Disease (VHL)	2-3	3p25: pVHL, a 232–amino acid protein that interacts with transcriptional factors that down-regulate HIF and VEGF	10%-17% (pNETs)	NF-pNETs: 98% Functional: 2%
Neurofibromatosis-1 (NF1, von Recklinghausen disease)	20-25	17q11.2: Neurofibromin, a 2484–amino acid protein that has Ras GTPase activity, binds microtubules, regulates mTOR growth, and induces cell cytoskeleton changes	0%-10% (duodenal carcinoids) Rare pNETs	SSomas
Tuberous sclerosis (Bourneville disease)	10	9q34 *(TSC1)* and 16p13 *(TSC2)*: Hamartin (1164–amino acid protein) and tuberin (1807–amino acid protein), which interact with the PI3K signaling cascade that regulates mTOR growth, GTPase activity affecting cell growth, energy regulation, response to hypoxia, and nutrients	Uncommon	NF-PETs > functional pNETs

GRF, Growth hormone-releasing factor; *GTP*, guanosine triphosphate; *HIF*, hypoxia-inducible factor; *mTOR*, mammalian target of rapamycin; *pNET*, pancreatic neuroendocrine tumor; *NF*, nonfunctional; *SS*, somatostatin; VEGF, vascular endothelial growth factor.

with an inherited (germline) mutation in one chromosome unmasked by a somatic deletion or mutation of the other normal chromosome, thereby removing the tumor suppressor effect of the normal gene product.[61,62] Numerous (>1300) different mutations have been described in *MEN1*, with over 75% of them being inactivating.[62]

Hyperparathyroidism is the most common clinical abnormality in patients with MEN-1 (Table 43.4).[61,67–69] Characteristically, hyperparathyroidism is the initial manifestation of MEN-1, usually presenting in the third decade of life, followed by the development of a pNET in the fourth to fifth decades.[61] Pituitary adenomas occur in roughly 20% of patients. Nonfunctional pNETs are nearly universal in patients with MEN-1, and pathology studies[12,61,68,70] have demonstrated that in almost every patient with MEN-1, the pancreas demonstrates diffuse microadenomatosis, with or without larger tumors. Among functional tumors, gastrinomas are most common (typically occurring in the duodenum). It is important to recognize when a patient with a pNET has MEN-1, because patients with and without MEN-1 differ in their clinical presentations, the need for family screening, the likelihood of surgical cure, and the clinical and diagnostic approach to the tumor.[61,71–73]

von Hippel–Lindau Disease

von Hippel–Lindau disease (VHL) is caused by a defect on chromosome 3p25 encoding for a 232–amino acid protein, pVHL, that forms a complex with a number of proteins that regulate ubiquitin-dependent proteolysis of large cell proteins and target the hypoxia-inducible factor (HIF)α.[74] VHL mutations result in altered transcriptional regulation, resulting in pathologic changes in angiogenic, growth, and mitogenic factors. Pancreatic lesions (primarily cysts) occur in 60% of VHL patients. pNETs are present in 10%–17% of patients with VHL. The pNETs are usually (>98%) asymptomatic and nonfunctional. The mean age at diagnosis of pNET in VHL is 29–38 years. Most patients have a single pNET that may be malignant.[75] Liver metastases occur in 9%–37% of VHL patients with pNETs.

Neurofibromatosis-1

NF1 is caused by a defect on chromosome 17q11.2 encoding for a 2845–amino acid protein, neurofibromin, which functions as a Ras signaling cascade inhibitor (see Table 43.3).[61,76] From 0% to 10% of NF1 patients develop a GI-NET (carcinoid), usually in the periampullary region of the duodenum.[61,77,78] These tumors frequently contain round calcium concretions (psammoma bodies) typical of somatostatinomas, although the somatostatinoma syndrome is rarely present. Metastases to liver and/or lymph nodes occur in 30%.[61,78]

Tuberous Sclerosis

Tuberous sclerosis is caused by mutations in either the 1164–amino acid protein, hamartin (TSC-1), or the 1807–amino acid protein, tuberin (TSC-2) (see Table 43.3).[61] These two proteins regulate the PI3K signaling cascade and the small guanosine triphosphatase–binding protein RHEB (Ras homolog enriched in brain), which play important roles in the regulation of protein translation and synthesis, growth, and proliferation, as well as maintenance of cellular energy levels. pNETs are present in 4% of patients with TSC-2.

FUNCTIONAL TUMORS

Insulinomas

Insulinomas are insulin-secreting pNETs that primarily originate in the pancreas and cause symptoms as a result of hypoglycemia (Table 43.5).

TABLE 43.4 Clinical Features of Patients With Multiple Endocrine Neoplasia Type I

Features	Frequency (%) [Range]
Hyperparathyroidism	97 [78-100]
Pancreatic endocrine tumor (any)	
• Any, including PPoma or nonfunctional	80-100
• Gastrinoma	54 [20-61]
• Insulinoma	18 [7-31]
• Glucagonoma	3 [1-6]
• VIPoma	1 [1-12]
• Somatostatinoma	0-1
• GRFoma	<1
Pituitary tumor	
• Any	60 [15-100]
• Prolactin-secreting	[15-46]
• Growth-hormone secreting	[6-20]
• ACTH-secreting (Cushing syndrome)	16
Adrenal cortical tumors	[27-36; symptoms <2]
Carcinoid tumor	
• Gastric (ECLoma)	[7-35; symptoms <5]
• Lung	[0-8]
• Thymus	[0-8]
Skin findings[a]	
• Angiofibroma	88
• Collagenoma	72
• Café-au-lait macules	38
• Lipomas	34
CNS tumor[a]	
• Meningioma	[0-8]
• Ependymomas and schwannomas	
Leiomyoma, leiomyosarcoma[a]	[1-7]
Thyroid adenoma[a]	5 [0-30]

[a]Symptomatic in <1%.

CNS, Central nervous system; *ECL*, enterochromaffin-like; *GRF*, growth hormone-releasing factor; *PP*, pancreatic polypeptide; *VIP*, vasoactive intestinal polypeptide.

Data modified from Jensen RT, Gardner JD. Gastrinoma. In: Go VLW, DiMagno E, Gardner JD, et al, eds. *The Pancreas: Biology, Pathobiology and Disease*. 2nd ed. New York: Raven Press; 1993:931–978; Jensen RT, Berna MJ, Bingham DB, et al. Inherited pancreatic endocrine tumor syndromes: advances in molecular pathogenesis, diagnosis, management, and controversies. *Cancer*. 2008;113:1807–1843; Thakker RV. Multiple endocrine neoplasia type 1. *Endocrinol Metab Clin North Am*. 2000;29:541–567; Gibril F, Schumann M, Pace A, et al. Multiple endocrine neoplasia type 1 and Zollinger-Ellison syndrome: a prospective study of 107 cases and comparison with 1009 cases from the literature. *Medicine (Baltimore)*. 2004;83:43–83; Gibril F, Jensen RT. Advances in evaluation and management of gastrinoma in patients with Zollinger-Ellison syndrome. *Curr Gastroenterol Rep*. 2005;7:114–121.

TABLE 43.5 Symptoms, Signs, and Laboratory Abnormalities in Patients With Insulinoma

	Frequency (%)
Anytime during the Clinical Course[a]	
Neuropsychiatric symptoms (loss of consciousness, confusion, dizziness, diplopia)	92
Confusion or abnormal behavior	80
Obesity	52
Amnesia or coma	47
Seizures (grand mal)	12
Cardiovascular symptoms, palpitations, tachycardia	17
GI symptoms (hunger, vomiting, abdominal pain)	9
During the First Attack[b]	
Neuroglycopenic symptoms	
• Visual disturbances (diplopia, blurred vision)	59
• Confusion	51
• Altered consciousness	38
• Weakness	32
• Transient motor defects, hemiplegia	29
• Dizziness	28
• Fatigue	27
• Inappropriate behavior	27
• Speech difficulty	24
• Headache	23
• Seizure	23
• Syncope	21
• Difficulty concentrating or thinking	19
• Paresthesia	17
• Memory loss	15
• Lethargy	12
• Amnesia	8
• Stupor	12
• Ataxia	4
• Disorientation	4
• Mental change	4
Adrenergic symptoms	
• Sweating	43
• Tremulousness	23
• Hunger, nausea	12
• Palpitations	10

[a]Data from Service FJ, Dale AJ, Elveback LR, et al. Insulinoma: clinical and diagnostic features of 60 consecutive cases. *Mayo Clin Proc*. 1976;51:417–429; Stefanini P, Carboni M, Patrassi N, et al. Beta-islet cell tumors of the pancreas: results of a study on 1,067 cases. *Surgery*. 1974;75:597–609.

[b]Data modified from Hirshberg B, Cochran C, Skarulis MC, et al. Malignant insulinoma: spectrum of unusual clinical features. *Cancer*. 2005;104:264–272.

Pathophysiology and Pathology

Insulinomas are almost always located in the pancreas.[12,28,31,39,79–81] Insulinomas are evenly distributed in the pancreas and are usually fairly small.[12,28,31,39,79–82] In one series, 39% were smaller than 1 cm and only 8% were larger than 5 cm.[82] Insulinomas occur as multiple tumors in only 2%–13% of patients,[28,82] in which case MEN-1 should be suspected.[61] Insulinomas are usually well encapsulated, firmer than normal pancreas, and highly vascular. Only 5%–16% of insulinomas are malignant.[83] Malignant insulinomas, generally large (average size, 6 cm in one series[84]), metastasize most often to the liver and/or regional lymph nodes.

Insulin is synthesized as preproinsulin by beta cells of the pancreatic islets in the rough endoplasmic reticulum. Proinsulin is liberated from preproinsulin and transferred to the Golgi apparatus.[32] Proinsulin, consisting of a 21–amino acid alpha chain and a 30–amino acid beta chain joined together by a 33–amino acid connecting peptide (C-peptide), is stored in beta cell secretory granules. Within these granules, a protease excises the C-peptide, and the C-peptide and the double-stranded insulin molecule are secreted in equimolar amounts.[32] Some proinsulin is also detected in normal subjects but represents less than 25% of total immunoreactive plasma insulin, whereas in almost all (>90%) patients with insulinomas, there are elevated proportions of proinsulin relative to total insulin.[85]

Clinical Features

Insulinomas usually occur in patients between 20 and 75 years of age; 60% are women.[10,12,28,31,39,79–81] Hypoglycemic symptoms are characteristically associated with fasting.[10,28,79–81] Symptoms may also occur during exercise. Hypoglycemia with fasting or exercise differs temporally from hypoglycemia that occurs after meals (postprandial hypoglycemia), which can be caused by many unrelated conditions.[86–91] The distinction between fasting hypoglycemia and postprandial (reactive) hypoglycemia can usually be made by a careful history.

Other less common causes of fasting hypoglycemia with hyperinsulinism from islet cell disease, besides insulinoma, include insulinomatosis, islet hyperplasia,[92] and nesidioblastosis.[93] In insulinomatosis, many macro and microadenomas expressing insulin are present with multiple small proliferative insulin-expressing mono-hormonal endocrine cell clusters.

Most symptoms of insulinomas[12,28,31,39,82] are caused by neuroglycopenia, because glucose is the main source of energy for the brain. Symptoms of hypoglycemia can also be caused by catecholamine release (adrenergic symptoms). Patients frequently learn to avoid symptoms by eating frequently, and obesity may result.[83] Neuroglycopenic symptoms can occur for several years before the diagnosis of insulinoma.[85]

Diagnosis

Keys to establishing the diagnosis of insulinoma are to suspect from the clinical history that the patient's symptoms could be caused by hypoglycemia and to establish a relationship of their symptoms to fasting.[10,12,28,31,39,79–81,90] Whipple triad, namely, hypoglycemic symptoms, hypoglycemia (blood sugar <50 mg/dL), and relief of symptoms following glucose ingestion, is not specific for insulinoma.[83] Following an overnight fast, fewer than 40% of patients with insulinoma have a blood glucose level below 50 mg/dL. However, if a fasting blood glucose determination is combined with a concomitant fasting plasma insulin level, this insulin level will be inappropriately elevated in 65% of patients with insulinoma.[12]

In patients lacking clear radiographic evidence of disease, an extended fast can be done, with blood glucose, plasma insulin, and C-peptide levels measured at 3–6-hour intervals.[10,12,28,31,39,79–81,90] Traditionally, a 72-hour fast is planned, but if at any point during the fast the patient becomes symptomatic, plasma insulin and glucose values should be determined before IV glucose is given and the test stopped. About 75%–80% of patients with an insulinoma will have symptoms and a blood sugar below 40 mg/dL within 24 hours of starting the fast, and almost 100% within 72 hours.[10,12,28,31,39,90] In healthy, nonobese fasted subjects, plasma insulin concentrations decrease to less than 6 μU/mL when blood glucose levels decrease to less than 40 mg/dL, and the ratio of plasma insulin (in μU/mL) to glucose (in mg/dL) remains less than 0.3. Thus a plasma insulin-to-blood glucose ratio over 0.3 is considered positive for insulinoma. In one study,[85] the most sensitive and specific criteria for diagnosing insulinoma during a 72-hour fast was the combination of a fasting glucose level below 45 mg/dL plus an elevated proinsulin level.

Multiple imaging studies can help localize insulinomas. These include multiphasic CT scans and EUS. Somatostatin receptor imaging, typically with the somatostatin receptor-2 analog Ga^{68} dotatate PET scan, is not routinely necessary unless metastases are suspected, or unless a suspected insulinoma cannot be detected using other methods. Invasive imaging studies using hepatic venous sampling after arterial calcium stimulation are rarely necessary to localize an occult insulinoma.

Treatment

Treatment of insulinoma consists of controlling symptoms of hypoglycemia, followed by tumor localization and resection. Tumor localization of all pNETs is discussed later, as is chemotherapy or other therapies directed at the tumor itself for the 5% –13% of patients with metastatic insulinoma.[84,94–97]

Medical Therapy

Hypoglycemia is controlled in most insulinoma patients by a combination of dietary and pharmacologic therapy.[10,12,28,31,39,83,97] Snack intake should not be restricted to rapidly absorbed carbohydrates, because their ingestion may occasionally stimulate insulin secretion from the tumor. More slowly absorbed forms of carbohydrates (starches, bread, potatoes, and rice) are preferable. During a hypoglycemic episode, however, rapidly absorbable carbohydrates such as fruit juices with glucose or sucrose are preferable. Occasionally, patients with severe hypoglycemia may require the use of a continuous IV infusion of glucose together with an increase in dietary carbohydrates.[12]

Diazoxide, a nondiuretic thiazide analog, has potent hyperglycemic effects.[10,12,96,98,99] It directly inhibits insulin release from beta cells through stimulation of α-adrenergic receptors and also has an extrapancreatic hyperglycemic effect that enhances glycogenolysis.[83] The GI side effects can be reduced by taking the diazoxide with a meal. Diazoxide should be initiated at an oral dose of 3–8 mg/kg/day, divided into 2 or 3 doses/day; if not effective, diazoxide can be increased to a maximum daily dose of 15 mg/kg. Adverse effects are dose related and may limit the ability to reach maximal doses. They include sodium retention/edema and GI symptoms such as nausea and hirsutism. Addition of a thiazide diuretic can correct the edema as well as augment the hyperglycemic effect of diazoxide. Somatostatin analogs (SSAs) can control symptoms of hypoglycemia in 40%–60% of patients with insulinoma. SSAs are thought to act primarily by interacting with somatostatin receptors on the tumor, especially subtypes 2 and 5.[100] The symptomatic response rate of insulinomas to octreotide is lower than that of other functional pNETs, because insulinomas generally have low levels of somatostatin receptors.[101] Because SSAs also decrease glucagon and growth hormone secretion, occasionally their administration may worsen the hypoglycemia.[94] Therefore closely monitored trials of short-acting octreotide are generally recommended prior to administration of long-acting depot formulations of octreotide or lanreotide. Everolimus, an mTOR inhibitor which causes hyperglycemia as a side effect, has been shown to be effective in controlling hypoglycemia in patients with metastatic insulinomas refractory to other therapies. Other cytotoxic systemic and liver-directed therapies (discussed later) can also control hypoglycemia in patients with metastatic insulinomas.[10,102]

Surgical Therapy

Because the large majority of insulinomas are localized,[103–105] surgical resection is curative in 70%–97% of patients.[12,98,106,107] Because insulinomas are almost invariably intrapancreatic and usually benign, insulinomas detected on imaging preoperatively are increasingly being resected successfully using a laparoscopic approach.[98,108,109]

GASTRINOMAS

ZES is caused by ectopic secretion of gastrin by a NET (gastrinoma), which causes excessive gastric acid secretion, characteristically causing peptic disease (often severe) and/or GERD.[110] This disease was first described in 1955 by Zollinger and Ellison in two patients with extreme acid hypersecretion and intractable PUD caused by a nonbeta cell tumor of the pancreas.

Pathophysiology and Pathology

Almost all the symptoms of ZES are caused by gastric acid hypersecretion (Table 43.6). PUD, GERD, and diarrhea disappear when gastric acid hypersecretion is controlled.[10,16,111,112] Parietal cell hyperplasia driven by hypergastrinemia increases the stomach's maximal acid secretory capacity, and the chronic hypergastrinemia also increases basal acid secretion, characteristic findings in ZES.[112] The high serum gastrin levels are trophic for the gastric mucosa, resulting in large gastric folds (Fig. 43.3) with not only parietal cell but also gastric EC-like (ECL) cell hyperplasia.[11,112–115] More than 99% of patients with ZES show some degree of ECL hyperplasia,[114–116] but the changes are generally much more advanced in the patients with MEN-1/ZES. Furthermore, type 2 gastric carcinoids (discussed later) are rarely seen in sporadic (non-MEN-1) ZES cases, whereas 23% of patients with MEN-1/ZES develop type 2 gastric carcinoid tumor(s).[116]

Increased gastric acid secretion results in diarrhea from direct acid damage in the small intestine. Furthermore, the low pH inactivates pancreatic lipase and can precipitate bile acids.[16] More than half of gastrinomas are found in the duodenum, with 56% of these occurring in the first portion and approximately 32%, 6%, and 4% in the second, third, and fourth portions of the duodenum, respectively.[71–73,81,111,117,118] Presently, 60%–90% of gastrinomas are found in the "gastrinoma triangle," an area formed by the junction of the cystic duct and bile duct posteriorly, the junction of the second and third parts of the duodenum inferiorly, and the junction of the pancreatic neck and body medially.[119] Gastrinomas rarely originate in a nonduodenal/nonpancreatic abdominal location.[120]

Lymph node primary gastrinomas are reported in up to 11% of sporadic cases of ZES.[81,111,121,122] Some patients with sporadic ZES remained normogastrinemic and apparently cured after a follow-up of 20 years following resection of only lymph node(s) containing gastrinoma. Based on lymph node or hepatic metastases, gastrinomas are malignant in 60%–90% of patients.[40,123] Bone metastases also occur in almost one-third of patients with tumors metastatic to the liver, most often to the pelvis, scapula, and ribs.[124]

Gastrinomas demonstrate two general growth patterns: aggressive disease (in 25%) and nonaggressive disease (in 75%).[27,110,125,126] In one study, predictors of hepatic metastases were a pancreatic (as opposed to a nonpancreatic) gastrinoma and a primary tumor size larger than 3 cm. Even among patients with gastrinomas that have metastasized to the liver, the tumor growth rate is highly variable.[127] Over 90% of duodenal gastrinomas are small (<1 cm), whereas only 8% of pancreatic gastrinomas are small. The difference in biological behavior and prognosis of duodenal and pancreatic gastrinomas has been used to support the hypothesis that they have different origins.[128]

TABLE 43.6 Clinical and Laboratory Features in Patients With ZES

	NIH	Range in Literature
Clinical Features		
Average age of onset (years)	41	41-53
Average duration of symptoms (years)	5.2	3.2-8.7
Male gender (%)	56	44-70
Abdominal pain (%)	75	26-98
Diarrhea (%)	73	17-73
History of confirmed PUD (%)	71	71-93
Heartburn (%)	44	0-56
Nausea (%)	30	8-37
Vomiting (%)	25	26-51
Bleeding (%)	24	8-75
MEN-1 (%)	22	10-48
Esophageal stricture (%)	4	4-6
GI perforation (%)	5	5-18
Laboratory Features (%)		
Fasting hypergastrinemia (%)	99	96-100
Positive secretin test (>120 pg/mL increase) (%)	94	94
BAO >15 mEq/h (no prior gastric surgery) or >5 mEq/h (prior gastric surgery) (%)	93	43-100

BAO, Basal acid output; *MEN-1*, multiple endocrine neoplasia type 1; *NIH*, National Institutes of Health.

Data from Gibril F, Schumann M, Pace A, et al. Multiple endocrine neoplasia type 1 and Zollinger-Ellison syndrome: a prospective study of 107 cases and comparison with 1009 cases from the literature. *Medicine (Baltimore)*. 2004;83:43–83; Osefo N, Ito T, Jensen RT. Gastric acid hypersecretory states: recent insights and advances. *Curr Gastroenterol Rep*. 2009;11:434–41; Berna MJ, Hoffmann KM, Serrano J, et al. Serum gastrin in Zollinger-Ellison syndrome: I. Prospective study of fasting serum gastrin in 309 patients from the National Institutes of Health and comparison with 2229 cases from the literature. *Medicine (Baltimore)*. 2006;85:295–340; Berna MJ, Hoffmann KM, Long SH, et al. Serum gastrin in Zollinger-Ellison syndrome: II. Prospective study of gastrin provocative testing in 293 patients from the National Institutes of Health and comparison with 537 cases from the literature. evaluation of diagnostic criteria, proposal of new criteria, and correlations with clinical and tumoral features. *Medicine (Baltimore)*. 2006;85:341–364; Gibril F, Jensen RT. Advances in evaluation and management of gastrinoma in patients with Zollinger-Ellison syndrome. *Curr Gastroenterol Rep*. 2005;7:114–21; Rogers A, Wang LM, Karavitaki N, et al. Neurofibromatosis Type 1 and pancreatic islet cell tumours: an association which should be recognized. *QJM*. 2015;108:573–576.

Clinical Features

The clinical features of ZES are summarized in Table 43.6.[129] Abdominal pain primarily caused by PUD remains the most frequent early symptom. Ulcer pain is clinically indistinguishable from that seen in patients with other forms of PUD.[40,111,129] The diagnosis may be suggested when ulcer-like symptoms become persistent, refractory to medication, or associated with complications (see Fig. 43.3).[10,130] Most patients with ZES have a typical duodenal ulcer at diagnosis. This is an important difference from older studies, where over 90% of patients presented with PUD, often with multiple ulcers or in atypical locations.[112,123,131] In older

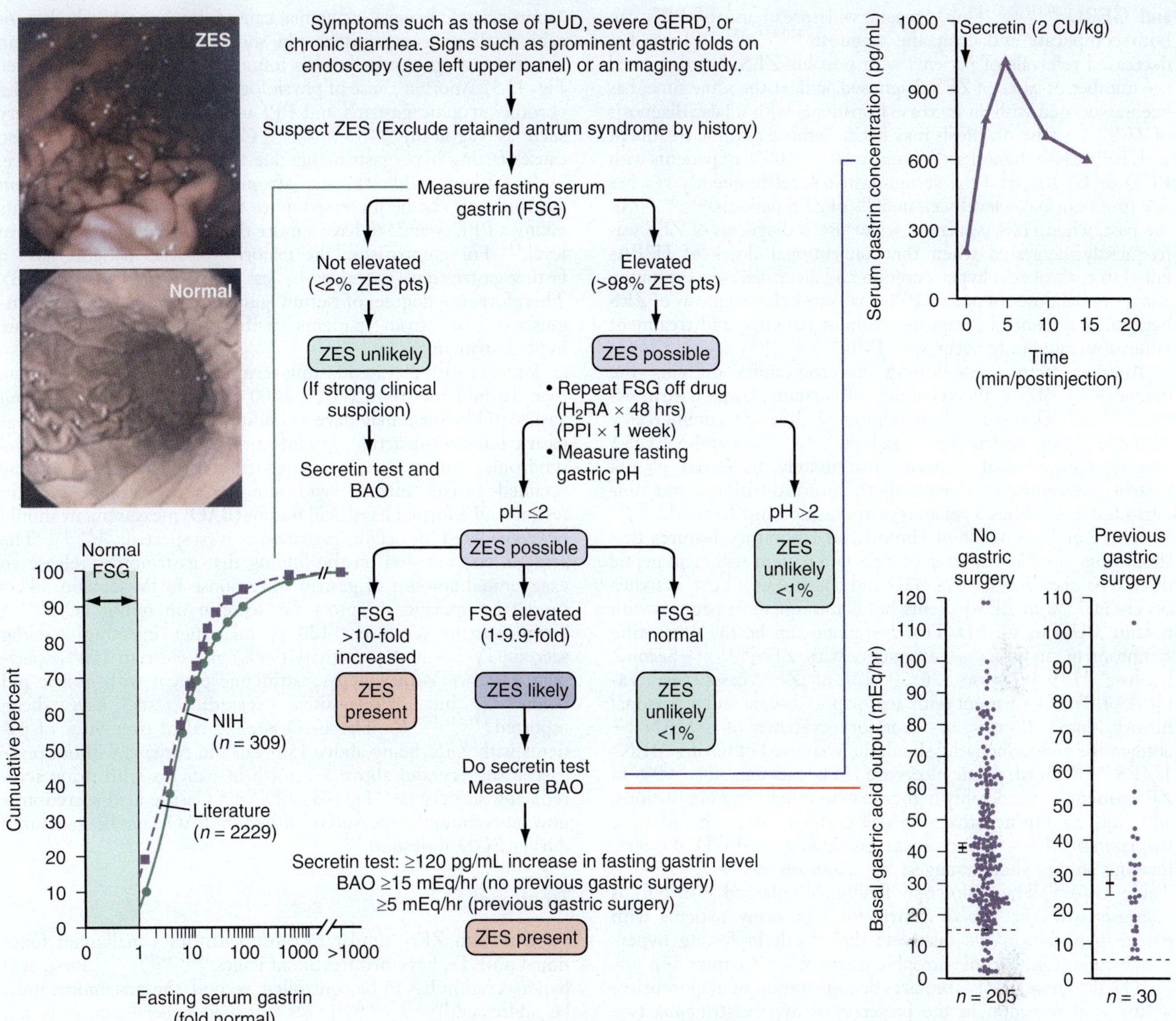

Fig. 43.3 Algorithm for the diagnosis of *ZES*. (*Right upper*) Typical *ZES* patient with a positive secretin test result (i.e., ≥120-pg/mL increase in fasting gastrin level). (*Right lower*) Marked elevations in mean basal acid output *(BAO)* with or without previous gastric acid–reducing surgery. The *dotted horizontal lines* show the proposed criterion of >15 or >5 mEq/h proposed to distinguish patients with ZE from those without ZES. (*Left upper*) Prominent gastric folds found on endoscopy in a ZES patient, compared with a normal subject. (*Left lower*) Fasting serum gastrin levels in ZES expressed as a multiple of the upper limit of normal on the horizontal axis. Very few patients had normal values; 60% had less than 10-fold serum gastrin increases.[40,73,130,142,150] *CU*, Clinical units.

studies, up to 100% of patients presented with, or developed, a complication of peptic disease (bleeding, perforation, obstruction, penetration, esophageal stricture). Presently, fewer than 30% of patients develop these complications, even though most have a confirmed history of PUD.[129]

Diarrhea occurs with abdominal pain in 28%–56% of cases and may be the only initial symptom in 10% of patients.[10,129] Nearly one in three patients presents with GERD as the initial manifestation, and approximately half of patients have GERD symptoms and/or esophageal pathology at initial evaluation.[129,132]

One in four patients with ZES has MEN-1, but the clinical presentation is similar to that of those with sporadic ZES.[61,68,73,133] Clues that should suggest the possibility of MEN-1/ZES as opposed to sporadic ZES include (1) a history of nephrolithiasis and/or renal colic (47% vs. 4%); (2) presentation at a younger age (mean, 34 vs. 43 years); and (3) personal or family history of certain endocrinopathies (see Table 43.4). In a review of patients with MEN-1/ZES,[68] close to 90% had hyperparathyroidism, 31%–60% pituitary disease, 6%–30% various other NETs (typically lung), and 6%–16% had other functional pNETs.[61,68]

Diagnosis

Despite the widespread availability of serum gastrin assays, diagnosis of ZES continues to be delayed by 4–6 years after onset of symptoms.[68,129,134] This delay occurs for many reasons. Because ZES is so rare (see Table 43.1), it is often not considered. Second, ZES is usually indistinguishable from other patients with PUD and GERD.[40,112,133] Third, recent widespread use of PPIs can both complicate and delay the diagnosis.[130,134–137] PPI use has decreased referrals of patients with possible ZES, has decreased the number of cases of ZES diagnosed, and, at the same time, has been associated with an increase in patients with a false diagnosis of ZES.[137] A false diagnosis may occur because chronic treatment with PPIs causes hypergastrinemia in 80%–100% of patients with PUD or GERD, and the serum gastrin level frequently reaches five times normal, a level seen in 60% of ZES patients.[130,134–136] In the past, when H2RAs were in wider use, a diagnosis of ZES was frequently suggested when the conventional doses of H2RAs failed to control acid hypersecretion and ulcer disease.[7] Presently, conventional doses of potent PPIs may mask the diagnosis of ZES because they control symptoms in most patients, and treatment failures uncommonly occur with PPIs.[10,129,134,138]

Another factor complicating and sometimes delaying the diagnosis of ZES is the reliability of current plasma gastrin assays.[134,139,140] One study[139] examining 12 different commercially available plasma gastrin kits (7 radioimmunoassays and 5 ELISA assays) reported that 7 assays inaccurately measured plasma gastrin concentrations, with both overestimations and underestimations. Thus a reliable gastrin assay must be used.[134,139]

There are a number of clinical and laboratory features that should suggest the diagnosis of ZES in a patient with acid peptic disease or diarrhea (see Fig. 43.3 and Table 43.6). First, diarrhea occurs in 73% of ZES patients but is infrequent in patients with routine PUD or GERD. Diarrhea alone can be the presenting symptom in up to 27% of patients with ZES.[40,112,129] Second, because MEN-1 causes 20%–25% of ZES cases (see Table 43.4),[61,68] any patient with acid peptic disease and a personal history, family history, or laboratory evidence of a MEN-1–compatible endocrinopathy should be suspected of having MEN-1/ZES.[68,134] Third, peptic ulcers are Hp negative in 50%–90% of ZES patients, considerably higher than in other ulcer populations, and thus an Hp-negative, NSAID-negative ulcer should raise suspicion of ZES.[10,141] Prominent gastric folds on EGD of gastric imaging studies should suggest the diagnosis (see Fig. 43.3 and Table 43.6).[129] The endoscopic finding of enlarged gastric folds contrasts with the loss of gastric folds in many patients with gastric hypochlorhydric disorders that result in fasting hypergastrinemia (e.g., chronic atrophic gastritis; see Chapter 54).

The diagnosis of ZES requires demonstration of inappropriate gastric acid secretion in the presence of hypergastrinemia (see Fig. 43.3).[10,40,118,131,134,136] Fasting hypergastrinemia occurs in 97%–99% of patients with ZES.[142] Hence, if the fasting serum gastrin level is normal, especially in repeated determinations, a diagnosis of ZES is very unlikely. Therefore the fasting serum gastrin should be the first study performed when ZES is suspected.[10,98,134,136,139,140] Because PPIs can elevate fasting serum gastrin levels, overlapping with plasma gastrin levels in the majority of ZES patients, it can be difficult to diagnose ZES when the patient is taking a PPI.[12,73,134–137,143,144] If the fasting gastrin level is elevated while taking a PPI, the general approach is to recommend that the measurement be repeated after stopping the PPI for at least a week (see Fig. 43.3).[12,134–136,143,144] However, if the patient has ZES, abruptly stopping a PPI can lead to rapid development of peptic complications. For this reason, one study suggested PPIs not be stopped and that the diagnosis of ZES be pursued by finding other signs of gastrinoma (e.g., a pNET on imaging) or by trying to taper the PPI dose in some fashion.[145] In rare circumstances, referral to a special center with experience in PPI drug withdrawal and its potential hazards is warranted.[98,134,136,146]

Achlorhydria, whether due to disease (e.g., chronic atrophic gastritis) or PPI use, is a far more common cause of fasting hypergastrinemia than ZES and can lead to a false-positive secretin test.[147] In one study of ZES patients,[131] 99% had a fasting gastric pH below 2. Therefore to exclude physiologic, "appropriate" hypergastrinemia caused by hypochlorhydria or achlorhydria) fasting gastric pH should be the next step if an elevated fasting gastrin level is found and ZES is suspected (see Fig. 43.3). Another cause of physiologic hypergastrinemia (besides chronic atrophic gastritis and PPI use) is acid-reducing surgery such as vagotomy.[10,40,98,130,134,136] Chronic kidney disease also causes fasting hypergastrinemia due to reduced gastrin clearance.

In patients with chronic atrophic gastritis, fasting serum gastrin levels can be increased more than 70-fold, and in patients taking a PPI, over 25% have a more than fourfold elevated gastrin level.[134] For comparison, the majority of ZES patients have a fasting gastrin level increased by less than 10-fold (see Fig. 43.3). Therefore no degree of serum gastrin elevation alone distinguishes ZES from patients with physiologic, appropriate hypergastrinemia.[134]

Patients with elevated fasting serum gastrin levels that are less than 10-fold increased (i.e., <1000 pg/mL) and with a fasting gastric pH below 2 may have a condition other than ZES, such as gastric outlet obstruction, Hp infection, renal failure, short bowel syndrome, antral G cell hyperfunction or hyperplasia, or the retained gastric antrum syndrome. In such patients, secretin testing and a formal basal acid output (BAO) measurement should be considered if occult gastrinoma is suspected.[134,142,148] The secretin test is based on the finding that gastrinomas release an exaggerated amount of gastrin in response to IV secretin, likely caused by specific receptors for secretin on tumor cells.[149] A serum gastrin increase >120 pg/mL after injecting 2 U/kg secretin IV has high sensitivity (94%) and close to 100% specificity (100%).[150] In a hypergastrinemic patient with gastric pH below 2, no false-positive secretin tests have been reported.[131,148,150–152] The BAO is elevated in over 90% of patients with ZES, being above 15 mEq/h in patients without prior gastric surgery and above 5 mEq/h in patients with prior acid-reducing surgery (see Fig. 43.3).[40,131,152] Gastric acid secretion is now uncommonly measured, although BAO can be measured during EGD if desired.[153]

Treatment

Patients with ZES, similar to those with other malignant functional pNETs, have two treatment issues.[10,73,94,98,146,152] First, acid hypersecretion has to be controlled; second, the gastrinoma must be addressed.[10,40,71,73,96,98,117,118,152] If acid hypersecretion is not controlled, life-threatening complications of peptic disease almost invariably occur, sometimes rapidly.[10,40,123,130,134,152,154] Even though most patients now receive some form of gastric antisecretory treatment prior to the diagnosis of ZES, almost 25% develop bleeding, 6%–7% experience ulcer perforations, and 8%–10% develop esophageal strictures.[12,129] With improved ability to control gastric hypersecretion medically, the natural history of the tumor is becoming the major determinant of long-term survival (Fig. 43.4).[110,126]

Control of Gastric Acid Hypersecretion

Because of their long duration of action and potency, PPIs allow once- or twice-daily dosing in most ZES patients (>95%) and are the drugs of choice.[10,40,73,152,155–157] All PPIs (omeprazole, lansoprazole, pantoprazole, esomeprazole, and rabeprazole) are effective.[10,152,155,156] H2RAs are also effective, although higher than conventional doses are usually required.[10,111,152]

For most ZES patients, a PPI is usually started at a dosage equivalent to 60 mg/day of omeprazole. Sufficient antisecretory drug needs to be given to reduce acid hypersecretion, measured during the hour prior to the next dose of drug, to less than 10 mEq/h in patients without prior gastric acid-reducing surgery or to less than 5 mEq/h in patients with prior gastric acid–reducing surgery. This degree of acid suppression allows peptic lesions to

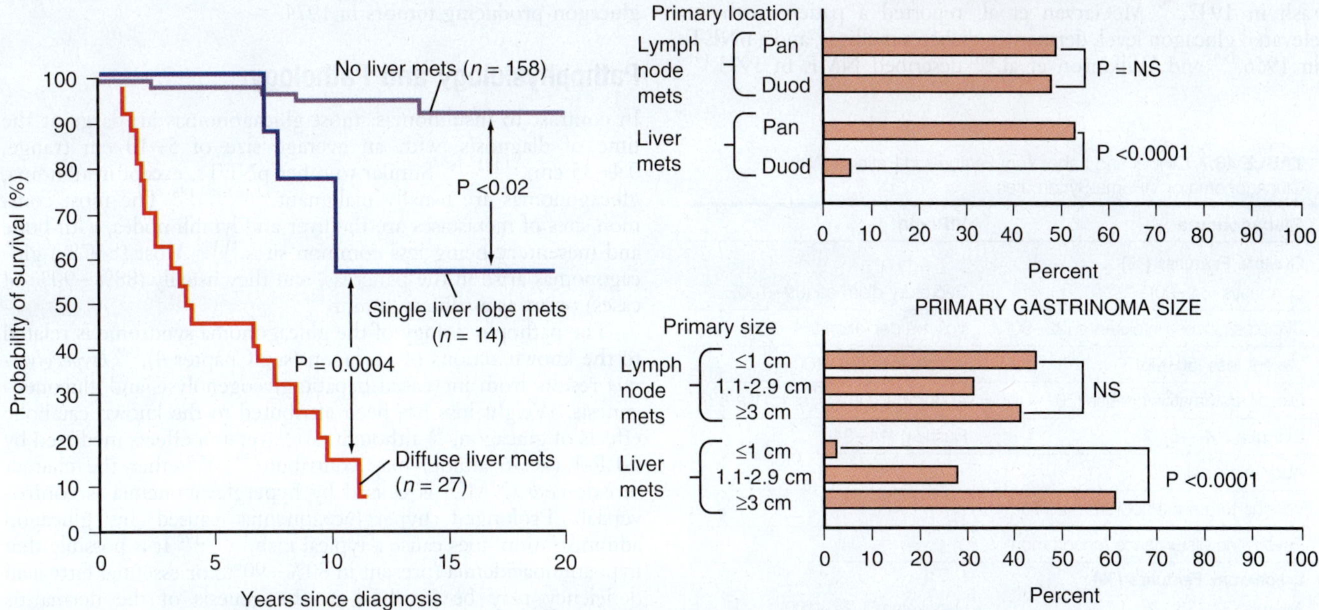

Fig. 43.4 Effects of gastrinoma extent on survival and of primary gastrinoma location and size on the development of lymph node or liver metastases (mets). (*Left*) Survival in patients with ZE syndrome, with or without liver metastases. *Right, upper part* shows the percentage of 83 patients with primary pancreatic or duodenal gastrinomas who developed lymph node or liver metastases. *Lower part* shows percentage of 118 patients with primary gastrinoma of varying diameter who developed lymph node or liver metastases. (*Left, adapted* from Yu F, Venzon DJ, Serrano J, et al. Prospective study of the clinical course, prognostic factors, causes of death, and survival in patients with long-standing Zollinger-Ellison syndrome. *J Clin Oncol.* 1999;17:615–30; (*Right,* adapted from Weber HC, Venzon DJ, Lin JT, et al. Determinants of metastatic rate and survival in patients with Zollinger-Ellison syndrome: a prospective long-term study. *Gastroenterology.* 1995;108:1637–49)

heal and prevents their recurrence. Although initial lower doses of PPIs are frequently used, these higher doses are recommended because of the desirability of rapidly controlling the acid hypersecretion in ZES patients.[158]

In some patients, such as those with MEN-1/ZES, severe GERD, or a previous Billroth II resection, a higher initial PPI dose equivalent to 60 mg twice daily of omeprazole is recommended.[98,132,152] Such patients require greater acid suppression, and antisecretory drugs should be increased to control symptoms and heal all mucosal lesions, which frequently require acid suppression to 1–2 mEq/h or even lower.[159] *Parathyroidectomy* in patients with MEN-1/ZES and hyperparathyroidism decreases fasting gastrin levels, decreases BAO, and increases sensitivity to antisecretory drugs.[40,134,160,161] This intervention is particularly important because, as mentioned earlier, patients with MEN-1/ZES with hyperparathyroidism can be relatively resistant to PPIs given the stimulatory effect of calcium on acid secretion.[152,156,157]

Long-term oral antisecretory treatment has remained effective for over 10 years without development of tachyphylaxis.[40,111,130,152,155,157] Concerns have been raised about the safety of PPIs,[162–167] but issues such as iron deficiency from iron malabsorption and increased risks of GI-NETs (carcinoid) have not been significant in clinical series. Vitamin B_{12} deficiency can occur on PPI therapy and should be monitored yearly.

Treatment of Localized Gastrinoma

Most authorities recommend surgical exploration of ZES patients for a possible curative resection as long as (1) diffuse metastatic disease to the liver is absent and (2) the patient does not have MEN-1.[72,73,98,117,146,168,169] In patients with sporadic (non-MEN-1) ZES, gastrinomas were found in 92%, and 51% of these resected patients were disease-free immediately after tumor resection; 34% were disease-free after 10 years.[72] This cure rate with surgery is much higher than rates reported in many earlier studies and is, in large part, the result of finding more small duodenal gastrinomas. Performing a duodenotomy routinely at surgery identifies more tumors than other commonly used methods.[111,117,170–172] The role of curative surgery in patients with MEN-1/ZES is controversial because the postresection, disease-free cure rate in such patients is below 5% if a more aggressive resection (e.g., pancreaticoduodenectomy) is avoided.[61,71,73,98,169,173,174] This unfavorable surgical outcome occurs because MEN-1/ZES patients have multiple duodenal gastrinomas and frequently have lymph node metastases at surgery.[175] The role of surgery is controversial in part because it is unclear whether early surgical resection will alter survival in MEN-1/ZES. Some recommend routine exploration in patients with MEN-1/ZES, others recommend medical therapy only and no exploration, and still others recommend exploration only if larger lesions (>2–3 cm) are found.[98,146,173,176] Although pancreaticoduodenectomy can cure a high proportion of MEN-1/ZES patients,[177] it is not generally recommended[98,146,178] because of adverse effects of the operation and the excellent long-term prognosis of unoperated patients with small pNETs (<2 cm).

GLUCAGONOMAS

Glucagonomas are rare NETs (almost always pNETs) that secrete excessive amounts of glucagon and cause a distinct syndrome characterized by weight loss, glucose intolerance, anemia, and a specific dermatitis known as *necrolytic migratory erythema*

(NME) (Table 43.7). Becker et al. described a pNET with a skin rash in 1942,[179] McGarvan et al. reported a patient with an elevated glucagon level, dermatitis, diabetes mellitus, and a pNET in 1966,[180] and Wilkinson et al.[181] described NME in 1973.[181] Finally, Mallinson et al.[5] established the association of NME with glucagon-producing tumors in 1974.

TABLE 43.7 Clinical and Laboratory Features in Patients With Glucagonoma or VIPoma Syndromes

Glucagonoma	VIPoma
Clinical Features (%)	
Dermatitis (54–90)	Secretory diarrhea (89–100)
Diabetes/glucose intolerance (22–90)	Volume depletion (44–100)
Weight loss (56–96)	Weight loss (36–100)
Glossitis/stomatitis/cheilitis (29–40)	Abdominal cramps, colic (10–63)
Diarrhea (14–15)	Flushing (14–34)
Abdominal pain (12)	
Venous thromboembolism (12–35)	
Psychiatric disturbance (uncommon)	
Laboratory Features (%)	
Anemia (34–85)	Hypokalemia (67–100)
Hypoaminoacidemia (26–100)	Hypochlorhydria (34–72)
Hypocholesterolemia (80)	Hypercalcemia (41–50)
Renal glycosuria (unknown)	Hyperglycemia (18–100)

VIP, Vasoactive intestinal polypeptide.

Glucagonoma data from Mallinson CN, Bloom SR, Warin AP, et al. A glucagonoma syndrome. *Lancet*. 1974;2:1–5; Jensen RT, Norton JA. Endocrine tumors of the pancreas and gastrointestinal tract. In: Feldman MFL, Brandt LJ, eds. *Sleisenger and Fordtran's Gastrointestinal and Liver Disease*. 8th ed. Philadelphia, PA: Saunders; 2006:625–666; Eldor R, Glaser B, Fraenkel M, et al. Glucagonoma and the glucagonoma syndrome—cumulative experience with an elusive endocrine tumour. *Clin Endocrinol (Oxf)*. 2011;74:593–598; Kindmark H, Sundin A, Granberg D, et al. Endocrine pancreatic tumors with glucagon hypersecretion: a retrospective study of 23 cases during 20 years. *Med Oncol*. 2007;24:340–347; Soga J, Yakuwa Y. Glucagonomas/diabetico-dermatogenic syndrome (DDS): a statistical evaluation of 407 reported cases. *J Hepatobiliary Pancreat Surg*. 1998;5:312–319; Guillausseau PJ, Guillausseau-Scholer C. Glucagonomas: clinical presentation, diagnosis, and advances in management. In: Mignon M, Jensen RT, eds. *Endocrine Tumors of the Pancreas: Recent Advances in Research and Management. Frontiers in GI Research*. Basel, Switzerland: S. Karger, 1995; Chastain MA. The glucagonoma syndrome: a review of its features and discussion of new perspectives. *Am J Med Sci*. 2001;321:302–306; van Beek AP, de Haas ER, van Vloten WA, et al. The glucagonoma syndrome and necrolytic migratory erythema: a clinical review. *Eur J Endocrinol*. 2004;151:531–537.

VIPoma data from Jensen RT, Norton JA. Endocrine tumors of the pancreas and gastrointestinal tract. In: Feldman MFL, Brandt LJ, eds. *Sleisenger and Fordtran's Gastrointestinal and Liver Disease*. 9th ed. Philadelphia, PA: Saunders; 2010:491–522; Matuchansky C, Rambaud JC. VIPomas and endocrine cholera: clinical presentation, diagnosis, and advances in management. In: Mignon MJR, ed. *Endocrine Tumors of the Pancreas: Recent Advances in Research and Management Frontiers in GI Research*. Basel, Switzerland: S. Krager; 1995:166–182; Song S, Shi R, Li B, et al. Diagnosis and treatment of pancreatic vasoactive intestinal peptide endocrine tumors. *Pancreas*. 2009;38:811–814; Adam N, Lim SS, Ananda V, et al. VIPoma syndrome: challenges in management. *Singapore Med J*. 2010;51:e129–e132; Soga J, Yakuwa Y. Vipoma/diarrheogenic syndrome: a statistical evaluation of 241 reported cases. *J Exp Clin Cancer Res*. 1998;17:389–400; Jensen RD, Doherty GM. Carcinoid tumors and the carcinoid syndrome. In DeVita Jr VT, Hellman S, Rosenberg SA, eds. *Cancer: Principles and Practice of Oncology*. 7th ed. Philadelphia, PA: Lippincott Williams and Wilkins; 2005:1559–1574.

Pathophysiology and Pathology

In contrast to insulinomas, most glucagonomas are large at the time of diagnosis, with an average size of 5–10 cm (range, 0.4–35 cm).[12,182–187] Similar to other pNETs, except insulinoma, glucagonomas are usually malignant.[12,182,183,188] The most common sites of metastases are the liver and lymph nodes, with bone and mesentery being less common sites.[11,182] Most (>97%) glucagonomas arise in the pancreas, and they usually (88%–90% of cases) occur as a solitary tumor.[185]

The pathophysiology of the glucagonoma syndrome is related to the known actions of glucagon (see Chapter 4).[189] *Hyperglycemia* results from increased hepatic glycogenolysis and gluconeogenesis. Weight loss has been attributed to the known catabolic effects of glucagon,[185] although taste aversion effects mediated by GLP-1 (7–36 amide) may contribute.[190] Whether the characteristic *rash* (NME) is caused by hyperglucagonemia is controversial. Prolonged hyperglucagonemia caused by glucagon administration does cause a typical rash.[12,191,192] It is possible that hypoaminoacidemia (present in 80%–90%) or essential fatty acid deficiency may be involved in the genesis of the dermatitis because, if these deficiencies are corrected, NME may improve without a change in plasma glucagon levels. The similarity of the skin lesions to those seen in zinc deficiencies has resulted in trials of zinc, with some responses. The rash may even resolve with volume repletion. Therefore there may be several contributing factors in different patients. Hyperglucagonemia may contribute to the *anemia* because treatment with glucagon decreases erythropoiesis in animals. The role of glucagon in causing *venous thromboembolism* and *psychiatric problems* is uncertain.[193]

Glucagon cell adenomatosis[194] may simulate the glucagonoma syndrome.[12,195,196] In glucagon cell adenomatosis, there are many microadenomas and hyperplastic islets that stain for glucagon. Also, a homozygous P86S mutation of the human glucagon receptor was, in a single case, associated with alpha cell hyperplasia, hyperglucagonemia, and NF-pNETs. This disorder, Mahvash disease, can be reproduced in mice deficient for the glucagon receptor.[196,197]

Clinical Features

Glucagonomas usually occur in individuals 50–70 years old.[12,90,182,184–186] NME is a common manifestation (Fig. 43.5; also see Table 43.7).[12,90,183–185,198,199] Dermatitis often precedes diagnosis of the syndrome for several years.[12,198] In 70% of patients, the skin lesion is the presenting sign of the disease and has been reported up to 3 years before the pNET is found.[200] Skin lesions may wax and wane and are often misdiagnosed.[200,201] Characteristically, the lesion starts as an erythematous patch, typically in periorofacial or intertriginous areas, such as the groin, buttocks, thighs, or perineum, and then spreads laterally. The lesions subsequently become raised, with superficial central blistering. The top of the bullae frequently detaches or ruptures, leaving eroded areas that crust. The lesions tend to heal in the center, whereas the edges continue to spread, with a crusting well-defined edge. Healing is associated with the development of hyperpigmentation. This entire sequence characteristically takes 1–2 weeks. The histopathology can be as varied as the clinical presentation.[11] In its classic form, early lesions demonstrate a superficial spongiosis and necrosis, with subcorneal and midepidermal bullae. Fusiform keratinocytes with pyknotic nuclei are often seen, as are mononuclear inflammatory infiltrates.[5,12,198,199]

Glucose intolerance or frank diabetes mellitus may precede diagnosis of glucagonoma by many years.[90,183–186] Profound hypoaminoacidemia (often less than 25% of normal, especially

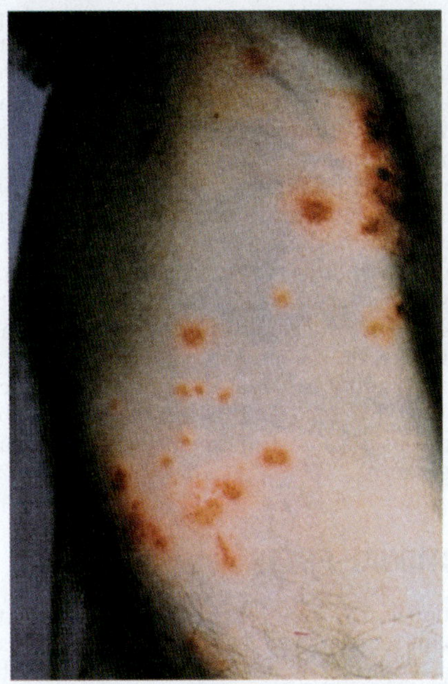

Fig. 43.5 Necrolytic migratory erythema (NME) in a patient with glucagonoma. NME is characterized by rapidly eroding superficial blisters. The lesions are usually localized to the buttocks, groin, perineum, elbows, hands, feet, and perioral area. (Courtesy Dr. Carl Grunfeld, San Francisco, CA.)

with glycogenic amino acids) is common,[5,11,90,184,186] and essential fatty acid deficiencies are also sometimes seen. Weight loss, often profound and associated with anorexia, occurs in most patients,[11,90,183–186] even with small, nonmetastatic tumors.[5,11,182]

Venous thromboembolism is more common in the glucagonoma syndrome than in other pNETs. Mild anemia, usually normocytic and normochromic with normal serum iron, folate, and vitamin B_{12} levels, can respond to successful tumor therapy.

Diagnosis

Glucagonomas are usually suspected because of the skin rash, NME (see Fig. 43.5).[90,176,177,179–187,195,198,202–205] The diagnosis of glucagonoma can be confirmed by demonstrating an increase in fasting plasma glucagon concentration (normal, less than 200 pg/mL). Most glucagonoma patients have a markedly elevated plasma glucagon level at presentation,[11,12,90,182,183,186,206] with a mean plasma glucagon concentration of 2110 pg/mL (range, 550–6600 pg/mL).[11] Mild hyperglucagonemia (200–500 pg/mL) also occurs in many other conditions, such as cirrhosis, chronic kidney disease, diabetic ketoacidosis, prolonged starvation, acute pancreatitis, acromegaly, Cushing, septicemia, severe burns, severe stress (trauma and exercise), celiac disease, danazol therapy, and familial hyperglucagonemia.[10,11,181,185] Provocative tests for glucagonoma have been described, but none are sufficiently reliable.

Treatment

Medical Treatment

Initial medical treatment is directed at relieving symptoms, restoring nutritional status, and controlling hyperglycemia as tumor localization studies (discussed later) are being performed. Glucagonoma patients are generally poor operative risks. The catabolic effects of glucagon combined with glucose intolerance and diabetes mellitus can markedly affect the nutritional status of these patients. Their heightened risk of venous thromboembolism increases postoperative morbidity.

SSAs have been useful in controlling symptoms in patients with glucagonoma.[182,183,185,207] The rash improves with SSA treatment in most patients, with disappearance in up to 30%. Plasma glucagon levels decrease in 80%–90% of treated patients, but into the normal range in only 10%–20%.

Surgical Treatment

Surgical resection should be considered in all patients with localized tumors.[208] Unfortunately, 50%–90% of patients with glucagonoma have metastases at the time of diagnosis.[182–184,209]

VIPomas

The VIPoma syndrome is caused by a NET that secretes excessive amounts of VIP. The syndrome is characterized by extreme watery diarrhea, hypochlorhydria, achlorhydria, and hypokalemia (see Tables 43.1 and 43.7).[4,210] Because of the resemblance of the diarrhea fluid to that seen in cholera, the term *pancreatic cholera* was proposed and the acronym WDHA (***w***atery ***d***iarrhea, ***h***ypokalemia, and ***a***chlorhydria) created.[211] VIP was suspected as the mediator of this syndrome, and the ability of VIP infusions to produce secretory diarrhea in humans at blood levels seen in patients with VIPomas was confirmed.[212]

Pathophysiology and Pathology

Most (80%–90%) VIPomas in adults are pNETs, with 42%–75% occurring in the tail of the pancreas[12,213,214]; VIP-producing SI NETs, lung cancers, or pheochromocytomas are rare.[12,211,213–217] VIPomas are almost always large, solitary tumors and are often metastatic at the time of diagnosis or surgery, similar to gastrinomas and glucagonomas. In young children (<10 years old) and, rarely, in adults (5% of adult cases), the VIPoma syndrome is caused by an extrapancreatic ganglioneuroma or ganglioneuroblastoma, tumors that are malignant in only 10% of patients.[11,211]

Almost half of VIPomas produce multiple hormones, including glucagon, somatostatin, insulin, and gastrin.[11,16]

VIP is the major mediator of the syndrome[11,16,211,218]; plasma VIP levels are usually elevated,[219] and a continuous IV infusion of VIP in normal human subjects, achieving plasma levels similar to those seen in patients with the VIPoma syndrome, produced watery diarrhea within 6–7 hours.[212] VIP interacts with specific receptors on intestinal epithelial cells, leading to intestinal electrolyte and fluid secretion (see Chapter 103).[11]

Flushing in patients with VIPoma has been attributed to the potent vasodilatory effects of VIP.[11] The finding that only a minority of patients with VIPoma syndrome flush, despite high plasma VIP levels, has been attributed to the fact that prolonged VIP infusions result in a gradual loss of flushing, suggesting tachyphylaxis. Severe hypokalemia is likely primarily caused by fecal K^+ loss; secondary hyperaldosteronism that results from volume depletion with renal K^+ loss and VIP stimulation of renin release may also contribute.[11] The pathogenesis of the achlorhydria or hypochlorhydria is not entirely clear but has been attributed to the inhibitory effect of VIP on gastric acid secretion. The mechanism of the hypercalcemia is also unclear. Hyperglycemia has been attributed to the glycogenolytic effect of VIP on the liver.

Clinical Features

The mean age for adults with VIPomas is 42–51 years (range, 32–81).[10,211,219–221] In children, the mean age is 2–4 years old (range, 10 months to 9 years). The cardinal features of the VIPoma syndrome are severe secretory diarrhea associated with hypokalemia and volume depletion (see Table 43.7).[10,211,219–221]

Diarrhea may be episodic[211,222] and exceed 1 L/day (usually >3 L/day).[11,16,213,214] The diarrheal fluid has the appearance of weak tea and persists during fasting.[11,16,218] Most (90%) patients have five or more bowel movements a day.

Laboratory abnormalities in patients with VIPoma are listed in Table 43.7.[10,211,219–221] Hypokalemia is often severe (<2.5 mmol/L) at some point in the course in over 90% of patients.[12,211,222] Tetany may occur and has been attributed to hypomagnesemia resulting from the diarrhea.[11] If measured, hypochlorhydria occurs in many cases.

Diagnosis

The diagnosis of the VIPoma syndrome requires large-volume secretory diarrhea that persists with fasting and demonstration of an elevated plasma concentration of VIP.[10,16,213,214,216,218] Diarrhea may be present for long periods prior to diagnosis. The diarrhea fluid is characteristic of a secretory diarrhea (see Chapter 17).

Other diseases can cause a chronic, large-volume secretory diarrhea with most of the clinical features of the VIPoma syndrome, except for a high plasma VIP level (pseudo-VIPoma syndrome). Such patients include individuals with gastrinoma,[16,40,129] chronic laxative abuse,[223] celiac disease,[224] AIDS enteropathy,[225] or idiopathic secretory diarrhea.[12,16,223,226–228] Elevated plasma VIP levels alone should not be the sole basis for making a diagnosis of VIPoma in a patient with diarrhea, because other conditions (e.g., prolonged fasting, IBD, small bowel resection, radiation enteritis, chronic kidney disease, and nesidioblastosis[229]) can occasionally elevate VIP levels.[11,16,230]

Treatment

Medical Treatment

The first objective is replenishment of fluid and electrolyte losses to correct the profound volume depletion, hypokalemia, and hyperchloremic metabolic acidosis (see Table 43.7). The patients may require 5 or more L/day of fluid[11] and over 350 mEq/day of potassium.[11,16,211,231] Hypokalemic nephropathy with severe renal failure may occur.[4] Fluid and electrolyte requirements should be carefully monitored. The diarrheal output should be controlled by use of SSAs.[10,12,16,98,146,207,232] Octreotide controls diarrhea in 78%–100% of patients.[10,207,220,232] Octreotide continued to be effective at 6 months in 56%–100% of patients, but 22% required an increase in dosage.[11,12] Plasma VIP concentrations decreased in 80%–89% of patients taking octreotide. Decreases in plasma VIP concentration with octreotide treatment did not always mirror clinical responses.[11,16,223] Treatment of metastatic VIPoma is discussed later.

Surgical Treatment

Once the fluid and electrolyte deficits are corrected, patients should undergo imaging studies (discussed later) to assess tumor resectability. After performing these imaging studies, surgical cure should be considered for all patients without metastatic disease.[10,98,105,208,214,222] Surgical resection of a pancreatic VIPoma relieves all symptoms in one-third of patients, and up to 30% of them are cured.[12,211,233] In children (and rare adults) with VIP-producing ganglioneuroblastomas,[12] surgical resection with control of all symptoms was possible in 78% of patients.

OTHER FUNCTIONAL PNETS

Less common pNETs are summarized in Table 43.1. ACTH-producing pNETs can cause Cushing syndrome. These tumors are often metastatic, aggressive, and refractory to treatment, including SSA therapy.[10,11,234,235]

pNETs secreting PTH-related peptide causing hypercalcemia are usually large and/or metastatic to the liver by the time of diagnosis. In addition to antitumor treatment, bisphosphonates can be used to control the hypercalcemia.[236] Serotonin-producing pNETs can cause the carcinoid syndrome and are rare, usually large, and predominantly malignant.[12,13,188]

The term "somatostatinoma" is sometimes used to describe rare pancreatic or duodenal tumors which secrete large amounts of somatostatin, resulting in relatively nonspecific symptoms such as diabetes mellitus, gallstones, diarrhea/steatorrhea, and weight loss. The term is also sometimes used to describe duodenal NETs which stain positively for somatostatin and are also characterized by psammoma bodies but do not necessarily secrete somatostatin. Such tumors are seen with increased frequency in NF1 patients. Due to the relatively subtle clinical manifestations of the somatostatinoma syndrome, this diagnosis is exceedingly rare.[237]

NONFUNCTIONAL PNETS

A nonfunctional pNET (NF-pNET) is a pNET that is not associated with secretion of a peptide/amine causing a functional syndrome, and whose symptoms are entirely caused by the local effects of the tumor itself.[12]

Clinical Features

The typical patient with a well-differentiated NF-pNET is 40–60 years old. The median time from initial symptoms to diagnosis varies from 6 months to almost 3 years. Increasingly, small NF-pNETs are diagnosed incidentally as patients undergo scans for unrelated reasons. Presenting symptoms/signs from the tumor include abdominal pain, jaundice, and weight loss.[10,25,29,67,238–240]

Treatment

Surgical resection is generally recommended for patients with localized, resectable NF pNETs. Future relapse is dependent on tumor size, grade, and lymph node positivity. The treatment of patients with small (<2 cm), sporadic, and incidentally diagnosed low-grade NF-PETs is controversial.[67] Several studies show high rates of disease stability in patients undergoing surveillance.[241] Certain radiographic features suggestive of indolent behavior include well-defined tumor borders and tumor homogeneity.[242] Ultimately, decisions regarding surgery versus surveillance need to factor in patient age, comorbidities, and willingness to undergo long-term surveillance.[67,243,244]

GI-NETS (CARCINOIDS)

GI-NETs (carcinoid tumors) comprise nearly 70% of all carcinoid tumors. Most of the others (roughly 25%) are found in the respiratory tract. GI-NETs most commonly occur in the small intestine, rectum, appendix, or stomach (Table 43.8).[245] Within the small intestine, the ileum is the most common site, followed by the duodenum and jejunum.[245] The incidence of GI-NETs is increasing, but not evenly so (see Fig. 43.1).[23] Survival is highly dependent on the tumor stage,[246] as shown for selected GI-NETs in Table 43.9.

Gastric NETs

Gastric NETs comprise 0.3% of all gastric tumors and 2%–6% of all carcinoid tumors in the United States. Their incidence has increased markedly over the last 30 years (see Fig. 43.1).[246–259] It is unclear whether this is a true increase in disease incidence or due to improved detection from increased use of EGD.[247] Thus gastric NETs are now often found by chance during EGD performed for some other reason.[118,249,250,252,256,257,259]

Gastric NETs are classified into three types (Table 43.10). For correct classification of gastric carcinoids into these types, the mucosa of the gastric antrum and the body/fundus should both be sampled, in addition to the removal or biopsy of the lesions.[146,247,249,259]

Type 1 gastric NETs, the most common type, are generally small and multiple and occur in patients (more often women) with chronic atrophic gastritis with or without pernicious anemia.[247–249,259] Type 1 gastric NETs occur in 1%–2% of patients with chronic atrophic gastritis (see Chapter 54).[252] At EGD, type 1 gastric NETs usually appear as polypoid lesions associated with mucosal atrophy (Fig. 43.6A).[252] If random mucosal biopsies are taken, additional intramucosal NETs will be found, though not seen at endoscopy.[252] Histologically, type 1 gastric NETs are well differentiated and always associated with varying degrees of gastric ECL cell hyperplasia. ECL hyperplasia is driven by hypergastrinemia caused by loss of the feedback inhibition by gastric acid on gastrin (G) cells (see Chapter 53).[248] Chronic hypergastrinemia, often profound, results in increasing degrees of ECL cell hyperplasia (diffuse, linear, and micronodular) and, in some cases, dysplasia and then neoplasia.[248] Type 1 gastric NETs are generally minimally invasive, with 27% limited to the mucosa and 64% limited to the submucosa; only 9% invade the muscularis propria.[256,259] Metastases to lymph nodes or liver are very uncommon.[22,247,260]

Type 2 gastric NETs are the least frequent type and occur almost exclusively in patients with MEN-1/ZES.[61,68,114,116,249,257] They occur in 23%–33% of patients with MEN-1/ZES, invariably with hyperparathyroidism.[61,68,116,160] Type 2 gastric NETs have only rarely been described in patients with the sporadic form of ZES.[68,114,116] Type 2 gastric NETs are, like type 1, generally multiple, but they tend to be larger, with only 35% smaller than 1 cm and as many as 20% larger than 2 cm (see Fig. 43.6B). Type 2 gastric NETs generally appear as polypoid lesions, although they too can be detected on blind biopsies as intramucosal tumors.[116,249] They are well-differentiated, always associated with ECL cell hyperplasia and a hyperplasic gastric mucosa.[114,116,249,257] Type 2 gastric NETs are somewhat more invasive than type 1, with 15% showing invasion limited to the mucosa, 60% extending into the submucosa, and 10% into the muscularis propria. Metastases are also more common in type 2 than type 1,[116,249,256,259] and the 5-year survival in patients with type 2 gastric carcinoids is lower than in type 1 (see Table 43.10). However, it is unclear whether this lower survival is due to the gastric NETs per se.[61,68,249]

Type 3 gastric NETs differ from the other two types in that they are not associated with hypergastrinemia or alterations in gastric acid secretion. They are solitary, sporadic NETs not associated with other diseases of the stomach (see Fig. 43.6C).[247,256,257,259] Endoscopically, type 3 gastric NETs are usually single, large, infiltrating lesions that in some cases are ulcerating (see Fig. 43.6C). Histologically, they are generally well-differentiated NETs (see Table 43.2a). Patients with type 3 gastric NETs may have signs of GI bleeding or advanced malignancy, prompting EGD.[259] At the time of diagnosis, most type 3 gastric carcinoids are already invasive. The 5-year survival rate is close to 50%, and 25%–30% of type 3 patients have a tumor-related death.[247,256,257,259]

The carcinoid syndrome (discussed later) occurs in a small percentage of patients with types 2 and 3 gastric NETs.[247,250,254] An atypical flush may occur in these patients because these gastric NETs may lack L-amino acid decarboxylase, and thus instead of producing serotonin, they secrete its unprocessed precursor, 5-hydroxytryptamine (5-HTP; Fig. 43.7).[247,250,255] The atypical flush is a prolonged red-purple flush involving the trunk and extremities.[247,255] The more typical carcinoid flush is shown in Fig. 43.8. Rare gastric NETs can also release histamine, which can result in bronchospasm, itching, cutaneous flushing, and lacrimation.[258]

The minimal laboratory evaluation in types 1 and 2 gastric carcinoids is an assessment of serum gastrin. In patients suspected to have type 1 gastric NETs with chronic atrophic gastritis, the clinician should consider ordering a complete blood count, parietal cell antibodies, serum B_{12} (see Chapters 53 and 54), and thyroid function tests (for possible associated autoimmune thyroiditis).[249] In patients with possible MEN-1/ZES, a full assessment for the features of MEN-1 should be performed. For all gastric NETs larger than 1 cm and for localized type 3 NETs, EUS should be performed to assess the depth of invasion prior to endoscopic removal.[247,249]

The overall 5-year survival rate for all types of gastric carcinoids in the U.S. SEER database is 49% (see Table 43.10), but these data include only primarily malignant tumors; therefore it is likely that many type 1 gastric carcinoids (with better survival) were not included.

Types 1 and 2 gastric NETs share many similar management aspects that differ markedly from the approach for type 3 carcinoids (see Table 43.10).

- Small (<1 cm) types 1 and 2 carcinoids should in most cases be treated endoscopically.[247] For type 1 or 2 gastric carcinoids that infiltrate to the submucosa, it is recommended that endoscopic mucosal resection (EMR) be considered, although many are still treated with traditional polypectomy.[247,253] EGD surveillance should be at least yearly. In one study[252] of patients with type 1 gastric carcinoids treated endoscopically, survival was 100% during the 46-month follow-up; no metastases occurred, a single patient developed a less differentiated tumor requiring surgery, and 64% had a recurrence after a median of 8 months, treated endoscopically. Thus endoscopic management was safe and effective.
- For types 1 and 2 gastric carcinoids 1–2 cm in size, there is not complete agreement on the best treatment.[247,253] Most commonly, after EUS assessment of depth, these lesions are removed endoscopically,[247,249,251,252,259] although some authors recommend surgical therapy.[247,248,259] In patients with high-risk tumors (e.g., size >2 cm, relatively high Ki-67 index), a surgical wedge resection can be considered.[247] Long-term treatment with an SSA may result in the disappearance of small (<1 cm) gastric carcinoids.[247,249,259] In patients with numerous type 1 gastric carcinoids, antrectomy eliminates the hypergastrinemia driving ECL cell growth and is effective in over 80% of patients.[259]
- Patients with type 3 gastric NETs require imaging for disease staging (discussed later). If distant metastases are not present, these patients should be managed surgically.[247,249,259] Some recommend that the rare small (<1 cm) type 3 gastric carcinoid without any risk factors may be treated conservatively by endoscopic mucosectomy.[261]

Patients with advanced metastatic gastric carcinoids of types 1 (rare), 2 (uncommon), or 3 require systemic antitumor therapies, as discussed later.

Poorly differentiated gastric NECs of the stomach comprise 3%–8% of all gastric neuroendocrine neoplasms.[247] They are generally solitary larger tumors (>2 cm); they are associated with metastases in 80%–100% of cases, and over 50% of patients have a tumor-related death.[247] These tumors are treated like other poorly differentiated GI-NECs in other locations (see later).[262,263]

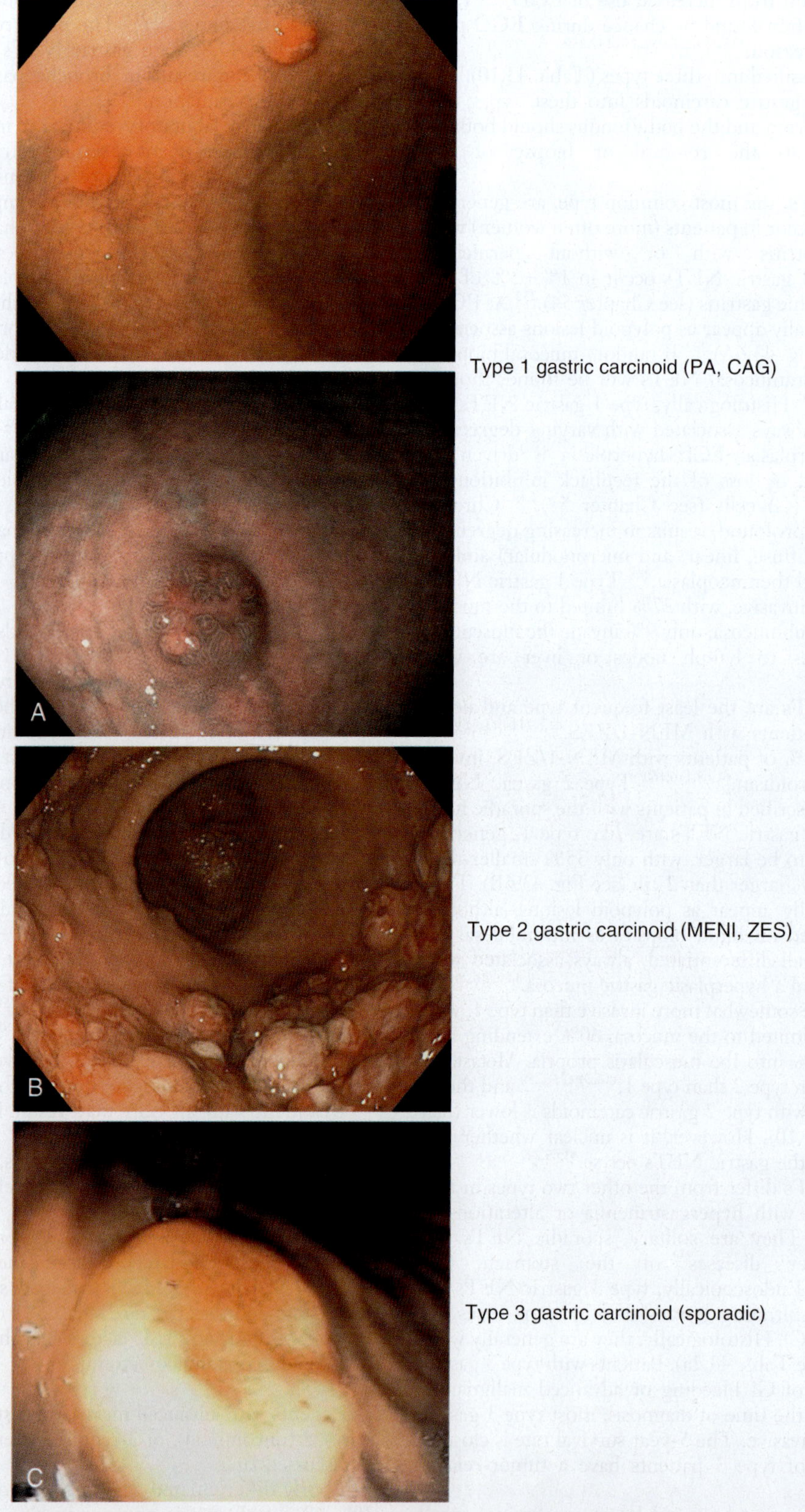

Fig. 43.6 Endoscopic images of the three types of gastric carcinoids. (A) Type 1, in patient with chronic atrophic gastritis (CAG) and pernicious anemia (PA). Note the atrophic mucosa and multiple small carcinoids with the typical appearance (raised with central small ulceration (1); narrow band image highlights the characteristic appearance (2). (B) Type 2, in a patient with *MEN-I/ZES*. Note the multiplicity of lesions with central ulceration and sparing of the antrum. (C) Type 3, which is characteristically solitary and often large. (Modified from Scherubl H, Cadiot G, Jensen RT, et al. Neuroendocrine tumors of the stomach [gastric carcinoids] are on the rise: small tumors, small problems? *Endoscopy*. 2010;42:664–71.)

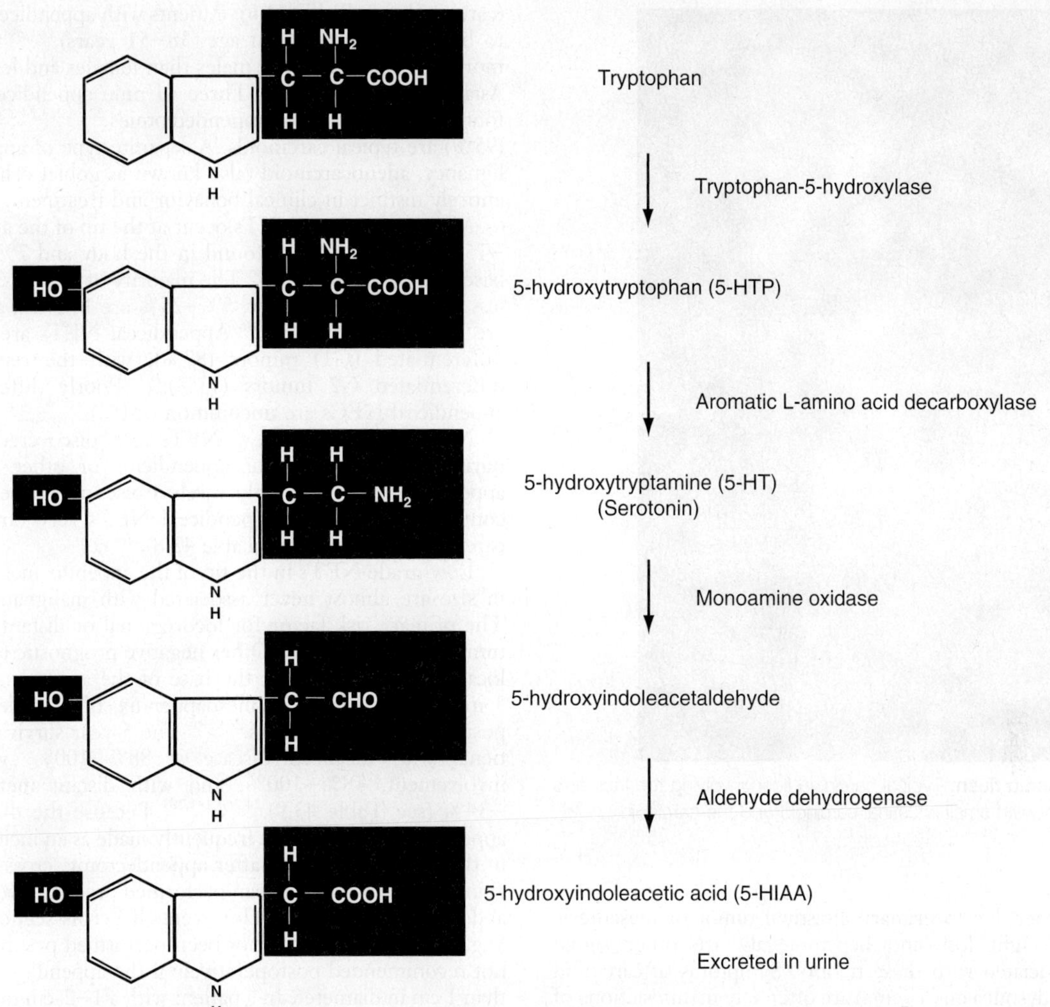

Fig. 43.7 Synthesis and degradation of serotonin [5-hydroxytryptamine (*5-HT*)]. Shown are the various enzymes that are important in the synthesis of serotonin from tryptophan and its degradation to 5-hydroxyindoleactic acid (*5-HIAA*), which is excreted in the urine.

Small Intestinal NETs (Jejunal/Ileal Carcinoid Tumors)

The incidence of SI NETs is increasing in the United States (see Fig. 43.1). SI NETs comprise more than half of all SI neoplasms.[264] In this chapter, we use the term SI NET to refer to jejunal and ileal NETs (also known as midgut NETs); duodenal NETs are discussed later.

The average age at presentation of patients with SI NETs is in the sixth decade of life.[265] These tumors occur less frequently in Asians and more frequently in African-Americans.[24] There are rare families with ileal NETs that appear to have autosomal dominant inheritance. Their tumors are clinically similar to sporadic cases and share frequent aberrations in chromosome 18.[266]

Many fewer NETs occur within the jejunum (9%–18%) than within the ileum (70%–87%), with 40%–70% of the latter occurring within 2 ft of the ileocecal valve.[245,265] SI NETs are generally small, with one-third less than 1 cm, another third 1–2 cm, and the final third larger than 2 cm (with 8% >5 cm).[22,265] Approximately 25% are multifocal.[223,267,268] SI NETs, although characteristically well differentiated, are often quite invasive: Only 28% are confined to the mucosal/submucosal, and 52% extend to the muscularis propria or are transmural. Metastases occur in the majority of patients with SI NETs (range, 20%–100%),[22,223,265,267] usually to the liver, lymph nodes, mesentery/omentum/peritoneum, lung, or bone.[22,30,265,269–277] Large central mesenteric lymph nodes, often with surrounding desmoplasia, are highly characteristic of SI NETs and generally indicative of a SI origin, even when the primary tumor is occult on scans.

SI NETs are thought to arise from EC cells. They are predominantly well-differentiated (G1) tumors, with 9%–19% of them G2 and 2% G3.[270] Numerous genetic/epigenetic changes have been reported in SI NETs, including loss of 3p13 (associated with better survival) and gain of chromosome 14 (associated with worse survival).[278]

Although SI carcinoids characteristically are diagnosed in the sixth decade of life,[265] the diagnosis is often delayed 4–5 years from symptom onset, and even much longer delays have been reported.[22,271] Most (>90%) patients present with symptoms that are either related to tumor or to carcinoid syndrome (discussed later). Tumor-related symptoms include abdominal pain, often intermittent, crampy. Recurrent cases of bowel obstruction may

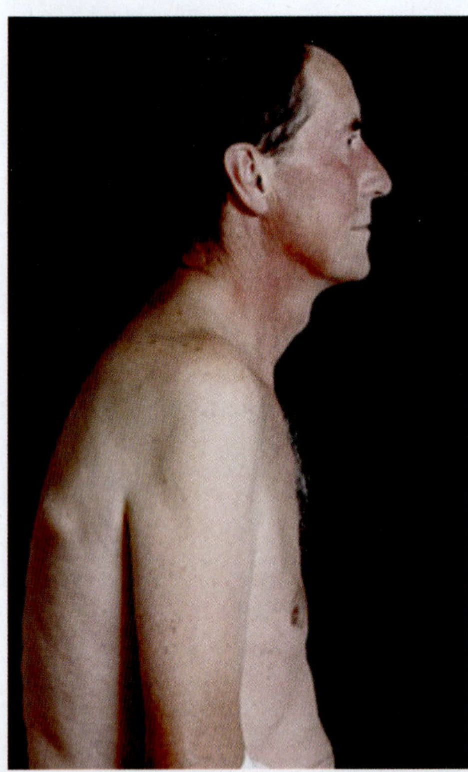

Fig. 43.8 Carcinoid flush. Typical carcinoid flush involving the face and neck in a patient with small intestinal carcinoid and the carcinoid syndrome.

also occur, either due to primary intestinal tumor or mesenteric metastases. Weight loss and hepatomegaly are other signs/symptoms associated with these tumors. Symptoms of carcinoid heart disease (dyspnea and edema) are often late manifestations of disease.[22,264,265,279,280]

Treatment of patients with SI NETs first requires staging the extent of disease by imaging studies and also determining whether the carcinoid syndrome is present (both discussed later).[105,264,281] Curative resection of the primary NET and adjacent lymph nodes improves the 5-year survival rates in patients with local or locoregional SI NETs.[276] Lymph node involvement around the superior mesenteric artery may require lymph node dissection.[264,281] Surgical resection of the primary NET, even in the presence of distant metastases, is often recommended (discussed later). At the time of surgery, a cholecystectomy is usually performed because many patients will subsequently be treated with SSAs that often cause biliary sludge and gallstones.[264,281]

The overall 5-year survival of patients with metastatic SI NETs is approximately 70%,[282] with a median survival of 8–9 years.[269,271,272] Survival is very much dependent on the stage of the disease (see Table 43.9). Prognostic factors for reduced survival in patients with SI NETs include male gender, older age, metastases, carcinoid syndrome (especially with carcinoid heart disease), and highly elevated urine 5-hydroxyindoleacetic acid (5-HIAA) levels.[22,269,271,273–275,277,283] In contrast to many other NETs, the size of the primary SI NET does not correlate well with biological activity. For example, about 46% of tumors smaller than 1 cm are associated with liver metastases.[22,271,277]

Appendiceal NETs (Carcinoids)

Appendiceal NETs comprise 32%–80% of appendiceal tumors and, in different series, represent 2%–38% of GI-NETs (carcinoid) (see Table 43.8). Patients with appendiceal NETs tend to be middle-aged (mean age, 38–51 years).[264,284,285] These tumors are less common in males than females and less common in Asians than other races. Three to nine appendiceal NETs are found for every 1000 appendectomies.[22,24,223,245,264,284,286] Most (95%) are typical carcinoids. A separate type of appendiceal malignancy, adenocarcinoid (also known as goblet cell carcinoid), is entirely distinct in clinical behavior and treatment.

Most appendiceal NETs occur at the tip of the appendix (60%–75%), with 5%–20% found in the body and 7%–10% at the base of the appendix.[264,286] The majority of them (60%–80%) are less than 1 cm in diameter, 5%–25% are 1–2 cm, and 2%–17% are larger than 2 cm.[264,286] Appendiceal NETs are usually well-differentiated (G1) tumors (87%), with the remainder well-differentiated G2 tumors (13%).[287] Poorly differentiated G3 appendiceal NECs are uncommon (<1%).[287]

Nearly all appendiceal NETs are discovered incidentally during appendectomy for appendicitis or other reasons. The appendiceal carcinoid only rarely causes the appendicitis.[264] In contrast to SI NETs, appendiceal NETs very rarely cause the carcinoid syndrome (see Table 43.8).[264]

Low-grade NETs in the tip of the appendix measuring <2 cm in size are almost never associated with malignant behavior.[288] The primary risk factor for locoregional or distant metastases is tumor diameter >2 cm. Other negative prognostic factors include location of the tumor at the base of the appendix, greater than 3 mm invasion into the mesoappendix, high-grade tumors, and positive resection margins.[264,281] The 5-year survival rate for patients with localized disease is 88%–100%; with regional involvement, 78%–100%; and with distant metastases, 12%–34% (see Table 43.9).[24,264,281,287] Because the diagnosis of an appendiceal NET is most frequently made as an incidental finding in the surgical specimen after appendectomy, cross-sectional imaging studies may have been performed preoperatively to evaluate abdominal pain.[105,264] However, if cross-sectional imaging (e.g., CT and MRI) had not been performed preoperatively, it is not recommended postoperatively if the appendiceal NET is less than 1 cm in diameter. In a patient with a 1–2-cm tumor, imaging studies can be considered to rule out the possibility of additional locoregional disease or distant metastases, even if the resection was complete.[264] Appendiceal NETs larger than 2 cm, with significant mesoappendiceal infiltration, and/or with vascular invasion require radiographic staging studies.[264,289] This same approach is also recommended in cases where completeness of resection is unclear or metastases are present.[264] Treatment of appendiceal NETs is primarily surgical, but the choice of operation depends on several factors:

For typical tumors 1 cm or smaller without gross metastases, with tumor invasion no deeper than the subserosa, with minimal (<3 mm) mesoappendiceal invasion, and with clear surgical margins, a simple appendectomy is sufficient.[264,281,286] Fortunately, these strict criteria apply to the majority of typical appendiceal NETs.[284] Of 103 such patients treated with a simple appendectomy and followed for at least 5 years (83 of them for 10–35 years), no patient developed a local recurrence or metastatic disease.[290] Patients with appendiceal NETs measuring 1–2 cm with high-risk features (e.g., lymphovascular invasion or mesoappendiceal invasion) have been considered possible candidates for completion right hemicolectomy due to the risk of locoregional lymph node involvement. However, a recent large database study with long-term follow-up indicated an absence of metachronous distant metastases among patients with appendiceal NETs measuring 1–2 cm regardless of risk factors or whether right hemicolectomy was performed.[291]

For appendiceal carcinoid tumors larger than 2 cm in diameter, most authorities,[264,286,290] but not all,[292] recommend a right hemicolectomy.

Treatment of patients with distant metastases is discussed later.

Rectal NETs (Carcinoids)

Rectal NETs are increasing in incidence (see Fig. 43.1).[24,293–296] It is unclear whether there is a true increased incidence of these tumors or simply better detection because of widespread use of lower GI endoscopy for cancer screening and other indications.[295] Earlier detection of rectal carcinoid tumors may explain the decreasing size of the typical rectal NET over the past decades.[295] Rectal carcinoids are found in 1 in every 1500–2500 proctoscopies/colonoscopies.[223,295] In the United States, rectal NETs are especially common in Asian-Americans and less common in Caucasian Americans, with African-Americans having an intermediate incidence.[245] In studies from Japan and other Asian countries, rectal NETs account for 60%–90% of all GI-NETs.[297,298]

Rectal NETs are often diagnosed in the sixth decade of life and are usually asymptomatic.[245,294,295,298–302] The carcinoid syndrome is very uncommon (0.7%) in patients with rectal NETs (see Table 43.8).[293,302]

Rectal NETs are characteristically small (mean diameter, 0.6 cm) polypoid lesions that occur on the anterior or lateral walls of the rectum 4–13 cm above the dentate line.[302] Most (98%) rectal carcinoids are well-differentiated NETs that are ENETS/WHO grade G1 (72%) or grade 2 (28%).[293,300,302] Nearly 80% of tumors invade no deeper than the submucosa, with some invading into the muscular layer (10%), transmurally (7%), or into neighboring structures (5%).[302] Metastases from rectal NETs are related to size: those that are less than 1 cm in diameter (the majority) rarely metastasize (2%–5%).[302] In contrast, the metastatic rate for tumors that are 1–2 cm is 5%–30%, and the metastatic rate jumps to 60%–80% for the 15% that exceed 2 cm.[245,302] The pooled incidence of metastases from rectal NETs in the United States is 22.6%, with lymph node, liver, bone, mesentery/omentum/peritoneum, and lung being the leading sites. Using AJCC TNM staging, 81% of rectal carcinoids are stage I, 5% stage II, 11.5% stage III, and 2.5% stage IV.[301] Overall 5-year survival with rectal NETs is 88%, with survival very much dependent on the stage of the disease (see Table 43.9).[245,293,299,300] Risk factors for more advanced disease and worse survival include larger primary tumor size (particularly >2 cm); increased depth of invasion; poor differentiation; elevated Ki proliferative index; neural, lymphatic, or vascular invasion; and nodal, hepatic, or distant metastases.[293,299,300]

If the rectal NET is relatively large (>2 cm), advanced stages are likely and cross-sectional imaging (CT or MRI) as well as somatostatin receptor imaging are indicated for staging.[293] Rectal EUS is also important for assessing tumor size, depth of invasion, and lymph nodes.[293,303]

Treatment of rectal NETs depends on their size, level of invasion, and stage[293,295,299]:

For tumors less than 1 cm in diameter that do not infiltrate into the muscularis propria or show lymphovascular invasion or lymph node metastases, endoscopic excision is recommended. Standard polypectomy can usually be performed, but if local mucosal/submucosal invasion is present, a more extensive endoscopic procedure may be appropriate (e.g., EMR or submucosal dissection).[293,295,299]

For rectal carcinoids 1–2 cm in diameter, the preferred treatment is a matter of dispute, with some recommending endoscopic removal and others more aggressive treatment.[293,295,304] These tumors have a metastatic rate of 10%–15% compared to 3% in patients with rectal carcinoids smaller than 1 cm.[245,293] Because some studies show no added benefit of more aggressive treatment, guidelines recommend that patients with 1–2-cm rectal NETs with a low mitotic rate and without invasion into the muscularis propria on EUS undergo local endoscopic resection.[118,249,293]

For rectal NETs greater than 2 cm in diameter, with their much higher metastatic risk of 60%–80%,[245,293] it is generally recommended that patients be treated like patients with rectal adenocarcinoma, especially if the neoplasm is a T3 or T4 lesion, the tumor is grade G3, or if locoregional lymph node involvement is present, with total mesorectal excision or abdominoperineal resection, depending on the distance from the tumor to the anal verge (see Chapter 127).[293,299]

Treatment of patients with metastatic disease is discussed in a later section.

Duodenal and Ampulla of Vater NETs (Carcinoids)

Duodenal NETs have an annual incidence of 0.19/100,000 in the United States.[24] They comprise 5% of all GI-NETs.[24,249] Their incidence is lower in England[296] and higher in Japan where they comprise 10% of all GI NETs and were found in almost 10% of autopsies.[118,305]

Most (>90%) duodenal NETs arise from the first or second part of the duodenum, with 18%–20% occurring in the periampullary region.[305,306] Duodenal somatostatinomas and gangliocytic paragangliomas show a preference for the ampullary region, and the former may be particularly associated with NF1 (see Table 43.3).[61,118] In fact, 25% of all ampullary NETs are associated with NF1.[307] Duodenal NETs are generally small, with a mean diameter of 1.2–1.5 cm; 75% of them are smaller than 2 cm.[305] Most (63%) are limited to the mucosa or submucosa, but they still can metastasize to lymph nodes (19%–60% of cases), although liver metastases occur in less than 10%.[118,249,295,299,305] Most duodenal carcinoids are solitary, but they are multiple in 9%–13%, particularly in patients with MEN-1, who comprise 6% of all patients with duodenal NETs.[118,249,306] For example, in MEN-1/ZES patients, 80%–90% of gastrinomas are in the duodenum, and they invariably are multiple.[61,68]

Duodenal NETs can be divided into five subtypes: duodenal gastrinomas, somatostatinomas, nonfunctioning NETs (i.e., not associated with a clinical syndrome), gangliocytic paraganglioma (<2%), and poorly differentiated NECs (<3%).[40,118,246] Many studies also differentiate NETs in the ampulla of Vater region or periampullary area from other duodenal NETs.[118,249,306] Carcinoid syndrome is almost never observed with duodenal NETs.[12]

Duodenal somatostatinomas may contain psammoma bodies.[118,305] Duodenal gangliocytic paragangliomas contain epithelial, ganglia, and spindle cells and stain for S-100 protein immunoreactive Schwann cells.[118]

The mean age at presentation is the sixth decade, with a slight male predominance.[118,249,305,306,308] Because the vast majority of duodenal NETs are not associated with a clinical syndrome, they are usually diagnosed during EGD for nonspecific symptoms.[118,249,305,306,309] The most frequent functional syndromes are ZES (10%) and carcinoid syndrome (4%); other syndromes (see Table 43.1) are rare (<1%).[249] Periampullary NETs most often (50%–60%) present with jaundice and may also cause pain, nausea/vomiting, and diarrhea.[118,249,307]

The 5-year survival rate in patients with well-differentiated duodenal NETs is 80%–95%. Five-year survival for those with duodenal gastrinomas is above 90%.[72,126] Poor prognostic factors include distant metastases, advanced stage, larger primary tumor size, depth of invasion into the muscularis mucosa or beyond, increased mitotic activity, and poorer differentiation.[246,305,306] Ampulla of Vater NETs may show different growth characteristics than other duodenal NETs, as the size of the ampullary NET does not correlate with the development of liver metastases.[246]

EGD with biopsies is the most common method to diagnose duodenal NETs, and it should be followed by EUS to assess the level of invasion.[249] For patients with suspected or proved advanced disease, CT (or MRI) and somatostatin-receptor imaging are indicated.

Treatment is based on size, location, and type of NET:

- Small (<1 cm) nonampullary duodenal NETs can be removed endoscopically if no metastases are present and tumor invasion is limited to the mucosa or submucosa.[118,246] However, if the duodenal NET is located in the ampullary region, surgical resection with lymphadenectomy is recommended.
- For intermediate-sized (1–2 cm) duodenal NETs, surgical treatment is generally recommended.[118,310–313]
- Large (>2 cm) duodenal NETs, or one of any size with lymph node involvement, should be treated by surgical resection.[246]
- For patients with sporadic (non-MEN-1) ZES and duodenal gastrinomas, surgical exploration with duodenotomy and resection, rather than endoscopic treatment, is recommended because the duodenal gastrinomas are almost always submucosal, and lymph node metastases are present in at least half of cases.[71,118,172]

For the minority of patients with a functional hormonal syndrome from a duodenal NET, specific therapy should be given to control symptoms, as discussed earlier.

Colonic NETs (Carcinoids)

Colonic NETs (excluding those in the rectum and the appendix) occur with an annual incidence of 0.06–0.19/1,000,000.[24,293,296] Colonic NETs represent 11% of all GI NETs.[245]

The majority of colonic NETs occur in the cecum, with the remainder arising in the ascending, transverse, descending, and sigmoid colon (11%, 8%, 4%, and 9%, respectively).[314] Cecal NETs belong to the "midgut NET" category and are often associated with carcinoid syndrome when metastatic. Colonic NETs tend to be large with more than half greater than 5 cm.[314] These tumors are often malignant, with metastases to lymph nodes (55%), liver (53%), mesentery/omentum/peritoneum (24%), lung (8%), and bone (4%) already present at the time of diagnosis.[293,299,314] Only 14% are limited to the mucosa/submucosa; another 10% have invasion into the muscularis propria. The remaining 76% have transmural invasion or involve adjacent structures.[314]

The overall 5-year survival rate of patients with colonic NETs is 33%–70%, and survival varies considerably by stage (see Table 43.9).[293,314] A worse prognosis is associated with older age, lymph node and/or distant metastases, poor tumor differentiation, larger tumor size, deeper tissue invasion, and histologic atypia.[293,314,315]

The mean age of presentation is 55–65 years with a slight male predominance.[293,314] Increasingly, colonic NETs are asymptomatic and found on cancer screening colonoscopy. Carcinoid syndrome occurs in 5%–12% of patients with colonic NETs, primarily originating in the cecum.[314,315]

Most localized colonic NETs should be treated surgically with appropriate lymphadenectomy. Exceptions are very small, superficial, and low-grade tumors.[293,315] Treatment of patients with distant metastases is discussed later.

CARCINOID SYNDROME

The carcinoid syndrome develops in approximately 8% of patients with GI-NETs (range, 2%–18%).[77,223,316–333] Its symptoms are summarized in Table 43.11, predominantly in patients with metastatic SI (midgut) NETs.

Pathophysiology

The carcinoid syndrome occurs when sufficient concentrations of hormonal products released by the tumor reach the systemic circulation. Its occurrence and severity are related to the tumor size in areas that drain into the systemic circulation. In more than 90% of cases, this syndrome occurs with metastatic disease, especially to the liver.[22,77,223,334–336]

Patients may develop a typical or an atypical carcinoid syndrome.[223,321,337] In the *typical* syndrome, hydroxylation of tryptophan to 5-hydroxytryptophan (5-HTP) is the rate-limiting step (see Fig. 43.7). Once formed, 5-HTP is converted rapidly to 5-hydroxytryptamine (5-HT; or serotonin) by aromatic L-amino acid decarboxylase. Serotonin is either stored in the tumor's neurosecretory granules or released into circulation, where most of it is taken up and stored by platelets. A small amount of 5-HT remains in the circulation, where most of it is converted to 5-HIAA by monoamine oxidase and aldehyde dehydrogenase. The 5-HIAA so produced is then excreted in urine.[223,321,338] In the *atypical carcinoid syndrome*, the tumor is thought to be deficient in aromatic L-amino acid decarboxylase. Thus the NET cannot convert 5-HTP to 5-HT (serotonin), and the 5-HTP is secreted into the circulation.[255,321,338] Plasma serotonin levels are normal in this situation, but urinary 5-HT levels are usually elevated because some of the circulating 5-HTP is decarboxylated to 5-HT in the kidney and excreted as 5-HT (or 5-HIAA). Patients with foregut NETs are more likely to excrete high levels of 5-HTP in the urine and present with the *atypical* carcinoid syndrome. However, there is considerable overlap in 5-HTP, 5-HT, and 5-HIAA urinary excretion from patient to patient with carcinoid syndrome.[338]

Originally, symptoms of the carcinoid syndrome were attributed to serotonin.[22,223,321] However, the role of serotonin in flushing remains unclear.[223,325] The cause of the flushing may differ depending on the tumor type. In patients with gastric NETs, the red, patchy, and pruritic flush is thought to be caused by histamine, because this type of flushing can be prevented by H_1 and H_2 antihistamines.[223,258,338] Other candidates for mediators of flushing include tachykinins (substance P, neurokinins) and other GI peptides.[12,325,339–341]

The pathogenesis of diarrhea in patients with carcinoid syndrome is also complex. Patients with the carcinoid syndrome have increased 5-HT-mediated colonic motility with a shortened intestinal transit time and, possibly, an alteration in intestinal secretion/absorption.[341,342] Serotonin overproduction is probably responsible for diarrhea in most patients.[16,223,325,341,342]

Serotonin (in combination with histamine) may be responsible for producing bronchospasm. With respect to the pathogenesis of carcinoid heart disease,[317,330,343] patients with heart disease have higher urinary 5-HIAA excretion and have higher plasma levels of tachykinins and other peptides than those without heart disease.[12,316,318,328,344,345] Serotonin may be the most important pathogenetic factor.[323,330,343,346] Carcinoid-like valvular plaques/fibrosis occurs in animals receiving serotonin long term, as well as in animals deficient in the serotonin transporter gene.[330] Furthermore, serotonin stimulates subendocardial cells in culture and collagen synthesis by heart valve interstitial cells.[317,330] The valvular heart disease caused by appetite suppressant drugs such as the serotonin agonist drug dexfenfluramine is indistinguishable from carcinoid heart disease. Serotonin may also be involved in other fibrotic reactions sometimes seen in the carcinoid syndrome, such as retroperitoneal fibrosis.[223,320,327]

Clinical Features and Diagnosis

The carcinoid syndrome is predominantly associated with midgut (SI) NETs. The most frequent symptoms are spontaneous cutaneous flushing (see Fig. 43.8) and diarrhea, followed by bronchospasm with wheezing and asthmatic symptoms and, later in the course of the disease, carcinoid heart disease with primarily right-sided heart failure (see Table 43.11).

The *typical* carcinoid flush is the sudden appearance of a deep red erythema of the upper part of the body, primarily the face and neck (see Fig. 43.8).[347,348] Flushes are often associated with an unpleasant feeling of warmth, occasionally with lacrimation, itching, palpitations, facial or conjunctival edema, and diarrhea. Flushes may be spontaneous or be precipitated by stress, alcohol, certain foods such as cheese, or exercise, or be pharmacologically induced by injections of catecholamines, calcium, or pentagastrin.[22,223] Flushes may be brief, lasting 2–5 minutes, especially initially, or may be prolonged for hours, especially later. With respiratory tract NETs, the flushes can be frequently prolonged (lasting for hours to days), reddish in color, and associated with salivation, lacrimation, diaphoresis, facial swelling, palpitations, deep furrowing of the forehead, diarrhea, and hypotension. The flushing with respiratory tract carcinoids has a greater tendency to cause diffuse body involvement, and after repeated flushing of this type, patients may develop a constant red or cyanotic coloration. The *atypical* flush associated with gastric NETs is also reddish in color but patchy in distribution over the neck and face. It is frequently provoked by food intake, with erythema associated with blotches and wheals with central clearing, frequently occurring around the neck and on the arms, and the lesions are frequently associated with pruritus.[22,223]

Diarrhea usually (85% of cases) occurs with flushing, but it may occur alone in 15% of cases.[16,321,343] The diarrhea is usually watery; less commonly it is frothy or the pale bulky stool of steatorrhea, with 2–30 stools/day. Most patients (60%) have fecal outputs less than 1 L/day.[16] Abdominal pain may be present with the diarrhea or independently.[16]

Carcinoid heart disease can be a late manifestation of carcinoid syndrome (Fig. 43.9; also see Table 43.11).[316,323,328] Fibrous deposits are diffuse and are found most commonly on the ventricular aspect of the tricuspid valve and the associated chordae, and less commonly on the pulmonary valve cusps.[223,317,323,330] Valvular lesions on the left side of the heart occur in 30% of autopsy cases, most frequently occur on the mitral valve, and are less extensive than in the right heart.[223] Tricuspid regurgitation is the most common result (90%–100%), followed by tricuspid stenosis (43%–59%), pulmonary regurgitation (50%–81%), and pulmonary stenosis (25%–59%).[318,323,332] At diagnosis, 27%–43% of patients with carcinoid heart disease are functional class I, 30%–40% are class II, 13%–31% class III, and 3%–12% class IV.[318,328] Carcinoid heart disease appears to be decreasing in frequency and severity.[22,318,330] This decrease has been attributed to widespread use of SSAs, which control the release of serotonin, tachykinins, and other biologically active agents thought to be important in the pathogenesis of carcinoid heart disease.[22,318,330]

Wheezing or asthma-like symptoms, pellagra-like skin lesions with hyperkeratosis and hyperpigmentation, arthritis/arthralgias, changes in mental state or confusion, ophthalmic changes during

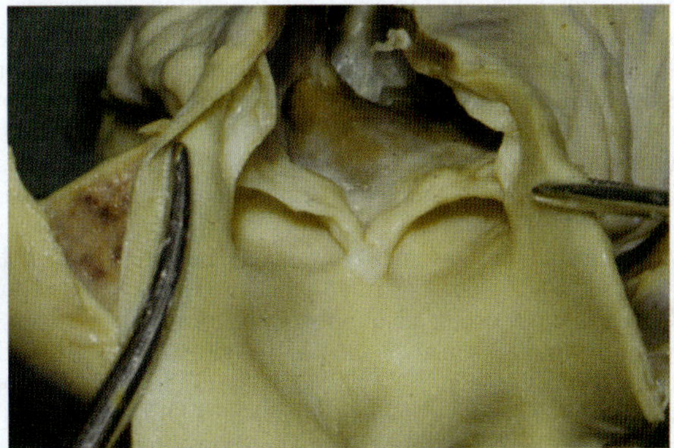

Fig. 43.9 Carcinoid heart disease. Note fibrotic thickening of the cusps of the pulmonary valve and the endocardium in a patient with small intestinal carcinoid tumor and liver metastases.

flushing, and cognitive impairment may also occur.[223,331] Furthermore, a variety of noncardiac problems caused by increased fibrous tissue have been reported in patients with carcinoid syndrome, including retroperitoneal fibrosis, Peyronie disease of the penis,[349] intra-abdominal fibrosis (especially with SI NETs), pleural and pulmonary fibrosis, skin fibrosis, and occlusion of the mesenteric arteries or veins.[320,327]

A serious complication of the carcinoid syndrome is a *carcinoid crisis*.[22,325] Carcinoid crises are usually precipitated during procedures such as surgery, anesthesia, chemotherapy, endoscopy, or interventional radiologic procedures (e.g., biopsies and hepatic tumor embolization).[22,322,324,326,333] Symptoms of crisis include extreme changes in blood pressure (usually hypotension, but sometimes hypertension), confusion, stupor, profound flushing, diarrhea, bronchospasm, hyperthermia, and cardiac arrhythmias.[22,325]

Carcinoid syndrome should be suspected in a patient with a carcinoid tumor if any of the typical symptoms are present (see Table 43.11). To confirm the syndrome, serotonin or one of its breakdown products is generally measured (see Fig. 43.7). In one study[350] of patients with carcinoids, urinary 5-HIAA/serotonin levels were elevated in 14%/18% of foregut, 76%/46% of midgut, and 0% of hindgut carcinoids.[350] A 24-hour urine 5-HIAA measurement is generally more specific than serum serotonin measurement. There is a very close correlation between a single plasma 5-HIAA determination and the 24-hour urinary 5-HIAA excretion,[351] raising the possibility that plasma measurements could replace the more inconvenient urinary collection that is currently the gold standard but that does not always yield reliable results because of incomplete and improper collection.[351]

False-positive urinary 5-HIAA results may occur if the patient is eating serotonin-rich foods, such as bananas, plantains, pineapple, kiwi fruit, walnuts, hickory nuts, pecans, and avocados.[352,353] Guaifenesin, acetaminophen, salicylates, and levodopa may also affect urinary 5-HIAA levels.[223,353,354] Elevations of urinary 5-HIAA can also occur in intestinal malabsorption and other conditions.[354] In foregut NETs that produce an atypical carcinoid syndrome with increased plasma 5-HTP levels (see Fig. 43.7), the urinary 5-HIAA may not be markedly increased. If one properly controls dietary and medication intake, the normal range for urinary 5-HIAA excretion is between 2 and 8 mg/day, although using a higher cutoff (15 mg/day) may reduce false-positive results.[354] Many patients with serotonin-secreting NETs have urinary 5-HIAA excretions in the 8–30-mg/day range. In one study, urinary 5-HIAA determinations had a 73% sensitivity and 100% specificity for the carcinoid syndrome.[340]

Diagnostic difficulties are common in patients who flush for reasons other than the carcinoid syndrome, who have the syndrome but do not flush, who have tumors such as foregut carcinoids where 5-HIAA may be normal or minimally elevated, or in rare patients who flush without metastatic disease.[336,355] The differential diagnosis of flushing is extensive and includes menopausal hot flashes, reactions to alcohol and glutamate, adverse effects to medications (e.g., chlorpropamide, calcium channel blockers, and nicotinic acid), chronic myelogenous leukemia, and systemic mastocytosis.[355] None of these flushing conditions causes increased urinary 5-HIAA excretion.

Treatment

SSAs are the first-line drugs of choice for treatment of carcinoid syndrome.[223,356,357] Use of somatostatin itself is limited by its short half-life (2.5–3 minutes).[223,358] With the development of the synthetic SSAs such as octreotide, subcutaneous treatment can be given every 6–12 hours.[223,358,359] Sustained-release formulations (octreotide LAR and lanreotide depot injection) allow control of carcinoid symptoms in the majority of patients with once-every-4-week administration.[360,361] Octreotide LAR is administered as an intramuscular injection, whereas lanreotide is administered as a deep subcutaneous injection. Both octreotide and lanreotide share a similar mechanism of action, binding avidly to somatostatin receptor subtype 2, and to a lesser extent with subtype 5.[362,363] Individual responses vary, and some patients require higher doses or more frequent dosing over time.[364–366] To prevent a carcinoid crisis, patients with carcinoid syndrome undergoing procedures should receive an additional SSA.[207,367] A supplementary subcutaneous bolus dose of 250–500 μg octreotide should be given within 1–2 hours before the procedure.[207] For emergency surgery in therapy-naïve patients, current guidelines recommend a 500–1000-μg IV bolus of octreotide or 500 μg subcutaneously 1–2 hours before the procedure,[207] although some use higher doses,[333] and others advise a continuous infusion of octreotide.[207]

Short-term adverse effects of SSAs are common, mild, and brief; most frequent are pain at the injection site, nausea, and diarrhea. Long-term side effects are usually mild and uncommonly lead to drug discontinutation.[94,223,232,357,368] These include biliary sludge/stones, steatorrhea, and deterioration in glucose tolerance.[94,223,364] The incidence of biliary disease in patients treated long term with octreotide is approximately 30%, with most patients developing sludge and 1%–10% developing symptomatic gallbladder disease.[94,223,232,365]

For a patient with severe refractory carcinoid syndrome and liver-dominant disease, hepatic artery embolization (discussed later) is palliative in most cases.[223,369–371]

Patients who develop refractory diarrhea while on standard doses of a SSA may benefit from treatment with telotristat ethyl, an oral tryptophan hydroxylase inhibitor. In the phase III TELESTAR trial, 135 patients with refractory diarrhea (defined as >4 bowel movements a day) were randomized to receive telotristat at two doses (250 and 500 mg tid) versus placebo (while continuing on a stable dose of SSA).[372] The primary endpoint was reduction in daily bowel movement frequency. After a 12-week double-blind duration, mean reductions in daily bowel movements were 0.81 for the 250 mg dose, and 0.69 for the 500 mg dose. Both doses of telotristat reduced levels of urine 5-HIAA by about 50%. As a result of this trial, the 250 mg tid dose of telotristat was approved for management of refractory diarrhea. The drug is relatively well tolerated with mild nausea and asymptomatic increases in serum GGPT observed in some patients. Constipation is a rare side effect.

In patients with symptomatic carcinoid heart disease, valve-replacement surgery is typically indicated.[317,328,330,343,373] With the improved ability to control the carcinoid syndrome preoperatively and perioperatively, cardiac valve surgery—associated mortality has decreased to 10%, and the median survival after surgery can be as long as 11 years.[317,373] The major indication for valve surgery is right heart failure.[343] Cardiac surgery is associated with a mortality reduction.[328,343]

TUMOR LOCALIZATION

Management of patients with NETS (pNETs and GI-NETs) requires determination of the tumor extent (stage) and, when possible, the site of the primary tumor.[12,22,98,367,374,375] Many tumor localization modalities are available.[12,22,98,367,375]

Endoscopy

As discussed earlier, endoscopy is essential for detection of primary gastroduodenal and colorectal NETs, as well as NETs originating in the terminal ileum adjacent to the ileocecal valve.[376] Occult primary SI NETs can sometimes be detected by capsule endoscopy or double-balloon enteroscopy, although routine use of these modalities is not routinely necessary or recommended. Typically, the presence of a typical mesenteric mass on cross-sectional imaging is indicative of a primary SI tumor.

Endoscopic Ultrasonography

EUS facilitates T staging (and possibly N staging) of gastric and rectal NETs.[12,246,249,259,299,377–379] EUS is also quite sensitive in detecting pNETs[98,178,380] and at providing histological confirmation of disease via FNA. EUS detects approximately 80% of insulinomas (range, 57%–92%), which is superior to conventional imaging studies.[12,71] EUS also detects approximately 70% of gastrinomas (range, 40%–100%).[12,377] In MEN-1 patients, EUS can detect pNETs not seen by other modalities and may prove particularly useful for serial assessments of the size of small lesions that are not resected when diagnosed.[12,379]

Computed Tomography and Magnetic Resonance Imaging

Abdominal CT and MRI are widely used to assess primary NET location and tumor staging.[22,374,375,380–383] Many SI NETs are too small to be seen on CT or MRI. Insulinomas and duodenal gastrinomas are also usually small (<1 cm), whereas most non-insulinoma pNETs present late in their course and are large (>4 cm) and more easily imaged.[12,101]

To enhance the conspicuity of liver metastases, three-phase CT imaging is recommended using arterial phase (roughly 20 seconds from contrast administration) as well as venous phase (roughly 70 seconds) and noncontrast imaging. Multiphasic imaging can also improve sensitivity of CT scans to detect small pancreatic NETs. MRI is even more sensitive than CT scans for detection of liver metastases. For patients undergoing gadolinium-based MRI scans, gadoxetate disodium (Eovist) contrast with hepatobiliary phase imaging improves conspicuity of small liver metastases.[384]

Somatostatin Receptor Imaging

Somatostatin-receptor imaging is useful both for optimal whole-body staging of disease as well as assessment of somatostatin-receptor expression. The latter function is important for assessing potential benefit of treatment with SSAs and radiolabeled SSAs (discussed later). In the past, somatostatin-receptor scintigraphy using ^{111}Indium-pentetreotide (OctreoScan) was the primary method of somatostatin-receptor imaging. More recently, ^{68}Gallium or ^{64}Cu dotatate PET imaging with CT fusion provides greater sensitivity and higher spatial resolution.[385,386] Studies have shown that an appropriately ordered dotatate scan can influence clinical decision-making in a substantial proportion of cases.[387] Although not routinely indicated for surveillance of disease, somatostatin receptor imaging should be performed at baseline in most patients with well-differentiated tumors, as well as prior to consideration of treatment with radiolabeled SSAs and prior to procedures such as surgery or liver embolization where optimal localization of tumors can be beneficial.

Other scanning methods for tumor localization in selected patients with GI-NETs have been described recently but are not widely available. Insulinomas overexpress receptors for GLP-1, and one study[388] demonstrated that a radiolabeled GLP-1 analog can detect occult insulinomas not localized by other imaging modalities.^{11}C and ^{18}F-labeled levodopa has been used to visualize NETs using PET[22,375]; ^{11}C-5-HTP has also been used.[22,380] PET using ^{18}F-deoxyglucose (FDG) may also be helpful in the subset of NETs with high proliferative rates and poor cell differentiation (discussed later).[375,389,390]

TREATMENT OF METASTATIC DISEASE

Because of the effectiveness of medical therapy (e.g., long-acting SSAs) for patients with carcinoid syndrome and functional pNETs, survival of these patients is increasingly being determined by the tumor's biology and growth pattern.[2,27,94,100,110,176,207,215–220,222–225,232,260,273,359,362,363,391–499] NETs can grow at different rates in different patients, and rate of growth is a prognostic factor. In general, metastatic NETs are relatively slow-growing compared with more common adenocarcinomas, although poorly differentiated NECs are highly aggressive.[24,126,441,500] Basic categories of treatment include cytoreductive hepatic surgery, liver-directed embolization therapies, and systemic treatments.

Cytoreductive Surgery

Removal of resectable metastatic tumor (cytoreductive surgery, debulking, and metastasectomy) is often considered, although there are no controlled studies to establish its value.[12,67,94,98,146,204,264,367,393,410,501] Hepatic cytoreductive surgery may be recommended if it is thought that more than 90% of liver metastases can be resected, with 5-year survival rates of 75%–80% and occasional cures,[12,67,94,146,204,264,367,393,410,465,501] but such a resection is possible in only 5%–15% of patients. Hepatic cytoreductive surgery may also be required in patients with functional NETs when other therapies cannot reduce plasma hormone levels sufficiently to control symptoms.[12]

Mesenteric adenopathy and/or fibrosis may develop in the mesenteric root in some patients with SI NETs, with resultant intestinal obstruction, abdominal pain, and other symptoms.[176,281,431] Some recommend that mesenteric disease should be debulked in such patients, even if they have liver metastases,[94,176,264,281,431,466,499] an approach that can relieve or prevent symptoms and may prolong survival.[94,176,264,431,466,499] At the time of cytoreductive surgery, prophylactic cholecystectomy is sometimes performed because of the risk of biliary sludge or stones from future long-term treatment with SSAs.[264,431,476]

Liver-Directed Nonsurgical Therapies

Several liver-directed therapies target hepatic metastases from NETs. Although they are widely used and mentioned in management guidelines, there are no completed randomized trials comparing them.[281,367,401,499] These liver-directed, nonoperative approaches are primarily considered in patients with unresectable NETs with metastases that are limited to the liver or liver-dominant, particularly in patients with functional syndromes in whom the hormone excess state cannot be well controlled by other modalities.[367,370,499]

Radiofrequency Ablation and Other Ablative Methods

Locally ablative techniques, RFA, microwave ablation, ethanol injection, and cryotherapy of hepatic metastases from NETs can be performed at the time of surgery or percutaneously using interventional radiologic techniques.[94,203,369,436,456,478,480,495] Microwave ablation is the most widely used, increasingly in combination with other techniques such as cytoreductive surgery.[203,369,436,456,478,480,495] Relative contraindications to ablation include large lesions (>3.5 cm), numerous lesions (>5), and metastases adjacent to vital structures.[51,367,369,436,456,478,480] Response rates are 80%–95%, with some responses lasting as long as 3 years.[203,369,436,495] Serious complications of RFA or microwave ablation include bleeding or abscess formation.[203,369,495] Although the value of ablation has not been established in a controlled trial, some guidelines endorse these techeniques as an effective therapy.[94,146,367]

Hepatic Artery Embolization and Chemoembolization

Most NETs are highly vascular, and interrupting their arterial supply can selectively damage the tumor; the uninvolved liver is less susceptible because it receives the majority of its blood from the portal vein (see Chapter 98).[94,369,433] Options include transarterial embolization (TAE) alone or combined with intra-arterial chemotherapeutic agents (TACE). The most common chemotherapy drugs used with TACE are doxorubicin, 5-fluorouracil (5-FU), cisplatin, mitomycin C, or streptozotocin.[94,369,433,438] Embolic particles include microembospheres, polyvinyl alcohol particles, or gel foam powder.[395,423,449]

Complete or relative contraindications to TAE or TACE include portal venous occlusion, significant liver dysfunction, involvement of greater than 50%–75% of the liver with tumor, surgical biliary reconstruction, and poor performance status.[94,203,369,395,398,433] From 60% to 100% of patients treated with TAE or TACE have symptomatic improvement, and 25%–86% have an objective tumor response for a highly variable period of time.[369,398,433,449] In patients with the carcinoid syndrome, TAE or TACE reduces symptoms in 64%–75%, and 5-HIAA excretion/tumor markers in 50%–70%.[484,502]

Five-year survival rates postembolizations are 30%–50% in patients with a metastatic GI-NET and 20%–35% in patients with a metastatic pNET.[94,369,438] Both TAE and TACE can lead to death (<6%) and to morbid complications (10%–80%), including a postembolization syndrome of abdominal pain, fever, and nausea/vomiting.[203,369,395,398,440,449] Serious complications are uncommon and include gallbladder necrosis, hepatic failure, liver abscess, and renal failure.[94,203,369,395,398,440,449] Recent guidelines concluded that, in centers with experience with the procedure(s), TAE or TACE should be considered for palliative treatment in patients with liver-dominant, metastatic NETs that are unresectable.[146,367] There are no completed prospective randomized studies comparing TAE with TACE.[353]

Hepatic Radioembolization

Another embolic option for patients with unresectable liver-dominant NETs is radioembolization using ^{90}Yttrium (^{90}Y) microspheres, referred to as *selective internal radiation therapy* (SIRT). Two types of ^{90}Y microspheres can be used: resin (SIR-Spheres, Sirtex Medical, Australia) and glass (TheraSpheres, Nordion, Canada).[94,394,486] Just prior to intra-arterial administration of ^{90}Y microspheres, a hepatic angiogram is performed to determine that the catheter tip is in the appropriate location and to avoid injection of the microspheres into duodenal or cystic arteries, which could result in duodenal ulceration or cholecystitis, respectively.[94,486] Another serious complication to avoid is radiation pneumonitis due to shunting of the ^{90}Y microspheres to the lung.[94,486] This latter complication can largely be prevented by confirming that the degree of lung shunting on scintigraphy is 10% or less and by adjusting the ^{90}Y dose.[94,442,454,486] A postembolization syndrome is common following SIRT.[353] Grade 2 constitutional side effects (weight loss, fatigue, fever) occur in 43% of patients, and GI side effects are common. Grade 3 short-term adverse effects are rare. However, long-term radiation-induced liver disease represents an important concern, particularly in patients with extensive bilobar metastases. The manifestations of this complication include jaundice, ascites, and a pseudo-cirrhotic appearance of the liver caused by damage to intrahepatic bile ducts.[503] The response rate to SIRT is 55% (range, 12%–89%); stable disease occurs in another 32%

(range, 10%–60%).[94,394] Symptom improvement, including improved quality of life, is seen in half of patients, with a mean survival of 30 months.[94,420,445,453]

Liver Transplantation

Liver transplantation is used in a small number of patients with metastatic GI-NETs, although its use is controversial.[94,367,419,437,443,444,463,470,504] In one review, the overall 5-year survival rate after transplantation was 52%, and disease-free survival was 30%. The surgical mortality rate is 10%–14%.[443,444] In the UNOS database, overall 1-, 3-, and 5-year survival rates were 81%, 65%, and 49%, respectively.[470] Factors predicting a poor outcome were a major resective surgery concurrent with the liver transplant, poor tumor differentiation, and hepatomegaly. With the recognition of these poor prognostic factors, the overall 5-year survival rate increased to 59% after the year 2000. Reanalysis for additional predictors of poor outcome identified age older than 45, hepatomegaly, and major or minor resective surgery concurrent with liver transplantation.[443] Additional adverse risk factors[94,437,444,463,470] may include a primary NET in the duodenum or pancreas,[444] extrahepatic metastases at the time of transplantation, extensive (>50%) liver involvement, and Ki-67 index above 10%.[94,463] Generally, guidelines restrict liver transplantation to patients with liver-only disease or to patients with minimal and resectable extrahepatic tumors (i.e., unresected primary sites).

Somatostatin Analogs

SSAs not only control hormone release from functional NETs but also have an inhibitory effect on tumor growth,[12,22,94,100,363,400,404,422,505] despite a negligible objective response rate. The precise mechanism for this antiproliferative effect is not clear. Except for insulinomas, over 90% of all well-differentiated GEP-NETs possess somatostatin receptors that can activate intracellular cascades that reduce cell proliferation. Somatostatin can also inhibit the release of growth factors from the NET or from adjacent cells and can have antigrowth effects on other cells that may contribute to cancer growth (e.g., vascular, stromal, and immune cells).[358,400,505]

Two pivotal phase III trials have established the inhibitory effects of SSAs on tumor growth. PROMID randomized 85 patients with well-differentiated, low-grade metastatic midgut NETs to receive octreotide LAR 30 mg every 4 weeks versus placebo. Median time to progression, the primary endpoint, improved from 6 months on placebo to 14.3 months with octreotide LAR ($P < .001$).[363] There was no significant effect on overall survival (OS), possibly because of the small number of patients who died during the study and the ability of patients receiving placebo to crossover to active drug after disease progression. In the CLARINET trial, 204 patients with enteropancreatic NETs (somatostatin receptor positive, Ki-67 index ≤10%) were randomized to receive lanreotide 120 mg every 4 weeks versus placebo.[362] The large majority of patients (96%) had stable disease prior to randomization. At the time of data analysis, median progression-free survival (PFS) was 18 months with placebo but had not been reached with lanreotide (HR 0.47; $P < .001$). Side effects of lanreotide included diarrhea, abdominal pain, and cholelithiasis.

As a result of the PROMID and CLARINET studies, both octreotide and lanreotide are recommended by various guidelines for management of somatostatin-receptor positive GEP-NETs. Due to similar mechanisms of action and outcomes, there are little data to favor use of one SSA versus the other, nor is there any data supporting use of one SSA after progression on the other.

Interferon-α

Similar to SSAs, interferon-α is effective at controlling symptoms of hormone excess states in functional GI-NETs and also has antiproliferative effects that primarily result in disease stabilization (30%–80%) rather than causing a decrease in tumor size (<15%).[94,406,428,506] The antiproliferative effect of interferon is thought to be mediated by several mechanisms: inhibiting DNA synthesis, blocking cell-cycle progression in G1 phase, stimulating an increase in bcl-2, inhibiting protein synthesis, inhibiting angiogenesis via decreased expression of VEGF/VEGFR, and inducing apoptosis.[94,428,498,506] Adverse effects of interferon include flu-like symptoms, anorexia, fatigue, myelosuppression, and hepatotoxicity. As a result of these side effects and lack of well-powered randomized trials confirming benefit, interferon-α is rarely used for management of GEP-NETs and considered controversial in guidelines (NCCN category 3).[367]

Everolimus

mTOR is a serine-threonine kinase that plays an important role in cell growth, proliferation, and apoptosis.[94,475,490,507] Activation of the mTOR cascade plays an important role in the growth of NETs, especially pNETs.[94,151,391,411,462,464,485,488,490,507] The oral mTOR inhibitor everolimus has been studied in three pivotal phase III trials, all of which evaluated PFS as the primary endpoint.

In the RADIANT-3 study, 410 patients with advanced progressive pNETs were randomized to receive everolimus (10 mg/day) or placebo, with crossover allowed upon progression on placebo. Everolimus prolonged median PFS from 4.6 to 11 months (HR 0.35, $P < .0001$).[151] The objective response rate was 5%. The most common grade 3 or 4 side effects were myelosuppression, diarrhea, stomatitis, or hyperglycemia, ranging in incidence from 3% to 7%; these side effects were generally manageable by dose reduction or drug interruption. Pneumonitis and infections were among other clinically important adverse effects. There was a nonsignificant trend toward improved OS.

The RADIANT 2 study randomized patients with progressive, unresectable, well-differentiated nonpancreatic NETs and history of carcinoid syndrome (primarily midgut NETs) to receive octreotide LAR (30 mg/month) with either everolimus (10 mg/day) or placebo. The results of this study were equivocal: The median PFS for the everolimus/LAR patients was 16.4 months compared to 11.3 months in the LAR/placebo group (HR 0.77; $P = .026$), a difference that did not reach the prespecified level of significance. OS analysis numerically favored the placebo group, although the results were not statistically significant. The RADIANT 2 study did not lead to approval of everolimus in this population of patients.[415]

The last phase III study, RADIANT 4, evaluated everolimus versus placebo in 302 patients with *nonfunctional* GI and lung NETs. As a result of the eligibility criteria, a diverse population of lung, gastroduodenal, and colorectal NETs were enrolled, with relatively few midgut NETs compared to RADIANT 2. No crossover was permitted in this study. This study met its primary endpoint, demonstrating improvement in median PFS from 3.9 months on placebo to 11.0 months with everolimus (HR 0.48, $P < .001$). Because of the RADIANT 4 study, everolimus was approved for treatment of nonfunctional GI and lung NETs.[508]

It is unclear whether tumor functional status (history of carcinoid syndrome) should be a determining factor in selection of everolimus for progressive GEP-NETs. In general, everolimus is appropriate for patients with clinically significant progression and is likely more appropriate in nonmidgut versus midgut NETs. Risks versus benefits need to be carefully weighed, particularly in patients who are older, frail, or have clinically significant comorbidities such as lung disease or diabetes.

Sunitinib

GEP-NETs are highly vascular tumors, expressing both VEGF and its receptor (VEGFR). Several antiangiogenic drugs have shown activity in single arm and small randomized studies, but only sunitinib is approved for use in patients with advanced pNETs.[367,492,509] Sunitinib is an orally active, small-molecule inhibitor of a number of tyrosine kinase receptors, including PDGFRs, VEGFR-1, VEGFR-2, c-KIT, and FLT-3.[477,509] In a placebo-controlled trial,[509] patients with progressive, unresectable, metastatic, and well-differentiated pNETs were randomly assigned to receive either oral sunitinib (37.5 mg/day) or placebo. Sunitinib increased median PFS from 4.5 to 11.4 months (HR 0.42; $P = .001$) and was associated with a trend toward OS benefit, outcomes that were very similar to those associated with everolimus in the RADIANT 3 trial.[509] Key adverse events included hypertension, myelosuppression, and palmar-plantar erythrodysesthesia (hand-foot syndrome).[509] Adverse effects were generally manageable with a dose reduction or drug discontinuation.[509] As with everolimus, it is not clear when sunitinib should be used relative to other therapies for patients with advanced progressive pNETs.[94,353]

Peptide Receptor Radionuclide Radiotherapy

^{177}Lutetium-Dotatate

Somatostatin receptors are highly expressed in most well-differentiated GEP-NETs, and treatment with radiolabeled SSAs allows targeted cytotoxic radiolabeled somatostatin receptor ligands to bind to the tumor.[396,397,447,493] This form of treatment is also known as peptide receptor radiotherapy (PRRT). Several radioisotopes coupled to SSAs have been evaluated, including ^{90}yttrium (^{90}Y) and ^{177}lutetium (^{177}Lu).[396,397,447,493] The most frequent SSAs used are octreotide or octreotate, an SSA with higher affinity to somatostatin receptor subtype 2; common chelators are DTPA or DOTA.[94,396,397,493] ^{90}Y is a beta-emitting isotope with a relatively long tissue penetration range of approximately 12 mm. In one study of 87 patients, objective radiographic responses observed with ^{90}Y-dotataoc were 28%. Another study, evaluating only patients with refractory carcinoid syndrome, demonstrated an objective response rate of only 4%, but a high rate of stable disease (70%).[510,511] One of the main toxicities involving ^{90}Y-based PRRT is renal insufficiency, a side effect that can be partially ameliorated with use of concurrent amino acid infusions, which inhibit glomerular reabsorption of the radioactive peptides.[512] In one large series of 1109 patients treated with ^{90}Y-based PRRT, 102 (9%) experienced severe renal toxicity. Long-term myelotoxicity (myelodysplastic syndrome or acute leukemia) occurs in roughly 2% of patients.[513]

^{177}Lu-based PRRT represents a new-generation radiolabeled SSA with a shorter particle range of roughly 2 mm. Studies using ^{177}Lu-dotatate have demonstrated objective response rates ranging from 18% to 44% with median PFS durations of approximately 30 months. With use of prophylactic amino acid infusions, rates of grade 3 or 4 nephrotoxicity have been <1%. Long-term rates of myelodysplastic syndrome/acute leukemia are approximately 2%.[514,515]

The NETTER-1 study, the first prospective phase III study of a radiolabeled SSA, included 231 patients with well-differentiated midgut NETs and evidence of progression on standard-dose octreotide LAR and evidence of somatostatin receptor expression on OctreoScan who were randomized to receive four cycles of ^{177}Lu-dotatate (200 mCi every 8 weeks) along with octreotide 30 mg versus high-dose octreotide (60 mg every 4 weeks). The primary endpoint was PFS by blinded central radiology review. The study demonstrated a clinically and statistically significant improvement in PFS, with a median PFS of 8.4 months on the high-dose octreotide arm of the study and median PFS not reached with ^{177}Lu-dotatate (HR 0.21; $P < .001$). The objective response rate with ^{177}Lu-dotatate was 18% compared to 3% with high-dose octreotide. There was also preliminary evidence of improved OS with ^{177}Lu-dotatate (HR 0.4; $P = .004$), which needs to be confirmed on planned final OS analysis.[516]

Based on results of the NETTER-1 study as well as a single-arm institutional registry data,^{177}Lu-dotatate was approved for treatment of advanced, progressive GEP-NETs. Appropriate selection of patients requires confirmation of somatostatin receptor expression on imaging studies (OctreoScan or ^{68}Ga-dotatate PET). There is evidence that degree of somatostatin receptor expression correlates with tumor response.[517] A standard treatment course consists of four cycles of ^{177}Lu-dotatate, although there is some controversy regarding the potential role of dosimetry in refining treatment dose and number of cycles. For patients who experience a prolonged duration of stable disease or response after an initial course of PRRT, subsequent retreatment is an option.[518] A total of eight individual treatment cycles (1600 mCi) are considered to be a lifetime maximum in some institutions, although some patients may be able to tolerate higher lifetime doses. There is no clear correlation between total treatment dose and risk of irreversible myelotoxicity.

Cytotoxic Chemotherapy

The role of cytotoxic chemotherapy in GEP-NETs is evolving. It is now evident that pNETs are substantially more sensitive to alkylating agent-based chemotherapy compared to midgut NETs. The role of chemotherapy in gastroduodenal and colorectal NETs is not well defined.[479]

Streptozocin-based regimens were tested extensively in NETs in the 1970s and 1980s and found to be active in pNETs. Two key randomized studies were performed. One reported objective response rates of 63% with streptozocin plus 5-FU versus 36% with streptozocin monotherapy.[519] Another study reported response rates of 69% with streptozocin plus doxorubicin versus 45% with streptozocin and 5-FU.[520] Neither study used strict radiographic response criteria, making the data difficult to apply in the context of modern treatment outcomes. A more recent retrospective analysis of a triple-drug regimen consisting of streptozocin, doxorubicin, and 5-FU demonstrated a response rate of 39% using objective radiographic parameters.[452]

Temozolomide is an oral alkylating agent with a more tolerable side effect profile compared to streptozocin. Several small phase II studies have evaluated temozolomide in combination with other agents.[399,481,521–525] A small study of temozolomide and thalidomide reported an objective response rate of 45% in 11 patients with pNETs (versus no responses in GI NETs).[525] Another study of temozolomide and bevacizumab reported a response rate of 33% and a median PFS of 14.3 months.[522]

The combination of capecitabine (an oral fluoropyrimidine) and temozolomide has been investigated in multiple retrospective series and in a recent prospective randomized clinical trial. In one institutional series of 30 chemotherapy-naïve patients with pNETs, a radiographic response rate of 70% and a median PFS of 18 months were observed.[399] Another institutional series consisting predominantly of pNETs reported a response rate of 61%.[526] Based on these data, a randomized phase II study was launched to compare capecitabine and temozolomide versus temozolomide monotherapy with patients with progressive well-differentiated pNETs. The results demonstrated a statistically significant improvement in PFS associated with the capecitabine/temozolomide combination: Median PFS was 22.7 months with the combination regimen versus 14.4 months with temozolomide monotherapy (HR 0.58; $P = .02$).[527] The regimen was well-tolerated with a 13% rate of grade 3/4 neutropenia and an 8% rate of grade 3/4 thrombocytopenia.[527] Rates of severe nausea are quite low when prophylactic ondansetron is used prior to temozolomide. Capecitabine/temozolomide is currently guideline recommended for the management of metastatic pNETs. There are conflicting data regarding the potential predictive value of methyl-guanine-methyl transferase expression.[528] Thus far, there are no completed studies comparing cytotoxic regimens to noncytotoxic drugs (everolimus or sunitinib) in the management of progressive pNETs.

Treatment of Poorly Differentiated Carcinomas

Poorly differentiated carcinomas comprise fewer than 5% of GEP-NETs.[94,260,262,263,403,408] Their recognition is important because of their aggressive course and their distinct treatment from well-differentiated tumors discussed earlier.[262,263,403,496] Poorly differentiated GI-NETs are characterized by their histologic features of aggressive growth (grade 3, with Ki-67 index >20%, and usually 50%–90%), necrosis, nuclear atypia, rapid growth, and poor clinical prognosis.[94,260,262,263,403,496] Histologically, they can be classified as small cell or large cell. These cancers generally contain few somatostatin receptors; therefore unlabeled or radiolabeled SSAs are rarely indicated. ^{18}FDG PET, CT, and MRI are frequently used to image these poorly differentiated NETs.[263] Because most patients with poorly differentiated NETs present with regional or distant metastases, surgery is rarely curative, although it still should be considered in the occasional patient with limited disease.[94,262,263,403,496]

In the typical patient with inoperable disease, chemotherapy with cisplatin (or carboplatin) plus etoposide is recommended. These agents induce remission in 14%–80% of patients, with a mean duration of response of less than 12 months.[262,263,367,403,460,461,479,496] The median survival with treatment is 4–16 months, and the average 5-year survival is only 11% (range, 0%–31%).[403] The chemotherapy regimens can be associated with significant toxicity, especially GI (nausea/vomiting), myelosuppression, and renal damage.[263,367,403,460,461,479]

Despite the absence of prospective data, patients with localized undifferentiated tumors undergoing surgical resection should generally receive adjuvant chemotherapy using cisplatin (or carboplatin) plus etoposide. Chemoradiation is another option for patients with local or locoregional poorly differentiated NEC and is the treatment of choice for locoregional small cell carcinoma of the esophagus.[529]

For platinum-resistant patients (defined as progression within 3–6 months of first-line or adjuvant platinum-based chemotherapy), there are few effective treatment options. Immunotherapy with the PD-1 inhibitor pembrolizumab has shown relatively low response rates compared to outcomes in small cell lung cancer.[530] Studies evaluating combination immunotherapy such as ipilumumab/nivolumab have shown more encouraging response rates, although most trials have been quite small.[531–535]

Full references for this chapter can be found at https://ebooks.health.elsevier.com.

44 Enterocolitis and Hepatitis Induced by Cancer Immunotherapy

Michael Dougan

IN THIS CHAPTER

INTRODUCTION

Immune checkpoint inhibitor (ICI) immunotherapy has transformed the treatment landscape for multiple malignancies over the past decade.[1] These drugs target three related immune regulatory pathways referred to as immune checkpoints: cytotoxic T lymphocyte antigen (CTLA)-4, lymphocyte activation gene (LAG)-3, and programmed death (PD)-1 or its ligand (PD-L1).[1,2] Inhibition of these immune checkpoints reinvigorates antitumor responses, largely through activation of effector memory CD8 T cells. These responses can lead to durable tumor regression, sometimes lasting for many years.[1,3]

Disabling key immune regulatory pathways to enhance antitumor responses comes at the cost of a wide spectrum of inflammatory toxicities that are collectively referred to as immune-related adverse events (irAEs).[3,4] These toxicities can involve any organ system in the body and typically resemble autoimmune diseases. The most common organs affected by these toxicities are those at barrier surfaces, including the skin, lungs, gastrointestinal tract, and liver.[4] Colitis, which can occur alone or in association with enteritis, is the most common gastrointestinal toxicity from ICI therapy, and is one of the most common toxicities overall, affecting up to 40% of patients on dual immunotherapy. Severe enterocolitis is less common, but still frequent, occurring in 10% on CTLA-4 inhibitors and 2%–5% of patients receiving PD-1 or PD-L1 inhibitors. Isolated clinically significant gastritis from immunotherapy is infrequent, though gastric inflammation often occurs in conjunction with enteritis.[5]

Hepatic toxicities occur in less than 10% of patients on single-agent immunotherapy, with toxicity more common in patients on CTLA-4 blockade (5%–10%) than in patients treated with PD-1/PD-L1 inhibitors (2%–5%).[6–11] Combination of CTLA-4 and PD-1 blockade has a substantially higher risk for hepatotoxicity with nearly a quarter of patients showing a rise in serum transaminases.[7,12] This risk is also elevated when immunotherapy is combined with other therapies such as tyrosine kinase inhibitors or chemotherapy.[13–16] These combination therapies are finding increasingly widespread clinical use.[1] Although most of the hepatotoxicity seen with these drugs is mild, approximately 1% of patients on single agent immunotherapy and nearly 10% of patients on combination therapy will develop severe hepatotoxicity, and acute liver failure has been reported.[6–12]

In the following chapter, we will discuss the mechanisms of gastrointestinal mucosal and hepatic toxicity from ICIs, the clinical features of these diseases, treatment options, and special circumstances related to these toxicities.

MECHANISM OF TOXICITY

ICIs disable immune regulatory pathways that are critical for maintaining peripheral tolerance and preventing autoimmunity; however, until recently, the effect of these inhibitors on the human immune system was studied almost exclusively in the context of antitumor responses.[4] ICIs are believed to primarily target T cells.[3,4] Activated T cells and regulatory T cells (Tregs) are high expressors of immune checkpoints, and expression increases upon repeated T-cell stimulation.[3,4] As a result, over time, T cells become increasingly resistant to further activation and enter a state often referred to as exhaustion or dysfunction where further stimulation does not occur under normal circumstances.[3] These cells can be reactivated, however, through the action of ICIs.[3,4]

In a subset of patients, ICIs can reactivate robust antitumor T-cell responses that can lead to durable remissions in multiple cancer types.[3,4] These productive responses are correlated with expansion of an effector memory CD8 T-cell population and production of interferon gamma (IFNγ).[3,17–20] Analyses of the side effects of ICIs have found evidence of lymphocytic inflammation in a variety of organs, including the colon and liver.[4,21–23] Although the immunologic drivers of these toxicities are not yet fully understood, detailed analyses of immune-related enterocolitis (irEC) have directly implicated IFNγ secreting–resident memory CD8+ T cells in the pathogenesis of this toxicity.[4,24,25] These cells are not only highly expanded in irEC in conjunction with an expansion of CD4+ IFNγ secreting cells, but inhibition of janus kinase (JAK) signaling downstream of the IFNγ receptor has shown evidence of therapeutic activity.[4,24–26] T cells with a similar phenotype have also been identified in immune-related thyroiditis, and JAK inhibitors have shown evidence of activity in immune-related myocarditis suggesting mechanistic similarities across toxicities.[27,28] Much less is known about the immune mechanisms driving hepatitis from ICIs (immune-related hepatitis or irH) at present and no detailed analyses have been reported beyond basic pathology and immunohistochemistry. In contrast to autoimmune hepatitis, plasma cells are not a substantial component of the inflammatory response in irH.[21] The infiltrate in irH mostly comprises T cells, though granulomatous hepatitis and a less inflammatory cholangitic hepatitis have also been described.[21,29,30]

ENTEROCOLITIS FROM IMMUNE CHECKPOINT INHIBITORS

Clinical Features

Diarrhea is the most common symptom associated with irEC, typically presenting as urgent, watery bowel movements without bleeding.[31] Nausea and vomiting are more common than with other causes of colitis, likely because of the high risk for upper gastrointestinal inflammation in these patients.[31,32] Bloody diarrhea, abdominal pain, cramping, and fevers are less common and are more likely to be associated with severe colitis.[31] Rapidly changing symptoms, often associated with immunotherapy infusions, are a common feature of ICI enterocolitis, setting it apart from most flares of inflammatory bowel disease (IBD). The rapidity of symptom change is particularly dramatic when patients are undergoing treatment with CTLA-4 inhibitors, where mild symptoms can become life-threatening within a few days.[31] This rapid escalation is one of the major reasons why expedited evaluation and treatment is so important in this patient population.

The severity of irEC is often rated using the common terminology criteria for adverse events (CTCAE) that grades toxicities on a scale from grade 1 (mild) to grade 5 (death). The CTCAE criteria have not been validated for irEC but are used widely in clinical trials and in most literature on the disease. Several studies have established that CTCAE-based severity scores correlate poorly with endoscopic severity, cross-sectional imaging, and, most importantly, treatment response.[31,33–35]

Diagnosis

Most patients with diarrhea on ICI therapy will ultimately be found to have inflammation in the upper or lower gastrointestinal tract.[32,36] The goal of diagnostic testing in these patients is to identify alternative causes of diarrhea in order to avoid unnecessary treatment with immunosuppressive therapy.

A focused history should include potential infectious exposures, other new medications that could be causing diarrhea, including chemotherapy and targeted therapies used in combination with ICIs, and timing of symptom onset in relation to ICI initiation. The specific ICI pathway that is inhibited in the patient (PD-1/PD-L1, CTLA-4 or LAG-3) is also important to know, as patients on CTLA-4 inhibitors are at higher risk for severe disease than are patients on other forms of immunotherapy.[31]

Although infectious causes of diarrhea are uncommon in these patients (representing less than 5% of total cases), stool cultures, and *Clostridioides difficile* testing should be sent on all patients with suspected ICI enterocolitis, given the risk of worsening an infectious colitis by starting immune suppression.[31] Ova and parasite testing should be reserved for patients who are determined to be at high risk based on their history.[31] Pancreatic insufficiency can also occur in patients on ICI therapy and should be considered in any patient whose initial diagnostic testing is unrevealing or who presents with steatorrhea.[37]

Blood tests are rarely helpful in determining the cause of diarrhea in patients on ICI therapy. Non-specific tests such as white blood cell counts or inflammatory markers, including C-reactive protein and erythrocyte sedimentation rate are even less specific in this patient population where inflammation can occur in multiple organs simultaneously, including in the tumor.

New onset or newly symptomatic Celiac disease occurs in a small fraction of these patients (1%–2%) and should be assessed serologically, given the accuracy of TTG-IgA testing in patients who have detectable serum IgA.[32] Thyroid function tests are collected as part of routine monitoring of all patients on ICI therapy, and hyperthyroidism should be considered as a potential etiology for new onset diarrhea, particularly when accompanied by other systemic symptoms.[38] Both hepatitis B serologies (surface antigen, surface antibody, and core antibody) and testing for latent tuberculosis should be sent in all patients who develop diarrhea on immunotherapy as many will require biologic immune suppression for management and rapid treatment escalation may be necessary as discussed below.[31]

Endoscopy has an important role in the diagnosis of ICI enterocolitis. Retrospective case series indicate that as many as 20% of patients with suspected ICI enterocolitis do not have any mucosal inflammation on biopsy, indicating an alternative etiology for their symptoms.[32,36] In many cases, these patients do not require systemic immune suppression. In addition to diagnostic accuracy, mucosal severity scores such as the Mayo Endoscopic Score more accurately correlate with treatment response than do the severity of symptoms, and the symptom severity has effectively no correlation with mucosal findings on endoscopy.[33] In addition, endoscopy is the only way to identify patients with microscopic colitis induced by ICI therapy, an important subgroup of patients.[36]

The best endoscopic exam for diagnosis of ICI enterocolitis is not fully yet established. The great majority of ICI colitis is pancolitis and thus can be diagnosed by flexible sigmoidoscopy as an alternative to a full colonoscopy.[23] Approximately 10%–20% of patients with diarrhea on ICI treatment will have isolated upper gastrointestinal tract inflammation and normal colons. As a result, esophagogastroduodenoscopy (EGD) should be considered a next diagnostic test in patients whose initial lower exam is normal.[32,36] Upper gastrointestinal symptoms such as nausea, vomiting, and early satiety do not reliably accompany enteritis, and therefore an EGD should be considered even in patients whose only symptom is diarrhea.

Precisely which patients with suspected ICI enterocolitis should undergo endoscopy has not been established, though in retrospective studies, endoscopy is correlated with improved treatment outcomes.[39] Generally, patients who are sick enough to require hospitalization or who have grade 3 or 4 symptoms on the CTCAE scale should be referred for endoscopic evaluation. Similarly, patients who are on concurrent medications that could be a competing cause of diarrhea should undergo endoscopy. When to perform an endoscopy on patients with milder symptoms (grade 1 or 2) is less clear. One possibility is to perform testing for fecal calprotectin or lactoferrin in order to risk strategy patients with mild symptoms, only endoscopically evaluating those patients with positive testing, though these tests have not been rigorously evaluated in ICI enterocolitis and may be less sensitive in patients with isolated enteritis.[31,40] When urgent endoscopy is available, evaluation prior to initiating immunosuppressive treatment is reasonable as this will confirm the diagnosis and help more accurately determine the severity of the inflammation. When endoscopy is not easily available, empiric treatment may be in the best interest of the patient given the potential risks of a delayed treatment initiation.[31]

Cross-sectional imaging is not helpful in the majority of patients with suspected ICI enterocolitis; the appearance by (CT) is indistinguishable from other forms of colitis. Retrospective studies have found sensitivities for abdominal CT ranging from 50%–85% and specificities ranging from 74%–78%, making CT scans relatively inaccurate as both rule-in and rule-out exams.[41,42] Cross-sectional imaging can be helpful in diagnosing extraluminal complications of ICI therapy such as perforation or abscess formation. Extraluminal complications should be considered in patients presenting with abdominal pain or fevers, both of which are uncommon in uncomplicated ICI enterocolitis.

Treatment

Data on the treatment of ICI enterocolitis is limited and mainly derived from clinical trials that were not specifically designed to evaluate this condition. Management guidelines rely on retrospective analyses and expert opinions and uniformly recommend systemic glucocorticoids as first line therapy.[31] ICI enterocolitis typically responds well to high doses of systemic glucocorticoids, though optimal dosing has not been rigorously studied, and patients are likely treated with higher doses than are necessary (Fig. 44.1).[31,43] Current guidelines recommend starting with 0.5–2 mg/kg of prednisone equivalent daily with a taper over 4–6 weeks.[31] For patients who are hospitalized with ICI enterocolitis, intravenous glucocorticoids are often used. Lower glucocorticoid doses or alternative treatments that spare glucocorticoids may ultimately prove beneficial in this population by reducing the risk of suppressing antitumor responses, though the importance of avoiding glucocorticoids in these patients remains unclear.[44]

Approximately, one-third of ICI enterocolitis patients do not respond adequately to initial glucocorticoid treatment, necessitating treatment with a secondary agent.[33,43] Second-line immune suppression should be considered in those who fail to respond to high-dose glucocorticoids within 72 hours of initiation, or who do not achieve a complete response within a week.[31] Furthermore, second-line immune suppression is generally appropriate in patients experiencing recurrent symptoms during the steroid taper or after completing a glucocorticoid course.[31] Colonic ulceration is the only identified predictive factor associated with the need for secondary immune suppression that has currently been identified; symptom severity as measured by CTCAE grading does not predict any response to glucocorticoids.[33–35] Identifying patients with ICI-associated diarrhea who have colonic ulceration is one of principle benefits of endoscopic evaluation.

Both infliximab and vedolizumab appear to be effective when used as second-line immune suppression at doses and with schedules adapted from the treatment of IBD.[33,45–48] Infliximab is typically administered intravenously at a dose of 5 mg/kg, given at weeks 0, 2, and 6, with some patients requiring longer term treatment.[31] Similarly, vedolizumab is given intravenously at a dose of 300 mg with the same infusion schedule.[31] Treatment responses are often rapid, typically occurring within a week. Although most cases of ICI enterocolitis will not recur unless the patient receives further ICI therapy, some patients may still require the full loading dose of infliximab or vedolizumab, and maintenance therapy is occasionally necessary.[31]

The choice between infliximab and vedolizumab should be based on other risk factors, as neither has demonstrated superiority in ICI enterocolitis treatment. These factors should include the risk of infection, underlying malignancy, comorbidities, and other concurrent irAEs. Infliximab should be avoided in patients with underlying hematologic malignancies due to the association

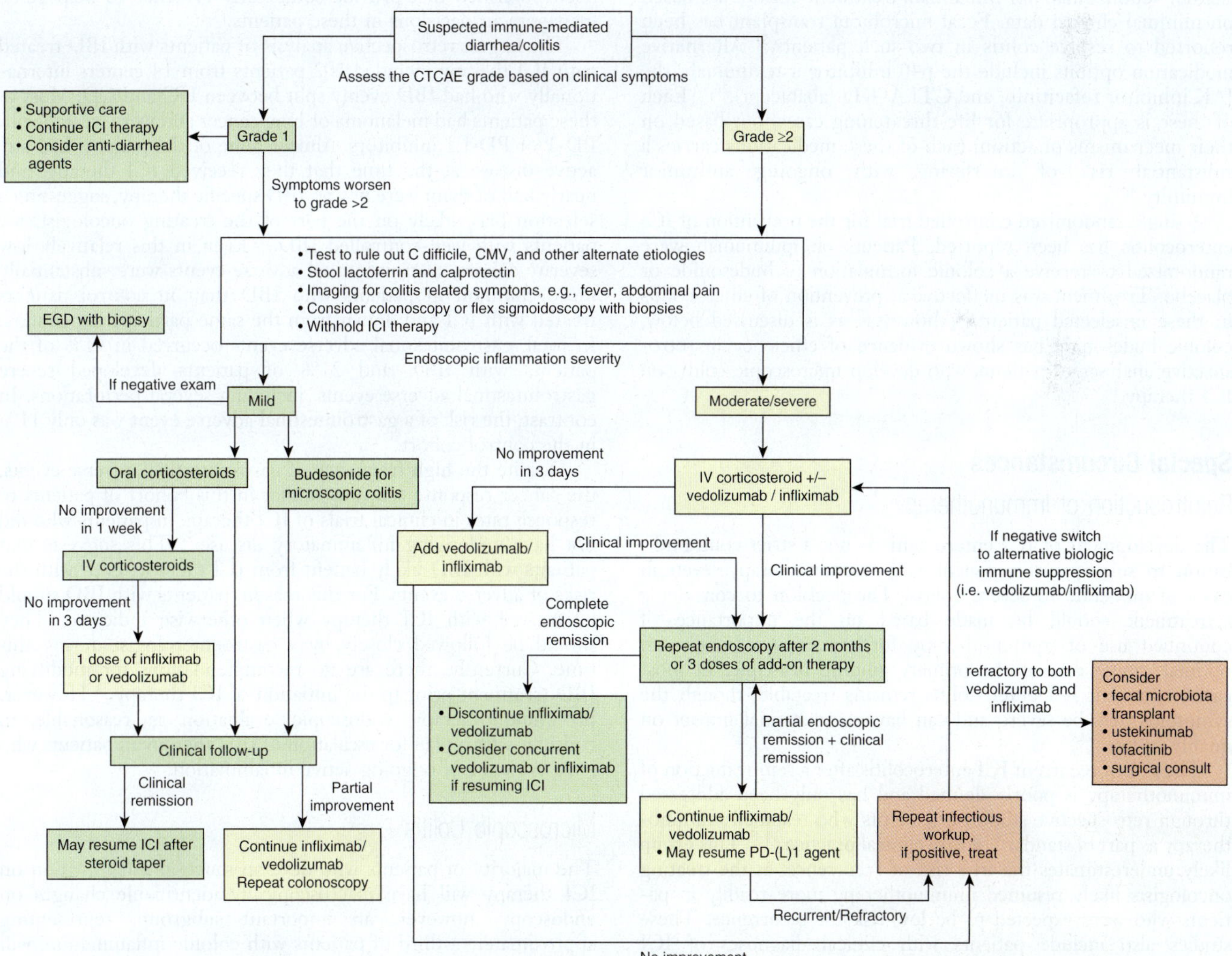

Fig. 44.1 Treatment algorithm for suspected ICI enterocolitis. (Image by Katherine Dougan. Adapted from Dougan M, Wang Y, Rubio-Tapia A, Lim JK. AGA clinical practice update on diagnosis and management of immune checkpoint inhibitor colitis and hepatitis: expert review. *Gastroenterology*. 2021;160(4):1384–1393.)

of TNF-α inhibitors with the development of rare lymphomas.[31] Additionally, caution should be exercised when using infliximab in patients with severe congestive heart failure.[31] A recent report suggests that infliximab might be associated with worse cancer outcomes; however, confounding factors such as glucocorticoid dose and duration were not adequately addressed in the analysis, making the validity of this finding less clear.[49] Infliximab can induce a rare form of hepatitis; consequently, it should be considered on a case-by-case basis for patients who have both ICI enterocolitis and hepatitis.[31] Vedolizumab may interfere with ongoing anti-tumor responses in the gastrointestinal mucosa, a particular problem for patients on ICI therapy who have primary gastrointestinal malignancies or gastrointestinal metastases. Neither therapy has yet been shown to substantially influence antitumor responses in a more general sense, though in retrospective analysis, these drugs are also used in combination with high dose glucocorticoids, making effects on antitumor immunity difficult to interpret.[50]

When patients do not respond to the initial choice of biologic therapy, switching to the alternative treatment class, either from infliximab to vedolizumab or vice versa, is recommended.[31,46] Waiting for a standard washout period is not recommended in these cases given the severity of ICI enterocolitis, and the next treatment should be initiated as soon as failure of the first agent becomes apparent. For patients who respond to neither vedolizumab nor infliximab, treatment options are based on minimal clinical data. Fecal microbiota transplant has been reported to resolve colitis in two such patients.[51] Alternative medication options include the p40 inhibitor ustekinumab, the JAK inhibitor tofacitinib, and CTLA-4-Ig (abatacept).[26,52] Each of these is appropriate for life-threatening cases, but based on their mechanisms of action, each of these medications carries a substantial risk of interfering with ongoing antitumor immunity.[4,50]

A single randomized controlled trial for the prevention of ICI enterocolitis has been reported. Patients on ipilimumab were randomized to receive a colonic formulation of budesonide or placebo. Treatment was ineffective at prevention of enterocolitis in these unselected patients[53]; however, as is discussed below, colonic budesonide has shown evidence of efficiency in retrospective analyses of patients who develop microscopic colitis on ICI therapy.[36]

Special Circumstances

Reintroduction of Immunotherapy

The development of ICI enterocolitis is not a strict contraindication to subsequent treatment with immunotherapy, even in cases of moderate to severe colitis. The decision to consider a retreatment should be made based on the importance of continued use of immunotherapy for cancer treatment, with optimal cancer care as the primary guiding principle. In most cases, recurrent ICI enterocolitis remains treatable, though the symptoms may be severe and can have a substantial impact on quality of life.[54,55]

The risk of recurrent ICI enterocolitis after a reintroduction of immunotherapy is poorly defined and has only been addressed through retrospective studies of patients who resumed immunotherapy as part of standard of care clinical practice.[54,55] This group likely underestimates the true risk of recurrence, as the treating oncologists likely resumed immunotherapy more readily in patients who were expected to be low risk for recurrence. These studies also include patients with clinical diagnoses of ICI enterocolitis without endoscopic or histopathologic confirmation, a group that we know includes a reasonably high proportion of patients who were misdiagnosed.[54,55]

The largest analysis of patients who resumed immunotherapy after developing ICI enterocolitis found that approximately a third of patients will develop colitis after restarting immunotherapy, with the highest risk in patients who resume ipilimumab.[54,55] The lowest risks are seen in patients who switch from CTLA-4 blockade to PD-1 blockade or from dual pathway immunotherapy to single agent PD-1 blockade. The risk of colitis recurrence in patients previously treated with a LAG-3 inhibitor has not yet been defined.[54,55]

Limited data suggest that maintenance therapy with either infliximab or vedolizumab may also be effective at reducing the risk of severe enterocolitis recurrence after restarting immunotherapy. This has been reported in two small case series, and a multicenter retrospective analysis.[48,54,56] The safety of this combination strategy remains to be established, and in particular, the effect on the antitumor response is unknown.

Immunotherapy in Patients With Underlying Inflammatory Bowel Disease

Patients with IBD have been excluded from the clinical trials of ICIs, as have other patients with underlying autoimmunity. For this reason, prospective, randomized data on the effect of these drugs in patients with ulcerative colitis (UC) and Crohn disease (CD) are not available. Retrospective case-control studies have been published that provide some early evidence to help guide management decisions in these patients.[31,57]

The largest retrospective analysis of patients with IBD treated with ICI therapy included 102 patients from 14 centers internationally who had IBD evenly split between UC and CD. Most of these patients had melanoma or lung cancer and were treated with PD-1 or PD-L1 inhibitors. Almost none of the patients had any active disease at the time that they received ICI therapy, and nearly half of them were not on IBD specific therapy, suggesting a selection bias, likely on the part of the treating oncologist, for patients with well-controlled IBD.[57] Even in this relatively low severity cohort, gastrointestinal adverse events were substantially more common in patients with IBD than in control patients treated with ICI and drawn from the same participating centers. In total, gastrointestinal adverse events occurred in 41% of the patients with IBD, and 21% of patients developed severe gastrointestinal adverse events, including several perforations. In contrast, the risk of a gastrointestinal adverse event was only 11% in the control cohort.[57]

Despite the high frequency of gastrointestinal adverse events, the cancer response rate was similar in this cohort of patients to response rates in clinical trials of ICI therapy in patients who did not have underlying inflammatory disease.[57] This suggests that patients with IBD likely benefit from ICI therapy, even with the risks of adverse events. For this reason, patients with IBD should be treated with ICI therapy when otherwise indicated. They should be followed closely by a gastroenterologist during this time. Currently, there are no recommendations for modifying IBD treatment prior to the initiation of ICI therapy.[31] However, pre-immunotherapy endoscopic evaluation is reasonable to consider with a plan for escalation of IBD therapy in patients who have evidence of ongoing active inflammation.

Microscopic Colitis

The majority of patients who develop mucosal inflammation on ICI therapy will have macroscopically identifiable changes on endoscopy; however, an important subgroup, representing approximately a third of patients with colonic inflammation, will develop a microscopic form of colitis.[36] This ICI-associated microscopic colitis is often indistinguishable from sporadic microscopic colitis on biopsy and has been associated with both a lymphocytic and a collagenous pattern on histology.[36] Limited retrospective data suggest that ICI-associated microscopic colitis responds to colonic formulations of budesonide and typically does not require treatment with systemic glucocorticoids. Many of these patients can resume their immunotherapy, while on budesonide, without a recurrence of their symptoms, although new inflammatory toxicities can still develop.[36]

Celiac Disease

New onset or newly symptomatic celiac disease is a rare complication of ICI therapy, representing approximately 1%–2% of patients who present with diarrhea on these agents.[32] Cases have been reported in patients treated with CLTA-4, PD-1, and PD-L1 inhibitors as well as combination therapy. As with sporadic cases, celiac disease associated with ICI therapy can be diagnosed through a combination of elevated IgA antibodies to tissue transglutaminase (TTG-IgA) and duodenal inflammation on biopsy. Symptomatically, these patients are indistinguishable from those with ICI enterocolitis, typically presenting with diarrhea. Nausea, vomiting, weight loss, and even life-threatening protein wasting can also occur.[32,58]

Unlike ICI enterocolitis, the great majority of cases of celiac disease associated with ICI therapy do not require the use of systemic immune suppression. Most patients will respond to a strict gluten–free diet and will be able to continue using immunotherapy as indicated for their cancer treatment.[32,58] For patients who do not respond to a gluten free diet, or who have colitis in addition to celiac disease, systemic glucocorticoids are generally effective therapy with secondary biologic immune suppression rarely necessary.[32]

Pancreatic Insufficiency

Damage to the exocrine pancreas is a rare but important cause of diarrhea associated with ICI therapy.[37,59] Although the precise prevalence of this complication is not known, it accounts for approximately 1% of cases of diarrhea on ICIs. Patients often do present with classic symptoms of steatorrhea precipitated by ingestion of high fat foods, though these features may be missed if not specifically addressed during a history. Often times, the diagnosis is made after ICI enterocolitis has been excluded endoscopically, or after empiric treatment with systemic immune suppression has failed to resolve diarrhea. Asymptomatic elevations in lipase are fairly common with ICI treatment, but the relationship between these elevations and pancreatic exocrine insufficiency is not currently clear. Some patients do present with apparent pancreatitis that is followed by rapid development of pancreatic exocrine deficiency, though most present with diarrhea and are otherwise asymptomatic. We currently have no evidence whether the systemic immune suppression can rescue the exocrine pancreas and restore normal function. Consequently, enzymatic replacement of lipase is the treatment of choice, and is generally effective.[37,59]

HEPATITIS FROM IMMUNE CHECKPOINT INHIBITORS

Clinical Features

Nearly all patients with irH present with asymptomatic elevations in transaminases (ALT and AST), which is typically detected through routine monitoring.[31] The level of elevation can vary from mild (1–5× ULN) to severe (>20× ULN) and is graded using a clinical trials grading system called the CTCAE (Table 44.1).[31] Although somewhat less common, irH can also present with a cholestatic pattern [elevated alkaline phosphatase (ALKP) and bilirubin] or a mixed pattern of laboratory abnormalities.[21,31,60] These elevations are most commonly detected in the first 2–3 months of ICI treatment, though irH can occur at any point on treatment.[61] Whether additional triggers contribute to the onset of irH in conjunction with ICI therapy is currently unknown.

Systemic symptoms associated with irH include fever, fatigue, and jaundice, though in most cases these symptoms can be attributed to other causes.[31] Many of these patients have other concomitant ICI toxicities or complications of their malignancy, including hepatic metastases, that can account for the observed symptoms.[31,61,62] Presentations of liver failure are exceptionally rare and are most common in patients who had underlying liver disease prior to initiation of ICIs.[31]

Diagnosis

irH is primarily a clinical diagnosis that is made after alternative diagnoses have been excluded.[31] irH should be suspected in any patient treated with ICI therapy regardless of the duration of treatment.[31] The differential diagnosis includes hepatic metastases, biliary compression, toxic ingestions such as alcohol, viral hepatitis, other drug-induced liver injury (for example acetaminophen), and ischemic or thrombotic injury.[31] Newly appreciated nonalcoholic steatohepatitis has also been reported in this population, though whether this is a rare direct side effect of ICIs, or is related to increased hepatic monitoring is still unclear.[21,29,31]

History should focus on identifying other potential causes of liver injury, including alcohol, other medications and supplements, the presence of hepatic or abdominal metastases, and risk factors for viral hepatitis. In addition, the specific class of immunotherapy used (e.g., PD-1 monotherapy, dual immunotherapy, or combination immunotherapy and targeted therapy) can greatly impact the risk of irH.[6–16] Any history of prior liver disease is also important to discuss, although any association between prior liver disease and irH remains incompletely understood.

Patients should be asked about symptoms including signs of obstruction such as pain, pruritus, and jaundice. Signs of systemic illness such as rash, fever, or arthralgia may indicate a concomitant ICI toxicity.[62] Weakness or muscle pain may indicate myositis, which may be an independent cause of transaminase elevation; as myositis can be associated with fatal myocarditis, this is a diagnosis that should not be missed.[28]

Physical examination should focus on signs of severe hepatitis (jaundice or scleral icterus) and chronic liver disease such as splenomegaly or ascites. irH is an acute hepatitis and the presence of signs of chronic liver disease should point to an alternative, potentially concomitant, diagnosis.[31,63] New muscle weakness should also be assessed.[28]

In addition to transaminases (AST and ALT), ALKP, and total bilirubin, which are routinely captured as part of surveillance monitoring in all patients on ICIs, patients with suspect irH should have testing for viral hepatitis, including hepatitis A (IgM and IgG), hepatitis B (surface antibody, surface antigen, and core antigen), and hepatitis C (antibody and RNA[31]). In some clinical circumstances, such as patients with underlying immune suppression, testing for EBV and CMV may also be appropriate.[31] Creatine kinase should be considered in all patients with elevated transaminases, but particularly in those with weakness.[28,31] INR should be measured in any patient where acute liver failure is suspected.[31]

In general, testing for autoimmune serologies is not helpful in the diagnosis of irH. Most patients with irH will not have any elevated antinuclear antibodies, anti-smooth muscle antibodies, or anti-mitochondrial antibodies, and the presence of these antibodies does not change current management recommendations, although this does remain an incompletely explored

TABLE 44.1 Common Terminology Criteria for Adverse Events (CTCAE)

Immune-Related Hepatitis Grade	Initial Workup	ICI Therapy	Treatment
Grade I: • AST/ALT elevated <3× ULN • Bilirubin elevated <1.5× ULN	• History to assess for the alternative etiologies of a liver injury • Rule out viral hepatitis • Discontinue potentially hepatotoxic medications/ supplements and alcohol • Monitoring of 1iver enzymes	Continue ICI therapy	Monitoring only
Grade II: • AST/ALT elevated up to 3 −5× ULN • Bilirubin elevated up to 1.5 −3× ULN	• Same as grade 1 • Consider a biliary imaging to exclude compression if primarily biliary pattern of injury • Consider imaging to exclude hepatic metastases • Consider a liver biopsy	Hold ICI therapy • Until resolution to grade 1	• 0.5–1 mg/kg oral prednisone or equivalent • Taper over 4–6 weeks after improvement to grade 1 • If no response by Day 3, treat as grade 3–4
Grade III-IV: • AST/ALT elevated >5× ULN • Bilirubin elevated >3× ULN	• Same as grade 1 • Consider a biliary imaging to exclude compression if primarily biliary pattern of injury • Consider imaging to exclude hepatic metastases • Consider a liver biopsy	Discontinue ICI therapy • If no other alternative treatments are available, resumption can be considered on a case-by-case basis after the normalization of liver chemistries	• 1–2 mg/kg oral prednisone or equivalent • Taper over 4–6 weeks after improvement to grade 1 • IV methylprednisolone for no response after 3 days or failure to drop by 1 grade level after 7 days • If no response to IV methylprednisolone after 3 days, biopsy and consider a secondary immune suppression
			• Secondary options include mycophenolate mofetil 500 −1000 mg BID, and tacrolimus 1 mg q12h

ICI, Immune checkpoint inhibitor.

question.[31] Whether patients with baseline elevated autoimmune serologies or a prior diagnosis of autoimmune hepatitis have an increased risk of irH is also unknown at this time. For many autoimmune diseases, use of ICI only marginally increases the risk of a flare, though this risk is considerably higher for patients with IBD.[4,57]

For the mildest grade of hepatitis (grade 1), additional testing beyond basic laboratory testing may not be indicated, and many patients can be safely observed without further diagnostics or treatment.[31] For patients with grade 2 or above irH, additional testing to exclude competing etiologies is warranted prior to initiation of hepatitis directed therapy.[31]

Abdominal imaging has an important role in the diagnosis of moderate to severe irH (grade 2 or greater), largely to exclude complications from the underlying malignancy.[31] Cross-sectional imaging, generally by CT, should be obtained for any patient who has not had recent (at least within the past month) imaging, and CT should be considered in all patients with known hepatic metastases or with tumors that have a high risk for hepatic spread.[31] Imaging findings of irH are typically nonspecific and can include mild hepatomegaly, attenuation of the liver parenchyma, periportal edema, and periportal lymphadenopathy.[64] For patients where the presentation could be consistent with Budd-Chiari (e.g., abdominal pain and distention), hepatic ultrasound with Doppler's may also be valuable.[31]

Patients with a cholestatic pattern of liver injury should have biliary imaging to exclude an obstruction.[31] Imaging options include magnetic resonance cholangiopancreatography, which has the highest sensitivity and specificity for bile duct disease, as well as biliary ultrasound and contrast-enhanced abdominal CT. Endoscopic retrograde cholangiopancreatography is not routinely used for diagnostic purposes, but may be indicated if an obstruction is detected on noninvasive imaging.

The role of liver biopsy in the diagnosis of grade 2 or higher irH is controversial.[31] In most scenarios, a clinical diagnosis of irH is considered sufficient to initiate treatment in patients with a hepatocellular pattern of liver injury and no identified alternative etiologies.[31] In this population, alternative causes of transaminases elevation are uncommon and liver biopsy has some associated procedural risk.[31,60]

Whether liver biopsy can distinguish irH from other drug-induced liver injuries is unclear as pathognomonic features of irH have not been identified.[21,29] Biopsy should be able to exclude noninflammatory causes of liver injury, including complications of the underlying malignancy.[21,29,31,60] Panlobular inflammation with milder portal involvement is the most common histologic finding in irH; in addition, fibrin ring granulomas can also be seen.[21,29,30] A primary biliary injury with portal mononuclear infiltrate around proliferating bile ductules represents an alternative pattern of irH injury.[21,29]

Much of the controversy surrounding the value of liver biopsy in this patient population is related to the interpretation of the competing risk of the biopsy and the risk of a misdiagnosis. In a retrospective cohort of 213 patients with grade 3 or 4 hepatitis on ICI cancer therapy, 107 of whom had a liver biopsy, liver biopsy was associated with delayed irH treatment.[60] A total of 12 patients had biopsy results that were inconsistent with a diagnosis of irH, including four cases of malignant biliary obstruction, four with a drug induced liver injury thought to be unrelated to ICI, two cases of infiltrating malignancy, and two cases without a clear cause.[60] Two patients had life-threatening complications of biopsy (hemothorax and splenic puncture).[60] In this cohort, the chance that a biopsy would detect unanticipated malignant infiltration of the liver was equivalent to the risk of a major procedural complication (~2%), and the chance that a biopsy would change the overall diagnosis was 11%.[60] Whether the risk of a misdiagnosis, and thus inappropriate initiation of irH therapy, justifies the risk of liver biopsy is the source of the current controversy; however, in most cases, treatment of irH without a confirmatory biopsy is standard practice as is recommended or considered reasonable in all major clinical guidelines.[31,65–67]

Several clinical scenarios should prompt consideration of a liver biopsy to confirm the diagnosis of irH.

Any patient who does not respond to first-line immunosuppressive therapy for irH (systemic glucocorticoids as discussed in the next section) should undergo a biopsy prior to escalation to second-line treatment.[31] These biopsies may be more likely to be non-diagnostic due to changes induced by glucocorticoid treatment but should still be able to eliminate infiltrating malignancy as an etiology.

Patients with an unclear diagnosis after initial history, serologic testing, and imaging should also be considered for liver biopsy.[31] Many of these patients will have a cholestatic pattern of liver injury without a discernable discrete biliary obstruction. In this group, infiltrating malignancy may be more common, increasing the diagnostic yield of a biopsy.[31]

Liver biopsy may be more useful in patients who have limited alternative therapeutic options. In this population, understanding whether their hepatitis was truly the result of their ICI therapy may have broader implications in subsequent treatment considerations, including whether to restart immunotherapy.

Treatment

Therapy for irH is generally guided by the severity of the laboratory abnormalities using the CTCAE grading scale (Table 44.1).[31,65–67] Prospective trials on irH treatment are lacking, and all current data are retrospective and largely guided by expert opinion. Systemic glucocorticoids are first-line immunosuppression therapy with alternative agents such as mycophenolate mofetil and tacrolimus as second-line therapy for glucocorticoid refractory disease.[31]

Grade 1 irH is typically monitored without an interruption in ICI therapy. Potentially contributing medications should be considered for a temporary hold, and liver tests should be monitored at least once weekly for evidence of worsening hepatitis.[31]

Grade 2 irH is managed by holding ICI therapy and discontinuing other potentially hepatotoxic medications.[31] Treatment with 0.5–1 mg/kg of prednisone or prednisone equivalent daily is often started after an initial workup as described above.[31] Alternatively, patients can be observed over the course of 1–2 weeks for evidence of hepatitis improvement after holding ICI therapy; glucocorticoids can then be considered in those patients whose hepatitis does not improve with the ICI therapy hold and the discontinuation of other hepatotoxic medications (e.g., concurrent targeted therapy).[31]

Grade 3 and 4 irH is managed by stopping ICI therapy alongside any potentially hepatoxic medications, and with prompt initiation of systemic glucocorticoids.[31] Although the dose of glucocorticoids used has not been well studied, doses of 1–2 mg/kg of prednisone or prednisone equivalent are typically used.[31] These patients should be treated by a hepatologist or a gastroenterologist familiar with irH.[31] For patients with grade 4 hepatitis or with rapidly escalating grade 3 hepatitis, admission can be considered for initiation of intravenous methylprednisolone.[31] Liver tests should be sent every 1–3 days for monitoring until the improvement to grade 2 is achieved, at which time the frequency of testing can be spaced out.[31]

For grades 2–4, patients who do not have any appreciable response to treatment within 3 days should be considered for an escalation of therapy.[31] Initial escalation options include increasing the glucocorticoid dose to 2 mg/kg of prednisone or prednisone equivalent and transition to intravenous methylprednisolone.[31] Patients who do not respond to glucocorticoid treatment within 1 week with a drop of at least 1 grade should be considered for initiation of secondary immune suppression.[31] Options for secondary immune suppression include mycophenolate mofetil 500–1000 mg BID, tacrolimus 1 mg q12h titrated to response, and azathioprine 1–2 mg/kg daily.[31] Secondary immune suppression can also be considered for patients who do not respond to initial management with glucocorticoids as an alternative to dose escalation.

After biochemical response is achieved, immune suppression should be continued until the irH is grade 1 or lower, and then a taper can begin.[31] Most tapering strategies decrease the dose of glucocorticoids by 10 mg/day every 5–7 days.[31] After completing a prednisone taper, secondary immune suppression can be tapered separately. Optimal timing for tapering of secondary immune suppression has not been studied, and it is generally discontinued over a period of 4–6 weeks depending on the difficulty of achieving irH remission. Patients whose liver tests worsen during a taper should be restarted on the last effective dose of immune suppression and should be considered for escalation of immune suppression with an additional agent.

The decision to hospitalize patients with irH should be done on a case-by-case basis since the benefits of hospitalization for this disease are not well established. The decision should depend on the ease of monitoring in an outpatient setting, the availability of diagnostic testing, and the perceived need for intravenous glucocorticoids. In addition, any patient with signs of hepatic failure associated with irH should be hospitalized for close monitoring; no defined treatment algorithm has been developed for these patients and all therapeutic approaches at this point are based on inference, expert opinion, and case report. Several theoretical considerations should guide management in patients with hepatic failure associated with irH. The majority of the evidence to date suggests that T cells secreting cytokines such as IFNγ play a central role in ICI toxicities.[4,24,25,68] Treatments that targeted T cells (anti-thymocyte globulin), T-cell activation (abatacept), or their cytokine products (JAK inhibitors) are likely to have efficacy, though definitive clinical data are lacking.[25,26,28,69–71] TNFα inhibitors are generally avoided because of the small risk of autoimmune hepatitis associated with this class of drugs, although they have been successfully used in patients who have irH and an alternative indication for anti-TNFα therapy such as immune-related enterocolitis.[31]

Special Circumstances

Reintroduction of Immunotherapy

The great majority of irH cases will resolve with appropriate therapy without any long-term sequelae of chronic liver disease. The appropriateness and timing of reintroduction of cancer immunotherapy then becomes an important decision, though evidence to guide this decision is currently minimal. In general the decision should be based on the severity of the hepatitis both in terms of the degree of transaminase elevation and its responsiveness to treatment, the importance of reinitiating cancer-directed therapy, and the availability of alternative treatment modalities. Changing classes of immunotherapy (switching from dual therapy to single agent PD-1 blockade, or switching from a CTLA-4 inhibitor to a PD-(L)1 inhibitor) is lower risk than continuing on the treatment that caused the irH, and is another important factor to consider.[72,73] At present, no treatments have been identified to mitigate the risk of irH.[72]

For grade 2 irH, most experts agree that a trial of reintroduction of immunotherapy is reasonable after biochemical resolution to grade 1 and tapering of glucocorticoids to 10 mg of prednisone daily or less.[31] For patients who have required secondary immune suppression to achieve biochemical remission, reintroduction of immunotherapy may be riskier.

For grade 3 and 4 irH, the reinitiation of immunotherapy should be considered on a case-by-case basis. Oncology guidelines generally recommend against restarting treatment though some of these patients likely can be restarted on immunotherapy safely.[31,65–67] Patients who change immunotherapy regimens or who have another likely inciting or contributing drug (such as concurrent targeted therapy) are reasonable candidates for restarting ICI therapy after resolution of grade 3 or 4 irH to baseline (generally normal liver biochemistries). For patients who will restart the same ICI treatment, the risk is influenced by the difficulty of controlling the initial irH. Patients who required secondary immune suppression or who had recurrence during their glucocorticoid taper are likely at the highest risk if ICIs are restarted; restarting ICI treatment in these patients should be considered only in cases of progressive metastatic disease and where no other good cancer-directed therapies are available.

Multi-Modality Therapies

Cancer immunotherapy is increasingly being used in combination with other cancer-directed treatments, including chemotherapy and targeted therapies.[1,13–16] These combination therapies have a higher risk of leading to elevations in liver biochemistries, though distinguishing between irH and more typical drug-induced liver injury is often complicated.[13–16] Although liver biopsies may be helpful in these patients, in the absence of clear histopathologic criteria to distinguish these two entities, biopsies are often insufficient.[14–16,21,29] Holding one or both classes of drugs followed by selective reintroduction of each agent is often the only way to definitively determine the drug responsive for elevated biochemistries in these situations. The long half-life and even longer receptor occupancy period for ICIs can reduce the diagnostic value of these selective reintroduction tests, however.

In practice, it is reasonable to treat combination liver toxicities as irH and then to reintroduce single modality treatment after resolution of the biochemistries to grade 1. For patients with clear evidence of responsiveness to immune suppression, an inflammatory component to the liver biochemistry elevation is likely, though even in these cases, many patients will tolerate single-agent reintroduction.

Immunotherapy in Patients With Underlying Liver Disease

Multiple ICI trials have included patients with underlying liver disease, primarily in the setting of hepatocellular carcinoma.[74–77] These patients do not appear to have a substantially elevated risk for irH, and most tolerated immunotherapy reasonably well compared to other patient populations.[74–77] Patients with underlying cirrhosis should be treated in conjunction with a hepatologist and should be monitored for signs of worsening liver disease.[31] As decompensation may occur at lower levels of biochemical changes, grade 1 toxicities should be managed similarly to grade 2 toxicities in these patients.

For patients with chronic hepatitis B or hepatitis C infections, antiviral therapy should be considered either before or concurrent with cancer therapy. These infections are not a contraindication to ICI therapy, and most tolerate the treatment well.[74–79] Enhanced immune responses to chronic hepatic infections have been observed, including substantial reductions in viral load, following ICI therapy.[78,79] These reactions can be confused with irH but do not appear to have a substantial risk for inducing hepatic failure.[78,79]

CONCLUDING THOUGHTS

As the indications for an ICI therapy for cancer continue to expand, irH and colitis are becoming increasingly common. These syndromes are important to recognize and treat early. As with most of the inflammatory toxicities associated with immunotherapy, irH and colitis can rapidly escalate and can become life-threatening. Perhaps more importantly, the development of these toxicities can lead to treatment delays and the discontinuation of immunotherapy, jeopardizing optimal cancer treatment. Our current understanding of the molecular and cellular immunology underlying irH is minimal, but we have an increasingly sophisticated understanding of immune-related colitis. Despite our growing understanding of the underlying immune mechanisms, treatment recommendations for both syndromes are based on a paucity of data, and are almost entirely reliant on expert opinion. This is an area where rigorous research is necessary to refine our treatment protocols and provide our patients with optimal care.

CONFLICT OF INTEREST

MD has received research funding from Eli Lilly; he has received consulting fees from Genentech, Partner Therapeutics, SQZ Biotech, AzurRx, Eli Lilly, Mallinckrodt Pharmaceuticals, Aditum, Foghorn Therapeutics, Palleon, Sorriso Pharmaceuticals, Generate Biomedicines, Asher Bio, Neoleukin Therapeutics, Alloy Therapeutics, Third Rock Ventures, DE Shaw Research, Agenus, Astellas, and Curie Bio; he is a member of the Scientific Advisory Board for Veravas, Monod Bio, Axxis Bio, and Cerberus Therapeutics.

Full references for this chapter can be found at https://ebooks.health.elsevier.com.

45 Anatomy, Histology, Embryology, and Developmental Anomalies of the Esophagus

James P. Callaway

IN THIS CHAPTER

ANATOMY AND HISTOLOGY

The esophagus acts as a conduit for the transport of food and liquids from the oral cavity into the stomach. To carry out this task safely and effectively, the esophagus is constructed as an 18–26-cm long hollow muscular tube with an innermost lining of stratified squamous epithelium, which shares similarities to the epidermal layer of the skin, although nonkeratinized (Fig. 45.1). Between swallows, the esophageal body is collapsed, but the lumen distends up to 2 cm anteroposteriorly and 3 cm laterally to accommodate a swallowed bolus. Structurally, the esophageal wall is composed of four layers: innermost mucosa, submucosa, muscularis propria, and outermost adventitia; unlike the remainder of the GI tract, the esophagus has no serosa.[1,2] These layers are depicted anatomically and as viewed by EUS in Fig. 45.2.

Musculature

The muscularis propria is responsible for carrying out the organ's motor function. The upper 5%–33% is composed exclusively of skeletal muscle, and the distal 50% is composed of smooth muscle. In between is a mixture of both types.[3] Proximally, the esophagus begins where the inferior pharyngeal constrictor merges with the cricopharyngeus, an area of skeletal muscle known functionally as the *upper esophageal sphincter* (UES) (Fig. 45.3A). The UES is contracted at rest and, hence, creates a high-pressure zone that prevents inspired air from entering the esophagus. Below the UES, the esophageal wall is

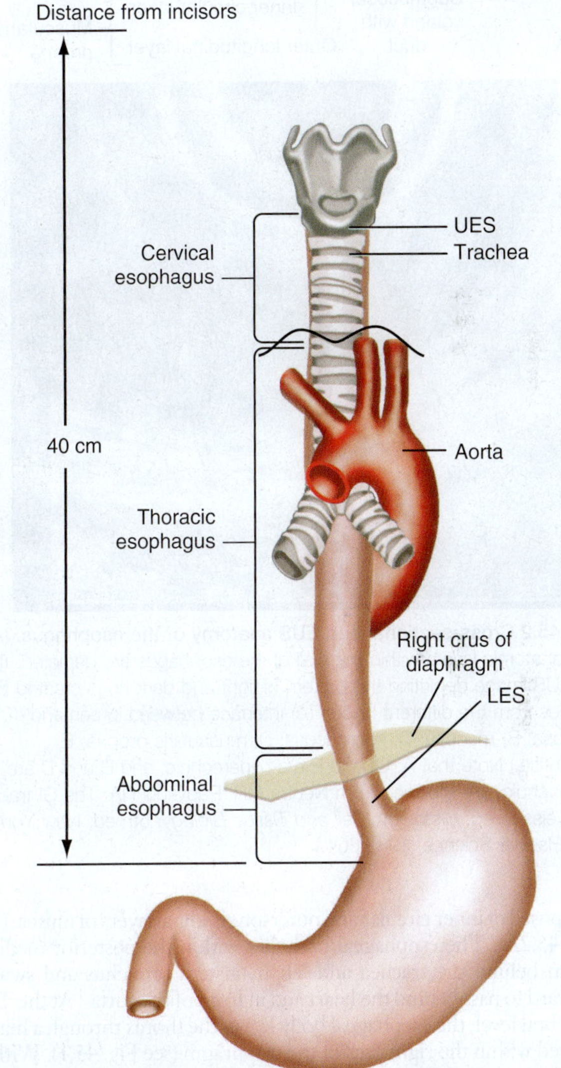

Fig. 45.1 Anatomy of the esophagus and its relationship to adjacent structure. The esophagus, approximately 25 cm in length, originates in the neck at the level of the cricoid cartilage, passes through the chest, and ends after passage through the hiatus in the right crus of the diaphragm by joining the stomach below. On barium esophagogram, adjacent structures may indent the esophageal wall, including the aortic arch, left mainstem bronchus, left atrium, and diaphragm. *LES*, Lower esophageal sphincter; *UES*, upper esophageal sphincter. (Modified from Liebermann-Meffert D. Anatomy, embryology, and histology. In: Pearson FG, Cooper JD, Deslauriers J, et al. eds. *Esophageal Surgery*. 2nd ed. Philadelphia, PA: Churchill Livingstone; 2002:8.)

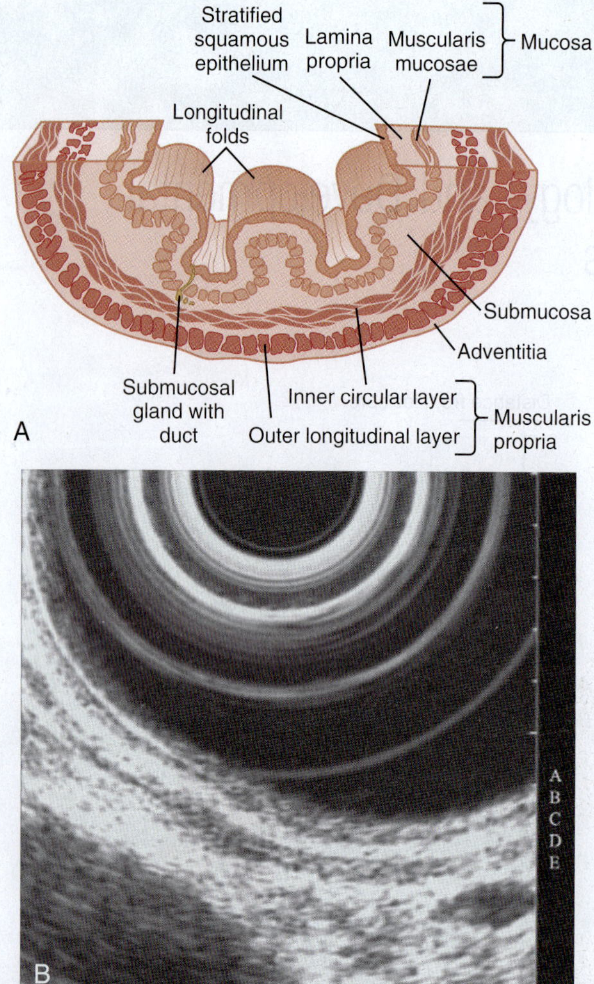

Fig. 45.2 **Cross-sectional and EUS anatomy of the esophagus.** (A) The anatomic layers within the wall of the esophagus are depicted. (B) An EUS image depicting the pattern of light and dark rings created by echoes from the different layers. (A, Interface between lumen and mucosa; B, mucosa; C, submucosa; D, muscularis propria; E, adventitia.) Note that A, C, and E are hyperechoic, and B and D are hypoechoic. ((A) Modified from Neutra MR, Padykula HA. The GI tract. In: Weiss L, ed. *Histology, Cell and Tissue Biology*. 5th ed. New York, NY: Elsevier Science; 1983:664.)

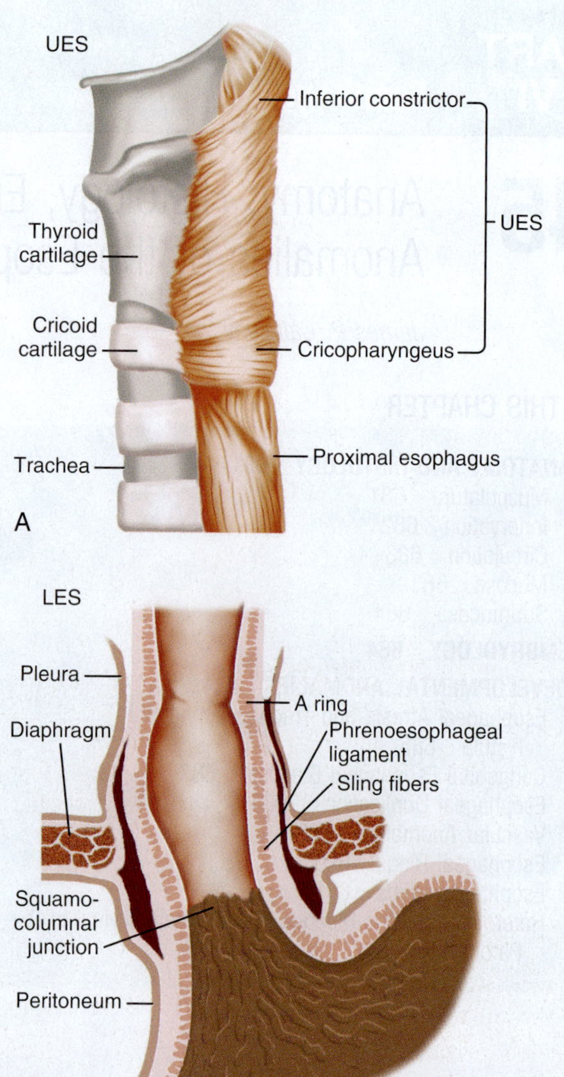

Fig. 45.3 (A) Anatomic detail of the *UES* and its relationship to adjacent structures. (B) Anatomic detail of the *LES* and its relationship to the diaphragm, phrenoesophageal ligament, and squamocolumnar junction. ((A) Modified from AGA Clinical Teaching Project. Esophageal disorders: Upper esophageal sphincter anatomy, slide 14, American Gastroenterological Association, 1995; (B) modified from Kerr RM. Hiatal hernia and mucosal prolapse. In: Castell DO, ed. *The Esophagus*. Boston, MA: Little, Brown & Company; 1992: 763.)

composed of inner circular and outer longitudinal layers of muscle (see Fig. 45.2A). The esophageal body lies within the posterior mediastinum behind the trachea and left mainstem bronchus and swings leftward to pass behind the heart and in front of the aorta.[1] At the T10 vertebral level, the esophageal body leaves the thorax through a hiatus located within the right crus of the diaphragm (see Fig. 45.1). Within the diaphragmatic hiatus, the esophageal body ends in a 2–4-cm length of asymmetrically thickened circular smooth muscle known as the *lower esophageal sphincter* (LES) (see Fig. 45.3B).[4] The phrenoesophageal ligament, which originates from the diaphragm's transversalis fascia and inserts on the lower esophagus, contributes to fixation of the LES within the diaphragmatic hiatus. This positioning is beneficial because it enables diaphragmatic contractions to assist the LES in maintenance of a high-pressure zone during exercise. The LES is contracted at rest, creating a high-pressure zone that prevents gastric contents from entering the esophagus. During swallowing, the LES relaxes to permit the swallowed bolus to be pushed by peristalsis from the esophagus into the stomach.

Innervation

The esophageal wall is innervated by parasympathetic and sympathetic nerves; the parasympathetics regulate peristalsis through the vagus nerve (Fig. 45.4). The cell bodies of the vagus nerve originate in the medulla. Those located within the nucleus ambiguus control skeletal muscle, and those located within the dorsal motor nucleus control smooth muscle. Medullary vagal postganglionic efferent nerves terminate directly on the motor endplate of skeletal muscle in the upper esophagus, whereas vagal preganglionic efferent nerves heading to smooth muscle in the distal esophagus terminate on neurons within Auerbach (myenteric) plexus, located between the circular and longitudinal muscle layers.[3] A second neuronal sensory network, Meissner plexus,

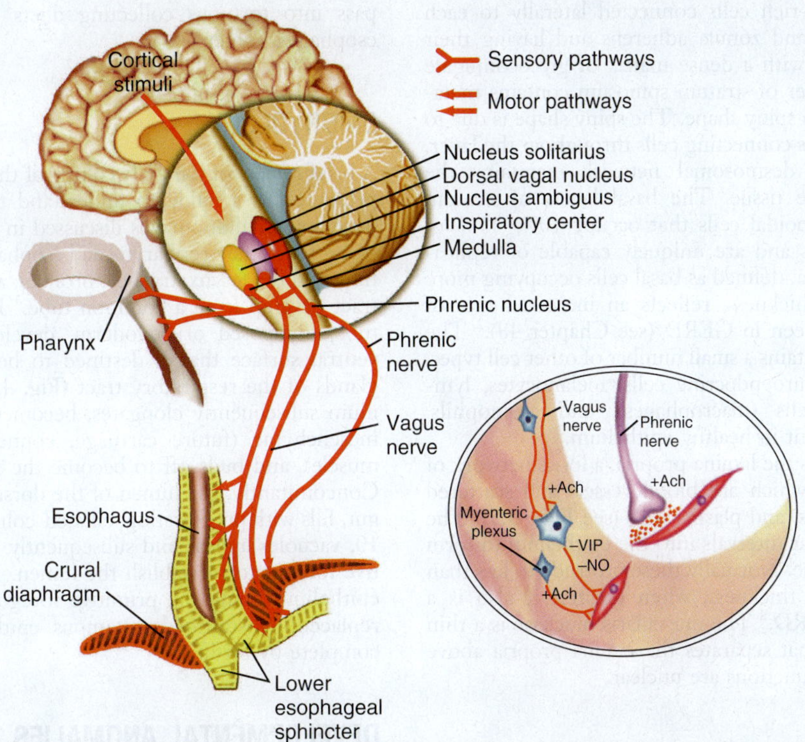

Fig. 45.4 Neural pathways of the esophagus. Extrinsic innervation is provided principally by the vagus nerve. Afferent vagal pathways carry stimuli to the nucleus solitarius, and efferent pathways originating in the dorsal vagal nucleus mediate esophageal peristalsis and LES relaxation. *Ach,* Acetylcholine; *NO,* nitric oxide; *VIP,* vasoactive intestinal peptide. (From Mittal RK, Balaban DH. The esophagogastric junction. *N Engl J Med*. 1997;336:924.)

located within the submucosa, is the site of afferent impulses within the esophageal wall. These are transmitted to the central nervous system through vagal parasympathetic and thoracic sympathetic nerves. Sensory signals transmitted via vagal afferent pathways travel to the nucleus tractus solitarius within the central nervous system (see Fig. 45.4); from there, nerves pass to the nucleus ambiguus and dorsal motor nucleus of the vagus nerve, where their signals may influence motor function.[5]

Pain sensation arising from the esophagus is typically triggered by stimulation of chemoreceptors in the esophageal mucosa or submucosa and/or mechanoreceptors in the esophageal musculature.[6] Central perception then occurs when these impulses are transmitted to the brain by sympathetic and vagal afferents. Sympathetic afferents travel through the dorsal root ganglia to the dorsal horn of the spinal cord, and vagal afferents travel through the nodose ganglia to the nucleus tractus solitarius in the medulla. Information from sympathetic/spinal afferents then proceeds via the spinothalamic and spinoreticular pathways to the thalamus and reticular nuclei before transmission to the somatosensory cortex for pain perception and limbic system for pain modulation. Information from vagal afferents in the medulla also travels to the limbic system and frontal cortex for pain modulation. Furthermore, because the esophageal neuroanatomic pathways overlap with those of the heart and respiratory system, in clinical practice, it may be difficult to discern the organ of origin for some chest pain syndromes.[6]

Circulation

The arterial and venous blood supply to the esophagus is segmental. The upper esophagus is supplied by branches of the superior and inferior thyroid arteries, the midesophagus by branches of the bronchial and right intercostal arteries and descending aorta, and the distal esophagus by branches of the left gastric, left inferior phrenic, and splenic arteries.[1–3] These vessels anastomose to create a dense network within the submucosa that probably accounts for the rarity of esophageal infarction. The venous drainage of the upper esophagus is through the superior vena cava, the midesophagus through the azygos veins, and the distal esophagus through the portal vein by means of the left and short gastric veins. The submucosal venous anastomotic network of the distal esophagus is important because it is where esophageal varices emerge in patients with portal hypertension.[1–3]

The lymphatic system of the esophagus is also segmental; the upper esophagus drains to the deep cervical nodes, the midesophagus to the mediastinal nodes, and the distal esophagus to the celiac and gastric nodes. However, these lymphatic systems are also interconnected by numerous channels, accounting for the spread of most esophageal cancers beyond the region at the time of their discovery.

Mucosa

During endoscopic evaluation, the normal esophageal mucosa appears smooth and pink. The normal esophagogastric junction appears as an irregular white Z-line (ora serrata), demarcating the interface between the lighter esophageal and the redder gastric mucosa. Histologically, the esophageal mucosa is a nonkeratinized, stratified squamous epithelium (Fig. 45.5). This multilayered epithelium consists of three functionally distinct layers: stratum corneum, stratum spinosum, and stratum germinativum. The most lumen-oriented stratum corneum acts as a permeability barrier between luminal content and blood by having layers of pancake-shaped glycogen-rich cells connected laterally to each other by tight junctions and zonula adherens and having their intercellular spaces filled with a dense matrix of glycoconjugate material.[7] The middle layer of stratum spinosum contains metabolically active cells with a spiny shape. The spiny shape is due to the numerous desmosomes connecting cells throughout the layer. Furthermore, this same desmosomal network maintains the structural integrity of the tissue. The basal layers of stratum germinativum contain cuboidal cells that occupy 10%–15% of the epithelium's thickness and are uniquely capable of replication.[2] Basal cell hyperplasia, defined as basal cells occupying more than 15% of epithelial thickness, reflects an increased rate of tissue repair, as is often seen in GERD (see Chapter 48).[2] The esophageal epithelium contains a small number of other cell types, including argyrophilic neuroendocrine cells, melanocytes, lymphocytes, Langerhans cells (macrophages), and eosinophils. Neutrophils are not present in healthy epithelium.[2]

Below the epithelium is the lamina propria, a loose network of connective tissue within which are blood vessels and scattered lymphocytes, macrophages, and plasma cells (see Fig. 45.5). The lamina propria protrudes at intervals into the epithelium to form rete pegs or dermal papillae. Normally these protrude to less than 50% of the epithelium's thickness; when greater, it also is a recognized marker of GERD.[8] The muscularis mucosae is a thin layer of smooth muscle that separates the lamina propria above from the submucosa. Its functions are unclear.

Submucosa

The submucosa comprises a dense network of connective tissue, within which are blood vessels, lymphatic channels, neurons of Meissner plexus, and esophageal glands (see Fig. 45.2A). These glands, which vary as to number and distribution along the esophagus, consist of cuboidal cells organized as acini.[9] They produce and secrete a lubricant, mucus, and factors such as bicarbonate and epidermal growth factor that are important for epithelial defense and repair. The secretions from these glands pass into tortuous collecting ducts that deliver them to the esophageal lumen.

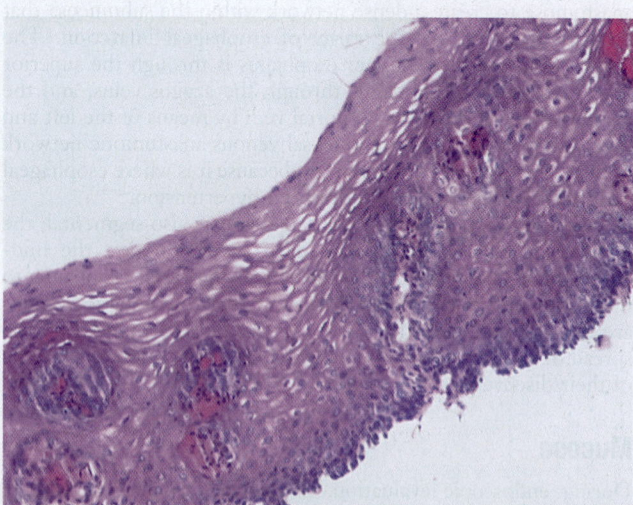

Fig. 45.5 Esophageal epithelium. The human esophagus, as shown on this biopsy specimen, is lined by nonkeratinized stratified squamous epithelium. The cells of the surface (*top*) are long and flat and have a small nucleus-to-cytoplasm ratio that contrasts with the cells of the basal layer (*bottom*), the density, cuboidal shape, and large nucleus-to-cytoplasm ratio of which account for their prominence. A subpopulation of these basal layer cells appears to have properties of esophageal stem cells.[7] Rete pegs, or dermal papillae containing elements of the lamina propria, normally extend into the epithelium about one-half the distance to the lumen. (Courtesy Pamela Jensen, MD, Dallas, TX.)

EMBRYOLOGY

A brief review of the embryology of the upper digestive system is presented as a guide to understand the origin of many of the developmental anomalies discussed in this chapter. In the developing fetus, the oropharynx and esophageal components of the GI tract and the larynx, trachea, bronchi, and lungs of the respiratory tract develop from a common tube.[3] By gestational week 4, this tube, composed of endoderm, develops a diverticulum on its ventral surface that is destined to become the epithelium and glands of the respiratory tract (Fig. 45.6A to D). This diverticulum subsequently elongates, becomes enveloped by splanchnic mesenchyme (future cartilage, connective tissue, and smooth muscle), and buds off to become the primitive respiratory tract. Concomitantly, the lumen of the dorsal tube, the primitive foregut, fills with proliferating, ciliated-columnar epithelium. By week 10, vacuoles appear and subsequently coalesce within the primitive foregut to reestablish the lumen. By week 16, the columnar epithelium lining the primitive foregut and future esophagus is replaced by stratified squamous epithelium, a process that is complete by birth.

DEVELOPMENTAL ANOMALIES

Congenital anomalies of the esophagus are relatively common and are due to either transmission of genetic defects or intrauterine

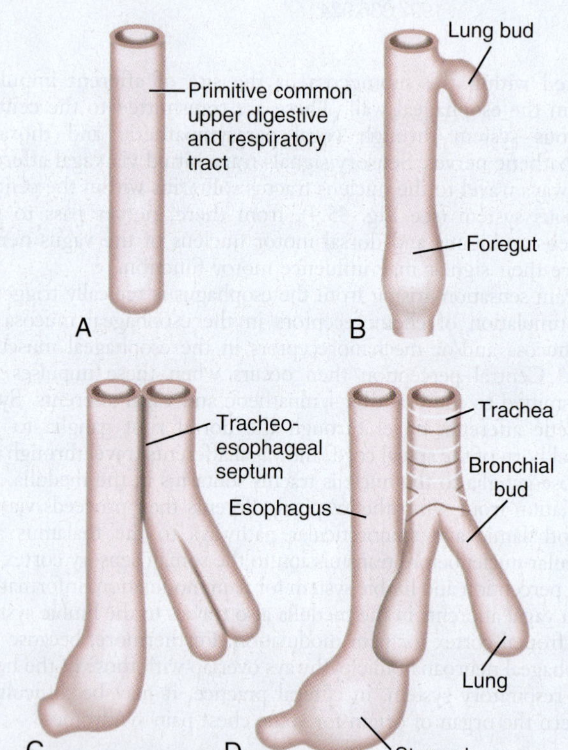

Fig. 45.6 Developmental stages in the formation of separate respiratory and digestive systems. These systems are derived from a common tube of endoderm during embryogenesis. (A) Single primitive tube. (B) Formation of a lung bud in the fourth week. (C) Elongation of the dorsal tube (primitive foregut) and lung bud and formation of a tracheoesophageal septum by 4–6 weeks. (D) Separation of the primitive foregut from the tracheobronchial tree at 6 weeks.

stress that impedes fetal maturation. Esophageal anomalies are common in premature infants, and 60% have other anomalies, reflected by the term *VACTERL* (formerly VATER), a mnemonic for the association of anomalies of the *v*ertebral, *a*nal, *c*ardiac, *t*racheal, *e*sophageal, *r*enal, and *l*imb systems. Common specific defects include patent ductus arteriosus, cardiac septal defects, and imperforate anus.[10]

Esophageal Atresia and Tracheoesophageal Fistula

Esophageal atresia, a loss of continuity between the upper and lower esophagus, and tracheoesophageal fistulas, abnormal connections between the trachea and esophagus, are the most common developmental anomalies of the esophagus (Figs. 45.7 and 45.8). The incidence of esophageal atresia and tracheoesophageal fistula is approximately 1 in 4000.[11] The former results from failure of the primitive foregut to recanalize and the latter from failure of the lung bud to separate completely from the foregut. Although the mechanisms are unclear, esophageal atresia and tracheoesophageal fistulas may result from genetic defects (Table 45.1).[12] Proper sonic hedgehog signaling is one of the pathways critical to achieve separation of the respiratory tract from the primitive foregut.[13] Experimental administration of the anticancer drug, Adriamycin (doxorubicin), into mouse or rat embryos commonly results in esophageal atresia and tracheoesophageal fistulas, as well as other anomalies that comprise the VACTERL group, by altering sonic hedgehog signaling.[14,15]

Esophageal atresia occurs as an isolated anomaly in only 7% of cases; the rest are accompanied by a form of tracheoesophageal fistula, most often (89%) a distal-type fistula (see Fig. 45.7B) and rarely (3%) the H-type fistula (see Fig. 45.7C).[16] In isolated atresia, the upper esophagus ends in a blind pouch, and the lower esophagus connects to the stomach (see Fig. 45.7A). The condition is suspected prenatally by the development of polyhydramnios (due to the inability of the fetus to swallow and so absorb amniotic fluid) and an absent or small stomach bubble.[17] The finding of a dilated proximal esophagus with a blind ending, also known as an esophageal pouch, during a prenatal US has high specificity for esophageal atresia, although the sensitivity of this finding is limited.[18] Distal fistulas can also be detected by prenatal ultrasound when targeted scanning techniques are utilized. [19] A distended fetal hypopharynx during US or MRI is an additional prenatal sign of esophageal atresia and has better sensitivity than an esophageal pouch. Prenatal MRI also provides images of the entire length of the esophagus and can be used to assist in the diagnosis of esophageal atresia and tracheoesophageal fistula (Fig. 45.9).[20] At birth, the combination of regurgitation of saliva and a scaphoid (gasless) abdomen strongly suggests isolated atresia without a distal tracheoesophageal fistula because no pathway exists for inspired or swallowed air to enter the bowel. At the first feeding, the high complete GI obstruction of esophageal atresia results in the rapid onset of choking, coughing, and regurgitation (Table 45.2). Once suspected, the diagnosis can be confirmed by failure to pass an NG tube into the stomach and by a concurrent chest radiograph with air contrast in the upper esophageal segment (the air being introduced through a catheter positioned within the upper esophageal segment). In some instances, the injection of 1 mL of water-soluble contrast into the obstructed segment helps with the diagnosis.

Tracheoesophageal fistula usually accompanies esophageal atresia. The most common type of tracheoesophageal fistula is the distal type associated with esophageal atresia (see Fig. 45.7B).[16] In this type, the atretic upper esophagus ends in a blind pouch, and the trachea communicates with the distal esophageal segment. The clinical presentation with this configuration is usually similar to isolated esophageal atresia, with the additional risk of aspiration pneumonia from refluxed gastric contents entering the trachea

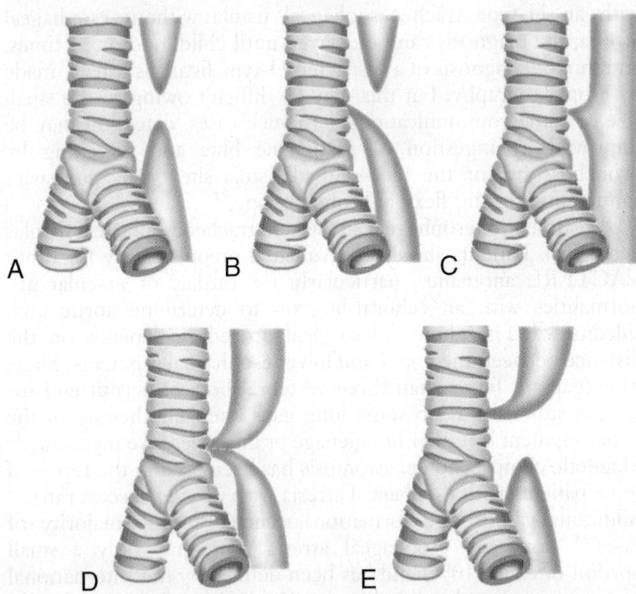

Fig. 45.7 Esophageal atresia (A) and tracheoesophageal fistulas TEF. In the most common TEF, the trachea communicates with the distal segment of the atretic esophagus (B). The next most common type is the H-type TEF, in which the trachea communicates with an otherwise normal esophagus (C). A TEF in which the trachea communicates with both upper and lower segments of an atretic esophagus (D) or only with the upper segment of an atretic esophagus (E) is rare. (Modified from The nonneoplastic esophagus. In: Fenoglio-Preiser CM, ed. *GI Pathology: An Atlas and Text*. 2nd ed. Philadelphia, PA: Lippincott-Raven; 1999:31.)

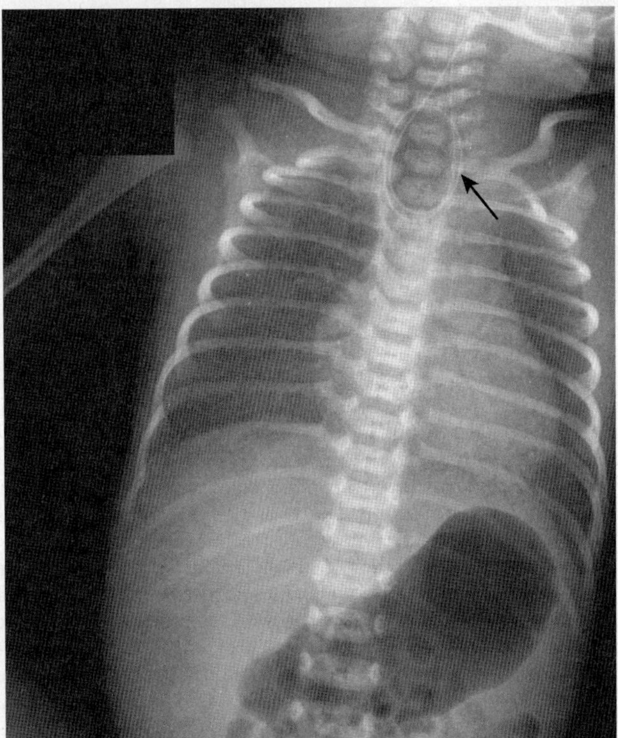

Fig. 45.8 Chest radiograph depicting tracheoesophageal fistula. A catheter is shown coiled in the esophagus (*arrow*) at the level of the second thoracic vertebra with air in the stomach. (From Forero Zapata L, Pappagallo M. Esophageal atresia and tracheoesophageal fistula. *N Engl J Med*. 2018;379(7):e11.)

TABLE 45.1 Syndromic Causes and Distinguishing Clinical Features of Tracheoesophageal Fistula and Esophageal Atresia

Syndrome	Gene	Clinical Features
Anophthalmia-esophageal-genital syndrome	*SOX2*	Anophthalmia/microphthalmia EA/TEF Urogenital anomalies
CHARGE syndrome	*CHD7*	Coloboma of the eye Cardiac anomalies Choanal atresia Intellectual disability Growth retardation Genital anomalies Ear anomalies Hearing loss EA/TEF
Feingold syndrome	*MYCN*	Esophageal/duodenal atresias Microcephaly Learning disabilities Syndactyly Cardiac defects
Fanconi anemia	>20 genes	Bone marrow failure Malignancies Short stature Abnormal skin pigmentation Radial ray defects Eye anomalies Renal anomalies Cardiac defects Abnormal ears Central nervous system anomalies Hearing loss Developmental delay Gastrointestinal anomalies including EA/TEF
VACTERL-H	*FANCB*	Vertebral anomalies Anal atresia Cardiac malformations TEF Renal anomalies Limb anomalies Hydrocephalus

EA, Esophageal atresia; *TEF*, tracheoesophageal fistula.
Adapted from Scott DA. Esophageal atresia/tracheoesophageal fistula overview. In: Adam MP, Ardinger HH, Pagon RA, et al., eds. *GeneReviews*. Seattle, WA: University of Washington; 1993.

through the fistula (see Table 45.2). Nonetheless, distinction between an isolated atresia and one associated with a distal tracheoesophageal fistula is straightforward because the communication between the trachea and the esophagus results in a gas-filled abdomen, as shown on plain radiographs (see Fig. 45.8). In some instances, the confirmation of the type of configuration is obtained by esophagography with or without bronchoscopy.

The three less common types of tracheoesophageal fistula occur when (1) the atretic upper esophagus communicates with the trachea, (2) both upper and lower segments of the atretic esophagus communicate with the trachea, and (3) an H-type fistula communicates with the trachea in a nonatretic esophagus (see Figs. 45.7E, D, and C, respectively). Because these types have in common the communication between upper esophagus and trachea, they all manifest clinically with signs and symptoms of recurrent (aspiration) pneumonia (see Table 45.2). Distinguishing among types, however, should not be difficult. Esophageal atresia accompanied by proximal tracheoesophageal fistula presents in infancy as recurrent pneumonia, and the presence or absence of

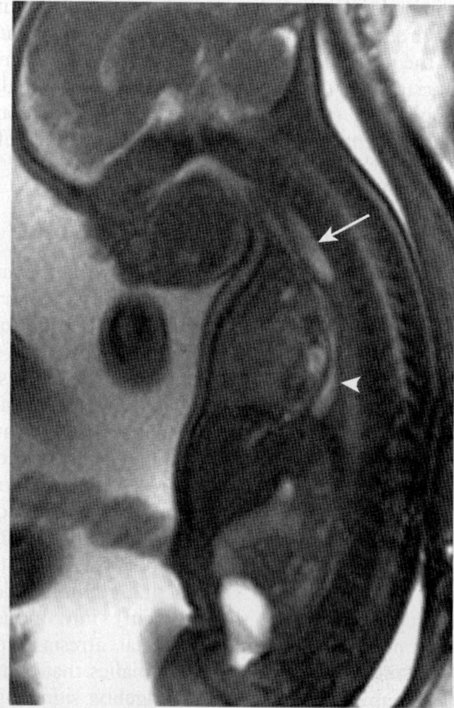

Fig. 45.9 Esophageal atresia is seen in a sagittal T2-weighted MRI sequence showing the proximal blind pouch (*arrow*) and the long distal esophagus (*arrowhead*). (From Cassart M. Fetal body imaging: When is MRI indicated? *J Belg Soc Radiol*. 2017;101(S1):3.)

bowel gas on a plain radiograph indicates whether an accompanying distal tracheoesophageal fistula exists. In contrast, in those with an H-type tracheoesophageal fistula without esophageal atresia, the diagnosis can be delayed until childhood or, at times, adulthood. Diagnosis of a suspected H-type fistula is usually made by esophagography, but this may be difficult owing to the small size of some communications.[21] In such cases, detection may be improved by ingestion of methylene blue and searching by bronchoscopy for the blue-stained fistula site or by guidewire cannulation during flexible bronchoscopy.[22]

Treatment of esophageal atresia and tracheoesophageal fistulas is surgical. Patients should be evaluated preoperatively for other VACTERL anomalies, particularly for cardiac or vascular abnormalities with an echocardiogram to determine aortic arch sidedness.[23] The choice of surgical procedure depends on the distance between the upper and lower esophageal segments. Short gaps (gaps of fewer than three vertebral bodies) permit end-to-end anastomosis, as do some long gaps after lengthening of the upper segment by either bougienage or intraoperative myotomy.[16] Magnetic compression anastomosis has been used in the repair of some patients with esophageal atresia with varying success rates.[24] Additionally, stricture formation occurred in the majority of cases.[24] Long-gap esophageal atresia represents only a small portion of cases (10%) and has been defined by the International Network of Esophageal Atresia (INoEA) as "any esophageal atresia that has no intra-abdominal air should be considered a long gap" and "all other types that technically prove to be difficult to repair."[25] If approximation of the two segments is not possible, primary reconstruction is undertaken, typically with a jejunal or colonic interposition or a gastric pull-up. Jejunal interposition is the preferred method as this graft grows at a similar rate as the child, and motility is preserved.[25] The gastric pull-up has an advantage of only requiring one anastomosis but has higher rates of gastroesophageal reflux compared to the jejunal interposition.[25]

TABLE 45.2 Clinical Aspects of Esophageal Developmental Anomalies

Anomaly	Age at Presentation	Predominant Symptoms	Diagnosis	Treatment
Isolated atresia	Newborns	Regurgitation of feedings Aspiration	Esophagogram[a] Plain film: gasless abdomen	Surgery
Atresia + distal TEF	Newborns	Regurgitation of feedings Aspiration	Esophagogram[a] Plain film: gas-filled abdomen	Surgery
H-type TEF	Infants to adults	Recurrent pneumonia Bronchiectasis	Esophagogram[a] Bronchoscopy[b]	Surgery
Esophageal stenosis	Infants to adults	Dysphagia Food impaction	Esophagogram[a] Endoscopy[b]	Dilation[c] Surgery[d] Peroral endoscopic myotomy[e]
Esophageal duplication cyst	Infants to adults	Dyspnea, stridor, cough (infants) Dysphagia, chest pain (adults)	EUS[a] MRI/CT[b]	Surgery
Vascular anomaly	Infants to adults	Dyspnea, stridor, cough (infants) Dysphagia (adults)	Esophagogram[a] Angiography[b] MRI/CT/EUS	Dietary modification[c] Surgery[d]
Esophageal ring	Children to adults	Dysphagia	Esophagogram[a] Endoscopy[b]	Dilation[c] Endoscopic incision[d]
Esophageal web	Children to adults	Dysphagia	Esophagogram[a] Endoscopy[b]	Dilation

[a]Diagnostic test of choice.
[b]Confirmatory test.
[c]Primary therapeutic approach.
[d]Secondary therapeutic approach.
[e]Novel therapeutic approach.
TEF, Tracheoesophageal fistula.

Colonic interposition is typically only used if the other options fail or are unfeasible.[25] The results of surgical correction of esophageal atresia are excellent when it exists as an isolated anomaly, with overall outcome determined principally by the severity of concomitant cardiac anomalies and by the birth weight of the infant.[26,27] Survival after successful repair of isolated esophageal atresia has steadily increased over the years and now approaches 100% in the absence of other major malformations.[28]

Despite dramatically improved survival rates over the last several decades, long-term complications are still common. In adult patients with esophageal atresia, gastroesophageal reflux disease, depending on the definition, occurs in between 26% and 75% of patients.[29–31] GERD with esophagitis occurs in 19%–40% of patients, with a 6% prevalence of Barrett esophagus.[32–34] The development of GERD is likely related to abnormalities of esophageal motility and impaired acid clearance following surgical repair.[35] Ineffective esophageal motility in the proximal esophagus is universal, and the motility may deteriorate with age.[31,36] Up to 45% of patients will undergo fundoplication for GERD at some point during their lives. Therapeutic success of fundoplication is lower in esophageal atresia patients compared to nonatresia patients, and sustained symptoms/complications are common.[37] The incidence of dysphagia may approach 85% in patients who survive to adulthood.[31,32,38] Adaptive eating habits were reported in 78% of adults.[39]Anastomotic strictures are common in both children and adults, with one series noting 42% of children having endoscopic evidence of strictures.[40] Treatment with esophageal balloon dilation is typically successful, but reports of the use of intralesional steroid injection, topical mitomycin C, and esophageal stenting have also been described for refractory cases.[41–44] Although the rates of reported Barrett esophagus in patients with esophageal atresia are higher than the general population, esophageal adenocarcinoma is rare. The prevalence of esophageal squamous cell carcinoma is estimated to be 100 times higher than the normal population, and as a result, endoscopic screening is typically recommended, although there is no consensus on timing and frequency.[30,34,45]

Congenital Esophageal Stenosis

Esophageal stenosis is a rare anomaly, occurring in only 1 in every 25,000–50,000 live births.[46] The stenotic segment varies from 2 to 20 cm in length and is usually located within the middle or lower third of the esophagus (Fig. 45.10A). The precise cause of the congenital stenosis is not entirely clear. Some patients (17%–33%) have other associated anomalies, the most common being esophageal atresia (see Fig. 45.10B) and tracheoesophageal fistula.[47] Three types of stenosis are recognized, based on histology: (1) ectopic tracheobronchial remnants (TBRs), which are sequestered respiratory tissue (hyaline cartilage, respiratory epithelium), suggesting its origin is incomplete separation of lung bud from primitive foregut[48]; (2) fibromuscular hypertrophy, associated with damage to the myenteric plexus with loss of the muscle-relaxing nitrinergic neural elements; and (3) membranous diaphragm, which is limited to the mucosa and does not involve the muscle layers.[49] A systematic review showed that congenital esophageal stenosis secondary to fibromuscular hypertrophy makes up 54% of cases; 30% of cases occur secondary to TBRs and 16% are secondary to membranous diaphragms.[50] Membranous diaphragms are typically found in the upper and middle esophagus, fibromuscular hypertrophy in the middle, and lower esophagus, and TBRs are primarily encountered in the lower third of the esophagus.[50] Roughly a quarter of cases are associated with esophageal atresia and tracheoesophageal fistula.[51]

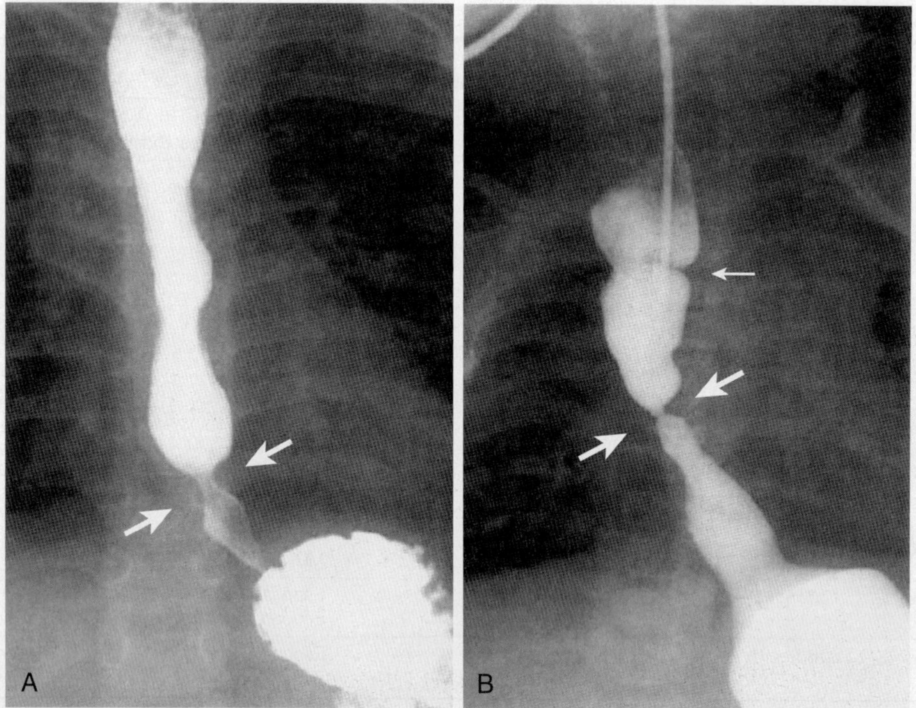

Fig. 45.10 Barium esophagograms in two patients with congenital esophageal stenosis. (A) Barium esophagogram with a tapered narrowing in the distal esophagus and dilatation of the proximal esophagus. (B) Barium esophagogram with an abrupt narrowing in the midesophagus (*large arrows*). The *small arrow* indicates the site of a previous repair for esophageal atresia. (A and B from Usui N, Kamata S, Kawahara H, et al. Usefulness of endoscopic ultrasonography in the diagnosis of congenital esophageal stenosis. *J Pediatr Surg*. 2002; 37:1744.)

Although tight stenoses are symptomatic in infancy, most stenoses present with dysphagia and regurgitation in childhood when more solid food is ingested (see Table 45.2). The stenosis is best demonstrated by esophagography, which may reveal either an abrupt or tapered stricture. Dilatation of the esophagus proximal to the stenosis is commonly noted (see Fig. 45.10). Endoscopy may be of value by demonstrating normal mucosa in the stenotic region, helping to exclude an acquired cause for the stenosis (e.g., GERD). EUS with a high-frequency mini-probe can show hyperechoic lesions with acoustic shadowing, which indicates the presence of cartilaginous structures in patients whose stenoses result from TBRs.[52] In cases where the stenosis may mimic achalasia, high-resolution esophageal manometry can be useful to differentiate.[53]

Some patients improve after endoscopic-guided bougienage or balloon dilation, although endoscopists should approach esophageal dilation carefully in these patients because chest pain and mucosal tears commonly occur. Perforation rates of 10%–44% following dilation have been reported.[54–56] Problematic stenoses may require surgical resection of the involved segment. One novel surgical approach to this lesion is circular myectomy, a technique that involves stripping of the esophageal muscle layers containing the TBRs, with preservation of the mucosal layer. This has the advantage of avoiding many of the potential complications associated with primary repair and end-to-end esophageal anastomosis.[57] In adults, the stenotic segment may also be amenable to treatment with peroral endoscopic myotomy (POEM).[58]

Esophageal Duplications

Congenital duplications of the esophagus occur in 1 in 8000 live births and represent roughly 20% of alimentary tract duplications.[2,59] The pathogenesis of esophageal duplications is uncertain, although they may develop as a result of aberrant vacuolization during organogenesis. Duplications are composed of both epithelial lining and a well-developed smooth muscular layer and maintain an attachment to the esophagus. Duplications can be either cystic, tubular, or diverticular in morphology. Cysts account for 80% of the duplications and are usually single, fluid-filled structures that typically do not communicate with the esophagus.[2] Most duplication cysts occur in the lower esophagus and are located within the posterior mediastinum, although intra-abdominal esophageal duplication cysts have been reported.[60] The majority of esophageal duplication cysts are diagnosed in childhood, with ~7% of cases presenting as symptomatic cysts in adulthood.[61] Some cysts are discovered while asymptomatic, manifesting as a mediastinal mass on a chest radiograph or a submucosal lesion on an esophagogram (Fig. 45.11A). Others manifest with symptoms from compression of structures adjacent to the tracheobronchial tree (cough, stridor, tachypnea, cyanosis, wheezing, or chest pain) and of structures adjacent to the esophageal wall (dysphagia, chest pain, or regurgitation) (see Table 45.2).[62]

The diagnosis of an esophageal duplication cyst is supported by the demonstration of a cystic mass on CT, MRI, or EUS (see Fig. 45.11B).[63] Duplication cysts appear as lesions that cause extrinsic compression of the true esophageal lumen with normal appearing mucosa. On EUS, duplication cysts can appear as homogeneous anechoic or hypoechoic masses with well-defined margins.[64] Peristalsis seen within a cyst is very specific (and is considered a diagnostic feature) of esophageal duplication cyst.[65] EUS-guided FNA of duplication cysts for pathologic diagnosis is controversial due to the significant risk of procedure-related infection.[64] Surgical removal is the preferred treatment of

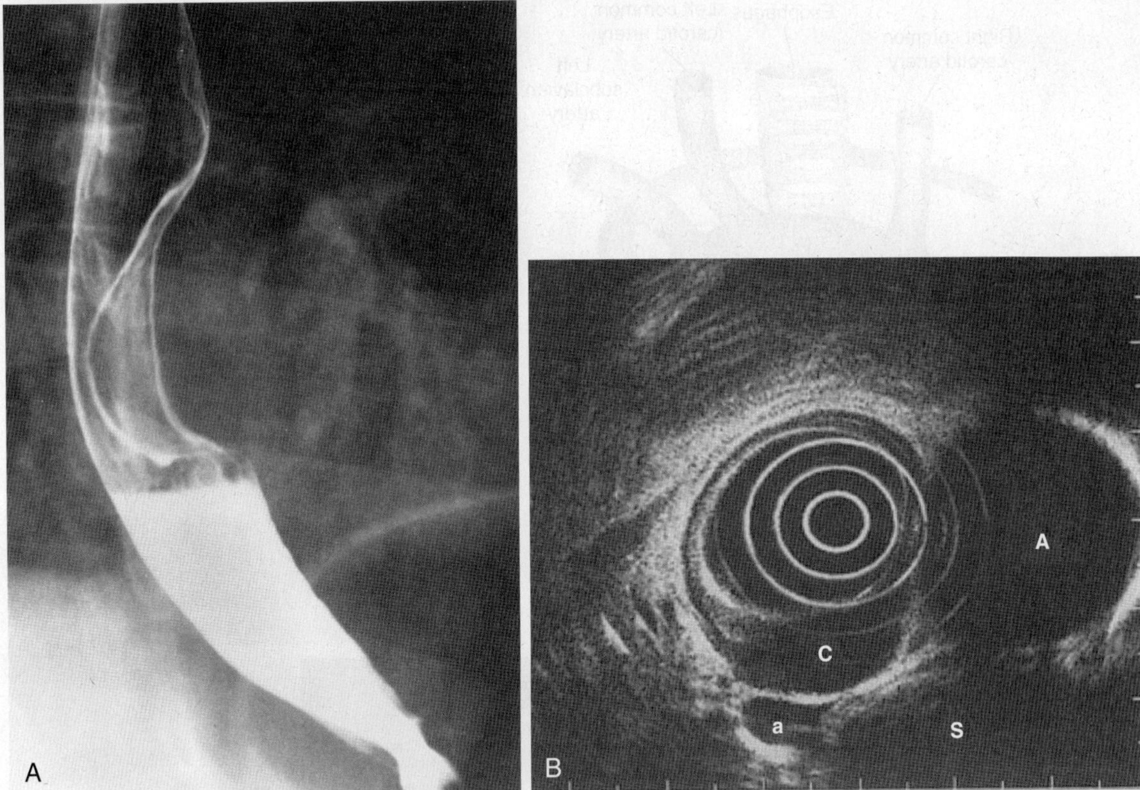

Fig. 45.11 Imaging studies showing an esophageal duplication cyst. (A) Barium esophagogram showing extrinsic compression of the wall of the esophagus. (B) EUS image showing the distortion of the esophageal wall created by the hypoechoic cyst (C) and the cyst's relationship to other hypoechoic areas created by the aorta (A), azygos vein (*a*), and spine (*S*). ((A) Courtesy David Ott, MD, Winston-Salem, NC; (B) from Kimmey MB, Vilman P. Endoscopic ultrasonography. In: Yamada T, ed. *Atlas of Gastroenterology*. 3rd ed. Philadelphia, PA: Lippincott Williams & Wilkins; 2003:1044.)

choice for confirmed cases of both symptomatic and asymptomatic duplication cysts.[64] Rarely, large duplication cysts can manifest with acute life-threatening respiratory symptoms. In this circumstance, emergent decompression can be achieved by radiologic- or endoscopically guided needle aspiration.

The tubular esophageal duplication is far less common than its cystic counterpart (20% of cases), and the diverticular type is rarely observed. The tubular type is usually located within the esophageal wall, parallels the true esophageal lumen, and, in contrast to duplication cysts, communicates with the true lumen at either or both ends of the tube.[62] Tubular duplications usually cause chest pain, dysphagia, or regurgitation in infancy, and the diagnosis is established by esophagography or endoscopy. Although some cases can be managed endoscopically, reconstructive surgery is indicated for most patients who are symptomatic.[62,66,67]

Vascular Anomalies

Intrathoracic vascular anomalies are present in 2%–3% of the population. Only rarely do they produce symptoms of esophageal obstruction despite evident vascular compression on an esophagogram. In infancy, most intrathoracic vascular anomalies manifest as respiratory symptoms from compression of the tracheobronchial tree. Later in childhood or adulthood, however, these same abnormalities can produce dysphagia and regurgitation, owing to esophageal compression (see Table 45.2).

Dysphagia lusoria is the term given for symptoms arising from vascular compression of the esophagus by an aberrant right subclavian artery (Fig. 45.12).[68] This condition results from defective development of the right-sided pharyngeal arch, which under normal circumstances transforms into the right subclavian artery. The right subclavian artery in *dysphagia lusoria* arises from the left side of the aortic arch and courses from the lower left to the upper right posterior to the esophagus. In 20% of cases, the artery courses anterior to the esophagus.[69] It is estimated that *arteria lusoria* is present in 0.7% of the general population on the basis of autopsy studies. Typically, the diagnosis is established by barium esophagogram, which shows the characteristic pencil-like indentation at the level of the third and fourth thoracic vertebrae (see Fig. 45.12B).[68] Confirmation is by CT, MRI, arteriography, or EUS (see Fig. 45.12C).[69] Given the considerable frequency with which such lesions are asymptomatic, endoscopy or esophageal manometry may be desirable to exclude other causes of dysphagia. During endoscopy, the right radial pulse may diminish or disappear from instrumental compression of the right subclavian artery. Esophageal manometry has demonstrated a pulsatile high-pressure zone at the location of the aberrant artery.[70] Functional luminal imaging probe (FLIP) panometry may also demonstrate obstructive physiology.[71] Symptoms usually respond to simple modification of the diet to meals of soft consistency and small size. When necessary, surgery relieves the obstruction by anastomosing the aberrant artery to the ascending aorta (see Fig. 45.12A).[70]

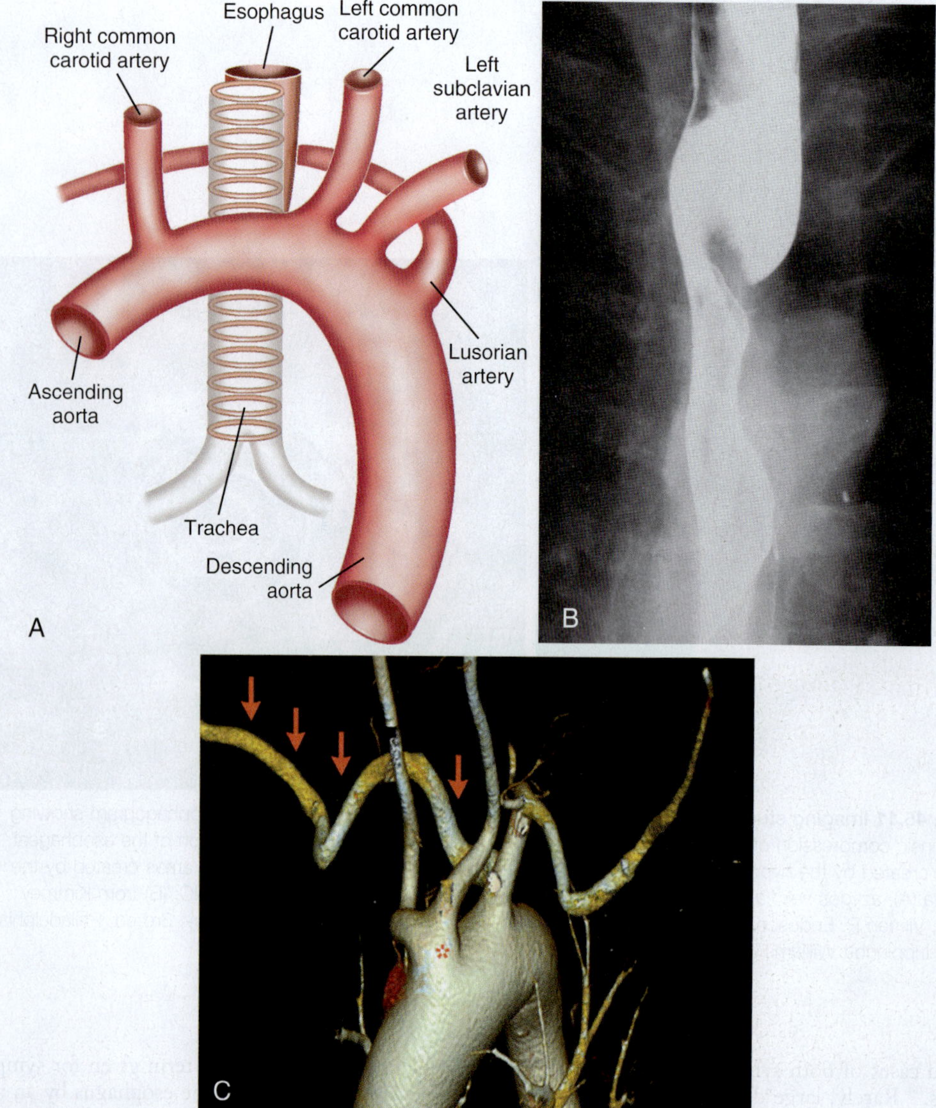

Fig. 45.12 **Dysphagia lusoria.** (A) Anatomic configuration of an aberrant right subclavian artery (lusorian artery) as it courses behind the esophagus from the aortic arch toward the right shoulder. (B) Barium esophagogram showing the characteristic diagonal indentation of the esophageal wall at the level of the third and fourth thoracic vertebrae. (C) CT with 3D reconstruction. ((A) From Janssen M, Baggen MG, Veen HF, et al. *Dysphagia lusoria*: clinical aspects, manometric findings, diagnosis, and therapy. *Am J Gastroenterol*. 2000;95:1411; (B) courtesy David Ott, MD, Winston-Salem, NC; (C) From Hudzik B, Gąsior M. *Dysphagia lusoria*. *N Engl J Med*. 2016;375(4):e4.)

Esophageal Rings

The distal esophagus may contain two "rings," the A and B (Schatzki) rings that demarcate anatomically the proximal and distal borders of the esophageal vestibule. The A (muscular) ring is located at the proximal border (see Fig. 45.3). It is a broad (4–5 mm) symmetrical band of hypertrophied muscle that constricts the tubular esophageal lumen at its junction with the vestibule. In this location, the A ring, which is covered by squamous epithelium, corresponds to the upper end of the LES.[72] The A ring is rare, and because it varies in caliber on esophagography depending on the degree of esophageal distention, it is generally asymptomatic. The A ring may have an association with gastroesophageal reflux.[73] Occasionally, an A ring is found in association with dysphagia for solids and liquids (see Table 45.2).[72] Symptomatic A rings can be treated by passage of a large-caliber esophageal dilator, injection of botulinum toxin, or by POEM.[74,75]

The B ring, otherwise known as the *mucosal* or *Schatzki ring*, is very common and found in 6%–14% of subjects having a routine upper GI series.[76] In a review of more than 10,000 upper endoscopies, a Schatzki ring was found in 4% of cases.[77] On barium study, it is always found in association with a hiatal hernia and is recognized as a thin (2-mm) membrane that constricts the esophageal lumen at the junction of the vestibule and gastric cardia (Fig. 45.13A). The Schatzki ring has squamous epithelium on its upper surface and columnar epithelium on its lower surface and so demarcates the squamocolumnar junction. The ring itself is composed of only mucosa and submucosa; there is no muscularis propria. Schatzki rings can be congenital or acquired, and a relationship to GERD is likely (see Chapter 48).[76]

Most B rings are asymptomatic, yet when the diameter of the esophageal lumen is narrowed to 13 mm or less, rings commonly are the cause of intermittent dysphagia for solids or unheralded acute solid-food impactions (see Table 45.2).[78,79] It is usually not

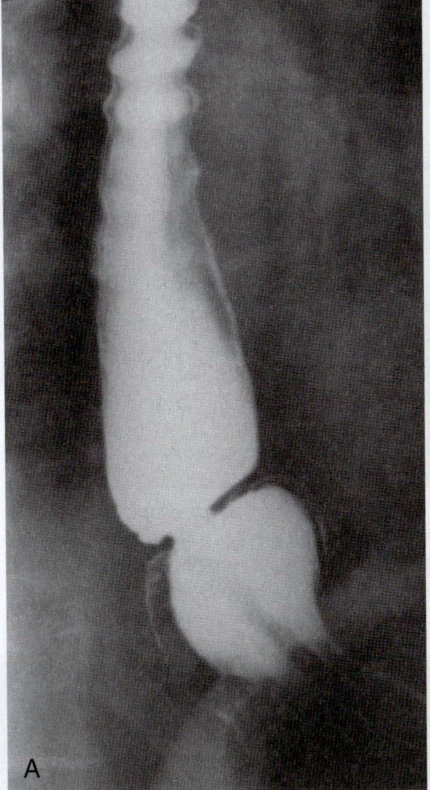

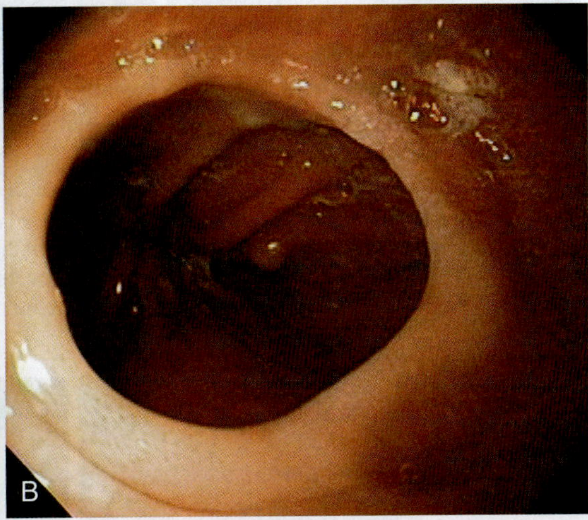

Fig. 45.13 Imaging studies showing an esophageal B (Schatzki) ring. (A) Barium esophagogram showing the ring of mucosa localized to the squamocolumnar junction. Below the B ring is a hiatal hernia. The hernia is visualized as a small sac between the B ring above and the diaphragm below. (B) Endoscopic view of the ring. ((A) Courtesy David Ott, MD, Winston-Salem, NC; (B) courtesy John D. Long, MD, Winston-Salem, NC.)

difficult to identify symptomatic rings on esophagography (see Fig. 45.13A) or endoscopy (see Fig. 45.13B), although attention should be paid to adequately distend the distal esophagus.[76] In some instances, the obstructing ring is best demonstrated radiographically by its ability to trap a swallowed marshmallow or a barium tablet, techniques that can also assist in determining the diameter of the ring.

Asymptomatic B rings require no treatment, and those producing dysphagia are effectively treated by passage of either a single, large dilator (balloon or bougie) or a series of such dilators of progressively larger diameter.[80] Early studies reported that 32% of patients required repeat dilation after 1 year.[76] More recent studies report much lower redilation rates (13%), perhaps due to the more routine use of both larger dilators and a course of postdilation antireflux therapy.[81] In 1 randomized placebo-controlled study of 44 patients with symptomatic Schatzki rings, maintenance therapy with omeprazole resulted in a 40% reduction in the need for redilation after a mean follow-up of 35 months.[82] A recent observational study demonstrated that complete Schatzki ring excision using four quadrant jumbo cold biopsy forceps was safe and effective in preventing recurrence.[83] Symptomatic rings that are refractory to dilation have been successfully treated by endoscopic means using electrocautery incision.[84] A randomized controlled trial of standard bougie dilation versus electrocautery incision for symptomatic Schatzki rings has demonstrated that the two therapies have comparable initial success rates but that endoscopic incision had a longer duration of symptom resolution.[85]

Esophageal Webs

Esophageal webs are developmental anomalies characterized by one or more thin horizontal membranes of stratified squamous epithelium within the upper (cervical) esophagus and mid-esophagus. Unlike rings, these anomalies rarely encircle the lumen but instead protrude from the anterior wall, extending laterally but not to the posterior wall (Fig. 45.14A and B). Webs are common in the cervical esophagus and are best demonstrated on an esophagogram with the lateral view. In up to 5% of cases, they are identified in an asymptomatic state, but when they are symptomatic, they cause dysphagia for solids (see Table 45.2).[86] Webs are fragile membranes and respond well to esophageal bougienage dilation.

As discussed in Chapter 47, an association in adults of cervical esophageal webs, dysphagia, and iron deficiency anemia has been described as the Plummer-Vinson or Paterson-Kelly syndrome.[86] The syndrome, although uncommon, occurs primarily in women. There may be an association between Plummer-Vinson syndrome and celiac disease.[87] The syndrome identifies a group of patients at increased risk for squamous carcinoma of the pharynx and esophagus.[86] Correction of iron deficiency in Plummer-Vinson syndrome may result in resolution of the associated dysphagia as well as disappearance of the web(s).[86]

Heterotopic Gastric Mucosa (Esophageal/Cervical Inlet Patch)

The *cervical inlet patch* refers to the appearance on endoscopy of a small (0.5–2 cm) distinctive, velvety-red island of heterotopic gastric mucosa amid a lighter pink squamous mucosa, generally localized immediately below the UES (Fig. 45.15A). They may be singular or multiple. When sought, an inlet patch can be detected in up to 10% of upper endoscopies, and biopsy specimens reveal gastric fundic- or antral-type mucosa (see Fig. 45.15B).[88,89] Identification can be aided by the intentional use of narrow-band imaging (NBI), which has become standard on most endoscopes.[90]

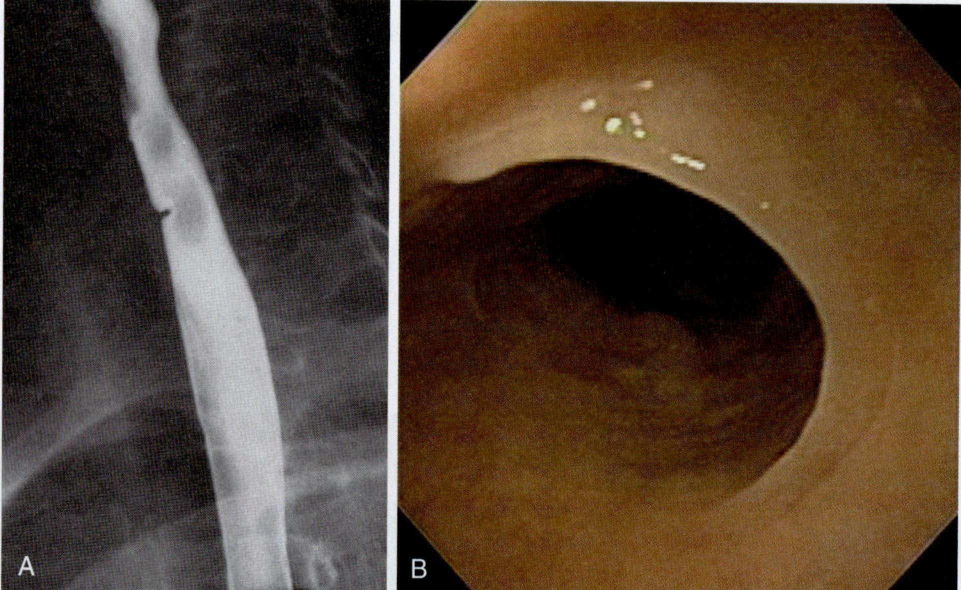

Fig. 45.14 Imaging studies of esophageal webs. (A) Barium esophagogram of a cervical esophageal web seen on the lateral view as a thin membrane protruding from the anterior esophageal wall. Webs, unlike rings, often incompletely encircle the esophageal lumen. (B) Endoscopic view of a cervical esophageal web. ((A) Courtesy David Ott, MD, Winston-Salem, NC; (B) courtesy John D. Long, MD, Winston-Salem, NC.)

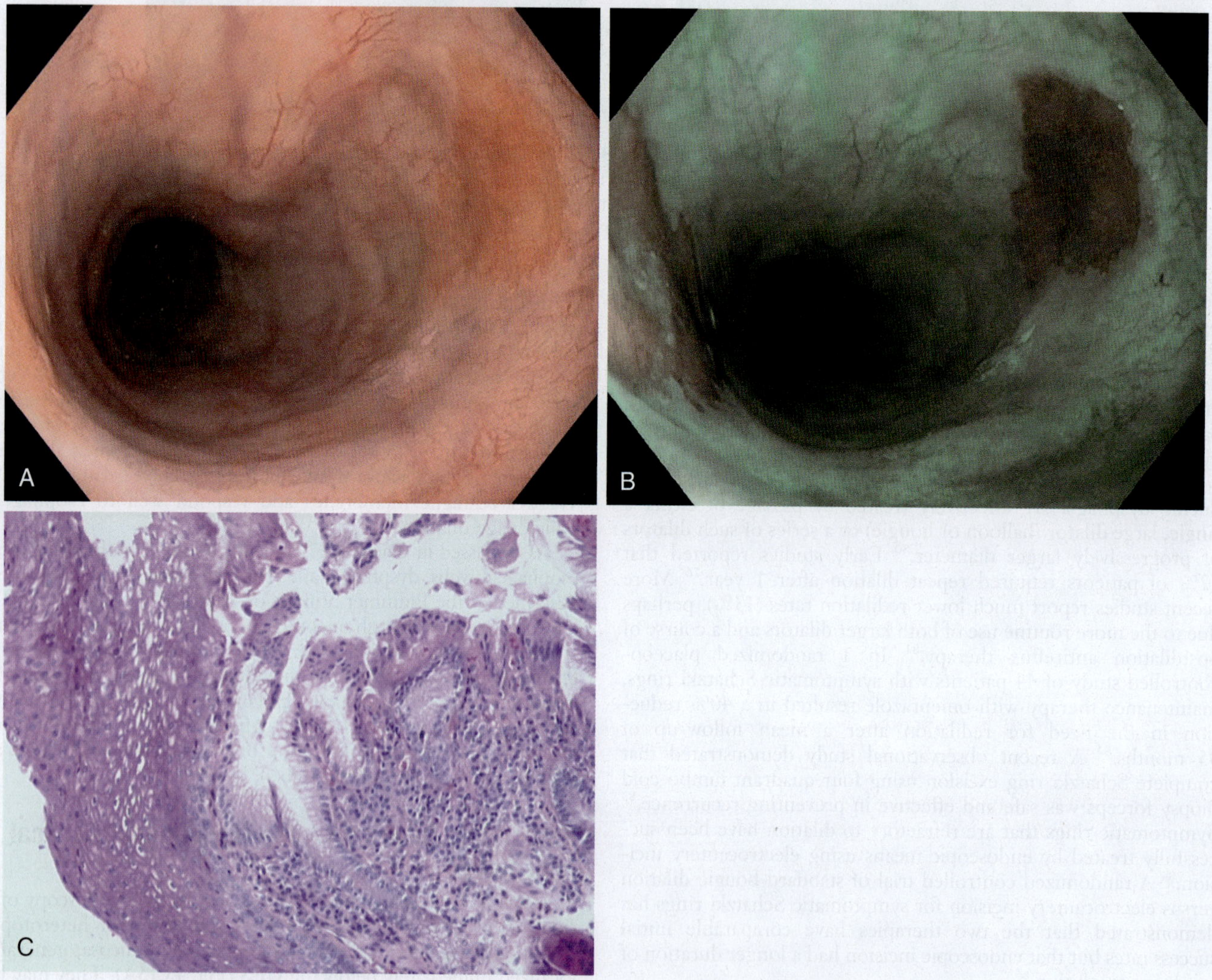

A

B

C

Fig. 45.15 Endoscopic images of an inlet patch. (A) Endoscopic view of heterotopic gastric mucosa in the cervical esophagus (inlet patch). (B) Endoscopic view of heterotopic gastric mucosa under narrow band imaging (NBI). Note the contralateral inlet patch that is now visible with virtual chromoendoscopy. (C) Photomicrograph view of an inlet patch showing glandular epithelium with parietal cells (*right*) adjacent to normal esophageal squamous epithelium (*left*). ((A and B, courtesy Lindsey Shipley, MD, Birmingham, AL. (C) Courtesy Pamela Jensen, MD, Dallas, TX.)

The fundic-type mucosa contains chief and parietal cells and, thus, in some specimens retains the capacity for acid secretion.[91,71] Similar to gastric mucosa in the stomach, the inlet patch may be infected with *Helicobacter pylori*.[92] However, inlet patches are usually asymptomatic and unassociated with disease and thus require no treatment. A possible association with globus pharyngeus was suggested in two studies in which this symptom was improved after ablation of inlet patches using argon plasma coagulation or radiofrequency ablation.[93,94] In rare instances, an inlet patch is found in association with an esophageal web or stricture[95] or ulcer, the latter resulting in bleeding or perforation.[89] Adenocarcinoma arising in an inlet patch is a rare complication, although there is a statistically significant association between inlet patches and proximal esophageal adenocarcinomas.[89,96] The necessity of surveillance endoscopy is controversial and a formal consensus has not been reached.

Full references for this chapter can be found at https://ebooks.health.elsevier.com.

46 Esophageal Neuromuscular Function and Motility Disorders

Dustin A. Carlson, C. Prakash Gyawali

IN THIS CHAPTER

The esophagus is a muscular tube with a sphincter at each end joining the hypopharynx to the stomach with the simple function of transporting food, fluid, and gas from the mouth to the stomach. The esophagus encompasses the anatomic and physiologic transition from the striated muscle oropharynx to the smooth muscle gut. Neurologically, the oropharynx is controlled by the cerebral cortex and medulla and capable of precise tactile sensation, while the distal esophagus is composed entirely of smooth muscle, controlled by the vagus nerve and enteric nervous system, and comparatively insensitive. Although there is a gradual transition from oropharynx to distal esophagus, motor and sensory function in the oropharynx and esophageal body are quite distinct, and the lower esophageal sphincter (LES) is composed entirely of smooth muscle. The ensuing discussion includes selected aspects of pharyngeal, gastric, and diaphragmatic function that are inextricably entwined with esophageal function.

MOTOR AND SENSORY FUNCTION

Oropharynx and Upper Esophageal Sphincter

Within the oral cavity, the lips, teeth, hard palate, soft palate, mandible, floor of the mouth, and tongue serve to form and contain food into a bolus suitable for transfer to the pharynx. Disorders of the oral phase of swallowing occur with many conditions characterized by global neurologic dysfunction, such as traumatic brain injury, brain tumors, or chorea. Detailed discussion of these conditions can be found in texts on swallow evaluation and therapy.[1]

The pharynx is divided into three segments: nasopharynx, oropharynx, and hypopharynx (Fig. 46.1). The nasopharynx extends from the base of the skull to the distal edge of the soft palate. Muscles in the nasopharynx elevate the soft palate during swallowing, seal the nasopharynx, and prevent nasopharyngeal regurgitation. The oropharynx extends from the soft palate to the base of the tongue. The inferior margin of the oropharynx is demarcated by the valleculae anteriorly and the mobile tip of the epiglottis posteriorly. The hypopharynx extends from the valleculae to the inferior margin of the cricoid cartilage and includes the upper esophageal sphincter (UES).

Musculature of the soft palate, tongue, and pharynx all participate during swallowing to collapse and shorten the pharyngeal lumen and then expel its contents into the esophagus. Additionally, extrinsic muscles elevate and pull the pharynx forward, thereby sealing the airway and opening the UES. Jaw-closing and jaw-opening muscles of mastication coordinate with each other to shift to the swallowing reflex when mastication ends and swallowing begins, under central control.[2] The intrinsic muscles of the pharynx, the superior, middle, and inferior pharyngeal constrictors (see Fig. 46.1), overlap and insert into a collagenous sheet, the buccopharyngeal aponeurosis. The inferior constrictor is composed of the thyropharyngeus (superior part) and the cricopharyngeus (inferior part). The thyropharyngeus arises from the thyroid cartilage, passes posteromedially, and inserts in the median raphe. The cricopharyngeus has superior and inferior components, each of which arises bilaterally from the sides of the cricoid lamina; the superior fibers course posteromedially to the median raphe whereas the inferior fibers loop around the esophageal inlet without a median raphe. Killian triangle, a triangular area of thin muscle, is formed posteriorly between these components and is the most common site of origin for pharyngeal pulsion diverticula.

The pharynx also contains five single or paired cartilages (see Fig. 46.1). The spaces formed between the lateral insertion of the inferior constrictor and the lateral walls of the thyroid cartilage are the pyriform sinuses that end inferiorly at the cricopharyngeus muscle, separating the pharynx from the esophagus. The larynx and trachea are suspended in the neck between the hyoid bone superiorly and the sternum inferiorly. A number of muscles, categorized as the laryngeal strap muscles, contribute to this suspension and, together with the intrinsic elasticity of the trachea, permit the larynx to be raised and lowered. The hyoid bone also serves as the base for the tongue that rests upon it. Laryngeal movement is crucial to the swallow response as the laryngeal inlet is both closed and physically removed from the bolus path in the course of a swallow. Failure to achieve this synchronized laryngeal movement can result in aspiration.

The pharyngeal muscles are densely innervated with motor fibers coming from nuclei of the trigeminal, facial, glossopharyngeal,

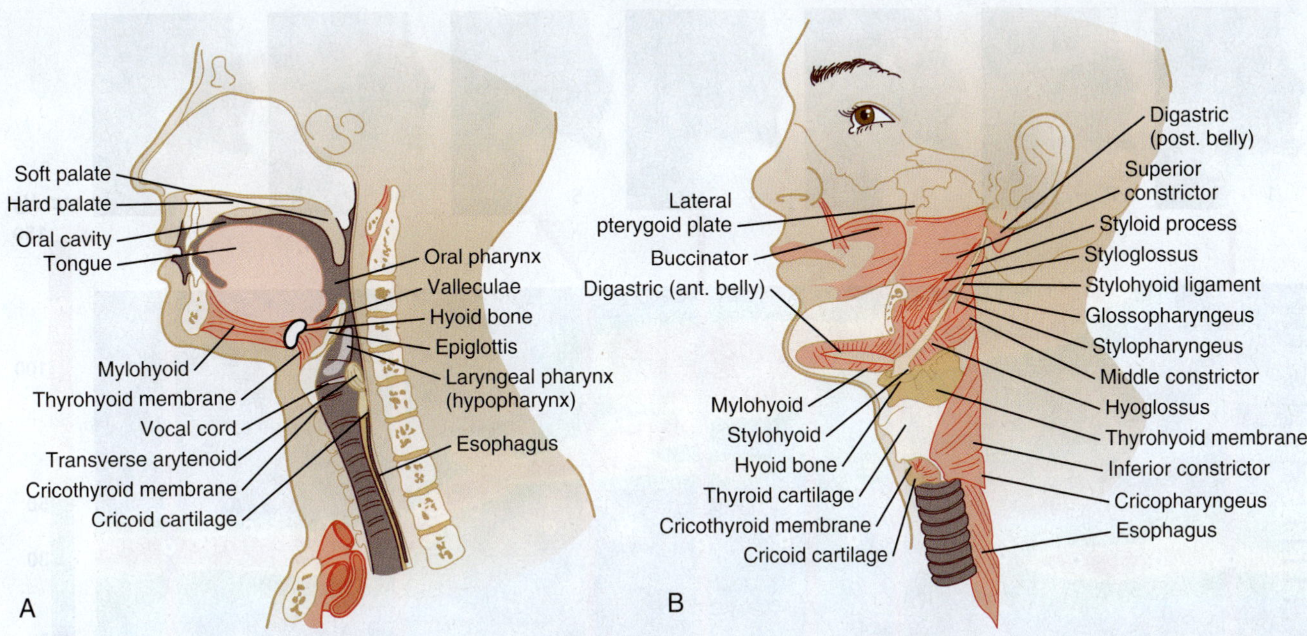

Fig. 46.1 Anatomy of the pharynx. (A) Sagittal view of the pharynx showing the musculoskeletal structures involved in swallowing. Note that the esophagus is collapsed and empty at rest. In the course of a swallow, the laryngeal inlet will be sealed and the mouth of the esophagus will be opened by highly coordinated muscular activity. (B) Cutaway view of the musculature of the pharynx. Note that the hyoid bone is positioned as a fulcrum and is instrumental in directing anterior, superior traction forces critical to closing the larynx and opening the esophageal inlet during a swallow. *ant.*, Anterior; *post.*, posterior. (Reprinted from Kahrilas PJ, Frost F. Disorders of swallowing and bowel motility. In: Green D, ed. *Medical Problems of the Chronically Disabled*. Rockville, MD: Aspen Publishers; 1990:11–37.)

and hypoglossal nuclei, as well as the nucleus ambiguus of the vagus and spinal segments C1 to C3. All motor neurons within nucleus ambiguus participate in swallowing, with those innervating the striated muscle esophagus situated rostrally and those innervating the pharynx and larynx more caudally.[3] The muscular components of the UES are the cricopharyngeus, adjacent esophagus, and adjacent inferior constrictor with the cricopharyngeus contributing the 1 cm zone of maximal pressure.[4] The closed sphincter has a slit-like configuration, with the cricoid lamina anterior and the cricopharyngeus lateral and posterior. Neural input via vagal trunks originating in the nucleus ambiguus maintains UES pressure and vagal transection abolishes this contractile activity.

Manometric evaluation of UES function is difficult because it is a short, complex anatomic zone that moves briskly during swallowing. Furthermore, UES pressure is heavily influenced by recording methodology, owing both to its marked asymmetry and to its reflexive contraction to pharyngeal and esophageal stimulation. The UES can move 2–3 cm during swallowing,[5] and the recording device itself may contribute to the measured pressure, with larger devices recording higher pressures.[6] Thus it is not possible to define a meaningful normal range of UES pressure.[7] UES relaxation during swallowing also poses substantial recording challenges, making for great variability in technique and interpretation. However, high-resolution manometry (HRM) using solid-state technology permits accurate tracking of UES relaxation and intrabolus pressure changes during swallowing (Fig. 46.2).

The UES maintains closure of the proximal end of the esophagus unless opening is required, necessitated for swallowing or belching. It also constitutes an additional barrier to refluxed material entering the pharynx from the esophagus and prevents air from entering the esophagus by contracting in synchrony with inspiration. Inspiratory augmentation is most evident during periods of low UES pressure and can be exaggerated in individuals experiencing globus sensation.[8] Balloon distension of the esophagus stimulates UES contraction,[9] with the effect being more pronounced with proximal balloon positions. However, when the distension pattern of gas reflux is simulated using a cylindrical bag or rapid air injection into the esophagus, UES relaxation rather than contraction occurs.[4] Belch-induced UES relaxation is also associated with glottic closure. Stress augments UES pressure, whereas anesthesia or sleep[10] virtually eliminates it. Neither experimental acid perfusion of the esophagus nor spontaneous gastroesophageal acid reflux alters continuously recorded UES pressure in either normal volunteers or in individuals with peptic esophagitis.

The Pharyngeal Swallow

The pharyngeal swallow is the largely subconscious coordinated contraction that transfers oral contents into the esophagus. A swallow can be volitionally initiated during eating or drinking, and involuntarily when saliva or respiratory secretions accumulate in the pharynx.[2] An average person swallows about 600 times a day, mainly while awake and during eating, and to a much lesser extent while asleep.[11] Afferent sensory fibers capable of triggering the pharyngeal swallow travel centrally via the internal branch of the superior laryngeal nerve (from the larynx) and the glossopharyngeal nerve (from the pharynx). These sensory fibers converge before terminating in the medullary swallow center, a network of neurons in the brainstem that form a swallowing pattern generator, which can produce sequential and rhythmic motor activity.[12] The swallowing pattern generator has complex connections to higher brain regions and to the motor nuclei of cranial nerves serving muscles along the swallowing pathway.

Although understood physiologically as the patterned activation of motor neurons and their corresponding motor units, swallowing is clinically evaluated in mechanical terms, and best

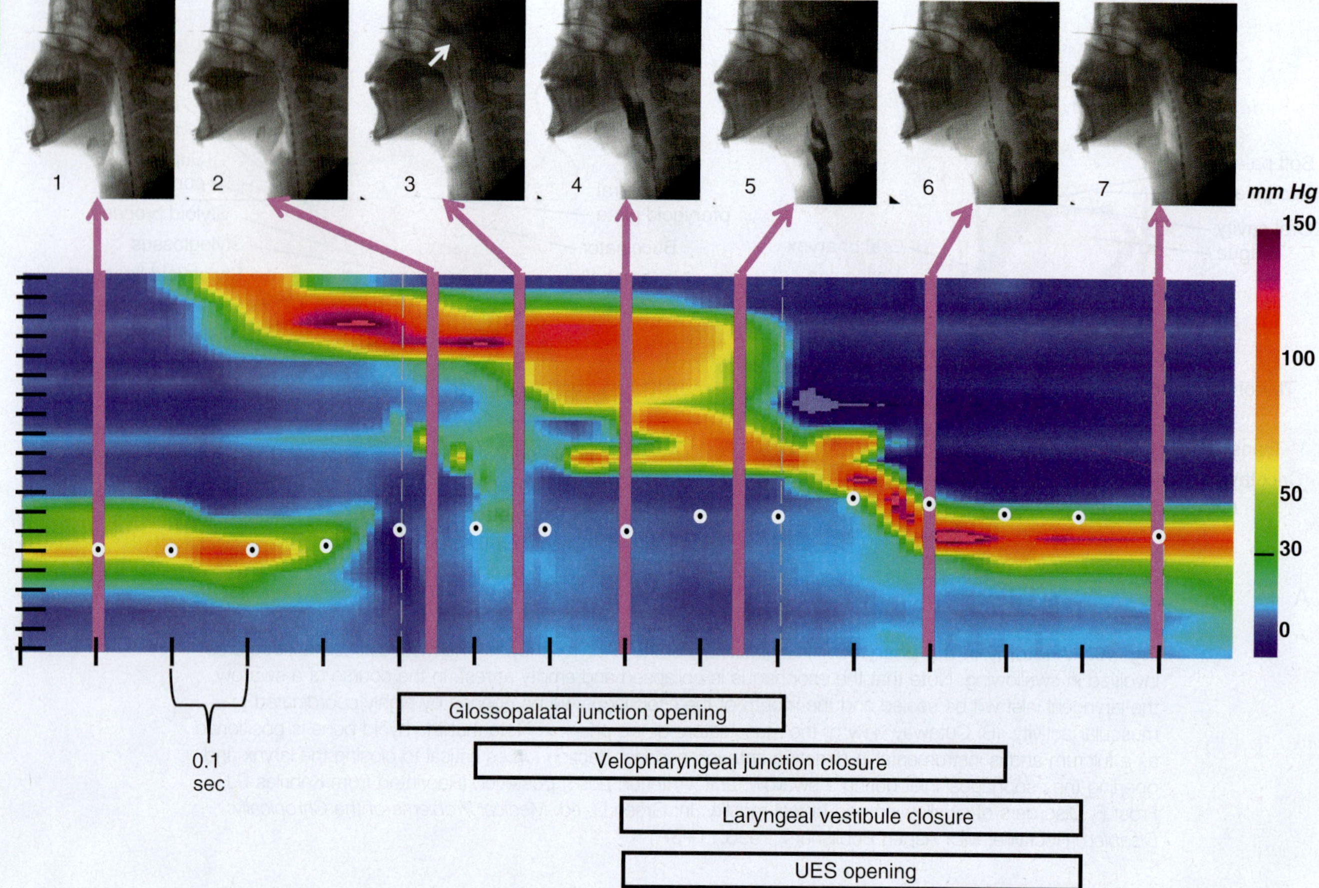

Fig. 46.2 Fluoroscopy combined with high-resolution manometry (HRM). The fluoroscopic images (*top*) are depicted at specific times demarcated on the HRM (*color panel by pink arrows*). The timeline illustrates the coordination and timing of events within the pharyngeal swallow on fluoroscopy. Each horizontal bar depicts the period during which one of the oropharyngeal valves is in its swallow configuration, as opposed to its configuration during respiration, and is correlated with the images on fluoroscopy: (1) baseline anatomy with bolus in the mouth; (2) glossopalatal opening occurring in synchrony with upper esophageal sphincter (UES) relaxation, which is typically to less than 10 mm Hg; (3) velopharyngeal junction closure, sealing off the nasopharynx to prevent regurgitation (note the elevation depicted by the *white arrow*); (4) laryngeal vestibule closure and UES opening occurring as the epiglottis inverts, closing the laryngeal vestibule as the bolus, led by air, is rapidly pushed through the UES; (5) continued bolus transit with the onset of the pharyngeal stripping wave; (6) bolus transfer to the esophagus is completed as the pharyngeal stripping wave traverses the UES while the laryngeal vestibule remains closed; (7) return of the pharynx to a respiratory configuration, with the laryngeal vestibule opened and the epiglottis back in its upright configuration. The *black dots* on the topography (HRM) plot represent the location of the proximal aspect of the UES at each time point. (With permission from the Esophageal Center at Northwestern.)

evaluated by videofluoroscopic or cineradiographic analysis. The pharyngeal swallow rapidly reconfigures pharyngeal structures from a respiratory to an alimentary pathway and then reverses this reconfiguration within 1 second. The pharyngeal swallow response can be dissected into several closely coordinated actions: (1) nasopharyngeal closure by elevation and retraction of the soft palate, (2) UES opening, (3) laryngeal closure, (4) tongue loading (ramping), (5) tongue pulsion, and (6) pharyngeal clearance. Precise coordination of these actions is an obvious imperative, and to some degree the relative timing of these events is affected either by volition or by the volume of the swallowed bolus (see Fig. 46.2).

The most fundamental anatomic reconfiguration required to transform the oropharynx from a respiratory to a swallow pathway is to open the inlet to the esophagus and seal the inlet to the larynx. These events occur in close synchrony, facilitated by laryngeal elevation, and anterior traction via the hyoid axis. It is critical to recognize the distinction between UES relaxation and UES opening. UES relaxation is due to cessation of excitatory neural input while the larynx is elevating. Once the larynx is elevated, UES opening results from traction on the anterior sphincter wall caused by contraction of the supra- and infra-hyoid musculature that also results in a characteristic pattern of hyoid displacement.

Bolus transport out of the oropharynx is facilitated by the tongue and pharyngeal constrictors. Tongue motion adapts to varied swallow conditions and propels most of the bolus into the esophagus prior to the onset of the pharyngeal contraction. On the other hand, the pharyngeal contraction is more stereotyped, functioning to strip the last residue from the pharyngeal walls. UES closure coincides with passage of the pharyngeal contraction. However, the contractile activity of the sphincter has an added dimension as well, exhibiting augmented contractility during laryngeal descent, resulting in a grabbing effect such that the sphincter and laryngeal descent complement each other to clear residue from the hypopharynx.[13] This clearing function probably acts to minimize the risk of postswallow aspiration by preventing residual material from adhering to the laryngeal inlet when respiration resumes.

Esophagus

The esophagus is a 20–22-cm tube composed of skeletal and smooth muscle. The proportion of each muscle type is species dependent, but in humans, the proximal 5% is striated, the middle 35%–40% is mixed with an increasing proportion of smooth muscle distally, and the distal 50%–60% is entirely smooth muscle. The outer longitudinal muscle arises from the cricoid cartilage with slips from the cricopharyngeus passing dorsolaterally to fuse posteriorly about 3 cm distal to the cricoid cartilage. This results in a posterior triangular area devoid of longitudinal muscle, Laimer triangle. Distal to Laimer triangle, the longitudinal muscles form a continuous sheath of uniform thickness around the esophagus. The adjacent, inner muscle layer is formed of circular or, more precisely, helical muscle also forming a sheath of uniform thickness along the length of the esophagus. There is a decreasing degree of helicity moving distally ranging from 60 degrees in the proximal esophagus to nearly 0 degrees at the LES.[14] Unlike the distal GI tract, there is no serosal layer to the esophagus.

The extrinsic innervation of the esophagus is via the vagus nerve with motor neurons in nucleus ambiguus (striated muscle portion) and the dorsal motor nucleus of the vagus (smooth muscle portion). Efferent vagal fibers reach the cervical esophagus by the pharyngoesophageal nerve, and synapse directly on striated muscle neuromuscular junctions. The vagus also provides sensory innervation; in the cervical esophagus, this is via the superior laryngeal nerve with cell bodies in the nodose ganglion, whereas in the remainder of the esophagus, sensory fibers travel via the recurrent laryngeal nerve or, in the most distal esophagus, via the esophageal branches of the vagus. Vagal afferents are strongly stimulated by esophageal distension.

The esophagus also contains an autonomic nerve network, the myenteric plexus, located between the longitudinal and circular muscle layers. Myenteric plexus neurons are sparse in the proximal esophagus, and their function is unclear because the striated muscle is directly controlled by nucleus ambiguus motor neurons, on the other hand, in the smooth muscle esophagus preganglionic neurons in the dorsal motor nucleus of the vagus synapse on relay neurons in the myenteric plexus ganglia. A second nerve network, the submucosal or Meissner's plexus, is situated between the muscularis mucosa and the circular muscle layer, but this is sparse in the human esophagus.

Esophageal Peristalsis

The esophagus is normally atonic and its intraluminal pressure closely reflects pleural pressure, becoming negative during inspiration. However, swallowing or focal distention initiates peristalsis. Primary peristalsis is initiated by a swallow and traverses the entire length of the esophagus; secondary peristalsis can be elicited in response to focal esophageal distention with air, fluid, or a balloon, beginning at the locus of distention. The mechanical correlate of peristalsis is of a stripping wave that milks the esophagus clean from its proximal to distal end. The propagation of the stripping wave corresponds closely with that of the manometrically recorded contraction such that the point of luminal closure seen fluoroscopically at each esophageal locus corresponds with the upstroke of the pressure wave on line tracings or the contractile wavefront on esophageal pressure topography (EPT) (Fig. 46.3). The likelihood of achieving complete esophageal emptying from the distal esophagus is inversely related to peristaltic amplitude, such that emptying becomes progressively impaired with peristaltic amplitudes of 30 mm Hg or less.[15] However, emptying is also modified by the pressure gradient across the esophagogastric junction (EGJ), and this interaction can have significant influence on both bolus transit and peristaltic contractility.

Another essential feature of peristalsis is deglutitive inhibition. A second swallow initiated while an earlier peristaltic contraction is still progressing in the proximal esophagus completely inhibits the contraction induced by the first swallow. Deglutitive inhibition in the distal esophagus is attributable to hyperpolarization of the circular smooth muscle and is mediated via inhibitory ganglionic neurons in the myenteric plexus. Deglutitive inhibition can be demonstrated experimentally in the esophagus by distending an intraluminal balloon, which stimulates esophageal contraction.[16] Once the high-pressure zone is established, deglutitive inhibition is evident after swallowing while recording intraluminal pressure between the balloon and the esophageal wall. Deglutitive inhibition can also be demonstrated during multiple swallows performed in rapid succession during esophageal manometry, during which complete inhibition of esophageal peristalsis and profound LES relaxation occur.[17,18]

The physiologic control mechanisms governing the striated and smooth muscle esophagus differ. The striated muscle receives exclusively excitatory vagal innervation, and its peristaltic contraction results from sequential activation of the musculature. These vagal fibers release acetylcholine (ACh) and stimulate nicotinic cholinergic receptors on the striated muscle cells. Striated muscle peristalsis is programmed by the medullary swallowing center in much the same way as is the pharyngeal swallow. The vagus nerves also exhibit control of primary peristalsis in the smooth muscle esophagus, but the mechanism of vagal control is more complex than that of the striated muscle because vagal fibers synapse on myenteric plexus neurons rather than directly on muscle cells. However, the myenteric plexus can also orchestrate peristalsis independently of vagal activation; secondary peristalsis can be elicited anywhere along the smooth muscle esophagus despite extrinsic denervation. In contrast, transection across the striated muscle esophagus does not inhibit peristaltic progression across the transection site or distally.

Regardless of central or ganglionic control, esophageal smooth muscle contraction is ultimately elicited by ganglionic cholinergic neurons. Less clear are the control mechanisms for the direction and velocity of peristalsis. Nerve conduction studies indicate that neural stimuli initiated by swallowing reach the ganglionic neurons along the length of the esophagus essentially simultaneously. However, the latency between the arrival of the vagal stimulus and muscle contraction progressively increases, moving aborally. In humans, the latent period is 2 seconds in the proximal smooth muscle esophagus and 5–7 seconds just proximal to the LES. The current hypothesis is that peristaltic direction and velocity result from a neural gradient along the esophagus, wherein excitatory ganglionic neurons dominate proximally and inhibitory ganglionic neurons dominate distally (Fig. 46.4). This organization is consistent with the demonstration of two subsegments within the smooth muscle segment with pressure topography plotting, the first of which is strongly reactive to cholinergic drugs.[19] The primary inhibitory neurotransmitter is nitric oxide (NO), produced from L-arginine by the enzyme NO synthase in myenteric neurons.[20] There is also evidence for a role of vasoactive intestinal polypeptide (VIP)-containing neurons mediating inhibition.[21]

Longitudinal Muscle

The longitudinal muscle of the esophagus also contracts during peristalsis, with the net effect of transiently shortening the structure by 2–2.5 cm. Similar to the pattern of circular muscle

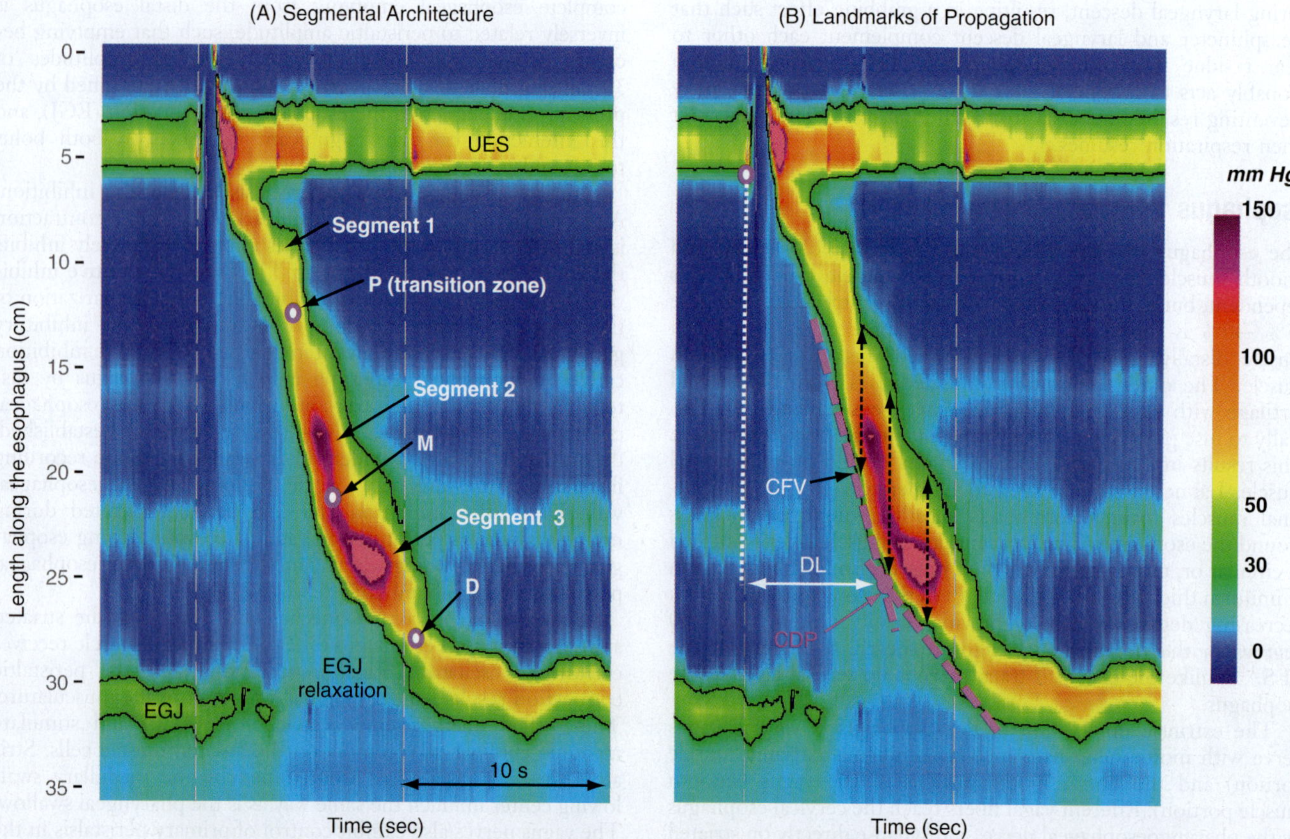

Fig. 46.3 Topographic depiction of esophageal peristalsis using high-resolution manometry showing the segmental architecture of peristalsis and landmarks of contractile propagation. (A) The 30-mm Hg isobaric contour plot (*black lines*) demonstrates that progression through the esophagus is not seamless. The proximal striated segment 1 and the distal smooth muscle esophageal contractile segments 2 and 3 are separated by a transition zone (P). The distal esophagus is also divided into two distinct contractile segments (2 and 3), separated by a pressure trough (M). The region of the esophagogastric junction (EGJ) is also distinguished by a distinct contractile segment that is separated from the adjacent esophagus by another pressure trough (D). (B) Same depiction with the topographic landmarks of peristalsis represented. The *pink circle* located within segment 3 localizes the contractile deceleration point (CDP), the point along the contractile wavefront at which velocity slows, demarcating the transition from peristalsis to sphincter reconstitution. The distal latency (DL), which is a manifestation of deglutitive inhibition, is measured from upper esophageal sphincter relaxation to the CDP. Contractile front velocity is measured by taking the best fit tangent from the CDP to the transition zone, P, of interest is the concept of concurrent esophageal contraction illustrated by the *vertical dashed arrows*. The length of the esophagus concurrently contracting, between the onset of the contractile front and the offset of contraction proximally, is, on average, 10 cm and maximizes in close approximation to the CDP. Following the CDP, the length of concurrent contraction lessens as the "rear" catches up with the slowed contraction front. (With permission from the Esophageal Center at Northwestern.)

contraction, longitudinal muscle contraction is propagated distally as an active segment at a rate of 2–4 cm/sec.[22] Central mechanisms control longitudinal muscle contraction during peristalsis with progressively increasing latency moving distally, similar to that seen with the circular smooth muscle. However, unlike the circular muscle, nerve stimulation studies suggest the longitudinal muscle to be free of inhibitory neural control.

Esophagogastric Junction

The anatomy of the EGJ is complex (see also Chapter 45). The distal end of the esophagus is anchored to the diaphragm by the phrenoesophageal ligament that inserts circumferentially into the esophageal musculature close to the squamocolumnar junction (SCJ). The esophagus then traverses the diaphragmatic hiatus and joins the stomach almost tangentially. Thus there are three contributors to the EGJ high-pressure zone: the LES, the crural diaphragm, and the musculature of the gastric cardia that constitutes the distal aspect of the EGJ. The LES is a 3–4-cm segment of tonically contracted smooth muscle at the distal extreme of the esophagus. Surrounding the LES at the level of the SCJ is the crural diaphragm, most commonly bundles of the right diaphragmatic crus forming a teardrop-shaped canal about 2 cm long on its major axis (Fig. 46.5).[23] The component of the EGJ high-pressure zone distal to the SCJ is largely attributable to the opposing sling and clasp fibers of the middle layer of gastric cardia musculature.[24] In this region, the lateral wall of the esophagus meets the medial aspect of the dome of the stomach at an acute angle, defined as the angle of His. Viewed intraluminally, this region extends within the gastric lumen, appearing as a fold that

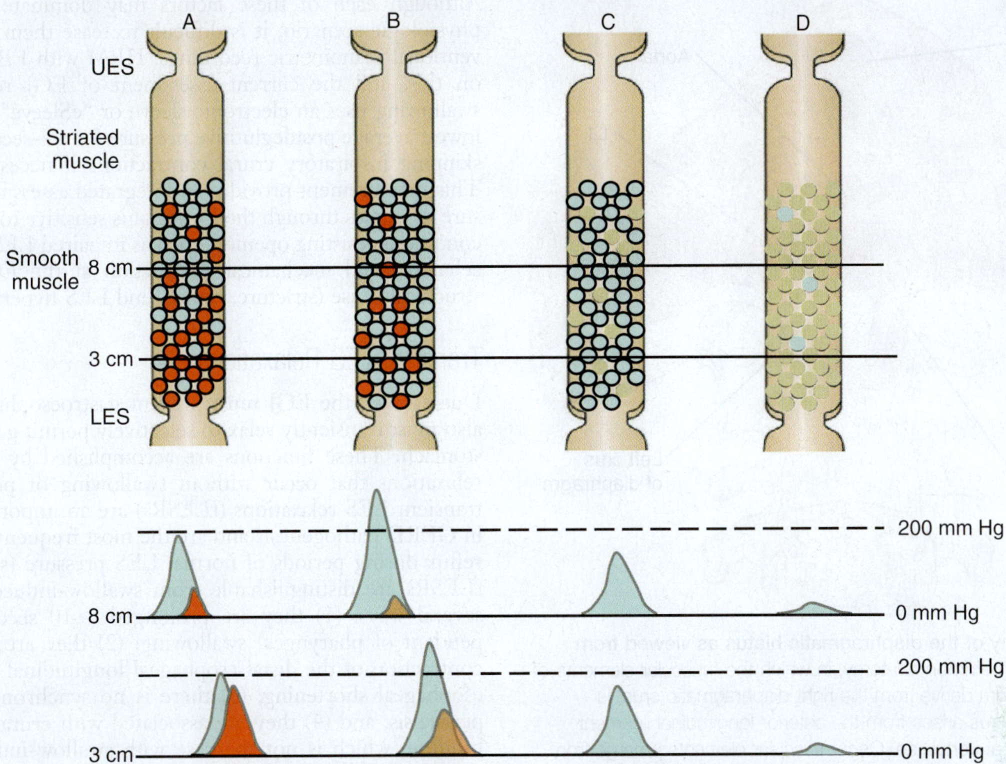

Fig. 46.4 Alterations in the balance and gradient of excitatory (cholinergic) and inhibitory (nitrergic) neurons in the distal esophagus as a pathophysiologic mechanism of esophageal motor disorders. The *upper panel* depicts the ganglionic constituents in the esophagus, and the *lower panel* illustrates manometric tracings at 3 and 8 cm above the LES. The *blue circles* represent excitatory neurons, and the *red circles* represent inhibitory neurons. (A) In normal subjects, cholinergic neurons are most dense proximally, becoming increasingly sparse distally. Conversely, inhibitory neurons are more prominent distally and relatively sparse proximally. This inverse neural gradient causes increasing latency of the contraction as it progresses distally. With simultaneous vagal stimulation of ganglia along the length of the esophagus, contraction first occurs proximally and propagates distally only as the effects of increasingly dense inhibition wear off. Thus pharmacologic manipulation can alter both contractile vigor and timing of propagation. Conceptually, esophageal motor pathophysiology can be explained by alterations in these neural gradients. (B) Patients with hypercontractility and normal (or fast) propagation may have a relative increase in excitatory neurons. (C) Patients with loss of inhibitory neurons will lose deglutitive inhibition, and contractions will occur simultaneously and prematurely. (D) Patients with loss of both excitatory and inhibitory neurons may present with absent or weak peristalsis that does not propagate. (Modified from Goyal R, Shaker R, GI Motility Online.)

has been conceptually referred to as a "flap valve" because increased intragastric pressure forces it closed, sealing off the entry to the esophagus.

Physiologically, the EGJ high-pressure zone is attributable to a composite of both the LES and the surrounding crural diaphragm extending 1–1.5 cm proximal to the SCJ and about 2 cm distal to it.[25] Resting LES tone ranges from 10 to 30 mm Hg relative to intragastric pressure, with considerable temporal fluctuation. With HRM, this is quantified as the EGJ contractile integral, and the normal value ranges from 28 to 125 mm Hg/cm.[26] The mechanism of LES tonic contraction is likely both myogenic and neurogenic, consistent with the observation that pressure within the sphincter persists after the elimination of neural activity with tetrodotoxin. Myogenic LES tone varies directly with membrane potential that leads to an influx of Ca^{2+}. Apart from myogenic factors, LES pressure is also modulated by intra-abdominal pressure, gastric distention, peptides, hormones, foods, and many medications. Large increases in LES pressure occur with the migrating motor complex; during phase III of the migrating motor complex, the LES pressure may exceed 80 mm Hg. Lesser fluctuations occur throughout the day, with pressure decreasing in the postprandial state and increasing during sleep.[27]

Superimposed on the myogenic LES contraction, input from vagal, adrenergic, hormonal, and mechanical influences will alter LES pressure. Vagal influence is similar to that of the esophageal body, with vagal stimulation activating both excitatory and inhibitory myenteric neurons. Thus the LES pressure at any instant reflects the balance between excitatory (cholinergic) and inhibitory (nitrergic) neural input, and altering the pattern of vagal discharge results in LES relaxation. The crural diaphragm is also a major contributor to EGJ pressure. Even after esophagogastrectomy, with consequent removal of the smooth muscle LES, a persistent EGJ pressure of about 6 mm Hg can be demonstrated during expiration. During inspiration, there is substantial augmentation of EGJ pressure attributable to crural diaphragm contraction. Crural diaphragm contraction is also augmented during abdominal compression, straining, or coughing.[28] On the other hand, during esophageal distension, vomiting, and belching, electrical activity in the crural diaphragm is selectively inhibited despite continued respiration, demonstrating a

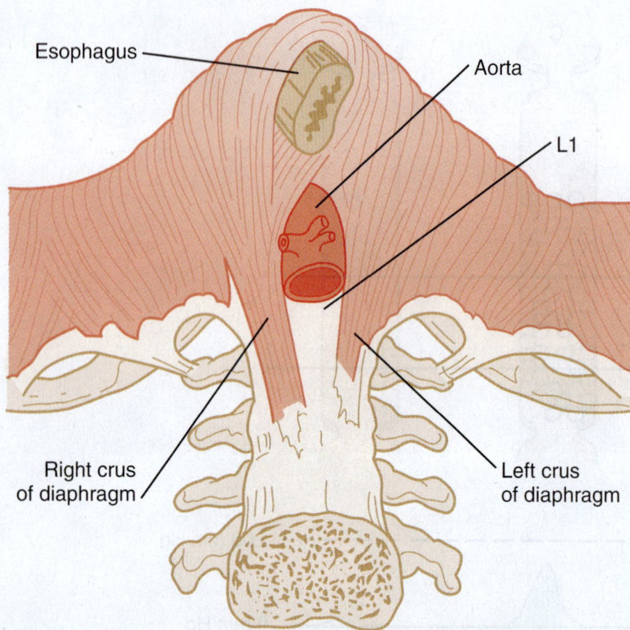

Fig. 46.5 Anatomy of the diaphragmatic hiatus as viewed from below. The most common anatomy, in which the muscular elements of the crural diaphragm derive from the right diaphragmatic crus, is shown. The right crus arises from the anterior longitudinal ligament overlying the lumbar vertebrae. Once muscular elements emerge from the tendon, two flat muscular bands form that cross each other in scissor-like fashion forming the walls of the hiatus and then merging with each other anterior to the esophagus. *L1*, First lumbar vertebrae. (Modified from Jaffee BM. Surgery of the esophagus. In: Orlando RC, ed. *Atlas of Esophageal Diseases*. 2nd ed. Philadelphia, PA: Current Medicine, Inc.; 2002:221–242.)

control mechanism independent of the costal diaphragm. This reflex inhibition of crural activity is eliminated with vagotomy.

LES Relaxation

LES relaxation can be triggered by distention from either side of the EGJ or swallowing. Relaxation induced by esophageal distention is an intramural process, unaffected by vagotomy. Relaxation is, however, antagonized by tetrodotoxin, proving that it is mediated by postganglionic nerves. Deglutitive LES relaxation is mediated by the vagus nerve, which synapses with inhibitory neurons in the myenteric plexus. NO, produced by NO synthase from the precursor amino acid L-arginine, is the main neurotransmitter in the postganglionic neurons responsible for LES relaxation. NO is released with neural stimulation in the esophagus, LES, and stomach, and NO synthase inhibitors block neurally mediated LES relaxation.[20,29] However, NO may not work alone. VIP-containing neurons have been demonstrated in the submucosal plexus, and VIP relaxes the LES by direct muscle action. It is thought that VIP acts on NO synthase–containing neural terminals as a prejunctional neurotransmitter, facilitating the release of NO and on gastric muscle cells to stimulate production of NO by the muscle.[30]

Another contributor to intraluminal pressure during bolus transit through the LES is the bolus itself. The LES relaxes during the initial phase of the swallow, but it does not actually open until the bolus enters the sphincter, thereby implicating intrabolus pressure. Hence EGJ opening is dependent on the balance of forces acting to open it (intrabolus pressure generated by peristalsis) and the forces resisting opening (LES tone and the mechanical properties of the esophageal wall and crural canal). Although each of these factors may dominate in a particular physiologic scenario, it is difficult to tease them apart with conventional manometric recordings. HRM with EPT has improved on this, and the current assessment of EGJ relaxation during swallowing uses an electronic sleeve or "eSleeve" to ascertain the lowest average postdeglutitive pressure for a 4-second time period, skipping inspiratory crural contractions if necessary (Fig. 46.6). This measurement provides an integrated assessment of the pressure dynamics through the EGJ that is sensitive to both pathologic conditions resisting opening, such as impaired LES relaxation with achalasia, and mechanical obstruction at the EGJ related to a structural cause (stricture, tumor, and LES hypertrophy).

Transient LES Relaxations

During rest, the EGJ must prevent gastroesophageal reflux, but also must transiently relax to selectively permit gas venting of the stomach. These functions are accomplished by prolonged LES relaxations that occur without swallowing or peristalsis. These transient LES relaxations (tLESRs) are an important mechanism in GERD pathogenesis and are the most frequent mechanism for reflux during periods of normal LES pressure (see Chapter 48). tLESRs are distinguishable from swallow-induced relaxation in several ways: (1) they are prolonged (>10 seconds) and independent of pharyngeal swallowing; (2) they are associated with contraction of the distal esophageal longitudinal muscle, causing esophageal shortening; (3) there is no synchronized esophageal peristalsis; and (4) they are associated with crural diaphragm inhibition, which is not the case with swallow-induced relaxation (Fig. 46.7).[31,32] tLESRs occur most frequently in the postprandial state during gastric distention. In the setting of the completely relaxed EGJ during tLESRs, even the minimal gastroesophageal pressure gradients observed with gastric distention (3–4 mm Hg) are sufficient to facilitate gas venting of the stomach. Thus tLESRs are the physiologic mechanism of belching.

Proximal gastric distention is the major stimulus for tLESR. Distention stimulates mechanoreceptors (intraganglionic lamellar endings) in the proximal stomach, activating vagal afferent fibers projecting to the nucleus of the solitary tract. The efferent limb of both swallow and nonswallow LES relaxations lies in the preganglionic vagal inhibitory pathway to the LES. Both types of relaxation can be blocked by bilateral cervical vagotomy, cervical vagal cooling, or NO synthase inhibitors. tLESRs triggered by gastric distention likely use NO and CCK as neurotransmitters, evident by increased tLESR frequency after IV CCK infusion and blockade by either NO synthase inhibitors or CCK-A antagonists. Finally, GABA-B agonists, such as baclofen, inhibit tLESRs, acting on both peripheral receptors and receptors located in the dorsal motor nucleus of the vagus.[33,34]

Owing to its significance in the pathogenesis of GERD, there has been substantial interest in modulating the tLESR reflex (see Chapter 44). The current concept is that vagal afferent endings terminating in intraganglionic lamellar endings located in the proximal stomach are primarily responsible for initiating the reflex, which is then mediated through the medulla and back to the esophagus and diaphragm via vagal efferents and the phrenic nerves. Pharmacologic and physiologic studies have demonstrated that the mechanotransduction properties of tension-sensitive vagal afferent fibers can be attenuated by the GABA-B receptor agonist baclofen, thereby reducing the frequency of tLESR. Glutamate receptors are also present in vagal and spinal sensory afferent fibers, and metabotropic glutamate receptor antagonists (especially mGluR5 antagonists) have also been shown to inhibit tLESR.[35]

Esophageal Sensation

The human esophagus can sense mechanical, electrical, chemical, and thermal stimuli, perceived as chest pressure, warmth, or pain,

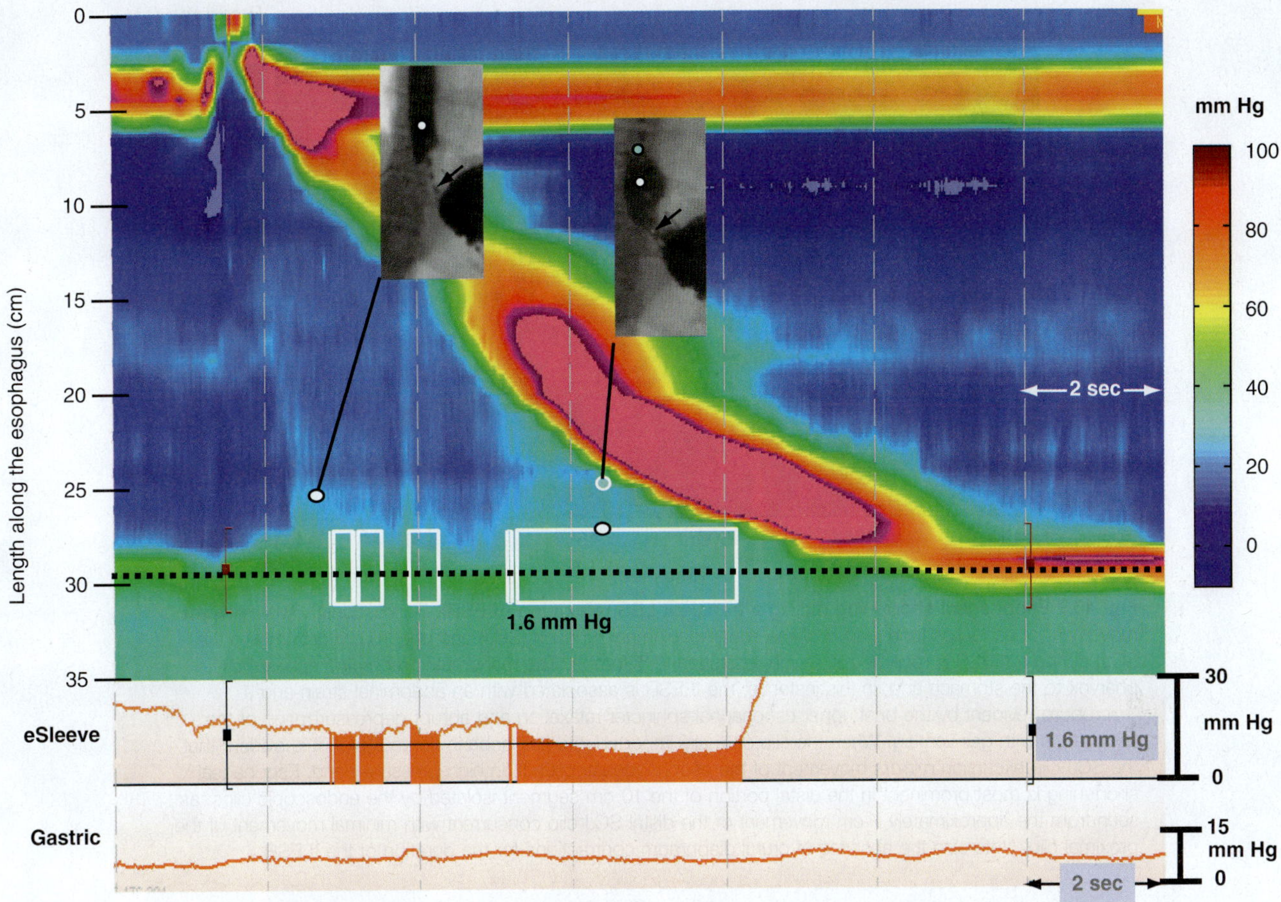

Fig. 46.6 Esophagogastric junction (EGJ) relaxation and bolus transit during swallowing. The integrated relaxation pressure (IRP) provides a pressure topography metric of the pressure dynamics across the EGJ during swallowing. The IRP is a complex metric because it involves accurately localizing the margins of the EGJ, demarcating the time window following deglutitive upper sphincter relaxation within which to anticipate EGJ relaxation, and then applying an eSleeve measurement within that 10-second time box (*delineated by the black brackets*). The eSleeve is referenced to gastric pressure and provides a measure of the greatest pressure across the axial domain of the EGJ at each time point and is plotted as a line tracing. The IRP is the mean value of the 4 seconds during which the eSleeve value is the lowest. The time intervals contributing to the IRP are indicated by the *white boxes* on the plot and by the *shaded red area* on the *red line* eSleeve tracing. In this example, the IRP is 1.6 mm Hg, which is normal. The EGJ is closed, and no flow occurs at the beginning of the swallow because the intrabolus pressure is insufficient to overcome EGJ pressure (*left fluoroscopic image*). Bolus transit occurs when the intrabolus pressure ahead of the contractile wavefront overcomes the resisting forces at the EGJ (*right fluoroscopic image*).

with substantial overlap in perception among stimuli.[36] Esophageal sensation is carried via both the vagal and spinal afferent nerves. The associated vagal neurons are located in the nodose and jugular ganglia, whereas the corresponding spinal neurons are located in thoracic and cervical dorsal root ganglia. Vagal afferents predominantly mediate homeostatic and secretory functions, whereas spinal afferents project centrally in a pattern characterized by overlap among spinal segments and convergence with somatic afferents. Consequently, esophageal pain tends to be poorly localized, accompanied by referred somatic pain and subject to viscerovisceral hyperalgesia.[37] Esophageal sensations are usually perceived substernally; in the instance of pain, radiation to the midline of the back, shoulders, and jaw is very analogous to cardiac pain. These similarities are likely due to convergence of sensory afferent fibers from the heart and esophagus in the same spinal pathways, even to the same dorsal horn neurons in some cases.

Esophageal afferents are predominantly activated by wall stretch, temperature, and acidity. When accompanied by mucosal injury, inflammatory mediators (prostaglandins, bradykinins, etc.) augment the response. The proximal esophagus is more sensitive than the distal esophagus, consistent with the observation that proximal stimuli such as reflux are more likely to be perceived.[38] Excessive proximal sensitivity has been associated with esophageal hypersensitivity and functional heartburn.[39]

With sensory endings concentrated deeply within the muscularis propria beneath a relatively impermeable mucosa, it seems unlikely that intraluminal acid can directly stimulate them. There is recent evidence suggesting a more superficial location of afferent sensory nerves in patients with esophageal hypersensitivity and nonerosive reflux disease.[38,40] These afferents easily respond to mucosally applied bile or capsaicin (a derivative of chili pepper), suggesting that these chemicals induce the release of an endogenous substance that in turn excites the afferents. These

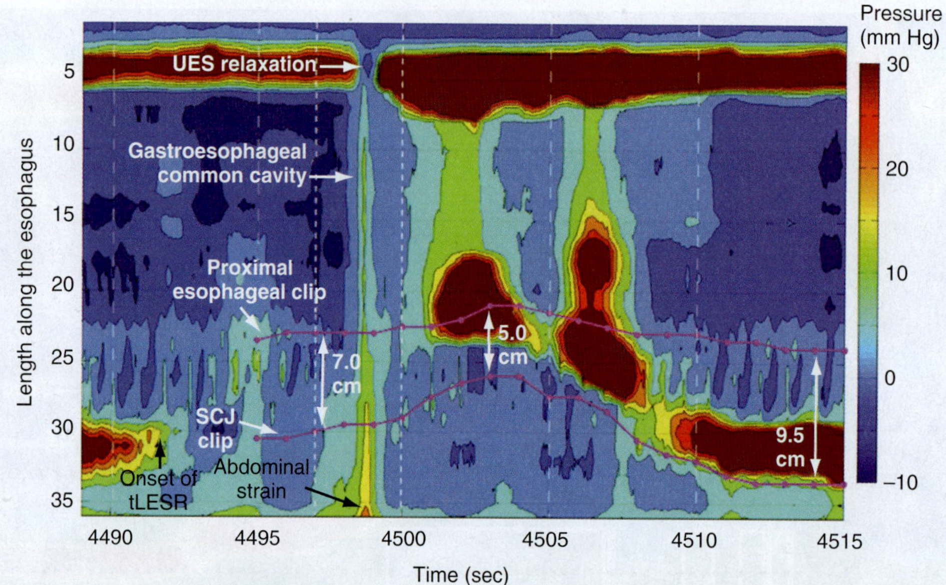

Fig. 46.7 Esophageal shortening during a transient LES relaxation (tLESR). Fluoroscopic visualization of movement of endoclips [one placed at the squamocolumnar junction (SCJ) and one 10 cm proximal to the SCJ] during a tLESR is recorded in a high-resolution EPT format. The manometric recording spans the pharynx to the stomach and, in this instance, the tLESR is associated with an abdominal strain and a "microburp" evident by the brief upper esophageal sphincter relaxation and abrupt depressurization of the esophagus with gas venting. When the clip data are imported into the isobaric contour plot, it is evident that the SCJ clip excursion mirrors movement of the esophagogastric junction high-pressure band. Esophageal shortening is most prominent in the distal portion of the 10-cm segment isolated by the endoscopic clips, as seen from the approximately 7-cm movement of the distal SCJ clip concurrent with minimal movement of the proximal clip. Note also the absence of crural diaphragm contractions for the duration of the tLESR.

responses are thought to be mediated by transient receptor potential vanilloid 1 (TRPV1) receptors and/or acid-sensing ion channels.[41,42] Consistent with this, current evidence suggests that chronic esophagitis increases mRNA expression of purinergic receptors accompanied by the upregulation of TRPV1 and neurotrophic factors mediating sensitization of the inflamed human esophagus.[43]

Recent investigations have also explored functional brain imaging, mainly functional magnetic resonance imaging, as a noninvasive assessment of brain function in visceral sensation and pain.[44] Although the results thus far are quite variable among research groups, the brain regions most consistently activated by esophageal stimuli are the anterior and posterior insula, cingulate cortex, primary sensory cortex, prefrontal cortex, and thalamus. Preliminary studies also suggest differences in functional magnetic resonance imaging activation patterns among subgroups of GERD patients and normal controls.[45]

ESOPHAGEAL MOTILITY DISORDERS

A working, albeit restrictive, definition of an esophageal motility disorder is: an esophageal disease attributable to neuromuscular dysfunction that causes symptoms referable to the esophagus, most commonly dysphagia, chest pain, or heartburn. Using this definition, the most important and profound primary esophageal motility disorder is achalasia. GERD could also fit this definition, and is clearly the most prevalent disorder within this category; fittingly, it is addressed in detail elsewhere in this text (see Chapter 48).

Dysphagia due to pharyngeal or UES dysfunction can also be included in a discussion of esophageal motor disorders, but this is usually as a manifestation of a more global neuromuscular disease process. Esophageal dysmotility can also be secondary phenomena, in which case esophageal dysfunction is part of a more global disease, such as in pseudoachalasia, Chagas disease, and systemic sclerosis (scleroderma). The major focus of this chapter will be on the primary motility disorders, particularly achalasia; proximal pharyngoesophageal dysfunction and secondary motility disorders will also be discussed.

Clinical Features

Dysphagia is a fundamental symptom of both oropharyngeal dysfunction and esophageal motility disorders. The patient history is crucial in the evaluation of dysphagia. Major objectives of the history are to differentiate oropharyngeal dysphagia from esophageal dysphagia, xerostomia (hyposalivation), or globus sensation. All are frequently confused with each other. Globus sensation, in particular, is frequently confused with dysphagia. Unlike dysphagia, which occurs only during swallowing, globus sensation is prominent among swallows. Patients relate the nearly constant sensation of having a lump in their throat or feeling a foreign object caught in their throat. In some instances, globus is associated with reflux symptoms, and in others with substantial anxiety. It is the linkage with anxiety that led to the older nomenclature "globus hystericus." Unfortunately, studies have failed to define an objective anatomic or physiologic cause for globus, and we are left with the crucial data being in the history; globus sensation persists regardless of the act of swallowing.[46]

Oropharyngeal dysphagia is suggested by the presence of associated aspiration, cough, nasopharyngeal regurgitation, drooling, pharyngeal residue following swallow, or co-occurring neuromuscular dysfunction (e.g., weakness, paresthesia, and slurred speech). On the other hand, the associated conditions of heartburn, regurgitation, chest pain, odynophagia, or intermittent esophageal obstruction suggest esophageal dysphagia. An important limitation of the patient history in esophageal dysphagia is that a patient's identification of the location of obstruction is of limited accuracy. Specifically, a distal esophageal obstruction caused by an esophageal ring, stricture, or achalasia will often be perceived as cervical dysphagia, and patients can correctly localize distal dysfunction only 60% of the time. Because of this subjective difficulty in distinguishing proximal from distal lesions within the esophagus, an evaluation for cervical dysphagia should encompass the entire length of the esophagus.

Another important consideration in patient management is that esophageal motility disorders are much less common than mechanical or inflammatory etiologies of dysphagia, such as tumors, strictures, rings, or esophagitis, be that peptic, pill-induced, eosinophilic, or infectious. Historical points suggestive of a motor disorder are difficulty with both solids and liquids, as opposed to only with solids, which is more suggestive of mechanical obstruction. However, the functional consequences of mechanical or inflammatory disorders can exactly mimic those of primary motility disorders. Thus as with the evaluation of oropharyngeal dysphagia, a motility disorder should be considered as an etiology for esophageal dysphagia only after exclusion of more common diagnoses by endoscopic, histologic, and/or radiographic examination.

Diagnostic Methods

Videofluoroscopy

Videofluoroscopy is particularly useful for a functional evaluation of the oropharyngeal phase of swallowing following an exam for anatomic explanations. Frequently referred to as a modified barium swallow, Logemann has described a protocol comprising a series of swallow tasks.[1] Images are obtained in a lateral projection, framed to include the oropharynx, palate, proximal esophagus, and proximal airway. These images are then evaluated with respect to four major categories of oropharyngeal dysfunction: (1) inability or excessive delay in initiation of pharyngeal swallowing, (2) aspiration, (3) nasopharyngeal regurgitation, and (4) bolus residue within the pharyngeal cavity after swallowing. Furthermore, the procedure allows for evaluation of the efficacy of various compensatory dietary modifications, postures, and swallowing maneuvers in compensating for observed swallowing dysfunction.

Endoscopy

Upper endoscopy should be the first test for evaluating new-onset esophageal dysphagia, because it combines the ability to detect most structural causes of dysphagia with the ability to obtain biopsies.[47] The increasing recognition of eosinophilic esophagitis (see Chapter 30) as a confounding clinical entity has increased the potential value of biopsies when performing upper endoscopy in the evaluation of dysphagia. The endoscopist should have a very low threshold for obtaining multiple esophageal mucosal biopsy specimens to evaluate for eosinophilic esophagitis in patients with dysphagia, even in patients with a normal-appearing esophageal mucosa.[48] Additionally, should a stricture or mucosal ring be detected, dilation can be accomplished in the same endoscopic session. However, even though upper endoscopy is an excellent tool for evaluating dysphagia, it has substantial limitations in assessing extraluminal structures and abnormal esophageal motility. It also has the potential to miss subtle obstructing lesions such as webs and rings.

Barium Esophagogram

Contrast studies of the esophagus are useful in assessing esophageal dysphagia if endoscopy is inconclusive. A barium esophagogram can also provide critical information regarding UES function, esophageal anatomy (e.g., dilatation, tortuosity, corkscrew configuration, and hiatus hernia) peristalsis, and bolus clearance through the EGJ. With advanced cases of achalasia (Fig. 46.8A) the findings are somewhat obvious, and it is only necessary clinically to differentiate between primary and secondary etiologies. However, with good technique, normal peristalsis can also be verified. Peristalsis is best evaluated in the prone position so that clearance does not occur by gravity.[49] Peristaltic abnormalities are inferred by retrograde escape of the bolus through the peristaltic wavefront, resulting in incomplete esophageal emptying. Normally the EGJ will become widely patent when the bolus reaches this area, and impaired relaxation can be inferred when either a smooth tapering is noted at the EGJ or bolus transit across the EGJ is impeded. Alternatively, fluoroscopy will occasionally

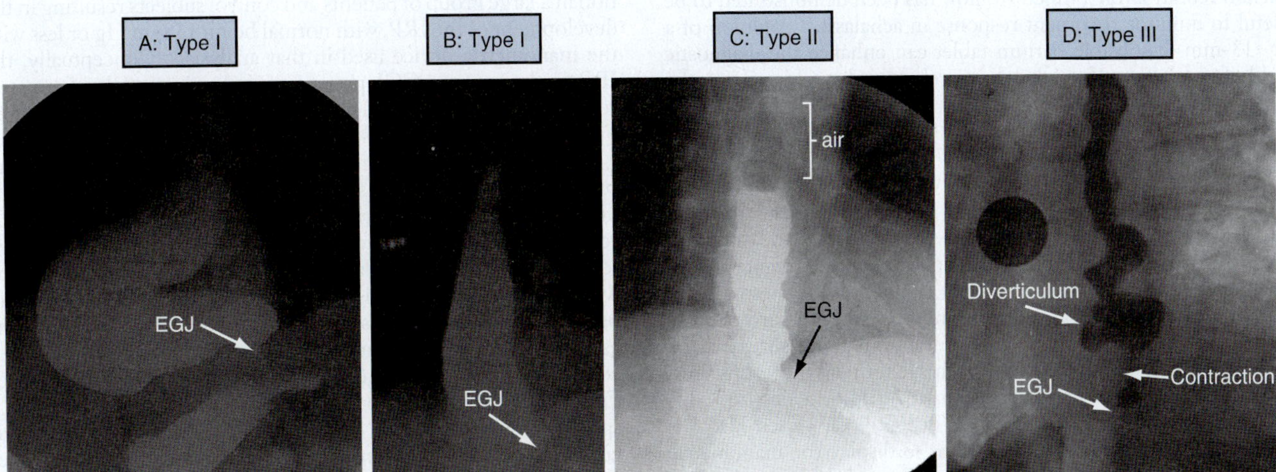

Fig. 46.8 Films from barium swallow studies in the three subtypes of idiopathic achalasia (see Table 46.2). Note esophageal dilatation with air-fluid levels (*left and center panels*) and the tapering at the esophagogastric junction (EGJ). Radiologic findings can be much more subtle in the early phases of the disease. The film in the *right* was taken during a timed barium esophagram, indicating that barium was still retained within the dilated esophagus at 5 minutes.

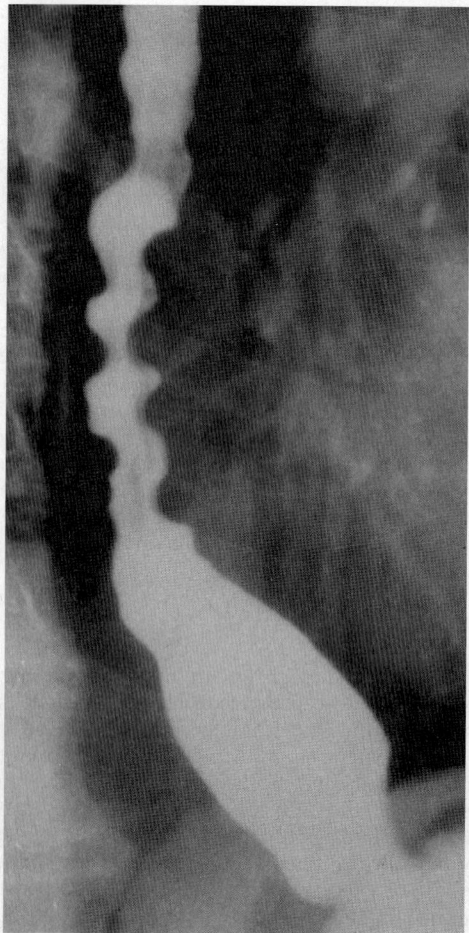

Fig. 46.9 Barium esophagogram showing a corkscrew esophagus in a patient with symptomatic distal esophageal spasm.

demonstrate spastic contractions, evident by a corkscrew appearance (Fig. 46.9). Utilization of a standardized "timed barium esophagram," that is, drinking 200 mL of thin barium in the upright position with images timed at 1, 2, and 5 minutes thereafter can provide an objective measure of esophageal retention.[50] Barium retention on a timed swallow has been demonstrated to be useful to monitor treatment response in achalasia.[51] Addition of a 12–13-mm dissolvable barium tablet can enhance the diagnostic yield of esophagram for achalasia or relevant obstruction when the tablet is retained in the esophagus.[52]

High-Resolution Manometry

Esophageal manometry is a test in which intraluminal pressure sensors are positioned within the esophagus to measure the contractile characteristics of the esophagus and segregate it into functional regions. The concept of high-resolution esophageal manometry is to use a sufficient number of pressure sensors within the esophagus such that intraluminal pressure can be monitored as a continuum along the length of the esophagus, much as time is viewed as a continuum in line tracings of conventional manometry, such as those in Fig. 46.3. When HRM is coupled with sophisticated algorithms to display the manometric data as pressure topography plots (Clouse plots), esophageal contractility is visualized with isobaric conditions among sensors indicated by isocoloric regions on the pressure topography plots. Fig. 46.3 depicts a normal swallow in a pressure topography plot encompassing both sphincters and the intervening esophagus; the relative timing of sphincter relaxation and segmental contraction as well as the position of the transition zone are all readily demonstrated.

HRM allows for the imaging of esophageal contractility as a continuum not only in time, but also along the length of the esophagus. Clouse et al. pioneered this technology, noting that peristalsis was not a seamless wave of pressurization, but rather a coordinated sequence of four contiguous contractile segments (see Fig. 46.3). A transition zone exists between the first and second segments, characterized by the nadir peristaltic amplitude, slightly delayed progression, and occasional failed transmission. The topographic analysis also reveals a segmental characteristic of peristaltic progression within the smooth muscle esophagus, with two contractile segments separated by a pressure trough, followed by the LES, which contracts with vigor and persistence quite dissimilar to the adjacent smooth muscle esophagus.[53] A distinct landmark along the wavefront is identified in the third segment, at which point contractile propagation slows dramatically (see Fig. 46.3).[54] This landmark, defined as the contractile deceleration point (CDP), has pathophysiologic significance because it is localized at the proximal aspect of the LES, and it is hypothesized that this represents the locus of termination of peristalsis.[55] Contraction beyond this point is more consistent with reconstitution of the LES that was relaxed, elongated, and effaced during peristalsis to form the phrenic ampulla.

To reflect advances in our understanding of HRM and esophageal motility disorders, a new classification was developed. The Chicago Classification of esophageal motor disorders was vetted and periodically updated by a group of international experts with the most recent version (version 4.0) published in 2021.[56] The Chicago Classification incorporates standardized metrics to quantify EGJ relaxation [integrated relaxation pressure (IRP)] and peristalsis [distal contractile integral (DCI) and distal latency (DL)] into an hierarchical algorithm to define esophageal motility disorders, with key distinction between disorders of EGJ outflow (including achalasia) and disorders of peristalsis (Fig. 46.10).[57]

The manometric evaluation of deglutitive EGJ relaxation is probably the most important measurement made during clinical esophageal manometry. Incomplete EGJ relaxation is an essential feature in the diagnosis of achalasia, and achalasia is the motor disorder with the most specific treatments. Despite this cardinal significance, there was no convention for defining incomplete deglutitive EGJ relaxation prior to the Chicago Classification. Key to the development of the Chicago Classification was a study comparing criteria for detecting impaired deglutitive EGJ relaxation in a large group of patients and control subjects resulting in the development of the IRP, with normal being 15 mm Hg or less with the manometric device used in that analysis.[58] Conceptually, the IRP is the average EGJ pressure for the 4 seconds of greatest relaxation within the 10-second period after a swallow (see Fig. 46.6).

HRM has been instrumental in defining a clinically relevant subclassification of achalasia.[59] A diagnosis of achalasia typically includes both absent peristalsis and impaired deglutitive EGJ relaxation. In its "classic" form (type I achalasia), this occurs in the setting of esophageal dilatation with negligible pressurization within the esophagus (Fig. 46.11A). However, despite lack of peristalsis, substantial pressurization remains possible within the esophagus. In fact, the most common pattern encountered is achalasia with panesophageal pressurization: type II achalasia (see Fig. 46.11B). The least common manometric pattern (type III) is spastic achalasia, where spastic and frequently nonperistaltic contraction occurs within the distal esophageal segment (see Fig. 46.11C). Several subsequent series, including a follow-up report on the European randomized controlled trial comparing laparoscopic Heller myotomy to pneumatic dilation,[60] confirmed the initial observation of that seminal study, that type II achalasia is the most responsive to treatment and type III the least responsive.

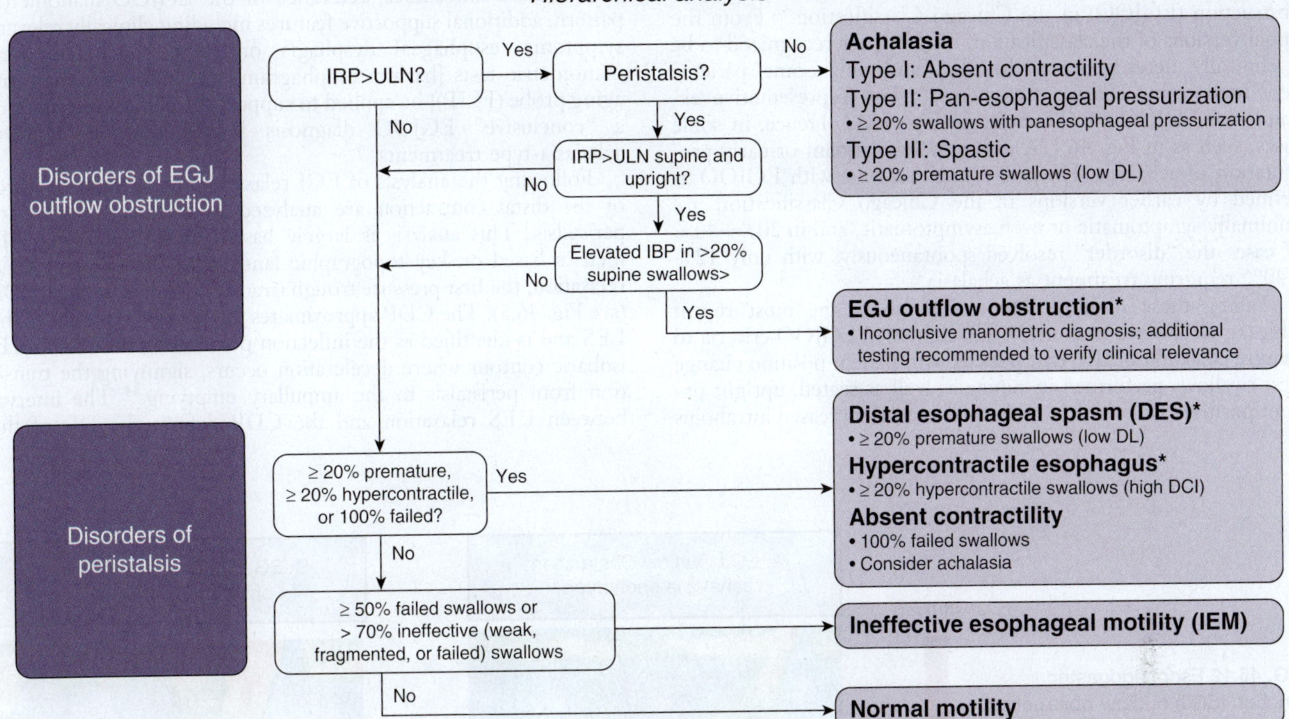

Fig. 46.10 Algorithm for applying the Chicago Classification of esophageal motor disorders. *DCI*, Distal contractile interval; *DL*, distal latency; *EGJ*, esophagogastric junction; *IBP*, intrabolus pressure; *IRP*, integrated relaxation pressure; *PEP*, panesophageal pressurization; *ULN*, upper limit of normal. *The presence of appropriate symptoms (esophageal dysphagia or chest pain) recommended to support a "conclusive" diagnosis. (See Table 46.2 for more detail.)

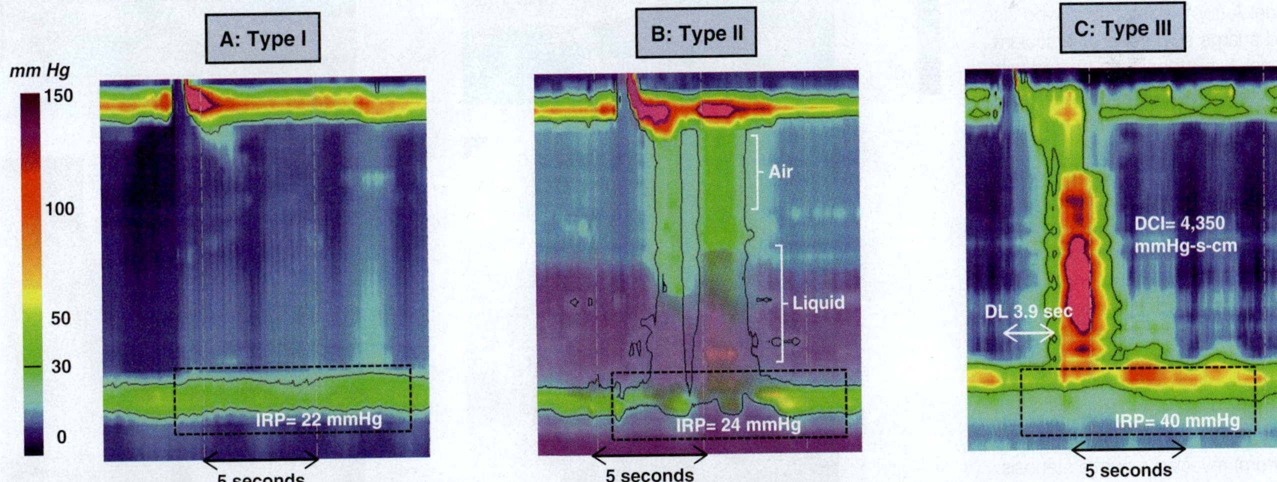

Fig. 46.11 Achalasia subtypes. The three subtypes are distinguished by distinct manometric patterns of esophageal body contractility. (A) In the patient with classic achalasia *(type I)*, there is no significant pressurization within the body of the esophagus and esophagogastric junction relaxation is impaired signified by the integrated relaxation pressure (IRP) greater than the upper limit of normal (15 mm Hg for this high-resolution manometry assembly). (B) A swallow from a patient with type II achalasia shows pan-esophageal pressurization of the fluid column trapped between the sphincters as the esophagus shortens. (C) The pressure topography plot in the type III achalasia patient is typical of spastic achalasia. Although this swallow is also associated with rapidly propagated and premature pressurization, the pressurization is attributable to an abnormal lumen-obliterating contraction. (With permission from the Esophageal Center at Northwestern.)

Patients with impaired EGJ relaxation, defined by an abnormal IRP with persistent peristaltic activity failing to meet diagnostic criteria for achalasia, are categorized as having EGJ outflow obstruction (EGJOO) in the Chicago Classification.[57] From the initial versions of the classification, EGJOO was recognized to be a clinically heterogeneous disorder, and only some patients benefitted from achalasia treatments.[61] Two representative examples of EGJOO are illustrated in Fig. 46.12. Hence, in some cases, such as in Fig. 46.12A, this may be a variant or early presentation of achalasia. However, many patients with EGJOO as defined by earlier versions of the Chicago Classification are minimally symptomatic or even asymptomatic, and in 20%–40% of cases the "disorder" resolved spontaneously, with only 12%–40% requiring treatment as achalasia.[62,63]

Taking these findings into consideration, the most recent Chicago Classification (version 4.0) tightened EGJOO criteria to require elevation in IRP that persists with patient position change (test swallows performed in supine as well as seated, upright patient positions) in addition to the presence of increased intrabolus pressurization (a supportive marker of EGJ obstruction). Additionally, Chicago Classification (version 4.0) recommended that due to uncertain clinical relevance of the EGJOO manometric pattern, additional supportive features including clinically relevant symptoms (esophageal dysphagia or chest pain) and non-manometric tests [barium esophagram or functional lumen imaging probe (FLIP)] be applied to support the clinical relevance of a "conclusive" EGJOO diagnosis before offering invasive, achalasia-type treatments.[56]

Following the analysis of EGJ relaxation, quantitative features of the distal contraction are analyzed to identify disorders of peristalsis. This analysis is largely based on the DCI and DL, metrics based on key topographic landmarks: the onset of UES relaxation, the first pressure trough (transition zone), and the CDP (see Fig. 46.3). The CDP approximates the proximal margin of the LES and is identified as the inflection point along the 30 mm Hg isobaric contour where deceleration occurs, signifying the transition from peristalsis to the ampullary emptying.[54] The interval between UES relaxation and the CDP defines the DL of the

A: EGJ Outflow Obstruction: achalasia phenotype

mm Hg
150
100
50
30
0

Locus of diverticulum above EGJ

IRP= 22.3 mm Hg

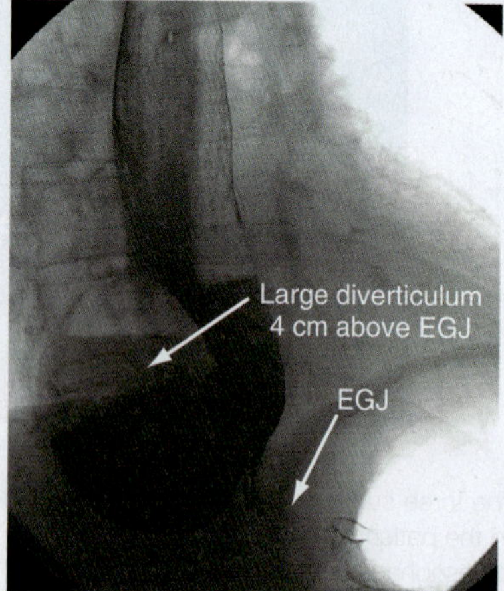

B: EGJ Outflow Obstruction: obstructing stricture

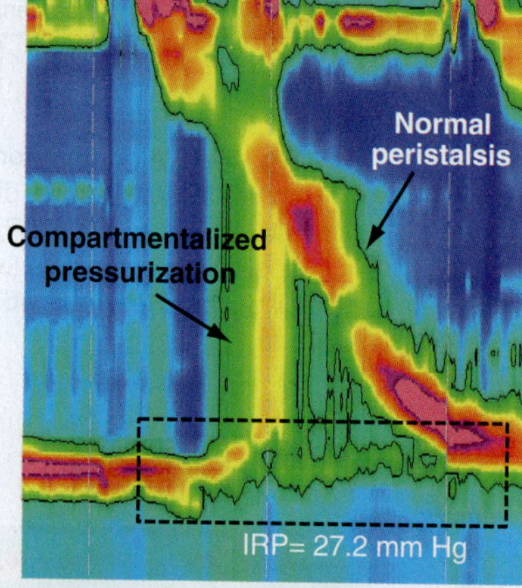

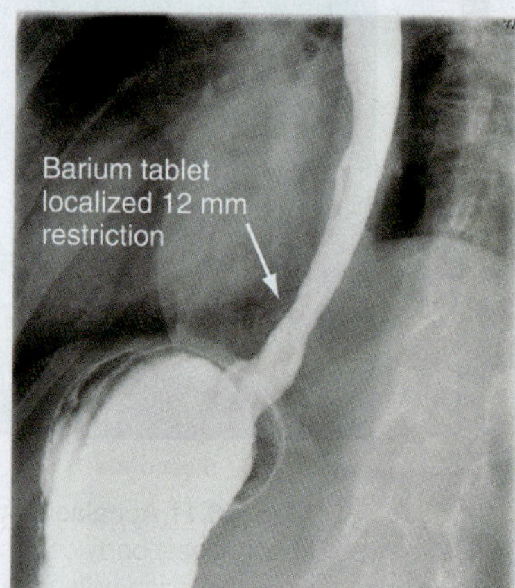

FIG. 46.12 Esophagogastric junction (EGJ) outflow obstruction. The criteria for EGJ outflow obstruction are an elevated integrated relaxation pressure (IRP) associated with some preserved weak or normal peristalsis, thereby not meeting the diagnostic criteria for types I, II, or III achalasia. Ultimately, this pattern may prove to be a phenotype of achalasia, as in Panel A (*top*). This patient, who also had a large epiphrenic diverticulum (Panel A, *bottom*), was treated with a laparoscopic myotomy and diverticulectomy with good result. Alternatively, EGJ outflow obstruction pattern can be associated with mechanical obstruction (Panel B). This patient had a patulous EGJ and a 9-mm endoscope passed with no resistance noted. However, the IRP was increased, and there was compartmentalized pressurization between the preserved peristaltic contraction and the EGJ (Panel B, *top*). The esophagogram (Panel B, *bottom*) revealed a subtle stenosis just proximal to the EGJ (*arrow*), where passage of a 12.5-mm barium tablet was delayed. The patient responded to 18-mm balloon dilation and therapy with a PPI. (With permission from the Esophageal Center at Northwestern.)

contraction, as illustrated in Fig. 46.3. DL values of less than 4.5 seconds define premature contractions, likely indicative of impaired inhibitory neuronal control. Hypercontractile swallows are defined by DCI >8000 mm Hg sec cm. Ineffective swallows include failed contractions (DCI <100 mm Hg sec cm), weak contractions (DCI 100–450 mm Hg sec cm), and fragmented contractions (DCI >450 mm Hg sec cm with peristaltic breaks >5 cm).[56]

Following analysis of individual swallows by the criteria outlined earlier, the component results are synthesized into a global manometric diagnosis by the criteria detailed in Table 46.2. The abnormalities encountered are described in specific functional terms, with the intent that these then be interpreted within the clinical context. The classification detailed in Table 46.2 represents the Chicago Classification (version 4.0) vetted with a consensus approach by the international HRM Working Group.[56]

Intraluminal Impedance Measurement

Intraluminal impedance monitoring was described more than two decades ago as a method to assess intraluminal bolus transit without using fluoroscopy. The technique uses an intraluminal catheter with multiple, closely spaced pairs of metal rings. An alternating current is applied across each pair of adjacent rings, and the resultant current flow between the rings is dependent on the impedance of the tissue and luminal content between the rings. Impedance decreases when the electrodes are bridged by liquid and increases when they are surrounded by air. Hence data from multiple impedance segments reveal the direction, content, and completeness of bolus transit. Validation data suggest that liquid bolus entry at the level of an electrode pair is indicated by a 50% drop in impedance. Return of the impedance tracing to 50% of baseline correlates with the passage of the tail of the bolus on fluoroscopy, also indicated by the contractile upstroke noted during manometry. Validation studies against videofluoroscopy have shown excellent concordance in ascertaining bolus transit.

Intraluminal impedance measurement has also been combined with manometry to assess the efficacy of esophageal emptying. With diminishing peristaltic amplitudes, the efficacy of emptying decreases. Currently, the main utility for combined HRM and impedance is in the assessment of esophageal transit abnormalities, particularly rumination and supragastric belching, and to assess the severity of esophageal retention in achalasia.[64]

Functional Lumen Imaging Probe

The FLIP is a catheter-based assembly with an infinitely compliant bag near the distal end that houses serially spaced impedance planimetry ring electrodes and a solid-state pressure sensor.[65] The FLIP can be positioned within the esophagus, typically during a sedated endoscopy. During volume-controlled filling of the bag (esophageal distension), FLIP measures the cross-sectional area at each impedance planimetry channel, concurrent intrabag pressure, and the relationship between luminal cross-section area and pressure (i.e., distensibility). Distensibility of the EGJ is quantified using a metric the EGJ-distensibility index (EGJ cross-sectional area divided by pressure) with values <2.0 mm^2/mm Hg (with EGJ diameter <12 mm) often observed in achalasia; Fig 46.13.[66] FLIP data can also be displayed as color-coded diameter topography plots (analogous to pressure topography of HRM) which facilitates evaluation of esophageal secondary peristalsis in response to the FLIP distension. Normal controls and patients with normal primary peristalsis on HRM generally have a FLIP contraction pattern of repetitive antegrade contractions (repetitive due to the sustained nature of the FLIP distension), whereas patients with nonspastic achalasia typically have an absent contractile response (Fig 46.13).[67] An approach applying the FLIP assessment of EGJ distensibility and secondary peristalsis pattern has been described akin to the Chicago Classification's approach to HRM, which particularly facilitates identification of achalasia at one extreme and normal esophageal motility at the other.[68] FLIP is recommended in the Chicago Classification as a useful test to help clarify inconclusive HRM diagnoses, such as EGJOO.[56]

Sensory Testing

Esophageal sensory nerves play a key role in determining symptoms of esophageal motor diseases, because the esophagus is sensitive to a variety of stimuli including mechanical (elicited by luminal distention or high-amplitude contractions), chemical (acid and/or other constituents of reflux), and temperature.[36] Typically, the visceral input is not perceived consciously, although some patients may experience symptoms attributed to hyperalgesia (exaggerated pain perception) or allodynia (perception of pain to a stimulus that is usually not painful).[37] Esophageal symptoms may be described as burning, pressing, pricking, or heat sensations. However, symptoms are not specific to a given stimulus, and substantial overlap in perception among stimuli is common.

Although the precise mechanism by which an esophageal stimulus causes pain or the perception of dysphagia is unclear, methodologies devised to evoke or stimulate pain by simulating physiologic events are available to assess the possible relationship between ongoing symptoms and suspected causes. These tests typically use forms of distention studies (balloon, barostat, impedance planimetry, or volume challenges) or direct mucosal stimulation (chemical, electrical, or thermal). Balloon distention studies have shown that esophageal distention can provoke chest pain and that patients with esophageal chest pain tend to have lower pain thresholds compared to controls.[36]

The standard test of chemosensitivity is the Bernstein test wherein 0.1 N HCl is perfused in the esophagus to reproduce chest pain or heartburn. Typically, acid infusion is alternated with saline perfusion in a blinded fashion to increase the objectivity of the test, but no standardized protocol exists. Beyond the Bernstein test, probes have been devised to test esophageal responsiveness to thermal challenges and transmucosal electrical nerve stimulation. However, although these tools have unquestionably been useful in improving understanding of the interaction between peripheral receptors and central pain perception, their clinical utility remains limited owing to the lack of protocol standardization and the somewhat cumbersome nature of the studies. Currently, use of these devices is limited to specialty centers, and further refinement will be required before mainstream clinical use can be advocated.

OROPHARYNGEAL DYSPHAGIA

Estimates of the prevalence of dysphagia among individuals older than 50 years range from 16%–22%, with most of this related to oropharyngeal dysfunction. Most oropharyngeal dysphagia is related to neuromuscular disease; the prevalence of the most common anatomic etiology, Zenker diverticulum, is estimated to range from a meager 0.01%–0.11% of the population in the United States, with peak incidence in men between the seventh and ninth decades.[69] The consequences of oropharyngeal dysphagia are severe: dehydration, malnutrition, aspiration, choking, pneumonia, and death. Within health care institutions, it is estimated that up to 13% of hospitalized patients and 60% of nursing home residents have feeding problems and, again, most are attributed to oropharyngeal dysfunction as opposed to

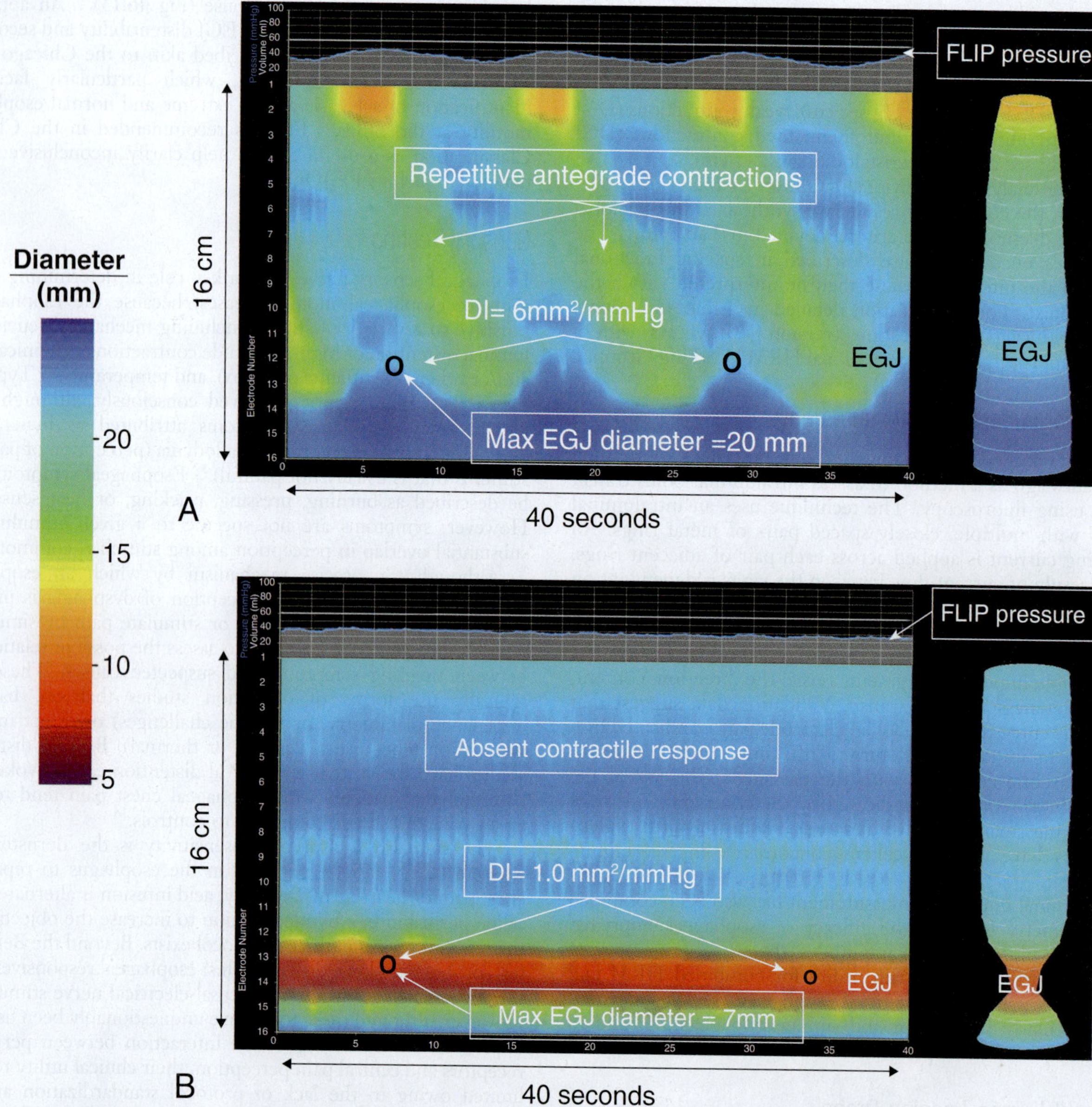

Fig. 46.13 Functional lumen imaging probe (FLIP). FLIP output from two patients (A and B) including 40 seconds of continuous FLIP data (*left panel*) and the 3D rendering of the esophageal lumen at the *right*. The esophagogastric junction (EGJ) can be appreciated as the narrowest segment of the distal portion of the FLIP. (A) The FLIP shows normal EGJ opening and a normal contractile response involving repetitive antegrade contractions. The patient had normal motility on high-resolution manometry (HRM). (B) The FLIP shows reduced EGJ opening and an absent contractile response. The patient had type II achalasia on HRM. *DI*, Distensibility index.

esophageal dysfunction. Mortality of nursing residents with dysphagia and aspiration can be as high as 45% over 1 year. As the U.S. population continues to age, oropharyngeal dysphagia will become an increasing problem associated with complex medical and ethical issues.

Pathogenesis

Obstructing lesions of the oral cavity, head, and neck can cause dysphagia. Structural abnormalities may result from trauma, surgery, tumors, caustic injury, congenital anomalies, or acquired deformities. The most common structural abnormalities of the hypopharynx associated with dysphagia are hypopharyngeal diverticula and cricopharyngeal bars.

If the etiology of oropharyngeal dysphagia is not readily apparent after an initial evaluation for anatomic disorders, evidence of functional abnormalities should be sought. Primary neurologic or muscular diseases involving the oropharynx are often associated with dysphagia. Whereas esophageal dysphagia usually results from esophageal diseases, oropharyngeal dysphagia frequently results from neurologic or muscular diseases, with oropharyngeal dysfunction being just one pathologic manifestation. Although the disease specifics vary, the net effect on swallowing can be analyzed according to the mechanical description of

TABLE 46.1 Mechanical Events of the Oropharyngeal Swallow, Evidence of Dysfunction, and Disease Association(s) in Patients with Oropharyngeal Dysphagia

Mechanical Event	Evidence of Dysfunction	Disease Association(s)
Nasopharyngeal closure	Nasopharyngeal regurgitation Nasal voice	Myasthenia gravis
Laryngeal closure	Aspiration during bolus transit	Stroke Traumatic brain injury
UES opening	Dysphagia Postswallow residue/aspiration Diverticulum formation	Cricopharyngeal bar Parkinson disease
Tongue loading and bolus propulsion	Sluggish misdirected bolus	Parkinson disease Surgical defects Cerebral palsy
Pharyngeal clearance	Postswallow residue in hypopharynx/aspiration	Polio or post-polio syndrome Oculopharyngeal dystrophy Stroke

the swallow outlined earlier. Table 46.1 summarizes the mechanical elements of the swallow, the manifestation and consequence of dysfunction, and representative pathologic conditions in which they are likely encountered. Neurologic examination may indicate cranial nerve dysfunction, neuromuscular disease, cerebellar dysfunction, or an underlying movement disorder. Functional abnormalities can be due to dysfunction of intrinsic musculature, peripheral nerves, or central nervous system control mechanisms. Of note, contrary to popular belief, the gag reflex is not predictive of pharyngeal swallowing efficiency or aspiration risk. The gag reflex is absent in 20%–40% of normal adults.[70]

Evident in Table 46.1, oropharyngeal dysphagia is frequently the result of neurologic or muscular diseases. Neurologic diseases can damage the neural structures requisite for either the afferent or efferent limbs of the oropharyngeal swallow. Virtually any neuromuscular disease can potentially cause dysphagia (see Chapter 35). As there is nothing unique to neurons controlling swallowing, their involvement in disease processes is usually random. Furthermore, in most instances, functions mediated by adjacent neuronal structures are concurrently involved. The following discussion will focus on neuromuscular pathologic processes most commonly encountered.

Stroke

Aspiration pneumonia has been estimated to inflict a 20% death rate in the first year after a stroke, and 10%–15% each year thereafter. It is usually not the first episode of aspiration pneumonia, but the subsequent recurrences over the years that eventually cause death. The ultimate cause of aspiration pneumonia is dysphagia leading to aspiration that can occur by a number of mechanisms: absence or severe delay in triggering the swallow, reduced lingual control, or weakened laryngopharyngeal musculature.[1] Conceptually, these etiologies can involve motor or sensory impairments. Cortical infarcts are less likely to result in severe dysphagia than brainstem strokes. Cortical infarcts are also more likely to demonstrate recovery from dysphagia. Of 86 consecutive patients who sustained an acute cerebral infarct, 37 (43%) experienced dysphagia when evaluated within 4 days of the event. However, 86% of these patients were able to swallow normally 2 weeks later, with recovery resulting from contralateral areas taking over the lost function.[71] Failure to recover was more likely among patients incurring larger infarcts or patients who had prior infarcts.

TABLE 46.2 Chicago Classification v4.0 of Esophageal Motility Disorders[56]

Diagnosis	Diagnostic Criteria
DISORDERS OF EGJ OUTFLOW	
Type I achalasia	100% failed peristalsis, median IRP > ULN
Type II achalasia	100% failed peristalsis and panesophageal pressurization with ≥20% of swallows; median IRP > ULN
Type III achalasia (spastic)	No normal peristalsis, premature contractions with ≥20% of swallows, median IRP > ULN
EGJOO[a]	Median IRPs (from swallows in both supine and upright positions) ≥ ULN; elevated IBP in ≥20% supine swallows; sufficient evidence of peristalsis such that criteria for achalasia are not met *All manometric diagnoses of EGJOO considered as clinical inconclusive (i.e., of unclear clinical relevance). Clinically relevant diagnoses should be confirmed by supportive symptoms (esophageal dysphagia or chest pain) and additional testing (e.g., timed barium esophagram or functional lumen imaging probe)
DISORDERS OF PERISTALSIS	
DES[a]	Median IRP < ULN; ≥20% premature contractions (distal latency <4.5 seconds) with DCI >450 mm Hg sec cm; some normal peristalsis may be present. Should be supported by clinically relevant symptoms (esophageal dysphagia or chest pain)
Hypercontractile esophagus[a]	Median IRP < ULN; ≥20% hypercontractile swallows (DCI > 8000 mm Hg sec cm)
Absent contractility	Median IRP < ULN (supine and upright swallows), 100% failed swallows (DCI < 100 mm Hg sec cm)
Ineffective esophageal motility	Median IRP < ULN; >70% ineffective swallows (weak, failed, or fragmented swallows) or ≥50% failed swallows

[a]Manometric patterns of unclear clinical significance in isolation. Clinical relevance should require supportive symptoms (i.e., esophageal dysphagia or chest pain) with additional supportive testing when indicated.

DCI, Distal contractile interval; *DES*, distal esophageal spasm; *DL*, distal latency; *EGJ*, esophagogastric junction; *EGJOO*, EGJ outflow obstruction; *IBP*, intrabolus pressure; *IRP*, integrated relaxation pressure; *ULN*, upper limit of normal (see text).

Amyotrophic Lateral Sclerosis

Amyotrophic lateral sclerosis is a progressive neurologic disease characterized by degeneration of motor neurons in the brain, brainstem, and spinal cord. Specific symptoms are dependent upon the locations of affected motor neurons and the relative severity of involvement. When the degenerative process involves the cranial nerve nuclei, swallowing difficulties ensue. Oropharyngeal dysfunction characteristically begins with the tongue and progresses to involve the pharyngeal and laryngeal musculature. Patients experience choking attacks, become volume depleted or malnourished, and incur aspiration pneumonia. The decline in swallowing function is progressive and predictable, invariably leading to gastrostomy feeding. Patients often die as a consequence of their swallowing dysfunction in conjunction with respiratory depression.[72]

Hypopharyngeal (Zenker) Diverticula and Cricopharyngeal Bar

Hypopharyngeal diverticula and cricopharyngeal bars are closely related disease entities in that it is a cricopharyngeal bar that can result in diverticulum formation. The most common type, Zenker diverticulum (Fig. 46.14), originates in the midline posteriorly at Killian dehiscence, a point of pharyngeal wall weakness between the oblique fibers of the inferior pharyngeal constrictor and the transverse cricopharyngeus muscle. Other locations of acquired pharyngeal diverticula include: (1) the lateral slit separating the cricopharyngeus muscle from the fibers of the proximal end of the esophagus, through which the recurrent laryngeal nerve and its accompanying vessels run to supply the larynx; (2) at the penetration of the inferior thyroid artery into the hypopharynx; (3) and at the junction of the middle and inferior constrictor muscles. The unifying theme of these locations is that they are sites of potential weakness of the muscular lining of the hypopharynx through which the mucosa herniates, leading to a "false" diverticulum. The best-substantiated explanation for the development of diverticula is that they form as a result of a restrictive myopathy associated with diminished compliance of the cricopharyngeus muscle. Surgical specimens of cricopharyngeus muscle strips from patients with hypopharyngeal diverticula demonstrated structural changes that would decrease UES compliance and opening.[73] The cricopharyngeus samples from these patients had "fibro-adipose tissue replacement and (muscle) fiber degeneration." Thus, although the muscle relaxes normally during a swallow, it cannot distend normally, resulting in the appearance of a cricopharyngeal indentation, or bar, during a barium swallow (Fig. 46.14). Diminished sphincter compliance necessitates increased hypopharyngeal intrabolus pressure to maintain *trans*-sphincteric flow through the smaller UES opening. The increased stress on the hypopharynx from the increased intrabolus pressure may ultimately result in diverticulum formation.

Parkinson Disease

Although only 15%–20% of patients with Parkinson disease complain of swallowing problems, more than 95% have demonstrable defects when studied videofluoroscopically.[74] This disparity suggests that patients compensate in the early stages of the disease and complain of dysphagia only when it becomes severe. Abnormalities include repetitive lingual pumping prior to initiation of a pharyngeal swallow, piecemeal swallowing, and oral residue after the swallow. Patients may also exhibit a delayed swallow response and a weak pharyngeal contraction, resulting in vallecular and pyriform sinus residue. Recent data suggest this to be related to the combination of incomplete UES relaxation and a weakened pharyngeal contraction.[74]

Vagus Nerve Disorders

Unilateral lesions of the vagus can result in hemiparesis of the soft palate and pharyngeal constrictors, as well as of the laryngeal musculature. The recurrent laryngeal nerves can be injured as a result of thyroid surgery, aortic aneurysms, pneumonectomy, primary mediastinal malignancies, or metastatic lesions to the mediastinum. Owing to its more extensive loop in the chest, the left recurrent laryngeal nerve is more vulnerable to involvement by mediastinal malignancy than the right laryngeal nerve. Unilateral recurrent laryngeal nerve injury results in unilateral adductor paralysis of the vocal cord. This defect can result in

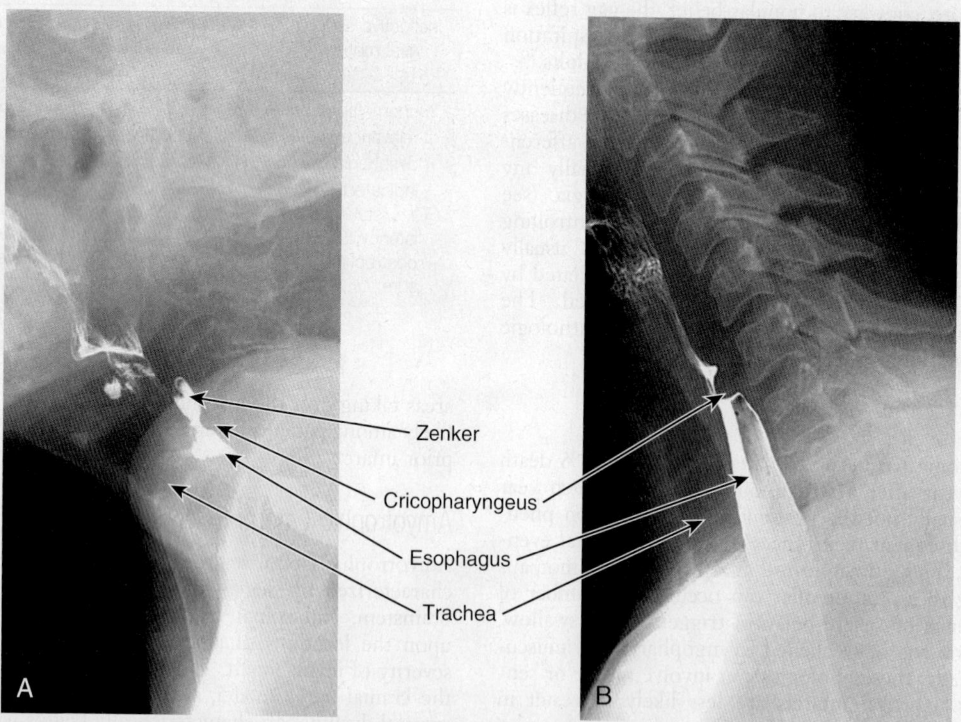

Fig. 46.14 Barium esophagram demonstrating Zenker diverticulum (A) and cricopharyngeal bar (B). (A) Small Zenker diverticulum. Although the point of herniation is midline posterior at Killian dehiscence, the diverticulum migrates laterally in the neck as it enlarges, because there is no potential space between the posterior pharyngeal wall and the vertebral column. (B) A cricopharyngeal bar in a patient with oropharyngeal dysphagia. The posterior indentation of the barium column is caused by a noncompliant cricopharyngeus muscle. (With permission from the Esophageal Center at Northwestern.)

aspiration during swallowing because of impaired laryngeal closure. It is, however, rare to have any primary pharyngeal dysfunction resultant from recurrent laryngeal nerve injury.

Oculopharyngeal Muscular Dystrophy

Oculopharyngeal muscular dystrophy is a syndrome characterized by ptosis and progressive dysphagia. In the past, afflicted patients reaching age 50 typically died of starvation resulting from pharyngeal paralysis. The disease is now known to be a form of muscular dystrophy and is inherited as an autosomal dominant disorder, with occurrences clustered in families of French-Canadian descent. Genetic studies of an afflicted family indicate linkage to chromosome 14, perhaps involving the region coding for cardiac alpha or beta myosin heavy chains. Oculopharyngeal dystrophy affects the striated pharyngeal muscles and the levator palpebrae. Although other forms of muscular dystrophy occasionally affect the pharyngeal constrictors, this is rarely a dominant manifestation. The first symptom of oculopharyngeal dystrophy is usually ptosis that slowly progresses and eventually dominates the patient's appearance. Dysphagia may begin after, concomitant with, or even before ptosis. The dominant functional abnormalities are of a weak or absent pharyngeal contraction, reduced cricopharyngeal opening, and hypopharyngeal stasis.[75] Dysphagia is slowly progressive, but may ultimately lead to starvation, aspiration pneumonia, or asphyxia.

Myasthenia Gravis

Myasthenia gravis is a progressive autoimmune disease characterized by high circulating levels of ACh receptor antibody and destruction of ACh receptors at neuromuscular junctions. Musculature controlled by the cranial nerves is almost always involved, particularly the ocular muscles. Dysphagia is prominent in more than a third of patients with myasthenia gravis and, in unusual instances, can be the initial and dominant manifestation of the disease. In mild cases, dysphagia may not be evident until after 15–20 minutes of eating. Classically, manometric studies reveal a progressive deterioration in the amplitude of pharyngeal contractions with repeated swallows. Peristaltic amplitude recovers with rest or following the administration of 10 mg edrophonium chloride, an acetylcholinesterase inhibitor. In more advanced cases, the dysphagia can be profound and associated with nasopharyngeal regurgitation and nasality of the voice, even to the extent of being confused with bulbar amyotrophic lateral sclerosis or brainstem stroke.[76]

Treatment

Management of oropharyngeal dysphagia is focused on four specific issues: (1) identification of an underlying disease, (2) characterization of a disorder amenable to surgery or dilation, (3) identification of specific patterns of dysphagia amenable to swallowing therapy, and (4) assessment of aspiration risk.

Identification of the Underlying Disease

A potential outcome of the evaluation is the identification of an underlying neuromuscular, neoplastic, or metabolic disorder that dictates specific management. For example, dysphagia can be the presenting symptom in patients with myopathy, myasthenia, thyrotoxicosis, motor neuron disease, or Parkinson disease. Whether or not treatment of the underlying disorder improves swallowing function depends on both the natural history of the specific disease and whether or not effective treatment exists.

Disorders Amenable to Surgery

The most common surgical treatment for oropharyngeal dysphagia is cricopharyngeal myotomy, but the efficacy of myotomy in neurogenic or myogenic dysphagia is variable. Most series evaluating the efficacy of myotomy in these circumstances are uncontrolled and lack validated (or even specific) outcome measures. Thus although an overall favorable response rate in excess of 60% is reported in this literature, there are no validated criteria for patient selection. Theoretically, the functional limitation faced by patients with neurogenic or myogenic dysphagia is of weak pharyngeal propulsion, and the potential benefit of myotomy is that circumstance is less obvious than in the case of obstruction at the level of the cricopharyngeus.

Patterns of Oropharyngeal Dysphagia Amenable to Swallow Therapy

Identifying potential treatments for oropharyngeal dysphagia begins with definition of the aberrant physiology, as categorized in Table 46.1. This is best accomplished with a videofluoroscopic swallowing study that first characterizes a patient's swallow dysfunction and then proceeds to test the effectiveness of selected compensatory or therapeutic treatment strategies. Compensatory treatments include postural changes, modifying food delivery or consistency, or the use of prosthetics. For instance, head turning can eliminate aspiration or pharyngeal residue by favoring the more functional side in patients with hemiparesis.[1] Similarly, diet modifications can reduce the difficulty of the swallow. Therapeutic strategies are designed to alter the physiology of the swallow, usually by improving the range of motion of oral or pharyngeal structures to the extent that that is possible using volitional control. Depending on the severity of the impairment, the level of motivation, and the global neurologic integrity, defective elements of the swallow can be selectively rehabilitated. For a detailed description of the techniques and limitations of swallow therapy, the reader is referred to treatises on the topic.[1,77]

Evaluating Aspiration Risk

Videofluoroscopy is considered the most sensitive test for detecting aspiration, reportedly detecting instances not evident by bedside evaluation in about 50% of patients. However, despite the logical association between deglutitive aspiration and the subsequent development of pneumonia, this sequence is not inevitable. Nonetheless, the balance of evidence suggests that detection of aspiration is a predictor of pneumonia risk, and that its detection dictates that compensatory swallowing strategies, nonoral feeding, or corrective surgery be instituted. Whether nonoral feeding eliminates the risk of aspiration is controversial, an issue raised by the provocative finding that among patients with radiographic aspiration, pneumonia, and death were more frequent among patients who received feeding tubes. This suggests that aspiration of oral secretions may be essential in controlling pneumonia risk and has led some to consider procedures such as tracheostomy to protect the airway.

Hypopharyngeal (Zenker) Diverticula and Cricopharyngeal Bar

The treatment of hypopharyngeal diverticula is cricopharyngeal myotomy with or without a diverticulectomy or diverticulopexy. Cricopharyngeal myotomy reduces both the resting sphincter tone and resistance to flow across the UES. Good or excellent results are reported in 80%–100% of Zenker patients treated by transcervical myotomy combined with diverticulectomy or diverticulopexy. There are instances in which a limited procedure would be adequate, but a definitive approach to the problem of pulsion diverticula should involve both diverticulectomy and myotomy. Diverticulectomy alone risks recurrence because the underlying stenosis at the level of the cricopharyngeus is not remedied.[77] Similarly, myotomy alone risks not solving the problem of food accumulation within the diverticulum, with attendant regurgitation and aspiration. Small diverticula may, however, disappear spontaneously following myotomy. A more recent trend is to treat Zenker diverticula via either rigid or flexible endoscopy. With both techniques, the principle is to divide the septum between the lumen of the diverticulum and the lumen of the esophagus. The division allows food and liquid to flow out of the diverticulum distal to the cricopharyngeus (which was within the septum) rather than to accumulate within the diverticulum. This procedure is achieved under general anesthesia, with a stapling device in the case of rigid endoscopy and under light sedation with a needle knife, argon plasma coagulation, or hot biopsy forceps in the case of flexible endoscopy. Controlled trials have not been done comparing the various procedures, but numerous case series suggest that each of them can be efficacious in skilled hands.[78]

Whether or not a cricopharyngeal bar in the absence of a Zenker diverticulum requires treatment is less clear. Certainly, if dysphagia exists and combined fluoroscopic/manometric analysis demonstrates reduced sphincter opening in conjunction with an elevated upstream intrabolus pressure, there is good rationale for treatment. One uncontrolled series suggests that in patients with symptomatic bars, dilation with a large-caliber bougie may be efficacious in relieving dysphagia, a reasonable treatment option prior to myotomy.[79]

ACHALASIA

Achalasia is the best-defined motor disorder of the esophagus. Modern estimates of the incidence of achalasia are about 2.9 per 100,000 population in the United States[80] and 2.6 per 100,000 in south Australia.[81] Achalasia usually presents between 25 and 60 years of age but can also occur in children or the elderly, and affects both genders equally.[49] Because achalasia is a chronic condition, its prevalence greatly exceeds its incidence; a recent estimate of achalasia prevalence in Chicago concluded that it may be as high as 76 per 100,000 population, given that the average age of diagnosis was 56 with an expected average survival of 26 years after diagnosis.[80] Reports of familial clustering of achalasia raise the possibility of genetic predisposition. However, arguing against a strong genetic determinant, a survey of 1012 first-degree relatives of 159 patients with achalasia identified no affected relatives. There is a rare genetic achalasia syndrome associated with adrenal insufficiency and alacrima. This syndrome is inherited as an autosomal recessive disease and manifests with the childhood onset of autonomic nervous system dysfunction including achalasia, alacrima, sinoatrial dysfunction, abnormal pupillary responses to light, and delayed gastric emptying.[82] It is caused by mutations in AAAS, which encodes a protein known as ALADIN.

Pathogenesis

Achalasia is characterized by impaired LES relaxation with swallowing and aperistalsis in the smooth muscle esophagus (types I and II achalasia). If there are premature, spastic contractions in the esophageal body, the disease is referred to as spastic (type III) achalasia.[59] These physiologic alterations result from damage to the innervation of the smooth muscle segment of the esophagus (including the LES) with loss of ganglion cells within the myenteric (Auerbach) plexus. Several observers report fewer ganglion cells and ganglion cells surrounded by mononuclear inflammatory cells in the smooth muscle esophagus of achalasics.[83] The degree of ganglion cell loss is thought to parallel the duration of disease, potentially progressing from EGJOO (i.e., impaired LES relaxation with some intact peristalsis) to type II achalasia, to type I achalasia, to end-stage achalasia.[83,84] Type III achalasia seems to have a unique pathogenesis, characterized by myenteric plexus inflammation and altered function, but not destruction.[83]

Physiologic studies in achalasia suggest dysfunction consistent with postganglionic denervation of esophageal smooth muscle potentially affect excitatory ganglion neurons (cholinergic), inhibitory ganglion neurons (NO ± VIP), or both (see Fig. 46.4). Muscle strips from the circular layer of the esophageal body of patients with achalasia contract when directly stimulated by ACh but fail to respond to ganglionic stimulation by nicotine, indicating a postganglionic excitatory defect. However, partial preservation of the postganglionic cholinergic pathway is suggested by the observations that in some cases of achalasia, LES pressure increases after administration of the ACh inhibitor edrophonium and decreases after administration of the muscarinic antagonist atropine. These are key observations for understanding why botulinum toxin may have some therapeutic benefit (see the "Treatment" section). Regardless of excitatory ganglion neuron impairment, it is clear that inhibitory ganglion neuron dysfunction is as an early manifestation of achalasia. These neurons mediate deglutitive inhibition (including LES relaxation) and the sequenced propagation of esophageal peristalsis; their absence offers a unifying hypothesis for the key physiologic abnormalities of achalasia: impaired LES relaxation and aperistalsis. Achalasia patients have been shown to lack NO synthase and have a marked reduction of VIP-staining neurons in the gastroesophageal junction.

There is substantial evidence of impaired esophageal postganglionic inhibitory innervation in achalasia. Muscle strips from the LES do not relax in response to ganglionic stimulation by nicotine as they do in normal controls. Furthermore, CCK, which normally stimulates the inhibitory ganglion neurons and thus reduces LES pressure, paradoxically increases LES pressure in achalasia.[85] Impaired inhibitory innervation of the smooth muscle esophagus above the LES has been more difficult to demonstrate because of the absence of resting tone in this region. However, in a clever experiment, Sifrim and coworkers used an intraesophageal balloon to create a high-pressure zone in the tubular esophagus that then relaxed with the onset of deglutitive inhibition. This deglutitive relaxation in the esophageal body was absent in early, nondilated cases of achalasia.[86]

The ultimate cause of ganglion cell degeneration in idiopathic achalasia remains uncertain, but there is increasing evidence pointing toward an autoimmune process in genetically susceptible individuals.[87] Analysis of the myenteric plexus infiltrate in achalasia patients revealed that the majority of inflammatory cells are either resting or activated cytotoxic T cells. Antibodies against myenteric neurons have been detected in sera of achalasia patients, especially in patients with specific HLA alleles. The trigger for initiating the autoimmune response leading to the development of achalasia remains controversial, but is suspected to be a chronic or latent human herpes virus 1 (HSV-1) infection.[87] Interestingly, HSV-1 was also detected in LES tissue from nonachalasic organ donors, suggesting that the development of achalasia is dependent on both the virus and a genetic predisposition.

Clinical Features

Clinical manifestations of achalasia may include dysphagia, regurgitation, chest pain, hiccups, halitosis, weight loss, and aspiration pneumonia. Nearly all patients have solid food dysphagia; and many also have variable degrees of liquid dysphagia. The onset of dysphagia is usually gradual, and often present for years at the time of presentation. The severity of dysphagia fluctuates but eventually plateaus. With long-standing disease, there is progressive esophageal dilatation, and regurgitation becomes frequent with recumbency. The regurgitant is often recognized as food that has been eaten hours, or even days, previously. It tends to be nonbilious, nonacid, and mixed with copious amounts of saliva. Patients often fail to recognize the slimy mucoid regurgitant as saliva, being unfamiliar with its visual consistency. Chest pain is a complaint early in the course of achalasia in approximately two-thirds of patients. Its etiology is unknown, but may be related to the occurrence of esophageal spasm. Treatment of achalasia is less effective in relieving chest pain than it is in relieving dysphagia or regurgitation. However, unlike dysphagia or regurgitation, chest pain may spontaneously improve or disappear over time.

With advanced achalasia, up to 10% of cases have bronchopulmonary complications as a result of regurgitation and aspiration; in some instances, it is these complications rather than dysphagia that prompts them to seek medical care. Another interesting, but fortunately rare, symptom of achalasia is airway compromise and stridor as a result of the dilated esophagus compressing the membranous trachea in the neck. This is hypothesized to occur because the neuromuscular apparatus facilitating UES relaxation as part of the belch reflex is compromised.[88]

It is paradoxical that many patients with achalasia may complain of heartburn even after the onset of dysphagia. Although reflux may be a common sequela of the treatments for achalasia, it seems physiologically inconsistent to simultaneously have dysphagia from impaired LES relaxation and reflux from excessive LES relaxation. In support of this skepticism, ambulatory 24-hour esophageal pH studies in achalasia have only shown periods of esophageal acidification caused by the bacterial fermentation of retained food in the esophagus, rather than discrete gastroesophageal reflux events.[89] Furthermore, incomplete tLESRs with crural inhibition, esophageal shortening, and profound after-contraction can occur in achalasia, but devoid of the LES relaxation element seen with traditional tLESRs.[90]

Differential Diagnosis

The differential diagnosis of achalasia includes other esophageal motility disorders and diseases of distinct pathophysiology that duplicate the functional consequences of achalasia. With respect to other motility disorders, there are similarities between distal esophageal spasm (DES) and achalasia, especially the subtype of spastic achalasia. In fact, the only distinction between these entities is the demonstration of incomplete LES relaxation in type III achalasia and there are case reports of DES evolving into spastic achalasia.[91] However, given the rarity of both conditions and the historical heterogeneity on how they are diagnosed, it seems likely that only a small minority of achalasia cases are part of a continuum with DES.

With respect to other diseases that duplicate the functional consequences of idiopathic achalasia, the main considerations are Chagas disease and pseudoachalasia that is associated with infiltrative diseases, malignancy, obstruction, or surgery.

Chagas Disease

Esophageal involvement in Chagas disease, which is endemic in areas of central Brazil, Venezuela, and northern Argentina, can be indistinguishable from idiopathic achalasia. An estimated 20 million South Americans are infected. Due to immigration, about 500,000 people in the United States are believed infected. Chagas disease is spread by the bite of a reduviid (kissing) bug that transmits the parasitic protozoan, *Trypanosoma cruzi*. An acute septicemic phase of the illness follows that varies in severity from going unnoticed to being fatal. The chronic phase of the disease develops up to 20 years after infection and results from destruction of autonomic ganglion cells throughout the body, including the heart, gut, urinary tract, and respiratory tract. Chronic cardiomyopathy with conduction system disturbances and arrhythmias are the most common cause of death. Within the digestive tract, the organs most commonly affected are the esophagus, duodenum, and colon. The severity of esophageal dysfunction is directly proportional to the degree of intramural ganglion cell loss; abnormal peristalsis is first detectable after 50% of ganglion cells are destroyed, and esophageal dilatation after 90% are destroyed. Paralleling this, the initial dysfunction is confined to the esophageal body, with LES dysfunction occurring late in the course of the disease. Neither the radiographic nor the manometric features of achalasia are specific for idiopathic achalasia or achalasia associated with Chagas disease. The most obvious clinical distinction between idiopathic achalasia and esophageal involvement in Chagas disease is evidence of additional tubular organ involvement (cardiomyopathy, megaduodenum, megacolon, megarectum, and megaureter) in Chagas disease.[92] With respect to esophageal pathology, the two are otherwise indistinguishable. The diagnosis of Chagas disease is made in the acute phase by visualizing the parasite in a blood smear. In the chronic phase, the diagnosis is confirmed by serologic tests using complement fixation or PCR. The treatment of the achalasia syndrome in Chagas disease is similar to that for idiopathic achalasia. Treatment of the infection itself is of limited efficacy in the acute phase and of no proved efficacy with chronic disease.

Pseudoachalasia

Tumor-related pseudoachalasia accounts for up to 5% of cases with manometrically defined achalasia. Adenocarcinoma of the EGJ accounts for more than half of tumor-associated pseudoachalasia cases, with a myriad of tumors (pancreatic, hepatocellular, prostatic, lung, esophageal, and lymphoma) accounting for the remainder.[49] These tumors produce an achalasia syndrome by infiltrating the wall of the esophagus at the EGJ, causing a malignant obstruction at the LES, with proximal esophageal dilatation. Similarly, pseudoachalasia can result from esophageal wall stiffness from an infiltrating disease (eosinophilic esophagitis and sarcoidosis), vascular obstruction, abdominal obesity, opiate effect, or surgery-related obstruction (as discussed later).[93] Although often discussed in the literature, an achalasic syndrome as a paraneoplastic syndrome without direct tumor involvement of the EGJ is rare.

Pseudoachalasia becomes more likely than idiopathic achalasia with advanced age (>50 years), abrupt and recent onset of symptoms (<1 year), and early weight loss in excess of 7 kg.[49,94] However, even though these criteria make pseudoachalasia more likely, they still have poor predictive value in the individual case. It is because of this potential pitfall that a thorough anatomic examination (including endoscopy) should be done as part of the diagnostic evaluation of every new case of achalasia. More than the slightest resistance of passage of the endoscope across the EGJ can be a clue to the presence of pseudoachalasia. In idiopathic achalasia, the endoscope should pop through with only gentle pressure required. Pseudoachalasia may manifest atypical or incomplete achalasia-like patterns on manometry.[94] If suspicion of pseudoachalasia is high, endoscopic biopsy, endoscopic ultrasound, or cross-sectional imaging (CT or MRI) should be considered for further evaluation, depending upon the individual circumstances.

Postsurgical Dysfunction

Dysphagia is common in the early period following fundoplication, and patients are advised to consume soft diets for the first 2–4 postoperative weeks. Dysphagia that persists longer than 4 weeks should be evaluated with an upper endoscopy or barium esophagogram to assess the integrity of the wrap and evaluate for possible paraesophageal hernia. Subjects without an overt mechanical disruption should be evaluated with manometry to assess peristaltic function, EGJ relaxation, and esophageal pressurization to determine whether the wrap is too tight or an underlying motility disorder, such as achalasia, exists. Diagnosing achalasia in the context of fundoplication can be difficult because the key manometric findings (aperistalsis and impaired EGJ relaxation) can be identical. Thus preoperative evaluation to exclude achalasia prior to antireflux surgery is essential, typically including manometry.

Bariatric surgery, especially laparoscopic adjustable gastric banding, can also be complicated by development of a pseudoachalasia syndrome.[95] A surgical report examined 121 patients 1 year postprocedure and found 14% of them to have esophageal dilatation in excess of 3.5 cm. Affected patients developed an achalasia-type syndrome with dysphagia and vomiting.[96] This form of pseudoachalasia is usually, but not always, reversible with removal of the gastric band.[97]

Treatment

Because the underlying neuropathology of achalasia cannot be corrected, the objectives of treatment are compensating for the poor esophageal emptying and preventing complications. In practical terms, this amounts to reducing LES pressure so that gravity along with whatever residual esophageal contractility exists promotes esophageal emptying. LES pressure can be reduced by pharmacologic therapy, forceful dilation, or surgical myotomy. Pharmacologic treatments, on the whole, are not very effective, making them most appropriate as temporizing maneuvers.

HRM allows the subtyping of achalasia into three distinct patterns: (type I) classic achalasia, (type II) achalasia with panesophageal pressurization, and (type III) spastic achalasia (see Fig. 46.11). From a conceptual vantage point, types I and II represent a continuum, with type II being early disease before the progression of esophageal dilatation characteristic of type I. Type III, on the other hand, is a subtype characterized by spasm of the distal esophagus. The significance of these disease subtypes is in how differently they responded to therapy. Until the past decade, the durable treatment options for achalasia were laparoscopic Heller myotomy or pneumatic dilation. An extensive literature has compared these treatments, culminating in a multicenter European randomized controlled trial, which concluded that both approaches were about 90% effective to achieve a symptom-based outcome with no statistically significant difference between them.[98,99] However, that, and all preceding trials, did not consider achalasia subtype in their design or in their assessment of treatment efficacy. Subsequently, a substantial amount of retrospective data and a reassessment of the European achalasia trial[60] suggest that achalasia subtype is of great relevance in determining treatment effectiveness. Indeed, in the European achalasia trial, the efficacy of pneumatic dilation for treating type II achalasia was 96% after 5 years, compared to only 88% for Heller myotomy ($P = .03$). In contrast, treatment success in type III achalasia was achieved in 48% and 86% of patients for pneumatic dilation and laparoscopic myotomy, respectively ($P = .09$).[99] Considering the low cost of pneumatic dilation compared to laparoscopic myotomy and that the risk of esophageal perforation between techniques is comparable (about 1%),[100] these findings argue for pneumatic dilation as the preferred initial treatment for type II achalasia.

The bulk of the literature pertinent to achalasia treatment is composed of uncontrolled case series using a variety of qualitative endpoints as indications of efficacy. As already noted, there has been minimal standardization as to the criteria for defining achalasia, disease severity, or the technical details of how the treatments are performed. Furthermore, some series were collected prospectively, some retrospectively, and some a combination. Given all of these limitations, there is little merit to embarking on a detailed comparison of outcomes among techniques. The existing treatment data can be summarized as follows.

Pharmacologic Therapy

Smooth muscle relaxants such as nitrates or calcium channel blockers, administered sublingually immediately prior to eating, can relieve dysphagia in achalasia by reducing the LES pressure. Amyl nitrite, sublingual nitroglycerin, theophylline, and β_2-adrenergic agonists have also been tried. The largest reported experience has been with isosorbide dinitrate and nifedipine. However, the side effects of nitrates, particularly headache, are common and the efficacy is very limited. Placebo-controlled trials have not been reported. With calcium channel blockers (mainly nifedipine) the limiting side effects are flushing, dizziness, headache, peripheral edema, and orthostasis. Sublingual nifedipine (30–40 mg/day) administered before meals was studied in 29 patients with early achalasia and was significantly better than placebo, with good results in 70% of achalasia patients followed for 6–18 months.[101] However, a subsequent placebo-controlled crossover trial of nifedipine found minimal benefit.[102]

Sildenafil is another smooth muscle relaxant that can decrease LES pressure in patients with achalasia by blocking phosphodiesterase type 5, the enzyme that metabolizes the cyclic guanosine monophosphate induced by NO. A double-blind placebo-controlled trial found that 50 mg of sildenafil significantly reduced LES pressure and LES relaxation pressure when compared to placebo.[103] The effect peaked at 15–20 minutes after administration and persisted for less than 1 hour. Although conceptually appealing, the practicality of using sildenafil clinically is limited by its cost and potential side effects.

Botulinum Toxin Injection

The initial landmark study of botulinum toxin in achalasia reported that intrasphincteric injection of 80 U of botulinum toxin decreased LES pressure by 33% and improved dysphagia in 66% of patients for a 6-month period.[104] Botulinum toxin irreversibly inhibits the release of ACh from presynaptic cholinergic terminals, effectively eliminating the neurogenic component of LES pressure. However, because this effect is eventually reversed by the growth of new axons, it is not a long-lasting therapy. The technique involves injecting aliquots of botulinum toxin into four quadrants of the LES with a sclerotherapy catheter. Side effects are rare but can include chest discomfort for several days and occasional rash. Although many patients initially experience a good response, there is minimal continued efficacy at 1 year.[105] Repeat injection can be effective, but the injections lead to a local inflammatory reaction and fibrosis, ultimately limiting that strategy. Doses greater than 100 U do not have increased efficacy.[106] Hence this option is best reserved for older adults or frail individuals who are poor risks for definitive treatments.

Pneumatic Dilation

Therapeutic dilation for achalasia requires distension of the LES to a diameter of at least 3 cm to effect lasting reduction of LES pressure, presumably by partially disrupting the circular muscle of the sphincter. Only dilators specifically designed to treat achalasia achieve adequate diameter for lasting benefit; dilation to a lesser diameter provides only very temporary benefit at best. Rigiflex dilators are available in 3.0-, 3.5-, and 4.0-cm diameters. These are long, noncompliant, cylindrical balloons that have radiopaque markings. They are designed to be passed over a guidewire and positioned across the LES fluoroscopically. Once positioned, the balloon is inflated to full diameter using a handheld manometer taking care to visualize the indentation of the sphincter on the balloon surface as it expands. Pneumatic dilation is commonly done on an outpatient basis with the patient under sedation as for endoscopy. However, the technique of pneumatic dilation is highly variable among practitioners in terms of patient preparation, parameters of balloon inflation, and postdilation monitoring.[107] In patients with substantial esophageal retention, it is useful to impose a clear liquid diet for 1 or more days prior to the procedure. Although there is minimal methodological consistency among authors, a cautious approach of beginning with a small-diameter dilator (3.0 cm) and progressing to larger diameters (3.5 and 4.0 cm) only when the smaller dilator proved ineffective is fairly universal. As for inflation pressures, these are of minimal relevance with modern noncompliant balloon dilators, because they do not distend beyond their specified diameter regardless of inflation pressure. Hence it is simply necessary to observe under fluoroscopy that the balloon is properly positioned to capture the LES, observed as the "waist" of the hourglass-shaped balloon silhouette, and that the waist fully effaces as the inflation proceeds.

The major complication of pneumatic dilation is esophageal perforation, with a reported incidence ranging between 0% and 5% and a global average of 1%.[100] With most perforations readily evident (or at least suspected) within an hour of the procedure because of persistent or severe chest pain, fever, or subcutaneous emphysema, patients should be observed for signs of an esophageal leak for at least 2 hours after pneumatic dilation. Alternatively, some practitioners routinely obtain a fluoroscopic examination of the esophagus following pneumatic dilation to ensure that perforation has not occurred. Usually, water-soluble contrast is given first, followed by barium. If a perforation appears small and is contained or intramural, conservative management consisting of hospitalization and close observation while maintaining the patient NPO, administering IV antibiotics is appropriate. Larger perforations can be closed with endoclips and endoscopic suture, or managed with endoluminal stent placement. However, if a perforation is substantial, or if worsening chest pain and fever occur, surgical repair should be pursued expediently. Patients with a perforation from pneumatic dilation that is recognized and promptly treated surgically (within 6–8 hours) have outcomes comparable to those of patients undergoing elective Heller myotomy.[108]

In instances of an unsatisfactory result following pneumatic dilation, it is reasonable to perform a subsequent dilation within a matter of weeks, using an incrementally larger dilator. If the benefit of the original dilation persisted for a year or more, it is common to repeat pneumatic dilation as necessary. The clinical efficacy reported for dilation ranges widely from 32% to 98%, likely because of the extreme variability in technique, methods for assessing treatment outcome, and the acceptability of performing repeated dilations over time.[107] Subsequent response to surgical myotomy is not influenced by the history of previous dilatations.

Heller Myotomy

Current surgical procedures for treating achalasia are variations on the esophagomyotomy described by Heller in 1913. Subsequently, this procedure was modified to an anterior myotomy via thoracotomy. The appeal of myotomy is that it offers a more predictable method of reducing LES pressure than does pneumatic dilatation. Although clearly efficacious, open Heller myotomy is associated with considerable morbidity related to the thoracotomy. However, adoption of the laparoscopic approach for achalasia surgery has largely mitigated this.

Published series of the efficacy of Heller myotomy in treating achalasia report good to excellent results in 62%–100% of patients, with persistent dysphagia in fewer than 10%. The laparoscopic approach is associated with similar efficacy, reduced morbidity, and shorter hospital stay compared to myotomy via thoracotomy, laparotomy, or thoracoscopy. In the past, post-myotomy gastroesophageal reflux could be particularly severe; however, with the use of PPIs, this is usually easily controlled. Thus laparoscopic Heller myotomy combined with a partial fundoplication (Toupet or Dor) has become the preferred surgical procedure for achalasia. An unsatisfactory result following Heller myotomy can result from incomplete myotomy, scarring of the myotomy, functional esophageal obstruction from the antireflux component of the operation, paraesophageal hernia, or severe esophageal dilatation.

In the European Achalasia Trial, a multicenter prospective randomized controlled trial that compared pneumatic dilation to laparoscopic Heller myotomy, 200 achalasia patients were randomized to laparoscopic myotomy with Dor fundoplication or pneumatic dilation, allowing for a maximum of three series of dilations in the pneumatic dilation group.[98,99] There was no difference in success rates after 2 or 5 years of follow-up: 92% and 82% for pneumatic dilation versus 87% and 84% for laparoscopic myotomy, respectively. Based on that evidence, laparoscopic myotomy and pneumatic dilation have comparable success rates, and cogent arguments can be made for each of these for treatments of type I and type II achalasia. Type III (spastic) achalasia had better symptomatic outcomes after laparoscopic Heller myotomy than pneumatic dilation. Overall, one should assess the available local resources, as well as patient preference, in selecting the initial therapy.

Peroral Endoscopic Myotomy

More recently, a hybrid technique has been developed for treating achalasia, essentially using endoscopy to achieve a surgical myotomy. This procedure, termed peroral endoscopic myotomy (POEM), requires making a transverse mucosal incision in the midesophagus, entering it, and creating a submucosal tunnel all the way to the gastric cardia using a forward-viewing endoscope with a transparent distal cap and a triangular dissection knife. Once the subcutaneous tunnel is complete, the endoscope is withdrawn and selective myotomy of the circular muscle accomplished with electrocautery tools for a variable length up the esophagus and 2 cm distal to the EGJ onto the gastric cardia. Endoclips are then used to seal the entry incision. Initial reports in prospective cohorts of achalasia patients treated with the POEM procedure reported success rates of greater than 90%, comparable to those of laparoscopic Heller myotomy. A systematic review and meta-analysis comparing outcomes of POEM (1958 patients) and laparoscopic Heller myotomy (5834 patients) found POEM to be more effective than laparoscopic Heller myotomy in relieving dysphagia in the short term (mean follow-up 16 months), but associated with a very high incidence of pathological reflux (odds ratio of 9.31 for erosive esophagitis).[109] Two multicenter randomized controlled trials involving POEM have been completed. One compared POEM with pneumatic dilation (the POEMA trial) and found the POEM procedure to be more efficacious in terms of therapeutic success, but also more likely to result in postprocedure reflux esophagitis. After 2 and 5 years, 92% and 81% (respectively) of the POEM patients ($n = 67$) were in clinical remission versus 54% and 40% (respectively) after pneumatic dilation ($n = 66$) ($P < .01$). A key difference between this trial and the European Achalasia Trial was that pneumatic dilation was only performed up to two times (30 mm, then 35 mm) with subsequent need for repeat pneumatic dilation considered as treatment failure. Finally, another multicenter randomized trial compared POEM ($n = 112$) and laparoscopic Heller myotomy with Dor fundoplasty.[110] Similar rates of treatment effectiveness (symptomatic outcome) were observed after 2 years with 83% success after POEM ($n = 112$) and 82% after Heller ($n = 109$); $P = .007$ for noninferiority of POEM. There again were greater rates of GERD after POEM with erosive esophagitis observed at 2 year endoscopy in 44% after POEM and 29% after Heller. Again, given the multiple effective treatment options for achalasia, initial treatment selection can be based off considerations of available local resources, as well as patient preference including potential need for repeat pneumatic dilation or ongoing treatment for GERD.

Treatment Failures

Persistent dysphagia after achalasia treatment suggests treatment failure and should be evaluated with some combination of endoscopy, HRM,[111] FLIP,[112] and fluoroscopic imaging. Endoscopy may detect esophagitis, stricture, paraesophageal hernia, or anatomic deformity. Impedance manometry may be useful to quantify persistent or recurrent sphincter dysfunction, distal spasm, or esophageal retention. FLIP study can identify a poorly distensive sphincter, even in cases that HRM suggests adequate relaxation.[113] Fluoroscopy is useful both to identify anatomic problems and to evaluate esophageal emptying using a timed barium swallow, a standardized method of measuring the height of the esophageal barium column 1 and 5 minutes after ingestion.[111] In some instances, these evaluations will lead to further intervention. This could potentially be either repeat dilation, POEM, or Heller myotomy. In patients who have already undergone myotomy, detection of a short myotomy or functional esophageal obstruction from the antireflux component of the surgery may require reoperation, but pneumatic dilation can be pursued as an alternative. Reoperation, in general, is less effective than an initial operation for any indication in achalasia.

Occasionally, patients fail to respond to optimally performed dilation or myotomy and require alternative treatment. In extremely advanced or refractory cases of achalasia, esophageal resection with gastric pull-up or interposition of a segment of transverse colon or small bowel may be the only option. Indications for this intervention include unresolvable obstructive symptoms, malnutrition, bleeding, chronic aspiration, cancer, and perforation during dilation. Although excellent long-term functional results can be achieved, the reported mortality of this surgery is about 4%, consistent with esophagectomy done for other indications.

Risk of Squamous Cell Cancer

Squamous cell carcinoma may develop in patients with achalasia. The tumors develop many years after the diagnosis of achalasia and usually arise in a greatly dilated esophagus with stasis esophagitis. Symptoms attributable to the cancer can be delayed, and the neoplasms are often large and advanced at the time of detection raising the issue of surveillance endoscopy. However, an analysis of a database encompassing the entire Swedish population of 1062 patients with achalasia suggests that after discounting incident carcinomas, the overall squamous cell cancer risk for achalasia was 17-fold compared with age-matched controls, resulting in a 0.15% cancer incidence. The authors calculated that if surveillance endoscopy was done annually, 406 exams would have to be done in men and 2220 in women before one potentially treatable tumor was found. However, even that calculation is optimistic, given that detection of a small cancer in a massively dilated esophagus with retained food and stasis esophagitis is far from assured. Consequently, the latest ASGE guidelines do not advocate routine endoscopic surveillance for achalasia patients. However, they also state that if surveillance was considered, it would be reasonable to begin 10–15 years after the onset of achalasia symptoms.[114]

Distal Esophageal Spasm

Although the diagnosis of DES is often invoked as a cause of esophageal chest pain, the entity is actually exceedingly rare with most cases of esophageal chest pain attributable to reflux disease, achalasia or a disorder of gut-brain interaction. Historically, the manometric criteria for diagnosing DES have been nonspecific, leading to overdiagnosis of the entity. This has been clarified somewhat with the Chicago Classification of HRM and the adoption of reduced DL of peristalsis as the cardinal abnormality in DES.[115]

There are no population-based studies on the incidence or prevalence of esophageal motility disorders other than achalasia. Thus the only way to estimate the incidence or prevalence of spastic disorders such as DES is to examine data on populations at risk and reference the observed frequency of spastic disorders to the incidence of achalasia, which, as detailed earlier, is about 2.75 per 100,000 population. Doing so, the prevalence of DES is much lower than that if modern restrictive diagnostic criteria are used. Populations at risk for motility disorders are patients with chest pain and/or dysphagia, so it is among these patients that extensive manometric data have been collected. Manometric abnormalities are prevalent among these groups, but in most cases the manometric findings are of unclear significance.[116]

Although DES is a disorder of peristalsis, the majority of afflicted patients exhibit normal peristaltic contractions most of the time. The neuromuscular pathology responsible for DES is unknown and there are no known risk factors. The most striking reported pathologic change is of diffuse muscular hypertrophy or hyperplasia in the distal esophagus with thickening of up to 2 cm. However, there are other well-documented cases in which esophageal muscular thickening was not found at thoracotomy, and still other instances of patients with muscular thickening not associated with DES symptoms.

Despite the absence of defined histopathology, physiologic evidence implicates myenteric plexus neuronal dysfunction in spasm because the latency of contraction along the smooth muscle esophagus is a function of postganglionic myenteric plexus neurons. Swallow-induced vagal impulses reach the entire smooth muscle segment of the esophagus simultaneously, and it is the balance of excitatory and inhibitory ganglionic neurons within the myenteric plexus that determine the timing of contraction at each esophageal locus. Furthermore, experimental evidence suggests heterogeneity among spasm patients, such that some primarily exhibit reduced inhibitory interneuron function, whereas in others the defect is of excess excitation.

Defining DES based on the latency of the postdeglutitive contraction puts it in a pathophysiologic continuum with achalasia, consistent with documented case reports of patients undergoing this evolution.[91] Furthermore, there are marked similarities between spastic achalasia and DES because both are characterized by rapidly propagated contractions in the distal esophagus. The differentiating features of vigorous achalasia are involvement of the LES and the absence of any normal peristalsis.

Clinical Features

The major symptoms attributed to DES are dysphagia and chest pain. Weight loss is rare. Dysphagia is usually intermittent and sometimes related to swallowing specific substances such as red wine or liquids at extreme hot or cold temperature. In some instances, patients experience episodes of esophageal obstruction while eating that persists until relieved by emesis.

Esophageal chest pain is very similar in character to angina, often described as crushing or squeezing in character, radiating to the neck, jaw, arms, or midline of the back. Pain episodes may last from minutes to hours, but continued swallowing is not always impaired. The mechanism producing esophageal pain is poorly understood. High-frequency intraluminal ultrasound data suggest that it may be related to sustained contraction of esophageal longitudinal muscle.[117]

Chest pain is also prevalent in patients subsequently found to have manometric abnormalities that are insufficient to establish a diagnosis of achalasia or DES. Among such individuals, there is a high prevalence of reflux and of psychiatric diagnoses, particularly anxiety and depression.[116]

Differential Diagnosis

The pain associated with DES can closely mimic that of angina pectoris. Given the potentially fatal consequences of myocardial ischemia, this must always be considered carefully in the differential diagnosis. Features suggesting an esophageal, as opposed to a cardiac, etiology of pain include: (1) prolonged nonexertional pain, (2) pain that interrupts sleep, (3) meal-related pain, (4) relief with antacids, and (5) additional accompanying esophageal symptoms, such as heartburn, dysphagia, or regurgitation. However, even these features can exhibit overlap with cardiac pain.

Furthermore, even within the spectrum of esophageal diseases, neither chest pain nor dysphagia is specific for DES; both symptoms are also characteristic of common esophageal disorders including GERD or esophagitis. Hence only after these more common diagnostic possibilities have been excluded by appropriate endoscopic evaluation, and a therapeutic trial of PPIs and/or ambulatory reflux monitoring, should DES be considered.

Treatment

Despite the dogma of treatment with smooth muscle relaxants, minimal controlled data exist regarding pharmacologic therapy of DES.[118] Long-term studies are not available; the basis for this therapy is generally anecdotal. Furthermore, most instances of esophageal chest pain are due to reflux rather than DES, and reflux symptoms will likely be made worse by treating with smooth muscle relaxants. Uncontrolled trials of small numbers of DES patients report clinical response to nitrates, calcium channel blockers, hydralazine, and anxiolytics.

Botulinum toxin injection is an appealing therapeutic approach for DES because it blocks cholinergic neural transmission. In a randomized controlled trial involving 22 patients with DES or nutcracker esophagus, 50% of patients responded to botulinum toxin injection, compared to 10% injected with saline ($P < .01$).[119] In a subsequent retrospective analysis of only the patients diagnosed with HRM, all six with DES had a positive response to botulinum toxin injection at 2 months and the response was sustained for more than 6 months in four patients.[120] However, another randomized, sham controlled trial of 23 patients with DES ($n = 4$), hypercontractile esophagus, and type III achalasia observed no difference in symptomatic outcome after 3 months between botulinum toxin and sham. Further, manometric resolution of spasm occurred in all three or three DES patients that completed HRM 3 months after the sham intervention. Additionally a case of fatal mediastinitis was reported in a DES patient who received botulinum toxin, so the procedure cannot be viewed as without risk.[121] Overall, the value of botulinum toxin for treatment of DES remains uncertain.

Until recently, surgery was rarely entertained in the treatment of DES because the options were of either a thoracotomy with a long myotomy or esophagectomy. However, since 2012, well-defined cases of DES have been successfully treated with POEM.[122] The unique advantage of POEM is that the length of myotomy can be extended to potentially involve the entire smooth muscle esophagus as gauged by HRM, esophageal wall thickening on EUS, or intra-operative FLIP. Supportive of this, a recent meta-analysis of uncontrolled POEM series reported a weighted pooled response rate of 88% (CI 61%–97%) in DES with the length of myotomy averaging 13.5 cm.[123]

Hypercontractile Esophagus

Vigorous esophageal contractions with normal DL, defined as esophageal hypercontractility in the Chicago Classification, can be associated with both dysphagia and chest pain.[56] A "jackhammer" pattern of hypercontractility is also described when there are repetitive, high amplitude esophageal body contractions (Fig. 46.15).[124] Hypercontractility is thought to be a manifestation of either excessive excitatory drive or a reactive compensation for outflow obstruction leading to myocyte hypertrophy.[125] Consistent with this, patients with hypercontractility demonstrate heightened sensitivity to cholinergic agonists such as edrophonium. Data supporting obstruction as an etiology of hypercontractility come from physiologic studies using an inflatable pressure cuff implanted around the distal esophagus of cats.[126] Small cuff inflation volumes augmented the amplitude of peristalsis, but with larger volumes there was complete disruption of the peristalsis. Repetitive and/or hypertensive contractions were also observed with an overinflation of laparoscopic adjustable gastric bands in humans.[127]

From a clinical perspective, the summary metric for quantifying distal esophageal contractility in HRM is the DCI. DCI values greater than 8000 mm Hg cm sec represent an extreme pattern of hypercontractility that is rarely seen in normal subjects and consistently associated with chest pain and dysphagia.[56] The current version of the Chicago Classification labels this condition

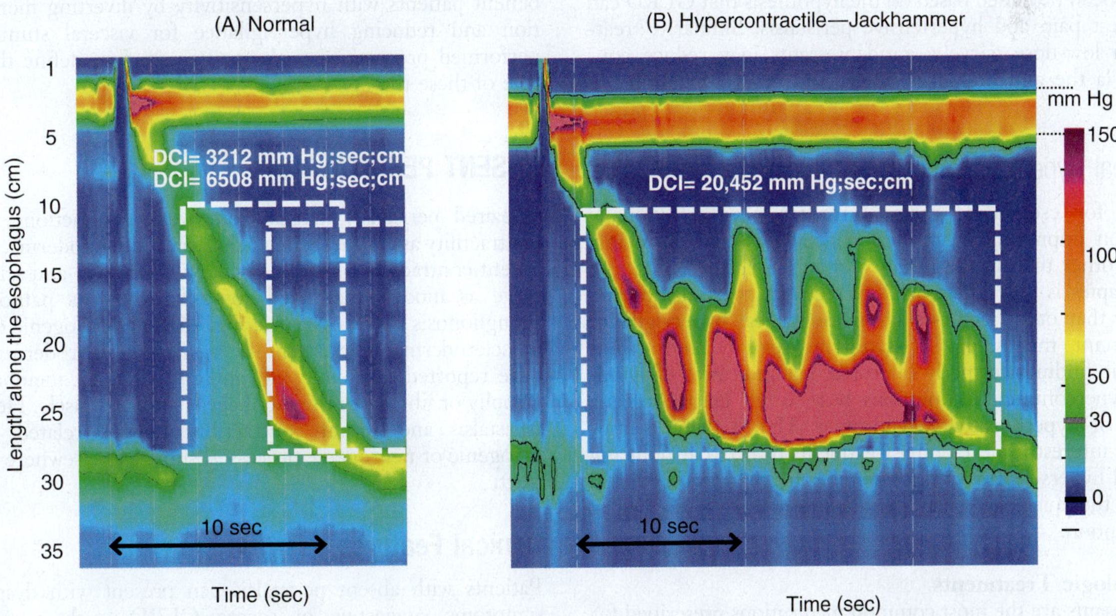

Fig. 46.15 Normal and abnormal contractile vigor. (A) A normal swallow with a distal contractile interval (DCI) of 3212 mm Hg sec cm, normal propagation, and a single uniform contraction. (B) Swallow with an extremely high DCI. This swallow exhibits repetitive contractions without evidence of an esophagogastric junction outflow obstruction. This is a hypercontractile or "jackhammer" pattern in the Chicago Classification (see Table 46.2). (With permission from the Esophageal Center at Northwestern.)

"hypercontractile esophagus" when $\geq$20% of 5 mL liquid test swallows demonstrate hypercontractile swallows during a manometric study.[56]

Clinical Features

The hypercontractile disorders also typically present with chest pain and dysphagia, although the dysphagia is less likely to involve impaired bolus transit. By definition, contractile latency is normal with hypercontractility; hence peristaltic progression and bolus transit are normal. However, the jackhammer pattern is associated with prolonged repetitive contractions that can persist long after bolus transit (Fig. 46.15B). The natural history of hypercontractility is unknown, but it is clear that at least in some cases jackhammer patients can have a prolonged and difficult clinical course.

Treatment

The same therapeutic options used for DES have also been advocated for patients with hypertensive (or hypercontractile) peristalsis. Smooth muscle relaxants such as calcium channel blockers and nitrates have been used for these disorders. Although they reduce peristaltic amplitude, neither has been shown to relieve chest pain or dysphagia in clinical trials. Sildenafil is an appealing alternative owing to its profound effect of reducing contraction amplitude and potentially reducing the occurrence of repetitive contractions.[128] Again, supportive clinical trial data do not exist. Similarly, botulinum toxin injection in the esophageal muscle, with or without EUS guidance, may be an option for patients with refractory symptoms. Finally, similar to the cases of spastic achalasia and DES, POEM has recently been proposed as a treatment for hypercontractility. The same meta-analysis of uncontrolled POEM series discussed above with respect to DES also analyzed data on jackhammer and reported a weighted pooled response rate of 72% (CI 55%–83%), notably less than the 92% response reported for type III achalasia.[123]

Because of the potential overlap between hypertensive peristalsis and GERD and the observation that many of these patients have coexistent psychological distress, therapies targeting acid secretion, visceral sensitivity, and stress have also been attempted. PPIs have been proposed based on the hypothesis that GERD can induce chest pain and hypertensive peristalsis. Similarly, treatment with low-dose tricyclic antidepressants may reduce contractions via the anticholinergic effect and may reduce visceral sensitivity.

Esophageal Hypersensitivity

Therapies for esophageal motor disorders have traditionally centered on improving esophageal contractility and emptying. However, other than in the instance of achalasia, the efficacy of these therapies is very limited. More recently, there has been a realization that other factors such as esophageal hypervigilance are important moderators of symptom severity and minor manometric findings formerly interpreted as indicative of symptomatic hypercontractile conditions were often epiphenomena indicative of hypersensitivity syndromes. Hence there is now substantial interest in developing treatments directed at reducing esophageal hypersensitivity, and a number of pharmacologic and behavioral therapies have been identified to modulate esophageal pain perception.

Pharmacologic Treatments

Antidepressants are the most common medications prescribed for visceral pain modulation or chest pain of esophageal origin. Among the antidepressants, the tricyclic antidepressants are the best studied. The mechanism of action for this therapeutic benefit is unknown, because these agents have multiple receptor targets, both centrally and peripherally. Proposed treatment with these agents is at lower doses than would be used for mood-altering effects and typical starting doses for antidepressants (amitriptyline and nortriptyline) are 10–25 mg at bedtime, with escalations of 10–25-mg increments to a target of 50–75 mg. However, as highlighted by a randomized controlled trial, it is difficult to differentiate the nonspecific effects of tricyclics from their effects on hypersensitivity.[129] In that trial of 43 functional heartburn and esophageal hypersensitivity patients randomized to treatment with 25 mg qhs imipramine and 40 randomized to matched placebo, the response rates, judged by a 50% reduction in reflux symptoms, were 37.2% and 37.5%, respectively. However, those treated with imipramine were more likely to experience improvement in quality of life as assessed by total SF-36 score, which is, after all, the main objective when treating functional disorders.

Experimental data also support the effectiveness of selective serotonin reuptake inhibitors in the treatment of esophageal hypersensitivity. Intravenous citalopram at a dose of 20 mg was found to significantly reduce both chemical (acid perfusion) and mechanical (balloon distention) esophageal sensitivity in a randomized double-blinded crossover study.[130] Although clinical trials are not yet available, mechanistic studies assessing other selective serotonin reuptake inhibitors have also yielded encouraging results. Along similar lines, there has been substantial interest in developing medications that influence serotonin (5-HT) pathways given their effects on gut motility and as treatments for nausea. Unfortunately, several of these medications have proved to have unacceptable risks related to cardiac arrhythmias or gut ischemia that led to their withdrawal.

Nonpharmacologic Treatments

Given the potential links among esophageal hypersensitivity, psychological factors, and psychiatric abnormalities, therapy focused on reassurance, behavioral modification, and relaxation techniques may be helpful. These therapies may benefit patients with comorbidities such as panic disorder, generalized anxiety, and depression. However, it is also possible that therapies using controlled breathing, relaxation techniques, or hypnotherapy may benefit patients with hypersensitivity by diverting mental attention and reducing hypervigilance for visceral stimuli. Well-performed prospective trials are necessary to define the clinical role of these therapies.

ABSENT PERISTALSIS

Impaired peristalsis ranges from weak contractions to absent contractility as can be seen in achalasia and scleroderma. Although absent contractility is often idiopathic, achalasia and scleroderma serve as models that shed some light on its pathogenesis—aganglionosis in achalasia (see Fig. 46.4) and myogenic disruption in scleroderma. Ultrastructure studies in scleroderma patients have reported thickening of capillary basement membranes and atrophy or fibrosis of the esophageal smooth muscle. Hence weak peristalsis and absent contractility can be related to either myogenic or neurogenic processes, similar to elsewhere in the GI tract.

Clinical Features

Patients with absent peristalsis can present with dysphagia or symptoms suggestive of severe GERD, such as heartburn, regurgitation, and chest pain. The severity of the presentation is to some degree dependent on the function of the EGJ; GERD symptoms are much worse when absent peristalsis is accompanied by gross EGJ incompetence. Alternatively, with an intact EGJ, absent peristalsis may be difficult to distinguish from achalasia, owing to the similar symptomatology and physiologic findings.[113]

Treatment

Although it is biologically plausible that treating an underlying disorder associated with absent peristalsis may improve esophageal motility, no medications have been identified that significantly improve peristalsis in the context of absent peristalsis. Consequently, treatments focus on minimizing potential complications using lifestyle modifications such as postural maneuvers to improve esophageal clearance and drinking liberally with meals to facilitate bolus transit. Patients with absent peristalsis and an incompetent EGJ (the "scleroderma pattern") will be vulnerable to severe GERD because they have both a reduced antireflux barrier and impaired esophageal clearance once reflux has occurred (see Chapter 48). These patients often require twice-daily PPI therapy. Additionally, these patients are vulnerable to pill esophagitis, and care should be taken to avoid potentially caustic medications and to convert medications to liquid formulation, sublingual, or smaller versions to prevent pill esophagitis.

INEFFECTIVE ESOPHAGEAL MOTILITY

Ineffective esophageal motility (IEM) manifests with ≥80% swallows (out of a complement of 10 swallows) with abnormal esophageal body contraction vigor (DCI 100–450 mm Hg cm sec), ≥5 cm breaks in peristaltic integrity or failure of peristalsis in the context of normal LES relaxation on HRM; additionally, ≥50% failed swallows can independently fulfill Chicago Classification 4.0 criteria for IEM.[56,131] IEM can be encountered in 10.0% of asymptomatic healthy individuals.[132] IEM is encountered more often in the context of reflux-related endoscopic changes including Barrett esophagus.[133,134] However, despite the frequent association of IEM and abnormal reflux monitoring, IEM is not pathognomonic for a diagnosis of GERD,[133] and does not reliably associate with reflux symptoms.[135–137] The perception of dysphagia is imperfect, and does not relate to abnormal bolus transit from weak or absent peristalsis.[136,138] In many instances, IEM does not impact quality of life and does not progress over time.[139]

Treatment

No pharmacologic intervention reliably restores esophageal smooth muscle contractility, or improves symptoms.[140] Conventional prokinetic agents (metoclopramide and domperidone) are not beneficial in esophageal hypomotility, and do not improve esophageal symptoms. Asymptomatic IEM does not require specific management. When GERD is identified, typical GERD treatments are instituted.

SUMMARY

Understanding the physiology of normal swallowing can help define the distinctions between oropharyngeal and esophageal dysphagia, and between structural and neuromuscular mechanisms of pathophysiology in both the oropharynx and in the tubular esophagus. Recurrent aspiration related to oropharyngeal dysfunction can be a cause of death after a stroke. Achalasia is the best-studied motility disorder of the tubular esophagus, and the only motility disorder that consistently improves with treatments directed at the LES or the smooth muscle esophagus. Achalasia should be suspected when absent contractility is associated with significant dysphagia and weight loss, and pseudoachalasia is suspected when symptoms and weight loss develop rapidly. Although dysphagia confirmed to be related to spastic disorders of the esophageal body (DES, hypercontractile esophagus) may improve after POEM, most patients with nonachalasia motility disorders benefit from symptomatic management and treatment of GERD.

Full references for this chapter can be found at https://ebooks.health.elsevier.com.

47 Esophageal Disorders Caused by Medications, Trauma, and Infection

David A. Katzka

IN THIS CHAPTER

MEDICATION-INDUCED ESOPHAGEAL INJURY

Medication-induced esophageal injury occurs at any age and from a variety of commonly used medications. Nevertheless, medication-induced esophageal injury is likely underdiagnosed in clinical practice for several reasons. First, common and more serious problems, such as acute coronary syndrome and pulmonary embolism, might be considered initially because of the severe chest pain, often pleuritic in nature, associated with pill-induced esophagitis. Second, patients may be assumed to be having a severe episode of acid reflux, a far more common condition than a medication-induced esophageal ulceration. Third, several of the medications that cause medication-induced esophagitis are over-the-counter medications (e.g., NSAIDs) or may have been taken safely for years (e.g., tetracycline) without injury and therefore are not considered by patients to be a possible contributor to their symptoms. Fourth, because it is not routinely reported or recognized, medication-induced esophageal injury is considered to be uncommon.[1,2] This underrecognition can be problematic as failure to recognize this entity can lead to failure to discontinue the offending agent and lead to extensive and erroneous evaluation and treatment of other conditions. Underrecognition may lead to failure to provide the patient proper instruction to avoid injury as well, because this chapter provides a detailed overview of medication-induced esophageal injury, with particular attention to suspecting this entity both by its symptoms and by the medications that are potentially culpable.

Mechanisms

Medications cause esophageal injury through several mechanisms. These can initially be divided into those that cause direct injury to esophageal mucosa because of their caustic nature or by facilitation of injury through other mechanisms such as induction of acid reflux (e.g., calcium channel antagonists). Medications directly damage the esophageal mucosa through one of four known mechanisms: (1) production of a caustic acidic solution (e.g., ascorbic acid and ferrous sulfate); (2) production of a caustic alkaline solution (e.g., alendronate); (3) creation of a hyperosmolar solution in contact with esophageal mucosa (e.g., potassium chloride); and (4) direct drug toxicity to the esophageal mucosa (e.g., tetracycline). For many medications, the mechanism of esophageal injury does not fall into any of these known categories. Other factors may influence the toxicity of the pill, particularly contact time, pills coated with gelatinous material,[3] sustained-release formulations, and a wax matrix form of the drug.[4] Cellulose fiber and guar gum pills may swell and lodge in the esophagus, causing complete obstruction because of their water-absorbing capacity. Finally, medications may cause esophageal injury through induction of a systemic reaction that affects the esophagus.[5]

It is commonly assumed that a predisposition to medication-induced esophageal injury is due to an anatomic or motility disorder of the esophagus or that the medication was taken incorrectly, in either case allowing for prolonged exposure of the medication to esophageal mucosa. For example, studies have shown that patients with left atrial enlargement,[6] esophageal strictures,[7] esophageal dysmotility,[8] and esophageal diverticula[9] (either Zenker or epiphrenic diverticula) have greater risk of pill-induced injury. Similarly, in the patient with normal esophageal function, the site of drug-induced injury most commonly occurs where there are areas of normal hypomotility or extrinsic compression, such as in the trough zone of the esophagus (where the smooth and skeletal muscle overlap) or at the level of the aortic or left bronchial impression on the esophagus.[10,11] These locations of relative stasis allow for a pill, when taken incorrectly, to cause injury. However, any part of the esophagus may be involved. Methods of taking a medication incorrectly that predispose to injury include ingesting a pill without enough water or assuming a recumbent position or sleeping immediately after pill ingestion, or both. The latter two factors are particularly problematic, by eliminating the help of gravity in esophageal transit and by reducing saliva production and frequent swallowing, which occur normally while awake. Importantly, however, many, if not most, patients who suffer pill-induced esophageal injury presumably have normal esophageal function and do not necessarily ingest their medication in a faulty manner. That pill-induced esophageal injury can occur under "normal" conditions is supported by data demonstrating prolonged radiographic retention of capsules in the esophagus by normal subjects even when taken with water in the upright position.[3,12] Capsules may have longer esophageal retention times than tablets.[13]

Clinical Features and Diagnosis

Patients typically note an acute onset of chest pain, which may radiate over the central chest and to the back. The pain is commonly accentuated with inspiration and may be accompanied by severe odynophagia, even to small sips of liquids. Some patients may complain of a severe acute onset of heartburn-type symptoms. This set of symptoms associated with ingestion of a potentially injurious medication taken incorrectly (particularly just before bedtime without enough water) strongly suggests the diagnosis. If objective confirmation of the diagnosis is necessary, endoscopy or radiography can be used, although endoscopy is considered more sensitive. Findings range from discrete ulcers to diffuse severe esophagitis with pseudomembranes, as may be seen with bisphosphonates[14] or with sodium polystyrene sulfonate suspension (Kayexalate), mimicking Candidal esophagitis.[15] A diffuse sloughing appearance of the mucosa, also known as *esophageal dissecans superficialis*, may also be identified.[16] Occasionally, severe inflammatory reactions causing stenoses and tumor-like appearances occur.[17,18] Similar findings may be seen radiographically, particularly when double-contrast radiography is used.[19,20] The range of findings described on esophagography may also include solitary or multiple ulcers; small or large ulcerations; ulcers with punctate, ovoid, linear, serpiginous, or stellate collections of barium; confluent ulcers; or areas of normal-appearing mucosa separating ulcers (Fig. 47.1).[10] The occurrence of multiple esophageal septa has also been described.[21] Rarely, severe complications of medication-induced injury occur such as esophagorespiratory fistula, esophageal perforation, hemorrhage secondary to ulceration, and chronic stricture formation. Pathologically, esophageal biopsies in affected areas reveal dilated intercellular spaces and a predominance of T lymphocytes and eosinophils in a pattern different from other causes of esophagitis.[22]

Prevention, Treatment, and Clinical Course

No specific treatments have been shown to be beneficial in altering the course of medication-induced injury. Treatment is aimed at symptom control, prevention of superimposed injury from acid reflux, maintenance of adequate hydration, and removal of the offending medication. Symptom control may be achieved topically by local anesthetics such as viscous lidocaine solution. Occasionally, narcotics are necessary. Prevention of superimposed reflux is best achieved with twice-daily proton pump inhibitors (PPIs), although no data show that prevention of acid reflux hastens symptomatic or pathologic improvement of pill-induced injury. For patients who have severe odynophagia prohibiting adequate oral intake, IV hydration may be necessary for a few days. Removal of the cause of injury is self-evident, although this is not always easily achieved. This is particularly true in clinical situations in which there may not be an adequate substitute such as in aspirin prophylaxis for cardiovascular disease, bisphosphonates for severe osteoporosis, or high-dose NSAIDs for pain from chronic inflammatory arthritides. No data address the question of whether rechallenge with a pill that induced prior esophagitis poses higher risk of recurrent injury if the pill is taken with better caution, with the possible exception of bisphosphonates. It is also unclear if patients with a theoretical underlying risk (e.g., esophageal dysmotility) have a greater risk of esophagitis with rechallenge. In the absence of stricture formation or catastrophic presentation, most patients have clinical resolution of symptoms within 2–3 weeks, and radiographic resolution has been described in 7–10 days.[19]

Because no treatment has been proved effective, it is hoped that proper administration of potentially injurious medications will help avoid occurrence of esophageal injury. On the basis of the sometimes normally slow transit of medications through the esophagus, particularly for gelatin capsules and larger tablets,[3] the following recommendations are made: (1) Medications should be swallowed with at least 8 ounces of a clear liquid, (2) patients should remain upright for at least 30 minutes following ingestion of the medication, and (3) in patients with potential underlying

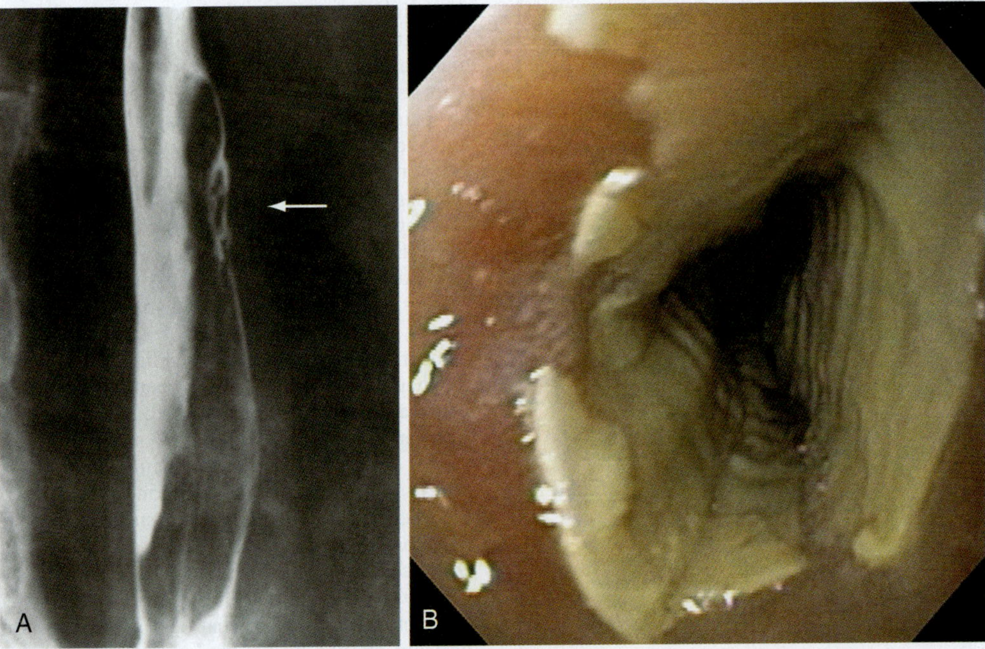

Fig. 47.1 (A) Barium esophagogram showing esophageal ulceration secondary to tetracycline, with the (*arrow*) pointing to an area of ulcerations. (B) Endoscopic image of a tetracycline-induced esophageal burn. ((A) Courtesy Dr. Marc Levine, Philadelphia, PA.)

increased risk for pill-induced injury (e.g., inability to follow the previous instructions, poor esophageal motility, anatomic compromise of the esophageal lumen), one should search for alternative safer medications or carefully weigh the risks and benefits of this medication against the disease for which this medication is necessary.

Specific Medications

Several broad categories of medication types cause esophageal injury. These include antibiotics, antivirals, NSAIDs, specific antiarrhythmic drugs, vitamins, and miscellaneous isolated drugs from varied categories.

Antibiotics

Tetracycline, doxycycline, and their derivatives are by far the most common causes of pill-induced esophagitis, with almost as many cases reported as all other cases combined (Box 47.1).[11] Its commonality of injury may be more a reflection of how frequently these drugs are used rather than a strong propensity of tetracycline to produce such injury. This relatively low incidence of esophageal ulceration from tetracycline for all users is suggested by a lack of any cases of esophageal injury seen in a recent survey of 491 Gulf War veterans treated with doxycycline.[2] Nevertheless, an increase in doxycycline-induced esophagitis was noted during the COVID epidemic.[23] The mechanism of injury is felt to be corrosive damage, because tetracycline dissolved in water produces a solution with a very low pH.[12] Symptoms may be acute in onset[24] and typically last several days to several weeks. Ulcerations may vary in appearance but are typically small and superficial, may have a "kissing" appearance, are located in the midesophagus just above the aortic arch or left mainstem bronchus,[10] and have a burn-like appearance (see Fig. 47.1). Stricture formation and mass appearance[25] are uncommon.

BOX 47.1 Medications Commonly Associated With Esophagitis or Esophageal Injury

ANTIBIOTICS

Clindamycin
Doxycycline
Penicillin
Rifampin
Tetracycline
Cloxacillin

ANTIVIRAL AGENTS

Nelfinavir
Zalcitabine
Zidovudine

BISPHOSPHONATES

Alendronate
Etidronate
Pamidronate

CHEMOTHERAPEUTIC AGENTS

Bleomycin
Cytarabine
Dactinomycin
Daunorubicin
5-Fluorouracil
Methotrexate
Vincristine
Crizotinib

NSAIDS

Aspirin
Ibuprofen
Naproxen

OTHER MEDICATIONS

Ascorbic acid
Ferrous sulfate
Lansoprazole
Multivitamins
Potassium chloride
Quinidine
Theophylline

Injury from other antibiotics is uncommon and mostly documented in case reports. These include clindamycin,[26,27] rifampin,[28] ciprofloxacin,[29] penicillins,[30,31] augmentin,[32] azithromycin,[33] and cloxacillin, but the incidence is still exceedingly low given their common use. If a history is compatible with pill-induced esophageal injury, any antibiotic currently being used should be considered a possible culprit, although rare.

Antiviral agents, particularly those used for treatment of HIV, also have been reported to cause medication-induced esophageal injury. These include zalcitabine,[34] zidovudine,[35] and nelfinavir.[36]

Bisphosphonates

The most rapidly emerging category of medication-induced esophagitis has been those injuries secondary to bisphosphonates used to treat osteoporosis. This class of medications has, in fact, become the most prevalent cause of medication-induced esophagitis.

To date, injury has been reported mostly with alendronate,[14,37–43] but also with etidronate[44] and pamidronate.[45] Although the overall incidence of injury is probably low (<100 cases reported)[11] when considering the millions of patients using the medication, injury can be serious and even fatal. Unfortunately, reflux-type symptoms are common and can be difficult to distinguish from medication-induced mucosal injury. Risedronate has low potential for causing esophageal injury, if at all.[46] Part of this might be explained by the rapid esophageal transit and subsequently minimal contact time of the drug with esophageal mucosa.[47] In 1 study prospectively following 255 patients treated with risedronate and undergoing endoscopy 8 and 15 days later, no patients developed esophageal ulceration. This study also underscored the overall safety of bisphosphonates in general in that only 3 of 260 patients receiving alendronate developed esophageal ulceration.[48]

Diagnosis is best made endoscopically, where marked exudates and inflammation are seen. Biopsies show an intense inflammatory exudate and granulation tissue that may contain polarizable crystals and multinucleated giant cells.[49] Stricture formation[50] occurs in up to one-third of patients,[11] and life-threatening hemorrhage,[41] Zenker diverticulitis (due to pill trapping),[51] and esophageal perforation[39] have been reported. Patients who sustain injury are commonly described to take the bisphosphonate not in accordance with directions (i.e., in the upright position with at least 8 ounces of beverage, remaining upright for at least 30 minutes). Still, as with other pill-induced esophagitis, patients taking the medication correctly may sustain esophageal injury. One question frequently answered anecdotally, but not clearly addressed scientifically, is whether patients with a history of GERD should avoid bisphosphonates. Furthermore, if GERD is a risk factor, it is unclear what degree of reflux constitutes risk. The decision should weigh the severity of osteoporosis and risk of fracture against the risk of esophagitis. Patients with GERD that predisposes to stasis, such as those with stricture or severe ineffective esophageal motility, should be particularly cautious.

NSAIDs

NSAIDs are another common cause of pill-induced esophageal injury. Similar to the other common causes of medication-induced esophageal injury, they occur in a small fraction of all NSAID users. Aspirin, naproxen, indomethacin, and ibuprofen account for the majority of cases,[11] but most other NSAIDs have been reported to cause esophageal injury in case reports. Not surprisingly, hemorrhage, which may be severe,[52] is a common complication of these esophageal ulcers, especially when compared with other medication causes of esophagitis. Bronchoesophageal fistula has also been reported.[53] Notably, it is over-the-counter use of NSAIDs that is most commonly associated with injury,[54] in keeping with their more commonly used venue.

In a study of 1122 patients hospitalized for GI bleeding, any dose of aspirin, including a low dose, was associated with increased risk of developing esophagitis.[55] Other studies have also identified NSAIDs in general as a risk factor for erosive esophagitis.[56] Whether the esophagitis in these studies is all directly due to these medications or whether they act synergistically with reflux-induced injury is unclear, although one study has suggested that aspirin makes the esophageal mucosa more sensitive to acid and pepsin.[57]

Other Medications

Potassium chloride (KCl) pills have been associated with esophageal injury. Injury can be severe, as documented by reports of esophageal stricture formation[58,59] or of perforation into the left atrium,[60] bronchial artery,[61] or mediastinum.[62] Patients who sustain esophageal injury from KCl pills commonly report associated conditions such as cardiac (including left atrial) enlargement or prior cardiac surgery.[63–65] Whether these processes truly predispose to pill stasis and injury because of extrinsic esophageal compression by the heart or because patients using KCl pills have a high prevalence of cardiac disease is still unclear.

Quinidine is another medication with the potential for severe esophagitis.[18] Endoscopically, quinidine may be associated with findings ranging from mild ulceration to a marked inflammatory response with edema suggesting carcinoma.[17,18] Ferrous sulfate,[66,67] theophylline,[68,69] oral contraceptives,[70] ascorbic acid,[30,71] mycophenolic acid,[72] and multivitamins[73] have caused esophageal ulceration. Numerous other medications have been reported to cause esophageal ulceration or perforation in single case reports. Examples include sildenafil,[74] phenytoin,[12] warfarin,[75] glyburide,[76] lansoprazole,[77] valproic acid,[78] chlorazepate,[79] captopril,[80] foscarnet,[81] deferasirox,[82] dabigatran,[83] paracetamol,[84] throat lozenges,[85,86] clopidogrel,[87] desloratadine,[88] calcium supplements,[89] and a caffeine pill.[90]

Chemotherapy-Induced Esophagitis

Dactinomycin, bleomycin, cytarabine, daunorubicin, 5-fluorouracil, methotrexate, vincristine, and chemotherapy regimens used in hematopoietic stem cell transplantation may cause severe odynophagia as a result of oropharyngeal mucositis, a process that can also involve the esophageal mucosa.[91] Esophageal damage is unusual in the absence of oral changes. Although mucositis is self-limited in most cases, some patients develop oral and esophageal damage that persists for weeks to months. Chemotherapy given months after thoracic irradiation to the esophagus, particularly doxorubicin, may cause a "recall" esophagitis. *Vinca* alkaloid drugs are neurotoxic, and dysphagia may complicate vincristine therapy.[92] Crizotinib, a tyrosine-kinase inhibitor used for non–small cell lung cancer, has been reported to cause severe ulcerative esophagitis similar to a more typical pill-induced esophagitis.[93–99] Finally, sharp-edged blister packs that contain medications have been reported to cause esophageal perforation.[100]

Esophageal Injury From Variceal Sclerotherapy

For many years, variceal sclerotherapy was the mainstay of therapy for endoscopic control of esophageal variceal bleeding. Although it is still an accepted form of therapy, it has been largely replaced by several other methods, including IV administration of octreotide, variceal banding, and transvenous intrahepatic portosystemic shunts. Nevertheless, its continued use by some physicians, as well as the occurrence of complications that may persist for several years, compels the gastroenterologist to recognize its various forms of potential esophageal injury.

Complications from variceal sclerotherapy can be divided into two main categories: gross structural injury and esophageal motility alterations. There is a wide range of gross injury from variceal injection. Injection of sclerosant into and around varices causes necrosis of esophageal tissues and mucosal ulceration; the risk is related to the number of injections and the amount of sclerosant. Small ulcers appear within the first few days after sclerotherapy in virtually all patients; larger ulcers develop in roughly one-half of patients. Other complications include intramural esophageal hematoma,[101] strictures,[102] and perforation.[103] Strictures occur in approximately 15% of patients undergoing sclerotherapy[102,104,105] and are usually amenable to Savary or balloon dilation. Unusual manifestations of sclerotherapy with deep needle penetration include pericarditis, esophageal-pleural fistula, pleural effusion, and tracheal obstruction due to compression by an intramural hematoma.[106,107] One case of squamous cell carcinoma of the esophagus was attributed to a course of variceal sclerotherapy 5 years earlier.[108]

Several studies have demonstrated abnormal esophageal motility after completed courses of sclerotherapy. These abnormalities may be related to wall injury or vagal dysfunction.[109] Specific motility abnormalities include delay in esophageal transit and decreased amplitude and coordination of esophageal contractions.[105,110] There is debate over whether these changes are reversible, with different studies demonstrating worsening[105] or resolution[111] of motility abnormalities over 4 weeks' time. Whether these motility changes reflect the effects of irreversible fibrosis or reversible inflammatory neuropathy is unclear. One potential consequence of motility dysfunction after sclerotherapy is the occurrence of pathologic gastroesophageal reflux, as documented by abnormal esophageal pH monitoring[112] and by abnormal scintigraphy and barium studies.[105] Other studies have also shown abnormal reflux following sclerotherapy that correlated with esophageal dysmotility and which did not occur in patients undergoing band ligation.[110] Furthermore, the amount of sclerosant injected paravariceally appears to correlate with increased acid reflux.[112]

The only agent that has been shown effective in preventing postsclerotherapy strictures and in healing ulcers is sucralfate, either alone or in combination with antacids and cimetidine.[113,114] Acid suppressive therapy alone, with either H2RAs or PPIs, has not been shown to be effective in preventing or healing post-sclerotherapy ulcers or strictures.[115,116]

ESOPHAGEAL INJURY FROM NASOGASTRIC AND OTHER NONENDOSCOPIC TUBES

NG tubes have long been recognized as a potential source of esophageal injury and stricture formation (Fig. 47.2). The putative mechanism is gastroesophageal reflux. In patients undergoing elective laparotomy, recent data have demonstrated an esophageal pH of less than 4 for nearly 9 of the first 24 hours compared with

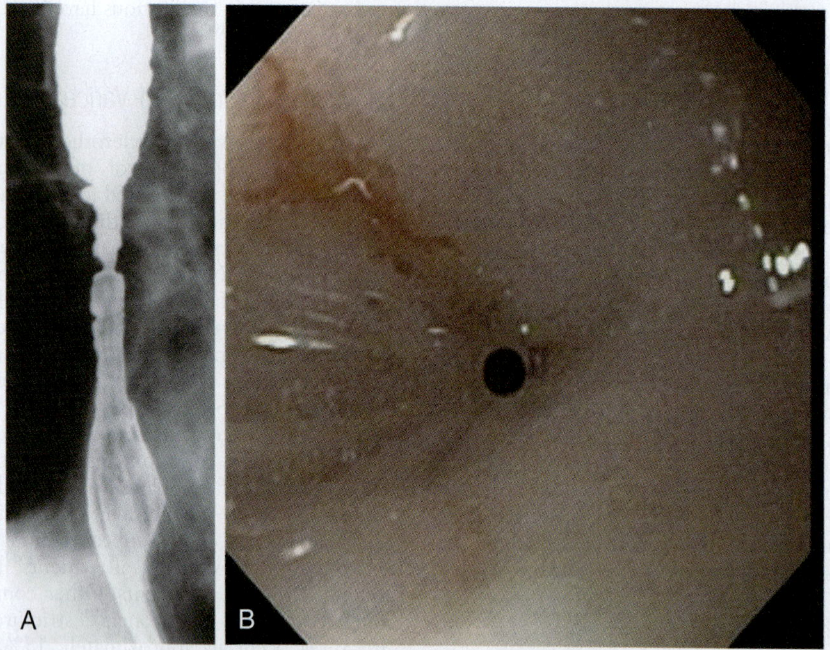

Fig. 47.2 (A) NG tube–induced stricture demonstrated by barium esophagography. (B) Endoscopic appearance of a tight NG tube–induced stricture. ((A) Courtesy Dr. Marc Levine, Philadelphia; (B) courtesy Dr. Gregory G. Ginsberg, Philadelphia, PA.)

less than 1.5 hours in a control group without tube placement.[117] One study demonstrated an increase in acid exposure even in normal volunteers undergoing NG tube placement.[118] When strictures occur, they are characteristically long, narrow, and difficult to manage endoscopically. Whether general use of potent acid-suppressing therapies has decreased the incidence of these strictures is unknown.

Respiratory luminal devices have also been reported as potential sources of esophageal trauma. Esophageal laceration with use of a Combitube,[119] tracheoesophageal fistula with a cuffed tracheal tube,[120] and esophageal perforation from a thoracostomy tube[121] or transesophageal echocardiography probes[122] have been reported.

More recently, several authors have reported the occurrence of an atrial-esophageal fistula complicating cardiac radiofrequency ablation procedures.[123–128] It is estimated to occur in 0.1% –0.25% of atrial fibrillation ablation procedures. This serious and often fatal complication has been described to occur anywhere from 10 days to 5 weeks after ablation. A shorter distance between the esophagus and the left atrium is associated with higher rates of esophageal thermal injury after radiofrequency ablation.[129] The initial presentation includes fever and neurologic abnormalities, the latter caused by air emboli to the brain from the esophagus through the fistula into the left heart. Laboratory studies may reveal leukocytosis and positive blood cultures. Imaging studies may reveal gas bubbles in the left atrium. Although generally fatal due to sepsis and upper GI hemorrhage, a recent report describes a patient who survived with surgical repair of the fistula,[126] suggesting that prompt recognition may reduce mortality. A case of intramural esophageal hematoma that resolved with conservative therapy has also been described.[130]

Finally, esophageal perforation may occur from probes used for transesophageal echocardiography.[131–133] Perforation may occur even without apparent resistance to passing the endoscope or a defined anatomic abnormality that would predispose to perforation.

ESOPHAGEAL INJURY FROM PENETRATING OR BLUNT TRAUMA

Noniatrogenic traumatic injury to the esophagus may occur through either penetrating or, less commonly, blunt injuries. Blunt trauma resulting in esophageal perforation is exceedingly rare; most cases have occurred in the cervical esophagus after motor vehicle accidents[134] and sometimes with delayed diagnosis.[135,136] Injury may result from the steering wheel,[137] seat belt,[138] or even from external vehicular impact.[139] Cervical esophageal transection due to shearing forces experienced with being thrown from a motorcycle has also been described.[140,141] Penetrating injuries to the esophagus are usually caused by gunshot or knife wounds, although cervical esophageal perforation secondary to cervical spine surgery has been well recognized.[142,143] In general, injuries from penetrating wounds are divided into those of the cervical and lower esophagus. Perforation of the cervical esophagus may be diagnosed initially by the finding of extramural air on radiographic studies such as lateral views of the neck or CT. Gastrografin contrast studies confirm the diagnosis, although this test is not always possible in patients with severe traumatic injuries. Although routine endoscopy is a relative contraindication in these patients, intraoperative endoscopy may be a valuable diagnostic tool for the diagnosis of perforation.[144] As with all esophageal perforations, an urgent treatment for blunt injuries improves survival.[145]

Cervical esophageal penetrating injuries are usually associated with concurrent tracheal, carotid, or spinal injury. One area of debate in the management of these injuries is whether surgical exploration is uniformly necessary. The concern in waiting is the development of sepsis, airway compromise, or tracheoesophageal fistulae,[146] estimated to occur in approximately 4% of penetrating esophageal wounds[147] and particularly in those patients undergoing tracheostomy for tracheal damage. Another downside of watchful waiting is the contamination of a previously sterile field. This may eliminate the option of primary closure and necessitate a two-step procedure, first with performance of a diverting cervical esophagostomy before definitive repair. As a result, some investigators continue to recommend an aggressive multimodal surgical approach.[142] In contrast, a recent study of 17 patients with cervical esophageal injury from knife or gunshot wounds suggested that conservative management with enteral feeding and antibiotics may allow for nonoperative healing.[148] A consensus seems to be that in those patients with contained small luminal cervical perforation, without sepsis and without the need for surgical exploration for other injuries, a conservative approach may be tried.[149]

For penetrating trauma to the more distal esophagus, similar principles apply but with some important differences. First, although diagnosis is often made by finding extraesophageal air on either chest radiographs or CT (or finding extravasation on contrast study of the esophagus), endoscopy may be performed, particularly for those unstable patients in whom contrast esophagography is not practical.[150] Some investigators feel that endoscopy should be the diagnostic test of choice.[144] Second, as opposed to a more contained perforation that occurs in the neck as dictated by its close tissue planes, perforation in the more distal esophagus may extend farther into the mediastinum and pleura. Also, there is a threat of coexistent injury to the aorta.

Third, because of the segmental and often variable esophageal blood supply (particularly in the distal esophagus), simple closure of a perforation is not often adequate owing to wound ischemia and consequent leakage.[151] As a result, esophageal resection with esophagogastric anastomosis is often necessary in these patients.[150] Fourth, because access to the esophagus through the mediastinum is so much more difficult than access through the neck, the consequences of perforation into the mediastinum, pleura, or aorta can be more devastating, and the surgery required for distal esophageal perforation may be much more extensive. As a result, the decision whether to operate is far more difficult. Despite these caveats, surgery is not only recommended in most patients[151,152] but must be performed in a timely fashion because there is significantly higher morbidity and mortality when surgery is delayed beyond 1–12 hours.[153] There may be a role for conservative management, with antibiotics and NG tube placement bypassing the perforation, in only a select group of patients. Finally, although metallic stents have been used successfully for nonoperative management of other causes of esophageal perforation,[154] their role in managing traumatic perforation of the esophagus is still evolving.

ESOPHAGEAL TEARS AND HEMATOMAS

Mallory-Weiss Syndrome

Mallory-Weiss (MW) syndrome (see Chapter 21) was originally described by Doctors Kenneth Mallory and Soma Weiss in 1929, who described patients with lacerations of the gastric cardia due to forceful vomiting.[155] The laceration is felt to result from shearing forces on the gastroesophageal junction and proximal stomach as it herniates through the diaphragm because of high intra-abdominal pressures due to forceful vomiting.[156,157] In accordance with Laplace's law, this shearing force has its greatest effect when there is a hiatal hernia, thereby exposing a relatively large-volume dilated sac to a high wall tension. Thus it is not surprising that the majority of patients who sustain a Mallory-Weiss tear have a hiatal hernia.[158] Although most tears will occur within 2 cm of the gastroesophageal junction, the likelihood of a more distal tear in the proximal portion of the stomach is increased when a larger hiatal hernia is present. Any bodily action that results in an abrupt increase in intra-abdominal pressure and gastric herniation may cause a Mallory-Weiss tear. Such actions include forceful coughing, straining, hiccupping,[159] retching during endoscopy, transesophageal echocardiography, and cardiopulmonary resuscitation.[156,160–165] Other factors that predispose to tearing include alcohol and aspirin use.[157,166,167]

Most patients present with hematemesis, but some present with melena alone. There is a tendency for MW tears to occur in middle-aged men.[168] Heavy drinking is a risk factor in men in contrast to underlying gastric disease in women.[169] Although a classic history includes vomiting or retching followed by hematemesis, up to a third of patients do not have an antecedent history of vomiting; hematemesis is their presenting symptom.[166,167] Iatrogenic tears have been reported after transesophageal echocardiography[170] and endoscopic submucosal dissection.[171] Typically, one laceration is seen at the time of endoscopy, most commonly along the lesser curve of the cardia, although more than one tear may occur in up to 10% of patients.[158] Bleeding is typically self-limited but may be massive in up to 10% of patients[158] and even fatal.[172] Endoscopy is also important not only for diagnosing a tear but also for ruling out other upper GI lesions that are found in more than a third of patients during the initial endoscopic evaluation. Such lesions include peptic ulcers, gastritis or gastropathy, erosive esophagitis, esophageal varices, and gastric outlet obstruction.

Treatment for Mallory-Weiss tear has usually been supportive because of the self-limited nature of the bleeding, along with attempts to reduce retching and vomiting. More recently, several methods of endoscopic therapy have been used. Thermal therapy has been used for some time. Injection of epinephrine and polidocanol and application of through-the-scope clips have been shown to significantly reduce bleeding and transfusion requirements and to shorten the hospital stay.[168,173] Endoscopic band ligation also has been shown to be efficacious[174,175] and in one trial was equivalent to injection therapy.[176] Endoscopic clip placement, an endoloop,[177,178] and endoscopic band ligation[179] have also been used as a therapeutic alternative for controlling bleeding from Mallory-Weiss tears.[180] For patients with persistent bleeding despite endoscopic therapy, angiographic embolization through the left gastric artery may be used.[181] The need for surgical intervention is rare.

Boerhaave Syndrome

A more extreme version of an esophageal tear that occurs from an acute increase in intra-abdominal pressure and accentuation of the intragastric-to-intrathoracic pressure gradient is Boerhaave syndrome. In this syndrome, a transmural tear with perforation occurs. The perforation specifically occurs at the margin of the contact between "clasp" and oblique esophageal fibers, typically at the left posterolateral wall of the distal one-third of the esophagus.[182] Similar to Mallory-Weiss syndrome, preceding symptoms, such as severe vomiting and retching, abdominal straining, blunt trauma, and coughing, may precipitate this perforation.[158] In addition to acute pressure changes at the gastroesophageal junction, some investigators have postulated that an abnormal esophageal mucosa may predispose to perforation. These conditions include reflux esophagitis,[183] Barrett esophagitis with ulceration,[184] infectious esophagitis,[185,186] and eosinophilic esophagitis.[187,188]

The clinical presentation is often catastrophic, with shock and sepsis due to a large esophageal perforation. Not surprisingly, death occurs in up to a third of patients.[189] Because of the acute presentation of severe chest pain, it is often confused with acute cardiac or pulmonary events, dissecting aortic aneurysm, or pancreatitis,[190] often leading to a delay in diagnosis and greater morbidity and mortality. Diagnosis is suggested by subcutaneous emphysema with crepitus and radiographic findings of pneumomediastinum and a left pleural effusion (that may contain salivary amylase, erroneously suggesting pancreatitis) or even a frank empyema. Perforation of the esophagus may be confirmed by esophageal contrast studies using Gastrografin. Management is generally surgical repair and drainage[191] with primary repair if treated early.[192] Successful nonoperative treatment with placement of a self-expandable covered metallic stent[193–196] and clip,[197,198] and in two patients, glue with chest drainage was used when detected early. Rarely, esophagectomy is needed.[199]

Spontaneous Esophageal Hematoma

Spontaneous esophageal hematoma is a rare entity in which an abrupt bleeding occurs between the mucosa and muscularis propria of the esophageal wall, often for a long length of the esophagus. The term *spontaneous* is somewhat of a misnomer as several underlying factors have been identified that predispose to hematoma formation. These include use of aspirin,[200–202] an underlying coagulopathy,[203] use of anticoagulants, including direct thrombin inhibitors,[204–206] preeclampsia,[207] or abrupt increases in the intra-abdominal-to-intrathoracic pressure gradient such as may occur with forceful vomiting, coughing, or sneezing,[208] and foreign body ingestion.[209] Not all cases have an obvious predisposing factor, however, and thus in essence, are spontaneous.[210] One-third of patients classically present with a triad of retrosternal chest pain, dysphagia, and hematemesis, and 50% present with at least two of these symptoms.[210] As in Boerhaave syndrome, there is often a delay in diagnosis because of the symptomatic overlap with more common cardiopulmonary catastrophes.[211] Interestingly, there may be a predisposition to this syndrome in middle-aged women, although this association is not uniform.[212–214] In one case, a Mallory-Weiss tear led to hemorrhagic shock from a large esophageal hematoma.[215]

Diagnosis can be made by several means. CT of the chest demonstrates a diffusely thickened esophagus and sometimes a "double barrel" appearance with obliteration of the esophageal lumen.[216] MRI also may be an accurate means of making the diagnosis.[217] Endoscopically, the obliteration of the esophageal lumen is seen with visualization of a long, deep, friable, blue submucosal mass with or without a visible tear.[209] Sometimes it may be difficult to distinguish hematoma from an esophageal malignancy.[218] Conservative treatment is the mainstay of treatment, maintaining the patient without oral intake and monitoring hemodynamic status,[209] usually taking up to several weeks to fully heal. Progress is monitored by repeated CT or endoscopy, usually at 1-week intervals. The need for surgical intervention is rare.

ESOPHAGEAL INFECTIONS IN THE IMMUNOCOMPETENT HOST

Esophageal infections are most common in immunocompromised patients, such as those infected with HIV (see Chapters 33 and 34) and those receiving chemotherapy or immunosuppressive therapies, particularly for hematologic malignancies or following organ transplantation (see Chapters 33 and 34) (Box 47.2). Nevertheless, there are some esophageal infections that occur in immunocompetent hosts. These include infections that (1) are more typically associated with immunodeficiency but are occasionally seen in patients with intact immune systems; (2) occur in patients with underlying esophageal diseases, particularly with those associated with prolonged stasis of luminal content; and (3) involve the esophagus because of a localized area of esophageal immune-compromise, such as with the use of inhaled topical steroids for respiratory disorders. The types of organisms found in these situations tend to be few in number, with *Candida* being the dominant organism.

BOX 47.2 Esophageal Infections in the Immunocompetent Host

TYPICALLY ASSOCIATED WITH IMMUNODEFICIENCY

HSV
- *Candida albicans*
- *Mycobacterium tuberculosis*

ASSOCIATED WITH ESOPHAGEAL STASIS (E.G., ACHALASIA AND SCLERODERMA)

Candida albicans

ASSOCIATED WITH USE OF GLUCOCORTICOID INHALERS

Candida albicans

OTHER ESOPHAGEAL INFECTIONS

Trypanosoma cruzi
Treponema pallidum
HPV

Candida albicans

Candidal organisms are the most common causes of esophageal infection in the immunocompetent host. Although several species of *Candida* have been implicated in esophageal infection, including *Candida tropicalis* and *Candida guilliermondii*,[219] *Candida albicans* accounts for the vast majority. In 1 large series of 933 patients in India with dysphagia or odynophagia, 56 were found to have candidal esophagitis of varying severity.[220] How many patients had clear motility disorders or *Candida* as a commensurate rather than a pathologic organism is not clear because *Candida* colonization of the esophagus in healthy ambulatory adults has a reported prevalence of approximately 20%.[221]

Although candidal esophagitis may occur rarely without a clear underlying mechanism, one should generally assume a predisposing condition, even in the immunocompetent host. The most common predisposing conditions are those associated with severe stasis such as achalasia or scleroderma (Fig. 47.3). In achalasia, infection seems related to severity, with those patients who have long-standing disease with marked esophageal dilation most at risk. These infections can be very difficult to treat medically without an effective achalasia therapy, and therefore the drainage of the esophagus is provided. *Candida* esophagitis is seen less often in scleroderma with esophageal involvement than in achalasia but, similarly, is usually seen in those patients with esophageal dilation and poor peristalsis. One risk factor for candidal infection in scleroderma might be acid suppression, as suggested by one study of patients with systemic sclerosis, in which the prevalence of *Candida* esophagitis was 44% (21 of 48 patients) for those on no acid suppression, compared with 89% (16 of 18 patients) among those on potent acid suppressive therapy.[222] Topical glucocorticoids (contained in inhalers for treatment of asthma) may lead to oropharyngeal and esophageal candidiasis in otherwise healthy adults.[223] Likewise, candidal esophagitis has been described and must be considered in patients with eosinophilic esophagitis treated with swallowed fluticasone.[224,225] Other medical illnesses that predispose to fungal esophagitis, albeit via impaired immune mechanisms, include diabetes mellitus, adrenal insufficiency, alcoholism, and advanced age.[226] Also, a rare condition known as *esophageal intramural pseudodiverticulosis* may be associated with candidal infection.[227] Diagnosis of candidal esophagitis can be made by its characteristic endoscopic appearance of white pseudomembranous or plaque-like lesions adherent to esophageal mucosa. Confirmation can be made by brushing the lesion, followed by cytology or biopsy, in which inflammation, hyphae, and masses of budding yeast are seen (not usually seen with colonization alone). The entity of the "black esophagus" (see later) has also been described with candidal esophagitis.[228] Although not as sensitive as endoscopy, candidal esophagitis may be diagnosed by double-contrast barium esophagography.[229] The characteristic findings are discrete plaque-like lesions oriented longitudinally,

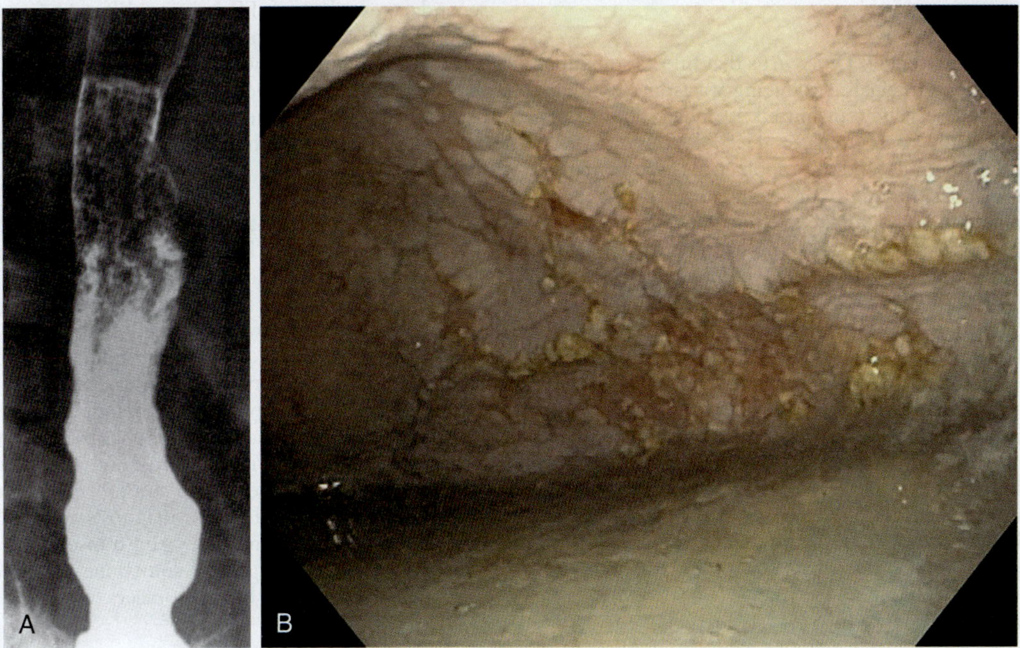

Fig. 47.3 (A) Achalasia with candidal infection demonstrated by barium esophagography. (B) Endoscopic photograph of a dilated esophagus with fluid, mucosal erosions, and *Candida* plaques in a patient with achalasia. ((A) Courtesy Dr. Marc Levine, Philadelphia, PA.)

with linear or irregular filling defects with distinct margins produced by trapped barium. Occasionally, mass-like lesions and strictures may be observed.

Treatment for most patients who have fungal esophagitis and have no immunologic deficiencies is with oral fluconazole or a topical antifungal agent. Fluconazole pills (100–200 mg/day) are commonly used because they are more convenient than topical therapy. The advantage of nonabsorbable topical agents is that they are virtually devoid of adverse effects and drug-drug interactions. Clotrimazole, a nonabsorbable imidazole, is well tolerated when delivered as a 10-mg buccal troche dissolved in the mouth 5 times daily for 1 week. Nystatin, a nonabsorbable polyene with a different mechanism of action and less palatability than clotrimazole, is also effective when used at a dose of 1 or 2 troches (each containing 200,000 units) 4 or 5 times daily for up to 14 days. There is some data to suggest that patients without immunocompromise and mild incidental candida colonization may not require a treatment.[230]

HSV

Herpes simplex esophagitis has been described in the immunocompetent host in a wide age range[231–235] and can represent either primary infection or, more commonly, a reactivation of latent virus in the distribution of the laryngeal, superior cervical, and vagus nerves. It may occur due to close physical contact or common exposure[236] and has been associated with eosinophilic esophagitis.[237,238] All ages are affected, and oropharyngeal lesions are found in only one in five cases. Severe odynophagia, heartburn, and fever are the dominant symptoms. Nausea, vomiting, and chest pain also may occur. The endoscopic appearance is characterized by diffuse friability, round or linear ulceration, and exudates, mostly in the distal esophagus. Classically, the earliest esophageal lesions are rounded 1–3-mm vesicles in the mid- to distal esophagus, the centers of which slough to form discrete circumscribed ulcers with raised edges. These lesions can also be appreciated radiographically. The appearance of a "black esophagus" has also been reported with HSV.[228,239] HSV esophagitis may be diagnosed by several methods. These include (1) characteristic viral cytopathic effect and/or demonstration of viral particles by electron microscopy on esophageal brushing or biopsy; (2) isolation by culture of HSV from mucosal biopsies; (3) HSV DNA detection in esophageal tissue by PCR; (4) demonstration of HSV through techniques of immunohistochemistry in esophageal tissue; and (5) isolation of HSV from oropharyngeal secretions in the setting of stomatitis and multiple esophageal ulcers.[240] Histologic stains of HSV-infected epithelial cells demonstrate multinucleated giant cells, ballooning degeneration, "ground glass" intranuclear Cowdry type A inclusion bodies, and margination of chromatin. Immunohistologic stains using monoclonal antibodies to HSV antigens or in situ hybridization techniques may improve the diagnostic yield in difficult cases by identifying infected cells that lack characteristic morphologic changes.

Most patients have self-limited disease paralleling concordant nasolabial herpes, if present, but upper GI bleeding and perforation have been reported.[231] Treatment for herpetic esophagitis is the same as other herpes simplex infections in the immunocompetent host, such as prompt initiation of a 7–10-day course of orally administered acyclovir or valacyclovir. Occasionally, severe odynophagia necessitates initial treatment with IV acyclovir, 250 mg/m^2 every 8 hours, and then changing to oral therapy when the patient can take oral medication. Given the relative rarity of esophageal involvement, however, no outcome data exist specifically on treating esophageal herpes simplex infection.

CMV

CMV is a member of the herpes virus family and is most commonly associated with esophageal infection in immunocompromised patients (see Chapters 33–35) including malignancy, steroid or chemotherapy use and organ or bone marrow transplantation[241] in addition to HIV infection. A recent case series, however, documented esophageal ulceration from CMV in four apparently immunocompetent patients.[242] All had a good response to antiviral therapy.

HPV

HPV is a small double-stranded DNA virus that infects squamous epithelium of healthy individuals, producing warts and condylomata. The virus can be sexually transmitted. Esophageal infections with HPV are typically asymptomatic. HPV lesions are most frequently found in the mid- to distal esophagus as erythematous macules, white plaques, nodules, or exuberant frond-like lesions.[243] In one patient, a papilloma developed at a sclerotherapy injection site.[244] The diagnosis is made by histologic demonstration of koilocytosis (an atypical nucleus surrounded by a ring), giant cells, or by immunohistochemical stains. Treatment is often not necessary, although large lesions have required endoscopic removal. Other treatments, such as those using systemic interferon (IFN)-α, bleomycin, and etoposide, have yielded varying results.[245] One patient had numerous lesions in the esophagus and upper airway that were unresponsive to all forms of therapy and was eventually fatal.[246]

HPV infection has been implicated as a risk factor for squamous cell carcinoma, particularly carcinoma of the uterine cervix. An association between HPV and squamous cell carcinoma of the esophagus has been demonstrated by PCR or in situ DNA hybridization in esophageal tumor specimens from South Africa, northern China, and Alaska.[247] In contrast, HPV DNA was not found in or near esophageal squamous cell carcinomas from continental Europe, the United States, Japan, or Hong Kong,[248,249] and its relation to esophageal cancer has been questioned.[250]

Other Infections

Trypanosoma cruzi

Chagas disease (see Chapter 115) is the result of progressive destruction of mesenchymal tissues and nerve ganglion cells throughout the body by *Trypanosoma cruzi*, a parasite endemic to South America. Abnormalities of the heart, esophagus, gallbladder, and intestines are the clinical consequence. Esophageal manifestations may appear 10–30 years after the acute infection and typically include difficulty swallowing, chest pain, cough, and regurgitation. Nocturnal aspiration is common. Esophageal manometric recordings are identical to findings in achalasia, although the lower esophageal sphincter pressure is lower in Chagas disease.[251] Manometric abnormalities of the esophagus can be found in asymptomatic seropositive patients.[252] The putative mechanism for disease is the development of antimuscarinic receptor antibodies in response to the infection.[253] A chagasic esophagus may be responsive to nitrates, balloon dilation, or, ultimately, myectomy at the gastroesophageal junction.[254] Patients who have intractable symptoms or pulmonary complications secondary to megaesophagus may be candidates for esophagectomy.[255] Those with long-standing stasis due to Chagas disease often have hyperplasia of esophageal squamous epithelia and are at increased risk for esophageal squamous cell cancer as in achalasia.

Mycobacterium tuberculosis

Most reports of esophageal *M. tuberculosis* infections are from areas of endemic TB. Esophageal manifestations of TB are almost exclusively a result of direct extension from adjacent mediastinal structures, but there are well-documented cases of primary esophageal TB.[256,257] The clinical presentation of secondary esophageal TB is quite different from those of most other causes of infectious esophagitis. Specifically, dysphagia is often accompanied by weight loss, cough, chest pain, and fever. Subsequent complications include bleeding, perforation, and fistula formation.[257] Choking on swallowing may be indicative of an underlying fistula between the esophagus and respiratory tract.

Other radiographic findings include displacement of the esophagus by mediastinal lymph nodes and sinus tracts extending into the mediastinum. The presentation may mimic cancer with an ulcerating mass lesion and paratracheal adenopathy on CT imaging.[258] Endoscopy is often necessary to confirm active TB; caution is advised to prevent infection of medical staff by aerosolized tubercle bacilli. Endoscopic findings include shallow ulcers, heaped-up lesions mimicking neoplasia, and extrinsic compression of the esophagus.[259] Lesions should be biopsied and brushed thoroughly, and specimens should be obtained for acid-fast stain, mycobacterial culture, and PCR, in addition to routine studies. When extrinsic compression is the only esophageal manifestation of TB, the diagnosis must be confirmed by bronchoscopy, mediastinoscopy, or transesophageal FNA cytologic evaluation.[260] Surgery is sometimes required to repair fistulas, perforations, and bleeding ulcers.

Treponema pallidum

Syphilis, which became increasingly prevalent in the United States in the 1990s, can rarely cause esophageal disease in immunocompetent individuals. Earlier literature described gummas, diffuse ulceration, and strictures of the esophagus in tertiary syphilis.[261] The diagnosis of syphilitic esophagus should be considered when a patient has an inflammatory stricture and other evidence of tertiary syphilis. Histologic evaluation may show perivascular lymphocytic infiltration; however, specific immunostaining should be done if this diagnosis is a possibility.

Rare Infections

Viral infections that rarely affect the esophagus in the immunocompetent adult include herpes zoster and EBV,[262,263] both of which may produce ulceration. Cytomegaloviral ulcerative esophagitis has also been described in an immunocompetent patient on glucocorticoids.[264] Rare fungal infections of the esophagus include blastomycosis, presenting as an esophageal mass,[265] and histoplasmosis, through direct extension of mediastinal adenopathy similar to TB.[266]

ACUTE ESOPHAGEAL NECROSIS

Acute esophageal necrosis (AEN, black esophagus) is a rare, poorly understood disorder. Ischemia, increased gastric acid exposure, and impaired mucosal barrier are thought to play a role in its pathogenesis,[267] though other etiologies suggested have included severe reflux and CMV.[268] Settings in which black esophagus have been described include diabetes mellitus, hematologic and solid organ malignancy, malnutrition, renal insufficiency, cardiovascular compromise, trauma, and hypercoagulation.[269] Treatment of the AEN is comprised of supportive management with intravenous fluids, PPI, sucralfate, parenteral nutrition, and antacids.[270]

Full references for this chapter can be found at https://ebooks.health.elsevier.com.

48 Gastroesophageal Reflux Disease

Joel E. Richter, Michael F. Vaezi

IN THIS CHAPTER

Gastroesophageal reflux (GER) is a physiologic process by which gastric contents move retrograde from the stomach to the esophagus. GER itself is not a disease and occurs multiple times each day without producing symptoms or mucosal damage. In contrast, GERD (GER disease) is considered to be a spectrum of disorders usually producing symptoms of heartburn and acid regurgitation. GERD is a consequence of the failure of the normal antireflux barrier to protect against frequent and abnormal amounts of refluxed material. Most patients have no visible mucosal damage at the time of endoscopy, whereas others have esophagitis, peptic strictures, or Barrett's esophagus. Other symptoms of GER may include chest pain or evidence of extraesophageal manifestations, such as pulmonary, ear, nose, or throat symptoms. GERD is a multifactorial process and one of the most common gastrointestinal diseases. In 2009 there were 8.9 million outpatient clinic visits for GERD in the United States, which was the leading diagnosis for all GI disorders.[1]

EPIDEMIOLOGY

Prevalence of Symptoms and GERD Complications

Accurate prevalence rates for GERD are difficult to ascertain with precision because many affected individuals, even those with Barrett's esophagus, have no symptoms. Furthermore, data based on objective tests, such as endoscopy (i.e., esophagitis) and esophageal pH testing, are impractical in large screening populations.[2]

On the basis of symptoms, the pooled prevalence of at least weekly GERD symptoms reported from population-based studies worldwide is approximately 13%, but there is considerable geographic variation (Fig. 48.1).[3] Heterogeneity in study designs makes it difficult to get an accurate measurement, but the prevalence of GERD is highest in South Asia and Southeast Europe (more than 25%) and lowest in Southeast Asia, Canada, and France (less than 10%). There are no prevalence data from Africa. The prevalence of at least weekly GERD in the United States is approximately 20%,[4] but prevalence estimates have ranged from 6% to 30% due to variability in questionnaires used, including the frequency and the duration of symptoms required to define GERD.[3] There are approximately 110,000 hospital admissions annually in the United States for GERD.[5] Importantly, the prevalence of GERD symptoms in North America, Europe, and Southeast Asia has increased by nearly 50% relative to the prevalence in the early-to-middle 1990s but has since plateaued.[4]

The predominant complications of GERD are reflux esophagitis, peptic strictures, Barrett's esophagus, and esophageal cancer. The true prevalence of esophagitis is very difficult to define because healthy subjects rarely undergo upper endoscopy. In three population-based studies of patients undergoing endoscopy regardless of symptoms, the prevalence of erosive esophagitis ranged from 6.4% in China to 15.5% in Sweden.[6–8] In asymptomatic subjects, the prevalence of erosive esophagitis ranged from 6.1% in China to 9.5% in Sweden. Erosive esophagitis may be a transient phenomenon—25% of subjects with nonerosive reflux disease at baseline had esophagitis on endoscopy 2 years later, and another study with similar designs found a 10% rate at 5 years.[9,10] Recurrent peptic strictures requiring repeat endoscopic dilation decreased from 16% in 1992 to 8% in 2000, possibly related to the increased use of PPIs.[11] From 2003 to 2006, there were approximately 10,570 hospital admissions annually for erosive esophagitis and 14,000 admissions for esophageal stricture.[5] Deaths are rare from erosive esophagitis, about 2.1 per million in 1988–1992.[5]

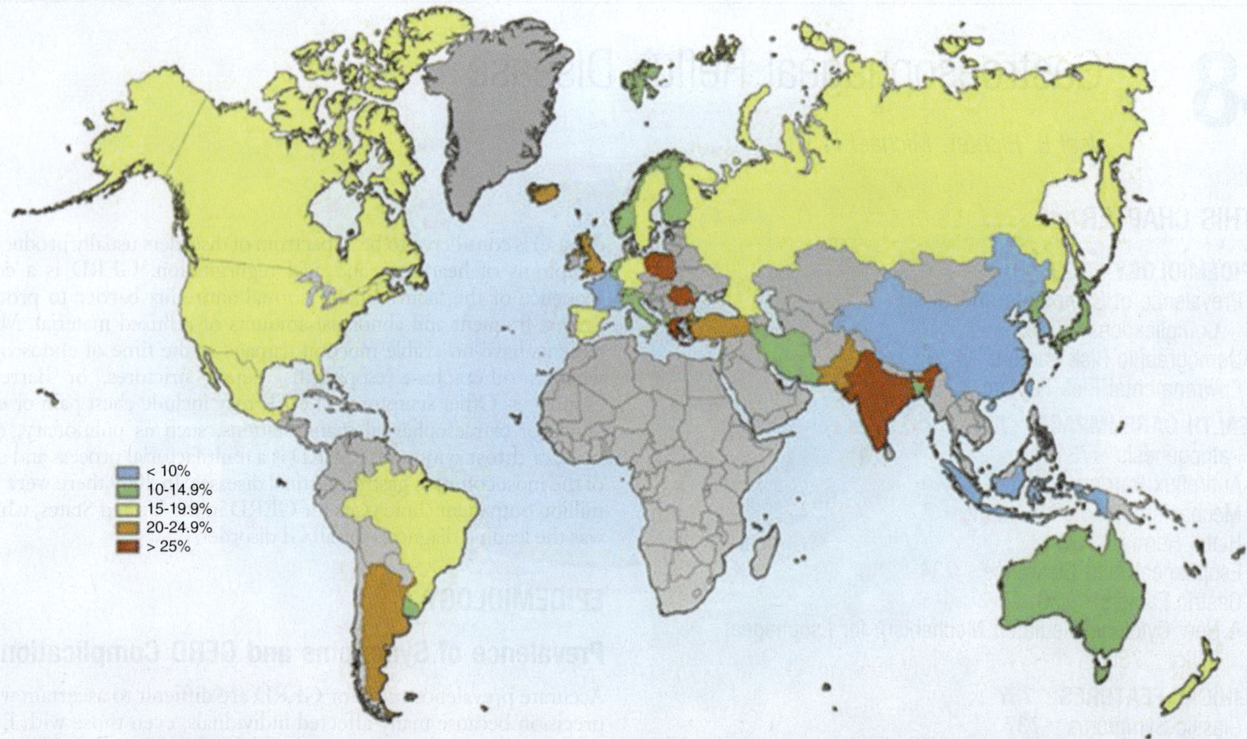

Fig. 48.1 Prevalence of weekly gastroesophageal reflux symptoms worldwide, based on symptoms at a frequency of once a week or more. Map lines delineate study areas and do not necessarily depict accepted national boundaries. (From Richter JE, Rubenstein JH. Presentation and epidemiology of gastroesophageal reflux disease. *Gastroenterology*. 2018;143:1179–1187.)

Demographic Risk Factors

There are a number of well-recognized risk factors for GERD and its complications. Gender is not a factor in North America and Europe, but women have a 40% higher rate of GERD symptoms compared with men in South America and the Middle East.[3] There is no clear association between gender and peptic stricture,[5] but men are at a greater risk of esophagitis, Barrett's esophagus, and adenocarcinoma than women.[12] Advancing age has been inconsistently associated with an increase in GERD symptoms but is strongly associated with complications of GERD, including esophagitis, esophageal stricture, and Barrett's esophagus with cancer.[3,5] In the United States, there appears to be a similar prevalence of GERD symptoms among different races,[12] but whites are at a greater risk for erosive esophagitis, Barrett's esophagus, and adenocarcinoma of the esophagus.

Environmental Risk Factors

The prevalence of GERD is increasing in Western countries,[4] and the two major factors likely to explain this trend are the obesity epidemic and decreasing prevalence of Hp-associated gastritis. Obesity is a major risk factor for GERD symptoms (odds ratio 1.73), erosive esophagitis (odds ratio 1.59), Barrett's esophagus (odds ratio, 1.24), and esophageal adenocarcinoma (odds ratio 2.45).[3,13] Central obesity, as measured by the waist-to-hip ratio, may be more important than BMI in association with complicated GERD.[13] Several mechanisms have been proposed to explain the association between central obesity and GERD: increased intragastric pressure that overwhelms the reflux barrier[14] and production by the visceral fat of a variety of cytokines, including interleukin-6 (IL-6) and TNF-α, which may modulate lower esophageal sphincter (LES) pressure, and contribute to insulin resistance.[15] Observational studies have shown that reducing the BMI by at least 3.5 kg/m^2 increased the odds for resolution of GERD symptoms by 1.5–2.4-fold.[16] Randomized trials have confirmed that weight loss, especially a decrease in waste circumference, results in improved GERD symptoms and decrease in esophageal acid exposure.[16]

In addition to the increasing prevalence of obesity, the falling prevalence of Hp gastritis might explain the trends in GERD and its complications (see Pathogenesis—Gastric Factors).[17] The gastric atrophy associated with Hp infection appears to be inversely related to erosive esophagitis,[18] Barrett's esophagus, and esophageal adenocarcinoma.[19,20] However, there is a much stronger inverse association in East Asia than in North America and equivocal association in Europe.

There are additional environmental exposures that are associated with GERD, but they are relatively weak and unpredictable across populations. Certain forms of physical activity may increase GER symptoms in susceptible individuals, such as stooped posture, bicycle riding, weight lifting, and swimming.[21] On the other hand, moderate, regular aerobic exercise has been inversely associated with GERD symptoms.[22] Tobacco use is weakly associated with GERD symptoms in cross-sectional studies (summary odd ratio, 1.26).[3] This relationship is supported by an 18-year longitudinal study in which decreased tobacco smoking was associated with a threefold decrease in GERD symptoms when compared with individuals who continued to smoke tobacco.[23] Similarly, in observational studies, alcohol use was not strongly associated with GERD symptoms (summary odds ratio, 1.11).[3] Although patients often report worse symptoms after red wine than white (perhaps related to the tannins in red wine), a randomized trial found that red wine had less effect on LES pressure and acid reflux than white wine.[24] Tobacco is an important risk factor for erosive esophagitis and esophageal adenocarcinoma, but there is no relationship between alcohol and erosive esophagitis or Barrett's esophagus.[2]

Along with environmental factors, the epidemiology of GERD may be affected by genetics. Family clustering of GERD and its complications, especially Barrett's esophagus, have been reported.[25,26] Two large case-control studies of twins from the United States and Sweden suggest the genetic liability for GERD in the range of 30%–45%.[27,28] The genetic mechanisms are unknown but may be related to a smooth muscle disorder associated with hiatal hernia, reduced LES pressure, and impaired motility.

HEALTH CARE IMPACT

Although rarely a cause of death, GERD is associated with considerable morbidity and complications, such as esophageal ulceration (5%), peptic stricture (4%–20%), and Barrett's esophagus (8%–20%).[2] Not surprisingly, the burden of GERD on health care is great. In 2009 GERD was the most common digestive disease diagnosis during ambulatory care visits.[1] For GI disorders, GERD was the 13th most common principal diagnosis at discharge, with an estimated total number per year of 66,000, a 2-day median length of stay, and a median cost of $4366.[1] As a secondary discharge diagnosis, it was the most common GI disorder and was listed 4.5 million times, threefolds higher than any other diagnosis.[1] During the years 2005–2010 in the United States, the indication for nearly one in four upper endoscopy exams was to evaluate reflux symptoms.[29] The total cost per patient in 2005 for PPI therapy in the United States was estimated to be $2040.[30] The economic burden may even be higher for patients with suspected extraesophageal GERD. During the initial first years, a Vanderbilt study found the direct costs were 5.6 times higher for extraesophageal GERD patients ($5154) than those reported for typical GERD ($971).[31]

An economic survey from Germany reported that 6% of individuals with established GERD missed at least 1 day of work per year due to this disorder; 61% of these patients visited their physician at least once in the previous year, and 2% were hospitalized specifically for GERD.[32] They estimated direct and indirect costs approximate $600 per patient per year. Data from the United States suggest that GERD has a relatively modest impact on work impairment.[1] A recent multinational survey revealed that workers with intense GERD symptoms miss an average of 2 hours of work per week as a direct result.[33]

GERD has been shown to significantly impair quality of life. Not surprisingly, GERD patients who fail to respond to antisecretory therapy have a lower quality of life, both mentally and physically, than responders.[34] GERD comorbidities are common and include irritable bowel syndrome and psychological distress in 36% and 41% of patients, respectively.[35] These comorbidities can potentiate the negative effect on quality of life seen with GERD and may affect the response to treatment with PPIs.

Pathogenesis

The pathogenesis of GERD is complex, resulting from an imbalance between defensive factors protecting the esophagus (antireflux barriers, esophageal acid clearance, and tissue resistance) and aggressive factors refluxing from the stomach (gastric acidity, volume, and duodenal contents).

Antireflux Barriers

The first tier of the 3-tiered esophageal defense against acid damage—the antireflux barriers—is an anatomically complex region, including the intrinsic LES, diaphragmatic crura, intra-abdominal location of the LES, the phrenoesophageal ligaments, and the acute angle of His.

The LES involves the distal 3–4 cm of the esophagus and at rest is tonically contracted.[36] It is the major component of the antireflux barrier, being capable of preventing reflux even when completely displaced from the diaphragmatic crura by a hiatal hernia.[37] The proximal portion of the LES is normally 1.5–2 cm above the squamocolumnar junction, whereas the distal segment, about 2 cm in length, lies within the abdominal cavity. Anatomic studies attribute this portion of the antireflux barrier to a fold-like function related to the opposing sling and clasp fibers of the gastric cardia. This location maintains gastroesophageal competence during intra-abdominal pressure excursions. Resting LES pressure ranges from 10 to 30 mm Hg, with a generous reserve capacity because only a pressure of 5–10 mm Hg is necessary to prevent GER.[38] The LES maintains a high-pressure zone by the intrinsic tone of its muscle and by cholinergic excitatory neurons.[39] There is considerable diurnal variation in basal LES pressure; it is lowest after meals and highest at night, and large increases occur with phase III of the migrating motor complex. It is also influenced by circulating peptides and hormones, foods (particularly fat), and a number of drugs.

The LES lies within the hiatus created by the right crus of the diaphragm and is anchored by the phrenoesophageal ligaments, which insert at the level of the squamocolumnar junction (Table 48.1). The hiatus is a teardrop shaped canal of about 2 cm along its major axis.

Developmentally, the crural diaphragm arises from the dorsal mesentery of the esophagus and is innervated separately from the costal diaphragm. It is inhibited by esophageal distention, by vomiting, and during transient LES relaxations (tLESRs), but not during swallowing. The crural diaphragm provides extrinsic squeeze to the intrinsic LES, contributing to resting pressure during inspiration and augmenting LES pressure during periods

TABLE 48.1 Modulators of Lower Esophageal Sphincter Pressure

	Increase LES Pressure	Decrease LES Pressure
Hormones/ peptides	Gastrin Motilin Substance P	CCK Secretin Somatostatin Vasoactive intestinal peptide
Neural agents	α-Adrenergic agonists β-Adrenergic antagonists Cholinergic agonists	α-Adrenergic antagonists β-Adrenergic agonists Cholinergic antagonists
Foods and nutrients	Protein	Chocolate Fat Peppermint
Other factors	Antacids Baclofen Cisapride Domperidone Histamine Metoclopramide Prostaglandin $F_{2\alpha}$	Barbiturates Calcium channel blockers Diazepam Dopamine Meperidine Morphine Prostaglandins E_2 and I_2 Serotonin Theophylline

LES, Lower esophageal sphincter.

of increased abdominal pressure, such as with coughing, sneezing, or bending.[39] Crural contractions impose rhythmic pressure increases of about 5–10 mm Hg on the LES pressure recording. During deep inspirations and some periods of increased abdominal straining, these changes may lead to pressures of 50–150 mm Hg.[40]

The oblique entrance of the esophagus into the stomach creates a sharp angle on the greater curve aspect of the gastroesophageal junction, the angle of His. This angle has been shown in cadavers to create a flap valve effect; however, the contribution to gastroesophageal junction competency remains unclear.[41]

Mechanisms of Reflux

Reflux usually occurs via four mechanisms: tLESR, low LES pressure, swallow-associated LES relaxation, and straining during periods of low LES pressure.[42]

Transient Lower Esophageal Sphincter Relaxations

tLESRs are the most frequent mechanism for reflux in patients with healthy sphincter pressures (Fig. 48.2). tLESRs occur independently of swallowing, are not accompanied by esophageal peristalsis, persist longer (>10 seconds) than swallow-induced LESRs, and are accompanied by inhibition of the crural diaphragm.[43] tLESRs account for nearly all reflux episodes in healthy subjects and 50%–80% of episodes in GERD patients, depending on the presence of hiatal hernia and severity of associated esophagitis (Fig. 48.3).[44] However, one study suggests that low basal LES pressure, rather than tLESRs, may be the primary mechanism of GER in patients with nonreducible hiatal hernias (see Fig. 48.3).[45]

tLESRs are not always associated with GER. In normal subjects, 40%–60% of tLESRs are accompanied by reflux episodes, compared with 60%–70% in GERD patients.[44,46] Possible factors

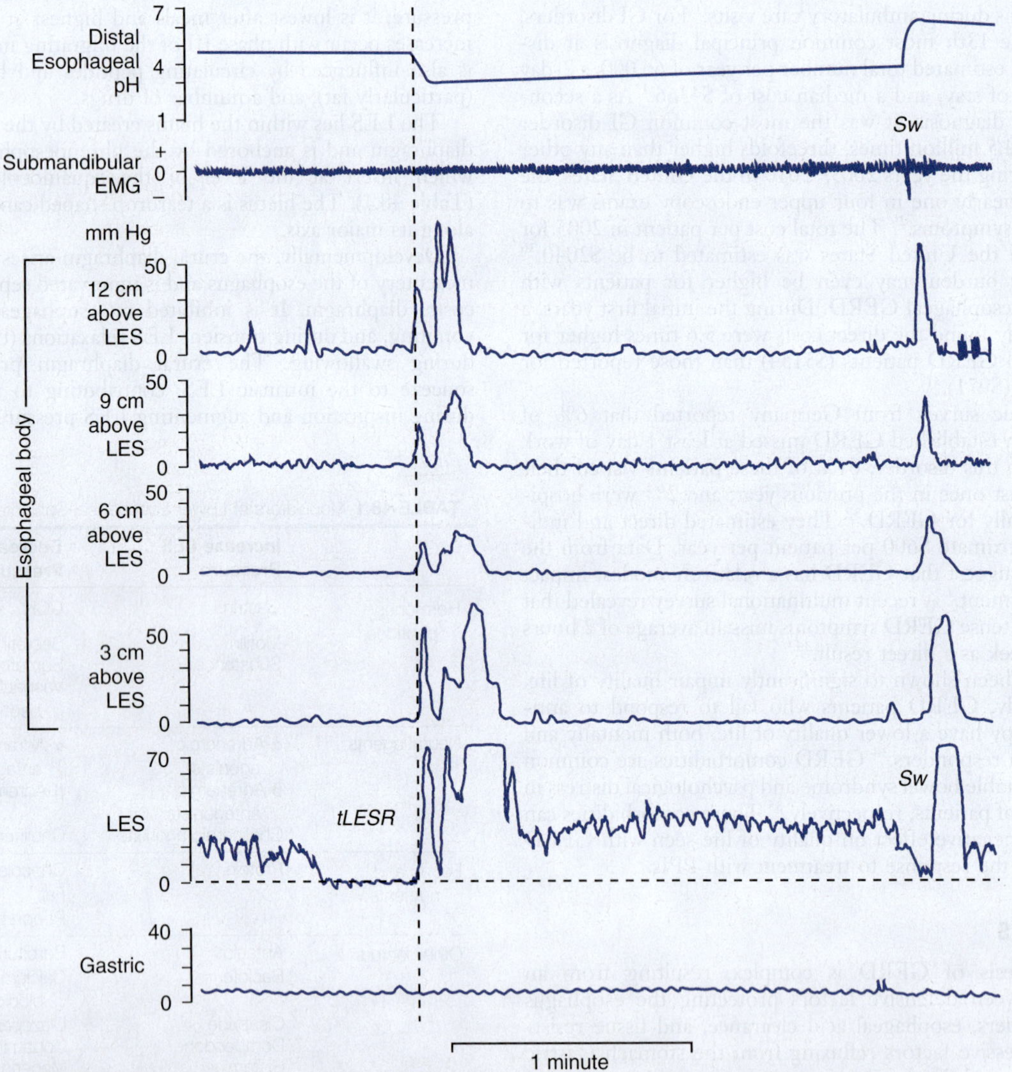

Fig. 48.2 Example of a transient lower esophageal sphincter relaxation (tLESR) on an esophageal manometry study. Lower esophageal sphincter (LES) pressure is referenced to gastric pressure, which is indicated by the *horizontal dashed line*. Note that the tLESR persisted for almost 30 seconds, whereas the swallow-induced LESR to the right (Sw) persisted for only 5 seconds. Moreover, note the absence of a submandibular electromyographic (EMG) signal during the tLESR, which indicates absence of a pharyngeal swallow. Finally, the associated esophageal motor activity is different in the two types of LESR: the swallow-induced relaxation is associated with primary peristalsis, whereas the tLESR is associated with a vigorous, repetitive "off contraction" throughout the esophageal body. (From Kahrilas PJ, Gupta RR. Mechanisms of reflux of acid associated with cigarette smoking. *Gut*. 1990;31:4.)

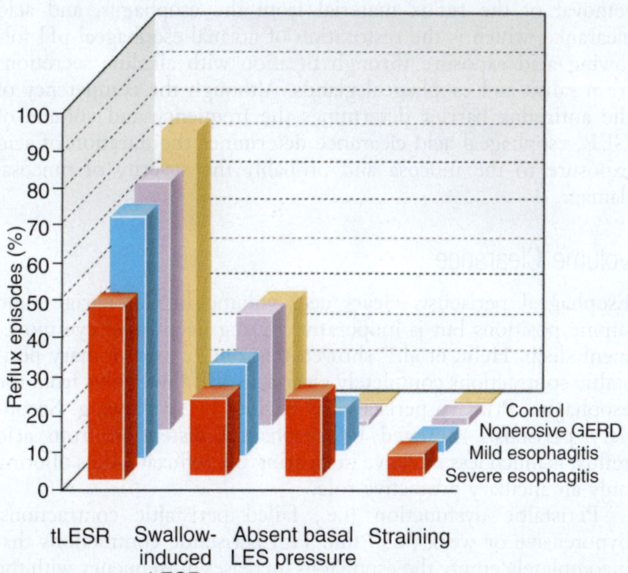

Fig. 48.3 Percentage of reflux episodes in control subjects and in patients with gastroesophageal reflux disease (GERD) occurring by the following mechanisms: transient lower esophageal sphincter relaxation (tLESR), swallow-induced LESR, absent basal lower esophageal sphincter (LES) pressure, and straining in the presence of low LES pressure. (From Holloway RH. The antireflux barrier and mechanisms of gastro-oesophageal reflux. *Ballieres Clin Gastroenterol.* 2000;14:681–699.)

determining whether reflux occurs include abdominal straining, the presence of a hiatal hernia, degree of esophageal shortening, and duration of tLESRs. The dominant stimulus for a tLESR is distention of the proximal stomach by either food or gas, which is not surprising given that a tLESR is the underlying mechanism of belching. Stretch receptors seem to be more relevant than tension receptors in triggering tLESRs.[39] More varying stimuli are dietary fat, stress, and subthreshold (for swallowing) stimulation of the pharynx.[47] Various drugs may reduce tLESRs, including CCK A (CCK-1) receptor antagonists, anticholinergic drugs, morphine, somatostatin, nitric oxide inhibitors, 5-hydroxytryptamine 3 antagonists, and γ-aminobutyric acid ($GABA_B$) agonists.[47]

The dominant stimulus for tLESRs is distension of the proximal stomach, which activates mechanoreceptors in the intraganglionic lamellar endings of vagal afferents.[48] These fibers project eventually to the brainstem and the dorsal motor nuclei of the vagus. These neurons project to the inhibitory neurons localized in the myenteric plexus of the distal esophagus. This results in an integrated motor response involving LES relaxation, longitudinal muscle contractions reducing esophagogastric junction (EGJ) obstruction and repositioning the LES above the crura, crural diaphragm inhibition, and contraction of the costal diaphragm.[49] Several neurotransmitters are involved in the control of tLESRs, including GABA, glutamate, and endocannabinoids.[50]

Swallow-Induced Lower Esophageal Sphincter Relaxations

About 5%–10% of reflux episodes occur during swallow-induced LESRs. Most episodes are associated with defective or incomplete peristalsis.[46] During a normal swallow-induced LESR, reflux is uncommon because (1) the crural diaphragm does not relax, (2) the duration of LESR is relatively short (5–10 seconds), and (3) reflux is prevented by the oncoming peristaltic wave (see right side of tracing in Fig. 48.2). Reflux during swallow-induced LESRs is more common with a hiatal hernia. This may be due to the lower compliance of the EGJ in hernia patients, permitting it to open at pressures equal to or lower than intragastric pressure, thereby allowing reflux of gastric juices accumulating in the hiatal hernia.[43,51]

Hypotensive Lower Esophageal Sphincter Pressure—Strained-Induced or Free Reflux

GER can occur in the context of a hypotensive LES by either strain-induced or free reflux.[45,52] Strain-induced reflux occurs when a relatively hypotensive LES is overcome by an abrupt increase in intra-abdominal pressure from coughing, straining, or bending over. This type of reflux is unlikely when the LES pressure is greater than 10 mm Hg, and there is no hiatal hernia.[42] Free reflux is characterized by a fall in intraesophageal pH without an identifiable change in intragastric pressure, usually occurring when LES pressure is less than 5 mm Hg. Reflux due to a low or absent LES pressure is uncommon, usually observed in patients with end-stage scleroderma or after myotomy for achalasia.[44] Mostly it occurs in patients with severe esophagitis, in whom it may account for up to 25% of reflux episodes; it rarely occurs in patients without esophagitis.[44]

These last three reflux mechanisms are nearly always seen in association with the presence of a hiatal hernia. These observations support the concept that the functional integrity of the EGJ depends on the intrinsic LES and extrinsic sphincter function of the diaphragmatic hiatus. In essence, GER requires two "hits" to the EGJ.[42] Patients with a normal EGJ require inhibition of the LES and crural diaphragm for reflux to occur (i.e., tLESRs). In contrast, when a hiatal hernia is present compromising the function of the crural sphincter, reflux can occur with only relaxation of the LES, during periods of LES hypotension, swallowing-induced relaxation, and straining.[51,52]

Hiatal Hernia

Many individuals demonstrate no evidence of GERD despite the presence of a hiatal hernia. Other individuals with no recognizable hernia have documented GERD due to other factors, such as excessive or prolonged tLESRs. Nevertheless, hiatal hernia occurs in 54%–94% of patients with reflux esophagitis, a rate strikingly higher than that in the healthy population.[53] Studies have also found that in individuals with reflux symptoms, the presence of hiatal hernia confers a significantly increased risk of erosive esophageal injury.[54] Recent epidemiologic data have confirmed the importance of hiatal hernia in patients with Barrett's esophagus and esophageal adenocarcinoma.[55]

The hiatal hernia promotes reflux through several mechanisms (Fig. 48.4). Proximal displacement of the LES from the crural diaphragm into the chest reduces basal LES pressure and shortens the length of the high-pressure zone; this is primarily due to loss of the intra-abdominal LES segment.[50] Hiatal hernia eliminates the increase of LES pressure that occurs during straining and increases tLESR frequency during gastric distention with gas.[56,57] Hiatal hernias serve as a persistent vestibule for gastric acid (the so-called acid pocket). Therefore there is an increased tendency for reflux to occur from the hernia sac during swallow-induced LESRs and tLESRs. Hiatal hernias that are large (≥3 cm) and nonreducible (hernias in which the gastric rugal folds remain above the diaphragm between swallows) are especially prone to reflux.[58]

Finally, increased EGJ compliance, especially in GERD patients with hiatal hernia, has been identified.[51] For the same degree of intragastric pressure, the esophageal junction opens at a lower pressure, and the cross-sectional area is greater and more symmetrical as intragastric pressure increases.

The etiology of a hiatal hernia remains unclear. Familial clustering of GERD suggests the possibilities of an inherited smooth muscle disorder.[27] Animal studies propose that reflux

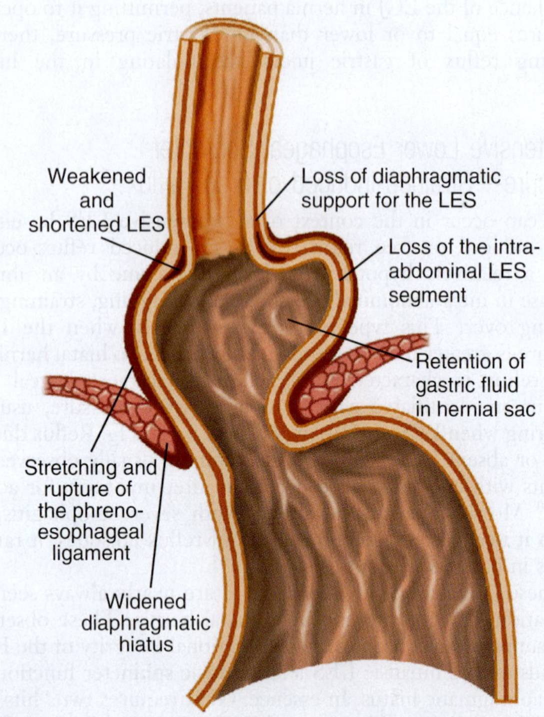

Fig. 48.4 Schematic diagram showing the effect of a hiatal hernia on the antireflux barrier. *LES*, Lower esophageal sphincter.

itself causes esophageal shortening, promoting the development of a hiatal hernia.[59] Other studies find an association with obesity[60] and heavy lifting,[61] raising the possibilities that over time, chronic intra-abdominal stressors may weaken the esophageal hiatus, causing the development of a hiatal hernia. This theory is attractive because it helps to reconcile the increased prevalence of hiatal hernias as the population grows older.[53]

The Acid Pocket

Gastric pH is usually around 2 in the fasting state. During meals, and for approximately 90 minutes thereafter, the pH remains elevated owing to the buffering effects of the food. Herein lies a paradox because most episodes of acid reflux occur immediately after a meal. This paradox is explained by the identification of a zone in the gastric cardia that remains unbuffered, now referred to as the *acid pocket*.[62,63] This pocket is postulated to be the source of acidic refluxate and has a pH considerably lower than the distal esophagus and remainder of the stomach after a meal. A subsequent study confirmed that this zone is poorly buffered by a meal in both normal subjects and those with symptomatic GERD.[64] In GERD patients, the presence of an acid pocket is more common than in controls and is larger as a result of extension more distally from the LES.[65] In GERD patients with hiatal hernia, the acid pocket is further enlarged because of the proximal migration of the LES. In addition, when the acid pocket is located above the diaphragm, especially in a hiatal hernia, more than 70% of the tLESRs were accompanied by acid reflux. In contrast, less than 20% of tLESRs were accompanied by acid reflux when the acid pocket was below the diaphragm.[58]

Esophageal Acid Clearance

The second tier of protection against reflux damage is esophageal acid clearance. This phenomenon involves two related but separate processes: volume or bolus clearance, which is the actual removal of the reflux material from the esophagus, and acid clearance, which is the restoration of normal esophageal pH following acid exposure through titration with alkaline secretions from saliva and esophageal glands. Although the competency of the antireflux barrier determines the frequency and volume of GER, esophageal acid clearance determines the duration of acid exposure to the mucosa and probably the severity of mucosal damage.

Volume Clearance

Esophageal peristalsis clears acid volume in the upright and supine positions but is inoperative during deep rapid eye movement sleep. Helm et al.[66] showed that one or two primary peristaltic contractions completely clear a 15-mL fluid bolus from the esophagus. Primary peristalsis is elicited by swallowing. Secondary peristalsis, initiated by esophageal distention from acid reflux, is much less effective in clearing the refluxate, thus offering only an ancillary protective role.

Peristaltic dysfunction [i.e., failed peristaltic contractions, hypotensive or weak (<30 mm Hg) peristaltic contractions that incompletely empty the esophagus increases in frequency with the severity of esophagitis. Savarino et al. found that increasing GERD severity was associated with decreased lower distal esophageal amplitude and an increased prevalence of ineffective esophageal motility.[67] Patients with erosive esophagitis had significantly impaired fluid bolus transit compared with patients with nonerosive reflux disease and functional heartburn.[67] Whether esophagitis per se leads to peristaltic dysfunction or whether an underlying smooth muscle motility disorder of the esophagus predisposes to the development of reflux disease is not clear. Animal studies have found that esophageal dysmotility associated with active esophagitis is reversible, but esophageal dysmotility associated with stricture or extensive fibrosis is irreversible. Clinical observations suggest that impaired motor function does not revert to normal following either effective medical or surgical therapies.

Hiatal hernia can also impair esophageal emptying. Concurrent pH recording and scintigraphy above the EGJ showed that impaired clearance was caused by re-reflux of fluid from the hernia sac during swallowing.[52] This impaired clearance was most compromised in patients with nonreducing hernia where retrograde flow of fluid from the hernia occurred even during deglutitive relaxation.

Gravity contributes to bolus clearance when reflux occurs in the upright position. At night when supine, this mechanism is not operative unless the head of the bed is elevated. This important lifestyle change markedly improves acid clearance time and is most beneficial in patients with aperistalsis (e.g., with scleroderma).

Salivary and Esophageal Gland Secretions

Saliva is the second essential factor required for normal esophageal acid clearance. The stimulus for salivation appears to be the presence of acid in the proximal esophagus (20 cm above LES).[68] The normal daily volume of saliva is 1.2 L, which may triple in response to persistent esophageal acidification.[69] Refluxed acid activates esophageal chemoreceptors, stimulating the salivary glands, and increases peristaltic activity through a neural reflex arc mediated by the vagus.[70] Saliva is a weak base with a pH of 6.4–7.8.[71] However, it easily neutralizes the small amount of acid remaining in the esophagus after several peristaltic contractions.[71]

Modulation of salivation may contribute to GERD. Decreased salivation during sleep is the reason that nocturnal reflux episodes are associated with markedly prolonged acid clearance times. Xerostomia is associated with prolonged esophageal acid exposure and esophagitis.[72] Cigarette smoking promotes GER. Originally attributed to nicotine's effect on lowering LES pressure, cigarette smokers have also hyposalivation, leading to prolonged esophageal acid clearance times.[73]

In addition to saliva, the aqueous bicarbonate-rich secretions of the esophageal submucosal glands dilute and neutralize residual esophageal acid.[74] Acid refluxing into the esophageal lumen stimulates these glands and helps neutralize the acid, even if swallowing does not occur.[75]

Tissue Resistance

Although clearance mechanisms minimize acid contact time with the epithelium, even healthy subjects have acid reflux during the day and sometimes at night. Nevertheless, only a few subjects experience symptomatic GER, and even fewer suffer GERD. This is due to a third tier for esophageal defense known as *tissue resistance*. Conceptually, tissue resistance can be subdivided into preepithelial, epithelial, and postepithelial factors, which act together to minimize mucosal damage from the noxious gastric refluxate.[76]

The *preepithelial defense* in the esophagus is poorly developed. There is neither a well-defined mucous layer nor buffering capacity by the surface cells to secrete bicarbonate ions into the unstirred water layer. Esophageal secretion of glycoconjugate (predominantly mucin) and prostaglandin E_2 may play a role in preepithelial defense.[77]

The *epithelial defenses* consist of structural and functional components. Structural components include the cell membranes and intercellular junctional complexes of the esophageal mucosa. This structure is a 25–30-cell-thick layer of nonkeratinized squamous epithelium functionally divided into a proliferating basal cell layer (stratum basalis), a midzone layer of metabolically active squamous cells (stratum spinosum), and a 5–10-cell-thick layer of dead cells (stratum corneum) on the mucosal surface. The esophageal mucosa is a relatively "tight" epithelium that resists ionic movement at the intercellular, as well as the cellular, level as the result of tight junctions and the matrix of lipid-rich glycoconjugates in the intercellular space.[78] Luminal acid attacks the epithelial defenses by damaging the intercellular junctions, allowing hydrogen ions to enter and acidify the intercellular space. As documented by transmission electron microscopy, the intercellular spaces expand, and eventually the buffering capacity of this space is overwhelmed, leading to acidification of the adjacent cytosol via the basolateral membrane.[76] The functional components of tissue resistance include the ability of the esophageal epithelium to buffer and extrude hydrogen ions. Intracellular buffering is accomplished by negatively charged phosphates and proteins, as well as bicarbonate ions. When the mucosal buffering capacity is exceeded and intracellular pH falls, the epithelium has the capacity to actively remove or neutralize H^+. This is possibly by the action of two transmembrane proteins, one Na^+/H^+ exchanger, and another Na^+-dependent Cl^-/HCO_3^- exchanger.[68,79] After reflux-induced cell acidification, these transporters restore the intracellular pH to neutrality by exchanging H^+ for extracellular Na^+ or by exchanging Cl^- for extracellular HCO_3^-, respectively. In addition, esophageal cells contain within their membrane an Na^+-independent Cl^-/HCO_3^- exchanger that extrudes HCO_3^- from the cytoplasm when the intracellular pH is too high.[68] When the epithelial cells are no longer able to maintain intracellular pH, they lose their ability to volume regulate, cell swelling occurs, balloon cells develop, and cell death follows. Additional contributors to the epithelial defense include salivary EGF, transforming growth factor-α, and prostaglandin E_2. These factors enhance epithelial cell turnover, enhance esophageal mucin production, and modulate bicarbonate secretion.[78] Upregulation of transcription of desmosomal proteins that support the epithelial cell cytoskeleton also occurs.[80]

Data suggest that dilated intercellular spaces are the earliest markers of esophageal epithelial cellular damage (Fig. 48.5).[76] These alterations arise with exposure to acid and pepsin during GER, but the exact pathway of damage to the intercellular junctions remains unclear.[81] One possibility is the proteolytic degradation of E-cadherin, a key molecule regulating tight junction permeability.[82] Other noxious contents of the refluxate, such as bile acids, are also harmful, and dilated intercellular spaces can be induced by acute psychological stress.[83] Dilated intercellular spaces can be assessed quantitatively with electron microscopy, but they are also recognizable with light microscopy.[76] In studies by Calabrese et al.,[84] all controls had intercellular spaces less than 1.69 μm. Symptomatic patients had a mean intercellular space value and a mean value of the maximum dilated intracellular space at least three times greater than controls. Statistical differences were not observed between esophagitis patients and nonerosive GERD patients. The authors speculated that increased paracellular permeability could partly explain the development of heartburn in the absence of overt esophagitis. This hypothesis is supported by the identification of vagal and spinal sensory afferent neurons superficially within the intercellular space.[85] Importantly, aggressive acid inhibition with PPIs leads to complete resolution of the dilated intercellular spaces in nearly all patients over 3–6 months. These changes correlated closely with the resolution of heartburn.[84]

The *postepithelial* defense is provided by the esophageal blood supply. Blood flow delivers oxygen, nutrients, and bicarbonate and removes H^+ and CO_2, thereby maintaining normal tissue acid-base balance. Blood flow to the esophageal mucosa increases in response to the stress of luminal acid.[86]

Gastric Factors

Gastric factors (volume and components of the gastric refluxate) are potentially important in the production of reflux esophagitis. Gastric acidity determines the degree of potential mucosal damage of the refluxate. Increases in gastric volume augment the rate of tLESRs, making gastric contents more likely to reflux.

Gastric Acid Secretion

Acid and pepsin are the key ingredients of the gastric refluxate producing esophagitis. In animal studies, acid alone causes minimal injury at a pH of less than 3, primarily by protein denaturation. However, acid combined with even small amounts of pepsin disrupts the mucosal barrier, resulting in increased H^+ permeability, histologic changes, and hemorrhage.[87] The degree of esophageal injury, from nonerosive GERD to Barrett's esophagus, parallels the increase in the frequency and duration of acid reflux ($pH < 4$).[88,89] Conversely, perfusing the esophagus of animals with a pepsin solution at pH 4–7.5 produces minimal mucosal disruption or change in mucosal permeability.[87] These observations are the cornerstone of acid inhibition therapy for the treatment of GERD-related esophagitis. However, reflux of weakly acidic gastric content may be a major factor in regurgitation, due to volume delivered into the esophagus and possibly heartburn and cough.[90]

Overall, gastric acid secretion is normal in patients with GERD.[91] On the other hand, the local distribution of acid rather than total gastric secretion may be more relevant to the pathogenesis of GERD. Data suggest that the gastroesophageal junction may escape the buffering effect of meals, remaining highly acidic compared with the body of the stomach. This proximal acid pocket, discussed earlier, extends from the cardia into the distal esophagus.

Hp infection, especially with the $CagA^+$ virulent strain, has the potential to raise or lower gastric acidity, depending on the site of infection. Acid output may be decreased by several mechanisms: (1) infection of the corpus, which can progress to multifocal atrophic gastritis; (2) increased gastric alkaline (bicarbonate) secretion, which returns to normal after Hp eradication; and

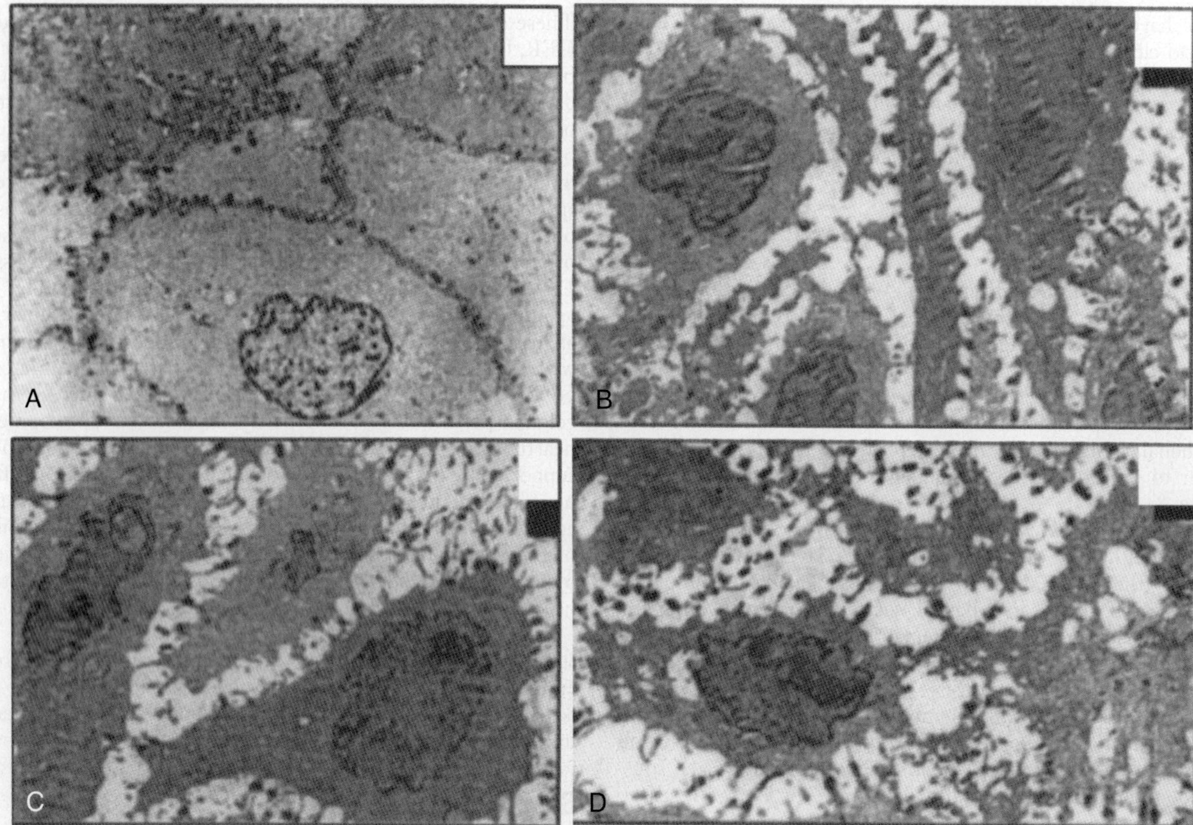

Fig. 48.5 Transmission electron micrographs of esophageal epithelium. Normal subjects (A) do not have dilated intercellular spaces. In contrast, patients with "bile" reflux (B), nonerosive gastroesophageal reflux disease (GERD) (C), and erosive GERD (D) have dilated intercellular spaces *(irregular white spaces)*. These dilations appear to be the earliest cellular marker of GERD and is independent of the degree of esophagitis. (From Calabrese C, Fabbri A, Bortolotti M, et al. Dilated intercellular spaces as a marker of oesophageal damage: comparative results in gastro-oesophageal reflux disease with or without bile reflux. *Aliment Pharmacol Ther*. 2003;18:525–532.)

perhaps (3) production of ammonia by the bacteria itself.[92] After eradication of Hp, the corpus mucosa can regenerate to normal, increasing acid secretion. In Asia, corpus-predominant gastritis is common, and eradication therapy in these patients may increase the risk of developing GERD. In a study from Japan, the cumulative prevalence of reflux esophagitis after Hp eradication was 26%, 33% in those with and 13% in those without corpus atrophic gastritis.[93] Conversely, Hp antrum-predominant gastritis has been shown to be associated with hypergastrinemia and gastric hypersecretion. Heartburn and regurgitation often improve significantly after eradication therapy in patients with antrum-predominant gastritis.[94]

Duodenogastric Reflux

Bile acids can alter the integrity of the mucosal barrier by disrupting cell function and damaging membrane structure. Animal studies demonstrate that conjugated bile acids produce their greatest injury in the presence of acid and pepsin, whereas deconjugated bile acids and trypsin are damaging in a more neutral environment.[95] Esophageal exposure to bile is always mixed with acid resulting in more severe grades of esophagitis. Analyses of the association of acid and bile reflux (quantified using bilirubin absorbances) with GERD support the hypothesis that the presence and severity of erosive esophagitis depend primarily on acid reflux, whereas Barrett's esophagus depends on exposure to both acid and bile.[96]

Delayed Gastric Emptying

The importance of delayed gastric emptying in the pathogenesis of GERD is controversial. Early studies suggested a rate as high as 50%, but more recent studies using a standardized 4-hour gastric emptying test found an overlap but in 8%–20% of patients.[97] Conceptually, impaired gastric emptying results in a greater volume of material in the stomach, which could be available to directly reflux into the esophagus due to distention of the proximal stomach. Recent studies with impedance-pH testing found that acid reflux values were not increased, but consistent with the reflux of the meal contents, the increase was in the postprandial liquid or mixed reflux events and non/weakly acid reflux.[98] Women and diabetics are more likely to have gastroparesis with secondary reflux. Complaints of abdominal bloating, pain, nausea, vomiting, and constipation should be helpful clues, and manometry often shows a normal LES pressure.

A New Cytokine-Mediated Mechanism for Esophageal Injury

Recent animal and human studies suggest a new paradigm for esophageal injury—refluxed gastric contents do not directly damage the esophagus but rather stimulates esophageal epithelial cells to secrete chemokines that mediate damage of esophageal tissue. Using a rat model with an esophagoduodenostomy, Souza et al.[99] removed the esophagus at various time points to analyze histologically the inflammatory changes. Reflux esophagitis started at postoperative Day 3 with lymphocytic infiltration of the submucosa that eventually progressed to the epithelial surface. Basal cell and papillary hyperplasia preceded the development of surface erosions—these findings are just the opposite of those expected from a caustic chemical injury. In another experiment in the same study, exposure of a human esophageal squamous cell line to acidified bile salts significantly increased the secretion of IL-8 and IL-1β, which triggered the migration of T cells and neutrophils.

In a preliminary study of 12 patients with a history of severe esophagitis healed with PPI therapy, the same group[100] observed that stopping antacid medications was associated with T lymphocyte predominant esophageal inflammation and basal cell and papillary hyperplasia. These changes occurred at 1 and 2 weeks after discontinuing PPIs, neutrophils and eosinophils were few or absent on biopsies, and there was not the loss of surface cells (i.e., erosions).

CLINICAL FEATURES

Classic Symptoms

Heartburn is the classic symptom of GERD, with patients generally reporting a burning feeling rising from the stomach or lower chest and radiating toward the neck, throat, and occasionally the back.[101] It usually occurs postprandially, particularly after large meals or after ingesting spicy foods, citrus products, fats, chocolates, and alcohol. The supine position and bending over may exacerbate heartburn. Sleep deprivation as well as psychological or auditory stress may lower the threshold for symptom perception.[102,103] Nighttime heartburn may occur after spontaneous conscious awakenings, leading to difficulty in returning to sleep. GERD is usually diagnosed symptomatically by the occurrence of heartburn two or more days a week, although less frequent symptoms do not preclude the disease.[101] Although an aid to diagnosis, the frequency and severity of heartburn do not predict the degree of esophageal damage.[101]

Heartburn symptoms can arise from acid reflux, weakly acidic reflux, bile reflux, and mechanical stimulation of the esophagus. The receptor that mediates the sensation of heartburn during acid perfusion has not been identified, although the capsaicin receptor, or vanilloid receptor 1 (TRPV1), is a leading candidate. TRPV1 is a cation channel that is expressed by sensory neurons, and its activation by heat, acid pH, or ethanol may trigger burning pain.[104] Weakly acidic reflux, as detected by combined pH and impedance technology, appears to produce symptoms when there is a large proximal extent reached by the refluxate, large reflux volumes, and prolonged acid-clearance times.[105] The mechanism that underlies bile acid–induced esophageal symptoms is unknown. Bile acids are postulated to induce the release of intracellular mediators via damage to lipid membranes.[106] In addition to acid-induced and bile acid–induced esophageal damage, pepsin can cause direct damage to the esophageal mucosa, leading to dilated intercellular spaces and increased esophageal mucosal permeability.[107] Esophageal distention and sustained esophageal contractions are other mechanisms proposed to explain the symptom of heartburn. Balaban and associates used high-frequency endoluminal US to demonstrate a correlation between spontaneous chest pain or chest pain induced by edrophonium chloride and sustained esophageal longitudinal muscle contractions.[108]

Regurgitation defined as the "perception of flow or refluxed gastric contents into the mouth or pharynx"[101] has been inconsistently described in clinical trials and epidemiologic studies of GERD. Among patients with daily regurgitation, LES pressure is often low; many patients have associated gastroparesis, and esophagitis is common, making this symptom more difficult to treat medically than classic heartburn.[109]

The lack of a gold standard for GERD diagnosis makes it difficult to define the accuracy of heartburn and/or regurgitation for GERD. The Diamond Study from the United Kingdom addressed this question by carefully evaluating 308 patients presenting to general physicians with suspected GERD.[110] GERD was present in 203 patients (66%) defined by endoscopic esophagitis and/or abnormal 24-hour pH test or positive symptom association. Only 49% of GERD patients recorded heartburn or regurgitation as their most troublesome symptom for a sensitivity and specificity of 63% and 63%, respectively. Reflux questionnaires did not perform any better. Nor could response of symptoms to PPI treatment (esomeprazole 40 mg for 2 weeks) increase diagnostic precision—a positive response to PPIs was observed in 69% of GERD patients and 51% of patients without GERD.[111] Similarly, a well-performed meta-analysis cast doubt of the PPI trial, finding that it identified GERD patients with 78% sensitivity and 54% specificity.[112]

Dysphagia is reported by more than 30% of individuals with GERD.[113] It usually occurs in the setting of long-standing heartburn, with slowly progressive dysphagia for solids. Weight loss is uncommon, and patients have good appetites. The most common causes are a peptic stricture or Schatzki's ring, but other etiologies include severe esophageal inflammation alone, peristaltic dysfunction, and esophageal cancer.

Less common symptoms associated with GERD include water brash, odynophagia, burping, hiccups, nausea, and vomiting.[114] *Water brash* is the sudden appearance in the mouth of a slightly sour or salty fluid. It is not regurgitated fluid but rather secretions from the salivary glands in response to acid reflux.[71] Odynophagia may be seen with severe ulcerative esophagitis. However, its presence should raise the suspicion of an alternative cause of esophagitis, especially infections or injury from impacted pills.

Some patients with GERD are asymptomatic. This is particularly true in older adults, perhaps because of decreased acidity of the reflux material in some or decreased pain perception in others. Many older adult patients present first with complications of GERD because of long-standing disease with minimal symptoms. For example, up to 40% of patients with Barrett's esophagus are insensitive to acid at the time of presentation.[2]

Extraesophageal Manifestations

GER may cause a wide spectrum of conditions, including noncardiac chest pain, asthma, posterior laryngitis, chronic cough, recurrent pneumonitis, dental erosions, and disordered sleep.[115] Some of these patients have classic reflux symptoms, but many are "silent refluxers," contributing to problems in making the diagnosis. Furthermore, it may be difficult to establish a causal relationship even if GER can be documented by testing (e.g., pH studies) because individuals may simply have two common diseases without a cause-and-effect relationship.

Chest Pain

GER-related chest pain may mimic angina pectoris, having a squeezing or burning quality, being substernal, and radiating to the back, neck, jaws, or arm. It frequently is worse after meals and may worsen during emotional stress. Reflux-related chest pain may last for minutes to hours, often resolves spontaneously, and may be eased with antacids. The mechanism for GERD-related chest pain is poorly understood and is probably multifactorial, related to the H^+ ion concentration, volume, and duration of acid reflux; secondary esophageal spasm; and prolonged contractions of the longitudinal muscles.[116,117] Chest pain episodes that occur in association with documented acid reflux events by pH testing usually respond well to acid antisecretory therapy.[118]

Asthma and Other Pulmonary Disorders

The estimated prevalence of GERD in asthmatics is between 34% and 89%, depending on the group of patients studied and how GERD is defined (e.g., symptoms or 24-hour pH monitoring).[119] Proposed mechanisms of reflux-induced asthma include aspiration of gastric contents into the lungs, with secondary bronchospasm and activation of a vagal reflex from the esophagus to the lungs causing bronchoconstriction. Animal[120] and human[121] studies report bronchoconstriction after esophageal acidification, but the response is mild and inconsistent. The reflux of acid into the trachea, as compared with the esophagus alone, predictably caused marked changes in peak expiratory flow rates in asthmatic patients.[122] Other pulmonary diseases associated with GERD include aspiration pneumonia, interstitial pulmonary fibrosis, chronic bronchitis, bronchiectasis, and lung transplantation complications.[296] In addition, GER may worsen the course of obstructive sleep apnea (OSA) in a subset of patients.[123]

Up to 30% of patients with GERD-related asthma have no esophageal complaints. Therefore there has been enthusiasm for empirical treatment for acid reflux even in asymptomatic patients with poorly controlled asthma. Data from randomized double-blind trials have failed to support this approach. One trial of adults with inadequately controlled asthma despite treatment with inhaled corticosteroids and with minimal or no symptoms of GER used either 40 mg of esomeprazole twice daily or matching placebo. Esomeprazole had no measurable impact on the frequency of poor asthma control events. The authors also found no effect of esomeprazole on pulmonary function, airway reactivity, nocturnal awakening, or quality of life. Even in the subgroup of poorly controlled asthmatics with an abnormal pH study, there was no benefit with acid suppression.[124] A more recent study using lansoprazole in children found similar results.[125] In addition, children treated with lansoprazole reported more respiratory infections.[126]

Ear, Nose, and Throat Diseases

Laryngeal inflammation may be associated with a variety of presenting symptoms, including hoarseness, globus sensation, frequent throat clearing, recurrent sore throat, and prolonged voice warm-up.[127] Ear, nose, and throat signs attributed to GERD include posterior laryngitis with edema and redness, vocal cord ulcers, granulomas, leukoplakia, and even carcinoma.[128] These changes are usually limited to the posterior third of the vocal cords and interarytenoid areas, both in proximity to the upper esophageal sphincter (Fig. 48.6). Animal studies find that the combination of acid, pepsin, and conjugated bile acids is very injurious to the larynx.[129] Human studies have confirmed that increased esophageal acid exposure is significantly more common in patients with laryngeal symptoms and signs than in the general population.[127] Although acid suppression is frequently recommended as an empirical treatment for chronic laryngeal symptoms, meta-analysis of results from controlled trials using PPI therapy failed to find objective improvement compared with placebo.[130]

GERD has been postulated to be a leading cause of chronic cough (after sinus problems and asthma).[131] GER increases the cough sensitivity reflex (i.e., reduces the cough threshold) in patients with chronic cough.[132] However, the importance of this association in humans has not been shown in treatment studies, which, in sum, have not demonstrated a superiority of PPIs over placebo.[133] Dental erosion, the loss of tooth structure by nonbacterial chemical processes, can be caused by GER, and acid suppressive therapy is helpful in counteracting progression of reflux related dental erosions.[134]

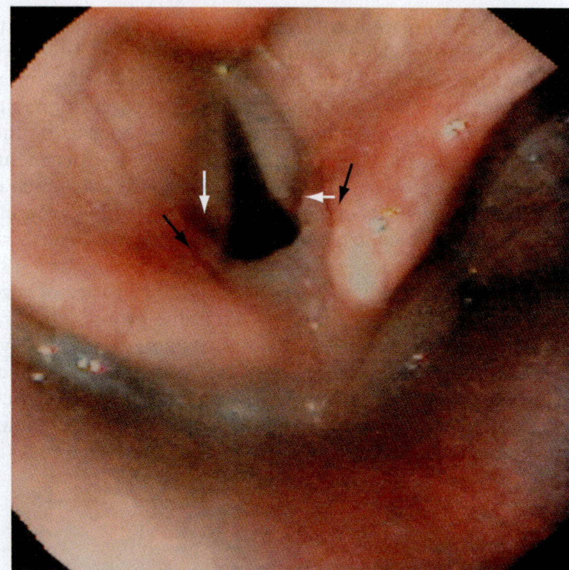

Fig. 48.6 Characteristic findings of "reflux laryngitis" in a 31-year-old man with hoarseness whose symptoms and signs resolved after PPI treatment for 3 months. *Black arrows:* erythema of the medial arytenoid walls. *White arrows:* red streaks on the true vocal folds. Reflux changes in the larynx are usually confined to the posterior portion nearest the upper esophageal sphincter (*bluish gray ridge behind the arytenoid complex*).

Sleep Disorders

Nocturnal GERD can lead to interruptions in sleep, leading to high rates of absenteeism from work and a reduced quality of life.[135] PPI therapy has demonstrated superiority over placebo in providing relief from nocturnal heartburn and in reducing GERD-related sleep disturbances, resulting in improvement in sleep quality and work productivity.[136] Epidemiologic studies have also found an association between nocturnal GERD and OSA.[137] This was confirmed in a study using pH-impedance, finding that OSA patients have more episodes of pathologic acid reflux than those without OSA.[125] The mechanism for this association remains unclear, although it appears that GERD is a consequence of OSA, not the converse. For example, a study found that patients with OSA had more tLESRs during sleep related to preceding sleep arousals and shallow sleep.[138]

DIFFERENTIAL DIAGNOSIS

Symptoms associated with GERD may be mimicked by other esophageal and extraesophageal diseases, including achalasia, eosinophilic esophagitis (EoE), Zenker's diverticulum, gastroparesis, gallstones, PUD, functional dyspepsia, and angina pectoris. These disorders usually can be identified by failure to respond to aggressive PPI therapy and appropriate diagnostic tests. Although GERD is the most common cause of esophagitis, other etiologies of esophagitis (pills, infections, or radiation injury) need to be considered in difficult-to-manage cases, older individuals, or immunocompromised patients.

ASSOCIATED CONDITIONS

Several medical and surgical conditions can predispose to GERD. The most common is pregnancy, in which 30%–80% of women complain of heartburn, especially in the first trimester (see Chapter 38). Pregnancy increases the risk for reflux by reducing

LES pressure due to the effects of estrogen and progesterone and possibly mechanical factors from the gravid uterus.[139] Although symptoms may be severe, esophagitis is uncommon, and this type of situational GERD is cured with childbirth. Up to 90% of patients with scleroderma (PSS or CREST syndrome) have GERD due to smooth muscle fibrosis causing low LES pressure and weak or absent peristalsis (see Chapter 35). Severe disease is common, with up to 38% of patients having esophagitis.[140] Acid hypersecretion and increased gastric volume are the major factors causing GERD in patients with ZES (see Chapter 53). In these patients, the esophagitis and complications are more difficult to treat than the ulcer disease.[141] After Heller myotomy or the more recent per-oral endoscopic myotomy for achalasia (see Chapter 46), 10%–39% of patients may develop GERD.[142] In patients undergoing bariatric surgery for morbid obesity (see Chapter 8), de novo symptoms of GERD may develop postoperatively.[143] Finally, prolonged NG intubation may cause reflux esophagitis, in part because acid tracks orad along the tube and because the tube mechanically interferes with the LES barrier function (see Chapter 47).[144]

DIAGNOSIS

A large number of tests are available for evaluating patients with suspected GERD.[145] Many times these tests are unnecessary because the classic symptoms of heartburn and acid regurgitation are sufficiently specific to identify reflux disease and begin medical treatment. However, this is not always the case, and clinicians must decide which tests to choose so as to make a diagnosis in a reliable, timely, and cost-effective manner depending on the information desired (Box 48.1).[145]

Empirical Trial of Acid Suppression

An empirical trial of acid suppression is the simplest method for diagnosing GERD and assessing its relationship to symptoms. With the advent of PPIs, it has become the first test used in patients with classic or atypical reflux symptoms without alarm complaints. Symptoms usually respond to a PPI trial in 1–2 weeks. If symptoms disappear with therapy and then return when the medication is discontinued, GERD has been established.

In empirical trials for heartburn, the initial PPI dose was high (e.g., omeprazole 40–80 mg/day), usually given for at least 2 weeks, and a positive response was defined as at least 50% improvement in heartburn. Using this approach, the PPI empirical trial has a sensitivity of 68%–83% but poor specificity for determining the presence of GERD.[146,147] However, these studies were enriched with GERD patients and may not represent the general population. For example, the PPI test was not as useful in a UK primary care setting with a large group of patients with a variety of UGI symptoms.[111] A positive response was observed in

BOX 48.1 Tests for Gastroesophageal Reflux Disease

- GERD Questionnaires (RDQ, GERD Q)
- PPI test
- Manometry
- Barium swallow
- Endoscopy
- Histology
- pH monitoring (catheter based or wireless)
- Intraluminal impedance-pH monitoring
- Mucosal impedance

64% of patients with well-documented GERD and in 51% of those without GERD—not much better than a coin toss.

An empirical PPI trial for diagnosing GERD offers many advantages: the test is office based, easily done, inexpensive, and available to all physicians and avoids many needless procedures. For example, Fass et al.[148] showed a savings of more than $570 per patient that was due to a reduction in the number of diagnostic tests performed for noncardiac chest pain. Disadvantages are few, including a placebo response and uncertain symptomatic end point if symptoms do not totally resolve with extended treatment; however, the false-positive rate may be higher in a general practice than previously anticipated.[111] Estimating the diagnostic test characteristics of successful PPI treatment with 24-hour pH monitoring as the reference standard, one study showed a combined estimates of sensitivity and specificity of 78% and 54%, respectively, for short-term PPI trial for diagnosing GERD.[112] However, the most recent consensus on diagnosis and treatment of GERD (Lyon Consensus 2.0) recommends against empiric PPI trial in patients without typical symptoms.[297]

Endoscopy

Upper endoscopy is the standard for documenting the presence and extent of esophagitis and excluding other etiologies for the patient's symptoms. However, only 20%–60% of patients with abnormal esophageal reflux by pH testing have esophagitis at endoscopy. Thus the sensitivity of endoscopy for GERD is low, but it has high specificity at 90%–95%.[149]

The earliest endoscopic signs of acid reflux include edema and erythema, but these findings are nonspecific and dependent on the quality of endoscopic visual images.[149] More reliable signs are friability, granularity, and red streaks. Friability (easy bleeding) results from the development of enlarged capillaries near the mucosal surface in response to acid. Red streaks extend upward from the esophageal junction along the ridges of the esophageal folds.[150] Erosions develop with progressive acid injury, characterized by a shallow break in the mucosa with a white or yellow exudate surrounded by erythema. Typically, erosions begin at the gastroesophageal junction, occurring along the tops of esophageal mucosal folds where acid injury is most prone; they may be single or multiple. Erosions can also be caused by NSAIDs, heavy smoking, and infectious esophagitis.[149] Ulcers reflect more severe esophageal damage, being deeper into the mucosa or submucosa and either isolated along a fold or surrounding the esophageal junction. The most thoroughly evaluated esophagitis classification is the Los Angeles (LA) system, which is now widely used throughout the world (Fig. 48.7 and Table 48.2).[151] The most recent GERD consensus, however, suggests that while LA grades B, C, and D are conclusive evidence of GERD, the diagnostic accuracy of grade A esophagitis[297] remains uncertain. Esophageal capsule endoscopy for the evaluation of reflux symptoms has thus far been disappointing. The capsule is 11 by 26 mm and acquires video images at 14 frames per second. After swallowing, images are transmitted to a portable receiver via digital radiofrequency. In a study, compared with standard upper endoscopy, the capsule had a sensitivity of only 50% for erosive esophagitis, 54% for the presence of a hiatal hernia, and 79% for the presence of Barrett's esophagus.[152]

Most patients with GERD are treated initially with PPIs and without endoscopy. The important exception is the patient experiencing "alarm" symptoms: dysphagia, odynophagia, weight loss, vomiting, and GI bleeding. Here, endoscopy should be performed early to diagnose complications of GERD (e.g., strictures) and to rule out other entities, such as infections, ulcers, cancers, or varices. Current guidelines by the American College of Physicians suggest the major role of endoscopy is to diagnose and treat GERD complications, especially peptic strictures, and to define Barrett's esophagus.[153] Other indications

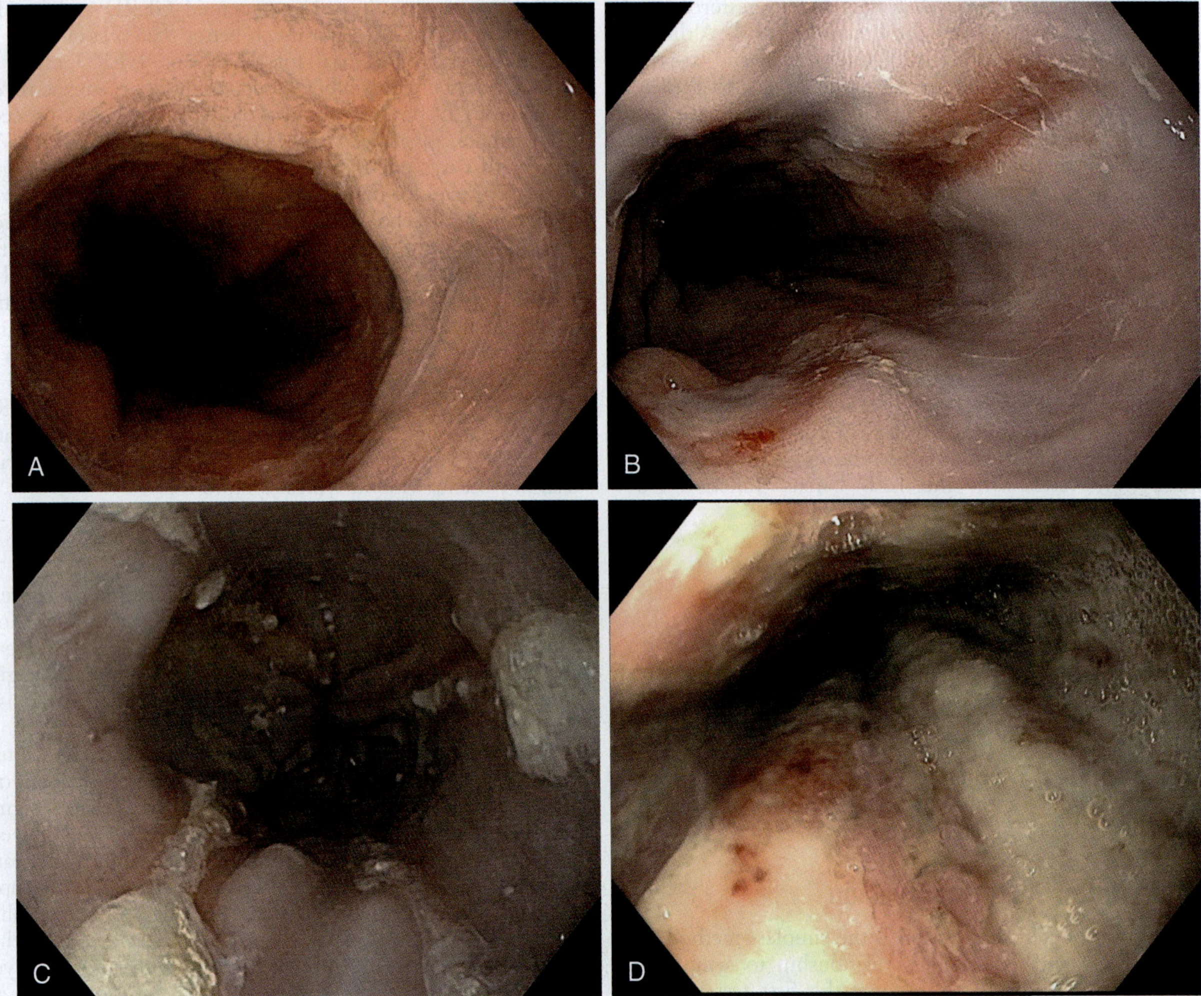

Fig. 48.7 Endoscopic photographs of the four grades of esophagitis (A–D) using the Los Angeles classification system (see Table 46.2).

TABLE 48.2 Los Angeles Endoscopic Classification System for Esophagitis

Grade A	One or more mucosal breaks confined to folds, ≤5 mm
Grade B	One or more mucosal breaks >5 mm confined to folds but not continuous between the tops of mucosal folds
Grade C	Mucosal breaks continuous between tops of two or more mucosal folds but not circumferential
Grade D	Circumferential mucosal break

include typical GERD symptoms that persist despite a 4–8-week trial of twice-daily PPI therapy and patients with severe esophagitis after a 2-month PPI course, to assess healing and rule out Barrett's esophagus.

Esophageal Biopsy

Like endoscopy, the role of esophageal biopsies in evaluating GERD has evolved over the years.[145] Microscopic changes of reflux may occur even when the mucosa endoscopically appears normal.[154] Classic changes of basal cell hyperplasia and increased height of the rete peg, both representing increased epithelial turnover of the squamous mucosa, are sensitive but not specific histologic findings for GERD.[155] Acute inflammation characterized by the presence of neutrophils and often eosinophils (Fig. 48.8) is very specific for esophagitis; however, the sensitivity is low, in the range of 15%–40%.[156] Thus there is little value for histologic examination of normal-appearing squamous mucosa to identify GERD. However, this dictum recently has been tempered by the need to differentiate EoE from GERD, particularly in patients complaining of dysphagia.[157] In young patients with dysphagia, especially food impaction, clinical suspicion for EoE is high requiring esophageal biopsies both in the distal and proximal esophagus. In patients with classic reflux esophagitis, biopsies are usually not taken except to exclude neoplasm, infection, or bullous skin disease. Therefore the current primary indication for esophageal biopsies is to define Barrett's epithelium and exclude EoE.[158] When Barrett's is suspected, biopsies are mandatory and best done when esophagitis is healed (see Chapter 49).

Esophageal Reflux Testing

Esophageal reflux monitoring has undergone substantial changes in the past 10 years.[145] Wireless pH capsules and the ability to measure all forms of reflux, both acid and nonacid, are important advances in the field of reflux testing. Ambulatory intraesophageal pH monitoring is still the standard for establishing pathologic acid reflux.[145,159,160] For catheter-based pH testing, the probe is passed

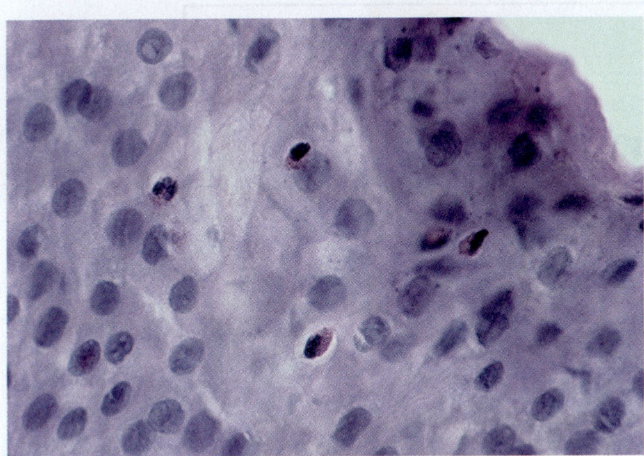

Fig. 48.8 Histopathology of gastroesophageal reflux disease. Inflammatory cells (eosinophils and neutrophils) are interspersed between squamous epithelial cells. (Courtesy Edward Lee, MD, Washington, DC.)

nasally, positioned 5 cm above the manometrically determined LES, and connected to a battery-powered data logger capable of collecting pH values every 4–6 seconds. An event marker is activated by the patient when symptoms, meals, and body position changes occur. Patients are encouraged to eat normally and engage in regular daily activities, with monitoring carried out for 18–24 hours. Reflux episodes are defined by a pH drop of less than 4. Conventionally measured parameters include percentage of total time when pH is less than 4, percentage of time upright and supine when pH is less than 4, total number of reflux episodes, duration of longest reflux episode, and number of episodes greater than 5 minutes. The percentage of total time pH is less than 4 is the most reproducible measurement for GERD, with reported upper limits of normal ranging from 4% to 5.5%.[159] The most recent Lyon consensus has suggested that acid exposure time (AET) of >6% is diagnostic of GERD, while AET between 4% and 6% is inconclusive.[297] Ambulatory pH testing discerns positional variations in GER, meal- and sleep-related episodes, and helps relate symptoms to reflux events.

The first of the three new technology advancements in reflux testing was the catheter-free system (Fig. 48.9, *upper panel*).[161] This system uses a wireless pH capsule that is affixed to the esophageal mucosa with a delivery system that drives a small needle into the epithelium. The capsule then transmits pH data to a portable receiver using radiofrequency signals. Catheter-free testing is now the preferred method of pH testing because monitoring can be extended beyond 24 hours (usually 48 hours), and limitations on normal daily activities and meals are negligible.[162] Because the capsule only accurately measures acid reflux (pH < 4), all studies must be performed off PPIs for at least 7 days.[163]

The second technology improvement combines impedance with pH testing, allowing the measurement of acid and nonacid reflux (see Fig. 48.9, *lower panel*). The latter is particularly important for patients on PPIs who continue to reflux, but now most episodes have pH higher than 4.[158] Nonacid reflux is measured by the detection of a retrograde bolus of ion-rich fluid in the esophagus. Refluxates that are a mixture of liquid and air are also readily detected. In a large group of normal subjects of PPIs, roughly 40% of reflux episodes were either weakly acidic (pH 4–6.5) or alkaline (pH > 6.5).[164] In a multicenter study using combined impedance-pH testing, 37% of patients experienced continued reflux symptoms despite twice-daily PPI therapy that was due to nonacid reflux.[165] Lyon consensus suggests that AET of >4% and >80% episodes of reflux by pH impedance monitoring tested on acid suppressive therapy is evidence for actionable refractory GERD.[297]

The most recent technologies for detecting GERD measure mucosal integrity alteration during endoscopy by detecting mucosal impedance changes or based on intraluminal impedance testing (nocturnal baseline impedance and post swallow-induced peristaltic wave index).[166–169] Mucosal impedance measurements have identified patients with GERD and EoE with a high degree of accuracy. It is too early to assess the clinical impact of this new technology, but the efficiency of diagnosing GERD without the need for prolonged ambulatory testing is promising. The role of nocturnal baseline impedance and post swallow-induced peristaltic wave is anticipated to be limited given need for catheter-based testing and complicated means of measuring both parameters. Finally, salivary pepsin testing and a catheter-based transoral pH monitoring are purported to help in the diagnosis of extraesophageal reflux; however, studies on their clinical benefit have shown mixed results.[145]

A critical limitation of esophageal pH monitoring is that there exists no absolute threshold value that reliably identifies GERD patients. Studies comparing patients with endoscopic esophagitis who underwent pH tests report sensitivities from 77% to 100%, with specificities from 85% to 100%.[145] However, esophagitis patients rarely need pH testing; rather, patients with normal endoscopy and suspected GERD might benefit most from this test. Unfortunately, data on these patients are less conclusive, with considerable overlap between controls and nonerosive refluxers.[159] Other drawbacks of pH testing include possible equipment failure, pH probe missing reflux events because the probe is buried in a mucosal fold, and false-negative studies due to dietary or activity limitations from poor tolerability of the nasal probe.

Ambulatory reflux pH monitoring is the only test that records and correlates symptoms with reflux episodes over extended periods of time. However, because only 10%–20% of reflux episodes are associated with symptoms, different statistical analyses have evolved, attempting to define a significant association between symptoms and reflux episodes, including the symptom index, symptom sensitivity index, and symptom association probability.[169] Unfortunately, no studies have defined the accuracy of these symptom scores in predicting response to therapy. Furthermore, validation studies were done only for heartburn, regurgitation, and chest pain with acid reflux; there were no studies with atypical reflux symptoms or nonacid reflux. More recent studies have questioned the validity of symptom association probability and have warned against its use, especially in those with normal reflux parameters.[170,171] Therefore pH testing can define an association between complaints and GER, but only treatment trials address the critical clinical issue of causality.

Clinical indications for ambulatory reflux monitoring are established.[145] Before fundoplication, pH testing should be done in patients with normal endoscopy to ensure the presence of pathologic acid reflux. After antireflux surgery, persistent or recurrent symptoms warrant repeat pH testing. In these situations, pH monitoring is performed with the patient off antireflux medications. Esophageal reflux testing is particularly helpful in evaluating patients with GERD-like symptoms who are resistant to treatment and who have normal or equivocal endoscopic findings. However, here there is controversy whether this should be done on or off PPIs.[160] For this indication, impedance-pH testing can be done on PPI therapy to define two populations: those with and those without continued abnormal acid or nonacid exposure times. The group with persistent GER needs intensified medical therapy, whereas patients with symptoms and good reflux control have another etiology for their complaints. The off-PPI approach is gaining popularity because 50%–60% of patients with poorly responding symptoms and normal endoscopy do not have GERD. A negative pH test off therapy is useful because it directs the diagnostic workup toward other causes and enables

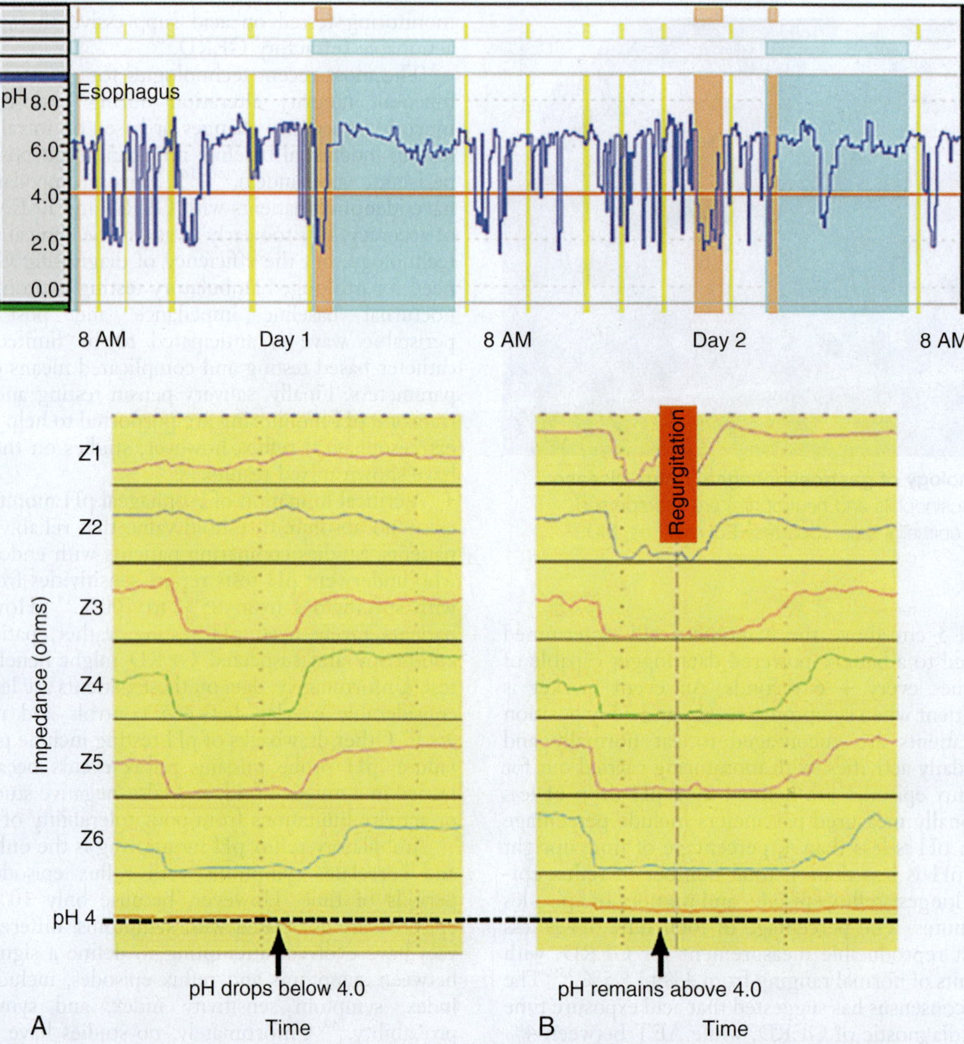

Fig. 48.9 Tracings from 48-hour esophageal pH and multichannel impedance-pH studies. *Top panel* is a 48-hour pH capsule study in a patient with gastroesophageal reflux disease. Meals/drinks are shown by the *yellow lines*, supine periods are shown in *blue*. The *orange bars* represent symptoms that were associated with acid reflux. The *bottom panels* are examples of acid and nonacid reflux detected by multichannel impedance-pH monitoring. (A) Acid reflux, with a typical pattern of sequential impedance drops in a retrograde direction, reaching the third impedance-measuring segment (Z3) and associated with an esophageal pH fall to less than 4.0. (B) Nonacid reflux in a patient on a PPI who reports an episode of regurgitation during this reflux episode, with a typical impedance pattern of retrograde flow reaching Z1 and despite esophageal pH remaining above 4.

cessation of unnecessary PPI therapy. However, a recent study[172] found that more than 42% of patients with negative tests for acid reflux still continued PPI therapy. Finally, ambulatory pH testing may help in defining patients with extraesophageal manifestations of GERD. However, its most important utility is in ruling out reflux as the cause for patients' persistent reflux. Initially most of these studies were done off antireflux medications to confirm the coexistence of GERD; however, this does not guarantee symptom causality. Therefore an approach is to first treat aggressively with PPIs, reserving pH testing for those patients not responding after 4–12 weeks of therapy.[158]

Barium Esophagogram

The barium esophagogram is an inexpensive, readily available, and noninvasive esophageal test.[173] It is most useful in demonstrating anatomic narrowing of the esophagus and assessing the presence and reducibility of a hiatal hernia. Schatzki's rings, webs, or minimally narrowed peptic strictures may only be seen with an esophagogram, being missed by endoscopy, which may not adequately distend the esophagus. Giving a 13-mm radiopaque pill or marshmallow along with the barium liquid can help to identify these subtle narrowings. The barium esophagogram allows good assessment of peristalsis and is helpful preoperatively in identifying a weak esophageal pump. The ability of barium esophagogram to detect esophagitis varies, with sensitivities of 79%–100% for moderate to severe esophagitis, whereas mild esophagitis is usually missed. Barium testing also falls short when addressing the presence of Barrett's esophagus. The spontaneous reflux of barium into the proximal esophagus is very specific for reflux, but it is not sensitive. Provocative maneuvers (e.g., leg lifting, coughing, Valsalva, and water siphon) can elicit stress reflux and improve the sensitivity of the barium esophagogram, but some argue that these maneuvers also decrease its specificity.[174]

Esophageal Manometry

As with reflux testing, the advent of multichannel high-resolution manometry has revolutionized this esophageal function test.[175] With 32–36 pressure transducers spanning the entire esophagus, manometry can now accurately assess LES pressure and relaxation, as well as peristaltic activity, including contraction amplitude, duration, and velocity. However, esophageal manometry is generally not indicated in the evaluation of the uncomplicated GERD patient because most have a normal resting LES pressure. Esophageal manometry to document adequate esophageal peristalsis and exclude variants of achalasia and scleroderma is traditionally recommended before antireflux surgery.[158] If the study identifies ineffective peristalsis (low amplitude or frequent failed peristalsis) or aperistalsis, then a complete fundoplication may be contraindicated. However, this assumption is challenged because reflux control was better, and dysphagia no more common, in patients with weak peristalsis after a complete, as opposed to a partial, fundoplication.[176] An improvement of traditional manometry, combining it with impedance testing, is helping to clarify this controversy. Using this technique, a study found that less than 50% of patients with ineffective peristalsis had a significant delay in esophageal bolus transit measured by impedance.[177] Therefore potentially only these patients with a significant physiologic defect in motility will require a modified fundoplication. Recently, functional lumen imaging probe is being employed during endoscopy to assess esophageal motility, especially in those suspected of having achalasia or when normal esophageal motility is suspected.[298] This technology measures motility through esophageal response to distension. Ongoing studies will clarify its role in those with dysphagia and how it compares to the traditional high-resolution manometry.

CLINICAL COURSE

The clinical course of GERD depends to a great extent on whether the patient has erosive or nonerosive disease. There is controversy as to whether GERD exists as a spectrum of disease severity or as a categorical disease in three distinct groups: erosive, nonerosive, and Barrett's esophagus. Patients tend not to cross over from one group to another; in follow-ups ranging from 6 months to longer than 22 years, less than 25% of patients with nonerosive disease evolved over time to having erosive esophagitis, nearly all to LA grade A/B disease, or to having complications of GERD.[10,178]

Nonerosive Disease

Early studies from tertiary referral centers suggested that the majority of GERD patients had esophagitis.[179] However, recent data suggest that up to 70% of GERD patients have a normal endoscopic examination.[180,181] Endoscopy-negative GERD patients are more likely to be female, younger, thin, and without hiatal hernia, and they have a higher prevalence of functional GI disorders.[182] Despite their mild mucosal damage, these patients demonstrate a chronic pattern of symptoms with periods of exacerbation and remission.[183] Nonerosive GERD is suspected in the patient with typical reflux symptoms and a normal endoscopy and confirmed by the patient's response to antisecretory therapy. Esophageal pH testing identifies three distinct subsets of nonerosive GERD patients. First are the patients with excessive acid reflux who usually respond to PPI therapy. Second are the patients with normal acid reflux parameters but a good correlation between their symptoms and acid reflux episodes. This group represents 30%–50% of nonerosive GERD patients and, based on recent Rome IV criteria, is classified as "reflux hypersensitivity."[184] These patients probably have heightened esophageal sensitivity to acid and are less likely to respond to antireflux therapy.[185] The third group is characterized by normal AETs and poor symptom correlation. This group is classified as "functional heartburn."[184]

Erosive Disease

Patients with erosive esophagitis tend to be male, older, and overweight and are more likely to have hiatal hernias.[182] The clinical course of these patients with erosive esophagitis is more predictable and associated with complications of GERD. Longitudinal studies have shown that up to 85% of patients with erosive GERD and given no maintenance reflux therapy will relapse within 6 months of stopping PPI therapy; the relapse rate is highest in patients with more severe grades of esophagitis (see Table 48.2).[186,187] Several studies confirm that erosive esophagitis patients are prone to reflux complications, including ulcers, strictures, and Barrett's esophagus. In a Finnish study, 20 patients with erosive GERD treated with lifestyle changes, antacids, and prokinetic drugs were followed for a median of 19 years. Fourteen patients continued to have erosions, and six new cases of Barrett's esophagus were detected.[178] In another more recent European study,[10] patients with LA grade C/D esophagitis developed Barrett's esophagus over 2 years at a rate of 5.8%, compared with only 1.4% for LA grade A/B and 0.5% for nonerosive GERD.

COMPLICATIONS

Hemorrhage, Ulcers, and Perforation

GERD-related noncancer deaths are rare (0.46 per 100,000 persons). The most common fatal causes are hemorrhagic esophagitis, aspiration pneumonia, ulcer perforation, and rupture with severe esophagitis.[188] Major hemorrhage and esophageal perforation are usually associated with deep esophageal ulcers or severe esophagitis.[189] Esophageal perforations are very rare in the PPI era but can result in mediastinitis and death. Clinically important hemorrhage has been reported in 7%–18% of GERD patients[190] and may result in iron deficiency anemia.

Peptic Esophageal Strictures

Strictures occur in 7%–23% of patients with untreated reflux esophagitis. They are commonly seen in older men[191] and linked to chronic NSAID use.[192] Stricture formation is complex, starting as reversible inflammation with edema, cellular infiltration, and vascular congestion, progressing to collagen deposition, and ending in irreversible fibrosis. As dysphagia progresses, heartburn often decreases, and reflecting the stricture acting as a barrier to further reflux. Dysphagia is usually limited to solids. Unlike malignant strictures, patients with peptic strictures have a good appetite, alter their diet, and lose little weight.

Peptic strictures are smooth-walled, tapered, circumferential narrowings in the lower esophagus, usually less than 1 cm long but occasionally extend to 8 cm (Fig. 48.10). In these unusual cases, the clinician should suspect a predisposing condition, such as ZES, pill esophagitis, or prolonged NG intubation.[191] A mid-to-upper esophageal stricture should raise concern for Barrett's esophagus or malignancy. Although once controversial, today a Schatzki's ring is considered a forme fruste of an early peptic stricture.[193] All stricture patients should undergo endoscopy to confirm the benign nature of the lesion and take biopsies to exclude EoE, cancer, and Barrett's esophagus.

Barrett's Esophagus

See Chapter 47.

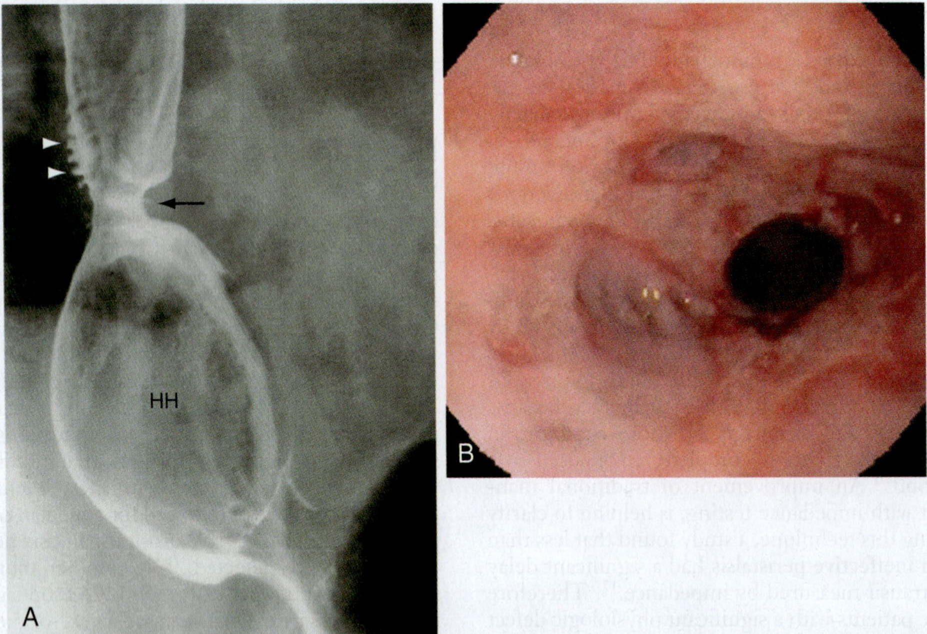

Fig. 48.10 Classic peptic esophageal stricture demonstrated by barium esophagogram (A) and endoscopy (B). The film shows a large hiatal hernia (HH) common to all gastroesophageal reflux disease strictures. *The black arrow* points to a short, thick fibrous stricture associated with multiple pseudodiverticula (*white arrowheads*). Although not seen on barium examination, the endoscopic view also demonstrates circumferential esophagitis (Los Angeles grade D).

TREATMENT OF UNCOMPLICATED DISEASE

The rationale for GERD therapy depends on a careful definition of specific aims.[194] In patients without esophagitis, the therapeutic goals are to relieve reflux symptoms and prevent frequent symptomatic relapses. In patients with esophagitis, the goals are to relieve symptoms and heal esophagitis while preventing further relapses and complications.

Nonprescription Therapies

Although GERD is common, many sufferers do not seek medical care, instead choosing to change their lifestyles and self-medicate with over-the-counter (OTC) antacid preparations. These observations have led to the "iceberg" model of the GERD population. Most heartburn suffers are invisible because they self-medicate and do not seek professional help; only those at the tip of the iceberg, typically patients with severe symptoms or reflux complications, are seen by physicians.[21]

Lifestyle Modifications

Selective lifestyle changes, carefully explained to the patient, should be part of the initial management plan and are especially helpful in those with mild, intermittent complaints. These include elevating the head of the bed, losing weight if overweight, restricting alcohol and smoking, making dietary changes, refraining from lying down after meals, and avoiding bedtime snacks. Physiologic studies show that these maneuvers enhance esophageal acid clearance, decrease acid reflux–related events, or ease heartburn symptoms.[195] However, a tailored approach to lifestyle modifications is recommended. Head-of-the-bed elevation can be done by using 6–8-in blocks or a foam wedge under the mattress to elevate the upper torso. This maneuver should be used in those who continue to have regurgitation likely due to mechanical defect, such as a hiatal hernia. Eating several hours before retiring and avoiding bedtime snacks keeps the stomach empty at night, thereby decreasing nocturnal reflux episodes. Losing weight aims to reduce the incidence of reflux by the "abdominal stress" mechanism. Targeted weight loss may be helpful, whereas discrete periods of weight gain can be associated with exacerbation of reflux symptoms.[196] Cessation of smoking and alcohol reduction are valuable because both agents lower LES pressure, reduce acid clearance, and impair intrinsic squamous epithelial protective functions.[21,73] Reducing meal size and avoiding fats, carminatives, and chocolate reduces reflux frequency by decreasing episodes of tLESRs, as well as lowering LES pressure.[21] In addition, some patients complain of heartburn after citrus drinks, spicy foods, tomato-based products, coffee, tea, or cola drinks. Stimulation of gastric acid secretion or esophageal sensitivity to low pH (or perhaps hyperosmolar solutions) may account for these symptoms.[197] However, indiscriminate food prohibition should be avoided but rather tailored to individual sensitivity to better promote compliance. Finally, patients should avoid, if possible, drugs that lower LES pressure (see Table 46.1) or promote localized esophagitis, such as certain bisphosphonates (see Chapter 45).

How good are the clinical studies assessing the efficacy of lifestyle changes? In an evidence-based review,[21] studies of smoking, alcohol, chocolate, fatty foods, and citrus products had sound physiologic data that their intake can adversely affect symptoms or promote reflux on esophageal pH tests. However, there was little convincing evidence that cessation of these products predictably improved reflux symptoms. Only elevation of the head of the bed, left lateral decubitus positioning, and weight loss were associated with GERD improvement in case-controlled studies.[21]

Over-the-Counter Medications

These drugs are used in treating mild, infrequent heartburn symptoms triggered by lifestyle indiscretions. Antacids increase

LES pressure but work primarily by buffering gastric acid, albeit for short periods. Heartburn symptoms are rapidly relieved, but patients may need to take antacids frequently, usually 1–3 hours after meals. Gaviscon, containing alginic acid and antacids, mixes with saliva to form a highly viscous solution that floats on the gastric pool, acting as a mechanical barrier. Recent studies found that the raft colocalized with the postprandial acid pocket and displaced it below the diaphragm, resulting in significant suppression of postprandial acid reflux.[198] A meta-analysis of OTC medications found that compared with placebo, antacids showed minimal symptomatic improvement [absolute benefit of 8%, number to treat (NNT) of 13], whereas Gaviscon was better (absolute benefit of 26%, NNT of 4).[199] However, these therapies do not heal esophagitis, and long-term trials suggest symptom relief in only 20% of patients.[200,201]

OTC H2RAs are available at doses usually one-half the standard prescription dose. Although onset of relief is not as rapid as with antacids, the OTC H2RAs relieve symptoms for 6–10 hours. Based on a meta-analysis of three studies, H2RAs given before a provocative meal were superior to placebo (absolute benefit of 11%–16%, NNT of 9–6) in symptom relief/improvement.[199] Therefore they are particularly useful when taken before potentially refluxogenic activities. Like antacids, OTC H2RAs are ineffective in healing esophagitis.[202]

The long-term safety and efficacy of PPIs led the FDA to approve omeprazole at full dose (20 mg) for OTC use in 2003. Drug labeling suggested daily use for only 2 weeks and recommended physician follow-up for persistent symptoms. Despite initial "real world" concerns of abusing this drug, early actual-use data support that consumers accurately self-select if OTC omeprazole is appropriate for use, comply with a 2-week regimen, and seek physician care for longer term management of frequent heartburn.[203]

Prescription Medications

Patients with frequent heartburn, esophagitis, or complications usually see a physician and receive prescription medications. Prokinetic drugs attempt to correct the GERD-related motility disorders associated with GERD. However, the most clinically effective drugs for short- and long-term reflux treatment are acid suppressive drugs.

Prokinetic Drugs

Until recently, three prokinetic drugs were available in the United States for treating GERD: bethanechol, a cholinergic agonist; metoclopramide, a dopamine antagonist; and cisapride, a serotonin (5-hydroxytryptamine 4) receptor agonist that increases acetylcholine release in the myenteric plexus. These drugs improve reflux symptoms by increasing LES pressure, acid clearance, or gastric emptying. However, none alters tLESRs, and their effectiveness decreases with disease severity.[204] Current prokinetics provide modest benefit in controlling heartburn, particularly in patients with delayed gastric emptying, but have unreliable efficacy in healing esophagitis unless combined with acid-inhibiting drugs.[204]

The current use of prokinetic drugs is greatly limited by their side-effect profile. Bethanechol commonly causes flushing, blurred vision, headaches, abdominal cramps, and urinary frequency. Metoclopramide, which crosses the blood-brain barrier, has a 20%–50% incidence of fatigue, lethargy, anxiety, and restlessness and rarely causes tremor, parkinsonism, dystonia, or tardive dyskinesia, especially in older patients. Side effects may be decreased by reducing the dosing regimen to twice a day, taking a larger single dose before dinner or at bedtime, or using a sustained-release tablet. Domperidone, another dopamine antagonist not crossing the blood-brain barrier, has fewer side effects, primarily hyperprolactinemia and nipple tenderness/discharge. It is not approved for GERD use in the United States but is readily available from Canada or compounding pharmacies. Cisapride was the best prokinetic drug for treating GERD but was withdrawn from the U.S. market in 2000 because of reports of serious cardiac dysrhythmias (ventricular tachycardia, ventricular fibrillation, torsades de pointes, and QT prolongation), with associated cardiac arrest and deaths related to possible drug interactions.[205]

European investigators are rejuvenating interest in prokinetic drugs for GERD with studies on macrolides such as azithromycin. This class of drugs increases gastric emptying, increases LES and proximal stomach tone, and, among patients with a small hiatus hernia, displaces the acid pocket below the diaphragm.[206] Small clinical studies found azithromycin decreased acid reflux episodes and total acid exposure in GERD patients with hiatal hernia[206] and lung transplant patients.[207]

Transient Lower Esophageal Sphincter Relaxation Inhibitors

Regulating the frequency of tLESRs is an attractive target for GERD treatment because of its pivotal role in all types of reflux episodes. Currently, the only medication available that decreases tLESRs is baclofen, a $GABA_B$ agonist used for many years to treat spasticity. Baclofen (5–20 mg three times daily) significantly reduces tLESRs, decreases both acid and duodenal reflux, and improves symptoms in GERD patients treated for 4 weeks to several months.[208,209] The critical issue with baclofen is tolerability. Side effects, including drowsiness, dizziness, nausea, and vomiting, require discontinuation in up to 20% of patients.[208] Other $GABA_B$ agonists with improved tolerability have been developed (lesogaberan, arbaclofen placarbil) but were abandoned mainly because of limited clinical efficacy. For example, lesogaberan as add-on therapy to PPIs in patients with refractory GERD symptoms resulted in a low, although significant, 16% remission rate compared with 8% remission for PPIs alone.[210] Among 150 patients with frequent heartburn and/or regurgitation, arbaclofen placarbil (20, 40, or 60 mg twice daily) was no better than placebo over 4 weeks in reducing heartburn events.[211] Finally, a negative allosteric modulator of mGluR5 receptor (ADX 10059) as monotherapy was shown to improve reflux symptoms and decrease reflux events but failed to demonstrate significant clinical efficacy in refractory GERD patients; further development of this component has been halted.[212]

H2RAs

These drugs (cimetidine, ranitidine, famotidine, and nizatidine) are more effective in controlling nocturnal than meal-stimulated acid secretion.[213] The four H2RAs are equally effective when used in proper doses, usually twice a day before meals. GERD trials find that heartburn can be significantly decreased by H2RAs when compared with placebo, although symptoms are rarely abolished. A comprehensive metaanalysis found that the overall esophagitis healing rates with H2RAs rarely exceeded 60% after up to 12 weeks of treatment, even when higher doses were used (Fig. 48.11B).[214] Healing rates differ in individual trials, depending primarily on the severity of esophagitis being treated: grade I and II esophagitis heal in 60%–90% of patients, whereas grades III and IV heal in only 30%–50% despite high-dose regimens.[214]

Although PPIs are more effective than H2RAs, nocturnal gastric acid breakthrough while on PPI therapy may cause reflux symptoms in some patients. H2RAs given at bedtime successfully eliminated this problem in a study, suggesting a new indication for H2RAs in the PPI era.[215] However, this study used only a single evening dose and did not account for the tolerance that frequently develops to H2RAs over weeks to months.[216] This tolerance impairs the effectiveness of chronic nocturnal dosing of H2RAs to

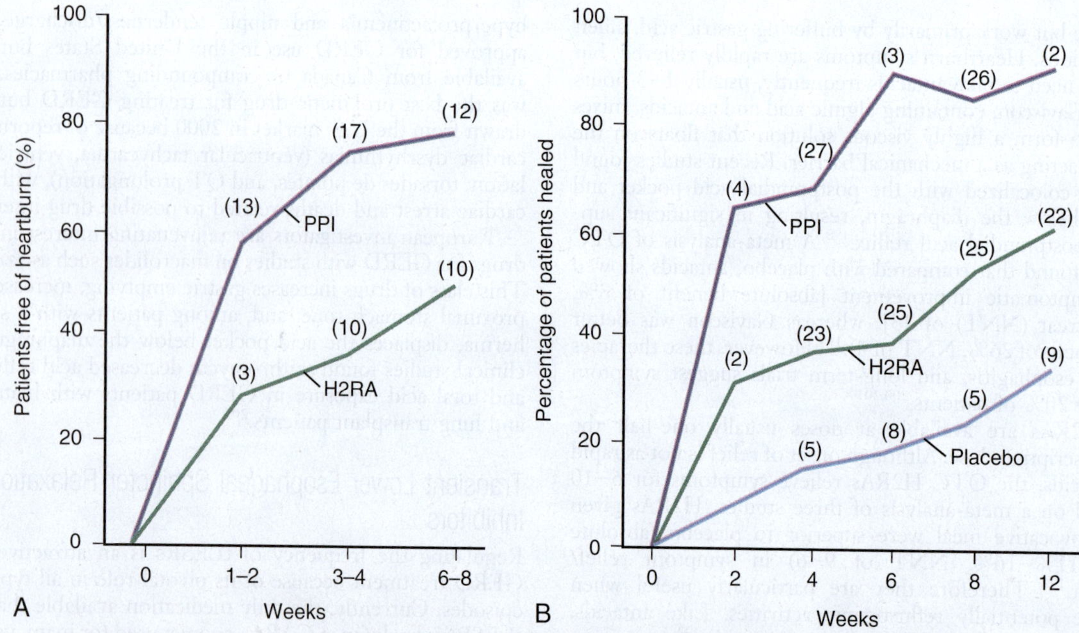

Fig. 48.11 (A) Symptom relief time curve over 8 weeks for a PPI or H2RA corrected for patients free of heartburn at baseline. More patients treated with a PPI for 2 weeks were asymptomatic as compared with those treated with an H2RA, even after a much longer duration of treatment with the H2RA. (B) Esophagitis healing time curve for PPI, H2RA, and placebo over 12 weeks. Treatment with a PPI for 4 weeks healed esophagitis in more patients than in the other two groups over 12 weeks, implying a substantial therapeutic gain. The numbers of studies included for each time point and treatment are shown in parentheses. (Data based on meta-analysis from Chiba N, Gara CJ, Wilkinson JM, Hunt RH. Speed of healing and symptom relief in grade II to IV gastroesophageal reflux disease: a meta-analysis. *Gastroenterology*. 1997;112:1798–1810.)

eliminate nocturnal acid breakthrough[217] but suggests a useful role in as-needed medications in situations in which lifestyle indiscretions may promote nocturnal complaints.

The H2RAs are very safe, with a side effect rate of about 4%, most of which are minor and reversible.[213] Serum concentrations of phenytoin, procainamide, theophylline, and warfarin are higher after the administration of cimetidine and, to a lesser degree, ranitidine, whereas these interactions are not reported with the other 2 H2RAs. H2RAs do not inhibit the antiplatelet effect of clopidogrel.

PPIs

PPIs inhibit meal-stimulated and nocturnal acid secretion to a significantly greater degree than H2RAs[218] but rarely render patients achlorhydric. After oral ingestion, acid inhibition is delayed because PPIs need to accumulate in the parietal cell secretory canaliculus to bind irreversibly to actively secreting proton pumps.[219] Therefore the slower a PPI is cleared from plasma, the more it is available for delivery to the proton pumps. PPIs should be taken before the first meal of the day, when most proton pumps become active. Because not all pumps are active at any given time, a single PPI dose will not inhibit all pumps. A second dose, if necessary, can be taken before the evening meal; however, this is an off-label indication. PPIs do not "cure" reflux disease, rather they treat GERD in an indirect way by decreasing the number of acid reflux episodes. In exchange, the weakly acidic (pH > 4) episodes are increased, while the total number of reflux episodes and proximal extent are not affected by PPI therapy.[162]

PPIs (omeprazole, lansoprazole, rabeprazole, pantoprazole, and esomeprazole) have superior efficacy compared with H2RAs on the basis of their ability to maintain an intragastric pH greater than 4 from 10 to 14 hours daily compared with approximately 6–8 hours daily with the H2RAs.[219,220] PPIs are superior to H2RAs in completely relieving heartburn symptoms in patients with severe GERD, usually within 1–2 weeks (see Fig. 43.11A).[214] PPI therapy has been shown in a Cochrane metaanalysis to be superior to placebo and H2RAs in nonerosive GERD and for undiagnosed reflux symptoms in primary care, although the effect is 20%–30% lower than in patients with esophagitis.[221,222] Unlike heartburn, the GERD symptom of regurgitation does not have a robust response to PPIs. In a recent review of 7 placebo-controlled trials, the therapeutic gain for regurgitation averaged only 17% relative to placebo and was at least 20% less than that observed for heartburn.[223]

Controlled studies and a large metaanalysis report complete healing of even severe ulcerative esophagitis after 8 weeks in more than 80% of patients taking PPIs, compared with 51% on H2RAs and 28% receiving placebo (see Fig. 43.11B).[214,224–226] In another recent Cochrane review,[227] PPIs were superior to H2RAs in healing esophagitis at 4–8 weeks (risk ratio, 0.47), with an NNT of 3. In patients not healing initially, prolonged therapy with the same dose or an increased PPI dose usually resulted in 100% healing.[228] Until recently, therapeutic efficacy among PPIs was similar. However, large studies have found esomeprazole 40 mg superior to omeprazole 20 mg and to lansoprazole 30 mg in healing esophagitis.[229,230] A metaanalysis of 10 randomized clinical trials[231] comparing esomeprazole to all other PPIs found the therapeutic advantage is minimal with LA grade A/B esophagitis (NNT of 50 and 33, respectively) and greater with severe LA grade C/D esophagitis (NNT of 14 and 8, respectively). This superiority is related to higher systemic bioavailability and less interpatient variability with esomeprazole. Despite their frequent use twice daily in treating GERD, only a recent Japanese study[232] documents the superiority of off-label dosing of twice-daily PPIs for healing esophagitis over 8 weeks compared with once-daily dosing. Healing rates were similar for rabeprazole 20 mg twice daily (77%) and 10 mg twice daily (78%) and significantly superior to rabeprazole 20 mg each morning (59%). Several PPIs are available in the United States for IV use.[233]

Recent approaches to enhance acid suppression with PPIs include immediate-release omeprazole and dexlansoprazole. The former contains nonenteric coated omeprazole and an antacid that protects the omeprazole from acid degradation in the stomach and allows for rapid absorption. Immediate-relief omeprazole can be dosed on an empty stomach at bedtime and provides more rapid control of nighttime gastric pH and nocturnal acid breakthrough than esomeprazole or lansoprazole.[234] Dexlansoprazole MR is the R-enantiomer of lansoprazole, with two distinct drug release periods (90 minutes and 4–5 hours after ingestion) that prolong the plasma concentration-time profile, thus extending the duration of acid suppression. Precise meal time may not be required for optimal efficacy.[235,236] In a recent placebo-controlled study among 178 patients receiving twice-daily PPIs, stepping down to once-daily dexlansoprazole 30 mg maintained excellent symptom relief over 6 weeks in 88% of patients.[237]

PPIs are well tolerated, with headaches and diarrhea being the most common side effects. Fasting serum gastrin levels increase with all the PPIs, but the elevations generally do not exceed the normal range and return to baseline values within 1–4 weeks of drug discontinuation. Omeprazole decreases the clearance of diazepam, warfarin, and clopidogrel owing to competition for the cytochrome P450 isoenzyme P2C19.[238]

Maintenance Therapies

GERD may be a chronic relapsing disease, especially in patients with low LES pressure, severe grades of esophagitis, and difficult-to-manage symptoms.[201] After esophagitis is healed, recurrence within 6 months of stopping medication occurs in more than 80% of patients with severe esophagitis and in 15%–30% of those with milder esophagitis.[186,239]

Cochrane reviews have identified the superiority of PPIs over H2RAs in maintaining the remission of esophagitis over 6–12 months.[240] Among 10 randomized trials, the relapse rate for esophagitis was 22% on PPIs versus 58% with H2RAs (NNT of 2.5). The FDA has approved all the PPIs, sometimes at one-half the acute dose, for maintenance therapy, but only ranitidine 150 mg twice a day among the H2RAs has maintenance indications for mild esophagitis. Many clinicians now place their patients with severe disease (daily symptoms, severe esophagitis, or complications) on chronic PPI therapy indefinitely. The efficacy of this approach is supported by open, compassionate-use data, primarily from the Netherlands and Australia.[241] In a study of 230 patients with severe esophagitis healed with 40 mg omeprazole, all subjects remained in remission for up to 11 years on maintenance omeprazole. More than 60% were maintained on omeprazole 20 mg a day, whereas higher doses of 60 mg or more were necessary in only 12% of patients, confirming a lack of tolerance to PPIs. Relapses were rare (1 per 9.4 years of follow-up), strictures did not occur, and Barrett's esophagus did not progress.

Although PPIs offer the best symptom relief and esophagitis healing, many patients do well long-term on lower dose treatments after having their complaints initially alleviated with PPIs. Using this "step-down approach," a Veterans Affairs study reported that 58% of 71 patients on chronic PPIs could be switched to H2RAs and/or prokinetics or taken off medication completely.[242] Younger age and severe heartburn symptoms predicted a PPI requirement. Overall, this approach saved money for the health care system. A similar study by the same investigators found that 80% of patients using multiple-dose PPIs could be stepped down to single-dose PPI, remaining symptom free for 6 months with considerable cost savings.[243] Hence the adage "once on a PPI, always on a PPI" is not true. Patients who continue to have symptoms despite PPI therapy likely have other etiologies for their symptoms than GERD.[244]

Safety of PPI Therapy

As a class, PPIs are very safe drugs. Owing to their efficacy and safety, the worldwide sales of PPIs approached 14 billion dollars in 2009.[1] The initial concerns about the development of gastric carcinoid tumors and colon cancer has not been confirmed.[245,246] More recently, the literature has been overwhelmed with reports raising concerns about potential adverse events from long-term acid suppression.[247] In the United States, such reports have led the FDA to issue a number of broad-based product warnings (black box warnings) including all the available PPIs, either prescription or OTC. However, these studies are all from retrospective case-control studies and demonstrate association, not causality.[247] No prospective, observational, or randomized trial can substantiate the concerns discussed as follows.

Fundic gland polyps are the most common gastric polyp found at endoscopy. Their association with chronic PPI use has been a topic of debate since these drugs were first described. A recent study evaluated 599 patients, of whom 322 used PPIs and 107 had fundic gland polyps.[248] Long-term PPI use was associated with up to a fourfold increase in the risk of fundic gland polyps. Low-grade dysplasia was found in one fundic gland polyp. These polyps arise because of parietal cell hyperplasia and parietal cell protrusions resulting from acid suppression.

Recent studies confirm that chronic acid suppression may be associated with an increased risk of community-acquired pneumonias and enteric infections. In a large Scandinavian population-based study,[249] the adjusted relative risk for pneumonia among current PPI users, compared with those who stopped using PPIs, was 1.89. Current users of H2RAs had a 1.63-fold increased risk of pneumonia compared with those who stopped. A significant positive dose-response relationship was observed in the PPI users. Likewise, systematic reviews and meta-analyses found an increased risk of enteric infections (*Salmonella*, *Campylobacter*, and *Clostridioides difficile*) and of spontaneous bacterial peritonitis[250,251] with acid suppression. The relationship with community- and hospital-acquired *C. difficile* interaction is particularly alarming, with PPI use beginning to approach antibiotics as a risk factor for this infection.

Chronic use of PPIs is purported to affect the absorption of calcium, vitamin B_{12}, magnesium, and iron. A nested case-controlled study from the United Kingdom among 13,556 patients found that the risk of hip fractures increased with chronic PPI use over 1 year (adjusted odds ratio, 1.44), especially patients receiving high-dose PPIs (adjusted odds ratio, 2.65). A smaller but still significant risk was observed in chronic H2RA users.[252] A large Canadian study[253] reached similar conclusions but found the risk for hip fractures became apparent only after 5 years of treatment (adjusted odds ratio, 1.62) and after 7 years for all osteoporotic fractures (adjusted odds ratio, 1.92). However, more recent cross-sectional, longitudinal, and prospective studies (even done by the same Canadian center[254]) do not support these earlier observations, suggesting issues of undetected biases and future need for randomized studies to address this issue.[247,255] It has been suggested that if PPIs cause osteoporosis, they may interfere with insoluble calcium absorption or possibly inhibit the osteoclastic proton transport system, potentially reducing bone resorption.

PPIs could retard the absorption of vitamin B_{12} by decreasing gastric acidity, reducing the release of cobalamin from dietary protein, or by promoting SIBO, thereby increasing luminal cobalamin consumption. However, cohort and case-control studies have not shown a convincing link between PPI use and vitamin B_{12} deficiency.[247]

Most recently a series of case reports (<50 cases) associate hypomagnesemia with long-term PPI use.[256] Symptoms were severe, requiring hospitalization; some were resistant to magnesium repletion, but all corrected with discontinuation of PPIs, and several cases relapsed when the PPIs were restarted. The mechanism for this magnesium loss is unknown; there was no identifiable GI or renal source of wasting.

Dietary iron is primarily nonheme iron and requires acid for absorption. Animal studies suggest iron absorption is impaired in a low acid state. Patients with hemochromatosis on chronic PPI therapy have a significant reduction in yearly volume of blood that has to be removed to keep iron studies at appropriate levels.[257] On the other hand, patients with gastric acid hypersecretion due to ZES who required long-term high-dose PPIs to reduce acid secretion had no evidence of iron deficiency over 4 years.[258]

PPIs have been implicated as a cause of acute intestinal nephritis. It appears to be a very rare idiosyncratic occurrence causing hypersensitivity inflammatory damage to the renal interstitium and tubules.[259] Chronic renal failure, dementia, and death have also been attributed to PPI use; however, the overwhelming concern about such associations is potential for confounding.[247]

In 2009 the FDA issued a warning regarding the potential for increased adverse cardiovascular events in patients using PPIs and clopidogrel, especially omeprazole, lansoprazole, and esomeprazole. The concern arose from the fact that the antiplatelet activity of clopidogrel requires conversion from a prodrug to an active metabolite by the CYP2C19 isoenzyme. This is the same pathway required for metabolism of some PPIs but not pantoprazole or dexlansoprazole. However, the data currently do not conclusively show a clinically significant drug-drug interaction. A recent metaanalysis (27 studies)[260] that focused on primary outcomes (myocardial infarction, stroke, stent occlusion, or death) and secondary outcomes (rehospitalization for cardiac events or revascularization procedures) found no consistent adverse interaction between PPIs and clopidogrel. The only large randomized trial demonstrated a significant reduction of GI bleeding events with combination clopidogrel-omeprazole therapy versus clopidogrel alone (hazard ratio: 0.34), with no significant cardiovascular morbidity (hazard ratio: 0.99).[261]

These ever-increasing reports of possible PPI interactions can be alarming to the public. Although the current data are relatively weak, they increase the obligation of all physicians to prescribe PPIs only for appropriate indications, to minimize the use of twice-daily PPIs when once-daily therapy will suffice, and to be vigilant about long-term continuous use of PPIs, substituting on-demand therapy for patients with symptomatic uncomplicated GERD. However, it is also important to recognize that most such associations are weak and do not suggest a causal link.[247] In fact, the most recent ACG guidelines for the management of GERD state that the studies suggesting association between PPI therapy and long-term safety "have flaws" and "are not considered definitive."[281]

Surgical Therapy

Only surgical fundoplication corrects the physiologic factors contributing to GERD and potentially eliminates the need for long-term medications. Antireflux surgery reduces acid and nonacid GER by increasing basal LES pressure, decreasing tLESRs, and inhibiting complete LES relaxation.[262] This is done by reducing the hiatal hernia into the abdomen, reconstructing the diaphragmatic hiatus, and reinforcing the LES. The two most popular procedures, performed laparoscopically through the abdomen, are the Nissen 360-degree fundoplication and the Toupet partial fundoplication (Fig. 48.12).[262] The former is a superior operation with better long-term durability, but it causes more postoperative dysphagia and gas bloat symptoms.[263] The typical hospital stay is 1–2 days, and many patients return to normal activity in 2 weeks. Patients with more severe disease and a short esophagus, suggested by a large nonreducible hiatus hernia, tight stricture, or long-segment Barrett's esophagus, will require a Collis lengthening procedure to create a 3–5-cm neoesophagus, allowing the fundoplication to be placed in the abdomen under minimal tension.[264]

Since the advent of the laparoscopic operation, the number of antireflux operations performed in the United States nearly

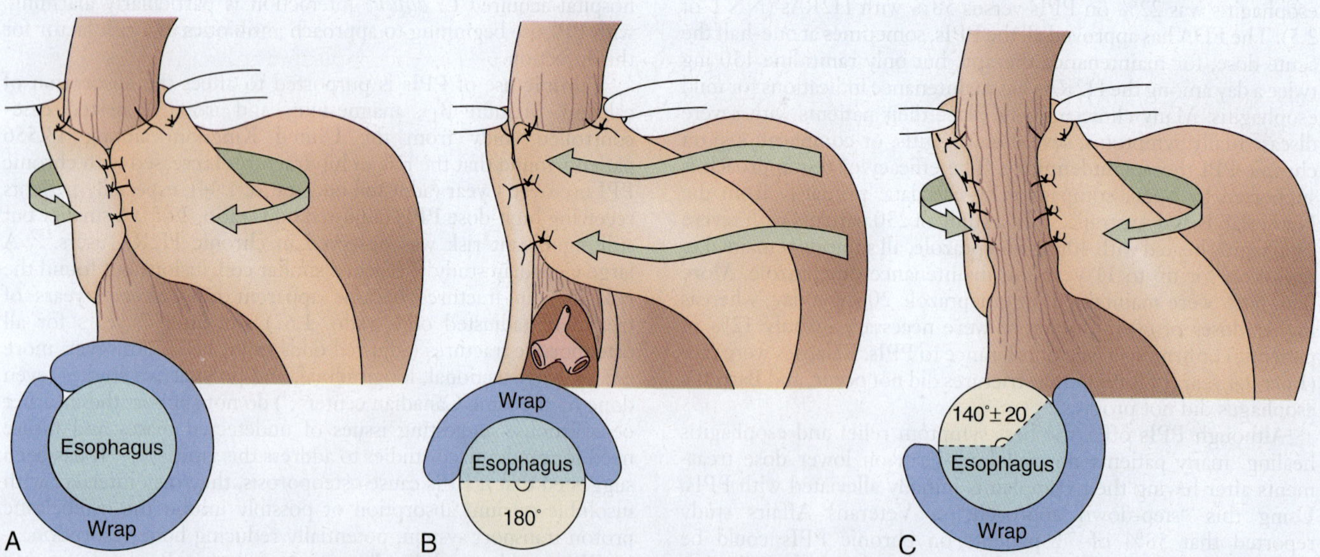

Fig. 48.12 Surgical fundoplications used during antireflux surgery. (A) The most popular worldwide is the 360-degree Nissen fundoplication. (B) An anterior wrap (e.g., Thal, Dor) is commonly used to prevent gastroesophageal reflux after a Heller myotomy for achalasia. The experience with this repair is limited in patients with classical gastroesophageal reflux disease. (C) The posterior wrap (Toupet) is popular in patients with poor esophageal motility, because postoperative dysphagia is less frequent than after the other operations. Toupet procedure entails is a 220 ± 20-degree wrap. (From Oelschlager BK, Eubanks TR, Pellegrini CA. Hiatal hernia and gastroesophageal reflux disease. In: Townsend CM, Beauchamp RD, Foshee JC, et al, eds. *Sabiston Textbook of Surgery: The Biological Basis of Modern Surgical Practice*. 18th ed. Philadelphia: Saunders; 2007.)

tripled from 11,000 per year in 1985 (open surgery) to a peak of nearly 32,000 in 1999, but leveled off at around 20,000 cases per year in 2006 and is continuing to gradually fall.[265,266] In a systematic review that identified 6 randomized controlled trials involving 449 patients that compared open and laparoscopic fundoplication,[263] there was no significant difference in recurrence rates between the procedures, and laparoscopic fundoplication was associated with lower operative morbidity (NNT of 8) and shorter hospital stay.

In the PPI era, symptom resolution on treatment helps predict the success of antireflux surgery for classic and atypical symptoms.[267] Antireflux surgery is a reasonable option in (1) healthy patients with typical or atypical GERD symptoms well controlled on PPIs, desiring alternative therapy because of drug expense, poor medication compliance, or fear of possible long-term side effects; (2) patients with volume regurgitation and aspiration symptoms not controlled on PPIs; and (3) recurrent peptic strictures in younger patients.[263] Patients recalcitrant to PPI therapy may well have another etiology for their complaints (e.g., pill esophagitis, gastroparesis, achalasia, and functional heartburn) and should be approached cautiously with surgery, especially those with extraesophageal complaints alone.[268]

Testing must be done before antireflux surgery. Endoscopy is necessary to exclude stricture, Barrett's esophagus, and dysplasia or carcinoma. A barium esophagogram helps define a nonreducible hiatal hernia, a shortened esophagus, and poor esophageal motility. Esophageal manometry combined with impedance will identify a weak esophageal pump and previously misdiagnosed achalasia or scleroderma. In patients with nonerosive GERD or those with esophagitis not responding to PPI therapy, esophageal pH testing is necessary. Gastric acid secretion measurements (if available), fasting serum gastrin assay, and gastric emptying tests may be indicated in selected patients. Careful testing will result in modification of the original operation or an alternative diagnosis in approximately 30% of patients.[269]

Antireflux surgery relieves reflux symptoms and reduces the need for stricture dilation in more than 90% of patients, but Barrett's esophagus rarely regresses, and the risk of developing esophageal cancer is unchanged.[270] In two large randomized studies,[271,272] open and laparoscopic antireflux surgery was not found to be superior to PPI therapy, especially when dose titration was permitted. For example, in the European LOTUS randomized study, the 5-year symptom remission rate was 92% (95% confidence interval, 89%–96%) in the esomeprazole group and 85% (95% confidence interval, 81%–90%) in the laparoscopic surgery group.[272] Mortality is rare (<1%) after antireflux surgery, but new postoperative complaints occur in up to 25% of patients, including dysphagia, gas bloat, diarrhea, and increased flatus.[273] Most symptoms improve over 1 year, but persistent complaints suggest too tight a wrap, a displaced fundoplication, or inadvertent damage to the vagus nerve. Successful antireflux surgery does not guarantee a permanent cure, but long-term studies suggest continued symptom relief for 20–30 years.[274,275] Best surgical results are obtained by experienced surgeons in high-volume centers, who report long-term symptom recurrence in only 10%–17% of patients.[262,273,276] However, many operations are performed in lower volume community hospitals where the results are more variable.[275] From long-term follow-up studies, 25%–62% of patients are back on some type of acid-suppressive medication 5–15 years after their antireflux surgery.[266,273,277] However, the evidence for recurrent GERD by pH testing is infrequent.

Tertiary specialized centers are seeing an increased rate of fundoplication failures. The most common reasons for failure are herniation of an intact fundoplication into the chest, "slipped" fundoplication with a recurrent hiatal hernia possibly due to a short esophagus, paraesophageal hernia through an intact fundoplication, too tight a fundoplication, and malpositioned fundoplication usually on the cardia of the stomach. Total breakdown of the fundoplication is now rare.[278] Revisional antireflux surgery must be performed by very experienced surgeons after thorough esophageal testing, because reoperation has increased morbidity and mortality compared with the initial operation.

Novel Endoscopic/Surgical Therapies

Since their introduction in the late 1990s, a series of endoscopic treatments for GERD (Stretta, Endocinch, Enteryx to name a few) have failed to show long-term efficacy. Moreover, side effects and complications, some fatal, were common with widespread use.[279] As a result in 2006, the American Gastroenterological Association Institute medical position statement recommended that "current data suggest that there are no definite indications for endoscopic therapy for GERD at this time."[280] Most of these devices have been removed, although the Stretta and magnetic sphincter augmentation (MSA) are still being employed. New attempts to endoscopically reconstruct a normal esophageal hiatus and competent LES continue. The newest approach is the transoral incisionless fundoplication which recreates at 200–270-degree value using polypropylene fasteners placed endoscopically.[282] Initial studies show symptom improvement, especially regurgitation and decrease use of PPIs. However, over time the fasteners tend to dislodge, with a systematic review reporting GERD symptom recurrence in 60% of patients with a similar rate back on PPIs although usually a lower dose than before treatment.[283]

Several novel surgical innovations, not altering the anatomy of the cardia, can potentially relieve reflux symptoms with minimal to no side effects. The first is the magnetic sphincter, which is a necklace of titanium beads with magnetic cores placed around the cardia, with minimal dissection of the hiatus. When the esophagus is at rest, the magnetic force augments the LES sufficiently to prevent reflux, yet is weak enough to allow peristalsis with swallowing to open the device. In a 3-year prospective study of 100 patients with GERD,[284] 64% normalized their acid reflux values, 93% reduced their PPI use by 50%, and 92% had significant improvement in quality of life. Dysphagia was frequent, occurring in 68% of patients postoperatively, 11% at 1 year, and 4% at 3 years. Six patients had the device removed, three because of severe dysphagia. This long-term efficacy has been maintained for up to 5 years with only 15% back on PPIs.[285] Device erosion into the esophagus or stomach is now being reported but seems to be rare. The ACG guidelines could not recommend the use of Stretta due to inconsistent and variable data but did suggest the use of MSA in patients with regurgitation who failed medical therapy as a potential alternative to antireflux fundoplication.[281]

The second surgical innovation is the use of electrical stimulation to the LES to improve LES pressure without interfering with LES relaxation.[286] This procedure was done laparoscopically by placing bipolar stitch electrodes in the muscularis propria of the LES, connected to an implantable pulse generation in a subcutaneous pocket on the anterior abdomen. A study from Chile[287] in 24 patients with GERD and small hiatal hernias (<2 cm) reported that over 6 months, electrical stimulation improved symptom scores by 75%; 91% of patients were off PPIs, and the median time that the esophageal pH was below 4 over a 24-hour period improved from 10.1% at baseline to 5.1% at 6 months. No patients complained of dysphagia, gas bloat, or inability to belch. An FDA randomized study with 1-year follow-up is ongoing in the United States. However, subsequent multicenter randomized controlled study did not show efficacy and the device development was halted.

To date, none of the new devices have been compared in randomized studies with the gold standard, Nissen fundoplication. For these reasons, many private insurers have been slow to adopt reimbursement guidelines on these new operations.[282]

TREATMENT OF PEPTIC ESOPHAGEAL STRICTURES

Dysphagia in patients with esophageal strictures and rings is related to stricture diameter and severity of esophagitis.[288] When the esophageal lumen diameter is less than 13 mm, dysphagia is common and esophageal dilation is required. Simple short strictures can be dilated by blind peroral passage of rubber Hurst (rounded ends) or Maloney (tapered ends) mercury-filled dilators of increasing sizes (16–60 Fr; 3 Fr = 1 mm). Complicated, longer, tighter, or more irregular strictures will require bougienage over a guidewire using hollow-centered, Savary, plastic-covered polyvinyl dilators, or balloon (Gruentzig) dilators.[289] The extensive use of PPIs has markedly impacted our treatment of peptic strictures and esophageal rings. PPIs are superior to H2RAs in relieving symptoms of heartburn and dysphagia experienced by stricture patients while reducing the frequency of repeat dilations and the cost for treating these patients.[290] Several studies in community and veterans' hospitals note an approximate 33% decline in the incidence of recurrent strictures. The timeline for this decrease parallels the marked increase in PPI use since 1995.[291] Another randomized study convincingly showed that in patients with symptomatic Schatzki's rings, maintenance PPI therapy after bougienage markedly decreases future relapses of the rings.[193] More recalcitrant strictures not responding to PPIs and dilation therapy may require intralesional injections of steroids or self-expanding plastic stents.[292] Intralesional steroids impede collagen deposition and enhance its breakdown, and this therapy potentially reduces scar formation. The usual dose is 40 mg/mL diluted 1:1 with saline and injected in 0.5-mL aliquots in all four quadrants in the most stenotic portion of the stricture.[293] Self-expanding plastic stents are removable and have higher expansive force than metal stents, thereby decreasing migration. In patients failing other therapies and prior to surgical intervention, large series show 100% success in proper placement and 80% short-term relief.[294] Stents are usually removed after 3 months. Stent migration, occurring in 1% of patients, is the most common complication. For selected patients, esophageal self-dilation may be an alternative, avoiding surgery and markedly decreasing health care utilization.[295]

Full references for this chapter can be found at https://ebooks.health.elsevier.com.

49 Barrett Esophagus

Swathi Eluri, Cary C. Cotton, Nicholas J. Shaheen

IN THIS CHAPTER

Barrett esophagus (BE) is a premalignant condition in which abnormal columnar epithelium that has both gastric and intestinal features replaces the stratified squamous epithelium that normally lines the esophagus.[1] This metaplastic transformation is associated with chronic GERD, which damages the esophageal squamous mucosa, such that 5%–12% of people with chronic GERD develop BE.[2,3] While highly associated with chronic GERD, BE causes no symptoms in and of itself and is of clinical importance solely because of its potential to develop into esophageal adenocarcinoma (EAC), a cancer associated with high morbidity and mortality and increasing in incidence over recent decades.[4,5]

DIAGNOSIS

Clinical guidelines define BE by endoscopic and histologic criteria: most commonly, salmon-colored mucosa extending 1 cm or more proximal to the top of gastric folds with intestinal metaplasia on biopsies.[6,7] Notable exceptions to these criteria are guidelines from the United Kingdom and Japan that require columnar mucosa but not necessarily intestinal metaplasia on the biopsies, a distinction discussed in greater detail in the pathogenesis section.[8] Proper identification of key endoscopic landmarks in the stomach and esophagus is critical for accurate diagnosis (Fig. 49.1). There must be salmon-colored mucosa at least 1 cm proximal to the top of gastric folds for a diagnosis of BE to be made; operationally, this means that the distance from the incisors to the top of the gastric folds minus the distance from the incisors to the top of the esophageal columnar epithelium must be 1 cm or more. A commonly used system for measuring the extent of the BE, the Prague criteria, reports both the maximal contiguous length of the BE (the Prague M measurement), and the length of the circumferential BE (the Prague C measurement).[9] Diagnosis of long segment BE, defined as BE extending at least 3 cm proximal from the top of gastric folds, is highly replicable, but interobserver agreement is worse among shorter segment lengths.[10]

While endoscopy with biopsies is the gold standard of BE diagnosis and remains the clinical norm, noninvasive testing is an area of significant interest and progress in research. The Cytosponge device (Fig. 49.2A) is a cytology sponge within a capsule, which is attached to a string for retrieval. The encapsulated sponge is swallowed and allowed to dwell in the stomach for 7 minutes, during which time the capsule dissolves and the sponge is released. The sponge is then retracted through the esophagus, collecting cells from the inner lining of the esophagus. Combined with histopathology for trefoil factor 3, the Cytosponge had a 73% sensitivity and 94% specificity compared to endoscopic diagnosis,[11] and had a 59% positive predictive value in a primary care setting among patients with long-term proton pump inhibitor (PPI) use.[12] A retrievable, inflatable cytology balloon, EsoCheck (Fig. 49.2B) also offers noninvasive esophageal tissue sampling where the operator can control the timing of inflation of the balloon, and thus can control the location of tissue sampling.[13] A robust blood-based test for BE does not exist, but serum adipokines and insulin levels have been correlated with BE diagnosis.[14,15]

SCREENING

There are no recommendations from clinical guidelines[6,16] or the United States or Canadian[17] Preventative Services Task Force for general population screening for BE. Current recommendations do support an upper endoscopy for detection of BE in certain high-risk groups. Screening has been recommended by U.S. societal guidelines for patients with a family history of BE or EAC,[16] which is both a strong risk factor for BE and for EAC.[18] Another U.S. guideline recommends a single screening endoscopy in patients with chronic gastroesophageal disease (GERD) symptoms and three or more additional risk factors for BE, which could include male sex, age 50 years or older, white race, tobacco smoking, obesity, and family history of BE or EAC in a first-degree relative.[6] Uptake of these recommendations in primary care, however, has been slow.[19] Screening has been recommended after sleeve gastrectomy based on high rates of erosive esophagitis and a cumulative incidence of BE greater than 5% at 5 years.[20]

It has been argued that without population-based screening it would be impossible to prevent the majority of EAC through a BE screening intervention because almost half of patients diagnosed with EAC do not report any history of chronic GERD symptoms.[21] However, significant barriers remain to population-based screening. Most cases of BE identified through screening are nondysplastic BE[22]; and, while the treatment of BE with dysplasia has proven benefit, it is unproven whether surveillance of nondysplastic BE prevents progression to EAC. Endoscopic testing for BE is costly and carries risks of harm,[23] a problem magnified by the relative rarity of EAC when compared to cancers where screening has proven benefit with evidence supported by randomized controlled trials, such as colorectal or breast cancer.[24]

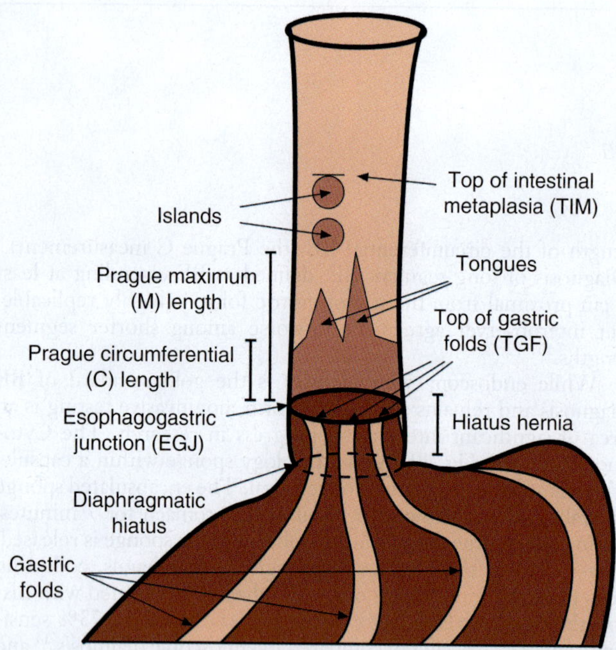

Fig. 49.1 Key anatomic landmarks in Barrett esophagus.

EPIDEMIOLOGY

BE is common in the populations of most economically developed countries (Fig. 49.3).[24–26] Much of the epidemiologic data in BE is limited by the fact that BE is usually asymptomatic and diagnosis generally cannot be made without invasive testing; therefore population-based estimates of prevalence and incidence would require performing endoscopy on substantial numbers of asymptomatic people.[8] A population-based, endoscopic prevalence study based in Sweden found a 1.6% prevalence of BE,[27] while reports in clinic-based and symptomatic populations find higher prevalence rates.[22] A symptomatic clinical population likely significantly concentrates risk for BE compared to the general population. At diagnosis, about 90% of patients with early EAC have concomitant BE, but only about one in six has a previous diagnosis of BE.[28] These studies suggest that a substantial proportion of patients with BE are not diagnosed. No studies have reported the incidence of BE in the general population.

GERD symptoms at least weekly are a strong risk factor for long-segment BE (≥3 cm), with a meta-analytic odds ratio (OR) of 6.3, but are less predictive of short-segment disease, with an OR of 1.3.[22] Given this finding, and the strong biological basis to think GERD is important in the pathogenesis of BE, several additional risk factors for BE may be mediated by GERD. Central adiposity is a strong risk factor for BE with an adjusted OR of 1.98 (Table 49.1) and this effect occurs independent of elevated BMI.[29] Obesity's causative role in GERD is through increased intra-abdominal pressure and the formation of a hiatus hernia,[30] although humoral effects of obesity may also promote BE. Hiatus hernia is a risk factor for BE with a meta-analytic OR of 2.7.[31] Tobacco smoking increases the risk of GERD by relaxation of the lower esophageal sphincter,[32] as well as deposition of proinflammatory byproducts on the esophageal mucosa. Smoking is associated with BE with an OR of 1.4, an effect size that appears insensitive to the amount of cumulative tobacco exposure (Table 49.1).[33] GERD is implicated in the associations of obesity and tobacco use with BE but may not be the only mediator of the associations.

Gastric sleeve surgery appears to have an increased risk of BE, with a 5.7% cumulative incidence at 5 years, accompanied by elevated rates of erosive esophagitis, suggesting that increased GERD is the mechanism.[34] On the other hand, Roux-en-Y gastric bypass may cause remission of BE as reported in some cases.[35] Lung transplant may also be a risk factor for the development of BE.[36]

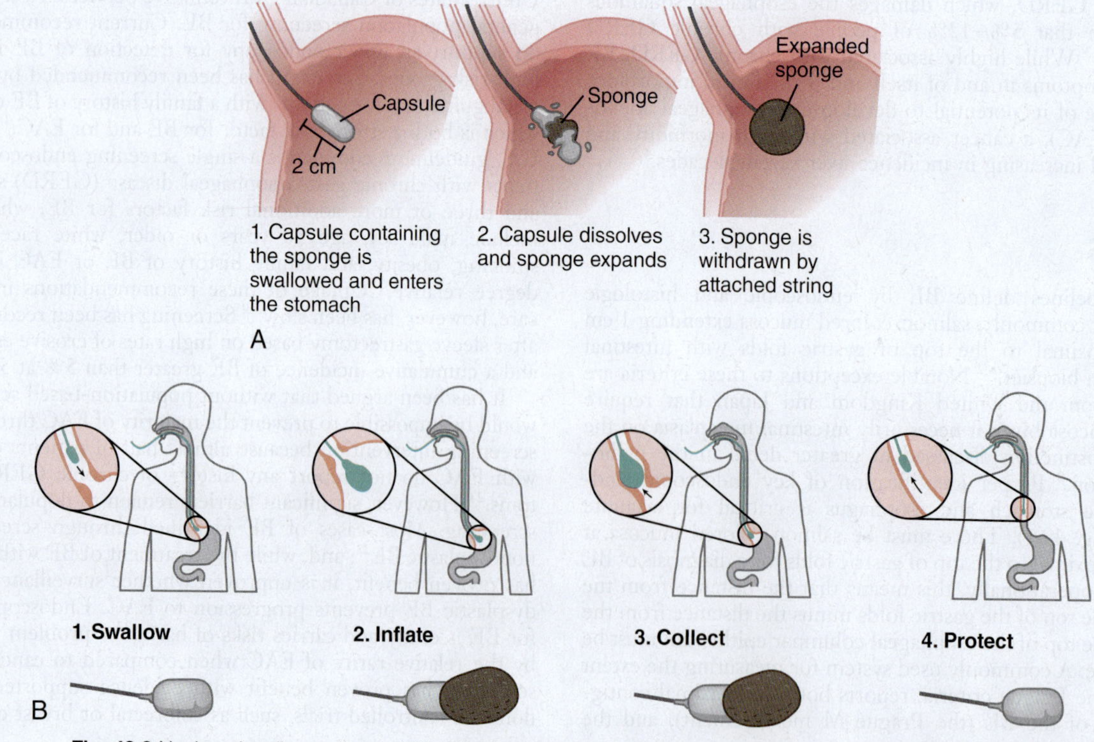

Fig. 49.2 Noninvasive diagnostic modalities for Barrett esophagus. A, Cytosponse device; B, EsoCheck inflatable cytology ballon.

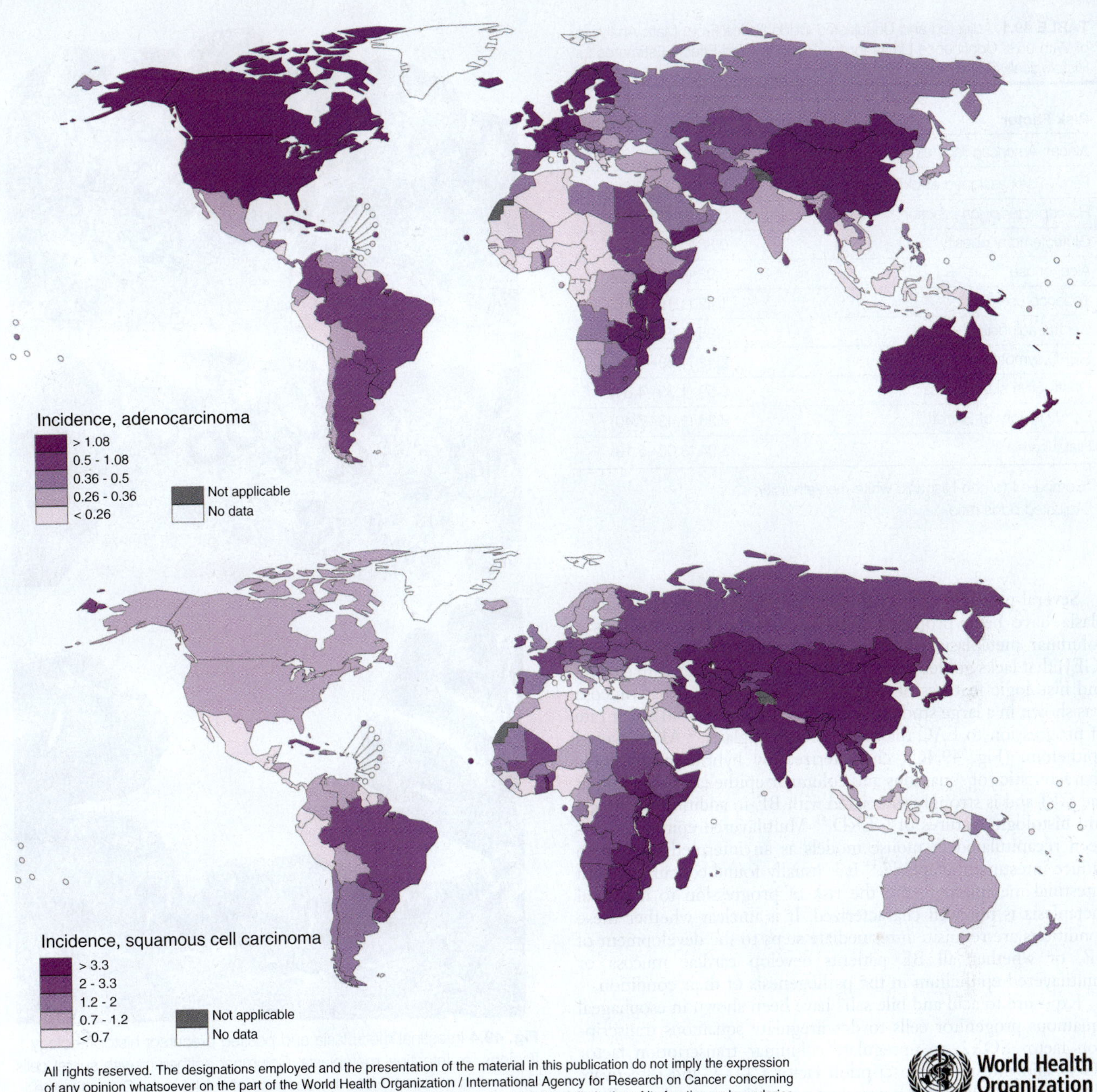

Fig. 49.3 GLOBOCAN estimated global incidence of esophageal adenocarcinoma in 2020.

Strong differences by race/ethnicity are observed in epidemiological studies of BE, with a greatly decreased prevalence of disease in populations of African Americans.[37] Access to high-quality health services among BE patients in the United States is heterogeneous across racial groups and this may affect rates of diagnosis in patients with prevalent BE,[38] but this does not fully explain the strikingly lower prevalence in African Americans. This decreased risk of BE is manifest by much lower rates of EAC in non-Hispanic black persons, who are at greater risk for squamous cell carcinoma of the esophagus.[39] While lower rates of EAC are found among non-Hispanic Asians, Pacific Islanders, and Hispanic whites compared to non-Hispanic white persons,[39] it has not been shown that a similar pattern holds for BE.

PATHOGENESIS AND RISK FACTORS FOR BE

Clinical guidelines in the United States[6] define BE by the endoscopic finding of 1 cm or more of salmon-colored mucosa in the distal esophagus, biopsies from which show intestinal metaplasia. Intestinal metaplasia describes the morphologic change from a normal stratified squamous epithelium to columnar epithelium with goblet cells that resembles normal intestinal mucosa (Fig. 49.4A).[40] GERD is central to theories of the pathogenesis of BE, but the mechanisms by which gastroesophageal reflux causes BE, and individual responses to reflux damage, with some severe reflux sufferers never developing BE, are matters of significant ongoing inquiry and debate.

TABLE 49.1 Adjusted and Unadjusted Odds Ratios From Meta-Analyses of With 95% Confidence Limits for the Pooled Mixed Effects Estimates for Histologically Confirmed Barrett Esophagus

Risk Factor	Odds Ratio (95% Confidence Limits)
African American race/ethnicity[37,a]	0.25 (0.20–0.33)
Female sex assigned at birth[51]	0.44 (0.30–0.65)
Helicobacter pylori infection[137]	0.53 (0.45–0.64)
Gluteofemoral obesity[138]	0.88 (0.81–0.96)
Alcohol use[139]	0.98 (0.62–1.34)
Tobacco use[33]	1.42 (1.15–1.76)
Central adiposity[29]	1.98 (1.52–2.57)[b]
GERD symptoms[22]	2.42 (1.59–3.68)
Obstructive sleep apnea[140]	2.59 (1.39–4.84)
Family history of Barrett[141]	3.26 (1.43–7.40)
Hiatal hernia[142]	3.94 (3.02–5.13)

[a]Compared to non-Hispanic white race/ethnicity.
[b]Adjusted odds ratio.

Several precursor histopathological lesions to intestinal metaplasia have been proposed. Cardiac mucosa (Fig. 49.4B) is a columnar metaplasia common at the gastroesophageal junction (GEJ) that lacks goblet cells and is strongly associated with clinical and histologic features of GERD but not BE.[41] Cardiac mucosa was shown in a large study to have more than a fivefold lower rate of progression to EAC than intestinal metaplasia.[42] Multilayered epithelium (Fig. 49.4C), characterized by hybrid morphologic characteristics of squamous and columnar epithelia, is common at the GEJ and is strongly associated with BE in addition to clinical and histologic features of GERD.[43] Multilayered epithelium has been recapitulated in mouse models as an intermediate step to induce intestinal metaplasia.[44] It is usually found concurrent with intestinal metaplasia,[45] and the risk of progression to intestinal metaplasia is not well characterized. It is unclear whether these conditions are requisite intermediate steps to the development of BE, or whether all BE patients develop cardiac mucosa or multilayered epithelium in the pathogenesis of their condition.

Exposure to acid and bile salts have been shown in esophageal squamous progenitor cells to downregulate squamous transcription factor SOX2, to upregulate columnar transcription factor SOX9 and intestinal transcription factor CDX2, and to activate Hedgehog signaling.[40] It is not clear where the progenitor cells of BE originate, and a translational study in humans and mice supports that transitional basal cells in the cardia that express p63, KRT5, and KRT7 may initiate intestinal metaplasia in a wound healing process with an intermediate multilayered epithelium, with these cells ultimately responding to acid and bile salts to express similar transcriptional changes to those described in the esophageal squamous basal cells.[44] Alternatively, esophageal submucosal glands, compact mucus glands, and blood-borne circulating progenitor cells have been studied as possible progenitor cells, with the molecular mechanisms of metaplasia incompletely understood.[40]

Genetic heterogeneity is estimated to account for about one-third of the heterogeneity in risk of BE, but gold standard twin studies have not been performed.[46] Investigators have described a large number of single nucleotide polymorphisms associated with a small increase in risk for BE[46] and a few rare germline mutations associated with a more significant risk of BE.[47] Similar genetic loci to those for BE have been identified as risk factors for EAC.[46] The genetic loci identified have mechanisms involved in risk of

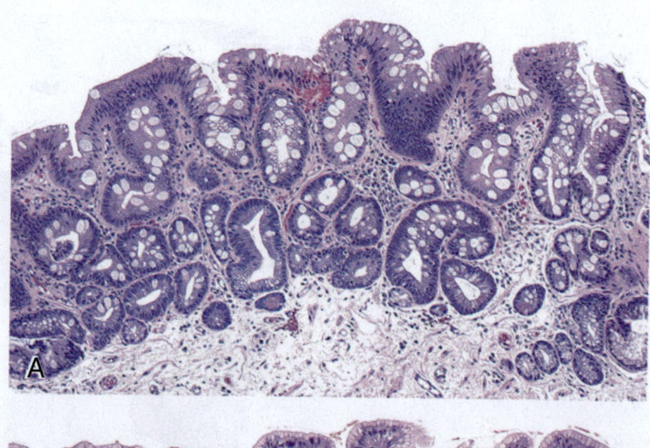

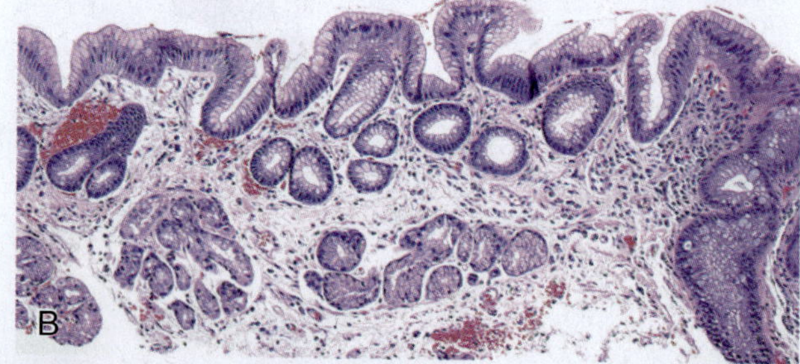

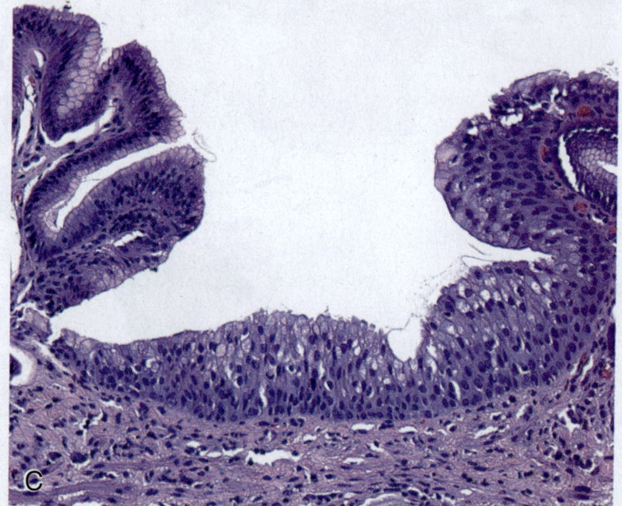

Fig. 49.4 Intestinal metaplasia and posited precursor histopathology findings. A, Intestinal metaplasia. Columnar epithelium with sublet cells. B, Cardiac mucosa. Note the absence of sublet cells. C, Multilayered epithelium. Note characteristics of both squamous and columnar epithelium.

smoking, abdominal adiposity, the response to inflammation, and control of tissue differentiation.[40,48]

CARCINOGENESIS AND RISK FACTORS FOR PROGRESSION OF BE TO EAC

The majority of BE identified in clinic- and population-based endoscopic studies lacks any dysplasia.[22,27] The rate of progression to EAC of nondysplastic BE (NDBE) was estimated in a meta-analysis at 0.3% per person-year.[49] In contrast, BE with dysplasia is less common but has a higher risk of neoplastic progression.

Segment length is a strong determinant of risk of progression, with long segment BE (3 cm or more) having more than three times the risk of progression of short segment BE (less than 3 cm;

TABLE 49.2 Odds or Hazard Ratios From Meta-Analyses With 95% Confidence Limits for the Pooled Mixed Effects Estimates for Progression of Nondysplastic Barrett Esophagus to Esophageal Adenocarcinoma

Risk Factor	Odds or Hazard Ratio (95% Confidence Limits)
Short-segment Barrett[a,50]	0.32 (0.18–0.57)
Female gender[51]	0.44 (0.30–0.65)
Age per additional year[52]	1.03 (1.01–1.05)
Ever smoking versus never[52]	1.47 (1.09–1.98)

[a]Less than 3 cm.

Table 49.2).[50] Longer segment length may increase risk of progression due to the larger surface area effected and at risk. Longer BE segments also have more significant exposure to gastroesophageal reflux, which may itself be a mediator of progression, and are more prone to sampling error during surveillance exams, given the smaller proportion of surface area sampled in longer segments of disease. Male sex,[51] advanced age,[52] and tobacco smoking[52] were additional risk factors identified in a meta-analysis for risk of progression of NDBE to EAC. However, when these clinically available risk factors were combined with low-grade dysplasia (LGD), they still had only a modest ability to discriminate the patients who would progress to high-grade dysplasia (HGD) or EAC, with area under the receiver-operator characteristic curve (AUC) of 0.7.[53]

The large number of persons with nondysplastic BE and the relative inability to determine which patients are at a clinically significant risk of progression to HGD or EAC has led to vigorous efforts to develop biomarkers that predict progression. Studies have consistently found abnormal p53 predicts progression of nondysplastic BE to dysplasia and cancer.[54,55] A panel of biomarkers, including p53, abnormal DNA content, cyclin A, and *Aspergillus oryzae* lectin in addition to LGD, had an AUC of 0.73 to discriminate the patients who would progress to HGD or EAC.[54] A combination of biomarkers, including p53, p16, HER2, CD68, COX2, and certain morphologic features on tissue histopathology, achieved an AUC of 0.75.[56] Of note, a commercially marketed, tissue systems biology approach using immunofluorescent staining of BE tissue combined with morphologic analysis has reported the ability to risk stratify BE with prediction for progression to dysplasia or cancer superior to readings by expert pathologists.[57]

LGD in BE is histologically characterized by relatively preserved crypts with mild nuclear atypia that extends from the base to the surface of each crypt.[58] Similar nuclear atypia isolated to the crypt bases is described as crypt dysplasia, and may imply a risk of progression as well, but less so than LGD.[59] High interobserver variability is found between pathologists in diagnosing LGD.[60] In the control arm of a European trial of endoscopic eradication therapy (EET) for LGD, where a confirmed diagnosis was required, 26% of LGD progressed to HGD or EAC over 3 years, but some cohorts in the United States have described a progression rate in LGD to be as low as 1.3% per year.[60] The heterogeneity in pathological interpretation of this lesion, as well as the disparate outcomes reported in cohorts with LGD, have hobbled efforts to study the condition and make it difficult to be dogmatic regarding recommendations for care of this cohort.

HGD is characterized by advanced changes in nuclear morphology or architectural morphology.[61] The rate of progression from HGD to EAC is estimated at 6.2% per year but has been reported in excess of 20% annually in some highly vetted studies.[62,63] Interobserver agreement among pathologists is higher for HGD at 71% compared to much lower rates of 42% seen in LGD.[64] Therefore having a second pathologist review on a diagnosis of dysplasia is imperative prior to treatment initiation.

MANAGEMENT

Endoscopic Surveillance for Dysplasia

Upon diagnosis of BE, endoscopic surveillance is recommended for patients with BE and no dysplasia, as well as selected patients with BE and LGD, at intervals based on the baseline degree of dysplasia.[6] The goal of endoscopic surveillance is the early-stage detection of dysplasia and carcinoma at a time when successful intervention can be achieved with EET or surgery. In order for surveillance exams to be effective, a careful endoscopic exam of the esophageal mucosa needs to be performed to identify any visible mucosal irregularities that have a higher chance of harboring neoplasia. However, subtle lesions can be missed even with careful examination with white-light endoscopy (WLE). Therefore adjunctive technologies, such as acetic acid or electronic chromoendoscopy, are recommended for use during routine surveillance of BE.

While currently rarely performed, chromoendoscopy has been demonstrated to be effective in the surveillance of BE patients. Acetic acid chromoendoscopy relies on loss of whitening of dysplastic Barrett mucosa for easier lesion identification and has been shown to have a pooled sensitivity of 0.92 (95% CI 0.83–0.97) and specificity of 0.96 (95% CI 0.85–0.99) for the detection of HGD and EAC in a meta-analysis of 1379 patients.[65] Methylene blue is another stain that is actively absorbed by the epithelium. While some early studies demonstrated increased dysplasia detection in BE with the use of methylene blue, a subsequent meta-analysis failed to show any incremental yield of dysplasia detection compared to WLE.[66,67]

Today, in most endoscopy labs equipped with endoscopes with this capability, electronic chromoendoscopy is commonly used for contrast endoscopy in BE, due to easier accessibility and evidence showing that use of narrow band imaging improves detection of dysplasia through identification of subtle mucosal and vascular irregularities (Fig. 49.5). A meta-analysis of 9 electronic chromoendoscopy studies comprising 625 patients showed that targeted biopsies guided by narrow band imaging had a pooled sensitivity of 94.2% (95% CI 83%–98%) and specificity of 94.4% (95% CI 81%–99%) for detecting dysplasia or neoplasia.[68] Furthermore, recent data have shown that use of electronic

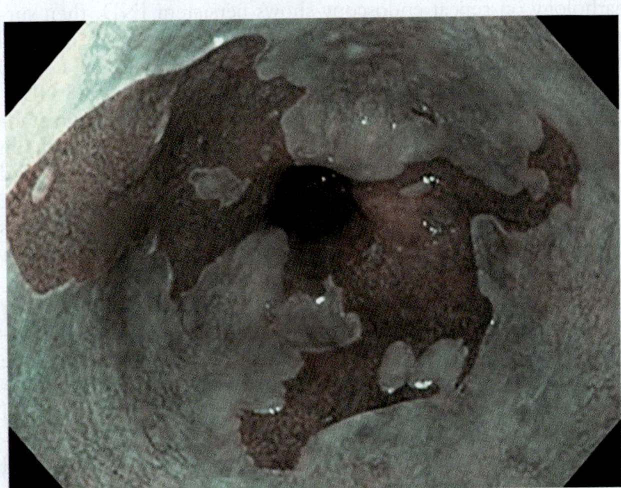

Fig. 49.5 Barrett mucosa with use of narrow band imaging (electronic chromoendoscopy).

chromoendoscopy improves the quality of surveillance exams by increasing dysplasia detection regardless of the expertise level of the endoscopist.[69,70]

In addition to chromoendoscopy, the adjunctive use of advanced imaging techniques such as confocal laser endomicroscopy and volume laser endomicroscopy has been studied.[71–73] However, these techniques are not recommended routinely due to the expense associated with them, limited availability, and the minimal incremental benefit in dysplasia detection during surveillance exams compared to a careful exam with WLE with narrow band imaging. Finally, while not yet optimized to be used in routine clinical care, the application of artificial intelligence-based software for detection of early neoplasia holds promise to improve Barrett surveillance by highlighting areas for targeted biopsies.[74] However at this current time, in addition to targeted biopsies of any visible abnormalities, standardized biopsies throughout the Barrett segment per the Seattle protocol, described below, are recommended during these exams.

The Seattle biopsy protocol consists of systematic biopsies in four quadrants obtained every 2 cm throughout the BE segment for patients with no history of dysplasia, or every 1 cm throughout the BE segment for those with a history of dysplasia, with additional separate biopsies from areas of visible mucosal irregularities. Biopsies obtained from each location should be placed in separate jars. The goal of a structured biopsy protocol during surveillance exams is to decrease sampling error, with data demonstrating increased dysplasia detection compared to random biopsies.[75] However, even with the application of the Seattle biopsy protocol, sampling error and nonadherence are important limiting factors.[53]

Currently, surveillance intervals for BE are determined by the segment length and baseline degree of dysplasia. While previously, it was recommended that all patients with nondysplastic BE endoscopic surveillance with a structured biopsy protocol every 3 years, most recent guidelines[6] recommend a 5-year surveillance interval for patients with short-segment BE and every 3 years for long-segment BE. This recommendation is supported by a large body of literature demonstrating that the annual rate of neoplastic progression is significantly higher in long-segment BE.[50,53] A meta-analysis showed progression to EAC was lower for short-segment than for long-segment BE: 0.06% versus 0.31% (OR 0.25; 95% CI 0.11–0.56; $P < .001$).[76] In patients with BE indefinite for dysplasia (IND) confirmed by a second pathologist, a surveillance exam should be performed after 6 months of high-dose PPI therapy. If repeat exam shows NDBE, the recommended surveillance interval for NDBE should be followed. If pathology on repeat endoscopy shows persistent IND, then surveillance intervals should occur annually, as data show a pooled annual incidence of HGD and/or EAC in IND to be 1.5/100 person-years (95% CI 1.0–2.0), which is similar to that of LGD.[77] In LGD patients who opt for surveillance over endoscopic eradication, surveillance exams are recommended every 6 months in the first year and annually thereafter. It is generally recommended to discuss cessation of surveillance at the age of 75 years in the absence of prior dysplasia or at a time when patient's overall status of comorbidities would not make them an ideal candidate for EET or other treatments for EAC.

Although it is common clinical practice to recommend regular endoscopic surveillance to prevent death from EAC for BE patients, there are no randomized controlled trials to demonstrate that surveillance confers a survival benefit in this group. A majority of the data suggesting a mortality benefit are observational studies susceptible to lead- or length-time bias.[78] However, evidence does support that BE patients enrolled in a screening and surveillance program do have detection of EAC in its earlier stages when it is amenable to endoscopic treatment, resulting in more favorable outcomes, when compared to patients with EAC presenting symptomatically. Furthermore, modeling data[79,80] suggest that surveillance is beneficial, and given the relatively low risks of endoscopy compared to the dire consequences of a missed opportunity for early detection of EAC, most major societies recommend surveillance despite the low quality of evidence supporting this practice.

Nonendoscopic Treatment

Treatment of GERD

It is recommended that patients with BE are maintained on at least once daily PPI therapy, with higher doses if the patient suffers from an inadequate control of GERD symptoms. This recommendation is based on multiple observational studies, which have shown an association between increased EAC risk and frequency and severity of GERD symptoms.[81–83] PPIs are recommended even in the absence of GERD symptoms due to indirect evidence suggesting that uncontrolled acid exposure promotes carcinogenesis in Barrett metaplasia, thus supporting the role of PPIs in chemoprevention.[84,85] A meta-analysis showed a 71% reduction in the risk of HGD or EAC (adjusted OR 0.29; 95% CI 0.12–0.79) in the setting of BE with PPI therapy.[83] Other cohort studies also demonstrate that PPI users were less likely to progress to HGD or EAC (aHR 0.32; 95% CI 0.15–0.67). However, a subsequent meta-analysis of 9 observational studies with 5712 Barrett patients did not show a statistically significantly decreased risk of esophageal neoplasia associated with PPI use (unadjusted OR 0.43, 95% CI 0.17–1.08); while interesting, this study was limited by the inclusion of heterogeneous studies.[86] While the theoretical risks of long-term PPI therapy do need to be taken into account, their overall safety have been demonstrated in randomized controlled trials, and most studies suggest that PPIs can reduce the risk of malignant progression in BE. Therefore, based on the current body of available evidence, it is prudent to maintain patients with BE on at least daily PPI therapy.

Surgical antireflux procedures have a well-demonstrated role in the treatment of medically refractory GERD but are not recommended as an alternative to PPIs for prevention of cancer in BE. Multiple studies, including a randomized controlled trial, have not demonstrated superiority of surgical management in decreasing the risk of progression to neoplasia.[87] These studies are limited by suboptimal methods of measuring adherence to PPI therapy, and inadequate power to detect small differences. Within the context of the existing data and given the complications associated with even low risk procedures such as laparoscopic fundoplication, taking into account the relatively small risk of neoplastic progression in NDBE, antireflux surgery should not be performed solely for cancer prevention in patients with BE.

Aspirin and Other Nonsteroidal Anti-Inflammatory Drugs (NSAIDs)

There is evidence suggesting that aspirin and other nonsteroidal anti-inflammatory drugs (NSAIDs) play a role in protecting against EAC through cyclooxygenase pathway that mediates inflammation and oncogenesis.[88] NSAIDs have been shown to decrease both Barrett related metaplasia and neoplasia in animal models.[89] A number of epidemiologic and observational studies have also suggested that NSAID use is associated with a decreased risk of developing EAC.[90] An RCT of BE patients, taking PPI twice a day and aspirin at a dose of 325 mg daily, demonstrated reduced levels of prostaglandin E2 in Barrett tissues.[81] The AspECT study evaluated the efficacy of high dose esomeprazole and aspirin for the combined endpoint of development of HGD, EAC, and all-cause mortality.[91] This study showed no statistically significant differences between the aspirin and no aspirin groups but did find that the combination of high-dose PPI with aspirin was superior to low-dose PPI without aspirin. Despite these findings, medical societies currently do not recommend the routine prescription for aspirin or other NSAIDs for chemoprevention in BE due to potential associated serious risks of gastrointestinal bleeding and cardiovascular side effects. Moreover, the endpoint that drove the differences between the two groups in the AspECT trial was all-cause mortality, not BE-related outcomes. Of course, many patients with BE are likely to be on aspirin for cardioprotection due to overlapping risk profiles between BE and other conditions associated with metabolic syndrome. In such cases, patients may derive additional benefits from the aspirin with respect to their BE.

Other Chemopreventive Agents

Statins have also been studied for chemoprevention in BE due to evidence from animal and human models demonstrating some efficacy in EAC prevention.[92] A meta-analysis[93] showed a 40% risk reduction of EAC (OR = 0.59; CI = 0.50–0.68) with statin use in BE patients and an 85% reduced EAC risk in a case control study using the SEER-Medicare database.[94] Although data have been promising pertaining to use of statins in BE, given their side effect profile and lack of prospective data, they are currently not recommended for solely chemopreventive purposes in BE. Metformin is another agent that has been studied given its antiproliferative properties seen in other cancers through both the adenosine monophosphate–activated protein kinase dependent and independent pathways.[95] However, both observational data[94] and a randomized trial[96] failed to support the use of metformin for chemoprevention in BE.

ENDOSCOPIC TREATMENT OF MUCOSAL NEOPLASIA

EET of Barrett associated dysplasia and early stage EAC is effective in disease eradication and plays a key role in management in averting the need for esophagectomy. EET consists of endoscopic resection of any visible lesions within the Barrett mucosa, followed by sessions of ablation with radiofrequency ablation (RFA) or cryotherapy every 2–3 months until a complete eradication of intestinal metaplasia (CEIM). Among the ablative modalities, RFA has the largest body of evidence demonstrating its safety, effectiveness, and efficacy, as well as the only level one evidence documenting cancer prevention, and is thus considered the first-line treatment.[63,97,98]

Endoscopic Resection

Endoscopic resection using either endoscopic mucosal resection (EMR) or endoscopic submucosal dissection (ESD) can provide both therapeutic and diagnostic benefits. Resection of irregular, raised, or nodular areas, which have higher rates of harboring malignancy, can provide a tissue specimen necessary to determine depth of invasion of neoplasia. Disease involvement of the submucosa is associated with an increased risk of lymph node metastases, so accurate staging is essential to direct future therapy. EUS has been shown to overestimate the depth of disease invasion and therefore is not recommended for staging in early EAC[99] but may be useful to allow evaluation and sampling of any enlarged periesophageal lymph nodes. In contrast to EUS staging, there is an excellent correlation between preoperative staging of early Barrett neoplasms using EMR and postoperative staging by examination of esophagectomy specimens.[100] In addition, resection specimens provide key prognostic information such as lymphovascular invasion, depth of invasion, grade of differentiation, and perineural invasion.[101]

EMR can be performed with a cap-assisted method with target mucosa treated with submucosal fluid injection and suctioned into the cap at the end of the endoscope, followed by resection using a polypectomy snare. An alternate method is multiband-EMR which deploys elastic bands around the suctioned mucosa, similar to variceal band ligation, followed by removal with a snare (Fig. 49.6). Both EMR techniques are comparable, but in head-to-head comparison studies, the band ligation method was less costly, more efficient, and resulted in fewer complications.[102] ESD is a technique to directly dissect within the submucosal layer. Compared to EMR, ESD allows for larger, en-bloc resections and provides information regarding disease involvement of the lateral margins. ESD may be preferable to EMR when treating large lesions, those concerning for submucosal invasion, lesions arising postablation, or those lesions that may be difficult to lift with EMR. One limitation to ESD is that it is more time consuming, complex, and technically more challenging than EMR, and should thus be performed in high volume centers. Complications of endoscopic resection techniques include bleeding, perforation, and a dose-dependent risk of stricture formation.

Following successful resection of any visible mucosal irregularities demonstrating dysplasia, ablation of the residual BE segment irrespective of the histology of the residual BE should be performed, due to high rates of metachronous dysplasia or recurrent incident dysplasia in the residual BE.[103] While stepwise, radical EMR of the entire BE segment results in high rates of eradication and duration of remission,[104] stricture rates are significantly higher compared to EMR followed by ablation.[103] A randomized controlled trial comparing combination therapy versus stepwise radical EMR of residual Barrett showed the

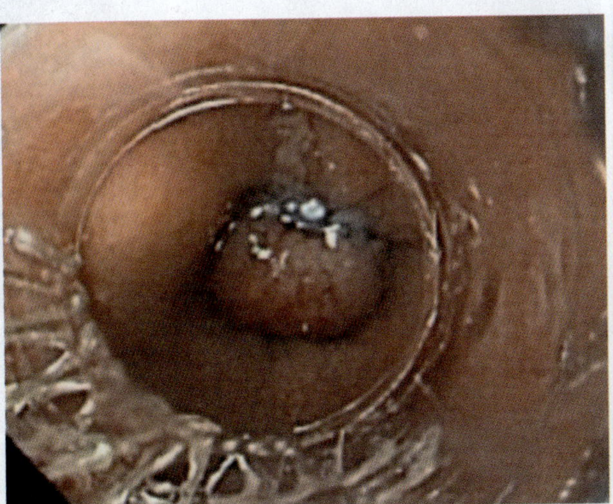

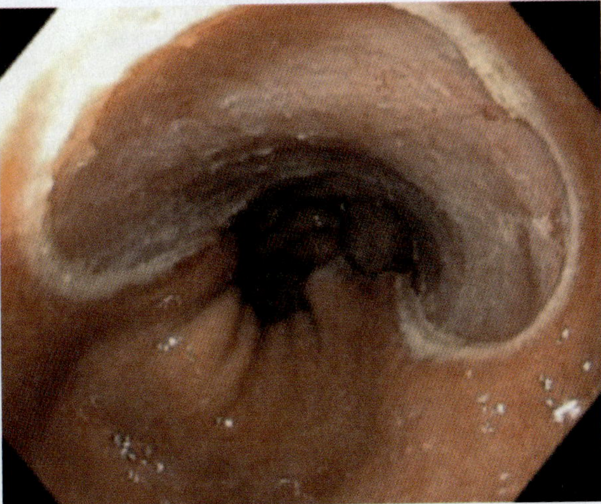

Fig. 49.6 Use of multiband-endoscopic mucosal resection technique for removal of target lesion in Barrett mucosa. An elastic band is deployed around the suctioned mucosa followed by resection with a snare.

ablation arm needed fewer treatments to attain CEIM, and suffered fewer complications, especially strictures, in doing so.[105]

Endoscopic Ablation

Endoscopic ablation is recommended for the treatment of residual Barrett after the resection of any mucosal irregularities. Endoscopic ablative therapy uses either coagulation, cryotherapy, or photochemical energy (photodynamic therapy) to destroy the Barrett epithelium. Heat can be delivered by laser, electrocoagulation, argon plasma coagulation (APC) or RFA. Cryotherapy consists of freezing the unwanted tissue through exposure to liquid nitrogen (LN) or carbon dioxide.

Of these ablation modalities, RFA has the greatest body of literature for safety and efficacy. In a multicenter, randomized, sham-controlled trial of RFA (the Ablation of Intestinal Metaplasia Dysplasia trial), 90.5% of patients with LGD and 81% of patients of HGD achieved a complete eradication of dysplasia.[63] CEIM was found in 77.4% of all patients in the ablation group, compared with 2.3% of those in the control group ($P < .001$). Overall 7% of the ablation group had complications, including one upper gastrointestinal bleed and five esophageal strictures. Significantly fewer treated patients progressed to EAC compared to the sham controls. In the European Surveillance versus Radiofrequency Ablation (SURF) trial in which 136 patients with confirmed LGD were randomized to RFA versus surveillance, progression to HGD or EAC was 1.5% in the ablation and 26.5% in the control group.[98] While the SURF trial was performed in a highly centralized and expert center, given the risk reduction in progression to HGD/EAC, RFA is considered the treatment of choice for dysplastic Barrett and early stage EAC. A study in the United States seeking to replicate the SURF study in a U.S. population, the SURVENT trial, is ongoing.[106]

RFA applies radiofrequency energy whose depth of thermal injury is controlled by a generator with adjustable power, density, and duration of energy applied. Radiofrequency energy is applied to the esophageal epithelium through an electrode attached to the end of the endoscope to treat short or noncircumferential segments of Barrett mucosa, as well as the mucosa around the GEJ (Fig. 49.7A). Focal ablation is performed with two sequential applications of 12 J/cm^2, with coagulum cleaned using the distal edge of the focal catheter, followed by an additional two applications of 12 J/cm^2, for a total of four treatments for each affected site. For circumferential lesions, an inflatable balloon with an array of closely spaced electrodes delivers uniform, circumferential thermal injury. Currently, self-sizing balloon-based catheters (Barrx 360 Express RFA balloon catheter, Medtronic, Minneapolis, MN) have replaced the older technology, which required that the luminal diameter to be measured by a sizing balloon prior to selecting a single-size catheter. The balloon-based catheter is placed over a guidewire under direct endoscopic visualization, and energy at 10 J/cm^2 is applied once to areas of Barrett mucosa sequentially throughout the total length of the BE, followed by cleaning of the coagulum, and then the delivery of a second treatment of 10 J/cm^2 to the same areas. Some studies that have evaluated the efficacy of a simplified RFA regimen consisting of 3×12 J/cm^2, without cleaning, versus the standard regimen showed an increased rate of stricture, and one RCT demonstrated noninferiority in efficacy but was inadequately powered.[107]

APC is another treatment modality using ionized argon gas to conduct electrical current for noncontact tissue coagulation for the treatment of dysplastic BE. Reported rates of CEIM with APC have varied from 57% to 99% with relatively poor durability of 19%–38%.[108–111] "Hybrid APC" is a newer method that uses mucosa lift prior to APC treatment with a single catheter, with prospective data showing rates of CEIM of 88%, an efficacy comparable to RFA, but with a worse durability of 66% at 2 years.[112] Reported adverse events with hybrid APC treatment include pain in 21%, with 4% developing strictures.

Cryotherapy is an alternate ablative modality that uses compressed carbon dioxide or liquid nitrous oxide that is applied by a spray catheter or balloon-based device.[113] Cryotherapy uses rapid tissue freezing and thawing to induce cell death by disrupting cell membranes, cellular apoptosis, and inducing secondary vascular injury. Currently available cryoablation modalities include LN spray cryotherapy (truFreeze; STERIS, Mentor, OH) that delivers LN at −196°C through a spray catheter (Fig. 49.7B).[114] A decompression tube is placed adjacent to the catheter, given expansion of LN to gas while spraying, to allow ventilation of nitrogen gas as the LN boils off. The C2 CryoBalloon Ablation system (Pentax Medical, Redwood City, CA) uses a balloon-based

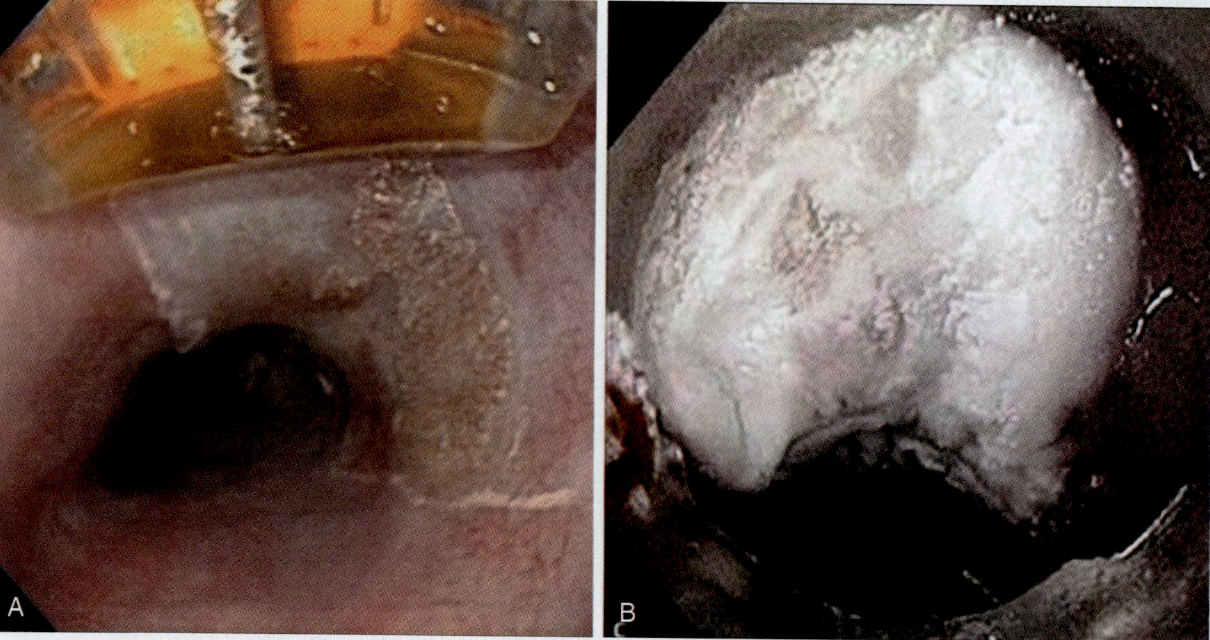

Fig. 49.7 (A) Radiofrequency ablation and (B) cryoablation of Barrett mucosa.

delivery system to deliver liquid nitrous oxide to the inside of a transparent balloon. This balloon is positioned in apposition to BE epithelium, such that energy transfers from the balloon to the epithelium.[115] Reported rates of CEIM with cryotherapy are slightly lower than that of RFA and range from 53% to 65%, with complete eradication of dysplasia of 81%−88%.[114,116] Cryotherapy is associated with a 9%−12% stricture rate. There is paucity of long-term prospective data and no comparative trials of RFA and cryotherapy. While RFA remains the first-line ablation modality, there is utility of cryotherapy for patients who are treatment refractory to RFA, with pooled estimates for CEIM ranging from 46% to 58% and CED of 76%−82%.[115,117]

Patient Selection for EET

Currently, EET is recommended for patients with confirmed HGD and intramucosal adenocarcinoma (IMC) over esophagectomy. A recent systematic review showed no difference in mortality and 5-year survival between patients undergoing EET and esophagectomy.[118] Esophagectomy is associated with a mortality of 3%−7%, and complications such as bleeding, infection, anastomotic leaks, and prolonged hospitalization in 40% or more of patients.[119] On the other hand, EET has proven efficacy, with comparable rates of eradication of HGD and IMC (RR 0.96, 95% CI 0.91−1.01) and a relatively low rate of complications.[120] Pooled adverse events associated with EET have been reported to be 5.6% (95% CI 4.2−7.4) for stricture, 1% (95% CI 0.8% −1.3%) for bleeding, and 0.6% (95% CI 0.4%−0.9%) for perforation.[120] Within this context, EET remains the treatment of choice for patients with BE harboring HGD and IMC. While EET is not recommended in the setting of submucosal invasion due to increased risk of lymph node metastases, observational data support that it may serve a role in the treatment of T1b EAC with superficial submucosal invasion (sm1—invasion into the upper third of the submucosa to a depth <500 μm) and low-risk features such as negative deep margins, well-to-moderate differentiation and no lymphovascular invasion.[121]

For patients with BE with LGD, endoscopic therapy is recommended, but surveillance is also considered a viable alternative. Due to the high interobserver variability among pathologists in the diagnosis of LGD, it is important that all patients with LGD have the diagnosis confirmed by expert pathology review.[122,123] Studies have estimated that the rate of disease progression in LGD is 1.73% −11.8% per patient-year with a higher rate in the first year after diagnosis.[98] In those with confirmed LGD, the decision to proceed with EET or endoscopic surveillance should be based on shared decision-making and taking into context patient comorbidities to assess fitness to undergo EET. Surveillance for LGD consists of endoscopies with biopsies every 6 months in the first year and then annually in those with persistent LGD. The most robust data in support for EET for LGD, the SURF trial described above, showed a marked reduction in progression to HGD/EAC in the ablation arm compared to surveillance. Lower rates of progression with EET were also reported in a systematic review and metaanalysis with 12.6% (95% CI 9.8−15.9) in the surveillance group and 1.7% (95% CI 1.1−2.6) in the RFA group progressing.[118] Despite data supporting EET for LGD, the studies are from expert centers, limiting generalizability of the results. Proponents of surveillance for LGD highlight the interobserver variability of LGD diagnosis, the possibility of regression of LGD on subsequent exams, the potential for detection of progression to HGD or IMC on surveillance exams allowing early intervention, and the adverse events related to EET.

Posttreatment Surveillance

CEIM is defined as the successful endpoint of EET. CEIM is considered to be attained on a surveillance endoscopy if there is no visible columnar epithelium and no IM in biopsies taken from the GEJ and the tubular esophagus. Following CEIM, it is important to recognize that risk of recurrence of intestinal metaplasia is substantial, at approximately 8% per patient-year, and reported to be as high as 9.6% per patient-year in a retrospective study of 218 patients.[124] Predictors of recurrence include higher dysplasia grade at baseline, longer segment length, older age, and treatment at low volume centers.[125,126] Recurrence is typically defined as detection of IM or dysplasia in the tubular esophagus, or dysplasia in the GEJ or high cardia of the stomach. The significance of nondysplastic IM in stomach cardia biopsies following otherwise successful ablation is unclear, with treatment of this lesion not resulting in lower rates of development of dysplasia.[127] Therefore IM of the cardia is generally not considered an actionable finding on surveillance biopsies. Nearly 75% of recurrences occur in the GEJ and a majority of these tend to be visible areas of mucosal irregularity.[128] The distal 3 cm of the tubular esophagus is the location with the highest recurrence rates. Therefore random biopsies of the neosquamous epithelium without mucosal abnormalities in areas of previous BE greater than 3 cm from the GE junction are likely low yield and thus not recommended.[129] Incidence of subsquamous intestinal metaplasia or "buried glands" as a complication of EET is also less prevalent than previously reported.[130] In a systematic review and meta-analysis of 39 studies on EET, the pooled incidence was 7.5 (95% CI 6.1−9.0)/100 patient-years for any recurrence, 4.8 (95% CI 3.8−5.9)/100 patient-years for intestinal metaplasia, and 2.0 (95% CI 1.5−2.5)/100 patient-years for dysplasia recurrence.[131] Recurrences of IM or dysplasia after CEIM may be greatest in the first year after CEIM, although not all studies support this finding, and appear to continue to increase in incidence to at least 5 years after CEIM.[128,129,132]

Given that the risk of recurrence after EET is not insignificant, surveillance endoscopy is recommended after CEIM at intervals dictated by baseline degree of dysplasia. Recent evidence-based surveillance guidelines have been developed from a modeling study utilizing recurrence data from the US RFA Registry and validated in the UK HALO Registry, using a threshold 0.1% risk of recurrent invasive EAC as the maximal acceptable risk.[133] According to these guidelines, surveillance is recommended in patients with LGD at 1 year after CEIM and every 2 years thereafter. In patients with baseline HGD or IMC, surveillance is recommended at 3, 6, and 12 months after CEIM and annually thereafter. Due to the ongoing risk of recurrence, cessation of post-CEIM surveillance is not recommended unless dictated by patient comorbidities. Surveillance exams after EET should consist of careful visual inspection of the tubular esophagus and GEJ under high-definition WLE as well as electronic chromoendoscopy. Any recurrences should be treated with EET, in a manner similar to that of the initial EET. If there is no visual evidence of recurrence, surveillance biopsies should be obtained from the distal 2−5 cm of the tubular esophagus, as well as four quadrant biopsies of the GEJ just below the squamocolumnar junction, placed in separate jars. Any visible mucosal irregularities should also be biopsied separately or treated with resection as deemed appropriate. During the post-CEIM surveillance period, patients continue to be maintained on twice a day PPI therapy to optimize acid suppression and minimize risk of recurrence. Patients desiring to decrease to once daily therapy may do so 2 months prior to a regularly scheduled surveillance examination, so that the presence of erosive esophagitis might be detected on that examination, with uptitration of PPI dosage to protect the neosquamous epithelium in that subgroup of patients.

Quality Metrics

Recently quality indicators have been established for endoscopic exams for BE screening and surveillance, as well as for the

TABLE 49.3 Ten-Step Approach to Endoscopic Examination of Barrett Esophagus[6]

Identify esophageal landmarks, including the location of the gastroesophageal junction, the squamocolumnar junction, and the diaphragmatic hiatus in the presence of hiatal hernia
Use of a distal attachment cap to help improve visualization especially in patients with known dysplasia
Clean mucosa well using a water jet channel and carefully suction the fluid
Use insufflation and desufflation
Spend adequate time inspecting the Barrett segment and gastric cardia in retroflexion
Examine the Barrett segment using high-definition and white-light endoscopy
Examine the Barrett segment using chromoendoscopy (including virtual chromoendoscopy)
Use the Prague classification to describe the circumferential and maximal Barrett segment length
Use the Paris classification to describe superficial neoplasia
Use the Seattle Protocol (in conjunction with electronic chromoendoscopy) with a partially deflated esophagus to sample the Barrett segment

performance of EET in those with dysplastic BE.[134,135] Quality indicators for screening and surveillance of BE focus on identifying and documenting landmarks and extent of BE, not obtaining biopsies in the setting of a normal-appearing squamocolumnar junction, utilizing the Seattle biopsy protocol, and performing surveillance endoscopy in patients with NDBE at 3–5 year intervals based on segment length. While increasing inspection time of Barrett mucosa has been correlated with an increased detection of dysplasia, it is currently not recommended as a quality metric. The most recent guidelines from the American College of Gastroenterology[6] outline a 10-step approach to the endoscopic exam of BE (Table 49.3), which includes techniques for optimal visualization, identification of landmarks, using the Prague and Paris classification for reporting BE extent and appearance, and biopsies per protocol. While not currently a quality indicator, postendoscopy esophageal cancer rate or PEEC, defined as the proportion of patients of developing an EAC within a year after an apparently normal upper endoscopy, will likely be implemented as an indicator in the future.[136] A recent systematic review and meta-analysis that included 52 studies and 145,726 patients showed that 21% (95% CI 13–31) had postendoscopy EAC and 26% (95% CI 19–34) had a combined endpoint of HGD/EAC in those who had an index exam with NDBE, LGD, or IND within the prior 1 year. Among patients developing EAC, 17% (95% CI 11–23) were found to have NDBE on an exam in the prior year. Therefore a meticulous endoscopic screening and surveillance exam is critical in BE to minimize risk of missed lesions.

Quality indicators for BE EET include factors such as the rate at which a dysplasia diagnosis is confirmed by a second pathologist, achievement of complete eradication of dysplasia within 18 months of the first treatment in those with baseline dysplasia or IMC, and documentation and tracking of adverse events that occur post-EET. All these quality metrics are likely to be implemented to assess quality of care delivery and quality of education in BE care in training programs.

RECOMMENDATIONS

- Screening for Barrett esophagus (BE) should be considered in patients with chronic GERD and at least three additional risk factors for BE including age >50 years, male sex, white race, tobacco smoking, and family history of BE or EAC in a first-degree relative.
- The diagnosis of BE is confirmed in the presence of at least 1 cm of columnar mucosa in the tubular esophagus on endoscopy with corresponding biopsies demonstrating intestinal metaplasia.
- Effective screening and surveillance exams for BE consists of adequate clearing, visualization, and inspection of the Barrett mucosa with both WLE and narrow band imaging, and obtaining systematic biopsies every 1–2 cm in four quadrants throughout the BE segment utilizing the Seattle protocol, with additional separate biopsies of targeted lesions.
- Endoscopic surveillance is recommended in BE patients without dysplasia and select patients with low-grade dysplasia (LGD) every 5 years in short-segment BE (<3 cm) and every 3 years for long-segment BE (≥3 cm).
- All diagnoses of dysplasia should be confirmed by a second expert pathology review prior to endoscopic eradication therapy (EET). EET is the treatment of choice for BE with dysplasia (LGD, HGD, and IMC). EET can be considered in superficial T1b lesions with favorable prognostic features.
- EET consists of resection of any visible lesions with EMR or ESD followed by an ablation of the residual Barrett mucosa performed at intervals every 2–3 months until a complete eradication of intestinal metaplasia (CEIM).
- Following CEIM, patients enter the surveillance phase of management with endoscopic exams with biopsies to detect recurrent disease at intervals dictated by the baseline degree of dysplasia.
- All BE patients are maintained on at least once daily PPI therapy for chemoprevention with twice a day dosing in those who undergo EET.

Full references for this chapter can be found at https://ebooks.health.elsevier.com

50 Esophageal Tumors

Hazem Hammad, Sachin Wani

IN THIS CHAPTER

CONFLICTS OF INTEREST AND ACKNOWLEDGEMENT

SW: Supported by the University of Colorado Department of Medicine Outstanding Early Scholars Program, Consultant—Medtronic, Boston Scientific. HH: Consultant—Medtronic. Neal C. Patel and Francisco C. Ramirez contributed to earlier versions of this chapter.

Esophageal cancer is the tenth most common cancer worldwide with an estimated 604,100 incident cases representing 3.1% of all cancer cases diagnosed annually. It is also the seventh leading cause of cancer mortality worldwide, accounting for approximately 544,000 deaths of all cancer deaths annually.[1,2] In 2018 it is estimated that there were 17,290 new cases and 15,850 deaths due to esophageal cancer in the United States.[3] The lifetime risk of esophageal cancer in the United States is ~1 in 125 men and ~1 in 400 women.[4] Esophageal cancer usually presents at an advanced stage, and thus curative treatment is limited and the prognosis is poor, with a mortality-to-incidence ratio of 0.88 (overall 5-year survival less than 20%).[2,5] Recent data suggest an improvement in 5-year survival rates, especially in patients with early and locally advanced cancers.[4,6] Esophageal cancer has two main subtypes—esophageal squamous cell carcinoma (ESCC) and esophageal adenocarcinoma (EAC); both subtypes are associated with distinct geographic distributions, time trends, and risk factors.[6,7]

CARCINOMAS

Esophageal Squamous Cell Carcinoma

ESCC is the most common form of esophageal cancer worldwide (Fig. 50.1). Although it is no longer the most common form of esophageal carcinoma in Western societies, ESCC continues to be the most prevalent type of esophageal cancer in the East, representing 90% of all cancers in most Asian, African, and Eastern European countries.[8] The areas of highest risk for ESCC are in two geographic belts: the Asian esophageal cancer belt across central Asia from the Caspian Sea to northern China and a belt on the eastern coast of Africa, from Ethiopia to South Africa (see Fig. 50.1).[9,10]

Recent data on the trend of ESCC incidence in the United States between 1999 and 2008 indicate substantial regional variations. The data reviewed covered 85% of the U.S. population and found that the national age-standardized incidence rate for ESCC was 4.93 per 100,000 in men and 2.30 per 100,000 in women. The incidence was highest in patients older than age 65. Over the study period, the incidence of ESCC in the United States fell by 3.41% and 3.13% per year in men and women, respectively. The majority (70.8%) of esophageal cancers diagnosed during the study period were EAC rather than ESCC.[11]

Although ESCC is more common in men than women, the ratio varies among low-risk areas like the United States (4:1) and high-incidence areas of China and Iran where the ratio is lower, approaching or even exceeding 1:1.[12] Environmental factors may be important in explaining the geographic variability in the incidence of ESCC. The etiologies and risk factors vary in low- and high-incidence areas.[13] A population-attributable risk of 89% using cigarette smoking, alcoholic beverage consumption, and low consumption of fruits and vegetables was reported in a study in the United States.[14] In contrast, a large cohort study conducted in China found that tobacco smoking played little role in ESCC risk.[15]

In industrialized countries, the two most important risk factors are tobacco use and excess alcohol consumption (Box 50.1).[16–19] Furthermore, these two independent risk factors have a synergistic effect on cancer incidence.[20] The risk of developing ESCC with active tobacco smoking increases three- to ninefold.[21,22] Although the highest risk has been reported with smoking cigarettes, other forms of tobacco use such as pipe, cigar, hookah smoking, chewing tobacco, and the Asian betel quid have also been linked to ESCC.[23] Exposure intensity and longer duration have been reported to be associated with the risk of ESCC.[24,25] Tobacco-specific nitrosamines and polycyclic aromatic hydrocarbons are thought to be the major carcinogenic substances in tobacco. Alcohol use has been reported to have a slightly lower

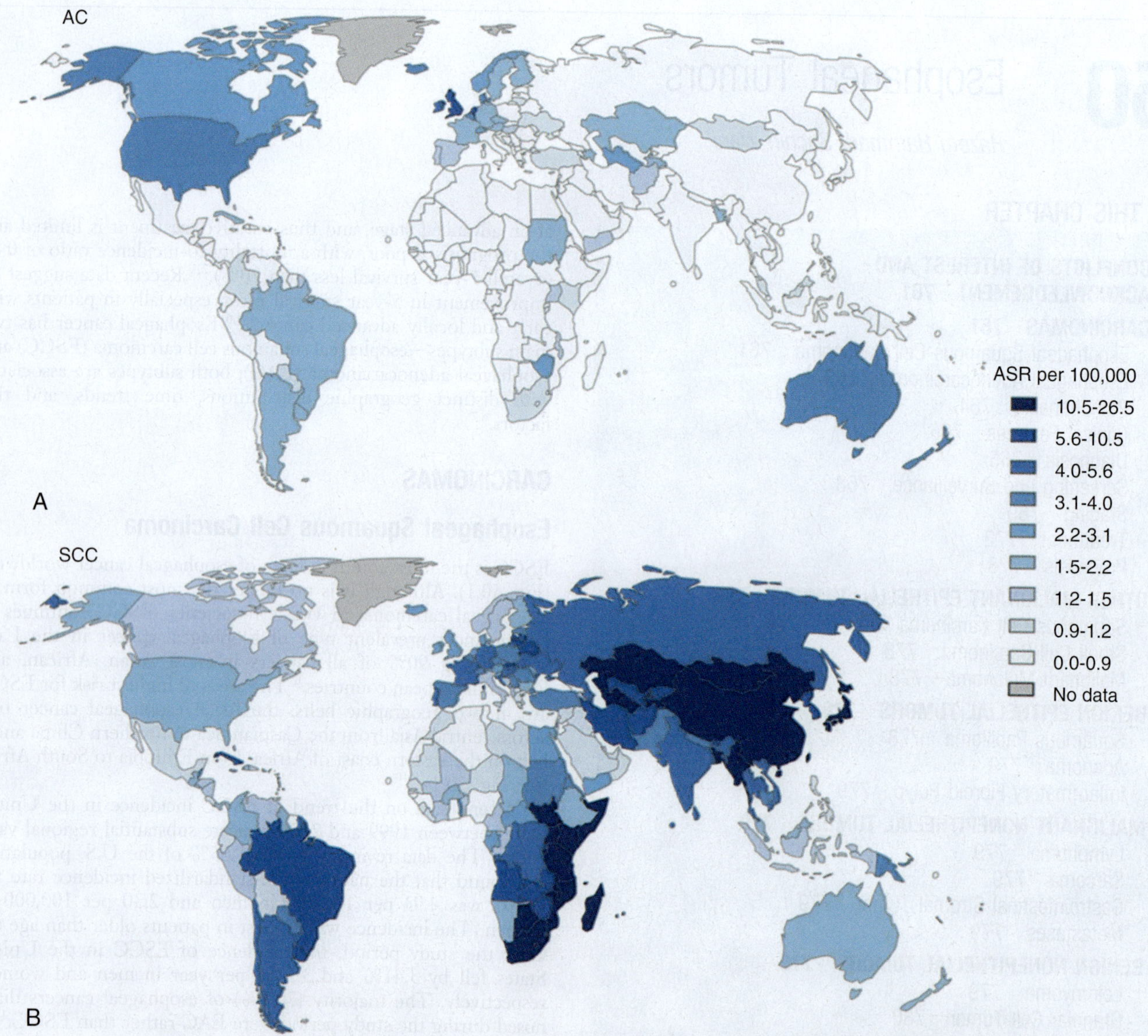

Fig. 50.1 Age-standardized incidence rate (ASR) per 100,000 men of esophageal adenocarcinoma (A) and squamous cell carcinoma in men (B). Map lines delineate study areas and do not necessarily depict accepted national boundaries. *AC*, Adenocarcinoma; *SCC*, squamous cell carcinoma. (From Rubenstein JH, Shaheen NJ. Epidemiology, diagnosis, and management of esophageal adenocarcinoma. *Gastroenterology*. 2015;149(2):302–317.e1.)

risk compared with tobacco, increasing risk of ESCC by three- to five-fold.[21] The risk increases significantly with alcohol intake above the maximum recommended U.S. dietary guidelines of 140 g/week.[18] Acetaldehyde, the first metabolite of ethanol metabolism, is a class I carcinogen.

In developing regions, factors such as nutritional deficiencies appear to have a stronger relation to the incidence of ESCC.[19,26] Although the exact mechanism is unclear, low socioeconomic status per se is a risk factor for ESCC, even after adjusting for tobacco, alcohol, age, and many potential risk factors.[7,27,28] Micronutrient deficiencies (such as vitamins A, C, and E) are also risk factors.[29,30] These vitamins are thought to have important antioxidant properties, preventing formation of free radicals and nitrosamines. However, a 6-year randomized trial conducted in China with 20-year follow-up showed that multivitamin supplementation did not reduce risk in a subpopulation of persons at high risk for ESCC.[31] Other nutritional deficiencies, such as folic acid, zinc, and selenium, have also been reported as risk factors for ESCC. Decreased intake and impaired metabolism of folate, mostly due to gene polymorphisms, have been proposed as risk factors for several GI malignancies, including ESCC.[32] In a case-control series, lower serum levels of folic acid were reported of patients with ESCC.[29] The trace elements zinc and selenium are protective against ESCC.[33–35] Zinc deficiency is thought to potentiate the carcinogenic effect of nitrosamines. Selenium supplementation is also thought to have chemo-preventive effects against ESCC. After a 10-year follow-up, a study showed that selenium supplements (along with β-carotene and vitamin E) reduced risk of esophageal cancer death by 17% among participants younger than 55 years old.[33,36] A systematic review of predominantly case-control studies demonstrated that higher intake of fruits and vegetables probably decreases the risk of esophageal cancer with each increment of 50 g/day of raw vegetables and fruit associated with a 31% and 22% decrease in risk of esophageal cancer, respectively.[14] Other dietary factors have also been theorized to increase the risk of ESCC. High-temperature beverage drinking has been associated with increased risk of ESCC in multiple studies, likely due to the chronic thermal injury.[37] Yerba

BOX 50.1 Risk Factors for ESCC and EAC

ESCC
- Tobacco
- Alcoholic beverages
- Low consumption of fruits and vegetables
- Low socioeconomic status
- Micronutrient deficiencies
- High-temperature foods
- Achalasia
- Lye ingestion
- Rare disorders (Plummer-Vinson syndrome, Fanconi anemia, and tylosis)

EAC
- Tobacco
- GERD
- Obesity

EAC, Esophageal adenocarcinoma; *ESCC*, esophageal squamous cell carcinoma.

mate, a hot herbal tea commonly consumed in South America, has been found to be a risk factor for ESCC.[38] Other previously reported risk factors, such as ingestion of *N*-nitroso compounds (animal carcinogens found in cured meat products and pickles) and *Fusarium verticillioides* (a fungus found on maize), have mixed evidence as risk factors for developing ESCC.[39,40]

Multiple studies have shown a possible association of ESCC and infection with HPV.[41] Recently, a large international consortium performed complex serological analysis for multiple HPV serotypes in ESCC cases and control subjects and found very limited evidence for an association of HPV with ESCC.[42] No definitive association can be proved at this time, and further investigation is necessary.[43]

Some esophageal disorders increase the risk of ESCC. As discussed in Chapter 46, it is estimated that the prevalence of ESCC among patients with achalasia is approximately 5%.[44] Between years 1 and 24 after diagnosis of achalasia, the risk is increased 16-fold, especially in men.[45] In fact, a large achalasia cohort from Sweden was shown to have an increased risk for both ESCC and EAC.[46] The mechanism is likely due to stasis of food material in the esophagus, leading to chronic inflammation. Similarly, as discussed in Chapter 28, patients with esophageal strictures from lye ingestion have an increased risk of ESCC occurring decades after the initial ingestion.[47] Patients with esophageal webs, such as those with Plummer-Vinson syndrome (iron deficiency anemia, dysphagia, and postcricoid webs) and with Fanconi anemia (an inherited bone marrow failure linked to several cancers), are also at increased risk for ESCC (see Chapter 45).[7,48]

Another rare condition associated with ESCC is tylosis, an autosomal-dominant disorder characterized by hyperkeratosis of the palms/soles and leukoplakia (see Chapter 25). The tylosis esophageal cancer gene *TOC (RHBDF2)* has been localized to chromosome 17q25.[49] Recent reports have suggested that this gene may be epigenetically silenced rather than mutated.[50] In one report, the risk of developing ESCC in those with this gene was 95% by the age of 65 years.[51]

Certain factors are protective for ESCC. These include obesity and frequent use of aspirin and NSAIDs.[52–55]

Esophageal Adenocarcinoma

EAC is the second most common form of esophageal carcinoma worldwide (see Fig. 50.1). The prevalence and incidence of EAC have not only changed over time but also geographically. ESCC used to be the most common type of esophageal cancer in both Western and Eastern countries. Based on surgical series, EAC of the esophagus was uncommon prior to 1978.[56] In Western countries, its incidence has markedly increased such that in 1994, EAC surpassed ESCC in prevalence in the United States. Today, EAC is the predominant type of esophageal cancer in the West. In the United States, its incidence among white men rose from 0.5 to 0.9/100,000 in the 1970s to 3.2 to 4.0/100,000 over the ensuing 2 decades.[57] This shift represents a 463% and 335% increase among white men and white women, respectively.[58] More recent population-based studies carried out from 2003 to 2007 estimated the incidence of EAC to be 5.3/100,000.[59] EAC was eight times more common in men than women and five times more common in Caucasians than African-Americans. Furthermore, this rapid increase in the incidence of EAC is not isolated to the United States; a similar trend has been noted in other Western countries such as the United Kingdom, Iceland, and Australia.[60–64] Furthermore, based on mathematical predictive models, the incidence of EAC is expected to continue to rise till 2030, at which point the predicted incidence of EAC will be 8.4–10.1 per 100,000 person-years.[65] The overall 5-year observed survival rates for EAC are strongly dependent on the stage at diagnosis and are among the lowest for all cancers. A recent analysis using the USA National Cancer Institute's Surveillance, Epidemiology, and End Results (SEER) registry showed that the proportion of EAC that had localized, regional, or distant stage disease remained relatively stable (40% of EAC patients diagnosed with distant stage disease). Recent data also suggest an overall improvement in 5-year survival rates with the greatest improvement in patients with localized disease reflecting improvements in curative treatment modalities.[4] The relationships between EAC of the distal esophagus and adenocarcinomas of the esophagogastric junction and the gastric cardia are discussed in Chapters 49 and 56.

This geographic change in EAC incidence over time is thought to be related to the significant increase in GERD (see Chapter 48) and, more importantly, obesity in Western societies. The epidemiologic gradient across both Western and Eastern countries may be related, in part, to socioeconomic status, because high socioeconomic status is more commonly seen in EAC, and low socioeconomic status is more commonly seen in ESCC.[27,58] However, other indicators of improved socioeconomic status, including per capita gross domestic product and level of education, have not correlated with the observed esophageal cancer gradient in different parts of the world.[58]

Because the rise in the incidence of EAC has been so dramatic, the possibilities of misclassification and/or overdiagnosis have been raised. A population-based study using data from SEER 9, which represented approximately 10% of the U.S. population between 1973 and 2001, found that reclassification of EAC to ESCC and adjacent gastric cardia cancer was unlikely to change the incidence of EAC. The anatomic distribution of esophageal cancer has shifted from the upper third of the esophagus to the lower third. The lower third of the esophagus, the location where adenocarcinoma usually arises, was the only esophageal location with an increased incidence. Because there had been minimal change in the rates of in situ or localized disease and the fact that the mortality of EAC had also increased significantly (sevenfold, from 2 to 15 deaths/million), overdiagnosis was unlikely to explain the marked increase in EAC incidence.[66] Furthermore, the possibility of heightened surveillance with EGD as a potential reason for the observed dramatic increase in the incidence of EAC was negated by showing that the rates of EAC increased in white men and women in all stages and age groups.[67]

In general, risk factors affecting EAC incidence are commonly seen in economically developed countries.[5] Similar to ESCC, tobacco is a risk factor for EAC (see Box 50.1).[13,17,18] Pooled data from the international Barrett and Esophageal Adenocarcinoma Consortium (BEACON) confirmed an association between smoking and EAC (OR 1.96, 95% CI 1.64%–2.34%). A dose-response relationship was also seen; heavy smokers had the highest risk of cancer. Furthermore, smoking cessation has been shown to be associated with reduced risk of cancer (smoking cessation ≥10 years associated with a 30% lower risk of EAC).[68] In contrast to ESCC, alcohol does not seem to be as strong a risk factor for EAC or Barrett esophagus (BE) as it is for ESCC.[69] Pooled analysis of 11 studies from BEACON showed no association between alcohol consumption and risk of EAC.[70] GERD is the most important risk factor for the development of EAC (see Chapters 46 and 49).[71] Although most of the large studies are in agreement over the increased risk, the reported risk has varied from four- to eightfold.[72–74] A study in Sweden showed that the risk of EAC in individuals with recurrent symptoms of GERD (at least weekly heartburn and/or regurgitation symptoms) was eightfold higher than individuals with less frequent symptoms (OR 7.7, 95% CI 5.3%–11.4%).[72] This study also showed that the risk of EAC was especially high among individuals with more severe and longer-lasting GERD symptoms (OR 43.5, 95% CI 18.3% –103.5%). A recent pooled analysis of individual-level data from five large population-based case-control studies in BEACON reported a strong dose-dependent relationship between frequency of GERD symptoms and EAC (at least weekly: OR 4.81, 95% CI 3.4%–6.8%; daily symptoms: OR 7.96, 95% CI 4.51%–14%).[75] Although GERD is a well-established risk factor for EAC, most patients with GERD never develop EAC. In fact, the majority of patients with EAC deny any substantial prior symptoms of GERD.[76] It is believed that, in predisposed individuals, GERD leads to distal esophageal injury resulting in an aberrant healing process resulting in BE. BE is the only identifiable premalignant condition for EAC and is defined by the replacement of the normal stratified squamous epithelium with a columnar-lined distal esophagus with intestinal metaplasia (see Chapter 49). BE is seen in ~7%–15% of individuals with GERD and is estimated to be present in 1%–2% of the general adult population.[77] BE patients have a 10- to 55-fold higher risk of EAC; however, progression to EAC from BE has been reported in a small percentage of patients (0.12%–0.3% per year).[77–79] Similarly, obesity is another strong risk factor for EAC, and this risk increases with higher BMI.[80–82] The increased risk of EAC in obesity has been estimated to be two- to fivefold.[83] In addition, abdominal obesity (independent of the BMI) has been shown to be associated with an increased risk of EAC.[84,85] A high intake of dietary calories and fat, by itself, is also a risk factor for EAC.[86] Obesity may increase the risk of hiatal hernia and GERD via increased intra-abdominal pressure.[71] However, abdominal obesity is associated with BE even after adjusting for GERD, and obesity is associated with EAC even in the absence of GERD symptoms.[83] In addition to its mechanical effect, abdominal obesity is also associated with alterations in circulating levels of peptides that are associated with BE and EAC.[10,87] Metabolic syndrome has been associated with BE and EAC.[88,89] In addition, studies have also found associations between insulin-like growth factor, leptin, and adiponectin with the progression of BE to EAC.[10]

The striking male predominance in esophageal cancer has raised the question as to whether sex hormones might play a role. When male-to-female ratios of EAC and ESCC, diagnosed between 1992 and 2006, were calculated, the highest male-to-female rate ratio was seen among Hispanics (20.5), followed by Caucasians (10.8) and African-Americans (7.0). In contrast, the male-to-female incidence rate ratios in ESCC were much lower. These findings supported the hypothesis that female sex hormone exposure might play a protective role in the development of EAC.[90] The differences in the risk of EAC among men may also be related to differences in use of tobacco or types of obesity.

Several factors have been reported to have a protective role against developing EAC. The prevalence of *Helicobacter pylori* infection (a known risk factor for gastric cancer) has been reported to be inversely associated with EAC.[91–93] This risk reduction has been estimated at 50%. The infection appears to decrease EAC risk by reducing gastric acidity. Also, as with ESCC, aspirin and NSAIDs use appears to be protective in EAC.[94–96] Observational studies have also shown that the use of PPIs reduces the risk of neoplastic progression among BE patients by 71% as shown in a systematic review and meta-analysis.[97] Similarly, statins have been shown to reduce the risk of EAC, especially in BE patients.[98] Finally, an inverse association between fruit and vegetable consumption and EAC has been shown.[71]

Pathogenesis

Human cancers occur in a multistep manner as a result of an accumulation of epigenetic changes and genetic alterations (see Chapter 1).[99,100] A combination of environmental factors, hereditary factors, and acquired genetic alterations are likely to be important risk factors in the development of esophageal cancer. In EAC, there is a gradual accumulation of somatic-cell genetic abnormalities that occur during the metaplasia-dysplasia-carcinoma sequence in the esophageal epithelium (see Chapters 1 and 49). The inflammatory microenvironment and somatic genomic alterations in stem cell populations are believed to mediate progression from BE to EAC.[101] An understanding of the sequence of these abnormalities may lead to a more accurate stratification of patients according to their individual cancer risk.[102] Because there is some evidence to suggest that only patients with a complete pathologic response to neoadjuvant therapy have a survival benefit (discussed later), a search is underway for prognostic and predictive genetic markers that would tailor a more efficacious multimodal therapy.[103–105] ESCC, on the other hand, is thought to arise from hyperproliferative epithelium that progresses to low-, intermediate-, and high-grade dysplasia (HGD) leading, ultimately, to invasive cancer.[106,107] Both concurrent genetic changes and epigenetic modifications, in the form of hypermethylation of tumor suppressor genes, occur frequently in both EAC and ESCC.[108–110]

Although most cases of BE and EAC are sporadic without a definite family history, there are several findings that suggest a genetic component. These findings include familial clustering, the fact that only a subset of patients with GERD develop BE, and that the amount of reflux is not an accurate predictor of BE development.[111–113] In these cases, the risk of developing BE is strongly influenced by gene-gene and gene-environment interactions (see Chapter 49).

Based on the description of the six essential components in human carcinogenesis,[114] molecular factors have been described for each of these six steps in esophageal cancer, as summarized below.[115]

1. *Self-sufficiency in growth signals.* Cancer cells can either make their own growth factors (autocrine effect; see Chapter 4) or alter their growth factor receptors and signaling pathways to free themselves from exogenous growth-limiting signals. For example, expression of the gene for EGF receptor 2 (*HER2/neu*) is a prognostic factor in esophageal cancer.[116–118] *HER2/neu* gene amplification correlates with shortened patient survival and independently predicts poor outcomes in patients with EAC.[119] Conversely, low expression of *HER2/neu* is associated with an improved response to neoadjuvant chemoradiotherapy than tumors with high *HER2/neu* expression.[120] Similar effects have been shown for ESCC.[121,122] Furthermore, in ESCC, expression of cyclin D1, a key cell cycle regulator (see Chapter 1), has been associated with shorter patient survival compared to cyclin D1-negative patients.[123]
2. *Insensitivity to antigrowth signals.* Inactivation of tumor suppressor genes is an important mechanism by which tumor cells become desensitized to antigrowth signals. This may happen

by mutation, loss of heterozygosity, or promoter hypermethylation.[115] Expression of the tumor-suppressor gene *TP53* in ESCC is an independent prognostic factor. Tumors with low p53 staining are associated with significantly longer survival than tumors with high p53 protein expression.[124,125] Also, p21 staining in ESCC has been associated with an improved survival,[126,127] and ESCC patients whose tumors had high levels of p16 had longer survival.[128]

3. *Avoidance of apoptosis.* Apoptosis (programmed cell death) puts a brake on expansion of the cell pool. A tumor's capability to expand is determined not only by its rate of cell proliferation but also by its avoidance of apoptosis. Some important regulators of apoptosis include Bax, Bcl-2, and Bcl-X. Expression of these proteins, alone or in combination, correlates with prognosis and response to neoadjuvant chemoradiation.[129,130] Survivin, another member of the inhibitor of apoptosis gene family, has been found to be a useful predictive factor in neoadjuvant therapy for esophageal cancer. Specifically, partial responders to neoadjuvant chemotherapy have lower survivin expression than nonresponders.[131] Thus future therapeutic strategies to reduce survivin expression or block survivin signaling pathways may increase histopathologic response rates and prognosis.[132]
4. *Uncontrolled replicative potential.* Malignant cells, by an overexpression of telomerase, destabilize mechanisms that limit their proliferative capacity, and they thus become resistant to cellular aging and death. Although there seems to be an increase in the expression of the human telomerase reverse transcriptase catalytic subunit in the pathogenesis of EAC, there are no studies showing any prognostic significance of the finding.[133–135]
5. *Sustained angiogenesis.* Sustained angiogenesis is crucial for the development, progression, and eventual metastasis of cancer. Angiogenesis factors such as vascular endothelial growth factor (VEGF), COX-2, and fibroblast growth factor receptor 1 have been suggested as potential prognostic factors in esophageal cancer. Of these, VEGF seems to be the most important.[132] High expression of VEGF is an independent, negative prognostic factor in ESCC, although a correlation in EAC has not been demonstrated.[136] COX-2 is known to increase progressively as the tissue progresses through Barrett metaplasia, to dysplasia, and to frank EAC.[132] In ESCC, COX-2 overexpression correlates with depth of tumor invasion, tumor stage, and reduced survival.[137] Amplification of fibroblast growth factor receptor 1 was shown to be an independent adverse prognostic factor in ESCC.[138] Expression of thymidine phosphorylase, another angiogenic factor, predicts an only partial response to chemoradiation in patients with ESCC.[139]
6. *Invasion and metastasis.* Abnormalities in cell-to-cell adhesion molecules (i.e., E-cadherin glycoproteins, catenins, and matrix metalloproteins) and their inhibitors are associated with poor histologic differentiation and greater tumor invasion and nodal metastasis.[140–142]

Clinical Features

Patients with EAC and ESCC have a similar clinical presentation despite the differences in demographics and risk factors. In the early stages, most patients are asymptomatic. However, as the disease progresses, progressive dysphagia and weight loss are the most common symptoms. The diagnosis is often delayed because patients experiencing dysphagia tend to avoid the foods causing the symptom and adjust their dietary intake. Dysphagia is initially with solids but progresses to liquids in the later stages of the disease. Solid food dysphagia typically occurs with an esophageal luminal diameter of 13 mm or less. The severity of dysphagia and concomitant weight loss from decreased oral intake is proportional to the degree of luminal obstruction. The point of difficulty with swallowing as localized by the patient is a poor predictor of the actual location of the mass. Odynophagia is a less common symptom and usually indicates the presence of an ulcerated lesion.

Other less common clinical presentations include iron deficiency anemia, palpable cervical lymphadenopathy, and/or chest pain. Chest pain, often radiating to the back, suggests the possibility of invasion into peri-esophageal structures. Tumor erosion can lead to an esophageal-respiratory fistula, which can present as refractory cough, recurrent pneumonia, or pleural effusions. A rare complication is esophageal-aortic fistula, which can cause massive upper GI hemorrhage and exsanguination. Hoarseness is another rare presentation due to recurrent laryngeal nerve injury from the tumor per se or associated lymphadenopathy. Metastatic lesions can be found not only in lymph nodes but also in lungs, liver, brain, and bone.

Diagnosis

Laboratory tests are nonspecific and can reveal anemia (iron deficiency or chronic disease type), hypoalbuminemia, and/or hypercalcemia (usually associated with osteolytic metastasis). Although paraneoplastic syndromes are rare with esophageal cancer, ESCC rarely can cause hypercalcemia due to tumoral production of a circulating parathyroid hormone-related protein.[143] There are no specific serologic markers for esophageal cancer.

The diagnosis of esophageal cancer is primarily made by endoscopic biopsies in a patient presenting with progressive dysphagia to solids (Fig. 50.2). The endoscopic appearance is similar between advanced ESCC and EAC; however, approximately three quarters of all EAC lesions are found in the distal esophagus, whereas ESCC is more frequent in the proximal to middle esophagus. Esophageal cancer can appear as a mass, raised nodule, ulceration, depression, stricture, or subtle irregularity in the mucosa. It is critical for endoscopists to spend adequate time inspecting the esophagus and documenting landmarks such as the gastroesophageal junction (GEJ), extent of BE using the Prague C (circumferential) and M (maximal extent) criteria, the presence or absence of extension into the stomach, and the exact location of the tumor.[144] These data points determine the surgical technique used in the management of patients with esophageal cancer. Clear description of morphologic features of tumors may also help in determining candidacy for endoscopic eradication therapies, therapies that have become standard of care in the management of early esophageal cancer (ESCC and EAC).

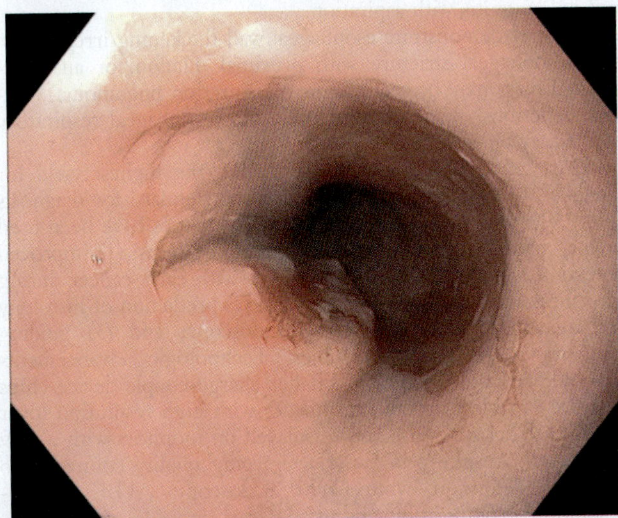

Fig. 50.2 Endoscopic image of a mass in the distal esophagus in the setting of Barrett esophagus, consistent with adenocarcinoma.

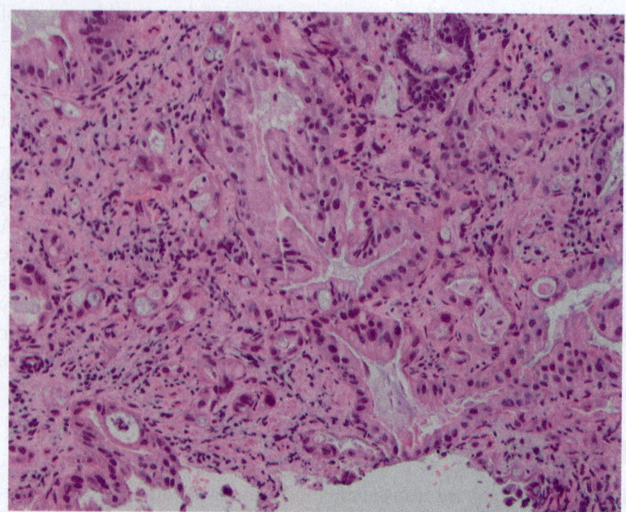

Fig. 50.3 Histopathology of esophageal adenocarcinoma specimen showing irregular, malignant glands with luminal mucin production involving esophageal mucosa, with inflammatory stromal response. A component of "signet ring" cells with large cytoplasmic vacuoles and eccentric nuclei is seen at the *left-center* of the image (200×). (Courtesy Dr. Michael Argyres, Denver, CO.)

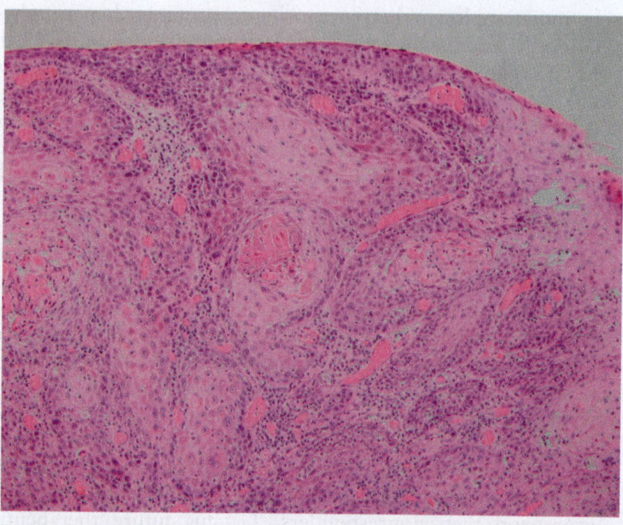

Fig. 50.4 Histopathology of esophageal squamous cell carcinoma showing nests of malignant keratinocytes with glassy cytoplasm, nucleoli, and keratin involving esophageal mucosa, with an inflammatory stromal response. A keratin "pearl" is seen at *center* of the image (100×). (Courtesy Dr. Michael Argyres, Denver, CO.)

Various other imaging modalities can aid in diagnosis. Routine chest radiography can reveal nonspecific findings such as aspiration pneumonia, a dilated esophagus with an air-fluid level (pseudo-achalasia), metastatic lesions in the lung parenchyma, pleural effusions, or signs of fistulas. Barium esophagogram can be helpful in diagnosis of esophageal cancer. A sign of early cancer with this modality is an abnormal esophageal mucosal lining, which can represent a plaque, polypoid lesion, ulceration, or nonspecific focal irregularity. Advanced tumors may be seen as overt masses, strictures with distinct shoulders, or luminal narrowing. Although it generally has fallen out of favor owing to widespread availability of endoscopy, barium esophagogram can be very useful prior to endoscopy in suspected esophageal-respiratory fistulas. When used for this concern, the endoscopist can have a "roadmap" of the anatomy prior to endoscopic stenting. Specific care should be taken to use barium as a contrast agent as opposed to hyperosmolar agents (diatrizoate meglumine and diatrizoate sodium), which carry a risk of severe pulmonary edema and pneumonitis with aspiration.

CT may demonstrate esophageal wall thickening/irregularity, focal esophageal stricture with proximal dilation, or an intraluminal mass may be seen. Signs of aspiration pneumonia, metastatic lesions, lymphadenopathy, and esophageal-respiratory fistula may be seen.

As stated, endoscopy with biopsy has the highest yield for diagnosis of esophageal cancer and is the standard for diagnosis (Figs. 50.3 and 50.4). Several imaging modalities have been used in the context of three major clinical applications: (1) improved detection and identification of patients with early cancer during screening and surveillance endoscopy; (2) prediction of histology and real-time diagnosis during endoscopy; and (3) guiding endoscopic eradication therapies. Technologic advancements have allowed the creation of smaller charge-couple device chips that are capable of producing images with high resolution (over 850,000 to 2.1 million pixels) displayed on monitors with a 16:9 aspect ratio resulting in superior imaging quality compared to standard definition white light endoscopy (WLE). High-resolution magnification endoscopes can optically magnify images up to 150 times (although not routinely available in the United States). High-resolution endoscopy, with or without magnification endoscopes, has been shown in several studies to increase the yield for detection of dysplasia and early cancer.[145–149] White-light endoscopy overall has a low sensitivity rate of 55%–63% in the detection of early ESCC.[150] The use of high-resolution WLE, where available, should be the minimum standard for evaluation of BE patients undergoing surveillance or being considered for endoscopic eradication therapy (EET) and for other subtle lesions in the esophagus (esophageal squamous dysplasia and early ESCC), a practice endorsed by GI society guidelines.[151,152] Endoscopic findings can vary from relatively normal-appearing mucosa (submucosal infiltrative pattern) to ulcers, nodules, and overt masses. Several other endoscopic techniques can also help identify areas of dysplasia and malignancy, including narrow-band imaging (NBI), chromoendoscopy (conventional or electronic), autofluorescence imaging (AFI), and confocal laser endomicroscopy (CLE). The chapter on BE discusses these imaging modalities in further detail (see Chapter 49).

Conventional chromoendoscopy involves the use of special stains to highlight subtle architectural changes to help direct biopsies and predict histology. Lugol's iodine, methylene blue, acetic acid, crystal violet, and indigo carmine are the most commonly used stains.[153,154] Lugol's iodine solution consists of a 0.5% to 3.0% aqueous solution of potassium iodide. Iodine stains glycogen-containing cells of the normal esophageal epithelium and is not taken up by dysplastic or malignant cells that are glycogen depleted (pink color sign). Chromoendoscopy with Lugol's iodine staining has become the standard of care for screening of ESCC in high-risk populations and has been shown to have a high sensitivity rate of 89%–100% with highly variable specificity rates due to false positive lesions.[150,155] In contrast, methylene blue, acetic acid, and indigo carmine staining are more useful in the detection of glandular abnormalities, as seen in EAC. These stains are sprayed in the esophagus with the intent of improving characterization of the mucosa resulting in selective uptake (vital staining—methylene blue) or enhancement of mucosal surface pattern (contrast staining—indigo carmine, acetic acid). Of importance, there are many limitations of conventional chromoendoscopy, including (1) dysplasia and inflammation (esophagitis) are not distinguishable from each other; (2) these techniques are generally cumbersome, time-consuming, and require dye spraying equipment; (3) difficulty in achieving complete and uniform coating of the mucosal surface with the dye; (4) inability to detect vascular patterns; (5) conflicting published data; (6) the need for magnification endoscopy; and (7) lack of standardized classification. Conventional chromoendoscopy has largely been replaced by optical chromoendoscopy (see below) while evaluating patients with BE and EAC.

Optical chromoendoscopy is another modality to detect signs of dysplasia and cancer by using selective light filters to highlight subtle architectural and vascular changes in the mucosa. This method avoids some of the concerns associated with conventional chromoendoscopy highlighted above. Several variations of electronic chromoendoscopy are available by different manufacturers, but most of the published studies have described the use of NBI (Olympus, Tokyo, Japan) in the setting of BE. NBI is an imaging technique that is based on the optical phenomenon that the depth of light penetration into tissue depends on the wavelength; the shorter the wavelength, the more superficial the penetration. Use of blue light with narrow-band filters enables detailed imaging of the mucosal and vascular surface patterns with a high level of resolution and contrast without the need for dye chromoendoscopy.[156] NBI is the most widely studied electronic chromoendoscopy technique to predict histology during surveillance, improve detection of dysplasia, and guide endoscopic eradication therapies. An international working group of experts recently established a classification system for BE using NBI.[157] A systematic review and meta-analysis showed that advanced imaging techniques (conventional and optical chromoendoscopy) increased dysplasia or cancer detection by 34% (95% CI 20%–56%).[158]

NBI without magnification has been evaluated in the detection of ESCC and squamous dysplasia. Endoscopically suspicious lesions for early ESCC appear as well-demarcated brown areas at NBI without magnification (Fig. 50.5). A prospective comparative study showed that NBI examination was reliable for the detection of early ESCC with sensitivity of 88% and specificity of 75%.[150,159]

AFI involves a technique that uses short-wavelength blue or ultraviolet light to stimulate biological fluorophores (e.g., collagen, porphyrins, flavins, and aromatic amino acids) in the esophagus. This technology has been mostly used in clinical trials for detecting BE-associated neoplasia. Pooled analysis from five prospective trials showed that AFI had little effect on the diagnosis of neoplasia with additional diagnostic value of 2% compared to WLE and with a high false-positive rate (78%).[160] Given this limited additional diagnostic and therapeutic value, AFI is not widely used clinically.

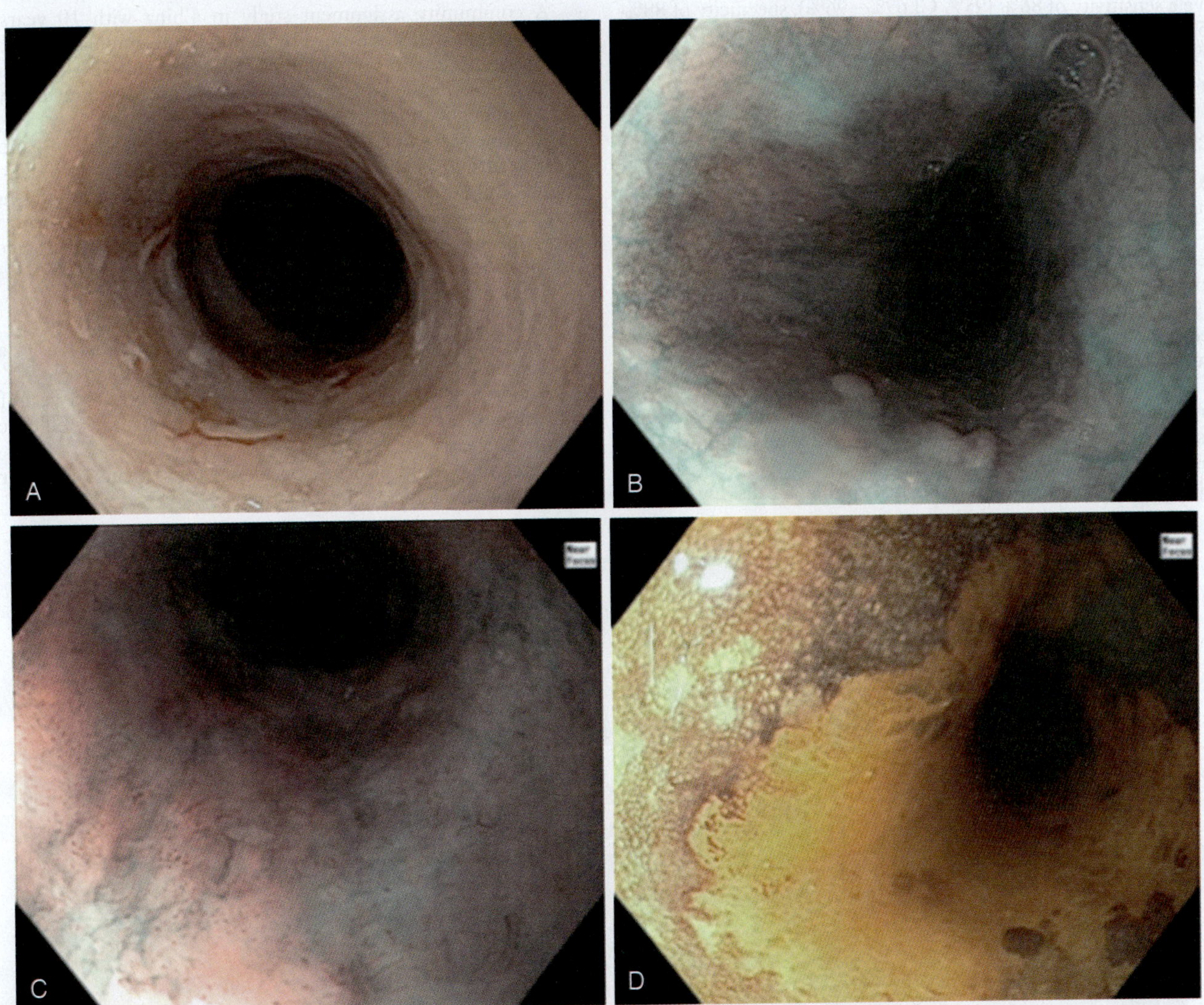

Fig. 50.5 (A) High-definition white light endoscopic image of esophageal squamous cell carcinoma showing subtle irregularities in the esophagus. (B) Narrow-band imaging (NBI) of the same area showing well-demarcated dark brown area. (C) Magnification NBI image showing abnormal intraepithelial papillary capillary loops pattern. (D) Lugol's chromoendoscopy with circumferential unstained lesion.

CLE allows real-time, in vivo microscopic imaging of the esophageal mucosa. It involves IV administration of a fluorescent dye (most commonly fluorescein sodium) that is taken up by normal mucosal cells. Fluorescent dye uptake is not seen in dysplastic cells, and thus they appear dark. This method creates magnification up to 1000 times. The only commercially available method currently for CLE is a probe-based instrument that can be passed through an accessory channel on the standard upper endoscope. Several prospective randomized controlled studies have reported that adding CLE to high-definition WLE significantly improves the diagnostic yield for BE-associated neoplasia.[161,162]

Optical coherence tomography emits near-infrared light to provide cross-sectional images of tissue, which also has the potential advantage of identifying submucosal lesions. Initial studies showed encouraging results for detecting dysplasia, but limitation for its use included small field of view and slow imaging processing.[163]

Volumetric laser endomicroscopy (VLE) is a second-generation optical coherence tomography technique that produces real-time cross-sectional images of large areas in the esophagus. NvisionVLE (NinePoint Medical Inc., Bedford, MA, United States) is approved by the Food and Drug Administration and is currently commercially available. This device has the ability of laser marking of suspicious areas for subsequent treatment. Using a diagnostic algorithm in a prospective cohort, VLE was shown to have a sensitivity of 86% (95% CI 69%–96%), specificity of 88% (95% CI 60%–99%), and diagnostic accuracy of 87% (95% CI 86%–88%) to detect BE-associated dysplasia.[164] This new technology is still not widely available.

Screening and Surveillance

EAC screening and surveillance are covered under BE (see Chapter 49). The histologic precursors of ESCC include dysplasia and carcinoma in situ (Fig. 50.6).[165] Given the time needed for dysplasia to develop into malignancy, screening and surveillance programs are designed to detect these early histologic precursors in an effort to improve survival. Early stage carcinoma is associated with a substantially improved survival rate (up to 86% at 5 years) when treated surgically.[166]

The primary screening strategy in areas of high ESCC incidence involves Lugol's chromoendoscopy, with endoscopic biopsies obtained from the unstained areas. Vital staining with Lugol's is based on the reversible chemical reaction between the iodine and glycogen present in normal epithelial cells. Dysplastic, cancerous, and inflammatory cells are usually devoid of stain (because of less abundant glycogen), and targeted biopsies can be obtained to confirm dysplasia/malignancy.[167] As mentioned above, Lugol's chromoendoscopy has a sensitivity and specificity of >90%.[155] Some studies showed low specificity of Lugol's solution to detect early ESCC that is likely secondary to difficulty differentiating between dysplasia/neoplasia and inflammation, but targeted biopsies should be helpful in this situation.[168] Vital staining with Lugol's solution, although simple and inexpensive, is associated with some limitations, including possible iodine allergy, risk of aspiration, or chest pain due to esophageal spasm.

NBI allows for clearer depiction of capillary networks and superficial mucosal patterns. Detailed classifications of these abnormalities have been proposed and validated in the identification and staging of squamous dysplasia and early ESCC (see Fig. 50.5).[169] A recent meta-analysis of 18 studies that included >1900 patients showed that NBI had a significantly improved specificity compared with chromoendoscopy with no difference in sensitivity.[168]

Cost-benefit studies have been carried out to assess esophageal cancer screening strategies.[170] One study found that a strategy of one-time screening at age 50 would be the best approach in underdeveloped high-risk areas, whereas a three-time screening strategy starting at age 40 (10-year intervals) would be preferable in areas with better health care resources.[171]

A community assignment study in China with 10 years of follow-up showed a one-third reduction in the cumulative ESCC-related mortality in communities where 40–69-year-old adults were screened once by Lugol's chromoendoscopy compared with communities without screening.[172]

Routine screening for ESCC is also recommended in patients with head and neck cancer. A retrospective study from Taiwan found a higher prevalence of secondary ESCC in head-and-neck cancer patients receiving routine endoscopies compared with the nonscreening group (4.5% vs. 3%, $P = .04$), with earlier stage at diagnosis ($P = .03$).[173]

The current screening guidelines include[9]:

1. One-time Lugol's chromoendoscopy for high-risk Asian and African populations beginning at the age of 40.
2. Endoscopy with Lugol's or NBI every 6 months to 1 year after completion of therapy for head and neck squamous cell cancer, for 10 years.
3. Screening could also be considered for patients at high risk (tylosis, achalasia, and caustic injury).

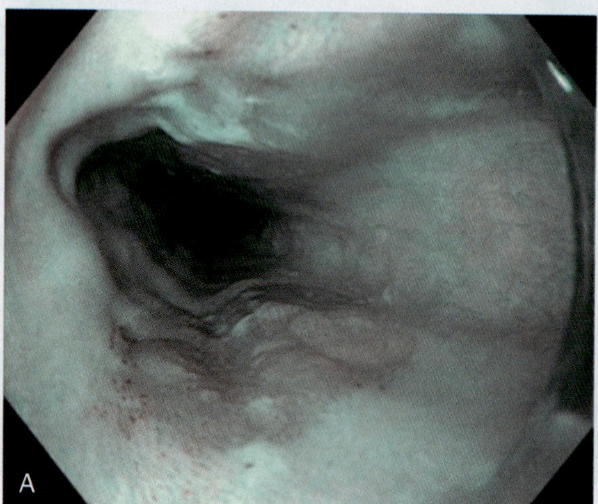

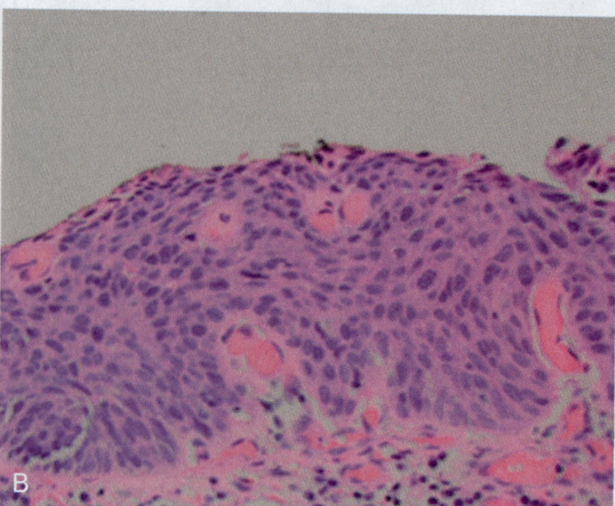

Fig. 50.6 (A) Subtle, well-demarcated nodularity in the upper esophagus at the 6 o'clock position concerning for early neoplasia. (B) Biopsies confirmed squamous high-grade dysplasia. (Courtesy Dr. Jeffrey Kaplan, Denver, CO.)

Other endoscopic techniques covered earlier, such as NBI and AFI, have also been evaluated as screening tools. NBI has been shown in multiple studies to detect early esophageal lesions based on superficial vasculature and surface pattern with excellent sensitivity and specificity but is still used in conjunction with Lugol's chromoendoscopy.[168] AFI is not sufficiently sensitive for lesions smaller than 10 mm, rendering it a less useful test for screening.[174]

Unsedated transnasal endoscopy (TNE) using an ultrathin endoscope has been shown to be safe and well tolerated.[175] A study of high-risk patients showed that TNE (with or without optical chromoendoscopy) has excellent specificity and sensitivity for early ESCC.[176] TNE is still not widely available but could be an important tool for ESCC screening.

Additional endoscopic techniques include endocytoscopy and high-resolution microendoscopy which allow for real-time pathological examination of the tissue. Limited initial data are promising, but these techniques are not widely available.[177,178]

Nonendoscopic methods for screening such as the use of peroral balloons and sponges have the advantage of being low cost and less invasive compared to endoscopy. However, these techniques have been shown to be inadequate owing to the poor sensitivities for dysplasia and even invasive carcinoma.[179] Combining nonendoscopic cytologic samples with biomarker (such as p53) may improve the sensitivity of the test.[180] Other noninvasive screening methods under investigation include breath markers (volatile organic compounds), antibodies to tumor-associated antigens, circulating microRNAs, and methylated DNA markers.

Staging

Staging of esophageal cancer is carried out using the American Joint Committee on Cancer staging system (Fig. 50.7), which was last updated in 2017 (8th edition).[181] This system not only separates staging for EAC and ESCC but also presents three classification systems separately for EAC and ESCC: the classic reference pathologic (pTNM) stage groups (Fig. 50.8), the newly introduced postneoadjuvant pathologic (ypTNM) stage groups (Fig. 50.9), and clinical (cTNM) stage groups (Fig. 50.10). This staging system recently revised the definition of the esophagogastric junction such that cancers involving it with epicenters no more than 2 cm into the gastric cardia are staged as EAC and those with >2 cm involvement of the gastric cardia are staged as gastric cancers.

The depth of tumor invasion (T stage) is an important factor because the rich lymphatic supply of the esophagus can provide a route of metastasis. Superficial cancers are defined as either carcinoma in situ (Tis) or T1 tumors. T1 is divided into T1a and T1b depending on whether the submucosa is spared or involved, respectively. Further classification for T1a includes M1 (intraepithelial cancer), M2 (invasion into the lamina propria), and M3

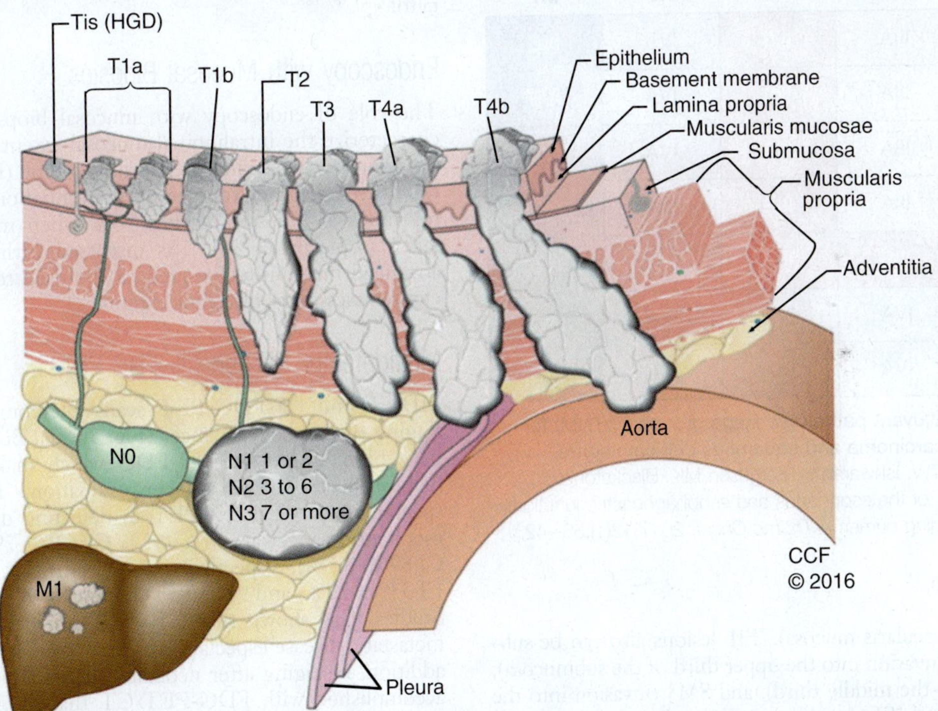

Fig. 50.7 American Joint Committee on Cancer (AJCC) TNM staging classification for carcinoma of the esophagus and esophagogastric junction. T is categorized as either Tis (high-grade dysplasia); T1 cancer that invades the lamina propria, muscularis mucosae, or submucosa and is subcategorized into T1a (cancer that invades the lamina propria or muscularis mucosae) and T1b (cancer that invades the submucosa); T2 cancer that invades the muscularis propria; T3 cancer that invades the adventitia; T4 cancer that invades the local structures, and is subcategorized as T4a (cancer that invades adjacent structures such as the pleura, pericardium, azygos vein, diaphragm, or peritoneum) and T4b (cancer that invades the major adjacent structures, such as the aorta, vertebral body, or trachea). N is categorized as N0 (no regional lymph node metastasis), N1 (regional lymph node metastases involving 1 or 2 nodes), N2 (regional lymph node metastases involving 3–6 nodes), and N3 (regional lymph node metastases involving 7 or more nodes). M is categorized as M0 (no distant metastasis) and M1 (distant metastasis). (From Rice TW, Ishwaran H, Ferguson MK, Blackstone EH, Goldstraw P. Cancer of the esophagus and esophagogastric junction: an eighth edition staging primer. *J Thorac Oncol*. 2017;12:36–42.)

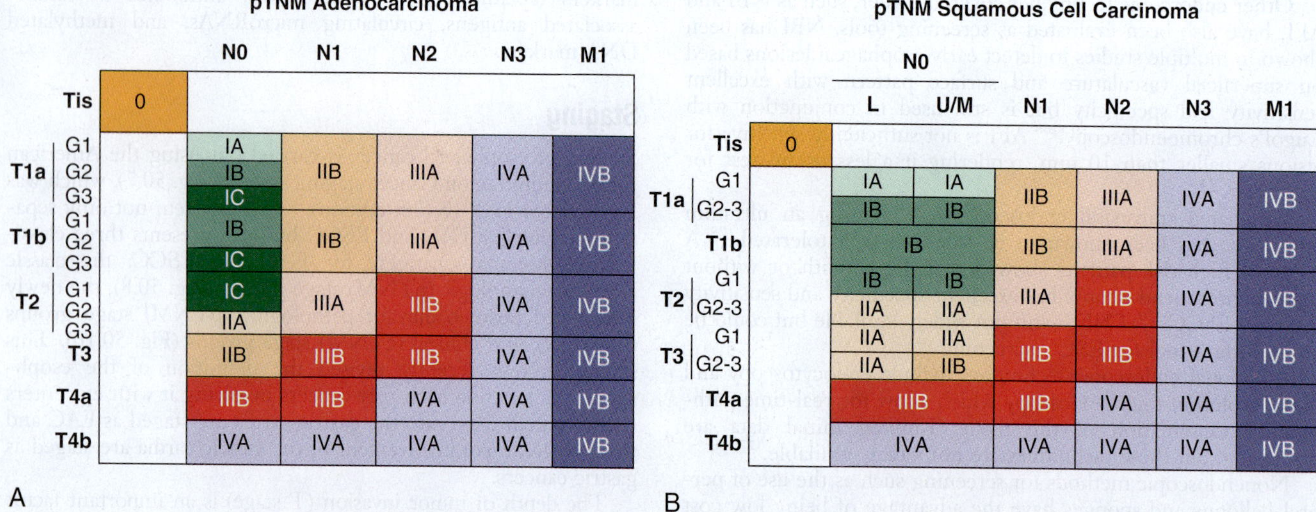

pTNM Adenocarcinoma

		N0	N1	N2	N3	M1
Tis		0				
T1a	G1	IA	IIB	IIIA	IVA	IVB
	G2	IB				
	G3	IC				
T1b	G1	IB	IIB	IIIA	IVA	IVB
	G2					
	G3	IC				
T2	G1	IC	IIIA	IIIB	IVA	IVB
	G2					
	G3	IIA				
T3		IIB	IIIB	IIIB	IVA	IVB
T4a		IIIB	IIIB	IVA	IVA	IVB
T4b		IVA	IVA	IVA	IVA	IVB

A

pTNM Squamous Cell Carcinoma

		N0 L	N0 U/M	N1	N2	N3	M1
Tis		0					
T1a	G1	IA	IA	IIB	IIIA	IVA	IVB
	G2-3	IB	IB				
T1b		IB		IIB	IIIA	IVA	IVB
T2	G1	IB	IB	IIIA	IIIB	IVA	IVB
	G2-3	IIA	IIA				
T3	G1	IIA	IIA	IIIB	IIIB	IVA	IVB
	G2-3	IIA	IIB				
T4a		IIIB		IIIB	IVA	IVA	IVB
T4b		IVA		IVA	IVA	IVA	IVB

B

Fig. 50.8 Pathologic stage groups (pTNM) for esophageal adenocarcinoma (A) and squamous cell carcinoma (B). (Modified from Rice TW, Ishwaran H, Ferguson MK, Blackstone EH, Goldstraw P. Cancer of the esophagus and esophagogastric junction: an eighth edition staging primer. *J Thorac Oncol.* 2017;12(1):36–42.)

ypTNM

	N0	N1	N2	N3	M1
T0	I	IIIA	IIIB	IVA	IVB
Tis	I	IIIA	IIIB	IVA	IVB
T1	I	IIIA	IIIB	IVA	IVB
T2	I	IIIA	IIIB	IVA	IVB
T3	II	IIIB	IIIB	IVA	IVB
T4a	IIIB	IVA	IVA	IVA	IVB
T4b	IVA	IVA	IVA	IVA	IVB

Fig. 50.9 Postneoadjuvant pathologic stage groups (ypTNM) for esophageal adenocarcinoma and squamous cell carcinoma. (Modified from Rice TW, Ishwaran H, Ferguson MK, Blackstone EH, Goldstraw P. Cancer of the esophagus and esophagogastric junction: an eighth edition staging primer. *J Thorac Oncol.* 2017;12(1):36–42.)

(invasion to the muscularis mucosa). T1b lesions also can be subdivided into SM1 (invasion into the upper third of the submucosa), SM2 (invasion into the middle third), and SM3 (invasion into the lower third). Tis and T1a lesions have a predicted lymph node metastasis rate of up to 8% compared to T1b lesions, which have up to a 56% lymph node metastasis rate.[182–184] In addition to the mediastinal nodes, lymph node metastases can occur in the neck and upper abdomen.[185] The risk of lymph node involvement is related to several factors (in decreasing order of frequency): grade III histology, SM3 invasion, lymphatic invasion, vascular invasion, SM2 invasion, and SM1 invasion. In ESCC, the best predictors of lymph node invasion are SM3 invasion and vascular invasion, whereas in EAC, the most important predictor is lymphatic invasion.[186] Fig. 50.11 shows correlation of survival and the T stage.

Staging can be performed by several methods: endoscopy with mucosal biopsies, endoscopic resection, multidetector CT (MDCT) with ^{18}F-fluoro-2-deoxy-D-glucose PET (^{18}F-FDG-PET), and EUS with fine-needle aspiration (FNA) for cytology.[187,188]

Endoscopy with Mucosal Biopsies

The role of endoscopy with mucosal biopsies in staging is to characterize the intraluminal mucosal extent of the tumor (location) and to determine the histologic type (ESCC or EAC) and the histologic grade (degree of differentiation).[189] The sensitivity for mucosal biopsies reaches 96% when multiple biopsies are taken (typically 6–8).[190] As discussed earlier, NBI and other advanced imaging techniques can be used to obtain a more accurate assessment of tumor extent.

Multidetector CT and ^{18}F-FDG-PET

MDCT and ^{18}F-FDG-PET scans are commonly used in the staging of esophageal cancer (Fig. 50.12). Both ESCC and EAC have high affinity for ^{18}F-FDG which makes PET scan very helpful in esophageal cancer evaluation. The sensitivity and specificity for ^{18}F-FDG-PET in detecting distant metastases in esophageal cancer are 71% (95% CI 62%–79%) and 93% (95% CI 89%–97%), respectively, whereas for CT, they are 52% (95% CI 33%–72%) and 91% (95% CI 86%–96%), respectively.[191,192] Studies have shown that CT-PET can identify 5%–28% with metastatic disease especially at sites not detected on CT alone. In addition, restaging after neoadjuvant therapy seems to be better accomplished with FDG-PET/CT than EUS-FNA or MDCT alone.[193]

EUS

EUS is increasingly used to assess the depth of tumor invasion and to distinguish T1 lesions from deeper infiltration. This distinction helps to choose candidates for stage-appropriate therapies. EUS is the only imaging modality that can clearly delineate the different esophageal wall layers. It is considered by most experts to be the best staging modality for T stage and locoregional lymph node (N) staging (Video 50.1). In a meta-analysis, the pooled sensitivity of EUS for T stages was 80%–90% with more than 90% specificity. The accuracy was higher for more advanced T stages. The

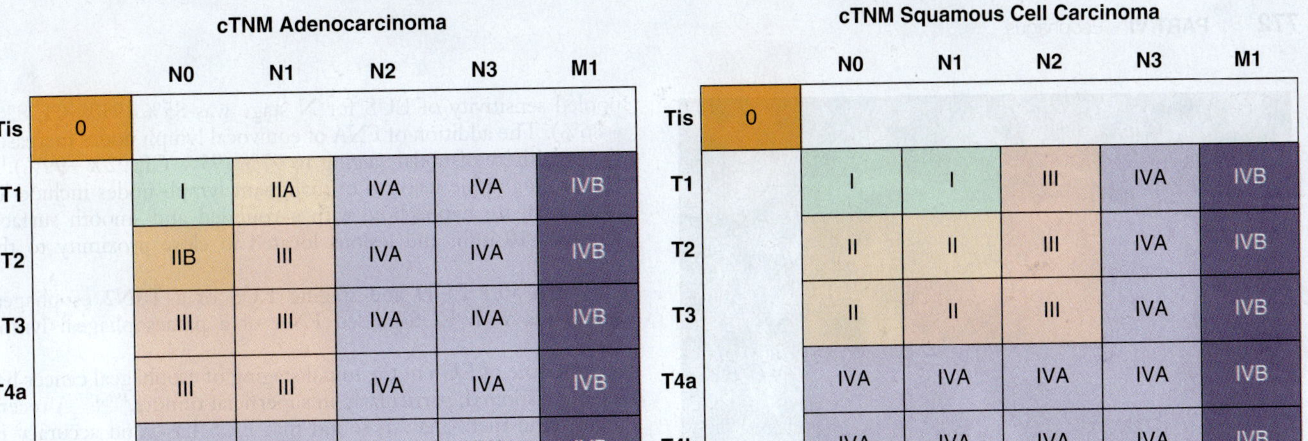

Fig. 50.10 Clinical stage groups (cTNM) for esophageal adenocarcinoma (A) and squamous cell carcinoma (B). (Modified from Rice TW, Ishwaran H, Ferguson MK, Blackstone EH, Goldstraw P. Cancer of the esophagus and esophagogastric junction: an eighth edition staging primer. *J Thorac Oncol*. 2017;12(1):36–42.)

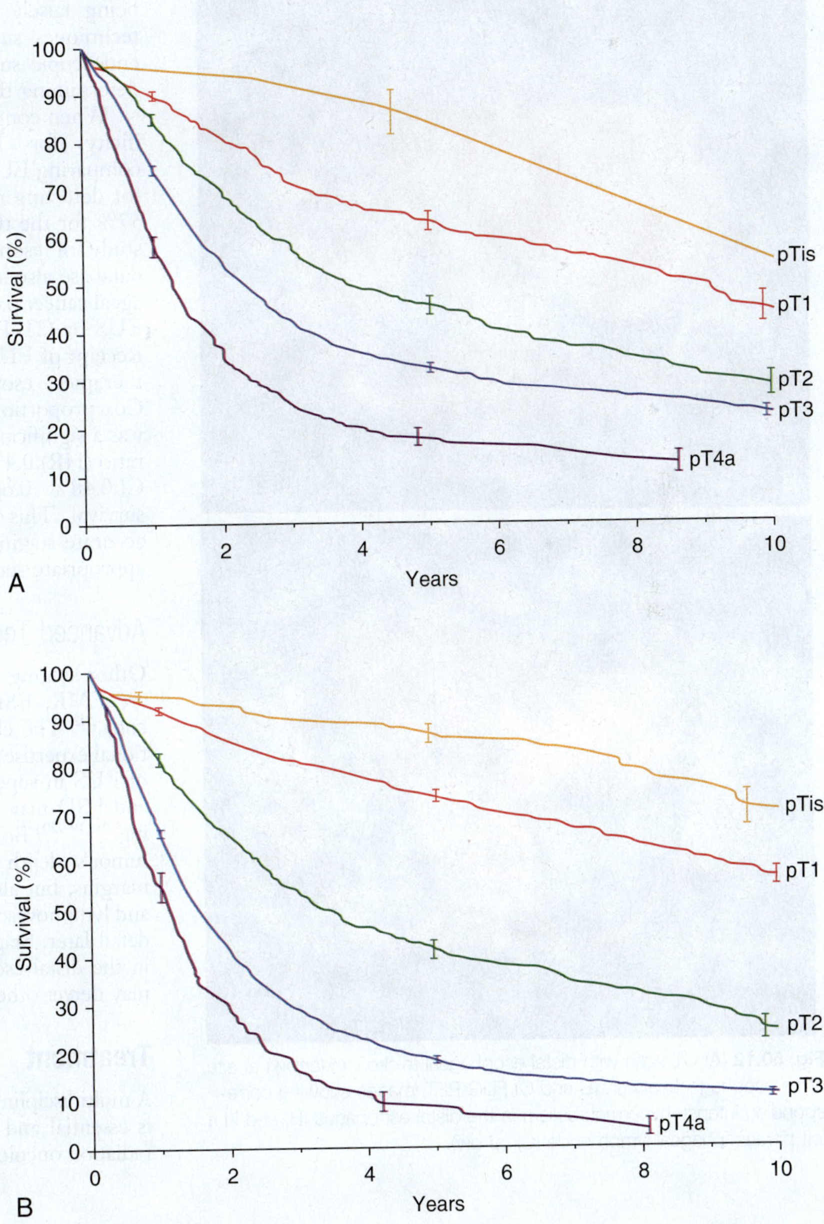

FIG. 50.11 Survival stratified by pT category. Kaplan-Meier estimates accompanied by vertical bars representing 68% confidence limits, equivalent to ±1 standard error. (A) Esophageal squamous cell carcinoma. (B) Esophageal adenocarcinoma. (Data from Rice TW, Chen LQ, Hofstetter WL, et al. Worldwide Esophageal Cancer Collaboration: pathologic staging data. *Dis Esophagus*. 2016;29(7):724–733.)

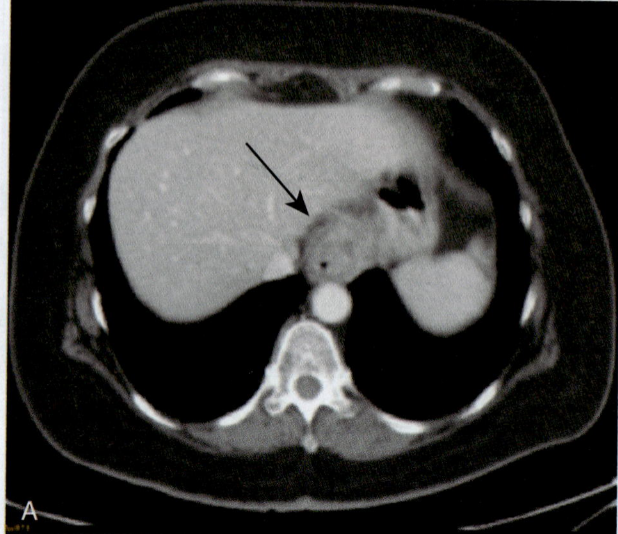

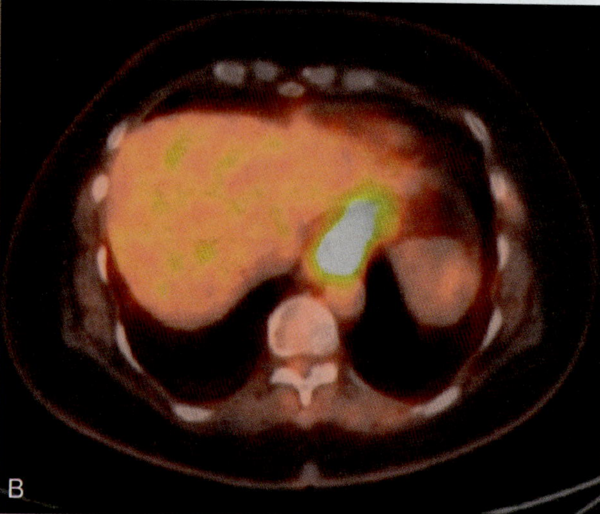

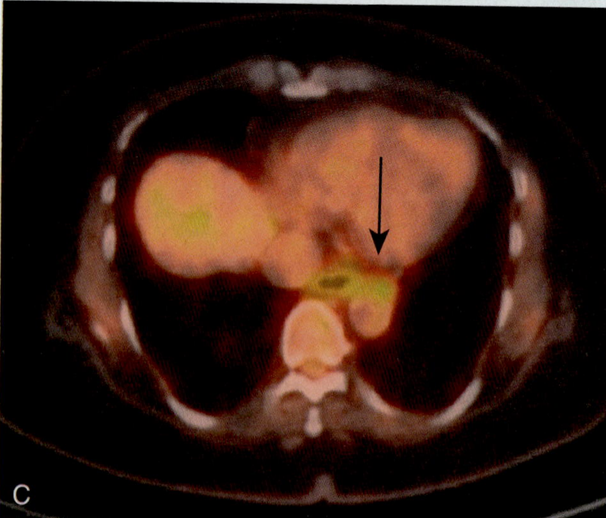

Fig. 50.12 (A) CT scan with distal esophageal thickening (*arrow*) at site of an esophageal cancer. (B and C) FDG-PET images showing corresponding intense hypermetabolism in the distal esophagus (B) and in a left paraesophageal lymph node (C) (*arrow*).

pooled sensitivity of EUS for N stage was 85% (95% CI, 82% −86%). The addition of FNA of equivocal lymph nodes increased the sensitivity of nodal staging to 97% (95% CI, 92%−99%).[194] Endosonographic features of malignant lymph nodes include lesions that are hypoechoic with a rounded and smooth surface, lesions >10 mm, and lesions located in close proximity to the tumor.[195]

Video 50.1 EGD and staging EUS of a T3N2 esophageal carcinoma with EUS-guided FNA of a paraesophageal lymph node.

The role of EUS in the initial staging of esophageal cancer has been questioned, particularly in superficial tumors.[196,197] A recent review and meta-analysis found that EUS has good accuracy in staging superficial esophageal cancers overall.[198] Factors such as location, histologic type of lesion, EUS method used, and the experience of the endosonographer may affect the diagnostic accuracy. Recent data from a systematic review and meta-analysis that assessed the false-positive rate of advanced disease on EUS exam at the tumor level (differentiating between T1a and T1b disease) showed that the use of EUS in patients with BE with dysplasia and early cancer resulted in a high proportion of patients being falsely overstaged and understaged.[199] Hence, advanced techniques such as endoscopic mucosal resection (EMR) and endoscopic submucosal dissection (ESD) play a pivotal role in determining the true extent of invasion.

When compared to CT, EUS has better sensitivity and specificity for locoregional metastasis.[195,200] A meta-analysis comparing EUS, CT, and FDG-PET showed pooled sensitivities for detecting regional lymph node metastasis of 80%, 50%, and 57% for the three modalities, respectively.[191] A recent case-only study of esophageal cancer using the SEER-Medicare linked database also showed an improved survival in a cohort of esophageal cancer patients undergoing EUS staging compared to the no EUS or CT-PET group, with the exception of stage 0 disease. Receipt of EUS increased the likelihood of receiving endoscopic therapies, esophagectomy, and chemoradiation. Multivariable Cox proportional hazards models showed that a receipt of EUS was a significant predictor for improved survival at 1 year [hazard ratio (HR) 0.49, 95% CI 0.39%−0.59%], 3 years (HR 0.57, 95% CI 0.48%−0.66%), and 5 years (HR 0.59, 95% CI 0.5%−0.68%) survival. This improvement in survival is most likely related to accurate staging of patients with esophageal cancer, resulting in appropriate stage-specific therapies.[201]

Advanced Techniques

Other staging modalities that are performed in selected centers are EMR, ESD, and minimally invasive staging using laparoscopy.[202] The choice and sequence are dependent on the institutional expertise and preference. Conflicting reports on the accuracy of EUS in superficial tumors have led some to believe that EMR and ESD may be more accurate methods for diagnosis and staging.[196,197,203] Both methods not only provide tissue for assessing the tumor's depth of invasion (T stage), and possibly tumor-free margins, but also provide information on grade of differentiation and lymphovascular invasion. EMR and ESD are discussed in more detail later. Staging laparoscopy is considered optional for tumors in the distal esophagus and at the esophagogastric junction, as it may detect otherwise radiologically occult metastasis.[204,205]

Treatment

A multidisciplinary approach to the treatment of esophageal cancer is essential and requires input from experts in surgical oncology, radiation oncology, medical oncology, gastroenterology, radiology, pathology, and often palliative care.[206] Tumor location, staging, histologic type, medical comorbidities, and patient preference are factors that must be considered for selecting the proper treatment. Some general principles can be summarized as follows[207]:

- Surgery is the standard treatment for a medically optimized surgical candidate with a localized, nonsuperficial tumor.
- For a patient with a localized tumor who is not a surgical candidate, definitive chemoradiation with curative intent may be considered.
- For all others (metastatic disease), palliation is recommended.

With a wide spectrum of treatment options for esophageal cancer, accurate staging is essential to selecting the appropriate treatment modality.[208] The primary objective is to identify those patients who may benefit from neoadjuvant therapy and those with widespread metastatic disease who are better candidates for palliation. Patient selection is another very important component of the management of esophageal cancer. The evaluation should include medical comorbidities and the patient's current performance status, nutrition, and cardiopulmonary function. Pulmonary complications, pneumonia in particular, are important determinants of early postoperative outcome and are associated with more than fourfold increase in mortality.[209–211] Interestingly, preoperative chemoradiation has been found to be a risk factor for postoperative pneumonia.[211] A scoring system involving spirometry results, age, and performance status is available to predict cardiopulmonary complications.[210] Selection based on mathematical scores may not be superior to a physician's clinical assessment; the two methods are complementary.[212] Importantly, the scores obtained may not be applicable to all institutions or populations. For example, patients with ESCC from Asia have a different risk profile (e.g., pulmonary and hepatic comorbidities from smoking and alcohol use) compared with patients in Western societies with EAC (e.g., cardiac risk factors or comorbidities).[213]

Patients with cervical or cervicothoracic esophageal tumors (<5 cm from the cricopharyngeus) are usually poor candidates for surgery because of limitations in surgical techniques.[214] These patients are typically treated with definitive chemoradiation, with an encouraging response rate in a recent study.[215]

Surgery

Resection of the esophagus with en bloc lymphadenectomy is the cornerstone of curative therapy for patients with locally advanced esophageal cancer.[216] In addition, according to the National Comprehensive Cancer Network (NCCN) guidelines, surgery alone is considered the standard of care and treatment of choice for T1b and T2 cancers without nodal involvement or distant metastasis. Surgery in conjunction with a multimodal approach is indicated for T1 to T4a tumors with lymph node metastases.[204] The final outcomes for patients undergoing esophagectomy are dependent not only on the patient's stage, comorbidities, and performance status but also on surgical team expertise and center volume. Esophagectomy has the potential for high perioperative morbidity (40%–50%) and mortality (3%–13%).[217–221] One recurrent theme in the surgical literature is that center volume of esophagectomy is a critical determinant of outcomes.[216,220,222] Thirty-day mortality is inversely related to the number of esophagectomies performed at the center. Treatment in high-volume centers with experienced surgeons along with the availability of ICU management and early detection of complications play significant roles in differential outcomes.

The mortality may increase to 20% in low-volume centers (<5 esophagectomies per year).[223–225] The operative mortality in high-volume centers (>20 per year) is estimated to be less than 2%.[226–228] In a review of quality-of-care indicators, patient selection and multidisciplinary team management were the most important factors influencing outcome in esophageal cancer surgery.[229]

Techniques

Several different variations on surgical technique have been described for esophagectomy in patients with esophageal cancer. The technique used can be influenced by surgical access site (transthoracic vs. transhiatal), extent of lymphadenopathy, type of anastomosis desired, type and method of preparation of the esophageal conduit, pyloric drainage procedure, and route of reconstruction. Most controversies are based on the type of surgical access and the extent of lymph node dissection.[230] The type of surgical access may not only influence the perioperative morbidity and mortality but also the ability to perform extensive lymph node dissection.[212]

Transthoracic approaches include Ivor Lewis esophagogastrectomy (right thoracotomy and laparotomy) and McKeown esophagogastrectomy (thoracotomy, laparotomy, and cervical anastomosis). Transhiatal approaches include laparotomy and cervical anastomosis.[231–236] The reported advantage of the transthoracic approach is better visualization of the mediastinum, which leads to decreased risk of adjacent organ injury, more complete cancer resection and lymph node retrieval, and more accurate staging.[234] Conversely, those in favor of a transhiatal approach note that cure of esophageal cancer is a rare phenomenon achieved in only very early tumors, making esophagectomy usually a palliative procedure. In this regard, a transhiatal approach has a shorter operative time with lower postoperative morbidity.[232] A large population-based study comparing transthoracic and transhiatal approaches found that the transhiatal esophagogastrectomy was associated with lower operative mortality rate (6.7% vs. 13.1%, $P = .009$), but the long-term survival was not different between the two approaches.[221]

Minimally invasive esophagectomy (MIE), which includes minimally invasive Ivor Lewis esophagogastrectomy (laparoscopy and limited thoracotomy or thoracoscopy) and minimally invasive McKeown esophagogastrectomy (thoracoscopy, limited laparotomy or laparoscopy, and cervical incision), has been gaining popularity recently.[237] It is aimed at minimizing surgical trauma and perioperative morbidity and mortality. The technique requires special training and expertise.[238] Minimally invasive surgery has been shown to have similar oncologic outcomes compared to conventional approach.[239] The advantages of minimally invasive surgery include less postoperative pain, a decreased length of hospital stay, lower need for intraoperative blood transfusion, and overall lower cost.[240–242] A recent prospective multicenter trial showed that MIE is safe and feasible with low perioperative morbidity and mortality (2.1%).[243] Despite encouraging results with MIE, recent population-based studies failed to demonstrate superiority of MIE over conventional approach.[244]

Lymph Node Dissection

Lymph node status is an independent predictor of survival in esophageal cancer.[245] For this reason, aggressive lymphadenectomy is thought to be essential to reduce locoregional recurrence, improve survival, and obtain a more accurate pathologic staging.[246,247] The number of lymph nodes removed during esophagectomy has been shown to be an independent predictor of survival.[248] In patients undergoing esophagectomy without neoadjuvant chemoradiation, the NCCN guidelines recommend that 15 or more lymph nodes be removed for adequate staging.[204] However, in patients who undergo neoadjuvant chemoradiation, the number of lymph nodes does not seem to correlate with increased survival.[249]

Outcomes

Measurement of short-term clinical outcomes after esophagectomy for esophageal cancer is difficult to compare among published reports because of the lack of standard methodology and other inconsistencies.[250] Moreover, outcomes after esophagectomy included in the largest thoracic surgical database in the United States are far better than the ones reported by other national clinical and administrative databases.[251] The most commonly reported complications are anastomotic leak and postoperative pneumonia.

A recent updated population-based study on esophageal cancer survival after surgery without neoadjuvant therapy has shown that the long-term survival has not improved since 2000. Rather, it has remained at 30.5% after 5 years. This survival rate in operated patients remained unchanged despite a decrease in the 30-day postoperative mortality from nearly 5%–2%.[252] The improved postoperative mortality probably reflects better ICU management of complications.[252,253] Thus improvements in surgical techniques have not translated into better long-term survival outcomes.

A substantial fraction of patients with potentially resectable tumors has a pathologic complete response after neoadjuvant chemoradiation (23% in EAC and 49% in ESCC).[254] Moreover, a recent study that compared surgery to definitive chemoradiation in patients with resectable ESCC showed that the 5-year overall survival was not different for patients with stage I (80% vs. 75.8%) and stage II disease (78.2% vs. 74.6%).[255] Another study showed similar outcomes between surgery and chemoradiation for stage I disease, but the risk of local recurrence (including metachronous lesions) was significantly higher in the chemoradiation group. Most recurrences in the chemoradiation group were intramucosal carcinoma and were cured after salvage therapy (mainly endoscopic), as discussed below.[256] Studies are currently underway to identify patients who can potentially avoid surgery.

Endoscopic Treatment

EET has revolutionized the management of BE-related dysplasia and early EAC (see Chapter 49) and esophageal squamous dysplasia and early ESCC. The role of endoscopic treatment of esophageal cancer can be either for curative intent or palliation. The former is reserved to mucosal tumors (T1a) confined to the mucosa (M1 or intraepithelial), the lamina propria (M2), or the muscularis mucosae (M3). These tumors have an extremely low chance of harboring lymph node metastasis. Submucosal tumors (T1b) are further classified into SM1 (superficial submucosal invasion), SM2 (invasion to center of submucosa), or SM3 (invasion into the deep submucosa). In contrast to T1a tumors, T1b tumors involving the submucosa have a higher risk of lymph node metastasis, up to 56% in SM3 tumors.[183,184]

Endoscopic Therapy With Curative Intent

Endoscopic resection techniques and endoscopic ablation therapy have been used for treatment of superficial esophageal carcinoma. Endoscopic resection has the added advantage of procuring large tissue specimens for pathologic diagnosis and accurate cancer staging (Fig. 50.13).[257,258] Both EMR and ESD allow targeted removal of tissue, such as nodular or flat Barrett epithelium with HGD and T1a cancers (Fig. 50.14). The effectiveness and safety of EET in eradicating Barrett-related neoplasia, maintaining remission, and preventing progression to invasive EAC (primary goal of EET) have been demonstrated in multiple studies.[259,260] The basic principles of EET with regard to management of Barrett-related dysplasia and early EAC are as follows: (1) resection of all visible lesions (these are lesions that harbor the highest grade of neoplasia); (2) eradication of the remaining BE to reduce the risk of metachronous neoplasia; (3) management of immediate adverse events such as bleeding, perforation, and long-term adverse events such as strictures and recurrence; and (4) enrollment in surveillance programs after achieving complete eradication.[261]

EET has now replaced esophagectomy as the standard of care for patients with Barrett-related HGD and early (mucosal) EAC.[262] Although there are no randomized controlled trials comparing esophagectomy with EET, results from population-based and observational studies have reported comparable outcomes (2- and 5-year EAC survival rates) after EET and esophagectomy, providing confidence in the contemporary management of BE-related neoplasia patients with EET. The most recent ASGE guideline document on the role of EET recommends against surgery and favors EET in BE patients with HGD and intramucosal cancer.[259]

The role of EMR as a staging and therapeutic tool in the management of BE-related neoplasia is well described. The staging superiority of EMR compared with biopsy specimens is related to a larger and deeper tissue specimen with limited distortion providing the ultimate proof of invasion depth along with improved interobserver agreement among pathology using EMR specimens.[258,263] A study that followed 1000 patients with T1a esophageal carcinoma for around 5 years showed that EMR was very effective, with 94% complete remission rate.[264] A SEER database analysis of 1458 patients between 1998 and 2008 with

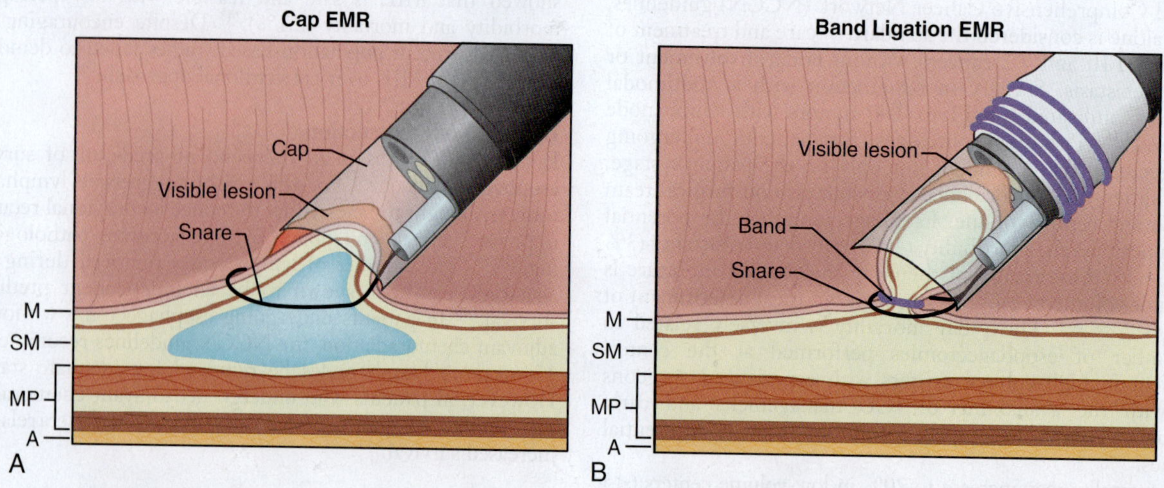

Fig. 50.13 Techniques for endoscopic mucosal resection. (A) Cap-assisted endoscopic mucosal resection (EMR). (B) Band-ligation EMR. *A*, Adventitia; *M*, mucosa; *MP*, muscularis propria; *SM*, submucosa.

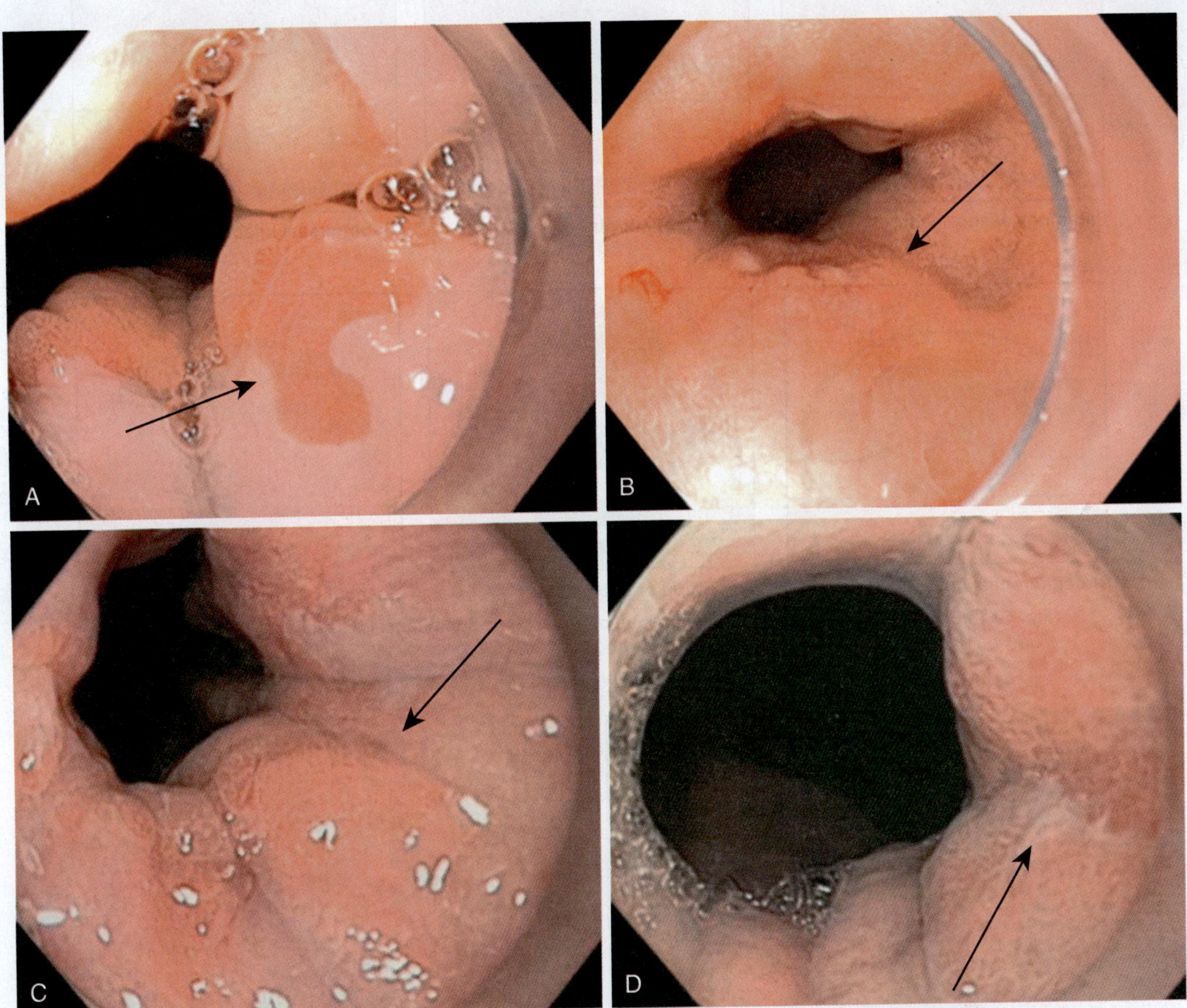

Fig. 50.14 (A–D) Examples of visible lesions detected at high-resolution endoscopy in patients with Barrett esophagus (*arrows*).

T1N0 esophageal cancer (ESCC and EAC) showed a similar overall survival between patients who underwent surgery (64.1%) and patients who underwent endoscopic therapy, including EMR with or without ablation (55.5%).[265] High rates of performance of EMR also appear to be a significant predictor for high eradication rates of BE.[266,267]

Complications of EMR include bleeding (up to 10%), perforation (<3%), and stricture.[257,268] Post-EMR strictures are, for the most part, responsive to endoscopic balloon dilation and are related to the circumference and length of mucosal resection.[269]

In light of the encouraging reports with EMR in early esophageal cancer, patient selection is crucial. Major limiting factors of EMR are lymph node involvement, presence of lymphovascular invasion, and multifocal disease.[270,271] Ultimately, the best disease-free results with EMR have been reported with nonulcerated or nodular mucosal lesions smaller than 20 mm in diameter, especially lesions that are well or moderately differentiated, intramucosal, and with no lymphovascular invasion.[272,273]

Early enthusiasm for endoscopic treatment led to new techniques for lesions extending into the submucosa. ESD can potentially increase the size of the en bloc local resection and remove submucosal tumors (Figs. 50.15 and 50.16).[274] However, these lesions have a significant risk of lymph node involvement, and thus ESD in this setting would be only diagnostic and not curative. Most of the ESD experience comes from Japan where en bloc resection rates in ESCC of 100% and curative resection rates of 80% have been reported.[275,276] When comparing ESD to EMR in esophageal mucosal cancers 20 mm or less, ESD has been found to provide an en bloc resection rate of 100%, whereas for EMR, it was for 87% (cap-assisted) and 71% (two-channel technique). The curative resection rate for ESD was 97%, significantly higher than either EMR technique (71% for cap and 46% for two-channel). Complications of ESD include perforation in 2%–5% and stricture in 5%–17%.[275–277]

The European Society of Gastrointestinal Endoscopy recommends that ESD is the preferred method of endoscopic resection of ESCC given higher en bloc resection rate and superior histological assessment. EMR can be used for lesions <10 mm if en bloc resection can be assured. For early EAC and HGD, EMR is still the mainstay method of endoscopic resection but ESD can be considered for lesions >15 mm, poor-lifting tumors, and lesions with high-risk features for submucosal invasion.[278]

Ablation can be achieved with radiofrequency ablation (RFA) or cryotherapy. Each method can be used alone or, more often, following EMR or ESD of visible nodules. Photodynamic therapy is rarely used in clinical practice currently due to high risk of adverse reactions (strictures and photosensitivity) and the availability of other ablative techniques.[279] RFA is being increasingly

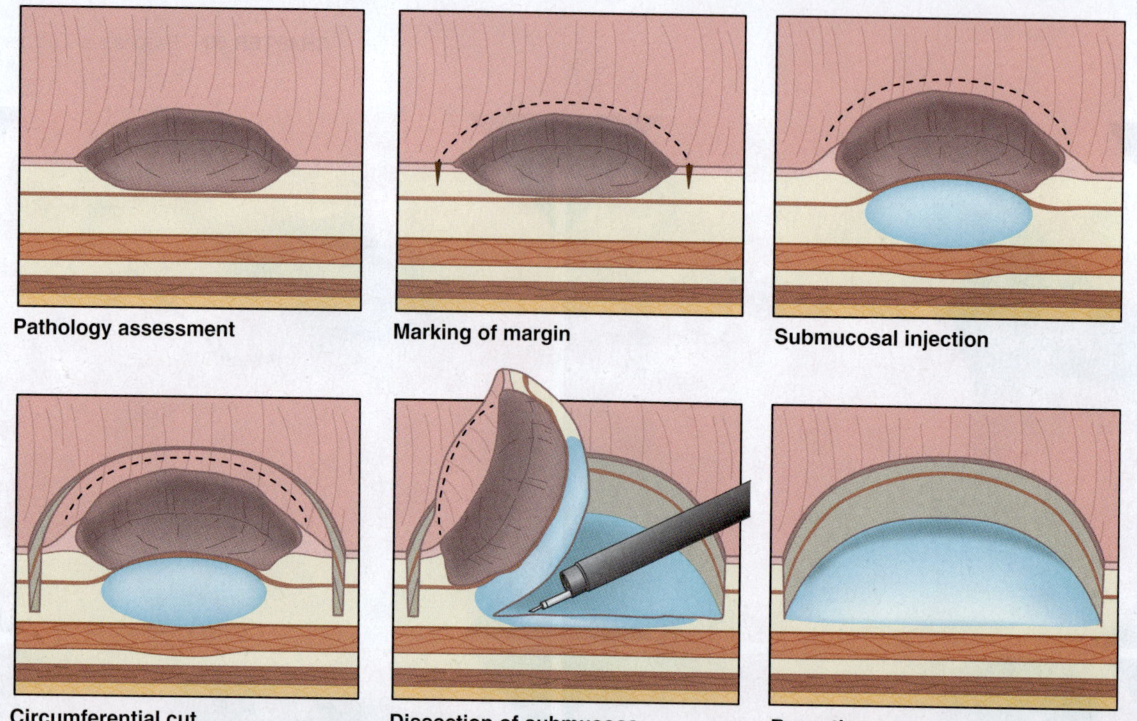

Fig. 50.15 **Schematic description of the technique of endoscopic submucosal dissection.** (Modified from *Current Gastroenterology Reports* 2014;16(5).)

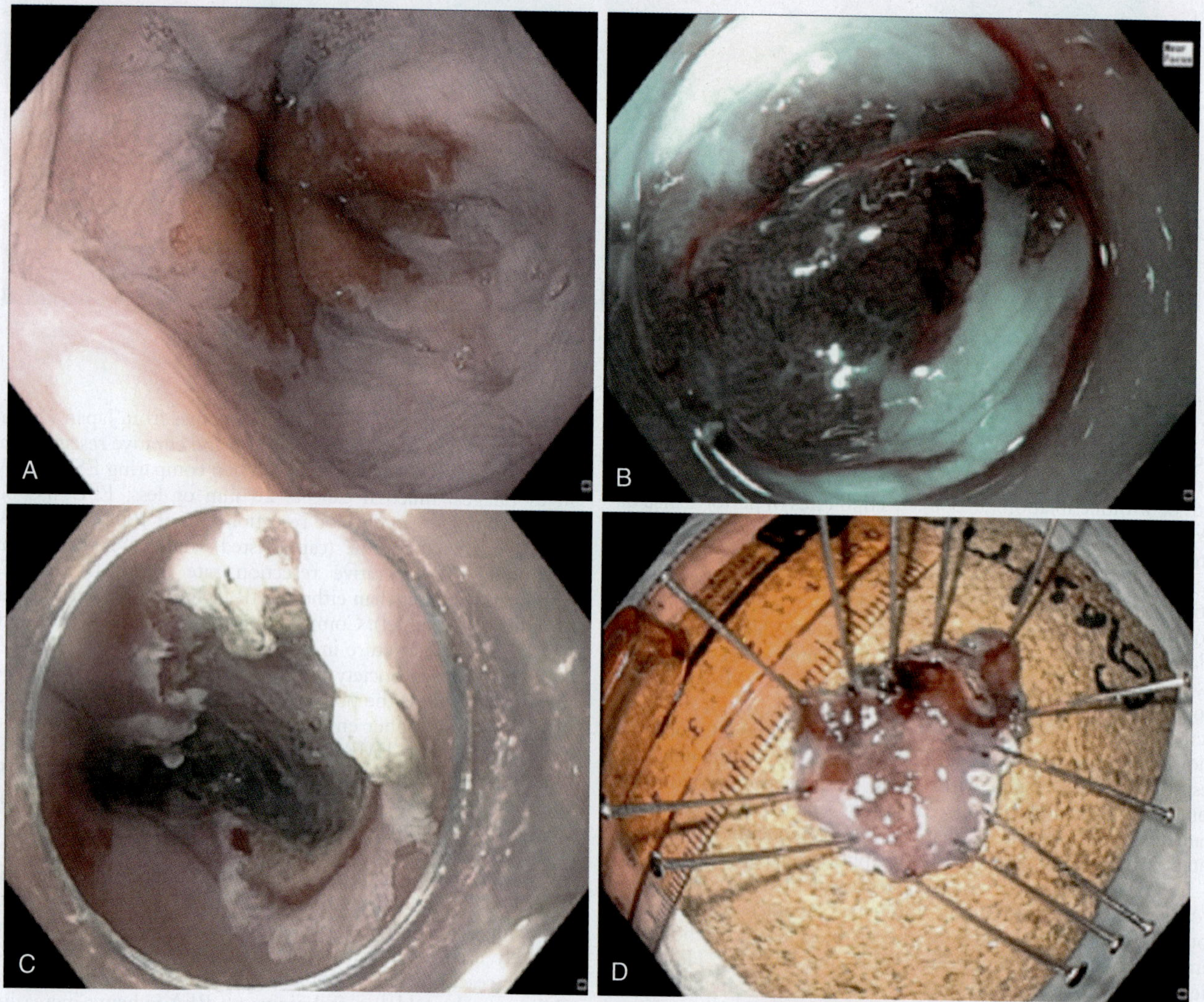

Fig. 50.16 (A) Distal esophageal nodule at the 1–3 o'clock position with biopsies consistent with adenocarcinoma. (B) Narrow-band imaging of the same area with irregular pit and vascular pattern. (C) Mucosal defect after endoscopic submucosal dissection (ESD) of the nodular area. (D) ESD specimen pinned on a cork board.

used in patients with BE-related HGD and low-grade dysplasia and mucosal EAC after EMR is performed for any visible lesion (see Chapter 49) and in adenocarcinoma in situ. In contrast to photodynamic therapy, RFA is associated with fewer complications and better preservation of esophageal function.[280–282] Based on data from randomized controlled trials and large observational studies, RFA is the most widely used technique in the management of BE-related neoplasia patients. RFA is not used as commonly in early ESCC, but a few recent reports demonstrated efficacy and safety of RFA for the treatment of early squamous cell neoplasia.[283] Although there is less evidence, cryotherapy also seems to be effective in early esophageal cancers.[284]

A major limitation of ablation therapy is that it does not provide tissue for further pathologic evaluation and staging.

Endoscopic Therapy With Palliative Intent

Endoscopic dilation can be performed for treatment of dysphagia. However, the effect is typically short-lived, and there is an increased risk of perforation.[285] Endoscopic placement of self-expandable metal stent can also be considered with excellent efficacy to alleviate dysphagia. The stents currently used are mostly covered stents due to better efficacy and less reintervention rate (Fig. 50.17).[286] Small-diameter (18 mm) and large-diameter (23 mm) stents seem to have the same efficacy.[287] Stents can also be used in combination with other modalities (chemotherapy, radiotherapy, or brachytherapy) to alleviate dysphagia.[288]

Endoscopic placement of gastrostomy or jejunostomy feeding tubes can help alleviate dysphagia and weight loss. Placement of gastrostomy tubes is not recommended in surgical candidates given that it may interfere with using the stomach as conduit. Moreover, using the pull technique for gastrostomy tube placement, metastatic seeding of the tube insertion site was reported. Direct gastrostomy tube placement may be favored to avoid this risk.[289] Covered self-expandable metal stent can successfully seal a tracheoesophageal fistula in up to 86% of patients with esophageal cancer.[290] Caution must be exercised when placing stents in the middle third of the esophagus because of the possible extrinsic compression of the airway, which lies just anteriorly.[291] The ASGE recommends placement of esophageal stents for fistulas because they provide durable and immediate relief.[292]

Chemotherapy and Radiation Therapy

Neoadjuvant Chemotherapy

Patients who receive preoperative chemotherapy and then undergo surgery and have no residual cancer have a better survival

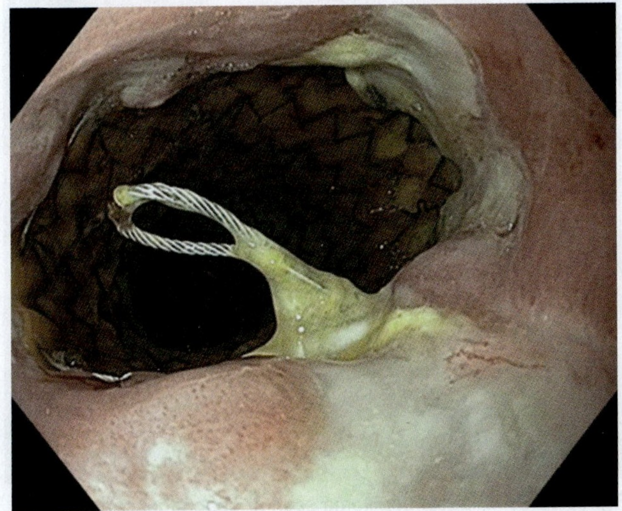

Fig. 50.17 Fully covered esophageal metal stent.

rate than those with residual or persistent cancer.[293–296] Results from North America and Europe have shown significant 3- and 5-year survival advantages of preoperative (and perioperative) chemotherapy compared to surgery alone.[297–299] These results were seen in both ESCC and EAC. A large meta-analysis also showed that neoadjuvant chemotherapy was associated with improved survival and higher rates of complete (R0) resection.[300] Although neoadjuvant chemoradiotherapy is the most common approach for locally advanced esophageal carcinoma, perioperative chemotherapy can be used as a treatment option for adenocarcinomas of the distal esophagus and GEJ.[301]

Neoadjuvant Chemoradiotherapy

Neoadjuvant chemoradiotherapy has become the standard of care for locally advanced esophageal cancer in many countries based on data from prospective trials and meta-analyses.[302,303] The CROSS study (Chemoradiotherapy for Oesophageal Cancer followed by Surgery Study) which included patients with esophageal cancer (75% with EAC and 23% with ESCC) randomized patients to neoadjuvant chemoradiation followed by surgery versus surgery alone. This study found that the combined modality arm had a longer median survival (49.4 vs. 24.0 months). Patients in the chemoradiation arm received perioperative weekly carboplatin, paclitaxel, and 41.4 Gy of radiotherapy followed by surgery. A lower proportion of patients had a local recurrence in the perioperative therapy group compared to the surgery-alone group (14% vs. 34%). Histologic tumor type did not affect survival; both EAC and ESCC benefited from neoadjuvant chemoradiation therapy.[103,304]

Neoadjuvant Radiation Therapy

In contrast to neoadjuvant chemotherapy and chemoradiotherapy just discussed, studies have not shown any benefit for preoperative radiation alone.[305] The NCCN recommends that radiation therapy alone should be used only for palliative purposes or for patients who are not candidates for chemotherapy.[204] Newer radiation therapy techniques are aimed at increasing dose delivery to the target tissue while reducing toxicity to the surrounding organs (heart, lungs, skin). These techniques, such as intensity-modulated radiation therapy and proton beam therapy, are still being evaluated for efficacy in esophageal cancer patients.[306,307]

Adjuvant Chemoradiotherapy

Compared to neoadjuvant chemoradiotherapy, adjuvant chemoradiotherapy does not appear to be effective, and a recent network meta-analysis showed no survival benefit when compared to surgery alone.[303] A retrospective study showed that adjuvant chemotherapy after neoadjuvant chemoradiotherapy and surgery was not effective in patients with no residual disease or with residual nonnodal disease but was associated with improved survival in patients with residual nodal disease.[308]

Targeted Therapy

Patients with EAC should be tested for human epidermal growth factor receptor 2 (HER2) on tumor biopsies. If high levels of expression are seen, HER2 antibodies such as trastuzumab and pertuzumab can be added to the chemotherapy regimen in patients with metastatic adenocarcinoma or locally advanced carcinoma where local therapy is not indicated.[309]

In a recent trial, VEGF receptor 2 antibodies, ramucirumab, showed promising results for patients with advanced GEJ adenocarcinomas refractory to standard chemotherapy regimen and were approved by the FDA for this indication.[310]

Immunotherapy

Another recently FDA-approved therapy is pembrolizumab, an antibody to programmed death ligand-1 (PD-L1). Pembrolizumab is approved for refractory adenocarcinomas that are PD-L1 positive or for tumors with microsatellite instability or that have DNA mismatch repair gene defects.[311]

Prognosis

The best predictors of esophageal cancer survival are depth of invasion (T stage) and lymph node involvement (N stage).[312,313] A retrospective study found that the N stage of esophageal cancer was an independent factor affecting overall and disease-free survival (N1 disease-free survival of 13.6%).[314] The 5-year survival at presentation for local, regional, and distant disease was 41%, 23%, and 5%, respectively.[315] The 5-year survival improved to above 90% when HGD (cancer in situ) or T1a cancer was diagnosed.[264] For those with locoregionally advanced disease at presentation (>50% of patients), however, their outcomes are poor, and most have a recurrence and die within 3–5 years of their diagnosis.[315] In addition to the depth of invasion and number of lymph nodes involved, histologic type, degree of differentiation, and location of the tumor also have an impact on the survival.[247] Despite the recent advances in treatment, the most recently reported overall 5-year survival rate is only 19%.[3]

Recent interest in brain metastases from esophageal cancer has been reported. Metastatic brain lesions are rare in esophageal carcinoma, with a recent report showing incidence of 3.8%.[316] Most of the reported cases are associated with EAC rather than ESCC.[316,317]

OTHER MALIGNANT EPITHELIAL TUMORS

Squamous Cell Carcinoma Variants

Verrucous carcinoma is a rare variant of ESCC, with less than 30 reported cases.[318] It is most commonly found in middle-aged individuals, and two-thirds of affected patients are men. Endoscopically, it presents with a papillary or warty appearance. The diagnosis requires a high index of suspicion and multiple biopsies because histology reveals well-differentiated hyperkeratosis and acanthosis with only a small column of neoplastic cells.[318] Despite the fact that these lesions are typically well differentiated and slow growing, they generally have a poor prognosis given the delay in diagnosis.

Another variant of ESCC is *carcinosarcoma* (also known as *pseudosarcoma*, *spindle cell carcinoma*, and *polypoid carcinoma*). This tumor presents with a polypoid appearance and can be solitary or multiple. Owing to the exophytic nature of the tumor(s), many patients will present with dysphagia or epigastric discomfort. Histologically, the tumors have a spindle cell component; they tend to have invaded the esophageal wall and spread to regional lymph nodes at the time of diagnosis and can metastasize. Therefore these tumors are associated with a poor prognosis (2-year survival of 25%).[319]

Small Cell Carcinoma

Small cell carcinoma of the esophagus is a rare entity, accounting for 0.8%–3.1% of all esophageal malignancies. The tumor is highly aggressive, with a very poor prognosis. The average age at diagnosis is 65 years, and two-thirds of affected patients are men. Dysphagia, weight loss, and epigastric pain are the presenting symptoms. There is usually a history of tobacco use (90%) and alcohol use (70%). The tumor is typically located in the middle third (52%) or lower third of the esophagus (35%). More than half of affected patients have extensive disease at the time of diagnosis.[320] The optimal management of these patients is not well established, but chemotherapy should always be a part of the multimodality treatment.[321] For a very select group of patients with limited disease, resection followed by chemotherapy may provide longer survival.[321] The median overall survival is only 11 months, with a 2-year survival of just 25%.[320]

Malignant Melanoma

Primary esophageal melanoma is rare, with just over 300 cases described.[322,323] Melanoma accounts for 0.1%–0.5% of all esophageal malignancies.[324] Primary esophageal melanoma metastasizes early and has a very poor prognosis. Melanocytosis at the basal layer of the epithelium caused by basal hyperplasia or chronic esophagitis is thought to play an important role in its pathogenesis.[325,326] Melanoma affects men twice as often as women; the average age of presentation is close to 60 years.[324] Dysphagia is the most common symptom. However, because of the soft nature of the tumor, symptoms can be delayed, and the size of the tumor at presentation is larger than 2 cm in over 90% of cases. The most common locations are the middle and distal thirds of the esophagus.[323] Endoscopic characteristics include a nonulcerated, pigmented tumor, although the color may vary depending on the amount of melanin, and an "amelanotic" variant has been described.[327] "Satellite" lesions occurring a few centimeters from the primary, larger lesion can be seen and are thought to be due to intramural metastasis. Histologically, melanoma can be misdiagnosed as poorly differentiated carcinoma owing to the lack of melanin granules, and immunohistochemistry may be necessary for establishing the correct diagnosis.[324] This is an aggressive disease and the incidence of regional lymph node and distant metastasis at presentation is high (40%–80%).[328] FDG-PET is currently the most accepted modality for detecting metastases. It is important to distinguish primary from metastatic melanoma, because metastatic melanoma (discussed later) can involve the esophagus in 4% of cases.[329] Radical resection combined with lymphadenectomy is the main treatment approach. The calculated 5-year survival rate for primary esophageal melanoma is 37%.[330] Age, stage, tumor location, and lymph node involvement are independent predictive factors of prognosis.[331]

BENIGN EPITHELIAL TUMORS

Squamous Papilloma

Esophageal papillomas are asymptomatic, benign epithelial tumors characterized endoscopically by a solitary, exophytic lesion in the lower third of the esophagus (Fig. 50.18). They tend to

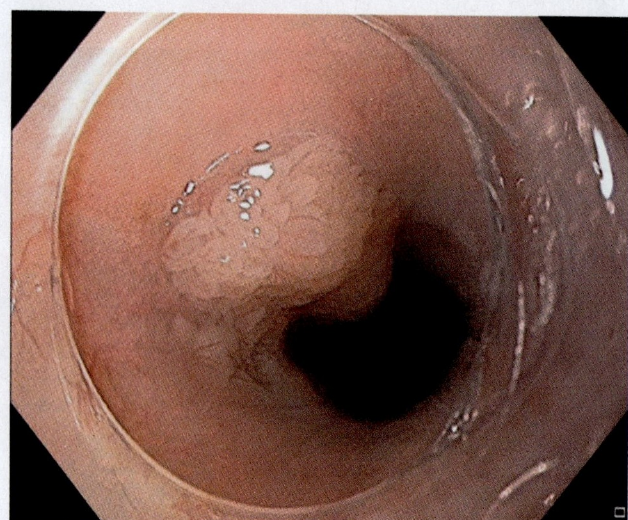

Fig. 50.18 Esophageal papilloma seen at esophagoscopy.

have a white or pink color. They have a soft consistency and a smooth or slightly rough surface. Histologically, they reveal finger-like projections of connective tissue lined by an increased number of squamous cells. The endoscopic differential diagnosis includes glycogenic acanthosis, verrucous border of squamous cell carcinoma, and verrucous carcinoma.[332] Squamous papillomas are rare, with a reported prevalence ranging from 0.01% to 0.43%.[332] Their pathogenesis is uncertain, but it has been hypothesized to be related to underlying inflammation (e.g., from GERD).[332] Another theory of pathogenesis is infection with HPV.[333] Papillomas are generally amenable to endoscopic resection, mostly using forceps given their small size or mucosectomy techniques. Recurrence after resection is uncommon. Malignant transformation has been reported in a few cases with multiple papillomas (esophageal papillomatosis), but cancer is rare in isolated lesions.[334,335]

Focal dermal hypoplasia (Goltz syndrome), a rare condition usually affecting females, is characterized by multiple abnormalities of ectodermal and mesodermal structures. Although dermatologic, ocular, and musculoskeletal manifestations dominate the clinical picture, esophageal papillomatosis may be present.[336,337] Caused by a mutation in *PORCN* on the X chromosome, Goltz syndrome has a dominant X-linked inheritance that is usually lethal in affected males. Goltz syndrome can be inherited or occur de novo.

Adenoma

Adenomas of the esophagus are rare and almost exclusively associated with Barrett metaplasia. Although adenocarcinoma is a much more frequently recognized lesion associated with Barrett, several cases of adenomas have also been reported.[338–340] They characteristically present as polypoid lesions within a segment of Barrett in the lower third of the esophagus. Histopathology shows dysplastic tubular glands covered by specialized intestinal epithelium. Similar to colonic adenomas, these are considered to be premalignant, and endoscopic resection is recommended for diagnosis and treatment.

Inflammatory Fibroid Polyp

Inflammatory fibroid polyp (also known as *inflammatory pseudopolyp* or *eosinophilic granuloma*) is characterized by a distinct histology. This includes a submucosal-based polypoid lesion with perivascular, concentric fibroblastic proliferation with an increase in eosinophils. Most polyps express CD34 and are negative for CD117. They most often are found incidentally in the stomach and large intestines, followed by the small intestine. The esophagus is a much less likely location (≈2% of cases).[341] They are nonneoplastic polyps and follow a benign course.

MALIGNANT NONEPITHELIAL TUMORS

Lymphoma

Lymphoma of the esophagus can be primary or secondary, with primary lymphoma being far less common. Primary esophageal lymphoma is defined as a lymphoma having predominantly esophageal involvement with only regional lymph nodes affected in the absence of disease in peripheral or mediastinal lymph nodes, spleen, or liver, and with a normal chest radiograph and WBC count.[342] Lymphoma accounts for less than 1% of esophageal malignancies.[343] Clinically, esophageal lymphoma can present with dysphagia, weight loss, GI bleeding, esophageal fistulas, and other nonspecific systemic symptoms (e.g., fevers, night sweats, and fatigue.). Endoscopically, the few cases that are reported describe a range of findings, including submucosal nodules, masses, ulcerations, and polypoid lesions. Esophageal lymphomas can be either the Hodgkin type or non-Hodgkin lymphoma (NHL). Diffuse large B-cell lymphoma is the most common subtype of NHL and has been associated with immunosuppressive states such as AIDS (see Chapter 32).[344]

Sarcoma

Sarcomas of the esophagus are rare mesenchymal tumors that include leiomyosarcomas, gastrointestinal stromal tumors (GISTs) (see later and Chapter 33), rhabdomyosarcoma, fibrosarcoma, liposarcoma, fibrous histiocytoma, Kaposi sarcoma, and choriocarcinoma. Leiomyosarcomas are the most common subtype and can be difficult to distinguish from benign leiomyomas. Tumors can be of intraluminal, polypoid, or infiltrative/invasive. Histologically, they consist of interlacing whorls of spindle cells with increased mitoses and marked pleomorphism. Mucosal biopsy is not a useful diagnostic tool in most cases, because these lesions are submucosal. On the other hand, EUS with FNA has been shown to be helpful for diagnosis. Lymph node involvement occurs in a third of cases. Esophagectomy with lymphadenectomy is the mainstay of treatment. Prognosis is poor, and the 5-year overall survival is 35%.[345]

Gastrointestinal Stromal Tumor

GISTs are the most common mesenchymal tumor of the GI tract and are discussed in detail in Chapter 42. GISTs occur in the esophagus in only 1%–3% of cases.[346,347] Typically they arise from the muscularis propria and, more specifically, the interstitial cells of Cajal. They typically present after the age of 40, and symptoms can include dysphagia, bleeding from ulceration, dyspepsia, and weight loss. Endoscopically, they are most often encountered as submucosal solitary masses in the distal third of the esophagus. GISTs are seen on CT scan as well-circumscribed, hypoattenuating masses.[348] EUS is the most accurate imaging modality and can even help predict malignant potential.[349,350] On histology, GISTs mostly show characteristic spindle-shaped cells with elongated nuclei that express CD117 encoded by the *KIT* gene. CD117 and DOG1 positivity are important differentiating characteristics because similar lesions, such as leiomyomas or other spindle-cell tumors, are typically CD117 and DOG1 negative.

As discussed in Chapter 35, the risk of malignant transformation of GISTs depends on the size of the GIST and its mitotic rate. Characteristics of GISTs with low malignant potential lesions include those smaller than 2 cm and a mitotic rate less than 5 per 50 high-power field.[351] Treatment of GISTs depends on size of lesion and stage. Recent reports indicate that ESD could become a more frequently used technique to resect small, nonadvanced lesions.[352] Otherwise, surgical resection is the traditionally preferred method of treatment. Tyrosine kinase inhibitors such as imatinib mesylate (Gleevec) are also an option as neoadjuvant therapy or for unresectable GISTs (see Chapter 35). CT and PET scans have been shown to be useful in monitoring patients after treatment.[353]

Metastases

Metastases to the esophagus are a rare occurrence. The two most common cancers to metastasize to the esophagus are melanoma and breast cancer. Typically, metastatic lesions cause extrinsic compression, with dysphagia a common symptom. EUS with FNA cytology can be helpful for diagnosis. Treatment most often consists of palliative endoscopic stenting.

BENIGN NONEPITHELIAL TUMORS

Leiomyoma

Leiomyomas are the most common benign esophageal tumors. They affect men twice as frequently as women.[354] The lesion is

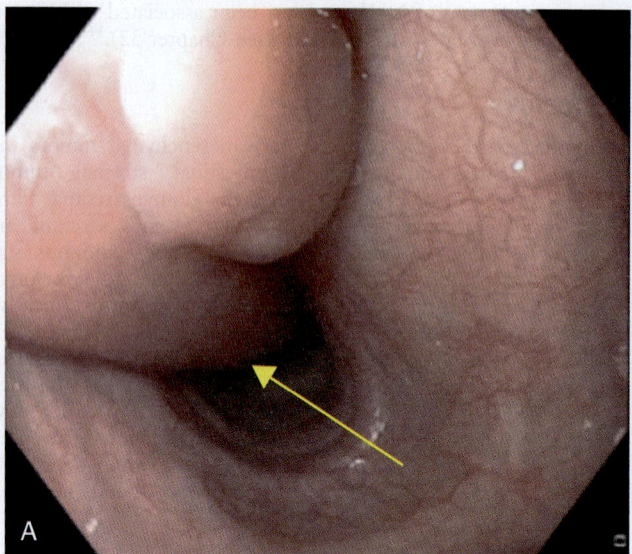

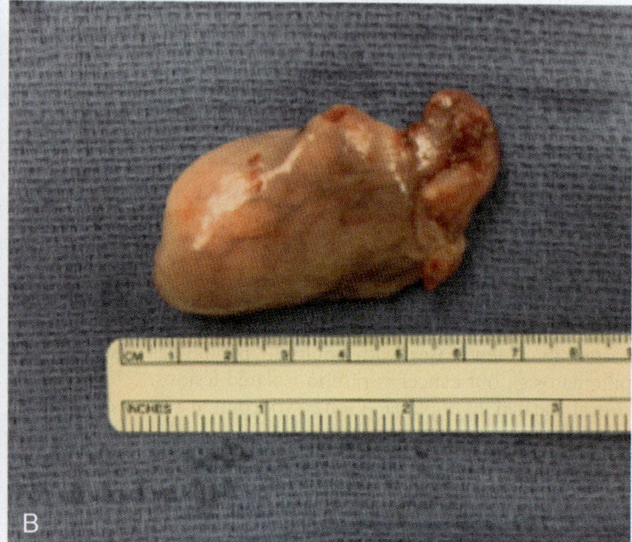

Fig. 50.19 (A) Endoscopic image of a giant fibrovascular esophageal polyp (*arrow*). (B) Polyp resected. (Courtesy Dr. Julie Goddard, Denver, CO.)

seen endoscopically as a submucosal solitary mass or masses in the middle or distal third of the esophagus. Biopsy is usually nondiagnostic because leiomyomas have normal overlying mucosa. EUS is the diagnostic test of choice; a leiomyoma is seen typically arising from the muscularis propria. Only large (>5 cm), symptomatic lesions require excision, which can be done endoscopically for smaller tumors (using ESD techniques) or surgically.[355]

Granular Cell Tumor

Granular cell tumors are most commonly located in the head and neck region (including in the oropharynx) and are less common in the GI tract. The most common site of GI involvement is the esophagus, accounting for 33% of cases. The endoscopic appearance, location within the esophagus, and number of lesions are variable.[356,357] Typically, granular cell tumors are solitary, submucosal lesions with a yellowish appearance, typically in the distal esophagus. They are mostly found incidentally on upper endoscopy, because most patients are asymptomatic. Histologically, granular cell tumors are composed of round or polygonal cells with abundant eosinophilic cytoplasm. The cells are periodic acid-Schiff positive and diastase resistant. They may have a neural crest origin, as evidenced by immunohistochemical expression of S-100 protein. Although a few cases of malignant transformation are reported, the majority of cases are benign.[358] Endoscopic resection is recommended, has been shown to be safe, and allows for a more accurate histologic diagnosis when required.[356]

Fibrovascular Polyp

Fibrovascular polyps are benign esophageal lesions (Fig. 50.19). They are almost exclusively seen in the cervical esophagus, likely because of the relatively loose submucosal tissue and redundant mucosa in this anatomic region.[359,360] They are typically pedunculated polyps consisting of blood vessels, adipose cells, and stroma covered by normal squamous epithelium. Although most cases are diagnosed incidentally, large polyps have been described to cause dysphagia and globus sensation. Peculiarly, prolapse of fibrovascular polyps out of the mouth has been described as fleshy tissue seen after vomiting or retching. Rarely, these polyps can cause fatal asphyxiation, and thus endoscopic or surgical removal is recommended. Some recommend EUS of larger polyps to determine the presence of large blood vessels prior to excision.

Hamartoma

Hamartomas are rare lesions in the esophagus. They are typically pedunculated polyps that can cause symptoms similar to fibrovascular polyps (i.e., dysphagia, globus sensation, polyp prolapse, and asphyxiation). Endoscopically, the two entities are indistinguishable. However, hamartomatous polyps are much less common and have a different histologic appearance. They often contain multiple tissue types, including cartilage, bone, adipose tissue, smooth muscle, and skeletal muscle. Endoscopic or surgical resection is recommended.[361]

Hemangioma

Hemangiomas of the esophagus are rare vascular malformations that can occasionally present with GI bleeding or dysphagia. There are two histologic types of esophageal hemangiomas: cavernous and capillary. Most lesions are of the cavernous type. Endoscopically, they are seen as blue- to red-colored submucosal nodules, which often will blanch with compression.[362] Interestingly, biopsy has not been associated with hemorrhage in reports.[363] Previously, surgical resection was the most common method of treatment, although endoscopic treatment is possible.[364]

Lipoma

Lipomas are rare benign tumors of the GI tract. Lipomas are more commonly found in the colon, small intestine, and stomach than in the esophagus. Almost all are asymptomatic and found incidentally on endoscopy as slightly yellowish, raised nodules in the proximal esophagus. Large, pedunculated esophageal lesions can cause dysphagia and asphyxiation. Often, esophageal lipomas exhibit the "pillow" sign—indentation or cushioning with "palpation." Superficial mucosal biopsies will usually be nondiagnostic. Deeper samples from the submucosa will reveal well-differentiated adipocytes. On EUS, a homogeneous, hyperechoic submucosal lesion with smooth outer margins is seen. Treatment of symptomatic lipomas is endoscopic or surgical resection.[365]

Full references for this chapter can be found at https://ebooks.health.elsevier.com.

PART VII Stomach and Duodenum

51 Anatomy, Histology, and Developmental Anomalies of the Stomach and Duodenum

Jessica B. Sarthi, Zachary M. Sellers

IN THIS CHAPTER

EMBRYOLOGY AND ANATOMY OF THE STOMACH

The stomach, as a J-shaped dilation of the alimentary canal, is continuous with the esophagus proximally and the duodenum distally. It functions as a digestive organ and as a reservoir to store large quantities of recently ingested food, allowing intermittent feedings, initiating the digestive process, and releasing its contents in a controlled fashion downstream to the smaller capacity of the duodenum. The stomach volume ranges from approximately 30 mL in a neonate to 1.5–2 L in adulthood.

The stomach is recognizable in the fourth week of gestation as a dilation of the distal foregut (Fig. 51.1).[1] As the stomach enlarges, the dorsal aspect grows more rapidly than the ventral aspect, therefore forming the greater curvature. Additionally, during the enlargement process the stomach rotates 90 degrees around its longitudinal axis, orienting the greater curvature (the dorsal aspect) to the left and the lesser curvature (ventral aspect) to the right. The combined effects of rotation and ongoing differential growth result in the stomach lying transversely in the mid- and left upper abdomen. The rotational events also explain the vagal innervation of the stomach: the right vagus nerve innervating the posterior stomach wall (the primordial right side) and the left vagus nerve innervating the anterior wall (the primordial left side).

The final location of the stomach is variable owing in part to its 2-point fixation at the esophagogastric and gastroduodenal junctions, allowing for considerable mobility. The esophagogastric junction generally lies to the left of the T10 vertebral body, 1–2 cm below the diaphragmatic hiatus. The gastroduodenal junction lies at L1 and generally to the right of the midline in the recumbent fasted individual. The gastroduodenal junction of a distended upright adult may be considerably lower. The left-

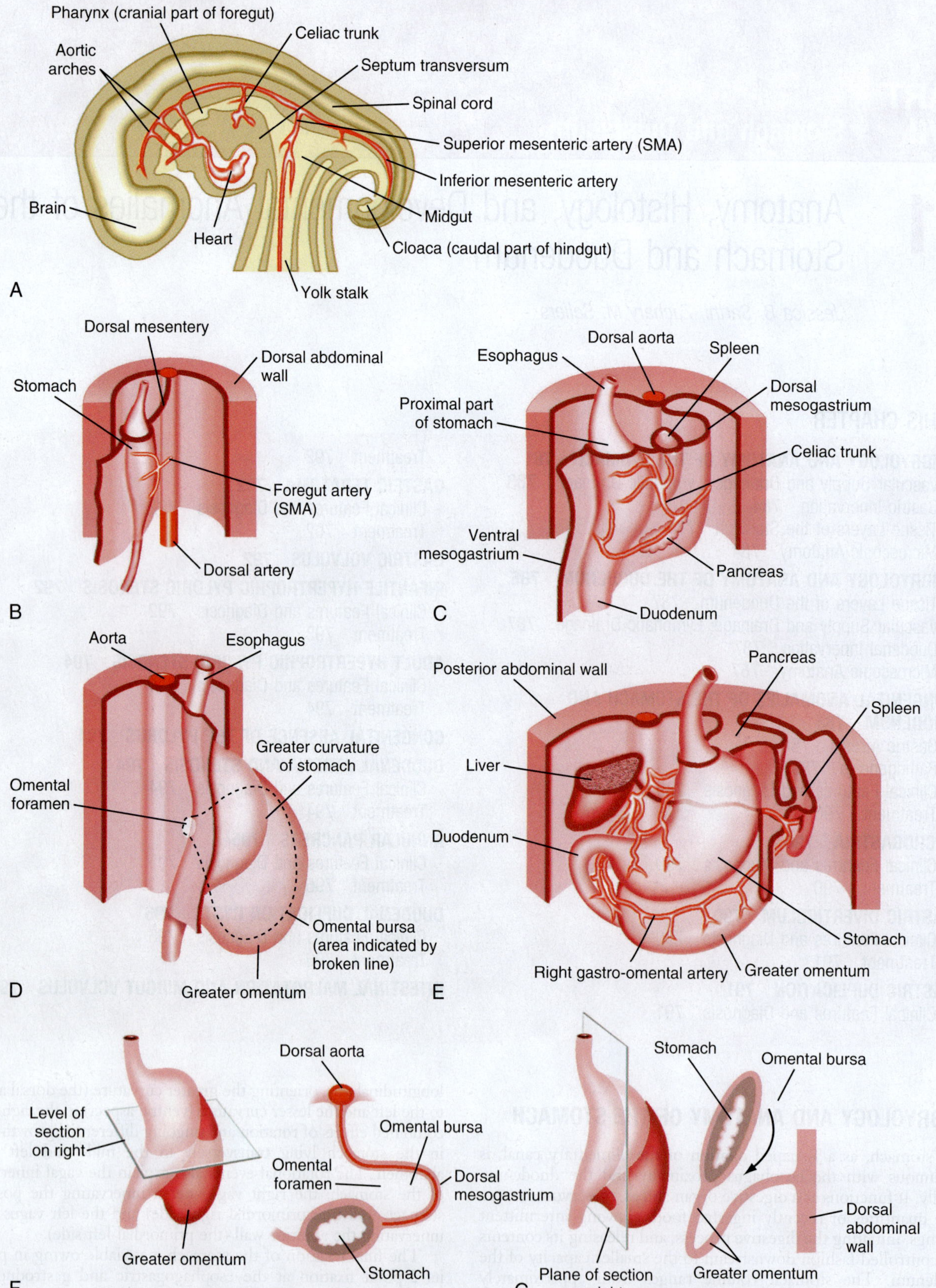

Fig. 51.1 Development of the stomach and duodenum and formation of the omental bursa (lesser sac) and greater omentum. (A) Median section of a 28-day embryo. (B) Anterolateral view of a 28-day embryo. (C) Embryo approximately 35 days old. (D) Embryo approximately 40 days old. (E) Embryo approximately 48 days old. (F) Lateral view of the stomach and greater omentum of an embryo at approximately 52 days. The transverse section shows the omental foramen and omental bursa. (G) Sagittal section showing the omental bursa and greater omentum. The embryology of the duodenum is discussed further in Chapters 57 and 98. (From Moore KL, Persaud TVN. *The Developing Human*. 7th ed. Philadelphia: WB Saunders; 2003:258.)

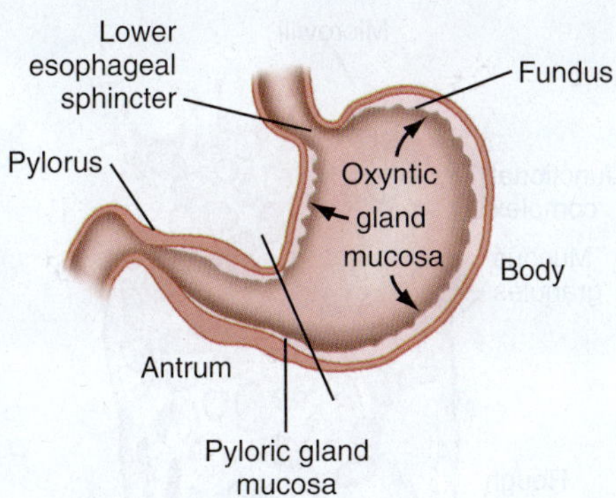

Fig. 51.2 Anatomic regions of the stomach. The line is drawn from the incisura angularis along the lesser curvature to an indistinct border between the gastric body and antrum along the greater curvature. (From Johnson LR. *Gastrointestinal Physiology*. 6th ed. St Louis: Mosby; 2001:76.)

sided and caudal greater curvature may extend below the umbilicus depending on the degree of distention, position, and gastric peristaltic phase.

The greater curvature forms the left lower stomach border, whereas the lesser curvature forms the right upper border. Posteriorly, portions of the pancreas, transverse colon, diaphragm, spleen, and apex of the left kidney and adrenal gland bound the stomach. The posterior wall of the stomach comprises the anterior wall of the omental bursa, or lesser peritoneal sac. Anteriorly, the liver bounds the stomach, whereas the inner aspect of the anterior abdominal wall bounds the anterior left lower aspect.

The stomach is completely invested by peritoneum, except for a small bare area at the esophagogastric junction. This peritoneum passes as a double layer from the lesser curvature to the liver as the gastrohepatic portion of the lesser omentum and then hangs down from the fundus and greater curvature as the greater omentum, extending to the transverse colon (as the gastrocolic ligament), spleen (as the gastrosplenic ligament), and diaphragm (as the gastrophrenic ligament).

The stomach is divided into four regions that can be defined by anatomic or histologic landmarks (Fig. 51.2).[2] Anatomically, the cardia is a small ill-defined area of the stomach immediately adjacent to its junction with the esophagus. This region of the stomach has been the focus of intense investigation. Controversy exists as to the nature, location, extent, and even existence of cardia mucosa. The fundus projects upward, above the cardia and esophagogastric junction. This dome-shaped area of the stomach is its most superior portion and is in contact above with the left hemidiaphragm and to the left with the spleen. The body, or corpus, which is the largest portion of the stomach, is located immediately below and continuous with the fundus. The incisura angularis, a fixed, sharp indentation two-thirds of the distance down the lesser curvature, marks the caudal aspect of the gastric body (Fig. 51.3). The gastric antrum extends from its indistinct border with the body to the junction of the pylorus with the duodenum. These gross anatomic landmarks correspond roughly with the mucosal histology because antral mucosa (pyloric gland mucosa) extends from an area on the lesser curvature above the incisura. The pylorus (pyloric channel) is a tubular structure joining the duodenum to the stomach and contains the palpable circular muscle, namely the pyloric sphincter. The pylorus is somewhat mobile owing to its enclosure between the peritoneum of the greater and lesser omenta but is generally located 2 cm to the right of midline at L1. Corresponding motor and secretory

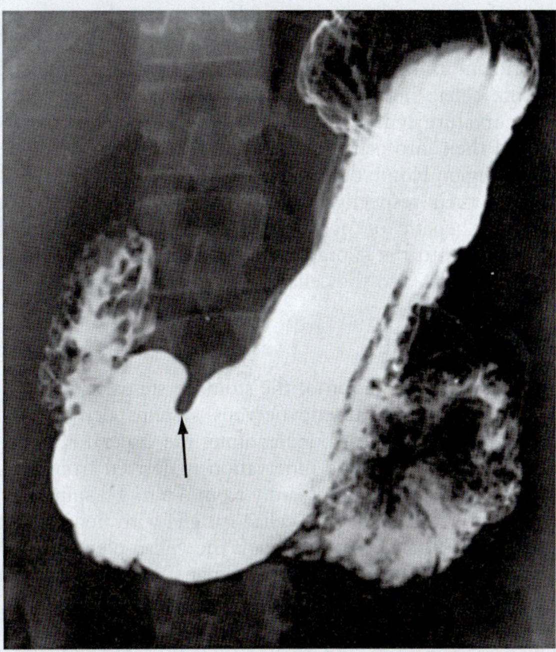

Fig. 51.3 Film from an UGIS demonstrating the incisura angularis (*arrow*) on the distal lesser curvature. (Courtesy James W. Weaver, MD.)

functions of these regions of the stomach are discussed in detail in Chapters 52 and 53.

Vascular Supply and Drainage; Lymphatic Drainage

The arterial blood supply to the stomach is derived from branches of the celiac artery—common hepatic, left gastric, and splenic arteries—that form two arterial arcades situated along the lesser curvature and the lower two-thirds of the greater curvature. The lesser curvature is supplied from above by the left gastric artery and from below by the right gastric artery, a branch of the common hepatic artery or gastroduodenal artery (which is a branch of the common hepatic artery). The greater curvature below the fundus is supplied from above by the left gastroepiploic artery (a branch of the splenic artery) and from below by the right gastroepiploic artery (a branch of the gastroduodenal artery). The right and left gastroepiploic arteries usually terminate by anastomosing, therefore completing the greater curvature arterial arcade; occasionally they end without anastomosis. The arterial supply to the gastric fundus and left upper aspect of the greater curvature is via the short gastric arteries, which arise from the splenic artery. The venous drainage of the stomach generally accompanies the arterial supply, emptying into the portal vein or one of its tributaries, the splenic or superior mesenteric veins. The left and right gastric veins drain the lesser curvature of the stomach. The left gastric vein is also known as the *coronary vein.* The right and left gastroepiploic veins drain the inferior aspect and a portion of the greater curvature of the stomach. The right gastroepiploic vein and several more distal veins become the gastrocolic veins, eventually terminating in the superior mesenteric vein. There is no gastroduodenal vein. The left gastroepiploic vein becomes the splenic vein and later receives the short gastric veins, therefore draining the fundus and upper great curvature of the stomach.

Most of the lymphatic drainage of the stomach eventually reaches the celiac nodes after passing through intermediary lymph nodes. Lymphatic channels anastomose freely in the gastric wall, with lymphatic flow directed through one-way valves into one of four groups of nodes. The inferior gastric region drains into subpyloric and omental nodes, then the hepatic nodes, terminating in the celiac nodes. The splenic or superior aspect of the greater curvature lymph initially drains into pancreaticosplenic nodes and then into celiac nodes. The superior gastric or lesser curvature region lymph drains into the left and right gastric nodes adjacent to their respective vessels and terminates in the celiac nodes. The hepatic or pyloric portion of the lesser curvature lymph drains into the suprapyloric nodes, then into the hepatic nodes, and finally into the celiac nodes.

Gastric Innervation

The autonomic innervation of the stomach stems from the sympathetic and parasympathetic nervous systems delivered via a complex tangle of nerves coursing along the visceral arteries.

The gastric sympathetic innervation is derived from preganglionic fibers arising predominantly from T6 to T8 spinal nerves, which synapse in the bilateral celiac ganglia with neurons whose postganglionic fibers course through the celiac plexus along the vascular supply of the stomach. Accompanying these sympathetic nerves are afferent pain-transmitting fibers from the stomach and motor fibers to the pyloric sphincter.

The parasympathetic innervation is via the right and left vagus nerves, which form the distal esophageal plexus, and gives rise to the posterior and anterior vagal trunks near the gastric cardia. The trunks contain preganglionic parasympathetic fibers, as well as afferent fibers from the viscera. Both trunks give rise to celiac and hepatic branches before continuing on within the lesser omentum slightly to the right of the lesser curvature as the anterior nerve of Latarjet and the posterior nerve of Latarjet. These nerves give rise to multiple gastric branches to the stomach wall, where the preganglionic fibers synapse with the ganglion cells in the submucosal (Meissner's) and myenteric (Auerbach's) plexuses. From these plexuses, postganglionic fibers are distributed to cells and glands and to smooth muscle.

Tissue Layers of the Stomach

The luminal surface of the gastric wall forms thick, longitudinally oriented folds, or rugae, that flatten with distention. Four layers make up the gastric wall: mucosa, submucosa, muscularis propria, and serosa. Mucosa lines the gastric lumen, appearing as a smooth, velvety, blood-filled lining. The mucosa of the cardia, antrum, and pylorus is somewhat paler than that of the fundus and body. It is within the fundic and body mucosa that most of the functional secretory elements of the stomach are located (see Chapter 53). The submucosa, immediately deep to the mucosa, provides the dense connective tissue skeleton of collagen and elastin fibers. Lymphocytes, plasma cells, arterioles, venules, lymphatics, and the submucosal plexus are also contained within the submucosa. The third tissue layer, the muscularis propria, is a combination of three smooth muscle layers: inner oblique, middle circular, and outer longitudinal. The inner oblique muscle fibers course over the gastric fundus, covering the anterior and posterior aspects of the stomach wall; the middle circular fibers encircle the body of the stomach, thickening distally to become the pyloric sphincter; and the outer longitudinal muscle fibers course primarily along the greater and lesser curvatures of the stomach. The final layer of the stomach is the transparent serosa, a continuation of the visceral peritoneum.

Microscopic Anatomy

The gastric mucosal surface is composed primarily of a simple layer of columnar epithelial cells 20–40 µm in height. These surface mucous cells (Fig. 51.4), which are similar throughout the stomach, contain basally located nuclei, prominent Golgi stacks, and dense cytoplasm with especially apically located, dense, mucin-containing membrane-bound granules. The cells secrete mucus in granules that are released via exocytosis, apical expulsion, and cell exfoliation. The primary role of mucus, along with bicarbonate, is luminal cytoprotection from "the elements": acid, pepsin, ingested substances, and pathogens. Cellular renewal time for a gastric surface mucous cell is approximately 3 days.

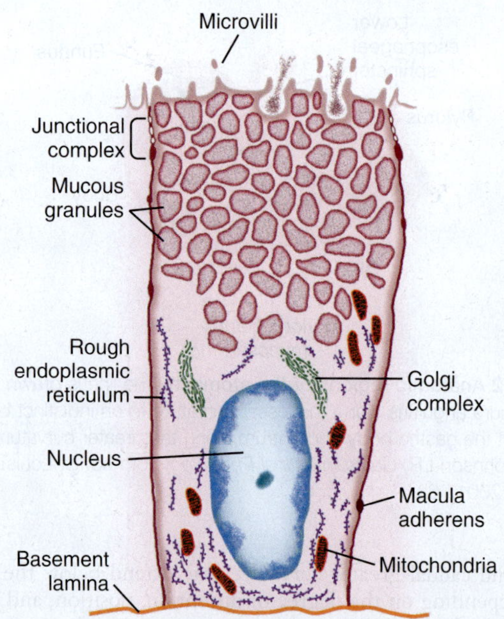

Fig. 51.4 **Schematic representation of a mucous surface cell.**

The surface epithelial lining is invaginated by gastric pits, or foveolae, that provide the gastric glands access to the gastric lumen, with a ratio of 1 pit to 4 or 5 gastric glands. The gastric glands of different anatomic regions of the stomach are lined with different types of specialized epithelial cells, allowing for differentiation of these regions by type of gastric gland (see Fig. 51.2). The first region, the cardia, is a small transition zone from esophageal squamous epithelium to gastric columnar epithelium. The cardia has been a controversial histologic area of discussion, with theories suggesting that its presence is pathologic. However, cardiac mucosa develops during gestation and is present at birth.[3] The cardiac glands have a branched and tortuous configuration and are populated by mucous, endocrine, and undifferentiated cells. There is a gradual transition from cardiac glands to the second region, the acid-secreting segment of the stomach. This region encompasses the gastric fundus and body and contains the parietal (or oxyntic or fundic) glands. Parietal, chief (also known as *peptic*), endocrine, mucous neck, and undifferentiated cells compose the oxyntic glands. The final region, corresponding to the antrum and pylorus, contains the pyloric glands, composed of endocrine cells, including gastrin-producing G cells and mucous cells.

By far the most numerous and distinctive gastric glands are the oxyntic glands (Fig. 51.5), responsible for the secretion of acid, intrinsic factor, and most gastric enzymes. These fairly straight and simple tubular glands are closely associated in the areas of gastric fundus and body. A typical gland is subdivided into three areas: the pit or foveolus (where surface mucous cells predominate), the isthmus that house the stem cells or progenitor cells, the neck (where parietal and mucous neck cells predominate), and the base (where chief cells predominate, along with some parietal and mucous neck cells). Endocrine cells, somatostatin-containing D cells, gastrin-producing G cells, and histamine-secreting enterochromaffin-like (ECL) cells (among others) are scattered throughout the oxyntic epithelium (see Chapter 53).

The principal cell type of the oxyntic gland is the parietal cell (Fig. 51.6), responsible for the oxyntic mucosal secretion of 3 × 10^4 hydrogen ions per second, at a final hydrochloric acid (HCl) concentration of approximately 150 mmol/L. Parietal cells bulge into the lumina of the oxyntic glands and, as the primary hydrogen secretors, have ultrastructural features different from other gastric cells, characterized by large mitochondria, microvilli lacking glycocalyx, and a cytoplasmic canaliculi system in contact with the lumen. In the nonsecreting parietal cell, a cytoplasmic tubulovesicular system predominates and short microvilli line the apical canaliculus. In the secreting state, the tubulovesicular system disappears, leaving an extensive system of intracellular canaliculi containing long microvilli. Mitochondria occupy approximately 30%–40% of the secreting parietal cell volume, providing energy required for acid secretion across apical microvilli (Fig. 51.6). Acid secretion, driven by the H^+, K^+-ATPase within the parietal cells, begins within 5–10 minutes of stimulation. Additionally, parietal cells are the site of intrinsic factor secretion via membrane-associated vesicle transport. Intrinsic factor is crucial for vitamin B_{12} absorption in the terminal ileum.

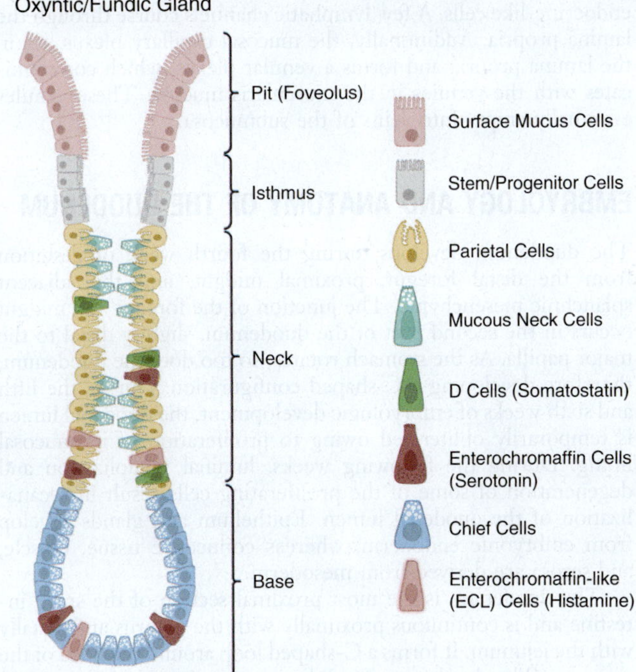

Fig. 51.5 Schematic representation of an oxyntic (gastric) gland divided into different regions—comprising of surface mucus cells (MSC) in the pit or foveolus, stem/progenitor cells in the isthmus, parietal and mucous neck cells (MNC) in the neck, chief cells at the base with enterochromaffin (EC) cells, somatostatin-containing D cells, and enterochromaffin-like (ECL) cells interspersed in the neck and base regions. (Created with BioRender.)

Closely associated with parietal cells are mucous neck cells, which appear singly close to parietal cells or in groups of 2 or 3 in the oxyntic gland neck or isthmus. Mucous neck cells differ from surface mucous cells in that the former are smaller and secrete acidic, sulfated mucus whereas the latter produce a more viscous neutral mucus. Additionally, mucous neck cells have basal nuclei and larger mucous granules around the nucleus, rather than apically located granules. Function of the two cell types appears different; the surface mucous cells are cytoprotective, whereas the mucous neck cells function as stem cell precursors for surface mucous, parietal, chief, and endocrine cells.

Chief cells, also known as *zymogen cells*, predominate in deeper layers of the oxyntic glands. These pyramid-shaped cells play a role in synthesis and secretion of pepsinogens I and II. The cytoplasm of chief cells has prominent basophilic staining owing to abundant ribosomes; these ribosomes are either free in the cytoplasm or in association with an extensive endoplasmic reticulum system. Zymogen granules lie in the apical cytoplasm; their contents are released into the gastric lumen following fusion of the granule membrane with the apical membrane. Once in the lumen, pepsinogens are converted to pepsin.

A variety of endocrine, or enteroendocrine, cells are scattered among the cells of the oxyntic glands (see Chapter 4). These cells vary in location, being either open or closed relative to the gastric

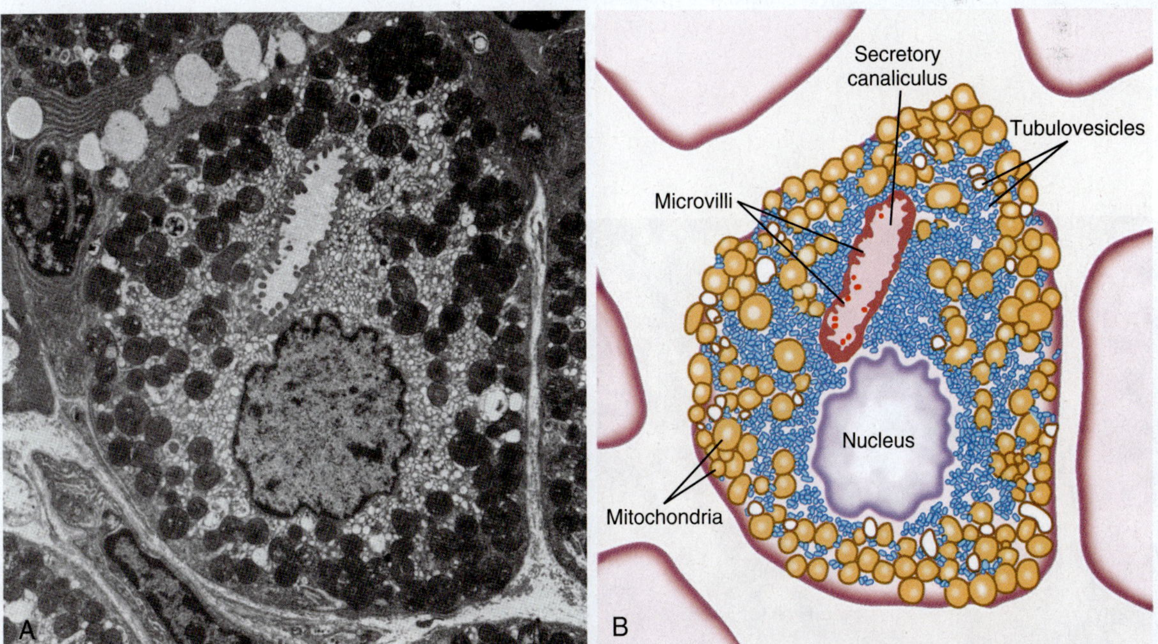

Fig. 51.6 Parietal cell. (A) Electron photomicrograph. (B) Schematic representation. (From Johnson LR. *Gastrointestinal Physiology*. 6th ed. St Louis: Mosby; 2001:78–79.)

lumen. Open endocrine cells have apical membranes containing receptors; these open cells discharge their contents by basilar exocytosis into the bloodstream, therefore exerting an endocrine effect. The closed endocrine cells contain several processes that terminate near its target cells, constituting a paracrine effect. The oxyntic gland model of the closed cell is the D cell, which secretes somatostatin via long processes reaching ECL, parietal, and chief cells.

Enteroendocrine cell (EEC) types have also been classified by their granular staining with silver or chromium. Those cells containing granules that reduce silver without pretreatment are called *argentaffin cells*. Argentaffin cells that stain with potassium dichromate are enterochromaffin (EC) cells; most ECs contain serotonin. Cells with granules staining with silver only in the presence of a reducing agent are called *argyrophilic*, or *ECL*, cells. Located primarily in the oxyntic glands, ECL cells are the only EECs containing histamine.

The final region of the stomach encompasses the antrum and pylorus and contains extensively coiled antral glands composed of endocrine and epithelial cells. The epithelial cells are predominantly mucous cells, as well as pepsinogen II—secreting mucous neck cells. Although small in number, gastrin-secreting (G) cells play a vital physiologic role and are the prototype of the open EEC. These cells, which occur either singly or in small clusters in the mid- to deep sections of antral glands (Fig. 51.7A), contain a basilar cytoplasm densely packed with gastrin-containing secretory granules (Fig. 51.7B). Gastrin release is stimulated by gastric distention, vagal stimulation, dietary amino acids, and peptides, with rapid appearance of the hormone into the bloodstream in the postprandial period (see Chapter 53). The apical or luminal surface of the G cell is narrowed into small microvilli thought to contain receptors responsible for amino acid and peptide stimulation of gastrin release. Significant quantities of gastrin are also secreted into the gastric lumen; gastrin is a known gastric growth and differentiation factor, mediated through upregulation of heparin-binding epidermal-like growth factor (HB-EGF) in gastric parietal cells.[4,5]

Antral enteroendocrine D cells, found in close association with G cells, manufacture somatostatin, a potent inhibitor of gastrin secretion. The D cells are present in small numbers in oxyntic glands. Somatostatin is thought to inhibit acid secretion through paracrine (direct action on ECL and perhaps parietal cells or indirect action on G cells) or endocrine effects (direct action on parietal cells) (see Chapter 53 for more details).

Immediately deep to the basement membrane of the gastric mucosa epithelial layer lies the lamina propria, which contains a variety of leukocytes (polymorphonuclear leukocytes, plasma cells, lymphocytes, and eosinophils), mast cells, fibroblasts, and endocrine-like cells. A few lymphatic channels course through the lamina propria. Additionally, the mucosal capillary plexus lies in the lamina propria and forms a venular plexus, which communicates with the venules in the muscularis mucosa. These venules eventually empty into veins of the submucosa.

EMBRYOLOGY AND ANATOMY OF THE DUODENUM

The duodenum develops during the fourth week of gestation from the distal foregut, proximal midgut, and the adjacent splanchnic mesenchyme. The junction of the foregut and midgut occurs in the second part of the duodenum, slightly distal to the major papilla. As the stomach rotates, so too does the duodenum, therefore developing a C-shaped configuration. During the fifth and sixth weeks of embryologic development, the duodenal lumen is temporarily obliterated owing to proliferation of its mucosal lining. During the following weeks, luminal vacuolization and degeneration of some of the proliferating cells result in recanalization of the duodenal lumen. Epithelium and glands develop from embryonic endoderm, whereas connective tissue, muscle, and serosa are derived from mesoderm.

The duodenum is the most proximal section of the small intestine and is continuous proximally with the pylorus and distally with the jejunum. It forms a C-shaped loop around the head of the pancreas. The duodenum in adults is approximately 30 cm or 12 inches in length, hence its name duodenum, Latin for "12 fingers." The duodenum is subdivided into four sections (commonly termed the *first*, *second*, *third*, and *fourth* parts), whose borders are delineated by angular course changes.

The first part of the duodenum is approximately 5 cm in length and courses rightward, upward, and backward from the pylorus. The proximal portion of the first part of the duodenum is also referred to as the *duodenal bulb* or *cap*. It is loosely attached to the

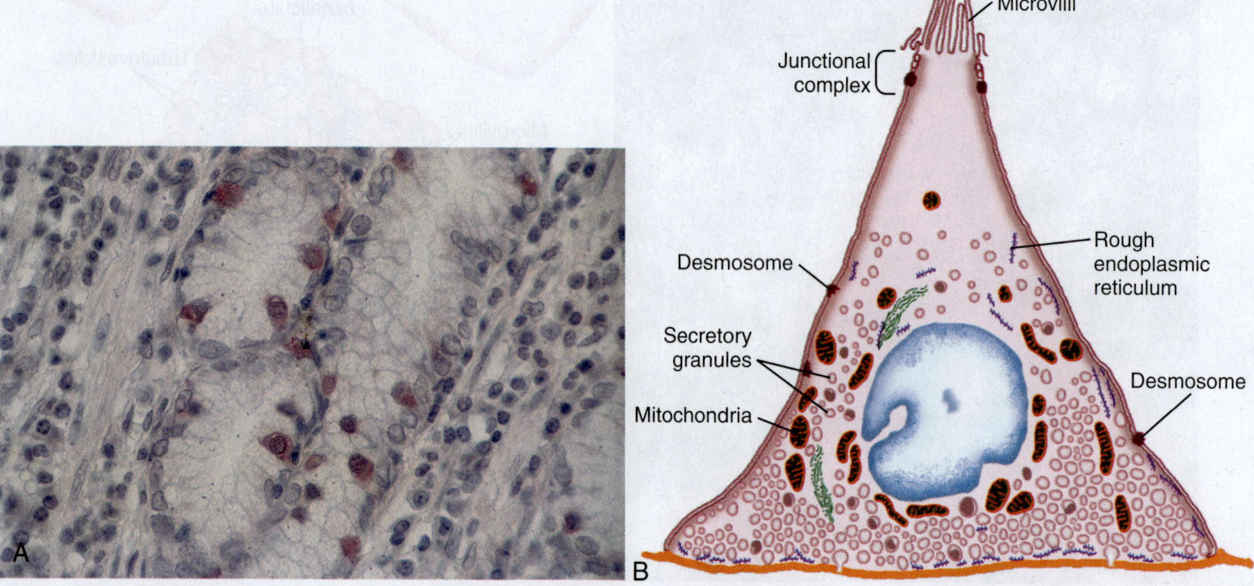

Fig. 51.7 Gastrin (G) cell. (A) Scattered G cells (*pink*) are evident in pyloric glands on this photomicrograph. (Immunoperoxidase stain). (B) Schematic.

liver by the hepatoduodenal portion of the lesser omentum and moves in response to the movement by the pylorus. The gastroduodenal artery, bile duct, and the portal vein lie posterior, whereas the gallbladder lies anterior to the first part of the duodenum. The second part of the duodenum, or the descending segment, is 7–10 cm in length, coursing downward, parallel, and in front of the hilum of the right kidney and to the right in contact with the pancreatic head. Slightly inferior to the midpoint of the second part of the duodenum on the posteromedial wall, the major duodenal papilla marks the location of the ampulla of Vater, through which the pancreaticobiliary ducts empty into the duodenum. On the same wall, approximately 2 cm proximal to the major papilla, there may be a minor duodenal papilla that forms the opening for the accessory pancreatic duct. The third part of the duodenum is approximately 10 cm in length and courses transversely from right to left, crossing the midline anterior to the inferior vena cava, spine, and aorta. The superior mesenteric artery and vein course anterior to the third part of the duodenum, generally to the right of midline. The fourth and final section of the duodenum, the ascending part, is 5 cm long and courses upward to the left of the aorta to reach the inferior border of the pancreas. The junction between the duodenum and the jejunum (duodenojejunal flexure) is fixed posteriorly by the ligament of Treitz.

Tissue Layers of the Duodenum

Similar to the stomach and rest of the gastrointestinal tract, the four layers of the duodenum from the luminal side are mucosa, submucosa, muscularis, and serosa. The duodenal wall is composed of outer longitudinal and inner circular smooth muscle layers. As is the case with the remainder of the small intestine, the luminal surface is lined with mucosa, forming circular folds known as the *plicae circulares* or *valvulae conniventes*. An exception to this is the duodenal bulb, distinguished radiographically and endoscopically by its smooth, featureless mucosa. The first few centimeters of the duodenum are shrouded by anterior and posterior elements of the peritoneum. The remainder of the duodenum lies posterior to the peritoneum and thus is retroperitoneal.

Vascular Supply and Drainage; Lymphatic Drainage

The arterial supply to the duodenum is rich and based on its embryonic origin, branches of the celiac trunk (as derived from foregut) supply the proximal duodenum, whereas the distal duodenum (as derived from midgut) is supplied by branches of the superior mesenteric artery. From the celiac trunk arises the common hepatic artery, from which arises the gastroduodenal artery. The gastroduodenal artery, in turn, branches into the superior pancreaticoduodenal artery, which gives off anterior and posterior branches to the duodenum. These branches anastomose with analogous anterior and posterior branches of the inferior pancreaticoduodenal artery, a branch of the superior mesenteric artery.

The venous drainage corresponds to the arterial supply, with the superior pancreaticoduodenal veins coursing between the duodenum and pancreatic head to enter the portal vein. Likewise, the inferior pancreaticoduodenal veins empty into either a jejunal vein or directly into the superior mesenteric vein.

The duodenal lymphatic drainage also corresponds to the vascular supply. Small anterior and posterior duodenal lymph channels drain into the pancreaticoduodenal nodes. From these nodes, lymph drains superiorly into the hepatic nodes or inferiorly into superior mesenteric nodes located at the origin of the superior mesenteric artery.

Duodenal Innervation

As in the case in the stomach, duodenal innervation is provided by the sympathetic and parasympathetic nervous systems. The preganglionic sympathetic nerves course through the celiac and superior mesenteric ganglia, with postganglionic neurons entering the duodenal intramural plexuses. Afferent fibers accompany the sympathetic neurons, primarily carrying fibers for visceral pain sensation. Parasympathetic fibers, supplied by the hepatic branch of the anterior vagus nerve and the mesenteric nerves, form a synapse with Meissner's and Auerbach's plexuses in the duodenal wall.

Microscopic Anatomy

The microscopic anatomy of the duodenum differs dramatically from the gastric mucosa, with the change from gastric glands and pits to a mucosa lined by columnar epithelial cells forming finger-like projections called villi that extend into the duodenal lumen surrounded by short intestinal glands called crypts of Lieberkühn that extend down towards the muscularis mucosae creating grooves between the villi (Fig. 51.8).[6] Thus the mucosa is extensively folded to maximize surface area for absorption. The villi and crypts are continuous however, distinct in cell types and function. The lamina propria portion of the mucosa lies underneath the mucosal epithelium and is rich in blood supply and lymphatic drainage. The submucosa underneath the mucosa muscularis contains characteristic Brunner's glands that secrete bicarbonate, which together with duodenal mucosal bicarbonate secretion and pancreatic bicarbonate secretion neutralize the acidic gastric contents. The villi in the proximal duodenum have a distorted appearance, thought to be related to its exposure to gastric acid. In contrast, the villi of the distal duodenum are tall, slender, and very regular, similar to those in the jejunum. The ratio of the length of villi to crypts in the distal duodenum is 4:1 or 5:1, like that of the jejunum.

A single layer of epithelial cells provides the interface between the duodenal lumen and mucosa in the areas of both villi and crypts. The duodenal epithelium consists of six different cell types, including, enterocytes, goblet cells, tuft cells, enteroendocrine, and microfold or M cells that arise due to differentiation of progenitors from intestinal stem cells (ISCs) residing in the base of the crypts.[7] Generally, proliferative (and relatively undifferentiated) cell types are located in the crypts and differentiated cell types are located in the villi, the exception being Paneth cells, which are terminally differentiated, but interspersed within the stem cells in the crypt base. The stem cell zone of the crypts consists of leucine-rich repeat containing G protein-coupled receptor 5 or *Lgr5*$^+$ cells that can self-renew and generate all the differentiated cell types of the epithelium. Above the stem cell zone is the highly proliferative transit amplifying zone that serves as a source of rapidly proliferating epithelial cells that aid in self-renewal of the intestinal epithelium. The absorptive enterocytes are the most abundant epithelial cell type, characterized by the presence of a brush border (microvilli) on the luminal surface of polarized columnar cells. Enterocytes are primarily involved in nutrient absorption, for example, ions, lipids, peptides, and water, as well as secretion of immunoglobulins. Contrary to earlier hypotheses that crypts are more secretory and villi are more absorptive in function, recent advances in intestinal physiology have led to reevaluation of this theory suggesting that villus enterocytes also have secretory functions.

Goblet cells are mucus secreting cells spread across the crypt-villus axis. Mucins present in the mucous play a role in neutralizing acids from the stomach, protecting the intestinal wall from damage as well as lubricating the luminal surface of the epithelium for easier passage of digested food.[8]

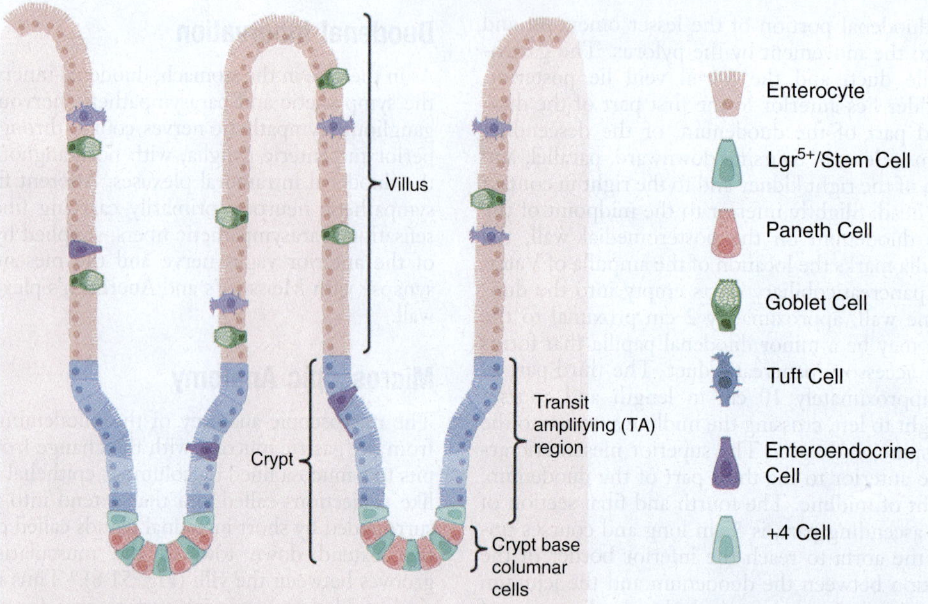

Fig. 51.8 Schematic representation of a duodenal crypt-villus cross-section. The crypts consist of crypt base columnar cells containing Lgr^{5+}/stem cells, arranged alternatively with Paneth cells followed by the +4 cells leading into the transit amplifying (TA) region of the crypt. The villus region follows the TA region and consists of secretory and absorptive enterocytes along with goblet cells, tuft cells and enteroendocrine cells. (Created with BioRender.)

EECs secrete various peptides and hormones such as somatostatin, and serotonin upon stimuli. EECs were originally termed *neuroendocrine* or *APUD* cells since they were thought to originate from neural crest cells; however, later studies showed that EECs in the gut arise from the same crypt stem cells that give rise to other duodenal epithelial cell types.[9] EECs are further subdivided into EC cells (secrete 95% of total serotonin), D cells (secrete somatostatin), and L cells (secrete peptides) based on their ultrastructural features as well as the peptide/amines present in their secretory vesicles.

Tuft cells are the more newly discovered cell types and get their name from the characteristic brush-border morphology on the neck of these flask-shaped cells that extend into the gut lumen. The microvilli on tuft cells are longer than neighboring cells.[10] Tuft cells are sentinels of the gastrointestinal tract and are involved in sensing luminal pathogenic metabolite via succinate as well as type-1 or *sweet taste receptors* and type-2 or *bitter taste receptors*.[11] In line with this, taste signal transduction genes such as *GNB1*, *GNG13*, *ITPR2*, and *TRPM5* are enriched in Tuft cells.[12] Tuft cells are primary responders to a host of luminal stimuli and communicate with the mucosal immune system as well as the nervous system and the neighboring EECs. Tuft cells synthesize a wide variety of paracrine and endocrine effector molecules, including IL-25, acetylcholine, eicosanoids, β-endorphins, and TSLP6.

Microfold or *M-cells* are found in the gut associated lymphoid tissue or Peyer's patches in the intestinal epithelium. M cells are mucosal immune surveillance cells that are involved in uptake and transport of luminal antigens to the underlying lymphoid cells to elicit a mucosal as well as a systemic immune response. M cells are closely associated with dendritic cells in the Peyer's patches and "hand-off" the luminal antigens to them for appropriate immune response, thus acting as antigen delivering cells.[13]

Finally, Paneth cells are the only long-lived differentiated cells with a lifespan of 3–6 weeks, in contrast to around 5 days for other differentiated epithelial cell types along the crypt-villus axis.[14] Paneth cells are interspersed within the crypt base columnar (CBC) stem cells forming a mosaic pattern and this close association is crucial to maintaining the stem cell niche. Mature Paneth cells secrete enzymes, antimicrobial peptides and growth factors. The antimicrobial peptides that Paneth cells secrete include α-defensins, C-type lectins, lysozyme, and phospholipase A_2 and thus serve as an additional line of defense against the luminal microbial antigens to protect the ISC-niche from bacterial invasion and regulate mucosal microbiota composition. Paneth cells also play an important role in epithelial cell self-renewal due to their strategic location in the stem cell niche and have been predicted to secrete Wnt, EGF, and Dll4, a Notch ligand, based on studies in mice. However, more detailed single-cell RNA sequencing analysis across the human intestine showed that Wnt3/11, EGF, and R-spondin (RSPO1) are not present in Paneth cells.[15]

Within the submucosa of the duodenum are the branched Brunner's glands, which secrete an alkaline and clear mucus containing bicarbonate, EGF, and pepsinogen II. Brunner's glands are most numerous in the proximal duodenum and decrease in number distally. Rather than emptying into the duodenum through their own duct system, they empty into the duodenum through adjacent intestinal glands.

CONGENITAL ANOMALIES OF THE STOMACH AND DUODENUM

The congenital anomalies of the stomach and duodenum are summarized in Table 51.1. Congenital anomalies of the stomach are among the least frequently encountered malformations of the GI tract. These lesions may present during the neonatal period or later in life, depending on the degree of gastric outlet obstruction.

Gastric Atresia

Gastric atresias generally occur in the antrum or pylorus in one of three forms: complete segmental defect, segmental defect bridged

TABLE 51.1 Anomalies of the Stomach and Duodenum

Anomaly	Incidence	Age at Presentation	Symptoms and Signs	Treatment
STOMACH				
Gastric, antral, or pyloric atresia	3/100,000, when combined with webs	Infancy	Nonbilious emesis	Gastroduodenostomy, gastrojejunostomy
Pyloric or antral membrane (web)	As above	Any age	Failure to thrive, emesis	Incision or excision, pyloroplasty
Microgastria	Rare	Infancy	Emesis, malnutrition	Continuous-drip feedings or jejunal reservoir pouch
Gastric diverticulum	Rare	Any age	Usually asymptomatic	Usually unnecessary
Gastric duplication	Rare; male:female, 1:2	Any age	Abdominal mass, emesis, hematemesis; peritonitis if ruptured	Excision or partial gastrectomy
Gastric teratoma	Rare	Any age	Upper abdominal mass	Resection
Gastric volvulus	Rare	Any age	Emesis, refusal to feed	Reduction of volvulus, anterior gastropexy
Pyloric stenosis (infantile hypertrophic and adult forms)	USA, 3/1000 (range, 1-8/1000 in various regions); male:female, 4:1	Infancy	Nonbilious emesis	Pyloromyotomy
Congenital absence of the pylorus	Rare	Childhood, adulthood	Dyspepsia, if symptomatic	Usually unnecessary
DUODENUM				
Duodenal atresia or stenosis	1/20,000	Newborn	Bilious emesis, upper abdominal distention	Duodenojejunostomy or gastrojejunostomy
Annular pancreas (see also Chapter 57)	1/10,000	Any age	Bilious emesis, failure to thrive	Duodenojejunostomy
Duodenal duplication cyst	Rare	Any age	GI bleeding, pain	Excision
Malrotation and midgut volvulus (also see Chapters 26, 27, and 100)	Rare	Any age	Bilious emesis, upper abdominal distention	Reduction, division of bands, possibly resection

by a remnant of a fibrous cord, or a membrane (also called a web, diaphragm, or septum). These lesions are uncommon, with a reported incidence of 1–3 per 100,000; membranes comprise the majority. Membranes consist of gastric mucosa, muscularis mucosa, and submucosa. In contrast, the fibrous cord generally lacks mucosal elements but contains normal serosal and muscular layers. Membranes may be complete (totally obstructive) or incomplete (perforate). For the sake of clarity, incomplete gastric membranes, which are by definition not atresias, are also considered here.

Pathogenesis

The cause of these lesions remains unknown, but the timing of a contrary developmental event may determine the type of atresia. For example, if there is fusion of redundant endoderm before 8 weeks' gestation (before muscle layer development), then discontinuity of gastric wall musculature would result in a segmental defect with or without a fibrous cord. On the other hand, if redundancy occurs after 8 weeks' gestation, when muscle layers are complete, a simple membrane develops. An alternative mechanism—focal ischemia at a critical time in development—has been proposed. Finally, failure of recanalization of the gastric lumen following temporary obstruction from mucosal proliferation has been suggested as a cause, but this is not a viable explanation because obstruction or recanalization does not occur in the stomach (unlike the esophagus and duodenum).[16] Total epithelial detachment of gastric mucosa, associated with $\alpha6\beta4$ integrin expression deficiency at the junction of epithelial cells and lamina propria, has been noted in a child with pyloric atresia.[17]

Genetic factors are also important. In addition to a familial form (autosomal recessive), gastric atresia is also associated with Down syndrome and junctional epidermolysis bullosa (JEB). In the case of epidermolysis bullosa—pyloric atresia—obstructive uropathy association, mutations in the $\alpha6$ and $\beta4$ integrin subunits of the hemidesmosome have been noted.[18,19] JEB (discussed in Chapter 25) is also known as the *JEB pyloric atresia syndrome*.[20] Other associated anomalies are intestinal malrotation, atrial septal defect, absent gallbladder, tracheoesophageal fistula, vaginal atresia, and absent extrahepatic portal vein.[21] In addition, gastric atresia may be associated with multiple intestinal atresias and immunodeficiency.[22]

Clinical Features and Diagnosis

In proximal GI obstruction, polyhydramnios is commonly noted during pregnancy. Newborn infants with any variant of gastric atresia have signs of gastric outlet obstruction including onset of forceful, nonbilious emesis following the first feeding. There may be drooling and respiratory distress. The abdomen is generally scaphoid unless gastric distention is present. When diagnosis is delayed, severe metabolic alkalosis, volume depletion, and shock occur; prolonged gastric distention may result in gastric perforation. Abdominal radiographs demonstrate gaseous distention of the stomach and a gasless intestine. Upper GI contrast study shows a complete obstruction of the stomach, generally at the level of the antrum or pylorus. The type of lesion (e.g., a membrane) can be determined only via surgical exploration. In the usual case of incomplete antral and pyloric membranes, the age of presentation depends on the degree of obstruction; symptoms may therefore develop at any age from infancy to adulthood.

These lesions, except for the presence of membrane perforations, are identical to the membranes of gastric atresia. Luminal narrowing is from the malformation itself as well as from local inflammation and edema. The primary symptom is vomiting, which in infants or children may result in failure to establish normal weight gain. In older children and adults, the symptoms may mimic those of peptic ulcer disease, with nausea, epigastric pain, and weight loss. Diarrhea has been observed, but its physiologic basis is unknown. The abdominal radiograph is typically normal, although gastric distention may be noted. Occasionally, prenatal diagnosis may be suggested by US findings of dilated stomach without polyhydramnios. Definitive diagnosis is established by contrast radiography, US, or EGD. Contrast radiography demonstrates the membrane as a thin, circumferential filling defect in the antrum or pylorus. Careful observation shows contrast material with delayed passage through a central defect in the membrane; overall gastric emptying is delayed. US may demonstrate the segmentation of the antrum, whereas on EGD a small, fixed opening in the antrum or pylorus may be evident, surrounded by a mucosa free of folds.

Treatment

Following patient stabilization with fluids, electrolytes, and gastric decompression, definitive treatment is surgical. Complete or incomplete antral membranes are treated by simple excision. Pyloric membranes require pyloroplasty. The presence of a concomitant duodenal atresia has been described [also known as *wind-sock diaphragm* (see Chapter 26)], and its presence or absence is verified by passage of a catheter distally into the duodenum intraoperatively. Endoscopic therapy using a snare, papillotome, laser, or dilation via balloon has also been described. In cases involving atretic gap, gastroduodenostomy is considered curative. An alternative approach is pyloric sphincter reconstruction via longitudinal pyloromyotomy, followed by end-to-end anastomosis of cul-de-sacs of gastric and duodenal mucosa.[23] Gastrojejunostomy is not recommended in children because of the risk of marginal ulcer. In a retrospective study, a mortality rate exceeding 50% was seen and attributed to the associated fetal anomalies and sepsis due to variety organisms (*Klebsiella*, *Pseudomonas*, and *Candida* species and methicillin-resistant *Staphylococcus aureus*). As previously mentioned, some of the patients had immune deficiency disorders.[24]

MICROGASTRIA

Microgastria is an extremely rare congenital anomaly of the caudal part of the foregut. A small, tubular or saccular, incompletely rotated stomach is associated with a megaesophagus. Varying degrees of the anomaly occur owing to arrested development during the fifth week of gestation in the differentiation of the greater curvature of the stomach such that neither rotation nor fusiform dilation of the stomach occurs.[25] A localized vascular insufficiency has been postulated to lead to the development of microgastria after the eighth week of gestation.[26] The etiology is unknown.

Fortunately, normal gastric histology is preserved. Microgastria may occur as an isolated anomaly but more commonly in association with other anomalies: duodenal atresia; nonrotation of the midgut; ileal duplication; hiatal hernia; asplenia; partial situs inversus; or renal, upper limb (microgastria—limb reduction anomaly), cardiac, pulmonary, skeletal, or spinal. In isolation, microgastria is not lethal, but other associated anomalies may be. It has been suggested that microgastria in association with limb reduction defects and central nervous system anomalies has a genetic basis, with an autosomal recessive pattern of inheritance.[27] Chromosome analysis is normal.

Clinical Features and Diagnosis

The infant typically presents with postprandial vomiting and malnutrition. There may also be diarrhea (a result of rapid gastric emptying) and dumping syndrome. Respiratory symptoms, including respiratory distress at birth and stridor, as well as recurrent pulmonary infections, have been reported. Anemia due to iron deficiency may occur because decreased gastric acid secretion may preclude adequate iron absorption; cobalamin (vitamin B_{12}) deficiency may follow hyposecretion of intrinsic factor. Prenatal US may detect a small stomach and polyhydramnios. Contrast radiography shows the megaesophagus and tubular or small stomach. The lower esophageal sphincter is poorly defined, and esophagogastric reflux is usually severe.

Treatment

The medical management of microgastria includes frequent small-volume feedings or continuous-drip feedings into the stomach. An alternative is nocturnal drip feedings via jejunostomy to supplement oral intake. Surgical creation of a double-lumen Roux-en-Y pouch anastomosed to the greater curvature of the stomach has been described. This Hunt-Lawrence jejunal pouch has allowed normal growth and development and prevented reflux and dumping syndrome.[28] One case report described gastric dissociation for the treatment of congenital microgastria with paraesophageal hiatal hernia.[29]

GASTRIC DIVERTICULUM

A gastric diverticulum is the rarest type of GI diverticulum. The true congenital diverticulum contains all gastric tissue layers and is located on the posterior wall of the cardia. The intramural (or partial) diverticulum projects into but not through the muscular layer, most commonly located along the greater curvature of the antrum. The false (or pseudo-) diverticulum is formed by mucosal and submucosal herniation through a defect in the muscular wall and lacks muscularis propria. Familial occurrence has not been described for any of these lesions.

Clinical Features and Diagnosis

Most congenital gastric diverticula are asymptomatic and are incidental findings on radiography or endoscopy, or at autopsy (see Chapter 26). Size varies from 1 to 11 cm. Contrast radiography shows a rounded, well-delineated mobile pouch, often with an air-fluid level. Emptying of the diverticulum may be delayed. On endoscopy, the diverticulum is seen as a well-delineated opening; distention by the scope may reproduce symptoms. Unfortunately, both upper GI radiologic studies and endoscopy may miss the diagnosis due to the typical location at the esophagogastric junction. Symptoms may be epigastric or lower chest pain, indigestion, bleeding, or nonbilious emesis. The differential diagnosis includes an acquired gastric diverticulum found in association with pancreatitis, gastric outlet obstruction, trauma, ulcer disease, or malignancy. Hiatal hernia and hypertrophic gastric folds may mimic a diverticulum on contrast studies. Radiology cannot distinguish between congenital and acquired diverticula.

Treatment

In the case of an incidentally discovered proximal gastric diverticulum, treatment is unnecessary. If symptoms are thought to be consistent with the diagnosis, the diverticulum may be amputated or invaginated. Because of the risk of malignancy associated with distal gastric diverticula, surgical treatment by amputation, invagination, or segmental resection has been recommended. Laparoscopic resection following gastroscopic localization has been described.

GASTRIC DUPLICATION

Approximately 20% of all GI duplications are gastric. Duplication of the stomach can occur in isolation, as a triplication (two gastric duplications in one individual), or combined with duplications of other structures in the GI tract such as the esophagus or duodenum. Location is contiguous with the stomach, generally along the greater curvature or posterior wall, and contains all layers of the gastric wall. Gastric and pancreatic mucosa lining the duplication are most clinically significant secondary to potential complications such as PUD and pancreatitis. The duplication rarely communicates with the stomach so for this reason, a tubular, fusiform, or spherical cystic mass develops. Infrequently, there may be a connection to the colon, pancreas, or pancreatic duplication; the connection may be the result of an acquired fistula from a penetrating peptic ulcer within the gastric duplication. Several embryologic defects have been proposed as etiologies for duplications, including errors in separation of notochord and endoderm, persistence of embryonic diverticula, and persistence of vacuoles within the epithelium of the primitive foregut.[30] Most duplications occur in women (65%) and are detected during infancy or childhood (80%), with no familial tendency. Aside from concurrent duplications, vertebral anomalies are the second most commonly linked abnormality.[31] Carcinomas arising in congenital duplications have been described in adults.

Clinical Features and Diagnosis

The clinical presentation of gastric duplication depends on factors such as size, location, and communicating structure (if any). Symptoms and signs vary and may include the following: colic, abdominal mass, epigastric pain, failure to gain appropriate weight, vomiting, occult or frank upper or lower GI bleeding secondary to peptic ulceration (the latter occurring via erosion into the colon), hematobilia via a communication with the intrahepatic bile duct, respiratory distress or hemoptysis (perforated cyst fistulized to lung),[32] pyloric obstruction, peritonitis secondary to rupture, pancreatitis, pancreatic pseudocyst, and acute abdomen. In early infancy, symptoms may mimic those of hypertrophic pyloric stenosis (HPS). Diagnosis is suggested by an abdominal radiograph showing displacement and extrinsic compression of gastric lumen. Contrast radiography may demonstrate the duplication via a mass effect on the stomach (Fig. 51.9A), or the cyst may be imaged directly when there is communication with the GI tract. US (see Fig. 51.8B) including prenatal US,[32] CT (Fig. 51.9C), MRCP, ^{99m}Tc-pertechnetate scanning, and EUS may also demonstrate the lesion. Peristalsis identified by EUS in a juxtaenteric cyst is

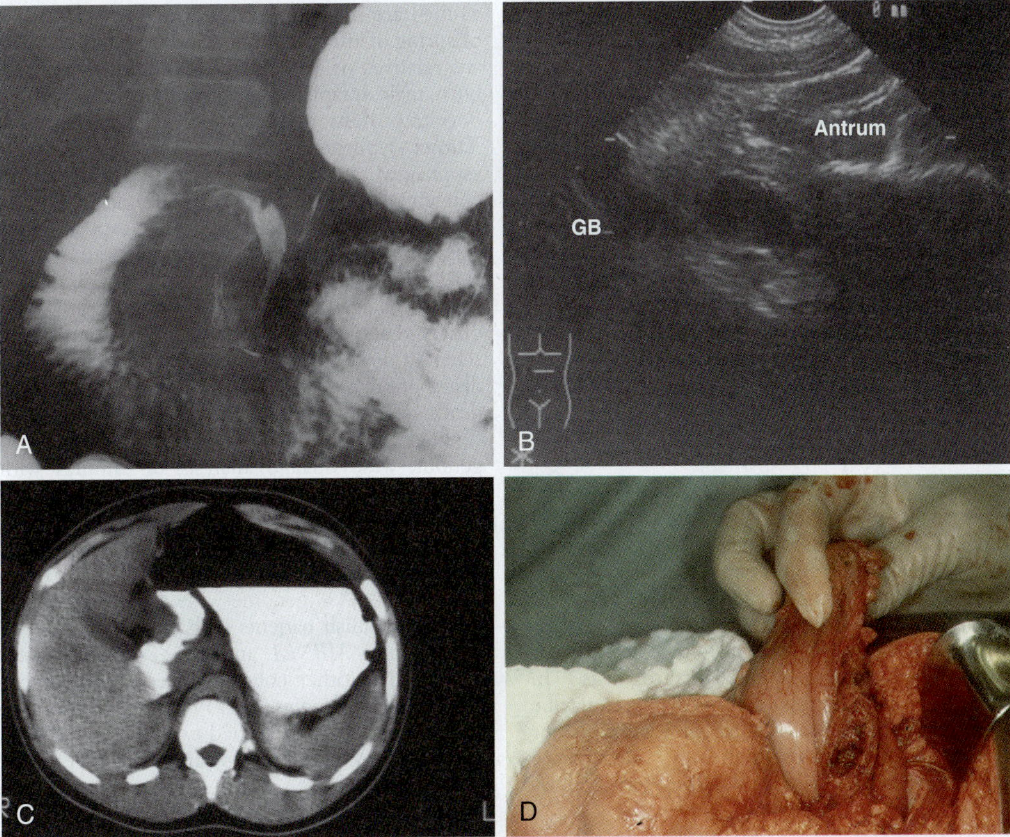

Fig. 51.9 Gastric duplication in a 12-year-old boy with a 1-year history of vomiting and intermittent abdominal pain. Physical examination and laboratory studies were normal. (A) A film from an UGIS shows an extrinsic mass displacing and compressing the antrum and duodenal C loop. (B) An US image shows a hypoechoic mass behind the gastric antrum and medial to the gallbladder (GB). (C) CT shows a circumferential soft-tissue thickening displacing and narrowing the antrum. (D) An intraoperative picture of the gastric duplication after dissection of the stomach and before resection.

specific for a duplication cyst and may be considered as a diagnostic feature of this condition.[33]

Treatment

Surgical excision is considered optimal therapy (Fig. 51.9D); laparoscopic resection has been described.[34] When complete excision is not possible, as may be the case when cyst and viscus have a common muscle layer, debulking, cyst-gastrostomy, or partial gastrectomy may be necessary. Additionally, mucosectomy or mucosal surface ablation should be considered because the development of malignancy in enteric duplications has been documented in adults.[35]

GASTRIC TERATOMA

Gastric teratomas are benign neoplasms of the stomach that occur almost exclusively in males. Gastric teratomas are rare, comprising only 1% of all childhood teratomas. These tumors may have their origins in pluripotential cells and contain all three embryonic germ cell layers. They are almost always diagnosed during infancy owing to their large size. Most are located along the greater curvature of the stomach and are extragastric, although intramural extension has been reported.[36] The immature type (which includes yolk cell tumor, germinoma, and embryonal carcinoma) may infiltrate regional structures, such as omentum, regional lymph nodes, and the left lobe of the liver, whereas the mature teratoma type does not. In virtually all cases, gastric teratoma is an isolated finding and is not associated with other tumors or malformations.[37]

Clinical Features and Diagnosis

The typical patient is a male infant with an abdominal mass; mean age at presentation is 3.2 months.[38] Vomiting may be present from intrinsic compression and GI bleeding due to transmural growth, and disruption of gastric mucosa can occur. Polyhydramnios may be noted prenatally from gastric obstruction by the mass. The newborn infant with a teratoma may be delivered prematurely or have respiratory distress due to increased abdominal pressure. Delivery may be difficult, putting the infant at risk for injuries such as shoulder dystocia. Gastric teratoma associated with gastric perforation, mimicking meconium peritonitis, has been described.[39] Noncontrast radiography demonstrates characteristic calcifications. US demonstrates solid and cystic areas, and CT or MRI confirms the diagnosis and evaluates regional infiltration.[38]

Treatment

Tumor excision with primary gastric repair is the procedure of choice and is curative. Partial or even total gastrectomy is required for intramural tumor extension. Premalignant changes and frank malignant transformation to adenocarcinoma have been reported,[40,41] and peritoneal gliomatosis has been observed. Fortunately, even those cases with malignant histologic features or extension into adjacent tissues have an excellent prognosis.[37] In the case of immature gastric teratomas, a serum AFP level may be useful, especially because of the possibility of recurrence or metastasis and the need for adjuvant chemotherapy.[42] Recurrence of gastric teratoma can occur after two decades, long-term follow-up is important.[43]

GASTRIC VOLVULUS

See Table 51.1 and Chapter 27.

INFANTILE HYPERTROPHIC PYLORIC STENOSIS

Infantile HPS (IHPS) is a form of gastric outlet obstruction caused by hypertrophy of circular muscle surrounding the pyloric channel. Correction of IHPS is the most common abdominal operative procedure during the first 6 months of life. Because the muscular hypertrophy and obstruction tend to be an evolving process during the postnatal period, IHPS is arguably not a true congenital defect.[44] The etiology of IHPS remains the subject of speculation. A localized lack of nitric oxide synthase, an enzyme associated with smooth muscle relaxation, or abnormal neuronal innervation associated with decreased muscle neurofilaments, nerve terminals, synaptic vesicle protein, and neural cell adhesion molecule has been implicated[45]; however, anatomic studies cannot determine whether nitric oxide synthase deficiency is a primary or secondary event,[46] and nitric oxide synthase deficiency is only notable in a subset of cases.[47] Pacemaker cells that regulate GI motility, the interstitial cell of Cajal (discussed in the next chapter), are observed only near the submucosa in IHPS instead of throughout the pylorus.[48,49] EGF and its receptors and HB-EGF are markedly increased in smooth muscle cells in IHPS,[50] but their triggers are unknown.

The incidence of IHPS in the U.S. is approximately 3 in 1000 live births but varies among ethnic groups and regions from 1 to 8 in 1000 live births. Incidence is highest among whites (especially northern Europeans), whereas incidence is lower among African-Americans and Africans and lowest among Asians. Males outnumber females by 4:1 or 5:1.

Familial clustering of IHPS is widely recognized, with autosomal dominant forms reported.[51] Approximately 50% of identical twins are affected, leading credence to the roles of both genetic and environmental factors. Male relatives of affected women are more likely to develop IHPS, such that siblings and offspring of affected women are more likely to develop IHPS than are relatives of affected men. Others at increased risk are first-born male infants, especially those with high birth weights or born to professional parents. IHPS also occurs in association with Turner syndrome, trisomy 18, Cornelia de Lange syndrome, esophageal atresia, Hirschsprung's disease, phenylketonuria, and congenital rubella syndrome. Multiple reports have described an association between early macrolide exposure in infants, including exposure through breast milk,[52] and the development of IHPS.[53–55] In addition, a recent decline in the incidence of IHPS that parallels that of sudden infant death syndrome has been observed and coincides with the recommendation of supine infant sleeping position; however, a study in Germany showed regional distribution of IHPS was different from that of sudden infant death syndrome.[56,57]

Five genetic loci have been identified with IHPS via genome-wide linkage analysis of families with two or more affected individuals: the gene for nitric oxidase synthetase, *NOS1* on chromosome locus 12q24.2–24.31; 2 loci, *IHPS2* (16p12–p13), and *IHPS5* (16q24.3) associated with autosomal dominant forms of the disease; *IHPS3* (11q14–q22); and *IHPS4* (Xq23–q24).[58] A genome-wide association study was performed on 1001 Danish patients with IHPS and 2401 healthy controls. Two genes, *MBNL1* and *NKX2-5*, were identified and then replicated in other cohort studies.[59] More recent genome-wide meta-analysis studies in 1395 surgery-confirmed IHPS cases, and 4438 controls identified two new loci, *BARX1* (9q22.32) and EML4-MTA3 (2p21), associated with IHPS.[60]

Clinical Features and Diagnosis

Infants with IHPS are typically asymptomatic until 3–4 weeks of age, although a small number may present as early as the first week of life. Initially, infants present with mild spitting, which progresses to projectile vomiting following feedings. Vomiting may be so forceful as to exit through the nostrils, as well as the mouth. Emesis may contain "coffee ground" material or small amounts of frank blood but is rarely bilious. Early in the course, the infant remains hungry following vomiting episodes but, with time, loses interest in feeding and may present wasted and severely volume depleted. Decreased urinary and stool output accompanies volume depletion. Marked metabolic alkalosis develops secondary to chloride loss in the vomitus. Infants may be misdiagnosed with formula allergy or gastroesophageal reflux.

On physical examination the infant with IHPS may appear malnourished and volume depleted, but the extent is variable and related to severity and duration of symptoms. The classic physical signs are a palpable pyloric mass and visible peristaltic waves. The palpable "olive" is most easily felt in an underweight patient, immediately following emesis or aspiration of the stomach. The location of the olive varies from the level of the umbilicus to near the epigastrium. The pyloric mass is palpable in 70%–90% of affected infants, depending on the experience and patience of the examiner. Emptying the stomach by nasogastric tube placement and palpation of the stomach with the infant in the prone position may enhance detection. Peristaltic waves are best observed during feeding of the naked infant while the infant is cradled in the mother's left arm. Many infants appear jaundiced due to an indirect hyperbilirubinemia related to volume depletion and, perhaps, malnutrition.

When the presentation is typical and the olive palpated, no studies are necessary. However, in the minority of infants with projectile vomiting, definitive diagnosis requires radiologic studies. Noncontrast radiography demonstrates a distended stomach with paucity of gas beyond the stomach. Diagnosis is confirmed by US of the pylorus, which has supplanted contrast radiography as the diagnostic study of choice for IHPS. Because volume depletion may affect the pyloric US measurements, ensuring an adequate fluid status may be prudent before US evaluation.[61] The length of the hypertrophied canal is variable and may range from as little as 14 mm to more than 20 mm. The numeric value for the lower limit of pyloric muscle thickness has varied in reports in the literature, ranging between 3 and 4.5 mm. This appears as a characteristic sonolucent "donut" (Fig. 51.10). Many consider the numeric value less important than the overall morphology of the canal and real-time observations. A negative US study hinges on an unequivocal diagnosis of a normal pyloric ring and a distensible antropyloric portion of the stomach.[62]

When the differential diagnosis includes IHPS, gastroesophageal reflux, or other upper GI disorders, contrast radiography may be the appropriate first test. Contrast radiography must be performed carefully, and gastric contents should first be aspirated. The infant is given barium and imaged in a semiprone position. Characteristic findings include an elongated narrow pylorus with the appearance of a "double channel." There is also indentation of the adjacent antrum and duodenum by the pyloric mass, producing the so-called shoulders (Fig. 51.11). The most common abnormality that mimics IHPS is pylorospasm. Diagnosis of IHPS by EGD has been described in which the pylorus appears as a cauliflower-like narrowing, through which a 7.8 mm (external diameter) endoscope cannot be passed[63]; however, another report on endoscopic diagnosis has refuted these claims.[64] EGD is also potentially beneficial to evaluate for eosinophilic gastroenteritis (see Chapter 30), which has been linked to pyloric stenosis.[65]

Treatment

The initial therapy for IHPS is fluid and electrolyte replacement to correct volume depletion and hypochloremic metabolic alkalosis. Depending on severity, fluid and electrolyte repletion can usually be accomplished within 24 hours. Definitive therapy is the Ramstedt pyloromyotomy, which entails a longitudinal incision through the hypertrophied pyloric muscle down to the submucosa on the anterior surface of the pylorus. After spreading the muscle,

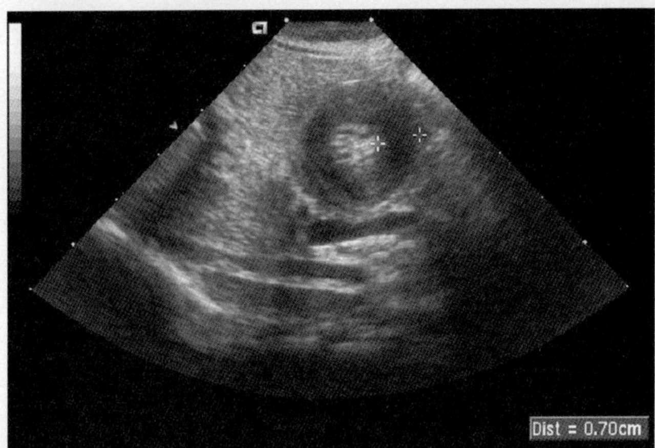

Fig. 51.10 Abdominal US image in a 1-month-old infant with idiopathic hypertrophic pyloric stenosis demonstrating the sonolucent "donut" of pyloric hypertrophy on cross-section. Crossbars measure an abnormal (7 mm) muscle thickness. (Courtesy Jeanne Joglar, MD.)

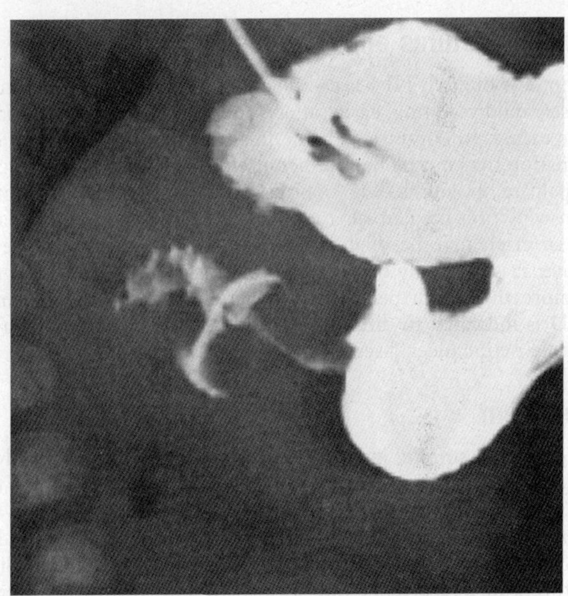

Fig. 51.11 Film from an UGIS in a 1-month-old infant with idiopathic hypertrophic pyloric stenosis, demonstrating an elongated pylorus and antral and duodenal "shoulders" secondary to a mass effect. (Courtesy Marcia Pritchard, MD.)

the intact mucosa bulges through the incision to the level of the incised muscle. An alternative operation is the pyloric traumamyoplasty, where the pylorus is grasped with a Babcock clamp that disrupts the hypertrophied circular muscles in two places.[66,67] Laparoscopic pyloromyotomy with its improved cosmetic results and reduced need for analgesics is becoming increasingly popular.[68,69] Although infants may continue to vomit for the first few days postoperatively, persistent vomiting is suggestive of inadequate surgery.

Nonoperative therapy consists of the use of anticholinergic medications[70] and paste-consistency feedings until such time that the muscle hypertrophy resolves.[71] Because of the high failure rate, the prolonged recovery period (compared with surgery), and the low risk of pyloromyotomy, the nonoperative approach is rarely used in the USA.

The prognosis following surgery is excellent, with the infant resuming normal growth and development. Although divergent gastric emptying rates have been observed for many years following the treatment of IHPS, gastric emptying by scintigraphy using radiolabeled liquids or solids was similar in patients treated surgically or conservatively versus controls.[63]

ADULT HYPERTROPHIC PYLORIC STENOSIS

HPS rarely occurs in adults; there are approximately 200 cases described in the literature. Adult HPS has anatomic features identical to the infantile type. In adults, pyloric thickening is generally associated with PUD, hypertrophic gastropathy,[72] or carcinoma. In a few cases, no etiology is determined; it is therefore unknown whether these are missed infantile cases or whether the hypertrophy occurred later in life. There is a family history of IHPS in some cases of adult HPS, again suggesting a role for genetic predisposition or missed infantile cases. In addition, 80% of adult HPS cases occur in men. The resected pylorus demonstrates normal mucosa and marked circumferential thickening of the muscularis propria.[73] Microscopically, there are variable degrees of inflammatory changes or edema, and degenerative changes in the ganglion cells of the myenteric plexus have been reported.[72]

Clinical Features and Diagnosis

Symptoms of adult HPS are similar to those observed in infancy: nausea, mild vomiting, early satiety, and epigastric pain, especially after eating. In contrast with the infantile form, the physical examination may not be helpful because the pyloric mass is difficult to palpate in adults. On contrast radiography, the elongated narrow pylorus is again apparent; gastric emptying is delayed, and the stomach may be dilated. US is the screening procedure of choice; it is generally considered abnormal if the pylorus is 1 cm or more thick with persistent elongation of more than 2 cm.[72] EGD is indicated to differentiate adult HPS from carcinoma or chronic peptic ulcer disease.

Treatment

Traditionally, surgical pyloromyotomy or resection of the involved region has been considered the procedure of choice. Because of the risk of a small focus of carcinoma, the surgical resection of the pylorus has been recommended. Endoscopic balloon dilation has also been efficacious in the management of adult HPS, but an 80% postprocedure recurrence rate within the first 6 months has been reported.[74] Palliation of pyloric stenosis caused by gastric cancer using an endoscopically placed stent has been described.[75]

CONGENITAL ABSENCE OF THE PYLORUS

In this very rare anomaly, the pylorus is closed off like a sac and the ostium of the gastric outlet is in an abnormal location along the incisura angularis of the lesser curvature (see Table 51.1).

DUODENAL ATRESIA AND STENOSIS

Duodenal atresia and stenosis are congenital defects characterized by complete and partial obstruction of the duodenum, respectively. Atresias occur in various anatomic configurations including a blind-ending pouch with no connection to the distal duodenum (least common), a pouch with a fibrous cord connecting to the distal duodenum, or a complete membrane obstructing the lumen (most common). Perforate membranes are also a cause of duodenal stenosis. All these lesions occur with greatest frequency near the ampulla of Vater, with most lesions (80%) occurring distal to this landmark. The overall incidence of the three anomalies combined is approximately 1 per 200,000 live births, with a slight predilection for girls. The etiology of these lesions may relate to failure to recanalize the duodenal lumen by vacuolization at 8–10 weeks' gestation. This is distinct from atresia or stenosis of the jejunum and ileum, which are caused by vascular accidents in utero.[76] Duodenal stenosis has been observed in sonic hedgehog (Shh)—mutant mice, therefore adding to our understanding that mutations in signaling pathways may play a role in this malformation.[77]

In two series of more than 100 cases,[78,79] more than 50% of affected patients had associated congenital defects including pancreatic defects, intestinal malrotation with congenital bands, esophageal atresia, Meckel's diverticulum, imperforate anus, congenital heart disease, central nervous system lesions, renal anomalies, and, rarely, biliary tract anomalies. Trisomy 21 is strongly associated with duodenal atresia/stenosis/web in that—anywhere from 25% to more than 50% of cases occur in infants and children with this chromosomal anomaly. Familial association is rare, although isolated case reports suggest a possible genetic association.[51,80] A report of father and son with periampullary obstruction due to duodenal stenosis and annular pancreas (in the father) and segmental duodenal atresia (in the son) serves as a reminder that with increased survival of affected infants, a genetic basis may be realized in the future.[81]

Clinical Features and Diagnosis

The diagnosis of duodenal atresia may be suspected prenatally when US demonstrates gastric and proximal duodenal dilation and polyhydramnios. Polyhydramnios is present in 33%–50% of cases of duodenal atresia. The absence of gastric and proximal duodenal dilation in the presence of polyhydramnios does not exclude the diagnosis, because intrauterine emesis may limit preobstructive dilation. High-frequency transvaginal transducers used in US may overdiagnose intestinal dilation, so longer scanning is recommended once obstruction is suspected.[82]

The infant with duodenal atresia is often born preterm and has early feeding intolerance characterized by vomiting and upper abdominal distention. Emesis is usually bilious because most lesions occur distal to the entry of the bile duct into the duodenum. Nonbilious emesis is seen in 15%–20% of cases secondary to more proximal obstruction. Any child with trisomy 21 and vomiting (especially bile-stained) requires further evaluation for duodenal stenosis. Duodenal stenosis or a partial membrane may present at any age, depending on the degree of obstruction. Infants and children present with vomiting, failure to gain weight adequately, and/or aspiration. Vomiting may be intermittent and of variable severity such that symptomatic lesions may remain undiagnosed for months to years. Occasionally, diagnosis is delayed until adulthood.

Noncontrast radiographs of the infant with duodenal obstruction classically demonstrate the presence of air in the stomach and in the first portion of the duodenum—the "double-bubble" sign (Fig. 51.12). The absence of air beyond the second bubble should be interpreted as probable duodenal atresia. Contrast radiography is generally effective in demonstrating atresias, stenosis, membranes, and other anomalies resulting in external compression of the duodenum (Fig. 51.13). In addition, normal or abnormal rotation and fixation of the bowel can be assessed. The ampullary sphincter has been noted to be incompetent in some cases. Reflux of contrast medium through the ampulla poses risks of developing cholangitis and pancreatitis. Occasionally, upper endoscopy is useful in diagnosing or defining a duodenal stenosis or membrane.

Treatment

A newborn infant suspected of duodenal obstruction should have a nasogastric tube placed for decompression, and fluid and electrolyte

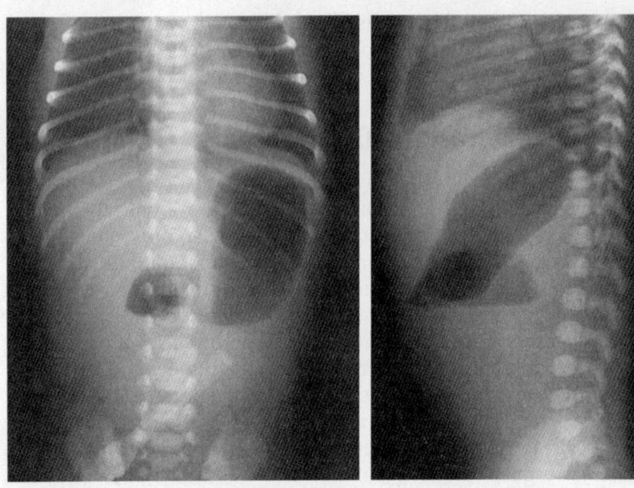

Fig. 51.12 Anteroposterior and lateral noncontrast films of an infant with duodenal atresia demonstrate the "double-bubble" sign. (Courtesy Marcia Pritchard, MD.)

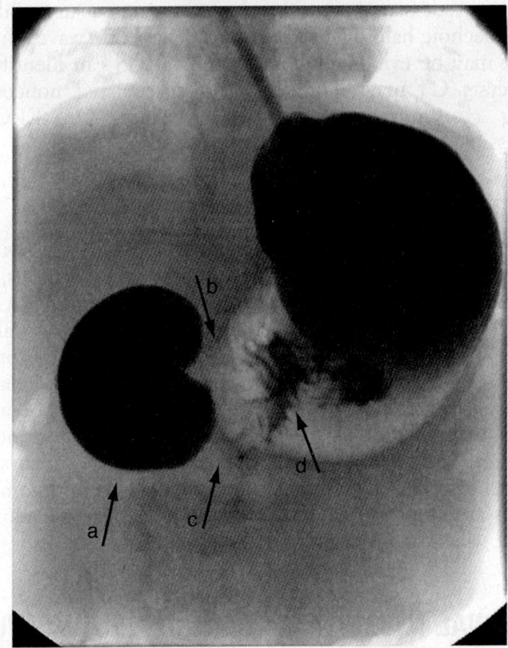

Fig. 51.13 Film from an UGIS in an infant with a duodenal membrane/web demonstrates dilatation (a) from the pylorus (b) to the third portion of the duodenum proximal to the webbed segment of duodenum (without contrast) (c) and a normal-caliber fourth portion of the duodenum (d). (Courtesy Korgun Koral, MD.)

abnormalities should be corrected. The surgical approach in the past was duodenojejunostomy, but duodenostomy is now preferred.[79] The operation has evolved from a side-to-side anastomosis to a proximal transverse to distal longitudinal ("diamond-shaped") anastomosis. Associated malrotation is corrected with a Ladd procedure. A catheter is passed into the distal duodenum to investigate for a second obstruction, which occurs in approximately 3% of cases. Membranes may be excised without anastomosis if the membrane was an isolated finding. Balloon dilation has been described for membranous duodenal stenosis.[83,84] Endoscopic laser resection of membranes has been reported; unfortunately, subsequent scar formation has resulted in stenosis and the need for surgery.[85] Complications that can plague patients months to years following primary repair include motility problems, megaduodenum, gastroesophageal reflux unresponsive to medications, gastropathy, adhesions, and PUD.[79] Proximal and distal segments in duodenal atresia may differ in the neural cells, musculature and distribution of the interstitial cells of Cajal, which may contribute to the onset of postoperative duodenal dysmotility.[86]

Approximately 12% of patients required revision or another intra-abdominal surgery over a 30-year follow-up period.[87] Two teenagers have presented with choledochal cyst.[78] Megaduodenum proximal to the obstruction, with abnormal peristalsis, is a common long-term issue, but most patients are asymptomatic. For symptomatic patients with megaduodenum, bowel plication may be indicated.[88]

ANNULAR PANCREAS

Annular pancreas is an unusual congenital malformation characterized by a thin ring of pancreatic tissue, most often encircling the second portion of the duodenum, contributing in variable degrees to obstruction (see Chapter 57). The lesion may present in the neonatal period, in childhood, or adulthood. It is the most common congenital anomaly of the pancreas presenting in children. Some cases remain asymptomatic and are discovered as an incidental finding during ERCP or at autopsy. The anomalous tissue is histologically normal and contains a moderately sized pancreatic duct. The pancreatic tissue may penetrate the muscularis of the duodenal wall or remain distinct from the duodenum. Several hypotheses exist regarding embryologic origin of annular pancreas. Evidence appears to favor Lecco's 1910 hypothesis that the ventral pancreatic anlage becomes fixed to the duodenal wall before rotation during the fifth week of gestation. With subsequent growth and fusion of the dorsal and ventral anlagen, a partial (75%) or complete (25%) ring of pancreatic tissue is formed.[16]

The incidence of the disorder is approximately 1 in 100,000 live births, but this figure does not account for cases found during adulthood, during ERCP (when it is usually noted as an incidental finding), or at autopsy. The true incidence may be as high as 1 per 250 live births. In infancy, the incidence is equal in male and female infants, whereas in adulthood, men outnumber women by 2:1. Infant and childhood cases are associated with other congenital anomalies in an estimated 40%–70% of cases, including trisomy 21, duodenal atresia, cardiac defects, anorectal malformations, Meckel's diverticulum, tracheoesophageal fistula, malrotation, genitourinary malformation, and situs inversus.[89] In adults, compared with children, it is more common to have malrotation, duodenal web, Shatzki's ring, duodenal atresia, tracheoesophageal fistula, and genitourinary abnormalities. Moreover, adults are at increased risk of pancreatobiliary neoplasia. In 13 adults with annular pancreas, 6 had pancreatobiliary neoplasia, including 2 with adenocarcinoma of the pancreas, 2 with ampullary adenoma, and 1 with adenocarcinoma of the gallbladder.[89] The finding of an annular pancreas in a woman and her child, as well as in two successive generations, suggests a possible hereditary link.[90] A case report showed that the 6q24.2 microduplication of the utrophin gene is a potential risk factor for the development of annular pancreas.[91]

Clinical Features and Diagnosis

Annular pancreas produces symptoms when tissue obstructs the duodenum or biliary tree. Controversy exists as to whether the annular pancreas actually plays a role in obstruction. The abnormally located pancreatic tissue is a visible indicator of an underlying duodenal abnormality that can range from minimal duodenal stenosis to atresia.[92] Infants may present with high-grade obstructive symptoms and signs such as bilious emesis and upper abdominal distention indistinguishable from duodenal atresia or malrotation with midgut volvulus. During childhood, intermittent bilious emesis and failure to thrive are common presenting symptoms, whereas during adulthood the most common symptom is abdominal pain. Other symptoms and signs in adults include nausea, vomiting, gastric outlet obstruction, pancreatitis, pancreatolithiasis, pancreas divisum, pancreatic mass, gastric or duodenal ulcer, or biliary obstruction resulting in jaundice. In the adult, symptoms peak in the third to fifth decades.

Noncontrast radiologic studies of the infant may demonstrate the double-bubble sign identical to that seen in duodenal atresia (see Fig. 51.10). Contrast radiography should be done to ensure that the obstruction is not due to midgut volvulus, which is a surgical emergency. In adults, transabdominal US, EUS, CT, or MRCP may diagnose annular pancreas. ERCP may demonstrate ductular structures consistent with annular pancreas, but in some cases it may not be technically feasible owing to duodenal obstruction proximal to the major ampulla. EUS is especially useful when prior gastric resection or duodenal obstruction precludes ERCP; in addition, a mass may be staged or undergo FNA at the time of EUS. The ability to evaluate for mass is a relatively new consideration, given reports of ampullary carcinoma in association with annular pancreas; hence jaundice should not be attributed to annular pancreas until carcinoma is ruled out.[93] MRCP, which allows spatial resolution of the entire pancreaticobiliary tree, can identify the annulus and the duct that surrounds the duodenum. Finally, intraoperative diagnosis at laparotomy is not unusual.

Treatment

The preferred operative therapy for annular pancreas includes duodenostomy or duodenojejunostomy. Prognosis postoperatively is excellent with either, and postoperative deaths among infants are generally due to associated anomalies. Division or dissection of the pancreatic tissue is not recommended owing to the high risk of complications, including pancreatitis, pancreatic fistula, and incomplete relief of symptoms due to intrinsic duodenal narrowing. An annular pancreas identified at the time of organ procurement has been transplanted along with a long segment of duodenum with good results, so that annular pancreas can be considered suitable for transplantation.[94]

DUODENAL DUPLICATION CYSTS

Duodenal duplication cysts are a rare anomaly, totaling only 7% of GI duplications. Most commonly located posterior to the first or second portion of the duodenum, these spherical or tubular cysts do not generally communicate with the duodenal lumen but do share blood supply with the duodenum. Histologic criteria for a duodenal duplication cyst include GI mucosa, a smooth muscle layer in the wall, and an association with the duodenal wall. The mucosa is typically duodenal, but in 15% of cases there is gastric mucosa and, very rarely, pancreatic tissue is found. Men and women are affected equally. Several embryologic theories have been postulated, but none explain the diversity of anatomic varieties.[95]

Clinical Features and Diagnosis

Duplications may be clinically silent for years before presentation. Presenting signs and symptoms of these cysts are typically that of partial gastric outlet obstruction and include vomiting, decreased oral intake, periumbilical tenderness, and abdominal distention. Conversely, an asymptomatic mass found on physical or radiologic examination may be noted first. If heterotopic gastric mucosa is present in the duplication, bleeding or perforation may be the initial presenting sign. In the neonate, duodenal obstruction due to a large duplication cyst has been reported. An infected duodenal duplication cyst has been noted as well.[96] Pancreatitis may occur if the cyst compresses or is in communication with the pancreatic duct. Finally, jaundice and duodenojejunal intussusception resulting in small bowel obstruction have been described.[97]

Noncontrast, as well as contrast, radiography may demonstrate obstruction or compression effect but, in general, findings are nonspecific and only suggestive of the diagnosis. US may show unilocular cystic structure with echogenic mucosa surrounded by thin hypoechoic halo of muscle layer.[96] Peristaltic waves through the cyst may be evident on US. Antenatal US can identify suspected cysts. CT may demonstrate an encapsulated, noncommunicating cyst posterior to the duodenum. On ERCP, a compressible periampullary mass may be seen.

Treatment

Surgical therapy should be individualized in accordance with the anatomy of the cyst. Because of potential complications, early neonatal resection, even for asymptomatic cysts, has been advocated.[98] Operations that have been performed include local excision and cystjejunostomy. Mucosal stripping of the common muscular wall and resection coupled with removal of free walls has been recommended.[99] This, however, may be complex because of the proximity of the cyst to the ampulla and biliary-pancreatic confluence. Endoscopic drainage, as well as removal, has been successful in adult and pediatric cases. As invasive carcinoma may occur in an adult with a duodenal duplication cyst, endoscopic drainage without resection may require reconsideration.

INTESTINAL MALROTATION AND MIDGUT VOLVULUS

See Table 51.1 and Chapter 100.

Full references for this chapter can be found at https://ebooks.health.elsevier.com.

52 Gastric Neuromuscular Function and Neuromuscular Disorders

Kenneth L. Koch

IN THIS CHAPTER

Gastric neuromuscular function refers to the contractions, relaxations, and peristaltic activities of the stomach.

The three major neuromuscular activities of the stomach are (1) receptive relaxation of the fundus, (2) recurrent peristaltic waves of the corpus and antrum, and (3) antral peristalsis with antropyloroduodenal coordination. These major neuromuscular activities of the stomach accomplish three key functions: (1) to receive the ingested food that we eat (receptive relaxation), (2) to mill (triturate) the ingested foodstuffs into a nutrient suspension termed *chyme*, and (3) to empty the chyme from the stomach through the pyloric sphincter into the duodenum in a highly regulated fashion. This sophisticated process is necessary to maximize further digestion and absorption of the nutrients in the small intestine. Neuromuscular dysfunction of the stomach results in nausea, early satiety, vomiting of chewed food, and dysregulation of the gastric emptying of solid and liquid nutrients.

These critical gastric neuromuscular activities and related functions are complexly modulated by the CNS, parasympathetic nervous system (PNS) and sympathetic nervous system (SNS), the interactions of the CNS and the activity of the enteric nervous system (ENS), the interstitial cells of Cajal (ICCs) that regulate the frequency of smooth muscle contractions and organize peristaltic waves, and the host of neurotransmitters that ultimately regulate the contraction and relaxation of gastric smooth muscle.

ELECTROPHYSIOLOGIC BASIS FOR NORMAL GASTRIC NEUROMUSCULAR FUNCTION

Extracellular Slow Waves and Plateau and Action Potentials

The stomach is a sophisticated hollow organ of smooth muscle organized into circular, longitudinal, and oblique muscle layers. *Slow waves* or *pacesetter potentials*, regulate, control, and pace gastric smooth muscle contractions.[1,2] In the normal human stomach the slow waves occur at approximately 3 cycles per minute (cpm) or between 2.5 and 3.7 cpm.[3,4] From the pacemaker region on the greater curvature of the stomach, between the fundus and the proximal corpus, slow waves propagate distally and circumferentially toward the pylorus every 20 seconds, with highest amplitude and velocity (approximately 7 mm/s) in the distal 2–4 cm of antrum (Fig. 52.1).[5] The gastric slow waves originate from the ICCs.[2,6]

The depolarization of the slow wave reduces the electrical threshold for circular smooth muscle contraction, and, in the appropriate situation, the amplitude of the circular smooth muscle contraction increases with the onset of the plateau potentials and action potentials.[7,8] The aboral propagation of slow waves linked to plateau potentials (with or without action potentials) is the electrophysiologic basis of gastric peristaltic waves (Fig. 52.2). Thus the slow waves linked with plateau or action potentials propagate through the corpus and antrum and create moving "ring contractions" that resolve in the antrum or at the pylorus in a terminal antral contraction. Gastric myoelectrical activity

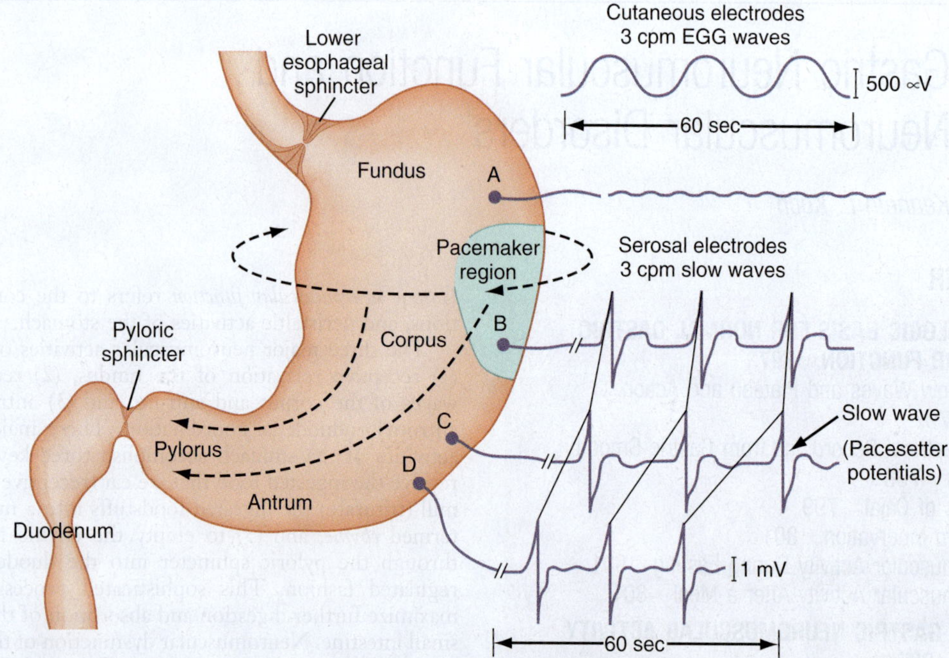

Fig. 52.1 Gastric electrical activity recorded from electrodes (A–D) positioned on the serosa of the stomach from the fundus to the antrum. Slow waves originate in the pacemaker region located at the juncture of the fundus and the corpus on the greater curvature. Note that the fundus does not have slow wave activity (electrode A). Slow waves propagate circumferentially and migrate distally to the pylorus approximately every 20 seconds, or 3 cpm *(dotted lines with arrowheads)*. Gastric myoelectrical activity (GMA) at 3 cpm can be recorded with cutaneous electrodes. The summed GMA recorded from electrodes positioned on the abdominal surface in the epigastrium is termed as electrogastrogram, and the normal rhythm is 3 cpm. (Modified from Koch KL. Electrogastrography. In: Schuster M, Crowel M, Koch, KL, eds. *Atlas of Gastrointestinal Motility*. Hamilton, ON: BC Decker; 2002:185–201.)

(GMA) is the summation of these electrocontractile events recorded from electrodes positioned on the serosa or skin. The pylorus provides an electrical barrier between the 3-cpm slow wave of the distal antrum and the 12–13-cpm slow wave of the duodenum.

Intracellular Electrical Recordings from Gastric Smooth Muscle Cells

Intracellular recordings from smooth muscle cells from the different regions of the stomach (fundus to the mid-corpus to the terminal antrum) illustrate the electrophysiologic characteristics that distinguish these regions (Fig. 52.3).[1] Key features are (1) regional differences in resting membrane potential, which range from −48 to −75 mV, (2) regional differences in threshold for contraction, which range from −52 to −40 mV, and (3) the occurrence of plateau potentials with or without spike potentials.[1] The fundic smooth muscle cells are unique because their resting membrane potential lies at or above the threshold for contraction (−50 mV), a situation that promotes sustained smooth muscle contraction and ongoing fundic tone. Inhibitory vagal input to the fundus increases during swallowing, however, and results in decreasing muscle tone associated with "receptive relaxation" and the gastric accommodation of swallowed foodstuffs.[9,10] Fundic muscle tone decreases in proportion to the intensity and duration of the inhibitory neural discharge.

In contrast to the fundus, intracellular recordings from the corpus indicate a lower resting membrane potential of −60 mV. The rapid upstroke depolarization in these cells is followed by a plateau potential that slowly returns to the baseline resting electrical potential. The plateau potentials are associated with circular muscle contraction activity in the corpus and antrum.[1] The plateau potential may be accompanied by action potentials in the corpus and antrum. Extrinsic stimuli such as release of acetylcholine or stretch of the stomach wall increases the amplitude and duration of the plateau potential and the occurrence of action potentials, resulting in contractions of varying force, as seen in the muscle of the terminal antrum. Depending on the excitatory neural stimuli and the amplitude of plateau potentials and the number of action potentials, peristaltic contraction waves of the circular muscle layer vary from very-low-amplitude contractions to high-amplitude lumen-occluding contractions. At the pylorus, the plateau potentials have long durations with superimposed action potentials that result in closure of the pyloric sphincter in conjunction with the terminal antral contraction.[1]

The membrane potential and the force of smooth muscle contraction also distinguish the fundus, corpus, and antrum (Fig. 52.4). The resting membrane potential of the fundus is approximately −50 mV and produces the sustained contraction and the resting tone of the fundus.[1] This fundic tone ensures a sensitive response to excitatory or inhibitory stimuli for relaxation or further contraction of the fundus. Receptive relaxation during ingestion of food is accomplished by these electrophysiologic attributes of smooth muscle in the fundus. In contrast, the resting membrane potentials of the corpus and antrum are −60 to −70 mV, respectively. In the presence of plateau potentials or action potentials, the membrane potential reaches −45 mV or less and smooth muscle contraction occurs. If the plateau potentials have higher amplitude, then contractions of larger amplitude or force occur. When the plateau potential and action potentials are linked to the propagating 3 cpm slow waves (Fig. 52.5), then the 3

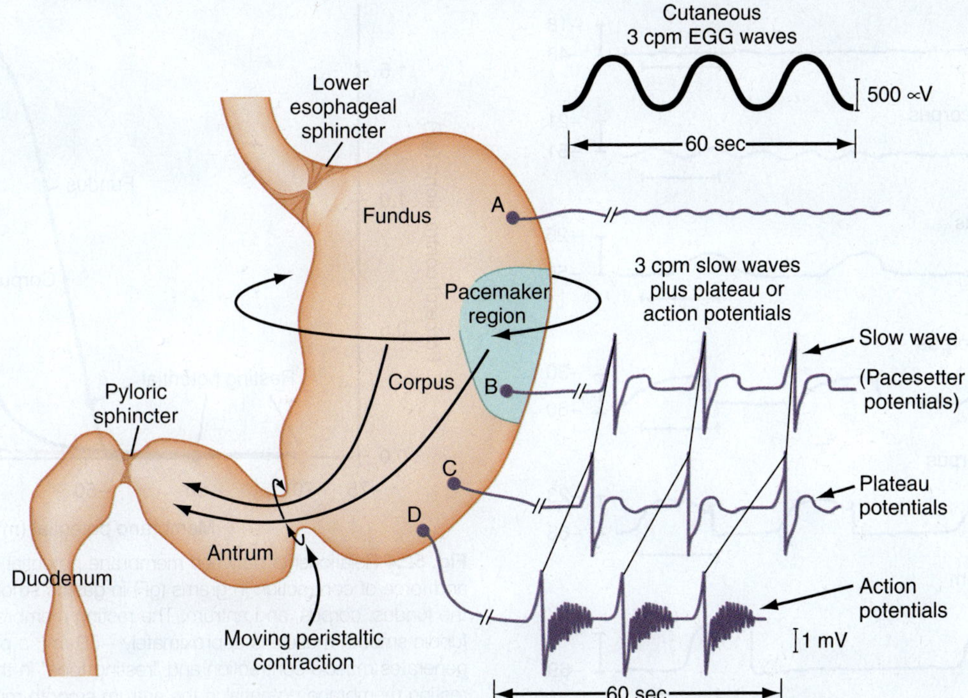

Fig. 52.2 Gastric slow waves linked with plateau potentials (or action potentials), the electrophysiologic basis of gastric peristaltic waves. The plateau and action potentials occur during circular muscle contractions. Peristaltic waves originate in the pacemaker area. The frequency (3 cpm) and the propagation velocity (≈14 mm/sec) of the gastric peristaltic waves are controlled by the slow wave, which leads the contraction from the proximal corpus to the distal antrum, as shown at electrodes (A)–(D). The *solid black lines* and *arrows* indicate the circumferential and distal propagation of the peristaltic wave, which forms a ring contraction (*small arrow*), indicating a moving peristaltic contraction. Peristaltic contractions occur three times per minute, the frequency of the gastric slow wave. The increased gastric myoelectrical activity of the plateau potentials and action potentials linked with the slow wave results in increased amplitude of the 3-cpm waves recorded in the electrogastrogram signal (*thick black lines*). The fundus does not participate in the gastric peristaltic contractions. (Modified from Koch KL. Electrogastrography. In: Schuster M, Crowel M, Koch, KL, eds. *Atlas of Gastrointestinal Motility*. Hamilton, Ontario BC Decker; 2002:185–201.)

cpm GMA reflects the 3 per minute gastric peristaltic "waves" migrating from corpus to pylorus.

In conjunction with terminal antral contractions, the pyloric sphincter contraction prevents emptying of gastric content into the duodenum and results in retention of solid foodstuffs in the stomach. Thus the peristaltic waves associated with terminal antral and pyloric sphincter contraction produce little or no emptying of the gastric contents from the stomach into the duodenum. In contrast, if the pylorus remains open during the gastric peristaltic wave, then an aliquot of nutrient chyme is emptied into the duodenum.

Interstitial Cells of Cajal

ICCs are the "pacemaker cells" that coordinate peristaltic contractions of the smooth muscle of the GI tract.[6,11,12] ICCs originate from c-Kit-positive mesenchymal cell precursors.[13] ICCs in the stomach are located in submuscular, intramuscular, myenteric, and subserosal layers of the gastric wall.[14–16] Fig. 52.6 shows the anatomic relationships between the ICCs in the myenteric plexus (MY-ICCs), the intramuscular ICCs (IM-ICCs), the enteric neurons, and the circular smooth muscle cells. MY-ICCs are located between the circular and longitudinal muscle layers of the stomach and are the ICCs responsible for the generation of the slow waves. These ICCs spontaneously generate slow waves that are conducted into adjacent smooth muscle cells and cause depolarization and contraction of the smooth muscle by activating voltage-dependent, dihydropyridine-sensitive (L-type) calcium channels.[16,17] The increased amplitude of the plateau potential correlates with increased amplitude of smooth muscle contraction. The slow waves propagate circumferentially and distally through the ICC network via gap junctions and entrain more distal ICCs with slower intrinsic frequencies to the higher slow wave frequency, the normal 3-cpm pacemaker frequency.

ICCs are also located within the layers of the circular smooth muscle (IM-ICCs), where they integrate and coordinate the spread of the slow wave and the smooth muscle contraction initiated by the MY-ICCs.[8] Slow waves are not regenerated in the smooth muscle cells because the ion channels needed to generate and propagate slow waves are not expressed by gastric smooth muscle. The generation of the 3 cpm slow wave rhythm originates in changing intracellular calcium fluxes in the ICCs.[17]

In the corpus and antrum, the MY-ICCs and IM-ICCs form a continuous lattice-like network of interconnections that extend from the pacemaker region circumferentially and aborally to the pylorus. The MY-ICCs establish the dominant pacemaker frequency, and IM-ICCs carry the slow wave into the circular smooth muscle bundles to coordinate circumferential and aboral propagation of the contraction wave associated with release of acetylcholine from enteric neurons.

The ICCs have innate rhythmicity that is based on their unique metabolism and fluxes in intracellular and extracellular

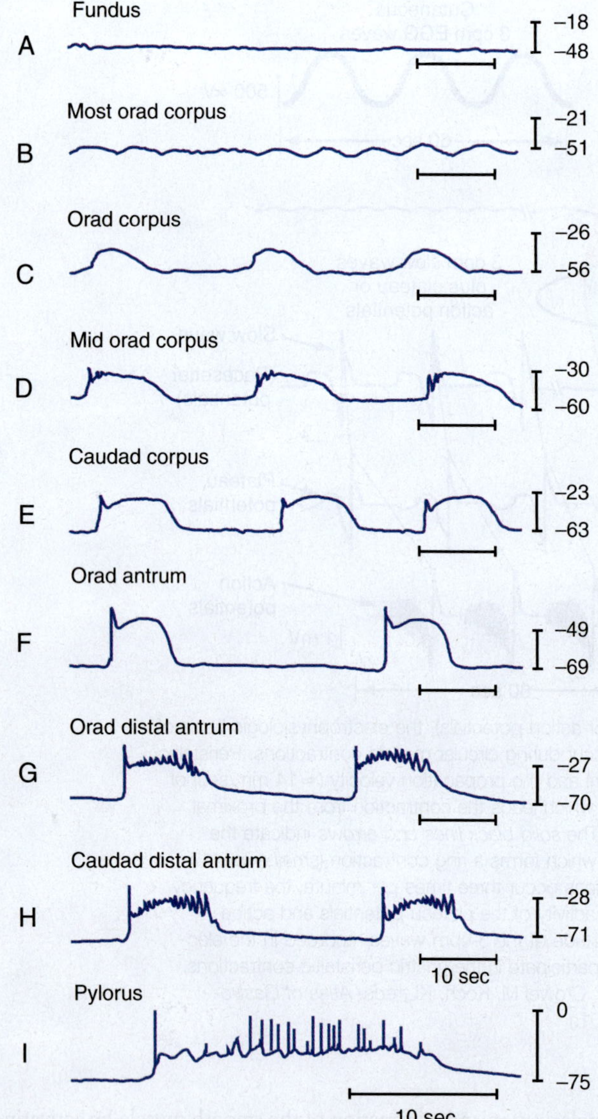

Fig. 52.3 Intracellular electrical recordings from smooth muscle from the fundus to the pylorus (A)–(I). Resting membrane potential in millivolts (mV) is shown on the vertical axis, and time is shown on the horizontal axis. Distinctive electrical characteristics in each region are shown: (A) Spontaneous electrical activity in the fundic smooth muscle is absent. (B–E) The resting membrane potential is less negative in the smooth muscle in the corpus compared with the antrum (F–H). Spontaneous upstroke depolarization is also recorded in the corpus and antrum, as well as in the pylorus (I). The upstroke depolarization in the smooth muscle is initiated by the interstitial cells of Cajal (see text). The upstroke depolarization is followed by the plateau potential and repolarization (D–I). The upstroke depolarization and plateau potentials are associated with contraction of the smooth muscle. Action potentials are superimposed on the plateau potentials in the terminal antrum and pylorus (G–I) and are associated with increased amplitude of smooth muscle contraction. (From Szurszewski JH. Electrophysiological basis of gastrointestinal motility. In: Johnson LR, ed. *Physiology of the Gastrointestinal Tract*. 2nd ed. New York: Raven Press; 1986:383.)

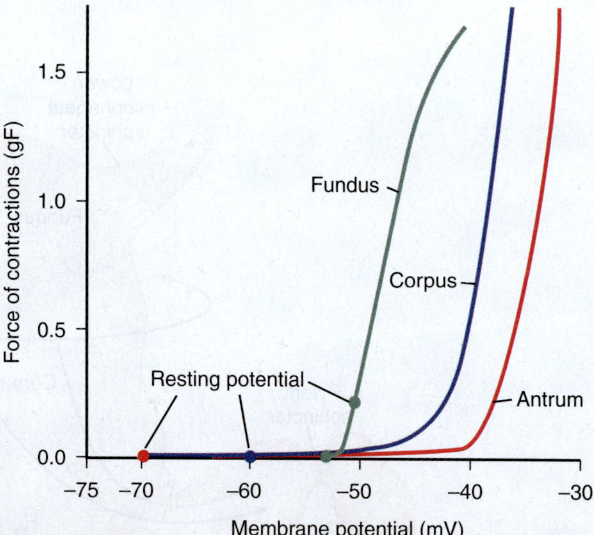

Fig. 52.4 Relationship between membrane potential in millivolts (mV) and force of contraction in grams (gF) in gastric smooth muscle from the fundus, corpus, and antrum. The resting membrane potential in fundic smooth muscle is approximately −50 mV, a potential that generates muscle contraction and "resting tone" in the fundus. The resting membrane potential in the antrum smooth muscle is −70 mV, almost 30 mV below the threshold for smooth muscle contraction. When the resting membrane potential reaches −40 or −35 mV, the steep slope of the voltage-contraction curve is observed in the corpus and antrum. (From Szurszewski JH. Electrophysiological basis of gastrointestinal motility. In: Johnson LR, editor. Physiology of the gastrointestinal tract. 2nd ed. New York: Raven Press; 1986. p 383.)

calcium ions.[17,18] The most active area of depolarization and repolarization of the ICCs is in the pacemaker area of the stomach located between the fundus and the proximal corpus (Fig. 52.1). The depolarization and repolarization of the ICCs is regenerated and propagated through the network of ICCs in a migrating wave front that moves from the pacemaker region on the greater curve through the corpus and antrum to the pylorus proscribing the pathway of 3 per minute gastric peristaltic contractions and 3 cpm GMA (Figs. 52.1 and 52.2). Excitatory input to the MY-ICC (e.g., cholinergic stimuli, stretch) results in opening of calcium channels and depolarization of the smooth muscle cells with IM-ICC activation to coordinate the contractions of the circular muscle cells in time and space. Thus the ICC networks provide the control of frequency and propagation velocity for the circular muscle contractions that comprise the GMA related to gastric peristalsis waves.

The fundus of the stomach lacks slow waves. The IM-ICCs in the fundus have a role in mechanoreception and act as sensory cells with interconnections to the vagal afferent neurons that innervate the fundus.[19] Fundic IM-ICCs are also innervated by inhibitory vagal neurons that regulate tone in the fundus.[19] Thus the ICCs also participate in the relaxation of fundic tone that occurs during accommodation.

Normal human corpus and antrum have more than 5 ICCs/high-power field (HPF).[20,21] Depletion of ICCs in the corpus-antrum and loss of CD206 macrophages are associated with diabetic gastroparesis (DGP) and idiopathic gastroparesis (IGP).[20–22] Severe depletion of ICCs is also associated with a variety of gastric dysrhythmias ranging from bradygastrias to tachygastrias and conduction defects.[21,23] Patients with DGP and loss of ICCs have more gastric electrical dysrhythmias (tachygastria), more upper GI symptoms, and poorer response to gastric electrical stimulation (GES) compared with patients with normal numbers of ICCs.[23] Interruption of ICC pathways from nondiabetic mechanisms also results in gastric dysrhythmias and ectopic pacemakers that are similar to gastric dysrhythmias found in patients with diabetes.[24] The loss of gastric ICCs in DGP in mice and humans

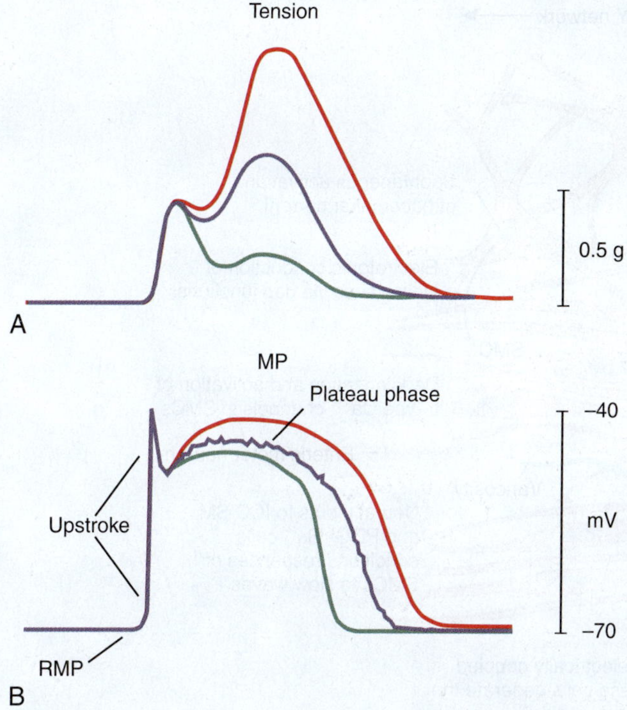

Fig. 52.5 Relationships between smooth muscle contraction (tension) and membrane potential (MP). In these intracellular recordings from antral smooth muscle, the upstroke potential is the rapid depolarization (upstroke) event, followed by the plateau phase. The plateau potentials are associated with the contraction of the smooth muscle cell, as shown in panel (A). Note that an increase in the amplitude of the plateau potentials [*red line* in panel (B)] is associated with greater contractility (tension). During redepolarization to the resting membrane potential (*RMP*), the contraction resolves. (Modified from Sanders KM, Ordog T, Koh SD, Ward SM. Properties of electrical rhythmicity in the stomach. In: Koch KL, Stern RM, eds. *Handbook of Electrogastrography*. New York: Oxford Press; 2004:13–36.)

is related to inflammatory infiltrates of M1 macrophages and increased production of inflammatory mediators such as interleukin-6, whereas M2 macrophages appear to protect ICCs.[25,26]

Nervous System Innervation

As reviewed earlier in Chapter 51, neurons of the ENS populate the stomach wall from the fundus to the pylorus.[27] These neurons are in the myenteric plexuses between the circular muscle and the longitudinal muscle layers. Neurons of the ENS are also located in submucosal and subserosal plexuses. The ENS provides local reflex circuits within the gastric wall as follows: (1) sensory afferent neurons located in the mucosa are linked to (2) interneurons in the myenteric plexus that are linked to (3) efferent neurons that innervate the smooth muscle and glands to perform the gastric secreto-muscular functions.[27] Release of excitatory neurotransmitters such as acetylcholine and substance P stimulates smooth muscle contractions, whereas inhibitory neurotransmitters such as nitric oxide and vasoactive intestinal polypeptide inhibit contractions. These enteric neural circuits within the gastric wall are programmed to modulate peristaltic contractions (in conjunction with ICC activity described earlier) by sequential inhibition of the distal smooth muscle segment and the contraction of the immediate proximal segment of the stomach wall.[28,29] Serotonin in the bowel wall has a primary role in initiating and controlling peristaltic events.[27,28]

Neurons of the ENS are in proximity to the MY-ICCs and IM-ICCs.[30] The ENS neurons provide additional control and modulation of contraction and relaxation of the gastric smooth muscle via cholinergic excitation and nitrergic inhibitory neurotransmission. Neurons of the ENS form gap junctions with MY-ICCs and IM-ICCs and provide crucial neural control that integrates slow wave activity and smooth muscle activity. Thus postganglionic excitatory and inhibitory neurons innervate MY-ICCs to modulate gastric neuromuscular contraction and relaxation and provide chronotropic effects on the slow waves. Ultrastructural abnormalities in gastric neural cell bodies and nerve endings occur in patients with IGP and DGP.[31]

The PNS and SNS modulate gastric neuromuscular activity. The vagus nerve provides the PNS input for the stomach, although approximately 80% of vagal fibers are afferent neurons. The afferent neurons respond to moment-to-moment contraction and relaxation (tone) of the stomach wall.[32] Efferent activity of the vagus nerve increases the release of acetylcholine, which increases the amplitude of gastric contractions and stimulates secretion of gastric acid and pepsin. The SNS innervates gastric smooth muscle with neurons that travel with the splanchnic vasculature. SNS activity generally elicits inhibitory action on the smooth muscle via effects on the myenteric neurons of the ENS.[33]

The release of various hormones, ranging from CCK to gastrin, affects the neuromuscular activity of the stomach. Gut hormones produce their effect on smooth muscle, ICCs, and ENS, as well as vagal efferent or afferent functions. These effects will be characterized under fasted and fed conditions and discussed in more detail later.

Gastric Neuromuscular Activity During Fasting

In the fasting state, electrical and contractile events of the corpus or antrum occur in a highly regular pattern termed the *migrating myoelectrical* (or "motor") *complex*, or MMC.[34] The three phases of the MMC, as described by changes in the pattern of intraluminal contractions, recur approximately every 90–120 minutes. Phase 1 is a period of quiescence wherein little or no contractile activity is recorded. In phase 2 random, irregular contractions occur. Phase 3 of the MMC is a burst of regular, high-amplitude phasic contractions that last from 5 to 10 minutes (Fig. 52.7A). Phase 3 contractions are also termed the "activity front." The activity front migrates from the antrum to the ileum, a journey of 90–120-minute duration. The 3 phases of the MMC occur regularly in the small intestine, although approximately 50% of the phase 3 activity fronts originate in the stomach and then migrate through the small intestine.[35] The MMCs that originate either in the stomach or duodenum travel through the small intestine and terminate in the distal ileum. If fasting continues, then another phase 3 activity front reappears in the antrum or duodenum at the 90–120-minute interval. The high-amplitude, 3-per-minute contractions of phase 3 that develop in the distal antrum empty nondigestible, fibrous foodstuffs that remain in the stomach.

Cyclic contractile activity associated with the onset of phase 3 also has been identified in the lower esophageal sphincter, the sphincter of Oddi, and the gallbladder. The phase 3 contractions correlate with rapid eye movement sleep and are related to a larger system of biological clocks.[36,37] MMCs develop after vagotomy, indicating that nonvagal mechanisms initiate and sustain MMC neuromuscular activity. Motilin is released during the intense phase 3 contractions that occur in the proximal duodenum.

Gastric Neuromuscular Activity After a Meal

Three basic gastric neuromuscular activities occur during and after ingestion of solid foods: (1) receptive relaxation to accommodate the ingested food, (2) trituration of the ingested solid food by

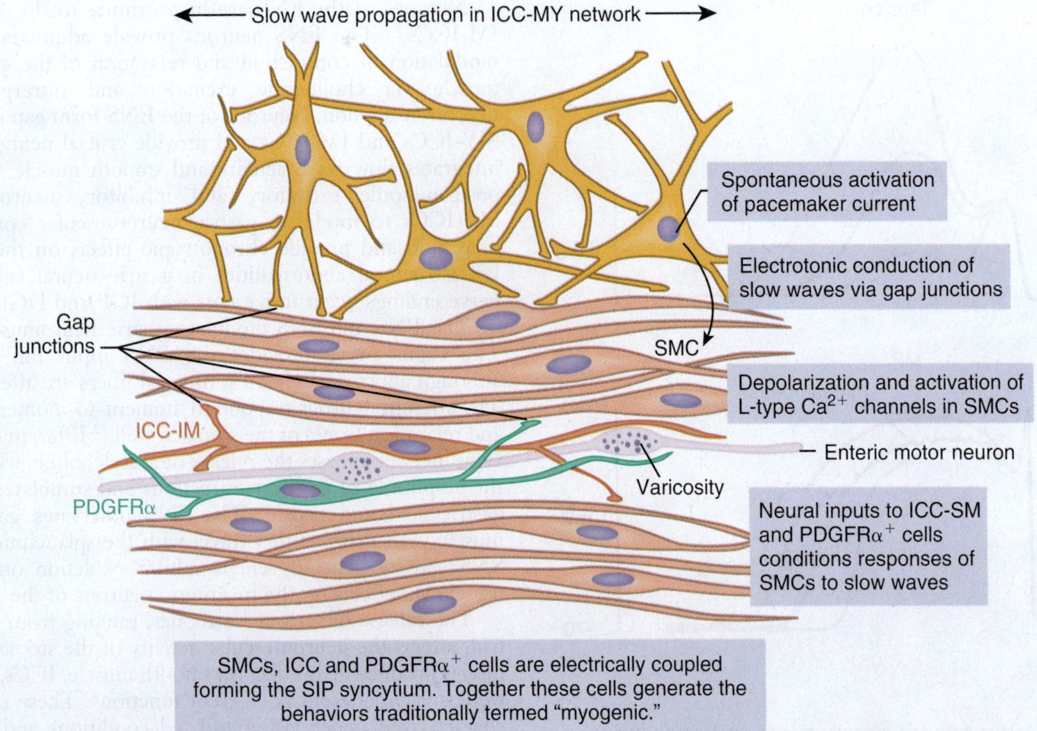

Fig. 52.6 Relationships among interstitial cells of Cajal (*ICCs*), platelet-derived growth factor receptor alpha-positive (*PDGFRα*$^+$) cells, smooth muscle cells (*SMC*) in the circular muscle layer, and motor neurons of the enteric nervous system. ICCs in the region of the myenteric plexus (*ICC-MY*) are pacemaker cells and spontaneously generate slow wave depolarizations. Slow waves conduct to adjacent SMCs via low-resistance junctions (gap junctions) as shown by the *curved arrow*. Depolarization of SMCs leads to activation of L-type calcium channels, Ca^{2+} entry, and contraction of the SMCs coordinated by ICC-intramuscular networks (ICC-IM). Thus slow waves organize the contractile pattern of gastric smooth muscles into a series of phasic and propagating contractions. SMCs do not possess the ionic mechanisms necessary to regenerate slow waves, so the amplitude of slow waves decreases as slow waves conduct from SMC to SMC in a muscle bundle. Active propagation of slow waves from the dominant (i.e., highest frequency) pacemaker along the greater curvature of the gastric corpus to the pyloric sphincter requires continuous coupled networks of ICC-MYs, ICC-IMs, and SMCs. ICC-IMs are ICCs that lie within the circular layer of smooth muscle bundles. The ICC-IMs appear to be important in mediating neurotransmission because they form very close synaptic connections (gap junctions) with the varicose terminals of enteric motor neurons (*short arrows*). Postjunctional neural responses can be conducted from IM-ICCs to muscle bundles. Thus the stimulation of excitatory enteric neurons leads to depolarization of ICC-IMs and increases the contractile responses of SMCs to slow wave depolarizations initiated by the ICC-MY. The stimulation of inhibitory enteric neurons causes hyperpolarization and stabilization of membrane potential and tends to inhibit contractile responses to slow wave depolarization. PDGFRα$^+$ cells are another class of ICCs with distribution similar to ICCs that appear to mediate purinergic neurotransmission and SMC responses. Thus these cells—the SMC, ICC, and PDGFRα$^+$—form a syncytium of SIPs that produces rhythmic, stationary, and propagative contractions (myogenic) events of the stomach.

recurrent corpus-antral peristaltic waves to produce chyme, and (3) antral peristalsis with antropyloroduodenal coordination to empty chyme in small aliquots into the duodenum in a controlled manner for optimal digestion and absorption of the nutrients.

Response to Ingestion of Solid Foods

The neuromuscular work of the stomach in mixing, milling, and emptying food depends upon the physical characteristics, volume, and the fat, protein, and carbohydrate content of the ingested food. For example, 240 minutes of neuromuscular work by the normal stomach is required to empty 90% of a 255-kcal low-fat, egg substitute sandwich.[38] In contrast, only 35 minutes of gastric neuromuscular work is required to empty 70% of a 20-kcal 500-mL soup broth meal that was consumed in 4 minutes.[38] Fig. 52.8 illustrates gastric neuromuscular activity required to receive, mix, and empty a solid meal. The spectrum of gastric work extends from fundic relaxation to gastric peristalsis to antropyloroduodenal coordination, the work that is needed to produce chyme and empty it into the duodenum. Ingestion of food abolishes the fasted state as regular 3-per-minute gastric peristalsis begins in the corpus and antrum to mix the food and then empty the chyme; in the fed state, a pattern of continuous small bowel contractions with short runs of peristalsis over distances of 2–4 cm optimize digestion and absorption of nutrients (see Fig. 52.7B).

Solid food delivered from the esophagus into the fundus is associated with a receptive relaxation of the fundus, the "work" of fundic muscle relaxation. As the fundic smooth muscle relaxes, larger amounts of solid or liquid food are accommodated in the fundus and proximal and distal corpus with little or no increase in intraluminal pressure. Liquids, in contrast, are immediately distributed throughout the antrum and corpus (emptying of liquids is discussed in the next section). Relaxation of the fundus in

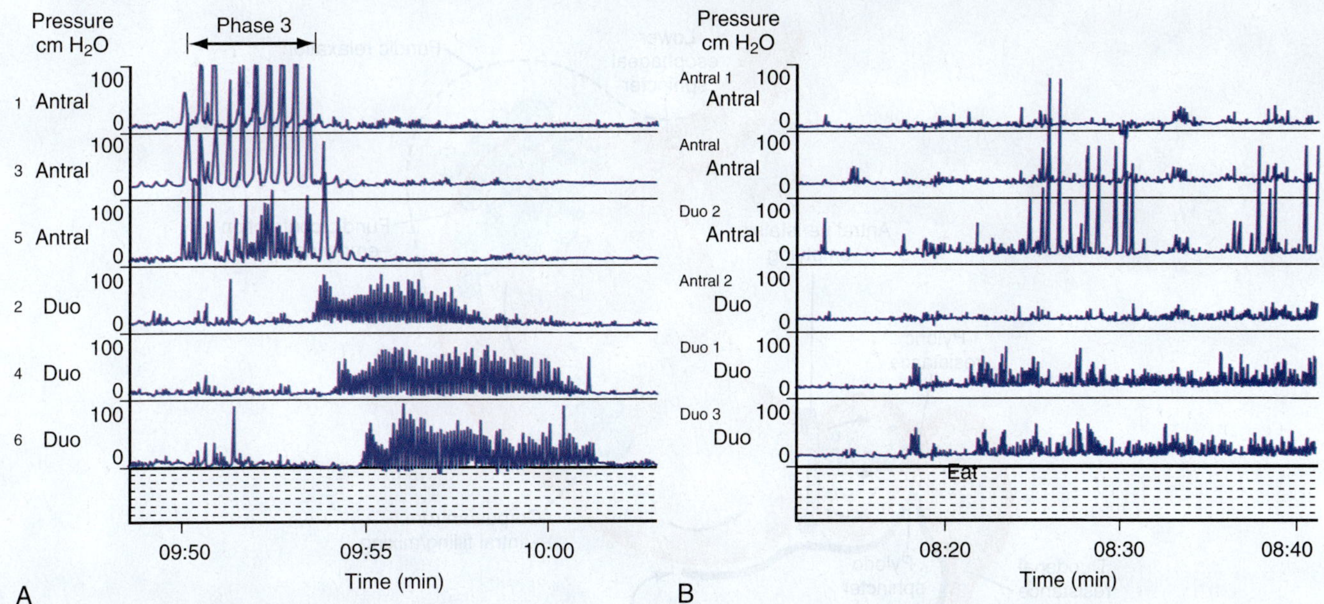

Fig. 52.7 Antroduodenal motor activity in a healthy subject. (A) *Fasted state:* Phase 3 contractions in the antrum (antral) and duodenum (Duo). Intraluminal contractions in the antrum (channels 1, 3, and 5) and the duodenum (channels 2, 4, and 6) are shown. A phase 3 activity front with 3-per-minute antral peristaltic contractions lasting almost 6 minutes is noted in channels 1, 3, and 5. The phase 3 activity front propagates distally and migrates past the duodenal recording ports. The frequency of contractions in the duodenum is approximately 11 or 12 per minute, the same as the frequency of the duodenal slow wave. After completion of the phase 3 contractions, the quiescence of phase 1 and lack of contractions are seen in the antrum. (B) *Fed state:* The subject ingested a standard liquid meal (Ensure). Contractions of variable amplitude are seen in the antrum and a series of relatively low-amplitude, irregular contractions are noted in the duodenum, all of which represent the fed state and are in marked contrast to phase 3 activity during the fasting state shown in panel A. (Modified from Koch KL. The stomach. Manometry. In: Schuster M, Crowell M, Koch KL, eds. *Atlas of Gastrointestinal Motility*. Hamilton, Ontario: BC Decker; 2002:135-150.)

response to ingestion of solid food occurs before the work of trituration in the corpus-antrum and is a vagal nerve–mediated event that requires nitric oxide.[39–41] Fig. 52.9 shows an example of the changes in intragastric volume during relaxation of the fundus and corpus-antrum in response to a liquid caloric meal.[39] Relaxation of the fundus and the stimulation of mechanoreceptors (stretch), mediated through IM-ICCs in the fundic wall, activate vagal afferent neurons and vasovagal reflexes. These reflexes involve the nucleus of the tractus solitarius and efferent neurons from the dorsal motor nucleus of the vagus. Vagal excitatory neurons are inhibited, and the vagal inhibitory neurotransmitters nitric oxide and vasoactive intestinal peptide are released to accomplish receptive relaxation.

Other factors influence the muscle tone of the fundus. Antral distention, duodenal distention, duodenal acidification,[42] intraluminal perfusion of the duodenum with lipid or protein, and colonic distention all decrease fundic tone through various reflexes. The gastric reflex is mediated through an arc initiated by capsaicin-sensitive afferent vagal nerves and is mediated by 5-hydroxytryptamine 3 (5-HT_3), gastrin-releasing peptide, and CCK_A receptors.[43]

Solid foods labeled with technetium are accommodated initially in the fundus and proximal corpus, and by obtaining frequent scintigraphic images, the distribution of the labeled solid meal can be followed over 4 hours using scintigraphic methods.[38] Fig. 52.10 shows that immediately after ingestion of this solid meal, the food is accommodated, and most of the meal is retained in the fundus and proximal corpus. Subsequently, contractions of the fundus press portions of the food into the corpus and antrum for trituration. This early postprandial period of accommodation and trituration that occurs before gastric emptying of the nutrients is termed the *lag phase*. The lag phase may last from 45 to 60 minutes for solid foods, but the duration of the lag depends on the thoroughness of chewing the food, the time required to ingest the meal, and the components of the meal. For a 255-kcal egg substitute test meal that is ingested in a 10-minute period, the lag phase is 30–45 minutes.

Once portions of the meal have been triturated into 1–2-mm particles suspended in gastric juice, a linear phase of gastric emptying of the chyme begins. Recurrent gastric peristaltic waves mix saliva, acid, and pepsin with the chewed food and then mill the food to produce chyme. The normal peristaltic waves occur every 20 seconds, generated by 3-cpm slow waves linked to plateau and action potentials. In healthy subjects approximately 60% of the egg substitute meal has emptied in 2 hours, and more than 90% has emptied at 4 hours (Fig. 52.11).[38]

During the linear phase of gastric emptying, each peristaltic wave empties from 3 to 4 mL of chyme through the open pylorus and into the duodenum.[44] Movement of chyme into the duodenum is usually, but not always, pulsatile due to the systole-like effect of antral peristaltic waves.[44] The volume of chyme delivered into the duodenum by each peristaltic wave is modulated by the configuration of the peristaltic wave (e.g., depth of contraction, length of the peristaltic wave), pressure within the stomach, and resistance to flow provided by the pyloric sphincter and duodenal contractions.[45,46] The gastric peristaltic wave delivers a larger "stroke volume" when the pylorus and the duodenum are relaxed to receive the aliquot of chyme, but the overall rate of calories delivered each minute to the duodenum is consistent at approximately 3–4 kcal/min.[43]

As time elapses after ingestion of the meal, the chewed/swallowed food is continually redistributed from the fundus to the

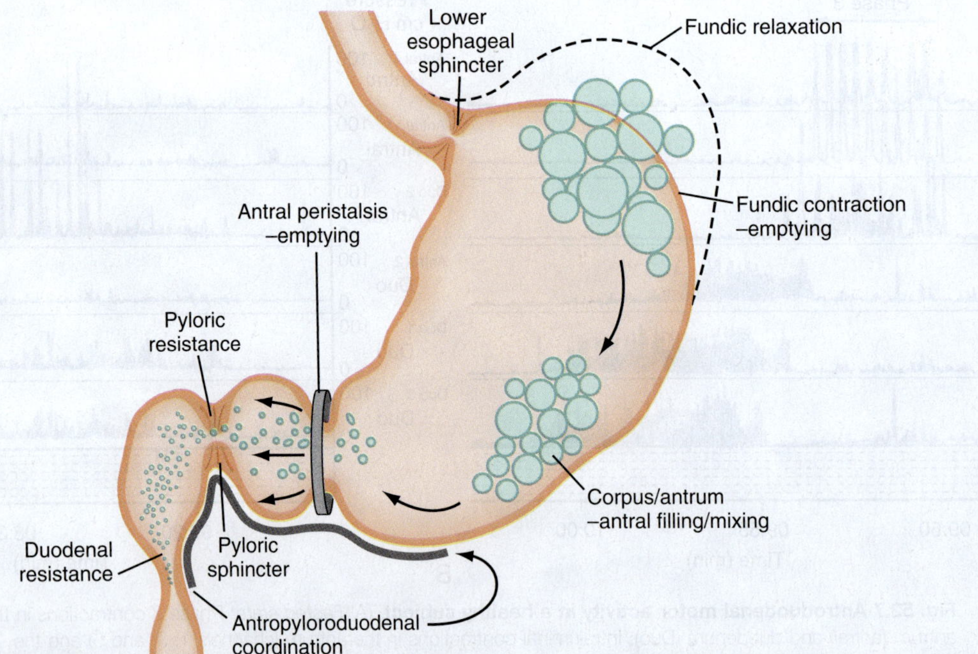

Fig. 52.8 The spectrum of gastric neuromuscular work after the ingestion of a solid meal. To receive the ingested solid foods and accommodate the volume of food without increasing intragastric pressure, the fundic smooth muscle relaxes (receptive relaxation). The fundus then contracts to empty the ingested solid food into the corpus and antrum for trituration and emptying. Recurrent corpus-antral peristaltic waves mill the solids into chyme, which is composed of 1–2-mm solid particles suspended in gastric juice. Antral peristaltic waves, indicated by the ring-like indentation in the antrum, empty 2–4 mL of the chyme through the pylorus and into the duodenal bulb at the slow wave frequency of 3 peristaltic contractions per minute. Antropyloroduodenal coordination indicates efficient emptying of chyme through the pylorus, which modulates flow of the chyme by varying sphincter resistance. Contractions in the duodenum also provide resistance to emptying. (Modified from Koch KL. Physiological basis of electrogastrography. In: Koch KL, Stern RM, eds. *Handbook of Electrogastrography*. New York: Oxford Press; 2004:37–67.)

antrum for trituration. Some gastric peristaltic waves end at various points in the antrum and others end with a terminal antral contraction associated with closure of the pylorus that prevents the emptying of larger food particles or indigestible solids. These terminal antral and pyloric contractions result in delayed emptying of the solid particles in the corpus and antrum. The terminal antrum, the 3–4 cm of antrum immediately proximal to the pylorus, is also where the slow waves have the greatest amplitude and velocity. In this manner, solid food particles that require further trituration are retained and subjected further to the milling effects of the recurrent peristaltic waves.

The intragastric pressure and intraluminal pH values recorded after a healthy subject ingested an egg substitute meal are shown in Fig. 52.12. Approximately 3.5 hours after the solid meal was ingested, high-amplitude contractions (>65 mm Hg) occur just before the pH suddenly increases from 1 to 6 as the wireless motility/pH capsule is emptied from the acidic antrum into the more alkaline environment of the duodenum. After the digestible components of the meal are emptied, strong antral contractions (phase 3–like contractions) empty the capsule from the stomach into the duodenum.[47] Thus fibrous and indigestible materials are emptied by high-amplitude antral contractions, whereas the digestible nutrients in the chyme are emptied earlier by the lower-amplitude peristaltic waves during the linear phase of emptying.[48]

The pylorus modulates the rate of gastric emptying by several mechanisms. Increased pyloric tone and isolated pyloric pressure waves prevent gastric emptying and promote the retention of food for further milling. Pyloric contractions associated with terminal antral contractions are common during the lag phase when trituration is occurring. Once the linear phase of emptying of solids begins, the numbers of isolated pyloric contraction waves diminish as chyme is available for emptying via the gastric peristaltic waves. Neuromuscular dysfunction of the pyloric sphincter is associated with gastroparesis, is more common than previously appreciated, and is reviewed later.

Response to Ingestion of Liquids

The gastric neuromuscular activity required to mix and empty liquids from the stomach is distinctly different from the emptying of solid foods.[39,49,50] Fig. 50.13 shows three-dimensional ultrasound (US) images of the stomach in a healthy subject during the fasting state and 10 minutes after the subject ingested 500 mL of soup.[39] The intragastric volume was approximately 40 mL during fasting and increased to 350 mL 10 minutes after ingestion of the soup, indicating the remarkable relaxation of the smooth muscle of the antrum and corpus (in addition to the fundic relaxation) that was required to accommodate this liquid volume. (In contrast, solid meals are initially accommodated and retained primarily in the fundus and proximal stomach.) Once accommodated, nutrient liquids are emptied into the duodenum in a controlled but more rapid rate compared with solid foods, which require trituration. Noncaloric liquid meals empty without the lag phase in a curve described as monoexponential emptying (Fig. 50.14).[50,51] Caloric-dense liquids, on the other hand, are retained for longer periods in the antrum and are emptied slower than noncaloric liquids. Liquids are emptied from the stomach by a combination of (1) pressure gradients between the stomach and the duodenum that

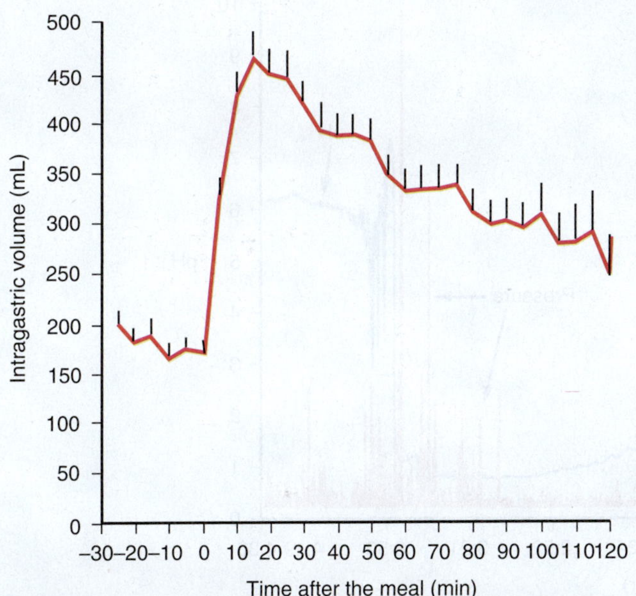

Fig. 52.9 Gastric accommodation of the fundus and proximal stomach in a healthy volunteer after a test meal. The intragastric volume, measured with a barostat balloon, increases from approximately 200 mL to approximately 450 mL during the 20 minutes after the meal is ingested. As the meal is emptied, the volume within the stomach slowly decreases over the 2-hour postprandial period. Relaxation of the proximal stomach and accommodation of the meal volume reflect vagal-mediated receptive relaxation. (From Tack J, Piessevuax H, Coulie B, et al. Role of impaired gastric accommodation to a meal in functional dyspepsia. *Gastroenterology*. 1998;115:1346–1352.)

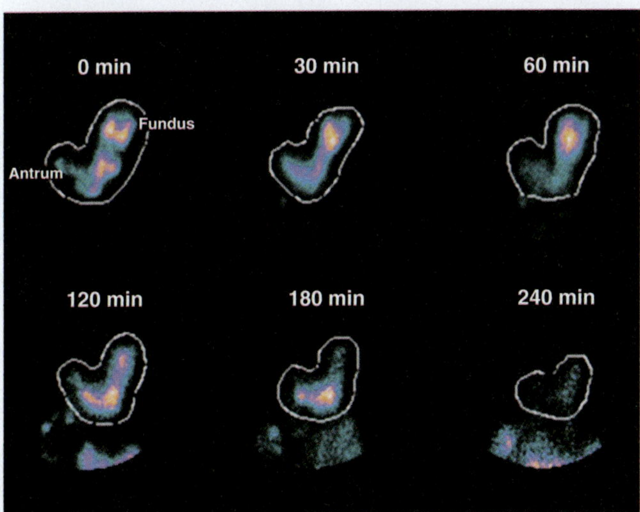

Fig. 52.10 Gastric emptying of an egg sandwich. One-minute scintigraphic images of a radiolabeled 255-kcal substitute egg meal in the stomach at time 0, 30, 60, 120, 180, and 240 minutes after ingestion are shown. The *yellow* and *pink* areas indicate regions of the stomach with higher isotope counts and more food than the other regions. Note the persistence of portions of the meal in the fundus at 120 minutes after ingestion. The meal is slowly redistributed from the fundus to the antrum for trituration and emptying. Only a small amount of the meal remains in the stomach by 240 minutes, and most of the labeled eggs are in the small intestine.

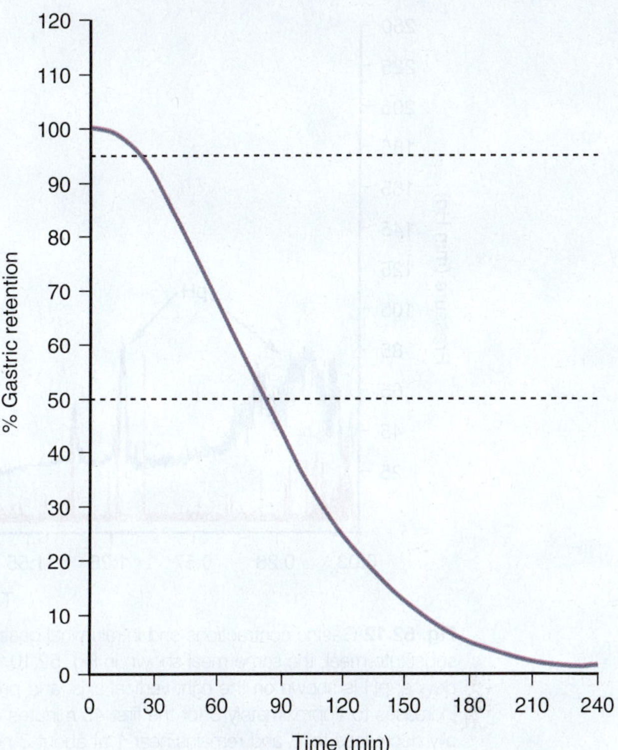

Fig. 52.11 Solid phase gastric emptying curve for 123 subjects after ingestion of a 255-kcal substitute egg meal. Note that only approximately 15% of the eggs are emptied in the first 45 minutes, the lag phase of gastric emptying of this meal. At 90 minutes, approximately 50% of the meal has been emptied and 50% is retained. By 240 minutes, more than 91% of the meal has been emptied. (Modified from Tougas G, Eaker EY, Abell TL, et al. Assessment of gastric emptying using a low fat meal: establishment of international control values. *Am J Gastroenterol*. 2000; 95:1456–1462.)

produce flow of liquid into the duodenum, (2) antral peristaltic contractions that produce a pulsatile pattern of emptying of liquids from the antrum into the duodenum, and (3) duodenogastric reflux events that modify gastric emptying rates.[43,44] From a GMA viewpoint, ingestion of water until the point of fullness induces a brief "frequency dip" followed by return of normal 3-cpm activity recorded noninvasively in the electrogastrogram (EGG) (Fig. 52.15).[52] The rate of gastric emptying of liquids is influenced by the volume, nutrient content, viscosity, and osmolarity of the ingested liquid.[39,45,46,51] These factors affect the neuromuscular activity of the stomach, which ultimately produces the rate of emptying. These factors are discussed later.

REGULATION OF GASTRIC NEUROMUSCULAR ACTIVITY AFTER A MEAL

Gastric emptying rates are regulated to achieve a consistent, regular presentation of calories in the form of chyme to the duodenum to optimize secretion of pancreatic enzymes and bile appropriate for the digestion of the contents of the chyme. Various gastric emptying rates are achieved by variations in the neuromuscular armamentarium of the stomach: fundic relaxation and contraction, the characteristics of gastric peristaltic

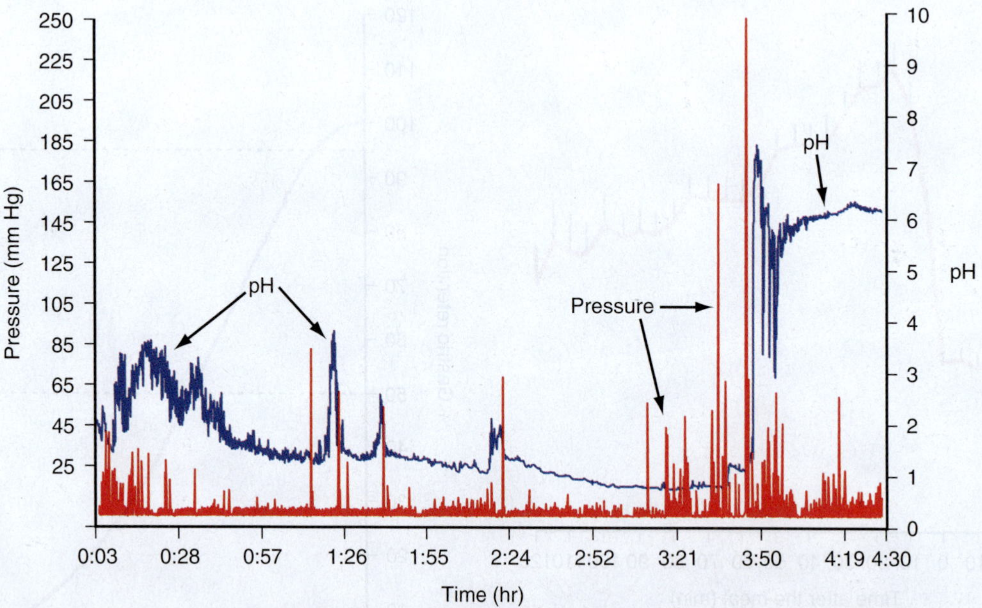

Fig. 52.12 Gastric contractions and intraluminal gastric pH recordings during the emptying of a 255-kcal egg substitute meal, the same meal shown in Fig. 52.10, recorded with an ambulatory capsule pH and motility device; pH is shown on the right vertical axis, and pressure in mm Hg is shown on the left vertical axis. The pH increases to approximately 3 for the first 45 minutes as gastric acid is buffered by the meal. The pH then gradually decreases to 1, and remains near 1 at about 3 hours after ingestion of the meal. Stomach contractions are generally of low amplitude, less than 10 mm Hg after ingestion of the meal. At approximately 3 hours and 40 minutes after the meal, the recorded pH increases abruptly to 7 and then decreases and remains stable at around 6. Prior to the abrupt increase in pH, there is a series of clustered, high-amplitude antral contractions (pressure). These antral contractions empty the capsule from the antrum (pH 1) into the duodenum, where the pH is 6 or more. The contractions that occurred during the 3 hours and 50 minutes required to empty the meal document the neuromuscular work required to triturate and empty this meal in a healthy subject.

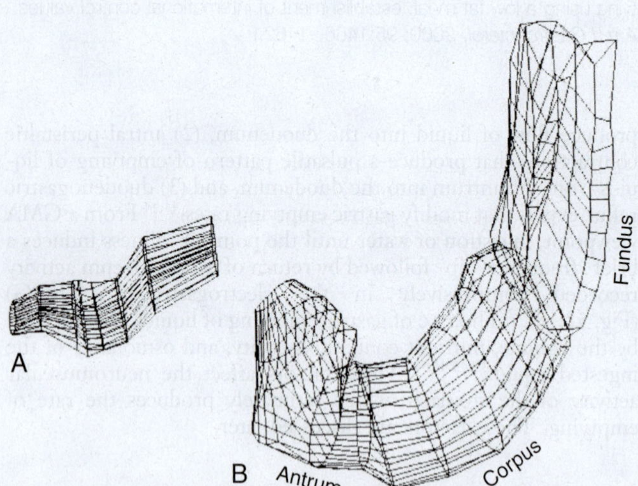

Fig. 52.13 Three-dimensional ultrasound reconstructed images from the stomach before and after a healthy subject ingested a 500-mL soup meal. (A) In the fasted state, the intragastric volume is approximately 38 mL. (B) Ten minutes after ingestion of the meal, the stomach volume is 350 mL. Note that the antrum, corpus, and fundus are now distended, indicating the marked relaxation of the smooth muscle required to accommodate this volume of liquid. (Modified from Gilja OH, Detmer PR, Jong JM, et al. Intragastric distribution and gastric emptying assessed by 3-dimensional ultrasonography. *Gastroenterology*. 1997;113:38–49.)

contractions, temporary suspension of 3-cpm slow waves and the onset of gastric dysrhythmias; the coordination of antropyloroduodenal contractions and duodenal contractions; pyloric sphincter contraction and relaxation; and duodenal contractions that promote duodenogastric reflux. The attributes of a specific meal stimulate the appropriate gastric neuromuscular responses that produce trituration and determine the rate of gastric emptying. Table 52.1 lists gastric neuromuscular factors, meal-related factors, and other factors that modulate the rate of gastric emptying. The rate of gastric emptying is decreased by the temporary occurrence of gastric dysrhythmias, modulation of the amplitude and the propagation distances of antral contractions, enhanced contractions of the pylorus, and reduced antropyloroduodenal coordination.

Meal-related factors that affect gastric emptying include the digestible components of the solids and liquids, fat content (nutrient density), viscosity, acid content, volume, osmolality, and indigestible foodstuffs. For example, foods with high fat content empty slower than foods with high protein or carbohydrate content. TGs are mixed with gastric lipase during the initial intragastric phases of digestion and are broken down to fatty acids and monoglycerides or diglycerides before emptying into the duodenum.[53] The duodenum is exquisitely sensitive to diet-derived fatty acids. Longer chain fatty acids (>C12) exposed to the mucosa of the duodenum result in the release of CCK. CCK relaxes fundic tone, decreases antral contraction, and increases pyloric tone, all of which result in delay in gastric emptying. In contrast, short- and medium-chain fatty acids (<C12) do not have these neuromuscular effects on gastric

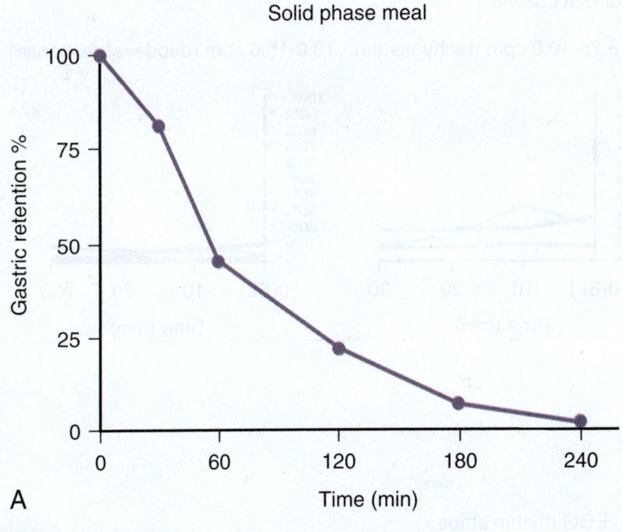

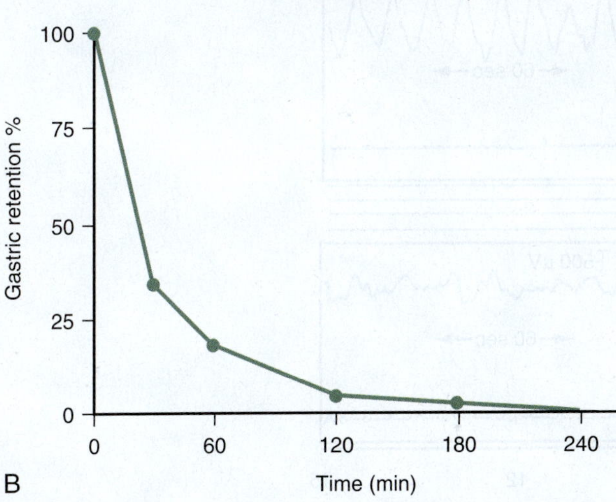

Fig. 52.14 Gastric emptying of a mixed liquid and solid meal in healthy subjects who ingested 300 mL of radiolabeled water with two radiolabeled eggs and toast. (A) Emptying rate for the solid phase of the meal. A short lag phase is noted before the linear phase of emptying, and by 60 minutes approximately 55% of the meal is emptied (45% is retained). The lag phase may be shortened if the subject has taken a relatively long time to eat the meal or the solids require little trituration. (B) Emptying rate for the liquid phase of the meal. Approximately 80% of the water is emptied (20% is retained) at 60 minutes, as the liquid is rapidly distributed throughout the antrum and corpus. This is considered a monoexponential liquid emptying curve. (Modified from Maurer AH, Parkman HP, Knight LC, Fisher RS. Scintigraphy. In: Schuster M, Crowel M, Koch, KL, eds. *Atlas of Gastrointestinal Motility*. Hamilton, Ontario: BC Decker; 2002:171–184.)

emptying rates.[46,54] CCK released from the duodenum also activates CCK_A receptors on vagal afferent neurons with synapses in the nucleus tractus solitaries.[55] Neurons from the nucleus tractus solitarius ascend to the periventricular nucleus of the hypothalamus that participate in mechanisms of satiation, and descending vagal efferent neurons from the dorsal motor nucleus of the vagus inhibit gastric emptying and maintain fundic relaxation. The sensitivity of the duodenal mucosa to fat and other nutrients led to the concept of duodenal tasting and duodenal brake, sensorimotor events that modulate gastric emptying of nutrients.[56,57]

TABLE 52.1 Factors That Modulate the Gastric Emptying Rate

Factors	Effect on Gastric Emptying Rate
Gastric Neuromuscular	
Tachygastria	Delay
Decreased fundic accommodation	Acceleration
Increased fundic accommodation	Delay
Antral hypomotility	Delay
Pylorospasm	Delay
Antroduodenal dyscoordination	Delay
Meal Related	
Volume	Proportional to meal volume
Increased acidity	Delay
Increased osmolarity	Delay
Nutrient density: fat > protein > carbohydrate	Delay
Tryptophan	Delay
Undigestible fibers	Delay
Small Intestinal	
Fatty acids in duodenum	Delay ("duodenal tasting," "duodenal brake")
Fatty acids in ileum	Delay "ileal brake"
Colonic	
Constipation, IBS	Delay
Other	
Hyperglycemia	Delay
Hypoglycemia	Acceleration
Illusory self-motion (vection)	Delay

Monosaccharides in the duodenum stimulate the release of incretins such as glucagon-like polypeptide-1, which promotes insulin secretion to match increasing postprandial blood glucose levels and decreases antral contractions.[58,59] To harmonize the relationships between glucose absorption, glycemia, and insulin secretion, the gastric emptying of carbohydrates is highly regulated.[60,61] Hyperglycemia decreases antral contractions and increases gastric dysrhythmias, a "physiologic" gastric dysrhythmia that decreases the rate of gastric emptying (Fig. 52.16).[62,63] Hyperglycemia increases fundic compliance and decreases sensations related to fundic distention.[64,65] Blood glucose levels greater than 220 mg/dL result in decreased antral contractions, decreased gastric emptying, and induced gastric dysrhythmias,[62] all of which are gastric neuromuscular activities that reduce gastric emptying and reduce further exposure of the duodenum to nutrients. Hypoglycemia episodes are also associated with delayed emptying in patients with insulin-dependent diabetes.[65]

The interaction between nutrients in the lumen and the regulation of the rate of gastric emptying continues in the later postprandial period as digestion and absorption of nutrients occur throughout the small intestine. For example, if diet-derived fatty acids or carbohydrates reach the lumen of the ileum, the so-called ileal break is activated, and gastric emptying is delayed. Infusion of nutrients into the lumen of the ileum delays gastric emptying.[66]

Regulation of stomach emptying also is achieved by vagus nerve and splanchnic nerve activity that modulates the neuromuscular activities of the stomach described earlier. Vagal afferent nerves "monitor" neuromuscular function in the stomach moment by moment, and interactions between afferent vagal nerve activity and the nucleus tractus solitarius and synapses with the efferent vagal nerve output from the dorsal motor nucleus produce an ongoing

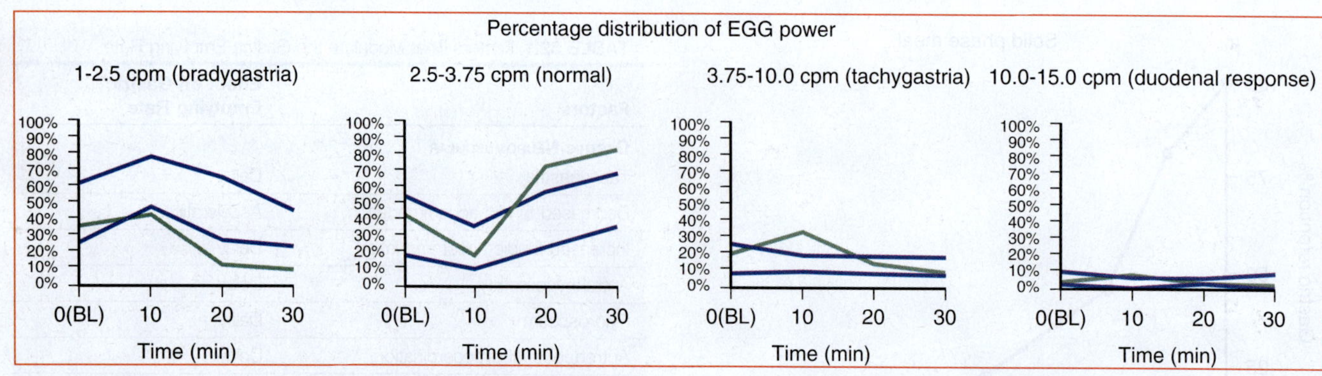

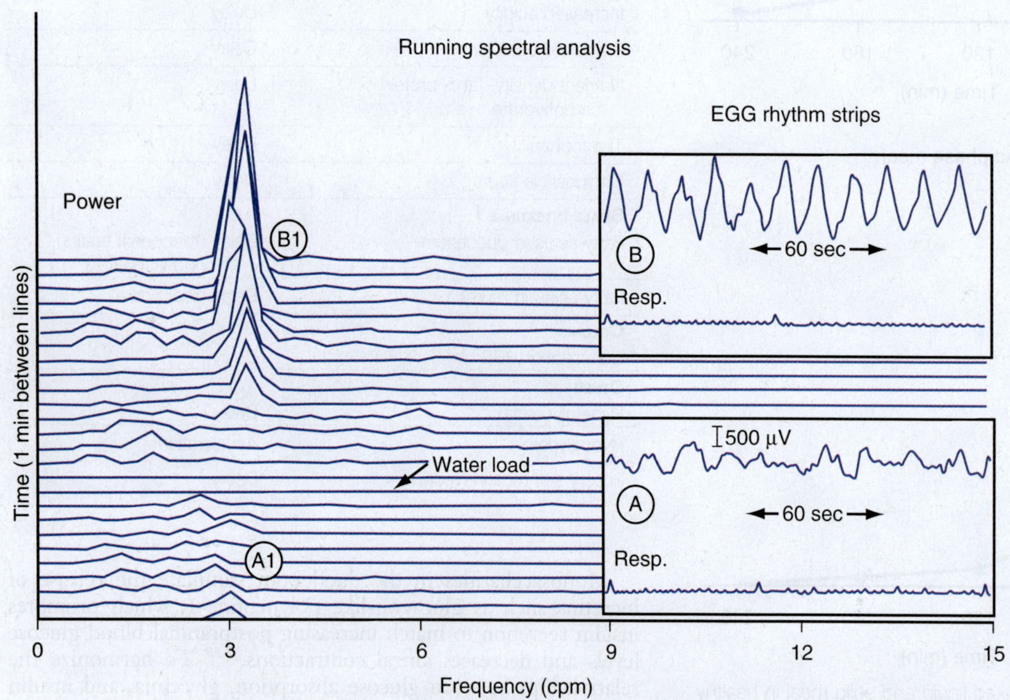

Fig. 52.15 Running spectral analysis of the electrogastrogram (EGG) signal and EGG rhythm strips before and after ingestion of a water load in a healthy subject. The X-axis shows the frequencies in the EGG signal in cycles per minute (cpm). The Y-axis indicates time, and the peaks (or Z-axis) indicate the power of the frequencies contained in the EGG signal. The baseline EGG rhythm strip (A) shows 3-cpm activity. The regularity and the amplitude of the 3-cpm EGG signal is increased (B) after the subject ingested 750 mL of water (*water-load arrow*) over a 5-minute period. The running spectral analysis shows relatively low-power 3-cpm peaks at baseline (A1). After ingestion of the water load, the peaks initially disappear (the frequency "dip"), and then 3-cpm peaks emerge and are prominent until the end of the 30-minute recording (B1). This is a normal gastric myoelectrical response to the filling of the stomach with water and the subsequent emptying of the water. The 4 graphs in the *insert* show the percentage distribution of EGG power in the 4 relevant frequency ranges during baseline (*BL*) and the 10, 20, and 30 minutes after the ingestion of the water by the subject (*green lines*). Normal ranges are shown by *blue lines*. Note the initial decrease in the percentage of normal EGG activity (2.5–3.75 cpm) 10 minutes after ingestion of the water (the frequency dip), followed by increased percentages in the 3-cpm normal range 20–30 minutes after ingestion of the water. *Resp*, Respiratory activity. (Modified from Koch KL. Physiological basis of electrogastrography. In: Koch KL, Stern RM, eds. *Handbook of Electrogastrography*. New York: Oxford Press; 2004:37–67.)

interaction of CNS excitatory and inhibitory effects on the stomach. Gastric emptying is delayed during stress. Corticotrophin-releasing factor plays a role in the mediation of stress and inhibits gastric emptying through central dopamine$_1$ and dopamin$_2$ and vasopressin pathways in the periventricular nucleus.[67] Other factors that affect the rate of gastric emptying not already mentioned include rectocolonic distention, nausea and vomiting of pregnancy, and vection-induced motion sickness.[68] Stimulation of various areas in the CNS affects gastric neuromuscular function. Illusory self-motion (vection) induces antral hypomotility, tachygastria, and decreased gastric emptying.[68,69] A series of studies using the experience of illusory self-motion, a unique CNS sensory stimulation, showed that the onset of nausea was associated with tachygastria and increased levels of plasma vasopressin.[69,70]

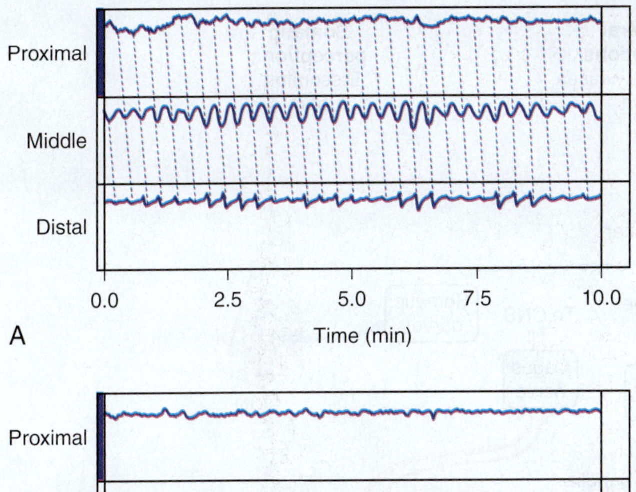

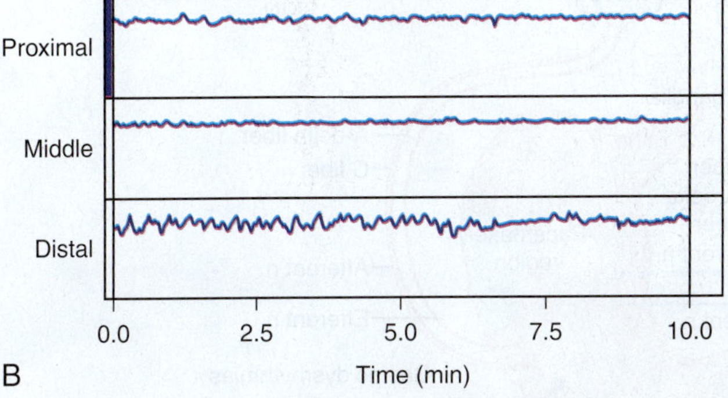

Fig. 52.16 Electrical recordings from electrodes secured to the mucosa of the proximal, middle, and distal antrum in a healthy subject. (A) 3-cpm electrical slow waves in the proximal, middle, and distal electrode leads. The slow waves are propagated in an aborad direction as indicated by the *dotted lines*. (B) Disruption of propagation and the onset of a 5–6-cpm tachygastria in the distal lead during hyperglycemia (glucose clamping), with a blood glucose level of 240 mg/dL. (Modified from Coleski R, Hasler WL. Coupling and propagation of normal dysrhythmic gastric slow waves during acute hyperglycemia in healthy humans. *Neurogastroenterol Motil.* 2009;21:492–499.)

Gender affects the gastric emptying rate of a standard meal. Gastric emptying is significantly slower in healthy women compared with men.[71] Gender differences in gastric emptying rates may be related to fluctuations in sex hormones, but phases of the menstrual cycle (variations in estradiol and progesterone concentrations) have not shown consistent relationships with emptying measurements.[72] The rate of gastric emptying increases as body mass index rises, a relationship that may be relevant to the onset and maintenance of obesity.

GASTRIC SENSORY ACTIVITIES

Free nerve endings in the stomach act as polymodal sensory receptors that respond to light touch or pressure, acid, and other chemical stimuli. Afferent neurons within the stomach are termed *intrinsic primary afferent neurons*, or IPANs.[73] Cell bodies of IPANs reside in the submucosal or the myenteric plexus areas of the stomach wall. IPANs may be activated by serotonin release from local enterochromaffin cells.[27,74] The afferent information in the IPANs is used in local reflexes and provides input to vagal and splanchnic afferent neurons for vagovagal and spinal reflexes, respectively, to subserve transmission of visceral sensory information to CNS centers. Vagal afferent neurons whose cell bodies reside in the nodose ganglia connect with the nucleus of the tractus solitarius and second-order neurons connect with a higher center of the hypothalamus, and some inputs reach the cortex, where they are consciously perceived as visceral sensations (stomach emptiness or fullness) or symptoms such as nausea or abdominal pain (Fig. 52.17).

From the SNS, splanchnic or spinal primary afferent neurons in the gastric wall mediate pain sensations. Cell bodies of these neurons lie in the dorsal horn of the spinal cord with second-order neurons that ascend via the spinothalamic and spinoreticular tracks in the dorsal columns. Sensory neurons are thin, myelinated A-delta or unmyelinated C fibers. Spinal afferents include a population of unmyelinated C fibers. Capsaicin-sensitive unmyelinated fibers contain neuropeptides such as calcitonin gene–related peptide, vasoactive intestinal peptide, somatostatin, substance P, and neurokinin A. These fibers are the primary route of transmission for various pain stimuli from the gut to the CNS. These nerve fibers may respond to inflammatory mediators that also awaken "silent" nociceptive fibers.[75]

In addition to interacting with IPANs, vagal afferent axons have multiple connections with the enteric neurons and innervate the circular muscle fiber bundles via connections with ICCs.[74] Vagal afferent neurons are also sensitive to chemostimuli via mucosal neurons and mechanosensitive neurons and ICCs in the muscle layers. CCK receptors on vagal afferent neurons are primarily activated by physiologic mechanical and chemical stimuli from the stomach during fasting and fed conditions. These vagal afferents mediate the sensory response to intraluminal acid and fat. Acid may have a direct action on the nerve endings themselves.[42]

Nausea is a common sensation that is often attributable to stomach neuromuscular dysfunction.[76] During the illusion of self-motion, gastric dysrhythmias develop as healthy individuals report nausea.[77] Plasma vasopressin levels increase in the subjects who develop nausea but do not increase in those who experience no nausea.[78] This brain-gut, gut-brain interaction during illusory self-motion illustrates the temporal relationships between the onset of gastric dysrhythmias in the periphery and the acute, severe nausea experience of the subject. Similarly, the acute distention of the antrum, but not the fundus, with a balloon induces nausea sensations and gastric dysrhythmias in healthy individuals.[79] These studies show that gastric dysrhythmias originate in the antrum in humans and that stretch of the antral wall is another mechanism that elicits gastric dysrhythmias and nausea sensations from the stomach. Distention of the gastric antrum and corpus by the water-load test (rather than a balloon) also elicits gastric dysrhythmias and nausea in patients with functional dyspepsia (FD).[52]

THE STOMACH AND THE REGULATION OF FOOD INTAKE, HUNGER, AND SATIETY

Hunger is a basic human drive, a stressful condition that is eliminated or reduced by the ingestion of food. Hunger is also described as an uncomfortable "emptiness" of the stomach. The ingestion of food elicits relaxation of the stomach musculature (receptive relaxation) and accommodation of the physical volume of the meal; as these gastric neuromuscular events occur, hunger disappears and the comfortable, postprandial sensations of stomach fullness are experienced.

The volume of food ingested suppresses hunger and stimulates the sense of fullness more than the calorie content of the meal.[80,81] Infusion of nutrients into the stomach induces a greater intensity of fullness or satiety compared with infusion of the same nutrients into the duodenum. The suppression of hunger is greater when nutrients are taken by mouth, indicating that CNS, oropharyngeal, and gastric neuromuscular factors are integrated to produce the comforts of normal postprandial stomach fullness.[82]

Healthy individuals usually eat until they are reasonably full. The physiologic attributes of postprandial fullness are not completely known, but the physical stretch on the stomach walls

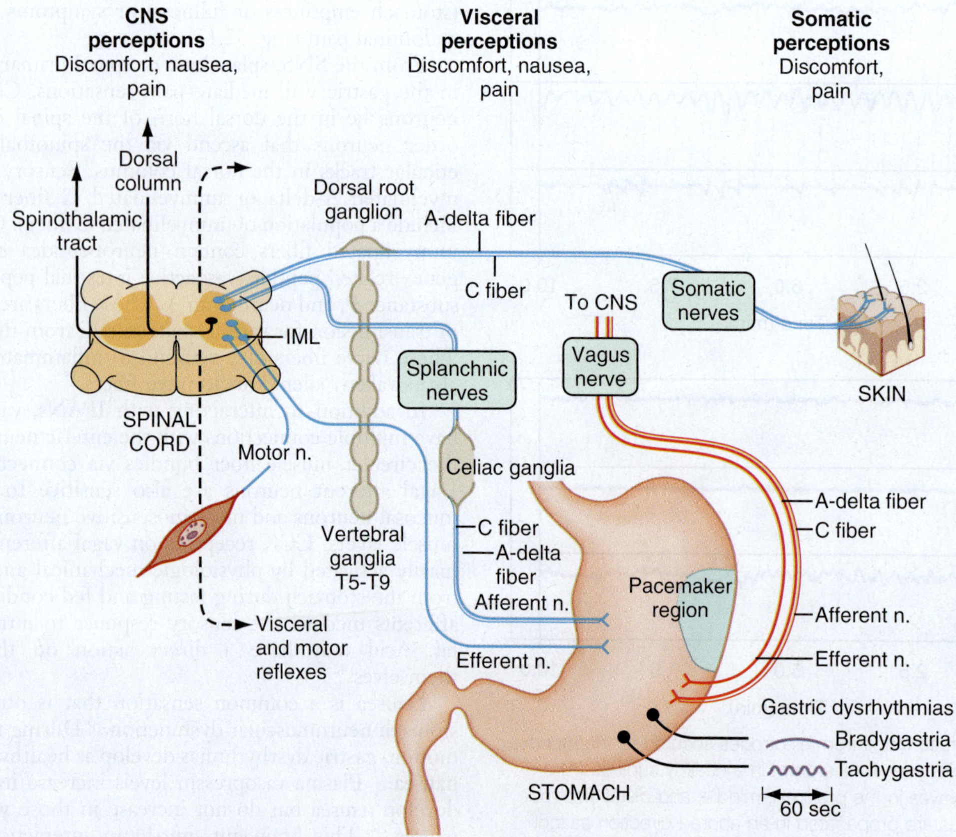

Fig. 52.17 Afferent and efferent neural connections between the stomach and CNS. The vagus nerve contains afferent nerves with A-delta and C pain fibers with cell bodies in the nodose ganglia and connections to the nucleus tractus solitarius (not shown). Low-threshold mechanoreceptors and chemoreceptors stimulate visceral sensations such as gastric emptiness or fullness and symptoms such as nausea and discomfort. These stimuli are mediated through vagal pathways and become conscious perceptions of visceral sensations if sensory inputs reach the cortex. The splanchnic nerves also contain afferent nerves with A-delta and C fibers that synapse in the celiac ganglia with some cell bodies in the vertebral ganglia (T5–T9). Interneurons in the white rami in the dorsal horn of the spinal cord cross to the dorsal columns and spinothalamic tracts and ascend to sensory areas of the medulla oblongata. These splanchnic afferent fibers are thought to mediate high-threshold stimuli for visceral pain. In contrast to visceral sensations, somatic nerves such as those from the skin carry sensory information via A-delta and C fibers through the dorsal root ganglia and into the dorsal horn and then through dorsal columns and spinothalamic tracts to cortical areas of somatic representation. Changes in gastric electrical rhythm, excess amplitude contractions, or stretch on the gastric wall are peripheral mechanisms that elicit changes in afferent neural activity (via vagal and/or splanchnic nerves) that may reach consciousness to be perceived as visceral perceptions (symptoms) emanating from the stomach. *IML*, Intermediolateral nucleus; *n*, nerve.

(and changes in intragastric pressure) induced by ingestion of food and the secretion of gastric juice are in part responsible.[80,81] Subjects experience a dramatic change from the sensation of stomach emptiness at baseline to the sensation of stomach fullness after ingesting water over a 5-minute period. The average volume of water ingested to achieve fullness is 600 mL; in contrast, patients with FD ingest, on average, only 350 mL to feel full, indicating a disturbance in stomach wall relaxation and/or wall tension.[52] Similarly, fullness and satiety can be achieved by ingesting a nutrient drink until achieving maximum tolerated satiety.[83] The presence of acid or nutrients in the duodenum or an elevated blood glucose level decreases the stomach wall tension.[84,85]

The ingestion of a solid meal initially elicits fundic relaxation, and little emptying of the food occurs during the lag phase. Sensations of fullness continue during the lag phase when the food is being triturated. Once the linear phase of gastric emptying begins, there is a progressive perception of decreasing stomach fullness and increasing stomach emptiness over time. Four or five hours after a solid meal, the stomach is indeed empty, and the healthy individual feels hungry once again.

The physiologic mechanisms of hunger and satiety (and stomach emptiness and fullness) are under intense investigation. In the fasting state plasma motilin levels increase during the phase 3 of the MMC, but correlations between the sensation of hunger and increases of motilin or onset of phase 3 have not been described. As discussed in Chapters 51 and 53, ghrelin is a 28-amino acid peptide secreted from endocrine cells of the oxyntic glands in the gastric fundus.[86] Ghrelin levels also increase in the plasma during fasting (hunger) and stimulate food intake, probably acting via vagal afferent nerves.[87] Orexins or appetite-stimulating peptides are synthesized by neurons in the lateral hypothalamus, promote food intake, and stimulate gastric contractility (in the rat) by actions on the dorsal motor nucleus of the vagus with projections to the gastric fundus and corpus.[88] After an ingestion of food, ghrelin levels decrease.[89]

Other hormones are candidates for important roles in the sensation of fullness or satiety, and these hormones are released after the ingestion of meals. CCK is released from the duodenal mucosa exposed to fatty acids. CCK receptors participate in fullness and nausea sensations elicited by intraduodenal lipid and gastric distention.[90,91] Leptin is synthesized in the stomach and released after food ingestion; circulating leptin reduces food intake via CNS regulation of the arcuate nucleus.[92] Glucagon-like polypeptide-1 enhances fullness after a standard meal, reduces antral motility, and increases gastric volume.[59,93] Apolipoprotein A-IV is released from the small intestine during absorption of TGs and decreases food intake and gastric motility, in part, via CCK and vagal afferent pathways.[94] Polypeptide-YY is released from the ileocolonic area after meals and is an important mediator of the "ileal brake" effect[98] and appetite suppression.[95,96]

DEVELOPMENTAL ASPECTS OF GASTRIC NEUROMUSCULAR FUNCTION

The brain and these gut hormones are clearly linked in the regulation of food intake and the regulation of gastric neuromuscular activity that produces stomach emptying.[59,97] The cephalic phase of gastric physiology is well known but has not been reexplored for many years. The sight, smell, and taste of food stimulate central vagal efferent activity that increases gastric acid secretion, gastric contractility, and increases 3-cpm GMA.[98–100] Sham feeding, during which the subject chews and spits out the test meal rather than swallowing it, elicits the cephalic-vagal reflex. Sham feeding a warm hot dog on a bun elicits enhanced 3-cpm activity on the EGG, whereas sham feeding a cold tofu dog, a food that the subjects considered disgusting, resulted in blunted or no increase in the normal 3-cpm myoelectrical activity (Fig. 52.18).[100] Thus sensory, and emotional attributes of food during the cephalic phase of ingestive behavior also affect the neuromuscular activity of the stomach.

DEVELOPMENTAL ASPECTS OF GASTRIC NEUROMUSCULAR FUNCTION

Gastric peristalsis appears between 14 and 23 weeks of gestation. Grouped or clustered peristaltic waves are evident by 24 weeks.[101] The neuroregulatory mechanisms responsible for the coordination of antropyloroduodenal motility in gastric emptying are well developed by 30 weeks of gestation.[102] EGG recordings show normal 3-cpm activity in preterm infants delivered at 35 weeks that are similar to EGG signals recorded in full-term infants.[103,104] On the other hand, EGG recordings from premature infants (<35 weeks' gestation) showed considerable tachygastria.[103] GMA matures further over the first 6–24 months of life and achieves full adult values by the end of the first decade.[105]

The development of ICCs has been studied intensely because of the interest in gastric electrical rhythmicity, smooth muscle contractions, and gastric dysrhythmias. Labels for the tyrosine kinase receptor (c-Kit) and the availability of knock-out mice lacking c-Kit have led to increased understanding of the development of ICCs.[106] The ICCs demonstrate differential development, with c-Kit expression on ICCs in the MY-ICCs developing before birth, whereas ICCs in the deep muscular plexus (IM-ICCs) develop after birth.[107] ENS and ICC networks are not fully developed and are poorly coupled at birth, but the progressive maturity of gastric rhythmicity and contractility occur during perinatal development.[103,104] The ENS and ICCs in the deep muscular plexus are closely related, whereas ICCs in the myenteric plexus can develop normally in the absence of the ENS.[107] Loss of ICCs in the pylorus is associated with a loss of the inhibitory neural activity that may contribute to the development of pyloric stenosis in infants (see Chapter ___).[108]

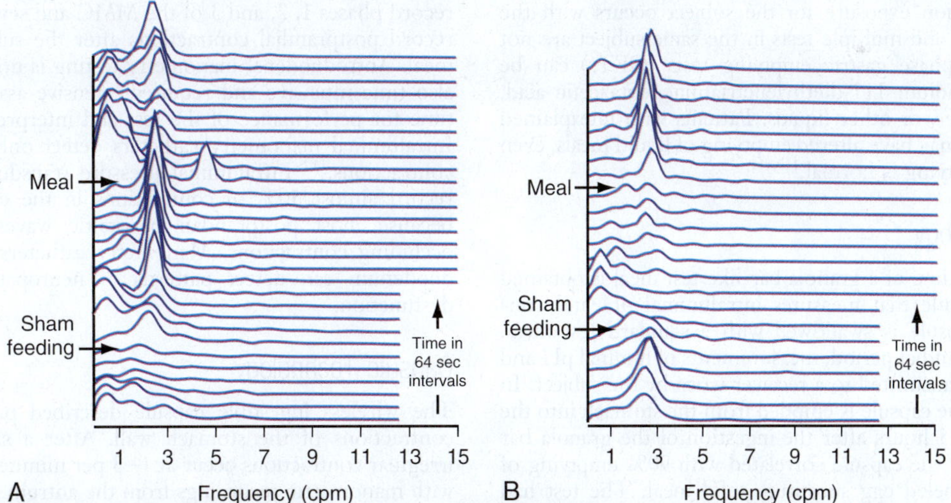

Fig. 52.18 Gastric myoelectrical response to sham feeding with tasty food (A) and "disgusting" food (B). (A) Running spectral analysis (RSA) of the electrogastrogram (EGG) signal recorded while a healthy subject chewed a warm hot dog and spit it out into a paper bag (sham feeding). The increase in amplitude of the peaks in the normal 3-cpm range during sham feeding is the normal response. "Meal" indicates the actual ingestion of a hot dog. (B) RSA of the EGG recorded while a healthy subject chewed a cold tofu dog and spit it out (sham feeding). The subject felt "disgusted" during the sham feeding effort. Note the lack in increase of 3-cpm peaks during sham feeding the tofu dog compared with (A). On both days, the subject then ingested a warm hot dog on a bun at "Meal"; note the subsequent increase in peaks at 3 cpm. (Modified from Stern RM, Crawford HE, Stewart WR, et al. Sham feeding. Cephalic-vagal influences on gastric myoelectric activity. *Dig Dis Sci*. 1989;34:521–527.)

ASSESSMENT OF GASTRIC NEUROMUSCULAR FUNCTION

Gastric Emptying Rate

Clinical tests currently approved by the FDA to assess gastric neuromuscular function are scintigraphy tests to measure the rate of gastric emptying, the capsule motility device to measure gastric emptying, and EGG devices to measure GMA before and after provocative test meals. These tests provide objective assessments of different aspects of the neuromuscular activity of the stomach in health and disease. Results of gastric emptying and GMA tests provide objective diagnoses of gastroparesis and gastric dysrhythmias and provide rational basis for treatments.

Scintigraphy

Test meals labeled with radioisotope are available to assess the rate of gastric emptying. The seminal solid phase gastric emptying protocol was a multinational study that used a 255-kcal technetium-99m (^{99m}Tc)-labeled egg substitute with bread and jam as the standard meal.[38] Scans were obtained for 1 minute immediately after ingestion of the meal and at 30, 60, 120, 180, and 240 minutes in 123 healthy individuals. Delayed gastric emptying was defined as greater than 60% retention of the meal at 120 minutes and greater than 9% retention at 240 minutes. The 4-hour emptying test was superior to the 2-hour test because almost 20% of patients with suspected gastroparesis had normal emptying at 2 hours but abnormal emptying at 4 hours.[109] This test remains the standard assessment of the rate of gastric emptying in clinical practice.

Pitfalls in the scintigraphic method for solid-phase gastric emptying studies include both improper binding of the isotope with the test meal, which results in rapid or normal emptying, and the continuance of medications that may stimulate (e.g., metoclopramide) or inhibit (e.g., narcotics, anticholinergic agents) gastric smooth muscle contractions. These medications should be stopped 5–7 days before all gastric neuromuscular tests, if possible. Radiation exposure for the subject occurs with the scintigraphic tests, and multiple tests in the same subject are not advisable. Liquid-phase gastric emptying tests (GETs) can be performed with indium 111-diethylenetriaminepentaacetic acid, ^{99m}Tc-labeled water, or other liquids. Patients with unexplained nausea symptoms may have altered emptying of liquid meals, even if solid phase emptying is normal.[110,111]

Capsule Technology

Gastric emptying time of a granola bar-like test meal is obtained from a small capsule that measures intraluminal pH and contractions. The capsule is swallowed with a standard test meal. During the postprandial period, measurements of luminal pH and contractions are transmitted to a receiver worn by the subject. In healthy subjects, the capsule is emptied from the stomach into the duodenum within 5 hours after the ingestion of the granola bar meal. Emptying of the capsule correlated with 90% emptying of the technetium-labeled egg substitute solid meal. The test had very good sensitivity and specificity in detecting gastroparesis.[112]

Breath Tests

Breath tests indirectly reflect gastric emptying of solid and liquid test meals. The solid meals are labeled with 13C and include 13C octanoic acid, 13C acetate, or 13C Spirulina platensis. The 13C octanoic acid breath test has been performed in many experimental protocols and is used widely in Europe for research and clinical studies.[113] The 13C-labeled food is emptied from the stomach and absorbed in the small intestine. The labeled nutrients are metabolized in the liver to $13CO_2$, excreted in the lungs, and detected in breath samples. Breath samples are collected 45, 90, 120, 150, and 180 minutes after the meal in the 13C Spirulina test. 13C is a stable isotope with no radiation risks. The 13C breath tests are generally comparable to scintigraphy.[114] Pitfalls include spurious results in patients with malabsorptive conditions, liver diseases, or lung diseases that may preclude normal oxidation and excretion of the 13C-labeled foods.

Ultrasound

Transabdominal US techniques are used to measure antral diameter and antropyloroduodenal function.[115] Three-dimensional US methods show the intragastric distribution of the test meal and regional variations in gastric volume.[39] The technique is ideal with a liquid meal. The clinical application is limited by the high level of expertise required by the US operators.

CT and MRI

These two techniques have been used to measure gastric emptying and demonstrate intragastric distribution of test meals. CT and MRI technologies offer unique anatomic and functional views of the stomach in the fasting and postprandial periods.[116] Sequential antral contractions can be visualized. Because of expense and availability, these techniques are not used in clinical practice.

Gastric Contractions

Antroduodenal Manometry

Antroduodenal manometry is an invasive technique wherein a solid-state catheter is placed either through the nose or the mouth and advanced to a position where the proximal transducers are in the distal antrum and the distal transducers are in the duodenum.[36] Placement of the catheter requires endoscopic or fluoroscopic aid. The recordings typically last for several hours to record phases 1, 2, and 3 of the MMC and several more hours to record postprandial contractions after the subject ingests a test meal. Antroduodenal manometry testing is not only invasive but also time intensive and requires extensive assistant or physician time for performance of the test and interpretation of the data. Intraluminal manometry catheters detect only lumen-occluding contractions.[117] Intraluminal pressure transducer devices fail to record almost 50% of contractions in the corpus and antrum because most postprandial peristaltic waves are not lumen-occluding contractions. Manometry catheters positioned in the duodenum can detect patterns of neuropathic or myopathic dysfunction.

Capsule Technology

The wireless ingestible capsule described previously measures contractions of the stomach wall. After a standard test meal, irregular contractions occur at 1–3 per minute and are consistent with manometric recordings from the antrum.[118] Several minutes of sustained high-amplitude, antral contractions occur prior to the emptying of the capsule into the duodenum and some patterns are consistent with phase 3–like contractions recorded by antroduodenal manometry. In patients with gastroparesis, capsule studies showed a decreased motility index during the 20–30 minutes before emptying of the capsule, but a normal motility index in the 10 minutes before the capsule was emptied into the duodenum. These studies suggest that normal terminal antral contractions may be maintained even in patients with gastroparesis, whereas antral contractility required for the trituration of digestible foodstuffs is abnormal.[119]

Gastric Myoelectrical Activity

GMA is recorded noninvasively using electrodes positioned on the abdominal surface.[4,120] The signal an EGG summates the ongoing GMA: the slow wave activity during fasting and the summation of slow wave activity linked to plateau and action potential activity during the postprandial period.[121] In response to a water load or a nutrient load, the amplitude of the EGG signal increases in the normal 2.5–3.7-cpm range, as determined by visual and computer analysis (e.g., an increase in the percentage of EGG power or in the postprandial power ratio in the normal frequency range).[52,122,123] Pitfalls for recording and analyzing EGGs include failure to identify artifact in the signal and harmonics in the computer analyses.[124]

Changes in the EGG frequency and amplitude are key measures. After ingestion of most solid- or liquid-meals, a so-called frequency dip occurs in the first 10–15 minutes after the meal. The frequency dip reflects changes resulting from marked gastric relaxation and the accommodation of the test meal related to the volume or the temperature of the meal.[125,126] Several minutes after the ingestion of the liquid test meals, the frequency of the EGG signal returns to the middle of the normal 2.5–3.7-cpm range.[125,126]

Gastric dysrhythmias are associated with symptoms of nausea in subjects with motion sickness,[78] nausea and vomiting of pregnancy,[127,128] FD,[52,129] and gastroparesis.[130–132] Gastric dysrhythmias include 0.5–2.5-cpm signals termed *bradygastrias* and 3.7–10-cpm signals termed *tachygastrias* (Fig. 52.19). Recordings that have combinations of tachygastria and bradygastrias are termed *mixed gastric dysrhythmias*.[121,133,134] GMA can also be recorded from serosal electrodes placed during surgery or with mucosal electrodes placed during endoscopy.[5,21,63,135] Multiple channel serosal recordings using up to 128 channels have shown 3-cpm myoelectrical signals, as well as a variety of gastric dysrhythmias with similarities to cardiac dysrhythmias.[136,137] The amplitude and velocity of the human slow wave are greatest in the terminal antrum, the 3–4 cm of antrum immediately proximal to the pylorus.[5] These same studies further confirm the normal human slow wave frequency ranges from 2.5 to 3.7 cpm. Slow frequencies are also present from 1 to 2 cpm (bradygastrias) and from 4 to 9 cpm (tachygastrias) in patients with nausea with or without gastroparesis.[21,138,139] Interest in normal and dysrhythmic GMA is increasing. A new multi-channel EGG machine records 3-cpm GMA after a solid-liquid caloric meal and the multiple channels allow the detection of propagation of the wavefronts.[140]

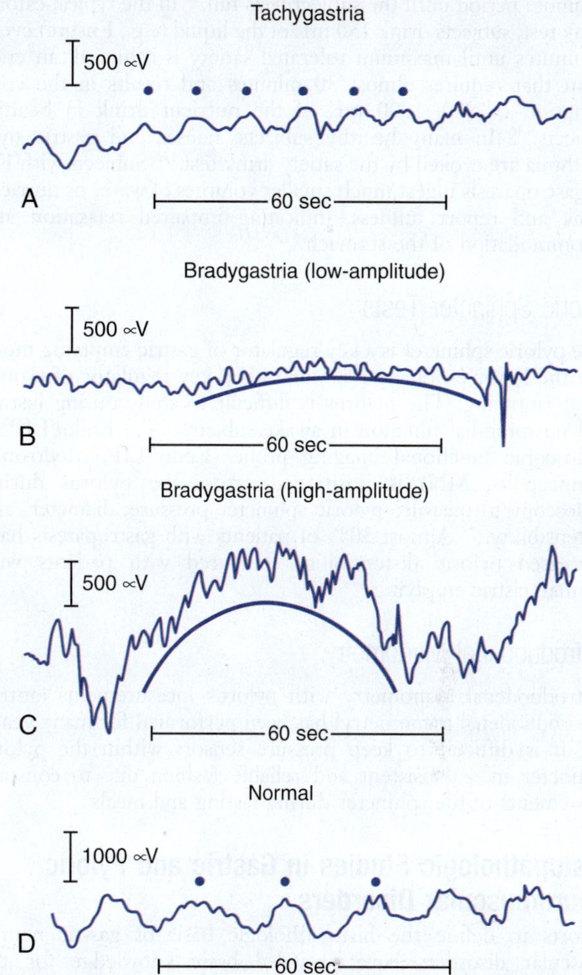

Fig. 52.19 Gastric dysrhythmias recorded with EGG methods. (A) Tachygastria, an abnormally rapid signal at 6 cpm, shown by *dots*. (B) and (C), Bradygastria at low- or high-amplitude 1-cpm wave, respectively. The 1-per-minute waves are indicated by the *solid curved lines*, and the smaller waves in the EGG signal represent respiratory activity. (D) Normal 3-cpm EGG signal is identified by *dots*.

Gastric Relaxation, Accommodation, and Volume

Barostat Tests

Due to the spherical shape of the fundus and the proximal stomach, standard manometric catheters are not useful in recording intraluminal pressures after meals. The barostat balloon was designed to measure changes in tone (or gastric relaxation) and volume in the more spherical areas of the proximal stomach.[41] Intraballoon pressure is maintained with infused air during the baseline or fasting period with the balloon slightly distended. As the fundus and proximal stomach relax in response to the test meal, more air is concomitantly infused into the balloon to maintain the established baseline intraballoon pressure.[141] The volume of air that is infused to maintain baseline pressure is an estimate of the increased gastric volume that occurs as the proximal stomach relaxes.

Barostat studies demonstrate abnormalities in fundic relaxation in almost 30% of patients with FD.[41] The failure of fundic relaxation correlates with early satiety. Failure of fundic relaxation has also been recorded in patients with gastroparesis.[41,142,143] Because the barostat method is invasive and uncomfortable for patients, these studies have been limited to the research laboratory.

Scintigraphy and Other Tests

Excessive or poor fundic relaxation in response to liquids and solids can be demonstrated with scintigraphy, US, and MRI. Single photon emission CT is a method that outlines the gastric wall before and after ingestion of a meal to determine changes in volume of the stomach. This method requires IV injection of ^{99m}Tc-pertechnetate to outline the gastric wall. The accommodation response can be identified with single photon emission CT.[144]

Nonnutrient Liquid and Nutrient Drink Satiety Tests

Nonnutrient liquids (the water-load satiety test) and nutrient drink tests are used to assess overall gastric volume or gastric capacity and visceral sensations, such as nausea, stomach fullness, or satiety in response to ingestion of these liquids,[52,83,145,146] often in conjunction with measures of GMA, accommodation, or emptying. In the water-load satiety test, water is consumed over a

5-minute period until the subject feels full.[52] In the typical caloric drink test, subjects drink 150 mL of the liquid (e.g., Ensure) every 5 minutes until maximum tolerated satiety is achieved, an endpoint that requires almost 30 minutes and results in the consumption of 800–1000 mL of the nutrient drink in healthy subjects.[146] In many healthy subjects, nausea and gastric dysrhythmia are evoked by the satiety drink test.[146] Subjects with FD or gastroparesis ingest much smaller volumes of water or nutrient drink and report fullness, indicating impaired relaxation and accommodation of the stomach.[52,83,133]

Pyloric Sphincter Tests

The pyloric sphincter is a key regulator of gastric emptying much like the lower esophageal sphincter is a key regulator of esophageal emptying. The pylorus is difficult to study during fasting and postprandial function in awake subjects. The EndoFLIP or endoscopic functional imaging probe (EndoFLIP, Medtronic, Minneapolis, MN) is positioned across the pylorus during endoscopy to measure pyloric sphincter pressure, diameter, and distensibility.[147] Almost 30% of patients with gastroparesis have decreased pyloric distensibility compared with patients with normal gastric emptying.[148]

Antroduodenal Manometry

Antroduodenal manometry with pylorus measurements (antropyloroduodenal manometry) has been performed for many years, but it is difficult to keep pressure sensors within the pyloric sphincter in a consistent and reliable fashion due to constant movements of the sphincter during fasting and meals

Histopathologic Studies in Gastric and Pyloric Neuromuscular Disorders

Efforts to define the histopathologic basis of gastric neuromuscular disorders have provided basic knowledge for the evolving field of neurogastroenterology. Most of the full-thickness specimens from the gastric wall and pylorus have been harvested during the placement of GES devices or the placement of jejunostomy feeding tubes in patients with severe gastroparesis. Endoscopic biopsy techniques have been explored that provide full-thickness specimens that contain elements of circular muscle, ENS neurons, and ICCs.[149,150] Histologic abnormalities in smooth muscle, neurons of the ENS, number or location of ICCs, and the distribution of key neural or muscular receptors represent the potential underlying mechanisms of disordered gastric smooth muscle relaxation, peristaltic contraction, and gastric slow wave activity.

Loss of gastric ICCs (MY-ICCs and IM-ICCs) was reported in patients with diabetes and IGP.[20,21,31] Interestingly, similar loss of ICCs was shown in diabetic mice, and the ICCs were restored with intense insulin therapy, suggesting that the ICCs are not entirely destroyed in diabetes but dedifferentiate into immature myoblasts during prolonged hyperglycemia.[151] Damage to ICCs, ENS, and smooth muscle can also be seen in inflammatory and neoplastic conditions.[152–155] Other studies in humans have shown fibrosis of smooth muscle layers but intact myenteric plexus and vagus nerve in patients with DGP, a loss of ICCs but minimal smooth muscle fibrosis, and inflammatory T lymphocyte infiltration in myenteric neurons.[156,157]

Full-thickness biopsies from patients with IGP and DGP showed marked depletion of ICCs, a range of mild- or minimal-injury to enteric nerve cell bodies and endings, and preserved smooth muscle.[20–23,31] Interestingly, more severe ICC depletion and enteric nerve injury were seen in the specimens from IGP patients compared with diabetics.[20,31] The gastric smooth muscles in these specimens were generally normal. Thus these disorders may be considered "Cajalopathies" or gastric enteric neuropathies or, more likely in most cases, combinations of both.

Further studies showed an immune infiltrate of CD204 macrophages was associated with decreased antral ICCs in patients with IGP and DGP.[22] The loss of ICCs appear to be more severe in the antrum compared with the corpus. The increase in CD204 macrophages was also associated with heme-oxygenase deficiency and loss of ICCs, whereas replacement of heme-oxygenase improved gastric emptying in mice.[158] However, a trial of hemin infusions in patients with DGP did not improve symptoms or gastric emptying.[159] Restoration of M2 macrophages in animals with gastroparesis resulted in increased numbers of ICCs and improved gastric emptying[160] and suggests novel therapeutic pathways to treat gastroparesis.

Finally, histochemical studies showed the pylorus in patients with gastroparesis contained decreased numbers of ICCs and increased fibrosis compared with control pyloric tissue.[161] These studies as well as physiologic studies of decreased distensibility of the pylorus in gastroparesis[147,148,162] suggest an important role of the pylorus in regulating the rate of gastric emptying and thus in the development of gastroparesis. Results from histochemical studies of full-thickness gastric and pyloric tissue also provide new directions for understanding the neuromuscular dysfunction of the stomach and stimulate ideas for novel therapeutic approaches.

NEUROMUSCULAR DISORDERS OF THE STOMACH

Gastric neuromuscular disorders encompass a continuum of electrical and contractile dysfunction. At the mild end of the spectrum are gastric dysrhythmias, which are subtle electrical disturbances associated with mild-to-severe nausea symptoms (Fig. 52.20). Studies showed these patients have a modest depletion of ICCs in the range of 3–5 ICCs/HPF.[139]Abnormalities in relaxation of the fundus are associated with early satiety. At the severe end of the spectrum of neuromuscular dysfunction spectrum, antral hypomotility, and delayed gastric emptying are present. However, the

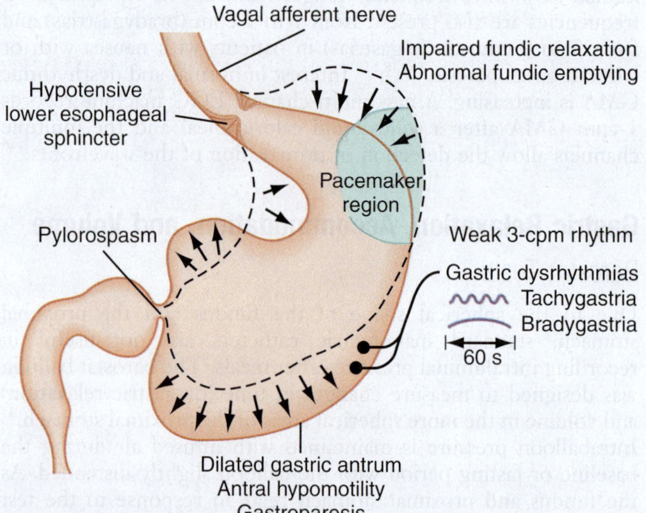

Fig. 52.20 The spectrum of gastric neuromuscular disorders. Gastric neuromuscular disorders range from abnormal fundic relaxation and emptying to gastric dysrhythmias and antral hypomotility and gastroparesis. Pyloric sphincter dysfunction, duodenal dysfunction, antroduodenal dyscoordination, and vagal hypersensitivity may all be present in some patients with gastric neuromuscular disorders. cpm, cycles per minute. See text for details. (Modified from Koch KL, Stern RM. Functional disorders of the stomach. *Semin Gastrointest Dis*. 1996;7:185–195.)

TABLE 52.2 Categories of Gastric Neuromuscular Disorders and Treatment Approaches Based on Gastric Emptying and Myoelectrical Test Results

Delayed Gastric Emptying		Normal Gastric Emptying	
Subtype 1	**Subtype 2**	**Subtype 1**	**Subtype 2**
Test results	**Test results**	**Test results**	**Test results**
Gastric dysrhythmia Hypo-normal 3-cpm GMA	Normal 3-cpm GMA	Gastric dysrhythmia	Normal 3-cpm GMA
Diagnosis	***Diagnosis***	***Diagnosis***	***Diagnosis***
Severe gastric myoelectrical-contractile disorder	Pylorospasm or fixed obstruction at the pylorus or duodenum (Electrocontractile dissociation?)	Gastric myoelectrical disorder	Visceral hypersensitivity Pylorospasm Nongastric causes
Treatment	**Treatment**	**Treatment**	**Treatment**
Nausea and vomiting diet[a] Prokinetic therapy Antinauseant therapy Gastrostomy tube/jejunostomy tube TPN Acustimulation Gastric electrical stimulation Gastric pacemaker	Endoscopic therapies[b] Botox/balloon dilation Surgery for fixed obstruction Nausea and vomiting diet[a]	Nausea and vomiting diet[a] Prokinetic therapy Antinauseant therapy	Nausea and vomiting diet[a] Antinauseant therapy Drugs for fundic/antral relaxation (Further workup for nongastric causes, such as atypical GERD, cholecystitis, IBS, or disorders of the central or autonomic nervous system) Antidepressant therapy

[a]See Table 52.6.
[b]See Table 52.5.
GP, Gastroparesis; *GERD*, gastroesophageal reflux disease; *GMA*, gastric myoelectrical activity, *cpm*, cycles per minute.
From Koch KL, Hasler WL, eds. *Nausea and Vomiting: Diagnosis and Treatment*. Switzerland: Springer International Publishing; 2017.

symptoms associated with gastroparesis are indistinguishable from the symptoms in patients with normal emptying and postprandial distress syndrome (PDS). [132,133] In patients with gastroparesis nausea and vomiting may be severe and weight loss and malnutrition develop and require enteral or parenteral nutritional support. These patients have severe depletion of ICCs (0–2 ICCs/HPF).[20–23] Patients with gastroparesis may also have multiple neuromuscular abnormalities: gastric dysrhythmias, dilated antrum, pyloric dysfunction, poor fundic relaxation, and gastric hypersensitivity or hyposensitivity due to vagal or splanchnic nerve dysfunction.[163,164] Symptoms associated with gastric neuromuscular disorders are summarized in Table 52.2.

The pyloric sphincter is a key pathophysiologic factor in over 30% of patients with gastroparesis.[165] In these patients, the GMA is 3-cpm and indicates normal numbers of ICCs in the corpus and antrum. Gastroparesis and normal or hypernormal 3-cpm GMA are found in patients with fixed obstruction at the pylorus[131] and in neuromuscular dysfunction of the pylorus.[147,148,166,167] Thus neuromuscular disorders of the stomach reflect a continuum of loss of ICCs but include obstructive gastroparesis.

In the normal corpus-antrum, there are five or more ICCs/HPF. In these healthy subjects the normal GMA is 3 cpm is present and test meals are emptied at the normal rate.[20–24,139] However, patients with chronic unexplained nausea and normal gastric emptying have decreased ICCs (3–4 ICCs/HPF) and a variety of gastric dysrhythmias ranging from tachygastrias to bradygastrias and various conduction defects (e.g., re-entrant rhythms, conduction blocks).[139] Subjects with nausea and vomiting and gastroparesis have more severe depletion of ICCs with 0–2/HPF and hyponormal 3-cpm GMA and a variety of gastric dysrhythmias from tachygastria to bradygastria.[20–24] Thus, as shown in Fig. 52.21 compared with 5 ICCs/HPF and normal 3-cpm GMA in healthy subjects, the histologic studies indicate a continuum of loss of ICCs that is associated with gastric dysrhythmias in FD and GP. A subtype of patients with GP, however, has normal 3-cpm GMA.

The subset of patients with gastroparesis and normal 3-cpm GMA has been studied.[131,133,166,167] These discordant findings (normal or hypernormal 3-cpm GMA and gastroparesis) indicate normal numbers of ICCs in the corpus/antrum but the gastric emptying is abnormal. This pattern associated with pyloric dysfunction.[131,133,167] In these patients, the gastroparesis may actually be due to (1) pyloric diseases such as peptic ulcer disease (PUD) with fibrous stenosis[131] or cancer obstructing the postpyloric duodenum,[166] or (2) pyloric neuromuscular dysfunction such as pylorospasm,[167] poor pyloric distensibility,[147,148] or abnormal antropyloroduodenal coordination.[168] The subgroup of patients with normal 3-cpm GMA and gastroparesis likely has normal numbers of ICCs, but this has not been established with full-thickness biopsies.

Gastroparesis

Gastroparesis means "paralysis" of the stomach, as defined by the delayed rate of emptying of a standard test meal from the stomach in the absence of mechanical obstruction. Approximately 90% of the patients with gastroparesis have either diabetic, postsurgical, or IGP, but fixed obstructive or functional obstructive gastroparesis subtypes are important to identify because they are reversible. Table 52.3 lists the differential diagnosis for gastroparesis.

The epidemiology of gastroparesis is just beginning to be understood. Data from Olmstead County, Minnesota, indicate an age-adjusted prevalence of definite gastroparesis of 9.6 per 100,000 persons for men and 37.8 per 100,000 for women. The incidence was 2.4 per 100,000 for men and 9.8 for women. The definite gastroparesis group was based on standard gastric scintigraphy results.[169] In diabetics, the incidence of gastroparesis was 1% in type 2 and nearly 5% in type 1, compared with 0.1% for nondiabetic subjects in the population of Olmstead County.[169] Gastroparesis evolves over time in patients with diabetes, usually appearing after a duration of 10 years or more. In a series from Olmstead County, Minnesota, 5.2% of patients with type 1

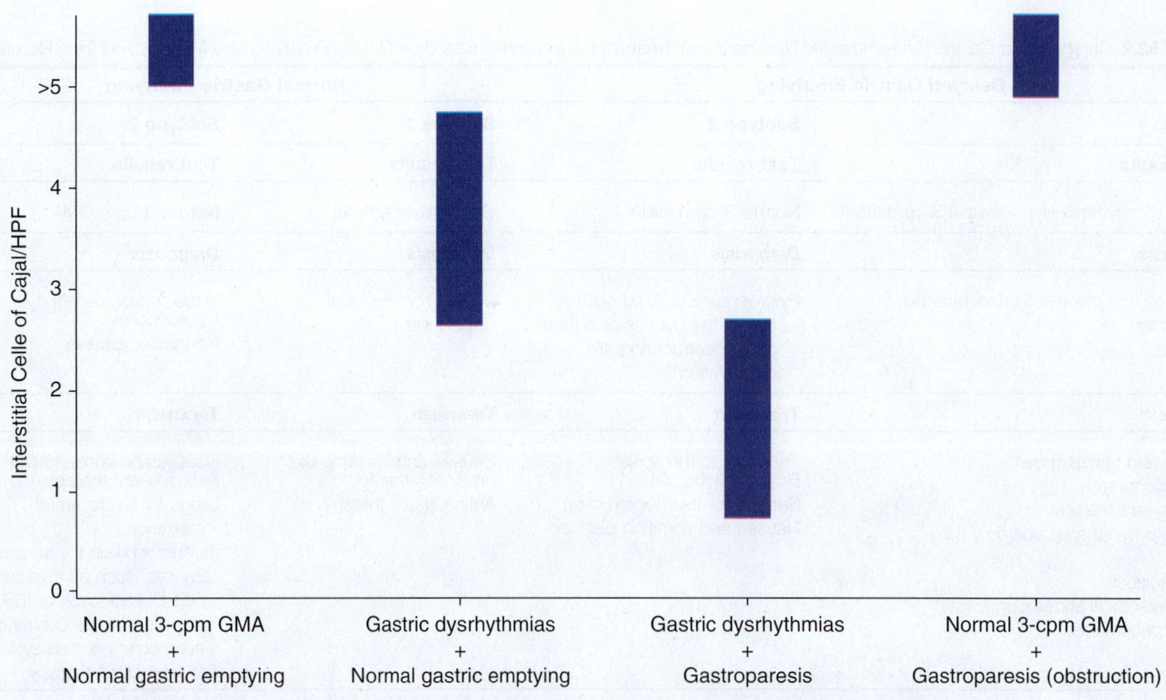

Fig. 52.21 Schematic of relationships among interstitial cells of Cajals (ICCs), gastric myoelectrical activity (GMA), and gastric emptying rates are shown. Numbers of ICCs are shown on the Y-axis [normal number of ICCs in antrum is >5/high-power field (HPF)] and related conditions are listed on the X-axis. Normal numbers of antral ICCs are associated with normal 3-cpm GMA and normal gastric emptying. Modest depletion of ICCs (3–4 ICCs/HPF) is associated with gastric dysrhythmias and normal gastric emptying, whereas severe ICC depletion (1–2 ICCs/HPF) is associated with gastric dysrhythmias and gastroparesis. In contrast, in the obstructive gastroparesis subtype, normal 3-cpm GMA is present, and reflects normal numbers of antral ICCs and presence of pyloric dysfunction.

TABLE 52.3 Causes of Gastroparesis

Diagnosis	Incidence (%)
Idiopathic gastroparesis[a] (20%–30% have obstructive gastroparesis)	40
Diabetic gastroparesis (type 1 and 2 diabetes mellitus) (20%–30% have obstructive gastroparesis)	35
Postsurgical gastroparesis (antrectomy, vagotomy, fundectomy, fundoplication)	20
Ischemic gastroparesis	<1
Miscellaneous causes	4

[a]Possibly postviral, drug-induced, degenerative, or inflammatory processes of enteric nerves, interstitial cells of Cajal, or smooth muscle.

diabetes and 1.0% of patients with type 2 diabetes developed gastroparesis over a 10-year period, whereas only 0.2% of control subjects developed gastroparesis.[170] In a community-based population of patients with type 2 diabetes mellitus, 6% of whites and 7% of African Americans had a moderate intensity of symptoms associated with gastroparesis.[171] In contrast, in referral centers, gastroparesis is present in almost 50% of patients with type 1 and 30% of patients with type 2 diabetes mellitus.[172,173]

Hospitalizations related to gastroparesis have increased markedly since 2000. Many of the admissions for gastroparesis were patients with DGP with problems of glycemic control or infections.[174] A portion of these admissions were also due to a surgical implantation of gastric stimulators for diabetic or IGP.[175]

Diabetic Gastroparesis

Many patients with long-standing type 1 diabetes mellitus develop DGP. These patients often have diabetes for more than 10 years, erratic and elevated glucose levels, peripheral neuropathy, nephropathy, and cardiovascular disease.[164,175–177] Patients with DGP have increased 5-year mortality compared with those without gastroparesis.[172,178] In a minority of patients the gastroparesis is the initial complication of their diabetes.

One important manifestation of gastric emptying dysfunction in patients with insulin-dependent diabetes is erratic glucose control, especially with unexpected hypoglycemic episodes in the postprandial period if the usual insulin doses are administered before meals. When postprandial insulin levels increase following insulin injection and yet gastric emptying is delayed, nutrient delivery into the duodenum and intestinal glucose absorption are delayed. Thus plasma glucose levels decrease in response to the insulin treatment and symptomatic hypoglycemia develops unexpectedly.[177]

Acute hyperglycemia (>220 mg/dL) is associated with tachygastrias and delayed gastric emptying in healthy subjects and in patients with diabetes.[63,179,180] Hyperglycemia is also associated with a loss of ICCs,[151] antral hypomotility,[181] isolated pyloric contractions,[182] gastric dysrhythmias,[63,179] and impaired prokinetic action of prokinetic drugs like erythromycin.[183] Relatively minor increases in the blood sugar level, even elevations within the physiologic range, delay gastric emptying in normal volunteers and diabetic patients.[180] Acute hyperglycemia produced by glucose clamp methodology elicits fullness, decreased antral contractility, gastric dysrhythmias, blunts the contractile pyloric response to intraduodenal lipid infusion, and modifies upper GI sensations.[63,179,180]

Gastric neuromuscular abnormalities documented in patients with type 1 diabetes include an abnormal intragastric distribution of food,[184] reduced receptive relaxation and accommodation,[185] reduced incidence of the antral component of the MMC, antral dilation, postprandial antral hypomotility,[181] and electrical dysrhythmias.[133,173,186] In patients with DGP, the ICCs are depleted and enteric nerve endings are abnormal,[20,21] pathologic findings that help explain the mechanism of gastric dysrhythmias and poor gastric contractile responses to test meals. Loss of the antral phase 3 contractions results in poor emptying of fibrous debris in the stomach and is the neuromuscular basis for the formation of bezoars (see Chapter 28). Thus the progressive neuromuscular dysfunction of the diabetic stomach reflects the effects of chronic hyperglycemia and superimposed, intermittent hyperglycemia episodes on the gastric ENS and ICCs.

Gastric smooth muscle dysfunction is another mechanism of delayed gastric emptying in some patients with diabetes. Gastric smooth muscle contractility in diabetic rats is reduced in response to electrical stimulation.[187] The inhibitory effect of hyperglycemia on stem cell factor has a role in the reduction in ICCs and smooth muscle contractility.[188] In humans with DGP, the smooth muscle is intact but has a thickened basal lamina.[20,21] Diabetic patients with gastroparesis were treated with insulin pump therapy with continuous glucose monitoring for 48 weeks. The Hgb A1C decreased significantly (by 1.1%) and the symptoms associated with gastroparesis recorded with the Gastroparesis Cardinal Symptoms Index decreased by 23% compared with baseline.[189] Thus aggressive insulin treatment in these patients helped glucose control and gastroparesis symptoms.[189]

Pylorospasm may cause a form of obstructive DGP.[167,190] In these cases the neuromuscular function of the corpus and antrum is intact, but functional obstruction at the pylorus due to pylorospasm or incomplete relaxation of the pylorus causes delayed emptying. These patients have normal or increased 3-cpm GMA, a discordant finding in patients with gastroparesis that suggests the possibility of gastric outlet obstruction from functional or mechanical causes at the pylorus. (Fig. 52.22A; see section on Obstructive Gastroparesis).[134,190]

Many patients with type 2 diabetes mellitus have unsuspected or subclinical gastroparesis. In tertiary centers, the incidence of gastroparesis in type 2 diabetes mellitus ranges from 30% to almost 50%.[191] Patients with type 2 diabetes differ significantly from patients with type 1 diabetes in that they have insulin resistance, the diabetes appears later in life, obesity is common, early satiety is more common, gastroparesis is less severe, and the hyperglycemia has been present longer before diagnosis compared with patients with type 1 diabetes.[191–194] In the early stages of type 2 diabetes mellitus, gastric emptying may be accelerated.[195] Patients with type 1 diabetes mellitus are younger, have more severe delays in gastric emptying, and have more hospitalizations compared with type 2 diabetes mellitus and gastroparesis. Type 2 diabetes mellitus patients with gastroparesis are older, have milder delays in gastric emptying, and more severe early satiety.[193,194]

Experimental diabetes in nonobese diabetic mice and in the type 2–like diabetes db/db mouse leads to gastroparesis. Neuronal nitric oxide synthase (nNOS) is reduced in the diabetic mouse stomach and is associated with antro-pylorus spasm and gastroparesis.[196] Notably, nNOS was decreased 40% in human stomach tissue from patients with DGP compared with control values.[20] Treatment with insulin or sildenafil restored NOS and was associated with reversal of the delay in gastric emptying in the diabetic mouse. Hypomotility of the fundus and hypercontractility of the pylorus were found in db/db mice.[197] In other studies of diabetic mice, the loss of ICCs was associated with electrical dysrhythmias, delayed gastric emptying, and reduced neurotransmission in gastric smooth muscle.[198]

Postsurgical Gastroparesis

Gastroparesis occurs in a subset of patients undergoing subtle or radical stomach operations that range from vagotomy to fundoplication to antrectomy. Truncal vagotomy produces complex effects on the neuromuscular function of the stomach. After vagotomy, the fundus fails to relax normally after meals, resulting in rapid filling of the antrum.[199] Vagotomy is also associated with

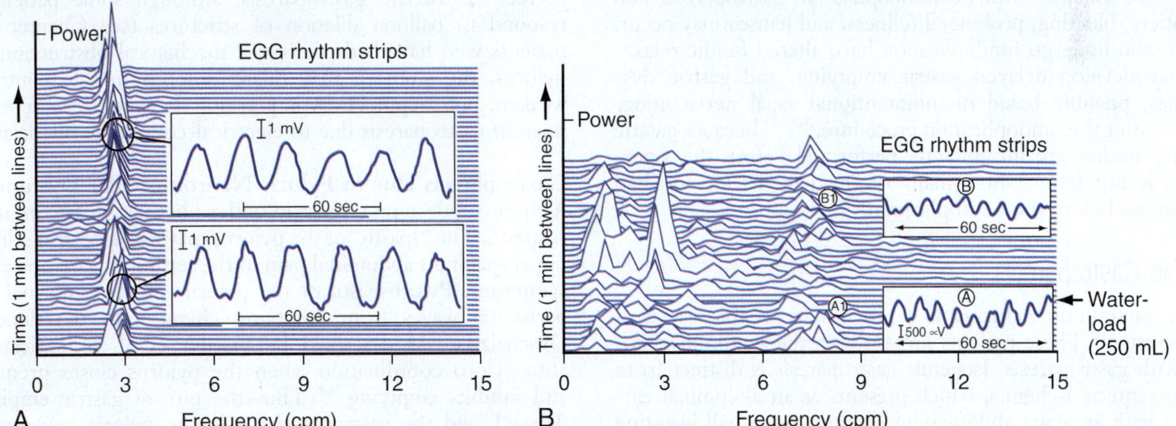

Fig. 52.22 RSA of the electrogastrogram (EGG) in patients with obstructive gastroparesis. (A) running spectral analysis (RSA) recording from a patient with gastroparesis due to mechanical obstruction at the pylorus secondary to chronic peptic ulcer disease. Note the persistent high-amplitude 3-cpm waves in the EGG rhythm strips and the uniform and unvarying peaks at 3 cpm in the RSA, findings that would not be expected in a patient with gastroparesis due to electrical and contractile dysfunction. (B) RSA and EGG rhythm strips. Recordings in a patient with IGP. Note that the EGG rhythm strips show a 7–8-cpm tachygastria before (B) and after (A) a water-load test. The RSA shows multiple peaks in the 7–8-cpm tachygastria range and few peaks in the normal 3-cpm range. This patient had electrical and contractile abnormalities of the stomach as documented by the tachygastria and gastroparesis. (Modified from Brzana RJ, Koch KL, Bingaman S. Gastric myoelectrical activity in patients with gastric outlet obstruction and idiopathic gastroparesis. *Am J Gastroenterol.* 1998;93:1803–1809.)

gastric dysrhythmias,[3] decreased antral contractions, and poor antropyloroduodenal coordination.[200] Truncal vagotomy performed during ulcer operations requires a pyloroplasty to reduce sphincteric resistance to antral outflow because antral contractions become weak, and peristalsis and emptying are then disrupted. Most patients recover from the effects of acute vagotomy. But in patients undergoing extensive resection of the antrum and corpus, prolonged symptoms and chronic gastric neuromuscular dysfunction are likely.

Lower esophageal resection for esophageal cancer includes resection of the fundus. The vagus nerves are transected and the fundic reservoir is lost. Pyloroplasty is performed to facilitate gastric emptying, but the loss of the fundus and variable amounts of the corpus (that may encompass the pacemaker region) often leads to chronic nausea, gastric dysrhythmias, and gastroparesis. Antral resections with Billroth I, Billroth II, or Roux-en-Y gastrojejunostomy for gastric tumors or PUD may lead to profound neuromuscular dysfunction of the stomach.[201,202] Critical amounts of the corpus-antrum (including unknown amounts of the gastric wall, containing the pacemaker region) required for normal gastric neuromuscular activity, may be removed, and the efficacy of trituration by the corpus and antrum may be markedly reduced. Ingested food is retained in the remnant fundus and fails to empty into the corpus[203]; the corpus fails to mix and empty gastric contents even though the anastomosis is widely patent. The Roux-en-Y gastroenterostomy operation may result in the Roux syndrome in which postprandial pain, bloating, and nausea develop. Delayed gastric emptying is due to "functional obstruction" by the Roux limb as the neuromuscular dyssynchrony within the Roux limb prevents emptying of the stomach.[204,205] After vagotomy and antrectomy, patients may develop the dumping syndrome described later. In the gastric "sleeve" resection for obesity, two-thirds of the stomach is removed including portions of the fundus, corpus, and antrum. The pylorus is retained. After the sleeve resection, gastric emptying of liquid is accelerated.[206] Sleeve gastrectomy in a mouse model disrupted ICC and postjunctional neuroeffector responses but over 4 months recovery ICC networks and neuromuscular responses normalized.[207]

Fundoplication is commonly performed to treat gastroesophageal reflux disease (GERD) that fails to respond to medical therapy (see Chapter 48). Postfundoplication gastroparesis and early satiety, bloating, prolonged fullness, and nausea may occur. Patients who undergo fundoplication have altered fundic relaxation, may develop delayed gastric emptying, and gastric dysrhythmias, possibly based on unintentional vagal nerve injury during or after the fundoplication procedure.[208,209] Because gastric emptying studies are infrequently performed before this operation, it is not known how many of the patients already had gastroparesis before the fundoplication.[209]

Ischemic Gastroparesis

Chronic mesenteric ischemia is a rare but reversible cause of gastroparesis.[210] These patients present with the symptoms associated with gastroparesis. Ischemic gastroparesis is distinct from acute mesenteric ischemia, which presents as an abdominal catastrophe with an acute abdomen and gangrenous small intestine (see Chapter 12). Chronic mesenteric ischemia is usually due to progressive atherosclerosis or hyperplasia of the intima of the arteries of the celiac, superior mesenteric, or inferior mesenteric artery. Collaterals of these obstructed arteries form over time so that neuromuscular function of the stomach is preserved, at least for some time. Bypass graft surgery or dilatation of the stenotic arteries results in resolution of symptoms, eradication of gastric dysrhythmias, and reversal of gastroparesis.[210] Thus ischemic gastroparesis is potentially a reversible form of gastroparesis and should be suspected in patients with gastroparesis, weight loss, and a history of peripheral vascular disease, cerebral vascular disease, or myocardial infarction. An abdominal bruit is present in approximately 50% of patients.

There are other rare forms of mesenteric vascular compromise (e.g., the median arcuate ligament syndrome) that may result in decreased blood flow to the stomach.[211] Release of the arcuate ligament and restoration of blood flow have been associated with improvement in gastric emptying in a case report.[211] On the other hand, superior mesenteric artery syndrome is not accepted as a cause of mechanical obstruction that leads to gastroparesis, nausea, and vomiting and other causes such as pyloric neuromuscular dysfunction should be investigated.

Patients with idiopathic (discussed below), diabetic, or postsurgical gastroparesis may have a subtype of gastroparesis—obstructive gastroparesis due to pyloric dysfunction. This subtype is important because endoscopic and surgical treatments are directed toward the pylorus.

Fixed Pyloric Obstruction

Fixed obstructive gastroparesis refers to delayed emptying due to mechanical obstruction at the pylorus or duodenal bulbar or postbulbar area by tumor, chronic peptic ulcer or inflammation, rings, or webs.[131,166] The obstructions may be distal to the duodenal bulb in the descending and transverse portions of the duodenum. These patients have gastroparesis and normal or hypernormal 3-cpm GMA.[131,166] Fig. 52.22A shows an example of high-amplitude 3-cpm GMA waves recorded in an EGG test in a patient with pyloric outlet obstruction due to chronic PUD and fixed narrowing of the pylorus. In these patients the smooth muscle, ENS, and numbers of ICCs in the corpus-antrum are normal, but the normal 3 per minute recurrent gastric peristaltic waves meet sustained resistance at the point of obstruction (the pylorus) and the emptying of solid food is delayed. In contrast, almost 2/3 of patients with IGP have bradygastria, tachygastria, or mixed gastric dysrhythmias indicating both electrical and contractile dysfunction (see Fig. 52.22B). However, if patients with IGP or DGP have 3-cpm GMA, then the obstructive causes for the gastroparesis should be considered. Gastroparesis may be due to pyloric stenosis or postduodenal bulb cancer.[131,166] Surgical correction of the fixed pyloric obstruction with resection and Billroth I or Billroth II gastrojejunostomy may be necessary to correct obstructive gastroparesis, although some patients may respond to balloon dilation of strictures (see Chapter 55) In patients who have had prolonged mechanical obstruction of the pylorus, the stomach may dilate, smooth muscle contractions weaken, but 3-cpm GMA is present, all which may represent a form of gastroparesis due to electrical-contractile dissociation.

Gastroparesis Due to Pyloric Neuromuscular Dysfunction

A more subtle type of gastric outlet obstruction occurs in pylorospasm. The "spasm" of the pylorus may cause postprandial right upper quadrant abdominal pain in the setting of gastroparesis-like symptoms. Pylorospasm of the pylorus prevents normal gastric peristaltic waves from emptying chyme into the duodenum. Dyschalasia was described by Fischer et al. to indicate poor antropyloro coordination when the pylorus closes prematurely and inhibits emptying.[168] Thus the rate of gastric emptying is delayed, and the gastroparesis is due to pyloric neuromuscular dysfunction. Almost 1/3 of patients with gastroparesis have normal 3-cpm GMA as recorded in the EGG in response to the water load satiety test.[133] The 3-cpm GMA indicates normal numbers of ICCs in the corpus-antrum and the cause of delayed emptying is pyloric neuromuscular dysfunction. In these patients dilatation of the pylorus with a 20-mm balloon for 2 minutes or botulinum toxin A injections into the pylorus decreased postprandial symptoms.[167] In patients with more than three successful endoscopic pyloric treatments, pyloroplasty was recommended and completed. All patients had improved symptoms and increased gastric emptying rates.[212] Finally and theoretically, some patients with obstructive gastroparesis may have normal 3-cpm EGG signals and poor gastric emptying based on "electromechanical dissociation." In this situation, it is possible that MY-ICCs or IM-ICCs that generate slow waves may be normal, but enteric neurons and/or smooth muscle dysfunction are present.

Idiopathic Gastroparesis

In more than one-third of patients, the gastroparesis is idiopathic (IGP).[213] Patients with IGP tend to have more abdominal pain compared with DGP, but nausea and vomiting are the dominant symptoms driving visits to gastroenterologists.[213] In 15% of these patients, an acute febrile illness preceded the diagnosis of gastroparesis by many months.[214] These "herald" illnesses are frequently described as flu-like with fever and nausea and vomiting. Patients often date the onset of their nausea from that point. Norwalk virus, HSV, and EBV infections have been documented in patients with sudden-onset gastroparesis and normal immune systems, whereas other patients are immunocompromised.[215] Postviral gastroparesis may resolve completely over 1–2 years. Nausea and vomiting and diarrhea occur in less than 10% of patients with COVID-19 infections[216] and long-term sequelae on gastrointestinal neuromuscular function are unknown. Histologic studies from the National Institutes of Health Gastroparesis Consortium indicate that patients with IGP have more severe depletion of ICCs and loss of enteric nerve endings compared with DGP.[20,31] Loss of ICCs in knock-out mice is associated with gastric dysrhythmias.[217] Gastric dysrhythmias are common in patients with IGP (see Fig. 52.22B) and indicate severe loss of ICCs in the corpus/antrum.[20–22] Other historical clues to the genesis of IGP are exposures to (1) multiple courses of antibiotics (e.g., treatments for chronic ear or sinus infections), (2) anesthetic agents for a variety of common operations, and (3) food poisoning–like illnesses of unknown cause. However, as discussed earlier, almost 30% of patients with IGP have normal 3-cpm GMA, the functional obstructive subtype of gastroparesis.

IGP is diagnosed in patients who have dyspepsia-like symptoms, delayed gastric emptying, and gastric dysrhythmias, but no primary causes of gastroparesis such as diabetes, ischemia, or gastric operations are present. Many other diseases and disorders, including intestinal pseudo-obstruction (discussed later), paraneoplastic diseases, autonomic nervous system abnormalities, thyroid and adrenal disease, or CNS diseases, may cause or are associated with gastroparesis. If these disorders are identified, then the gastroparesis may be secondary to these specific diseases.

Gastric Neuromuscular Dysfunction Associated With Other GI Disorders

Functional Dyspepsia

FD symptoms include epigastric discomfort or pain, early satiety, fullness, nausea, and vomiting in the setting of normal upper endoscopy and normal routine laboratory tests. FD is divided into an epigastric pain syndrome and PDS, the latter comprising 80% of the FD patients.[218] One of the dominant symptoms that patients with FD have been recurrent and unexplained nausea and vomiting. This is a debilitating symptom with a large differential diagnosis (Box 52.1), and these disease categories should be considered in the evaluation of the patient with nausea and vomiting. If the patient has one of these disorders, then FD is not the diagnosis. Importantly, postprandial distress symptoms of FD and symptoms associated with gastroparesis are indistinguishable.[219]

The gastric pathophysiologic mechanisms that drive FD symptoms remains an area of intensive investigation (see Chapter 5). If endoscopy is normal, then FD symptoms may be caused by several neuromuscular disorders of the stomach. For example,

BOX 52.1 Differential Diagnosis of Chronic Nausea and Vomiting

- Mechanical GI tract obstruction (pylorus, cystic duct, bile duct, small intestine, colon)
- Mucosal inflammation
- Peritoneal irritation
- Carcinomas (e.g., gastric, ovarian, renal, bronchogenic)
- Metabolic/endocrine disorders (diabetic mellitus, hypothyroidism, hyperthyroidism, adrenal insufficiency, uremia)
- Medications (anticholinergics, narcotics, L-dopa, progesterone, calcium channel blockers, NSAIDs, antidysrhythmia agents, lubiprostone, glucagon-like peptide-1 receptor agonists, metformin, amylin analogs)
- Gastroparesis (see Table 52.2)
- Gastric dysrhythmias (tachygastria, bradygastria, mixed)
- CNS disorders (tumors, migraine, seizures, stroke, orthostatic intolerance)
- Psychogenic disorders (anorexia nervosa, bulimia nervosa)

81% of patients with IGP have symptoms like those defining PDS.[133,219] The diagnosis in these patients is IGP with associated symptoms. Seventeen to 40% of patients with FD have gastroparesis, and 40%–62% have gastric dysrhythmias.[52,133] Treatments designed to address the several pathophysiologic abnormalities of FD such as poor gastric accommodation and dysrhythmic GMA are needed.

Studies show patients with FD or gastroparesis-like symptoms have the same symptoms and same severity of symptoms as patients with gastroparesis.[219] Patients with FD and IGP or DGP also have the same incidence of gastric dysrhythmias and normal 3-cpm GMA (135). Improvement in gastric dysrhythmia and FD symptoms was reported in patients treated with cisapride.[220–222] Thus gastric dysrhythmias are potential pathophysiologic mechanisms of FD symptoms and are a therapeutic target.[223] In patients with chronic nausea with normal or delayed gastric emptying treated with aprepitant, nausea symptoms and tachygastria decreased significantly compared with placebo.[224]

In other patients with FD, both gastric emptying and GMA are normal. Abnormalities in gastric accommodation (relaxation) or gastric hypersensitivity to distention may account for FD symptoms in these patients.[225–227] Thus a variety of neuromuscular dysfunctions in different regions of the stomach may be present in patients with FD symptoms. Treatments aimed at correcting gastric dysrhythmias, improving 3-cpm GMA and accommodation are needed.

Gastroesophageal Reflux Disease

Many patients with typical GERD have additional symptoms of early satiety, postprandial fullness, and nausea (see Chapter__?). Approximately 30% of patients with GERD also have FD.[228] Overall, 20%–30% of patients with GERD have delayed gastric emptying.[228,229] Symptoms associated with gastroparesis improved and gastric dysrhythmias reverted to normal 3-cpm GMA after treatment of the lower esophageal sphincter with radiofrequency ablation (RFA).[230] In some patients, nausea is a subtle, atypical symptom of esophageal acid reflux and nausea improves after aggressive acid suppression therapy.[231]

Lower esophageal sphincter abnormalities, including increased numbers of transient lower esophageal sphincter relaxation, may contribute to inefficient gastric emptying and gastric dysrhythmias reported in these patients.[232,233] GERD patients also tended to retain solids and liquids in the proximal stomach compared with control subjects,[234] an abnormality that may stimulate excessive transient lower esophageal sphincter relaxations. RFA treatment at the lower esophageal sphincter region in patients with heartburn and dyspepsia improved heartburn, gastric emptying rates, and gastric dysrhythmias.[230] These data suggest in some patients with GERD and gastroparesis, treatments of GERD by RFA or fundoplication improves the gastric electrical rhythms and the rate of gastric emptying.

Constipation, IBS, and Pseudo-Obstruction

Gastroparesis, gastric dysrhythmias, GERD, and IBS are all present in some patients and indicate diffuse or pan-GI neuromuscular dysfunction.[235] Gastroparesis occurs in 60% of patients with constipation-predominant IBS. In a study of 350 patients with IGP, 89% were taking proton pump inhibitors and 64% had IBS.[214] These patients represent another overlap syndrome of GI neuromuscular disorders (see Chapter 35).

Patients with intestinal pseudo-obstruction syndromes often have GERD, gastroparesis, small bowel dysmotility, and colonic inertia have the most severe form of generalized GI neuromuscular disorders.[235,236] Pseudo-obstruction secondary to progressive systemic sclerosis (scleroderma) commonly involves the esophagus and stomach but may also cause small bowel dysmotility and subsequent bacterial overgrowth.[237] Intestinal pseudo-obstruction may be due to idiopathic degenerative or inflammatory processes involving the smooth muscle or ENS.

A variety of neurologic diseases may also involve the stomach or other regions of the digestive tract and cause pseudo-obstruction-like symptoms. These neurologic disorders include Ehlers-Danlos syndrome,[238] postural orthostatic tachycardia syndrome,[239,240] spinal cord and head injuries, amyotrophic lateral sclerosis, myasthenia gravis, a variety of muscular dystrophies, and Parkinson disease (see Chapter 35).

Miscellaneous Conditions

Patients with gastroparesis-like symptoms and cirrhosis with portal hypertension,[241] chronic kidney disease,[242] chronic pancreatitis,[243] advanced HIV infections[244] may have underlying gastroparesis. Patients with the Rett syndrome, which includes lack of development, autistic behavior, ataxia, and dementia in young girls, frequently have failure to thrive and significant gastroparesis and esophageal contraction abnormalities.[245] A variety of cancers may have local and systemic effects on the stomach neuromuscular apparatus that result in gastroparesis.[246,247] The neoplastic and paraneoplastic neuropathic syndromes and the effects of cytotoxic chemotherapy and radiation may result in gastroparesis and affect the patient's nutrition and intravascular volume status.

Hp infection does not affect the rate of gastric emptying. On the other hand, abnormal GMA has been reported in patients with Hp gastritis, and the dysrhythmias disappeared after eradication of Hp.[248] Gastric emptying is delayed in patients with anorexia nervosa[249] but is normal in patients with bulimia.[250] Cyclic vomiting syndrome is an unusual entity in that days of profound and unremitting nausea and vomiting (that often requires hospitalization) are followed by many days or months with virtually no GI symptoms.[251] Cyclic vomiting syndrome occurs in adults as well as in infants.[251,252] Some patients with orthostatic intolerance present with nausea and symptoms of gastroparesis and reflect autonomic nervous system dysfunction and gastric neuromuscular dysfunction.[240,253,254]

Dumping Syndrome and Rapid Gastric Emptying

Dumping syndrome is well-described in patients who have had vagotomy and pyloroplasty or Billroth I or Billroth II gastrojejunostomy.[254] In these patients, the ingested foods are not accommodated and retained in the fundus because of poor fundic relaxation. In addition, the foods are not normally triturated by peristaltic waves if the antrum, corpus, and pylorus have been resected. Thus liquid, and solid nutrients are rapidly emptied or "dumped" into the duodenum or jejunum.

Dumping syndrome can occur in patients who have no history of gastric operations. Thus idiopathic dumping syndrome may be overlooked as a diagnosis by many physicians.[257] Symptoms associated with dumping syndrome can mimic the symptoms associated with gastroparesis and FD. The dumping syndrome symptoms include nonspecific abdominal discomfort, bloating, and nausea and vomiting. These symptoms are usually experienced in the first hour after ingestion of foods. Sweating and lightheadedness, however, may occur and be followed by abdominal cramps and diarrhea that occur 2–4 hours after the meal and are additional clues to the dumping syndrome. Early symptoms are due to the distention of the small bowel by rapidly emptied solids and liquids from the stomach, whereas symptoms that occur later are due to rapid absorption of carbohydrates and hyperglycemia that is poorly matched in time with secretion of insulin. This mismatch of plasma glucose and insulin can result in symptomatic hypoglycemia. The rapid small bowel transit and poor absorption of the ingested nutrients lead to an osmotic form of diarrhea.[255]

Patients with no history of gastric operations may also have rapid gastric emptying (idiopathic dumping syndrome),[254] including patients with FD.[255] Rapid gastric emptying is present when more than 30% of the test meal (a low-fat egg substitute meal) is emptied in 30 minutes, or more than 70% is emptied at 60 minutes.[38] Rapid gastric emptying is associated with early stages of type 2 diabetes mellitus (see earlier), Zollinger-Ellison syndrome and the variety of gastric surgeries described earlier. Almost 50% of patients with idiopathic rapid emptying have gastric dysrhythmias and the majority have diabetes mellitus.[255]

DIAGNOSIS OF GASTRIC NEUROMUSCULAR DISORDERS

History

Patients with gastric neuromuscular dysfunction ranging from accommodation defects to gastric dysrhythmias to frank gastroparesis have similar dyspepsia-like symptoms. Most patients with gastric neuromuscular disorders have few upper GI symptoms when they are fasting. However, the ingestion of meals stimulates the disordered gastric neuromuscular apparatus, and early satiety, prolonged epigastric fullness, epigastric discomfort, or pain, mild-to-severe nausea, and vomiting are then experienced.[218] The multiple symptoms are related to neuromuscular disorders of various regions of the stomach (Table 52.4). The symptoms of postprandial fullness, nausea, distention, and vomiting are symptoms like FD, postprandial distress with nausea, or gastroparesis-like symptoms.

Patients with IGP have more abdominal pain compared with DGP.[214] Patients with type 2 diabetes mellitus and gastroparesis have more bloating than patients with type 1 diabetes mellitus with gastroparesis. Pain is a dominant symptom in 20%–30% of patients with IGP.[214] Nausea and vomiting are the symptoms that lead to medical evaluation in over 85% of patients with gastroparesis. Vomitus that contains undigested, chewed food is strong evidence for gastroparesis. Prolonged postprandial fullness, weight loss, and female gender are predictive factors for gastroparesis.[256] Bloating is also an important symptom related to gastroparesis but may also be due to small bowel or colonic dysmotility.[257,258] Patients learn to reduce these postprandial symptoms by adjusting their diet and carry on for months or years before they seek medical attention, or their physicians recognize the possibility of gastroparesis.

TABLE 52.4 Disorders of Gastric Neuromuscular Activity: Physiology, Pathophysiology, and Symptoms

Neuromuscular Activity	Physiologic Effects	Pathophysiologic Consequence(s)	Pathophysiologic Abnormality	Symptoms
Receptive relaxation	Fundic accommodation	Excess or poor accommodation	↓nNOS Vagotomy	ES
Antral peristalsis	Trituration Gastric emptying	Weak peristalsis Gastroparesis	↓ICCs ↓Enteric neurons Vagotomy	PF
Normal 3-cpm slow wave	Normal peristalsis and Gastric emptying	Gastric dysrhythmia (e.g., tachygastria)	↓ICCs Vagotomy	Nausea
Antropyloro-duodenal coordination	Normal trituration Gastric emptying	Pylorospasm Pyloric stenosis	↓nNOS PUD	ES, PF, nausea, vomiting
Normal vagus, ANS and CNS function	Normal gastric neuromuscular function	Fundic dysfunction, gastric dysrhythmias aperistalsis	↓Vagus function ANS imbalance	ES, PF, nausea, vomiting

ANS, Autonomic nervous system; *CNS*, central nervous system; *cpm*, cycles per minute; *ES*, early satiety; *ICCs*, interstitial cells of Cajal; *n*, nerves; *nNOS*, neuronal nitric oxide synthetase; *PF*, prolonged fullness; *PUD*, peptic ulcer disease.

The Gastroparesis Cardinal Symptom Index is used in research to quantify gastroparesis symptoms.[259] Persistent nausea is one of the most noxious symptoms of the gastric neuromuscular disorders. A thorough review of the causes of nausea and vomiting is required (see Chapter 16), and an appropriate differential diagnosis should be considered (see Box 52.1).[76,260] Unexplained nausea and vomiting due to gastric neuromuscular disorders must be distinguished from atypical GERD, regurgitation, and rumination syndrome. Atypical GERD may present as unexplained nausea, because these patients report little or no heartburn.[232] Regurgitation is the gentle delivery of gastric content into the esophagus and pharynx (and the content is sometimes reswallowed), whereas vomiting is the forceful ejection of gastric contents from the mouth. *Rumination* refers to the effortless return of ingested liquids and solid foods into the mouth without burning, bitter taste, or nausea. Patients with rumination have impaired gastric accommodation and a more sensitive relaxation of the lower esophageal sphincter pressure in response to gastric distention.[261] Rumination occurs in healthy adolescents and young adults but was previously recognized among children with neural and developmental disorders.

Abdominal pain, in contrast to the abdominal discomfort of bloating and nausea, is severe in approximately 30% of patients with gastroparesis.[262–264] Any recurrent abdominal pain syndrome in patients must be worked up extensively because the nausea and vomiting may be secondary to the specific cause of the pain, for example, epigastric pain associated with nausea and vomiting may be due to erosive esophagitis. Once the esophagitis is diagnosed and treated, the pain and nausea disappear. A specific pain syndrome may suggest diagnoses such as cholecystitis or pancreatitis. On the other hand, the epigastric discomfort or pain in some gastroparesis patients may originate from the stomach. Potential causes of pain from the stomach include excessive muscle tone of the fundus, high-amplitude antral contractions, pylorospasm, or hypersensitivity of the corpus-antrum to stretch.[264] Recurrent retching and vomiting often result in abdominal pain, which may be due to abdominal muscle and rib tenderness or the abdominal wall syndrome.[265–267]

Physical Examination

The general examination may be normal or reveal signs of volume depletion, weight loss, and poor nutrition. Orthostatic changes may suggest dehydration or postural orthostatic tachycardia syndrome.[268] Almost 40% of patients with gastroparesis are overweight or obese.[269] Inspection of dentition may show an erosion of enamel associated with chronic GERD or bulimia. Abdominal examination may detect masses, organomegaly, and areas of tenderness. A succussion splash is rarely present in gastroparesis. Auscultation over the epigastrium may detect bruits that indicate stenoses of the celiac or superior mesenteric arteries. Pain and tenderness that are precisely localized to healed abdominal incisions and increase when the head is flexed and anterior abdominal muscles are contracted (positive Carnett sign) suggest the pain is from an abdominal wall syndrome and not the stomach or other abdominal organs.[265–267] Joint laxity may reflect the presence of Ehlers-Danlos syndrome.[238] Neurologic examination may reveal nystagmus, facial weakness, ataxia, or other abnormalities, which point to primary neurologic diseases.

Standard Tests

Common causes of nausea and vomiting and postprandial distress symptoms are excluded by routine laboratory studies, standard endoscopy, and CT of the abdomen and head. Gastric cancers are detected in less than 1% of these patients who undergo endoscopy.[270] If these standard tests are normal and symptoms persist, the gastric neuromuscular disorders should be considered.

Noninvasive Tests

An objective diagnosis of neuromuscular disorders of the stomach can be established by the results of GETs and EGG with water load satiety test. GETs and EGG are complementary in defining different aspects of gastric neuromuscular disorders (see Table 52.3).[52,132,260] By combining the results of GETs and EGG, pathophysiologic categories of gastric neuromuscular function can be defined, and rational treatment approaches designed. The categories are (1) gastroparesis with gastric dysrhythmia, (2) gastroparesis with normal 3-cpm gastric electrical rhythm, (3) normal gastric emptying with gastric dysrhythmia, and (4) normal gastric emptying with normal 3-cpm gastric electrical rhythm. The four categories provide a conceptual framework for understanding the spectrum of gastric neuromuscular disorders and providing an approach to therapy (see Table 52.2).

Regarding patients with gastroparesis, there are two subtypes: Subtype 1 patients have severe neuromuscular dysfunction with gastroparesis on GETs and gastric dysrhythmias such as tachygastria. These patients may have diabetic, idiopathic, or postsurgical gastroparesis. Patients in category 1 often have more severe symptoms, require many drugs, and may require venting gastrostomies, enteral feeding, and gastric pacing, as discussed later (Fig. 52.22).

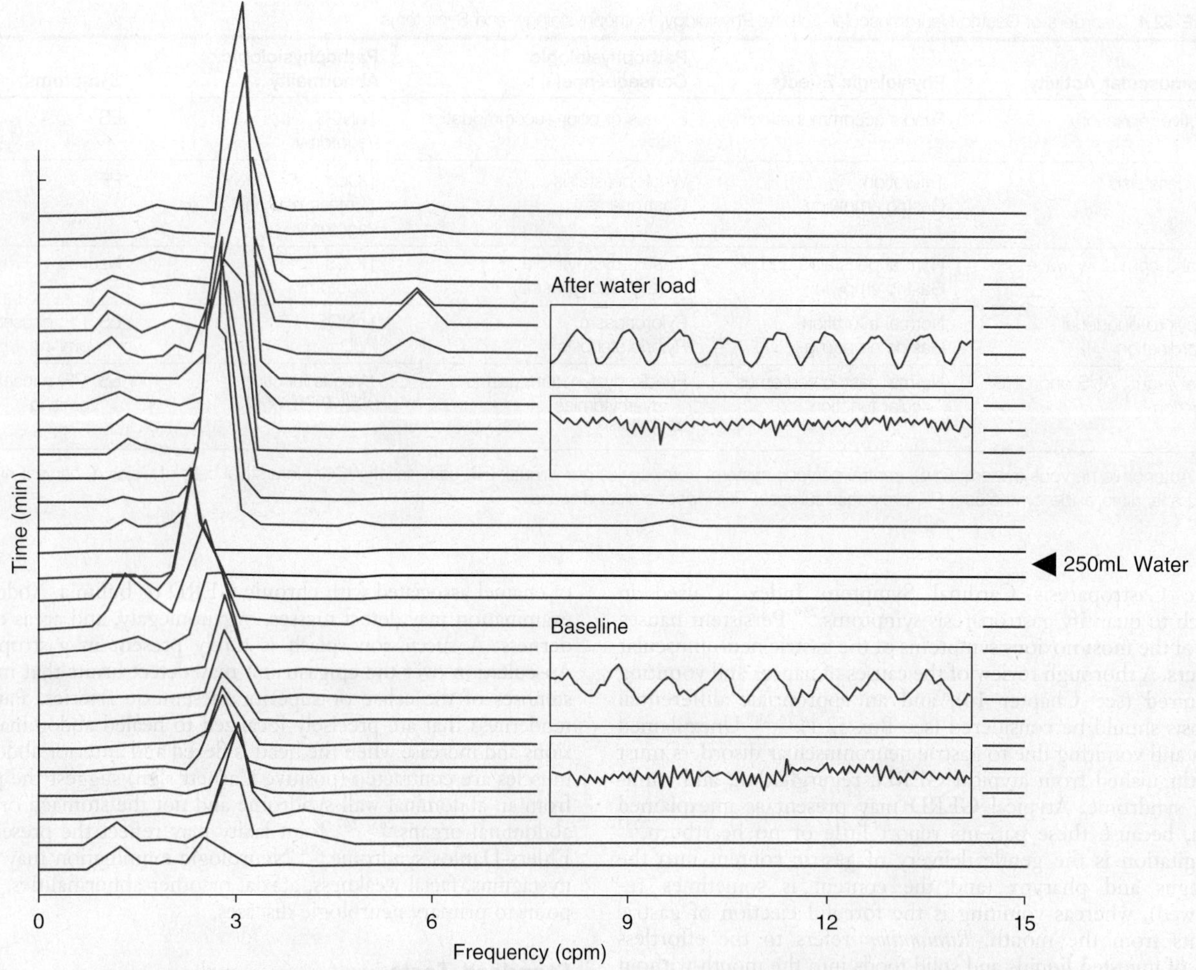

Fig. 52.23 Electrogastrogram (EGG) rhythm strips from baseline and 30 minutes after the water load test from a patient with idiopathic gastroparesis. The X-axis indicates frequencies in the EGG signal, the Y-axis indicates time, and the Z-axis indicates the power of the frequencies represented in the peaks. Clear 3-cpm waves are seen in the rhythm strips (*right*) and reflect normal slow waves and numbers of interstitial cells of Cajals. Computer analysis of the EGG recording (*left*) shows regular 3-cpm peaks in the running spectral analysis. This is the obstructive subtype of gastroparesis with gastroparesis and normal 3-cpm gastric myoelectrical activity. Mechanical obstruction at the pylorus was excluded at endoscopy. Neuromuscular dysfunction at the pylorus is the likely cause of the delayed gastric emptying.

Subtype 2 patients have gastroparesis and normal or high-amplitude 3-cpm EGG signals. (Fig. 52.23). These patients may have fixed mechanical obstructions of the pylorus or duodenum that are reversible with operation[131] or more often have normal endoscopy and have pyloric neuromuscular dysfunction that responds to endoscopic therapies and pyloroplasty.[167,212] Electromechanical dissociation is also a pathophysiologic possibility.

Regarding patients with FD or gastroparesis-like symptoms and normal gastric emptying, there are two subtypes: Subtype 1 patients have normal gastric emptying and hyponormal GMA and gastric dysrhythmias.[52] Two-thirds of patients with FD-postprandial distress symptoms had gastric dysrhythmias.[133] Category 1 patients had a significantly better response to the prokinetic agent cisapride than patients with normal 3-cpm EGG recordings.[221,223]

Category 2 patients have symptoms but normal gastric emptying and normal 3-cpm GMA. One-third of patients with FD had normal 3-cpm GMA in response to the WLST.[133] The gastroparesis-like symptoms may be due to poor gastric relaxation or gastric visceral hypersensitivity in response to distension with the water load. It is possible some of these patients have pyloric neuromuscular dysfunction. Diagnoses of nongastric disorders should also be considered as causes of symptoms in this patient group with normal endoscopy, normal 3-cpm GMA and water load test. Atypical GERD may cause nausea, and a 24-hour pH study will confirm the relationship.[232] A CCK-stimulated gallbladder emptying study may document rapid gallbladder dysfunction in the absence of cholelithiasis.[271] If postprandial abdominal discomfort/pain and disturbed bowel function are present, then IBS should be considered. CNS diseases and orthostatic intolerance as causes of nausea also should be assessed as outlined in Table 52.1.

TREATMENT

If delayed gastric emptying is confirmed, then the causes of gastroparesis should be reviewed (see Table 52.3). The reversible obstructive causes of gastroparesis due to fixed pyloric stenosis or functional pylorospasm and ischemic gastroparesis due to chronic mesenteric ischemia must be excluded because these entities are reversible. The rate of gastric emptying does not correlate well with symptoms associated with gastroparesis so new treatments are needed for other gastric neuromuscular dysfunction like dysrhythmic GMA or accommodation dysfunction.

If gastric emptying is normal, then gastric dysrhythmia and gastric accommodation disorders also may be the neuromuscular disorders that are relevant to the symptoms in these patients. By grouping patients based on GET and EGG test results, the pathophysiologic findings can help in the understanding of symptoms and in developing approaches to treatment (see Table 52.2). Treatments listed in Tables 52.5 and 52.6 reflect the broad but limited armamentarium that ranges from prokinetic agents to endoscopic and electrical therapies to diet counseling.

Drug Therapy

Prokinetic Agents for Corpus and Antrum

Drugs with prokinetic effects on gastric contractility and antiarrhythmic effects on gastric dysrhythmias are prescribed for patients with gastroparesis and those with normal emptying, gastric dysrhythmias (see Table 52.5). Patients who have gastroparesis and tachygastria have severe electrical and contractile abnormalities of the stomach. The treatment includes prokinetics, antinauseant therapies, and dietary counseling.[164,260]

Erythromycin is a macrolide antibiotic and motilin-like molecule that increases gastric emptying by stimulating strong phase 3–like antral contractions.[272,273] Erythromycin, however, often increases nausea and vomiting symptoms. Metoclopramide, a substituted benzamide related to procainamide, is a useful prokinetic antiemetic but has a "black box" warning. The drug is approved only in the United States for use for 2–8 weeks in gastroparesis, and meticulous follow-up is needed because metoclopramide may cause depression, extrapyramidal side effects, and irreversible tardive dyskinesia.[274,275] Domperidone is a dopamine antagonist that decreases nausea, corrects gastric dysrhythmias, and increases gastric emptying rates.[276] Domperidone may be obtained through a compassionate use drug application process with the FDA. Cisapride was not approved for gastric emptying disorders but increased gastric emptying rates and decreased dyspepsia symptoms in some patients.[277]

Prorelaxant Agents for Fundus and Pylorus

Few drugs relax the fundus. Sumatriptan, a 5-HT_1 antagonist, decreases fundic tone but was not better than placebo in reducing symptoms in patients with FD.[278] Buspirone relaxes the fundus and may decrease postprandial fullness.[279] Trials of dicyclomine or calcium channel blockers to decrease fundic tone have not been reported. Botulinum toxin relaxes the pyloric sphincter pressure and is described later in endoscopic therapy.

Antinausea Therapy

Nonspecific approaches to treating nausea and vomiting due to gastric neuromuscular disorders include serotonin (5-HT_3) receptor antagonists such as ondansetron and granisetron (see Table 52.5).[280] These agents, as well as the phenothiazines and antihistamines, such as promethazine, dimenhydrinate, and cyclizine, are often used for these symptoms, but there are no controlled trials in patients with gastric neuromuscular disorders. Lorazepam or alprazolam or other antianxiety medications reduce nausea in some patients.[175,176,280] Dronabinol and mirtazapine are other drugs used for nausea, but no controlled trial data are available for use in gastroparesis. An uncontrolled trial of tricyclic antidepressants alleviated nausea in approximately 70% of patients with unexplained nausea,[281] but a placebo-controlled trial showed that one tricyclic compound, nortriptyline, was no better than placebo in reducing symptoms of gastroparesis.[282] Aprepitant is a neurokinin-1 antagonist that significantly decreased nausea and decreased tachygastria in patients with normal or delayed gastric emptying and chronic nausea.[224]

Electrical Therapy

Acustimulation

Acustimulation (mild electrical stimulation of acupuncture points) reduces nausea of pregnancy, nausea due to chemotherapy agents, postoperative nausea, and the nausea of motion sickness[283,284] and symptoms related to gastroparesis.[285]

Gastric Electrical Therapies

Three different methods are being investigated to treat gastroparesis: (1) GES with high-frequency (e.g., 12 cpm) and short-duration (300 microseconds) stimulation, (2) gastric pacing with low-frequency (e.g., 3 cpm) and long-duration (300 milliseconds) stimulation, and (3) sequential neural electrical stimulation with multiple pairs of electrodes positioned on the corpus-antrum.

Gastric Electrical Stimulation

GES at 12 cpm during a 12-month period of continuous treatment significantly decreased nausea and vomiting in patients with refractory, idiopathic, diabetic, or postsurgical gastroparesis.[286–289] Stimulating the stomach at 12 cpm (four times the normal slow wave frequency) resulted in improvement in nausea and vomiting in patients with gastroparesis.[290] A 12-week placebo-controlled cross-over study of GES in DGP improved daily vomiting episodes compared to baseline but was not different than placebo; however, patients with open-label GES had a significant decrease in symptoms at 12 months compared with baseline and gastric emptying rates improved.[292] Uncontrolled studies from several centers indicate that 50%–70% of patients with IGP or DGP treated with GES report a decrease in their chronic nausea and vomiting symptoms.[287–289] Gastroparesis patients with normal 3-cpm EGG patterns and more ICCs on gastric biopsies had significantly better symptom response to GES compared with patients with tachygastria and fewer ICCs.[23] Patients with DGP had similar symptom improvement compared with patients with IGP.[286–289] Temporary gastric stimulation may help identify GES responders.[291] Intraoperative measurement of gastric slow waves showed tachygastrias, bradygastrias, and aberrant initiation and conduction abnormalities in 11 of 12 patients with gastroparesis, and may help direct pacing and stimulator treatments.[21] Complications of GES include a 10% incidence of infections in the subcutaneous pocket where the device is positioned. There is also a small incidence of fracture of the electrode wires.

Gastric Pacing

Low-frequency gastric stimulation using a 3-cpm stimulus to pace or entrain the normal slow wave rhythm in patients with gastroparesis seeks to stimulate 3 gastric peristaltic contractions per minute and improve gastric emptying.[292] In 13 patients, electrical stimulation at a frequency up to 10% higher than the normal 3 cpm, at an amplitude of 4 mÅ and a pulse width of 300 milliseconds, was used to entrain and pace the slow waves. Gastric dysrhythmias were eradicated in some patients. In a similar study of nine additional patients, electrical stimulation was used to entrain the slow wave, and tachygastria was converted to normal 3-cpm rhythms in two patients.[293] After 1 month of gastric pacing treatment, gastric emptying was significantly improved; symptoms of gastroparesis were significantly reduced. Adverse events due to gastric pacing devices are discomfort at the site of electrical stimulation and fracture or dislodgement of the electrodes. This methodology has not advanced to clinical application.

TABLE 52.5 Drug and Nondrug Therapies Used to Treat Symptoms in Patients With Gastric Neuromuscular Disorders

Therapy	Mechanisms and Sites of Action	Dose	Adverse Effects
PROKINETIC DRUGS			
Macrolides			
Erythromycin	Motilin receptor agonist	125–250 mg four times daily	Nausea, diarrhea, abdominal cramps, rash
Substituted Benzamides			
Metoclopramide	D_2 receptor antagonist; 5-HT_3 receptor antagonist; 5-HT_4 receptor agonist	5–20 mg before meals and at bedtime	Extrapyramidal symptoms, dystonic reactions, anxiety, depression, hyperprolactinemia, tardive dyskinesia
Domperidone	D_2-receptor antagonist (peripheral)	10–20 mg before meals and at bedtime	Hyperprolactinemia, breast tenderness, galactorrhea
Serotonin Agonists			
Cisapride[a]	5-HT_4 receptor agonist	5–20 mg before meals	Cardiac dysrhythmias, diarrhea, abdominal discomfort
Ghrelin-agonist			
PRORELAXANT DRUGS			
Dicyclomine	Muscarinic antagonist	10–20 mg before meals	Drowsiness, dry mouth
Buspirone	5-HT_{1a} agonist	7.5–15 mg two times daily	Dizziness, headache, nausea
Botulinum toxin (Botox)	See Endoscopic Therapies		
ANTINAUSEA DRUGS			
Serotonin Antagonists			
Ondansetron	5-HT_3 receptor antagonist	4–8 mg two to four times daily, either orally or IV	Headache, increased liver enzymes
Granisetron	5-HT_3 receptor antagonist	2 mg once daily or 3.1 mg/24-hours patch	Headache, increased liver enzymes
Phenothiazines			
Prochlorperazine	CNS	5–10 mg three times daily	Hypotension, extrapyramidal symptoms
Antihistamines			
Promethazine	CNS, H_1 receptor antagonist	25 mg twice daily	Drowsiness
Dimenhydrinate	H_1 receptor antagonist	50 mg four times daily	Drowsiness
Cyclizine	H_1 receptor antagonist	50 mg four times daily	Drowsiness
Butyrophenones			
Droperidol	Central dopamine receptor antagonist	2.5–5 mg IV every 2 hours	Sedation, hypotension
Antidepressants	CNS sites		
Amitriptyline		25–100 mg at bedtime	Constipation
Nortriptyline		10–75 mg at bedtime	Constipation
Mirtazapine		15 mg at bedtime	Weight gain
Benzodiazepines/Cannabinoids	CNS		
Lorazepam		0.5–1 mg four times daily	Drowsiness, lightheadedness
Alprazolam		0.25–0.5 mg three times daily	Drowsiness, lightheadedness
Dronabinol		5–10 mg two times daily	Sedation
Substance P Agonists			
Aprepitant	Substance P antagonist	15 mg/day	Tiredness, hiccups
ELECTRICAL THERAPIES			
Acupressure and acustimulation/ acupuncture	Spinal/vagal afferents? Endorphins	Variable N/A	Local tenderness

TABLE 52.5 Drug and Nondrug Therapies Used to Treat Symptoms in Patients With Gastric Neuromuscular Disorders—cont'd

Therapy	Mechanisms and Sites of Action	Dose	Adverse Effects
Gastric electrical stimulation	Vagal afferents?	12 cpm, 330 milliseconds, 5 mÅ	Pocket infection
Gastric pacing	Control dysrhythmias, improve gastric emptying	3 cpm, 300 microseconds, 4 mÅ	Pocket infection
Endoscopic Therapies			
Botox injection into the pylorus	Relax pyloric muscle	25–50 units per quadrant	None
Balloon dilation of the pylorus	Stretch pyloric muscle	20 mm balloon, 2 minutes	Abdominal pain after dilation
Radiofrequency ablation at LES	Reduce gastroesophageal reflux, improve gastric myoelectrical activity	N/A	Transient dysphagia
Diet Therapies			
Gastroparesis diet	Diet based on gastric emptying physiology	See Table 52.6	None
High-protein drinks	Decreases gastric dysrhythmias	Unknown	None
Gastrostomy	Venting paretic stomach	N/A	See Chapter 7
Jejunostomy	Enteral nutritional support	N/A	See Chapter 7
TPN	Bypass paretic stomach	As needed	Sepsis, thrombosis of central veins

[a]Compassionate clearance use only.
Botox, Botulinum toxin; *cpm*, cycles per minute; *D2*, dopamine-2; *5-HT*, 5-hydroxytryptamine; H_1, histamine-1; *N/A*, not applicable.

TABLE 52.6 Dietary Therapies of Nausea and Vomiting in Patients with Gastric Neuromuscular Disorders Step-Wise Approach

Diet	Goal	Foods to Avoid
Step 1: Sports Drinks and Bouillon		
For severe nausea and vomiting: Small volumes of salty liquids, with some caloric content to avoid volume depletion Chewable multiple vitamin	1000–1500 mL/day in multiple servings (e.g., 12 120-mL servings over 12–14 hours) Patient can sip 30–60 mL at a time to reach ≈120 mL/h	Citrus drinks of all kinds; highly sweetened drinks
Step 2: Soups and Smoothies		
If Step 1 is tolerated: Soup with noodles or rice and crackers Smoothies with low-fat dairy Peanut butter, cheese, and crackers in small amounts Caramels or other chewy confection Ingest above foods in at least 6 small-volume meals/day Chewable multiple vitamin	≈1500 calories/day to avoid volume depletion and maintain weight (often more realistic than weight gain)	Creamy, milk-based liquids
Step 3: Starches, Chicken, and Fish		
If Step 2 is tolerated: Noodles, pastas, potatoes (mashed or baked), rice, baked chicken breast, fish (all easily mixed and emptied by the stomach) Ingest solids in at least 6 small-volume meals/day Multiple vitamin (liquid or dissolvable)	Common foods that the patient finds interesting and satisfying and that provoke minimal nausea/vomiting symptoms	Fatty foods that delay gastric emptying; red meats and fresh vegetables that require considerable trituration; pulpy fibrous foods that promote formation of bezoars

From Koch KL, Hasler WL, Eds. *Nausea and Vomiting: Diagnosis and Treatment*. Switzerland: Springer International Publishing; 2017.

Sequential Neural Electrical Stimulation

Sequential neural electrical gastric stimulation is gastric pacing that uses a microprocessor to sequentially activate a series of electrodes that encircle the distal two-thirds of the stomach. The stimulation sequence induces propagated contractions that cause a forceful emptying of the gastric content.[294] This methodology has not advanced to clinical application.

Endoscopic Therapy

Endoscopic therapies refer to drug or device therapies delivered to the relevant regions of the stomach via endoscopes. The injection of botulinum toxin A into the pylorus to decrease sphincter pressure and to improve gastric emptying and nausea and vomiting in patients with gastroparesis produced results similar to placebo injections.[295–297] However, 33 patients with gastroparesis selected on the basis of normal 3-cpm GMA (functional gastric outlet obstruction) underwent balloon dilation of the pylorus or injection of botulinum toxin and symptoms improved in symptoms in 78% of them.[167] Patients with two or more successful endoscopic pyloric therapies were offered pyloroplasty for more durable treatment, and all had improved symptoms and six had normal gastric emptying when retested 6 months after the operation.[212] Pyloroplasty performed for patients undergoing GES also improved GE and symptoms.[298] Gastric-peroral endoscopic myotomy is an advanced endoscopic procedure during which a pyloromyotomy is performed for the treatment of gastroparesis. Early studies with gastric-peroral endoscopic myotomy indicate symptoms and gastric emptying improve after treatment.[299,300] Normal 3-cpm GMA and GP appears to define this subset of patients with functional gastric outlet obstruction due to pylorospasm or dyschalasia.[167,212] Assessment of pyloric distensibility with Endo-FLIP may help further define gastroparesis subgroups.[148] RFA treatment applied to the lower esophageal sphincter area in patients with GERD and dyspepsia improves GERD but also gastric dysrhythmias and gastric emptying.[231]

Diet Therapy

Dietary Counseling

Many patients with acute or chronic nausea and vomiting from gastric neuromuscular disorders do not know what to eat and will benefit from dietary counseling.[260,301] Only one-third of patients with gastroparesis have had a dietary consultation.[270] In the Nausea/Vomiting (Gastroparesis) Diet, liquid and solid foods that are easy for the stomach to mix and empty are prescribed.[301–303] This diet is based on gastric emptying principles and is a 3-step diet that requires minimal neuromuscular work of the stomach as the diet is advanced (see Table 52.6).

Step 1 is primarily electrolyte solutions that are consumed in small amounts over a 24-hour period to avoid volume depletion. Liquids require less gastric neuromuscular work to empty than solid foods. If patients tolerate Step 1, then Step 2 may be tried next. Step 2 diet includes soups containing noodles or rice. Milk-based creamy soups are avoided. Step 3 emphasizes starches and chicken and turkey breast. These solid foods require less gastric work to mix and empty compared with fresh vegetables or red meats. Fried and greasy foods are avoided because fats delay gastric emptying. A chewable multiple vitamin is taken daily in all the three Steps. Small particle diets like those described in Step 3 decrease symptoms in patents with gastroparesis.

Nutraceuticals

Liquid protein meals with or without ginger decrease nausea associated with motion sickness and gastric dysrhythmias, nausea of pregnancy, and delayed nausea after chemotherapy.[303–306] These protein-based meal therapies have not been formally evaluated in patients with gastroparesis or gastric dysrhythmias.

Other Approaches

For patients with chronic nausea and vomiting, percutaneous endoscopic gastrostomy (PEG) tubes may be placed for periodic venting gastric contents to avoid frequent vomiting episodes and to improve quality of life.[307] The venting PEG does not treat the underlying gastric neuromuscular disorder, but it allows the patients to empty the stomach rather than suffer repeated episodes of emesis and discomfort. Hospitalizations are reduced.[175] Medications and some nutritional liquids may be tolerated when given through the gastrostomy tube. However, for most patients with severe gastroparesis use of stomach to empty nutrients brings on too many symptoms. Jejunal feeding tubes for enteral nutrition may be needed to provide basic caloric support for patients with severe nausea and vomiting from gastric neuromuscular disorders. A PEG with J-tube extension usually fails because a single vomiting episode may propel the extension tube into the stomach. Techniques to anchor the feeding tube in the jejunum with clips should be considered. In some cases, a J-tube placed endoscopically or surgically will be required.[307] TPN via central IV catheters should be avoided if at all possible because of the development of line sepsis and venous thrombosis.

Full references for this chapter can be found at https://ebooks.health.elsevier.com.

53 Gastric Secretion

Ellie Chen, Hidekazu Suzuki, Jonathan D. Kaunitz

IN THIS CHAPTER

As discussed in Chapters 51–52, the stomach is an active reservoir that stores, grinds, and slowly dispenses partially digested food to the intestine for further digestion and absorption. Its main secretory function is the production of hydrochloric acid.[1] Gastric acid secretion is present on the first day of life and increases as infants become more mature.[2] By 2 years of age, acid secretion is similar to that of adults when corrected for body weight.[3] Most studies indicate that the rate of acid secretion changes little after the second decade of life unless there is coexisting disease of the acid-secreting glandular mucosa, such as infection with Hp or atrophic gastritis.[4–7]

Acid facilitates the digestion of protein by converting the proenzyme pepsinogen to the active proteolytic enzyme pepsin. It also facilitates the absorption of nonheme iron, vitamin B_{12}, certain medications (e.g., thyroxin), and calcium, as well as prevents bacterial overgrowth, enteric infection, and possibly spontaneous bacterial peritonitis (SBP).[8–22]

The stomach also secretes lipase, intrinsic factor (IF), electrolytes [e.g., bicarbonate (HCO_3^-), K^+, and Cl^-], and mucins in addition to a variety of neurocrine, paracrine, and hormonal agents (Fig. 53.1). Neurocrine agents are released from nerve terminals and reach their targets via synaptic diffusion [e.g., acetylcholine (ACh), gastrin-releasing peptide (GRP), vasoactive intestinal peptide (VIP), nitric oxide (NO), and pituitary adenylate cyclase–activating polypeptide (PACAP)]. Paracrine agents are released in proximity to their targets and reach them via diffusion (e.g., histamine and somatostatin). Hormones are released into the circulation and reach their targets via the bloodstream (e.g., gastrin) (see Chapter 4).

Gastric mucosal integrity depends on a delicate balance between secretion of aggressive (e.g., acid and pepsin) and defensive (e.g., bicarbonate and mucin) substances (Fig. 53.2).[23] When mucosal defense mechanisms are overwhelmed, ulceration may occur. To gain the benefits of acid without untoward effects, gastric exocrine and endocrine secretion is precisely regulated. This is accomplished by a highly coordinated interaction among a multitude of neural, paracrine, and hormonal pathways.

FUNCTIONAL ANATOMY

As discussed in Chapter 51, the stomach consists of 3 anatomic (fundus, corpus or body, and antrum) and 2 functional (oxyntic and pyloric gland) areas (Fig. 53.3). The oxyntic gland area, the hallmark of which is the oxyntic cell (*oxys*, Greek for acid), or parietal cell, comprises 80% of the organ (fundus and corpus). The pyloric gland area, the hallmark of which is the G or gastrin cell, comprises 20% of the organ (antrum). The human stomach contains approximately 1×10^9 parietal cells and 9×10^6 gastrin cells.[24] There is debate as to whether the cardia, a transition zone of 0–9 mm between the squamous mucosa of the esophagus and the oxyntic mucosa of the stomach, exists as a normal anatomic structure or develops as a result of abnormal reflux (see Chapters 45, 48, and 49). Autopsy and endoscopic studies suggest that cardiac mucosa is absent in more than 50% of the general population.[25]

The glandular area is organized in vertical tubular units that consist of an apical pit region, an isthmus, and the actual gland region that forms the lower part of the unit; the latter consists of a neck and a base (Fig. 53.4). The progenitor cell of the gastric unit, located in the isthmus, gives rise to all gastric epithelial cells. In the oxyntic gland area, the mucus-producing pit cells migrate upward from the progenitor cell toward the gastric lumen. Six acid-producing parietal cells are produced in one isthmus each month and migrate downward to the middle and lower regions of the gland[26]; as the cells migrate downward, they become more senescent and are less active acid secretors. The turnover time for parietal cells is 54 days in mice and 164 days in rats.[24] Besides hydrochloric acid, parietal cells produce IF, transforming growth factor (TGF)-α, amphiregulin, heparin-binding EGF, sonic hedgehog, hepcidin, and leptin.[27–29] Chief (zymogenic) cells predominate at the gland base and secrete pepsinogen and leptin.[30] Several distinct neuroendocrine cell types are contained within the gland, but only some of their products have been assigned physiologic functions (see Chapter 4). The cells include D cells (somatostatin and amylin), enterochromaffin-like (ECL) cells (histamine and parathyroid hormone–like hormone), enterochromaffin (EC) cells [atrial natriuretic peptide (ANP), serotonin, and adrenomedullin], and A-like or Gr cells (ghrelin and obestatin).[31–37] Somatostatin-containing D cells possess neural-like cytoplasmic processes that terminate in the vicinity of parietal and ECL cells (see Fig. 53.4). The functional correlate of this anatomic coupling is a tonic paracrine restraint exerted by somatostatin on acid secretion directly as well as indirectly by inhibiting histamine secretion (Fig. 53.5).[38–40] ECL cells are the dominant neuroendocrine cell type in oxyntic mucosa. They constitute 66% of the neuroendocrine cell population in rats and 30% in humans. Like somatostatin-containing D cells, ECL cells may also possess cytoplasmic processes that terminate in close proximity to parietal cells.[41]

Somatostatin-containing D cells are also present in the pyloric gland area (see Figs. 53.4 and 53.5) where they exert a tonic paracrine restraint on gastrin secretion from G cells.[42,43] The pyloric gland also

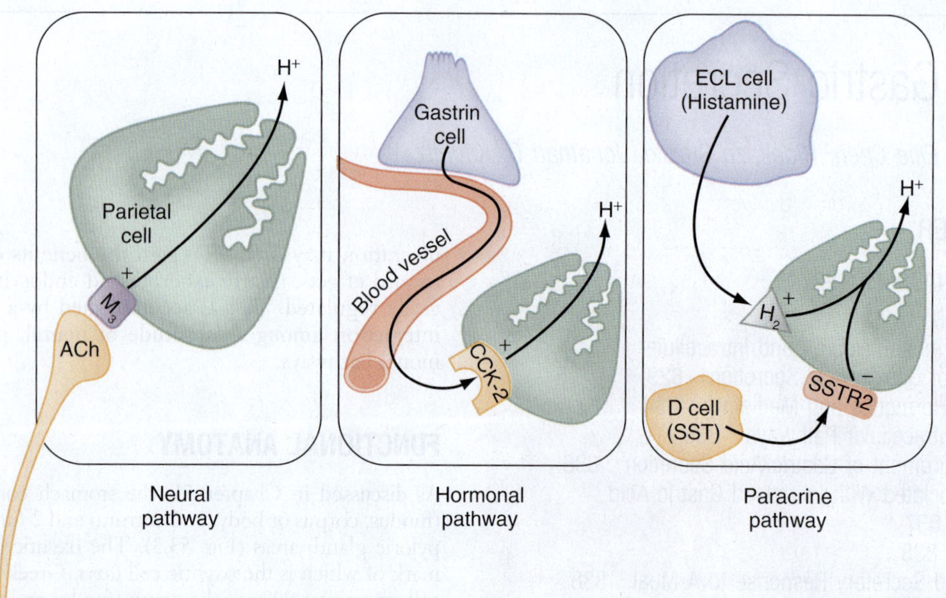

Fig. 53.1 Neural, hormonal, and paracrine pathways directly regulating parietal cell acid (H^+) secretion. *Left,* Acetylcholine (ACh) released from postganglionic enteric neurons within the oxyntic mucosa, stimulates the parietal cell directly via M_3 receptors coupled to release of intracellular calcium. *Center,* Gastrin released from antral G cells, travels in the circulation to reach the parietal cell and directly activates *CCK* subtype 2 (CCK-2) receptors which are coupled to release of intracellular calcium. *Right,* Histamine released from oxyntic *ECL* cells, diffuses to the parietal cell and directly activates histamine subtype 2 (H_2) receptors, which are coupled to the generation of cyclic adenosine monophosphate. Somatostatin *(SST),* released from oxyntic D cells, diffuses to the parietal cell and directly activates *SSTR2,* which are coupled to the inhibition of acid secretion. ACh, gastrin, and SST have also important indirect actions affecting acid secretion not shown here. +, Stimulatory; −, inhibitory.

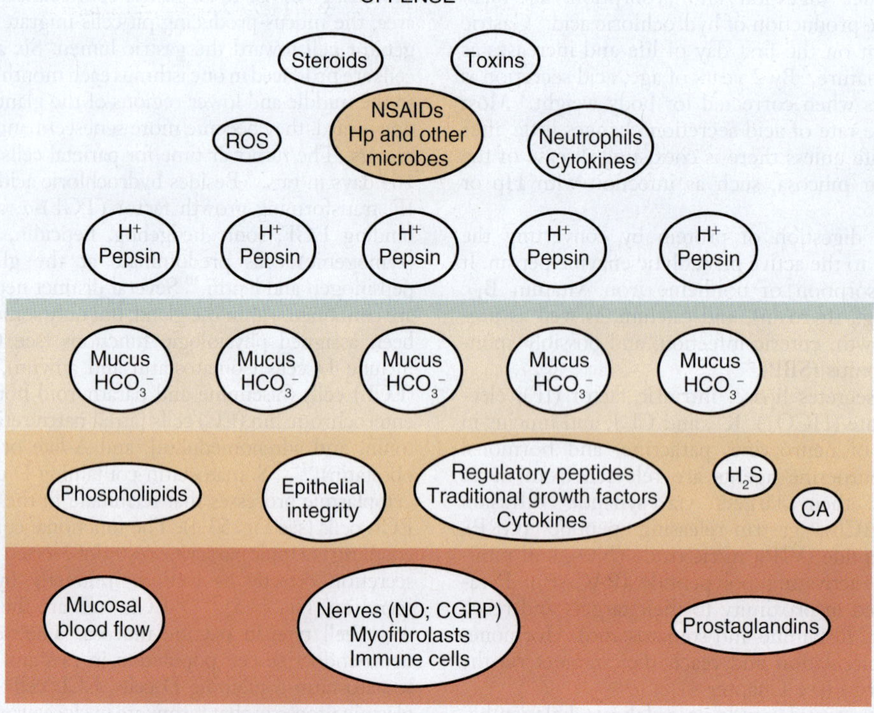

Fig. 53.2 Gastroduodenal offense and defense. Mucosal integrity depends on a delicate balance between aggressive and defensive factors. When mucosal defense mechanisms are overwhelmed, ulceration may occur. *CA,* Carbonic anhydrase; *CGRP,* calcitonin gene–related peptide; *H_2S,* hydrogen sulfide; *HCO_3–,* bicarbonate; *NO,* nitric oxide; *ROS,* reactive oxygen species.

contains EC cells (ANP and serotonin), A-like or Gr cells (ghrelin and obestatin), and endocrine cells containing orexin.[33,44,45]

Chromogranin A (CgA), an acidic glycoprotein, is contained within most neuroendocrine cells and, as discussed in Chapter 43, serum CgA has been used as a sensitive marker for the diagnosis of neuroendocrine tumors (NETs; e.g., carcinoid and gastrinoma).[46] The bulk of "normal" blood CgA is derived from gastric ECL cells. Hence elevated circulating CgA concentrations are also observed in patients with ECL hyperplasia caused by hypergastrinemia as a result of atrophic gastritis or treatment with proton pump inhibitors (PPIs) for as short as 5 days.[47] After a discontinuation of PPI therapy, serum CgA gradually declines with a half-life of 4–5 days.[48]

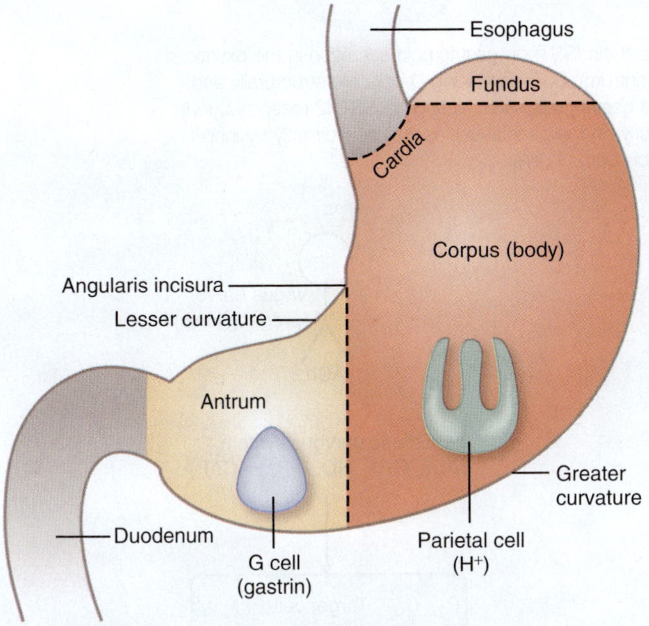

Fig. 53.3 Functional gastric anatomy. The stomach consists of 3 anatomic (fundus, corpus or body, and antrum) and 2 functional (oxyntic and pyloric gland) areas. The hallmark of the oxyntic gland area is the parietal cell. The hallmark of the pyloric gland area is the G or gastrin cell.

The stomach is innervated by a neural network, the enteric nervous system (ENS), which contains intrinsic neurons (i.e., neurons whose cell bodies are contained within the gastric wall) (Figs. 53.6–53.8). The ENS, the third division of the autonomic nervous system (the other two being the sympathetic and parasympathetic), is often referred to as the "little brain" because it contains as many neurons ($\approx 10^6$) as the spinal cord and can function autonomous of central input (see Fig. 53.6).[49] Nevertheless, the ENS receives input from and sends input to the central nervous system via sympathetic and parasympathetic neurons. In rats and guinea pigs, most of the intrinsic neural innervation of the stomach originates in the myenteric plexus, located between the circular and longitudinal muscle layers; the submucosal plexus in these species contains only a small number of neurons. Humans, in contrast, have a clearly defined submucosal plexus that regulates gastric secretion and contains a variety of neurotransmitters (see Figs. 53.7 and 53.8).

The vagus nerve is predominantly afferent, containing 80%–90% afferent fibers and 10%–20% efferent fibers. The efferent fibers arise from the dorsal motor nucleus in the medulla. They are preganglionic and do not directly innervate parietal or neuroendocrine cells but rather synapse with neurons of the ENS. The enteric neurons contain a variety of transmitters, including ACh, GRP, NO, VIP, and PACAP (see Fig. 53.8).[50] In the stomach, afferent nerve fibers containing calcitonin gene–related peptide (CGRP) are of extrinsic origin, with the cell bodies located outside the stomach wall.[51] Neurons of the ENS regulate acid secretion directly, as is the case for ACh, and/or indirectly by modulating the secretion of gastrin from G cells, somatostatin from D cells, and possibly histamine from ECL cells (see Fig. 53.8).

ACID SECRETION

Paracrine, Hormonal, Neural, and Intracellular Regulation of Gastric Acid Secretion

Primary Secretagogues

Parietal cells secrete hydrochloric acid at a concentration of approximately 160 mM or pH 0.8. Acid is thought to gain access

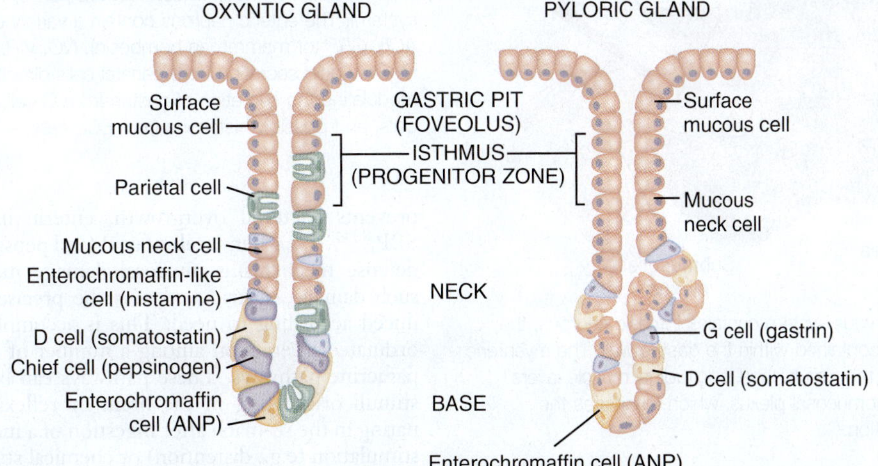

Fig. 53.4 Gastric gland anatomy. Somatostatin-containing D cells contain cytoplasmic processes that terminate in the vicinity of acid-secreting parietal and histamine-secreting ECL cells in the oxyntic gland area (fundus and corpus) and gastrin-secreting G cells in the pyloric gland area (antrum). The functional correlate of this anatomic coupling is a tonic paracrine restraint on acid secretion by somatostatin that is exerted directly on the parietal cell, as well as indirectly by inhibiting histamine and gastrin secretion. *ANP*, Atrial natriuretic peptide. (From Schubert ML, Peura DA. Control of gastric acid secretion in health and disease. *Gastroenterology*. 2008;134:1842–1860.)

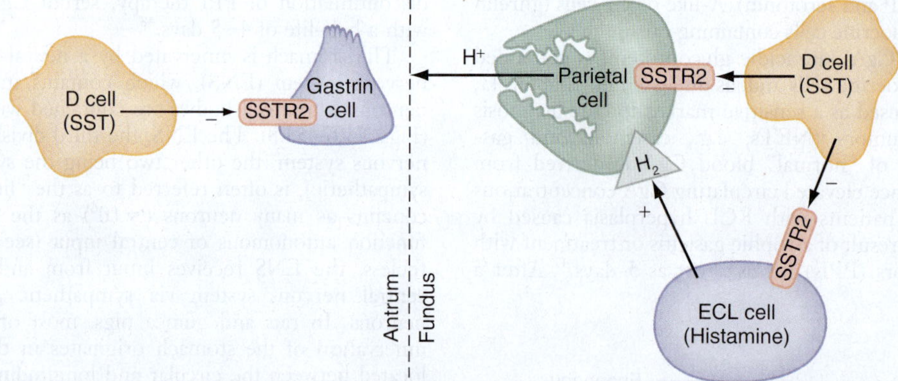

Fig. 53.5 Model illustrating the inhibitory actions of somatostatin (*SST*) on gastric acid secretion in the oxyntic gland area (fundus and body) and the pyloric gland area (antrum). SST-containing D cells are structurally and functionally coupled to their target cells: parietal, *ECL*, and gastrin cells. SST, acting via *SSTR2* receptors, tonically restrains acid secretion. This restraint is exerted directly on the parietal cell as well as indirectly by inhibiting histamine secretion from ECL cells and gastrin secretion from G cells.

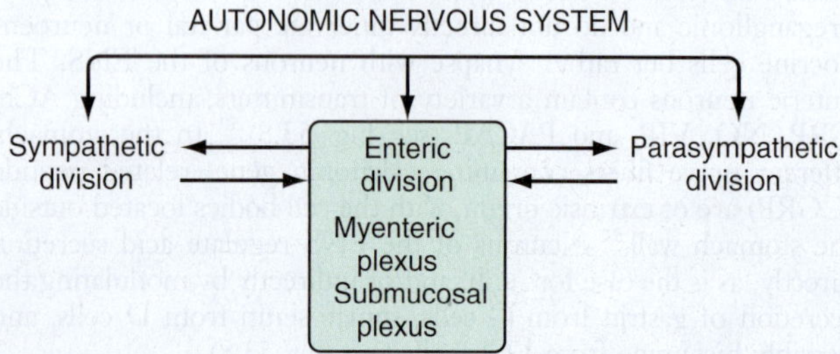

Fig. 53.6 The autonomic nervous system consists of sympathetic, parasympathetic, and enteric divisions. The enteric division consists of the myenteric plexus, which primarily regulates motility, and the submucosal plexus, which primarily regulates secretion. Although the enteric division can function autonomously, it receives input from and sends projections to the other divisions.

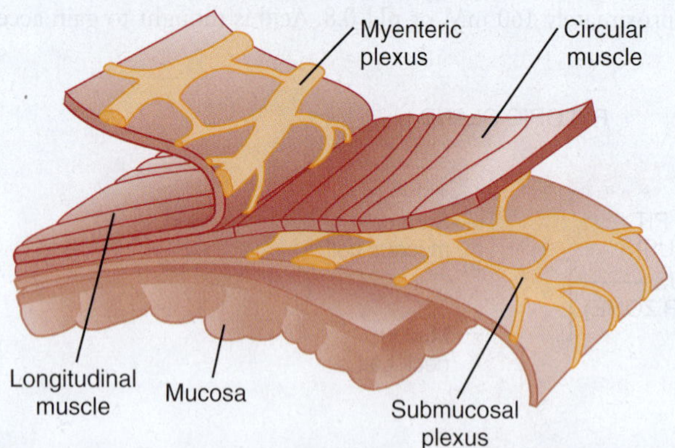

Fig. 53.7 The enteric nervous system contains intrinsic neurons, the cell bodies of which are contained within the gastric wall. The myenteric plexus, which innervates the circular and longitudinal muscle layers, regulates motility. The submucosal plexus, which innervates the mucosa, regulates secretion.

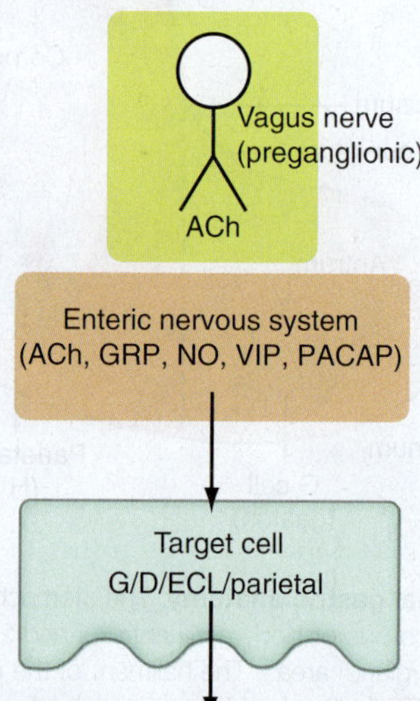

Fig. 53.8 Functional neural anatomy. The vagus nerve contains preganglionic neurons that synapse with enteric nerves (i.e., neurons within the wall of the stomach that are part of the enteric nervous system). The enteric neurons contain a variety of transmitters, including *ACh*, *GRP* (or mammalian bombesin), *NO*, *VIP*, and *PACAP*, that regulate acid secretion from parietal cells directly and/or indirectly by modulating the secretion of gastrin from G cells, somatostatin from D cells, and possibly histamine from *ECL* cells.

to the lumen via channels in the mucus layer created by the relatively high intraglandular hydrostatic pressures generated during secretion, about 17 mm Hg.[52]

Although acid facilitates the digestion of protein and absorption of nonheme iron, calcium, and vitamin B_{12}, as well as prevents bacterial overgrowth, enteric infection, and possibly SBP,[8–14,18–22] when levels of acid (and pepsin) overwhelm mucosal defense mechanisms, mucosal damage may occur. To prevent such damage, gastric acid must be precisely regulated and produced according to need. This is accomplished by a highly coordinated interaction among a number of neural, hormonal, and paracrine pathways. These pathways can be activated directly by stimuli originating in the brain or reflexively by stimuli originating in the stomach after ingestion of a meal, such as mechanical stimulation (e.g., distention) or chemical stimulation (e.g., protein and acid).

The principal stimulants of acid secretion are ACh, released from gastric enteric neurons (neurocrine); gastrin, released from antral G cells (hormonal); and paracrine [histamine, released from oxyntic ECL cells (Fig. 53.9); also see Fig. 53.1]. These agents interact with specific G protein–binding receptors (M_3,

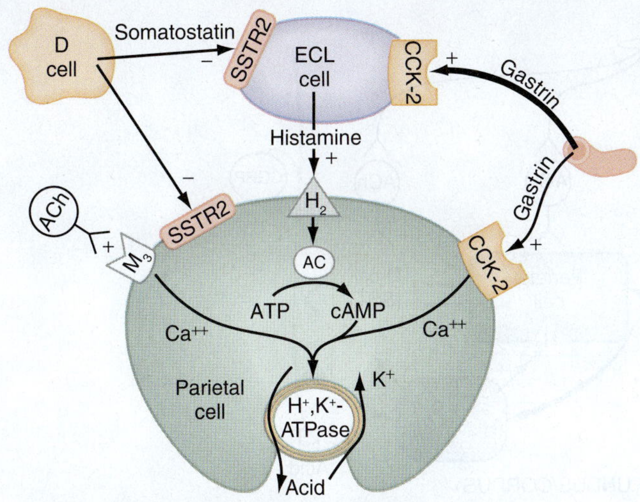

Fig. 53.9 Model illustrating parietal cell receptors and transduction pathways. The principal stimulants of acid secretion at the level of the parietal cell are histamine (paracrine), gastrin (hormonal), and *ACh* (neurocrine). Histamine, released from *ECL* cells, binds to H_2 receptors that activate adenylate cyclase *(AC)* and generate adenosine 3′,5′- *cAMP*. Gastrin, released from G cells, binds to CCK subtype 2 *(CCK-2)* receptors that activate phospholipase C (not shown) to induce the release of cytosolic calcium (Ca^{2+}). Gastrin stimulates the parietal cell directly and, more importantly, indirectly by releasing histamine from ECL cells. ACh, released from intramural enteric neurons, binds to muscarinic type 3 (M_3) receptors that are coupled to an increase in intracellular calcium. The intracellular cAMP- and calcium-dependent signaling systems activate downstream protein kinases, ultimately leading to fusion and activation of H^+,K^+-ATPase, the proton pump. Somatostatin, released from oxyntic D cells, is the principal inhibitor of acid secretion. Somatostatin, acting via the *SSTR2* receptor, inhibits the parietal cell directly as well as indirectly by inhibiting histamine release from ECL cells. +, Stimulatory; −, inhibitory.

CCK-2, and H_2, respectively) that are coupled to two major signal transduction pathways: intracellular calcium in the case of ACh and gastrin, and adenylate cyclase or adenosine 3′,5′-cyclic monophosphate (cAMP) in the case of histamine (see Fig. 53.9). There is evidence for potentiation (or synergism) between histamine and either ACh or gastrin, probably as a result of post receptor interaction between the two signaling pathways.[53] Caffeine stimulates acid secretion via bitter taste receptors (taste type 2 bitter receptors; TAS2Rs) localized to parietal cells.[54] The main inhibitor of acid secretion is somatostatin, released from oxyntic and antral D cells (paracrine) (see Figs. 53.1, 53.5, and 53.9). Each of these agents acts directly on the parietal cell as well as indirectly by modulating the secretion of neuroendocrine cells (Fig. 53.10).

Histamine

Histamine, produced in ECL cells by decarboxylation of L-histidine by histidine decarboxylase (HDC), stimulates the parietal cell directly by binding to H_2 receptors coupled to activation of adenylate cyclase and generation of cAMP (see Fig. 53.9).[55] Histamine also stimulates acid secretion indirectly by binding to H_3 receptors that inhibit somatostatin release from oxyntic D cells (see Fig. 53.10).[56,57] Gastrin, PACAP, VIP, and ghrelin stimulate, whereas somatostatin, CGRP, prostaglandins (PGs), peptide YY (PYY), and galanin inhibit histamine secretion.[58,59] As discussed later, gastrin also exerts a direct proliferative effect on ECL cells. ACh has no direct effect on histamine secretion.[60–62]

Gastrin

Gastrin, the primary stimulant of acid secretion during and following meal ingestion, is produced in G cells of the gastric antrum and, in much lower and variable amounts, in the proximal small intestine, colon, and pancreas. Gastrin is synthesized as a large precursor molecule of 101 amino acids, which is converted to progastrin (80 amino acids) by cleavage of the N-terminal signal peptide. Progastrin is further processed to yield peptides with C-terminal glycine (i.e., G34gly and G17gly). The final processing step involves amidation to yield G34amide and G17amide. In humans, more than 95% of secreted gastrins are amidated, and about half are tyrosyl-sulphated.[63] Of the amidated peptides, approximately 85% are G17, 5%–10% are G34, and the remainder, a mixture of bigger and smaller peptides (G71, G-52, G14, and G6). The plasma half-life of G34amide is 30 minutes, and that of G17amide is 3–7 minutes; they are metabolized primarily by the kidney and, in smaller amounts, by the intestine and liver.[64–66] Because the metabolism of G17 is much faster than that of G34, most gastrin in the circulation during fasting is G34, whereas after a meal it is G17. In patients with renal insufficiency or massive small bowel resection, fasting blood levels of G17 and G34 are elevated.[67,68] The test substance pentagastrin is not a naturally occurring peptide but rather is a manufactured analog that contains the biologically active C-terminus sequence Trp-Met-Asp-Phe-NH_2.

Gastrin and CCK belong to the same family of peptides and possess an identical carboxyl-terminal pentapeptide sequence (-Gly-Trp-Met-Asp-Phe-NH_2). Two main classes of gastrin/CCK receptors have been characterized: CCK-1 (formerly, CCK-A) and CCK-2 (formerly, CCK_B or CCK_B/gastrin). CCK-1 receptors are specific for CCK, whereas CCK-2 receptors recognize both CCK and gastrin with high affinity. Sulfated and unsulfated G17 and G34 possess similar affinities for the CCK-2 receptor that is a classical G protein-coupled receptor. The binding of gastrin to the receptor activates phospholipase C, which hydrolyzes phosphatidylinositol 4.5 bisphosphate to inositol 1,4,5-trisphosphate (IP_3) and diacylglycerol.[69] IP_3 mobilizes calcium from intracellular stores, and diacylglycerol activates protein kinase C isoforms. Gastrin, acting via CCK-2 receptors, stimulates the parietal cell directly and, more importantly, indirectly by releasing histamine from ECL cells (see Figs. 53.9–53.11).[70,71] Gastrin regulates the secretion and synthesis of histamine in a biphasic manner. The first phase involves a release of stored histamine. The second phase relates to the replenishment of histamine stores and involves an increase in HDC activity followed by an increase in HDC gene transcription.[72] H_2 receptor-, HDC-, and CCK-2 receptor knockout mice manifest decreased acid secretion, especially in response to gastrin.[73–75]

Although amidated gastrins had been thought to be the only forms with biological activity, glycine-extended gastrins may regulate the capacity of the parietal cell to respond to secretagogues, release histamine from ECL cells, and stimulate proliferation of colonic mucosa and colorectal cancers.[76,77] N-terminal progastrin fragments (e.g., progastrin fragments 1–35 and 1–19) have been reported to inhibit acid secretion in humans. ACh, GRP, PACAP, secretin, β_2/β_3-adrenergic agonists, serotonin, calcium, protein, amino acids, amines, capsaicin, and alcoholic beverages produced by fermentation stimulate gastrin secretion, whereas somatostatin, galanin, bradykinin, menin, and adenosine inhibit gastrin secretion. In addition, at least two negative-feedback pathways, mediated via release of somatostatin, regulate gastrin secretion. The first is activated by luminal acidity and involves sensory CGRP neurons (see Fig. 53.10). Low intragastric pH (high intragastric acidity) activates CGRP neurons that, via an axon reflex, stimulate somatostatin cells and thus inhibit gastrin secretion (see Fig. 53.10).[78–80] Conversely, when intragastric pH rises (low intragastric acidity)—for example, by administrating

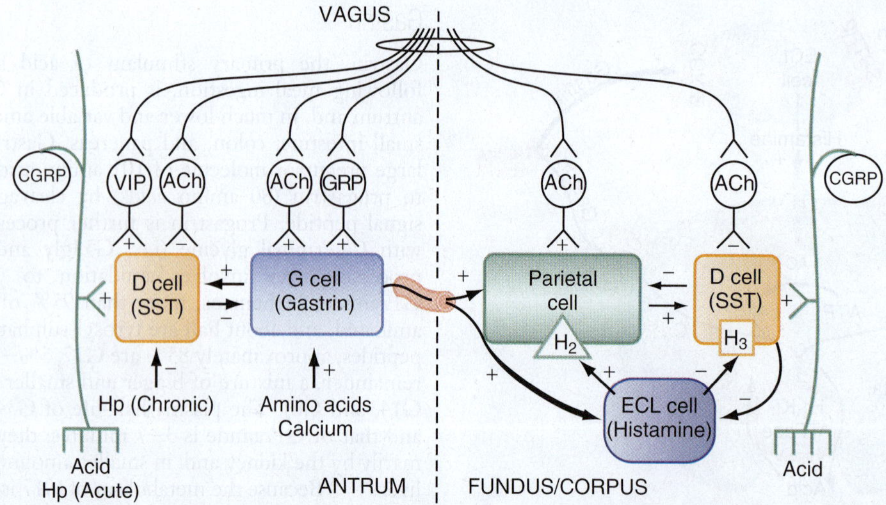

Fig. 53.10 Model illustrating the neural, hormonal, and paracrine regulation of gastric acid secretion in health and disease. Efferent vagal fibers synapse with intramural enteric cholinergic (*ACh*) and peptidergic (*GRP* and *VIP*) neurons. In the fundus (oxyntic mucosa), ACh neurons stimulate acid secretion directly as well as indirectly by inhibiting somatostatin (*SST*) secretion, thus eliminating its restraint on parietal cells and histamine-containing *ECL* cells. In the antrum (pyloric mucosa), ACh neurons stimulate gastrin secretion directly as well as indirectly by inhibiting SST secretion, thus eliminating its restraint on gastrin-containing G cells. GRP neurons, activated by luminal protein, also stimulate gastrin secretion. Amino acids and calcium may directly stimulate gastrin secretion. VIP neurons, activated by low-grade gastric distention, stimulate SST and thus inhibit gastrin secretion. Dual paracrine pathways link SST-containing D cells to parietal cells and to ECL cells in the fundus. Histamine released from ECL cells acts via H_3 receptors to inhibit SST secretion. This serves to accentuate the decrease in SST secretion induced by cholinergic stimuli and thus augments acid secretion. In the antrum, dual paracrine pathways link SST-containing D cells to gastrin cells. Release of acid into the lumen of the stomach activates extrinsic CGRP sensory neurons that act to restore SST secretion in both the fundus and antrum. Acute infection with Hp also activates CGRP neurons to stimulate SST and thus inhibit gastrin (and acid) secretion; inhibition of acid facilitates colonization and infection. In patients with duodenal ulcer who are chronically infected with Hp, the organism or cytokines released from the inflammatory infiltrate inhibit SST and thus stimulate gastrin (and acid) secretion. +, Stimulation; –, inhibition.

antisecretory medications, such as PPIs or by the development of gastric atrophy—somatostatin secretion is not stimulated, and patients develop hypergastrinemia (see Fig. 53.11).[81] There is some evidence that bacterial overgrowth induced by hypochlorhydria may also contribute to hypergastrinemia.[82] The second negative-feedback pathway involves a paracrine action whereby gastrin directly stimulates somatostatin and thus attenuates its own secretion (see Fig. 53.10).[83]

Gastrin also functions as a trophic hormone to stimulate mucosal proliferation. CCK-2 receptors are localized to the progenitor zone in oxyntic glands, and chronic hypergastrinemia induces proliferation of ECL and parietal cells directly as well as indirectly via the autocrine or paracrine action of growth factors, such as heparin-binding EGF, amphiregulin, TGF-α, metalloproteinases, and regenerating islet-derived 1 (see Fig. 53.11).[84,85] Rats rendered hypergastrinemic by PPI administration demonstrate a 5-fold increase in the number of ECL cells and a 1.5-fold increase in the number of parietal cells.[86] Gastrin acts directly on ECL cells in rodents to induce hyperplasia, dysplasia, and eventually neoplasia (carcinoids) (see Fig. 53.11),[87] whereas humans rarely develop carcinoid tumors in response to hypergastrinemia unless other factors are present, such as chronic atrophic gastritis or gastrinoma associated with multiple endocrine neoplasia type I [*MEN-I* (see Chapter 43)].[88] This may be due to the lesser degree of gastrin elevation and the many decades of mild hypergastrinemia that may be necessary to induce carcinoid tumors in humans. Since ECL cells contain somatostatin subtype 2 receptors (SSTR2), somatostatin scintigraphy with ^{111}indium-diethylenetriamine pentaacetic acid octreotide is the preferred imaging method to detect carcinoid tumors (see Chapter 43).[89,90]

Recent studies have implicated gastrin in carcinogenesis.[91,92] Gastrin and its receptor have been identified in several human gastrointestinal adenocarcinomas, including those of the esophagus, stomach, pancreas, and colon.[93–96,398,399]

Acetylcholine

ACh, released from postganglionic enteric neurons, stimulates the parietal cell directly as well as indirectly by inhibiting somatostatin secretion (see Fig. 53.10). The parietal cell muscarinic receptor is of the M_3 subtype.[97–99] Like CCK-2 receptors, M_3 receptors are coupled to the activation of phospholipase C, with a generation of inositol trisphosphate and release of intracellular calcium (see Fig. 53.9).[97–99] Alcoholic beverages produced by fermentation stimulate gastric acid secretion, and this effect may be mediated via activation of M_3 receptors.[100] ACh also stimulates acid secretion indirectly by activating M_2 and M_4 receptors on D cells coupled to the inhibition of somatostatin secretion, thus removing the tonic restraint exerted by this peptide on gastrin, ECL, and parietal cells (see Fig. 53.10).

Other Secretagogues

Miscellaneous Peptides

There are several minor peptides that increase gastric acid secretion. Since most of the reported studies were conducted with experimental animals or in vitro preparations, and since some of their effects on acid secretion are conflicting, their overall contribution to the regulation of human gastric acid secretion is not firmly established.

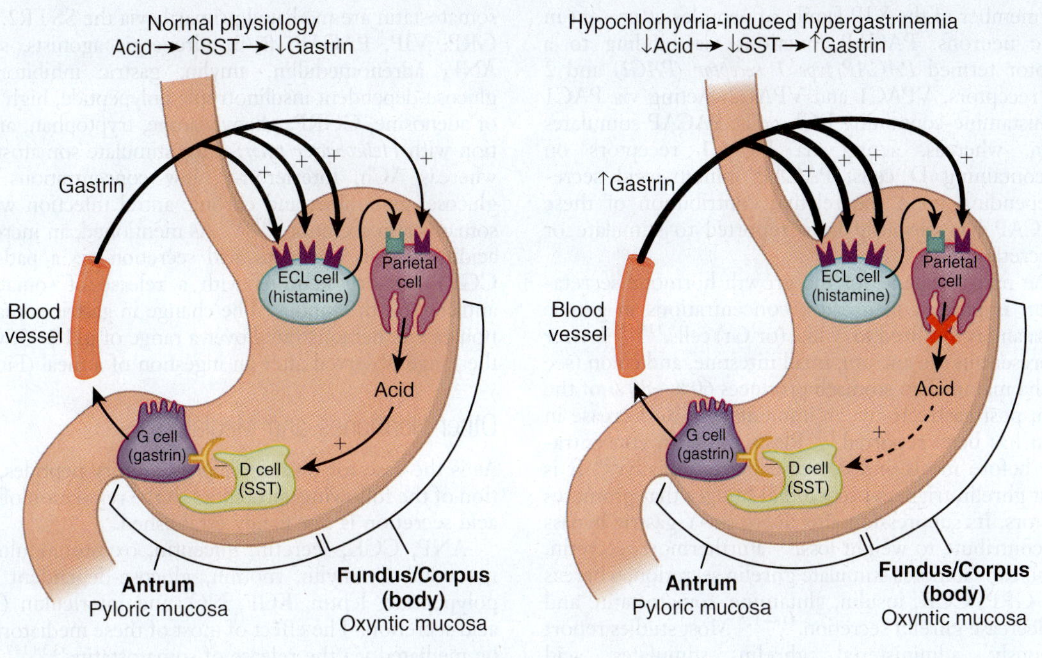

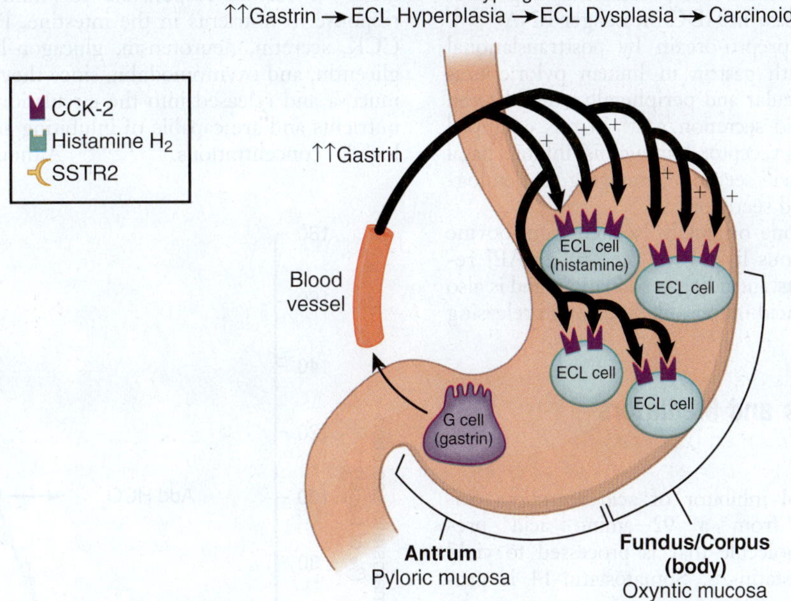

Fig. 53.11 Model illustrating the function and mechanism of gastrin as a secretagogue and trophic hormone in the stomach. *Left Panel (Normal Secretory Physiology)*: Gastrin, secreted into the local circulation by G cells of the gastric antrum (pyloric mucosa), is the main hormonal stimulant for acid secretion. Acting via CCK-2 receptors, gastrin stimulates the parietal directly and, more importantly, indirectly by releasing histamine from *ECL* cells. Histamine diffuses to neighboring parietal cells (paracrine pathway) where it binds to histamine H_2-receptors coupled to generation of cyclic adenosine monophosphate and subsequent activation of the acid proton pump, H^+/K^+-ATPase. Somatostatin *(SST)*, secreted by D cells in the antrum, binds to SST2 receptors on G cells and exerts a tonic inhibitory paracrine restraint on gastrin secretion. During the interdigestive state, a local feedback pathway is activated whereby unbuffered luminal acid [acting via release of CGRP from sensory neurons (see Fig. 53.10)] stimulates somatostatin and, thus, inhibits gastrin secretion, maintaining acid secretion at economically low levels. *Middle Panel (Hypochlorhydria-induced Hypergastrinemia)*: When acid secretion is suppressed (e.g., by potent antisecretory medications or gastric oxyntic atrophy), there is lesser stimulation of somatostatin secretion with a reciprocal increase in gastrin secretion; patients develop hypergastrinemia. *Right Panel (Chronic Hypergastrinemia)*: As gastrin is also a trophic hormone, especially to the oxyntic mucosa, chronic hypergastrinemia, acting via CCK-2 receptors, induces hyperplasia of ECL cells. Increased number of histamine-secreting ECL cells is responsible for rebound gastric acid secretion observed after abrupt withdrawal of PPIs. In susceptible individuals, chronic hypergastrinemia-induced ECL hyperplasia may progress to dysplasia and, eventually, carcinoid tumor.

PACAP, a member of the VIP family of peptides, is present in gastric enteric neurons. PACAP functions via binding to a PACAP receptor termed *PACAP type 1 receptor (PAC1)* and 2 types of VIP receptors, VPAC1 and VPAC2. Acting via PAC1 receptors on histamine-containing ECL cells, PACAP stimulates acid secretion, whereas, acting via VPAC1 receptors on somatostatin-containing D cells, PACAP inhibits acid secretion.[111,112] Depending upon the relative contribution of these pathways, PACAP has variously been reported to stimulate or inhibit acid secretion.[113]

Ghrelin, the natural ligand for the growth hormone secretagogue receptor, is present in greatest concentrations in gastric oxyntic mucosa and is localized to A-like (or Gr) cells.[114,115] Lesser amounts are present in the antrum, small intestine, and colon (see Chapter 4). The mammalian stomach produces 60%–80% of the body's ghrelin; post gastrectomy, an immediate 75% decrease in plasma ghrelin has been reported.[116] Plasma ghrelin concentrations increase before meals and decrease postprandially.[116] It is postulated that ghrelin triggers preprandial hunger that promotes feeding behaviors. Its suppression after Roux-en-Y gastric bypass may, in part, contribute to weight loss.[117] Furthermore, secretin, endothelin, and cannabinoids stimulate ghrelin secretion, whereas Hp infection, GRP, CCK, insulin, glutamine, somatostatin, and interferon-γ decrease ghrelin secretion.[118–120] Most studies report that exogenously administered ghrelin stimulates acid secretion.[121–123,400] The stimulatory effect appears to involve the vagus nerve and histamine, because it is abolished by vagotomy and is associated with an increase in HDC messenger RNA.[123,124]

Orexin-A, derived from prepro-orexin by posttranslational processing, is colocalized with gastrin in human pyloric mucosa.[122,125] Intracerebroventricular and peripherally administered orexin-A stimulate gastric acid secretion.[125,126] In rats equipped with a gastric fistula, an orexin receptor 1 antagonist inhibits basal and pentagastrin-stimulated acid secretion, implying that endogenous orexin-A stimulates acid secretion.[125,126]

Apelin is a peptide hormone originally isolated from bovine stomach that is the endogenous ligand for the orphan APJ receptor. Apelin has many effects, including vasodilation, and is also reported to stimulate gastric acid output, likely through releasing histamine.[401,402]

Antisecretory Hormones and Mediators

Somatostatin

Somatostatin is the principal inhibitor of acid secretion. Somatostatin is synthesized from a 92–amino acid preprosomatostatin precursor molecule that is processed to yield somatostatin-14 and somatostatin-28. Somatostatin-14 is predominantly found in the stomach, pancreas, and enteric neurons, whereas somatostatin-28 is the major form in the small intestine. The half-life of somatostatin-14 is 1–3 minutes, and the half-life of somatostatin-28 is about 15 minutes.

In the stomach, somatostatin is expressed almost exclusively in mucosal D cells, which are closely coupled to their target cells (gastrin cells in the antrum, parietal and ECL cells in the fundus/body) either directly via cytoplasmic processes or indirectly via the local circulation.[39,101] The functional correlate of this anatomic coupling is a tonic restraint exerted by somatostatin on acid secretion from the parietal cell, histamine secretion from the ECL cell, and gastrin secretion from the G cell (see Figs. 53.5 and 53.10).[39–43,102,103] Removing this restraint (i.e., disinhibition or elimination of the influence of an inhibitor) by activation of cholinergic neurons is an important physiologic mechanism for stimulating acid secretion (see Fig. 53.10). The biological activity of somatostatin is mediated via 6 G-protein-coupled receptors termed SSTR1-SSTR5; the SSTR2 receptor has two splice variants, termed SSTR2A and SSTR2B. In the stomach, the actions of somatostatin are mediated primarily via the SSTR2.[104–106] Gastrin, GRP, VIP, PACAP, β_2/β_3-adrenergic agonists, secretin, CCK, ANP, adrenomedullin, amylin, gastric inhibitory peptide or glucose-dependent insulinotropic polypeptide, high concentrations of adenosine, CGRP, phenylalanine, tryptophan, and acute infection with *Helicobacter pylori* (Hp) stimulate somatostatin secretion, whereas ACh, interferon-γ, low concentrations of adenosine, glucose, glutamine, and chronic antral infection with Hp inhibit somatostatin secretion.[107–109] As mentioned, an increase in luminal acidity acts to attenuate acid secretion via a pathway involving CGRP sensory neurons with a release of somatostatin in the antrum and the fundus. The change in gastric somatostatin secretion can be demonstrated over a range of pH 3–5, which is within the range observed after an ingestion of a meal (Fig. 53.12).[110]

Other Hormones and Mediators

As is the case for the minor prosecretory peptides, the contribution of the following substances to the regulation of human gastric acid secretion is not firmly established.

ANP, CCK, secretin, glicentin, oxyntomodulin, PYY, adrenomedullin, amylin, motilin, glucose-dependent insulinotropic polypeptide, leptin, EGF, NO, and interleukin (IL)-1β inhibit acid secretion. The effect of most of these mediators is believed to be mediated via the release of somatostatin.[33,38,127,403–405]

The term *enterogastrone* has been used to describe the intestinal factor or factors responsible for inhibiting acid secretion in response to nutrients in the intestine. Prime candidates include CCK, secretin, neurotensin, glucagon-like peptide 1 (GLP-1), glicentin, and oxyntomodulin, since they are present in intestinal mucosa and released into the circulation in response to luminal nutrients and are capable of inhibiting acid secretion at "physiologic" concentrations.[128–132,406] Although it is likely that

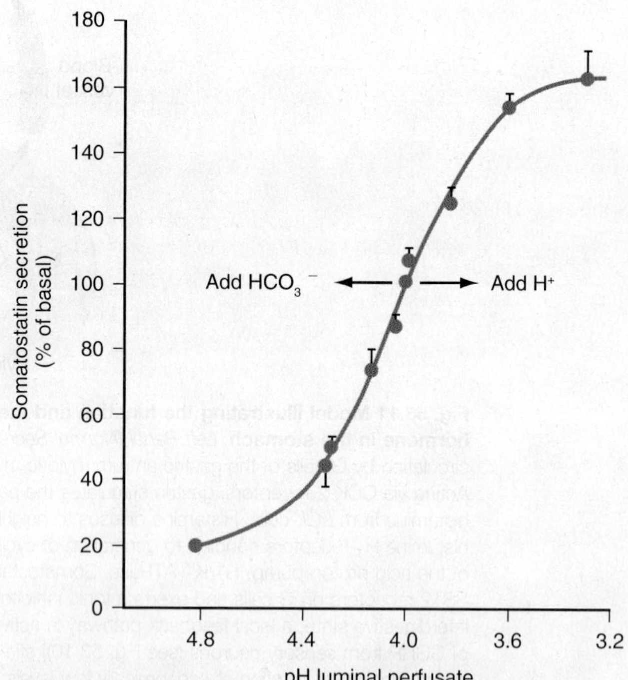

Fig. 53.12 Relationship between luminal pH and gastric somatostatin secretion. In the isolated mouse stomach, addition of bicarbonate (HCO_3^-) to neutralize basal acid secretion or HCl to augment luminal acidity causes a corresponding change in somatostatin secretion. (From Schubert ML, Edwards NF, Makhlouf GM. Regulation of gastric somatostatin secretion in the mouse by luminal acid: a local feedback mechanism. *Gastroenterology*. 1988;94:317–22.)

enterogastrone activity represents the combined influence of several of these peptides, the strongest evidence favors CCK (acting via somatostatin). CCK, produced in I cells in the proximal small intestine, is released by luminal protein and fat. The acid-inhibitory response to intraduodenal fat is abolished, in dogs, by pretreatment with a CCK-1 receptor antagonist and, in mice, by a knockout of the CCK-1 receptor.[133–136]

Parietal Cell Intracellular Pathways

In parietal cells, acid secretion is increased by activation of intracellular cAMP- and calcium-dependent signaling pathways that activate downstream protein kinases, ultimately leading to fusion and activation of H^+,K^+-ATPase (the proton pump), with concomitant activation of luminal membrane conductances for K^+ and Cl^- (Fig. 53.13; also see Fig. 53.9).[137] The H^+,K^+-ATPase actively pumps out H^+, as hydronium ions, against an immense concentration gradient (cell interior pH 7.4 or 40 nM; acid secreted at pH 0.8 or 160 million nM) in exchange for luminal K^+. The energy required comes from ATP produced by the parietal cell's extensive mitochondrial network. The H^+,K^+-ATPase consists of an α-subunit that carries out the catalytic and transport function of

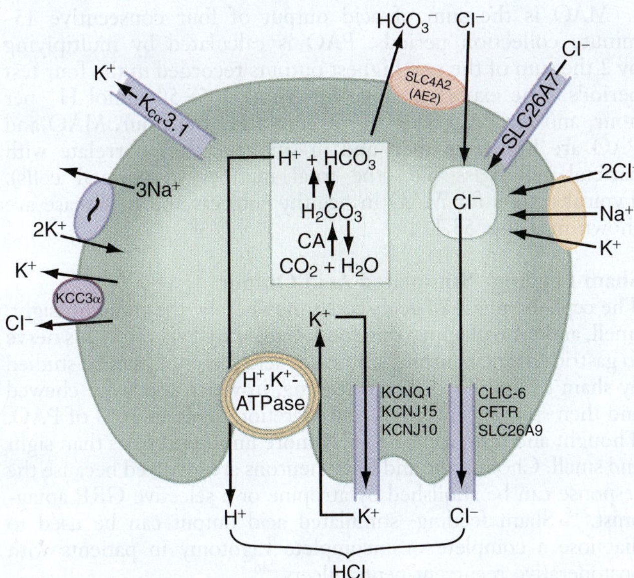

Fig. 53.13 Model illustrating ion transport and generation of hydrochloric acid (*HCl*) in the parietal cell. Acid secretion requires a functional H^+,K^+-ATPase as well as apical and basolateral K^+ and Cl^- channels, transporters, and exchangers. Acid is produced from the hydration of CO_2 to form H^+ and HCO_3^-, a reaction catalyzed by cytoplasmic carbonic anhydrase (*CA*). In the presence of luminal K^+, H^+,K^+-ATPase pumps H^+ into the lumen in exchange for K^+. Apical K^+ channels (KCNQ1, KCNJ15, and/or KCNJ10) provide the K^+ required for the functioning of the H^+,K^+-ATPase. The source of intracellular K^+ is the basolateral Na^+,K^+-ATPase (shown as ~) and the NKCC1. For each H^+ secreted, an HCO3 exits the cell across the basolateral membrane via an anion exchanger (SLC4A2, or AE2). Concurrently with H^+, Cl^- is extruded across the luminal membrane via the chloride intracellular channel-6 (*CLIC-6*), cystic fibrosis transmembrane regulator, and/or SLC26A9, resulting in electroneutral HCl secretion. The source of intracellular Cl– is the basolateral cotransporter NKCCl, exchanger SLC4A2 (AE2), and chloride channel SLC26A7. Recently, 2 K^+ exporters have been identified on the basolateral membrane that negatively regulate acid secretion: the electroneutral K^+, Cl^- cotransporter KCC3a and the intermediate Ca^{2+}-activated K^+ channel, Kca3.1. (From Chu S, Schubert ML. Gastric secretion. *Curr Opin Gastroenterol.* 2012;28:587–593.)

the enzyme[138] and a heavily glycosylated β-subunit that protects the enzyme from degradation.[139] Both subunits are necessary for trafficking to the apical membrane, and targeted knockout of either subunit results in achlorhydria.[140]

In the resting, unstimulated state, H^+,K^+-ATPase activity is sequestered within cytoplasmic tubulovesicles. On stimulation, there is a dramatic morphologic transformation as the vesicles translocate and fuse with the apical plasma membrane, resulting in a 6–10-fold increase in the membrane and the formation of the canalicular system (Fig. 53.14). Translocation of the H^+,K^+-ATPase into the canalicular membrane together with the presence of luminal K^+ activates the enzyme.[141] On cessation of secretion, the H^+,K^+-ATPase is retrieved from the apical membrane, and the tubulovesicular compartment is reestablished. Though the precise mechanisms regulating H^+,K^+-ATPase trafficking are unknown, data support the involvement of vesicular proteins (e.g., clathrin), actin-based microfilaments, actin-binding proteins (e.g., ezrin), small G proteins of the Rab family (e.g., Rab10, Rab11, Rab25, and Rab27b), soluble *N*-ethylmaleimide-sensitive factor attachment protein receptor proteins (e.g., VAMP-2 and syntaxin 1, 2, 3, and 4), and secretory carrier membrane proteins.[142–145]

Acid secretion requires not only a functional H^+,K^+-ATPase but also apical K^+ and Cl^- channels and basolateral HCO_3^- and Cl^- exchangers.[146] Acid is produced from the hydration of CO_2 to form H^+ and HCO_3^-, a reaction catalyzed by cytoplasmic carbonic anhydrase (see Fig. 53.13). Since the H^+,K^+-ATPase is unable to pump H^+ into the lumen without a parallel uptake of K^+, sufficient quantities of K^+ must be delivered to the lumen. This K^+ recycling is accomplished by the putative luminal potassium channels KCNQ1/KCNE2, KCNJ10 (Kir4.1), and KCNJ15 (Kir4.2).[147,148] KCNQ1 is a voltage-activated K^+ channel that, when modified by the small regulatory subunit KCNE2, becomes voltage insensitive, constitutively open, and acid activated.[149,150] The concentration of K^+ in gastric juice (8–12 mM) exceeds plasma K^+ by two to four folds. The basolateral membrane of the parietal cell may contain potassium exporters that negatively regulate acid secretion (i.e., the electroneutral K^+-Cl^- cotransporter, KCC3a, as well as the intermediate Ca^{2+}-activated K^+ channel, $K_{ca}3.1$).[151,152]

For each H^+ secreted, an HCO_3^- ion exits the cell across the basolateral membrane via SLC4A2, the anion exchanger 2 (AE2; see Fig. 53.13).[153] As a result of this HCO_3^-/Cl^- exchange, the pH within the parietal cell remains only slightly alkaline during acid secretion.[154] Rapid entry of HCO_3^- from parietal cells into the blood has been referred to as the *alkaline tide*. Some of this HCO_3 may be taken up and secreted by gastric surface epithelial cells.

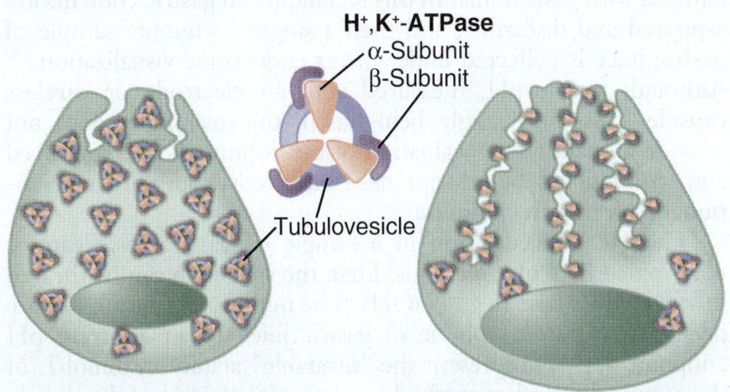

Fig. 53.14 Model illustrating the translocation and activation of H^+,K^+-ATPase. In the resting state, H^+,K^+-ATPase is sequestered within cytoplasmic tubulovesicles and is inactive. On stimulation, the tubulovesicles move to and fuse with the apical membrane, forming an extensive canalicular system. Translocation of H^+,K^+-ATPase into the canalicular membrane together with the presence of luminal K^+ activates the enzyme.

Concurrently with H^+, Cl^- is extruded across the luminal membrane via an apical chloride channel, possibly the chloride intracellular channel-6, cystic fibrosis transmembrane regulator, and/or SLC26A9 (see Fig. 53.13).[155] Chloride enters the cell via the basolateral anion exchanger 2 (SLC4A2), the SLC26A7 channel, and sodium-2 chloride potassium-cotransporter-1 (NKCC1) (see Fig. 53.13).[156–158]

Clinical Measurement of Gastric Acid Secretion

Indications

Gastric secretory testing assesses the basal and maximal capacity of the stomach to produce acid. Increased gastric acid secretion is seen in the majority of patients with duodenal ulcer disease and in virtually all patients with gastrinoma (Zollinger-Ellison syndrome; ZES), whereas very low or absent acid secretion is seen in chronic atrophic gastritis, pernicious anemia (PA), and gastric adenocarcinoma. Clinically, the utility of gastric secretory testing has diminished, but it may assist in the diagnosis and management of patients with hypergastrinemia (e.g., gastrinoma) and the diagnosis of incomplete vagotomy in patients with postoperative recurrent peptic ulcer. Demonstrating fasting acid secretion or an acidic fasting gastric pH excludes achlorhydria as a cause of an elevated fasting serum gastrin concentration. Patients with gastrinoma have hypergastrinemia with elevated basal acid output (BAO) (see Chapter 43). Gastric secretory testing may also be useful in assessing the inhibitory effect of new antisecretory medications and, perhaps, in modifying treatment in recalcitrant gastrointestinal reflux disease (GERD) and dyspeptic patients.

Methods

Aspiration of gastric juice was formerly the most widely used method for measuring acid secretion in humans. Traditionally, this is performed by positioning an NG tube into the most dependent portion of the stomach of a fasted individual. Proper positioning may be verified fluoroscopically or by recovery of more than 90 mL after injection of 100 mL water. Gastric juice is collected by suction. When the tube is properly positioned, only 5%–10% of gastric juice escapes collection and enters the duodenum. Neutralization by bicarbonate and diffusion of tiny amounts of acid back into the mucosa result in a small underestimation of the true rate of secretion. More recently, an endoscopic technique has been described to measure acid secretion in patients with gastrinoma. In this technique, all gastric contents are aspirated and discarded, and then a single 15-minute sample of gastric juice is collected under direct endoscopic visualization.[240] Although gastric pH, measured with an electrode or wireless capsule.[408] is increasingly being used, this technique does not provide a quantitative evaluation of the volume of acid produced and, consequently, does not necessarily correlate with conventional aspiration techniques.

The H^+ concentration in a sample of gastric juice can be determined by 1 of 2 methods. First, the specimen can be titrated in vitro with a base (e.g., NaOH). The millimoles (mmol) of base needed to titrate a volume of gastric juice to an arbitrary pH endpoint (e.g., 7) represent the "titratable" acidity in mmol/L of the sample. The other method is to measure the pH of the sample with an electrode. Because pH electrodes measure H^+ activity and not concentration, it is necessary to convert activity to concentration using a table of activity coefficients for H^+ in gastric juice.[241] Once the H^+ concentration of the sample in mmol/L is determined by either of these methods, it is multiplied by the volume of the sample in liters to determine the acid output during the collection period (e.g., mmol/hour or mmol/kg of body weight per hour).

Clinically Useful Measures of Gastric Acid Output

Basal Acid Output

BAO estimates resting acid secretion in the absence of intentional and avoidable stimulation. It is expressed as the sum of the measured acid output, expressed as mmol H^+ per hour, for four consecutive 15-minute periods. The upper limit of normal for BAO is about 10 mmol H^+ per hour in men and 5 mmol H^+ per hour in women (Table 53.1).[242] BAO fluctuates from hour to hour in the same person. The lowest BAO occurs between 6 and 11 AM, and the highest occurs between 2 and 11 PM. Variation is also related to cyclic gastric motor activity, with increased BAO in late gastric phase III (migrating motor complex).[243]

Maximal Acid Output and Peak Acid Output

Maximal acid output (MAO) and peak acid output (PAO) estimate the acid secretory response to an exogenous secretagogue, such as pentagastrin (subcutaneous or intramuscular at 6 μg/kg or continuous IV infusion at 6 μg/kg/h). Pentagastrin is a manufactured analog of gastrin that contains the biologically active C-terminus sequence. Possible side effects include flushing, nausea, abdominal pain, dizziness, and palpitations. Unfortunately, pentagastrin is no longer available in many countries.

MAO is the sum of acid output of four consecutive 15-minute collection periods. PAO is calculated by multiplying by 2 the sum of the two highest outputs recorded in the four test periods. The expected range for MAO is 5–50 mmol H^+ per hour, and for PAO, it is 10–60 mmol H^+ per hour. MAO and PAO are higher in men and in smokers; they correlate with parietal cell mass (i.e., the total number of parietal cells). Typical results for MAO in healthy subjects and in disease are shown in Table 53.1.

Sham Feeding–Stimulated Acid Output

The cephalic phase of acid secretion, whereby the thought, sight, smell, and taste of appetizing food, transmitted via the vagus nerve to gastric enteric neurons, stimulates acid secretion, can be studied by sham feeding.[175,244] Sham feeding, in which foods are chewed and then spit out, increases acid secretion to about 50% of PAO. Thought and taste appear to play more important roles than sight and smell. Cholinergic and GRP neurons are involved because the response can be abolished by atropine or a selective GRP antagonist.[245] Sham feeding–stimulated acid output can be used to diagnose a complete or incomplete vagotomy in patients with postoperative recurrent peptic ulcers.[246]

TABLE 53.1 Typical Results of Gastric Secretory Testing in Health and Disease

	Basal Acid Output (mmol H^+/hour)		Maximal Acid Output (mmol H^+/hour)	
	Average	**Range**	**Average**	**Range**
Healthy Subjects				
Men	2.5	0–10	25	7–50
Women	1.5	0–5	15	5–30
Duodenal Ulcer				
Men	5.0	0–15	40	15–60
Women	3.0	0–15	30	10–45
Gastric Ulcer				
Men	1.5	0–8	20	5–40
Women	1.0	0–5	12	3–25
Gastrinoma				
Both sexes	40.5	10–90	65	30–120

Meal-Stimulated Acid Output

Continuous in vivo intragastric titration is a research tool used to measure acid secretion in response to food in the stomach.[247,248] It measures the gastric and intestinal phases of acid secretion. A double-lumen tube is placed in the most dependent part of the stomach, and a homogenized meal buffered to pH 5.5 or 5 is infused into the stomach. Small volumes of gastric contents are sampled from one lumen, the pH is measured, and the contents are returned to the stomach. The second lumen is used to infuse sodium bicarbonate to maintain gastric pH at the meal pH. The amount of bicarbonate required to keep the pH of gastric contents constant is a measure of the postprandial acid secretory response. Rates of gastric acid secretion after eating increase rapidly and approach the PAO.

Diseases Associated With Increased Gastric Acid Secretion

Peptic Ulcer

Duodenal ulcer patients, as a group, manifest increased basal and stimulated gastrin and acid production (see Table 53.1).[249] Most cases of duodenal ulcer are due to antral-predominant infection with Hp (see Chapter 52), for which the perturbations in acid secretion observed in these patients have been attributed. Pentagastrin-stimulated PAO, an indicator of functional parietal cell mass, is increased in Hp-infected duodenal ulcer patients, as is GRP-stimulated PAO, an indicator of the stomach's functional response to endogenous gastrin.[234,250,251] Suppression of somatostatin secretion by the infection may be the underlying cause for these changes (see Figs. 53.10 and 53.15). Eradication of Hp both restores somatostatin secretion and lowers basal and stimulated gastrin and acid secretion over time to normal levels in most individuals, thus providing a permanent cure for duodenal ulcer disease.[233,234,250,252–254]

In contrast to duodenal ulcer patients, gastric ulcer (GU) patients, as a group, exhibit normal or decreased basal and stimulated acid production (see Table 53.1), even though they, too, are often infected with Hp. This suggests that altered gastric mucosal defense may be of primary pathophysiologic importance. GUs have been classified according to their location and concomitant association with duodenal ulcer.[255] Type I ulcers occur in the gastric body and are generally characterized by low acid secretion. These findings may reflect a greater degree and more generalized mucosal inflammation of the oxyntic mucosa with reduced functional parietal cell mass. Type II ulcers occur in the antrum and are characterized by low, normal, or high acid secretion. Type III ulcers occur within 3 cm of the pylorus, commonly accompany duodenal ulcers, and are characterized by high acid output. Type IV ulcers occur in the gastric cardia and are characterized by low acid secretion.[256] Accordingly, the more distant a GU is from the pylorus, the more likely acid secretion will be low.

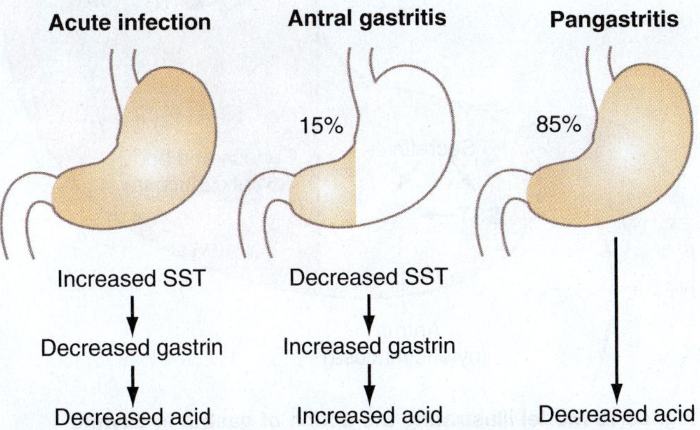

Fig. 53.15 Model illustrating the consequences of Hp infection on gastric acid secretion. Acute Hp infection is associated with increased somatostatin *(SST)* and, thus, decreased gastrin and acid secretion. Chronic infection may be associated with either decreased or increased acid secretion depending on the severity and distribution of gastritis. Most patients chronically infected with Hp manifest a pangastritis and exhibit decreased acid secretion. A minority of chronically infected patients manifest an antral-predominant gastritis; these patients, who are predisposed to duodenal ulcer, produce increased amounts of acid as a result of reduced antral SST secretion and a subsequent reciprocal increase in gastrin secretion. (From Schubert ML, Peura DA. Control of gastric acid secretion in health and disease. *Gastroenterology.* 2008;134:1842–1860.)

Other Diseases

A number of uncommon conditions are marked by gastric acid hypersecretion and subsequent peptic ulceration (also see Chapters 43 and 55). In patients with systemic mastocytosis, high histamine levels, as a result of increased numbers of mast cells, continuously stimulate parietal cells to secrete acid.[257] When a portion of the gastric antrum is retained inadvertently in the afferent remnant after antrectomy with Billroth II anastomosis, it is bathed in alkaline secretions, decreasing somatostatin secretion with consequent hypergastrinemia, increased acid production, and anastomotic ulceration.[80,110,258] Acid hypersecretion can also result from chronic hypercalcemia of any cause since calcium directly stimulates gastrin secretion from G cells and acid secretion from parietal cells.[259,260]

The best characterized acid hypersecretory condition is ZES,[261–263] as discussed in Chapter 43. The BAO is almost always higher than 15 mmol/h, and the BAO/PAO ratio, if measured, is usually 0.6 or greater (see Table 53.1). Gastrin, synthesized by the tumor, is secreted into the bloodstream, where it binds to CCK-2 receptors exptressed on acid-producing parietal and histamine-producing ECL cells to induce acid secretion as well as mucosal proliferation. The clinical correlates of mucosal proliferation are parietal cell and ECL cell hyperplasia are rugal hypertrophy with prominent gastric folds. Although healthy individuals primarily secrete G17 followed by G34, ZES patients mostly secrete G34 followed by G17, as well as increased concentrations of the larger gastrins.

Diagnosis and treatment of gastrinoma are discussed in detail in Chapter 43. The basis of the secretin test to diagnose gastrinoma is that normally somatostatin cells in the antrum tonically restrain gastrin secretion from G cells. Secretin activates the G cell directly and, at the same time, inhibits the G cell indirectly by stimulating somatostatin secretion; the effect of the latter usually dominates since gastrin is not stimulated to a significant degree by secretin (Fig. 53.16). Since the gastrinoma does not contain functionally coupled somatostatin cells, secretin solely stimulates gastrin release from the tumor.[264–266] Since almost all gastrinomas also contain somatostatin receptors, somatostatin receptor scintigraphy using ^{111}Indium-diethylenetriamine pentaacetic acid-D-phe1-octreotide (^{111}In-DTPA-Phel-Octreotide) is considered the initial localization study of choice, with a 71% sensitivity and 86% specificity for primary tumors and 92% detection for metastatic disease.[267,268] PPIs are currently the antisecretory therapies of choice since they are able to control acid secretion and prevent complications in most ZES patients[269] although potassium-competitive acid blockers (P-CABs) may prove to be an effective alternative.

Approximately 25% of patients with ZES have *MEN-I*, an autosomal dominant disorder characterized by pancreatic endocrine tumors, along with hyperparathyroidism and pituitary adenoma (see Chapters 43). *MEN-I* is caused by a mutation in the *MEN-I* gene that encodes for the nuclear protein, menin, a peptide present in G cells that inhibits gastrin gene expression.[270]

For a discussion of other diseases associated with gastric hypersecretion such as esophagitis, duodenitis, and gastritis and an in-depth discussion of peptic ulcer disease.

Hp Infection

After centuries of searching, Barry Marshall and Robin Warren published a landmark paper in published 1973 that provided the first conclusive proof that spiral bacteria that had long been observed in the gastric mucosa contributed to the pathogenesis of peptic ulcer disease.[409,410] Following this discovery, which along with the subsequent release of PPIs, greatly enlivened the field of gastroenterology in the 1980s and was followed by furious investigation of the mechanisms by which Hp infection exerted its pathologic effects. Acute infection with Hp results in hypochlorhydria,[202–206] whereas chronic infection results in either hypo- or hyperchlorhydria (Figs. 53.10 and 53.15), depending upon the severity and anatomic site of infection. Appreciation of the pathways discussed earlier provides some insight into the mechanisms whereby Hp colonizes the stomach and may lead to ulceration.

The decrease in acid secretion during acute Hp infection is thought to facilitate survival of the organism and its colonization of the stomach.[207] The mechanism whereby Hp inhibits acid secretion is multifactorial and includes *direct* inhibition of the parietal cell (and perhaps ECL cell) by a constituent of the bacterium (e.g., vacuolating cytotoxin, lipopolysaccharide, or acid-inhibitory factor) and *indirect* inhibition of parietal cell function as a result of changes in cytokines as well as hormonal, paracrine, and neural regulatory mechanisms.[208–211] Hp itself interferes with the transcription and translation of human H^+,K^+-ATPase, as well as its insertion into the parietal cell apical membrane.[212,213] It also elicits a secretion of at least 2 cytokines by the host (IL-1β and TNF-α) that directly inhibit parietal cell secretion.[214] Acute administration of Hp to rat gastric mucosa activates CGRP sensory neurons coupled to stimulation of somatostatin and thus inhibition of gastrin, histamine, and acid secretion (see Fig. 53.10).[206,215] Activation of neural pathways may offer an explanation as to how an initial patchy superficial colonization of the stomach by Hp induces hypochlorhydria.

Chronic infection with Hp, on the other hand, may be associated with either decreased or increased acid secretion depending on the severity and distribution of gastritis (see Fig. 53.10).[216] Most patients chronically infected with Hp manifest a pangastritis (see Chapter 54) and produce less-than-normal amounts of acid.[217] Reduced acid secretion, initially, is due to functional inhibition of parietal cells by either products of Hp itself or, more likely, products of the inflammatory process, as discussed earlier for acute infection[218,219]; this process is usually reversible with eradication of the organism.[220–222] In such patients, Hp may protect against GERD, Barrett's esophagus, and esophageal adenocarcinoma, as well as augment the antisecretory effect of PPIs.[223,224] In Hp-negative patients, discontinuance of long-term (i.e., >8 weeks) PPI therapy may result in rebound acid hypersecretion that may unleash or exacerbate GERD, particularly in patients with large hiatal hernias.[225,226] Acid hypersecretion following the discontinuation of long-term PPI therapy persists for at least 8 weeks and appears to be due to hypergastrinemia-induced increases in parietal and ECL cell masses.[227] The reason that this phenomenon does not occur in Hp-infected individuals who discontinue PPIs may be due to the observation that Hp, as well as the cytokines produced by the inflammatory infiltrate, inhibit acid secretion and thus mask the rebound. With time, atrophy of oxyntic glands with loss of parietal cells may occur in patients chronically infected with Hp, resulting in irreversible achlorhydria (see Chapter 54).

Autoimmune gastritis, also discussed in Chapter 54, is an inflammatory disorder of the oxyntic mucosa characterized by autoantibodies directed against the parietal cell H^+,K^+-ATPase, with a subsequent loss of parietal cells.[228,229] Since H^+,K^+-ATPase is a major autoantigen in a subset of patients infected with Hp, these antibodies may contribute to the subsequent development of atrophic gastritis. Antibodies are acquired due to molecular mimicry between Hp lipopolysaccharide and H^+,K^+-ATPase, both of which contain Lewis epitopes.[230] The prevalence of autoimmune gastritis is approximately 2% in the general United States population but increased three- to fivefolds in patients with other autoimmune disorders, such as type 1 diabetes, thyroid disease, and PBC.[231]

Only 10%–15% of patients chronically infected with Hp exhibit increased acid secretion. These patients have antral-predominant inflammation and are predisposed to duodenal ulcer (see Chapters 54 and 55). Increased acid secretion is thought to occur as a result of reduced antral somatostatin content with elevated basal and stimulated gastrin secretion (see Fig. 53.16).[232–235] The precise mechanism by which somatostatin secretion is decreased is not known but may involve cytokines induced by the inflammation and/or the production of N^α-methyl histamine, a selective H_3-receptor agonist, by Hp.[236,237] One may speculate that the H_3-receptor agonist could diffuse across the antral mucosa to interact with H_3 receptors on antral somatostatin cells, causing inhibition of somatostatin secretion and, thus stimulation of gastrin secretion.[57] In addition, IL-8 and platelet-activating factor are upregulated in Hp-infected mucosa and are capable of stimulating gastrin release from isolated G cells.[238,239]

Integrated Acid Secretory Response to A Meal

Stimuli originating inside and outside the stomach converge on gastric enteric neurons that are the primary regulators of acid

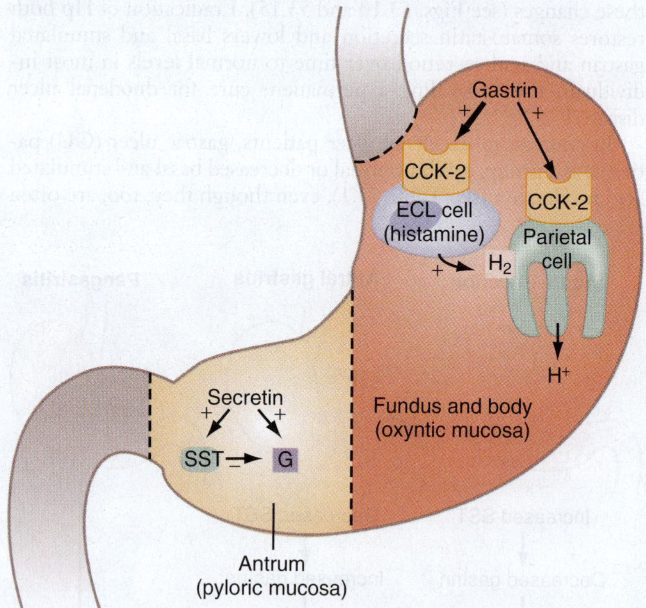

Fig. 53.16 Model illustrating the action of gastrin in oxyntic mucosa and secretin in pyloric mucosa of stomach in patients with ZES. Gastrin, synthesized and secreted by the gastrinoma into the bloodstream, acts via *CCK-2* receptors on acid-secreting parietal and histamine-secreting *ECL* cells to increase acid secretion and induce cell proliferation. In the antrum, exogenous secretin [i.e., secretin stimulation test (see text and Chapter 34)] normally stimulates gastrin secretion directly and concomitantly inhibits gastrin secretion by stimulating somatostatin (*SST*) secretion, resulting in little or no gastrin release. However, in patients with ZES, because the gastrinoma does not contain functionally coupled SST cells, the effect of secretin is solely to stimulate gastrin secretion from the tumor. (From Hung PD, Schubert ML, Mihas AA. Zollinger-Ellison syndrome. *Curr Treat Options Gastroenterol*. 2003;6:163–170.)

secretion. The effector neurons comprise cholinergic (ACh) and peptidergic (i.e., GRP and VIP) neurons. Although NO and PACAP neurons are present in gastric mucosa, their precise physiologic roles as regulators of acid secretion are not known. The effector neurons act on target cells directly as well as indirectly by regulating the secretion of gastrin, somatostatin, and possibly histamine (see Figs. 53.8 and 53.10).

During the basal state, acid secretion is maintained at an economically low level by the continuous inhibitory restraint exerted by somatostatin on the ECL (histamine) and parietal (acid) cells in the fundus/body (oxyntic mucosa) and on the G (gastrin) cell in the antrum (pyloric mucosa; see Figs. 53.5, 53.9, and 53.10). During ingestion of a meal, maximal acid secretion, approximately 10-fold above the basal fasting rate, is achieved by removing the inhibitory influence of somatostatin while at the same time directly stimulating acid and gastrin secretion. This is accomplished, in large part, by activation of cholinergic enteric neurons (see Fig. 53.10). The thought, sight, smell, and taste of food contribute up to 50% of total postprandial acid secretion.[175] Anticipation of a meal activates central neurons whose input is relayed via the vagus nerve to gastric cholinergic enteric neurons in oxyntic as well as pyloric mucosa.[176] The components of the central nervous system include the dorsal motor nucleus of the vagus, the nucleus tractus solitarius, and the hypothalamus. In the fundus/body, ACh released from cholinergic enteric neurons stimulates the parietal cell directly as well as indirectly by eliminating the inhibitory paracrine influence of somatostatin on parietal and ECL cells.[56,102] The resultant increase in histamine stimulates acid secretion directly via H_2 receptors on the parietal cell and indirectly via H_3 receptors that mediate suppression of somatostatin secretion (see Fig. 53.10).[56,177] Thus histamine, acting via H_3 receptors, amplifies the ability of secretagogues to stimulate acid secretion by suppressing somatostatin secretion. The net effect of cholinergic neurons is suppression of all paracrine inhibitory influence (i.e., somatostatin) and enhancement of paracrine stimulatory influences (i.e., histamine acting via H_2 receptors) on parietal cells. There is some evidence that PACAP enteric neurons may participate in the regulation of acid secretion, perhaps by stimulating histamine secretion from ECL cells, but its precise physiologic role is not known.[111–113,178–181]

In the antrum, cholinergic enteric neurons activated by anticipation of the meal stimulate gastrin secretion directly as well as indirectly by suppressing somatostatin secretion (see Fig. 53.10).[42,43,182–194] In physiologic concentrations, gastrin stimulates parietal cells directly and, more importantly, indirectly by enhancing the secretion of histamine.[195,196]

As the meal enters the stomach, the same cholinergic neurons are further activated mechanically by high distention and chemically by protein components of the food.[191,192,197,198] Initially, the ingested meal acts as a buffer of secreted acid. The resultant decrease in acidity (i.e., increase in pH) further inhibits somatostatin secretion and thus increases gastrin secretion. Luminal protein activates GRP neurons that directly stimulate gastrin secretion (see Fig. 53.10).[101,192] The calcium-sensing receptor and the L−amino acid receptor (GPRC6A) have been identified on G cells, suggesting that G cells may be capable of directly sensing luminal proteins and their breakdown products (see Fig. 53.10).[199–201] Suppression of somatostatin secretion facilitates an optimal gastrin response.

As the meal empties from the stomach, a number of paracrine and neural pathways are activated to restore the inhibitory influence of somatostatin in the fundus/body and antrum, and hence restrain acid secretion (see Fig. 53.10). First, a stimulatory paracrine pathway linking gastrin to antral somatostatin cells is activated that acts to restore antral somatostatin secretion after release of gastrin.[83] Second, there is less activation of cholinergic neurons by anticipation of the meal as well as by protein and distention. Third, as distention decreases, VIP neurons are preferentially activated that stimulate somatostatin secretion.[191] Fourth, as the buffering capacity of the meal is lost, antral and fundic somatostatin cells (via sensory CGRP neurons) become exposed to the full stimulatory effect of luminal acid. Fifth, enterogastrones released from the small intestine, such as CCK, stimulate somatostatin secretion. The resultant increase in fundic and antral somatostatin secretion attenuates acid and gastrin secretion and restores the basal interdigestive state. This state is marked by the continuous restraint exerted on ECL (histamine), parietal (acid), and G (gastrin) cells by contiguous somatostatin cells (see Figs. 53.9 and 53.10). A decrease in this restraint is sufficient to again initiate acid secretion.

Pharmacological Antisecretory Agents

Introduction

For centuries, symptoms such as abdominal pain, heartburn, and foregut mucosal injury, including peptic ulcer disease and esophagitis, have been attributed to excessive secretion of gastric acid. Until the 1980s the principal therapy for these symptoms and conditions consisted primarily of metallic alkaline salts such as calcium carbonate, sodium bicarbonate, bismuth subsalicylate, magnesium or aluminum salts, anticholinergic drugs, the hourly consumption of a bland diet consisting of "...milk, cream, eggs, cereal, and vegetable purées..." accompanied by frequent measurement of gastric juice acidity, and several weeks of bed rest.[415] In extreme cases of intractable ulcer, uncontrollable hemorrhage, or pyloric obstruction, surgery such as vagotomy and antrectomy was indicated.[411–414] In all cases, it was recognized early on that ulcer healing only occurred when gastric acidity was controlled for most of the day for at least several weeks. A study by Burget et al. reported that the degree, duration, and length of acid suppression were highly correlated with mucosal healing, with a threshold of 3, above which the authors stated was maximally effective.[416] This study also highlighted the superior acid suppression by the PPI omeprazole in comparison with the H2RAs cimetidine, ranitidine, and famotidine; the PG enprostil; and the cholinergic antagonist pirenzepine.

Basic studies of the paracrine and endocrine regulation of gastric secretion combined with the discovery of the structure and function of the gastric H^+,K^+-ATPase enabled the development of pharmacologic agents designed to specifically inhibit either the paracrine pathways that stimulant acid secretion or the H^+,K^+-ATPase itself. In the following sections, we will describe the three major classes of antisecretory drugs: the selective H2 receptor antagonists (H2RA), the PPIs, and the P-CABs.

H_2 Receptor Agonists

Background

The approval of the H2RA cimetidine in 1976 was a watershed occurrence in the field of gastroenterology since this represented the first well-tolerated, safe, and potent antisecretory drug available for clinical use, revolutionizing the therapy of clinical conditions attributed to acid-peptic injury.[417]

H2RAs, by antagonizing the H_2 receptor expressed on parietal cells, effectively impair the prosecretory signals from histamine while interrupting the synergy among endocrine signals from Ach and endocrine signals from gastrin as discussed in the prior section (Functional Anatomy); Fig. 53.9.[417] Although antihistamines were developed in the 1930s, they failed to inhibit gastric secretion even though histamine was known as a prosecretory hormone.[418] Further studies by James Black revealed that a second class of histamine receptors existed that he termed the H_2 receptors. This research eventuated in the first recognized H2RA burimamide that suppressed gastric acid secretion in a paradigm-shifting publication[419] that laid the foundation for modern pharmacotherapy of acid-peptic diseases, recognized by the awarding of the Nobel Prize for Physiology or Medicine to Sir James Black in 1988 for the discovery and development of propranolol and the H2RAs. Further development and testing led to the development of cimetidine, the first clinically approved H2RA.

Experimentally, cimetidine and its related H2RA ranitidine inhibited human gastric acid secretion stimulated by histamine, gastrin, or vagal stimulation, supporting the hypothesis of the interaction of these prosecretory pathways.[420,421]

Clinical Utility

Cimetidine, followed by its successors ranitidine, famotidine, and nizatidine, has proven useful for the therapy of acid-peptic diseases such as GU, duodenal ulcer, and reflux esophagitis, although their effectiveness is less than that of the PPIs, likely due to the inferior magnitude and duration of acid suppression,[422] decreasing their popularity for the treatment of these diseases. Due to their relative safety, low cost, rapid-onset of action, and activity independent of meal ingestion or parietal cell activation, this class of drugs has found a niche for nocturnal symptoms between doses of PPI,[422,424] for the treatment of functional and quasifunctional diseases, such as functional dyspepsia and nonerosive reflux disease,[425] possibly for the prophylaxis of mucosal injury in patients with cardiovascular disease taking dual-antiplatelet therapy,[426] and other indications in which an inexpensive, relatively safe, and rapidly-acting antisecretory is useful. Please note that since the data supporting these indications are mostly of low quality, these are not considered clinical recommendations.

Safety

A recent systematic "umbrella" review of 46 meta-analyses addressing the safety and efficacy of H2RAs concluded that H2RA therapy may increase the risk of infections such as pneumonia, peritonitis, necrotizing enterocolitis, *Clostridioides difficile* colitis, gastric and liver cancer, hip fracture, and asthma, although these conclusions are tempered by the overall very low quality of the data analyzed. These conclusions must be weighed against the more than 30 years of global use of billions of doses of these drugs, for which no unequivocal severe adverse effect associations have emerged. Furthermore, the ECL cell hyperplasia and rare carcinoid tumors are less likely than with the more potent antisecretory drugs discussed below due to the inferior acid suppression with less elevated serum levels of gastrin.[427,428]

Conclusions

As the first antisecretory drugs in widespread clinical use, H2RAs are not only of historical interest but also have emerged as useful in niche indications where PPIs are inferior. Although their low cost and longstanding over-the-counter status preclude much pharma interest, these drugs merit a careful evaluation for discrete indications for which they could prove to be a safe, inexpensive, and efficacious alternative to PPIs and P-CABs.

Proton Pump Inhibitors

Mechanism of Action

PPIs are acid-activated prodrugs that irreversibly inhibit the action of the parietal cell H^+,K^+-ATPase (also termed the proton pump) by covalently binding to the luminal surface of the ATPase. PPIs consist of 2 heterocyclic moieties, a pyridine and a benzimidazole ring, connected by a methylsulphinyl group (Fig. 17). They are weak bases (pK_a 4 or 5) that concentrate in acidic spaces within the body that have a pH less than 4. The pK_a of a molecule is based on a logarithmic scale such that a compound with a pK_a of 5 is 10-fold more basic than a compound with a pK_a of 4. When a compound is in an environment with a pH equal to its pK_a, half the molecules will be protonated and half will be nonprotonated. PPIs are membrane permeant in their nonprotonated form and relatively impermeant in their protonated form. If a compound, such as a PPI with a pK_a of 4, is placed in an environment with a pH <1, >99.9% of the molecules will be protonated and will not readily pass through biological membranes. In blood (pH 7.4), PPIs are predominantly nonprotonated and thus pass readily into cells (time to reach peak plasma concentration, ≈2 hours; elimination half-life, ≈1 hour), diffuse through the cytoplasm, and then become protonated and trapped, probably as sulfenamides or sulfenic acid, in the acidic environment of the secretory canaliculus.[159]

As a consequence of the basic pK_a of PPIs and "ion trapping," the concentration of PPIs in the secretory canaliculus is up to one millionfold higher than in the blood. The sulfenamide rapidly reacts with cysteines on the luminally exposed α-subunit of the H^+,K^+-ATPase to form a covalent (electrochemical) disulfide bond (see Figs. 53.17 and 53.18).[160] Whereas all PPIs bind to cysteine 813 of the α-subunit, omeprazole also binds to cysteine 892, lansoprazole to cysteine 321, and pantoprazole to cysteine 822.

Since only the apical-membrane inserted H^+,K^+-ATPase is susceptible to blockade by PPIs and an acidic environment (pH <4) is necessary for trapping and converting the PPI to its reactive species, the potency of PPIs is increased when the parietal cell is stimulated postprandially.[429,430] Since the number of H^+,K^+-ATPase pumps expressed on the parietal cell plasma membrane is greatest when the gastric luminal pH is increased,[431] it is recommended that PPIs should be taken 30–60 minutes before the first meal of the day. The rationale for this dosing is that a meal will typically raise the gastric luminal pH, activating acid sensors that release gastrin, which in turn activates ECL cells that then release histamine that activates histamine-2 (H_2) receptors expressed on the parietal cell.[432] The activated parietal cell recruits the H^+,K^+-ATPase to the parietal cell apical secretory membrane, increasing its capacity for acid secretion.[433] This process is estimated to take about 30–60 minutes (dependent on PPI type and dose), about the same time frame that orally ingested PPIs are converted and maximally concentrate in the secretory canaliculus.[434] If greater inhibition is needed, an additional dose should be taken before dinner.[435] Since PPIs irreversibly inhibit the H^+K^+-ATPase recovery from inhibition of acid secretion occurs by de novo synthesis of pump protein (54 hours in rats), although an endogenous mechanism whereby glutathione reduces of the cysteine disulfide bonds that adhere the sulfenamide to the H^+,K^+-ATPase, reactivating the pump, may exist, at least in theory.[434,436]

Consequences of Potent Acid Suppression

The principal physiologic consequence of acid suppression, whether by a PPI or through destruction of parietal ceils by surgery or by autoimmune mechanisms, is hypergastrinemia. Gastrin is not only a secretagogue but also exerts growth-promoting effects in normal and neoplastic tissues. In the

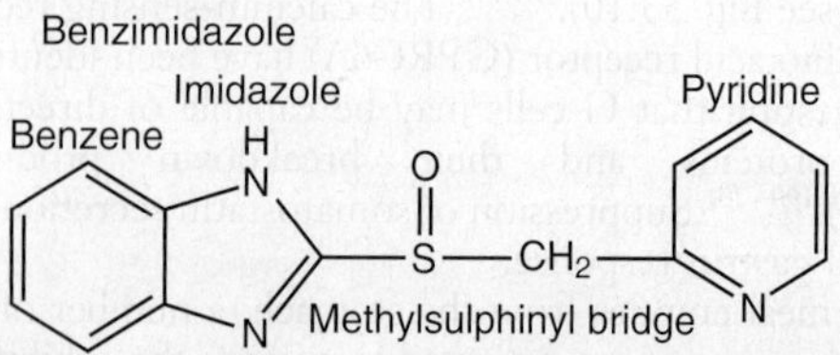

Fig. 53.17 Structure of PPIs. PPIs consist of 2 heterocyclic moieties, a benzimidazole ring and a pyridine, connected by a methylsulphinyl bridge. PPIs are weak bases (pKa 4-5) that accumulate and activate in acidic spaces within the body that have a pH less than 4. Once activated within the parietal cell canaliculus, the PPI binds covalently with certain cysteine residues within the α-subunit of the inserted H^+,K^+-ATPase.

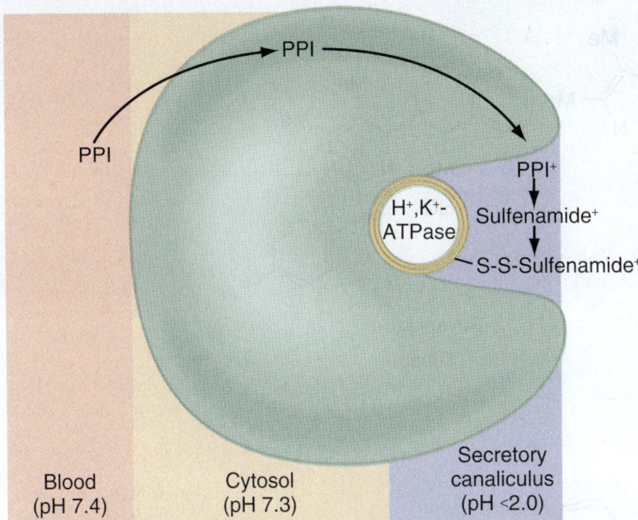

Fig. 53.18 Model illustrating the mechanism of action of PPIs. PPIs reach the parietal cell from the bloodstream, diffuse through the cytoplasm, and accumulate in the acid environment of the secretory canaliculus. In the canaliculus, the PPI becomes protonated and trapped as a sulfenic acid followed by dehydration to a sulfenamide. The sulfenamide binds covalently by disulfide bonds to one or more cysteines of the H^+,K^+-ATPase to inhibit the enzyme. Although all PPIs bind to cysteine 813, omeprazole also binds to cysteine 892, lansoprazole to cysteine 321, and pantoprazole to cysteine 822.

stomach, hypergastrinemia results in parietal and ECL cell hyperplasia, which persists for 2–3 months after stopping the PPI.[437] Endoscopically, chronic PPI use is associated with distinct mucosal features such as fundic gland polyps, hyperplastic polyps, multiple White and flat elevated lesions, cobblestone-like mucosa, or Black spots that histologically appear as parietal cell protrusion into the gland lumen, cystic dilation of gastric fundic glands, and foveolar epithelial hyperplasia (Fig. 53.19).[438] After discontinuation of long-term PPIs, rebound acid secretion occurs, presumably as a consequence of parietal or ECL cell hyperplasia,[439,440,441] that may induce dyspeptic symptoms in healthy individuals, exacerbate reflux symptoms in patients with GERD, and provoke symptoms in patients with peptic ulcers.[437,442] In patients with chronic severe hypergastrinemia, PPI-induced ECL hyperplasia may rarely progress to dysplasia and development of NET.[443–446] The incidence of NETs has increased more than fivefold over the past 25 years, and gastric carcinoid, derived from histamine-containing ECL cells, is the most frequent NET of the stomach (see Chapter 43).

Currently Available Drugs

Current FDA approved PPIs are dexlansoprazole, esomeprazole, lansoprazole, omeprazole, pantoprazole, and rabeprazole. Although omeprazole, esomeprazole, and lansoprazole are widely available over the counter, dexlansoprazole, pantoprazole, and rabeprazole require prescriptions (see Fig. 53.20 for their common chemical structure).[447] In healthy humans, the plasma half-life of PPIs is 1–2 hours,[434] though this has little bearing on its acid inhibition, since the key measure is the binding of the sulfenamide to the H^+,K^+-ATPase as discussed earlier. Thus despite the relatively short serum half-life, the duration of acid inhibition can be up to 48 hours due to the irreversible binding of the H^+K^+-ATPase. The oral bioavailability for PPIs is high, around 70%–90%.[448] Based on percentage time the gastric luminal pH is pH >4 over a 24-hour period, pantoprazole is the most potent PPI, followed by lansoprazole, omeprazole, esomeprazole, and rabeprazole.[435,449] Unlike other PPIs, dexlansoprazole, as the (*R*)-(+)-enantiomer of lansoprazole, releases drug at two points in time, with 25% of the drug released at pH of 5.5 and 75% of the drug released at pH of 6.8, facilitating once-daily administration for those who would usually require twice a day dosing.[450]

PPIs are predominantly metabolized by hepatic cytochrome P450 isoenzyme 2C19 (CYP2C19) and to a lesser extent by isoenzyme 3A4 (CYP3A4).[447,451] Genetic polymorphisms of the CYP2C19 enzyme include genotypes that are classified into rapid, intermediate, and poor metabolizer groups. Plasma PPI levels and intragastric pH values during PPI treatment are lowest in the rapid, intermediate in the intermediate, and highest in the poor metabolizer group. Genetic testing for CYP2C19 is currently commercially available, though few data support its clinical utility. Therefore the routine use of the CYP2C19 genotype-guided dosing of PPIs is not currently recommended by major gastroenterology society guidelines.[451,452]

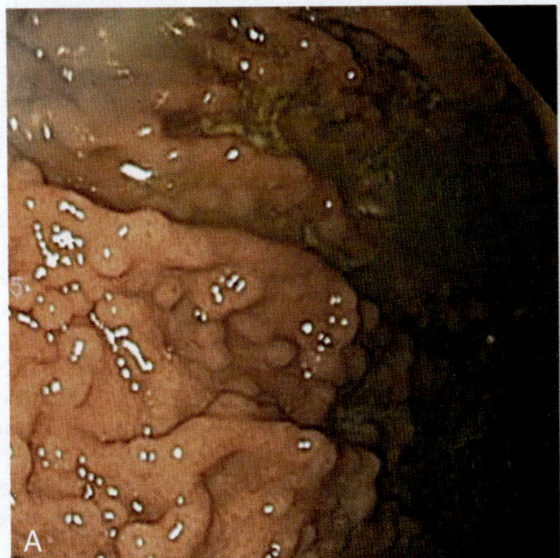

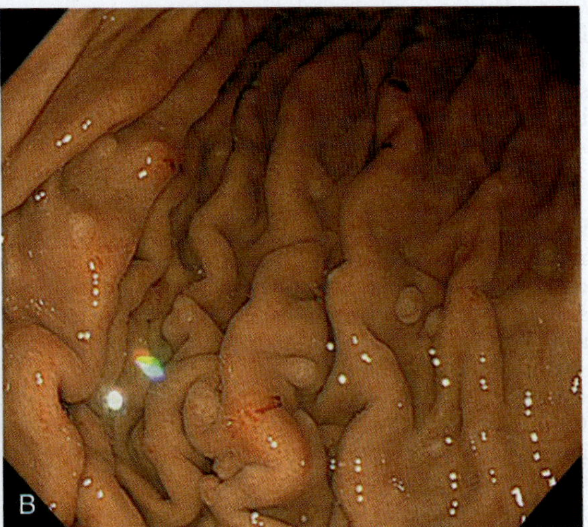

Fig. 53.19 Endoscopic view of fundic gland polyposis, a condition ucommonly associated with hypergastrinemia. (A) During PPI therapy. (B) Six months after cessation of PPI therapy.[495] (Reprinted from: Hamada K, Takeuchi Y, Akasaka T, Iishi H. Fundic gland polyposis associated with proton-pump inhibitor use. *Eur J Case Rep Intern Med.* 2017;4(5):000607 with permission from Commons Attribution Noncommercial 4.0 License.)

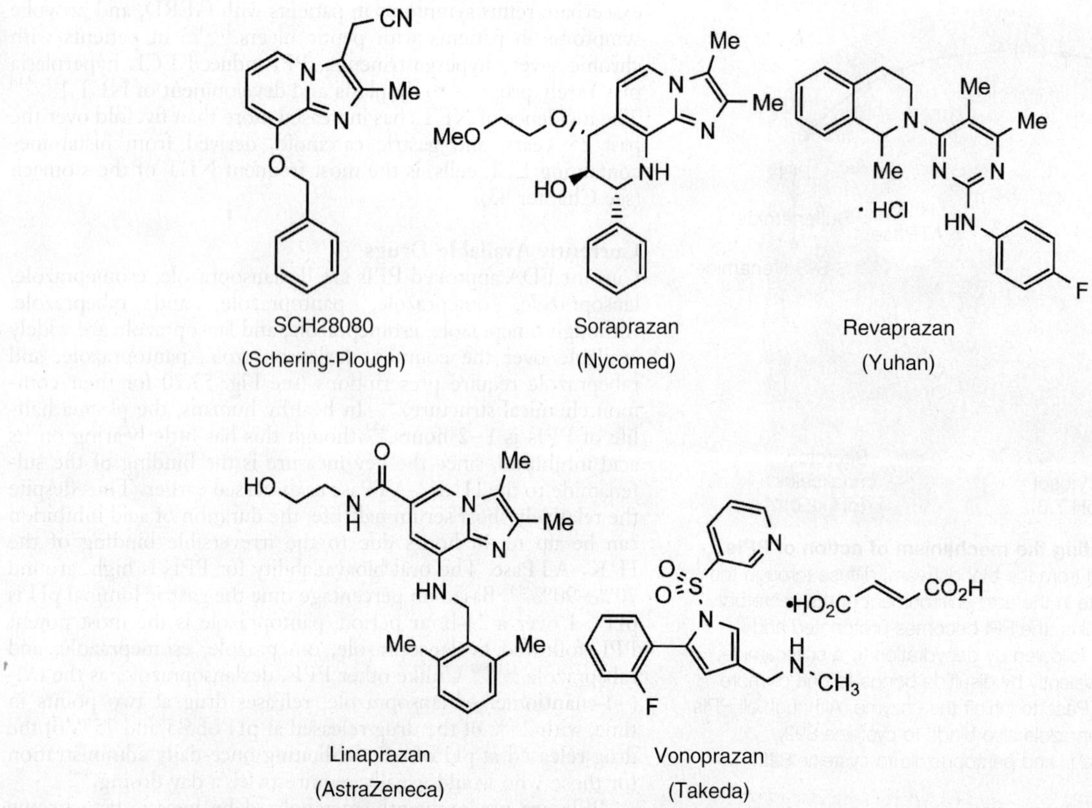

Fig. 53.20 Chemical structures of potassium-competitive acid blockers. (Reprinted from Inatomi N, Matsukawa J, Sakurai Y, Otake K. Potassium-competitive acid blockers: advanced therapeutic option for acid-related diseases. *Pharmacol Ther.* 2016;168:12–22.)

PPIs are one of the most commonly-prescribed medications in the United States with the use doubling from 1999 to 2012. In 2015 esomeprazole was reported to have $5 billion in sales worldwide.[453,454] The FDA-approved indications for PPIs in adults include healing of erosive esophagitis, maintenance of healed erosive esophagitis, treatment of GERD, risk reduction for GU associated with nonsteroidal anti-inflammatory drugs (NSAIDs), *Hp* eradication, pathological hypersecretory conditions, including ZES, and short-term treatment and maintenance of duodenal ulcers. No difference in efficacy exists between PPIs at similar doses.[435,455] The choice of which PPI to use is up to the provider and the patient based on preference, availability, price, pharmacy policy, and insurance coverage.

Safety

Recently, safety issues surrounding PPI therapy have attracted widespread media attention, with gastroenterologists often questioned by their patients regarding their long-term safety profile. Many adverse consequences of long-term PPI have been reported, including dementia, myocardial infraction, subcutaneous lupus erythematous, interstitial nephritis, *C. difficile* infection, microscopic colitis, bone fracture, small intestinal bacterial overgrowth (SIBO), hepatic encephalopathy, and cardiac QTc prolongation (Fig. 53.21).[172] Given the plethora of these purported adverse events, few are supported by high-quality data, with many studies flawed by inconsistencies, confounding factors, bias, and low absolute excess risks (Tables 53.2 and 53.3). In a randomized, controlled trial of over 1700 patients, there was no difference in safety outcomes of stroke, MI, pneumonia, fracture, diabetes, CKD, dementia, chronic obstructive pulmonary disease, and gastric atrophy between patients receiving pantoprazole 40 mg versus placebo, though enteric infections were more frequent in the pantoprazole group compared with the placebo group. The number needed to harm for enteric infections was 301 (95% CI, 152–9190) after a median of 3 years of PPI use.[456] Furthermore, in a large prospective cohort study following over 70,000 subjects over 13.8 years, long-term PPI use was not associated with excess all-cause mortality nor mortality due to cancer, cardiovascular diseases, respiratory disease, or digestive diseases after a lag-time adjustment was applied. (Lag-time was used to minimize the influence of protopathic bias, which is when a pharmaceutical agent is prescribed for an early manifestation of a disease, which then appears to cause the disease when it is eventually diagnosed). PPI use was associated with an increased mortality from renal disease despite applying lag-time of 2, 4, and 6 years.[457] Fig. 53.22 summarizes the quality of evidence behind PPI associated adverse events. There is evidence to support causal relationship between PPI use and acute kidney injury, structural and functional changes in the gastric mucosa, and enteric infections. There is low evidence to support causality for *C. difficile* infection, vitamin B_{12} deficiency, and hypomagnesemia or hypocalcemia. Nevertheless, there is insufficient evidence to support causality for chronic kidney disease, dementia, gastrointestinal malignancies, cardiovascular events, pneumonia, osteoporosis, or SIBO.[453] Development of fundic gland polyps is common and generally not of clinical significance. PPI discontinuation may resolve the lesions (Fig. 53.23).

Indications and Clinical Use

When PPIs are prescribed appropriately, their benefits greatly outweigh potential adverse effects. The latest American Gastrointestinal Association clinical practice update recommend that

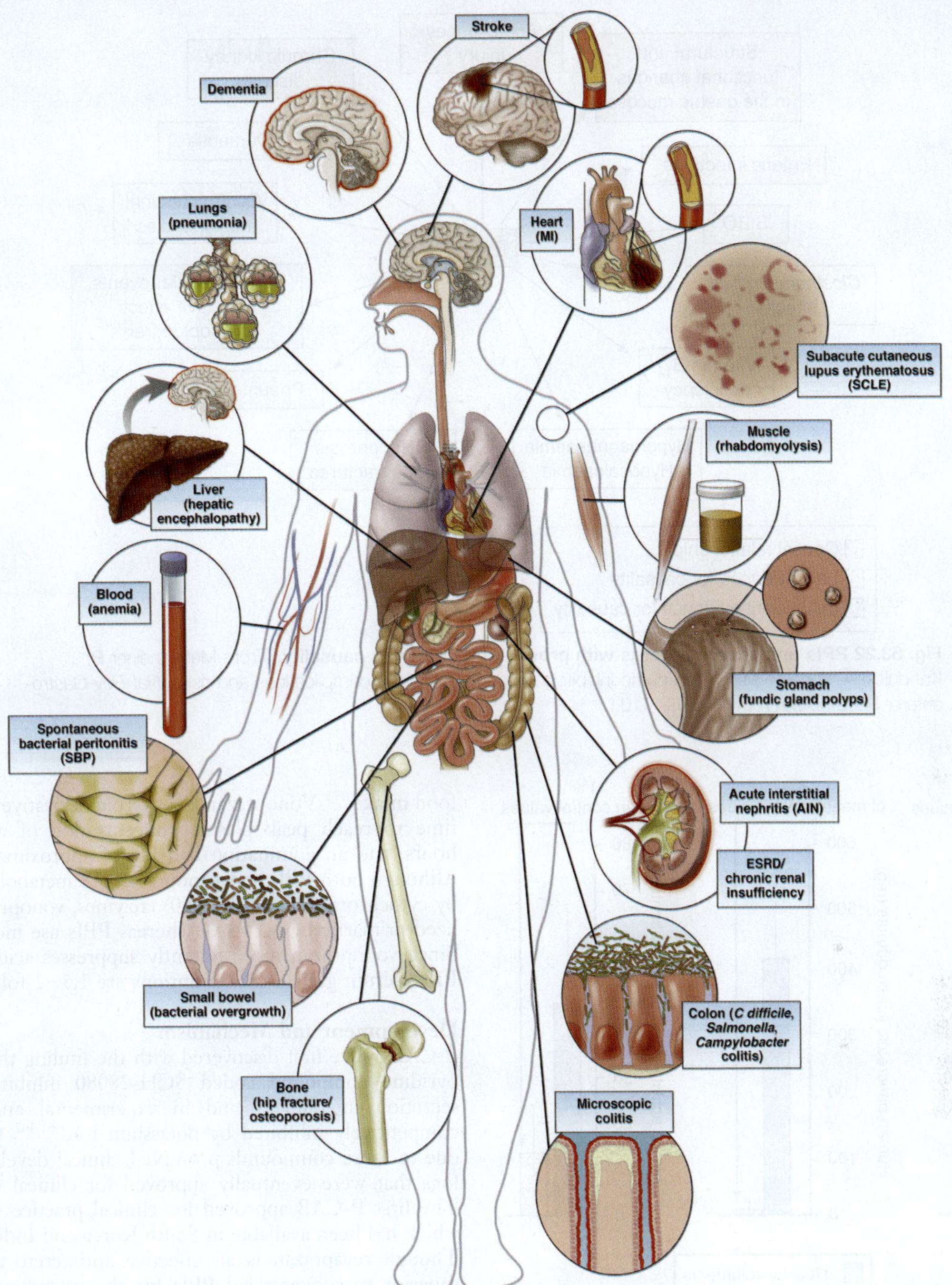

Fig. 53.21 Adverse consequences of long-term PPI therapy. The reported side effects include a variety of conditions involving multiple organ systems. (From Vaezi MF, Yang YX, Howden CW. Complications of proton pump inhibitor therapy. *Gastroenterology*. 2017;153(1):35–48.)

PPIs should be prescribed for patients with complicated GERD, especially those with erosive esophagitis and strictures, for patients with Barrett's esophagus, eosinophilic esophagus, ZES, or idiopathic pulmonary fibrosis, and for patients with increased risk of ulcer-related bleeding from NSAIDs, aspirin, and dual antiplatelet therapies. In patients without a definitive indication for chronic PPI therapy, a trial of PPI withdrawal should be considered. When prescribed in the long-term, PPIs should be used at the lowest effective doses, and their needs periodically reassessed. The decision to discontinue PPI should be based only on the lack of an indication for PPI use and not due to the concern for PPI associated adverse events.[458]

Potassium-Competitive Acid Blockers

Introduction

P-CABs (such as vonoprazan and revaprazan) potently inhibit the action of the parietal cell H^+,K^+-ATPase.[459,460] presumably by competitively blocking the apical membrane potassium channel (such as KNCQ1) that is the major site for potassium influx, as

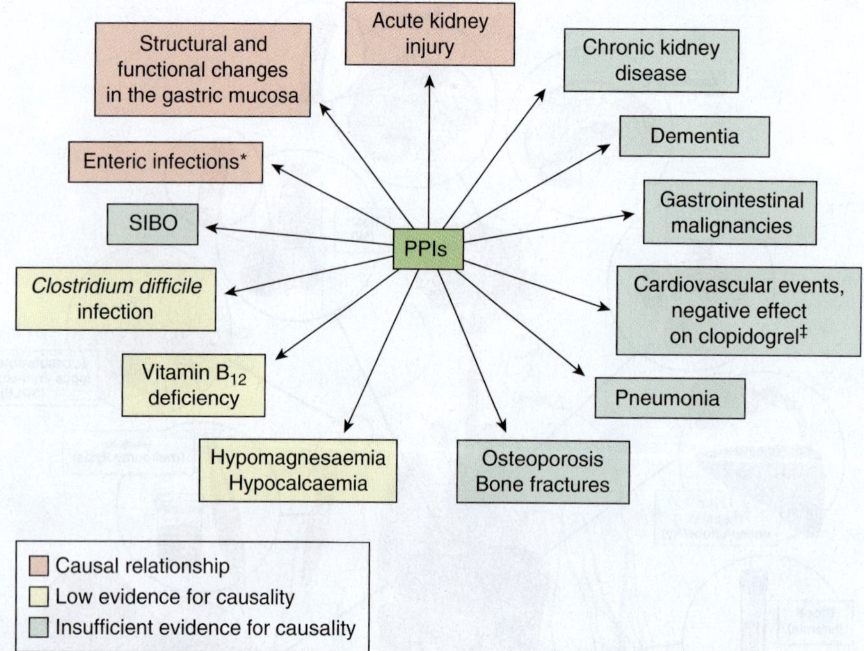

Fig. 53.22 PPIs and adverse events with proven and unproven causality. (From Malfertheiner P, Kandulski A, Venerito M. Proton-pump inhibitors: understanding the complications and risks. *Nat Rev Gastroenterol Hepatol*. 2017;14(12):697–710.)

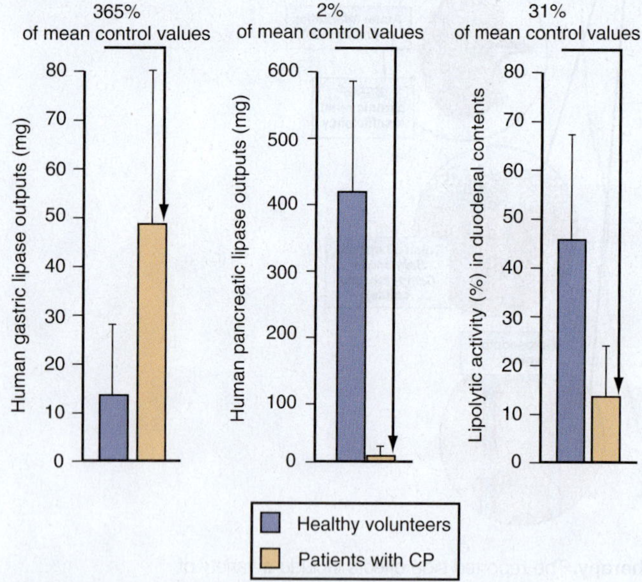

Fig. 53.23 Relative outputs of human gastric lipase *(left graph)*, human pancreatic lipase *(middle graph)*, and lipolytic activity in duodenal contents *(right graph)* in healthy volunteers and patients with chronic pancreatitis with exocrine insufficiency (*CP*). Note that despite the increase of human gastric lipase output in patients with CP, the overall magnitude of the rise is insufficient to fully correct the reduction in duodenal lipolytic activity. (From Carrière F, Grandval P, Renou C, et al. Quantitative study of digestive enzyme secretion and gastrointestinal lipolysis in chronic pancreatitis. *Clin Gastroenterol Hepatol*. 2005;3:28–38.)

discussed in the prior section. Compared with PPIs, acid-catalyzed activation is not necessary, the onset of action is more rapid, usually with on 1 day, and bioavailability is unaffected by food intake.[173] Vonoprazan is a pyrrole derivative with a pK_a of 9, time to reach peak plasma concentration of approximately 2 hours, and an elimination half-life of approximately 7 hours.[174] Although both PPIs and vonoprazan are metabolized in the liver by cytochrome P450 (CYP450) enzymes, vonoprazan is metabolized primarily by CYP3A4 whereas PPIs use mostly CYP2C19. Since vonoprazan more potently suppresses acid secretion than PPIs, serum gastrin concentrations are 1.5–2-fold higher.

Development and Mechanism

P-CABs were first discovered with the finding that the imidazopyridine compound coded SCH-28080 inhibited gastric acid secretion in humans and in experimental animals that was competitively inhibited by potassium ion.[461,462] Clinical toxicity due to these compounds prompted clinical development of analogs that were eventually approved for clinical development.[463] The first P-CAB approved for clinical practice was revaprazan, which has been available in South Korea and India since 2007.[464] Though revaprazan is an effective antisecretory,[465] it was not superior to conventional PPIs for the treatment of endoscopic submucosal dissection-induced ulcers[466] with no data suggesting that revaprazan is more effective than PPIs for the other gastric acid-related conditions. Vonoprazan, the second P-CAB available in the Japanese market, was released in Japan in 2015 and is now available in the Philippines, Singapore, Thailand, Malaysia, and China. Tegoprazan was approved as a treatment for GERD in South Korea since 2018. Other P-CABs (YH4808, DWP14012, and KFP-H008) are still being tested in clinical trials.[467–470] The chemical structures of the four P-CABs are depicted in Fig. 53.20.

The therapeutic efficacy of conventional PPIs is limited by instability in acidic conditions requiring enteric-coated formulation for clinical use, high pharmacokinetic variability due to genetic polymorphisms of cytochrome P450 (CYP) 2C19 metabolism, a relatively slow onset of pharmacological action that may require several days to achieve optimal acid suppression and symptom relief, and lack of stable suppression of gastric acid secretion over 24 hours.

TABLE 53.2 Summary of Evidence for Potential Proton Pump Inhibitor (PPI)-Associated Adverse Effects

Potential Adverse Effect	Types of Studies	Threats to Validity	Overall Quality of Evidence
Kidney disease	• Observational only	• Modest effect size • Residual confounding would bias toward harm • Absence of dose-response effect	Very low
Dementia	• Observational only	• Modest effect size • Residual confounding would bias toward harm	Very low
Bone fracture	• Observational only	• Inconsistent results • Modest effect size • Residual confounding would bias toward harm	Low or very low
Myocardial infarction	• Observational • RCT	• Results differ between RCTs and observational studies • Secondary analysis of RCT data • Modest effect size • Residual confounding would bias toward harm	Very low
Small intestinal bacterial overgrowth	• Observational • Crossover	• Sparse data • Residual confounding would bias toward harm • Protopathic bias	Low
Spontaneous bacterial peritonitis	• Observational only	• Modest effect size • Residual confounding would bias toward harm	Very low
Clostridium difficile infection	• Observational only	• Modest effect size • Residual confounding would bias toward harm	Low
Pneumonia	• Observational • RCT	• Results differ between RCTs and observational studies • Secondary analysis of RCT data • Modest effect size • Absence of dose-response effect • Residual confounding would bias toward harm • Protopathic bias	Very low
Micronutrient deficiencies	• Observational only	• Inconsistent results • Modest effect size • Absence of dose-response effect • Residual confounding would bias toward harm	Low or very low
Gastrointestinal malignancies	• Observational RCT	• Results differ between RCTs and observational studies • RCTs use surrogate outcomes • Modest effect size • Residual confounding would bias toward harm • Confounding by indication and protopathic bias	Very low

Note. Assessments regarding the quality of evidence are based on the methodology of the GRADE Working Group (see inset).
From Freedberg DE, Kim LS, Yang YX. The risks and benefits of long-term use of proton pump inhibitors: expert review and best practice advice from the american gastroenterological association. *Gastroenterology*. 2017;152(4):706–715.

Vonoprazan fumarate is a novel P-CAB developed to resolve the above limitations of conventional PPIs. Vonoprazan exhibited rapid, strong, and continuous gastric acid suppression.[459] Vonoprazan has a high solubility and stability over a broad pH range in aqueous conditions.[471] Furthermore, vonoprazan has a more potent and longer-lasting acid suppression effect than the conventional PPI, lansoprazole.[471] Preclinical pharmacokinetic studies have shown that vonoprazan is accumulated and retained in the stomach for more than 24 hours, even after it is eliminated from the plasma.[471]

Due to the potent gastric acid suppression, vonoprazan effectively treated *H. pylori* infection, GERD, and low-dose aspirin (LDA)-associated peptic ulcers.[459,472] From a pharmacological standpoint, there are several advantages to using vonoprazan over conventional PPIs. It is rapidly absorbed in the small intestine where it accumulates in the canalicular membranes of parietal cells[474] displaying a superior acid-inhibitory effect than those of esomeprazole and rabeprazole, as observed from the first day of administration.[474] It has also a longer duration of action with the ability to keep intragastric pH <4 significantly longer than for esomeprazole and rabeprazole.[474] It does not require acid activation, whereas PPIs are acid-activated prodrugs that require conversion to a protonated, impermeant form for activity (see previous section). Moreover, vonoprazan has a pK_a (>9) higher than PPIs (~4), facilitating protonation in the parietal cell canaliculi, achieving large concentration ratios.[434,459] As such, vonoprazan is more stable in an acidic environment than PPI.[475] Furthermore, vonoprazan has consistent acid suppressive capabilities irrespective of CYP2C19. It is metabolized to its inactive form mainly by CYP3A4, and partially also by CYP2B6, CYP2C19, CYP2D6, and SULT2A1, whereas most PPIs are mainly metabolized by CYP2C19.[476]

Tegoprazan is another potent and highly selective inhibitor of gastric H^+,K^+-ATPase. Interestingly, tegoprazan evoked a gastric phase III contraction of the migrating motor complex in a canine model.[467] YH4808 had a faster onset than esomeprazole and can maintain an intragastric acidity of pH <4 for a greater time than any PPI healthy volunteers.[468] DWP14012 showed rapid and sustained suppression of gastric acid secretion in healthy volunteers.[470] KFP-H008 showed a more effective, potent, and longer-lasting inhibitory action than that of lansoprazole in a rat model.[464]

TABLE 53.3 Absolute and Relative Risks for Adverse Effects Associated With Long-Term Proton Pump Inhibitors (PPIs)

Potential Adverse Effect	Relative Risk	Reference for Risk Estimate	Reference for Incidence Estimate	Absolute Excess Risk
Chronic kidney disease	10%–20% increase	Lazarus et al.[48]	Lazarus et al.48	0.1%–0.3% per patient/ year
Dementia	4%–80% increase	Haenisch et al.[90]	Haenisch et al.[90]	.07%–1.5% per patient/ year
Bone fracture[1]	30% to 4-fold increase	Yang et al.[27]	Yang et al.[27]	0.1%–0.5% per patient/ year
Myocardial infarction	No association in RCTs	–	–	–
Small intestinal bacterial overgrowth	2–8-fold increase	Lo et al.[91]	None available	Unable to calculate
Campylobacter or *Salmonella* infection	2–6-fold increase	Bavishi et al.[26]	Crim et al.[92]	.03%–0.2% per patient/ year
Spontaneous bacterial peritonitis	50% to 3-fold increase	Xu et al.[93]	Fernandez et al.[94]	3%–16% per patient/ year
Clostridium difficile infection'	No risk to 3-fold increase	Furuya et al.[95]	Lessa et al.[96]	0%–09% per patient/ year
Pneumonia	No association in RCTs	–	–	–
Micronutrient deficiencies'	60%–70% increase	Lam et al.[87]	Bailey et al.[98]	0.3%–0.4% per patient/ year
Gastrointestinal malignancies	No association in RCTs			

Reprinted from Vaezi MF, Yang YX, Howden CW. Complications of proton pump inhibitor therapy. *Gastroenterology*. 2017;153(1):35–48. https://doi.org/10.1053/j.gastro.2017.04.047 with permission from Elsevier.

Clinical Use

P-CAB and Gastroesophageal Reflux Disease

Vonoprazan is a candidate first-line drug for GERD treatment. In CYP2C19 EM patients of erosive esophagitis, 90.0% treated with vonoprazan (20 mg/day) achieved mucosal healing at 2 weeks compared with the 79.3% that were treated with lansoprazole ($P < .01$).[477] Similarly, at 4 and 8 weeks, the proportion of patients with healed erosive esophagitis tended to be higher in the vonoprazan group than in the lansoprazole group (at 4 weeks 96.1% vs. 90.9%, $P < .05$, at 8 weeks 98.9% vs. 94.5%, $P < .03$).[477] Moreover, vonoprazan was more effective for severe erosive esophagitis (LA Classification Grades C/D) than lansoprazole (at 8 weeks 98.7% vs. 87.5%, $P < .01$) and had more rapid effectiveness (at 2 weeks 88.0% vs. 63.9%, $P < .01$, at 4 weeks 96.0% vs. 80.6%, $P < .03$).[477] Therefore vonoprazan is highly effective for patients with more severe erosive esophagitis and CYP2C19 EM patients. Even in whole patients, vonoprazan is more effective than lansoprazole at each time point (at 2 weeks 90.7% vs. 81.9%, $P < .01$, at 4 weeks 96.6% vs. 92.5%, $P < .01$, at 8 weeks 99.0% vs. 95.5%, $P < .01$). On the other contrary, no data showed that P-CAB was effective to relieve the symptoms of mild esophagitis and NERD. A nonrandomized, controlled trial reported that 4-week treatment with vonoprazan (20 mg/day) was effective to relieve symptoms in 66.7% of NERD patients and 53.8% of PPI-resistant NERD patients.[477] In summary, 4-week treatment with vonoprazan (20 mg/day) was effective as initial therapy for severe erosive esophagitis; 4-week treatment with vonoprazan and 8-week treatment with a PPI were recommended as initial therapies for mild erosive esophagitis and NERD. Vonoprazan is effective for PPI-resistant reflux esophagitis.[478] Of the 24 subjects with PPI-resistant GERD enrolled, 58.3% had severe erosive esophagitis. In total, 87.5% of the subjects and 85.7% with severe erosive esophagitis patients achieved endoscopic healing 4 weeks after changing from PPI to vonoprazan (20 mg/day).[478] Furthermore, GERD symptoms were significantly improved starting the day after drug change.[478] Vonoprazan (40 mg/day) rescue therapy may also be useful for PPI-resistant reflux esophagitis.[479]

Continuous administration of vonoprazan (10 or 20 mg/day) is more efficacious than lansoprazole (15 mg/day) in maintaining healed erosive esophagitis.[480] Therefore, at present, the optimal maintenance strategy for erosive esophagitis is the continuous administration of vonoprazan at 10 mg/day. Umezawa et al. showed that on-demand therapy using vonoprazan is more effective than continuous PPI treatment as an alternative maintenance therapy for patients with mild erosive esophagitis.[477]

P-CAB and H. pylori *Eradication*

Potent acid inhibition stimulates the growth of the gastric resident pathogen *H. pylori*, enhancing the bactericidal effect of amoxicillin and presumably other antibiotics, underscoring the importance of antisecretory therapy in the eradication of *H. pylori*.[482] A meta-analysis revealed that high-dose PPIs are more effective than standard-dose in the eradication of *H. pylori* infection.[483] CYP2C19 polymorphisms are associated with the efficacy of PPI-based *H. pylori* eradication therapy, supporting the importance of acid suppression. The eradication rates for omeprazole and lansoprazole-based triple therapies were lower in for the extensive metabolizer CYP2C19 EM polymorphism than in the other groups.[484,485] Eradication regimens involving esomeprazole, rabeprazole, and newer generation PPIs achieved superior overall *H. pylori* eradication rates (especially those in CYP2C19 EM patients) than for those involving omeprazole, lansoprazole, and pantoprazole.[486]

Vonoprazan-amoxicillin-clarithromycin triple regimen considerably improved the eradication rate of first-line *H. pylori* treatment. The eradication rate was 92.6% with vonoprazan-based triple therapy versus 75.9% with lansoprazole-based triple therapy.[487] The eradication rate was significantly higher with vonoprazan compared with lansoprazole in those patients infected with clarithromycin-resistant strains (82.0% vs. 40.0%, $P < .01$).[487] In

CYP2C19 EM patients, the eradication rate of vonoprazan-based triple therapy was significantly higher than that of lansoprazole-based triple therapy (92.9% vs. 75.0%, $P < .01$).[487] In CYP2C19 PM patients, there was no significant difference, although the eradication rate of vonoprazan-based triple therapy was higher than the rate of lansoprazole-based triple therapy (90.9% vs. 81.3%, $P =$ N.S.). Conversely, the rate of the second-line metronidazole and amoxicillin-based triple therapy did not differ significantly between the PPI and vonoprazan groups (96.8% vs. 90.5%, $P =$ N.S.).[488] A meta-analysis showed that vonoprazan and conventional PPI-based therapies are equally effective in eradicating clarithromycin-susceptible *H. pylori* strains (95.4% vs. 92.8%, $P = .23$), and that vonoprazan-based triple therapy was significantly superior to PPI-based therapy in treating patients infected with clarithromycin-resistant *H. pylori* strains (82.0% vs. 40.0%, $P < .01$).[489] According to real-world data from Japan, vonoprazan was an independent factor for successful eradication in not only first-line but also second-line eradication.[490] Ono et al. showed that a clarithromycin-metronidazole-vonoprazan regimen had greater efficacy than clarithromycin-metronidazole-PPI regimen for penicillin allergy patients (92.9% vs. 54.6%, $P < .01$).[491]

P-CAB and Low-Dose Aspirin (LDA) or Nonsteroidal Antiinflammatory Drug (NSAID)-Associated Peptic Ulcers

Recently, vonoprazan was reported to have equivalent efficacy to lansoprazole in preventing LDA-associated ulcer recurrence (Farrington and Manning test: margin 8.7%, significance level 2.5%). At the same time, peptic ulcer recurrence rates were significantly lower with vonoprazan 10 mg than with lansoprazole 15 mg, as shown by the results of the *post-hoc* analyses of the extension study (log-rank test, $P = .039$).[492] The 24-week peptic ulcer recurrence rate was 2.8% and 0.5% in the lansoprazole (15 mg) and vonoprazan (10 mg) groups, respectively. With regard to NSAID-associated peptic ulcers, vonoprazan had superior efficacy.[493] The proportion of patients with endoscopically-confirmed recurrent NSAID-associated peptic ulcers within 24 weeks was 3.3%, 3.4%, and 5.5% for vonoprazan (10 and 20 mg) and lansoprazole (15 mg), respectively.[493]

Safety Considerations

P-CABS, in particular vonoprazan, due to their potent antisecretory effect, may also be subject to safety issues as discussed in the prior section for PPIs, in particular due to the hypergastrinemia that occurs as a consequence of the lack of feedback inhibition of G-cell mediated gastrin release due to potent inhibition of acid secretion. Longstanding hypergastrinemia and hypochlorhydria can cause in ECL hyperplasia, SIBO, and alteration of the composition of the gut microbiome. Although meta-analyses of clinical trials suggest that P-CABs are either noninferior or superior to PPIs in the treatment of acid-peptic disorders (as discussed above) with a similar safety profile,[494] there are few reports of large-scale real-world experience with these drugs that would provide a fairer comparison with PPIs and H2RAs. Vonoprazan, unlike PPIs, inhibits the renal H^+,K^+-ATPase in the medullary collecting ducts, though the significance of this finding is unknown.

Conclusions

The P-CABs are a promising class of antisecretory drugs that potently suppress gastric acid secretion. Since they have been used almost exclusively in patient populations in East Asia, it is difficult to generalize these data to the rest of the world. Nevertheless, they show promise, in particular where rapid and near complete acid suppression is beneficial, such as with high-grade erosive esophagitis and with Hp eradication, especially in the face of antibiotic resistance. Further studies, especially in populations outside of East Asia, and for indications, such as ulcer hemorrhage, postendoscopic surgery, Barrett's esophagus, eosinophilic esophagus, ZES, idiopathic pulmonary fibrosis, and acid-peptic-mediated mucosal damage resistant to therapy with PPIs, in addition to the aforementioned indications, are needed before definitive therapeutic recommendations can be made.

NONACID GASTRIC SECRETIONS

Pepsinogen

Pepsinogens, which belong to a family of enzymes called *gastric aspartic proteases*, are inactive polypeptide proenzymes known as *zymogens*. They are synthesized primarily in chief cells but also in mucous neck cells. Pepsinogens are converted in the gastric lumen by gastric acid to pepsins, which contain two active-site aspartate residues. Once this reaction begins, pepsins can autocatalyze the conversion of pepsinogens to pepsins.[271] Pepsins are optimally active at pH 1.8–3.5, reversibly inactivated at pH 5, and irreversibly denatured at pH 7. Gastric acid not only provides an optimum pH for peptic activity but also itself denatures dietary protein, making it more susceptible to peptic hydrolysis. Thus acid and pepsin work in concert to promote digestion of dietary protein. As discussed, partially digested protein stimulates gastrin and thus acid secretion.[272] More recent data suggest that pepsins may also be important for killing ingested bacteria.[17,273]

Pepsinogens have been separated into seven isozymogens. The five fractions (pepsinogen 1 to pepsinogen 5) that electrophoretically migrate toward the anode most rapidly at pH 5 are similar immunologically and referred to as *group I pepsinogens* (PG I; old term, "pepsinogen A").[274] PG I is expressed in chief and mucous cells of the oxyntic mucosa. Migrating slightly behind the PG I are 2 immunologically similar isozymogens, pepsinogen 6 and pepsinogen 7, that are referred to as *group II pepsinogens* (PG II; old term, "pepsinogen C"). PG II, which represents approximately 20% of total pepsin content, is expressed in oxyntic and pyloric mucosa as well as in duodenal Brunner glands.

The most important physiologic stimulant for pepsinogen secretion is ACh released from cholinergic enteric neurons. ACh, acting via M_1 and M_3 muscarinic receptors on chief cells, increases cytosolic calcium concentrations.[275] Calcium, in turn, activates cytosolic kinases, phosphatases, and NO synthase that induce pepsinogen secretion.[276] Other agents capable of stimulating pepsinogen secretion from chief cells via the calcium signaling pathway include CCK, gastrin, and GRP.[277–280] Agents that increase cAMP within chief cells, such as isoproterenol, secretin, VIP, and histamine, also augment pepsinogen secretion, as do agents that activate tyrosine kinase, such as EGF and TGF-α.[279] Moreover, stomach distention increases pepsinogen secretion through a cholinergic pathway coupled with NO secretion into the gastric lumen.[281] Inhibitors of pepsinogen secretion include somatostatin, neuropeptide Y, PYY, and IL-1β. Thus eradication of Hp, a bacterium that promotes a host inflammatory response with production of IL-1β, can restore pepsinogen secretion.[282] Optimal pepsinogen secretion also requires a functional sodium-2 chloride-potassium cotransporter (NKCCl).[157]

Serum concentrations of PG I correlate with MAO; serum pepsinogens are increasingly being used to noninvasively diagnose gastric atrophy (see Chapter 54).[283,284] A linear correlation exists between the loss of chief cells in patients with oxyntic atrophy and serum PG I.[285,286] Thus a serum PG I less than 30 μg/L or a serum PG I/PG II ratio of 3.0 or less has been used as noninvasive tests to detect oxyntic atrophy.[287,288] Because hypergastrinemia is a physiologic response to achlorhydria, a fasting serum gastrin concentration more than 400 pg/mL may also suggest the presence of gastric atrophy. Serum PG I, PG II, PG I/PG II, and gastrin measurements in a large Japanese population were analyzed using receiver operating curve analysis to show that the diagnostic accuracy is further increased by stratifying into Hp positive and negative status.[289] Therefore PG I, PG II, their ratio, and fasting gastrin have been used as serological markers to assess atrophy.[285–288]

Serum PG I is increased in humans treated with PPIs, and serum PG II is increased in patients infected with Hp.[290–292] PG I and PG II are both filtered and metabolized by the kidney, but serum PG I concentration is increased more than PG II concentration in patients with renal insufficiency.[293,294] Furthermore, differences may exist between Western and Asian populations with regard to PG I and PG II concentrations in relation to acid secretion.

Because PGs are secreted by the stomach, their presence in nongastric tissues can signify pathology. For example, the presence of pepsin in the esophagus can indicate the presence of GERD; its presence in the airway may signify laryngopharyngeal reflux. Some data support the uptake of pepsin by epithelial cells in the aerodigestive tract, with possible involvement in carcinogenesis.[295]

Gastric Lipase

Gastric lipase, secreted by chief cells of the oxyntic mucosa, facilitates the digestion of dietary TGs by hydrolyzing them to free fatty acids, diglycerides, and 2-monoglycerides. The properties of gastric lipase are quite distinct from those of pancreatic lipase. Gastric lipase has a pH optimum of 4.5–5.5 (compared with 6.5–7.4 for pancreatic lipase) and does not require colipase. Furthermore, protection from peptic proteolysis by an *N*-glycosylated asparagine at residue 308 permits gastric lipase to retain its activity in acidic gastric juice (pH 2) despite high gastric juice peptic activity.[296,297]

Stimulants and inhibitors of gastric lipase are similar to those for pepsinogen secretion. Aging has been reported to decrease gastric lipase secretion, although data are controversial.[298] In humans, increasing the lipid content of the diet causes a corresponding increase in gastric lipase secretion.[299] The amount of gastric lipase secreted after a meal is small compared to that of pancreatic lipase. Nevertheless, the specific activity of gastric lipase is equal to or greater than that of pancreatic lipase. Thus gastric lipase is capable of digesting 10%–25% of dietary TG.[300] In patients with exocrine pancreatic insufficiency, gastric lipase secretion is increased three- to fourfold and can partly, but incompletely, compensate for loss of pancreatic lipase (Fig. 53.23).[301] A feedback mechanism exists whereby fat in the small intestine inhibits gastric lipase secretion by a hormonal pathway, with GLP-1 the prime candidate as mediator.[302]

Intrinsic Factor

IF a 50-kd glycoprotein secreted by human parietal cells and, to a lesser degree, chief cells, is necessary for the optimal absorption of cobalamin (vitamin B_{12}).[303]

Although all stimulants (e.g., gastrin, histamine, and ACh) and inhibitors (e.g., somatostatin) of gastric acid secretion discussed previously have similar effects on IF secretion, secretion of IF is not specifically coupled to acid secretion. PPIs, for example, inhibit acid secretion but have no significant effect on basal or stimulated IF secretion.[304] Several reports indicate, however, that chronic use of PPIs may decrease serum cobalamin concentrations, probably as a result of impaired acid-facilitated peptic release of cobalamin from food proteins.[305,306] The recommended daily allowance of cobalamin is only 2 μg/day; total body stores are around 2500 μg. Cobalamin deficiency due to antisecretory therapy is therefore rare, owing to incomplete acid suppression by PPIs combined with high overall body stores.[12,307,308]

The delivery of cobalamin from food to tissues begins with the release of cobalamin from dietary protein by the pH-dependent activity of pepsin, followed by the binding of cobalamin to 2 binding proteins that are secreted into gastric juice: IF and haptocorrin (R binder).[309,310] Haptocorrin, also secreted in saliva and bile, binds cobalamin more avidly than IF in the acidic gastric lumen, and therefore most cobalamin initially binds to haptocorrin. In the duodenum, cobalamin is released from haptocorrin by pancreatic trypsin, and the free cobalamin then binds to IF. IF-cobalamin complexes are resistant to pancreatic proteolysis and eventually bind to a specific receptor on the distal ileal mucosa. This receptor, cubilin, is expressed in clefts between microvilli and mediates endocytosis of the IF-cobalamin complex.[311] Once within the ileal enterocyte, IF is degraded by lysosomal enzymes, and cobalamin binds to transcobalamin. The cobalamin-transcobalamin complex is released into the circulation and enters cells by receptor-mediated endocytosis. Once within cells, cobalamin is dissociated from its transport protein and converted to its active forms, methylcobalamin and 5-deoxyadenosyl cobalamin. The active forms serve as coenzymes for methionine synthase and methylmalonyl–coenzyme A mutase, enzymes involved in methylation of homocysteine to methionine and the catabolism of branched-chain amino acids and odd-chain fatty acids in mitochondria, respectively.[312]

When radiolabeled cobalamin is administered orally after a large dose of nonradioactive cobalamin is given parenterally, patients with IF deficiency excrete much lower amounts of radioactive cobalamin in a 24-hour urine collection than do normal controls (Schilling test, part I). If IF is administered orally together with radioactive cobalamin to IF-deficient patients, urinary radioactive cobalamin excretion normalizes (Schilling test, part II). In addition to lack of IF, cobalamin deficiency may result from achlorhydria or hypochlorhydria (reduced peptic hydrolysis of cobalamin from food protein), bacterial overgrowth (cobalamin competed for by bacteria), pancreatic insufficiency (impaired tryptic cleavage of haptocorrin-cobalamin complex), ileal receptor defect (cubilin mutation), and ileitis or ileal resection (absent IF-cobalamin absorptive site).[313–315]

Secretion of IF far exceeds the amount necessary for cobalamin absorption. Thus in most patients with hypochlorhydria, continued IF secretion in low amounts is sufficient to prevent cobalamin deficiency. Patients with PA do develop cobalamin deficiency. PA affects 2% of individuals older than the age of 60.[316] The pathology of autoimmune metaplastic atrophic gastritis (see Chapter 54) involves a chronic inflammatory, mainly lymphocytic, infiltrate of the oxyntic mucosa accompanied by loss of parietal and chief cells. The pathogenesis involves proinflammatory Th1 $CD4^+$ T lymphocytes directed toward the α- and β-subunits of the parietal cell H^+,K^+-ATPase, accompanied by circulating autoantibodies directed against H^+,K^+-ATPase or IF.[317–321] Chronic infection with Hp may substantially contribute to the immunologic response in some patients. Hp-induced inflammation may decrease tolerance for self-antigens such as H^+,K^+-ATPase in genetically susceptible individuals, or those antibodies are acquired due to molecular mimicry between Hp lipopolysaccharide and H^+,K^+-ATPase, both of which contain Lewis epitopes.[228,230,322] Antibodies directed against H^+,K^+-ATPase are present in 90% of patients with PA, although their prevalence may decrease to approximately 55%–80% with progression of autoimmune gastritis, presumably because of the disappearance of Hp and the loss of antigenic drive.[317–322] Genetic factors, such as a Glu → Arg (Q5R) mutation in the IF gene, may also predispose individuals to PA.[323]

Treatment of cobalamin deficiency due to chronic atrophic gastritis is with B_{12}, either as a monthly injection of 1 mg or high daily oral doses of 1–2 mg. High oral doses are effective because a small amount of cobalamin can be passively absorbed without the requirement for IF.[1,324]

Bicarbonate

Regulation of gastric bicarbonate (HCO_3^-) secretion has been studied much less intensively than has duodenal HCO_3^- secretion.

The precise function of gastric HCO_3^- secretion is uncertain given the overwhelming simultaneous secretion of H^+. Nevertheless, HCO_3^- secretion has been implicated in the formation of a protective preepithelial alkaline layer (see Fig. 53.2).

Measurement of gastric HCO_3- secretion has been impeded by the presence of considerable H^+ secretion, necessitating the use of potent antisecretory compounds to eliminate as much acid as possible[325] or by using measurement methods unaffected by the presence of acid. One means of measuring bulk HCO_3- secretion is with the use of inline pH and CO_2 electrodes, in which HCO_3^- concentration is calculated using the Henderson-Hasselbalch equation.[326,327]

Gastric HCO_3^- secretion is an energy-dependent process. The finding that there is virtually no change in gastric electrical potential difference during HCO_3^- secretion suggests that HCO_3^- transport takes place via an electroneutral ion exchange mechanism, probably an exchange of HCO_3^- for Cl^-.[328] Although several candidate anion exchangers, solute carriers, and anion transporters have been localized to gastric cells, including AE2, AE4, SLC4A2, SLC4A4, SLC26A6, SLC26A9, and PAT1, there is little evidence that gastric surface cells actually secrete HCO_3^-.[329–335] The precise cell responsible for HCO_3^- secretion is not known, but the source of some of the HCO_3^- secreted during H^+ secretion may actually be the parietal cell. As discussed previously, for each H^+ secreted, a HCO_3^- ion exits the parietal cell across the basolateral membrane via the anion exchanger, SLC4A2 (see Fig. 53.13).[153] This HCO_3^- may alkalinize the blood that perfuses surface epithelial cells, be taken up by sodium bicarbonate cotransporters (NBC1 and NBC2), and then be secreted by epithelial cells in an effort to protect them from luminal acid.[333] The parietal cell may not be the only source of HCO_3^- for surface cells, however, because marked inhibition of gastric H^+ secretion by PPIs does not significantly diminish gastric HCO_3^- secretion in patients with duodenal ulcer.[334]

PG E_2 analogs stimulate gastric HCO_3^- secretion,[335,336] and blockade of endogenous PG synthesis reduces gastric HCO_3^- secretion.[337] In mice and rats, the PG E receptor subtype involved in stimulation of gastric HCO_3^- secretion is EP1.[338–340] PG-stimulated HCO_3^- secretion in response to focal epithelial damage apparently is dependent upon the anion transporter SLC26A9, because it is abolished in SLC26A9 knockout mice.[341] Gastric mucosal PG synthesis and HCO_3^- secretion decline in older adults.[342–344] More recently, the gaseous mediators NO and hydrogen sulfide along with PGs and capsaicin-sensitive afferent nerves have been implicated in the regulation of gastric HCO_3^- secretion.[345,346]

Mucus

A firmly adherent viscous mucus gel overlies the gastric surface. It is composed of 95% water and 5% extensively cross-linked mucin glycoproteins that are products of MUC genes.[347,348] Ultrastructural studies reveal alternating layers of two distinct mucin classes, MUC5AC (secreted by surface and pit area epithelial cells) and MUC6 (secreted from neck and gland cells). Observations that the gastroprotective compound geranylgeranylacetone increases MUC6 expression in rat gastric mucosa[349] and the gastroprotective compounds lafutidine and rebamipide increase mucus thickness and mucin content in humans[350,351] suggest that the mucus gel may contribute to mucosal defense. Furthermore, Hp inhibits MUC1 secretion and accumulates within and disrupts the MUC5AC-enriched gel layer.[352,353] MUC5AC secretion is increased in first-degree relatives of subjects with gastric cancer infected with Hp, suggesting that mucus secretion may be a marker for a more severe inflammatory response to the organism.[354]

Mucus gel thickness is dynamic (Fig. 53.24). It can be measured continuously and noninvasively in living rodents either

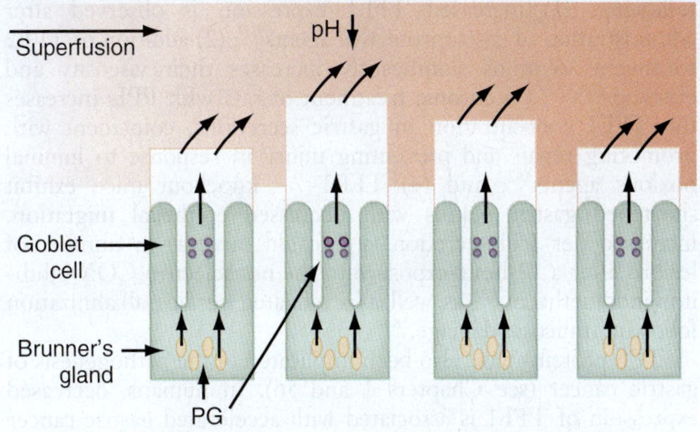

Fig. 53.24 Dynamic regulation of duodenal mucus gel thickness in response to luminal acid. In the *left panel*, alkaline mucus secretion and the rate of sloughing into the lumen are balanced. Luminal acid creates a sudden exocytotic burst of mucus secretion from goblet cells and Brunner glands, which thickens the gel (*2nd panel*). The newly secreted mucus sloughs into the lumen at a higher rate, resulting in a new steady-state gel thickness (*3rd and 4th panels*).[397] (Adapted from Kaunitz JD, Akiba Y. Luminal acid elicits a protective duodenal mucosal response. *Keio J Med*. 2002;51:29–35.)

by alternately focusing between fluorescently labeled surface epithelial cells and the mucus gel surface, as delineated by carbon particles or by fluorescent microspheres, or by measuring the vertical travel of micropipettes between the luminal mucus surface and epithelial cell surface.[355–358]

A pH gradient at the gastric mucosal surface has been observed in a variety of species, including humans.[356] In most cases, the gradient is relatively alkaline at the tissue surface and gradually more acidic at distances further from the surface. The gradient is dependent on active epithelial bicarbonate secretion.[359] Although most measurements using microelectrodes have reported pH values near neutrality at the gastric mucosal surface, more recent measurements using pH-sensitive fluorescent dyes coupled with ex vivo confocal microscopy report a surface pH near pH 4 in guinea pigs and frogs.[360,361] The observation that the steady-state surface pH gradient extends beyond the thickness of the mucus gel layer suggests that the unstirred layer formed at the interface between the mucus and the aqueous lumen or the interface between the epithelial surface and the luminal contents may also enhance mucosal defense by restricting convective mixing within the unstirred layer.[356] Little data support the hypothesis that the overlying mucus is a significant diffusion barrier to protons.[362–365] Physical study of the gastric mucus layer with fluorescent beads revealed that gastric mucus has a firmly adherent inner layer, in contrast to intestinal mucus.[366] Proteomic analysis of the mucin core proteins has confirmed that gastric mucus is primarily composed of the gene product of MUC5AC, with marked differences of *O*-glycan patterns between mucins of the gastric mucosa and mucins secreted by other segments of the GI tract.[367,368]

Trefoil factor (TFF) peptides are cosecreted with mucins.[369] These are 7–12-kd peptides sharing a common structure of 3 internal disulfide bonds that yield the signature "trefoil" structure of 3 internal loops and are designated TFF1, TFF2, and TFF3. TFFs are pepsin resistant and able to survive intact in the gastric lumen.[370] TFF1 is stored in gastric pit and surface mucous cells, TFF2 in gastric gland mucous cells, and TFF3 in intestinal goblet cells.[371–375] The concentration of TFF2 in rat gastric mucus is approximately 10 μM.[371,376]

The localization and coordinated secretion of trefoil peptides with mucins suggest that they too may be involved in mucosal defense.[373,377,378] Evidence to support this notion includes the following: (1) increased TFF1 expression is observed after administration of gastroprotective agents[379]; (2) addition of TFF2 to mucin solutions significantly increases their viscosity and elasticity[380,381]; (3) chronic treatment of rats with PPIs increases the TFF2 concentration in gastric secretions, coincident with promoting repair and preventing injury in response to luminal noxious agents[382]; and (4) TFF2−/− knockout mice exhibit shortened gastric glands with decreased epithelial migration, increased net acid secretion, a fourfold increase in number of lesions after a 12 hour-exposure to the nonselective COX inhibitor indomethacin,[383] as well as attenuated surface alkalinization following mucosal damage.[384]

TFF proteins have also been implicated in the pathogenesis of gastric cancer (see Chapters 1 and 56). In humans, decreased expression of TFF1 is associated with accelerated gastric cancer progression and poor survival.[385] In mice, knockout of TFF1 increased susceptibility to premalignant and malignant gastric lesions.[386] The effect of Hp infection on TFF expression is uncertain, with 1 report showing increased and another decreased expression of TFF2.[387,388]

The clinical significance of the different mucin types has also been studied in subjects with constipation, in which decreased gastric mucus secretion rate and viscosity were reported.[389]

Gastric Cancer Biomarkers

The advent of newer technologies such as reverse transcriptase polymerase chain reaction-based measurement of noncoding RNAs such as microRNAs (miRs) and long-noncoding RNAs (lncRNAs) in combination with mass and infrared spectroscopy, gas chromatography, and other analytical methods has opened up a new field of gastric analysis, where minute amounts of substances can be quantified and used diagnostically in clinical diagnosis or as biomarkers.

Studies have been published describing the test characteristics of lncRNAs, miRs, and tryptophan metabolites in the diagnosis of gastric cancer.[390–394] These studies were performed using small samples of gastric juice collected during a diagnostic endoscopy. The expression level among lncRNA in plasma, tumor tissue, and gastric juice correlated well, as did the alteration of gastric juice lncRNA expression with tumor stage. In one study, in vitro studies were used to test the hypothesis that lncRNA-RMRP (RNA component of mitochondrial RNA processing endonuclease) acted as a "sponge" for miR-206, an miR involved in cyclin-mediated cellular proliferation.[393] Alteration of tryptophan metabolites was reported in a study of gastric juice obtained endoscopically from gastric cancer and gastritis patients. The authors attributed the observed alterations to upregulation of the kynurenine pathway, speculating that metabolic alterations of this nature may form the basis for biomarker identification.[391] Because PG expression is associated with gastric cancer, the PG I/II in gastric juice combined with gastric juice concentrations of melanoma-associated gene[395] has high specificity and sensitivity for gastric cancer detection.[396]

Full references for this chapter can be found at https://ebooks.health.elsevier.com.

54 Gastritis and Gastropathy

Sameer Al Diffalha, Colin W. Howden

IN THIS CHAPTER

DEFINITIONS

Patients, clinicians, endoscopists, and pathologists often define gastritis differently. Some define it as a symptom complex, others as an abnormal endoscopic appearance of the stomach, and still others use the term to connote microscopic inflammation of the stomach, usually its mucosa. This last definition of gastritis is preferred and is used in this chapter. Other noninflammatory conditions of the stomach are referred to as gastropathies.

There is a weak relationship between histologic gastritis and symptoms. In fact, many patients with gastritis are asymptomatic. The relationship between microscopic and gastroscopic abnormalities is also imprecise. In a study of 400 patients, histologic gastritis was present despite a normal gastroscopic examination in 14%; another 20% had an abnormal gastroscopic examination without gastritis.[1] The latter patients (abnormal gastroscopy without gastritis) often have reactive gastropathy (discussed later).

Gastric biopsies must be obtained to diagnose gastritis. Gastroscopic biopsies should be obtained when EGD is performed in patients with dyspepsia.[2] They should also be obtained when EGD identifies gastric erosion(s) or ulcer(s), thick gastric fold(s), gastric polyp(s) or mass(es), and for the diagnosis of *Helicobacter pylori* (*H. pylori*) infection (discussed later). Two biopsies should be taken from the antrum (lesser and greater curvatures), one from the incisura angularis,[3] and two more from the gastric body (lesser and greater curvatures). The density of *H. pylori* can vary at different sites, possibly leading to sampling error, and the sensitivity of histology may decrease in patients taking a proton pump inhibitor (PPI). The updated Sydney system recommends taking five biopsy specimens from different sites. However, if this is not possible, the greater curvature of the gastric body could be a better site to detect current *H. pylori* infection, especially in the presence of peptic ulcer bleeding, atrophic gastritis, and intestinal metaplasia (IM) or gastric cancer. In the presence of peptic ulcer bleeding, histology is also the most reliable test. PPI treatment can reduce the sensitivity of histology; ideally, that PPI should have been stopped 2 weeks before testing. The biopsy samples from different areas should be placed in separate containers, and the locations of biopsy sites should be identified for the pathologist on the accompanying form. Every biopsy represents an excellent opportunity for the clinician and pathologist to communicate to correlate clinical data, endoscopic findings, and histopathology. Errors may occur when the pathologist attempts to interpret biopsies without clinical input.

The Sydney classification system attempted to unify terminology for endoscopic and histologic gastritis and gastropathy.[4] However, the complexity of the Sydney system and the frequent failure of endoscopists to obtain adequate numbers of biopsies have precluded its widespread use outside of clinical research studies. This chapter provides an etiology-based classification of gastritis and gastropathies.

ACUTE GASTRITIS

Acute gastritis, characterized by dense infiltration of the stomach with neutrophilic leukocytes, is rare. This rarity is in distinction to the much more common chronic active gastritis, where neutrophils can be present along with chronic inflammatory cells (lymphocytes, plasma cells), as in *H. pylori*–related gastritis (see later). Most forms of acute neutrophilic gastritis are due to infections with invasive organisms.

Phlegmonous (suppurative) gastritis is an infection of the gastric submucosa and muscularis propria, often sparing the mucosa.[5–20] Many types of invasive microorganisms have been identified, including Gram-negative bacilli, anaerobes, Gram-positive cocci, including group A streptococci, and fungi (e.g., mucormycosis; see later). The gastric phlegmon may simulate a mass. The esophagus may also be involved or even be the apparent source of the infection. Infection may spread to the adjacent liver and spleen with abscess formation. Acute phlegmonous/necrotizing gastritis has been associated with a variety of conditions, including recent large intake of alcohol, respiratory tract infection, and AIDS and other immunocompromised states, including liver transplantation.

An especially severe form of phlegmonous gastritis is *emphysematous gastritis*, due to gastric infections with gas-producing organisms, such as *Clostridium perfringens*. In this condition, gas is often present in the wall of the stomach and in the portal venous system (Fig. 54.1). Imaging studies (plain films, CT) show gas bubbles conforming to the contour of the stomach, often in the form of cystic gas pockets. Although full recovery from phlegmonous or emphysematous gastritis may occur, the condition may progress to gastric (and esophageal) gas gangrene and death. Risk factors for emphysematous gastritis include recent gastroduodenal surgery, ingestion of corrosive materials, gastroenteritis, or GI infarction.

Patients with phlegmonous or emphysematous gastritis are typically very ill with sepsis and are likely to present with acute upper abdominal pain, fever, hypotension, peritonitis, and purulent ascitic fluid. Preoperative diagnosis is possible with abdominal x-ray, US, or CT. Gastroscopy with or without biopsy and culture of gastric contents may establish the diagnosis.

Grossly, the stomach wall appears thick and edematous with multiple perforations, and the mucosa may demonstrate a granular, green-black exudate. Microscopically, the edematous submucosa reveals an intense polymorphonuclear infiltrate and numerous Gram-positive and/or Gram-negative bacteria, as well as vascular thrombosis. The mucosa may demonstrate extensive areas of necrosis.

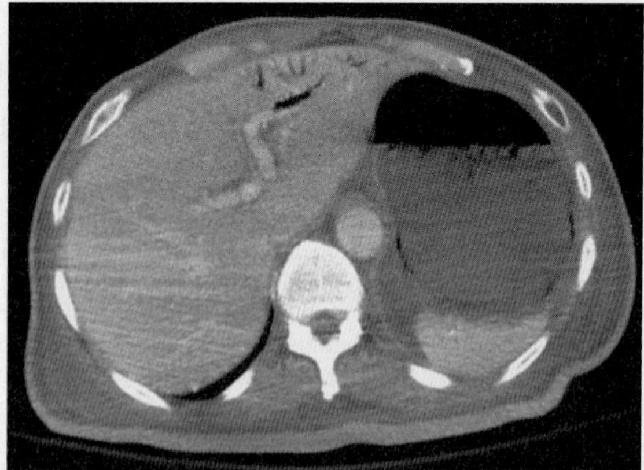

Fig. 54.1 CT of emphysematous gastritis. Abdominal CT image in a 67-year-old male diabetic with coronary artery disease and prior stroke who was admitted from his nursing home with sudden onset of nausea, vomiting, and abdominal pain. Physical examination showed diffuse tenderness throughout the abdomen. CT shows curvilinear air in the posterior wall of the fluid-filled stomach, as well as portal venous gas. He was treated successfully with broad-spectrum antibiotics, with resolution of the emphysema documented on a repeat scan 2 weeks later. (Courtesy T. Ynosencio, MD, Baylor University Medical Center, Dallas, TX.)

The mortality rate of phlegmonous gastritis is ~70%, probably because it is so rare and difficult to diagnose and because treatment is initiated too late. The definitive treatment is either gastric resection or drainage combined initially with systemic broad-spectrum antibiotics directed against the most common organisms (*Escherichia coli* and other Gram-negative bacilli, anaerobic and group A streptococci, and *Staphylococcus aureus*). Vancomycin and piperacillin/tazobactam is one empiric regimen that has been used.

Paradoxically, acute phlegmonous gastritis can also be associated with both granulocytic leukemia and with neutropenia. Although not as common as neutropenic cecitis (typhlitis) or enterocolitis, neutropenic gastritis can be an isolated finding.

Other forms of acute gastritis are discussed later (see "Infectious Gastritis").

CHRONIC GASTRITIS

Chronic gastritis is much more common than acute gastritis, although it may be clinically silent. Its prevalence is declining in developed countries.[21] The major importance of chronic gastritis (including *H. pylori*–related gastritis) relates to the fact that it is a risk factor for peptic ulcer disease, gastric adenocarcinoma, and gastric mucosa-associated lymphoid tissue (MALT) lymphoma, discussed in detail in other chapters. Chronic gastritis unrelated to *H. pylori* infection is increasingly recognized; its cause is usually unknown. In a predominantly male U.S. veteran population, chronic *H. pylori*-negative gastritis was less common in African Americans than in other races and was associated with use of PPIs.[22]

Three types of chronic gastritis are recognized: diffuse antral gastritis that is usually due to *H. pylori* infection, environmental metaplastic atrophic gastritis (EMAG), and autoimmune metaplastic atrophic gastritis (AMAG; Figs. 54.2 and 54.3).

H. pylori-Related Gastritis

H. pylori is a Gram-negative helical- or spiral-shaped, flagellated bacterium. Infection typically causes diffuse antral gastritis (see Fig. 54.3A). *H. pylori*–related gastritis initially affects the superficial layers of the mucosa. In some instances, particularly in childhood, the infection is short-lived but more typically results in chronic active gastritis, which is essentially a lifelong condition if not treated. Chemokines induced by *H. pylori* infection lead to a persistent acute inflammatory infiltrate with neutrophils and other cells (active inflammation) coexisting with lymphocytes, plasma cells, and macrophages characteristic of chronic inflammation. Despite this robust host immune response, the bacteria persist in most people who are infected.[23] Host factors that result in clearance of *H. pylori* in some cases of acute infection remain largely unknown.[24,25]

One form of *H. pylori*–related gastritis is characterized by mucosal infiltration by plasma cells that contain Russell bodies (Russell body gastritis).[26,27] Another form that can be recognized endoscopically is nodular gastritis, which may resolve following eradication of infection.[28–30] Nodular gastritis/gastropathy, which is recognized endoscopically by its "chicken skin" appearance, can be seen in other conditions, including Crohn disease, syphilitic gastritis, lymphocytic (varioliform) gastritis, collagenous gastritis (all discussed later), and AA-amyloidosis.[31]

Epidemiology, Risk Factors, and Transmission

H. pylori infection is the most common chronic bacterial infection of humans. Over 50% of the world's population is infected with the bacterium, with prevalence rising to 70%–80% in developing nations. Genetic sequence analysis suggests that humans have

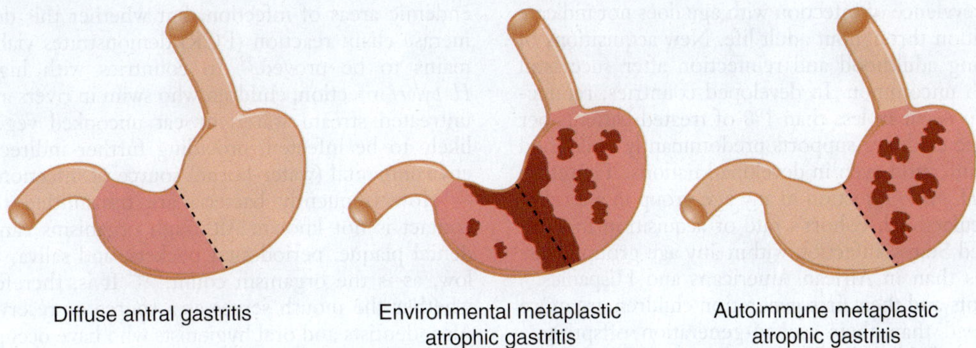

Fig. 54.2 Topographic patterns of chronic gastritis. The *darker areas* in the schematic of environmental metaplastic atrophic gastritis and autoimmune metaplastic atrophic gastritis represent areas of focal atrophy and intestinal metaplasia.

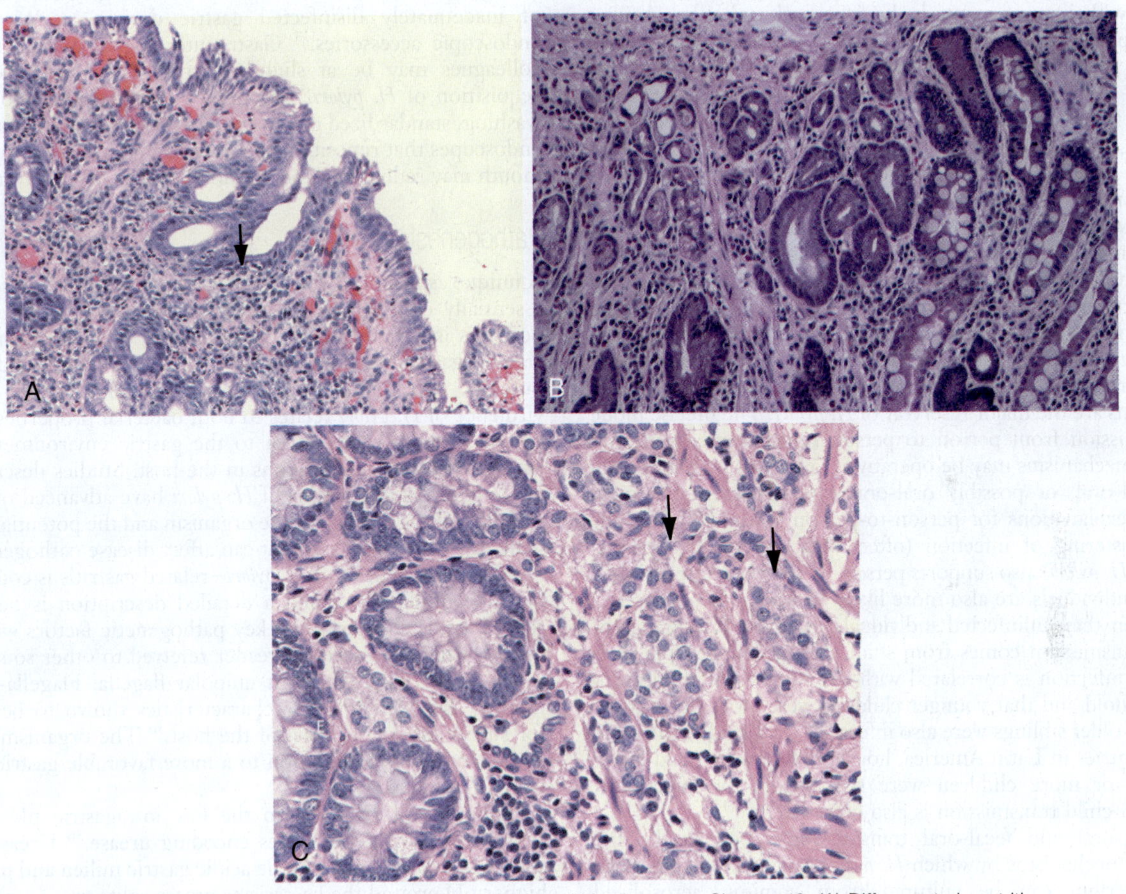

Fig. 54.3 Histopathology of chronic gastritis. For normal histology, see Chapter 49. (A) Diffuse antral gastritis. Chronic inflammation within the lamina propria and neutrophils infiltrating the gastric pit epithelium. This lesion is characteristic of Hp infection (H&E, ×400). (B) Environmental metaplastic atrophic gastritis. Note several glands lined by goblet cells (*arrow*) (H&E, ×200). (C) Autoimmune metaplastic atrophic gastritis, with goblet cell metaplasia and nests of enterochromaffin-like cells (*arrows*) (H&E, ×400).

been infected for more than 60,000 years, corresponding to the time when they first migrated from Africa.[32]

A key risk factor for infection is socioeconomic status during childhood. Infection is commonly acquired at an early age, particularly in developing countries where most children become infected before the age of 10.[33,34] During early childhood, spontaneous clearance of the infection is common, but often with subsequent reinfection. In older children and adults, infection usually persists so that its prevalence can exceed 80% by ages 20–30 in developing countries. Young children also acquire *H. pylori* in developed countries, including the United States. However, with spontaneous clearance, there is a lower chance of reinfection; consequently, persistent infection is less frequent.[34,35] In fact, serologic evidence of *H. pylori* infection is uncommon in children before age 10 but rises to 10% between 18 and 30 years of age and further increases to 50% in those aged 60 or older.[34]

This increasing prevalence of infection with age does not indicate continuing acquisition throughout adult life. New acquisitions of the infection during adulthood and reinfection after successful treatment are both uncommon. In developed countries, reinfection is estimated to occur in less than 1% of treated patients per year. Epidemiologic evidence supports predominantly childhood acquisition of the infection even in developed nations. Therefore the prevalence of *H. pylori* infection in any age group in a locality reflects that particular birth cohort's rate of acquisition in early life.[34] In the United States, infection within any age group is less common in whites than in African Americans and Hispanics.[36] Hispanic immigrants and their first-generation children are more likely to be infected than their second-generation offspring.[37] These differences probably relate to factors early in life that are linked to acquiring infection.

Housing density, crowded conditions in the home, number of siblings, bed sharing, and poor sanitation have all been linked to higher rates of infection.[34,38] In Japan, the declining prevalence of *H. pylori* infection has paralleled the nation's postwar economic progress with improvements in hygiene and sanitation. Among Japanese born before 1950, more than 70% are infected compared with 45% born between 1950 and 1960, and 25% born between 1960 and 1970.[39] Currently, childhood infection in Japan is uncommon. A similar declining prevalence is being observed in the United States, suggesting that infection-related illnesses, such as peptic ulcer, will decrease as current birth cohorts in developed countries reach older age.[40]

Twin studies support some degree of genetic susceptibility to *H. pylori* infection because monozygotic twins who were raised in different households have a greater concordance of infection than dizygotic twins raised separately.[41] However, twins growing up together have a higher concordance for the infection than twins growing up separately, suggesting that environmental factors are also important for childhood acquisition.

Humans are the major reservoir of *H. pylori*. The precise mode of transmission from person to person remains uncertain, and multiple mechanisms may be operative. Transmission *via* gastric-oral, fecal-oral, or possibly oral-oral exposure seem the most probable explanations for person-to-person spread.[33,42] Within-family clustering of infection (often with genetically identical strains of *H. pylori*) also supports person-to-person transmission.[34] Infected individuals are also more likely to have infected spouses or children than uninfected individuals. Support for sibling-to-sibling transmission comes from studies reporting that the likelihood of infection is correlated with the number of children in the household and that younger children were more likely to be infected if older siblings were also infected.[34] In a study conducted in six countries in Latin America, household crowding and living with four or more children were risk factors for infection.[18] Mother-to-child transmission is also quite likely.[35,43]

Gastric-oral and fecal-oral transmission appear to be the dominant mechanisms by which *H. pylori* gains access to its host. The bacterium can be cultured from vomitus, aerosolized vomitus, and diarrheal stools, suggesting the potential for transmission.[44] Organism loads are 100-fold higher in vomitus when compared with feces and saliva; organisms are also present in aerosolized vomitus for up to 1.2 m shortly after vomiting. Exposure to an infected family member during an acute GI illness, especially with vomiting, appears to be a risk factor for infection.[45] Natural transmission could occur through contact with infected vomitus during an acute illness[45] or with regurgitated material from an infected child. Such contact could explain the higher concordance of maternal/child infection and the presumed child-to-child transmission that occurs in infant daycare settings.[46]

Especially in developing countries, *H. pylori*–contaminated water might serve as an environmental source of infection, because the organism can remain viable in water for several days.[47] *H. pylori* DNA can be found in samples of municipal water from endemic areas of infection, but whether this detection by polymerase chain reaction (PCR) demonstrates viable organisms remains to be proved.[32] In countries with high prevalence of *H. pylori* infection, children who swim in rivers and streams, drink untreated stream water, or eat uncooked vegetables are more likely to be infected, providing further indirect evidence of an environmental (water-borne) source of infection.

How frequently bacteria are transmitted through oral-oral contact is not known. Although organisms can be identified in dental plaque, periodontal pockets, and saliva, the prevalence is low, as is the organism count.[48,49] It is, therefore, questionable whether the mouth serves as a source or reservoir for *H. pylori*. Also, dentists and oral hygienists who have occupational exposure to dental plaque, periodontal pockets, and oral secretions do not have increased prevalence of *H. pylori* infection.[28] In developed countries, oral-oral transmission of infection to spouses also appears to be uncommon.

Infected gastric juice may serve as a source of transmission.[50,51] Iatrogenic infection has also occurred during the use of a variety of inadequately disinfected gastric devices, endoscopes, and endoscopic accessories.[33] Gastroenterologists and their nursing colleagues may be at slightly increased risk for occupational acquisition of *H. pylori*.[52] Mandated universal precautions, hand washing, standardized disinfection of equipment, and use of video endoscopes that reposition the instrument channel away from the mouth may reduce such occupational and iatrogenic transmission.

Pathogenesis

A unique aspect of *H. pylori* is that it confers disease despite being essentially confined to the stomach. However, gastric infection per se is insufficient to fully explain the wide spectrum of associated gastroduodenal diseases. Pathogenicity and clinical outcome depend on both bacterial and host factors. Thus the virulence of *H. pylori* relates to both bacterial properties allowing colonization and adaptation to the gastric environment and to pathophysiological alterations in the host. Studies describing the genome of distinct strains of *H. pylori* have advanced our understanding of the ecology of the organism and the potential bacterial gene expression patterns that can affect disease pathogenesis.[53–55]

The pathogenesis of *H. pylori*–related gastritis is complex and not fully understood, and a detailed description is beyond the scope of this chapter. Only key pathogenetic factors will be discussed, with the interested reader referred to other sources.[56–78]

H. pylori has six to eight unipolar flagella. Flagella-mediated motility is one of the few characteristics shown to be required for successful colonization of the host.[56] The organism's flagella allow for its rapid migration to a more favorable gastric location below the mucus layer.

Exposure of *H. pylori* to the low intragastric pH increases expression of bacterial genes encoding urease.[56] Urease activity allows *H. pylori* to adapt to the acidic gastric milieu and produces a higher pH around the bacteria as urease splits urea into CO_2 and ammonia (NH_3), with the NH_3 reacting with H^+ to produce ammonium ions (NH_4^+).[57]

H. pylori shows strict tropism for gastric-type mucosa, including in extragastric regions of the GI tract (i.e., where there is gastric metaplasia). Conversely, *H. pylori* does not colonize gastric epithelium that has IM (see later), possibly because antimicrobial factors produced by host metaplastic epithelium select against colonization. This is supported by the finding that *H. pylori* only rarely colonizes deeper portions of the gastric glandular mucosa, where antimicrobial *O*-glycans are found.[58] Metaplasia may also be associated with hypochlorhydria/achlorhydria, encouraging overgrowth of the stomach with other bacteria.

Toll-like receptors (TLRs) are a family of pattern recognition receptors with specificity for various bacterial molecules.[44,64]

TLRs are components of the host's innate immune system.[45] Lipopolysaccharide from *H. pylori* stimulates gastric epithelial cell and monocyte responses via TLR4 and TLR2.2.[65–67,79]

A key interaction between *H. pylori* and the gastric epithelium is mediated by a segment of bacterial DNA referred to as the cag (cytotoxin-associated gene) pathogenicity island (cag PAI). Genes within the cag PAI encode for a Type 4 secretion apparatus, cagE that allows other bacterial macromolecules, such as cagA to be delivered directly into the host cell.[54,68] The cag PAI plays an important role in the pathogenesis of chronic *H. pylori*–related gastritis.[54,69] *H. pylori* strains bearing the cag PAI are associated with increased interleukin (IL)-8 expression, mucosal inflammation, peptic ulceration, and apoptosis compared with cag PAI-negative strains.[70,71] Mongolian gerbils infected with mutated *H. pylori* strains that lack cagE exhibit less severe gastritis, fewer peptic ulcers, less IM, and less gastric cancer than gerbils infected with the wild-type strain.[72] Different cagA proteins from distinct geographic populations of *H. pylori* appear to be tyrosine phosphorylated by host cells in different manners, resulting in variable effects on intracellular signaling.[80–87] Such heterogeneity in cagA may lead to different host responses that could account for some of the geographic differences seen in *H. pylori*–associated disease. Although tyrosine phosphorylation of the cagA protein may be important, it is not the only mechanism whereby this molecule regulates the host response.[88,89]

All strains of *H. pylori* possess the *vacA* gene, and more than half of strains produce the vacuolating cytotoxin (VacA) that it encodes.[54,74] VacA attaches to host epithelial cells *via* an interaction with cellular protein-tyrosine phosphatases.[73] Thus mice deficient in a protein-tyrosine phosphatase do not develop gastric ulceration when exposed to *H. pylori* that secretes VacA.[75] Different *vacA* alleles have been detected in the five signal region (s-region) and in the middle region (m-region) of the *vacA* gene.[76] The s-region is present as allele s1 (which can be further distinguished as s1a, s1b, s1c) or as allele s2, whereas the m-region is present as allele m1 or m2. Production of VacA is designated by the allelic combinations (e.g., s1/m1, s1/m2, s2/m1, s2/m2). Specific vacA alleles (s1 and m1) are associated with peptic ulceration[76] and the induction of host epithelial cell apoptosis.[77]

Other bacterial virulence factors have also been associated with a putative increased risk of gastric adenocarcinoma. However, studies showing direct cancer causation for any of these bacterial factors in isolation have proved unfruitful. These findings support the notion that any bacterial or host factors that increase the host inflammatory response to infection may increase the risk of gastric cancer and that the degree of mucosal inflammation, cell injury, and gastric atrophy is the best determinant of cancer risk in an individual patient.[78]

Gastric epithelial cells play an integral part in the host response to *H. pylori* infection, in addition to being the target of infection. Epithelial cell responses to *H. pylori* include changes in their morphology,[90] disruption of their tight junctional complexes,[91] production of cytokines,[68] increased proliferation, enhanced cell death *via* apoptosis, and induction of numerous host genes associated with the cellular stress that accompanies infection.[24]

Expression of genes by epithelial cells infected with *H. pylori* is regulated by transcription factors, particularly nuclear factor-kappa B (NF-κB). As discussed in Chapter 2, NF-κB regulates expression of a wide variety of proinflammatory cytokines and cellular adhesion molecules in response to infection or the local cytokine milieu. Enhanced gastric epithelial cell NF-κB activity correlates with the intensity of neutrophil infiltration and mucosal IL-8 levels. [49,68] This pathway is of particular interest given that certain polymorphisms in the IL-8 gene[92] are linked to increased mucosal IL-8 expression, inflammation, and other premalignant changes associated with gastric cancer. *H. pylori* appears to activate NF-κB in gastric epithelial cell lines through various signaling mechanisms, including mitogen-activated protein kinases.[50,67,69,93] The mitogen-activated protein kinase cascades regulate a wide range of cell functions, including proliferation, inflammatory responses, and cell survival.[70,94–96]

Oxidative stress also regulates host gene expression during *H. pylori* infection.[97,98] Oxidation of host DNA by reactive oxygen species such as hydroxyl radicals (•OH) is thought to play a causal role in malignant transformation through the induction of DNA damage. For this reason, there is growing interest in the role of antioxidants in cancer prevention or treatment. *H. pylori* infection is associated with decreased levels of ascorbic acid, a tissue antioxidant scavenger. Moreover, there is evidence that diets high in antioxidants[99] or "nutraceuticals" of the isothiocyanate group, such as sulforaphane,[100] may antagonize oxidative stress and protect the host from gastric cancer, perhaps by decreasing inflammation and attenuating bacterial load. In vitro and in vivo studies in Mongolian gerbils show that an *N*-acetylcysteine, a precursor to the antioxidant compound glutathione, reduces *H. pylori*–related gastritis if administered soon after infection.[101] However, whether this compound would reduce carcinogenesis is uncertain.

Strains of *H. pylori* that express outer membrane inflammatory protein A (OipA) are associated with increased bacterial density, higher mucosal IL-8 levels,[102] and neutrophil infiltration, as well as more severe clinical consequences.[103]

Peptidoglycan (murein) from the cell wall of *H. pylori* can translocate into gastric epithelial cells *via* the cagE encoded by the cag PAI. Once inside the host cell, nucleotide-binding oligomerization domain-1 recognizes this murein, providing a novel mechanism of bacterial sensing.[104] Binding of murein to nucleotide-binding oligomerization domain-1 can lead to activation of NF-κB and the subsequent expression of various host genes encoding proinflammatory molecules, as discussed earlier.

H. pylori neutrophil-activating protein promotes neutrophil adhesion to endothelial cells and stimulates chemotaxis of neutrophils and monocytes, nicotinamide adenine dinucleotide phosphate hydrogen oxidase complex assembly at the plasma membrane, and the subsequent production of reactive oxygen intermediates.[88,105] Within the inflammatory environment present in *H. pylori*–related gastritis, the effects of *H. pylori* neutrophil-activating protein on neutrophils can be potentiated by TNF-α and interferon (IFN)-γ. After epithelial cells undergo apoptosis, phagocytes remove the dead cells. Engulfment of necrotic epithelial cells by phagocytes may be another important mechanism by which *H. pylori* can activate a host response.[2,24]

Recruitment and activation of neutrophils and macrophages cause the release of other inflammatory mediators. Increased expression of inducible nitric oxide synthase occurs in the gastric mucosa during *H. pylori* infection.[24] The nitric oxide (NO) produced reacts with superoxide anion (O_2^-) produced by infiltrating neutrophils to form peroxynitrite ($ONOO^-$), a potent oxidizing and nitrating agent. NO and $ONOO^-$ have antimicrobial effects, but uncontrolled or inappropriate production could also play a role in the gastric mucosal cell damage observed during infection. Furthermore, catabolism of urea by *H. pylori*'s urease produces NH_3 and CO_2, with the latter rapidly neutralizing the bactericidal activity of the peroxynitrite by reacting with it to form the intermediate $ONOOCO_2^-$ and then nitrate. Urease, thus, may favor *H. pylori* colonization by neutralizing some host cell responses, but this mechanism also enhances the nitration potential of $ONOO^-$ and may favor mutagenesis of host cell DNA.

Cytokines induced in macrophages by bacterial urease include TNF-α and IL-6,[91,106] and IL-6 is also induced by heat shock protein 60.[107] Cytokines secreted by epithelial cells complement those released by inflammatory cells in the lamina propria. Intact bacteria can induce the production of chemokines that recruit T cells,[93,108] as well as IL-12[94,95,109,110] and IL-18,[96,111] cytokines that favor the selection of Th1 cells, with their characteristic patterns of cytokine secretion. Th1 cells promote cell-mediated immune responses through the production of IFN-γ and TNF-α, whereas Th2 cells produce IL-4, IL-5, IL-10, and transforming growth factor-β (TGF-β). Th2 cells can promote mucosal IgA or IgE responses to helminths and other parasites, as well as diminish the inflammation caused by Th1 cytokines. Previous studies suggest that the *H. pylori*–infected gastric mucosa is preconditioned to favor Th1 development over Th2 cell development.[94,109]

Th1 cell activation by *H. pylori* infection may contribute to more severe inflammation and risk of gastroduodenal diseases. Increased levels of IL-17 (a cytokine produced by activated $CD4^+$ T lymphocytes) are found in the mucosa of infected patients.[112,113] IL-17, in turn, induces IL-8 expression by gastric epithelial cells, thereby enhancing neutrophil recruitment. Activation of transcription factors by IL-17 may also contribute to the increased levels of numerous other proinflammatory cytokines and enzymes observed during *H. pylori* infection, such as IL-1β, TNF-α, and COX-2. IFN-γ and TNF-α produced by Th1 cells can increase the expression of many genes in the epithelium, including IL-8. These cytokines also enhance bacterial binding[67] and may also increase bacterial load.[114] In animal models, Th1 cells increase epithelial cell apoptosis[39] as well as inflammation, glandular atrophy, and a tendency toward dysplasia.[115] TNF-α, IFN-γ, and IL-1β also upregulate gastric epithelial cell Fas antigen expression.[116] Because Th1 cells express higher levels of Fas ligand (FasL) than Th2 cells, the relative increase in Th1 cells during *H. pylori* infection may induce epithelial cell death through Fas-Fas ligand (FasL) interactions.[116,117] This notion is substantiated by the observation that H^+, K^+-ATPase-specific Th1 cells in the gastric mucosa kill target epithelial cells via Fas-FasL interactions and may act as effector cells in autoimmune gastritis (discussed later).[118]

IgA antibodies, normally produced in the GI tract (see Chapter 2), are highly adapted for mucosal protection, conferring protective immunity without activating the complement cascade and causing deleterious amounts of cell damage and inflammation. The number of IgA-producing plasma cells is increased in *H. pylori* infection. However, increased numbers of IgG- and IgM-producing plasma cells are also detected, along with activated complement. Monoclonal antibodies that recognize *H. pylori* can cross-react with human and murine gastric epithelial cells.[119,120] Transfer of these antibodies to recipient mice induces gastritis,[119] as does the transfer of B cells that recognize heat shock proteins from individuals with MALToma.[121]

With few exceptions, infection with *H. pylori* persists for the life of the host unless it is successfully treated. This observation has led to investigations as to whether immunologic tolerance impairs immunity. Several bacterial factors, including urease and catalase, thwart innate host responses to infection.[23] Furthermore, production of arginase by *H. pylori* inhibits NO production and may favor bacterial survival,[122] whereas virulent strains of *H. pylori* impair phagocytosis[123] and mucus production.[124] The VacA toxin can impair bacterial antigen presentation by macrophages through inhibition of the antigen presentation pathway.[125] Moreover, *H. pylori* produces molecules that mimic host molecules, such as Lewis antigens. Theoretically, these could stimulate T cells to release cytokines that help to avoid autoimmune reactions. However, as already discussed, the cytokine profile associated with *H. pylori* infection is not one that would be expected to occur in a tolerant environment. For example, IL-4, IL-10, and TGF-β (which could mediate an anti-inflammatory effect) are not expressed to the same levels as proinflammatory Th1 cytokines such as IFN-γ and TNF-α.[24] Because the infected gastric mucosa is characterized by chronic active inflammation, tolerance, if it has occurred, may favor persistent infection even though it cannot prevent the chronic inflammatory response.

Genetic heterogeneity in the regions of the host genome that controls the magnitude of inflammation is associated with gastric cancer development (see Chapter 54).[126] Polymorphisms in the regions controlling IL-1[127] are associated with an increased incidence of hypochlorhydria and gastric cancer in infected individuals and decrease duodenal ulcer recurrence.[128] Increased IL-1 expression may not only drive inflammation but may also lead to a physiologic change known to precede gastric cancer development because IL-1 potently inhibits gastric acid secretion (see Chapter 51). Other genes that regulate the magnitude of the inflammatory response to *H. pylori*, including IL-10, TNF-α, and IL-8, have also been associated with the sequence of events leading to cancer.[129,130]

BOX 54.1 Some Components of Hp That Are Involved in the Pathogenesis of Gastritis

Cag pathogenicity island (PAI), including cagA and CagE
Flagella
HP neutrophil-activating protein (HP-NAP)
Lipopolysaccharide
Outer inflammatory protein A (Oip A)
Peptidoglycan (murein)
Urease
Vacuolating toxin A (VacA)

Elevated fasting and meal-stimulated serum gastrin levels are well documented in individuals with *H. pylori* infection.[4] However, the net effect of *H. pylori* infection on gastric acid secretion in an infected individual depends on the duration and distribution of the infection and the presence or absence of atrophy of the oxyntic glandular mucosa (see Chapters 51 and 53). *H. pylori* infection also reduces gastric mucin secretion and mucosal hydrophobicity; these abnormalities can be reversed after eradication of infection. Epithelial barrier function is altered during *H. pylori* infection as a consequence of both direct effects of the infection and the accompanying inflammatory responses that collectively increase epithelial cell proliferation and programmed cell death.[24]

Bacterial factors involved in the pathogenesis of *H. pylori*–related gastritis in the host discussed earlier are summarized in Box 54.1. Environmental factors can have a moderating role in the *H. pylori*-host interactions. Such factors as smoking, a high salt diet, and various environmental mutagens can heavily influence both the degree and rate of progression of mucosal injury. In Japan, for example, the incidence of gastric cancer fell by 60% between 1965 and 1995 despite no change in the virulence of the most common strain of *H. pylori*. This dramatic drop has been attributed to societal changes such as refrigeration (as opposed to preservation with salt), Westernization of the diet, and smoking reduction.[78]

Diagnosis

Both endoscopic and nonendoscopic tests are available to diagnose *H. pylori* infection. Such techniques may detect *H. pylori* directly (gastric histology, stool bacterial antigen, culture) or indirectly (urease detection or antibody response).[131,132] The appropriate method to choose depends on the clinical situation, likely prevalence of infection in the population, the pretest probability of infection, local availability of testing methods, and cost. Recent use of antibiotics or PPIs can influence the results of certain tests.[133] The commonly used diagnostic tests and their advantages and disadvantages are summarized in Table 54.1.

Endoscopic tests. It is neither necessary nor appropriate to perform EGD and biopsy solely for the diagnosis of *H. pylori* infection. When EGD is clinically indicated, *H. pylori* infection

TABLE 54.1 Tests for Hp Infection

Endoscopic Tests	Advantages	Disadvantages
Biopsy urease	Rapid results Accurate in patients not using PPIs or antibiotics No added pathology cost	Requires endoscopy Less accurate after treatment or in patients using PPIs
Histology	Excellent sensitivity and specificity, especially with special immunostaining Provides additional information about gastric mucosa	Expensive (endoscopy and pathology costs) Some interobserver variability Accuracy affected by PPI and antibiotic use
Culture	Specificity ≈ 100% Allows antibiotic sensitivity testing	Difficult culture protocol Not widely available Expensive
Nonendoscopic Tests		
Serology (qualitative or quantitative IgG)	Widely available Inexpensive Good NPV	Poor PPV if Hp prevalence is low Not useful after treatment
Urea breath (^{13}C or ^{14}C)	Identifies active infection Accuracy (PPV, NPV) not affected by Hp prevalence Useful both before and after treatment	Availability and reimbursement inconsistent Accuracy affected by PPI and antibiotic use Small radiation dose with ^{14}C test
Stool antigen	Identifies active infection Accuracy (PPV, NPV) not affected by Hp prevalence Useful both before and after treatment	Fewer data available Accuracy affected by PPI and antibiotic use

can be diagnosed from gastric biopsy specimens by urease testing, histology, next-generation sequencing (NGS), or culture. The choice of method depends on the clinical situation, cost, availability, and test accuracy.[127] As discussed above, biopsies should be obtained from both the antrum and corpus.

Biopsy urease testing is efficient, relatively inexpensive, and generally accurate.[133,134] Gastric biopsy material is tested for urease activity by placing the specimen in a medium containing urea and a pH reagent such as phenolphthalein. Since the healthy human stomach is devoid of urease, any detectable urease activity in a gastric biopsy specimen can be assumed to be from *H. pylori*. Its urease hydrolyzes urea to produce NH_3 and CO_2. NH_3 production results in an increase in pH and a resultant color change of the phenolphthalein test medium.[131] Test results can be positive within minutes to hours. Several urease test kits are commercially available, differing only regarding medium (agar gel or membrane pad) and testing reagents.[131] Although these kits are generally inexpensive, there may be added costs associated with obtaining gastric tissue samples in Western centers (e.g., upcoding of a diagnostic endoscopy). Nevertheless, biopsy urease testing is less expensive than histology. Sensitivity and specificity of biopsy urease tests are 90%–95% and 95%–100%, respectively.[131,135] Accuracy can be negatively affected by blood in the stomach[136] or by use of antibiotics, bismuth-containing compounds, or PPIs.[137] Therefore a negative urease test does not exclude *H. pylori* infection in an individual taking a PPI. Unfortunately, this is a fairly common scenario in patients referred for EGD. Biopsy urease testing should be performed at least 2 weeks after stopping the PPI, and biopsy samples should be obtained from both the antrum and corpus. Histamine H_2-receptor antagonists in standard dose should not influence the sensitivity of the biopsy urease test. Therefore it is acceptable for patients previously on a PPI to use these agents in preparation for the biopsy urease test.

Gastric mucosal histology assessment is generally unnecessary to diagnose *H. pylori* infection, but it can provide information regarding the severity of mucosal inflammation (see Fig. 54.3A) and can also detect *H. pylori*–associated precancerous lesions such as metaplastic (chronic) atrophic gastritis (discussed later) and dysplasia.[131] Histologic examination had been considered the gold standard for identifying infection, with reported sensitivity and specificity as high as 95% and 98%, respectively.[138] However, the distribution and density of organisms can vary within the stomach, with the potential for sampling error, particularly in patients taking a PPI. Detection of organisms is common with standard H&E staining but is improved with special stains such as Giemsa, silver, Genta, or specific immunohistochemical stains (Fig. 54.4).[132,138,139]

Culture of mucosal biopsies is difficult because *H. pylori* is fastidious and slow growing, requiring specialized media and growth environment.[131,132] It is not routinely available in contemporary U.S. practice. When culturing gastric mucosal biopsies for *H. pylori*, tissue should be obtained before biopsy forceps are exposed to formalin. Tissue should then be placed in a container with only a few drops of saline or appropriate media to preserve the specimen during transport to a local or offsite microbiology facility.[132] Although mucosal culture is not generally recommended, culture with antibiotic sensitivity testing can guide subsequent treatment in patients with refractory infection, with the understanding that in vitro sensitivity testing does not always predict treatment outcome.[132,140]

NGS for *H. pylori* can be performed on fresh or stored gastric mucosal biopsy specimens. This can also be performed on fecal samples, so avoiding an endoscopy.[141,142] This offers the future prospect of a rapid diagnostic test for *H. pylori* followed (when positive) by reflexive testing for antimicrobial susceptibility and resistance.

Nonendoscopic tests. Serology remains a popular noninvasive test in clinical practice, used mainly for its convenience and relatively low cost. However, based on its relatively poor performance characteristics, some payors no longer reimburse for serological testing. In general, noninvasive tests of active infection (see below) are preferred over serology. As described earlier, infection incites a systemic immune response, and enzyme-linked immunosorbent assay technology can detect serum IgG antibodies to a variety of bacterial antigens.[131,132] Tests for IgA and IgM antibodies are less reliable, and their use is discouraged.[131] In adult practice, there is no justification for measuring IgM antibodies to *H. pylori*. Office-based kits that test whole blood can provide results within 30 minutes and permit "point of service" testing. Although serology is relatively inexpensive, noninvasive, and suited to a primary care setting, the population prevalence of *H. pylori* infection influences its accuracy.[133] The sensitivity of

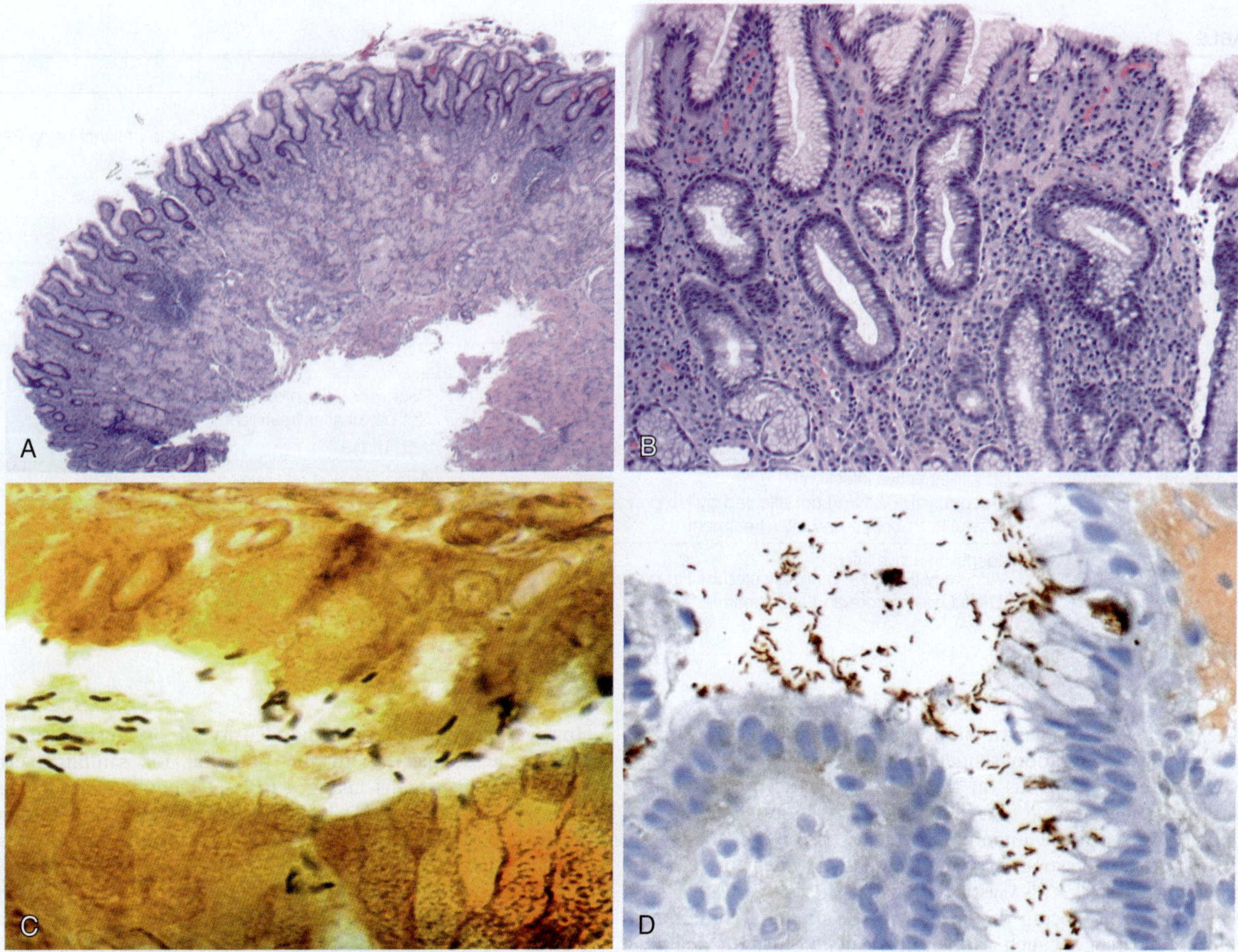

Fig. 54.4 Histopathology of *Helicobacter pylori* (Hp) gastritis. (A) Active chronic gastritis with diffuse band-like lymphoplasmacytic inflammation in the upper third of the mucosa (H&E, ×20). (B) Higher magnification showing diffuse lymphoplasmacytic inflammation in the lamina propria and neutrophils infiltrating the gastric pit epithelium (H&E, ×100). (C) Silver special stain highlights Hp microorganisms (silver stain, ×600). (D) Immunohistochemistry for Hp showing organisms along the gastric epithelial surfaces (IHC, ×400).

serology is generally quite high (90%–100%), but its specificity is variable (76%–96%). Therefore in populations where the prevalence of the infection is relatively low (including much of the United States), the positive predictive value is low, with many false-positive results. A positive serological test is not adequately reliable as the sole basis for initiation of treatment for *H. pylori* infection. Instead, a confirmatory test of active infection, such as a urea breath test or stool antigen test (discussed later), is recommended before embarking on treatment. Conversely, the negative predictive value of serology is high in low prevalence populations. A negative serological test reliably excludes active *H. pylori* infection. Among infected individuals, serology can remain positive for months or longer even after successful treatment of infection. Therefore serology should never be used to determine *H. pylori* status after treatment for the infection. Although seroconversion (i.e., a change from a positive to a negative result) demonstrated months after treatment can indicate successful eradication, it is an impractical means of testing for eradication.[143]

Urea breath testing (UBT) detects active *H. pylori* infection and may be used for making the initial diagnosis and for documenting eradication.[133] The UBT relies on bacterial hydrolysis of orally administered urea in which the carbon atom of atomic weight 12 has been replaced by another isotope, either nonradioactive ^{13}C or radioactive ^{14}C (Fig. 54.5). Hydrolysis of urea generates ammonia and either $^{13}CO_2$ or $^{14}CO_2$, which can be detected in exhaled breath.[144] The nonradioactive ^{13}C test is generally preferred over the radioactive ^{14}C test. The radiation dose with the ^{14}C test is around 1 μC (equivalent to 1 day of background radiation exposure). The specificity of the UBT exceeds 95%, making false-positive results uncommon. The sensitivity of the test is 88%–95%, with false-negative results in patients taking PPIs, bismuth compounds, or antibiotics. To improve diagnostic accuracy, PPIs, bismuth salts, and antibiotics should be stopped for 2 weeks before UBT. UBT is not accurate in patients who have had partial gastric resection.

Stool antigen testing is an immunoassay that detects *H. pylori* antigens and is the other principal noninvasive modality to diagnose active infection and to confirm eradication following treatment. Overall, sensitivity and specificity are comparable to the UBT (94% and 97%, respectively). A rapid stool antigen test allows for testing during a clinic visit, but it is slightly less accurate than a traditional laboratory-based stool test.[145] The sensitivity of stool testing is also reduced by PPIs, bismuth salts, and antibiotics, which can decrease bacterial load; thus similar precautions as described for UBT are recommended.

PCR is a sensitive method to detect *H. pylori* and to detect antibiotic resistance genes.[146] It is useful for testing for antibiotic resistance genes.

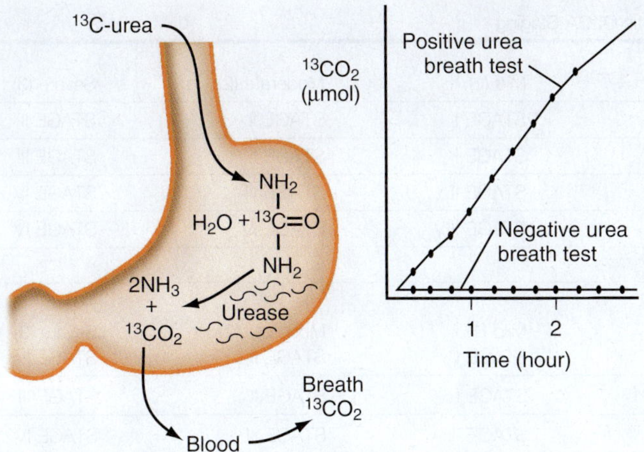

Fig. 54.5 The urea breath test (see text for a more complete description). (From Walsh JH, Peterson WL. Drug therapy: the treatment of *Hp* infection in the management of peptic ulcer disease. *N Engl J Med*. 1995;333:984–991.)

Following treatment of *H. pylori* infection, it is essential to check for successful eradication. Unless EGD is clinically indicated, this should be performed with either a UBT or stool antigen test—the choice being largely dependent upon local availability. USA treatment guidelines (discussed later) state that all individuals should undergo testing to confirm successful eradication of infection after treatment.[147,148] Posttreatment endoscopy with biopsy is only appropriate if a repeat procedure is clinically indicated. In such patients, sampling multiple areas of the stomach is important to avoid missing persistent infection due to alteration of the bacterial density and distribution by recent antibiotic or PPI use. Tests for eradication should not be performed sooner than 8 weeks after completion of treatment, because earlier testing might yield false-negative results. Also, medications that could affect test results, such as PPIs, should be discontinued for at least 2 weeks before testing to improve accuracy. The chronic inflammation associated with *H. pylori* infection may take months to resolve following eradication of the organism, so its presence in biopsy material should not be interpreted as persistent infection.

Chronic Atrophic Gastritis (Gastric Atrophy)

As discussed in Chapter 51, the gastric mucosa has a rapid rate of turnover, with new cells derived from progenitor (stem) cells replacing cells that are shed into the lumen or destroyed. This process maintains the thickness and the varied cell population of glands comprising the oxyntic and antral mucosa. In chronic gastritis, the rate of cell loss may exceed the ability of the stem cells to replace lost cells, leading to thinning of the mucosa. This is often accompanied by metaplasia of this epithelium derived from isthmus-located stem cells.[149] This thinning of the mucosa and accompanying metaplasia (most often intestinal, but sometimes pseudopyloric, pancreatic, squamous, or ciliated) is termed *chronic atrophic gastritis*, or *gastric atrophy* if associated with chronic inflammation. Chronic atrophic gastritis may be regional or diffuse and is often patchy (see Fig. 54.2). It is an important risk factor for dysplasia and gastric cancer (see Chapter 54).[150,151]

In chronic atrophic gastritis (gastric atrophy),[152–172] loss of parietal and chief cells within gastric glands leads to a reduction or absence of their secreted products, including intrinsic factor, hydrochloric acid (hypochlorhydria or achlorhydria), and pepsinogen, with an increased risk of adverse consequences such as vitamin B_{12} malabsorption, gastric bacterial overgrowth, and enteric infections.

An international group of gastroenterologists and pathologists (the Operative Link for Gastritis Assessment [OLGA]) attempted to stage the risk of progression from chronic atrophic gastritis to gastric cancer.[173] OLGA stages 0 through IV are recognized (Table 54.2). The OLGA system is based on the assumption that gastric cancer risk is related to the degree of gastric glandular atrophy.[174–177] Others have proposed that IM, easier to recognize by pathologists than gastric atrophy, can be used in place of gastric atrophy (OLGIM).[178,179] However, focusing on IM rather than the degree of gastric atrophy may be less sensitive in identifying patients at high risk of gastric cancer.[180] The Kyoto classification system is also used to assess cancer risk, especially in Japan.[181] Subtyping of IM into complete (small intestinal) or incomplete (colonic) is of uncertain prognostic value, although a literature review suggested a higher cancer risk with the incomplete (colonic) type, especially if the intestinal goblet cells contain predominantly sulfomucins as opposed to sialomucins.[182]

The two types of chronic atrophic gastritis are EMAG, also called *multifocal atrophic gastritis*, and AMAG, also called *diffuse corporal atrophic gastritis* (Figs. 54.2 and 54.3B and C). At the two ends of the spectrum, these can be distinguished using clinical, laboratory, endoscopic, and histologic features (Table 54.3). However, in many cases, the distinction between EMAG (usually due to chronic *H. pylori* infection) and AMAG (usually due to autoreactive T and B/plasma cells against various antigens of the parietal cell) is blurred because of overlapping features. For example, in EMAG, *H. pylori* may have disappeared from the stomach over time as the gastric epithelium has been replaced by metaplastic intestinal epithelium, although serum IgG antibodies to *H. pylori* may persist as a marker of prior infection. Likewise, through molecular mimicry, antibodies to *H. pylori* may cross-react with parietal cell antigens such as the α and β chains of H^+, K^+-ATPase (the proton pump) to result in a form of AMAG.[183,184] The sequence of IM, dysplasia, and gastric cancer, first popularized by Correa, is now well accepted and is discussed in Chapter 54. The role of endoscopic surveillance in patients with gastric IM is controversial but has been advocated by some.[151,185] U.S. guidelines gave a strong recommendation for testing for *H. pylori* in patients with gastric IM and treatment to eradicate the infection—but only conditional recommendations for endoscopic follow-up surveillance.[186] Gastric metaplasia and dysplasia may be detected during gastroscopy, particularly if enhanced imaging methods, such as narrow band imaging and chromoendoscopy, are used (Fig. 54.6).[151]

EMAG

EMAG is characterized by involvement of both the gastric antrum and corpus with glandular atrophy and IM (Fig. 54.3B). At least two biopsies should be obtained from the antrum, one from the incisura angularis, and two from the gastric body in order for the pathologist to be able to render a diagnosis of EMAG. Atrophic gastritis involving the corpus may be associated with pseudopyloric metaplasia, in which the mucosa resembles antral mucosa but lacks gastrin stain positivity that is normally present in the antrum but instead stains for pepsinogen I (PGI), a proenzyme normally expressed in corpus mucosa. Other types of metaplasia (pancreatic, squamous, and ciliated) may also occur.

Gastroscopy may show a pale mucosa, shiny surface, and prominent submucosal vessels due to mucosal thinning (see Fig. 54.6). However, endoscopy is neither sensitive nor specific in diagnosing chronic atrophic gastritis.[152] Magnifying endoscopy and autofluorescence imaging video endoscopy may be more sensitive in detecting atrophy.[150,151]

The pathogenesis of EMAG is multifactorial, but *H. pylori* infection plays the most important role and has been incriminated in about 85% of patients. EMAG can occur early in life in *H. pylori*–infected individuals. Genetic and environmental factors,

TABLE 54.2 OLGA and OLGIM Classifications of Cancer Risk in Chronic Gastritis OLGA Staging

Corpus (Body, Fundus)					
ATROPHY		None (0)	Mid (1)	Moderate (2)	Severe (3)
ANTRUM*	None (0)	STAGE 0	STAGE I	STAGE II	STAGE II
	Mid (1)	STAGE I	STAGE I	STAGE II	STAGE III
	Moderate (2)	STAGE II	STAGE II	STAGE III	STAGE IV
	Severe (3)	STAGE III	STAGE III	STAGE IV	STAGE IV
OLGIM Staging					
Corpus (Body, Fundus)					
ANTRUM	INTESTINAL METAPLASIA (IM)	None (0)	Mild (1)	Moderate (2)	Severe (3)
	None (0)	STAGE 0	STAGE I	STAGE II	STAGE II
	Mild (1)	STAGE I	STAGE I	STAGE II	STAGE III
	Moderate (2)	STAGE II	STAGE II	STAGE III	STAGE IV
	Severe (3)	STAGE III	STAGE III	STAGE IV	STAGE IV

*Antrum includes the biopsy result from the incisura angularis.

Modified from Rugge M, Correa P, Di Mario F, et al. OLGA staging for gastritis: a tutorial. *Dig Liver Dis*. 2008;40:650–658; Capelle LG, de Vries C, Haringsma J, et al. The staging of gastritis with the OLGA system by using intestinal metaplasia as an accurate alternative for atrophic gastritis. *Gastrointestinal Endosc*. 2010;71:1150–1158.

TABLE 54.3 Spectrum of AMAG and EMAG

AMAG ↔ AMAG/EMAG	**Overlap ↔ EMAG**
Antibodies to intrinsic factor, parietal cell	Hp gastritis (Current, past)
Other autoimmune disorders	Potentially reversible (Hp Rx)
Antral sparing	Antral involvement
↓Serum PGI and ↓PGI/PGII ratio	Serum PG levels more variable
Hypergastrinemia (can be marked)	Normal or slight increase in serum gastrin
Gastric neuroendocrine tumors	

PG, Pepsinogen.

especially diet, are also important. Certain population groups are predisposed to EMAG, including African Americans, Scandinavians, Asians, Hispanics, Central and South Americans, Japanese, and Chinese. In China, a model has been developed based on gender, general health, family history of cancer, and diet/alcohol use to stratify the risk of gastric cancer in patients with EMAG and to determine the need for screening gastroscopy.[153] IM is a risk factor for dysplasia and gastric cancer, usually of the intestinal type (see Chapter 54). The incidence of gastric neoplasia (dysplasia, cancer) in intestinal metaplastic lesions of the stomach has been estimated to be 1% per year, although most of these incident lesions were dysplastic rather than invasive cancers.[155] IM of the gastric mucosa can be classified into three subtypes depending on the morphology of the epithelium and the types of mucins produced.[182]

AMAG

AMAG, also called *diffuse corporal atrophic gastritis*, is an autoimmune destruction of glands in the gastric corpus. AMAG is the pathologic process underlying pernicious anemia, an autoimmune disorder that typically occurs in patients of northern European or Scandinavian background and in African Americans. It may be associated with other autoimmune disorders, especially autoimmune thyroiditis. Although some patients with AMAG are asymptomatic, many complain of dyspepsia with postprandial distress.[187]

Patients with AMAG exhibit achlorhydria or hypochlorhydria, hypergastrinemia with antral G-cell hyperplasia secondary to low or absent gastric acid, and low serum PGI concentrations with low ratios of serum PGI/PGII.[188,189] Affected patients often have circulating antibodies to parietal cell antigens and to IF. Antibodies to IF are less sensitive for AMAG but more specific, whereas antibodies to parietal cell antigens are more sensitive but less specific. Autoreactive T cells and subsequent production of autoantibodies against the α and/or β chains of the H^+, K^+-ATPase (ATP4A and ATP4B) by B/plasma cells are thought to play a role in the pathogenesis of AMAG.[190] Pseudopyloric metaplastic (sometimes called spasmolytic polypeptide-expressing metaplasia) and metaplastic pancreatic acinar cells are also a feature of AMAG.[191]

Histologically, atrophic glands with extensive IM are confined to the corpus mucosa (Fig. 54.3C).[192] Atrophy is usually focal and the preserved islands of relatively normal oxyntic mucosa may appear polypoid endoscopically or radiologically (pseudopolyps). Rarely, AMAG progresses to diffuse (complete) gastric atrophy. Hypergastrinemia, a consequence of achlorhydria, is associated with enterochromaffin-like cell hyperplasia and gastric neuroendocrine tumors,[156] discussed in more detail in Chapter 43.

Antibodies to parietal cell antigens, most notably H^+, K^+-ATPase, are frequently present in patients with AMAG. These antibodies can also be detected in patients with various other autoimmune diseases, including type 1 diabetes mellitus[158–160] and autoimmune thyroid diseases,[161,162] explaining the association of these conditions with pernicious anemia. The risk of AMAG is increased 3- to 5-fold in individuals with type 1 diabetes. Some authors have suggested screening those with type 1 diabetes with gastroscopy and mucosal biopsy. AMAG has also been associated with autoimmune pancreatitis, as well as celiac disease/dermatitis herpetiformis.[166,193]

In patients with AMAG, a proportion of the $CD4^+$ lymphocytes present in the chronic inflammatory infiltrate within the gastric mucosa proliferate in response to H^+, K^+-ATPase. Most $CD4^+$ cells secrete Th1 cytokines, such as IFN-γ and TNF-α, provide help for B cell immunoglobulin production, and enhance

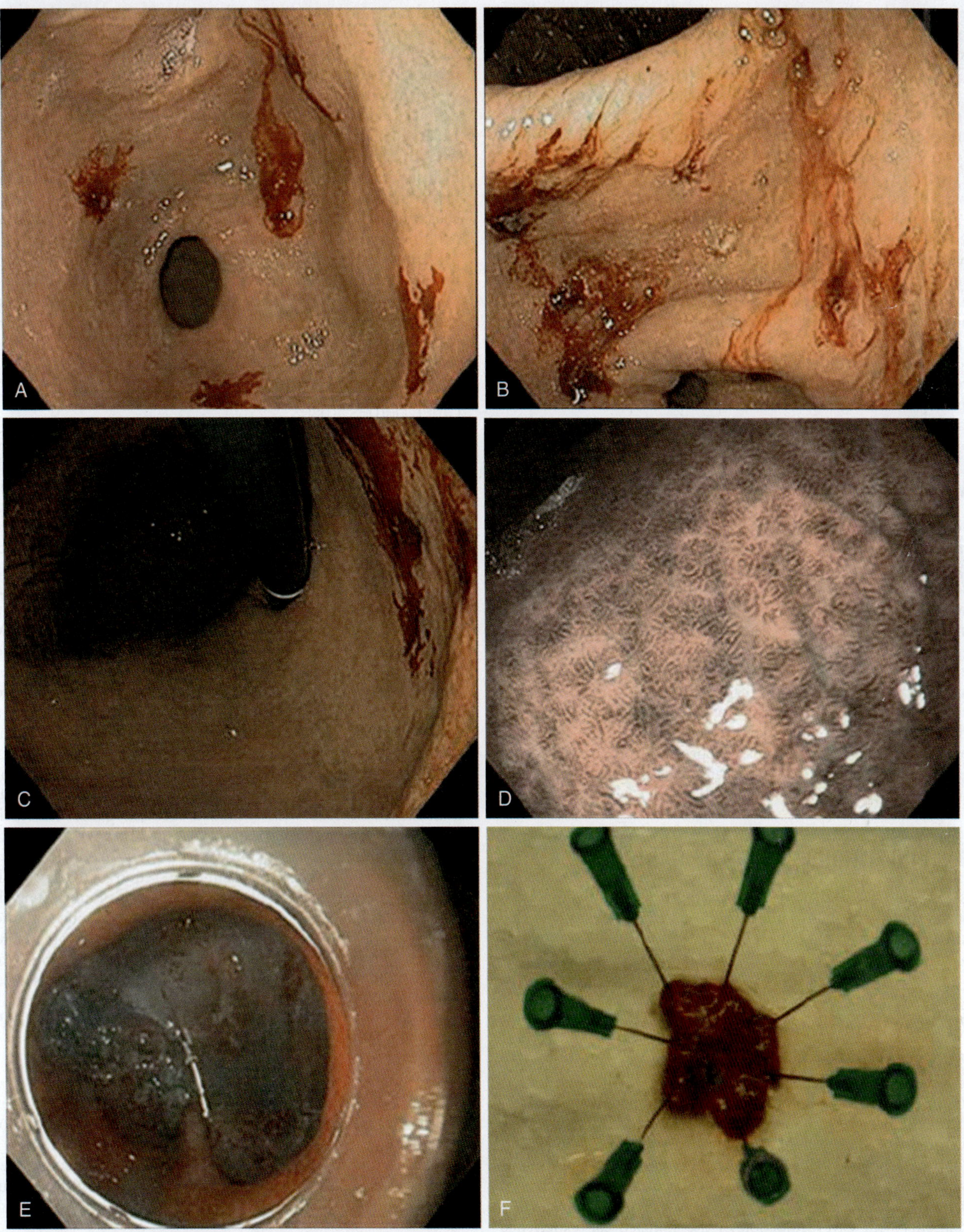

Fig. 54.6 EGDs in patients with metaplastic atrophic gastritis. (Left) Note paucity of folds in the antrum (panel A), at the incisura (panel B), and along the lesser curvature in the gastric body (panel C). Biopsy sites are shown with local bleeding. Narrow-band imaging (panel D), which highlights the mucosal vascular pattern, did not suggest dysplasia, nor did 0.8% indigo carmine staining (not shown). (Right) Note 2.5 cm area of dysplastic epithelium in the antrum (panel E); the dysplastic area has been marked in anticipation of endoscopic submucosal resection (panel F). (From Gomez JM, Wang AY. Gastric intestinal metaplasia and early gastric cancer in the west: a changing paradigm. *Gastroenterol Hepatol*. 2014;10:369–378, with permission.)

perforin-mediated cytotoxicity, as well as Fas-Fas ligand-mediated apoptosis. These factors in combination may contribute to gland destruction in AMAG.

Many patients with AMAG have circulating antibodies to *H. pylori* and/or have *H. pylori* detectable in the oxyntic mucosa of the stomach. Thus *H. pylori* may play a role in the pathogenesis of AMAG.[194] Strains that produce both cagA and VacA may be most likely to cause AMAG. These particular strains of *H. pylori* are often of the s1m1 VacA subtype that also expresses Lewis blood group antigens X and Y.[195] Lewis antigens on *H. pylori* may help to camouflage the organism since they are also present on human gastric epithelial cells. When antibodies to Lewis antigens X and Y from *H. pylori* develop, they may cross-react with similar antigens on epithelial cells, resulting in AMAG (i.e., molecular mimicry). If such patients develop chronic atrophic gastritis with IM, the prevalence of active *H. pylori* infection will then decrease.

Immune checkpoint inhibitors that block programmed death receptors (e.g., PD-1) are being increasingly used in cancer patients. One such agent, nivolumab, has been reported to cause an autoimmune hemorrhagic gastritis.[196]

CARDITIS

There is often a small rim of gastric glands in the cardia of the stomach just below the squamocolumnar junction (see Chapter 49). In an endoscopic study in healthy subjects, most had cardiac-type mucosa in this region; the remainder had oxyntic mucosa with its specialized parietal and chief cells.[197] Inflammation of cardiac-type mucosa (carditis) has been attributed to both *H. pylori* infection and to GERD. Carditis found in healthy subjects is mainly due to infection with *H. pylori*. However, in patients found to have carditis during a diagnostic endoscopy, *H. pylori* was present in only 11%. Severity of carditis in this diagnostic endoscopy population was more closely related to 24-hour acid exposure of the lower esophagus.[198] Chronic atrophic carditis with IM may be a precursor of adenocarcinoma at the gastroesophageal junction (see Chapters 46–48 and 54).

OTHER INFECTIOUS CAUSES OF GASTRITIS

Besides *H. pylori*–related gastritis and acute phlegmonous gastritis, there are many other infectious forms of gastritis that lead to morbidity.

Viral

CMV

CMV is a member of the viral family known as herpesviruses, Herpesviridae, or human herpesvirus (HHV5). Although gastric CMV infection may occur in an immunocompetent host, infection usually occurs in the immunocompromised.[199] Patients with solid organ or hematopoietic cell transplants (see Chapter 34), AIDS (see Chapter 33), cancer, or those who are taking immunosuppressive drugs (especially glucocorticoids) are at increased risk.

Patients with CMV infection of the stomach can experience epigastric pain with fever and atypical lymphocytosis.[200] Gastric imaging may reveal marked thickening of gastric folds and a rigid and narrowed gastric antrum suggestive of an infiltrating neoplasm. Gastroscopy may reveal thickened hemorrhagic folds with a congested and edematous antral mucosa, covered with multiple ulcerations, suggestive of gastric malignancy, submucosal antral mass, or peptic ulcer. A hypertrophic and/or polypoid type of gastritis resembling Ménétrier's disease (discussed later) with protein-losing gastropathy may occur, especially in children, including one case with CMV/*H. pylori* coinfection.[201]

Examination of mucosal biopsy specimens varies between near normal to ulcerated mucosa with granulation tissue formation. Enlarged cells infected with CMV show inclusion bodies indicative of active infection (Fig. 54.7-IA). "Owl-eye" intranuclear inclusions are the hallmark of CMV infection in routine H&E histologic preparations and may be found in vascular endothelial cells, mucosal epithelial cells, and connective tissue stromal cells. Multiple granular, basophilic cytoplasmic inclusions may also be present (see Fig. 54.7-IB). When typical inclusions are hard to find in H&E-stained sections, immunohistochemical stain for CMV may be helpful. Usual treatment is with IV ganciclovir or foscarnet, along with reducing immunosuppression, if feasible. In patients with AIDS, antiretroviral therapy is required to prevent relapse of CMV infection.

Other Herpesviruses

Gastritis from HSV-1 (HHV1) or *varicella-zoster* virus (HHV3) is rare.[202,203] Infected individuals typically experience the initial infection at an early age, and the virus then remains dormant until reactivation, which has been related to cancers (including lymphoma) and to radiation therapy and/or cancer chemotherapy agents. The typical immunocompromised patient with herpesvirus gastritis may experience nausea, vomiting, abdominal pain, fever, chills, fatigue, and weight loss. Air-contrast barium radiographs may show a cobblestone pattern, shallow ulcerations with a ragged contour, and an interlacing network of crevices filled with barium corresponding to areas of ulceration. Gastroscopy reveals multiple, small, raised, ulcerated plaques or linear, superficial ulcers in a crisscrossing pattern, giving the stomach a cobblestone appearance. Brush cytology and biopsies should be performed. Brush cytology has the advantage of sampling a wider area of mucosa. Grossly, the ulcers are multiple, small, and of uniform size. Microscopically, cytological smears and biopsy specimens show nonspecific active inflammation containing scattered multinucleated cells with smudged (ground glass) intranuclear inclusions (see Fig. 54.7-II). HHV1 and HHV3 show identical histology. Immunohistochemistry, viral culture, or PCR of an appropriate swab or tissue specimen is required to differentiate these infections.[203] Treatment with acyclovir is of unproven value.

EBV (HHV4) is not present in normal gastric mucosa but can be present in the stomach in almost half of the patients with gastritis.[204] Whether EBV is a cause of the gastritis in these cases is uncertain. EBV infection has been linked to gastritis cystica profunda (GCP; discussed later) and with gastric cancer.[205] Infectious mononucleosis due to acute EBV infection may lead to gastric lymphoid hyperplasia with atypical lymphocytes.[206]

Measles

Measles, caused by rubeola virus, has many GI manifestations, including gastritis. The characteristic histologic pattern is of numerous multinucleated giant cells (Warthin-Finkeldey cells) within gastric epithelial and stromal cells, with mild background chronic inflammation.[207]

Bacterial

Mycobacteria

Gastric infection with *Mycobacterium tuberculosis* is rare.[208] Patients typically present with abdominal pain, nausea and vomiting, GI

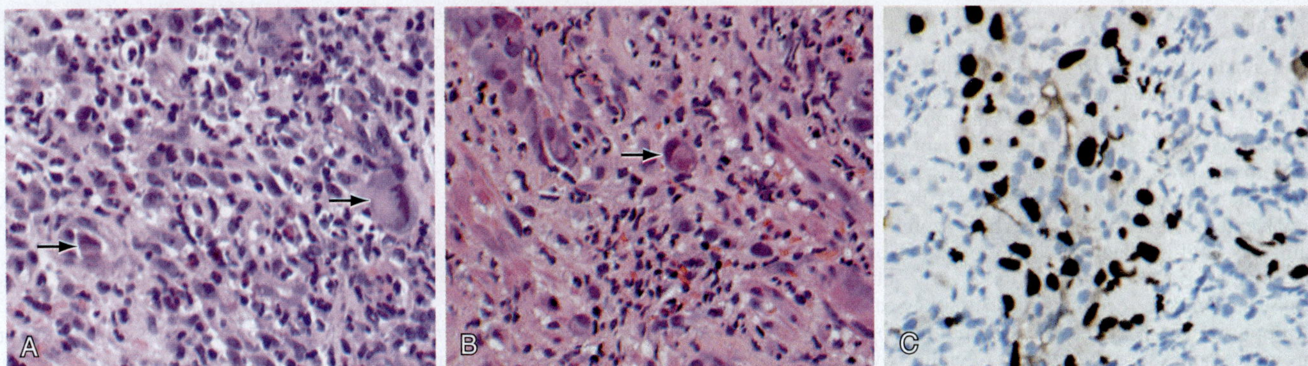

Fig. 54.7-I Histopathology of CMV gastritis. (A) Gastric ulcer with granulation tissue containing several CMV inclusions (*arrows*) (H&E, ×600). (B) Classic CMV-infected cell with cytomegaly, well-formed Cowdry type A nuclear inclusion, and granular cytoplasmic inclusions (H&E, ×600). (C) Immunohistochemical stain highlights CMV-infected cells (CMV IHC, ×400).

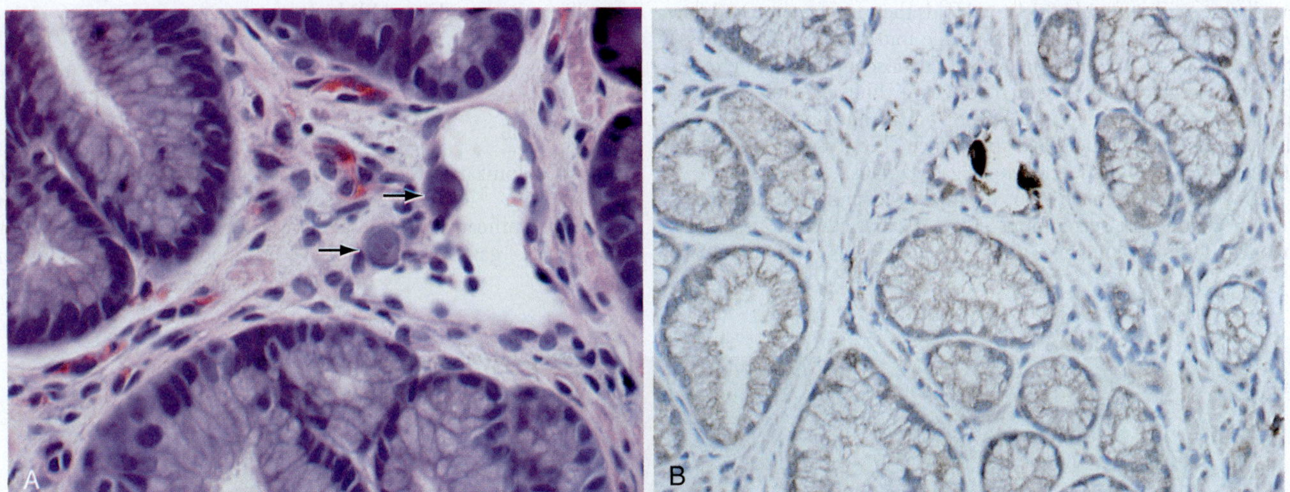

Fig. 54.7-II Histopathology of HSV gastritis. (A) Biopsy specimen shows nonspecific inflammation, containing scattered multinucleated cells with smudged (*ground glass*) intranuclear inclusions (*arrows*) (H&E, ×600). (B) Immunohistochemical stain highlights the positive HSV-infected cells (HSV1/2 IHC, ×400).

bleeding from tuberculous gastric ulcer(s), anemia, fever, and weight loss. Gastric tuberculosis may also be associated with gastric outlet obstruction. Imaging studies reveal an enlarged stomach with a narrowed, deformed antrum and prepyloric ulcerations. Upper endoscopy may demonstrate ulcers, masses, or gastric outlet obstruction. Duodenal tuberculosis can also cause gastric outlet obstruction.[209] Grossly, the stomach may demonstrate multiple small mucosal erosions, ulcers, an infiltrating mass (hypertrophic form), sclerosing inflammatory disease, or pyloric obstruction either by extension from peripyloric nodes or by invasion from other neighboring organs. Biopsies show caseating granulomas containing Langhans giant cells and rare tiny bacilli, seen only with an acid-fast stain. Treatment is discussed in Chapter 86.

Infection with the *Mycobacterium avium* complex (*M. avium, M. intracellulare, M. chimaera*) is a common opportunistic infection among patients with AIDS (see Chapter 35), but the stomach is only rarely involved. Microscopically, the gastric mucosa demonstrates numerous foamy histiocytes containing many acid-fast bacilli. Treatment is with a macrolide (clarithromycin or azithromycin) plus rifampicin and ethambutol.

Actinomycosis

Primary gastric actinomycosis is a rare, chronic, progressive, suppurative disease characterized by formation of multiple abscesses, draining sinuses, and abundant granulation and dense fibrous tissue.[210] The presenting features may include fever, epigastric pain, epigastric swelling, abdominal wall abscess with fistula, and upper GI bleeding. Radiographic studies frequently suggest a malignancy or a gastric ulcer. Endoscopy may be suggestive of a circumscribed and ulcerated gastric carcinoma, and the diagnosis can be made with endoscopic biopsy.

Grossly, the resected stomach demonstrates a large, ill-defined, ulcerated mass in the wall. Microscopically, multiple abscesses show the infective agent, *Actinomyces israelii*, a Gram-positive filamentous anaerobic bacterium that normally resides in the mouth. A biopsy of a mass containing pus, or a biopsy of a draining sinus, may reveal actinomycosis. If the disease is recognized only by histologic examination, the prognosis is good. Prolonged (6–12 months) high-dose antibiotic treatment with penicillin or amoxicillin/clavulanic acid is recommended.

Syphilis

The incidence of primary and secondary syphilis is increasing in the United States, with a 17.6% increase between 2015 and 2016.[211] Case reports and small case series emphasize the importance of the gastroenterologist and pathologist remaining alert to the protean manifestations of syphilis and being familiar with the histopathologic pattern of the disease.[212,213] Gastric involvement in secondary or tertiary syphilis is rarely recognized clinically, and its diagnosis by examination of endoscopic biopsy specimens has been reported infrequently. The features of gastric syphilis should be recognized because they can provide a window of opportunity for effective antibiotic therapy before the disease progresses and causes permanent disability. Syphilitic gastritis can occur in conjunction with hepatitis and proctitis.[212] Gastric syphilis can occur in the setting of HIV infection.

Patients typically present with symptoms of peptic ulcer, often with upper GI bleeding. Diseases that may mimic gastric syphilis include peptic ulcer, gastric adenocarcinoma, gastric lymphoma, tuberculosis, and Crohn disease. The acute gastritis of early secondary syphilis produces the earliest radiologically detectable signs of the disease, with diffusely thickened folds that may become nodular, with or without ulcers. Strictures in the mid-stomach ("hourglass" stomach) may be present (Fig. 54.8A). Endoscopy shows numerous shallow, irregular ulcers with overlying white exudate and surrounding erythema (see Fig. 54.8B). The surrounding mucosa may also demonstrate a nodular appearance. Gastroscopy may also demonstrate prominent, edematous gastric folds.

Grossly, the stomach may be thickened and contracted and may show multiple serpiginous ulcers. Partial gastrectomy specimens may show compact, thick, mucosal folds, and numerous small mucosal ulcers. Microscopically, biopsies show severe gastritis with a dense plasma cell infiltrate in the lamina propria, a characteristic finding, varying numbers of neutrophils and lymphocytes, gland destruction, vasculitis, and granulomas. Warthin-Starry silver stain or modified Steiner silver impregnation stain reveals numerous spirochetes. Serum Venereal Disease Research Laboratory and *Treponema* immunofluorescence studies may be positive, and PCR may detect the *Treponema pallidum* gene. Treatment with penicillin is highly effective (see Fig. 54.8C).

Other Bacteria

Helicobacter heilmannii is a spiral bacterium and an infrequent cause of chronic active gastritis; this infection may be a risk factor for gastric MALToma.[214] These organisms, originally known as *Gastrospirillum hominis*, are longer than *H. pylori* and have a different morphology with multiple spirals. One of these *H. heilmannii* species, *Helicobacter bizzozeronii*, has been isolated from human gastric mucosa.[215] *Campylobacter hyointestinalis* is another organism that, like *H. pylori*, can stain with the Giemsa reagent.[216] The clinical significance of these non-*H. pylori* curved bacilli remains to be established.

Fungal

Candidiasis

Fungal colonization of gastric ulcers with *Candida* species is not uncommon.[217] There is debate whether such colonization has any clinical significance or whether the organisms may aggravate and perpetuate gastric ulceration. Endoscopically, gastric ulcers

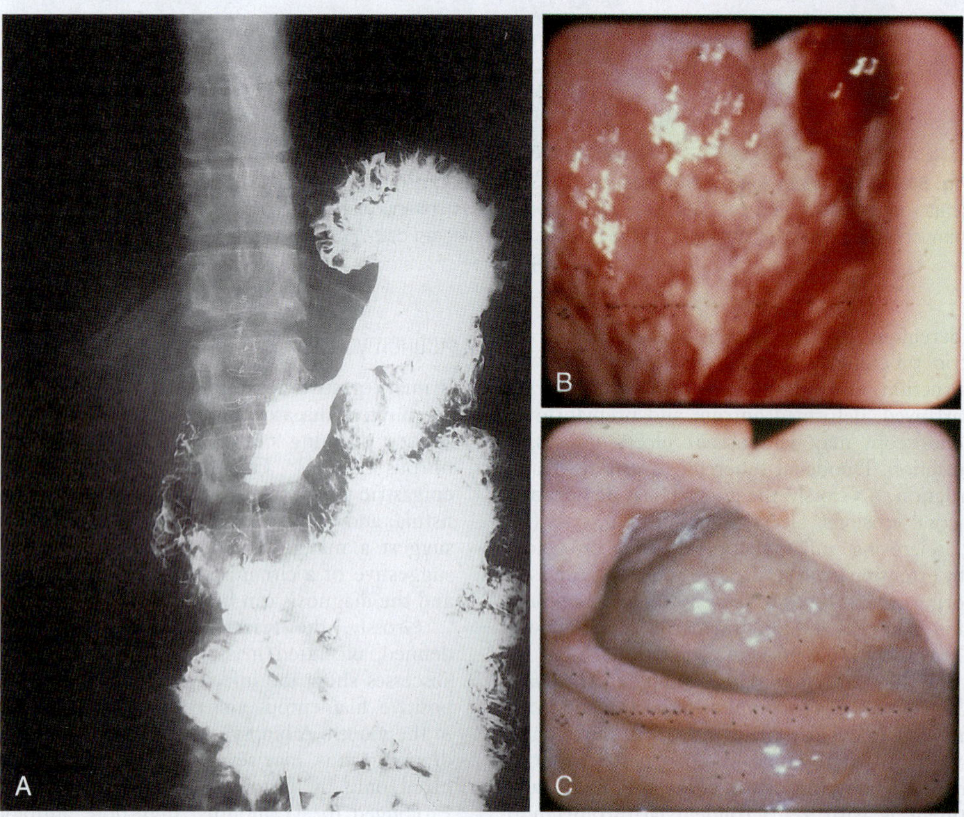

Fig. 54.8 Gastric syphilis (syphilitic gastritis). Film from an upper GI series (A) showing a stricture in the mid-stomach (hourglass stomach), with antral deformity. Endoscopic appearance before (B) and 4 weeks after (C) penicillin therapy in another patient with gastric syphilis. (Courtesy Mark Feldman, MD, Dallas, TX.)

associated with *Candida albicans* colonization tend to be larger in diameter and are more often suspected to be malignant than typical gastric ulcers. Diffuse superficial erosions may also be noted. The earliest detectable radiographic change in gastric candidiasis may be tiny aphthoid erosions. Aphthoid ulcers may progress to deep linear ulcers.

Fungal colonization of the GI tract, frequent in patients with underlying malignancy and in immunocompromised patients who have been treated with antibiotics or glucocorticoids, may also occur in immunocompetent patients. Massive growth of yeast organisms in the gastric lumen (yeast bezoar) is a potential complication of some gastric surgical procedures. *Candida* infection of the stomach may also occur in alcoholic patients.

Grossly, the gastric mucosa demonstrates tiny erosions, widespread punctate, linear ulcerations, or gastric ulcers. Microscopically, the layer of necrotic fibrinoid debris demonstrates yeasts or pseudohyphae. The organisms can be seen with H&E staining; however, special stains such as periodic acid-Schiff-diastase stain or Gomori methenamine silver stain may be required. Treatment for the Candida *per se* is usually not necessary. However, if symptomatic candidiasis is suspected, fluconazole is reasonable but of unproven efficacy.

Histoplasmosis

Progressive disseminated histoplasmosis is rare, occurring most frequently in the very young, older adults, or in those with immunodeficiency. Disseminated histoplasmosis can involve any portion of the GI tract,[218] although gastric involvement is uncommon.[219] Gastric histoplasmosis may be associated with hypertrophic gastric folds, a mass mimicking gastric adenocarcinoma, or gastric ulceration. Radiographic studies may demonstrate an annular infiltrating lesion of the stomach. Endoscopy may demonstrate enlarged and reddened gastric folds. Biopsy specimens show noncaseating granulomas within a mixed chronic inflammatory infiltrate. Gomori methenamine silver stains will highlight numerous small (2–5 μm) round-to-oval yeast forms with occasional budding, compatible with *Histoplasma capsulatum*. Treatment with IV liposomal amphotericin B followed by itraconazole for ≥12 months is appropriate.[220]

Mucormycosis

Gastric mucormycosis (also called *zygomycosis* or *phycomycosis*) is a rare and highly lethal fungal infection.[221] Risk factors include malnutrition, immunosuppression, antibiotic therapy, and severe metabolic acidosis, usually diabetic ketoacidosis. Most patients present with upper GI bleeding and/or gastric ulceration.[222] Gastric mucormycosis can be classified as invasive or noninvasive (i.e., colonization). Deep invasion of the stomach and blood vessel walls by the fungus characterizes the former (see the "Acute Gastritis" section). Abdominal pain is the most frequent presenting complaint. In the noninvasive type, the fungus colonizes the superficial mucosa without causing an inflammatory response.

Grossly, surgical specimens from affected patients reveal hemorrhagic necrosis involving the mucosa and gastric wall. Microscopically, nonseptate 10–20-μm hyphae branched at right angles are present in the tissue and infiltrating into blood vessel walls. Treatment is resection of the affected necrotic portion of the stomach. Invasive gastric mucormycosis is almost always fatal.

Aspergillosis

Acute *Aspergillus* gastritis is rare and can be highly invasive.[223]

Cryptococcosis

The stomach and duodenum may be involved in immunocompromised hosts, including patients with AIDS in conjunction with cryptococcal meningitis.[224]

Monascus Ruber

This form of fungal gastritis is acquired by eating dried, salted fish and can result in invasive fungal infection.[225]

Parasitic

Cryptosporidiosis

Cryptosporidiosis may rarely involve the stomach (see also Chapter 115).[226]

Giardiasis

Giardia lamblia can rarely infect the stomach.[227] An association of infection with trophozoites with chronic atrophic gastritis and its associated hypochlorhydria has been suggested.

Strongyloidiasis

The stomach is rarely affected by *Strongyloides stercoralis*.[228] The organism may colonize the intact gastric mucosa and may also be associated with bleeding peptic ulcer. Most patients are immunocompromised. There may be peripheral eosinophilia. Diagnosis can be confirmed by endoscopic biopsy, examination of stools, or examination of a duodenal aspirate. Disseminated strongyloidiasis (hyperinfection) can be rapidly fatal. Treatment consists of ivermectin and reducing immunosuppression, if feasible (see Chapter 114).

Anisakidosis

Invasive anisakidosis (formerly, anisakiasis) may occur after the ingestion of raw marine fish containing nematode larvae of the genus *Anisakis*. Most cases have been diagnosed in Japan. The parasite may migrate into the wall of the stomach, small intestine, or colon.[229] Patients may present with sporadic epigastric pain or may be asymptomatic. Gastric perforation due to chronic gastric anisakidosis may occur. Some patients exhibit mild peripheral eosinophilia. Endoscopy may show firm, yellowish submucosal masses with erosions. Imaging studies may reveal notched-shadow defects suggestive of a gastric tumor.

Grossly, the stomach demonstrates multiple erosive foci with hemorrhage and small 5–10-mm gastric lesions. Microscopically, sections of the stomach show a marked eosinophilic granulomatous inflammatory process with intramural abscess formation and granulation tissue. The eosinophilic abscess may contain a small worm measuring 0.3 mm in diameter, which is the larval form. If the larvae are not detected at endoscopy, the diagnosis may be confirmed serologically. Treatment is endoscopic removal of the nematode, followed by albendazole. Successful relief of acute dyspeptic symptoms, which can be quite severe, has been reported with an over-the-counter medicine containing wood cresolate.[230]

Ascariasis

Although gastric ascariasis is rare, *Ascaris lumbricoides* may cause chronic, intermittent gastric outlet obstruction.[231] Gastric ascariasis has also been associated with upper GI hemorrhage; endoscopy may show several *Ascaris* in the stomach and duodenum. Treatment is endoscopic removal, followed by mebendazole or albendazole (see Chapter 114).

Necatoriasis

Endoscopic discovery, capture, and removal from the stomach of the hookworm *Necator americanus* have been reported.[232]

Capillariasis

Eosinophilic gastritis from capillariasis has been reported, perhaps linked to ingestion of raw fish.[233]

GRANULOMATOUS GASTRITIS

A variety of granulomatous diseases can affect the stomach.[234,235] In children, the most common is Crohn disease (Fig. 54.9-I), discussed later and in Chapters 117 and 118. In adults, sarcoidosis (see Chapter 35) and Crohn disease are the most common causes. Infection with spirochetes (e.g., *T. pallidum*), mycobacteria (e.g., *M. tuberculosis*), fungi, parasites, and the bacterium *Tropheryma whipplei* (see Chapter 111) can also cause granulomatous gastritis, as can xanthogranulomatous gastritis (XGG; discussed later), foreign bodies, lymphoma, Langerhans cell histiocytosis (gastric eosinophilic granuloma), eosinophilic granulomatosis with polyangiitis (formerly Churg-Strauss syndrome), chronic granulomatous disease of childhood, and, very rarely, granulomatosis with polyangiitis (see Chapter 35).

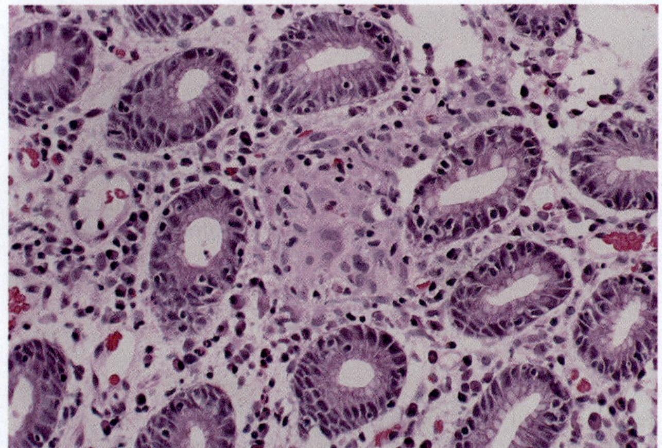

Fig. 54.9-I Histopathology of granulomatous gastritis in a patient with Crohn disease. (A) Noncaseating granuloma is present within the lamina propria (H&E, ×200).

Isolated idiopathic granulomatous gastritis may be "idiopathic," but some may eventually evolve into Crohn disease or sarcoidosis. Other cases of "idiopathic" granulomatous gastritis appear to be due to *H. pylori* infection and may resolve slowly following appropriate treatment, sometimes leaving a mucosal discoloration.[236]

Sarcoidosis

Sarcoidosis is a systemic granulomatous disease, sometimes involving the GI tract, liver, and spleen (see Chapter 35). The gastric antrum is the most common site in the GI tract to be affected in sarcoidosis, being involved in approximately 10% of cases.[237] A diagnosis of sarcoid gastritis cannot be made with confidence in the absence of granulomatous disease in other organs.

Affected patients, usually in the third to fifth decades of life, typically present with epigastric pain, nausea, vomiting, and weight loss. Occasionally they present with massive GI hemorrhage. Gastric sarcoidosis may result in pyloric outlet obstruction, achlorhydria, and vitamin B_{12} deficiency with anemia. Radiographically, gastric sarcoidosis may mimic the diffuse form of gastric adenocarcinoma (linitis plastica) or Ménétrier's disease.

Endoscopy may reveal a narrow distal stomach with multiple prepyloric ulcers or erosions, atrophy, thick gastric folds with a diffuse cobblestone appearance, or normal mucosa associated with microscopic granulomas. Surgical specimens from patients with gastric sarcoidosis show a thickened stomach wall with foci of erosions and ulcers. Microscopically, mucosal biopsies typically show multiple noncaseating granulomas, although these may be necrotizing.[238] As the presence of granulomas in GI tissue is nonspecific, special stains should be performed to rule out granulomatous infections, particularly tuberculosis. In some cases, it may be difficult to differentiate gastric sarcoidosis from gastric Crohn disease or from isolated idiopathic granulomatous gastritis (Fig. 54.9-II).

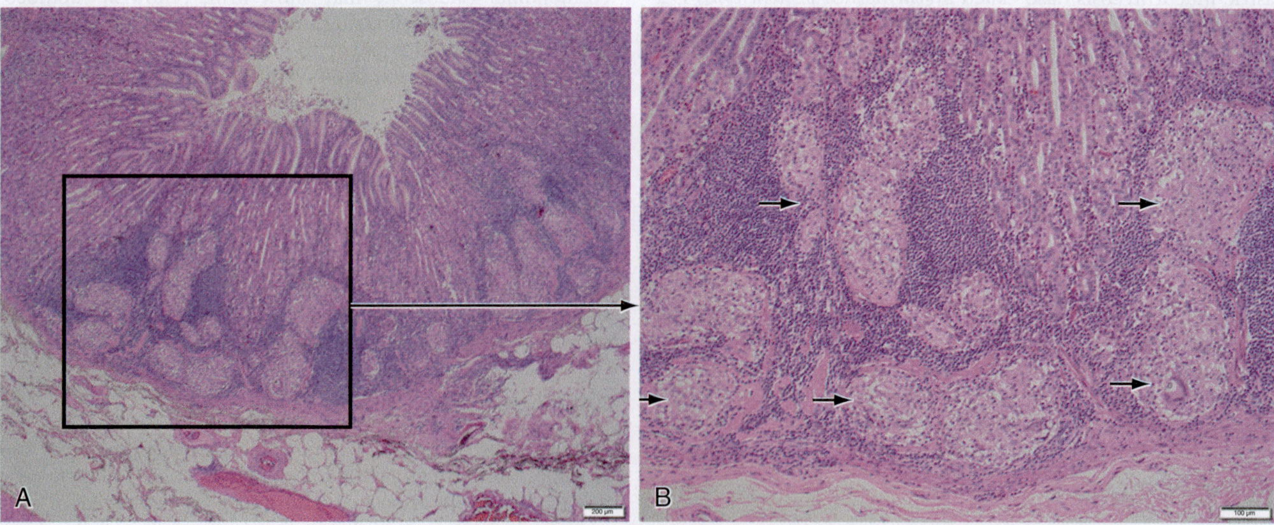

Fig. 54.9-II Histopathology of granulomatous gastritis in a patient with sarcoidosis. (A and B) Noncaseating granuloma is present within the lamina propria (H&E, ×40 and ×100, respectively). The granulomas are small-medium in size, back-to-back with small rime of lymphocytes.

Glucocorticoid therapy is the cornerstone of treatment for gastric sarcoidosis (see Chapter 37). Subtotal gastric resection is reserved for patients with obstruction and severe hemorrhage.

Xanthogranulomatous Gastritis

This is a rare form of gastritis, with fewer than 15 reported cases worldwide. XGG is characterized by marked proliferation of foamy histiocytes mixed with acute and chronic inflammatory cells, multinucleated giant cells, and fibrosis. The destructive inflammatory and fibrotic process may extend into adjacent organs and simulate, or coexist with, a gastric neoplasm.[239–241] An association of XGG with gastric actinomycosis has been reported.[242]

DISTINCTIVE CAUSES OF GASTRITIS

Collagenous Gastritis

This is rare and can be associated with collagenous duodenitis, collagenous colitis, lymphocytic colitis, celiac disease, and/or autoimmune disorders.[243–249] It has also been reported in children and adolescents, where it is usually an isolated phenomenon. In one series, two clinical patterns were identified. In children and young adults, the presenting features of anemia and epigastric pain were attributed to the gastritis *per se*. In adults aged 35–77, the presenting symptom was often diarrhea due to coexisting celiac disease or collagenous colitis.[248]

Barium radiography may demonstrate an abnormal mucosal surface with a mosaic-like pattern in the body of the stomach, corresponding to mucosal nodularity. Endoscopy may reveal multiple diffusely scattered, discrete submucosal hemorrhages, gastric erosions, and coarse folds of the body of the stomach along the greater curvature. Biopsy specimens from the body and antrum reveal a patchy, chronic, superficial gastritis, focal atrophy, and irregular deposition of collagen 20–75-μm thick in the subepithelial region of the lamina propria often containing entrapped capillaries (Fig. 54.10). Tiny erosions of the surface epithelium are often present, and the inflammatory infiltrate consists mainly of plasma cells, intraepithelial lymphocytes, and eosinophils, together with marked hypertrophy of the muscularis mucosa. Little is known about the etiology, natural history, and proper treatment of this condition.

Lymphocytic Gastritis

This[79] is characterized by a dense lymphocytic infiltration of surface and pit gastric epithelium (Fig. 54.11-IA). Lymphocytic gastritis is related to an endoscopic form of gastritis known as *varioliform gastritis*, characterized by nodules, thickened folds, and erosions.[250] Lymphocytic gastritis in adults is typically seen in association with *H. pylori* infection. Eradication of *H. pylori* in such patients causes significant improvement in the gastric intraepithelial lymphocytic infiltrate, corpus inflammation, and dyspeptic symptoms. The relationship between lymphocytic gastritis and gastric lymphoid hyperplasia, which is also associated with *H. pylori* infection, is not clear. Patients with gastric MALToma have a significantly increased prevalence of lymphocytic gastritis due to *H. pylori* infection. Thus lymphocytic gastritis may be a precursor of gastric MALToma in patients with *H. pylori* infection (see Chapters 41 and 56).

There is compelling evidence that lymphocytic gastritis may occur as a manifestation of celiac disease and also be a marker of a more severe and earlier onset form of celiac disease (see Chapter 109).[250,251] Following institution of a gluten-free diet, the lymphocytic gastritis slowly resolves in these patients. Other etiologic associations of lymphocytic gastritis include HIV infection, Crohn disease, common variable immunodeficiency, and medication.[252]

Endoscopy in lymphocytic gastritis shows thick mucosal folds, nodularity, and aphthous erosions (varioliform gastritis).[250,253] Gastric biopsies show expansion of the lamina propria with plasma cells, lymphocytes, and rare neutrophils. These findings may be seen only in the antral or body mucosa, or both. The surface and superficial pit epithelium shows a marked intraepithelial infiltrate with CD3+ T lymphocytes, with flattening of the epithelium and loss of apical mucin secretion.

Lymphomatoid gastropathy[254,255] is due to $CD56^+$ natural killer lymphocytic infiltration of the stomach, simulating a gastric lymphoma. Most cases have been reported in Japan, where there is routine endoscopic screening of healthy individuals for cancer. In a series of 10 adults, the lesions appeared as approximately 1-cm elevated nodules. Dyspeptic symptoms were absent. Most lymphomatoid lesions resolved without therapy, although sometimes recurred. Deaths have not been reported.

Chronic active gastritis can also occur in X-linked lymphoproliferative disease.[256]

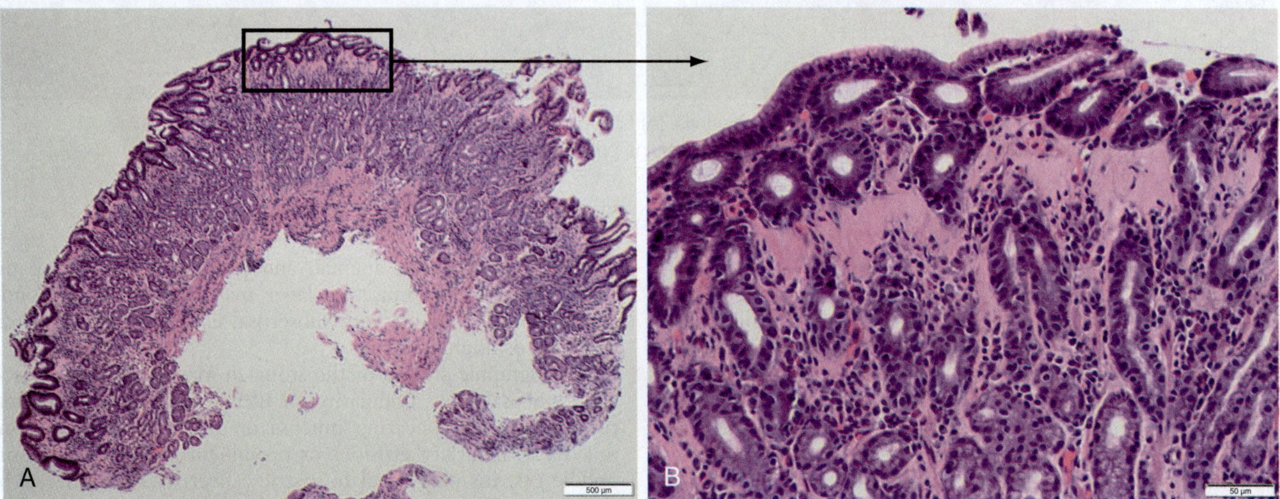

Fig. 54.10 Histopathology of collagenous gastritis [(A and B) H&E, ×20 and ×200, respectively)]. The subepithelial thickening of the collagen band is apparent.

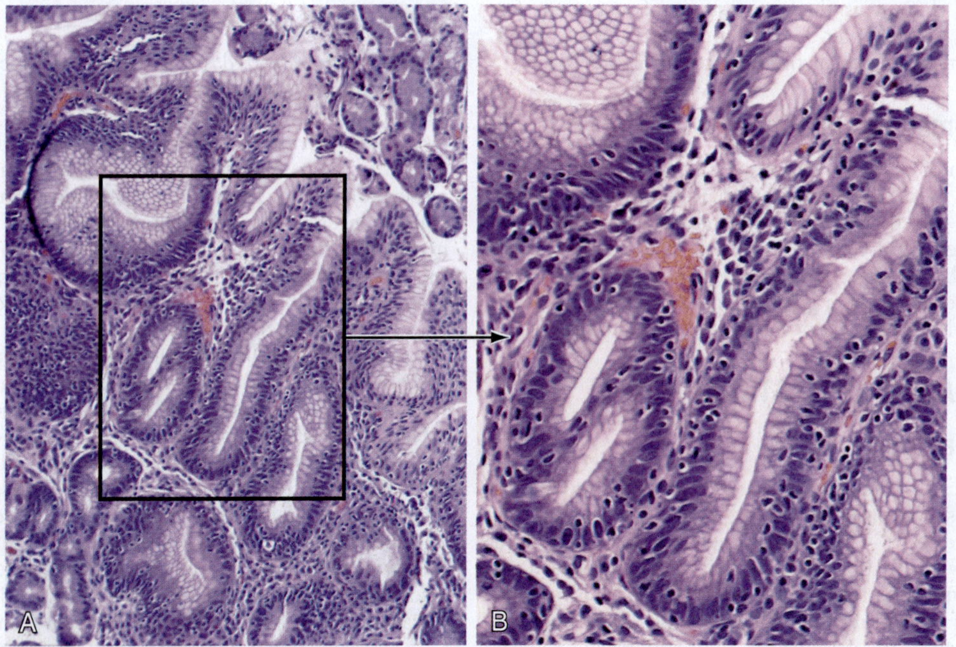

Fig. 54.11-I Histopathology of lymphocytic gastritis. (A) Low-power view of the antral mucosa and (B) high-power view show numerous dark-staining mononuclear cells with striking intraepithelial lymphocytosis (H&E, ×200 and ×400, respectively).

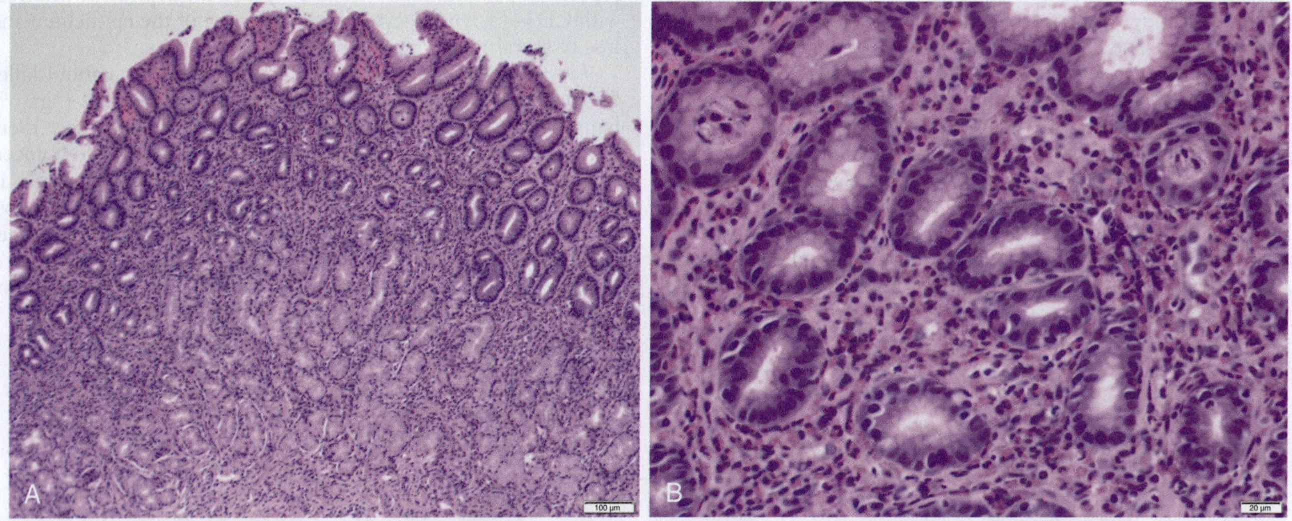

Fig. 54.11-II Histopathology of eosinophilic gastritis. (A) Low-power view of the antral mucosa and (B) high-power view show numerous eosinophils within the lamina propria, the walls, and lumens of the gastric glands (H&E, ×100 and ×400, respectively).

Eosinophilic Gastritis

This is a frequent component of eosinophilic gastroenteritis,[257–259] a condition of unknown etiology characterized by eosinophilic infiltration of the GI tract, peripheral eosinophilia, and GI symptoms in the absence of known causes of eosinophilia (e.g., parasitic infections, cow's milk protein allergy) or other inflammatory GI diseases (e.g., IBD). Eosinophilic gastroenteritis is discussed in more detail in Chapter 30.

Eosinophilic gastritis, like eosinophilic gastroenteritis, is classified according to the layer(s) of the stomach involved (i.e., mucosal disease, muscle disease, and subserosal disease). Gastric mucosal involvement may result in abdominal pain, nausea, vomiting, weight loss, anemia, and protein-losing gastropathy. Involvement of the muscular layer may produce gastric outlet obstruction.[258] Patients with subserosal eosinophilic disease may develop eosinophilic ascites.

Radiographic studies of the stomach may demonstrate thickened mucosal folds, nodularity, or ulcerations. Gastroscopy may reveal a normal-appearing mucosa or a hyperemic, edematous mucosa with surface erosions or prominent gastric folds. Eosinophilic gastritis may simulate gastric cancer. Gastric mucosal biopsies are critical to the diagnosis and show marked eosinophilic infiltration, eosinophilic pit abscesses, necrosis with numerous neutrophils, and epithelial regeneration (see Fig. 54.11-II). Abnormal eosinophilic infiltration, defined as at least 20 eosinophils per high-power field, can be either diffuse or multifocal. A diagnosis of eosinophilic gastritis has been proposed for cases in which eosinophils infiltrate the surface, foveolar epithelium, the deeper mucosa or submucosa, or are associated with other features of mucosal damage (e.g., foveolar hyperplasia or architectural distortion with significant chronic or active inflammation).[257] Full-thickness biopsy is necessary to diagnose muscle disease. Paracentesis can be performed to diagnose serosal disease.

As discussed in Chapter 30, patients with eosinophilic gastritis associated with disabling GI symptoms can be effectively treated with glucocorticoids after other systemic disorders associated with peripheral eosinophilia have been excluded (e.g., eosinophilic granulomatosis with polyangiitis, hypereosinophilic syndrome, parasitic infections). Preliminary studies suggest some effectiveness of an anti-Siglec eight antibody.[260] Endoscopic therapy (e.g., balloon dilation) or surgical intervention may be required in patients with gastric outlet obstruction.

GASTRITIS IN INFLAMMATORY BOWEL DISEASE

Gastritis is increasingly recognized in adults and children with Crohn disease or ulcerative colitis (UC).[261–263] The most common histologic abnormalities in IBD-associated gastritis are chronic inactive and chronic active gastritis. Focally enhanced gastritis and *H. pylori*–related gastritis are less common in these patients. Focally enhanced gastritis is characterized by tiny collections of lymphocytes and macrophages (histiocytes) surrounding gastric pits and glands, often also with infiltrates of neutrophils (Fig. 54.12). Focally enhanced gastritis can sometimes be seen in Crohn disease, but not commonly in UC.

Crohn Disease

Crohn disease involving the stomach is uncommon[264] and usually occurs with concomitant intestinal involvement (see Chapters 117 and 118). Although rare cases may be isolated to the stomach and/or duodenum, a diagnosis of isolated Crohn disease of the stomach should be made with caution.[265] Close follow-up of such patients is indicated for the subsequent development of either Crohn disease in the lower GI tract or of other granulomatous diseases, such as sarcoidosis.

Symptoms of gastric Crohn disease are nonspecific and include nausea and vomiting, epigastric pain, anorexia, and weight loss. Radiologic contrast studies of the stomach may show antral fold thickening, antral narrowing, shallow ulcers (aphthae), or deeper ulcers. Involvement of the stomach from adjacent disease segments in the small intestine or colon is best examined radiologically. Endoscopy allows better examination of mucosal defects and is characterized by reddened mucosa, irregularly shaped ulcers, and erosions in a disrupted mucosal pattern. Nodular lesions occur and often have erosions on the top of nodules. An atypical cobblestone pattern may be associated with nodules surrounded by fissure-like ulceration. The edematous folds, traversed by linear furrows or erosive fissures, have been referred to as "bamboo-joint like."[266] Gastric ulcers or erosions associated with Crohn disease are most commonly located in the antrum and prepyloric region. In contrast to peptic ulcer disease, where the ulcers tend to be round or oval, the ulcerations and erosions of Crohn disease are frequently serpiginous or longitudinal.

The microscopic features of mucosal biopsy or surgical specimens of gastric Crohn disease can resemble those in the ileum or colon (see Chapters 115 and 116). They include granulomatous inflammation (see the "Granulomatous Gastritis" section), transmural chronic inflammation, serpiginous or longitudinal ulcers, and marked submucosal fibrosis (see Fig. 54.9-I). Granulomas may be present in endoscopically normal antral mucosa. As mentioned earlier, focally enhanced gastritis characterized by tiny collections of lymphocytes and macrophages (histiocytes) surrounding gastric pits and glands, often also with infiltrates of neutrophils, is also common (Fig. 54.12). Focally enhanced gastritis can sometimes be seen in Crohn disease, but not commonly in UC.

Treatment of gastritis in Crohn disease should be driven by symptoms and not solely by demonstration of gastritis on mucosal biopsy. Double-blinded, randomized, controlled clinical trials of pharmacologic agents for gastric and duodenal Crohn disease are lacking. PPI therapy should be the first approach for symptomatic patients. Glucocorticoids, aminosalicylates, immunosuppressants (such as azathioprine), and biologic agents (such as anti-TNF-α drugs) have not yet been demonstrated to be effective in controlled clinical trials, but there are reports of success with infliximab.[265] Gastric outlet obstruction refractory to medical and endoscopic therapy can be treated by gastroenterostomy, ideally performed laparoscopically. Treatment of Crohn disease is discussed in more detail in Chapters 117 and 118.

Ulcerative Colitis

The prevalence of gastritis is lower in UC than in Crohn disease, particularly the prevalence of focally enhanced gastritis, but it is greater than in controls without IBD.[261,262] In approximately 5% of patients with UC, the endoscopic appearance of the stomach is abnormal and similar to the appearance of the rectum and colon (see Chapters 117 and 118). Such patients with "ulcerative

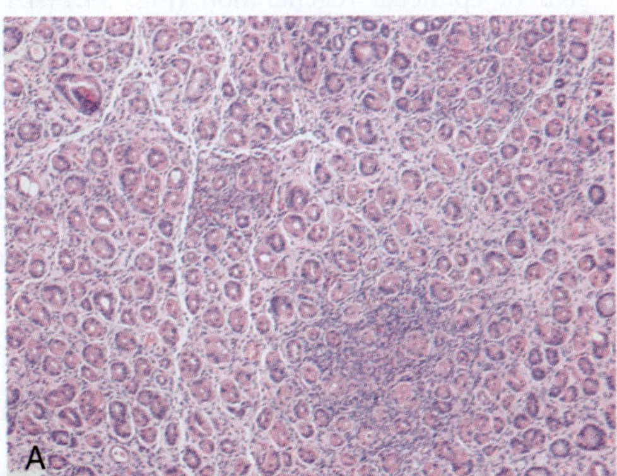

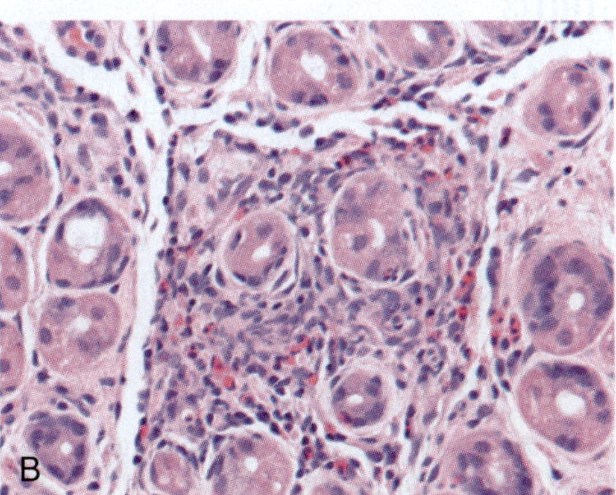

Fig. 54.12 Histopathology of focally enhanced gastritis. (A) Low-power view of gastric mucosa showing ill-defined nodules of inflammatory cells (H&E, ×100). (B) High-power view shows a mixed infiltrate of lymphocytes, eosinophils, and neutrophils focally impinging on the glandular epithelium (H&E, ×400). (Courtesy Jonathan Baker, MD, and Pamela Jensen, MD, Dallas, TX.)

gastritis" are characterized by gastric histopathology similar to colonic histopathology, little or no response to acid-reducing medications, and response to standard treatment for UC. All patients with UC who have ulcerative gastritis either had pancolitis or had had a proctocolectomy; many of the latter also had pouchitis.[267–269] Anti-inflammatory drugs such as glucocorticoids may treat and thus mask the ulcerative gastritis in some patients.

GASTRITIS CYSTICA PROFUNDA

GCP is a rare pseudotumor of the stomach characterized by cystically dilated gastric glands extending through the muscularis mucosa into the submucosa.[270–277] This lesion can occur as a complication of partial gastrectomy with gastrojejunostomy for peptic ulcer disease, typically occurring at the site of the gastroenterostomy. GCP may also develop in an unoperated stomach and be associated with Ménétrier's disease[270] or gastric cancer.[271–274] Inverted hyperplastic gastric polyp may be a variant of GCP, which may also be iatrogenic after attempted gastric polypectomy.[275]

Targeted deletion of the β subunit of the apical K^+ efflux channel of the parietal cell leads to a GCP-like lesion in mice with invasive gastric cancer.[276]

Injury and inflammation within the mucosa may lead to breaks in the muscularis mucosa and migration of epithelium into the submucosa.[277] If present, symptoms in GCP are nonspecific. Gastric imaging and endoscopy typically demonstrate multiple exophytic gastric masses that may simulate malignancy. Endoscopic ultrasound may assist in the diagnosis by demonstrating the cystic nature of the lesions. A diagnosis of GCP should lead to a thorough examination for gastric cancer. Whether GCP patients without gastric cancer require endoscopic surveillance for subsequent cancer development is not clear.

GCP can be removed by snare polypectomy after submucosal injection to elevate the lesion(s). Endoscopic submucosal dissection of GCP has also been reported, with removal of coexistent early gastric cancer.[271] In some cases, surgical resection will be required.

Grossly, the gastric mucosal surface demonstrates multiple nodules and exophytic masses. On section, the gastric wall is thick, and multiple cysts are present. Microscopically, the mucosa shows foveolar hyperplasia with cystic glands extending through a disrupted muscularis mucosa into the submucosa and, rarely, into the muscularis propria (Fig. 54.13). There is associated chronic inflammation, and splayed muscle bundles lie between the dilated glands.

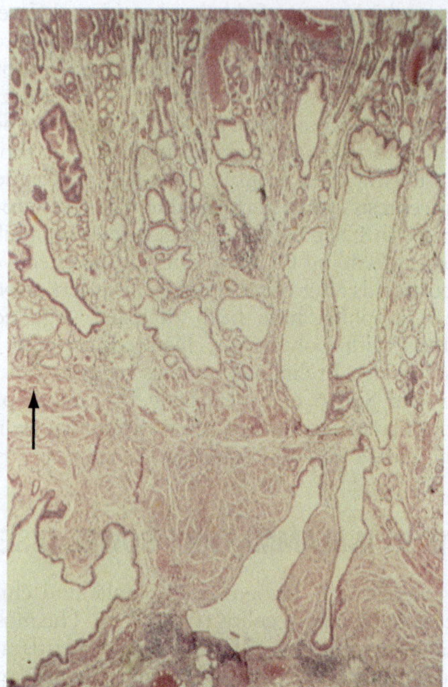

Fig. 54.13 Histopathology of gastritis cystica profunda. Note the cystic dilatation of numerous gastric glands that extend through the muscularis mucosae (*arrow*), simulating a gastric carcinoma (H&E stain).

ALLERGIC GASTRITIS

Infants allergic to cow's milk protein may manifest hematemesis and melena with a wide spectrum of gastritis and gastropathy at gastroscopy (see also Chapter 10).[278] Gastric mucosal biopsy in such infants may show neutrophilic or eosinophilic gastritis with mucosal hemorrhage. In contrast, children diagnosed with food allergies by an open elimination challenge test have no higher incidence of gastritis than children without food allergy.[279]

REACTIVE GASTROPATHIES

The epithelial cells of the gastric mucosa may be damaged by a variety of mechanisms that do not produce a significant inflammatory infiltrate. This injury leads to rapid epithelial restitution (resurfacing) and to cell regeneration with foveolar hyperplasia. Because of the paucity of inflammatory cells, the mentioned lesions are better referred to as *reactive gastropathy*, although the older term "acute erosive gastritis" is still sometimes used. Reactive gastropathy is present in approximately 15% of endoscopic biopsies of the gastric mucosa. Its incidence increases with age and, ironically, with inflammatory conditions elsewhere in the GI tract.[280]

The endoscopic appearance of the gastric mucosa of patients who exhibit reactive gastropathy demonstrates a spectrum of reddish streaks,[281] subepithelial hemorrhages, mucosal erosions, and even acute ulcers. Acute erosions and ulcers are frequently multiple, and the base of these lesions often stains dark brown owing to exposure of hemoglobin to gastric acid.

Grossly, most gastric erosions and acute gastric ulcers appear as well-defined hemorrhagic lesions 1–2 mm in diameter. If the insult is severe, the mucosa between the lesions can be intensely hemorrhagic. Microscopically, an erosion demonstrates superficial lamina propria necrosis. An acute ulcer is an area of necrosis that extends to the muscularis mucosa. Foveolar hyperplasia, a sign of epithelial regeneration (Fig. 54.14-IA and B), is often associated with glands that have atypical nuclei that can be misdiagnosed as dysplasia or even carcinoma. The diagnosis of neoplasia in a background of mucosal necrosis, cellular debris, and granulation tissue should be made with utmost caution. The biopsy procedure itself may induce tissue hemorrhage; thus subepithelial hemorrhage should involve more than one-fourth of a biopsy specimen to be considered significant. In some patients with reactive gastropathy, the stomach may "light up" during PET scanning.[282]

GASTRIC ANTRAL VASCULAR ECTASIA

Although the most common cause of reactive gastropathy is acute erosive gastritis. It can also be seen in gastric antral vascular ectasia (GAVE). This is usually seen in patients with portal hypertension. Endoscopy typically reveals features of "watermelon stomach." The biopsy from GAVE patients shows reactive

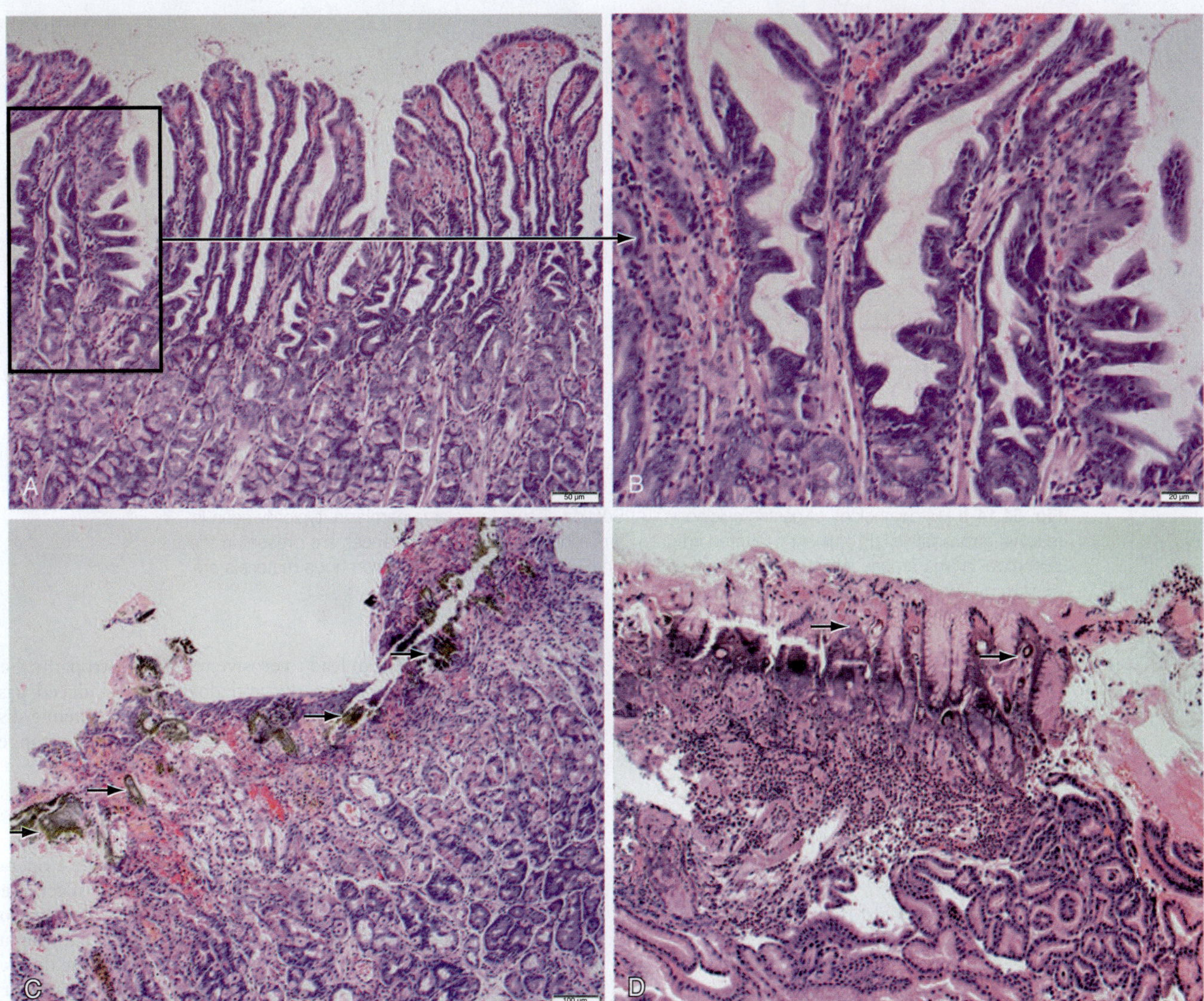

Fig. 54.14-I Histopathology of foveolar hyperplasia, typically seen in reactive gastropathies. (A and B) The gastric pits show an elongated, corkscrew appearance (H&E stains ×100 and ×200, respectively). (C) Iron pill gastritis. The mucosa is eroded and showed amorous martials (*arrows*) representing iron deposition (H&E ×100). (D) Doxycycline-induced gastric injury. Section shows erosive mucosa with distinctive capillary degeneration (*arrows*) (H&E ×200).

gastropathy with associated fibrin thrombi in the lamina propria Fig. 54.15.

Medications, Toxins, and Illicit Drugs

Ingestion of aspirin and/or nonaspirin nonsteroidal anti-inflammatory drugs (NSAIDs), including COX-2-selective inhibitors, are very common causes of reactive gastropathy.[269] The relationship between NSAID gastropathy and peptic ulcer is discussed in Chapter 53. Other medications that can injure the stomach are listed in Table 54.4.[283–290] Lanthanum carbonate (Fosrenol) is a phosphate binder used in patients with end-stage renal disease; the lanthanum phosphate produced can deposit in the gastric mucosa (Fig. 54.16), causing whitish spots and tissue histiocytosis.[290]

TABLE 54.4 Some Medications, Toxins, and Illicit Drugs That May Cause Reactive Gastropathy

Medications	Toxins and Illicit Drugs
Aspirin, other NSAIDs, and COX-2 inhibitors	Caustic/corrosive agents (see Chapter 28)
Bisphosphonates (e.g., alendronate)	Cocaine
Bromazepam (a schedule IV benzodiazepine)	Ethyl alcohol
Cancer chemotherapy drugs	Heavy metals (e.g., mercury sulfate)
Fluorides	Ketamine (inhaled for recreational use)
Iron supplements	Selenium
Sodium phosphate (bowel preps)	

NSAIDs, Nonsteroidal anti-inflammatory drugs.

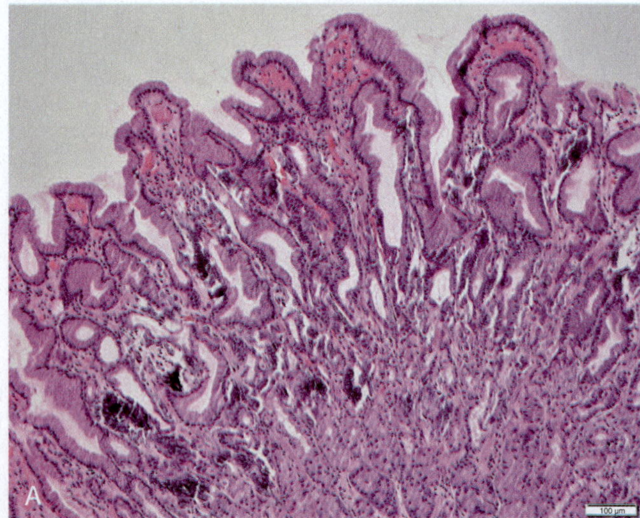

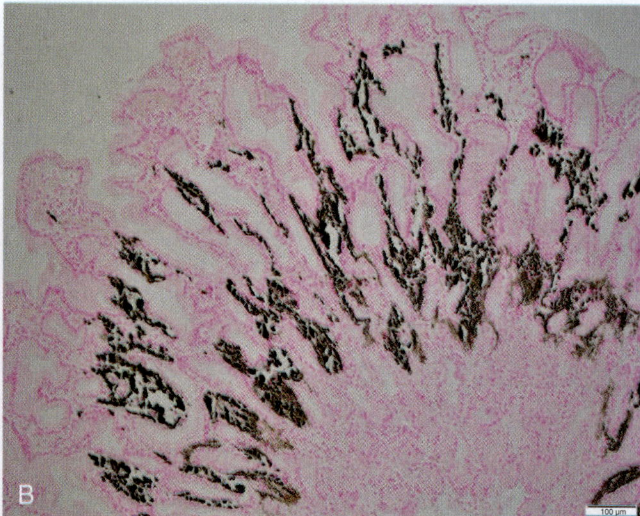

Fig. 54.14-II Histopathology of gastric calcinosis. (A) Section shows foveolar hyperplasia, typically seen in reactive gastropathies. Prominent scattered irregular, amorphous basophilic substances are present in the superficial lamina propria, abutting the gastric epithelium (H&E ×100). (B) These amorphous materials are positive by von Kossa special stain (von Kossa ×100).

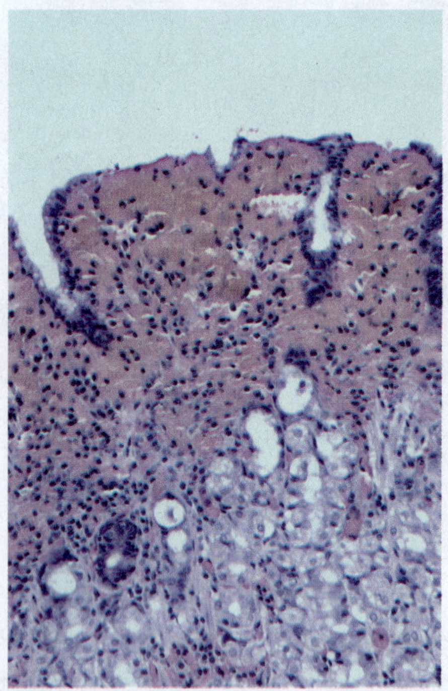

Fig. 54.15 Histopathology of alcoholic gastropathy. Hemorrhage is confined to the superficial portion of the mucosa, with a paucity of inflammatory cells (H&E stain).

Numerous toxins and illicit drugs can damage the stomach, with ethanol being the most common. After[291] acute ethanol ingestion, subepithelial hemorrhages can be seen at endoscopy, typically without prominent mucosal inflammation on biopsy specimens (Fig. 54.15). The combined effect of alcohol and aspirin (and/or NSAID) is associated with more gastric mucosal damage than that caused by either agent alone. Hemorrhage, gastric ulceration, and pyloric or prepyloric perforation due to crack cocaine use are well described.[292] Some other causes of toxin-induced reactive gastropathy are listed in Table 54.4.

Other medications can lead to erosive reactive gastropathy. See Fig. 54.14-I for iron gastropathy and doxycycline-induced gastropathy and gastric calcinosis in Fig. 54.18. Some systemic diseases such as amyloidosis can also lead to reactive changes (Fig. 54.19).

Bile Reflux

Reflux of bile into the stomach is common after surgical operations on the stomach, including those for peptic ulcer (see Chapter 53), gastric cancer, or obesity.[293–295] Bile reflux gastropathy may also occur after procedures that allow continuous exposure of the duodenum to bile with the potential for duodenogastric bile reflux, including cholecystectomy[296] or biliary sphincterotomy.

Bile reflux gastropathy can also be found in patients who have not had surgery.[282,297] For example, adult patients with dyspeptic symptoms, who are found to have reddish streaks at gastroscopy and reactive gastropathy histologically, often have bile in their stomachs.[282] Children with proven bile reflux are mainly characterized as having foveolar hyperplasia.[297] Bile reflux gastropathy may eventually result in IM.[296]

Diagnosis of bile reflux gastropathy can be challenging because many patients with bile in their stomach have no symptoms. Thus a combination of clinical, endoscopic, and histologic findings is required. There are no universally agreed criteria for diagnosis. A bile reflux index has been proposed based on histology (the presence of IM and tissue edema and the absence of *H. pylori* and chronic inflammation). Using this index, patients with GERD were found to have a higher prevalence of bile reflux gastropathy than controls.[298] A more direct approach has been to assess the bilirubin concentration in the stomach (Bilitec 2000),[299] but this is a test for duodenogastric reflux rather than gastropathy.

Endoscopy in patients with bile reflux gastropathy shows edema, redness, erosions, and bile staining of the gastric mucosa. It is uncertain whether, in patients with prior gastrectomy, coexisting *H. pylori*–related gastritis worsens or lessens the endoscopic abnormalities.[300,301] Biopsy specimens show foveolar hyperplasia, dilated cystic glands, atypical glands that may be misdiagnosed as dysplasia or carcinoma, and a paucity of acute and chronic inflammatory cells. IM[296] and even gastric atrophy can result and may increase the risk of carcinoma in the gastric remnant (see Chapter 54). Bile-diverting procedures performed because of severe bile gastropathy do not reverse IM or gastric atrophy. It may, therefore, be worthwhile, at the time of the original gastric surgery performed for gastric cancer or peptic ulcer, to construct a 30-cm Roux-en-Y limb or perform a 10–12-cm isoperistaltic jejunal interposition to try to prevent bile gastropathy and subsequent metaplastic and atrophic changes.

Treatment of bile reflux gastropathy in the intact or operated stomach is challenging and is not based on a large number of controlled clinical trials.[302–306] In one randomized trial in bile reflux gastropathy following cholecystectomy, the PPI rabeprazole (20 mg daily), the antacid hydrotalcite (1 g three times daily), and especially their combination improved symptoms and gastric histopathologic abnormalities and also reduced bile reflux as assessed by Bilitec 2000 monitoring.[306] Sucralfate has also been used successfully in some studies, but this has not been consistent.[303,305] In most clinical trials, placebo was not given; instead, medications were compared to observation alone. Other medical therapies for bile reflux gastropathy include ursodiol and cholestyramine.[302,304] A nonrandomized study found that ursodiol appeared to be superior to a PPI.[305]

In patients who fail medical therapy, surgery is recommended for severe symptoms. For patients with bile reflux gastropathy or esophagitis following truncal vagotomy and gastrojejunostomy, it has been recommended that the gastrojejunostomy be dismantled. For patients with prior Billroth II gastrectomy and gastrojejunostomy, a Roux-en-Y diversion can be performed. Long-term results of Roux-en-Y biliary diversion in previously unoperated and in unoperated patients are good.[307,308]

Stress

Erosions and acute ulcers of the gastric mucosa may occur rapidly after major physical or thermal trauma, shock, sepsis, or head injury. These are often referred to as *stress ulcers* and are discussed in Chapter 53.

Radiation

Injury to the stomach from external ionizing radiation can be classified as acute (<6 months) or chronic (>1 year) (see Chapter 39).[309,310] The tolerance level for radiation-induced gastropathy is approximately 4500 cGy. With a gastric dose of ≥5500 cGy, most patients will develop clinical evidence of gastropathy and/or gastric ulcer formation. Long term, vascular ectasias may be seen. Selective internal radiation therapy with yttrium-90 microspheres infused into the hepatic artery to treat hepatocellular carcinoma (see Chapter 98) can also lead to reactive gastropathy. Radiation-induced gastric ulcers are usually solitary, 0.5–2 cm in diameter, and located in the antrum. Massive hemorrhagic gastropathy requiring endoscopic therapy for control of bleeding has been reported.

Graft-Versus-Host Disease

This most often occurs after allogeneic bone marrow transplantation and is less common after solid organ transplantation (see Chapter 34). Acute GVHD occurs between posttransplant Days 21 and 100, whereas chronic GVHD occurs after Day 100. The GI tract (especially the intestine) is commonly affected in acute GVHD.

Gastric GVHD is characterized by nausea, vomiting, and upper abdominal pain without diarrhea. EGD in GVHD may show mucosal loss, erosions, or edema. Gastric mucosal biopsies may be necessary to diagnose GVHD in patients without diarrhea and in patients with or without diarrhea but with normal rectosigmoid biopsy specimens, especially if these patients have upper GI symptoms. In general, however, rectosigmoid biopsies are more sensitive than gastric (or duodenal) biopsies in diagnosing acute GVHD.[311] The basic pathologic lesion of gastric GVHD consists of necrosis of single cells (apoptotic bodies) in the neck region of the gastric mucosa (Fig. 54.20). The necrosis consists of an intraepithelial vacuole filled with karyorrhectic debris and fragments of cytoplasm. A 2014 NIH conference updated the histopathologic diagnostic criteria for the major organ systems affected by acute and chronic GVHD. Within the stomach, the diagnosis is confirmed with greater than or equal to one focus of apoptosis per biopsy piece. Long-standing GVHD is marked by gland destruction, ulceration, and/or submucosal fibrosis. Inflammation is typically minimal.[312]

Ischemia

Histologic changes consistent with a reactive gastropathy may be demonstrated in patients with chronic mesenteric ischemia (see Chapter 36).[313] Chronic ischemic reactive gastropathy as well as chronic ischemic gastric ulcers may occur secondary to chronic mesenteric insufficiency or in association with atheromatous embolization.[314,315] Athletes involved in intense physical activity, especially long-distance running, may experience recurrent ischemic gastropathy and chronic GI bleeding with anemia.[316]

Prolapse

The mucosa of the gastric cardia may prolapse into the esophageal lumen during retching and vomiting and become injured.[317] Barium studies and endoscopy may demonstrate the prolapsed gastric mucosa. The prolapsed, congested mucosa may show erosions and superficial ulcerations. One study showed a high incidence of pathologic gastroesophageal acid reflux in patients with prolapse gastropathy.[318]

HYPERPLASTIC GASTROPATHIES, INCLUDING MÉNÉTRIER'S DISEASE

Hyperplastic gastropathy is a rare condition characterized by giant gastric folds associated with epithelial hyperplasia.[319] Two clinical syndromes have been identified: Zollinger-Ellison syndrome (ZES), which is discussed in Chapter 55, and Ménétrier's disease and an even rarer variant of it referred to as *hyperplastic, hypersecretory gastropathy*. Fig. 54.16-A and B demonstrates enlarged gastric folds in these conditions. The enlarged gastric folds in Ménétrier's disease are due to foveolar cell hyperplasia, edema, and variable degrees of inflammation.

Ménétrier's disease is often associated with protein-losing gastropathy (see Chapter 31) and hypochlorhydria, whereas its rare hyperplastic, hypersecretory variant is associated with increased or normal acid secretion and parietal and chief cell hyperplasia, with or without excessive gastric protein loss. Ménétrier's disease has been associated with infection with *H. pylori*, CMV, or HIV.[320–322]

Other conditions more common than Ménétrier's disease and ZES can also cause enlarged gastric folds,[319] including gastric malignancy (adenocarcinoma and lymphoma), granulomatous gastritis, gastric varices, and eosinophilic gastritis. Furthermore, pachydermoperiostosis (primary hypertrophic osteoarthropathy) has been reported to cause a type of hypertrophic gastropathy akin to Ménétrier's disease,[323,324] as has primary Sjögren's syndrome.[325]

Patients with Ménétrier's disease may present with weight loss, epigastric pain, vomiting, anorexia, dyspepsia, hematemesis, and positive fecal occult blood tests. Ménétrier's disease may be self-limited and may completely resolve in patients younger than 10 years of age or when it occurs in the postpartum period. CMV infection can cause Ménétrier's disease of childhood.[201]

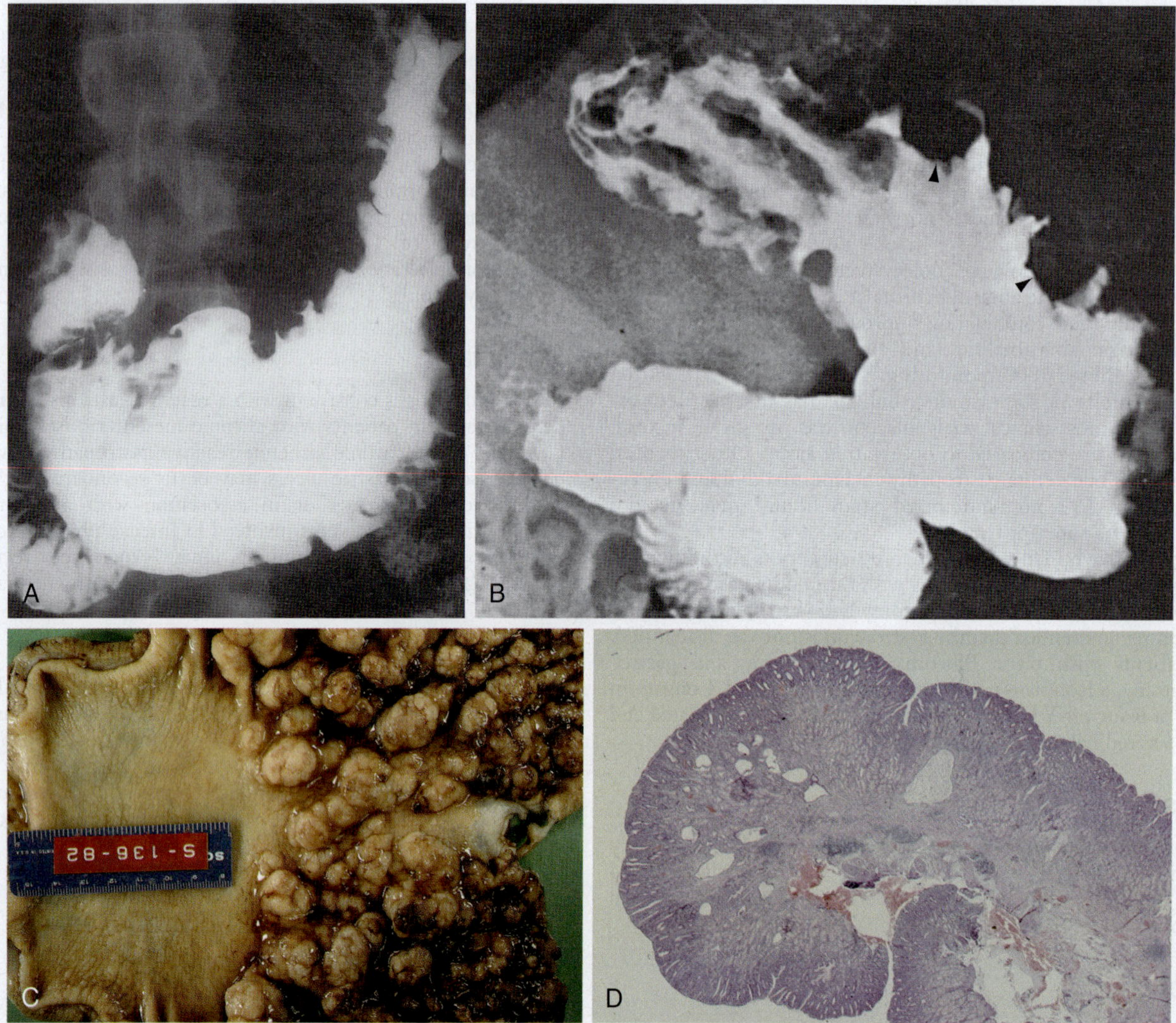

Fig. 54.16 Radiologic and histopathologic examples of hyperplastic gastropathy with giant gastric folds. (A) Film from an upper GI series in a patient with ZES. (B) Film from an upper GI series in a patient with Ménétrier's disease. (C) Total gastrectomy specimen in a patient with Ménétrier's disease (right: body, revealing hyperplastic mucosa and cerebriform folds; left: antrum, with relative sparing). (D) Histopathology of Ménétrier's disease showing enlarged folds with foveolar hyperplasia, cystically dilated glands, and minimal gastritis.

The risk of gastric cancer appears to be increased in Ménétrier's disease (see Chapter 56).[326] A fibrosing variant of the disease can mimic *linitis plastica* in the diffuse form of gastric cancer.[327]

The mucosa of patients with Ménétrier's disease demonstrates irregular hypertrophic folds that involve the entire gastric corpus. The mucosa also demonstrates an edematous, spongy appearance subdivided by creases, creating a picture like cerebral convolutions. Ménétrier's disease can be suspected when endoscopic ultrasound shows thickening in the second layer of the gastric wall (deep mucosa, normally hypoechoic) and can be confirmed histologically by endoscopic mucosal resection.[328,329] A polypoid variant of Ménétrier's disease that resembles multiple hyperplastic gastric polyps has been described.

Gastric resection specimens from patients with Ménétrier's disease typically show large polypoid gastric folds or large cerebriform gastric folds with antral sparing (see Fig. 54.21). In the absence of a gastrectomy, a full-thickness gastric mucosal biopsy is required to adequately assess the gastric histology in patients with hyperplastic gastropathy. The predominant microscopic feature of Ménétrier's disease and hyperplastic, hypersecretory gastropathy is foveolar hyperplasia with cystic dilation (see Fig. 54.22). The parietal and chief cells may be decreased and replaced by mucous glands in typical Ménétrier's disease.

The etiology of Ménétrier's disease is unknown, although some cases have undoubtedly been caused by infection with CMV or *H. pylori*. Concurrence of the disorder in identical twin men, who presented at ages 29 and 35, suggests a genetic component.[330] A germline mutation in *SMAD4* associated with juvenile polyposis can lead to a mixed hypertrophic/polypoid gastropathy.[331] Hyperplasia of surface mucous cells may be due to enhanced EGF signaling in the gastric mucosa due to local overproduction of TGF-α.[332] A unifying working hypothesis for juvenile polyposis syndrome and Ménétrier's disease has been proposed.[331] The authors hypothesized a mechanism that involves TGF-β-SMAD4 pathway inactivation and TGF-α overexpression related to *H. pylori* infection.[332] An association between UC and Ménétrier's disease has been proposed.[333]

Ideal treatment of hyperplastic gastropathy is unclear because the condition is so rare and controlled trials are lacking. Spontaneous resolution may occur, especially in children. Ganciclovir has been used in children with Ménétrier's disease associated with

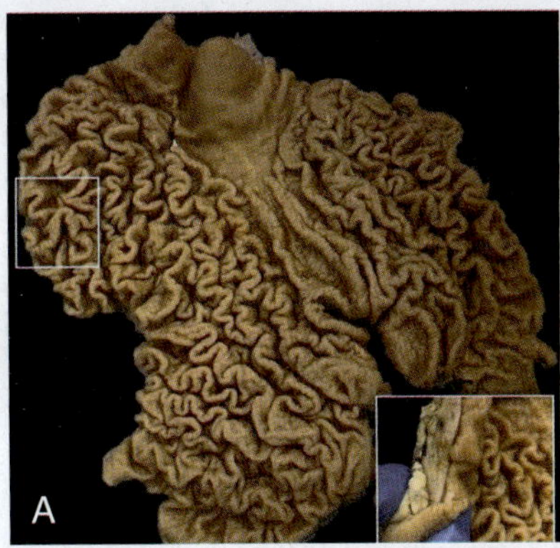

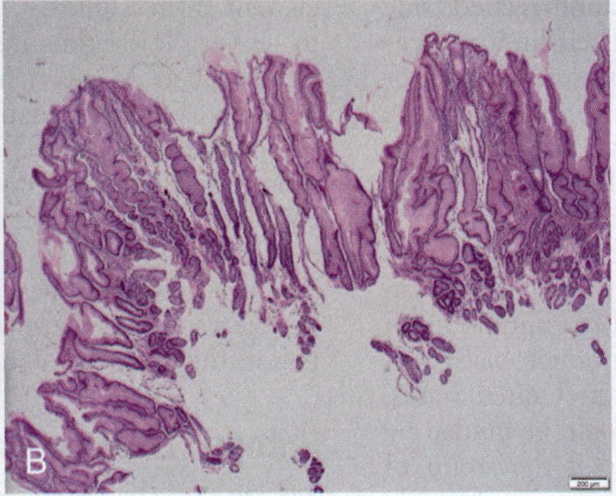

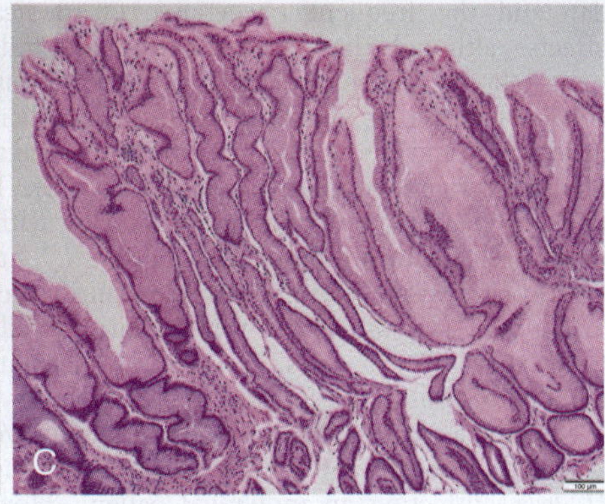

Fig. 54.16-II (A) Total gastrectomy specimen in a patient with Ménétrier's disease. Body is revealing hyperplastic mucosa and cerebriform folds. *Inlet* image shows side aspect of gastric-wall thickness. Lower part of the gastrectomy shows antrum with relative sparing. (B and C) Histopathology of Ménétrier's disease showing foveolar hyperplasia and minimal gastritis (H&E ×40 and ×100, respectively).

TABLE 54.5 Effect of Intravenous Cetuximab on the Course of Ménétrier's Disease in Seven Patients Treated at One Institution[333,349]

Patient	Duration of Cetuximab (Months or Cycles)	Most Recent Histology	Posttreatment Status
1	18	Minimal FH	Off treatment
2	15	Minimal FH	Off treatment
3	40	Minimal FH	Still on treatment
4	9	Normal	Gastrectomy
5	24	Dysplastic lesion 12 mo after therapy stopped	Gastrectomy
6	9	FH	Gastrectomy
7	8	FH	Gastrectomy

FH, Foveolar hyperplasia.

CMV gastritis. *H. pylori* infection should be sought and treated, if present. Symptoms may improve with antisecretory agents,[334] especially if the patient has ZES or the normogastrinemic hyperplastic, hypersecretory variant of Ménétrier's disease. Gastric antisecretory drugs may reduce gastric protein loss by strengthening intercellular tight junctions.

Some patients with Ménétrier's disease have responded to infusions of cetuximab,[333] a monoclonal antibody against the EGF receptor (Table 54.5). Others have responded to the somatostatin analog octreotide.[335,336] Partial or total gastric resection is reserved for severe complications, including refractory or recurrent bleeding, obstruction, severe hypoproteinemia, and dysplasia or cancer development.

PORTAL HYPERTENSIVE GASTROPATHY

This condition represents an important cause of GI blood loss in patients with portal hypertension. Gastric mucosal biopsies show vascular ectasia and congestion without significant inflammatory infiltrate or reactive gastropathy (see Chapters 21 and 94).

DIFFERENTIAL DIAGNOSIS

The most important disorders that can simulate gastritis and gastropathy are gastric polyps (neoplastic and nonneoplastic) and gastric malignancy (see Chapters 41 and 54). Although CT criteria have been useful in distinguishing gastritis/gastropathy from gastric malignancy,[337] endoscopy and gastric biopsy with review by an expert pathologist are the most useful diagnostic procedures. Increased fluoro-deoxyglucose uptake by the stomach, especially its proximal half, is occasionally seen during PET scanning in patients with reactive gastropathy (acute erosive gastritis) and should not be confused with neoplasia.[282] Demonstration of B cell clonality (e.g., by immunostaining) can also help distinguish gastric marginal zone lymphomas from chronic lymphocytic gastritis or lymphomatoid gastropathy.

TREATMENT

H. pylori Infection

The most recent recommendations on the treatment of *H. pylori* infection come from the Toronto consensus conference, an updated guideline from the American College of Gastroenterology (ACG), and the Maastricht VI/Florence consensus report.[147,148,338]

The treatment of *H. pylori* infection varies worldwide, although certain principles of treatment are generally agreed upon. Specific recommendations in different parts of the world generally reflect availability and resistance patterns to antimicrobial agents and local concerns about certain outcomes of infection, such as gastric cancer. Major guidelines for management reflect general management concordance, with regional differences.[339–369] Historically, recommended treatment regimens for *H. pylori* infection generally included a PPI plus two antibiotics given together for 10–14 days. However, recent recommendations have moved toward a standard 14-day treatment duration, as shorter treatment durations are associated with reduced effectiveness. However, some flexibility in treatment duration is offered in view of insufficient evidence from randomized controlled trials to support a strong recommendation for a specific treatment duration. Furthermore, some quadruple combinations of a PPI and three antimicrobial agents are now generally recommended.[148]

Adherence to treatment can be problematic because of the requirement to take multiple medicines at different times of the day and the frequent occurrence of medication-related side effects—although these are generally mild and self-limiting. Patients should be counseled in advance about expected minor adverse effects (e.g., diarrhea and taste disturbance) that they may experience and about the importance of taking all prescribed medicines together for the complete course. Treatment success rates vary among countries and regionally within countries, primarily related to antibiotic resistance.[342,343] From a study from Houston, resistance rates to five antibiotics are shown in Table 54.6. *H. pylori* strains were sensitive to all five antibiotics in fewer than 50% of cases.[359] Table 54.7 lists antimicrobial resistance rates from different studies performed in the United States.

Ideally, a personalized treatment regimen would be guided by knowledge of the antibiotic resistance pattern of the strain of *H. pylori* infecting an individual patient. However, as of early 2023, such information is still difficult to obtain in contemporary U.S. practice because relatively few commercial laboratories routinely offer this service. However, this is changing with the growing availability of NGS that can be performed on gastric biopsy material or on a fecal sample. In the future, the increased availability of NGS should simplify practice as it will become much simpler to determine a patient's *H. pylori* status and—if positive—to design a treatment regimen based on the results of reflexive testing for antimicrobial resistance and susceptibility. However, and until then, it is important to determine an individual patient's personal antibiotic history and to have some understanding of local antibiotic resistance patterns.[344] Patients who have a history of macrolide use (for any reason) should not be prescribed clarithromycin as part of a regimen for treating *H. pylori* infection. Similarly, patients with a history of fluoroquinolone use should not receive levofloxacin. As will be evident from Table 54.7, resistance rates to amoxicillin continue to be very low—thus making amoxicillin a valuable agent in the treatment of *H. pylori* infection. Patients with a true allergy to penicillin (e.g., an anaphylaxis-type reaction) clearly cannot be prescribed amoxicillin. However, many patients have a much more questionable history of penicillin "allergy" (e.g., a rash in childhood). Such patients are unlikely to be truly allergic to penicillin. The 2017 update on the management of *H. pylori* infection from the ACG recommended that such patients should be referred to an allergist to determine if they are truly allergic.[147] If not, they can be safely treated with amoxicillin.

TABLE 54.6 Antimicrobial Drug Resistance in 135 Hp Strains Isolated From Patients in Houston

Antimicrobial Drug	% of Strains Resistant (95% CI)
Amoxicillin	0
Clarithromycin	16% (10%–23%)
Levofloxacin	31% (23%–39%)
Metronidazole	20% (13%–27%)
Tetracycline	1% (0%–2%)

From Shiota S, Reddy R, Alsarra A, et al. Antibiotic resistance of *Helicobacter pylori* among male United States veterans. *Clin Gastro Hepatol*. 2015;13:1616–1624.

Primary Treatments

The 2017 update of the ACG's practice guideline included several regimens as possible primary treatments for *H. pylori* infection.[147] The strength of recommendation and quality of evidence given to each regimen are summarized in Table 54.8. A variety of "primary" treatments were suggested so that clinicians would have some flexibility in choosing the best regimen for an individual patient, assuming some knowledge of the patient's prior antibiotic history. Strong recommendations were made for only a small number of primary treatment regimens. Although not all currently available PPIs are approved by the U.S. FDA as part of treatment regimens for *H. pylori* infection, there is little difference within this class of drugs with respect to efficacy in the treatment of *H. pylori* infection.

Clarithromycin triple therapy comprises the twice-daily combination of clarithromycin 500 mg, amoxicillin 1000 mg, and a PPI in standard dose taken for 14 days. Patients who are genuinely allergic to penicillin should receive metronidazole 500 mg three times daily in place of amoxicillin. Although clarithromycin triple therapy remains frequently used, it has fallen into disfavor because of rising rates of clarithromycin resistance. In general, clarithromycin should not be used in the treatment of *H. pylori* infection unless there is evidence from antimicrobial sensitivity testing that the strain is clarithromycin-susceptible. Clarithromycin should not be given to patients for the treatment of *H. pylori* infection if they have previously received it or any other macrolide (such as azithromycin) for any indication. Clarithromycin resistance is best considered an absolute phenomenon that cannot be overcome by increasing the dose of clarithromycin.

Bismuth-based quadruple therapy is another recommended primary treatment option. It consists of the combination of a bismuth salt (e.g., bismuth subsalicylate or bismuth subcitrate),

TABLE 54.7 Resistance Rates (%) of *H. pylori* to Specific Antibiotics as Reported in U.S.-Based Studies

References	Years of study	CLA	MET	AMOX	TET	LEVO	RIF
1	2009–2013	16	20	0	1	31	NR
2	2000–2016	30	43	2	<1	14	NR
3	2009–2019	43	42	NR	NR	69	NR
4	2017–2018	17	17	6	3	58	0
5	2018–2019	30	30	1	<1	30	<1
6	2019–2021	22	22	2	NR	NR	NR

1 Shiota et al. *Clin Gastroenterol Hepatol*. 2015;13:1616.
2 Mosites et al. *J Glob Antimicrob Resist*. 2018;15:148.
3 Kumar et al. *GastroHep*. 2020;2:6.
4 Hulten et al. *Gastroenterology*. 2021;161:342.
5 Argueta et al. *Gastroenterology*. 2021;160:2181.
6 Mégraud et al. *Am J Gastroenterol*. 2023;in press. (Note that the study by Kumar et al. was conducted among patients with previous failed attempts at cure of *H. pylori* infection—thereby accounting for the particularly high resistance rates.)
AMOX, Amoxicillin; *CLA*, clarithromycin; *LEVO*, levofloxacin; *MET*, metronidazole; *NR*, not reported; *RIF*, rifabutin; *TET*, tetracycline.

tetracycline, metronidazole, and a PPI for 10–14 days. Because this regimen contains neither clarithromycin nor amoxicillin, it is an appropriate choice for patients who have previously used macrolides, who reside in areas with high (≥15%) macrolide resistance, and for those who are truly penicillin-allergic. The presence of clarithromycin resistance does not influence the effectiveness of bismuth-based quadruple therapy. A combination capsule containing bismuth subcitrate 140 mg, metronidazole 125 mg, and tetracycline 125 mg may help to simplify bismuth-based quadruple therapy for patients. In two separate studies, patients treated with three of these combination capsules four times daily and a PPI twice daily for 10 days had comparable eradication rates compared with standard 10-day clarithromycin triple therapy (88% vs. 83%),[353] and significantly higher efficacy when compared with 7-day clarithromycin triple therapy.[354,355] However, and as noted above, treatment of *H. pylori* infection is generally recommended to last 14 days. In a nonrandomized study from Brown University, Rhode Island, bismuth-based quadruple therapy was the most efficacious regimen employed—and the only one to achieve successful eradication in close to 90% of patients treated.[370] Substituting doxycycline for tetracycline was associated with lower eradication rates.

Concomitant therapy (also known as nonbismuth-based quadruple therapy) is the quadruple combination of clarithromycin, amoxicillin, metronidazole (or tinidazole), and a PPI. Although it was one of the recommended primary treatments in the 2017 ACG guideline, there have been no U.S.-based clinical trials assessing its effectiveness. Optimal duration of treatment is uncertain. It is no longer generally recommended because of its use of three antibiotics, which makes it almost inevitable that some patients (e.g., those with a clarithromycin-susceptible strain) would receive one unnecessary antibiotic (in this case, metronidazole).

Except for bismuth-based quadruple therapy, all the regimens listed earlier include clarithromycin. In view of the problem of clarithromycin resistance, regimens that replace clarithromycin with an alternative antimicrobial have been developed for first-line treatment. The most frequently evaluated alternative to clarithromycin has been levofloxacin. Regimens have usually combined it with a PPI and amoxicillin. Levofloxacin triple therapy has not been formally evaluated as a first-line treatment in North America. However, studies from around the world indicate that it has similar efficacy as clarithromycin triple therapy but that local rates of antimicrobial resistance limit its effectiveness.

Treatment-related adverse effects can occur in as many as 50% of patients taking one of the treatment regimens described in Table 54.8, but generally these are mild and do not require discontinuation of therapy. Some of the more common adverse effects include taste alteration and GI upset with metronidazole and clarithromycin, and diarrhea with amoxicillin. In addition, tetracycline should not be prescribed to children or women of childbearing potential. Adverse effects of treatment regimens for *H. pylori* infection have been extensively reviewed.[345,346]

TABLE 54.8 Summary of First-Line Treatment Regimens as Recommended in the 2017 ACG Clinical Guideline on the Treatment of Hp Infection

First-Line Regimen	Components	Duration (Days)	Recommendation	Level of Evidence	Comments
Clarithromycin triple therapy	PPI, clarithromycin 500 mg, and amoxicillin 1000 mg, each twice daily (or, if penicillin allergic, metronidazole 500 mg 3 times daily in place of amoxicillin)	14	Conditional	Low (for duration, moderate)	Avoid in patients with prior macrolide exposure. Avoid in areas where local clarithromycin resistance rate is 15%
Bismuth-based quadruple therapy	PPI twice daily, bismuth subcitrate or subsalicylate four times daily, tetracycline 500 mg four times daily, and metronidazole 250–500 mg three or four times daily	10–14	Strong	Low	Particularly recommended for patients with prior macrolide exposure or proven penicillin allergy
Concomitant therapy	PPI, clarithromycin 500 mg, and amoxicillin 1000 mg, and a nitroimidazole 500 mg, each twice daily	10–14	Strong	Very low	Nitroimidazole may be metronidazole or tinidazole
Sequential therapy	PPI and amoxicillin 1000 mg, both twice daily PPI, clarithromycin 500 mg, and a nitroimidazole 500 mg, each twice daily	5–7 5–7	Conditional	Low (for duration, very low)	Nitroimidazole may be metronidazole or tinidazole
Hybrid therapy	PPI and amoxicillin 1000 mg, both twice daily PPI, clarithromycin 500 mg, amoxicillin 1000 mg, and a nitroimidazole 500 mg, each twice daily	7 7	Conditional	Low (for duration, very low)	Nitroimidazole may be metronidazole or tinidazole
Levofloxacin triple therapy	PPI twice daily, levofloxacin 500 mg once daily, and amoxicillin 1000 mg twice daily	10–14	Conditional	Low (for duration, very low)	–
Levofloxacin sequential therapy	PPI and amoxicillin 1000 mg, each twice daily PPI and amoxicillin 1000 mg, each twice daily, levofloxacin 500 mg once daily, and a nitroimidazole 500 mg twice daily	5–7 5–7	Conditional	Low (for duration, very low)	Nitroimidazole may be metronidazole or tinidazole

Modified from Checchi S, Montanaro A, Pasqui L, et al. l-Thyroxine requirement in patients with autoimmune hypothyroidism and parietal cell antibodies. *J Clin Endocrinol Metab*. 2008;93:465–469.

Counseling patients to expect minor adverse effects is likely to improve adherence rates.[348]

Since the publication of the 2017 ACG practice guideline on the management of *H. pylori* infection, additional regimens have been evaluated in U.S.-based clinical trials and subsequently approved by the FDA. The first comprises a fixed-dose triple combination of omeprazole, rifabutin, and amoxicillin (Talicia; RedHill Biopharma, Raleigh, NC). In a randomized trial comparing it to the dual combination of omeprazole and amoxicillin (given in the same doses as Talicia but without the rifabutin component), intent-to-treat (ITT) eradication rates were 83.8% for Talicia and 57.7% for omeprazole and amoxicillin ($P < .0001$). Among patients with demonstrated adherence to study medications, corresponding rates were 90.3% and 64.7%, respectively ($P < .0001$).[371] The total daily dose of rifabutin in this regimen is 150 mg. Since this is given for only 14 days, the risk of myelotoxicity is probably minimal. In the clinical trial cited here, there was no prevalent or incident resistance to rifabutin documented.

Potassium-competitive acid blockers (P-CABs) are novel gastric antisecretory drugs that act on H^+, K^+-ATPase in a manner different to the PPIs.[372] One such agent—vonoprazan—has been evaluated in combination with one or two antibiotics for the treatment of *H. pylori* infection in a randomized clinical trial in the United States and Europe.[373] A 14-day dual regimen (vonoprazan 20 mg twice daily and amoxicillin 1000 mg three times daily) and a 14-day triple regimen (vonoprazan 20 mg, clarithromycin 500 mg, and amoxicillin 1000 mg—all given twice daily) were compared with the triple combination of lansoprazole 30 mg, clarithromycin 500 mg, and amoxicillin 1000 mg—all given twice daily. ITT eradication rates among patients with strains of *H. pylori* that were sensitive to both clarithromycin and amoxicillin were 84.7% for the vonoprazan triple regimen, 78.5% for the vonoprazan dual regimen, and 78.8% for the lansoprazole triple regimen. Both vonoprazan-based regimens were noninferior to the lansoprazole regimen in that analysis. Both vonoprazan-based regimens were statistically significantly superior to the lansoprazole regimen among patients with clarithromycin-resistant strains of *H. pylori* and in the entire patient population (i.e., those with either resistant or susceptible strains). Both vonoprazan-based regimens were approved by the U.S. FDA in 2022.

Neither the rifabutin-based regimen nor the vonoprazan-based regimens were included in the 2017 ACG practice guideline as no information was available on them at the time of its preparation. The Maastricht VI/Florence consensus statement did consider the role of P-CABs in the treatment of *H. pylori* infection.[338] The authors concluded that combinations of a P-CAB and antimicrobials were either noninferior or superior to PPI-based triple regimens for the treatment of *H. pylori* infection—and superior among patients with antimicrobial-resistant strains.

Rescue Treatments

Initial treatment of *H. pylori* infection fails in many patients. The most important predictors of failure of treatment are antibiotic resistance and poor adherence to treatment. Because patients' upper GI symptoms after treatment are an unreliable guide to its success or failure, all patients should be retested after treatment.[147] Posttreatment testing should be with a test of active infection such as the urea breath test or fecal antigen test; serologic testing should always be avoided after treatment of the infection. Only by the implementation of a program of routine posttreatment testing can clinicians get some understanding of the success rates of eradication treatments in practice. Patients who fail treatment with a first-line regimen should be retreated with a rescue regimen. Patients should not be treated with a clarithromycin or levofloxacin if these have been used before.

For patients with persistent infection following treatment with a clarithromycin-based primary regimen, retreatment with either bismuth-based quadruple therapy or levofloxacin-based triple therapy is recommended. Table 54.9 summarizes recommendations about rescue treatment regimens. The American Gastroenterological Association (AGA) has issued recommendations for the management of refractory *H. pylori* infection.[374] However, this is a rapidly evolving field. Given the progressive rise in antibiotic resistance rates and the development and introduction of additional treatment regimens, it is likely that there will be further refinements and updates related to this.

Primary resistance to antibiotics that are used to treat *H. pylori* infection varies widely throughout the world. For the most recently reported resistance rates in the United States, see Table 54.7. In a meta-analysis of 19 studies performed in the United States between 2011 and 2021, pooled resistance rates were 31.5% for clarithromycin, 42.1% for metronidazole, 37.6% for levofloxacin, 2.6% for amoxicillin, 0.9% for tetracycline, and 0.2% for rifabutin. Overall, 11.7% of strains were resistant to both clarithromycin and metronidazole.[375] Metronidazole and clarithromycin resistance may increase with patient age and are more common in women than in men. The low rates of resistance to amoxicillin, tetracycline, and rifabutin underscore the importance of these antibiotics in the treatment of *H. pylori* infection. Unlike the case with clarithromycin and levofloxacin, it is permissible to include amoxicillin in a rescue treatment even if it has been part of the initial failed regimen. However, this also

TABLE 54.9 Summary of Rescue Treatment Regimens as Recommended in the 2017 ACG Clinical Guideline on the Treatment of Hp Infection

Rescue Regimen	Duration (Days)	Recommendation	Level of Evidence	Comments
Bismuth-based quadruple therapy (see Table 54.8)	14	Strong	Low	Appropriate for patients who failed initial treatment with a clarithromycin-based regimen
Levofloxacin triple therapy (see Table 54.8)	14	Strong	Moderate (for duration, low)	Appropriate for patients who failed initial treatment with a clarithromycin-based regimen
Concomitant therapy (see Table 54.8)	10–14	Conditional	Very low	
Rifabutin triple therapy	10	Conditional	Moderate (for duration, very low)	PPI twice daily, rifabutin 300 mg once daily, and amoxicillin 1000 mg twice daily
High-dose dual therapy	14	Conditional	Low (for duration, very low)	PPI and amoxicillin 750 mg, each four times daily

Modified from Checchi S, Montanaro A, Pasqui L, et al. l-Thyroxine requirement in patients with autoimmune hypothyroidism and parietal cell antibodies. *J Clin Endocrinol Metab*. 2008;93:465–469.

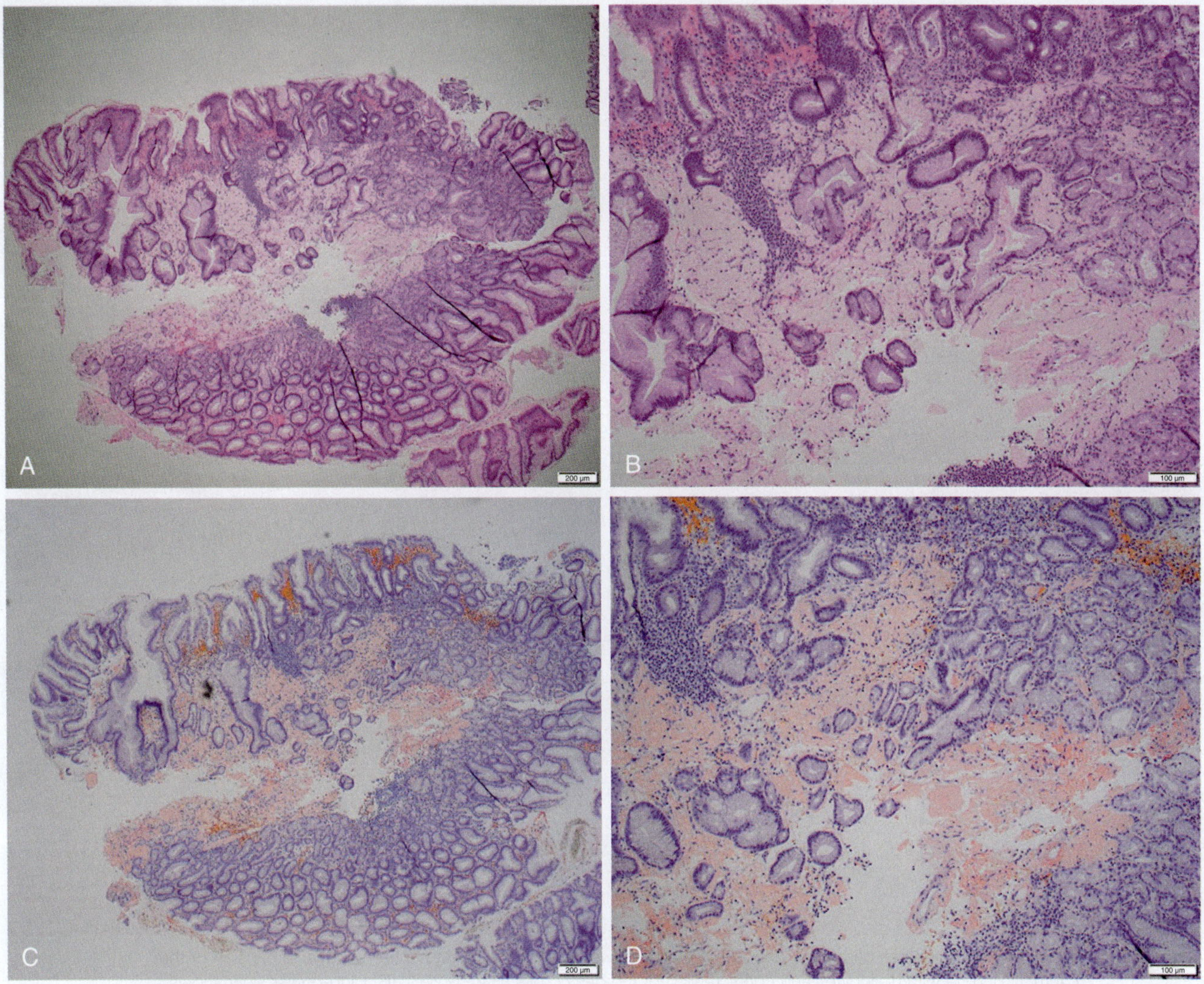

Fig. 54.17 (A and B) Biopsy shows amorphous, eosinophilic materials present in lamina propria, submucosa, and around blood vessels (H&E ×40 and ×100, respectively). (C and D) Congo red special stain demonstrates red staining (Congo red ×40 and ×100, respectively). Congo red stain will reveal apple green birefringence under polarization.

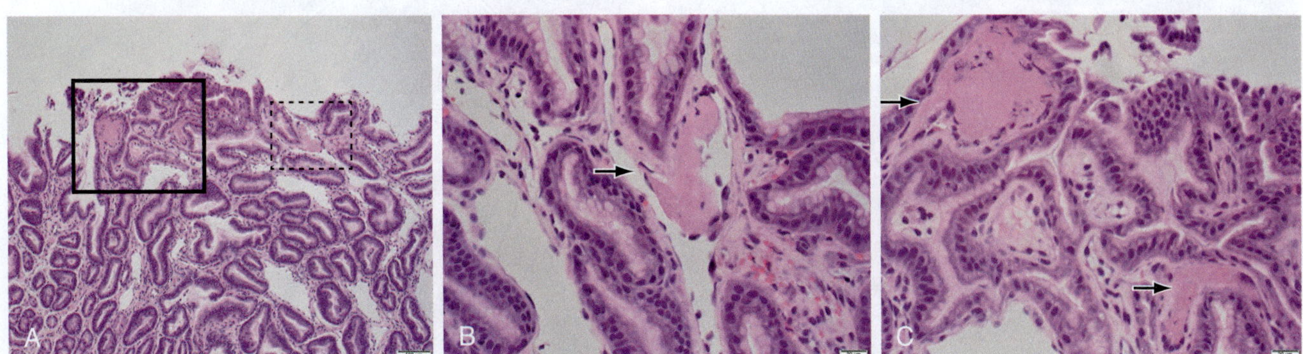

Fig. 54.18 Gastric antral vascular ectasia. (A) Section shows antral mucosa with increase in blood vessel number and diameter. It is usually associated with reactive foveolar epithelial changes and resembles reactive gastropathy (H&E ×100). (B and C) Higher power magnification shows dilated blood vessels in the lamina propria with associated fibrin thrombi (H&E ×400).

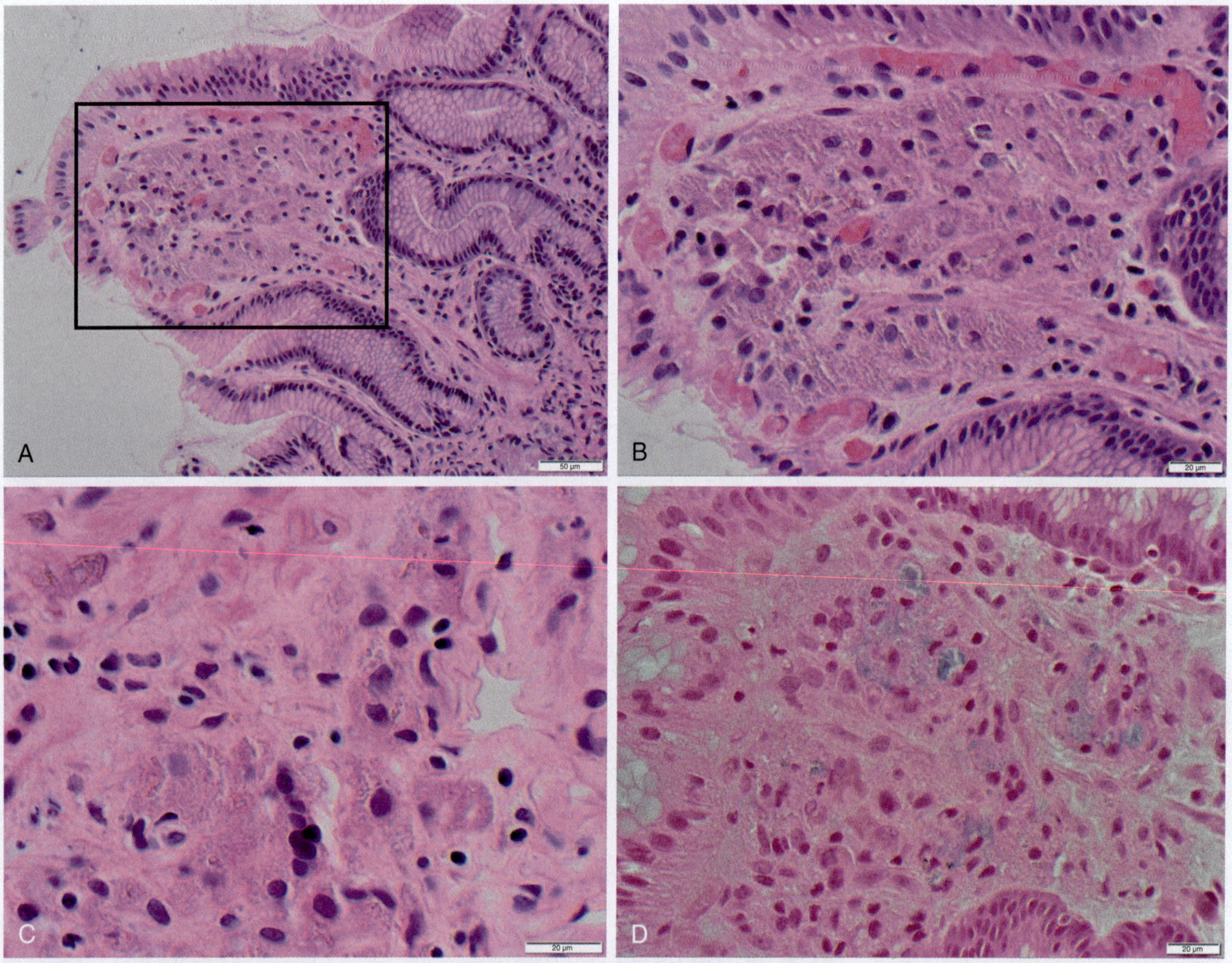

Fig. 54.19 Lanthanum carbonate deposits. (A) Low-power view of the gastric antrum shows expansion of the lamina propria with histiocytes and corkscrewing of the gastric pits (H&E ×200). (B) High-power view shows histiocytes forming a vaguely round aggregate (H&E ×400). (C) The granular amorphous material in histiocytes that appears light brown to purple (H&E ×600). (D) Some of these deposits variably stain with Prussian blue stain (iron stain) may cause confusion with iron-therapy-related gastric injury, although in that condition, the deposits usually appear as yellow to brown coarse extracellular deposits in the superficial lamina propria that stain strongly with Prussian blue stain (Iron stain ×400).

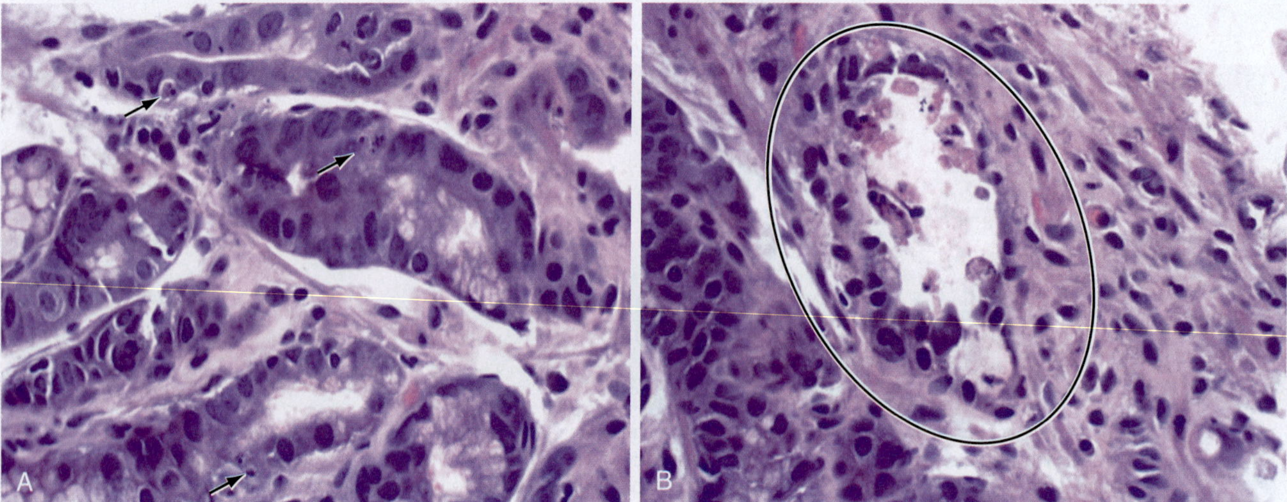

Fig. 54.20 Graft versus host disease (GVHD). (A) Sections mild lymphoplasmacytic inflammation with scattered eosinophils in the lamina propria. Apoptotic bodies are seen (*arrows*) as the main feature of GVHD, although not specific (H&E ×400). (B) It may have severe gland or crypt distortion/destruction (circle) (H&E ×400).

highlights the problem of amoxicillin "allergy" in contemporary U.S. clinical practice. Up to 10% of the adult U.S. population may claim to be allergic to penicillin(s), which would ordinarily preclude the use of amoxicillin as part of a treatment regimen for *H. pylori* infection. However, up to 90% of those will have negative skin testing for penicillin allergy,[376] indicating the absence of a true sensitivity. Therefore patients who fail first-line treatment for *H. pylori* infection and who give a history of penicillin "allergy" should ideally be referred to an allergist for formal allergy testing. If found to be nonallergic, an amoxicillin-based rescue treatment (see Table 54.9) can be used safely.

Antibiotic resistance significantly affects the success of clarithromycin-based triple therapy but is less important with bismuth-based regimens. Clarithromycin resistance consistently affects treatment outcomes, whereas metronidazole resistance appears to be more of an in vitro than an in vivo phenomenon when metronidazole is used in an appropriate regimen. Resistance to clarithromycin appears to be absolute and cannot be easily overcome by increasing the dose. One of three bacterial point mutations within its conserved loop of 23S strand of ribosomal RNA (A2143G, A2142G, and A2142C) can interfere with ribosomal macrolide binding and lead to clarithromycin resistance.[133] The A2143G mutation appears to have the greatest adverse effect on treatment and is probably the major reason for failure of a clarithromycin-based regimen. Because testing for specific mutations is not yet widely clinically available, it is essential that clarithromycin is not included in any regimen if clarithromycin resistance is suspected or confirmed by culture and sensitivity testing. In contrast, resistance to metronidazole appears to be a relative phenomenon that can be overcome in most instances by using a higher dose (500 mg) or combining the drug with a bismuth preparation. A bacterial point mutation(s) that prevents reduction of metronidazole to its active metabolite is responsible for drug resistance.[133,342]

Recurrence of *H. pylori* infection includes both reinfection (new strain) and recrudescence (original strain). Recrudescence tends to dominate in the first year after therapy and true reinfection thereafter. Recrudescence may be associated with a false-negative posttreatment diagnostic test result at 6–8 weeks. In a critical review of the global literature, the overall annual *H. pylori* recurrence risk ranged from 3.4% (95% CI, 3.1–3.7) in developed countries to 8.7% (95% CI, 8.8–9.6) in developing countries.[366] In the United States and Western Europe, adult reinfection is probably less than 1% annually. Reinfection tends to be more common in children and is also reported to be higher in adults living in areas of the world with high *H. pylori* prevalence.[367] In seven Latin American communities, the overall 1-year recurrence rate was 11.5%, with a range from 6.8% to 18.1% among sites.[368,369]

Over the past few decades, there have been reported associations of *H. pylori* infection with several nongastroduodenal diseases,[377] including immune thrombocytopenic purpura (ITP)[378,379] and iron deficiency with or without anemia.[380] The American Society of Hematology recommends testing adults with ITP for *H. pylori* infection and treating them for it if positive. An AGA Clinical Practice Guideline has recommended that patients with iron deficiency anemia and no identifiable cause after colonoscopy and EGD should have noninvasive testing for *H. pylori*—followed by treatment, if positive.[381]

Prevention of *H. pylori* Infection

A three-dose oral vaccine using the B-subunit of *H. pylori*'s urease (fused with the B subunit of *E. coli* heat-labile enterotoxin as an adjuvant) reduced naturally acquired *H. pylori* infection by 72% in the first postvaccine year among 4000 initially uninfected Chinese children aged 6–15. The efficacy of this vaccine waned to approximately 55% in the 2nd and 3rd postvaccine years.[382] This oral vaccine had a similar adverse effect profile to placebo vaccine. Other vaccine trials in geographic areas with a high prevalence of *H. pylori* infection are anticipated.

A case-control study, also performed in China in a region with a very high prevalence of chronic gastritis and gastric cancer, found that ingestion of green tea reduced the risk of both gastritis and gastric cancer by close to 50%.[383]

Acknowledgment

The authors thank Mark Feldman and Pamela J. Jensen, who previously contributed to parts of this chapter.

Full references for this chapter can be found at https://ebooks.health.elsevier.com.

55 Peptic Ulcer Disease

Ivan S.F. Lau, Francis K.L. Chan, James Y.W. Lau

IN THIS CHAPTER

An ulcer in the GI tract can be defined as a 5 mm or larger break in the lining of the mucosa, with appreciable depth at endoscopy or with histologic evidence of submucosal extension. An erosion is a break less than 5 mm. The distinction between an ulcer and an erosion is somewhat arbitrary. The term PUD is used to include ulcerations and erosions in the stomach and duodenum from a number of causes. These lesions are called "peptic" because the enzyme pepsin, proteolytic at an acidic pH (see Chapter 53), plays a major role in causing the mucosal breaks, regardless of the inciting agent.

Decades of research focused on the role of gastric acid secretion and the effects of stress, personality type, and genetics in the pathogenesis of PUD. The discovery of the histamine-2 (H_2) receptor and development of H2RAs,[1] and subsequently PPIs, led to major changes in the management of PUD. The discovery of Hp and its role in PUD (see Chapter 54) transformed PUD from a chronic, recurrent disease to a curable one.[2] Hp infection remains an important cause of PUD in the world. In developed countries, frequent use of NSAIDs, including low-dose aspirin for cardiovascular indications, has emerged as a leading cause of PUD, especially among the aging population.

EPIDEMIOLOGY

The epidemiology of PUD has undergone remarkable changes in the last two centuries. The risk of developing PUD and dying from PUD increased in successive cohorts born between 1840 and 1890 and then declined thereafter.[3] There was a peak in the incidence of GU in the first half of the 19th century and a subsequent peak in the incidence of DU in the second half of the 19th century. Sonnenberg proposed a birth-cohort effect to explain the peaks in the incidence of, and mortality from, peptic ulcers. Hp infection acquired during childhood or adolescence became manifested as peptic diseases in later years. As Hp infection gradually declined in the population over time, the prevalence of infection also gradually shifted from a younger toward older age groups. The incidence of DU and GU has declined in parallel with the decline in the prevalence of Hp infection, likely a result of improved sanitary conditions and a safer food and water supply.

Based on physicians' diagnoses, the annual incidence of PUD ranges from 0.14% to 0.19% in developed countries. Based on hospital diagnoses, the incidence is lower: 0.03%–0.17%. The prevalence of PUD ranges from 0.12% to 4.7% for physician-diagnosed and from 0.1% to 2.6% for hospital-diagnosed case series.[4] There is a wide geographic variation in the prevalence of PUD. In an endoscopic series involving 1022 volunteers from Shanghai, China (average age, 48 years), the prevalence of PUD was 17.2%, of whom 93% were infected with Hp.[5]

The most frequent complication from PUD is bleeding; the reported annual incidence of bleeding among populations varies from 19 to 57 per 100,000 individuals (≈0.02%–0.06%). Peptic ulcer perforation (PULP), less frequent than bleeding, has reported incidences of 4–14 per 100,000 individuals (0.004%–0.014%).[6] Along with a decline in uncomplicated PUD cases, there is a similar decline in the incidence of ulcer complications in recent years. Laine et al.[7] used a national inpatient database to calculate the annual incidence of, and mortality from, GI complications during 2001–2009. During this time period, the incidence of peptic ulcer bleeding fell from 48.7 to 32.1 per 100,000. Over the same period, the age- and sex-adjusted case fatality rates from UGI bleeding decreased from 3.8% to 2.7%. In 2009, the case fatality rate for UGI bleeding (2.45%) was considerably lower than for UGI perforation (10.7%). In a nationwide population-based cohort study of 403,567 Taiwanese patients, hospitalizations for complicated peptic ulcers decreased significantly over a 10-year period[8]; thus the annual incidence of hospitalizations for bleeding DU or for perforated DU fell from 108 to 40 and from 9.8 to 5.8 per 100,000, respectively. A similar decline was evident for bleeding and perforated GUs (from 117 to 61 and from 11 to 6 per 100,000, respectively).

ETIOLOGY AND PATHOGENESIS

The principal risk factors for PUD are Hp infection and NSAID use (Fig. 55.1), and as will be discussed, many patients with PUD have both of these risk factors. On the other hand, PUD patients may have neither of these risk factors (Hp-negative, NSAID-negative ulcers); some of these latter patients will have another

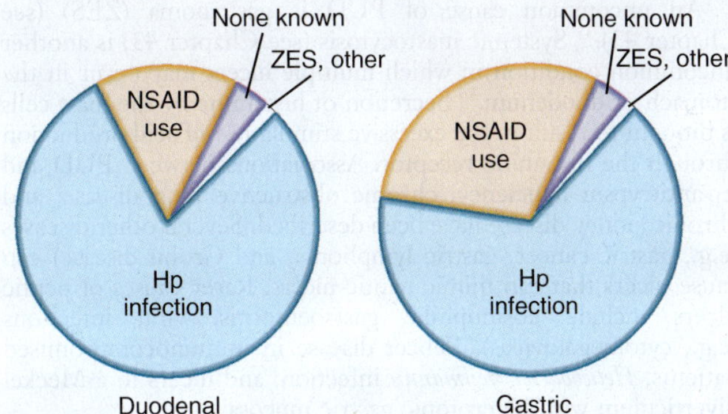

Fig. 55.1 Pie charts depicting conditions associated with PUD. The percentages shown are rough approximations based on studies from Western countries. The relative contributions of Hp infection and NSAID use to peptic ulcer vary considerably among different populations and, within populations, vary with age and socioeconomic status. Also, the separation depicted in this figure is somewhat artificial because NSAID use and Hp infection often coexist.

cause of ulcer such as gastrinoma (ZES; see Chapter 43), whereas others will have ulcers that are idiopathic.

Hp Infection

The prevalence of Hp infection varies widely among countries in the world (see Chapter 54).

In a systematic review and meta-analysis of Hp infection between 1970 and 2016, the prevalence of infection ranged from 18.9% to 87.7%, depending on the country. The lowest prevalence was observed in Oceania and Northern America (24.4% −37.1%). The highest prevalence was observed in Africa, Latin America, the Caribbean, and Asia (70.1−79.1). In general, since the 21st century, the rate of Hp infection has declined in the Western world, whereas prevalence has plateaued at a high level in developing and newly industrialized countries.[9] Feinstein and colleagues studied hospital discharge records for PUD in the United States between 1998 and 2005.[10] In parallel with a decline in annual hospitalization rates for PUD, from 71.1 to 56.5 per 100,000, there was a decrease in hospitalization due to Hp-related disease, from 35.9 to 19.2 per 100,000. The prevalence of Hp infection in patients with bleeding ulcers remains high. Sanchez-Delgado and colleagues compiled 71 studies containing 8496 patients with bleeding peptic ulcers and found an Hp infection rate of 72%. The use of an Hp diagnostic test after the index bleed was associated with high Hp prevalence.[11]

As discussed in Chapters 53 and 54, Hp causes an antrum-predominant gastritis in 10%−20% of infected patients, which results in high gastric acid secretion and an increased risk of DU. The increased acid output from the stomach results in increased acid load to the duodenum that can result in gastric metaplasia in the duodenal bulb.[12] Some believe that the metaplastic epithelium then becomes infected with Hp from the stomach, resulting in focal "duodenitis" (technically, gastritis), sometimes followed by erosion and ulcer formation.

Most patients with Hp infection have a pan-gastritis involving both the antral and fundic mucosa that lowers gastric acid secretion[13] and predisposes to GU formation. In these individuals, it is proposed that weakened mucosal defense mechanisms (see Chapter 53), rather than high acid secretion, are what predisposes to gastric ulceration. The role of Hp's genes and their protein products in the pathogenesis of PUD is discussed in Chapter 54.

Use of Aspirin and Other NSAIDs

Aspirin is increasingly used on a regular basis for the prevention of cardiovascular events, either alone or in combination with a platelet adenosine diphosphate inhibitor such as clopidogrel (dual antiplatelet therapy). NSAIDs are used on a regular basis by approximately 11% of the U.S. population. Regular use of NSAIDs increases the odds of GI bleeding up to five- to sixfold.[14] Serious ulcer-related complications often leading to hospitalization occur in 1%−4% of NSAID users.[15] NSAID users who also take aspirin are at an especially high risk for complications. In a population-based study from Denmark, the odds ratio (OR) for GI bleeding in people taking low-dose aspirin alone was 2.6, and this ratio increased to 5.6 in patients who were also taking an NSAID.[16] In a national study of mortality associated with a hospital admission for adverse GI events related to NSAID use in Spain, the death rate attributed to NSAID/aspirin use was 15.3 per 100,000 population compared to 2.5 per 100,000 of the general population.[17]

The gastric and duodenal mucosa have several defense mechanisms protecting them from digestion by acid and pepsin (see Chapter 53). NSAIDs cause mucosal damage through disruption of mucus phospholipids, cell membranes and by uncoupling mitochondrial oxidative phosphorylation, but most evidence suggests that NSAIDs damage the gastric and duodenal mucosa by suppression of prostaglandin synthesis.[18] COX isoforms, COX-1 and COX-2, are responsible for the synthesis of prostaglandins. COX-1 is expressed in the stomach and helps maintain the integrity of gastric epithelium and the mucous barrier. COX-2 is not expressed in the healthy stomach but is rapidly expressed in response to the cytokines generated by inflammatory processes. Conventional NSAIDs such as ibuprofen inhibit the COX-1 and the COX-2 isoenzymes more or less equally. COX-1 inhibition reduces prostaglandin synthesis, which leads to a reduction in mucosal defense. Animal experiments have found that neutrophil adherence to the gastric microcirculation plays a critical role in initiating NSAID injury. Neutrophil adherence liberates oxygen-free radicals, releases proteases, and obstructs capillary blood flow. Inhibition of neutrophil adherence has been shown to reduce NSAID-induced damage. In addition, two gaseous mediators, nitric oxide (NO) and hydrogen sulfide (H_2S), contribute to maintaining the gastric mucosal barrier. NO and H_2S increase mucosal blood flow, stimulate mucus secretion, and inhibit neutrophil adherence.[19] NO-releasing and H_2S-releasing derivatives of NSAIDs have been shown to protect against gastric damage when compared to the parent drugs. Gastric acid plays a secondary but important role by turning superficial mucosal lesions into deeper injury, interfering with platelet aggregation, and impairing ulcer healing.[20]

Hp infection appears to influence the risk of PUD in patients receiving NSAIDs. A meta-analysis showed that Hp infection raised the risk of peptic ulcer bleeding more than sixfold in patients receiving long-term NSAIDs, whereas Hp alone and NSAID use alone raised the risk by 1.79- and 4.85-fold, respectively.[21] An updated meta-analysis showed similar findings.[22] Among patients who are about to start NSAID therapy, eradication of Hp reduces the subsequent risk of ulcer development.[23,24] A systematic review has shown that testing for (and eradication of) Hp lowers the risk of peptic ulcers among NSAID users[25]; however, eradication of Hp infection alone is insufficient to prevent peptic ulcer bleeding in NSAID users at high ulcer risk.[26,27]

There is also evidence that Hp infection increases the risk of PUD in patients receiving low-dose aspirin. Among Hp-infected patients with recent ulcer bleeding who continued to take low-dose aspirin, successful eradication of Hp infection resulted in a very low risk of recurrent ulcer bleeding, similar to that seen with aspirin/omeprazole cotherapy.[26] This low risk of ulcer rebleeding after eradication of Hp was not seen in patients with bleeding ulcers who continued to take NSAIDs. In a long-term prospective cohort study,[28] Hp-infected low-dose aspirin users (≤160 mg/day) with bleeding ulcers who resumed their aspirin had a low risk of recurrent ulcer bleeding after eradication of Hp, a risk that was not significantly different from the risk in new aspirin users with no history of ulcer disease (<1 bleed per 100 patient-years). In contrast, aspirin users with bleeding ulcers but without Hp infection (past or present) were at high risk of recurrent ulcer bleeding with continued enteric-coated aspirin treatment (>5 bleeds per 100 patient-years). For patients starting aspirin as primary prevention, the American College of Gastroenterology guidelines advocate for Hp eradication in view of bleeding risks.[29] A large-scale double-blind randomized control trial in the United Kingdom demonstrated Hp eradication protects against aspirin-associated peptic ulcer bleeding in the older population (study population mean age 73.6 years old).[30] As primary prevention, Hp eradication reduced time to hospitalisation or death secondary peptic ulcer bleeding. However, in this study, the effect was lost after 2.5 years. The number needed to treat was 238 patients. Importantly, there were no significant differences in thrombotic cardiovascular episodes, and the reported side effects were similar to those already known.

Other Causes of Ulcers and Idiopathic Ulcers

Deep ulcers and perforations of the stomach and duodenum have been described in cocaine and methamphetamine users, presumably due to mucosal ischemia.[31] Bisphosphonate therapy has also been associated with gastroduodenal ulceration,[32] although esophageal injury with bisphosphonates is clinically more of a concern. There is little, if any, risk for PUD in patients taking glucocorticoids.[33] In combination with NSAIDs, however, glucocorticoids increase the risk of PUD above the risk with NSAIDs alone.[34] There is also a weak association between use of selective serotonin reuptake inhibitor antidepressants and PUD, especially in those with concurrent NSAID use.

Smoking, stress, type A personality, and excessive alcohol use are some of the risk factors implicated for PUD. Although these factors can contribute to PUD, none has emerged as a sole cause of the disease. Hp infection is a confounder that was not addressed in earlier studies.

An uncommon cause of PUD is gastrinoma (ZES) (see Chapter 43).[35] Systemic mastocytosis (see Chapter 43) is another uncommon condition in which multiple ulcers may occur in the stomach or duodenum.[36] Secretion of histamine by the mast cells is thought to result in the excessive stimulation of acid production through the histamine receptor. Associations between PUD and α_1-antitrypsin deficiency, chronic obstructive lung disease, and chronic kidney disease have been described. Several other diseases (e.g., gastric cancer, gastric lymphoma, and Crohn disease) can cause ulcers that can mimic peptic ulcers. Rarer causes of peptic ulcers include eosinophilic gastroenteritis, viral infections (e.g., cytomegalovirus), Behçet disease in immunocompromised patients, *Helicobacter heilmannii* infection, and ulcers in a Meckel diverticulum with heterotopic gastric mucosa.

With a global decline in the prevalence of Hp infection, the proportion of patients with idiopathic ulcers has been increasing. Studies in North America have shown that more than 10% of peptic ulcers are not associated with Hp infection or the use of NSAIDs. Whether the incidence of idiopathic ulcers is increasing or not is controversial. It has been argued that only the relative proportion, but not the true incidence, of idiopathic ulcers has increased as a result of a falling incidence of *Hp* ulcers. However, there are prospective data showing that the absolute incidence of idiopathic bleeding ulcers has increased by fourfold. Importantly, patients with a history of idiopathic bleeding ulcers have a fourfold increased risk of recurrent ulcer bleeding and more than twofold increase in mortality compared to patients with history of *Hp* ulcers.[37]

CLINICAL FEATURES AND DIAGNOSIS

The predominant symptom of patients with uncomplicated PUD is epigastric pain. Pain is typically associated with hunger, occurs at night, and is often relieved by food and antacids. Often patients complain of dyspeptic symptoms such as a bloated sensation and fullness. Some patients complain of heartburn that may or may not be accompanied by erosive esophagitis. Chronic NSAID users, typically older adult patients, can present with ulcer bleeding or perforation without prior ulcer symptoms.

EGD is the procedure of choice for diagnosis of uncomplicated PUD (Fig. 55.2A and B). EGD is more sensitive and specific than radiologic studies, such as UGI series with barium.

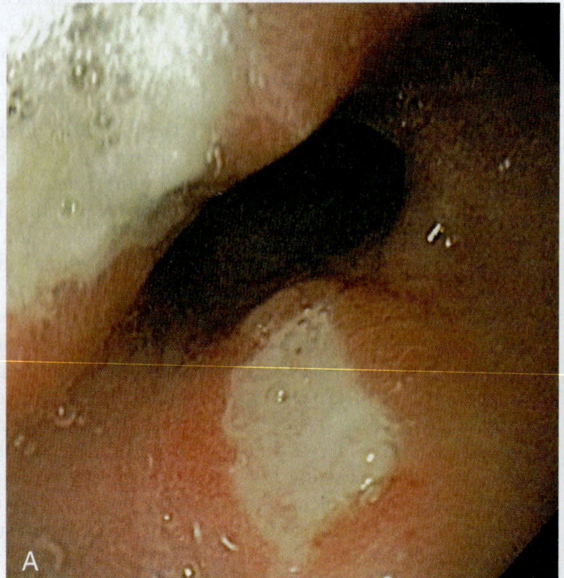

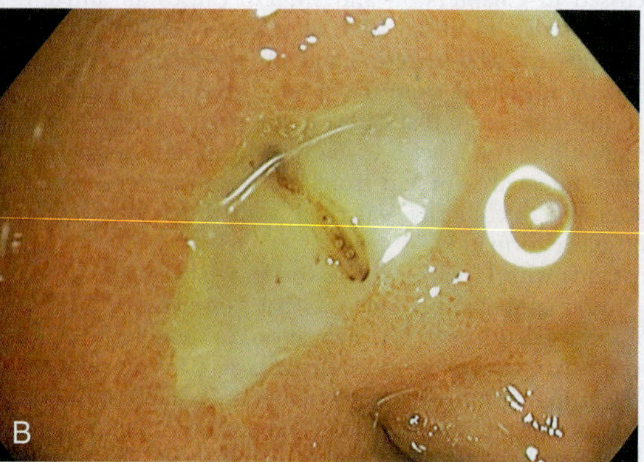

Fig. 55.2 (A) Endoscopic view of a clean-based antral GU in a patient taking an NSAID. Tests for infection with Hp were negative. (B) Endoscopic view of a DU in a patient with a positive rapid urease test for Hp. There was no history of NSAID use.

Nevertheless, endoscopy is expensive and has the potential for complications (see Chapter 40). Therefore the decision to perform endoscopy in a patient suspected of having PUD is based on several factors. As discussed later in this chapter and in Chapter 40, patients presenting with acute GI bleeding need endoscopic evaluation to allow an accurate diagnosis and for the administration of endoscopic therapy. Furthermore, patients with epigastric pain suggestive of PUD but also with "alarm" features such as weight loss or recurrent vomiting may prompt concern for gastric malignancy as well as require EGD (Box 55.1). If a DU or GU is found during EGD, gastric mucosal biopsies should be obtained for a rapid urease test to diagnose Hp infection (see Chapter 54). Biopsies should also be taken from the edges of GUs because of risk of gastric cancer. Customarily, if the GU biopsies are benign, EGD is repeated 8 weeks later to confirm healing of the GU, because up to 4% of apparently benign GUs at initial endoscopy are subsequently found to be malignant.[38,39]

BOX 55.1 Alarm Features in Patients With UGI Symptoms*

- Age older than 55 years with new-onset dyspepsia
- Family history of UGI cancer
- GI bleeding, acute or chronic, including unexplained iron deficiency
- Jaundice
- Left supraclavicular lymphadenopathy (Virchow node)
- Palpable abdominal mass
- Persistent vomiting
- Progressive dysphagia
- Unintended weight loss

*These features should prompt EGD and often other testing to establish a definitive diagnosis (see Chapter 15).

Dyspeptic upper abdominal symptoms consisting of pain or discomfort in the upper abdomen are common in clinical practice, accounting for 2%–5% of visits to family practitioners (see Chapter 15).[40] Owing to the high cost and impracticality of subjecting all dyspeptic individuals to prompt endoscopy, two other nonendoscopic strategies (besides UGI series, with its inherent lower sensitivity and specificity for PUD) have been proposed as an initial step in the management of suspected PUD (Fig. 55.3). The strategies are (1) "test-and-treat," based on a noninvasive diagnosis of Hp infection and subsequent eradication therapy when Hp is detected, and (2) empirical antisecretory therapy, usually with a PPI.

Gisbert and Calvet[41] reviewed the literature and concluded that the Hp test-and-treat strategy will cure most cases of PUD and prevent most cases of gastroduodenal disease. A small proportion of patients with Hp-related functional dyspepsia would also improve in their symptoms. The test-and-treat strategy has been compared with endoscopy-directed diagnosis in eight randomized controlled trials (RCTs). These trials differed in how Hp

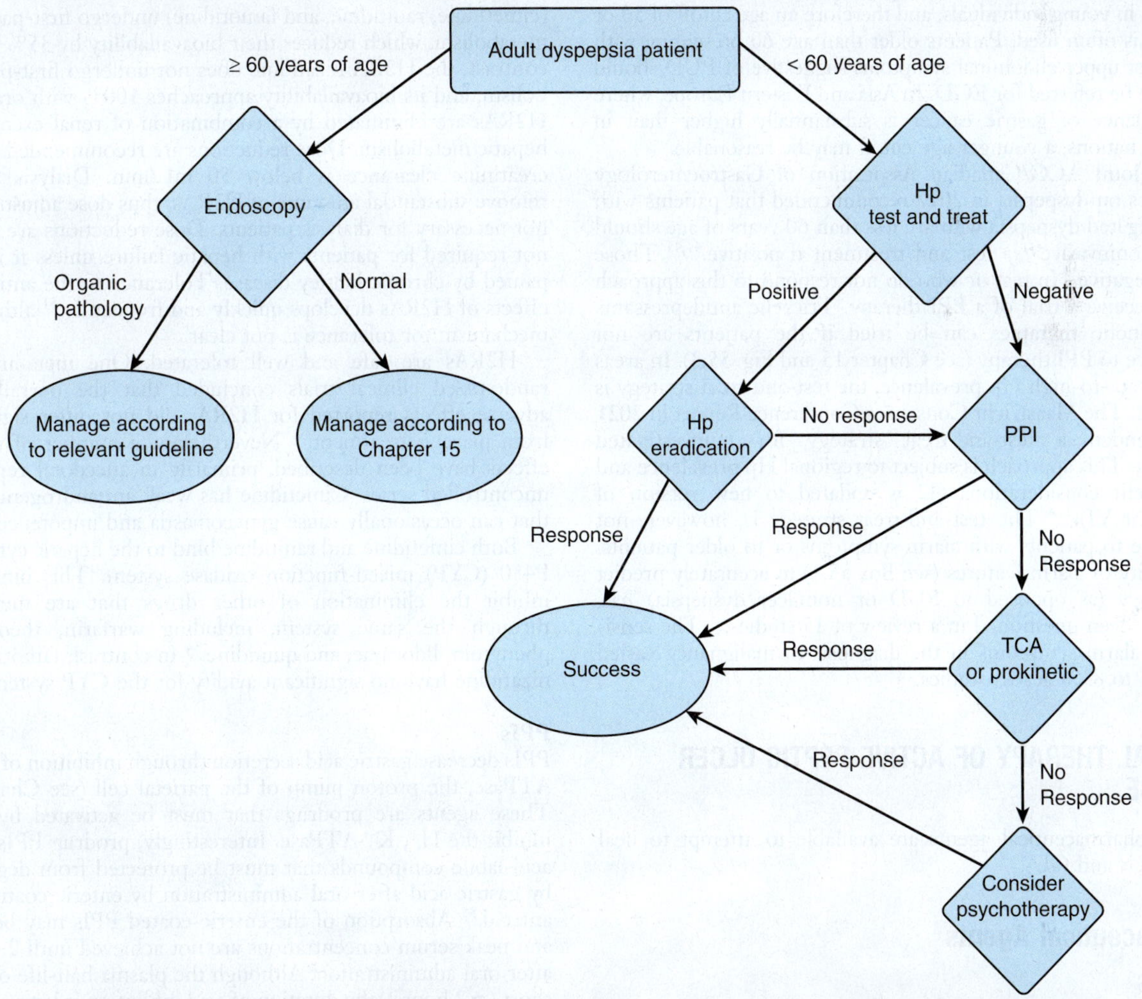

Fig. 55.3 ACG and Canadian Association of Gastroenterology (CAG) guideline algorithm for the management of undiagnosed PUD. This is also the current management approach for patients with suspected PUD. *TCA*, Tricyclic antidepressant. (Adapted from Moayyedi P, Lacy BE, Andrews CN, et al. ACG and CAG clinical guideline: management of dyspepsia. *Am J Gastroenterol*. 2017;112:988–1013.)

was diagnosed, and the upper age cutoff varied from 45 to 55 years. In some studies, serology was used for diagnosis of infection, which is less specific than[13] C urea breath testing (see Chapter 53). The background Hp prevalence in the study populations ranged from 23% to 53%. After a 12-month follow-up, the prevalence of dyspeptic symptoms was similar in the two groups. In seven of the eight trials, cost data were reported, and the test-and-treat strategy was less expensive because of the many endoscopies avoided. Ford and colleagues performed a meta-analysis of 5 RCTs involving 1924 patients and found a slight benefit at 12 months of prompt EGD on dyspeptic symptoms over test-and-treat [risk ratio, 0.95; 95% confidence index (CI), 0.92–0.99], possibly because a normal EGD may have had a reassuring effect in some patients.[42]

According to a joint ACG/Canadian Association of Gastroenterology guideline, it was recommended that patients with uninvestigated dyspepsia who are less than 60 years of age should have a noninvasive test for Hp and provide treatment if positive. Those with a negative test or do not respond to this approach should receive a trial of PPI therapy. Tricyclic antidepressants or prokinetic therapies can be tried if they are not responsive to PPI therapy. The incidence of UGI malignancies, including gastric cancer, rises with age, and, thus, current nonendoscopic management strategies are generally reserved for younger patients with upper abdominal symptoms. The age after which prompt EGD should become routine is debated and, to a substantial degree, depends on the epidemiology of UGI cancer in the population under consideration. In Western populations, UGI cancer is uncommon in young individuals, and therefore an age cutoff of 50 or 55 years is often used. Patients older than age 60 presenting with new-onset upper abdominal symptoms suggestive of PUD should therefore be referred for EGD. In Asia and Eastern Europe, where the incidence of gastric cancer is substantially higher than in Western nations, a younger age cutoff may be reasonable.

The Joint ACG/Canadian Association of Gastroenterology guidelines on dyspepsia in 2017 recommended that patients with uninvestigated dyspepsia who are less than 60 years of age should have a noninvasive *Hp* test and treatment if positive.[41,43] Those with a negative Hp test or who do not respond to this approach should receive a trial of a PPI therapy. Tricyclic antidepressants or prokinetic therapies can be tried if the patients are not responsive to PPI therapy (see Chapter 15 and Fig. 55.3). In areas of moderate-to-high Hp prevalence, the test-and-treat strategy is preferred. The Maastricht Consensus Conference Report in 2021 recommended a test-and-treat strategy for uninvestigated dyspepsia. This approach is subject to regional Hp prevalence and cost-benefit considerations (42 is updated to new version of Maastricht VI).[42,44]The test-and-treat strategy is, however, not applicable to patients with alarm symptoms or to older patients. The ability of alarm features (see Box 55.1) to accurately predict malignancy (as opposed to PUD or nonulcer dyspepsia) has, however, been questioned in a review of 15 studies.[45] The sensitivity of alarm symptoms in the diagnosis of malignancy varied from 0% to 83% across studies.

MEDICAL THERAPY OF ACTIVE PEPTIC ULCER DISEASE

Several pharmaceutical agents are available to attempt to heal active DUs and GUs.

Pharmaceutical Agents

Antacids

Antacids neutralize gastric acid, but their ability to heal ulcers is poor. Most physicians do not use antacids as primary therapy to heal ulcers but instead recommend their use to relieve dyspeptic symptoms. The most common adverse effect of magnesium-containing antacids is diarrhea. In contrast, aluminum- and calcium-containing antacids may cause constipation. All antacids must be used with caution, if at all, in patients who have chronic kidney disease, in whom magnesium-containing agents can cause hypermagnesemia, calcium-containing antacids hypercalcemia, and aluminum-containing antacid neurotoxicity.[46]

Antisecretory Agents

Antisecretory therapy is not routinely required for patients with uncomplicated Hp ulcers in whom ulcers heal after successful eradication of Hp even without antisecretory therapy; however, antisecretory drugs play an important role in the management of patients with PUD not associated with Hp. The role of antisecretory drugs in the management of gastrinoma (ZES) is discussed in Chapter 43.

H2Ras

H2RAs are competitive inhibitors of histamine-stimulated acid secretion (see Chapter 53) and markedly suppress basal and meal-stimulated acid secretion.[47] When administered in the evening, H2RAs are effective in suppressing nocturnal acid output.[48] H2RAs are well absorbed after oral dosing, and their absorption is not affected by food. Peak blood levels are achieved within 1–3 hours after an oral dose. H2RAs cross the blood-brain barrier and the placenta.[49,50] After oral administration, several H2RAs (cimetidine, ranitidine, and famotidine) undergo first-pass hepatic metabolism, which reduces their bioavailability by 35%–60%. In contrast, the H2RA nizatidine does not undergo first-pass metabolism, and its bioavailability approaches 100% with oral dosing. H2RAs are eliminated by a combination of renal excretion and hepatic metabolism. Dose reductions are recommended when the creatinine clearance is below 50 mL/min. Dialysis does not remove substantial amounts of H2RAs; thus dose adjustments are not necessary for dialysis patients. Dose reductions are generally not required for patients with hepatic failure unless it is accompanied by chronic kidney disease. Tolerance to the antisecretory effects of H2RAs develops quickly and frequently,[51] although the mechanism for tolerance is not clear.

H2RAs are safe and well tolerated. One meta-analysis of randomized clinical trials concluded that the overall rate of adverse effects reported for H2RAs did not differ significantly from placebo treatment.[52] Nevertheless, a number of untoward effects have been described, primarily in anecdotal reports and uncontrolled series. Cimetidine has weak antiandrogenic activity that can occasionally cause gynecomastia and impotence.[53]

Both cimetidine and ranitidine bind to the hepatic cytochrome P450 (CYP) mixed-function oxidase system. This binding can inhibit the elimination of other drugs that are metabolized through the same system, including warfarin, theophylline, phenytoin, lidocaine, and quinidine.[54] In contrast, famotidine and nizatidine have no significant avidity for the CYP system.

PPIs

PPIs decrease gastric acid secretion through inhibition of H^+, K^+-ATPase, the proton pump of the parietal cell (see Chapter 53). These agents are prodrugs that must be activated by acid to inhibit the H^+, K^+-ATPase. Interestingly, prodrug PPIs are also acid-labile compounds that must be protected from degradation by gastric acid after oral administration by enteric coating or an antacid.[55] Absorption of the enteric-coated PPIs may be erratic, and peak serum concentrations are not achieved until 2–5 hours after oral administration. Although the plasma half-life of PPIs is short ($\approx$2 hours), the duration of acid inhibition is long as a result of covalent binding of the active metabolite of the prodrug to the H^+, K^+-ATPase. PPIs undergo significant hepatic metabolism, but dose adjustments are not required in patients with significant renal or hepatic impairment. There is genetic polymorphism in CYP2C19, one of the isoenzymes involved in PPI metabolism. Approximately 25% of Asians and 3% of Caucasians have deficient CYP2C19 activity. This polymorphism leads to substantially higher plasma levels of omeprazole, lansoprazole, and pantoprazole, but not rabeprazole.[38,39,56]

PPIs, as a result of their requirement for concentration and activation in acidic compartments, bind predominantly to those proton pumps that are actively secreting acid. With meal stimulation, 60%–70% of the proton pumps actively secrete acid; thus PPIs are most effective if they are administered immediately before meals. For once-daily dosing, it is recommended that PPIs be taken immediately before breakfast.[57] Unlike H2RAs, tolerance to the antisecretory effects of PPI therapy has not been seen.

PPIs, by raising the gastric pH, can affect the absorption of a number of drugs. However, this pH effect rarely has clinically important effects, except when the PPIs are given with ketoconazole or digoxin.[57–59] Ketoconazole requires gastric acid for absorption, and this antifungal drug may not be absorbed effectively if PPIs have also been prescribed. If a patient requires both a PPI and antifungal therapy, it is recommended that an agent other than ketoconazole be chosen. Conversely, an elevated gastric pH facilitates absorption of digoxin, resulting in higher plasma digoxin levels. For patients treated concomitantly with PPIs and digoxin, clinicians should consider monitoring plasma digoxin levels.

Because PPIs are metabolized by the CYP system, they have the potential to alter the metabolism of other drugs that are eliminated by CYP enzymes. The potential interaction between PPIs and clopidogrel has drawn widespread attention. Clopidogrel, a nonaspirin antiplatelet prodrug, is activated by hepatic CYP2C19 and other CYPs to its active metabolite. PPIs reduce the antiplatelet effect of clopidogrel through competitive inhibition of CYP2C19. Meta-analysis of observational studies reported a significant increase in major adverse cardiovascular events, including cardiovascular deaths, among patients receiving concomitant PPIs and clopidogrel.[60,61] However, an association between PPI and clopidogrel use has not been confirmed by prospective studies and a large-scale RCT.[62,63] Despite the inconsistent findings, regulatory authorities in the United States and Europe have issued warnings against the use of certain PPIs in patients receiving concomitant clopidogrel.

There are other concerns about the safety of long-term use of PPIs. To date, PPI use has been implicated in many conditions, including osteoporosis, hypomagnesaemia, gastric cancer, enteric infections, interstitial nephritis, pneumonia, dementia, and NSAID-enteropathy. Currently, there is no definite evidence to suggest that these conditions are attributable to PPI use.[64] It is possible that new evidence will emerge to indicate a causal relationship. In the meantime, long-term use of PPI without a strong indication should be discouraged.

Potassium-Competitive Acid Blocker

Potassium-competitive acid blocker (P-CAB) therapy competes with potassium to inhibit H^+, K^+-ATPase in parietal cells at the final stage of the acid secretory pathway (see Chapter 53).[65] Unlike PPIs, a P-CAB is acid stable and does not require an acidic environment for activation (i.e., a prodrug is not required). To date, vonoprazan is the only P-CAB commercially available in Japan and some other countries. Vonoprazan exerts a near-maximum inhibitory effect from the first dose, and its effect lasts for 24 hours.[65] Owing to this unique characteristic, it has a promising role in Hp infection eradication. In a meta-analysis of 10 studies comprising of retrospective cohort studies from Japan, vonoprazan-based triple therapy was superior to PPI-based triple therapy, without compromise in safety and tolerance.[66] In 2021 another retrospective cohort meta-analysis demonstrated that vonoprazan-based therapy was most effective as second-line therapy, particularly as it has high rates of eradication in clarithromycin-resistant Hp strains.[67] Similar results were replicated in United States and European phase 3 RCTs.[68]

Additionally, P-CAB may also be an alternative for preventing and healing PUD. In two phase 3 RCTs, vonoprazan (20 mg once daily) was not inferior to lansoprazole (30 mg once daily) for the healing of GUs and DUs.[69,70] Two other randomized trials showed that vonoprazan (10 and 20 mg) was as effective as lansoprazole (15 mg) in preventing ulcer recurrence associated with long-term use of NSAIDs and low-dose aspirin.[71]

Mucosal Protective Agents

Sucralfate is a complex aluminum salt of sulfated sucrose. When exposed to gastric acid, the sulfate anions can bind electrostatically to positively charged proteins in damaged tissue.[72,73] Sucralfate (1 g four times daily) is equally effective to H2RAs in healing DUs and is approved by the FDA in the United States for this indication. Very little (<5%) of sucralfate is absorbed owing to its poor solubility, and the drug is excreted via the enteral route. Because of its lack of systemic absorption, sucralfate appears to have no systemic toxicity. The effect on the accumulation of aluminum in the body has not been adequately studied in patients with chronic kidney disease treated with sucralfate, and sucralfate is best avoided in this population. Important drug interactions appear to be rare and can be avoided if sucralfate is administered at a time separate from other medications.

Colloidal bismuth preparations, such as colloidal bismuth subcitrate and bismuth subsalicylate (e.g., Pepto-Bismol), have modest efficacy in healing peptic ulcers, but the mechanism is unclear.[74] The bismuth salts form complexes with mucus that appear to coat ulcer craters. Bismuth-induced increased mucosal prostaglandin synthesis and bicarbonate secretion have also been proposed. Bismuth salts have antimicrobial activity against Hp, and bismuth has been approved in the United States by the FDA for use, in combination with other agents, for the treatment of Hp infection (see Chapter 54). Bismuth is largely unabsorbed and excreted in the feces. Colonic bacteria convert bismuth salts to bismuth sulfide, which turns the stools black. Trace amounts of bismuth are absorbed in the UGI tract, with the bismuth then slowly excreted in the urine for 3 months or longer. Short-term, standard-dose therapy with bismuth appears to carry little risk of toxicity; however, there is the potential for bismuth encephalopathy with neuropsychiatric symptoms if the agent is given for extended periods in high dosage, especially in patients with chronic kidney disease.

Misoprostol is a prostaglandin E_1 analog approved by the FDA for the prevention of NSAID-induced PUD.[75] The drug not only enhances mucosal defense mechanisms but also inhibits gastric acid secretion through inhibition of histamine-stimulated cyclic 3′,5′-cyclic adenosine monophosphate production.[76] Well absorbed after oral administration, the plasma misoprostol concentration peaks after approximately 30 minutes, with a serum half-life of approximately 1.5 hours. The drug has no effect on hepatic CYP450. Misoprostol metabolites are excreted in the urine, but dose reductions are unnecessary in patients with chronic kidney disease. Dose-related diarrhea is the most common adverse effect, occurring in up to 30% of patients and limiting the usefulness of misoprostol. Diarrhea is related to prostaglandin-induced increases in intestinal electrolyte and water secretion and/or acceleration of intestinal transit time. Administration of misoprostol with food may reduce diarrhea. Misoprostol also stimulates uterine smooth muscle and is therefore contraindicated in women who may be pregnant.

Hp-Associated Ulcers

Treatment of Hp infection is discussed in detail in Chapter 53. It is well established that curing Hp infection not only heals peptic ulcers but also prevents ulcer relapses and complications.[77–80] Because Hp infection accounts for 80%–90% of DU cases, testing for the infection in patients with DU is mandatory. If the diagnosis of DU is made endoscopically, gastric biopsy specimens should be taken to detect Hp infection. There is good evidence that a 10- to 14-day course of Hp eradication therapy is sufficient to heal DUs such that additional antisecretory therapy is not usually required. Follow-up endoscopic examination to document healing and perform testing to document Hp eradication following antibiotic therapy is not recommended routinely in patients with uncomplicated DUs. However, noninvasive tests, such as the urea breath test, can be used to confirm Hp eradication. Whether antisecretory therapy is required after a 7- to 14-day course of Hp eradication therapy in patients with GU is somewhat controversial. One week of antibacterial therapy without acid suppression effectively heals Hp-related GUs.[77] In a meta-analysis of GU healing trials, treatment with Hp eradication therapy produced similar outcomes to treatment with an ulcer-healing drug[78]; however, in patients with large or complicated GUs, additional antisecretory therapy can facilitate ulcer healing. Follow-up endoscopy is recommended in patients with large or complicated GUs to document healing, exclude malignancy, and confirm successful Hp eradication.

NSAID Ulcers

H2RAs

Conventional doses of H2RAs are more effective in healing NSAID-related DUs than GUs. There are limited data on the efficacy of H2RAs in healing peptic ulcers if patients continue to receive NSAIDs. Therefore H2RAs are not preferred agents in patients with ulcers who require uninterrupted NSAID therapy.

PPIs

Current evidence[81–83] indicates that PPIs are superior to standard-dose H2RAs in healing NSAID-induced peptic ulcers. In a randomized comparison of esomeprazole (20 or 40 mg/day) and ranitidine (150 mg twice daily) in ulcer patients who continued to take NSAIDs, ulcer healing at 8 weeks occurred in 85% and 86% of patients given esomeprazole and in 76% of those given ranitidine.[83] In another study of patients with NSAID-associated GUs who continued to use NSAIDs, ulcer healing at 8 weeks occurred in 69% and 73% of patients given lansoprazole (15 or 30 mg/day) but in only 53% of those given ranitidine (150 mg twice daily).[82]

Misoprostol

In ulcer patients who continued their NSAID, misoprostol healed the ulcers in 67% of patients at 8 weeks, compared with only 26% of patients treated with placebo.[84] However, misoprostol is not as effective as PPI therapy in healing NSAID-associated ulcers. One randomized trial compared full-dose misoprostol (200 μg four times daily) with omeprazole (20 or 40 mg daily) in DU or GU patients who continued NSAID treatment.[85] After 8 weeks, DUs had healed in 89% of patients receiving either dose of omeprazole and in 77% of those receiving misoprostol. Similarly, GUs had healed in 87% of those receiving 20 mg of omeprazole, 80% of those receiving 40 mg of omeprazole, and 73% of those receiving misoprostol. Although misoprostol is seldom used for treatment or prevention of peptic ulcer nowadays, two randomized trials have shown that misoprostol is effective for the healing of small bowel ulcers and erosions in patients with obscure bleeding taking NSAIDs and low-dose aspirin.[86,87]

Other Causes of Ulcers and Idiopathic Ulcers

When the cause of a peptic ulcer can be identified as other than Hp or NSAID use (e.g., gastrinoma), the underlying disorder should be treated (see Chapter 43). The treatment of idiopathic, non-Hp, non-NSAID ulcers relies on acid antisecretory therapy, usually a PPI, which is often given long term (maintenance therapy), much as antisecretory therapy is used long term to prevent NSAID-induced ulcers in moderate- and high-risk patients (see later).

REFRACTORY ULCERS

Most peptic ulcers heal within 8 weeks of initiation of antisecretory therapy. Nevertheless, in a small but considerable minority of patients, the ulcers persist despite conventional treatment. Such ulcers can be considered refractory. There is no standardized definition for refractory peptic ulcer, making comparisons among studies difficult. In some patients with refractory ulcers, symptoms of ulcer disease persist and may be severe. In others, the refractory ulcer becomes asymptomatic and is only detected at endoscopy (e.g., at the 8-week follow-up endoscopy to assess healing of a GU).

For the patient whose ulcer does not heal despite a trial of conventional therapy, the clinician should ask the following questions:

- Has the patient complied with the prescribed treatment?
- Is the ulcer penetrating the pancreas, liver, or other organ?
- Is there Hp infection? If antibiotic therapy had already been prescribed, the patient should be tested to confirm that the infection has indeed been eradicated. If no attempt had been made to diagnose and treat Hp infection, it should be made now. False-negative test results for Hp should be considered (see Chapter 54).
- Is the patient still taking an NSAID? NSAID use may be surreptitious. A careful history regarding the use of over-the-counter NSAIDs (including low-dose aspirin) should be obtained, and NSAIDs should be stopped if possible.
- Does the patient smoke cigarettes? If so, he or she should be counseled strongly to discontinue cigarettes.
- Has the duration of ulcer treatment been adequate? Large ulcers require a longer duration of therapy than small ulcers to heal. A large ulcer (e.g., >2 cm) probably should not be considered refractory until it has persisted beyond 12 weeks of antisecretory therapy.
- Is there evidence of a hypersecretory condition? A family history of gastrinoma or MEN type I or a personal history of chronic diarrhea, hypercalcemia caused by hyperparathyroidism, or ulcers involving the postbulbar duodenum or proximal jejunum suggest a diagnosis of ZES (see Chapter 43).
- Finally, is the ulcer indeed peptic? Primary or metastatic neoplasms, infections (e.g., cytomegalovirus), cocaine use, eosinophilic gastroenteritis, and Crohn disease can cause ulcerations of the stomach and duodenum that can mimic peptic ulcers. These disorders should be considered and excluded appropriately.

Treatment options for truly refractory peptic ulcers include a more prolonged course of antisecretory therapy, often at double the prior PPI dose. Although uncommon nowadays, elective ulcer surgery may be necessary to attempt to heal a symptomatic refractory or penetrating ulcer. Surgical options are discussed later in this chapter.

PREVENTION OF ULCER DISEASE

Most studies of ulcer prophylaxis have used endoscopy endpoints (rather than clinical endpoints) to assess the effectiveness of various regimens. An "endoscopic ulcer" has been arbitrarily defined as a circumscribed mucosal defect having a diameter of 5 mm or more with a perceivable depth.[88] However, many studies have loosened this criterion to include flat mucosal breaks with a diameter of 3 mm or more as ulcers. The distinction between small ulcers and erosions is arbitrary and is prone to interobserver bias. The clinical relevance of these minor endoscopic lesions is uncertain. It is assumed that endoscopic findings roughly correlate with clinical outcomes in subjects at low-to-average risk for ulcer complications. It is unclear if results of endoscopic studies can be generalized to high-risk patients. Because there are few prospective outcome trials to evaluate the true clinical efficacy of ulcer prophylactic agents, clinical judgment relies on data largely using endoscopic endpoints.

Hp ulcers do not require ulcer prophylaxis if the organism can be eradicated from the stomach (see earlier and Chapter 54). Most use of ulcer prophylaxis regimens is, therefore, related to prevention of NSAID ulcers in patients at moderate-to-high ulcer risk. The risk factors for NSAID-induced ulcers are listed in Table 55.1. Pharmaceutical agents that may reduce the development of NSAID-induced ulcers are discussed later. Ulcer prophylaxis is also frequently used in patients with idiopathic ulcers. Among the agents listed, only the antisecretory agents are commonly used in the prevention of idiopathic ulcers.

Antacids

Many clinicians prescribe antacids as cotherapy for patients taking NSAIDs, both to relieve dyspeptic symptoms and to (hopefully) prevent ulcers; however, antacids have no proved efficacy in the prevention of NSAID-induced ulcers. Antacids may mask dyspeptic symptoms, thereby creating a false sense of ulcer protection and increasing the risk of silent ulcer complications with prolonged NSAID therapy. Coprescription of antacids in patients taking NSAIDs who are at risk for ulcer should be discouraged.

H2RAs

Standard doses of H2RAs are ineffective in preventing NSAID-induced GUs,[89,90] and, as already mentioned, may be harmful. A systematic review[90] of randomized trials in NSAID users concluded that using twice the standard daily dose of H2RA significantly reduces the risk of endoscopic NSAID-induced DUs and GUs. However, whether high-dose H2RAs prevent NSAID-induced ulcer complications is unknown. In contrast, H2RAs appear to be more effective for prevention of ulcers associated with low-dose aspirin than with NSAIDs. In a 12-month, multicenter, randomized trial of low-dose aspirin users at risk for recurrent ulcer bleeding, there was no significant difference in the incidence rates of recurrent bleeding between patients receiving a PPI and patients receiving an H2RA.[91]

TABLE 55.1 Risk Factors for NSAID Ulcers[a]

Risk Factor	Risk Ratio
History of complicated ulcer	13.5
Use of multiple NSAIDs (including aspirin, COX-2 inhibitors)	9
Use of high doses of NSAIDs	7
Use of an anticoagulant	6.4
History of an uncomplicated ulcer	6.1
Age >70 years	5.6
Hp infection	3.5
Use of a glucocorticoid	2.2

[a]Not all NSAIDs pose the same risk.

Misoprostol

The efficacy of misoprostol in preventing NSAID-induced ulcers has been assessed in RCTs.[92,93] A systematic review of these trials indicated that all doses of misoprostol studied (400–800 μg/day) reduce the risk of NSAID-induced endoscopic ulcers.[90] However, only full-dose misoprostol (800 μg/day) reduces ulcer complications.[92] In a randomized double-blind trial in patients with rheumatoid arthritis who received NSAIDs, misoprostol (200 μg four times daily) lowered the rate of GI complications by 40% (from 0.95% in the placebo group to 0.57% in the misoprostol group). However, up to 30% of misoprostol-treated patients in this trial experienced GI upset, thereby limiting its clinical use. Even though endoscopic studies had suggested that lower doses of misoprostol, such as 200 μg two or three times daily, can prevent NSAID-induced ulcers with fewer adverse effects than the full dose,[92] such low doses of misoprostol fail to prevent ulcer complications.[94]

PPIs

PPIs significantly reduce the risk of endoscopic duodenal and GUs.[90] The efficacy of PPIs has been compared with that of H2RAs and with misoprostol in patients who received NSAIDs. Two 6-month studies compared omeprazole 20 mg once daily with either standard-dose ranitidine (150 mg twice daily) and half-dose misoprostol (200 μg twice daily).[81,85] Omeprazole was more effective than standard-dose ranitidine and comparable with half-dose misoprostol in preventing endoscopic ulcers. The superiority of omeprazole over ranitidine in preventing NSAID-related ulcer was due to a greater reduction in endoscopic DUs. A post hoc analysis revealed that most of the added protection attributable to omeprazole over ranitidine occurred among those with Hp infection. Another endoscopic study compared high-dose misoprostol (200 μg four times daily) with two doses of lansoprazole (15 and 30 mg daily) for the prevention of ulcers in long-term NSAID users without Hp infection and with a history of GU.[94] Misoprostol was more effective than either dose of lansoprazole in preventing GU, but there was no practical advantage of misoprostol over lansoprazole because of the high withdrawal rate in the misoprostol group. In a head-to-head endoscopic ulcer prevention study comparing two doses of pantoprazole with 20 mg/day of omeprazole in patients with rheumatoid arthritis receiving NSAIDs, the 6-month probabilities of remaining ulcer free were 91%, 95%, and 93% for pantoprazole 20 mg, pantoprazole 40 mg, and omeprazole 20 mg, respectively.[91]

Two identical multicenter randomized clinical trials compared esomeprazole (20 or 40 mg) with placebo in the prevention of ulcers in patients taking NSAIDs or COX-2 inhibitors over a 6-month period. Patients in both studies were Hp negative, older than age 60, and had a history of GU or DU. Overall, the rates of ulcers were 17.0%, 5.2%, and 4.6% in the groups receiving placebo, esomeprazole 20 mg, and esomeprazole 40 mg, respectively.[95]

Whether PPIs can reduce the risk of NSAID-associated peptic ulcer bleeding is largely based on observational studies and one randomized trial in high-risk patients. A large-scale, case-control study found that PPI therapy was associated with a significant reduction in risk of UGI bleeding among chronic NSAID users (relative risk, 0.13; 95% CI, 0.09–0.19).[96] The randomized trial compared long-term (6 months) omeprazole therapy to 1 week of Hp eradication therapy for the prevention of recurrent ulcer bleeding in Hp-infected patients with a recent history of NSAID-related ulcer bleeding who continued to use naproxen.[97] Recurrent ulcer bleeding occurred in 18.8% of patients undergoing eradication therapy compared with only 4.4% of patients receiving omeprazole.

COX-2 Inhibitors (In Place of NSAIDs)

COX-2 inhibitors offer the hope of minimizing GI toxicity of NSAIDs while preserving their therapeutic effects.[98–102] In a systematic review of randomized trials, when compared with nonselective NSAIDs, the COX-2 inhibitors led to significantly fewer gastroduodenal ulcers (relative risk, 0.26; 95% CI, 0.23–0.30) and ulcer complications (relative risk, 0.39; 95% CI, 0.31–0.5), as well as fewer withdrawals caused by GI symptoms[99]; however, the sparing effect of COX-2 inhibitors on ulcer development is negated by concomitant use of low-dose aspirin.[61]

Current evidence indicates that COX-2 inhibitors are as effective as a combination of nonselective NSAIDs combined with a PPI in patients at risk for ulcers. In a randomized comparison of the NSAID diclofenac plus omeprazole versus celecoxib for secondary prevention of ulcer bleeding in patients who either were Hp negative or had undergone Hp eradication,[100] a similar proportion of patients had recurrent bleeding in 6 months (6.4% in the diclofenac/omeprazole group and 4.9% of patients in the celecoxib group). Although the two treatments were comparable in terms of the incidence of ulcer bleeding, a subsequent follow-up endoscopic study showed that 20%–25% of patients receiving either treatment developed recurrent endoscopic ulcers at 6 months. These findings suggest that neither treatment can eliminate the risk of recurrent bleeding in very high-risk patients. In a 13-month, double-blind randomized trial comparing celecoxib alone with celecoxib/esomeprazole in patients with a history of NSAID-associated ulcer bleeding, 8.9% of the celecoxib-alone group had recurrent ulcer bleeding compared with none of the combined therapy group ($P = .0004$).[101]

Despite the improved gastric safety profile of COX-2 inhibitors, the cardiovascular risk associated with this new class of NSAIDs has been a subject of much concern. In the VIGOR study,[102] the incidence of acute myocardial events, although low, was four times higher among patients receiving rofecoxib than among patients receiving naproxen. Whether this observed difference in myocardial infarction rates was related to an antiplatelet property of naproxen or to a pro-thrombotic effect of rofecoxib was debated. Further data regarding the cardiovascular hazards of COX-2 inhibitors were derived from two long-term studies of colon polyp prevention, using either rofecoxib [the Adenomatous Polyp Prevention on Vioxx (APPROVE) study][103] and celecoxib [the Adenoma Prevention with Celecoxib (APC) study].[104] In APPROVE, interim data at 18 months indicated that patients who had received 25 mg rofecoxib a day had twice the risk of serious cardiovascular events compared with patients who received placebo. In 2004 rofecoxib was voluntarily withdrawn from worldwide markets in light of this unexpected finding. In the APC study, interim data at 33 months showed that serious cardiovascular events were significantly more frequent with celecoxib at the high dose of 400 mg twice a day (hazard ratio, 1.9; 95% CI, 1 to 3.3). The MEDAL program was a prespecified pooled analysis of cardiothrombotic events from three trials in which patients with osteoarthritis or rheumatoid arthritis were randomly assigned to etoricoxib (60 or 90 mg daily) or diclofenac (150 mg daily). After an average treatment of 18 months, rates of cardiothrombotic events were similar between the two treatment groups.[105]

Current evidence suggests that not only COX-2 inhibitors but also nonselective NSAIDs, except for full-dose naproxen (1000 mg/day), increase cardiothrombotic risk. In a meta-analysis of randomized trials of COX-2 inhibitors (data mostly derived from rofecoxib and celecoxib), all COX-2 inhibitors increased the cardiothrombotic risk compared with placebo (risk ratio, 1.42; 95% CI, 1.13 to 1.78). This was largely attributable to an increased risk of myocardial infarction, with little difference in other vascular outcomes. A dose-dependent increase in cardiothrombotic events was observed with celecoxib. Importantly, there was no significant difference in cardiothrombotic risk between COX-2 inhibitors and nonselective NSAIDs, with naproxen (500 mg twice daily) the only exception. In a meta-analysis of observational studies, high-dose rofecoxib (≥25 mg a day), diclofenac, and indomethacin were associated with an increase in cardiothrombotic events, whereas celecoxib did not significantly increase the cardiothrombotic risk, although an increased risk could not be excluded with doses greater than 200 mg/day.[106] In a large-scale, randomized, noninferiority trial of celecoxib versus naproxen and ibuprofen in patients with arthritis (mostly osteoarthritis) and with increased cardiovascular risk,[107] more than 24,000 patients were recruited with a mean treatment duration of 20 months and a mean follow-up period of 34 months. Celecoxib (on average approximately 200 mg/day) was found to be noninferior to ibuprofen (approximately 2000 mg/day) or naproxen (approximately 850 mg/day) with regard to cardiovascular safety. Patients treated with celecoxib had a significantly lower risk of adverse GI events than with naproxen or ibuprofen. The risk of adverse renal events was also significantly lower with celecoxib than with ibuprofen; however, the proportion of patients continued on concomitant low-dose aspirin during the study period was unclear, and very few patients had a history of GI bleeding. It is, therefore, unclear whether the advantage of celecoxib over naproxen or ibuprofen can be extrapolated to patients on concomitant aspirin with high risk of GI bleeding. In another 18-month randomized trial of patients at high risk of both cardiovascular and GI adverse events who required concomitant low-dose aspirin and an NSAID, celecoxib plus a PPI was found to be superior to naproxen plus a PPI in reducing the risk of recurrent ulcer bleeding.[108,109]

Assessing Risk and Choice of Agent(s)

Safe prescription of NSAIDs should be based on assessment of an individual patient's GI and cardiovascular risks. In patients with low cardiovascular risk, the therapeutic approach can be stratified according to their levels of GI risk as follows (Table 55.2):

- Low ulcer risk: No risk factors. Patients without risk factors (see Table 55.1) are at very low risk of ulcer complications with NSAID use (≈1% per year). Rational use of NSAIDs, including avoidance of high doses of NSAIDs and use of a less ulcerogenic NSAID (e.g., ibuprofen, diclofenac) at the lowest effective dose, is a cost-effective approach.
- Moderate ulcer risk: One or two risk factors. These patients should receive combination therapy with an antiulcer agent (a PPI or misoprostol) and an NSAID. Alternatively, substitution with celecoxib alone is as effective as the combination therapy mentioned earlier.
- High ulcer risk: Three or more risk factors, history of ulcer complications, or concomitant use of low-dose aspirin, glucocorticoids, or anticoagulant therapy. In general, NSAIDs should be avoided in these patients, not only because of the high risk of ulcer complications but also owing to the serious consequences of ulcer complications in the presence of comorbidities. Glucocorticoid therapy (without NSAID) can be considered if short-term anti-inflammatory therapy is required for acute, self-limiting arthritis (e.g., gout), because glucocorticoids alone do not increase the risk of ulcer. If regular anti-inflammatory therapy is required for chronic arthritis, the combination of celecoxib and a PPI offers the best GI protection.

TABLE 55.2 Recommendations for Reducing the Risk of NSAID Ulcers as a Function of GI and Cardiovascular Risk

	GI Risk[a]		
	Low	**Moderate**	**High**
Low CV risk	NSAID at the lowest effective dose	NSAID plus a PPI, or celecoxib alone	Celecoxib plus a PPI
High CV risk[b]	Naproxen or celecoxib, plus a PPI	Naproxen or celecoxib, plus a PPI	Celecoxib plus a PPI if simple analgesics failed

[a]*Low GI risk* denotes no risk factors (see Table 55.1); *moderate GI risk* denotes one or two risk factors; *high GI risk* denotes ≥three risk factors, prior complicated ulcer, or concomitant use of low-dose aspirin or anticoagulants. All patients with a history of ulcer who require NSAIDs should be tested for Hp, and if infection is present, eradication therapy should be given (see Chapter 54).

[b]*High CV risk* denotes the requirement for prophylactic low-dose aspirin for primary or secondary prevention of serious CV events.

CV, Cardiovascular.

Defining patients with high cardiovascular risk remains arbitrary. The American Heart Association recommends that aspirin should be considered in all apparently healthy men and women whose 10-year risk for a cardiovascular event is 10% or above.[110] We consider patients with arthritis to have significant cardiovascular risk if they are already on aspirin for secondary prophylaxis or if they require aspirin for primary prophylaxis according to the American Heart Association guidelines. Because the potential cardiovascular hazards of COX-2 inhibitors and most nonselective NSAIDs, patients with high cardiovascular risk should avoid using these drugs, if possible. Ibuprofen can attenuate the cardioprotective effect of aspirin, possibly through competitive binding to platelet COX-1, and concomitant use of ibuprofen and low-dose aspirin, therefore, should be avoided. If an NSAID is deemed necessary in patients at high cardiovascular risk, current evidence suggests that either celecoxib at moderate dose (200 mg/day) or naproxen can be considered. One major drawback of concomitant use of NSAIDs such as naproxen and low-dose aspirin is that the combination will markedly increase the risk of ulcer complications; thus combination of celecoxib and low-dose aspirin may be the best available option for patients with high GI and high cardiovascular risk who require NSAIDs for long term.

Because Hp infection increases the risk of ulcer complications in NSAID users, patients with a history of PUD who require NSAIDs for long term should be tested for Hp, and, if present, the infection should be eradicated.

COMPLICATIONS AND THEIR TREATMENT

Bleeding

Acute UGI bleeding, the most common complication of PUD, is discussed in detail in Chapter 21. PUD remains the leading cause of acute UGI bleeding.[111] Consensus groups have recommended a multidisciplinary approach to the care of patients presenting with UGI bleeding.[112] Patients with acute UGI bleeding should be assessed promptly on presentation. Volume resuscitation should take priority and precede endoscopy. Features of liver disease should call attention to the possibility of bleeding from esophagogastric varices rather than an ulcer. This distinction has prognostic as well as management implications. Variceal hemorrhage carries a higher death rate than ulcer bleeding. The possibility of variceal hemorrhage calls for specific measures prior to endoscopy, such as the use of vasoactive drugs (e.g., octreotide) and antibiotics (e.g., cefotaxime) as prophylaxis against infective complications such as spontaneous bacterial peritonitis (see Chapters 94 and 95).

Endoscopic Therapy

Urgent and early endoscopy is generally defined as EGD performed within 6–12 and 24 hours, respectively, after a patient's presentation. In patients with signs of active UGI bleeding, urgent endoscopy establishes a diagnosis and offers a possible intervention. However, urgent endoscopy may not necessarily improve outcomes.

In patients at high risk for re-bleeding, whose condition could be stabilized after initial resuscitation, an RCT demonstrated early endoscopy was not inferior to urgent endoscopy in patients with acute UGIB. Urgent endoscopy required more frequent endoscopic treatment, which however, did not translate into a lower incidence of further bleeding or 30-day mortality.[113]

In patients with PUD bleeding, urgent endoscopy without adequate resuscitation may actually lead to harm. In a prospective cohort study of 12,601 patients from Denmark, urgent endoscopy in hemodynamically unstable patients was associated with an increased in-hospital and 30-day mortality compared to early endoscopy. In hemodynamically stable patients with significant comorbidities, in-hospital mortality was lowest with endoscopy at 12–36 hours after admission.[114] The above illustrates the importance of hemodynamic resuscitation and optimization of comorbidities prior to consideration of endoscopic therapy. In patients at low risk for re-bleeding, RCTs demonstrated that early endoscopy allowed early hospital discharge, reduced resource utilization, and facilitated management as outpatients.[109,115,116] Meta-analysis of 18 clinical trials that compared endoscopic therapy to pharmacotherapy alone showed that endoscopic therapy was superior with regard to the rates of further bleeding (OR 0.35; 95% CI, 0.27–0.46), surgery (OR 0.57; 95% CI, 0.41–0.81), and, importantly, mortality (OR 0.57; 95% CI, 0.37–0.89).[117]

An international consensus group[110] recommended the use of a prognostic score to guide patient management. The Rockall scoring system is a composite score using pre-endoscopy and postendoscopy clinical parameters to predict mortality. The score was derived from data gathered from the first National UK Audit.[116] The Glasgow Blatchford score (GBS), on the other hand, uses only clinical parameters to predict the need for intervention and is calculated from patient's Hgb level and blood urea concentration, pulse, and systolic blood pressure on admission, the presence or absence of melena or syncope, as well as evidence of cardiac or hepatic failure.[117] The GBS has been the most widely validated score and correlates with clinical outcomes.

In a multicentre prospective study[118] of 3012 patients, the GBS score was the best of the four at predicting the need for intervention or death with an area under the receiver operating curve (AUROC) of 0.86. A GBS score of 1 appears to be the threshold for outpatient management. The GBS score, however, does not define a cutoff value above which urgent endoscopy becomes mandatory. A significant proportion of patients at low-to-median scores require endoscopic treatment.

At the time of EGD, endoscopic stigmata of bleeding in an ulcer not only pinpoint PUD as the source of bleeding but are themselves prognostic for patient outcomes (see Chapter 21). The commonly used nomenclature is a version modified from Forrest and Finlayson's[119] original description. Laine and Jensen[120] summarized rates of further bleeding, surgery, and mortality associated with stigmata of bleeding in prospective trials without endoscopic therapy.

- Type I: Active bleeding:
  Ia: Spurting hemorrhage (Fig. 55.4)
  Ib: Oozing hemorrhage (see Fig. 55.4)
- Type II: Stigmata of recent hemorrhage:
  IIa: Nonbleeding visible vessel (see Fig. 55.4)
  IIb: Adherent clot (see Fig. 55.4)
  IIc: Flat pigmentation (see Fig. 55.4)
- Type III: Clean-base ulcers

Actively bleeding ulcers and ulcers with nonbleeding visible vessels ("protuberant discoloration" or a "sentinel clot") warrant endoscopic therapy (see Chapter 21).

Endoscopic therapy of ulcers with "adherent clots" had been controversial. The definition of adherent clot varies with the vigor in endoscopic washing. Two randomized controlled studies[121,122] and a meta-analysis compared medical therapy to endoscopic treatment in ulcer patients with "adherent clots" and concluded that clot removal followed by endoscopic treatment of the vessel underneath lowers the risk of recurrent bleeding from 30% to 5%.

The term *sentinel clot*, is often used synonymously with *visible vessel*.[124] It represents a fibrin clot, which plugs the rent in an eroded artery. As the ulcer begins to heal, the clot resolves, leaving a flat pigmentation to the ulcer base, which eventually disappears from the ulcer floor. This evolution of a bleeding vessel usually takes less than 72 hours. Ulcers with a flat pigmentation or a clean base do not warrant endoscopic therapy.

Recently, a group from UCLA reported their experience with the use of an endoscopic Doppler probe to interrogate the ulcer base. In a prospective cohort of 163 patients with bleeding ulcers and varying endoscopic stigmata or recent hemorrhage, Doppler signals were found in ulcers with minor stigmata (adherent clots, 68.4%, and flat pigmentations, 40.5%).[125] In a subsequent RCT of 148 patients with bleeding peptic ulcers, Jensen and associates[126] compared Doppler endoscopic probe–guided hemostasis to standard endoscopic hemostasis. The 30-day re-bleeding rate was lower with the use of a Doppler probe to guide the treatment endpoint (11.1% vs. 26.3%, $P = .02$).

Endoscopic therapeutic modalities are discussed in more detail in Chapter 21, and the methods used are discussed briefly here.

Injection Methods

Endoscopic injection of diluted epinephrine into a bleeding peptic ulcer works by volume tamponade and local vasoconstriction. The technique is easy to learn and is not damaging to tissues. Diluted epinephrine, however, does not induce vessel thrombosis. Recurrent bleeding after injection with diluted epinephrine alone occurs in 20%–30% of patients. Injection with diluted epinephrine allows a clear view of the bleeding vessel and should then be combined with application of either thermal-coagulation or clips. In a meta-analysis,[127] addition of a second modality after epinephrine injection significantly reduced the rate of recurrent bleeding (RR 0.57, 0.43–0.76), emergency surgery (RR 0.68, 0.5–0.93), and mortality (RR 0.64, 0.39–1.06). Improved outcomes are more evident in ulcers with active bleeding (Forrest type I ulcers). Injection with diluted epinephrine alone should no longer be considered an adequate treatment. A second treatment to induce arterial thrombosis should be added.

Thermal Methods

Thermal methods include contact and noncontact methods. Contact thermal methods are more often used. Commonly used

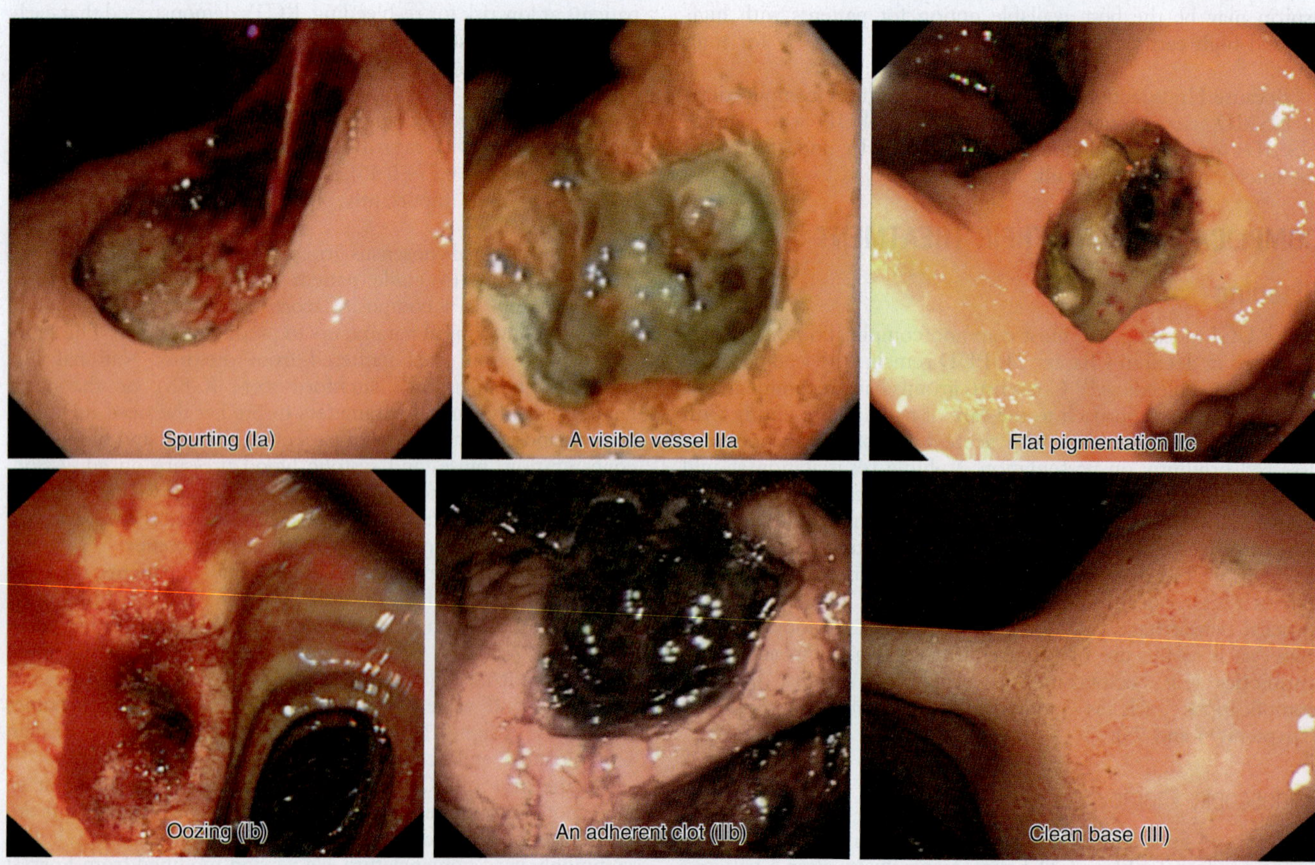

Fig. 55.4 Endoscopic appearances of bleeding peptic ulcers using the Forrest classification.[152]

contact thermal probes are the heater probe and bipolar probes. The term *coaptive thermal-coagulation* emphasizes the need for firm mechanical compression of the vessel. Cessation of blood flow by compression reduces the "heat-sink" effect when heat energy is generated, welding the arterial lumen. The main noncontact method is argon plasma coagulation (see Chapter 21).

Mechanical Methods

The mechanical method of hemoclipping is widely used. Tangential applications of clips in treating bleeding posterior duodenal bulbar or lesser curvature ulcers with the endoscope in a retroflexed position can be technically difficult. In meta-analyses comparing endoscopic treatment modalities, hemoclips were superior to injection alone in rate of hemostasis and comparable to thermal coagulation.[109,128]

Recently, a multicenter RCT compared the use of over-the-scope clips (OTSC) to standard through-the-scope clips and thermal methods in 66 patients with refractory bleeding ulcers.[129] The use of OTSC was associated with a reduced rate of further bleeding (15.2% vs. 57.6%). OTSCs are made of shape memory nitinol of up to 13 mm in diameter, capable of strong tissue compression over a wider area. The current standard is the use of either through-the-scope hemoclips or thermal-coagulation with or without preinjection of epinephrine. OTSC appears to be a useful rescue when other modalities fail.

Antisecretory Therapy

The rationale for antisecretory therapy in bleeding PUD is based on the fact that both pepsin activity and platelet aggregation are pH dependent. An ulcer stops bleeding when a fibrin or platelet plug blocks the rent in a bleeding artery. When gastric pH exceeds 4, pepsin is inactivated, preventing enzymatic digestion of blood clots. A gastric pH of 6 or greater is critical for clot stability and hemostasis. Labenz and associates[130] studied gastric pH in patients with GU or DU who were receiving either a high dose of omeprazole (IV bolus 80 mg, followed by 8 mg/h) or a high dose of ranitidine (IV bolus 50 mg, followed by 0.25 mg/kg/h). The gastric pH exceeded 6 with omeprazole 99.9% of the time, but less than 50% of the time in patients receiving ranitidine (46% of the time in GU patients and 20% of the time in DU patients). The PUB study was an international multicenter study that enrolled 764 patients with ulcer bleeding. It evaluated use of high-dose esomeprazole after endoscopic hemostasis in bleeding peptic ulcers. The PPI reduced the rate of recurrent bleeding over 30 days from 11.6% to 6.4%. In addition, fewer patients given the PPI needed further endoscopic therapy, blood transfusion, and surgery.[131]

A Cochrane systematic review of randomized trials that compared PPI use to placebo or an H2RA concluded that the use of PPI therapy significantly reduces rates of recurrent bleeding and surgery but not overall mortality.[132] In a subgroup analysis among patients with active bleeding or with a nonbleeding visible vessel, a significant reduction in mortality was observed with use of PPI (OR 0.53; 95% CI, 0.31–0.91).

The optimal PPI dose to use and the routine use of PPI administration continue to be controversial. A meta-analysis of RCTs that compared low- to high-dose PPI use after endoscopic hemostasis consisted of trials that included bleeding ulcers with minor stigmata of bleeding and clean-based ulcers.[133] The majority of studies were underpowered to declare equivalence between low- and high-dose PPI. An international consensus group has continued to endorse the use of a high-dose PPI, especially in high-risk patients.[110] RCTs, however, have demonstrated PPI therapy after endoscopic hemostasis significantly reduced further bleeding and mortality.[134–137] The typical therapy consists of 80 mg bolus followed by 8 mg/h infusion for 72 hours.[104,138,139]

Pre-emptive use of an IV PPI infusion prior to endoscopy was studied in a large-scale randomized study.[140] Patients with overt signs of UGI bleeding were randomized to receive either a high-dose PPI infusion or placebo. Most (60%) of the patients in this cohort were found at EGD to be bleeding from a peptic ulcer. The study demonstrated that early PPI infusion downstaged endoscopic bleeding stigmata in patients with peptic ulcers and thereby reduced the need for endoscopic therapy; thus there were fewer ulcers with active bleeding or with major stigmata of recent hemorrhage observed during the following morning's EGD in the PPI group. PPI infusion starts ulcer healing, and significantly more clean-based ulcers are seen the next day. The study has cost-saving implications, with less endoscopic therapy required with the preemptive use of an IV PPI. In patients awaiting endoscopy, it is reasonable to start PPI therapy.

Surgical Therapy

Effective endoscopic intervention and improved pharmacotherapy have greatly reduced the need for emergency ulcer surgery. In the United States, the incidence of surgery to control ulcer bleeding has continued to decline (from 13.1% in 1993 to 9.7% in 2006), while there was an increase in the use of endoscopic treatment (12.9%–22.2%).[141] In an UK National Audit in 2006, only 2.3% of 4478 patients who presented with UGI bleeding required surgery. Mortality after surgery was 29%.[142] Surgery is indicated in patients with bleeding not controlled during endoscopy or with further bleeding refractory to endoscopic therapy. Independent predictors for recurrent bleeding after endoscopic hemostatic therapy include hemodynamic instability, comorbid illnesses, active bleeding at endoscopy, large ulcer size, posterior DU, or lesser curvature ulcer.[143] Often, an attempt at further endoscopic control is indicated. An RCT that compared endoscopic retreatment to surgery suggested that the former can secure bleeding in 75% of cases and is associated with less procedure-related morbidities.[144]

The type of emergency operation to be performed for ulcer bleeding is controversial. Some surgeons maintain that oversewing of ulcers alone, combined with acid-suppression therapy, is safer than "definitive" surgery using either gastrectomy or vagotomy. Hp eradication and PPIs have provided incentives for surgeons to perform the minimum operation.

Two RCTs that compared minimal with definitive surgery were published before the era of endoscopic hemostasis and PPI infusion.[145,146] A United Kingdom multicenter study compared minimal surgery (oversewing the vessel or ulcer excision alone plus IV H2RA therapy) with a definitive ulcer operation (vagotomy and pyloroplasty or partial gastrectomy) in patients with bleeding GUs or DUs. The trial was aborted because of the high rate of fatal recurrent bleeding in those assigned to minimal surgery (7 in 62 patients, with 6 deaths). Of the 67 patients who received definitive ulcer surgery, 4 re-bled and none died.[145] In a trial conducted by the French Association of Surgical Research, patients with DU were randomized to receive oversewing plus vagotomy and drainage or partial gastrectomy.[146] After oversewing and vagotomy, recurrent bleeding occurred in 10 of 60 patients (17%); conversion to a Billroth II gastrectomy was required in 6 of the 10 patients with recurrent bleeding. In the group of 60 patients assigned to undergo partial gastrectomy, only 2 (3%) had re-bleeding, and both recovered with conservative treatment. With an intention-to-treat analysis, no differences in overall mortality rates or duodenal leak rates were seen. These two RCTs suggest that simple oversewing with or without vagotomy is associated with a higher rate of recurrent bleeding. Exclusion of an ulcer or, in the case of GUs, ulcer excision is important in preventing recurrent bleeding. In a review of data from the American College Surgeons National Surgical Quality Improvement Program, 30-day mortality was higher in patients who underwent a simple oversewing or ulcer excision (106/498, 21.3%) when compared to that after vagotomy with resection or drainage (39/283, 13.8%). There was obvious bias in this retrospective analysis.[147]

Angiographic Therapy

Angiographic embolization of bleeding arteries is a nonoperative alternative to surgery in patients with bleeding peptic ulcer. In a pooled analysis of six retrospective studies comparing angiography and surgery, a higher re-bleeding rate was observed after angiographic treatment (51/178, or 29% vs. 36/241, or 15%; RR 1.82; 95% CI, 1.20–2.67).[148] Mortality was not significantly different (17% vs. 23%). When radiology skills are available, angiography is often attempted before surgery. A recent RCT that compared added embolization to standard treatment after endoscopic hemostasis did not confirm a mortality benefit of prophylactic embolization.[149] In a per protocol analysis, the rate of further bleeding was lower after added embolization (6/96, or 6.2% vs. 14/123, or 11.4%). In a subgroup analysis of ulcers of 15 mm or more in size, embolization reduced bleeding from 23.1% to 4.5%. The authors suggested that for larger ulcers with significant bleeding, angiographic embolization should be considered after endoscopic hemostasis.

Perforation

Perforation of a GU or DU (Fig. 55.5) is a surgical emergency that may be the initial manifestation of PUD, especially in patients using NSAIDs. Ulcer perforation is associated with a mortality approaching 30%. Older adults with significant comorbid illnesses and a delay in performing surgery have the worst prognosis. The clinical presentation is one of peritonitis, but clinical signs can be obscured in older and immunocompromised patients (see Chapter 37).

Medical Therapy

It has been suggested that a standardized perioperative management protocol can improve outcomes. In a Danish multicenter study ($n = 2619$),[150] the PULP trial group showed that with aggressive and specific treatment of sepsis and, importantly, surgery within 6 hours, mortality was 17% in 117 hospitals with strict management protocols and was 27% in 512 hospitals without protocols. Other measures include goal-directed fluid therapy, general respiratory and circulatory support, intravenous broad-spectrum antibiotics, and insertion of a double-barreled NG tube and a urinary catheter. An intravenous PPI is given routinely after surgery.

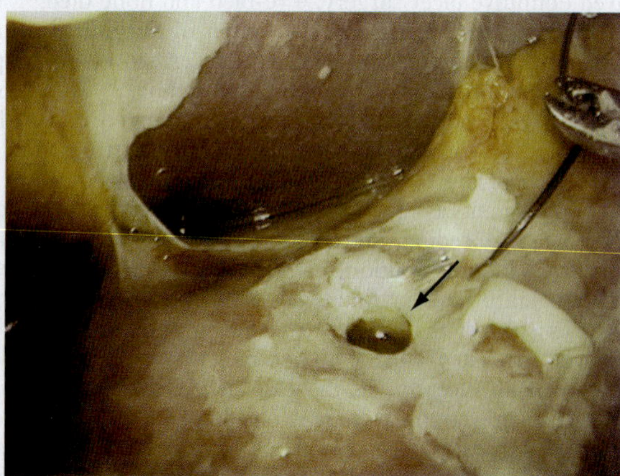

Fig. 55.5 Laparoscopic view of a perforated DU (*arrow*) with fibrinous exudate on the adjacent peritoneum.

Nonoperative management of ulcer perforation should seldom be practiced. It involves NG suctioning, parenteral antibiotics, and IV fluids. In an RCT, Crofts and associates[151] assigned patients with the presumptive diagnosis of perforated peptic ulcers to either conservative treatment or prompt surgery. Overall, morbidity and mortality rates (5%) were low and similar in the medical and surgical groups. Of the 40 patients assigned to conservative treatment, 11 showed no improvement within 12 hours and underwent operation. Three of these 11 patients were found to have perforated carcinomas (2 gastric and 1 sigmoid colon). Findings of the study highlight common objections to the use of nonoperative management: uncertainty of the site of perforation, the possibility of a perforated GI tumor, and atrophic momentum making spontaneous sealing unlikely. Older adults tolerate sepsis poorly. Any delay in definitive treatment leads to poor outcomes.

Surgical Therapy

Perforated gastroduodenal ulcer carries a high mortality rate. In a review of surgery for perforated ulcers between 2011 and 2013 in Denmark, the 90-day mortality was 25.5% among 726 patients. Re-operation was required in 124 patients (17.1%), approximately one-third of them caused by persistent leaks.[152]

Boey and associates[153] identified preoperative shock, major medical illnesses, and perforation longer than 12 hours as important adverse prognostic factors. The PULP score was recently developed from a cohort of 2668 patients who received surgery in 11 hospitals across Denmark. Variables included were age greater than 65 years, active malignant disease or acquired immunodeficiency, cirrhosis, glucocorticoid use, perforation more than 24 hours, shock, raised serum creatinine level, and American Society of Anesthesiologists score greater than 1. The PULP score was accurate in predicting mortality from ulcer perforation (AUROC of 0.83).[154] The score, however, has not been validated in centers outside Denmark.

The controversies in the operative management of perforated peptic ulcers have revolved around the choice between laparoscopic and open repair and the need for a definitive ulcer operation after closure of the perforation (and which definitive operation to perform). Treatment also differs for duodenal and gastric perforations. Simple closure of a perforated duodenal or a juxta-pyloric ulcer with the use of an omental patch is widely practiced.

Meta-analyses of three RCTs (two from Hong Kong and the Dutch LAMA study) that compared laparoscopic to open surgical treatment of perforated peptic ulcers tend to favor laparoscopic repair with respect to rates of abdominal septic complications (OR 0.66; 95% CI, 0.3–1.47), and pulmonary complications (OR 0.43; 95% CI, 0.17–1.12)[155]; thus laparoscopic repair should, at the least, be considered not inferior to open repair. There may, however, have been selection bias in these RCTs. Poor risk patients (those with delayed presentations, shock, and with significant comorbidities) may be better suited for a laparotomy. Large perforations (>10 mm) suggest sizable ulcerations and should also be managed by laparotomy; often, gastric resections are required in such patients.

GU accounts for approximately 20% of perforated peptic ulcers. Epidemiologic data suggest a rising proportion of GUs among perforated ulcers, especially in older adult patients who use NSAIDs. Patients with perforated GUs are more likely to be older and to have significant comorbid illnesses, making their prognosis less favorable. As with perforated DUs, there has been a debate regarding the choice of surgery for perforated GUs. Simple closure should be offered to small perforations at the prepyloric area. The optimal treatment of an angular notch GU along the lesser curvature should entail an antrectomy and lesser curve ulcer excision, followed by either a Billroth type I or II reconstruction. The role of vagotomy is unclear. The advocates for primary resection in perforated GUs argue that mortality rates after gastrectomy are not increased and that the rate of postoperative ulcer-related complications is reduced. The arguments for primary resection also include the possibility that the ulcer is malignant. Malignancy is seen in approximately 6% of perforated GUs.[156] In a retrospective series comprising 287 perforated GUs, death occurred in 21.5% of patients who underwent patch closure alone and in 24.3% of those who underwent gastric resections.[157]

In Hp-associated ulcers, Hp eradication reduces the relapse of ulceration after patch repair. In an RCT from Hong Kong, 99 patients after patch repairs for perforated ulcers were assigned to Hp eradication or a course of PPI. At 1 year, there were fewer relapses in those given Hp eradication (4.8% vs. 38.1%).[158] A meta-analysis of five RCTs that compared simple closure plus Hp eradication to closure alone in patients with perforated DU showed that the pooled incidence of ulcer relapse in the year after Hp eradication was 5.2% compared to 35.2% in those without eradication. These data support the use of simple closure in the majority of perforated DUs.[159]

Obstruction

Gastric outlet obstruction is now an infrequent complication of PUD. Its clinical manifestations—nausea and postprandial vomiting, abdominal fullness, pain, and early satiety—are discussed in Chapter 15, as is the diagnostic approach to patients presenting with possible gastric outlet obstruction. Gastric outlet obstruction should alert clinicians to possible malignancy (see Chapter 56).

Medical Therapy

Patients with obstructing peptic ulcers are often volume depleted. The loss of fluid, hydrogen ions, and chloride ions in the vomitus leads to hypochloremic, hypokalemic metabolic alkalosis. The patient should be volume resuscitated with normal saline followed by potassium replacement once urine output is adequate. In severely malnourished patients, parenteral nutrition should be considered. Decompression of the stomach by a large-bore NG tube relieves vomiting, helps to monitor fluid loss, and allows the stomach to regain its tone. A high-volume, non–bile-stained aspirate can help distinguish gastric outlet obstruction from a high small bowel obstruction. Use of an IV PPI reduces gastric acid output, making fluid and electrolyte management easier. PPI therapy also initiates ulcer healing, ameliorates inflammatory edema, and assists in resolving obstruction. Approximately half of patients respond to this management. Improvement is especially noticeable in patients with active ulceration and edema. Surgery is, therefore, deferred until after an adequate trial of conservative management. Other factors that may influence the decision to proceed to surgery are chronicity, a history of previous ulcer complication, and the patient's age and general medical condition. Furthermore, many authorities argue for initial endoscopic dilation before surgery.

Endoscopic Therapy

Endoscopic balloon dilation has been used successfully in patients with gastric outlet obstruction from PUD (Fig. 55.6).[160–162] During endoscopic examination, the stenosis is traversed by means of a biliary-type guidewire with a flexible tip. A low-compliance through-the-scope balloon is then passed over the guidewire, and dilation can be seen through the endoscope. The use of a balloon is preferred because its inflation produces a uniform radial force, which has a theoretical advantage over the longitudinal shearing force associated with the use of conventional dilators. The procedure is typically performed with fluoroscopic guidance. A regimen of gradual dilation over two or three sessions seems sensible. The targeted diameter is unclear; many authorities recommend dilation to 15 mm, which is often associated with relief of symptoms. The presence of gastric atony also contributes to symptoms. The risk of perforation increases with the size of balloon. Endoscopic series reported immediate relief of obstruction in 78%–100% of cases. In a small series of Hp-infected patients, balloon dilation followed by Hp eradication led to sustained symptom relief.[163]

Surgical Therapy

A variety of operations have been described for obstructing DUs, pyloric channel ulcers, and prepyloric ulcers. They include vagotomy with either a drainage procedure (gastrojejunostomy or pyloroplasty) or an antrectomy. In the unusual event of an

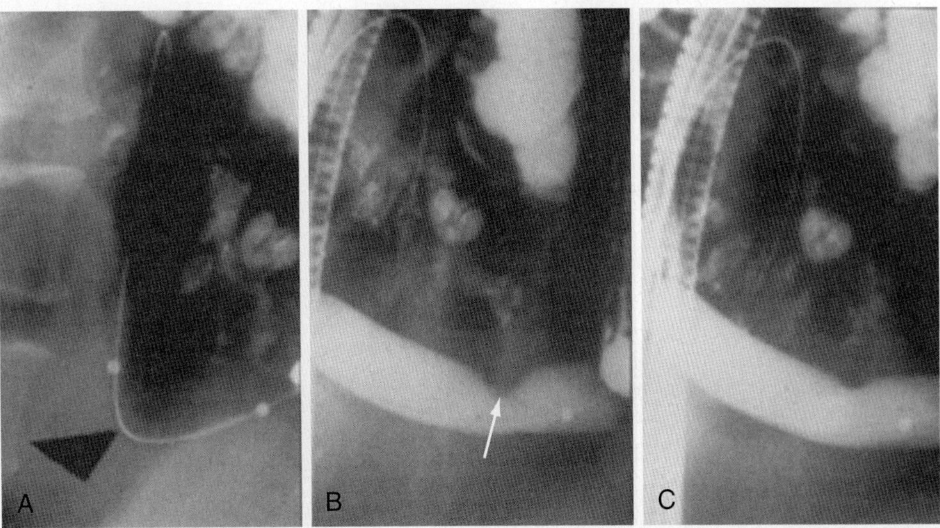

Fig. 55.6 A through-the-scope dilation of an obstructed pylorus caused by an ulcer. The procedure was performed under fluoroscopic guidance. A dual-channel endoscope with a 3.7 mm therapeutic channel was used. (A) The stricture was first traversed with a biliary-type guidewire *(arrowhead)*. A through-the-scope balloon was passed over the guidewire across the stricture. (B) A waist, representing the stricture *(arrow)*, was observed and was nearly abolished on balloon inflation (C).

obstructing prepyloric GU, an antrectomy followed by a Billroth type I gastroduodenostomy is the procedure of choice.

STRESS ULCERS

Stress-related gastric and duodenal mucosal injury (stress ulcers) is an illness of the critically ill who are typically cared for in an ICU. The etiology of stress ulceration is probably related to mucosal ischemia and splanchnic hypoperfusion from shock or low cardiac output. Fortunately, only a small proportion of patients with stress-related mucosal lesions have clinically overt GI bleeding. In a cohort study[164] of 2252 ICU patients, only 1.5% developed clinically important bleeding. Respiratory failure (OR 15.6) and coagulopathy (OR 4.3) were independent predictive factors for bleeding stress ulcers. In 2015 a prospective study[165] of 1034 patients admitted to ICUs was published; clinically important GI bleeding occurred in 2.6% of patients. Those with three or more comorbid illnesses, liver disease, receiving renal replacement therapy, and with a high organ failure score were at risk. Patients in the ICU with traumatic brain injuries and burns also belong to a high-risk group of developing GI bleeding. Across different studies, there appear to be different candidate predictors for bleeding. The use of enteral nutrients buffers acid and protects against bleeding.

PPI, H2RA, and sucralfate are drugs used for stress ulcer prophylaxis. In a network meta-analysis of 57 RCTs ($n = 7293$), Alhazzani and associates[166] showed that PPIs were more effective for preventing clinically important bleeding than H2RA (OR 0.38), sucralfate (OR 0.30), or placebo (OR 0.24). PPIs, however, increased the risk of nosocomial pneumonia compared with H2RA (OR 1.27), sucralfate (OR 1.65), and placebo (OR 1.52). There is concern that acid suppression predisposes patients to nosocomial infection probably linked to gut dysbiosis.[167]

A European multicenter study randomized 3298 ICU patients to receive 40 mg of intravenous PPI or placebo and found that deaths by 90 days were similar between groups (31.1% vs. 30.4%). The rate of composite adverse events (gastrointestinal bleeding, *Clostridium difficile* infection, pneumonia, or myocardial ischemia) was comparable (21.9% vs. 22.6%). There were fewer clinically important bleeding events in the PPI group (2.5% vs. 4.2%).[168]

Full references for this chapter can be found at https://ebooks.health.elsevier.com.

56 Adenocarcinoma of the Stomach and Other Gastric Tumors

Michael Quante, Jan Bornschein

IN THIS CHAPTER

Gastric cancer remains a major cause of cancer-related mortality in the world, despite declining rates of incidence in many industrialized countries. In this chapter, we mainly discuss gastric adenocarcinoma, which makes up most of gastric malignancies.

EPIDEMIOLOGY

Gastric cancer is the fourth leading cause of cancer mortality in the world,[1] although the overall incidence is declining.[2] The estimate in 2020 was of about 1 million new cases and 769,000 deaths worldwide.[1] In Western countries, the incidence of gastric cancer has decreased significantly over the past century; in the United States, gastric cancer mortality has decreased 87% since 1950 with a similar trend being reported in Europe.[3] In the United States, the incidence of gastric cancer has diminished to approximately 7.6 cases per 100,000 people,[4] whereas as recently as 1945, gastric cancer was the leading cause of cancer mortality in men.[5]

There is marked geographic variation in gastric cancer incidence, with the highest incidence rates in the Far East—and almost half of all cases occurring in China (Fig. 56.1).[6] Globally, the age-standardized incidence rate of stomach cancer is reported as 15.4 per 100,000 population, with an age-standardized death rate of 11.0 per 100,000 population. Eastern Europe and Central and South America also have high incidence rates, with the lowest incidence rates observed in North America, North Africa, South Asia, and Australia.[6] Although gastric cancer was common in industrialized countries in the past, the latest data indicate that more than 70% of new cases occur in developing countries,[1,6] Countries with implemented early detection programs, such as Japan and Korea, show significantly better survival rates.[485]

In the United States, the median age of diagnosis is 68 years.[4] In Japan, a country with a high incidence of gastric cancer, the mean age of diagnosis is roughly a decade earlier, likely reflecting lead-time bias due to widespread screening. The incidence of gastric cancer in males is approximately twice that in females (Table 56.1).[1] The incidence of gastric cancer in blacks in the United States is nearly double that in whites. Native Americans and Hispanics also have a higher risk of developing gastric cancer than whites.

In contrast to the pattern seen with nonjunctional gastric cancers, the incidence rates of adenocarcinomas at the esophagogastric junction (EGJ, formerly "cardia cancer") are rising,[2] According to the U.S. Surveillance, Epidemiology, and Ends Results (SEER) database, junctional cancers represent 27% of gastric cancers in the United States, up from just 10% in 1975.[4] Ethnic background contributes to the individual risk. Junctional cancers account for about 35.6% of all stomach cancers in non-Hispanic whites, whereas for less than 15% in the Hispanic, black, and Asian-Pacific U.S. population.[486]

There are numerous dietary, environmental, and genetic risk factors for gastric adenocarcinoma (Box 56.1). The dominant risk

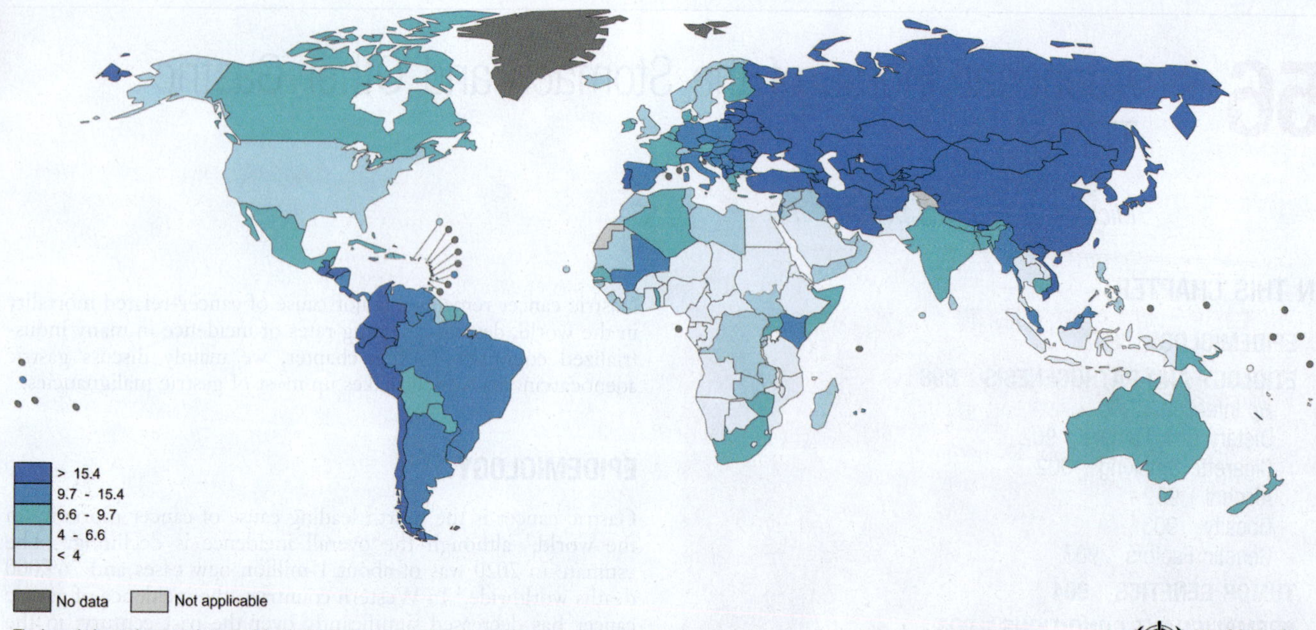

> 15.4
9.7 - 15.4
6.6 - 9.7
4 - 6.6
< 4
No data
Not applicable
The boundaries and names shown and the designations used on this map do not imply the expression of any opinion whatsoever on the part of the World Health Organization concerning the legal status of any country, territory, city or area or of its authorities, or concerning the delimitation of its frontiers or boundaries. Dotted and dashed lines on maps represent approximate border lines for which there may not yet be full agreement.
Data source: GLOBOCAN 2012
Map production: IARC
World Health Organization

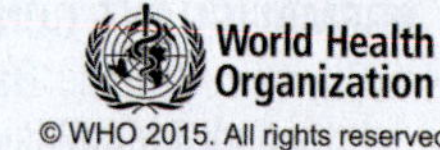

World Health Organization
© WHO 2015. All rights reserved

Fig. 56.1 Worldwide incidence per 100,000 population of gastric cancer in men in 2012 (WHO).

TABLE 56.1 Gastric Cancer Incidence and Mortality Rates per 100,000 Population (Age-Adjusted) in 2012

	Incidence		Mortality	
	Male	**Female**	**Male**	**Female**
Developed countries	15.6	6.7	9.2	4.2
Developing countries	18.1	7.8	14.4	6.5

Data from Torre LA, Bray F, Siegel RL, et al. Global cancer statistics, 2012. *CA Cancer J Clin*. 2015;65:87–108. Available from http://www.ncbi.nlm.nih.gov/pubmed/25651787

factor remains, however, infection with *Helicobacter pylori* (*Hp*) and the associated chronic-active inflammation of the gastric mucosa (see Chapter 54).

ETIOLOGY AND PATHOGENESIS

Gastric cancer can be subdivided using the Laurén classification into two distinct histologic subtypes with different epidemiologic and prognostic features (Fig. 56.2).[7] The *intestinal type* of cancer is characterized by the formation of gland-like tubular structures with features reminiscent of intestinal glands. This type of gastric cancer is more closely linked to environmental and dietary risk factors, tends to be the predominant form in regions with a high incidence of gastric cancer, and is the form of cancer that is now declining worldwide. The *diffuse type* of cancer lacks glandular structure and consists of poorly cohesive cells that infiltrate the wall of the stomach. It is found at the same frequency throughout the world, occurs at a younger age, and is associated with a worse prognosis than the intestinal form. Extensive involvement of the stomach by the diffuse type can result in a rigid and thickened stomach, a condition referred to as *linitis plastica*. Another key feature of diffuse type cancers are signet-ring cells, special mucin-filled cells that are not present in intestinal type adenocarcinomas. There are also mixed phenotypes that contain heterogenous areas that feature predominantly either intestinal- or diffuse-type characteristics.

Adenocarcinoma of the stomach is also classified into proximal tumors (EGJ and gastric cardia) and distal or nonjunctional tumors (fundus, body, and antrum of the stomach). Junctional cancers can be further classified according to the Siewert classification by the location of the main tumor mass into type I (1–5 cm above the EGJ), type II (from 1 cm above to 2 cm below the junction), and type III (2–5 cm below the junction) tumors.[8] There is no clear distinction between the genetic and cellular origin of adenocarcinomas of the distal esophagus, the EGJ, and a subgroup of nonjunctional distal gastric cancers.[9]

Precision medicine in this case allows by genomic analysis to realize that otherwise indistinguishable tumors indeed have discrepant biology and require distinct therapies. Although there are distinct molecular subtypes in EAC and GC (as there are within colorectal adenocarcinoma), these cancers in the future should be viewed as the single entity: gastroesophageal adenocarcinoma (GEAC), with therapeutic approaches guided less by location and more by their distinct molecular profiles.

Interestingly, with the decreasing incidence of *Hp* infection, the incidence of nonjunctional tumors has declined, while the number of more proximal tumors has increased. In a mouse model, it has even been postulated that Barrett esophagus-related esophageal cancer and cancer of the EGJ both have their origins in the gastric cardia.[10] Emerging data from gene expression profiling suggest that differences in pathologic appearance and clinical behavior may be due to the presence of unique molecular phenotypes. Characterization of the gastric cancer genomic

BOX 56.1 Risk Factors for Gastric Adenocarcinoma

DEFINITE

Adenomatous gastric polyps*
Chronic atrophic gastritis
Cigarette smoking
Dysplasia*
EBV
History of gastric surgery (esp. Billroth II)*
Hp infection
Intestinal metaplasia

GENETIC FACTORS

Family history of gastric cancer (first-degree relative)*
Familial adenomatous polyposis (with fundic gland polyps)*
Hereditary nonpolyposis colorectal cancer*
Juvenile polyposis*
Peutz-Jeghers syndrome*

PROBABLE

High salt intake
History of gastric ulcer
Obesity (adenocarcinoma of the cardia only)
Pernicious anemia*
Regular aspirin or other NSAID use (protective)
Snuff tobacco use

POSSIBLE

Diet high in nitrates
Heavy alcohol use
High ascorbate intake (protective)
High intake of fresh fruits and vegetables (protective)
Low socioeconomic status
Ménétrier disease
Statin use (protective)

QUESTIONABLE

High green tea consumption (protective)
Hyperplastic and fundic gland polyps

*Surveillance for cancer is recommended in patients with this risk factor.

landscape reveals the presence of multiple alterations in the expression of tyrosine kinase receptors, which in conjunction with their ligands and downstream effector molecules represent potential pathways for future drug development.

The Cancer Genome Atlas (TCGA) consortium suggested[4] gastric cancer subtypes based on the genomic profile of about 300 gastric cancers.[11] This classification correlated well with the clustering of high throughput data of different platforms, including epigenome, transcriptome, and proteome analysis. So far, there are only little data to support the biological relevance of this proposed classification. Previous transcriptome analyses of gastric cancers, on the other hand, have demonstrated phenotypic clusters with either distinct prognostic outcomes or different response to systemic treatment.[12,13]

It is believed that the development of intestinal-type gastric cancer occurs through a multistep process in which the normal mucosa is sequentially transformed into a hyperproliferative epithelium, followed by metaplastic processes leading to glandular atrophy, dysplasia, and then carcinoma. In colon cancer, the evidence is strong that each step in the transition is associated with a specific gene mutation,[14] but the evidence that gastric cancer follows a comparable sequence of genetic events has been lacking. However, in both the intestinal-type gastric cancer and colorectal cancer, it does appear that DNA mutations are established over time in stem cells in the normal human stomach, and that in intestinal metaplasia (IM), these mutations spread through the stomach through a process involving crypt fission and monoclonal conversion of glands.[15] The contention that the pathogenesis of intestinal-type gastric cancer is a multistep process is supported mainly by the observation that both chronic atrophic gastritis and IM are found in higher incidences in patients with intestinal-type cancer and in countries with a high incidence of gastric cancer (see Chapter 54).[16,17]

This multistep model of intestinal-type gastric cancer, developed in large part by Pelayo Correa et al.,[18] postulates that there is a temporal sequence of preneoplastic changes that eventually lead to the development of gastric cancer. A common feature of the initiation and progression to intestinal-type gastric cancer is chronic inflammation of the gastric mucosa. *Hp* infection is the primary cause of gastric inflammation and the leading etiologic agent for gastric cancer (see Chapter 54). In a subset of patients,

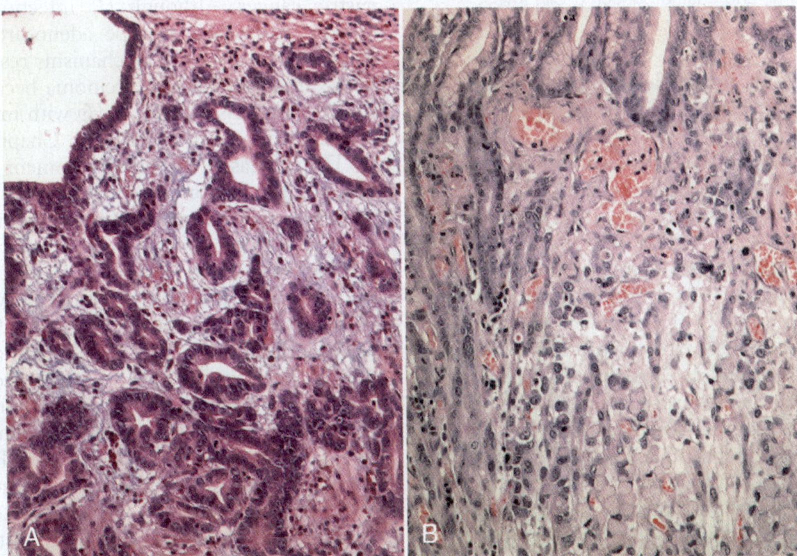

Fig. 56.2 Histopathology of the two types of gastric cancer. (A) The intestinal type of gastric adenocarcinoma is characterized by the formation of gland-like tubular structures mimicking intestinal glands. (B) The diffuse type of gastric cancer contains singly invasive tumor cells that frequently contain abundant mucin and that lack any glandular structure (H&E stains). (Courtesy Rhonda K. Yantiss, MD, Boston, MA, United States.)

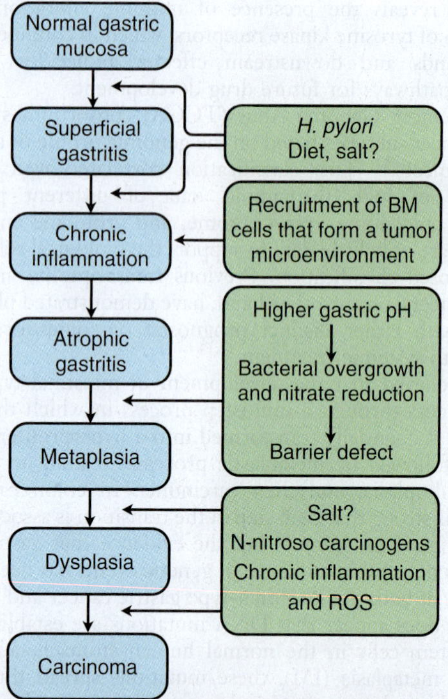

Fig. 56.3 Proposed Correa pathway of pathologic events in gastric adenocarcinoma. In well-differentiated, intestinal-type gastric cancer, histopathologic studies indicated that chronic *Hp* infection progresses over decades through stages of chronic gastritis, atrophic gastritis, intestinal metaplasia, dysplasia, and cancer. The development of cancer has been attributed to alterations in DNA caused by chronic inflammation, which is associated with the recruitment and of bone marrow-derived immune and mesenchymal cells (BM cells) that form a microenvironment that favors tumorigenesis. An imbalance between epithelial cell proliferation and apoptosis and, in a milieu of atrophy and achlorhydria, gastric colonization by enteric bacteria with nitrate reductase activity facilitating formation of carcinogenic nitrosamines allow the accumulation of oncogenic genetic alterations. Corpus-predominant atrophy, or the loss of specialized glandular cell types, such as parietal and chief cells, appears to be the critical initiating step in the progression toward cancer. *ROS*, Reactive oxygen species. (From Fox JG, Wang TC. Inflammation, atrophy, and gastric cancer. *J Clin Invest.* 2007;117:60–69.)

the inflammatory process leads to the development of atrophic gastritis (with loss of glandular tissue) followed by progression to IM, dysplasia, early gastric cancer (EGC), and, eventually, advanced gastric cancer (Fig. 56.3). Although animal models suggested that all stages prior to the development of high-grade dysplasia are potentially reversible, there is still ongoing debate what defines the "point of no return" for humans from which further progression of neoplasia can no longer be prevented.[19,20] Eradication of *Hp* has the potential to prevent gastric cancer as shown in recent meta-analyses.[21,22] The preventive effect of eradication is more evident if there are no preneoplastic conditions of the gastric mucosa (glandular atrophy, IM) at the time of intervention.[23] *Hp* eradication can prevent further progression of preneoplastic conditions, and even a certain degree of regression can be documented.[24] Although it is currently assumed that presence of IM is most likely to mark the *point of no return*, there is even an effect of *Hp* eradication if advanced lesions are present (e.g., after endoscopic resection of an EGC).[25]

Unlike the situation observed with colon cancer, the precise genes involved in each step of this progression are still not defined. Nevertheless, next-generation sequencing techniques have shown that there is more heterogeneity in genetic alterations in gastric cancer and cancer of the EGJ than in colon cancer.[26,27] Furthermore, the premalignant stages of gastric cancer are not as readily identifiable during endoscopy as those of colon cancer, and many gastric carcinomas are very heterogeneous, containing a large percentage of stromal cells. These stromal cells, which also include cancer-associated fibroblasts (CAFs) known to promote tumor growth, have been reported to show distinct genetic and epigenetic changes that may confound tumor analysis.[28,29] This feature makes characterization of the timing of specific gene mutations in gastric cancer difficult at best. Currently, the role of chronic inflammation in the diffuse type of gastric cancer, as well as the similarities if any to the proposed pathway in Fig. 56.3 for the intestinal type of cancer, remain to be clarified. One common factor that is related to both histological subtypes is a strong association with *Hp* infection, which has shown to directly modify genes involved in DNA damage repair (DDR) pathways.[30] Modifications of DDR-related genes are a common event in gastric carcinogenesis.[31]

Hp Infection

Hp is a gram-negative microaerophilic bacterium that infects nearly half the world's population and is recognized as the primary etiologic agent for gastric cancer (see also Chapter 54). Indeed, *Hp* has been classified as a class I (or definite) carcinogen by the International Agency for Research on Cancer, a branch of the WHO. Infection with *Hp* has been found in every population studied, although the prevalence is higher in developing countries and most parts of East Asia.[32,33]

The natural history of chronic *Hp* infection includes three possible outcomes[34]: (1) simple gastritis, where patients often remain asymptomatic; (2) duodenal ulcer phenotype, which occurs in 10%–15% of infected subjects; and (3) gastric ulcer/gastric cancer phenotype. The risk for gastric cancer development varies with the type of background gastritis, but in general, corpus-dominant gastritis resulting in a low acid state is mainly associated with an increased risk. *Hp*-induced duodenal ulcer disease is associated with a high gastric acid output as well as a reduced risk for developing gastric cancer.[35] Studies suggest that *Hp*-infected patients develop chronic atrophic gastritis at a rate of 1%–3% per year of infection.[18,36,37] Thus those patients who are genetically predisposed to developing atrophic gastritis in response to *Hp* infection are likely to be also predisposed to gastric cancer. Although *Hp* infection is associated with both diffuse- and intestinal-type adenocarcinomas, we focus in this chapter mainly on the mechanisms responsible for the formation of intestinal-type adenocarcinoma because they have been better studied. The association of *Hp* with mucosa-associated lymphoid tissue lymphoma is discussed in Chapter 41.

The increased risk of development of gastric adenocarcinoma due to *Hp* infection depends on multiple factors, including host genetic factors, the strain of bacteria (including bacterial virulence factors), the duration of infection, and the presence or absence of other environmental risk factors (e.g., poor diet, smoking). In a Japanese cohort, only those infected with *Hp* developed gastric adenocarcinoma during follow-up (2.9% vs. 0%; $P < .001$).[38] Additional cohort studies from China and Taiwan have reported similar findings.[39,40] In Western countries, the association between *Hp* and gastric cancer appears to be confined to non-junctional tumors.[41] There are data, however, that *Hp* is likely to be also associated with Siewert type III junctional cancers as well as potentially a subgroup of type II tumors.[42,43]

A combination of a virulent bacterial strain, a genetically permissive host, and a favorable gastric environment may be necessary for cancer to occur. Currently, genetic susceptibility factors of the human host are studied based on individual genes, but new technologies, such as next-generation sequencing, will enhance the identification of host genetic factors. Nevertheless, the most important factor appears to be the induction of chronic inflammation by *Hp* infection. This leads to an impairment of the epithelial barrier function of the gastric mucosa, thereby increasing the impact of other pathogenic factors (e.g., diet). Several aspects of the inflammatory milieu have been implicated as carcinogens; they include increased oxidative stress and the formation of oxygen free radicals, leading to DNA damage, increased CD4+ T cells and myeloid cells, and elevated proinflammatory cytokine production, all leading to accelerated cell turnover, reduced apoptosis, and the potential for faulty or incomplete DNA repair.[44] Indeed, recent studies suggest that animals with deficient DNA repair mechanisms display more severe gastric dysplasia after chronic infection with *Hp*.[45] As mentioned earlier, *Hp* is capable of directly modifying DDR-related genes and their function.[30] Thus evidence to date clearly indicates that the most important cofactor in the induction of *Helicobacter*-related disease is the host immune response. Indeed, chronic inflammation has been linked to a large number of nongastric cancers.

Chronic inflammation of the gastric mucosa appears necessary for the progression through atrophy to gastric cancer. Disease mechanisms are difficult to study in human infection, and therefore, much of our understanding of the immune response to *Helicobacter* organisms comes from work performed in a mouse model. Different inbred strains of mice respond to infection with varying degrees of disease susceptibility, and several knockout models have helped to elucidate the roles of individual components of the immune response in disease.

Genetic manipulation of the C57BL/6 susceptible murine strain has facilitated detailed study and has thus led to a deeper understanding of genetic factors that promote murine gastric cancer, and particularly, the role of the adaptive immune response. For example, gastric *Helicobacter* infection in mice deficient in lymphocytes does not result in tissue damage, cell lineage alterations, or the metaplasia-dysplasia-carcinoma sequence.[46,47] In contrast, infection in B cell–deficient mice (which retain a normal T-cell response) results in severe atrophy and metaplasia identical to that seen in infected wild-type mice.[47] Taken together, these studies underscore the crucial role of CD4+ T lymphocytes in orchestrating gastric neoplasia.

Although the composite immune milieu most likely dictates disease manifestations, there may be a role for individual cytokines in both the predisposition to and protection from disease. During *Helicobacter* infection, the Th1 cytokine IFN-γ can promote or inhibit inflammation-driven cancer of the stomach, suggesting that a more specific immune response is responsible for cancer promotion or surveillance. Although studies in the past have suggested that IFN-γ might promote the development of gastric preneoplasia,[52] IFN-γ overexpression in the stomach at low levels was recently shown to be able to suppress gastric cancer in models of IL-1β– and *Helicobacter felis*–dependent carcinogenesis.[53] In addition, IFN-γ was shown to counteract the development of Th17 cells.[53] Thus different composition of the same cells and cytokines in the tumor microenvironment can contribute to a constellation that favors or inhibits carcinogenesis. On the other hand, mice lacking IL-10, a cytokine that acts to dampen an immune response, demonstrate severe atrophic gastritis in response to infection.[46–50] More recently, genetic murine models have illustrated the importance of the IL-6/IL-11 family of cytokines in the development of gastric cancer.[54]

Manipulation of the immune response within wild-type strains confirms the central role of the Th1/Th2 response in producing disease. For example, infection with the intestinal helminth *Heligmosomoides polygyrus* skews the immune response toward Th2 polarization and protects the C57BL/6 host from *Helicobacter*-induced atrophy and metaplasia.[55] This mouse model mimics both the parasitic infection status and the paradoxical low gastric cancer-high *Hp* infection rates seen in areas of Africa, potentially explaining this apparent inconsistency. These observations in mice led to human studies in Africa and Latin America that confirmed that geographic regions with low gastric cancer rates had much higher Th2/Th1 immune responses to *Hp*.[56,57] In general, the increased Th2-type responses were found in areas where serum IgE levels were high and the prevalence of intestinal parasitism by helminthes is above 50%. These findings further stress the importance of the host response to infection and suggest the possibility that manipulation of the genetically predetermined host cytokine profile in response to environmental challenges may lessen or exacerbate the disease process.

Studies on human tissue have also demonstrated that the degree of colonization with *Hp* depends on various factors, such as the presence and activity of regulatory T-cells (Treg), or the initial (naive) parietal cell mass (which reflects the acid-secreting capacity of the gastric body).[58–60] Tregs are associated with increasing bacterial colonization,[61] chronic inflammatory changes,[62] and the expression of immunosuppressive cytokines, such as IL10, IL17, and TGF-β.[59,63] In the case of gastric cancer, Tregs are increased both in the gastric mucosa and the peripheral blood.[64–66] The ratio of Th1/Th2-derived cytokines is the highest in asymptomatic gastritis, showing a steady decrease in gastric atrophy, IM and intraepithelial neoplasia progression to gastric adenocarcinoma. This is associated with a concomitant increase of the Treg cell compartment in the peripheral blood as well as persistence of CagA positive strains that favors a Treg-mediated chronic inflammation.[67] Whereas *Hp* infection has been unequivocally linked to gastric cancer, the development of dysplasia and invasive cancer tends to occur at a time when *Hp* colonization has either dramatically declined or, in some cases, has disappeared from the stomach altogether. Gastric cancer almost always occurs in the setting of prolonged gastric atrophy and hypochlorhydria, a condition that predisposes to enteric bacterial overgrowth. Although antibiotic eradication therapy targeting *Hp* delays and inhibits development of gastric cancer in mice,[20,68] antibiotics eradicate not only *Hp* but also other microorganisms that colonize the atrophic, hypochlorhydric stomach. Indeed, the infection of otherwise germ-free INS-GAS mice with *Hp* resulted in delayed progression to gastric cancer compared to *Hp*-infected INS-GAS mice colonized with conventional flora.[69] Thus *Hp* may represent simply the initial, or the most prevalent, microbial factor responsible for gastric cancer progression. Ferreira et al. reported recently that the gastric microbiota of patients with gastric adenocarcinomas is significantly different from patients with chronic gastritis.[70] The dominant gastric dysbiosis is characterized by reduced microbial diversity and reduced *Hp* abundance as well as an overrepresentation of bacterial genera that include intestinal commensals. With regard to these findings, it is also of interest that *Hp*—when present—dominates the otherwise much more diverse gastric microbiome in humans, as well as mice, prior to cancer development.[71]

There is a great deal of genetic diversity between strains of *Hp* owing to point mutations, insertions, deletions, and base-pair substitutions within the genome. Several strains may infect a single individual, and existing strains can undergo mutations and change over time.[72,73] Despite this genetic diversity, several genes are recognized as risk factors for gastric carcinoma, including the *cag* pathogenicity island, the *vacA* gene, and the *babA2* gene, being the most relevant and most extensively studied thus far among other factors.

The *Hp* genome is 1.65 million base pairs and codes for approximately 1500 genes, two-thirds of which have been assigned biological roles.[74] The function of the remaining one-third of the genome remains obscure, but genome-wide analyses using DNA microarray or whole-genome sequencing technology will give a broad view of the genome of *Hp* in the near future. Factors that contribute to carcinogenesis include those that enable the bacteria to effectively colonize the gastric mucosa, those that incite a more aggressive host immune response, and those that affect host cell-growth signaling pathways.

Motility toward epithelial cells of the stomach is a vital feature of *Hp* survival tactics. This is ensured by several factors. Spiraling movement is mediated by the FlaA and FlaB proteins, which are designed to navigate the thick gastric mucus. In addition, *Hp* produces *HP1069*, a putative collagenase, which modifies the extracellular matrix and mucus layer, thus decreasing viscosity and allowing bacterial penetration.[75,76] In addition, *Hp* expresses a variety of genes that contribute to buffering of stomach acid to maintain a relatively neutral pH. This includes a urease gene cluster consisting of seven genes, of which UreA/UreB complex (comprising the urease enzyme) codes for 10% of the protein of *Hp* and is vital for its survival.

The *cag* pathogenicity island is approximately 40 kb and contains 31 genes. The terminal gene of this island, *cagA*, is often used as a marker for the entire *cag* locus. Compared with cagA-negative (cagA−) strains, cag-positive (cagA+) strains are associated with more severe inflammation, higher degrees of atrophy, and a greater chance of progressing to gastric adenocarcinoma.[77–80] The estimated relative risk (RR) has ranged from 2 to as high as 28.4.[34] However, many of the genes adjacent to *cagA* code for a type 4 secretion system (TFSS), often viewed as a molecule needle that injects bacterial proteins (e.g., cagA) into host cells. The remarkable finding that CagA is injected into host cells, where it is phosphorylated by Src- and c-Abl kinases, has raised the possibility that CagA could directly promote growth, migration, and transformation. Indeed, the transgenic expression of *Hp* CagA induces both GI and hematopoietic neoplasms in mice.[81] Other genes within the pathogenicity island are also believed to be important for disease (*cagE* or *picB*, *cagG*, *cagH*, *cagI*, *cagL*, *cagM*) because they appear to be required for in vitro epithelial cell cytokine release, although they do not seem to have as great an effect on immune cell cytokine activation.[82–84] These findings may explain the attenuated inflammatory response and lower cancer risk with cagA− strains in vivo.[85–88]

Intracellular phosphorylation of CagA occurs at certain glutamate-proline-isoleucine-tyrosine-alanine (EPIYA) motifs. Four distinct EPIYA motifs are described (EPIYA-A, -B, -C, and -D), whose prevalence varies by geographical region.[89,90] The motifs further influence the CagA-induced immune response as well as the related cancer risk. The odds ratio (OR) for gastric cancer is close to 7.3 in the case of 1 EPIYA-C segment and can be up to 51 in case of 2 or more segments.[91,92] Moreover, genetic variations in further cagPAI-related genes have been demonstrated to be associated with gastric cancer.[93]

All strains of *Hp* carry the *vacA* gene, which codes for a pore-forming, vacuolating toxin, but expression differs according to allelic variation. Approximately, 50% of *Hp* strains express the *vacA* protein, which has been shown to be a very powerful inhibitor of T cell activation in vitro.[94] Although vacA and *cagA* map to different loci within the *Hp* genome, the vacA protein is commonly expressed in cagA+ strains. There are various forms of vacA, and the s1m1 strains are highly toxigenic. Other bacterial virulence factors, such as *cagE*, may play a role in the modulation of apoptosis and the host inflammatory response, thereby contributing to disease manifestations. Indeed, "virulent strains" (cagA+, cagE+, and VacA+ s1m1) appear to be more potent inducers of proinflammatory mediators than "nonvirulent strains" (cagA−, cagE−, and VacA−), possibly explaining the higher association of cagA+ strains with gastric cancer.[95]

Dietary Risk Factors

Numerous dietary factors have been implicated as risk factors for gastric cancer. The decline in gastric cancer rates has coincided with the widespread use of refrigeration and the concomitant higher intake of fresh fruits and vegetables and lower intake of pickled and salted foods. Use of refrigeration for more than 10–20 years has been associated with a decreased risk of gastric cancer.[18] Lower temperatures reduce the rate of bacterial, fungal, and other contaminants of fresh food, as well as the bacterial formation of nitrites. In addition, high intake of highly preserved foods may be associated with increased gastric cancer risk,[96] potentially due to higher contents of salt, nitrates, and polycyclic aromatic amines.

Much attention has been given to the effects of high nitrate intake. When nitrates are reduced to nitrite by bacteria or macrophages, they can react with other nitrogenated substances to form *N*-nitroso compounds that are known *mitogens* and *carcinogens*. In rats, *N*-nitroso compounds have been shown to cause gastric cancer. However, studies trying to link *N*-nitroso exposure to gastric cancer risk have been inconclusive, perhaps reflecting the fact that nitrate intake does not necessarily correlate with nitrosation levels.[97] A Swedish cohort study found a nearly two-fold increased risk of gastric cancer associated with high dietary nitrate intake.[96] However, separate large cohort studies from Europe did not demonstrate an association between nitrate intake and risk of gastric cancer.[98,99]

Another factor implicated in the development of gastric cancer is a diet high in salt (pickled foods, soy sauce, dried and salted fish, and meat). High salt intake has been associated with higher rates of atrophic gastritis in humans and animals in the setting of *Helicobacter* infection and increases the mutagenicity of nitrosated food in animal models.[18,100] High-salt diets are associated with a roughly a 1.5–2-fold increased risk of gastric cancer.[101] Cohort and case-control studies have also found an increased risk of gastric cancer associated with processed meat intake.[96,102] Possible mechanisms include higher bacterial loads, upregulation of *Hp* cagA expression, and increased cell proliferation and p21 expression.[100,103,104] There is a clear interaction between *Hp* infection and dietary risk factors for gastric cancer leading to a disproportional risk increase for *Hp*-positive subjects with high intake of red or processed meat compared to individuals in whom only one of these risk factors is present.[105]

Epidemiologic studies have had inconsistent findings with regard to fruit and vegetable consumption and risk of gastric cancer.[106–109] Other foods or dietary factors that have been implicated as potential risk factors for gastric cancer are high intake of fried food, foods high in fat, high intake of red meat, and aflatoxins.[102,110–112] Diets with a high intake of fresh fish and antioxidants may be protective (also see later).[111,113–115] However, there are insufficient data to make definitive conclusions regarding these factors.

Cigarette Smoking

Tobacco has long been established as a carcinogen, and numerous epidemiologic studies have demonstrated an association between cigarette smoking and gastric cancer.[116] Several large cohort studies from Europe and Asia have reported a significantly increased risk of gastric cancer among smokers.[117–119] A recent meta-analysis found that, compared to never smokers, current smokers had a 1.5–2-fold increased risk of gastric cancer, both for the cardia and noncardia region.[120] The authors also reported an increased association with greater amounts of smoking.

Moist snuff is a smokeless tobacco product promoted as an alternative to cigarettes that has reportedly reduced levels of carcinogenic nitrosamines. Nevertheless, results of a Swedish cohort study demonstrated a 1.4-fold increased risk of noncardia gastric cancer among regular snuff users.[121] Snuff exposure also increases the rate of gastric carcinogenesis in *Hp*-infected mice.[122]

Alcohol

Most epidemiologic studies have failed to demonstrate an association between alcohol consumption and cardia or noncardia gastric cancer.[119,123,124] However, several meta-analyses suggest a small but significant association between heavy alcohol use and gastric cancer risk (RR, 1.16–1.87 in selected subgroups).[125–128] Although some of these analyses suggest that the risk is higher for junctional cancers than more distal gastric cancer, some authors state the opposite effect. Overall, the risk increase seems to be moderate and influenced by multiple factors (including tobacco consumption and physical activity). Interestingly, alcohol intake may increase the risk of gastric cancer in patients with certain polymorphisms of the alcohol dehydrogenase gene.[129]

Obesity

Obesity is a recognized risk factor for numerous GI malignancies.[130] Increased BMI is associated with a mild to moderate increased risk of gastric cardia cancer, but not noncardia cancer.[131–134] Results of the National Institutes of Health-American Association of Retired Persons (NIH-AARP) Diet and Health Cohort Study demonstrated that morbid obesity (defined as a BMI $\geq$ 35) as well as large waist circumference were associated with a two- to threefold increased risk of gastric cardia cancer, but not noncardia cancer.[135] A separate cohort study from the Netherlands also found an increased risk of cardia cancer with increasing BMI.[131] In a recent analysis of the EPIC cohort data from 391,456 individuals with 124 incident esophageal and gastric adenocarcinomas, neither 193 cardia cancers nor 224 noncardia gastric cancers were associated with BMI.[136] The possible association between obesity and cardia cancer risk is likely mediated by proinflammatory cytokines and adipokines produced by intraabdominal visceral fat.[137]

Genetic Factors

As is true for most malignancies, both genetic and environmental factors play important roles in the pathogenesis of gastric cancer. Generally, intestinal-type gastric cancer is considered largely due to environmental causes (i.e., *Hp* infection), whereas diffuse gastric cancer is considered a primarily genetic malignancy. In the case of intestinal-type gastric cancer, however, assigning relative values to environmental and genetic contributions is complex, given that the major environmental factor, *Hp*, also tends to exhibit familial clustering. Nevertheless, in the future, gastric cancer types might rather be classified by genetic alterations and grouped to molecular subgroups with distinct carcinogenic mechanisms as well as clinical behavior, than to a histologic phenotype.[138]

Overall, 10% of cases of gastric cancer appear to exhibit familial clustering,[139] and family history is likely an independent risk factor even after controlling for *Hp* status.[140,141] In a cohort study of relatives of patients with gastric cancer, siblings had a twofold increased risk of gastric cancer, adjusted for *Hp* infection.[142] In a case-control study from Japan, a positive family history was associated with a significantly increased odds of gastric cancer in women (OR, 5.10), but not in men.[143] A study from Scandinavia showed that having a twin with gastric cancer conferred a markedly higher RR for the disease (RR, 9.9 for monozygotic twins and 6.6 for dizygotic twins), leading the researchers to calculate that heritable factors accounted for 28% of gastric cancers, compared with 10% for shared environmental factors and 62% for nonshared environmental factors.[144] A recent meta-analysis of 32 studies, including more than 80,000 individuals reported an increased pooled RR of 2.35 (95% CI, 1.96–2.81) for subjects with a positive family history of gastric cancer; the risk was even higher (RR 2.71; 95% CI, 2.08–3.53) if first-degree relatives had a gastric cancer diagnosis.[145]

Some of the familial clustering seen with intestinal-type gastric cancer may be related to genetic factors that play a role in the host immune response to *Hp* infection. Data from South Korea indicate that individuals with a family history of gastric cancer more frequently have both *Hp* infection and associated atrophic gastritis or IM.[146] In a case-control study from Scotland, relatives of patients with gastric cancer had a higher prevalence of atrophy and hypochlorhydria, but a similar prevalence of *Hp* infection, compared with controls.[147] The greater prevalence of atrophy was confined to those patients with *Hp* infection, suggesting the possibility these individuals were perhaps exhibiting a more vigorous immune response to *Hp*. In a number of model systems, the development of gastric atrophy has been linked to a strong Th1 immune response.[50,55,148] Thus it was postulated that candidate disease-susceptibility genes for gastric atrophy and cancer might be genes that participate in the innate and adaptive immune responses to *Hp* infection. Inflammation is modulated by an array of pro- and antiinflammatory cytokines, and several genetic polymorphisms have been described that influence cytokine response. With the recently started next-generation sequencing approaches, we may be able to determine whether families with increased gastric cancer incidence have a genetic predisposition for a more carcinogenic immune response.

One such factor is IL-1β, an important proinflammatory cytokine and a powerful inhibitor of acid secretion. Indeed, there is an association between proinflammatory IL-1 gene cluster polymorphisms (*IL-1B* encoding IL-1β, and *IL-1RN* encoding its naturally occurring receptor antagonist, IL-1RA) and neoplastic progression in the setting of *Hp* infection. Individuals with the *IL-1β-31*C* or *-511*T* and *IL-1RN*2/*2* genotypes were shown in the study to be at higher risk for developing *Hp*-dependent hypochlorhydria and gastric cancer.[149] The increased risk of progression to cancer with these genotypes was in the two- to threefold range compared with noninflammatory genotypes. The initial report was confirmed in other studies.[150–154] Subsequently, Hwang et al.[155] demonstrated that carriers of the *IL-1B-511T/T* genotype or the *IL-1RN*2* allele had higher mucosal IL-1β levels than noncarriers and also confirmed the association between the *-511T/T* genotype and severe gastric inflammation and atrophy. The importance of IL-1β carcinogenesis has now been demonstrated in a transgenic study, where stomach-specific expression of human IL-1β in transgenic mice led to spontaneous gastric inflammation and cancer that correlated with early recruitment of myeloid-derived suppressor cells to the stomach.[156] Of note, in a mouse model of Barrett esophagus and esophageal and EGJ tumors, IL-1β expression in the esophageal squamous epithelium also led to esophagitis and expansion of cardia stem cells forming gastroesophageal tumors, supporting the hypothesis that Barrett's-associated adenocarcinoma arises from the gastric cardia resembling a gastric cancer phenotype.[10]

Additional associations with gastric cancer risk have been reported for genetic polymorphisms in TNF-α and IL-10. Proinflammatory genotypes of TNF-α and IL-10 were each associated with a twofold higher risk of noncardia gastric cancer. When combined with proinflammatory genotypes of *IL-1B* and *IL-1RN*, patients with three or four high-risk genotypes showed a 27-fold greater risk of gastric cancer.[157] Additional studies have shown that polymorphisms of the Toll-like receptor-4 (*TLR-4*) gene also increases the risk of gastric cancer. Carriers of the *TLR4*+896G polymorphism had an 11-fold increased OR for hypochlorhydria, and significantly more severe gastric atrophy and inflammation.[158] Accumulated evidence suggests that the genetic predisposition to gastric cancer may be largely determined by the TLR and cytokine responses to chronic *Helicobacter* infection. Polymorphisms in the TLR1 seem to protect against gastric cancer development (OR 0.4; 95% CI, 0.22–0.72) and are furthermore related to alterations of downstream cytokine signaling.[159,160]

The best described form of hereditary gastric cancer is the diffuse type gastric cancer that is seen in the presence of a germline mutation in the gene *CDH1*, which encodes the cell adhesion molecule E-cadherin. A large New Zealand kindred was found to have a germline mutation in the E-cadherin gene, and similar mutations have been reported in several additional kindreds, all with diffuse-type gastric cancer.[161–164] The age of onset of gastric cancer in individuals with *CDH1* mutations is less than 40 years but can be highly variable, and the estimated lifetime risk of gastric cancer is close to 70%.[165,166] Germline *CDH1* mutations are also associated with familial lobular breast cancer.[167,168]

A small part of the familial clustering of gastric cancer can be attributed to other cancer syndromes. Patients with familial adenomatous polyposis have a prevalence of gastric adenomas ranging from 35% to 100%, and their risk of gastric cancer is close to 10-fold higher than that of the general population.[169] Dysplastic lesions in this specific group of patients frequently arise from fundic gland polyps and develop at an early age.[170,171] Fundic gland polyps do not otherwise tend to progress toward dysplasia. Patients with hereditary nonpolyposis colorectal cancer (HNPCC) syndrome have an approximately 11% risk of developing gastric cancer, predominantly of the intestinal type, with a mean age at diagnosis of 56 years.[172] Patients with juvenile polyposis also have a 12%–20% incidence of gastric cancer.[173,174]

In addition to the germline genetic alterations described earlier, next-generation sequencing techniques, such as exome sequencing, have led to the detection of new molecules and mechanisms that are involved in gastric carcinogenesis. In 8%–10% of the gastric cancer patients, somatic mutations were identified in the *ARID1A* gene (also called *BAF250a*, *SMARCF1*, or *OSA1*), an accessory subunit of the SWI-SNF chromatin remodeling complex that is involved in processes of DNA repair, differentiation, and development.[175–178] Notably, cancers with EBV infection showed mutations of *ARID1A* in 73% of the cases. In addition, *ARID1A* mutations were negatively associated with mutations in *TP53* and occurred together with *PIK3CA* mutations. Patients with *ARID1A* alterations had longer recurrence-free survival, suggesting that these cancers belong to a molecular subgroup with distinct carcinogenic mechanisms as well as clinical behavior.[175–178] Analysis of somatic copy number aberrations have additionally shown significantly amplified genes, including therapeutically targetable kinases, such as *ERBB2*, *FGFR1*, *FGFR2*, *EGFR*, and *MET*, in gastric and gastroesophageal cancers.

TUMOR GENETICS

Although atrophy and IM correlate with gastric cancer risk, direct cell progression through these stages has not been conclusively shown. Indeed, gastric cancer most likely arises from stem or progenitor cells present within the gastric mucosa rather than directly from terminally differentiated metaplastic cells. For several decades, investigators have sought to unravel the mutations responsible for gastric cancer initiation and progression to uncover a logical sequence of acquired mutations akin to what is seen in colorectal cancer. However, gastric cancer does not follow a pattern like the adenoma-carcinoma sequence in colorectal carcinoma progression, there is no clear-cut linear sequence of mutations in gastric cancers, and there is an even greater heterogeneity in genetic alterations.

Although initial studies on large high throughput data focused mainly on transcriptome analyses,[179–181] the advent of more advanced genomic sequencing enabled genome-wide analyses of the mutational landscape of gastric cancer.[182–184] The combined efforts of multiple research groups in international consortia enabled a more comprehensive integrative analysis of multilevel *omics*-data from large cohorts.[9,13,138] TCGA consortium presented comprehensive data on five different platforms for about 300 gastric cancers. They demonstrated a good correlation of clustering between different levels of genomic data as well as epigenetic changes and transcriptome and even proteome analyses.[138] Based on their cluster analysis, the authors suggested a 4-group classification of gastric cancers, with the first group (EBV) being related to EBV infection, showing a dominant epigenetic hypermethylation profile (EBV). The second group [microsatellite instability (MSI)] was positive for MSI, similar to the MSI subgroup of colorectal cancers. The remaining tumors were divided into a group with a low mutation rate and low frequency for copy number aberrations, called the "genomically stable" (GS) subtype and a group with high mutation rates and further related genomic changes, called the "chromosomally instable" (CIN) type. It is of note the GS group comprised predominantly diffuse-type tumors, whereas CIN tumors represented more intestinal-type cancers. There were some differences in the distribution of these subtypes with regard to location, with CIN tumors showing higher proportions with more proximal location, which was later also confirmed for esophageal adenocarcinomas.[487] The Asian Cancer Research Group followed a similar approach in their cohort of 300 gastric cancers, although putting more focus on transcriptome data than the TCGA.[13] Thus Cristescu et al. presented a similar four-group classification, also reporting properties as prognostic predictors for their groups.[13] This classification was validated in several independent cohorts, including the group of TCGA patients. The actual genomic changes described in these comprehensive studies are in line with results that have been published previously. Other approaches focus more on transcriptome profiling, with a recent study showing a distinct prognostic outcome in three transcriptome-based gastric cancer subgroups that could be verified in four independent cohorts.[488] Interestingly, the distribution of the respective subgroups did not depend on tumor location within the stomach, with the cohorts, including junctional cancers.

With regards to the actual genetic changes reported in gastric cancer, aneuploidy is common (60%–75%), but cytogenetic studies have failed to identify any consistent chromosomal abnormality.[185]

The most commonly mutated gene in gastric cancer is *TP53* (60%–70%). Mutations in *Ras*, *APC*, and *Myc* are rare.[186,187] Loss of heterozygosity at the APC locus occurs more commonly. Genes that inhibit entry into the cell cycle, such as *p16* and *p27*, show diminished expression in nearly one-half of gastric cancers and are often associated with prognosis.[188–193] Diminished expression of these genes often occurs secondary to hypermethylation.[192]

Multiple tumor suppressor and mismatch repair genes have been shown to be methylated in gastric cancers. Emerging evidence suggests that these epigenetic changes, including global hypomethylation and promoter hypermethylation, occurs quite early in gastric carcinogenesis with the former being associated with poor prognosis. In addition, it appears that DNA methylation changes also occur in the tumor-associated stromal fibroblasts, suggesting an important role for the tumor microenvironment. *Hp* infection is a factor that can contribute to hypermethylation with changes showing a dynamic response to eradication treatment.[489] While some of these epigenetic changes can return to a regular methylation pattern, *Hp*-induced hypermethylation can remain stable in areas adjacent to early neoplastic lesions.[490]

Overexpression or amplifications with genes of a number of growth factors and related pathways has been described, including *COX-2* (70%), hepatocyte growth factor/scatter factor (*HGF/SF*) (60%), vascular endothelial growth factor (*VEGF*) (50%), *c-met* (50%), amplified in breast cancer-1 (*AIB-1*) (40%), and β-catenin (25%) (Table 56.2).[195] Approximately 15% of gastric cancers overexpress both EGF and the EGF receptor (EGFR), consistent with an autocrine mechanism. Mutations in *PIC3A*, a gene that codes for a catalytic subunit of phosphatidylinositol 3-kinase (PI3K), have been found in up to 25% of gastric cancers.[196] In addition, mutations in genes encoding human protein tyrosine phosphatases were found in 17% of gastric cancers.[197]

TABLE 56.2 Genetic Abnormalities in Gastric Adenocarcinoma

Abnormalities	Approximate Gene Frequency (%)
Microsatellite instability	15–50
DNA aneuploidy	60–75
Deletion/Suppression	
p53	60–70
FHIT (fragile histidine triad gene)	60
APC (adenomatous polyposis coli gene) loss of heterozygosity	50
DCC (deleted in colorectal cancer gene) loss of heterozygosity	50
Decreased Expression Due to Hypermethylation	
p16	≈50
TFF1 (human trefoil factor 1 gene)	≈50
p27	<50
MLH1 (human mutL homolog 1 gene)	15–20
E-cadherin	50
Amplification/Overexpression	
COX-2	70
HGF (hepatocyte growth factor)	60
VEGF (vascular endothelial growth factor)	50
c-met	50
AIB-1 (amplified in breast cancer-1)	40
Beta-catenin	25
EGFR (EGF receptor gene)	15
Mutations	
PI3K (phosphatidylinositol 3-kinase gene)	25
PTPRT (protein-tyrosine phosphatase receptor type gene)	17

Loss of *TFF1* has been described in around 50% of gastric carcinomas, and *TFF1* knockout mice develop spontaneous gastric antral tumors. Mutations of the *TFF1* gene can enhance gastric cancer cell invasion through signaling pathways that include PI3-kinase and phospholipase-C.[200] TFF1 expression is repressed by STAT-3, and activation of STAT-3 is another key gene involved in that leads to gastric cancer development.[54] RUNX3 is altered in 82% of gastric cancers and most likely suppresses gastric epithelial growth by inducing p21 and Bim, attenuating Wnt signaling.[201]

MSI in dinucleotide repeats secondary to defects in DNA mismatch repair genes, such as *MLH1* and *MLH2* (mutL homologs 1 and 2), have been mainly implicated in the development of colorectal cancer, and in particular the HNPCC syndrome. Patients with HNPCC have an 11% incidence of gastric cancer, suggesting that MSI may also play a role in the development of gastric cancer.[172] MSI is found in 15%–50% of sporadic gastric cancers, with a higher prevalence in intestinal type of cancers.[202–207] Low-level microsatellite activity (e.g., MSI-low) can be found in 40% of areas of IM in patients with gastric cancer[207] and in 14%–20% of adenomatous polyps.[205,207,208] MSI-H occurs in only 10%–16% of gastric cancers. MSI is associated with less frequent occurrence of *TP53* mutations, well-to-moderately differentiated histology, and distal location of the cancer in the stomach. Studies that have examined the effect of MSI on patient survival have shown inconsistent results.[208,209] When the findings are taken together, it would appear that MSI does play a role in the pathogenesis of gastric cancer, likely even prior to the development of IM (see Fig. 56.3), and is most commonly due to methylation of the *MLH1* promoter.

Most families with hereditary diffuse gastric cancer carry a germline mutation in the E-cadherin gene (*CDH1*).[161–163,210,211] However, mutations in *CDH1* are also a dominant feature in sporadic diffuse-type gastric cancer. Further evidence supporting a role for E-cadherin in the pathogenesis of gastric cancer comes from studies showing that suppression of E-cadherin expression occurs in 51% of gastric cancers, with a higher percentage found in diffuse-type cancers.[212] Overall, *CDH1* mutations in gastric cancer are rare. Thus the decreased expression of E-cadherin seen in gastric cancer is likely secondary to hypermethylation of the *CDH1* promoter, which occurs in 50% of gastric cancers and 83% of diffuse-type gastric cancers.[215] E-cadherin is a transmembrane protein that connects to the actin cytoskeleton through α- and β-catenins to establish cell polarity and mediates homophilic cellular interactions.[216,217] Decreased expression of E-cadherin is believed to promote dissociation of cancer cells from their cell matrix, enhancing the migration and invasion of gastric cancer cells. Expression of α-catenin is also decreased or absent in 68% of gastric cancers.[218] Therefore E-cadherin appears to act as a tumor suppressor gene that may be important in the pathogenesis of diffuse gastric cancer. E-cadherin underexpression is associated with higher rates of lymph node metastases and reduced survival.[213,214] Other alterations that commonly occur in diffuse type gastric carcinoma are alterations in Wnt-related genes as well as changes in the Ras homolog gene family, Member A gene (*RHOA*), which seems to be exclusive to this histological subtype.[184]

Perhaps as important as the genetic alterations acquired during the progression to gastric adenocarcinoma is the question, "In what target cells do these changes occur?" For a cell to accumulate the quantity of genetic changes necessary for autonomous growth, it must be long lived. For these reasons, the current thinking is that a resident tissue stem cell is the most likely target of genetic mutations and becomes the "cancer stem cell"—capable of autonomous growth and with metastatic potential. Several elegant genetic lineage-tracing studies in mice established markers that allow the distinction of two different types of GI stem cells. Crypt base columnar (CBC) cells are fast-cycling stem cells expressing Lgr5 and CD[133] (Prom-1).[219,220] A villin transgene has allowed the identification of a multipotent progenitor located in the lower third of a subset of antral gastric glands,[221] whereas multiple intestinal stem cell markers could also be identified in the antrum. Interestingly, Lgr5 shows lineage labeling in some antral gastric glands and in the gastric cardia.[220] Slower cycling cells, which are usually found at the +4 position of the crypts of the antrum (i.e., the fourth epithelial cell in the crypt, counting from the bottom of the crypt upward), are characterized by a pronounced expression of Bmi1 and Tert.[222,223] Although these two types of cells are functionally interconnected,[224] their exact hierarchical relationship remains to be identified. Sigal et al. demonstrated a direct CagA-dependent activation of Lgr5-positive gastric stem cells, thus reporting a further mechanism by which *Hp* infection induces gastric carcinogenesis.[225] The same group also suggested orchestration of epithelial hyperproliferation and gland hyperplasia as a response to the infection by cells of the stromal compartment, mainly myofibroblasts involving *Hp*-induced Wnt signaling.[226]

In the gastric oxyntic glands, the proliferative zone with the gastric stem cell has been localized to the isthmus, the middle portion of the tubule, and cells are thought to migrate bidirectionally to supply gastric surface mucus cells that coat the gastric pits, and gastric parietal and zymogenic cells that comprise the base of the gland.[227] The gastric corpus stem cell has not yet been identified; none of the markers discussed earlier labels any specific cells within the gastric isthmus. Recently, progenitor cells (e.g., Krt19+ and TFF2+ cells) have been shown through lineage tracing studies to label different gastric progenitor cells.[228,229] Typically, columnar metaplasia is positive for TFF2 and Krt19. Given that IM arises in the gastric mucosa and in the esophagus, it is plausible that a similar stem cell gives rise to both. Regardless of their localization (CBC or +4 position) or their function, GI stem cells depend on signals from the stem cell niche, such as pericryptal myofibroblasts, and neighboring differentiated epithelia.[230] Important signaling pathways required for stem cell maintenance and proliferation comprise the Wnt, Notch, bone morphogenetic proteins, and Hedgehog pathways.[231]

There is increasing knowledge on the interaction of the local stromal microenvironment with the epithelium. A regulator of the biological behavior of gastric cancer cells are CAFs that have been shown to modify TGFβ-dependent signaling, increasing cellular motility, and, therefore, invasiveness.[232,233] The density of tumor-infiltrating lymphocytes and their vicinity also modifies the tumor's aggressiveness and therefore has an impact on the prognostic outcome in patients with adenocarcinomas in the stomach or at the EGJ.[234,235] This factor is partly reflected by the level of systemic inflammation.[236] Systemic inflammation can be partly mediated by the visceral adipose tissue and it has been demonstrated that omental adipocytes enhance the invasiveness of gastric cancer by activation of PI3K-Akt signaling in the tumor cells.[237]

Besides the valuable data from in vitro and ex vivo models, approaches for "virtual microdissection" of next generation high throughput and sequencing data are promising to enhance our understanding of the network of different cellular components and its impact on tumor initiation, promotion, and progression (including invasive and metastasizing behavior) (Fig. 56.4).

More recently, advances in the field of single cell analyses allowed much more detailed understanding of the factors that drive tumor behavior, especially in view of local invasion and metastases. Studies demonstrate focal molecular tumor heterogeneity as well as the impact of the organ-specific microenvironment on the cellular structure of metastases.[491,492] Single-cell analysis helps not only to dissect individual cancer cell lineages, but also the interaction of different tumor subtypes with the mesenchymal compartment of the adjacent gastric mucosa.[493] Patrick Tan's group demonstrated a step-wise accrural of CAFs by plasma-cell enriched diffuse type cancers. Similarly, a focal interaction of tumor and immune cells delivers explanations for the impairment of different immune checkpoints that are now amenable to systemic treatment.[494]

PREMALIGNANT CONDITIONS

Chronic Atrophic Gastritis

Chronic atrophic gastritis, which is defined as the loss of specialized glandular tissue in its appropriate region of the stomach, is an established change that occurs along the morphological sequence toward the development of gastric cancer.[238] The presence of atrophic gastritis has an annual incidence of progression to gastric cancer of approximately 0.1%–1.0%.[239–243] The extent of atrophic gastritis within the stomach correlates with risk of progression to cancer,[244–246] and large studies have demonstrated that only patients with extensive mucosal atrophic changes at baseline develop gastric adenocarcinoma during long-term follow-up.[247]

There are two forms of atrophic gastritis (see Chapter 54). The more common is environmental, multifocal atrophic gastritis (MAG), which is associated with *Hp* infection and more likely to be associated with metaplasia. The presence of *Hp* infection results in an approximately 10-fold increased risk of atrophic gastritis.[248] There is considerable regional variation in the prevalence of atrophic gastritis in *Hp*-infected individuals, with a roughly threefold increase in Asia compared to Western countries.[248,249] The second form of atrophic gastritis, autoimmune metaplastic atrophic gastritis, is associated with antiparietal cell and/or antiintrinsic factor antibodies. This form of atrophy is confined to the body and fundus of the stomach. Autoimmune metaplastic atrophic gastritis is associated with pernicious anemia and an increased gastric cancer risk, albeit not as high as that seen with *Hp*-induced MAG, owing most likely to a lesser degree of inflammation.[240,250]

Mechanisms underlying the increased risk of gastric cancer in the setting of gastric atrophy may be related to low acid output (hypo- or achlorhydria), which predisposes to increased bacterial overgrowth with non-*Helicobacter* organisms, greater formation of *N*-nitroso compounds, and diminished ascorbate secretion into the gastric lumen.[251] In addition, circulating gastrin levels increase in response to the reduced acid output. Gastrin is a known growth factor for gastric mucosal cells, and sustained elevations of gastrin may contribute to abnormal growth and increased risk of neoplastic progression.[252,253]

Intestinal Metaplasia and Dysplasia

IM can be subdivided into three categories, as classified by Filipe's group.[254] *Type I* (complete) IM contains goblet cells that secrete sialomucins and mature, nonsecretory absorptive cells. Type I IM is not a risk factor for gastric cancer. *Type II* (incomplete) IM contains few if any absorptive cells, columnar "intermediate" cells in various stages of differentiation secreting neutral or acidic sialomucins, and goblet cells secreting sialomucins and/or occasionally sulfomucins. *Type III* (incomplete) is less differentiated than type II, with the intermediate cells secreting mainly sulfomucins and the goblet cells secreting sialo- and/or sulfomucins. *Type II* and *III* IM is associated with an approximately 20-fold increased risk of gastric cancer.[255,256] EGC develops in 42% of patients with *type III* IM within 5 years of follow-up, suggesting that IM represents a precursor lesion for the intestinal form of gastric cancer.[256] A large nationwide cohort study from the Netherlands on 92,250 individuals identified a 0.25% annual progression rate toward cancer in patients with gastric IM.[243] Similar rates were confirmed for advanced atrophy.[495] Long-term follow-up has demonstrated that the risk for progression is significantly higher in patients with *Hp* persistence.[496] The risk for progression is further associated with age, male gender and non-White ethnicity.[497] However, whether cancer arises from areas of IM or whether IM simply represents a marker for higher gastric cancer risk remains unclear, mainly due to the focal and patchy appearance of this condition. As is the case with atrophic gastritis, the prevalence of IM in *Hp*-infected individuals is higher in Asia (≈40%) compared to the West.[248,249] Although it is generally accepted that IM is associated with an increased risk for the intestinal type gastric cancer, patients with diffuse type tumors also show a high prevalence of IM in the nontumorous gastric mucosa.[257,258]

As mentioned above, a number of studies have revealed that IM is not the only possible metaplastic precursor of gastric cancer. Although controversy exists as to the sequence and connection of mucosal lineage changes associated with increased risk for gastric cancer, there is a general agreement that the loss of acid-secreting parietal cells, also known as *oxyntic atrophy*, is a prerequisite for induction of metaplasia. Antralization of the fundus, or the presence of metaplastic glands in the fundus with a general phenotype similar to that of the antral or pyloric glands (also known as *pseudopyloric metaplasia*), is frequently associated with intestinal-type adenocarcinoma. This phenotype has also been called *spasmolytic polypeptide-expressing metaplasia* (SPEM)[259] and is characterized by the presence of trefoil factor 2 (TFF2, or spasmolytic polypeptide) immunoreactive cells in the gastric fundus, with morphologic characteristics resembling those of deep antral gland cells. SPEM was observed in association with more than 90% of resected gastric cancers in three studies in the United States, Japan, and Iceland.[259–261] Data from mice demonstrate that

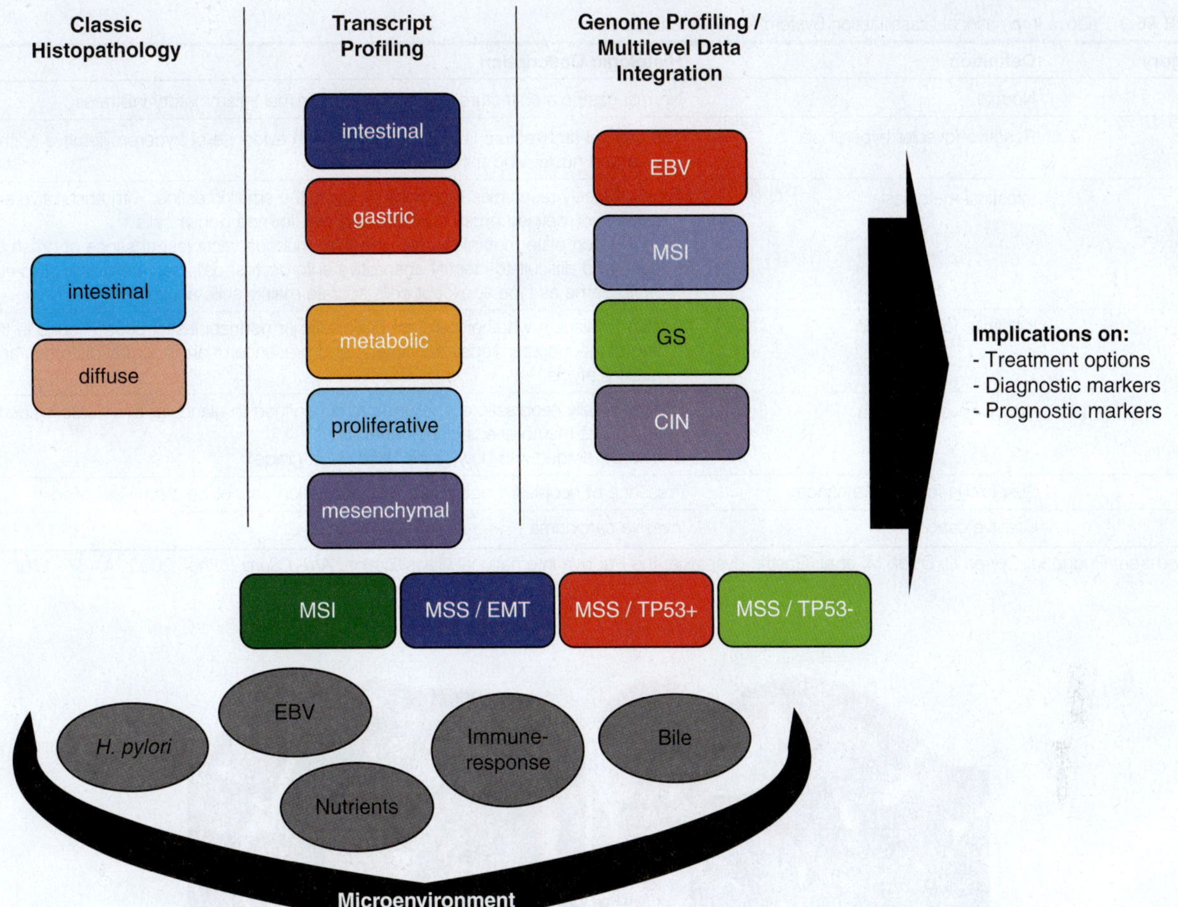

Fig. 56.4 Molecular stratification of gastric cancer. Displayed is an overview of recent concepts of gastric cancer subtyping. These classifications emerged from data gathered by transcript profiling high throughput study as well as next generation sequencing and transcend the classic histopathological classification (*left*). Early transcriptome data suggested dichotomous groups that showed similar features to the classic Lauren types (*middle, top*), before more functional interpretation was enabled by pathway analyses (*middle, bottom*). Recent concepts are usually based on multilevel data integration but still originate mainly from genome data like The TCGA approach (*EBV*; *MSI*, microsatellite instability positive cancer; *GS*, genomically stable cancer; *CIN*, chromosomal instability cancer) or from transcriptome data like the Asian Cancer Research Group (ACRG) approach (*MSI*, microsatellite instability positive cancer; *MSS/EMT*, microsatellite stable with transcript signature for epithelial mesenchymal transition; *MSS/TP53+*, microsatellite stable with TP53 mutation; *MSS/TP53-*, microsatellite stable with wild-type TP53). A special interest lies in the understanding of factors that drive each phenotype, mostly the interaction with the tumor microenvironment.

Helicobacter-induced expression of TFF2 are associated with CD44+ cancer stem cell in the same compartment of the gastric mucosa, therefore possibly facilitating further malignant progression. SPEM and IM might share equal importance as putative preneoplastic lesions in the stomach. Nevertheless, it remains to be determined whether either or both these metaplasias can progress to dysplasia or neoplasia. Alternatively, IM may potentially reflect a further benign attempt by the mucosa to increase repair in the face of chronic infection and inflammation.

Numerous studies have confirmed that the risk of progression towards dysplastic and neoplastic, invasive lesion increases with the extent of atrophy and/or IM in the stomach. A popular system to stratify risk groups is the OLGA system (Operative Link on Gastritis Assessment) classifying risk groups according to the degree of glandular atrophy, or OLGIM, respectively, assessing IM instead.[498,499] Long-term follow-up studies have shown that only patients with extensive mucosal changes are at risk to develop cancer.[500,501] These patients should undergo further endoscopic surveillance to facilitate early cancer detection (see later).[502]

Histologic assessment of gastric dysplasia and adenocarcinoma is based on the Vienna classification, the result of an international consensus conference of GI pathologists in 2000 (Table 56.3).[262] The prevalence of gastric dysplasia ranges from as low as 0.5% in low-risk areas[263] to 20% in high-risk areas.[264] Prospective studies have shown that low-grade dysplasia may regress in up to 60% of cases, whereas 10%–20% progress to high-grade dysplasia (Fig. 56.5).[265–267] High-grade dysplasia rarely regresses and is associated with a 2%–6% annual incidence of progression to gastric cancer.[267,268] In a prospective cohort study from the Netherlands, the presence of high-grade dysplasia was associated with a 40-fold increased risk of progression to gastric cancer. High-grade dysplasia is often associated with synchronous cancer and can be uni- or multifocal.[269]

Gastric Polyps

The prevalence of gastric polyps in the general population is approximately 0.8%–2.4%.[270,271] Gastric polyps consist

TABLE 56.3 Padova International Classification System for Gastric Dysplasia

Category	Definition	Histologic Description
I	Normal	Normal gastric architecture with absent or minimal inflammatory infiltrates
	Reactive foveolar hyperplasia	The general architecture is well preserved, with evidence of hyperproliferative epithelium, enlarged nuclei, and mitotic figures
	Intestinal metaplasia	*Type I.* Closely resembles the morphology of the small intestine, with absorptive enterocytes, well-defined brush borders, and well-formed goblet cells *Type II.* Incomplete metaplasia with irregular mucous vacuoles, absence of brush borders, and difficult-to-identify absorptive enterocytes; cells secrete mainly sialomucins *Type III.* Same as type II, except cells secrete mainly sulfomucins
II	Indefinite for dysplasia	Unable to discern whether cells are neoplastic or nonneoplastic; usually found in the setting of inadequate biopsy specimens and presence of architectural distortion and nuclear atypia
III	Noninvasive neoplasia	Phenotypically neoplastic epithelium that is confined to glandular structures inside the basement membrane; includes adenomas Should be divided into "low-grade" and "high-grade"
IV	Suspicious for invasive cancer	Presence of neoplastic epithelium where invasion cannot be clearly identified
V	Invasive cancer	Invasive carcinoma

Adapted from Rugge M, Correa P, Dixon M, et al. Gastric dysplasia: the Padova International Classification. *Am J Surg Pathol.* 2000;24:167–176.

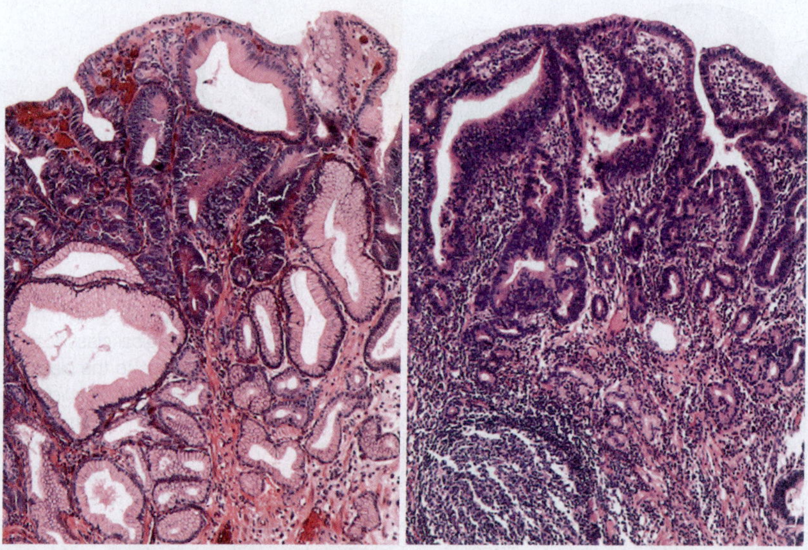

Fig. 56.5 Histopathology of gastric dysplasia. (*Left*) Low-grade dysplasia is characterized by a proliferation of neoplastic epithelial cells with nuclear pseudostratification and hyperchromasia in the absence of architectural changes. (*Right*) High-grade dysplasia has more severe cytologic abnormalities with abnormal architectural features, including irregular fused or cribriform glands and papillae (H&E stains).

predominantly of fundic gland polyps (≈50%), hyperplastic polyps (≈40%), and adenomatous polyps (≈10%).[271,272]

The clinical course of fundic gland polyps is generally benign, and they are detected with increasing frequency in the era of PPI use. In a series of 599 consecutive patients who underwent upper endoscopy, use of PPIs for more than 5 years was associated with a nearly fourfold increased risk of fundic gland polyps.[273] The rate of malignant transformation of these polyps is generally quite low (≈1%) and confined to polyps larger than 1 cm.[274] One notable exception to the benign nature of fundic gland polyps is in familial adenomatous polyposis (Video 56.1). In this group, the prevalence of fundic gland polyps ranges from 51% to 88%, with dysplasia present in over 40% of cases.[170,171]

Hyperplastic polyps are generally benign, often multiple, and are typically observed in the setting of chronic inflammatory conditions (e.g., chronic atrophic gastritis), pernicious anemia, chronic antral gastritis, adjacent to ulcers and erosions, and especially at sites of a gastroenterostomy. Over time, the polyps may regress, remain stable, or increase in size, and they often regress following *Hp* eradication. Men and women are equally affected, and the polyps typically appear in mid- to late-adult life.[275] The rare hyperplastic polyps that undergo malignant transformation often contain focal dysplasia or IM and typically form a well differentiated intestinal-type cancer.[274]

In contrast to other polyps of the stomach, gastric adenomas undergo malignant transformation at a high rate. When gastric adenomas were followed by serial endoscopy with biopsy, progression through dysplasia to carcinoma in situ developed within 4 years in approximately 11% of cases.[276] Endoscopic biopsy of gastric polyps can be associated with significant sampling error.[277] The British Society of Gastroenterology updated their guidelines regarding the management of gastric polyps in 2019.[278] Among the recommendations were: (1) gastric polyps and other fundic gland polyps should be biopsied; (2) the number, location, and the size of gastric polyps should be documented; (3) all gastric adenomas, polyps >1 cm, symptomatic polyps (or those causing complications), and polyps with dysplasia should be removed; and (4) the gastric background mucosa of patients with hyperplastic or adenomatous polyps should be investigated for atrophy, IM and *Hp*.

Previous Gastrectomy

It has been reported by several groups that gastric surgery for benign conditions can predispose patients to a higher risk of gastric cancer, beginning 20 years after the surgery.[279–282] The risk is greatest for those who underwent surgery before the age of 50 years, perhaps reflecting the long lag period necessary between the operation and the development of cancer.[281] The cancers tend to occur at or near the surgical anastomosis on the gastric side; only rarely do they reside on the intestinal side of the anastomosis.[283]

Numerous theories have been proposed to explain the increased propensity for cancer to form at the surgical anastomosis site. They include hypochlorhydria resulting in bacterial overgrowth with increased production of nitrites, chronic enterogastric reflux of bile salts and pancreatic enzymes (which are potent gastric irritants), and atrophy of the remaining fundic mucosa due to low levels of antral hormones, including gastrin.[18,284,285] The Billroth II operation with gastrojejunostomy predisposes to the development of cancer at a fourfold higher rate than a Billroth I procedure with gastroduodenostomy, suggesting that bile reflux may be a significant predisposing factor.[280] *Hp* and associated IM are found less frequently in postgastrectomy gastric cancers as compared to distal gastric cancers in the nonoperative stomach.[286] It is unclear whether screening for gastric cancer in this population of patients in areas of low cancer incidence would be cost-effective. With the advent of *Hp* eradication therapy as well as PPIs, the number of gastric resections for peptic ulcer disease has decreased dramatically, significantly reducing the impact of the postgastrectomy state as a risk factor for gastric cancer.

PUD

Large epidemiologic studies have demonstrated a consistently increased risk of gastric cancer in patients with a history of a gastric ulcer (see also Chapter 55). In a cohort study, Swedish adults who were followed for an average of 9 years, a history of gastric ulcer was associated with a 1.8-fold increased risk of gastric cancer.[287] Interestingly, a history of duodenal ulcer was associated with a reduced risk of gastric cancer. These findings were replicated in a case control study of U.S. veterans.[288] The associations were confined to noncardia gastric cancer; there was no association between history of gastric ulcer and cardia cancer.[288] It is unclear whether gastric ulcers per se predispose to the development of cancer. The increase risk may be mediated by infection with *Hp*, which can lead to atrophic gastritis, IM, and cancer.

Ménétrier Disease

In a review of case reports, 15% of patients with Ménétrier disease had associated gastric cancer,[289] including several cases that documented a progression from dysplasia to cancer (see also Chapter 54).[290,291] Because of the rarity of Ménétrier disease, it has been difficult to study its relationship with gastric cancer in any controlled fashion, and no recommendations regarding endoscopic surveillance can be made.

SCREENING AND SURVEILLANCE

The majority of the literature regarding screening for gastric cancer comes from East Asia, where the prevalence of this disease is among the highest in the world.[292] Since 1960 the Japanese have performed mass screening using upper GI barium studies followed by endoscopy if any suspicious lesions are found. However, direct upper endoscopy is now the most widely used screening test for gastric cancer in Asia.[295]

Not surprisingly, studies from Japan have shown that screening results in diagnosis of gastric cancer at earlier stages, with one study reporting more than half of screened cases diagnosed as stage I.[296] Long-term follow-up data from the Japanese Public Health Center cohort showed that subjects who underwent screening had a nearly 50% reduced risk of death from gastric cancer.[297] A separate cohort study from Japan found a 25%–35% risk reduction in death from gastric cancer among those who participated in gastric cancer screening.[298] A large population-based cohort study from China confirmed this effect in a cohort of 375,800 individuals of which 14,670 underwent endoscopic screening. Individuals that were ever screened showed an overall benefit of disease specific (and overall) survival (RR 0.18; 95% CI, 0.13–0.25) with a risk reduction of gastric cancer mortality by two thirds (RR 0.33; 95% CI, 0.20–0.56).[503] Similar data on a cohort from Korea (n = 46,701) showed an HR for death by gastric cancer of 0.36 (95% CI, 0.34–0.37) in patients who have been screened by endoscopy.[504] The effect was less pronounced for those who were screened by upper GI radiology series (HR 0.69; 95% CU, 0.67–0.73). The inferiority of radiology testing compared to endoscopy was confirmed in several further studies and a recent meta-analysis.[505,506] Survival further increased for those who were screened more than once.[507]

The serum pepsinogen (PG) test is increasingly used to screen for patients at highest risk for having preneoplastic gastric lesions. The stomach produces two types of PGs: PGI and PGII. In chronic atrophic gastritis, production of PGI is reduced due to reduction of the number of gastric chief cells, whereas PGII levels remain relatively constant or can sometimes even be raised in response to inflammation (see Chapter 54). Therefore both low serum PGI levels (<70 mg/L) and a low PGI/II ratio (<3.0) are useful for the identification of patients with atrophic gastritis.[292] Large prospective cohort studies have shown that baseline PGI, PGI/II, and *Hp* antibody levels combined can successfully identify patients at highest risk for developing gastric cancer for whom referral to endoscopy might be appropriate.[299–302,506]

Prescreening by such blood tests can be considered in low incidence areas where population-based endoscopic screening is not feasible. Screening with upper endoscopy is only cost-effective in high-incidence areas such as Japan.[508] In Western countries, vulnerable individuals with a higher risk should be targeted rather than using a population-based approach.[509,510] The selection criteria should include factors like age, gender, and ethnic background.[511,512] An additional group for screening are patients with genetic predispositions for gastric neoplasia, such as Lynch syndrome or FAP.[513–515] Further options to increase cost-effectiveness of screening in low incidence areas are the combination of stomach assessment with colorectal cancer screening that has been shown to be feasible in several cohorts.[516–518]

European consensus guidelines recommend endoscopic surveillance in patients in whom extensive atrophy of the gastric mucosa has been diagnosed—an approach that has now been adopted by several national guidelines in Europe.[304,519–521] Gastroscopy is recommended every 3 years in these patients. Initial analyses that such an approach can be cost-effective, and prospective randomized trials are currently underway to support this strategy.[305,306] A recent meta-analysis from the United States suggests that this strategy can only be cost-effective in low-incidence Western countries when applied to selected individuals with further risk factors.[307]

PREVENTION

Given the lethal nature of gastric cancer and its link to chronic infection and inflammation, much attention has been paid to the possibility of "chemoprevention" of gastric neoplastic lesions. The approach most studied has been *Hp* eradication, but consideration has also been given to supplementation with antioxidants and the use of NSAIDs and COX-2 inhibitors.

Eradication of *Hp*

Eradicating *Hp* leads to a decrease of the subsequent risk of gastric cancer. There is little question that chronic inflammation in a variety of organ systems can lead to malignancy and that *Hp* eradication can reduce or alleviate gastric inflammation. *Hp* eradication can lead to decreased oxidative stress and cell proliferation.[308] In addition, limited studies involving eradication of gastric *Helicobacter* organisms in Mongolian gerbils suggest that eradication of infection can partially reverse atrophy and metaplasia and inhibit progression to gastric cancer.[309] Studies in mice confirm the reversibility of metaplasia and prevention of gastric cancer with early eradication. With later eradication, cancer progression was slowed and cancer mortality dramatically decreased.[19]

Nevertheless, definite proof of the cancer-preventing effect of *Hp* eradication by prospective randomized trials in humans is lacking. This is partly due to the need for high numbers of at-risk patients to be included to achieve adequate power with regard to the rare endpoint of incident gastric cancer, and partly due to ethical concerns to randomize patients into a study arm that would leave them untreated with a class I carcinogen. One approach to tackle the first issue has been to examine the effect of *Hp* eradication on premalignant conditions, such as gastric atrophy and IM. Thus a majority of studies have shown a beneficial effect in preventing progression of gastric disease.[310–314] In a randomized, placebo-controlled trial from China of 587 patients with *Hp* infection, assignment to eradication was associated with a significantly reduced risk of progression of IM (OR, 0.63).[314] In contrast, a randomized placebo-controlled trial of Mexican adults did not demonstrate a benefit of *Hp* eradication for the prevention of histologic progression.[313]

A prospective, randomized placebo-controlled trial in 1630 "healthy" *Hp*-positive individuals sought to determine whether *Hp* eradication in a high-risk population in China would reduce the incidence of gastric cancer. Although no overall group benefit was seen in the group receiving *Hp* eradication, there was a reduction in gastric cancer incidence in the subgroup of patients who did not already have precancerous lesions (gastric atrophy, IM, or dysplasia) at study initiation. It is possible that some of the patients in the eradication arm had passed the earlier mentioned "point of no return," when cellular alterations had sufficiently accumulated to promote cancer.[315] A meta-analysis of randomized trials found that *Hp* eradication is associated with a significant 35% reduction in the risk of gastric cancer.[22]

There may even be benefit to *Hp* eradication after treatment of EGC in light of the high rate of associated multifocal dysplasia. In an open-label randomized controlled trial of patients with resected EGC by Fukase et al., *Hp* eradication was associated with a reduction in the risk of development of metachronous gastric cancer (OR, 0.35; 95% CI, 0.0161−0.775). Although there are conflicting results, recent meta-analyses support the initial findings of Fukase et al.[316,317]

In Western countries, gastric cancer prevention has not been extensively pursued due to the lower prevalence of *Hp* infection and decreasing incidence of gastric cancer. However, a cost-effectiveness model by Parsonnet et al.[318] suggested that screening and treatment of *Hp* infection would be potentially cost-effective in the prevention of gastric cancer, particularly in high-risk populations, if it was assumed that treatment of *Hp* infection prevented 30% of attributable gastric cancers. Using a more conservative 10% reduction in gastric cancer risk, an analysis from the United Kingdom also concluded that *Hp* eradication was cost-effective.[319]

An alternative option would be population-based vaccination against *Hp* infection. But development of an effective vaccine as well as definition of the right timepoint for vaccination have demonstrated to be difficult. Despite a recent study showing promising results, it is not clear yet if a clinically applicable vaccine will be available in the near future.[320]

Aspirin and Other NSAIDs, Including COX-2 Inhibitors

Among other effects, aspirin and other NSAIDs inhibit cyclooxygenases. COX-1 is constitutively expressed in the GI tract. COX-2 expression is generally not observed in normal GI mucosa, but is induced in multiple epithelial malignancies, including gastric cancer.[321,322] COX-2 expression is associated with aggressive cell growth in both human and mouse models of cancer[323–326] and has been found to be overexpressed in 70% of gastric cancers.[327] In this setting, COX-2 could potentially promote the growth of tumors, inhibit apoptosis, and increase angiogenesis. COX-2 expression has been reported to be elevated in preneoplastic lesions, including both IM and dysplasia, and COX-2 expression appears to diminish after *Hp* eradication.[328]

Multiple epidemiologic studies have demonstrated a consistent association between NSAID use and reduced risk of gastric cancer.[329–332] In a case-control study from Los Angeles County, NSAID use for more than 5 years was associated with a reduced risk of noncardia gastric cancer (OR, 0.61), and there was a significant NSAID dose-related effect.[330] A nested case-control study using the General Practitioners Research Database in the United Kingdom found that long-term users of nonaspirin NSAIDs had a decreased risk of gastric cancer (OR, 0.65), although there was no effect of aspirin use on the risk of gastric cancer.[332] This study was in contrast to a recent study in two UK cohorts from England and Scotland on 3833 patients with gastric cancer and 4654 patients with esophageal cancer.[333] In these cohorts, long-term aspirin use was not associated with cancer-specific mortality after diagnosis of gastric cancer (pooled adjusted HR, 1.06; 95% CI, 0.85−1.32). On the other hand, recent meta-analyses reported a significant association between any NSAID use and reduced risk of gastric cancer (RR: 0.78, 95% CI, 0.72−0.85), with broadly similar findings for both acetylsalicylic acid (aspirin) (ASA) and non-ASA NSAIDs and a slightly more pronounced effect for noncardia gastric cancer.[334]

In a randomized controlled trial of *Hp*-negative patients with IM, there was no difference in the rate of regression of IM after 2 years between patients receiving the COX-2 selective inhibitor rofecoxib and placebo.[335] This trial was limited by the relatively short follow-up period and use of premalignant endpoints. In a separate randomized controlled trial in patients with *Hp* and histology showing chronic atrophic gastritis (or worse), both *Hp* eradication and 24 months of the COX-2 selective inhibitor celecoxib resulted in histologic regression, although no additive effect was observed.[336] In a summary analysis of randomized trials of aspirin versus no aspirin for various outcomes, those studies with 10−20 years' follow-up reported a reduced risk of gastric cancer in those assigned to aspirin (OR, 0.42).[337] Further trials in high-risk patients are warranted to determine if NSAIDs are effective for gastric cancer prevention.

Statins

Statins, the widely prescribed class of HMG CoA-inhibiting cholesterol-lowering drugs, have been found in numerous epidemiologic studies to be associated with decreased risks of various malignancies. In addition to their cholesterol-lowering properties, statins also have antiproliferative and proapoptotic effects.[338] A population-based case-control study from Taiwan found a significantly reduced risk of gastric cancer in patients prescribed statins (OR, 0.68), with greater risk reduction observed among those with the highest cumulative statin use.[339] In a separate case-control study of diabetics from South Korea, a history of statin use was associated with an 80% reduced likelihood of gastric cancer.[340] A pharmacy database study from the Netherlands found a significant association between statin use and a decreased risk of cancer of any type; however, there was no significant association with gastric cancer, although the number of cases was relatively small.[341] meta-analyses agree on an overall favorable profile of statins with regards to gastric cancer risk, showing a risk reduction that ranges between 32% and 44%.[342,343] Interestingly, there was no statistically significant difference between Western or Asian cohorts with regards to this effect.

Future randomized controlled trials of various statins in patients at high risk for gastric cancer will help define the role of this class of drugs as chemopreventive agents.

Antioxidants

Chronic inflammatory states, such as *Hp* gastritis, can result in the generation of free radicals derived from oxygen and nitrogen.[344] These free radicals can promote carcinogenesis via numerous different means, including direct DNA damage and inhibition of DNA repair mechanisms, inhibition of apoptosis, and activation of cellular proliferation pathways. Antioxidants, such as carotenoids and vitamins C and E, bind with reactive oxygen and nitrogen species to neutralize their damaging effects.

Epidemiologic data support a relationship between increased antioxidant intake and reduced risk of gastric cancer.[345–349] In a nested case-control study from Japan, low plasma beta carotene levels were associated with an increased risk of gastric cancer.[347] A case-control study from Korea found that elevated nitrate/antioxidant intake ratios were associated with increased risk of gastric cancer.[348] In a Swedish cohort study, high levels of vitamin A, retinol, and alpha and beta carotene intake were associated with a 50% risk reduction in gastric cancer.[349] A recent meta-analysis on the impact of alpha and beta carotene intake analyzed data from 13 case-control and 8 cohort studies and reported inconsistency of the respective results between case-control and cohort studies.[350]

Randomized controlled trials have shown inconsistent effects of antioxidant supplementation on gastric cancer risk. In a randomized placebo-controlled trial of antioxidants (either vitamin A, C, or E) in patients with precancerous gastric lesions (nonatrophic or atrophic gastritis, IM, or dysplasia), antioxidant supplementation did not result in either reduced histologic progression or increased histologic regression.[351] A randomized controlled trial in China also found no effect of combined vitamin C, E, and selenium supplementation on the prevalence of a combined endpoint of atrophic gastritis, IM, dysplasia, or cancer.[352] In a 10-year follow-up of the General Population Nutrition Intervention Trial in China, subjects who received a combination of selenium, vitamin E, and beta carotene were found to have reduced mortality from gastric cancer.[353] Interestingly, Li et al. reported in a systematic analysis of the data available in 2013 that although high dietary intake of vitamin C, vitamin E, and alpha and beta carotene resulted in a reduced risk for gastric cancer, the actual blood levels of these factors were not associated with gastric cancer risk.[354] Given a lack of convincing chemopreventive effect as well as the results of the Beta Carotene and Retinol Efficacy Trial, in which subjects who received beta carotene and vitamin A had an increased risk of lung cancer,[355] antioxidant supplementation for the prevention of gastric cancer cannot yet be recommended. This is in line with a recent Cochrane meta-analysis on the effect of selenium supplementation on cancer prevention.[356] Although there are some data from observational studies suggesting a minor decrease in the site-specific risk for stomach cancer, studies are heterogeneous and prospective randomized controlled trials would be needed to support this hypothesis.

Other Dietary Factors

Green tea is widely consumed in Asian countries and is hypothesized to have protective effects against cancer of the upper digestive tract. Polyphenols and other metabolites present in green teas, such as epigallocatechin-3-gallate (EGCG) and other catechins, have a variety of antitumor effects, including induction of apoptosis, inhibition of tumor cell growth and proliferation, and reduction in COX-2 expression.[357–359] EGCG also has antioxidant properties and may have antiinflammatory properties as well.[360,361] Although case-control studies have shown an inverse association between the risk of gastric cancer and the consumption of green tea, cohort studies have largely failed to show an association.[362,363] One cohort study from Japan did report a reduced risk of gastric cancer in women with high green tea consumption, but no change in risk among men.[364] A recent meta-analysis of observational studies suggested a slightly decreased risk by long-term high-dose green tea intake,[365] but in the absence of prospective controlled trials, green tea cannot be recommended as chemoprevention for gastric cancer. Similar results are available on the effect of garlic consumption.[366]

Adherence to a Mediterranean diet has the potential to reduce gastric cancer risk and related mortality by nearly 30% (RR 0.72; 95% CI, 0.60–0.86).[367] A recent model calculation predicted that increasing fruit and vegetable intake would prevent a relatively high proportion of gastric cancer cases by 2025, mostly in developing countries.[368]

CLINICAL FEATURES

EGCs are asymptomatic in up to 80% of cases. When symptoms do occur, they tend to mimic peptic ulcer disease. With advanced gastric cancer, the most common symptoms are weight loss (≈60% of patients) and abdominal pain (≈50%).[369] Other presenting symptoms include nausea, vomiting, anorexia, dysphagia, melena, and early satiety. Pyloric outlet obstruction can occur with tumors of the antrum and pylorus, and tumors of the cardia can cause dysphagia due to involvement of the lower esophageal sphincter and development of pseudoachalasia (see Chapter 46).[370] Rarely, paraneoplastic syndromes occur. There have been reports of thrombophlebitis (Trousseau sign), neuropathies, nephrotic syndrome, and DIC.[371–373] Dermatologic paraneoplastic syndromes are also uncommon and include hyperpigmented patches in the axilla (acanthosis nigricans; see Chapter 25) and the sudden onset of seborrheic dermatosis (senile warts) and pruritus (sign of Leser-Trélat).[374]

The physical exam is usually unremarkable. Cachexia and signs of bowel obstruction are the most common abnormal findings. Occasionally, it is possible to detect an epigastric mass, hepatomegaly, ascites, and lower extremity edema.[375] Laboratory studies are generally unrevealing until the cancer reaches advanced stages. Anemia and a positive test result for fecal occult blood may occur from chronic bleeding of an ulcerated mass.

Hypoproteinemia can occur. Liver enzyme values, particularly serum alkaline phosphatase levels, can be elevated secondary to hepatic metastases.

Gastric cancer is metastatic at the time of diagnosis in 33% of cases.[376] The most common sites of metastasis are the liver (40%) and peritoneum.[377] Other sites of spread include periumbilical lymph nodes (Sister Joseph nodule), left supraclavicular sentinel nodes (Virchow node), the pouch of Douglas (rectal shelf of Blumer), and the ovaries (Krukenberg tumor). Gastric cancer has also been reported to metastasize to the kidney, bladder, brain, bone, heart, thyroid, adrenal glands, and skin.[375] There are reports of unusual presentations of metastatic disease, such as shoulder-hand syndrome from bone metastasis, diplopia and blindness from orbital and retinal metastases, and virilization due to Krukenberg tumors.[378–381]

DIAGNOSIS

Endoscopy

EGD with biopsies is currently the procedure of choice for the diagnosis of gastric cancer (Fig. 56.6A). When a nonhealing gastric ulcer is found, at least 6–8 biopsy specimens from the edge and base of the ulcer are recommended.[382] The American Gastroenterological Association recommendeds that an upper endoscopy should be performed in patients older than 55 years with new-onset dyspepsia and in patients younger than 55 years who present with "alarm" symptoms (weight loss, recurrent vomiting, dysphagia, evidence of bleeding, and anemia).[383] Dyspeptic patients in whom an empirical trial of PPIs and eradication of *Hp* (following a positive test result) do not relieve symptoms should undergo prompt endoscopic evaluation as well.[522] The basis for these recommendations is the low incidence of gastric cancer in individuals younger than 55 years. The yield of upper endoscopy for the detection of gastric cancer in patients with occult bleeding and a normal colonoscopy varies, based on the patient's baseline risk of gastric cancer.

In Japan and other areas of high gastric cancer prevalence, chromoendoscopy, magnification endoscopy, and virtual chromoendoscopy modalities (e.g., narrow band imaging) are used alone or in combination as aids in the detection of EGC (see Fig. 56.6B). Distinct irregular mucosal surface and vascular patterns correlate with the presence of dysplasia and carcinoma.[384] Virtual chromoendoscopy enhances lesion recognition compared to standard white light endoscopy.[523,524] Several recent studies on the use of linked-color imaging confirm that there is a benefit for both expert and nonexpert endoscopists, especially in case of lesions that are more challenging to detect.[525,526] There are ongoing investigations into the utility of further techniques, such as autofluorescence and confocal microendoscopy, for the diagnosis of early gastric neoplasia.[385,386] In the past, barium studies have been reported to have 60%–70% sensitivity and 90% specificity for the detection of advanced gastric cancer.[387] Nevertheless, upper GI series has been largely replaced by upper endoscopy as the initial test of choice for the diagnosis of gastric cancer.

A classification system has been developed for EGC based on endoscopic appearance,[388] the purpose of which is to assess early lesions for risk of submucosal invasion as well as risk of lymph node spread (Fig. 56.7). The three types include superficial polypoid (types 0–I), superficial flat/depressed (types 0–IIa–c), and superficial excavated (types 0–III) lesions. The most commonly observed subtype is 0–IIc, the nonpolypoid depressed lesion.[388] This classification system is used most often in Japan, where endoscopic mucosal resection (EMR) and submucosal dissection are frequently performed for early gastric neoplasia.

There is increasing interest in the application of artificial intelligence systems in endoscopic assessment of the upper GI tract.[527] Overall detection of EGC reaches high accuracy with sensitivity and specificity reaching close to 90%.[528] Most promising are systems applying convolutional neural network-based image analysis—if the modules are well trained in the first place.[529] Application includes not only the reduction of possible blind spots during first assessment, but also estimation of the depth of invasion of early lesions.[530,531]

CT Gastrography

Since CT colonography has gained significant attention for its potential role as a screening modality for colon polyps and colon cancer, CT gastrography has also been studied for the diagnosis of EGC. In a study from South Korea of 39 patients with EGC, CT

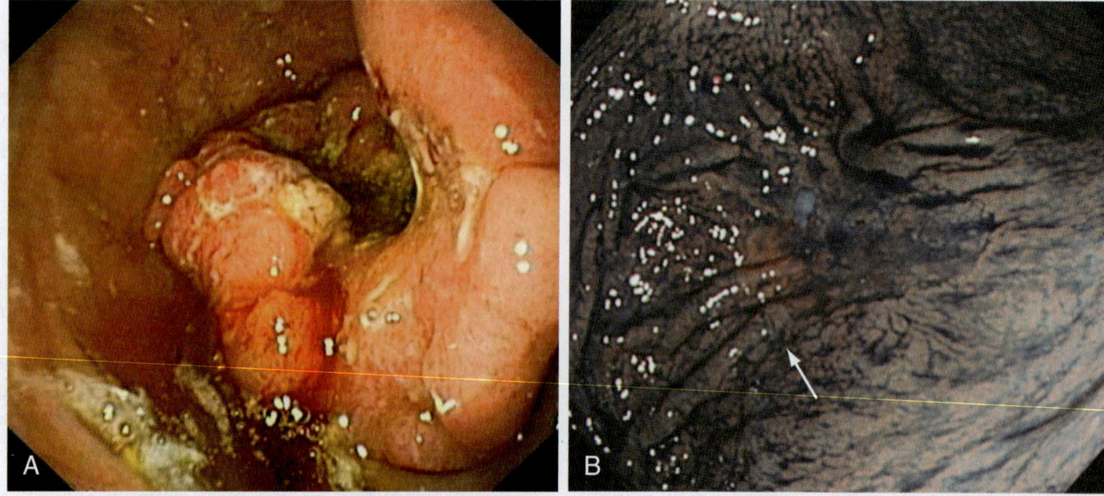

Fig. 56.6 Endoscopic examples of gastric cancer. (A) Ulcerated gastric adenocarcinoma mass lesion. (B) Chromoendoscopic view of a superficial depressed gastric cancer, highlighted with indigo carmine (*arrow*). ((A) With permission from the Gastrolab Endoscopy Archives. *The Wasa Workgroup on Intestinal Disorders*. 2008. Accessed 14 Oct 2008, at http://www.gastrolab.net/pa-269.htm; (B) from Toyoda H, Tanaka K, Hamada Y, et al. Endoscopic diagnosis of hypopharyngeal, esophageal and gastric neoplasm. *Dig Endosc.* 2006;18:S41–S43.)

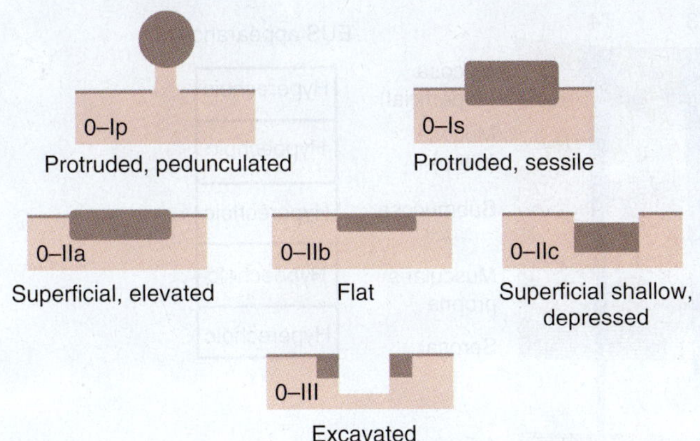

Fig. 56.7 Schematic representation of the major variants of type 0 neoplastic lesions of the stomach: polypoid (Ip and Is), nonpolypoid (IIa, IIb, and IIc), nonpolypoid and excavated (III). (From the Paris endoscopic classification of superficial neoplastic lesions: esophagus, stomach, and colon: November 30 to December 1, 2002. *Gastrointest Endosc*. 2003;58:S3–43.)

gastrography had a sensitivity of 73%–76% and good interobserver reliability ($\kappa = 0.84$).[389] Only small studies have been performed thus far using this imaging modality, and CT gastrography cannot yet be recommended for screening outside of the research setting.

Serum Markers

To date, no reliable serum marker has been identified with high sensitivity and specificity for the diagnosis of gastric cancer. Low serum PGI levels, low ratios of PGI to PGII, and hypergastrinemia have been reported in patients with atrophic gastritis and IM, but the results for the detection of gastric cancer have been mixed.[390,391] In a study of 17,000 Japanese males, a positive PG test (defined as PGI < 50 μg/L, and PGI/II < 3.0) in combination with upper GI series identified gastric cancer in only 0.28% of subjects; however, 88% of these cancers were early cancers.[392] In addition, 89% of the cancers identified by the PG test alone were EGCs. The major limitation of this test is the low specificity for the diagnosis of gastric cancer.[393] Therefore assessment of serum PG is currently rather used to identify patients with preneoplastic conditions that benefit from further diagnostic testing (i.e., by endoscopy).[532]

Serum CEA and carbohydrate antigen (CA) 19-9 have both been extensively studied for the diagnosis of gastric cancer. The sensitivities of these markers are especially low for EGC,[394] and elevated levels are also seen in other epithelial malignancies. These tumor markers are frequently elevated in recurrent gastric cancer, especially in patients who had elevated levels prior to surgical resection.[395] The diagnostic quality of these markers remains low and they might rather have a role as prognostic indicators instead, with both CEA and CA19-9 being associated with unfavorable clinical-pathological characteristics and poor outcome for gastric cancer patients.[396,397] Among other targets, studies have identified, TGF-β1, CA 72-4, tumor M2-pyruvate kinase, and hepatocyte growth factor as potential markers for gastric cancer,[398–401] but as for CEA and CA19-9, these might rather serve as prognostic indicators, particularly for recurrence after surgical treatment.[402]

Apart from classic serum markers, a recent research focus has been placed on so-called liquid biopsies, mainly the assessment of circulating tumor cells and circulating tumor DNA, as well as RNA components. Recent advancements in enrichment and sequencing approaches enables the analysis of these factors which can deliver information on mutational profile and tumor heterogeneity even without the need for invasive tissue sampling.[403] Although data on diagnostic accuracy and value as prognostic markers are still inconsistent, the potential use to guide targeted therapy becomes more interesting. A prominent example is the assessment for Her2 amplification by analysis of circulating plasma DNA.[404,405] This approach has the potential to overcome problems of tissue analyses with tumor heterogeneity and sampling error.[406]

Another modality that is under investigation for its potential application as noninvasive screening methods is the assessment of volatile markers in the exhaled breath.[533] While initial results are promising, this is far from clinical application yet.

CLASSIFICATION AND STAGING

Several classification systems exist to further define gastric cancer and predict prognosis. As mentioned earlier (see Fig. 56.2), gastric cancers can be subdivided into intestinal and diffuse types. Gastric cancer can also be divided into early and advanced lesions. *EGC* is defined as a cancer that does not invade beyond the submucosa, regardless of lymph node involvement. This form of cancer has a much higher prevalence in the Far East, especially Japan, and carries a very favorable prognosis, with 5-year survival rates greater than 90% being reported in Asia and greater than 80% in Western countries.[407–410]

The most commonly used clinical staging classification system for gastric cancer is the TNM system, used by the International Union Against Cancer and the American Joint Committee on Cancer.[411,412] In the TNM staging system, T (Tumor) indicates the depth of penetration (Fig. 56.8): T1a denotes a tumor that invades the lamina propria or mucosa, T1b denotes invasion of the submucosa, T2 denotes invasion of the muscularis propria, T3 denotes invasion of the subserosal connective tissue, T4a denotes invasion of the serosa (visceral peritoneum), and T4b denotes invasion into adjacent organs or structures. N (Nodes) indicates the degree of lymph node invasion: N0 denotes no lymph node involvement, N1 denotes involvement of 1–2 lymph nodes, N2 denotes involvement of 3–6 lymph nodes, and N3 denotes involvement of 7 or more lymph nodes. M (Metastasis) indicates the presence of distant metastases, with M0 denoting no metastases and M1 denoting distant metastases, including positive peritoneal cytology (Table 56.4). In the American Joint Committee on Cancer staging manual, cardia cancer (tumors within 2 cm of and crossing the GE junction) is classified together with esophageal and GE junction tumors.[412] Recent studies have investigated reclassification of gastric cancer based on biological characteristics. The prospect of incorporating tumor biology into staging classification systems is intriguing, although future validation studies are required for this to occur.

EUS

EUS allows the visualization of the five layers of the gastric wall. The superficial gastric mucosa is represented by an echogenic first layer, and the deeper mucosa by a hypoechogenic second layer; the submucosa is represented by an echogenic third layer, the muscularis propria as a hypoechogenic fourth layer, and the serosa as an echogenic fifth layer. EUS can also identify and biopsy submucosal lesions, such as gastric lymphomas and stromal tumors. These lesions typically involve thickening of the submucosa and muscularis propria and may appear as gastric fold thickening on barium studies or endoscopy.

Based on the results of a meta-analysis of EUS for gastric cancer staging, EUS has sensitivity of 86% and specificity of 91% to distinguish T1-2 versus T3-4 tumors.[413] Intramucosal lesions (T1a) are identified with 83% sensitivity and 79% specificity.

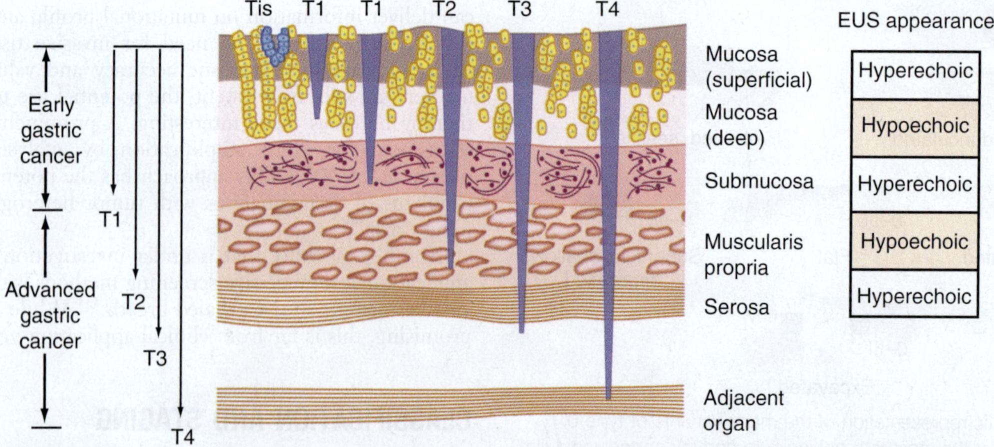

Fig. 56.8 Classification of gastric adenocarcinoma by depth of invasion (T classification). In the TNM classification, T denotes depth of invasion: Tis designates carcinoma in situ; T1 tumors are confined to the mucosa (T1a) and submucosa (T1b); T2 tumors invade the muscularis propria but not the serosa; T3 tumors penetrate the subserosal connective tissue without involving the visceral peritoneum or contiguous structures; and T4 tumors invade the serosa (visceral peritoneum) and may involve adjacent organs and tissues. In early gastric cancer, the disease is confined to the mucosa and submucosa (T1), regardless of nodal involvement.

TABLE 56.4 Clinical Staging of Gastric Cancer Based on the TNM Classification

	N0	N1	N2	N3	M1 (Any N)
Tis	0	–	–	–	–
T1	IA	IB	IIA	IIB	IV
T2	IB	IIA	IIB	IIIA	IV
T3	IIA	IIB	IIIA	IIIB	IV
T4a	IIB	IIIA	IIIB	IIIC	IV
T4b	IIIB	IIIB	IIIC	IIIC	IV

is, in situ; *M*, metastases; *N*, node involvement; *T*, tumor.
From Brierley JD, Gospodarowicz MK, Wittekind C, editors. *TNM Classification of Malignant Tumours*. 8th ed. Hoboken, NJ: Wiley-Blackwell; 2017.

EUS may be particularly useful for identifying EGC lesions amenable to EMR or submucosal dissection[414] (Fig. 56.9). It is of note that the diagnostic quality of CT for T-staging has caught up with EUS during recent years now achieving similar results.[534] In terms of N staging, the rate of detection of perigastric nodes with EUS is comparable to staging with CT.[415,416] However, EUS is slightly less accurate in the assessment of nodal status as compared to depth of tumor invasion, with 69% sensitivity and 84% specificity to distinguish positive from negative lymph node status.[413] A particular difficulty with N staging lies in the fact that many small lymph nodes can also harbor metastases, and thus understaging can occur. The need for EUS as a staging tool complementary to CT should be determined based on local expertise and availability as well as patient-dependent factors.

CT and PET

Advances in imaging technology have greatly improved the ability of CT to stage gastric tumors.[535] Although not as extensively studied as EUS, multidetector row CT (MDCT), by which the wall of the stomach can be seen as three layers (an inner layer corresponding to the mucosa, an intermediate layer corresponding to the submucosa, and an outer layer of slightly higher attenuation corresponding to the muscularis propria and serosa), appears to have comparable accuracy to EUS in terms of both T and N staging. The loss of fat planes between the gastric mass and an adjacent organ suggests tumor invasion. The accuracy of MDCT for overall T staging ranges from 77% to 91%, and discriminates serosal involvement with an accuracy of 83%–100%.[417,418] Accuracy with respect to N staging may be as high as 89% with MDCT.[419,420] As with all other imaging modalities, CT has difficulty discerning metastases in lymph nodes smaller than 5 mm. It is not yet clear whether EUS or MDCT (or the combination) is superior for T and N staging in gastric cancer, and the underlying technology continues to evolve and improve.

PET scanning alone is not recommended as a sole imaging test for gastric cancer staging, largely because most gastric adenocarcinomas have low F-18 fluorodeoxyglucose uptake and there are false-positives as well (see Chapter 54).[421] However, in patients initially staged as having localized gastric cancer, combined PET/CT increases the detection of metastatic disease by 10%, thus having a potential impact on clinical management.[422] A recent meta-analysis estimated that this leads to an actual change in the clinical management of the patient in 3%–29%, with the actual impact being under debate.[536]

Laparoscopy With Peritoneal Lavage

Similarly, staging laparoscopy is considered an important adjunct modality for initial staging. Approximately half of gastric cancer patients with metastatic disease have cancer involving the peritoneum.[377] EUS and CT have limited ability to detect peritoneal dissemination. In fact, up to one-third of patients with seemingly resectable disease will have evidence of peritoneal spread at the time of staging laparoscopy.[423] National Comprehensive Cancer Network guidelines recommend consideration of laparoscopy with peritoneal lavage for patients with seemingly resectable disease in whom neoadjuvant chemotherapy is being considered.[424] Although considered to be generally cost-effective, the United States has been slow to adopt this practice; a study using SEER-Medicare data found that only 8% of gastric cancer patients who had any surgery underwent laparoscopy.[425,537] Introduction of both PET-CT and staging laparoscopy to standard care pathways in the Netherlands did not change the rate of patients who remain on curative pathways, although the impact of laparoscopy results is generally deemed to be more relevant than those of PET-CT.[538,539]

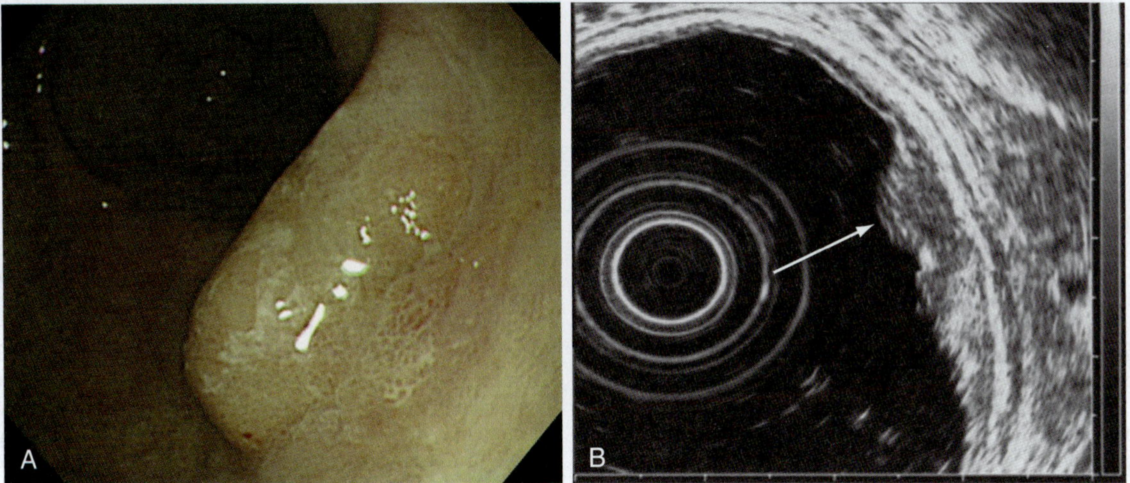

Fig. 56.9 Gastric cancer staging. (A) Endoscopic image of an early gastric cancer showing a 25-mm protruding mass located on the posterior wall of the antrum. (B) EUS image of the lesion, showing the hypoechoic mucosal mass (*arrow*) with an intact submucosal layer. (From Kim JH, Song KS, Youn YH, et al. Clinicopathologic factors influence accurate endosonographic assessment for early gastric cancer. *Gastrointest Endosc.* 2007;66:901–908.)

Other Imaging Modalities

MRI with gadolinium has also been used for gastric cancer staging. It is similar to CT in its advantages (ability to find distant metastases) and weaknesses (need for adequate gastric distention). The accuracy of MRI ranges from 90% to 93% for T staging and from 91% to 100% for N staging.[417] However, given the small number of studies and the potential for image artifacts in routine conditions outside clinical studies, MRI cannot yet be advocated as the test of choice for staging gastric cancer.

Restaging after Neoadjuvant Treatment

The accuracy of restaging gastric cancer after neoadjuvant chemotherapy decreases considerably. EUS has less than 50% accuracy for both T and N restaging, and similarly disappointing results have been reported for posttreatment staging with CT.[426] However, the use of preoperative clinical staging to assess response to neoadjuvant chemoradiation may correlate well with both overall and disease-free survival.[427] Restaging is therefore primarily used to rule out distant metastasis as part of the assessment for surgical resectability.

PROGNOSIS AND TREATMENT

Overall, the 5-year survival rate in the United States from gastric cancer is 27% (compared with 64% for colon cancer).[4] The TNM classification is used to stratify disease into four clinical stages (I–IV) to predict prognosis in patients treated with gastrectomy (see Table 56.4). There are data to suggest that large tumor size (>5 cm) may be independently associated with worse survival, independent of nodal status or overall tumor stage.[429]

In general, neoadjuvant, adjuvant and additive procedures are available. In principle, therapy is based on prognostic factors, the general condition of the patient, and the possibility of R0 resection. Crucial for the assessment of resectability is the T stage. Peri- and preoperative approaches offer advantages over postoperative therapies, at least conceptually, for three reasons: First, compliance is significantly better with neoadjuvant concepts, that is, the required therapy is more likely to be applied. Second, tumor downsizing often occurs with neoadjuvant therapy, increasing the chances of complete (R0) resection. Third, neoadjuvant chemotherapy is the earliest way to target systemic seeding of tumor cells. This seeding is a cause of the limited long-term prognosis.

Surgery

Surgical resection remains the primary curative treatment for gastric cancer. However, survival after surgery alone is poor (20% –50% at 5 years), necessitating efforts to improve the outcomes for this group of patients using perioperative chemotherapy or postoperative (adjuvant) chemoradiotherapy. In addition, surgical resection often provides the most effective palliation of symptoms, particularly those of obstruction. In some cases, surgery is required for diagnosis, as in cases of nonhealing gastric ulcers with negative biopsy results and persistent pyloric outlet obstruction suggesting an antral carcinoma. Surgery should be attempted in most cases of gastric cancer. However, in the presence of extensive involvement of diffuse-type cancer (or *linitis plastica*), bulky metastatic disease, retroperitoneal invasion, or peritoneal carcinomatosis, or if the patient has severe comorbid illnesses, the prognosis may be sufficiently poor to make the value of resection questionable.

Surgery, and laparoscopy in particular, can be useful in the staging of cancer. Laparoscopy can help identify primary tumor resectability, peritoneal deposits, and appropriate candidates for neoadjuvant therapy. Laparoscopic peritoneal lavage has been used to detect intraperitoneal free cancer cells. A positive peritoneal lavage correlates significantly with eventual development of overt peritoneal metastases.[430]

In general, total gastrectomy is performed for proximal gastric tumors and for diffuse gastric cancer, and partial gastrectomy is reserved for tumors in the distal stomach. Large, randomized multicenter trials in France and Italy comparing subtotal with total gastrectomy for adenocarcinoma of the antrum found no differences in 5-year survival rates or operative mortality.[431,432] Some centers have argued for performing a complete splenectomy with gastrectomy. However, several retrospective and prospective studies found that concurrent splenectomy increased morbidity and had either no effect on or worsened survival.[433,434]

Open gastrectomy remains the preferred surgical treatment for gastric cancer worldwide. In high-volume, experienced centers, however, laparoscopic gastric resection (and more recently robotic gastrectomy though data with this are more limited) provides an alternative that offers patients a faster recovery and fewer complications while recovering a similar number of lymph nodes compared with open surgery.[540] Long-term oncologic data from several prospective randomized trials are expected. Today, laparotomy is an acceptable approach to achieve total or partial gastrectomy with D2 lymphadenectomy for gastric cancer. A laparoscopic approach may be selectively proposed in expert hands. Robot-assisted gastrectomy has shown similar oncological outcomes in terms of survival and lymph node yield compared with conventional laparoscopic gastrectomy. With technical advances, future gastric cancer surgery will most likely become increasingly minimally invasive and will probably take advantage of the rapidly developing robotic technologies.

Given the apparent impact of D2 lymphadenectomy on disease-specific survival, most major cancer centers are performing a D2, as compared with a D1, dissection. Treatment guidelines recommend that gastric cancer resection include the regional lymphatics, including perigastric (D1) nodes as well as those along the left gastric artery, common hepatic artery, celiac artery, splenic hilum, and splenic artery (D2 lymph nodes), with the goal of examining 15 or more lymph nodes. As long as it is carried out in specialized, high-volume centers with appropriate surgical expertise and postoperative care, a pancreas- and spleen-preserving D2 lymphadenectomy provides superior staging information and may provide a survival benefit while avoiding excess morbidity. The optimal extent of lymph node dissection, however, remains an area of significant discussion in surgical circles.[400,433,435,436] There are two main arguments against the routine use of an extended lymphadenectomy: the higher associated morbidity and mortality (particularly if splenectomy is performed to achieve extended lymphadenectomy) and the lack of a survival benefit for extended lymphadenectomy in most large randomized trials.

Endoscopic Mucosal Resection and Submucosal Dissection

Advances in endoscopic techniques have permitted EMR and endoscopic submucosal dissection (ESD) to be used as curative therapies for select EGCs (Video 56.2). This technique has been used widely for intestinal-type cancers in Japan and South Korea, where studies have shown that only 3.5% of patients with EGCs smaller than 2–3 cm have lymph node involvement, making these lesions amenable to local therapy. Lesions larger than 4.5 cm have a greater than 50% chance of spread into the submucosa, are associated with "positive" nodes, and are therefore less likely to be endoscopically resectable.[438]

The following criteria have been suggested for EMR in gastric cancer: (1) the cancer is located in the mucosa and the lymph nodes are not involved, as indicated by EUS examination; (2) the maximum size of the tumor is less than 2 cm when the lesion is slightly elevated (type IIa) and less than 1 cm when the tumor is flat or slightly depressed (type IIb or IIc) without an ulcer scar; (3) there is no evidence of multiple gastric cancers or simultaneous abdominal cancers; and (4) the cancer is of the intestinal type.[439] Despite these guidelines, it is generally not possible to remove lesions larger than 1.5–2.0 cm en bloc by EMR, and piecemeal removal of EGC is associated with decreased rates of curative resection.[440]

ESD is a technique developed in Japan and permits en bloc resection of larger EGCs, as well as selected tumors with submucosal invasion. With ESD, submucosal injection is performed, followed by use of endoscopic electrosurgical knives to resect the entire tumor (Fig. 56.10).[441] Endoscopic prediction of EGC T stage is less accurate than in the colon and lesion margins are less distinct. Moreover, unlike in the colon, lymphatics are found within gastric mucosa and gastric lesions do not follow the adenoma-carcinoma sequence of transformation. As a result of these differences, en bloc resection by ESD affords the best chance of accurate histological staging and potential cure for EGC. In addition to an R0 resection, ESD allows for more precise histopathologic assessment of depth of invasion and lymphovascular involvement and permits appropriate assessment for risk of lymph node metastasis. If preprocedure evaluation does not reveal regional lymph node involvement, much larger superficial lesions can be resected. The Japanese have developed expanded criteria for ESD for EGC: (1) mucosal intestinal-type cancer of any size without ulceration, (2) mucosal intestinal-type cancer less than 3 cm with ulceration, and (3) submucosal intestinal-type cancer less than 3 cm and with submucosal invasion less than 500 μm.[442,443] As experience with this ESD has increased, en bloc resection rates are now reported to be over 90%, with local recurrence rates lower than 3%.[441] Owing to the large size of some of the lesions being resected, the risk of gastric perforation is relatively high (2%–6%).[444,445] However, perforations recognized early can generally be treated conservatively with closure using endoscopic clipping.[441]

Western guidelines for gastric ESD include both absolute and expanded criteria depending on lesion size and morphology. Recent gastric ESD studies from Western centers have shown comparable outcomes to that of Eastern centers, particularly in critical endpoints, such as R0 resection and complications. In a prospective observational study of 191 EGC resected by ESD from a single Western referral center, en bloc and R0 resection rates of 98.4% and 90.2% (for lesions meeting guideline criteria) and 89.0% and 73.6% (for lesions meeting expanded criteria), respectively, were seen. For patients with EGC but higher risk of lymph node involvement and who are poor candidates for surgical gastrectomy, combination ESD with laparoscopic lymph node dissection may be an alternative approach.[446] There are no published randomized clinical trials comparing surgery to endoscopic resection for EGC.

By precisely determining the depth of extension in the ESD specimen individualized, risk-adapted therapy planning can be performed, depending on the histopathologically assessed depth of infiltration of the tumor. Histologic findings of stage T1m (mucosal carcinoma) or T1sm1 (tumors infiltrating the first third of the submucosa) do not require further surgical therapy, as lymph node metastasis is highly unlikely in these stages. Thus today's endoscopic procedures are no longer to be considered purely diagnostic but can certainly be used with definitive, curative intent if indicated.[541]

Chemotherapy

In Western countries, approximately 75% of patients with gastric cancer have disease that has spread to the perigastric lymph nodes or have distant metastases at the time of diagnosis.[447] Patients presenting at early stages should be treated with surgery in combination with perioperative chemotherapy with curative intent. Numerous clinical trials have been performed evaluating the role of adjuvant chemotherapy after curative resection for gastric cancer.[448] The majority of the studies were inconclusive, but a series of meta-analyses of these trials suggested a 15%–20% reduction in the risk of death in patients who received adjuvant chemotherapy.[449–452]

Neoadjuvant chemotherapy shows a clear benefit in patients with resectable disease. In the UK MAGIC trial, 503 patients with gastric, gastroesophageal, or distal esophageal cancer were randomly assigned to undergo surgery alone or surgery following neoadjuvant epirubicin, cisplatin, and 5-fluorouracil (5FU). Compared to surgery alone, the neoadjuvant group had significantly improved 5-year (36% vs. 23%), progression-free, and overall survival (OS).[454] As a result, preoperative (neoadjuvant)

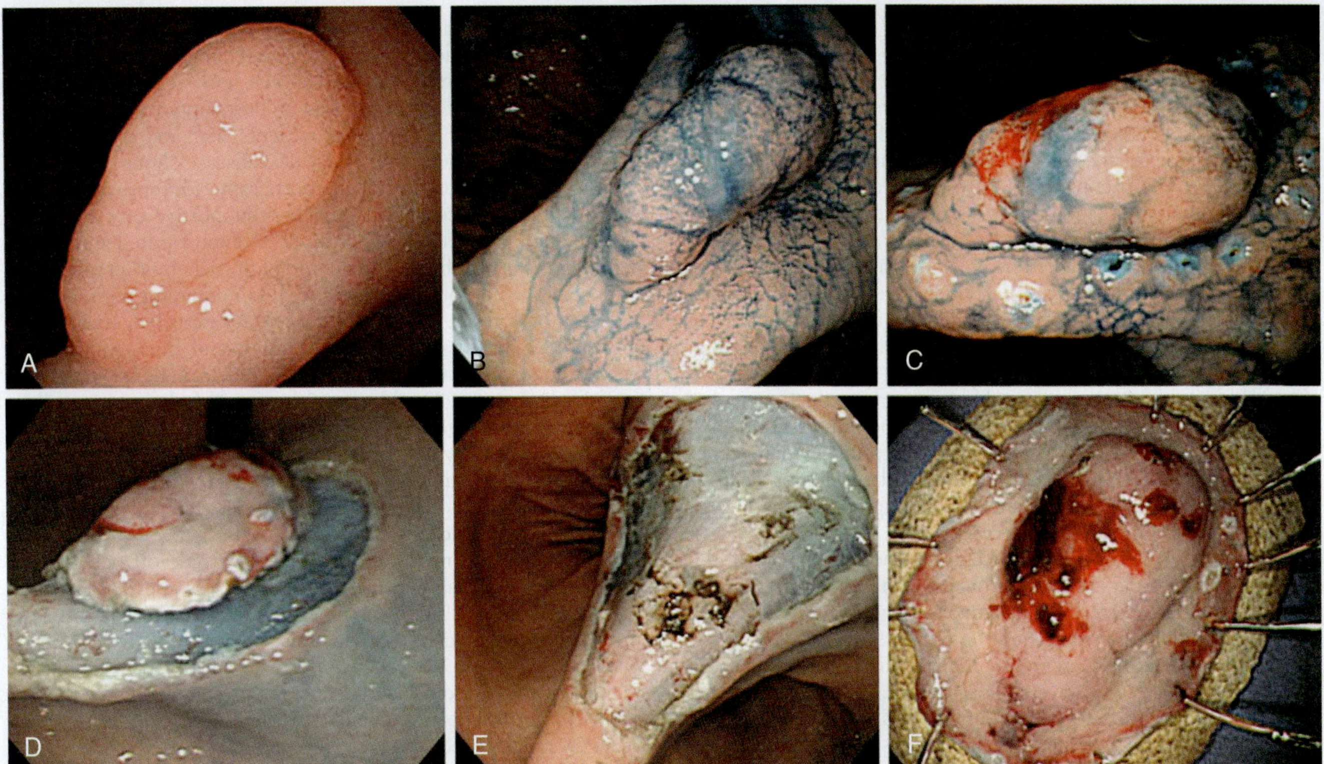

Fig. 56.10 Endoscopic submucosal dissection for early gastric cancer (EGC). (A) Conventional endoscopic view showing an EGC type 0–Ip at the angularis. (B) Endoscopic view after indigo carmine spraying to enhance the lesion margin. (C) Normal tissue surrounding the lesion has been marked with a needle knife. (D) A circumferential cut around the marking dots has been made with an insulated-tip electrosurgical knife. (E) The base after en bloc submucosal dissection of the lesion has been performed. (F) The specimen stretched and pinned on a wood plate before immersion in formalin. (From Lee IL, Wu CS, Tung SY, et al. Endoscopic submucosal dissection for early gastric cancers: experience from a new endoscopic center in Taiwan. *J Clin Gastroenterol*. 2008;42:42–47.)

chemotherapy is now considered and the standard treatment option prior to surgery for gastric cancer. In the recent FLOT4-A10 trial, perioperative chemotherapy with docetaxel, oxaliplatin, and fluorouracil/leucovorin (FLOT) significantly improved progression-free survival (PFS) and OS among patients with resectable gastric cancers compared with epirubicin, cisplatin, and fluorouracil or capecitabine (ECF/ECX). Thus FLOT is the new standard in perioperative therapy of patients with adenocarcinomas of the stomach or gastroesophageal junction (GEJ). Alternatively, treatment can be given according to the FLO or the FOLFOX regimen. Regarding the value of perioperative chemotherapy with the addition of trastuzumab and pertuzumab in patients with resectable Her2neu-positive adenocarcinoma of the stomach and AEG tumors, data from clinical trials are expected in the near future. Further efforts are currently directed towards testing the additional efficacy of immunotherapeutic approaches.

Chemoradiation

Combined chemoradiation after surgical resection appears to be effective at improving progression-free and OS in gastric cancer. The Intergroup Trial 0116 randomized 603 patients with gastric or gastroesophageal cancer to undergo surgery alone or surgery followed by 5FU, leucovorin, and radiation therapy. Subjects in the surgery alone group had a shorter median survival time (27 vs. 36 months) and a worse overall and relapse-free survival.[455] Following publication of the results of this study, adjuvant chemoradiation became the standard of care in the United States, although the optimal chemotherapy regimen is not yet clear. Early studies of the use of neoadjuvant chemoradiation as well as recent as yet unpublished trials have also shown promising results.[456]

Intraperitoneal Chemotherapy

Because systemic chemotherapy is largely ineffective for peritoneal metastasis, intraperitoneal (IP) chemotherapy can be considered in patients whose tumors are resected for cure but have a high likelihood of microscopic residual disease. In a randomized trial of 248 patients with gastric cancer, postoperative hyperthermic IP chemotherapy was associated with improved OS compared to surgery alone.[457] The treatment benefits were most pronounced in patients with stage III and IV disease, serosal invasion, and lymph node metastases. Although a second clinical trial reported similar results,[458] other studies have failed to demonstrate a benefit of hyperthermic IP chemotherapy.[459,460] A meta-analysis of studies of IP chemotherapy for patients with resectable gastric cancer reported a significantly reduced risk of death in patients who received hyperthermic IP chemotherapy (OR, 0.60).[461] At present, the use of hyperthermic IP chemotherapy should be confined to patients enrolled in clinical trials. According to data presented at the 2018 Gastrointestinal Cancers Symposium in San Francisco, undergoing cytoreductive surgery plus hyperthermic intraperitoneal chemotherapy in 180 patients treated in 19 French centers between 1989 and 2014 resulted in improved OS compared with resection alone for 97 patients with gastric cancer with peritoneal carcinomatosis.

Unresectable Disease

In the presence of distant metastases, curative therapy is no longer possible in most cases. Patients have an average survival time of 6 months. It is, therefore, important to focus on palliation. Extensive tumor stenoses lead to a significant reduction in the quality of life. Endoscopic procedures, such as bougienage, laser ablation, or stent implantation, are available for treatment. Surgically, palliative resections or placement of feeding tubes (jejunocath/PEG) can be used. The goal of palliative measures is generally intervention for the purpose of treating local complications with minimal risk while maintaining maximum quality of life, such as in the case of otherwise unstoppable tumor bleeding, complete stenosis, or tumor perforation. In the era of effective chemotherapeutic agents, surgical tumor mass reduction is not useful, as confirmed in an international randomized controlled trial (REGATTA). However, there is increasing evidence that patients with stable disease or tumor response under chemotherapy may benefit from resection, including all metastatic sites in case of limited metastasis.

Regarding chemotherapy concepts, adenocarcinomas of the esophagus and cardia are often grouped with gastric carcinomas, as molecular characterizations increasingly demonstrate the molecular similarity of these tumors[542] (Fig. 56.11).

Therapy should be increasingly individualized not only on the basis of tumor histology, grading, localization, stage of spread, and general condition of the patient, but also taking into account the molecular characteristics of the tumor. First-line platinum-based doublet chemotherapy is the standard of care, with the addition of trastuzumab in human epidermal growth factor receptor-2 (HER2)-positive and/or additional immunotherapy (see below).

The optimal chemotherapy regimen for first-line chemotherapy has yet to be clearly established. Unfortunately, up to one-third of patients with gastric cancer will have unresectable disease at the time of diagnosis.[376] Chemotherapy for locally advanced gastric cancer without distant metastases can result in shrinking of the tumor to the point where successful curative resection is possible.[462,463] Even when curative surgery is not possible, chemotherapy has been shown both to improve survival as well as quality of life compared to best supportive care in this group of patients.[464] Therefore patients with inoperable locally advanced and/or metastatic (stage IV) disease should be considered for systemic treatment (chemotherapy) to improved survival and quality of life compared with best supportive care alone.

A meta-analysis by Wagner et al.[465] demonstrated a small but significant survival benefit for combination chemotherapies, with a median survival of 8.3 months with combination regimens and 6.7 months for single-agent therapies. As expected, toxicity was increased in the combination schedules, and thus, combination chemotherapy should only be considered in patients with good performance status. Doublet combinations of platinum and fluoropyrimidines are generally used, and there remains controversy regarding the utility of triplet regimens.

Whether a 3-drug regimen is more effective than a potentially less toxic doublet is a point of controversy. The FLOT regimen showed good efficacy (RR 57.7%, PFS 5.2 months, OS 11.1 months) with moderate toxicity.[543] A trade-off between the undoubted statistical gain in survival (which is approximately 1–2 months) and the significant increase in toxicity that this buys must be made on a case-by-case basis and according to "remission pressure."

Cisplatin has traditionally been a mainstay of palliative therapy for AEG but has been gradually replaced by oxaliplatin in recent years. A randomized phase II trial confirmed the benefit of cisplatin 50 mg/m^2 to weekly administration of 5-FU (2000 mg/m^2 over 24 hours) and folinic acid (500 mg/m^2) (PLF regimen) in terms of response rates and median survival. Cisplatin therapy carries the risk of several toxicities, including nephrotoxicity and ototoxicity, but may also result in cumulative neuropathies. Studies with alternative platinum derivatives showed excellent results for oxaliplatin: The REAL-2 trial, powered as a non-inferiority trial, used a 2 × 2 factorial design to examine the place

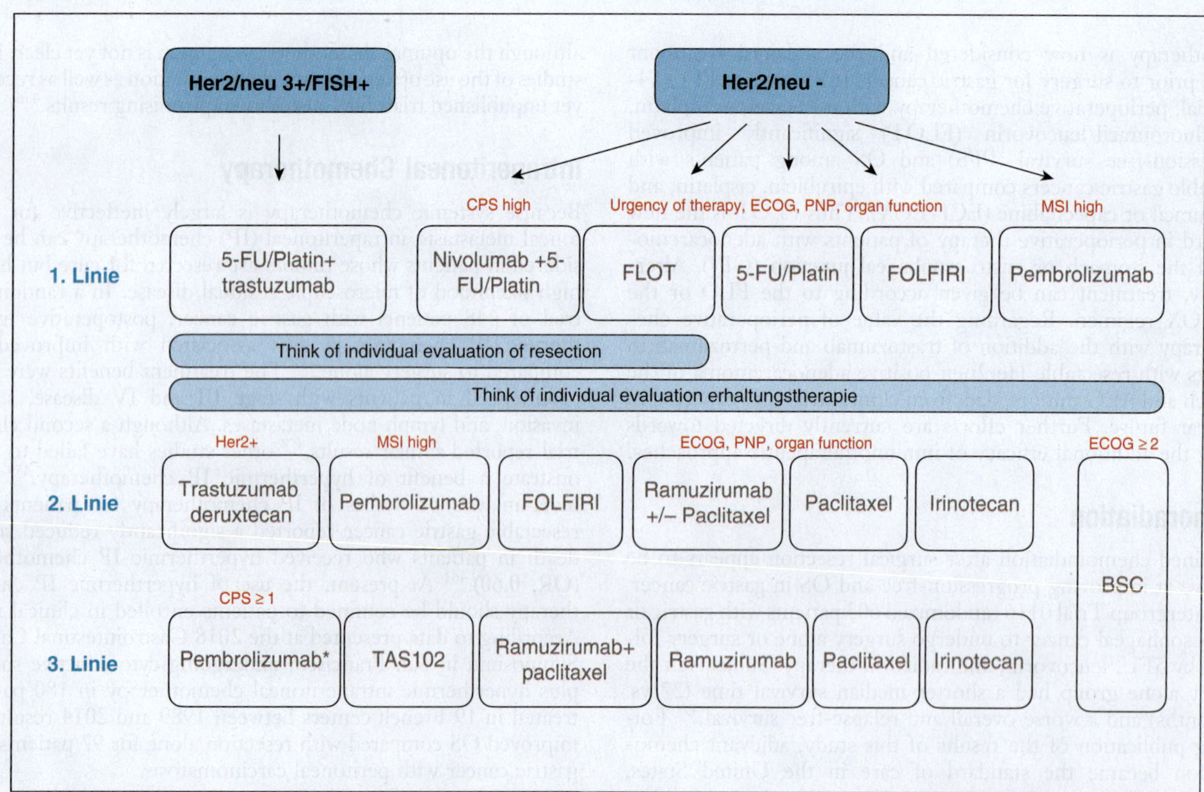

Fig. 56.11 A flowchart outlines treatment pathways for gastric cancer based on staging, surgical options, and chemotherapy.

of oxaliplatin versus cisplatin and capecitabine versus 5-FU in the ECF protocol. Here, patients in the EOX (epirubicin, oxaliplatin, capecitabine) arm experienced a significantly prolonged OS of 11.2 versus 9.9 months compared with ECF ($P = .020$).[544] While the FOLFOX-6 protocol showed good efficacy but less than satisfactory tolerability, the FLO variant with lower oxaliplatin dose and without the 5-FU bolus benefitted mainly elderly patients. In summary, oxaliplatin can, therefore, be considered at least an equivalent but better tolerated alternative to cisplatin in combination protocols in gastric cancer.

Although there is no single standard of care in advanced gastric cancer, there is some evidence coming from meta-analyses. Drugs related to increased survival in phase III trials are cisplatin, docetaxel, and trastuzumab, a monoclonal antibody that interferes with the HER2/neu receptor. HER2 is amplified and is a key driver of tumorigenesis in 7%–34% of gastric cancers. In the ToGA phase III multicenter randomized study, patients with gastric cancer and HER2 overexpression received chemotherapy and trastuzumab, resulting in a median OS of 13.8 months, compared with 11.1 months in those treated with chemotherapy alone.[466] Further manipulation of this pathway using the novel anti-HER2-directed agents pertuzumab and T-DM1, in addition to dual EGFR/HER2 blockade with lapatinib, may yield positive results. Consequently, tumor assessment for HER2 over-expression should be performed, and the addition of trastuzumab to palliative chemotherapy should be considered for every patient with HER2+ gastric adenocarcinoma (Fig. 56.12). In contrast, targeting of the epidermal growth factor receptor (EGFR) pathway in combination with chemotherapy in unselected patients has not been fruitful to date. Similarly, use of the antiangiogenic monoclonal antibody bevacizumab was not successful in a large global randomized trial.[467–471] Careful selection of patient subsets will become a key factor in future clinical trials.

Several randomized clinical trials have demonstrated efficacy of multidrug cisplatin-based regimens.[472,473] A newer clinical trial using the EOX regimen [*e*pirubicin, *o*xaliplatin, and capecitabine (*X*eloda)] was found to be noninferior to cisplatin-based regimens, and had a median survival of 11.2 months.[474] The benefit of the EOX regimen is the substitution of oxaliplatin and capecitabine for cisplatin and 5-FU, respectively, resulting in greater convenience, ease of administration, and potentially fewer side effects. Second-line chemotherapy may also be superior to best supportive care, but again no standard regimens have been defined. Monotherapy with docetaxel or irinotecan has been shown to be superior to best supportive care,[475–477] and a recent study showed no superiority of irinotecan over weekly paclitaxel. Thus monotherapy with irinotecan or taxanes, such as paclitaxel, can be considered an option in advanced gastric cancer patients as a second-line treatment.[478] The anti-VEGFR-2 monoclonal antibody ramucirumab has shown activity in two randomized phase III trials. As a single agent, it is associated with a survival benefit comparable to cytotoxic chemotherapy in the second-line setting, whereas ramucirumab, in addition to paclitaxel, is associated with a survival benefit compared with paclitaxel alone.

Patients with advanced gastric cancer of the distal antrum or pylorus are at risk for developing gastric outlet obstruction. Traditionally, surgical gastrojejunostomy was performed for relief of symptoms and to allow continued enteral nutrition. With the advent of endoscopic stents, duodenal stenting across the obstructing tumor has emerged as a nonsurgical alternative for palliation. The results of a literature review of studies evaluating gastrojejunostomy versus stenting found no differences in rate of technical success (96%–100%), early and late complications, and persistent symptoms.[479] Recurrent obstructive symptoms were more common with stenting. Both gastrojejunostomy and endoscopic stenting are acceptable options for the relief of malignant gastric outlet obstruction. The decision should be based on the individual clinical scenario as well as the availability of appropriate surgical or endoscopic expertise.

Precision oncology including broad sequencing analysis will define modern therapy strategies in upper GI-cancers. Nevertheless, it will be as important to understand the basic biology of these cancers. Analysis of EAC and gastric adenocarcinoma could not clearly distinguish these two cancers. In addition, research

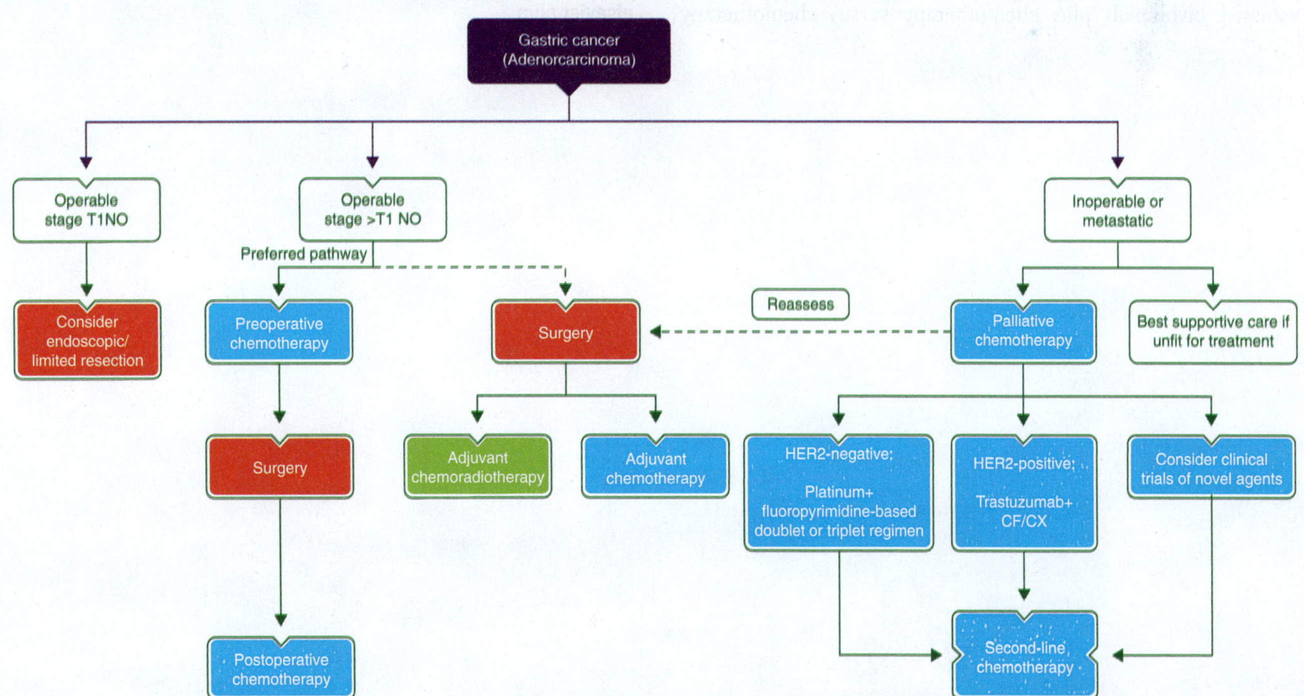

Fig. 56.12 Algorithm for the treatment of gastric cancer. (From Smyth EC, Verheij M, Allum W, et al. Gastric cancer: EMSO clinical practice guidelines for diagnosis, treatment, and follow-up. *Ann Oncol*. 2016; 27(suppl 5):v38–v49.)

from a preclinical mouse model and distinct human studies suggests that gastric progenitor cells give rise to EAC.[545] Thus medical treatment does not depend so much on the localization of the tumor (esophageal vs. gastric) but more on the histology (adenocarcinoma vs. squamous cell carcinoma), arguing against a combination of EAC and ESCC in clinical trials, as unfortunately still done in ongoing phase III drug approval studies. In terms of precision oncology, there are distinct molecular subtypes in EAC and GC[546,547] with the need to be treated with respect to their molecular profile (i.e., MSI, CIN, EBV, genomic stability, PDL-1, Her2/neu). The distinct genetic and epigenetic profiles of gastroesophageal adenocarcinomas (EAC and GC) in comparison to ESCC strongly argue against any combining of EAC and ESCC patients in clinical trials, as has occurred commonly in past and in some ongoing phase III drug approval studies. EAC and ESCC are distinct in their lineage, epigenetic and key molecular drivers, thus necessitating separate clinical trials. The FDA has already allowed the grouping of GEJ EAC and GC as a common entity in recent immunotherapy approval.

Immunotherapy

Reliable detection of novel therapeutic targets in tumor tissue is a major challenge in the development of effective targeted therapies. Immunotherapy with anti-PD-L1 antibodies to block the PD-1 checkpoint (programmed death receptor-1 and its ligand PD-L1) promises a new therapeutic option. Immune checkpoint inhibition is gaining ground not only in melanoma, renal cell carcinoma, bladder cancer, and nonsmall cell lung cancer, but also in gastrointestinal carcinoma. Cancer cells create an immunosuppressive environment and regulatory T cells depend on the activity of CTLA-4, PD-1 and PD-L1 to induce immunosuppression. By overexpressing PD-L1 on the cancer cell surface or inducing PD-L1/CTLA-4 expression on immune cells, cancer cells utilize the PD-1/PD-L1 and CTLA-4 signaling pathway, leading to immune escape and tumor growth. Drugs that block the checkpoint proteins PD-1, PD-L1, CTLA-4 reactivate and enhance the antitumor T cell–mediated immune response by blocking these inhibitory signals. The CheckMate 649 trial evaluated nivolumab plus chemotherapy versus chemotherapy alone as first-line treatment in patients with non-HER-2 positive advanced gastric cancer.[548]

In summary, randomized phase III trials show consistent benefit of checkpoint inhibition in a subset of gastroesophageal cancers, providing a new treatment option. In the first-line setting, a clear change in our standard of care is emerging, where patients with high PD-L1 expression are candidates for immune checkpoint inhibitors plus chemotherapy. However, more data are needed on the subgroups that benefit from treatment (e.g., PD-L1 CPS groups and MSI). In later lines of therapy, checkpoint inhibitors have also shown relevant activity in PD-L1 expressing tumors and tumors with EBV association. Therefore determination of MSI, PD-L1, and EBV should already be performed at initial diagnosis. MSI-high, PD-L1 CPS, and EBV can serve as predictive biomarkers, but further refinement and harmonization of biomarker scoring is needed. Patients with MSI-H gastric cancer have high response rates and excellent long-term outcomes when treated with anti-PD-1 monotherapy.[549] Enhancement of the effect of anti-HER-2 therapy in combination with immune checkpoint blockade is investigated in the Keynote-811 trial and is already approved in the United States based on early PFS and tumor response (ORR) data, and will certainly soon be a relevant therapy adjunct in Europe.[550]

MISCELLANEOUS GASTRIC TUMORS

Gastric lymphomas, GISTs, and neuroendocrine (carcinoid) tumors are covered in Chapters 41–43. Metastatic disease to the stomach can occur with primary tumors of the breast, melanoma, lung, ovary, liver, colon, and testicular cancers, with breast cancer being the most common.[480] Other rare malignant tumors that can involve the stomach are Kaposi sarcoma (see Chapter 33), myenteric schwannoma, glomus tumor, small cell carcinoma, and parietal cell carcinoma.[481–484] Miscellaneous benign tumors of the stomach include lipomas (see Video 54.2), as well as pancreatic rests (see Chapter 57), xanthelasma, and fundic gland cysts.

Full references for this chapter can be found at https://ebooks.health.elsevier.com.

PART VIII Pancreas

57 Anatomy, Histology, Embryology, and Developmental Anomalies of the Pancreas

Sohail Z. Husain, Megha S. Mehta

IN THIS CHAPTER

HISTORY OF THE PANCREAS

Although the identity of the pancreas has been known for some time, its critical digestive functions were only recently appreciated.[1,2] The first description of the pancreas was made by the Greek physician Herophilos at around 300 BCE. In the late 1st century CE, another Greek authority, Rufus of Ephesus, named the organ the "pancreas." The term literally means "all flesh or meat," which distinguished it from bone or cartilage. Unfortunately, the name "kalikreas," meaning "beautiful flesh," given to the organ by Galen around the same time or shortly after Rufus, was not adopted. Nonetheless, Galen thought the pancreas served to support and protect overlying blood vessels. In the Talmud, the central text of Jewish law, the pancreas was referred to as the "finger of the liver." Vesalius considered the organ a mere cushion for the stomach. In 1642 Wirsung characterized the pancreatic ducts of humans, and in 1664, de Graaf discovered pancreatic secretions from the pancreatic fistula of dogs.

The digestive action of pancreatic secretions was discovered almost 200 years later. Eberle in 1834, Purkinje and Pappenheim in 1836, and Valentin in 1844 observed that pancreatic juice emulsified fat, proteolyzed proteins, and digested starch, respectively. Bernard subsequently demonstrated the combined digestive action of pancreatic juice using secretions from pancreatic fistula preparations. In 1876 Kuhne introduced the term "enzyme" and was the first to isolate trypsin. The concept of enzymes quickly led to the identification of pancreatic amylase and lipase. In 1889 Chepovalnikoff, a student of Pavlov, discovered enterokinase in the duodenal mucosa, an enzyme that is essential for activating trypsin and the subsequent cascade of other digestive proteases. In 1895 Dolinsky, another of Pavlov's students, stimulated pancreatic secretion by instilling acid into the duodenum. This led to the discovery of secretin in 1902 by Bayliss and Starling, which was the first hormone ever to be identified.[3]

The histologic structure of the pancreas was first described in 1869 by Langerhans. Shortly thereafter, Heidenhain found that as the granular region of pancreatic acinar cells disappeared after feeding, enzymatic activity in pancreatic juice inversely increased; he correctly concluded that the granules contained digestive enzyme precursors, or zymogens. In 1875 Friedreich wrote the first systematic description of pancreatic diseases, followed by a classic account by Fitz on acute pancreatitis in 1889.[4]

The pancreas first came to the attention of the Nobel Committee in 1905, when Ivan Pavlov was awarded the prize for his work on the physiology of digestion, with particular emphasis on neural control of the stomach and pancreas. In 1923 Canadians Frederick Banting and John Macleod were awarded the prize for successfully purifying insulin from the pancreas of dogs. It is notable that a medical student, Charles Best, was a codiscoverer and shared the prize money with Macleod. In 1946 John Northrop coshared the Nobel Prize for his work on purifying enzymes in their crystalline form. Among the pancreatic enzymes, he managed to crystallize trypsin, chymotrypsin, and carboxypeptidase. In 1958 Frederick Sanger received his first Nobel Prize for determining the structure of insulin. Sanger, however, is best known for his second Nobel Prize, in 1980, for developing a signature method for sequencing DNA. In 1974 George Palade, along with Albert Claude and Christian de Duve, received the Nobel Prize for making seminal discoveries in cell biology. Palade used the pancreatic acinar cell, in combination with newly developed techniques of differential centrifugation, electron microscopy, and pulse-chase, to describe the role of ribosomes along the endoplasmic reticulum (rough ER) in synthesizing proteins and the transit of proteins through the Golgi apparatus into secretory pathways.[5] In 1977 Rosalyn Yalow received the prize for the development of radioimmunoassays of peptide hormones, in which the prototype was insulin. She worked with Solomon Berson, but he unfortunately died before the Nobel Prize was awarded. More recently, Günter Blobel won the prize in 1999 for his work using pancreatic acinar cells to discover signal peptides, which govern intracellular protein transport and localization. These awards demonstrate how the study of the pancreas continues to advance major scientific development.

ANATOMY

The pancreas is a soft, elongated, flattened gland that is 12–20 cm in length.[6] The adult gland weighs between 70 and 110 g. The pancreas is coarsely lobulated and covered with fine connective tissue, without a true capsule. It is primarily retroperitoneal, lying approximately at the level of the L1–L2 lumbar vertebrae. The head of the pancreas is on the right, lying within the curvature of the duodenum, and the remainder of the pancreas lies obliquely in the posterior abdomen, with the tail extending as far as the gastric surface of the spleen (Fig. 57.1).

The anterior surface of the head of the pancreas is adjacent to the pylorus, the first part of the duodenum, and the transverse colon. The posterior surface abuts the hilum and medial border of the right kidney, the inferior vena cava and the right renal vessels, the right gonadal vein, and the right crus of the diaphragm.

The uncinate process (lingula) is a prolongation of pancreatic tissue that projects off the lower part of the pancreatic head, extending upward and to the left. The uncinate process lies anterior to the aorta and inferior vena cava and is covered superiorly by the superior mesenteric vessels that emerge below the neck of the pancreas. There is much variation in the size and shape of the uncinate process, and it may even be absent altogether.

The neck of the pancreas is a constricted part of the gland, extending from the head of the pancreas toward the left to connect the head with the body of the pancreas. It is 1.5–2 cm long and 3–4 cm wide. Posterior to the neck of the pancreas lies the confluence of the portal vein with the superior mesenteric and splenic veins. Anteriorly it is covered in part by the pylorus and peritoneum of the lesser sac. The neck extends to the right as far as the anterosuperior pancreaticoduodenal artery from the gastroduodenal artery.

The body of the pancreas runs toward the left side, anterior to the aorta. It is retroperitoneal and held against the aorta by the peritoneum of the lesser sac. The anterior surface of the body is covered by peritoneum of the omental bursa, which separates the stomach from the pancreas. The antrum and body of the stomach and the transverse mesocolon contact the body anteriorly. Posterior to the body of the pancreas are the aorta, the origin of the superior mesenteric artery, the left crus of the diaphragm, the left kidney, the left adrenal gland, and the splenic vein. The midline part of the body overlies the lumbar spine, which makes this area of the pancreas most vulnerable to abdominal trauma. The body passes laterally and merges with the tail of the pancreas, without a discernible junction point. The tail is relatively mobile, with its tip usually reaching the hilum of the spleen. It is defined somewhat arbitrarily, beginning halfway from the distance of the left border of the mesenteric vessels and extending to the tip of the pancreas. The tip of the tail is intraperitoneal, lying between layers of the splenorenal ligament. The relationship of the pancreas to important structures in the posterior abdomen is seen in Fig. 57.2.

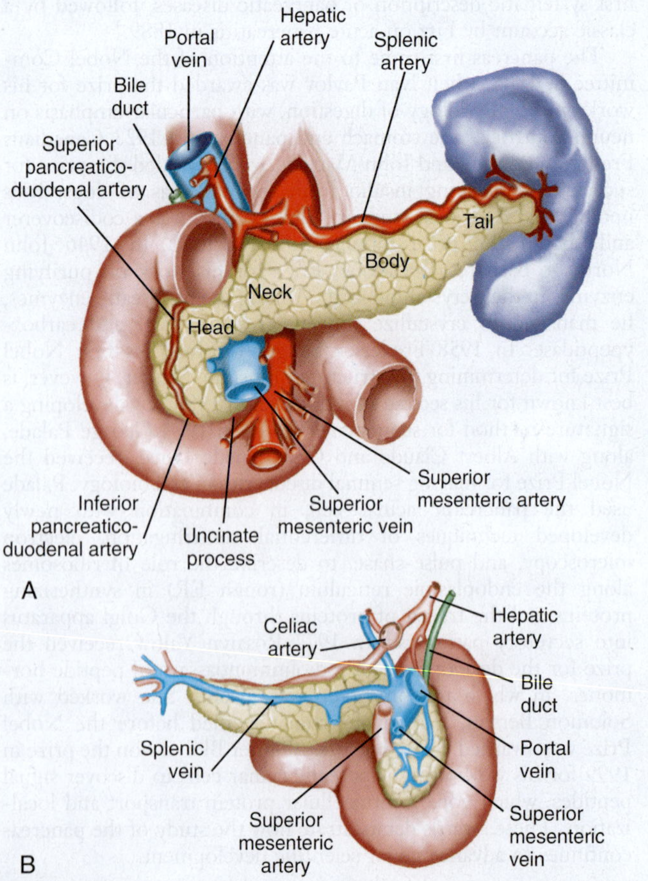

Fig. 57.1 Anatomic relationships of the pancreas: (A) anterior view and (B) posterior view.

Ductal Structures

The main pancreatic duct (of Wirsung) begins near the tail of the pancreas. It is formed from anastomosing ductules draining the lobules of the gland. It courses left to right and is enlarged by additional ducts. Through the tail and body, the duct lies midway between the superior and inferior margins and slightly posterior. The main duct turns caudal and posterior on reaching the head of the pancreas. At the level of the major papilla, the duct turns horizontally to join in most cases with the bile duct (Fig. 57.3A).

The duct of Wirsung and the common bile duct empty into the duodenum obliquely via the major papilla. The ampulla of Vater is the common pancreaticobiliary channel within the papilla where the two ducts come together, separated by common adventitia. The length of the common channel (when present) averages 4.5 mm, with a range of 1–12 mm.[7,8] Three circular muscle bundles, collectively called the sphincter of Oddi, encircle each duct as well as the ampulla of Vater. The relationship of the

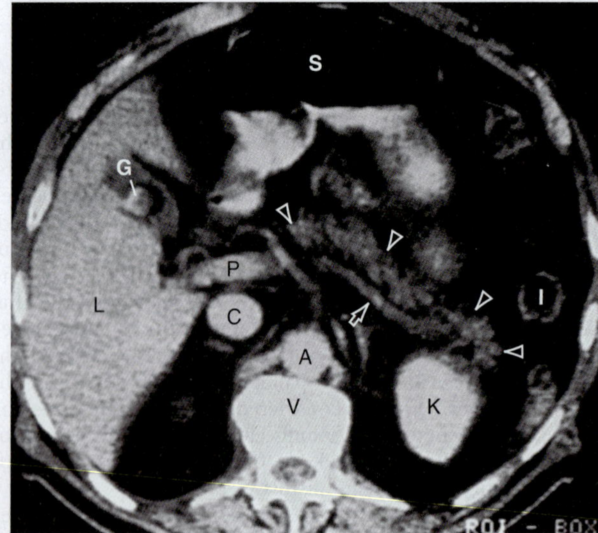

Fig. 57.2 CT showing the normal anatomic relation of the pancreas with other intra-abdominal structures. The borders of the pancreas are indicated by *arrowheads*. The splenic vein is indicated by an *arrow*. *A*, Aorta; *C*, vena cava; *G*, incidental gallstone; *I*, small intestine; *K*, left kidney; *L*, liver; *P*, portal vein; *S*, stomach; *V*, vertebra. (Courtesy M.P. Federle, MD.)

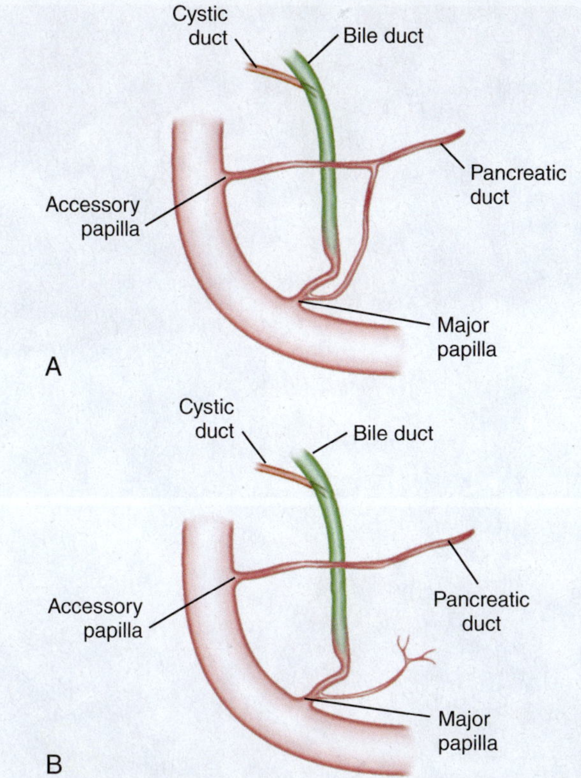

Fig. 57.3 Anatomic arrangements of the pancreatic duct system. (A) The most common arrangement. Most of the pancreatic secretion empties into the duodenum along with bile through the major papilla. The proximal portion of the embryonic dorsal pancreatic duct remains patent in about 70% of adults and empties through the accessory papilla. (B) Pancreas divisum. The embryonic dorsal and ventral ducts fail to fuse. Most of the pancreatic secretion empties through the accessory papilla. Only pancreatic secretions from the uncinate process and part of the head of the pancreas (which are derived from the embryonic ventral pancreas) drain through the major papilla.

bile duct and the duct of Wirsung at the papilla is complex.[9–11] By autopsy and ERCP studies, it appears that about two-thirds to three-quarters of the general population has a common channel, whereas about one-fifth have completely separate openings and just under one-tenth have an interposed sputum that separates the two ducts. Long common channels, due to *pancreaticobiliary malunion*, can predispose to pancreatitis or biliary cancer.

Approximately 70% of the general population has a patent accessory duct (of Santorini), which is also known as the *minor duct* (see Fig. 57.3A).[12] The accessory duct lies anterior to the bile duct and drains into the minor papilla, which lies proximal to the major papilla, but is also located in the second portion of the duodenum. Up to 10% of people have an interruption between the major papilla and the main duct, with drainage into the duodenum occurring via the minor papilla; this variant is called *pancreas divisum* (PD) (see Fig. 57.3B, discussed later). A number of other variations in the ducts are encountered.

The main pancreatic duct is widest at the head of the pancreas, and the duct gradually tapers as it progresses to the tail.[13] Upper limits of normal for the pancreatic duct diameter in the head (5 mm), body (4 mm), and tail (3 mm) are generally accepted, although there are variations based on age in pediatric patients (Table 57.1).[14–17] It is important to know the normal size range of the pancreatic duct to discern abnormal ductal dilation or narrowing, as in chronic pancreatitis.

TABLE 57.1 Average Age-Related Pediatric Pancreatic Duct Size, Based on US

Age (Years)	PD Duct Size at Body (mm) (Avg ± SD)
1–3	1.13 ± 0.15
4–6	1.35 ± 0.15
7–9	1.67 ± 0.17
10–12	1.78 ± 0.17
13–15	1.92 ± 0.18
16–18	2.05 ± 0.15

Data from Chao HC, Lin SJ, Kong MS, et al. Sonographic evaluation of the pancreatic duct in normal children and children with pancreatitis. *J Ultrasound Med*. 2000;19:757–763.

Circulation

The pancreas has a rich circulation that is derived from branches of the celiac and superior mesenteric arteries.[6] The head of the pancreas and surrounding duodenum are supplied by 2 pancreaticoduodenal arterial arcades. They are formed by the anterior and posterior superior pancreaticoduodenal arteries from the hepatic branch of the celiac artery that join a second pair of anterior and posterior inferior pancreaticoduodenal arteries branching from the superior mesenteric artery. All of the major pancreatic arteries lie posterior to the ducts.

The course of the splenic artery is posterior to the body and tail and loops above and below the superior margin of the pancreas. It gives off the dorsal pancreatic artery, which usually joins one of the posterior arcades after giving off the inferior pancreatic artery.

The caudal pancreatic artery arises from the left gastroepiploic artery or from a splenic branch at the spleen. It joins with branches of the splenic and great pancreatic arteries and other pancreatic arteries. The rich circulation allows the pancreas to expeditiously carry out its key endocrine functions of maintaining glucose homeostasis by sensing blood glucose concentrations and controlling the release of other hormones from the islets.

In general, the venous drainage of the pancreas is similar to the arterial blood supply. It flows into the portal venous system, which is formed by the joining of the superior mesenteric and splenic veins at the confluence behind the neck of the pancreas. The portal vein lies behind the pancreas and in front of the inferior vena cava. The common bile duct lies anterior to the portal vein with the hepatic artery to the left of the common bile duct. The splenic vein originates at the hilum of the spleen and curves behind the tail of the pancreas and below the splenic artery, to the right along the posterior surface of the pancreas. The pancreatic veins drain the neck, body, and tail of the pancreas and join the splenic vein. The pancreaticoduodenal veins lie close to their corresponding arteries and empty into the splenic or portal veins. Because of the close anatomic relationship of the splenic vein with the pancreas, inflammatory or neoplastic diseases involving the pancreatic body and tail can lead to splenic vein occlusion. This in turn can result in retrograde venous drainage toward the splenic hilum and then, by way of flow through the short gastric and left gastroepiploic veins, can create gastric varices.

Lymphatic Drainage

The lymphatics, in general, drain the surface network of lymph toward regional nodes and are formed near the larger blood vessels.[18] They begin as small periacinar and perilobuar capillary networks that drain into larger ducts alongside pancreatic blood vessels. The superior lymphatic vessels run along the upper border of the pancreas closely with the splenic blood vessels, whereas inferior lymphatic vessels run with the inferior pancreatic artery. Superior and inferior lymphatic vessels draining the left pancreas, including the tail of the pancreas and left half of the body empty into nodes in the splenic hilum. The superior lymphatic vessels draining the right pancreas including the neck and right half of the body empty into nodes near the upper border of the head of the pancreas. These nodes also receive tributaries from the anterior and posterior pancreatic surfaces. The remaining regions of the neck and body drain toward the right. Overall, the extensive network of blood vessels and lymphatics, as well as the ability of tumors to induce angio- and lymphangiogenesis, provide ample avenues for pancreatic cancer to metastasize.[19]

Innervation

The visceral efferent innervation of the pancreas is through the vagus and the splanchnic nerves by way of the hepatic and celiac plexus. The efferent fibers of the vagus pass through this plexus without synapsing and terminate in parasympathetic ganglia found in the interlobular septa of the pancreas. The postganglionic fibers innervate acini, islets, and ducts. The bodies of the preganglionic neurons of the sympathetic efferent nerves originate in the lateral gray matter of the thoracic and lumbar spinal cord. The bodies of the postganglionic sympathetic neurons are in the great plexus of the abdomen. Their postganglionic fibers innervate only blood vessels. The autonomic fibers, both efferent and afferent, are located in proximity to the blood vessels of the pancreas. The vagus also carries some visceral afferent fibers.

HISTOLOGY AND ULTRASTRUCTURE

The pancreas is a compound, finely nodular gland that in its contour bears resemblance to the salivary glands. The lobules are visible on gross examination and are connected by connective tissue septa that contain the ducts, blood vessels, lymphatics, and nerves. The basic subunit of the exocrine portion is the acinus, which has at one end a spherical mass consisting of dark-staining secretory cells called *acinar cells* (Fig. 57.4). The spherical acinus connects to a goblet-shaped neck that is composed of tubular cells called *ductal cells*. The inner lumen of the acinus forms the terminal portion of the secretory duct.

Corrosive casts of the ductular system formed by retrograde injection of latex demonstrate that there is an extensive network of ducts of increasing size that drain pancreatic secretions from the acinar lumen, through intralobular, interlobular, interlobar, and finally into the main pancreatic duct (Fig. 57.5).[20]

The pancreatic ductal system is nonstriated and lined by columnar epithelium. Goblet cells and occasional argentaffin cells are also present. The larger ducts have a thick wall consisting of connective tissue and elastic fibers. The endocrine portion consists of the islets of Langerhans, which on H&E staining are spherical clusters of light-staining cells. Each of the main parenchymal cells of the pancreas reveals remarkable structure-function relationships.

By light microscopy, acinar cells are tall pyramidal or columnar epithelial cells, with their broad bases on a basal lamina and their apices converging on a central lumen. In the resting state, numerous eosinophilic zymogen granules fill the apical portion of the cell. The basal portion of the cells consists of 1 or 2 spherical nuclei and basophilic cytoplasm. The Golgi complex lies between the nucleus and zymogen granules and can be seen as a clear, nonstaining region.

Electron microscopy provides vivid detail of the subcellular structure of the acinar cells (Fig. 57.6). The most prominent feature is the dense zymogen granules that are concentrated at the apical pole. Tight junctions form a belt-like band around the

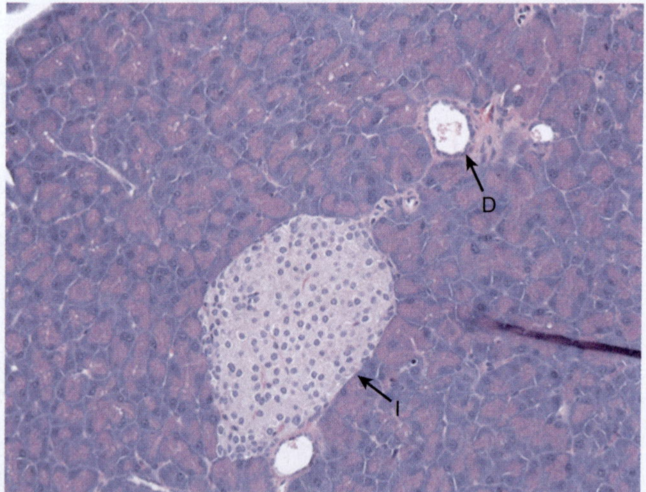

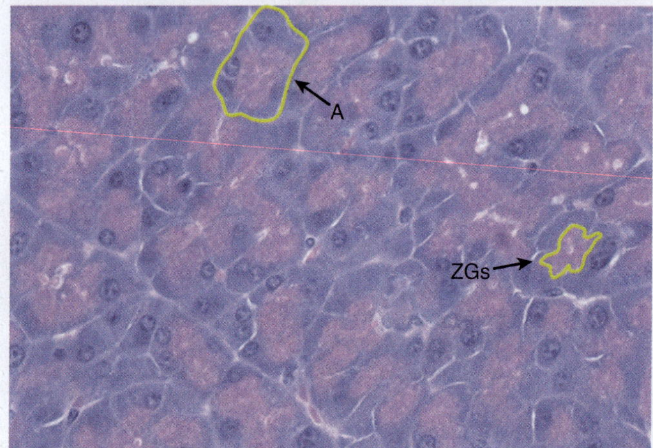

Fig. 57.4 Histology of the pancreas. (Top) Low-power histologic section of the pancreas showing a ductule (D) and islet (I) (H&E). (Bottom) A higher-power section, showing numerous acini (A), which contain eosinophilic zymogen granules (ZGs). (Courtesy Abrahim I. Orabi.)

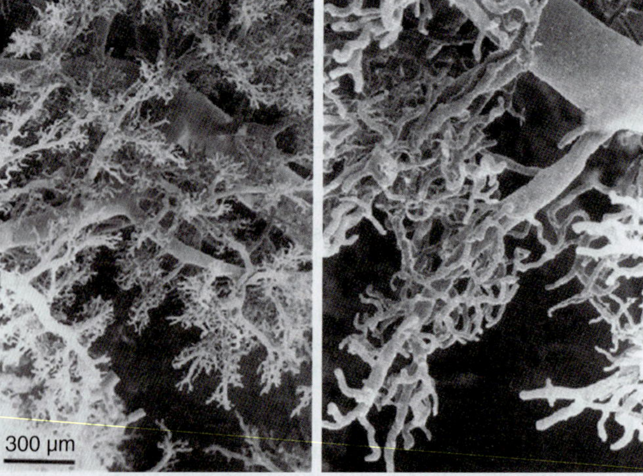

Fig. 57.5 Scanning electron micrographs of the exocrine pancreatic ductal system obtained after filling the pancreatic duct with latex and digesting away the pancreatic tissue. The smallest radicles of the ductal system are connected to acini. The *right panel* is a magnified image. (From Ashizawa N, Watanabe M, Fukumoto S, et al. Scanning electron microscopic observations of three-dimensional structure of the rat pancreatic duct. *Pancreas*. 1991;6:542–550.)

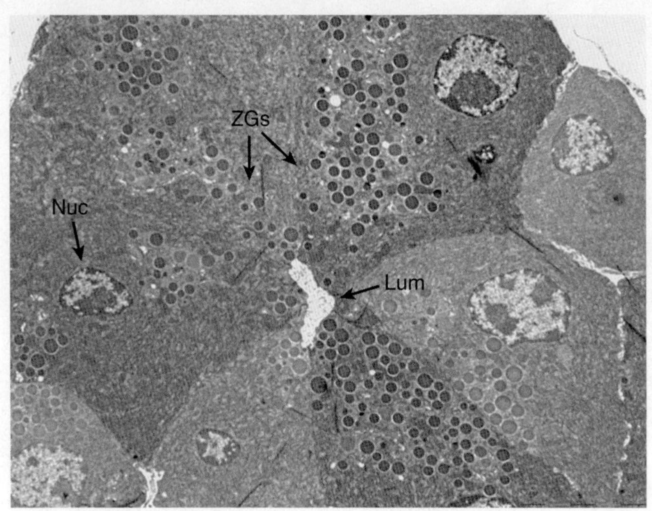

Fig. 57.6 Electron micrograph of a pancreatic acinus showing acinar cells surrounding a central lumen (Lum). The acinar cell nucleus (Nuc) and (ZGs) are easily identified (×3200). (Courtesy Abrahim I. Orabi.)

apical end of the cell and are produced by the apposition of the external membrane leaflets of neighboring cells. These junctions prevent the reflux of secreted substances from the apical lumen into the intercellular space.[21] Gap junctions, which permit intercellular flow of small molecules, are distributed on the lateral cellular membranes and are formed by the apposition of larger, disk-shaped membrane plaques.

Mitochondria are elongate cylindrical structures that appear oval in cross-section and contain well-developed cristae and matrix granules (Fig. 57.7). They are concentrated in several parts of the acinar cells, including as a belt around the zymogen granules, the nucleus, and the basolateral membrane.[22] Rough ER occupies about 20% of the cell volume.[23] It takes up most of the basal region of the acinar cells as well as interdigitates with the zymogen granules in the apical region. This abundance of rough ER allows the acinar cell to synthesize more protein than any other parenchymal cell in the body.[24] The Golgi complex consists of flattened, membranous saccules, as well as small vesicles that contain flocculent electron-dense material. The Golgi conducts the transport of secretory proteins and the formation of zymogen granules from maturing condensing vacuoles.

Studies of the chemical composition of the zymogen granules have shown that they contain 12 to 15 different digestive enzymes, which make up about 90% of the granule protein.[25] The acinar cells undergo cyclic changes in morphology in response to meals.[26] After a large meal, the zymogen granules are quickly emptied into the acinar duct lumen by a specialized form of regulated secretion called *sequential compound exocytosis*.[27,28] In this scenario, there is an initial fusion of zymogen granules with the apical plasma membrane, followed by sequential granule-granule fusion events that connect together multiple vesicles to the apical lumen in a beads-on-a-string formation. This process solves the problem of rapidly emptying large amounts of granule contents from a relatively small region of the cell.

The apical membrane of the acinar cell constitutes only a small portion of total plasma membrane, but its surface area is expanded by several short, slender microvilli that are about 0.2 µm in length and extend into the lumen of the acinus (Fig. 57.8). Thin

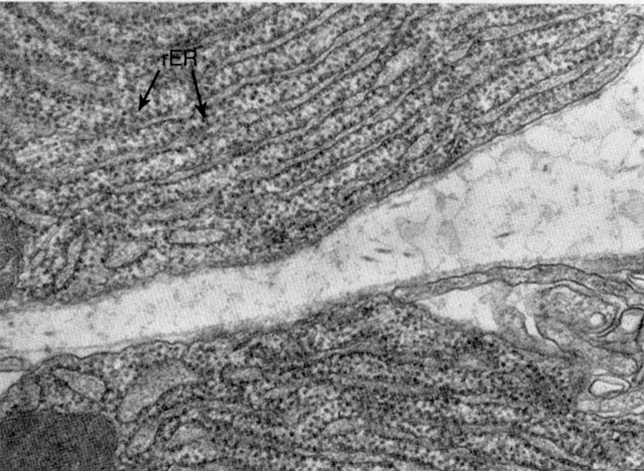

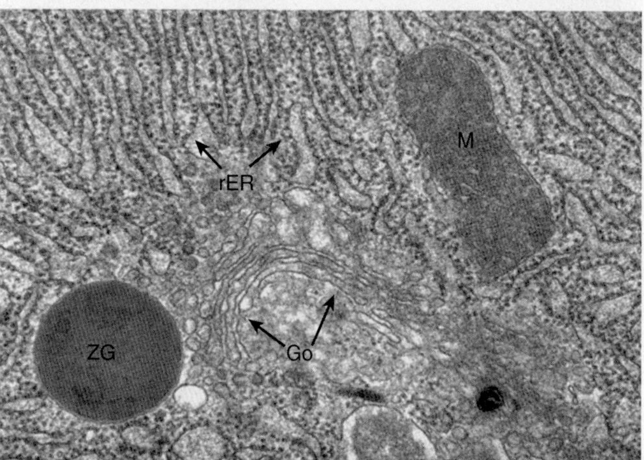

Fig. 57.7 Electron micrograph of portions of an acinar cell. The *top panel* represents a basolateral region showing sheets of rough endoplasmic reticulum (rER). The *bottom panel* also shows a Golgi complex (Go), mitochondria (M), and a *ZG* (×43,000). (Courtesy Abrahim I. Orabi.)

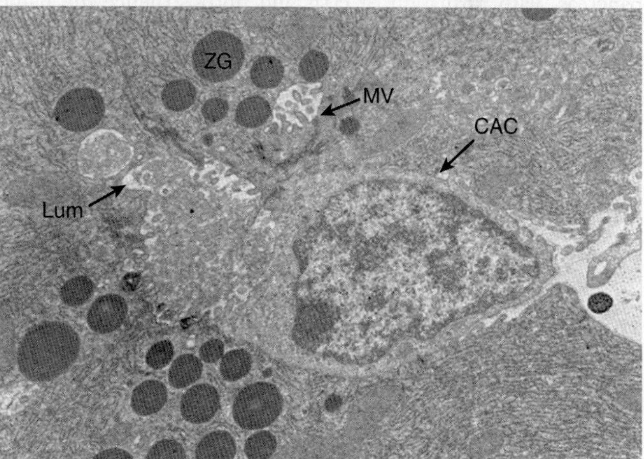

Fig. 57.8 Electron micrograph of a centroacinar cell (CAC) and acinar cells surrounding a central lumen (*Lum*) (×9000). *MV*, Microvilli; *ZG*, zymogen granule. (Courtesy Abrahim I. Orabi.)

filaments form the axis of the microvilli as well as a network beneath the apical plasmalemma. The lumen typically contains flocculent electron-dense material that represents the secreted digestive enzymes. Morphologically distinct cells, called *centroacinar cells*, bridge acinar cells with the ductal epithelium. These centroacinar cells are pale-staining on H&E staining and smaller than the acinar cells.

Along the basal surface of the acinar cells, but not extending between adjacent cells, is a thin basal lamina, below which are collagen fibers and a rich capillary network. Efferent nerve fibers, derived from the sympathetic and parasympathetic systems, penetrate the basal lamina adjacent to the acinar cells. The collagen fibers and other extracellular matrix proteins are secreted by a less common resident cell type, the pancreatic stellate cell (PSC).[29] In the quiescent state, the PSC has baseline functions of maintaining the pancreatic microarchitecture and facilitating acinar cell secretion. In its activated state during pancreatic injury and inflammation, however, it transforms into myofibroblast-like cells that replenish the matrix necessary for proper recovery. With persistent injury, it can also cause harm by inducing fibrosis due to the increased deposition of extracellular matrix proteins, and lead to chronic pancreatitis (see Chapter 59). The PSC can also provide abundant stromal environment around pancreatic adenocarcinoma, which can limit the effect of cancer therapies. Finally, PSCs can also accompany cancer cells to metastatic sites to facilitate cancer progression.[30]

The ductal cells have electron-lucent cytoplasm containing few cytoplasmic organelles.[31] They are, however, endowed with an abundance of mitochondria, which are necessary for allowing the ductal cells to carry out their primary function of active ion transport.[32] Whereas the acinar cells secrete small amounts of sodium chloride–rich fluid, the net function of ductal cells is to secrete bicarbonate and water, which makes up the bulk of the fluid in pancreatic juice. The bicarbonate-rich pancreatic juice enters the intestine, neutralizes gastric acid, and generates an optimally buffered pH for digestive enzyme function. Several enzymes and a multitude of ion channels within the ductal cells orchestrate this net bicarbonate and water secretion. They include carbonic anhydrase and the cystic fibrosis transmembrane conductance regulator (CFTR). The former enzyme can be used to label ductal cells. Severe defects in CFTR cause pancreatic duct plugging during pancreas development and intrauterine destruction of the exocrine pancreas, with formation of cysts and fibrosis; hence the name coined for the disorder is "cystic fibrosis" (see this chapter).

The islets of Langerhans number about 1 million in the human pancreas. Islets consist of anastomosing cords of polygonal endocrine cells (see Fig. 57.4). Each islet is approximately 0.2 mm in diameter, much larger than a single acinus, and separated from the surrounding exocrine tissue by fine connective tissue fibers that are continuous with those of the exocrine gland. Each islet is surrounded and penetrated by a rich network of capillaries that are lined by a fenestrated endothelium. The capillaries are arranged in a portal system that conveys blood from the islets to the acinar cells (Fig. 57.9). This islet-acinar portal axis consists of afferent arterioles that enter the islet, form a capillary glomerulus, and leave the islet as efferent capillaries passing into the exocrine tissue.[33–35] This microportal system permits islet hormones, especially insulin, to exert a localized effect on the exocrine pancreas. An additional parallel arterial system supplies blood directly to the exocrine pancreas. Acinar cells surrounding the islets of Langerhans (peri-insular acini) are morphologically and biochemically different from acini situated farther away (teleinsular acini). Peri-insular acini have a larger size of acinar cells, nuclei, and zymogen granule regions, and different proportions of some of the digestive enzymes. Peri-insular acini may be conferred with special properties that have evolved to receive trophic cues from the islets, such as insulin, and, conversely, they may be protective to the islets.

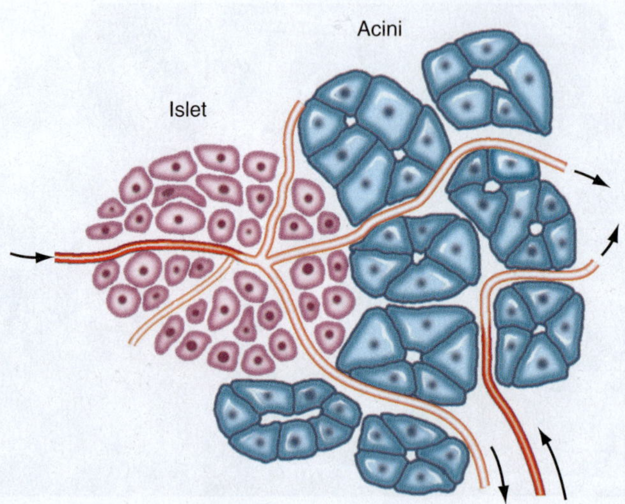

Fig. 57.9 Schematic diagram of the insuloacinar portal system illustrating the dual blood supply to the exocrine pancreas. (From Goldfine ID, Williams JA. Receptors for insulin and CCK in the acinar pancreas: Relationship to hormone action. *Int Rev Cytol.* 1983;85:1.)

There are 5 major cell types in the endocrine pancreas. *Beta cells* are the most numerous, constituting about 50% to 80% of the islets. They secrete insulin and amylin. *PP cells*, also known as *F cells*, make up 10% to 35% and secrete pancreatic polypeptide and adrenomedullin. *Alpha cells* make up 5% to 20% and secrete glucagon. The remaining 5% consists of *delta cells*, which secrete somatostatin, and *epsilon cells*, which secrete ghrelin. Other rarer subpopulations of islet cells make additional hormones such as galanin.

DEVELOPMENT OF THE PANCREAS

Embryonic and Fetal Development

The pancreas arises from posterior foregut endoderm.[36] Two buds form: one dorsal and the other bilobed ventral. About a month into gestation, the foregut evaginates into a condensation of overlying mesenchyme to form the first morphologic evidence of the dorsal bud. About a week later, a ventral bud forms as an outpouching of hepatic diverticulum. The ventral bud has a bilobed origin, of which the left ventral bud gradually regresses.[37] Both dorsal and ventral buds undergo elongation of a stalk region and branched morphogenesis. At 37–42 days into gestation, as the duodenum grows, the ventral pancreas rotates around the duodenum and fuses with the dorsal pancreas (Fig. 57.10).

The dorsal pancreas forms the tail, body, and superior portion of the pancreatic head. It also contains the dorsal duct, which forms the distal portion of the main pancreatic duct (of Wirsung) and the entire minor accessory duct (of Santorini). The ventral pancreas forms the uncinate process and the inferior part of the head. It also contains the ventral duct, which forms the proximal portion of the main pancreatic duct (of Wirsung). As mentioned earlier, the two ductal systems corresponding to the ventral and dorsal buds fail to fuse in up to 10% of the general population. In this situation, *PD*, the accessory duct functions as the main conduit for drainage of pancreatic juice. The clinical significance of PD is discussed later. Failure of the ventral pancreas to fully rotate around the duodenum, or persistence of the left ventral bud, can lead to an *annular pancreas*, also discussed later.

After the pancreatic buds fuse, the cellular architecture of the pancreas rapidly expands. Notably, all three functionally distinct

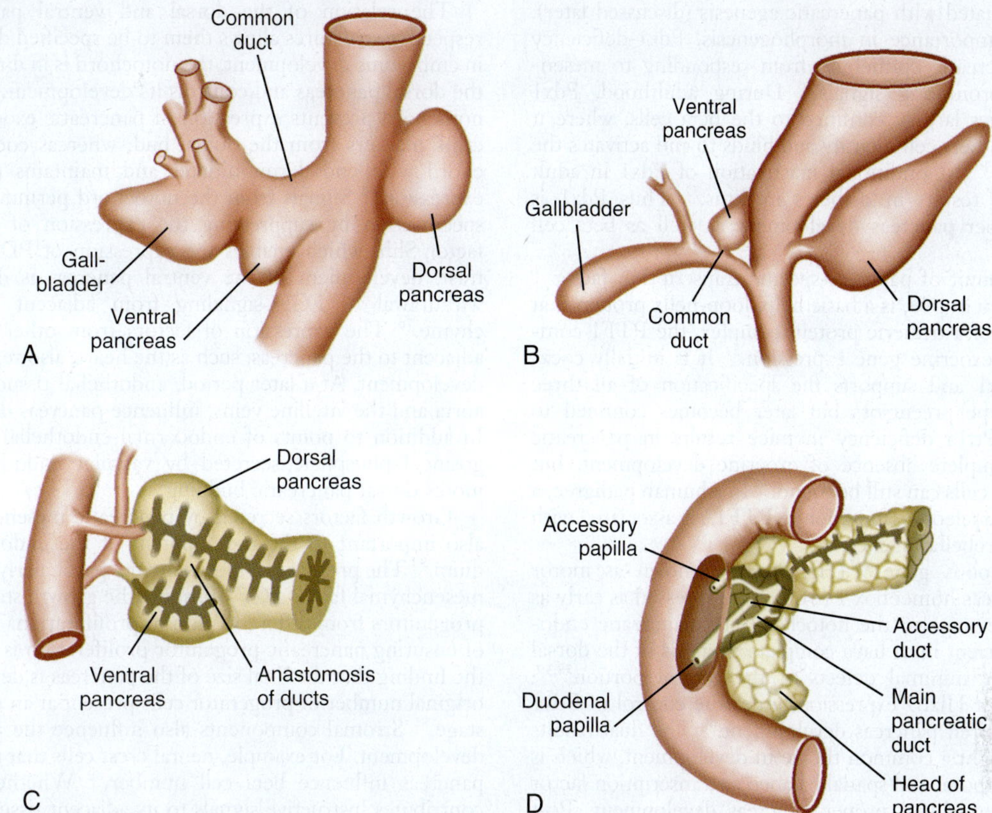

Fig. 57.10 Stages in the embryonic development of the pancreas. (A) At about 4 weeks of gestation, dorsal and ventral buds are formed from the foregut. (B) At about 6 weeks the ventral pancreas extends toward the larger dorsal pancreas. (C) By about 7 weeks, fusion of the dorsal and ventral pancreas has occurred and ductular anastomosis is beginning. (D) At birth, the pancreas is a single organ, and ductular anastomosis is complete. (Modified from Arey LB. *Developmental Anatomy: A Textbook and Laboratory Manual of Embryology*. 7th ed. Philadelphia, PA: WB Saunders; 1974.)

parenchymal cell types—acinar, duct, and islet cells—differentiate from a common pancreatic progenitor lineage. Classic studies by Rutter et al. have divided pancreatic differentiation into two distinct phases.[38] The first, termed the *primary transition*, is defined as the conversion of predifferentiated cells to a protodifferentiated state in which low levels of pancreas-specific proteins are present. The second phase, or the *secondary transition*, is marked by a dramatic rise in pancreatic cell number and pancreas-specific protein synthesis, as well as an acceleration in both exocrine and endocrine differentiation. The pancreatic acinar cells at this stage develop their characteristic abundance of endoplasmic reticulum and dense apically localized zymogen granules.[39] Both the dorsal and ventral pancreas appear to exhibit simultaneous exocrine differentiation according to the two phases.[40]

In the ontogeny of endocrine cells, glucagon-positive alpha cells initially predominate; after the secondary transition, however, insulin-positive beta cells outnumber all other endocrine cell types.[41] In addition, a remarkable morphologic transformation occurs in the endocrine lineage. Although they start off as epithelial cells, it is thought that at this point in development, instead of dividing parallel to the basement membrane, they begin to divide perpendicular to it and eventually develop into islet units.[39] The newly oriented cell descendants lose their tight junctions and connections to the lumen. The endocrine lineage ultimately undergoes a complete epithelial-to-mesenchymal transformation, which is a process that to this day ranks among the great wonders in developmental biology and at the same time offers clues to mechanisms underlying metastasis in cancer biology.[42]

Transcription Factors and Extrinsic Signals

The sequence and signaling factors that guide pancreas development are strikingly similar across vertebrate species, differing mostly in the time to organ formation. Indeed, much of our knowledge base is derived from descriptions of mouse development and the ability to perform lineage tracing experiments by exploiting transgenic mice. Nonetheless, there is a perpetual need to confirm animal models of development using observations of the human condition.[43]

The morphologic changes in the pancreas and the cellular growth, expansion, and differentiation of pancreatic progenitors are orchestrated by hierarchical signals from two distinct sources: from *within the genome* of the cells of the pancreas, notably by a host of transcription factors,[44] and from *tissues and structures adjacent to the forming pancreas*. Each will be discussed.

Transcription factors are proteins that bind to specific DNA sequences.[45] They function to either activate or suppress the recruitment of RNA polymerases that are required for transcription. Transcription factors are classified according to their DNA binding domains. A summary of a few of the key transcription factors in pancreas development is provided.

Pancreatic and duodenal homeobox 1 (Pdx1), also known as *insulin promoter factor 1* (Ipf1) or *islet/duodenum homeobox 1* (Idx1), is the earliest pancreas-specific transcription factor, detected at 5 weeks of development, before bud formation.[46,47] Thus Pdx1 is used as a marker of early pancreatic progenitors. Studies of pancreas development frequently target the Pdx1 gene promoter for pancreas-specific expression. Deletion of Pdx1 in both mice[48] and humans[49] is associated with pancreatic agenesis (discussed later), highlighting its importance in morphogenesis. Pdx1-deficiency prevents the pancreatic epithelium from responding to mesenchymal growth-promoting signals.[50] During adulthood, Pdx1 expression becomes largely confined to the beta cells, where it serves to maintain beta cell identity and binds to and activates the insulin promoter.[46,51] Conditional inactivation of Pdx1 in adult mouse beta cells results in diabetes mellitus.[52] Thus Pdx1 is required for proper pancreas development as well as beta cell function.

The alpha subunit of pancreas-specific transcription factor 1 (Ptf1a), also known as p48, is a basic helix-loop-helix protein that functions as part of a trimeric protein complex, the PTF1 complex, to regulate exocrine gene expression.[53] It is initially coexpressed with Pdx1 and supports the specification of all three pancreatic cell type precursors but later becomes confined to acinar cells.[54,55] Ptf1a deficiency in mice results in pancreatic agenesis with complete absence of exocrine development, but ectopic endocrine cells can still be found.[56] In a human pedigree, a truncating single nucleotide mutation in PTF1A is associated with pancreatic and cerebellar agenesis.[57]

Human homeobox gene 9 (Hlxb9), also known as motor neuron and pancreas homeobox 1 (Mnx1), is expressed as early as the eighth somite stage in the notochord and pancreatic endoderm. Hlxb9-deficient mice have complete agenesis of the dorsal pancreas but only minimal defects of the ventral portion[58,59]; however, persistent Hlxb9 expression under the control of Pdx1 also leads to impaired pancreas development.[60] The dual results with Hlxb9 highlight a common theme in development, which is that a delicate temporal and spatial balance of transcription factor expression is essential for proper pancreas development. Post development, Hlxb9 expression within the pancreas is maintained only in beta cells.[58,59]

Neurogenin3 (Ngn3) is a basic helix-loop-helix transcription factor that heralds the differentiation of Pdx1-expressing progenitor cells into an endocrine lineage.[61] Interestingly, Ngn3 expression is downregulated after endocrine differentiation starts. Mice completely deficient in Ngn3 lack pancreatic endocrine cells.[62] In comparison, patients with a hypomorphic mutation in Ngn3 (NEUROG3), meaning that they have a partial loss of gene function, develop a profound congenital diarrhea that is associated with an absence of enteroendocrine cells, but they do not succumb to neonatal diabetes.[63] Taken together, the results suggest that low levels of Ngn3 expression are required for endocrine differentiation.[64]

Gata4 and Gata6 are part of a family of zinc-finger transcription factors that regulate cell proliferation and differentiation in several endodermal organs.[65] Mutations in GATA4 or GATA6 are associated with pancreatic agenesis in humans. Gata6 is expressed in multipotent stem cells. In addition, mice models demonstrate the role of Gata4/6 in maintaining pancreas identity; knockouts drive the ventral and dorsal buds toward intestinal or stomach lineages due to loss of Gata4/6-mediated inhibition of Sonic hedgehog (Shh).[66] There is also a role for Gata6 in beta cell differentiation.[67]

Additional transcriptions factors involved in exocrine specifications include Mist1 for acinar cells and Sox9 for ductal cells. Transcription factors for endocrine pathways are MafA, Isl-1, Brn-4, NeuroD, Nkx6.1, Nkx2.2, Pax4, Pax6, and Arx.

In addition to the critical role of transcription factors expressed from within the developing pancreas, fluctuating levels of signaling proteins from adjacent tissues and structures also control pancreas development. Early on, pancreas specification from endoderm requires the suppression of Wnt (see Chapter 1) and fibroblast growth factor 4 (FGF4) signaling from adjacent mesoderm.[68,69] In addition, mesodermal retinoic acid signals refine the anterior-posterior position in which the pancreas can develop.[70–72]

The relation of the dorsal and ventral pancreas to their respective structures allows them to be specified differently. Early in embryonic development, the notochord is in direct contact with the dorsal pancreas and controls its development. Removal of the notochord prevents expression of pancreatic exocrine and endocrine markers from the dorsal bud, whereas coculture of notochord with endoderm initiates and maintains pancreatic gene expression.[73] Signals from the notochord permit dorsal pancreas specification by suppressing the expression of anti–pancreatic factor Shh, which enables the expression of PDX1.[74,75] In contrast, development of the ventral pancreas is dependent upon withdrawal of FGF signaling from adjacent cardiac mesenchyme.[76] The expression of factors from other nascent organs adjacent to the pancreas, such as the heart, also regulates pancreas development. At a later period, endothelial tissue, such as dorsal aorta and the vitelline veins, influence pancreas development.[77,78] In addition to points of endodermal-endothelial contact, sphingosine-1-phosphate secreted by vascular endothelial cells promotes dorsal pancreatic budding.[79]

Growth factors secreted by pancreatic mesenchymal cells are also important to the development of the endodermal primordium.[80] The presence of mesenchyme, particularly the presence of mesenchymal factor FGF-10, shifts the growth state of pancreatic progenitors from differentiation to proliferation. The importance of ensuring pancreatic progenitor proliferation is underscored by the finding that the final size of the pancreas is determined by the original number of progenitor cells present at an early embryonic stage.[81] Stromal components also influence the pancreas during development. For example, neural crest cells that migrate into the pancreas influence beta cell number.[82] Whether the pancreas contributes instructive signals to its adjacent tissues has not been well studied.

Reemergence of Embryonic Factors During Pancreatic Injury

Several features of pancreas development are recapitulated in two clinically relevant conditions. In the first scenario, during recovery from pancreatic injury (e.g., after a bout of acute pancreatitis), several embryonic transcription factors reemerge from within the remaining acinar cells to form new ductular complexes called *acinar-to-ductal metaplasia*. They precede the onset of recovery and regeneration of the pancreas.[83] In the second scenario, pancreatic ductal adenocarcinoma and its noninvasive precursor lesion, pancreatic intraepithelial neoplasia, develop from a similar process of acinar-to-ductal metaplasia, in addition to forcing the transcription of embryonic genes, such as *Notch* (in the setting of active pancreatic *Kras* mutations),[84] or by offsetting pathways, such as β-catenin.[85] Thus understanding pancreas development will be important toward devising strategies for enhancing pancreatic recovery and understanding how pancreatic cancer can arise.

Another area of intense interest related to pancreas development is the search for stem cell niches or progenitor pancreatic cells that contribute to pancreatic renewal and regeneration.[86] Although it is known that acinar cells can divide during a process termed *adaptive growth*,[87] several studies have suggested that some of the remaining acinar cells undergo acinar-to-ductal metaplasia and that this new ductular complex functions as progenitors for the neogenesis of the other pancreatic cell types. Some groups maintain that primary ductal cells are the facultative progenitor.[88,89] Alternatively, isolated centroacinar cells, expressing the marker ALDH1 (aldehyde dehydrogenase), were shown to differentiate into both exocrine and endocrine cells.[90] Others have suggested that an altogether new gland seen by electron microscopy as an outpouching from the pancreatic duct, called the *pancreatic duct gland*, functions as a stem cell niche.[91] As mentioned earlier, there are even suggestions that mesenchymal cells, such as the PSC, can become a progenitor cell. These new insights point to the complex environment of factors and cells within the pancreas that maintains its integrity and allows for renewal and regeneration beyond the initial period of development.

DEVELOPMENTAL ANOMALIES

Annular Pancreas

Annular pancreas is a congenital anomaly in which a portion of the pancreas forms a thin band around the preampullary portion of the duodenum, leading to complete or partial bowel obstruction (Fig. 57.11). The incidence of annular pancreas is estimated to be between 1 in 1000[92–94] and 3 in 20,000[95,96] based on retrospective studies of patients undergoing abdominal imaging and autopsy, respectively.

Strong evidence suggests that genetic factors are involved in the pathogenesis of annular pancreas. There are reports of annular pancreas occurring in siblings[97] and identical twins,[98] and a microduplication on chromosome 6q24.2 encompassing the utrophin gene (*UTRN*) was detected in a mother and her child, both of whom were diagnosed with annular pancreas.[99] Annular pancreas has also recently been reported in alveolar capillary dysplasia with misalignment of pulmonary veins, annular pancreas, and intestinal malrotation due to FOX1 mutation.[97,98]

Moreover, annular pancreas is more common in patients with other congenital anomalies, such as trisomy 21, cardiac defects, malrotation, duodenal atresia, genitourinary anomalies, and tracheoesophageal fistula.[99,100] A recent study found 5.3% of VATER/VACTERL patients had annular pancreas in a large German cohort.[101] The role of *Hh* genes in pancreatic organogenesis is discussed earlier in this chapter. *Shh* and *Ihh* gene defects have shown a 42%–85% incidence of annular pancreas in mouse models.[102,103]

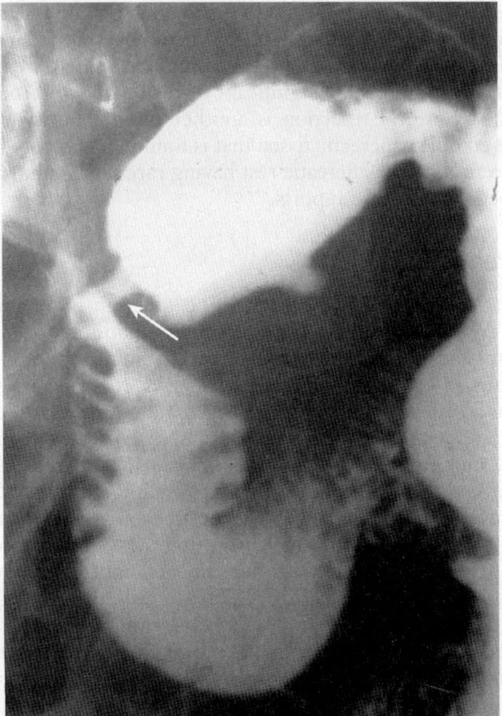

Fig. 57.11 A film from a barium contrast upper GI series demonstrating a mid-duodenal stricture (*arrow*) with proximal dilatation, findings compatible with an annular pancreas. An annular pancreas was identified on CT scan and confirmed during surgery. (Courtesy Michael Federle, MD.)

Although annular pancreas is often diagnosed prenatally or during infancy, it is erroneous to consider it solely a disease of infancy. A second peak of detection occurs in the fourth through seventh decades of life,[100] with symptoms differing dramatically in adults compared to children. Pediatric patients not identified by prenatal US tend to present with nonbilious emesis and feeding intolerance. In contrast, adults present with abdominal pain, pancreatitis, evidence of biliary obstruction, or with nausea, vomiting, and bloating.[100] Diagnosis in children is suspected by findings on abdominal radiographs, US, or upper GI series. In adults, CT scan, MRCP, or ERCP may be more commonly used. Not infrequently, the diagnosis of annular pancreas is made at laparotomy.

Duodenoduodenostomy appears to be an effective surgical treatment for bowel obstruction in these cases and is considered the treatment of choice in children and in some adult patients. Complex pancreatic surgery is more likely to be required in adults compared with children.[99,100] Following surgical repair, there appears to be an increased risk of acute and recurrent pancreatitis into adulthood.[100,104] The risk of pancreaticobiliary neoplasia is significantly increased in adults with annular pancreas,[102,105] and an association with duodenal carcinoma has been reported as well.[106] Thus ongoing cancer screening and surveillance should be considered in this population.

Pancreas Divisum

PD results from a failure of the dorsal and ventral pancreatic ducts to fuse during embryogenesis (Fig. 57.12), resulting in primary drainage of exocrine secretions through the relatively smaller dorsal duct of Santorini and minor papilla. There are three types of PD identified.[107] Classic or complete divisum, in which there is complete failure of fusion between the dorsal duct (Santorini) and ventral duct (Wirsung), occurs in 70% of patients with PD such that the body and tail primarily drain from minor accessory duct (of Santorini), whereas most of the head and the uncinate process drain from the major pancreatic duct (of Wirsung). The second type of PD is incomplete PD, in which there remains a small communication between the ventral and dorsal ducts, occurs in approximately 15% of patients. The last type, reverse PD, occurs

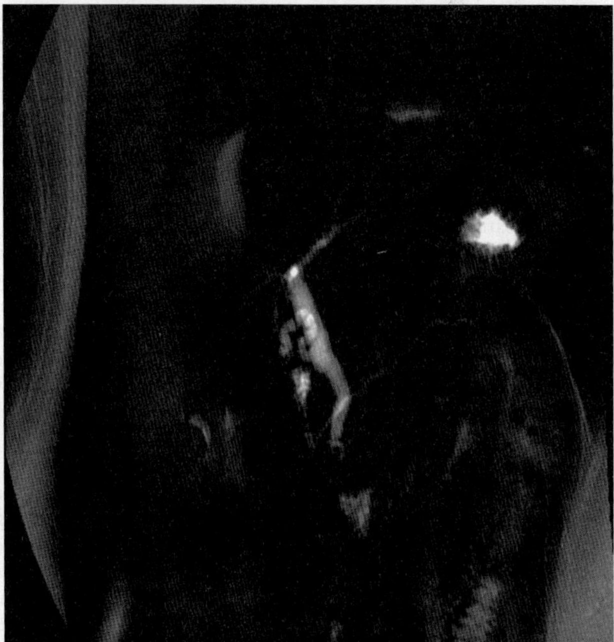

Fig. 57.12 MRCP imaging of a child with recurrent pancreatitis, pancreas divisum, and a type 1 choledochal cyst.

when the minor accessory duct (of Santorini) does not communicate with the main pancreatic duct (of Wirsung) such that a small component of the dorsal pancreas remains isolated with drainage through the minor accessory duct. This variant behaves similarly to normal pancreas but may be more susceptible to increased severity in biliary pancreas, as the lack of communication prevents overflow drainage through the minor accessory duct.

PD has been detected in 5%–10% of the population in autopsy studies and in a similar percentage of patients undergoing ERCP.[108–110] Several decades ago, Cotton reported that 26% of adult patients undergoing ERCP for evaluation of recurrent acute pancreatitis were found to have PD,[111] suggesting a causative link. A 2011 cross-sectional study concluded that PD should be considered a predisposing factor for chronic and recurrent pancreatitis, based on MRI.[112] However, recent papers have shown an association between genetic mutations in *SPINK1* and *CFTR* and PD in symptomatic patients suggesting PD in association with other risk factors for pancreatic disease has an additive effect in the development of pancreatic disease.[113,114] Moreover, a recent systematic review found no clear correlation between PD and pancreatic disease.[115] It remains unclear whether PD is a cause or a cofactor in the development of pancreatic disease, and perhaps it is more appropriate to consider it as one of many risk factors for pancreatic disease. A possible carcinogenic role has also been described in a case report of ampullary cancer associated with PD in 2011, followed by a retrospective review of MRCP imaging finding 7.8% of patients with PD had pancreaticobiliary tumors.[116,117]

PD can be diagnosed by endoscopic retrograde pancreatography, EUS, abdominal CT, or MRCP. Although endoscopic retrograde pancreatography is considered the gold standard in diagnosing PD, secretin-enhanced MRCP has emerged as a potential tool, with a recent study[118] showing a sensitivity of 73.3% and a specificity of 96.8%; MRCP without secretin was nondiagnostic. Although only a minority of patients with PD develop symptoms due to their abnormal anatomy, it appears that endoscopic or surgical therapy can relieve symptoms in some patients with recurrent acute pancreatitis and chronic pancreatitis (see Chapter 59). In 2008 a retrospective database study of 57 patients with PD undergoing minor papilla endotherapy revealed clinical improvement in 76% with recurrent acute pancreatitis, in 42% with chronic pancreatitis, and in 33% with pain alone after a median follow-up of 20 months.[119] Long-term outcomes were again assessed in a 2009 database study of 145 patients with PD who underwent minor papilla endotherapy. Clinical improvement was achieved in 53% of patients with recurrent acute pancreatitis, 18% of patients with chronic pancreatitis, and 41% of patients with pancreatic-type pain, at median follow-up of 43 months.[120] Kanth et al. found endotherapy to be an effective treatment option for patients with acute recurrent pancreatitis in a systematic review of 528 patients.[121] Another recent systematic review in 2017 examined the role of both endoscopic and surgical therapy and concluded that while both modalities resulted in symptom improvement, surgical therapies led to superior outcomes (72% vs. 62.3% symptom improvement).[122] Ongoing prospective studies may be able to better assess the role of endoscopic therapy.

Ectopic Pancreatic Tissue

Ectopic (heterotopic) pancreatic tissue, often referred to as a *pancreatic rest*, occurs in 0.6%–13.7% of the population according to autopsy material. This tissue lacks a physical connection to the pancreas and has an independent blood supply. Pancreatic rests are most commonly found in the stomach (Fig. 57.13), duodenum, and proximal jejunum. Less frequently, it can be found in a Meckel diverticulum (6%), esophagus, ileum, or even the umbilicus, bile duct, gallbladder, splenic hilum, colon, appendix, or mesentery.[123,124] Although rarely clinically significant, ectopic pancreatic tissue has resulted in pancreatitis,[125] ulceration and bleeding,[126] obstruction,[124] intussusception,[127] and malignancy.[128,129] On imaging, pancreatic rests appear as a smooth, broad-based submucosal mass with about 45% having a classic central umbilication. On CT, pancreatic rests can present as a small intramural mass with microlobulated margins and endoluminal growth. Acinar dominant lesions have a rich vascular supply and will homogenously enhance with IV contrast, whereas duct dominant lesions are less vascular with more heterogenous enhancement. EUS has been used for accurate preoperative differentiation between GISTs and pancreatic rests,[130] and typical features on EUS include antral location, mucosal dimple, three to four layers, and lesional duct.[131] When necessary, endoscopic band ligation with snare polypectomy can safely resect the lesion(s) if symptoms are significant or histologic confirmation is needed.[132] Surgical resection is another option, but whether to remove ectopic pancreatic tissue that is found incidentally remains controversial, with pancreatic rest having rare malignant potential described only in case reports.[133]

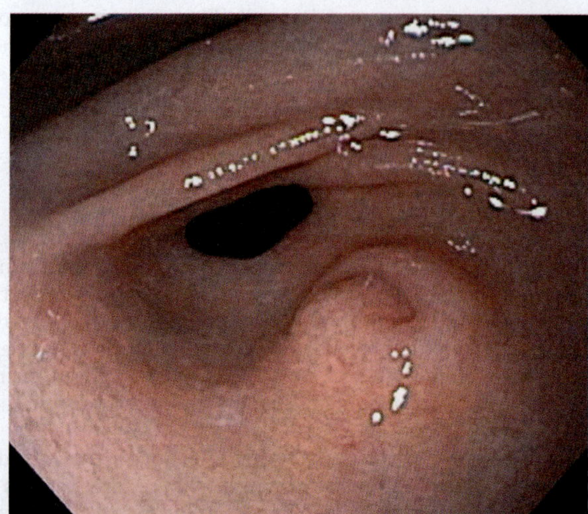

Fig. 57.13 Endoscopic view of a pancreatic rest in the gastric antrum of an 8-year-old boy. Note the central umbilication.

Pancreatic Agenesis

Pancreatic agenesis is a rare condition that can be complete or partial. Mice homozygous for a targeted mutation in the insulin-promoter-factor 1 gene (*IPF1*) are born without a pancreas,[48] and mutations in *PDX1* and *PTF1A* have been reported in humans with pancreatic agenesis.[49,57,134] *GATA6* mutations were identified in 15 of a cohort of 27 subjects with pancreatic agenesis.[135] Finally, mutations in *CNOT1* are associated with HPE12 (holoprosencephaly 12 with or without pancreatic agenesis).[136,137]

Complete pancreatic agenesis is mostly fatal because infants are stricken with diabetes and malabsorption, as well as intrauterine growth retardation due to lack of insulin, an important intrauterine growth factor.[138,139] Partial pancreatic agenesis, or agenesis of the dorsal pancreas, may be less significant clinically owing to the presence of some functioning pancreatic tissue. Also known as *congenital short pancreas*, agenesis of the dorsal pancreas is associated with polysplenia and intestinal malrotation,[140] renal anomalies,[141] and heterotaxy.[142] A recent study has also described a new phenotype associated with maturity onset diabetes of the young due to variants in *PDX1*.[143] Pancreatic agenesis should be suspected based on clinical findings and can be confirmed with MRI.

Congenital Cysts

Congenital cysts of the pancreas are rare and may be diagnosed at any age, even prenatally by routine US.[144,145] The cysts may be solitary or multiple and are distinguished from pancreatic fluid collections by the presence of an epithelial lining. They are thought to form due to anomalies in the development of the pancreatic ductal system. Typically, the embryonic duct regresses as permanent ducts develop; however, if the embryonic ducts persist, they can become obstructed and fluid filled resulting in congenital cysts.[146]

The clinical presentation is variable, ranging from an incidental finding on an imaging study to an abdominal mass, with or without vomiting, biliary obstruction, or acute pancreatitis. Solitary pancreatic cysts are often enteric duplications that may be located entirely within the pancreatic parenchyma and may communicate with the pancreatic duct.[147] Multiple pancreatic cysts tend to occur in patients with associated anomalies and may be seen in systemic disorders such as von Hippel-Landau syndrome, Ivemark II syndrome, or polycystic kidney disease.[148,149] In a review of 15 cases of congenital pancreatic cysts, most presented before the age of 2 years, and associated anomalies were found in 30% of cases.[150] Congenital pancreatic cysts are more often located in the body and tail (62%) of the pancreas than in the head (32%).[151] Surgical therapy consists of total excision when possible. Cysts in the pancreatic head may be addressed using endoscopic or surgical drainage procedures, when necessary.

Pancreaticobiliary Malunion

Pancreaticobiliary malunion (PBM), also called anomalous pancreaticobiliary union, is a congenital malformation in which a common channel for bile and pancreatic fluid is formed, owing to the absence of a septum between the ducts (Fig. 57.14). A classification for PBM has been proposed by dividing it into three types: *pb type*, in which the pancreatic duct appears to join the bile duct; *bp type*, in which the insertion of the bile duct is into the pancreatic duct; and *Y type*, in which there is a long common channel measuring greater than 15 mm in length.[152,153] In large series, the *bp* and *pb* types have each been reported to be the most common type of PBM.[154,155] PBM is diagnosed by traditional cholangiography (ERCP, intraoperative cholangiography, or percutaneous cholangiography), MRCP, or helical CT scan. Traditional cholangiography remains the gold standard.

Bile duct dilation may accompany PBM. Choledochal cysts are almost universally associated with PBM (94% and 100% in two series).[154,155] The abnormal union occurs outside the duodenal wall; thus, the influence of the sphincter of Oddi is lost, allowing reflux of pancreatic exocrine secretions into the biliary system and bile into the pancreatic duct. Recent data have suggested that a markedly elevated amylase concentration can be detected in the bile of patients with a common channel of 5 mm or greater.[156] Biliary stasis, intermixed with refluxed pancreatic secretions, increases risk for biliary neoplasms that manifest in adulthood.[157] Conversely, biliary reflux into the pancreas increases risk for acute pancreatitis.

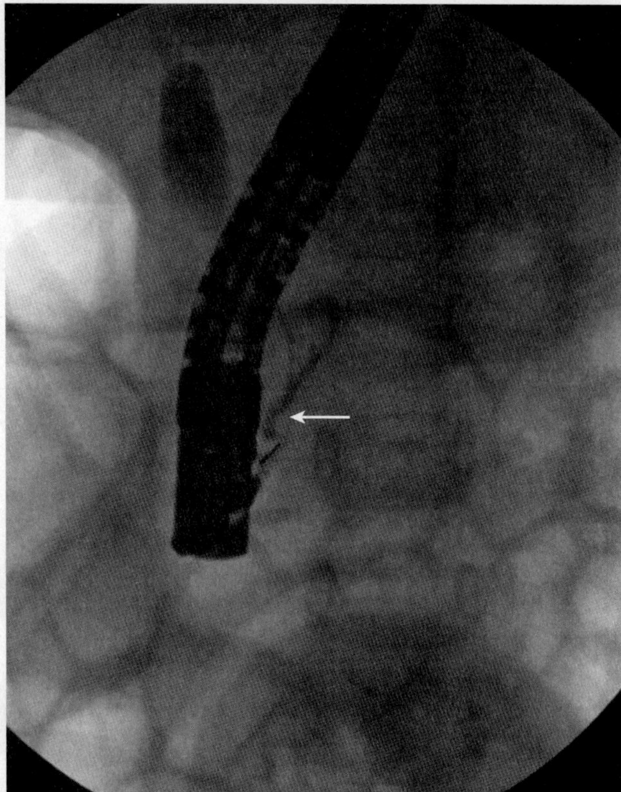

Fig. 57.14 Choledochal cyst and long common channel visualized by ERCP in a 4-year-old female. The common bile duct narrows crossing through the head of the pancreas secondary to acute and chronic pancreatitis.

The increased risk of biliary tract malignancy in patients with PBM is well documented. Malunions were seen in 62.5% of adults with gallbladder cancer, in 50% of patients with gallbladder adenomyomatosis, and in 33.3% of patients with bile duct cancer.[154] Moreover, the incidence of biliary cancer is 15–20 years earlier in patients with PBM in comparison to patients without PBM.[157] In Japan, high incidences of gallbladder carcinomas were seen in patients with PBM, with and without cystic dilation of the bile duct.[158] Conversely, cystic dilation of bile duct is associated with increased risk of bile duct neoplasm (32.1% vs. 7.3% in patients without biliary dilation).[159] Patients with PBM have increased cellular proliferative activity of the gallbladder mucosa, even in early childhood.[160] Although there is controversy concerning management of PBM among patients of various ethnic groups,[161–163] given the cancer risk for the patient with this anomaly, consideration for cholecystectomy, resection of the bile duct, and hepaticojejunostomy may be advised.[158,164]

Full references for this chapter can be found at https://ebooks.health.elsevier.com.

58 Exocrine Pancreatic Secretion

Stephen J. Pandol, Sohail Z. Husain

IN THIS CHAPTER

The exocrine pancreas has been of considerable interest to physiologists and other scientists for quite some time; in fact, the first demonstration of a hormone action around the turn of the 20th century was in the pancreas.[1] The pancreas has also been the major organ used to demonstrate general mechanisms of synthesis and transport for exportable proteins,[2] ion and water secretion,[3,4] and their related signaling pathways.[5] This chapter presents a concise description of the current understanding of exocrine pancreatic physiology.

FUNCTIONAL ANATOMY

The functional unit of the exocrine pancreas is composed of an acinus and its draining ductule (Fig. 58.1).[6] The ductal epithelium extends to the lumen of the acinus, with the centroacinar cell situated as an extension of the ductal epithelium into the acinus (see Chapter 57). The centroacinar cell plays a key role in providing progenitor cells for pancreatic cell lineages.[7,8] The ductule drains into interlobular (intercalated) ducts, which, in turn, drain into the main pancreatic ductal system.

The acinus (from the Latin term meaning "berry in a cluster") can be spherical or tubular, as shown in Fig. 58.1, or can have an irregular form.[6] The acinar cells are specialized to synthesize, store, and secrete digestive enzymes. On their basolateral membrane are receptors for hormones and neurotransmitters that stimulate secretion of digestive enzymes.[5] The basal aspect of the cell contains the nucleus as well as abundant rough endoplasmic reticulum (RER) for protein synthesis (Fig. 58.2, left). The apical region of the cell contains zymogen granules, the storage site of digestive enzymes. The apical surface of the acinar cell also possesses microvilli. Within the microvilli and in the cytoplasm underlying the apical plasma membrane is a filamentous actin meshwork that is involved in exocytosis of the contents of the zymogen granules.[9] Secretion is into the lumen of the acinus. Tight junctions between acinar cells form a band around the apical aspects of the cells and act as a barrier to prevent passage of large molecules such as the digestive enzymes.[10] The junctional complexes also provide for the paracellular passage of water and ions.

Another intercellular connection between acinar cells is the gap junction. This specialized area of the plasma membrane between adjacent cells acts as a pore to allow small molecules (molecular weight 500–1000 Da) to pass between cells. The gap junction allows chemical and electrical communication between cells. For example, calcium signaling is coordinated between the cells of an acinus through gap junctions and has effects on digestive enzyme secretion.[11,12]

The duct epithelium consists of cells that are cuboidal to pyramidal and contain the abundant mitochondria necessary for energy products needed for ion transport (see Fig. 58.2, right). The duct cells as well as the centroacinar cells contain carbonic anhydrase, which is important for their ability to secrete bicarbonate.[3]

COMPOSITION OF EXOCRINE SECRETIONS

Inorganic Constituents

The principal inorganic components of exocrine pancreatic secretions are water, sodium, potassium, chloride, and bicarbonate (Fig. 58.3). The purposes of the water and ion secretions are to deliver digestive enzymes to the intestinal lumen and to help neutralize gastric acid emptied into the duodenum. The primary mediator of water and ion secretion from ductal and acinar cells is the hormone secretion, which is released into the circulation from specialized enteroendocrine cells along the intestinal epithelium called S cells. Pancreatic juice secreted during stimulation with secretin is clear, colorless, alkaline, and isotonic with plasma. As a result of this stimulation, the flow rate ramps ups from an average rate of 0.2 or 0.3 mL/min in the resting (interdigestive) state to 4.0 mL/min during postprandial stimulation. The total daily volume of secretion is 2.5 L. The osmolality of pancreatic juice is independent of the flow rate. However, when the pancreas is stimulated by secretin, bicarbonate, and chloride concentrations change reciprocally (see Fig. 58.3).

Secretin stimulates secretion by binding to its receptor on the basolateral membrane of the duct cell, thus activating adenylate cyclase and increasing cyclic adenosine monophosphate (cAMP).[3] The initial events with secretin stimulation involve cAMP- and Ca^{2+}-dependent chloride (Cl^-) channel activation on the luminal membrane as well as K^+ channel activation on the basolateral membrane (Fig. 58.4).[3,13] The cAMP-dependent luminal Cl^- channel is the cystic fibrosis transmembrane conductance regulator (CFTR).[13,14] Activation of this channel by cAMP leads to Cl^- secretion into the lumen, where it is coupled to a Cl^-/HCO_3^- exchanger, resulting in an exchange of Cl^- for HCO_3^- in the lumen. Evidence suggests that CFTR is also directly involved in HCO_3^- secretion when the luminal bicarbonate concentration exceeds a certain threshold. This phenomenon is mediated

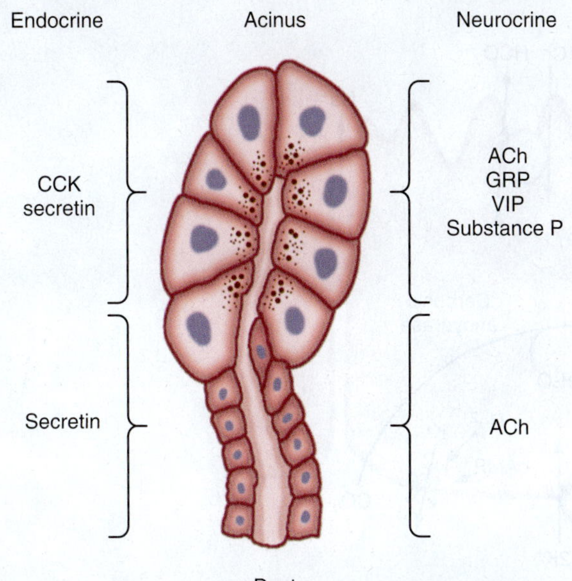

Fig. 58.1 Regulation of exocrine pancreatic secretion during the intestinal phase of digestion. Exocrine secretions are regulated by endocrine and neurocrine pathways. In addition, the endocrine and neurocrine mediators regulate secretion from the acinus and the duct differently. For the acinus, *CCK*, secretin, acetylcholine (*ACh*), gastrin-releasing peptide (*GRP*), vasoactive intestinal polypeptide (*VIP*), and substance P regulate secretion. Signaling mechanisms [second messengers] are shown in Fig. 58.6. Secretin and ACh are the major regulators of pancreatic bicarbonate secretion from the duct. (Transporters involved in ductal secretion are illustrated in Fig. 58.4.) (Adapted from Gorelick F, Pandol SJ, Topazian M. *Pancreatic Physiology, Pathophysiology, Acute and Chronic Pancreatitis*. Gastrointestinal Teaching Project, American Gastroenterological Association; 2003.)

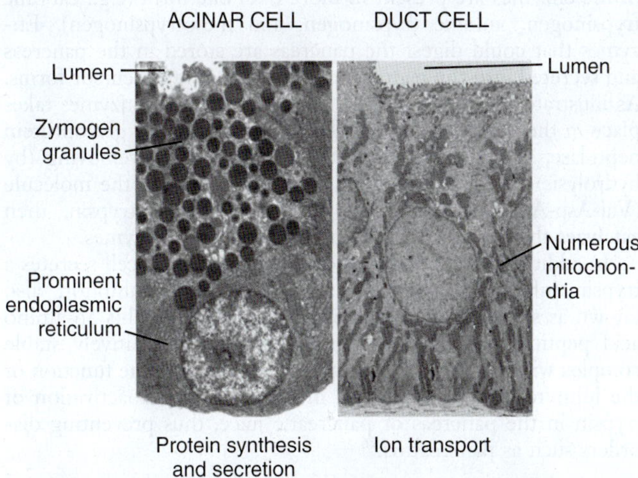

Fig. 58.2 Ultrastructure of exocrine cells. The ultrastructure of exocrine cells reflects their specialized function. The pancreatic acinar cell (*left*) and duct cell (*right*) are both polarized, with clearly defined apical (luminal), lateral, and basal domains. The pancreatic acinar cell has prominent basally located rough endoplasmic reticulum for synthesis of digestive enzymes and apically located zymogen granules for storage and secretion of digestive enzymes. The pancreatic duct cell contains numerous mitochondria for energy generation needed for its ion transport functions. (Adapted from Gorelick F, Pandol SJ, Topazian M. *Pancreatic Physiology, Pathophysiology, Acute and Chronic Pancreatitis*. Gastrointestinal Teaching Project, American Gastroenterological Association; 2003.)

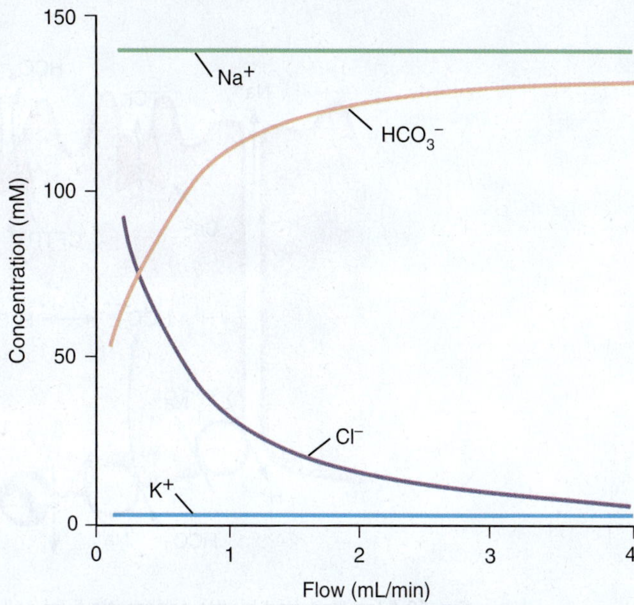

Fig. 58.3 Secretion of pancreatic bicarbonate and other electrolytes. With stimulation (i.e., a meal), there is an increase in the flow of pancreatic secretions. Furthermore, with rising flow rates, there are dramatic changes in the concentrations of chloride and bicarbonate in pancreatic juice. The increase in bicarbonate concentration results in an alkaline secretion. The bicarbonate comes from pancreatic ductal epithelial cells. In contrast to acinar cells, the ducts secrete a large volume of fluid with a high concentration of bicarbonate. The volume of secretion from the acinar cells is believed to be small compared with ductal secretion, and with increasing stimulation of the pancreas, the concentration of ions approaches that of the ductal secretions. Of note, the alkaline secretions from the pancreas, the biliary system, and the duodenal mucosa neutralize the acid secretion delivered to the duodenum from the stomach. This pH-neutral environment is important for optimal digestive enzyme and intestinal mucosal function. (Adapted from Gorelick F, Pandol SJ, Topazian M. *Pancreatic Physiology, Pathophysiology, Acute and Chronic Pancreatitis*. Gastrointestinal Teaching Project, American Gastroenterological Association; 2003.)

through WNK signaling.[3,4,15,16] On the basolateral surface of the duct cell is a Na^+–H^+ exchanger, a Na-HCO_3^- cotransport, 2 ATPases (H^+-ATPase and Na^+, K^+-ATPase), and a K^+ channel. In combination, these various transporters facilitate HCO_3^- secretion at the apical surface as well as maintain a neutral pH within the duct cell.[17] Na^+ and water are secreted into the ductal system to counter the electrical and osmotic forces resulting from the HCO_3^- secretion. Of importance, mutational alterations with complete lack of CFTR function result in destruction of the exocrine pancreas in childhood (i.e., in cystic fibrosis), whereas mutations with partial function can lead to pancreatitis later in life.[18] Also, recent studies show that alcoholism and smoking cause inhibition of CFTR function, which could play a role in causing pancreatitis.[19,20] These disorders result in pancreatic disease because the lack of fluid flow from pancreatic ducts prevents movement of thick protein-containing secretions from acinar tissue. This results in blocking the ductal system, secondary injury, inflammation, and cell death in acinar tissue.

Organic Constituents

The human pancreas has a large capacity for synthesizing protein (mostly digestive enzymes).[21–24] Box 58.1 lists the major proteolytic, amylolytic, lipolytic, and nuclease digestive enzymes. Some

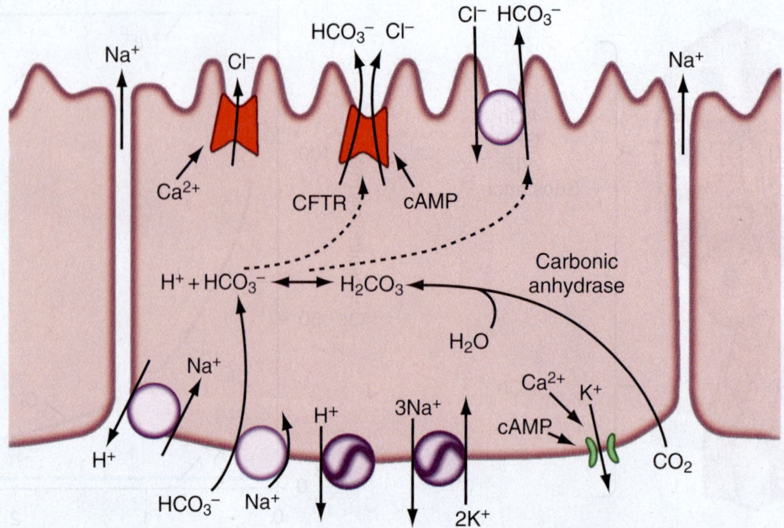

Fig. 58.4 Ion transport by the pancreatic duct cell. HCO_3^- is delivered for ultimate secretion by two mechanisms. In one, membrane-diffusible CO_2 is catalytically converted to HCO_3^- and H^+ by the action of carbonic anhydrase, which hydrates CO_2, thereby forming H_2CO_3, which then dissociates to HCO_3^- and H^+. The duct cell is rich in carbonic anhydrase. In the other Na^+ and HCO_3^- are cotransported on the basolateral membrane. The HCO_3^- is then available for apical secretion by both the cystic fibrosis transmembrane conductance regulator (*CFTR*) and Cl^--HCO_3^- anion exchange. Na^+ and H_2O are delivered to the lumen through intercellular junctions. H^+ is removed from the cell by a basolateral Na^+, H^+ antiport and a H^+-ATPase to maintain a constant intracellular pH. Secretion is activated by increased permeability of apical Cl^- and HCO_3^- channels and basolateral K^+ channels through agonists (i.e., secretin and acetylcholine) that increase cellular cyclic AMP (*cAMP*) levels (secretin) and calcium levels (acetylcholine). (Adapted from Gorelick F, Pandol SJ, Topazian M. *Pancreatic Physiology, Pathophysiology, Acute and Chronic Pancreatitis*. Gastrointestinal Teaching Project, American Gastroenterological Association; 2003.)

BOX 58.1 Pancreatic Acinar Cell Secretory Products

PROENZYMES*

Anionic trypsinogen
Cationic trypsinogen
Chymotrypsinogen (A, B)
Kallikreinogen
Mesotrypsinogen
Procarboxypeptidase A (1, 2)
Procarboxypeptidase B (1, 2)
Proelastase
Prophospholipase A_2

ENZYMES

Amylase
Carboxylesterase
DNase
Lipase (TG lipase)
RNase
Sterol esterase

*Proenzymes listed are stored in the pancreas and secreted into the duodenal lumen as inactive proenzyme forms. If these enzymes were active in the pancreas, they would digest the pancreatic gland. Other enzymes, such as amylase and lipase, are stored and secreted in their active forms.

Adapted from Gorelick F, Pandol SJ, Topazian M. *Pancreatic Physiology, Pathophysiology, Acute and Chronic Pancreatitis*. Gastrointestinal Teaching Project, American Gastroenterological Association; 2003.

of the enzymes are present in more than one form (e.g., cationic trypsinogen, anionic trypsinogen, and mesotrypsinogen). Enzymes that could digest the pancreas are stored in the pancreas and secreted into the pancreatic duct as inactive precursor forms. As illustrated in Fig. 58.5, the activation of these enzymes takes place in the intestinal lumen, where a brush-border glycoprotein peptidase, enterokinase, activates trypsinogen by removing (by hydrolysis) an *N*-terminal hexapeptide fragment of the molecule (Val-Asp-Asp-Asp-Asp-Lys).[21] The active form, trypsin, then catalyzes the activation of the other inactive proenzymes.

In addition to the digestive enzymes, the acinar cell secretes a trypsin inhibitor, pancreatic secretory trypsin inhibitor, also known as serine protease inhibitor Kazal type 1. This 56-amino acid peptide inactivates trypsin by forming a relatively stable complex with the enzyme near its catalytic site.[25] The function of the inhibitor is as a protective mechanism for autoactivation of trypsin in the pancreas or pancreatic juice, thus preventing disorders such as pancreatitis.[26]

FUNCTIONS OF THE MAJOR DIGESTIVE ENZYMES

Amylase

The pancreas and salivary gland each secrete a specific isoform of amylase, and both have identical enzymatic activity in digesting starch and glycogen in the diet. However, they differ in molecular weight, carbohydrate content, and electrophoretic mobility.[27] Salivary amylase initiates digestion in the mouth and may account for a significant portion of starch and glycogen digestion because

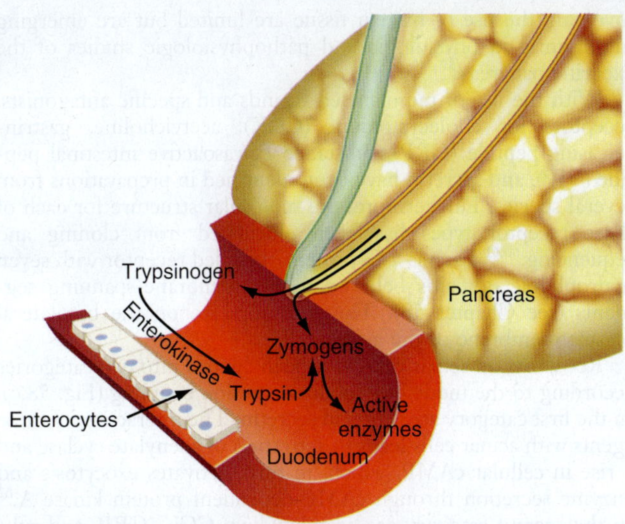

Fig. 58.5 Site of zymogen activation. Trypsinogen, chymotrypsinogen, proelastase, procarboxypeptidase, and prophospholipase A_2 are stored in the pancreas and secreted into the duodenal lumen as inactive proenzyme forms. Other enzymes, such as amylase and lipase, are stored and secreted in their active forms. The active forms of these latter enzymes have no effect on the pancreas because it does not contain starch or triglyceride (TG). Activation of the inactive proenzymes takes place in the duodenal lumen. There, the brush-border enzyme enterokinase converts secreted trypsinogen to trypsin. Trypsinogen and the other proenzymes are then converted to active forms by proteolytic cleavage by trypsin. (Adapted from Gorelick F, Pandol SJ, Topazian M. *Pancreatic Physiology, Pathophysiology, Acute and Chronic Pancreatitis*. Gastrointestinal Teaching Project, American Gastroenterological Association; 2003.)

it is transported with the meal into the stomach and small intestine, where it continues to hydrolyze its substrates. In the stomach, the amylase activity is protected from secreted gastric acid by buffering from the meal and by the alkaline environment of salivary and gastric mucus. The action of both salivary and pancreatic amylase is to hydrolyze 1,4-glycoside linkages at every other junction between carbon 1 and oxygen. The products of amylase digestion are maltose and maltotriose (2- and 3-α-1,4–linked molecules, respectively) and α-dextrins containing 1,6-glycosidic linkages, because 1,6-glycosidic linkages in starch cannot be hydrolyzed by amylase. The brush-border enzymes of the enterocyte complete the hydrolysis of the end products of amylase digestion to the monosaccharide glucose, which is thereafter transported across the intestinal absorptive epithelial cell by a Na^+-coupled transport (see Chapter 58).[28]

Lipases

The pancreas secretes three triglyceride (TG) lipases: pancreatic triglyceride lipase (PTL) and its family members, pancreatic lipase-related protein 1, and pancreatic lipase-related protein 2 (see Box 58.1). Salivary (or lingual) and gastric lipases also contribute to fat digestion but in a minor fashion (see Chapter 58).

PTL binds to the oil-water interface of the TG oil droplet, where it acts to hydrolyze a TG molecule to two fatty acid molecules released from carbons 1 and 3 and a monoglyceride with a fatty acid esterified to glycerol at carbon 2.[21,29] Bile acids as well as colipase facilitate the full activity of lipase. Bile acids aid in the emulsification of TG to enlarge the surface area for lipase to act on, and they form micelles with nonesterified fatty acids and monoglyceride products of lipase, thus removing them from the oil-water interface. Colipase is believed to form a complex with lipase and bile acids. This ternary complex anchors lipase and allows it to act in a more hydrophilic environment on the hydrophobic surface of the oil droplet.

Other lipid-digesting enzymes secreted from the pancreas include phospholipase A_2 and carboxylesterase. Phospholipase A_2 catalyzes the hydrolysis of the fatty acid ester linkage at carbon 2 of phosphatidylcholine.[23] This cleavage leads to the formation of nonesterified fatty acid and lysophosphatidylcholine. Carboxylesterase has broad specificity and will cleave cholesterol esters, lipid-soluble vitamin esters, TGs, diglycerides, and monoglycerides. Carboxylesterase is also facilitated by bile acids.[30]

Proteases

The pancreas secretes a variety of proenzyme proteases that are activated in the duodenum by trypsin (see Box 58.1). Of these, trypsin, chymotrypsin, and elastase are endopeptidases that cleave at specific peptide motifs away from the ends of the protein primary structure.[21] Another type of protease found in pancreatic juice is the carboxypeptidases, which are exopeptidases that cleave peptide bonds at the carboxyl terminus of proteins.

The combined actions of gastric pepsin and the pancreatic proteases result in the formation of oligopeptides and free amino acids. The oligopeptides can be further digested by enterocyte brush-border enzymes (see Chapter 58). Free amino acids and oligopeptides are transported across the intestinal mucosa by a group of Na^+- and H^+-coupled transporters.[31] It is interesting that only certain amino acids (mostly essential amino acids) are detectable in the lumen during digestion, indicating that the combined action of the proteases is not random and that the products result from the combined specificities of the individual proteases. These free amino acids in the lumen also exert a more potent effect on stimulating pancreatic secretion, inhibiting gastric emptying, regulating small bowel motility, and causing satiety. Thus the distinct products of the pancreatic digestive proteases can modulate the function of several organs in the GI tract.

DIGESTIVE ENZYME SYNTHESIS AND TRANSPORT

Synthesis of digestive enzymes takes place in the internal space of the RER (see Fig. 58.2, left).[2,32] The mechanism for translation of the cell's messenger RNA (mRNA) into exportable protein is explained by the signal hypothesis. The main feature of the hypothesis is that ribosomal subunits attach to mRNA and initiate synthesis of a hydrophobic "signal" sequence on the NH_2-terminal of nascent proteins. This complex then attaches to the outer surface of the endoplasmic reticulum, and the signal sequence targets the protein being synthesized into the lumen of the RER.

Newly synthesized proteins can undergo posttranslation modifications in the endoplasmic reticulum, including disulfide bridge formation, phosphorylation, sulfation, and glycosylation.[33] Conformational changes resulting in tertiary and quaternary structures of the protein also take place in the endoplasmic reticulum. Important conformational specificities are required for appropriate function and transport of proteins between compartments. These conformational specificities are facilitated by proteins that include *chaperones* and *foldases*. When there is increased demand on the RER for protein synthesis or in the setting up of cellular stress causing unfolding of proteins, the RER responds by invoking the unfolded protein response, which increases synthesis of chaperones and foldases, ceases synthesis of the proteins, and even degrades unfolded proteins.[33] By keeping proteins in their appropriate conformation, the unfolded protein response (UPR) maintains the normal transport of proteins between compartments of the cell. Importantly, recent studies show that one of the mechanisms by which excessive alcohol drinking and smoking mediate pancreatitis is through alterations of protein folding in the RER combined with inhibition of the UPR.[34–36]

Processed proteins in the RER are transported to the Golgi complex where further posttranslational modification and concentration occur.[37] The Golgi complex also serves the important function of sorting and targeting newly synthesized proteins into various cell compartments. Digestive enzymes are transported to the zymogen granules, whereas lysosomal hydrolases are sorted to the lysosome.[32,38,39] The mechanisms for sorting to the lysosome are much better understood compared to those for the zymogen granule. For the lysosomal pathway, mannose-6-phosphate groups are added as oligosaccharide chains to the proteins destined for lysosomal delivery during their presence in the Golgi complex. The mannose-6-phosphate groups serve as a recognition site for their cognate receptor (i.e., mannose-6-phosphate receptor). The interaction of the lysosomal enzyme-mannose 6-phosphate with its receptor leads to formation of vesicles that transport this complex to the lysosome, delivering the lysosomal enzymes. In the lysosome, the enzymes dissociate from the mannose-6-phosphate receptor, which, in turn, cycles back to the Golgi complex.

Secretion of digestive enzymes occurs by a coordinated process of exocytosis.[2] Exocytosis consists of movement of the secretory granule to the apical surface, the recognition of a plasma membrane site for fusion, and the fission of the granule membrane-plasma membrane site after fusion. The cellular machinery that is necessary for exocytosis includes actin-myosin,[40–43] the SNARE (soluble *N*-ethylmaleimide–sensitive factor attachment protein receptor) proteins,[44,45] and guanosine triphosphate-binding proteins.[42,46,47] Of note, the SNARE family represents a large group of proteins that mediate vesicle-fusion steps in both endocytic and secretory pathways.

Regulation of Protein Synthesis

The mechanisms involved in regulating expression of digestive enzymes in the exocrine pancreas have been partially elucidated. The investigations have addressed the following two questions: First, what accounts for the specific expression of digestive enzymes in the pancreas? Second, how do alterations in dietary nutrients change the synthesis of specific digestive enzymes? For the answer to the first question, genes for digestive enzymes, such as amylase, chymotrypsin, and elastase, contain enhancer regions in their 5′ flanking nucleotide sequences that regulate the transcription of their mRNAs, termed the *pancreas consensus element*.[48–51] A transcription factor, pancreas transcription factor-1 (PTF-1), is present selectively in the exocrine pancreas, binds to this region, and is essential for expression of these digestive enzymes.[52,53] Thus PTF-1 represents at least one of the differentiation-regulated factors that accounts for digestive enzyme expression in the pancreas. Regarding the second question, numerous studies have demonstrated that the relative synthesis rates of specific digestive enzymes change as a function of dietary intake. For example, a carbohydrate-rich diet results in an increase in synthesis of amylase and a decrease in that of chymotrypsinogen,[54] a lipid-rich diet enhances lipase expression,[55] and an alcohol-rich diet decreases amylase expression.[56] Several studies have also demonstrated that amylase gene expression is regulated by insulin and diet.[56] The mechanisms responsible for this adaptation are only partially understood and include both transcriptional and posttranscriptional regulation.[54]

CELLULAR REGULATION OF ENZYME SECRETION

The mechanism of neurohumoral stimulation of the acinar cell has been demonstrated with the use of in vitro preparations of dispersed acinar cells and acini from small animals. Studies involving the use of human tissue are limited but are emerging importantly in physiologic and pathophysiologic studies of the exocrine pancreas.[57–59]

With the use of radiolabeled ligands and specific antagonists, receptors for cholecystokinin (CCK), acetylcholine, gastrin-releasing peptide (GRP), substance P, vasoactive intestinal peptide (VIP), and secretin have been identified in preparations from several species. Furthermore, the molecular structure for each of these receptor types has been elucidated from cloning and sequencing.[60,61] Each is a G-protein–coupled receptor with seven hydrophobic domains believed to be membrane-spanning segments (see Chapter 58). The receptors are on the basolateral plasma membrane of the acinar cell.

Receptors on acinar cells have been divided into two categories according to the mode of stimulus-secretion coupling (Fig. 58.6). In the first category are VIP and secretin. The interaction of these agents with acinar cells leads to activation of adenylate cyclase and a rise in cellular cAMP, which, in turn, activates exocytosis and enzyme secretion through cAMP-dependent protein kinase A.[62] In the second category are acetylcholine, CCK, GRP, and substance P. The actions of these agonists include stimulating cellular metabolism of membrane phosphoinositides and raising intracellular free calcium concentrations ($[Ca^{2+}]i$) from mobilization of intracellular stores.[63,64] Specifically, the agonist-receptor interaction leads to a phospholipase C–mediated hydrolysis of phosphatidylinositol 4,5-bisphosphate to 1,2-diacylglycerol and inositol 1,4,5-triphosphate (IP_3). IP_3, in turn, releases calcium from endoplasmic reticulum stores. The calcium release into the cytosol causes a rapid rise in the concentration of free calcium that mediates the secretory response.[65] Calcium release into the cytosol is also mediated by ryanodine receptors and by signals interacting with the ryanodine receptor, such as calcium and fatty acid–coenzyme A esters.[66,67] Other molecules involved in intracellular calcium release are cyclic adenosine diphosphate–ribose and nicotinic acid adenine dinucleotide phosphate.[68,69]

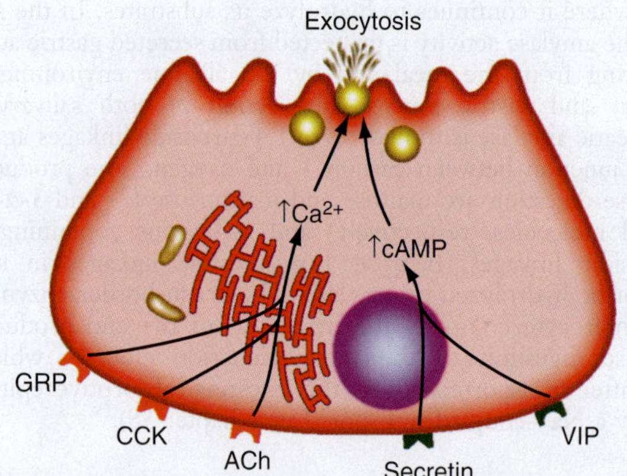

Fig. 58.6 Receptor-mediated secretion. Pancreatic acinar cell agonists that stimulate digestive enzyme secretion act through two separate pathways. In one pathway, agonists such as gastrin-releasing peptide (*GRP*), cholecystokinin (*CCK*), and acetylcholine (*ACh*) mediate secretion through increases in cellular calcium (Ca^{2+}). In the other pathway, agonists such as vasoactive intestinal polypeptide (*VIP*) and secretin mediate secretion through increases in cellular cyclic adenosine monophosphate (*cAMP*). Simultaneous increases in both cellular calcium and cAMP after stimulation with a combination of agonists have a synergistic effect on secretion. That is, the observed response is greater than would be expected from the additive responses of the individual agonists acting alone. (Adapted from Gorelick F, Pandol SJ, Topazian M. *Pancreatic Physiology, Pathophysiology, Acute and Chronic Pancreatitis*. Gastrointestinal Teaching Project, American Gastroenterological Association; 2003.)

The mechanism by which increases in intracellular [Ca^{2+}] mediate secretion is not established but involves calmodulin-dependent protein kinases and actin-myosin interactions, SNARE proteins, and guanosine triphosphate-binding proteins, as discussed earlier. The continued stimulation of enzyme secretion by these agents also depends on the influx of extracellular calcium.[70] The influx mechanisms involve a complex interplay between the internal endoplasmic reticulum and its stores of calcium and a set of scaffolding proteins connected to a plasma membrane channel.[71] The plasma membrane channel necessary for influx of calcium is composed of subunits of Orai-1.[72] The importance of Orai-1 channels is emerging in therapeutics for pancreatitis, as this channel is highly activated in experimental pancreatitis, and inhibition of Orai-1 decreases pancreatitis severity.[73]

The intracellular mechanism of enzyme secretion may also be regulated by 1,2-diacylglycerol and protein kinase C,[74] as well as arachidonic acid.[75] Specific phosphorylation and dephosphorylation of cellular proteins also occur with cAMP agonists and calcium-phosphoinositide agonists.[76] The exact roles of these events in secretion are not established.

ORGAN PHYSIOLOGY

Human exocrine pancreatic secretion occurs constitutively during the fasting (interdigestive) state and is further stimulated after ingestion of a meal (digestive). The interdigestive pattern of secretion begins when the upper GI tract is cleared of food. In an individual who eats three meals per day, the digestive pattern begins after breakfast and continues until late in the day, after the evening meal is cleared from the upper GI tract.

Interdigestive Secretion

The interdigestive pancreatic secretory pattern is cyclic and follows the pattern of the migrating myoelectric complex (MMC; see Chapter 58).[77,78] The patterns recur every 60–120 minutes, with bursts of enzyme secretion temporally associated with the periods of increased motor activity in the stomach and duodenum (i.e., phases II and III). In addition to pancreatic enzyme secretion, the secretion of bicarbonate and bile (secondary to partial gallbladder contraction) into the duodenum is increased during phases II and III of the MMC (see Chapter 58). The underlying mechanism involves the cholinergic nervous system as well as the hormones motilin and pancreatic polypeptide.[78,79] The pancreatic secretion during the interdigestive phase is integral to the "housekeeping" function of the MMC (see Chapter 58).

Digestive Secretion

The digestive phase, exocrine pancreatic secretion that occurs with the ingestion of a meal, is divided, similar to gastric secretion, into three phases: cephalic, gastric, and intestinal. The cephalic phase involves stimuli coming from a meal before swallowing; the gastric phase involves stimuli emanating from the meal in the stomach; and the intestinal phase from the meal in the intestine.

The *cephalic phase* of the exocrine secretion is mediated by the vagal nerves. The extent of cephalic stimulation of exocrine pancreatic secretion in humans has been evaluated through measurement of exocrine secretions stimulated by sham feeding (chewing and spitting out the food). One study[80] indicated that sham feeding stimulated pancreatic enzyme secretion at up to 50% of the maximal secretory rate, with no increase in pancreatic bicarbonate secretion when acidic gastric secretions were prevented from entering the duodenum. When gastric secretions were allowed entry into the duodenum, however, the rate of pancreatic enzyme secretion rose to about 90% of maximal, and bicarbonate was also secreted. These results suggest that cephalic stimulation specifically increases pancreatic acinar secretion, while gastric stimulation during the cephalic phase results in acid secretion entering the duodenum, augments acinar secretion as well as causes ductal bicarbonate secretion. The augmentation of acinar secretion results because acetylcholine (from cephalic vagal innervation) and increased circulating secretin coming from acid delivery to the duodenum are known to act synergistically.

The *gastric phase* of pancreatic secretion results from meal stimuli acting in the stomach. The major stimulus is gastric distention, which causes predominantly secretion of enzymes with little secretion of water and bicarbonate ductal secretion. Balloon distention of either the gastric fundus or the antrum results in a low-volume, enzyme-rich secretion by way of a gastropancreatic vagovagal reflex.[81]

Acetylcholine strongly mediates cephalic phase pancreatic secretion because cholinergic antagonists greatly reduce and, in some cases, abolish sham feeding–stimulated pancreatic secretion in humans.[82,83] In addition, nerve endings containing the peptides VIP, GRP, CCK, and enkephalins have been identified in the pancreas. There are further data to support the role of VIP and GRP in the cephalic phase.[84,85] Both are released into the pancreatic venous effluent with vagal stimulation in animals. Furthermore, as discussed earlier, acinar cells have receptors for GRP and VIP that mediate enzyme secretion (see Fig. 58.6). The ductal epithelium also responds to VIP with the secretion of water and bicarbonate.[85]

The *intestinal phase* begins when chyme first enters the small intestine from the stomach. When gastric juice and contents of a meal enter the duodenum, a variety of intraluminal stimulants can act on the intestinal mucosa to stimulate pancreatic secretion through neural and humoral mechanisms. The stimulants include gastric acid and early meal gastric digestion products (i.e., gastric pepsin and lipase) coming from the stomach.

The intestinal phase is mediated by hormones and enteropancreatic vagovagal reflexes. In contrast to the cephalic and gastric phases, there is significant ductal secretion during the intestinal phase. Ductal secretion is initiated by hydrogen ions in the intestinal lumen from gastric acid. Secretin is released from enteroendocrine S cells in the duodenal mucosa when the pH of the lumen is less than 4.5.[86,87] The quantity of secretin released, as well as the volume of pancreatic secretion, depends on the load of titratable acid delivered to the duodenum. Immunoneutralization of secretin with a specific antisecretin antibody decreases meal-stimulated pancreatic volume and bicarbonate secretion by as much as 80%.[88] The antisecretin antibody also inhibits meal-stimulated enzyme secretion by as much as 50%, suggesting that secretin also has a role in enzyme secretion, possibly by potentiating the action of agonists such as acetylcholine as mentioned earlier.

During the intestinal phase, the pancreatic secretion of digestive enzymes is mediated in rank order by intraluminal fatty acids that are more than eight carbons in length, monoglycerides of these fatty acids, peptides, amino acids, and, to a small extent, carbohydrates and glucose.[89] The most potent amino acids for stimulating pancreatic secretion in humans are phenylalanine, valine, methionine, and tryptophan.[90] The pancreatic response to peptides and amino acids is related to the total load perfused into the intestine rather than the concentration.[91,92]

The mediators of the enzyme secretory response from intestinal stimuli are coordinated through neural and humoral circuits (Fig. 58.7). On a neural level, truncal vagotomy and atropine markedly inhibit the enzyme (and bicarbonate) responses to low intestinal loads of amino acids and fatty acids, as well as to infusion of physiologic concentrations of CCK.[93,94] This finding reinforces the role of vagovagal reflexes in mediating enzyme secretion and augmenting bicarbonate secretion stimulated by secretin.

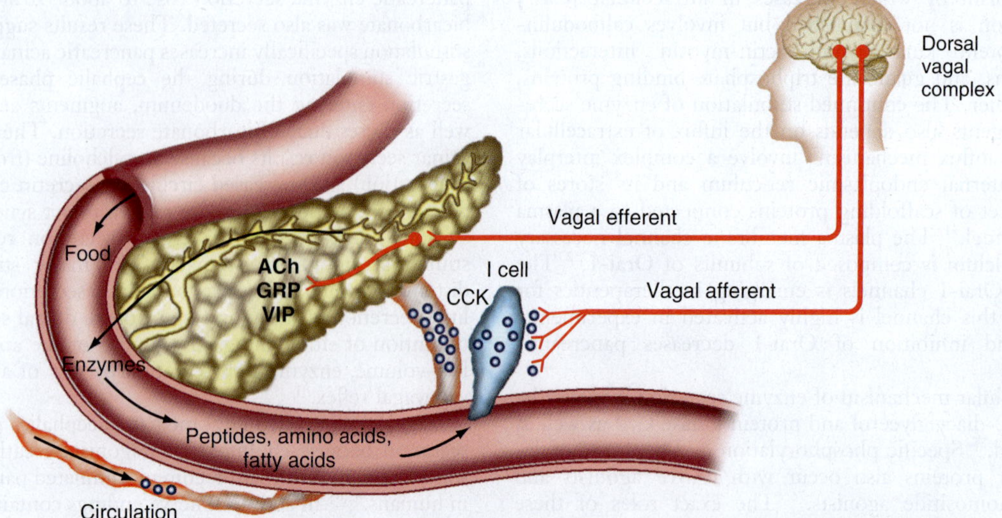

Fig. 58.7 Diagram illustrating the several neural and hormonal pathways that mediate meal-stimulated pancreatic secretion that involve cholecystokinin (*CCK*). First, meal nutrients such as peptides, amino acids, and fatty acids delivered into the duodenum stimulate the local release of CCK from the CCK-containing I cell to the area around the basolateral surface of the I cell. The released CCK activates vagal afferent neurons that transmit the signal to the dorsal vagal complex, where the sensory information is integrated and vagal efferents are activated. Vagal efferents synapse with neurons in the pancreatic ganglia. In turn, via the neurotransmitters acetylcholine (*ACh*), gastrin-releasing peptide (*GRP*), and vasoactive intestinal polypeptide (*VIP*), effector neurons arising in the pancreatic ganglia activate secretion by pancreatic parenchymal cells. In addition to activating the neural pathway, CCK released by the I cell enters the general circulation and may act as a hormone on the pancreatic acinar cells to cause secretion. (Adapted from Gorelick F, Pandol SJ, Topazian M. *Pancreatic Physiology, Pathophysiology, Acute and Chronic Pancreatitis*. Gastrointestinal Teaching Project, American Gastroenterological Association; 2003.)

On a humoral level, CCK is the major humoral mediator of meal-stimulated enzyme secretion during the intestinal phase. The circulating concentration of CCK rises with a meal,[89] and the main circulating form is 58 amino acids in size (CCK-58).[95] CCK is released from the upper small intestinal mucosa by digestion products of fat and protein and, to a lesser extent, by starch digestion products.[89] CCK activates afferent neurons in the duodenal mucosa.[96] These afferent neurons activate a vagovagal reflex acetylcholine that causes pancreatic enzyme secretion, as illustrated in Fig. 58.7.

During the intestinal phase, the magnitude of stimulation varies as a function of type of nutrients and site of delivery of the nutrients.[97–100] For example, delivery of an elemental diet (protein as amino acids) causes less pancreatic enzyme secretion compared to a standard meal, and delivery of nutrients to the jejunum causes less pancreatic secretion than delivery to the duodenum. Such information could be useful for strategies to provide nutrients to patients with pancreatic disorders such as acute or chronic pancreatitis. With acute pancreatitis, the traditional view is that high levels of stimulation of the pancreas can exacerbate the severity of the disease; and in chronic pancreatitis, stimulation of the pancreas can exacerbate pain.[101]

Feedback Regulation

In animals, diversion of pancreatic juice from the intestine results in augmented pancreatic secretion.[102] On the other hand, intraluminal digestive enzymes have been found to inhibit pancreatic digestive enzyme secretion in both animals and humans[103,104]; CCK is involved in this regulation,[104] leading to the concept that intraluminal factors regulating enzyme secretion include the digestive enzymes. After the meal, trypsin and other digestive enzymes are free in the lumen of the intestine and inhibit intestinal CCK release and pancreatic enzyme secretion. One example of how this feedback occurs involves a protein called *monitor peptide* that is secreted by the pancreas.[103] Another is called *luminal CCK-releasing factor* secreted by intestinal lining cells.[105] Monitor peptide and luminal CCK-releasing factor stimulate CCK release from its luminal endocrine cell. It is believed that trypsin, described earlier, causes proteolytic degradation of monitor peptide and CCK-releasing factor when trypsin is free and not bound to meal proteins. Thus, when the amount of trypsin is in excess of its needs for digestion, monitor peptide and CCK-releasing factor are available for stimulation of CCK release. On the other hand, when little trypsin is available, there is less CCK release and pancreatic secretion.

PANCREATIC SECRETORY FUNCTION TESTS

Various tests have been devised to measure the secretory function of the pancreas to diagnose primary exocrine pancreatic insufficiency (EPI) or secondary disorders of EPI due to chronic pancreatitis and pancreatic cancer (Table 58.1).[106–108] EPI occurs when there is insufficient secretion of pancreatic enzymes to digest a meal. Of importance is the fact that there may be pancreatic disease (i.e., chronic pancreatitis) with little effect on function as measured by the tests described here.

Measurements of pancreatic functions have been adapted to use with endoscopic procedures and may include measurements of proteins and protein modifications in pancreatic juice.[109–111] The function tests fall into two general categories: direct (stimulating) and indirect (nonstimulating). Direct tests of pancreatic secretory function involve collection of pancreatic secretions after pancreatic stimulation of one or more secretagogues, a standardized meal (Lundh) and a newer Stallings test, or ingestion of labeled

TABLE 58.1 Pancreatic Secretory Function Tests

Test	Description	Advantages	Disadvantages	Clinical Indications
DIRECT				
Secretin	Measurements of volume and HCO_3^- secretion into the duodenum after IV secretin	Provide the most sensitive and specific measurements of exocrine pancreatic function	Require duodenal intubation and IV administration of hormones; not widely available	Detection of mild, moderate, or severe exocrine pancreatic dysfunction
CCK	Measurements of duodenal outputs of amylase, trypsin, chymotrypsin, and/or lipase after IV CCK			
Secretin and CCK	Measurements of volume, HCO_3^-, and enzymes after IV secretin and CCK			
INDIRECT (REQUIRING DUODENAL INTUBATION)				
Lundh test meal	Measurement of duodenal trypsin concentration after oral ingestion of a test meal	Does not require IV administration of hormones	Requires duodenal intubation, a test meal, and normal anatomy, including small intestinal mucosa; not widely available	Detection of moderate or severe exocrine pancreatic dysfunction when a direct test cannot be done (e.g., due to limited availability)
INDIRECT (TUBELESS)				
Fecal fat	Measurement of fat in the stool after ingesting meals with a known amount of fat	Provides a quantitative measurement of steatorrhea	Requires sufficient dietary fat intake and collection of stool; only detects severe pancreatic dysfunction	Detection of severe exocrine pancreatic dysfunction and steatorrhea
Fecal chymotrypsin	Measurement of chymotrypsin or elastase1 in the stool	Do not require IVs, tubes, or administration of oral substrates	Insensitive for detecting mild or moderate dysfunction	Detection of severe exocrine pancreatic dysfunction
Fecal Elastase 1				
NBT-PABA	Oral ingestion of NBT-PABA or fluorescein dilaurate with a meal, followed by measurements of PABA or fluorescein in serum or urine	Provide simple measurements for severe pancreatic dysfunction	Do not detect mild or moderate dysfunction; results may be abnormal in patients with small intestinal mucosal disease	Detection of severe exocrine pancreatic dysfunction
FLUORESCEIN DILAURATE				

CCK, Cholecystokinin; *NT-PABA*, *N*-benzoyl-L-tyrosyl-para-aminobenzoic acid.

compounds. Indirect tests of pancreatic secretory function are tests of constitutive nonstimulated secretion. They include measurements of pancreatic enzymes in the stool and plasma concentrations of hormones or other markers that are altered in pancreatic insufficiency states.

Which pancreatic function test should be used depends on the clinical question and the characteristics and availability of the test. The exocrine pancreas has a very large functional reserve. Maldigestion and malabsorption do not occur until the functional capacity, as measured by CCK-stimulated digestive enzyme secretion, is reduced to 5%–10% of normal.[112,113] Thus many tests relying on the conversion of an ingested substrate by digestive enzymes to a measurable product will be insensitive in pancreatic disease unless moderate to severe pancreatic insufficiency is present. Therefore the measurement of duodenal secretory products after the IV administration of pancreatic secretagogues provides the greatest sensitivity and specificity. The major drawbacks to the direct tests are the requirements for duodenal intubation and the fact that not all centers are proficient in performing the studies properly. Furthermore, improved imaging techniques for diagnosing pancreatic disease have greatly decreased the use of the tests. On certain occasions, however, direct pancreatic function tests may be helpful for diagnosing pancreatic disease. Importantly, despite advances in imaging, there are still difficulties in making the diagnosis of chronic or recurrent acute pancreatitis, making use of function still relevant and the development of new measurements (for example, inflammatory biomarkers) in pancreatic juice as important potential advances.[110,114,115]

Direct Tests

Direct tests provide a gold standard for measurement of pancreatic function. Stimulation of secretion has been described most commonly with secretin, CCK, or the two combined. The combination provides complete information about acinar and ductular cell secretions. In the classic description, the stomach and duodenum are intubated. The gastric intubation is required to remove gastric secretions that would interfere with the ability to measure water and bicarbonate secretion from the pancreas. Low pH may also alter pancreatic enzyme activity. The duodenal tube is used for infusion of a nonabsorbable marker and collection of pancreatic secretions. The use of a nonabsorbable marker such as cobalamin or polyethylene glycol allows the quantitation of secretions without the need for complete aspiration of secretions.

The direct function tests are based on the principle that maximal water, bicarbonate, and enzyme secretion are related to the functional mass of the pancreas. Historically, the secretin test (IV administration of secretin, with volume and bicarbonate measurement) provided information about the function of the pancreas in various clinical settings.[106–108] Administration of CCK and the measurement of digestive enzyme secretion also have been used successfully to demonstrate pancreatic enzyme insufficiency.[116] Currently, the preferred test is based on administration of secretin IV and measurement of the peak bicarbonate concentration in pancreatic fluid over a 45–60 minute interval using endoscopic suctioning of the pancreatic secretions.[111,117–119] The dose of synthetic secretin (SecroFlo, ChiRhoClin, Inc.) is 0.2 μg/kg injected over 1 minute. Measurements of bicarbonate concentrations are made in collections over 15-minute periods for 1 hour. Amylase, trypsin, chymotrypsin, and lipase can also be measured.[116,120–122] Development of measures on inflammatory markers will likely be valuable to determine the presence or absence of inflammation in the pancreas when function is normal.

Adaptations of direct secretory tests to upper endoscopy also have been described.[101,109,110] At the time of endoscopy, either secretin, CCK, or the combination is administered IV, and pancreatic secretions are collected via the endoscope positioned in the duodenum.

Of note, historically, administration of a defined meal called the Lundh test meal[123] followed by aspiration from the intubated duodenum for measurement of digestive enzyme concentration was used for investigating pancreatic function. This method has been supplanted by the direct tests listed above.

Measurement of Fecal Fat

Steatorrhea occurs when stimulated lipase output drops to less than 5%–10% of normal.[112] Thus measurement of fat in the stools collected for 72 hours in a subject ingesting a diet adequate in fat (70–100 g/day) is considered an effective means of diagnosing steatorrhea. Normally 7% or less of ingested fat appears in the stool. A simple qualitative microscopic examination of a single stool for oil is almost as sensitive as quantitative measurements for fat.[106,124]

Measurement of Fecal Chymotrypsin and Elastase 1

Fecal chymotrypsin measurements have been used as an indirect test of pancreatic function for many years, especially to establish pancreatic insufficiency in patients with CF.[106,108] Such measurements are about 85% sensitive in patients with advanced pancreatic dysfunction but are relatively insensitive in patients with mild to moderate disease.

Fecal pancreatic elastase 1 measurement is widely used in clinical practice and is abnormal in patients with pancreatic insufficiency. Of note, fecal elastase 1 measurements correlate with fecal fat output only in severe pancreatic exocrine insufficiency[125]; and may be normal in patients with mild or moderate pancreatic disease from chronic pancreatitis.[126–128]

Other Tests

Other indirect (nonstimulating) tests have been developed for measuring efficacy of digestion by orally administering substrates that yield measurable products in the blood or urine after ingestion. Two listed in Table 58.1 are NBT-PABA and fluorescein dilaurate. As indicated in Table 58.1, these tests only detect severe EPI.

In sum, several of the tests described here are able to detect severe pancreatic disease with pancreatic exocrine insufficiency and steatorrhea. However, only the direct tests have the capability of identifying patients with milder forms of pancreatic disease. Recent endoscopic adaptations allow improvements in direct function testing. Moreover, advances will be made in specific measurements of inflammatory proteins and protein modifications that occur in pancreatitis.

Full references for this chapter can be found at https://ebooks.health.elsevier.com.

59 Genetic Disorders of the Pancreas and Pancreatic Disorders in Childhood

David C. Whitcomb

IN THIS CHAPTER

BACKGROUND

Clinical implications: Acute pancreatitis (AP), recurrent AP (RAP), chronic pancreatitis (CP), and complications of fibrosis, exocrine pancreatic insufficiency (EPI), diabetes mellitus, chronic pain syndromes, and pancreatic cancer (PC) are strongly influenced by genetic variants. Mendelian disorders such as hereditary pancreatitis (HP) and cystic fibrosis (CF) are rare. The vast majority of cases are "complex" with combinations of factors affecting susceptibility, severity, and progression. The key concepts are that (1) AP is very hard to predict, (2) the majority of management decisions should be made after the onset of the **first** (sentinel) AP event (SAPE) using genetics and other factors, and (3) the goals are to determine which specialized cell types (e.g., acinar cell, duct cell, and islet cell) are genetically dysfunctional and require targeted treatment to prevent ongoing injury and progression to end-stage CP with complications that cannot be reversed. The process of breaking a complex chronic disease down into the component parts, determining the underlying cause of pathogenic signs and symptoms, and focusing treatment on the causative problem rather than downstream symptoms is called "precision medicine."

The new paradigm of *precision medicine* provides a robust framework for understanding pancreatic diseases and leads to new insights into disease mechanisms. This framework has resulted in a series of breakthroughs in clinical and translational sciences, primarily related to rare diseases (e.g., CF) and cancer (focusing on tumor genetics). Little progress has been made in the practical application of precision medicine to manage complex chronic diseases—except for pancreatitis.

The first step in addressing the problem of CP was to change the definition. The new, internationally accepted *mechanistic definition* of CP that facilitates precision medicine is that it defines the essential process of the disorder rather than just describing end-stage features.[1] Waiting until the "pathologic" diagnosis of irreversible disease provides little guidance for targeted treatments and leaves only supportive therapies aimed at replacing lost function (e.g., giving oral pancreatic digestive enzymes to treat maldigestion and insulin for diabetes).[2] Thus a new paradigm is required to improve management of pancreatic diseases by making an early diagnosis of the CP process and targeting the underlying mechanisms to *maintain* normal function and *prevent* end-stage disease.

This chapter focuses on genetics as a key component of precision medicine and is predicated on the mechanistic definition of CP. It highlights both Mendelian disorders and complex genetic conditions affecting the pancreas focusing on which specialized cells are affected and which systems are within the cells. The rapidly expanding genetic information has been organized into systems and models and linked to clinical management considerations when possible. This chapter will outline current knowledge of many key genes and genetic syndromes that are known to influence human health. When possible, the discussion will go beyond genetics to discuss principles of precision medicine for pancreatic diseases and to guide the clinician in using genetic data for patients with established, suspected, early, or complex pancreatic diseases.

HISTORY OF PANCREATIC DISEASE DIAGNOSIS AND MANAGEMENT BASED ON MEDICAL PARADIGMS

The traditional (20th century, Western medicine) paradigm was based on the germ theory of disease, where one and *only* one factor causes a specific disease. A specific disease is defined in the germ theory model using clinicopathologic criteria. A disease may be further classified as a *syndrome*, consisting of a group of signs and symptoms that typically occur together to characterize and diagnose the disease. Defining a disease as a syndrome does not require knowing or addressing the causes, the mechanism, the natural course, or the effects of interventions. An international effort to define pancreatitis, and specifically CP, occurred in 3 "Marseille Symposia" between 1963 and 1989.[3–5] Because pancreatic tissue is challenging to obtain in living patients, a more pragmatic clinical approach was developed in 1984 using imaging criteria as a surrogate of fibrosis, known as the Cambridge Score.[6] CP was defined as "a continuing inflammatory disease of the pancreas, characterized by irreversible morphological change, and typically causing pain and/or permanent loss of function."[6] Subsequent definitions and diagnostic criteria followed this approach. However, a clinicopathologic approach provides little insight into the underlying mechanism of CP. Thus after 100 years of research using the "scientific method" as prescribed in the germ theory paradigm (e.g., Koch's postulates),[7] it was conceded in 1995 that CP "remains an enigmatic process of uncertain pathogenesis, unpredictable clinical course, and unclear treatment."[8]

The 1996 discovery that a mutation in the cationic trypsinogen gene (*PRSS1*) caused HP, with phenotypes of RAP and CP that were similar to common pancreatic inflammatory diseases,[9,10] introduced the concept of genetics to inflammatory diseases of the pancreas. However, this concept did not fit into the traditional definition of CP nor the diagnostic criteria of demonstrating irreversible fibrosis. The discovery of additional genetic risk variants in other disease-associated genes further challenged the clinicopathologic framework for pancreatic disorders. These facts, plus new observations described later, indicate that the traditional approach to complex disorders like pancreatitis is inadequate.

Health care professionals and patients recognized many of the shortcomings of the traditional approaches to pancreatitis based on tissue fibrosis detected by imaging procedures such as ERCP or CT. First, the time between the onset of symptoms and disease diagnosis is often 5–10 years or more.[11,12] During this time, the patient may suffer from RAP and progressive pain, undergo multiple costly and invasive diagnostic tests, and may seek radical treatments that may not be in their long-term interest.[2] Second, diagnosis of "early" CP is impossible using imaging alone because the sensitive findings for early fibrosis are nonspecific for CP.[2,13,14] Third, the clinical course, including disease trajectory, complications, and outcomes, using clinicopathologic assessments, is unpredictable.[8,15] Fourth, treatment tends to be symptom-based and not targeted at the underlying problem so that the disease typically continues to progress even while under treatment.[2,7] Because CP is a complex disorder affecting multiple pathways, selecting "fibrosis" as the primary biomarker to define the disease and measure progression is problematic. Specifically, imaging features of fibrosis do not correlate well with pain,[16] exocrine pancreatic function,[17–22] diabetes mellitus,[13,23] or disease prognosis[14,15]—which are the primary clinical concerns of these patients.

A new paradigm is needed for early diagnosis and ongoing management of syndromes such as pancreatitis that are *complex*.[7] Complex disorders require that two or more independent factors interact to cause a disease while the individual factors are neither necessary nor sufficient to cause disease alone. A precision medicine paradigm is required for complex disorders such as pancreatitis because multiple etiologies result in the same pathology, the same pathology results in variable outcomes, and the treatment effects are unpredictable. Precision medicine for pancreatic diseases focuses on underlying mechanisms (rather than case-control associations in populations defined by clinicopathologic criteria), disease modeling, and simulation of disease progression and complications. This new approach relies on understanding the biology underlying a disease, requires the use of disease models that incorporate the relevant biological mechanism within specialized cell types as well as patient-specific variants that may disrupt normal function or response, and seeks to predict the effects of multiple interacting variables under defined conditions rather than seeking to identify a single causative factor to explain everything. Although the integration of useful models into relevant models for applying precision medicine to many diseases remains a futuristic concept, precision medicine for pancreatic diseases is now possible.

The pancreas serves as an important use-case for precision medicine because the pancreas is a simple gland affected by only a few environmental and metabolic factors.[7] The pancreas has only three types of specialized cells: acinar, duct, and islet. Each cell type has one primary function, and the molecular mechanisms are well described. Furthermore, the pancreas is protected from direct contact with most environmental insults because of its retroperitoneal location (somewhat protected from trauma), sphincter-protected duct system (protected from direct contact with the gut luminal environment), and its blood supply (protected from the portal venous blood coming from the intestine). It is also generally protected from most toxic compounds because it does not play a major role in xenobiotic detoxification or clearance of waste products. The lack of strong, independent environmental factors or other agents to directly cause complex inflammatory diseases of the pancreas, such as CP, highlights the importance of other factors such as pathogenic genetic variants and disease modifiers, alone or in combination. Knowledge of the molecular mechanisms, including the proteins, the genes that code for them, and regulatory mechanism(s) within the context of a patient's existing conditions and environment, provides the basis for precision medicine. The importance of genetic testing for multiple genes in idiopathic RAP and CP in adults and children is clinically indicated for diagnosis and management of these disorders.[24–27] Additional benefit comes with the integration of simple and complex genetic findings with clinical symptoms, biomarkers, and progressive stages into clinical practice using new tools and approaches. Precision medicine also goes beyond genetics to consider the individual's exposure to the environment (internal and external) and lifestyle.[28,29] It endeavors to redefine our understanding of disease onset and progression, treatment response, and health outcomes through the more precise measurement of potential contributors.[28,29] Although there remains a number of hurdles to widespread adoption and utilization of precision medicine for most diseases,[30] the new mechanistic definition of CP and associated models now makes precision medicine possible for inflammatory diseases of the pancreas.

Some remaining challenges include the large number of genetic variants to be considered, including disease modifiers, and the expertise of genetic laboratory directors who generate clinical reports for complex non-Mendelian and noncancerous conditions and who are trained in anatomical or laboratory pathology or Mendelian genetics rather than patient care. Because most patients with RAP and/or early CP do not have a single etiology, a strong family history, distinguishing familial features, or pathology, the traditional context for defining and diagnosing the disorder, or for providing guidance in clinical management, is lacking. New integrative approaches and useful tools are needed to benefit more fully from the new opportunities of precision medicine.

DEFINITIONS AND TERMINOLOGY

Precision medicine: Precision medicine, also called personalized or individualized medicine, is defined here as the discipline of deciphering the origin of disorders that lead to a disease and using targeted therapies to minimize dysfunction, improve health, and save money. For complex diseases, a *disorder* is defined as the disruption of the regular or normal functions, whereas a *disease* is a pathologic condition that impairs normal function of an organ or system and is typically manifested by distinguishing signs and symptoms. Acquired diseases of the pancreas indicate that the organ, or system, functions sufficiently for a period without disease despite the underlying disorder. However, the existence of pathogenic germline mutations within protein-coding genes or regulatory regions indicates lifetime existence of an underlying functional *disorder* within specific biological systems that are normally required to perform a biological function under specific conditions. With injury or stress, a system may be pushed beyond a tolerated threshold, and the cell or gland can no longer compensate for the *disorder* and pathologic consequences develop. The more "pathogenic" the variant, the lower the threshold for pathology. The pathologic consequences of the combination of disease-associated genetic variants, metabolic conditions, environmental stressors, or injuries initiate and drive the pathogenic process to *disease*. Thus in the *absence of disease*, the pathogenic genetic variants represent *risk*, whereas in the *presence of disease*, pathogenic genetic variants help define the *disease mechanism* and *disease etiology*.

Inflammatory diseases of the pancreas: The majority of clinically significant pancreatic disorders are complex inflammatory conditions classified as AP,[31,32] RAP,[24,25] and CP.[1,24,33] In addition, there are rare Mendelian syndromes that affect the pancreas in different ways (e.g., EPI), but the stages and management of these genetic disorders generally follow the approach to the more common pancreatic disorders.

AP: AP represents an *event* triggered by sudden pancreatic injury that is followed by sequential inflammatory responses (see Chapter 60). RAP has been defined as a syndrome of multiple distinct acute inflammatory responses originating within the pancreas in individuals with genetic, environmental, traumatic, morphologic, metabolic, biologic, and/or other risk factors who experienced two or more episodes of documented AP, separated by at least 3 months.[25]

CP: CP is a *process* with persistent and progressive pathologic stages that usually begins as AP or RAP and ends with immune system-mediated destruction of the pancreas and widespread glandular fibrosis and atrophy.[6,24,33–35] In older patients, CP may develop without a clinically recognized SAPE. The new mechanistic definition of CP includes the previously well-described *characteristics* of established and advanced CP, including "pancreatic atrophy, fibrosis, pain syndromes, duct distortion and strictures, calcifications, pancreatic exocrine dysfunction, pancreatic endocrine dysfunction, and dysplasia."[1] In addition, the *essence* of CP is defined for the first time as "a pathologic fibro-inflammatory syndrome of the pancreas in individuals with genetic, environmental, and/or other risk factors who develop persistent pathologic responses to parenchymal injury or stress."[1] This definition is linked to a progressive model (Fig. 59.1) that covers a patient's lifetime.[1] The definition also links CP specifically to variations in the normal injury → inflammation → resolution → regeneration sequence of the acinar or duct cells to injury or stressors, providing specificity as to the disorders of RAP and leading to CP. The new definition is linked with a progressive model that includes AP as the SAPE[36,37] and RAP as an important proximal risk factor for progressing to CP. The progressive model also anticipates early CP, which *cannot* be diagnosed by traditional definitions of CP.[2,38] Thus the processes leading to CP can potentially be detected early in patients with RAP and/or early CP *before* the common features of well-established and advanced CP emerge

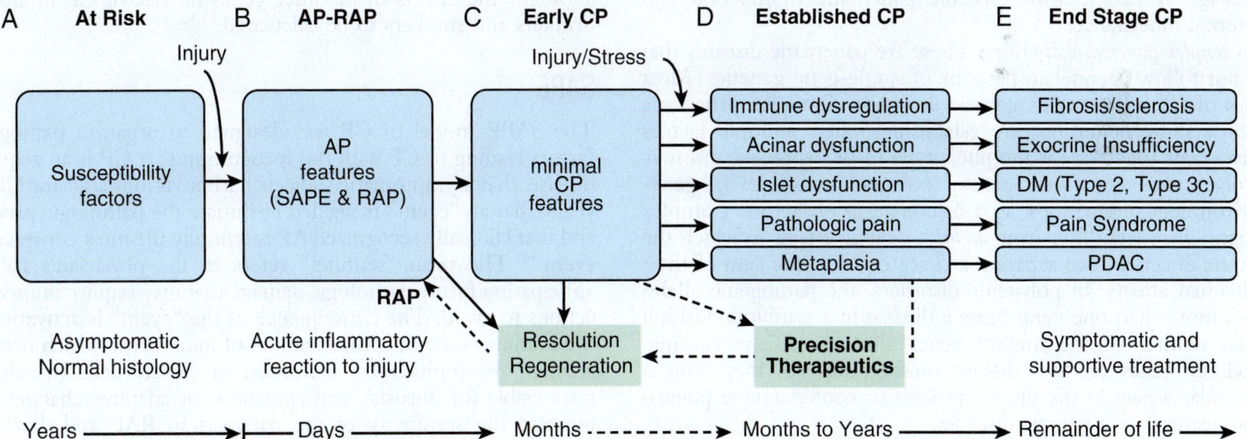

Fig. 59.1 Progressive model of the clinical stages of pancreatitis. Five clinical stages of pancreatitis (A–E) are defined by clinical symptoms and biomarkers of disease. The process reflects normal and abnormal response to the injury → inflammation → resolution → regeneration sequence. The risk of recurrent symptoms within a stage and progression to the next stage is determined by genetic and environmental risk factors linked to recurrent injury or stress. Stage (C), early CP, cannot be diagnosed by traditional imaging criteria, but the likelihood of CP can be calculated using a precision medicine approach that integrates the patient's clinical condition, risk levels, and relevant biomarkers.[2] Stages (D) and (E) reflect persistent (possibly permanent) damage and dysfunction to specific cell types, including chronic inflammatory cells such as stellate cells producing excessive fibrosis, acinar cells, duct cells, islet cells, nerve cells, and metaplasia of regenerating cells. Because the cell types have different levels of risk for dysfunction, the features of CP vary between cases. Preventative and therapeutic approaches are aimed at Stages (C) and (D) (*dashed lines*) where normal function can be salvaged. Stage (E) reflects loss of function and requires symptomatic (e.g., pain management) or replacement therapy (e.g., PERT and insulin). *AP-RAP*, AP and recurrent acute pancreatitis; *CP*, chronic pancreatitis; *DM (T3c)*, diabetes mellitus type IIIc or pancreatogenic diabetes mellitus; *PDAC*, pancreatic ductal adenocarcinoma; *PERT*, pancreatic enzyme replacement therapy; *SAPE*, sentinel acute pancreatitis event. (From Whitcomb DC, Frulloni L, Garg P, et al. Chronic pancreatitis: an international draft consensus proposal for a new mechanistic definition. *Pancreatology*. 2016;16:218–224.)

and when earlier management is most likely to be effective.[2] The new definitions of RAP[25] and CP[1] are not mutually exclusive, and *both* syndromes can be present at the same time.[39] Furthermore, early CP remains an enigma using the modern Western medicine approaches but is the most important stage in precision medicine where risk factors are determined and analyzed so that a rational management plan can be instituted to prevent progression to an untreatable end-stage.

HP: HP refers to RAP or CP in an individual from a family in which the pancreatitis phenotype appears to be inherited through a disease-causing gene mutation expressed in an autosomal dominant pattern.[40,41] Individuals with pancreatitis who carry a gene mutation that causes autosomal dominant pancreatitis (e.g., *PRSS1* p.N29I, p.R122H) but who do not have a clear family history also have HP.

Familial pancreatitis: This term refers to pancreatitis from *any* cause that occurs in a family with an incidence that is greater than would be expected by chance alone, given the size of the family and incidence of pancreatitis within a defined population. Familial pancreatitis may or may not be caused by a genetic defect.

Tropical pancreatitis (TP): TP was previously defined as a form of early age-onset, nonalcoholic CP occurring in tropical regions[42] that is often clustered among family members and that may have a complex genetic basis.[43,44] With growing knowledge of complex genetics, the term "tropical pancreatitis" may become obsolete.

Mendelian syndromes involving the pancreas: These diseases are pancreatic disorders following classic Mendelian inheritance patterns, which are recognized as autosomal dominant (e.g., HP; see earlier) or autosomal recessive (e.g., CF) genetic disorders. They often affect multiple organs outside the pancreas as illustrated by CF, Shwachman-Diamond syndrome (SDS), Johanson-Blizzard syndrome, and others. Pearson marrow-pancreas syndrome is a rare mitochondrial DNA (mtDNA) breakage syndrome with exocrine pancreatic dysfunction and maternal inheritance.

Complex pancreatic disorders: These are pancreatic diseases that do not follow Mendelian patterns of single-gene genetics. Most cases of CP are complex genetic disorders. Complex pancreatic disorders, by definition, are established when multiple factors must occur together for the phenotype to be expressed and may involve two or more genes (polygenic disorders), gene-environment interactions, or a combination of factors. Complex genetic disorders differ from *additive* genetic effects in which the genetic effects at two separate loci are equal to the sum of their individual effects. In polygenic disorders, the pathogenic alleles from more than one gene cause a disease in a symbiotic fashion when neither of the mutant genes alone is disease causing. Modifier genes are not disease causing; instead, they alter a particular aspect of the disease process or confer unique phenotypic features to a genetic disorder.

Models of Pancreatic Biology and Disease

Fig. 59.1 shows a progressive model of CP that organizes genetic and environmental risks and modifying factors, clinical features, biomarkers, and complications in response to dysfunction of the injury → inflammation → resolution → regeneration sequence.[1] Some patients develop evidence of CP without going through all of the steps, but the model still allows for the complex risk profile and probabilities of progression to be calculated in most patients. The model is agnostic to the mechanism of injury or progression through the various stages as long as it includes significant injury and/or stress and inflammation. The later complications of fibrosis, pancreatic exocrine insufficiency, diabetes mellitus, various chronic pain syndromes, and cancer risk are not surrogates of each other but represent disease features of different cell types or systems linked to the pancreas.

There are many independent and combined risk factors for CP, which become pathogenic once the inflammatory process has been initiated (see Fig. 59.1, Stage A). TIGAR-O is an acronym for classes of etiological factors, including toxic-metabolic, idiopathic, genetic, autoimmune, recurrent acute or severe AP, and obstructive causes.[33] An updated TIGAR-O list (Box 59.1) organizes the major etiological factors found in an individual recognizing that most patients have multiple risk factors. The TIGAR-O approach is also integrated into the M-ANNHEIM classification system using a modified acronym.[45]

Alcohol and Smoking

Alcohol use and smoking are important qualitative and quantitative risk factors for AP, RAP, and CP in adults. Alcohol and smoking use alone are not sufficient to cause RAP or CP, but they significantly increase risk of disease severity and progression in the context of pancreatitis—both at the time of symptom onset or diagnosis and going forward from that point in time. Alcohol can be modeled in subjects having or not having alcoholism, by drinks per day/drinking days per week, by a 3-point scale (<2, 2–5, or >5 drinks/day), or by other standardized scales, and modeled over a lifetime.[46,47] Smoking can be classified as never (smoked <100 cigarettes in a lifetime) or ever (smoked >100 cigarettes) and past or current smokers, and quantified by packs per day and pack-years of smoking.[46,47] Use of this approach in the North American Pancreatitis Study II (NAPS2)[48–50] demonstrated that the risk of CP occurs only at or above the threshold of five alcoholic drinks/day and that smoking is associated with risk of CP in a dose-dependent fashion that is independent of alcohol use. Thus the effects of alcohol and smoking are additive and/or multiplicative. The effect of alcohol and smoking differs between men and women, and between people of European and African ancestries.[46,47] Furthermore, the quantification and timing of exposure allow for the effects of modifier genes on risk of CP in alcohol drinkers and smokers to be calculated.[51,52]

SAPE

The SAPE model of CP was designed to organize pathogenic factors leading to CP with the recognition that CP is an acquired disease, that asymptomatic subjects harbor various risks for CP for years, that an "event" is needed to initiate the pathologic process, and that clinically recognized AP is typically the most conspicuous event.[36] The term "sentinel" refers to the physician's role in anticipating future pathologic damage that may require immediate actions to avoid. The consequence of the "event" is activation of the immune system, with attraction of monocytes (which become resident macrophages),[53] activation of stellate cells (which are responsible for fibrosis), and epigenetic or adaptive changes that increase the sensitivity of the pancreas to RAP and drive the pathologic processes resulting in the characteristic findings of CP.[54] The SAPE model was proposed[48–50] as an alternative to the necrosis-fibrosis model of CP,[55] because most patients with CP never had AP with significant pancreatic necrosis. Furthermore, the mechanism of disease in HP[9,10] was incompatible with the protein-plug/lithiasis model of CP.[56] The SAPE model therefore acts as a framework to analyze the effects of multiple etiologies and progressive stages of RAP and CP, as well as investigating differences in pathogenic factors between patients with CP who do or do not have a history of AP.

Multiple cohort studies demonstrate that the SAPE model is applicable to the majority of CP patients.[57] The risk of progression from AP to CP is further defined by environmental and genetic factors.[51,58–61] Thus the SAPE model serves an important role within the progressive model to organize the timing and nature of pancreatitis within the context of pancreatic diseases.

BOX 59.1 TIGAR-O Version 2 Classification of Pancreatitis Etiologies

TIGAR-O version 2 risks classification. The list updates version 1 proposed in 2001 by Etemad and Whitcomb[33] to reflect new discoveries and clarification of older categories. Patients typically have *multiple* risk factors from the list that contribute to recurrent acute and chronic pancreatitis. All contributing etiologies should be documented in each patient. Major changes to the 2001 version include risk stratification according to alcohol and smoking exposure, further definition of hypertriglyceridemia to include genetic risk, limiting idiopathic to age of onset (making *tropical pancreatitis* a historical category), updating the genetic profile to focus on inflammatory disorders that are Mendelian and complex, and specifying modifier genes, celiac disease genes, and hypertriglyceridemia genes. The autoimmune disease classification was updated. The *RAP Severe AP* categories were updated by separating out *Injury subtypes* to specifically include biliary pancreatitis and other extra-acinar cell and extra-duct cell etiologies. See text for abbreviations used. *NOS,* Not otherwise specified.

TOXIC-METABOLIC

- Alcohol-associated
  - 1–2 drinks/day (low risk)
  - 3–4 drinks/day (intermediate risk)
  - 5 or more drinks/day (high risk)
  - >occasional—high risk for progression
- Tobacco smoking
  - Past smoker (intermediate risk)
  - Current smoker (high risk for susceptibility and progression)
- Hypercalcemia
  - Hyperparathyroidism
  - Other NOS
- Hypertriglyceridemia
  - Clinical diagnosis—sporadic or genetics unknown (see below)
- Chronic renal failure
- Medications (see Box 59.2 and Chapters 60 and 61)
- Toxins
  - Oxidative stress-generating
  - Organotin compounds (e.g., DBTC)
  - Other, NOS
- Other
  - Postirradiation
  - Other, NOS

IDIOPATHIC

- Early onset (<35 years of age)
- Late onset (≥35 years of age)
- Tropical (obsolete)
  - Tropical calcific pancreatitis
  - Fibrocalculous pancreatic diabetes
  - Other, NOS

GENETIC

- Suspected (No or limited genotyping available)
- Autosomal dominant (Mendelian inheritance)
  - *PRSS1* mutations (hereditary pancreatitis)
  - Carboxyl ester lipase (*CEL*)—MODY 8 phenotype
  - Other, NOS
- Autosomal recessive (Mendelian inheritance)
  - *CFTR,* 2 severe variants in *trans* (cystic fibrosis)
  - *CFTR,* <2 severe variants in *trans* (CFTR-RD)
  - *SPINK1* 2 pathogenic variants in *trans*
  - Other, NOS
- Complex genetics—any disease mechanism not included above:
  - with pathogenic calcium-sensing receptor *(CASR)* variants
  - with pathogenic *CEL* variants (non-MODY 8)
  - with pathogenic *CFTR* variants
  - with pathogenic *CTRC* variants
  - with pathogenic *SPINK1* variants
  - Other, NOS
- Modifier genes (pathogenic-linked variants)
  - *CLDN2*
  - *SLC26A9*
  - *GGT1*
  - *ABO*—B blood type
  - Celiac disease-associated pathogenic variant
  - Other, NOS
- Hypertriglyceridemia syndromes (pathogenic-linked variants)
  - *LPL*—lipoprotein lipase deficiency
  - *APOC2*—Apolipoprotein C-II deficiency
  - Other familial chylomicronemia syndrome (FCS)
  - Multifactorial chylomicronemia syndrome (MCS)
  - Other, NOS
- Rare, nonneoplastic pancreatic genetic variant-associated syndromes
  - Shwachman-Diamond syndrome
  - Johanson-Blizzard syndrome
  - Mitochondrial, including Pearson marrow-pancreas syndrome
  - Other, NOS

AUTOIMMUNE PANCREATITIS (AIP) AND IMMUNE DISEASES-ASSOCIATED

- Isolated autoimmune chronic pancreatitis
  - AIP type I (isolated to pancreas)
  - AIP type II
- Immune system disorders associated with pancreatitis
  - IgG4-related disease (including AIP type I).
  - Crohn disease–associated pancreatitis
  - Ulcerative–associated pancreatitis

RECURRENT AND SEVERE ACUTE PANCREATITIS

- Recurrent acute pancreatitis
- Postnecrotic (severe acute pancreatitis)
- Injury subtypes
  - Biliary pancreatitis
  - Traumatic—*with* pancreatic necrosis
  - Ischemic or perioperative
  - Vascular diseases
  - Undetermined, or NOS

OBSTRUCTIVE

- Pancreas divisum
- Sphincter of Oddi dysfunction or stricture
- Main duct pancreatic stones
- Widespread pancreatic calcifications
- Localized mass (excluding desmoplastic reactions)
- Duct strictures—including traumatic without pancreatic necrosis
- Preampullary duodenal wall cysts
- Other, NOS

(Modifications by Whitcomb, 2018).

The Acinus: An Exocrine Pancreas Functional Unit Model

Although physicians typically view the exocrine pancreas as a unit, the etiology and mechanism of pancreatitis generally begin within either the acinar cell or duct. The distinction is important for targeting treatments and developing management plans.

The acinar and duct cells are organized in functional units called acini (the plural of acinus) (see Chapter 57). A simplified model of the acinus and duct is given in Fig. 59.2. An acinus (top) is a local organization of acinar cells with the apical membrane facing the lumen at the most upstream part of the pancreatic duct. The duct (bottom) is an organization of duct cells to form a tube that extends from the center of each acini to the lumen of the duodenum. The nerves, blood vessels, islets, immune cells, and supportive tissue, which are important for various aspects of complex pancreatic disease, are not shown here because the initiation of AP originates within the context of Fig. 59.2. Many of these factors affecting the acinar cell or duct interact with each other as a complex, disease susceptibility mechanism with different combinations of risk factors in different subjects.

Acinar Cell Dysfunction and Disease

The acinar cells make up the bulk of the parenchymal mass and are responsible for most of the inflammatory diseases of the pancreas, either directly or indirectly, as their products are the primary contributor to duct content. The principal function of the pancreatic acinar cell is to synthesize and secrete pancreatic digestive enzymes (see Chapter 58). The process includes the synthesis of a range of pancreatic proenzyme proteins (zymogens) in the rough endoplasmic reticulum (RER), transportation of the properly folded proteins to the Golgi apparatus for sorting and packaging in zymogen vesicles, vesicular trafficking of the zymogens to the apex, and apical secretion of the zymogens into the pancreatic ducts (Fig. 59.3). The process requires large amounts of energy for protein synthesis and transport of ions, such as calcium, from one compartment to another.

The maintenance of low calcium concentrations within the acinar cells is critical to protecting them from premature trypsinogen activation. Acinar cell calcium can rise through neurohormonal hyperstimulation[62,63]; high extracellular calcium concentrations[64]; bile acid reflux, which opens apical membrane calcium pathways[65,66]; prolonged, high-dose alcohol consumption, which lowers the threshold for stimulation-induced AP[67]; mitochondrial damage[68]; and other factors that regulate intracellular calcium.[69] Any process that increases acinar cell calcium will predispose to AP through a calcium-dependent trypsinogen activation and stabilization mechanism.[69]

Trypsin-Dependent Pancreatitis Pathway

AP can be triggered and driven to CP from within the acinar cell by several mechanisms.[70] Trypsinogen is synthesized in the pancreatic acinar cell as an inactive pancreatic digestive enzyme

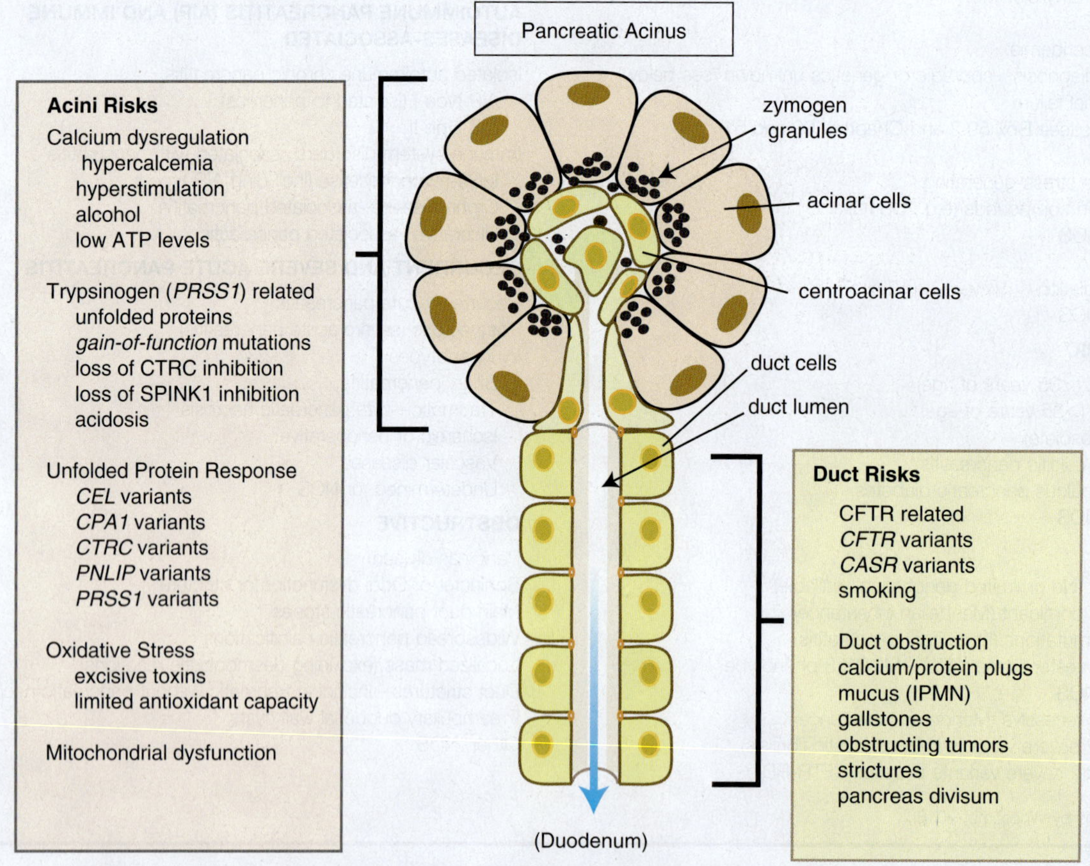

Fig. 59.2 Pancreatic acinus. A model acinus is outlined demonstrating the relationship between the individual acinar cells with zymogen granules at the apical membrane, and the duct cells forming the ducts that eventually lead to the duodenum. Centroacinar cells have duct-cell physiology but reside within the acini. Pancreatitis risk can generally be assigned to the acini (*left side list*) or duct (*right side list*). *IPMN*, Intraductal papillary mucinous neoplasm; for other abbreviations, see text. (Illustration courtesy David C Whitcomb.)

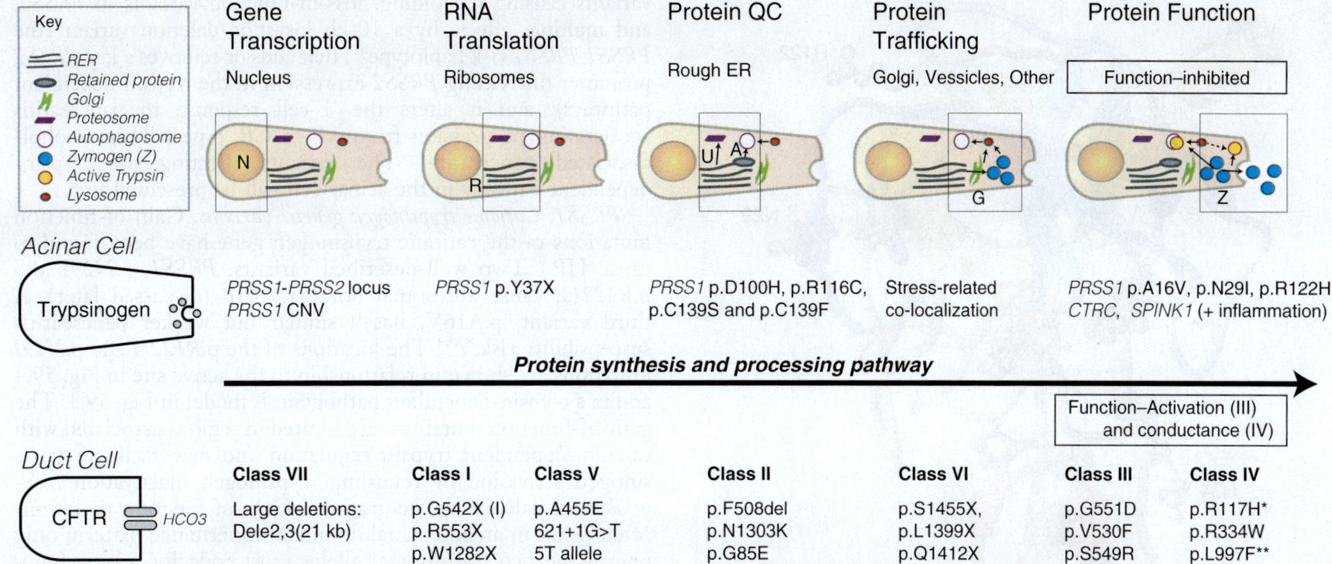

Fig. 59.3 Trypsinogen and CFTR synthesis in acinar and duct cells, respectively, with locations of gene mutation effects. *Key*; subcellular compartments. *Top row*: General cell processes occurring within specific compartments. *Second row*: Depiction of an acinar cell indicating the subcellular location of various compartments and activities that are paralleled in the duct cell (not shown). *Third row*: Acinar cell biology. *Gene transcription* generates RNA. *PRSS1-PRSS2* promoter variant decreases gene transcription, whereas copy number variants (*CNV*) increase the number of transcripts. *Gene translation* occurs in the ribosomes (*R*) and rough endoplasmic reticulum (*RER*). Truncation mutations (*X*) result in failed translation of RNA to protein in the RER. *Protein quality control (Protein QC)* detects defective or unfolded proteins that are ubiquitinated (*U*) and transferred to the proteasome for recycling into amino acids. If the proteins form complex aggregates that obstruct the RER, the obstructed section of RER is excised and undergoes autophagy (*A*). Protein trafficking begins in the Golgi and continues with zymogen granules (*Z*). Trypsinogen can be activated to trypsin with missorting of molecules, fusion of zymogen granules with lysosomes (*L*), or stress conditions, especially with gain-of-function *PRSS1* mutations [active trypsin (*yellow* vacuole) within a zymogen granule or mixed compartment]. CTRC and SPINK1 are synthesized and sorted with trypsinogen and provide protection from trypsin. SPINK1 is upregulated with stress to provide additional protection. *Protein function* is normally delayed until the zymogens are released from the acinar cell and transported to the duodenum. *Fourth row*: Duct cell biology. *CFTR* variants are organized by function groups (classes I–VII) rather than the subcellular location of altered processing. A new class VII was recently proposed[199] for variants resulting in no (or reduced) RNA transcription. Nonsense and splice site variants disrupt translation into functional proteins either completely (class I) or partially (class V). Nonsynonymous amino acid substitutions causing misfolding and clearance from the RER are typically class II. Some variants alter aspects of trafficking and retention on the apical membrane as class VI variants. Some variants result in CFTR molecules on the apical surface that are either nonfunctional (class III) or have diminished function to anion conductance in general, bicarbonate (**), or both (*). (Illustration courtesy David C. Whitcomb.)

(zymogen). Trypsinogen is activated by cleaving a small "trypsin activation peptide" from the N-terminus of the protein which normally happens after the zymogens are delivered to the duodenum, but pathologically it can be activated inside the pancreas. **Trypsin is a key to triggering AP**. Trypsin is the master digestive enzyme because it activates itself and all the other zymogens to their active form (see Chapter 58). Activation of digestive enzymes within the pancreas leads to autodigestion, the release of immune-activating molecules, and direct cross-activation of components of the immune system further amplifying the immune response to injury.[37,71] The importance of trypsin in causing AP is illustrated by genetically engineered trypsin "knockout" mice that are resistant to experimental AP.[72] Thus minimizing generation of uncontrolled trypsin activity within the pancreas is critical to protecting the patient from AP. Determining the etiology and preventing recurrence is a key to managing patients with AP and potentially RAP.[70]

Cationic trypsinogen (*PRSS1*) is the major form of trypsinogen (≈65%) followed by anionic trypsinogen (*PRSS2*, ≈30%) and mesotrypsin (*PRSS3*, ≈5%). The trypsinogen molecule has two globular domains linked by a single connecting chain (Fig. 59.4). Activation of trypsinogen normally occurs when enterokinase or trypsin cleave an 8 amino acid peptide, the trypsinogen activation peptide (not shown), from trypsinogen to form trypsin.

Trypsinogen also has two sites that allow it to be digested by proteolytic enzymes. Trypsin can be digested by cleavage at the Arg122-Val123 peptide bond by another trypsin molecule or at the Leu81-Glu82 peptide bond by another digestive enzyme, chymotrypsin C (CTRC).[73,74]

The trypsinogen molecule also has two calcium-binding pockets that determine if the trypsinogen molecule will be activated by trypsin (in high calcium concentrations) or destroyed by trypsin (in low calcium concentrations). Thus local calcium concentrations serve as a critical switch between trypsin activation and inactivation.[75]

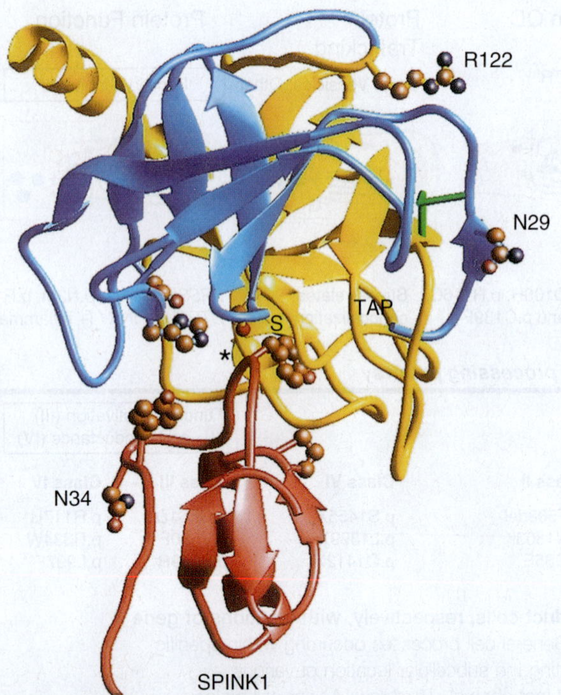

Fig. 59.4 X-ray crystallography-based model of cationic trypsinogen (PRSS1) and pancreatic secretory trypsin inhibitor (*SPINK1*). The cationic trypsinogen molecule contains two globular domains (*blue and yellow*) joined by a connecting side chain (*top of drawing*). Trypsinogen is activated to trypsin with cleavage of trypsinogen activation peptide (*TAP*), allowing a 3D conformational change, opening of the specificity pocket (S), and high-efficiency enzyme activity at the active site (*). The locations of the two major *PRSS1* mutations (*N29, R122*) associated with hereditary pancreatitis are illustrated. Note the location of R122 in the side chain connecting the two (*blue and yellow*) globular domains of trypsinogen. The SPINK1 molecule (*red*) is shown bound to trypsin. The location of the major *SPINK1* mutation associated with idiopathic and familial pancreatitis, N34, is illustrated. (Courtesy Drs. Andrew Brunskill and William Furey.)

Trypsinogen can be prematurely activated to trypsin by autoactivation (facilitated by elevated calcium and lower cell pH), by another trypsin, by other enzymes in other cellular compartments (e.g., lysosomes), and/or other mechanisms.[76–78] Furthermore, multiple mechanisms of controlling trypsin activity in the wrong place at the wrong time have been deduced based on studies of humans with idiopathic RAP, cell biology studies, animal models, and in vitro experiments.

AP occurs when more trypsin is generated inside the pancreas than the protective mechanism can control. Deficiency in any of the protective mechanism makes it easier for an injury or intracellular stress to cause pancreatitis. The genetic variants that either increase trypsin activation or retard inactivation are grouped into the trypsin-dependent pancreatitis pathway.[37,79–81] One group of factors normally controls trypsin inside the acinar cell, while another controls trypsin inside the duct. Here we focus on the acinar cell mechanisms (see Fig. 59.3).

While uncontrolled intrapancreatic trypsin is clearly the proximal cause of AP, the genetics of the human genome containing trypsin genes *PRSS1* and *PRSS2* is complex, and genetic variants in this region of chromosome 7 (that also contains the T-cell receptor beta chain gene complex, *TRB*) can alter risk for AP and CP through at least five ways: gain-of-function variants in *PRSS1*, copy number variants in *PRSS1* increasing trypsinogen expression, endoplasmic reticulum (ER) stress-generating protein variants causing misfolding, loss-of-function variants in *PRSS2*, and multiple effects by a 10-kb insertion/deletion variant (the *PRSS1-PRSS2* risk haplotype[82]) that adds or removes a key *PRSS2* promoter (increasing *PRSS2* expression in the trypsin-dependent pathways), and it alters the T-cell response to pancreatitis accelerating progression from AP to CP, especially in alcohol-associated pancreatitis. The variants affecting the trypsin-dependent pathway in the acinar cell will be presented first.

PRSS1: Cationic trypsinogen genetic variants. Gain-of-function mutations in the cationic trypsinogen gene have been found to cause HP.[9] Two well-described variants, *PRSS1*, p.N29I and p.R122H, cause autosomal dominant HP (discussed later). A third variant, p.A16V, has a similar but weaker pancreatitis susceptibility risk.[83,84] The locations of the p.*R122H* and p.*N29I* mutations are shown in relationship to the active site in Fig. 59.4 and in a trypsin-dependent pathogenesis model in Fig. 59.3. The gain-of-function mutations are located in regions associated with calcium-dependent trypsin regulation and may facilitate trypsinogen activation or retarding trypsinogen inactivation *independent* of calcium concentrations. Gain-of-function mutations often result in an autosomal dominant inheritance pattern; only one of the two trypsinogen alleles must code for a superfunctional trypsin to cause pancreatitis, thus manifesting the phenotype.

Three additional lines of genetic evidence illustrate the importance of trypsin in the development of RAP and CP. First, duplication of the *PRSS1* locus results in copy number variants that also predispose to HP through a dose effect.[85,86] Second, a noncoding promoter region variant in the *PRSS1–PRSS2* locus diminishes trypsinogen expression and is protective from RAP and CP from a variety of etiologies that are linked to the trypsin-dependent pathways, including alcoholic RAP and CP.[51,87–89] Third, comprehensive evaluation of genetically engineered mice models (GEMMs) demonstrates the phenotypic AP and CP effects of manipulating the human *PRSS1* gene.[90,91]

PRSS2: Anionic trypsinogen genetic variants. Anionic trypsinogen (*PRSS2*) is a form of pancreatic trypsinogen that is usually expressed at about half the amount as cationic trypsinogen, although this ratio may change in some cases. *PRSS2* p.G191R is associated with protection from pancreatitis.[92,93] The mutation introduces an arginine (R) into a surface loop of *PRSS2*, making it a target for immediate trypsin-mediated degradation. Susceptibility to the destruction of PRSS2 even in high calcium concentrations, which protects the natural autolysis site, likely reduces total trypsin levels and is therefore protective. *PRSS2* p.T8I (p.Thr8Ile, rs62473563) may have a pathogenic role as it is associated with meconium ileus in CF patients, suggesting a more severe pancreatitis phenotype. It is not clear if this variant is functional or if it is linked to the high-risk *PRSS1–PRSS2* haplotype since it is also an expression quantitative trait locus for *PRSS2*.[94]

Asparaginase-induced AP. Asparaginase-induced AP develops in 5%–10% or more of patients treated for acute lymphoblastic leukemia and non-Hodgkin lymphoma.[95–98] Since the rate is not 0% or 100%, there must be specific variables that put some patients at high risk. Some clear risk factors for AP include higher doses/exposure, age >10 years, and obesity.[96,97,99–101] However, multiple studies suggest that underlying genetic risk factors are also important.[96,98,102–105] The most consistent finding has been the *PRSS1-PRSS1* risk haplotype (discussed below).

The pathophysiology of asparaginase-induced AP involves the activation of trypsin (by default) but the mechanisms are not clear. Leukemic cells depend on exogenous asparagine (Asn) for survival, and depletion of Asn by asparaginase results in cell death. The pancreas may be at high risk for asparaginase treatment as Asn, needed for protein synthesis, is depleted.[106] Amino acid deficiency causes ER stress with the pancreatic acinar cells activating the unfolded protein response (UPR) and the amino acid response with upregulation of asparagine synthetase to generate Asn from aspartic acid and glutamine (Gln).[106] Pancreatic digestive enzymes are rich in both Asn and Gln making a rich upstream supply of these amino acids essential to exocrine function. Although the pancreas has the highest expression of asparagine synthetase of all organs, ongoing depletion of Asn and Gln may be a key factor in triggering pancreatitis, especially with the depletion of antioxidants such as glutathione as retinoids and vitamin A.[106–108] Furthermore, asparaginase-associated AP usually does not occur at the first round of therapy, but after several courses suggesting that depletion of key amino acids and antioxidant defense pools must be depleted before AP develops.[109]

SPINK1: Pancreatic secretory trypsin inhibitor gene mutations. The most common genetic variants affecting *SPINK1* are regulatory elements and reduced protein expression. *SPINK1* variants are often associated with a worse prognosis for RAP and CP. Pancreatic secretory trypsin inhibitor [pancreatic secretory trypsin inhibitor {*PSTI* or serine protease inhibitor, Kazal type 1 (*SPINK1*)}] is a 56–amino acid peptide that is a suicide inhibitor of trypsin, which irreversibly blocks the active site (see Fig. 59.4). SPINK1, synthesized by pancreatic acinar cells along with trypsinogen, colocalizes with trypsinogen in zymogen granules. Within the pancreas, SPINK1 serves as one of the most important lines of defense against prematurely activated trypsinogen.[9,110]

SPINK1 expression is independent of trypsinogen expression. SPINK1 is an acute-phase reactant, and serum concentrations markedly rise with systemic inflammation.[111,112] Under normal conditions in the pancreas, trypsinogen expression levels are among the highest of all genes in the pancreas, whereas SPINK1 levels are very low, resulting in a very limited inhibitory potential.[113] With pancreatic inflammation, the expression of SPINK1 is dramatically increased to several times higher than trypsinogen,[113] potentially resulting in marked reduction in free trypsin activity.

The *SPINK1* p.N34S variant is present in 1%–4% of most populations throughout the United States, Europe, and South Asia.[110,114] The variant results in loss of SPINK1 function. The p.N34S amino acid substitution itself is benign but marks a complex haplotype that reduces gene expression.[115] Several other variants of the *SPINK1* gene also have been described.[116] For instance, the *SPINK1* IVS3 + 2T>C pathogenic variant causes exon skipping[117] and is most commonly found in individuals of Eastern Asian ancestry.[118–120]

SPINK1 variants are common in early onset RAP and CP in children,[110,121] in familial pancreatitis,[114] TP,[43,44] and alcoholic CP[122,123] and are often a feature of polygenic pancreatitis–associated genotype.[61,124–126] Thus pathogenic *SPINK1* variants may be relevant to any etiology of pancreatitis that goes through a trypsin-dependent pancreatitis pathway. This hypothesis was tested using multiple meta-analyses on *SPINK1* variant frequencies in subjects classified by different proximal etiologic risk.[127] The strongest effect of *SPINK1* p.N34S was in pancreatitis etiologies that were linked (high odds ratio, or OR) with the trypsin-dependent pathway [idiopathic CP (OR 15) and tropical CP (OR 19)], with weaker effects in other etiologies [e.g., alcohol-associated pancreatitis (OR 5)]. Mutant *SPINK1* will therefore fail to prevent trypsin-associated *recurrent* pancreatic injury. Thus *SPINK1* mutations in an unaffected individual are of minimal importance, whereas the effect of a *SPINK1* mutation in a subject with RAP, and especially when associated with *PRSS1* or *CFTR* mutations, is very important.

There is debate whether *SPINK1* is a CP susceptibility gene or modifier gene, because *SPINK1* variants are relatively common and become pathogenic in the context of other trypsin-activating genetic variants. However, some individuals have homozygous or compound heterozygous pathogenic *SPINK1* genotypes without other obvious pathogenic factors. In these cases, the effects of compound pathogenic *SPINK1* variants appear to be causative (see the "Isolated Enzyme and Other Digestive Enzyme-Associated Defects" section).

CTRC: Chymotrypsinogen C variants. CTRC is a calcium-dependent serine protease that is synthesized along with other zymogens in the pancreatic acinar cell. Functional studies on CTRC[73,74,128] demonstrate that CTRC serves a major role in trypsin degradation and that loss-of-function mutations in *CTRC* disrupt this mechanism. Rosendahl et al.[73] conducted a candidate gene analysis of the *CTRC* gene and identified multiple, rare, loss-of-function mutations that were more common in patients with CP than controls. Importantly, they demonstrated that *CTRC* variants p.R29Q, p.G214R, and p.S239C impaired function.[129] These variants are rare and seldom seen in clinical settings.[52]

The first genome-wide association study (GWAS) on pancreatitis identified a strong association between the *CTRC* gene locus and pancreatitis in patients from the United States.[51] The effect was not within the CTRC protein itself, although the complex haplotype included a p.G60G synonymous variant in the coding region.[52] Although the high-risk c.180C>T (p.G60G) allele is common in the general population (~11% of alleles), it was significantly associated with concurrent pathogenic *CFTR* variants or *SPINK1* p.N34S [combined 22.9% vs. 16.1% (10.2% with no alcoholism), OR = 1.92, 95% CI = 1.26–2.94, $P = .0023$] and with alcoholic versus nonalcoholic CP etiologies (20.8% vs. 12.4%, OR = 1.9, 95% CI = 1.30–2.79, $P = .0009$).[52] A very high prevalence of *CTRC* p.G60G variants is also seen in CP patients from Poland,[130] France,[131] and India.[132] These findings suggest that the high-risk complex haplotype interferes with the normal and important role of CTRC in degrading intrapancreatic trypsin, possibly by altering gene expression.[52]

The effect of the *CTRC* p.G60G haplotype in alcoholic pancreatitis was especially important. Alcohol and smoking generally occurred together, but the frequency of *CTRC* c.180T (p.G60G) in CP, but not RAP, was higher among never drinkers–ever smokers (22.2%) than ever drinkers-never smokers (10.8%), suggesting that *smoking* rather than alcohol may be the driving factor in this association.[52]

The trypsin-dependent pancreatitis pathway also affects children. The fraction of patients with major genetic mutations is much higher in children than adults in the United States.[133,134] The most common etiologies are genetic mutation affecting the trypsin-dependent pathways, including *PRSS1* gain-of-function mutations, *CTRC* expression, and *SPINK1* expression variants.[61] In Poland, the high-risk *CTRC* p.G60G haplotype is very high prevalent and penetrant size with a minor allele frequency (MAF) of 32% (vs. 10% in controls) and an OR of 23 ($P < .001$).[130] Although antioxidant treatment shows promise in preliminary studies,[135] and a diet high in fruits and vegetables and low in red meat or processed meat may be protective,[136] new well-designed clinical studies of target-specific therapy are needed.[39,137,138]

Other aspects of the trypsin-dependent pancreatitis pathway. Patients harboring pancreatitis-associated gene mutations do not have pancreatitis all the time (with the possible exception of CF where inflammation starts *in utero*). Key factors in triggering trypsin activation include high intracellular calcium[62,63,69,139] and low intra-acinar cell pH.[140–142] Alcohol, at high doses, is also an important risk factor for AP and CP,[59,143,144] but recent genetic epidemiology studies reveal that nearly 40% of patients with light-to-moderate or heavy alcohol use have significant pancreatitis-associated genetic variants.[145,146] The mechanism of biliary AP is also linked to intrapancreatic trypsin activation through a combination of blocking trypsinogen/trypsin flushing, increasing intraductal pressure, and/or reflux of bile acids.[65,147,148]

Protein Misfolding-Dependent Pancreatitis Pathway

The acinar cell is a secretory protein factory. Disruption in the production pipeline by misfolded proteins, or stress from misdirected proteins, leads to cell stress from the UPR.[149] The state of cell activation, level of gene expression, degree of misfolding, and propensity to aggregate within the RER all influence activation and perpetuation of the UPR.[150–153] Since this pathway does not include premature activation of trypsin, the patient may develop CP without major episodes of AP and RAP.

Background on protein quality control mechanisms. Protein synthesis is one of the highest resource-using processes of cells, especially in protein-secreting cells. Eukaryotic cells require a huge, complex, and highly regulated system to monitor protein synthesis, increasing or decreasing global protein synthesis based on availability of required nutrients and cell stress.[154–156] Special proteins called chaperones ensure that newly synthesized proteins fold properly, do not aggregate, and go to the right subcellular compartment. Chaperones were first identified as "heat-shock proteins" because they were markedly upregulated after thermal stress, which denatures proteins and triggers synthesis of more protein-folding support molecules. Complex protein degradation systems are also maintained, including the ubiquitination-proteosome system that degrades specific misfolded proteins and the autophagy system that degrades larger protein aggregates and cellular debris. Conditions that increase the amount of unfolded proteins in the RER trigger the UPR that consists of a coordinated translational and transcriptional program aimed at decreasing protein synthesis rates, increasing heat-shock proteins synthesis, and priming the cell for autophagy and apoptosis.

One of the key molecules in the protein quality control system is *UBR1*, a cytoplasmic and nuclear "garbage collector" of mislocalized and misfolded proteins of the secreted protein motif. [157] The UBR1 protein is an E3 ubiquitin ligase that identifies misfolded/unfolded proteins or proteins misdirected to the cytoplasm by recognition of an N-terminal signal and then links them to ubiquitin via E2 and E1 ligases where they are either directed to the proteasome to be hydrolyzed to amino acids or, if they represent larger aggregates of insoluble proteins, directly to the autophagosome for hydrolysis by lysosomal enzymes.[157,158] Genetic testing of *UBR1* as a "pathogenic" independent gene causing pancreatitis finds minimal association.[159] Instead, risk variants in *UBR1* are enriched in patients with mutations in *PRSS1*, *CPA1*, and *CEL* with the co-occurrence rate increasing from AP to RAP to CP.[157] These data suggest that in most cases, the pancreas can tolerate the effects of some mutations in *PRSS1*, *CPA1*, and *CEL* as long as the compensatory protein quality control systems are fully operational.

Recent work on the pancreatic acinar cell demonstrates that unregulated trypsin activity (from a Spink3 knockout mouse[160]), a strong UPR response, dysfunction in the autophagy pathway, and/or acinar cell mitochondrial dysfunction all contribute to impaired autophagy and are major contributors to the pathogenesis of AP and CP for multiple proximal etiologies.[78,156,160,161] Thus microreductionist approaches to specific sites in specific molecules lose the greater picture of pancreatitis pathogenesis arising from milder risk variants and subclinical stress becoming pathogenic when the back-up control systems do not work.

Clinically important variants in the protein misfolding-dependent pathway. In general, the overall amount of UPR stress on the pancreatic acinar cells depends on the amount of the mutant protein produced, the tendency of the unfolded proteins to form large complexes, and the capacity of the defense systems within the UPR system.

Some *PRSS1* gene mutations cause CP through misfolding, complex formation, and retention in the RER. Examples include p.D100H, p.C139F, p.K92N, p.S124F, and p.G208A.[162] This mechanism is shared by other zymogen misfolding variants.

This includes rare mutations in carboxypeptidase A1 (*CPA1*),[153,163] *CTRC*,[164] pancreatic triglyceride lipase (*PNLIP*),[165,166] CEL (below), and others.[149,151] Not all protein sequence variants cause misfolding and UPR. Functional studies are required to characterize this specific type of dysfunction in cultured cells and other models. By knowing the pathogenic mechanism of these specific types of variants, it allows for early detection and possibly repurposing drugs developed for other diseases caused by unfolded proteins.

CEL: Carboxyl ester lipase variants and CEL-CELP fusion proteins. CEL is a pancreatic digestive enzyme that causes pancreatic pathology through several complex processes related to its unique structure and adjacent pseudogene (*CELP*). Two Norwegian kindreds with diabetes mellitus (MODY7) and exocrine pancreas dysfunction were found to have mutations in exon 11 of the *CEL* gene.[167] Studies in tissue culture suggest that the *CEL* variants form intracellular aggregates that trigger a maladaptive UPR leading to apoptotic cell death as the pathophysiology underlying the development of CP.[151,168–170]

About 1% of adults have a recombined allele of *CEL* and its pseudogene, *CELP*. The hybrid gene encodes a predicted chimeric protein of the proximal region of *CEL* and the distal end of *CELP*, including the variable number of tandem repeat region of *CELP*.[171] The hybrid allele is more than fivefold enriched in a population of Northern Europeans with idiopathic CP indicating that it is a genetic risk variant for CP. The recombined allele was not present in three Asian populations.[172] Technical challenges in DNA sequencing have made screening for these variants challenging.

Other mechanism of CP risk linked to the acinar cells.

PRSS1-PRSS2 locus. This is a very important group of genetic variants that are linked together as a unit and affect pancreatitis risk in several ways. Two synonymous mutations in *PRSS1*, p.Asp162 = (rs6666) and p.Asn246 = (rs6667), are in very high linkage with this pancreatitis risk haplotype initially identified in the first pancreatitis GWAS as rs10273639T>C.[82] Ongoing research reveals that the risk haplotype includes a 10.6 kb tandem duplication expanding the GRCh38 reference genome from a three-gene sequencing that includes *PRSS1*, *PRSS3P1*, and *PRSS2* (chr7:142746720-142778572), to that of the alternate contig with trypsinogen genes *PRSS1*, *PRSS3P1*, *PRSS3P2*, *TRY7*, and *PRSS2*, a *PRSS2* promoter site plus many *TRB* genes (chr7_KI270803v1_alt:7 49 409-8 01 557).[94,173] Important implications include highly unreliable next-generation sequencing results using the GRCh38 three-gene contig in patients with the five-gene genome,[173] and frequent miscalls of *PRSS1* rs111033566A>T p.N29I (p.Asn29Ile) HP mutations using the GRCh37 contigs where *PRSS2* (wild-type p.Ile29) was not included in the initial reference contig[94] resulting in incorrect alignment of the shotgun sequences of *PRSS2* exon 2 to *PRSS1* that was interpreted as an HP-causing missense mutation [note false global MAF estimates in ALPHA of T=0.18408, and ExAC of T=T=0.475109 (from dbSNP, https://www.ncbi.nlm.nih.gov/snp/rs111033566, accessed 22.03.23)]. The marked increased expression of *PRSS2* in the five-trypsin gene risk haplotype (which contains a *PRSS2* promoter[94]) is predicted to increase risk of pancreatitis through the trypsinogen activation pathway. Furthermore, the rs10273639 C risk haplotype is associated with highly significant change in expression of 173 TRB transcripts, including *TRBV29-1* levels in the pancreas.[115] The fact that the phenotype is of an aggressive immune response to ongoing pancreatic injury and that the inflammatory response is accelerated by alcohol suggests that the effects are more likely on the immune response than the trypsin-pathway of injury alone.[115] The *PRSS1-PRSS2* haplotype is not "pathogenic" (disease causing) but is a risk factor for asparaginase-associated pancreatitis (above) and markedly influences the likelihood of progressing from AP to CP, especially in patients who continue to smoke and drink alcohol.

CLDN2 (-*MORC4*) Risk Haplotype

Claudin 2 is a tight junction molecule that is coded for by *CLDN2*. Claudins seal the space between epithelial cells, mark the transition between the apical and basolateral membrane, and control the paracellular flux of water and electrolytes. The human genome has up to 27 claudins, which are generally divided into "tight" sealing claudins (e.g., 1, 3, 5, 11, 14, and 19) and "leaky" pore-forming claudins (e.g., 2, 10, 15, and 17).[174] Claudin 2, which is inserted into the tight junction in exchange for "sealing" claudins (e.g., claudin 4) during active secretion/absorption or with inflammation, forms pores so that the tight junction becomes leaky to sodium and water through self-assembling pores.[174–176]

The first GWAS identified a strong association between a large complex haplotype at the *CLDN2* locus that extended from the *TBC1D8B-RIPPLY* genes across *CLDN2* and the *MORC4* genes defined by rs7057398 and rs12688220.[51] The risk allele is prevalent in the control population (about 26% in European, 36% in Asian, and 2% in African ancestries), suggesting that it may be a disease severity modifier. The association with this locus and risk of pancreatitis has been replicated in multiple studies in multiple non-African ancestral groups.[87–89,177] Claudin 2 is expressed in the pancreatic duct and acinar cells and upregulated in AP.[51,178] No mutations in the coding region of *CLDN2* link with disease risk.[51,179] *MORC4* is a CW-type zinc finger protein and possible transcription factor expressed at low levels in most cells, but in high levels in testis and placenta.[180,181] *MORC4* expression in the pancreas does not appear to change in pancreatitis,[51] but further research is needed to determine possible pathogenicity in pancreatic diseases. *RIPPLY1* and *TBC1D8B* are not known to be expressed in the pancreas.[51]

The *CLDN2* locus (also known as the *CLND2-MORC4* locus) requires separate analysis of populations by sex because it is located on the X chromosome. Males possess one chromosome (hemizygous genotype), and females possess 2 (homozygous or heterozygous genotypes). Using the NAPS2 cohort, Whitcomb et al.[51] modeled male risk allele carriers as homozygous (male hemizygote frequency is 0.26) and females who are truly homozygous for the risk allele (female homozygote frequency is 0.07) and suggested that this may help explain a higher risk of CP for males than females. Giri et al. calculated an OR for homozygous and heterozygous rs12688220 risk alleles at 14.62 and 1.51, respectively.[89] Comparing CP subsets by alcohol and nonalcohol etiology, the *CLDN2* high-risk haplotype was shown to be strongly associated with alcohol ($P = 4 \times 10^{-7}$), with the high-risk allele haplotype seen in 26% of controls, 32% of nonalcohol-related etiologies, and 43% of alcohol-related pancreatitis,[51] and with a stronger effect in men (OR 2.66) compared with women (OR 1.71).[87]

The importance of *CLDN2* in precision medicine stems from the high frequency of the allele in most populations and the strong interaction of the risk allele with alcohol. Although further work needs to be done to better understand the underlying mechanisms, these data are useful for risk stratification and counseling of patients with pancreatitis and alcohol use.

Acinar Cell Dysfunction/Failure Without Pancreatitis

SDS gene mutations (SBDS): SDS is an autosomal recessive, multisystem Mendelian disorder characterized by EPI rather than pancreatitis, cyclic neutropenia, bone malformation, and other features.[182,183] A previously uncharacterized causative gene was discovered and named the Shwachman-Bodian-Diamond syndrome gene (*SBDS*).[182] The gene product participates in ribosome maturation, a process critical to many cell types. In addition, mutations in other genes such as *DNAJC21*, *SRP54*, *EFL1*, and others appear to cause a similar syndrome.[184–187] The molecular mechanism of disease and clinical syndrome will be discussed later.

Johanson-Blizzard syndrome (UBR1): Johanson-Blizzard syndrome is an autosomal recessive, multisystem Mendelian characterized by pancreatic exocrine destruction beginning in utero, although milder cases may present later in life.[188,189] Johanson-Blizzard syndrome is a recessive disorder due to severe mutations in *UBR1*,[190] which encodes one of the E3 ubiquitin ligases that is normally involved in removing and degrading various cytosolic digestive enzymes from the cell through the proteasome[154] as discussed above. The clinical spectrum of Johanson-Blizzard syndrome is further described later.

Duct Cell—Related Pancreatitis Mechanisms

The pancreatic duct system serves two important functions. First, it connects every acinus to the duodenum for delivery of pancreatic digestive enzymes to the duodenum. Second, it generates large volumes of sodium bicarbonate to neutralize gastric hydrochloric acid. The alkaline pancreatic juice also protects the pancreas from premature activation of pancreatic digestive enzymes, and likely other protective functions.

There are two general pathologic conditions that link the duct to pancreatitis (see Fig. 59.2). The first is failure of the duct cells to generate sufficient bicarbonate-rich fluid on demand. The second is duct obstruction (see Fig. 59.2 and Box 59.1). Reduction in flow can therefore be caused by low head pressure, high distal resistance, or a combination of both.

Overview of Duct Cell Physiology and Duct-Associated Pancreatitis

Proximal (upstream) duct cells and duct-like centroacinar cells secrete a bicarbonate-rich fluid into the duct lumen to flush the zymogens out of the pancreas and into the duodenum. Gastric acid in the duodenum releases the hormone secretin that stimulates pancreatic duct cells to open CFTR and start secreting bicarbonate. Fluid secretion continues until duodenal pH normalizes and secretin is no longer released completing a negative feedback loop (see Chapters 4 and 58). Duct cell bicarbonate secretion appears to be further regulated by protease-activated receptors on the duct cell as well as by calcium sensors (*CASR*) and other activation mechanisms linked to injury and inflammation (including CFTR trafficking).

Bicarbonate secretion is an energy-dependent anion (chloride and/or bicarbonate) transport system with entry on the basolateral membrane of the duct cell and exit on the apical membrane where bicarbonate is secreted into the duct (Fig. 59.5). Fluid secretion is linked to positively charged sodium cations being pulled into the duct lumen through claudin 2 changes to neutralize the negatively charged bicarbonate (and some chloride) anions.[191–193] The addition of sodium and chloride/bicarbonate increases solute concentration, and the high osmotic pressure draws water into the duct as well. The duct is a *cul-de-sac*, and with increasing hydrostatic pressure, the solution is forced out of the acinus, ducts, and pancreas and into the duodenum.

AP and CP can be triggered when the duct flushing mechanism fails, trypsin is generated, other zymogens are activated, and ensuing injury begins. The best known example of this failure is obstruction of the pancreatic duct with a gallstone causing biliary AP. In addition to obstruction, the pancreas becomes susceptible to AP with diminished secretion that occurs with mutations in *CFTR* or failure to activate CFTR and flush the duct when conditions favoring trypsin activation are present. Environmental factors such as cigarette smoking also diminish duct cell function and reduce fluid secretion, in part by causing internalization of CFTR.[194,195] Cigarette smoking and other environmental factors may also cause mucin accumulation or protein plugging.[56,196]

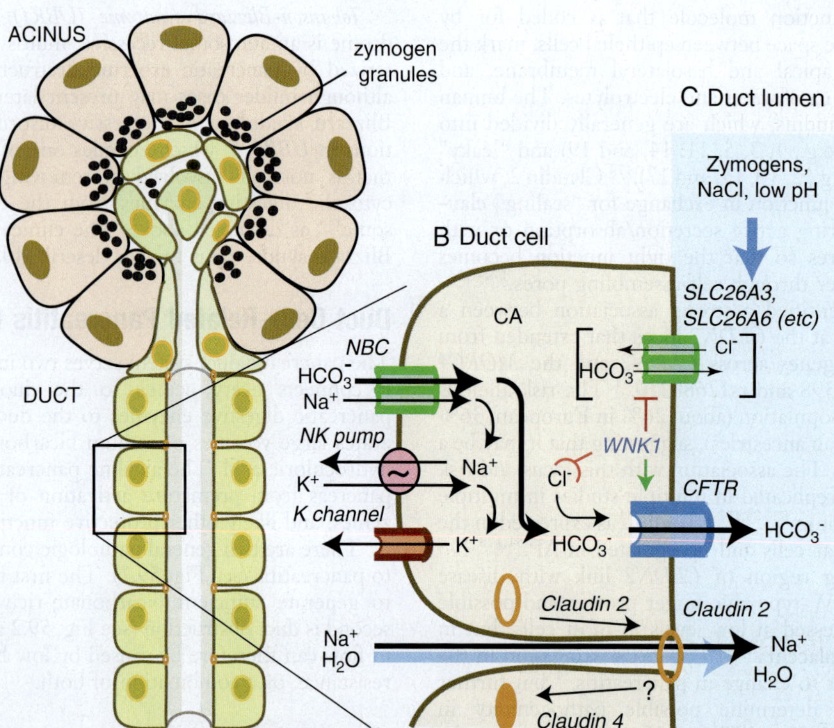

Fig. 59.5 Duct cell and bicarbonate secretion. (A) Pancreatic acinus demonstrating the anatomical location of the duct and duct cells. (B) Expanded view of a single duct cell with key transporters and channels required for pancreatic sodium bicarbonate secretion. Bicarbonate (HCO_3^-) is primarily pulled into the duct cell against an electrical gradient using the sodium-bicarbonate cotransporter (*NBC*). The sodium (N^+) gradient is maintained by the sodium-potassium pump (*NK pump*), whereas the membrane potential is regulated by potassium (K^+) channels. With duct cell activation, CFTR opens and both chloride (Cl^-) and bicarbonate begin moving across the apical membrane (junction of Panels B and C) based on the electrochemical gradients to reach steady-state concentrations. Because the membrane potential is negative (e.g., −60 mV) and both Cl^- and HCO_3– are anions (negative charge), the initial direction of ion flux is cell to luminal. At the same time, it is likely that at the tight junction claudin 4 is replaced by claudin 2, forming paracellular channels for Na^+ and H_2O. Addition of anions into the narrow lumen increases ion concentration and negative charges, drawing sodium and water into the lumen and forcing the fluid out of the duct and into the duodenum. As the upstream fluid is replaced by sodium and bicarbonate, the chloride concentration drops. With loss of intracellular chloride, WNK1 (an intracellular chloride concentration detector) interacts with CFTR to transform it into a bicarbonate-conducting channel and inhibits the SLC26A6 chloride-bicarbonate exchanger to limit further chloride loss. When CFTR closes, the system reverts to resting state. (Illustration courtesy David C Whitcomb.)

Taken together, disorders of the duct produce a "plumbing" problem and require different management strategies from acinar cell-associated mechanisms.

CFTR Genetic Variants

Clinically, genetic variants are important to identify in patients with RAP or early CP since they specifically affect the duct system and can be treated with CFTR-specific therapies. [70] The type of *CFTR* variant and diplotype is therefore important both for CF and CFTR-related disorders.

The *CFTR* gene is the most important molecule for regulating pancreatic duct cell function. Loss of functional CFTR molecules from biallelic severe pathogenic genetic mutations results in CF, which is the only known major Mendelian (autosomal recessive) genetic disorder of the duct cells. The human proximal (upstream) pancreatic duct cells use CFTR to secrete bicarbonate, and there is no alternative—so loss of CFTR results in damage to the pancreas so that phenotype correlates *directly* with genotype. The pancreas is also the first organ to fail in CF patients, and the early CP with pseudocyst and fibrosis resulted in the name "cystic fibrosis of the pancreas," now simply referred to as CF. Milder mutations and complex genotypes that include mutations in CFTR cause CF-like diseases limited to one or more organs and are called CFTR-related disorders, or CFTR-RD.

The CFTR molecule forms a regulated ion channel expressed on epithelial cells in the respiratory system, sweat glands, digestive tract mucosa, biliary epithelium, pancreatic duct cells, and other locations. The primary anions conducted through CFTR under physiologic conditions are chloride and, under some conditions, bicarbonate. The *CFTR* gene contains 24 exons and 3 splice variants that code for a single protein of 1480 amino acids. The CFTR molecule has 12 membrane-spanning domains, 2 nucleotide-binding domains (NBD1 and NBD2), and a regulatory domain (R domain) with multiple phosphorylation sites (Fig. 59.6). Genetic variants causing amino acid substitutions

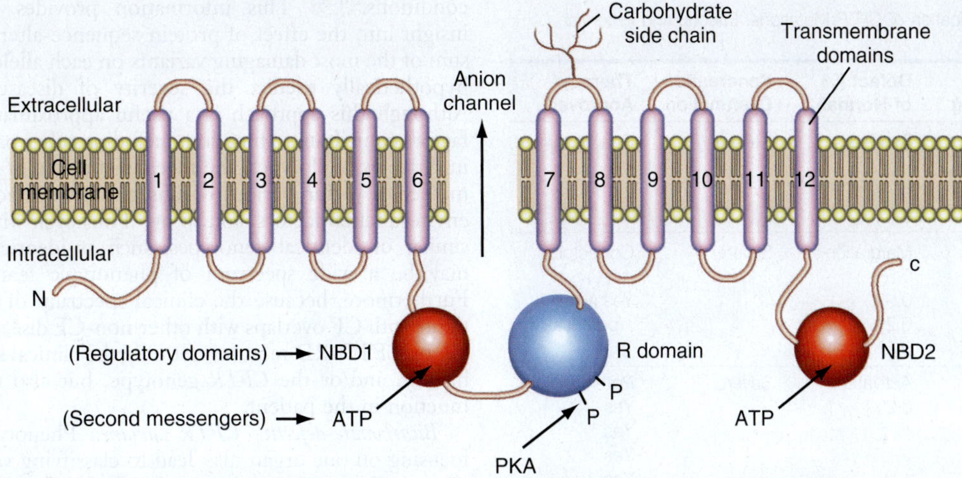

Fig. 59.6 CFTR structural domains. The CFTR molecule is a single peptide that forms a regulated anion channel through the apical cell membrane of the pancreatic duct cell. CFTR exists in at least two conformations (single channel and double channel). The molecule is positioned in the cell membrane by 12 transmembrane domains (numbered *1* through *12*). There are at least three major regulatory domains, including nucleotide binding domain 1 and 2 (*NBD1, NBD2*) and a regulatory domain (*R domain*). Several second-messenger systems interact directly with these three regulatory domains, including ATP and PKA. Calcium, intracellular glutamate, and other second messenger systems or factors (not shown) also regulate various aspects of CFTR. *CFTR*, CF transmembrane conductance regulator; *PKA*, protein kinase A.

within the various domains determine different types of dysfunction, which are further divided into different classes (described later).

CFTR-mediated pancreatic fluid secretion is stimulated when the duct cell is activated by secretin or vasoactive intestinal peptide acting on basolateral receptors that increase intracellular cyclic adenosine monophosphate (see Chapter 58). The cyclic adenosine monophosphate activates protein kinase A–mediated phosphorylation of various sites in the R domain, followed by increased anion conductance (e.g., chloride and bicarbonate) through the CFTR channel. Duct cell stimulation by cholinergic agents or other agonists that increase intracellular calcium also potentiates anion secretion.

CFTR genetic variant classes: CFTR genetics plays a major role in disorders of CFTR function, with clinical disease features reflecting the effect of other factors such as sex, modifier genes, environmental factors, metabolic states, lifestyles, and comorbidities. Although about 2000 *CFTR* variants are known (www.cftr2.org), less than 100 comprise the vast majority of clinical cases of CF or CFTR-RD. In populations with a Northern European ancestry, only about 20 variants have a MAF above 0.1% and with only p.F508del, p.G551D, p.W1282X, and p.N1303K having a MAF greater than 1%.[197] Other populations have much lower allele prevalences for the top variants seen in CF patients, including the United States where MAF in the ExAC and TOPMed databases has the variant associated with p.F508del (rs113993960) at 0.004–0.007, pG542X (rs113993959) at 0.0003–0.0004, pG551D (rs75527207) at 0.0001–0.0003, p.W1282X (rs77010898) at 0.0003–0.0004, p.N1303K (rs80034486) at 0.001–0.002, p.R5553X (rs74597325) at 0.0001, and p.R117H (rs78655421)—important in CFTR-RD at 0.0015–0.0016 (with variable severity depending on linkage with the 5T allele). *CFTR* variants are classified according to their impact on the patient phenotype as severe, mild-variable, borderline, or benign. *CFTR* variants are also organized into one of seven mechanistic classes according to their effect on protein production, stability, and channel function (Table 59.1). Class I variants include premature stop codons that result in a truncated, nonfunctional protein. Class II variants cause defective processing, including p.F508del, due to protein misfolding or other features. Class III variants alter CFTR channel regulation and are considered gating mutations, as the channel fails to open or stay open. Class IV variants affect CFTR channel conductance so that the ion flux through the channel occurs, but at a significantly reduced level. Class V variants alter the amount of functional CFTR on the cell surface due to exon skipping (e.g., the IVS8-T5 allele causing a high rate of exon skipping) or causing decreased stability. Additional classes include class VI that affects protein stability[198] and perhaps a class of germline mutations that produce no RNA (e.g., large deletions and altered regulatory elemets). Classes I–III are functionally severe, and no or minimal functional CFTR protein reaches the cell surface. Classes IV and V are functionally mild-variable and borderline because CFTR protein reaches the plasma membrane but does not function adequately. A class VI category has been proposed that represents rapid molecule turnover at the cell membrane and class VII for variants that impact generation of mRNA.[199] The organization of the functional classes along the protein synthesis and processing pathway is highlighted in Fig. 59.3 (bottom row).

CFTR genotypes: The genotype is a combination of the two alleles at the CFTR locus that define the overall function of CFTR in cells, with one allele being inherited from the father and the other from the mother. *CFTR* variants can be on one or both alleles, and functionally severe variants must be on both alleles to cause CF. If a severe variant is on one allele, then the person is typically asymptomatic and considered a carrier—even though cellular CFTR function is reduced approximately 50%. If a person has three or more *CFTR* gene variants, then at least two of them must be on the same allele (known as complex alleles). Variants that are on the same allele are said to be in *cis*, whereas those on opposite alleles are in *trans*. If there are multiple pathogenic *CFTR* variants that are all in *cis*, then the person is a *CFTR* variant carrier and will be asymptomatic unless there are unidentified variants on the *trans* allele (e.g., class VII) or if they have a complex disorder involving other genes and environmental factors.

CFTR functional phenotypes: Many of the organs that are affected in patients with CF have alternative pathways and

TABLE 59.1 Classification of *CFTR* Mutations, Effects, and Potential Therapy

Class	Mutation (Examples)	Defect (% of Normal)	Pancreatic Dysfunction	Therapy/ Approved
I	W1282X G542X R553X R1162X	Synthesis	Severe	Readthrough
II	F508del A561E N1303K G85E	Maturation 0.5% 0.0% 0.2% 0.5%	Severe	Correctors (+) Yes (with potentiator)
II	G551D S549R S549N G1244E G1349D	Activation 3.2%	Severe	Potentiators Yes Yes Yes Yes Yes
IV	R117H R334W R347H R347P A455E	Conductance 20.0% 3.9% 1.0% 5.6%	Mild	Potentiators Yes Yes Yes
V	A455G 3849+ 10kbC >T 2789+5G >A 621+3A >G 711+3A >G	Abundance	Mild	Potentiators Yes Yes
VI	A455G 3849+ 10kbC >T 2789+5G>A 621+3A>G 711+3A>G	Stability	Mild	Stabilizers
VII	Del2,3(21kb) 1717-1G>A 1898+1G>A	No Protein	Severe	Unrescuable

Examples to illustrate variants in each CFTR functional class and approved therapy in the United States. New therapies and expanded indications are in a continuous development and approval pipeline so therapeutic decisions should be based on the most current updates.

protective mechanisms that minimize the impact of complete loss of CFTR function. The pancreas and sweat gland are two exceptions, where there is good genotype-phenotype correlation. Because complete loss of one CFTR copy has no phenotype, the relative severity of biallelic pathogenic *CFTR* variants is defined by the least severe variant. Thus a person with two severe *CFTR* genotypes will likely have classic, early onset CF with pancreatic insufficiency (PI), whereas a person with one severe and one mild-variable *CFTR* genotype may have a milder form of CF, later age on onset, and pancreatic sufficiency (PS).[200] However, the pancreas is not easily studied, and therefore testing CFTR function in an individual is typically done by sweat chloride testing.

Measures of variant CFTR function: Of the approximately 2000 *CFTR* variants, a clear majority are tentatively classified as severe, mild-variable, borderline, or benign based on the patient phenotype when the unclassified variant is in *trans* with a known, severe variant. The most accurate measure of CFTR protein function is to perform site-directed mutagenesis and test the permeability and conductance characteristics of the mutant *CFTR* in an optimized cell system under a variety of experimental conditions.[201,202] This information provides direct functional insight into the effect of protein sequence-altering variants. The sum of the most damaging variants on each allele (in *trans*) should hypothetically predict the severity of disease in the patient. Although this approach is a useful approximation, many other factors contribute to function, including other pathogenic variants in complex haplotypes, the mechanistic role of CFTR and other molecules within various organs, modifying factors, epigenetics, environmental factors, and so on. Thus even within patients with similar or identical genotypes, such as identical twins,[203] there may be a wide spectrum of phenotypic features or severity. Furthermore, because the clinical spectrum of symptoms in patients with CF overlaps with other non-CF diseases, a diagnosis of CF or CFTR-RD requires not only the clinical setting, the family history, and/or the *CFTR* genotype, but also testing of CFTR function in the patient.

Bicarbonate-defective CFTR variants: Phenotyping diseases by focusing on one organ may lead to classifying variants as benign, whereas they are strongly associated with disease in other organs. Such is the case of a class of *CFTR* variants that are associated with pancreatitis but classified as benign by investigators seeing patients referred for lung disease. Epithelial cells have an internal chloride concentration monitoring receptor called WNK1 that regulates the activity of multiple ion channels, transporters, and pumps.[204] WNK1 directly regulates CFTR, dynamically changing the permeability and conductance characteristics from a chloride-type channel to a bicarbonate-type channel.[205] LaRusch et al.[202] demonstrated the critical role of CFTR-dependent bicarbonate secretion in the human pancreas based on this paradigm and previous mathematical modeling.[191] They screened 984 well-phenotyped pancreatitis cases from the NAPS2 study for candidate mutations in CFTR with bicarbonate-defective conductance (CFTR-BD) from among 81 previously described *CFTR* variants in pancreatitis patients. Nine variants (CFTR p.R74Q, p.R75Q, p.R117H, p.R170H, p.L967S, p.L997F, p.D1152H, p.S1235R, and p.D1270N) not associated with typical CF were associated with pancreatitis (OR 1.5, $P = .002$). The variants were cloned and tested for chloride and bicarbonate conductance in EK 293T cells, and although chloride was normal, bicarbonate permeability and conductance were significantly diminished in the presence of WNK1. A 3D model suggests that defective bicarbonate conductance may be caused by at least four mechanisms (Fig. 59.7). Molecular dynamics simulations suggest physical restriction of the CFTR channel and altered dynamic channel regulation. Because several other organs use CFTR to secrete bicarbonate, the NAPS2 cohort was further evaluated for chronic sinusitis (because bicarbonate is needed for mucus hydration), and male infertility because bicarbonate is necessary for vas deferens development (avoiding congenital bilateral absence of the vas deferens; CBAVD) and sperm survival. *CFTR-BD* variants significantly increased risk for rhinosinusitis (OR 2.3, $P < .005$) and male infertility (OR 395, $P < .0001$). Furthermore, heterozygous *CFTR-BD* variants plus *SPINK1* p.N34S variant genotypes were strongly associated with pancreatitis without the sinus or infertility effects.[125,202]

Sweat chloride testing: Sweat chloride testing remains the most reliable, standardized, and widely available functional test of CFTR function, because normal sweat gland function is directly dependent on CFTR function and because most of the other glands and organs linked to the morbidity of CF disease are relatively inaccessible.[206] The sweat gland is composed of a secretory coil (eccrine gland) that generates an isotonic salt solution and a sweat duct connecting the gland to the skin surface. CFTR and epithelial sodium channels are expressed in both the eccrine gland and especially the duct, where they absorb chloride and sodium resulting in a hypotonic (low sodium and chloride concentrations) solution (sweat) that evaporates to provide body cooling, without the loss of electrolytes. Normally, the

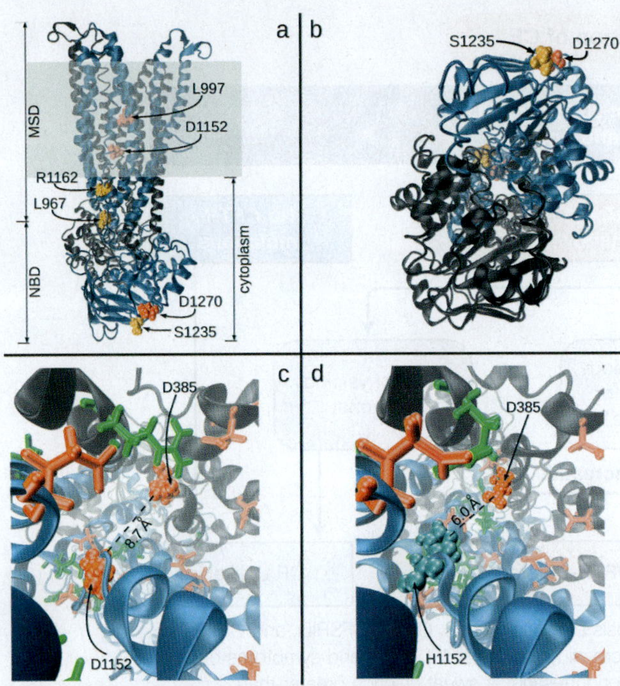

Fig. 59.7 CFTR structure—bicarbonate variants (CFTR-BD). Panels (A) and (B) display the CFTR molecule from the side and bottom with residues 1–859 in *black*, residues 860–1480 in *blue*, the CFTR-BD variants are in *red*, and the *shaded region* indicates the location of the plasma membrane. The various locations of the CFTR-BD variants suggest multiple mechanisms, including obstruction of the channel, altered interactions of the NBDs, altered intracellular signaling, and/or other mechanisms. Panel (C) is the predicted location of wild-type p.D1152 viewed by looking down the barrel of the channel. Panel (D) is the predicted location of the pathogenic variant p.H1152. Panels (C) and (D) illustrate the effect of CFTR p.D1152H on bicarbonate conductance through physical obstruction of the pore for the larger bicarbonate ion. The charge distribution around p.D1152H is highlighted with negatively charged residue in *red* and positively charged residues in *green*. The variant residue in Panel (D), H1152 (*cyan*), can move toward the center of the channel, thus leading to a constriction in the channel diameter. *Å*, Channel diameter at the location of wild-type and variant residues measured in Ångströms; *MSD*, membrane-spanning domains; *NBD*, nucleotide-binding domains. (From LaRusch J, Jung J, General IJ, et al. Mechanisms of CFTR functional variants that impair regulated bicarbonate permeation and increase risk for pancreatitis but not for cystic fibrosis. *PLoS Genet*. 2014;10(4):e1004376.)

concentration of chloride in sweat is less than 20 mmol/L, but levels increase with increasing rates of secretion and can reach nearly 60 mmol/L in some people.[206]

In CF, the concentrations of chloride are three to five times higher than normal, with resting concentrations above 60 mmol/L and stimulated chloride levels approaching 120 mmol/L. Subjects who are heterozygous for severe, CF-causing mutations typically have nearly normal sweat chloride testing.[206] Of note, extensive genetic testing of some patients with clinical CF and with a very abnormal sweat chloride test have only one identifiable pathogenic *CFTR* variant (i.e., they appear to be heterozygous), suggesting that other important factors that strongly affect CFTR function are yet to be identified. Current clinical guidelines for the diagnosis of CF include a sweat chloride of ≥60 mmol/L as well as clinical features consistent with CF (including positive newborn screening, NBS) and/or a positive family history.[207] Patients with features of CF and intermediate sweat chloride test results of 30–59 mmol/L may still have CF.[207] Patients with *CFTR* variants that only affect bicarbonate conductance may be missed by sweat chloride testing.

Sweat chloride testing may also be important in the evaluation of symptomatic patients who may have undiagnosed CF or CFTR-RD. CFTR-RD includes RAP and CP, CBAVD, disseminated bronchiectasis, and sclerosing cholangitis, alone or in combination with other features.[208–210] When a patient with unexplained RAP and/or early CP is found to have likely pathogenic *CFTR* variants, the clinically validated functional test to determine if they have CF or CFTR-RD is the sweat chloride test. The importance of diagnosing CF or CFTR-RD is highlighted by the availability of new therapies that specifically target CFTR function (described later). Although secretin-stimulated pancreatic function testing also measures CFTR function, the interpretation of the results is confounded by the diminished bicarbonate concentrations in pancreatic juice in progressive pancreatic disease and by environmental factors such as smoking.[211–213]

The Cystic Fibrosis Foundation Clinical Care Guidelines suggest further evaluation of intermediate sweat chloride levels as outlined in Fig. 59.8. The algorithm begins with "clinical presentation of CF," which may include patients with elevated immunoreactive trypsinogen levels during NBS in the United States, but who have intermediate sweat chloride test results.[214] This approach may also be useful with CFTR-RD affecting only the pancreas, but the utility of this approach in an adult RAP or CP population has not yet been reported.

Newborn CF screening—CRMS/CFSPID: The vast majority of infants with NBS and an intermediate sweat chloride test result remained disease free for an indeterminate time. These infants have therefore been classified as CF transmembrane conductance regulator-related metabolic syndrome in the United States (the "metabolic syndrome" reflected a billing code issue rather than any metabolic feature) and CF screen positive, inconclusive diagnosis (CFSPID) in other countries.[214] A new unified definition by a U.S./European consensus group defines CRMS/CFSPID as a feature in an infant who has a positive NBS test for CF and either (1) a sweat chloride less than 30 mmol/L and 2 *CFTR* mutations, at least 1 of which has unclear phenotypic consequences, or (2) an intermediate sweat chloride value (30–59 mmol/L) and 1 or 0 CF-causing mutations.[214] The CF-causing mutations are generally defined in the CFTR2 database (www.cftr2.org) with other variants classified as mutations of varying clinical consequence (MVCC, e.g., class IV or V), non-CF-causing mutation when the mutation in *trans* with another CF-causing mutation will not result in CF (which does not exclude the possibility that the mutation may contribute to CF-like clinical characteristics resembling mild CF or CFTR-RD), variants of unknown significance, or benign.[210] Genetic counseling and follow-up clinical evaluations by qualified physicians and further testing are recommended.[214]

CFTR disease mechanism: The medical approach to CF is presented later, whereas the mechanism of CFTR in disease is discussed here. Severe mutations in both CFTR alleles leading to total or near-total loss of CFTR function result in CF. The molecular consequences of CF include inability to adequately hydrate mucus and other macromolecules, leading to accumulation of viscid material and inspissated glands. This condition results in progressive organ destruction of the pancreas and respiratory system, and dysfunction of the liver, intestine, sweat glands, and other sites where epithelial cell secretion plays an important physiologic role. As noted earlier, the pancreas incurs a double risk because most of its proteins are zymogens and trypsin activation will lead to recurrent injury and eventually destruction of the pancreas through progressive fibrosis. Trypsin-mediated injury and destruction of the pancreas in children with CF are consistent with this model because the pancreatic pathology in CF is pseudocyst formation and fibrosis rather than atrophy alone (as

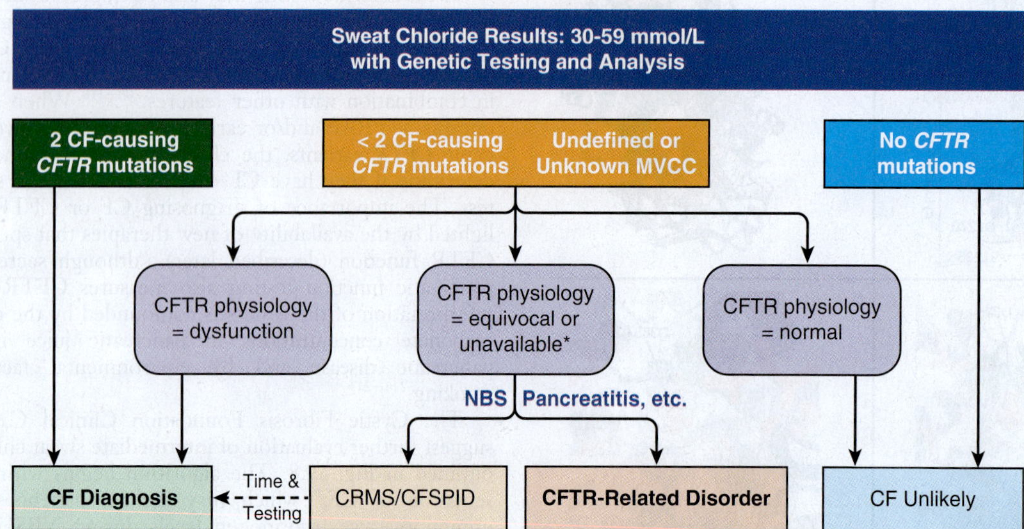

Fig. 59.8 CF and CFTR-RD diagnostic guidelines. Diagnosis of cystic fibrosis, CRMS/CFSPID, and CFTR-RD. Clinical manifestations of CF include positive newborn screening results (*NBS*), signs and symptoms of CF, and/or family history of CF. Evaluation begins with sweat chloride testing. A sweat chloride greater than 60 mmol/L is diagnostic of CF, and less than 29 mmol/L makes CF unlikely (not shown). Sweat chloride of 30–59 mmol/L (*blue bar*) represents an intermediate range and extended *CFTR* gene analysis and/or functional analysis should be considered. If the *CFTR* genetic testing identifies one pathogenic *CFTR* variant and/or MVCCs and/or undefined variants, then CFTR physiology testing (NPD or ICM) is needed to define a final classification of CF, CRMS/CFSPID (in infants), CFTR-related disorder (typically older children or adults), or another disorder that is not CF. Note that CRMS/CFSPID category (*light yellow box*) does not exclude an eventual CF diagnosis because clinical features may develop with time or further testing (*dashed arrow*). The *dashed arrow* is one-way because a diagnosis of CF is almost impossible to erase in the minds of patients and their families. Patients with complex genotypes that include one *CFTR* variant plus another pathogenic variant (e.g., in SPINK1 and CTRC) may be at high risk of pancreatitis but are at low risk of CF and may have close to normal CFTR physiology by NPD or ICM because this measures overall genotype rather than the function of each allele product (classified as CF Unlikely, *light blue box*). *CRMS/CFSPID*, Cystic fibrosis-related metabolic syndrome/cystic fibrosis screen positive inclusive diagnosis; *ICM*, intestinal current measurement; *MVCC*, mutations of varying clinical consequence; *NPD*, nasal potential difference. *See text for clinical signs and symptoms of the CF syndrome. (Modified from Farrell PM, White TB, Ren CL, et al. Diagnosis of cystic fibrosis: consensus guidelines from the Cystic Fibrosis Foundation. *J Pediatr*. 2017;181S:S4–S15.e1. Illustration courtesy David C Whitcomb.)

expected with duct obstruction).[215] It appears that pancreatic gland injury in CF children roughly parallels the expression of trypsinogen in the developing acinar cells, which begins at 16 weeks' gestation and gradually increases in concentration until birth and through the first 6 months of life when levels markedly rise.[216,217] The resulting histology has many of the features of end-stage CP that develops in children and adults but also has striking expanded ducts that appear as multiple protein-filled cysts (Fig. 59.9).

The overall clinical picture in an individual with pathogenic *CFTR* variants depends on the nature of the combined CFTR mutations, the genetic background in which the defective genes operate (e.g., modifier genes), and environmental factors.[210,215,218] About 70%–90% of non-Hispanic white patients with CF have p.F508del. Distinct mutations are common to other ethnic and ancestral groups, including 3120 + 1G > A which is the second most frequent CF allele in African-Americans (9.5%–12.3%),[219] the p.R334W mutation which is common in Hispanics, and the p.W1282X in Ashkenazi Jews (~45%).[210,220,221]

Patients with 2 CFTR^{severe} mutations in *trans* typically develop classic features of CF, with elevated chloride levels in sweat glands, PI, recurrent and chronic pulmonary infections, and CBAVD in males. Complicating manifestations of severe CF can also include meconium ileus, distal intestinal obstruction syndrome (DIOS), gallbladder dysfunction, liver cirrhosis, and other GI problems.

Patients with one severe *CFTR* mutation (classes I–III, e.g., p.F508del) and one mild-variable *CFTR* mutation (class IV or V, e.g., p.*R117H* or p.*R334W*) typically have CF with PS-CF due to incomplete loss of CFTR function, partially reduced chloride and/or bicarbonate conductance, and subsequent residual duct cell function, resulting in acinar cell survival.[191,200] This residual pancreatic parenchyma with abnormal CFTR function leaves a PS-CF patient at high risk for AP and RAP, with an incidence of 22%.[200] These patients are more likely to have only a subset of organs expressing CFTR affected, and presenting symptoms may occur later in life (teens or 20s).

Environment and modifier gene variants: Many of the features of CF cannot be explained by variations in CFTR sequence. Instead, these features are caused by specific environmental factors or modifier genes.[210,215] Environmental factors, such as bacterial colonization of the respiratory system, tobacco smoke, poor nutritional status,[222] *and environmental allergens*,[223] contribute to the severity of lung disease. The other major factors are modifier

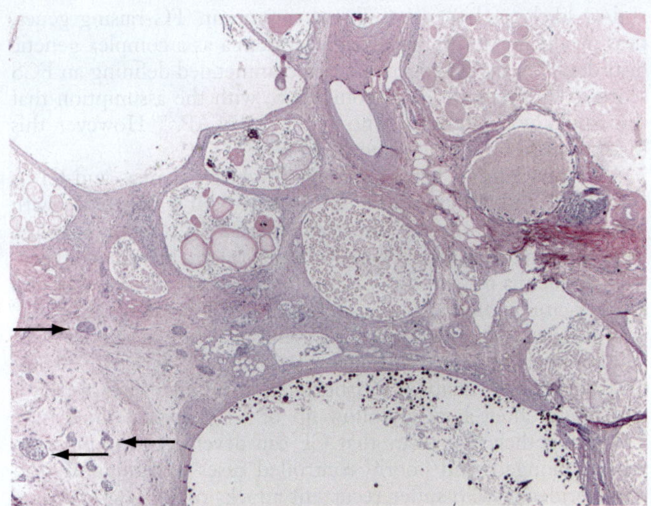

Fig. 59.9 Histopathology of the pancreas from an autopsy of a child with severe features of CF. There are no residual normal ducts or acini. Instead, dilated ducts and "cysts" with inspissated material are seen. Other cases of CF span the spectrum between this image and chronic pancreatitis seen with other forms of pancreatitis, with acinar atrophy, fibrosis, and chronic inflammation. *Arrows* demonstrate residual islets. (From Whitcomb DC. Cystic fibrosis–associated pancreatitis. In: Beger HG, Warshaw A, Buchler MW, et al., eds. *The Pancreas: An Integrated Textbook of Basic Science, Medicine and Surgery*. Oxford: Blackwell; 2008.)

genes that strongly contribute to the wide range of clinical features in patients with apparently identical *CFTR* genotypes.[210,221,224]

In 1998 two groups[225,226] demonstrated that pathogenic *CFTR* variants were also very common in idiopathic and alcoholic CP, suggesting that *CFTR* mutations may be part of a more complex trait.[125,227] Because heterozygous pathogenic *CFTR* variants are common in populations with European ancestry, and because the parents of CF children (obligate *CFTR* mutation carriers without CF) do not appear to have an increased incidence of AP or CP compared with the normal population,[228] it is likely that a second factor that specifically targets the pancreas is required.[37,227] In early onset idiopathic pancreatitis, this second factor may be a genetic variant in *SPINK1*, *CTRC*, or *CASR*, an anatomical factor like pancreatic divisum, an environmental factor, or other mechanism.[120,124–126,202,229] Although high-quality treatment trials for these patients are still needed, the problem is one of "plumbing" and methods to restore lost CFTR function and/or reduce resistance to pancreatic juice flow should be considered.

Calcium-Sensing Receptor Gene (*CASR*) Variants

Calcium plays multiple roles in pancreatic physiology and pathophysiology. On one hand, the regulation of intra-acinar cell calcium is critical for the prevention of pancreatic injury,[139,230] whereas increasing concentrations of calcium in the pancreatic duct increases the risk of sustained trypsin activation and precipitation as calcium-containing stones. The calcium-sensing receptor gene (*CASR*) is a membrane-bound member of the G-protein-coupled receptor superfamily. *CaSR* plays an important role in calcium homeostasis, as is reflected in its expression by cells of the parathyroid gland and renal tubules that are involved in the calcium homeostasis. *CaSR* has been identified in human pancreatic acinar and ductal cells, as well as in various nonexocrine tissues,[231] although its functional significance in the pancreas has not yet been determined. A possible role of the *CaSR* in the pancreatic duct is plausible by extension of duodenal physiology, noting that CaSR is coexpressed with CFTR in bicarbonate-secreting epithelial cells.[232] CaSR activation dose-dependently raises intracellular calcium levels which causes calcium-dependent CFTR bicarbonate secretion as well as modulating other molecules involved in the process.[232] More than 170 functional mutations (activating and inactivating) have been described in the *CASR* related to familial hypocalciuric hypercalcemia, neonatal severe primary hyperparathyroidism, autosomal dominant hypocalcemia, and related hypercalcemic or hypocalcemic disorders.[233] The common *CASR* variants p.R990G, p.A986S, and p.Q1011E are strongly associated with urolithiasis and hypercalcuria in various populations.[234]

In 2003 Felderbauer[235] investigated a kindred with familial pancreatitis and the *SPINK1* p.N34S variant. However, only two of these family members had CP, and both were found to have a novel *CASR* c.518T>C mutation that was linked to hypercalcemia. An association between additional *CASR* variants, with or without *SPINK1* mutations, was subsequently identified in patients in India with TP,[236] as well as in the United States in sporadic and alcoholic CP in which the *CASR* p.R990G (rs1042636) variant doubles and triples the relative risk, respectively[237] (the rs number is given because the amino acid number may change based on the CASR transcript used). Multiple rare *CASR* variants were also identified in a French cohort[238] and the p.A986S variant (rs1801725) in multiple Chinese pancreatitis patients.[239] CASR p.Q1011E (rs1801726) is also widely studied, but a clear role in pancreatic disease has not been established. The finding of different CASR polymorphisms in different populations is intriguing, but it appears that the presumed mild hypercalcemia is a cofactor for pancreatitis rather than an independent risk factor, as seen in animal models of hypercalcemia,[64,240] or as part of complex functional genotypes with *SPINK1* or *CFTR* or other factors. *CASR* variants that reduce CaSR function may also contribute to pancreatic disease because CaSR also serves as an amino acid receptor in the duodenum, linking luminal nutrients with release of cholecystokinin that subsequently stimulates pancreatic enzyme secretion.[241]

γ-GLUTAMYL TRANSPEPTIDASE (GGT1)

GGT is an extracellular enzyme that is primarily expressed and secreted by ducts and tubule epithelia (biliary, gallbladder, kidney, epididymis, and prostate) and the small intestine where it salvages glutamate, cysteine (Cys), and glycine from glutathione in the ductal or intestinal fluids.[242,243] It plays critical role in the pancreatic duct to provide the precursors of glutathione for phase II detoxification pathway. Genetic association studies linked risk for CP and PC to *GGT1* regulatory elements altering gene expression.[244,245] Single-cell RNA sequencing links *GGT1* expression to pancreatic duct cells (Whitcomb, unpublished results), and co-occurrence analysis shows that in patients with AP, RAP, and CP, a combination of *GGT1* variants and *CFTR* variants occurs together more often than expected by chance alone.[157] Thus GGT plays an important role in the duct cell response to stress (e.g., caused by *CFTR* variants), and loss of GGT expression diminishes protection and enhances pathogenesis.

Genes that Modify Inflammation, Progression to Chronic Pancreatitis and Modifier Phenotypes

A number of pathogenic genetic variants have been identified in genes that are associated with the response to injury and inflammation. The pathogenic effects of these variants do not appear to be through causing injury, but rather in altering the response to injury or inflammation caused by other etiologies. See *PRSS1–PRSS2* and *CLDN2* genetic variants above.

Hypertriglyceridemia-Associated Gene Variants

Hypertriglyceridemia is a risk factor for AP, for AP severity, and for CP. Pathogenic variants in the lipoprotein lipase gene (LPL) serve as a prototype for hypertriglyceridemic disorders associated with pancreatitis. Triglycerides (TGs) themselves are not directly toxic, but their hydrolysis by lipases (including pancreatic lipases) produces saturated and unsaturated fatty acids that are proinflammatory and toxic at high levels to the pancreas and other organs.[246,247]

Patients are classified by fasting serum TG levels.[248] The *normal* levels are less than 150 mg/dL (1 mmol = 88.6 mg/dL) with hypertriglyceridemia either *mild* (150–199 mg/dL), *moderate* (200–999 mg/dL), *severe* (1000–1999 mg/dL), or *very severe* (≥2000 mg/dL).[248] The lifetime risk of pancreatitis in patients with severe hypertriglyceridemia is about 5% and very severe about 10%–20%, which is significantly higher than the general population lifetime risk of about 0.5%–1%.[249] While the risk of developing AP is primarily seen with severe or very severe hypertriglyceridemia (see Chapter 60), in practice, the serum TG levels vary markedly with diet, and outpatient levels do not correlate well with levels seen in patients with TG levels seen early in AP.[250]

TG levels directly correlate with severity and complications of AP.

In a single-site study of 400 AP patients from Pittsburgh, Pennsylvania, United States, the rate of persistent organ failure increased proportionally to TG levels, with 17% at less than 150 mg/dL, 30% at 150–199 mg/dL, 39% at 200–999 mg/dL, and 48% at greater than 1000 mg/dL.[251] On multivariate analysis, risk of persistent organ failure increased by OR 2.6 and 4.9 for TGs of 200–999 mg/dL and greater than 1000 mg/dL, respectively.[251] A similar trend was seen among 1539 AP patients in Nanchang, Jiangxi, People's Republic of China.[252] The risk of hypertriglyceridemia AP is associated with untreated/poorly controlled diabetes mellitus, alcohol abuse, pregnancy, many medications, and genetic factors.[249] Thus hypertriglyceridemic AP represents a complex gene-environment and variable risk complex with the potential of being managed through precision medicine evaluation and targeted treatment.

The genetics of hypertriglyceridemia involves a few familial syndromes with TG levels in the thousands, and more complex situations requiring a combination of genetic and environmental conditions. Familial hyperlipidemias, previously classified as Fredrickson types I, V, and IV, are often associated with RAP. Type 1 hyperlipoproteinemia is now known as *familial chylomicronemia syndrome* (FCS) and is an autosomal recessive disorder associated with pathogenic variants in *LPL* or other genes.

LPL: Lipoprotein lipase deficiency[253–255] from mutations in *LPL*[256] causes about 80% of the cases of FCS. The diagnosis of LPL deficiency is supported by the presence of markedly elevated serum TG concentrations and chylomicrons and can be confirmed with an intravenous heparin test[255] performed when the patient is *not* having an attack of AP.

Other dyslipidemia genes: FCS can also be seen with loss-of-function mutations in other genes such as apolipoprotein C-II (*APOC2*),[254] *APOA5*, glycosylphosphatidylinositol-anchored high-density lipoprotein-binding protein 1 (*GPIHBP1*), and lipase maturation factor 1 (*LMF1*), and in the presence of circulating inhibitors to the LPL enzyme.[257,258] In addition, Johansen et al.[259] conducted a GWAS of patients with dyslipidemia/hypertriglyceridemia and identified common variants with strong disease associations in several genes, including *APOA5*, *GCKR*, *LPL*, and *APOB*.

It is now clear that many patients with familial or sporadic hypertriglyceridemia have a complex syndrome, termed *multifactorial chylomicronemia syndrome* (MCS). Patients with MCS may have a combination of a heterozygous loss-of-function mutation and/or likely pathogenic frequent variants in TG-raising genes, thus producing severe hypertriglyceridemia as a complex genetic disorder.[260] A recent expert panel recommended defining an FCS score to differentiate FCS from MCS, with the assumption that this would help determine who was at risk of AP.[260] However, this hypothesis has not been adequately tested.

The relationship between familial hyperlipidemias and CP is complex and represents a subset of patients with hypertriglyceridemic AP. In the NAPS2-CV cohort of 521 well-phenotyped patients with CP, physicians identified hypertriglyceridemia to be the primary etiology in 4% of the cases, and a risk factor in another 13%, indicating an increased risk of CP with hypertriglyceridemia to be about twofold to sixfold.[49] In another study of 121 AP patients with serum TG levels ≥500 mg/dL from the University of Pittsburgh, CP was identified in 16.5% of patients after a mean follow-up of 64.7 ± 42.8 months.[261] Taken together, it appears that CP can develop in the most severe, prolonged, and poorly controlled cases of familial hypertriglyceridemia who suffer recurrent attacks of AP (e.g., patients with genetic LPL deficiencies) as well as patients with complex hypertriglyceridemia and AP.

SLC26A9: CF Disease Severity Modifier

The role of genetic modifiers in pancreatic diseases is well defined in CF. Genetic association studies in patients with CF have identified a number of modifier genes associated with worse pancreatic disease during newborn screening for CF and CF-related diabetes (CFDM), as discussed later.[262,263] One of the strongest modifying genes in CF is the Solute Carrier Family 26 member 9 gene *(SLC26A9)*, a multifunctional ion transporter that functions as a Cl^-/HCO_3^- exchange, chloride channel, and sodium chloride cotransport[264] that was originally identified as the primary CFDM modifier in a GWAS study.[262]

SLC26A9 is expressed in high concentrations in the salivary glands, stomach, and lung, with lower levels in the kidney, duodenum, pancreas, and other organs. SLC26A9 is not critical to pancreatic function; the primary phenotype of knockout mice is complete loss of gastric acid secretion rather than pancreas dysfunction, indicating an essential role of this channel/transporter in gastric acid secretion.[264] However, SLC26A9 cooperates with CFTR in many fluid-secreting epithelial cells, and loss of both CFTR function and reduction in SLC26A9 function results in a much worse CF phenotype.[262,263,265,266] Patients with CF and high-risk *SLC26A9* genetic variants have worse pancreatic disease,[263,265,267] as well as a much higher risk of meconium ileus,[263] lung dysfunction,[266] and other effects.[265,268] Furthermore, patients carrying pathogenic *SLC26A9* variants are at high risk of DM, as GWAS studies identified *SLC26A9* SNPs with the highest association between CF and DM of all loci in the human genome.[262] Although it is clear that other solute carrier family genes and other genes also modify CF, other syndromes, and diseases with defining pathologic features, *SLC26A9* represents a prototype of genetic variants that are not associated with a specific human disease but make a variety of dysfunctional cell and organs systems worse. The opportunity to target these modifiers to improve patient disease severity is a goal of future research.

CF-Related Diabetes Risk

In non-CF pancreatic diseases, diabetes mellitus (DM) represents a common, variable, and potentially severe complication that likely has multiple genetic and environmental risks, as well as anatomical mechanisms. A nontype 1, nontype 2 DM due to severe, end-stage destruction of the pancreas in CP, or surgical removal of some or all the pancreatic parenchyma with obligate reduction of the islet cell mass, has been called type 3cDM. However, 20%–30% of patients with RAP or earlier stage CP also have DM, possibly due to modifiers or other factors rather than loss of the entire islets. To investigate the nongenetic risk factors for DM, researchers used the NAPS2 cohort to compare demographic and disease characteristics from CP patients with or without DM.[23] The risk profile was similar to population controls with type 2 DM, being more likely if the patient had a family history of DM, was of African ancestry, overweight (OR 1.62), or obese (OR 2.8). Severity of CP also affected risk as measured by calcifications, atrophy, and prior pancreas surgery, with EPI also a significant risk (OR 1.9).[23] The fact that ancestry and family history significantly affected risk suggests that genetic modifiers contribute to DM in CP.

INTEGRATION OF GENETICS AND PATIENT MANAGEMENT

A precision medicine approach adds to the multidisciplinary training and care of the health care industry through the use of new technologies. The first technical advance is the organization and standardization of health care information for detailed tracking of all features, tests, and biomarkers of a patient's disease journey, framed and compared with other patients with overlapping or distinct diseases and outcomes.[269,270] To be fully useful, this information must be readily available to the patient and various health care providers.[30] The second is advancing imaging technology, providing structural and functional evidence of disease pathology and disease stage. Third is the "omics" revolution, where millions of analytes can be measured in a patient within a specific clinical context. Foremost among these "omics" is deciphering the patient's entire genome, which does not change throughout their life and contains powerful predictive implications on how specific genes, protein products, cell types, and biological systems are likely to work under different conditions. Fourth, the availability of research and population data sets linked to new computational and analysis tools is needed to provide context and comparisons for the rich data sets to advance biomedical discovery.[269–271] Fifth, simple and sophisticated disease models are needed to organize the variables within a single patient, and determine the disease drivers, disease stage, disease activity, complication susceptibilities, and targets for treatment.[1,2,7] Fortunately, simple models such as pancreatic duct secretory deficits linked to mutations in *CFTR* can be readily detected by genetic testing, and effective targeted treatment strategies have been demonstrated.[272] Finally, the "smart phone" and other devices allow the patient to track and record their condition and response to therapies continually and to more fully participate in their health care.[30] Because unique combinations of risk and features of uncommon disorders are few, novel approaches are also required to parse the features of these complex disorders, such as *N*-of-one trials, to collect, organize, and evaluate the evidences as to whether specific interventions are effective under defined conditions.[39,273]

Consensus recommendations for managing pancreatic disease include early diagnosis and structured longitudinal care.[2,274,275] No consensus exists for diagnosing early CP, although there is agreement that it exists and is important.[2,38] Because the diagnosis of early, mild, noncalcific, or minimal change CP is challenging, some experts suggest that patients should be followed using a "place-holder" diagnosis of probable CP, or "insufficient evidence."[276] Clinical data collection and recording should be standardized during evaluation and follow-up of patients with suspected or proven CP.[274] Tracking the function of each component of pancreatic diseases is important because imaging, exocrine function, endocrine function, pain, and cancer risk do not correlate well with each other.

The initial evaluation for suspected or documented pancreatitis patients should address the risk factors (family history and genetics, environmental exposures, and clinical setting such as prior episodes of AP), differential diagnosis, signs and symptoms, and baseline measures of nutrition and pancreatic structure and function. The family history (preferably using a standardized family tree) should include pancreatitis, PC, diabetes mellitus, and hypertriglyceridemia, and previous genetic testing results should be considered. If no genetic testing, or an inadequate panel of variants, was performed, then an extended genetic panel should be ordered after appropriate genetic counseling. Alcohol and smoking history should be quantified. Anthropomorphic measures, including height, weight, blood pressure, and heart rate, should be documented. High-quality imaging of the pancreas with standardized techniques and reporting is required,[277] and better methods of standardizing and reporting structure and physical features, such as fibrosis with elastography or functional with secretin-stimulated magnetic resonance cholangiopancreatography (sMRCP), are emerging.[24,278–280] Laboratory tests should include serum levels of fat-soluble vitamins (A, D, E, and K), vitamin B_{12}, minerals, and trace elements; a baseline bone mineral density, and screening for diabetes mellitus (e.g., fasting glucose, hemoglobin A1c, and referral if abnormal).[274,281] Common measures of nutrition and inflammation include total protein, albumin, ionized calcium, prealbumin, osteocalcin, selenium, C-reactive protein, and a lipid panel.[282] Pancreatic exocrine function testing should be included as well. Although there is no consensus on the best method, human fecal elastase-1 testing (in formed stool), secretin-stimulated pancreatic function test (in the absence of *CFTR* mutations), or serum trypsinogen levels (in patients without a painful flair) are often used. Pain assessment should use multidimensional scales measuring its intensity, nature and location, frequency, and pain's impact on mood or activity level.[275]

As part of a baseline evaluation, the patient should have counseling about genetic testing if this has not previously been provided. Genetic testing for Mendelian disease has utility for identifying the disease-causing variant in affected family members, clarifying etiology and prognosis, and providing information for at-risk family members and family planning. However, additional considerations are required for complex genetic disorders, and the role of a qualified genetic counselor in the evaluation process is different than with Mendelian disorders.[283] Genetic testing for risk variants may also clarify disease etiology, outcomes, and management strategies. These are particularly important to interpret in the context of other risk factors. Patients should be specifically counseled prior to testing so that they understand the benefits, risks (e.g., life insurance), and limitations and provide informed consent.[283] Patients should also be counseled after testing so that they understand what was identified and what it means for them and their family (and provided their test results). Many genetic testing companies provide this service.

Patients should be evaluated at least annually, with assessment and documentation of changes in pancreatitis-related symptoms or interval hospitalizations, development of new symptoms (particularly those that may suggest cancer), functional abnormalities (exocrine and/or endocrine insufficiency), morphological changes on imaging (if performed), and laboratory testing.[274,284] Patients should be asked for symptoms suggestive of EPI, including abdominal bloating, distention, frequent bowel movements (particularly after eating), weight loss, and the presence of steatorrhea.[274] Patients with CP should be screened for nutritional deficiencies in fat-soluble vitamins, minerals, and trace elements on at least an annual basis and be monitored for bone density and treated based on assessment of fracture risk.[274] Although there is insufficient data to recommend routine PC screening for patients with CP, clinicians should track for new-onset diabetes mellitus, painless jaundice, weight loss, or new abdominal pain radiating to the back.

The emergence of new and established drugs and therapies that can be repurposed and used in pancreatic diseases continues to be examined and applied to specific problems.[39,272] The systematic collection of recommended measures of individual patients over time will allow the use of these therapies to be studied and optimized.

PANCREATITIS IN CHILDREN

Once considered uncommon, the incidence of pancreatic disease in children appears to be increasing. Increased physician awareness appears to account for most of the increase.[285] AP occurs in all pediatric age groups, including infants.[286,287] Common causes of AP in adults—excessive alcohol use and gallstones—are less often seen in children. The majority of cases of RAP and CP in children have a structural or genetic basis (Box 59.2).[61,121,288] The genetic factors predisposing to AP appear to be similar to those associated with CP and are discussed in detail in the following sections.

Acute Pancreatitis

Etiology: AP (defined earlier) is a sudden inflammatory disease of the pancreas with multiple etiologies (see Box 59.2). The most common known causes in children are biliary tract disease (10%–30%), medications (25%), systemic disease (33%), trauma (10%–40%), metabolic disease (2%–7%), and HP (5%–8%); 13%–34% of cases are idiopathic.[289] Much of the variation in incidence results from studies done at a time when AP was underdiagnosed in children. Some of these cases occur in children with high-risk genetic alterations, especially pancreatic-specific combinations of *SPINK1* and *CFTR* mutations.[290] Genetic testing, discussed later, is usually performed after recurrent episodes and when other common causes have been excluded.

Trauma: Trauma is a cause of AP even though the pancreas is well protected from minor injury by its retroperitoneal location. The trauma is usually blunt, associated with injuries to other abdominal viscera, and becomes evident soon after the injury, although injury may apparently precede the manifestation or recognition of pancreatitis by several weeks. Injury to the pancreas is often not considered in a severely injured or battered child.

Structural abnormalities: Structural abnormalities are being recognized earlier as imaging techniques such as MRI and MRCP improve. Pancreas divisum is the most common anatomic aberration, although a wide variety of other structural abnormalities of the bile and pancreatic duct also have been observed (see Chapter 57).

Post-ERCP pancreatitis has been a significant cause of pancreatitis in several series,[291,292] and this etiology is seen wherever ERCP is performed in children. The widespread availability of MRCP has drastically reduced the use of diagnostic ERCP, although ERCP remains invaluable for therapeutic intervention (see Chapter 63).

Biliary tract disease: Gallstone pancreatitis is less common in children than in adults and is probably a reflection of the relative infrequency of cholelithiasis before puberty.[61] However, this diagnosis must be considered, regardless of age.

Medications: Medications remain a frequent cause of AP in children, although the disease underlying the prescription must also be considered in the differential diagnosis.[293,294] Recent studies identified valproate as the most frequent drug associated

BOX 59.2 Causes of Acquired Pancreatitis in Children

TRAUMA

ERCP

Medications

α-Methyldopa
Antimony (pentavalent)
Azathioprine
Azodisalicylate
Cimetidine
Cytosine arabinoside
Didanosine
Erythromycin
Estrogen
Furosemide
Glucocorticoids
Isoniazid
IV lipid emulsion
Lamivudine
L-Asparaginase
6-Mercaptopurine
Mesalamine
Metronidazole
Pentamidine
Procainamide
Rifampin
Sulfasalazine
Sulfonamides
Sulindac
Tetracycline
Valproic acid
Zalcitabine

INFECTIONS

AIDS/HIV-associated
Ascariasis
Coxsackie B virus
Echovirus
Enterovirus
EBV
HAV
Herpesviruses
Influenza A
Leptospirosis
Malaria
Measles
Mumps
Mycoplasmosis
Rabies
Rubella
Typhoid fever

BILIARY TRACT DISEASE

Pancreas Divisum

Metabolic Disorders

CF
Hypercalcemia
Hypertriglyceridemia
Protein-calorie malnutrition
Reye syndrome

FAMILIAL DISORDERS

Miscellaneous Causes

Congenital partial lipodystrophy
Diabetic ketoacidosis
Henoch-Schönlein purpura
Tropical pancreatitis
Kawasaki disease
Perforated duodenal ulcer
SLE

with pancreatitis in children, followed by L-asparaginase, prednisone, or 6-mercaptopurine.[291,292,295,296] The development of persistent abdominal pain in a child receiving any medication should suggest the possibility of drug-induced pancreatitis. This is confirmed only by documentation of pancreatic disease, improvement on drug withdrawal, and return of disease when the drug is reintroduced.

Infections: Infections, particularly with viruses,[297] are frequently associated with childhood pancreatitis. Enteroviruses, particularly coxsackievirus, are associated with idiopathic AP.[298] Pancreatitis has been reported in children with EBV infections.[299] Pancreatitis in children is often attributed to mumps virus on the basis of abdominal pain and an elevated serum amylase value with parotitis.[300] Mycoplasma pneumoniae infection and AP, sometimes developing a week or 2 later, have been documented in multiple cases reports.[297] Although uncommon in the United States, ascariasis is among the most frequent causes of pancreatitis in children in regions such as South Africa and India; worms can be found within the pancreatic duct. Pancreatitis was common in patients with HIV/AIDS, possibly due to medications and associated with hyperlipidemia and/or mitochondrial toxicity (see Boxes 59.1 and 59.2, and Chapter 33).

Systemic diseases: Hemolytic uremic syndrome was the most common systemic cause of AP in two studies.[291,292] The mechanism is unknown and likely multifactorial although uremia from any cause is a risk factor for pancreatic injury. SLE[301] and Kawasaki disease[302] have been associated with pancreatitis. AP should be considered in the ICU when the child is not responding to other therapies or appears to have an unexplained acute inflammatory process. AP is also common after organ transplantation (see Chapter 34). Pancreatitis is occasionally observed in diabetic ketoacidosis[291,292,303] and various inborn errors of metabolism.[304]

Acquired metabolic derangements: The most common metabolic derangement associated with development of pancreatic disease in children is protein-calorie malnutrition. In severely malnourished children, pancreatic enzyme secretion is often compromised, whereas volume and bicarbonate secretion are preserved. Recovery of pancreatic function is said to occur more promptly after kwashiorkor than after marasmus, but in either case, the pancreatic disease may contribute to malabsorption during convalescence. Vigorous early refeeding of malnourished children has been associated with the development of clinically significant pancreatitis. Malnutrition was considered a major contributing factor to TP, but this has now been questioned because TP is observed primarily in well-nourished patients, often with genetic mutations.[42,44,305]

Clinical features: The diagnosis of AP is based on the syndrome of sudden onset of typical abdominal pain with elevation of serum amylase or lipase to at least three times the upper limit of normal levels (see Chapter 60).[31,306,307] The pain is usually supraumbilical, worsens with eating, and may be accompanied by nausea, vomiting, and occasionally jaundice. A transient fever is often present. In infants and toddlers, vomiting, fever, irritability, and abdominal distention can be presenting symptoms.[286] Normal serum amylase values increase with age, which is explained perhaps by the delayed appearance of pancreatic isoamylase, which is usually not present before the age of 3 months and often not detected until the age of 11 months; even then it is not present at adult levels until the age of 10 years. Salivary isoamylase appears and matures much sooner.

After the initial episode of AP, RAP is seen in about 10% of children.[292] The most common diagnoses in patients with RAP are structural abnormalities, or familial pancreatitis or complex genetic risk.[61,121,292] A careful evaluation aimed at identifying or ruling out reversible causes should be undertaken to prevent further attacks and to reduce the risk for developing CP and its complications.[284]

Recurrent Acute Pancreatitis and Chronic Pancreatitis

Once thought to be rare, numerous children with RAP and CP are being reported. Improvement in abdominal imaging, physician awareness, and possible change in prevalence demonstrated that CP is a major medical problem in children with very high costs.[308]

A recent multinational cross-sectional study of RAP and CP in children (International Study Group of Pediatric Pancreatitis: In Search for a CuRE; INSPPIRE) provides new insights into this complex of pediatric pancreatic disorders beyond CF.[121] Among 301 cases in the initial cohort, the mean and standard deviation of the children's ages was 11.9 ± 4.5 years, with 57% female. CP was documented in 146 patients, and 84% of them reported prior recurrent episodes of AP. Hispanic children were more likely to have RAP than CP. At least one gene mutation in pancreatitis-related genes was found in 48% of patients with RAP versus 73% of patients with CP ($P < .001$). Children were more likely to present with CP than with RAP if they had pathogenic variants in *PRSS1* (OR 4.2) or *SPINK1* (OR 2.30).[121] Pancreatitis-related abdominal pain was a major symptom in 81% of children with RAP or CP within the previous year, with emergency department visits, hospitalizations, and medical, endoscopic, and surgical interventions being more common in the CP group.[121]

Children have less exposure to environmental risk factors for AP and CP than adults, especially long-standing alcohol use and smoking. Demographic and clinical information on children with RAP or CP in the INSPPIRE cohort was evaluated for risk factors according to age.[61] Among 342 cases, 38% of the children were less than 6 years of age at first diagnosis, 32% were 6–11 years of age, and 30% were ≥12 years of age. Early onset disease was significantly associated with pathogenic genetic variants in *PRSS1* and *CTRC*, a family history of AP or CP, biliary cysts, or chronic renal failure.[61] Later-onset RAP and CP were associated with hypertriglyceridemia, ulcerative colitis, autoimmune diseases, or medication use.[61] Children with later-onset disease also were more likely to visit the emergency department ($P < .05$) or have diabetes mellitus ($P < .01$).[61]

Recommendations for the evaluation of patients with new-onset AP, RAP, and CP continue to evolve. The INSPPIRE consortium recently made a series of recommendations for the causal evaluation of RAP and CP.[284] Systematic evaluation of anatomical, metabolic, and genetic causes is recommended, including a sweat chloride test or *CFTR* genetic testing (even if newborn screening for CF was negative), *PRSS1*, *CTRC*, and *SPINK1* genetic testing and for screening for celiac disease.[284] Testing for EPI and related vitamin and nutritional deficiencies, diabetes, and complications should also be evaluated annually.[284]

CLINICAL MANAGEMENT OF MENDELIAN DISORDERS OF THE PANCREAS

Several genes that are critical to pancreatic function manifest genetic variations and polymorphisms that lead to Mendelian pancreatic disorders, usually with multisystem involvement (Table 59.2).

Cystic Fibrosis

CF is the most common lethal genetic defect of white populations, seen in 1/2500–1/3200 live births. Compared to children of European ancestry, the incidence of CF is lower in children of African, Native American, Asian, East Indian, or Middle Eastern backgrounds.[309] Prognosis has dramatically improved, with the predicted median survival of CF patients extending beyond age 47 years.[310] Still, the median age at death is

TABLE 59.2 Hereditary and Congenital Disorders of the Exocrine Pancreas and the Associated Gene

Disorder	Defective Gene or Protein (Inheritance)
Exocrine Pancreatic Insufficiency	
Pancreatic agenesis (see Chapter 57)	*PDX1* or *PTF1A* (recessive)
CF	$CFTR^{sev}/CFTR^{sev}$ (recessive)
Shwachman-Diamond syndrome	*SBDS* (recessive)
Johanson-Blizzard syndrome	*UBR1* (recessive)
Pearson marrow-pancreas syndrome	Mitochondrial DNA (mitochondrial)
Isolated enzyme deficiency	See text
Pancreatitis	
Hereditary	*PRSS1* (autosomal dominant)
	CEL
Familial	*SPINK1/SPINK1* (autosomal recessive)
	$CFTR^{sev}$ or $CFTR^{bl}/SPINK1$ (complex)
CFTR-RD	$CFTR^{sev}/CFTR^{m\text{-}v}$ (recessive)
Sporadic	*CTRC* (complex)
	CASR (complex)
Modifiers	*CLDN2*
	SLC26A9 (CFTR-associated)
Hypertriglyceridemia	Lipoprotein lipase (dominant)
	Apolipoprotein C-II

TABLE 59.3 Frequency of Selected GI Manifestations in CF[a]

Organ	Manifestation	Frequency in All Patients (%)	Frequency in Adults (%)
Pancreas	Total achylia	85–90	85–90[a]
	Abnormal glucose tolerance	20–30	20–30
	Partial or normal function	10–15	10–15
	Pancreatitis	1–2 (all CF) 22% (PS-CF)	2–3
	Diabetes mellitus	4–7	4–7
Intestine	Meconium ileus	10–25	
	Rectal prolapse	1–2	
	Distal intestinal obstruction syndrome	3	18
	Intussusception	1	1–2
Liver	Fatty liver	7	20–60
	Focal biliary cirrhosis	2–3	11–70
	Portal hypertension	2–3	28
Biliary tract	Gallbladder abnormal, nonfunctional, or small	25	5–20
	Gallstones	8	10–25
	Bile duct strictures	1–20	1–20
Esophagus	GERD	Unknown	80

[a]Frequency may depend on the genotype.
PS-CF, CF with pancreatic sufficiency.

about 30 years. Here we focus on manifestations of *CFTR* gene mutations on the pancreas, with briefer discussions of intestinal, hepatobiliary, and nutritional problems also seen by gastroenterologists (Table 59.3).

Clinical features: Over 60% of CF patients are diagnosed by newborn screening in the United States.[310] In 2016 the median age at diagnosis for all patients was 4 months and 67% were diagnosed in the first year of life. Around 10% of all patients were diagnosed after age 10, and a few were diagnosed after age 40.

Most infants identified by newborn screening are minimally symptomatic or asymptomatic when screened. Of the infants who screen positive for CF, most are easily confirmed after demonstration of elevated sweat chloride concentrations (Table 59.4) or demonstration of an abnormal nasal bioelectrical response in specific testing protocols that also reflect abnormal CFTR function. When performed appropriately, these tests are reliable. However, false-positive as well as false-negative results may be observed in newborns, in patients with malnutrition, with some medications, or if inadequate sweat is obtained (see Table 59.4). Thus most experts insist on using the standardized methods performed at CF centers that use these testing methods frequently.

Because of the explosion of new phenotypic and genotypic information in patients with CF, the CF Foundation selected an international consensus committee to provide recommendations on the diagnosis of CF,[207] in large part by recognition that many patients have *CFTR*-associated abnormalities but do not have CF.[311] The panel concluded that a presumptive diagnosis of CF can be made in a patient with a positive newborn screen and two

TABLE 59.4 Sweat Test (Quantitative Pilocarpine Iontophoresis): Indications and Conditions with High Sweat Electrolyte Levels

Indications	Conditions With High Sweat Electrolyte Levels
Siblings with CF	CF
Chronic pulmonary symptoms	Ectodermal dysplasia
Persistent cough	Glycogen storage disease, type 1
Recurrent respiratory infection	Adrenal insufficiency
Bronchitis	Familial hypoparathyroidism
Bronchiectasis	Fucosidosis
Lobar atelectasis	Pitressin-resistant diabetes insipidus
Failure to thrive (stunting of growth)	Mucopolysaccharidosis
Rectal prolapse	Familial cholestasis syndrome
Nasal polyposis	Environmental deprivation syndrome
Intestinal obstruction of newborn	Acute respiratory disorders (croup, epiglottitis, viral pneumonia)
Meconium ileus	Chronic respiratory disorders (bronchopulmonary dysplasia)
Jaundice in early infancy	α_1-Antitrypsin deficiency
Cirrhosis in childhood or adolescence	
Portal hypertension	
Adult males with aspermia or azoospermia	
Heat stroke	
Hypoproteinemia	
Hypoprothrombinemia	

CF mutations from the *CFTR2* mutation list (http://cftr2.org/) or signs and symptoms of CF or meconium ileus, but the diagnosis must be confirmed with a positive sweat chloride test (>60 mmol/L). The guidelines classified patients who did not have CF into two groups: *CFTR*-related metabolic syndrome (CRMS) and *CFTR*-related disease (*CFTR*-RD), as described earlier.

The clinical features of CF are listed in Box 59.3, and frequencies of the various GI manifestations of CF are listed in Table 59.3. The early clinical features are those of maldigestion or other pancreatic and intestinal manifestations of *CFTR* mutations (discussed later). The phenotype-genotype relationship between some childhood disorders and *CFTR* mutations is often striking, with severe *CFTR* mutations detected in more than 85% of all children presenting with PI and in the majority of infants presenting with meconium ileus.[218]

Pulmonary function is normal in patients with CF at birth but accounts for much of the morbidity and almost all of the mortality associated with CF beyond the neonatal period. The severity of lung disease depends on known and unknown factors. Genetic and environmental factors contribute proportionally to pulmonary function variation in CF,[312] demonstrated by a wide variation in the severity of lung disease among patients with identical *CFTR* genotypes. Environmental factors may include chronic infection with *Pseudomonas aeruginosa*, nutritional status, tobacco smoke, and environmental allergens,[223] whereas genetic factors include variants in inflammatory response genes[313,314] and modifier genes.[315–317]

Pancreatic pathology: Most (85%–90%) patients with CF present with evidence of exocrine pancreatic dysfunction.[200,318] Although pancreatic dysfunction in an infant with CF may initially appear minimal, it usually progresses to pancreatic exocrine failure. When severely affected, the pancreas is shrunken, cystic, fibrotic, and fatty. Histologically, hyperplasia and eventual necrosis of ductular and centroacinar cells, together with inspissated secretions, lead to blockage of pancreatic ductules and subsequently encroach on acini, causing flattening and atrophy of the epithelium (see Fig. 59.9). Cystic spaces are filled with calcium-rich eosinophilic concretions. A mild inflammatory reaction may be present around obstructed acini, and progressive fibrosis gradually separates and replaces the pancreatic lobules. The islets of Langerhans are spared in most cases until late in the process and become concentrated in the shrinking pancreas. Calcification, although rare, may be apparent on radiographs. US, MRI, and CT can document progression of pancreatic disease. The pancreas can appear normal, have incomplete or complete lipomatosis (most common), be cystic or macrocystic, or appear as an atrophic pancreas.[319] Correlation of abnormalities with the degree of exocrine dysfunction is poor.[2]

Exocrine pancreas dysfunction and pancreatitis: Patients with CF are usually PI, a problem compounded by intestinal pathology, high caloric demands, and poor appetite. Fat and protein maldigestion with fecal losses are the primary pancreatic manifestations of CF, although there may be considerable variation in severity from one patient to another. Steatorrhea and azotorrhea are generally greater with PI than with mucosal malabsorption. EPI may be recognized only when the secretion of lipase and trypsin falls to below 10% of normal.[320] Most patients with CF exhibit this pattern of PI. RAP may complicate the course of CF in patients who do not experience complete loss of pancreatic function in infancy. Pancreatitis tends to be more problematic in older patients.[200]

Endocrine pancreas dysfunction and diabetes mellitus: Glucose intolerance has been reported in 30%–75% of patients with CF, and clinically significant diabetes mellitus occurs in up to 10% of young patients. CF-related diabetes mellitus (CFRD) develops with increasing age. At 20 years of age, 30% of CF patients will require insulin and 40% require insulin by age 30.[321] The development of CFRD differs in etiology and presentation from typical type 1 diabetes mellitus or type 2 diabetes mellitus (T2DM) and may reflect destruction of the islets of Langerhans similar to what is observed in other forms of CP. However, the severity of the endocrine deficiency lags behind the exocrine

BOX 59.3 Clinical Manifestations of CF

UPPER RESPIRATORY

Sinusitis
Mucous membrane hypertrophy, nasal polyposis

LOWER RESPIRATORY

Atelectasis
Emphysema
Infections
Bronchitis, bronchopneumonia, bronchiectasis, lung abscess
Respiratory failure, right-sided heart failure

GI

Bile salt deficiency
Pancreatic insufficiency
GERD
PUD
Meconium ileus
Volvulus
Peritonitis
Ileal atresia
Distal intestinal obstruction syndrome
- Fecal masses
- Intussusception

Rectal prolapse

PANCREATIC

Pancreatitis
Nutritional failure
Diabetes mellitus
Calcification
Maldigestion with steatorrhea and azotorrhea
Vitamin deficiencies

HEPATOBILIARY

Mucus hypersecretion
Gallstones, atrophic gallbladder
Focal biliary cirrhosis
Portal hypertension ± esophageal varices
Hypersplenism

REPRODUCTIVE

Females: increased viscosity of vaginal mucus, decreased fertility
Males: sterility; absent ductus deferens, epididymis, and seminal vesicles

SKELETAL

Retardation of bone age
Demineralization
Hypertrophic pulmonary osteoarthropathy

OPHTHALMOLOGIC

Venous engorgement
Retinal hemorrhage

OTHER

Salt depletion through excessive loss of salt through skin
Heat stroke
Hypertrophy of apocrine glands

deficiency because the islets are relatively spared until later in the course of pancreatic destruction (see Fig. 59.9). CFRD is associated with deterioration in both respiratory and nutritional status, the development of late microvascular complications, and increased mortality.[322] Experts emphasize the need for a multidisciplinary team approach, use of a high-energy diet (>100% of the recommended daily intake), and appropriate adjustment of insulin doses.[322] Overnight enteral feedings may be necessary to maintain adequate nutrition. The choice of therapies should also be carefully considered for maximizing endogenous incretins, optimizing metabolism, preserving beta cell function, and reducing risk of PC.[281]

Treatment of Pancreatic Dysfunction

Pancreatic enzyme supplements: Nutrition is a major challenge in CF (see the "Nutritional Management" section). Treatment of maldigestion from pancreatic exocrine failure in CF requires delivery of active digestive enzymes to the proximal small intestine with meals (see Chapter 61). Numerous pancreatic preparations are available, but enzyme activities vary considerably from one product to another, and reduced activity of lipase remains a problem for some CF patients. Enteric-coated minimicrospheres are the preferred form of replacement because they protect the digestive enzymes from destruction by gastric acid ($pH < 4$) and are effective. The size of the microspheres must be considered. If the majority of the spheres are too large (>1 mm), emptying of the spheres/enzymes can be delayed until after food is well into the small intestine. H2RAs or PPIs, together with uncoated or enteric-coated pancreatic enzyme supplements, also should be considered, especially because the pancreatic and duodenal bicarbonate transport systems that help neutralize gastric acid are disrupted. In contrast with other forms of PI, bicarbonate secretion within the duodenum and biliary tree is also impaired in CF, resulting in a significantly lower-than-normal duodenal pH.[323,324] Thus without acid suppression, the uncoated enzymes are susceptible to inactivation by gastric acid, and enteric-coated products may not release their contents.[323] The use of antacids containing calcium carbonate or magnesium hydroxide should be avoided because they may interfere with the pancreatic enzyme supplements.

Initial therapy for pancreatic exocrine insufficiency in CF includes pancreatic enzyme replacement at doses ranging from 500 to 2000 U of lipase activity per kilogram of body weight per meal, given just before a meal and with snacks.[325] The amount is usually advanced to 1000–2500 U of lipase activity per kilogram, with final dosage depending on the age, the degree of PI, the amount of fat ingested, and the commercial preparation chosen. Adequacy of treatment is typically determined on clinical grounds. Frequent, bulky, and fatty stools; excessive bloating and flatus; and excessive appetite or inadequate growth velocity are signs of inadequate treatment. Even with optimized treatment, fat absorption may not return to normal. In large part, inability to normalize fat absorption may reflect decreased uptake of fatty acids by the abnormal intestinal mucosa.[326]

Pancreatic enzyme replacement commonly causes perioral and perianal irritation in infants, although less commonly with microsphere preparations. Because of the high purine content of pancreatic extracts, hyperuricosuria may develop in some patients taking large doses of enzyme preparations. Colonic strictures and fibrosing colonopathy were reported with very high-dose administration of pancreatic enzymes and led to a withdrawal of all the high-dose formulations of enzymes. Fibrosing colonopathy, first recognized in 1994,[327] had nearly disappeared by 1996.[328]

Vitamin supplements: Fat-soluble vitamin deficiencies (A, D, E, and K) may develop in CF as a consequence of fat maldigestion and malabsorption.[282,329] Vitamin A deficiency in CF rarely manifests with clinical abnormalities or causes eye and skin problems, whereas excessive levels of vitamin A can harm the respiratory and skeletal systems in children and interfere with the metabolism of other fat-soluble vitamins.[330] However, because there are no randomized, controlled studies on retinoid supplementation, no conclusion on the supplementation of vitamin A in people with CF can be made.[330] Vitamin D deficiency may occur, affecting calcium homeostasis, bone mineralization, inflammation, mood, and other extraskeletal effects. Vitamin D levels are affected by dietary intake, sunlight exposure, and genetics, and deficiencies are more complex than intake alone.[282,331,332] Supplementation can be effective, and replacement has been recommended for individual patients based on serum measurements.[333,334] Vitamin E deficiency is common in CF children and can cause a host of conditions such as hemolytic anemia, cerebellar ataxia, and cognitive difficulties.[335] Although treatment such as water-soluble vitamin E can significantly improve serum vitamin E levels compared with control, studies have not yet demonstrated clinical benefit to therapy.[335] Vitamin K deficiency with coagulopathy may occur at any age. Its manifestations vary from mildly increased bruising or purpura to catastrophic hemorrhage and affect bone formation. Supplementation of 1 mg vitamin K/day appears to improve osteocalcin levels, a marker of bone metabolism, and no harm was identified with vitamin K supplementation in a systematic review.[336]

All CF patients should receive a multivitamin preparation daily, and many require vitamin A, D, E, and K supplements, plus pancreatic enzyme replacement therapy (PERT) for patients with EPI.[282,288] Annual monitoring of the serum concentrations of fat-soluble vitamins is important in children with CF and is recommended.[288]

Intestinal Manifestations

Because CFTR is expressed at the apical membrane of enterocytes, CF significantly affects the GI tract.[337] Distal ileal obstruction syndrome, intussusception, appendicitis, chronic constipation, colonic wall thickening, fibrosing colonopathy, pneumatosis intestinalis, GERD, and PUD have been described.[319]

Pathology: The mucosal glands of the small intestine of patients with CF may contain variable quantities of inspissated secretions within the lumen but rarely have increased numbers of goblet cells. The appendix is often involved and may rarely cause appendicitis or intussusception.[338] Brunner glands may show dilation, flattening of epithelial lining cells, and stringy secretions within their lumens. The small intestinal mucosa in older CF patients often shows widely dilated crypts packed with mucus; the mucus frequently appears laminated or may extrude from a gaping crypt. Bulging goblet cells seem to crowd out the intervening columnar epithelium. Variable cellular infiltration may be present in the lamina propria. Mucus in CF is more abundant, stains more intensely, and contains more weak acid groups and protein.

Radiologic features: Radiographic features of the GI tract vary widely in CF.[319] Radiographic examination is typically done in response to specific symptoms, and both CF-related and non-CF-related pathologies can be detected. Meconium ileus in infants and DIOS in children and adults (described later) are exceptions and have clear radiographic appearances.[319,339,340]

Intestinal pathophysiology: The changes in small bowel mucosa cause physiological dysfunction of the intestine. Various studies have demonstrated absorption defects that are apparently unexplained by EPI or that persist after adequate pancreatic replacement therapy.

Basal and stimulated duodenal bicarbonate secretion is largely dependent on functional CFTR. The same abnormalities in duodenal bicarbonate secretion are also present in CF patients, which partially explains the decrease in postprandial pH in the proximal duodenum of CF patients, even after pancreas stimulation.[324] Unlike the small bowel and respiratory tract, the CFTR defect in the colon cannot be compensated by any other chloride channel.[341] Therefore the defect in colonic function closely relates to the *CFTR* genotype.

Lactase deficiency with lactose malabsorption in patients with CF merely reflects a normal ethnic- and age-related phenomenon. However, patients with adult-type hypolactasia and lactose malabsorption may have decreased bone mineral density.[342]

Meconium ileus: Meconium ileus can be uncomplicated or complicated. Complicated meconium ileus includes intestinal obstruction with segmental volvulus, atresia, necrosis, perforation, meconium peritonitis (generalized), and giant meconium pseudocyst formation.[343,344] Uncomplicated meconium ileus characteristically demonstrates a narrow distal ileum with a beaded appearance caused by waxy, gray pellets of inspissated meconium, beyond which the colon is unused. As many as half of the cases of meconium ileus are complicated by volvulus, atresia, or meconium peritonitis from extravasation of meconium into the peritoneal cavity after intestinal perforation; this may manifest clinically merely as intra-abdominal calcifications, a meconium pseudocyst, generalized adhesive meconium peritonitis, or meconium ascites. Fetal volvulus and vascular compromise may cause atresia.

Characteristic radiologic findings are unevenly distended loops of bowel with absent or scarce air-fluid levels.[319,339,340,345] Small bubbles of gas trapped in the sticky meconium may be scattered throughout the distal small bowel.[346] Barium enema demonstrates a microcolon and may outline the obstructing meconium mass in the distal ileum (Fig. 59.10). Abdominal calcification reflects meconium peritonitis, and a meconium pseudocyst may displace loops of bowel.

Meconium ileus classically manifests with signs of intestinal obstruction within 48 hours of birth in an infant who is otherwise well; complicated meconium ileus manifests even earlier, and infants appear much sicker. Hydramnios is a common prenatal finding. When feedings are initiated, bilious emesis occurs with or without abdominal distention. The infant with meconium peritonitis often presents with additional signs of abdominal tenderness, fever, and shock.[346] A family history of CF is helpful in establishing the diagnosis. Dilated, firm, rubbery loops of bowel may be visible and palpable through the abdominal wall, particularly in the right lower quadrant.

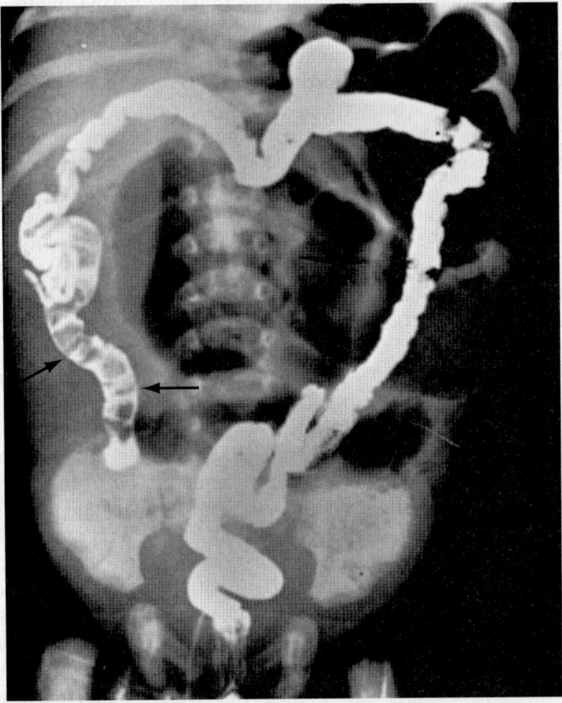

Fig. 59.10 Film from a barium enema examination in an infant with meconium ileus demonstrating a microcolon as well as meconium in the distal ileum (*arrows*). Distended small bowel loops are also noted.

Genetic screening for *CFTR* variants should be performed in patients with abnormal prenatal ultrasonographic evidence of meconium ileus such as hyperechoic bowel or peritoneal calcifications.[346] If the results indicate normal *CFTR* genotypes, genetic counseling should focus on limits of testing and an expanded differential diagnosis, whereas detection of pathogenic CFTR alleles in one or more parents or the child should lead to more focused counseling on CF.[346]

Meconium ileus was considered invariably fatal until 1948, when the first patients were successfully treated by surgery. More recent reports indicate a very low operative mortality, and long-term survival approaches 90% for uncomplicated meconium ileus.[346] Complicated meconium ileus requires surgical therapy.[347]

Various irrigating solutions have been used during the operation and postoperatively to dissolve and dislodge the abnormal meconium. *N*-acetylcysteine (Mucomyst), which reduces the viscosity of mucoprotein solutions by cleaving disulfide bonds in the mucoprotein molecule, and polysorbate 80 (Tween 80), a mild industrial detergent and preservative, are now generally recognized as safe and effective. For most infants with uncomplicated meconium ileus, nonoperative relief of bowel obstruction by enema administration using diluted diatrizoate (Gastrografin, Hypaque) or full-strength Omnipaque or Cysto-Conray II reduces the length of hospitalization and early respiratory complications.[343,346] These enemas are hyperosmolar (1900 mOsm/L) and work by hydrating the contents of the colon by drawing water out of the infant's body.[343] Reflux of the enema into the terminal ileum is critical for the bowel obstruction to be relieved.[343] However, water-soluble hypertonic enemas may cause dangerous fluid and electrolyte shifts, especially in small, sick infants, and they can cause colonic perforation. In addition, more recent case series suggest that uses of Gastrografin enemas only have success rates of 36%–39%.[343] A diagnostic barium enema should precede a therapeutic Gastrografin enema. Infants with CF and meconium ileus who survive beyond 6 months of age have the same prognosis as any patient with CF and do not tend to have more severe disease.

DIOS: The DIOS is complete or incomplete intestinal obstruction by viscid fecal material in the terminal ileum and proximal colon in patients with CF.[348,349] The incidence and prevalence of DIOS among CF patients is less than 3%. Recent incidence estimates in Europe are 5–12 episodes/1000 patient-years.[349,350] The European Society for Pediatric Gastroenterology and Nutrition CF Working Group defined DIOS as "a short history (days) of abdominal pain and/or distension and a fecal mass in ileocecum, but without signs of complete obstruction."[350] In contrast to DIOS, constipation in CF was defined as "abdominal pain and/or distension or a decline in the frequency of bowel movements in the last few weeks to months and/or increased consistency of stools in the last few weeks or months, while the symptoms are relieved by the use of laxatives."[350]

Reduced fluid secretion and hydration of the intestinal contents and delayed or inadequate fat and nutrient digestion contributes to DIOS, possibly through slow intestinal transit induced by nutrient-mediated release of ileal break hormones such as peptide YY.[351] Other risk factors for DIOS include a severe genotype, dehydration, history of meconium ileus or DIOS, organ transplantation, and CFRD.[348,349] The possible role of modifier genes causing meconium ileus has not been fully addressed in DIOS. Intussusception and, less frequently, volvulus may complicate DIOS.

DIOS may be the presenting symptom of CF. A clinical spectrum from partial or complete obstruction of the bowel by abnormal intestinal contents occurs in DIOS: (1) recurrent and cramping abdominal pain caused by constipation or fecal impaction; (2) soft, palpable cecal masses that may eventually pass spontaneously; and (3) complete obstruction of the bowel by firm, putty-like fecal material in the terminal ileum, right colon, or both. Acute onset of vomiting of bilious material with progressive, colicky abdominal pain and/or fluid levels in the small intestine on abdominal radiography are signs of DIOS with complete intestinal obstruction.[348] The fecal bolus can be identified on barium enema but may have to be differentiated from a cecal neoplasm or appendiceal abscess. Abdominal-pelvic CT typically shows significant proximal small bowel dilation with inspissated fecal material in the distal ileum.[348] The differential diagnosis of DIOS includes constipation, appendicitis, appendicular abscess or mucocele, intussusception, Crohn's disease, adhesions, volvulus, fibrosing colonopathy, and malignancy.[348]

Treatment of DIOS is largely empirical.[348,350,352] Once a surgical issue, uncomplicated DIOS now usually responds to medical management, with less than 5% of patients now requiring surgery.[349,353] A stepwise approach with therapeutic trials of more than one modality should be attempted in each patient before a consideration of surgery.[352] Vigorous medical therapy includes regular oral doses of pancreatic enzymes and stool softeners, including polyethylene glycol,[353] oral or rectal administration of 10% *N*-acetylcysteine, and Gastrografin enemas if necessary, although high-quality evidence from randomized trials for prevention or treatment is lacking.[354] Maintenance treatment with oral doses of *N*-acetylcysteine, increased doses of pancreatic enzymes, and lactulose has been used successfully to prevent recurrent episodes of the syndrome. Treatment of this disorder with balanced intestinal lavage solutions may also be beneficial. Maintenance therapy with polyethylene glycol continues to grow in popularity because it is effective and there are few side effects.

Liver and Biliary Manifestations

CF liver disease (CFLD) covers a number of liver abnormalities seen in patients with CF, including hepatic steatosis, elevated serum transaminase levels, cholangiopathy, neonatal cholestasis, multilobular cirrhosis, and focal biliary cirrhosis.[355,356] Liver disease accounted for 2.7% of deaths in CF in 2016.[310] In a large French cohort, the incidence of CFLD increased by approximately 1% every year, reaching 32.2% by age 25 years.[357] In addition, the incidence of severe CFLD increased only after the age of 5, reaching 10% by age 30.[357] Risk factors for CFLD and severe CFLD are male sex, neonatal liver disease, severe *CFTR* genotypes, pancreatic exocrine insufficiency, a history of meconium ileus, and modifier genes.[265,357–359] Additional risk factors may predispose CF patients to development of hepatobiliary problems, and some features overlap with non-CF patients who have nonalcoholic steatosis.[359]

One study of children with CFLD suggested that these patients had a more severe CF phenotype than age- and gender-matched controls without liver disease.[360] In 2016 gallstones (0.6%), cirrhosis (2.8%), noncirrhotic liver disease (3.9%), acute hepatitis (0.1%), hepatic steatosis (0.4%), and other liver disease (2.0%) were reported.[310] Another study found cirrhosis in 28% of adults with CF, two-thirds of whom had associated portal hypertension.[361] The prevalence of liver abnormalities in CF patients with PS is markedly lower.

Liver injury tests may be moderately elevated and fluctuate over the course of the illness. Up to 20% of CF patients with PI have elevated serum ALT values, and 40%–50% of patients have intermittently increased serum aminotransferase levels. Fasting bile acid levels are elevated in many CF patients, and this may be among the more sensitive measures of liver function in this disease.

Bile acid metabolism is disturbed in patients with CF and EPI. Fecal bile salt losses are high, often approaching those of patients with ileal resection (see Chapter 66). Pancreatic enzyme replacement improves fat absorption, thereby reducing fecal bile acid excretion and steatorrhea. The fractional turnover rate of the bile acid pool is increased and the total bile acid pool size diminished in the absence of pancreatic enzymes,[362] whereas the biliary lipid composition and saturation index approach those of patients with cholelithiasis.[363] Treatment with pancreatic supplements returns abnormal biliary lipid values toward normal.

Gallbladder and biliary tract: The gallbladder and biliary tract are abnormal in approximately 25% of patients with CF, independent of age, clinical course, or hepatic pathology. Microgallbladders are found in 23% and stones or sludge in 8% of patients. Data from the Cystic Fibrosis Registry suggest that only about 0.3% of individuals with CF eventually require gallbladder surgery.[310]

Small gallbladders are commonly found, characteristically containing thick, colorless "white bile." Mucus is present within the epithelial lining cells, and numerous mucus-filled cysts may exist immediately beneath the mucosa. The cystic duct may be atrophic or occluded with mucus. Obstruction of the hepatic or bile ducts by mucous plugs does not occur, but intraductal stones sometimes cause obstructive symptoms and predispose to cholangitis.

Other Manifestations

Genital abnormalities in male patients: Although male reproduction is not a digestive system complication, infertility is among the most sensitive phenotypes associated with severe or mild *CFTR* variants and overlaps with *CFTR*-associated pancreatitis, including bicarbonate-defective conductance variants (described earlier).

The most striking changes in the male genital tract occur in the epididymis, the vas deferens, and the seminal vesicles. The rete testes are intact. Multiple histologic sections of the spermatic cord rarely show patency at more than one level. In addition to these defects, there is a striking increase in abnormalities associated with testicular descent, such as inguinal hernia, hydrocele, and undescended testes. Approximately 97% of males with CF are sterile as a result of these changes. These defects may be found in male infants shortly after birth and may be useful in supporting the diagnosis of CF in atypical cases.

Evaluation of patients with congenital absence of the vas deferens who are not clinically suspected of having CF reveals a high frequency of *CFTR* mutations.[364] Up to 70% of men with the sole finding of congenital absence of the vas deferens have a detectable mutation in at least one allele of *CFTR*. Alterations in RNA transcription also may be associated with this defect, inasmuch as a mutation, 5T, which reduced functional messenger RNA transcripts of wild-type *CFTR*, is found in high frequency in men with congenital absence of the vas deferens.[364] Secretion of bicarbonate through CFTR is critical to sperm, and infertility can occur in men with *CFTR-BD* variants.[202] This group of men, without other manifestations of CF, is classified as CFTR-RD.[208]

Cancer risk: With CF patients reaching older ages, a higher risk of cancer is being recognized. Cancer tended to occur in the third decade of life and involved the esophagus, small and large intestines, stomach, liver, biliary tract, pancreas, or rectum.[365,366] A recent 20-year study in the United States of almost 42,000 patients demonstrated an increased risk of digestive tract cancer, especially after transplantation.[367] This same study also found an increased risk of lymphoid leukemia and testicular cancer but a decreased risk of melanoma. The pathogenesis is uncertain, but an increased risk of PC[366,368] has also been seen in CF patients as well as patients with CP from other causes.[369,370] This heightened cancer risk should be kept in mind as the survival of persons with CF continues to increase. Adolescents and adults with unexplained complaints, especially relating to the abdominal organs, should be evaluated for occult malignancy. A recent consensus panel on colorectal cancer screening in CF patients recommended colonoscopy at age 40 years with follow-up screening as indicated by individual findings.[371] Organ transplant recipients should be screened for colorectal cancer starting at 30 years of age.

Nutritional Management

Nutrition goals: In the routine clinical setting, the nutritional management of patients with CF is based on an assessment of nutritional requirements (see Chapter 7), considering age, height, weight, and anthropometrics for age in children and BMI in adults, the severity of lung disease, as well as anorexia, PI, and mucosal dysfunction.[288,372] Ideally, an age-appropriate diet that is 1.1–2 times the reference calorie intake for healthy populations should be encouraged, with adequate PERT provided (and with gastric acid suppression, if indicated) to achieve as normal a fat balance as possible.[288] High-calorie, high-fat, and liberal salt diets are also encouraged by many CF centers. The role of nutrition is important in lung function, as patients with a BMI $\geq$ the 50th percentile tend to have pulmonary function (FEV_1) within 80% of normal.[288,372]

In 2005 the Cystic Fibrosis Foundation revised the nutrition classification guidelines to eliminate the use of percentage of ideal body weight to define nutritional failure. The guidelines were reviewed and updated in 2008.[372] For children younger than age 2, weight-for-length percentile should be maintained at or above the 50th percentile. Up to age 20, BMI $\geq$ the 50th percentile was recommended. It was also recommended that women should have a BMI of 22 kg/m^2 or greater, and men 23 kg/m^2 or greater. Similar recommendations were given in the *ESPEN-ESPGHAN-ECFS* guidelines on nutrition care for infants, children, and adults with CF in 2016.[288]

Malnutrition in CF can result from a variety of factors that increase nutrient loss, reduce energy intake, and increase energy expenditure. Increased losses are primarily related to underlying PI but are also influenced by conditions such as poorly controlled diabetes mellitus, vomiting and/or regurgitation, excess intestinal mucus, and inadequate bile salt secretion. Energy intake can be affected both by disease complications and by psychosomatic issues, psychosocial issues, stress, and treatment noncompliance, especially in children and adolescents.[288] Severe respiratory symptoms can be accompanied by anorexia, nausea, and vomiting. GI symptoms or complications such as abdominal pain, GERD with chest pain, anorexia, and vomiting can lead to reduced caloric intake. In some patients, clinical depression, physical fatigue, a disordered sense of smell (food is unappetizing), and altered body image can lead to reduced food intake. Increased energy expenditure also frequently accompanies the severe respiratory disease of CF and is likely related to variables, including chronic infections, fever, increased work of breathing, and bronchodilator medications.[288]

The optimal dietary intake for a CF patient is greater than the RDA of healthy children and adults. To prevent or delay onset of nutritional deficits, the *ESPEN-ESPGHAN-ECFS guidelines on nutrition* recommend advising patients on macronutrient balance in the diet, with attention to protein and fat intake that is sufficient to prevent or delay loss of muscle mass and function. In general, intake of energy should be age-appropriate and support normal weight, noting a wide interindividual range from about 1.1 to 2 times the reference intake for healthy populations. Advice on dietary intake of electrolytes, with supplementation as needed; supplementation of fat-soluble vitamins; and prescription of PERT for individuals with PI is also recommended.[288]

The use of PERT in CF is lifesaving, but the dosing is more empiric and may not translate well to recommendations for adult patients with CP and EPI. A recent consensus recommendation for CF patients who are infants (up to 12 months) was: 2000–4000 U lipase/120 mL formula or estimated breast milk intake and approximately 2000 U lipase/g dietary fat in food.[288] For children 1–4 years, use 2000–4000 U lipase/g dietary fat, increasing the dose upward as needed (maximum dose 10,000 U lipase/kg/day).[288] For children more than 4 years and adults, start at 500 U lipase/kg/meal, titrating upward to a maximal dose of 1000–2500 U lipase/kg/meal, or 10,000 U lipase/kg/day, or 2000–4000 U lipase/g dietary fat taken with all fat-containing meals, snacks, and drinks.[288] This would equate to 70,000–175,000 U lipase/meal for a 70-kg patient with CF, which is similar to a dose of 72,000 U lipase/meal shown to be effective in improving the coefficient of fat absorption in a double-blind, randomized, placebo-controlled, parallel-group trial of pancreatin capsules (3 Creon 24,000).[373]

Enteral tube feeding: Even without supporting evidence from randomized trials, enteral tube feeding remains a frequent therapy for malnutrition in CF. About 10% of CF patients require supplemental tube feeding.[310] A recent retrospective Belgian CF registry study of enteral tube feeding demonstrated that enteral tube feeding improved BMI *z*-score and stabilized the FEV_1.[374] The finding is in line with prior studies showing an association between nutritional status and pulmonary function.[372] Importantly, the registry study found that tube feedings were not started until patients already had significantly worse nutritional and pulmonary status than the CF cohort as a whole. This observation implies that better anticipatory planning and early markers of pending nutritional failure are needed.

The presence and severity of GERD symptoms may influence the decision on the preferred route for tube feeding. Some adolescents learn to pass soft silastic feeding tubes nightly to administer nasogastric feedings. Gastrostomy feedings may be preferred by some families and patients, especially in younger children. Gastrostomy or jejunostomy feedings are instituted at the first sign of nutritional failure. Standard formulas are usually well tolerated. Nocturnal infusion is encouraged to promote normal eating patterns during the day. Initially, 30%–50% of the estimated caloric needs should be provided overnight. Very low-fat, elemental formulas may be used without enzyme supplements for patients with an enteral feeding tube and should be given by continuous infusion.[375] For standard formulas, the approach to providing PERT during the feeds is variable. A novel in-line cartridge containing immobilized lipase offers another attractive option.[376,377] Patients receiving enteral feedings should be monitored for carbohydrate intolerance on at least two separate nights by measuring blood glucose levels 2–3 hours into the feeding and at the end of the feeding. Insulin may be required to prevent hyperglycemia, with adjustment of the insulin dosage during acute illness, glucocorticoid therapy, or other changes in health status. In some cases, parenteral nutrition may be necessary, but it should be reserved for acute support with a return to some form of enteral nutrition as soon as possible.

Treatment of CFTR functional variants with targeted drug therapy: After considerable effort to treat CF by increasing functional CFTR in the lung through delivery of DNA or protein failed to provide long-lasting improvement in humans, efforts turned toward recovering function of endogenous CFTR.[378] Using high-throughput screens with thousands of small molecules, investigators identified compounds that improved endogenous, mutant CFTR function.[379] The first targeted therapy with one of these compounds, VX-770 or ivacaftor (Kalydeco), was directed at the third most common CF-causing mutation, p.G551D. VX-770 improves function of p.G551D CFTR by altering the gating function of mutant CFTR to increase the probability of channel opening, thereby increasing Cl^- secretion.[380] In phases II and III clinical trials, VX-770 improved predicted FEV_1, decreased sweat chloride concentration, and decreased the frequency of pulmonary exacerbations.[381,382] Follow-up of a subset of subjects who did not have an early response to treatment showed they had long-term clinical benefits.[383] VX-770 was FDA-approved for use in patients with a variety of mutations that cause gating dysfunction in CFTR.[384–386] This population does not include patients carrying the most common disease-causing variant, *CFTR* p.F508del. That variant causes multiple defects in CFTR folding, trafficking, membrane stability, and chloride channel activity. The issue was approached by combining VX-770 with VX-809 (lumacaftor), a small molecule that facilitates CFTR folding. The combination results in a partial rescue of p.F508del CFTR function.[387] Clinical trials of the combination therapy showed improved clinical outcomes in patients homozygous for p.F508del CFTR, and the therapy was approved by the FDA.[388] However, it appears that, in general, the effects of CFTR enhancers and correctors are not mutation specific. Instead, the magnitude of drug response is highly correlated with residual CFTR function for the potentiator ivacaftor, the corrector lumacaftor, and ivacaftor-lumacaftor combination therapy, and the effects are additive.[389] About half of eligible CF patients take the combination of ivacaftor and lumacaftor.[310] Other small molecule combinations are in development or trials, and improvements in efficacy will likely result.[390]

Prognosis: Survival statistics estimated from data in national CF registries are often confusing because different groups use different methods and terminology when reporting survival data.[391] The latest estimate of median predicted survival for patients born between 2012 and 2016 in the United States is 42.7 years of age.[310] For patients who attain 40 years of age, the median predicted survival is almost 60 years of age. Still, for the 373 people who died from CF in 2016, their median age was only 29.6 years. Most of the morbidity and mortality is related to chronic pulmonary disease; respiratory or cardiorespiratory disease contributes to 67% of deaths.[310] The relative roles of nutritional support, pancreatic enzyme replacement, and aggressive treatment of pulmonary disease in improving the quality and duration of life remain under study. CF patients with PS have better pulmonary status than those with PI, suggesting that the disease is heterogeneous and that survival is improved with better nutrition and treatment.

As survival improves, the problems facing CF patients will likely change and begin to spill over into the domain of caretakers predominantly focused on the issues of CF adults. These medical problems will include such entities as pancreatitis, malnutrition, cirrhosis with portal hypertension, diabetes mellitus with its long-term complications, osteopenia, and reproductive issues, as well as all of the more common problems seen in childhood. In the 2016 report from the Cystic Fibrosis Registry, the prevalence of bone disease, GERD, sinus disease, asthma, anxiety, and depression is higher in older patients. CF-related diabetes is more common in adults than in children (35.1% vs. 6.4%). Pulmonary disease is more severe in adults than in children, and malnutrition continues to be a problem in adults with CF although nutritional outcomes are improving overall.[310] Increasingly, these patients will require evaluation for potential malignancies of the digestive tract and evaluation for liver disease or other complications that will necessitate the specialized attention of a gastroenterologist.

Hereditary Pancreatitis

HP is a syndrome of RAP, often leading to CP, that develops in an individual from a family in which the pancreatitis phenotype appears to be inherited through a disease-causing gene mutation expressed in an autosomal dominant pattern.[9,392] The most common cause is a gain-of-function mutation in the cationic trypsinogen gene (*PRSS1*) that alters the regulatory domains usually controlled by calcium (see Fig. 59.4). Most kindreds with *PRSS1* mutations are from the United States and Europe, with a few from Japan, South America or Southern Asia. Most (65%–81%) but not all kindreds with an autosomal dominant-appearing inheritance pattern of pancreatitis have *PRSS1* mutations.[393,394]

Clinical features: The phenotypic features of HP caused by *PRSS1* mutations are confined to the pancreas because the pancreas is the primary site of trypsinogen expression. The primary phenotype is RAP, with a subset of patients progressing to CP with all of the complications shared with other forms of CP.

AP: An attack of AP typically signals the onset of disease in patients with HP. The median age for the first diagnosis of pancreatitis in a family/cohort of 181 symptomatic *PRSS1* mutation carriers in the United States was 7 years of age (interquartile range, 3–16; range <1–73).[12] In France, median onset of symptoms was 10 years (range 1–73),[395] and was 10 years for *PRSS1* p.R122H and 14 years for *PRSS1* p.N29I in the EUROPAC study.[393] AP and RAP are diagnosed and managed as with other types of pancreatitis (see Chapter 60). The severity of attacks varies. Some families appear to have more severe attacks and complications than others.[10,396] The vast majority of attacks lasted less than 7 days; affected patients averaged 2 (p.R122H) or 1.4 (p.N29I) attacks per year. The hospital admission rate was significantly greater with p.R122H (0.33 per year) than with p.N29I mutations (0.19 per year).[393] Uncommonly, prolonged, persistent, or smoldering AP for which the patient may remain hospitalized for weeks or months may occur.

The penetrance of the pancreatitis phenotype in gene mutation carriers is incomplete (≈80%).[12,393,395,397] The apparent incomplete penetrance and variable expression appear to be determined by both genetic and environmental factors.[398] For example, earlier age of onset and a more severe clinical course are seen in patients with additional mutations (e.g., *PRSS1* plus *SPINK1*).[399]

The first episode of AP (SAPE) signals the beginning of a cycle of RAP that may end in CP. There are not specific preventative treatments in patients with HP to stop progression or minimize severity of attacks. Multiple small meals, avoidance of high-fat meals, and use of antioxidants and vitamins are generally recommended. Both alcohol and smoking must be avoided. In a study of 14 HP patients with CP, there was a significantly higher serum level of superoxide dismutase and lower serum level of vitamin E and selenium than in other family members, population controls, or in seven children with non-HP.[400] A small open-label trial using antioxidants and vitamins appeared to reduce the number of days of pain attacks in an HP family.[401] In another pilot study of the calcium channel blocker amlodipine, the four treated patients had a reduction in analgesic use and symptom score.[402]

CP: The onset of CP is currently difficult to determine, but the time between the onset of symptoms (usually those of AP) and exocrine/endocrine failure has been estimated in HP (Fig. 59.11). In the EUROPAC study, the cumulative risk of pancreatic exocrine failure was 2.0% at age 10 years, 8.4% at age 20, 33.6% at age 40, and 60.2% at age 70.[393] Similar findings were observed in France and the United States.[12,395]

Pain: Pain is among the most distressing and debilitating features of HP. The pain experience is highly variable, suggesting the presence of multiple modifying factors.[275,403] Of note, in a North American Study, pain did not correlate with imaging studies based on Cambridge criteria, suggesting other risk factors for pain.[404] The severity of pain may be affected by depression and/or anxiety,[405,406] possibility with genetic predisposition.[407–409] In general, patients with constant pain in the context of either RAP or CP typically have more pain-related disability/unemployment and significantly lower quality-of-life scores.[410,411] Persistent pancreatic pain signals can lead to pain centralization and a chronic pain syndrome that is debilitating for the patient

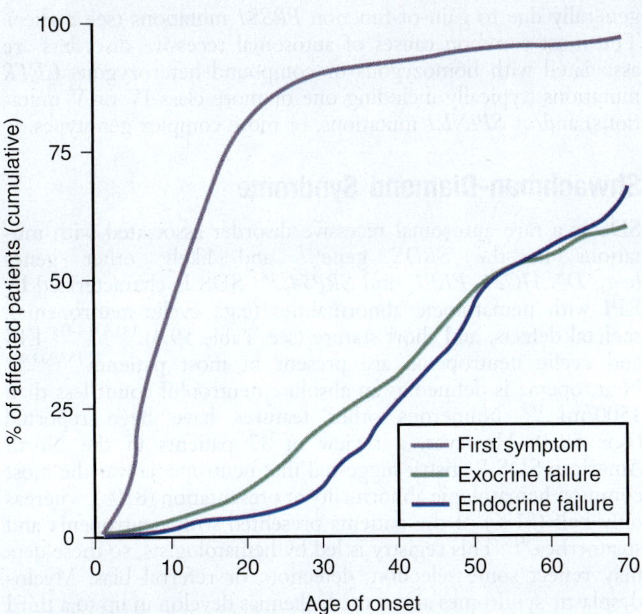

Fig. 59.11 Age of symptom onset in patients with hereditary pancreatitis (HP). Subjects with HP due to *PRSS1* R122H mutations usually have an early age of onset (before age 20), although first symptoms can occur at older ages. A subset of subjects develops exocrine and/or endocrine failure, usually 20–30 years after the first symptoms. *PRSS1*, Protease, serine 1 (trypsin 1). (From Howes N, Lerch MM, Greenhalf W, et al. Clinical and genetic characteristics of hereditary pancreatitis in Europe. *Clin Gastroenterol Hepatol*. 2004;2:252–261.)

and linked with high health resource use.[403,410,412,413] Patients with severe neuropathic pain may also have surgical findings of nerve hypertrophy and increased neural density as seen in patients with pancreatitis from other etiologies[414,415] that is highly resistant to medical therapy. In cases where intractable pain in patients with impaired quality of life due to CP or RAP in whom medical, endoscopic, or prior surgical therapy have failed, total pancreatectomy with islet autotransplantation (TPIAT) should be considered a potentially effective therapy.[416] Of note, patients with *PRSS1* variants that undergo a TPIAT have better outcomes if they are younger and have shorter duration of disease, likely because of less fibrosis and better islet yield.[417] In expert centers, patients with TPIAT had highly significant improvement in average health-related quality of life, based on data from the Medical Outcomes Study SF-36 in both mean physical component summary score and mental component summary.[418] Although further work is being done to identify environmental and genetic factors associated with pain and targeted therapy, current evidence suggests that earlier surgery helps reduce the likelihood of central pain.[403]

Diabetes mellitus: In the EUROPAC study, the cumulative risk of endocrine failure was 1.3% at age 10 years, 4.4% at age 20, 8.5% at age 30, and 47.6% by age 50 (see Fig. 59.11).[393] Likewise, 26% of French HP patients developed diabetes mellitus, with a median age of onset of 38 years.[395] The cumulative incidence of endocrine failure (diabetes) continues to increase after age 50, especially in those with the p.N29I variant in at least one study.[393]

At least two studies highlight high-risk factors for diabetes mellitus in pancreatitis. First, among patients with RAP or CP from all causes, diabetes was associated with African ancestry, overweight, or obese, a family history of diabetes, imaging studies demonstrating pancreatic calcifications with atrophy, prior pancreas surgery and EPI.[23] Many of these risk factors overlap with T2DM. A genetic study was conducted to polygenic risk scores (PRSs) for T2DM between patients with RAP/CP with or without diabetes. The PRS in for T2DM was high in patients with pancreatitis and diabetes and normal in patients with pancreatitis without diabetes.[419] Thus inflammation of the exocrine pancreas can affect risk for T2DM. Early recognition of risks for T2DM should lead to early involvement of endocrinologist to help minimize other risk factors to delay the development and severity of T2DM in these patients.

PC: The incidence of PC in patients with HP is dramatically increased.[12,393,420,421] PC appears to develop about 30–40 years after the onset of pancreatitis.[420,422,423] The initial estimated cumulative risk of PC by age 70 was 40% (95% CI, 9%–71%).[420,424] In France, the cumulative risk of PC at ages 50 and 75 years was 11% and 49% for men and 8% and 55% for women.[421] However, two additional studies with older, larger cohorts identified a lower cumulative risk at age 70 years—18.8% in the EUROPAC study[393] and 7.2% in the United States.[12]

The reasons for the high incidence of PC are unknown. The *PRSS1* gene does not appear to play a role in sporadic PC,[425] and our current knowledge of trypsin biology provides no rationale for how trypsin may act as an oncogene or other cancer-related factor. Rather, the recurrent pancreatic injury caused by unregulated trypsinogen activation, and subsequent inflammatory response appears to provide an environment that is oncogenic in nature.[423,426] However, although pancreatic intraepithelial neoplasia (PanIN) lesions occur frequently and early in patients with HP, they do not appear to correlate with extent of calcification, fibrosis, or inflammation.[427] PC is caused by germline mutations, and it is assumed that patients with other mutations that alter DNA repair mechanisms will be at higher risk.

Treatment options for PC are limited, and the prognosis remains poor despite some recent advances. The most effective approach is prevention, with the recognition that early onset pancreatitis is one of the strongest known risk factors for PC. The most effective lifestyle target is tobacco smoking, which doubles the risk for PC.[370] This doubling of risk becomes critically important in individuals with HP, who already have an underlying risk of PC that is 50-fold the risk of the general population. Indeed, the age- and sex-adjusted OR for individuals with HP is doubled by tobacco smoking, and the median age of diagnosis of PC is 20 years earlier in smokers.[420] In addition to smoking, diabetes mellitus appears to be a risk factor of PC in patients with HP.[421]

Although HP families have a high cancer risk, no effective screening methods have been established. Early detection of PC in the anatomically distorted gland of a pancreatitis patient is difficult. For this reason, the consensus guidelines of an expert panel suggest that if an individual in the PC risk age range is contemplating pancreatic surgery, a total pancreatectomy should be considered.[428] Younger patients may be offered a TPIAT, but due to the risk of transplanting malignant cells, the role of islet autotransplantation in older adult patients with long-standing CP is uncertain.[416,429]

Diagnosis: Prior to 1996 the diagnosis of HP was based purely on clinical criteria, including examination of the family pedigree. The discovery of the cationic trypsinogen gene mutations *PRSS1* p.R122H and p.N29I opened the door to molecular diagnosis.[9,227] Although the majority of kindreds with an autosomal dominant pattern of RAP and CP (and/or diabetes mellitus or PC) will have gain-of-function *PRSS1* mutations, up to 20% of families with HP will not have an identifiable *PRSS1* mutation.[12,393,395] *PRSS1* duplication variants are also associated with HP.[85,86,430] The diagnosis requires both clinical signs of otherwise idiopathic AP or RAP and either a strong family history or *PRSS1* variants associated with HP.[41]

Genetic testing: Genetic testing results remain unchanged throughout the life of the patient, have implications for future descendants and other family members, and may affect social and reproductive choices, employment, and insurability.[41,431] Thus the clinician must fully comprehend the implications of testing, be prepared to provide pre- and posttest genetic counseling to the patient (or refer the patient to a genetic counselor), and ensure that informed consent is obtained before testing.[41,431]

Reasons for *PRSS1* mutation testing include verification of a clinical suspicion, helping a patient understand or validate his or her condition, and assisting individuals to assess their risk of pancreatitis and eventually PC. Genetic information may also be useful in making life decisions to minimize risk of disease (e.g., reproduction, diet, alcohol, and smoking). Identification of an established pancreatitis-associated gene mutation can be valuable in expediting an expensive and prolonged evaluation of RAP in children and may preclude further evaluation of elusive causes of pancreatitis in adults.

The positive and negative predictive value of a genetic test in identifying specific mutations is almost perfect with properly applied modern techniques.[283,432] Interpretation of test results and explanation of their meaning to the patient continue to be pivotal issues. Prognosis can be outlined in general terms from the clinical discussion earlier, noting that there is significant variability and that the effectiveness of future treatments in preventing adverse outcomes is unknown. Finally, the mutation-positive individual has a 50% chance of passing on the mutation to each child.

A positive test result in a clinically unaffected person is interpreted as an increased risk of pancreatitis, with this risk *possibly* diminishing with age. A negative test result in a family with a known mutation in the *PRSS1* gene essentially eliminates the risk of this genetic form of pancreatitis. If a mutation has *not* been previously identified in the family, a negative test result in an *unaffected* person is considered noninformative because one cannot distinguish whether the tested individual is free from genetic risk or whether he or she has inherited a different pancreatitis-predisposing gene mutation. Up-to-date information should always be available through the commercial genetic testing laboratory. Genetic counseling information can be found through the National Society of Genetic Counselors or the American Board of Genetic Counseling.[432]

Genetic testing of children raises unique issues.[432] Unlike an adult patient, a child legally cannot provide informed consent. Thus the decision for a child is essentially left to the parents or legal guardian. For children age 7 and older, a parent or legal guardian may provide consent for genetic testing, although these older children should also provide assent to the testing. The primary reason for testing children for *PRSS1* gene mutations is to assist in determining the cause of unexplained pancreatitis or to confirm suspected pancreatitis in a child at risk for HP, thereby limiting further investigations. The testing of asymptomatic children is strongly discouraged because currently there is no clear medical benefit in identifying carriers at a young age. Because alcohol consumption, fatty foods, and emotional stress have been reported to precipitate pancreatitis attacks, and because smoking increases the risk of pancreatitis and PC, testing for the purpose of encouraging mutation-positive older children to avoid these excesses is advocated by some caregivers. However, avoidance of fatty foods, alcohol, and tobacco represents excellent general health advice for all children and, therefore, provides no compelling reason for testing. In either case, the personal desires of older children to postpone testing or to proceed with testing to relieve their own anxieties and learn more about their own health must also be carefully considered.

Familial Pancreatitis

Familial pancreatitis, in which the initial symptoms occur at a young age (e.g., <20 years), is more likely associated with a strong genetic risk. Autosomal dominant inheritance patterns are generally due to gain-of-function *PRSS1* mutations (see earlier). The most common causes of autosomal recessive disorders are associated with homozygous or compound heterozygous *CFTR* mutations (typically including one or more class IV or V mutations) and/or *SPINK1* mutations, or more complex genotypes.

Shwachman-Diamond Syndrome

SDS is a rare autosomal recessive disorder associated with mutations in the *SBDS* gene[182] and likely other genes (e.g., *DNAJC21*, *ELF1*, and *SRP54*).[183] SDS is characterized by EPI with hematologic abnormalities (e.g., cyclic neutropenia), skeletal defects, and short stature (see Table 59.4).[183,433–435] EPI and cyclic neutropenia are present in most patients.[183,433,435] Neutropenia is defined as an absolute neutrophil count less than 1500/mL.[183] Numerous other features have been reported (Box 59.4). However, a review of 37 patients in the North American SDS Registry suggested that neutropenia was the most common hematologic abnormality at presentation (81%), whereas only half (51%) of the patients presented with neutropenia and steatorrhea.[436] This registry is led by hematologists, so these data may reflect some selection, detection, or referral bias. Myelodysplastic syndromes and acute leukemias develop in up to a third of patients.

Severe cases of SDS present in infancy with malabsorption, failure to thrive, or recurrent infections. Because of the variable expression of pancreatic, hematologic, and other features, diagnosis in mild cases may be delayed.[433,436,437] Several hundred

BOX 59.4 Clinical Features of Shwachman-Diamond Syndrome (Frequency, in %)

PANCREATIC

Exocrine pancreatic hypoplasia (91%–100%)
Steatorrhea (55%–88%)

HEMATOLOGIC

Neutropenia (88%–100%)
Elevated fetal Hgb level (80%)
Leukopenia (52%)
Anemia (42%–66%)
Pancytopenia (44%)
Thrombocytopenia (24%–34%)
Myelodysplastic syndromes (8%–33%)
Leukemia (12%)

SKELETAL

Metaphyseal dysostosis (44%)
Thoracic dystrophy (32%)
Long-bone tubulation defects (?)
Short or flared ribs (?)
Others (<5%)

GROWTH

Short statue with normal growth velocity (common)

OTHER

Psychomotor delay (common)
Abnormal liver biochemical test levels (common)
Myocardial abnormalities (50% at autopsy)
Mental retardation (33%)
Diabetes mellitus (<5%)
Hepatomegaly (<5%)
Renal tubular dysfunction (?)
Dental abnormalities (?)
Ichthyosis (?)

families, most with a single affected member, have been identified.[434]

SDS genetic defects: The primary gene linked to SDS is the *SBDS* gene. This gene has 5 exons and encodes a predicted protein of 250 amino acids and participates in ribosomal maturation and related systems.[438] The genetic defect in most cases of SDS is caused by gene conversion between the normal *SBDS* gene and a nonfunctional pseudogene designated *SBDSP* that results in a dysfunctional protein product.[182,438] The *SBDSP* pseudogene DNA code is 97% identical to *SBDS* gene code. Fourteen distinct mutations were initially identified in the original kindreds, with the most common being the conversion mutations 183-184TA → CT and 258 + 2T → C; 183-184TA → CT introduces a premature stop codon, p.K62X, whereas 258 + 2T → C disrupts a donor splice site. More than 40 novel genetic variants in *SBDS* have now been found as compound heterozygous genotypes with one of the common gene conversion alleles.[438] No homozygotes for the p.K62X variant have been described, indicating that a functional SBDS protein is required for survival. Fewer than 10% of patients with clinical features of SDS do not have mutations in *SBDS*. Some of these individuals have biallelic genetic variants in *DNAC21*, the protein product of which aids maturation of the 60S ribosomal subunit.[184]

SBDS encodes a highly conserved and widely expressed protein of 29 kd. Along with guanosine triphosphatase elongation factor 6 from the 60S ribosomal subunit, SBDS functions to initiate translation.[439–441] In addition, SBDS likely participates in regulating telomerase recruitment to telomeres and, thereby, aids in maintaining telomer length.[442] The genetic defect results in a pancreatic acinar cell defect with markedly reduced zymogen synthesis and PI rather than susceptibility to pancreatitis. Lack of SBDS expression also affects myeloid differentiation and increases risk for bone marrow failure and acute myeloid leukemia.[436] A mouse model of SBDS deficiency shows that the protein is required for pancreatic development and function.[443] Human embryonic stem cells and induced pluripotent stem cells with defects in SBDS manifest deficits in exocrine pancreatic and hematopoietic differentiation in vitro, enhanced apoptosis, and elevated protease levels in culture supernatants; the deficits could be reversed by restoring SBDS protein expression through transgene rescue or by supplementing culture media with protease inhibitors suggesting that protease-mediated autodigestion contributes to the pathogenesis of SDS.[444] Ataluren, a drug that suppresses nonsense mutations originally developed to treat CF, restored SBDS expression and stimulated myeloid differentiation in hematopoietic cells obtained from patients with SDS.[445]

Clinical features: The clinical features of SDS are pancreatic and hematologic. A wide range of features and degrees of severity can now be confirmed by integrating the genotype and phenotype in high-risk families.

PI: The clinical features of SDS usually become evident in the first year of life.[217,433,437,446] Severe PI, steatorrhea, and failure to thrive are frequent presenting symptoms but are not always present or necessary to make a diagnosis.[433,436,437,447] A normal sweat chloride concentration (or other normal measure of CFTR function) can help distinguish SDS from CF[217] if genetic testing is not diagnostic.[448] The pancreatic lesion appears to begin with developmental failure of the pancreatic acini in utero.[217] Macroscopically, the pancreas appears fatty and may be small or normal size. The extensive lipomatous changes result in characteristic changes during abdominal imaging by CT (Fig. 59.12), MRI, or US,[449,450] *but these imaging findings are not always present*.[436] The main pancreatic ducts and islets are normal; there is extensive fatty replacement of the pancreatic acinar tissue.[217] Serial assessments of exocrine pancreatic function reveal persistent deficits of enzyme secretion, but nearly half of patients showed moderate age-related improvements after age 4, resulting in PS,[433,437] with some pancreatic enzymes (e.g., trypsin) returning more than others (e.g., amylase).

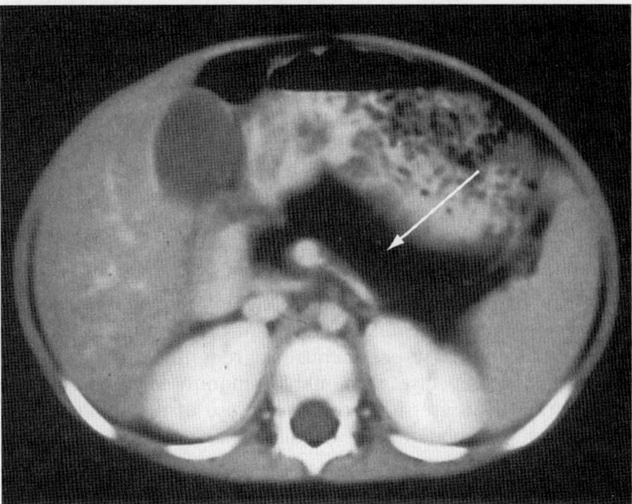

Fig. 59.12 CT appearance of the pancreas in a patient with Shwachman-Diamond syndrome. Note that the pancreas (*arrow*) retains a typical size and shape, but it is highly fatty and therefore appears as a very low-density structure. (Image courtesy Professor Peter Durie.)

Hematologic manifestations: Neutropenia-related infections are also an early and potentially serious problem in SDS. The neutropenia occurs in a cyclical fashion in two-thirds of patients, and when tested, the neutrophils appear to have impaired migration and chemotaxis,[451] *although they can still form abscesses*.[183] SDS patients are susceptible to a variety of bacterial, viral, and fungal infections beyond that expected in patients with neutropenia.[183,435] Common infections include otitis media, sinusitis, pneumonia, osteomyelitis, urinary tract infections, skin and soft tissue infections, and lymphadenitis.[183,452] Normochromic, normocytic anemia occurs in up to 80% of patients.[183] Thrombocytopenia is sometimes present. Patients with pancytopenia have the worst prognosis.[433] Whereas the median age of survival for all SDS patients is 35 years, patients with pancytopenia have a median life expectancy of only 24 years. Pancytopenia appears at a mean age of 6 years and occurs in 10%–25% of patients.[452] Up to a third of SDS patients develop a myelodysplastic syndrome, and approximately 10%–25% develop leukemia, usually acute myeloid leukemia.[433,435,437,451]

Growth and development: The birth weight of children with SDS is typically low (2.9 ± 0.5 kg, 25th percentile),[433] and by 6 months of age, the mean heights and weights are characteristically below the 5th percentile. Thereafter, growth velocity appears normal.[433] The short stature is independent of nutrition.[217,435] Some clinically evident skeletal abnormalities may be present. For example, metaphyseal chondrodysplasia and dysostosis may be evident in 44% of patients, especially in the femoral head and proximal tibia.[183,217] Thoracic dystrophy, such as pectus, asphyxiating thoracic dystrophy, flared ribs, and other skeletal abnormalities also have been described.[183,217,433,453] Most patients remain below the 3rd percentile for height and weight, although some adults reach the 25th percentile for height.[217] Males and females are probably affected equally, but males are more likely to undergo thorough investigation for short stature than females, leading to a mild ascertainment bias.[434,437]

Treatment: The treatment of pancreatic exocrine deficiency is more straightforward with SDS than with CF, because bicarbonate secretion in the pancreas and duodenum is spared. Pancreatic enzyme replacement should be initiated with an expectation of diminished steatorrhea and improved weight gain. Fat-soluble vitamins, medium-chain TGs, and other high-calorie supplements may be needed, as discussed for CF.

Patients with SDS are typically followed by multidisciplinary teams led by a hematologist. During periods of granulocytopenia, febrile episodes should be evaluated and treated with appropriate antimicrobial drugs. Patients with severe neutropenia or those suspected to have severe infections should be hospitalized and treated with intravenous antibiotics until they improve.[435] Chronic use of G-CSF should be considered for recurrent invasive bacterial and/or fungal infections in the presence of severe neutropenia.[435] Patients may respond to an intermittent schedule with low doses of G-CSF (e.g., 2–3 μg/kg every 3 days) or may require higher doses continuously.[435] Hematopoietic stem cell transplant remains the only curative therapy for SDS individuals with severe aplastic anemia or malignant transformation.[183] Episodes of bleeding or severe anemia may require blood or platelet transfusion.[435] Hip disease should be monitored, with surgical intervention if progression occurs. The use of recombinant human growth hormone in this condition has not been systematically investigated, but anecdotal reports have shown efficacy in accelerating growth.

RARE GENETIC SYNDROMES WITH PANCREATIC PATHOLOGY

Johanson-Blizzard Syndrome

Johanson-Blizzard syndrome is a rare autosomal recessive syndrome linked to mutations in the ubiquitin-ligase E3 *(UBR1)* gene.[190,454,455] The pancreatic component of the syndrome is characterized by EPI and growth restriction, with lipomatous transformation of the pancreas rather than AP. Most mutations in *UBR1* are nonsense, frameshift, splice-site mutations, or small in-frame deletions that result in an inactive protein.[455] Some patients have missense mutations or small in-frame deletions that result in a milder phenotype.[188,455,456] A recent study identified exon deletions or duplications of *UBR1* in patients with Johanson-Blizzard syndrome, thereby extending the genotype of this disorder.[457]

Ubiquitin-ligase E3 belongs to the N-end rule pathway of an intracellular protein degradation system. Digestive serine proteases, which are known to trigger autodigestion during pancreatitis, are specific substrates of UBR1 and are upregulated in the pancreas when UBR1 is defective due to loss-of-function mutations.[190,455] The predominant and most consistent human phenotype, pancreatic exocrine insufficiency, is a consequence of intrauterine pancreatitis, resulting in complete gland destruction although this is not always the case. The pancreatic involvement in Johanson-Blizzard syndrome may be mild and not apparent until later in life.[189] The murine knockout of *UBR1* exhibits features that are very similar to the human phenotype, with restricted growth, craniofacial abnormalities, and pancreatic exocrine insufficiency. The murine acinar cells have impaired cholecystokinin receptor–stimulated excitation-secretion coupling and are more susceptible to experimental pancreatitis than wild-type animals and to a more severe systemic inflammatory response in the disease course. These findings are consistent with intracellular failure to degrade various cytosolic digestive enzymes.

Patients with Johanson-Blizzard syndrome have preservation of ductular output of fluid and electrolytes, like patients with SDS and unlike patients with CF.[458] They also have decreased acinar secretion of trypsin, colipase, and total lipase, and low serum immunoreactive trypsinogen levels, consistent with a primary acinar cell defect.[458] Histologically, the pancreatic ducts and islets are preserved but are surrounded by connective tissue and a total absence of acini. In addition to pancreatic acinar cell defects with malabsorption, the syndrome is characterized by aplastic alae nasi, deafness, hypothyroidism, dwarfism, absent permanent teeth, cardiac anomalies, genitourinary malformations, midline ectodermal scalp defects, and imperforate or anterior anus.[189,455,457] There are no hematologic abnormalities as in SDS.[458] Thus far, the association of variants in *UBR1* with CP continues to be investigated.[455,459]

Pearson Marrow-Pancreas Syndrome

Pearson marrow-pancreas syndrome is a rare autosomal dominant mtDNA breakage syndrome characterized by refractory sideroblastic anemia with vacuolization of marrow precursors, often with exocrine pancreatic dysfunction.[460,461] Other affected organ systems include the kidney (tubulopathy, aminoaciduria, and Fanconi syndrome), liver (hepatomegaly, cytolysis, and cholestasis), endocrine glands (diabetes mellitus, adrenal insufficiency), neuromuscular system, and heart.[461–463] Biochemical features include lactic acidosis, low levels of plasma citrulline and arginine, and urine with elevated citrulline, lactic/pyruvic aciduria, increased citric cycle intermediates, and, occasionally, ketonuria consistent with loss of key enzymes in the citric acid cycle and other mitochondrial functions.[461]

Patients with this syndrome may have transfusion-dependent macrocytic anemia in infancy, but all of the bone marrow cell lines otherwise appear to be normal. The PI results from pancreatic fibrosis rather than fatty replacement of the acinar cells, as in SDS, and is more likely to be associated with diabetes mellitus. The syndrome has a high-mortality rate in early childhood; patients who survive develop progressive involvement of multiple systems, including the liver, kidney, gut, and skin, all of which have abnormal mitochondria.

The molecular defect in Pearson marrow-pancreas syndrome was initially identified as a 4977–base pair deletion of mtDNA encompassing portions of the genes coding for NADH dehydrogenase, cytochrome oxidase, and ATPase.[464] A variety of other mitochondrial defects have now been identified,[462,465] and these deletions appear to be flanked with nucleotide repeats.[465] Cherry et al.[466] demonstrated that pluripotent stem cells with the high burden of deleted mtDNA had differences in growth, mitochondrial function, and hematopoietic phenotype when cultured in vitro compared with control pluripotent stem cells. The clinical features and severity of disease appear to correlate with the organ distribution and proportion of abnormal mtDNA.[462,467] Patients who survive may develop features of other mtDNA deletion syndromes. No specific treatment to correct these abnormalities is yet known.

Pancreatic Agenesis

Agenesis of the pancreas is extremely rare and is discussed in detail in Chapter 57.[468,469] Cardiac malformations, gallbladder agenesis, and gut malformations are also common in these patients. Intestinal malrotation typically results in aplasia of the uncinate process of the pancreas, likely as a developmental problem associated with duodenal rotation.[470]

The differential diagnosis of pancreatic agenesis includes transient diabetes mellitus of the newborn, pancreatic hypoplasia, CF, SDS, Johanson-Blizzard syndrome, and other rare disorders. However, in pancreatic agenesis, the profound endocrine and exocrine deficiencies persist, serum C-peptide and glucagon levels are undetectable, and the pancreas is absent on imaging studies (e.g., MRI). These children are managed as having type 1 diabetes mellitus (treated with insulin) and severe EPI (treated with pancreatic enzyme supplementation). Survival is possible with proper diagnosis and treatment.

Partial pancreatic agenesis of the dorsal pancreas is also extremely rare (see Chapter 57). Unlike complete agenesis of the pancreas, patients may be asymptomatic or may present with bile duct obstruction, pancreatitis, or diabetes.[471] Agenesis and hypoplasia of the ventral pancreas are also extremely rare. The lack of the ventral and dorsal pancreas has been described in patients carrying mutations in the gene-encoding hepatocyte nuclear factor 1 homeobox B (HNF-1B).[472]

Other Rare Syndromes

Other rare syndromes have been identified that affect the pancreas. Examples include asplenia with cystic liver, kidney, and pancreas (Iverson syndrome); "dysplasia" (in the sense of disturbed development) of the kidney, liver, and pancreas occurs without other abnormalities.[473] Histologically, the pancreas has dilated, large, irregular-shaped ducts surrounded by concentric loose mesenchyme and prominent areas of fibrosis and atrophy of its parenchyma.[473]

Isolated Enzyme and Other Digestive Enzyme-Associated Defects

Lipase: Congenital absence of pancreatic lipase is a rare disorder accompanied by variable preservation of other enzymes.[474–476] No mutations had been identified in this gene in patients suspected of having lipase deficiency until recently when two brothers with a novel mutation in *PNLIP* were reported.[477,478] Both males and females are affected. The earliest and most characteristic manifestation of this disease seems to be the passage of stool with an unusual amount of readily separable oil, which is often responsible for soiling. Failure to thrive is only occasionally noted, and systemic manifestations are absent. The two brothers with a known mutation in *PNLIP*, p.Thr221Met, had clinical evidence of CP.[478] The mechanism of disease appears to be protein misfolding and RER stress.[165]

Pancreatic lipase activity within duodenal contents in these patients is low to absent. Trypsin and amylase activity are somewhat diminished in some patients, but other parameters of exocrine function (including colipase and phospholipase A activities, bicarbonate, and volume secretion) are usually normal. Any residual lipase activity has been presumed to be a result of lingual or gastric lipase activity.

In addition to its functional absence, no immunologically reactive lipase can be detected,[474] suggesting either the complete absence of pancreatic lipase or the occurrence of a major structural change affecting both immunogenicity and function. The response to exogenous pancreatic enzyme therapy is suboptimal, and limitation of dietary fat is often necessary to avoid oily stools and incontinence.

Colipase: Colipase deficiency has been described in male offspring of consanguineous and nonconsanguineous marriages.[479,480] These patients present with loose stools and steatorrhea, but growth and development are normal. Colipase activity is markedly reduced, with otherwise normal pancreatic enzyme secretion. Fat absorption improves dramatically with the intraduodenal instillation of purified colipase. In studies of patients with exocrine pancreatic insufficiency associated with CF and SDS, steatorrhea occurs only when lipase and colipase secretion are diminished to less than 2% and less than 1% of mean normal values, respectively.[481] To date, no genetic variants in *CLPS* have been associated with colipase deficiency.

Serine protease inhibitor Kazal type 1 (SPINK1) deficiency: Two patients with homozygous variants of *SPINK1* presented with infantile EPI.[482] Both patients had loss-of-function genetic variants in *SPINK1*. One patient had a complete deletion of *SPINK1*, and the other had an inverted Alu element inserted into 3′-untranslated region of *SPINK1* resulting in undetectable levels of mRNA encoding SPINK1. Each patient's pancreas showed diffuse lipomatosis. Apparently, diabetes was not a feature of the syndrome because both patients did well on pancreatic enzyme replacement alone. *Spink3* (the mouse homolog of *SPINK1*) deficient mice had normal pancreas development until 15.5 days after coitus.[160] They then had progressive loss of pancreatic acinar cells until death by age 14.5 days, presumably from malnutrition. Together these findings suggest that SPINK1 and Spink3 have critical functions in the survival or regeneration of pancreatic acinar cells separate from their more well-known function to inhibit trypsin.

Enterokinase deficiency: Although few reports of congenital absence of enterokinase (enteropeptidase) have appeared since the original description in 1969,[483] a familial nature was suggested by its documentation in siblings.[484] DNA sequencing of two families revealed compound heterozygosity for nonsense mutations in two affected siblings and for a nonsense mutation and a frameshift mutation in the patient from the second family.[485] These patients presented with malabsorption, hypoproteinemia, and severe growth restriction. Evaluation included normal amylase and lipase activities but very low trypsin activity in the duodenum, with normal concentrations of sweat electrolytes. Luminal trypsinogen could be activated by the addition of exogenous enterokinase. Small intestinal morphology and disaccharidase levels were normal. Congenital enterokinase deficiency is recognized in 1%−2% of infants undergoing evaluation of suspected PI although there have been no recent reports of new patients.[484] Follow-up into adulthood shows that the poor weight gain present in infancy resolves, and the patients do not have GI symptoms even without PERT.[485]

The steatorrhea associated with enterokinase deficiency may be related to a secondary deficiency of phospholipase, the activation of which requires trypsin, which in turn is activated by enterokinase. Patients with CF and SDS have increased intraluminal but normal mucosal enterokinase activity.[484] Enterokinase levels and activity may also theoretically decline with significant small intestinal mucosal injury. However, even in untreated celiac disease, normal mucosal and normal intraluminal enterokinase activities have been reported.[486]

FAMILIAL METABOLIC SYNDROMES ASSOCIATED WITH RECURRENT ACUTE AND CHRONIC PANCREATITIS

Familial Hyperparathyroidism With Hypercalcemia

Hypercalcemia is associated with AP, RAP, and CP. [487,238,488] The etiology of pancreatitis is intra-acinar cell trypsinogen activation.[64] Most causes are due to major metabolic disturbances such as primary hyperparathyroidism, malignancies such as multiple myeloma, vitamin D toxicity, sarcoidosis, total parenteral nutrition, and infusions of perioperative high-dose calcium during cardiopulmonary bypass.[489–493] For CP, calcium levels were also associated with CP in a recent Mendelian randomization study (OR 2.20; CI, 1.30, 3.72).[488]

Genetic risk for hypercalcemic AP has been studied. Research into the *CASR* gene suggests that a combination of *CASR*, *SPINK1*, and/or *CFTR* variants, plus alcohol or other factors are required to target the pancreas as a complex disease resulting in RAP and CP because *CASR* mutations alone are not sufficient.[235–237,494] A woman with a loss-of-function mutation in *CYP24A*, a gene that encodes a mitochondrial 24-hydroxylase that inactivates 1,25$(OH)_2$ D, developed hypercalcemia, nephrolithiasis, nephrocalcinosis, and AP during pregnancy,[495] although episodes of AP do not appear to be common in patients with this syndrome.[496]

Chylomicronemia Syndromes

The FCS and MCS were discussed earlier.

Acknowledgment

The authors would like to acknowledge the contribution of Mark Lowe MD, PhD, for his contributions to the previous edition of this chapter.

Full references for this chapter can be found at https://ebooks.health.elsevier.com.

60 Acute Pancreatitis

Peter J. Lee, Georgios I. Papachristou

IN THIS CHAPTER

INCIDENCE AND BURDEN OF ACUTE PANCREATITIS

The incidence of acute pancreatitis (AP) has been increasing worldwide, and it remains one of the most common reasons for hospitalization with a gastrointestinal condition.[1,2] Many studies demonstrate a variable worldwide incidence, generally in the range of 20–70 per 100,000 person-years.[1] This trend is significantly driven by the increasing AP incidence in North America and Europe, while in Asia its incidence has been stable in recent decades.[1] Both alcoholic and biliary etiologies—the two most common causes of AP—have shown an increase in their incidence. In 2018 AP was the 11th most common principal diagnosis for emergency department visits in the United States and the third most common GI-related principal diagnosis with almost 500,000 total annual admissions.[2] The health care cost was 2.6 billion dollars. In the same year, there were 5678 deaths contributed to by AP in the United States, making it the 12th most common cause of death due to a GI disease (up from 14th in 2012).

The overall mortality of AP has been decreasing. Age-standardized mortality rate is estimated to be approximately 1.4 per 100,000, a statistically significant decline from 1.7 per 100,000 from 1990.[3] Based on population-based cohort studies, globally, AP is the most common pancreatic disease, whereas pancreatic cancer is the most lethal.[4] A large increase in pediatric cases also accounts for the rising increase in the incidence of AP. This increase is presumably—as in adults—due to the rise in obesity-associated cholelithiasis. However, true incidence is difficult to ascertain because mild cases may not be captured [e.g., a patient with recurrent AP who opts to stay home instead of presenting to the endoplasmic reticulum (ER)]. Furthermore, epidemiologic studies rely on international classification of diseases codes to identify AP cases, which are subject to misclassification bias (e.g., patients with nonpancreatic diseases with elevated pancreatic enzymes can be misdiagnosed as having AP).[5]

The following sections are written with the focus on clinical management for practicing gastroenterologists and trainees based on recent evidence-based literature.

DEFINITIONS

AP is best defined physiologically as an acute inflammatory process of the pancreas with variable involvement of other regional or remote organ systems. The most widely accepted diagnosis of AP is based on meeting at least two of the following three criteria: (1) symptoms (e.g., acute onset epigastric and/or left upper quadrant pain, often radiating to the back) consistent with pancreatitis, (2) a serum amylase or lipase level greater than three times the upper limit of the laboratory's reference range, and (3) radiologic imaging consistent with pancreatitis, usually using computerized tomography (CT) or magnetic resonance imaging (MRI). It is worth noting that using abdominal pain with biochemical elevation of pancreatic enzymes alone as diagnostic criteria can fail to diagnose up to a quarter of patients with true AP and falsely diagnose patients with AP up to 1 in 10 patients when they have an alternative diagnosis (see "Laboratory Diagnosis" section).[6]

Limitations in the diagnostic performance of biochemical elevation of pancreatic enzymes are attributable to their diminished ability to capture AP patients presenting days after the onset of pain when the biochemical enzymes, mostly cleared by the kidney, have fallen to the normal range[6,7] (false negative). Furthermore, a host of nonpancreatic diseases can cause abdominal pain and elevated pancreatic enzymes (false-positive). On the other hand, imaging manifestations of AP may significantly lag symptom onset; so, relying on imaging studies alone can miss AP patients presenting early in their disease course. As such, having three diagnostic criteria facilitates capturing patients who present both early and late in the disease course.

Pancreatitis is classified as acute unless there are findings on CT, MRI, endoscopic ultrasound (EUS), or endoscopic retrograde cholangiopancreatoscopy (ERCP) suggestive of chronic pancreatitis. If such findings are present, pancreatitis is classified as chronic pancreatitis, and any further episode of AP is considered an exacerbation of or acute on chronic pancreatitis (see Chapter 61).

Once the diagnosis of AP is established, patients can be classified based on disease severity. The Revised Atlanta Criteria (RAC) 2012 (Box 60.1) classified severity as mild, moderately severe, or severe. The underlying classification principle of RAC is based on factors that determine in-hospital morbidity (e.g., length of hospitalization, need for intensive care unit admission, and need for a pancreatic intervention) and mortality.

Mild severity: Most AP episodes are mild, which, has no associated organ failure, local or systemic complications, and usually resolve within the first week. As expected, mild AP is associated with a short length of hospitalization, negligible need for ICU admission, and diminutive mortality.[8] Mild pancreatitis accounts for nearly 75%–80% of all cases. On contrast-enhanced CT scan, the pancreas is perfused well, without any nonperfused, low attenuation areas but appears edematous. Such an appearance is typically labeled as "interstitial pancreatitis."[9] The terms *mild* and *interstitial* pancreatitis can be used interchangeably if there are no local complications (e.g., peripancreatic or pancreatic fluid collections), organ failure, or exacerbation of comorbid conditions during an episode of AP.

Moderate severity: The moderately severe category includes patients forecasted to have high-morbidity and low-mortality. Its defining criteria include development of transient organ failure (lasting <48 hours), exacerbation of an existing comorbid condition (such as congestive heart failure or chronic obstructive pulmonary disease), and/or the development of local complications.[9] Local complications include acute (peri)pancreatic fluid collections, acute necrotic collections (pancreatic and peripancreatic necrosis, sterile or infected), pseudocysts, and walled-off necrosis (WON; sterile or infected; Figs. 60.1 and 60.2). The distinguishing hallmarks between these different local complications

BOX 60.1 2012 Atlanta Classification Revision of Acute Pancreatitis

MILD ACUTE PANCREATITIS

No organ failure
No local or systemic complications

MODERATELY SEVERE ACUTE PANCREATITIS

Transient organ failure (<48 hours) and/or
Local or systemic complications[a] without persistent organ failure

SEVERE ACUTE PANCREATITIS

Persistent organ failure (>48 hours)—single organ or multiorgan

[a]Local complications are peripancreatic fluid collections, pancreatic necrosis and peripancreatic necrosis (sterile or infected), pseudocyst, and walled-off necrosis (sterile or infected).

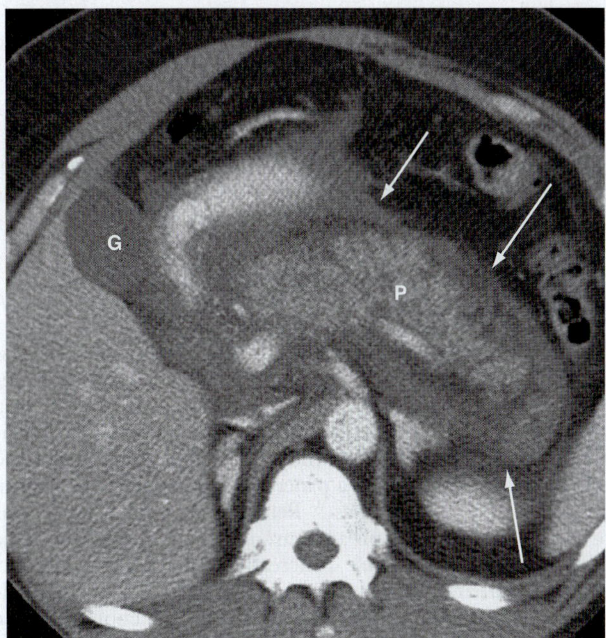

Fig. 60.1 CT showing acute interstitial pancreatitis with diffuse swelling of the pancreas (P) and peripancreatic inflammatory changes (*arrows*). The pancreas was well perfused without evidence of necrosis. G, Gallbladder.

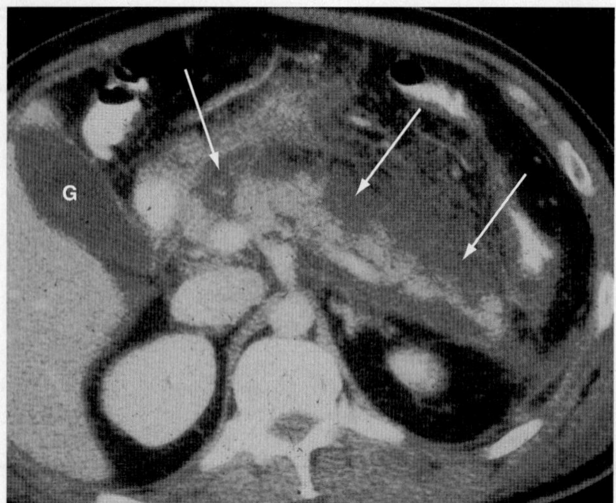

Fig. 60.2 CT showing acute pancreatic necrosis with focal areas of decreased perfusion in the pancreatic parenchyma (*arrows*) and surrounding peripancreatic inflammation. The necrosis was estimated to involve less than 30% of the pancreas. *G*, Gallbladder.

are the presence or absence of necrotic debris within the collection and the collections' chronicity (i.e., how long has the collection been present?).

Acute Necrotic Collections and Walled-Off Pancreatic Necrosis

Necrotizing pancreatitis according to the revised Atlanta classification[9] includes both pancreatic and/or peripancreatic necrosis. Approximately 45% of all cases of necrotizing pancreatitis involve both pancreatic parenchyma and peripancreatic fat tissue, with another 45% of cases being isolated peripancreatic necrosis. Pure pancreatic necrosis is seen only in about 5%–10% of the cases.[10] Peripancreatic fluid collections are seen as low attenuation areas around the pancreas. Necrotic collections, which can be pancreatic and/or peripancreatic, develop a wall after 4 weeks and are then referred to as walled-off pancreatic necrosis (WON). If these collections become infected, they are referred to as infected acute necrotic collection and infected walled-off pancreatic necrosis, respectively. The most specific sign of an infected necrotic collection is the presence of gas within the collection on the CT scan. However, the absence of gas within a collection does not rule out the infection status. Infected necrosis can be entertained as a diagnosis when a patient with necrotizing pancreatitis develops persistent fevers in the setting of a bloodstream infection without an alternative source of infection. Procalcitonin level of 1.8 ng/mL for 2 consecutive days has also a high diagnostic accuracy.[11,12] Alternatively, fine-needle aspiration can be considered when infection is suspected, but this is not commonly done in clinical practice.[13]

Acute Nonnecrotic Fluid Collections and Pseudocysts

Approximately 30%–50% of cases of AP develop acute peripancreatic fluid collections, which typically resolve within weeks. After a period of 4 weeks, if the acute peripancreatic fluid collections persist and develop a wall, then they are called "pseudocysts." Because most of these collections resolve, true pseudocysts are uncommon after an AP episode. Pseudocysts are typically located within or adjacent to pancreatic parenchyma. At times, these enzyme-rich fluid-filled cysts can be found remotely in the pelvis or chest.

Why Distinguish Between Necrotic and Nonnecrotic Collections?

This distinction becomes especially important, if an intervention is being considered for patients with symptomatic fluid collection(s). Draining noninfected necrotic collections early (before 4 weeks) is not recommended, because the necrotic debris is typically thick, often with the consistency of rubber.[14,15] Thus simple drainage of acute necrotic collections early in the course of the disease will usually result in superimposed infection of the necrotic collection, which can worsen a patient's course. After 4 weeks, symptomatic necrotic collections can be drained with a minimally invasive approach either surgically, endoscopically, or percutaneously. A necrotic collection is considered symptomatic when the patient experiences persistent abdominal pain, nausea, vomiting, and inability to tolerate oral diet and/or failure to thrive. A decline in the clinical course [usually manifesting in systemic inflammatory response syndrome (SIRS) with organ failure] with the development of fevers can be suggestive of infected necrosis. Most WON require debridement, whereas pseudocysts typically resolve with drainage alone (see Chapter 63). Pancreatic debridement can be achieved with minimally invasive surgery or endoscopically. Direct endoscopic necrosectomy typically requires multiple sessions based on the amount of necrotic debris and the WON size.

Severe AP: Important distinction between severe AP and nonsevere AP (i.e., mild and moderately severe) is its association with mortality.[9,16,17] Severe AP patients not only experience a highly morbid course but also, importantly, death occurs between 20% and 50% in this category.[8,18] Historically, there has been much debate on what determines mortality in AP, and the best available evidence indicates that the development of persistent organ failure is the key determinant.[9] Therefore its sole defining criterion is the presence of persistent organ failure (lasting >48 hours). The organ systems included in the RAC include the lungs, heart, and kidneys because they are most commonly involved. Organ failure is defined based on Modified Marshall Score of at least 2.[19] It is important to note that the presence of pancreatic necrosis *without* persistent organ failure is not a qualifying criterion for severe AP, because the mortality rate among patients with pancreatic necrosis without organ failure is substantially lower than those with persistent organ failure.[8,18]

CLINICAL COURSE OF ACUTE PANCREATITIS

First (early) phase: Local pancreatic inflammation may become systemic and lead to a cytokine storm and the SIRS. Fever, tachycardia, tachypnea, and leukocytosis are typically related to SIRS and represent the four criteria assessed to calculate the SIRS score (Box 60.2). SIRS typically develops early within the first week of presentation. Dysfunction of the respiratory, circulatory, and renal systems is usually associated with persistent SIRS (i.e., SIRS lasting for 48 hours or longer) and overall patient's physical condition. Approximately 40% of patients with persistent SIRS develop end-organ failure.[20] Infectious complications are relatively less common in the early phase, but in patients with necrotizing pancreatitis, it can still occur in between 5% and 22% of AP patients.[21] GI bleeding, liver failure, and coagulation disturbances have been included in some older studies as systemic complications, but the revised Atlanta classification did not include any of them because they are rare, and data regarding these complications is sparse. Between 65% and 90% of organ failure occurs during the first 2 weeks of the disease driven by the end-organ effects of the cytokine storm and other systemic events

BOX 60.2 Factors Associated With Severe Acute Pancreatitis

PATIENT CHARACTERISTICS

Age >55 years
Obesity (BMI > 30 kg/m^2)
Altered mental status
Comorbid disease
Systemic inflammatory response syndrome (SIRS)
 Two or more of the following (SIRS criteria)
 Pulse >90/min
 Respirations >20/min or $PaCO_2$ < 32 mm Hg
 Temperature >38°C or <36°C
 WBC count >12,000 or <4000/mm^3 or >10% band forms

LABORATORY FINDINGS

BUN > 20 mg/dL or rising BUN level
Elevated serum creatinine level
Hematocrit >44% or rising hematocrit

IMAGING FINDINGS

Pleural effusion(s)
Pulmonary infiltrate(s)
Multiple or extensive extrapancreatic fluid collections

in response to the acinar cell injury and necrosis (see section "Pathophysiology").[18,22,23]

The initial state of local pancreatic inflammation evolves dynamically, with the variable degrees of pancreatic and peripancreatic edema and ischemia toward either resolution, the development of acute collections in and around the pancreas, and/or irreversible necrosis. The extent of the pancreatic and peripancreatic injury is usually proportional to the severity of extrapancreatic organ failure. However, organ failure may rarely develop independent of pancreatic necrosis.[18] Conversely, patients with pancreatic necrosis may have no evidence of organ failure.[16]

Second (late) phase: Approximately 70%–80% of patients with AP have a resolution of the disease process (interstitial pancreatitis) and are discharged from the hospital within a week. However, in ~20% of patients, a more protracted course develops, typically related to the necrotizing process (necrotizing pancreatitis) lasting weeks to months. Mortality in this late phase is related to a combination of factors, including organ failure secondary to sterile necrosis, infected necrosis, locoregional complications (e.g., bleeding complication from pseudoaneurysm) from the necrotic process, or complications from surgical/minimally invasive intervention.

Historically, two-time peaks for mortality were described in AP: the first peak during the early phase due to end-organ failure from the cytokine storm and the second peak during the late phase driven by infected pancreatic necrotic collections. However, recent evidence suggests that the second peak in mortality has dampened largely due to the development of effective minimally invasive treatments for infected WON.[24] Recent studies in the United States and Europe reveal that most deaths occur within the first or second week because of persistent multiorgan failure.[18] In a large international prospective study that enrolled more than 1500 subjects, 85% of all deaths occurred from severe pancreatitis developing within the first 2 weeks of presentation.[18] In another large multicenter European study exclusively, including patients with necrotizing AP, 65% of all deaths occurred exclusively in the group that develop concomitant persistent organ failure (meaning severe pancreatitis) during the first 2 weeks of presentation.[23] Patients who are older with comorbid illnesses that lack the physiologic reserves have a substantially higher mortality rate than younger healthier patients for both in-hospital mortality and postdischarge death.[25–27] The most vulnerable period following discharge appears to be the first 90 days, when AP-related sepsis and heart failure are common causes of death.[25] In those who survive their illness, emerging evidence suggests that endocrine and exocrine pancreatic function may diminish with the development of diabetes and exocrine pancreatic insufficiency.[28,29] Furthermore, patients after an index AP episode (especially those with alcoholic or hypertriglyceridemic etiology) are at risk of developing recurrent AP attacks and subsequently chronic pancreatitis, with all of its complications (see Chapter 59).

PATHOGENESIS AND PATHOPHYSIOLOGY

There have been significant advancements in our knowledge of pathogenesis and natural history of AP from animal models (Figs. 60.3 and 60.4). Investigators have uncovered important cellular, locoregional, and systemic mechanisms and processes that elucidate how varying conditions predispose to the development of AP (Box 60.3), as well as can guide the development of new drugs or repurpose existing drugs for testing. For example, after discovery of the central importance of intra-acinar calcium overload and its downstream effects on the development of AP, a calcium channel inhibitor (targeting intracellular calcium overload) has been tested in a pilot setting with promising results. This medication is currently undergoing a multicenter phase 2b randomized clinical trial.[30] Despite these advancements, it is important to recognize that findings in animal models have uncertain applications to humans. For example, cerulein and taurocholate, commonly used to induce pancreatitis in animal models, do not cause human pancreatitis.

The current mechanistic evidence suggests that when the magnitude of pancreatic injury overwhelms the restorative homeostatic and compensatory capacity of the pancreas, injury progresses to cell death, and promotes a proinflammatory host response toward the pancreas that ultimately results in acute inflammation of the pancreas. A variety of behavioral factors (e.g., excessive alcohol drinking, cigarette smoking, and possibly dietary habits),[31–35] gene mutations (e.g., PRSS1, PSINK1, and CFTR mutations), medical conditions (e.g., hypertriglyceridemia and acute choledocholithiasis), and procedures/surgeries (e.g., ERCP, EUS with FNA, and cardiac surgery) can inflict varying degrees of pancreatic injury through several mechanisms.[22] Once clinically evident AP ensues, there are multiple self-perpetuating pathways (e.g., calcium overload, diminished ATP production, and activation of immune system) that interact with various host related baseline risk factors (e.g., male sex, pancreatic and peripancreatic fat content, genetic predisposition to SIRS, and organ dysfunction) that can lead to disease progression.[36] It is, therefore, helpful to think of the pathophysiology of AP in the framework of *initiating cellular events that inflict pancreatic injury*, *host response* (immune and locoregional response), and *systemic injury* (see Figs. 60.3 and 60.4). The resulting clinical phenotype and outcome depend on the degree of progression from the inciting pancreatic injury.

INITIATING CELLULAR EVENTS

Premature Digestive Enzyme Activation

Among the earliest events in the pathogenesis of AP is conversion of trypsinogen to trypsin within the acinar cells in sufficient quantities (seen within 10 minutes of initiation of AP) to overwhelm normal compensatory mechanisms of active trypsin clearance (see Fig. 59.3). Trypsin, in turn, catalyzes the conversion of different proenzymes, including trypsinogen and inactive

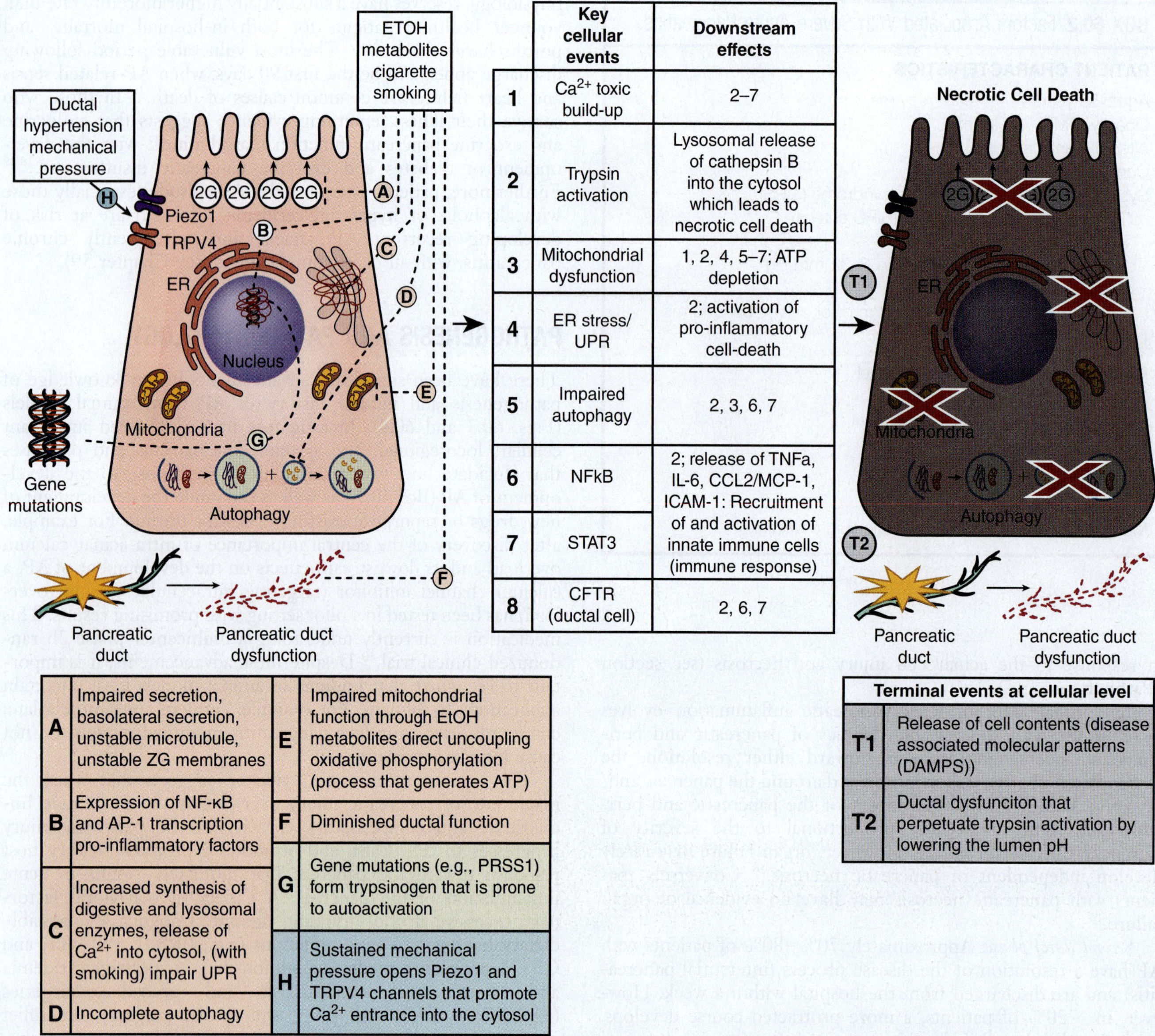

Ductal hypertension mechanical pressure
ETOH metabolites cigarette smoking
Piezo1
TRPV4
ER
Nucleus
Mitochondria
Gene mutations
Autophagy
Pancreatic duct
Pancreatic duct dysfunction
Key cellular events
Downstream effects
1 Ca2+ toxic build-up 2–7
2 Trypsin activation Lysosomal release of cathepsin B into the cytosol which leads to necrotic cell death
3 Mitochondrial dysfunction 1, 2, 4, 5–7; ATP depletion
4 ER stress/ UPR 2; activation of pro-inflammatory cell-death
5 Impaired autophagy 2, 3, 6, 7
6 NFkB
7 STAT3
2; release of TNFa, IL-6, CCL2/MCP-1, ICAM-1: Recruitment of and activation of innate immune cells (immune response)
8 CFTR (ductal cell) 2, 6, 7
Necrotic Cell Death
T1
T2
Terminal events at cellular level
T1 Release of cell contents (disease associated molecular patterns (DAMPS))
T2 Ductal dysfunciton that perpetuate trypsin activation by lowering the lumen pH
A Impaired secretion, basolateral secretion, unstable microtubule, unstable ZG membranes
B Expression of NF-κB and AP-1 transcription pro-inflammatory factors
C Increased synthesis of digestive and lysosomal enzymes, release of Ca2+ into cytosol, (with smoking) impair UPR
D Incomplete autophagy
E Impaired mitochondrial function through EtOH metabolites direct uncoupling oxidative phosphorylation (process that generates ATP)
F Diminished ductal function
G Gene mutations (e.g., PRSS1) form trypsinogen that is prone to autoactivation
H Sustained mechanical pressure opens Piezo1 and TRPV4 channels that promote Ca2+ entrance into the cytosol

Fig. 60.3 Pathogenesis of acute pancreatitis: starting from mechanisms of cellular injury to progression to systemic injury and organ failure.

precursors of elastase, phospholipase A_2 (PLA_2), and carboxypeptidase, to active enzymes (see Chapter 58). Trypsin also activates the complement and kinin systems. Activated zymogens within the acinar cells autodigest the pancreas and initiate a vicious cycle of active enzyme release. Normally, small amounts of trypsinogen are spontaneously activated within the pancreas, but protective intrapancreatic mechanisms quickly remove the activated trypsin. Pancreatic secretory trypsin inhibitor (now called SPINK1) binds and inactivates about 20% of the trypsin activity. Additional protective mechanisms are the sequestration of pancreatic enzymes inside intracellular compartments during their synthesis and transport within the acinar cells. Moreover, the separation of the digestive enzymes from lysosomal hydrolases as they pass through the Golgi apparatus, which is important because cathepsin B can activate trypsinogen to trypsin. Low intra-acinar cell calcium concentrations also prevent further autoactivation of trypsin. In support of the role of premature trypsin activation in AP initiation, the trypsin activated peptide (TAP), which is produced when trypsinogen is activated to trypsin, is found in plasma, urine, and ascites of subjects with AP, and its levels correlate with the severity of the pancreatic inflammatory response.[37,38] The trypsin-centric theory helps explain how mutations in the trypsin gene in patients with hereditary pancreatitis (usually a R122H or a N29I mutation) can cause episodes of AP. Certain mutations result in trypsin being resistant to degradation or cause premature trypsinogen activation (gain-of-function mutation), leading to autodigestion of the pancreas. Another genetic abnormality associated with pancreatitis that involves the trypsin activation is mutations of the *SPINK1* gene. As already noted, *SPINK1* protects the pancreatic acinar cell by inhibiting prematurely activated trypsin. *SPINK1* mutations limit its activity leading to increased trypsin activity (Chapter 59).[39]

In nonhereditary pancreatitis models where spontaneous autoactivation of trypsinogen is not expected as the initial cellular event (i.e., models with intact *PRSS1* and *SPINK1* genes), toxic cytosolic build-up of calcium (Ca^{2+}; see below) plays a key role in premature trypsinogen activation. Cytosolic build-up of Ca^{2+} within acinar cells activates the phosphatase calcineurin, which, in

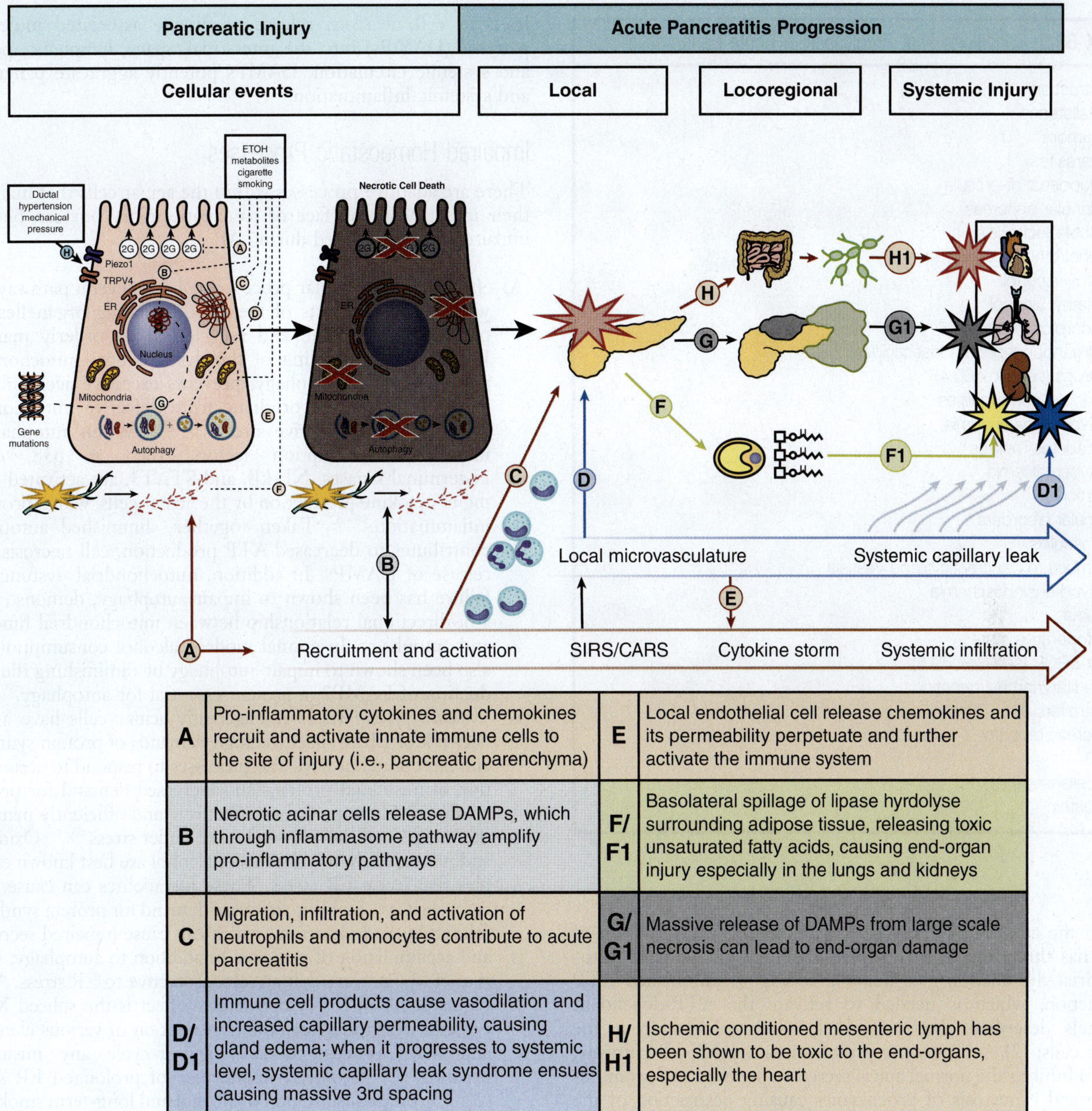

A	Pro-inflammatory cytokines and chemokines recruit and activate innate immune cells to the site of injury (i.e., pancreatic parenchyma)	E	Local endothelial cell release chemokines and its permeability perpetuate and further activate the immune system
B	Necrotic acinar cells release DAMPs, which through inflammasome pathway amplify pro-inflammatory pathways	F/ F1	Basolateral spillage of lipase hyrdolyse surrounding adipose tissue, releasing toxic unsaturated fatty acids, causing end-organ injury especially in the lungs and kidneys
C	Migration, infiltration, and activation of neutrophils and monocytes contribute to acute pancreatitis	G/ G1	Massive release of DAMPs from large scale necrosis can lead to end-organ damage
D/ D1	Immune cell products cause vasodilation and increased capillary permeability, causing gland edema; when it progresses to systemic level, systemic capillary leak syndrome ensues causing massive 3rd spacing	H/ H1	Ischemic conditioned mesenteric lymph has been shown to be toxic to the end-organs, especially the heart

Fig. 60.4 Pathogenesis of acute pancreatitis: starting from mechanisms of cellular injury to progression to systemic injury and organ failure.

turn, mediates premature trypsinogen activation, as well as activation of the proinflammatory nuclear factor-κB (NF-kB) pathway.[40] Trypsinogen activation also occurs through colocalization of zymogen granules and lysosomes containing cathepsin B following exposure to injurious agents (e.g., bile acids).[41–44] The engulfment of dead acinar cell molecules at the site of pancreatic injury can also activate trypsinogen within the macrophages leading to activation of the NF-kB pathway.[45] In summary, while intrapancreatic trypsinogen activation likely plays an important role in the initiation of AP, there are additional trypsin-independent mechanisms that mediate progression of injury and systemic injury.[41,46]

Cytosolic Calcium Overload

Calcium signaling is critical for maintaining homeostasis of the functional units within the pancreas, especially for its secretory function. In a physiologic state, Ca^{2+} levels oscillate in a localized area within the acinar cells, mediate ATP production in the mitochondria, and initiate exocytosis and secretion of inactive zymogens at the acinar cell apex.[47] Increases in cytosolic Ca^{2+} levels are mediated through entry of calcium into the cytosolic space from within the ER upon stimulation via ACh and cholecystokinin. Reduction of cytosolic Ca^{2+} is achieved through the activity of ATP-dependent channels located in the smooth ER that move Ca^{2+} back into the ER and in the plasma membrane that move Ca^{2+} out of the acinar cells.[22] However, certain toxins (i.e., bile acids and metabolites of alcohol such as fatty acid ethanol esters) result in release of stored Ca^{2+} from the ER into the cytosol in an unregulated fashion. When the Ca^{2+} stores are depleted within the ER, then Ca^{2+}-release activated Ca^{2+} channels open to promote additional Ca^{2+} entry from the extracellular space with concurrent failure of mechanisms to move Ca^{2+} out of the cytosol. The resulting event is a sustained Ca^{2+} level build-up

BOX 60.3 Conditions That Predispose to Acute Pancreatitis

- Obstruction
  - Gallstones
  - Tumors
  - Parasites
  - Duodenal diverticula
  - Annular pancreas
  - Choledochocele
- Alcohol/other toxins/drugs
  - Ethyl alcohol
  - Methyl alcohol
  - Scorpion venom
  - Organophosphorus insecticides
  - Drugs (see Box 60.4)
- Metabolic abnormalities
  - Hypertriglyceridemia
  - Diabetes mellitus
  - Hypercalcemia
- Infection
- Vascular disorders
  - Vasculitis
  - Emboli to pancreatic blood vessels
  - Hypotension/ischemia
- Trauma
- Postoperative state
- Post-ERCP (see Box 60.5)
- Hereditary/familial/genetic
- Controversial
- Pancreas divisum
- SOD
- Miscellaneous
- Idiopathic

within the acinar cell. This excessive cytosolic concentration of Ca^{2+} has three important downstream effects: (1) Causes mitochondrial dysfunction (see below), leading to diminished ATP production, which is needed to activate the ATP-dependent channels described above that help clear calcium from the acinar cells; (2) Activates the proinflammatory NF-kB pathway; and (3) Inhibits the normal apical secretory pathway and promotes basolateral exocytosis of proenzymes causing destruction of the interstitial space.[41,48–51] This recently discovered mechanism of toxic cytosolic Ca^{2+} build-up involves the pressure sensitive Ca^{2+} channels, Piezo1, and TRPV4.[52,53] These channels have been shown to mediate Ca^{2+} entry from outside the cell upon sensing of increased pancreatic duct pressure (e.g., when the ampulla becomes edematous during ERCP causing intraductal pressure build-up) leading to the same toxic cytosolic build-up of Ca^{2+} when the intraductal pressure/trauma is sustained.

Mitochondrial Dysfunction

Mitochondrial dysfunction, resulting from calcium overload, leads to a sequence of events that amplify the inflammatory response. Excessive reactive oxygen species are produced by dysfunctional mitochondria, which in turn promote the NF-kB pathway. NF-kB mediates proinflammatory proteins to recruit and trigger local inflammation. In addition, mitochondrial dysfunction leads to activation of caspases, which in turn lead to activation of potent proinflammatory cytokine, interleukin-1β.[49,50,54–56] Sustained increase in cytosolic Ca^{2+} ultimately leads to opening of the mitochondrial permeability transition pore that uncouples oxidative phosphorylation. This, ultimately, results in ATP depletion and leads to cell necrosis, release of disease associated molecular patterns (DAMPs) into the interstitial, space, lymphatic, portal, and systemic circulation. DAMPs potently aggravate pancreatic and systemic inflammation.

Impaired Homeostatic Processes

There are adaptive processes within the acinar cells that maintain their integrity in the face of pancreatic injury but can become impaired and disordered during AP.

(A) *Autophagy* is a cellular process involving several pathways, by which different parts of the cells, including organelles, are processed, discarded, and recycled in an orderly manner. For example, recycling of the dysfunctional mitochondria, which is called mitophagy, prevents excessive accumulation of free radicals that originate from defective mitochondria and can cause oxidative stress.[41,55,57,58] When autophagy is inhibited, transcription factors, such as p38, c-Jun N-terminal kinases, NF-kB, and STAT3, are activated leading to cytokine production by the acinar cells, which promote inflammation.[59–62] Taken together, diminished autophagy contributes to decreased ATP production, cell necrosis, and release of DAMPs. In addition, mitochondrial dysfunction/failure has been shown to impair autophagy, demonstrating a bi-directional relationship between mitochondrial function and autophagy. In animal models, alcohol consumption has also been shown to impair autophagy by diminishing the production of LAMP2, a protein essential for autophagy.[59]

(B) *Unfolded protein response:* Pancreatic acinar cells have a rich network of ER to meet the high demands of protein synthesis and secretion, but have also processes to respond to accumulation of misfolded proteins and increased demand for protein synthesis. These processes effectively and efficiently maintain the integrity of the ER machinery under stress.[63–65] Oxidative and nonoxidative metabolites of alcohol are best known examples that cause ER stress. These metabolites can cause toxic cytosolic Ca^{2+} build-up, increase demand for protein synthesis, microtubular dysfunction, which can cause impaired secretion and accumulation of proteins. In addition to autophagy, UPR is a set of pathways that are cytoprotective to ER stress. A key regulator of UPR's cytoprotective effect is the spliced XBP1 protein, which increases the transcription of various elements and helps process, discard, and recycle any misfolded proteins.[65–67] However, in the case of prolonged ER stress (e.g., chronic consumption of alcohol and long-term smoking), the cellular capacity to respond to ER stress becomes overwhelmed. Then, a different pathway, the PERK/ATF4 pathway, is activated in a sustained manner, which promotes inflammation and cell death.[65,67,68] Prolonged ER stress, impairment of the UPR pathway and inhibition of autophagy are most relevant to alcoholic pancreatitis.

HOST RESPONSE

Immune Response

Acinar cell injury and necrosis activate the inflammatory response through the release of proinflammatory signals (e.g., IL-6, TNF-α, IL-1β, and chemokines) and DAMPs, respectively (Fig. 60.4). Recent evidence has confirmed the ability of human acinar cells to secrete proinflammatory cytokines and chemokines in response to pathologic stimuli.[61] DAMPs are "sterile" intracellular contents that evoke a proinflammatory immune response. Examples include high mobility group box 1 DNA binding protein, ATP, S100 protein, and nuclear components, such as histones. Some DAMPs bind to the receptor $P2X_7$ (e.g., sRAGE and HMGB1) and others to Toll-like receptors 4 and 9 (DNA).[69,70] The resulting downstream events include DAMP sensing cell's release of IL-1β and IL-18, followed by IL-6. Toll-like receptors 4 and 9 are expressed on the pancreatic ductal cells, endothelial cells, and tissue macrophages, which then amplify the proinflammatory signals.

Leukocyte Migration and Activation

When monocytes are activated by cytokines, they release several molecules that promote migration of the peripheral inflammatory cells toward the pancreas. These molecules are the intercellular adhesion molecule-1 (ICAM-1 or CD54), vascular cell adhesion molecule-1 (VCAM-1), E-selectin, integrin alpha L (CD11a), and integrin alpha M (CD11b). ICAM-1 mediates neutrophils' adhesion to endothelial and epithelial cells, and its levels are increased in serum, pancreatic, and lungs in animal models of AP.[71,72] When neutrophils migrate, they expel neutrophil extracellular traps (NETs) that are composed of nuclear DNA and histones, which can promote organ injury. NETs can also induce trypsinogen and STAT3 activation.[73] Similarly, monocytes also migrate to the local site of injury. Signals that recruit and activate monocytes include the chemokines C-C motif ligand 2 (a.k.a monocyte chemokine protein 1), CCL3, and CCL5, which are then amplified by the activated monocytes. These early signals, such as IL-1, IL-6, and ICAM-1, are further amplified not only in the pancreas but also in the lungs, liver, and kidneys. Macrophages in the peritoneum and alveoli appear to play a key role in the migration of leucocytes to the pulmonary system and abdomen contributing to organ dysfunction. Taken together, leucocyte trafficking, migration, and amplification of proinflammatory signals culminate in pancreatic inflammation and, in some cases, progression to systemic injury.[74] Other innate immune cells, such as dendritic cells and mast cells, are not as well studied. Existing evidence suggests dendritic cells may have a regulatory role in AP by suppressing inflammation, clearing byproducts of tissue injury, antigens, and necrotic cell contents.[58] Mast cells, on the other hand, can disrupt the endothelial barrier function in the pancreas and other end-organs.

Pancreatic Microcirculation

In the animal models, the pancreas has been shown to be particularly vulnerable to hypovolemia, where compensatory mechanisms to sustain perfusion are less robust compared to the small intestine. Microcirculatory changes, including vasoconstriction, capillary stasis, decreased local oxygen saturation, and progressive ischemia, occur early in experimental AP. Early proinflammatory cells and molecules increase capillary permeability and promote "capillary leak." These include neutrophils that adhere to postcapillary venules, substance P (a neuropeptide), platelet-activating factor released from endothelial, mast cells, and macrophages, bradykinin, and thromboxane A2.[75] Heterogeneous distribution of vasoconstriction causes shunting and ischemia in some areas and edema in others. NETs, formation of intravascular thrombi, also contribute to microcirculatory disturbances and subsequently pancreatic necrosis.[51,73] Ischemia and severe inflammation of the pancreatic parenchyma can lead to disruption of the main pancreatic duct and side branches, leading to local pancreatic fluid release within and surrounding the pancreas that can eventuate into acute pancreatic fluid collections.

Intestine and the Lymphatic System

Preservation of intestinal barrier is critical in preventing translocation of gut flora. AP can cause barrier dysfunction, and in patients with hypotension, ischemia-reperfusion injury can have several downstream consequences. Pancreatic microcirculation can be impaired, promotes translocation of gut flora by barrier failure, conditions the mesenteric lymph to become toxic (to the cardiovascular system), and microvascular dysfunction leading to fluid leak and obstruction of the capillaries.[76] However, clinical trials have not demonstrated benefits of intestinal barrier preservation strategy, such as early feeding in predicted severe AP.[77] Gut-lymph model suggests that ischemic gut conditioned lymph may contain mediator(s) of organ failure, and it is supported by promising preliminary evidence.[76,78]

Systemic Injury and End-Organ Dysfunction

The pathogenesis of systemic injury in AP is incompletely understood.[74] Current hypotheses of the pathways involved in organ failure involve the vascular leak syndrome, which refers to systemic capillary leak from vascular endothelial dysfunction,[79–81] unrestrained activation of the immune system with cytokine storm,[82,83] and lipolysis with release of toxic free fatty acids.[84–86] It is likely that all four proposed mechanisms mediate end-organ dysfunction in an interlinked way. Based on translational studies in severe AP, DAMPs, such as S100 proteins, high-mobility group box1, and histones,[87–89] proinflammatory adipokines, such as resistin and visfatin, and cytokines, IL-6, IL-1β, IL-8, MCP-1, angiopoietin-2, and TNF-α,[83,90–94] have been associated with the development of end-organ dysfunction. In a mouse model of severe AP, the inflammasome pathway drives the SIRS, which further supports the key role of DAMPs.[69]

However, extensive clinical evidence suggests that while an excessive degree of pancreatic necrosis (a process that would release large amounts of DAMPs) correlates with the development of organ failure, a large proportion of AP patients with necrosis do not develop organ failure.[17,95] This observation suggests that there are additional pathways at play than massive necrosis with the release of DAMPs and the inflammasome as the sole mediating events to organ failure. Immune cells, such as neutrophils, monocytes, and proinflammatory cytokines, have been linked to the development of organ failure, especially in the lungs. For example, neutrophil infiltration into the alveoli via chemoattractants may mediate acute lung injury.[96] Furthermore, elevated levels of P- and E-selectin, which mediate neutrophil infiltration, are found in AP patients with acute lung injury.[97] Additionally, angiopoietin-2, IL-1β, IL-6, IL-8, MCP-1, and TNF-α are well-studied cytokines linked to severe AP. However, components of the immune system have pleiotropic effects that include protective effects, and further work is required to fully characterize the immune pathways that mediate systemic injury in SAP.

There is accumulating evidence on the role that visceral fat (intra- and peripancreatic) lipolysis pathway in mediating organ failure.[74,98–102] Lipolysis of fat tissue occurs from basolateral release of lipase that catabolizes the triglycerides within the adipose tissue. Lipolysis results in an increase in unsaturated fatty acids, such as linoleic and arachidonic acid, which can inhibit mitochondrial function by affecting complexes I and V and injure renal tubules and the lungs.[101]

Another conceptual model to explain systemic injury in severe AP is the capillary leak syndrome.[79] This hypothesis suggests that due to the severe endothelial dysfunction[80,81,97,103] that occurs during AP, there is a massive amount of fluid redistributed in the third-space due to leakage of oncotic proteins that promote flow of fluid from within the vessels to the interstitial space. This results in pulmonary congestion, hypovolemia with acute tubular necrosis, circulatory failure, and potentially death. In support of this hypothesis, angiopoetin-2, a key regulator of endothelial permeability, is strongly associated with severe AP, and its serum levels staying elevated during the first week in severe AP patients when compared with nonsevere AP patients.[104] This hypothesis is also supported by clinical observations that markers of diminished intravascular volume, such as hemoconcentration, blood urea nitrogen, and serum creatinine elevations, are also strongly associated with organ failure.[105] What remains unclear though, it is the mechanism that determines which patients develop capillary leak syndrome.

Pancreatic infection (infected pancreatic and WON) can occur from the hematogenous route or by translocation of bacteria from the colon into the lymphatics. Under normal circumstances bacterial translocation does not occur, because there are complex immunologic and morphologic barriers to it.[106] However, during AP, these barriers can break down. Penetration of the gut barrier by enteric bacteria is likely due to gut ischemia secondary to hypovolemia and pancreatitis-induced arteriovenous shunting in the gut. In canine experimental pancreatitis, luminal *Escherichia coli* translocate to mesenteric lymph nodes and to distant sites.[107] In feline experimental pancreatitis, enclosing the colon in impermeable bags prevents translocation of bacteria from the colon to the pancreas.[108]

PREDISPOSING CONDITIONS

Obstruction

Biliary Sludge, Microlithiasis, and Gallstones

The most common obstructive process leading to pancreatitis is gallstones (see Chapter 67), which cause approximately 40%–60% of cases of AP. Gallstone pancreatitis is more common in women than men because gallstones are more frequent in women.[109] AP occurs more frequently when stones are less than 5 mm in diameter (odds ratio, 4–5), because small stones are more likely than large stones to pass from the gallbladder through the cystic duct in the distal common bile duct and cause ampullary obstruction.[110] Cholecystectomy and clearing the bile duct of stones via ERCP prevent recurrence, confirming the cause-and-effect relationship.[111,112] AP is rare in pregnancy, occurring most commonly in the third trimester, and gallstones are the most common cause.

Biliary sludge is a viscous suspension in the gallbladder, and biliary microlithiasis means calculi ≤5mm (in diameter).[113] The distinct definition for the two terminologies was established via consensus recently to promote standardization for studies investigating sludge and microlithiasis.[113] On the ultrasound (US), sludge exhibits hyperechogenicity without shadowing and it forms sediments in the most dependent part of the gallbladder. Biliary microlithiasis exhibits hyperechoic material with acoustic shadowing sized 5 mm or less. Biliary sludge is usually composed of cholesterol monohydrate crystals or calcium bilirubinate granules. Sludge may develop from functional bile stasis, such as that associated with prolonged fasting or TPN, or from mechanical stasis, such as occurs in distal bile duct obstruction. In addition, the third-generation cephalosporin antibiotic, ceftriaxone, can result in sludge formation within the biliary system when its solubility in bile is exceeded; this process rarely causes stones, and the sludge resolves after stopping the drug.

The causative association between biliary sludge and AP is suggested by the results of two uncontrolled studies, demonstrating that biliary sludge can lead to pancreatitis. In these two studies, the incidence of biliary sludge in presumed idiopathic pancreatitis was 67% and 74%, respectively.[112,114] Treatment choices include cholecystectomy that targets elimination of its site of accumulation, ERCP with biliary sphincterotomy that facilitates the passage of sludge through the ampulla, and ursodeoxycholic acid (ursodiol) therapy, which prevents its formation and will reduce the risk of recurrent attacks of AP. In patients in whom surgical risk is acceptable, cholecystectomy is associated with superior efficacy in secondary prevention of AP.[111,115,116]

Tumors

Pancreatic tumors may infrequently cause acute and recurrent AP, presumably by obstructing the PD, especially in individuals older than age 40 (see Chapter 62). Pancreatic cancer was found to be the cause for AP in 1.4% of a recent series of 1609 patients. In this series, when the CA 19-9 was higher than 200 U/L, then pancreatic cancer was present in 15.8% of patients with AP.[117] The most common tumor that presents in this manner is intraductal papillary mucinous neoplasm (IPMN). Suggested mechanism by which IPMN causes AP is obstruction of the main pancreatic duct by mucin plugs; thus some advocate pancreatic sphincterotomy for secondary prevention of AP largely based on uncontrolled case series.[118–120] Metastases to the pancreas from other cancers (lung, breast, and kidney) have also caused pancreatitis. Large ampullary adenomas can likewise occasionally be the cause of obstructive pancreatitis (see Chapter 71).

Other Causes

Other obstructive conditions, rarely associated with AP, are discussed in other chapters and include choledochoceles,[121] duodenal diverticulae,[122] annular pancreas,[123] and parasitic diseases of the pancreaticobiliary system, such as ascariasis or clonorchiasis.[124,125]

Ethyl Alcohol and Other Toxins

Ethyl Alcohol

Alcohol is the second most common cause of AP after gallstones and causes at least 30% of the cases.[3,126] Prolonged alcohol consumption (more than 4–5 drinks per day for at least 5 years) is required to increase the risk of AP, but still the lifetime risk of AP in such drinkers is only 2%–5%.[127] Recent evidence suggests that there may be gender disparities in the vulnerabilities to alcohol consumption and the risk of AP.[128] While there is a linear dose-response relationship between the dose of alcohol consumption and the risk of AP in men; in women, doses of less than 40 g/day are protective of AP, and there is a precipitous increase in the risk of AP for doses more than 40 g/day. This highlights the complex pathophysiology of alcoholic pancreatitis.[128]

Other Toxins

Methyl alcohol,[129] organophosphorus insecticides,[130] and the venom of the Trinidad scorpion[131] have been reported to induce AP. The mechanism of the latter two toxins is thought to be by hyperstimulation of the pancreas and perhaps sphincter of Oddi spasm with scorpion venum. Cigarette smoking has also been shown to be an independent risk factor for AP in studies, including multiethnic cohorts, studies from Europe, and the United States.[132,133] Interestingly, these results were not reproduced in a study from Taiwan, which reported that smoking was not associated with an increased risk of AP.[134]

Drugs

Medications represent a relatively uncommon but important cause of AP. There are reports suggesting that drug-induced AP accounts for 1%–4% of all cases in adults.[135] More than 120 drugs have been implicated, mostly from anecdotal case reports, which suffer from a combination of inadequate criteria for the diagnosis of AP, failure to rule out more common causes, or a lack of a rechallenge trial with the medication. In addition, many case reports inappropriately implicate drugs when the latter have been administered for long periods (>6 months) before the onset of AP. Given these inappropriate causal inferences, it is likely that true drug-induced pancreatitis likely accounts for <1% of all AP. Drug-induced pancreatitis tends to occur within 4–8 weeks of starting a drug. In the absence of well-designed clinical trials, clinicians largely rely on these published case reports for the determination that a drug may have caused AP. As an example, statins, long regarded as a class I cause of drug-induced pancreatitis, have been found to have protective effects against the development of AP in several large epidemiologic studies.[136,137] Corticosteroids, on the other hand, even though regarded as class III, recent epidemiologic studies support a strong association with the risk being highest 4–14 days after drug dispensation.[138]

Drug-induced pancreatitis rarely is accompanied by clinical or laboratory evidence of a drug reaction, such as rash, lymphadenopathy, or eosinophilia. Although a positive rechallenge with a drug is the best evidence available for cause and effect, it is not 100% proof because many patients with idiopathic pancreatitis or biliary microlithiasis have recurrent attacks of AP. Despite the lack of a rechallenge, a drug may be strongly suspected when there is a consistent latency between initiating the drug and the onset of AP among the case reports. Box 60.4 shows the drugs with strong evidence for causing AP in published case reports, those with rechallenge evidence, or with a relatively predictable latency. Some drugs have been implicated as causing AP through reporting to the FDA Adverse Event Reporting System. However, the Adverse Event Reporting System largely depends on clinicians submitting MedWatch reports and is plagued by reporting bias. In a population-based study from Sweden, increased use of AP-associated drugs, did not have any major impact on the observed epidemiological changes in occurrence, severity, or recurrence of AP.[139]

There are several potential pathogenic mechanisms for drug-induced pancreatitis. The most common is a hypersensitivity reaction. This tends to occur 4–8 weeks after starting the drug and is not dose related. On rechallenge with the drug, pancreatitis recurs within hours to days. Examples of drugs that may operate through this mechanism are 5-aminosalicylates, metronidazole, and tetracycline. The second mechanism is the presumed accumulation of a toxic metabolite that may cause pancreatitis, typically after several months of use. Examples of drugs in this category are valproic acid and didanosine (DDI). Drugs that induce hypertriglyceridemia (e.g., thiazides, isotretinoin, and tamoxifen) are also included in this category. Finally, a few drugs may have intrinsic toxicity wherein an overdose of them can cause pancreatitis (erythromycin and acetaminophen).

There has been significant literature in recent years about the risk of AP due to dipeptidyl peptidase-4 inhibitors, which are used with increasing frequency to treat type 2 diabetes.[140–143] The published reports were conflicting about the risk. A recent meta-analysis of 13 studies revealed a marginally higher risk of AP with dipeptidyl peptidase-4 inhibitors.[143] However, this risk was not observed in cohort studies.[144] Thus further clinical trials are required to confirm this finding. In a population with type 2 diabetes at high cardiovascular risk, there were numerically fewer events of AP among patients treated with liraglutide (a GLP-1 receptor agonist) regardless of previous history of pancreatitis than in the placebo group.[145] Liraglutide was associated, however, with increases in serum lipase and amylase, which were not predictive of an event of subsequent AP.[145]

In general, drug-induced pancreatitis tends to be mild and self-limited. The diagnosis should be entertained after other causes have been exhaustively ruled out. Some medications have been shown to cause AP in randomized trials at relatively high frequencies (e.g., 6-mercaptopurine in 3%–5% and DDI in 5%–10%),[146] but in many drugs the assigned causation is less evident based on evidence.

BOX 60.4 Drugs Associated With Acute Pancreatitis[a]

Acetaminophen
5-Aminosalicylic acid compounds (sulfasalazine, azodisalicylate, and mesalamine)
L-Asparaginase
Azathioprine
Benazepril
Bezafibrate
Cannabis
Captopril
Carbimazole
Cimetidine
Clozapine
Codeine
Cytosine arabinoside
Dapsone
Didanosine
Dexamethasone
Enalapril
Erythromycin
Estrogen
Fluvastatin
Furosemide
Hydrochlorothiazide
Hydrocortisone
Ifosfamide
Interferon-α
Isoniazid
Lamivudine
Lisinopril
Losartan
Meglumine
Methimazole
Methyldopa
Metronidazole
6-Mercaptopurine
Nelfinavir
Norethindrone/mestrol
Pentamidine
Pravastatin
Procainamide
Pyritinol
Simvastatin
Sulfamethazine
Sulfamethoxazole
Stibogluconate
Sulindac
Tetracycline
Trimethoprim/sulfamethoxazole
Valproic acid

[a]Class 1 and class 2 drugs only are listed. Class 1 drugs: 2 or more case reports published, absence of other causes of acute pancreatitis, rechallenge documented in at least 1 report. Class 2 drugs: 4 or more case reports published, absence of other causes of acute pancreatitis, consistent latency in at least 75% of cases published.

From Badalov N, Baradarian R, Iswara K, et al. Drug induced acute pancreatitis: an evidence based approach. *Clin Gastroenterol Hepatol.* 2007;101:454–476.

Metabolic Disorders

Hypertriglyceridemia

Hypertriglyceridemia is the third most common identifiable cause of AP, after gallstones and alcoholism, accounting for anywhere from 2% to 5% to 20% of cases.[1,3] A systematic review of 31 studies comprising 1340 patients with hypertriglyceridemic AP reported that this condition accounts for 9% of all cases of AP and that 14% of patients with significant hypertriglyceridemia will develop AP.[147] Hypertriglyceridemia is also implicated in more than half of cases of gestational pancreatitis. Serum triglyceride concentrations above 1000 mg/dL (11 mmol/L) may precipitate attacks of AP.

The pathogenesis of hypertriglyceridemic pancreatitis is unclear, but the local release of free fatty acids by pancreatic lipase may damage pancreatic acinar cells or endothelial cells. Release of free fatty acids that induce free radical damage can directly injure cell membranes.

Most adults with hyperchylomicronemia have a mild form of genetically inherited type 1 or type 5 hyperlipoproteinemia and an additional acquired condition known to raise serum lipids [e.g., alcohol abuse, obesity, diabetes mellitus, hypothyroidism, Cushing syndrome, pregnancy, nephrotic syndrome, and drug therapy (estrogen or tamoxifen, glucocorticoids, thiazides, or beta adrenergic blockers)]. Typically, three types of patients develop hypertriglyceridemia-induced pancreatitis. The first is a poorly controlled diabetic patient with a history of hypertriglyceridemia. The second is alcoholic patients with hypertriglyceridemia detected on hospital admission. The third (15%–20%) is nondiabetic, nonalcoholic, nonobese subjects who have drug- or diet-induced hypertriglyceridemia. Drug-induced disease is more likely to occur when there is an underlying hypertriglyceridemia prior to drug exposure.

Most subjects who abuse alcohol have moderate but transient elevations of serum triglyceride levels. This condition is likely an epiphenomenon and not the cause of their pancreatitis, because alcohol itself not only damages the pancreas but also may increase serum triglyceride concentrations in a dose-dependent manner. Alcoholic patients with severe hypertriglyceridemia often have a coexisting primary genetic disorder of lipoprotein metabolism.

There is some evidence that hypertriglyceridemic pancreatitis may portend worse prognosis. For example, a meta-analysis of 15 studies (1564 patients) found a worse prognosis compared with nonhypertriglyceridemia causes.[147] The likely mechanism underlying this observation is through the lipolysis pathway (see Pathogenesis under "Systemic Injury"). The serum amylase and/or lipase levels may not be substantially elevated at presentation in patients with hypertriglyceridemic pancreatitis (see later).

Diabetes Mellitus

Diabetes has historically been treated as a risk factor for developing AP (see Chapter 35).[148] For example, epidemiologic studies have shown the increased risk of AP in the diabetic population and possibly greater risk for developing severe AP. However, it is difficult to disentangle its independent risk from other common confounders, such as obesity, cholelithiasis, and hypertriglyceridemia. In a large study of type 2 diabetic patients (LEADER, Liraglutide Effect, and Action in Diabetes: Evaluation of Cardiovascular Outcome Results), nearly 25% had elevated serum lipase or amylase levels without symptoms of AP.[144] The clinicians must take these data into account when evaluating abdominal symptoms in type 2 diabetic patients. Patients with diabetes tend to develop gallstones due to common concurrent dyslipidemia that can lead to cholesterol-supersaturated bile and precipitation of cholesterol crystals (see Chapter 65). Moreover, patients with long-standing diabetes often develop bile stasis in the gallbladder, leading to the precipitation of cholesterol crystals and formation of gallstones.

Hypercalcemia

Hypercalcemia of any cause is rarely associated with AP. Proposed mechanisms include deposition of calcium salts in the PD lumen and calcium activation of trypsinogen to trypsin within the pancreatic parenchyma. The low incidence of AP in chronic hypercalcemia suggests that mechanisms other than the serum calcium level per se are responsible for pancreatitis (e.g., acute elevations of serum calcium). Acute calcium infusion into rats leads to conversion of trypsinogen to trypsin, hyperamylasemia, and dose-dependent morphologic changes of AP.

Primary hyperparathyroidism represents less than 0.5% of all cases of AP, and the incidence of AP in patients with hyperparathyroidism varies from 0.4% to 1.5% (Chapter 37).[149] Rarely, pancreatitis occurs with other causes of hypercalcemia, including metastatic bone disease, TPN, sarcoidosis, vitamin D toxicity, and infusion of calcium in high doses during cardiopulmonary bypass.

Infections

Although many infectious agents have been proposed as causing AP, these published reports often do not clearly establish a causal relationship. The diagnosis of AP caused by an infection requires evidence of an active infection at the time of AP diagnosis with the absence of other common causes of AP. AP has been associated with viruses, especially in children (mumps, coxsackievirus, hepatitis A, B, and C, and several herpesviruses, including cytomegalovirus, varicella-zoster, herpes simplex, and EBV); the vaccine that contains attenuated measles, mumps, and rubella viruses; bacteria (*Mycoplasma*, *Legionella*, *Leptospira*, *Salmonella*, TB, and brucellosis); fungi (*Aspergillus*, *Candida*); and parasites (*Toxoplasma*, *Cryptosporidium*, *Ascaris lumbricoides*, *Clonorchis sinensis*). *C. sinensis* and *A. lumbricoides* can cause pancreatitis by obstructing the main PD. In patients with AIDS (see Chapter 33), infectious agents causing AP include cytomegalovirus, *Candida* species, *Cryptococcus neoformans*, *Toxoplasma gondii*, and possibly *Mycobacterium avium* complex.[150]

VASCULAR DISEASE

Rarely, pancreatic ischemia causes AP. In most cases, it is mild, but fatal necrotizing pancreatitis may occur. Ischemia may result from vasculitis (e.g., SLE[151] and polyarteritis nodosa[152]), atheromatous embolization of cholesterol plaques after transabdominal aortography,[153] intraoperative hypotension,[154] hemorrhagic shock, ergotamine overdose, and during transcatheter arterial catheter embolization for hepatocellular carcinoma.[155] Moreover, ischemia is one possible explanation for pancreatitis after cardiopulmonary bypass. In pigs, cardiogenic shock induced by pericardial tamponade causes vasospasm and selective pancreatic ischemia due to activation of the renin-angiotensin system.[156] AP in long-distance runners may also be of ischemic etiology.[157]

Trauma

Either penetrating trauma (gunshot or stab wounds) or blunt trauma can injure the pancreas.[158] Blunt trauma results from compression of the pancreas by the spine, such as in an automobile accident with compression by the steering wheel. In blunt trauma, it is important to determine preoperatively whether there is injury to the pancreas because, depending on the severity of pancreatic injury, it will be necessary to include the pancreas in the surgical plan. Second, even in the absence of serious injury to adjacent organs, surgery or endoscopic therapy may be necessary to treat a pancreatic ductal injury.

The diagnosis of traumatic pancreatitis is difficult and requires a high degree of suspicion. Trauma can range from a mild contusion to a severe crush injury or transection of the gland; the latter usually occurs at the point where the gland crosses over the spine. Transection injury can cause acute duct rupture and pancreatic ascites. It is impossible to determine based on the characteristics of the abdominal pain and tenderness whether the pancreas has been injured as opposed to adjacent intra-abdominal structures. Serum amylase or lipase activity may be increased in patients with abdominal trauma regardless of the pancreas been injured or not.

Diagnosis of pancreatic trauma is highly dependent on CT, MRI, or magnetic resonance cholangiopancreatography (MRCP), which may show enlargement of a portion of the gland caused by a contusion or subcapsular hematoma, pancreatic inflammatory changes, or fluid within the anterior pararenal space if there is ductal disruption. CT may be normal during the first 2 days despite significant pancreatic trauma. When there is a strong clinical suspicion of pancreatic injury with equivocal cross-sectional imaging, ERCP is required to define whether there is PD injury. If the PD is intact and there are no other significant intra-abdominal injuries, surgery is not required. However, if ERCP reveals duct transection with extravasation of contrast on pancreatogram and there are no other intra-abdominal injuries, stenting of the PD across the leak, when technically feasible, may be curative.[159] Serious injuries to the pancreas are treated surgically. Associated injuries to the duodenum or bile duct can be treated by biliary diversion, gastrojejunostomy, and feeding jejunostomy. External pancreatic fistulas occur in approximately one-third of patients after surgery for pancreatic trauma. Octreotide may be beneficial after pancreatic injury to decrease pancreatic secretion.[160]

The prognosis in patients with pancreatic trauma is favorable if there is no serious injury to other structures (regional blood vessels, liver, spleen, kidney, duodenum, and colon). However, duct injuries can scar and cause a stricture of the main PD, resulting in obstructive chronic pancreatitis.

Post-ERCP

AP is the most common complication of ERCP, associated with substantial morbidity (see Chapter 40). Clinical AP occurs in approximately 10% of all ERCPs and up to 25% in high-risk patient groups, such as those with suspected sphincter of Oddi dysfunction (SOD) or with a history of post-ERCP pancreatitis (PEP).[161–164]

A recent systematic review of 145 randomized controlled trials (RCTs) with 19,038 patients in the placebo or no-stent arms reported an overall cumulative incidence of PEP of 10.2%, and the mortality rate was 0.2%. Severity of PEP was reported at 2.6% for moderately severe and 0.5% for severe AP. The incidence of PEP in 3733 high-risk patients was 14.1% (severe in 0.8%, respectively, with a 0.2% mortality rate). Overall, the incidence of PEP was 10.4% in North American RCTs.[165]

The mechanisms that lead to PEP are complex and not fully understood. Rather than a single pathogenesis, PEP is believed to be multifactorial, involving a combination of chemical, hydrostatic, enzymatic, mechanical, and thermal factors. Although there is some uncertainty in predicting which patients will develop PEP, a number of risk factors acting independently or in concert have been proposed as predictors of PEP (Box 60.5). Identification of these risk factors for PEP is essential to recognize cases in which ERCP should be avoided when not clearly indicated. For example, in a multicenter prospective cohort study with more than 1000 patients, women with suspected choledocholithiasis and normal serum bilirubin, who underwent a sphincterotomy but without the presence of a bile duct stone, were at greatest risk with 27% developing PEP.[166] MRCP and EUS are the preferred modalities in the initial evaluation of patients with suspected choledocholithiasis.

The three major modalities shown to reduce the risk are PEP include placement prophylactic pancreatic stents, periprocedural intravenous fluids, and rectal administration of nonsteroidal anti-inflammatory drugs (NSAIDs).

BOX 60.5 Factors That Increase the Risk of Post-ERCP Pancreatitis

PATIENT-RELATED

Young age, female gender, suspected SOD, history of recurrent pancreatitis, history of post-ERCP pancreatitis, normal serum bilirubin level

PROCEDURE-RELATED

Pancreatic duct injection, difficult cannulation, pancreatic sphincterotomy, precut access, and balloon dilation

OPERATOR- OR TECHNIQUE-RELATED

Trainee (fellow) participation, nonuse of a guidewire for cannulation, failure to use a pancreatic duct stent in a high-risk procedure

Nonsteroidal Anti-inflammatory Drugs

There has recently been a substantial body of evidence to support the use of NSAIDs for prevention of PEP among both high-risk patients and patients with native papilla without a risk factor undergoing ERCP.[161] Therefore rectal NSAID administration is the standard of care for prevention of PEP in patients with native papilla.[161] A landmark multicenter, double-blind, placebo-controlled RCT of 602 high-risk patients undergoing an ERCP demonstrated a significant reduction of the incidence of PEP and moderately severe or severe PEP when patients were given rectal indomethacin after the procedure.[167] There have been many studies published on patient cohorts with different risk stratification, types of NSAID (e.g., diclofenac vs. indomethacin), and timing of rectal administration (i.e., prior to the procedure or after the procedure based on the endoscopic interventions). In a network meta-analysis which included 55 randomized clinical trials evaluating 20 interventions in 17,062 patients, NSAIDs, given either rectally or intramuscularly (in the case of diclofenac) led to significant reduction in incidence of PEP when compared with placebo (RR range 0.24–0.60).

Pancreatic Duct Stent Placement

Placement of PD stents has become a standard practice for patients who are thought to be at high risk for pancreatitis after the procedure (see Box 60.5). PD stent placement is effective, presumably by preventing PD obstruction and reducing intraductal hypertension, which mediate AP.[52,53,168] The rationale behind this is the spasm and edema of the ampulla after ERCP because of cannulation and cautery can result in obstruction of the pancreatic duct that can lead to the development of AP. Several studies and meta-analyses have confirmed the benefit of prophylactic pancreatic ductal stents in patients at high risk of PEP.[161] Prophylactic PD stents can be either a three French (1 mm) or five French (1.67 mm) in diameter, 3 cm or greater than 7 cm in length and placed temporarily to cover the 2- to 3-day period of ampullary edema.[169–173] When a radiograph after 1–2 weeks suggests the PD stent has not migrated out, then it needs to be removed with a repeat endoscopy, because when left in place for a prolonged period, it may cause chronic ductal injury.

Cannulation Technique

Guidewire cannulation, whereby the biliary or pancreatic duct is initially cannulated by a guidewire inserted through the cannula or sphincterotome under fluoroscopic guidance but without injection of contrast, has been shown to decrease the risk of PEP with comparable high levels (~98%) of cannulation success (see Box 60.5).[174] A technique, frequently used when the guidewire initially enters the pancreatic duct, is to leave the guidewire in the PD and attempt biliary cannulation with a second guidewire, which is called double guidewire technique. A meta-analysis in patients with difficult biliary cannulation during ERCP showed that the double guidewire technique appears to increase the risk of PEP without any superiority in achieving biliary cannulation compared with other techniques.[175] Therefore prophylactic PD stenting is recommended when the double guidewire technique is used. The effect of complementary NSAID administration when a PD is placed is unclear. Recently a large-scale, multicenter RCT to address whether NSAID administration alone is noninferior to dual intervention (PD stenting AND NSAID administration) has concluded enrollment and is awaiting analysis.[172]

Extending the observation that adequate intravenous fluid administration with lactated Ringer (LR) solution critical in the early management of AP (discussed later), several pilot studies showed beneficial effects of periprocedural intravenous fluid administration in preventing PEP. The timing of such administration differed in studies, starting before the procedure or during the procedure and continuing for variable times in the post-procedure period.[169,176,177] These initial promising reports culminated in a recent RCTs.[178] This trial randomized a total of 826 patients to receive either aggressive IV hydration (20 mL/kg bolus followed by 3 mL/kg for 8 hours) with rectal indomethacin or controlled IV hydration (1.5 mL/kg for 8 hours) and found no incremental benefit of adding aggressive IV hydration to rectal indomethacin in preventing PEP.[178]

Postoperative State

Postoperative AP can occur after thoracic or abdominal surgery. Pancreatitis can occur in 0.4%–7.6% of patients undergoing cardiopulmonary bypass operations.[179,180] Overall, 27% of patients undergoing cardiac surgery develop hyperamylasemia, and 1% develop necrotizing pancreatitis. Significant risks for AP after cardiopulmonary bypass are preoperative renal insufficiency, postoperative hypotension, and administration of calcium chloride perioperatively. AP occurs in 6% of patients undergoing liver transplantations.[181] Contributors to the morbidity and mortality of postoperative AP can be delay in diagnosis, hypotension, medications (e.g., azathioprine/perioperative calcium chloride administration), infections, and comorbidities. Postoperative AP is also recognized as a complication after pancreatic surgery.[182]

Hereditary and Genetic Disorders

Hereditary pancreatitis, an autosomal dominant genetic disorder with variable penetrance and clinical course, is discussed in Chapter 59.

Miscellaneous Causes

Inflammatory bowel disease (IBD): AP has been rarely associated with IBD. A recent case-control study from Denmark found a fourfold increase in AP incidence in patients with concurrent Crohn disease and a 1.5-fold increase in patients with ulcerative colitis.[183] This increase in IBD patients has been partially attributed to the use of drugs, such as 5-aminosalicylates/sulfasalazine and thiopurines (azathioprine/6-mercaptopurine; see Box 60.4). Theories to support a putative relationship between idiopathic IBD and AP include that pancreatitis represents an extraintestinal manifestation of IBD, duodenal Crohn disease can cause obstruction to the flow of pancreatic juice, granulomatous inflammation in Crohn disease may involve the pancreas, or that there is associated autoimmune pancreatitis in IBD patients. A database of patients with Crohn disease from Canada reported that 6.2% of patients taking thiopurines developed AP.[183]

Celiac disease has also been described to be association with AP, but the relationship remains uncertain.[184] It has been suggested that abnormalities in the normal barrier of the small bowel seen in patients with celiac disease may allow excessive absorption of amylase from the intestinal lumen, leading to hyperamylasemia. In the setting of abdominal pain in a patient with celiac disease, it is not uncommon to find elevations in the serum amylase and/or lipase in the absence of AP.[185]

Autoimmune pancreatitis (discussed in the next chapter in more detail): Episodes of AP or recurrent AP resulting from autoimmune pancreatitis are rare, seen with type 2 disease, and associated with granulocyte epithelial lesions. Investigators have also described patients with autoimmune recurrent pancreatitis, especially younger women, often without the classic elevation of serum IgG4.[186,187] Two defining criteria for diagnosis of autoimmune pancreatitis are imaging features and histopathologic features.[186,187] In patients without imaging features of autoimmune pancreatitis, IgG4 levels alone are insufficient for diagnosis.[188] Additionally, pancreatic malignancy is more common than autoimmune pancreatitis, and the two can be extremely difficult to distinguish even in expert centers[189]—thus preemptive steroids treatment without supporting histopathology is strongly discouraged outside the context of a pancreatic center of excellence.

Penetrating duodenal or gastric ulcers can involve the pancreas and cause AP that may be fatal (see Chapter 55). Though uncommon nowadays, a penetrating ulcer as the cause of pancreatitis should be considered in the appropriate clinical setting.

Controversial Causes

Pancreas Divisum

Pancreas divisum is the most common anatomical variation of the pancreas, occurring in 5%–10% of the general population. Pancreas divisum occurs in development when the ventral bud and dorsal bud of the pancreas fail to fuse. This results in the body and tail of the pancreas to drain through the dorsal pancreatic duct, also called accessory or duct of Santorini, rather than ventral PD, also called main or duct of Wirsung. The vast majority of subjects with pancreas divisum never develop pancreatitis (see Chapter 57). Controversy continues to surround the issue as to whether pancreas divisum alone is a cause of recurrent AP. The presumed mechanism of action in those who develop AP is that there is relative obstruction to the flow of pancreatic juice through the minor papilla. Arguments in favor of attributing recurrent AP to pancreas divisum include: (1) various series from ERCP referral centers showed that patients referred with recurrent AP have a higher frequency of pancreas divisum than would be expected from the general population[190,191]; (2) multiple observational series report that performing ERCP with endoscopic sphincterotomy or placing a stent across the minor papilla reduces the rate of recurrent pancreatitis[190,191]; and (3) a small randomized controlled study suggesting that patients with pancreas divisum and recurrent AP who underwent stenting of the minor papilla had a lower frequency of attacks of pancreatitis over the following year compared to those not stented.[192] Arguments against the association include: (1) other studies supporting the incidence of AP in pancreas divisum subjects to be the same as the general population[193]; (2) recurrent AP is a disease of great variability in its natural history; and (3) the above single randomized study was flawed in that it was not blinded, included only 19 patients, and some of these patients may had already progressed to chronic pancreatitis.[192]

The prevalence of genetic abnormalities in patients with pancreas divisum and recurrent AP is either the same or higher than expected in the general population or population of patients with AP of other etiologies, suggesting a possible genetic contribution. For example, there appears to be a higher incidence of *CFTR* mutations in patients with pancreas divisum who develop recurrent AP. Because several authors have reported associations of *SPINK-1* and *CFTR* mutations in patients with AP and pancreas divisum, experts suggest that pancreatitis (either acute or recurrent acute) in patients with pancreas divisum is likely associated with genetic abnormalities and is not solely due to pancreas divisum.[194–196] Taking into consideration the controversial evidence and the high risk of PEP in these patients, the risk-benefit ratio of treating pancreas divisum endoscopically with minor papilla sphincterotomy and stenting is considered unfavorable by some experts. To address this clinical equipoise, a double-blinded, randomized clinical trial examining the role of endoscopic minor sphincterotomy in reducing the risk of recurrent AP in subjects with pancreas divisum is underway[197] (NCT: 03609944).

Sphincter of Oddi Dysfunction

SOD is also considered a controversial cause of AP (see Chapter 63). Investigators who study patients with recurrent AP report that pancreatic SOD (usually defined as a basal pancreatic sphincter pressure >40 mm Hg during ERCP with sphincter of Oddi manometry) is the most common abnormality discovered, occurring in approximately 35%–40% of patients.[198] The main argument in favor of this entity as a cause of AP is many observational series that reported endoscopic pancreatic sphincterotomy or surgical sphincteroplasty to reduce recurrent attacks of pancreatitis.[199] The arguments against pancreatic SOD as a cause of AP include: (1) the lack of any prospective controlled blinded trials in the treatment of this disorder; (2) the short duration of follow-up in the observational reports; (3) the high risk of AP (25%–35%) associated with ERCP, sphincter of Oddi manometry, and pancreatic sphincterotomy in patients with suspected SOD; (4) the extremely variable natural history of idiopathic recurrent AP, which may mask the minimal effects of therapy; and (5) the relative dearth of data determining the normal range of pancreatic sphincter pressure that is the basis for the pathogenesis of SOD.

Traditionally, large numbers of patients with abdominal pain after cholecystectomy but no objective evidence of biliary or pancreatic disease were subjected to ERCP, sphincter of Oddi manometry, and biliary and/or pancreatic sphincterotomy with a diagnosis of type 3 SOD. However, this endoscopic practice has changed over the last decade based on the results of a large rigorously conducted multicenter RCT in patients with type 3 SOD, the EPISOD trial.[200] The trial concluded that in patients with abdominal pain after cholecystectomy undergoing ERCP with manometry, sphincterotomy did not reduce disability due to pain when compared to the sham group (no sphincterotomy). Thus these findings do not support performing ERCP, manometry, and sphincterotomy in patients with type 3 SOD. Encouragingly, since 2013 when the EPISOD trial was published, there has been a significant and sustained decrease in rates of endoscopic sphincterotomy for patients with newly-diagnosed SOD type 3.[201]

CLINICAL FEATURES OF AP

It is difficult to diagnose AP by history and physical examination because its clinical features are similar to those of other acute abdominal illnesses (Box 60.6).

History

Abdominal pain is present at the onset of most attacks of AP. Biliary pain may herald or progress to AP. Pain in pancreatitis usually involves the entire upper abdomen. However, it may be epigastric, in the right upper quadrant, or, infrequently, confined to the left side. Pain in the lower abdomen may arise from the rapid spread of pancreatic exudation to the left colon.

BOX 60.6 Differential Diagnosis of Acute Pancreatitis

Biliary pain
Acute cholecystitis
Perforated hollow viscus (e.g., perforated peptic ulcer)
Mesenteric ischemia or infarction
Intestinal obstruction
Myocardial infarction
Dissecting aortic aneurysm
Ectopic pregnancy

Onset of pain is rapid but not as abrupt as that of a perforated viscus. Usually, it is at maximal intensity in 10–20 minutes. Occasionally, pain gradually increases and takes several hours to reach maximum intensity. Pain is steady and ranges in intensity from moderate to very severe. There is little pain relief with changing position. Frequently, pain is unbearable, steady, and boring. Band-like radiation of the pain to the back occurs in half of patients. Pain that lasts only a few hours and then disappears suggests a disease other than pancreatitis, such as biliary pain or peptic ulcer. Pain is absent in 5%–10% of AP episodes (often in postsurgical ischemic pancreatitis), and a painless presentation can be a feature of serious fatal disease.[202]

Most patients develop nausea and vomiting. Vomiting may be severe, last for hours, be accompanied by retching, and may not alleviate pain. Vomiting may be related to severe pain or to inflammation involving the posterior gastric wall.

Physical Examination

Physical findings vary with the severity of an AP episode. Patients with mild pancreatitis may not appear acutely ill. Abdominal tenderness may be mild and abdominal guarding absent. In severe pancreatitis, patients appear severely ill and often have abdominal distention, which is due to gastric, small bowel, or colonic ileus. Almost all patients are tender in the upper abdomen, which may be elicited by gently shaking the abdomen or by gentle percussion. Guarding is more marked in the upper abdomen. Tenderness and guarding can be less than expected, considering the intensity of abdominal discomfort. Abdominal rigidity, as occurs in diffuse peritonitis, is unusual but can be present, and differentiation from a perforated viscus may be challenging in these instances. Bowel sounds are reduced and may be absent.

Additional abdominal findings may include ecchymosis in one or both flanks [Gray Turner sign (Fig. 60.5A)], or in the periumbilical area [Cullen sign (Fig 60.5B)], owing to extravasation of hemorrhagic exudate to these areas. These signs occur in less than 1% of cases and are associated with a poor prognosis. Rarely there is a brawny erythema of the flanks caused by extravasation of pancreatic exudate to the abdominal wall. A palpable epigastric mass may appear during the disease from a large acute peripancreatic fluid collection or a large inflammatory mass.

The general physical examination may uncover markedly abnormal vital signs when there are third-space fluid losses and systemic toxicity. Commonly, the pulse is 100–150 bpm (sinus tachycardia). Blood pressure can be initially higher than normal (due to pain) and then lower than normal with third-space losses and hypovolemia. Initially the temperature may be normal, but within 1–3 days it may increase to 101°F–103°F, owing to severe local inflammatory process and/or the SIRS.

Tachypnea with shallow respirations may be present if the subdiaphragmatic inflammatory exudate causes painful breathing. Dyspnea may accompany pleural effusions, atelectasis, ARDS, or

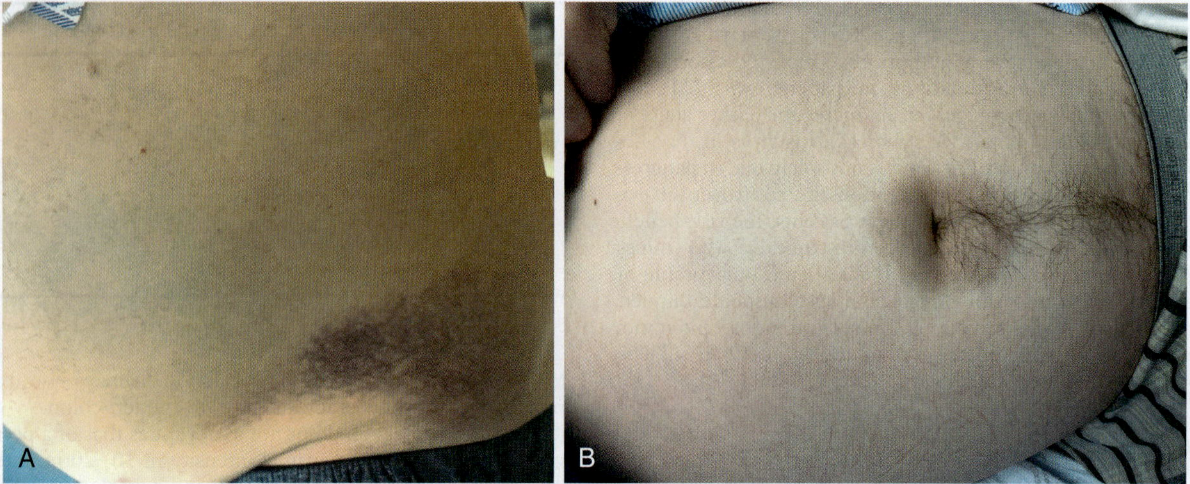

Fig. 60.5 (A) Grey Turner sign. Ecchymosis in the left flank of a 57-year-old man with a 1-week history of epigastric pain secondary to acute biliary necrotizing pancreatitis. (B) Cullen sign: Ecchymosis and subcutaneous edema in the periumbilical area of a 40-year-old man with alcoholic pancreatitis. (Courtesy Dr. Shilpa Sannapaneni, Dallas, TX.)

heart failure. Chest examination may reveal limited diaphragmatic excursion when abdominal pain causes splinting of the diaphragm or dullness to percussion and decreased breath sounds at the lung bases when there is a pleural effusion. There may be neurologic symptoms, such as disorientation, hallucinations, agitation, or coma, which may be due to alcohol withdrawal, hypotension, and electrolyte imbalance, such as hyponatremia, hypoxemia, fever, or toxic effects of pancreatic enzymes on the central nervous system. Conjunctival icterus, when present, may be due to bile duct obstruction from choledocholithiasis in gallstone AP, edema in the head of the pancreas, or from coexistent liver disease.

Uncommon physical findings in AP include panniculitis with subcutaneous nodular fat necrosis that may be accompanied by polyarthritis (PPP syndrome; see Chapter 25).[203] Subcutaneous fat necroses appear as 0.5- to 2-cm tender red nodules that usually involve the distal extremities but may occur over the scalp, trunk, or buttocks. They occasionally precede the abdominal pain or may occur without abdominal pain, but usually they appear during a clinical episode and disappear with clinical improvement.

Certain physical findings point to a specific etiology of AP. Hepatomegaly, spider angiomas, and thickening of palmar sheaths favor alcoholic pancreatitis. Eruptive xanthomas and lipemia retinalis suggest hyperlipidemic pancreatitis. Parotid pain and swelling are features of mumps. Band keratopathy (an infiltration on the lateral margin of the cornea) occurs with hypercalcemia. Microembolization in the retina can lead to typical fundus findings associated with visual disturbances, including blindness. This is known as Purtscher retinopathy and can be seen in a variety of conditions besides AP.

DIFFERENTIAL DIAGNOSIS

The abdominal pain of biliary origin, especially in symptomatic choledocholithiasis, may simulate AP. It is frequently severe and epigastric, precipitated by food ingestion, especially fatty meals, but it typically lasts for several hours rather than several days (see Chapter 65). The pain of a perforated peptic ulcer is sudden, becomes diffuse, and precipitates a rigid abdomen; movement aggravates pain. Nausea and vomiting occur but disappear soon after onset of pain (see Chapter 55). In mesenteric ischemia or infarction, the clinical setting often is an older person with atrial fibrillation or atherosclerotic vascular disease who develops sudden pain out of proportion to physical findings, bloody diarrhea, nausea, and vomiting. Abdominal tenderness may be mild to moderate, despite severe pain (see Chapter 118). In intestinal obstruction, pain is cyclical, abdominal distention is prominent, vomiting persists and may become feculent, and peristalsis is hyperactive and often audible (see Chapter 125). Other conditions that consider in the differential diagnosis of AP are listed in Box 60.6.

LABORATORY DIAGNOSIS

Pancreatic Enzymes

In general, the diagnosis of AP relies on at least a threefold elevation of amylase or lipase in the blood.

Serum Amylase Level

In healthy persons, the pancreas accounts for 40%–45% of serum amylase activity with the salivary glands accounting for the rest. Simple analytic techniques can separate pancreatic and salivary amylases. Because pancreatic diseases increase serum pancreatic (P) isoamylase, measurement of P-isoamylase can improve diagnostic accuracy. However, this test is rarely used due to its cost.[204]

The total serum amylase test is most frequently ordered to diagnose AP because it can be measured quickly and cheaply. It rises within 6–12 hours of AP onset and is cleared fairly rapidly from the blood (half-life, 10 hours).[204] Less than 25% of serum amylase is removed by the kidneys. It is uncertain what other processes clear amylase from the circulation. The serum amylase is usually increased on the first day of symptoms, and it remains elevated for 3–5 days in uncomplicated attacks. Sensitivity is at least 85%. The serum amylase may be normal or only minimally elevated in severe necrotizing pancreatitis,[204] during a mild AP episode, or an attack superimposed on chronic pancreatitis (because the pancreas has little remaining acinar tissue), or during recovery from AP as amylase is cleared from the circulation. The level may return to normal quickly, in just a few days. Serum amylase may also be falsely normal in hypertriglyceridemia-associated pancreatitis because an amylase inhibitor may be associated with triglyceride elevations. In this case, a serial dilution of serum often reveals an elevated serum amylase.

Hyperamylasemia is also not specific for pancreatitis; it occurs in many conditions. In fact, one-half of all patients with an elevated serum amylase level may not have pancreatic disease. In AP, the serum amylase concentration is usually more than three times the upper limit of normal; it is usually less than this with other causes of hyperamylasemia. However, this level is not an absolute discriminator. Thus an increased serum amylase level supports rather than confirms the diagnosis of AP. In addition, there are some individuals who have persistent hyperamylasemia without clinical symptoms. This has been reported to be due to macroamylasemia (discussed later) or pancreatic hyperamylasemia on a familial basis. Nonpancreatic diseases that lead to hyperamylasemia include pathologic processes in other organs that normally produce amylase (e.g., salivary glands and fallopian tubes). Furthermore, mass lesions, such as papillary cystadenocarcinoma of the ovary, benign ovarian cysts, and carcinoma of the lung, can cause hyperamylasemia because they produce and secrete salivary (S-type) isoamylase. Leakage of P-type isoamylase across the intestine with peritoneal amylase absorption probably explains hyperamylasemia in patients with intestinal infarction or GI tract perforation. Renal failure can increase serum amylase up to four to five times the upper limit of normal because of decreased renal clearance of this enzyme. Patients on hemodialysis tend to have higher serum amylase levels than those on peritoneal dialysis. In patients with chronic kidney disease, there is not a clear inverse correlation between the creatinine clearance rate and serum levels of amylase, and about one-third of patients with marked renal insufficiency (low creatinine clearance) have normal pancreatic enzyme levels.[205]

Chronic elevations of serum amylase (without amylasuria) occur in macroamylasemia.[206] In this condition, normal serum amylase is bound to an immunoglobulin or abnormal serum protein to form a complex that is too large to be filtered by renal glomeruli and, thus, has a prolonged serum half-life. Macroamylasemia may lead to a false diagnosis of pancreatic disease, but it has no other clinical consequence. The urinary amylase-to-creatinine clearance ratio (ACCR) increases from approximately 3%–10% in AP. However, even moderate renal insufficiency interferes with the accuracy and specificity of the ACCR. Other than to diagnose macroamylasemia, which has a low ACCR, urinary amylase measurements and the ACCR are not used clinically.

In the emergency room, computer order set de-selection of amylase when using lipase was an effective tool to reduce nonvalue-added testing and reduce cost while maintaining quality patient care and physician choice in patients presenting with abdominal pain.[207] The rapid and easy-to-operate amylase assay may have potential application in the fields of point-of-care clinical diagnosis, particularly in rural and remote areas where lab equipment may be limited.

Serum Lipase Level

The sensitivity of serum lipase for the diagnosis of AP is similar to that of serum amylase and is at least 79%.[6,208,209] Lipase may have greater specificity for pancreatitis than amylase, however. Serum lipase is normal when serum amylase is elevated in nonpancreatic conditions such as salivary gland disease, amylase-producing tumors, gynecologic conditions such as salpingitis, and macroamylasemia. Serum lipase always is elevated on the first day of illness and remains elevated longer than does the serum amylase, providing a slightly higher sensitivity.[6] Combining amylase and lipase does not improve diagnostic accuracy and increases cost.

Specificity of lipase can suffer from some of the same problems as those of amylase, however. In the absence of pancreatitis, serum lipase may increase less than twofold above normal in renal insufficiency.[210] With acute GI conditions that resemble AP, serum lipase increases to levels less than threefold above normal, presumably by absorption through an ischemic, inflamed, or perforated intestine.[211] Rarely, a nonpancreatic abdominal condition, such as small bowel obstruction, can raise the serum lipase (and amylase) above three times normal. Some believe that serum lipase measurement is preferable to that of serum amylase because it is at least as sensitive as amylase measurement and more specific, whereas others find no clear advantage of one over the other.

Many normal persons have elevations of serum amylase and/or lipase of little clinical significance. Diabetics appear to have higher median lipase compared with nondiabetic patients.[144] In this prospective study, it was shown that 16.6% of type 2 diabetics had an elevated serum lipase, and 1.2% had a serum lipase of more than threefold elevation despite the absence of symptoms. However, when evaluating serum amylase, 11.8% of type 2 diabetics were found to have an elevated level, and 0.2% had more than threefold elevation. Although the ramifications of these findings are unclear, there is a recent study that suggested that these low-level elevations in pancreatic enzymes may be associated with ductal changes in the pancreas consistent with chronic pancreatitis. In outpatients with diabetes and elevated pancreatic enzymes without symptoms, extensive investigations should be avoided. Nevertheless, a one-time cross-sectional imaging study may be reasonable to rule out potential neoplastic causes of pancreatic enzyme elevations (e.g., pancreatic cancer, acinar cell carcinoma, and metastatic gastric cancer).[211]

It is also possible to analyze serum lipase subtypes, such as the pancreatic fraction of the lipase. However, in the small study it was found that such subtype estimation is not superior to a regular lipase assay but can be used as an add-on test if required. Given that the pancreatic lipase is present at 100 times greater concentration than other isoforms of hepatic, endothelial, and lipoprotein lipase, analyzing serum lipase subtype is not necessary.[204] Lipase levels should not be used to predict severity. The most common primary diagnoses in non-AP patients with elevated lipase included shock, cardiac arrest, and malignancy.[211] Elevated serum lipase levels can have nonpancreatic origins, with liver and renal failure being the most frequent. Lipase should replace amylase as the first-line laboratory investigation for suspected AP.

In summary, neither lipase nor amylase has ideal diagnostic test performance characteristics. A Cochrane systematic review looked at the diagnostic accuracy of serum amylase, serum lipase, urinary trypsinogen-2, and urinary amylase, either alone or in combination, in the diagnosis of AP in people with the acute onset of a persistent, severe epigastric pain or diffuse abdominal pain, and found a false-negative rate of 25% and a false-positive rate of 10%.[6] This is one of the reasons the society guidelines' diagnostic criteria to include imaging findings to optimize accurate diagnosis of AP.

Other Pancreatic Enzyme Levels

During acute pancreatic inflammation, pancreatic digestive enzymes other than amylase and lipase leak into the systemic circulation and have been used to diagnose AP. They include trypsin/trypsinogen, trypsinogen activation peptide (TAP), urinary and serum trypsinogen-2, carboxypeptidase A, phospholipase A_2, carboxylester lipase, colipase, ribonuclease, and elastase. None—alone or in combination—are diagnostically superior to serum amylase or lipase, and most are not available on a routine basis.

Standard Blood Tests

The white blood cell (WBC) count frequently is elevated, often markedly so in subjects with SIRS and does not generally indicate infection. The blood glucose may also be high and associated with high levels of serum glucagon. Serum aspartate aminotransferase (AST), alanine aminotransferase (ALT), alkaline phosphatase, and direct and total bilirubin may also increase, particularly in gallstone pancreatitis. Presumably, calculi in the bile duct account for these abnormalities. However, inflammation of the pancreatic head per se may partially obstruct the distal bile duct in AP. Serum aminotransferases may help distinguish biliary from alcoholic pancreatitis (see later). The decrease in serum calcium often seen in patients with AP is mainly related to the decreased serum albumin. As will be discussed later, the decrease in calcium is a marker of severity because it is carried bound to albumin-rich intravascular fluid that extravasates to the peritoneum. Another mechanism is through binding to nonesterified fatty acid elevation, which is elevated during severe AP and other critical illnesses.[212]

DIAGNOSTIC IMAGING

Abdominal Plain Film

Findings on a plain radiograph range from no abnormalities in mild AP to localized ileus of a segment of small intestine (sentinel loop) or the colon cutoff sign in more severe disease. In addition, an abdominal plain film helps exclude other causes of abdominal pain, such as bowel obstruction and perforation. Images of the hollow GI tract on an abdominal plain radiograph depend on the spread and location of pancreatic exudate. Gastric abnormalities are caused by exudate in the lesser sac producing anterior displacement of the stomach, with separation of the contour of the stomach from the transverse colon. Small intestinal abnormalities are due to inflammation in proximity to small bowel mesentery and include ileus of one or more loops of jejunum (the sentinel loop). Generalized ileus may occur in severe disease. The descending duodenum may be displaced and stretched by an enlarged head of the pancreas. In addition, spread of exudate to specific areas of the colon may produce spasm of that part of the colon and either no air distal to the spasm (the colon cutoff sign) or dilated colon proximal to the spasm. Other findings on plain radiography of the abdomen may give clues to etiology or severity, including calcified gallstones (gallstone pancreatitis), pancreatic stones, or calcification (acute exacerbation of chronic pancreatitis).

Chest Radiography

Abnormalities visible on the chest x-ray occur in 30% of patients with AP, including the elevation of a hemidiaphragm, pleural effusion(s), basal or plate-like atelectasis secondary to limited respiratory excursion, and pulmonary infiltrates. Pleural effusions may be bilateral or confined to the left side; rarely they are only on the right side.[213,214] Patients with AP found to have a pleural effusion and/or pulmonary infiltrate on admission are more likely to progress to severe disease. In patients with severe disease, signs of ARDS or heart failure may be seen later in the clinical course. Pericardial effusions are rare.

Abdominal Ultrasound (US)

Abdominal US is used during the first 24 hours of hospitalization to search for gallstones, dilation of the bile duct due to choledocholithiasis, and ascites. Owing to overlying gas, the diagnosis of cholelithiasis and choledocholithiasis may be obscured during the acute attack but may be found after bowel gas has receded. Ascites is common in patients with moderate to severe AP as protein-rich fluid extravasates from the intravascular compartment to the peritoneal cavity. When the pancreas is visualized by US (bowel gas obscures the pancreas 25%–35% of the time), it is usually diffusely enlarged and hypoechoic. Less frequently, there are focal hypoechoic areas. There may also be US evidence of chronic pancreatitis, such as intraductal or parenchymal calcification(s) and dilation of the PD. Abdominal US is not as accurate in evaluating extrapancreatic spread of inflammation or pancreatic necrosis and consequently is not useful to ascertain severity of pancreatitis.

Endoscopic Ultrasound and Endoscopic Retrograde Cholangiopancreatography

Imaging of the pancreas by EUS during an attack of AP, and for weeks following an episode, reveals abnormal signals that are typically hypoechoic and indistinguishable from chronic pancreatitis and malignancy. EUS is useful at an early stage in AP to assess for concurrent common bile duct stones and guide the indication for ERCP at the same session, thus avoiding ERCP when the bile duct does not contain stones.[215] While EUS done at an early stage in AP can reliably detect pancreatic necrosis, the role of EUS remains with patients in whom choledocholithiasis is suspected. Clinical utility of an urgent EUS is limited. In a recent multicenter study, an urgent EUS performed within 24 hours of admission in predicted severe biliary pancreatitis to guide the need for an urgent ERCP with sphincterotomy did not improve outcomes, such as major complications or death.[216] In idiopathic AP, recent guidelines and reviews recommend obtaining EUS after a period of 8 weeks to look for causes like microlithiasis in the common bile duct, small tumors near the PD causing obstruction, chronic pancreatitis presenting as an AP attack, and some anatomical abnormalities missed on CT scan, such as pancreas divisum or annular pancreas.[113,217,218] In a recent meta-analysis comparing MRCP and EUS in the evaluation of idiopathic AP, EUS had a higher diagnostic accuracy than MRCP (64% vs. 34%) in establishing an etiology of pancreatitis.[217,219]

Computerized Tomography

Abdominal CT is an important imaging test modality for the diagnosis of AP and its intra-abdominal complications. The two main indications for a CT in AP are to (1) exclude other serious intra-abdominal conditions (e.g., mesenteric infarction or a perforated peptic ulcer) and (2) determine whether locoregional complications of pancreatitis are present (e.g., development of pancreatic necrosis, involvement of the GI tract or nearby blood vessels, and organs, including the liver, spleen, and kidney). Helical CT is the most common technique. When IV contrast is given, normal perfusion of the pancreas indicates interstitial pancreatitis (see Fig. 60.1) whereas pancreatic necrosis manifests as perfusion defects after IV contrast injection (see Fig. 60.2). CT scan is able to quantify the extent of pancreatic necrosis and whether there is concomitant or isolated peripancreatic necrosis.

It has been suggested that administration of IV contrast media early in the course of AP might increase the risk of pancreatic necrosis based on experimental AP studies in rats.[220] However, data in humans are conflicting with a lack of high-level evidence.[221–223] Society guidelines unanimously discourage contrast-enhanced CT scan in the early (i.e., first 72 hours) period of AP because of its lack of clinical utility.[217,218,224,225] First, when AP diagnosis is in question early in the course, a *noncontrast* CT is adequate to confirm the diagnosis or ascertain an alternative diagnosis (e.g., perforated ulcer and small bowel obstruction). Second, pancreatic necrosis may not fully exhibit its enhancement patterns until 72 hours of illness.[217,218,224] Third, early diagnosis of pancreatic necrosis does not usually impact management. Despite the society guidelines, the overutilization of early CT scans in AP continues to be an issue from health care cost standpoint.[226,227]

The severity of locoregional injury in AP on imaging studies can be classified into five grades (A to E) based on findings on unenhanced CT (discussed later). The extent of locoregional injury as detected on cross-sectional imaging determines the morbidity, but not mortality of AP patients. The presence of gas

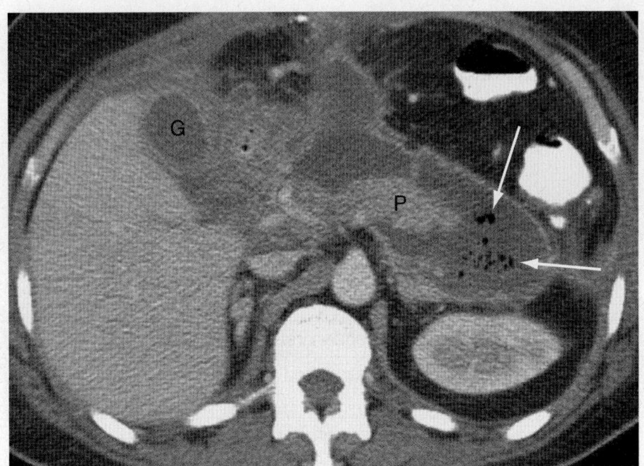

Fig. 60.6 CT showing acute necrotizing pancreatitis. The pancreas (P) is surrounded by peripancreatic inflammation that contains bubbles of air (*arrows*) due to sterile necrosis. The patient was not clinically ill, and therefore an abscess was not considered likely. *G*, Gallbladder.

in the pancreas suggests pancreatic infection with a gas-forming organism or necrosis (Fig. 60.6) with a microperforation of the gut or "autofistulization" of the pancreatic fluid collection to surrounding gastrointestinal tract.

Magnetic Resonance Imaging

An abdominal MRI provides similar information regarding the intra-abdominal extent and complications of AP, as does the CT scan. However, MRI is more accurate to CT in assessing the necrotic debris within (peri)pancreatic fluid collections. A special type of MRI that gives detailed images of the pancreas and biliary tree called MRCP is frequently ordered in patients with AP because it is more accurate than CT scan, but comparable to EUS in detecting concurrent choledocholithiasis. However, EUS has a higher diagnostic accuracy for CBD stones sized 4 mm in diameter or less.[228,229] MRCP has also the advantage over CT scan in better delineating the pancreatic duct and detecting any PD disruption and disconnection. Additionally, the use of IV secretin prior to MRCP allows a better visualization of the pancreatic duct.[230] This has been shown to be particularly useful in the evaluation of patients with idiopathic pancreatitis and recurrent pancreatitis. Whereas MRI has a definite role in the management of AP, the limitations of this modality need to be recognized. MRI is less accessible, more expensive, and requires subjects to remain still for a much longer period compared to CT scan.

DISTINGUISHING ALCOHOLIC FROM GALLSTONE PANCREATITIS

Differentiation between alcoholic and gallstone AP is important because eliminating these etiologies may prevent further attacks of pancreatitis but it can be challenging. This challenge is attributable to the fact that less than 5% of heavy alcohol consumers develop AP[127,231] and cholelithiasis, a criterion by which biliary etiology is determined[216,232,233] can be concurrently present in a patient with a history of alcohol abuse. To complicate the matter further, there is strong epidemiologic evidence that moderate alcohol intake in females decreases the risk of symptom development in patients with cholelithiasis, whereas heavy users increase the risk.[128] Therefore clinicians should be careful not to assign etiology without supporting evidence. The following paragraph summarizes parameters that are helpful in ascertaining these etiologies.

It is important to remember that the first clinical episode usually occurs after 5–10 years of heavy alcohol consumption (~40 g of alcohol/day) so taking a careful history to ascertain patient's drinking history and prior complications of alcoholism is paramount. Laboratory tests may also help distinguish between these two disorders. Mean corpuscular volume is often elevated in chronic heavy drinkers and is seen in up to 86% of female alcoholics and 63% in male alcoholics.[234] However, vitamin B_{12}/folate deficiency, liver disease, and hypothyroidism, which are alternative causes of macrocytosis, need to be ruled out first before using MCV as a parameter to support chronic alcohol use.[234] The more accurate biomarkers of recent alcohol consumption are now available, including phosphatidylethanol, which has excellent diagnostic performance and it should be ordered in every patient where the etiology is unclear.[235] The main disadvantage of PeTH is its turnaround time of 1–2 weeks but it is nevertheless useful for patients who will be seen in outpatient clinic for evaluation of idiopathic pancreatitis or for patients with recurrent visits to the ER with AP. Additionally, approximately 39% of alcoholic AP patients have coexisting alcoholic liver disease often manifesting in evidence of cirrhosis with/without portal hypertension.[236]

The specificity of a serum ALT concentration greater than 150 IU/L (≈3-fold elevation) for gallstone pancreatitis has been estimated at 96% with a high positive predictive value of 95%, but the sensitivity is only 48%.[237] The serum AST concentration is nearly as useful as the ALT, but the total bilirubin and alkaline phosphatase concentrations are not as helpful to distinguish gallstone pancreatitis from alcoholic and other etiologies. The presence of sludge, microlithiasis, and/or stones in the gallbladder in a patient with AP where other predisposing conditions have been ruled out—is usually adequate to establish biliary as the cause of AP. There are differing reports as to whether a high serum lipase-to-amylase ratio can differentiate alcoholic from other causes of pancreatitis, but its diagnostic performance has been suboptimal. In landmark clinical trials on biliary pancreatitis, the determining criteria include the presence of gallstones, sludge, or microlithiasis on imaging, dilated common bile duct (>8–9 mm in ≤75 years or >10–11 mm in patients when older than >75 years), or ALT > two times the upper limit of normal.[23,111,232,233] For this reason, conventional abdominal US should be performed in every patient with a first attack of AP to search for gallstones in the gallbladder, common duct stones, or signs of extrahepatic biliary tract obstruction. Presence of concurrent choledocholithiasis clearly supports biliary etiology but most stones pass during the acute attack.

PREDICTORS OF DISEASE SEVERITY

Despite a large body of literature, none of the existing prediction models have optimal performance.[90,238] Most predictors have a very high negative predictive value but low positive predictive value and this can be partially explained because a significant proportion of the patients with AP do not develop moderately severe or severe disease.[126] From two prospectively collected cohorts, it was reported that the existing scoring systems seem to have reached their maximal efficacy in predicting persistent organ failure in AP.[238] Sophisticated combinations of predictive rules are more accurate but cumbersome to use and therefore of limited clinical use. Our ability to predict the severity of AP cannot be expected to improve unless we develop new approaches. The most recent AGA technical review on early management of AP found no studies using a predictive tool that improved clinical outcomes. Hence it is recommended using clinical judgment in combination with as simple predictive tool in clinical practice.[239] Thus many of the predictors will be listed below briefly, with added information on some predictors that were widely studied.

Scoring Systems

The acute physiology and chronic health evaluation (APACHE II) score has been the most validated system in the literature and showed only moderate accuracy in predicting severe AP.[240] APACHE II is also cumbersome (like most of the systems) and is very rarely used in clinical practice. Most studies used a score of 8 or more as severe AP. Ranson et al. identified 11 signs that had prognostic significance during the first 48 hours.[241] The original list was analyzed in patients who primarily suffered from alcoholic pancreatitis and was then modified 8 years later for those with gallstone pancreatitis. A score of 3 or more is considered to accurately predict severe AP. The Imrie or Glasgow score is a slightly simplified list (eight criteria) that is used commonly in the United Kingdom. Analyzing a large database including almost 37,000 patients from more than 200 hospitals, including a validation study, a simpler scoring system that included only five variables.[242] The scoring system, referred to as *BISAP* (Bedside Index for Severity in AP), assigns each parameter 1 point: ***B***UN greater than 25 mg/dL, ***I***mpaired mental status, ***S***IRS, ***A***ge older than 60 years, and ***P***leural effusion, for a possible total of 5 points. A BISAP score of 4 or 5 is associated with a 7–12-fold increased risk of developing organ failure. BISAP is not superior to APACHE II. Other scoring systems include the harmless AP score, the Japanese AP severity score, and the PANC 3 score.

The simple SIRS score has been commonly used in more recent observational studies and clinical trials in AP. SIRS is defined by two or more of the following four criteria: pulse >90 bpm, rectal temperature <36°C or >38°C, WBC count <4000/mm^3 or >12,000/mm^3, and a respiratory rate greater than 20/minute or an arterial PCO_2 <32 mm Hg (see Box 60.2). SIRS is cheap, easy to calculate with parameters readily available at the time of admission and as accurate as any of the more complex scoring systems. The presence of SIRS at admission and persistence of SIRS at 48 hours significantly increases the morbidity and mortality rate in AP. In one study, death occurred in 25% of patients with persistent SIRS, in 8% with transient SIRS, and in less than 1% without SIRS.[18,20,243]

Computed Tomography

The findings of extensive fluid collections and/or extensive pancreatic necrosis on CT scan have been correlated with severe disease in AP. Balthazar et al. developed a CT severity index (CTSI) reported that among AP patients with a score of 0–6, only 3.8% died as compared to 18% with scores of 7–10 (Table 60.1).[244,245] The CT grading scores correlate better with the moderately severe (pancreatic necrosis and acute fluid collections) than the development of organ failure. There is controversy in the literature as to whether the extent of necrosis on CT predicts organ failure. A modified CTSI has been found to be more useful where a simplified assessment of inflammation and necrosis, as well as the assessment of extrapancreatic complications, were included. As with the other scoring systems discussed above, their modest predictive performance and uncertain impact on clinical outcomes have limited the usefulness of CT-based grading systems.

Chest Radiography

A pleural effusion documented within 72 hours of admission by chest radiography (or CT) correlates with severe disease.

TABLE 60.1 CT Grading System of Balthazar and the CT Severity Index (CTSI)

Balthazar Grades	Definition	Points
A	Normal pancreas consistent with mild pancreatitis	0
B	Focal or diffuse enlargement of the gland, including contour irregularities and inhomogeneous attenuation but without peripancreatic inflammation	1
C	Grade B plus peripancreatic inflammation	2
D	Grade C plus associated single fluid collection	3
E	Grade C plus 2 or more peripancreatic fluid collections or gas in the pancreas or retroperitoneum	4
CTSI = Balthazar Grade Points Plus Necrosis Score[a]		
	Necrosis score	**Points**
	Absence of necrosis	0
	Necrosis of up to 33% of the pancreas	2
	Necrosis of 33%–50%	4
	Necrosis of >50%	6

[a]Highest attainable CTSI score: 4 (Balthazar grade E) + 6 (necrosis of >50%) = 10 points.

NOVEL BIOMARKERS

Given the limitations of existing scoring systems and laboratory parameters, such as BUN, creatinine, and hematocrit, an extensive number of novel biomarkers and radiomics have been studied to find *the* one with optimal predictive performance.[91,246–258] These investigations are mostly informed by findings of the mechanistic studies of severe AP that established important roles of DAMPs, unregulated immune response, leucocyte infiltration into end-organs, visceral adiposity in the pancreatic and peripancreatic region, endothelial integrity, and gut barrier in mediating organ dysfunction.[74,79,83,99,259–263] Therefore the principal domains of investigation included components of the immune system (cytokines, DAMPs, and genetic polymorphisms in toll-like receptors), measures of inflammation (acute phase proteins), measures of volume of adiposity (adipokines, CT and/or MRI quantification of visceral adipose tissue), and measures of endothelial dysfunction & leucocyte migration/trafficking. The list of the studied biomarkers is extensive, and it continues to grow. However, none of these parameters are routinely available for use in clinical practice and require further validation.

TREATMENT

Initial Management During the First 2 Weeks

There is no specific drug therapy to treat AP, and thus, treatment guidelines focus on supportive care and the treatment of complications once they develop (Fig. 60.7). Due to improving the efficiency of supportive care, including ICU care and treatment of pancreatic necrosis and other complications, the mortality in AP has decreased.[24,264] Therefore the central management principle during the early phase of AP is one of *do no harm* by avoiding unnecessary antibiotics administration, avoiding fluid overload, and avoiding potentially harmful invasive interventions

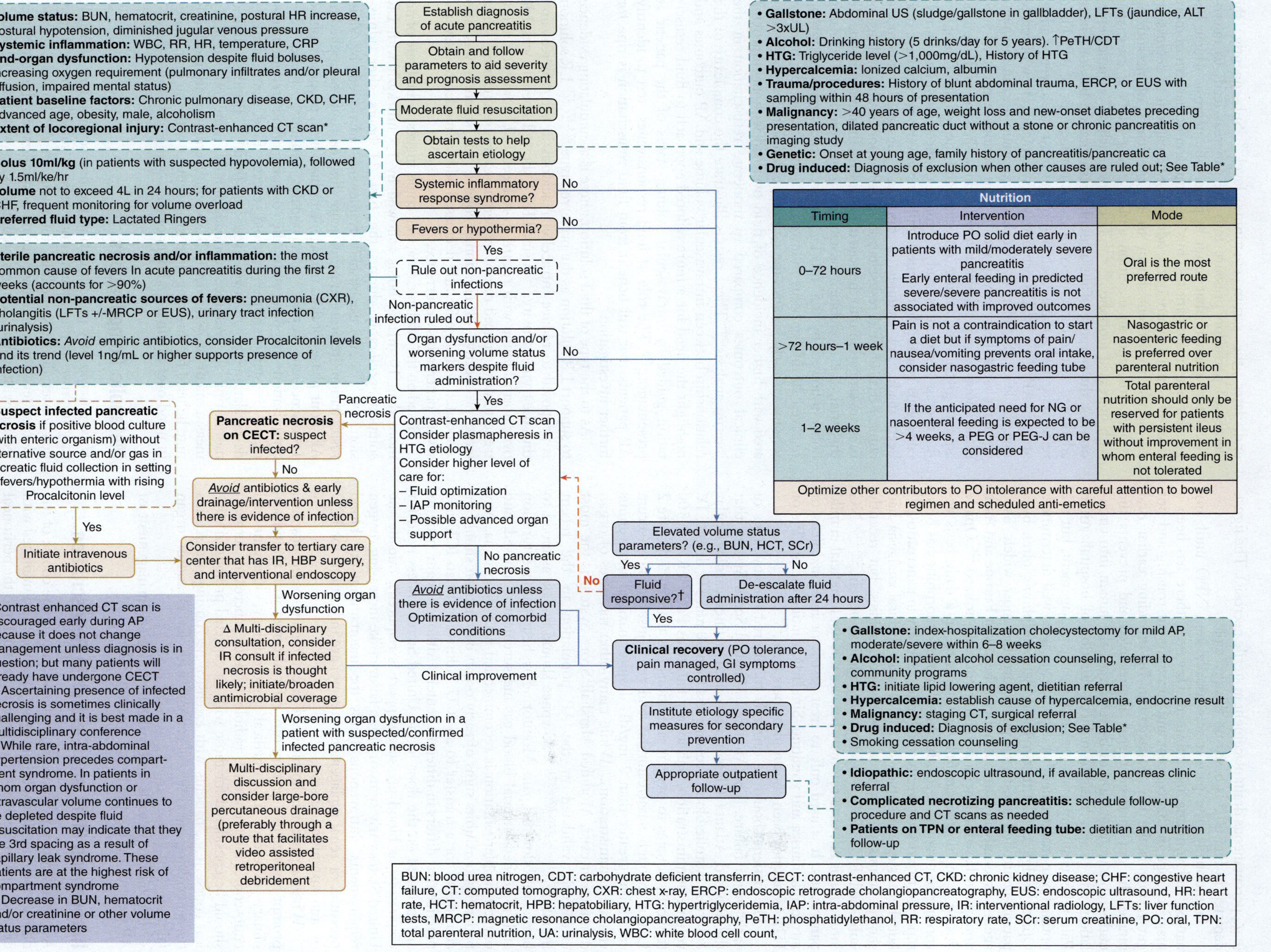

Fig. 60.7 Algorithm for the management of acute pancreatitis during the first 2 weeks.

(e.g., percutaneous drain placement in sterile necrosis). The figure depicted in Fig. 60.5 is based on this principle.

Traditionally, the patient was usually kept NPO until any nausea and vomiting has subsided. However, there has been a major change in this concept and currently gut rousing and not gut resting is the key management. By providing earlier oral intake, the gut mucosal barrier is preserved and prevents the undesirable translocation of bacteria from the lumen into circulation, and it also leads to reduced duration of hospitalization. Pain relief is an important area in the early management, but the optimal pain management strategy has not been well determined. Opiate analgesics like fentanyl and hydromorphone, often by a patient-controlled anesthesia pump, are the most widely used agents, especially in North America, whereas in Europe and Asia, nonopioid based analgesia is more frequently utilized.[126] Opiate dosing is monitored carefully and adjusted on a daily basis according to ongoing needs. In animal models, morphine has been reported to worsen severity and hinder recovery in pancreatitis,[265] but there is sparse human data. Thoracic epidural analgesia had shown promising results in observational studies, but recently published RCT failed to show any clinical benefit.[266,267] NG intubation is not used routinely because it is not beneficial in mild pancreatitis. It is used only to treat gastric or intestinal ileus or intractable nausea and vomiting. Similarly, routine use of PPIs or H2RAs has not been shown to be beneficial.[268]

The patient should be carefully monitored for any signs of early organ failure. The Modified Marshall Score System that the Revised Atlanta Classification used defines cardiovascular failure as systolic blood pressure less than 90 mm Hg despite IV volume administration, pulmonary failure as $PaO_2/FiO_2 < 300$ (typically equates to oxygen saturations less than 96% despite 2 L/min through nasal cannula), and renal insufficiency (serum creatinine greater than 2 mg/dL despite maximal intravenous volume administration).[9] While many other measures of organ dysfunction exist, Modified Marshall Score System is the most extensively validated in the AP population in the recent literature.[8,18,105,126,269–271] Tachypnea should not be assumed to be due to abdominal pain. Monitoring oxyhemoglobin saturation and, if needed, arterial blood gas measurement is advised, and oxygen supplementation is recommended with hypoxemia. Any patient who exhibits signs of early organ dysfunction should be considered for a transfer to an ICU. Admission to an ICU is a practice that differs in different centers. Although many patients are managed on the floor in the United States (unless need for respiratory or blood pressure support is required), outside the United States early signs of organ failure (like increasing oxygen requirements, intravenous fluids for maintaining the blood pressure, or renal replacement therapy) are indications for ICU or step-up unit admission.

When a patient is hospitalized in community-based hospital, prompt transfer to a tertiary care referral center with multidisciplinary expertise (i.e., medical pancreatology, interventional endoscopy, interventional radiology, and pancreatic surgery) should be considered for those with an expected prolonged clinical course [e.g., patients with extensive necrotizing pancreatitis (large evolving necrotic collections) with fevers and/or organ failure].

Fig. 60.5 represents a flow diagram to guide management of AP patients during the first 2 weeks of illness.

Intravenous Fluid and Electrolyte Resuscitation

As the inflammatory process progresses early in the course of the disease, the endothelial cell integrity may become diminished with extravasation of protein-rich intravascular fluid into the peritoneal cavity and retroperitoneum. This phenomenon is called vascular leak syndrome resulting in hemoconcentration and decreased renal perfusion with the associated elevation in the BUN level and, later, the serum creatinine level.[79] Subsequently, the decreased perfusion pressure into the pancreas leads to microcirculatory changes that result in pancreatic necrosis which, begets further inflammation. Thus an admission hematocrit of more than 44% and a failure of the admission hematocrit to decrease at 24 hours have been shown to be predictors of necrotizing pancreatitis, and an elevation and/or rising BUN is associated with increased mortality.[105,272] Therefore early IV volume repletion for the purpose of intravascular resuscitation has long been advocated as the centerpiece of early management of AP. Fluid resuscitation in AP has been one of the most extensively studied areas in AP.[269,273–282] Unfortunately, a systematic review observed that the level of evidence of such an important area in the management is at best very poor.[283] The various aspects of such intravenous volume administration include the type of fluid, total amount given, rate, timing, duration, and the weight to monitor the therapy. Since this study,[283] much of these identified knowledge gaps remain, but some significant advancements have also been made. For example, a rigorously designed randomized clinical trial of fluid resuscitation in AP reported the findings of their investigation into the role of aggressive fluid resuscitation. In this trial, the moderate resuscitation group received 10 mL/kg bolus followed by 1.5 mL/kg, whereas the aggressive group received 20 mL/kg bolus followed by 3 mL/kg, but the trial was terminated early because the aggressive resuscitation was associated with higher incidence of fluid overload without improving clinical outcomes compared to moderate resuscitation in the interim analysis.[269] These results illustrate the complexity of the relationship between intravascular volume and AP outcomes and highlight the need for a more tailored approach to fluid resuscitation guided by intravascular volume status of the patient at presentation.[284] The role of fluid responsiveness test to identify AP patients that will benefit from fluid resuscitation is ripe for further investigation.[276]

As to the type of fluid solution, there is accumulating evidence to support LR solution as the preferred type.[273,277,279] LR solution is proposed to reduce intracellular acidosis in the pancreas and thus the tryptic activity.[212] A small RCT showed a benefit with LR over normal saline with regard to reduced ICU admission and a trend toward reduced risk of moderate/severe pancreatitis.[277] In a large prospective observational cohort, LR solution was also associated with significantly decreased odds of moderately severe/severe pancreatitis occurrence.[273]

Based on the available data, one could suggest a fluid rate of no more than 10 mL/kg bolus followed by 1.5 mL/kg/h with LR solution, preferably during the first 24 hours after admission.[225,269,285] An established framework advocated by fluid resuscitation literature in other acute illnesses could be applied to AP. Four phases of fluid management have been proposed: phase 1—rescue—to restore intravascular volume, phase 2—optimization—to determine the ongoing fluid requirements, phase 3—stabilization—to avoid excess fluid, and phase 4 de-escalation—to remove excessive fluid.[286] Besides clinical monitoring for volume overload, hourly urine output, daily measurement of hematocrit, BUN, and serum creatinine levels may be used for directing fluid management with the four phases in mind over the first 72 hours of AP.

Metabolic Complications

Hyperglycemia may present during the first several days of AP. It may improve as the inflammatory process subsides or persist as new onset diabetes mellitus following an AP episode. Blood glucose levels may fluctuate during hospitalization thus are better treated with insulin administered cautiously with a sliding scale.

Hypocalcemia is mainly due to a low serum albumin levels. Serum albumin is lost as albumin-rich intravascular fluid extravasates into peritoneum and retroperitoneum, as well as the negative phase reactant effect on reducing albumin synthesis during the acute illness phase. This albumin loss causes a decrease in the calcium normally bound to the albumin. Because this loss is nonionized, hypocalcemia is largely asymptomatic and requires no specific therapy. However, reduced ionized serum calcium levels may also occur and need to be replaced because they can cause neuromuscular irritability. If *hypomagnesemia* coexists, it inhibits the release of parathyroid hormone; magnesium replacement should restore serum calcium to normal in such instances. Causes of magnesium depletion include the loss of magnesium in the urine, stool, or vomitus or deposition of magnesium in areas of fat necrosis. Once the serum magnesium levels are normal, signs or symptoms of neuromuscular irritability may require administering IV calcium gluconate. Serum potassium levels need to be followed as well since administration of intravenous calcium increases the binding of calcium to myocardial receptors, which displaces potassium and may induce a serious dysrhythmia.

ANTIBIOTICS

Empiric antibiotic use is strongly discouraged in patients with AP, especially during the first 2 weeks of illness when sterile systemic inflammation dominates the course and both pancreatic and extrapancreatic infection typically occur late (i.e., after 2 weeks).[287] Approximately 30%–40% of (peri)pancreatic necrosis will become infected (infected pancreatic necrosis) and it is associated with increased morbidity and mortality and needs to be treated.[288,289] The role of antibiotics in established infection of the pancreas or extrapancreatic sites is well established. Imipenem, fluoroquinolones (ciprofloxacin, ofloxacin, and pefloxacin), and metronidazole have emerged as the drugs that achieved the highest inhibitory concentrations in the pancreatic tissue. However, their prophylactic role in predicted moderately severe or severe AP or in established necrotizing pancreatitis is where significant controversy exists and there is inadequate evidence to support antibiotics prophylaxis. Therefore the society guidelines do not recommend the use of prophylactic antibiotics.[15,217,290] Despite the guidelines' recommendations against its use, inappropriate use of antibiotics in AP is still prevalent. In a systematic review, the frequency of antibiotic use in all AP patients ranged between 31% and 82% (with a higher proportion among patients with pancreatic necrosis). Elevated WBC, c-reactive protein, and the presence of fever were identified as the most common reasons for initiating antibiotics despite their lack of significant association with an active infection.[291] Emerging data suggest the role of procalcitonin as a biomarker of infected pancreatic necrosis to guide appropriate antibiotic use.[292] Furthermore, application of clinical protocols can reduce the overutilization of antibiotics in AP.[293] However, in a recent study where a procalcitonin level of $\geq$1.0 ng/mL was used as a cutoff, antibiotics were still administered in 45% of all AP patients. Such rates of antibiotic use are extremely high when the incidence of infected pancreatic necrosis is estimated not to exceed 5% of all AP patients.[109,250,293–295] In addition to high procalcitonin levels, infected necrosis should be considered the cause of acute clinical deterioration (i.e., development of organ failure) requiring ICU level of care.[15,296,297]

URGENT ENDOSCOPIC RETROGRADE CHOLANGIOPANCREATOGRAPHY (ERCP)

The question of early removal of a possibly impacted common bile duct stone in improving the outcome of gallstone pancreatitis has been a controversial issue. Because the obstruction by a stone at the level of ampulla is the main mechanism postulated in acute biliary pancreatitis, it is appealing to remove the stone by ERCP to help the patient recover. However, most stones pass spontaneously so early ERCP is unnecessary, and as an intervention could potentially cause more harm. ERCP in a patient with biliary pancreatitis can be urgent or elective before cholecystectomy. Urgent ERCP has been variously defined as within 24, 48, or 72 hours from presentation. A recent randomized clinical trial evaluated the role of urgent ERCP in predicted severe biliary pancreatitis on outcomes of AP.[232] In this study, urgent ERCP with sphincterotomy did not reduce the composite endpoint of major complications or mortality compared with conservative treatment. A recent AGA technical review reported a meta-analysis on 8 RCTs of urgent ERCP in acute biliary pancreatitis, comprising 935 patients.[239] This report found no benefit of urgent ERCP in acute biliary pancreatitis regarding single organ failure or multiple organ failure, infected peripancreatic necrosis, occurrence of necrotizing pancreatitis, or mortality. In the only study available with small number of cholangitis patients, there was no difference with urgent ERCP. Most recent studies try to exclude patients with proven cholangitis, as ERCP is the standard of care in those patients. However, the definition and description of cholangitis varied among the studies, making interpretation difficult. Most recently, the Dutch Group evaluated the role of EUS in patients with predicted severe pancreatitis to guide selection for ERCP.[216] In this study of 83 patients undergoing urgent EUS within 24 hours of presentation, gallstones or sludge was found by EUS in 58% of patients all of whom underwent urgent ERCP. However, no difference in the primary outcome of mortality was found compared to a historical conservative treatment group.

The latest society guidelines on management of cholangitis, while recognizing very low level of evidence on the matter, recommends an ERCP within 48 hours for patients with cholangitis citing reduced length of stay, possibly improved survival as potential benefits to be gained without increase in harm.[298] For mild biliary AP, same-admission laparoscopic cholecystectomy is the standard therapy, which reduces recurrence and is cost-effective.

Nutritional Support

For decades, keeping patients NPO for several days was the established practice in the management of patients with AP. However, several well-designed trials have recently supported early feeding in patients with AP. Mechanistically, fasting adversely affects the gut mucosal barrier and facilitates translocation of bacteria from the gut lumen to extraluminal tissues, including the inflamed pancreas, with a resultant increase in infectious complications, morbidity, and mortality. Thus the concept of gut rousing by oral nutrition and not gut resting by fasting has now become the recommended practice.[21,288,299,300]

In mild AP, RCTs reported that it is possible to feed patients immediately, even with a full solid diet without standard practice of NPO initially, and others reporting that feeding can be with low fat solid diet versus clear liquids or soft diet versus clear liquids, immediately without waiting for the pain to subside or the enzymes to normalize. Even in severe AP, patients who were fed early with low volume oral feeds had significantly less infection, need for intervention, and ICU and hospital stay. Based on 11 RCTs, an AGA technical review, and AGA guidelines recommended early feeding (usually within 24 hours) for all patients with AP (mild, moderately severe, and severe) as tolerated by the patient.[239] However, if there is significant nausea and vomiting or ileus, then one may have to wait until they subside.

What Is the Role of Parenteral Nutrition in AP?

In predicted severe and in established moderately severe, severe, and necrotizing pancreatitis, as well as in some cases of mild AP,

TPN has been studied with an intention to put the bowel to rest. The meta-analysis of 11 RCTs revealed increased harm with TPN compared with enteral or oral feeding with regard to single and multiple organ failure and infected necrosis, and AGA guidelines gave a strong recommendation based on moderate quality of evidence, which in AP enteral nutrition is preferred to TPN if the patient is not able to tolerate oral feeding for prolonged period.[239] Thus currently TPN is indicated in AP in those who are not able to take oral diet for a long time and if enteral feeding is not possible or not tolerated. Even in established necrotizing pancreatitis or predicted severe AP, it has been shown that it is possible to feed them orally very quickly without the need for any artificial nutrition. Some reports suggested in predicted severe or established necrotizing pancreatitis starting enteral nutrition early on, preferably in the first 24 hours, may be beneficial. However, an RCT did not support the superiority of such immediate enteral nutrition in predicted severe AP compared with on-demand enteral nutrition after 3 days.[77]

When Is Enteral Feeding Indicated in AP?

Diagnosis of moderately severe or severe AP usually takes 3–5 days to firmly establish, and at that time if oral feeding is not possible, enteral feeding either via nasogastric or nasojejunal route may be considered. It is very clear that nasogastric and nasojejunal feeds are equally effective: a meta-analysis of five RCTs did not show any difference between the two modalities of enteral nutrition.[301] There are some theoretical advantages of nasojejunal feeding, particularly in that it provides more rest to the pancreas via the ileal break mechanism. Hence at this time the current guidelines recommend either nasogastric or nasojejunal feeding (and NOT TPN) for patients with AP if oral intake is not possible for prolonged periods.

In summary, in patients with AP regardless of severity, one can initiate a clear liquid diet immediately when vomiting is not pronounced. Advancing to a low-fat diet can be instituted quickly if eating does not exacerbate pain or cause vomiting. For those patients who can do not tolerate anything by mouth due to vomiting and/or worsening pain after 3–5 days, a low-fat diet given by nasogastric tube and, if not tolerated, a postpyloric feeding should be given. One should rarely require TPN.

Other Noninterventional Treatments

Alcohol counseling that begins during the admission with view to be continued as an outpatient intervention should be administered in all alcoholic pancreatitis patients. In an RCT, a brief 30-minute intervention consisting of education and counseling, followed by 6 monthly repeated intervention versus single intervention during hospitalization, led to significantly reduced recurrent episodes (5 vs. 15 episodes; $P = 0.02$) at 2 years superior to subsequent outpatient counseling in terms of reduction in overall admissions.[302] The need for continued outpatient intervention is highlighted by another study that suggested that the brief intervention during hospitalization, while reduces 30-day readmission rate, does not affect 1-year readmission rates.[303] Young individuals with high Alcohol Use Disorders Identification Test scores that indicate heavy alcoholism are at greatest risk of recurrence, and resources should be allocated to focus on this group.[304] Along the same lines, smoking cessation counseling is important given its strong and independent association with AP.[132]

Interventional Treatments

Cholecystectomy

The recurrence of further attacks of AP is estimated at 18% in 6 weeks if cholecystectomy is not performed at the time of index attack of biliary pancreatitis.[305] In the past, surgeons were hesitant to operate on the gallbladder during an attack of AP due to concerns about inflammation in the abdomen at the time of surgery. However, in patients with mild, interstitial pancreatitis, the experience with cholecystectomy evolved, and more recent guidelines recommend same-admission cholecystectomy for cases of mild biliary pancreatitis because it is cost-effective and leads to a significant risk reduction with eight same-admission cholecystectomies preventing one recurrence.[111,306]

When Is the Best Time to Perform the Same-Admission Cholecystectomy?

While some advocate for cholecystectomy within 24 hours of admission for mild biliary AP citing reduced cost and length of stay as their rationale, such approach should be taken with great caution.[307] As described earlier, pancreatic necrosis may take up to 72 hours to fully manifest and there is currently no reliable tool to rule out moderately severe/severe pancreatitis at an early stage.[239] A recent report observed that in patients who underwent same-admission cholecystectomy with a mistaken diagnosis of mild, interstitial pancreatitis, the subsequent evolution of their necrotizing pancreatitis had worse outcomes (e.g., infected pancreatic necrosis) compared with age- and sex-matched necrotizing pancreatitis patients who had not undergone such same-admission cholecystectomy.[308]

For patients with moderately severe to severe (necrotizing) biliary pancreatitis early cholecystectomy (defined as cholecystectomy within 14 days of admission) is associated with increased risk of morbidity and mortality, especially among older and fragile patients (mortality: early cholecystectomy 15.6% compared to delayed cholecystectomy of 1.2%).[309] Therefore recent observational data support the optimal timing of cholecystectomy in high-risk patients with necrotizing pancreatitis to be at 8 weeks because the risk of recurrent pancreatitis significantly increases after 8 weeks from hospital discharge [risk ratio 0.14 (95% CI, 0.02–1.0), $P = .02$].[115]

Interventions for Pancreatic Fluid Collections

Acute pancreatic fluid collections appear to become more demarcated and develop a wall, usually by 4 weeks. As acute nonnecrotic pancreatic fluid collections usually resolve by that time, those that persist and become encapsulated usually contain necrotic debris and represent WON rather than purely fluid-filled pseudocysts (Fig. 60.8). The mere presence of these local complications is not an indication for intervention. Decision to intervene, intervention modality, strategy, and follow-up plan need to be carefully devised via multidisciplinary discussion. Approximately two-thirds of patients with necrotizing pancreatitis will recover without any interventions.[310,311] The indications for minimally invasive drainage or debridement of WON include development infected (peri)pancreatic necrosis, obstruction of the GI or biliary tract, persistently unwell state with loss of weight and debility, and disconnected PD syndrome.[15,217] Out of these indications, best level of evidence for infected necrosis for informing treatment strategy exists for infected necrosis.[312] Historically, pancreatic necrotic fluid collections were treated by open necrosectomy in those with signs of infection of such collections or whose clinical condition was worsening. Subsequently, an RCT demonstrated that operating early (within 2 weeks) increases mortality and morbidity, and subsequent recommendations emphasized operating later in the course after the infected necrotic fluid collections develop a wall, which is usually around 4 weeks.[313] This recommendation is based on a wealth of observational data that suggested delaying interventions for necrotizing pancreatitis is associated with improved outcomes, including mortality.[314]

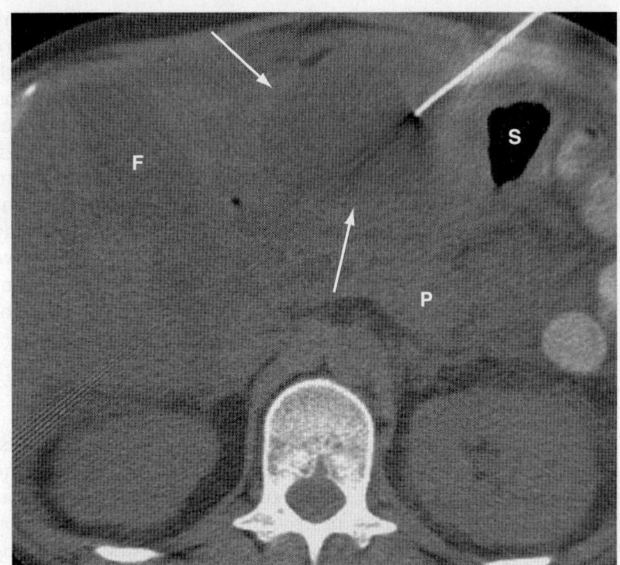

Fig. 60.8 CT showing walled-off pancreatic necrosis. A 5.4-cm pus-filled fluid collection (*arrows*) with the tip of an aspirating needle in its lumen is seen. The infected necrosis is anterior to the pancreas (P) and medial to the stomach (S). A right subhepatic fluid collection (F) is present.

What is the Best Type of Intervention for WON?

A large RCT showed that a step-up minimally invasive approach starting with a percutaneous drain followed by a video-assisted retroperitoneal approach when needed resulted in better clinical outcomes compared to open surgical necrosectomy.[182] One RCT showed superiority of the minimally invasive step-up approach with percutaneous drainage initially and later video-assisted retroperitoneal drainage over surgical necrosectomy.[297] This was followed by another RCT by the same group that demonstrated the superiority of endoscopic intervention over surgical necrosectomy.[315] The most recent RCT by the same group compared endoscopic intervention to videoscopic retroperitoneal intervention and demonstrated reduced complications like fistula and hospital stay with endoscopic intervention, with similar mortality and other major complications.[316] It has to be emphasized that all three RCTs were conducted in patients with suspected or confirmed infected walled-off pancreatic necrosis (collections that are 4 weeks or older). In comparison, there is very limited data available to inform the right strategy for patients with symptomatic sterile necrosis, even though sterile necrotic collections are more common than infected necrosis.

Disconnected PD syndrome is an entity when a significant amount of pancreatic body necrosis disconnects the PD in the proximal and distal segments. The diagnosis is made usually by necrosis of the middle part of the pancreas initially, a persistent fluid collection in the area of necrosis, complete cutoff of the PD on ERCP in the same region, and a viable enhancing distal segment of the pancreas. Following the initial reports that this complication needs long-term pigtail catheter drainage (transgastric or transduodenal) into the fluid collections, recent reports have confirmed this recommendation.[14,317–319] A recent large series of 167 patients reported that these patients more often required hybrid interventions (EUS-guided multigate/dual modality technique, endoscopic/percutaneous sinus tract necrosectomy) when compared with patients without disconnected PD.[318] Although an EUS-guided cystenterostomy with the placement of a lumen apposing metal stent (LAMS) can be the initial drainage approach that can facilitate direct endoscopic debridement, subsequently (in 3–4 weeks) LAMS are exchanged to plastic pigtail stents, which can be left in the collection indefinitely.

For pseudocysts, EUS-guided transmural drainage is usually effective. Due to the safety of EUS-guided technique with comparable efficacy to surgical cystogastrostomy, EUS-guided transmural drainage has become the preferred method. However, in certain scenarios, surgical cystogastrostomy may be the better option. For example, in a patient with biliary pancreatitis in whom cholecystectomy has been deferred and needs a symptomatic pseudocyst drained, surgery offers a one-stop solution for both problems. Barring exceptional circumstances, endoscopic drainage is preferred and this is supported by an RCT of endoscopic drainage versus surgical cyst gastrostomy for symptomatic pseudocysts in AP, which found that surgical cyst gastrostomy was not superior to endoscopic therapy; however, endoscopic therapy was associated with shorter hospital stay, better mental and physical health of the patient, and reduced costs.[320]

Other Complications

Abdominal Compartment Syndrome

Abdominal compartment syndrome (ACS) is defined as a sustained intra-abdominal pressure (IAP) greater than 20 mm Hg (typically determined by a pressure-recording catheter in the urinary bladder) that is associated with the development of organ dysfunction or failure (see Chapter 11).[321] The incidence of ACS in AP may be attributable to the widespread use of aggressive IV volume repletion, allowing more fluid to sequestrate into the peritoneum. Studies that correlate intra-abdominal volume with IAP suggest that when a critical intra-abdominal volume is reached, IAP increases exponentially.[322] When ACS develops, mortality is as high as 49%, and morbidity can be up to 90%.[321] Intervention options include percutaneous drainage and decompressive laparotomy and some authors advocate for these interventions citing their potential mortality benefit.[323–325] The best available guidance comes from the World Society of the ACS consensus definitions and clinical practice guidelines, which gives a GRADE 2C recommendation to consider percutaneous decompression in patients with intraperitoneal fluid with symptomatic IAH or ACS and a GRADE 1C recommendation for surgical decompression in ACS when other treatment options are unsuccessful.[326] It also gives a GRADE 1C recommendation to consider presumptive decompression in patients who demonstrate multiple risk factors for IAH and ACS which include obesity, positive fluid balance, ileus, and increased APACHE-II/SOFA score all of which are often present in severe AP.[326]

Gastrointestinal Bleeding

Gastrointestinal bleeding may arise from lesions not directly related to the local inflammatory aspects of AP, such as peptic ulcer or Mallory-Weiss tear. Alternatively, bleeding can be due to the inflammatory aspects of the pancreatitis (Box 60.7). The latter is thought to occur from the irritative effects of liberated activated enzymes on vascular structures or pressure necrosis of inflammatory debris or fluid collections on surrounding structures. Acute and chronic inflammatory processes of the pancreas can lead to thrombosis of the adjacent splenic vein, which can lead to gastric varices, with or without esophageal varices. These varices can rupture, leading to massive bleeding (see Chapters 21 and 94). Treatment of variceal rupture can be endoscopic, with banding of varices or splenectomy, which is curative. Necrotizing pancreatitis complicated by pseudoaneurysm formation, which can usually be seen by dynamic contrast-enhanced CT (Fig. 60.9). If these bleed, arteriography with embolization is the treatment of choice. Pseudoaneurysms are also being increasingly found in necrotizing pancreatitis before an episode of GI bleeding occurs. When a

BOX 60.7 Complications of Acute Pancreatitis

LOCAL

Pseudocyst
Sterile necrosis (peripancreatic, pancreatic, or both)
Infected necrosis (peripancreatic, pancreatic, or both)
Abscess
GI bleeding
- Pancreatitis-related
  - Splenic artery rupture or splenic artery pseudoaneurysm rupture
  - Splenic vein rupture
  - Portal vein rupture
  - Splenic vein thrombosis leading to gastroesophageal variceal bleeding
  - Pseudocyst or abscess hemorrhage
  - Postnecrosectomy bleeding
- Nonpancreatitis-related
  - Mallory-Weiss tear
  - NSAID gastropathy
  - Stress-related mucosal gastropathy
- Splenic complications
  - Infarction
  - Rupture
  - Hematoma
  - Splenic vein thrombosis
- Fistulization to or obstruction of the small intestine or colon
- Hydronephrosis

SYSTEMIC

Respiratory failure
Renal failure
Shock
Hyperglycemia
Hypocalcemia
DIC
Fat necrosis (subcutaneous nodules)
Retinopathy
Psychosis

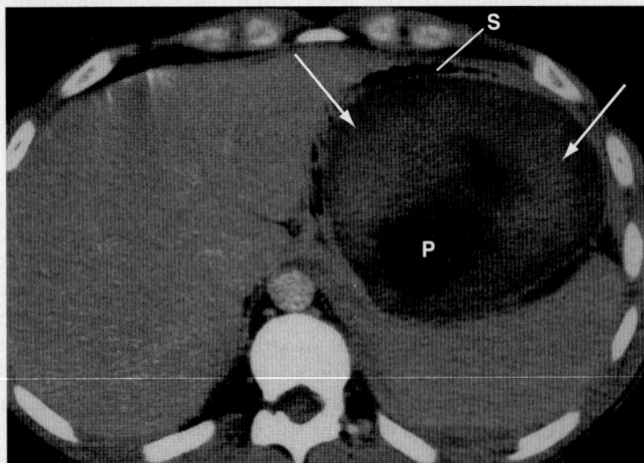

Fig. 60.9 CT showing a pancreatic pseudocyst with acute hemorrhage. A 10-cm pancreatic pseudocyst (P) containing high-density (45 Hounsfield units) material (*arrows*) representing acute blood is seen. The pseudocyst is compressing the stomach (S). These findings were confirmed at surgery.

pseudoaneurysm is detected, it is important to treat before any bleeding occurs, because all three layers of an intact artery are lacking, and hence likely to rupture with high frequency. A high degree of success with interventional radiology and embolization has been reported.[327] If this is not successful, percutaneous thrombin injection is also a possibility before resorting to open surgery which is done very rarely nowadays. Rarely, bleeding into the PD occurs (hemosuccus pancreaticus), but this is more common in chronic pancreatitis (see Chapter 59). Postnecrosectomy bleeding is common and can be caused by overly aggressive debridement or the placement or the use of noncompliant drainage tubes next to vascular structures or long-term use of metallic stents.[14,328,329]

Splenic Complications

Splenic complications of pancreatitis include splenic pseudocysts, splenic vein thrombosis, splenic infarction and necrosis of the spleen, splenic rupture, and hematoma. Some of these complications can be life-threatening and require emergency splenectomy (see Box 60.7). Splanchnic venous thrombosis occurs in approximately 7% of patients with AP.[330–332] Anticoagulation is safe in patients without bleeding complications, but it is unclear if it improves recanalization rates and improves outcomes.[330] Recommendations to anticoagulate acute splanchnic vein thrombosis are based on extrapolation of findings of benefits from clinical trials performed in cirrhotic populations with acute splanchnic vein thrombosis.[333] The cited goals of anticoagulation are recanalization and prevention of intestinal ischemia/infarction. Use of anticoagulation is recommended for a period of 3–6 months if there are no underlying hypercoagulable conditions.[333]

Bowel Compression or Fistula Formation

Pressure necrosis from inflammatory debris from the tail of the pancreas can obstruct or fistulize into the small or large bowel. In two large studies, colonic complications of ischemia, perforation, and fistulization occur in up to 10% of patients with necrotizing pancreatitis.[334,335] Treatment is frequently surgical for patients with colon involvement but remain conservative in patients with gastric or duodenal involvement.[334]

Long-Term Sequelae of Acute Pancreatitis

Exocrine and endocrine insufficiency after an attack of AP is common. A systematic review found that 15% of patients with AP developed new onset diabetes mellitus within 12 month period after the acute event and the risk increased significantly at 5 years.[336] Pancreatic exocrine insufficiency occurs in 40% of individuals with newly diagnosed prediabetes or diabetes mellitus after AP.[337] A recent meta-analysis revealed that 10% of patients after the first episode of AP and 36% of those with recurrent AP develop subsequent chronic pancreatitis.[338]

Miscellaneous Complications

Pancreatic encephalopathy consists of a variety of central nervous system symptoms occurring in patients with AP, including agitation, hallucinations, confusion, disorientation, and coma.[339] A similar syndrome may be due to alcohol withdrawal, and other causes are possible, such as electrolyte disturbances (e.g., hyponatremia) or hypoxia. *Purtscher retinopathy* (discrete flame-shaped hemorrhages with cotton wool spots) can cause sudden blindness.[340] It is thought to be due to microembolization in the choroidal and retinal arteries.

Pancreatic panniculitis denotes inflammation of the subcutaneous fat, which has been described in AP patients in case reports and case series.[341–343] Histopathology shows lobular panniculitis, fat necrosis, and adipocytes with absent nuclei surrounded by thick cell membranes, frequently described "ghost adipocytes."[343] Physical examination usually reveals tender edematous pink plaques, which sometimes also exhibit a central eschar. It is uncommon, and it has been described in other benign and malignant pancreatic diseases as well as, present in 0.3%–3% of all patients with underlying pancreatic disease.[341–344] Other structures can be involved, including periarticular adipocytes and bone marrow fat which can cause lytic lesions on radiologic imaging which can be mistaken for manifestations of multiple myeloma.[345]

Full references for this chapter can be found at https://ebooks.health.elsevier.com.

61 Chronic Pancreatitis

Anna Evans Phillips, Vikesh Singh

IN THIS CHAPTER

Chronic pancreatitis (CP) is a progressive fibro-inflammatory syndrome of the pancreas resulting from a variety of etiologies and leading to irreversible scarring, accompanied by clinical manifestations, including abdominal pain, endocrine and exocrine dysfunction, and sometimes complications and sequelae such as pseudocysts or pseudoaneurysms.

The traditional definition of CP has been based on histology, wherein evidence of fibrosis, chronic inflammation and destruction of ductal, exocrine (acinar cell), and endocrine (islets of Langerhans) pancreatic tissue is seen under the microscope (Fig. 61.1). This histologic definition is of limited clinical utility as pancreatic tissue is rarely available to clinicians. Some patients may have histologic evidence of CP and yet have no symptoms or complications from the disease. In addition, the histologic features of CP are often focal, and sampling error may result in missing the disease. Finally, the histologic features that are seen in CP are not unique and may be seen in other conditions (such as normal aging, social use of alcohol, smoking, and long-standing diabetes). CP may also be defined based on clinical features [abdominal pain, exocrine insufficiency (steatorrhea), or endocrine insufficiency (diabetes mellitus)] or on imaging techniques including ultrasound (US), computed tomography (CT), endoscopic US (EUS), magnetic resonance imaging or cholangiopancreatography (MRI or MRCP), and endoscopic retrograde cholangiopancreatography (ERCP). Defining CP based on imaging studies also has significant limitations, as many of these modalities may not reveal changes in the early part of the clinical course. Early diagnosis of CP, at a time when a preventive therapy might be administered, is therefore often difficult or impossible.[1] Diagnostic criteria are largely based on consensus agreements that rely on a mixture of diagnostic and staging criteria simultaneously determining both presence and severity of disease.

Acute and CP commonly exist within a spectrum of disease in which acute pancreatitis is an event.[2] Progression along the spectrum of disease occurs in a single direction toward the disease state of CP. Not all patients progress, however, and those that do so progress at a variable pace. Many patients will experience recurrent attacks of acute pancreatitis that lead to irreversible scarring of the organ and eventual CP. A minority of patients receive an incidental diagnosis of CP without having had a preceding episode of acute pancreatitis.[3] CP is best conceptualized as a syndrome, with a constellation of features including exposure to known risk factors, genetic background, symptoms, derangements in pancreatic exocrine or endocrine function, structural changes visible on imaging studies, and histology if a tissue sample is available. A single feature is insufficient for diagnosis, and the combination of features differs significantly between patients.

EPIDEMIOLOGY

CP can be demonstrated in up to 5% of autopsies though the utilization of this figure alone to estimate prevalence would be misleading as many of these individuals may not have had symptoms of CP during life.[4,5] Similar, though less pronounced, histologic features are seen even more commonly.[6,7] Long-standing alcohol use, even in moderate amounts, can lead to histologic changes of CP without symptoms or clinical features of

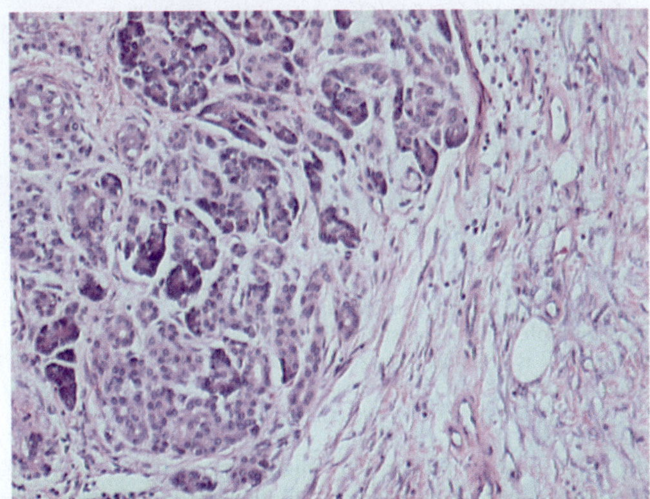

Fig. 61.1 Histology of chronic pancreatitis. Pictured here is the destruction of acinar tissue, replaced by extensive fibrosis with relative sparing of pancreatic islets (Hematoxylin and eosin).

CP.[8–10] Similarly, aging, smoking, chronic kidney disease, and long-standing diabetes mellitus can induce histologic changes within the pancreas that are difficult to distinguish from those of CP.[6,7,11]

Estimates of annual incidence of CP in several retrospective studies range from 5 to 12 cases per 100,000 population.[12–17] In the United States, the incidence rate is approximately 5–8/100,000[15,18,19] and appears to be increasing over time.[20] The prevalence of CP is about 50/100,000.[15–19,21,22] In many studies, alcohol abuse accounts for one-half or more of all cases of CP.[15] These epidemiologic data demonstrate substantial geographic variation.[15,19,22] While variation may partly be due to differences in alcohol consumption in different populations, it may also reflect different diagnostic approaches and different diagnostic criteria.

CP is more common in men and is mostly diagnosed in patients above the age of 40.[15–18] CP accounts for substantial morbidity and health care costs. Approximately 37,000 hospital admissions to nonfederal hospitals with a first-listed diagnosis of CP occur yearly; in more than 190,000 yearly admissions, CP is listed as one of the discharge diagnoses.[15,21,23–26,14,19,21–24] The prognosis of CP is variable and is driven largely by the presence of ongoing alcoholism in persons with chronic alcoholic pancreatitis and equally by concomitant tobacco use.[15,18,21] One can estimate prognosis from such features as need for medical care or hospitalization or from the development of complications, reduced quality of life, or mortality.

Mortality in patients with CP is heavily influenced by the presence of tobacco and alcohol abuse.[15,18] In fact, the cause of death in patients with CP usually is not the pancreatitis itself; rather mortality is secondary to other medical conditions commonly associated with smoking, continued alcohol abuse, pancreatic carcinoma, and postoperative complications.[15,27,28] In one large multicenter study, the standardized mortality ratio was 3.6:1 (i.e., those with a diagnosis of any form of CP died at 3.6 times the rate of age-matched controls), and older subjects, those who smoked, and those with alcoholic CP had the most significant reduction in survival. Continuing alcohol use raised mortality risk by an additional 60%. Similar rates of increased mortality have been observed in other studies.[17,32] Sarcopenia has also been associated with a decrease in survival.[18,28] Overall, 10-year survival in patients with CP is about 70%, and 20-year survival is approximately 45%.

PATHOLOGY

The different etiologies of CP usually produce similar pathologic findings (see Fig. 61.1), particularly as the disease progresses. In early CP, the damage is variable and uneven. Areas of interlobular fibrosis are seen, with the fibrosis often extending to the ductal structures. Infiltration of the fibrotic area and lobules with lymphocytes, plasma cells, mast cells, and macrophages is seen.[29,30] The ducts may contain eosinophilic protein plugs. In affected lobules, acinar cells are surrounded and replaced by fibrosis. The islets are usually less severely damaged until very late in the course of the disease. Features of acute pancreatitis also may be seen, such as edema, acute inflammation, and acinar cell or fat necrosis. As the disease progresses, fibrosis within the lobules and between lobules becomes more widespread. The pancreatic ducts become more abnormal with progressive fibrosis, stricture formation, and dilation. The ductal protein plugs may calcify and obstruct major pancreatic ducts. Ductal epithelium may become cuboidal, may develop atrophy or squamous metaplasia, or may be replaced by fibrosis entirely. Activated pancreatic stellate cells may be identified in close association with fibrosis.

Many of these histologic features, in particular perilobular fibrosis and ductal metaplasia, are commonly seen in patients of advanced age without CP and in patients with long-standing diabetes mellitus.[6,7,11] Obstructive CP that is secondary to a tumor or stricture can differ slightly in that the histologic changes are limited to the gland upstream of the obstruction and protein precipitates and intraductal stones are not as commonly seen.[30]

Autoimmune CP can demonstrate several unique histological patterns.[31–34] In one form (type 1), a more robust lymphoplasmacytic infiltrate, including plasma cells, is seen, and these are usually positive when stained for immunoglobulin G subtype 4 (IgG_4). Obstructive phlebitis affecting the major and minor veins and a whorled (storiform) fibrosis pattern are also characteristic, a pattern termed lymphoplasmacytic sclerosing pancreatitis. Type 1 autoimmune pancreatitis (AIP) is considered a manifestation of IgG_4-related disease.[35] A second pattern (type 2) termed idiopathic duct-centric CP is characterized by neutrophilic infiltration and the absence of IgG_4-positive plasma cells.[37] A third type of autoimmune injury can happen in the setting of immune-checkpoint inhibitor therapy administered for treatment of malignancy. In this type of AIP (type 3), immune T-cells densely infiltrate the pancreatic parenchyma in an increased $CD8^+/CD4^+$ ratio and drive cytotoxic effects that may result in pancreatic inflammation and subsequent atrophy.[33,36] With time, each of these patterns may assume a more end-stage CP appearance following inflammation and then atrophy, subsequently becoming indistinguishable in many ways histologically from other forms of CP.

PATHOPHYSIOLOGY

The pathophysiology of CP remains incompletely understood. The study of mechanisms of disease is hampered by the difficulty of obtaining tissue in humans and the relative lack of animal models of CP, as opposed to acute pancreatitis.[40] The pathophysiologic processes must ultimately account for the features of CP, including loss of parenchymal cells, self-sustaining chronic inflammation, and fibrosis. Any proposed mechanism must therefore include explanations for cellular necrosis or apoptosis, initiation and maintenance of inflammatory cell activation, and fibrogenesis by pancreatic stellate cells.[2] The pancreas, like all other organs, has a limited repertoire of responses to injury, and although it is not likely that all of the various etiologies share a similar pathophysiology, the end histologic result is similar.[37]

Alcoholic CP has been most extensively studied.[38–41] No single theory explains adequately why fewer than 5% of heavy alcohol users develop CP.[15,42] Genetic differences may certainly play an important role. Alcohol is metabolized by the liver and the pancreas. In the liver, the main end product of oxidative alcohol metabolism is acetaldehyde. In the pancreas, an alternative pathway produces fatty acid ethanol esters (FAEEs). Alcohol and its metabolites, like FAEE, have direct injurious effects on pancreatic acinar cells.[43] Increased membrane lipid peroxidation, a marker of oxidative stress and free radical production, can be seen in animal models and human alcoholic CP. In addition, FAEEs are able to induce sustained elevations in cytosolic calcium in acinar cells, a mechanism shared by other experimental causes of pancreatitis.[37] Alcohol may also lead to pathologic increases in acinar cell sensitivity to physiologic stimuli such as cholecystokinin (CCK)[37] or to other pathologic exposures such as smoking.[42,44] The interaction of smoking and alcohol exposure is an increasingly recognized risk factor for CP.[15,42] Chronic alcohol ingestion in animal models also alters expression of multiple genes in acinar cells, which could increase the sensitivity to physiologic stress and upregulate the expression and activity of enzymes involved in cell death. Alcohol can promote the inflammatory responses involved in pancreatitis.[38,39] These multiple effects of alcohol on the acinar cell are complemented by alcohol injury to ductal cells. Finally, alcohol and its metabolites appear to stimulate the pancreatic stellate cell.[38,42,45–47] These cells, as in the liver, appear to be the final common pathway for fibrosis.[46,47]

Pancreatic stellate cells are found in association with the acini. They are typically found in the periacinar space, with long cytoplasmic processes extending to the acini themselves, but are also present in smaller numbers in association with blood vessels and ducts. Quiescent pancreatic stellate cells are recognized by the presence of vitamin A lipid droplets in the cytoplasm. When activated, they assume a stellate or myofibroblastic appearance, express smooth muscle actin, and lose their lipid droplets. This activation is necessary for the cell to begin to secrete extracellular matrix and produce fibrosis within the gland. Activation of pancreatic stellate cells can occur by alcohol or one of its metabolites but also occurs in response to both inflammatory cytokines that are released following pancreatic acinar cell necrosis and to reactive oxygen species.[45–47] In addition, growth factors (platelet-derived growth factor, transforming growth factor-β1), hormones, intracellular signaling molecules, transcription factors, and angiotensin II can activate pancreatic stellate cells. Activated pancreatic stellate cells are found in areas of extensive necrosis and inflammation in acute pancreatitis, in human as well as animal tissues. These activated pancreatic stellate cells produce autocrine factors that maintain the activated cell phenotype. In addition to their role in secretion and modulation of the extracellular matrix, pancreatic stellate cells can proliferate in response to stimulation, migrate to areas of inflammation, and participate in phagocytosis. Activation of pancreatic stellate cells is likely occurring through multiple mechanisms in alcoholic (and other forms of) CP.

Chronic alcohol ingestion may produce CP by additional mechanisms. Longtime alcohol use leads to the secretion of a pancreatic juice rich in protein and low in volume and bicarbonate. These characteristics favor the formation of protein precipitates, which are present early in the evolution of alcoholic CP. These precipitates may calcify, leading to the formation of pancreatic ductal stones and producing further ductal and parenchymal injury upstream from these stones. In most patients, however, these protein precipitates and ductal stones do not appear to cause the initial pancreatic injury (PI) but may facilitate disease progression.

There have been several hypotheses for the pathophysiology of CP that attempt to interweave these observations into a coherent paradigm. One hypothesis focuses on the concept that ductal obstruction (from strictures or stones) is the cause rather than the effect of CP; however, this is not consistent with most clinical and experimental evidence and, with few exceptions is not applicable to human CP. A second paradigm, the toxic-metabolic hypothesis, focuses primarily on the role of alcohol and its metabolites (or smoking or other toxins) and their ability to damage the pancreas and activate pancreatic stellate cells. A third model that has been proposed is the necrosis-fibrosis hypothesis, which holds that the occurrence of repeated or severe episodes of acute pancreatitis with cellular necrosis or apoptosis eventually leads to the development of CP as the healing process replaces necrotic tissue with fibrosis. This last hypothesis has significant supporting evidence from some natural history studies that document the more common development of CP in patients with more severe and more frequent acute attacks of alcoholic pancreatitis.[48–51] The concept that multiple clinical or subclinical attacks of acute pancreatitis lead to CP is certainly being reinforced by observations in both animal models[37] and in humans.[1,2]

Although heavy alcohol use is a risk factor for CP, not all heavy users develop disease for reasons that remain unclear.[15] Some of the many possible explanations might include the presence of important co-toxins, differences in the genetic or epigenetic background, or differences in the microenvironment in the pancreas. Tobacco use is one very important cofactor for the development of alcoholic CP.[1,2,15,52–58] There are also unexplained racial differences in the rates of alcoholic CP.[14,59,60] Multiple mutations have been identified in several forms of CP, suggesting a complex genetic background that provides the relative predisposition to develop CP. Mutations in the cystic fibrosis transmembrane conductance regulator (*CFTR*), cationic trypsinogen gene (*PRSS1* gene), serine protease inhibitor Kazal Type 1 (*SPINK1*, a trypsin inhibitor), chymotrypsin C, calcium-sensing receptor gene, carboxypeptidase A-1 (*CPA1*), caryl ester lipase, claudin-2 (*CLDN2/MORC*), and many others have been identified.[61,62] These mutations and the many more yet to be identified may be adequate in and of themselves to produce pancreatitis or may only predispose to disease. This paradigm of underlying genetic abnormalities conceptualizes a predisposition to disease.[1,2,63,64] This genetic background may include mutations in genes that code for digestive enzymes, protease-enzyme inhibitors, ion channels, tight-junction proteins, and a variety of others including genes that affect the metabolism of environmental toxins (e.g., tobacco, alcohol), genes that have a role in inflammation or fibrosis, and others yet to be discovered. Only one mutation (*PRSS1* gain-of-function mutation seen in families with hereditary pancreatitis) is sufficient to produce pancreatic damage in most or all who carry it, but even this causes variable disease severity. The majority of mutations identified provide only a predisposition to disease.[62] On this complex, polygenic background is overlaid some environmental insult, such as chronic alcohol use, smoking, or some trigger for an initial episode of pancreatitis (e.g., gallstones, hypertriglyceridemia). This applies physiologic stress to the acinar, ductal, and stellate cells. This stress may be insufficient to produce injury or may produce cellular injury, necrosis, or apoptosis. The initiating event for necrosis appears to be the premature activation of digestive enzymes within the acinar cell, either by the toxic effect of the environmental insult or the underlying etiology. Inflammation follows the necrosis, and this necro-inflammatory process may progress or resolve. This event is essentially an episode of acute pancreatitis, although it may or may not be symptomatic. In some individuals, the situation may never progress beyond this stage, and the process resolves. In others, continued cell metabolic and oxidative stresses (a second hit) or some other trigger could produce continuing or repeated acinar and ductal cell injury with necrosis. This explains the high risk for CP in those with repeated episodes of acute pancreatitis.[65] This process, as is the case in the liver, would be associated with the activation of stellate cells and the production of extracellular matrix, with the ultimate formation of fibrosis. Fibrosis could start a vicious circle by causing additional acinar cell ischemia and continuing to drive the process.

This type of hypothesis could theoretically explain many forms of CP. This framework seems to fit the developing experimental and clinical data and is a useful way in which to think about the pathophysiology of CP: as a disease associated with a variety of different genetic predispositions, a variety of disease triggers, multiple intervening modifiers, and a similar final common pathway producing PI and fibrosis, ultimately with organ failure. These genetic predispositions, environmental triggers, and modifiers are individually neither necessary nor required for disease development but work in concert in individual patients to produce disease.[66]

ETIOLOGY

Alcohol

In Western countries, alcohol causes upwards of 50% of all cases of CP (Box 61.1).[15,17,42,57,58,67–70] The risk of alcoholic CP increases logarithmically with rising alcohol use, but there is no true threshold value below which the disease does not occur.[15,42] Men are more likely than women to develop alcoholic CP, possibly due to increased alcohol usage or perhaps to other genetic factors.[62] Alcohol accounts for approximately 40% of the attributable risk for CP and appears to increase the risk of PI from other causes of CP.[15,65,70] In countries with widespread alcohol consumption, it may be difficult to determine with certainty whether alcohol contributed to disease. In nearly all patients with alcoholic CP, at least 5 years (and in most patients more than 10 years) of intake exceeding 4–5 drinks per day are required before the development of CP.[15,57,58] One study found that individuals with daily or almost daily intake of ≥5 drinks per day had a 2.61 times higher risk of developing CP than individuals who never drank alcohol.[71] Only 2%–5% of heavy drinkers ultimately develop CP, suggesting important cofactors.[15,42] Potential cofactors include genetic polymorphisms and mutations,[62,72] a diet high in fat and protein,[73,74] the type of alcohol or manner of ingestion,[15,71,74–76] an associated relative deficiency of antioxidants or trace elements,[77,78] and smoking.[15,53–58,79,80] Of these, smoking appears to be the strongest association. In some studies, 90% of those who develop alcoholic CP are also chronic smokers.[15,55–58,79,80] Smoking also appears to predispose to more rapid development of pancreatic calcification.[81,82] There are also racial differences in the risk for development of alcoholic pancreatitis, perhaps suggesting some difference in the ability to detoxify environmental toxins or alcohol or other genetic or epigenetic factors. Although the risk of alcoholic CP is higher in blacks, data from self-reported surveys of alcohol use find that the proportion of blacks who drink alcohol or smoke is similar to that in whites.[15,59,60]

Many patients with alcohol-induced CP have an early phase of recurrent attacks of acute pancreatitis.[65] A systematic review and meta-analysis evaluating the progression from acute to CP found that the prevalence of CP in those with a single episode of acute pancreatitis was approximately 10%; in those that had recurrent attacks of acute pancreatitis, the prevalence was 36%.[83] The same study showed that alcohol and tobacco use were the two most significant modifiable risk factors that affect the progression of disease. A separate retrospective study investigating the progression from acute to CP showed that the combination of alcohol and tobacco use produces the highest cumulative risk of progression to CP.[84] Stopping alcohol does seem to reduce the chance of recurrent attacks of acute alcoholic pancreatitis in those who have not yet developed obvious CP.[85] Cessation of alcohol use after the onset of alcoholic pancreatitis appears to diminish the rate of progression to exocrine insufficiency and endocrine insufficiency but does not halt it.[15] Alcoholic CP is not always preceded by acute pancreatitis. It is necessary to note that rarely patients may present with chronic pain in the absence of antecedent acute pain. In the population of approximately 10% of CP patients with painless disease, approximately one-third have been estimated to have disease secondary to alcohol etiology.[86] Rarely, patients may present with exocrine or endocrine insufficiency even in the absence of abdominal pain.[15,67–69]

The prognosis of alcoholic CP is relatively poor, and mortality is generally greater than that seen in CP of other etiologies.[15,18,28,87] Alcohol etiology of CP has been independently associated with a lower quality of life.[88] Pain generally continues for years, although rarely it may spontaneously remit.[89] Exocrine and/or endocrine insufficiency develops in many patients: In one large natural history study, exocrine insufficiency developed in 48% of patients at a median of 13.1 years after presentation, whereas endocrine insufficiency developed in 38% after a median of 19.8 years after presentation.[68] Diffuse pancreatic calcifications developed in 59% at a median of 8.7 years after diagnosis. Other studies have noted more rapid and more frequent development of calcifications, exocrine insufficiency, and endocrine insufficiency.[67]

Tobacco

Tobacco smoking is an independent risk factor for susceptibility to CP and progression of disease.[83,90] Exposure to tobacco smoke has been seen to induce pancreatic damage in animals.[37,44] The risk of CP is more than threefold for smokers of more than one pack per day.[15,52–58] Smoking may account for up to 25% of the attributable risk for CP and is particularly injurious in those who also drink alcohol.[15,56,58,79,80,84] The lifetime prevalence of tobacco smoking in CP patients is high—in one large cohort, it was estimated to be as high as 51%.[91] Smoking is associated with an increased risk for pancreatic calcifications, and smoking cessation after the clinical onset of CP reduces the risk of subsequent calcifications.[15,52,57,58,81,82,92] Smoking has been independently associated with worse quality of life in CP.[93] Smoking is also associated with a much higher rate of secondary pancreatic cancer and overall mortality in patients with CP.[15–19,28,87]

Tropical Pancreatitis

Tropical pancreatitis is a common form of CP in Southwest India, although its incidence is decreasing as the incidence of other forms of idiopathic CP appears to be increasing.[94,95] It has been rarely reported from a number of other geographic areas, including Africa, Southeast Asia, and Brazil. Tropical pancreatitis is generally a disease of youth and early adulthood, with a mean age at onset of 24 years.[96–101] More than 90% of patients have the illness before 40 years. The overall prevalence from surveys in an endemic area (Southern India) is 1 in 500 to 1 in 800 population.[98] Tropical pancreatitis used to account for about 70% of all cases of CP in Southern India, whereas alcohol is a more dominant cause in the North. Recent reports have noted that there is a shift toward older age at presentation, less malnutrition, and less severe diabetes.[99–101] Most recent reviews also now note that alcohol and smoking are gradually becoming the most common cause of CP in India.[99–101]

Tropical pancreatitis classically manifests as abdominal pain, severe malnutrition, and exocrine or endocrine insufficiency. One striking feature is the propensity to diabetes, and endocrine insufficiency appears to be an inevitable consequence of tropical CP (often classified as a specific cause of diabetes called fibrocalculous pancreatic diabetes).[102] Exocrine insufficiency is also very common. Large pancreatic calculi develop in more than 90% of patients. The pathology is characterized by these large intraductal calculi along with marked dilation of the main pancreatic duct and gland atrophy.

The pathophysiology of tropical pancreatitis is unknown, but recent analyses point to a strong genetic component, with mutations in the *SPINK1*, *CFTR*, *CTRC*, *CLDN2/MORC*, and *CASR*

BOX 61.1 Classification of Contributors to Chronic Pancreatitis

TOXIC-METABOLIC

Alcohol
Tobacco
Hypercalcemia
Hypertriglyceridemia
Chronic renal failure

IDIOPATHIC

Tropical calcific pancreatitis
Early-onset idiopathic
Late-onset idiopathic

GENETIC

Autosomal dominant
Hereditary pancreatitis (*PRSS1* mutations)
Autosomal recessive or modifier genes (known)
- *CFTR* mutations
- *SPINK1* mutations
- Chymotrypsin C mutations
- Claudin mutations
- Calcium-sensing receptor gene
- Carboxy ethyl lipase

AUTOIMMUNE PANCREATITIS

IgG4-related systemic disease, type 1
Type 2 autoimmune pancreatitis
Immune-checkpoint inhibitor-associated pancreatitis (type 3 autoimmune pancreatitis)

RECURRENT AND SEVERE ACUTE PANCREATITIS

Postnecrotic (after severe necrotizing pancreatitis)
Vascular disease/ischemia

OBSTRUCTIVE

Benign pancreatic duct obstruction
- Traumatic stricture
- Stricture after severe acute pancreatitis

Ampullary obstruction
- Sphincter of Oddi stenosis
- Celiac disease
- Crohn's disease
- Pancreas divisum

Malignant pancreatic duct obstruction
- Ampullary carcinoma
- Duodenal carcinoma
- Pancreatic ductal adenocarcinoma
- Intraductal papillary mucinous neoplasm

IgG_4, Immunoglobulin G; *PRSS1*, protease serine 1 gene; *SPINK1*, serine protease inhibitor, Kazal type 1 gene.

genes being most common.[95,103,104] Results from a recent molecular dynamics study of the *CASR* gene in tropical pancreatitis suggest that genetic variants result in structural changes in the CaSR protein structure, rendering it functionally impaired and unable to complete its normal interactions with other molecules.[105] Environmental triggers for the disease that have been proposed include protein-calorie malnutrition, deficiencies of trace elements and micronutrients coupled with oxidative stress (via xenobiotics, industrial pollutants, diet, or nutritional deficiency), cyanogenic glycosides present in cassava (tapioca—a main dietary component), viral and parasitic infections, and others.

Genetic

Only one type of mutation appears sufficient to cause CP: mutations in *PRSS1* in families with hereditary pancreatitis.[62,63,66,104] All other identified mutations and polymorphisms should be considered cofactors, mutations that predispose to disease by increasing susceptibility to environmental toxins, or as modifier genes that increase the pace or severity of disease. It is likely that mixtures of polymorphisms and mutations work together to determine the susceptibility to disease. The most identified mutations occur in the *PRSS1* (cationic trypsinogen), *SPINK1* (trypsin inhibitor), and *CFTR* genes, with others identified less frequently, including chymotrypsin C, *CPA1*, carboxy ethyl lipase, and claudin-s (*CLDN2/MORC*). Several studies have suggested that certain less severe *CFTR* gene mutations and *SPINK1* mutations may be associated with "idiopathic" CP. *CFTR* gene mutations have been identified in up to half of patients with idiopathic CP.[62,106] This proportion is far greater than expected within this population. Analysis of these data has suggested that the combination of a more severe *CFTR* mutation on one chromosome with a mild mutation on the other is particularly associated with CP. The mechanisms by which these mutations cause or contribute to CP are thought to involve several potential pathways,[107,108] including trypsin-dependent pathways leading to activation of digestive enzymes within the acinar cells (e.g., PRSS1, SPINK1); ductal obstruction through inadequate fluid and bicarbonate flow (e.g., CFTR); and protein misfolding leading to ER stress (e.g., CPA1). Genetic testing for these mutations and others is commercially available.

Autoimmune Pancreatitis

AIP refers to three different chronic inflammatory and fibrosing diseases of the pancreas.[31–39,104,109–110] (Box 61.2). The pancreas in patients with type 1 AIP is densely infiltrated with immune cells, including CD4-positive T cells and plasma cells, many of which express IgG_4 on their surface (Figs. 61.2A and 61.3). Elevations in serum levels of IgG_4 can also be seen in many patients with type 1 AIP. IgG_4 is unable to crosslink antigens and does not activate the classical complement cascade, and no specific target of the IgG_4 has been consistently identified. It is not clear that the IgG_4 is involved in the pathogenesis of disease, and some data suggest it may be anti-inflammatory in patients with AIP and the related condition of IgG_4-related disease.[111] Experimental evidence suggests a complex mechanism involving both humoral and cellular immunity.[31,35,109] Fibrosis, sclerosis, and obliterative phlebitis are characteristically seen in the pancreas in association with the dense chronic inflammatory infiltrate in type 1 AIP.[31–34] Although this inflammatory infiltrate is present in the pancreas, similar infiltrates may be seen in the bile duct, salivary glands, retroperitoneum, lymph nodes, kidney, prostate, ampulla, and occasionally organs.[35,109,112–114] More than 10 IgG_4-positive plasma cells per high-power field in biopsy specimens of the pancreas are consistent with the diagnosis of type 1 AIP,[32–34,109,114] but this number varies depending on the organ that is biopsied. The fibrosis is usually storiform or present in a whirling pattern resembling the spokes of a wheel. Venous channels are obliterated by the dense inflammatory infiltrate. This pattern has been termed lymphoplasmacytic sclerosing pancreatitis.

61

BOX 61.2 Characteristics of Type 1, Type 2, and Type 3 Autoimmune Pancreatitis

Feature	Type 1 AIP	Type 2 AIP	Type 3 AIP
Histologic features	Lymphoplasmacytic infiltration Dense periductal infiltrate without damage to ductal epithelium Storiform fibrosis Obliterative phlebitis Abundant (>10 cells/HPF) IgG4-positive cells Fibroinflammatory process may extend to peripancreatic region	Lymphoplasmacytic and neutrophilic infiltration around ducts Destruction of duct epithelium by neutrophils (granulocytic epithelial lesion) Obliterative phlebitis is rare No IgG4-positive cells	T-cell mediated inflammatory response, with $CD3^+$ lymphocyte infiltration in healthy parts of pancreas and elevation in $CD8^+/CD4^+$ ratio in 'unhealthy' parts of pancreas
Average age at presentation	60–70 years	40–50, but may present in young adults and even children	*See gender predominance
Gender predominance	Male	Equal	Immune-related adverse events are more common in Caucasian men in their sixth decade of life, though in type 3 AIP there is no current clear gender or age predominance
Usual clinical presentations	Obstructive jaundice (75%) Acute pancreatitis (15%)	Obstructive jaundice (50%) Acute pancreatitis (33%)	Asymptomatic pancreatic enzyme elevation (majority) Acute pancreatitis (minority)
Pancreatic imaging	Diffuse pancreatic enlargement (40%) Focal pancreatic enlargement (60%)	Diffuse pancreatic enlargement (15%) Focal pancreatic enlargement (85%)	Diffuse pancreatic enlargement (56%) Focal pancreatic enlargement (44%)
IgG4	Elevated in serum (≈2/3 of patients) Positive in staining of involved tissues	Not associated	Not associated
Other organ involvement	Biliary strictures Sialoadenitis Retroperitoneal fibrosis Pseudotumors Kidney Lung Others	Not associated	Immune checkpoint inhibitor toxicity can affect any organ system
Associated diseases		IBD	Malignancy treated with immune checkpoint inhibitors
Long-term outcome	Frequent relapses	Rare or no relapse	Pancreatic atrophy, increased risk of development of diabetes

Type 1 AIP may occur in an isolated pancreatic form but is more commonly associated with extrapancreatic manifestations in the diagnosis of IgG_4-related disease (Fig. 61.2).[4,35,57,109,112–114] The most common extrapancreatic conditions identified include biliary strictures, hilar lymphadenopathy, sclerosing sialadenitis, retroperitoneal fibrosis, and tubulointerstitial nephritis.[113,114] Biopsies of these organs will reveal a similar inflammatory infiltrated rich in IgG_4-positive plasma cells. Involvement of other organs occurs in at least 60% of patients with type 1 AIP[109,113,114] and may occur before, after, or at the same time as the pancreatic disease. A number of conditions are now included as a manifestation of IgG_4-related disease, including Mikulicz syndrome (in which a massive IgG_4-positive mononuclear infiltrate is seen in the salivary and lacrimal glands), Küttner tumor (submandibular glands), Riedel thyroiditis, eosinophilic angiocentric fibrosis (orbits and upper respiratory tract), multifocal fibrosclerosis, inflammatory pseudotumors, mediastinal and retroperitoneal fibrosis, periaortitis, inflammatory aortic aneurysm, and idiopathic hypocomplementemic tubulointerstitial nephritis.[35,112–114]

A second form of AIP, termed type 2, is characterized by a different histologic pattern termed idiopathic duct-centric pancreatitis. Type 2 AIP is more common in Western countries but remains overall less common than type 1, accounting for less than 20% of all cases of AIP.[109] Type 2 AIP demonstrates neutrophilic infiltration in the pancreas with microabscesses (granulocyte-epithelial lesions), and obliterative phlebitis is rare (Table 61.1).[32,33] Type 2 AIP is limited to the pancreas and is not associated with an infiltration of IgG_4-positive plasma cells in the pancreas nor with elevations in serum levels of IgG_4. Type 2 AIP may, however, be seen in association with underlying IBD (15%–30% of patients with type 2 AIP).

Type 1 AIP is seen more commonly in men (2:1) and usually manifests in middle age or beyond.[35,109] More than 85% of patients present after the age of 50 years, and the mean age of presentation is 70. Type 2 AIP presents at a younger age and may even present in young adults and children. The most common initial presentation for both types 1 and 2 AIP is painless obstructive jaundice due to obstruction of the intrapancreatic bile duct (see Fig. 61.2B). Jaundice may occur from compression of the bile duct by the enlarged pancreas or by infiltration of the biliary tree (IgG_4 cholangitis). A less common initial presentation is acute pancreatitis, and this is most common in those with type 2 AIP. Additional symptoms may include weight loss, vomiting, and glucose intolerance. Although pain is not frequently present, abdominal and referred back pain may occur. These clinical features, coupled with imaging studies demonstrating diffuse or focal

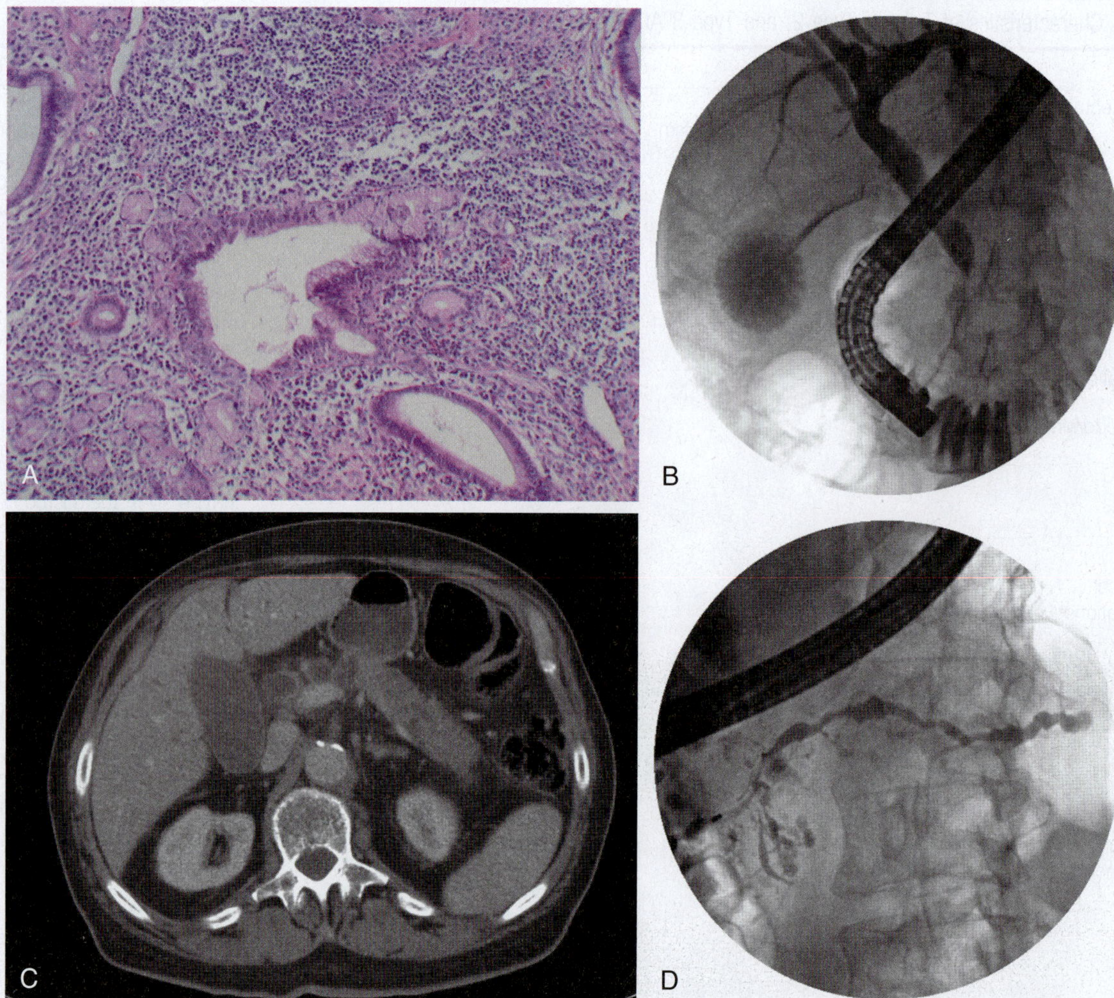

Fig. 61.2 Autoimmune pancreatitis. (A) Histopathology of a pancreatic resection specimen demonstrating a robust lymphoplasmacytic infiltrate involving the larger pancreatic ducts (Hematoxylin and eosin). (B) Cholangiogram demonstrating a smooth stricture involving the intrapancreatic portion of the bile duct. (C) CT shows a dilated pancreatic duct without pancreatic parenchymal atrophy. (D) Pancreatogram reveals a moderately dilated pancreatic duct with diffuse areas of irregularity and alternating areas of stenosis and dilatation. There is an area of more dominant stricture in the pancreatic head. (Courtesy of C. Mel Wilcox, MD, Orlando, FL.)

pancreatic enlargement (see Fig. 61.2C), often raise the suspicion of pancreatic adenocarcinoma. In studies in patients who underwent pancreatic resection for presumed pancreatic carcinoma but were found to have no malignancy in the resected specimen, up to 10% show evidence of AIP.[115,116] In type 1 AIP, jaundice or cholestasis may also occur due to additional strictures of the proximal biliary tree. A pattern similar to that seen in PSC is seen, with a predilection for involvement of the hilar region. The pattern may mimic not only PSC but also cholangiocarcinoma. The disease, unlike classic PSC, is not typically associated with inflammatory bowel disease and is steroid-responsive. Additional common clinical manifestations of type 1 AIP include a sclerosing sialadenitis (usually presenting as bilateral symmetrical swelling of the salivary glands), retroperitoneal fibrosis (most commonly presenting as hydronephrosis due to entrapment of the ureters), renal mass, tubulointerstitial nephritis, lymphadenopathy (particularly mediastinal, cervical, and abdominal), prostatitis, sclerosing cholecystitis, interstitial pneumonia, and pseudotumors of the liver, lung, prostate, and pituitary.[109,114]

The radiographic features of the pancreas are similar for types 1 and 2 AIP. Abdominal US usually shows a diffusely enlarged and hypoechoic pancreas. The appearance on EUS is similar. CT most commonly reveals a diffusely enlarged sausage-shaped pancreas (see Fig. 61.2C) in which enhancement with the intravenous contrast agent is delayed and prolonged[31,34,109,115,117] some patients may have a capsule-like low-density rim around the pancreas in delayed images. Focal swelling can also occur, mimicking a pancreatic mass. Additional CT findings, such as contiguous fibrosis and inflammation extending into the retroperitoneum or surrounding the retroperitoneal vessels, can also raise a suspicion of carcinoma. MRI of the pancreas also may reveal this diffuse pancreatic enlargement, typically with decreased T1-weighted intensity and increased T2-weighted intensity.[109,117] MRCP can be very helpful in identifying the biliary strictures and in visualizing the pancreatic duct, which is also abnormal in AIP.[34,114,117,118] EUS may demonstrate a diffusely enlarged and hypoechoic gland.[119] The use of EUS-guided fine-needle aspiration of the gland is usually not diagnostic,[120]

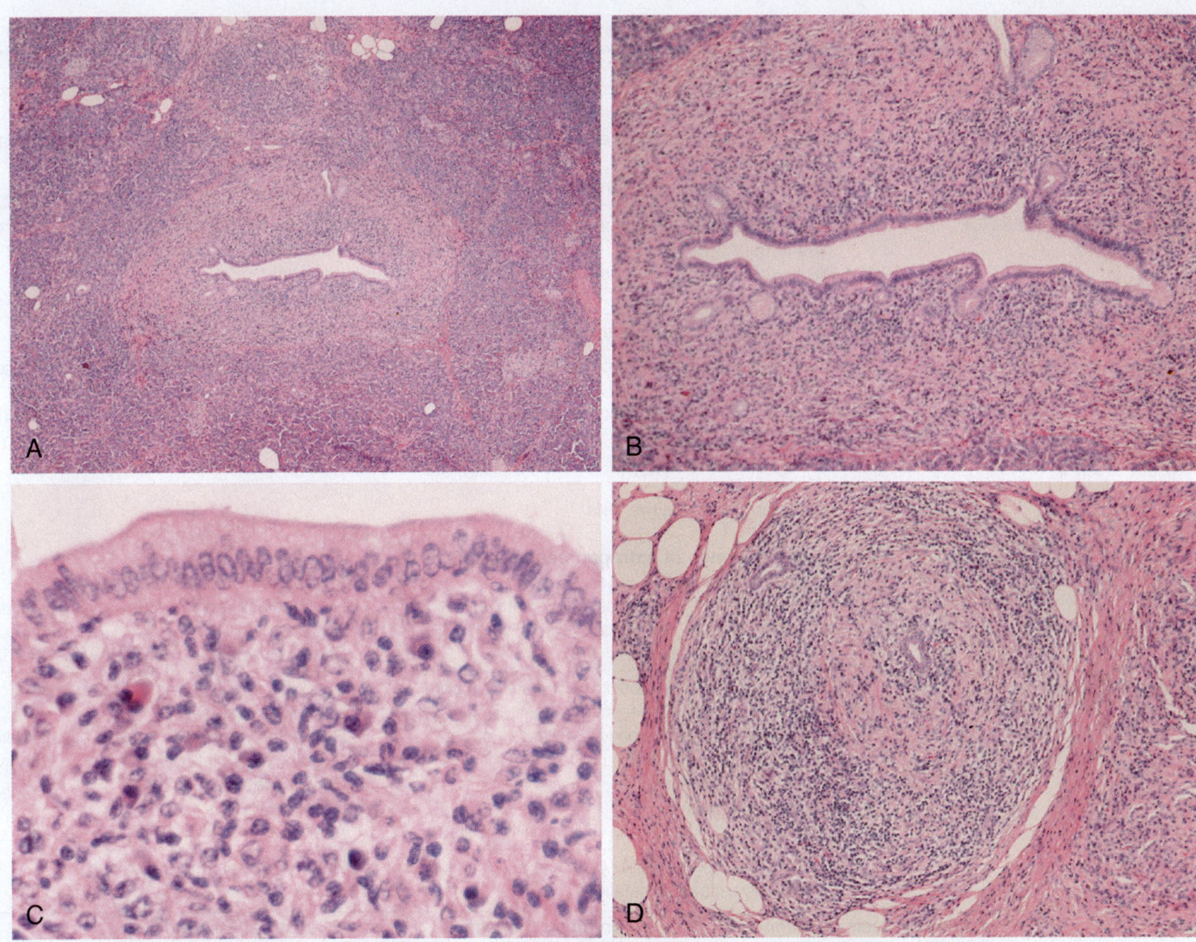

Fig. 61.3 Lymphoplasmacytic sclerosing pancreatitis, the most common form of autoimmune pancreatitis. (A) Cuff-like periductal lymphoplasmacytic infiltration with normal surrounding pancreatic parenchyma (H&E, ×20). (B) Prominent periductal infiltrate (H&E, ×200). (C) Plasma cell-rich, mixed infiltrate around bile ducts (H&E, ×200). (D) Another example of a cuff-like infiltrate with periductal fibrosis (H&E, ×20). (Courtesy Dr. Pamela Jensen, Dallas, TX.)

although there are case reports of EUS-guided core biopsy being diagnostic.[121]

One of the hallmarks of both types of AIP is diffuse or segmental irregularity and narrowing of the pancreatic duct (see Fig. 61.2D). The duct may be diffusely narrowed and thread-like or may instead demonstrate alternating areas of stricture and normal caliber or dilated duct.[34,109,117,122] MRCP is often able to identify the pancreatic duct abnormalities but may not be able to visualize the duct if it is thread-like and diffusely affected. ERCP is better able to visualize the pancreatic duct[122] but carries more risk and cost than MRCP. Some patients may have a more focal segmental or isolated area of pancreatic duct narrowing, in a pattern more suggestive of malignancy. Some studies in which a second ERCP has been performed note progression from a segmental form to diffuse form in the absence of glucocorticoid treatment. With time, and particularly in those with untreated or relapsing disease, the disease may burn out and lead to pancreatic gland atrophy and calcification. At that point, it is indistinguishable from other forms of CP. Studies from Japan note that up to 6% of all patients evaluated for CP have AIP, and the overall prevalence is estimated to be 4.6 per 100,000 persons.[35,123] Very few other epidemiologic estimates exist.

AIP—both types 1 and 2—are usually suspected based on clinical and imaging features. In type 1 AIP, laboratory evaluation may reveal elevations in serum immunoglobulins, seen in one-half to two-thirds of cases, especially in IgG_4. Although various cutoffs have been used, current consensus diagnostic guidelines use levels of IgG_4 more than two times the upper limit of normal.[34,109] Elevation in serum IgG_4 is not specific for AIP and may also be seen in occasional patients with pancreatic adenocarcinoma. A variety of other autoantibodies have also been reported, including antinuclear antibodies, antilactoferrin antibodies, anticarbonic anhydrase II antibodies, antismooth muscle antibodies, rheumatoid factor, and antimitochondrial antibody. These autoantibodies do not have the sensitivity of IgG_4 and hence are inferior for diagnostic purposes. These serologic markers of disease are absent in those with type 2 AIP.

There are several systems for diagnosis of type 1 AIP. An international consensus conference developed criteria (seen in Table 61.1) that are now widely used across the world.[34] There are five criteria, including imaging of the pancreas and pancreatic duct, serology, other organ involvement, histology (if available), and response to steroid trial. This system allows patients to be categorized as definitive or probable type 1 AIP, depending on the mix of criteria present. It should be noted that whereas type 1 AIP can be diagnosed with reasonable accuracy without a pancreatic biopsy, the diagnosis of type 2 AIP almost always requires pancreatic biopsy or resection. Making an accurate diagnosis of AIP requires that it be differentiated from pancreatic cancer.[115,116,124–126] This is particularly important, as

TABLE 61.1 International Consensus Diagnostic Criteria for Type 1 Autoimmune Pancreatitis

Criteria	Level 1 Evidence	Level 2 Evidence
P: Parenchymal imaging	Typical imaging: Diffuse enlargement of pancreas with delayed enhancement With or without rim-like enhancement or pancreas	Indeterminate imaging: Segmental or focal enlargement of pancreas With delayed enhancement
D: Ductal imaging (ERCP or MRCP)	Long (>1/3 of the length of pancreatic duct) stricture, or Multiple strictures without upstream dilation of pancreatic duct	Segmental or focal narrowing of pancreatic duct Without marked (>5 mm) upstream dilation of pancreatic duct
S: Serology	IgG4 >2 × upper limit of normal	IgG4 1–2 × upper limit of normal
OOI: Other organ involvement	Histology of extrapancreatic organ involvement (at least 3 of 4 below) Marked lymphoplasmacytic infiltration with fibrosis Storiform fibrosis Obliterative phlebitis Abundant IgG4-positive cells OR **Imaging evidence of extrapancreatic organ involvement (any)** Segmental/multiple proximal or proximal and distal bile duct strictures Retroperitoneal fibrosis	Histology of extrapancreatic organ involvement, including bile duct or ampullary biopsies Marked lymphoplasmacytic infiltration and Abundant IgG4-positive cells OR Physical or radiologic evidence Symmetrically enlarged salivary or lacrimal glands Renal involvement consistent with AIP
H: Histology of pancreas	Lymphoplasmacytic sclerosing pancreatitis on core biopsy or resection specimen (at least 3) Periductal lymphoplasmacytic infiltrate without granulocytic infiltration Obliterative phlebitis Storiform fibrosis Abundant (>10 cells/HPF) IgG4-positive cells	Lymphoplasmacytic sclerosing pancreatitis on core biopsy (at least 2) Periductal lymphoplasmacytic infiltrate without granulocytic infiltration Obliterative phlebitis Storiform fibrosis Abundant (>10 cells/HPF) IgG4-positive cells
Rt: Response to steroids	Rapid (2 week) radiologically demonstrable resolution or marked improvement in pancreatic/extrapancreatic manifestations	

Diagnosis	Primary Basis of Diagnosis	Imaging Evidence	Collateral Evidence
Definitive type 1 AIP	Histology	Typical/indeterminate	
	Imaging	Typical	Any non-D level 1/level 2
		Indeterminate	Two or more from level 1
	Response to steroids	Indeterminate	Level 1 S/OOI or level 1 D +level 2 S/OOI/H
Probable type 1 AIP		Indeterminate	Level 2 S/OOI/H + Rt

The diagnosis of type 2 AIP requires typical imaging with either histologic confirmation or both the presence of IBD and a response to steroids.
AIP, Autoimmune pancreatitis; *IgG_4,* immunoglobulin G subtype 4.
From Chari ST, Kloeppel G, Zhang L, et al. Histopathologic and clinical subtypes of autoimmune pancreatitis: the Honolulu consensus document. *Pancreatology*. 2010;10:664–672; Shimosegawa T, Chari ST, Frulloni L, et al. International consensus diagnostic criteria for autoimmune pancreatitis: Guidelines of the International Association of Pancreatology. *Pancreatology*. 2011;40:352–358.

pancreatic cancer is far more common than AIP. Features that are especially concerning for malignancy include a dilated pancreatic duct, a single high-grade pancreatic duct stricture with upstream atrophy of the gland, or a low-density focal mass on CT imaging. These imaging features are unfortunately not highly sensitive and specific, and making the distinction between AIP and pancreatic cancer may require a pancreatic core biopsy, a trial of steroids, or a pancreatic resection. Prior to initiating a trial of glucocorticoid therapy, vigorous efforts should be made to exclude malignancy.

Autoimmune CP can progress within months in some patients from initial symptoms to end-stage CP. There is some evidence that early therapy with glucocorticoids can result in symptom resolution and radiographic abnormalities and may also prevent subsequent disease complications.[109,127] A treatment algorithm has been provided by an international consensus of expert providers, offering a structured approach to therapy.[128] Between 30% and 50% of patients with type 1 AIP experience a relapse after glucocorticoid therapy.[109,127] Patients with type 2 AIP relapse very rarely, if at all. Relapse in type 1 AIP may be managed by a repeat course of glucocorticoids followed by maintenance at a low dose of prednisone (e.g., 5–10 mg/day). Immunomodulators, such as azathioprine, have been used with variable success in steroid-dependent patients as steroid-sparing therapy.[127] In those that relapse on azathioprine or in those who cannot tolerate it, continuing steroids is often effective and rituximab may be used in especially refractory cases.[109,114,127] Glucocorticoid therapy may improve not only the structural abnormalities of the pancreas but also exocrine and endocrine pancreatic function (and salivary function if it is affected). Improvement in function is variable, depending on the level of fibrosis and atrophy already established when therapy is initiated. Clinical relapses after resection (e.g., pancreaticoduodenectomy) are rare.

An additional type of autoimmune PI—type 3 AIP—has been identified as an immune-related adverse event in patients receiving immune checkpoint inhibitor (ICI) therapy as treatment for malignancy.[129] ICI-induced ICI-PI may manifest as an asymptomatic lipase elevation or acute pancreatitis meeting standard criteria (≥2 of three typical abdominal pain, amylase or lipase more than two to three times upper limit of assay normal, and findings on cross-sectional imaging); a recent publication has proposed reclassifying type 3 AIP into these two categories to better understand what may be two distinct entities.[130] The diagnosis is made by temporal association with ICI therapy and exclusion of other causes of PI. The pathophysiology of this phenomenon remains incompletely understood, though it is suggested to result from T-cell mediated response with influx of specific subtypes into different areas of the gland (Box 61.2). Risk of ICI-PI is higher with combination ICI therapy than with monotherapy. The incidence of endocrine toxicity has been noted to be particularly severe in this patient population, with suspicion that in some individuals there may be selective attack on islet cells.[131,132] Glucocorticoid therapy has been utilized in ICI-PI, though its effects remain unclear.[133] Cessation of ICI therapy—at least temporarily—is the mainstay of treatment in this disorder, though the risk is for progression of malignancy.

Obstructive

Mechanical obstruction of the main pancreatic duct by tumors, scars, ductal stones, duodenal wall cysts, or stenosis of the papilla of Vater or the minor papilla can produce CP in the parenchyma upstream of the obstruction. Obstruction of the branched pancreatic ducts may contribute to another phenotype of CP termed "small duct disease" (i.e., obstruction of small or large ductal branches by protein precipitates in alcohol-induced CP). Obstructive CP in this discussion, however, refers to a distinct entity thought of as "large duct disease" produced most frequently by a single dominant narrowing or stricture of the main pancreatic duct. A number of entities can produce obstructive CP. Acquired strictures of the main pancreatic duct can occur because of tumor obstruction from adenocarcinoma, islet cell tumor, intraductal papillary mucinous tumors, or ampullary neoplasms. Benign strictures may also develop after a severe attack of acute pancreatitis or following blunt and penetrating trauma to the pancreas.

Pancreas divisum is a common normal variant, occurring in approximately 4%–11% of the population. In rare patients with this anomaly, the size of the minor papilla may be inadequate to allow for free flow of pancreatic juice into the duodenum, resulting in recurrent attacks of acute pancreatitis. Pancreas divisum, however, is not considered a primary cause of CP. Large natural history studies have failed to identify a clear link between pancreas divisum and either acute or CP. Patients with pancreas divisum who do develop pancreatic disease often have coexistent underlying genetic mutations that may explain the pancreatitis, rather than the effect of divisum alone.[134,135] Dysfunction of the sphincter of Oddi, like pancreas divisum, is also often proposed as a cause of acute or recurrent acute pancreatitis rather than CP. The response to sphincter ablation in patients with CP and presumed sphincter of Oddi dysfunction or pancreas divisum is unpredictable, but generally poor, and neither surgical nor endoscopic techniques are commonly recommended given a lack of proven efficacy.

Miscellaneous

Recurrent or Severe Acute Pancreatitis

CP can develop after a severe attack of acute pancreatitis, usually with associated pancreatic necrosis and additional complications. Recurrent milder episodes of acute pancreatitis or a smoldering course of acute pancreatitis secondary to any etiology may also eventually lead to the development of a chronic inflammatory response within the pancreas, the activation of pancreatic stellate cells, and CP. One example of this is hypertriglyceridemia. Elevations of serum triglyceride values greater than 1000 mg/dL can produce acute pancreatitis, which is often severe. Many of these patients will have repeated clinical and subclinical attacks of acute inflammation, and some will ultimately develop CP.[136,137]

It appears that after an initial attack of acute pancreatitis, approximately 10% of patients will be diagnosed with CP.[15,50,83] Predictors of CP include multiple relapsing attacks, smoking, and alcohol use with the last two being the strongest predictors.[15,48–51,83] In patients with any etiology of severe acute pancreatitis complicated by substantial pancreatic necrosis, features of CP may also develop.[15,138–141]

Asymptomatic Pancreatic Fibrosis

There are several situations in which histologic evidence of CP and specifically fibrosis may be observed in the absence of clinical CP. This is differentiated here from patients with painless CP who present with symptoms or features of the disease in the absence of pain.[86] Older adults may develop histologic changes within the pancreas that resemble CP.[4–7] ERCP may also demonstrate changes in the pancreatic duct consistent with CP in these patients.[142,143] These structural changes do not usually correspond to functional disturbances of pancreatic function or to clinical features of CP.[143] Chronic alcohol users who do not have clinical CP commonly have histologic evidence of CP.[8,9]

The incidence of acute pancreatitis is increased in patients undergoing hemodialysis, and some evidence suggests that CP may also be seen with greater frequency in this population. Imaging and autopsy data note changes consistent with CP in up to one in five individuals in the absence of clinical symptoms.[133,134,144,145] Chronic renal failure appears to frequently produce asymptomatic pancreatic fibrosis. Changes in pancreatic morphology and function are also common in patients with long-standing diabetes.[11] The pancreas is smaller than normal, particularly in patients with type 1 diabetes.[11,146] The pancreatic duct is abnormal in 40%–50% of diabetic patients when studied by ERCP, with abnormalities suggestive of CP.[147,148] Pancreatic function, as defined by fecal elastase measurements[11,149] or by more formal direct pancreatic function testing,[150] is abnormal in 40%–50% of patients. The reason for these associations is not clear, whether the diabetes is causing the changes in the pancreas or vice versa. Because insulin is a trophic factor for the exocrine pancreas, and because diabetes can produce microvascular angiopathy, insulin deficiency, and long-standing diabetes together could explain the pancreatic damage. Although these measures of pancreatic structure and function may be present, they are usually not responsible for symptoms and these patients do not routinely merit treatment with pancreatic enzymes.[11] Smoking is a strong risk factor for CP, and autopsy studies reveal that smoking also produces pancreatic fibrosis,[151] particularly intralobular fibrosis.

These observations may be combined to suggest that a wide variety of disease states and normal wear and tear (e.g., normal aging, chronic alcohol ingestion, and smoking) on the pancreas may produce damage that by histologic criteria resembles CP but is not sufficient to cause symptoms and is not severe enough to cross the diagnostic threshold of labeling that patient as having this disease.

Idiopathic

Idiopathic pancreatitis accounts for 10%–30% of all cases of CP,[15,57,60,152,153] but this varies depending on the population and location. Idiopathic disease is particularly common in women; in some studies, it is the most common etiology in women.[152] However, many patients are probably mislabeled as having idiopathic disease. Given that there is no reliable method of determining alcohol ingestion and that there is not an absolute threshold of ingestion for pancreatitis, some of these patients certainly suffer from at least some toxicity from alcohol. Similarly, some of these idiopathic cases occur in patients with known and unknown genetic abnormalities,[95,104,106–108,154,155] particularly those with onset in young adulthood.[155] Some of what was formerly labeled idiopathic is instead autoimmune. In many previous studies, smoking was not included as a potential etiologic agent, and so smoking may also account for a significant proportion of these patients. Interpreting the literature on idiopathic CP is therefore difficult because most studies of this entity are probably dealing with cases with several different etiologies.

Idiopathic CP appears to occur in two forms, an early-onset type that manifests in the late second or third decade of life and a late-onset form that appears in the sixth or seventh decade of life.[68,153] Early-onset idiopathic CP has a mean age at onset of around 20 years. There appears to be an equal gender distribution. Pain is the predominant feature of this disease, occurring in up to 96% of patients, a higher rate than in either alcoholic or late-onset CP. Pancreatic calcifications, exocrine insufficiency, and endocrine insufficiency (i.e., diabetes) are extremely rare at presentation (<10%) and develop very slowly thereafter. The mean time to calcification in this group is 25 years, to exocrine insufficiency 26 years, and to endocrine insufficiency 27.5 years.[68] Complications of CP (pseudocyst, abscess, biliary obstruction, and duodenal obstruction) occur in about 20% of patients, whereas surgery (primarily for abdominal pain) is ultimately needed in 60%. Thus early-onset idiopathic CP is a disease characterized by severe pain but much delayed development of structural (calcifications) or functional (exocrine or endocrine insufficiency) evidence of CP. The delay may make diagnosis quite difficult because most available diagnostic tools rely on these structural or functional abnormalities.

Late-onset idiopathic CP manifests less commonly as pain. In the best documented series,[68] only 54% of patients presented with pain, although 75% ultimately experienced pain. The median age of onset is 56 years, and the disease occurs equally in men and women. Exocrine insufficiency (22%) and endocrine insufficiency (22%) were present not infrequently at the time of diagnosis, ultimately occurring in 46% and 41% of cases, respectively. The median time to development of exocrine insufficiency and endocrine insufficiency was 16.9 and 11.9 years, respectively. Life-table analysis suggested that with very long follow-up (>30 years), exocrine insufficiency will ultimately develop in 75%, endocrine insufficiency in 50%–60%, and diffuse pancreatic calcifications in 90% of patients.[68,156] The disease therefore tends to be one of a comparatively painless course associated with the frequent development of pancreatic calcifications, exocrine insufficiency, and endocrine insufficiency. Aging itself can be associated with the development of structural changes within the pancreatic parenchyma and duct that are indistinguishable from those seen in late-onset CP,[143] so the distinction between normal aging and late-onset idiopathic CP may not always be clear.

CLINICAL FEATURES

Abdominal Pain

Abdominal pain affects over 80% of patients during the course of their disease and is the main driver of morbidity in CP.[157] Intractable pain is the most common reason for hospitalization, endoscopic intervention, and surgery in patients with CP. Abdominal pain in CP is associated with lower quality of life and with higher rates of psychiatric comorbidity.[158] Most commonly, patients describe epigastric abdominal pain, sometimes radiating to the back; however, there is not just one pattern of pain.[159–165] Postprandial pain can result in decreased oral intake, contributing to weight loss, malnutrition, and further sequelae, including sarcopenia. Constant severe pain leads to a dramatic reduction in quality of life,[159–165] loss of social functioning, the potential for addiction to narcotic analgesics,[166,167] and increased rates of suicide.[168] In the United States, about half of all patients with CP are treated with opioids.[166]

The natural history of abdominal pain in CP varies and is difficult to predict. Classically, pain phenotypes have been divided into two main groups: one with episodes of pain interspersed with long pain-free periods and the other with chronic constant pain, punctuated by exacerbations of more severe pain.[169] More recent work has shown that pain patterns are quite dynamic for patients, and rather than fitting solely into one category or the other, patients exhibit significant changes in their pain pattern over time.[170] The judgment of therapeutic efficacy for any treatment for CP must consider this extremely variable natural history of pain.[171–173]

The proposed causes of pain in CP are numerous; however, overall they can largely be included in one of two overarching categories: (1) increased pressure, ischemia, and inflammation in the pancreas and (2) injury to and alterations in function of peripheral and central nociceptive nerves. In many chronic pain conditions, including CP, one can also classify pain as nociceptive pain (due to actual or threatened damage to nonneural tissue and the activation of nociceptors) and neuropathic pain (pain caused by a lesion or disease of the somatosensory nervous system).[171,174–176]

Increased Pressure With Ischemia and Inflammation

One proposed mechanism of pain is tissue ischemia, driven by increased pressure within the pancreatic duct or parenchyma. Several lines of clinical and experimental evidence point to increased pressure within the pancreatic duct or parenchyma as being important in the genesis of pancreatic pain. Pancreatic ductal and tissue pressures are usually elevated in patients with CP undergoing surgery for chronic pain.[177–179] Elevations in pancreatic ductal pressure measured during ERCP have also been documented in some patients with painful CP.[180,181] Surgical drainage of the pancreatic duct leads to a reduction in pressure to normal levels and is associated with pain relief.[177–179] However, pancreatic duct pressures may not be different in those with and without pain,[181] and a reduction in pressure after endoscopic stenting does not correlate with pain relief.[182]

Increased pressure within the pancreatic duct would be expected to be related to obstruction of the pancreatic duct, either in the main duct or in side branches. The presence of a pancreatic duct stricture and upstream pancreatic duct dilation might be an accurate indicator of a group of patients with increased pressure and therefore pain. However, there is not a relationship between pancreatic duct strictures or ductal dilation and pain.[171,175,183,184] Nonetheless, it is believed that patients with a dilated pancreatic duct or pancreatic duct stricture are most likely to experience pain relief from endoscopic or surgical therapy.

The mechanism by which increased pressure could cause pain is speculative but may be related to pancreatic tissue ischemia. In animal models of CP, increased pancreatic pressure is associated with reductions in pancreatic blood flow, tissue oxygen tension, and interstitial pH. In these models, pancreatic secretagogues lead to a further decrease in pancreatic blood flow (rather than the normally expected increase), decreased capillary filling, and worsening tissue ischemia. These observations are consistent with those seen in a compartment-type syndrome.[178] Small studies in humans with CP undergoing surgery also demonstrate lower pancreatic tissue pH than patients without CP.[185] Pancreatic blood flow, measured at ERCP with the use of platinum electrodes, is also lower in patients with CP compared with controls.[186] Tissue ischemia that is worsened by secretory stimulation of the pancreas may therefore be the mechanism by which elevations in tissue pressure cause pain.

Inflammation in the pancreas, with the release of inflammatory mediators, also likely contributes to pain. In particular, trypsin released from damaged acinar cells and tryptase released from resident mast cells can activate proteinase-activated receptor 2 (PAR-2) and sensitize the response of transient receptor vanilloid active fibers, releasing substance P as a key molecule in pain signaling.[175,176] It is noteworthy that during painful flares in patients with CP, there may not be elevations in serum levels of lipase or amylase or imaging evidence of acute pancreatic inflammation. Ongoing evaluations of neuroinflammatory biomarkers are attempting to identify a biochemical signature for different types of nerve inflammation leading to specific pain patterns in CP.[174]

Alterations in Peripheral and Central Nociceptive Nerves

The perception of pain requires signaling through nociceptive neurons. Morphologic studies in patients with CP demonstrate increases in the diameter and number of intrapancreatic nerves, foci of inflammatory cells associated with nerves and ganglia, and damage to the perineural sheath.[175,176,187,188] The disruption of the perineural sheath may allow inflammatory mediators to gain access to the neural elements. Regardless of the local events in and around the pancreas causing pain, perception of the pain message requires communication with the central nervous system. The innervation of the pancreas is complex, with both visceral somatic and autonomic nerves. Dendrites of the pancreatic nociceptive sensory afferents travel with sympathetic nerves from the pancreas and reach the celiac ganglia, although no synapse is made there. These dendritic fibers continue, bundled as the left and right greater splanchnic nerves, to the sympathetic trunk ganglia, before reaching the first cell body, located in the dorsal root ganglia in spinal cord segments T5 through T9-T10. Projections of these dorsal root neurons often traverse upward and downward for several spinal segments before entering the dorsal horn of the spinal cord. Afferent pain fibers may cross the midline in several of these connections, accounting for the midline perception of pancreatic pain. Axons from the first-order dorsal root ganglion cell bodies have two distinct pathways. Some project to the dorsal horn of the spinal cord and may release a variety of mediators, including substance P, calcitonin gene-related peptide, and glutamate, onto second-order neurons that project to the thalamus via the spinothalamic white matter columns. These may then synapse with third-order neurons that project to the somatosensory cortex (for cognitive integration of pain) and to the limbic system and hypothalamus (for affective and autonomic integration of pain). A second pathway for projections involves synapses within the same level of the spinal cord with sympathetic efferent cell bodies that project back down the splanchnic nerves to the celiac plexus, with second-order sympathetic neurons projecting back to the pancreas. Vagal afferents may also carry noxious stimuli from the pancreas (especially for stretch).

Noxious stimulation of these pathways can occur through a variety of mechanisms. Pressure, ischemia, inflammation, heat, and other classic stimuli can activate these pathways. The accumulation of inflammatory mediators and nerve injury can sensitize the nerve, making it hyperresponsive.[175,176,189] There is an increase in nociceptive neurotransmitters (e.g., substance P, calcitonin gene-related peptide) in interlobular and intralobular nerve bundles in patients with CP.[176,189] The close spatial relationship between intrapancreatic nerves and inflammatory cells supports the additional mechanism of neuroimmune interaction. Expression of nerve growth factor and one of its receptors (TrkA) is seen in patients with painful CP and in animal models of CP.[189,190] Nerve growth factor is one of the key molecules involved in sensitization.[189,190] Endogenous proteases, like trypsin, can also activate and sensitize sensory neurons in the pancreas, a process mediated through the PAR-2. Another activator of PAR-2 is tryptase, a mast cell product.[176,189] Interestingly, mast cells are seen commonly in pancreatic tissue specimens from patients with CP. The exact mechanisms by which the inflammatory cells and their products and intrapancreatic neurons interact in CP remain to be fully clarified, although the data suggest that the production of sensitizing factors near pancreatic nerves alters sensory neuron form and function.

In addition, there is substantial evidence from studies of other types of chronic pain that chronic peripheral nerve injury or inflammation leads to changes in nociceptive processing that involve both the spinal cord and central nervous system. Chronic pain can produce a centrally sensitized pain state in which elimination of the original source of pain may not relieve pain.[175,176,191,192] In this situation, pain may occur in response to innocuous or physiologic stimuli (allodynia) or may respond in an exaggerated fashion to stimuli that are painful (hyperalgesia). These phenomena depend on changes at both the spinal cord level and the brain. A number of studies document changes in central nervous system structure and function in patients with CP.[175,176,193,194] These changes include altered central processing of nociceptive inputs, altered pain thresholds, and altered brain micro- and macrostructure. Some examples of these changes in patients with CP compared to normal healthy controls include reorganization of the insula, secondary somatosensory cortex, and cingulate cortex, with abnormal neuronal excitability of these neural networks.[176] Numerous structural changes can also be documented, including reduced thickness of cortical volume in areas of visceral pain processing, abnormal EEGs, and abnormal functional MRI of the brain.[175,176] The central nervous system reorganization and plasticity underlying hyperalgesia and allodynia are likely major factors limiting the effectiveness of treatments for pain. Nowhere is this fact made more obvious than in the patient who continues to have pancreatic pain after a total pancreatectomy. Pancreatic quantitative sensory testing (P-QST), an emerging bedside neurosensory testing technique, offers an opportunity to assess nociceptive phenotypes and classify patients according to the degree of their altered sensitization.[195,196] To date, this technique has facilitated the assessment of pain phenotypes with clinical and demographic factors. Pain is complex, and no single mechanism is likely to be present in all patients. P-QST has allowed for the assessment of hyperalgesia as an independent contributing factor to the pain experience in CP.[197] The overlapping presence of hyperalgesia with additional pain-associated factors (ductal obstruction, psychiatric comorbidity) is shown to be associated with an increase in pain severity and interference with everyday activities, as well as a linear decrease in quality of life.[198] The complexity of the pain experience seen in CP naturally implicates that short of a cure for the disease, no single therapy will be effective.

Other Causes of Pain

In addition to these two main mechanisms, a variety of other contributors to pain should be considered. Complications of CP may also cause pain. These complications include duodenal obstruction, bile duct obstruction, a pseudocyst, and secondary pancreatic carcinoma. These usually have specific therapy. Hyperstimulation of the pancreas via CCK has also been postulated as a potential cause of pain because serum levels of CCK may be elevated in CP, and stimulation of the pancreas by CCK could increase pressure within the gland or facilitate basolateral rather than apical secretin of enzymes. Reducing serum CCK levels is the proposed mechanism for the use of nonenteric-coated pancreatic enzymes to reduce pain.

Steatorrhea (Exocrine Pancreatic Insufficiency)

The human pancreas has substantial exocrine reserve, and true exocrine insufficiency manifesting with steatorrhea has long been considered to occur only when pancreatic lipase secretion is reduced to less than 10% of the maximum output.[199] A more contemporary understanding of exocrine pancreatic insufficiency acknowledges that there may be nuanced or gradual loss of pancreatic enzyme secretion in accordance with progressive scarring of the gland, or in an episodic fashion with periods of inflammation or other unknown causes. Often, the gradual decline of pancreatic exocrine function remains unrecognized until it reaches an extreme. Steatorrhea is a feature of far-advanced CP, in which most of the acinar cells have been injured or destroyed but may also be seen with blockage of the pancreatic duct, after pancreatic surgery, and after an attack of necrotizing acute pancreatitis. With advanced CP, maldigestion of fat, protein, and carbohydrates will occur. Azotorrhea (protein maldigestion) also occurs when secretion of proteases is severely impaired. Affected patients may present with diarrhea and weight loss. Some patients may note bulky, foul-smelling stools or may even note the passage of frank oil droplets. Unlike in small bowel diseases associated with malabsorption, watery diarrhea, excess gas, and abdominal cramps are less common in patients with CP. This difference may be due to better preserved carbohydrate absorption and small bowel and colonic function in patients with CP and exocrine insufficiency than in those with small intestinal diseases such as celiac disease. Even when there is significant loss of fat in stool, most patients pass only three or four stools daily and some may pass only one.

In general, fat maldigestion occurs earlier and is more severe than protein or carbohydrate maldigestion. There are several explanations for this phenomenon. First, fat digestion depends primarily on pancreatic lipase and colipase, although gastric lipase can hydrolyze up to 20% of dietary fat. Second, lipase output decreases earlier and more substantially as CP progresses compared with the secretion of other pancreatic enzymes such as trypsin or amylase. Third, lipase is more sensitive to acid destruction than other pancreatic enzymes. As bicarbonate secretion decreases in CP and duodenal pH drops, lipase is inactivated. Fourth, in addition to lipase inactivation, the low duodenal pH also predisposes to precipitation of bile salts, thereby preventing the formation of mixed micelles and further interfering with lipid digestion and absorption. Fifth, lipase is more sensitive to digestion and degradation by pancreatic proteases than other digestive enzymes.

The median time to development of exocrine insufficiency in CP has been reported to be as low as 5 years,[67] but most studies report longer duration of disease prior to development of steatorrhea. In one large natural history study, the median time to development of exocrine insufficiency was 13.1 years in patients with alcoholic CP, 16.9 years in patients with late-onset idiopathic CP, and 26.3 years in patients with early-onset idiopathic CP.[68] With very long follow-up, approximately 50%–80% of patients with CP eventually have exocrine insufficiency.[67–69,156]

Significant weight loss may occur in the setting of maldigestion, but additional causes should be investigated as simultaneous contributors since exocrine pancreatic insufficiency is unlikely to occur in isolation.[200–205] It is noted that resting energy expenditure is generally increased in patients with CP. Weight loss may be commonly seen during painful flares that prevent adequate oral intake because of pain, nausea, or vomiting. Weight loss may also occur as a result of the development of a concomitant disease such as small bowel bacterial overgrowth or pancreatic or extrapancreatic malignancy. Finally, weight loss may occur in patients who develop financial difficulties, suffer from chronic severe alcoholism, or lose social support because these may contribute to inadequate caloric and protein intake.

Deficiencies of fat-soluble vitamins develop in patients with CP and steatorrhea.[201–206] Significant vitamin D deficiency and osteopenia and osteoporosis occur in patients with CP.[204–208] Deficiencies of water-soluble vitamins and micronutrients are less common and generally seen only as a consequence of inadequate intake. Even though vitamin B_{12} absorption requires intact pancreatic function to degrade R-factor from dietary cobalamin, vitamin B_{12} deficiency is quite rare in patients with CP. The presence of exocrine insufficiency, in addition to the metabolic consequences noted above, is also associated with increased overall mortality in patients with CP.[209,210]

Osteopathy

Osteopathy is highly prevalent in patients with CP. This has long been described in retrospective studies, but more recent, prospectively collected evidence shows this finding to be even more pronounced.[207] In one large prospectively enrolled North American cohort of CP patients, cross-sectional analysis showed that over half of included subjects were diagnosed with osteopathy, with 39% having osteopenia and 17% having osteoporosis.[211] Risk factors for osteopathy seen on multivariable analysis included female sex, white race, and underweight body mass, but of interest was the new finding that one-third of patients <50 years of age were affected. This suggests that all CP patients, even those with the diagnosis at young age, should be screened for osteopathy to assess their baseline risk for traumatic or spontaneous fracture.

Diabetes Mellitus (Pancreatic Endocrine Insufficiency)

Like exocrine insufficiency, endocrine insufficiency is a consequence of long-standing CP and is especially common after pancreatic resection and in tropical (fibrocalcific) pancreatitis. Islet cells appear to be relatively resistant to destruction in CP (see Fig. 61.1).[212] When diabetes develops, the mechanism is more complex than just a simple loss of beta cells due to the progressive destruction of islets.[213–217] Various factors make diabetes due to CP (and pancreatic cancer) different than either classic type 1 or type 2 diabetes, and pancreaticogenic diabetes is defined as type 3c diabetes.[217] Type 3c diabetes is characterized by low levels of insulin and counter-regulatory hormones (particularly glucagon and pancreatic polypeptide), rare ketosis, and frequent treatment induced hypoglycemia.[213–217] About half of patients with CP who develop diabetes will require insulin.[215] Unlike type 1 diabetes, insulin-producing beta cells and glucagon-producing alpha cells are both injured. This combination increases the risk of prolonged and severe hypoglycemia with overvigorous insulin treatment, owing to the lack of a compensatory release of glucagon.[214,218]

Diabetes mellitus appears to be almost as common as steatorrhea in patients with far-advanced CP. In one study, the median times to development of diabetes in patients with alcoholic, late-onset idiopathic, and early-onset idiopathic CP were 19.8, 11.9, and 26.3 years, respectively.[68] Other studies have noted shorter median times of 6–10 years.[67,69,219,220] Ultimately with long-term follow-up, 40%–80% of patients with CP have diabetes, depending on etiology.[67,68] Those with CP who undergo pancreatic surgery have higher rates of both exocrine and endocrine insufficiency.[221–223] Microangiopathic complications are as common in patients with diabetes associated with CP as in patients with type 1 diabetes with similar duration of disease.[214,224]

PHYSICAL EXAMINATION

There are very few physical examination findings diagnostic or specific for CP. Patients may appear undernourished with sarcopenia and may demonstrate mild to moderate abdominal tenderness. In those with more advanced disease, weight loss and malnutrition may be more evident. Rarely, a palpable mass is found, indicating a pseudocyst. Jaundice may be observed in the presence of coexistent alcoholic liver disease or bile duct compression within the head of the pancreas. A palpable spleen may also rarely be found in patients with thrombosis of the splenic vein and sinistral portal hypertension because of CP or in patients with portal hypertension due to coexistent chronic liver disease. In some patients with AIP, evidence of a coexistent autoimmune feature, such as salivary gland enlargement or lymphadenopathy, may be found.

DIAGNOSIS

A variety of diagnostic tests for CP are available. These diagnostic tests are usually separated into those that are designed to detect abnormalities of pancreatic function and those that detect abnormalities of pancreatic structure (Table 61.2). Before considering these tests in more detail, it is useful to remember that in almost all patients, CP is a slowly progressive disease. In the early stages within the pancreas, chronic inflammation, cellular necrosis and apoptosis, and activation of pancreatic stellate cells have all developed, but these features of CP remain visible only on histology. With progressive fibrosis and loss and destruction of tissue, the disease becomes more evident. Abnormalities of pancreatic structure or function may take years or even decades to develop or may not develop at all.[1,2,66–69,110,225] All available diagnostic tests are most accurate in far-advanced disease, when obvious functional or structural abnormalities have developed. Conversely, to greater or lesser degrees, all diagnostic tests are less accurate in less advanced or early CP.

Functional abnormalities in CP include exocrine insufficiency (maldigestion and steatorrhea) and endocrine insufficiency (type 3c diabetes mellitus). In addition, some diagnostic tests measure maximum stimulated secretory capacity of the pancreas, which appears to become abnormal before there is failure of exocrine or endocrine function.[225,226] Structural abnormalities that can be diagnostic include changes within the main pancreatic duct (dilation, strictures, irregularity, pancreatic ductal stones), side branches of the pancreatic duct (dilation, irregularity), or pancreatic parenchyma (lobularity of the gland, alterations in echogenicity, cysts, stones, atrophy, and others). Patients with alcoholic CP, hereditary CP, tropical pancreatitis, and late-onset idiopathic CP are most prone to development of these abnormalities of function or structure, although the process may still take several years. These changes develop particularly slowly, and sometimes not at all, in patients with early-onset idiopathic CP.[1,66,68,225]

TABLE 61.2 Available Diagnostic Tests for Chronic Pancreatitis[a]

Tests of Pancreatic Structure	Tests of Pancreatic Function
EUS	Direct hormonal stimulation (with pancreatic stimulation by secretin or cholecystokinin or both): Using oroduodenal tube Using endoscopy
MRI with MRCP, with or without secretin stimulation	Fecal elastase
CT	Serum trypsinogen (trypsin)
ERCP	Fecal chymotrypsin
Abdominal US	Fecal fat
Plain abdominal x-ray	Blood glucose level

[a]Ranked in estimated order of decreasing sensitivity for each category.
CT, Computed tomography; *ERCP*, endoscopic retrograde cholangiopancreatography; *EUS*, endoscopic ultrasound; *MRCP*, magnetic resonance cholangiopancreatography; *MRI*, magnetic resonance imaging.

The determination of the sensitivity, specificity, and accuracy of any of these diagnostic tests requires that the test result be compared with some gold standard, a test that gives reliable and certain evidence as to the presence or absence of disease. In the case of CP, this gold standard has been pancreatic histology (see Fig. 61.1). Unfortunately, the histologic changes are not uniform throughout the gland,[29] so findings in a biopsy specimen may be misleading. Even more important, obtaining pancreatic tissue carries risk and is seldom performed solely for diagnosis. In addition, similar histologic findings may be encountered in patients without clinical features of CP, such as with aging, social alcohol use, smoking, and diabetes.[5–11,143] Given the lack of a functional gold standard, substitutes for the gold standard include other diagnostic tests or long-term follow-up. Most studies have not monitored patients diagnosed with early CP or possible early CP (patients in whom diagnostic tests are not unequivocally positive) for long enough to establish the presence or absence of CP with certainty. Another potential substitute for the gold standard is some other diagnostic test, and in fact, new diagnostic tests are often compared with such modalities as ERCP, EUS, CT, MRI, and pancreatic function tests, or composites of these.

In patients with definite CP and far-advanced structural or functional abnormalities, little else can mimic these abnormalities, and essentially all diagnostic tests are accurate. The situation is quite different in patients with early or less advanced or minimal-change CP, and even more so in patients with suspected or possible CP, in whom these easily identifiable structural or functional abnormalities are lacking.[1,225,227] In this situation, only tests of maximum sensitivity have a chance of enabling a diagnosis, and the lack of a gold standard can lead to diagnostic confusion and difficult decision-making. In addition to choosing a diagnostic test based on sensitivity and specificity, clinicians must consider the availability, cost, and risk of each of these tests to maximize diagnostic information and minimize risk.

Tests of Pancreatic Function

Tests of pancreatic function can be divided into those that directly measure pancreatic function by measuring the output of digestive enzymes or bicarbonate from the pancreas and those that measure the released enzymes indirectly (through their action on a substrate or its level in blood or stool).

Direct Tests

Direct hormonal stimulation tests are believed to be the most sensitive function tests for CP.[1,225–228] These tests require placement of a tube or endoscope in the duodenum, stimulation of pancreatic secretions (usually with secretin, but in some cases with CCK), and collection of pancreatic secretions for analysis (bicarbonate concentration in the case of secretin infusion, enzyme secretion in the case of CCK). A few studies have compared the results of these hormonal stimulation tests with pancreatic histology with overall sensitivities ranging from 67% to 88%.[229–231]

While direct pancreatic function tests do appear in general to be more sensitive than ERCP, it is important to note that several small studies have shown discordant results between the two studies in both directions.[230–235] In addition, several small studies followed patients with a diagnosis of CP based solely on an abnormal hormonal stimulation test result and found that on long-term follow-up, 90% of them eventually developed classic signs of CP, suggesting that in situations where the two tests are discordant, direct pancreatic function testing may be slightly more sensitive.[236–238]

Some experts have suggested that the pancreas has such reserve that 30%–50% damage to the gland is necessary before direct pancreatic function tests yield reliably positive results. A direct pancreatic function test is most useful in patients with presumed CP in whom easily identifiable structural and functional abnormalities have not been demonstrated on more widely available diagnostic modalities such as CT or MRI, or when these imaging studies are equivocal. Despite their theoretical advantages, direct pancreatic function tests have several limitations. First, they have not been well standardized across institutions offering the test. Second, they are available at only a very few referral centers and so are not available to most clinicians seeing patients with CP. Third, it can be difficult for patients to tolerate unsedated placement of an oroduodenal tube for the hour or more required for the test. Fourth, accurate measurement of bicarbonate concentrations or enzyme output may be challenging. False-positive results have been reported in patients who have undergone Billroth II gastrectomy, in patients with diabetes, celiac disease, and cirrhosis, and in patients recovering from a recent attack of acute pancreatitis, making it difficult to generalize across the population.

There are variations of direct pancreatic function tests that may be easier for patients to tolerate (by sedating them) and might be able to be made more widely available. One variation is to collect pancreatic secretions at the time of ERCP by placement of a catheter directly in the pancreatic duct (the so-called intraductal secretin test). This test typically samples pancreatic output for only 15 minutes to minimize the likelihood of ERCP-induced pancreatitis. It is not standardized and does not appear to be as accurate as standard direct pancreatic function testing.[239] Another common variation of pancreatic function testing is to use sedation and a standard upper endoscope to take the place of the usual oroduodenal tube, with analysis of bicarbonate output using the regular hospital laboratory. This endoscopic variation appears to be nearly, although not quite, as accurate as standard direct pancreatic function testing.[226,240–243] Another variation of the test is to measure lipase output rather than bicarbonate output, with CCK as the secretagogue.[244] This variation appears to be less accurate than secretin-based pancreatic function testing. Like traditional pancreatic function testing, endoscopic-based pancreatic function tests have been compared to alternative diagnostic tests like ERCP,[245] with an overall agreement in 86% of patients and a high negative predictive value for endoscopic pancreatic function testing. The value of pancreatic function tests, whether traditional or endoscopic, lies in their high sensitivity and consequent ability to rule out CP.[225,240,243,246]

Indirect Tests

The desire to develop indirect tests of pancreatic function is an outgrowth of the complexity, discomfort, and limited availability of direct pancreatic function testing. Indirect tests generally measure pancreatic enzymes in blood or stool.

Pancreatic Enzymes in Stool

Fecal elastase-1 is the most used indirect measure of pancreatic function at this time. Levels less than 200 μg/g of stool are considered abnormal and suggestive of exocrine pancreatic insufficiency. Levels less than 100 μg/g of stool are considered evidence of exocrine pancreatic insufficiency. The test is reasonably accurate to detect pancreatic exocrine insufficiency in more advanced CP; however, it exhibits both low sensitivity and specificity in patients with indeterminate pancreatic disease or without history of pancreatic disease.[210,227,247,248] The major limitation of fecal elastase-1 is that it can be falsely low due to dilution in other diseases causing diarrhea, such as short bowel syndrome and small bowel bacterial overgrowth. This results in frequent false-positives among patients who have no history of pancreatic disease but diarrhea from other causes. The test should be performed on a solid or semisolid stool specimen that can be collected randomly. Fecal elastase measurement is widely available and can be performed through a home stool collection, which can then be delivered to a reference or commercial laboratory at numerous locations throughout the United States.

Fecal chymotrypsin is another substance that can be measured in random stool sample and is low in most patients with CP and steatorrhea. Low concentrations of either chymotrypsin or elastase in stool can reflect inadequate delivery of these pancreatic enzymes to the duodenum. Fecal chymotrypsin is also available from commercial laboratories. Like fecal elastase, false-positive results have been reported in other malabsorptive conditions (celiac disease, Crohn disease), in diarrheal diseases in which the stool is diluted, and in severe malnutrition. Because the test is usually normal in patients without steatorrhea, it is reliably positive only in advanced CP. It is notable that fecal elastase-1 has significant advantages over fecal chymotrypsin in that it is much more stable in passage through stool and is easier to measure.

Serum Trypsinogen

Serum trypsinogen (often called serum trypsin) can be measured in blood and provides a rough estimation of pancreatic function. Abnormally low levels of serum trypsinogen can be seen in patients with advanced CP with steatorrhea.[249] Serum trypsin is not decreased in patients with other forms of steatorrhea, but low levels of serum trypsinogen may be seen in patients with pancreatic ductal obstruction, including malignant obstruction. The test is available through commercial laboratories, but each has different normal ranges.

Fecal Fat Excretion

Maldigestion of fat is detectable when pancreatic lipase secretory capacity is quite impaired. An evaluation of pancreatic lipase action is the measurement of fecal fat excretion during a 72-hour collection of stool. Although theoretically quite simple, the test is difficult to perform in practice. The patient must follow a diet containing 100 g/day of fat for at least 3 days before the test and the 3 days after the test, and complete collection of the sample is difficult to achieve. In health, less than 7 g of fat (7% of the ingested dose) should be present in stool. Measuring fecal fat requires that the dietary content of fat be known exactly, which is difficult to ascertain for most patients in the outpatient setting. A qualitative analysis of fecal fat can also be performed with a Sudan III stain of a random specimen of stool. The finding of more than six globules per high-power field is considered a positive result, but as with fecal fat excretion, the patient must be ingesting adequate fat to allow measurable steatorrhea. Sudan III staining of stool is positive only in patients with substantial steatorrhea.[227,228]

Tests of Pancreatic Structure (Imaging)

Plain Abdominal Radiography

The finding of diffuse (but not focal) pancreatic calcifications on plain abdominal films is quite specific for CP. Focal calcifications may be seen in cystic and islet cell tumors of the pancreas and in peripancreatic vascular calcifications. Calcifications occur late in the natural history of CP and may take from 5 to 25 years to develop.[68,69,156] Calcifications are most common in alcoholic, late-onset idiopathic, hereditary, and tropical pancreatitis and far less common in early-onset idiopathic pancreatitis. Accelerations of the clinical course of CP and subsequent calcifications are particularly common in patients who smoke.[51–56,85,92,250]

Abdominal Ultrasound

US has been widely studied as a diagnostic tool for CP. This modality is limited in that the pancreas (and particularly the pancreatic head) cannot be adequately visualized in many patients owing to overlying bowel gas or body habitus. Ultrasonographic findings indicative of CP include dilation of the pancreatic duct, shadowing pancreatic ductal stones, gland atrophy, irregular gland margins, pseudocysts, and changes in the parenchymal echotexture (see Table 61.2). Most studies suggest a sensitivity of 50%–80% with a specificity of 80%–90%.[251] In a study directly comparing transabdominal ultrasonography with CT, ERCP, and EUS, the accuracy of US was 56%.[252] In this study, some abnormality (such as changes in parenchymal echotexture) was noted on US in 40% of patients who had a normal pancreas as defined by the other diagnostic tests. A large screening study of transabdominal US in Japan encompassing 130,000 examinations found increased echogenicity, mild dilation of the pancreatic duct, small cystic cavities, and even ductal calcification in the absence of clinical features of CP.[253] The majority of these abnormalities could not be attributed to CP and were instead attributed to aging. These studies suggest that there is a large spectrum of ultrasonographic findings in normal individuals and that it can be difficult to distinguish normal (or age-related) variability from CP if the visualized changes are mild. Although relatively inexpensive and safe, transabdominal US is not generally useful in the evaluation of patients with suspected CP. The finding of a normal pancreas or moderate to marked changes of advanced CP can be diagnostic, but mild changes of CP are less specific and must be interpreted in light of the clinical history and the patient's age. US can be useful in screening for complications of CP (e.g., pseudocyst or bile duct obstruction) and in evaluating for other conditions that might mimic the symptoms of CP (i.e., biliary tract disease).

Computed Tomography

The overall sensitivity of CT for CP is between 75% and 90%, with a specificity of 85% or more.[251,252,254] CT is able to image the pancreas in essentially all patients and hence has a substantial advantage over US. Table 61.3 outlines the diagnostic abnormalities seen on CT in CP. Like all diagnostic tests, CT is most accurate in advanced CP after substantial structural changes have developed (Fig. 61.4). Although CT is more expensive than US and exposes the patient to ionizing radiation, it is more sensitive and more specific. One finding of unknown significance seen on CT is the presence of fatty replacement of the pancreas.[255,256] This condition, variously termed fatty pancreas, pancreatic lipodystrophy, nonalcoholic fatty pancreas disease, and others, may be related to metabolic syndrome, obesity, aging, or other unknown factors and is in itself not a specific finding of CP. While it has been associated with numerous other pancreatic and extrapancreatic conditions, its contribution to causation or pathophysiology of pancreatic disease remains unknown.[257]

Magnetic Resonance Imaging

MRI, coupled with MRCP, is as accurate, and probably more so, than CT in patients with CP.[251,254,258] MRCP results agree with ERCP results in about 90% of cases.[240,243] Agreement between MRCP and ERCP is less common in areas where the pancreatic duct is small (tail of pancreas and side branches) or when the ductal changes are more subtle. Improved visualization of the pancreatic duct can be achieved by administering secretin.[251,258–261] In addition, signal intensity (usually on T1 imaging) and arterial enhancement ratios can be obtained using gadolinium as a contrast agent, which may improve the ability to image the gland.[258,262] Finally, a qualitative or semiquantitative assessment of fluid output from the pancreas to the duodenum can be made during MRCP after secretin injection (S-MRCP), which may allow estimation of pancreatic secretory function.[258,263,264]

TABLE 61.3 Grading of Chronic Pancreatitis by US or CT

Grade	US or CT Findings
Normal	No abnormal findings on a good-quality study visualizing the entire gland
Equivocal	One of the following: Mild dilatation of the pancreatic duct (2–4 mm) in the body of the gland Gland enlargement less than or equal to twofold normal
Mild-moderate	One of the preceding findings plus at least one of the following: Pancreatic duct dilatation (>4 mm) Pancreatic duct irregularity Cavity (ies) <10 mm Parenchymal heterogeneity Increased echogenicity of duct wall Irregular contour of the head or body Focal necrosis or loss of parenchyma
Severe	Mild/moderate features plus one or more of the following: Cavity (ies) >10 mm Intraductal filling defects Calculi/pancreatic calcification Ductal obstruction (stricture) Severe duct dilatation or irregularity Contiguous organ invasion

CT, Computed tomography; *US*, ultrasound.
Adapted from Sarner M, Cotton PB. Classification of pancreatitis. *Gut*. 1984;25:756.

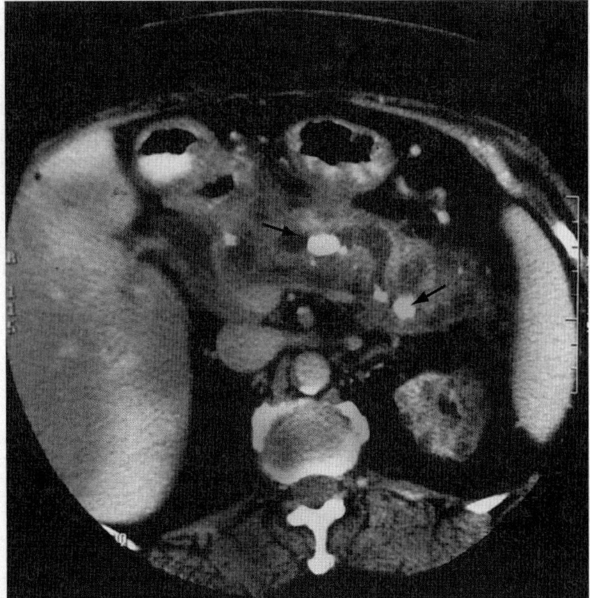

Fig. 61.4 CT demonstrating several large, densely calcified stones (*arrows*) within a markedly dilated pancreatic duct in long-standing chronic pancreatitis.

Secretin-MRCP has been compared with endoscopic-based pancreatic function testing.[264] Abnormalities on MRCP were seen in 8/23 patients with a normal pancreatic function test, suggesting secretin-MRCP may have a significant false-positive rate. Some analyses suggest that just measuring volume after secretin stimulation, instead of bicarbonate concentration, is too inaccurate to be clinically useful.[265] One study also compared MRI findings with histology in a group of patients undergoing total pancreatectomy for noncalcific CP.[266] Using a cutoff of ≥2 MRI features only reached 65% sensitivity and 89% specificity; the strongest predictors of CP were pancreatic duct irregularity, T1-weighted signal intensity, and duodenal filling after secretin. T1-weighted signal intensity has continued to show promise in recent studies both as a solo marker and in combination with other markers as a marker of the presence and severity of CP.[267,268] It is important to remember as a limitation of this modality that although MRI is widely available, not all centers have the capacity to perform high-quality MRCP or S-MRCP.

Endoscopic Retrograde Cholangiopancreatography

Pancreatography has been considered the most specific and sensitive test of pancreatic structure. It also has the advantage over all previously discussed tests in that therapy (e.g., pancreatic duct stenting, stone extraction) may be administered. The disadvantage, however, is that ERCP is the riskiest diagnostic test, with complications occurring in at least 5% of patients (in as many as 20% of certain subgroups) and a mortality rate of 0.1%–0.5%. In most studies in patients with CP, the sensitivity of ERCP is between 70% and 90%, with a specificity of 80%–100%.[251,252,269] Thus CP can exist in the absence of any visible changes within the pancreatic duct.[1,229,238,245,251,269–271]

The diagnostic features of CP on ERCP are well established (Table 61.4).[272,273] The diagnosis is based on abnormalities seen in the main pancreatic duct and the side branches. ERCP is highly sensitive and specific in patients with advanced disease. The appearance of a massively dilated pancreatic duct with alternating strictures (the chain-of-lakes appearance) is a classic appearance of advanced CP (Fig. 61.5). Less dramatic pancreatographic changes are less definitive and specific, and nuance is required to place these changes within the clinical context to make the diagnosis (Fig. 61.6). The accurate interpretation of an ERCP requires a study of adequate quality (filled to the second generation of the side branches and without significant movement artifact) and the capability to obtain radiographic images of high resolution. Many pancreatograms do not meet these criteria for an adequate study.[269] An underfilled pancreatic duct can appear to have an irregular duct margin (leading to overdiagnosis of CP) or might not delineate changes within the inadequately filled side branches (leading to underdiagnosis of CP).

TABLE 61.4 Cambridge Grading of Chronic Pancreatitis on Endoscopic Retrograde Pancreatography

Grade	Main Pancreatic Duct	Side Branches
Normal	Normal with filling of duct to side branches	Normal
Equivocal	Normal	<3 Abnormal
Mild	Normal	≥3 Abnormal
Moderate	Abnormal	≥3 Abnormal
Severe	Abnormal with at least 1 of the following: Large cavity (>10 mm) Obstruction or stricture Filling defect(s) Severe dilatation or irregularity	≥3 Abnormal

Adapted from Axon ATR, Classen M, Cotton PB, et al. Pancreatography in chronic pancreatitis: international definitions. *Gut*. 1984;25:1107–1112.

The pancreatic duct abnormalities characteristic of CP can be seen in other conditions. The most common is the effect of aging on the pancreatic duct. Although pancreatic function is well preserved in normal aging, impressive abnormalities may develop in the pancreatic duct. They include focal or diffuse dilatation of the main pancreatic duct and its side branches, the development of cystic cavities, and even ductal calculi.[142,143,269,274,275] In the large screening US study mentioned previously, 50% of all calcification and more than 80% of ductal dilation and cystic lesions seen were

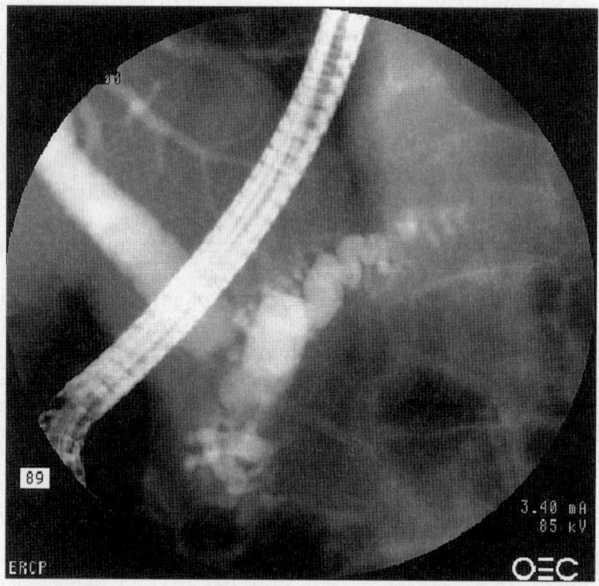

Fig. 61.5 Endoscopic retrograde pancreatogram showing a markedly dilated pancreatic duct with alternating strictures and dilatation. This "chain-of-lakes" appearance is diagnostic of chronic pancreatitis.

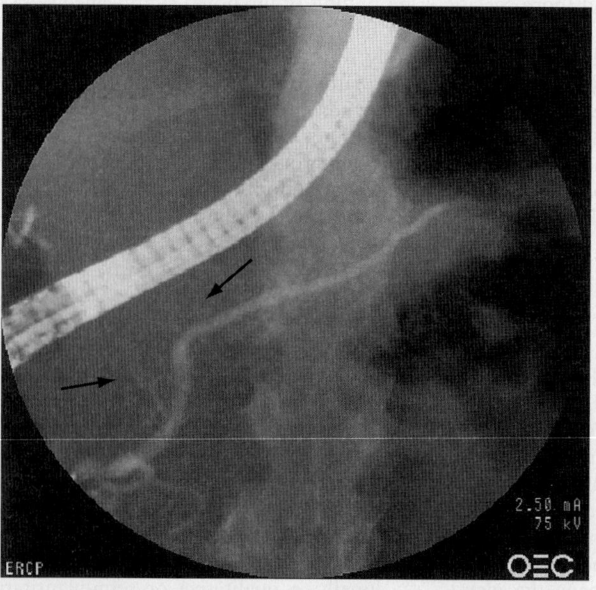

Fig. 61.6 Endoscopic retrograde pancreatogram demonstrating subtle changes limited to the side branches (*arrows*) in a patient in whom a direct pancreatic function (secretin) test indicated chronic pancreatitis. These subtle findings are generally not sufficient for a definitive diagnosis of chronic pancreatitis.

believed to be attributable to aging, not CP.[253] Whether these changes represent the consequences of the normal wear and tear on the pancreas during life is not known. Temporary changes in the pancreatic duct may also occur after an episode of acute pancreatitis and may take months to resolve.[269] Pancreatic carcinoma may produce changes within the pancreatic duct that resemble those of CP. Finally, the placement of pancreatic duct stents can produce new abnormalities within the pancreatic duct that mimic CP and that may not entirely resolve after stent removal.[269,276,277] Pancreatic stents are placed to prevent post-ERCP pancreatitis. These temporary, very small-caliber stents used for these purposes appear to rarely produce these ductal changes.[278]

There is significant potential for substantial interobserver and intraobserver variability in the interpretation of ERCP.[269] Some abnormalities, such as a dilated pancreatic duct, abnormal duct contour, and abnormal side branches, are very clear, but there is subjective interpretation of images, and there are no absolute criteria to differentiate normal from abnormal or normal variant.[273] Much of the intraobserver and interobserver variability in ERCP evaluations is related to the interpretation of mild or subtle pancreatographic changes rather than dramatic abnormalities.[142,279] This is the most substantial clinical problem related to ERCP as a diagnostic tool; subtle or minor abnormalities of the pancreatic duct are quite nonspecific and are not reliable markers of CP.

Given the risk of ERCP and the availability of alternative methods to image the pancreatic duct (MRCP or EUS), ERCP should be used only when therapy is planned and not used as a diagnostic tool in patients with presumed CP.

Endoscopic Ultrasound

EUS allows a highly detailed examination of pancreatic parenchyma and the pancreatic duct by overcoming the imaging problems in transabdominal US (such as intervening gas in the bowel lumen). The traditional diagnostic system (MST or minimal standard terminology) is based on the presence of abnormalities in the pancreatic duct and the parenchyma (Table 61.5). These features may be individually classified as none, minimal, moderate, or extensive but in practice are generally only graded as present or absent, and the total number of features is used as the score. The sensitivity and specificity of the test are determined by the threshold total score used to define CP. A large range of threshold scores has been used, ranging from 1 to 6. Most studies have used the presence of three or more features to define a positive result.[251,270,280–282] A second diagnostic system termed the Rosemont criteria is also used for EUS diagnosis of CP (see Table 61.5). This was developed through expert consensus and includes major and minor criteria, with an attempt to provide semiquantification of severity. Despite the development of this new scoring system, interobserver agreement still remains a limitation of this modality for diagnosis of CP, especially at early stages of the disease.[254,270,280–285] Intraobserver agreement seems to be high, unlike ERCP.[286]

EUS has been compared with pancreatic histology in a limited number of patients. One study compared EUS features with histology in 71 patients who underwent surgical therapy for presumed CP.[287] Utilizing a cutoff of more than 3 EUS criteria, the sensitivity of EUS was 83% and the specificity was 57%. In a subgroup with more advanced histologic evidence of CP by histology, the sensitivity was 83% and specificity 80%. No single EUS criteria predicted fibrosis better than any other, but there was a general correlation between the number of EUS criteria and the histologic severity of disease. Another study in 42 patients who underwent EUS prior to pancreatic surgery (largely for carcinoma) determined a cutoff of more than 4 EUS criteria had a sensitivity of 90% and specificity of 86%.[288] A study in 25 patients noted that pancreatic fibrosis correlated with the EUS score and that an abnormal EUS (≥4 criteria) had a sensitivity of 84%.[289] A study of 50 patients with chronic abdominal pain undergoing total pancreatectomy for

TABLE 61.5 Diagnosis of Chronic Pancreatitis on EUS

Standard MST EUS Grading System		**Rosemont Criteria for EUS Diagnosis**	
Parenchymal abnormalities	Hyperechoic foci Hyperechoic strands Lobularity of contour Cysts	Major features	Hyperechoic foci with shadowing (Major A) Main pancreatic duct calculi (Major A) Lobularity with honeycombing (Major B)
Ductal abnormalities	Main duct dilatation Main duct irregularity Hyperechoic ductal walls Visible side branches Calcification	Minor features	Lobularity without honeycombing Hyperechoic foci without shadowing Stranding Cysts Irregular main pancreatic duct contour Main pancreatic duct dilation Hyperechoic duct margin Dilated side branches
In the standard EUS system, each finding counts equally and the score is the total number of findings. In the Rosemont system, the diagnostic strata are as follows:			
Most consistent with chronic pancreatitis		1 Major A feature and ≥3 minor features or 1 Major A feature and 1 Major B feature or 2 Major A features	
Suggestive of chronic pancreatitis		1 Major A feature and <3 minor features or Major B feature and ≥3 minor features or ≥5 minor features	
Indeterminate for chronic pancreatitis		3–4 minor features or Major B feature with <3 minor features	
Normal		≤2 minor features	

EUS, Endoscopic ultrasound; *MST*, minimal standard terminology.

noncalcific CP compared Rosemont criteria to histology.[290] There was noted to be relatively close correlation between MST and Rosemont systems, but rather poor correlation of either system with histology. In the analysis, more than half of those with a normal Rosemont score had histologic evidence of CP, whereas 80% of those with "indeterminate" features had CP, and almost all of those with "suggestive" features had CP. A study using EUS-guided Tru-cut biopsy of the pancreas noted poor agreement between EUS and histology, but the histologic specimens obtained were small and likely not representative of the entire gland.[291]

EUS and ERCP agree in about 80% of patients.[251,269,270,292–296] EUS has also been compared with standard and intraductal direct pancreatic function testing. The agreement between these tests varies widely in these studies, ranging from 10% to 90%.[243,269,270,295–297] This variability is partly related to the severity of disease and spectrum bias. The agreement is best in those with more advanced disease. In one study the sensitivity of EUS for advanced CP (classic findings on ERCP and an abnormal pancreatic function test) was good (sensitivity of 73% and specificity of 81% using more than 3 criteria), but the sensitivity for less advanced CP was only 10%.[297]

In the majority of instances in which EUS findings disagree with results of other diagnostic tests, it is the EUS findings that are abnormal when the other tests are normal.[298] This speaks to the question of the specificity of EUS. Specificity is determined by the cutoff chosen, and in this instance, it is degraded by other conditions that can mimic the EUS findings of CP. This may be a substantial conundrum, because EUS changes of CP are frequently encountered. The edema associated with a recent episode of acute pancreatitis can make duct margins and intralobular septa more apparent, which will reduce specificity.[270] Age-related changes can be observed in the pancreas by EUS that mimic the changes of CP.[299] Chronic alcohol and tobacco use can produce similar changes, in the absence of clinical CP.[270,300–302] In one study, 39% of patients with unexplained dyspepsia had five or more EUS features of CP, and 34% of controls had three or more features.[303] It is unlikely that CP is present or will develop in all or even most of these patients.

The diagnosis of CP by EUS is based on the interpretation of sonographic images. It remains unclear as to whether the presence of three or four (or fewer) EUS features, in the absence of corroborating information from other diagnostic tests, is adequate for a conclusive diagnosis of CP to be made.[243,269,298,304,305] Resolution of this issue will require long follow-up of patients, given the lack of a useful gold standard, and some studies show limited ability of EUS to predict the ultimate development of clear-cut CP.[298] Advances in EUS imaging, including the use of contrast, digital image analysis, and EUS elastography, are being studied but have not yet been shown to improve diagnostic accuracy,[305] and these techniques may have the most applicability to assessing mass lesions in the pancreas.[116]

EUS is highly accurate in patients with advanced CP (Fig. 61.7). An EUS score of greater than 5 (using MST criteria) is relatively specific for CP. A completely normal or near normal EUS (0–2 criteria) makes CP unlikely.[304,305] EUS scores of 3 or 4 should be considered indeterminate and should be interpreted in light of the patients' clinical features and with recognition of the effect of alcohol, tobacco, age, and other associated conditions (diabetes, chronic kidney disease) that can mimic the changes of CP.

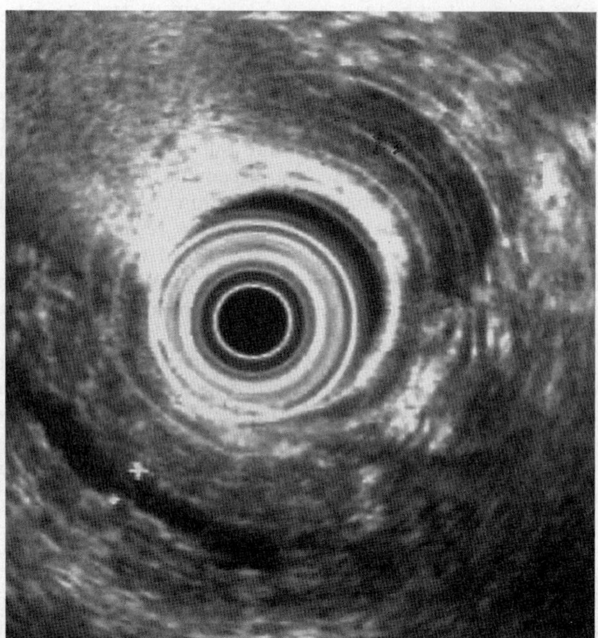

Fig. 61.7 EUS image of the pancreatic body in a patient with chronic pancreatitis. The markers on the dilated pancreatic duct demonstrate hyperechoic margins, one of the diagnostic features of chronic pancreatitis. The parenchyma surrounding these markers demonstrates hyperechoic strands and foci, additional features of chronic pancreatitis.

DIAGNOSTIC STRATEGY

The diagnosis of CP is most often suspected due to the presence of an abdominal pain syndrome and less commonly due to a suspicion of exocrine (diarrhea, steatorrhea, weight loss) or endocrine insufficiency (diabetes mellitus). In the subgroup with suspected exocrine or endocrine insufficiency, the disease is likely to be long-standing, and most available diagnostic tests will be able to detect this relatively far-advanced disease. Because other conditions may mimic CP (pancreatic malignancy, intraductal papillary mucinous neoplasms, cystic neoplasms), a high-quality cross-sectional imaging test is necessary to rule out these other possible diseases. A high-quality CT scan using multidetector technology and a pancreatic protocol or an MRI with MRCP are the best initial diagnostic tests.[243,269,304,305] Many of these patients may have already had a routine abdominal CT (often through an emergency department) but have not had a high-quality CT with contrast administered at phases specifically timed to evaluate the pancreas (or MRI with MRCP), so it may be worthwhile to repeat them if the previous studies are of low quality. If the CT or MRI does not demonstrate CP, then tests of maximum sensitivity should be used next. Because direct pancreatic function tests are not widely available, EUS is the most reasonable next step. Hormonal stimulation pancreatic function testing, if available, could logically be used next if EUS findings are equivocal.[1,269,304] This may require referral of the patient to a center performing function tests. ERCP should not be used for diagnostic purposes. If the diagnosis remains in doubt, follow-up over time with periodic reassessment may be the best diagnostic approach. In some patients, a system such as the M-ANNHEIM multiple risk factor classification system may help to assess the risk factors at play and even track the natural history of disease as it evolves or declares itself.[306] New diagnostic biomarkers are needed, and large studies are underway to identify predictors of the development of CP and its complications.[307]

TREATMENT

Abdominal Pain

Abdominal pain is the most debilitating symptom of CP and affects over 80% of patients over the course of their disease.[308] It is also the major driver of morbidity in the disease and moves patients to seek care, including both medical and invasive interventions that hold promise of potential pain relief.

It should be highlighted that there exists no cure for CP, nor medication or intervention to truly slow or stop progression. Treatment is therefore limited to symptom management, and numerous consensus guidelines have been agreed upon, aiming to standardize the progression of treatment strategies in this challenging patient population.[171,175,309,310] Similar to other chronic pain conditions, the first step is to quantify the severity, character, and temporal nature of pain and the impact on quality of life. Recent development of disease-specific tools such as the Comprehensive Pain Assessment Tool for CP has streamlined this process and has the potential to shed light on triggers, efficacy of current treatment, and burden of pain.[311] Any contributing factors to disease progression should be addressed as a foundation of therapy, including alcohol and tobacco abstinence and therapy for metabolic factors, including uncontrolled hypertriglyceridemia, hyperglycemia, or hypercalcemia. In concordance with the World Health Organization analgesic ladder, an attempt at medical therapy utilizing low-potency analgesics should be tried first. The addition of pancreatic enzyme supplementation and antioxidants as part of medical therapy may be tried, although the data supporting their effectiveness in reducing pain is limited. In those with an inadequate response, more potent narcotic analgesics coupled with an adjunctive agent (such as a gabapentinoid, SSRI, or SNRI) should be considered. If this is ineffective, the next therapeutic decision hinges on whether the pancreatic duct is dilated. In those with a dilated pancreatic duct, endoscopic or surgical therapy should be considered. The choice of endoscopic or surgical therapy and the type of surgical therapy depends on patient choice, available expertise, and pancreatic anatomy, including degree of ductal dilation. In those with a nondilated pancreatic duct, continued medical therapy is appropriate, with consideration of total pancreatectomy and islet cell auto-transplantation only for very selected patients with refractory pain symptoms. It is noted that the placebo response in CP pain trials has been found to be at least 20%.[312]

Cessation of Alcohol and Tobacco

Continued alcohol abuse in patients with alcoholic CP hastens the development of pancreatic dysfunction and increases mortality.[15,18,87,313] While complete abstinence alone does not prevent progression of disease,[313] many studies have documented a decrease in pain or painful relapses in patients who stop drinking alcohol.[314,315] Tobacco smoking has been associated with a lower quality of life in CP patients, making cessation a clear priority in this population with high smoking prevalence.[91,93] Cessation of smoking appears to have even more benefits, in both preventing tobacco-induced illness and in reducing the risk of secondary pancreatic carcinoma.[15,18,50–53,316] Strategies and treatments offered to individual patients for tobacco cessation have taken numerous forms but are largely unsuccessful; policy changes appear to have had the biggest impact on smoking cessation in this population.[317,318]

Medical Therapy

Analgesics

The majority of patients with CP require some form of analgesia to treat pain from their disease.[166] Some patients' pain may be managed with acetaminophen or nonsteroidal anti-inflammatory medications, but many require more potent analgesia, including opioid agents. While efforts to minimize opioid use are appropriate, they should not be withheld in patients with severe pain. An escalating analgesic pain ladder concept can be used to describe the progressive analgesic escalation in CP.[319] Over half of CP patients in the United States are maintained on chronic opioid therapy.[166]

If nonopioid agents have failed to control pain, it is appropriate to begin with lower-potency opioid agents like tramadol. Tramadol is a dual-action analgesic with mu-opioid agonistic and monoaminergic properties. High dosages of tramadol are equivalent to oral morphine in treating CP, with fewer effects on gut motility.[175,227,320] In the situation where gradual increase in opioid dosage is needed to control pain, it is important to focus the patient on the goal of pain control at an acceptable level rather than complete relief of pain. There is a risk of addiction associated with opioid use. Although the risk has not been well defined, awareness and recognition of the potential for opioid use disorder and treatment as well as selection of alternative analgesic agents are important aspects of pain control in this population.[166,321]

Adjunctive agents are a critical part of therapy. Neuropathic pain is a significant contributor to the pain experience in CP for many patients,[174] Gabapentin and pregabalin (α_2d subunit voltage-gated N-type calcium channel inhibitors) have been effectively used in CP to reduce pain and should be considered in patients where a neuropathic component to pain is suspected.[171,175] In one randomized trial in patients with CP requiring narcotics for pain control, pregabalin reduced pain at a dosage of up to 300 mg twice daily.[322] Side effects of gabapentinoids, including dizziness and a feeling of being intoxicated, are common, and dosing should be adjusted to avoid these.

Additional psychotropic medications as adjunctive agents have not been rigorously studied, but they are commonly used in patients with continued severe pain from CP to improve pain control and minimize the dosage and potency of narcotics. Concomitant symptoms of anxiety and depression are common in CP, and the presence of these symptoms has been associated with higher pain severity, higher pain interference with daily activities, and a higher CP symptom burden.[158] A genetic basis for this association may exist: genetic loci for depression have been associated with constant, severe pain in CP, adding another dimension to the clinical association that has been well described.[323] Tricyclic antidepressants can be useful adjuncts, not only by treating depression and potentially modulating central pain perception but also because they have direct effects on pain and potentiate the effect of narcotics. Other antidepressants such as serotonin reuptake inhibitors (SSRIs) and combined serotonin and norepinephrine reuptake inhibitors (e.g., duloxetine) may also have this effect.[171,175] There is little data on the effect of marijuana or its components as adjunctive treatment for pain. A single retrospective study evaluating patients enrolled in a state-monitored therapeutic cannabis program in New Hampshire showed decreased mean daily opioid use, hospitalization rates, and emergency department visit rates compared with patients not enrolled in the program, though these reductions were not statistically significant.[324] A phase 2 study of tetrahydrocannabinol in a mixed cohort of patients with chronic pain secondary to surgery or CP showed no statistically difference from placebo in pain reduction at 50 days from enrollment.[325] Additional studies are needed to better understand the potential and limitations of marijuana and its components for painful CP.

Antioxidants

Damage by free radicals is one mechanism for pancreatic damage in alcoholic and other forms of CP. Patients with CP (particularly alcoholic) have evidence of oxidant stress and reduced antioxidant capacity.[66,106,175,326] Oxidant stress is also a strong activator of pancreatic stellate cells.[45–47] In one large study from India,[327] a significant reduction in number of painful days/month was seen in the antioxidant group (7.3 fewer days per month, compared to 3.2 fewer in the placebo group). This trial recruited subjects who were relatively young, underweight, and suffered from mainly idiopathic or tropical pancreatitis. The trial used a combination of selenium, beta-carotene, vitamin C, vitamin E, and methionine. A randomized, double-blinded, placebo-controlled trial of combination antioxidant therapy plus pregabalin after clearance of an obstructed pancreatic duct enrolled 87 patients and showed significant pain reduction in pain intensity in the treatment group that persisted even at 6 months after intervention.[328]

A trial from the United Kingdom[329] used higher dosages of the same antioxidants as in the first Indian trial but recruited a population that was older, not malnourished, and suffered from CP mainly due to alcohol and smoking. This trial demonstrated no benefit from antioxidant therapy, despite improvements in serum levels of these antioxidants. A review of all the available evidence noted a slight reduction in overall pain score.[330] The overall effect of antioxidants is therefore limited, and they are not widely used in the United States.[167]

Pancreatic Enzyme Therapy

Pancreatic secretion is under feedback control by the presence of pancreatic proteases and nutrients in the duodenum. The use of pancreatic enzymes to reduce pain is based on the ability of these agents to activate this feedback control system in a way to reduce pancreatic secretion. Delivering proteases to the duodenum or very proximal jejunum can suppress pancreatic secretion. This action is due to the ability of the proteases in this segment of small bowel to reduce CCK release, by destroying an intestinal CCK-releasing factor, which is one of the primary stimulants of CCK release in the presence of nutrients. In patients with CP, the lack of delivery of proteases to the duodenum could allow more CCK-releasing factor to escape denaturing. As a result, one would expect higher levels of CCK-releasing factor within the duodenum and higher serum levels of CCK. Higher levels of circulating CCK could stimulate the pancreas to secrete, with this stimulation potentially leading to pancreatic pain by raising pancreatic duct or tissue pressure or by forcing digestive enzymes into the interstitium if secretion is occurring against pancreatic ductal obstruction. The oral administration of pancreatic enzymes could restore normal feedback suppression of pancreatic secretion by providing active serine proteases in the duodenum, which could again denature the CCK-releasing factor, thereby reducing the hyperstimulation and relieving pain.

As described in Chapter 58, pancreatic secretion of volume and bicarbonate is not controlled by the presence of proteases within the duodenum. Also, pancreatic secretion is under humoral as well as neural control. Therefore, suppressing pancreatic enzyme release by administering oral enzyme supplements is not likely to produce complete suppression of secretion, and the magnitude of the effect on secretion could vary from patient to patient. The presence of this feedback control system, which can control pancreatic enzyme secretion, is well documented in humans without CP as well as in some patients with CP.[331] One marker of this disordered feedback system might be elevations in serum CCK in patients with CP, particularly those with pain. Elevations in serum CCK are seen in only some patients with CP. It is likely that this disordered feedback, as in all presumed causes of pain, is potentially only important in a subgroup of patients.

Several small randomized, prospective, double-blind trials have attempted to delineate the effectiveness of orally administered pancreatic enzymes to decrease pain in patients with CP. Two studies using enzymes in nonenteric-coated (tablet) form reported a benefit.[332,333] Four other studies using enteric-coated microsphere preparations showed no benefit.[334–337] The difference between these studies may reflect patient selection but may also reflect the different choice of enzyme preparations (Table 61.6). The feedback-sensitive part of the small bowel appears to be the most proximal portion, and enteric-coated preparations may not release most of their proteases until they reach the more distal small bowel. Nonenteric-coated enzymes might therefore be needed for adequate delivery of serine proteases to the duodenum. Analyses of these studies combining the two enzyme types concluded that enzymes do not reduce pain,[338,339] but the combined analysis methodology may not be appropriate in this instance given the proposed mechanism just discussed. Nonetheless, enzymes are used widely to treat pain in these patients.[167] Because nonenteric-coated enzymes can be inactivated by gastric acid, the concomitant use of an agent to suppress gastric acid or neutralize acid is suggested. In the two studies that demonstrated effectiveness, patients with less advanced disease (without a dilated pancreatic duct, calcifications, and steatorrhea), women, and patients with idiopathic CP had the best response. There is only one nonenteric-coated preparation in the United States. A dosage of approximately 150,000 units of protease 4 times daily (2 tablets of Viokace 20,800 4 times daily with meals and at night) is used. A trial of enzymes for pain is rarely successful in those with advanced CP with diffuse calcifications or a dilated pancreatic duct, although these patients often need enzyme replacement for pancreatic exocrine insufficiency.

Endoscopic Therapy

The primary goal of endoscopic therapy is to improve drainage of the pancreatic duct by relieving ductal obstruction (see Chapter 63). Endoscopic therapy is limited to a subgroup of patients with amenable pancreatic ductal anatomy. These are generally patients with a dilated pancreatic duct (>5 mm) with a single or dominant stricture or an obstructing stone in the head of the pancreas, with dilation of the pancreatic duct upstream of the obstruction. It is important to remember, however, that some patients with pancreatic duct dilation have little or no clinical symptoms,[184] and that a dilated duct does not necessarily correlate with elevations in duct pressure. Strictures and calculi in the upstream body or tail of the gland are not generally amenable to endoscopic therapy as they are too far from the tip of the endoscope to allow therapy. Specific endoscopic therapies that have been studied are pancreatic sphincterotomy, stent placement, and stone extraction (sometimes coupled with lithotripsy). The individual contribution of each of these therapies is difficult to quantify because they are usually performed together.

Pancreatic Duct Sphincterotomy

Pancreatic duct sphincterotomy is required for larger-caliber pancreatic stent placement and for pancreatic duct stone

TABLE 61.6 Enzyme Products for the Treatment of Chronic Pancreatitis

Product	Formulation	Lipase Content/Pill or Capsule (USP Units)
Creon	Enteric-coated porcine capsule	3000, 6000, 12,000, 24,000, 36,000
Zenpep	Enteric-coated porcine capsule	3000, 5000, 10,000, 15,000, 20,000, 25,000, 40,000
Pancreaze	Enteric-coated porcine capsule	4200, 10,500, 16,800, 21,000
Pertzye	Enteric-coated porcine with bicarbonate	4000, 8000, 16,000
Viokase	Nonenteric-coated porcine tablet[a]	10,440, 20,880

[a]Nonenteric-coated agents require co-treatment with a histamine-2 receptor antagonist or proton pump inhibitor to avoid denaturation of enzymes by gastric acid.

The total dosage of lipase per meal should be titrated based on response but usually requires 40,000–90,000 units of lipase per meal and one-half that amount with snacks. The dosage should be split equally during the meal.

extraction. This may be performed with a pull-type sphincterotome or with a needle-knife sphincterotome over a small-caliber pancreatic duct stent.[340] Both techniques are used depending on local preferences. Major papilla pancreatic sphincterotomy alone as a therapy would be applicable only in patients in whom longstanding cicatricial stenosis of the sphincter has produced obstructive CP, a form of CP that is exceedingly rare. There is no evidence to support sphincter of Oddi dysfunction as a cause or contributor to CP,[341] and its contribution to acute relapsing pancreatitis remains controversial.[342–344] There are no data to support the performance of sphincter of Oddi manometry and manometry-guided therapy in patients with CP. Very rarely, patients with pancreas divisum present with marked upstream dilation of the dorsal pancreatic duct and CP. Sphincterotomy of the minor papilla over a stent in this setting may be useful, but minor papilla sphincterotomy for chronic pain in the absence of dorsal pancreatic ductal dilation is ineffective. In addition, patients with symptomatic pancreatitis and pancreas divisum often have underlying genetic mutations that explain the pancreatitis,[134,135] making the role and effect of endoscopic therapy even more difficult to define.

Stent Placement

Stent placement in the pancreatic duct, discussed in detail in Chapter 63, is most often performed to dilate and bypass an obstructing stricture (Fig. 61.8). A number of retrospective case series of stent therapy from expert centers report endoscopic success (successful placement of the stent) in close to 90% and pain improvement in about one-half to two-thirds of patients.[345–347] The high rates of endoscopic success reflect the high degree of expertise from these centers and the stringent patient selection, but successful endoscopic therapy may not lead to pain relief. In the largest multicenter report involving more than 1000 patients, 57% of patients with a single dominant stricture in the head of the pancreas who underwent stenting had significant improvement in pain at a mean follow-up of 4.9 years, with an additional 19% noting significant pain improvement but still requiring ongoing endoscopic therapy.[346] Complications of stent therapy occur in about 20% of patients, with a mortality rate of 0.6%.[345–347] The most commonly reported complications are clogging of stents (producing recurrent pain, attacks of acute pancreatitis, or pancreatic sepsis), inward stent migration (which may require surgical extraction), and ductal perforation. New stent-induced strictures of the pancreatic duct occur in these patients but are generally not of clinical significance (unlike those who develop these strictures in a normal preexisting duct).

One might assume that patients with pain relief after stent placement would be those with high pancreatic duct pressures and that stent therapy reduced this pressure. In one study that measured pain relief and pancreatic duct pressure after stenting, three of nine patients with normal pressure at the end of the stenting period still had pain, whereas none of four patients with continued high pressure in the pancreatic duct still had pain.[181] Pain improvement is similar whether pancreatic duct diameter (a surrogate marker for a decrease in pancreatic duct pressure) decreased or not after stenting, and pain relief may not be affected by occlusion of the stent.[182] It does not seem that the response to stent therapy is predictable from measurements of intraductal pressure or by the initial duct diameter. The decision to remove the stents entirely is therefore most often based on symptoms rather than changes in duct diameter of drainage. Even in expert centers, about one in four patients requires surgery for failure of endoscopic therapy.[182,345–347] Symptoms recur in one-third to one-half of patients after an initial clinical response.

Pancreatic Duct Stone Removal

The endoscopic removal of pancreatic duct stones can be difficult and is possible in only a subset of patients. Multiple stones, large stones, stones in the body and tail of the gland, stones in side branches, impacted stones, or stones behind a tight pancreatic duct stricture are generally not manageable with endoscopic techniques. The removal of large or impacted stones requires lithotripsy, using extracorporeal shock-wave lithotripsy (ESWL) primarily, or intraductal lithotripsy devices. There is no close correlation between the presence of pancreatic duct stones and pain, and many patients with pancreatic ductal stones have no pain. Most retrospective case series report success rates in carefully selected patients in whom endoscopic stone extraction seems feasible. In an analysis of 27 published studies on ESWL encompassing 3189 patients, complete duct clearance ranged from 16% to 88%,[348] with an average of about 71%. Partial duct clearance occurred in an additional 22%, and stones reformed in

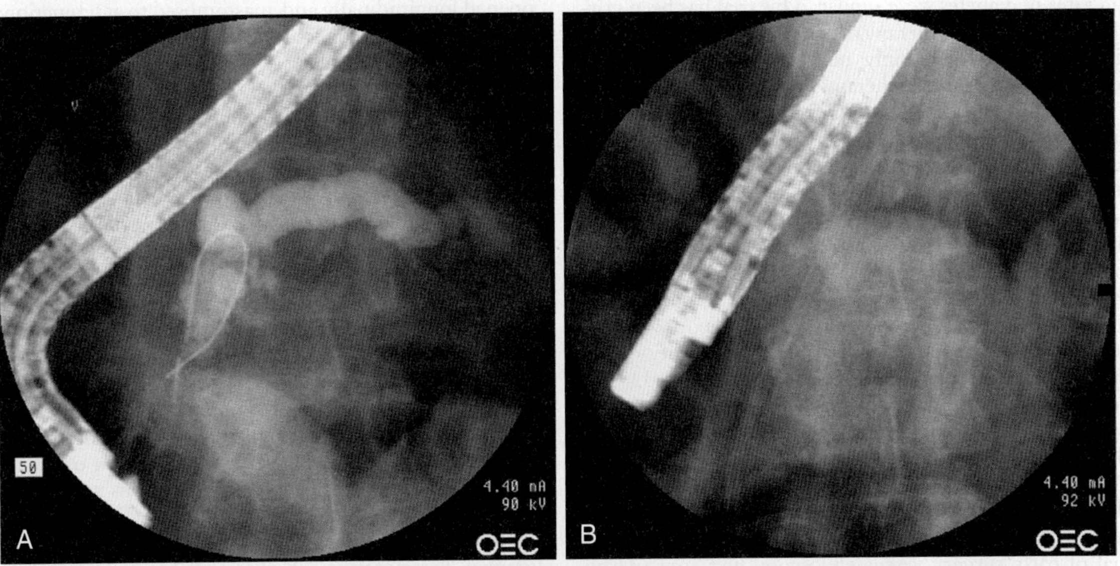

Fig. 61.8 Endoscopic retrograde cholangiopancreatography in a patient with chronic pancreatitis. (A) A dilated pancreatic duct with a single dominant stricture in the head of the pancreas and upstream dilatation is seen. (B) A stent has been placed across the stricture.

around 20% over follow-up.[348] Pain relief was measured with variable metrics in the studies analyzed, with 53% being pain-free at follow-up, 33% having improved but moderate pain at follow-up, and 10% having ongoing severe pain. The rate of symptom improvement is thus greater than the rate of complete stone clearance. In a randomized trial comparing ESWL alone to ESWL followed by endoscopic removal of stones, pain relief was similar in both groups.[349] In this trial, pain relapse during 2 years of follow-up was 38% in the ESWL arm and 45% in the ESWL plus endoscopy arm. Treatment costs were three times higher in the ESWL plus endoscopy group. These data suggest that ESWL may be able to reduce the size of stones to the point that they are not obstructing, or that there is some other effect on pancreatic pain separate from the ability to fragment pancreatic stones. Some guidelines recommend ESWL alone as an appropriate therapy for pancreatic ductal stones greater than 5 mm in patients with painful CP.[175,305] Complications of lithotripsy are infrequent, occurring in less than 10%.[348] Devices now also exist to perform pancreatoscopy with small scopes and perform lithotripsy under direct visualization. Limited data exist on the effectiveness of this approach,[350] though a recent single-center retrospective study comparing this technique to ESWL directly suggested increased efficiency and fewer total procedures with intraductal lithotripsy and comparable rates of successful stone clearance and adverse events to conventional ESWL.[351] An ongoing clinical trial is designed to directly compare the two techniques.[352]

Combined Endoscopic Therapy

Although the endoscopic therapies just discussed were presented as separate endoscopic techniques, a combination of these therapies is usually needed to manage patients with CP. These patients are those with amendable ductal anatomy and hence represent only a subset of patients with CP. In large case series, endoscopic therapy is successful in about two-thirds of patients, using variable measures of pain relief.[175,305,346,347,353] There are small randomized trials comparing endoscopic with surgical therapy for CP with amenable ductal anatomy. One trial randomized 72 patients to endoscopic therapy (pancreatic sphincterotomy, stent therapy, or stone removal) or surgical therapy (pancreatic duct drainage or pancreatic resection).[354] At 1 year of follow-up, rates of pain relief were similar. However, at 5 years of follow-up, partial pain relief or absence of pain was seen in 86% of the surgical group and 61% of the endoscopic group. In addition, the surgical group had gained more weight, and rates of diabetes were similar. This trial has been criticized in that the endoscopic therapy may have been less aggressive than optimal (some patients only underwent pancreatic duct sphincterotomy) and the surgical therapy was more aggressive than might be typical (80% underwent pancreatic resection), as well as for several methodological weaknesses. This trial used pseudo-randomization and was not analyzed on an intention to treat analysis. A second randomized trial compared a more aggressive endoscopic approach (including ESWL as needed) to a more routine surgical procedure (pancreaticojejunostomy or modified Puestow operation).[355,356] This trial was stopped early when only 39 patients were entered, due to better outcomes in the surgical group. At a median follow-up of 2 years, patients randomized to surgery had a lower pain score and better physical health on quality-of-life measurement. Complete or partial pain relief was seen in 32% of the endoscopic group and 75% of the surgical group. At 5 years of follow-up 68% of the patients in the endoscopy group required additional endoscopic or surgical therapy for pain relief, compared to 5% in the surgery group[356] with continued advantage in pain relief in the surgery group. Quality of life and residual pancreatic function were comparable between groups. A recent randomized clinical trial of early surgery versus endoscopy-first approach in patients with painful CP evaluated 88 patients total across the two arms. Complete or partial pain relief over the 18 months of follow-up was achieved in significantly more patients in the surgery arm than the endoscopy-first arm.[357] However, it is important to note that when comparing those in the endoscopic group who achieved ductal clearance with the surgical group, pain outcomes were similar. These data together suggest that surgical therapy is somewhat more effective and more durable than endoscopic therapy,[358] although further study is still needed to clarify the findings and understand what additional factors are influencing outcome. These data should be discussed with patients who are considering these options. Many patients will still choose endoscopic therapy out of a desire to avoid surgery. Only a subset of patients with CP and specific ductal anatomy are candidates for endoscopic therapy, including a dilated pancreatic duct (usually >5 mm) and an obstructing stricture or stone in the head of the pancreas. The endoscopic treatment of complications such as bile duct strictures and pseudocysts is discussed later and in Chapter 61.

Surgical Therapy

Surgical therapy in CP is commonly considered for intractable abdominal pain for which medical therapy has failed. Other indications for surgery in these patients are complications involving adjacent organs or structures (duodenal, splenic venous, or biliary complications), failure of endoscopic or radiologic management for pseudocysts, internal pancreatic fistulas, and exclusion of malignancy despite an extensive evaluation. Surgical options for pain are pancreatic ductal drainage, resection of all or part of the pancreas, and both. The choice of surgical procedure depends in large part on the ductal anatomy, presumed pathogenesis of pain, and associated complications as well as local surgical preferences and expertise.[305,359–361]

Ductal drainage procedures are the least technically demanding and preserve the most pancreatic parenchyma. The rationale for these procedures is to relieve ductal obstruction and reduce pancreatic pressures, thereby relieving pain. Pancreatic ductal drainage procedures generally require dilation of the pancreatic duct to more than 5 mm, a diameter that allows relatively easy identification and anastomosis.[359] This operation is considered in patients with a dilated pancreatic duct but without an inflammatory mass in the head of the pancreas. The most commonly performed procedure is the lateral pancreaticojejunostomy or Partington-Rochelle modification of the Puestow procedure. In this procedure the pancreatic duct is opened longitudinally and anastomosed to a defunctionalized limb of small bowel, which is connected with a Roux-en-Y anastomosis. This limb also can be used to decompress any coexisting pseudocysts. At the time of the operation, ductal strictures can be incised, and stones can be readily removed as needed. The procedure also can be performed in the absence of a dilated pancreatic duct (normal duct Puestow procedure or "V-plasty"), but the efficacy for relieving pain is believed to be less.[360] The procedure can be performed laparoscopically. The operative mortality for a modified Puestow procedure is extremely low.[359]

No randomized trials comparing a modified Puestow procedure with other surgical therapies have been conducted. Immediate pain relief is seen in approximately three-quarters of carefully selected patients.[359–361] With long-term follow-up, about half continue to experience pain relief. The explanation for this decline in effectiveness is unknown but may reflect closure of the anastomosis, pain originating in the undrained segments of the head of the pancreas, or the development of other sources of pain (neural inflammation, central nervous system sensitization, duodenal or bile duct obstruction, etc.). There is thus a tradeoff between the simplicity and low risk of this procedure and the gradual deterioration of pain relief over time. Exocrine and endocrine functions are generally unaffected by this surgical procedure per se but appear to continue to deteriorate as in unoperated patients.

In an attempt to overcome the modest early and substantial late failure rates of simple drainage procedures, approaches combining resection of the pancreas with drainage of the pancreatic duct have been developed. These have focused particularly on the head of the pancreas because this is felt to be the pacemaker of the disease by many surgeons. A routine longitudinal pancreaticojejunostomy does not completely decompress the ducts in the head of the gland, the duct of Santorini, and the small ducts draining the uncinate process. Some patients may have an associated inflammatory mass of the head of the pancreas, making drainage of the pancreatic duct within the head of the pancreas more difficult. In addition, resection of the head of the pancreas may be necessary in patients with a large inflammatory mass of the head that compresses and obstructs the duodenum or the bile duct. Options to deal with these problems include resection of the head of the pancreas [pancreaticoduodenectomy (Whipple operation), duodenum-preserving Whipple operation, or duodenum-preserving pancreatic head resections (DPPHR)] and combinations of ductal drainage with local resection of all or part of the pancreatic head.[361] It should be noted that improved pain relief after these surgical procedures involving pancreatic resection may be partially explained by the denervation of visceral pancreatic afferent nerves during more extensive dissection rather than better drainage of the pancreatic ducts in the head of the pancreas.

Whipple resection or duodenum-preserving Whipple resection produces pain relief in 65%–95% of patients.[305,359] Whipple operations are generally considered in patients with disease limited to the head of the pancreas, particularly those with a large inflammatory mass of the pancreas in whom malignancy is also being considered. Associated biliary or duodenal obstruction, seen more commonly in these patients with inflammatory masses of the head of the pancreas, can also be treated at the time of the resection. These operations have higher morbidity and mortality than simple ductal drainage operations. Although the mortality in high-volume centers is less than 3%, early postoperative complications (primarily disruptions of normal motility and pancreatic duct leaks) can occur in up to half of cases. Surgical mortality is higher if the inflammatory mass occludes or compresses major arteries or veins.

Several procedures have been developed to resect all or part of the head of the pancreas without the disruptions of GI physiology seen with traditional Whipple operations and to limit the amount of pancreatic tissue removed. The DPPHR, variant developed by Beger, is performed by resecting the pancreatic head but sparing the duodenum and covering the site with a defunctionalized Roux-en-Y jejunal limb to allow drainage of pancreatic and biliary secretions.[362] Modifications of this procedure were subsequently developed to avoid dissecting around the portal and superior mesenteric veins (and the associated bleeding risk) and to limit the amount of pancreatic tissue (in particular islet cells) that is removed. In one modification, developed by Frey, less of the head of the pancreas is cored out, leaving the bile duct and peripancreatic vessels undisturbed.[363] This approach is coupled with a longitudinal incision of the pancreatic duct in the body and tail of the pancreas and the overlaying of a long jejunal anastomosis covering both the opened duct and the cored-out head. A third operation, termed the Berne procedure, uses a pancreatic head resection without longitudinal duct incision but leaves a narrow layer of pancreatic tissue against the duodenum and retropancreatic vessels.[364]

There have been several randomized trials and meta-analyses comparing one of the Whipple operations with DPPHR (either the Frey or Beger procedure).[359,365,366] In short-term follow-up, these procedures appear to have equivalent efficacy in relieving pain, with more diabetes seen in those undergoing Whipple procedures. In long-term follow-up this advantage of a DPPHR may be lost. Randomized trials comparing the Beger with the Frey operations, however, show similar rates of postoperative complications, efficacy, and long-term quality of life. Postoperative complications are more common than with a simple modified Puestow procedure, but both short- and long-term pain relief is superior. In the United States, a limited number of surgeons are trained in these variations of DPPHR. Laparoscopic and robotic-assisted approaches are possible for most of these operative approaches for both benign and malignant pancreatic diseases.[367,368] The complications occurring after surgery for CP vary with the operation chosen. They include pancreatic fistula, wound infection, delayed gastric emptying, intra-abdominal abscess, pancreatitis, cholangitis, and bile leak.

The optimal timing of surgery is not known. In the past, surgery was considered a last option and considered when other therapy (medical and endoscopic) has failed to provide sufficient pain relief. Some analyses have suggested earlier surgery, before patients have developed hyperalgesia and/or opiate dependence, would be preferable.[369,370] The recently completed randomized clinical trial of early surgery versus endoscopy-first approach suggested that early surgery showed overall benefit in terms of pain relief measured by an integrated pain score over 18 months.[357] However, differences between the early surgery and endoscopy-first groups disappeared when the analysis was adjusted for ductal clearance, suggesting that this question requires additional study.

The surgical therapy of CP may also involve some less commonly used operations. In some patients with disease limited to the body and tail of the pancreas, typically after trauma to the pancreatic duct in the body of the pancreas with upstream obstructive CP, resection of the body and tail may be considered. Total or near-total pancreatectomy with concomitant islet cell auto-transplantation is being performed more frequently. It is most commonly considered in patients with intractable pain and a nondilated main pancreatic duct. It is imperative that these patients be accurately diagnosed as having CP, as they often do not have clear-cut imaging evidence of CP prior to surgery.[240,246,266,290] Islet cell auto-transplantation, if successful, can salvage sufficient islets to avoid diabetes. In practice, insulin independence is achieved in about 40% of patients, with pain relief in 80% of patients.[371,372] The risk of postoperative diabetes is dependent on the yield of islet cells at the time of the pancreatectomy. Islet yields are reduced in those patients with previous pancreatic surgery.[371–373] Total pancreatectomy with islet cell auto-transplantation is also used in pediatric pancreatitis (particularly genetic forms). At the current time, it remains mainly a salvage operation for patients with overwhelming pain, in whom other options have failed. A prospective observational study is ongoing to better understand and eventually help optimize patient selection, timing of procedure, quality of life, diabetes outcomes, and cost-effectiveness.[374]

In caring for patients who have undergone surgery for CP, it is important to remember that exocrine insufficiency and endocrine insufficiency can develop as a consequence of the surgery as well as the ongoing disease process. Exocrine insufficiency in particular may escape detection because symptoms may be mild. Steatorrhea can develop in 30%–40% of patients undergoing simple drainage procedures and in up to two-thirds of those undergoing pancreatic resections.[210,375] The use of pancreatic enzyme supplements after pancreatic surgery leads to better absorption of nutrients and should be considered for most (or all) patients after surgery for CP. The development of endocrine insufficiency (diabetes) after surgery for CP is also common but not invariable, occurring because of pancreatic resection and progressive disease.

Nerve Blocks and Neurolysis

The celiac plexus transmits visceral afferent impulses from the upper abdominal organs, including the pancreas. The greater, lesser, and least splanchnic nerves travel from the celiac plexus and then pass through the diaphragm to reach the spinal cord. Attempts to block the transmission of nociceptive stimuli have met with limited success. Celiac plexus block (usually using a combination of a glucocorticoid and a long-acting local anesthetic like bupivacaine) and celiac plexus neurolysis (using an injection of absolute alcohol) can be administered by CT- or EUS-guided techniques, but EUS guidance is safer, more effective, and more long-lasting than that delivered under CT guidance.[376–378] Despite that advantage, EUS-guided celiac plexus block is used infrequently due to the unpredictable response and short-lived effect.[379] Celiac plexus neurolysis has been used in pancreatic carcinoma but is not recommended for patients with CP. Current guidelines do not recommend celiac plexus block or neurolysis for painful CP.[175,227,305]

Interfering with nerve transmission through the splanchnic nerves might also block central perception of nociceptive inputs. This generally involves sectioning the greater splanchnic nerve on one or both sides. This can be performed through a thoracoscopic approach. Pain relief after thoracoscopic splanchnicectomy averages about 50% at 1 year and drops to 25% with longer follow-up.[380,381] The lack of response might be explained by the multiple spinal levels that receive input from the splanchnic nerves and the tremendous variation in the number of splanchnic roots, which makes complete neurotomy difficult. This therapy is rarely performed.

Another approach to minimizing nociception focuses on the central nervous system and pain perception. This has included therapy with centrally acting agents like SSRIs and gabapentinoids as discussed above, but also spinal cord stimulation and *trans*-cranial magnetic stimulation of pain centers in the brain.[175,382,383] These are novel approaches, but their overall effectiveness remains to be determined.

The Role of Central Sensitization in Painful Chronic Pancreatitis

Central sensitization is a phenomenon of heightened pain perception due to neuropathic and neuroplastic changes in the peripheral and central nervous systems. Chronic pancreatic pain can lead to abnormal spinal cord gating in nociceptive neurons, a centrally sensitized pain state, with hyperalgesia and allodynia.[175,189–192] Alterations in nociception in the setting of chronic visceral afferent signaling from the pancreas are thought to contribute in CP. Central sensitization is believed to account for at least some part of the variability in pain response to otherwise technically successful interventions or medical therapies administered to relieve pain. To date, there has been no clinical biomarker developed to identify the presence of central sensitization in any painful condition. P-QST is a research beside neurosensory evaluation that uses a standardized set of stimulations as a nociceptive proxy to assess for patterns of response suggesting central sensitization in pancreatic disease.[195] In a cross-sectional evaluation of 179 CP patients, widespread hyperalgesia suggestive of central sensitization was seen in 38 (21%), and segmental hyperalgesia suggestive of neural changes mainly involving the pancreatic viscerotome and not the central nervous system was seen in 50 (27.9%).[196] These phenotypes did not associate with the presence of psychiatric comorbidity, suggesting that the presence of anxiety or depression symptoms alone did not account for the differences seen in nociceptive experience. The presence of hyperalgesia suggestive of central sensitization has been associated with higher rates of constant pain, higher pain intensity, and higher pain interference compared to patients with no hyperalgesia.[196] In trying to tease out the roles of psychiatric comorbidity and hyperalgesia in the CP pain experience, it has also been shown that presence of hyperalgesia associates with past or current experience of pain, but psychiatric comorbidity persists only with current pain, suggesting that relief of pain in this disease has the potential to relieve symptoms of anxiety and depression even if nociceptive changes persist.[384] Hyperalgesia has been shown to have significant overlap with both psychiatric comorbidities and evidence of ductal obstruction in patients with CP.[198] The cumulative effects of each of these overlapping factors have been associated with a linear increase in pain severity and interference, and a linear decrease in quality of life, potentially explaining some of the phenomena seen clinically in this patient population that was previously unexplained.[198] Quantitative sensory testing has previously been used to predict outcome of therapy with pregabalin and may have the potential to predict outcome for additional invasive therapies. An ongoing clinical trial is assessing the capability of P-QST to predict outcomes of invasive therapies for painful ductal obstruction. The identification of central sensitization through P-QST has the potential to help reshape the understanding of the CP pain experience. In addition, it could help to improve patient selection for specific treatments, including therapies to relieve ductal obstruction in patients without central sensitization and centrally acting neural agents for patients with underlying central sensitization. Chronic pancreatic pain can lead to abnormal spinal cord gating in nociceptive neurons, a centrally sensitized pain state, with hyperalgesia and allodynia.[175,189–192]

Maldigestion and Steatorrhea

Although patients with CP may maldigest fat, protein, and carbohydrates, it is fat maldigestion that is the principal clinical problem. It has been estimated that 90,000 USP units of lipase delivered to the intestine with each meal should be sufficient to eliminate steatorrhea.[199,210,227] This corresponds to approximately 10% of the normal lower limit of pancreatic output of lipase. A number of factors limit the effectiveness of commercially available enzyme supplements. Pancreatic enzyme supplements vary in enzyme content. The lipase content of commercially available preparations ranges from 3000 to 40,000 USP units of lipase per pill or tablet. Five brand-name products are currently available (see Table 61.6), and generic forms of pancreatic enzymes are not available.

Much of the lipase may not reach the small bowel in an active form, being denatured by gastric acid or destroyed by proteases. Most commercially available enteric-coated enzyme preparations use a microsphere size that is too big to empty from the stomach in synchrony with the food. These enteric-coated microspheres may also not release their enzyme contents until they reach the distal jejunum or ileum, too distal for efficient fat digestion and absorption. Finally, the enzyme preparations are of relatively low potency, so many pills or tablets must be taken with each meal and snack. This requirement can have a major negative influence on compliance. Finally, these are costly agents and can cost patients up to $2000/monthly. These factors all interfere with the effective treatment of steatorrhea. Even in clinical studies, correction of fat digestion to normal levels is uncommon.[385]

The goal of managing steatorrhea is to assure that at least 90,000 USP units of lipase are present with each meal in the prandial and postprandial phases. It may not be necessary to administer that amount in every patient, as many patients still have some residual pancreatic secretion and because gastric lipase may partially compensate for the loss of pancreatic lipase.[386] A starting dose of 40,000–50,000 is common, with upward titration based on effect. Many patients are undertreated,[210,387–389] including those who are at highest risk after pancreatic surgery or resection for CP.[375] If the nonenteric-coated preparation is chosen, concomitant suppression of gastric acid with a histamine-2 receptor antagonist or proton pump inhibitor is necessary. The effectiveness of enzyme supplementation is generally gauged by clinical parameters, including improvement in stool consistency, loss of visible fat in the stool, and gain in body weight. Performing a 72-hour fecal fat analysis before the start of and during therapy, to prove effectiveness, is rarely needed but can be considered in those who do not show the expected response. It is important to periodically evaluate for deficiencies of fat-soluble vitamins, particularly vitamin D, and to assess for the presence of osteopenia or osteoporosis with a bone mineral density test.[201–210,227,389] Appropriate enzyme therapy improves nutritional status, body weight, quality of life, and possibly mortality.[209] There are numerous dietary recommendations for CP, usually using very low-fat diets. There is no evidence that these diets are less likely to cause pain than other diets, and very low-fat diets may lead to worsening fat-soluble vitamin deficiencies. A heart-healthy or Mediterranean diet is reasonable, with avoidance of foods that cause symptoms.

There are several potential explanations for failure of enzyme therapy for steatorrhea. The most common is inadequate dose, often due to patient noncompliance with the number of pills, or the cost of pills, that must be taken. Changing to a more potent preparation to reduce the number of pills taken can be helpful. It is also important to make sure that acid suppression has been prescribed and is being used by patients on the nonenteric-coated preparation. The enteric-coated preparations are not typically coadministered with an agent to reduce gastric acid. In some patients, the enteric-coated preparations may release enzymes in the mid or distal small bowel, and this delayed release may not be sufficient to effectively treat steatorrhea. Adding an agent to suppress gastric acid can force these enteric-coated preparations to open more proximally in the small intestine and improve fat digestion in some patients and can be considered in those that are not responding to therapy. The enzymes should be taken spread out over the course of the meal.[210,389] It is occasionally useful to change from one formulation to another (e.g., changing from enteric-coated preparations to a combination of a nonenteric-coated preparation plus an agent to suppress acid) or to raise the dose higher than 90,000 USP units of lipase per meal, if the response is still not satisfactory. If all these measures fail to achieve the desired effect, it is appropriate to search for alternative diagnoses that could also produce malabsorption, such as celiac disease or small intestinal bacterial overgrowth (SIBO), which may be a particular problem in these patients.[390,391] The mechanism of SIBO in these patients is unknown but is likely related to abnormalities in small bowel motility (induced by the disease or by narcotic analgesics); the common use of proton pump inhibitor therapy, which facilitates bacterial overgrowth in the stomach; previous pancreatic and intestinal surgery; and possibly a decrease in the bactericidal capacity of pancreatic juice. Finally, if all these measures fail, one can replace dietary fat with medium-chain triglycerides, which do not require lipolysis (and hence lipase) for absorption.

Diabetes Mellitus

Periodic monitoring for the development of diabetes is appropriate in patients with CP. A yearly fasting glucose level and hemoglobin A1c are appropriate.[214,227] Residual functional β-cell mass can be estimated by measuring C-peptide levels. Although many patients may have diabetes because of islet destruction, about half of the risks of diabetes in these patients are typical risk factors for type 2 DM.[392] Diabetes mellitus is an independent predictor of mortality in patients with CP. Morbidity and mortality due to diabetes mellitus may occur from progressive microangiopathic complications or from more dramatic complications, such as treatment-induced hypoglycemia (in those with inadequate glucagon reserve and particularly in those who are malnourished).[213–216] Ketoacidosis is unusual. Some patients show response to the use of an oral hypoglycemic, such as a sulfonylurea, thiazolidinedione, metformin, or other agents. Metformin is preferred, as there is circumstantial evidence that it may lower the risk of secondary pancreatic carcinoma.[215] Insulin is often needed, however, and patients with CP tend to have lower insulin requirements than patients with type 1 diabetes mellitus.[215,216] Overvigorous attempts at tight control of blood glucose value may be associated with disastrous complications of treatment-induced hypoglycemia.[218] Attempts at tight control of blood glucose value are indicated in one subgroup, however—patients with hyperlipidemic pancreatitis—in whom the diabetes is usually a primary illness and tight control of blood glucose makes control of serum lipids possible. In long-standing diabetes, appropriate monitoring for nephropathy, retinopathy, and neuropathy is indicated.

COMPLICATIONS

Pseudocyst

Pseudocysts are fluid-filled and walled-off cavities containing pancreatic fluid. They occur in about 25% of patients with CP and are most commonly seen in alcoholic CP.[393–396] The most common symptom associated with a pseudocyst is abdominal pain, which occurs in the majority of symptomatic patients. Less common manifestations are a palpable mass, nausea and vomiting (due to compression of the stomach or duodenum in the setting of a large collection of fluid), jaundice (due to compression of the bile duct), and bleeding. Some patients are asymptomatic. Elevations in serum lipase and amylase values are found in at least one-half of patients, and a persistent elevation in serum lipase or amylase can be a clue to the presence of a pseudocyst. The diagnosis of pseudocyst is generally made through imaging studies, including US, CT, MRI, and EUS. The advantages of CT and MRI in this setting are visualization of the capsule of the pseudocyst, which can be used to gauge the maturity of the collection, and determination of the relation of the pseudocyst to the stomach and duodenum, which can be useful in the choice of therapy. MRI can also give some additional information on the character of the contents of the collection, in particular whether it is mainly fluid or a mixture of fluid and solid material. Pseudocysts occur outside the pancreas and contain very little solid material.[397] This differentiates them from walled-off necrosis, containing fluid and solid material and replacing the normal pancreas. ERCP is not required for diagnostic purposes, although around 70% of pseudocysts communicate with the pancreatic duct.[394,395] ERCP is associated with an approximately 15% chance of infection of a previously uninfected pseudocyst, so this procedure should be undertaken only after antibiotics have been administered and therapy is imminent.

The natural history of pseudocysts in CP is not fully defined. Overall, complications of pseudocysts occur in 20%–40% of cases. Complications include compression of large peripancreatic vessels, stomach, or duodenum; infection; hemorrhage; and development of a fistula. Many pseudocysts will remain without symptoms or complications. Unlike fluid collections and pseudocysts associated with acute pancreatitis, those occurring in a background of CP resolve far less commonly. Despite that, treatment is not necessary in all patients. Patients who have minimal or no symptoms and no complications should be managed conservatively.[394,395,398] Symptomatic or complicated pseudocysts require therapy. Pseudocysts occurring in the setting of CP are generally mature at the time of their diagnosis (they have a visible capsule of granulation tissue surrounding them on CT or MRI), and a delay in therapy is not needed to allow the pseudocyst capsule to mature.

Therapy for symptomatic, complicated, or rapidly enlarging pseudocysts can be surgical, percutaneous, or endoscopic. Percutaneous tube drainage of pseudocysts is possible if a safe tract to the collection can be identified. Percutaneous drainage of pancreatic pseudocysts complicating CP is discouraged owing to the widely held view that such cysts are frequently associated with ductal obstruction downstream from the fluid collection, making the risks of fistula formation along the tract and of pseudocyst recurrence or chronic fistula after removal of the tube unacceptably high. The long-term success of percutaneous drainage is still unknown but is certainly relatively low. Re-accumulation of the collection after tube removal is the rule. Complications, which occur in less than 10%–15% of cases, include bleeding, infection of the cavity, and formation of a draining fistula along the tube tract.

Endoscopic therapy of pseudocysts is possible if the fluid collection can be accessed through the papilla or through the wall of the stomach or duodenum. The route chosen depends on the location of the pseudocyst. Transpapillary drainage is possible for smaller pseudocysts in the head of the gland that communicate with the pancreatic duct. All others that are amenable to endoscopic therapy are better managed with endoscopic cystogastrostomy or cystojejunostomy, depending on their location. Success rates of 80%–90% are routinely reported.[398–401] Many centers use endoscopic therapy as first-line therapy, and the use of lumen-apposing metal stents has become common.[402] The complication rate is about 10%.[398–401] Most complications are related to transmural stent placement and include bleeding (which may occasionally be massive), perforation, and infection of previously uninfected collections. Using EUS to assess for large vessels between the gut lumen and the pseudocyst, and a direct EUS-guided puncture to avoid nearby vessels reduces complications. Antibiotic coverage and readily available surgical backup are essential if endoscopic therapy is undertaken. Typically, stents are left in place for several weeks, or longer, to allow the pseudocyst to decompress. Most, but not all, pseudocysts are amenable to endoscopic therapy. The long-term success rate of endoscopic therapy is not well defined but appears to be as good as surgical techniques.

Surgical therapy usually involves cyst decompression into a loop of small bowel or stomach, often coupled with a pancreatic ductal drainage procedure (e.g., modified Puestow procedure). Surgical therapy has a long-term success rate of around 90% and an operative mortality of less than 3%.[403] Although pseudocysts recur after surgery in only about 10% of cases, pain may return in up to one-half with long-term follow-up. This is true of all therapies for pseudocysts, in that pain from the underlying CP may also occur in the absence of a pseudocyst. Surgical therapy is also necessary in patients who experience severe complications of less-invasive endoscopic or percutaneous treatments. Cystogastrostomy and cystojejunostomy can be performed with laparoscopic techniques.[403] One small prospective randomized trial compared EUS-guided pseudocyst drainage to open surgical cystogastrostomy and found no difference in pseudocyst recurrence and that endoscopic therapy was associated with shorter hospital stays, better quality of life, and lower costs.[404] No studies have directly compared laparoscopic with endoscopic techniques.[405,406]

It has been noted that failure of percutaneous drainage of pseudocysts is often associated with a stricture of the pancreatic duct downstream (toward the duodenum) from the pseudocyst or a significant disruption of the duct. These features predict prompt recurrence after the tubes are removed. Endoscopic therapy is prone to a similar problem unless these anatomic problems are dealt with. MRCP can be used to identify patients with pancreatic duct strictures or major disruptions who are at increased risk of recurrence. Although not a routine practice at all centers, performance of ERCP in association with (immediately before or after) EUS-guided pseudocyst drainage may be considered.[400,401] The goal of the ERCP is to identify a pancreatic duct stricture or large duct disruption and treat this with a bridging stent. This might reduce the risk of pseudocyst recurrence after removal of the transenteric pseudocyst stents. In some patients in whom this is not possible, *trans*-enteric stents have been left in place indefinitely,[399–401] but the long-term safety of this approach is not known.

Pseudocysts account for 90% of all cystic collections associated with the pancreas. Areas of walled-off pancreatic necrosis (in the setting of acute pancreatitis) can appear cystic on CT scans but have a different therapeutic approach than a pseudocyst.[397] A number of other cystic collections can mimic the appearance of a pseudocyst, in particular cystic neoplasms (Box 61.3, and see Chapter 62).

GI Bleeding

GI bleeding in the setting of CP may develop from a variety of causes. Some are not related to CP, such as bleeding from a Mallory-Weiss tear, esophagitis, peptic ulcer disease, and varices from concomitant alcoholic cirrhosis. Others occur as a direct result of the pancreatitis, most notably bleeding from a pancreatic pseudocyst, pseudoaneurysm, and portal or splenic vein thrombosis.

Bleeding may occur from the wall of a pseudocyst. Bleeding occurs from small vessels (venous, capillary, or arteriole) in the wall, which can lead to expansion of the pseudocyst and further rupture of these small vessels.[407] Blood may remain in the pseudocyst or may reach the gut via a spontaneous pseudocyst decompression into the GI lumen or into the pancreatic duct (hemosuccus pancreaticus).[408] Bleeding from small vessels in the wall of the pseudocyst is generally of low volume but is often associated with increased abdominal pain due to expansion of the pseudocyst.

Pseudoaneurysm

Pseudoaneurysms form as a consequence of enzymatic and pressure digestion of the muscular wall of an artery by a pseudocyst. The pseudoaneurysm may rupture either into the pseudocyst (converting the pseudocyst into a larger pseudoaneurysm) or directly into an adjacent viscus, peritoneal cavity, or pancreatic duct. Pseudoaneurysmal bleeding may complicate 5%–10% of all

BOX 61.3 Cystic Collections Within the Pancreas

Pseudocyst (70%–90%)	
Cystic neoplasms (10%–15%)	Mucinous cystadenoma and cystadenocarcinoma
	Intraductal papillary mucinous neoplasm
	Serous cystadenoma
	Serous cystadenocarcinoma
	Solid pseudopapillary tumor
	Acinar cell cystadenocarcinoma
	Choriocarcinoma
	Teratoma
	Islet cell tumors with cystic degeneration
	Pancreatic ductal adenocarcinoma
True cysts (rare)	Polycystic disease of the pancreas (isolated or associated with polycystic disease of the kidneys)
	von Hippel-Lindau disease
	Simple true cyst
	Dermoid cyst
Miscellaneous cystic lesions (very rare)	Lymphoepithelial cyst
	Endometrial cyst
	Macrocyst associated with cystic fibrosis
	Retention cyst
	Parasitic cyst (*Echinococcus granulosus or Taenia solium*)

cases of CP with pseudocysts, although pseudoaneurysms may be seen in up to 21% of patients with CP undergoing angiography.[407,409,410] Pseudoaneurysms are also seen after pancreatic surgery. Many visceral arteries may be involved, the splenic artery being most common, followed by gastroduodenal or pancreaticoduodenal arteries. Once bleeding occurs, the mortality is at least 40%, being related both to the severity of the blood loss and to the presence of coexisting conditions. Although death from a pseudocyst is rare, more than half the overall mortality of pseudocysts is due to hemorrhage.

Bleeding from a pseudoaneurysm may be slow and intermittent or acute and massive. Common presentations are abdominal pain (due to the enlargement of the pseudocyst), unexplained anemia, and overt GI bleeding (if the blood can reach the gut lumen through the pseudocyst or through the pancreatic duct). In many cases, an initial self-limited bleed occurs (so-called sentinel bleed), followed hours or days later by a massive exsanguinating hemorrhage. The initial self-limited nature of the bleed may be due to transient tamponade of the bleeding within the confines of the pseudocyst. The presence of unexplained blood loss or any amount of GI bleeding in a patient with pancreatitis or a known pseudocyst should immediately raise the possibility of a pseudoaneurysm. If a pseudoaneurysm is suspected in the setting of upper GI blood loss, an urgent upper endoscopy should be undertaken. If no obvious bleeding site is seen, pseudoaneurysm formation should be considered. Rarely, blood may be seen issuing from the ampulla (hemosuccus pancreaticus), but the absence of this finding does not rule out pseudoaneurysm.

The next step in the evaluation should be an emergency CT scan with intra-arterial contrast. The finding of high-density material within a pseudocyst on the initial noncontrast images is highly suggestive of a pseudoaneurysm, as is a circular opacifying structure within the low-attenuation pseudocyst after the administration of contrast agent (Fig. 61.9). It is prudent to avoid oral administration of a contrast agent so that it will not interfere with invasive angiography if required. In most centers, such a CT finding is followed immediately by invasive angiography to define and embolize the pseudoaneurysm. Once a pseudoaneurysm has been identified, it should be treated regardless of whether or not it has caused bleeding. Angiographic embolization or stent-graft placement has largely replaced primary surgery,[409,410] which is reserved for cases in which these therapies have failed.

Variceal Bleeding From Splenic Vein Thrombosis

Variceal bleeding may complicate CP because of either associated alcoholic cirrhosis or thrombosis of the splenic (and, less commonly, portal) vein. Thrombosis of the splenic vein is most common and produces a segmental or left-sided portal hypertension.[411] Decompression of splenic venous outflow occurs through the short gastric veins to the coronary vein, producing prominent variceal channels in the gastric cardia and fundus. Depending on the venous anatomy, esophageal varices may also be produced, although they are generally smaller than the gastric varices. The natural history of gastric varices in this setting is not known, but the overall risk of bleeding is less than with esophageal varices due to cirrhosis.[407] The risk of gastric variceal bleeding is around 10% or less.[411] Therapy is therefore not required in the absence of bleeding. Should bleeding occur, splenectomy is curative, though rarely performed. Endoscopic control of bleeding is possible with gastric varices, utilizing cyanoacrylate injection or other techniques. Endovascular approaches such as balloon-assisted retrograde transvenous obliteration or placement of a transjugular intrahepatic portosystemic shunt have been well described, though the optimal treatment remains to be established.

Bile Duct Obstruction

The distal bile duct is enclosed within the posterior portion of the head of the pancreas. Inflammatory and fibrotic conditions of the head of the pancreas, as well as cancer or a pseudocyst in this location, can compress this intrapancreatic bile duct, leading to abnormal liver chemistry values, jaundice, biliary pain, or cholangitis. Symptomatic bile duct obstruction occurs in about 10% of patients. The ductal stricture can be suspected from cholestatic liver chemistry values, CT or US findings of biliary ductal dilation, or both. ERCP characteristically demonstrates a long tapered stenosis of the distal bile duct (Fig. 61.10).

The occurrence of cholangitis is an absolute indication for therapy. The presence of abnormal liver chemistry values or jaundice is not so straightforward because those most affected are alcoholic patients, and alcoholic (and other intrinsic) liver disease can also produce substantial abnormalities in liver chemistry values. The clinical, biochemical, and even radiologic features are not always sufficient to distinguish biliary stenosis from intrinsic liver disease.[412]

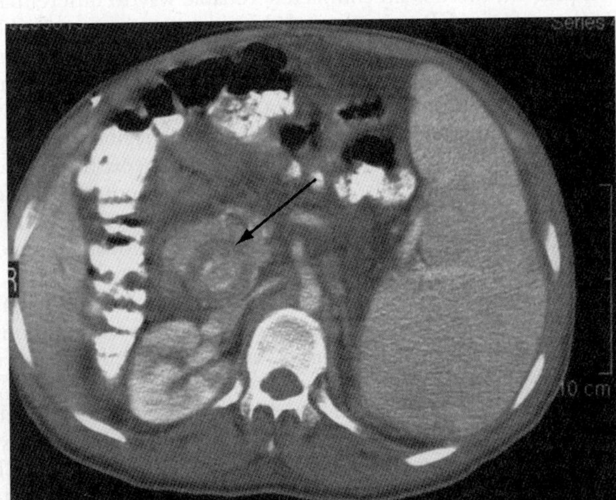

Fig. 61.9 CT scan demonstrating a pseudocyst containing a pseudoaneurysm (*arrow*) that is opacified following intravenous injection of contrast agent.

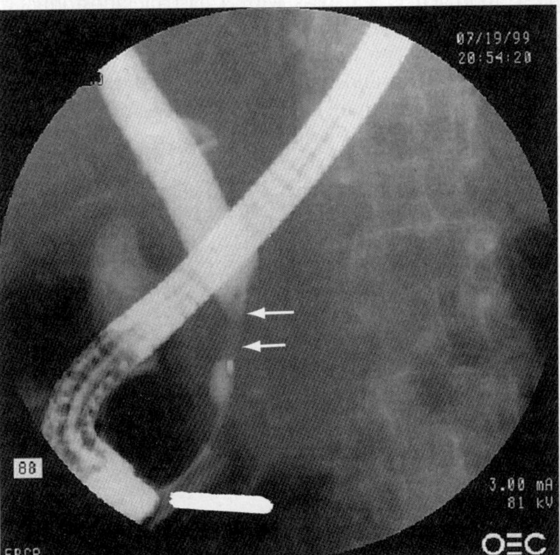

Fig. 61.10 A retrograde cholangiogram showing a smooth stricture of the bile duct (*arrows*) as it passes through the head of the pancreas in a patient with chronic pancreatitis.

Liver biopsy may be necessary to determine the choice of therapy. An asymptomatic stenosis of the intrapancreatic bile duct, in the absence of symptoms, jaundice, or progressive abnormalities in liver chemistry values, can often be followed conservatively. If there is a concern about the development of secondary biliary cirrhosis, a liver biopsy should be performed. In patients with jaundice or biliary pain, in the absence of alternative explanations (i.e., intrinsic liver disease), therapy should be undertaken. Definitive therapy of bile duct obstruction usually involves surgical biliary bypass with choledochojejunostomy or choledochoduodenostomy. Many of these patients may have a large inflammatory mass of the head of the pancreas and undergo concomitant resection (Whipple operation or duodenum preserving pancreatic head resection). One study suggested that hepatic fibrosis due to chronic biliary obstruction may actually decrease after successful surgical decompression.[413] Although endoscopic plastic stent therapy for biliary obstruction due to CP is generally temporarily effective, (see Chapter 63), the long-term success is relatively low.[414] Placement of one or more plastic stents to treat bile obstruction is relatively simple, but the long-term management is complicated by the need for multiple stent exchanges over many months to years, and stent migration and obstruction are common. Long-term endoscopic stent therapy usually requires the use of either multiple plastic stents or a fully covered metal stent, with treatment times of 6–12 months.[415,416] Long-term response is far less than surgical biliary bypass. The development of a bile duct stenosis in a patient with CP may also signal the development of a pancreatic malignancy.[116] EUS is useful in this setting to attempt to differentiate benign from malignant strictures.

Duodenal Obstruction

Approximately 5% of patients with CP experience symptomatic duodenal stenosis. Fibrosis in the head of the pancreas, often associated with an inflammatory mass, is the most common explanation. Pancreatic malignancy superimposed on CP can present in the same manner.[116] Symptoms of duodenal obstruction include nausea, vomiting, weight loss, and abdominal pain. Coexistent obstruction of the bile duct may occur. The diagnosis is best made with CT using oral contrast or an upper GI barium study, because the extent of duodenal stenosis is often underestimated at the time of endoscopy. Because the degree of stenosis may improve with resolution of some of the inflammation, a trial of conservative therapy may be worthwhile. Surgical therapy is required for those in whom conservative management fails. The simplest approach is a bypass with a gastrojejunostomy, which may be performed with laparoscopic techniques. This may be coupled with drainage of the bile duct and/or pancreatic duct (lateral pancreaticojejunostomy). Resection of the head of the pancreas with a duodenum preserving pancreatic head resection or Whipple procedure may also be considered in select patients with a large inflammatory mass of the head of the pancreas,[359–361] or in those in whom malignancy is also being considered.

Pancreatic Fistulas

External Fistulas

External pancreatic fistulas occur most commonly as a consequence of surgical or percutaneous therapy for CP or pseudocyst.[417,418] It has been estimated that perhaps half of such fistulas heal with complete bowel rest and parenteral hyperalimentation. The most common complications are abscess and bleeding. There is some evidence that the addition of octreotide, in a dosage of 100 μg subcutaneously every 8 hours, can hasten closure of such fistulas. Successful medical treatment, even with octreotide, can take many weeks. The placement of an endoscopic stent across the site of ductal disruption is effective at closing the fistula rapidly. Up to 75% of pancreaticocutaneous fistulas may be effectively treated with endoscopic techniques,[417,418] although this approach may need to be coupled with percutaneous drainage of intra-abdominal fluid collections. In patients in whom endoscopic therapy fails or cannot be performed, surgical treatment can involve pancreatic resection (if the fistula is in the tail) or a fistulojejunostomy, in which the fistula tract is "capped" with a defunctionalized limb of jejunum.[417]

Internal Fistulas

Internal pancreatic fistulas occur mainly in the setting of CP after rupture of a pseudocyst or after pancreatic trauma. The fluid may track to the peritoneal cavity (pancreatic ascites) or into the pleural space (pancreatic pleural effusion) or rarely to an adjacent hollow organ (stomach or duodenum or colon) or even pericardium. The site and track of the fistula can usually be appreciated on MRCP. Affected patients may not complain of symptoms of CP but may instead note abdominal distention or shortness of breath, depending on the site of fluid accumulation. Although such fistulas occur in advanced CP, there may not be a clear-cut history of recent symptomatic pancreatitis. The diagnosis can be established through documentation of high levels of amylase within the respective fluid, typically more than 4000 U/L.

Conservative treatment, consisting of complete bowel rest, parenteral hyperalimentation, paracentesis or thoracentesis, and octreotide, is effective in some internal pancreatic fistulas.[417] If the leak is in the body or head of the pancreas, a pancreatic duct stent covering the fistula site is highly effective. In some cases, merely bridging the ampulla with a short pancreatic duct stent may be enough to heal the fistula. Endoscopic therapy is less effective but sometimes still worthwhile if the leak is from the tail. It is ineffective if the leak is present upstream from a complete blockage of the pancreatic duct (excluded pancreatic tail syndrome). In this situation, resection or surgical drainage of the distal pancreas is required, and MRCP is used preoperatively to delineate the ductal anatomy for surgical planning.

Malignancy

The risk of pancreatic cancer is higher with all forms of CP (see Chapter 60). The lifetime risk for pancreatic cancer in patients with CP may be as high as 4%, with an estimated relative risk of 13.[15,28,87,419] The risk of pancreatic cancer is highest in patients with hereditary pancreatitis (though more recent studies suggest that this is lower than previously estimated), as well as those who smoke and those who have coexistent diabetes.[15,217,419–423]

At present, there is no completely reliable way to differentiate CP alone from CP complicated by adenocarcinoma.[116] The symptoms and signs may be similar (abdominal pain, weight loss, jaundice). In the absence of widespread metastases, imaging studies such as CT, US, and even ERCP may be unable to establish the diagnosis. EUS is most accurate, but finding a small hypoechoic tumor within a diseased gland with preexisting altered echotexture can be difficult. However, EUS is superior to CT for detection of coexistent malignancy, particularly when the lesion is small. EUS also has the substantial advantage of allowing directed tissue biopsy of any suspicious lesions.

Tumor markers may be helpful in attempting to differentiate CP from cancer. CA 19-9, the tumor marker most commonly used for pancreatic adenocarcinoma, is elevated in the serum in 70%–80% of patients with adenocarcinoma of the pancreas.[424] Biliary obstruction and cholangitis can also raise CA 19-9 levels. The use of any of these techniques for surveillance is not cost-effective in the general population of patients with CP, although they may be useful in families with hereditary pancreatic cancer and hereditary pancreatitis. In some patients, laparoscopy or laparotomy is required to determine the presence or absence of coexistent pancreatic carcinoma. In those with a benign pseudotumor who undergo resection to rule out malignancy, a variant of autoimmune CP is often found.[34,116]

Extrapancreatic cancers are also increased in patients with CP, These cancers, particularly those of the upper digestive tract and lungs, are probably related to the effect of concomitant tobacco use.[15,18,28,87]

Dysmotility

Gastroparesis and antroduodenal dysmotility are seen in patients with CP,[425,426] as a consequence of perigastric inflammation, hormonal changes associated with CP (e.g., increases in plasma CCK), pancreatic surgery with reconstruction, or a side effect of narcotic analgesics. Gastroparesis is clinically important because it may produce symptoms occasionally indistinguishable from those of the disease and may interfere with the effective delivery of pancreatic enzymes.[426] Gastroparesis should be considered in patients with early satiety, nausea, vomiting, and weight loss.

Small Intestinal Bacterial Overgrowth

In addition to or potentially as an added consequence of altered motility of the gastrointestinal tract in CP, there can be significant changes to the microbiome. Prevalence estimates of SIBO in CP vary widely due to differences in SIBO diagnostic techniques and heterogeneity of the populations studied. It is important to note that there exists no gold standard test for SIBO. A recent systematic review and meta-analysis included studies with prevalence estimates ranging from 14% to 92% based on breath testing; a pooled prevalence estimate was 36%.[427] A small prospective case–control study of nonsurgical CP patients with EPI and age- and sex-matched controls using a glucose hydrogen breath test revealed a lower prevalence of approximately 15% in this carefully defined population.[390] Prior gastrointestinal surgeries, gut dysmotility and changes in gut immune function all predispose patients to SIBO. In CP, decreased pancreatic enzyme secretion, fat malabsorption in the setting of EPI, diabetic neuropathy, and loss of physiologic synchrony in the interdigestive process may further facilitate bacterial overgrowth.[390] In CP patients, especially those who have EPI and inadequate response to PERT, testing for SIBO in the setting of nonspecific but persistent gastrointestinal symptoms can be considered part of a thorough diagnostic workup.

Full references for this chapter can be found at https://ebooks.health.elsevier.com.

62 Pancreatic Cancer, Cystic Neoplasms, and Other Tumors

S. George Barreto, Kjetil Soreide, John A. Windsor

IN THIS CHAPTER

PANCREATIC CANCER

Pancreatic cancer (PC) is the second most common gastrointestinal malignancy in most countries around the world. While there are many types of PC, pancreatic duct adenocarcinoma (PDAC) is the most common. In the United States, approximately 64,050 new cases are expected to be diagnosed in 2023.[1] Despite its relatively low incidence compared with other malignancies, it represents the fourth leading cause of cancer death in men and women (50,550 deaths expected in 2023 in the United States), and it is projected to become the second leading cause of cancer-related death by 2030.[2] Overall, PC carries devastating prognosis with an overall median survival of just 7.4 months.[3] The 5-year relative survival rate for localized disease is 44% and for distant disease, it is 12%.[1] Improvements in outcome have been slower than for all other solid cancers. In part, this is because of the challenges of late presentation with delayed diagnosis. While the safety of surgical resection has dramatically improved over the last few decades, it is unlikely that further improvements in outcome will come from surgery, but rather from more effective systemic therapy.

Epidemiology

Incidence

The overall incidence rate for PC has increased by 1% per year since the late 1990s in both sexes in the United States. The incidence of PC rises sharply over the age of 50, but the incidence among those under 50 has risen steadily over the last three decades.[4,5] The global age-standardized incidence rate for males and females are 5.5 and 4.0/100,000,[6] respectively. The incidence rates also vary with ethnicity and social deprivation. In Australia, PC incidence among the First Nations people is reported to be 10–21/100,000 depending on the location within the country.[7] This is 1.6 times higher than the rest of the nation's population. Reports from Aotearoa New Zealand depict the same trend of a higher incidence of PC among the Māori peoples in comparison to non-Indigenous people of the country.[8]

Populations at Risk

There are a number of risk factors associated with the development of PC. The nonmodifiable risk factors include age, gender, ethnicity, race, and family history. Other risk factors are potentially modifiable, including alcohol, obesity, smoking, and chronic pancreatitis.

While the vast majority of PCs are sporadic, up to 10% are inherited. Familial PC is defined as those with 2 or more first-degree relatives (FDRs) with PC. The risk of PC is increased 6.4-fold with 2 affected FDRs and 32-fold with 3 FDRs.[9] The risk of PC also depends on the actual gene mutations and whether this is part of a recognizable familial PC syndrome. Patients with a familial PC syndrome tend to be younger at diagnosis.[10] Table 62.1 summarizes some of the genetic syndromes associated with an increased risk of PC. The most frequent inherited gene mutations associated with inherited PC are *PALB2*, *STK11*, *PRSS1*, and *SPINK2*. *CDKN2A* and *BRCA2* are, with BRCA2 mutations representing the most common gene mutation.[10,11] Lynch syndrome is associated with a number of inherited gene mutations: *BRCA2*, *CDKN2A*, *ATM*, and mismatch repair enzyme instability. Familial atypical multiple mole melanoma (FAMMM) is an autosomal dominant condition defined by a mutation of tumor suppressor gene *CDKN2A*. Normally, *CDNKN2A* encodes the *p16* protein preventing phosphorylation and activation of the retinoblastoma gene. Patients with FAMMM are at risk of both melanoma and PC.[12] Hereditary pancreatitis (see Chapter 57), commonly caused by an autosomal dominant mutation in the PRSS gene, is associated with a near 50% incidence of PC by age 74.[13] Patients with other, nonhereditary forms of chronic pancreatitis also have a higher likelihood of developing PC.[14] Smoking and alcohol use are synergistic risk factors that increase the risk of PC in patients with chronic pancreatitis.[15] Individuals with Peutz-Jeghers syndrome with *STK11* gene mutations, discussed in Chapter 126, have a cumulative risk of PC by age 65–70 of 11%–36%.[16]

Screening is the best way of identifying these people at high risk of PC but there are challenges because of the low incidence of disease, cost, low accuracy of imaging modalities, and expertise necessary for imaging. Currently, family history and the presence of defined gene mutations represent the most effective way of identifying the high-risk populations.[17] The recent International Cancer of the Pancreas Screening consortium agreed that FDRs in a kindred with at least two affected FDRs, patients with Peutz-Jeghers syndrome (irrespective of the patient's family history), and any of the above-mentioned mutation carriers with at least one affected FDR are candidates for screening.[18] Germline *ATM* mutation carriers with one affected FDR have now been added to the recommended surveillance list.[18] Initial screening should be MR/MRCP scanning and/or endoscopic ultrasonography (EUS), if this is available. In general, pancreas cancer screening in

TABLE 62.1 Historical Features and Genetic Syndromes Associated With an Increased Risk of Pancreatic Cancer

History	Mutated Gene	Relative Risk	Individual Risk by Age 70
None	None	1	0.5%
Breast cancer	*BRCA2*	3.5–10	5%
	BRCA1	2	1%
FAMMM syndrome	*TP16 (CDKN2A)*	20–34	10%–17%
≥3 FDRs with PC	Unknown	32	16%
Hereditary pancreatitis	*PRSS1*	50–80	25%–40%
Peutz-Jeghers syndrome	*STK11/LKB1*	132	30%–60%
HNPCC syndrome	*MLH1*, *MSH2*, others	Unknown	<5%
Young age-onset PC	*FANC-C*, *FANC-G*, others	Unknown	Unknown
Family X	Palladin	Unknown	Unknown

FAMMM, Familial atypical multiple mole melanoma; *FDRs*, first-degree relatives; *HNPCC*, hereditary nonpolyposis colorectal cancer; *X*, a single family in which familial pancreatic cancer was studied.
Modified from Hruban R, Pitman M, Klimstra D. *Ductal Adenocarcinoma. AFIP Atlas of Tumor Pathology. Tumors of the Pancreas*. Washington, D.C: American Registry of Pathology; 2007:111–164.

high-risk individuals should begin at age 50 years, or 10 years younger than the initial age of familial onset. And this should be adjusted 10 years earlier if the person is a smoker. The current recommendation for surveillance of patients with hereditary pancreatitis is recommended at 40 years of age, or 20 years following the first attack of pancreatitis.[18] Screening should be initiated at age 35 years in the setting of Peutz-Jeghers syndrome.[19]

The outcome from screening has been reported. Screening that utilizes imaging in groups at high familial risk has been shown to be useful in detecting PC (18 cases detected in 1156 high-risk adults, compared to 0 cases in 161 patients deemed to be of average risk). The evidence of harm resulting from this detection is limited.[20] One registry of 309 asymptomatic at-risk relatives over age 35 offered participants MRCP followed by EUS if lesions were found. Out of the 109 relatives who had completed at least initial screening, 9 had a significant abnormality confirmed by EUS, with an overall diagnostic yield of 8.3% in at-risk relatives (Fig. 62.1).[21]

Various strategies have been explored for the diagnosis of early PC and precancerous lesions, including the use of blood biomarkers as screening tools, but with varying success.[22] These “liquid biopsies” are designed to detect genetic material associated with cancer, such as extracellular vesicles, circulating tumor cells, DNA, and abnormally expressed microRNAs,[23,24] alone,[25] or in combination with existing tumor markers, for example, CA 19-9.[26,27] Commercially available tools are becoming available. CancerSEEK developed as a panel of biomarkers to screen for multiple cancers and uses DNA assays and protein biomarkers. For PC, it has a 99% specificity and 72% sensitivity.[28] The IMMray PanCan-d assay combines eight-plex biomarkers with CA19-9 specifically to distinguish PC stages I and II. It has a 99% specificity and 89% sensitivity after exclusion of Lewis-null individuals.[29]

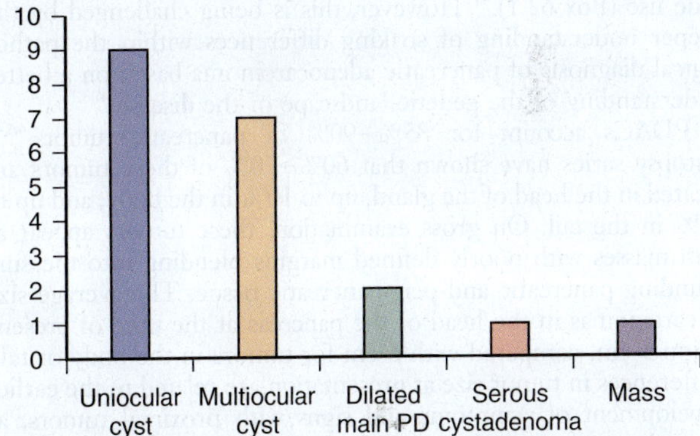

Fig. 62.1 Distribution of positive findings on initial cross-sectional pancreatic imaging in asymptomatic, at-risk relatives of patients with pancreatic cancer over age 35. Six relatives underwent surgical resection; two had IPMN, two had carcinoma in situ (PanIN 2 in one and PanIN 3 in another), one had a T3N0 PC, and one had a serous cystic neoplasm. *IPMN*, Intraductal papillary mucinous tumor; *PanIN*, pancreatic intraepithelial neoplasia; *PD*, pancreatic duct. (Modified from Ludwig E, Olson SH, Bayuga S, et al. Feasibility and yield of screening in relatives from familial PC families. *Am J Gastroenterol*. 2011;106:946–954.)

Environmental Risk Factors

The most significant and only established environmental risk factor for PC is cigarette smoking. Meta-analysis data have demonstrated that smoking is associated with a 1.7 relative risk of developing PC. The risk for PC remains elevated for up to 10 years after cessation of smoking. The risk appears to be dose dependent, with risk rising with every five cigarettes smoked daily.[30] Smoking is likely a contributing cause in 20%–25% of all PCs.[31]

There is a two-way relationship between diabetes mellitus and PC as diabetes mellitus is both a risk factor[32] and a consequence of PC.[33] Diabetes mellitus and glucose intolerance are present in approximately 85% of patients at diagnosis and are diagnosed in 55%–85% within the 2 years before PC diagnosis.[34,32] Glucose tolerance sometimes improves in patients who have undergone tumor resection.[35] Approximately 20% of asymptomatic patients with PC develop new-onset diabetes mellitus at a median of 6.5 months prior to the diagnosis of PC offering an avenue for early detection.[36] While longstanding diabetes, greater than 10 years, has been associated with an increased risk of PC, a causal relationship remains unproven. Cohort analysis has demonstrated an eight-fold increased risk of PC compared with age-matched patients without diabetes mellitus.[37] GLP-1 mimetic drugs (e.g., exenatide) and inhibitors of GLP-1 metabolism (DPP4 inhibitors, e.g., sitagliptin) which are used to treat type 2 diabetes mellitus, have been associated with a nearly three-fold increased risk of PC, unlike other classes of oral antidiabetic agents.[38]

Obesity is also a risk factor for PC. The 2012 World Cancer Research Fund Panel directly linked increased body mass, abdominal girth, and abdominal weight to PC.[39] There is a stepwise increase in risk of PC with an increase in BMI.[40]

Dietary constituents appear to have less influence as environmental risk factors for PC than previously reported. There is some evidence that a high intake of red or processed meat may increase the risk of developing PC.[41] A protective effect of dietary folate has not been supported by recent analysis.[42] There is some limited evidence from case-control studies supporting a protective effect of fruit and vegetable consumption on risk of developing PC.[43–45]

Pathology

As reviewed in Chapter 57, there are different epithelial cell types in the normal pancreas: (1) acinar cells, which account for approximately 80% of the gland volume; (2) ductal cells, comprising 10%–15%; and (3) endocrine (islet) cells, comprising approximately 1%–2%. More than 95% of the malignant neoplasms of the pancreas arise from the exocrine elements of the gland (ductal and acinar cells), and while many demonstrate features consistent with adenocarcinoma, there are a number of different exocrine PCs. Endocrine neoplasms account for only 1% –2% of pancreatic tumors and are discussed in Chapter 43. Nonepithelial pancreatic malignancies are exceedingly rare.[46] The WHO classification of pancreatic exocrine tumors remains in wide use (Box 62.1).[47] However, this is being challenged by the deeper understanding of striking differences within the pathological diagnosis of pancreatic adenocarcinoma based on a better understanding of the genetic landscape of the disease.[48]

PDACs account for 85%–90% of pancreatic tumors.[46,47] Autopsy series have shown that 60%–70% of these tumors are located in the head of the gland, up to 10% in the body, and up to 15% in the tail. On gross examination, these tumors appear as firm masses with poorly defined margins blending into the surrounding pancreatic and peri-pancreatic tissue. The average size of carcinomas in the head of the pancreas at the time of presentation 3 cm, compared with 6 cm for tumors in the body or tail. Differences in tumor size at presentation are related to the earlier development of symptoms and signs with proximal tumors, as with obstructive jaundice, than with distal neoplasms.

BOX 62.1 WHO Classification of Primary Tumors of the Exocrine Pancreas

I. Benign
   i. Serous cystadenoma
   ii. Mucinous cystadenoma
   iii. Intraductal papillary mucinous adenoma
   iv. Mature cystic teratoma
II. Borderline (uncertain malignant potential)
   i. Mucinous cystic tumor with moderate dysplasia
   ii. Intraductal papillary mucinous tumor with moderate dysplasia
   iii. Solid pseudopapillary tumor
III. Malignant
   i. Ductal adenocarcinoma
   ii. Osteoclast-like giant cell tumor
   iii. Serous cystadenocarcinoma
   iv. Mucinous cystadenocarcinoma (noninvasive or invasive)
   v. Intraductal papillary mucinous carcinoma (noninvasive or invasive)
   vi. Acinar cell carcinoma
   vii. Pancreatoblastoma
   viii. Solid pseudopapillary carcinoma
   ix. Miscellaneous carcinomas

Data from Hruban R, Pitman M, Klimstra D. *Ductal Adenocarcinoma. AFIP Atlas of Tumor Pathology. Tumors of the Pancreas*. Washington, DC: American Registry of Pathology; 2007:111–164.

Tumors in the head of the pancreas usually arise from and obstruct the pancreatic duct and grow to obstruct the distal bile duct. Ductal obstruction of these structures can result in jaundice and symptoms of chronic pancreatitis (including steatorrhea and pain), respectively. Pancreatic duct dilatation and fibrous atrophy of the pancreatic parenchyma commonly occur proximal to the PC. Local invasion of a PC in the head can also involve the duodenum, ampulla of Vater, and hepatic flexure of the colon. Extra-pancreatic extension into the retroperitoneum is common at the time of diagnosis and can result in encroachment, narrowing, and invasion of the portal vein and superior mesenteric vessels. In contrast, PC's of the body and tail of the pancreas almost never present with obstructive jaundice from biliary obstruction, unless there are prominent portal node metastases. Extra-pancreatic extension of proximal tumors can invade the spleen, stomach, splenic flexure of the colon, and/or left adrenal gland. In patients with advanced disease, metastases to the lymph nodes, liver, and peritoneum are common; the lung, pleura, and bone are less commonly involved.[49]

Microscopically, PDACs are graded as well, moderately, or poorly differentiated.[46] Well-differentiated tumors show irregular tubular neoplastic glands with mild cellular atypia, low mitotic activity, and significant mucin production. Loss of differentiation is evidenced by lack of cellular arrangement into glandular structures, increases in cellular atypia and mitotic activity, and cessation of mucin production. Several studies using multivariate analysis have demonstrated that histologic grading correlates with survival after resection.[50]

PDACs elicit a strong desmoplastic reaction,[51] especially at the interface with normal pancreas. In contrast with chronic pancreatitis, intraductal calcifications are not a recognized feature of PC. Pancreatic ducts away from the PC can demonstrate the potential for multifocal disease with *pancreatic intraepithelial neoplasia* (PanIN) (see below) with malignant potential, but ductal papillary hyperplasia or mucinous cell hypertrophy are of uncertain significance. Perineural invasion (PNI) is said to be a common, if not ubiquitous, feature of PDAC. Microscopic invasion of lymphatic vessels is also a common feature. Metastasis of tumors in the head of the pancreas to first-echelon lymph nodes in the pancreaticoduodenal basin is common but less frequent to celiac and para-aortic lymph nodes.

Several immunohistochemical markers are useful with mucin-producing PCs, including PDAC. Among the better-known markers are CA 19-9, MUC1, MUC3, MUC4, carcinoembryonic antigen (CEA), DuPan 2, and CA 125.[46] These markers are particularly useful in separating neoplastic from nonneoplastic changes in the pancreatic duct and in distinguishing ductal from acinar or neuroendocrine tumors. But they are not able to differentiate between neoplasms of pancreatic and extra-pancreatic origins, limiting their usefulness in the evaluation of liver metastases of unknown primary. Cytokeratins are other useful markers in differentiating between acinar, ductal, and islet cell tumors. Although all PDACs stain for cytokeratins 7, 8, 18, and 19, most acinar and neuroendocrine tumors do not stain for cytokeratin 7.[46]

Molecular Pathology and Genetic Alterations

Pancreatic tumorigenesis is the result of a complex series of events, likely combining the effects of multiple intracellular genetic mutations as well as epigenetic influences on cellular behavior and kinetics[52] with an altered inflammatory extracellular microenvironment. PC is thought to develop in a stepwise manner from a nonmalignant precursor lesion, referred to as PanIN, through progressive cellular and nuclear atypia to invasive adenocarcinoma (82% of PCs are associated with PanINs). This histopathologic progression is mediated through a series of potentially inherited and acquired genetic alterations over time (Table 62.2).[53] PanINs share some specific characteristics, including an increase with age, multicentricity, location in the pancreatic head, is more frequently encountered in familial PC

TABLE 62.2 Commonly Affected Signaling Pathways and the Most Commonly Affected Genes From These Pathways in Pancreatic Cancer

Signaling Pathway	Affected Gene(s) (Chromosomal Region)
Apoptosis	*TP53* (17p)
DNA damage repair	*TP53* (17p)
G1/S phase transition	*CDKN2A/p16* (9p) *CCND1* (11q13)
Cell-cell adhesion	
Regulation of invasion Integrin signaling Homophilic cell adhesion	*CDH1* (16q22)
Embryonic signaling Notch pathway Hedgehog pathway Wnt pathway	—
MAPK signaling c-Jun N-terminal kinase ERK TGF-β signaling	*K-ras2* (12p) *SMAD4/DPC4* (18q)

Adapted from Ottenhof N, de Wilde R, Maitra A, et al. Molecular characteristics of pancreatic ductal adenocarcinoma. *Pathol Res Int.* 2011;2011:620601.

kindreds, is more common in association with other pathologies, is three times more commonly associated with PC, and is frequently associated with lobular parenchymal atrophy, which can often be detected by EUS.

Recently, gene sequencing of PDACs has revealed changes in the SWI/SNF chromatin remodeling complex, specifically the subunit BRG1. The association of this with *KRAS* has been implicated in the development of intraductal papillary mucinous neoplasia (IPMN) and invasive adenocarcinoma.[54]

KRAS is an oncogene where activating mutations represent the most common gene mutation present in PDACs. An activating mutation in *KRAS* is detected in approximately 30% of early neoplasms and 95% of advanced malignancy.[53] Mutations in *KRAS* allow for constitutive activation and dysregulation within the mitogen-activated protein kinase and AKT pathways leading to uncontrolled cellular proliferation and survival.[55] *KRAS* codon 12 mutations have been demonstrated to be an early acquired mutation in the transition from normal tissue through nonmalignant neoplastic lesions (PanIN) to invasive adenocarcinoma.[56] Due to their relatively common prevalence in pancreatic neoplasia, *KRAS* targets represent a potential early detection test as well as a possible target for treatment.

CDKN2A, a tumor-suppressor gene, is an acquired mutation generally found in advanced rather than early Pan-IN mutations. Loss of the *CDKN2A* gene product, *p16*, has been associated with uncontrolled cyclin D1 activation. Loss of the *p16* gene product has been associated with progressive histologic dysplasia.[57] Mutations in the tumor-suppressor genes *SMAD4* and *TP53* are found almost exclusively in high-grade PanIN lesions. The *TP53* protein product, *p53*, is integral in DNA repair and apoptosis. Loss of *TP53* leads to uncontrolled cell growth of potentially damaged cells.[58]

Progression of neoplastic cells to invasive malignancy often occurs via clonal evolution through the acquisition of mutations. As detailed earlier, there are a number of mutations that occur concomitantly with *KRAS* mutations, including *CDKN2A/p16*, *TP53*, and *SMAD4*. Genetically engineered mouse models have experimentally recapitulated this spectrum of lesions, confirming their importance. For example, progression of PanIN lesions from grade 1 to grade 3 to invasive carcinoma has been linked to a

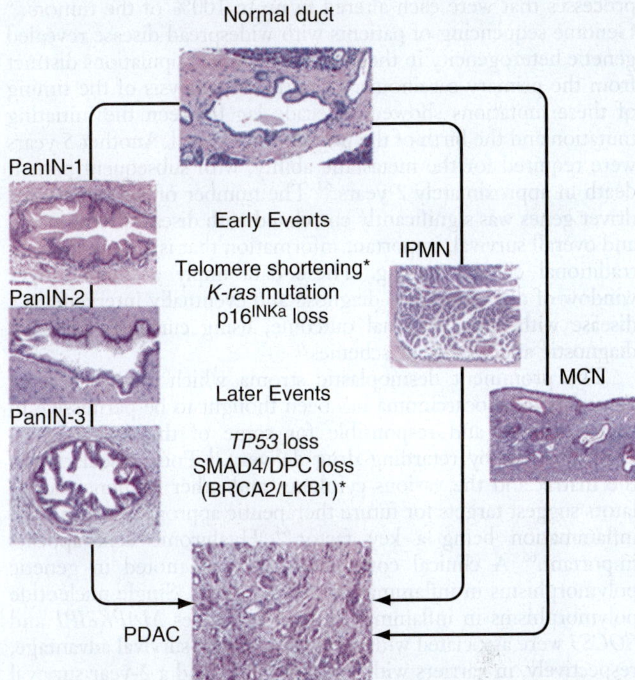

Fig. 62.2 Pancreatic precursor lesions and genetic events involved in pancreatic progression to adenocarcinoma. Pictured are three known human pancreatic ductal adenocarcinoma (PDAC) precursor lesions: PanIN, MCN, and IPMN. The PanIN grading scheme is shown on the *left*; increasing grades (1 through 3) reflect increasing atypia, eventually leading to frank PDAC. The *right side* illustrates the potential progression of MCN and IPMN to PDAC. The genetic alterations documented in pancreatic adenocarcinomas also occur in PanIN, and to a lesser extent in MCN and IPMN, in an apparent temporal sequence, although these alterations have not been correlated with the acquisition of specific histopathologic features. The various genetic events are listed and divided into those that occur predominantly early or late in PDAC progression. *Asterisks* indicate events that are not common to all precursor lesions (e.g., telomere shortening and *BRCA2* loss are documented in PanIN, and *LKB1* loss is documented in a subset of PDACs and IPMNs). *IPMN*, Intraductal papillary mucinous neoplasm; *MCN*, mucinous cystic neoplasm; *PanIN*, pancreatic intraepithelial neoplasia. (From Hezel AF, Kimmelman AC, Stanger BZ, et al. Genetics and biology of pancreatic ductal adenocarcinoma. *Genes Dev.* 2006;20:1218–1249. Copyright © 2006, Cold Spring Harbor Laboratory Press.)

stepwise presence of an increasing number of genetic mutations (Fig. 62.2).[59] Better understanding of the cascade of events requires analysis of not only individual cellular alterations but also cell-cell interactions and microenvironmental forces. Sequencing the PC genome has allowed an integrated histologic-molecular classification system to emerge. An integrated genomic expression analysis of 456 PDACs convincingly demonstrated 4 distinct molecular subtypes: squamous, pancreatic progenitor, aberrantly differentiated endocrine exocrine, and immunogenic types.[60] Recent evidence has found that the squamous molecular subtype[60] represents a more aggressive tumor biology with poor outcomes following surgery irrespective of the presence of a favorable pathological stage and negative margin status.[61] This is an example of how genetic profiling will transform the classification of PCs based on biological behaviors and will increasingly provide the basis for tumor-specific systemic treatments.

Global genomic sequencing of human pancreatic adenocarcinoma reveals the extreme complexity of tumor genetics and identified a core set of 12 cellular signaling pathways and processes that were each altered in up to 100% of the tumors.[56] Genome sequencing of patients with widespread disease revealed genetic heterogeneity in the metastatic clonal populations distinct from the primary carcinoma. Quantitative analysis of the timing of these mutations showed a decade lag between the initiating mutation and the birth of the primary cancer cell. Another 5 years were required for the metastatic ability, with subsequent patient death in approximately 2 years.[62] The number of the four major driver genes was significantly correlated with disease-free survival and overall survival, important information that is independent of traditional clinical staging. These data imply a much longer window of opportunity to diagnose and eventually intervene in a disease with such a dismal outcome, using currently available diagnostic and treatment schemes.[63]

The prominent desmoplastic stroma which is a feature of pancreatic adenocarcinoma has been thought to be permissive to tumor growth and responsible for some of the resistance to chemotherapy by retarding drug delivery.[51] Poor vascularity of the matrix and the various cytokines and other immune modulators suggest targets for future therapeutic approaches, with local inflammation being a key factor.[64] Hyaluronic acid appears important.[65] A clinical correlation has been noted in genetic polymorphisms in inflammatory-related genes. Single nucleotide polymorphisms in inflammatory pathway genes *MAPK8IP1* and *SOCS3* were associated with a 10- or 6-month survival advantage, respectively, in carriers with 1 minor allele, and a 2-year survival advantage if both minor alleles are present.[66]

Clinical Features

Most patients with PC experience symptoms relatively late in the course of disease. The lack of early and specific symptoms leads to delays in diagnosis, and most patients present with unresectable and/or metastatic disease.[67] Tumors of the head of the pancreas produce symptoms earlier in the course of disease, because of the proximity of the bile duct, ampulla of Vater, and duodenum. In contrast, tumors of the distal gland are characterized by their "silent" presentation, or lack of symptoms (Table 62.3).[68]

Tumors of the pancreas often present with signs of biliary obstruction such as jaundice, dark urine, light/clay-colored stool, pruritis, scleral icterus, pancreatitis, and cholangitis. Patients with concomitant obstruction of the pancreatic duct, which is common with PDAC may also show clinical evidence of pancreatic exocrine insufficiency in the form of steatorrhea, abdominal pain, flatulence, and weight loss.[69]

Pain can be a major symptom in patients with PC, although this is not common in patients with smaller cancers. Pain is thought to be due to either pancreatic duct obstruction, pancreatic inflammation, and/or invasion of the celiac or superior mesenteric arterial neural plexi.[70] The latter pain tends to be of low intensity, dull, and vaguely localized to the upper abdomen with radiation localized to the middle and upper back. In contrast, an obstructed main pancreatic duct can cause postprandial pain. This pain and associated nausea and anorexia can lead to accelerated weight loss. Pancreatic duct obstruction by tumor can lead to hyperlipasemia, often mild clinical acute pancreatitis, and should raise clinical suspicion in an older adult patient who presents with acute pancreatitis without another clear etiology. Thus in patients over the age of 50 years[71] with idiopathic acute pancreatitis, it is essential to perform cross-sectional imaging upon resolution of the acute episode to rule out an underlying malignancy as a cause.

Duodenal invasion with stenosis may lead to increased duodeno-gastric and gastro-esophageal reflux, nausea, and vomiting. As presented above in more detail, diabetes and pancreatitis of varying severity can occur in PC. Very rarely, patients with invasion of the colon (hepatic or splenic flexure) can have a degree of concomitant colonic obstruction.

TABLE 62.3 Demographic Features and Presenting Symptoms and Signs in Patients With Unresectable (Palliated) and Resectable (Resected) Pancreatic Cancer

	Palliated (N = 256)	Resected (N = 512)
Demographic Features		
Age, average (year)	64.0	65.8
Men/women	57%/43%	55%/45%
Race	91% White	91% White
Symptoms and Signs (%)		
Abdominal pain	64	36[a]
Jaundice	57	72[a]
Weight loss	48	43
Nausea/vomiting	30	18[a]
Back pain	26	2[a]

[a]P = .001 versus palliated group.
Modified from Sohn T, Lillemoe K, Cameron J, et al. Surgical palliation of unresectable periampullary adenocarcinoma in the 1990s. *J Am Coll Surg*. 1999;188:658–666.

Investigation and Diagnosis

Ultrasonography and Computerized Tomography

Transabdominal US is a useful first investigation in many patients with PC who present with obstructive jaundice, as it determines whether it is due to gallstone disease (e.g., choledocholithiasis or Mirizzi's syndrome) and allows measurement of the extrahepatic bile duct diameter. A dedicated pancreatic computerized tomography (CT) scan is the preferred approach to determining whether there is a pancreatic mass, and if so, to stage it.[72] Overall sensitivity of CT for PC is 86%–97%, but sensitivity for lesions less than 2 cm is 77%.[34] The pancreatic CT protocol consists of dual-phase scanning using IV and oral contrast agents. The first, early arterial phase scan is obtained at 25 seconds after IV contrast injection and offers visualization of the arterial anatomy for surgery.[73] The second, arterial (pancreatic) phase scan is obtained 40 seconds after administration of IV contrast agent. At this time, maximum enhancement of the normal pancreas is obtained, allowing identification of non- or less-enhancing neoplastic lesions (Fig. 62.3A). The third, portal venous phase scan is obtained 70 seconds after injection of IV contrast agent and allows accurate detection of liver metastases and assessment of tumor involvement of the portal and mesenteric veins (see Fig. 62.3B). Thus the early phase delineates the tumor, whereas the late phase enhances the vascular relationships and liver metastases.[74]

Although there are minor variations between multiple guidelines, the CT criteria for unresectability of a pancreatic tumor are[75] as follows: (1) presence of distant metastasis (e.g., to liver, peritoneum, or other sites), (2) encasement of the celiac axis or superior mesenteric artery (>180° of the circumference), and/or (3) unreconstructible portal vein or superior mesenteric vein due to tumor involvement or occlusion. The increasing use of venous and arterial resection (and very rarely resection of oligometastatic disease) means that these criteria are no longer considered absolute. Notably, these criteria are reliant on CT scanning, and yet the outcome for patients is not just related to the anatomic disposition of the tumor but also to the tumor biology and the patient's physiological reserve.[76] The detection of vascular invasion is accomplished with a sensitivity of 55%–97% and specificity of 91%–100%. The determination of resectability is accomplished with a sensitivity of 76%–92% and specificity of 82%–100%.[34]

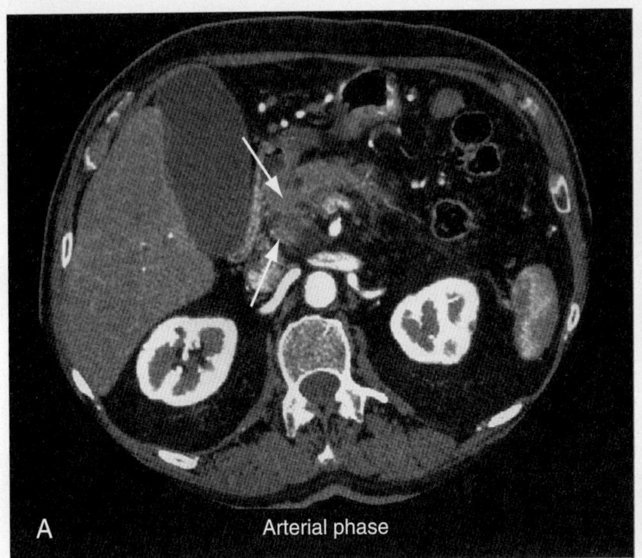

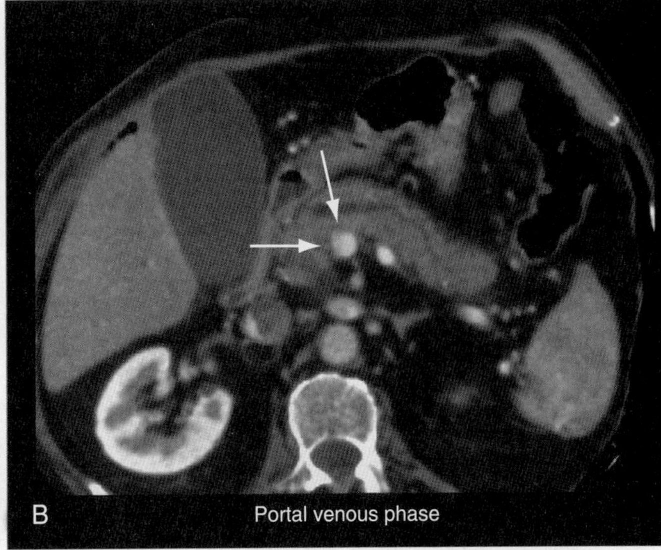

Fig. 62.3 Pancreatic protocol CT in a patient with pancreatic cancer. (A) Arterial phase showing a nonenhancing lesion in the head of the pancreas (*arrows*). (B) Venous phase showing a noninvolved fat plane around the portal vein (*arrows*).

Magnetic Resonance Imaging

Magnetic resonance imaging (MRI) is increasingly used to evaluate pancreatic tumors, and several recent studies have shown results that rival those of CT.[77] High field strengths greater than 1.5 T, liver-specific contrast agents, and diffusion-weighted imaging have all contributed to improved imaging. MRI offers greater soft tissue contrast compared with CT, leading to a greater sensitivity in detection of noncontour deforming lesions.[78]

PC typically has the appearance of an ill-defined mass with varying intensity. The tumor is typically hypointense on fat-suppressed T1, with variable intensity on T2-weighted images. Multiple acquisition sequences are required for full assessment of both the primary tumor and any distant disease.[79] MRI offers better assessment of CT isoattenuating lesions, small tumors, hypertrophied pancreatic head, and focal infiltration of the parenchyma.[78] Lesions that are isoattenuating on CT may show only secondary signs such as gland atrophy or pancreatic duct dilation, yet may be seen with 79.2% sensitivity on MRI.[80] MRI with MRA techniques using gadolinium contrast enhancement can demonstrate vascular involvement by tumor, with sensitivity equal to CT in assessing resectability.[77] Unlike CT, MRI does not involve radiation and uses an iodine-free contrast agent that cannot be used in the setting of renal insufficiency but has rare renal toxicity.

MRCP can also be obtained at the time of MRI. MRCP uses heavily T2-weighted images that emphasize fluid-containing structures such as ducts, cysts, and peripancreatic fluid collections. Images obtained are highly comparable with those obtained with endoscopic retrograde cholangiopancreatography (ERCP) and readily demonstrate pancreatic ductal obstruction, ectasia, and calculi. In contrast to ERCP, MRCP is noninvasive and does not require injection of contrast into the pancreaticobiliary tree, avoiding possible complications such as allergic reaction, pancreatitis, or infection. No therapeutic or diagnostic intervention can be performed with MRCP, and patients requiring endoscopic therapy or biopsy will require ERCP.

Positron Emission Tomography/Computerized Tomography Scanning

Hybrid positron emission tomography/CT (PET/CT) is a noninvasive imaging tool that provides metabolic and semiquantitative data and tumor morphology, the latter being the contribution on CT scanning which contributes enhanced spatial interpretation. The method is based on greater uptake and metabolism of radio-labeled glucose by tumor cells compared with normal pancreatic parenchyma. The radioactive glucose analog ^{31}F-FDG is administered intravenously, followed by detection of FDG uptake by the PET scanner. The normal pancreas is not usually visualized by PET scan. In contrast, pancreatic carcinoma appears as a focal area of increased uptake in the pancreatic bed. Hepatic metastases and nodal metastases also appear as "hot spots." A recent study showed no improvement in detection rate by PET/CT when compared to contrast-enhanced multidetector CT, [81] but the NCCN guidelines recommend the performance of PET/CT in patients at high risk of metastases.[75] PET/CT can also be useful in assessing tumor recurrence after pancreatic resection, when scar tissue or postoperative changes may be difficult to differentiate from recurrent carcinoma.[82] Finally, PET/CT can be of benefit in assessing tumor response to primary or neoadjuvant chemotherapy, which may lead to alteration in clinical management.[83]

Endoscopic Retrograde Cholangiopancreatography

ERCP is a key tool in the diagnosis of various tumors of the periampullary region.[84] ERCP allows direct visualization of ampulla of Vater and duodenal invasion, and with contrast injection, the delineation of both the pancreatic and biliary ducts. This allows detection of choledocholithiasis and delineation of biliary strictures, helping to distinguish benign from malignant causes of obstruction. A "double-duct sign" on ERCP (and cross-sectional imaging), representing strictures of both biliary and pancreatic ducts, which is usually due to PDAC, but can be found in patients with chronic pancreatitis with benign strictures of both ducts (Fig. 62.4). A malignant-type biliary stricture without concomitant pancreatic duct obstruction is usually due to a cholangiocarcinoma.

ERCP can also provide a pathological diagnosis by biliary brushings (for cytology) or biopsy forcep (for histology or genetic analysis).[85] Direct visualization of the stricture for directed biopsy is now possible with small caliber flexible scopes "Spyglass" passes through the working channel of the duodenoscope used for ERCP. Most experts recommend a combined approach, both brushings and biopsy, to increase sensitivity of diagnostic ERCP.[73]

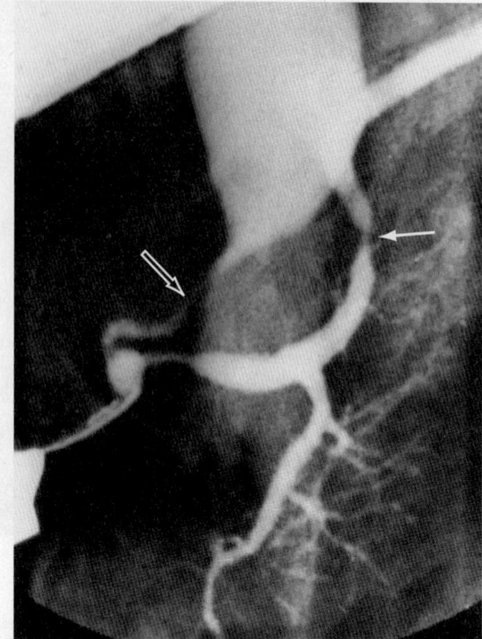

Fig. 62.4 ERCP showing strictures of the bile duct (*open arrow*) and pancreatic duct (*closed arrow*) in a patient with pancreatic cancer. The bile duct is markedly dilated proximal to the bile duct stricture.

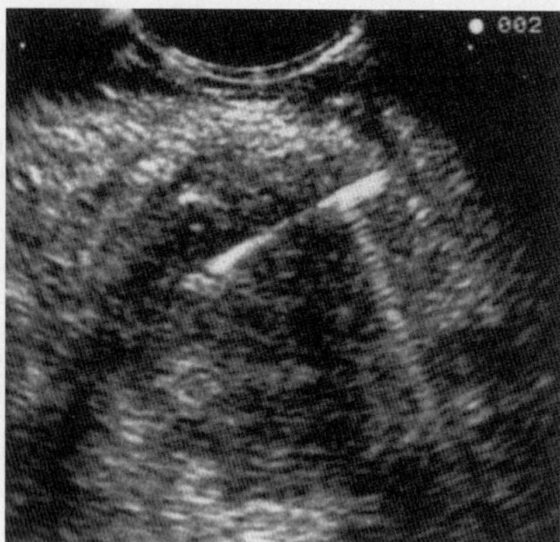

Fig. 62.5 EUS image of pancreatic cancer showing the needle during biopsy of the tumor. *EUS*, Endoscopic ultrasonography.

Endoscopic Ultrasonography

EUS has become the most accurate single test for the diagnosis of PC[86] but it is highly operator dependent and demands significant experience before reaching user proficiency.[87] EUS offers visualization of the pancreas via the stomach and the duodenum, with numerous studies showing a higher specificity and sensitivity than CT for detecting pancreatic masses (Fig. 62.5). Retrospective and prospective observational data have demonstrated superior accuracy using EUS in the diagnosis of PC compared with CT scanning,[88,89] especially for the detection of tumors <3 cm.[90] As such, EUS demonstrates significant advantage in small, potentially resectable lesions and when suspicion of PC is high but MDCT fails to detect a mass.[91] EUS is complementary to cross-sectional imaging because it cannot provide information regarding metastatic disease for complete pretreatment staging of disease.

FNA cytology of the pancreas has been one of the major advances in the management of patients with pancreatic tumors. CT-guided biopsy was used for more than 30 years and is regarded as a safe, reliable procedure, with a reasonable sensitivity and virtually no false-positive results. EUS-guided FNA achieves similar results. Even in patients with a mass without obstructive jaundice, a diagnostic accuracy of 97.6% can be achieved.[92] When a patient is considered to have unresectable or metastatic PC, CT- or EUS-guided FNA biopsies are indicated for histologic confirmation of disease, unless a palliative surgical procedure is required, at which time a biopsy can be obtained. Even if the diagnosis of chronic pancreatitis has been ruled out, proof of malignancy may exclude other rare benign diseases of the pancreas, such as tuberculosis and sarcoidosis. FNA cytology and immunohistochemistry can usually distinguish between adenocarcinoma and other pancreatic tumors, such as neuroendocrine tumors and lymphomas, and may lead to a different treatment plan.

Historically, tissue diagnosis was not considered a prerequisite to proceeding with surgery in most patients with appropriate clinical and CT findings and potentially resectable tumors. However, with the increasing use of neoadjuvant treatment and the value of molecular subtyping, tissue diagnosis is required for virtually all patients, including patients for palliative systemic therapy. Pretreatment tissue diagnosis is best obtained by EUS-guided biopsy (rather than CT-guided biopsy) because of better diagnostic yield, safety, and potentially lower risk of peritoneal seeding when compared with the percutaneous approach.[75] It is important to note that while EUS-FNA has a low false-positive rate, the false-negative rate can be as high as 25%[93] meaning that a negative FNA result does not exclude malignancy. The smaller and potentially curable tumors are more likely to be missed by CT-guided FNA or EUS-FNA.

There are other situations where EUS can be helpful. When there is uncertainty about a vascular margin on cross-sectional imaging, EUS can be helpful in examining the margin (especially of the portal vein) to help with the decision about whether a PC is resectable, or not.[94] As we move into the era of tailoring treatment for individual patient PC subtypes and especially in the context of treatment trials, it is becoming essential to obtain tissue from patients for molecular markers. For this, EUS will play an increasingly important role.[94]

Serum Tumor Markers

A wide variety of tumor markers have been proposed for diagnosis, prognosis, and monitoring of PC and its treatment. In practice only serum CA 19-9 has found a role in clinical practice, but not as a screening tool. For diagnosing PC, the sensitivity and specificity of CA 19-9 vary with the threshold values used in different jurisdictions. One of the major limitations of this tumor marker is a low positive predictive value, especially in asymptomatic individuals. One study demonstrated that a level of 37 units/mL was the most accurate cutoff for differentiating benign from malignant pancreatic disease. At this level, the reported sensitivity and specificity were only 77% and 87%, respectively.[95] A very high CA 19-9 can be found in the presence of jaundice due to benign causes and especially with cholangitis, in the absence of malignancy (false-positive results). In addition, up to 10% of patients have a negative Lewis blood group phenotype (Le[a−], Le[b−]) and do not express the CA 19-9 antigen (so-called nonsecretors) resulting in false-negative results.[96]

CA19-9 levels have prognostic value in the setting of resectable disease. High levels of preoperative CA 19-9 are associated with higher potential for occult metastatic disease.[97] A study of 260 PC patients who underwent resection found that patients with normalization of CA 19-9 within 6 months had twice the mean survival of those with persistent elevations (29.9 vs. 14.8 months; $P = .0004$). It has been found that patients with postresection levels above 90 U/mL did not benefit from adjuvant chemotherapy.[98] A chemotherapy trial in patients with metastatic disease found that decreases in CA 19-9 correlated with an increased response rate, progression-free survival, and overall survival.[83] Similarly, CA 19-9 response rates and time to nadir following neoadjuvant therapy may provide valuable information on response to treatment, optimal time of surgery, and eventual survival.[99,100]

Staging

The eighth edition of the American Joint Committee on Cancer staging system for PC Table 62.4[101] proposed cutoff points for T-stage (based on tumor diameter) and N-stage (based on the number of positive lymph nodes). Tumor diameter is a variable that is more reproducible between institutions and pathologists. The nodal groups, too, have been found to correlate with survival estimates. Both these changes enable a better stratification of patients with resected tumors according to their lymph node involvement without compromising their prognostic accuracy.[102]

While staging is based on TNM a further categorization of patients has been introduced to help with decision-making around resectability and chemotherapy. There are multiple definitions (Table 62.5)[103–109] based on solely anatomic criteria around the relationship between the tumor and subjacent vessels. More recently it is being accepted that the decision about proceeding to resection is one that is also dependent on the biology of the tumor (for which satisfactory markers, other than CA 19-9 are still awaited) and the physiological reserve or condition of the patient.[76] These criteria define four patient categories, but they are likely to have less clinical importance when future treatment decisions are based on molecular and genetic markers rather than anatomic criteria. The first category is patients with "metastatic" disease, and treatment is palliative chemotherapy. The second category is patients with "locally advanced" disease but without demonstrable metastases. These patients rarely benefit from neoadjuvant chemoradiation and, according to their treatment response, may rarely be candidates for subsequent surgical exploration and would usually require venous and/or arterial resection.[110] The third category is patients with "borderline-resectable" disease, and treatment is neoadjuvant therapy followed by surgery (if occult metastatic disease has not become apparent) and adjuvant chemotherapy.[111] The fourth category is patients with "resectable" disease for whom prompt surgical treatment has been traditionally offered. While the data are not yet convincing, neoadjuvant treatment for resectable disease is being offered in a number of centers as treatment failure in these patients is most often due to occult metastatic disease.

TABLE 62.4 TNM System and American Joint Committee on Cancer Staging of Pancreatic Cancer

Primary Tumor (T)	
TX	Primary tumor cannot be assessed
T0	No e/o primary tumor
Tis	Carcinoma in situ
T1	Maximum tumor diameter <2 cm
T2	Maximum tumor diameter >2≤4 cm
T3	Maximum tumor diameter >4 cm
T4	Tumor involves the celiac axis or the superior mesenteric artery (unresectable primary tumor)
Regional Lymph nodes (N)	
NX	Regional lymph node(s) cannot be assessed
N0	No regional lymph nodal metastasis
N1	Metastasis in 1–3 regional lymph nodes
N2	Metastasis in ≥4 regional lymph nodes
Distant Metastases (M)	
M0	No distant metastases
M1	Distant metastases
Anatomic Stage	
Stage 0	Tis—N0—M0
Stage IA	T1—N0—M0
Stage IB	T2—N0—M0
Stage IIA	T3—N0—M0
Stage IIB	T1-3—N1—M0
Stage III	Any T—N2—M1
Stage IV	T4 Any N M0
	Any T Any N M1

From Kakar S, Pawlik T, Allen P. Exocrine pancreas. Pancreatic adenocarcinoma. In: Amin M, ed. *AJCC Cancer Staging Manual*. 8th ed. New York: Springer-Verlag; 2016.

Staging for a patient with PC includes a physical examination and cross-sectional imaging of the chest, abdomen, and pelvis. As discussed earlier, multiphase contrast CT and MRI/MRA are comparable and accurate in identifying unresectable disease.[77,80] In borderline-resectable tumors and in planning for preoperative therapy, EUS is important to provide a tissue diagnosis and additional assessment of vascular margins. CT has been shown to predict an R0 resection rate in resectable, borderline resectable, and unresectable PC at the rate of 73%, 55%, and 16%, respectively.[112] The CT also has a limitation of resolution (~4–6mm) meaning that it misses small pancreatic masses and is unable to detect small lesions on the peritoneal surfaces of the liver, abdominal wall, stomach, intestine, or omentum. Published data demonstrate that approximately 25% of patients in whom localized disease is demonstrated by CT also have unsuspected metastases.[111]

The role of staging laparoscopy is important in patients with ascites CT scan and in those suspected to have peritoneal disease. It identifies a further 5%–15% of resectable patients with features of unresectability.[113] These patients do not benefit from surgical exploration, and their identification by preoperative imaging remains a challenge. The staging procedure adds only a few minutes to planned surgery and consists of a simple diagnostic laparoscopy with biopsy of suspicious nodules. Enthusiasm for peritoneal washings for cytologic analysis has waned because a positive lavage does not predict survival in patients with locally advanced disease or in those with visible metastases,[114] although this may change as neoadjuvant approaches are explored.

The combination of CT scan and selective staging laparoscopy has improved the accuracy of identifying metastatic, localized unresectable, and resectable PC and has helped in stratifying patients to different treatment protocols. A current algorithm for the diagnosis and staging of PC should include laparoscopy for all patients with tumors in the body and tail of the pancreas (in which the frequency of unsuspected metastases approaches 50%) and for patients with tumors larger than 2 cm in the head of the pancreas, because the yield of laparoscopy is proportional to the size of the primary tumor.[113] Staging laparoscopy has also been shown to be of value in patients with borderline-resectable PC by detecting occult metastases in about 10% of patients. The potential for these patients to receive palliative systemic chemotherapy exceeds that of patients who underwent a laparotomy (76.9% vs. 30.0%, $P = .040$) and in whom occult metastases were found.[115]

Serum CA 19-9 whilst not useful as a marker of diagnosis, may help predict the biological behavior of the tumor, especially in patients with borderline-resectable disease.[76] In patients with borderline resectable, or locally advanced PC, normalization of CA 19-9 levels after neoadjuvant therapy may help in guiding further therapy, for example, early surgery over further therapy.[116,117] Normalization of CA 19-9 levels postsurgical resection is predictive of better disease-free survival.[118]

Treatment

It is now well accepted that PC presents with systemic disease in the vast majority of patients, which is reinforced by the overall

TABLE 62.5 Variations in the Definition of Borderline-Resectable PC

	MD Anderson Cancer Centre	American Hepatopancreatobiliary Association, Society for surgery of the Alimentary Tract, the Society of Surgical Oncology	National Comprehensive Cancer Network	Intergroup trial (Alliance A021101)	American Pancreatic Association[a]
SMV/PV	Short segment occlusion of SMV PV, or SMV-PV confluence with suitable option for vascular reconstruction available because of a normal SMV below and normal PV above area of tumor involvement	Tumor abutment with or without impingement and narrowing of lumen or encasement of SMV/PV, or short segment venous occlusion resulting from either tumor thrombus or encasement but with suitable vessel proximal and distal to vessel involvement, allowing for safe resection and reconstruction	Abutment with impingement or narrowing	Interface between primary tumor and ≥180° of the circumference of SMV-PV and/or short segment occlusion of SMV-PV with normal vein above and below the level of obstruction amenable to resection and venous reconstruction	Tumor contact of >180° with SMV or PV tumor contact of ≤180° with contour irregularity of the vein or thrombosis ot the vein but with suitable vessel proximal and distal to site of involvement allowing for safe and complete resection and reconstruction
SMA	Tumor abutment with ≤180° of circumference	Tumor abutment not to exceed >180° of circumference	Abutment	Interface between tumor and <180° of the circumference of artery wall	Tumor contact of ≤180°
GDA	–	Encasement	–	–	
CHA/HA	Short segment encasement amenable to resection and reconstruction	Either short segment encasement or direct abutment	Abutment or short segment encasement	Short segment interface (of any degree) between tumor and HA with normal artery proximal and distal to the interface amenable to resection and arterial reconstruction	Contact with CHA or HA bifurcation allowing for safe and complete resection and reconstruction
Coeliac trunk/axis	No extension	No extension	No abutment or encasement	Interface between tumor and <180° of the circumference	No extension
IVC	–	–	–	–	Tumor contact
Vascular anomalies	–	–	–	–	Tumor contact with variant arterial anatomy (e.g., accessory or replaced RHA or replaced CHA)

[a]Adopted by National Comprehensive Cancer Network.

SMV, Superior mesenteric vein; *SMA*, superior mesenteric artery; *PV*, portal vein; *RHA*, right hepatic artery; *CHA*, common hepatic artery; *HA*, hepatic artery; *GDA*, gastroduodenal; *IVC*, inferior vena cava.

Reproduced with permission from Barreto SG, Windsor JA. Justifying vein resection with pancreatoduodenectomy. *Lancet Oncol*. 2016;17:e118–e124.

5-year survival of less than 10%. As a result, surgery has a role in the minority of patients. The approach to treatment of many other common solid cancers (e.g., breast, colon, stomach, and esophagus) has changed to recognize the primacy of systemic therapy and with level 1 evidence the establishment of neoadjuvant chemotherapy as standard of care. This paradigm shift is only now happening for the treatment of PC.[119]

Surgical Treatment

Only about a quarter of patients are offered surgical resection which in combination with chemotherapy offers the best chance of long-term survival.[120,111,121,122] Unfortunately, even in the most optimal situation, the median survival rate of a resected PC treated with adjuvant chemotherapy ranges from 20 to 23 months.[123] The most important prognostic factors are negative margins (R0), absence of lymph node metastases, and low volume tumor.[124,125] The addition of neoadjuvant therapy (esp. FOLFIRINOX/***fol***inic acid, ***f***luorourcil, ***irin***otecan, ***ox***aliplatin) prior to surgery has, however, demonstrated the promise of improved survival in patients with borderline-resectable PDAC.[126]

The decision to offer surgical resection should be made with multidisciplinary input, including medical oncologists. Patients with resectable disease are usually offered upfront surgery, but this is changing. While further evidence is required, it stands to reason that if patients with borderline-resectable disease are candidates for neoadjuvant therapy, the same should apply to those with resectable disease.[127] That most patients develop recurrence or metastases after surgery emphasizes the primary importance of effective systemic therapy. As the effectiveness of neoadjuvant therapeutic agents and combinations continues to improve, it is expected that more patients will become candidates for surgery due to downstaging.

Indications for resection in locally advanced disease are debated, although the goal of any surgical resection should be an *R0* resection.[128] Relative contraindications to resection include encasement or occlusion of the superior mesenteric vein or portal vein, or direct extension of disease to the celiac axis, superior mesenteric artery, vena cava, or aorta. Vascular resection and reconstruction are being performed more often because *R0* resections can be achieved in selected cases[103] if direct extension to the vein is the only barrier to complete resection of borderline resectable or locally advanced disease.[129]

Routine preoperative ERCP and biliary duct stenting to relieve jaundice has not been shown to decrease postoperative morbidity and mortality, and the procedure may increase the likelihood of surgical infectious complications.[130,131] Therefore routine preoperative biliary stenting in patients with resectable tumors (as assessed by CT) cannot be recommended as standard practice.[132] The role of ERCP and placement of biliary stents is reserved for patients presenting with deep jaundice and cholangitis, with or without renal impairment, in those unfit for surgery in whom optimization prior to surgery is essential, patient with jaundice embarking on neoadjuvant therapy, or as a definitive procedure for biliary obstruction in patients with an unresectable lesion.[133] In patients too frail to withstand an operation or with unresectable disease, endoscopic biliary stenting, preferably with expandable metal stents, offers excellent palliation.[134,135]

The most common operation for PC is pylorus-sparing pancreatoduodenectomy (Fig. 62.6), which removes primarily the head of the pancreas *en bloc* with the duodenum, distal bile duct, and proximal jejunum, with pancreatico-jejunal anastomosis.[136,137] There has been a trend towards total pancreatectomy for patients with hereditary PC, in patients with associated IPMN, in patients deemed to be at a high risk for a postoperative pancreatic fistula

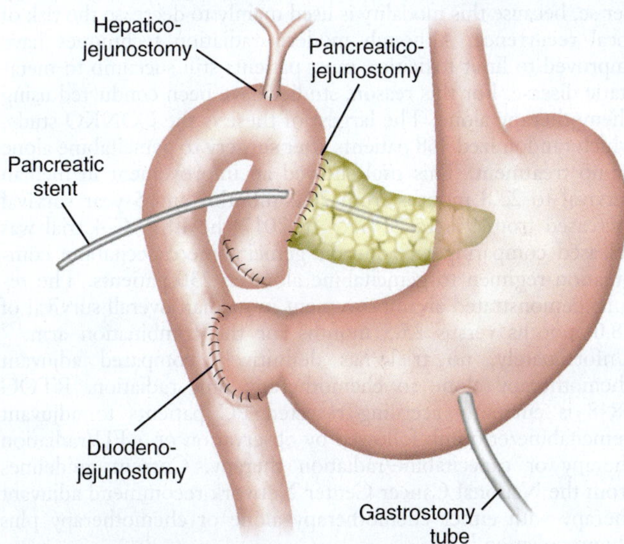

Fig. 62.6 Diagram of the pylorus-preserving pancreatoduodenectomy. A pancreatic stent is shown in the pancreatic duct. (From Jimenez RE, Fernandez-del Castillo C, Rattner DW, et al. Outcome of the pancreaticoduodenectomy with pylorus preservation or with antrectomy in the treatment of chronic pancreatitis. *Ann Surg*. 2000;231:293–300.)

(POPF), especially in the situation where a vascular resection and reconstruction is necessitated, and to ensure the likelihood of achieving an *R0* resection margin.[138] The historical concerns about "brittle" diabetes and the challenges of maintaining excellent glucose tolerance after total pancreatectomy have been partially offset by overall improvements in diabetes management.

Other extensions to the standard Whipple's procedure, such as addition of extended retroperitoneal lymphadenectomy, have shown no significant survival benefit. The decision to extend the resection beyond the traditional anatomic border of the pancreatic neck, based on intraoperative frozen section, has also been evaluated. Even when an initial *R1* margin proves to be R0 on final histology report, the additional resection produced no improvement in survival compared to patients with an *R1* resection and no additional resection.[139] Multiple randomized clinical trials demonstrated prolonged surgical time, increased bleeding, and postoperative mortality, but no survival benefit.[140–145]

Previously, pancreatoduodenectomy (Whipple's procedure) was associated with high morbidity and mortality rates. Many contemporary large series now consistently show mortality rates of under 3%.[146] Despite the significant improvements in surgical resection and perioperative care, postoperative morbidity rates are 30%–60%.[147] POPF, historically the most common complication after the Whipple's procedure, is seen in approximately 22% –26% of patients.[148] Numerous potential endogenous and surgical risk factors have been evaluated as causes of POPF, including age, gender, body mass index, diabetes, cardiovascular factors, disease site, pancreatic remnant fibrosis, size of the pancreatic duct, anastomotic technique, and intraoperative blood loss. A high index of suspicion is required for the early diagnosis of POPF, and the deterioration of a patient or departure from the expected clinical course is often associated with increase in abdominal pain, nausea, and ileus and a systemic inflammatory response, confirmed with a leucocytosis and elevate C-reactive protein. The level of amylase and/or lipase in fluid effluent from drains can help confirm the suspicion of POPF, although concomitant acute pancreatitis can be the explanation.[149,150] A CT scan is indicated in these patients, and a collection associated with the anastomosis can confirm a pancreatic leak, especially if there is speckled gas within it.

Treatment of POPF consists of source control by ensuring optimal percutaneous drainage of the intra-abdominal collection(s), the judicious use of antibiotics, enteral nutrition whenever feasible,[151] (but adding parenteral nutrition if required), and early detection of hemorrhagic complications (usually seen as an index bleed into an abdominal drain). An index bleed should prompt selective angiography for stenting or embolization if the source of bleeding is identified, especially in the presence of pseudoaneurysm. Surgery for completion pancreatectomy is often fatal and should be a treatment of last resort.

Improved outcomes are found in centers of excellence for pancreatic surgery, where surgeons have greater experience and expertise, although it is known that lower volume surgeons can deliver equivalent results. Individual surgeon experience, rather than annual institutional or surgeon volume, may drive outcomes.[152] A study using the Medicare database from the 1990s showed a fourfold increase in mortality when comparing pancreatoduodenectomy performed in hospitals with low volume (<1 case/year) to higher-volume (>5 cases/year) hospitals.[153] Controversy continues over the role of institutional volume as an independent predictor of mortality for pancreatoduodenectomy. The relationship between outcome and volume is complex as there are many factors that contribute to improved outcomes, including 24 hours specialist care, access to interventional radiology, enhanced recovery programs and a culture of active clinical surveillance. Overall, the most important determinant of institutional outcomes is the ability to rescue patients who develop complications. "Failure to rescue" is now recognized as a key factor linking volume to outcome.[154] Other determinants of mortality are age, performance status, and malnutrition and have been shown to be more important than hospital.[155] Minimally invasive and robotic surgery have been introduced but have not made a significant difference to mortality or morbidity after pancreatoduodenectomy. To date, they have equivalent morbidity and mortality, with slightly shorter length of stay offset by higher readmission rates. The prolonged operative time (427 vs. 360 minutes) and costs have not yet been offset by decreased rates of fistula formation or delayed gastric emptying.[156]

The implementation of minimally invasive and robotic techniques has increased operative times, and the American College of Surgeons National Surgical Quality Improvement Program has found that longer operative time is independently associated with worse perioperative outcomes. All morbidities increased in a stepwise manner with increasing operative time, independent from known preoperative risk factors.[157]

Despite improving outcomes and better patient selection, surgery for PC appears to be underutilized. A cohort study of patients with early-stage PC using the National Cancer Data Base up to 2004 identified that 38.2% of patients with potentially resectable disease were not offered surgery.[122] Surgery was less likely to be offered to patients who were older than 65 years, Black, of low socioeconomic status, less educated, or had cancer involving the head of the pancreas. The study also reported differences in outcomes between patients with stage I disease who underwent pancreatectomy versus those not offered surgery, with median survivals of 19.3 months versus 8.4 months, respectively.[158] These data may reflect both a nihilistic attitude toward the effectiveness of pancreatic surgery and disparities in availability of health care options.

Ultimately, prognosis for PC remains poor, even after potentially curative surgery in appropriately selected patients. Five-year survival rates after resection remain approximately 25%,[159] with median survival between 12.7 and 24.1 months based on stage.[160] These are improving with newer approaches to chemotherapy, especially in borderline-resectable patients.[119] Despite decreases in procedure-associated early mortality and improved short-term survival, long-term survival has not improved much over three decades.[161] Recent advances in surgical technique and perioperative care have likely approached their maximum survival benefit.[162] Surgery alone is limited by the biological behavior of the tumor and the anatomic boundaries for complete resection.[163] Microscopic margins may be a marker of tumor biology more than a reflection of surgical inadequacy.[164,165] Major improvements in long-term outcomes await concerted efforts with multimodal therapy, likely driven by immunotherapy and the rapidly evolving molecular targeted therapies.[64,66]

Adjuvant and Neoadjuvant Therapy

For the 15%–20% of patients who have resectable tumors, survival remains poor, with 5-year survival rates of 10%–30%. Survival may be improving over time with better surgical techniques, improved postoperative care, and adjuvant therapy. Risk factors for recurrent disease include positive margins, lymph node involvement, high-grade tumors, and primary tumor size greater than 2.5 cm.[166,167] Adjuvant therapy is defined as treatment given after surgery to prevent cancer recurrence. PCs most commonly recur with distant metastatic disease, with only 15% of recurrences isolated to the local tumor bed.[168] This has led to an ongoing debate about the role of adjuvant radiation therapy in addition to chemotherapy.

From 1980 to 2000, adjuvant chemoradiation, chemotherapy given concurrently with radiation, was the standard of care after potentially curative PC resection. These recommendations were based on the results of a small study conducted by the Gastrointestinal Tumor Study Group (GITSG) between 1974 and 1982.[169] The study randomized 43 patients after surgery to either observation alone or chemoradiation with 4000 cGy of external beam radiation, with a concurrent bolus of 5-fluorouracil (5-FU) as a radiosensitizer. Median survival in the treated group was 21 months, which was significantly longer than the 11-month median survival in the untreated group. The GITSG study was criticized for its small sample size and lack of statistical power. A separate study by the Norwegian PC Trial group showed similar results and supported a survival benefit for adjuvant treatment.[170]

In 1999 the results of a study by the European Organization for Research and Treatment of Cancer (EORTC) questioned the value of adjuvant chemoradiation in PC.[171] Similar to the study design by the GITSG, the EORTC randomized 114 patients after surgery to observation or chemoradiation (4000 cGy external beam radiation and concurrent continuous-infusion 5-FU). The median survival was only 4.5 months longer in the treatment group than in the observation group (17.1 vs. 12.6 months, respectively), and this difference was not statistically significant. Likewise, the projected 2-year survival was not significantly different between the 2 groups (37 vs. 23 months, respectively).

Further controversy ensued after the results of a larger 289-patient study by the European Study Group for PC (ESPAC-1 trial) were released in 2001.[172] The ESPAC-1 study had a complicated design that randomized patients after surgery to four groups: observation, chemotherapy, chemoradiation, or chemoradiation plus chemotherapy. The results showed no difference in median survival between patients receiving chemoradiotherapy and those who did not (15.5 vs. 16.1 months). Even for patients with positive resection margins, thought to be the most appropriate candidates for adjuvant chemoradiation, this treatment did not have a survival impact. In a subset analysis of those patients who received chemotherapy only, the 2-year survival was 30%, which suggested a benefit of chemotherapy alone.

Gemcitabine has been shown to be a more effective drug for treating PC than 5-FU, used in the earlier adjuvant studies. RTOG 9704 evaluated the use of gemcitabine given prior to 5-FU–based chemoradiation, followed by additional gemcitabine. This trial showed a trend toward improved 5-year survival (22% vs. 18%) with the addition of gemcitabine, but this difference was not statistically significant.[173]

Many have questioned the role of adjuvant radiation therapy per se, because this modality is used mainly to decrease the risk of local recurrence. Although modern radiation techniques have improved to limit toxicities, most patients still succumb to metastatic disease. For this reason, studies have been conducted using chemotherapy alone. The largest of these is the CONKO study, which randomized 368 patients after surgery to gemcitabine alone or no treatment. This trial showed an improvement in median survival to 22.8 months from 20.2 months, and 5-year survival increased from 9% to 21%.[123] In 2017 the ESPAC-4 trial was released comparing an adjuvant gemcitabine/capecitabine combination regimen to gemcitabine alone in 730 patients. The results demonstrated an improvement in median overall survival of 28.0 months versus 25.5 months for the combination arm.[174] Unfortunately, no trial has definitively compared adjuvant chemotherapy alone to chemotherapy plus radiation. RTOG 0848 is currently accruing resected PC patients to adjuvant gemcitabine/erlotinib followed by observation or 5-FU/radiation therapy or capecitabine/radiation therapy. Current guidelines from the National Cancer Center Network recommend adjuvant therapy with either chemotherapy alone or chemotherapy plus chemoradiation.[175]

There has been notable emerging interest in neoadjuvant therapy[119] which is now considered standard of care in patients with borderline-resectable PC and those at high risk for margin-positive resection. Borderline-resectable disease is localized disease that is unlikely to be resected with an *R0* resection due to proximity or direct involvement of venous and/or arterial vasculature.[104] For borderline-resectable PC, NCCN recommends avoidance of upfront surgery and multimodality therapy with neoadjuvant chemotherapy and/or chemoradiation.[75] In recent years there have been numerous randomized trials exploring the role of neoadjuvant chemotherapy (predominantly gemcitabine and FOLFIRINOX) or chemoradiotherapy compared to upfront surgery in patients with borderline resectable and locally advanced PC.[176–181] Options for neoadjuvant therapy include radiation, chemotherapy, sequential therapy, concurrent therapy, or a blended regimen. The findings of the studies have uniformly confirmed a survival advantage for neoadjuvant therapy.[176,178–180] Neoadjuvant therapy increases the likelihood that patients with resectable disease receive chemotherapy and has the aim to downstage disease to increase the likelihood of a negative (*R0*) margin resection.[75] And this also potentially avoids surgery in patients harboring subclinical metastatic disease on presentation and treats micrometastatic disease. However, the randomized trials were divided in terms of the benefits of chemotherapy[178,179] or chemoradiation therapy[176,180] in the neoadjuvant setting. While the choice of optimal regimen, chemotherapeutic agents, the number of cycles, assessment of response, etc., needed to guide management are in a state of evolution the early evidence supports the use of neoadjuvant therapy in borderline resectable and locally advanced PC prompting the NCCN and ASCO guidelines to consider a regimen of neoadjuvant therapy for borderline disease a reasonable treatment option.

Palliative Procedures

Patients with unresectable PC are candidate for palliative care, but not all are suitable for palliative procedures. Frailty and advanced age often prohibit intervention especially as the goal is quality and not necessarily quantity of life.[182] Historically, surgical biliary-enteric bypass was standard practice for patients presenting with obstructive jaundice. This fell out of favor because of the high risk of gastro-duodenal obstruction.[183] Over the last decade, endoscopic and percutaneous approaches to stenting have come to the fore (see Chapters 63 and 72). As a result, the use of palliative surgical double bypass has dramatically declined, but also because improved preoperative imaging has reduced the frequency of exploration to determine resectability and therefore fewer subclinical unresectable disease patients are going to surgery.[184] It is worth noting that this is still often required after neoadjuvant therapy for borderline-resectable PC where re-staging by cross-sectional imaging is difficult to interpret. Palliative endoscopic procedures are well tolerated and performed on an outpatient basis. In experienced hands, endoscopic biliary and duodenal stent placement has a success rate of greater than 90%, with a low procedure-related morbidity and mortality.[185] And decreased survival between patients palliated endoscopically versus those treated surgically for obstructive jaundice probably reflects greater comorbidities and worse functional status in patients treated endoscopically.[186]

Two types of biliary stents are available: plastic and self-expandable metallic stents. The plastic stents are preferred for short-term use and require exchange every 3 months to prevent complications from stent occlusion or cholangitis. Self-expandable metal stents and covered stents have improved long-term patency rates when compared with plastic stents and are more durable for longer-term applications, such as when patients receive neoadjuvant chemoradiation.[187,188]

Historically, duodenal obstruction was treated by surgical gastrojejunostomy. A comparison of outcomes in asymptomatic patients who were unresectable and either had a prophylactic surgical bypass or no bypass demonstrated that the former was associated with decreased risk of late gastric outlet obstruction, with no difference in postoperative complications or length of hospital stay.[189] The use of expandable metallic stents to relieve malignant duodenal obstruction has shown some success and is increasingly used in preference to palliative surgical bypass.[185,190] A stent can be inserted if and when duodenal obstruction occurs. Readmission for biliary or duodenal stent-related complications is more common than readmission for failed surgical bypass, but the total number of inpatient days was not reduced in the surgically bypassed patients.[191] Prior surgical bypass makes subsequent endoscopic stenting, if it fails, more difficult.

Pain in inoperable PC is a common problem, with 80% of affected patients experiencing severe pain.[192] This pain difficult to control with opioid administration and celiac plexus neurolysis with EUS is sometimes required. Not all patients benefit, and one study chemical neurolysis by EUS was 73% effective in improving pain,[193] and a single injection is usually adequate.[194] Thoracoscopic splanchnicectomy is an alternative approach to neurolysis,[195] but the efficacy is only moderate. While this study showed significant pain relief, there was no significant decrease in morphine consumption, improvement in quality of life, or increase in survival (see Chapter 61).[196]

Treatment of Advanced Disease

Distant Metastatic Disease

Single-agent chemotherapy has been the mainstay of therapy for metastatic PC. Gemcitabine alone has historically been the standard of care for metastatic PC; however, response rates are low at 6%–10%.[197,198] Gemcitabine was approved based on a landmark trial that showed decreased disease-related symptoms, including pain and weight loss.[199] For years after this trial, studies of other combinations with chemotherapy, targeted therapy, or immunotherapy did not show a statistically significant improvement in survival. In 2007 a randomized phase 3 study of gemcitabine, alone or with erlotinib, showed a statistically significant survival advantage for combination therapy over gemcitabine alone.[200] Median survival improved from 5.91 to 6.24 months in favor of the addition of erlotinib. Many questioned whether a 10-day increase in median survival was a clinically meaningful benefit. The next step forward in treatment came with the publication of a study randomizing patients to receive combination therapy with FOLFIRINOX versus gemcitabine.[201] This trial showed a marked improvement in survival, from 6.8 to 11.1 months, in favor of the combination regimen (Fig. 62.7). Toxicities with this regimen were significantly higher than with gemcitabine alone. An alternative is combining gemcitabine and albumin-bound paclitaxel (nab-paclitaxel) which also improved survival from 6.8 to

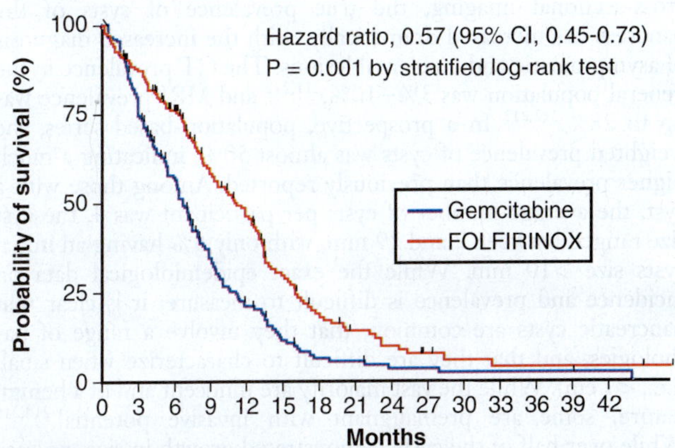

Fig. 62.7 Kaplan-Meier estimates of overall survival rates in patients with metastatic pancreatic cancer according to treatment with gemcitabine or FOLFIRINOX. (Modified from Bilimoria K, Bentrem DJ, Ko CY, et al. National failure to operate on early-stage pancreatic cancer. *Ann Surg*. 2007;246:173–180.)

8.5 months with the combination compared with gemcitabine alone.[202] Current recommendations for treatment of patients with metastatic disease include combination therapy with either FOLFIRINOX or with gemcitabine plus nab-paclitaxel for those patients with a good performance status who can tolerate combination therapy, or gemcitabine alone for those who cannot. Data on the benefit of immunotherapy in patients with disease progression but who remain in good performance status are limited but offer some promise.

Unresectable Disease

Autopsy series have demonstrated that 30% of patients die due to complications from local disease rather than distant metastatic disease.[168] A number of studies have used chemotherapy, chemoradiotherapy or sequential therapy as modalities to control local disease. These studies generally had heterogeneous older study populations and used less efficacious chemotherapy regimens.[203] Higher response rates have been obtained with gemcitabine/nab-paclitaxel or FOLFIRINOX regimens. The real benefits of radiotherapy have not been well established. The American Society of Oncology recommends induction chemotherapy for locally advanced disease, with a consideration for subsequent concurrent chemoradiotherapy for those who do not progress after induction therapy.[204] Newer treatment modalities, including better definition of treatment fields and "dose sculpting" by intensity-modulated radiation therapy,[205] have allowed improvement in toxicity while maintaining dose intensity. Historically, nodal drainage basins are usually included in the radiation field due to the approximate 30% risk of nodal spread,[206] but to minimize toxicity, current studies tend to avoid elective nodal irradiation.[207] Stereotactic body radiation therapy (SBRT) has demonstrated promise and uses high doses per fraction given over limited doses in a conformal fashion, with phase II data demonstrating high local control rates with well-controlled toxicity.[208] Emerging evidence has suggested that SBRT may achieve similar disease control outcomes as compared to IMRT, with the additional benefit of reduced acute toxicity. These findings present SBRT as an attractive technique for pancreatic radiotherapy owing to the convenience and tolerability given the equivalent efficacy.[209]

PANCREATIC CYSTIC NEOPLASMS

Historically, cystic neoplasms of the pancreas have been considered relatively uncommon, accounting for less than 10% of pancreatic cystic neoplasms.[210] However, with the increased use of cross-sectional imaging, the true prevalence of cysts of the pancreas has increased dramatically, with the increased diagnosis of asymptomatic and incidental lesions. The CT prevalence in the general population was 3%–10%,[211,212] and MRI prevalence was up to 28%.[212,213] In a prospective, population-based series, the weighted prevalence of cysts was almost 50%, indicating a much higher prevalence than previously reported. Among those with a cyst, the average number of cysts per participant was 4, the cyst size ranged between 2 and 29 mm, with only 6% having an initial cysts size >10 mm. While the exact epidemiological data on incidence and prevalence is difficult to measure, it is clear that pancreatic cysts are common, that they involve a range of pathologies, and that they are difficult to characterize when small (i.e., <1 cm). While the vast majority are innocent and of a benign nature, some are premalignant with invasive potential.[214,215] While over half of the cysts demonstrated growth in size, no case of PC was detected during 5-year follow-up in a prospective German cohort.[216]

The clinical management of pancreatic cysts has become a major theme in pancreatic units and has created a considerable workload.[217]

Pancreatic Cysts and Risk of Malignancy

The WHO guidelines for digestive tumors include 27 different types of pancreatic cysts (Table 62.6), including neoplasia that can present with a cystic component, such as pancreatic adenocarcinoma and neuroendocrine tumors. At detection of an incidental pancreatic cyst, the most important distinction to be made is between mucinous and nonmucinous cysts (Fig. 62.8). The importance of mucinous cysts lies in their definite malignant potential, while this is nearly negligible for nonmucinous cysts. Of note, over 80% of resected cystic lesions are mucinous [IPMN and mucinous cystic neoplasm (MCN)] and nonmucinous (SCN).[218] Accurate preoperative diagnosis is important to reduce the risks associated with resection of benign lesions, even when they have malignant potential.[218,219] Accurate recognition of these lesions is also important because of their ability to masquerade as pancreatic pseudocysts, and also because surgical treatment is usually curative (see Chapter 62). As many of the cysts are too small (<1 cm) at the time of detection to be characterized, they labeled "undesignated cyst" requiring surveillance scans (Fig. 62.9).[217]

Some of the distinguishing features of the most common pancreatic cystic neoplasms are summarized in Table 62.7. Note there is considerable overlap in patients' demographic and clinical presentation that may occur among cyst types. Consensus work on the classification of cysts has guided a more unified understanding and reporting of pancreatic cystic neoplasms.[220–222]

TABLE 62.6 Proposed WHO List of Cystic Lesions of the Pancreas

Epithelial Neoplastic	Epithelial Nonneoplastic
Intraductal papillary mucinous neoplasm (IPMN)	Lymphoepithelial cyst
Mucinous cystic neoplasm (MCN)	Mucinous nonneoplastic cyst
Serous cystic neoplasm (SCN)	Enterogeneous cyst
Serous cystadenocarcinoma	Retention cyst/dysontogenic cyst
Cystic neuroendocrine tumor	Periampullary duodenal wall cyst
Acinar cell cystadenoma	Endometrial cyst
Cystic acinar cell carcinoma	Congenital cyst
Solid pseudopapillary neoplasm (SPN)	
Accessory-splenic epidermoid cyst	
Cystic hamartoma	
Cystic teratoma (dermoid cyst)	
Cystic ductal adenocarcinoma	
Cystic pancreatoblastoma	
Cystic metastatic epithelial neoplasm	
Others	
Nonepithelial neoplastic	**Nonepithelial nonneoplastic**
Benign nonepithelial neoplasm (e.g., Lymphangioma)	Pancreatitis associated pseudocyst
Malignant nonepithelial neoplasms (e.g., sarcomas)	Paracitic cyst

The list may not be exhaustive as there are cystic variants of solid neoplasms.
From *WHO Classification of Tumors*, 5th ed. Digestive system tumours.

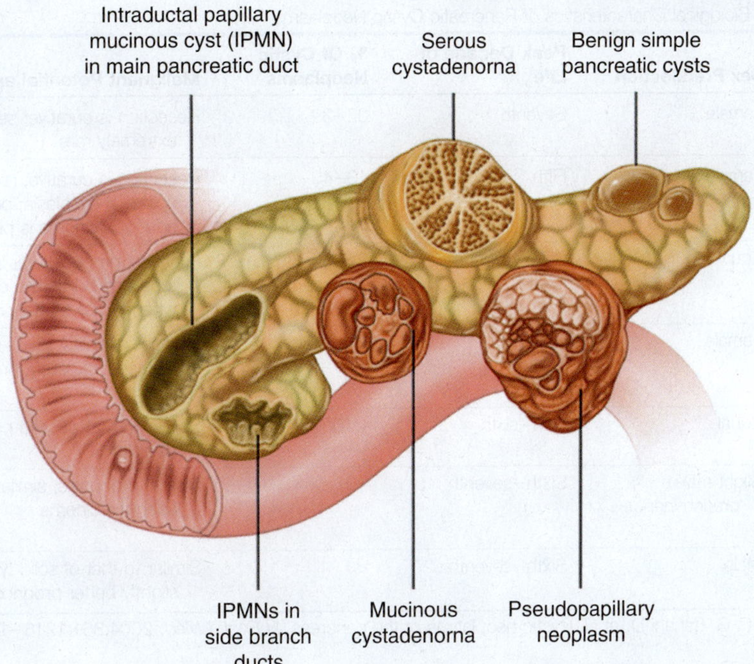

Fig. 62.8 Illustration of the most common mucinous and nonmucinous cystic lesions of the pancreas. Mucinous lesions consist of IPMN, either main duct (MD) mixed type (MT) or branch duct (BD) IPMNs or mucinous cystic neoplasia (MCN). Typical nonmucinous cystic lesions are represented by SCN, SPN and pseudocysts. (Reproduced and modified with permission from Aunan JR, Al-Saiddi MS, Stutchfield B, Jamieson NB, Søreide K. Pancreatic cystic lesions and risk of cancer. In: Søreide K, Stättner S, eds. *Textbook of Pancreatic Cancer: Principles and Practice of Surgical Oncology*. Cham: Springer International Publishing; 2021:777–797.)

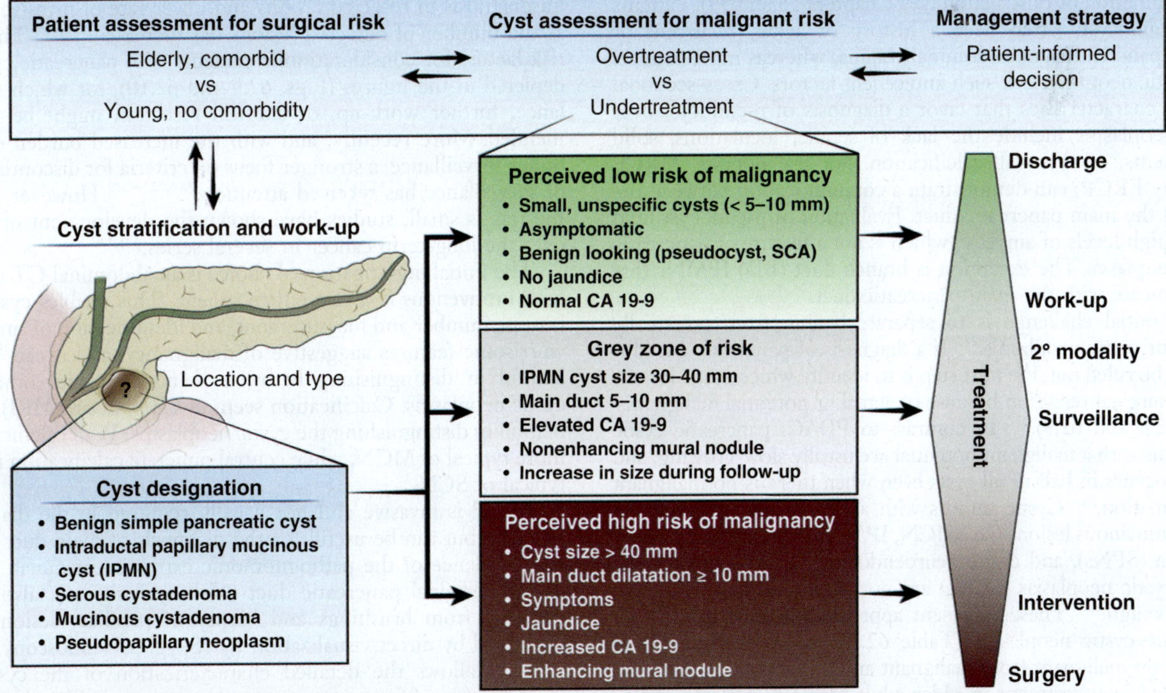

Fig. 62.9 The incidental pancreatic lesions. The pancreatic lesion, usually presenting as an undesignated cyst, requires further designation for both etiology and perceived risk. The clinical factors must be weighted in along with the patient's expressed wish before a decision plan can be made according to the lesion and risk at hand. The cyst risk factors vary slightly among current guidelines, with risk for over- and undertreatment, yet the majority will be considered in a gray area for which further surveillance is recommended. (Reproduced with permission from Søreide K, Marchegiani G. Clinical management of pancreatic premalignant lesions. *Gastroenterology*. 2022;162(2):379–384, under the creative commons CC-BY license.)

TABLE 62.7 Epidemiologic and Biological Characteristics of Pancreatic Cystic Neoplasms

Neoplasm	Sex Predilection	Peak Decade of Life	% Of Cystic Neoplasms	Malignant Potential and Natural History
Serous cystadenoma	Female	Seventh	32–39	Resection is curative; serous cystadenocarcinoma is extremely rare
Mucinous cystic neoplasm	Female	Fifth	10–45	Resection is curative, regardless of the degree of epithelial dysplasia; poor prognosis when invasive adenocarcinoma is present
Intraductal papillary mucinous neoplasm	Equal	Sixth–seventh	21–33	Excellent prognosis for lesions showing only adenomatous and borderline cytologic atypia; poor prognosis when invasive adenocarcinoma is present
Solid pseudopapillary neoplasm	Female	Fourth	<10	Indolent neoplasm with rare nodal and extranodal metastases; excellent prognosis when completely resected
Cystic endocrine neoplasm	Equal	Fifth–sixth	<10	Similar to that of solid neuroendocrine neoplasm (see Chapter 33)
Ductal adenocarcinoma with cystic degeneration	Slight male predominance	Sixth–seventh	<1	Dismal prognosis, similar to that of solid adenocarcinoma
Acinar cell cystadenocarcinoma	Male	Sixth–seventh	<1	Similar to that of solid type; aggressive neoplasm with slightly better prognosis than ductal adenocarcinoma

Modified from Brugge W, Lauwers G, Sahani D, et al. Cystic neoplasms of the pancreas. *N Engl J Med*. 2004;351:1218–1226.

Initial Diagnostic Work-Up of Pancreatic Cystic Neoplasms

After discovery of a cystic lesion of the pancreas, the initial effort should be directed towards excluding a pancreatic pseudocyst, by history and investigation. In contrast to cystic neoplasms, pseudocysts lack an epithelial lining and represent collections of pancreatic secretions that have extravasated from a duct disrupted by inflammation or obstruction (see Chapters 58 and 59). Patients with pseudocysts often have a history of acute, recurrent or chronic pancreatitis, or abdominal trauma, whereas most patients with cystic neoplasia lack such antecedent factors. Cross-sectional imaging characteristics that favor a diagnosis of pseudocyst over cystic neoplasms include the lack of septae, loculations, solid components, or cyst wall calcification. For pseudocysts, MRCP (or rarely ERCP) can demonstrate a communication between the cyst and the main pancreatic duct. Evaluation of pseudocyst fluid reveals high levels of amylase, which is not a feature of pancreatic cystic neoplasia. The exception is branch duct (BD) IPMNs that communicate with the main pancreatic duct.

The initial challenge is to separate benign from potentially malignant cystic neoplasms.[217] If a diagnosis of pancreatic pseudocyst can be ruled out, the next step is to identify which cystic lesions require surgical resection because of actual or potential malignancy (Figs. 62.8 and 62.9).[217] In contrast to PDAC, pancreatic cystic neoplasms with a malignant potential are usually slow-growing, and growth occurs in half of all cysts even when there is no malignant transformation.[216] Cystic tumors with a clear malignant potential include mucinous lesions (i.e., MCN, IPMN), solid pseudopapillary neoplasia (SPNs), and cystic neuroendocrine tumors. In contrast, serous cystic neoplasias (SCNs) are not mucinous and are almost always benign.[223] These represent approximately one-third of all pancreatic cystic neoplasms (Table 62.7). A key challenge is to separate premalignant from malignant and invasive neoplasia. This is to avoid overtreatment in older-adult high-risk patients and to focus surveillance imaging in a cost-effective manner to facilitate a safe nonoperative strategy.[217,224,225]

Currently, five guidelines related to the management of pancreatic cystic lesions are available. These are the American Gastrointestinal Association guidelines, the American College of Gastroenterology guidelines, the American College of Radiology recommendations, the European evidence-based guidelines, and the International Association of Pancreatology (also referred to as Fukuoka) guidelines.[226–230] While several inconsistencies in recommendations are found between these guidelines,[225,226] the definition of lesions with a malignant potential (MCN and IPMN) is agreed as target lesions for decision-making. Early studies suggested a high rate of malignant transformation in resected lesions, while more recent data suggest a high rate of misdiagnosis in resected lesions and lower rate of invasive cancer as the number of detected lesions has increased.[218,219] The main risk factors for consideration in patients with pancreatic cysts are depicted in the figures (Figs. 62.9 and 62.10), for which surveillance, further work-up, or surgical resection might be recommended. More recently, and with the increased burden of cysts under surveillance, a stronger focus on criteria for discontinuation of surveillance has received attention.[224,227–230] However, even if the risk is small, studies have shown the development of cancer over the long-term cancer in several series.[231,232]

The initial investigation of choice is an abdominal CT or MRI with intravenous contrast enhancement. This enables cyst localization, number and measurement, and identification of sinister or worrisome features suggestive of malignancy, and it can be very helpful in distinguishing between pseudocysts and other true cystic neoplasms. Calcification seen on CT (but not MRI) can be helpful in distinguishing the cystic neoplasms. Wall calcification is more typical of MCN, while central punctate calcification is more typical of SCN.

ERCP is invasive and not usually required in the diagnostic work-up but can be useful for the diagnosis of main duct IPMN with evidence of the pathognomonic extrusion of mucin from a dilated terminal pancreatic duct ("fish-eye" sign). It also allows cytology from brushings and biopsy of papillary lesions, now facilitated by direct visualization by "Spyglass" endoscopy.

EUS allows the detailed characterization of the cyst wall, identification of fine structures (such as septa, papillary lesions, or wall nodules) (Fig. 62.11), confirmation of sinister or worrisome features such as asymmetric wall thickening or the wall nodules and several novel techniques for tissue sampling.[233–235] Additionally, EUS-guided FNA or biopsy of the cyst contents is important for cyst fluid analysis[236–238] (Table 62.8) and molecular profiling to differentiate cyst types, respectively.[234,239,240]

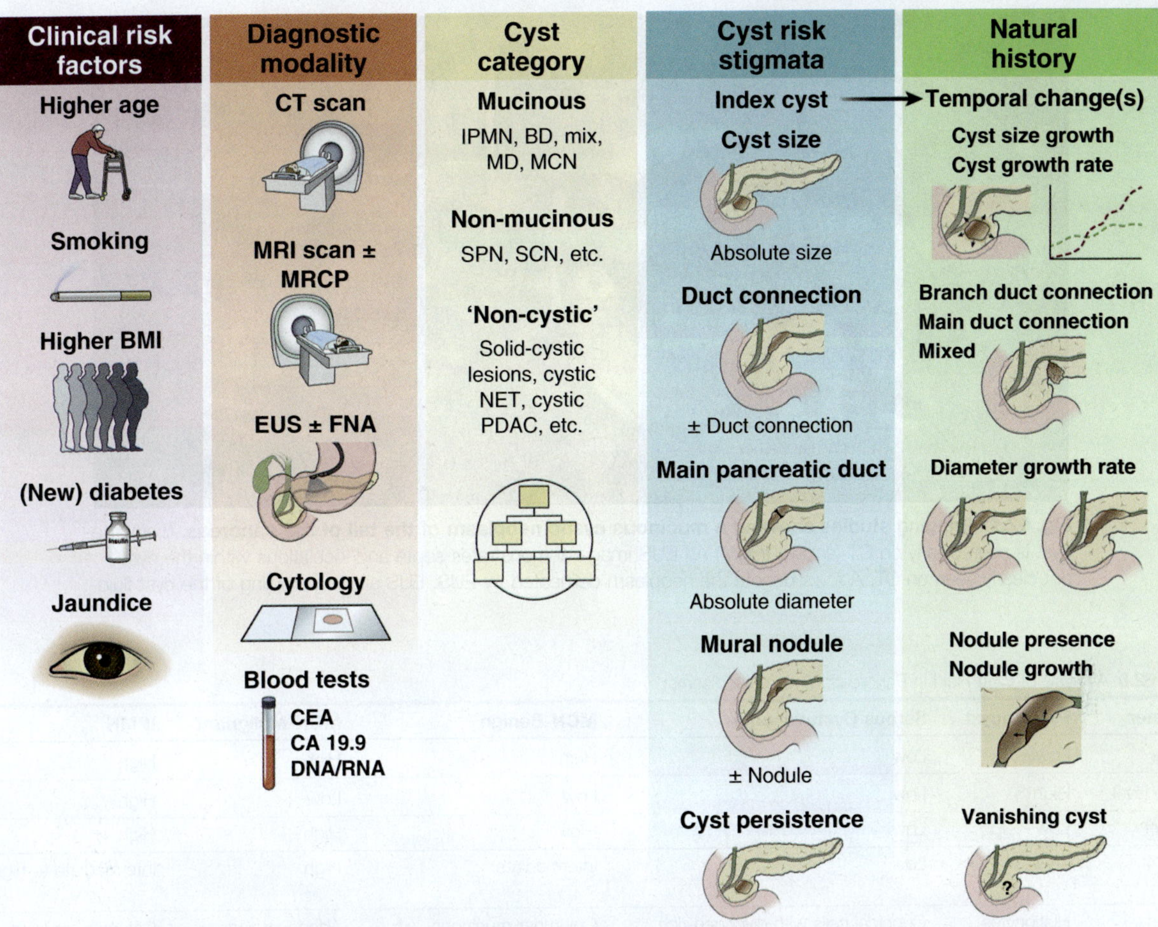

Fig. 62.10 Several clinical risk factors need a combined and multidisciplinary approach. Clinical factors are considered in relation to diagnostic findings and further need for endoscopy with evaluation of cystic fluid content. Designation into cyst category may be difficult in smaller lesions. Presence of cyst risk stigmata (variably defined across guidelines) should be considered at presentation and during surveillance to add the likely unchanged or developing natural history to the clinical information. Very rarely, cysts may disappear. *BD*, Branch duct; *BMI*, body mass index; *CA19.9*, carbohydrate antigen 19.9; *FU*, follow up; *MCN*, mucinous cystic neoplasia; *MD*, main duct; *NET*, neuroendocrine tumor; *SCA*, serous; *SCN*, serous cystic neoplasia; *SPN*, solid pseudopapillary neoplasia. (Reproduced with permission from Søreide K, Marchegiani G. Clinical management of pancreatic premalignant lesions. *Gastroenterology*. 2022;162(2):379–384, under the creative commons CC-BY license.)

In a meta-analysis the diagnostic accuracy for cyst fluid biomarkers found that mutations in *KRAS* and/or *GNAS* allowed identification of mucinous cysts with a sensitivity of 79% and specificity of 98%.[237] Mutational analyses exceeded the performance of the traditional biomarker CEA that had a sensitivity of 58% and specificity of 87%. Mutations in VHL were specific for serous cystadenomas (SCAs), with a reported sensitivity 56% and specificity 99% and helped to exclude mucinous cysts. Mutations in *CDKN2A*, *PIK3CA*, *SMAD4*, and *TP53* each had high specificities of 97%, 97%, 98%, and 95%, respectively, to identify high-grade dysplasia (HGD) or PDAC in mucinous cysts. However, DNA-based cyst fluid analyses are not routinely used in most pancreatic centers.

Management Strategies for Pancreatic Cystic Neoplasms

After diagnostic work-up, a management plan must be made for the pancreatic cystic neoplasm at hand. In principle, this may involve any of three strategies: discharge, surveillance, or surgical resection. Discharge from any further evaluation or surveillance is appropriate for lesions that are clearly defined as benign, small, in elderly patients or obviously unfit for surgery. Notably, much controversy consists regarding criteria for discharge or discontinuation of surveillance for those who are fit for surgery or have lesions with a very low (but not negligible) risk. Hence, many lesions, and probably far too many, will continue under surveillance. This includes BD IPMN, a lesion known to harbor very low risk,[241] but for which current guidelines till propose long-term (even life-long) surveillance.[230,231,242] Surveillance strategies, intervals, and duration are currently being scrutinized, with emerging data suggesting further groups of low or no risk to be discontinued from active surveillance. In one study, discontinuation from surveillance could be justified after 5 years of stability in patients older than 75 years with cysts <30 mm, and in patients 65 years or older who had cysts ≤15 mm, as the risk of cancer is negligible.[228]

Surgery may be indicated (by absolute or relative criteria) in patients with symptoms (such as jaundice) or those with one or more worrisome features or high-risk stigmata.[243–245] Worrisome features differ across guidelines, but the Fukuoka guidelines[246] define these as cyst size ≥3 cm, thickened or enhancing cyst walls,

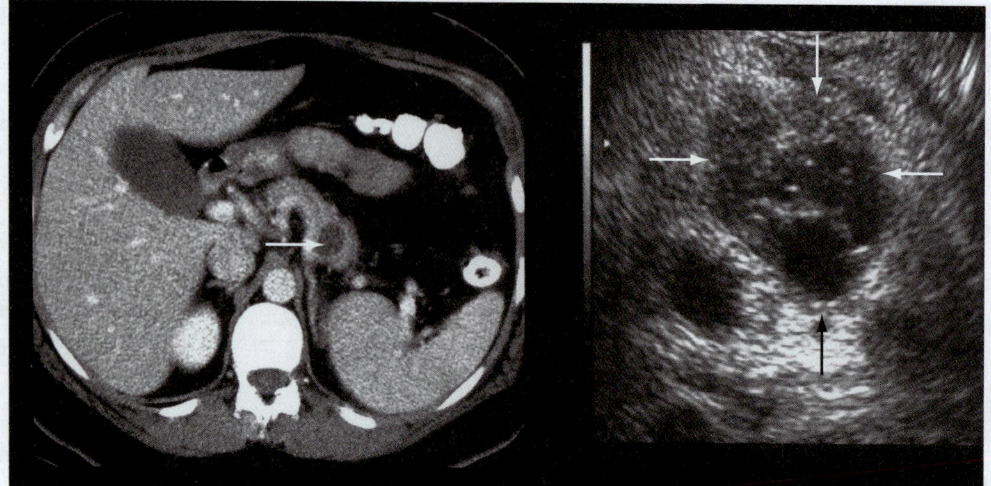

Fig. 62.11 Imaging studies showing a mucinous cystic neoplasm of the tail of the pancreas. (*Left*) The cyst is seen clearly on CT (*arrow*). (*Right*) An EUS image demonstrates septa and loculations within the cyst not clearly seen on CT. *Arrows* denote the neoplasm delineated by EUS. EUS allows sampling of the cyst fluid.

TABLE 62.8 Analysis of Cyst Fluid in Pancreatic Cystic Neoplasms

Parameter	Pseudocyst	Serous Cystadenoma	MCN-Benign	MCN-Malignant	IPMN
Viscosity	Low	Low	High	High	High
Amylase level	High	Low	Low	Low	High
CEA level	Low	Low	High	High	High
CA 72–4 level	Low	Low	Intermediate	High	Intermediate to high
Cytologic findings	Histiocytes	Cuboidal cells with glycogen-rich cytoplasm	Columnar mucinous epithelial cells with variable atypia	Adenocarcinoma cells	Columnar mucinous epithelial cells with variable atypia

IPMN, Intraductal papillary mucinous neoplasm; *MCN*, mucinous cystic neoplasm.

main duct size 5–9 mm, nonenhancing mural nodules, an abrupt change in pancreatic duct caliber with distal pancreatic atrophy, pancreatitis, and lymphadenopathy. High-risk stigmata are referred to as obstructive jaundice, enhancing mural nodule, or main pancreatic duct diameter >10 mm. Accumulation of worrisome features or high-risk stigmata increases the risk of invasive cancer in the final pathology of the resected specimen (even if not visible on preoperative imaging).[244,245] Surgery should be performed with the first objective to remove all tissue at risk (e.g., HGD without cancer) to prevent cancer development and the second objective is offer curative treatment for early stage cancer and the chance of long-term survival. The type of pancreatic surgery depends on the location of the lesion, either as a pancreatoduodenectomy or distal pancreatic resection. Total pancreatectomy is reserved for those cases with the entire gland affected (e.g., main duct IPMN) but can be avoided with judicious evaluation of the remaining/remnant duct by perioperative pancreaticoscopy (Spyglass).[247]

Mucinous Cystic Neoplasms

Most MCNs consist of thick-walled cysts with occasional septations that are filled with thick mucus that is sometimes hemorrhagic (Fig. 62.12; also see Fig. 62.11). MCNs are very female predominant (almost 95% are women) and are most often confined to the body and tail of the pancreas. The mean age at presentation is 50 years. In the past, most patients were diagnosed based on symptoms of abdominal pain or a palpable mass. However, the wide availability of CT and MRI scanning has led to an increasing percentage of tumors being identified as incidental findings.

MCNs are solitary, mucin-containing, multilocular, or unilocular lesions.[248] MCNs display a histologic spectrum ranging from benign to malignant behavior, with the vast majority (in particular those <4 cm in size) of a benign nature.[249] Current pathologic classification of MCN distinguishes between low-grade dysplasia (LGD), HGD, and invasive cancer.[220] The histologic presence of ovarian-type stroma within the tumor is a key criterion for establishing the diagnosis of MCN and distinguishes it from an IPMN. These are recognized as 2 distinct neoplasms with different genetics, biological behaviors, and prognosis.[220,249]

An MCN should be suspected when a CT or MRI of the abdomen shows a cyst within the body or tail of the pancreas in a middle-aged woman. The cyst might involve peripheral mural calcification in contrast to central calcification with SCN. There is no communication between the main pancreatic duct and the MCN, which distinguishes it from branch-duct IPMN. EUS is indicated when clinical and imaging characteristics are uncertain and deviate from this classic pattern. EUS can identify septations and cyst wall nodules in more detail than MRI or CT, and allows cyst wall biopsy and cyst fluid aspiration, and more recently genetic analysis. Cyst fluid analysis from an MCN generally reveals viscous or mucoid material, low fluid amylase, elevated tumor markers (CEA), and mucinous epithelial cells on cytology. These findings may help in differentiating MCN from SCAs (low fluid CEA) and IPMN (high fluid amylase) (see Table 62.8).

Owing to the inherent potential for malignancy in MCNs, surgical resection is advocated for many, but not all, MCNs.[249,250] MCNs are probably more indolent lesions than was previously thought.[249,251] Of note, in presumed MCN (prior to surgery), up to 1 in 5 may be misdiagnosed[250] and represent other lesions. On preoperative imaging, the presence of mural nodules, size >50 mm and enhancing wall features were predictive of malignant MCNs.[250,252]

Five-year survival rates are excellent for benign or borderline MCNs, where the reported cure rate is 100%. Long-term surveillance is not required for patients with resected noninvasive tumors, as no synchronous or recurrence are reported.[249] For invasive MCNs, 5-year survival rates range from 30% to 63% in resected tumors.[249]

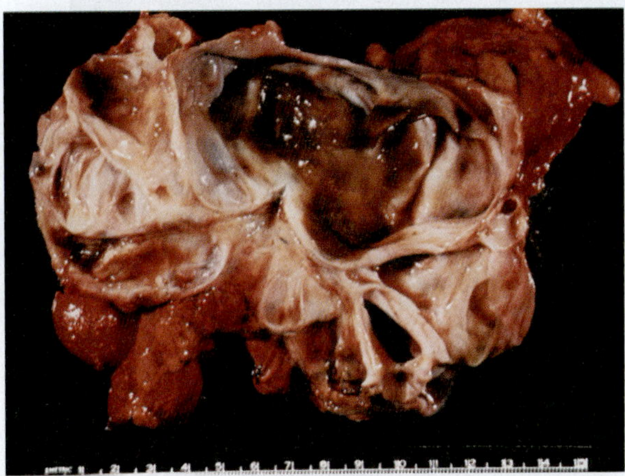

Fig. 62.12 Multiloculated mucinous cystic neoplasm of the tail of the pancreas.

Serous Cystic Neoplasms

Serous cystic neoplasms (SCNs) are generally considered benign tumors with an extremely low risk of malignant behavior,[223,253] even if rare cases have been reported.[254] The clinical presentation of SCNs is similar to that of MCNs, occurring mostly in the body or tail of the pancreas in women (75%), with a mean age of 50–60 years at diagnosis. An association with von Hippel-Lindau disease has been noted.[255] Historically, most patients present with vague abdominal pain or discomfort, sometimes associated with a palpable mass, when the tumor has attained a large size (10–25 cm). Currently, the majority of SCNs are incidental, asymptomatic tumors detected incidentally during imaging for other unrelated conditions.

Macroscopically, SCAs are well-circumscribed with numerous tiny cysts separated by delicate fibrous septa, often giving them a honeycomb appearance (Fig. 62.13).[253] The cysts are filled with clear watery fluid and are often arranged around a central stellate scar that may be calcified. The pathognomonic CT image is that of a spongy mass with central calcification, but this finding occurs in only 10% of patients with SCN (Fig. 62.14A). As most SCNs are incidental, small, and difficult to diagnose, they are often "undesignated pancreatic cysts" at first presentation. EUS can allow better resolution of the honeycomb structure than CT (Fig. 62.14B). Macrocystic variants occur, and tumors may undergo cystic degeneration, leading to diagnostic confusion with pseudocysts or MCNs. Cyst fluid analysis characteristically reveals low viscosity, low levels of CEA, and negative cytology (Table 62.8).

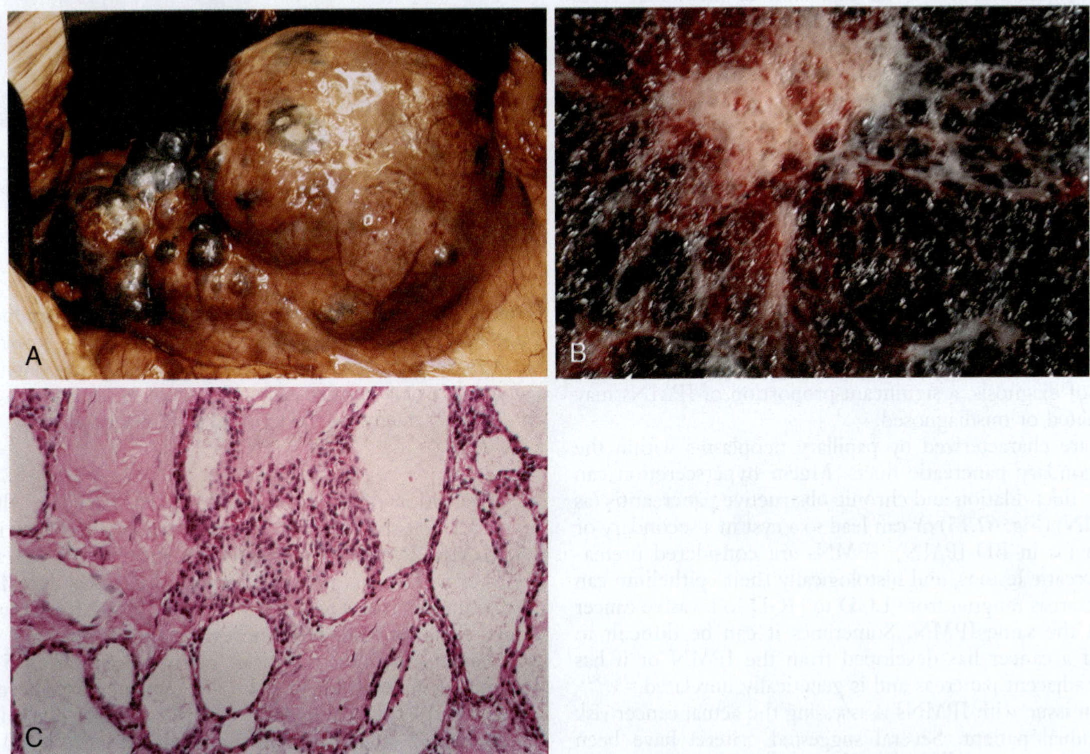

Fig. 62.13 Serous cystadenoma of the tail of the pancreas. (A) At surgery, most of the pancreatic parenchyma has been replaced by a cystic neoplasm. (B) Cut surface shows multiple cysts and a central fibrotic scar. (C) Histopathology showing cysts containing serous fluid and lined by bland cuboidal cells rich in glycogen (H&E).

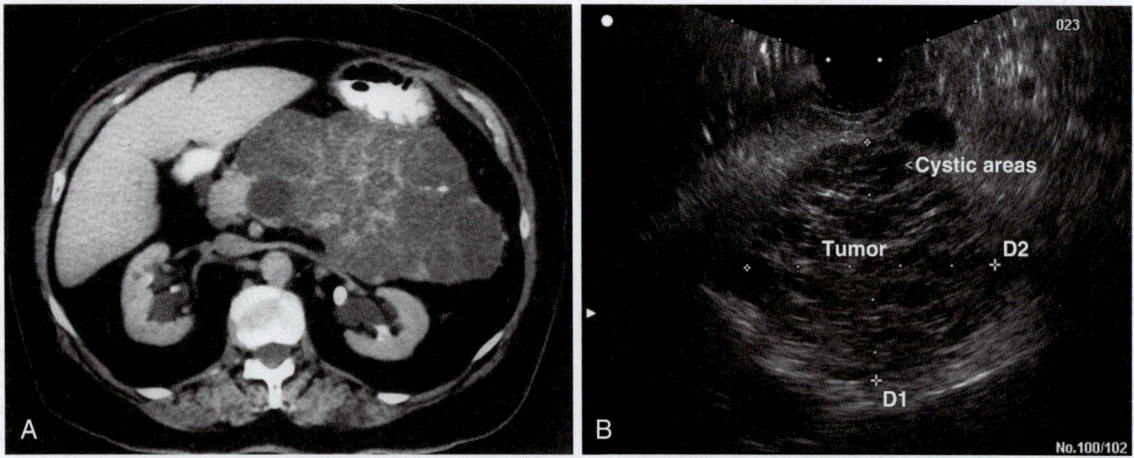

Fig. 62.14 Imaging studies showing a serous cystadenoma of the body and tail of the pancreas. (A) CT showing its spongy appearance and calcification. (B) EUS shows the honeycomb appearance of a 4.5 × 4.8 cm serous cystadenoma. (Courtesy Michael Nunez, MD, Dallas, TX.)

SCNs are considered benign tumors and are not recommended for routine surveillance.[256] Surveillance is only indicated where there is diagnostic doubt, where there has been growth or compression of other organs. However, most lesions remain asymptomatic. Symptomatic SCNs warrant resection, and with confirmation of benign histology, discharged from follow-up.

Intraductal Papillary Mucinous Neoplasms

The IPMN is the most important cystic neoplasm of the pancreas, due to its high prevalence and its significance as a defined premalignant lesion.[217] Increased awareness about IPMN, differentiation from chronic pancreatitis, and widespread high-quality diagnostic imaging has led to an explosion of incidental cases being recognized and reported.[257]

Clinically, IPMNs occur with equal frequency in men and women, with a mean age at diagnosis of 65 years. Most patients are asymptomatic with IPMN diagnosed on cross-sectional imaging performed for other indications. When presenting with symptoms, abdominal pain and weight loss are the most common complaints. A history of recurrent pancreatitis is given by 20% of patients, and acute pancreatitis is found in up to 25% at presentation. Malignant variants of IPMNs are difficult to diagnose but are more likely to be in older patients and in those who present with jaundice or new-onset diabetes.

There are three IPMN variants: 70% are BD IPMNs, with the remainder being either main-duct IPMNs (MD-IPMN) or mixed-type (IPMN) (Fig. 62.8). Because they are relatively small at the time of diagnosis, a significant proportion of IPMNs may be undesignated or misdiagnosed.

IPMNs are characterized by papillary neoplasms within the main or secondary pancreatic ducts. Mucin hypersecretion can lead to main duct dilation and chronic obstructive pancreatitis (as in MD-IPMN) (Fig. 62.15) or can lead to a cyst in a secondary or branch duct (as in BD-IPMN). IPMNs are considered premalignant pancreatic lesions, and histologically their epithelium can demonstrate areas ranging from LGD to HGD to invasive cancer even within the same IPMN. Sometimes it can be difficult to determine if a cancer has developed from the IPMN or if has arisen from adjacent pancreas and is genetically unrelated.[258,259]

The main issue with IPMNs is assessing the actual cancer risk in an individual patient. Several suggested criteria have been proposed to identify risk,[228,229,260–262] with inconsistencies across the various existing guidelines.[225,226]

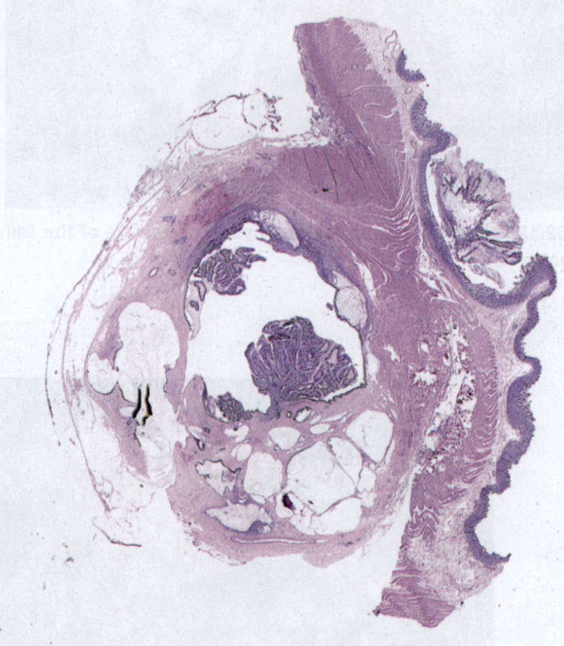

Fig. 62.15 Histopathologic view of a malignant intraductal papillary mucinous neoplasm. A papillary tumor is growing within the pancreatic duct. Note the surrounding lakes of mucin in the pancreas. At the *right* of the picture is the duodenum, which is focally invaded by the mucinous tumor at the top right (H&E low power).

Evaluation of patients includes MRI/MRCP of the pancreas with EUS ± ERCP[256,263] if further characterization is required. MRI/MRCP often demonstrates dilation of the pancreatic duct, with or without an associated cystic mass. Focal duct dilation may be so impressive as to mimic MCNs (Fig. 62.16). However, most duct dilatations are less impressive and uncertainty with intermediate main duct dilatation (often ranging from 5–9 mm in diameter) and the likely risk of malignancy.[264] There is a more defined risk of malignancy when the main duct dilatation is >10 mm.[265] In a two-center model, cyst size >3.0 cm, solid component/mural nodule, pain symptoms, and weight loss were significantly associated with HGD or invasive cancer.[266] MRI

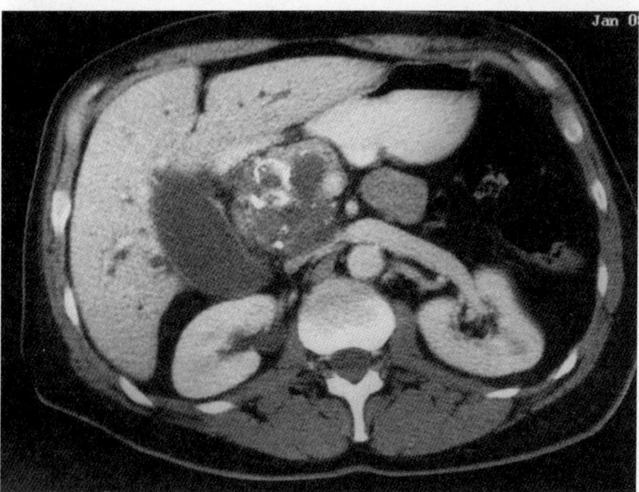

Fig. 62.16 CT showing an intraductal papillary mucinous neoplasm (IPMN) affecting the head of the pancreas.

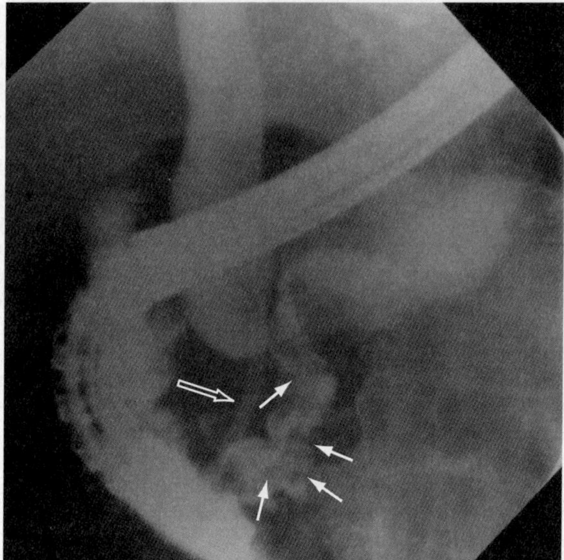

Fig. 62.17 ERCP showing an intraductal papillary mucinous neoplasm. Multiple filling defects are seen in the proximal pancreatic duct (*solid arrows*). Bile duct obstruction, treated with a stent, can also be seen (*open arrow*).

finds mural nodules (60% vs. 4%) and wall enhancement (74% vs. 21%) more frequently in malignant IPMNs.

Evaluation by ERCP typically shows a patulous ampulla of Vater with extruding mucus "fish eye," a finding that is pathognomonic for IPMNs but found in less than a third of patients. Other findings during pancreatography include main duct dilation, filling defects due to viscid mucus or papillary tumor nodules (Fig. 62.17), and communication between cystic areas and the main pancreatic duct.

Pancreatic resection is required in patients with features associated with cancer or high risk of malignant transformation. The current challenge lies in distinguishing these lesions from benign cysts with the risk of both under- and overtreatment. Once an invasive cancer has developed from an IPMN, the prognosis is similar to PDAC, with high risk of systemic recurrence and poor overall survival.[267] This should not surprise since both arise from pancreatic ductal cells. It is important to consider the potential for multifocality with the diagnosis of MD-IPMN. When present total pancreatectomy is indicated. Preoperative imaging is not accurate for diagnosing multifocal MD-IPMN, and intraoperative pancreaticoscopy ± biopsy of the remnant pancreas should be performed before deciding on the extent of resection.[247,268]

Prognosis after resection of IPMN is related to the presence or absence of invasion, stage, margin status, and CA 19-9 levels.[269,270] Factors associated with worse outcome in patients with invasive histology include lymph node metastases, lymphovascular invasion, PNI, and positive margins.[270] Disease recurrence in the pancreatic remnant is not rare after resection of PNIIPMNs and may occur in 14%–25% depending on IPMN type and grade of dysplasia.[271–273] Risk of subsequent new HGD or invasive cancer underscores the importance of continuing surveillance after resection for IPMN.[274,275] Patients with recurrent disease localized to the pancreas should be considered for completion pancreatectomy.[271,276–278]

Solid Pseudopapillary Neoplasms

Solid pseudopapillary neoplasms (SPNs) of the pancreas account for less than 2% of tumors of the pancreas.[279] Because they are sometimes cystic, they need to be considered in the differential diagnosis of pancreatic cystic neoplasms. Women are more frequently affected than men, with over 85% of SPNs reported in women in a large systematic review of almost 1400 patients.[279] In general, this is a disease of young women in their 30s,[279] with very few cases (5%) reported in adults older than 50 years.[279–283] Several pediatric series can be found in the literature, and these patients (ranging from 1 to 18 years) account for at least 20% of all known cases.[280,281]

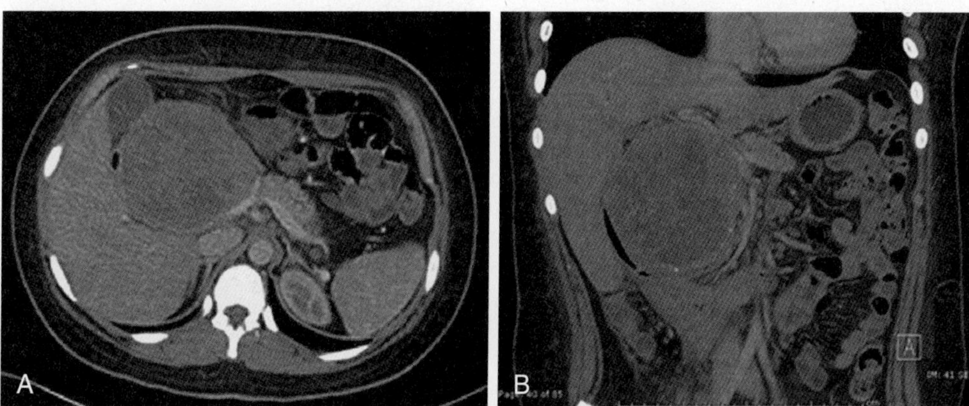

Fig. 62.18 Cross-sectional image (A) and coronal CT image (B) showing an extensive solid pseudopapillary tumor of the pancreas in a 16-year-old female. An R0 resection was obtained after a common femoral vein graft was used to replace a long segment of portal vein and superior mesenteric vein involvement.

The most common clinical presentation is abdominal pain, found in over half of all of patients.[279] The second most common finding is a large abdominal mass, which is the principal complaint in 35% of patients. Cross-sectional imaging is done less frequently in younger people, which may explain the increased rate of symptomatic presentation. As a result only 15% of SPNs are discovered incidentally.[283] As for other cystic lesions of the pancreas, evaluation with either CT or MRI (Fig. 62.18) and consideration for EUS-FNA provide sufficient information to direct clinical management.

Most (60%) SPNs are found in the body and tail of the pancreas. The tumors can be quite large at presentation, with 34% of patients having SPNs larger than 10 cm in diameter. Grossly, small tumors are relatively solid, whereas larger variants show significant cystic degeneration. Microscopically, a mixture of solid, pseudopapillary, and hemorrhagic pseudocystic areas is observed. Uniform neoplastic tumor cells are seen separated by vascular hyalinized stroma.

Although most SPNs demonstrate benign behavior, these tumors are considered to be lesions with a malignant potential. A large meta-analysis of published series found a 3% frequency of distant or lymph node metastasis in solid pseudopapillary neoplasia, while the accumulated rate was 13% in a series from the National Cancer Data Bank.[281,283] Current criteria for the diagnosis of malignancy include PNI, vascular invasion, invasion of adjacent tissues, or metastases.[281] The most common site of metastasis is the liver, and metastatic disease is observed in up to 13% of patients at presentation.[281]

Despite their female predominance, no association to estrogen receptors has been identified in SPNs. Other common mutated genes in pancreatic carcinogenesis, such as *K-ras* and *TP53*, are also absent in these tumors. In one series investigating the molecular features of SPN, a total of 28 driver genes were detected with mutations in at least 2 tumor samples, and the top 3 frequently mutated genes were CTNNB1, ATRNL1, and MUC16.[284]

Overall, SPNs are very slow-growing neoplasms, with overall survival better than 98%.[279] Complete resection is the treatment of choice, and resection of synchronous or interval metastases is also recommended when technically feasible. Prolonged survival has also been reported, even in the presence of metastatic disease. In one large series of 390 resected SPNs, only 4% experienced recurrence or distant metastasis in the follow-up.[284]

Data on adjuvant treatment of SPNs are scarce, but these lesions do not appear to be chemosensitive based on registry reports.[281] In patients with tumors <4 cm and no clinical suspicion of involved lymph nodes, the risk of metastases is very low. In patients who are poor surgical candidates, close surveillance can be considered given the risks of pancreatic surgery.[285]

OTHER PANCREATIC TUMORS

Other nonendocrine tumors of the pancreas include acinar cell carcinomas, lymphomas, and sarcomas. Acinar cell carcinomas are extremely rare, representing 1%–2% of PCs. Clinical presentation is usually indistinguishable from PDAC. CTs of acinar cell carcinomas have several features that can differentiate them from PDAC, including a large size without biliary or pancreatic duct obstruction, exophytic morphology, and an enhancing capsule.[286] A minority of these patients (up to 15%) may present with the *lipase hypersecretion syndrome*, with high serum lipase levels and peripheral fat necrosis observed clinically.[287] The lipase hypersecretion syndrome is more often present in the setting of liver metastases and is considered an unfavorable prognostic factor. Overall, acinar cell carcinomas are considered an aggressive malignancy, and 50% of cases present with liver metastasis; however, prognosis appears to be better than for PDAC. In a recent study of acinar cell carcinomas using the Surveillance, Epidemiology, and End Results database, 5-year survival was 22% for patients with unresectable disease and 72% for those with resectable disease.[288] In patients with limited metastatic disease, an aggressive approach including synchronous and metachronous liver resection had equal survival to those patients with localized disease.[289]

Primary pancreatic lymphoma represents less than 0.7% of all pancreatic malignancies, and less than 1% of all extra-nodal non-Hodgkin's lymphomas (see Chapter 41).[290] Non-Hodgkin lymphoma with secondary pancreatic involvement is more common. Patients with primary pancreatic lymphoma have no peripheral or mediastinal lymphadenopathy, no hepatic or splenic involvement, and a normal WBC count.[291] EUS FNA biopsy with flow cytometry is highly accurate in establishing the diagnosis.[292] Identification of primary pancreatic lymphoma is important because treatment is primarily nonsurgical (see Chapter 41). Treatment usually consists of a combination of chemotherapy and radiation therapy, and cure rates near 30% are reported in the literature.[293] A few patients with small tumors, thought to represent carcinomas, have been treated with surgery alone and have had excellent survival.

Full references for this chapter can be found at https://ebooks.health.elsevier.com.

63 Endoscopic Treatment of Pancreatic Disease

Ji Young Bang, Shyam M. Varadarajulu

IN THIS CHAPTER

Since the first report of ERCP and endoscopic biliary sphincterotomy in 1974, there have been numerous advances in ERCP techniques. Less invasive diagnostic modalities, including EUS, CT, and MRCP, have replaced diagnostic ERCP. However, therapeutic ERCP remains useful for the treatment of pancreatic diseases, and continually evolves. This chapter reviews the endoscopic treatment of acute pancreatitis and its complications, as well as the endoscopic treatment of recurrent acute pancreatitis, chronic pancreatitis, pancreatic cancer, and pancreatic cysts.

ACUTE PANCREATITIS

When a patient presents with acute pancreatitis, the role of endoscopy is limited to two situations: first, those patients with gallstone-induced pancreatitis (see Chapters 60, 67, and 72) and, second, to provide nutritional support via enteric feeding (see Chapter 6). Gallstone pancreatitis is caused by transient or sustained impaction of sludge or a stone within the common channel of the ampulla of Vater. ERCP and biliary sphincterotomy are used to improve the outcome of gallstone pancreatitis by removal of an impacted stone and subsequent relief of pancreatic ductal obstruction. Early studies of patients with acute gallstone pancreatitis suggested that ERCP and sphincterotomy within 72 hours of admission improved outcomes in patients with clinically severe acute pancreatitis.[1] Meta-analyses have not, however, demonstrated that early routine ERCP significantly affects mortality and local or systemic complications of pancreatitis, regardless of predicted severity. However, there is support for current recommendations that early ERCP should be considered in patients with coexisting cholangitis or biliary obstruction.[2] Thus ERCP is best reserved for patients with suspected biliary obstruction, based on hyperbilirubinemia and evidence of clinical cholangitis, because it is unlikely that the ampulla is obstructed in the presence of a normal serum bilirubin.[3–6] Less invasive imaging modalities that can evaluate bile duct stones in patients with severe biliary pancreatitis include MRCP[7] and EUS.[8,9] These tests can help select patients for ERCP if bile duct stones are identified and prevent unnecessary ERCP and the risk of potential adverse events.[10,11] If bile duct stones are not identified during ERCP performed for acute gallstone pancreatitis, there are no data to guide whether an empiric biliary sphincterotomy should be performed. Sphincterotomy can reduce the risk of recurrent acute pancreatitis and cholangitis prior to cholecystectomy.[12] In patients with mild gallstone pancreatitis, cholecystectomy within 24 hours of admission has been shown to reduce rate of ERCPs, time to surgery, and hospital length-of-stay.[13] Indeed, early cholecystectomy is considered the standard of care.[14] In severe acute biliary pancreatitis, data are limited and, based on observational studies, it is recommended that cholecystectomy is performed once peripancreatic collections and local complications have resolved, generally beyond 6 weeks, to minimize the risk of infection in the peripancreatic collection.[15] In those patients who do not undergo cholecystectomy, ERCP with biliary sphincterotomy reduces the risk of recurrent gallstone pancreatitis.[16]

Evidence supports early enteral feeding for patients with severe acute pancreatitis, based on randomized prospective studies. Lower cost and fewer infectious complications are seen with enteral feeding as compared to parenteral nutrition (see Chapter 6). NG feeding appears to be as effective as tubes placed beyond the ligament of Treitz,[17]although the latter are preferred in patients who do not tolerate NG feeding owing to gastric retention from severe duodenal edema. There are a variety of endoscopic techniques for placing nasojejunal feeding tubes in the setting of acute pancreatitis, including transnasal endoscopy.[18–23]

LOCAL COMPLICATIONS OF ACUTE PANCREATITIS

There are a variety of local complications that can arise as a complication of acute pancreatitis with defined nomenclature (also see Chapter 60).[24] These include peripancreatic fluid collections, pancreatic and peripancreatic necrosis (sterile or infected), and pseudocyst and walled-off necrosis (WON; sterile or infected). Patients with well-demarcated symptomatic and/or infected collections that are in close proximity (apposition) to the gastric or duodenal wall can be treated with endoscopic drainage.[25] Acute peripancreatic fluid collections form early in the course of acute pancreatitis and usually resolve without therapy. Acute pseudocysts arise as a sequela of acute pancreatitis, require at least 4 weeks to encapsulate, and are devoid of significant solid debris. Acute pancreatic pseudocysts usually form as a result of a pancreatic ductal leak (Fig. 63.1A,B). Alternatively, areas of pancreatic and peripancreatic fat necrosis may liquefy over time and become a pseudocyst.[26] Despite the requirement of at least 4 weeks for a pseudocyst to encapsulate, it is important to realize that in some patients with significantly early acute pancreatic necrosis (>30% necrosis), the pancreatic and peripancreatic necrosis may evolve into a collection that radiographically resembles a pseudocyst.[27] These collections contain significant solid debris, and endoscopic treatment of them using typical pseudocyst drainage methods often results in infectious complications because of contamination and inadequate removal of solid debris.[28–30]

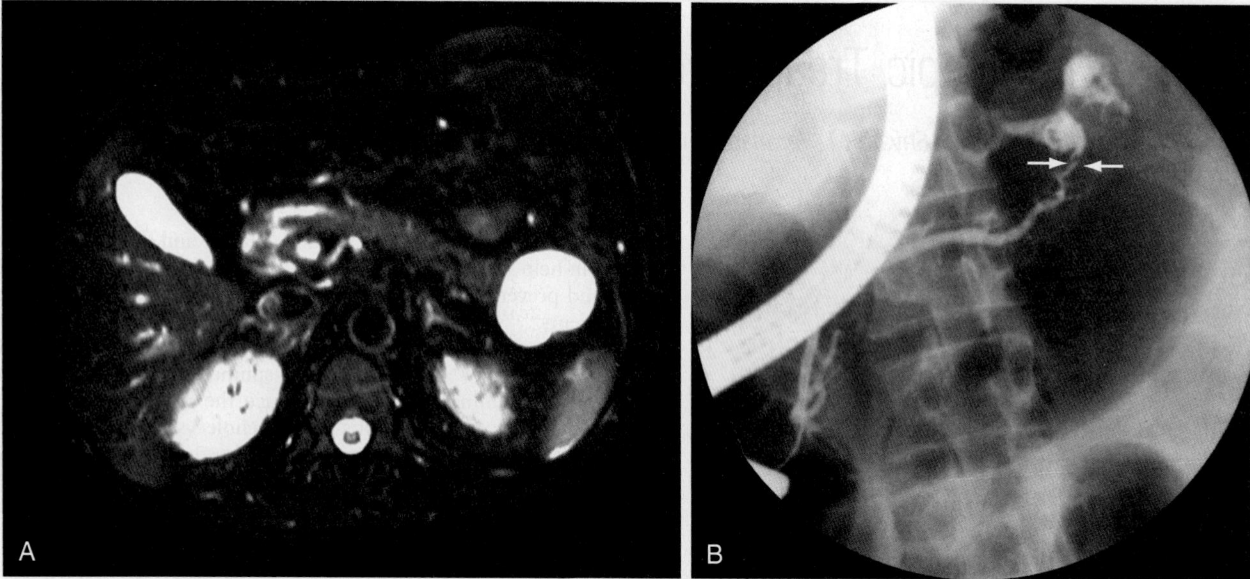

Fig. 63.1 (A) MRI of the abdomen reveals a pseudocyst in the tail of pancreas. (B) Pancreatogram reveals a duct leak (*arrows*) in the tail of pancreas.

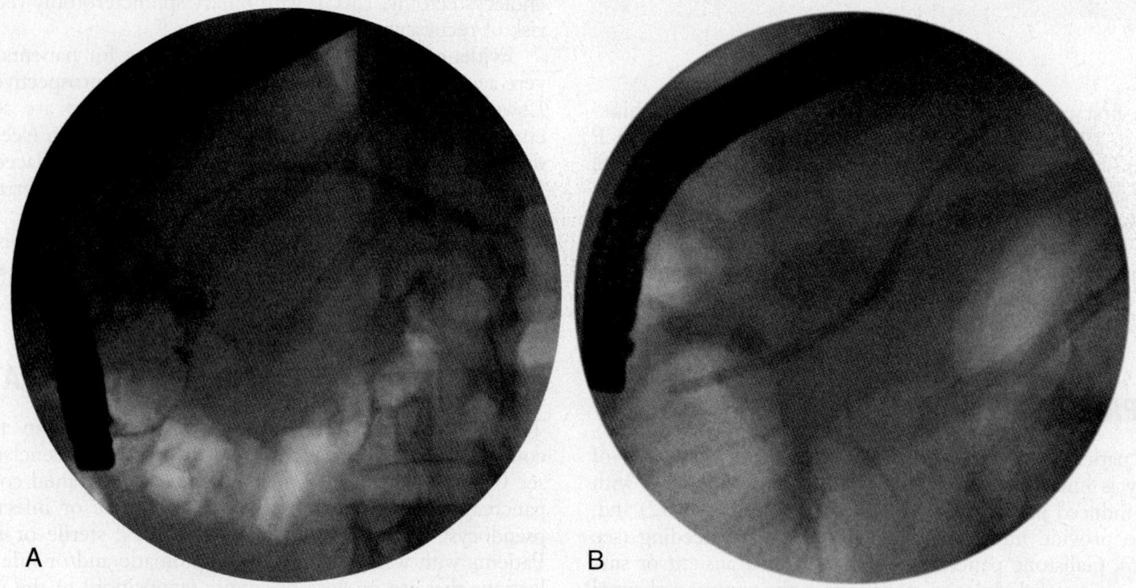

Fig. 63.2 (A) Pancreatogram reveals a leak in the neck of the pancreas with upstream opacification of the main pancreatic duct. (B) A stent was placed bridging the leak to restore ductal continuity.

Pseudocysts

Drainage is indicated for the treatment of symptomatic pseudocysts that may or may not be infected[31] and for progressive enlargement on imaging studies. Symptoms and signs from an acute pseudocyst include abdominal pain (often exacerbated by eating), weight loss, gastric outlet obstruction, obstructive jaundice, and pancreatic duct leakage, which may result in pancreatic ascites or pancreatic fistulae.[32] Pseudocysts may be drained through the papilla (transpapillary), through the gastric or duodenal wall (transmurally), or by using a combination of these modalities.[33,34]

Transpapillary Drainage

If the pseudocyst communicates with the main pancreatic duct, the placement of a pancreatic duct stent with or without pancreatic sphincterotomy is effective, especially for smaller pseudocysts (<5–6 cm) that are not otherwise approachable transmurally.[35,36] The proximal end of the stent (toward the pancreatic tail) may directly enter the pseudocyst, bridge the area of leak into the pancreatic duct upstream from the leak, or lie completely downstream to the leak. Bridging the leak is the preferred approach because it restores ductal continuity and appears to be more effective (Fig. 63.2A,B).[37,38] Transpapillary drainage avoids bleeding or perforation that may occur with transmural drainage. However, pancreatic stents may induce scarring of the main pancreatic duct in patients with a normal duct.[39]

Transmural Drainage

There is no standardized approach to transmural pseudocyst drainage. Transmural drainage is performed by entering the collection using a needle without electrocautery or using an electrocautery device [e.g., needle knife, cystotome, and cautery-enhanced lumen-apposing metal stent (LAMS)].[40] EUS-guided drainage is preferred over non-EUS-guided drainage to prevent adverse events such as bleeding and perforation.[41] Although the superiority of EUS-guided versus non-EUS-guided drainage has not been clearly demonstrated,[42] data support its routine use during transmural drainage,[42–45] especially when non-EUS-guided drainage fails.[46] EUS-guided entry is successful in more than 95% of patients and has low adverse event rates.[47–50] Traditionally, once the pseudocyst cavity is successfully entered, the transmural tract is balloon dilated to 8–10 mm in diameter to allow the placement of 1 or 2 double pigtail 7- or 10-French plastic stents (Fig. 63.3A–C).[51] A novel LAMS has been recently developed to mitigate many of the limitations of traditional drainage techniques using plastic stents.[52] The LAMS stents are much larger in diameter (8–20 mm) and can be deployed over an electrocautery-aided platform as a single-step method without the need for predilation of the transluminal tract (Fig. 63.4A,B). Therefore stent placement is technically easier and the fluid collection can be more rapidly drained as compared to plastic stents.

Following uncomplicated attempted endoscopic drainage, a follow-up CT is obtained 4–6 weeks after the procedure. All internal stents are endoscopically removed after documented radiographic pseudocyst resolution. Success rates, recurrence rates, and adverse event rates of endoscopic drainage of pancreatic pseudocysts are variable, likely because many published reports are heterogeneous, including patients with both acute and chronic pseudocysts, as well as necrotic collections erroneously classified as pseudocysts. Nonetheless, cumulatively, successful drainage is achieved in greater than 85%, with adverse event rates of about 5% and pseudocyst recurrence rates of 0% to 25%.[53–55]

Walled-Off Necrosis

Pancreatic necrosis is nonviable pancreatic parenchyma, usually associated with peripancreatic fat necrosis. Its earliest form is detected on contrast-enhanced CT by demonstrating areas of

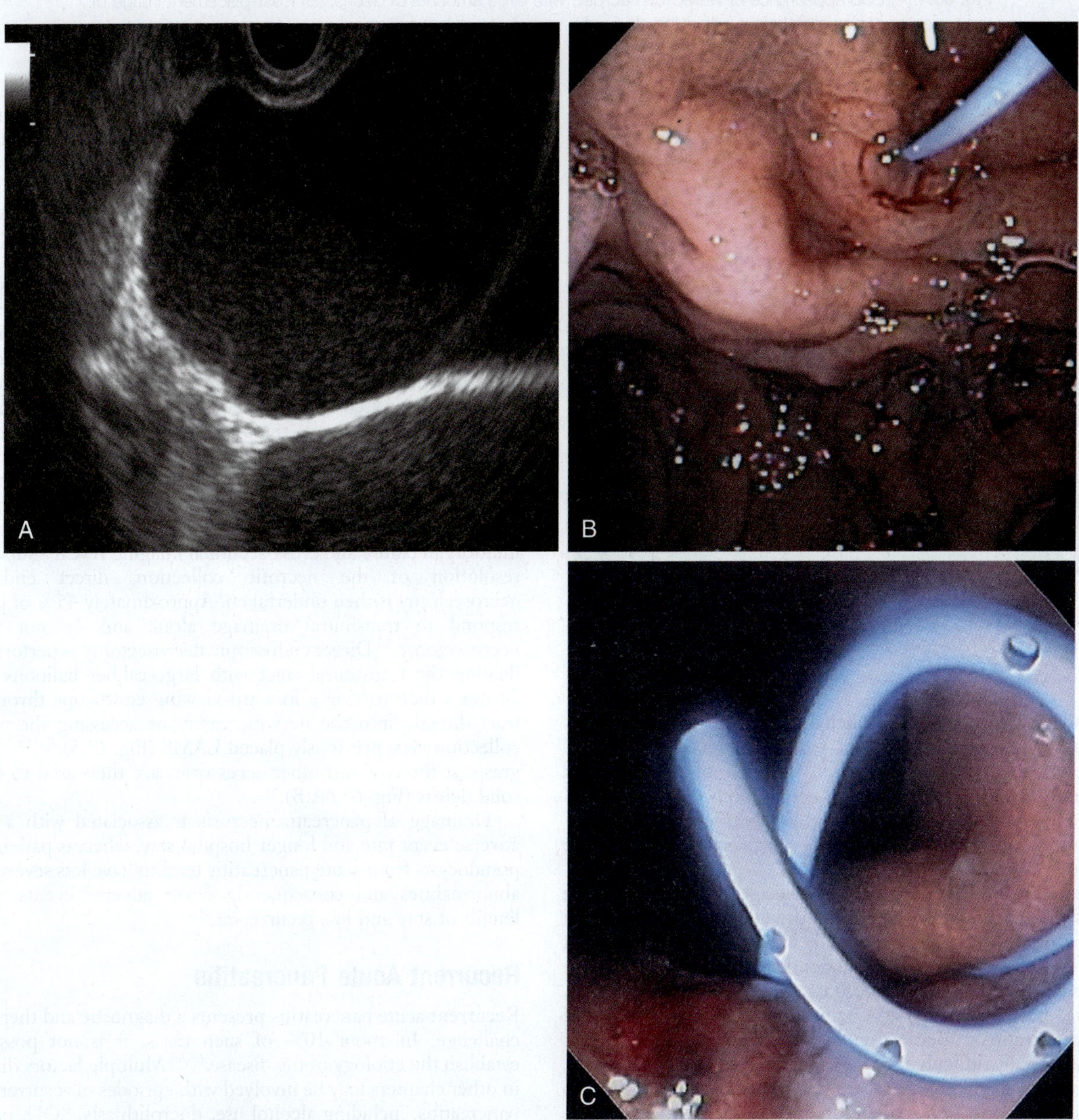

Fig. 63.3 (A) EUS appearance of a pancreatic pseudocyst. (B) The pseudocyst was entered and a guidewire coiled into the cyst. (C) After dilation a double pigtail plastic stent has been placed into the cyst.

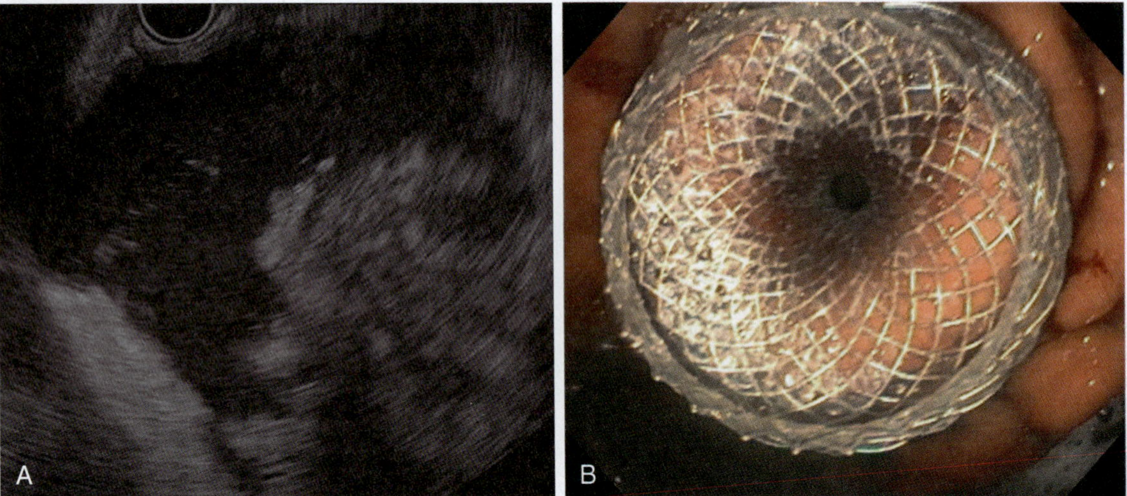

Fig. 63.4 (A) EUS appearance of walled-off necrosis with large amounts of debris. (B) Post-placement image of the lumen-apposing metal stent within the stomach.

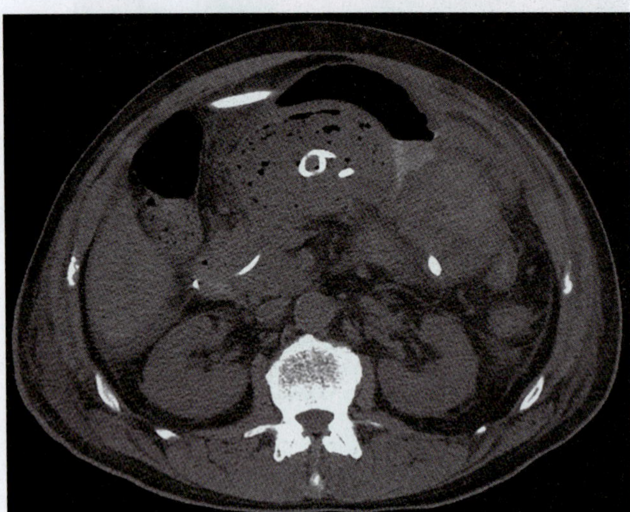

Fig. 63.5 CT of the abdomen revealing a large encapsulated necrotic fluid collection with gas consistent with infected walled-off necrosis. A indwelling plastic stent is seen within the collection.

nonenhancing pancreatic parenchyma. Pancreatic necrosis is frequently accompanied by major pancreatic ductal disruptions. Over the course of several weeks, the area of necrosis may continue to evolve and expand, containing both liquid and solid debris, and is commonly referred to as WON (Fig. 63.5). The CT appearance of WON may be mistaken as an acute pseudocyst.[27,30,56,57]

The indications for and timing of drainage of sterile WON are controversial. Endoscopic drainage should not be undertaken until the process becomes organized. Indications for drainage of sterile WON are refractory abdominal pain, gastric outlet obstruction, or failure to thrive (i.e., continued systemic illness, anorexia, and weight loss) at 4 or more weeks after the onset of acute pancreatitis.[58] Because endoscopic drainage of WON is more technically difficult, it carries a higher rate of adverse events, and tends to involve more severely ill patients. The decision to endoscopically intervene when the process is sterile must be carefully considered.[30,59] On the other hand, infection is an absolute indication for endoscopic drainage of WON. Alternative management options to endoscopic drainage include nutritional support with parenteral or enteral jejunal feeding and non-endoscopic drainage methods such as percutaneous and surgical drainage, including minimally invasive surgical techniques.[58] The management option selected is usually based on local expertise and severity of comorbid medical illnesses. Ideally, these patients are best managed by a multidisciplinary approach.

Because of the need to evacuate solid material, the endoscopic approach to drainage of WON differs from drainage of pseudocysts and the procedural techniques have evolved significantly. In general, the transpapillary approach alone is inadequate because it does not allow the removal of solid debris. The transmural approach is most commonly used, as it allows for the drainage of liquefied contents and removal of solid debris. The most commonly favored approach is to first place a 15 or 20 mm LAMS, as the wide diameter enables spontaneous drainage of liquid and semisolid contents. If patients are persistently symptomatic with ongoing sepsis, systemic inflammatory response or multiorgan failure and cross-sectional imaging reveal a suboptimal resolution of the necrotic collection, direct endoscopic necrosectomy is then undertaken. Approximately 45% of patients respond to transmural drainage alone and do not require necrosectomy.[60] Direct endoscopic necrosectomy is performed by dilating the transmural tract with large-caliber balloons (up to 20 mm), then passing a forward-viewing endoscope through the tract directly into the necrotic cavity or accessing the necrotic collection via a previously placed LAMS (Fig. 63.5).[30,61,62] Snares, grasping forceps, and other accessories are then used to remove solid debris (Fig. 63.6A,B).[63]

Drainage of pancreatic necrosis is associated with a higher adverse event rate and longer hospital stay, whereas patients with pseudocysts from acute pancreatitis tend to have less severe ductal abnormalities and consequently fewer adverse events, shorter length of stay and less recurrence.[64]

Recurrent Acute Pancreatitis

Recurrent acute pancreatitis presents a diagnostic and therapeutic challenge. In about 10% of such cases, it is not possible to establish the etiology of the disease.[65,66] Multiple factors discussed in other chapters may be involved with episodes of recurrent acute pancreatitis, including alcohol use, microlithiasis, SOD, pancreas divisum, hereditary pancreatitis, CF and other gene mutations, choledochocele, annular pancreas, anomalous pancreaticobiliary

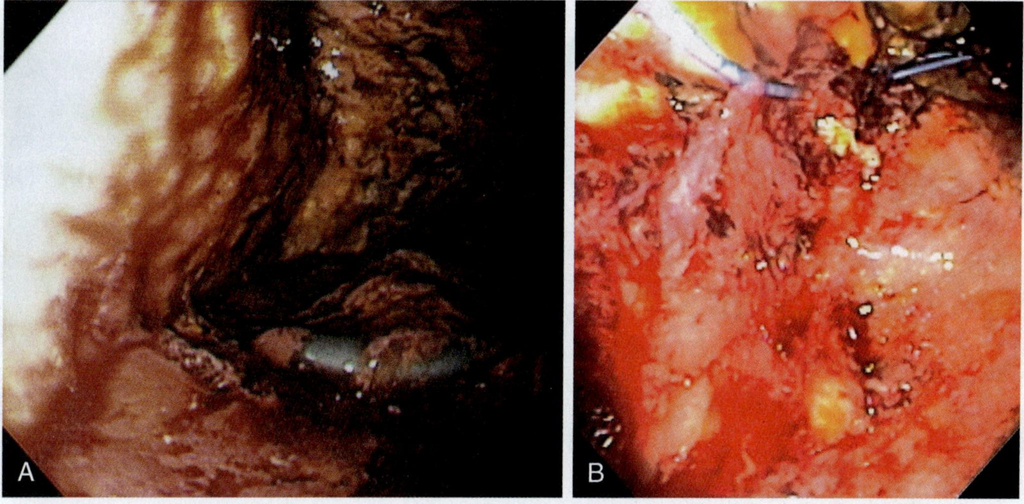

Fig. 63.6 Direct endoscopic necrosectomy performed in the patient depicted in Fig 63.5. (A) Endoscopic view from inside the necrotic cavity; an indwelling pigtail stent is seen with surrounding necrotic debris. (B) After endoscopic necrosectomy the cavity is devoid of debris and is covered with health granulation tissue.

junction, ampullary lesions, pancreatic tumors, and autoimmune pancreatitis.

EUS is considered an important tool for evaluating for possible causes of recurrent acute pancreatitis.[67] EUS allows the detection of gallstones, sludge, and microlithiasis[68] within the pancreaticobiliary system that can direct treatment toward cholecystectomy or therapeutic ERCP. In addition, a diagnosis of autoimmune pancreatitis can be suspected based on imaging findings and confirmed by EUS-FNA or core biopsies.[69,70] In patients with otherwise unexplained recurrent acute pancreatitis after exhaustive clinical and laboratory evaluation and EUS, the measurement of pancreatic sphincter pressure by ERCP with pancreaticobiliary manometry can allow the diagnosis of pancreatic SOD.[71,72] Subsequent biliary and pancreatic sphincterotomy (when elevated sphincter pressures are identified) may prevent recurrent attacks of pancreatitis. It should be noted, however, that the role of pancreatic SOD as a cause of recurrent pancreatitis is highly controversial.

Pancreas divisum is present in up to 10% of the population (see Chapter 57) and results from failure of the dorsal and ventral pancreatic ducts to fuse.[73] The role of pancreas divisum as a cause of pancreatitis is controversial[74] but may contribute in a subset of patients as the minor papilla produces functional obstruction to the flow of pancreatic secretions. Pancreas divisum can be diagnosed by CT, MRI, or EUS.[75] Secretin MRCP may predict which patients have functional minor papilla obstruction.[76] Pancreas divisum is confirmed by cannulation of the minor papilla, which can be facilitated by IV administration of secretin. Endoscopic minor papilla sphincterotomy in properly selected patients without extensive changes of chronic pancreatitis may prevent further attacks of acute pancreatitis.[77–79]

CHRONIC PANCREATITIS

A variety of endoscopic interventions can be performed in patients with symptomatic chronic pancreatitis (Box 63.1) (see also Chapter 61).[80]

Pancreatic Ductal Endotherapy

Pancreatic duct strictures and pancreatic duct stones frequently coexist, cause obstruction to the main pancreatic duct, and may contribute to abdominal pain and episodes of acute pancreatitis superimposed on chronic pancreatitis. Endoscopic therapy of pancreatic duct strictures is performed with balloon or catheter dilation followed by placement of one or more plastic pancreatic stents (Fig. 63.7A–D).[80,81] Stents are exchanged and remain in place for a variable period of time.

BOX 63.1 Endoscopic Therapies for Chronic Pancreatitis

- Pancreatic sphincterotomy
- Extraction of pancreatic duct stones
- Dilation of pancreatic duct strictures
- Dilation of biliary strictures
- Treatment of pancreatic duct leaks resulting in ascites or pleural effusions
- Drainage of pancreatic pseudocysts
- Placement of biliary and pancreatic stents

In adults, pancreatic sphincterotomy and stone removal can rarely be successfully performed using standard biliary stone removal techniques, because the stones are calcified and usually impacted within side branches and pancreatic duct strictures. Extracorporeal shock-wave lithotripsy, if available, can be used to fragment stones prior to, or without, endoscopic removal[80,82–84] and is essential if large, obstructive stones are to be removed. Intraductal lithotripsy (laser or electrohydraulic) under pancreatoscopic guidance has also been used to fragment and remove obstructing stones.[85] Pancreatic endotherapy has a high rate of initial technical success.[86] In some series, long-term clinical success has been achieved in two-thirds of patients without need for surgery and with a significant reduction in the annual rate of hospitalizations for pain.[82,87]

Two prospective randomized studies comparing endotherapy and surgery for patients with painful obstructive chronic pancreatitis have been conducted.[88,89] Endotherapy was associated with a higher number of procedures, and pain improvement was seen more often in the surgical groups. However, there were limitations to endotherapy in both the studies—namely, lack of availability of extracorporeal shock-wave lithotripsy in one study and less aggressive endoscopic stricture therapy in another.[90]

In cases where transpapillary approaches are not possible for treatment of pancreatic duct obstruction because of impassable

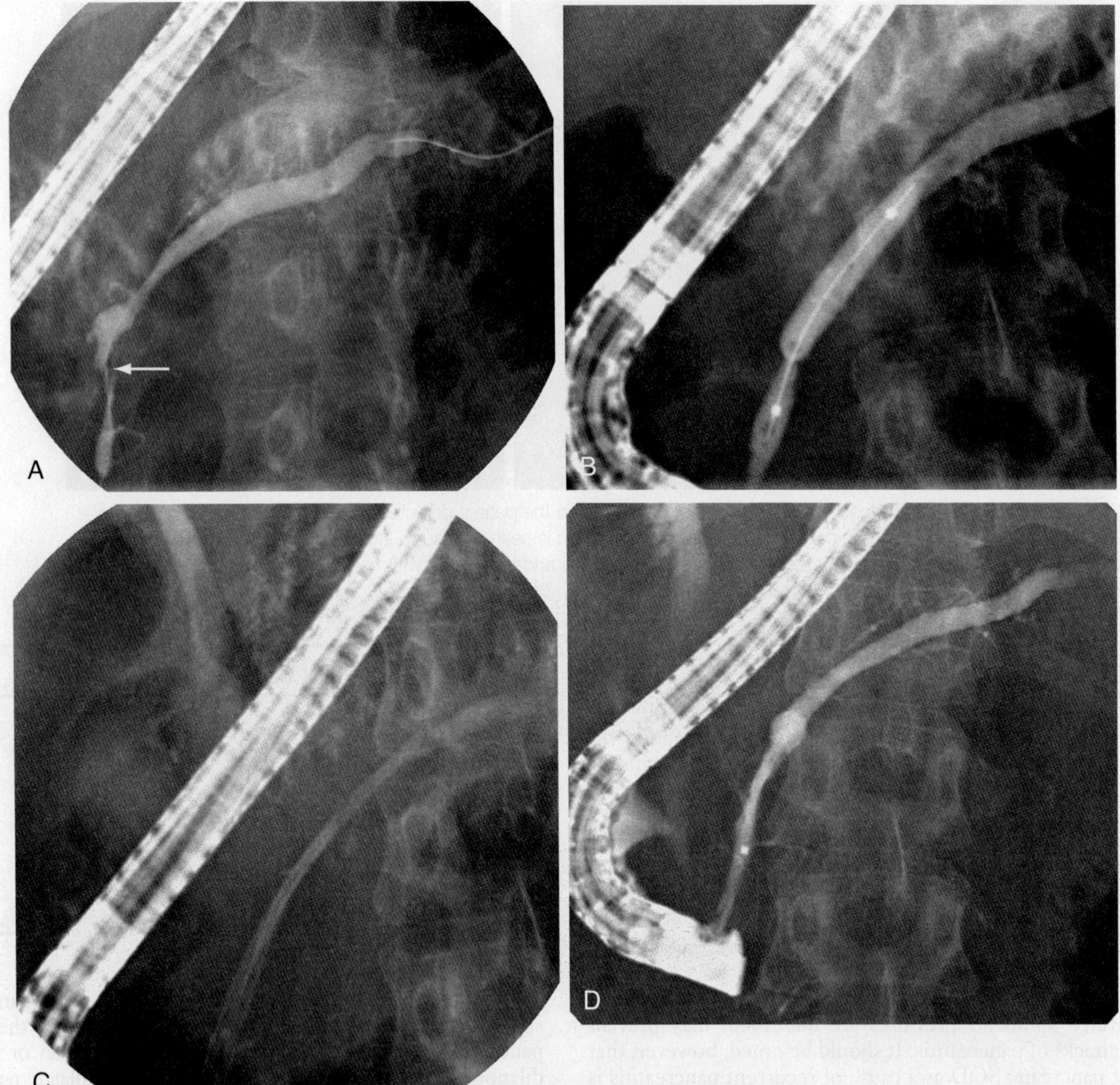

Fig. 63.7 Endoscopic treatment of a pancreatic duct stricture. (A) Initial pancreatogram showing a stricture in the head of the pancreas (*arrow*) with upstream ductal dilatation. (B) Balloon dilation of the stricture (note the waist). (C) Placement of two side-by-side plastic stents. (D) A follow-up pancreatogram showing improvement in the stricture.

stones or strictures within the pancreatic head, EUS-guided transgastric or transduodenal pancreatic duct puncture can be performed.[91] This can facilitate a rendezvous access or enable transgastric or transduodenal ductal stent placement.[92,93]

Pseudocysts

The mechanism of formation of a chronic pseudocyst is different than an acute pseudocyst. As discussed in Chapter 61, chronic pseudocysts arise as a sequela of chronic pancreatitis and downstream pancreatic ductal obstruction from fibrotic strictures or stones.[94] This results in a pancreatic ductal blowout (leak) and accumulation of pancreatic fluid. These collections do not contain solid debris and usually do not arise as a result of acute inflammatory processes. The endoscopic approach to chronic pancreatic pseudocysts is similar to that described earlier for acute pseudocysts. The main difference is that the underlying ductal abnormalities may lead to recurrences if left untreated.[95,96]

Biliary Strictures

The fibrosing process within the pancreatic head can encase the distal bile duct and result in formation of a biliary stricture. Possible sequelae include hepatic fibrosis (secondary biliary cirrhosis) and cholangitis. Balloon dilation and endoscopic insertion of multiple side-by-side plastic stents or a fully covered self-expandable metal stent (SEMS) across the biliary stricture may result in stricture resolution.[81,97–99] Endoscopic insertion of biliary stents can be used for treatment of benign biliary strictures due to chronic pancreatitis in several situations: (1) preoperative placement for relief of jaundice or cholangitis, (2) temporary placement when biliary obstruction occurs following recent acute pancreatitis superimposed on chronic pancreatitis, and (3) long-term therapy of refractory strictures.[100] Placement of fully covered SEMS for up to 12 months has resulted in the resolution of biliary strictures that were due to chronic pancreatitis in up to 75% of patients at 24-month follow-up.[101] Uncovered SEMS should not be used in the setting of a benign biliary stricture secondary to chronic pancreatitis.

PANCREATIC DUCT LEAKS

Pancreatic duct leaks and pancreatic duct disruptions may occur as sequelae of acute or chronic pancreatitis (see Chapters 60 and 61), as well as after pancreatic surgery (Fig. 63.8A and B) and trauma. Leaks can arise from the tail, body, or head of the pancreas. Fluid can then track laterally (toward the spleen), medially toward the duodenum or bile duct, into the lesser sac, or into the mediastinum or abdomen, with resultant pleural effusions and ascites, respectively.

External leaks (pancreaticocutaneous fistulas) usually occur following pancreatic surgery or percutaneous drainage of pancreatic fluid collections. External fistulae are identified by output of high amylase fluid.

Most pancreatic leaks that occur after pancreatic surgery are already controlled by in-dwelling surgical drains. Many of these leaks will close over time, and endoscopic therapy is generally reserved for persistent or refractory leaks.[102,103] In the absence of a surgical drain, endoscopic therapy is performed to treat leaks that are associated with clinical deterioration or if symptoms require intervention.[104]

Endoscopic intervention for pancreatic duct leaks is similar to that described for pancreatic pseudocysts and necrosis. In the setting of a large pancreatic fluid collection, transmural drainage of the collection may be undertaken, with or without concomitant transpapillary therapy. This will control the leak internally. In the absence of a pancreatic fluid collection, the treatment is transpapillary pancreatic duct stent placement to promote internal drainage.[32,105,106]

Transpapillary therapy is performed with the intent of crossing the site of the leak,[37] although it is not feasible when leaks follow pancreatic tail resection or are located in the pancreatic tail. In this situation, the tip of the stent is positioned downstream to the site of leakage (Fig. 63.9A–D).

In patients with external drains in whom endoscopic therapy is being performed to allow drainage removal, success depends on the size of the external drain as compared with the size of the internal stent. Downsizing, clamping, or removing the external drain after successful endoscopic stent placement can promote internal drainage and fistula closure. A variety of gluing agents have been used to seal pancreatic fistula and leaks,[107] although these agents are not FDA approved and have the potential for occlusion of the main pancreatic duct.

PANCREATIC CANCER

Endoscopic treatment of pancreatic cancer primarily involves the palliation of malignant biliary obstruction via placement of transpapillary biliary stents at ERCP (see Chapters 62 and 72). In select patients, placement of a stent into the pancreatic duct can relieve abdominal pain from pancreatic ductal obstruction.[108] In addition, some pancreatic cancer patients with pancreatic ductal obstruction will develop pseudocysts or leaks; endoscopic pancreatic duct stent placement across the pancreatic duct stricture can be useful. Pancreatic cancer can produce gastric outlet obstruction due to duodenal invasion by tumor in 15%–20% of patients.[109,110] Endoscopic placement of an uncovered SEMS is an effective palliative method, with more rapid return of per oral intake but with an increased risk of occlusion and need for reintervention as compared with surgical bypass.[111,112] EUS-guided gastroenterostomy, whereby the stomach is anastomosed to the duodenum or jejunum using a LAMS is a newer nonsurgical intervention for the palliation of gastric outlet obstruction.[113] Combined palliation of malignant biliary and duodenal obstruction is also feasible.[93,114–116] Pancreatic cancer pain can be treated by EUS-guided celiac plexus block using ethanol to allow a permanent ablation of the ganglion. This treatment appears to be effective and sustainable.[117] EUS-guided fiducial placement can be used in patients undergoing radiation therapy for the treatment of pancreatic cancer. Gold fiducials are placed at several locations at the tumor margin to aid in localization during image-guided radiation therapy.[118]

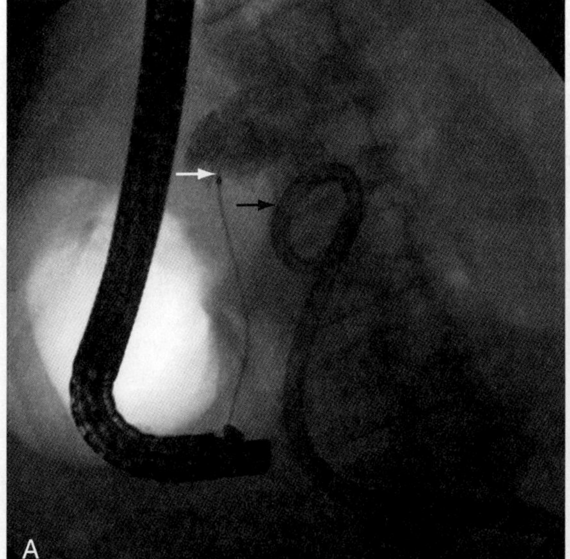

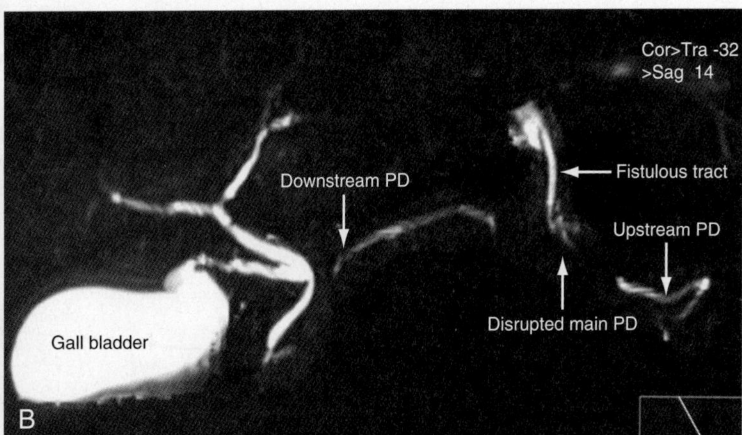

Fig. 63.8 (A) Pancreatogram in a patient with external pancreatic fistula: complete pancreatic duct disruption with contrast extravasation (*white arrow*). Pancreatic duct upstream to disruption is not visualized. Percutaneous catheter is noted (*black arrow*). (B) MRCP in the same patient demonstrating upstream PD, disrupted PD, and a fistulous tract from upstream duct.

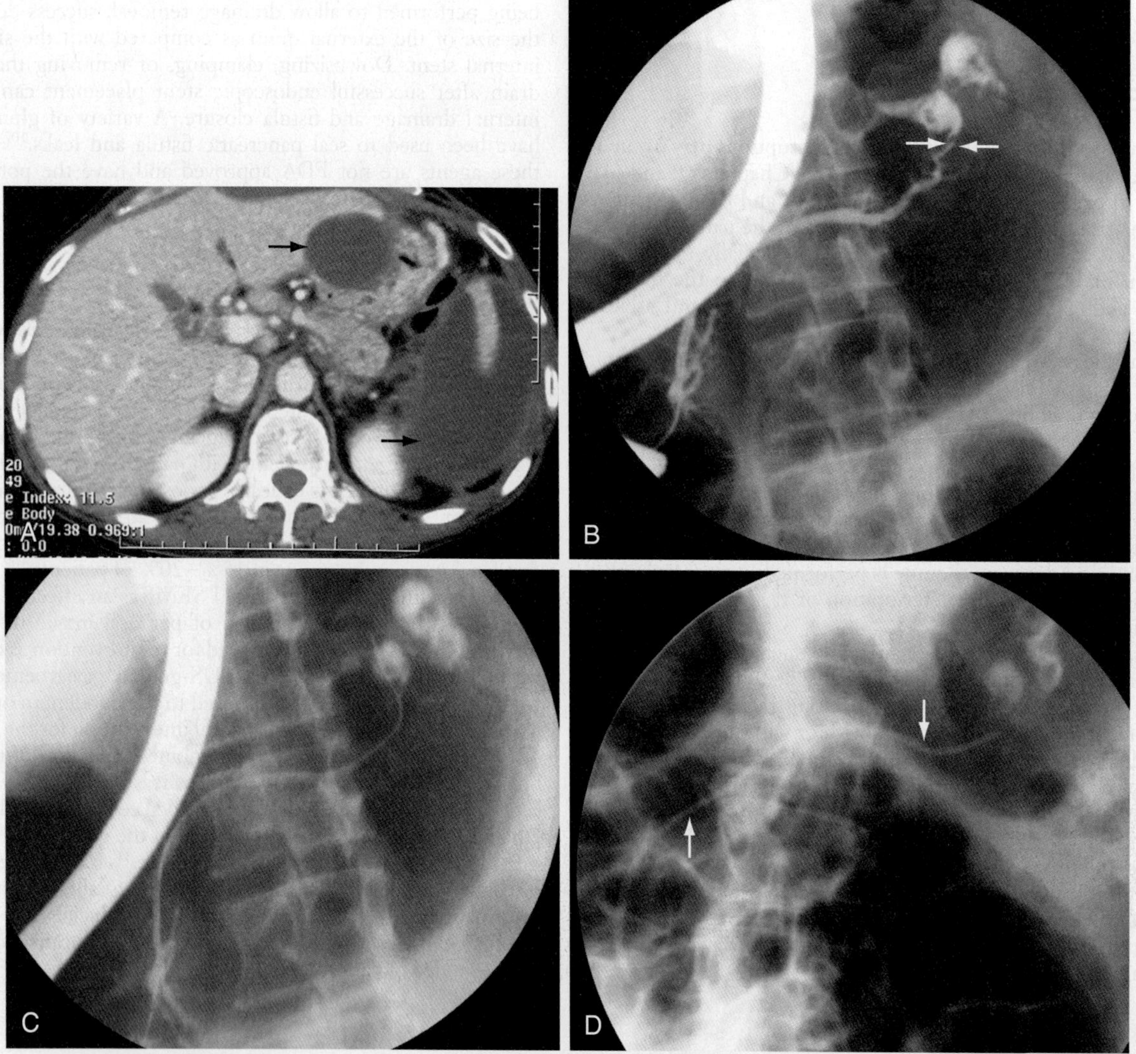

Fig. 63.9 (A) CT abdomen of patient with chronic pancreatitis, perihepatic and perisplenic pseudocysts (*arrows*). (B) Pancreatogram revealing mildly dilated main pancreatic duct, irregular side branches and disruption at terminal most part of tail end (*arrows*). (C) At ERCP, guidewire is negotiated into disruption. (D) A 5-Fr 15 cm pancreatic stent was placed at site of disruption (*arrows*).

PANCREATIC CYSTS

There are a wide variety of pancreatic cysts and cystic neoplasms, as discussed in Chapter 62. CT, MRI, and EUS allow differentiation and direction of management toward observation or surgery.[119,120] Increasing data suggest that an EUS-guided injection of chemotherapeutic agents into specific types of cysts may be a useful nonsurgical alternative in the future.[121]

Full references for this chapter can be found at https://eBooks.Health.Elsevier.com.

PART IX Biliary Tract

64 Anatomy, Histology, Embryology, Developmental Anomalies, and Pediatric Disorders of the Biliary Tract

Frederick J. Suchy, Jr., Cara L. Mack

IN THIS CHAPTER

In this chapter, the embryologic and anatomic characteristics of the bile ducts and gallbladder are reviewed, with a focus on information useful for diagnosing and treating biliary tract disease and understanding the anomalies and congenital malformations of these structures. Biliary tract disease in infants and children is considered because many of the disorders that occur early in life are due to abnormal morphogenesis or adversely affect the process of development.

EMBRYOLOGY OF THE LIVER AND BILIARY TRACT

The human liver is formed from 2 primordia (Fig. 64.1): the liver diverticulum and the septum transversum (see also Chapter 73).[1,2] The proximity of cardiac mesoderm, which expresses fibroblast growth factors (FGFs) 1, 2, and 8, and bone morphogenetic proteins, causes the foregut endoderm to develop into the liver. The liver diverticulum forms through the proliferation of endodermal cells at the cranioventral junction of the yolk sac with the foregut and grows into the septum transversum in a cranioventral direction. Surrounding mesoderm and ectoderm participate in the hepatic specification of the endoderm to hepatoblasts, via signaling from mesodermal tissues, including ligands of bone morphogenic protein, Wnt, and FGF families of proteins.[1] In humans, after their specification and migration into the septum transversum, hepatoblasts undergo proliferation and migration between 26 and 32 days of gestation in the process of forming an organ bud.[1,3] The homeodomain transcription factors hematopoietically expressed homeobox (Hhex) and Prospero homeobox protein 1, in the anterior endoderm and hepatic diverticulum, are required for the migration of hepatoblasts into the septum transversum that precedes liver growth and morphogenesis.[3–5] Another homeodomain protein, Hlx, is necessary for hepatoblast proliferation. At the 5-mm stage, a solid cranial portion (hepatic) and a hollow caudal portion of the diverticulum can be clearly distinguished. The large hepatic portion differentiates into proliferating cords of hepatocytes and the intrahepatic bile ducts. Hepatocyte nuclear factor (HNF)4α expression drives further hepatocyte differentiation and epithelial transformation into the characteristic sinusoidal architecture.[6]

Bipotential hepatoblasts express alpha fetoprotein and markers for hepatocytes such as albumin and cytokeratin (CK19) for cholangiocytes. In mice, the transcription factor sex-determining region Y-box 9 (SOX9) is the earliest specific biliary marker detected in endodermal cells that line the hepatic diverticulum. Its expression disappears as soon as hepatoblasts invade the septum transversum but reappears in cells of the biliary lineage throughout the development.[1] This early change occurs on the eighteenth day of gestation and corresponds to the 2.5-mm stage of the embryo. The homeobox gene *Hhex* is essential for proper hepatoblast differentiation and bile duct morphogenesis.[5] Members of the transforming growth factor (TGF)-β, Wnt, FGF, Hippo, GATA, FOXA, ONECUT2, and HNF3/forkhead transcription factor families and HNF6 are also required for formation and differentiation of gut endoderm tissues.[3,4] The septum transversum consists of mesenchymal cells and a capillary plexus formed by the branches of the two vitelline veins. At the 3- to 4-mm stage, between the third and fourth weeks of gestation, the growing diverticulum projects as an epithelial plug into the septum transversum.

The intrahepatic and extrahepatic biliary systems develop separately, requiring distinct transcriptional and signaling mechanisms. Critical mechanistic observations have come from the mouse models. Bile duct morphogenesis begins around gestational Day 45 in humans and embryonic Day 14.5 in mice.[1–4]

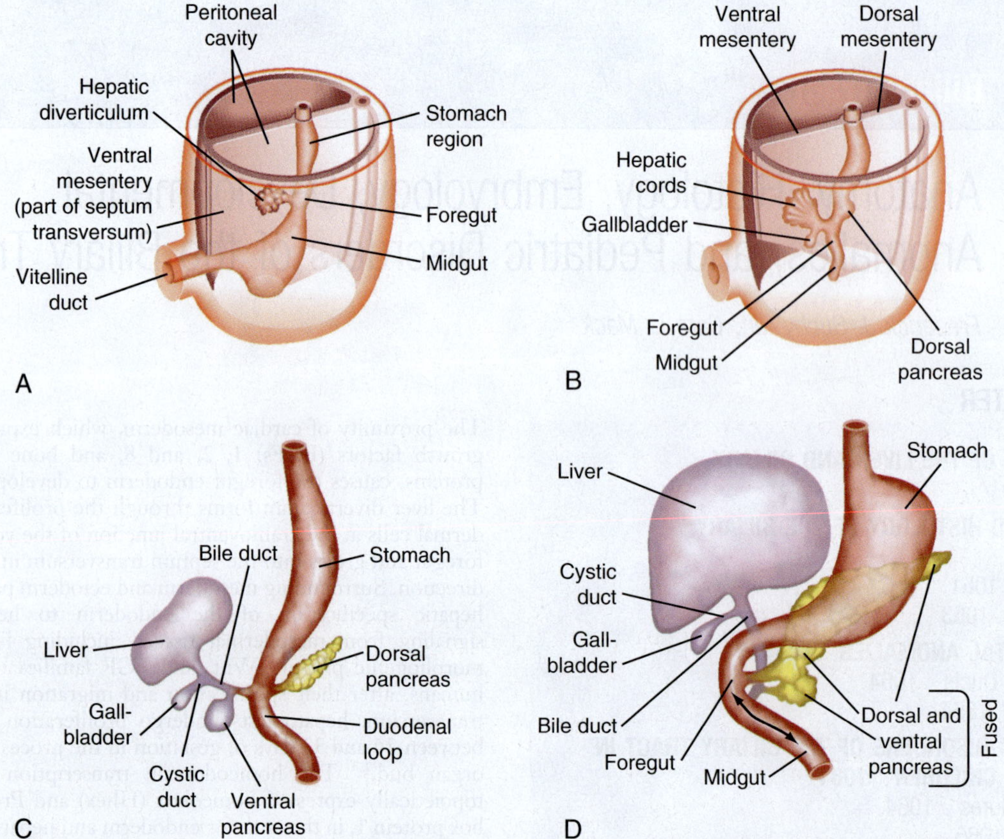

Fig. 64.1 Stages in embryologic development of the liver, gallbladder, extrahepatic ducts, pancreas, and duodenum. (A) 4 weeks. (B) and (C) 5 weeks. (D) 6 weeks. (From Moore KL. *The Developing Human*. Philadelphia, PA: WB Saunders; 1973.)

The intrahepatic bile ducts develop from primitive hepatocytes around branches of the portal vein.[2,4] The process is initiated near the hilum of the liver and progressively asymmetrically toward the periphery through a series of remodeling stages.[5,6] Cholangiocytes are associated with the basement membrane throughout bile duct development, suggesting that cholangiocytes receive morphogenic signals from components of the extracellular matrix, including laminin and type IV collagen.[7,8] A ring of hepatocytes in proximity to the portal vein branches first transforms into bile duct-type cells. A second layer of primitive hepatocytes is similarly transformed and produces a circular cleft around the portal vein that is lined on both sides by bile duct epithelial cells.[9] This double-walled cylinder with a slit-like lumen, the ductal plate, can be detected at 9 weeks of gestation. Thus the entire network of interlobular and intralobular bile ductules develops from the limiting plate. The periportal mesenchyme secretes TGF-β and produces a portal-to-parenchymal gradient of TGF-β signaling, with the highest activity near the mesenchyme.[10] The mesenchyme also produces Jagged1, which via cell-cell contacts induces Notch2-mediated signaling in the differentiating biliary cells. TGF-β and Notch signaling, in cooperation with other signaling pathways, stimulate sequential differentiation of the two layers of biliary cells (ductal plate) to induce asymmetrical tubulogenesis.[10] Secreted factors of the Wnt family also regulate differentiation of hepatoblasts to biliary cells. Bile ducts develop according to the two axes: ducts mature along their radial axis, and they also grow in length according to an axis that extends from the hilum of the liver to the periphery of the liver lobes.

In sections of the 10-mm embryo, many of the liver cords are traversed by double-walled canals that branch and are morphologically indistinguishable from bile capillaries of the adult. These structures differ from those of the adult in that they are bounded by six or more liver cells instead of two. The process of differentiation of bile ductular epithelial cells (cholangiocytes) from primitive hepatocytes has been documented in humans using immunohistochemical staining with several anticytokeratin antibodies. During the phenotypic shift toward bile duct–type cells, hepatocytes first display increased reactivity for CKs 8 and 18 and express CK19 at 20–25 weeks' gestation.[10] Cholangiocyte-mesenchymal cell interaction is important for the formation of bile ducts. During the transition from ductal plates to bile ducts, portal myofibroblasts expand significantly and surround newly formed bile ducts. Periportal connective tissue, corticosteroid hormones, and basal laminar components may play important roles in the differentiation of bile ducts. The ductal plate structure requires extensive remodeling through a process of reabsorption, possibly through apoptosis, to yield the characteristic anastomosing system of biliary channels that surround the portal vein. Proteins that appear to have a role in the promotion of apoptosis, specifically Fas antigen and c-Myc, are consistently detected in primitive intrahepatic ductal cells.[11] Lewis antigen, which is expressed in damaged and apoptotic cells, is also present. Bcl-2 protein, an inhibitor of apoptosis, is not found in early stages of intrahepatic bile duct cell development but becomes detectable later. Computed three-dimensional (3D) reconstruction of the developing ductal plate has shown that the ductal plate remodeling process starts at the porta hepatis at approximately 11 weeks' gestation and progresses toward the periphery of the liver.[10] The process is in large part completed at term, but even at 40 weeks' gestation, some of the smallest portal vein branches may not be accompanied by an individual bile duct and may still be surrounded by a (discontinuous) ductal plate. Ductal plate malformation is a common feature of pediatric biliary disorders and may be initiated at distinct stages of bile duct morphogenesis, owing to defects in ductal plate remodeling, abnormal differentiation of hepatoblasts into ductal plate cells, or abnormal maturation of primitive ductal structures.[10,12]

The extrahepatic bile ducts, bile duct (common bile duct), cystic duct, and gallbladder arise from a region of ventral foregut proximate to the liver and ventral pancreas and share a common origin with the ventral pancreas but not the liver.[3] Development of the extrahepatic biliary system precedes that of intrahepatic bile ducts. The extrahepatic system (but not intrahepatic bile ducts) are derived from a progenitor cell expressing the transcription factor pancreatic-duodenal homeobox 1 (Pdx1).[3,13] The Sox17 transcription factor is an important determinant of how cells within the Pdx1 domain are assigned to the two different fates of pancreas or extrahepatic biliary system. Appropriate segregation of extrahepatic biliary system and ventral pancreatic lineages is also regulated by hairy and enhancer of split-1 (Hes1), a transcriptional effector of Notch signaling.[1]

In neonatal mice there are several important differences in the structural and functional properties of extrahepatic bile ducts that may predispose to injury, including a lack of a protective apical glycocalyx, immature and potentially leaky tight junctions, and an underdeveloped supporting submucosal matrix related to decreased deposition of collagen and elastin.[14]

The primitive extrahepatic bile duct maintains continuity with the ductal plate, from which intrahepatic bile ducts are eventually formed.[7] Contrary to long-held concepts of biliary development, no "solid stage" of endodermal occlusion of the bile duct lumen is found at any time during gestation. However, it is unknown how the intra- and extrahepatic ducts join. At 16 mm, the cystic duct and proximal gallbladder are hollow, but the fundus of the gallbladder is still partially obstructed by remnants of the epithelial plug. The gallbladder is patent by the third month of gestation. Further development until birth consists primarily of continued growth. The characteristic folds of the gallbladder are formed toward the end of gestation and are moderately developed in the neonate. Bile secretion starts at the beginning of the fourth month of gestation; thereafter, the biliary system continuously contains bile, which is secreted into the gut and imparts a dark green color to the intestinal contents (meconium).

ANATOMY AND HISTOLOGY OF THE BILIARY TREE

Bile is an alkaline, yellow-green fluid (7.5–8.1 pH) secreted by hepatocytes (600–1000 mL/day), further modified by the absorptive and secretory systems in cholangiocytes, and is rendered acidic (5.2–6.0 pH) when stored and concentrated in the gallbladder.[14] Bile is ~95% water and contains 0.7% bile salts, 0.2% bilirubin, 0.51% fats (cholesterol, fatty acids, and phospholipids), and 200 meq/L inorganic salts. Variable quantities of exogenous drugs, xenobiotics and environmental toxins may also be present.

Bile Ducts

The adult human liver has more than 2 km of bile ductules and ducts. Cholangiocytes that line bile ducts constitute ~3% of total parenchymal liver cell volume.[14] Quantitative computer-aided 3D imaging has estimated the volume of the entire macroscopic duct system of human liver to be a mean of 20.4 cm.[14,15] In these studies, the mean internal surface of 398 cm^2 is magnified approximately 5.5-fold by the presence of microvilli and cilia at the apical surfaces of cholangiocytes that play an important role in the regulation of cholangiocyte functions. These structures are far from being inert channels; they are capable of modifying biliary flow and composition significantly in response to hormones such as secretin.[16,17] A general feature of bile ductules is their anatomic intimacy with portal blood and lymph vessels, which potentially allows selective exchange of materials between compartments. No major ultrastructural differences exist between cholangiocytes lining small and large bile ducts, but the functional properties of cholangiocytes are heterogeneous.[17] For example, large, but not small, intrahepatic bile ducts are involved in secretin-regulated bile ductal secretion.[18] Correspondingly, the secretin receptor and chloride-bicarbonate exchanger messenger RNAs have been detected in large, but not small, intrahepatic bile duct units.[17]

Bile secretion begins at the level of the bile canaliculus, the smallest branch of the biliary tract.[19] Its boundaries are formed by a specialized membrane of adjacent apical poles of liver cells. The canaliculi form a meshwork of polygonal channels between hepatocytes with many anastomotic interconnections.[19] Bile then enters the small terminal channels (the canals of Hering), which have a basement membrane and are lined partly by hepatocytes and partly by cholangiocytes.[15] The canals of Hering provide a conduit through which bile may traverse the limiting plate of hepatocytes to enter the larger perilobular or intralobular ducts.[20,21] These smallest of biliary radicles are less than 15–20 μm in diameter, with lumens surrounded by cuboidal epithelial cells. At the most proximal level, one or more fusiform-shaped ductular cells may share a canalicular lumen with a hepatocyte; gradually, the ductules become lined by 2–4 cuboidal epithelial cells as they approach the portal canal.[19] Bile flows from the central lobular cells toward portal triads (from zone 3 to 1 of the liver acinus) (see Chapter 73). The terminal bile ductules are thought to proliferate as a result of chronic extrahepatic bile duct obstruction.[21]

The interlobular bile ducts form a richly anastomosing network that closely surrounds the branches of the portal vein.[22–24] These bile ducts (Fig. 64.2) are initially 30–40 μm in diameter and are lined by a layer of cuboidal or columnar epithelium that displays a microvillar architecture on its luminal

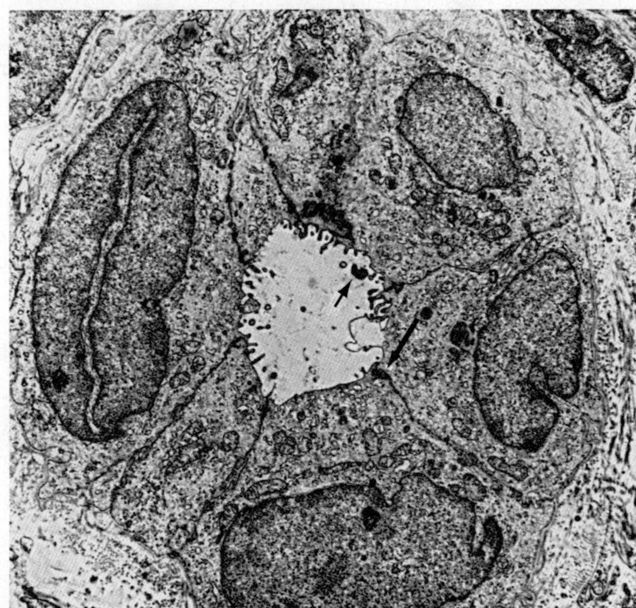

Fig. 64.2 Ultrastructure of an interlobular bile duct. The duct is lined by a layer of cuboidal epithelial cells that are joined by tight junctions (*long arrow*) and demonstrate a microvillar architecture on their luminal surface (*short arrow*). (From Jones AL, Springer-Mills E. The liver and gallbladder. In: Weiss L, ed. *Modern Concepts of Gastrointestinal Histology*. New York: Elsevier; 1984:740.)

surface.[19] The cells have a prominent Golgi apparatus and numerous vesicles that likely participate in the exchange of substances among cytoplasm, bile, and plasma through the processes of exocytosis and endocytosis.[19] These ducts increase in caliber and possess smooth muscle fibers within their walls as they approach the hilum of the liver. The muscular component may provide the morphologic basis for the narrowing of the ducts at this level, as observed on cholangiography.[24] Because the ducts become progressively larger, the epithelium becomes thicker, and the surrounding layer of connective tissue grows thicker and contains many elastic fibers. These ducts anastomose further to form the large hilar intrahepatic ducts, which are 1–1.5 mm in diameter and give rise to the main hepatic ducts.

The common hepatic duct emerges from the porta hepatis after the union of the right and left hepatic ducts, each of which is 0.5–2.5 cm long (Fig. 64.3).[25,26] The confluence of the right and left hepatic ducts is outside the liver in some 95% of cases; uncommonly, the ducts merge inside the liver, or the right and left hepatic ducts do not join until the cystic duct joins the right hepatic duct.[26] Because the hepatic ducts leave the porta hepatis, they lie within the two serous layers of the hepatoduodenal ligament. This sheath of fibrous tissue binds the hepatic ducts to the adjacent blood vessels. In the adult, the common hepatic duct is about 3 cm long and is joined by the cystic duct, usually at its right side, to form the common bile duct (or simply bile duct).[26] The length and angle of junction of the cystic duct with the common hepatic duct are variable. The cystic duct enters the common hepatic duct directly in 70% of patients; alternatively, the cystic duct may run anterior or posterior to the bile duct and spiral around it before joining the bile duct on its medial side.[25] The cystic duct may also course parallel to the common hepatic duct for 5–6 cm and enter it after running posterior to the first portion of the duodenum.

In humans, the large intrahepatic bile ducts at the hilum (1–1.5-mm diameter) have many irregular side branches and pouches (150–270-μm diameter) that are oriented in one plane, corresponding anatomically to the transverse fissure.[19] Smaller pouches of the side branches are also found. Many side branches end as blind pouches, but others, particularly at the hilum, communicate with each other. At the bifurcation, side branches from several main bile ducts connect to form a plexus. The functional significance of these structures is unknown. The blind pouches may serve to store or modify bile, whereas the biliary plexus provides anastomoses that may allow exchange of material between the large bile ducts.

The anatomy of the hepatic hilum is particularly important to the surgeon (see also Chapter 73). A plate of fibrous connective tissue in the hepatic hilum includes the umbilical plate that envelops the umbilical portion of the portal vein, the cystic plate in the gallbladder bed, and the Arantian plate that covers the ligamentum venosum.[26] Histologic examination of the sagittal section of the hilar plate reveals abundant connective tissue, including neural fibers, lymphatic vessels, small capillaries, and small bile ducts. The bile ducts in the plate system correspond to the extrahepatic bile ducts, and their lengths are variable in every segment.[26]

Similar to the intestine, the cystic, common hepatic, and bile ducts possess mucosa, submucosa, and muscularis.[24] The ducts are lined by a single layer of columnar epithelium. Mucus-secreting tubular glands can be found at regular intervals in the

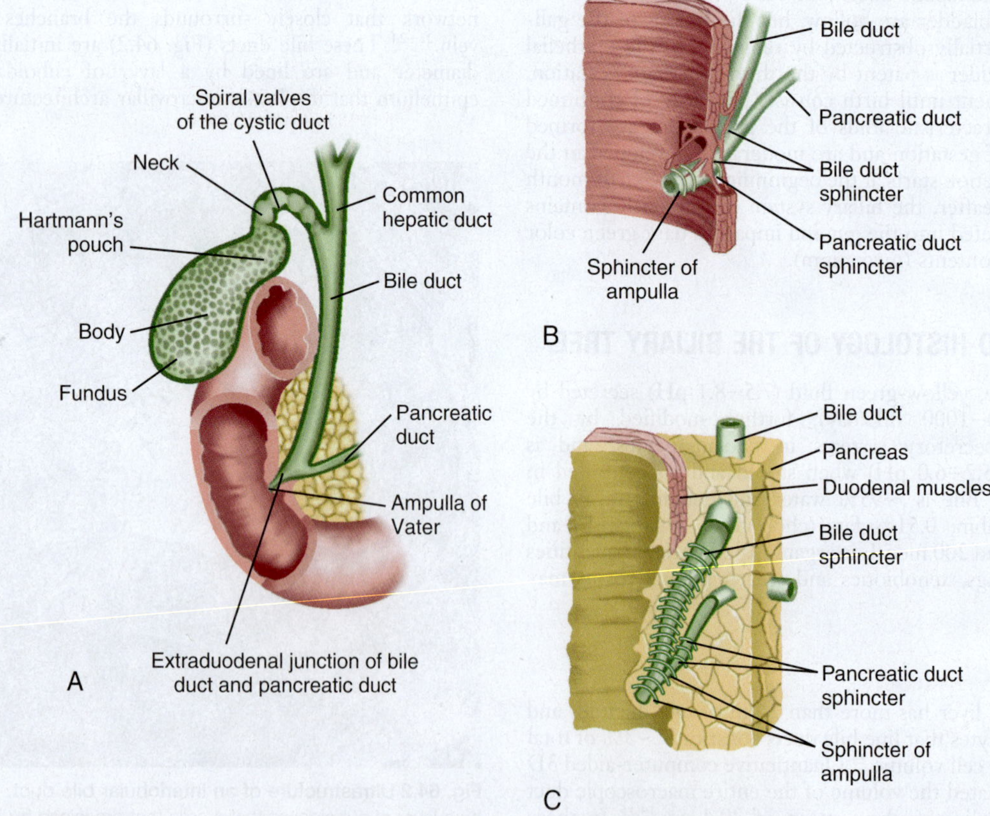

Fig. 64.3 Schematic representation of the gallbladder, extrahepatic biliary tract, and choledochoduodenal junction (A) with enlarged views of the junction of the bile duct and pancreatic duct (B) and the sphincter of Oddi (C). (From Lindner HH. *Clinical Anatomy*. East Norwalk, CT: Appleton & Lange; 1989, copyright McGraw-Hill.)

submucosa, with openings to the surface of the mucosa. The common bile duct is 6.0–8.0 cm long, runs between layers of the lesser omentum, and lies anterior to the portal vein and to the right of the hepatic artery.[26] The bile duct is normally 0.5–1.5 cm in diameter.[21] The wall of the extrahepatic bile duct is supported by a layer of connective tissue with an admixture of occasional smooth muscle fibers. The smooth muscle component is conspicuous only at the neck of the gallbladder and at the lower end of the bile duct. The bile duct passes retroperitoneally behind the first portion of the duodenum in a notch on the back of the head of the pancreas and enters the second part of the duodenum. The duct then passes obliquely through the posterior medial aspect of the duodenal wall and joins the main pancreatic duct to form the ampulla of Vater (see Fig. 64.3).[25] The mucous membrane bulge produced by the ampulla forms an eminence, the duodenal papilla. In 10%–15% of patients, the bile and pancreatic ducts open separately into the duodenum. The bile duct tapers to a diameter of 0.6 cm or less before its union with the pancreatic duct.[26]

As they course through the duodenal wall, the bile and pancreatic ducts are invested by a thickening of both the longitudinal and circular layers of smooth muscle (see Fig. 64.3) of the sphincter of Oddi (see also Chapter 65).[27] There is considerable variation in this structure, but it is usually composed of several parts: (1) the sphincter choledochus—circular muscle fibers that surround the intramural portion of the bile duct immediately before its junction with the pancreatic duct; (2) the sphincter pancreaticus, which is present in approximately one-third of persons and surrounds the intraduodenal portion of the pancreatic duct before its juncture with the ampulla; (3) the fasciculi longitudinales—longitudinal muscle bundles that span intervals between the bile and pancreatic ducts; and (4) the sphincter ampullae—longitudinal muscle fibers that surround a sparse layer of circular fibers around the ampulla of Vater.[24] The sphincter choledochus constricts the lumen of the bile duct and, thus, prevents bile flow. Contraction of the fasciculi longitudinales shortens the length of the bile duct and, thus, promotes the flow of bile into the duodenum. The contraction of the sphincter ampullae shortens the ampulla and approximates the ampullary folds to prevent reflux of intestinal contents into the bile and pancreatic ducts. When both ducts end in the ampulla, however, contraction of the sphincter may cause reflux of bile into the pancreatic duct.[27]

The intrahepatic and extrahepatic bile ducts are highly dependent on arterial blood supply for oxygenation. An abundant anastomotic network of blood vessels from branches of the hepatic and gastroduodenal arteries supplies the bile duct.[22,24,28] The supraduodenal portion of the duct is supplied by vessels running along its wall inferiorly from the retroduodenal artery and superiorly from the right hepatic artery. Injury to these blood vessels can result in bile duct ischemia and stricturing.[25]

The surface of the intrahepatic and extrahepatic bile ducts is drained by fine venous plexuses that communicate with each other.[21,22] A fine reticular epicholedochal venous plexus lies on the surface of the bile ducts, and a paracholedochal venous plexus lies outside the bile ducts and courses parallel to the ducts.

An extraordinarily rich plexus of capillaries surrounds bile ducts as they pass through the portal tracts.[22,28] Blood flowing through this peribiliary plexus empties into the hepatic sinusoids via the interlobular branches of the portal vein. The peribiliary plexus may modify biliary secretions through the bidirectional exchange of proteins, inorganic ions, and bile acids between blood and bile. Because blood flows in the direction (from the large toward the small ducts) opposite to that of bile flow, the peribiliary plexus presents a countercurrent stream of biliary-reabsorbed substances to hepatocytes.

The intrahepatic arteries, veins, bile ducts, and hepatocytes are innervated by adrenergic and cholinergic nerves. In the autonomic nervous system, there are a number of regulatory peptides, such as neuropeptide tyrosine, calcitonin gene-related peptide, somatostatin, vasoactive intestinal polypeptide, enkephalin, and bombesin. Neuropeptide tyrosine-positive nerves present in extrahepatic bile ducts may serve to regulate bile flow by autocrine or paracrine mechanisms.

The lymphatic vessels of the hepatic, cystic, and proximal portions of the bile duct empty into glands at the hilum of the liver.[24] Lymphatics draining from the lower portion of the bile duct drain into glands near the head of the pancreas.

Gallbladder

The gallbladder (see Fig. 64.3) is a storage reservoir that allows bile acids to be delivered in a high concentration and in a controlled manner to the duodenum for the solubilization of dietary lipid (see Chapter 66).[14,24,29] It lies in a fossa on the undersurface of the right lobe of the liver.[29] This distensible pear-shaped structure is 3 cm wide and 7 cm long in the adult and has a capacity of 30–50 mL.[29] The gallbladder has a thin muscular layer with the smooth muscle cells largely oriented around the circumference of the gallbladder. The absorptive surface of the gallbladder is enhanced by numerous prominent folds. The gallbladder is covered anteriorly by an adventitia that is fused with the capsule of the liver. On its posterior aspect and at the apex, it is covered by the visceral peritoneum. The portions of the gallbladder are the fundus, body, infundibulum, and neck.[24] The anterior portion of the fundus is located at the level of the right lateral border of the musculus rectus abdominis and the ninth costal cartilage. The posterior aspects of the fundus and body lie close to the transverse colon and duodenum, respectively; with perforation of the gallbladder, gallstones can readily penetrate these structures.[29,30] The infundibulum is an area of tapering between the gallbladder body and neck. Hartmann pouch is a bulging of the inferior surface of the infundibulum that lies close to the neck of the gallbladder. Gallstones can become impacted in Hartmann pouch, thereby obstructing the cystic duct and producing cholecystitis.[29] Extensive inflammation in Hartmann pouch can lead to an obstruction of the adjacent common hepatic duct (Mirizzi syndrome) (see Chapter 67).

The gallbladder is connected at its neck to the cystic duct, which empties into the bile duct (see Fig. 64.3).[29] The cystic duct is about 4 cm long and maintains continuity with the surface columnar epithelium, lamina propria, muscularis, and serosa of the gallbladder. The mucous membrane of the gallbladder neck forms the spiral valve of Heister, which is involved in regulating flow into and out of the gallbladder.

The gallbladder is supplied by the cystic artery, which usually arises from the right hepatic artery.[29,31] The artery divides into two branches near the neck of the gallbladder: a superficial branch that supplies the serosal surface and a deep branch that supplies the interior layers of the gallbladder wall. Variations in the origin and course of the cystic artery are common.[29] Because the cystic artery is an end artery, the gallbladder is particularly susceptible to ischemic injury and necrosis that result from inflammation or interruption of hepatic arterial flow.

The cystic vein provides venous drainage from the gallbladder and cystic ducts and commonly empties into the portal vein and occasionally directly into the hepatic sinusoids.[24,29] The lymph vessels of the gallbladder are connected with the lymph vessels of Glisson capsule. Subserosal and submucosal lymphatics empty into a lymph gland near the neck of the gallbladder.[24] Sympathetic innervation of the gallbladder originates from the celiac axis and travels with branches of the hepatic artery and portal vein. Visceral pain is conducted through sympathetic fibers and is frequently referred to the right subcostal, epigastric, and right scapular regions. Branches of both vagus nerves provide parasympathetic innervation that likely contributes to the regulation of gallbladder motility.[24]

The gallbladder is lined by a mucosa that manifests multiple ridges and folds and is composed of a layer of columnar epithelial cells. The gallbladder wall consists of a mucosa, lamina propria, tunica muscularis, and serosa.[32] The tunica muscularis is thick and invested with an interlocking array of longitudinal and spiral smooth muscle fibers. Tubuloalveolar glands are found in the region of the neck of the gallbladder and are involved in mucus production.[29,32] The Rokitansky-Aschoff sinuses are invaginations of the surface epithelium that may extend through the muscularis.[24] These structures can be a source of inflammation, most likely as a result of bacterial stasis and proliferation within the invaginations. The ducts of Luschka may be observed along the hepatic surface of the gallbladder and open directly into the intrahepatic bile ducts rather than into the gallbladder cavity. These structures are thought to represent a developmental anomaly, and when they are present in the gallbladder bed may be a source of a bile leak after cholecystectomy.[29]

DEVELOPMENTAL ANOMALIES

Extrahepatic Ducts

Accessory bile ducts are aberrant ducts that drain individual segments of the liver; they may drain directly into the gallbladder, cystic duct, right and left hepatic ducts, or bile duct.[25,33] In rare cases, the right hepatic duct may connect to the gallbladder or cystic duct. These anomalies must be recognized on cholangiography to prevent inadvertent transection or ligation of bile ducts during surgery.

Complete duplication of the bile duct occurs rarely. In most cases, separate ducts drain the right and left hepatic lobes and open into the duodenum.[25]

Variation in the drainage and course of the cystic duct is common.[25] Duplication of the cystic duct may also be encountered. The cystic duct is absent in most cases of agenesis of the gallbladder (see later); rarely, the duct alone may be absent, and the gallbladder empties directly into the common hepatic duct.

Gallbladder

Most structural anomalies of the gallbladder are of no clinical importance, but occasionally the abnormal gallbladder may be a predisposing factor for bile stasis, inflammation, and formation of gallstones.[25,33] Gallbladder disease in an anomalous or malpositioned gallbladder may cause diagnostic confusion.

Agenesis of the gallbladder may be an isolated anomaly or occur in association with other congenital malformations.[33] The abnormality has a frequency at autopsy of 0.04%–0.13% and likely reflects a lack of development of the gallbladder bud or failure of the normal process of vacuolization. Incomplete vacuolization of the solid endodermal cord during development can result in congenital strictures of the gallbladder or cystic duct. Ectopic tissues of foregut endodermal origin, including gastric, hepatic, adrenal, pancreatic, and thyroid tissues, may be found within the gallbladder wall.

A double gallbladder is another rare malformation that occurs in 1–5 per 10,000 persons in the general population.[25,33,34] The two gallbladders may share a single cystic duct, forming a Y-shaped channel, or each may have a distinct cystic duct that enters the bile duct separately.[25] *Vesica fellea* triplex, or triplication of the gallbladder, is another rare congenital anomaly.[35] Multiple gallbladders are usually discovered because of cholelithiasis, sludge, cholecystitis, or neoplasia. Bilobed gallbladders and gallbladder diverticula are other rare anomalies. A single gallbladder may be divided by longitudinal septa into multiple chambers, probably secondary to incomplete vacuolization of the solid gallbladder bud during morphogenesis.[34] Diverticula and septations of the gallbladder may promote bile stasis and gallstone formation.

Various malpositions of the gallbladder have been described.[25,34] Rarely, the gallbladder lies under the left lobe of the liver, to the left of the falciform ligament. This defect likely results from migration of the embryonic bud from the hepatic diverticula to the left rather than to the right.[25] Some researchers have proposed that a second gallbladder may develop independently from the left hepatic duct, with a regression of the normal structure on the right. In other cases, a caudal bud that advances farther than the cranial bud may become buried within the cranial structure, creating an intrahepatic gallbladder. It is thought that if the caudal bud lags behind the movement of the cranial bud, a floating gallbladder results. In this setting, the gallbladder is covered completely with peritoneum and suspended from the undersurface of the liver by mesentery to the gallbladder or cystic duct; the gallbladder is abnormally mobile and prone to torsion. Rarely, gallbladders have been found in the abdominal wall, falciform ligament, and retroperitoneum.[34]

Several forms of "folded" gallbladders have been described. In one variant, the fundus appears to be bent, giving the appearance of a "Phrygian cap."[34] The gallbladder is usually located in a retroserosal position, and the anomaly is thought to result from aberrant folding of the gallbladder within the embryonic fossa. Aberrant folding of the fossa during the early stages of development can result in kinking between the body and the infundibulum of the gallbladder. Kinked gallbladders probably do not lead to clinical symptoms but may be a source of confusion in the interpretation of imaging studies.[34]

APPROACH TO DISORDERS OF THE BILIARY TRACT IN INFANTS AND CHILDREN

General Features

Cholestatic liver disease results from processes that interfere with either bile formation by hepatocytes or bile flow through the intrahepatic and extrahepatic biliary tract. A number of these disorders are due to defective ontogenesis or a failure of postnatal adaptation to the extrauterine environment. Box 64.1 provides a list of disorders that affect the biliary tract and occur in both

BOX 64.1 Biliary Tract Disorders in Infants and Children

DISORDERS OF THE BILE DUCTS

Allograft rejection
Biliary atresia
Biliary helminthiasis
Caroli disease
Choledochal cyst
Cystic fibrosis
Graft-versus-host disease
Idiopathic bile duct stricture (possibly congenital)
Inspissated bile syndrome
Paucity of intrahepatic bile ducts (syndromic and nonsyndromic)
Post-traumatic bile duct stricture
Sclerosing cholangitis (primary, immunodeficiency-related, neonatal)
Spontaneous perforation of bile duct
Tumors intrinsic and extrinsic to the bile duct

DISORDERS OF THE GALLBLADDER

Acalculous cholecystitis
Acute cholecystitis
Acute hydrops of the gallbladder
Anomalies
Cholelithiasis
Chronic cholecystitis
Tumors

TABLE 64.1 Relative Frequencies of Various Disorders of Neonatal Cholestasis

Disorder	Frequency (%)
Extrahepatic biliary atresia	25–40
Idiopathic neonatal hepatitis	20
α_1-Antitrypsin deficiency	10–20
Alagille syndrome	2–14
Other genetic diseases (PFIC, inborn error of metabolism, storage diseases, mitochondropathies, other)	~10
Endocrinopathy (panhypopituitarism)	5
Infectious hepatitis (CMV, HSV, others)	3–5
Choledochal cyst	2–4
Bacterial sepsis	2

infants and older children; they are discussed later in this chapter. There is a particular emphasis on neonatal cholangiopathies and the unique aspects of biliary disease in the older child. The general features of the many cholestatic liver diseases of the neonate are similar, and a central problem of pediatric hepatology is differentiating intrahepatic from extrahepatic cholestasis (Table 64.1).[36] The treatment of metabolic or infectious liver diseases and the surgical management of biliary anomalies require early diagnosis. Even when effective treatment is not possible, infants and children with progressive liver disease benefit from optimal nutritional support and medical management of chronic liver disease before they are referred for LT.

Because of the immaturity of hepatobiliary function, the number of distinct disorders that exhibit cholestatic jaundice may be greater during the neonatal period than at any other time of life (see Box 64.1).[37,38] Genomic sequencing is identifying new defects that were previously labeled as idiopathic neonatal hepatitis. Liver dysfunction in the infant, regardless of the cause, is commonly associated with bile secretory failure and cholestatic jaundice. Although cholestasis may be traced to the level of the hepatocyte or the biliary apparatus, in practice there may be considerable overlap among disorders with regard to the initial and subsequent sites of injury. For example, damage to the biliary epithelium is often a prominent feature of neonatal hepatitis due to CMV infection. Mechanical obstruction of the biliary tract invariably produces liver dysfunction and in the neonate may be associated with abnormalities of the liver parenchyma, such as giant cell transformation of hepatocytes. Whether giant cells—a frequent nonspecific manifestation of neonatal liver injury—reflect the noxious effects of biliary obstruction or whether the hepatocytes and the biliary epithelium are damaged by a common agent during ontogenesis, such as a virus with tropism for both types of cells, is unknown. Another common histologic variable that often accompanies neonatal cholestasis is bile ductular paucity or a diminution in the number of interlobular bile ducts.[39] This finding may be of primary importance in patients with Alagille syndrome and may also occur as an occasional feature of many other disorders, including idiopathic neonatal hepatitis, congenital CMV infection, and α_1-antitrypsin deficiency.

Diagnosis

In most infants with cholestatic liver disease, the condition appears during the first few weeks of life. Differentiating conjugated hyperbilirubinemia from the common unconjugated physiologic hyperbilirubinemia of the neonate or the prolonged jaundice occasionally associated with breastfeeding is essential.[40] The

BOX 64.2 Evaluation of the Infant With Cholestasis

HISTORY AND PHYSICAL EXAMINATION

Details of family history, pregnancy, presence of extrahepatic anomalies, hepatomegaly, splenomegaly and stool color

TESTS TO ESTABLISH THE PRESENCE AND SEVERITY OF LIVER DISEASE

Fractionated serum bilirubin analysis
Liver biochemical tests (AST, ALT, alkaline phosphatase, GGTP)
Tests of liver function (prothrombin time, partial thromboplastin time, serum albumin level, serum ammonia level [as indicated], serum cholesterol level, blood glucose)

TESTS FOR INFECTION

CBC
Bacterial cultures of blood, urine, and other sites if indicated
CMV urine culture or blood PCR
Serologic tests as indicated based on history or symptoms (HBsAg, TORCH, EBV, parvovirus B19, HIV, others)

METABOLIC AND GENETIC STUDIES

α_1-Antitrypsin level and phenotype
Metabolic screen (urine and serum amino acids, urine organic acids)
Urine for reducing substances
Red blood cell galactose-1-phosphate uridyl transferase activity
Serum iron and ferritin levels
Sweat chloride analysis
Thyroid-stimulating hormone (evaluation of hypopituitarism as indicated)
Urine and serum analysis of bile acids and bile acid precursors
Genetic studies as indicated for Alagille syndrome, progressive familial intrahepatic cholestasis, other genetic causes of cholestasis (consider cholestasis genetics panel)

IMAGING STUDIES

US of liver and biliary tract (first)
Hepatobiliary scintigraphy-rarely indicated
MRCP
Radiography of long bones and skull for congenital infection, and of chest for lung and cardiac disease
Percutaneous gallbladder cholangiography (rarely indicated)

PROCEDURES

Percutaneous liver biopsy (for light and electron microscopic examination)
Paracentesis if ascites
Exploratory laparotomy and intraoperative cholangiography

HBsAg, Hepatitis B surface antigen; *TORCH*, toxoplasmosis, other, rubella CMV, herpes.

possibility of liver or biliary tract disease must be considered in any neonate older than 14 days with jaundice (see also Chapter 79). The stools of a patient with well-established biliary atresia are acholic, but early in the course of incomplete or evolving biliary obstruction, the stools may appear normal or only intermittently pigmented. Life-threatening but treatable disorders such as bacterial infection and a number of inborn errors of metabolism must be excluded. Success of surgical procedures in relieving the biliary obstruction of biliary atresia or a choledochal cyst depends on early diagnosis and surgery.

The approach to evaluation of an infant with cholestatic liver disease is outlined in Box 64.2. The initial assessment should promptly establish whether cholestatic jaundice is present and assess the severity of liver dysfunction. A more detailed investigation may be required and should be guided by the clinical features of the case. All relevant diagnostic tests need not be performed in every patient. US may promptly establish a diagnosis of a choledochal cyst in a neonate with jaundice and, thus, obviate the need to exclude infectious and metabolic causes of liver disease. Numerous routine and specialized biochemical tests and imaging procedures have been proposed to distinguish intrahepatic from extrahepatic cholestasis in infants and thereby avoid unnecessary surgical exploration.[40,41] Standard liver biochemical tests usually show variable elevations in serum direct bilirubin, aminotransferases, alkaline phosphatase, and lipid levels. Unfortunately, no single test has proved to have satisfactory discriminatory value, because at least 10% of infants with intrahepatic cholestasis have bile secretory failure sufficient to lead to an overlap in diagnostic test results with those suggestive of biliary atresia.[42] The presence of bile pigment in stools is sometimes cited as evidence against biliary atresia, but coloration of feces with secretions and epithelial cells that have been shed by the cholestatic patient may be misleading.

US can be used to assess the size and echogenicity of the liver. Even in neonates, high-frequency real-time US can usually define the presence and size of the gallbladder, detect stones and sludge in the bile ducts and gallbladder, and demonstrate cystic or obstructive dilatation of the biliary system. Extrahepatic anomalies can also be identified. A triangular cord or band-like periportal echogenicity (≥3 mm in thickness), which represents a cone-shaped fibrotic mass cranial to the portal vein, appears to be a specific ultrasonographic finding in the early diagnosis of biliary atresia, but is dependent on the technical expertise of the ultrasonographer.[43,44] CT provides information similar to that obtained by US but is less suitable in patients younger than 2 years of age because of exposure to radiation, the paucity of intra-abdominal fat for contrast, and the need for heavy sedation or general anesthesia.[45] MRCP, performed with T2-weighted turbo-spin echo sequences, is widely used to assess the biliary tract in all age groups, including neonates. In some patients with biliary atresia, nonvisualization of the bile duct and demonstration of a small gallbladder have been characteristic MRCP findings. Another study found that MRCP is 82% accurate, 90% sensitive, and 77% specific for depicting biliary atresia. Contrary to previous reports, false-positive and false-negative findings occur with MRCP. Differentiation of severe intrahepatic cholestasis from biliary atresia may be difficult because the ability of MRCP to delineate the extrahepatic biliary tract depends on bile flow.[46] MRCP can accurately define choledochal cysts and has emerged as the procedure of choice in the diagnosis of PSC.

The use of hepatobiliary scintigraphic imaging agents such as ^{99m}Tc-iminodiacetic acid derivatives has limited utility in differentiating biliary atresia from other causes of neonatal jaundice.[45] A 1997 study showed that in 50% of patients who had a paucity of interlobular bile ducts but no extrahepatic obstruction, biliary excretion of radionuclide was absent.[47] In patients who had idiopathic neonatal hepatitis, 25% also demonstrated no biliary excretion. Nevertheless, the modality remains useful for assessing cystic duct patency in patients with a hydropic gallbladder or cholelithiasis.

ERCP may be useful in evaluating children with extrahepatic biliary obstruction and has been performed successfully in cholestatic neonates.[41] Considerable technical expertise is required of the operator to complete this procedure in infants. Percutaneous transhepatic cholangiopancreatography may be of value in visualizing the biliary tract in selected patients,[48] but the technique is more difficult to perform in infants than in adults because the intrahepatic bile ducts are small and because most disorders that occur in infants do not result in dilatation of the biliary tract. Interventional ERCP is commonly used to dilate biliary strictures and to remove common bile duct stones in children.

Percutaneous liver biopsy is particularly valuable in evaluating cholestatic patients and can be undertaken in even the smallest infants with only sedation and local anesthesia.[49] When doubt about the diagnosis persists, the patency of the biliary tract can be examined directly by a minilaparotomy and operative cholangiography. In a meta-analysis of various diagnostic methods used in 11 studies involving 646 patients, the accuracy rate of percutaneous liver biopsy was better than that of all noninvasive methods, with a pooled sensitivity of 98% (95% CI 96%–99%), specificity of 93% (95% CI 89%–95%), a positive predictive value of 93.0%, and a negative predictive value of 97.7%.[50] Liver biopsy is also valuable in demonstrating bile duct paucity or biliary damage from medications or viruses.

PEDIATRIC DISORDERS OF THE BILE DUCTS

Biliary Atresia

Biliary atresia is characterized by complete obstruction of bile flow as a result of the destruction of all or a portion of the extrahepatic bile ducts.[51] As part of the underlying disease process or as a result of biliary obstruction, concomitant injury and fibrosis of the intrahepatic bile ducts also occurs to a variable extent.[52]

Epidemiology

The disorder occurs in 1 in 10,000–15,000 live births in the United States and accounts for approximately one-third of cases of neonatal cholestatic jaundice (see Table 64.1). It is the most frequent indication for referral for LT in children (~50% of all cases).[53] The cause of biliary atresia is unknown. The disease is not inherited, reports of familial cases have been rare and there have been several reports of dizygotic and monozygotic twins discordant for biliary atresia. In a study of 461 patients in France, seasonality, time clustering, and time-space clustering could not be demonstrated.[54] In the multistate case-controlled National Birth Defects Prevention Study conducted between 1997 and 2002, babies born to non-Hispanic black mothers were at greater risk than those born to non-Hispanic white mothers.[55]

Etiology and Pathogenesis

Several mechanisms have been proposed to account for the progressive obliteration of the extrahepatic biliary tract.[56] There is no evidence that biliary atresia results from a failure in morphogenesis or recanalization of the bile duct during embryonic development or from an ischemic origin of extrahepatic bile duct injury. Support for potential toxin-induced injury is based on the finding that ingestion of a plant isoflavonoid was associated with the development of biliary atresia in livestock and in a zebrafish model.[57] Congenital infections with CMV, group C rotavirus, EBV, and reovirus 3 occasionally have been implicated.[56] In one study, 56% of patients with biliary atresia had significant increases in interferon (IFN)-γ-producing liver T cells in response to CMV, suggesting perinatal CMV infection as a plausible initiator of bile duct damage.[58]

Genome-wide association and other genomic studies have identified *GPC1* as a biliary atresia susceptibility gene.[59] This gene encodes glypican 1, a heparan sulfate proteoglycan, which regulates Hedgehog signaling and inflammation. Liver samples from patients with biliary atresia had reduced levels of apical GPC1 in cholangiocytes, compared with samples from controls. Another genome-wide association study identified a susceptibility locus for biliary atresia on locus 10q24.2 that had a strong association with X-prolyl aminopeptidase P1(XPNPEP1) and *ADD3*.[59] XPNPEP1 is expressed in biliary epithelia and is involved in the metabolism of inflammatory mediators. *ADD3* encodes adducin, a membrane skeletal protein that functions in regulating epithelial cell-cell adhesions and is highly expressed in fetal livers.

Oligonucleotide-based gene chip analysis of complementary RNA from livers of infants with biliary atresia has demonstrated a coordinated activation of genes involved in lymphocyte differentiation and inflammation.[60] There is increasing evidence for the roles of autoimmunity and dysregulated cellular, humoral, and innate immunity in a mouse model and in patients with biliary atresia (see Chapter 2).[61] Prenatal viral infection likely causes cholangiocyte apoptosis, release of antigens, and aberrant MHC class II expression in extrahepatic and intrahepatic bile ducts in a genetically susceptible host.[56] Viral, native, or altered bile duct antigens are phagocytosed and processed by macrophages or dendritic cells and presented to naïve T cells. Activated $CD4^+$ T cells, $CD8^+$ T cells, and macrophages release cytotoxic inflammatory mediators that contribute to cholangiocyte injury through apoptotic or necrotic pathways (see Chapters 1 and 74). The regulatory T cell (Treg) subset of $CD4^+$ T cells, responsible for controlling T cell-mediated immune responses to pathogens, is deficient in infants with biliary atresia, and this deficiency may exacerbate bile duct injury.[56] Hepatic stellate cells (myofibroblasts) and fibroblasts are activated, thereby causing fibrosis of the intra- and extrahepatic bile ducts. How these events are coordinated, why the disease occurs only in the first few months of life, why a minority of infants with prenatal viral infections develop biliary atresia, and why the disease does not recur in a transplanted liver are unanswered questions.

Circulating markers of inflammation persist in biliary atresia and are largely unaffected by portoenterostomy (see later), with clear progressive elevation in both type 1 T helper (Th1) effectors interleukin-2 and IFN-γ, some type 2 T helper (Th2) effectors (interleukin-4), as well as a macrophage marker (TNF-α). Increased expressions of the soluble cell adhesion molecules, sICAM-1 and sVCAM-1, are also found and likely reflect ongoing recruitment of circulating inflammatory cells into the liver and biliary system.[62] Whether this immune response is induced by a viral infection or reflects a genetically programmed response to an infectious or environmental exposure remains unknown.

Extrahepatic anomalies occur in ~15% of patients and include cardiovascular defects, polysplenia, malrotation, situs inversus, and bowel atresias.[63,64] In the setting of splenic defects, this subtype of biliary atresia is also known as "biliary atresia splenic malformation syndrome (BASM)." Some patients who have heterotaxia and biliary atresia have been found to have loss-of-function mutations in the *CFC1* gene.[65,66] This gene encodes a protein called CRYPTIC, which is involved in establishing the left-right axis during morphogenesis. In contrast, limited studies of infants with biliary atresia and heterotaxia have not found mutations in the *INV* gene, which is also involved in determining laterality.[67] Whole exome sequencing of 67 BASM subjects identified five subjects with biallelic variants in the polycystin 1-like 1 (*PKD1L1*) gene, a gene associated with ciliary calcium signaling, and laterality determination.[68] *Jagged1* (the gene defective in Alagille syndrome [see later]) missense mutations have been identified in 9 of 102 patients with biliary atresia and are associated with a poor prognosis.[69]

Pathology

Histopathologic findings on initial liver biopsy specimens are of great importance in the management of patients with biliary atresia.[51,53] Early in the course, hepatic architecture is generally preserved, with a variable degree of bile ductular proliferation, canalicular and cellular bile stasis, and portal tract edema and fibrosis (Fig. 64.4).[53] The presence of bile plugs in portal tract bile ducts is highly suggestive of large-duct obstruction. Furthermore, bile ductules show varying injury to the biliary epithelium, including swelling, vacuolization, and even sloughing of cells into the lumen. Portal tracts have variable amounts of infiltrating inflammatory cells, and in approximately 25% of patients, giant cell transformation of hepatocytes may be seen to a degree observed more commonly in neonatal hepatitis. Bile ductules occasionally may assume a ductal plate configuration, suggesting that the disease has interfered with the process of ductular remodeling that occurs during prenatal development.[70] Biliary cirrhosis may be present initially or may evolve rapidly over the first few months of life, with or without successful restoration of bile flow.[71]

The morbid anatomic characteristics of the extrahepatic bile ducts in biliary atresia are highly variable. Kasai proposed a useful classification of the anatomic variants.[72] Three main types have been defined based on the site of the atresia. Type I is atresia of the common bile duct with patent proximal ducts. Type II atresia involves the hepatic duct, with cystically dilated bile ducts at the porta hepatis. In type IIa atresia, the cystic and bile ducts are patent, whereas in type IIb atresia, these structures also are obliterated. These forms of biliary atresia have been referred to as "surgically correctable" but unfortunately account for less than 10% of all cases. Overall, 90% or more of patients have type III atresia, involving obstruction of the common hepatic, right and left hepatic, and common bile duct, without cystically dilated hilar ducts. The entire perihilar area is in a cone of dense fibrous tissue. The gallbladder is also fibrotic in the majority of cases. The type III variant has been characterized as "noncorrectable," in that there are no patent hepatic or dilated hilar ducts that can be readily used for a biliary-enteric anastomosis.

Complete fibrous obliteration of at least a portion of the extrahepatic bile ducts is a consistent feature found on microscopic examination of the fibrous remnant.[72] Other segments of the biliary tract may demonstrate lumens with varying degeneration of bile duct epithelial cells, inflammation, and fibrosis in the periductular tissues (see Fig. 64.4). In most patients, bile ducts within the liver that extend to the porta hepatis are patent during the first weeks of life but are destroyed progressively, presumably by the same process that damaged the extrahepatic ducts and by the effects of biliary obstruction.

Clinical Features

Most infants with biliary atresia are born at term after a normal pregnancy and have a normal birth weight.[73] Female infants are affected more commonly than male infants. The perinatal course is typically unremarkable. Postnatal weight gain and development usually proceed normally. Jaundice is observed by the parents or the physician after the period of physiologic hyperbilirubinemia. Prolonged jaundice may be erroneously attributed to breastfeeding.[74] The possibility of liver or biliary tract disease must be considered in any neonate older than 14 days with jaundice. The stools of a patient with well-established biliary atresia are acholic, but early in the course the stools may appear normally pigmented or only intermittently pigmented. Screening for biliary atresia in Taiwan by the use of a stool color card given to parents has decreased the number of late referrals for evaluation of cholestasis.[75]

The liver is typically enlarged, with a firm edge palpable 2–6 cm below the right costal margin.[53] The spleen is usually not enlarged early in the course but becomes enlarged as portal hypertension develops. Ascites and edema are not present initially, but coagulopathy may result from vitamin K deficiency.

Laboratory studies initially reveal evidence of cholestasis, with a serum total bilirubin level of 6–12 mg/dL, at least 50% of which is conjugated.[53] A study in 2011 showed that over one-half of patients with biliary atresia have elevated direct bilirubin levels shortly after birth, suggesting a prenatal onset of disease.[76] Serum aminotransferase, GGTP, and alkaline phosphatase levels are moderately elevated.

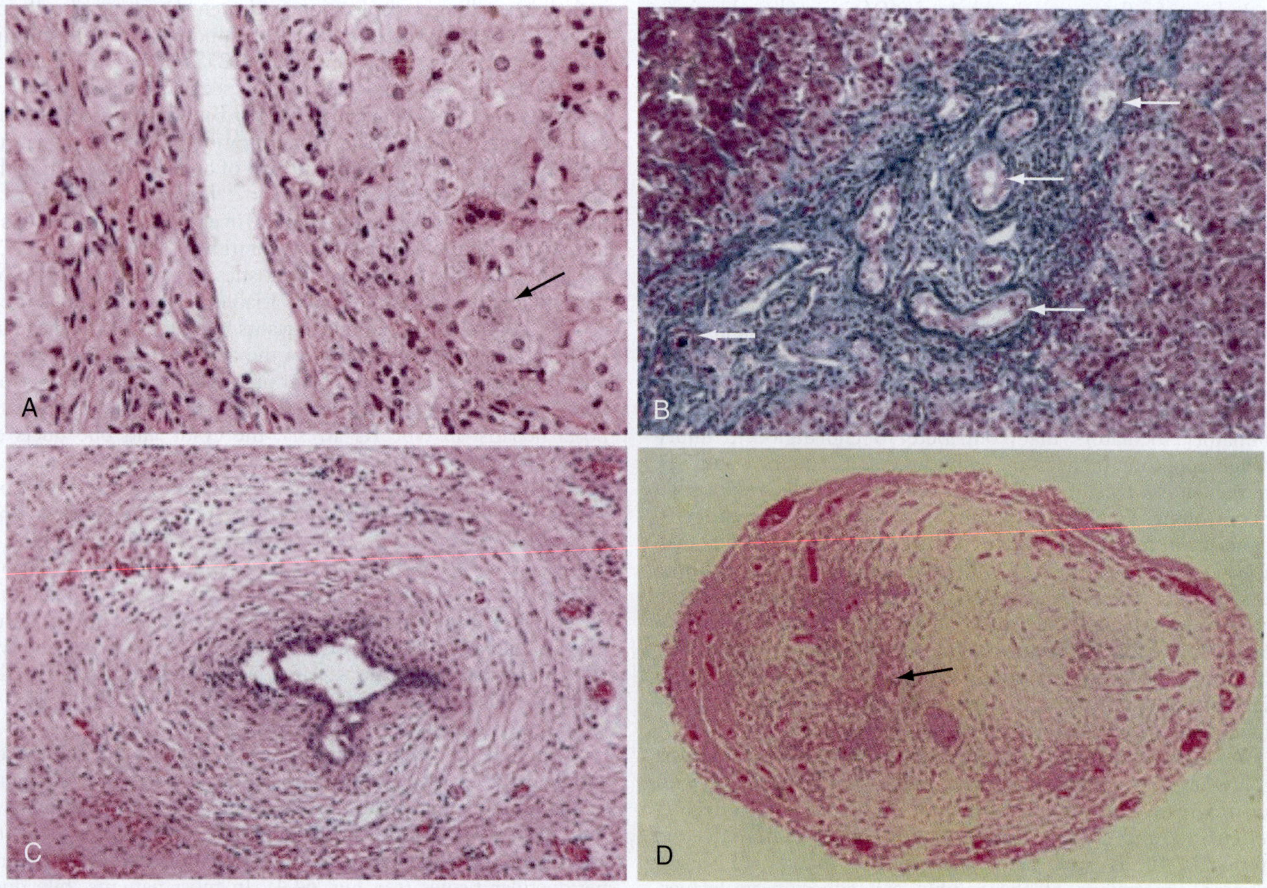

Fig. 64.4 Histology of the liver and extrahepatic bile duct in biliary atresia. (A) Hepatocellular and canalicular cholestasis, multinucleated giant cells (*arrow*), and portal tract inflammation (H&E, ×400). (B) Expanded portal tract with portal fibrosis, bile ductular proliferation (*thin arrows*), and a bile plug in the bile duct (*thick arrow*) (Masson trichrome, ×250). (C) Proximal common hepatic duct in the porta hepatis, with sloughing of biliary epithelium, concentric fibrosis of the bile duct wall, lymphocytic infiltration around the duct, and a narrowed but patent lumen (H&E, ×150). (D) Remnant of a bile duct with complete obliteration of the lumen (*arrow*) and concentric fibrosis of the duct wall (H&E, ×40). (From Sokol RJ, Mack C, Narkewicz MR, Karrer FM. Pathogenesis and outcome of biliary atresia: current concepts. *J Pediatr Gastroenterol Nutr.* 2003;37:4–21. Used with permission.)

Treatment

The initial workup for biliary atresia usually includes percutaneous liver biopsy to assess for histologic evidence of biliary obstruction (bile duct proliferation, bile duct plugs, and portal tract fibrosis). When the possibility of biliary atresia has been raised by clinical, pathologic, and imaging findings, exploratory laparotomy and operative cholangiography are necessary to document the site of obstruction and direct attempts at surgical treatment.[52,77] In most patients who have obliteration of the proximal extrahepatic biliary tract, the preferred surgical approach is the hepatoportoenterostomy procedure developed by Dr. Kasai (Fig. 64.5).[78,79] The distal bile duct is transected, and the fibrous bile duct remnant is dissected to an area above the bifurcation of the portal vein.[80] The dissection then progresses backward and laterally at this level, and the fibrous cone of tissue is transected flush with the liver surface, thereby exposing an area that may contain residual microscopic bile ducts. The operation is completed by the anastomosis of a Roux-en-Y loop of jejunum around the bare edge of the transected tissue to provide a conduit for biliary drainage. Multiple attempts at reexploration and revision of nonfunctional conduits should be avoided.[81] Adjuvant therapy with glucocorticoids and UDCA as a choleretic agent may be prescribed postoperatively,[82,83] but in a prospective double-blind randomized placebo-controlled trial, glucocorticoids did not reduce the need for LT after a Kasai portoenterostomy.[84]

Prognosis

The prognosis of untreated biliary atresia is extremely poor; death from liver failure usually occurs within 2 years.[85] In the largest report of over 1000 children with biliary atresia, the 5- and 30-year survival rates with the native liver were 41% and 22%, respectively. Furthermore, the earlier the age at Kasai, the better the survival rates (Fig. 64.6).[86] Several series from Europe, Japan, and the United States have demonstrated similar results.[87–90] The Childhood Liver Disease Research Network, a multicentered consortium to study biliary atresia in the United States and Canada, reported on 219 children with biliary atresia who were alive with their native livers approximately 10 years after the Kasai portoenterostomy. Over 98% of these patients had clinical or biochemical evidence of chronic liver disease.[89] Therefore children with biliary atresia derive long-term benefit from the Kasai portoenterostomy procedure, although most have persisting liver

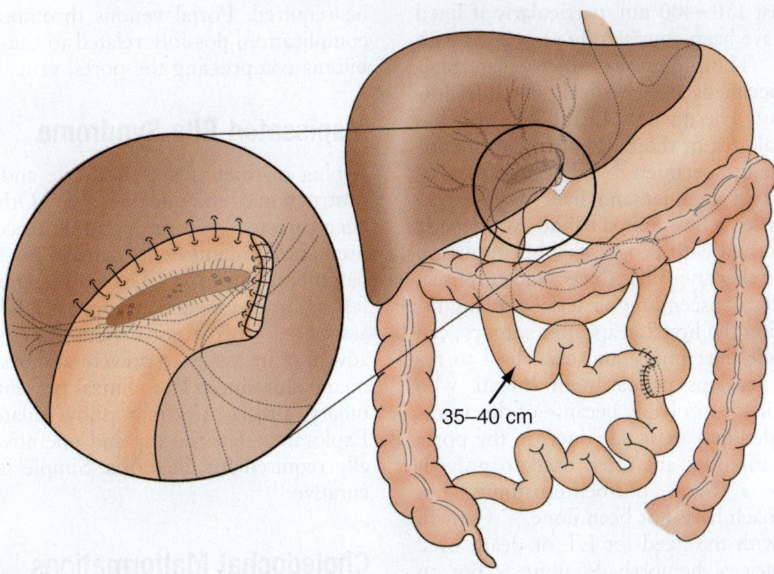

Fig. 64.5 The Kasai operation for biliary atresia. A 35- to 40-cm Roux-en-Y anastomosis is made to the porta hepatis after surgical excision of the atretic extrahepatic biliary tract and a cone of fibrous tissue from the porta hepatis. Multiple small but patent bile ducts may be uncovered by this dissection and drained into the Roux loop. An enlarged depiction of the anastomosis of the jejunal loop to the porta hepatis is shown on the left. (Figure drawn and kindly provided by Dr. Frederick Ryckman, Cincinnati, OH.)

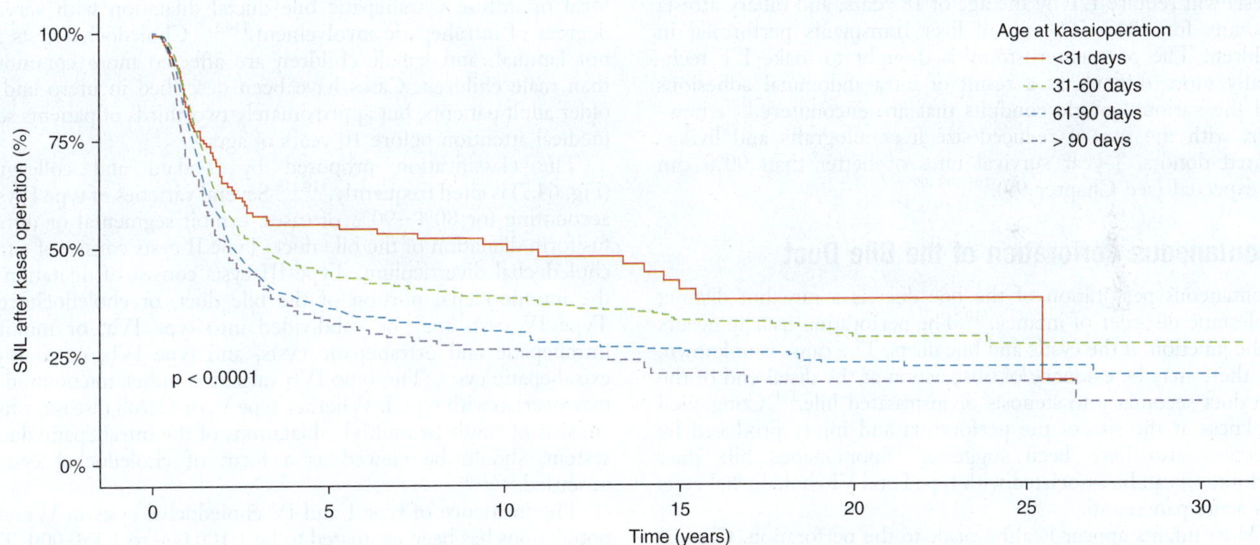

Fig. 64.6 Survival with native liver (SNL) according to age at Kasai portoenterostomy. (From Fanna M, Masson G, Capito C, et al. Management of biliary atresia in France 1986 to 2015: Long-term results. *JPGN*. 2019;69:416–424.)

dysfunction. Progressive biliary cirrhosis may result in death from hepatic failure or the need for LT despite an apparently successful restoration of bile flow.

Several factors have been found to contribute to the varying outcome after hepatic portoenterostomy. The age of the patient at the time of surgery is most critical.[86–88,91] In several series, bile flow was reestablished in ~80% of infants who were referred to for surgery within 60 days of birth.[87,92] Resolution of jaundice may still occur with diagnoses after 90 days of age, but long-term survival is compromised even in the era of LT.[91] In a prospective US study of 244 infants, the risk of transplantation or death was increased in patients with porta hepatis atresia, a nonpatent common bile duct, BASM, ascites, and a nodular liver.[93] Independent prognostic factors for overall survival in a large French study were performance of the Kasai operation and age less than 45 days at surgery[88]; complete atresia of extrahepatic bile ducts and BASM were associated with a less favorable outcome. The experience of the surgical center was also important.[88]

Prognostic factors include the level of the serum total bilirubin at 3 months post-Kasai portoenterostomy. If the total bilirubin is ≤2 mg/dL at 3 months post-Kasai procedure, then one can predict that the patient will not need LT in the first 2 years of life. If the total bilirubin is ≥6 mg/dL at that time point, then there is a high likelihood of the need for LT within 2 years.[94–96] Prehilar bile duct structures of at least 150–400 μm, particularly if lined with columnar epithelium, have been consistently associated with an unfavorable prognosis.[94,97] The presence of ductal plate malformation on liver biopsy specimens also predicts poor bile flow after hepatoportoenterostomy. The quantity of the bile flow has been correlated with the total area of the biliary ductules identified in the excised porta hepatis specimen.[98,99] The rate of progression of the underlying bile ductular and liver disease also limits survival.[51,100] The disorder is not limited to the extrahepatic biliary tract and can be associated with progressive inflammation and destruction of the intrahepatic bile ducts and eventual cirrhosis.[51] Recurring episodes of ascending bacterial cholangitis, which are most frequent during the first 2 years after surgery, can contribute to the ongoing bile duct injury and even lead to re-obstruction.[101] Cholangitis develops primarily in infants who have some degree of bile drainage, probably because of the access to ascending infection provided by patent bile ducts in the porta hepatis. Prophylactic oral antibiotics are often used to prevent recurrent cholangitis after a Kasai portoenterostomy, but controlled trials of this approach have not been done.[102] Growth failure has been associated with the need for LT or death by 2 years of age. Esophageal variceal hemorrhage alone is not an absolute indication for urgent LT in patients with good bile drainage and preserved liver synthetic function.[103,104]

LT is essential in the management of children in whom portoenterostomy does not successfully restore bile flow, referral is late (probably at 120 days of age or later), and end-stage liver disease develops despite bile drainage.[88,105,106] In the United States, approximately 80% of patients with biliary atresia will require LT by the age of 18 years, and biliary atresia accounts for 40%–50% of all liver transplants performed in children. The portoenterostomy is thought to make LT technically more difficult as a result of intra-abdominal adhesions and the various enteric conduits that are encountered[107]; however, with the use of reduced-size liver allografts and living-related donors, 1-year survival rates of better than 90% can be expected (see Chapter 99).[105,108,109]

Spontaneous Perforation of the Bile Duct

Spontaneous perforation of the bile duct is a rare but distinct cholestatic disorder of infancy.[110] The perforation usually occurs at the junction of the cystic and bile ducts. The cause is unknown, but there may be evidence of obstruction at the distal end of the bile duct secondary to stenosis or inspissated bile.[111] Congenital weakness at the site of the perforation and injury produced by infection also have been suggested. Spontaneous bile duct perforation can be associated with type I and VI choledochal cysts and acute pancreatitis.

Most infants appear healthy prior to the perforation. Clinical signs, including jaundice, acholic stools, dark urine, and ascites, typically occur during the first months of life.[111] The infant also may experience vomiting and lack of weight gain. Progressive abdominal distention is a usual feature; bile staining of fluid within umbilical or inguinal hernias may be observed.

Mild-to-moderate conjugated hyperbilirubinemia with a minimal elevation of serum aminotransferase levels is typical. Abdominal paracentesis reveals clear, bile-stained ascitic fluid, which usually is sterile. US reveals ascites or loculated fluid in the RUQ; the biliary tract is not dilated. Hepatobiliary scintigraphy demonstrates the free accumulation of isotope within the peritoneal cavity.[111]

Operative cholangiography is required to demonstrate the site of the perforation.[112] Surgical treatment may involve simple drainage of the bilious ascites and repair of the site of the perforation.[112] If the perforation is associated with obstruction of the bile duct, however, drainage via a cholecystojejunostomy may be required. Portal venous thrombosis has been reported as a complication, possibly related to the irritative effects of bile or a biloma compressing the portal vein.

Inspissated Bile Syndrome

A plug of thick, inspissated bile and mucus also may cause the obstruction of the bile duct.[113,114] Otherwise, healthy infants have been affected, but the condition occurs more commonly in ill premature infants who cannot be fed and require prolonged parenteral nutrition. The pathogenesis may involve bile stasis, fasting, infection, and an increased bilirubin load. The cholestasis associated with massive hemolysis is now infrequent with the advent of measures to prevent and treat Rh and ABO blood group incompatibilities. The clinical presentation may resemble that of biliary atresia. US may show dilated intrahepatic bile ducts. Exploratory laparotomy and operative cholangiography are usually required for diagnosis. Simple irrigation of the bile duct is curative.[115]

Choledochal Malformations

Epidemiology and Classification

Choledochal malformations are not cysts as they have commonly been referred to, because they are not enclosed epithelialized structures. These congenital anomalies will continue to be referred to as choledochal cysts for historical reasons but are likely heterogeneous in etiology and have in common a spectrum of focal or diffuse extrahepatic bile ductal dilatation with varying degrees of intrahepatic involvement.[116,117] Choledochal cysts are not familial, and female children are affected more commonly than male children. Cases have been described in utero and in older adult patients, but approximately two-thirds of patients seek medical attention before 10 years of age.

The classification proposed by Todani and colleagues (Fig. 64.7) is cited frequently.[118,119] Several varieties of type I cysts, accounting for 80%–90% of cases, exhibit segmental or diffuse fusiform dilatation of the bile duct. Type II cysts consist of a true choledochal diverticulum. Type III cysts consist of dilatation of the intraduodenal portion of the bile duct, or choledochocele. Type IV cysts may be subdivided into type IVa, or multiple intrahepatic and extrahepatic cysts, and type IVb, or multiple extrahepatic cysts. The type IVb variant is either uncommon or may overlap with type I. Whether type V, or Caroli disease, which consists of single or multiple dilatations of the intrahepatic ductal system, should be viewed as a form of choledochal cyst is unsettled.[119,120]

The incidence of type I and IV choledochal cysts in Western populations has been estimated to be 1:100,000 to 1:150,000. The incidence may be as high as ~1:10,000 in some Asian countries. Choledochal diverticula (type II cysts) and choledochoceles (type III cysts) are much less common (~1:1,000,000).[116,117]

Etiology

The cause of choledochal malformations has not been established.[117] Congenital weakness of the bile duct wall, a primary abnormality of epithelial proliferation during embryologic ductal development, and congenital obstruction of bile ducts have been suggested.[116,121] A relationship to other obstructive cholangiopathies (e.g., biliary atresia) has been proposed but not proved. In a gene sequencing study of 33 patients with choledochal malformations, no single-gene defects were detected, but 21 potentially damaging de novo pathogenic variants were found that could affect developmental processes of the hepatobiliary tract even in a compound heterozygote state.[122] A high frequency

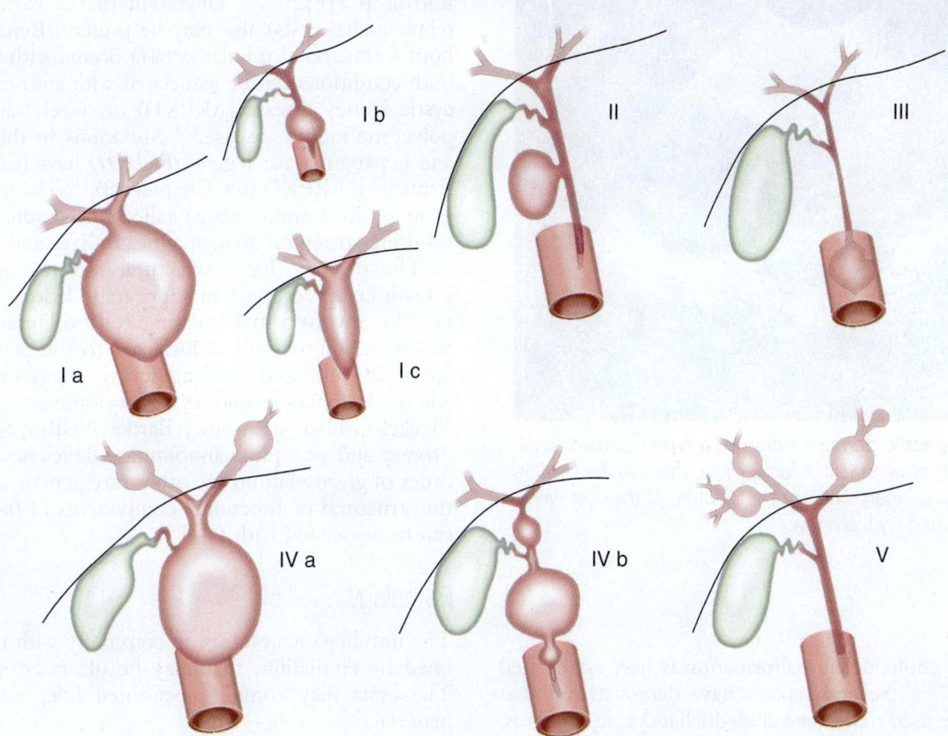

Fig. 64.7 Classification of choledochal malformations according to Todani and colleagues.[119] *Ia*, Common type; *Ib*, segmental dilatation; *Ic*, diffuse dilatation; *II*, diverticulum; *III*, choledochocele; *IVa*, multiple cysts (intra- and extrahepatic); *IVb*, multiple cysts (extrahepatic); *V*, single or multiple dilatations of the intrahepatic ducts (Caroli disease). (From Savader SJ, Benenati JF, Venbrux AC, et al. Choledochal cysts: classification and cholangiographic appearance. *AJR*. 1991;156:327–331.)

(40%) of pancreaticobiliary malunion (anomalous union of the pancreatic and bile ducts), which may allow the reflux of pancreatic secretions into the biliary tract, has been described (see Chapter 57).[123] This process may result in progressive injury to the developing ductal system, with subsequent weakness and dilatation. Choledochal cysts may be associated with other developmental anomalies, including colonic atresia, duodenal atresia, imperforate anus, pancreatic arteriovenous malformation, multiseptate gallbladder, ventricular septal defect, aortic hypoplasia, pancreatic divisum, pancreatic aplasia, focal nodular hyperplasia of the liver, and congenital absence of the portal vein. Choledochal cysts have also been found in some patients with autosomal recessive polycystic renal disease (see Chapter 98).[123,124] Chromosomal anomalies, including chromosomal duplications and microdeletions in 17q12, and a de novo 2p15p16.1 microdeletion, have been identified in several patients. Trio-based whole exome-sequencing has identified potentially damaging de novo variants that could contribute to disease pathogenesis.[123]

Pathology

The dilated biliary segments are composed of a fibrous wall; there may be no epithelial lining or a low columnar epithelium.[117] Mild chronic inflammation may be present. Complete inflammatory obstruction of the terminal portion of the bile duct is common in infants who have a choledochal cyst.

Liver biopsy specimens in the affected neonate show features typical of large-duct obstruction.[117] Findings may mimic those observed in extrahepatic biliary atresia. Portal tract edema, bile ductular proliferation, and fibrosis may be prominent. A pattern of biliary cirrhosis may be observed in older patients with long-standing biliary obstruction. Carcinoma of the cyst wall may occur by adolescence (see Chapter 71).[125,126]

Clinical Features

The infantile form of choledochal cyst disease must be distinguished from other forms of hepatobiliary disease of the neonate, particularly biliary atresia.[116] The disorder often appears during the first months of life, and as many as 80% of patients have cholestatic jaundice and acholic stools.[117] Vomiting, irritability, and failure to thrive may occur. Examination reveals hepatomegaly, and in about half of patients an abdominal mass is palpated. In a series of 72 patients diagnosed postnatally, 50 (69%) exhibited jaundice that was associated with abdominal pain in 25 or with a palpable mass in 3; 13 (18%) had abdominal pain alone, and 2 (3%) had a palpable mass alone. In a 2008 series, adults were more likely to exhibit abdominal pain (97% vs. 63%; $P < .001$), and children were more likely to experience jaundice (71% vs. 25%, $P = .001$).[126] In older patients, epigastric pain may be due to pancreatitis. Intermittent jaundice and fever may result from recurrent episodes of cholangitis. The classic triad of abdominal pain, jaundice, and a palpable abdominal mass is observed in less than 20% of patients.[126] Biliary tract malignancy may be a presenting feature in older patients.[127]

Choledochal cysts may undergo spontaneous perforation, particularly when bile flow is obstructed. Progressive hepatic injury can occur during the first months of life as a result of biliary obstruction caused by poor bile flow, sludge, protein plugs, and stones composed of fatty acids and calcium.[127]

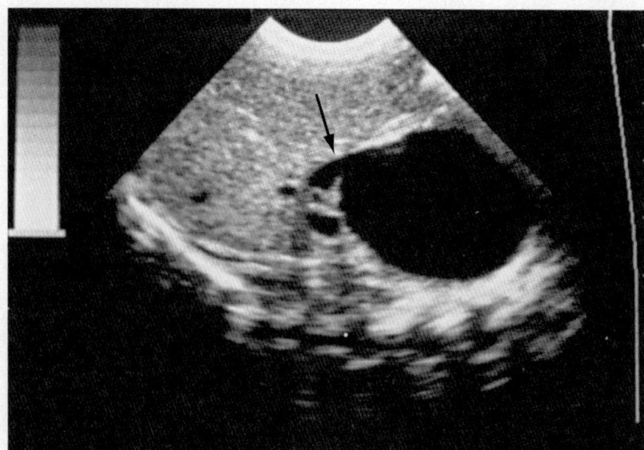

Fig. 64.8 Ultrasonographic demonstration of a type I choledochal cyst in an infant with cholestasis. A large cystic mass in the RUQ is shown on this transverse scan. The point of juncture of the cyst with the bile duct is delineated by the *arrow*.

Diagnosis

The diagnosis of a choledochal malformation is best established by US (Fig. 64.8).[45,128] Several reports have demonstrated that antenatal US can be used to detect a choledochal cyst in the fetus. Sequential ultrasonographic examinations have allowed the study of the evolution of choledochal cysts during pregnancy. In the older child, percutaneous transhepatic cholangiography or ERCP may help define the anatomic features of the cyst; its site of biliary origin, including an anomalous arrangement of the pancreaticobiliary junction; and the extent of both extrahepatic and intrahepatic disease, including the presence of intraductal strictures and calculi.[128] MRCP is used to evaluate the extent of the cyst and defects within the biliary tract and to detect pancreaticobiliary malunion.[129] MRCP has been less effective than ERCP for detecting minor ductal abnormalities and small choledochoceles in adults.[130] In practice, most pediatric surgeons rely on an operative cholangiogram to define the extent of intrahepatic and extrahepatic disease.[117]

Treatment

The preferred treatment is surgical excision of the cyst with the reconstruction of the extrahepatic biliary tract.[117,119] Laparoscopic surgery is feasible in many cases. Biliary drainage is usually accomplished by a choledochojejunostomy with a Roux-en-Y anastomosis. Excision of the cyst reduces bile stasis and the risk of cholangitis and cholangiocarcinoma. The overall risk of cancer has been reported to be 10%–15%, is greatest in types I and IV forms, and increases with age. Simple decompression and internal drainage should be done only when the complicated anatomic characteristics do not allow complete excision. Long-term follow up is essential because recurrent cholangitis, lithiasis, anastomotic stricture, and pancreatitis may develop years after the initial surgery. In 45 surgically treated patients (19 followed for more than 10 years), no patients developed malignancy during follow-up.[127]

Hepatic Fibrocystic Disease

Nonobstructive saccular or fusiform dilatation of the intrahepatic bile ducts is a rare congenital disorder.[131,132] In the pure form, known as *Caroli disease*, dilatation is classically segmental and saccular and associated with stone formation and recurrent bacterial cholangitis. A more common type, *Caroli syndrome*, is associated with a portal tract lesion typical of congenital hepatic fibrosis (CHF).[132–134] Dilatation of the extrahepatic bile ducts (choledochal cysts) also may be present. Renal disease occurs in both forms, renal tubular ectasia occurs with Caroli disease, and both conditions can be associated with autosomal recessive polycystic kidney disease (ARPKD) or, rarely, autosomal-dominant polycystic kidney disease.[135] Mutations in the polycystic kidney and hepatic disease 1 gene *(PKHD1)* have been identified in patients with ARPKD (see Chapter 98).[136] The gene encodes a large protein (4074 amino acids) called fibrocystin to reflect the main resulting structural abnormalities in liver and kidney.

The protein shares structural features with the hepatocyte growth factor receptor and appears to belong to a superfamily of proteins involved in regulating cell proliferation, adhesion, and repulsion. Fibrocystin is localized to the primary cilia of renal epithelial cells and cholangiocytes, suggesting a link between ciliary dysfunction and cyst development. Joubert syndrome, Meckel-Gruber syndrome, Bardet-Biedl syndrome, Jeune syndrome, and phosphomannomutase-deficiency (a congenital disorder of glycosylation) are other rare genetic disorders that affect the structural or functional components of the primary cilia and can be associated with CHF.

Pathology

The intrahepatic cysts are in continuity with the biliary tract and lined by epithelium that may be ulcerated and hyperplastic.[131] The cysts may contain inspissated bile, calculi, and purulent material.

Liver biopsy specimens may reveal normal tissue or features of acute or chronic cholangitis. Portal tract edema and fibrosis may be present. In cases associated with CHF, findings associated with the ductal plate malformation can be expected; the lumen of the portal bile duct forms an epithelium-lined circular cleft surrounding a central vascularized connective tissue core, or a series of bile duct lumens are arranged in a circle around a central fibrous tissue core.

Clinical Features

Patients usually seek medical attention during childhood and adolescence because of hepatomegaly and abdominal pain.[135,136] The disorder appears in the neonate as renal disease or cholestasis.[136] The saccular or fusiform dilatation of bile ducts predisposes to stagnation of bile, leading to the formation of biliary sludge and intraductal lithiasis. Fever and intermittent jaundice may occur during episodes of bacterial cholangitis. Hepatosplenomegaly is found in cases associated with CHF; affected patients may bleed from esophageal varices.[131] Polycystic kidneys may be palpable.

CHF may take several forms. A portal hypertensive presentation is most common with esophageal variceal hemorrhage in childhood. A cholangitic form is characterized by cholestasis and recurrent cholangitis. Patients may also display a mixed phenotype with features of both portal hypertension and cholangitis. Biliary disease may be very subtle or even latent, and not easily defined by liver biochemical testing or imaging.

In a prospective study of 73 patients with CHF and ARPKD (age, 1–56 years; mean, 12.7 years), initial symptoms related to the liver occurred in 26.[133] Splenomegaly was observed early in life and was present in 60% of children younger than 5 years of age. The platelet count was the best predictor of the severity of portal hypertension. Biliary abnormalities were present in 70% (40% with Caroli syndrome, 30% with isolated dilatation of the common bile duct). The variability in severity of liver and kidney was not explainable by the specific PKHD1 mutation. In a review of hepatic complications of ARPKD compiled from the literature, portal hypertension was documented in 45% and recurrent cholangitis in 54% of 788 patients.[134] Owing to the abnormal biliary tract in CHF, cholangitis can occur even in the absence of Caroli syndrome.

Liver biochemical tests may have normal results or show mild-to-moderate elevations of serum bilirubin, alkaline phosphatase, and aminotransferase levels.[132–134] Liver synthetic function is well preserved, but repeated episodes of infection and biliary obstruction within the cystic bile ducts eventually may lead to hepatic failure. A reduced maximal concentrating capacity is the most frequently abnormal renal function test finding; variable elevations of blood urea nitrogen and serum creatinine levels reflect the severity of the underlying kidney disease.[136]

Diagnosis

US, MRCP, and CT are of great value in demonstrating the cystic dilatation of the intrahepatic bile ducts.[133,137,138] Increased liver echogenicity reflects the underlying fibrosis in this condition. Renal cysts or hyperechogenicity of papillae may be detected. Percutaneous or endoscopic cholangiography (Fig. 64.9) usually demonstrates a normal bile duct with segmental saccular dilatations of the intrahepatic bile ducts.[139] Rarely, the process may be limited to one lobe of the liver. Liver biopsy is rarely required for diagnosing CHF.

Prognosis and Treatment

The clinical course is often complicated by recurrent episodes of cholangitis[136,139]; sepsis and liver abscess may occur. The prognosis in the setting of persistent or recurrent infection is poor. Calculi frequently develop within the cystically dilated bile ducts and can complicate the treatment of cholangitis. Patients who have extensive hepatolithiasis may experience intractable abdominal pain. Removal of stones by surgery, endoscopy, or lithotripsy usually is not feasible. Hepatic resection is indicated for disease limited to a single lobe.[140] Surgical drainage procedures generally are not effective and may complicate later LT. Therapy with UDCA has been used successfully to dissolve intrahepatic stones. Cholangiocarcinoma may develop within the abnormal bile ducts, owing to bile stasis and recurrent cholangitis.[141] Portal hypertension and variceal bleeding may predominate in patients with CHF and Caroli disease.[136] End-stage renal disease develops in some patients who have associated polycystic kidney disease. LT is an option in patients who have extensive disease and frequent complications, including refractory cholangitis.[142] Genotype-phenotype correlations in a group of 304 patients identified several enhancing and mitigating *PKHD1* variants that impacted on the primary endpoint of survival without substantial hepatic complications.[137]

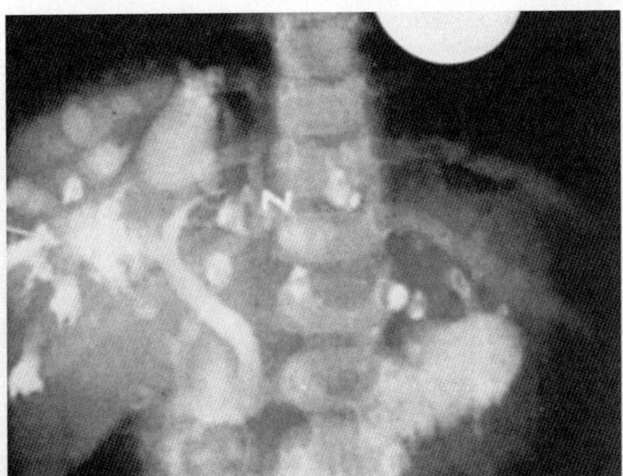

Fig. 64.9 Cholangiographic findings in Caroli disease. Percutaneous cholangiography reveals multiple cystic lesions throughout a markedly enlarged liver. Cystic lesions are in continuity with bile ducts. The extrahepatic bile ducts are normal. (From Kocoshis SA, Riely CA, Burrell M, Gryboski JD. Cholangitis in a child due to biliary tract anomalies. *Dig Dis Sci*. 1980;25:59–65.)

Nonsyndromic Paucity of the Interlobular Bile Ducts

A paucity of interlobular bile ducts may be an isolated and unexplained finding in infants and children with idiopathic cholestasis or a feature of a heterogeneous group of disorders that include congenital infections with rubella and CMV and genetic disorders such as α_1-antitrypsin deficiency and inborn errors of bile acid metabolism.[143,144] Bile duct paucity has been observed in some cases of Williams Syndrome, Noonan Syndrome, and Trisomy 21.[145,146] Paucity of interlobular bile ducts has been defined as a ratio of the number of interlobular bile ducts to the number of portal tracts of less than 0.4.[10,147] At least 10 portal tracts should be examined on a liver biopsy specimen to be confident that bile duct paucity is present. Cases may arise from true biliary dysgenesis but more often result from active injury and loss of bile ducts.[10,147] Bile duct paucity may occur without associated developmental anomalies and without a documented intrauterine infection or genetic disorder, but this idiopathic form of nonsyndromic bile duct paucity is likely to be heterogeneous in cause, with extremely variable clinical features and prognosis.[144] Cholestasis typically develops early in infancy and may be associated with progressive liver disease.

The development of bile duct paucity beyond the neonatal period is often referred to as the vanishing bile duct syndrome. Liver damage may be progressive, leading to death or LT. This disorder is heterogeneous in etiology, which includes infection, ischemia, adverse drug reactions, autoimmune diseases, chronic allograft rejection, and malignancy. Amoxicillin-clavulanic acid and trimethoprim/sulfamethoxazole are drugs associated with vanishing bile duct syndrome in children (see Chapter 90).[148]

Syndromic Paucity of the Interlobular Bile Ducts (Alagille Syndrome, or Arteriohepatic Dysplasia)

Syndromic paucity of interlobular bile ducts (Alagille syndrome or arteriohepatic dysplasia) is the most common form of familial intrahepatic cholestasis. This disorder is characterized by chronic cholestasis, a decreased number of interlobular bile ducts, and a variety of other congenital malformations.[149,150]

Etiology

An autosomal-dominant mode of transmission with incomplete penetrance and variable expressivity has been established from family studies.[151] A partial deletion of the short arm of chromosome 20 was detected in some patients and led to identification of the Alagille syndrome gene. Mutations in the *Jagged1 (JAG1)* gene have been identified in approximately 94% of affected patients and include total gene deletions as well as protein truncating, splicing, and missense mutations.[152] *JAG1* encodes a ligand in the Notch signaling pathway that is involved in cell fate determination during development.[153] Mutations in the gene encoding the Notch2 receptor have been found in patients with Alagille syndrome who are negative for *JAG1* mutations.[154] Similar to patients with *JAG1* mutations, patients with Notch2 receptor gene mutations demonstrate highly variable expressivity of the affected systems but generally have liver disease. *THBS2*, which encodes thrombospondin 2, has been identified in a genome-wide association study as a candidate genetic modifier for severe liver disease. Thrombospondin 2 is expressed in bile ducts and periportal regions of mouse liver and affects Jag-Notch signaling.[155]

There appears to be no phenotypic difference between patients with the deletion of the entire *JAG1* gene and those with intragenic mutations. The disorder may affect only one family member; such cases may represent spontaneous mutations of the *JAG1* gene. Alternatively, it is possible that the variability in gene expression is so great that minimally affected family members are not diagnosed. A 1994 analysis of 33 families collected through 43 probands corroborated the autosomal-dominant inheritance and concluded that the rate of penetrance is 94% and that 15% of cases are sporadic; however, expressivity was variable, and 26 persons (including 11 siblings) exhibited minor forms of the disease.[156]

Pathology

The hallmark of this condition is a paucity of interlobular bile ducts.[147] Paucity may be defined as a significantly decreased ratio of the numbers of interlobular portal bile ducts to portal tracts (<0.4).[148] The histologic features during the first months of life may overlap with those of neonatal hepatitis, in that there can be ballooning of hepatocytes, variable cholestasis, portal inflammation, and giant cell transformation. Often the number of interlobular bile ducts is not decreased on initial liver biopsy specimens, but bile duct injury consisting of cellular infiltration of portal tracts contiguous to interlobular bile ducts, lymphocytic infiltration and pyknosis of biliary epithelium, and periductal fibrosis may be evident. Serial biopsy specimens from an individual patient may initially show bile duct proliferation, followed later in life by a paucity of bile ducts (Fig. 64.10).[157] Paucity of interlobular bile ducts is usually apparent after 3 months. The extrahepatic bile ducts are patent but usually narrowed or hypoplastic. Ultrastructural studies have demonstrated the accumulation of bile pigment in the cytoplasm near lysosomes and vesicles of the outer convex space of the Golgi apparatus. The bile canaliculi most often appear to be structurally normal, but in some cases, they may appear to be dilated, with blunting and shortening of microvilli.

Pathogenesis

The mechanisms involved in the pathogenesis of bile duct paucity and cholestasis are unsettled. Also unknown is how the hepatobiliary disease relates to the multiplicity of congenital anomalies found in other organ systems. Mice homozygous for the *Jag1* mutation die of hemorrhage early during embryogenesis and exhibit defects in remodeling of the embryonic and yolk sac vasculature.[158] The strong *JAG1* expression during human embryogenesis, both in the vascular system and in other mesenchymal and epithelial tissues, implicates abnormal angiogenesis in the pathogenesis of Alagille syndrome and particularly the paucity of interlobular bile ducts. In human embryos, *JAG1* is expressed in the distal cardiac outflow tract and pulmonary artery, major arteries, portal vein, optic vesicle, otocyst, branchial arches, metanephros, pancreas, and mesocardium; around the major bronchial branches; and in the neural tube.[159] All these structures are affected in Alagille syndrome. Many of the *JAG1* mutations generate premature termination codons, and many of these mutations produce a truncated protein that exerts a dominant-negative effect on Notch signaling.[160] Although a vascular basis for the anomalies in Alagille syndrome seems possible, the precise mechanisms leading to bile duct paucity remain unknown. Notch signaling has an important role in the differentiation of biliary epithelial cells and is essential for their tubular formation during intrahepatic bile duct development.[161] There is evidence that a lack of branching and elongation of bile ducts during postnatal liver growth contributes to peripheral bile duct paucity and cholestasis.[162]

It is of great interest to note that profound cholestasis can occur in this disorder during the neonatal period, even when the interlobular bile ducts are not decreased in number. By contrast, later in life when cholestasis may be less severe as judged by clinical and biochemical criteria, interlobular bile ducts may be undetectable on liver biopsy specimens.

Clinical Features

Chronic cholestasis of varying severity affects 95% of patients.[151,163] Jaundice and clay-colored stools may be observed during the neonatal period and become apparent in most patients during the first 2 years of life. Intense pruritus may be present by 6 months of age.[149] The liver and spleen are often enlarged. During the first years of life, xanthomata appear on the extensor surfaces of the fingers and in the creases of the palms and popliteal areas. Dysmorphic facies (Fig. 64.11) are usually recognized during infancy and become more characteristic with age.[150] The forehead is typically broad, the eyes are deeply set and widely spaced, and the mandible is somewhat small and pointed,

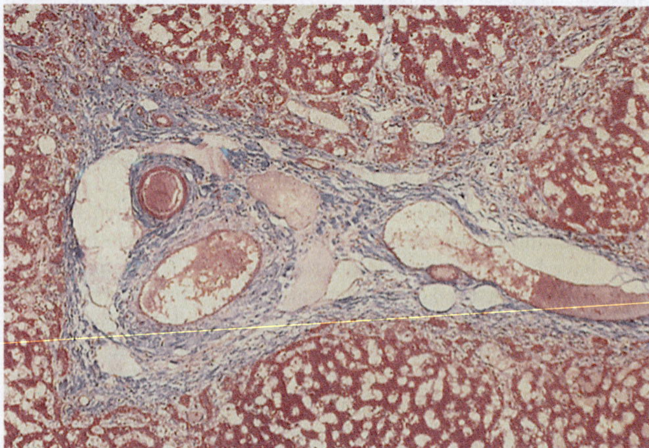

Fig. 64.10 Histologic features of syndromic paucity of interlobular bile ducts. A portal triad in the liver, with a distinct artery and vein but with no bile duct, is shown in this low-power photomicrograph. (Masson trichrome stain.) (From Portmann BC, Roberts EA. Developmental abnormalities and liver disease in childhood. In: Burt AD, Portmann BC, Ferrell LD, eds. *MacSween's Pathology of the Liver*. 6th ed. London: Churchill Livingstone Elsevier; 2012:121.)

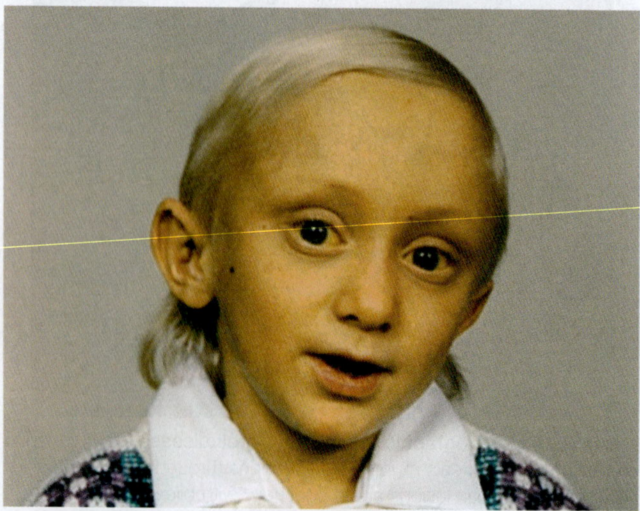

Fig. 64.11 Facial appearance in syndromic paucity of the intrahepatic bile ducts. (Photograph courtesy Dr. Binita Kamath, Philadelphia, PA.)

imparting a triangular appearance to the face. The malar eminence is flattened, and the ears are prominent. Extrahepatic anomalies have been described with this syndrome, but the phenotypic expression varies considerably. In a 1999 series of 92 patients, cholestasis occurred in 96%, cardiac murmur in 97%, butterfly vertebrae in 51%, posterior embryotoxon (mesodermal dysgenesis of the iris and cornea) in 78%, and characteristic facies in 96% of patients.[163] Short stature is a regular feature but is only partially due to the severity of chronic cholestasis. Growth hormone insensitivity associated with elevated circulating levels of growth hormone–binding protein has been described in these patients.[164] Mild-to-moderate mental retardation affects 15%–20% of patients. Congenital heart disease occurs in most patients, and peripheral pulmonic stenosis is observed in about 90%.[163,165] Systemic vascular malformations are widespread and associated with a risk of intracranial bleeding. Osseous abnormalities include a decreased bone age, variable shortening of the distal phalanges, and vertebral arch defects (e.g., butterfly vertebrae, hemivertebrae, and decrease in the interpedicular distance). Ophthalmologic examination may reveal eye anomalies, including posterior embryotoxon, retinal pigmentation, and iris strands. Renal abnormalities and hypogonadism also have been described.[151,164]

Laboratory studies reveal an elevation of total serum bilirubin levels (usually 2–8 mg/dL) during infancy and intermittently later in life.[163,166] Approximately 50% of the total serum bilirubin is conjugated. Serum alkaline phosphatase and GGTP levels may be extremely high and correlate somewhat with the degree of cholestasis. Serum aminotransferase levels are mildly to moderately increased. Serum cholesterol levels are often 200 mg/dL or higher, and serum triglyceride concentrations may range from 500 to 1000 mg/dL. Total serum bile acid concentrations are markedly elevated, but the bile acid profiles in serum, urine, and bile do not differ qualitatively from those seen in other cholestatic disorders.

Prognosis and Treatment

The clinical course is marked by varying degrees of cholestasis, sometimes worsened by intercurrent viral infections. Morbidity may result from pruritus, cutaneous xanthomata, and neuromuscular symptoms related to vitamin E deficiency. Treatment involves providing an adequate caloric intake, preventing or correcting fat-soluble vitamin deficiencies, and symptomatic measures to relieve pruritus (see Chapters 22 and 93). Partial external biliary diversion may be effective for treating severe pruritus and hypercholesterolemia in patients without cirrhosis who do not respond to medical therapy.[167,168] The long-term prognosis depends on the severity of the liver disease and associated malformations.[165] Factors that contributed significantly to mortality were hepatic disease or transplantation (25%), complex congenital heart disease (15%), and intracranial hemorrhage (25%)[163] HCC may occur.[169] A serum total bilirubin level above 6.5 mg/dL, conjugated bilirubin above 4.5 mg/dL, and cholesterol above 520 mg/dL in children younger than 5 years of age are likely to be associated with severe liver disease in later life.[170] In a retrospective review of 268 patients, vascular anomalies such as intracranial aneurysms accounted for 34% of the mortality.[171] An international study of the natural history of Alagille syndrome in 1443 patients found 10 and 18 year survival with native liver rates of 54% and 40%, respectively.[172] Survival and candidacy for LT may be limited by the severity of associated cardiovascular anomalies. Of the 467 children in the UNOS database transplanted for Alagille syndrome, 1- and 5-year patient survival rates were significantly lower in patients with Alagille syndrome than in those with biliary atresia (82.9% and 78.4% vs. 89.9% and 84%, respectively). Death from graft failure, neurologic disease, and cardiac complications was significantly more frequent in patients with Alagille syndrome than in those with biliary atresia.[173,174]

Primary Sclerosing Cholangitis

PSC is a rare progressive disease of the biliary tract characterized by inflammation and fibrosis of the intrahepatic and extrahepatic biliary ductal systems, leading eventually to biliary cirrhosis.[175,176] Epidemiologic studies report a PSC prevalence in children of 15 cases per million children in North America.[177] Only aspects of PSC that are of particular importance to infants and children are discussed here (see Chapter 70 for a detailed discussion of PSC). PSC in children is usually associated with IBD, as seen in adults. In children, the clinical presentation is variable, with ~50% of children being asymptomatic; the most common symptoms are abdominal pain, jaundice, and lethargy.[176,177] Physical examination sometimes reveals hepatomegaly, which may be associated with splenomegaly, and rarely jaundice or ascites.

A multicentered analysis of 781 children with PSC revealed that 61% were male, 76% had IBD, 33% had overlap with autoimmune hepatitis, and 13% had small-duct PSC. Portal hypertension and biliary complications developed in 38% and 25%, respectively, after 10 years of disease.[178] The IBD-related bowel symptoms can precede, occur simultaneously with, or appear years after the diagnosis of PSC. As in adults, treatment of the bowel disease, including colectomy, does not influence the progression of PSC. Celiac disease has also been associated with PSC.[179]

The onset of PSC has also been reported in the neonatal period[180]; in such cases, cholestatic jaundice and acholic stools have been observed within the first 2 weeks of life. The presenting features are virtually identical to those of extrahepatic biliary atresia, but percutaneous cholecystography discloses a biliary system that is patent and exhibits rarefaction of segmental branches, stenosis, and focal dilatation of the intrahepatic bile ducts. The extrahepatic bile ducts may be involved. Jaundice subsides spontaneously within 6 months, but later in childhood, biliary cirrhosis and portal hypertension may develop.[180] In contrast to PSC in adults and older children, PSC in neonates has not been associated with intestinal disease.

Neonatal ichthyosis and sclerosing cholangitis is a distinct syndrome caused by mutations of *CLDN1* encoding claudin-1, a tight-junction protein. In this disorder, cholestasis is proposed to be due to the absence of claudin-1, leading to increased paracellular permeability and bile duct injury secondary to paracellular bile regurgitation.[181] LT does not affect the cutaneous manifestations of this disease and should be reserved for progressive liver disease. Another genetic link with neonatal sclerosing cholangitis is the *DCDC2* gene; biallelic variants in DCDC2 result in a ciliopathy that can also be associated with global developmental delays.[182]

Secondary sclerosing cholangitis may occur in association with other disorders, including Langerhans cell histiocytosis, immunodeficiency, psoriasis, and CF. Lesions similar to those of PSC have been defined by cholangiography in Langerhans cell histiocytosis, but the process is caused by histiocytic infiltration and progressive scarring of portal tracts, with resulting distortion of intrahepatic bile ducts. Cholestasis can occur before the diagnosis of Langerhans cell histiocytosis has been established but most often is found later.[183] Children with Langerhans cell histiocytosis may have involvement of multiple organs, with diabetes insipidus, bone lesions, skin lesions, lymphadenopathy, and exophthalmos. Chemotherapy does not affect the course of the biliary tract disease. LT has been successful in several children who experienced progression to end-stage liver disease.[184]

Secondary sclerosing cholangitis appears to develop in some children with a variety of immunodeficiencies, both cellular and humoral. Cryptosporidia and CMV have been found concurrently in the biliary tract in some of these patients, as well as in adults with AIDS (see Chapter 33).[185] Treatment of the associated infection has no proven effect on the biliary tract disease.

Immunoglobulin (Ig) G4-related sclerosing cholangitis associated with elevated serum IgG4 levels is the biliary manifestation of a multisystem fibroinflammatory disorder in which affected organs have a characteristic lymphoplasmacytic infiltrate of IgG4-positive cells (see Chapter 70). It has rarely been reported in children and usually in association with autoimmune pancreatitis (see Chapter 59 and 61). In contrast to PSC, the disorder is not associated with IBD, commonly presents with obstructive jaundice, and responds to therapy with glucocorticoids.[186] There is no definitive diagnostic test for PSC; the diagnosis is based on a combination of biochemical, histologic, and imaging data. The serum alkaline phosphatase and GGTP levels are often elevated in children with PSC, and serum aminotransferase levels may be mildly elevated.[187,178] Hyperbilirubinemia is seen in less than half of pediatric patients. Serum autoantibodies, including ANA and smooth muscle antibodies, may be found in some patients.[187] Atypical ANCA with perinuclear fluorescence may be detected in two-thirds of children.

On liver biopsy specimens, the histologic findings may be suggestive of PSC, but usually are not diagnostic. Characteristic concentric periductal ("onion skin") fibrosis may be present later in the course of the disease, but more often only neoductular proliferation and fibrosis are found.[188]

Differentiating PSC from autoimmune hepatitis, particularly in the presence of circulating nonorgan-specific autoantibodies and hepatic features on liver biopsy specimens, may be difficult.[178] In 25%–30% of cases, an overlap syndrome may occur in children, with both hepatic and cholestatic serum liver biochemical test results and with histologic features of autoimmune hepatitis and PSC (see Chapter 92).[175] Serologic findings include the presence of ANA, smooth muscle antibodies, and anti-liver-kidney microsome type 1 antibodies and perinuclear ANCA.[189]

The diagnosis of PSC is established by cholangiography.[190] MRCP is the method of choice for visualizing the intrahepatic and extrahepatic bile ducts and is comparable to ERCP findings and significantly less invasive than ERCP.[190] Irregularities of the intrahepatic and extrahepatic ducts can be found, including alternating strictures and areas of dilatation that produce a beaded appearance. Occasionally, a dominant stricture of the extrahepatic ducts or papillary stenosis is found. Small-duct PSC with a normal cholangiogram but histologic features of PSC occurs in 10%–15% of children.[178,191]

The prognosis of PSC in children is guarded.[176,178] The clinical course of the disorder is variable but usually progressive. In a 1994 series of 56 children, the median survival from onset of symptoms was approximately 10 years, similar to that reported in adults.[192] In another study of 52 children, the median survival free of LT was 12.7 years.[176] A risk-stratification tool to predict liver-related outcomes in children with PSC has been developed using a cohort of 1333 patients at 51 centers. Total bilirubin, serum albumin, gamma glutamyltransferase, platelet count and cholangiography were effective in predicting a primary outcome of liver transplantation or death and a secondary outcome of hepatobiliary complications.[193] HCC also may occur, but cholangiocarcinoma, an important complication of adult PSC, has rarely been reported in children.[178]

The treatment of PSC in children is unsatisfactory.[194] No controlled trials have shown convincingly that any medical therapy improves histologic characteristics and prolongs survival. Therapy with UDCA in adults and children has led to an improvement in clinical symptoms and in liver biochemical test abnormalities, but a long-term benefit of treatment on survival has not been demonstrated and high doses have been detrimental in adults with PSC.[177,194] In limited studies, oral vancomycin has been an effective treatment for concomitant PSC and IBD in children, possibly related to its effect as an antibiotic and its immunomodulatory properties.[195] Endoscopic dilation of a dominant stricture may be required.

LT is an important option for patients who experience progression to end-stage liver disease, recurrent bacterial cholangitis, or intractable pruritus. Long-term results in children appear to be comparable to those for age-matched children who undergo transplantation for other indications.[196] PSC recurs after transplantation in 10%–27% of patients.[176,196]

Medical Management of Chronic Cholestasis

Cholestatic liver disease in children adversely affects nutritional status, growth, and development, and these adverse effects contribute to morbidity and mortality. In a child with chronic cholestatic liver disease, efforts should be directed to promoting growth and development and minimizing discomfort.[197]

Protein-energy malnutrition leading to growth failure is an inevitable consequence of chronic liver disease in 60% of children.[197–199] Steatorrhea is common in children with cholestasis, as a result of impaired intraluminal lipolysis, solubilization, and intestinal absorption of long-chain triglycerides. Medium-chain triglycerides do not require solubilization by bile salts before intestinal absorption and, thus, can provide needed calories when administered orally in one of several commercial formulas or as an oil supplement.

Morbid conditions resulting from fat-soluble vitamin deficiencies can be prevented in large part in cholestatic children.[200] The liquid multiple fat-soluble vitamin preparation made with tocopheryl polyethylene glycol-1000 succinate to promote absorption has been studied prospectively in infants with biliary atresia because of ease of administration and presumed efficacy. However, biochemical fat-soluble vitamin insufficiency is observed commonly in infants with biliary atresia and persistent cholestasis despite administration of this preparation. Individual vitamin supplementation and careful monitoring are warranted in infants with biliary atresia, especially those with total serum bilirubin levels greater than 2.0 mg/dL.[201]

Because metabolic bone disease, manifesting as rickets and pathologic fractures, can result from vitamin D deficiency, vitamin D should be provided as D_2 (up to 8000 IU/day) or as 25-hydroxycholecalciferol (3–5 μg/kg/day). Supplements of elemental calcium (50–100 mg/kg/day) and phosphorus (25–50 mg/kg/day) also may be required. Bone mass can be reduced in cholestatic children even with normal serum 25-hydroxyvitamin D levels, possibly related to impaired insulin-like growth factor I production by the liver.[202]

Xerophthalmia, night blindness, and thickened skin have been reported in patients who have vitamin A deficiency. Oral supplements of vitamin A, 5000–25,000 IU/day, should be administered.[200]

Vitamin K deficiency and associated coagulopathy may be treated initially with an oral water-soluble supplement administered in doses of 2.5–5 mg twice weekly to as much as 5 mg daily. Children who do not respond or who have serious bleeding require intramuscular injections of vitamin K (see Chapter 96).[203]

Chronic deficiency of vitamin E may produce a disabling degenerative neuromuscular syndrome characterized by areflexia, ophthalmoplegia, cerebellar ataxia, peripheral neuropathy, and posterior column dysfunction.[200] The onset can be observed within the first 2 years of life. Because serum vitamin E levels may be elevated spuriously in the presence of hyperlipidemia, the ratio of serum vitamin E to total serum lipids is most useful in monitoring the patient's vitamin E status; deficiency in a child younger than 12 years of age, for example, is indicated by a ratio of less than 0.6. The child may not respond to massive doses of standard vitamin E preparations (150–200 IU/kg/day) and the water-soluble form of vitamin E, *d*-alpha-tocopherol polyethylene glycol-1000-succinate (15–25 IU/kg/day), is an effective alternative.[200]

Xanthomata and pruritus may cause substantial discomfort. Pruritus may be observed by 3 months of age.[204] The success of most therapies for pruritus depends on the presence of patent bile ducts that allow bile acids and other biliary constituents to reach the intestinal lumen. Biliary diversion has been used as a successful alternative to relieve intractable pruritus in some patients with intrahepatic cholestasis.[204,205] The antibiotic rifampin, through upregulation of pathways for biotransformation and biliary excretion, and the choleretic bile acid UDCA have been used for the treatment of pruritus, with varying degrees of success.[206–208] Because of evidence that a component of pruritus may be of central neurogenic origin mediated by the opiate receptor system, opioid receptor antagonists such as naltrexone have been effective in some patients with severe pruritus unresponsive to other agents; however, side effects, withdrawal symptoms, and the lack of experience in children limit the general use of these medications. The nonabsorbable anion exchange resin cholestyramine may be used to bind bile acids, cholesterol, and presumably other potentially toxic agents in the intestinal lumen.[206–208] This medication may lower serum lipid levels and bind the substances involved in the pathogenesis of pruritus. A dose of 0.25–0.5 g/kg/day is administered before breakfast or in divided doses before meals to relieve severe pruritus and xanthomata.[204] Cholestyramine is relatively unpalatable, however, and carries modest risks of intestinal obstruction due to inspissation of the drug, as well as hyperchloremic acidosis. The bile acid–binding efficacy of colesevelam, a novel bile acid sequestrant that is taken in a more palatable tablet form, is superior to cholestyramine,[209] but its use in cholestatic liver disease has been limited (see Chapter 66 and 93). Maralixibat and odevixibat are orally administered, small-molecule ileal bile acid transporter (IBAT) inhibitors that have been approved and are effective for treatment of cholestatic pruritus in infants with Alagille syndrome.[209a]

TABLE 64.2 Risk Factors for the Development of Gallstone Disease in Children

Risk Factor	Example
Hemolytic disease	Hereditary spherocytosis Sickle cell disease Thalassemia
Neonatal or congenital condition	Choledochal cyst Necrotizing enterocolitis Parenteral nutrition Prematurity
Genetic disorder	*ABCB4* mutations (MDR3 deficiency) *ABCB11* mutations *ABCG5/G8* mutation CF Gilbert syndrome Trisomy 21
Nutritional condition	Insulin resistance Obesity
Systemic disorder	Crohn's disease Liver disease and cirrhosis Sepsis
Medication	Cephalosporins Diuretics
Surgery	Cardiac surgery (hemolysis on cardiopulmonary bypass) Ileal resection Neonatal bowel resection
Miscellaneous	Biliary dyskinesia Cancer or leukemia therapy

ABC, ATP-binding cassette; *MDR*, multidrug resistance.
Modified from Svensson J, Makin E. Gallstone disease in children. *Semin Pediatr Surg*. 2012;21:255–65.

PEDIATRIC DISORDERS OF THE GALLBLADDER

Cholelithiasis

Epidemiology

Cholelithiasis is uncommon in otherwise healthy children and usually occurs in patients who have a predisposing condition.[210–213] An ultrasonographic survey of 1570 persons (aged 6–19 years) detected gallstones in only two female subjects, aged 13 and 18 years.[214,215] None of those in the study population had undergone cholecystectomy. The overall prevalence of gallstone disease was 0.13% (0.27% in females). Most cases come to light near the time of puberty, but gallstones have been reported at any age, including during fetal life. Pigmented gallstones predominate in infants and children.[212] Conditions associated with an increased risk of cholelithiasis are listed in Table 64.2. Analysis of data combined from two large series of 605 pediatric patients is informative[216,217]; 53% of patients reported symptoms, and 18% presented with a complication (e.g., pancreatitis, choledocholithiasis, acute calculous cholecystitis) as the first indication of cholelithiasis. An underlying condition or risk factor could be identified in 60% of patients.[216,217] The metabolic syndrome, which is linked to obesity and nonalcoholic fatty liver disease, is also associated with cholesterol gallstone formation.[218]

Pathogenesis

An in-depth discussion of the pathogenesis of gallstones can be found in Chapter 67; certain factors may assume greater importance during infancy and childhood.[213,219] An increased frequency of calculous cholecystitis is reported in sick premature infants, who often undergo a period of prolonged fasting without frequent stimulation of gallbladder contraction and who require periods of prolonged parenteral nutrition. Many of these patients have complicated medical courses that include frequent blood transfusions, episodes of sepsis, abdominal surgery, and use of diuretics and narcotic analgesics. Limited analyses of gallstones in such cases generally have shown the presence of mixed cholesterol-calcium bilirubinate stones. In the critically ill infant, there may be a continuum from the common occurrence of an enlarged, distended gallbladder filled with sludge to the eventual development of cholelithiasis. As in adults, because of an interruption of the enterohepatic circulation of bile acids, the incidence of gallstones is increased in children with ileal disease or after resection of the terminal ileum. In a 2007 series, 24% of 30 children with gallstones had calcium carbonate stones, which previously were considered rare.[220]

Black pigment gallstones commonly occur in patients who have chronic hemolytic disorders such as sickle cell disease and hereditary spherocytosis.[221] These stones are predominantly composed of calcium bilirubinate, with substantial amounts of crystalline calcium carbonate and phosphate. In sickle cell disease, the risk of gallstones increases with age and occurs in at least 14% of children younger than age 10 and 36% of those between age 10 and 20 (see Chapter 35).[222] The polymorphism in the promoter of the uridine diphosphate–glucuronyl transferase 1A1 *(UGT1A1)* gene that underlies Gilbert syndrome, a chronic form of unconjugated hyperbilirubinemia (see Chapter 22), appears to be a major genetic risk factor, increasing the frequency and leading to an earlier age of onset of gallstones in patients with sickle cell disease.[223]

The genetic factors that lead to cholelithiasis have not yet been defined in children. Polymorphisms in genes encoding the biliary cholesterol transporter ATP-binding cassette G5/G8 and the phospholipid transporter *(ABCB4)* have been limited to gallstone disease in adults (see Chapter 67). The nuclear receptor subfamily 1, group H, member 4 *(NR1H4)* gene, which encodes the nuclear bile salt receptor farnesoid X receptor, is another candidate gene for cholesterol gallstone susceptibility. Low phospholipid–associated cholelithiasis occurs in association with *ABCB4* mutations (multidrug resistance 3 deficiency) and low biliary phospholipid concentrations that lead to symptomatic and recurring cholelithiasis. Patients may show intrahepatic lithiasis, sludge, or microlithiasis along the biliary tract.[224]

Obstructive jaundice in infants can also be caused by brown pigment cholelithiasis.[225,226] Brown pigment stones are composed of varying proportions of calcium bilirubinate, calcium phosphate, calcium palmitate, cholesterol, and organic material. Unconjugated bilirubin accounts for a large percentage of the total bile biliary pigments. In several cases, bile has had high β-glucuronidase activity and on culture has grown an abundant population of several bacteria. Pigment gallstones are postulated to have formed spontaneously in these infants who had bacterial infections of the biliary tract.

Patients who have no identifiable cause of cholelithiasis are more likely to be female, older, and obese; have a family history of gallbladder disease; and have a greater likelihood of adult-like symptoms. Gallstones were detected in 10 of 493 obese children (2%; 8 girls, 2 boys).[227] Cholesterol gallstones predominate in these patients. Insights into the pathogenesis of gallstones have been gained through careful studies of Pima Indians, who have an extraordinarily high prevalence of cholesterol gallstones. Highly saturated bile has not been detected among Pima Indians younger than age 13 years, but bile saturation increases significantly in both sexes during pubertal growth and development.[228] In this population, the sex-related difference in the size of the bile acid pool begins during puberty; young men show a significant rise in the size of the bile acid pool with age, whereas young women show only a slight rise. Because cholesterol gallstones are associated with smaller bile acid pools, the divergence in bile acid pool size between the two sexes also may account for the sex-related difference in the frequency of gallstones that begins during adolescence.

Prolonged use of high-dose ceftriaxone, a third-generation cephalosporin, has been associated with the formation of calcium-ceftriaxone salt precipitates in the gallbladder. The process, also called *biliary pseudolithiasis*, is observed in 30%–40% of children treated with the drug for severe infections.[229] Patients may complain of abdominal pain and exhibit signs of intrahepatic cholestasis. Biliary sludge and gallbladder precipitates are found on US. The problem generally resolves spontaneously with discontinuation of the drug.

Clinical Features

Most gallstones are found in the gallbladder. Children have a lower incidence of bile duct stones than adults. Most patients are asymptomatic; the gallstones are discovered either incidentally during investigation of another problem or during screening because the patient has a condition associated with a high risk of cholelithiasis.[213] Patients may complain of intermittent abdominal pain of variable severity; the pain may be localized to the RUQ in older children but is generally poorly localized in infants. The physical examination findings are usually unremarkable. Tenderness in the RUQ suggests cholecystitis, as occurs when a stone migrates to the neck of the gallbladder and obstructs the cystic duct. Infants may exhibit irritability, cholestatic jaundice, and acholic stools.[213]

Liver biochemical test results are usually normal.[213] Plain films of the abdomen may reveal calculi, depending on the calcium content of the stone. Cholesterol stones are radiolucent and, therefore, are not visible on an abdominal radiograph US is considered the most sensitive and specific imaging technique for demonstrating gallstones. Hepatobiliary scintigraphy is a valuable adjunct; failure to visualize the gallbladder provides evidence of acute cholecystitis (see later).

Treatment

Cholecystectomy remains the treatment of choice in patients who have symptoms or a nonfunctioning gallbladder.[213] Laparoscopic cholecystectomy is done frequently in children and infants as young as 10 months.[230] Operative cholangiography and exploration of the bile duct may be indicated on the basis of clinical imaging and operative findings. If choledocholithiasis is demonstrated prior to laparoscopic cholecystectomy in the older child and adolescent, then endoscopic sphincterotomy and stone extraction may be done first.

In asymptomatic patients without biochemical abnormalities ("silent gallstones"), management poses a more difficult problem. Epidemiologic studies and radiocarbon dating of gallstones in adults indicate a lag time of more than a decade between initial formation of a stone and development of symptoms.[231] In patients who have underlying disorders such as hemolysis or ileal disease, cholecystectomy may be carried out at the same time as another surgical procedure. To prevent the potential complications of cholecystitis and choledocholithiasis, elective laparoscopic cholecystectomy has become the norm in children with chronic hemolytic anemias and asymptomatic cholelithiasis.[232] In cases associated with hepatic disease, severe obesity, or CF, the surgical risk of cholecystectomy may be substantial, and clinical judgment must be applied. In these cases, the patient should be counseled about the nature of the disease and the symptoms that may develop. Spontaneous resolution of cholelithiasis and even bile duct stones has been reported in infants. In a study with ultrasonographic follow-up, resolution of gallstones occurred in 16.5% of symptomatic children and in 34.1% of infants.[216] Because recurrence of lithiasis is rare in infants, cholecystectomy may not be required; however, patients with obstructive cholestasis are at risk of sepsis and cholangitis and should undergo surgery.[213]

Biliary microlithiasis and associated clinical symptoms may occur in children. Biliary imaging studies are typically normal. EUS may demonstrate microlithiasis of the gallbladder. Laparoscopic cholecystectomy is usually curative.[233]

Little experience with alternative therapies for gallstones (e.g., medical dissolution with oral bile acid administration, shock-wave lithotripsy) has been reported in children. UDCA therapy is of no value in treating the predominantly pigment stones found in this age group but may be of value in patients with multidrug resistance 3 deficiency.[224] UDCA failed to dissolve radiolucent gallstones in 10 children with CF.[234]

Calculous Cholecystitis

Cholelithiasis may be associated with acute or chronic inflammation of the gallbladder (see Chapter 67).[210,211,213] Acute cholecystitis is often precipitated by the impaction of a stone in the cystic duct. A progressive increase in pressure in the gallbladder secondary to fluid accumulation, the presence of stones, and the chemical irritant effects of bile acids can lead to progressive inflammation, congestion, and vascular compromise. Infarction, gangrene, and perforation can occur. Proliferation of bacteria within the obstructed gallbladder lumen can contribute to the process and lead to biliary sepsis.

Chronic calculous cholecystitis is more common than acute cholecystitis. It may develop insidiously or after several attacks of acute cholecystitis. The gallbladder epithelium commonly becomes ulcerated and scarred.

Clinical Features

The acute onset of RUQ pain is a constant feature of acute cholecystitis.[235] The pain may be poorly localized in infants. Nausea and vomiting are frequent. Children have a higher frequency of jaundice (50%) than do adults. The patient may appear acutely ill with shallow respirations and may be febrile, particularly if bacterial infection is superimposed. Guarding of the abdomen is common, and palpation usually elicits RUQ tenderness; Murphy's sign may be present.

The onset of chronic cholecystitis is usually more indolent. The clinical course may be marked by recurrent episodes of upper abdominal discomfort. Older patients may experience intolerance to fatty foods. Episodes of RUQ pain may develop in 64% of children with cholelithiasis and no cystic or bile duct obstruction and is most likely due to chronic cholecystitis. Physical examination may yield negative findings or disclose local tenderness over the gallbladder and a positive Murphy's sign.

In acute cholecystitis, the white blood cell count is often elevated, with a predominance of polymorphonuclear leukocytes.[213] Serum bilirubin and alkaline phosphatase levels may be increased. Serum aminotransferase levels may be normal, but high elevations, suggestive of hepatocellular disease, can occur early with acute obstruction of the bile duct.

In patients with chronic cholecystitis, results of a complete blood count and liver biochemical tests are usually normal. In patients with an acute or chronic presentation, a plain film of the abdomen may demonstrate calcifications in the RUQ.[213] Abdominal US is extremely useful in detecting stones in the gallbladder, may show thickening of the gallbladder wall, and may demonstrate the dilatation of the biliary tract secondary to obstruction of the bile duct by a stone that has migrated from the gallbladder. MRCP may demonstrate similar findings but usually requires general anesthesia in infants and young children.[236] Hepatobiliary scintigraphy is rarely necessary in the acutely ill patient but may be of value in demonstrating a malfunctioning gallbladder in patients with chronic cholecystitis.

Treatment

The acutely ill patient should be treated with intravenous fluids, analgesics, and broad-spectrum antibiotics. Cholecystectomy should be performed as soon as fluid deficits are corrected and infection is controlled.[237] High-risk acutely ill patients may benefit from percutaneous drainage via a transhepatic cholecystostomy; surgical results are excellent (see Chapter 68). Care should be taken to exclude bile duct stones by operative cholangiography and, if necessary, exploration of the duct. Laparoscopic bile duct exploration for choledocholithiasis can be safely performed in children at the time of cholecystectomy and can clear all bile duct stones in most patients.[238]

Cholecystectomy is also the treatment of choice for patients with chronic calculous cholecystitis. Laparoscopic cholecystectomy is the preferred approach for most patients.[239,240]

Acalculous Cholecystitis

Acalculous cholecystitis is an acute inflammation of the gallbladder without gallstones (see Chapter 69).[241] The disorder is uncommon in children but has been associated with infection or severe systemic illness, resulting from dysfunction or hypokinesis of gallbladder emptying.

Pathogens have included streptococci (groups A and B); *Leptospira interrogans*; Gram-negative organisms such as *Salmonella* and *Shigella* species and *Escherichia coli*; and parasitic infestations with *Ascaris* species or *Giardia lamblia* and can be early manifestation of COVID-19 infection. The disorder may occur rarely in infections with HAV or HEV. In immunocompromised patients, pathogens such as *Isospora belli*, CMV, *Cryptosporidium*, *Aspergillus*, and *Candida* species should be considered.[242] Acalculous cholecystitis may follow abdominal trauma and has been observed in patients with systemic vasculitis, including polyarteritis nodosa, systemic lupus erythematosus, Henoch-Schönlein purpura, Churg-Strauss vasculitis, and Kawasaki disease; however, in these conditions, gallbladder distention without inflammation also may occur. Congenital narrowing or inflammation of the cystic duct or external compression by enlarged lymph nodes has been associated with the disorder in children.

The pathogenesis of acalculous cholecystitis is multifactorial. Biliary stasis and localized ischemia damage the gallbladder mucosa and may lead to gallbladder gangrene, empyema, and perforation.

Clinical features of acute acalculous cholecystitis include RUQ or epigastric pain, nausea, vomiting, fever, and occasionally jaundice.[243] RUQ guarding and tenderness are present; a tender gallbladder is sometimes palpable. The findings may be less apparent in infants or critically ill patients, because the presentation may be obscured by the underlying illness.

Laboratory evaluation may reveal elevated serum levels of alkaline phosphatase and conjugated bilirubin. Leukocytosis may occur. US discloses an enlarged, thick-walled gallbladder that may be distended with sludge but contains no calculi.[243] Pericholecystic fluid and intramural air may also be seen.

Some children may present with chronic symptoms of RUQ pain and nausea or vomiting.[241] The WBC count and results of liver biochemical tests are usually normal. Most patients demonstrate abnormal gallbladder function on radionuclide hepatobiliary scanning. These patients generally have chronic inflammation in the gallbladder and require cholecystectomy.

Many patients with acalculous cholecystitis respond to nonoperative management with nasogastric suction, intravenous fluids, and antibiotics with resolution of clinical and imaging finding. Cholecystectomy will be required in cases associated with increasing gallbladder wall thickening and distension and with persistence of the nonshadowing echogenic materials or sludge in the gallbladder and of pericholecystic fluid.[241,243] The diagnosis is confirmed at laparotomy. The gallbladder is usually inflamed, and cultures of bile may yield positive results for the offending bacteria or contain parasites. The gallbladder may become gangrenous. Percutaneous cholecystostomy drainage may be an alternative approach in critically ill patients except in cases of gallbladder perforation or gangrene.

Acute Hydrops of the Gallbladder

Acute noncalculous, noninflammatory distention of the gallbladder may be observed in infants and children.[244,245] The gallbladder is not acutely inflamed, and cultures of the bile are usually sterile. The absence of gallbladder inflammation and generally benign prognosis distinguish acute hydrops from acute acalculous cholecystitis. There may be a generalized mesenteric adenitis of lymph nodes near the cystic duct without mechanical compression. A temporal relationship to other infections, including scarlet fever and leptospirosis, has been observed in some cases.[246] Acute hydrops has been associated with Kawasaki disease and Henoch-Schönlein purpura.[247] Similar to acalculous cholecystitis, the disorder can occur in children on prolonged parenteral nutrition. In some cases, a cause is not identified.

Acute hydrops is associated with the acute onset of cramping abdominal pain, and often nausea and vomiting.[247] Fever and jaundice may be present. The RUQ is usually tender, and the distended gallbladder may be palpable.

Liver biochemical test levels may be mildly elevated. The WBC count may be elevated. Some of these changes can be due to associated disorders such as scarlet fever or Kawasaki disease. US reveals an enlarged, distended gallbladder without calculi.

The diagnosis of acute hydrops is confirmed in many patients at laparotomy.[247] Cholecystectomy obviously is required if the gallbladder appears gangrenous. Pathologic examination of the gallbladder wall usually shows edema and mild inflammation. Bile cultures are usually sterile. These benign findings have led some surgeons to treat acute hydrops by a simple cholecystostomy instead of a cholecystectomy,[247] but treatment of gallbladder hydrops is frequently nonsurgical, with a focus on supportive care and management of the intercurrent illness. In most patients, particularly in children on total parenteral nutrition in whom enteral feeding has been initiated, the process subsides spontaneously. US has been useful in establishing the diagnosis and following the spontaneous resolution of gallbladder distention. The prognosis is excellent. Gallbladder function can be expected to return to normal in most cases.[247]

Gallbladder Dyskinesia

Gallbladder, or biliary dyskinesia is recognized as a cause of chronic abdominal pain in children.[249] The diagnosis is suggested by the presence of postprandial abdominal pain, the absence of cholelithiasis, and an abnormal ejection fraction on cholecystokinin-stimulated hepatobiliary scintigraphy. In a recent multicenter study involving 16 institutions and 678 patients, right upper quadrant pain was reported in 76.7% and postprandial pain in 71.4% of pediatric patients with a diagnosis of biliary dyskinesia.[250] Gallbladder ejection fractions of less than 35%–50% have sometimes been considered abnormal and an indication for surgery (see Chapters 65 and 69). However, there is no consensus regarding diagnostic criteria for biliary dyskinesia in children, and symptoms often overlap with functional dyspepsia.[249]

Gallbladder dyskinesia was the most common indication for surgery in 62 (58%) of 107 children who underwent cholecystectomy in one experience.[250] In another published report of 51 children who underwent laparoscopic cholecystectomy for gallbladder dyskinesia after exclusion of more common GI disorders, 27 of 38 (71%) patients available for follow up experienced complete relief of symptoms.[251] Pain relief after cholecystectomy has been variable in several reports.[248] In the previously cited large multicenter study persistent symptoms were seen in 48.5% of patients but with significant variability between centers.[250] The presence of nausea, upper abdominal pain, and a gallbladder ejection fraction of less than 15% most reliably predicted benefit from cholecystectomy (positive predictive value of 93%). Histologic evidence of chronic cholecystitis was found in only 10 of 27 (41%) children with complete relief of symptoms and was not an independent predictor of a successful outcome. The presence of chronic inflammation in these patients suggests they may have had an acalculous cholecystitis rather than gallbladder dysmotility.

Full references for this chapter can be found at https://ebooks.health.elsevier.com.

65

65 Biliary Tract Motor Function and Dysfunction

Amy E. Hosmer, B. Joseph Elmunzer

IN THIS CHAPTER

ANATOMY AND PHYSIOLOGY

The gallbladder is a distensible pear-shaped reservoir, the function of which is to store bile and deliver it to the duodenum for digestion (see Chapter 64). It is located along the undersurface of the liver and composed of 3 regions: the fundus, body, and neck. Gallbladder filling and emptying occur in both the interdigestive and postprandial periods. Emptying of bile into the duodenum in response to the presence of food in the upper GI tract is regulated primarily by cholecystokinin (CCK).

The sphincter of Oddi (SO) is composed of layers of smooth muscle that are embedded in, but functionally separate from, the muscle of the duodenal wall and that serve as a 4–10-mm high-pressure zone (see also Chapter 64). The SO comprises three parts: a small segment (sphincter ampullae) that covers the common channel formed by the union of the bile and pancreatic ducts (when a common channel is present); a second small portion (sphincter pancreaticus) that surrounds the beginning of the main pancreatic duct; and the largest portion (sphincter choledochus) that covers the distal bile duct (Fig. 65.1). In addition, the fasciculi longitudinales are muscle bundles that span intervals between the bile and pancreatic ducts. The SO functions primarily as a resistor, with tonic contraction that limits bile flow during the interdigestive period. It also serves as a pump, with phasic contractions that facilitate the flow of bile into the duodenum, perhaps serving a housekeeping function for the distal bile duct. The SO participates in the migrating motor complex, with motilin-induced increases in the frequency and amplitude of sphincter contractions shortly before and during bursts of intense duodenal contractions.

The complex neurohormonal control of biliary motility involves sympathetic, parasympathetic, spinal, and enteric nerves.[1] Almost every neurotransmitter in the enteric nervous system has been identified in the biliary tract. Reflex pathways between the gallbladder and SO coordinate the flow of bile.[2]

DYSFUNCTIONAL GALLBLADDER DISORDER

Although acalculous gallbladder pain has been attributed to dysmotility, the correlation is far from perfect. Gallbladder stasis clearly predisposes to sludge and stone formation, but whether gallbladder dysfunction (or dyskinesia)—delayed emptying of the gallbladder in the absence of stones or sludge—causes biliary symptoms remains unclear. Based on a single small randomized controlled trial (RCT) and several observational studies, delayed gallbladder emptying has been reported to predict pain relief after cholecystectomy[3–6]; however, this finding remains controversial.[7,8] Delayed gallbladder emptying occurs in normal asymptomatic persons and is even more common in patients with other disorders of gut-brain interaction (DGBI; formerly functional GI disorders).[9–11] It also appears to be associated with many unrelated diseases such as obesity and diabetes mellitus. Additionally, gallbladder hyperkinesia—markedly increased ejection fraction—has been implicated as a cause of biliary pain that responds to cholecystectomy and also merits further study.[12] There may be a correlation between dysmotility and gallbladder inflammation, which is present in many resected acalculous specimens, but the confirmation of a gallbladder source of symptoms based on histologic diagnosis of chronic cholecystitis has been disputed.[13]

A meta-analysis of 9 studies[7] and a systematic review of 23 studies[8] concluded that existing evidence does not support gallbladder ejection fraction as a predictor of symptom relief after cholecystectomy (see Chapter 69). Other smaller meta-analyses, however, have demonstrated a statistically significant benefit associated with cholecystectomy in symptomatic patients with gallbladder dysfunction.[14–16] Despite the controversial nature of this diagnosis, gallbladder dysfunction is the primary indication

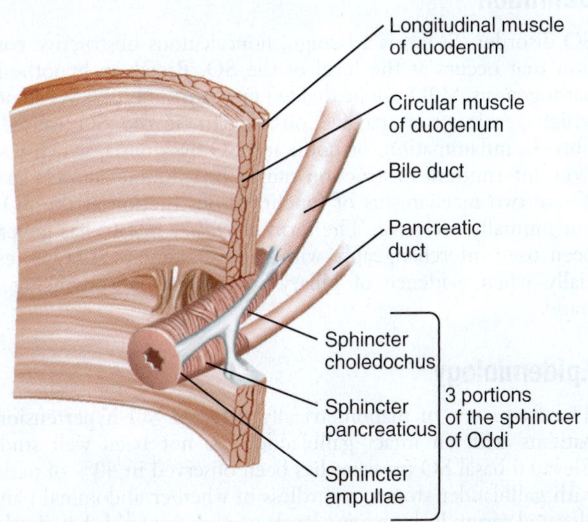

Fig. 65.1 Anatomy of the sphincter of Oddi. Note the three portions of the sphincter of Oddi: the sphincter ampullae (surrounding the short common channel), the sphincter pancreaticus, and the sphincter choledochus (the largest portion).

for cholecystectomy in up to 20% of adults and 50% of pediatric patients in the United States.[17,18] Indeed, cholecystectomy for acalculous biliary pain is 3.5 times more frequent in the United States than in other developed countries, suggesting that it is overused.[19]

Patients who experience typical biliary pain but have no evidence of gallstones on transcutaneous US should undergo endoscopic ultrasonography (EUS) to look for microlithiasis and sludge. If the result of EUS is negative, but the clinical history is classic for biliary-type abdominal pain, no further evaluation is needed, because many patients with biliary pain, no stones on US, and normal gallbladder motility experience symptomatic improvement after cholecystectomy.[20] If the pain history is atypical, the patient is likely to have a more classic DGBI, and surgery should not be offered. If the clinical history is neither classic nor atypical, then gallbladder emptying may be assessed with scintigraphic imaging during intravenous infusion of CCK, although, as mentioned earlier, the ability of this test to predict response to cholecystectomy remains highly controversial.

A multidisciplinary consensus panel unanimously agreed that a large, multicenter RCT comparing surgery with conservative management in patients with typical biliary pain, a normal gallbladder ultrasound result, and abnormal CCK cholescintigraphy is necessary.[21] Although the most natural role for this test may be in the evaluation of patients with neither classic nor atypical symptoms, the panel recommended that if CCK cholescintigraphy is considered, it should be reserved for patients with typical biliary pain (i.e., those meeting Rome IV Consensus Committee criteria [see Chapters 13, 15, 23, and 69]) who are not experiencing symptoms or hospitalized at the time of the test. Indeed, a prospective study of 93 subjects with a low gallbladder ejection fraction showed that patients with typical biliary pain had a substantially higher likelihood of responding to cholecystectomy than those with atypical symptoms (odds ratio 22.3, $P < .001$).[22] Conversely, some studies have demonstrated spontaneous symptom improvement without cholecystectomy in patients with atypical symptoms.[23] The panel also recommended against making clinical decisions based solely on the provocation of pain by CCK infusion.[21]

SPHINCTER OF ODDI DISORDERS

Definition

SO disorder (SOD) is a benign, noncalculous obstructive condition that occurs at the level of the SO. Based on hypothesized pathogenesis, SOD can be divided into two subtypes: SO stenosis, which results from passive obstruction at the SO caused by fibrosis, inflammation, or both; and SO dyskinesia, which results from intermittent obstruction caused by sphincter muscle spasm. These two mechanisms of functional obstruction at the SO are not mutually exclusive. The term *ampullary stenosis* has generally been used interchangeably with the SO stenosis subtype, especially when evidence of biliary obstruction is convincing and static.

Epidemiology

The frequency of manometrically detected SO hypertension in patients with an intact gallbladder has not been well studied. Elevated basal SO pressure has been observed in 40% of patients with gallbladder stones, regardless of whether abdominal pain or elevated serum liver enzyme levels were present.[24] It has also been reported that 70% of 81 patients with biliary-type pain and an intact gallbladder, but no gallstones, had delayed gallbladder emptying, SOD, or both.[25] By contrast, a basal SO pressure elevation of greater than 30 mm Hg was not found in 50 asymptomatic volunteers without gallstones.[26]

TABLE 65.1 Clinical Associations With SOD

Probable	Biliary-type pain after cholecystectomy
	Biliary-type pain in a patient with an intact gallbladder
Possible	After LT
	After RYGB
	AIDS-associated viral and protozoal infections
	Chronic pancreatitis
	Hyperlipidemia
	Idiopathic recurrent acute pancreatitis
	Opium use

The frequency of SO hypertension in postcholecystectomy patients with persistent or recurrent biliary-type pain has been better studied but depends on the criteria for patient selection. Pain resembling preoperative biliary pain occurs in 10%–20% of postcholecystectomy patients.[27] The most common explanation for this pain is that the preoperative symptoms were not caused by gallbladder disease. The most likely diagnosis in this group of patients is another DGBI such as IBS or functional dyspepsia. SOD has been reported in 9%–14% of patients evaluated for postcholecystectomy pain.[28] When other causes of postcholecystectomy pain have been excluded and SO manometry (SOM) has been performed in a more carefully screened group, the frequency of SOD has been reported to be 30%–60%.[29]

Clinical Features

SOD is most commonly implicated in acalculous biliary-type pain in patients with or without a gallbladder and in recurrent idiopathic (unexplained) pancreatitis. SOD generally occurs spontaneously but has also been described with increased frequency in patients who have undergone liver transplantation,[30] have acquired immunodeficiency syndrome,[31] are chronic opium users,[32] have hyperlipidemia,[33] and perhaps after Roux-en-Y gastric bypass[34,35] (Table 65.1).

Although biliary SOD has been diagnosed in all age groups, it is most common in middle-aged women. The female preponderance varies from 75% to 90%. The pain is typical of biliary pain; it is severe and occurs in the epigastrium or the RUQ and may radiate to the back or right shoulder blade. The pain is generally episodic, lasts more than 30 minutes, and occurs at least once a year.[36] The Rome Consensus Committee has proposed diagnostic criteria for SO disorder, based predominantly on expert opinion (https://theromefoundation.org/rome-iv/rome-iv-criteria/).[37] Although these criteria may be helpful in selecting patients who are most likely to benefit from intervention, they require prospective validation.

Because endoscopic retrograde cholangiopancreatography (ERCP) remains the only reliable diagnostic and therapeutic intervention for SOD and brings with it substantial risks, defining the clinical characteristics that reliably predict the presence of SOD and the response to sphincter ablation is of paramount importance. Limited data suggest that patients are more likely to respond if their pain is intermittent, accompanied by nausea and vomiting, and absent for at least 1 year after cholecystectomy.[38] Transient elevations of serum aminotransferase levels during attacks of pain support the diagnosis of SOD.[39] A poor response to sphincterotomy (see later) has been associated with delayed gastric emptying, daily opioid use, and age less than 40 years.[40] These predictors, however, have not been rigorously validated and, with the exception of elevated liver biochemical test levels, do not appear to play a clear role in clinical practice. An ongoing multicenter prospective cohort study (The RESPOnD Study) aims to rigorously characterize patients with suspected SOD who undergo ERCP with the ultimate objective of defining clinical and procedural characteristics associated with response to therapy.

Classification

Patients with suspected biliary SOD have historically been classified into three categories based on diagnostic criteria, which have undergone modification, known as the Milwaukee classification system. This system was embraced in clinical practice because of its perceived ability to predict the outcome of biliary sphincter ablation.

According to the modified Milwaukee classification system, type I SOD is diagnosed in patients with biliary-type pain, serum liver enzyme (aminotransferase or alkaline phosphatase) elevations [more than 1.1 times the upper limit of normal (ULN)], and bile duct dilatation to a diameter greater than 9 mm. Type II SOD is defined as biliary-type pain and either elevated liver enzyme levels or a dilated bile duct. Type III SOD is defined as biliary-type pain without any of the other objective abnormalities. This classification system does not require that the liver enzyme elevations correlate with attacks of pain, although such an association may be a predictor of response to treatment.[39]

A similar classification system for possible pancreatic SOD has been proposed (see later).[41] Patients with pancreatic SOD type I have pancreatic-type pain, a serum amylase or lipase level of at least 1.1× the ULN on one occasion, and pancreatic duct dilatation (>6 mm in the head and >5 mm in the body); those with pancreatic SOD type II have pain and one of the other two criteria; and those with pancreatic SOD type III have pancreatic-type pain only. However, no evidence exists to support this classification system, and a diagnosis of pancreatic SOD is nowadays generally only considered in the setting of unexplained recurrent pancreatitis.

The diagnosis and classification of SOD in clinical practice will likely be impacted by novel data providing more precise estimates of the normal range for pancreaticobiliary duct size.[42] A large population-based study of healthy asymptomatic individuals undergoing abdominal MRI determined that the age-dependent upper reference limit of bile duct diameter is 8 mm in persons <65 years and 11 mm in those ≥65 years; this ULN increases to 13 and 14 mm after cholecystectomy in the 2 age groups, respectively. The pancreatic duct upper reference diameter is 3 mm in individuals <65 years and 4 mm in those ≥65 years. Approximately 20% of healthy volunteers in this analysis would have been considered to have abnormal ductal dilation according to the conventional reference standard. Although the effect of this new reference range on predicting response to sphincterotomy will require prospective validation, the findings of this study may have significant implications for the diagnosis and classification of SOD and consequently in selecting patients for ERCP. For example, according to the new reference standard, a 68-year-old patient with abdominal pain and a prior cholecystectomy with bile duct diameter of 10 mm would not meet diagnostic criteria for SOD, although this patient would have been classified as type 2 SOD in the past.

A landmark multicenter RCT published in 2014 (the EPISOD trial) and its long-term follow-up analysis published in 2018 demonstrate no medium- or long-term benefit associated with ERCP and sphincterotomy in patients with suspected type III SOD.[43,44] On the basis of this study as well as the overall evidence, the traditional classification of SOD subtypes has been abondoned.[45] In particular, type III SOD has been eliminated because it does not represent a sphincter disorder. Abnormal small bowel interdigestive motor activity[46] and duodenal visceral hyperalgesia in response to duodenal (but not rectal) distention[47] in this group of patients suggests the presence of a different DGBI, which should be managed as such.

Under the new paradigm, the term *biliary SOD* is applied to all patients with biliary-type pain and at least transient evidence of biliary obstruction. Most of these patients experience intermittent *SO spasm* as the underlying physiologic abnormality; however, some, with a chronically dilated duct, may have a concurrent element of sphincter stenosis. A subgroup of patients with static elevation of liver enzyme levels and a dilated bile duct are considered to have a mechanical obstruction or tonic contraction at the level of the SO, and the term *SO stenosis (or ampullary stenosis) is applied.* This new framework better represents our current state of understanding but requires clarification regarding the overlap between SO stenosis and spasm.

Diagnosis

Noninvasive Tests

Evaluation of patients in whom SOD is suspected is initiated with liver biochemical testing, serum amylase and lipase measurements, and often abdominal imaging with either abdominal US, CT, or magnetic resonance cholangiopancreatography (MRCP). Physical examination findings are usually normal, although mild RUQ or epigastric tenderness may be present. Standard evaluation, including routine endoscopic and imaging studies and therapeutic trials for more common causes of abdominal pain, such as GERD, NAFLD, and IBS, has usually been undertaken as well.

Noninvasive diagnostic tests for SOD include biliary scintigraphy; fatty meal, CCK, or secretin-stimulated US; secretin-stimulated MRI; and secretin-stimulated EUS. The performance characteristics of these tests have largely been validated by SOM, which has been recognized increasingly as an inadequate gold standard (see later),[43,48] thereby limiting their applicability to clinical practice.

Biliary scintigraphy can be used to assess the flow of bile into the duodenum and has been proposed as a safe screening test before SOM.[49] Although scintigraphy findings are usually positive in patients with dilated bile ducts and high-grade biliary obstruction, the modality lacks sufficient sensitivity in patients with lower-grade or intermittent obstruction of the SO.[50] After a lipid-rich (fatty) meal or intravenous administration of CCK, the bile duct may dilate under pressure if the SO is dysfunctional, and this change can be detected on transcutaneous US. Compared with SOM in postcholecystectomy patients, fatty meal US has a sensitivity of 21% and a specificity of 97% for SOD.[51] Similarly, after stimulation by intravenously administered secretin, the pancreatic duct may dilate, and this test, therefore, can be used to assess pancreatic sphincter dysfunction (see later). Compared with SOM, secretin-stimulated US testing has a sensitivity of 88% and a specificity of 82% for SOD in patients with recurrent acute pancreatitis.[52]

Secretin-stimulated magnetic resonance pancreatography has also been used to assess pancreatic outflow obstruction in patients with idiopathic acute recurrent pancreatitis. Preliminary reports have shown high specificity but low sensitivity rates compared with SOM.[53,54] Similarly, in one study, secretin-stimulated EUS showed limited sensitivity in the evaluation of patients with recurrent pancreatitis and manometrically proved SOD.[55]

Therefore noninvasive diagnostic tests for SOD lack sufficient accuracy to drive clinical decision-making and do not yet play a clear role in the diagnostic algorithm for this condition.

Invasive Tests

ERCP remains the gold standard for the diagnosis and treatment of SOD, although patients in whom this diagnosis is suspected have the highest rates of procedural complications. Such patients have a threefold increase in the risk of post-ERCP pancreatitis, with absolute rates exceeding 25% if prophylactic interventions are not implemented.[56] Although the prophylactic placement of a temporary pancreatic stent and administration of an NSAID rectally reduce the risk of post-ERCP pancreatitis,[57–59] substantial morbidity and occasional mortality still occur in patients who undergo ERCP for SOD. Therefore ERCP should be reserved for persons who have severe or debilitating symptoms in whom the risk-benefit ratio is most favorable. Although alternative biliary imaging methods, such as MRCP and EUS, are safer than ERCP for excluding stones, tumors, and pancreas divisum, they cannot diagnose (or be used to treat) SOD. Occasionally, an intraampullary neoplasm may mimic SOD. If there appears to be excess tissue in the ampulla after endoscopic sphincterotomy, biopsy specimens of the area should be obtained.[60]

Sphincter of Oddi Manometry

SOM had traditionally been considered the gold standard for the diagnosis of SOD based primarily on small RCTs in patients with type 2 biliary SOD in whom manometric findings correlated strongly with response to sphincterotomy.[61,62] However, based on more recent evidence, the diagnostic value of SOM has been increasingly questioned, and as a result, SOM has largely been abandoned in clinical practice.[63] Some uncontrolled studies have suggested that more easily measurable criteria, such as elevated liver enzyme levels and biliary dilatation, are superior in predicting a response to sphincter ablation.[64] Other studies have suggested that manometry is highly specific for diagnosing SOD but may lack sensitivity; lack of sensitivity may account for the 42% symptom response rate to sphincterotomy in patients with biliary SOD type II and normal manometric results. The lack of sensitivity may also explain the relatively low rate of abnormal SOM results (65%–85%) in patients with type I biliary SOD, in whom the response rate to sphincterotomy is greater than 90%.[65] Another possible explanation for the insensitivity of SOM is that short-term observation of sphincter pressure may not detect intermittent spasm that is not occurring at the time of the procedure. Two studies have shown that a second SOM may be abnormal in 40%–60% of persistently symptomatic patients with an initially normal SOM result.[66,67] Manometry was not reproducible or predictive of any outcome in the aforementioned EPISOD trial.[43,48] Some practitioners still use SOM for diagnosing traditional type II SOD or pancreatic SOD (see later) or for assessing the presence of residual sphincter muscle in patients with recurrent symptoms after a prior sphincterotomy, although the evidence base to support this practice remains weak.

Other ERCP-Based Diagnostic Interventions

Placement of a pancreatic or biliary stent on a trial basis to predict a response to subsequent sphincterotomy and injection of botulinum toxin into the SO has been proposed as alternative methods of diagnosing SOD.[68,69] Although preliminary data have suggested utility of diagnostic stent placement, the need for multiple procedures, with their attendant risks, and the risk of stent-induced pancreatic ductal damage limit their widespread application. Botulinum toxin injection into the SO was shown in an exploratory prospective study to reduce the incidence of clinically significant postoperative fistula after distal pancreatectomy, implicating sphincter hypertension in the pathogenesis of this important complication and suggesting that temporary paralysis of the SO can have a favorable therapeutic effect.[70,71] Whether this observation can be inferred to the diagnosis and treatment of SOD requires further study. Additional research is necessary to define the role of these approaches, if any, in the diagnostic algorithm for SOD.

Treatment

Medical Therapy

Dietary and medical therapy for suspected or documented SOD has undergone minimal study. Some providers recommend a low-fat diet to reduce pancreaticobiliary stimulation, although no data are available to substantiate this approach. Nifedipine, nitrates, octreotide, antispasmodics, phosphodiesterase type 5 inhibitors, transcutaneous nerve stimulation, and electroacupuncture have been shown to lower basal SO pressure, although consistent clinical outcomes data are lacking. Two short-term, placebo-controlled crossover studies showed that 75% of patients with suspected or documented SOD experienced statistically less pain with use of oral nifedipine.[72,73] A subsequent study, however, demonstrated that slow-release nifedipine provided no clinical benefit but increased cardiovascular side effects compared with placebo.[74] A prospective study of nitrates in SOD published in abstract form revealed reduction in pain, but therapy was also limited by side effects.[75] Another prospective study demonstrated that the combination of trimebutine (an antispasmodic) and nitrates (sublingual or transdermal) improved pain associated with SOD at rates comparable with that for sphincter ablation.[76] Additional studies are clearly necessary to establish the role of pharmacotherapy for SOD; however, in light of the benign nature of SOD, medical therapy should be considered in all patients with less severe manifestations of SOD before sphincter ablation is offered. A trial of antispasmodics, low-dose tricyclic antidepressants (to reduce visceral hypersensitivity), and other neuromodulators should be attempted in such patients. Patients with biliary SOD and more severe pain are less likely to respond to medical therapy and can be considered for an initial trial of endoscopic therapy.

Sphincterotomy

The most common scenario in which the diagnosis of SOD is considered is biliary-type pain in a postcholecystectomy patient. When SOM is performed in this patient population and the findings are abnormal, abdominal pain is relieved after sphincterotomy in 90%–95% of patients with traditional type I biliary SOD and 85% of those with traditional type II SOD. When the SOM result is normal, pain relief after sphincterotomy still occurs in 90%–95% of patients with type I biliary SOD. Because SOM findings may be misleading in these cases (they are normal in 14%–35% of patients), SOM is not clinically indicated for patients with type I biliary SOD. Rather, endoscopic sphincterotomy should be performed empirically.

Pain relief after sphincterotomy occurs in 35%–42% of patients with type II biliary SOD and normal SOM results. Although this response rate is similar to that in sham-treated controls, a true clinical response likely occurs in a few patients. Therefore although sphincterotomy is indicated in patients with type II SOD and abnormal SOM findings, whether SOM is truly required to justify sphincterotomy in this group has been increasingly challenged. Based on the aforementioned data pertaining to the performance characteristics of SOM, most authorities now advocate empirical biliary sphincterotomy in patients with traditional type II SOD. This strategy has the advantage of providing therapy to those patients with a normal SOM result who respond to sphincterotomy, but this advantage comes at the expense of potential additional procedure-related complications, such as bleeding and perforation. A decision analysis model revealed that a strategy of empirical sphincterotomy by an experienced biliary endoscopist in patients meeting criteria for type II SOD is cost-effective compared with an SOM-driven strategy.[77]

The treatment of patients with former type III SOD has always been controversial. Many therapeutic endoscopists have traditionally avoided ERCP with manometry in this patient population because of the perceived unfavorable risk-benefit ratio. The findings of the EPISOD trial affirmed the sentiment that ERCP has no role in the management of patients with post-cholecystectomy pain and no objective findings. Long-term follow-up of enrolled patients confirmed findings of the original trial—that sphincterotomy is no more successful than sham intervention at 5 years.[44] As a result, trends in the utilization of sphincterotomy are changing substantially. A recent study utilizing a large electronic health record–based dataset demonstrated that despite an increase in the incidence rate of SOD from 2010 to 2019, not only was SOM infrequently utilized, but a parallel reduction in rates of biliary sphincterotomy was observed (34.3% −24.5%).[78] As the highly anticipated RESPOnD Study (see earlier) looks to estimate the benefit of ERCP with sphincterotomy when performed for SOD, baseline characteristics of those enrolled are also changing. The RESPOnD cohort suggests that ERCP and sphincterotomy are more frequently reserved for those with dilated bile ducts or liver biochemical abnormalities.[79]

Few studies have addressed SOD in patients with biliary-type pain, an intact gallbladder, and no gallstones. Whether cholecystectomy is pathophysiologically responsible for the development of SOD or whether patients with SOD are simply more likely to have undergone cholecystectomy because of the nature of their symptoms, is unclear. Cholecystectomy has been postulated to unmask preexisting subclinical SOD by removing the reservoir that serves to decompress the extrahepatic biliary system during SO spasm.[80] Further, nerves that travel from the gallbladder to the SO via the cystic duct are severed during cholecystectomy, potentially leading to altered SO motility.[81] Limited data, however, suggest that SOD may occur in patients with an intact gallbladder. A small case series of patients with documented SO hypertension and an intact gallbladder who were treated with sphincterotomy demonstrated that 43% had long-term pain relief; some additional patients eventually improved following cholecystectomy.[82]

FAILURE OF RESPONSE TO BILIARY SPHINCTEROTOMY

Possible explanations for a lack of response to biliary sphincterotomy in patients with SOD are listed in Box 65.1. The most likely explanation is that the pain was not of pancreaticobiliary origin but was caused instead by altered intestinal motility or visceral hypersensitivity.[47] Alternatively, the biliary sphincterotomy may have been inadequate, or restenosis may have occurred.[83]

Patients who experience recurrent symptoms reminiscent of their original SOD pain following a period of significant relief after sphincterotomy may benefit from repeat ERCP to determine whether the sphincter is adequately ablated and to exclude restenosis, although the initial response in some of these patients was likely due to the sham (placebo) effect.[84] The role of residual pancreatic sphincter hypertension as a source of continuing pain in the absence of pancreatic abnormalities is dubious. Some experts advocate initial dual sphincterotomies to prevent this problem, although the reintervention rate for persistent or recurrent pain has not been different from that for historical controls in whom a single sphincterotomy (of one duct) was performed.[85]

Finally, some patients in whom SOD is suspected and who have shown no response to biliary sphincterotomy may have "minimal-change" chronic pancreatitis. EUS may demonstrate parenchymal and ductal changes associated with chronic pancreatitis in these patients (see Chapter 61).[86]

BOX 65.1 Possible Causes for Failure to Achieve Pain Relief After Biliary Sphincterotomy in Patients With Presumed SOD

- Nonpancreaticobiliary pain, especially another disorder of gut-brain interaction
- Inadequate initial sphincterotomy
- Occurrence of restenosis
- Minimal change chronic pancreatitis

SPHINCTER OF ODDI DYSFUNCTION IN PANCREATITIS

Idiopathic Recurrent Acute Pancreatitis

Impaired flow through the SO can result in transient or sustained elevation of pancreatic duct pressure, leading to parenchymal inflammation and subsequent injury. Although pancreatic duct obstruction due to a stone or tumor can cause acute pancreatitis, whether SO stenosis or spasm can serve as the obstructive process in a first attack of idiopathic pancreatitis is unknown. For repeated episodes of pancreatitis, it is possible that the index episode of idiopathic pancreatitis leads to sphincter fibrosis and/or inflammation that induces or contributes to subsequent attacks. Regardless of whether it was truly the inciting cause, SO hypertension has been identified in 31%–78% of patients with idiopathic recurrent acute pancreatitis (IRAP).[41,87,88]

ERCP is commonly offered at referral centers for the evaluation and treatment of patients with IRAP that is unexplained despite standard evaluation and EUS and/or MRCP. Observational data suggest that ERCP-based interventions may eliminate or reduce future attacks of pancreatitis in 50%–60% of patients.[87,89,90] This benefit, however, has not been rigorously proved and must be weighed against the significant risks of the procedure. A single attack of unexplained pancreatitis, or even two attacks separated by several years, is not sufficient to warrant ERCP, because many patients will not have further episodes.[88]

Patients referred for endoscopic therapy, however, generally experience crippling symptoms and are desperate and eager to undergo ERCP. Given the vulnerable nature of this patient population and the costs and risks of the intervention, a methodologically rigorous RCT of ERCP versus sham endoscopy (EUS) for IRAP is much needed to guide clinical decision-making.

When ERCP is performed in patients with IRAP, the technical approach to the procedure varies among experts and is based on weak evidence. Strategies have traditionally included dual biliary and pancreatic manometry (followed by selective sphincterotomy), empirical biliary sphincterotomy and pancreatic manometry, or empiric dual sphincterotomy (given the diagnostically equivocal nature of manometry). A randomized trial suggested that biliary sphincterotomy alone (which also reduces pancreatic duct pressure by ablating the common sphincter) yields results equivalent to those for dual sphincterotomy in patients with abnormal pancreatic manometry.[87] Although this study was underpowered, its findings are appealing because pancreatic sphincterotomy carries a higher risk of acute and long-term complications, including papillary restenosis (which can occasionally lead to a course that is worse than the original problem). Therefore many endoscopists have adjusted their practices toward empirical biliary sphincterotomy alone at the time of the index ERCP and reserve pancreatic endotherapy for an inadequate response to biliary therapy. Clearly, additional research is necessary, and any randomized trial of ERCP for IRAP should compare biliary and dual sphincterotomy.

EUS should be performed before considering the diagnosis of pancreatic SOD in the 10%–30% of acute pancreatitis cases that remain unexplained despite initial evaluation to assess for anatomic abnormalities in the pancreaticobiliary system that may predispose to or cause acute pancreatic inflammation, such as occult stones or sludge in the gallbladder or bile duct, an unrecognized pancreatic or ampullary neoplasm, a pancreatic ductal abnormality (pancreas divisum, anomalous pancreaticobiliary union), or chronic pancreatitis. In aggregate, existing studies suggest that EUS may uncover a definitive or potential etiology of IRAP in 30%–80% of patients with a previously negative workup, depending in part on how many attacks the patient has experienced and whether the gallbladder is present.[91,92]

For the patient with an intact gallbladder and frequent episodes of unexplained pancreatitis, options include biliary sphincterotomy or empirical cholecystectomy, with the implication that microlithiasis is the likely cause (see Chapters 60 and 67).[93] Given the accuracy of EUS for excluding microlithiasis, however, biliary sphincterotomy has been favored because it addresses both SOD and biliary crystal disease that may be undetected by EUS.

Chronic Pancreatitis

SOD has been described in 40%–87% of patients with chronic pancreatitis.[94] Whether SOD is the result of chronic inflammation or independently plays a role in the pathogenesis of chronic pancreatitis is not known. Uncontrolled studies suggest that endoscopic pancreatic sphincterotomy improves pain in approximately 50% of patients with chronic pancreatitis and documented pancreatic hypertension.[95,96] In the absence of solid evidence, however, whether ERCP should be offered to patients with chronic pancreatitis and recurrent episodes of acute inflammation or with chronic pain alone, or not at all, remains to be determined. In some cases, pancreatic sphincterotomy must be performed to facilitate other therapeutic maneuvers, such as pancreatic ductal stone extraction and stricture dilation. Overall, the role of SOD in chronic pancreatitis remains limited.

Full references for this chapter can be found at https://ebooks.health.elsevier.com.

66 Bile Formation and Bile Acid Cycling in Health and Disease

Peter Fickert, Paul A. Dawson

IN THIS CHAPTER

Bile formation is essential for intestinal lipid digestion and absorption, cholesterol homeostasis, and hepatic excretion of lipid-soluble xenobiotics, drug metabolites, and heavy metals.[1] The process of bile formation depends on hepatic synthesis and canalicular secretion of bile acids, the predominant organic anions in bile, and maintenance of hepatic bile formation is essential for normal liver function. Bile acids also undergo an efficient enterohepatic circulation, with most of the bile acids in bile having previously transited the small intestine and been returned to the liver for secretion by hepatocytes. As a result, alterations in the synthesis, biliary secretion, intestinal absorption, or gut microbial metabolism of bile acids have profound effects on bile formation and hepatic and gastrointestinal physiology. Identification of the enzymes, transporters, regulatory factors, and mechanisms responsible for the biosynthesis, metabolism, and enterohepatic cycling of bile acids has advanced our understanding of genetic and acquired disorders of bile formation and secretion.[2] In addition, the recognition that bile acids act as hormones that signal via nuclear and G-protein-coupled receptors has provided new insights into the pathogenesis of and potential treatments for bile acid–related disorders. This chapter reviews the current knowledge of bile acids and their function, synthesis, secretion, and cycling. Available bile acid–based therapies are also discussed.

Bile is a complex, lipid-rich micellar solution that is isosmotic with plasma and composed primarily of water, inorganic electrolytes, and organic solutes such as bile acids, phospholipids [mostly phosphatidylcholine (PC)], cholesterol, and bile pigments (Table 66.1). Bile also contains extracellular vesicles, which carry hepatocyte- or cholangiocyte-derived proteins, lipids, and RNA molecules.[3] The relative proportion of the major organic solutes in bile is illustrated in Fig. 66.1. The volume of hepatic bile secreted is estimated to range from 500 to 600 mL/day, and bile acids are the most abundant organic components. In healthy humans, active canalicular bile acid secretion is efficient and remarkably concentrative; the intracellular monomeric concentration of bile acids is estimated to be in the low micromolar range in the hepatocyte and more than 1000 µmol/L in canalicular bile. After canalicular secretion, bile acids travel down the biliary tract and are stored and concentrated in the gallbladder. In response to a meal, the gallbladder contracts and empties its contents into the duodenum. The bile acids then travel down the length of the small intestine, where they facilitate the digestion and absorption of fats, activate intestinal receptors, stimulate the production of gut hormones, and interact with the gut microbiome. Bile acids undergo passive absorption down the length of the small intestine and colon and are actively absorbed in the terminal ileum. Bile acids are then returned to the liver in the portal circulation, transported across the hepatocyte sinusoidal membrane, and resecreted across the canalicular membrane into bile.[4]

The physiologic functions of bile acids in the liver and GI tract are multiple. (1) Bile acids induce bile flow and hepatic secretion of biliary lipids (phospholipid and cholesterol). The vectorial movement of bile acids from blood into bile concentrates bile acids in the canalicular network and promotes ductular water secretion as a major determinant of bile flow.[1,5] (2) Bile acids facilitate the digestion of dietary fats and are essential for the intestinal absorption of cholesterol and fat-soluble vitamins. They also aid intestinal absorption by solubilizing dietary lipids and lipid digestion products as mixed micelles to promote their aqueous diffusion and delivery to the intestinal mucosa. Fat-soluble vitamins (A, D, E, and K) are poorly absorbed in the absence of bile acid micelles, and disturbances in the synthesis, hepatic secretion, or cycling of bile acids lead to fat-soluble vitamin deficiency. Along with their major role in dietary lipid absorption, bile acids may also facilitate intestinal assimilation of protein by accelerating protein denaturation and its subsequent digestion by pancreatic proteases. (3) Bile acids play an integral role in maintaining cholesterol homeostasis. Bile acids are essential for the absorption of biliary and dietary cholesterol from the small intestine. Conversely, bile acids promote cholesterol

TABLE 66.1 Composition of Hepatic Bile

Component	Concentration
Electrolytes and Minerals (mmol/L)	
Sodium	140–160
Potassium	3–8
Chloride	70–120
Bicarbonate	20–50
Calcium	1–5
Phosphate	1–2
Metals (μmol/L)	
Magnesium	1–3
Iron	18–52
Copper	12–21
Organic Constituents (mmol/L)	
Bile acids	5–50
Bilirubin (total)	1–2
Phospholipid (lecithin)	0.5–20.0
Cholesterol	0.5–1.0
Glutathione	3–5
Glucose	0.2–1.0
Urea	2.2–6.5
Protein (g/dL)	0.2–3.0

Values obtained from measurements of human bile are drawn from Albers CJ, Huizenga JR, Krom RA, et al. Composition of human hepatic bile. *Ann Clin Biochem*. 1985;22:129–32; Keulemans YC, Mok KS, de Wit LT, et al. Hepatic bile versus gallbladder bile: a comparison of protein and lipid concentration and composition in cholesterol gallstone patients. *Hepatology*. 1998;28:11–16; Ho KJ. Biliary electrolytes and enzymes in patients with and without gallstones. *Dig Dis Sci*. 1996;41:2409–2416.

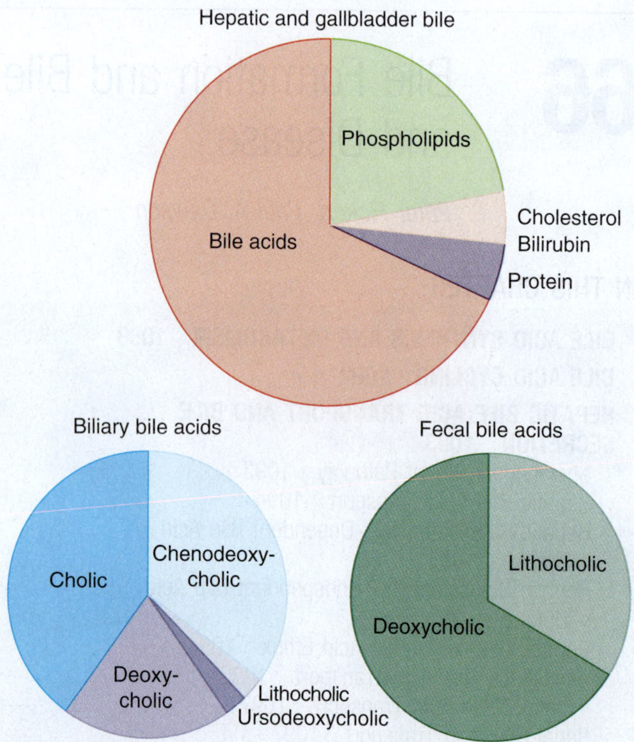

Fig. 66.1 (*Top*) **Typical solute composition of hepatic and gallbladder bile in healthy humans.** Bile acids are the primary solute in bile, constituting approximately 67% of bile. Phospholipids account for approximately 22%, cholesterol 4%, bilirubin 0.3%, and protein 4.5% of bile. Biliary bile acid composition is shown in the *bottom left*. Cholic acid, chenodeoxycholic acid, and deoxycholic acid constitute more than 95% of the biliary bile acids, and virtually all the biliary bile acids are in conjugated form. The proportion of biliary lithocholic acid and UDCA varies but rarely exceeds 5%. The majority of lithocholic acid in bile is present in sulfated form. When administered in therapeutic doses, the proportion of UDCA in bile may rise to as much as 40%. Fecal bile acid composition is shown in the *bottom right*. Fecal bile acids are almost entirely unconjugated because of microbial deconjugating enzymes in the intestine and colon and consist primarily of the dehydroxylated bile acids, deoxycholic acid, and lithocholic acid, and their "iso" and esterified derivatives.

elimination from the body by several different mechanisms. First, cholesterol conversion to bile acids balances fecal bile acid loss, and this accounts for almost half of the cholesterol excreted each day. Second, bile acids facilitate hepatic biliary secretion of cholesterol, thereby promoting its passage into the intestinal lumen for elimination, and function as cholesterol acceptors in the intestinal lumen to promote direct transintestinal cholesterol excretion.[6] (4) Bile acids function to shape the structure of the gut microbiome and in turn are actively metabolized and biotransformed by the gut bacteria. The effects of bile acids on the gut microbiome include direct bile acid bacteriostatic actions and bile acid signaling in the gut to induce production of antimicrobial factors and enhance mucosal barrier integrity, thereby reducing small bowel bacterial translocation and inflammation.[7] Gut microbial metabolism of bile acids significantly alters the physicochemical and signaling properties of the bile acid pool. These gut microbiota-bile acid interactions have been linked to the regulation of host metabolism and immunity as well as host disease complications or progression in pathophysiologic conditions such as metabolic syndrome, MASLD, MetALD, and hepatic cirrhosis.[8–10] (5) Bile acids function as hormones that signal through nuclear and G-protein-coupled receptors to regulate their cycling and metabolism. In addition, bile acid signaling contributes to the regulation of hepatic metabolism, gut motility, and fat, glucose, protein, and energy homeostasis.[11–13] (6) Conjugated bile acids are fully soluble as calcium salts and prevent formation of insoluble calcium precipitates that promote development of gallstones in the biliary tract and gallbladder. Bile acids also protect against development of kidney stones by preventing enteric hyperoxaluria.[14]

BILE ACID SYNTHESIS AND METABOLISM

Bile acids are synthesized from cholesterol in pericentral hepatocytes of the hepatic acini. In this process, cholesterol, a lipophilic compound, is converted into a water-soluble product. In humans, the newly synthesized bile acids are cholic acid (CA), a trihydroxy-bile acid with hydroxy groups at the C-3, C-7, and C-12 positions, and chenodeoxycholic acid (CDCA), a dihydroxy-bile acid with hydroxyl groups at the C-3 and C-7 positions (Fig. 66.2). The newly synthesized bile acids are termed *primary* bile acids to distinguish them from the products of bacterial metabolism, which are termed *secondary* bile acids. The kinetics of bile acid synthesis and turnover in humans is summarized in Table 66.2. Under normal physiologic conditions, hepatic bile acid synthesis ranges from 0.2 to 0.6 g/day but can be induced to

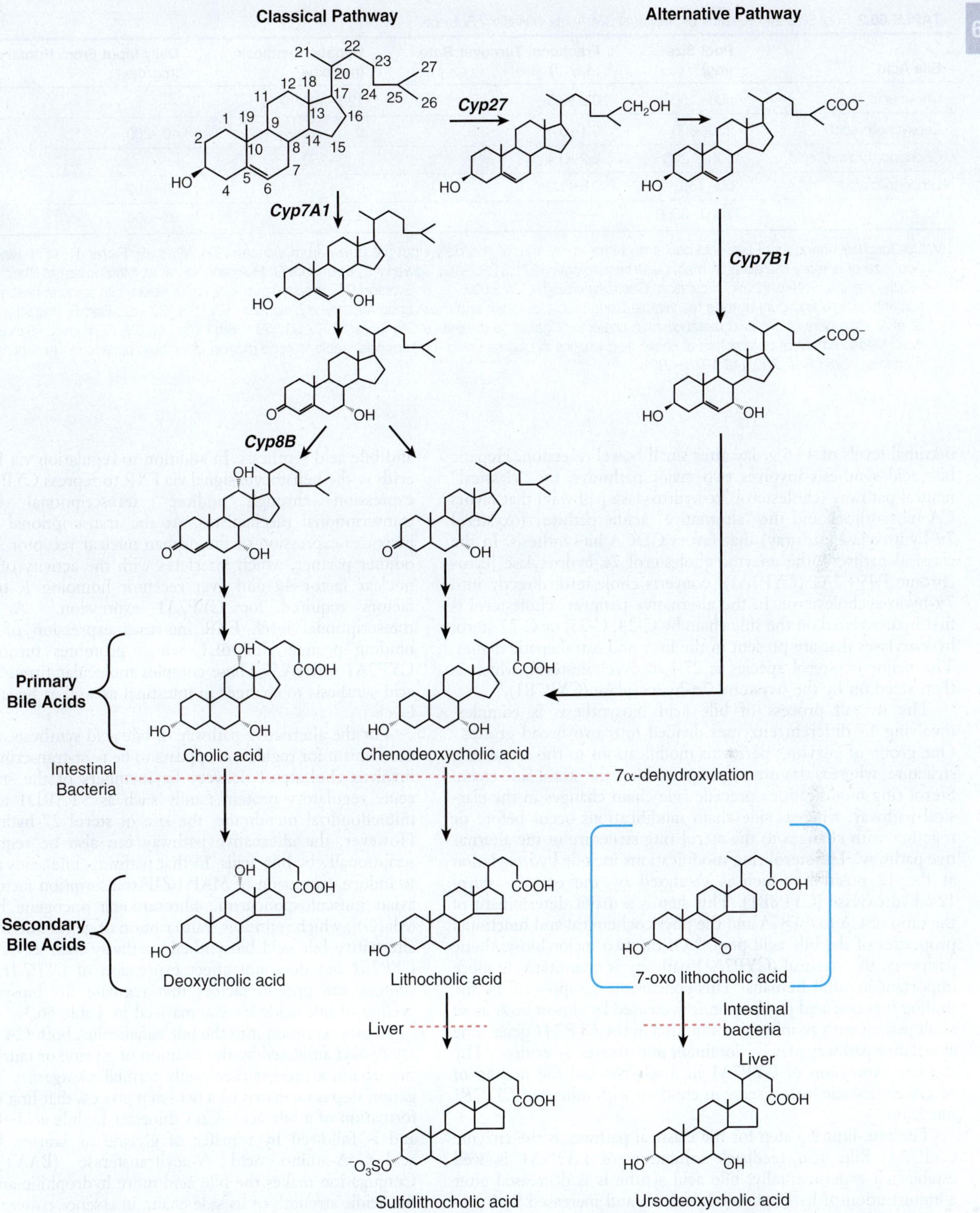

Classical Pathway

Alternative Pathway

21 22 23 27 20 12 18 17 24 25 26 11 13 16 1 19 9 14 15 2 10 8 HO 3 5 7 4 6

Cyp27

CH_2OH

COO^-

Cyp7A1

HO OH

Cyp7B1

COO^-

O OH

HO OH

Cyp8B

Primary Bile Acids

COOH

Cholic acid

Chenodeoxycholic acid

Intestinal Bacteria

7α-dehydroxylation

Secondary Bile Acids

Deoxycholic acid

Lithocholic acid

7-oxo lithocholic acid

Liver

Intestinal bacteria

Liver

O_3SO

Sulfolithocholic acid

Ursodeoxycholic acid

Fig. 66.2 Bile acid synthesis and metabolism. The primary bile acids are synthesized from cholesterol in the liver by 2 major pathways, the "classical" neutral pathway (*CYP7A1/CYP8B1* pathway) that favors cholic acid and the "alternative" acidic (*CYP27A1/CYP7B1*) pathway that favors chenodeoxycholic acid. Secondary metabolism of bile acids includes 7α-dehydroxylation by the intestinal flora, deconjugation by the intestinal flora, epimerization of the 3α- and 7α-hydroxyl groups by the intestinal flora, hepatic reduction of the 7-oxo derivative of chenodeoxycholic acid to 7-oxo lithocholic acid, and hepatic re-epimerization of 3β-hydroxy bile acids. Bile acids are also sulfated primarily at the C-3 position by the liver and kidney. *CYP*, Cytochrome P450; *CYP7A1*, cholesterol 7α-hydroxylase; *CYP7B1*, oxysterol 7α-hydroxylase; *CYP8B1*, sterol 12α-hydroxylase; *CYP27A1*, sterol 27-hydroxylase. (Adapted with permission from Dawson PA. Bile formation and the enterohepatic circulation. In: Johnson LR, Ghishan FK, Kaunitz JD, et al., eds. *Physiology of the Gastrointestinal Tract*. 5th ed. London: Academic Press; 2012:1466.)

TABLE 66.2 Pool Size and Kinetics of Individual Bile Acids in Healthy Subjects

Bile Acid	Pool Size (mg)	Fractional Turnover Rate (day^{-1})	Hepatic Synthesis (mg/day)	Daily Input From Primary Bile Acids (mg/day)
Cholic acid	500–1500	0.2–0.5	120–400	–
Deoxycholic acid	250–800	0.1–0.4	0	40–200
Chenodeoxycholic acid	500–1200	0.2–0.4	100–250	–
Lithocholic acid	50–150	0.8–1.0	0	50–100
Total	1300–3650	–	220–650	90–300

Values for measurements of bile acid pool size, turnover, synthesis, and daily input are drawn from Vlahcevic ZR, Miller JR, Farrar JT, et al. Kinetic and pool size of primary bile acids in man. *Gastroenterology*. 1971;61:85–90; Cowen AE, Korman MG, Hofmann AF, et al. Metabolism of lithocholate in healthy man. II. Enterohepatic circulation. *Gastroenterology*. 1975;69:67–76; Everson GT. Steady-state kinetics of serum bile acids in healthy human subjects: single and dual isotope techniques using stable isotopes and mass spectrometry. *J Lipid Res*. 1987;28:238–52; Berr F, Pratschke E, Fischer S, et al. Disorders of bile acid metabolism in cholesterol gallstone disease. *J Clin Invest*. 1992;90:859–868; Hulzebos CV, Renfurm L, Bandsma RH, et al. Measurement of parameters of cholic acid kinetics in plasma using a microscale stable isotope dilution technique: application to rodents and humans. *J Lipid Res*. 2001;42:1923–1929.

maximal levels of 4–6 g/day after small bowel resection. Hepatic bile acid synthesis involves two major pathways, the "classical" neutral pathway (cholesterol 7α-hydroxylase pathway) that favors CA biosynthesis and the "alternative" acidic pathway (oxysterol 7α-hydroxylase pathway) that favors CDCA biosynthesis. In the classical pathway, the enzyme cholesterol 7α-hydroxylase [cytochrome P450 7A1 (CYP7A1)] converts cholesterol directly into 7α-hydroxycholesterol. In the alternative pathway, cholesterol is first hydroxylated on the side chain by C-24, C-25, or C-27 sterol hydroxylases that are present in the liver and extrahepatic tissues. The major oxysterol species is 27-hydroxycholesterol, which is then acted on by the oxysterol 7α-hydroxylase (CYP7B1).[15]

The overall process of bile acid biosynthesis is complex, involving 17 different enzymes divided into two broad groups.[2] One group of enzymes performs modifications to the sterol ring structure, whereas the other group modifies the sterol side chain. Sterol ring modifications precede side chain changes in the classical pathway, whereas side chain modifications occur before or together with changes to the sterol ring structure in the alternative pathway. The sterol ring modifications include hydroxylation at the 12 position, which is catalyzed by the enzyme sterol 12α-hydroxylase (CYP8B1). This step is a major determinant of the ratio of CA to CDCA and the physicochemical and functional properties of the bile acid pool.[16] Of the two major biosynthetic pathways, the classical (CYP7A1) pathway is quantitatively more important in adult humans. This conclusion is supported by the finding that bile acid production is decreased by almost 90% in an adult patient with an inherited mutation in the *CYP7A1* gene. The alternative pathway may be dominant in neonates, as evidenced by the low expression of CYP7A1 in newborns and the finding of severe cholestatic liver disease in children with inherited *CYP7B1* mutations.

The rate-limiting step for the classical pathway is the enzyme CYP7A1. Bile acid feedback inhibition of CYP7A1 is well established experimentally; bile acid synthesis is decreased after administration of hydrophobic bile acids and increased by interruption of the enterohepatic circulation following ileal resection or administration of bile acid sequestrants.[15] The molecular mechanisms responsible for the negative feedback regulation of the CYP7A1 pathway involve the liver and small intestine and have been elucidated. For the major pathway, bile acids act as ligands for the farnesoid X receptor (FXR) in ileal enterocytes to induce synthesis of an endocrine polypeptide hormone, fibroblast growth factor-19 (FGF19; rodent ortholog is FGF15). FGF19 is secreted into the portal circulation and acts on hepatocytes through its cell surface receptor, a complex of the β-klotho protein and FGF4-receptor (FGFR4), to repress CYP7A1 expression and bile acid synthesis. In addition to regulation via FGF19, bile acids in the hepatocyte signal via FXR to repress CYP7A1 mRNA expression through indirect transcriptional and post-transcriptional mechanisms. At the transcriptional level, FXR increases expression of the orphan nuclear receptor small heterodimer partner, which interferes with the activity of hepatocyte nuclear factor 4α and liver receptor homolog 1, transcription factors required for CYP7A1 expression.[17] At the post-transcriptional level, FXR increases expression of the RNA-binding protein ZFP36L1, which promotes turnover of the CYP7A1 mRNA.[18] These complex molecular titrations link bile acid synthesis to changes in intestinal as well as hepatic bile acid levels.

For the alternative pathway of bile acid synthesis, the primary mechanism for regulation appears to be post-transcriptional. This involves cholesterol delivery by members of the steroidogenic acute regulatory protein family such as STARD1 to the inner mitochondrial membrane, the site of sterol 27-hydroxylation.[19] However, the alternative pathway can also be regulated transcriptionally by bile acids. In that pathway, bile acids act via FXR to induce expression of MAP bZIP transcription factor G [v-maf avian musculoaponeurotic fibrosarcoma oncogene homolog G (MafG)], which represses transcription of genes important for the alternative bile acid biosynthetic pathway such as *CYP27A1* and *CYP7B1* but does not affect expression of *CYP7A1*.[20] The receptors and protein factors that regulate the biosynthesis and cycling of bile acids are summarized in Table 66.3.

Before secretion into the bile canaliculus, both CA and CDCA are *N*-acyl amidated by the addition of glycine or taurine on their side chain, a process commonly termed *conjugation*. This conjugation step is mediated by a two-step process that first involves the formation of a bile acid–CoA thioester by bile acid–CoA ligases and is followed by transfer of glycine or taurine by the bile acid–CoA-amino acid *N*-acyltransferase (BAAT) enzyme. Conjugation makes the bile acid more hydrophilic and increases the acidic strength of its side chain, in essence converting a weak acid ($pK_a \approx 5.0$ for the unconjugated bile acid) to a strong acid ($pK_a \approx 3.9$ for the glycine conjugate; $pK_a \approx 2.0$ for the taurine conjugate). A major function of conjugation to glycine or taurine is to decrease the passive diffusion of bile acids across cell membranes during their transit in the enterohepatic circulation. As a result, efficient uptake and export of conjugated bile acids requires the presence of specific membrane carriers. Compared with unconjugated bile acids, conjugated bile acids are also more soluble at acidic pH and more resistant to precipitation in the presence of high concentrations of calcium. The net effect of conjugation is to maintain high intraluminal concentrations of bile acids in the

TABLE 66.3 Genes Involved in the Regulation of Bile Acid Synthesis and Cycling

Protein (*Gene*)	Description and Function
CAR (*NR1I3*)	Xenobiotic-activated nuclear receptor involved in detoxification of secondary bile acids
FGF19 (*FGF19*)	Protein growth factor; secreted by ileum, liver, and gallbladder in response to bile acids; regulator of hepatic bile acid synthesis via the FGFR4:β-klotho complex
FGFR4 (*FGFR4*)	Membrane receptor; negative feedback regulator of CYP7A1 and hepatic bile acid synthesis
FXR (*NR1H4*)	Bile acid–activated nuclear receptor; regulation of bile acid synthesis, transport, and metabolism
HNF4α (*NR2A1*)	Nuclear receptor; positive regulator of CYP7a1 expression and hepatic bile acid synthesis
β-Klotho (*KLB*)	Membrane coreceptor protein associated with FGFR4; confers liver specificity to FGFR4–FGF19 pathway; negative feedback regulator of CYP7A1 and hepatic bile acid synthesis
LRH-1 (*NR5A2*)	Nuclear receptor; positive regulator of CYP7a1 expression and hepatic bile acid synthesis
MafG (*MAFG*)	Transcription factor; negative regulator of bile acid synthesis and transport
MALRD1	Intestinal protein involved in ileal enterocyte secretion of FGF19
PXR (*NR1I2*)	Bile acid and xenobiotic-activated nuclear receptor involved in detoxification of secondary bile acids
SHP (*NR0B2*)	Nuclear receptor; negative feedback regulation of hepatic bile acid synthesis by antagonizing HNF4α and LRH-1; regulation of bile acid transport and metabolism
STAR (*STARD1*)	Intracellular cholesterol transfer protein; mediates cholesterol trafficking to the inner mitochondrial membrane for bile acid synthesis via the alternative pathway
TGR5 (*GPBAR1*)	Bile acid–activated G-protein-coupled receptor; mediates the systemic actions of bile acids; regulates intestinal motility, metabolism
VDR (*NR1I1*)	Vitamin D and bile acid–activated nuclear receptor; involved in detoxification of LCA
ZFP36L1 (*ZFP36L1*)	RNA-binding protein; negative regulator of CYP7a1 expression and hepatic bile acid synthesis

CAR, Constitutive androstane receptor; *FGF19*, fibroblast growth factor-19; *FGFR4*, fibroblast growth factor receptor 4; *FXR*, farnesoid X-receptor; *HNF4α*, hepatocyte nuclear factor 4 alpha; *LCA*, lithocholic acid; *LRH-1*, liver receptor homolog 1; *MafG*, MAF bZIP transcription factor G (v-maf avian musculoaponeurotic fibrosarcoma oncogene homolog G); *MALRD1*, MAM and LDL Receptor Class A Domain containing 1; *PXR*, pregnane X-receptor; *SHP*, small heterodimer partner; *STAR*, steroidogenic acute regulatory protein; *TGR5*, Takeda G-protein-coupled receptor; *VDR*, vitamin D receptor; *ZFP36L1*, zinc finger protein 36-like 1.

biliary tract, gallbladder, and small intestine to facilitate lipid solubilization, digestion, and absorption. The physiologic significance of this bile acid modification is illustrated by the finding that patients with inherited defects in bile acid conjugation present with fat-soluble vitamin malabsorption and steatorrhea and respond favorably to therapeutic administration of conjugated bile acids.[21,22]

Metabolism of bile acids by the gut microbiota begins in the small intestine and continues in the colon. Although most of the conjugated bile acids secreted into the small intestine are efficiently absorbed intact, gut bacteria-derived bile salt hydrolases will remove the glycine or taurine group from ≈15% of the bile acids in the small intestine. These deconjugated bile acids can be passively absorbed in the small intestine and returned to the liver, where they are reconjugated to glycine or taurine and resecreted into bile along with newly synthesized bile acids. This process of intestinal deconjugation and hepatic reconjugation is a normal part of bile acid metabolism. A fraction of the circulating bile acid pool escapes absorption from the small intestine and passes into the colon, where deconjugation continues almost to completion and additional gut microbial metabolism occurs. Those gut microbial reactions include bile acid dehydroxylation, epimerization of the hydroxyl groups to form "iso" bile acids, oxidation and reduction to form "allo" bile acids, secondary side chain conjugation to leucine, tyrosine, phenylalanine, or other amino acids, and esterification to fatty acids. Among the most important of those biotransformations is removal the hydroxyl group at the C-7 position (7α-dehydroxylation), thereby converting CA to deoxycholic acid (DCA), a dihydroxy bile acid with hydroxyl groups at the C-3 and C-12 positions, and converting CDCA to lithocholic acid (LCA), a monohydroxy bile acid with a hydroxyl group at position C-3 (see Fig. 66.2).[23] Although other gut microbiome-catalyzed bile acid modifications such as deconjugation, epimerization, oxidation, and secondary amino acid conjugation can be reversed by host enzymes, bile acids are not rehydroxylated at the C-7 position in humans.[24] Therefore this bacterial reaction is particularly important for shaping the composition and properties of the bile acid pool. Microbial epimerization of bile acid α-hydroxyl groups generates their corresponding β-hydroxy derivatives ("iso" bile acids), such as isolithocholic acid and isodeoxycholic acid, which are present in cecal or colonic contents.[25,26] The 7α-hydroxy group of CDCA is also epimerized by the gut microbiota to form the 3α,7β-dihydroxy bile acid UDCA. After being absorbed from the intestine, UDCA is conjugated to glycine or taurine in the liver and circulates as a minor component, normally less than 5%, of the bile acid pool. However, UDCA is also administered therapeutically for forms of cholestatic liver disease such as primary biliary cholangitis and becomes a major component of the bile acid pool in those patients (see Chapter 93).[27,28]

The colon absorbs about 50% of the DCA as well as a portion of the LCA formed. After returning to the liver, DCA is reconjugated to glycine or taurine and circulates with the primary bile acids, whereas LCA is reconjugated and sulfated.[29] Hepatic reconjugation of bile acids returning from the intestine is extremely efficient, so virtually all the endogenous bile acids (primarily CA, CDCA, DCA, and UDCA) secreted into bile are in conjugated form. Bacterial deconjugation and dehydroxylation of bile acids in the colon is also efficient, so the feces contain primarily unconjugated secondary bile acids and only small amounts (<15%) of other bile acid species (see Fig. 66.1).

Several pathways exist for host metabolism of secondary bile acids, including hepatic re-epimerization of β-hydroxy iso-bile acids, hepatic reduction of 7-oxo-lithocholate to form CDCA or UDCA, and hydroxylation, glucuronidation, or sulfation of bile acids (see Fig. 66.2).[29] The modification of bile acids by sulfation or glucuronidation blocks their intestinal and renal reabsorption, and these sulfated or glucuronidated species are rapidly lost from the circulating pool of bile acids. Sulfation is particularly significant for metabolism of LCA. Unmodified LCA is intrinsically hepatotoxic, and sulfation of LCA at the 3α-hydroxy position hastens its elimination from the body, thereby playing an important hepatoprotective role.[30] In addition to sulfation or glucuronidation, bile acids can be hydroxylated at other sites on their sterol rings, including the C-1, C-2, C-4, or C-6 positions. Under normal physiologic conditions in adults, these polyhydroxylated bile acids are typically present at only very low levels. However, these unusual bile acid species are present at higher levels in newborns, in patients after bariatric surgery, and in patients with cholestatic liver disease. Expression of the hepatic phase 1 and phase 2 enzymes responsible for hydroxylation and sulfation of bile acids is induced by LCA or agents such as rifampin by a transcriptional mechanism involving the xenobiotic-sensing nuclear receptors pregnane X receptor and constitutive androsterone receptor (see also Chapter 90).

BILE ACID CYCLING

The anatomic components of the bile acid circulation include the liver, biliary tract, gallbladder, small intestine, colon, portal venous circulation, kidney, and systemic circulation (Fig. 66.3). At a fundamental level, the circulation of bile acids can be considered to consist of a series of storage chambers (gallbladder and small intestine), valves (sphincter of Oddi and ileocecal valve), mechanical pumps (hepatic canaliculi, small intestine), and chemical pumps (hepatocyte, cholangiocyte, ileal enterocyte, and renal proximal tubule cell).

Efficient intestinal reabsorption and hepatic extraction of bile acids enable an effective recycling and conservation mechanism that largely restricts bile acids to the intestinal and hepatobiliary compartments. During fasting, bile acids move down the biliary tract and are concentrated approximately 10-fold in the gallbladder, resulting in lower levels of bile acids in the small intestine, portal vein, systemic circulation, and liver. However, basal rates of hepatic bile acid secretion are maintained, and cycling continues for that portion of the bile acid pool that is not sequestered in the gallbladder. In response to a meal, cholecystokinin is released from the intestinal mucosa and acts on the biliary tract to relax the sphincter of Oddi and stimulate gallbladder contraction. A concentrated solution of mixed micelles (bile acids, phospholipids, and cholesterol) in gallbladder bile then passes via the bile duct into the small intestine. In the intestinal lumen, these micelles facilitate fat digestion and absorption by stimulating the action of pancreatic lipase on triglyceride, solubilizing the hydrolytic products such as long-chain saturated fatty acids, and shuttling these hydrophobic lipids across the unstirred water layer to the mucosal surface. During digestion of a large meal, the gallbladder remains contracted, and bile acids secreted by the liver bypass the gallbladder and empty directly into the duodenum. During this period, the intraluminal bile acid concentration in the small intestine is 5–10 mmol/L, well above the threshold concentration of approximately 1.5 mmol/L that is required for micelle formation. During the interdigestive period, the sphincter of Oddi contracts and the gallbladder relaxes, causing a larger fraction of the bile acids secreted into bile to enter the gallbladder for storage. This is controlled in part by bile acids, which act directly by activating the G-protein-coupled receptor

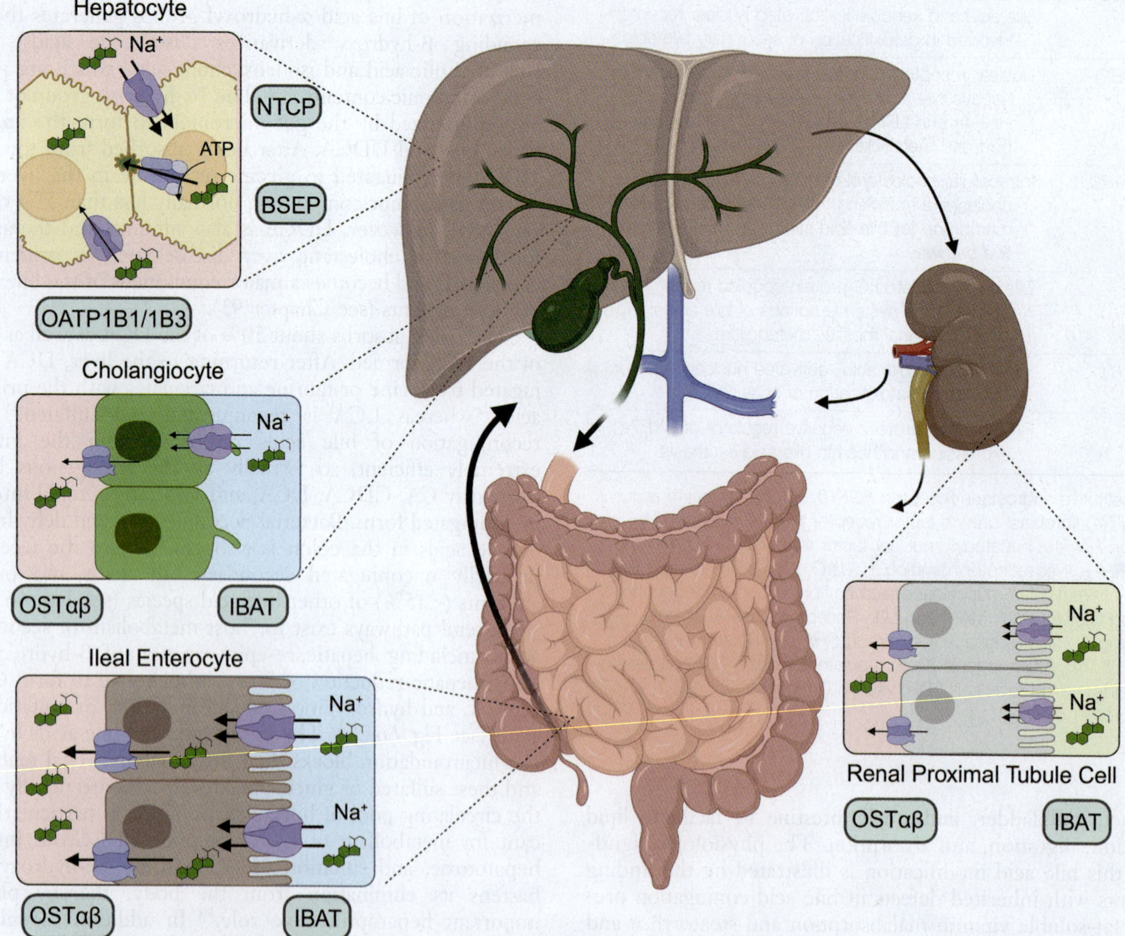

Fig. 66.3 Bile acid circulation showing the individual transport proteins responsible for transport across epithelia of various cells, including hepatocytes, cholangiocytes, ileal enterocytes, and renal proximal tubule cells. *IBAT* (*SLC10A2*), Ileal bile acid transporter; *BSEP* (*ABCB11*), bile salt export pump; *NTCP* (*SLC10A1*), Na+-taurocholate cotransporting polypeptide; *OATP*, organic anion-transporting polypeptide; *OST*, organic solute transporter. (Created with BioRender.com.)

called TGR5 and indirectly by stimulating the ileal synthesis and release of FGF19, a polypeptide hormone that induces gallbladder relaxation.[31] In general, the cycling of bile acids accelerates during digestion and slows between meals and during overnight fasting. This pulsatile rhythm of bile acid secretion is maintained even after cholecystectomy. When the gallbladder is absent, bile acids are stored in the proximal small intestine during fasting, with the intestinal migrating motor complex driving the distal movement of the intraluminal bile acid pool (see Chapter 101). Following ingestion of a meal, small intestinal contractions accelerate and propel the stored bile acids to the distal ileum, where they are actively reabsorbed and carried back to the liver for resecretion into bile.

The cycling of bile acids is extremely efficient; less than 10% of the bile acids secreted into the intestine escape reabsorption and are eliminated in the feces. Bile acids are absorbed by passive absorption down the length of the intestine and colon and by active transport in the terminal ileum. In adult humans, the bile acid circulation maintains a pool size of approximately 2–4 g. The bile acid pool cycles two to three times per meal, and the intestine may reabsorb between 10 and 30 g of bile acid per day. Approximately 0.2–0.6 g of bile acid escapes reabsorption and is eliminated in the stool each day.[32] Hepatic conversion of cholesterol to bile acid balances fecal excretion to maintain the bile acid pool size. The kinetics of bile acid turnover in humans is summarized in Table 66.2.

An active recirculation of bile acids is advantageous because it results in the accumulation of a large mass of detergent molecules that can be used repeatedly during digestion of a single meal or multiple meals throughout the day. The presence of an ileal active transport system and bile acid circulation dissociates hepatic bile acid secretion from de novo bile acid synthesis, thereby improving the efficiency of intestinal nutrient digestion and absorption. Because bile acids induce bile flow, maintenance of the bile acid circulation also promotes continuous secretion of bile. The dissociation of bile acid biosynthesis from intestinal delivery is also aided by the presence of a gallbladder because the availability of a concentrative storage reservoir permits bile acids to be delivered in a controlled fashion at high concentrations to the duodenum. The ileal bile acid transporter (IBAT) and gallbladder are complementary rather than redundant, and they function together to conserve bile acids. In the absence of an active IBAT, the bile acids secreted into the intestine are not efficiently reabsorbed. Emptying of the gallbladder contents would necessarily be followed by a refractory period during which the supply of bile acids is insufficient to promote lipid digestion and absorption. This refractory period would last until hepatic synthesis restores the bile acid pool. Conversely, removal of the gallbladder has few effects on bile acid homeostasis or intestinal fat absorption when active ileal bile acid transport is intact.

HEPATIC BILE ACID TRANSPORT AND BILE SECRETION

Bile formation involves the secretion of inorganic and organic solutes into the canalicular space and biliary tract lumen by hepatocytes and the biliary epithelial cells (cholangiocytes) and was originally studied using metabolically inert markers such as mannitol or erythritol. In the current model, hepatocyte canalicular bile formation is considered a mechano-osmotic process involving significant contributions by both canalicular secretion of osmotically active solutes and bile canaliculi peristalsis. Traditionally, canalicular bile secretion was divided into two components: bile acid–dependent bile flow (bile flow relating to bile acid secretion predominantly by periportal hepatocytes) and bile acid–independent flow (bile flow attributed to active secretion of inorganic electrolytes and other solutes by pericentral hepatocytes), which is thought to account for approximately 60% and 40%, respectively, of spontaneous basal bile flow.[1,33] Hepatic ATP–dependent carriers actively secrete bile acids into the canalicular lumen, where they form aggregates and mixed micelles that are too large to diffuse back across the tight junctions that line the canaliculi. Compounds such as the conjugated bile acids that are actively pumped across the canalicular membrane are termed *primary solutes*. Besides bile acids, primary solutes include glutathione (GSH), conjugated bilirubin, heavy metals, and conjugates of various metabolites and xenobiotics. The ATP-dependent canalicular secretion of GSH and GSH conjugates via the multidrug resistance–associated protein 2 (MRP2) is important at several levels. In addition to being secreted at high concentrations into bile, intraluminal catabolism of GSH by GGTP and dipeptidases raises the solute concentration and contributes to the osmotic driving force for canalicular bile formation. The choleretic activity of each primary solute is defined as the volume of bile flow induced per amount of solute secreted. For natural bile acid species, the choleretic activity ranges from 8 to 40 μL of bile flow induced per micromole of bile acid secreted. Newly secreted hepatic canalicular bile is significantly modified during its transit through the biliary tract via the action of cholangiocytes. The ductular modifications to canalicular bile include (1) the absorption of solutes such as glucose, amino acids, and bile acids; (2) the movement of water through specific channels (aquaporins) and paracellularly; and (3) the secretion of solutes such as bicarbonate and chloride. The ATP-independent secretion of bicarbonate via the HCO_3^-/Cl^- anion exchanger AE2 is particularly important for bile flow. The majority of this HCO_3^- secretion occurs at the level of the bile duct epithelial cells in response to stimulation by biliary constituents such as bile acids, ATP, and a variety of hormones and neuropeptides, such as secretin, vasoactive intestinal peptide, and histamine. The contribution of this ductular secretion to bile formation is considerable and estimated to account for 40% or more of total daily bile secretion in humans. This may be an underestimate since very recent studies using high resolution confocal and intravital microscopy have questioned the contribution of canalicular versus ductular water flow to bile formation. These studies suggested that hepatocellular secretion of bile acids and other solutes drives bile flow by acting at the level the bile duct epithelium rather the canalicular space.[5]

Cholehepatic Shunt Pathway

The term *cholehepatic shunt* was coined by Alan Hofmann to describe the cycle whereby unconjugated dihydroxy bile acids in bile are passively absorbed by cholangiocytes and returned via the venous drainage directly to the hepatocyte for uptake and resecretion into bile. This cycle was proposed to explain the increased bile flow and biliary bicarbonate secretion observed after administration of therapeutic doses of unconjugated C-24 dihydroxy bile acids such as UDCA or unconjugated side chain–shortened C-23 bile acid analogs such as the UDCA analog norucholic acid.[34,35] Although the proposal is conceptually sound and in general agreement with existing data, the intrahepatic location and passive nature of the cholehepatic shunt cycle have made it difficult to study or prove. In addition, because ductal bile normally contains almost all conjugated bile acids under normal physiologic conditions, the contribution of cholehepatic shunting of endogenous biliary bile acids to bile flow was originally thought to be negligible. The subsequent discovery that the biliary epithelium expresses the IBAT (also called the ASBT, apical sodium-dependent bile acid transporter; gene symbol *SLC10A2*) and the organic solute transporter OSTα–OSTβ (gene symbols *SLC51A* and *SLC51B*) offered a potential mechanism for active cholehepatic shunting of conjugated bile acids. However, the physiological role and therapeutic significance of the cholangiocyte bile acid transporters or the cholehepatic shunt pathway in humans still remain elusive.[36] Indeed, the role of IBAT in the biliary epithelium may be to permit cholangiocytes to sample biliary bile acid concentrations to activate cellular signaling pathways and stimulate bicarbonate secretion rather than to reabsorb significant quantities of bile acids from the biliary tract.[36,37]

Hepatic Bile Acid Transport

More than 90% of the bile acids secreted into bile are derived from the recirculating pool. To maintain this process, hepatocytes must transport bile acids efficiently from the portal blood into bile. This vectorial *trans*-hepatocellular movement of bile acids is a concentrative transport process that is driven by a distinct set of primary (ATP-dependent), secondary (Na^+ gradient dependent), and tertiary (OH^-- or HCO_3^--dependent anion exchange) transport systems at the sinusoidal and canalicular plasma membranes. Bile acid flux through the liver and the number of participating hepatocytes vary under physiological conditions. In the fasting state, uptake of bile acids is highest in the periportal hepatocytes (closest to the portal venules), whereas during feeding, more distal hepatocytes in the liver acinus are recruited to participate. Conversely, production and secretion of newly synthesized bile acids is highest in pericentral hepatocytes (closest to the central vein). In this fashion, the periportal hepatocytes transport a larger fraction of the bile acid pool.

The concentration of bile acids in the portal blood of healthy humans is 20–50 μmol/L. Uptake by the liver is typically expressed as fractional extraction, or first-pass extraction, and represents the percentage of bile acids removed during a single passage through the hepatic acinus. The fractional extraction of bile acids from sinusoidal blood ranges from 50% to 90% and remains constant irrespective of systemic bile acid concentrations. The hepatic fractional extraction is related to bile acid structure and albumin binding and is highest (80%–90%) for hydrophilic-conjugated bile acids such as conjugated CA and lowest (50%–60%) for unconjugated hydrophobic protein-bound bile acids such as CDCA. Due to the rapid differential hepatic clearance, the concentration of total bile acids in the systemic circulation is low, averaging 2–5 and 5–15 μmol/L in the fasting and fed states, respectively, and the bile acid composition in the systemic circulation does not strictly mirror that of the other compartments in the body.[38] The major transport proteins that function to maintain the circulation of bile acids have been identified and are shown in Figs. 66.3 and 66.4. The general properties of these carriers are listed in Table 66.4. Because of their importance for bile secretion, the bile acid transporters are highlighted; however, the hepatocyte sinusoidal and canalicular membranes also express specialized transport proteins for a wide spectrum of endogenous and exogenous compounds.[39,40]

Hepatic Sinusoidal Na^+-Dependent Bile Acid Uptake

The uptake of conjugated bile acids at the sinusoidal (basolateral) membrane is predominantly mediated (>80%) by a secondary active Na^+-dependent transport system, which is driven by the basolateral Na^+,K^+-ATPase that maintains the prevailing out-to-in Na^+ gradient. Although important for conjugated bile acids, Na^+-dependent transport accounts for less than half of the uptake of unconjugated bile acids such as CA and UDCA. The major transporter responsible for hepatocytic Na^+-coupled uptake of bile acids is the Na^+-taurocholate cotransporting polypeptide (NTCP; gene symbol *SLC10A1*). Inherited defects in the NTCP gene are associated with greatly elevated (25- to 100-folds) plasma levels of conjugated bile acids in the absence of jaundice, pruritus, or other signs of liver disease.[41,42] In addition to being the major hepatic bile acid uptake transporter, NTCP has been identified as a cell surface receptor on hepatocytes for the binding and entry of HBV and HDV (see Chapters 81 and 83).[43] A naturally occurring variant in NTCP, which converts a serine at position 267 to a phenylalanine (c.800C>T; rs2296651; p.Ser267Phe), leads to nearly complete loss of bile acid transport activity. This variant, which is prevalent in Asian populations (minor allele frequency ranging from 3.1% to 9.2%) has an attenuated ability to support viral entry and is associated with increased resistance to HBV infection.[44] These findings stimulated efforts to design viral entry inhibitors targeting NTCP to block de novo infection or reduce viral load in HDV-infected patients, culminating in the clinical development of bulevirtide for the treatment of chronic hepatitis D in patients with hepatitis B virus and hepatitis D virus coinfection.[45,46]

Hepatic Sinusoidal Na^+-Independent Bile Acid Uptake

In liver, unconjugated bile acids such as CA are taken up predominantly in an Na^+-independent fashion by members of the organic anion-transporting polypeptide (OATP) gene family (gene symbol *SLCO*, in which "SLC" and "O" are designations for solute carrier and OATP, respectively). Unlike the Na^+-cotransporters such as NTCP and IBAT, the molecular transport mechanism and driving force for OATP-mediated solute uptake are not well understood and potentially include facilitative diffusion and electroneutral exchange that couple solute transport to bicarbonate or GSH efflux.[40] Human OATP1B1 (gene symbol *SLCO1B1*; original protein name OATP-C) and OATP1B3 (gene symbol *SLCO1B3*; original protein name OATP8) are expressed primarily in liver and account for the majority of hepatic Na^+-independent bile acid clearance. OATP1B1 and OATP1B3 transport both conjugated and unconjugated bile acids but play only a minor role in hepatocellular clearance of conjugated bile acids as compared to NTCP. However, OATP1B1 and OATP1B3 play an important role in hepatocellular clearance of nonbile acid metabolites, drugs, and xenobiotics. OATP1B1 and OATP1B3 transport a wide variety of organic anions and solutes, including bilirubin glucuronides (see Chapter 22), steroid metabolites (such as estradiol-17β-glucuronide, dehydroepiandrosterone-3-sulfate, and estrone-3-sulfate), arachidonic acid products [such as prostaglandin E_2, thromboxane B_2, and leukotriene C_4, diagnostic dyes {such as bromosulfophthalein and indocyanine green (ICG)}], and drugs (such as rifampin, statins, digoxin, and fexofenadine). Notably, combined loss of *SLCO1B1* and *SLCO1B3*, which are adjacent genes on human chromosome 12, causes Rotor syndrome, a rare and benign hereditary conjugated hyperbilirubinemia distinct from Dubin-Johnson syndrome.[47] Although the plasma clearance of unconjugated bile acids has not been measured in human subjects deficient in OATP1B1/OATP1B3, mice deficient in the orthologous Oatp1a/1b genes show defective hepatic clearance of unconjugated but not conjugated bile acids.[47] Moreover, the loss of OATP1B3 alone is sufficient to delay ICG clearance, thereby yielding an abnormal ICG retention test result in subjects with otherwise normal laboratory values and normal liver biopsy specimens.[48] Inherited polymorphisms in the OATP genes influence drug metabolism and contribute to some forms of drug toxicity.[49]

Hepatic Sinusoidal Bile Acid Efflux

Under cholestatic conditions, unconjugated, conjugated, or modified (sulfated, glucuronidated, and polyhydroxylated) bile acids are effluxed from the hepatocyte interior across the basolateral (sinusoidal) membrane into the space of Disse by the heteromeric organic solute transporter, OSTα-OSTβ, members of the MRP family including MRP3 (gene symbol *ABCC3*) and

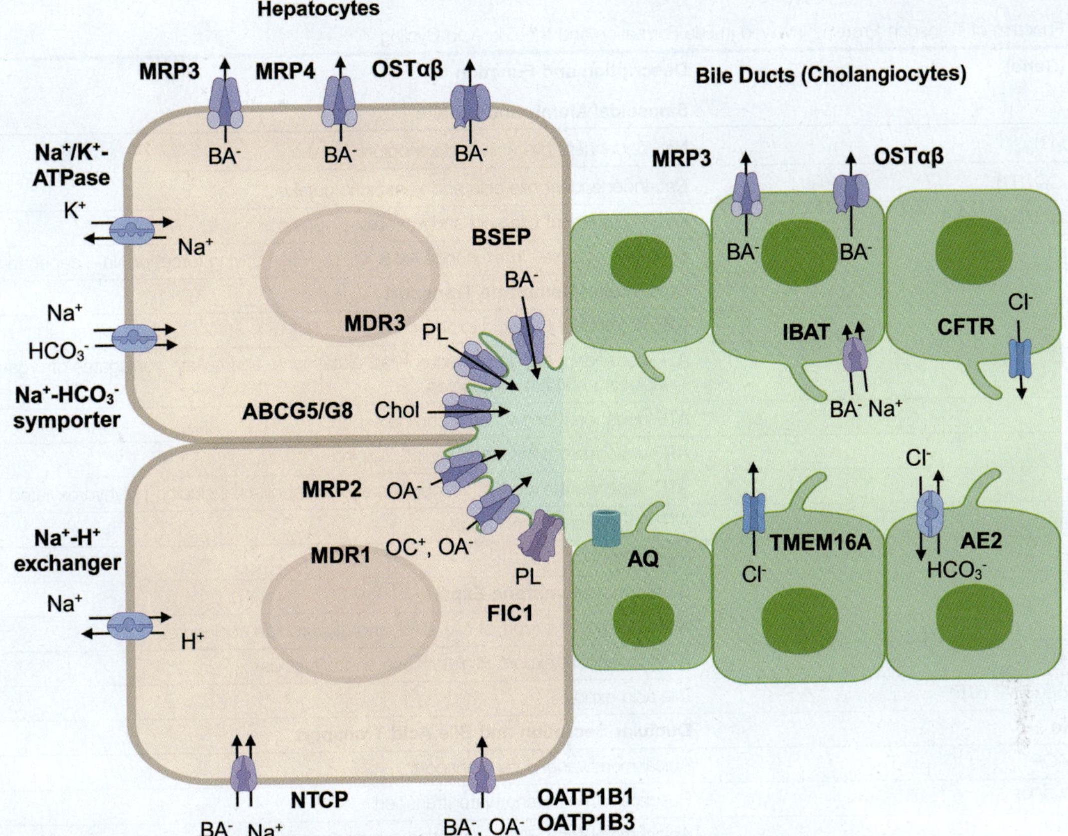

Fig. 66.4 Hepatocyte and cholangiocyte transporters are important for bile acid secretion. At the sinusoidal membrane of hepatocytes, the Na^+-taurocholate cotransporting polypeptide (NTCP; gene symbol *SLC10A1*) mediates the uptake of conjugated bile acids. Sodium-dependent uptake of bile acids through the NTCP is driven by an inwardly directed sodium gradient generated by the Na^+/K^+-ATPase. The Na^+-independent bile acid uptake is mediated by the organic anion-transporting polypeptides OATP1B1 (*SLCO1B1*) and OATP1B3 (*SLCO1B3*). The sinusoidal membrane also contains a sodium-hydrogen exchanger and a sodium-bicarbonate cotransporter (symporter). At the canalicular membrane, bile acids are secreted via the bile salt export pump (*ABCB11*), whereas sulfated and glucuronidated bile acids are secreted via the multidrug resistance–associated protein 2 (MRP2; *ABCC2*). The canalicular membrane also expresses ATP-dependent export pumps that transport phospholipid (multidrug resistance protein 3, MDR3; *ABCB4*), cholesterol and plant sterols (*ABCG5/ABCG8*), and drug metabolites (MDR1; *ABCB1*) into bile. FIC1 (*ATP8B1*) is a P-type ATPase and phospholipid flippase that is mutated in progressive familial intrahepatic cholestasis type 1. Within the cholangiocytes of the large bile ducts, conjugated bile acids are absorbed by the ileal bile acid transporter (IBAT; *SLC10A2*). Bile acid then exits at the basolateral surface into the hepatic arterial circulation via the heteromeric transporter OSTαβ (*SLC51A-SLC51B*) or an ATP-dependent carrier, MRP3 (*ABCC3*). Cholangiocytes also express a variety of other carriers important for modifying bile, including the chloride channels TMEM16 and CFTR, AE2 for secretion of bicarbonate, and numerous aquaporin (*AQ*) isoforms to facilitate water movement. *BA*⁻, bile acid anion; *Chol*, cholesterol; *OA*⁻, organic anion; *OC*⁺, organic cation; *PL*, phospholipid. (Created with Biorender.com.)

MRP4 (gene symbol *ABCC4*), and possibly other carriers. After their efflux, the unconjugated, conjugated, or modified bile acids are carried in sinusoidal blood to more pericentral hepatocytes for reuptake and secretion into bile.[50] This process dynamically recruits additional hepatocytes from the more pericentral zones 2 and 3 within the liver lobule to participate in the clearance and secretion of bile acids into bile, thereby safeguarding vulnerable zone 1 periportal hepatocytes. In addition, the polyhydroxylated, glucuronidated, and sulfated bile acids generated by hepatocyte phase 1 or phase 2 metabolism and effluxed across the sinusoidal membrane can escape hepatic clearance and pass into the systemic circulation, where they are filtered by the kidney and excreted in urine. These hepatoprotective mechanisms, which also include downregulation of the major liver bile acid uptake transporters, are an important part of the adaptive response to conditions of bile acid overload.[51]

Canalicular Bile Acid Transport

Because bile acids are potent detergents, their hepatocellular uptake and export must be carefully balanced to avoid intracellular accumulation and cytotoxicity. Circulating bile acids returning to the liver as well as newly synthesized bile acids are shuttled to the hepatocyte canalicular membrane for secretion into bile by the

TABLE 66.4 Function of Transport Proteins Involved in Bile Formation and the Bile Acid Cycling

Transporter (*Gene*)	Description and Function
Hepatocyte	**Sinusoidal Membrane Uptake**
NTCP (*SLC10A1*)	Na^+-dependent bile acid and xenobiotic uptake
OATP1B1 (*SLCO1B1*)	Na^+-independent bile acid and xenobiotic uptake
OATP1B3 (*SLCO1B3*)	Na^+-independent bile acid and xenobiotic uptake
Na^+,K^+-ATPase	Secretion of 2 Na^+ in exchange for 3 K^+; provides driving force for Na+-dependent uptake
Hepatocyte	**Canalicular Membrane Transport**
BSEP (*ABCB11*)	ATP-dependent bile acid export
MRP2 (*ABCC2*)	ATP-dependent export of glucuronide, glutathione, and sulfate conjugates of organic solutes, including bilirubin conjugates
MDR3 (*ABCB4*)	ATP-dependent phosphatidylcholine export
FIC1 (*ATP8B1*)	ATP-dependent aminophospholipid flipping
MDR1 (*ABCB1*)	ATP-dependent export of xenobiotics and metabolites, including polyhydroxylated bile acids
ABCG5/ABCG8	ATP-dependent sterol export
NPC1L1	Sterol import
Hepatocyte	**Sinusoidal Membrane Export**
MRP3 (*ABCC3*)	ATP-dependent export of bile acids and glucuronide conjugates
MRP4 (*ABCC4*)	ATP-dependent export of glutathione and bile acids
OSTα-OSTβ (*SLC51A, 51B*)	Bile acid export
Cholangiocyte	**Ductular Secretion and Bile Acid Transport**
Aquaporin 1 (*AQP1*)	Apical membrane water transport
Aquaporin 4 (*AQP4*)	Basolateral membrane water transport
AE2 (*SLC4A2*)	Apical membrane HCO_3^- secretion in exchange for Cl^-
CFTR (*ABCC7*)	Apical membrane Cl^- secretion
IBAT (*SLC10A2*)	Apical membrane bile acid uptake (cholehepatic shunt)
OSTα-OSTβ (*SLC51A, 51B*)	Basolateral membrane bile acid export
MRP3 (*ABCC3*)	Basolateral membrane ATP-dependent export of bile acids and glucuronide conjugates
Ileal Enterocyte	
IBAT (*SLC10A2*)	Apical membrane bile acid uptake
IBABP (*FABP6*)	Cytosolic transport of bile acids
OSTα-OSTβ (*SLC51A, 51B*)	Basolateral membrane bile acid export
MRP3 (*ABCC3*)	Basolateral membrane ATP-dependent export of bile acids and glucuronide conjugates
Renal Proximal Tubule Cell	**Kidney Tubule Bile Acid Absorption**
IBAT (*SLC10A2*)	Apical membrane bile acid uptake
OSTα-OSTβ (*SLC51A, 51B*)	Basolateral membrane bile acid export
Renal Proximal Tubule Cell	**Kidney Tubule Bile Acid Secretion**
OAT3 (*SLC22A8*)	Basolateral membrane sulfated bile acid sulfate uptake
MRP2 (*ABCC2*)	ATP-dependent export of glucuronide, glutathione, and sulfate conjugates of organic solutes, including bile acid conjugates
MRP4 (*ABCC4*)	ATP-dependent export of glutathione and bile acids

ABC, ATP-binding cassette; *AE2*, chloride-bicarbonate anion exchanger isoform 2; *AQ*, aquaporin; *BSEP*, bile salt export pump; *FIC1*, P-type ATPase mutated in progressive familial intrahepatic cholestasis type 1; *IBABP*, ileal bile acid binding protein; *IBAT*, ileal bile acid transporter; *MDR*, multidrug resistance protein; *MRP*, multidrug resistance–associated protein; *NPC1L1*, Niemann-Pick C1 Like 1; *NTCP*, Na^+-taurocholate cotransporting polypeptide; *OAT*, organic anion transporter; *OATP*, organic anion-transporting polypeptide; *OST*, organic solute transporter; *SLC*, solute carrier.

ATP-dependent bile salt export pump (BSEP; gene symbol *ABCB11*). The role of BSEP as the major canalicular membrane bile acid transporter was confirmed by identification of *ABCB11* mutations in patients with progressive familial intrahepatic cholestasis type 2 (PFIC2), a hepatic disorder characterized by impaired biliary bile acid secretion (see Chapter 79).[52] Although conjugated bile acids are the major physiologic substrate, a variety of other compounds can interact with BSEP as nonsubstrate inhibitors to potentially impede bile acid export. This list of compounds includes drugs such as cyclosporin, rifampin, troglitazone, bosentan, and glibenclamide. The direct inhibition of BSEP may be an important mechanism underlying some forms of drug-induced hepatoxicity (see Chapter 90).[53] In contrast to conjugated bile acids, sulfated, glucuronidated, or polyhydroxylated bile acids are poor substrates for BSEP and exported into bile by other canalicular membrane transporters. If not effluxed across the hepatocyte sinusoidal membrane, sulfated and glucuronidated bile acids are secreted across the canalicular membrane into bile by the multidrug resistance–associated protein (MRP2; gene symbol *ABCC2*), whereas canalicular membrane export of polyhydroxylated bile acids is mediated by MRP2 and the multidrug resistance protein 1 (MDR1; gene symbol *ABCB1*).

Intestinal Bile Acid Transport

Numerous observations indicate that the terminal ileum is the major site of bile acid reabsorption. For example, there is little drop in intraluminal bile acid concentrations prior to the ileum, and bile acid malabsorption occurs after ileal resection. Studies using in situ perfused intestinal segments to measure bile acid absorption demonstrated that ileal bile acid transport is a high-capacity system and sufficient to account for the biliary output of bile acids. Ileal active transport is the major route of conjugated bile acid uptake, particularly for the more hydrophilic- and taurine-conjugated species. In the proximal small intestine, a fraction of the glycine-conjugated bile acids become protonated and uncharged when the intraluminal pH becomes transiently acidic during digestion and can be absorbed by nonionic passive diffusion. In addition, gut microbiota metabolism of conjugated bile acids starts in the small intestine and continues in the colon to generate unconjugated hydrophobic bile acids, which are weak acids and are passively absorbed if they remain in solution.

Renal Bile Acid Transport

A fraction (10%–50%) of the bile acids returning in the portal circulation escapes hepatic first-pass extraction and spills into the systemic circulation. The binding of bile acids to plasma proteins reduces glomerular filtration and urinary excretion of bile acids. In healthy humans, the kidney filters approximately 100 μmol of bile acids each day. Remarkably, only 1–2 μmol are excreted in the urine because of highly efficient tubular reabsorption. Even in patients with cholestatic liver disease, in whom plasma bile acid concentrations are significantly elevated, the 24-hour urinary excretion of nonsulfated bile acids is much less than the quantity that undergoes glomerular filtration. Subsequent studies have shown that the conjugated bile acids that are not sulfated or glucuronidated in the glomerular filtrate are selectively reabsorbed from the renal proximal tubules, and this process contributes to the rise in serum bile acid concentrations in patients with cholestatic liver disease. As in the ileum, the renal proximal tubule epithelium expresses a Na^+ gradient–driven transporter that functions as a salvage mechanism to conserve bile acids. In contrast, urinary clearance of plasma-modified (sulfated and glucuronidated) bile acids in cholestatic patients can be 100-fold higher than for conjugated bile acids, with the increase in urinary bile acid excretion overwhelming in the sulfated versus nonsulfated fraction. Mechanistically, this involves (1) increased glomerular filtration coupled with an absence of sulfated/glucuronidated bile acid reabsorption from the proximal tubule lumen into blood and (2) direct renal tubule secretion of sulfated bile acids from blood into the tubule lumen for urinary excretion.

Molecular Mechanisms of Intestinal and Renal Bile Acid Transport

Bile acids are transported actively across the ileal brush-border membrane by the well-characterized IBAT. The relationship among the hepatic, biliary, ileal, and renal Na^+–bile acid cotransport systems was resolved with the cloning of the bile acid carriers from those tissues. The hepatocyte expresses the related Na^+–bile acid cotransporter, NTCP, whereas the ileal enterocyte, renal proximal tubule cell, and cholangiocyte all express IBAT. The driving force for IBAT-mediated bile acid uptake across the ileal apical brush-border membrane includes the negative intracellular potential, as well as the inwardly directed Na^+ gradient and paracellular flow of Na^+ from the intestinal submucosa back into the lumen.[54] IBAT transports all the major species of bile acids but does not appear to transport most modified bile acids such as sulfated or glucuronidated bile acids or unrelated solutes. The finding that *SLC10A2* mutations are responsible for primary bile acid malabsorption, a disorder associated with intestinal bile acid malabsorption and steatorrhea, demonstrated that intestinal conjugated bile acid absorption in humans is mediated by IBAT.[55] The ileal bile acid binding protein (IBABP; gene symbol *FABP6*) is a member of the fatty acid binding protein family and an abundant cytosolic protein in ileal enterocytes. Although not essential for bile acid transport, IBABP likely functions to protect the ileal enterocyte against bile acid–induced injury and participates in the transcellular transport of bile acids, as evidenced by a partial impairment of ileal bile acid absorption in IBABP-deficient mice.[56] The transporter responsible for bile acid export across the basolateral membrane of the ileal enterocyte, cholangiocytes, and renal proximal tubule cells has been identified. The heteromeric organic solute transporter, OSTα-OSTβ, is expressed on the basolateral membrane of ileal enterocytes, hepatocytes, cholangiocytes, and renal proximal tubule cells and transports bile acids as well as a variety of organic anions and drugs. Inherited loss-of-function mutations in the human OSTα (*SLC51A*) or OSTβ genes (*SLC51B*) cause congenital chronic diarrhea in agreement with the proposed critical role of OSTα-OSTβ in intestinal bile acid absorption. These pediatric patients also exhibited features of cholestatic liver disease, underscoring an important functional role for OSTα-OSTβ in human hepatocytes and cholangiocytes.[57,58]

DISORDERS OF THE BILE FORMATION AND BILE ACID CIRCULATION

Disorders of the bile acid circulation include bile acid diarrhea (BAD) and cholestasis. BAD is caused by primary defects in intestinal bile acid absorption and, more commonly, by dysregulation of bile acid homeostasis leading to elevated colonic bile acid levels. Cholestasis is defined as interruption of the normal process of bile formation and is classically subdivided into *intrahepatic cholestasis*, a functional defect in bile formation at the level of the hepatocyte and intrahepatic bile ductules, and *extrahepatic cholestasis*, an obstruction to bile flow within the biliary tract. Impaired hepatic transport of bile acids and other organic solutes is a prominent feature of both inherited and acquired forms of cholestatic liver disease. Disorders of the bile formation and bile acid cycling are classically divided into the following four categories: (1) defects in bile acid formation (synthesis and conjugation), (2) defects in membrane transport of bile acids (uptake and secretion), (3) disturbances involving bacterial transformation (deconjugation and dehydroxylation), and (4) disturbances in movement through or between organs (bile acid circulation).[59,60]

Traditionally, specific diagnosis of rare inherited bile acid biosynthetic defects were made by analysis of body fluids (urine, blood, and bile) using methods such as fast atom bombardment ionization-mass spectrometry and electrospray ionization-tandem mass spectrometry.[2,61] The biosynthetic disorders present with markedly reduced or complete absence of CA and CDCA and greatly elevated concentrations of atypical bile acids in bile, serum, and urine. Elevated fasting serum bile acids have also been noted as an early marker of intrahepatic cholestasis of pregnancy (ICP). However, with the exception of ICP, measurement of total serum bile acid concentrations alone without profiling the individual bile acids and bile acid intermediates appears to offer little additional benefit over conventional liver biochemical tests in the diagnosis or management of most forms of liver disease or bile acid malabsorption. For pediatric forms of liver disease, targeted sequencing panels or whole exome sequencing are becoming widely available and are increasingly being used to diagnose inherited disorders of bile acid synthesis and transport that are associated with liver disease.[62]

Bile Acid Synthesis Defects

Bile acid synthesis from cholesterol is required to maintain the bile acid pool. Although inherited biosynthetic defects are rare, these disorders serve to illustrate the importance of bile acids for normal hepatic and intestinal function. The effects of a block in bile acid synthesis include depletion of the bile acid pool by fecal excretion, loss of bile acid–stimulated bile flow, decreased biliary excretion of cholesterol and xenobiotics, malabsorption of fat and fat-soluble vitamins, and cellular accumulation of cytotoxic bile acid biosynthetic intermediates in liver and extrahepatic tissues. Inherited defects in 10 of the enzymes and 1 transporter involved in bile acid biosynthesis have been reported. The list includes cholesterol 7α-hydroxylase (*CYP7A1*), sterol 27-hydroxylase (*CYP27A1*), oxysterol 7α-hydroxylase (*CYP7B1*), 3β-hydroxy-Δ5-C_{27}-steroid oxidoreductase (*HSD3B7*), Δ4-3-oxosteroid 5β-reductase (*AKR1D1*), 2-methylacyl-coenzyme A racemase (*AMACR*), acyl-CoA oxidase 2 (*ACOX2*), D-bifunctional protein (*HSD17B4*), sterol carrier protein X (*SCP2*), bile acid–CoA ligase (*SLC27A5*), bile acid coenzyme A:amino acid *N*-acyl-transferase (*BAAT*), and the peroxisomal ATP-binding cassette (ABC) transporter (*ABCD3*).[2,61] In addition to these specific defects, disorders that disrupt peroxisome biogenesis such as Zellweger syndrome also affect bile acid synthesis because the bile acid side chain modification steps occur in the peroxisome (see Chapter 79).

A single enzyme defect is usually not sufficient to block production of all bile acids, because multiple biosynthetic pathways exist. Clinically, patients with bile acid synthesis defects typically present with steatorrhea, growth retardation, sequelae associated with fat-soluble vitamin malabsorption, and mild to severe liver disease. Although serum GGTP levels are elevated in some other forms of cholestasis, GGTP levels are typically normal in the cholestatic patient with a bile acid biosynthesis defect because the block occurs prior to canalicular secretion. Depending on the step in the pathway and the nature of the mutation, the consequences of bile acid biosynthesis defects can vary, with the most severe producing neonatal cholestatic liver disease or neurologic disease later in life. For example, cerebrotendinous xanthomatosis (CTX) is a rare, inherited disease caused by mutations in the mitochondrial enzyme sterol 27-hydroxylase (*CYP27A1*). CYP27A1 is expressed by the liver and extrahepatic tissues. In CTX, the alternative pathway for bile acid synthesis is blocked, and the production of bile acids via the classical pathway is diminished but not eliminated. CTX can present with cholestatic liver disease in early infancy but is generally characterized by progressive neurologic disturbances, premature atherosclerosis, cataracts, and tendinous xanthomas later in life. The most reported defect in bile acid synthesis is 3β-hydroxy-Δ5-C_{27}-steroid oxidoreductase (*HSD3B7*) deficiency, which affects both the classical and alternative pathways for bile acid biosynthesis. The disease is characterized by progressive intrahepatic cholestasis and accumulation of abnormal bile acids. Clinical manifestations include unconjugated hyperbilirubinemia, jaundice, serum aminotransferase elevations, steatorrhea, fat-soluble vitamin deficiency, pruritus, and poor growth. The progression of disease is variable but ultimately results in cirrhosis and hepatic failure in a high proportion of affected persons. Administration of bile acids such as CA and CDCA beginning early in life is efficacious for the treatment of patients with bile acid biosynthetic defects and in some patients with Zellweger spectrum disorders (see also Chapter 79).[63,64]

Membrane Transport of Bile Acids and Biliary Lipids

A growing number of disorders have been found to be associated with mutations in genes important for bile acid or solute transport.[60] These disorders are summarized in Table 66.5 and include PFIC, ICP, low phospholipid-associated cholelithiasis (LPAC), cystic fibrosis, Dubin-Johnson syndrome, Rotor syndrome, sitosterolemia, primary bile acid malabsorption, and forms of congenital diarrhea.

PFIC type 1 (PFIC1; also called ATP8B1 deficiency and formerly called Byler disease) manifests primarily as chronic intrahepatic cholestasis and coarse granular bile in patients with *low or normal serum GGTP* levels. The gene defect in patients with PFIC1 was mapped to chromosome 18 in the same region where a similar but milder disease phenotype (termed benign recurrent intrahepatic cholestasis; BRIC) had been localized. A combined search identified a P-type ATPase, designated FIC1 (gene symbol *ATP8B1*), as the defective gene product responsible for PFIC1, some forms of BRIC, and Greenland familial cholestasis. P-type ATPases are distinct from ABC transporters and constitute a large family that includes ion pumps such as the Na^+/K^+-ATPase, the Ca^{2+}-ATPase, and the copper-transporting Wilson disease gene product. An analysis of the spectrum of *ATP8B1* mutations in patients with PFIC1 and BRIC revealed that mutation type and location in the gene generally correlate with clinical severity. More innocuous *ATP8B1* missense mutations are common in BRIC, whereas nonsense, frame-shifting, and large deletion mutations are more common in PFIC1.[65,66] FIC1 is an aminophospholipid (phosphatidylserine) flippase that functions to help maintain the asymmetric distribution of lipids between the inner and outer leaflets of the plasma membrane, and its activity requires the coexpression of an accessary protein, CDC50A (also called TMEM30A), which promotes the trafficking of FIC1 to the plasma membrane.[67] In humans, the FIC1 protein is expressed in many tissues, including the pancreas, small intestine, urinary bladder, adrenal, stomach, prostate, and inner ear. Loss of FIC1 activity in these tissues is likely associated with the high frequency of diarrhea, pancreatitis, bacterial pneumonia, sweat electrolyte abnormalities, and hearing loss in PFIC1 patients and the persistence of these extrahepatic symptoms following LT.[68,69] Although the mechanisms responsible for cholestasis associated with FIC1 deficiency remain to be fully elucidated, results from the *ATP8B1* mutant mouse indicate that loss of aminophospholipid flippase activity makes the canalicular membrane more susceptible to damage from hydrophobic bile acids. Medical management options for PFIC1 and the associated pruritis include UDCA, IBAT inhibitors, rifampin, and supplementation with fat-soluble vitamins. Surgical management is indicated for patients who do not respond to medical therapy, and partial external biliary diversion (PEBD) is recommended. In those patients who have not developed cirrhosis, PEBD improves growth and liver function, while reducing pruritus and slowing progression of hepatic fibrosis. LT leads to the resolution of cholestasis in PFIC1 patients but does not improve and may even worsen hepatic steatosis.[66,70]

PFIC2 (also called BSEP deficiency) is associated with low bile acid secretion, progressive cholestasis, *low or normal serum GGTP levels*, lobular and portal fibrosis, hepatic giant cell transformation, and the lack of bile duct proliferation on examination of liver histology. The disease had been mapped to chromosome 2q24, and the defective gene (*ABCB11*) was shown to encode the canalicular BSEP protein. The mutations in *ABCB11* impact BSEP protein synthesis, cellular trafficking, or stability, and the

TABLE 66.5 Inherited Disorders of Bile Formation and Bile Acid Cycling

Disorder	Defect	Protein(s) (*Gene*)	Features
PFIC			
PFIC1	Aminophospholipid membrane transport	FIC1 (*ATP8B1*)	Progressive cholestasis, elevated serum bile acid levels, pruritus, pancreatitis, intestinal malabsorption, hearing loss, low or normal serum GGTP, high serum bile acids
PFIC2	Bile acid export	BSEP (*ABCB11*)	Progressive cholestasis, jaundice, giant cell formation, lobular and portal fibrosis, hepatobiliary malignancy, low or normal serum GGTP, high serum bile acids
PFIC3	Phosphatidylcholine secretion into bile	MDR3 (*ABCB4*)	Cholestasis, extensive bile duct proliferation and periportal fibrosis, high serum GGTP, normal serum bile acids
PFIC4	Tight junction disorder	TJP2	Progressive bland cholestasis; increased risk of hepatobiliary malignancy; low or normal serum GGTP; high serum bile acids
PFIC5	Altered bile acid signaling; impaired bile secretion, altered hepatic synthetic function	FXR (*NR1H4*)	Giant cell hepatitis, rapid progressive cholestasis with ductular reaction; low or normal GGTP; high serum bile acids low or normal serum GGTP; high serum bile acids
PFIC6	Intracellular trafficking; transporter targeting to the canalicular membrane	MYO5B	May present in patients with intestinal microvillous inclusion disease (MVID) or as isolated cholestatic liver disease
LPAC			
LPAC	Phosphatidylcholine secretion into bile	MDR3 (*ABCB4*)	Cholelithiasis, intrahepatic hyperechoic foci, biliary cirrhosis, high serum GGTP levels
ICP			
ICP	Phosphatidylcholine secretion into bile	MDR3 (*ABCB4*)	Cholestasis in third trimester of pregnancy, fetal loss and prematurity, high serum GGTP levels
ICP	Bile acid export	BSEP (*ABCB11*)	Cholestasis in third trimester of pregnancy, fetal loss and prematurity, normal serum GGTP levels
Dubin-Johnson Syndrome			
	Organic anion conjugate export	MRP2 (*ABCC2*)	Jaundice, benign conjugated hyperbilirubinemia
Rotor Syndrome			
	Sinusoidal membrane organic anion uptake; bilirubin glucuronide reuptake	OATP1B1 (*SLCO1B1*) OATP1B3 (*SLCO1B3*)	Jaundice, benign conjugated hyperbilirubinemia, delayed clearance of cholephilic anions such as BSP and ICG
Sitosterolemia			
	Cholesterol and phytosterol export	*ABCG5*, *ABCG8*	Xanthomas, hypersterolemia, coronary artery disease
Hypercholanemia (NTCP-deficiency)			
	Hepatocyte Na^+-dependent bile acid uptake	NTCP (SLC10A1)	High serum bile acids in the absence of jaundice, pruritus, or other signs of liver disease
Primary Bile Acid Malabsorption			
	Ileal apical membrane $Na+$-dependent bile acid uptake	IBAT (*SLC10A2*)	Chronic diarrhea, steatorrhea, fat-soluble vitamin malabsorption; elevated hepatic bile acid synthesis; low serum bile acids
	Basolateral membrane bile acid export in liver and intestine; altered bile acid signaling	OSTα (*SLC51A*) OSTβ (*SLC51B*)	Chronic diarrhea, steatorrhea, fat-soluble vitamin malabsorption; decreased hepatic bile acid synthesis; features of cholestatic liver disease; high serum GGTP; low serum bile acids
Cystic fibrosis			
	Channelopathy affecting Cl^- conductance in multiple tissue, including biliary tract and small intestine	CFTR (*ABCC7*)	Cholestasis with bile duct proliferation and inflammation; elevated serum GGTP; meconium ileus

ABC, ATP-binding cassette; *BSEP*, bile salt export pump; *BSP*, bromosulfophthalein; *CFTR*, cystic fibrosis transmembrane conductance regulator; *FIC1*, P-type ATPase mutated in progressive familial intrahepatic cholestasis type 1; *IBAT*, ileal bile acid transporter; *ICG*, indocyanine green; *ICP*, intrahepatic cholestasis of pregnancy; *LPAC*, low-phospholipid-associated cholelithiasis; *MDR*, multidrug resistance protein; *MRP*, multidrug resistance–associated protein; *MYO5B*, myosin V type protein; *OST*, organic solute transporter; *PFIC*, progressive familial intrahepatic cholestasis; *TJP2*, tight junction protein 2.

absence of BSEP protein or canalicular membrane expression correlates with increased disease severity and poorer treatment outcomes.[52,71]

Patients with PFIC2 present as infants with high serum bile acid levels, intractable pruritus, intestinal malabsorption, failure to thrive, and cholestasis, and they ultimately develop fibrosis and end-stage liver disease before adulthood. In addition to cholestasis, severe BSEP deficiency significantly increases the risk for hepatobiliary malignancy, including HCC and cholangiocarcinoma.[56,57] The treatment of PFIC2 is similar to that for PFIC1 and includes nutritional support, IBAT inhibitors, UDCA, rifampin, fat-soluble vitamin supplementation, and PEBD, with biliary diversion procedures such as PEBD showing long-term benefit in PFIC2 patients with mild BSEP mutations.[71] Ultimately, LT is required for most patients with severe forms of BSEP deficiency. However, recurrent low-GGTP cholestasis has been reported in PFIC2 patients following LT, as a result of the development of inhibitory antibodies to BSEP.[72,73] Beyond PFIC2, BSEP mutations associated with milder disease may also confer increased risk of ICP and drug-induced liver injury.[74]

PFIC3 (also called MDR3 deficiency) is quite distinct from the other PFIC subtypes. Serum *GGTP levels are markedly elevated* in these patients, and liver histologic examination shows extensive bile duct proliferation and portal and periportal fibrosis.[75] The most common clinical presentation includes cholestasis, pruritus, jaundice, hepatomegaly, splenomegaly, and portal hypertension, and PFIC3 may be associated with an increased risk of cholangiocarcinoma. The defect in PFIC3 lies in MDR3 (gene symbol *ABCB4*), a canalicular membrane ABC transporter that is responsible for PC secretion into bile.[76] In PFIC3, hepatic bile acid secretion is not directly impaired, but biliary PC transport is greatly diminished. In bile, PC normally forms mixed micelles with bile acids and acts to buffer their cytotoxic detergent properties. In the absence of biliary phospholipid, the hydrophobic bile acids are toxic and cause cholestatic liver damage.[51] In addition to the early and severe clinical presentation of children with PFIC3, homozygous or heterozygous genetic variants in *ABCB4* are also associated with a milder phenotype that may be asymptomatic until adulthood. For example, heterozygous or less severe mutations in *ABCB4* are associated with LPAC and ICP (see Table 66.5 and Chapter 66). Medical treatment for PFIC3 includes UDCA and rifampin but is not satisfactory as long-term therapy for those PFIC3 patients with more severe disease, for whom LT is curative. IBAT inhibitors are approved for use as a nonsurgical treatment for PFIC; however, as of 2023, clinical data are still limited regarding the long-term response of PFIC3 patients to treatment.[77]

Many of the forms of PFIC that have been characterized involve the hepatocyte canalicular membrane transporters described earlier. Mutations in other genes that result in a PFIC-like presentation have also been identified.[60] The affected gene products and the associated clinical presentations include (1) the tight junction protein (*TJP2*), which results in *low or normal GGTP*-associated cholestasis; (2) the bile acid–activated nuclear receptor FXR, which results in neonatal cholestasis and end-stage liver disease; (3) myosin 5B (*MYO5B*), which cause microvillus inclusion disease but can also present with *a low or normal GGTP*-associated cholestasis in the absence of recurrent diarrhea; and (4) UNC-45 myosin chaperone A (*UNC45A*), which interacts with MYO5B and causes Aagenaes syndrome/lymphedema cholestasis syndrome 1.[78,79]

Bile Acid Biotransformation (Deconjugation and Dehydroxylation)

Gut microbiota–mediated bile acid deconjugation begins in the small intestine and is increased in patients with small intestinal stasis and bacterial overgrowth. The unconjugated bile acids are less soluble than their glycine or taurine conjugates and precipitate in the gut lumen or are absorbed passively if they remain in solution. As a result, extensive small intestinal bacterial deconjugation reduces the intraluminal concentration of bile acids available to form micelles with dietary lipids in the small intestine, resulting in malabsorption and diarrhea (see Chapter 107). In healthy humans, bile acid deconjugation continues in the colon. The unconjugated bile acids can undergo 7α-dehydroxylation to yield DCA and LCA and other microbiome-catalyzed metabolism. The level of DCA in bile varies considerably among individuals, ranging from almost undetectable levels to more than half of the biliary bile acids. The production of DCA is controlled by colonic levels of the bile acid 7α-dehydroxylating bacteria and by the colonic transit time, which can be affected by diet and factors that alter gut motility. Beyond disorders of bile formation and bile acid cycling, alterations in gut microbial metabolism of bile acids have been implicated in an increasing number of digestive and metabolic diseases.[8–10]

Bile Acid Circulation

Biliary Obstruction and Biliary Fistula

Biliary obstruction caused, for example, by a gallstone or cholangiocarcinoma leads to retention of hepatic bile acids, which may cause hepatic necrosis or apoptosis. A portion of the retained bile acids undergoes phase 2 metabolism (sulfation/glucuronidation), and the modified as well as unmodified bile acids are regurgitated from hepatocytes back into the systemic circulation. Despite increased urinary excretion of bile acids, particularly for sulfated species, plasma concentrations of bile acids rise as much as 20-fold. When biliary obstruction is complete, bile acids are not secreted into the small intestine, and intestinal malabsorption of fat-soluble vitamins and steatorrhea results. Secondary bile acids are not formed, and fecal bile acid output diminishes.

In a patient with a biliary fistula, bile acids are diverted from entering the small intestine. Because bile acid biosynthesis is controlled by negative feedback, bile acid synthesis rises markedly, up to 20-fold. Hepatic function is not impaired, although the flux of bile acids through the liver is decreased substantially because maximal bile acid synthesis (4–6 g/day) is less than the normal flux in the presence of an intact bile acid circulation (12–18 g/day). As in biliary obstruction, lower bile acid concentrations in the small intestine result in malabsorption of fat-soluble vitamins. Absorption of dietary fats, especially dietary triglycerides that contain long-chain saturated fatty acids, is also decreased.

Cholecystectomy

Despite removal of an important site for storing and concentrating bile acids, the overall effect of cholecystectomy on biliary bile acid secretion is small, and bile acid homeostasis is not altered substantially.[80] In the absence of a gallbladder, the bile acid pool is stored in the small intestine during the fasting state. After ingestion of a meal, the bile acid pool moves to the terminal ileum, where it is actively absorbed and returned to the liver via the portal circulation. Increased dehydroxylation of CA to DCA has been reported and may be secondary to increased bile acid cycling in the fasting state. Diarrhea is one of the most common symptoms after cholecystectomy.[81] In a subset of these patients, the changes in bile acid cycling may overwhelm ileal transport or the gut-liver signaling mechanisms that control hepatic bile acid synthesis, thereby leading to BAD. The affected patients generally respond to administration of a bile acid sequestrant.[82]

Ileal Resection

Resection of the terminal ileum causes intestinal bile acid malabsorption. If the resection is short (<100 cm), the effect on bile acid metabolism is minimal because increased hepatic bile acid biosynthesis balances fecal loss. Excess amounts of unabsorbed bile acids enter the colon and act to inhibit water absorption or induce secretion, thereby resulting in mild, watery diarrhea.[83] Symptomatic response is obtained with the administration of a bile acid sequestrant. When 100 cm or more of ileum is resected, including the ileocecal valve, hepatic bile acid secretion diminishes because maximal synthesis is considerably less than the normal hepatic secretion rate. The bile acid pool becomes progressively depleted during the day, and intestinal fat malabsorption appears because of the lack of micelles and loss of intestinal mucosal surface. The increased transit of fatty acids into the colon inhibits water absorption and results in severe diarrhea that responds poorly to bile acid sequestrants. If the diarrhea is of sufficiently large volume and accompanied by malabsorption of other nutrients, the patient may be diagnosed as having short bowel syndrome. Therapy is complex. In some patients, fecal weight and frequency are reduced by elimination of fat from the diet. Other therapies include administration of glutamine and growth factors such as analogs of glucagon-like peptide-2.[84]

Bile Acid Diarrhea

Under normal physiological conditions, the bile acid circulation functions to conserve bile acids efficiently and limit their fecal loss. However, a variety of pathophysiological conditions can lead to excess concentrations of dihydroxy bile acids in the colon, which alters colonocyte function, accelerates colonic transit, and disrupts the regulation of intestinal electrolyte and fluid balance.[83,85] Bile acids play a role in colonic water transport apparently by increasing chloride secretion in the perfused colon via an inositol 1,4,5-triphosphate and calcium-dependent mechanism.[83] Trihydroxy bile acids and hydrophilic bile acids such as UDCA have no effect. However, hydrophobic dihydroxy bile acids induce net fluid secretion at high concentrations and block absorption of fluid and water at low concentrations. To induce net secretion, bile acids must (1) have an appropriate structure (hydrophobic dihydroxy bile acids such as DCA or CDCA); (2) be present in high concentrations (>1.5 millimolar) in the aqueous phase; and (3) exist in an environment with the appropriate alkaline pH (fecal pH > 6.8).

BAD is subdivided into three types based on etiology.[82] *Type 1* is the most common subtype of BAD, resulting from impaired intestinal absorption of bile acids, and is caused by ileal resection or diseases involving the ileum such as Crohn disease. *Type 2* (idiopathic or primary BAD) is a common and likely underdiagnosed cause of diarrhea-predominant Irritable Bowel Syndrome (IBS) and functional diarrhea.[86] Evidence suggests that the BAD is secondary to hepatic overproduction of bile acids rather than defective intestinal absorption and involves alterations in the FXR-FGF19 gut-liver signaling pathway for the regulation of hepatic bile acid synthesis. Also included in the type 2 subgroup of BAD are mutations in the IBAT gene, which are responsible for a rare form of congenital or primary bile acid malabsorption. These patients present early in infancy with chronic diarrhea, steatorrhea, fat-soluble vitamin malabsorption, and poor growth.[55] *Type 3* is associated with conditions such as cholecystectomy, chronic pancreatitis, celiac disease, diabetes mellitus, cystic fibrosis, small intestinal bacterial overgrowth, and the use of NSAIDs, which can damage the ileal mucosa. BAD can be diagnosed using a selenium-75 labeled homotaurocholic acid (^{75}SeHCAT) nuclear medicine imaging test, measurements of the fasting levels of serum 7α-hydroxy-4-cholesten-3-one (C4; a biomarker for hepatic bile acid synthesis) and FGF19, or measuring fecal bile acids.[87]

BILE ACID–BASED THERAPY

Bile Acid Replacement Therapy

Bile acid replacement therapy is used to correct a bile acid deficiency, which may be caused by rare inborn errors of bile acid biosynthesis or depletion of the bile acid pool. In patients with impaired bile acid biosynthesis and normal bile acid conjugation (amidation), the administration of unconjugated CA suppresses the synthesis of cytotoxic bile acid precursors, restores the input of primary bile acids into the enterohepatic circulation, and provides long-term benefit.[63,64] However, in those rare patients with inherited defects in bile acid conjugation, the administration of conjugated bile acids, such as glycocholic acid, is required for treatment.[22] Although used for other indications, the administration of UDCA alone is not recommended in this setting because it does not suppress endogenous synthesis of the cytotoxic bile acid precursors. In patients with severe bile acid malabsorption or short bowel syndrome, bile acid replacement therapy partially corrects the impairment of micellar solubilization and absorption of fat in the small intestine.[88,89]

UDCA and norUDCA

Because of its safety and lack of hepatotoxicity, UDCA remains the most widely used form of bile acid therapy.[35] After oral administration, UDCA accumulates and ultimately constitutes up to 40% of the circulating bile acid pool, displacing the more hydrophobic endogenous bile acids. UDCA was originally administered and approved by the FDA for gallstone dissolution but was not widely used for that purpose because of the success of laparoscopic cholecystectomy. However, the use of UDCA to prevent gallstones has undergone a mild resurgence to treat the symptomatic cholelithiasis observed after bariatric surgery as the number of these procedures continues to increase.[90] The FDA has also approved the use of UDCA for treatment of PBC (see Chapter 93). UDCA appears to stimulate biliary bicarbonate secretion to protect against bile acid–induced ductular damage. Administration of UDCA has been shown to delay the progression of fibrosing cholangiopathy, reduce the need for LT, and improve survival in a significant fraction of PBC patients.[28,35,91] UDCA therapy also has some benefit for ICP and favorable effects in other conditions such as LPAC.[92,93] Moreover, combination therapy with the lipid-lowering agent bezafibrate or the FXR agonist obeticholic acid (see later) has been shown to improve cholestasis in patients with PBC with an inadequate response to UDCA alone.[94–96]

Norucholic acid (norursodeoxycholic acid) is a chemical analog of UDCA with one less carbon atom in its side chain. As a result of this modification, norucholic acid is resistant to conjugation with taurine or glycine and undergoes significant cholehepatic shunting. Norucholic was superior to UDCA in treating peribiliary fibrosis in the MDR2/Abcb4 knockout mouse, an animal model of sclerosing cholangitis, and has shown benefit in a phase 2 clinical trial in patients with PSC.[97]

Bile Acid Receptor Agonists

Identification of the regulators of bile acid homeostasis together with the design of potent bile acid receptor ligands has led not only to the development of novel drugs for cholestatic liver diseases (e.g., obeticholic acid) but also to interest in the therapeutic uses of steroidal and nonsteroidal FXR agonists to modulate fat, glucose, protein, and energy homeostasis to treat MASLD and MASH (see Chapter 89).[98] The FXR agonist obeticholic acid was conditionally approved for second-line therapy in patients with PBC who have shown only a partial response to UDCA, although not in patients with decompensated cirrhosis (see Chapter 93).[96]

BILE ACID SEQUESTRANTS AND BILE ACID TRANSPORTER INHIBITORS

Bile acid sequestrants are positively charged polymeric resins that bind bile acids in the intestinal lumen to decrease the aqueous concentration and the efficiency of intestinal conservation of bile acids. In patients with mild BAD, bile acid sequestrants provide symptomatic relief by lowering the concentration of free bile acids in the colon.[99] Bile acid sequestrants also are used to decrease pruritus in patients with cholestasis, presumably by reducing the concentration of bile acids or other anionic biliary constituents in the systemic circulation. In addition to the older preparations, cholestyramine and colestipol, more potent sequestrants with superior bile acid–binding properties have been developed. Colesevelam is a newer bile acid sequestrant approved by the FDA for the treatment of hypercholesterolemia and for the improvement of glycemic control in adults with type 2 diabetes mellitus. However, the clinical evidence supporting the efficacy of bile acid sequestrants as a treatment for cholestatic pruritus is limited.[100,101] An alternative to luminal sequestration of bile acids with binding resins is direct inhibition of the IBAT with gut-restricted IBAT inhibitors. This design mimics features of surgical interruption of the enterohepatic circulation of bile acids, which has efficacy in pediatric cholestasis patients.[70,102,103] Gut-restricted IBAT inhibitors have shown clinical benefit in cholestatic patients[77,104,105] and received FDA approval as nonsurgical treatments for children with PFIC and Alagille syndrome.

Full references for this chapter can be found at https://ebooks.health.elsevier.com.

67 Gallstone Disease

David Q.-H. Wang, Nezam H. Afdhal

Dedicated to the Memory of Dr. David Wang

IN THIS CHAPTER

Cholesterol cholelithiasis is one of the most prevalent and costly digestive diseases in Western countries. At least 20 million Americans (≈12% of adults) have gallstones.[1–11] The prevalence of gallstones appears to be rising due to the epidemic of obesity, associated with insulin resistance and the metabolic syndrome. Each year, roughly 1 million new cases are discovered.[12–14] Although many gallstones are "silent," about one-third eventually cause symptoms and complications.[15] In the United States, annually 893,000 cholecystectomies are performed for gallbladder disease and related medical expenses for the treatment of gallstones exceed $6 billion annually.[2] In addition, unavoidable complications of gallstones result in 3000 deaths (0.12% of all deaths) per year.[1] In the United States, persons with gallstone disease have increased cardiovascular disease, cancer, and overall mortality.[10]

TYPES OF GALLSTONES

Based on chemical composition and macroscopic appearance, gallstones are divided into three types: *cholesterol*, *pigment*, and *rare stones*.[3,4,16] The majority (≈75%) of gallstones in the United States and Europe are cholesterol stones,[15] which consist mainly of cholesterol monohydrate crystals and precipitates of amorphous calcium bilirubinate, often with calcium carbonate or phosphate in one of the crystalline polymorphs. These stones are usually subclassified as either pure cholesterol or mixed stones that contain at least 50% cholesterol by weight. The remaining gallstones are pigment stones that contain mostly calcium bilirubinate and are subclassified into 2 groups: black pigment stones (≈20%) and brown pigment stones (≈4.5%). Rare gallstones (≈0.5%) include calcium carbonate stones and fatty acid–calcium stones. Gallstones also are classified by their location as *intrahepatic*, *gallbladder*, and *bile duct (choledocholithiasis) stones*. Intrahepatic stones are predominantly brown pigment stones. Gallbladder gallstones are mainly cholesterol stones, with a small group of black pigment stones. Bile duct stones are composed mostly of mixed cholesterol stones.

EPIDEMIOLOGY

Investigations of gallstone prevalence are more common than those of gallstone incidence because of the nature of the statistical analyses. *Prevalence* is often defined as the number of cases of gallstones at any one point or period of time divided by the population at risk of forming stones. *Incidence* is usually defined as the number of new cases of gallstones occurring in a time period divided by the population at risk of forming stones. Therefore the determination of incidence requires that investigation for

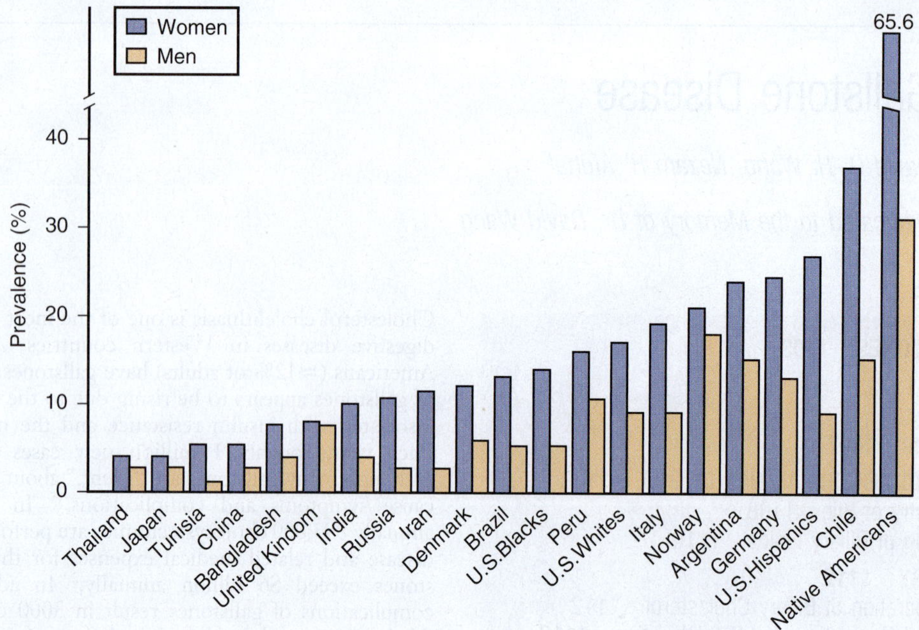

Fig. 67.1 Prevalence rates of cholesterol gallstones by gender in 18 countries based on US surveys.

gallstones be performed at a minimum of two different times—that is, at the beginning and at the end of an interval of time. By contrast, prevalence can be determined by sampling at only one point in time—for example, at ultrasound (US) screening or autopsy.

Although determining the true incidence of gallstones in a given population is not straightforward, a large study of the incidence of gallstones in the Danish population has been performed.[17] The 5-year incidence of gallstones was 0.3%, 2.9%, 2.5%, and 3.3% for Danish men, and 1.4%, 3.6%, 3.1%, and 3.7% for Danish women ages 30, 40, 50, and 60, respectively. Women have a higher incidence than men at ages 30 and 40 years, but the difference declines with increasing age. These incidence rates may reflect an interaction between genetic and environmental factors on gallstone formation in the specific populations studied because they are in accordance with estimated prevalence rates reported for Denmark and other populations.[18] In a major Italian study, the incidence of gallstones was obtained at 10 years' follow-up in an originally gallstone-free cohort in the town of Sirmione.[19] This study revealed that new cases of gallstones developed at a rate of 0.5% per year. Although age, female gender, parity, obesity, and hypertriglyceridemia were associated with gallstones in the cross-sectional prevalence study of Sirmione, multivariate analysis of risk factors for the formation of gallstones in the longitudinal study identified only age and obesity as risk factors.

Differences in the incidence of gallstone formation among different populations are striking, suggesting that genetic factors play a crucial role in the pathogenesis of cholesterol gallstones. Pathogenic factors are likely to be multifactorial and to vary among populations. Most relevant studies have found that the prevalence of gallstones in women ranges from 5% to 20% between the ages of 20 and 55 years and from 25% to 30% after the age of 50 years. The prevalence in men is approximately half that of women of the same age.

US screening or autopsy data are often used to estimate the prevalence of gallstone disease in different populations, as illustrated in Fig. 67.1. Although US screening cannot be used to distinguish cholesterol from pigment stones, 70%–80% of detected gallbladder gallstones are assumed to be cholesterol stones.

The prevalence of gallstones in American Pima Indians was investigated by oral cholecystography (OCG).[20] The well-studied Pima Indians in southern Arizona exhibit a high prevalence of gallstones, which occur in 70% of the women after the age of 25 years. Subsequently, real-time US was used for screening in nationally representative samples of Mexicans, Hispanic white Americans, non-Hispanic white Americans, and non-Hispanic black Americans of both genders ages 20–74. The cross-sectional prevalence rates of gallstones were found to be highest in certain tribes of Native Americans (e.g., Pima Indians), higher in Hispanic Americans than in whites, and lowest in black Americans.[14]

Fig. 67.2 shows the world distribution of cholesterol gallstones. American Pima Indians are an extremely high-risk population. Other high-risk populations include Native American groups in North and South America and Scandinavians, of whom 50% develop gallstones by age 50. By contrast, African populations show the lowest risk of gallstones. The prevalence of gallstones in Asian populations is intermediate. Within a given population, first-degree relatives of index cases of persons with gallstones are 4.5 times more likely to form gallstones as matched controls, thereby underscoring the importance of genetic predisposition.

Risk Factors

Age and Gender

Epidemiologic and clinical studies have found that cholesterol gallstones occur infrequently in childhood and adolescence, and the prevalence of cholesterol gallstones increases linearly with age in both genders and approaches 50% at age 70 years in women.[21,22] Furthermore, older adults are at higher risk for complications of gallstones, and mortality from surgery is often unacceptably high in patients older than 65 years. Cholesterol saturation of bile is significantly higher in older Swedes and Chilean women than in younger controls, and age correlates positively with an increased hepatic secretion rate of biliary cholesterol.[23,24] In animals, aging has been shown to be associated with increased cholesterol gallstone formation as a result of increased biliary secretion and intestinal absorption of cholesterol, decreased hepatic synthesis and secretion of bile salts, and reduced gallbladder contractility.[25]

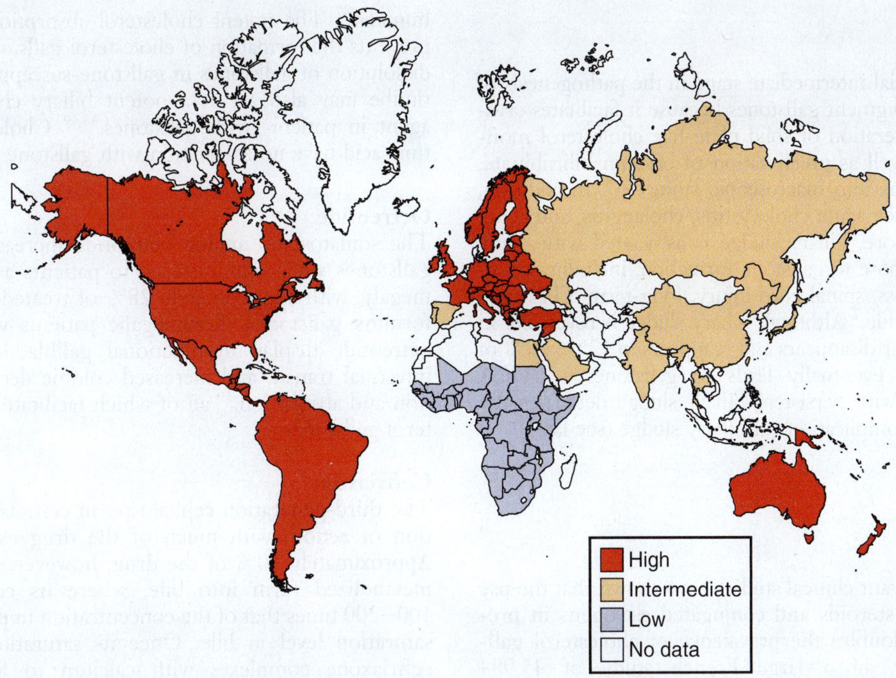

Fig. 67.2 Prevalence of cholesterol gallstones around the world. Map lines delineate study areas and do not necessarily depict accepted national boundaries.

Epidemiologic investigations have found, and clinical studies have confirmed, that at all ages, women are twice as likely as men to form cholesterol gallstones. The difference between women and men begins during puberty and continues through the childbearing years because of the effects of female sex hormones[15] and differences between the sexes in metabolism of cholesterol by the liver in response to estrogen. Human and animal studies have shown that estrogen increases the risk of cholesterol gallstones by augmenting hepatic secretion of biliary cholesterol, thereby leading to an increase in cholesterol saturation of bile.[26–29]

Diet

Epidemiologic investigations have shown that cholesterol cholelithiasis is prevalent in populations that consume a Western diet consisting of high amounts of total calories, cholesterol, saturated fatty acids, refined carbohydrates, proteins, and salt, as well as a low amount of fiber. The prevalence of cholesterol gallstone disease is significantly higher in North and South Americans as well as European populations than in Asian and African populations.[3,31] Several clinical studies have found an association between the increased incidence of cholesterol gallstones in China and Westernization of the traditional Chinese diet.[30] In Japan, cholesterol cholelithiasis was once rare, but since the 1970s, the adoption of Western-type dietary habits has led to a markedly increased incidence.[31]

Pregnancy and Parity

Pregnancy is a risk factor for the development of biliary sludge and gallstones.[32] During pregnancy, bile becomes more lithogenic because of a significant increase in estrogen levels, which results in increased hepatic cholesterol secretion and supersaturated bile. In addition, gallbladder motility is impaired, with a resulting increase in gallbladder volume and bile stasis. These alterations promote the formation of sludge and stones in the gallbladder.[33] Increased progestogen concentrations also reduce gallbladder motility. Because plasma concentrations of sex hormones, especially estrogen, increase linearly with duration of gestation, the risk of gallstone formation is high in the third trimester of pregnancy. Increasing parity is probably a risk factor for gallstones, especially in younger women.

Rapid Weight Loss

Rapid weight loss is a well-known risk factor for the formation of cholesterol gallstones.[34] As many as 50% of obese patients who undergo gastric bypass surgery form biliary sludge and eventually gallstones within 6 months after surgery. Gallstones also develop in 25% of patients who undergo strict dietary restriction. Furthermore, about 40% of these patients display symptoms related to gallstones within the same 6-month period. The mechanisms by which rapid weight loss causes gallstone formation include enhanced hepatic secretion of biliary cholesterol during caloric restriction, increased production of mucin by the gallbladder, and impaired gallbladder motility. Gallstones may be prevented in this high-risk population by prophylactic administration of UDCA, which, in a dose of 600 mg/day, has been reported to reduce the prevalence of gallstones from 28% to 3% in obese patients on a very-low-calorie diet (see later).[35]

TPN

TPN is associated with the development of cholelithiasis and acalculous cholecystitis. As early as 3 weeks after initiation of TPN, biliary sludge often forms in the gallbladder because of prolonged fasting. In addition, the sphincter of Oddi may fail to relax, leading to preferential flow of bile into the gallbladder. Approximately 45% of adults and 43% of children form gallstones after 3–4 months of TPN.[36,37] Because patients who receive TPN often have serious medical problems and are not good candidates for abdominal surgery, prophylactic treatment to prevent gallstones should be prescribed if no contraindication exists. CCK octapeptide administered twice daily via an IV line to patients on long-term TPN has proved to be safe and cost-effective[38] and should be used routinely in TPN-treated patients.

Biliary Sludge

Biliary sludge is a crucial intermediate stage in the pathogenesis of both cholesterol and pigment gallstones because it facilitates crystallization and agglomeration of solid plate-like cholesterol monohydrate crystals, as well as precipitation of calcium bilirubinate, and ultimately develops into macroscopic stones.[39,40] In addition, biliary sludge can induce acute cholecystitis, cholangitis, and acute pancreatitis. Furthermore, biliary sludge is associated with many conditions that predispose to gallstone formation, including pregnancy, rapid weight loss, spinal cord injury, long-term TPN, and treatment with octreotide.[3] Although biliary sludge is reversible in most cases, it persists or disappears and reappears in 12%–20% of affected persons and eventually leads to gallstones.[41] UDCA treatment of patients with persistent biliary sludge decreases the frequency of clinical complications of biliary sludge (see later).

Drugs

Estrogens

Most, but not all, relevant clinical studies have shown that the use of oral contraceptive steroids and conjugated estrogens in premenopausal women doubles the prevalence of cholesterol gallstones.[15,42] Moreover, in a large French study of 45,984 postmenopausal women, use of hormone replacement therapy was associated with an increased risk of cholecystectomy [hazard ratio (HR), 1.10]; the increase in risk was limited to women who received unopposed estrogen (HR, 1.38).[43]

Administration of estrogen to postmenopausal women and estrogen therapy to men with prostatic carcinoma has similar lithogenic effects.[42,44] Therefore estrogen has been proposed to be an important risk factor for the formation of cholesterol gallstones. In mice, the hepatic estrogen receptor α, but not β, plays a crucial role in cholesterol gallstone formation in response to estrogen.[28] The hepatic estrogen receptor α, which is activated by estrogen, interferes with the negative feedback regulation of cholesterol biosynthesis by stimulating the sterol-regulatory element binding protein-2 (SREBP-2) pathway, with the resulting activation of the SREBP-2–responsive genes in the cholesterol biosynthetic pathway.[29] These alterations lead to increased hepatic secretion of newly synthesized cholesterol and supersaturation of bile, thereby predisposing to precipitation of solid cholesterol monohydrate crystals and formation of gallstones. Moreover, genetic analysis in mice reveals that the G protein–coupled receptor 30 (GPR30), a novel estrogen receptor, is a gallstone gene named *Lith18*. GPR30 exerts a synergistic lithogenic action with estrogen receptor α to enhance estrogen-induced gallstone formation.[45] In addition, estrogen induces a decrease in plasma LDL cholesterol levels and an increase in plasma HDL cholesterol concentrations. The decrease in plasma LDL levels is a result of increased expression of the hepatic LDL receptor, which increases the clearance of plasma LDL. The increased uptake of LDL by the liver may also result in increased secretion of cholesterol into bile. High levels of estrogen may induce gallbladder hypomotility and consequently bile stasis.

Lipid-Lowering Drugs

Lipid-lowering drugs may influence the formation of gallstones because they regulate key pathways in cholesterol and bile salt metabolism. Clofibrate is a lipid-lowering drug associated with gallstone formation. Clofibrate induces cholesterol supersaturation in bile and diminishes bile salt concentrations by reducing the activity of cholesterol 7α-hydroxylase (the rate-limiting enzyme in the classical pathway of bile salt synthesis) (see Chapter 66).[46] The 3-hydroxy-3-methylglutaryl coenzyme A (HMG-CoA) reductase inhibitors (statins) reduce the biliary cholesterol saturation index (CSI), but their role in the prevention or therapy of gallstone disease requires further investigation in humans.[47] The potent cholesterol absorption inhibitor ezetimibe prevents the formation of cholesterol gallstones and facilitates the dissolution of gallstones in gallstone-susceptible C57L mice. Ezetimibe may also act as a potent biliary cholesterol-desaturating agent in patients with gallstones.[48,49] Cholestyramine and nicotinic acid have no association with gallstone formation.

Octreotide

The somatostatin analog octreotide increases the prevalence of gallstones when administered to patients as treatment for acromegaly, with approximately 28% of treated acromegalic patients forming gallstones. Acromegalic patients who are treated with octreotide display dysfunctional gallbladder motility, sluggish intestinal transit, and increased colonic deoxycholic acid formation and absorption,[50] all of which facilitate formation of cholesterol gallstones.

Ceftriaxone

The third-generation cephalosporin ceftriaxone has a long duration of action, with much of the drug excreted in the urine. Approximately 40% of the drug, however, is secreted in an unmetabolized form into bile, where its concentration reaches 100–200 times that of the concentration in plasma and exceeds its saturation level in bile. Once its saturation level is exceeded, ceftriaxone complexes with calcium to form insoluble salts, thereby resulting in formation of biliary sludge. Up to 43% of children who receive high doses of ceftriaxone (60–100 mg/kg/day) have been reported to form biliary sludge, and about 19% of these patients experience biliary symptoms.[51] The sludge usually disappears after ceftriaxone is discontinued.

Glucagon-like peptide receptor-1 Agonists (GLP1-RA)

GLP1-RA utilization for diabetes and more recently obesity has increased over the last few years. Several clinical trials suggested a higher rate of gallbladder events in patients randomized to GLP1-RA versus placebo.[322–324].

This initial finding was recently confirmed in a meta-analysis of 76 randomized controlled trials involving 103,371 patients (mean [SD] age, 57.8 (6.2) years; 41 868 [40.5%] women). GLP1-RA treatment was associated with increased risk of gallbladder or biliary diseases (RR, 1.37; 95% CI, 1.23–1.52), specifically, cholelithiasis (RR, 1.27; 95% CI, 1.10–1.47), cholecystitis (RR, 1.36; 95% CI, 1.14–1.62), and biliary disease (RR, 1.55; 95% CI, 1.08–2.22). Both higher doses and longer duration of treatment were associated with increased risk of biliary disease.[325]

Farnesoid X Receptor Agonists (FXR agonists)

The FXR agonist obeticholic acid (OCA) is approved for the treatment of primary biliary cholangitis and is under clinical investigation for metabolic dysfunction-associated steatotic liver disease (MASLD). In a recent clinical report,[326] subjects were administered OCA for 3 weeks prior to scheduled cholecystectomy. The study showed that OCA increased the CSI, increased the gallbladder bile hydrophobicity index, and decreased cholesterol solubility. Taken together, this combination of biophysical changes increases the lithogenicity of bile and promotes gallstone or bile stone/sludge formation.

This increase in lithogenic bile resulted in an increased incidence of gallstone or bile duct stones/sludge and related complications observed in the OCA-treated subjects relative to placebo. Events of gallstones and bile duct sludge/stones led to more invasive procedures, including cholecystectomy and endoscopic retrograde cholangiopancreatography (ERCP) in the OCA-treated subjects relative to placebo-treated subjects.

Lipid Abnormalities

Epidemiologic investigations have shown that plasma HDL cholesterol levels are inversely correlated with the prevalence of cholesterol gallstones.[52] By contrast, hypertriglyceridemia is positively associated with an increased prevalence of gallstones.[53] These seemingly independent variables are actually interrelated because high plasma TG levels tend to increase with increasing body mass and are inversely correlated with plasma HDL levels. Interestingly, high plasma total and LDL cholesterol levels are not likely to be risk factors for the formation of gallstones.

Systemic Diseases

Obesity and Insulin Resistance

Obesity is a well-known risk factor for cholelithiasis, and the prevalence of gallstones is rising with the worldwide obesity epidemic and the increasing incidence of insulin resistance.[54,55] A large prospective study of obese women demonstrated a strong linear association between body mass index (BMI) and the prevalence of cholelithiasis.[56] In this study, the risk of gallstones was sevenfold higher in women with the highest BMI (>45 kg/m^2) than in nonobese control women. Obesity is associated with increased hepatic secretion of cholesterol into bile, possibly because of higher enzymatic activity of HMG-CoA reductase and increased cholesterol synthesis in the liver. As a result, gallbladder bile is more lithogenic in obese than in nonobese persons, and a higher ratio of cholesterol to solubilizing lipids (bile acids and phospholipids) is observed in the former group. These alterations predispose to cholesterol crystallization and gallstone formation. Gallbladder motility is often impaired in obese persons, thereby promoting mucin secretion and accumulation, as well as cholesterol crystallization. The effect of pronucleating and antinucleating factors on cholesterol crystallization and gallstone formation in gallbladder bile warrants further investigation in both obese and nonobese subjects.

Diabetes Mellitus

Patients with diabetes mellitus have long been considered to be at increased risk of developing gallstones because hypertriglyceridemia and obesity are associated with diabetes mellitus and because gallbladder motility is often impaired in patients with diabetes mellitus.[57] Proving that diabetes mellitus is an independent risk factor for gallstones has been difficult, however. Mice with hepatic insulin resistance induced by liver-specific disruption of the insulin receptor are markedly predisposed to formation of cholesterol gallstones.[58] Hepatic insulin resistance promotes hepatic secretion of biliary cholesterol by increasing expression of the hepatic cholesterol transporters Abcg5 and Abcg8 through the forkhead transcription factor FoxO1 pathway. Insulin resistance also reduces expression of the bile salt synthetic enzymes, particularly oxysterol 7α-hydroxylase, thereby resulting in a lithogenic bile salt profile.

Diseases of the Ileum

Disease or resection of the terminal ileum has been found to be a risk factor for gallstone formation. For example, intestinal bile salt absorption is often impaired in patients with Crohn disease, who are at increased risk of gallstones.[59] The loss of specific bile salt transporters [e.g., ileal apical sodium-dependent bile acid transporter (ASBT)] in the terminal ileum may result in excessive bile salt excretion in feces and a diminished bile salt pool size, presumably with a consequent increase in the risk of cholesterol gallstones. These changes may also lead to the formation of pigment gallstones because increased bile salt delivery to the colon enhances the solubilization of unconjugated bilirubin, thereby increasing bilirubin concentrations in bile.[60]

Spinal Cord Injuries

Spinal cord injuries are associated with a high prevalence of gallstones, which have been reported in some 31% of such patients, who have an annual rate of biliary complications of 2.2%. Although the complication rate associated with gallstones in patients with spinal cord injuries is at least twofold higher than the rate of gallstones in the general population, the relative risk is still low enough that prophylactic cholecystectomy is probably not justified. The mechanisms responsible for the association between spinal cord injuries and gallstone formation remain unclear. Gallbladder relaxation is impaired in these patients, but gallbladder contraction in response to a meal is normal. Therefore the increased risk of gallstones is unlikely to be due to biliary stasis alone.

Metabolic-Associated Steatotic Liver Disease (Formerly Known as NAFLD)

Both gallstone disease and MASLD are highly prevalent in the general population and often coexist in the same populations (see Chapter 89). These epidemiologic and clinical studies raise the possibility that both disorders could be causally related or that similar risk factors influence the natural history of MASLD and gallstone disease. Although many clinical studies have investigated the association between MASLD and gallstone disease, the results have been variable.[61–66] The relationship among insulin resistance (evaluated with the homeostatic model assessment), liver fibrosis, MASH, and gallstone disease has been studied in morbidly obese patients with MASLD before bariatric surgery.[65] The prevalence of MASH is 18% in a morbid obese population with gallbladder disease. The third large U.S. National Health and Nutrition Examination Survey (NHANES) between 1988 and 1994 investigated 12,232 subjects by US and reported an association between gallstone disease, with a prevalence of 7.4% for gallstones and 5.6% for cholecystectomy, and MASLD, with a prevalence of 20.0%.[61] The prevalence of MASLD was significantly higher in the group that underwent cholecystectomy (48.4%) and in the gallstone group (34.4%) than in the gallstone-free group (17.9%). These findings suggest that both conditions are tightly associated with metabolic disturbances such as obesity, insulin resistance, dyslipidemia, and the metabolic syndrome.

Celiac Disease

Celiac disease is a chronic, small intestinal, autoimmune enteropathy caused by an intolerance to dietary gluten in genetically predisposed individuals (see Chapter 109). Clinical studies have found that, because of defective CCK release from the proximal small intestine caused by enteropathy in patients with celiac disease before they start a gluten-free diet, gallbladder emptying in response to a fatty meal is impaired.[65–70] Lack of CCK markedly enhances susceptibility to cholesterol gallstones via a mechanism involving dysmotility of both the gallbladder and the small intestine.[71] Because a gluten-free diet can significantly improve celiac enteropathy, early diagnosis and therapy in celiac patients is crucial for preventing the long-term impact of CCK deficiency on biliary and intestinal function. When gluten is reintroduced in the diet, clinical and histologic relapse often occurs in patients with celiac disease. Moreover, some patients do not respond well to a gluten-free diet. Patients with celiac disease should routinely undergo US to determine whether gallbladder motility function is preserved and whether biliary sludge (a precursor to gallstones) is present in the gallbladder. Impaired intestinal CCK secretion is the link between celiac disease and cholesterol gallstone disease.[72] Because neither epidemiologic investigations of gallstone prevalence rates in patients with celiac disease nor clinical studies of the impact of celiac disease on the pathogenesis of gallstones have been reported, whether celiac disease is an independent risk factor for gallstone disease remains largely unknown.

Protective Factors

Statins

Use of statins has been associated with a decreased risk of gallstone disease in two large case-control studies. The first study compared 27,035 patients with gallstone disease who required cholecystectomy with 106,531 matched controls and showed a benefit to long-term statin use (>20 prescriptions filled and use of statins for >1.5 years)[73]; statin use was associated with a decreased risk of gallstone disease requiring cholecystectomy [adjusted odds ratio (OR), 0.64]. Similar results were observed in a population study from Denmark of 32,494 patients with gallstone disease matched with 324,925 controls.[74] The ORs of having gallstone disease in current and prior users of statins (>20 prescriptions filled) were 0.76 and 0.79, respectively, compared with controls.

Ascorbic Acid

The observation that deficiency of ascorbic acid (vitamin C) is associated with the development of gallstones in guinea pigs prompted investigation of the relationship between ascorbic acid levels and gallstones in humans. Serum ascorbic acid levels have been correlated with clinical or asymptomatic gallstones in 7042 women and 6088 men who were enrolled in the third NHANES.[75] Among women, but not men, each standard deviation increase in serum ascorbic acid levels was associated with a 13% lower prevalence rate of clinical gallbladder disease.

Coffee

In a 10-year follow-up of 46,000 male health professionals, subjects who consistently drank 2 to 3 cups of regular coffee per day were approximately 40% less likely to develop symptomatic gallstones.[76] Drinking 4 or more cups per day was even more beneficial (relative risk 0.55), but there was no benefit to drinking decaffeinated coffee. A similar benefit to regular coffee was noted in a cohort study involving 81,000 women.[77]

COMPOSITION AND ABNORMALITIES OF BILE

Physical Chemistry of Bile

Chemical Composition of Bile

Cholesterol, phospholipids, and bile salts are the three major lipid species in bile, and bile pigments are minor solutes. Cholesterol accounts for up to 95% of the sterols in bile and gallstones; the remaining 5% of the sterols are cholesterol precursors and dietary sterols from plant and shellfish sources.

Concentrations of cholesteryl esters are negligible in bile and account for less than 0.02% of total sterols in gallstones. The major phospholipids are lecithins (phosphatidylcholines), which account for more than 95% of total phospholipids; the remainder consists of cephalins (phosphatidylethanolamines) and a trace amount of sphingomyelin. Phospholipids constitute 15%–25% of total lipids in bile. Lecithins are insoluble amphiphilic molecules with a hydrophilic zwitterionic phosphocholine head group and hydrophobic tails that include two long fatty acyl chains. Biliary lecithins possess a saturated C-16 acyl chain in the *sn*-1 position and an unsaturated C-18 or C-20 acyl chain in the *sn*-2 position. The major molecular species of lecithins (with corresponding frequencies) in bile are 16:0–18:2 (40%–60%), 16:0–18:1 (5%–25%), 18:0–18:2 (1%–16%), and 16:0–20:4 (1%–10%). Lecithins are synthesized principally in the endoplasmic reticulum of the hepatocyte from diacylglycerols through the cytidine diphosphate-choline pathway. The common bile salts typically contain a steroid nucleus of four fused hydrocarbon rings with polar hydroxyl functions and an aliphatic side chain conjugated in amide linkage with glycine or taurine. In bile, more than 95% of bile salts are 5β,C-24 hydroxylated acidic steroids that are amide-linked to glycine or taurine in an approximate ratio of 3:1. Bile salts constitute approximately two-thirds of the solute mass of normal human bile by weight. The hydrophilic (polar) areas constitute approximately of bile salts are the hydroxyl groups and conjugated side chain of either glycine or taurine, and the hydrophobic (nonpolar) area is the ringed steroid nucleus. Because they possess both hydrophilic and hydrophobic surfaces, bile salts are highly soluble, detergent-like, amphiphilic molecules. Their high aqueous solubility is due to their capacity to self-assemble into micelles when a critical micellar concentration is exceeded.

The primary bile salts are hepatic catabolic products of cholesterol and are composed of cholate (a trihydroxy bile salt) and chenodeoxycholate (a dihydroxy bile salt) (see Chapter 66). The secondary bile salts are derived from the primary bile salt species by the action of intestinal bacteria in the ileum and colon and include deoxycholate, ursodeoxycholate, and lithocholate. The most important of the conversion reactions is 7α-dehydroxylation of primary bile salts to produce deoxycholate from cholate and lithocholate from chenodoxycholate. Another important conversion reaction is the 7α-dehydrogenation of chenodeoxycholate to form 7α-oxo-lithocholate. This bile salt does not accumulate in bile but is metabolized by hepatic or bacterial reduction to form the tertiary bile salt chenodeoxycholate (mainly in the liver) or its 7β-epimer ursodeoxycholate (primarily by bacteria in the colon).

Bile pigments are minor solutes and are formed as a metabolic product of certain porphyrins. They account for roughly 0.5% of total lipids in bile by weight. They are mainly bilirubin conjugates with traces of porphyrins and unconjugated bilirubin. Bilirubin can be conjugated with a molecule of glucuronic acid, which makes it soluble in water. In human bile, bilirubin monoglucuronides and diglucuronides are the major bile pigments. Other bile pigments are monoconjugates and diconjugates of xylose, glucose, and glucuronic acid and various homoconjugates and heteroconjugates of them.

Proteins and inorganic salts are also found in bile. Albumin appears to be the most abundant protein in bile, followed by immunoglobulins G and M, apolipoproteins AI, AII, B, CI, and CII, transferrin, and α_2-macroglobin. Other proteins that have been identified but not quantitated in bile include EGF, insulin, haptoglobin, CCK, lysosomal hydrolase, and amylase. Inorganic salts detected in bile include sodium, phosphorus, potassium, calcium, copper, zinc, iron, manganese, molybdenum, magnesium, and strontium.

Physical States of Biliary Lipids

Cholesterol is nearly insoluble in water, and the mechanism by which cholesterol is solubilized in bile is complex because bile is an aqueous solution. The two main types of macromolecular aggregates in bile are *micelles* and *vesicles*, which greatly enhance the solubilization of cholesterol in bile.

Bile salts are soluble in an aqueous solution because they are amphiphilic, in that they have both hydrophilic and hydrophobic areas. This unique property of bile salts is dependent on the number and characteristics of the hydroxyl groups and side chains, as well as the composition of the particular aqueous solution. When bile salt concentrations exceed the critical micellar concentration, their monomers can spontaneously aggregate to form *simple micelles*. The simple micelles (≈3 nm in diameter) are small, disk-like, and thermodynamically stable aggregates that can solubilize cholesterol. They can also solubilize and incorporate phospholipids to form *mixed micelles* that are capable of solubilizing at least triple the amount of cholesterol compared with that solubilized by simple micelles. Mixed micelles (4–8 nm in diameter) are large, thermodynamically stable aggregates composed of bile salts, phospholipids, and cholesterol. Their size depends on the relative proportion of bile salts and phospholipids. The mixed micelle is a lipid bilayer with the hydrophilic groups of the bile salts and phospholipids aligned on the "outside" of the bilayer, interfacing with the aqueous bile, and the hydrophobic groups on the "inside." Therefore cholesterol molecules can be solubilized on the inside of the bilayer away from the aqueous areas on the outside. The amount of cholesterol that can be solubilized is dependent on the relative proportions of bile salts, and the maximal solubility of cholesterol occurs when the molar ratio of phospholipids to bile salts is between 0.2 and 0.3. Furthermore, the solubility of cholesterol in mixed micelles is enhanced when the concentration of total lipids in bile is increased.

When model and native biles are examined by quasielastic light-scattering spectroscopy and electron microscopy, it is found that, besides micelles, vesicles solubilize cholesterol in bile. Biliary vesicles are unilamellar spherical structures that contain phospholipids, cholesterol, and little if any bile salts. Vesicles are substantially larger than either simple or mixed micelles (40–100 nm in diameter) but much smaller than liquid crystals ($\approx$500 nm in diameter) that are composed of multilamellar spherical structures. Because vesicles are present in large quantities in hepatic bile, they could be secreted by hepatocytes. Unilamellar vesicles are often detected in freshly collected samples of unsaturated bile and are physically indistinguishable from those identified in supersaturated bile. Dilute hepatic bile, in which solid cholesterol crystals and gallstones never form, is always supersaturated with cholesterol because vesicles solubilize biliary cholesterol in excess of what could be solubilized in mixed micelles. Cholesterol-rich vesicles are remarkably stable in dilute bile, consistent with the absence of cholesterol crystallization in hepatic bile. The unilamellar vesicles can fuse and form large multilamellar vesicles (also known as *liposomes* or *liquid crystals*). Solid cholesterol monohydrate crystals may nucleate from multilamellar vesicles in concentrated gallbladder bile.

Vesicles are relatively static structures that are affected by several factors, including biliary lipid concentrations and the relative ratios of cholesterol, phospholipids, and bile salts. The relative concentrations of these three important lipids in bile are influenced by their hepatic secretion rates, which vary with fasting and feeding. For example, during the fasting period, hepatic output of biliary bile salts is relatively low. As a result, the ratio of cholesterol to bile salts is increased, and more cholesterol is carried in vesicles than in micelles. By contrast, with feeding, hepatic output of biliary bile salts is increased, and more cholesterol is solubilized in micelles than in vesicles. In addition, when the concentration of bile salts is relatively low, especially in dilute hepatic bile, vesicles are relatively stable, and only some vesicles are converted to micelles. By contrast, with increasing bile salt concentrations in concentrated gallbladder bile, vesicles may be converted completely into mixed micelles. Because relatively more phospholipids than cholesterol can be transferred from vesicles to mixed micelles, the residual vesicles are remodeled and may be enriched in cholesterol relative to phospholipids. If the remaining vesicles have a relatively low ratio ($<$1) of cholesterol to phospholipids, they are relatively stable, but if the ratio of cholesterol to phospholipids in vesicles is greater than 1, vesicles become increasingly unstable. These cholesterol-rich vesicles may transfer some cholesterol to less cholesterol-rich vesicles or to micelles or may fuse or aggregate to form larger ($\approx$500 nm in diameter) multilamellar vesicles (i.e., liposomes or liquid crystals). Liquid crystals are often visible by polarizing light microscopy as lipid circular droplets with characteristic birefringence in the shape of a Maltese cross. Liquid crystals are inherently unstable and may form solid plate-like cholesterol monohydrate crystals, a process termed *cholesterol nucleation*. Therefore nucleation of cholesterol monohydrate crystal results in a decrease in the amount of cholesterol contained in vesicles but not in micelles, and vesicles may serve as the primary source of cholesterol for nucleation.

Under normal physiologic conditions, bile is concentrated gradually within the biliary tract so that the bile salt concentration approaches its critical micellar concentration. When this occurs, bile salts begin to modify the structure of phospholipid-rich vesicles that are secreted into bile by hepatocytes. These interactions signify the start of a complex series of molecular rearrangements that ultimately lead to formation of simple and mixed micelles. In supersaturated bile, two pathways result in formation of cholesterol-rich vesicles from phospholipid-rich vesicles at the canalicular membrane of hepatocyte. Because bile salts solubilize phospholipids more efficiently than cholesterol, cholesterol-rich vesicles may form when bile salts preferentially extract phospholipid molecules directly from phospholipid-rich vesicles. The alternative pathway is the rapid dissolution of phospholipid-rich vesicles by bile salts with the production of unstable mixed micelles that contain excess cholesterol. Structural rearrangements of these unstable micellar particles result in the formation of cholesterol-rich vesicles.

Phase Diagrams and Cholesterol Solubility in Bile

In the 1960s Small et al. defined the maximal solubility (saturation) limits for cholesterol in model quaternary bile systems that consisted of varying proportions of cholesterol, phospholipids, bile salts, and water.[78–80] The relative proportions (as molar percentages) of the three lipids in bile play a critical role in determining the maximal solubility of cholesterol. When the relative proportions of the three lipids at a fixed total lipid concentration are plotted in a triangular coordinate, the solubility of cholesterol for any given solute concentration can be determined.[75] The triangular coordinate diagram also illustrates the physical phases of cholesterol in bile. For example, the phase diagram shown in Fig. 67.3 is specific for a total lipid concentration of 7.5 g/dL, which is typical of human gallbladder bile.[81,82] For hepatic bile, with a typical total lipid concentration of 3 g/dL, the phase boundaries would be different, with a smaller micellar zone, all phase boundaries shifted to the left, and an expanded 2-phase zone on the right (i.e., region E in Fig. 67.3). The effect of total lipid concentration on cholesterol solubilization in the micellar zone explains why hepatic bile tends to be more saturated with cholesterol than is gallbladder bile in the same subject. Because hepatic bile contains a large number of cholesterol-phospholipid vesicles that are relatively stable, solid plate-like cholesterol monohydrate crystals never occur in hepatic bile.

Equilibrium phase diagrams can also be used to predict the phases in which solid cholesterol crystals can be found at equilibrium.[9] Although the equilibration process starts after hepatic bile is secreted from hepatocytes and flows into the biliary tract, the evolution to cholesterol monohydrate crystals occurs only in gallbladder bile. For example, in unsaturated bile, all cholesterol can be solubilized in both simple and mixed micelles, and relative biliary lipid compositions are located in the micellar zone of the phase diagram. By contrast, in supersaturated bile, cholesterol cannot be completely solubilized by simple and mixed micelles, and relative biliary lipid compositions are located outside the micellar zone of the phase diagram. Under these circumstances, high vesicular cholesterol concentrations and high total lipid concentrations in bile can work together to produce the solid crystalline phase. Therefore with typical physiologic lipid ratios, at equilibrium, cholesterol monohydrate crystals are present with saturated simple and mixed micelles or with saturated micelles plus vesicles that have become multilamellar liquid crystals. The final physical state of bile is also influenced by the ratio of the concentration of bile salts to that of phospholipids and the overall hydrophilic-hydrophobic balance of both bile salt and phospholipid species.

Within the micellar zone (see Fig. 67.3), bile is a visually clear, stable solution that is considered *unsaturated* because all cholesterol can be solubilized in thermodynamically stable simple and mixed micelles. At the boundary line of the micellar zone, bile is *saturated* because all the solubilizing capacity for cholesterol is used, and no further cholesterol can be carried in micelles.

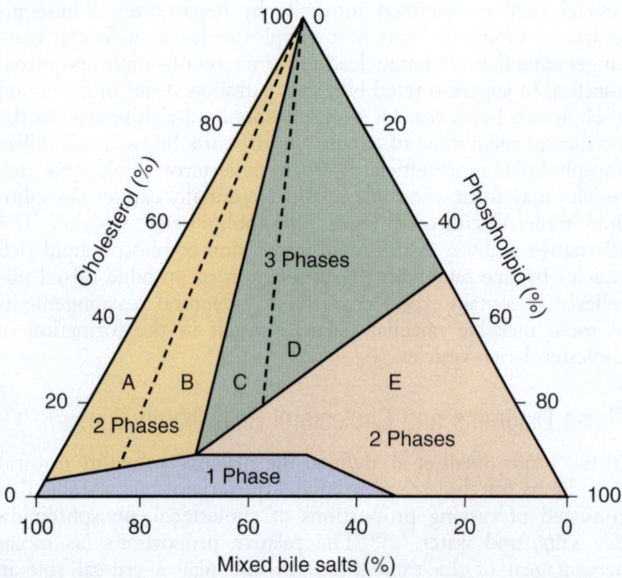

Fig. 67.3 Equilibrium phase diagram of a cholesterol–phospholipid (lecithin)–mixed bile salt system (37°C, 0.15 M NaCl, pH 7.0, total lipid concentration 7.5 g/dL) showing positions and configuration of crystallization regions. Components are expressed in moles percent. The 1-phase micellar zone at the bottom is enclosed by a *solid angulated line*, and above it, two *solid lines* divide the 2-phase zones from a central 3-phase zone. Based on the solid and liquid crystallization sequences present in the bile, the left 2-phase and central 3-phase regions are divided by *dashed lines* into regions A–D. The number of phases represents the equilibrium state. The phases are cholesterol monohydrate crystals and saturated micelles for crystallization regions A and B; cholesterol monohydrate crystals, saturated micelles, and liquid crystals for regions C and D; and liquid crystals of variable composition and saturated micelles for region E. Of note is that decreases in temperature (37°C → 4°C), total lipid concentration (7.5 g/dL → 2.5 g/dL), and bile salt hydrophobicity (3α,12α→3α,7α→3α,7α,12α→3α,7β-hydroxylated taurine conjugates) progressively shift all crystallization pathways to lower phospholipid contents, retard crystallization, and reduce micellar cholesterol solubilities. These changes generate a series of new condensed-phase diagrams with an enlarged region E. (Reproduced with permission from Wang DQ, Carey MC. Complete mapping of crystallization pathways during cholesterol precipitation from model bile: influence of physical-chemical variables of pathophysiologic relevance and identification of a stable liquid crystalline state in cold, dilute, and hydrophilic bile salt–containing systems. *J Lipid Res.* 1996;37:606–630.)

Outside the micellar zone, bile is *supersaturated* because excess cholesterol cannot be solubilized by micelles[80,83] and exists in more than 1 phase (micelles, liquid crystals, and solid monohydrate crystals); the solution is visually cloudy. Obviously, relatively stable unilamellar cholesterol-phospholipid vesicles solubilize a significant proportion of cholesterol outside the micellar zone. The term *metastable zone* refers to the area in the phase diagram (above but near the micellar zone) in which bile is supersaturated with cholesterol but may not form solid cholesterol monohydrate crystals even after many days. The diagram also suggests that when the quantity of cholesterol in bile exceeds that which can be solubilized by the available bile salts and phospholipids, solid plate-like cholesterol monohydrate crystals precipitate in bile. Furthermore, the proportional distance outside the micellar zone directed along an axis joined to the cholesterol apex is often calculated as the CSI (or lithogenic index).[83] Therefore the degree of saturation of bile with cholesterol can be quantitated. A CSI for a sample of bile can be estimated directly from the diagram or calculated by using a formula. The CSI is the ratio of the actual amount of cholesterol present in a bile sample to the maximal amount of cholesterol that can be dissolved in it. Bile that has a CSI of 1 is saturated; bile with a saturation index less than 1 is unsaturated; and bile with a saturation index greater than 1 is supersaturated. The degree of saturation can also be expressed as percent saturation by multiplying the saturation index by 100. For example, at the boundary of the micellar zone, bile is saturated, and the CSI is 100%. Supersaturated bile has a CSI above 100%, and unsaturated bile has a CSI below 100%. The CSI values are also useful for predicting the proportion of lipid particles and the metastable and equilibrium physical states in bile.

Hepatic Secretion of Biliary Lipids

Source of Lipids Secreted in Bile

The supply of hepatic cholesterol molecules that can be recruited for biliary secretion depends on the balance of input and output of cholesterol and its metabolism in the liver (Fig. 67.4) (see also Chapters 66 and 74). Input is related to the amount of cholesterol (both unesterified and esterified) taken up by the liver from plasma lipoproteins (LDL > HDL > chylomicron remnants) plus de novo hepatic cholesterol synthesis. Output is related to the amount of cholesterol disposed of within the liver by conversion to cholesteryl ester (to form new VLDL and for storage) minus the amount of cholesterol converted to primary bile salts. An appreciable fraction of cholesterol in bile may also be derived from the diet via apolipoprotein E–dependent delivery of chylomicron remnants to the liver. Under low or no dietary cholesterol conditions, bile contains newly synthesized cholesterol from the liver and preformed cholesterol that reaches the liver in several different ways. Approximately 20% of the cholesterol in bile comes from de novo hepatic biosynthesis, and 80% is from pools of preformed cholesterol within the liver. De novo cholesterol synthesis in the liver uses acetate as a substrate and is mainly regulated by the rate-limited enzyme HMG-CoA reductase. This enzyme can be up- or downregulated depending on the overall cholesterol balance in the liver. An increase in the activity of this rate-limiting enzyme leads to excessive cholesterol secretion in bile. The major sources of preformed cholesterol are hepatic uptake of plasma lipoproteins (mainly HDL and LDL through their receptors on the basolateral membrane of hepatocytes). Consistent with their central role in reverse cholesterol transport, HDL particles are the main lipoprotein source of cholesterol that is targeted for biliary secretion. Under conditions of a high cholesterol diet, dietary cholesterol reaches the liver through the intestinal lymphatic pathway as chylomicrons and then chylomicron remnants, after chylomicrons are hydrolyzed by plasma lipoprotein lipase and hepatic lipase. The synthesis of new cholesterol in the liver is reduced and comprises only about 5% of biliary cholesterol. Overall, the liver can systematically regulate the total amount of cholesterol within it, and any excess cholesterol is handled efficiently.

Although biliary phospholipid is derived from the cell membranes of hepatocytes, the composition of biliary phospholipid differs markedly from that of hepatocyte membranes. The membranes of hepatocytes contain phosphatidylcholines (lecithins), phosphatidylethanolamines, phosphatidylinositols, phosphatidylserines, and sphingomyelins. The major source of phosphatidylcholine molecules destined for secretion into bile is hepatic synthesis. A fraction of biliary phosphatidylcholines may also originate in the phospholipid coat of HDL particles. From 10 to 15 g of phospholipids are secreted into bile each day in humans.

More than 95% of bile salt molecules, after secretion into bile, return to the liver through the enterohepatic circulation by absorption mostly from the distal ileum via an active transport

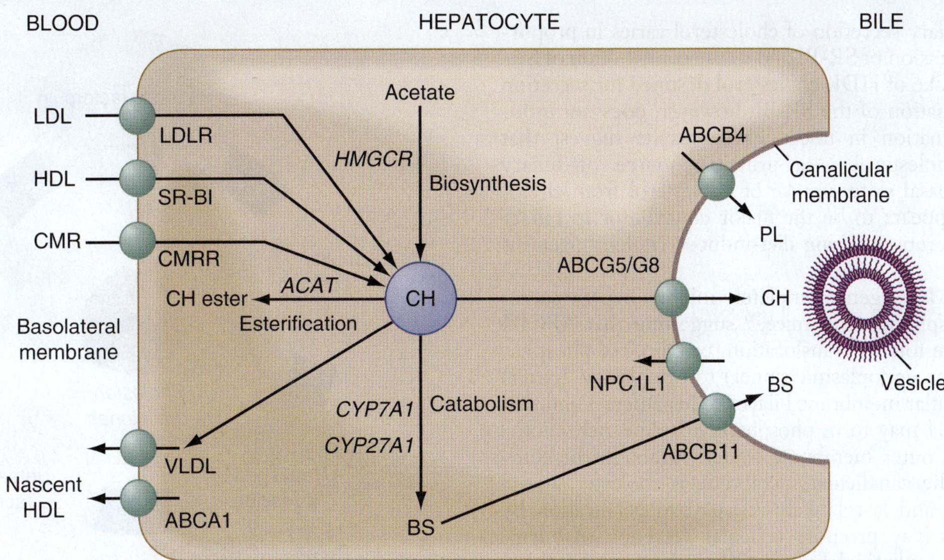

Fig. 67.4 Uptake, biosynthesis, catabolism, and biliary secretion of cholesterol at the hepatocyte level. Hepatic uptake of cholesterol is mediated by the *LDL* receptor (*LDLR*), by scavenger receptor class B type I (*SR-BI*) for HDL, and by the chylomicron remnant receptor (*CMRR*) for chylomicron remnants (*CMR*). Biosynthesis of hepatic cholesterol (*CH*) from acetate is regulated by the rate-limiting enzyme 3-hydroxy-3-methylglutaryl-coenzyme A reductase (*HMGCR*). Part of the cholesterol is esterified by acyl-coenzyme A:cholesterol acyltransferase (*ACAT*) for storage in the liver. Some of the cholesterol is used for the formation of *VLDL*, which is secreted into the blood. The ABC transporter *ABCA1* may translocate, either directly or indirectly, cholesterol and phospholipids to the cell surface, where they appear to form lipid domains that interact with amphipathic α-helices in apolipoproteins. This interaction solubilizes these lipids and generates nascent HDL particles that dissociate from the cell. A proportion of cholesterol is used for synthesis of bile salts (*BS*) via the classical and alterative pathways, as regulated by two rate-limiting enzymes, cholesterol 7α-hydroxylase (*CYP7A1*) and sterol 27-hydroxylase (*CYP27A1*), respectively. Hepatic secretion of biliary cholesterol, bile salts, and phospholipids (*PL*) across the canalicular membrane is determined by three lipid transporters, *ABCG5/G8*, *ABCB11*, and *ABCB4*, respectively. The Niemann-Pick C1-like 1 (*NPC1L1*) protein may have a weak role in taking cholesterol back from hepatic bile to the hepatocyte. A vesicle is shown in the canaliculus.

system such as ASBT and organic solute transporters α and β (OSTα and β) (see Chapter 66). Consequently, newly synthesized bile salts in the liver contribute only a small fraction (<5%) to biliary secretion and compensate for bile salts that escape intestinal absorption and are lost in feces. Fecal excretion of bile salts is increased when the enterohepatic circulation of bile salts is partially or completely interrupted by surgery, disease states, or drugs (e.g., bile salt-binding resins such as cholestyramine). Complete interruption of the enterohepatic circulation results in upregulation of bile salt synthesis in the liver, which restores bile salt secretion rates to approximately 25% of their usual values. Cholesterol from two sources serves as substrate for bile salt synthesis: cholesterol that is newly synthesized in the smooth endoplasmic reticulum and cholesterol that is preformed outside the smooth endoplasmic reticulum. The first step in this process is catalyzed by cholesterol 7α-hydroxylase. In the basal state, bile salt synthesis uses principally newly synthesized cholesterol as a substrate. When de novo cholesterol biosynthesis is suppressed by long-term therapy with an HMG-CoA reductase inhibitor such as a statin, preformed cholesterol originating from plasma lipoprotein substitutes for newly synthesized cholesterol.

Biliary Lipid Secretion

Bile salts have been shown to stimulate hepatic secretion of vesicles, which are always detected in freshly collected hepatic bile.[84,85] When cultured under specified conditions, rat hepatocytes form couplets with isolated "bile canaliculi" at the interface between adjoining cells. With the use of laser light-scattering techniques, vesicle formation can be observed within these bile canaliculi after exposure to bile salts. In addition, rapid fixation techniques and electronic microscopy have provided direct morphologic evidence of vesicle formation and secretion at the outer surface of the canalicular membrane of hepatocytes.[86,87] Most, if not all, bile salts are thought to enter canalicular spaces as monomers, whereas biliary phospholipids and cholesterol enter as unilamellar vesicles (see Fig. 67.4). A study on the molecular genetics of sitosterolemia (see Chapter 66) has shown that efflux of biliary cholesterol from the canalicular membrane of the hepatocyte is a protein-mediated process. Two plasma membrane proteins—ATP-binding cassette (ABC) sterol transporters ABCG5 and ABCG8—promote cellular efflux of cholesterol. The significance of this process for bile formation has been examined in genetically modified mice in which overexpression of the human *ABCG5* and *ABCG8* genes in the liver was shown to increase the cholesterol content of gallbladder bile.[88–92] Despite a reduced prevalence of gallstones, formation of gallstones is still observed in *Abcg5/g8* double-knockout mice, as well as in *Abcg5* or *Abcg8* single-knockout mice fed a lithogenic diet.[88–92] These findings strongly support the existence of an ABCG5/G8-independent pathway for hepatic secretion of biliary cholesterol and its role in formation of cholesterol gallstones. The Niemann-Pick C1-like 1 (NPC1L1) protein is expressed in the canalicular membrane of hepatocytes as well as the apical membrane of enterocytes; however, its expression levels are significantly lower in the liver than in the small intestine in humans. These observations suggest that hepatic NPC1L1 may have a weak role in the regulation of biliary cholesterol secretion.[93] In addition, scavenger receptor class B type I (SR-BI) is localized in sinusoidal and possibly canalicular membranes of hepatocytes, and in transgenic and knockout mice fed a chow diet, biliary secretion of cholesterol varies in proportion to hepatic expression of SR-BI and to the contribution of SR-BI to sinusoidal uptake of HDL cholesterol destined for secretion into bile.[94,95] Attenuation of the SR-BI, however, does not influence gallstone formation in mice. These results suggest that although HDL cholesterol is a principal source of biliary cholesterol in the basal state, uptake of cholesterol from chylomicron remnants appears to be the major contributor to biliary cholesterol hypersecretion during diet-induced cholelithogenesis in the mouse.[94]

Deletion of the *Abcb4* gene completely inhibits hepatic secretion of biliary phospholipids in mice,[96] suggesting that ABCB4 could be responsible for the translocation, or "flip," of phosphatidylcholine from the endoplasmic (inner) to ectoplasmic (outer) leaflet of the canalicular membrane bilayer of hepatocytes and that the action of ABCB4 may form phosphatidylcholine-rich microdomains within the outer membrane leaflet. Although the ectoplasmic leaflet of the canalicular membrane is cholesterol- and sphingomyelin-rich and is relatively resistant to penetration by bile salts, bile salts may promote vesicular secretion of biliary cholesterol and phosphatidylcholine. Bile salts may partition preferentially into these areas to destabilize the membrane and release phosphatidylcholine-rich vesicles because detergent-like bile salt molecules within the canalicular space could interact with the canalicular membrane. Mutations of the *ABCB4* gene in humans result in the molecular defect underlying type 3 progressive familial intrahepatic cholestasis, as well as low phospholipid-associated cholelithiasis (see Chapter 79).[97,98]

Biliary bile salts include those that are newly synthesized in the liver and those that undergo enterohepatic cycling. The precise molecular mechanism of bile salt secretion is not known, although it involves ABCB11, a bile salt export pump (see Chapter 66).[99–101] Although hepatic secretion of biliary bile salts directly affects cholesterol-phospholipid vesicle secretion, whether bile salt secretion is coupled to cholesterol and phospholipid secretion at a molecular level remains unknown. The relationship between bile salt secretion and cholesterol secretion is curvilinear: At low bile salt secretion rates (usually <10 µmol/h/kg), more cholesterol is secreted per molecule of bile salt than at higher rates. Although bile salt secretion rates are not low in normal subjects, they may diminish during prolonged fasting, during the overnight period, and with substantial bile salt losses, as occur with a biliary fistula or ileal resection when the liver cannot compensate sufficiently by increasing bile salt synthesis. At high bile salt secretion rates, for example, during and after eating, biliary cholesterol saturation is less than that during interprandial periods. In laboratory animals, biliary secretion of organic anions does not influence bile salt secretion but does inhibit hepatic secretion of phospholipids and cholesterol into bile because organic anions bind bile salts within bile canaliculi and prevent interactions with the canalicular membrane of hepatocytes.

PATHOPHYSIOLOGY

Fig. 67.5 shows interactions of 5 primary defects that lead to formation of cholesterol gallstones: (1) certain genetic factors, including *LITH* genes, (2) hepatic hypersecretion of biliary cholesterol, (3) gallbladder hypomotility, (4) rapid phase transitions of cholesterol, and (5) certain intestinal factors. These defects act together to facilitate cholesterol nucleation and crystallization and ultimately promote formation of cholesterol gallstones.

Hepatic Hypersecretion of Biliary Cholesterol

Hepatic hypersecretion of biliary cholesterol plays a primary role in the pathogenesis of cholesterol gallstone formation. By

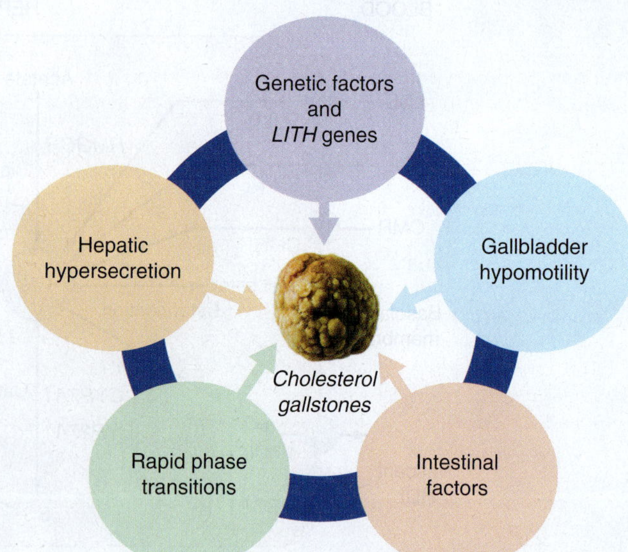

Fig. 67.5 Five primary defects work together to promote formation of cholesterol gallstones. The 5 defects are genetic factors and *LITH* (gallstone) genes, hepatic hypersecretion of cholesterol, gallbladder hypomotility, rapid phase transitions, and intestinal factors. The hypothesis proposed is that hepatic hypersecretion of biliary cholesterol is the primary defect and is the outcome, in part, of a complex genetic predisposition. Downstream effects include gallbladder hypomotility and rapid phase transitions (see Fig. 67.3). A major result of gallbladder hypomotility is alteration in the kinetics of the enterohepatic circulation of bile salts (intestinal factors). Alterations in intestinal factors result in increased cholesterol absorption, as well as reduced bile salt absorption, that lead to abnormal enterohepatic circulation of bile salts and a diminished biliary bile salt pool size. Not only does gallbladder hypomotility facilitate cholesterol nucleation and crystallization, but it also allows the gallbladder to retain solid plate-like cholesterol monohydrate crystals. Although a large number of candidate LITH genes have been identified in mouse models and many human LITH genes have been discovered, their contributions to gallstone pathogenesis require further investigation (see Table 67.1).

definition, supersaturated bile contains cholesterol that cannot be solubilized at equilibrium by bile salts and phospholipids. Cholesterol supersaturation could result from (1) excessive hepatic secretion of biliary cholesterol, (2) decreased hepatic secretion of biliary bile salts or phospholipids with relatively normal cholesterol secretion, or (3) a combination of hypersecretion of cholesterol and hyposecretion of the solubilizing lipids. With the passage of time and in the presence of heterogeneous pronucleating agents (usually mucin gel), cholesterol supersaturation leads to the precipitation of solid plate-like cholesterol monohydrate crystals in bile, followed by agglomeration and growth of the crystals into mature and macroscopic stones.

Rapid Cholesterol Nucleation and Crystallization

Cholesterol nucleation and crystallization is a process by which solid plate-like cholesterol monohydrate crystals precipitate from supersaturated bile. The crystals can be detected by polarizing light microscopy in a sample of bile previously rendered crystal-free "isotropic."[102] Bile from patients with cholesterol gallstones and from certain normal controls is supersaturated with cholesterol, and the degree of cholesterol supersaturation is not a reliable predictor of gallstones. On the other hand, rapid in vitro cholesterol nucleation and crystallization from the isotropic phase of gallbladder bile distinguishes the lithogenic bile of patients with cholesterol gallstones from cholesterol-supersaturated bile of nongallstone control subjects.[102] The phase diagram of cholesterol, phospholipids, and bile salts discussed earlier (see Fig. 67.3) is often used to study the phase transitions where metastable intermediates form. Five crystallization pathways can be identified on the basis of the phospholipid-to-bile salt ratio, total lipid concentration, bile salt species (hydrophilic and hydrophobic properties), temperature, and CSI.[81,103] Furthermore, these crystallization pathways have been confirmed in fresh human and mouse gallbladder biles.[81,103,104] In Fig. 67.3, which shows the cholesterol-phospholipid–mixed bile salt model bile system, the five distinct crystallization pathways are designated A to E, with each representing a different sequence of phase transitions, including an anhydrous cholesterol pathway and a liquid crystalline pathway that leads to formation of solid plate-like cholesterol monohydrate crystals.[81,103] Transient arc-like crystals appear in some of the pathways and are consistent with crystalline anhydrous cholesterol.[105,106] Why anhydrous cholesterol crystals should precipitate in an aqueous environment is unknown, but they are characteristic of the pathways that seem to originate from unilamellar, as opposed to multilamellar, vesicles. In these pathways, the critical nucleus may be a unilamellar vesicle that could contain liquid anhydrous cholesterol molecules in its core, possibly reflecting internal nucleation. In essence, these early vesicular "nuclei" may already have initiated the nucleation cascade by the time bile enters the gallbladder. The current paradigm for cholesterol nucleation and crystallization, based principally on observations from video-enhanced polarized light microscopy, suggests that biliary vesicles must fuse or at least aggregate to form crystalline cholesterol monohydrate. Because cholesterol nucleation and crystallization are apparently initiated in vesicles, the stability of the vesicle determines the stability of bile. Unstable vesicles can fuse, aggregate, and grow into multilamellar liquid crystalline structures (liposomes) in which cholesterol crystallizes out of solution. Furthermore, evidence from quasielastic light-scattering spectroscopy shows that nucleation of solid cholesterol crystals may occur directly from supersaturated micelles in conjugated deoxycholate-rich bile in vitro without an intervening vesicle or liquid crystalline phase.

In bile with the lowest phospholipid content (region A in Fig. 67.3), arc-like crystals with a density (d = 1.030 g/mL) consistent with anhydrous cholesterol appear first and evolve via helical and tubular crystals to form plate-like cholesterol monohydrate crystals (d = 1.045 g/mL).[81,105,106] With higher phospholipid contents (region B), cholesterol monohydrate crystals appear earlier than arc-like crystals and other transitional crystals. With typical physiologic phospholipid contents (region C), early liquid crystals (d = 1.020 g/mL) are followed by cholesterol monohydrate crystals; subsequently, arc-like and other intermediate crystals appear. With still higher phospholipid contents (region D), liquid crystals are followed by cholesterol monohydrate crystals only. At the highest phospholipid mole fractions (region E), liquid crystals are quite stable, and no solid crystals form. Decreases in temperature (37°C → 4°C), total lipid concentration (7.5 g/dL → 2.5 g/dL), and bile salt hydrophobicity ($3\alpha,12\alpha \rightarrow 3\alpha,7\alpha \rightarrow 3\alpha,7\alpha,12\alpha \rightarrow 3\alpha,7\beta$-hydroxylated taurine conjugates) progressively shift all crystallization pathways to lower phospholipid contents, reduce micellar cholesterol solubilization, and retard crystallization.[81,103]

Cholesterol crystallization pathways and sequences in human gallbladder bile are identical to those of model bile samples matched for appropriate physical-chemical conditions, and in the physiologic state, three of the five sequences observed in model bile samples are found in human and mouse gallbladder biles.[103] Notably, the kinetics of all these phase transitions are faster in lithogenic human bile than in identically patterned model bile samples, most likely a result in part of the combined influences of increased levels of cholesterol, secondary bile salts, and mucin glycoproteins.[82] In addition, biliary lipid, inorganic salt, and protein factors may be important in stabilizing supersaturated bile. Nonprotein factors that retard cholesterol nucleation and crystallization include (1) a total lipid concentration less than 3 g/dL, (2) reduced hydrophobicity of the bile salt pool, (3) low bile salt-to-phospholipid ratios, (4) low cholesterol-to-phospholipid ratios in vesicles, and (5) low total calcium ion concentrations. The states opposite to these conditions accelerate cholesterol nucleation and crystallization.[107]

Imbalance of Pronucleating and Antinucleating Factors

Cholesterol crystallization is significantly more rapid in the gallbladder bile of patients with gallstones than in that of control subjects even though CSI values are similar. These findings imply that lithogenic bile may contain pronucleating agents that accelerate crystallization or that normal bile may contain antinucleating agents that inhibit crystallization. Furthermore, bile may contain both accelerators and inhibitors of crystallization, and imbalances between them can induce rapid cholesterol crystallization in gallbladder bile in patients with cholesterol gallstones.[108,109]

Mucin was the first biliary protein shown to promote cholesterol crystallization.[110] The mucin-producing cells of the gallbladder secrete mucin that serves as a protective layer over the mucosa in the normal physiologic state. Mucin or mucin glycoproteins are large molecules that consist of a protein core and many carbohydrate side chains.[111] An important property of mucin is its ability to form a gel phase in higher concentrations, and the gel has greatly increased viscosity compared with the sol (soluble) phase.

Gallbladder mucins, a heterogeneous family of *O*-linked glycoproteins, are divided into two classes: epithelial and gel-forming mucins.[112] The epithelial mucins, which are produced by mucin gene 1 (*MUC1*), *MUC3*, and *MUC4*, are not able to form aggregates and are integral membrane glycoproteins located on the apical surface of epithelial cells.[113–116] The gel-forming mucins MUC2, MUC5AC, and MUC5B, which are secreted by specialized gallbladder mucin-producing cells, provide a protective coating on the underlying mucosa.[113–116] They form disulfide-stabilized oligomers or polymers, a phenomenon that accounts for their viscoelastic properties. Mucins from different organs vary in carbohydrate side chain, protein composition, and charge but generally have similar properties. Mucins have hydrophilic domains to which many water molecules bind. They have an overall charge and are capable of binding other charged species such as calcium. Hydrophobic domains in the mucin molecule (on the nonglycosylated regions of the polypeptide core) allow binding of lipids such as cholesterol, phospholipids, and bilirubin.

Gallbladder mucins play an important role in the early stages of gallstone formation and are a potent pronucleating agent for accelerating cholesterol crystallization in native and model biles. Indeed, hypersecretion of gallbladder mucins is a prerequisite for gallstone formation, and increased amounts of gallbladder mucins are consistently observed in gallbladder bile of several animal models of gallstones.[104,110,117] Mucins are also found within gallstones, where they act as a matrix for stone growth.[118] The mucins in gallstones have been found to extend from the amorphous center to the periphery in either a radial or laminated fashion. Mucins are also a major component of sludge in the gallbladder, and sludge has been shown to be a precursor of gallstones. Therefore two roles in the formation of gallstones have been proposed for mucins: (1) a pronucleating agent for accelerating the nucleation and crystallization of cholesterol from saturated bile and (2) a scaffolding for the deposition of solid cholesterol monohydrate crystals during the growth of stones.

The synthesis of mucin glycoproteins that are secreted by the mucin-producing cells of the gallbladder and bile ducts may be regulated by mucosal prostaglandins derived from arachidonic acid–containing biliary phospholipids.[111] During gallstone formation, the gallbladder hypersecretes mucins, mostly as a result of stimulation by some components of saturated bile. Then, the carbohydrate groups of the polymers of mucins avidly bind water to form gels. The hydrophobic polypeptides in the core of mucin glycoproteins can also bind bilirubin and calcium in bile. The resulting water-insoluble complex of mucin glycoproteins and calcium bilirubinate provides a surface for nucleation of cholesterol monohydrate crystals and a matrix for the growth of stones.

Mucin secretion and accumulation in the gallbladder are determined by multiple mucin genes. Targeted disruption of the *Muc1* gene reduces MUC1 mucin in the gallbladder of mice, thereby leading to a decrease in susceptibility to cholesterol gallstone formation.[119] Also, expression levels of the gallbladder *Muc5ac* gel-forming mucin gene are significantly reduced in *Muc1*-knockout mice in response to a lithogenic diet. As a result, cholesterol crystallization and the development of gallstone formation are significantly retarded. These findings suggest that gene-gene interactions between the *Muc1* and *Muc5ac* genes might affect mucin secretion and accumulation in the gallbladder. Furthermore, increased gallbladder epithelial MUC1 mucin enhances cholelithogenesis, mostly by promoting gallbladder cholesterol absorption and impairing gallbladder motility in mice that are transgenic for the human *MUC1* gene; this lithogenic mechanism is completely different from that associated with the gel-forming mucins.[120] Collectively, these findings support the concept that inhibition of the secretion and accumulation of not only the gel-forming mucins but also the epithelial mucins in the gallbladder may completely prevent formation of cholesterol gallstones.

Many glycoproteins that bind reversibly to concanavalin A–Sepharose also speed up cholesterol crystallization.[121] These glycoproteins include aminopeptidase N, immunoglobulins, α_1-acid glycoprotein, phospholipase C, fibronectin, and haptoglobin. Other pronucleating agents are the amphipathic anionic polypeptide fraction/calcium-binding protein, albumin-lipid complexes, and group II phospholipase A_2. Nonprotein components of bile also expedite cholesterol crystallization. Calcium bound to micelles and vesicles in bile may accelerate cholesterol crystallization by promoting fusion of cholesterol-rich vesicles. Precipitation of calcium salts in bile that is supersaturated with calcium salts and cholesterol may lead to rapid cholesterol crystallization, an effect enhanced by the presence of mucins. The rapidity of cholesterol crystal formation also varies in proportion to the deoxycholate content of bile and is related to the effect of deoxycholate on the equilibrium phase relationships of biliary lipids. The degree of cholesterol supersaturation of bile may also be a determinant of rapid crystallization of cholesterol.

Several inhibitors of cholesterol crystallization have been identified, including apolipoproteins AI and AII, a 120-kd glycoprotein, a 15-kd protein, and secretory immunoglobulin A and its heavy and light chains.[122–124] Apolipoproteins AI and AII may prolong the crystal detection time of supersaturated model bile. Apolipoproteins AI and AII are present in a fraction of human bile that may inhibit cholesterol nucleation and crystallization. Precholecystectomy treatment with the hydrophilic bile acid UDCA for 3 months prolongs the crystal detection time of bile in patients with cholesterol gallstones, thereby suggesting that UDCA could be an antinucleating factor.[81,125–127] UDCA may exert its effect by stabilizing vesicles, perhaps by enhancing the incorporation of apolipoprotein AI into (or onto) the vesicles. In addition, a potential antinucleating factor from normal human gallbladder bile is detected by lectin affinity chromatography and high-performance liquid ion-exchange chromatography and found to be a slightly acidic glycoprotein with an apparent molecular size of 120 kd. The protein may inhibit the growth of solid cholesterol crystals by attaching to the most rapidly growing microdomains on a crystal face and interfering with further solute attachment. It is still uncertain whether only 1 or several antinucleating factors exist and how they may inhibit the initiation of cholesterol crystal formation, but unilamellar vesicles have been proposed to be the key sites of action.

In summary, although many biliary proteins besides mucin gel have been proposed as either pronucleating or antinucleating factors influencing cholesterol nucleation and crystallization in bile, their in vivo roles (if any) in the pathogenesis of cholesterol gallstone formation remain unclear. Furthermore, proteolysis of soluble biliary glycoproteins does not influence the detection time of cholesterol monohydrate crystals either in normal or abnormal gallbladder and hepatic biles, and soluble biliary proteins may not play an important pathophysiologic role in cholesterol crystallization.

Gallbladder Dysfunction

Under normal physiologic conditions, frequent gallbladder contractions occur throughout the day. Between meals, the gallbladder stores hepatic bile (with an average fasting volume of 25–30 mL in healthy subjects). Following a meal, depending on the degree of neurohormonal response, the gallbladder discharges a variable amount of bile.[128] Studies using a combination of cholescintigraphy and US have found that after a meal, the gallbladder empties immediately and refills repeatedly.[128] By contrast, an increased fasting gallbladder volume, as well as incomplete emptying and high residual gallbladder volume, is often observed in patients with cholesterol gallstones, regardless of whether they have tiny or large stones or simply lithogenic bile. In patients with cholesterol gallstones and gallbladder motility abnormalities, inflammation in the gallbladder wall is usually mild and cannot account for the impaired dynamics of the gallbladder. Furthermore, the poor interdigestive gallbladder filling is consistent with the delivery of a greater percentage of lithogenic bile from the liver directly into the small intestine, leading to the augmentation of the enterohepatic effects of increased recycling and bile salt hydrophobicity. These observations show that emptying and filling of the gallbladder are affected in patients with gallbladder hypomotility.[128,129] Clinical investigations have confirmed that gallbladder hypomotility is associated principally with the formation of cholesterol gallstones, although a milder degree of gallbladder dysmotility, in the absence of an enlarged gallbladder in the fasting state and any gallbladder inflammation, is also found in patients with pigment gallstones.[130] In patients with cholesterol gallstones, impaired gallbladder motility persists in the stone-free gallbladder following successful extracorporeal shock-wave lithotripsy and oral bile acid dissolution therapy (see later).[131,132] The degree of impairment of gallbladder emptying has been found to increase in proportion to the cholesterol content of gallbladder bile, even in healthy subjects without gallstones. These findings imply that excess cholesterol molecules in the gallbladder wall may act as myotoxic agents.

In vitro studies have found that compared to that in control subjects, gallbladder function in patients with cholesterol gallstones shows abnormalities in the binding of agonists such as CCK to plasma membrane CCK-1 receptors (CCK-1R), alterations in the contraction of isolated smooth muscle cells, and decreased contractility of isolated smooth muscle strips and whole gallbladder preparations. In particular, signal transduction in response to binding of agonists is impaired. Defects in contractility associated with cholesterol gallstones are reversible at an early stage and are mainly due to accumulation of excess biliary cholesterol in the membranes of gallbladder smooth muscle cells. This mechanism appears to explain why gallbladder emptying is impaired before gallstones are formed in animal models at a time when bile is supersaturated with cholesterol. In addition, the intracellular mechanisms of smooth muscle contraction seem to be intact in human gallbladder muscle cells from patients with cholesterol gallstones. These findings support the hypothesis that increased absorption of cholesterol from the gallbladder lumen is associated with gallbladder smooth muscle dysfunction. This alteration may induce stiffening of sarcoplasmic membranes secondary to an increase in cholesterol content of the membranes. As a result, when CCK binds to its receptor on smooth muscle cells of the lithogenic gallbladder, G proteins are not activated, and gallbladder motility is impaired.[133,134]

Gallbladder hypomotility could precede gallstone formation. Gallbladder stasis induced by the hypofunctioning gallbladder could provide the time necessary to accommodate nucleation of cholesterol crystals and growth of gallstones within the mucin gel in the gallbladder.[135,136] Furthermore, the viscous mucin gel that forms in the gallbladder lumen may contribute to hypomotility by impairing gallbladder emptying mechanically, possibly at the level of the cystic duct. In particular, sludge contains calcium, pigment, bile salts, and glycoproteins and could serve as a nidus for nucleation and crystallization of cholesterol or precipitation of calcium bilirubinate. The high prevalence of cholelithiasis in patients receiving long-term TPN (see earlier) highlights the importance of gallbladder stasis in the formation of gallstones.[137] For example, 49% of patients with Crohn disease who are on TPN have gallstones, whereas only 27% of patients with Crohn disease alone have gallstones. During TPN, the gallbladder does not empty completely because the stimulus (ingestion of meals) for CCK release is eliminated. As a result, bile stagnates and sludge develops in the gallbladder, thereby enhancing gallstone formation. Daily IV administration of CCK can completely prevent gallbladder dysmotility and eliminate the inevitable risk of biliary sludge and gallstone formation. In addition, slow emptying and increased volume of the gallbladder, as measured by US, often occur during pregnancy and during administration of oral contraceptives, two conditions that predispose to formation of gallstones (see earlier).[27,28]

Concentration of bile by the gallbladder increases cholesterol solubility but also enhances cholesterol nucleation and crystallization in bile and may thereby contribute to gallstone formation.[138,139] In addition to concentrating bile, the normal gallbladder can acidify bile. Acidification increases the solubility of calcium salts (e.g., bilirubinate, carbonate), which may be promoters of nucleation and crystallization of cholesterol; therefore defective acidification may promote the formation of gallstones.

Differential absorption rates of cholesterol, phospholipids, and bile salts by the gallbladder epithelial cells may reduce cholesterol saturation of bile in normal subjects; however, the gallbladder epithelium of patients with cholesterol gallstones loses the capacity for selective absorption of biliary cholesterol and phospholipids.[140,141] Impaired lipid absorption by the gallbladder may contribute to gallstone formation by sustaining cholesterol supersaturation of bile during storage.[142] The physical-chemical fate of cholesterol absorbed by the gallbladder may be similar to that which occurs during the development of an atherosclerotic plaque. In all likelihood, cholesterol molecules are absorbed continuously by the gallbladder mucosa from supersaturated bile,[143] and the unesterified cholesterol molecules diffuse rapidly to the muscularis propria because the gallbladder lacks an intervening muscularis mucosae and submucosa. Because the gallbladder apparently does not synthesize lipoproteins for exporting cholesterol to plasma, excess unesterified cholesterol molecules are removable from gallbladder mucosa and muscle only by esterification and storage or back diffusion into bile.[144] In the lithogenic state, back diffusion of cholesterol molecules into bile is blocked because gallbladder bile is continuously saturated. As a result, gallbladder mucosal acyl-coenzyme A:cholesterol acyltransferase (ACAT) esterifies most, but not all, cholesterol molecules. As in an atherosclerotic plaque, mucosal and muscle membranes apparently become saturated with cholesterol and coexist with stored cholesteryl ester droplets. Furthermore, the unesterified cholesterol molecules become intercalated within the membrane bilayer of muscle cells, a process that may alter the physical state of phospholipid molecules, as reflected by their increased rigidity. Consequently, gallbladder motility function is impaired because signal transduction in response to CCK is markedly diminished. In addition, excess cholesterol molecules absorbed from the lithogenic bile may be direct stimulants to proliferative and inflammatory changes in the mucosa and lamina propria of the gallbladder.[128]

Intestinal Factors

The high efficiency of intestinal cholesterol absorption correlates significantly with the prevalence of cholesterol gallstones in inbred strains of mice, and gallstone-susceptible C57L mice display significantly higher intestinal cholesterol absorption than do gallstone-resistant AKR mice.[145] These observations show that high dietary cholesterol intake and high efficiency of intestinal cholesterol absorption are two independent risk factors for cholesterol gallstone formation. Differences in the metabolism of chylomicron remnant cholesterol between C57L and AKR mice may account for lithogenic bile formation in the former, and the cholesterol absorbed from the small intestine provides an important source for biliary cholesterol hypersecretion in mice fed a lithogenic diet.[146]

Altered intestinal motility also may have a role in gallstone formation. Delayed or impaired small intestinal transit is associated with enhanced intestinal cholesterol absorption, biliary cholesterol secretion, and gallstone formation in CCK-1 receptor-knockout mice.[146] The association of impaired colonic motility with increased biliary deoxycholate levels is found in some patients with cholesterol gallstones. Evidence for a causal relationship among impaired intestinal motility, deoxycholate formation, and bile lithogenicity comes from studies in humans and mice. Clinical studies have found that acromegalic patients treated with octreotide [a known risk factor for cholesterol gallstone disease (see earlier)] display a prolonged colonic transit time, high levels of biliary deoxycholate concentration, and rapid precipitation of cholesterol crystals.[147–150] Furthermore, higher levels of biliary deoxycholate are associated with increased amounts of Gram-positive anaerobic bacteria and increased activity of 7α-dehydroxylase in the cecum of patients with cholesterol gallstones compared with control subjects who have no stones.[151] Biliary deoxycholate and cholesterol concentrations can be lowered by antibiotic treatment that reduces fecal 7α-dehydroxylation activity. Compared with resistant AKR mice, gallstone-susceptible C57L mice also have higher biliary levels of deoxycholate, which are associated with cholesterol supersaturation and gallstone formation.[104,112] Chronic intestinal infection has been proposed to be a potential risk factor in the pathogenesis of cholesterol gallstones. A mouse study has shown that distal intestinal infection with a variety of enterohepatic *Helicobacter* species (but not Hp) is essential for nucleation and crystallization of cholesterol from supersaturated bile.[152,153] These *Helicobacter* species also have been identified in the bile and gallbladder tissue of Chilean patients with chronic cholecystitis.[154] Whether chronic intestinal infection has a direct pathogenic role in the formation of cholesterol gallstones requires further investigation.

In patients with Crohn disease and those who have undergone intestinal resection or total colectomy, gallbladder bile is supersaturated with cholesterol, and cholesterol crystals are prone to precipitate and form gallstones.[155] The enterohepatic circulation of bile salts is probably impaired in these patients, so hepatic secretion of biliary bile salts is greatly reduced and the solubilization of cholesterol in bile is decreased. Moreover, Crohn disease may lead to impaired enterohepatic cycling of bilirubin, with increased biliary bilirubin levels and precipitation of calcium bilirubinate, thereby providing a nidus for cholesterol nucleation and crystallization.[60,156]

Growth of Gallstones

Findings in patients who have cholesterol crystals but no gallstones in the gallbladder suggest that the growth of cholesterol crystals into gallstones does not always follow crystallization. Stone growth may represent a second critical stage in gallstone formation that results from delayed emptying of the gallbladder. When multiple gallstones are found in the gallbladder, they often are equal in size, indicating that cholesterol crystallization for this family of stones occurred simultaneously and the stones grew at the same rate. By contrast, stones of unequal size could represent different generations. The amorphous material in the center of stones contains bilirubin, bile salts, mucin glycoproteins, calcium carbonate, phosphate, copper, and sulfur, which could have provided a required nidus for cholesterol nucleation and crystallization. Solid plate-like cholesterol monohydrate crystals could assemble about this nidus. Formation of a nidus and subsequent stone growth could be determined by mucins, other biliary proteins, and the cholesterol saturation of bile. The growth of stones is likely a discontinuous process punctuated by deposition of rings of calcium bilirubinate and calcium carbonate. Because cholesterol monohydrate crystals often aggregate randomly in amorphous groupings and layer radially and concentrically, cholesterol stones consist of radially or horizontally oriented cholesterol crystals embedded within an organic matrix. In the outer portion of stones, cholesterol monohydrate crystals are oriented perpendicularly to the surface.[157] Throughout the formation of gallstones, mucins could provide a matrix on which gallstone growth occurs. Furthermore, concentric pigmented rings separate layers of cholesterol monohydrate crystals that have different axial orientations. The chemical composition of these rings often resembles the center of gallstones, and the rings may reflect cyclic deposition of calcium bilirubinate, other calcium salts, and mucin glycoproteins.

GENETICS

Evidence for a genetic component of cholesterol gallstone disease in humans is mostly indirect and based on geographic and ethnic differences, as well as on family and twin studies.[20,158–165] A genetic predisposition is clearly present in the Pima and certain other North and South American Indians, who display the highest prevalence rate (≈48%) of gallstones in the world.[20,158–165] By contrast, the overall prevalence of gallstones in white American and European populations is about 20%. The lowest rates (<5%) are observed in African populations, and intermediate rates are found in Asian populations (5% to 20%), as shown in Figs. 67.1 and Fig. 67.2. Although some independent risk factors (e.g., aging, gender, parity, obesity, insulin resistance, some drugs, and rapid weight loss) for gallstone formation have been found,[25,29,58,166–168] none can explain the striking differences in the prevalence of gallstones among different populations, thereby suggesting a genetic contribution to the etiology of the disease.[5,6]

Gallstones are more frequent by a ratio of 3:1 in siblings and other family members of affected persons than in spouses or unrelated controls.[160] Using US to detect gallstones in first-degree relatives of index patients, Gilat et al.[162] found a 21% prevalence rate in first-degree relatives compared with 9% in matched controls. Sarin and coworkers[163] also observed a prevalence that was five times higher in relatives than in controls. Furthermore, cholesterol supersaturation is higher in fasting duodenal bile of older sisters of patients with cholesterol gallstones than in controls.[164] Cholesterol synthesis rates, bile saturation levels, and gallstone prevalence rates are also significantly higher on pair-wise correlations in monozygotic than in dizygotic male twins.[165] Despite these observations, a mode of inheritance that fits a Mendelian pattern cannot be shown in most cases.

Study of populations with different incidence rates of gallstones but living in the same environment should provide insights into genetic mechanisms of the disease. Unfortunately, intermarriages between two populations result in a rapid loss of the original genetic background within a few generations and make such studies impossible. With the use of pedigree data to explore the genetic susceptibility to symptomatic gallbladder disease in a Mexican-American population of 32 families, heritability (i.e., the proportion of the phenotypic variance of the trait that is due to genetic effects) has been estimated to be 44%.[169] A variance component analysis in 1038 persons from 358 families in the United States has determined the heritability of symptomatic gallbladder disease to be 29%.[170] A large study of 43,141 twin pairs in Sweden has provided conclusive evidence for the role of genetic factors in the pathogenesis of cholesterol gallstones.[171] In this study, concordance rates were significantly higher in monozygotic twins than in dizygotic twins, with genetic factors accounting for 25% of the phenotypic variation between twins.

Evidence that human gallstones may be caused by a single gene defect came initially from a study by Lin et al.,[172] who reported that among 232 Mexican-Americans, a variant of the cholesterol 7α-hydroxylase (*CYP7A1*) gene was associated with gallstones in men but not in women. *CYP7A1* is an attractive candidate gene because it encodes the rate-limiting enzyme in hepatic bile salt synthesis of the classical pathway and because bile salts are essential for forming bile and for keeping cholesterol molecules solubilized in simple and mixed micelles in bile. Pullinger et al. found a link between another single gene defect of *CYP7A1* and cholesterol gallstones associated with hypercholesterolemia resistant to HMG-CoA reductase inhibitors in two male homoyzgotes.[173]

Missense mutations in the *ABCB4* gene, which encodes the phosphatidylcholine transporter in the canalicular membrane of hepatocytes, are the basis of a particular type of cholelithiasis.[96,173] The disorder is characterized by intrahepatic sludge, gallbladder cholesterol gallstones, mild chronic cholestasis, a high cholesterol-to-phospholipid ratio in bile, and recurrent symptoms after cholecystectomy.[174–176] Lack of biliary phospholipids caused by the *Abcb4* deletion in the liver is a critical risk factor for cholesterol gallstone disease in mice by significantly reducing cholesterol solubility in bile through disruption of the liquid crystalline pathway, whereas it leads to more rapid cholesterol crystallization via the anhydrous crystalline pathway.[177] These findings provide novel insights into the pathophysiologic mechanisms by which cholesterol gallstones are rapidly formed in patients with the *ABCB4* mutations, thereby leading to low phospholipid-associated cholelithiasis, a rare biliary disease caused by a single-gene mutation. Moreover, in patients with hepatolithiasis, a common disease in Asia, low expression of *ABCB4* and low levels of phosphatidylcholine transfer protein occur together, with markedly reduced phospholipid concentrations in bile (see Chapter 68).[178] Additionally, HMG-CoA reductase activity is increased and CYP7A1 activity is reduced in patients with gallstones compared with control subjects. In this disorder, the formation of cholesterol-rich intrahepatic stones could be induced by decreased hepatic secretion of biliary phospholipids in the setting of increased cholesterol synthesis and decreased bile salt synthesis.

Because gallbladder hypomotility favors gallstone formation, the genes for CCK and the CCK-1R, which regulate gallbladder motility, are attractive candidates.[134,167] Genetic variation in CCK-1R is associated with gallstone risk, and an aberrant splicing of

CCK-1R, which is predicted to result in a nonfunctional receptor, has been found in a few obese patients with gallstones.[179,180] A search for mutations or polymorphisms in the *CCK-1R* gene in patients with gallstones has been unsuccessful, however.[181]

Some studies have reported that certain polymorphisms of the apolipoprotein *(APO)E* and *APOB* genes and the cholesteryl ester transfer protein, all of which are involved in carrying cholesterol in plasma, are associated with gallstone formation. The *APOE* polymorphisms are the most extensively studied polymorphisms in patients with gallstones, but reports concerning the protective role of the *ε4* allele against gallstones have been inconsistent.[182–186] The *ε2* allele appears to protect against gallstones, and the degree of dietary cholesterol absorption in the intestine varies with the APOE isoform ($\varepsilon 4 > \varepsilon 3 > \varepsilon 2$). Also, the fecal excretion of cholesterol tends to be higher in persons with the APOE2 phenotype than in those with the APOE3 or APOE4 phenotypes.[187] In a study of polymorphisms at the *APOB, APOAI*, and cholesteryl ester transfer protein gene loci in patients with gallbladder disease, a polymorphism of the cholesteryl ester transfer protein gene, in relation to another HDL-lowering factor, was found to be associated with cholesterol gallstones.[188] Also, a link was found between the *X+* allele of the *APOB* gene and an increased risk of cholesterol gallstones.[189] A genome-wide association study in a large cohort of patients with gallstones from Germany[190] and a linkage study in affected sibling pairs[191] identified a common variant (D19H) of the sterol transporters ABCG5 and ABCG8 on the canalicular membrane of hepatocytes as a risk factor for gallstones. Subsequently, many studies have shown that ABCG8 variants (T400K, D19H, A632V, M429V, C54Y) and ABCG5 variants (Q604E) may be important risk factors for gallstone formation in European, Asian, and Chilean Hispanic populations.[192–198]

Table 67.1 summarizes progress in identifying *LITH* genes and the major classes of candidate genes for cholesterol and pigment gallstones in humans.[199] Although some candidate genes have been found in humans, their roles in cholelithogenesis merit further investigation. In general, genes that contribute to cholesterol gallstone formation include those that encode (1) hepatic and intestinal membrane lipid transporters, (2) hepatic and intestinal lipid regulatory enzymes, (3) hepatic and intestinal intracellular lipid transporters, (4) hepatic and intestinal lipid regulatory transcription factors, (5) hepatic lipoprotein receptors and related proteins, (6) hormone receptors in the gallbladder, and (7) biliary mucins.

Based on mouse and human studies, the concept has been proposed that hepatic hypersecretion of biliary cholesterol is induced by multiple *LITH* genes, with insulin resistance as part of the metabolic syndrome interacting with cholelithogenic environmental factors to cause the phenotype.[5,200,201] These studies strongly suggest that cholesterol gallstone disease is determined by multiple *LITH* genes and that the susceptibility to gallstones is a dominant trait not only in mice but also in humans.

Changes in the expression and function of one of several ABC transporters in the canalicular membrane may influence gallstone formation by inducing an alteration of biliary lipid secretion and bile composition. In addition, mutations in genes that encode several lipoprotein receptors and related proteins that determine the uptake of HDL and LDL and in several intracellular proteins that transport biliary lipids through the cytosol of hepatocytes, as well as transcription factors that regulate hepatic cholesterol and bile salt metabolism and biliary lipid secretion, may cause formation of cholesterol gallstones. Mutations in genes that affect CCK, the CCK-1R (see earlier), and the secretion and properties of mucin may also play a role in the pathogenesis of gallstones. A large case-control study[202] has found that increased hepatic biosynthesis and fecal excretion of cholesterol may precede cholesterol gallstone formation and may be key metabolic features in some ethnic groups at high risk of gallstones. This study strongly suggests that inhibiting both hepatic synthesis and intestinal absorption of cholesterol to reduce biliary output of cholesterol may be a therapeutic strategy for genetically defined subgroups of persons at high risk for gallstones.[203]

The factors that regulate intestinal membrane lipid transporters, lipid regulatory enzymes, intracellular lipid transporters, and lipid regulatory transcription factors may influence the amount of cholesterol of intestinal origin that contributes to biliary secretion by the liver. Direct evidence for the role of intestinal factors in mouse gallstones comes from a study of ACAT2-knockout mice.[204] Because of the deletion of the *Acat2* gene, the lack of cholesteryl ester synthesis in the small intestine significantly reduces intestinal cholesterol absorption and leads to complete resistance to diet-induced cholesterol gallstones. Furthermore, the potent cholesterol absorption inhibitor ezetimibe prevents gallstones by effectively reducing intestinal absorption and biliary secretion of cholesterol and protects gallbladder motility by desaturating bile in mice.[48,205] Moreover, ezetimibe significantly reduces biliary cholesterol saturation and retards cholesterol crystallization in bile of patients with gallstones.[48] Therefore reduced intestinal absorption of cholesterol or hepatic uptake of chylomicron remnants may induce a decrease in biliary cholesterol secretion and saturation. In addition, reduced expression levels of the genes that encode the ileal ASBT, the cytosolic ileal lipid binding protein, and OSTα and β may contribute to gallstone formation by decreased ileal bile acid reabsorption and an altered bile acid pool and composition in female and nonobese patients with gallstones compared with control subjects (see Chapter 66).[206,207] The single nucleotide polymorphism rs9514089 in the ASBT gene (gene symbol *SLC10A2*) has been identified as a susceptibility variant for cholelithiasis in humans,[208] although the effect of *rs9514089* genotype on gallstone risk was not replicated in Sorbs.[209] Further analyses in larger cohorts are required to evaluate the role of genetic variants of *SLC10A2* as a risk factor for gallstone formation.

PIGMENT STONES

Although the pathogenesis of black and brown pigment gallstones is not as well understood as that of cholesterol gallstones, and each type of stone probably has a distinctive pathogenesis, both types of pigment stones result from abnormalities in the metabolism of bilirubin and are pigmented as a result of bilirubin precipitation.[210–212] In general, the bile of patients with either type of pigment stones contains an excess of unconjugated bilirubin, analogous to the saturation of bile with cholesterol in patients with cholesterol stones.[213] Also, both types of pigment stones are composed primarily of bile pigment and contain a matrix of mucin glycoproteins. In black stones, however, the pigment is predominantly an insoluble highly cross-linked polymer of calcium bilirubinate, whereas in brown stones, the main pigment is monomeric calcium bilirubinate. The two types of pigment stones also differ in radiodensity, location within the biliary tract, and geographic distribution.

Results of studies of susceptibility genes for pigment stones are summarized in Table 67.1. Several candidate genes enhance the formation of pigment stones by increasing enterohepatic cycling of bilirubin. Persons with Gilbert syndrome have mild, chronic, unconjugated hyperbilirubinemia in the absence of liver disease or overt hemolysis because of reduced expression of bilirubin uridine diphosphate glucuronyl transferase 1 (gene symbol *UGT1A1*), which is due to an abnormality in the promoter region of the gene for this enzyme (see Chapter 22).[214] A genome-wide association study has identified a variant of the *UGT1A1* gene as a major risk factor for gallstone disease in humans.[215] The *UGT1A1* promoter variant increases the susceptibility to pigment stone formation in

TABLE 67.1 Human Gallstone (*LITH*) Genes and Gene Products That Have Been Identified as of 2019

Gene Symbol	Gene Name	Chromosome Location	Gene Variants	Inheritance pattern: Rare Monogenic	Familial Oligogenic	Common Polygenic	Potential Mechanism(s)
CHOLESTEROL STONES							
Lipid Membrane Transporters							
ABCG5/G8	ATP-binding cassette transporters G5/G8	2p21	ABCG8 p.D19H (rs1188753)	–	–	+	↑ Biliary cholesterol secretion
ABCB4	ATP-binding cassette transporter B4	7q21.1	Multiple	–	+	–	↓ Biliary phospholipid secretion
ABCB11	ATP-binding cassette transporter B11	2q24	Multiple	+	–	–	↓ Biliary bile salt secretion
SLC10A2 (IBAT)	Solute carrier family 10, member 2 (Ileal sodium-dependent bile salt transporter)	13q33	c.378–105A>G (rs9514089)	–	+	+	↓ Intestinal bile salt absorption
SLCO1B1 (OATP1B1)	Solute carrier organic anion transporter family, member 1B1	12p12	p.P155Thr (rs11045819)	–	–	+	↓ Intestinal bile salt absorption
TM4SF4	Transmembrane 4	3q25.1		–	TBD	TBD	Superfamily member 4
Lipid Regulatory Enzymes							
CYP7A1	Cholesterol 7α-hydroxylase (Cytochrome P450 7A1)	8q11-q12	Promoter SNP–204A>C	+	–	+	↓ The rate-limiting enzyme for bile salt biosynthesis in the classical pathway
UGT1A1	Bilirubin UDP-glucuronyl transferase	2q37	Promotor A(TA) 7TAA	–	–	+	↑ Hepatic bilirubin conjugation
SULT2A1	Sulfotransferase	19q13.33	rs2547231	–	–	+	? Sulfate conjugation and detoxification of bile salts family 2A, member 1
GCKR	Glucokinase	2p23.3	rs1260326	–	–	+	↑ Altered glucose homeostasis, ↑ cholesterol synthesis regulatory protein
Intracellular Lipid Regulatory Transporter							
CETP	Cholesteryl ester transfer protein	16q12–q21	RFLP	–	–	+	↑ Hepatic cholesterol uptake from increased HDL catabolism
Lipid Regulatory Transcription Factor							
NR1H4 (FXR)	Nuclear receptor 1H4 (Farnesoid X receptor)	12q23.1	Promoter SNPs –1G>T and –20647T>G, IVS7–31 A>T	–	–	+	↓ Conversion of cholesterol into bile salts ↑ Biliary cholesterol secretion
Lipoprotein Receptors and Related Genes							
APOA1	Apolipoprotein A1	11q23–q24	–75G>A, RFLP	–	–	+	↑ Biliary cholesterol secretion secondary to increased reverse cholesterol transport

TABLE 67.1 Human Gallstone (*LITH*) Genes and Gene Products That Have Been Identified as of 2019—cont'd

Gene Symbol	Gene Name	Chromosome Location	Gene Variants	Inheritance pattern: Rare Monogenic	Inheritance pattern: Familial Oligogenic	Inheritance pattern: Common Polygenic	Potential Mechanism(s)
APOB	Apolipoprotein B	2p24–p23	c.2488C>T, c.4154G>A	+	–	+	↑ Biliary cholesterol secretion secondary to reduced hepatic VLDL synthesis ↑ Intestinal cholesterol absorption
APOC1	Apolipoprotein C1	19q13.2	RFLP	–	–	+	↑ APOC1 remnant-like particle cholesterol
LRPAP1	LDL receptor–related protein-associated protein 1	4p16.3	Intron 5 insertion/deletion (rs11267919)	–	–	+	↑ Hepatic cholesterol uptake from chylomicron remnants via LRP
Hormone Receptors							
CCK1R (CCKAR)	Cholecystokinin 1 receptor (CCK A receptor)	4p15.1–p15.2	RFLP	+	–	+	↓ Gallbladder and small intestinal motility
ESR2 (ERβ)	Estrogen receptor 2	14q23.2	c.1092+3607(CA)n	–	–	+	↑ Hepatic cholesterol biosynthesis
AR	Androgen receptor	Xq12	c.172(CAG)n	–	–	+	↓ Gallbladder motility
ADRB3	β3-Adrenergic receptor	8p12	p.R64W (rs4944)	–	–	+	↓ Gallbladder motility
Black Pigment Stones							
ANK1	Ankyrin 1	8p11.1	Multiple	–	+	–	Spherocytosis → hemolysis
CFTR (ABCC7)	CF transmembrane regulator	7q31.2	Δq31	+	–	–	↑ Enterohepatic bilirubin circulation ↓ Bile pH ↑ Fecal bile salt excretion
G6PD	Glucose-6-phosphate dehydrogenase	Xq28	Multiple	+	+		↑ Hemolysis
GPI	Glucose-6-phosphate isomerase	19q13.1	p.Leu339Pro		TBD		TBD
PKLR	Pyruvate kinase	1q21	p.R510Q		TBD		TBD
HBA1/2	Hemoglobin alpha chain complex	16p13.3	HbH	–	+	+	α-Thalassemia/β-thalassemia intermediate/minor/sickle cell disease → hemolysis
HBB	Hemoglobin beta chain complex	11p15.5	p.E26K (HbE) p.E6V (HbS)		TBD		TBD
UGT1A1	Bilirubin UDP-glucuronyl transferase	2q37	Promotor A(TA)7TAA	–	–	+	↑ Hepatic bilirubin conjugation
Biliary Tract Stones							
COMT	Catechol-O-methyltransferase	22q11.21	Exon4–76C>G (rs4818)	–	–	+	↑ Estrogen levels
CXCR2	Chemokine (C-X-C motif) receptor 2	2q35	c.811C>T (rs2230054) c.1235T>C (rs1126579)	–	–	+	TBD

Continued

TABLE 67.1 Human Gallstone (*LITH*) Genes and Gene Products That Have Been Identified as of 2019—cont'd

Gene Symbol	Gene Name	Chromosome Location	Gene Variants	Inheritance pattern			Potential Mechanism(s)
				Rare Monogenic	Familial Oligogenic	Common Polygenic	
IL8	Interleukin-8	4q13–q21	−351A>T (rs4073)	–	–	+	↑ IL8 expression → inflammation
NOS2	Nitric oxide synthase 2	17q11.2–q12	Exon16+14C>T (rs2297518)	–	–	+	TBD
RNASEL	Ribonuclease L	1q25	Exon1−96A>G (rs486907)	–	–	+	TBD

LRP, Low-density lipoprotein receptor-related protein; *RFLP*, restriction fragment length polymorphism; *SNP*, single nucleotide polymorphism; *TBD*, to be determined; *UDP*, uridine diphosphate.

Adapted with permission from Krawczyk M, Wang DQ, Portincasa P, et al. Dissecting the genetic heterogeneity of gallbladder stone formation. *Semin Liver Dis*. 2011;31:157–172.

patients with sickle cell disease or cystic fibrosis (CF).[216–218] A regression analysis has shown that serum bilirubin levels and the prevalence of gallstones are strongly associated with the number of *UGT1A1* promoter [TA] repeats in patients with sickle cell disease, with each additional repeat correlating with an increase in serum bilirubin levels of 21% and in cholelithiasis risk of 87%.[219] Moreover, *UGT1A1* gene variants in linkage disequilibrium with the variant are associated with the risk of developing cholesterol gallstones. These findings imply that the supersaturation of bile with bilirubin may be a risk factor for the formation of both pigment and cholesterol gallbladder stones. As discussed earlier, increased biliary bilirubin levels and enhanced precipitation of calcium bilirubinate in bile provide a critical nidus for cholesterol nucleation and crystallization.

The frequency of gallstones in patients with CF is 10%–30% compared with less than 5% in age-matched control subjects, but biliary cholesterol saturation does not differ between patients with and without gallstones. In fact, gallstones in patients with CF are generally black pigment stones (i.e., composed of calcium bilirubinate with an appreciable cholesterol admixture) but rarely cause symptoms. In a mouse (ΔF508 mutant) model of CF, increased fecal bile salt loss induces more hydrophobic bile salts in hepatic bile and augments enterohepatic cycling of bilirubin.[220] These alterations lead to hyperbilirubinbilia and significantly higher levels of all bilirubin conjugates and unconjugated bilirubin, followed by hydrolysis and precipitation of divalent metal salts of unconjugated bilirubin in bile. In addition, lower gallbladder bile pH values and elevated levels of calcium bilirubinate ion products in bile increase the likelihood of supersaturating bile with bilirubin and forming black pigment gallstones. The pancreatic duodenal homeobox gene-1 (*Pdx1*) is required for proper development of the major duodenal papilla, peribiliary glands, and mucin-producing cells in the bile duct and for maintenance of the periampullary duodenal epithelial cells during the perinatal period (see Chapter 64). Loss of the major duodenal papilla allows duodenobiliary reflux and bile infection, resulting in the formation of brown pigment stones in *Pdx1*-knockout mice, and treatment with antibiotics significantly reduces the frequency of brown pigment stones.[221]

Black Stones

Black pigment stones are formed in uninfected gallbladders, particularly in patients with chronic hemolytic anemia (e.g., β-thalassemia, hereditary spherocytosis, sickle cell disease), ineffective erythropoiesis (e.g., pernicious anemia), ileal diseases (e.g., Crohn disease) with spillage of excess bile salts into the large intestine, extended ileal resections, and liver cirrhosis. These alterations promote formation of black pigment stones because higher colonic bile salt concentrations enhance the solubilization of unconjugated bilirubin, thereby increasing bilirubin concentrations in bile.[222] The resulting unconjugated bilirubin is precipitated as calcium bilirubinate to form stones.[223] This type of stone is composed of either pure calcium bilirubinate or polymer-like complexes consisting of unconjugated bilirubin, calcium bilirubinate, calcium, and copper. Mucin glycoproteins account for as much as 20% of the weight of black pigment stones. A regular crystalline structure is not present in this type of stone.

For hepatic secretion, bilirubin is first mono- or diglucuronidated by UGT1A1 and subsequently secreted by ABC transporter C2 (ABCC2), also called *multidrug-resistance associated protein 2* (MRP2) (see Chapters 66 and 79). Under normal physiologic conditions, unconjugated bilirubin is not secreted into bile. Although bilirubin glucuronides are hydrolyzed by endogenous β-glucuronidase, unconjugated bilirubin constitutes less than 1% of total bile pigment, primarily because the activity of the enzyme is inhibited by β-glucaro-1,4-lactone in the biliary tract.[224,225] The unifying predisposing factor in black pigment stone formation is hepatic hypersecretion of bilirubin conjugates (especially monoglucuronides) into bile. In the presence of hemolysis, hepatic secretion of these bilirubin conjugates increases 10-fold. Unconjugated monohydrogenated bilirubin is formed by the action of endogenous β-glucuronidase, which coprecipitates with calcium as a result of supersaturation. A 1% hydrolysis rate may give rise to high concentrations of unconjugated bilirubin that often greatly exceed the solubility of bilirubin in bile. A defect in acidification of bile may also be induced by gallbladder inflammation or the reduced buffering capacity of sialic acid and sulfate moieties in the mucin gel. The reduction in buffering capacity facilitates supersaturation of calcium carbonate and calcium phosphate that would not occur at a more acidic pH. Gallbladder motility defects are not observed in patients with black pigment stones.

Brown Stones

Brown pigment stones are composed mainly of calcium salts of unconjugated bilirubin, with varying amounts of cholesterol, fatty acids, pigment fraction, and mucin glycoproteins, as well as small amounts of bile salts, phospholipids, and bacterial residues. Brown pigment stones may be easily distinguished grossly from black pigment stones by their reddish brown to dark brown color and lack of brightness. Their shape is irregular or molded and occasionally spherical. Most of the stones are muddy in consistency, and some show facet formation. Brown pigment stones are either smooth or rough without any surface luster and are soft, fragile, and light in comparison with other gallstones. The cut surface is generally a stratified structure (lamellation) or is amorphous without the radiating crystalline structure seen in cholesterol stones. Almost invariably, brown pigment stones have a lamellated cross-sectional surface with calcium bilirubinate-rich layers alternating with calcium palmitate-rich layers.

Brown pigment stones are formed not only in the gallbladder but also commonly in other portions of the biliary tract, especially in intrahepatic bile ducts. Formation of brown pigment stones requires the presence of structural or functional stasis of bile associated with biliary infection, especially with *Escherichia coli*.[226] These stones are quite prevalent in Asia, where *Clonorchis sinensis* and roundworm infestations are common, and parasitic elements have been considered to be kernels of brown pigment stone formation (see Chapter 86).[227] Bile stasis predisposes to bacterial infection as well as accumulation of mucins and bacterial cytoskeletons in the bile ducts. Bile stasis may be induced by bile duct stenosis and bacterial infection caused by infestation of parasites and their ova.[228] As the incidence of biliary infections has decreased in Asian populations prone to development of brown pigment stones, the ratio of cholesterol stones to pigment stones has also changed in these populations. The percentage of brown pigment stones in Japan has fallen from 60% to 24% since the 1950s, and similar changes have been reported from other Asian countries.[229–231]

Enteric bacteria produce β-glucuronidase, phospholipase A_1, and conjugated bile acid hydrolase. Activity of β-glucuronidase results in the production of unconjugated bilirubin from bilirubin glucuronide; phospholipase A_1 liberates palmitic and stearic acids from phospholipids; and bile acid hydrolases produce unconjugated bile salts from glycine or taurine-conjugated bile salts. Partially ionized saturated fatty acids, unconjugated bilirubin, and unconjugated bile salts may precipitate as calcium salts. Mucin gel can trap these complex precipitates and facilitate their growth into macroscopic brown pigment stones. Fig. 67.6 shows the postulated mechanisms underlying the formation of brown pigment stones. Under normal physiologic conditions, bilirubin in bile exists mainly as bilirubin glucuronide, which is soluble in aqueous media. Bile also contains β-glucuronidase of tissue origin, the activity of which is inhibited by β-glucaro-1,4-lactone, which is also formed in the liver. If infection with *E. coli* occurs, the concentration of bacterial β-glucuronidase increases significantly and exceeds the inhibitory power of β-glucaro-1,4-lactone. As a result, bilirubin glucuronide is hydrolyzed to produce unconjugated bilirubin and glucuronic acid; the former is water-insoluble and combines with calcium to form calcium bilirubin at its carboxyl radical, thereby leading to the formation of brown pigment gallstones.

NATURAL HISTORY

The natural history of gallstones is typically described in two separate groups of patients: those who have symptoms and those who are asymptomatic. Autopsy studies clearly show that the vast majority of patients with gallstones are asymptomatic and remain so. Ascertaining the true frequency of complications in persons with asymptomatic stones (as well as those with symptomatic stones) is critical to providing rational, cost-effective recommendations regarding therapy (see later). Unfortunately, the information available on the natural history of gallstones has been sparse and somewhat varied.[232–234]

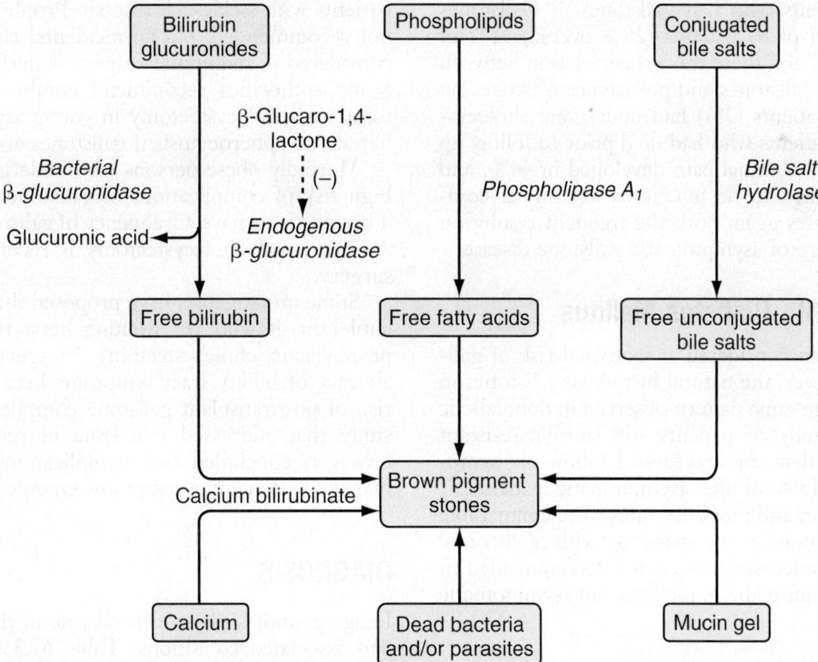

Fig. 67.6 Proposed mechanisms for the pathogenesis of brown pigment stones. Under normal physiologic conditions, unconjugated bilirubin is not secreted into bile. Although modest hydrolysis of bilirubin glucuronides by endogenous β-glucuronidase occurs, unconjugated bilirubin constitutes less than 1% of total bile pigment, mostly because the activity of β-glucuronidase is inhibited by β-glucaro-1,4-lactone in the biliary system. The presence of excess bacterial β-glucuronidase, however, overcomes the inhibitory (–) effect of β-glucaro-1,4-lactone, which results in hydrolysis of bilirubin glucuronide into free bilirubin and glucuronic acid. Free bilirubinate combines with calcium to yield water-insoluble calcium bilirubinate. In addition, phospholipase A1 liberates free fatty acids such as palmitic and stearic acids from phospholipids, and bile salt hydrolases produce unconjugated bile salts from glycine or taurine-conjugated bile salts. Dead bacteria and/or parasites could act as nuclei that accelerate precipitation of calcium bilirubinate. The mucin gel in the gallbladder can trap these complex precipitates and facilitate their growth into macroscopic stones.

Asymptomatic Stones

The study that changed our understanding of the course and appropriate therapy of gallstone disease was performed by Gracie and Ransohoff.[232] They monitored 123 University of Michigan faculty members for 15 years after they had been found to have gallstones on routine screening US. At 5, 10, and 15 years of follow-up, 10%, 15%, and 18% of the patients, respectively, had become symptomatic, and none had experienced serious complications. The investigators suggested that the rate at which biliary pain develops in persons with asymptomatic gallstones is about 2% per year for 5 years and then decreases over time. Biliary complications developed in only three patients in this study, and all complications were preceded by episodes of biliary pain. In fact, biliary pain, not a biliary complication, is the initial manifesting symptom in 90% of people with previously asymptomatic gallstones.[232] Therefore in patients with asymptomatic stones, the frequency of complications is low, and prophylactic cholecystectomy is not necessary.

Subsequent studies have reported slightly higher rates of biliary pain and complications in patients with initially asymptomatic gallstones,[233] but only one was a long-term and prospective study.[239] The Group for Epidemiology and Prevention of Cholelithiasis (GREPCO) in Rome reported the courses of 151 subjects with gallstones, 118 of whom were asymptomatic on entering the study. In those who were initially asymptomatic, the frequency of biliary pain was 12% at 2 years, 17% at 4 years, and 26% at 10 years, and the cumulative rate of biliary complications was 3% at 10 years.[234]

In a 1987 study, incidental gallstones were discovered in 285 (21%) of 1371 patients from Norway who had not had a cholecystectomy.[235] Twenty-four years later, a follow-up study included 134 of the patients who had gallstones.[236] Gallstones were present on US in 25 of 89 patients (28% overall, 31% of women, and 25% of men), and there was no correlation between initial size and number of gallstones and persistence of stones on follow-up. Nine of 134 patients (7%) had undergone cholecystectomy, as had 5 of 91 patients who had died prior to follow up (6%). During follow-up, abdominal pain developed in 44%, and 29% had what were deemed to be functional abdominal complaints. This study illustrates again both the frequent resolution and relatively benign nature of asymptomatic gallstone disease.

Stones in Patients With Diabetes Mellitus

Diabetic patients have been considered at increased risk of gallstone complications; however, the natural history of gallstones in diabetic patients follows the same pattern observed in nondiabetic persons. A prospective study of patients with insulin-resistant diabetes mellitus showed that after 5 years of follow-up, symptoms had developed in 15% of the asymptomatic patients.[237] Moreover, the complication and mortality rates were comparable to those in studies of nondiabetic patients with gallstones. Therefore prophylactic cholecystectomy is not recommended in patients with insulin-resistant diabetes mellitus and asymptomatic gallstones.

Symptomatic Stones

The cardinal symptom of gallstones is biliary pain "colic," which is described as pain in the RUQ often radiating to the back, with or without nausea and vomiting. The pain is usually not true colic (see Chapter 12) and is almost never associated with fever. The natural history of symptomatic gallstones has a more aggressive course than that of asymptomatic stones. The U.S. National Cooperative Gallstone Study showed that in persons who had an episode of uncomplicated biliary pain in the year before entering the study, the rate of recurrent biliary pain was 38% per year.[238] Other investigators have reported a rate of recurrent biliary pain as high as 50% per year in persons with symptomatic gallstones.[239] As noted earlier, biliary complications are also more likely to develop in persons with symptomatic gallstones. The risk of biliary complications is estimated to be 1% to 2% per year and is believed to remain relatively constant over time.[240] Therefore cholecystectomy should be offered to patients after biliary symptoms develop. In patients with high operative risk, an alternative approach is close observation, because 30% will have no further episodes of biliary pain.

Special Patient Populations

The clinical manifestations of gallstones are shown schematically in Fig. 67.7 and summarized in more detail in Table 67.2.[241–245] Biliary pancreatitis is discussed in Chapter 60. Although the standard approach to asymptomatic gallstones is observation, some patients with asymptomatic gallstones may be at increased risk of complications and may require consideration of prophylactic cholecystectomy.

An increased risk of cholangiocarcinoma and gallbladder carcinoma has been associated with certain disorders of the biliary tract and in some ethnic groups (e.g., Native Americans) (see Chapter 71). Risk factors include choledochal cysts, Caroli disease, pancreaticobiliary malunion (also referred to as anomalous union of the pancreatic and biliary ducts, in which the pancreatic duct drains into the bile duct), large gallbladder adenomas, and porcelain gallbladder (see Chapters 57, 64, 69 and 67). Patients at increased risk of biliary cancer may benefit from prophylactic cholecystectomy. If abdominal surgery is planned for another indication, an incidental cholecystectomy should be performed.

Pigment gallstones are common and often asymptomatic in patients with sickle cell disease. Prophylactic cholecystectomy is not recommended, but an incidental cholecystectomy should be considered if abdominal surgery is performed for other reasons. Some authorities recommend combined prophylactic splenectomy and cholecystectomy in young asymptomatic patients with hereditary spherocytosis if gallstones are present.

Morbidly obese persons who undergo bariatric surgery are at high risk of complications of gallstones (see Chapters 8 and 9). These patients have a frequency of gallstones of greater than 30%. An incidental cholecystectomy is recommended at the time of surgery.

Some investigators have proposed that patients with incidental cholelithiasis who are awaiting heart transplantation undergo a prophylactic cholecystectomy irrespective of the presence or absence of biliary tract symptoms because they are at increased risk of posttransplant gallstone complications.[246] A retrospective study that addressed this issue in renal transplant recipients, however, concluded that complications of gallstones could be managed safely after symptoms emerged.[247]

DIAGNOSIS

Imaging studies play a central role in the diagnosis of gallstones and associated conditions. Table 67.3 shows the wide array of imaging techniques available to evaluate the biliary tract.[248–251] Each modality has its strengths and limitations, and the methods vary widely in relative cost and risk to the patient. With the possible exception of US, none of the modalities should be ordered routinely in the evaluation of a patient with suspected gallstone disease; rather, the diagnostic evaluation should proceed in a rational stepwise fashion based on the individual patient's symptoms, signs, and results of laboratory studies (see later).

Notably absent from the list of imaging studies of the biliary tract is the plain abdominal film. Although useful on occasion for evaluating patients with abdominal pain, plain abdominal films are

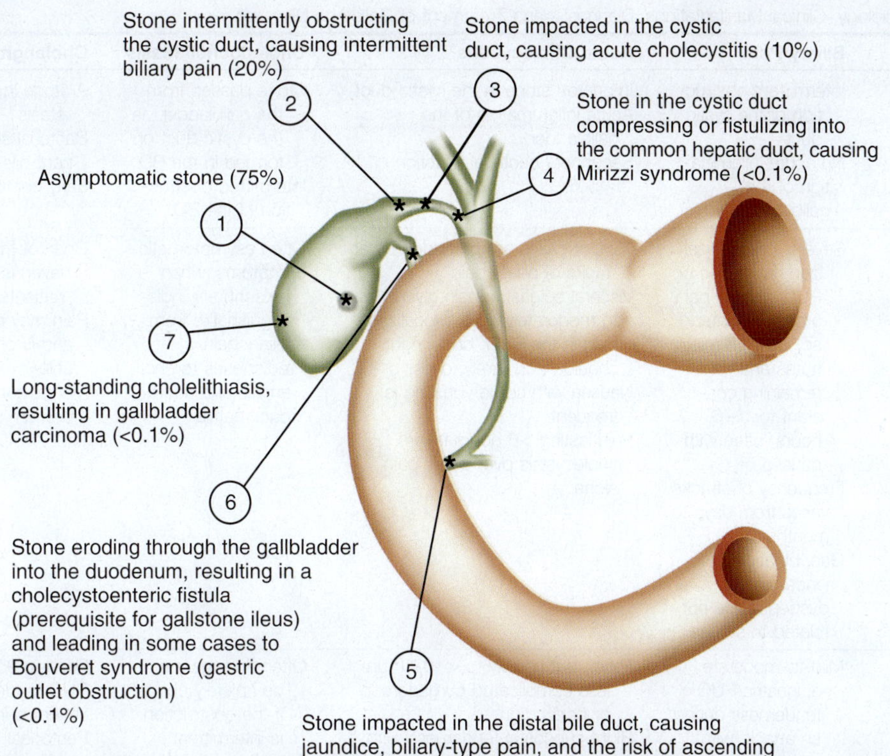
Stone intermittently obstructing the cystic duct, causing intermittent biliary pain (20%)
Stone impacted in the cystic duct, causing acute cholecystitis (10%)
Stone in the cystic duct compressing or fistulizing into the common hepatic duct, causing Mirizzi syndrome (<0.1%)
Asymptomatic stone (75%)
1
2
3
4
5
6
7
Long-standing cholelithiasis, resulting in gallbladder carcinoma (<0.1%)
Stone eroding through the gallbladder into the duodenum, resulting in a cholecystoenteric fistula (prerequisite for gallstone ileus) and leading in some cases to Bouveret syndrome (gastric outlet obstruction) (<0.1%)
Stone impacted in the distal bile duct, causing jaundice, biliary-type pain, and the risk of ascending cholangitis or acute biliary pancreatitis (5%)

Fig. 67.7 Schematic depiction of the natural history and complications of gallstones. Percentages indicate approximate frequencies of complications that occur in persons with gallstones, based on natural history data. The most frequent outcome is for the patient with a stone to remain asymptomatic throughout life (1). Biliary pain (2), acute cholecystitis (3), cholangitis (5), and pancreatitis (5) are the most common complications. Mirizzi syndrome (4), cholecystoenteric fistula (6), Bouveret syndrome (6), and gallbladder cancer (7) are uncommon. (The sum of percentages is >100% because patients with acute cholecystitis generally have had prior episodes of biliary pain.)

limited by a lack of sensitivity and specificity. Only 50% of pigment stones and 20% of cholesterol stones contain enough calcium to be visible on a plain abdominal film. Because 80% of gallstones in the Western world are of the cholesterol type, only 25% of stones can be detected by simple radiographs. Plain abdominal films have their greatest usefulness in evaluating patients with some of the unusual complications of gallstones (e.g., emphysematous cholecystitis, cholecystenteric fistula, gallstone ileus) or in detecting a porcelain gallbladder (see later).

Ultrasound

Since its introduction in the 1970s, US examination of the biliary tract has become the principal imaging modality for the diagnosis of cholelithiasis. US requires only an overnight or 8-hour fast, involves no ionizing radiation, is simple to perform, and provides accurate anatomic information. It has the additional advantage of being portable and thus available at the bedside of a critically ill patient.[233]

The diagnosis of gallstones relies on detection of echogenic objects within the lumen of the gallbladder that produce an acoustic shadow (Fig. 67.8A). The stones are mobile and generally congregate in the dependent portion of the gallbladder. Modern US can detect stones as small as 2 mm in diameter routinely. Smaller stones may be missed or may be confused with biliary sludge (layering echogenic material that does not cast an acoustic shadow).[252]

The sensitivity of US for detection of gallstones in the gallbladder is greater than 95% for stones larger than 2 mm.[253] The specificity is greater than 95% when stones produce acoustic shadows. Rarely, advanced scarring and contraction of the gallbladder around gallstones make locating the gallbladder or the stones impossible, raising the possibility of gallbladder cancer. The contracted gallbladder filled with stones may give a "double-arc shadow" or "wall-echo shadow" sign, with the gallbladder wall, echogenic stones, and acoustic shadowing seen in immediate proximity. If the gallbladder cannot be identified ultrasonographically, then a complementary imaging modality such as OCG or abdominal CT is warranted.

US is the standard for the diagnosis of stones in the gallbladder but is distinctly less sensitive for the detection of stones in the bile duct (common bile duct).[254] Because of the proximity of the distal bile duct to the duodenum, luminal bowel gas often interferes with the US image, and the entire length of the bile duct cannot be examined.[255] As a result, only about 50% of bile duct stones are actually seen on US.[249] The presence of an obstructing bile duct stone, however, can be inferred when a dilated duct is found in the absence of cholecystectomy. Because ERCP has uncovered a rising frequency of falsely negative US results, the upper limit of normal of the diameter of the bile duct has declined from 10 mm to 6 mm. Even so, inferring choledocholithiasis from a dilated bile duct on US has a sensitivity of only 75%.

US is quite useful for diagnosing acute cholecystitis.[256] Pericholecystic fluid (in the absence of ascites) and gallbladder wall thickening to more than 4 mm (in the absence of hypoalbuminemia) are suggestive of acute cholecystitis (see Fig. 67.8B). Unfortunately, in the critical care setting, these nonspecific findings are seen frequently in patients with no other evidence of

TABLE 67.2 Pathophysiology, Clinical Manifestations, Diagnosis, and Treatment of Gallstone Disease[a]

	Biliary Pain	Acute Cholecystitis	Choledocholithiasis	Cholangitis
Pathophysiology	Intermittent obstruction of the cystic duct No acute inflammation of the gallbladder	Impacted stone in the cystic duct Acute inflammation of the gallbladder Secondary bacterial infection in ≈50%	Stone passed from the gallbladder via the cystic duct or formed in the BD Intermitted obstruction of the BD	A stone in the BD causing bile stasis Bacterial superinfection of stagnant bile Early bacteremia
Symptoms	Severe, poorly localized, epigastric or RUQ visceral pain growing in intensity over 15 minutes and remaining constant for 1–6 hours, often with nausea Frequency of attacks varies from days to months Gas, bloating, flatulence, and dyspepsia are not related to stones	75% of cases are preceded by attacks of biliary pain Visceral epigastric pain gives way to moderately severe localized pain in the RUQ, back, right shoulder, or, rarely, chest Nausea with some vomiting is frequent Pain lasting >6 hours favors cholecystitis over biliary pain alone	Often asymptomatic Symptoms (when present) are indistinguishable from biliary pain Predisposes to cholangitis and acute pancreatitis	Charcot triad (pain, jaundice, and fever) is present in 70% of patients Pain may be mild and transient and is often accompanied by chills Mental confusion, lethargy, and delirium suggest sepsis
Physical findings	Mild-to-moderate epigastric/RUQ tenderness during an attack, with mild residual tenderness lasting days Often, findings are normal	Fever, but usually to <102°F unless complicated by gangrene or perforation Right subcostal tenderness with inspiratory arrest (Murphy sign) Palpable gallbladder in 33% of patients, especially those having their first attack Mild jaundice in 20%; higher frequency in older adults	Often findings are completely normal if the obstruction is intermittent Jaundice with pain suggests stones; painless jaundice and a palpable gallbladder favor malignancy	Fever in 95% RUQ tenderness in 90% Jaundice in 80% Peritoneal signs in 15% Hypotension and mental confusion (forming Reynolds pentad in combination with Charcot triad) coexist in 15% and suggest Gram-negative sepsis
Laboratory findings	Usually normal Elevated serum bilirubin, alkaline phosphatase, or amylase levels suggest coexisting BD stones	Leukocytosis with band forms is common Serum bilirubin level may be 2–4 mg/dL, and aminotransferase and alkaline phosphatase levels may be elevated even in the absence of a BD stone or hepatic infection Mild serum amylase and lipase elevations are seen even in the absence of pancreatitis If serum bilirubin is >4 mg/dL or amylase or lipase is markedly elevated, a BD stone should be suspected	Elevated serum bilirubin and alkaline phosphatase levels are seen with BD obstruction Serum bilirubin level >10 mg/dL suggests malignant obstruction or coexisting hemolysis A transient "spike" in serum aminotransferase or amylase (or lipase) levels suggests the passage of a stone	Leukocytosis in 80%, but the remainder may have a normal WBC count with or without band forms Serum bilirubin level is >2 mg/dL in 80% Serum alkaline phosphatase level is usually elevated Blood cultures are usually positive, especially during chills or a fever spike; two organisms are grown in cultures from half of patients
Diagnostic studies (see Table 67.3 for details on imaging studies)	US Oral cholecystography Meltzer-Lyon test (see Chapter 69)	US Hepatobiliary scintigraphy Abdominal CT	ERCP EUS MRC Percutaneous THC	ERCP Percutaneous THC
Natural history	After the initial attack, 30% of patients have no further symptoms Symptoms develop in the remainder at a rate of 6% per year, and severe complications at a rate of 1%–2% per year	50% of cases resolve spontaneously in 7–10 days without surgery Left untreated, 10% of cases are complicated by a localized perforation and 1% by a free perforation and peritonitis	The natural history is not well defined, but complications are more common and more severe than for asymptomatic stones in the gallbladder	A high mortality rate if unrecognized, with death from septicemia Emergency decompression of the BD (usually by ERCP) improves survival dramatically

TABLE 67.2 Pathophysiology, Clinical Manifestations, Diagnosis, and Treatment of Gallstone Disease[a]—cont'd

	Biliary Pain	Acute Cholecystitis	Choledocholithiasis	Cholangitis
Treatment (see Chapters 68 and 72)	Elective laparoscopic cholecystectomy, possibly with IOC ERCP for stone removal or BD exploration if IOC shows stones	Laparoscopic cholecystectomy, possibly with IOC if feasible; otherwise open cholecystectomy BD exploration or ERCP for stone removal if IOC shows stones	Stone removal at the time of ERCP, followed in most cases by early laparoscopic cholecystectomy	Emergency ERCP with stone removal or at least biliary decompression Antibiotics to cover gram-negative and possibly anaerobic organisms and Enterococcus spp. Subsequent cholecystectomy

[a]See Chapter 60 for a discussion of biliary pancreatitis.
BD, Bile duct; *IOC*, intraoperative cholangiography; *MRC*, magnetic resonance cholangiography; *THC*, transhepatic cholangiography.

TABLE 67.3 Imaging Studies of the Biliary Tract

Technique	Condition Tested For	Findings/Comments
US	Cholelithiasis	Stones manifest as mobile, dependent echogenic foci within the gallbladder lumen with acoustic shadowing Sludge appears as layering echogenic material without shadows Sensitivity >95% for stones >2 mm Specificity >95% for stones with acoustic shadows Rarely, a stone-filled gallbladder may be contracted and difficult to see, with a "wall-echo-shadow" sign Best single test for stones in the gallbladder
	Choledocholithiasis	Stones are seen in the BD in only ≈50% of cases but can be inferred from the finding of a dilated BD (>6 mm diameter), with or without gallstones, in another ≈25% of cases Can confirm, but not exclude, BD stones
	Acute cholecystitis	Sonographic Murphy sign (focal gallbladder tenderness under the transducer) has a positive predictive value of >90% in detecting acute cholecystitis when stones are seen Pericholecystic fluid (in the absence of ascites) and gallbladder wall thickening to >4 mm (in the absence of hypoalbuminemia) are nonspecific findings but are suggestive of acute cholecystitis
EUS	Choledocholithiasis	Highly accurate for excluding or confirming stones in the BD Concordance of EUS with the ERCP diagnosis ≈95%; many studies suggest slightly higher sensitivity rates for EUS than for ERCP Specificity ≈97% Positive predictive value ≈99%, negative predictive value ≈98%, accuracy ≈97% With experienced operators, EUS can be used in lieu of ERCP to exclude BD stones, particularly when the clinical suspicion is low or intermediate Considered for patients with low to moderate clinical probability of choledocholithiasis
Oral cholecystography[a]	Cholelithiasis	Stones manifest as mobile filling defects in an opacified gallbladder Sensitivity and specificity exceed 90% when the gallbladder is opacified, but nonvisualization occurs in 25% of studies and can result from multiple causes other than stones Opacification of the gallbladder indicates cystic duct patency May be useful in the evaluation of acalculous gallbladder diseases such as cholesterolosis and adenomyomatosis (see Chapter 69)
Cholescintigraphy (hepatobiliary scintigraphy; hydroxyiminodiacetic acid or diisopropyl iminodiacetic acid scan)	Acute cholecystitis	Assesses patency of the cystic duct A normal scan shows radioactivity in the gallbladder, BD, and small bowel within 30–60 minutes A positive result is defined as nonvisualization of the gallbladder, with preserved hepatic excretion of radionuclide into the BD or small bowel Sensitivity is ≈95% and specificity is ≈90%, with false-positive results seen in fasted critically ill patients With cholecystokinin stimulation, the gallbladder "ejection fraction" can be determined and may help evaluate patients with acalculous biliary pain (see Chapter 69) A normal scan result virtually excludes acute cholecystitis

Continued

TABLE 67.3 Imaging Studies of the Biliary Tract—cont'd

Technique	Condition Tested For	Findings/Comments
ERCP	Choledocholithiasis	ERCP is the standard diagnostic test for stones in the BD, with sensitivity and specificity of ≈95% Use of ERCP to extract stones (or at least drain infected bile) is lifesaving in severe cholangitis and reduces the need for BD exploration at the time of cholecystectomy Recommended for patients with a high clinical probability of choledocholithiasis
	Cholelithiasis	When contrast agent flows retrograde into the gallbladder, stones appear as filling defects and can be detected with a sensitivity rate of ≈80%, but US remains the mainstay for confirming cholelithiasis
MRCP	Choledocholithiasis	A rapid, noninvasive modality that provides detailed bile duct and pancreatic duct images equal to those of ERCP Sensitivity ≈93% and specificity ≈94%, comparable with those for ERCP Useful for examining nondilated ducts, particularly at the distal portion, which often is not well visualized by US Adjacent structures such as the liver and pancreas can be examined at the same time Recommended for patients with low to moderate clinical probability of choledocholithiasis
CT	Complications of gallstones	Not well suited for detecting uncomplicated stones but excellent for detecting complications such as abscess, perforation of gallbladder or BD, and pancreatitis Spiral CT may prove useful as a noninvasive means of excluding BD stones; some studies suggest improved diagnostic accuracy when CT is combined with an oral cholecystographic contrast agent

*Performed infrequently.
BD, Bile duct.

gallbladder disease.[256] A more specific finding is the so-called sonographic Murphy sign, in which the ultrasonographer elicits focal gallbladder tenderness under the US transducer. Eliciting a sonographic Murphy sign is somewhat operator dependent and requires an alert patient. Presence of the sign has a positive predictive value of greater than 90% for detecting acute cholecystitis if gallstones are present.[257] US may help localize other abdominal diseases, such as abscesses or pseudocysts, that may be in the differential diagnosis.

EUS

EUS is highly accurate for detecting choledocholithiasis. More invasive and more expensive than standard US, EUS has the advantage of being able to visualize the bile duct from within the GI lumen and is comparable to ERCP in this respect. Intraluminal imaging provides several advantages over transabdominal US, including closer proximity to the bile duct, higher resolution, and lack of interference by bowel gas or abdominal wall layers (Fig. 67.9). In several studies, EUS had a positive predictive value of 99%, negative predictive value of 98%, and accuracy rate of 97% for the diagnosis of bile duct stones compared with ERCP.[258,259] If bile duct stones are found on EUS, endoscopic removal of the stones is necessary, and it can be argued that ERCP should be the initial study if choledocholithiasis is strongly suspected. Nevertheless, several studies that compared EUS with ERCP have found both techniques to be accurate for confirming or excluding choledocholithiasis, with EUS having advantages in both safety and cost.[260–262]

EUS has also been found to be superior to MRCP (or simply magnetic resonance cholangiography [MRC]) in detecting the presence or absence of bile duct stones (see later). The major benefit of EUS in patients with a clinical suspicion of choledocholithiasis is the ability to avoid unnecessary ERCP and sphincterotomy, which is not without risk. Use of EUS to determine if ERCP is indicated may avoid a significant number of ERCPs and result in fewer complications. A systematic review of randomized controlled trials compared EUS-guided ERCP with ERCP alone for detection of bile duct stones.[263] Patients randomized to EUS were able to avoid ERCP in 67% of cases and had lower rates of complications and pancreatitis compared with those randomized to ERCP alone (OR, 0.35 and 0.21, respectively). EUS failed to detect bile duct stones in only 2 of 213 patients (0.9%). Therefore EUS is considered an appropriate modality for excluding bile duct stones, especially if the pretest probability of finding stones is low to intermediate.

Oral Cholecystography

Once the mainstay of imaging studies of the gallbladder, OCG now has limited application as a secondary approach to identifying stones in the gallbladder.[249] The only useful clinical indications for OCG are the evaluation of patients in whom medical dissolution of stones or lithotripsy is being considered (see Chapter 68)[264] and the evaluation of patients for unsuspected gallbladder disease, such as adenomyomatosis or cholesterolosis, when US has been nondiagnostic (see Chapter 67).

Cholescintigraphy

Cholescintigraphy (hepatobiliary scintigraphy) is a radionuclide imaging test of the gallbladder and biliary tract that is most useful for evaluating patients with suspected acute cholecystitis.[265] By demonstrating patency of the cystic duct, cholescintigraphy can exclude acute cholecystitis rapidly (within 90 minutes) in a patient who presents with abdominal pain.[266,267] The procedure can be performed on an emergency basis in a nonfasting patient after IV administration of gamma-emitting ^{99m}Tc-labeled hydroxyl iminodiacetic acid or diisopropyl iminodiacetic acid (DISIDA), which is taken up rapidly by the liver and secreted into bile.[249] As shown in Fig. 67.10, serial scans after injection normally should show radioactivity in the gallbladder, bile duct, and small intestine within 30–60 minutes.[211] In the past, imaging of jaundiced patients with this technique was limited, but use of DISIDA may

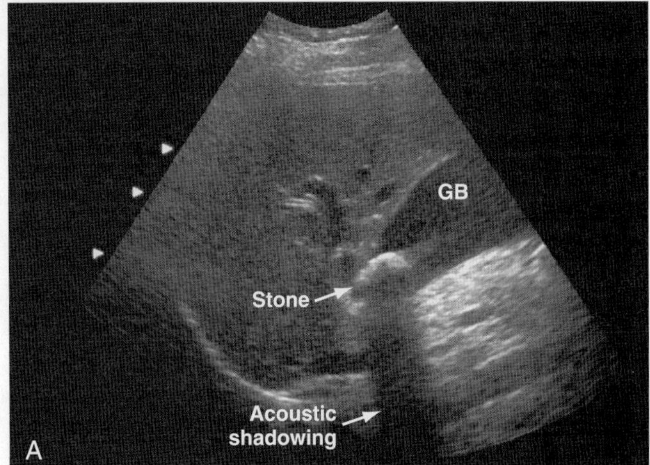

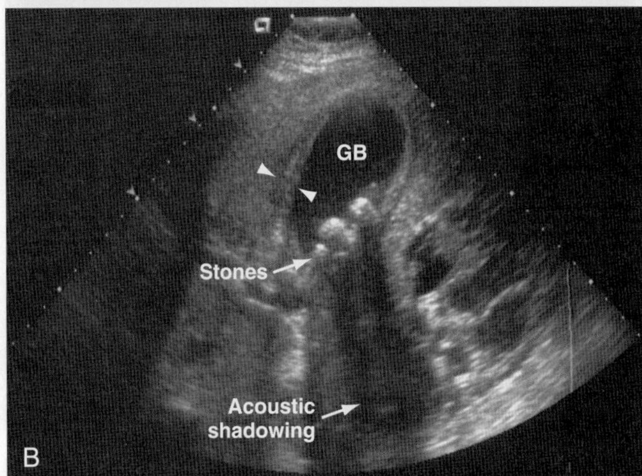

Fig. 67.8 (A) Typical ultrasonographic appearance of cholelithiasis. A gallstone is present within the lumen of the gallbladder (GB), with acoustic shadow behind it. With repositioning of the patient, stones will move, thereby excluding the possibility of a gallbladder polyp. (B) Cholelithiasis in the setting of acute cholecystitis. Multiple gallstones can be seen within the gallbladder lumen, with associated acoustic shadowing. In addition, the gallbladder wall is thickened (*arrowheads*). (Courtesy Julie Champine, MD, Dallas, TX.)

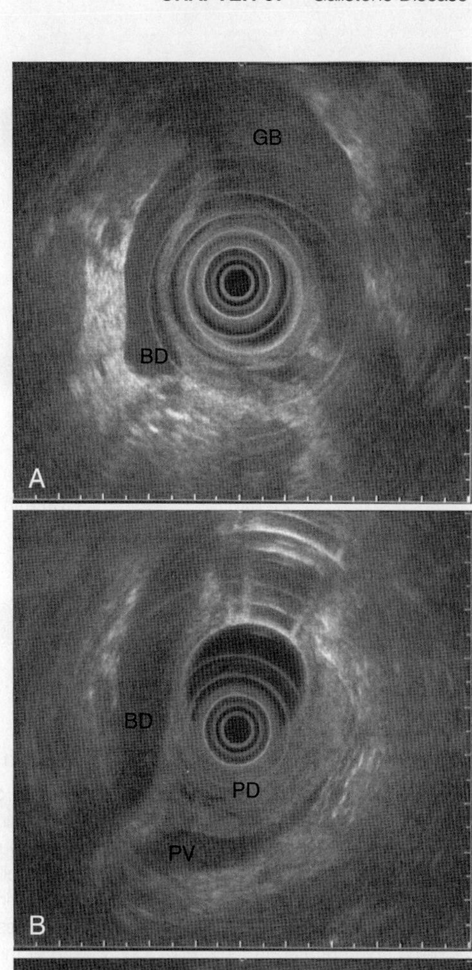

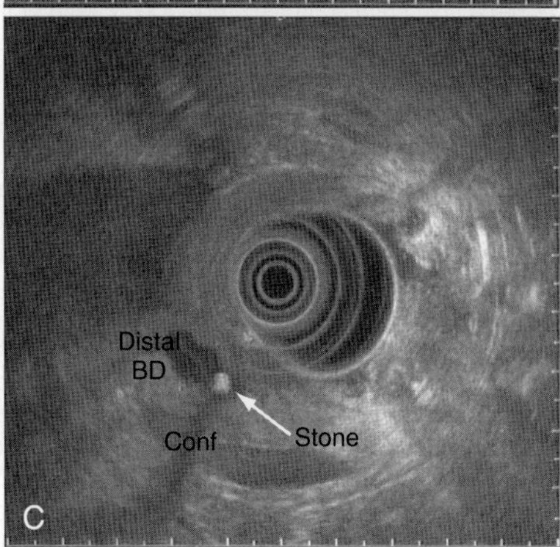

Fig. 67.9 EUS with a radial sector scanning endoscope, demonstrating choledocholithiasis. The bile duct (*BD*) is shown extending to the level of the gallbladder (*GB*) (top) and distally (A and B). The greatest diameter of the BD is 12 mm (B), and the duct tapers distally to a diameter of 7 mm (C). Within the distal BD, a gallstone is clearly visualized (C). Note the proximity of adjacent structures to the BD and the ease with which these structures are resolved by EUS. *Conf*, Confluence of portal and splenic veins; *PD*, pancreatic duct; *PV*, portal vein.

allow imaging of the biliary tract in a patient with a serum bilirubin value as high as 20 mg/dL.

An abnormal, or "positive," scan result is defined as nonvisualization of the gallbladder, with preserved excretion into the bile duct or small intestine. The accuracy of the test for detecting acute cholecystitis is 92%, superior to that for US. False-positive results occur primarily in fasting or critically ill patients, in whom gallbladder motility is decreased. The reduction in gallbladder motility leads to greater water resorption, which results in a gelatinous bile. In critically ill patients, cholestasis and hepatocyte dysfunction result in reduced clearance of radionuclide imaging agents. Although nonvisualization of the gallbladder because of cystic duct obstruction is the hallmark of acute cholecystitis, pericholecystic hepatic uptake of radionuclide is a useful secondary sign.[268]

In some patients (e.g., those with chronic cholecystitis, liver disease, or choledocholithiasis), imaging of the gallbladder by radionuclide scanning is delayed for several hours, and scanning must be repeated in 4 or more hours to confirm the absence of acute cholecystitis. This delay in visualization of the gallbladder is problematic in the acutely ill patient but has largely been overcome with the administration of IV morphine sulfate to patients in whom the gallbladder fails to be visualized within 60 minutes. Morphine raises the pressure within the sphincter of Oddi, thereby leading to the preferential flow of bile into the gallbladder if the cystic duct is not obstructed. Another scan is obtained 30 minutes after injection of morphine, and if the gallbladder is visualized, cystic duct obstruction, and hence acute

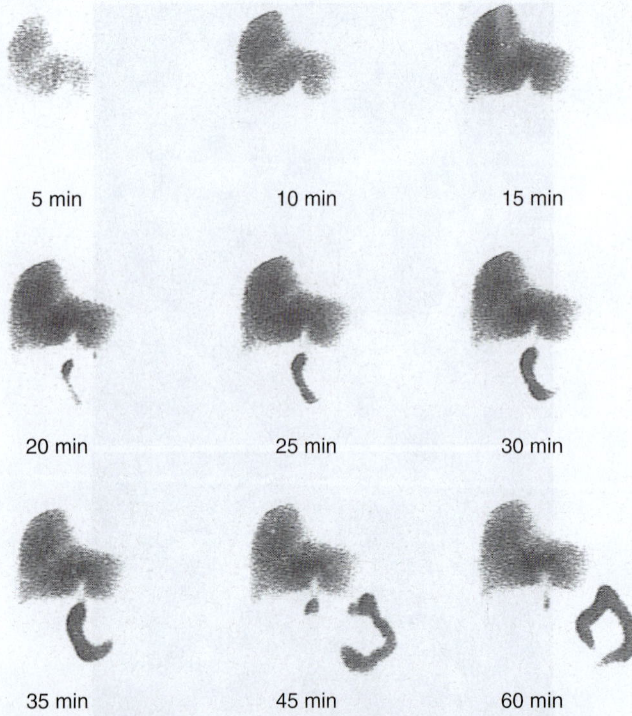

Fig. 67.10 Cholescintigraphy demonstrating an obstructed cystic duct characteristic of acute cholecystitis. The gamma-emitting radioisotope diisopropyl iminodiacetic acid is injected intravenously, rapidly taken up by the liver (at 5 minutes), and excreted into bile (at 20 minutes). Sequential images show the isotope quickly entering the duodenum (at 45 minutes) and passing distally in the small intestine without ever being concentrated in the gallbladder. Failure of the gallbladder to be visualized as a hot spot within 30–60 minutes constitutes a positive result and implies obstruction of the cystic duct.

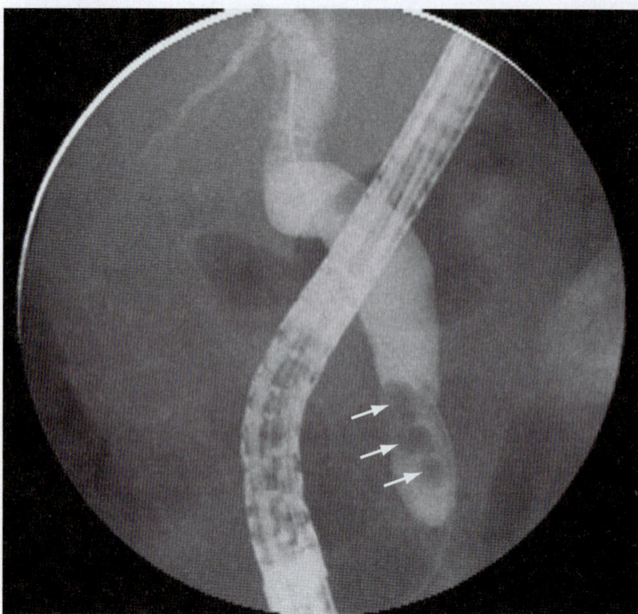

Fig. 67.11 ERCP demonstrating choledocholithiasis with dilatation of the bile duct to 15 mm and 3 filling defects representing stones (*arrows*).

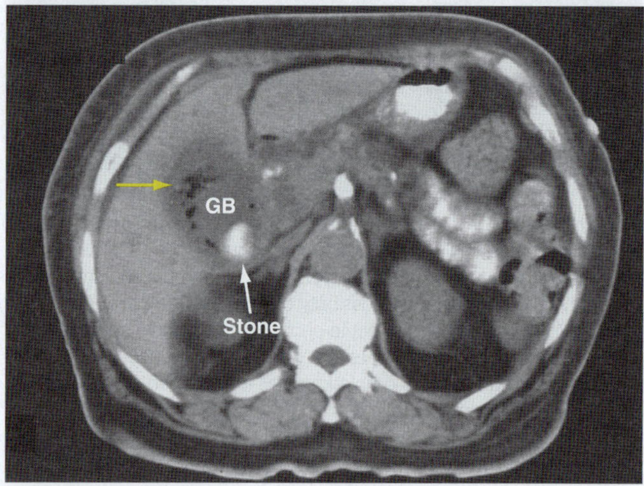

Fig. 67.12 Abdominal CT demonstrating emphysematous cholecystitis with associated cholelithiasis. Pockets of gas (*yellow arrow*), resulting from a secondary infection with gas-forming organisms, are present within the wall of the gallbladder (*GB*). (Courtesy Julie Champine, MD, Dallas, TX.)

cholecystitis, is excluded. The gallbladder may not be visualized in approximately half of critically ill patients even after injection of morphine, thereby leading to false-positive cholescintigraphy results.

Although primarily a tool for evaluating acutely ill patients with suspected acute cholecystitis, cholescintigraphy after administration of CCK may be useful in identifying patients with chronic acalculous biliary pain who are likely to benefit from empirical cholecystectomy (see Chapter 67). An additional important role for cholescintigraphy is the noninvasive detection of bile leakage from the cystic duct as a complication of cholecystectomy (see Chapter 68).[269]

Endoscopic Retrograde Cholangiopancreatography

ERCP is one of the most effective modalities for detecting choledocholithiasis.[270] The technique is discussed in more detail in Chapter 72. Stones within the bile duct appear as filling defects and can be detected with a sensitivity of around 95% (Fig. 67.11).[271] Care should be taken to avoid inadvertent injection of air into the biliary tract,[272] because bubbles may mimic gallstones. The specificity of ERCP for the detection of bile duct stones is approximately 95%.

The therapeutic applications of ERCP have revolutionized the treatment of patients with choledocholithiasis[273] and other bile duct disorders (see Chapter 72). As the use of EUS and MRC has increased, the role of ERCP in the diagnosis of choledocholithiasis has changed considerably. A National Institutes of Health consensus conference has recommended the use of ERCP only when the clinical probability of choledocholithiasis is high (i.e., when the need for therapeutic intervention is likely). For diagnosis of choledocholithiasis alone, EUS and MRC are equal in accuracy to ERCP.[274]

CT and MRI

In patients with cholelithiasis or choledocholithiasis, CT has been used principally for detecting complications such as pericholecystic fluid in acute cholecystitis, gas in the gallbladder wall (suggesting emphysematous cholecystitis), gallbladder perforation, and abscesses (Fig. 67.12). Helical (or spiral) CT cholangiography (CTC) with use of an oral cholecystographic contrast

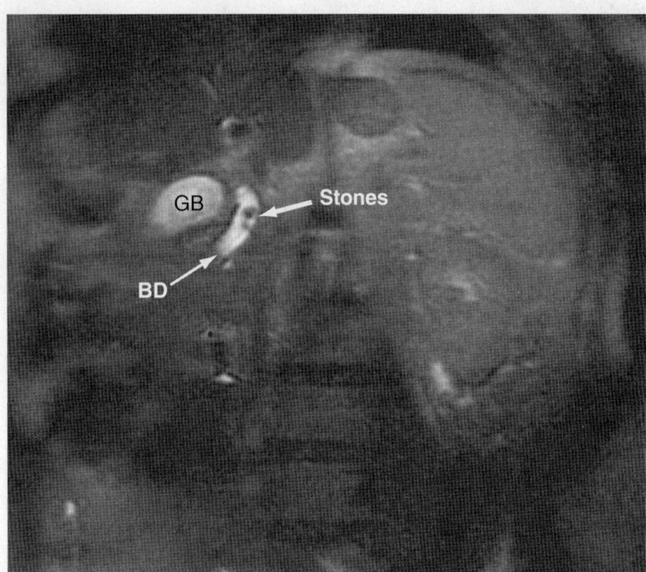

Fig. 67.13 MRCP demonstrating choledocholithiasis. Within the bile duct (*BD*) are 2 filling defects representing gallstones. *GB*, Gallbladder. (Courtesy Charles Owen, III, MD, Dallas, TX.)

agent has been studied for the detection of choledocholithiasis.[275,276] Although CTC is still inferior to ERCP imaging for detecting bile duct stones, it may reveal other surrounding pathologic abnormalities.[277]

MRC is highly useful for imaging the bile duct and detecting gallstones. This modality is especially useful for detecting abnormalities in the most distal extrahepatic portion of the bile duct when the duct is not dilated; this region is often not well visualized by transabdominal US.[234] With the advent of laparoscopic cholecystectomy, an easy, quick, and preferably noninvasive method of excluding bile duct stones is needed. MRC permits construction of a three-dimensional image of the bile duct with a high sensitivity for detecting bile duct stones (Fig. 67.13).[261,262] In a systematic review that compared MRC with diagnostic ERCP for detection of choledocholithiasis, MRC had a sensitivity of 93% and a specificity of 94%.[263]

CLINICAL DISORDERS

Biliary Pain and Chronic Cholecystitis

Biliary pain is the most common presenting symptom of cholelithiasis, and about 75% of patients with symptomatic gallstone disease seek medical attention for episodic abdominal pain. In patients who present with a complication of gallstones, such as acute cholecystitis, a history of recurrent episodes of abdominal pain in the months preceding the complication is often elicited.

Pathogenesis

Biliary pain (conventionally referred to as biliary "colic," a misnomer) is caused by intermittent obstruction of the cystic duct by one or more gallstones. Biliary pain does not require that inflammation of the gallbladder accompany the obstruction. The term "chronic cholecystitis" to describe biliary pain should be avoided because it implies the presence of a chronic inflammatory infiltrate that may or may not be present in a given patient. Indeed, the severity and frequency of biliary pain and the pathologic changes in the gallbladder do not correlate.[278] The most common histologic changes observed in patients with biliary pain are mild fibrosis of the gallbladder wall with a chronic inflammatory cell infiltrate and intact mucosa. Recurrent episodes of biliary pain can also be associated with a scarred, shrunken gallbladder and Rokitansky-Aschoff sinuses (intramural diverticula). Bacteria can be cultured from gallbladder bile or gallstones themselves in about 10% of patients with biliary pain, but bacterial infection is not believed to contribute to the symptoms (see Chapter 67).

Clinical Features

Biliary pain is visceral in nature and thus poorly localized.[279] In a typical case, the patient experiences episodes of upper abdominal pain, usually in the epigastrium or RUQ, but sometimes in other abdominal locations. Ingestion of a meal often precipitates pain, but more commonly no inciting event is apparent. The onset of biliary pain is more likely to occur during periods of weight reduction and marked physical inactivity such as prolonged bed rest than at other times.

The term "biliary colic," used in the past, is a misnomer because the pain is steady rather than intermittent, as would be suggested by the word *colic*. The pain increases gradually over a period of 15 minutes to an hour and then remains at a plateau for an hour or more before slowly resolving. In one-third of patients, the onset of pain may be more sudden, and on rare occasions, the pain may cease abruptly. Pain lasting more than 6 hours suggests acute cholecystitis rather than simple biliary pain (see Chapter 12).

In order of decreasing frequency, biliary pain is felt maximally in the epigastrium, RUQ, LUQ, and various parts of the precordium or lower abdomen. Therefore the notion that pain not located in the RUQ is atypical of gallstone disease is incorrect. Radiation of the pain to the scapula, right shoulder, or lower abdomen occurs in half of patients. Diaphoresis and nausea with some vomiting are common, although vomiting is not as protracted as in intestinal obstruction or acute pancreatitis. Like patients with other kinds of visceral pain, the patient with biliary pain is usually restless and active during an episode.

Complaints of gas, bloating, flatulence, and dyspepsia, which are common in patients with gallstones, are probably not related to the stones themselves. These nonspecific symptoms are found with similar frequencies in persons without gallstones. Accordingly, patients with gallstones whose only symptoms are dyspepsia and other nonspecific upper GI tract complaints are not candidates for cholecystectomy. Physical findings are usually normal, with only mild to moderate gallbladder tenderness during an attack and perhaps mild residual tenderness lasting several days after an attack.

Diagnosis

In a patient with uncomplicated biliary pain, laboratory parameters are usually normal. Elevations of serum bilirubin, alkaline phosphatase, or amylase levels suggest coexisting choledocholithiasis.

In general, the first, and often the only, imaging study recommended in patients with biliary pain is US of the RUQ. Despite the impressive diagnostic accuracy of US, a clinically important stone is occasionally missed, and the correct diagnosis is delayed because of the large number of patients who undergo US for any reason.[250] Given the relatively benign natural history of biliary pain, patients with suspected gallstones but a negative US result can safely be observed, with further diagnostic testing reserved for those in whom symptoms recur.[280]

Differential Diagnosis

The differential diagnosis of recurrent episodic upper abdominal symptoms includes reflux esophagitis, peptic ulcer, pancreatitis, renal colic, diverticulitis, carcinoma of the colon, IBS, radiculopathy, and angina pectoris (see Chapter 12). Usually a carefully taken history assists in narrowing the differential diagnosis. In a study of 1008 patients who underwent cholecystectomy for gallstones, clinical features associated with biliary pain "episodic gallbladder pain" were episodic pain (usually once a month or less), pain lasting 30 minutes to 24 hours, pain during the evening or at night, and the onset of symptoms 1 year or less before presentation.[281] Xanthogranulomatous cholecystitis is a rare aggressive variant of chronic cholecystitis characterized by grayish-yellow nodules or streaks, representing lipid-laden macrophages, in the gallbladder wall; it may present as acute jaundice.

Treatment

Patients with recurrent uncomplicated biliary pain and documented gallstones are generally treated with elective laparoscopic cholecystectomy (see Chapter 68). Acute biliary pain improves with administration of meperidine, with or without ketorolac or diclofenac. Aspirin taken prophylactically has been reported to prevent gallstone formation as well as acute attacks of biliary pain in patients with gallstones, but long-term use of other NSAIDs does not prevent gallstone formation.[275,276]

Acute Cholecystitis

Acute cholecystitis is the most common complication of gallstone disease. Inflammation of the gallbladder wall associated with abdominal pain, RUQ tenderness, fever, and leukocytosis is the hallmark of acute cholecystitis. In approximately 90% of cases, the underlying cause is obstruction of the outlet of the gallbladder by a gallstone in the cystic duct, gallbladder neck, or Hartmann pouch.[282] In the remaining 10% of cases, cholecystitis occurs in the absence of gallstones [*acalculous cholecystitis* (see Chapter 67)]. Acute cholecystitis caused by gallstones is a disease of young, otherwise healthy women and generally has a favorable prognosis, whereas acute acalculous cholecystitis occurs more commonly in critically ill patients and is associated with high morbidity and mortality rates.

Pathogenesis

Acute cholecystitis generally occurs when a stone becomes embedded in the cystic duct and causes chronic obstruction, rather than transient obstruction as in biliary pain.[282] Stasis of bile within the gallbladder lumen results in damage of the gallbladder mucosa, with the consequent release of intracellular enzymes and activation of a cascade of inflammatory mediators.

In animal studies, if the cystic duct is ligated, the usual result is gradual absorption of the gallbladder contents without the development of inflammation[283]; the additional instillation of a luminal irritant (e.g., concentrated bile or lysolecithin) or trauma from an indwelling catheter is required to cause acute cholecystitis in an obstructed gallbladder. Phospholipase A is believed to be released by gallstone-induced mucosal trauma and converts lecithin to lysolecithin. Although normally absent from gallbladder bile, lysolecithin is present in the gallbladder contents of patients with acute cholecystitis.[284] In animal models, installation of lysolecithin into the gallbladder produces acute cholecystitis associated with increased protein secretion, decreased water absorption, and evidence of WBC invasion associated with elevated production of prostaglandins E and $F_1\alpha$. Administration of indomethacin, a COX inhibitor, has been shown to block this inflammatory response. Studies of human tissue obtained at cholecystectomy have demonstrated enhanced prostaglandin production in the inflamed gallbladder. Additionally, administration of IV indomethacin and oral ibuprofen to patients with acute cholecystitis has been shown to diminish both luminal pressure in the gallbladder and pain.[284]

Supporting evidence for the role of prostaglandins in the development of acute cholecystitis comes from a prospective study in which patients who presented with biliary pain were randomized to receive diclofenac (a prostaglandin synthetase inhibitor) or placebo.[285] Ultimately, acute cholecystitis developed in 9 of 40 patients who received placebo, whereas episodes of biliary pain resolved in all 20 patients who received diclofenac. These data suggest a chain of events in which obstruction of the cystic duct in association with 1 or more intraluminal factors damages the gallbladder mucosa and stimulates prostaglandin synthetase. The resulting fluid secretion and inflammatory changes promote a cycle of further mucosal damage and inflammation.[285]

Enteric bacteria can be cultured from gallbladder bile in roughly one-half of patients with acute cholecystitis.[286] Bacteria are not believed to trigger the actual onset of acute cholecystitis, however.

Pathology

If examined in the first few days of an attack of acute cholecystitis, the gallbladder is usually distended and contains a stone embedded in the cystic duct.[287] After the gallbladder is opened, inflammatory exudate and, rarely, pus are present. Later in the attack, the bile pigments that are normally present are absorbed and replaced by thin mucoid fluid, pus, or blood. If the attack of acute cholecystitis is left untreated for a long period but the cystic duct remains obstructed, the lumen of the gallbladder may become distended with clear mucoid fluid, a condition known as *hydrops of the gallbladder*.

Histologic changes range from mild acute inflammation with edema to necrosis and perforation of the gallbladder wall. Surprisingly, the severity of histologic changes correlates little with the patient's symptoms.[287] If the gallbladder is resected for acute cholecystitis and no stones are found, the specimen should be carefully examined histologically for evidence of vasculitis or cholesterol emboli, because these systemic disorders may manifest as acalculous cholecystitis (see Chapter 35).

Clinical Features

Approximately 75% of patients with acute cholecystitis report prior attacks of biliary pain (see Table 67.2).[288] Often, such a patient is alerted to the possibility that more than simple biliary pain is occurring by the prolonged duration of the pain. If biliary pain has been constant for more than 6 hours, acute cholecystitis should be suspected.

In contrast to uncomplicated biliary pain, the physical findings can, in many cases, suggest the diagnosis of acute cholecystitis. Fever is common, but body temperature is usually less than 102°F unless the gallbladder has become gangrenous or has perforated (Fig. 67.14). Mild jaundice is present in 20% of patients with acute cholecystitis and 40% of older adult patients. Serum bilirubin levels are usually less than 4 mg/dL.[289] Bilirubin levels above this value suggest the possibility of bile duct stones, which may be found in 50% of jaundiced patients with acute cholecystitis. Another cause of pronounced jaundice in patients with acute cholecystitis is Mirizzi syndrome, which is associated with inflammatory obstruction of the common hepatic duct (see later).

The abdominal examination often demonstrates right subcostal tenderness with a palpable gallbladder in a third of patients; a palpable gallbladder is more common in patients having a first attack of acute cholecystitis. Repeated attacks usually result in a scarred, fibrotic gallbladder that is unable to distend. For unclear reasons, the gallbladder is usually palpable lateral to its normal anatomic location.

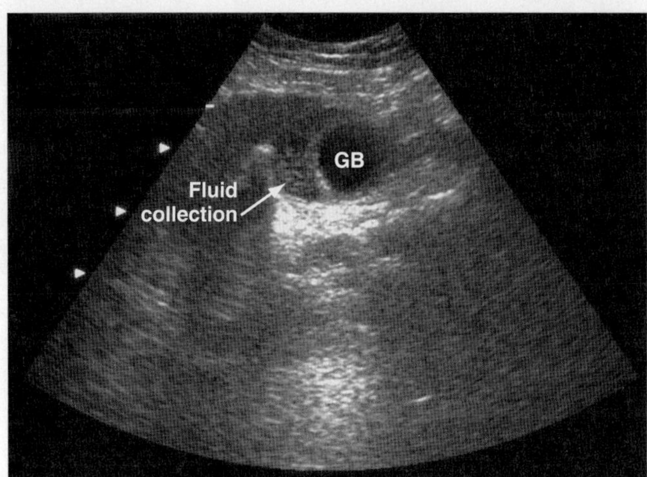

Fig. 67.14 US demonstrating a complex fluid collection adjacent to the gallbladder (*GB*), consistent with gallbladder perforation. (Courtesy Julie Champine, MD, Dallas, TX.)

A relatively specific finding of acute cholecystitis is a *Murphy sign*.[288] During palpation in the right subcostal region, pain and inspiratory arrest may occur when the patient takes a deep breath that brings the inflamed gallbladder into contact with the examiner's hand. The presence of a Murphy sign in the appropriate clinical setting is a reliable predictor of acute cholecystitis, although gallstones should still be confirmed by US.

Natural History

The pain of untreated acute cholecystitis generally resolves in 7–10 days.[290] Not uncommonly, symptoms remit within 48 hours of hospitalization. One study has shown that acute cholecystitis resolves without complications in about 83% of patients but results in gangrenous cholecystitis in 7%, gallbladder empyema in 6%, perforation in 3%, and emphysematous cholecystitis in fewer than 1%.[291]

Diagnosis

Perhaps because it is so common, acute cholecystitis is often at the top of the differential diagnosis of abdominal symptoms and is actually overdiagnosed when clinical criteria alone are considered. In a prospective series of 100 patients with RUQ pain and tenderness and suspected acute cholecystitis, this diagnosis was correct in only two-thirds of cases. The clinician must therefore use laboratory and imaging studies to confirm the presence of acute cholecystitis, exclude complications such as gangrene and perforation, and look for alternative causes of the clinical findings.

Table 67.3 shows the most common laboratory findings in acute cholecystitis.[290] Leukocytosis with a shift to immature neutrophils is common. Because a diagnosis of bile duct stones with cholangitis is usually in the differential diagnosis, attention should be directed to results of liver biochemical tests.[289] Even without detectable bile duct obstruction, acute cholecystitis often causes mild elevations in serum aminotransferase and alkaline phosphatase levels. As noted earlier, the serum bilirubin level may also be mildly elevated (2–4 mg/dL), and even serum amylase and lipase values may be elevated nonspecifically. A serum bilirubin value above 4 mg/dL or amylase value above 1000 U/L usually indicates coexisting bile duct obstruction or acute pancreatitis, respectively, and warrants further evaluation.

When the level of leukocytosis exceeds 15,000/mm^3, particularly in the setting of worsening pain, high fever (temperature >102°F), and chills, suppurative cholecystitis (empyema) or perforation should be suspected, and urgent surgical intervention may be required. Such advanced gallbladder disease may be present even if local and systemic manifestations are unimpressive.

US is the single most useful imaging study in acutely ill patients with RUQ pain and tenderness. It accurately establishes the presence or absence of gallstones and serves as an extension of the physical examination. The presence of a *sonographic Murphy sign*, defined as focal gallbladder tenderness under the transducer, has a positive predictive value greater than 90% for detecting acute cholecystitis if gallstones are also present, the operator is skillful, and the patient is alert.[292] Additionally, US can detect nonspecific findings suggestive of acute cholecystitis, such as pericholecystic fluid and gallbladder wall thickening greater than 4 mm. Both findings lose specificity for acute cholecystitis if the patient has ascites or hypoalbuminemia.[250,293]

Because the prevalence of gallstones is high in the population, many patients with nonbiliary tract diseases that manifest as acute abdominal pain (e.g., acute pancreatitis and complications of peptic ulcer) may have incidental and clinically irrelevant gallstones. The greatest usefulness of cholescintigraphy in these patients is its ability to exclude acute cholecystitis and allow the clinician to focus on nonbiliary causes of the patient's acute abdominal pain.[243] A normal cholescintigraphy result shows radioactivity in the gallbladder, bile duct, and small intestine within 30–60 minutes of injection of the isotope. With rare exceptions, a normal result excludes acute cholecystitis due to gallstones. Several studies have suggested that the sensitivity and specificity of scintigraphy in the setting of acute cholecystitis are approximately 94% each. However, sensitivity and specificity are reduced considerably in patients who have liver disease, are receiving parenteral nutrition, or are fasting. These conditions can lead to a false-positive result, defined as the absence of isotope in the gallbladder in a patient who does not have acute cholecystitis. If a positive result is defined as the absence of isotope in the gallbladder, then a false-negative result is defined as the filling of the gallbladder with isotope in the setting of acute cholecystitis, a situation that virtually never occurs. Therefore scintigraphy should not be used as the initial imaging study in a patient with suspected cholecystitis but rather should be used as a secondary imaging study in patients who already are known to have gallstones and in whom a nonbiliary cause of acute abdominal pain is possible.[294]

The greatest usefulness of abdominal CT in patients with acute cholecystitis is to detect complications such as emphysematous cholecystitis and perforation of the gallbladder. At the same time, CT can exclude other intra-abdominal processes that may engender a similar clinical picture. For example, abdominal CT is highly sensitive for detecting pneumoperitoneum, acute pancreatitis, pancreatic pseudocysts, hepatic or intra-abdominal abscesses, appendicitis, and obstruction or perforation of a hollow viscus. Abdominal CT usually is not warranted in patients with obvious acute cholecystitis, but if the diagnosis is uncertain or the optimal timing of surgery is in doubt, CT may be invaluable.

Differential Diagnosis

The principal conditions to consider in the differential diagnosis of acute cholecystitis are appendicitis, acute pancreatitis, pyelonephritis or renal calculi, peptic ulcer, acute hepatitis, pneumonia, hepatic abscess or tumor, and gonococcal or chlamydial perihepatitis. These possibilities should be considered before a cholecystectomy is recommended.

Treatment

The patient in whom acute cholecystitis is suspected should be hospitalized. The patient is often hypovolemic from vomiting and poor oral intake, and fluid and electrolytes should be administered intravenously. Oral feeding should be withheld, and an NG tube should be inserted if the patient has a distended abdomen or persistent vomiting.

In uncomplicated cases of acute cholecystitis, antibiotics need not be given. Antibiotics are warranted if the patient appears toxic or is suspected of having a complication such as perforation of the gallbladder or emphysematous cholecystitis. Broad-spectrum antibiotic coverage is usually indicated to cover Gram-negative organisms and anaerobes, with multiple possible regimens. The most commonly used regimens include piperacillin-tazobactam, ceftriaxone plus metronidazole, or levofloxacin plus metronidazole.

Definitive therapy of acute cholecystitis consists of cholecystectomy. The safety and effectiveness of a laparoscopic approach in the setting of acute cholecystitis have been demonstrated (see Chapter 68).[295]

Choledocholithiasis

Choledocholithiasis is defined as the occurrence of stones in the bile ducts. Like stones in the gallbladder, stones in the bile ducts may remain asymptomatic for years, and stones from the bile duct are known to pass silently into the duodenum, perhaps frequently. Unlike stones in the gallbladder, which usually become clinically evident as relatively benign episodes of recurrent biliary pain, stones in the bile duct, when they do cause symptoms, tend to manifest as life-threatening complications such as cholangitis and acute pancreatitis (see Chapter 60). Therefore discovery of choledocholithiasis generally should be followed by an intervention to remove the stones (see Chapter 72).

Etiology

Gallstones may pass from the gallbladder into the bile duct or form de novo in the duct. Generally, all gallstones from one patient, whether from the gallbladder or bile duct, are of one type, either cholesterol or pigment. Cholesterol stones form only in the gallbladder, and any cholesterol stones found in the bile duct must have migrated there from the gallbladder. Black pigment stones, which are associated with old age, hemolysis, alcoholism, and cirrhosis, also form in the gallbladder but only rarely migrate into the bile duct. The majority of pigment stones in the bile duct are the softer brown pigment stones. These stones form de novo in the bile duct as a result of bacterial action on phospholipid and bilirubin in bile (see earlier).[296] They are often proximal to a biliary stricture and are frequently associated with cholangitis. Brown pigment stones are found in patients with hepatolithiasis and recurrent pyogenic cholangitis (see Chapter 70).[297]

Fifteen percent of patients with gallbladder stones also have bile duct stones. Conversely, of patients with ductal stones, 95% also have gallbladder stones.[298] In patients who present with choledocholithiasis months or years after a cholecystectomy, determining whether the stones were overlooked at the earlier operation or have subsequently formed may be impossible. In fact, formation of pigment stones in the bile duct is also a late complication of endoscopic sphincterotomy.[299] In a study of the long-term consequences of endoscopic sphincterotomy in more than 400 patients, the cumulative frequency of recurrent bile duct stones was 12%; all the recurrent stones were of the brown pigment type, irrespective of the chemical composition of the original gallstones. This observation suggests that sphincterotomy permits chronic bacterial colonization of the bile duct that results in deconjugation of bilirubin and precipitation of pigment stones.

Stones in the bile duct usually come to rest at the lower end of the ampulla of Vater. Obstruction of the bile duct raises bile pressure proximally and causes the duct to dilate. The pressure in the bile duct is normally 10–15 cm H_2O and rises to 25–40 cm H_2O with complete obstruction. When the pressure exceeds 15 cm H_2O, bile flow decreases, and at 30 cm H_2O, bile flow stops.

The bile duct dilates to the point that dilatation can be detected on either US or abdominal CT in about 75% of cases. In patients who have had recurrent bouts of cholangitis, the bile duct may become fibrotic and unable to dilate. Moreover, dilatation of the duct is sometimes absent in patients with choledocholithiasis because the obstruction is low-grade and intermittent.

Clinical Features

The morbidity of choledocholithiasis stems principally from biliary obstruction, which raises biliary pressure and diminishes bile flow. The rate of onset of obstruction, its extent, and the amount of bacterial contamination of the bile are the major factors that determine resulting symptoms. Acute obstruction usually causes biliary pain and jaundice, whereas obstruction that develops gradually over several months may manifest initially as pruritus or jaundice alone.[300] If bacteria proliferate, life-threatening cholangitis may result (see later).

Physical findings are usually normal if obstruction of the bile duct is intermittent. Mild to moderate jaundice may be noted when obstruction has been present for several days to a few weeks. Deep jaundice without pain, particularly with a palpable gallbladder (Courvoisier sign), suggests neoplastic obstruction of the bile duct, even when the patient has stones in the gallbladder. With longstanding obstruction, secondary biliary cirrhosis may result, leading to physical findings of chronic liver disease.

As shown in Table 67.2, the results of laboratory studies may be the only clue to the presence of choledocholithiasis.[301] With bile duct obstruction, serum bilirubin and alkaline phosphatase levels both increase. Bilirubin accumulates in serum because of blocked excretion, whereas alkaline phosphatase levels rise because of increased synthesis of the enzyme by the canalicular epithelium. The rise in the alkaline phosphatase level is more rapid and precedes the rise in bilirubin level.[302] The absolute height of the serum bilirubin level is proportional to the extent of obstruction, but the height of the alkaline phosphatase level bears no relation to either the extent of obstruction or its cause. In cases of choledocholithiasis, the serum bilirubin level is typically in the range of 2–5 mg/dL[237] and rarely exceeds 12 mg/dL. Transient "spikes" in serum aminotransferase or amylase levels suggest passage of a bile duct stone into the duodenum. The overall sensitivity of liver biochemical testing for detecting choledocholithiasis is reported to be 94%; serum levels of GGTP are elevated most commonly but may not be assessed in clinical practice.[302]

Natural History

Little information is available on the natural history of asymptomatic bile duct stones. In many patients, such stones remain asymptomatic for months or years, but available evidence suggests the natural history of asymptomatic bile duct stones is less benign than that of asymptomatic gallstones.[300,303]

Diagnosis

US actually visualizes bile duct stones in only about 50% of cases,[254] whereas dilatation of the bile duct to a diameter greater than 6 mm is seen in about 75% of cases. US can confirm, or at least suggest, the presence of bile duct stones but cannot exclude choledocholithiasis definitively. EUS, although clearly more invasive than standard US, has the advantage of visualizing the bile duct more accurately. EUS can exclude or confirm choledocholithiasis with sensitivity and specificity rates of approximately 98% as compared with ERCP.[258]

ERCP is the standard method for diagnosis and therapy of bile duct stones,[304] with sensitivity and specificity rates of about 95%. When the clinical probability of choledocholithiasis is low, however, less invasive studies such as EUS and MRCP should be performed first (see earlier).[274]

Percutaneous transhepatic cholangiography (THC) is also an accurate test for confirming the presence of choledocholithiasis. The procedure is most readily accomplished when the intrahepatic bile ducts are dilated and is performed primarily when ERCP is unavailable or has been technically unsuccessful.

Laparoscopic US may be used in the surgical suite immediately before mobilization of the gallbladder during cholecystectomy. Laparoscopic US may be as accurate as surgical cholangiography in detecting bile duct stones and may thereby obviate the need for the latter.[305]

Differential Diagnosis

Symptoms caused by obstruction of the bile duct cannot be distinguished from those caused by obstruction of the cystic duct. Therefore biliary pain is always in the differential diagnosis in patients with an intact gallbladder. The presence of jaundice or abnormal liver biochemical test results strongly points to the bile duct rather than the gallbladder as the source of the pain.

In patients who present with jaundice, malignant obstruction of the bile duct or obstruction from a choledochal cyst may be indistinguishable clinically from choledocholithiasis (see Chapters 64 and 71). AIDS-associated cholangiopathy[306] and papillary stenosis should be considered in HIV-positive patients with RUQ pain and abnormal liver biochemical test results (see Chapter 33).

Treatment

Because of its propensity to result in serious complications such as cholangitis and acute pancreatitis, choledocholithiasis warrants treatment in nearly all cases.[307] The optimal therapy for a given patient depends on the severity of symptoms, presence of coexisting medical problems, availability of local expertise, and presence or absence of the gallbladder.

Bile duct stones discovered at the time of a laparoscopic cholecystectomy present a dilemma to the surgeon. Some surgeons may attempt laparoscopic exploration of the bile duct. In other cases, the operation can be converted to an open cholecystectomy with bile duct exploration, but this approach results in greater morbidity and a more prolonged hospital stay. Alternatively, the laparoscopic cholecystectomy can be carried out as planned, and the patient can return for ERCP with removal of the bile duct stones. Such an approach, if successful, cures the disease but runs the risk of necessitating a third procedure, namely, a bile duct exploration, if the stones cannot be removed at ERCP. In general, the greater the expertise of the therapeutic endoscopist, the more inclined the surgeon should be to complete the laparoscopic cholecystectomy and have the bile duct stones removed endoscopically.[307]

In especially high-risk patients, endoscopic removal of bile duct stones may be performed without cholecystectomy. This approach is particularly appropriate for older adult patients with other severe concurrent illnesses.[308] Cholecystectomy is required subsequently for recurrent symptoms in only 10% of patients. Surgical management and endoscopic treatment of gallstones are discussed in detail in Chapters 68 and 72, respectively.

Cholangitis

Of all the common complications of gallstones, the most serious and lethal is acute bacterial cholangitis. Pus under pressure in the bile ducts leads to rapid spread of bacteria via the liver into the blood, with resulting septicemia. Moreover, the diagnosis of cholangitis is often problematic (especially in the critical early phase of the disease) because clinical features that point to the biliary tract as the source of sepsis are often absent.[32] Table 67.2 delineates the symptoms, signs, and laboratory findings that can aid in an early diagnosis of cholangitis.

Etiology and Pathophysiology

In approximately 85% of cases, cholangitis is caused by a stone embedded in the bile duct, with resulting bile stasis.[309] Other causes of bile duct obstruction that may result in cholangitis are neoplasms (see Chapters 62 and 71), biliary strictures (see Chapters 70 and 72), parasitic infections (see Chapters 70 and 86), and congenital abnormalities of the bile ducts (see Chapter 64). This discussion deals specifically with cholangitis caused by gallstones in the bile duct.

Bile duct obstruction is necessary but not sufficient to cause cholangitis. Cholangitis is relatively common in patients with choledocholithiasis and nearly universal in patients with a post-traumatic bile duct stricture but is seen in only 15% of patients with neoplastic obstruction of the bile duct. It is most likely to result when a bile duct that already contains bacteria becomes obstructed, as in most patients with choledocholithiasis and stricture but in few patients with neoplastic obstruction. Malignant obstruction is more often complete than obstruction by a stricture or a bile duct stone and less commonly permits reflux of bacteria from duodenal contents into the bile ducts.[310]

The bacterial species most commonly cultured from the bile are *E. coli*, *Klebsiella*, *Pseudomonas*, *Proteus*, and enterococci. Anaerobic species such as *Bacteroides fragilis* and *Clostridium perfringens* are found in about 15% of appropriately cultured bile specimens. Anaerobes usually accompany aerobes, especially *E. coli*. The fever and shaking chills of cholangitis are due to bacteremia from bile duct organisms. The degree of regurgitation of bacteria from bile into hepatic venous blood is directly proportional to the biliary pressure and, hence, the degree of obstruction.[294] For this reason, decompression alone often effectively treats the illness.

Clinical Features

The hallmark of cholangitis is *Charcot triad*, consisting of RUQ pain, jaundice, and fever (see Table 67.2). The full triad is present in only 70% of patients.[310] The pain of cholangitis may be surprisingly mild and transient but is often accompanied by chills and rigors. Older adult patients in particular may present solely with mental confusion, lethargy, and delirium. Altered mental status and hypotension in combination with Charcot triad, known commonly as *Reynolds pentad*, occur in severe suppurative cholangitis.

On physical examination, fever is almost universal, occurring in 95% of patients, and usually greater than 102°F. RUQ tenderness is elicited in about 90% of patients, but jaundice is clinically detectable in only 80%. Notably, peritoneal signs are found in only 15% of patients. The combination of hypotension and mental confusion indicates gram-negative septicemia. In overlooked cases of severe cholangitis, intrahepatic abscess may manifest as a late complication (see Chapter 86).

Laboratory study results are often helpful in pointing to the biliary tract as the source of sepsis. In particular, the serum bilirubin level exceeds 2 mg/dL in 80% of patients. When the bilirubin level is normal initially, the diagnosis of cholangitis may not be suspected.[305] The WBC count is elevated in 80% of patients. In many patients who have a normal WBC count, examination of the peripheral blood smear reveals a dramatic shift to immature neutrophil forms. The serum alkaline phosphatase level is usually elevated, and the serum amylase level may also be elevated if pancreatitis is also present.

In the majority of cases, blood culture results are positive for enteric organisms, especially if culture specimens are obtained during chills and fever spikes. The organism found in the blood is invariably the same as that found in the bile.

Diagnosis

The principles of imaging diagnosis of cholangitis are the same as those for choledocholithiasis. Stones in the bile duct are seen ultrasonographically in only about 50% of cases[186] but can be inferred by detection of a dilated bile duct in about 75% of cases (see Table 67.3). Normal US findings do not exclude the possibility of choledocholithiasis in a patient in whom the clinical presentation suggests cholangitis.[294]

Abdominal CT is an excellent test for excluding complications of gallstones such as acute pancreatitis and abscess, but standard abdominal CT is not capable of excluding bile duct stones. EUS and MRC, as noted earlier, have a much higher accuracy rate than CT for detecting and excluding stones in the bile duct.

ERCP is the definitive test for the diagnosis of bile duct stones and cholangitis. Moreover, the ability of ERCP to establish drainage of infected bile under pressure can be lifesaving. If ERCP is unsuccessful, percutaneous THC can be performed (see Chapter 72).

Treatment

In cases of suspected bacterial cholangitis, blood culture specimens should be obtained immediately and therapy started with antibiotics effective against the likely causative organisms.[311] In mild cases, initial therapy with a single drug (e.g., cefoxitin 2.0 g IV every 6–8 hours) is usually sufficient. In severe cases, more intensive therapy (e.g., gentamicin, ampicillin, and metronidazole or a broad-spectrum agent such as piperacillin-tazobactam 3.375 g IV every 6 hours or, if resistant organisms are suspected, meropenem 1 g IV every 8 hours) is indicated.

The patient's condition should improve within 6–12 hours, and in most cases, the infection comes under control within 2–3 days, with defervescence, relief of discomfort, and a decline in WBC count. In these cases, definitive therapy can be planned on an elective basis. If, however, after 6–12 hours of careful observation, the patient's clinical status declines, with worsening fever, pain, mental confusion, or hypotension, the bile duct must be decompressed immediately.[311] If available, ERCP with stone extraction, or at least decompression of the bile duct with an intrabiliary stent, is the treatment of choice. Controlled studies in which ERCP and decompression of the bile duct were compared with emergency surgery and bile duct exploration have shown dramatically lower morbidity and mortality rates in patients treated endoscopically.[307] The surgical treatment and endoscopic management of cholangitis are discussed in detail in Chapters 68 and 72, respectively.

UNCOMMON COMPLICATIONS

Table 67.4 describes the clinical manifestations, diagnosis, and treatment of several uncommon complications of gallstone disease.

TABLE 67.4 Uncommon Complications of Gallstone Disease

Complication	Pathogenesis	Clinical Features	Diagnosis/Treatment
Emphysematous cholecystitis	Secondary infection of the gallbladder wall with gas-forming organisms (*Clostridium welchii*, *Escherichia coli*, and anaerobic streptococci). More common in older adult diabetic men; can occur without stones (see Chapter 67)	Symptoms and signs similar to those of severe acute cholecystitis	Plain abdominal films may show gas in the gallbladder fossa US and CT are sensitive for confirming gas Treatment is with IV antibiotics, including anaerobic coverage, and early cholecystectomy High morbidity and mortality rates
Cholecystoenteric fistula	Erosion of a (usually large) stone through the gallbladder wall into the adjacent bowel, most often the duodenum, followed in frequency by the hepatic flexure, stomach, and jejunum	Symptoms and signs similar to those of acute cholecystitis, although sometimes a fistula may be clinically silent Stones >25 mm, especially in older adult women, may produce a bowel obstruction, or "gallstone ileus"; the terminal ileum is the most common site of obstruction Gastric outlet obstruction (Bouveret syndrome) may occur rarely	Plain abdominal films may show gas in the biliary tract and/or a small bowel obstruction in gallstone ileus, as well as a stone in the RLQ if the stone is calcified Contrast UGIS may demonstrate the fistula A fistula from a solitary stone that passes may close spontaneously Cholecystectomy and bowel closure are curative Gallstone ileus requires emergency laparotomy; the diagnosis is often delayed, with a resulting mortality rate of ≈20%
Mirizzi syndrome	An impacted stone in the gallbladder neck or cystic duct, with extrinsic compression of the common hepatic duct from accompanying inflammation or fistula	Jaundice and RUQ pain	ERCP demonstrates dilated intrahepatic ducts and extrinsic compression of the common hepatic duct and possible fistula Preoperative diagnosis is important to guide surgery and minimize the risk of BD injury
Porcelain gallbladder	Intramural calcification of the gallbladder wall, usually in association with stones	No symptoms attributable to the calcified wall per se, but carcinoma of the gallbladder is a late complication in ≈20% (see Chapter 69)	Plain abdominal films or CT show intramural calcification of the gallbladder wall Prophylactic cholecystectomy is indicated to prevent carcinoma

BD, Bile duct.

Emphysematous Cholecystitis

Patients who have emphysematous cholecystitis present with the same clinical manifestations as patients with uncomplicated acute cholecystitis, but in the former, gas-forming organisms have secondarily infected the gallbladder wall. Pockets of gas are evident in the area of the gallbladder fossa on plain abdominal films, US, and abdominal CT (see Fig. 67.13).[312] Emphysematous cholecystitis often occurs in diabetic persons or older men who do not have gallstones, in whom atherosclerosis of the cystic artery with resulting ischemia may be the initiating event (see Chapter 67). Emergency antibiotic therapy with anaerobic coverage and early cholecystectomy is warranted because the risk of gallbladder perforation is high.

Cholecystoenteric Fistula

A cholecystoenteric fistula occurs when a stone erodes through the gallbladder wall (usually the neck) and into a hollow viscus. The most common entry point into the bowel is the duodenum, followed in frequency by the hepatic flexure of the colon, the stomach, and the jejunum. Symptoms are initially similar to those of acute cholecystitis, although at times the stone may pass into the bowel and may be excreted without causing any symptoms.[313] Because the biliary tract is decompressed, cholangitis is not common, despite gross seeding of the gallbladder and bile ducts with bacteria. The diagnosis of a cholecystoenteric fistula is suspected from imaging evidence of pneumobilia and may be confirmed by barium contrast studies of the upper or lower GI tract; often the precise anatomic location of the fistula is not identified until surgery.

If the gallstone exceeds 25 mm in diameter, it may manifest (especially in older adult women) as a small intestinal obstruction *(gallstone ileus);* the ileocecal area is the most common site of obstruction.[314] In such cases, a plain abdominal film may show the pathognomonic features of pneumobilia, a dilated small bowel, and a large gallstone in the right lower quadrant. Unfortunately, the diagnosis of a gallstone ileus is often delayed, with a resulting mortality rate of approximately 20%. *Bouveret syndrome* is characterized by gastric outlet obstruction resulting from duodenal impaction of a large gallstone that has migrated through a cholecystoduodenal fistula.[315]

Mirizzi Syndrome

Mirizzi syndrome is a rare complication in which a stone embedded in the neck of the gallbladder or cystic duct extrinsically compresses the common hepatic duct, with resulting jaundice, bile duct obstruction, and in some cases a fistula.[316,317] Typically the gallbladder is contracted and contains stones. ERCP usually demonstrates the characteristic extrinsic compression of the common hepatic duct. Treatment is traditionally by an open cholecystectomy, although endoscopic stenting and laparoscopic cholecystectomy have been performed successfully. Preoperative diagnosis of Mirizzi syndrome is important so that bile duct injury can be avoided (see Chapter 68).[318]

Porcelain Gallbladder

Strictly speaking, *porcelain gallbladder*, defined as intramural calcification of the gallbladder wall, is not a complication of gallstones but is mentioned here because of the remarkable tendency of carcinoma to develop as a late complication of gallbladder calcification (specifically, a gallbladder with focal rather than diffuse wall calcification).[319] The diagnosis of a porcelain gallbladder can be made with a plain abdominal film or abdominal CT, which shows intramural calcification of the gallbladder wall. In occasional persons, hypersecretion of calcium into bile results in a "milk of calcium" or "limy" bile that can mimic the imaging features of porcelain gallbladder. Prophylactic cholecystectomy, preferably through a laparoscopic approach, is indicated to prevent subsequent development of carcinoma, which may otherwise occur in up to 20% of cases (see Chapter 71).[320]

Acknowledgment

The authors acknowledge the contributions of Drs. Jeffrey D. Browning and Jayaprakash Sreenarasimhaiah to this chapter in previous editions of the book as well as the contributions of colleagues in the gallstone field. This work was supported in part by research grants DK54012, DK73917, DK101793, DK106249, DK114516, and AA025737 (D.Q.-H.W.) from the National Institutes of Health (U.S. Public Health Service).

Full references for this chapter can be found at https://ebooks.health.elsevier.com

68 Treatment of Gallstone Disease

Robert E. Glasgow

IN THIS CHAPTER

Many options are available for the treatment of patients with symptomatic gallstone disease. Improvements in endoscopic, radiologic, and chemical therapies for gallstones have enhanced the overall management of these patients. Nevertheless, surgery remains the most important therapeutic option. Laparoscopic cholecystectomy is the standard method for the management of patients with biliary pain and complications of gallstone disease, such as acute cholecystitis, gallstone pancreatitis, and choledocholithiasis (see also Chapter 67).

MEDICAL TREATMENT

Medical treatment of gallstone disease was first proposed by Schiff in Italy in 1873.[1] Dabney of Virginia first reported the effective treatment of gallstones with bile acids in 1876, an observation later confirmed by Rewbridge of Minnesota in 1937.[2,3] Despite these initial reports, the use of medical dissolution treatment did not gain acceptance until large clinical series were reported in the 1970s. Contact dissolution of gallstones with solvents and percutaneous cholecystolithotomy techniques also have been reported, but these modalities have not proved superior to oral dissolution, shock-wave lithotripsy, or laparoscopic cholecystectomy and have been abandoned. The mainstay of current nonsurgical treatment of gallstone disease is oral dissolution with UDCA, with or without extracorporeal shock-wave lithotripsy.

Although nonsurgical treatment of gallstones has proved effective in carefully selected patients, only a limited number of patients are candidates for this treatment option. Nonsurgical treatments are effective only in patients with small, radiolucent cholesterol gallstones. Significant admixtures of pigment or calcium salts make stones indissoluble. In addition, long-term success with medical treatment of gallstones occurs only in patients in whom the lithogenic disturbance that led to gallstone formation is transient. For most patients, gallstone formation represents an imbalance in biliary lipid excretion, gallbladder stasis, or infection of the bile (see Chapter 67). In these patients, successful dissolution is followed by recurrence of gallstones in 30%–50% of patients within 5 years.[4–6] Therefore the proper choice of treatment must take into account the type and severity of symptoms, physical characteristics of the stones, gallbladder function, and characteristics and preference of the patient.

Dissolution Therapy

The rationale for oral dissolution therapy is the reversal of the condition that led to formation of cholesterol gallstones, namely, the supersaturation of bile with cholesterol (see Chapter 67). Cholesterol stones dissolve if the surrounding medium can solubilize the cholesterol in the stones. Both chenodeoxycholic acid and UDCA dissolve gallstones by decreasing biliary cholesterol secretion and desaturating bile. These agents encourage the removal of cholesterol from stones via micellar solubilization, formation of a liquid crystalline phase, or both. Chenodeoxycholic acid was the first bile acid used for gallstone dissolution but has been abandoned because of side effects, including diarrhea and increased serum aminotransferase and cholesterol levels. UDCA is well tolerated and is currently used in oral dissolution regimens. In randomized comparisons, UDCA was just as effective as chenodeoxycholic acid alone or in combination with UDCA.[6–8]

The rate of stone dissolution is a function of (1) thermodynamic forces, including the degree of bile desaturation and concentration of UDCA in bile; (2) kinetic forces, including stirring of bile; and (3) the surface-to-volume ratio of the stones. Oral dissolution targets the thermodynamic forces.[9] Because small stones have a smaller surface-to-volume ratio, they respond more quickly and reliably to oral dissolution therapy. The use of oral dissolution therapy does not address the problem of gallbladder stasis.[10] Although prokinetic agents, including α-adrenergic antagonists, clarithromycin, and domperidone, have been shown to increase gallbladder motility, their use in preventing and treating gallstones has been shown to be ineffective.[11–13]

Patient Selection

Selection of patients for oral dissolution therapy is a function of the stage of gallstone disease, gallbladder function, and characteristics of the stones. Selection criteria are summarized in Box 68.1. Oral dissolution therapy should be considered for patients with uncomplicated gallstone disease, including those

BOX 68.1 Selection Criteria for Oral Bile Acid Dissolution Therapy

STAGE OF GALLSTONE DISEASE

Symptomatic (biliary pain) without complications

GALLBLADDER FUNCTION

Opacification of gallbladder on oral cholecystography (patent cystic duct)
Normal result of stimulated cholescintigraphy (normal gallbladder emptying)
Normal result of functional US (normal gallbladder emptying after a test meal)

STONE CHARACTERISTICS

Radiolucent
Isodense or hypodense to bile and absence of calcification on CT
Diameter ≤10 mm (<6 mm optimal)

with mild, infrequent biliary pain. Patients with asymptomatic gallstones should not be treated with either dissolution therapy or surgery because the natural history of most asymptomatic stones is to remain asymptomatic. Patients with severe or frequent biliary pain and patients with complications of gallstones, including cholecystitis, pancreatitis, and cholangitis, should not be treated with oral dissolution therapy; these patients should be referred for surgery as soon as possible (see later). In addition, the gallbladder must function, and the cystic duct must be patent to allow unsaturated bile and stones to clear from the gallbladder. The patency of the cystic duct has generally been evaluated by oral cholecystography. More recently, stimulated cholescintigraphy and functional US have been used. These latter modalities assess cystic duct patency as well as gallbladder function.

The characteristics of the stones play an important role in determining the efficacy of dissolution treatment. Oral dissolution therapy works only on cholesterol stones. Although verifying the composition of gallstones can be difficult, the appearance of stones on plain films or CT images can be useful. Cholesterol stones are radiolucent on plain films, and they are hypodense or isodense to bile and lack stone calcification on CT images.[14] During oral cholecystography, the specific gravity of cholesterol stones is less than or equal to that of contrast-enriched bile, thereby resulting in stone buoyancy. The number of stones does not influence the success of oral dissolution therapy; however, only patients with stones that occupy less than half of the gallbladder volume should be considered for treatment. Although oral dissolution therapy has been effective in stones up to 10 mm in diameter, results are best in stones less than 5 mm in size.[15,16] The ideal stones for oral dissolution treatment are shown in Fig. 68.1.

Therapeutic Regimens

UDCA (ursodiol) is the preferred drug for oral dissolution treatment. It is taken in a dose of 10–15 mg/kg of body weight per day. Nighttime dosing is more effective and is associated with better patient adherence than mealtime dosing.[17] Unlike chenodeoxycholic acid (chenodiol), UDCA is well tolerated and has no important side effects. Treatment should continue until stone dissolution is documented by two consecutive negative ultrasonograms at least 1 month apart. Treatment should be stopped if the patient does not tolerate the drug or experiences a complication of gallstones during therapy or if the stones fail to dissolve after 6 months or dissolve only partially after 6 months with lack of progression to complete dissolution by 2 years.

Efficacy

With UDCA, complete dissolution is achieved in 20%–70% of patients. The variability in the reported response rates is a function of differences in patient selection, doses of bile acid, treatment times, and diagnostic techniques used to document stone dissolution. A meta-analysis of all randomized trials of dissolution treatment showed stone dissolution in 37% of patients.[8] The frequency of stone dissolution was 29% for stones larger than 10 mm, 49% for stones smaller than 10 mm, and 70% for stones less than 5 mm. The time to resolution varies among patients, with a median rate of 0.7 mm/month.[9] Improvement in symptoms occurs before stones have dissolved completely. In addition, long-term treatment has been reported to decrease the risk of biliary pain and acute cholecystitis, independent of gallstone dissolution.[16] Despite initial dissolution of stones in properly selected patients, the rate of gallstone recurrence after oral dissolution therapy is 50% after 5 years, with most recurrences within the first 2 years.[5,18] This observation illustrates that other factors relevant to gallstone formation, such as gallbladder stasis and superinfection, are not addressed by dissolution treatment. The risk of recurrence is lower in patients with a solitary stone than in those with multiple stones.

Extracorporeal Shock-Wave Lithotripsy

The rationale for shock-wave lithotripsy is to diminish the surface-to-volume ratio of a stone, thereby increasing the efficacy of oral dissolution therapy and decreasing stone size to allow small stones and debris to pass directly from the gallbladder into the intestine without causing symptoms. The technique involves the delivery of focused high-pressure sound waves to gallstones. Four types of lithotripters have been developed: underwater spark-gap, piezoelectric crystal, electromagnetic membrane, and, most recently, laser lithotriptors. Regardless of the energy source, the shock waves from the lithotriptor are delivered from an underwater source to the soft tissue. Passage of the shock wave through the soft tissue does not diminish the energy wave significantly. Passage of the shock wave through the anterior and posterior walls of the stone liberates compressive and tensile forces and causes cavitation at the anterior surface of the stone, thereby leading to stone fragmentation. Factors that influence fragmentation include the size, microcrystalline structure, and architecture of the stone. Although the composition of the stone does not influence successful lithotripsy, only cholesterol stone fragments are dissolved effectively by bile acid therapy, which can be used in combination with lithotripsy.

Patient Selection

Because shock-wave lithotripsy is usually combined with oral dissolution therapy, patient selection criteria for shock-wave lithotripsy are similar to those for oral dissolution treatment and are summarized in Box 68.2. Gallbladder function and cystic duct patency are required and are demonstrated by oral cholecystography, functional US, or stimulated cholescintigraphy. Lithotripsy should be considered only for patients with mild, uncomplicated biliary pain. Pregnant patients and patients on anticoagulants should not undergo lithotripsy. In patients with a solitary stone, shock-wave lithotripsy is reserved for patients with a stone measuring less than 2 cm in size.[19,20] Because only cholesterol stones are reliably cleared by the addition of oral dissolution therapy, stones should have imaging features, such as radiolucency, suggestive of cholesterol stones.

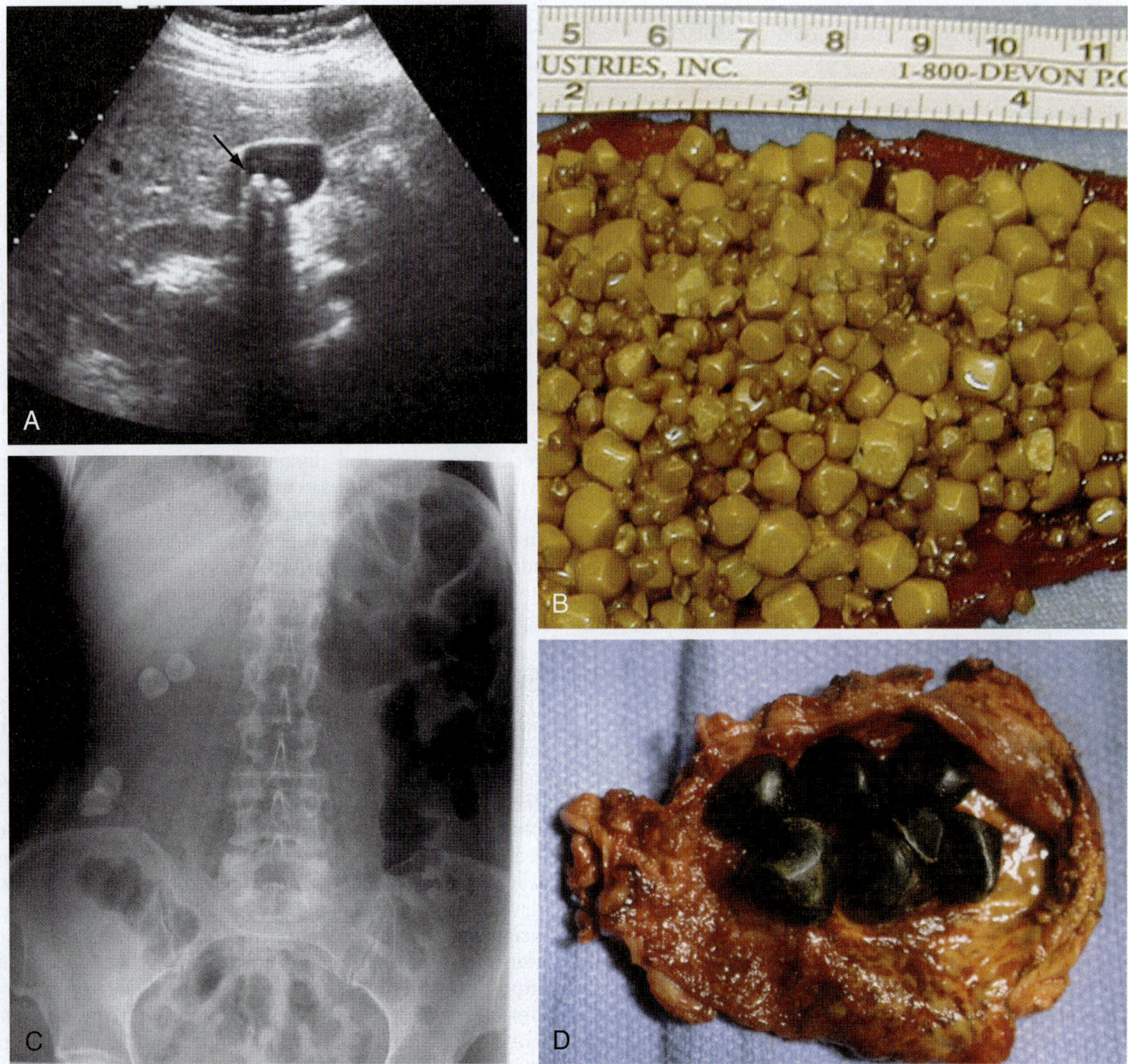

Fig. 68.1 (A and B) Gallstones for which oral dissolution therapy is appropriate. (A) US showing small gallstones (*arrow*); (B) multiple small cholesterol stones. (C and D) Gallstones for which oral dissolution therapy is inappropriate: (C) radiopaque gallstones on a plain film; (D) large pigmented gallstones.

BOX 68.2 Selection Criteria for Extracorporeal Shock-Wave Lithotripsy

STAGE OF GALLSTONE DISEASE

Symptomatic (biliary pain) without complications

GALLBLADDER FUNCTION

Opacification of gallbladder on oral cholecystography (patent cystic duct)

Normal result of stimulated cholescintigraphy (normal gallbladder emptying)

Normal result of functional US (normal gallbladder emptying after a test meal)

STONE CHARACTERISTICS

Radiolucent

Isodense or hypodense to bile and absence of calcification on CT

Single

Diameter <20 mm

Therapeutic Approach

Patients are usually given sedatives and analgesics or anesthetized and placed in the prone position to minimize the distance between the energy source and the stones and to eliminate interference from intestinal gas and the costal margin. Targeting and monitoring for fragmentation are accomplished with US.[21] Multiple treatment sessions are often required to achieve maximum pulverization. Factors that predict the success of lithotripsy include the degree of fragmentation and gallbladder emptying.[22–24] Fragmentation depends on stone characteristics and the dose of the shock wave. Important stone characteristics include the size and number of stones as well as their structure and the presence of calcification.[25] The energy of shock waves, number of shock waves per session, and number of sessions also influence the success rate.[26,27] UDCA is administered orally to dissolve stone fragments, especially when residual stone fragments are larger than 2 mm in size, gallbladder function is poor, or the gallbladder has not cleared small fragments within 3–6 months of lithotripsy. An example of successful combined treatment is shown in Fig. 68.2.

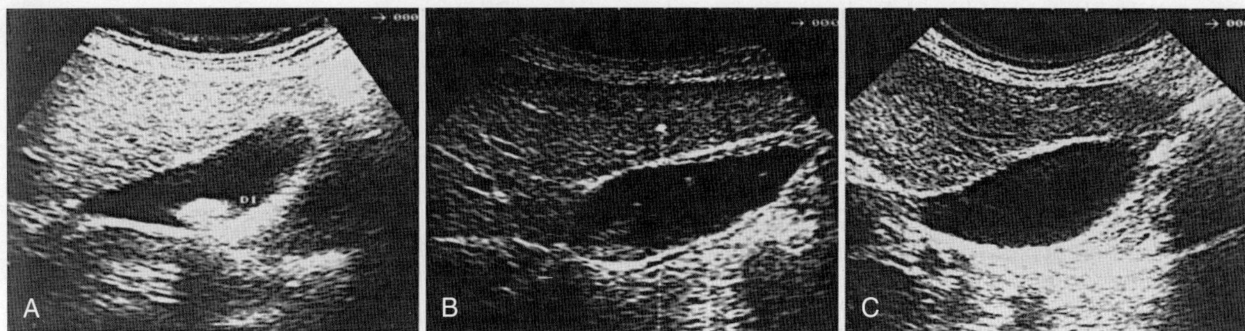

Fig. 68.2 US of a gallbladder with a single stone before (A), 1 day after (B), and 6 weeks after (C) extracorporeal shock-wave lithotripsy. Multiple small stone fragments seen 1 day after lithotripsy (B) have disappeared 6 weeks after lithotripsy (C).

Efficacy

The percentages of patients who are free of stones after 6 and 12 months are 47%–77% and 68%–84%, respectively.[20,22,28–32] Follow-up data reveal cumulative recurrence rates of 27%, 41%, and 54% at 3, 5, and 10 years, respectively.[33] Recurrence is most often related to the presence of lithogenic bile and gallbladder dysmotility, rather than patient variables such as gender, age, and weight. Factors that predict higher rates of treatment failure include stone size larger than 16 mm, multiple stones, and stones with a CT density greater than 84 Hounsfield Units (HU).[34] Recurrent stones are usually small and multiple and cause recurrent biliary pain. Maintenance therapy with UDCA after lithotripsy has not been shown to be effective.[35]

Side effects of lithotripsy include petechiae of the skin at the site of shock-wave delivery (8%), hematuria (4%), and liver hematomas (<1%). No long-term liver biochemical abnormalities have been noted. Biliary pain develops in approximately one-third of patients; cystic duct obstruction develops in 5%; and complications of stone passage, such as biliary pancreatitis, develop in less than 2%.[22]

Lithotripsy is more cost-effective in older adults than in the young and less cost-effective in patients with multiple stones than in those with a single stone. When combined with UDCA, lithotripsy is at least as cost-effective as open cholecystectomy for patients with small stones and less cost-effective for those with large stones.[36,37] When lithotripsy is compared with laparoscopic cholecystectomy, patients who undergo laparoscopic cholecystectomy experience a greater incremental improvement in quality of life at 6 months, whereas those who undergo lithotripsy have higher rates of recurrent stones and biliary symptoms.[38]

Bile Duct Stones

Extracorporeal shock-wave lithotripsy has also been used in the management of choledocholithiasis. Intracorporeal electrohydraulic lithotripsy has been shown to be effective in this setting as well. These treatment options are reserved for patients who fail conventional endoscopic measures (see Chapter 72), mechanical lithotripsy, or surgical treatment of choledocholithiasis (see later). Appropriate indications for shock-wave lithotripsy are large stones impacted in the bile duct that are not amenable to endoscopic extraction, intrahepatic stones, stones above a biliary stricture, cystic duct remnant stones, and bile duct stones associated with Mirizzi syndrome (compression of the common hepatic duct) (see Chapter 67). Selection of patients for shock-wave treatment of bile duct stones is similar to that for treatment of uncomplicated gallbladder gallstones.

The success rate for treatment of bile duct stones is 70%–90%.[39–44] Most patients require endoscopic extraction of large stone fragments following treatment. Mild, transient hemobilia occurs in 10% of patients, and biliary sepsis develops in 4% following the procedure. Other complications are similar to those seen after lithotripsy for gallbladder stones. Because of the potential for septic complications, preprocedure endoscopic, nasobiliary, or percutaneous biliary drainage is performed. Antibiotics are given to minimize the risk of biliary sepsis.

SURGICAL TREATMENT

Approximately 700,000 cholecystectomies are performed for gallstone disease in the United States each year; the vast majority are performed using laparoscopic techniques. For example, 7,888 cholecystectomies were performed in Utah in 2005; 96% of these operations were laparoscopic cholecystectomies, and 4% were open procedures. A review of the National Hospital Discharge Database from 1997 to 2006 showed that 12% of cholecystectomies were performed by an open approach.[45] Of those procedures done laparoscopically, the rate of conversion to open cholecystectomy is 5%–10%.[46,47] Patients with complicated gallstone disease, including acute cholecystitis, gallstone pancreatitis, and choledocholithiasis, are more likely than those with uncomplicated disease to require an open cholecystectomy or conversion from a laparoscopic to an open approach.[46] Despite the increased reliance on minimally invasive techniques in the care of these patients, open cholecystectomy continues to play an important role in the management of complications of gallstones.

Open Cholecystectomy

Carl Langenbuch, a surgeon in Berlin, is credited with performing the first cholecystectomy in 1882. Since then, cholecystectomy has remained the main therapeutic option for the management of patients with gallstones, largely because of its remarkable success in relieving symptoms and its low morbidity. In prospective studies, 90%–95% of patients who undergo cholecystectomy experience substantial or complete relief of their symptoms.[48,49] Cholecystectomy is more effective in relieving biliary pain than in relieving nonspecific GI symptoms, including dyspepsia and flatulence.

Technique

The technique of open cholecystectomy has not changed substantially since its first description. With the surgeon standing on the patient's right side, a right subcostal (Kocher) incision is made two fingerbreadths below the right costal margin. Alternatively, a midline incision may be used. After exploring the abdomen and taking down any adhesions to the gallbladder, the gallbladder is dissected from the gallbladder fossa in a retrograde fashion, from the fundus down to the infundibulum. When the gallbladder has been mobilized, the cystic artery and duct are readily identified. A cholangiogram may be performed to look for bile duct stones or to confirm the anatomy. The cystic duct and artery are ligated and divided. An alternative approach is to perform a dissection of the triangle of Calot structures, as is done during laparoscopic cholecystectomy (see later), prior to removing the gallbladder from the liver. The triangle of Calot is the space bordered by the cystic duct, cystic artery, and inferior edge of the gallbladder. Dissection and identification of these structures permits safe division of the cystic duct and minimizes the chance of bile duct injury. The abdominal incision is then closed. Closed suction drains are rarely indicated after cholecystectomy.

Results

The risk of open cholecystectomy has declined over the years. The overall mortality rate of cholecystectomy in 35,373 patients operated on before 1932 was 6.6%.[50] This rate decreased to 1.8% by 1952.[51] Since then, the overall mortality rate for cholecystectomy has averaged about 1.5%. The mortality rate is considerably lower in patients operated on electively for biliary pain, with an average of less than 0.5% (Table 68.1).[52–54] The risk of death is several-fold higher when cholecystectomy is performed as an emergency for acute cholecystitis and when bile duct exploration is required (see Table 68.1). In addition, the mortality rate is directly proportional to the patient's age (Fig. 68.3). In a report of the entire Danish experience with cholecystectomy from 1977 to 1981, patients under 50 years of age had a risk of death of 0.028% from elective cholecystectomy[53]; the rate rose to 5.56% in patients older than 80 years of age. The experience in the United States has been similar. Of 11,808 patients who underwent cholecystectomy at the New York Hospital-Cornell Medical Center between 1932 and 1978, the risk of death from elective cholecystectomy for chronic cholecystitis was 0.1% in patients less than 50 years of age and 0.8% in those 50 years of age or older.[54] In a later series, the overall mortality rate of 42,474 patients who underwent cholecystectomy in 1989 in California and Maryland was 0.17%.[55] In this series, the mortality rate in patients less than 65 years of age was 0.03%, compared with more than 0.5% in patients 65 years of age and older. Likewise, the morbidity rate, mean length of hospital stay, and average hospital charges were significantly higher in the older patients than in the younger group. Most mortality following cholecystectomy is related to cardiac disease, particularly myocardial infarction.

Major complications after open cholecystectomy are infrequent. In a large survey of 28,621 patients who underwent cholecystectomy in the 1960s, complications occurred in 4.0%.[52] Subsequent studies have confirmed a 4.0%–5.0% rate of perioperative morbidity.[56–58] Most complications are relatively minor, such as wound infections or seromas, urinary retention or infection, and atelectasis. Complications related specifically to cholecystectomy include bile leaks, bile duct injury, and acute pancreatitis. Of these complications, bile duct injury is the most serious and often requires endoscopic therapy and, in some cases, complicated and technically difficult surgical repair. Alternatively, bile duct injury can lead to benign biliary stricture formation and bile duct obstruction with secondary biliary cirrhosis and liver failure. The rate of bile duct injury during open cholecystectomy is not known precisely but has been estimated to be 1 in 200–600 cases.[59,60] In general, bile duct injuries are preventable complications and are commonly the result of inadequate surgical training, unrecognized variations in bile duct anatomy, or misidentification of normal anatomy. Unusual amounts of bleeding, severe inflammation, and emergency operations do not play as great a role in these injuries as might be supposed.

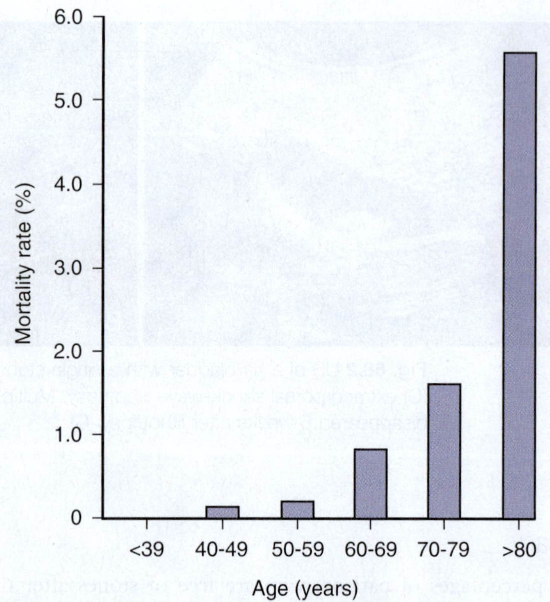

Fig. 68.3 Relationship between age and mortality from open cholecystectomy. Data include all patients operated on in Denmark between 1977 and 1981. (Data from Bredesen J, Jorgensen T, Andersen TF, et al. Early postoperative mortality following cholecystectomy in the entire female population of Denmark, 1977-1981. *World J Surg.* 1992;16:530–535.)

Laparoscopic Cholecystectomy

After the first reports in the late 1980s, laparoscopic cholecystectomy rapidly gained acceptance as the technique of choice for the management of the patient with biliary pain and complications of gallstones. The benefits of this minimally invasive approach compared with open cholecystectomy, including lower

TABLE 68.1 Mortality Rates for Open Cholecystectomy as a Function of the Clinical Setting

			Clinical Setting of Cholecystectomy (% Mortality)		
References	Years	No. of Patients	Biliary Pain	Acute Cholecystitis	Bile Duct Exploration
52	1962–1966	28,621	1.5	3.5	N/A
53	1977–1981	13,854	0.4	1.6	2.3
54	1932–1978	11,808	0.5	2.9	3.5
55	1989	42,474	0.02	0.26	N/A

N/A, Not available.

overall morbidity and mortality and quicker return to normal activities, are well established. Historically, laparoscopic cholecystectomy was an outgrowth of diagnostic laparoscopy and the early efforts of gynecologists at operative laparoscopy. The development of laparoscopic cholecystectomy was predicated on technical advances in miniaturized video cameras and other specialized equipment. Advances in instrument and equipment design and manufacture have led to significant improvements in the safety and utility of minimally invasive surgery in the treatment of most GI diseases, especially gallstone disease.

Technique

Laparoscopic cholecystectomy is performed under general anesthesia. Prophylactic antibiotics are not administered routinely to patients with uncomplicated gallstone disease, including biliary pain.[61] Patients with potential infectious complications of gallstones, including acute cholecystitis and cholangitis, and patients with long-standing symptoms or advanced age should receive antibiotics if these agents have not been started already before surgery. Sequential compression stockings are used to reduce the risk of lower extremity thromboembolism.

To view the abdominal contents and provide room for instruments, a space is developed by inducing a pneumoperitoneum with carbon dioxide, which is a nonflammable, physiologically benign gas. Pneumoperitoneum is achieved by either a closed technique in which a Veress needle is inserted into the peritoneum through a small incision, followed by placement of an operating trocar, or by a direct, open technique in which the operating trocar is placed directly into the abdomen under direct visualization through a small incision. After the pneumoperitoneum has been established, a trocar is placed at the umbilicus and a laparoscope is introduced. Three additional trocars are placed in the upper abdomen under direct vision for inserting operating instruments and retractors.

The current technique of laparoscopic cholecystectomy is best described as "the critical view of safety" approach,[62] as summarized in Fig. 68.4. In this approach, the entire hepatocystic triangle is dissected, exposing the cystic duct and artery, infundibulum of the gallbladder, and junction of the gallbladder and cystic duct, before a cholangiogram is performed or the cystic duct and artery are divided. The assistant retracts the gallbladder fundus cephalad, anterior to the liver, and the infundibulum laterally. The surgeon, operating through the epigastric port, identifies and dissects the cystic duct and artery circumferentially. Special care must be taken to identify the junction of the cystic duct and gallbladder, to ensure that the bile duct has not been isolated inadvertently. Cholangiography is performed via cannulation of the cystic duct. If the cholangiogram shows normal anatomy and no evidence of choledocholithiasis, the cholangiocatheter is removed and the cystic duct and artery are divided between small metal clips. The gallbladder is then dissected out of the liver bed with cautery and delivered through the umbilical incision, usually with a specimen retrieval bag to minimize contamination of the epigastric port wound. Care is taken to avoid perforation of the gallbladder during its dissection from the liver because the spillage of gallstones and bile has been shown to increase the risk of postoperative fever and intra-abdominal abscess formation.[63] The operation concludes with evacuation of the pneumoperitoneum and closure of the incisions.

Laparoscopic cholecystectomy has been performed by some surgeons using a single-incision approach in which the operating surgeon introduces the laparoscope and surgical instruments into the abdomen via a single operating port placed at the umbilicus. This technique has the advantage of improved cosmetics over the traditional 4-port laparoscopic approach. The single-incision laparoscopic surgery procedure has not gained wide acceptance because of longer operating times, higher cost, a higher rate of wound complications and hernias, and, possibly, a higher rate of bile duct injury.[64–66]

A robotic approach to minimally invasive laparoscopic surgery has recently gained enthusiasm across a wide spectrum of surgical specialties and procedures. This is despite limited supporting evidence of a clinical benefit over conventional laparoscopic approaches for most procedures.[66a] Robotic cholecystectomy has been shown to have similar safety and perioperative outcomes compared to laparoscopic cholecystectomy but is associated with significantly increased cost and duration of surgery.[66b] An advantage of robotic surgery for procedures such as cholecystectomy over a laparoscopic approach has not been demonstrated.

Rationale for Cholangiography

Cholangiography during laparoscopic cholecystectomy has two main purposes. First, the cholangiogram may detect unsuspected bile duct stones. Second, the cholangiogram confirms the surgeon's impression of the anatomy of the biliary tract. In the era before laparoscopic cholecystectomy, the value of routine cholangiography during cholecystectomy was debated, with some surgeons arguing in favor of its selective use.[67] This debate continues in the laparoscopic era. Routine cholangiography has been criticized because of its relatively low yield, failure to identify all retained stones, occasional false-positive results, cost, and risk. Nevertheless, 8%–16% of all patients with cholelithiasis harbor bile duct stones with higher rates seen in patients experiencing a prior history of common duct stone-related complications such as gallstone pancreatitis. Routine use of operative cholangiography detects unsuspected bile duct stones in about 5% of patients who undergo cholecystectomy and detects anatomic ductal abnormalities in 12%.[68] During laparoscopic cholecystectomy, the two-dimensional video image and inability to palpate structures of the porta hepatis make identification of the cystic duct–bile duct junction problematic. Cholangiography plays an especially important role in delineating bile duct anatomy prior to division of any important structures. Large population studies from Australia and Sweden have demonstrated the importance of routine intraoperative cholangiography in decreasing the frequency of major bile duct injuries.[69,70] The rate of bile duct injury during laparoscopic cholecystectomy when routine cholangiography is performed is 0.2%–0.4%, compared with 0.4%–0.6% when cholangiography is not performed routinely.[71] Routine cholangiography is cost-effective when the cost associated with bile duct injuries is considered.[72] In addition, routine cholangiography permits earlier identification of intraoperative bile duct injuries, if they occur,[73] and thereby improves the rate of repair.

Despite these observations in favor of routine cholangiography, the low frequency of unsuspected bile duct stones and low rate of bile duct injury serve as the basis for most surgeons adopting a selective approach to using cholangiography. Cholangiography is done when the history is suggestive of possible bile duct stones (e.g., pancreatitis, cholangitis, elevated liver biochemical test levels, and bile duct stones seen on preoperative imaging) or when intraoperative confirmation of ductal anatomy is aided by the addition of cholangiography.

Results

Several large series have described experiences with laparoscopic cholecystectomy (Table 68.2).[74–83] A review of the experience with laparoscopic cholecystectomy in the United States showed an operative mortality rate of 0.06%. Internationally, operative mortality rates have ranged from 0% to 0.15%. Conversion to an open procedure was required in 2.2% of patients in the United States and 3.6%–8.2% internationally, generally because of inflammation that precludes safe dissection of the porta hepatis. Major morbidity occurred in approximately 5% of patients, and bile duct injuries occurred in 0.14%–0.5%. Operating time ranged from 1 to 2 hours, with most patients undergoing same-day surgery and

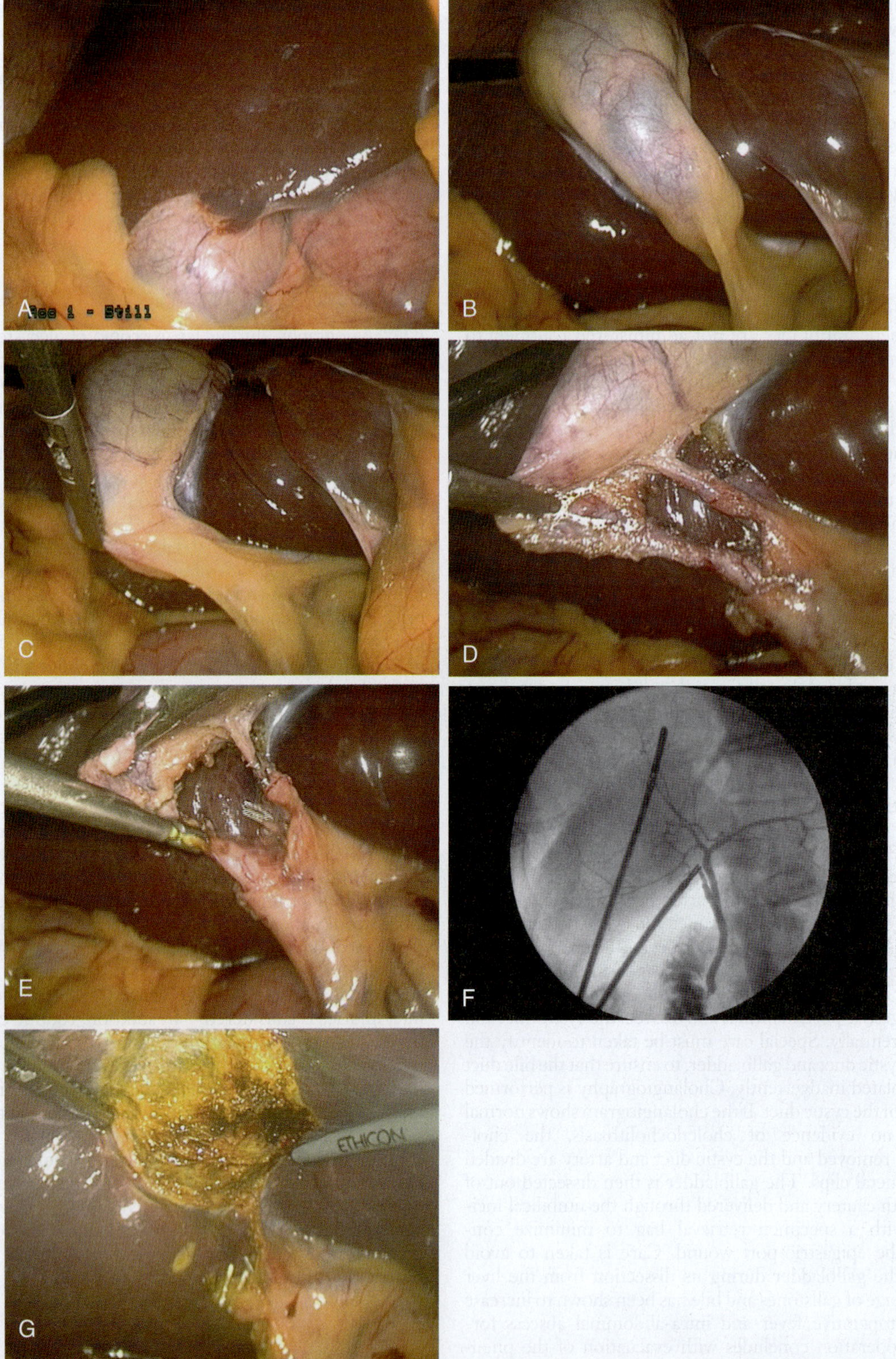

Fig. 68.4 Laparoscopic cholecystectomy. (A) Gallbladder in situ. (B) Cephalad retraction of the fundus toward the right shoulder exposes the infundibulum of the gallbladder. (C) Retraction of the infundibulum toward the right lower abdominal quadrant opens the hepatocystic triangle, which is the area bordered by the cystic duct, gallbladder edge, and liver edge. (D) Division of the peritoneum overlying the anterior and posterior aspects of the hepatocystic triangle exposes "the critical view of safety." (E) Cholangiogram catheter in the cystic duct. (F) Normal cholangiogram. (G) Gallbladder removed from the gallbladder fossa with electrocautery.

TABLE 68.2 Outcomes of Laparoscopic Cholecystectomy

Reference	No. of Patients	Morbidity Rate (%)	Mortality Rate (%)	Bile Duct Injury (%)	Conversion[a] Rate (%)
74	3319	6.7	0.15	0.33	5.2
75	6076	4.3	0.12	0.86	6.8
76	13,833	4.3	0.14	0.59	5.3
78	2201	4.3	0	0.14	4.3
79	114,005	5.4	0.06	0.5	2.2
80	33,563	8.5	0.09	0.2	3.5
81	56,591	N/A	N/A	0.42	N/A
82	3285	10.1	0.2	0.25	3.6
83	22,953	14.6	0.3	0.3	5.3

[a]To open cholecystectomy.

TABLE 68.3 Cholecystectomy-Related Mortality in Maryland Before (1989) and After (1992) the Introduction of Laparoscopic Cholecystectomy

Variable	1989	1992	% Change
Number of cholecystectomies	7416	9993	+35
Crude rate of cholecystectomies per 1000 population	1.57	2.04	+30
Operative mortality rate (%)	0.84	0.56	−33
Number of deaths	62	56	−10

Data from Steiner CA, Bass EB, Talamini MA, et al. Surgical rates and operative mortality for open and laparoscopic cholecystectomy in Maryland. *N Engl J Med*. 1994;330:403–408.

outpatient surgery in elective cases. Most patients return to full activities, including work, within 1 week.

No randomized prospective trials have compared the results of laparoscopic cholecystectomy with those of open cholecystectomy in the United States, nor are any likely. Patient enthusiasm for the laparoscopic approach and the rapid acceptance of the procedure by surgeons have made direct, controlled comparison of the two procedures difficult. Nonrandomized data from the United States and small, randomized trials from other countries support the contention that the laparoscopic approach is superior to the open approach.[52,84–88] In these analyses, the main benefits of the laparoscopic approach have included a shortened hospital stay, decreased pain, reduced disability, quicker return to normal physical and social activity, and lower costs. Population studies have shown a substantial decline in cholecystectomy-related mortality rates following the introduction of the laparoscopic technique (Table 68.3).[89]

Against the perceived benefits of laparoscopic cholecystectomy over the open approach is concern about unacceptably high complication rates, especially for bile duct injury. Although the exact frequency of bile duct injury around the world is not known, two lines of evidence suggest that the rate has declined. First, regional studies have demonstrated a decrease in the rate of bile duct injury as overall experience with laparoscopic cholecystectomy has increased (Fig. 68.5).[90,91] Curiously, however, the frequency of bile duct injury does not continue to fall with increasing experience of the individual surgeon, but rather plateaus.[91–93] Although bile duct injuries are more common early in an individual surgeon's experience, they still occur in the hands of seasoned surgeons, albeit at a lower rate. As overall experience has increased, the rate of bile duct injury for laparoscopic cholecystectomy has approximated that seen with open cholecystectomy. Second, the number of patients with bile duct injury treated at tertiary referral medical centers has declined since the early days of laparoscopic cholecystectomy.[94] Introduction of laparoscopic cholecystectomy in the United States was rapid and may have exceeded the capability of the medical educational

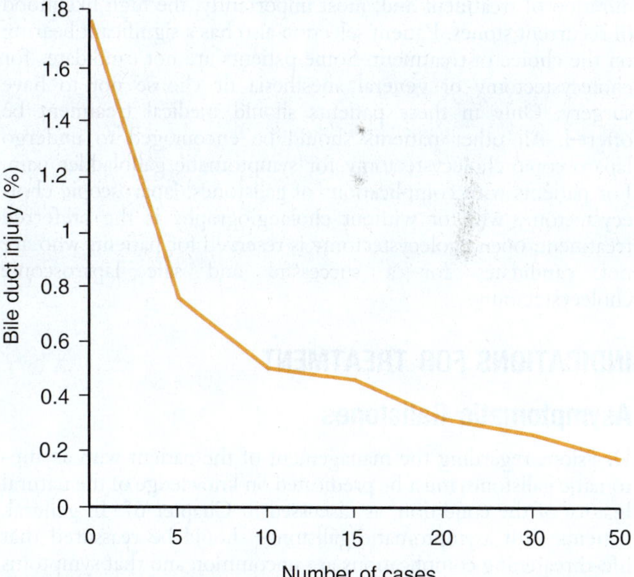

Fig. 68.5 Effect of a surgeon's experience on the risk of bile duct injury during laparoscopic cholecystectomy. The dramatic decline in risk as experience is gained has been attributed to a "learning curve." (Data adapted from Moore MJ, Bennett CL. The learning curve for laparoscopic cholecystectomy. The Southern Surgeons Club. *Am J Surg*. 1995;170:55–59.)

system to train all practitioners adequately. The initial relatively high rate of bile duct injury has been ascribed to a "learning curve" and is a cautionary example for other new technologies that may be introduced into medical practice.

Concern has been raised about the increased use of laparoscopic cholecystectomy for gallstone disease when compared with historical rates for open cholecystectomy. In a defined health maintenance organization population in Pennsylvania, the rate of cholecystectomy increased from 1.35 per 1000 enrollees in 1988, just before the introduction of the laparoscopic approach, to 2.15 per 1000 enrollees in 1992, just after its introduction.[95] No contemporaneous changes in the rates of herniorrhaphy or appendectomy were observed. Similarly, statewide data from Maryland showed that the rate of cholecystectomy rose from 1.69 per 1000 residents in 1987–1989 to 2.17 per 1000 residents in 1992,[89] and Scottish nationwide data showed a 20% increase in the age-standardized rate of cholecystectomy.[96] The reasons for the increases in use are not yet clear but most likely include expanding indications for cholecystectomy to include nonstone gallbladder disease (see Chapter 69). The consensus of experts in the field is that selection of patients for cholecystectomy should not be altered by the availability of the laparoscopic approach.

CHOICE OF TREATMENT

Several factors influence the choice of treatment for symptomatic gallstone disease, including the stage of gallstone disease, characteristics of the stone, gallbladder function, and preference of the patient. For patients with uncomplicated biliary pain, treatment options include surgery and oral dissolution with or without lithotripsy. Surgery has the advantage of dealing with the underlying causes of gallstones—stasis and lithogenic bile—regardless of the number, size, and type of stones. Although oral dissolution therapy is effective in treating selected patients, the low morbidity rate associated with laparoscopic cholecystectomy negates any potential advantages of nonsurgical treatment. In addition, nonsurgical treatment is less desirable because of the duration of treatment and, most importantly, the high likelihood of recurrent stones. Patient selection also has a significant bearing on the choice of treatment. Some patients are not candidates for cholecystectomy or general anesthesia or choose not to have surgery. Only in these patients should medical treatment be offered. All other patients should be encouraged to undergo laparoscopic cholecystectomy for symptomatic gallbladder pain. For patients with complications of gallstones, laparoscopic cholecystectomy with or without cholangiography is the preferred treatment; open cholecystectomy is reserved for patients who are not candidates for a successful and safe laparoscopic cholecystectomy.

INDICATIONS FOR TREATMENT

Asymptomatic Gallstones

Decisions regarding the management of the patient with asymptomatic gallstones must be predicated on knowledge of the natural history of the condition, as discussed in Chapter 67. In general, patients with asymptomatic gallstones should be reassured that life-threatening complications are uncommon and that symptoms related to the stones develop in only a minority of patients.[97–101] In the event that an asymptomatic patient becomes symptomatic, the initial presentation is most often with uncomplicated biliary pain. In fact, most patients in whom complications of gallstones develop have antecedent biliary pain.[102] Decision analysis calculations suggest that the risks of cholecystectomy in the asymptomatic patient approximate the potential benefit in preventing future serious sequelae of gallstones.[103] These calculations were based on historical data regarding the outcome of open cholecystectomy; the rate of serious sequelae of gallstones was determined from long-term follow-up of a group of male faculty members at a major midwestern university. Whether these data are applicable to the more common female patient considering laparoscopic cholecystectomy today is not known. Nevertheless, the strategy of prophylactic cholecystectomy in all asymptomatic patients probably has no major advantage over the recommendation that cholecystectomy be limited to symptomatic patients.[104,105] In addition, studies that have analyzed health-related quality of life do not support cholecystectomy for asymptomatic patients.[106]

In certain subgroups, the benefits of prophylactic cholecystectomy for asymptomatic gallstones may outweigh the risks. Native Americans, for example, appear to have a rate of gallstone-associated gallbladder cancer high enough to justify prophylactic cholecystectomy.[106] In recipients of heart and lung transplants, complications of gallstone disease carry a high morbidity rate, and prophylactic cholecystectomy may be indicated.[107,108] Curiously, kidney transplant patients with asymptomatic gallstones have a low risk of complications related to gallstone disease and, therefore, should not be considered for prophylactic cholecystectomy (see later).[109,110] The risks of complications of gallstone disease in children may outweigh the risk of cholecystectomy (see later). Incidental cholecystectomy is not indicated in asymptomatic patients undergoing bariatric or other types of abdominal surgery.[111]

Diabetic persons have been thought to be particularly prone to gallstone formation and to complications from the stones. Morbidity and mortality rates for diabetic patients who undergo emergency operations for complications of gallstone disease have also been thought to be excessive. These perceptions have not been borne out, however, when confounding variables, such as hyperlipidemia, obesity, cardiovascular disease, and chronic kidney disease are taken into account.[112] Therefore prophylactic cholecystectomy in an asymptomatic diabetic patient with gallstones is not warranted.[113] Data do support early intervention in diabetic patients in whom symptoms develop because these patients are at an increased risk of developing gangrenous cholecystitis.[114] Therefore the severity of complications may be higher when complications of gallstones arise in diabetic than in nondiabetic patients.

Biliary Pain and Chronic Cholecystitis

Patient Selection

Most operations for biliary tract disorders are performed to relieve symptoms related to intermittent obstruction of the cystic duct by gallstones. This constellation of symptoms, including intermittent epigastric or RUQ pain, nausea, and vomiting has been termed *biliary pain* ("biliary colic" in the past) (see Chapters 13 and 67). Histologically, gallbladders from patients experiencing repeated attacks of biliary pain usually, but not always, show fibrosis and mononuclear cell infiltration that are characteristic of chronic cholecystitis. Furthermore, patients with biliary pain are more likely than patients with asymptomatic stones to experience complications of gallstones. Cholecystectomy is indicated in these symptomatic patients. As with any operation, the potential benefits in terms of relief of symptoms and prevention of future complications must be weighed against the risk of surgery. Fortunately, the physiologic stress of cholecystectomy is minimal, and the operation may be undertaken safely even in older adults and the infirm. In the poorly compensated cirrhotic patient, the risk of cholecystectomy is substantially higher.[115] Surgery in this setting is justified only if the symptoms are severe, complications arise, or the cirrhosis is well compensated[116,117] (see Chapter 76). When cholecystectomy is performed for uncomplicated biliary pain, routine perioperative antibiotics are seldom indicated.[118]

Evaluation

The diagnosis of biliary pain is generally suspected from the clinical history (see Chapter 67). Few important findings specific to gallstone disease are elicited on physical examination; most patients with uncomplicated biliary pain have no tenderness between episodes of pain. Few preoperative laboratory tests are routinely necessary, although liver biochemical tests should be

TABLE 68.4 Early Versus Delayed Open or Laparoscopic Cholecystectomy for Acute Cholecystitis: Combined Results From Seven Randomized Trials

Timing of Cholecystectomy	No. of Patients	Mortality Rate (%)	Bile Duct Injuries	Total Mean Hospital Stay (Days)	Failure of Regimen[a]
Early[b]	378	0	0	9.6	N/A
Delayed[c]	364	2.0	0	17.8	26%

[a]Failure is defined as a worsening of acute symptoms requiring early surgery.
[b]Within days of presentation.
[c]After 6–8 weeks.
N/A, Not applicable.
Data from Johansson M, Thune A, Nelvin L, et al. Randomized clinical trial of open versus laparoscopic cholecystectomy in the treatment of acute cholecystitis. *Br J Surg*. 2004;92:44–49. Jarvinen HJ, Hastbacka J. Early cholecystectomy for acute cholecystitis: a prospective randomized study. *Ann Surg*. 1980;191:501–505. Lahtinen J, Alhava EM, Aukee S. Acute cholecystitis treated by early and delayed surgery. A controlled clinical trial. *Scand J Gastroenterol*. 1978;13:673–678. Linden WVD, Sunzel H. Early versus delayed operation for acute cholecystitis. A controlled clinical trial. *Am J Surg*. 1970;120:7–13. Lo CM, Liu CL, Fan ST, et al. Prospective randomized study of early versus delayed laparoscopic cholecystectomy for acute cholecystitis. *Ann Surg*. 1998;227:461–467. McArthur P, Cuschieri A, Sells RA, Shields R. Controlled clinical trial comparing early with interval cholecystectomy for acute cholecystitis. *Br J Surg*. 1975;62:850–852. Lai PB, Kwong KH, Leung KL, et al. Randomized trial of early versus delayed laparoscopic cholecystectomy for acute cholecystitis. *Br J Surg*. 1998;85:764–767.

performed to screen for unsuspected choledocholithiasis if the surgeon does cholangiography on selected patients rather than routine cholangiography on every patient. Imaging evaluation can be limited to US in most patients with biliary pain. US has a high sensitivity (95%) and specificity (98%) in this setting and is also useful for detecting gallbladder inflammation—which is suggested by thickening of the gallbladder wall and pericholecystic fluid—and dilatation of the bile ducts. Ancillary tests, including oral cholecystography, MRCP, ERCP, or CCK scintigraphy, are useful for confirming the diagnosis in the unusual patient in whom gallstones are suspected but US is negative or in evaluating patients suspected of having complicated gallstones. In patients with atypical symptoms, EGD, CT, or both, may be performed to exclude other disorders such as esophagitis, PUD, or an occult neoplasm.

Acute Cholecystitis

Management of the patient with acute cholecystitis begins with IV hydration and restoration of tissue perfusion and electrolyte balance. IV antibiotics are indicated because bile or gallbladder wall cultures are positive for bacteria in more than 40% of patients.[119] A cephalosporin, such as cefoxitin, is satisfactory for mildly to moderately ill patients, but in more severe cases, broad-spectrum antibiotics, such as piperacillin-tazobactam or a third-generation cephalosporin with metronidazole, should be given. If gangrenous or emphysematous cholecystitis is suspected, an agent effective against anaerobic organisms should be included. If source control is achieved with surgery, postoperative antibiotic therapy is not indicated in patients with mild-to-moderate cholecystitis.[119] For patients with severe infection, intraoperative perforation of an infected purulent gallbladder, or gangrenous cholecystitis, antibiotics should be continued postoperatively.

Subsequent management depends on the certainty of the diagnosis, severity of the attack, and general condition of the patient. If cholecystitis is severe and complications such as perforation appear imminent, cholecystectomy should be undertaken urgently. If the nature of the symptoms is uncertain, surgery may be indicated to establish the diagnosis. Conversely, the older adult patient with concurrent illnesses such as heart failure may benefit from an initial nonoperative approach.

In the past, the timing of cholecystectomy for the typical patient with acute cholecystitis was controversial. Multiple prospective randomized controlled clinical trials have compared the strategies of early (within 3 days of presentation) and delayed (after 6–8 weeks) surgery for acute cholecystitis (Table 68.4).[85,120–126] A meta-analysis of these trials has shown that, for the average patient, early operation is preferable because the total length of hospitalization and costs are reduced, morbidity is less, and deaths related to progressive acute cholecystitis are prevented.[127] Early operation does not appear to increase the major risks of cholecystectomy, such as bile duct injury, substantially.

Despite initial concerns as to its safety in acute cholecystitis, laparoscopic cholecystectomy is feasible in most cases. Technical problems are encountered occasionally in patients with severe inflammation that obscures identification of the structures of the hepatocystic triangle or with coagulopathy. In these settings, an alternative approach to total cholecystectomy, such as laparoscopic subtotal fenestrating or reconstituting cholecystectomy or use of an open approach, may be necessary.[128] Cholangiography is particularly valuable in patients with acute cholecystitis to confirm the ductal anatomy. The benefits of laparoscopic cholecystectomy in patients with biliary pain, including decreased incisional pain, shortened hospital stay, and more rapid return to work, also apply to patients with acute cholecystitis.

For the high-risk patient with severe concurrent illnesses, such as liver, pulmonary, or heart failure, cholecystostomy (gallbladder drainage) is preferable to cholecystectomy. Operative cholecystostomy has been superseded by a percutaneous approach in most patients. After the patient has recovered from the attack of acute cholecystitis, laparoscopic cholecystectomy should be performed if the patient's overall condition permits it. Alternatively, residual stones can be removed via the cholecystostomy tube, and the patient may be managed expectantly. Recurrent biliary symptoms develop in approximately half of all patients treated with a cholecystostomy.[129] An example of a patient best managed by percutaneous cholecystostomy is shown in Fig. 68.6. The indication for a percutaneous cholecystostomy is the patient's high surgical risk rather than the severity of the acute cholecystitis or appearance of the gallbladder on an imaging study. More recently, endoscopic transmural gallbladder drainage has shown to be as effective as percutaneous drainage in decompressing the gallbladder in patients deemed to be unfit for surgery.[130] In this procedure, the gallbladder is drained by placing an endoluminal stent connecting the gallbladder to the viscera, usually the duodenum. Patients should not undergo endoscopic transmural drainage if there is a possibility they may become candidates for surgery in the future, because surgery would then entail repairing a hole in the duodenum in addition to the removal of the gallbladder.

Acute cholecystitis in diabetic patients is associated with a significantly higher frequency of infectious complications, such as sepsis, compared with nondiabetic patients.[131] Cholecystectomy should be performed expeditiously in this group of patients.

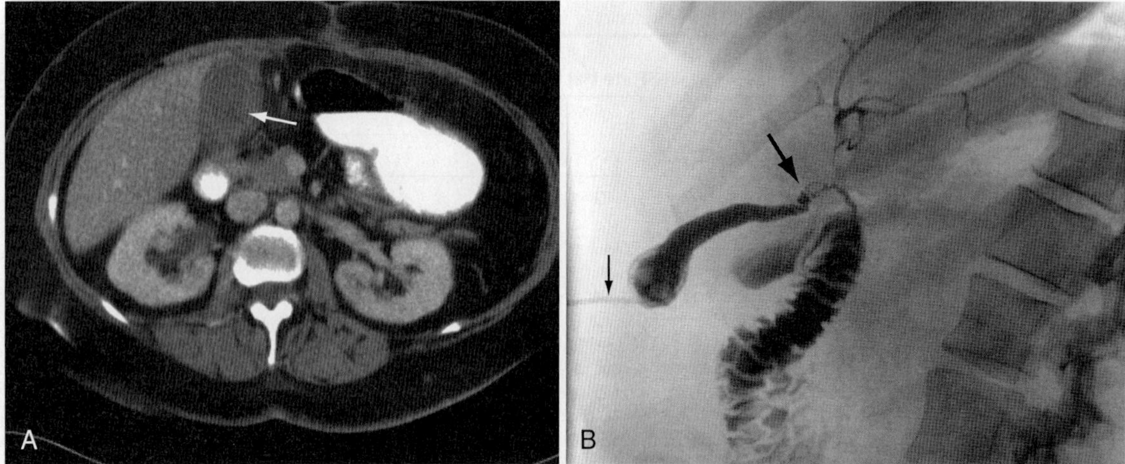

Fig. 68.6 Imaging studies in a 47-year-old woman with severe acute cholecystitis complicating a prolonged ICU stay for multisystem organ failure after surgery for a perforated viscus. (A) CT showing acute cholecystitis with gallbladder wall thickening and pericholecystic fluid (*arrow*). (B) Cholangiogram via a percutaneous cholecystostomy (*small arrow*) showing a gallstone impacted at the neck of the gallbladder (*large arrow*). A cholecystostomy tube was left in place, and the patient improved clinically.

Similarly, acute cholecystitis in older adults may have a deceptively benign clinical presentation but is associated with high rates of occult severe acute cholecystitis, including empyema and gangrene. Factors associated with gangrenous or emphysematous cholecystitis include male gender, diabetes mellitus, cardiovascular disease, and an initial WBC count in excess of 15,000/mm^3. As with diabetic patients, early cholecystectomy is warranted in older adult patients to ensure prompt control of infection. The routine use of surgical drainage catheters after laparoscopic cholecystectomy for acute cholecystitis is not warranted and may be deleterious.[131]

Acalculous Cholecystitis

Acute cholecystitis that occurs in the absence of gallstones is termed *acalculous cholecystitis* (see Chapter 69). Most commonly, acalculous cholecystitis occurs in a patient hospitalized for other serious illnesses, such as trauma, burns, or major surgery. It may develop in outpatients, among whom older adult male patients with peripheral vascular disease appear to be at highest risk.[132] Acalculous cholecystitis may also complicate the treatment of patients with AIDS (see Chapter 33).[133]

The pathophysiology of acalculous cholecystitis is unclear, but biliary stasis caused by fasting, alterations in gallbladder blood flow, activation of factor XII, prostaglandins, and endotoxin all may play roles (see Chapter 69). Sludge is generally present in the gallbladder and may obstruct the cystic duct. Gangrene, empyema, and perforation of the gallbladder complicate the course of acalculous cholecystitis more commonly than they complicate the course of acute cholecystitis caused by gallstones. In some series, the frequency of these complications has approached 75%.[134]

Cholecystectomy has been the mainstay of therapy for acalculous cholecystitis. Prompt removal of the gallbladder is particularly important when gangrene or empyema is suspected and when perforation is imminent. In some patients, however, the risk of surgery is high because of the severity of their underlying illness. These patients may be managed initially with placement of a percutaneous tube cholecystostomy under ultrasound guidance. Most patients treated with tube cholecystostomy recover. Those in whom evidence of intra-abdominal sepsis develops or persistent obstruction of the cystic duct is seen on cholangiography require cholecystectomy.

Emphysematous Cholecystitis

Emphysematous cholecystitis is an uncommon condition characterized by infection of the gallbladder wall by gas-forming bacteria, particularly anaerobes (see Chapter 69). Diabetes mellitus has been cited as a risk factor. Gangrene and perforation commonly complicate the course of emphysematous cholecystitis. The treatment of emphysematous cholecystitis is prompt laparoscopic cholecystectomy after restoration of fluid and electrolyte balance. Antibiotics are indicated, with coverage directed against Gram-negative rods and anaerobic bacteria.

Gallstone Pancreatitis

The pathophysiology and clinical presentation of patients with gallstone pancreatitis are discussed in Chapters 60 and 67. Initial management of patients with gallstone pancreatitis includes fluid resuscitation, bowel rest, and monitoring for complications. Most patients have a relatively mild illness that resolves clinically within 1 week with conservative management.

The presence of cholelithiasis should be determined by US early in the course of the treatment of a patient with acute pancreatitis. If cholelithiasis is present, laparoscopic cholecystectomy generally should be performed prior to the patient's discharge from the hospital. In the past, cholecystectomy early in the course of gallstone pancreatitis carried significant risk. For that reason, the timing of cholecystectomy was delayed for 1–2 months to allow resolution of the inflammatory process. A major disadvantage of this delayed approach was that up to one-half of patients had further attacks of pancreatitis during the observation period. It is now recognized that cholecystectomy may be performed safely during the same hospitalization when the clinical signs of pancreatitis have resolved.[135,136] This approach shortens the total duration of illness and hospitalization.[136] In addition, it prevents recurrent pancreatitis. Cholangiography should be performed during the cholecystectomy to exclude residual bile duct stones, as recommended by the International Association of Pancreatology.[137]

In patients with severe or necrotizing pancreatitis, cholecystectomy is delayed for several weeks to allow (1) patients to recover from the sequelae of pancreatitis; (2) inflammation of the hepatoduodenal ligament to decrease, thereby permitting safe dissection; and (3) identification of the small subset of patients in whom pancreatic pseudocysts develop and may require additional surgical treatment. In patients with concomitant cholangitis or with persistent cholestasis complicating severe pancreatitis, endoscopic sphincterotomy and clearance of the bile duct is indicated.[138] This approach is less morbid than early surgery with bile duct exploration (see Chapter 72).

Special Problems

Gallstone Disease During Pregnancy

Occasionally, gallbladder disease is first noted or becomes more troublesome during pregnancy. The most common clinical presentations in this setting are worsening biliary pain and acute cholecystitis. Jaundice and acute pancreatitis caused by choledocholithiasis are rare. Imaging evaluation of symptoms suggestive of biliary tract disease can nearly always be limited to US. The potential teratogenic effects of conventional radiography and radionuclide scanning make these techniques unjustified in the pregnant patient.

In the past, cholecystectomy during pregnancy was discouraged because of the fear of complications such as spontaneous abortion and preterm labor in operated women in the first and third trimesters of gestation, respectively. In addition, pregnancy was formerly considered an absolute contraindication to laparoscopic surgery because of concern about potential trocar injury to the uterus and the unknown effects of pneumoperitoneum on the fetal circulation. Improvements in anesthesia and tocolytic agents appear to have made abdominal surgery safer during pregnancy. Several large case series have suggested that cholecystectomy may be undertaken during pregnancy with minimal fetal and maternal morbidity.[139,140] Even though proved safe, laparoscopic cholecystectomy is performed during pregnancy only when necessary. Indications include complicated gallstone disease, including acute cholecystitis and pancreatitis, when the underlying disease poses a threat to the pregnancy or when the mother is unable to maintain adequate nutrition. In these scenarios, the risk to the pregnancy from the underlying disease exceeds the risk to the pregnancy of surgery. Surgery is probably safest during the second trimester, when the risk of fetal loss and teratogenicity that may occur in the first trimester and the risk of preterm labor that may occur in the third trimester are both low.

Gallstone Disease During Childhood

Gallstone disease in the pediatric population appears to be increasing in frequency. Chronic hemolysis leading to pigment gallstones is the cause in about 20% of patients.[141] A history of prolonged fasting with total parenteral nutritional support is an increasingly important risk factor. Ileal disorders or previous bowel resection increase the risk of gallstone development. Management of childhood cholelithiasis must take into account the type of stone (pigment or cholesterol), the presence or absence of symptoms, and underlying risk factors such as TPN. Cholecystectomy is indicated in all symptomatic patients with gallstones. The management of asymptomatic gallstones is less clear. Gallstones in infants who are receiving total parenteral nutrition occasionally resolve following reinstitution of oral feedings. Therefore observing the asymptomatic infant in this setting for up to 12 months seems reasonable. Persistent gallstones and asymptomatic pigment stones (which do not resolve spontaneously) are best treated with laparoscopic cholecystectomy.

Mirizzi Syndrome

Mirizzi syndrome refers to common hepatic duct obstruction resulting from compression by a gallstone impacted in the cystic duct. Two types of Mirizzi syndrome were originally described.[142] In type I, the hepatic duct is compressed by a large stone impacted in the cystic duct or Hartmann pouch. Associated inflammation may contribute to the obstruction and formation of a stricture in the central section of the extrahepatic bile duct. In type II, the calculus has eroded into the common hepatic duct to produce a cholecystocholedochal fistula. Mirizzi syndrome is rare, occurring in about 1% of all patients who undergo cholecystectomy. Most patients present with repeated bouts of pain, fever, and jaundice. US generally reveals gallstones with a contracted gallbladder and moderate intrahepatic ductal dilatation with normal extrahepatic biliary anatomy. MRCP and ERCP are useful in delineating the hepatic duct anatomy. The typical findings are a dilated intrahepatic biliary tract, with a normal-sized bile duct, secondary to obstruction at the level of the cystic duct insertion into the common hepatic duct. The appearance of the obstruction and surrounding inflammation may be confused with a Klatskin tumor (see Chapter 71).

The possibility of Mirizzi syndrome should be considered during a difficult cholecystectomy. Management of type I Mirizzi syndrome includes cholecystectomy with or without bile duct exploration. In the presence of severe inflammation, in which identification of the anatomy is difficult, partial cholecystectomy with postoperative endoscopic sphincterotomy to ensure clearance of bile duct stones is preferable. Management of type II Mirizzi syndrome is based on the extent of compromise of the common hepatic duct and bile duct. To guide surgical treatment, type II Mirizzi syndrome has been reclassified as types II, III, and IV. Type II is present when less than one-third of the bile duct is involved by the fistula, type III when one-third to two-thirds is involved (Fig. 68.7), and type IV when more than two-thirds is involved. Types II and III Mirizzi syndrome can be treated with partial cholecystectomy, removal of the calculus, and choledochoplasty as needed. Roux-en-Y hepaticojejunostomy is required to repair a large defect as seen in type IV Mirizzi syndrome.[142]

Gallstone Ileus

Gallstone ileus is an uncommon form of intestinal obstruction caused by impaction of a large gallstone in the intestinal lumen. Bouveret syndrome refers to impaction of a gallstone in the distal duodenum or at the pylorus with resulting symptoms of gastric outlet obstruction. Gallstone ileus represents a true mechanical obstruction rather than a defect in motility, as the name "ileus" would suggest. The median age of affected patients is more than 70 years. Most are women. Gallstone ileus is the cause of intestinal obstruction in less than 1% of patients younger than 70 years in age but nearly 5% of those 70 years of age or older.[143] Symptoms are typical of mechanical intestinal obstruction and include cramping abdominal pain, vomiting, and abdominal distention. Only a minority of patients have symptoms suggestive of acute cholecystitis, but half are known to have a history of gallstones.[144] Liver biochemical test levels are elevated in 40% of patients, but overt jaundice is rare. Plain abdominal films reveal an intestinal gas pattern compatible with intestinal obstruction in most patients. Pneumobilia is present in about half of all patients, and the aberrant gallstone is visible in a minority. Upper or lower GI barium studies may occasionally identify the site of obstruction or the fistula, but these tests are unnecessary in most cases. US is useful for confirming the presence of cholelithiasis and may allow visualization of the fistula.

The pathophysiology of gallstone ileus involves erosion of a gallstone, generally over 2.5 cm in diameter, into the intestinal lumen via a cholecystoenteric fistula. The fistula occurs most commonly in the duodenum and less often in the colon. As the gallstone is passed down the length of the intestine, it obstructs the lumen intermittently. Characteristically, complete obstruction occurs in the ileum, where the lumen is narrowest. The

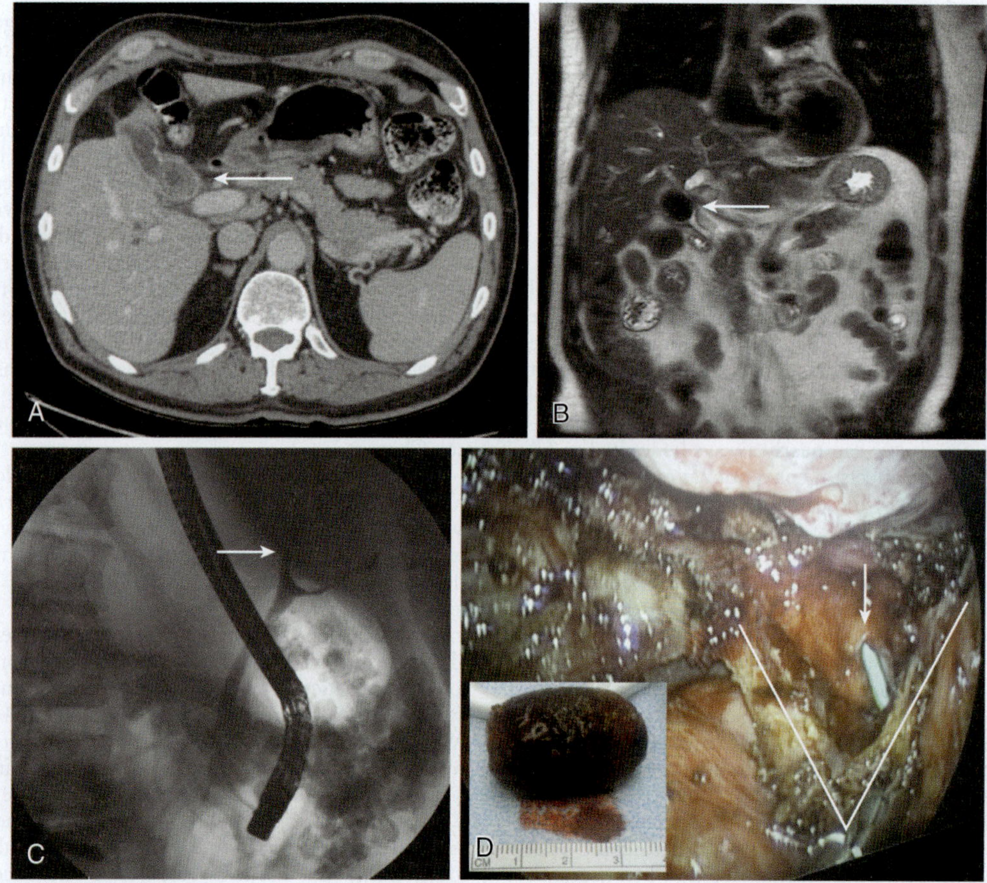

Fig. 68.7 Type III Mirizzi syndrome. (A) CT showing a large gallstone impacted in the infundibulum of the gallbladder (*arrow*). (B) MRCP showing a large gallstone impacted in the infundibulum of the gallbladder (*arrow*). (C) ERCP showing obstruction of the common hepatic duct by a large intraluminal gallstone consistent with a cholecystocholedochal fistula (*arrow*). (D) Intraoperative photograph of the anterior wall of the gallbladder removed with the edge of the remaining medial gallbladder wall highlighted by *white lines*. A fistula (containing a blue biliary stent placed during ERCP) between the common hepatic duct and the medial wall of the gallbladder infundibulum is seen (*arrow*), with 50% disruption of the common hepatic duct integrity, consistent with type III Mirizzi syndrome. The inset shows the causative 3-cm gallstone.

obstruction has been described as "tumbling" because the symptoms wax and wane during the passage of the stone.

Management should be directed initially at restoration of fluid and electrolyte balance, followed by exploratory laparotomy. A laparoscopic approach is technically feasible and effective. Removing the stone via a small enterotomy relieves the intestinal obstruction. A search should be made for additional stones. Bowel resection is necessary only when perforation or intestinal ischemia has occurred. Cholecystectomy with closure of the cholecystoenteric fistula, the connection between the gallbladder and adjacent duodenum, is not necessary because the gallbladder decompresses itself of stones through the fistula. More importantly, surgery may be technically difficult and morbid, and many fistulas close spontaneously with time.[144] Mortality rates in this high-risk patient population are high, averaging 15%–18%. Gallstone ileus recurs in about 5% of patients.

Incidental Cholecystectomy

Occasionally, gallstones are identified unexpectedly before or during another operation. When this happens, incidental cholecystectomy should be considered at the time of the original, planned, procedure and discussed during the informed consent process. The rationale for incidental cholecystectomy is to prevent later development of symptomatic gallstone disease, including early postoperative acute cholecystitis. Another justification often cited is that some operations make subsequent endoscopic or surgical intervention to treat gallstone-related complications difficult, as is the case with gastrectomy or gastric bypass for obesity (see Chapter 9). As expected, addition of a cholecystectomy increases the risk of postoperative complications. The decision to proceed with an incidental cholecystectomy is based on an assessment of the expected benefits and risks.

As discussed previously, the typical patient with gallstones tends to remain asymptomatic. On long-term follow-up, symptoms develop in 18%–35% of these initially asymptomatic persons.[97,103,104] Certain groups, however, are at higher risk. Patients with large (>2.5 cm) gallstones and those with calcification of the gallbladder wall (porcelain gallbladder) have an increased risk for the development of acute cholecystitis, gallstone ileus, and gallbladder cancer. In these patients, incidental cholecystectomy is warranted.[145–147] In patients with sickle cell disease, who are at risk for the development of pigment gallstones because of chronic hemolysis, distinguishing the clinical presentation of a sickle cell crisis from acute cholecystitis may be difficult, and incidental cholecystectomy is indicated in these patients.[148] Similarly, patients with other hemolytic anemias, such as β-thalassemia, are at high risk for the development of gallstones, and a high proportion of them become symptomatic.[149] Cholecystectomy appears warranted for asymptomatic patients with stones if splenectomy is undertaken for the hemolytic anemia. Finally, laparotomy for reasons other than cholecystectomy is associated with a high frequency of postoperative biliary symptoms if a gallbladder that contains stones is left in situ. Of 68 asymptomatic patients with stones who underwent laparotomy in one study, 54% became symptomatic postoperatively, and 22% required cholecystectomy within 30 days.[150,151]

The risk of adding incidental cholecystectomy to another abdominal procedure appears to be low.[152] If the patient is in otherwise reasonable health, the primary operation has proceeded smoothly, and operative exposure is adequate, incidental cholecystectomy can be done safely at the time of another operation, including colectomy. The risk does not appear to be increased in older adults. The risk of postoperative wound infections, however, may be increased in some cases by the addition of an incidental cholecystectomy.[153]

CHOLEDOCHOLITHIASIS

Choledocholithiasis may be detected when gallbladder stones are discovered during an evaluation for biliary tract symptoms, during cholecystectomy, or after a cholecystectomy. Several management options are available, including oral dissolution therapy, interventional radiologic and endoscopic techniques, and surgery (see Chapter 72). Which management strategy is most appropriate for a given patient depends on the clinical situation in which the stones have been identified (jaundice, cholangitis, pancreatitis, or absence of symptoms), status of the gallbladder, and age and general condition of the patient. Additional factors to consider are the expertise of the available surgical, endoscopic, and radiologic specialists.

Choledocholithiasis Known Preoperatively

When choledocholithiasis is known to be present preoperatively, an acceptable approach is to clear the bile duct by endoscopic sphincterotomy and then proceed with laparoscopic cholecystectomy. An alternative approach is an open or laparoscopic cholecystectomy with bile duct exploration. In the era of laparoscopic cholecystectomy and endoscopic stone retrieval, laparoscopic bile duct exploration has been performed less commonly than open bile duct exploration was performed during the open cholecystectomy era.[154] Laparoscopic bile duct exploration via either a transcystic duct approach or direct incision of the bile duct is a technically demanding procedure. When performed by an experienced surgeon, however, the success rate for clearing the duct of stones ranges from 83% to 97%.[155–157] Decision analyses and randomized trials have shown that laparoscopic cholecystectomy with bile duct exploration via either a transcystic or transcholedochal approach results in lower rates of morbidity and mortality as well as a shorter hospital stay, quicker return to health, and lower number of procedures than preoperative endoscopic retrieval followed by laparoscopic cholecystectomy.[154,155,158] The decision to proceed with the surgery-only approach depends greatly on the experience and technical skill of the surgeon and his or her team. If a surgeon lacks adequate training or appropriately trained staff and equipment, a two-stage (surgical and endoscopic) approach is preferable.

Choledocholithiasis Identified During Cholecystectomy

If unsuspected choledocholithiasis is identified by cholangiography during laparoscopic cholecystectomy, the following three options are available: (1) conversion to an open operation with bile duct exploration; (2) laparoscopic bile duct exploration; and

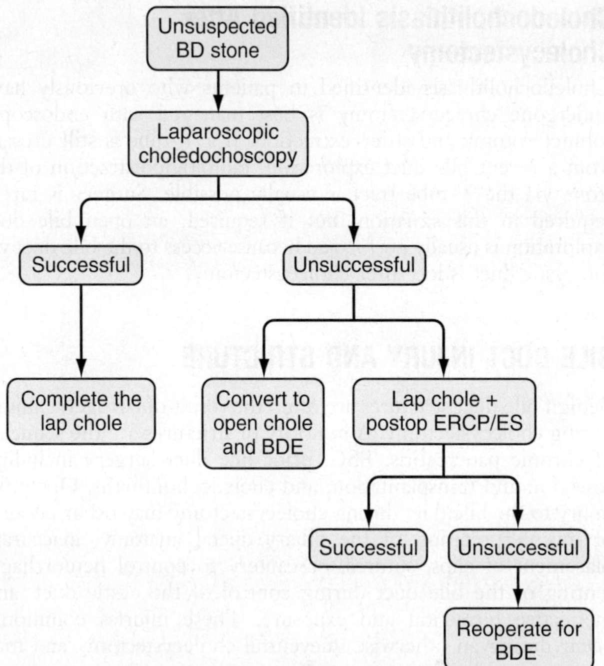

Fig. 68.8 Suggested algorithm for the management of bile duct (BD) stones found unexpectedly during laparoscopic cholecystectomy (lap chole). *BDE*, Bile duct exploration; *ERCP/ES*, ERCP/endoscopic sphincterotomy; *postop*, postoperative.

(3) completion of the laparoscopic cholecystectomy with postoperative endoscopic sphincterotomy and stone extraction. An algorithm of these options is shown in Fig. 68.8. Factors that influence this decision include the number and location of bile duct stones, presence of associated ductal pathology, and skill and experience of the surgeon and endoscopist. Completion of the laparoscopic cholecystectomy with postoperative endoscopic sphincterotomy is satisfactory for most patients and has the advantage of preserving the minimally invasive approach. Endoscopic sphincterotomy may be technically unsuccessful, however, in 5%–10% of patients—even in the hands of a skilled endoscopist—and complete clearance of stones from the bile duct is possible in only 84%–89% of patients.[156] In such patients, a second attempt may be required. Increasing experience has shown that laparoscopic bile duct exploration is safe and effective. Stone clearance rates average 95%, with an operative mortality rate of 0.5%.[155,156,159,160] Laparoscopic bile duct exploration compares favorably with endoscopic sphincterotomy in terms of efficacy, cost, and safety.[161]

As with open bile duct exploration, laparoscopic bile duct exploration is done preferably through a transcystic approach, in which the bile duct is explored, and stones are removed via an incision in the cystic duct. On rare occasions in which the stones are too large or located above the insertion of the cystic duct into the bile duct, a transcholedochal approach is needed. This approach involves exploration of the bile duct and removal of stones via an incision directly into the bile duct. The incision in the bile duct must be closed with sutures, often over a T-tube to prevent stricturing of the bile duct, especially when the duct is small and suture closure in the absence of a T-tube may lead to a stricture that is difficult to dilate. Therefore a small bile duct is a contraindication to direct transcholedochal exploration. T-tubes are also left in the bile duct when evacuation of stones is incomplete to allow biliary decompression and percutaneous stone extraction by an interventional radiologist.

Choledocholithiasis Identified After Cholecystectomy

Choledocholithiasis identified in patients who previously have undergone cholecystectomy is best managed with endoscopic sphincterotomy and stone extraction. If a T-tube is still present from a recent bile duct exploration, radiologic extraction of the stone via the T-tube tract is usually possible. Surgery is rarely required in this situation, but if required, an open bile duct exploration is usually performed because access to the bile duct via the cystic duct is lost after cholecystectomy.

BILE DUCT INJURY AND STRICTURE

Benign bile duct strictures are often the result of iatrogenic injury during cholecystectomy. A minority of strictures are the sequelae of chronic pancreatitis, PSC, prior bile duct surgery including resection and transplantation, and choledocholithiasis. Operative injury to the bile duct during cholecystectomy may occur because of misinterpretation of the biliary ductal anatomy; inaccurate placement of clips, sutures, or cautery to control hemorrhage; tenting of the bile duct during control of the cystic duct; and ineffective retraction and exposure. These injuries commonly occur during an otherwise uneventful cholecystectomy and may be unnoticed by the surgeon.

Bile duct injury presents in one of three patterns. In the first pattern, the bile duct has been completely occluded, and jaundice develops rapidly in the early postoperative period after cholecystectomy. In the second pattern, the injury is manifested by the development of bile ascites that results from transection of an extrahepatic bile duct, ineffective placement or dislodgement of cystic duct ligatures, or a bile leak from the gallbladder fossa as a result of a divided cystohepatic duct or duct of Luschka. A bile leak is often associated with an infected bile collection in the subhepatic space. In the third pattern, partial bile duct obstruction leads to intermittent episodes of pain, jaundice, or cholangitis, usually within 2 years of the cholecystectomy. The three patterns of injury are illustrated in Fig. 68.9.

In the early postoperative period following laparoscopic cholecystectomy, the clinician should suspect the possibility of bile duct injury in any patient with persistent abdominal pain, nausea, and fever. The differential diagnosis of bile duct obstruction in a patient with a history of cholecystectomy, whether in the early postoperative period or remote from surgery, consists mainly of bile duct stricture and choledocholithiasis. Stricture and choledocholithiasis may be difficult to differentiate on clinical grounds because the symptoms, signs, and liver biochemical test levels may be identical.

The imaging evaluation of a patient with suspected bile duct injury and/or stricture usually begins with US to identify dilated ducts or a subhepatic fluid collection or biloma. In the early postoperative period, a technetium-labeled radionuclide scan may expeditiously and noninvasively demonstrate patency of the biliary tract and exclude a bile leak. If these studies suggest bile duct injury, ERCP is indicated to define the lesion. The initial goals of management include control of subhepatic infection, usually via percutaneous drainage of any fluid collection, and biliary drainage, either via an endoscopic or transhepatic route (see Chapter 72). Following the control of infection and biliary drainage, complete cholangiography, by ERCP transhepatic cholangiography, is necessary to define the anatomy and plan reconstruction.

Most patients with a bile duct injury or benign postoperative biliary stricture are best managed with surgical repair. Although numerous operations have been described, the best results are obtained with resection of the damaged duct and an end-to-side Roux-en-Y choledochojejunostomy or hepaticojejunostomy. The principles of a successful repair include a complete dissection of the injured or strictured segment, creation of a tension-free anastomosis, accurate mucosa-to-mucosa approximation of the anastomosis with fine absorbable suture material and unscarred proximal ductal tissue, and preservation of the ductal blood supply. The mortality rate of operations to correct benign biliary strictures averages 0%–2%. The risk of surgery is related directly to the presence of risk factors such as cirrhosis, renal failure, uncontrolled cholangitis, age, and malnutrition. The long-term results of biliary reconstruction for a benign bile duct stricture are good, with cure achieved in 85%–98% of patients.[162–165] Results are worse in patients with high strictures or cirrhosis. In those with high strictures, special techniques may be necessary to obtain healthy ductal tissue that is uninvolved in the inflammatory process for anastomosis; liver resection may be required. Recurrent strictures pose technical difficulties, but satisfactory results are still achieved in about 75% of patients.[166]

Postoperative strictures may be treated with endoscopic or percutaneous balloon dilation with or without stent placement provided the remaining duct has not been disrupted. Benign postoperative strictures often can be managed endoscopically with the placement of plastic, removable stents. Although several endoscopic procedures are often required, good results can be achieved in appropriately selected patients (see Chapter 72). No randomized prospective trials have compared surgical, endoscopic, and radiologic approaches. In one nonrandomized trial, long-term bile duct patency was achieved in 88% of patients treated with hepaticojejunostomy compared with 55% of those who underwent balloon dilation, but stents were not used.[167] No procedure-related mortality was observed. In view of the excellent long-term results and low mortality rate of hepaticojejunostomy in experienced hands, surgery should be offered as the initial treatment to all fit patients with a bile duct stricture. Nonoperative management is best reserved for patients with biliary cirrhosis, significant comorbid illness, or high recurrent strictures.

POSTCHOLECYSTECTOMY SYNDROME

Postcholecystectomy syndrome refers to the occurrence of abdominal symptoms that often resemble biliary pain following cholecystectomy (see also Chapters 65 and 67). The term is misleading because it encompasses a wide spectrum of biliary and nonbiliary disorders that are rarely related to the operation itself. The frequency of such symptoms following cholecystectomy ranges from 5% to 40%.[49,168–171] The most common postoperative symptoms are dyspepsia, flatulence, and bloating, which usually antedate the cholecystectomy. Other patients have persistence of RUQ or epigastric abdominal pain. A small percentage of patients with postcholecystectomy symptoms present with severe abdominal pain, jaundice, or emesis; investigation is much more likely to reveal a distinct, treatable cause in this group of patients than in those with mild or nonspecific symptoms. If the symptoms arise early in the postoperative period, bile peritonitis secondary to iatrogenic biliary injury must be suspected.

The differential diagnosis of symptoms after cholecystectomy includes extraintestinal disorders such as cardiac ischemia, nonbiliary GI conditions such as PUD, biliary disorders such as choledocholithiasis, functional illnesses such as IBS, and psychiatric diseases (Box 68.3). The clinician must carefully consider the possibility of nonbiliary causes of pain and direct the evaluation appropriately.

Choledocholithiasis

Bile duct stones are the most common cause of postcholecystectomy symptoms. They may be residual stones overlooked at the time of cholecystectomy or, less frequently, stones that have formed primarily in the bile duct. The natural history of

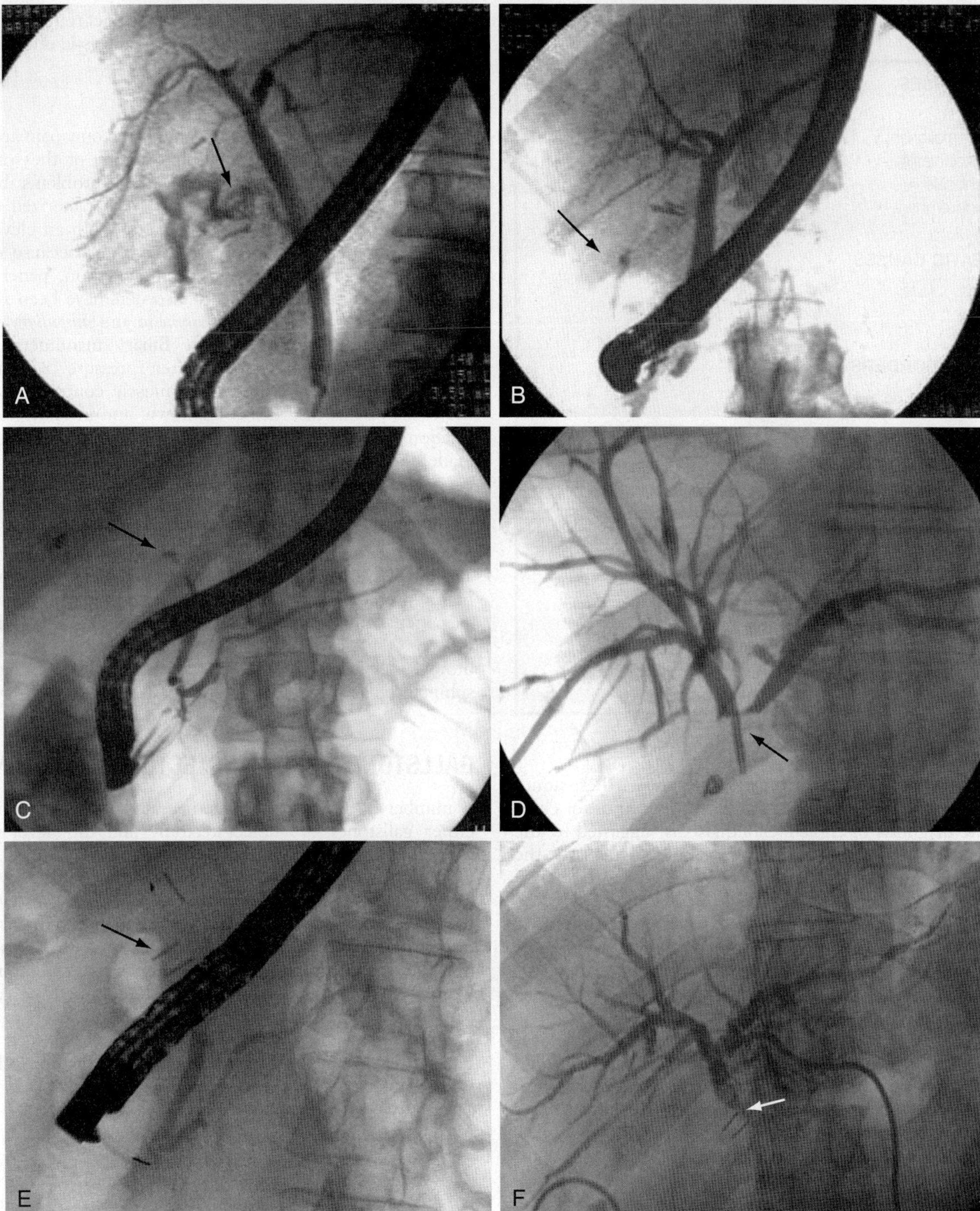

Fig. 68.9 Three common patterns of bile duct injury during laparoscopic cholecystectomy. With the first pattern (A and B) the patient may present with a biloma or bile ascites from a cystic duct stump leak (*arrow* in A) or a bile leak from a duct of Luschka (*arrow* in B). With the second pattern (C and D), the patient presents with jaundice, with or without a bile leak, as a result of excision of the bile duct secondary to misinterpretation of the bile duct for the cystic duct. These problems usually involve injury to the confluence of the hepatic ducts and to the right hepatic artery as well. (C) An ERCP showing surgical clips occluding the bile duct (*arrow*); (D) the corresponding transhepatic cholangiogram demonstrating excision of the hepatic duct confluence (*arrow*). With the third pattern (E and F) the patient presents with jaundice caused by a stricture resulting either from a surgical clip placed on the bile duct instead of the cystic duct or from a thermal injury. (E) An ERCP showing a stricture from a surgical clip (*arrow*); (F) the corresponding transhepatic cholangiogram showing the bile duct stricture (*arrow*).

BOX 68.3 Causes of Abdominal Pain After Cholecystectomy

BILIARY CAUSES

Biliary stricture
Biliary tract malignancy
Choledocholithiasis
Choledochocele
Cystic duct remnant
SOD

PANCREATIC CAUSES

Pancreatitis
Pseudocyst
Malignancy

OTHER GI DISORDERS

Esophageal motor disorders
GERD
IBS
Intestinal malignancy
Intra-abdominal adhesions
Mesenteric ischemia
PUD

EXTRAINTESTINAL DISORDERS

Coronary artery disease
Intercostal neuritis
Neurologic disorders
Psychiatric disorders
Wound neuroma

choledocholithiasis is not known, but in some patients, these stones clearly can cause biliary-type pain, jaundice, pancreatitis, or cholangitis. The diagnosis of choledocholithiasis is suggested by the clinical picture. Liver biochemical test values, particularly the alkaline phosphatase level, may be elevated. US may show a dilated bile duct, but visualization of the stone is uncommon. MRCP and ERCP may confirm the presence of ductal stones and exclude other possibilities such as a bile duct stricture or tumor. Endoscopic sphincterotomy with stone extraction is curative in most patients.[172]

Cystic Duct Remnant

In some patients, the cause of postcholecystectomy symptoms has been attributed to pathology in the cystic duct remnant (or stump) or small retained portion of the gallbladder.[173,174] Abnormalities that have been described include cystic duct stones, fistulas, granulomas, and neuromas. Associated bile duct stones are common. Although the existence of such a syndrome has been controversial, in one randomized trial, complete excision of the cystic duct during cholecystectomy was associated with fewer postoperative sequelae than a standard operative technique in which a portion of the cystic duct was left in situ.[175] In the era of laparoscopic cholecystectomy, the cystic duct is divided closer to its origin from the gallbladder to minimize the risk of bile duct and right hepatic artery injury that may arise from dissection at the insertion of the cystic duct into the common hepatic duct; as a result, the frequency of cystic duct remnant syndrome may be higher.[176] MRCP and ERCP are useful for delineating the biliary anatomy in patients with suspected cystic duct remnant pathology. Treatment is with surgical excision of the cystic duct remnant.

SOD

Up to 10% of patients with postcholecystectomy pain are found to have a structural or functional abnormality of the sphincter of Oddi (see Chapter 65).[177,178] Structural problems have been referred to as *sphincter stenosis*, which is characterized by a fixed narrowing of the sphincter in association with an elevated basal sphincter pressure. The stenosis may occur because of trauma such as passage of gallstones, instrumentation, pancreatitis, or infection. Functional or motility disorders have been referred to as *biliary* or *sphincter of Oddi dyskinesia* and *ampullary spasm* and more recently *sphincter disorder*. Biliary manometry in these patients reveals elevated sphincter pressure resulting from abnormal tonic or phasic smooth muscle contractions. Because the cause of this disorder is unknown, and in many cases a distinction between a structural or functional process cannot be made, the generic term *sphincter of Oddi dysfunction* is preferred.

Clinical manifestations of SOD include biliary-type pain, jaundice, and pancreatitis. ERCP findings of a dilated bile duct and delayed (>45 minutes) drainage of contrast medium from the bile duct are typical. The combination of biliary-type pain, abnormal liver biochemical test levels, and a dilated bile duct is highly predictive of a response to endoscopic sphincterotomy.[179] In patients in whom the diagnosis is not as clear, biliary manometry is indicated. Treatment is with endoscopic sphincterotomy. Selected patients may require transduodenal sphincteroplasty and septoplasty (see Chapter 65).[180]

GALLSTONES, CHOLECYSTECTOMY, AND CANCER

A number of reports have demonstrated an association between either gallstones or cholecystectomy and the development of cancers in organs as diverse as the gallbladder, bile ducts, stomach, colon, breast, and uterus. Whether a causal relationship exists between gallbladder disease or its treatment and the development of these malignancies is unclear. Common environmental factors, perhaps dietary, may influence the rates of all these diseases. On the other hand, alterations in the composition of bile in patients with gallstones could influence the development of carcinoma. Moreover, cholecystectomy increases the enterohepatic circulation of bile acids, which increases mucosal exposure to potentially carcinogenic secondary bile acids such as deoxycholic acid (see Chapter 66).

Biliary Tract Cancer

The strongest association between gallstones and cancer is with cancers of the biliary tract itself, particularly gallbladder carcinoma (see Chapter 71). Most patients with gallbladder cancer have gallstones, and epidemiologic data show a strong relationship between the two diseases. The risk of gallbladder cancer is greater in patients with large gallstones than in those with small gallstones, in those with multiple gallstones than a single gallstone, and in Native Americans.[181–183] Calcification of the gallbladder wall, or porcelain gallbladder, is also associated with gallbladder cancer.[184] A weaker statistical association exists between gallstones and cholangiocarcinoma, and a causal relationship is suggested by the finding that the risk is lower in patients who undergo cholecystectomy than in those whose gallstones are untreated.[185,186]

Colorectal Cancer

Studies from the early 1980s identified a statistical association between cholecystectomy and the subsequent development of colorectal cancer, particularly in the right colon.[187–189] The magnitude of the risk of colorectal cancer, although statistically significant, was low (relative risk 1.5–2.0). Subsequent studies have disputed the association, attributed it to the gallstones rather than cholecystectomy, or shown that the increased frequency of colon cancer occurs too soon following cholecystectomy to be causal (see Chapter 129).[190,191] These findings should not represent a deterrent to cholecystectomy in a patient with a clear indication for the procedure.

Full references for this chapter can be found at https://ebooks.health.elsevier.com

69 Acalculous Biliary Pain, Acute Acalculous Cholecystitis, Cholesterolosis, Adenomyomatosis, and Gallbladder Polyps

Karin L. Andersson, Lawrence S. Friedman

IN THIS CHAPTER

The majority of cholecystectomies are performed for treatment of symptomatic gallstone disease[1] but a consistent 15% of these operations are performed in patients without gallstones.[2] In these patients, the majority of cholecystectomies are performed as treatment for one of two distinct clinical syndromes: acalculous biliary pain and acalculous cholecystitis. As shown in Table 69.1, acalculous biliary pain is generally a disorder of young, predominantly female, ambulatory patients and mimics calculous biliary pain. Acute acalculous cholecystitis is typically a disease of immobilized and critically ill older men with coexisting vascular disease. Because the clinical features and prognosis of these two entities are quite different, they are considered separately in this chapter. Three typically asymptomatic conditions of the gallbladder—cholesterolosis, adenomyomatosis, and gallbladder polyp—are also reviewed.

ACALCULOUS BILIARY PAIN

Definition and Clinical Features

Biliary pain (or biliary "colic") is typically characterized by intense epigastric or right upper quadrant pain that starts suddenly, rises in intensity over a 15-minute period, and continues at a steady plateau for 30 minutes or more before slowly subsiding. The localization of pain to the right hypochondrium or radiation to the right shoulder suggests a biliary tract origin.[3] The attacks of pain are frequently precipitated by an ingestion of a meal and may be accompanied by restlessness, nausea, or vomiting. Between attacks, the physical findings are usually normal, with the possible exception of residual upper abdominal tenderness.

When a patient presents with such a history and US confirms the presence of gallstones, the management is straightforward—namely, elective cholecystectomy. In comparison, the management of *acalculous biliary pain* represents a significant challenge. Patients with acalculous biliary pain have clinical features and biliary-type pain similar to those of patients with cholelithiasis, but a normal gallbladder on US and normal serum levels of liver and pancreatic enzymes.[4,5] Acalculous biliary pain may stem from a spectrum of overlapping disorders, including chronic acalculous cholecystitis and gallbladder dysmotility or functional gallbladder disorder (FGBD), which share symptomatology but differ in the pathologic findings of the resected gallbladder. In patients with acalculous biliary pain, symptomatic improvement following cholecystectomy is variable.

Epidemiology and Pathophysiology

US-negative biliary pain is common in population studies, with reported frequencies of approximately 7% in men and 20% among women.[6] Acalculous biliary pain is predominantly a disorder of young women. In one series of more than 100 patients, 83% were female, and the mean age was approximately 30 years.[5]

The cause of the acalculous biliary pain syndrome is not known, but indirect evidence suggests that several different etiologies may culminate in the same clinical presentation. Stimulated duodenal bile from patients with acalculous biliary pain is more dilute with respect to both bile acids and phospholipids than bile from patients with gallstones or from control women without biliary symptoms.[7] The low bile acid concentration may be related to the sluggish or incomplete gallbladder contraction that has been observed in patients with acalculous biliary pain. The lower molar percentage of phospholipids supports the hypothesis that biliary phospholipids are hydrolyzed to free fatty acids, which incite inflammation.

TABLE 69.1 Comparison of Acalculous Biliary Pain and Acute Acalculous Cholecystitis

	Acalculous Biliary Pain	Acute Acalculous Cholecystitis
Epidemiology	Female preponderance (80%) Young to middle-aged ambulatory patient Risk factors are similar to those for cholelithiasis (i.e., obesity and multiparity)	Male preponderance (80%) A critically ill older adult patient in an ICU Risk factors are preexisting atherosclerosis, recent surgery, and hemodynamic instability
Clinical features	Episodic RUQ or epigastric pain identical to calculous biliary pain Physical findings are usually normal Laboratory findings are usually normal	Unexplained sepsis with few localizing signs; rapid progression to gangrene and perforation Physical examination may show fever; RUQ tenderness is present in only 25% Leukocytosis and hyperamylasemia may be present
Diagnostic tests	US shows no stones and usually a normal gallbladder Stimulated cholescintigraphy using CCK to measure the GBEF may identify patients who are likely to improve after cholecystectomy	See Table 69.2
Treatment	Elective cholecystectomy may be considered for patients with classic biliary pain or a GBEF <35% or >81% and persistent symptoms not suggestive of underlying functional GI disease	Urgent cholecystostomy or emergency cholecystectomy for gangrene or perforation
Prognosis	Good; attacks resolve spontaneously or with cholecystectomy	Poor; mortality rate of 10%–50% related to underlying comorbid diseases

GBEF, Gallbladder ejection fraction.

The striking preponderance of young, fertile women among patients with acalculous biliary pain closely parallels the epidemiology of cholelithiasis, suggesting that the two conditions have similar risk factors. Some studies have shown that up to half of patients with acalculous biliary pain have microscopic cholelithiasis in resected gallbladder specimens,[8] indicating that the original US was falsely negative. Several studies have shown that a small subset of patients with acalculous biliary pain have histologic evidence of cholesterolosis in their resected gallbladders (see later).[9] Although usually an incidental pathologic finding, cholesterolosis of the gallbladder may, in some patients, disrupt normal gallbladder contraction and result in biliary pain. In other patients, the resected gallbladder demonstrates significant inflammation, characteristic of chronic acalculous cholecystitis.[10]

Finally, acalculous biliary pain is listed as a functional GI disorder, designated DGBI, by a multinational working committee of GI investigators [Rome IV classification (see Chapter 124)], with the implication that a pathologic lesion is not required for the diagnosis.[4] In patients with a histologically normal gallbladder, a lack of coordination between gallbladder contraction and sphincter of Oddi relaxation or duodenal hyperalgesia may cause biliary pain (see Chapter 65). The strong link between acalculous biliary pain and other functional bowel disorders suggests that visceral hypersensitivity may be a common cause of biliary pain in patients with a normal gallbladder.[6]

Diagnosis and Treatment

As described earlier, the symptoms of acalculous biliary pain may be indistinguishable from those of cholelithiasis. A careful review of the patient's complaints should confirm that the symptoms are genuinely suggestive of biliary pain rather than dyspepsia, heartburn, cramping abdominal pain, or flatulence.[3] If the symptoms are consistent with biliary pain, a detailed review of the US results with a radiologist is warranted. Although gallstones greater than 2 mm are unlikely to be missed (the sensitivity of US for detecting stones exceeds 95%), other US evidence of gallbladder disease may be overlooked if the primary focus is to exclude stones. In patients with typical biliary symptoms and a negative US result, further assessment of the biliary tract with EUS, MRCP, or secretin-enhanced MRCP may be of benefit.[11] Patients with abnormalities such as gallbladder adenomyomatosis or polyps may also have biliary pain that is relieved by cholecystectomy (see later). Determining when and in whom to pursue cholecystectomy for patients with biliary pain and normal imaging presents a challenge (see Chapter 65).

Stimulated Cholescintigraphy

A possible, but controversial, approach to determining which patients with acalculous biliary pain are likely to benefit from cholecystectomy involves calculation of a gallbladder ejection fraction (GBEF) using cholescintigraphy (see also Chapter 65). An IV-administered radiolabeled hepatobiliary agent (e.g., ^{99m}Tc-diisopropyl iminodiacetic acid) is concentrated in the gallbladder, and a computer-assisted gamma camera measures activity before and after stimulation of gallbladder contraction with a slow IV infusion of CCK over 30 minutes. The GBEF is defined as the change in activity divided by the baseline activity. Studies in healthy volunteers have shown that normal GBEF averages 75% and virtually always exceeds 35%.[5] Fatty meal cholescintigraphy is a less costly alternative to the CCK-stimulated test and uses oral fat intake (typically half-and-half milk) to stimulate gallbladder contraction physiologically; normal values for GBEF tend to be lower than those for CCK-stimulated cholescintigraphy.[12,13]

Fewer than one-half of patients with acalculous biliary pain have a depressed GBEF, but most of those who do have a depressed GBEF continue to have symptoms when followed for as long as 3 years. In these patients, the gallbladder may have abnormal findings, including histologic evidence of chronic cholecystitis in approximately 90%, cystic duct narrowing in 80%, and cholesterolosis in 30%.[12] Long-term symptom relief following cholecystectomy may occur in more than 50% of patients with an abnormal GBEF[5,14,15]; however, up to 50% of patients managed without surgery also experience symptom relief.[16] In one study of patients with a GBEF less than 35% and atypical symptoms, 30% experienced spontaneous resolution of symptoms, whereas 57% of those with persistent symptoms experienced symptom resolution following cholecystectomy.[17,18] In the single randomized, controlled trial of cholecystectomy as treatment for biliary pain in 21 patients with a depressed GBEF, the 11 patients who underwent cholecystectomy reported resolution (n = 10) or improvement (n = 1) of their symptoms over an average follow-up period of 54 months. The 10 patients in the group randomized to no surgery continued to experience symptoms.[5] A 2023 retrospective study suggested a similar benefit to CCY in patients with a hyperkinetic gallbladder, defined as a GBEF possibly >81%. In this study, 78% of patients with a GBEF in this range experienced symptom relief after CCY, as compared with 60% of those with a normal GBEF.[18a]

Patients with acalculous biliary pain and a normal GBEF also have a variable, although generally benign, course. Some are found to have a nonbiliary cause of the symptoms, and in others the pain resolves with time. Cholecystectomy has not typically been recommended for patients with acalculous pain and a normal GBEF, although the frequency of symptom relief following cholecystectomy in this population may be equivalent to that of patients with a depressed or hyperkinetic GBEF who undergo cholecystectomy.[19] As a result, although the GBEF is used commonly to evaluate patients with acalculous biliary-type pain, it is not a reliable predictor of the response to cholecystectomy. As a general rule, typical biliary pain tends to resolve more reliably following cholecystectomy than do atypical symptoms such as bloating or dyspepsia. This observation raises the question as to whether surgery should be recommended based on symptoms, without scintigraphy, and suggests a period of observation or medical management to allow for symptoms to resolve without surgery.

As stimulated cholescintigraphy has been used earlier in the evaluation of patients with biliary pain (sometimes immediately after US fails to demonstrate gallstones), patients with nonbiliary or self-limiting diseases have not been weeded out, and the positive predictive value of the test has declined.[20] A low GBEF is not specific for functional gallbladder disease and can occur in asymptomatic, healthy persons, those with IBS, and persons taking medications that affect GI motility, including calcium channel blockers, oral contraceptives, and H_2RAs. The test should be used when there is a high pretest probability of gallbladder-related symptoms and after other diagnoses have been ruled out. Experts recommend that patients with biliary pain and normal US undergo serum liver biochemical testing, pancreatic enzyme measurement, and upper endoscopy to exclude other causes of the symptoms.[21] If these tests fail to provide an alternative explanation, the patient should be observed for several months to allow the possibility of spontaneous resolution of symptoms before undergoing cholescintigraphy. In patients with atypical symptoms or other functional GI complaints, the treatment of visceral hypersensitivity should be considered (see Chapters 13, 15, 25, and 124).

When cholecystectomy is performed for symptomatic gallstone disease, 30%–40% of patients experience nonbiliary pain postoperatively.[22,23] Patients with functional GI disorders are more likely to experience abdominal pain after cholecystectomy. For individuals with suspected visceral hypersensitivity, preoperative counseling should highlight the possibility of persistent symptoms after surgery. An apparent consequence of the diagnostic uncertainty associated with acalculous biliary pain is a dramatic increase in the rate of cholecystectomy for acalculous biliary pain, particularly in young and insured persons and since the advent of laparoscopic surgery. The rate of cholecystectomy for gallstone disease has declined in the same population.[24]

ACUTE ACALCULOUS CHOLECYSTITIS

Definition

Acute acalculous cholecystitis is acute inflammation of the gallbladder in the absence of stones. Acute cholecystitis resulting from calculi is discussed in Chapter 67. The term *acalculous cholecystitis* may incorrectly suggest that the disease is simply cholecystitis without stones. Instead, the term *necrotizing cholecystitis* has been proposed to reflect the distinct etiology, pathology, and prognosis of the disease but is not widely used.[25]

Epidemiology

Acute acalculous cholecystitis accounts for 5%–10% of cholecystectomies performed in the United States. In fact, of the cholecystectomies performed in postoperative or hospitalized patients recovering from trauma or burns, more than half are for acalculous disease.[26] In one series, acalculous cholecystitis occurred in 0.19% of surgical ICU admissions and accounted for 14% of all cases of acute cholecystitis.[27]

Less commonly, acute acalculous cholecystitis may occur in the absence of antecedent trauma or stress, especially in children,[28] older adult patients with coexisting vascular disease,[29] bone marrow transplant recipients, patients receiving chemotherapy,[30] and patients with AIDS.[31] In some cases, specific infectious causes can be identified, such as *Salmonella* spp.,[32] *Staphylococcus aureus*,[33] CMV, and Zika virus[34] in immunocompromised patients, EBV in children,[28] and possibly as a consequence of SARS-CoV-2 systemic infection.[35] Systemic vasculitides such as polyarteritis nodosa, SLE, Henoch-Schönlein purpura, and eosinophilic granulomatosis with polyangiitis (Churg-Strauss syndrome) may manifest as acute acalculous cholecystitis caused by ischemic injury to the gallbladder.[36] Several cases of acute acalculous cholecystitis have been observed during alemtuzumab therapy for multiple sclerosis.[37] Finally, acute acalculous cholecystitis has been recognized increasingly in otherwise healthy people without any risk factors.[38,39] As a group, patients with acute acalculous cholecystitis are more likely to be older men, in contrast to patients with cholecystitis caused by calculi, cases of which cluster in younger women.[27]

Pathogenesis

Most cases of acute acalculous cholecystitis occur in the setting of prolonged fasting, immobility, and hemodynamic instability. The gallbladder epithelium, although normally a robust tissue, is exposed continuously to one of the most noxious agents in the body: a concentrated solution of bile acid detergents. In the course of a normal day, the gallbladder empties the concentrated bile several times and is replenished with dilute (and presumably less noxious) hepatic bile. With prolonged fasting, the gallbladder is not stimulated by CCK to empty, and concentrated bile stagnates in the gallbladder lumen.[40] In addition, the gallbladder epithelium has relatively high metabolic energy requirements to absorb electrolytes and water from the bile. Therefore, in an immobile, fasting patient with splanchnic vasoconstriction (often resulting from septic shock in a patient in an ICU), ischemic and chemical injury to the gallbladder epithelium may occur.[41] A study that compared the microcirculation of gallbladders removed for gallstone disease with those removed for acute acalculous cholecystitis showed that the capillaries barely filled in gallbladders associated with acalculous cholecystitis, indicating that disturbed microcirculation and ischemia may play an important role in its pathogenesis.[42]

Inappropriate activation of factor XII (demonstrated to initiate gallbladder inflammation in animals)[43] and local release of prostaglandins in the gallbladder wall[44,45] have also been implicated in the tissue injury associated with acalculous cholecystitis. In animal models, tissue destruction can be attenuated by inhibiting prostaglandin synthesis with indomethacin. Expression of tight junction proteins in the gallbladder epithelium of patients with acute acalculous cholecystitis differs from that in patients with calculous cholecystitis, perhaps reflecting the role of increased gallbladder wall permeability in the systemic inflammatory response.[46] Infection of the gallbladder mucosa with bacteria, usually Gram-negative enteric organisms and anaerobes,[47] is thought to be a secondary event in acute acalculous cholecystitis, following rather than causing the initial injury.

One postulated explanation for the rising incidence of acute acalculous cholecystitis, particularly in younger patients, is obesity and the accompanying increase in gallbladder wall fat, which has been demonstrated to interfere with gallbladder emptying in animal models. In one study, 16 patients with acute acalculous cholecystitis had significantly more gallbladder wall fat than normal subjects without cholecystitis.[48]

Clinical Features

The clinical features of acute acalculous cholecystitis often differ from those of acute cholecystitis caused by stone disease. Although RUQ pain, fever, localized tenderness overlying the gallbladder, and leukocytosis may be evident in classic presentations, such as those of younger outpatients, some or all of these features are commonly lacking in older adult postoperative patients.[49] Symptoms or signs referable to the RUQ are initially absent in 75% of cases. Unexplained fever, hypotension, leukocytosis, or hyperamylasemia may be the only warning signs.

Compared with the clinical course of typical calculous cholecystitis, that of acute acalculous cholecystitis is more fulminant. By the time the diagnosis has been made, at least half of the patients have experienced a complication of cholecystitis, such as gangrene or a confined perforation of the gallbladder.[50,51] Empyema of the gallbladder and ascending cholangitis may further complicate cases in which bacterial superinfection of the gallbladder has occurred. Because the disease often occurs in debilitated patients and complications occur rapidly, the mortality rate of acute acalculous cholecystitis is high, ranging from 10% to 50%, as compared with a 1% mortality rate in patients with calculous cholecystitis. Such high mortality rates have led some investigators to propose that empirical cholecystostomy be considered in gravely ill patients in the ICU in whom no source of sepsis can be found.[52]

Diagnosis

The rapid development of complications in acute acalculous cholecystitis makes early diagnosis critical for avoiding excessive mortality. Unfortunately, the lack of specific clinical findings that point to the gallbladder, combined with a confusing clinical picture related to antecedent surgery or trauma, makes early diagnosis difficult. For older adult patients at risk, a high index of suspicion for biliary tract sepsis is the best hope for early recognition and treatment. Table 69.2 delineates several diagnostic criteria for acute acalculous cholecystitis.

TABLE 69.2 Diagnostic Criteria for Acute Acalculous Cholecystitis

Technique	Findings
Clinical evaluation	RUQ tenderness, if present, supports the diagnosis but is lacking in 75% of cases Unexplained fever, hypotension, leukocytosis, or hyperamylasemia is frequently the only finding
US	Thickened gallbladder wall (>4 mm) in the absence of ascites and hypoalbuminemia (serum albumin <3.2 g/dL) Sonographic Murphy's sign (maximum tenderness over the US-localized gallbladder) Pericholecystic fluid collection *Bedside availability is a major advantage*
CT	Thickened gallbladder wall (>4 mm) in the absence of ascites and hypoalbuminemia Pericholecystic fluid, subserosal edema (in the absence of ascites), intramural gas, or sloughed mucosa *The best test for excluding other intra-abdominal diseases but requires moving the patient to a scanner*
Hepatobiliary scintigraphy	Nonvisualization of the gallbladder with normal excretion of radionuclide into the bile duct and duodenum indicates a positive result for acute cholecystitis Results in critically ill, immobilized patients may be falsely positive because of viscous bile *Better at excluding than confirming acute cholecystitis*

US

In the evaluation of patients with suspected acute acalculous cholecystitis, US offers the distinct advantage of being widely available and easily transportable to the bedside.[53] Three US findings indicative of gallbladder disease are a (1) thickened gallbladder wall (defined as >4 mm) in the absence of ascites or hypoalbuminemia, (2) sonographic Murphy's sign (defined as maximum tenderness over the US-localized gallbladder), and (3) pericholecystic fluid collection. A thickened gallbladder wall (Fig. 69.1) is not specific for cholecystitis but in the proper clinical setting is suggestive of gallbladder involvement and should prompt further evaluation. A sonographic Murphy's sign is operator dependent and requires a cooperative patient but, when present, is a reliable indicator of gallbladder inflammation.[54] A pericholecystic fluid collection indicates advanced disease. Sensitivity rates of US for detecting acute acalculous cholecystitis have been reported to range from 67% to 92%, with a specificity of more than 90%.[53]

Investigators have proposed a US scoring system to improve the diagnostic accuracy of US in critically ill patients.[55] Two points are given for distention of the gallbladder or thickening of the gallbladder wall, and one point each is given for "striated" thickening (alternating hypoechoic and hyperechoic layers) of the gallbladder wall, sludge, and pericholecystic fluid. Scores of 6 or higher accurately predict acalculous cholecystitis.

One group evaluated the routine use of US for early detection of acalculous cholecystitis in the ICU. In a group of 53 mechanically ventilated patients, three men were diagnosed with acute acalculous cholecystitis by US findings and clinical features; however, gallbladder abnormalities were also detected in 30% of patients without acalculous cholecystitis. US should be performed in patients with a high pretest probability of acute acalculous cholecystitis.[56]

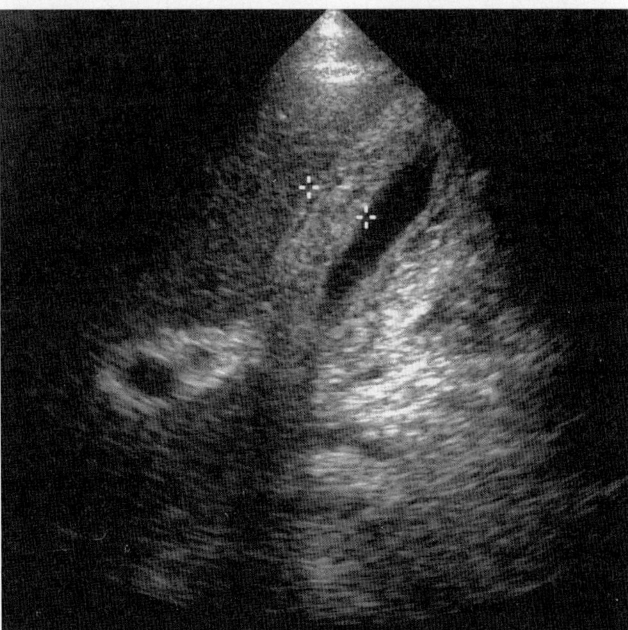

Fig. 69.1 US demonstrating thickening of the gallbladder wall to 17 mm (*denoted by asterisks*) characteristic of acute acalculous cholecystitis. Point tenderness was noted when the transducer was pressed onto the abdomen over the gallbladder (sonographic Murphy's sign). The diagnosis was confirmed at surgery. (Courtesy David Hurst, MD, Dallas, TX.)

CT

CT findings suggestive of cholecystitis are similar to US findings and include gallbladder wall thickening (>4 mm), pericholecystic fluid, subserosal edema (in the absence of ascites), intramural gas, and sloughed gallbladder mucosa. The sensitivity and specificity of these findings for predicting acute acalculous cholecystitis at surgery exceed 95%. CT is also superior to US in detecting other intra-abdominal sources of fever, hypotension, or abdominal pain.[57] An obvious disadvantage of CT is that it cannot be performed at the bedside, as is necessary in many critically ill patients. Several investigators have emphasized that CT is complementary to US and may detect gallbladder disease in high-risk patients with normal US findings.

Hepatobiliary Scintigraphy

Hepatobiliary scintigraphy may be useful for excluding cystic duct obstruction in patients with clinical features suggestive of acute cholecystitis. Under normal conditions, IV-administered radionuclide is taken up by the liver, secreted into bile, concentrated in the gallbladder (where it produces a "hot spot" on a scan), and emptied into the duodenum. A positive scan result for cystic duct obstruction is defined as failure of filling of the gallbladder despite the normal passage of radionuclide into the duodenum. In suspected calculous cholecystitis, the pathogenesis of which involves obstruction of the cystic duct by a stone, filling of the gallbladder on scintigraphy virtually excludes cholecystitis as the cause of the patient's symptoms.[58]

Hepatobiliary scintigraphy is less precise in acute acalculous cholecystitis. Gallbladder and cystic wall edema can cause an obstructive picture similar to that of calculous cholecystitis on scintigraphy. Patients with acute acalculous cholecystitis have often fasted for prolonged periods, a state that can result in concentrated, viscous bile that flows poorly through the cystic duct and causes a false-positive hepatobiliary scan result. Most patients with acute acalculous cholecystitis (in contrast to those with calculi) do not have an obstructed cystic duct; hence, hepatobiliary scans can be falsely negative as well.[59] The sensitivity of the test may exceed 90%, but the lack of specificity in fasted, critically ill patients limits the usefulness of the test primarily to excluding acute acalculous cholecystitis rather than confirming the diagnosis. A study in which US and cholescintigraphy were performed in critically ill patients found cholescintigraphy to be useful for the early diagnosis of acute acalculous cholecystitis, whereas US alone did not permit an early decision regarding the need for surgery.[60]

In an effort to improve the accuracy of biliary scintigraphy, investigators have proposed the use of *morphine-augmented cholescintigraphy*, in which morphine sulfate is administered IV (0.05–0.1 mg/kg) to increase resistance to the flow of bile through the sphincter of Oddi and, hence, "force fill" the gallbladder if the cystic duct is patent to reduce the likelihood of a false-positive result.[61] Although this test may exclude cholecystitis as a cause of sepsis, it is difficult to perform in critically ill patients.

Treatment

In light of the rapid progression of acute acalculous cholecystitis to gangrene and perforation, early recognition and intervention are required. Supportive medical care should include the restoration of hemodynamic stability as well as antibiotic coverage for Gram-negative enteric organisms and anaerobes if biliary tract infection is suspected.

Surgical Cholecystectomy and Cholecystostomy

In the past, the definitive therapeutic approach to acute acalculous cholecystitis was emergency laparotomy and cholecystectomy (see Chapter 68). Subsequently, laparoscopic cholecystectomy became the standard surgical approach. More recently, radiographically guided percutaneous cholecystostomy or endoscopic gallbladder drainage has been used more frequently because patients are often too unstable to tolerate surgery.[62,63] If necessary, definitive cholecystectomy can be undertaken after cholecystostomy when the patient is stable. In one retrospective study, the long-term outcome of acute acalculous cholecystitis treated by nonsurgical management was similar to that for cholecystectomy, with a higher incidence of posttreatment complications in the surgical group.[64]

Percutaneous Cholecystostomy

Several investigators have reported favorable results with the US-guided percutaneous transhepatic placement of a cholecystostomy drainage tube, coupled with IV administration of antibiotics, as definitive therapy in patients in whom surgery poses a high risk.[52,65,66] This approach controls acute acalculous cholecystitis in 85%–90% of patients and has a complication rate of approximately 10%. The short-term mortality rate of patients undergoing cholecystostomy is high but reflects the high mortality of the underlying disease rather than that of the procedure. Most patients with acute acalculous cholecystitis can be treated with percutaneous drainage; if the postdrainage cholangiogram is normal, the catheter can be removed, and subsequent cholecystectomy is unlikely to be necessary.[65,66] This is the preferred approach for an unstable or critically ill patient in the ICU.

Transpapillary or Transmural Endoscopic Cholecystostomy

Some critically ill patients with suspected acute acalculous cholecystitis are poor candidates for US-guided percutaneous cholecystostomy, typically because of ascites or uncorrectable coagulopathy. Such patients may benefit from an endoscopic approach in which the cystic duct is selectively cannulated during ERCP with an obliquely angled guidewire that tracks along the lateral wall of the bile duct and facilitates cannulation of the cystic duct. If the wire can negotiate the spiral valves within the cystic duct successfully, a pigtail stent is deployed in the gallbladder, and the other end is brought out through a nasobiliary catheter or left to drain internally into the duodenum (a "double-pigtailed" stent).[67] The risk of bleeding is low if a sphincterotomy is not performed. Because the gallbladder is in close proximity to the GI tract, EUS-guided transmural placement of a covered, self-expandable, lumen-apposing metal stent is also used as a treatment for acalculous cholecystitis, with reported success rates of 97%.[68] This approach is used most often in patients with advanced liver disease and ascites; it may be associated with less pain than a percutaneous procedure.

Successful intubation of the gallbladder via ERCP can be achieved in 90% of attempts, and drainage and lavage of the viscous black bile and sludge from the gallbladder result in clinical resolution in most of these critically ill patients. The endoscopic techniques may be more cumbersome and expensive than US-guided placement of a cholecystostomy tube and should be reserved for patients who would not tolerate a percutaneous approach or who have coagulopathy.[69]

CHOLESTEROLOSIS

Definition

Cholesterolosis is an acquired histologic abnormality of the gallbladder epithelium characterized by excessive accumulation of cholesteryl esters and TG within epithelial macrophages (Fig. 69.2).[70] Clinicians generally encounter the lesion only as an incidental pathologic finding after surgical resection of the

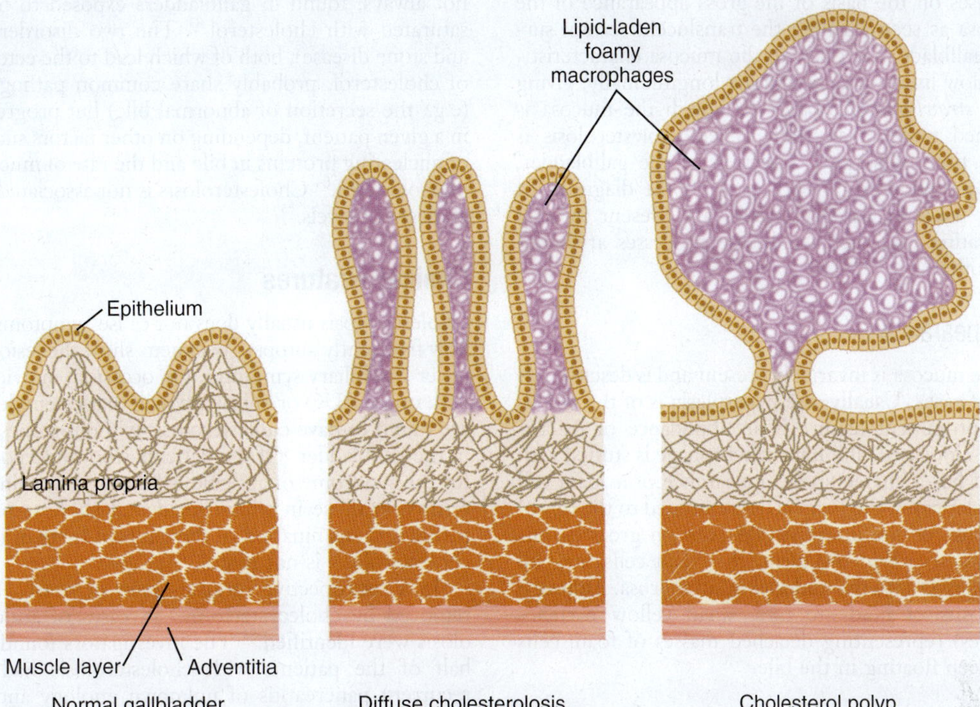

Fig. 69.2 Schematic representation of a normal gallbladder, diffuse cholesterolosis, and a cholesterol polyp. Note the distribution of lipid-laden foamy macrophages in cholesterolosis and the cholesterol polyp. The diffuse form of cholesterolosis (*center*; see also Fig. 69.3) accounts for 80% of cases and generally causes no symptoms. Cholesterol polyps (*right*), present in 10% of cases of cholesterolosis, are typically small, fragile excrescences that have a tendency to ulcerate or detach spontaneously from the mucosa. Combined diffuse cholesterolosis and cholesterol polyps account for 10% of cases. Although usually asymptomatic, these polyps have been associated with biliary pain and even acute pancreatitis.

gallbladder, although the diagnosis may be suspected in certain patients before surgery.

Cholesterolosis, as well as adenomyomatosis of the gallbladder (see later), has been classified as one of the "hyperplastic cholecystoses," a term introduced in 1960 to describe several diseases of the gallbladder thought to share the common features of mucosal hyperplasia, hyperconcentration and hyperexcretion of dye on cholecystography, and absence of inflammation.[71] The proponents of this concept believed that biliary pain, in the absence of gallstones, could be explained by the presence of one of the hyperplastic cholecystoses. However, because of the lack of a common etiology and the nonspecificity of the clinical features, the term hyperplastic cholecystoses should be abandoned.

Epidemiology

Depending on whether gross or microscopic criteria are used for diagnosis, the frequency of cholesterolosis in autopsy specimens has ranged from 5% to 40%. A large autopsy series involving more than 1300 cases in which each gallbladder was examined microscopically found the frequency of cholesterolosis to be 12%.[72] When surgically resected gallbladders were examined, the frequency was, not surprisingly, about 50% higher (18%) than that found in autopsy material.[73,74] The incidence of cholesterolosis has not been calculated because its onset is rarely known.

The epidemiology of cholesterolosis is analogous to that of cholesterol gallstone disease,[75] in that similar groups of persons are predisposed; however, the two lesions occur independently and do not necessarily coexist in the same person. Like gallstone disease, cholesterolosis is uncommon in children and shows a marked predilection for women until the age of 60 years. After that, the gender differences are less pronounced. No racial, ethnic, or geographic differences in prevalence have been described, although if the analogy with cholesterol gallstone disease is extended, the prevalence would be expected to be higher in Western than non-Western societies. Obesity also appears to be a risk factor for cholesterolosis; a frequency of 38% has been observed in gallbladders resected during weight loss surgery.[76]

Pathology

Cholesterolosis is defined pathologically by the accumulation of lipid (cholesteryl esters and TG) within the gallbladder mucosa. The four patterns of lipid deposition are as follows[70]:

Diffuse: The lipid is distributed throughout the epithelial lining of the gallbladder and ends abruptly at the cystic duct. This pattern accounts for 80% of all cases.

Cholesterol polyps: The excess lipid is confined to one or more areas of the epithelium that eventually form excrescences into the lumen of the gallbladder. Isolated cholesterol polyps in the absence of diffuse cholesterolosis account for about 10% of the total cases.

Combined diffuse cholesterolosis and cholesterol polyps: Cholesterol polyps occur on a background of diffuse cholesterolosis. This pattern accounts for about 10% of cases.

Focal cholesterolosis: Excess lipid deposition is limited to a small area of the mucosa.

Gross Appearance

When the gallbladder is inspected visually at the time of laparotomy or laparoscopy, a diagnosis of cholesterolosis can be made in 20% of the cases on the basis of the gross appearance of the gallbladder mucosa as seen through the translucent serosal surface. When the gallbladder is opened, the mucosa characteristically has pale, yellow linear streaks running longitudinally, giving rise to the term *strawberry gallbladder* (although the mucosa is usually bile stained rather than red). When cholesterolosis is diagnosed at the time of surgical resection of the gallbladder, gallstones are also present in 50% of cases. If the diagnosis of cholesterolosis is made at autopsy, stones are present in only 10%,[72] demonstrating that the two disease processes are independent of each other.

Microscopic Appearance

Hyperplasia of the mucosa is invariably present and is described as marked in 50% of cases. Usually, the hyperplasia is of the villous type. The most prominent feature is an abundance of macrophages within the elongated villi. Each macrophage is stuffed with lipid droplets and has a characteristic appearance of a foam cell (Fig. 69.3). In milder cases, the foam cells are limited to the tips of the villi (accounting for the linear streaks seen on gross examination); with more severe involvement, the foam cells may fill entire villi and spill over into the underlying submucosa. Although extracellular deposits of lipid are rare, small yellow particles (lipoidic corpuscles) representing detached masses of foam cells are occasionally seen floating in the bile.

Pathogenesis

The cause of the accumulation of cholesteryl esters and TG in cholesterolosis remains obscure.[77] Postulated mechanisms are that the cholesterol is derived from the blood[78] or that mechanical factors that impede emptying of the gallbladder lead to local deposition of lipid.[79] Data have shown unequivocally that the gallbladder epithelium is capable of absorbing cholesterol from the bile, as might be expected in epithelium that is embryologically and histologically similar to intestinal absorptive cells.[80,81] Moreover, the cholesterol in gallbladder bile is already in the ideal physical state for absorption (i.e., a mixed micelle). The question remains as to why, in some patients, resorbed biliary cholesterol is esterified and then stored in foamy macrophages as cholesterolosis.[82] Like cholesterol stones, cholesterolosis is frequently, but not always, found in gallbladders exposed to bile that is supersaturated with cholesterol.[83] The two disorders (cholesterolosis and stone disease), both of which lead to the ectopic accumulation of cholesterol, probably share common pathogenic mechanisms (e.g., the secretion of abnormal bile) but progress independently in a given patient, depending on other factors such as the presence of nucleating proteins in bile and the rate of mucosal esterification of cholesterol.[84] Cholesterolosis is not associated with high serum cholesterol levels.[75]

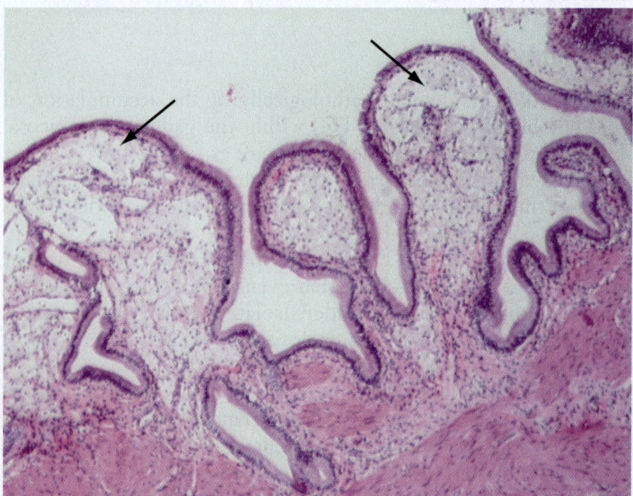

Fig. 69.3 Histopathology of diffuse cholesterolosis. Note the hyperplastic, elongated villi, and the foamy macrophages (*arrows*) (H&E). (Courtesy Pamela Jensen, MD, Dallas, TX.)

Clinical Features

Cholesterolosis usually does not cause symptoms, as is evident by how frequently autopsy specimens show the lesion in patients who never had biliary symptoms. On occasion, individual patients have dull, vague RUQ or epigastric pain that resembles biliary pain and are found to have cholesterolosis without stones or inflammation in the gallbladder. Of the patients who undergo cholecystectomy for the syndrome of acalculous biliary pain, pain is more likely to resolve in those in whom incidental cholesterolosis is found on pathologic examination of the gallbladder than in those in whom cholesterolosis is not found.[9]

In a retrospective surgical series of nearly 4000 gallbladders removed by cholecystectomy, 55 cases of acalculous cholesterolosis were identified.[85] The investigators found that nearly one-half of the patients with cholesterolosis had presented with recurrent pancreatitis of unknown etiology and speculated that small cholesterol polyps had detached from the gallbladder wall and transiently obstructed the sphincter of Oddi, thereby provoking the acute pancreatitis. In 5 years of postoperative follow-up, pancreatitis did not recur. These investigators[85] and others[86,87] have suggested that cholesterolosis (or, more specifically, cholesterol polyps) should be considered in the differential diagnosis of idiopathic pancreatitis. A retrospective review of 6868 patients who underwent cholecystectomy, of whom 18% (1053) had cholesterolosis, has challenged this theory: when patients with gallstones were excluded from this population, not a single patient had experienced pancreatitis.[73]

Diagnosis

Diffuse cholesterolosis (which, as noted earlier, constitutes 80% of cases) is only rarely detectable by either US or oral cholecystography. In the polypoid form, however, polyps of sufficient size have a characteristic appearance on US as single or multiple, nonshadowing, fixed echoes that project into the lumen of the gallbladder.[88] Most of the polyps are small (2–10 mm). The polyps can be identified accurately as cholesterolosis polyps by EUS, which demonstrates a characteristic aggregation of hyperechoic spots.[89] On oral cholecystography, the polyps appear as small, round radiolucencies in the lumen of the opacified gallbladder and are best demonstrated after the gallbladder has emptied partially and abdominal compression has been applied.

Treatment

Because cholesterolosis is only rarely diagnosed before resection of the gallbladder, treatment is usually not a consideration. In the rare case of polypoid cholesterolosis diagnosed on US or cholecystography, the absence of biliary tract symptoms argues against any intervention. If the patient has symptoms consistent with biliary pain or pancreatitis, a cholecystectomy is indicated.[85] Symptom resolution following cholecystectomy may be higher for those with cholesterolosis as compared to chronic cholecystitis on histologic evaluation.[9] There is no medical therapy for cholesterolosis.

ADENOMYOMATOSIS

Definition

Adenomyomatosis (an unwieldy term that obscures its meaning) of the gallbladder is an acquired, hyperplastic lesion characterized by an excessive proliferation of surface epithelium with invaginations into the thickened muscularis or even more deeply.[90] The literature on this condition is complicated by the use of a number of different terms to describe the same lesion, the most common of which are adenomyoma (used when the lesion is localized to the gallbladder fundus), Rokitansky-Aschoff sinuses (familiar but anatomically incorrect), and adenomyosis.[91] Despite the prefix *adeno-*, the lesion is generally benign and unrelated to adenomatous epithelia elsewhere in the GI tract. Simple adenomyomatosis is not thought to have the potential for malignant transformation.

Epidemiology

The prevalence of adenomyomatosis of the gallbladder varies greatly according to the criteria used for diagnosis and whether resected gallbladders or autopsy specimens are examined. In a large series of more than 10,000 cholecystectomy specimens, Shepard and associates[92] found only 103 cases of adenomyomatosis, for a frequency of about 1%. The lesion is more common in women than men by a 3:1 ratio, and the prevalence rises with age. Neither ethnic nor geographic differences in prevalence have been described.

Pathology

A review of the normal histologic architecture of the gallbladder and Rokitansky-Aschoff sinuses is useful for understanding the pathology of adenomyomatosis (Fig. 69.4). Unlike the small intestine, the gallbladder has no muscularis mucosa, and the lamina propria abuts directly on the muscular layer. In childhood, the epithelial layer is cast up into folds and supported by the lamina propria. As the gallbladder ages, the valleys of the epithelial layer may deepen so that they penetrate into the muscular layer and form Rokitansky-Aschoff sinuses. These sinuses are acquired lesions present in about 90% of resected gallbladders. If Rokitansky-Aschoff sinuses are deep and branching and are accompanied by thickening (hypertrophy) of the muscular layer, a diagnosis of adenomyomatosis can be made.[90] Rupture of Rokitansky-Aschoff sinuses is thought to underlie the rare entity *xanthogranulomatous cholecystitis*, in which the gallbladder is involved in an inflammatory process with lipid-laden macrophages (see Chapter 67).

Gross Appearance

Adenomyomatosis may involve the entire gallbladder (diffuse or generalized adenomyomatosis) or, more commonly, may be localized to the gallbladder fundus, in which case the lesion is often termed *adenomyoma*. On rare occasions, the process may be limited to an annular segment of the gallbladder wall (segmental adenomyomatosis) and may give rise to luminal narrowing and a "dumbbell-shaped" gallbladder (Fig. 69.5). In any case, the involved portion of the gallbladder wall is thickened to 10 mm or more, and the muscle layer is three to five times its normal thickness. On cut sections, cystic dilatations of the Rokitansky-Aschoff sinuses are evident and may be filled with pigmented debris or calculi.

Microscopic Appearance

Hyperplasia of the muscle layer is invariably present, and the epithelial lining occasionally undergoes intestinal metaplasia. Mild chronic inflammation is often present.

Pathogenesis

The pathogenesis of adenomyomatosis is unknown. Increased intraluminal pressure in the gallbladder from mechanical obstruction (e.g., an obstructing calculus, kink in the cystic duct, and congenital septum) has been postulated to result in cystic dilatation of the Rokitansky-Aschoff sinuses, subsequent hyperplasia of the muscle layer, and adenomyomatosis.[90] Like pressure-related colonic diverticula, Rokitansky-Aschoff sinuses are most likely to be found where the muscle layer is weakest (at the site of a penetrating blood vessel). Nevertheless, evidence of outflow

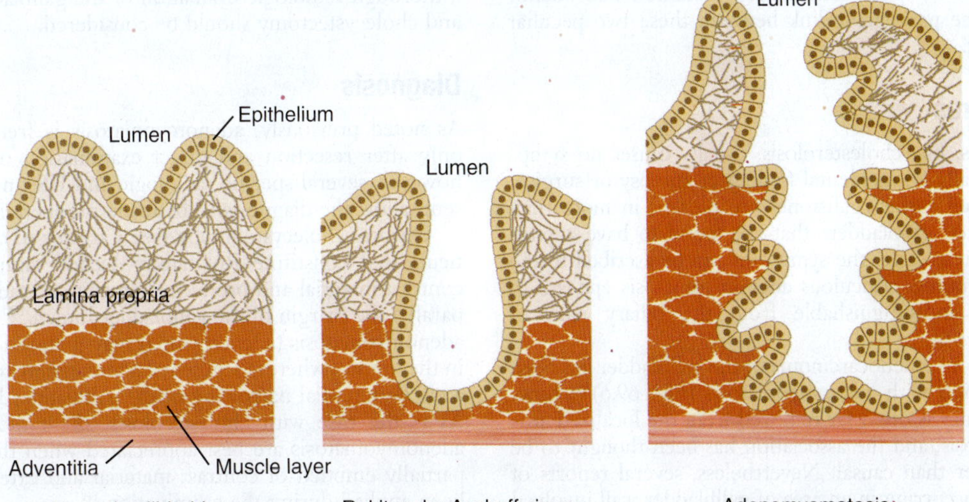

Fig. 69.4 Schematic representation of a normal gallbladder, a Rokitansky-Aschoff sinus, and adenomyomatosis. Rokitansky-Aschoff sinuses, which are present in about 90% of resected gallbladders, consist of invaginations of the epithelium into the muscle layer to produce tiny intramural diverticula. By themselves, they have no clinical significance. A histologic diagnosis of adenomyomatosis requires that the Rokitansky-Aschoff sinuses be deep, branching, and accompanied by hypertrophy of the muscle layer.

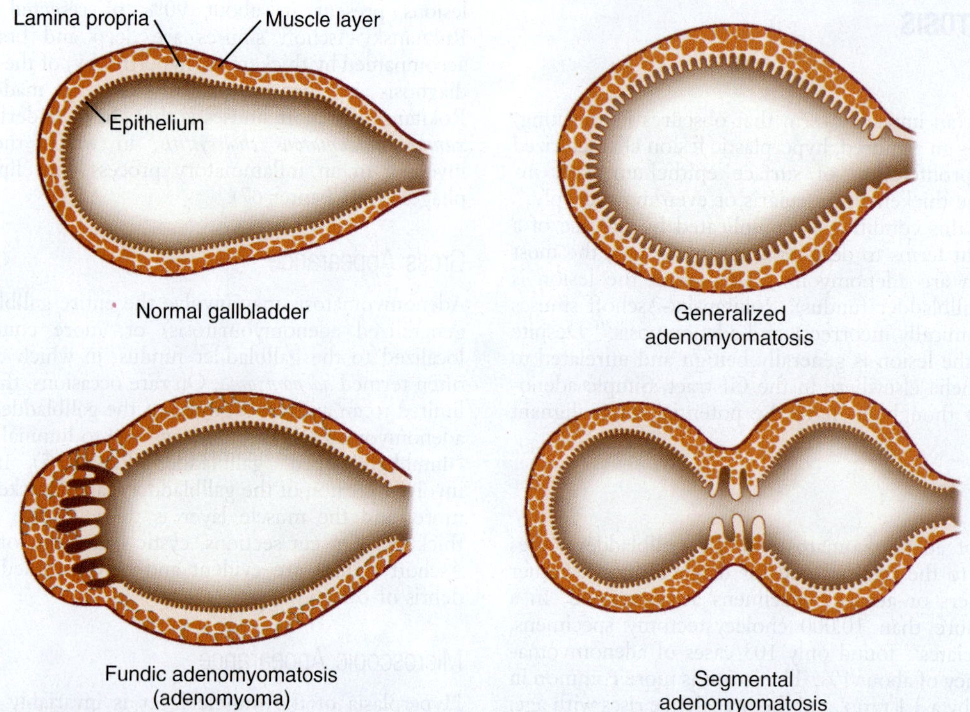

Fig. 69.5 Schematic representation showing the different patterns of adenomyomatosis. Most of the cases are localized to the fundus of the gallbladder (in which case the lesion is termed an *adenomyoma*); generalized and segmental patterns are much less common. An adenomyoma is usually 10–20 mm in diameter and may be largely confined to the wall or may project into the lumen to produce a polypoid lesion.

obstruction of the gallbladder is not always found; for example, calculi are present in only about 60% of cases of adenomyomatosis.[91] Some investigators have proposed that adenomyomatosis is a consequence of chronic inflammation,[92] but inflammation is not always present, particularly when the lesion is localized to the fundus.[93] Finally, several investigators have noted an association between adenomyomatosis and pancreaticobiliary malunion (anomalous pancreaticobiliary ductal union) (see Chapters 57 and 64). In one study, one-half of the patients with adenomyomatosis had pancreaticobiliary malunion,[94] and in another study, one-third of patients with pancreaticobiliary malunion had adenomyomatosis.[95] The pathogenic link between these two peculiar entities is unclear.

Clinical Features

Adenomyomatosis, like cholesterolosis, usually causes no symptoms and is typically an incidental finding at autopsy or surgical resection. As noted earlier, gallstones are present in more than half of the resected gallbladders that are found to have adenomyomatosis; in these cases, the symptoms can be ascribed to the stones.[91] Uncommonly, acalculous adenomyomatosis appears to cause symptoms indistinguishable from the biliary pain of cholelithiasis.

On rare occasions, adenocarcinoma of the gallbladder has been found in association with adenomyomatosis (Fig. 69.6)[96]; however, the malignancy is often far removed from the localized area of adenomyomatosis, and the association has been thought to be coincidental rather than causal. Nevertheless, several reports of adenocarcinoma occurring in an area of gallbladder wall involved with adenomyomatosis have created diagnostic uncertainty on US or cholecystography.[97] A retrospective review of more than 3000 resected gallbladders revealed a significantly higher frequency (6.4%) of gallbladder cancer in gallbladders with the segmental form of adenomyomatosis than would have been expected by chance alone. The investigators proposed that segmental adenomyomatosis should be considered a potentially premalignant lesion.[98] A second review of gallbladder cancers associated with segmental adenomyomatosis revealed a spectrum of cytologic atypia in the specimens ranging from hyperplastic to malignant epithelium, suggestive of neoplastic progression.[99]

When simple adenomyomatosis of the gallbladder is discovered incidentally, the lesion is likely to be benign. If there is any suspicion of an associated mass lesion, particularly one greater than 10 mm, or if segmental adenomyomatosis is found, however, a thorough radiologic evaluation of the gallbladder is warranted, and cholecystectomy should be considered.

Diagnosis

As noted previously, adenomyomatosis is frequently diagnosed only after resection and direct examination of the gallbladder; however, several specific radiologic and US findings may, if present, allow the diagnosis to be made preoperatively.

On oral cholecystography (see Chapter 67), the mural diverticula that constitute Rokitansky-Aschoff sinuses may fill with contrast material and produce characteristic radiopaque dots that parallel the margin of the gallbladder lumen.[100] Localized, fundal adenomyomatosis (adenomyoma) may manifest as a filling defect in the fundus, whereas segmental adenomyomatosis may appear as a circumferential narrowing of the gallbladder lumen (Fig. 69.7). As is the case with cholesterolosis, the radiologic findings in adenomyomatosis are best appreciated when the gallbladder has partially emptied of contrast material and external pressure has been applied during the examination.[100]

Although US has largely replaced oral cholecystography in the evaluation of the gallbladder, the US findings in adenomyomatosis are less specific. A thickened gallbladder wall (>4 mm) is not specific for adenomyomatosis and can also be seen in many other conditions such as liver disease with ascites.[101] Carefully performed

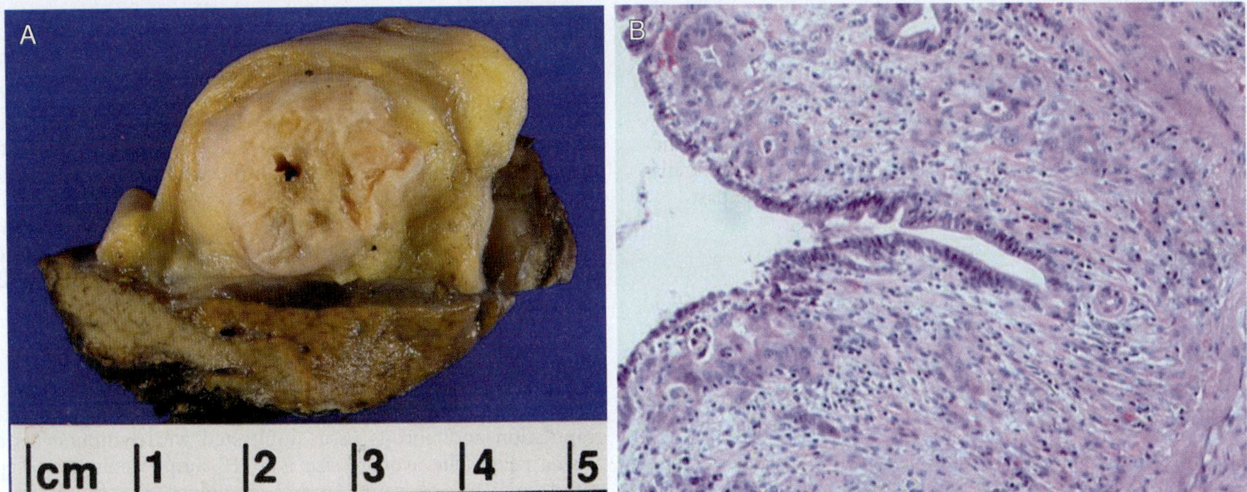

Fig. 69.6 Adenocarcinoma of the gallbladder associated with adenomyoma. (A) Gross pathologic appearance of a gallbladder adenomyoma involved by adenocarcinoma. (B) Histopathology shows a moderately differentiated adenocarcinoma of the gallbladder undermining the mucosa of the adenomyoma (H&E). (Courtesy Aviva Hopkowitz, MD, Dallas, TX.)

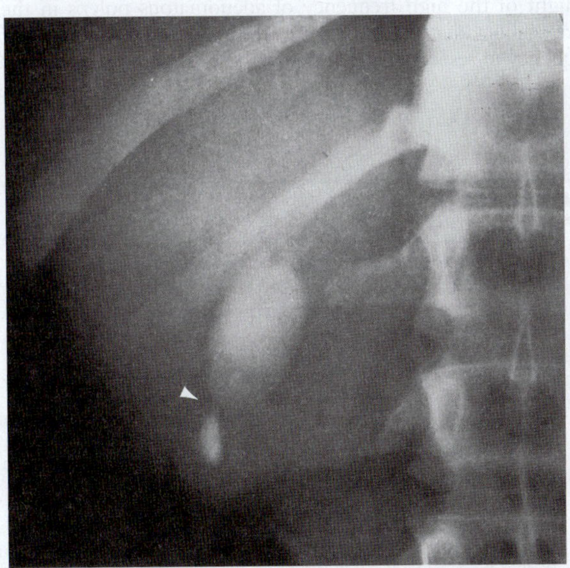

Fig 69.7 Oral cholecystogram showing segmental adenomyomatosis in a 28-year-old man with postprandial epigastric pain radiating through to the back. The film demonstrates an annular segment of the gallbladder wall (*arrowhead*) involved with adenomyomatosis, which has produced a constriction of the lumen. Although no gallstones were present, a cholecystectomy was performed, and the patient's symptoms were relieved. (Courtesy W. J. Kilman, MD, Dallas, TX.)

studies in which radiologic and US findings of adenomyomatosis were correlated with pathologic findings have shown that diffuse or segmental thickening of the gallbladder wall in association with intramural diverticula (seen as round anechoic foci) accurately predicts adenomyomatosis.[102] If the intramural diverticula (dilated Rokitansky-Aschoff sinuses) are filled with sludge or small calculi, the lesions may appear echogenic with acoustic shadowing or a reverberation artifact.[103] Contrast-enhanced US has greater sensitivity for characterizing adenomyomatosis.[104] The presence of intramural cystic spaces on high-resolution US has a high accuracy for differentiating adenomyomatosis from gallbladder cancer.[105] Similarly, EUS may demonstrate the characteristic finding of multiple microcysts, corresponding to the proliferated Rokitansky-Aschoff sinuses.[89] CT and MRI findings in adenomyomatosis include differential enhancement of gallbladder wall layers,[106] detection of Rokitansky-Aschoff sinuses within a thickened gallbladder wall,[107] and subserosal fatty proliferation.[108] In a study of 20 patients with surgically proved adenomyomatosis who underwent preoperative US, helical CT, and MRI, the diagnostic accuracies of the three modalities were 66%, 75%, and 93%, respectively.[109] In patients in whom the diagnosis is uncertain, MRI is the most accurate modality for differentiating adenomyomatosis from a malignant gallbladder lesion.[110] In one case report, an adenomyoma without histologic evidence of cancer was the cause of a false-positive finding on 18-fluorodeoxyglucose PET, likely because of the associated inflammatory activity.[111]

Treatment

In the absence of biliary tract symptoms, adenomyomatosis requires no treatment. If the patient has biliary pain and radiographic or US evidence of adenomyomatosis with calculi, a cholecystectomy is indicated. A more difficult clinical problem arises when a patient is symptomatic and has suspected adenomyomatosis but no stones.[97] In such cases, the more extensive or severe the adenomyomatosis appears to be, the more likely that the symptoms are related to the lesion and that the patient will benefit from cholecystectomy. Fear of malignant transformation is not a reason to operate, unless imaging suggests a possible mass or perhaps shows the segmental form of adenomyomatosis.

GALLBLADDER POLYPS

Definition

The term *polyp of the gallbladder* is used to describe any mucosal projection into the lumen of the gallbladder.[112] The vast majority of gallbladder polyps are the result of lipid deposits or inflammation, rather than a neoplasm. Because the nature of a polyp cannot be defined without histologic evaluation, however, clinicians must decide whether concern about malignancy is sufficient to recommend cholecystectomy based on indirect information such as the imaging appearance of the polyp, patient demographics, and symptoms.

Epidemiology

The frequency of gallbladder polyps defined either pathologically or radiologically[113] ranges from 1% to 4% but may be as high as 5%–10% in some populations. Often, a gallbladder polyp is an incidental finding at the time of cholecystectomy. With the increasing use of imaging in clinical practice, incidental gallbladder polyps are detected more frequently than in the past.

Pathology

Polyps of the gallbladder may be classified as shown in Table 69.3 as either nonneoplastic (95% of all gallbladder polyps) or neoplastic.[114]

Cholesterol Polyps

Cholesterol polyps are the most common type of gallbladder polyp. They are variants of cholesterolosis that result from infiltration of the lamina propria with lipid-laden foamy macrophages. The pathogenesis of cholesterol polyps is discussed in the section on cholesterolosis (see earlier). Cholesterol polyps are typically small (<10 mm in diameter), pedunculated polyps that are attached to the mucosa by a thin, fragile stalk.[114] Frequently, detached tiny cholesterol polyps are found floating in the bile when the gallbladder is opened after cholecystectomy.[115] Although they may be solitary in 20% of cases, the mean number of cholesterol polyps present in one series was 8.[116] A multiplicity of polyps generally indicates cholesterol polyps and predicts benignity.

Adenomyomas

Adenomyomatosis of the gallbladder localized to the fundus may produce a hemispheric projection into the lumen that resembles a polyp. Such a lesion has come to be known as an *adenomyoma*, although it is not neoplastic in origin. The pathogenesis of an adenomyoma is discussed in the section on adenomyomatosis (see earlier). The lesion is usually approximately 15 mm in size, and its bulk is confined to the muscular wall of the gallbladder.[114]

Inflammatory Polyps

Inflammatory polyps are small sessile lesions that consist of granulation and fibrous tissue infiltrated with lymphocytes and plasma cells. The average size is 5–10 mm. A solitary polyp is found in 50% of cases, and 2–5 polyps are found in the remainder.[114] When discovered at the time of cholecystectomy, an inflammatory polyp is almost always an incidental finding.

Adenomas

In light of the high frequency of adenomatous polyps in the GI tract, gallbladder adenomas are surprisingly uncommon. Their frequency in resected gallbladder specimens is only about 0.15%.[117]

TABLE 69.3 Types of Gallbladder Polyps

Histologic Type	Relative Frequency (%)	Neoplastic	Size Range (mm)	Number of Polyps	Comments
Cholesterol polyp (a polypoid form of cholesterolosis)	60	No	2–10	Multiple (average of 8)	May detach and behave clinically as a stone; may cause biliary pain, bile duct obstruction, or pancreatitis Surgery is not required unless the patient is symptomatic
Adenomyoma (a localized form of adenomyomatosis)	25	No	10–20	1	Always localized to the gallbladder fundus Forms a hemispheric projection into the lumen with the bulk confined to the muscular wall Surgery is not required unless the patient is symptomatic or a neoplasm cannot be excluded
Inflammatory polyp	10	No	5–10	1 in half of cases; 2–5 in the remainder	Consists of granulation tissue and fibrous tissue with lymphocytes and plasma cells that infiltrate the lamina propria Surgery is not required
Adenoma	4	Yes	5–20	1 in two-thirds of cases; 2–5 in the remainder	A rare lesion, found in only 0.15% of resected gallbladders Usually is pedunculated and coexists with stones in one-half of cases The only polyp in the gallbladder with a premalignant potential; the frequency of progression from adenoma to carcinoma is much lower than that for colon polyps Virtually all adenomas with a focus of carcinoma are >12 mm in diameter; lesions <10 mm may generally be monitored with US For lesions 10–18 mm in size, laparoscopic cholecystectomy should be considered in good surgical candidates For lesions >18 mm in size, open rather than laparoscopic cholecystectomy should be considered because invasive cancer is more likely and extended resection may be required
Miscellaneous neoplasms	<1	Yes	5–20	1	Extremely rare lesions (see text), with frequencies of <0.10% of polyps

Adenomas are typically solitary, pedunculated masses from 5 to 20 mm in diameter. They may occur anywhere in the gallbladder. When multiple, as they are in approximately one-third of cases, 2–5 polyps are usually present. Histologically, they are classified as either papillary or nonpapillary. The former type consists of a branching, tree-like skeleton of connective tissue covered with tall columnar cells, whereas the latter consists of a proliferation of glands encased by a fibrous stroma. On rare occasions, the entire gallbladder mucosa may undergo adenomatous transformation that results in innumerable tiny mucosal polyps termed *multicentric papillomatosis*. Notably, gallstones are present in half of cases of adenomatous polyps.[114]

Unlike the colon, in which adenomas are much more common than adenocarcinomas, the gallbladder is affected less commonly by adenomas than by carcinomas (by a 1:4 ratio). The frequency of progression from adenoma to adenocarcinoma is not well defined. In a series of more than 1600 consecutive cholecystectomies from Japan, 18 of the operated patients were found to have gallbladder adenomas.[118] Seven of the adenomas contained foci of carcinoma. In the same series, 79 cases of invasive carcinoma were found; 15 (19%) of the lesions were thought to have residual adenomatous tissue within the cancer, suggesting that the initial lesion may have been an adenoma. Notably, all the adenomas that contained foci of carcinoma were larger than 12 mm—a finding that suggests that large adenomas may represent premalignant lesions.

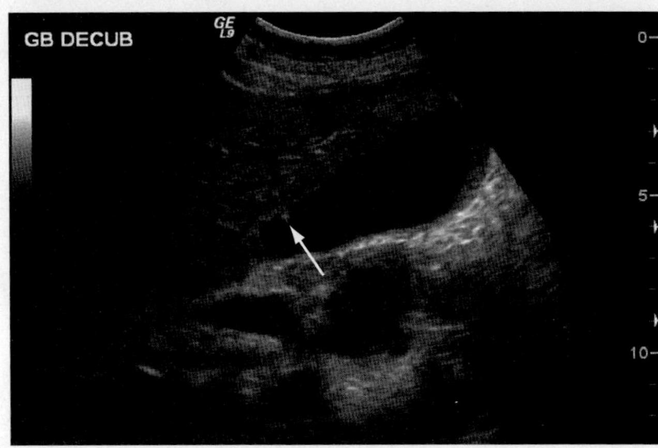

Fig. 69.8 US (*right longitudinal view*) showing a gallbladder polyp in a 55-year-old woman with mild biliary pain. A 4-mm luminal filling defect is demonstrated (*arrow*). It does not cast an acoustic shadow and is fixed to the gallbladder wall. The findings are consistent with a gallbladder polyp, although the histology cannot be predicted from the ultrasonogram. A cholecystectomy demonstrated multiple cholesterol polyps, one of which was unusually large. (Courtesy R. S. Harrell, MD, Dallas, TX.)

Miscellaneous Polyps

Although a wide variety of benign lesions may manifest as polyps in the gallbladder, these lesions are rare. Fibromas, leiomyomas, and lipomas of the gallbladder are extraordinarily rare, particularly considering how commonly they are found elsewhere in the GI tract. Neurofibromas, carcinoids,[119] and heterotropic gastric glands occur even less frequently.[120] Taken together, the combined frequency of nonadenomatous neoplastic polyps of the gallbladder is considerably less than 1 per 1000 resected specimens.[114]

Clinical Features and Diagnosis

Polyps of the gallbladder typically do not cause symptoms. They are often noted as an incidental finding during cholecystectomy for gallstones or by imaging studies performed for other indications. In the exceptional case in which a polyp (without gallstones) is identified radiographically because of symptoms, the clinical symptomatology may resemble that of biliary pain, although classic features (e.g., intense epigastric or RUQ pain starting suddenly, rising in intensity over a 15-minute period, and continuing at a steady plateau for several hours before slowly subsiding) may be absent. Rare instances of acute acalculous cholecystitis as well as hemobilia have been ascribed to benign gallbladder polyps.[121]

The accuracy of US for the detection of gallbladder polyps is generally reported to be 80%, with higher accuracy rates when gallstones are not present; however, as many as one-third of patients with gallbladder polyps identified on US have no polyp in the gallbladder at cholecystectomy. In one study of 213 patients undergoing cholecystectomy for the question of a gallbladder neoplasm on US, 83% of lesions measuring 5 mm or less on imaging were not present on pathologic examination.[122] Another study evaluated 108 patients who underwent cholecystectomy for gallbladder polyps with a mean polyp diameter of 11 mm. On pathologic examination no abnormality was found in 44%, 4.7% had cholesterolosis, and only three patients had adenomas.[123]

The histologic types of gallbladder polyps cannot be distinguished on clinical grounds alone. US and cholecystographic findings do not predict histology reliably (Fig. 69.8).[101] Although the sensitivity of transabdominal US may be as high as 80% for detecting polyps, its accuracy in characterizing the type of polyp may be as low as 20%.[124,125] EUS is a more sensitive and specific method for diagnosing gallbladder polyps. One study comparing transabdominal US and EUS found that the diagnostic accuracy of EUS for differentiating polyp types exceeded 90%.[126] Several studies have shown that an EUS scoring system that incorporates the size, number, shape, and echogenicity of polyps and polyp margins may predict the neoplastic potential of gallbladder polyps; color Doppler flow on EUS may also predict malignancy.[126–129] Several cases in which preoperative 18-fluorodeoxyglucose PET accurately predicted the presence of malignant tumor of the gallbladder in patients with gallbladder polyps have been reported.[130]

A 2024 study evaluated EUS elastography in characterizing gallbladder polyps. In this study, the strain ratio of elastography differed significantly among malignant polyps, benign neoplastic polyps, and non-neoplastic polyps. Elastography might be used as an adjunctive assessment of risk for intermediate-sized gallbladder polyps or for large polyps in patients with a high surgical risk.[129a]

Other studies have evaluated clinical and imaging predictors of malignancy. Aside from polyp size (>10 mm), patient age above 60 years is the strongest predictor of neoplastic disease. Other risk factors for malignancy include PSC, Asian ethnic background, and a sessile polypoid lesion with focal gallbladder wall thickening of more than 4 mm.[131] The presence of concurrent gallstones is also associated with a higher risk of malignancy.[132] Single polyps and symptomatic polyps may be more likely to be malignant than multiple polyps and asymptomatic polyps, respectively.

Natural History

The few studies that have attempted to define the natural history of untreated gallbladder polyps highlight the benign nature of most polyps and support a "watch and wait" approach in most cases.[133] On the basis of records at the Mayo Clinic, one study identified approximately 200 patients in whom cholecystograms demonstrated gallbladder polyps and immediate cholecystectomy was not performed.[134] After 15 years of follow-up, symptoms sufficient to warrant surgery developed in fewer than 10% of the patients, and none of the patients available for follow-up had evidence of gallbladder cancer.

One group of investigators performed annual or semi-annual US for a 5-year period on 109 patients with polyps smaller than 10 mm. During this time, no patient developed gallbladder cancer, and more than 88% of patients experienced no polyp growth.[135] Another study identified 224 patients with gallbladder polyps, 95% of which were predicted to be cholesterol polyps on the basis of the US appearance and the remainder of which were classified as "polypoid lesions of uncertain benignity."[136] After an average follow-up of 9 months, all the polyps thought initially to be benign remained the same size or were proven to be benign at cholecystectomy. Two-thirds of the polypoid lesions in which a benign nature was uncertain were found to be adenomas or carcinomas when the gallbladder was resected. These findings suggest that most gallbladder polyps are benign, and that high-risk polyps often have an identifiable characteristic such as larger size.

Other studies have suggested that the 10-mm diameter cut-off value for cholecystectomy may be too high, because premalignant or malignant gallbladder lesions may rarely be found in persons with polyps that were initially 6–9 mm in size.[137,138] A study from China of 1446 patients with US-detected polyps who subsequently underwent cholecystectomy examined predictors of malignancy.[139] In this group, the frequencies of polyp types were as follows: cholesterol polyps 87.1%; benign, noncholesterol polyps 11.2%; and malignant polyps 1.7%. Most of the benign, noncholesterol polyps were adenomas, and more than half were less than 10 mm in size. The investigators found that age over 50 years, symptoms, size greater than 10 mm, and gallstones were independent predictors of a malignant polyp. A single polyp that was 8 mm in size proved to be malignant, but the majority of malignant polyps (83%) were larger than 15 mm. These data suggest that large, symptomatic gallbladder polyps, particularly when associated with gallstones, should be managed with cholecystectomy; however, application of these data to the management of small, asymptomatic polyps in a low-risk population is complicated. The investigators recommend regular imaging surveillance for 5 years for patients who have polyps without high-risk characteristics, with the frequency of surveillance depending on polyp size.

Another large study evaluated 1204 patients with gallbladder polyps on imaging who subsequently underwent cholecystectomy ($n = 194$) or surveillance ($n = 1010$).[140] The mean polyp size was 6.9 mm. In 28% of patients, polyps grew during the 2 years of follow-up. Malignant polyps were significantly larger than benign lesions, with a mean size of 27.5 mm versus 12.3 mm, respectively. Of concern, 5% of malignant lesions were only 3–5 mm in size, and 8% were 5–10 mm in size. The authors concluded that surgery should be considered as definitive treatment for patients with polyps that are 3–10 mm in size; however, the patients in this study were selected for surgery based on risk, including polyp growth or suspicion for malignancy, so the relatively high risk of malignancy (20%) may have been anticipated. The study also included symptomatic patients and those with gallstones, so there may have been other known predictors of risk for malignancy and indications for cholecystectomy.

Treatment

Patients with biliary pain and US evidence of both polyps and stones in the gallbladder should undergo elective cholecystectomy. The decision is more complicated for patients in whom gallbladder polyps without concurrent gallstones are discovered. For these patients, the decision to operate depends on the severity of symptoms, confidence of the clinician that the symptoms are biliary in origin, and US features (particularly the size) of the polyp.

Because polyps 10 mm in size or larger have a greater likelihood of being cancerous, elective laparoscopic cholecystectomy should be considered in acceptable surgical candidates with asymptomatic polyps of this size.[141–143] In a patient who is a poor surgical risk with a polyp that is 10 mm or larger, periodic monitoring for polyp growth (perhaps every 6 months) with US or additional characterization with EUS may be reasonable.[141,143] Polyps larger than 18 mm in diameter pose a significant risk of malignancy and should prompt cholecystectomy, if possible. One study found that lesions of this size often contain advanced, invasive cancer that involves the serosal surface of the gallbladder and requires a more extensive dissection than can be accomplished by laparoscopy.[144] As a result, the investigators advocate open cholecystectomy for these large polypoid lesions of the gallbladder.

How best to manage patients with polyps that are 6–9 mm in size is debated. In this generally low-risk population, periodic surveillance for polyp growth or change may be prudent. One group of investigators has recommended transabdominal US evaluation 3–6 months after the initial discovery of such polyps to exclude a rapidly growing tumor, followed by ongoing surveillance at 6–12-month intervals. The optimal duration of surveillance is unknown. Other investigators have advocated cholecystectomy for polyps of this size (particularly for individuals with one or more risk factors for malignancy, including age over 60, Asian ethnicity, origin from a region endemic for gallbladder carcinoma, PSC, or sessile polypoid lesion), given the small but definite risk of neoplasia, but this approach is aggressive.[131,145,146,146a]

Many experts now recommend no routine surveillance for asymptomatic polyps smaller than 5–6 mm because polyps of this size have been demonstrated to be benign in large studies.[146] Historically, experts have recommended repeating US in 6–12 months after the diagnosis, followed by repeat examination at intervals of 6–12 months for 1–2 years to confirm stability in polyp size for all polyps smaller than 10 mm.[147] More recent guidelines suggest performing US surveillance at 6 months, 1 year, and 2 years for polyps 6–9 mm in size, or for polyps 5 mm or smaller in patients with risk factors for malignancy. Other guidelines published in 2022 suggest that no follow-up is needed for low-risk polyps less than 6 mm in size but recommend surveillance US in 1 year for polyps 7–9 mm in size.[148] The recommended surveillance for asymptomatic gallbladder polyps smaller than 10 mm is summarized in Table 69.4.

The purpose of surveillance is to detect growth, a possible predictor of malignant risk. Unfortunately, guidance as to how to manage enlarging subcentimeter polyps also varies. One guideline suggests that cholecystectomy be considered for appropriate surgical candidates if a polyp grows by 2 mm, whereas another recommends surgery when polyp growth exceeds 4 mm during

TABLE 69.4 Recommended Surveillance for Asymptomatic Gallbladder Polyps <10 mm[a]

Predictors of Malignancy[b]	Polyp Size (mm) <5	Polyp Size (mm) 6–9
Absent	No surveillance	US at 6 months, 1 year, and 2 years[c]
Present (at least one)	US at 6 months, 1 year, and 2 years[c]	Consider cholecystectomy or continued close surveillance

[a]Cholecystectomy is generally recommended for polyps >10 mm.
[b]Age >60 years, Asian ethnicity, origin from a region endemic for gallbladder carcinoma, PSC, gallbladder wall thickness >4 mm, sessile lesion.
[c]Surveillance may be stopped if there is no growth by the second year.

surveillance. Nevertheless, polyp growth is not always a cause of concern. In 1 health plan study of more than 600,000 adults, including 35,000 (6%) with gallbladder polyps, approximately half of gallbladder polyps enlarged slowly over the surveillance period.[149] Growth exceeding 2 mm occurred in 66%, and approximately half of the subcentimeter polyps grew to exceed the 1 cm cut-off for surgery. For these higher-risk polyps, 32.2% underwent cholecystectomy, and no cancers were found. Moreover, the rate of gallbladder cancer was similar in those with and without gallbladder polyps, thus highlighting the challenges of assessing the true malignant risk of small, asymptomatic gallbladder polyps.

The best practice for gallbladder polyp surveillance needs clarification. A cost-benefit analysis in the United Kingdom has reported an estimated cost of $9.7 million over 20 years to survey all patients with gallbladder polyps by US every 6 months. US surveillance might save an estimated 5.4 lives per year, assuming all neoplastic polyps become malignant (a course that is not well proved). Given the rarity of gallbladder cancer, the cost of universal gallbladder polyp surveillance may not be justifiable; the cost-effectiveness might be improved by limiting surveillance to polyps between 5 and 10 mm in size.[150]

The recommendations for following small gallbladder polyps expectantly may not apply to patients with PSC, in whom the risk of malignancy in polypoid lesions of the gallbladder may be as high as 60% (see Chapter 70).[151] In this high-risk population, cholecystectomy for polyps smaller than 10 mm should be considered.

Full references for this chapter can be found at https://ebooks.health.elsevier.com.

70 Primary and Secondary Sclerosing Cholangitis

Christopher L. Bowlus, Cynthia Levy

IN THIS CHAPTER

Sclerosing cholangitis encompasses a spectrum of cholestatic conditions that are characterized by patchy inflammation, fibrosis, and destruction of the intrahepatic and extrahepatic biliary tracts. These conditions are typically chronic, progressive disorders in which persistent biliary damage may lead to biliary obstruction, biliary cirrhosis, and hepatic failure, with associated complications. The first description of sclerosing cholangitis is credited to Delbet[1] and has been attributed to be the cause of Beethoven's diarrhea and cirrhosis from which he died in 1827 at the age of 57 years.[2] Although sclerosing cholangitis had been considered for many years to be a rare disorder, the advent of ERCP in the 1970s and magnetic resonance cholangiography has allowed an improved understanding of the true prevalence of this disorder and facilitated careful study of its natural history. Nevertheless, many aspects of sclerosing cholangitis remain poorly understood or lacking, most notably a detailed knowledge of its etiology and medical therapy with proven effectiveness.

Many distinct conditions may lead to the cholangiographic appearance of *sclerosing cholangitis*, a diffuse stricturing and segmental dilatation of the biliary system. The most common and best described is primary sclerosing cholangitis (PSC), a disorder that usually occurs in association with inflammatory bowel disease (IBD), either ulcerative colitis (UC) or Crohn's colitis. PSC may also be associated with a wide variety of fibrotic, autoimmune, and infiltrative disorders, although whether such associations imply a common pathogenesis or represent epiphenomena is unclear. The term *secondary sclerosing cholangitis* (SSC) refers to a syndrome that is similar to PSC but develops as a consequence of a known disease or injury (Table 70.1).

PRIMARY SCLEROSING CHOLANGITIS

The original description of PSC was of an "obliterative cholangitis" of the extrahepatic biliary tract with diffuse thickening of the wall and narrowing of the lumen.[3] Early descriptions noted the predominance of men in the third and fourth decades of life and the association with UC. However, increasingly the features of PSC have been seen in a variety of clinical settings with variable subphenotypes.[4,5] The classic form of PSC, often referred to as *large-duct PSC*, with segmental biliary strictures and proximal dilations, occurs predominantly in men (male:female ratio 3:2), is coexistent with IBD in 60%–80% of cases, and typically presents with cholestasis. The IBD typically is a mild and asymptomatic pancolitis or right-sided colitis with ileitis and rectal sparing. The association between PSC and IBD appears to be greater in Northern latitudes, although even there the frequency of non-IBD PSC is increasing. The natural history of large-duct PSC ranges from rapidly progressive to indolent. The mean liver transplant-free survival has been reported to be from 12 (in earlier reports) to more than 20 years.[6–11]

Small-duct PSC is a term used to describe a small group of patients who present with clinical, biochemical, and histologic features compatible with PSC but who lack the typical cholangiographic findings of PSC, yet frequently have biliary enhancement on MR imaging.[12] These patients account for 5%–20% of all patients with PSC.[13–16] In some series, but not others, IBD has been required for the diagnosis. Persons with small-duct PSC without IBD have different HLA haplotypes from those with large-duct PSC, suggesting that the entities are distinct.[17] In the past, many of these patients may have been labeled as AMA-negative PBC or autoimmune cholangiopathy. In studies with extended follow-up of patients with small-duct PSC, 12% to more than half of patients progressed to classic large-duct PSC.[12–15,18] Cholangiocarcinoma did not develop in any patient over a median follow-up of 63–126 months, and survival in the small-duct PSC group was better than that of matched control patients with classic PSC.[13–15]

Depending on the criteria used, from 1% to 53.8% of patients with PSC may be diagnosed with overlapping features of autoimmune hepatitis (AIH). With use of a standardized scoring system for the diagnosis of AIH (see Chapter 92), 7.5% of patients with PSC are characterized as "definite" or "probable" AIH, but there remain no universally accepted diagnostic criteria for PSC-AIH overlap.[19,20] These patients may present with significant elevations of serum aminotransferase levels and histologic findings consistent with AIH, or they may present as a typical case of AIH that subsequently becomes cholestatic with the development of sclerosing cholangitis. In some cases, PSC-AIH overlap may respond to immunosuppressive treatment. Importantly, autoantibodies, including antinuclear (ANA) and smooth muscle antibodies (SMA), are frequently present in patients with PSC without evidence of AIH. In addition, 10% or more of patients with AIH may have cholangiographic features consistent with PSC on magnetic resonance cholangiopancreatography (MRCP).[21,22]

Epidemiology

Determination of the true incidence and prevalence of PSC is complicated by the variable presentation of the disease, inconsistent diagnostic criteria, and referral bias inherent in many published studies.[9] In addition, case ascertainment may have been limited in early studies before the widespread use of MRI and MRCP. Further, a specific International Classification of Disease code was only assigned to PSC in 2018 (K83.01).

Data from large cohorts of patients suggest that the incidence of PSC in North America and Northern Europe is approximately

TABLE 70.1 Causes of Secondary Sclerosing Cholangitis

Pediatric	Benign	Malignant
Biliary atresia Cystic fibrosis Congenital bile duct abnormalities Histiocytosis X Ichthyosis with sclerosing cholangitis Neonatal sclerosing cholangitis Primary and secondary immunodeficiency Progressive familial intrahepatic cholestasis type 3 Sickle cell disease	***Autoinflammatory*** IgG4-related sclerosing cholangitis Eosinophilic cholangitis Mast cell cholangitis Sarcoidosis ***Infectious*** Recurrent pyogenic cholangitis HIV-related cholangiopathy SARS-CoV2 ***Vascular*** Intra-arterial chemotherapy Iatrogenic bile duct injury Portal cavernoma cholangiopathy Vasculitis ***Other*** Biliary inflammatory pseudotumor Chronic pancreatitis	Cholangiocarcinoma Lymphoma Metastatic cancer

1 to 1.5 cases per 100,000 person-years, with a prevalence of 6–16 cases per 100,000.[23–26] Estimates of the prevalence of PSC in other parts of the world are limited, but the frequency of PSC among patients with IBD in Southeast Asia has been reported to be similar to those observed in European and North American cohorts.[27–30] This is in contrast to a single report from India in which only 48 cases of PSC were identified among 12,216 patients with IBD.

Although PSC has been diagnosed in neonates and as late as the eighth decade of life, most patients present between the ages of 25 and 45 years, with a median age of diagnosis ranging from 36 to 39 years.[7,8,24,31] Approximately two-thirds of patients with PSC are men, but in the subset of patients without IBD, the male-to-female ratio is lower.[31] Women with PSC are generally older at diagnosis. PSC is also associated with nonsmoking, but whether this effect is independent of IBD remains controversial.[32–34] Coffee consumption and, among women, the use of hormone therapy have been associated with a reduced risk of PSC.[35,36]

Populations of special interest include children and non-Caucasian persons with PSC. PSC in children appears to have many of the same features as PSC in adults, namely, a male predominance and strong association with IBD.[17] Children with PSC appear to have a higher rate of biochemical response to medical treatment (see later) and higher frequency of overlap with AIH, but survival appears to be similar to adults.[37] Most studies of PSC have been performed in Northern European populations or populations of Northern European descent, leading some to conclude that PSC is a disease of Caucasians. However, the incidence and prevalence of PSC among African Americans appears to be at least as great as those of Caucasians.[38–40] In African Americans, the male predominance is less striking, and the rate of IBD is lower. HLA-DR3, which is strongly associated with PSC in European populations, is rare among African Americans and is not associated with PSC in African American patients listed for LT, although an association with HLA-B8 is shared between both Caucasian and African American patients.[39]

Etiology and Pathogenesis

The etiology and pathogenesis of PSC remain poorly understood. Genetic, environmental, and immunologic factors appear to play key roles in disease susceptibility, and progression of disease may be dependent on cholestasis. Currently, the most attractive model of disease pathogenesis postulates that PSC represents an immunologic reaction that develops in genetically susceptible persons who are exposed to an environmental or toxic trigger, such as bacterial cell wall products. Any theory of the pathogenesis of PSC must explain the strong association with IBD and address the unique relationship between the intestinal tract and the liver as well as the role of fibrosis, bile acids, and immune cells (Fig. 70.1)

Genetic Factors

The importance of genetic factors in the pathogenesis of PSC was demonstrated by a 9- to 39-fold increase in the risk of the disease among siblings and an association with specific HLA haplotypes.[41] Early studies identified strong associations with HLA B8 and DR3, and subsequent studies have led to the identification of additional disease genes on the basis of genome-wide association studies in several thousand patients.[42–50] Over 20 risk genes have been identified with sufficient validation, but they account for only a fraction of the estimated PSC susceptibility. The majority of identified loci have been associated with other immune-mediated diseases, including UC and Crohn disease.[47,51] In addition, 33 genes have been implicated at a lower level of significance based on an a priori assumption that there is an overlap in the genetic associations between PSC and other immune-mediated disease, so-called pleiotropy.

Despite these advances, the HLA haplotype associations remain the most significant. These findings are not explained simply by the association between PSC and IBD because HLA-B8 and DR3 are not overrepresented in patients with IBD without PSC.[52] The subsequent development of molecular genotyping demonstrated that the extended HLA haplotypes that are most strongly associated with PSC are as follows[39,50,53–55]:

B*08:01;
DRB1*03:01-DQA1*05:01-DQB1*02:01;
DRB1*13:01-DQA1*01:03-DQB1*06:03;
DRB1*15:01-DQA1*01:02-DQB1*06:02; and
DRB1*01:01-DQA1*01:01.

Haplotypes associated with protection from PSC include the following:

DRB4*01:03-DRB1*04:01-DQA1*03-DQB1*03:02;

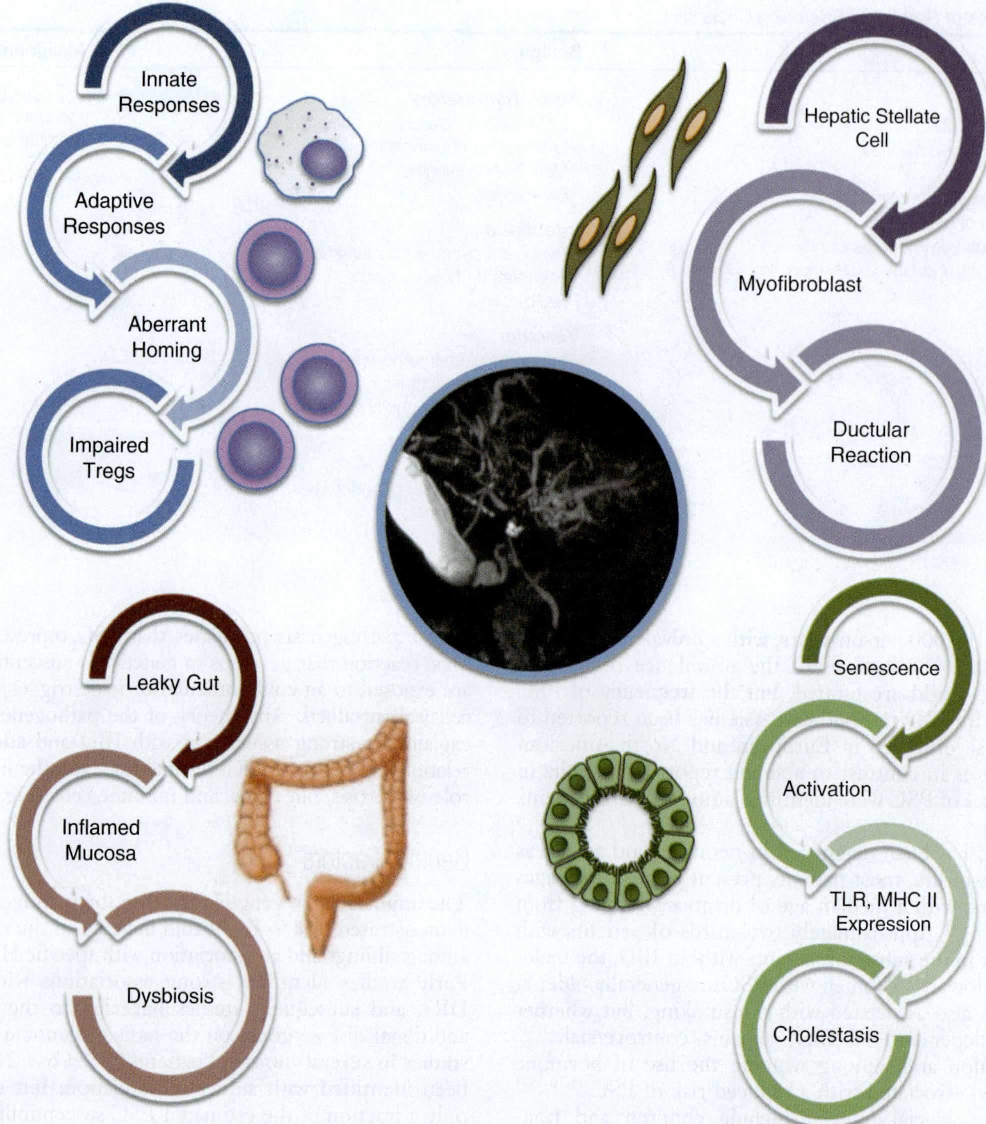

Fig. 70.1 The current model of the pathogenesis of primary sclerosing cholangitis involves an altered microbiome, inflamed mucosa, and impaired intestinal barrier (*bottom left*) resulting in intestinal lymphocytes, microbial products, and/or metabolites translocating to the liver, activating innate and adaptive immune responses (*top left*). Biliary epithelial cells are activated, which can perpetuate inflammatory responses (*bottom right*). Peribiliary mesenchymal cells acquire a myofibroblast phenotype, leading to large duct fibrosis (*top right*).

DRB4*01:03-DRB1*07:01-DQA1*02:01-DQB1*03:03; and DRB4*02:02-DRB1*11:01-DQA1*05:01-DQB1*03:01.

HLA-B*08 and DRB1*13:01 have been associated with small-duct PSC only in patients who also have IBD, suggesting that small-duct and large-duct PSC are genetically related.[17] However, unique HLA associations, including HLA-B*07 and HLA-DRB1*15, have been associated with PSC patients with elevated immunoglobulin (Ig)G4 levels.[56]

Identifying the causative gene or genes responsible for the HLA association in PSC remains challenging. Fine mapping of the region and modeling of the effects of variants on the HLA-DR peptide binding groove have implicated changes in residues 37 and 86 in the HLA-DRβ chain that affect the binding of peptide antigens to be presented by class II molecules.[54] Other studies have implicated HLA-C and HLA-B variants that have been associated with PSC and can act as inhibitory ligands for killer immunoglobulin receptors on natural killer (NK) cells.[57,58] Further, an HLA-independent association with the *NOTCH4* gene in the class III region has been reported.[53] Notably, genetic studies to date have been limited to Northern European populations. In African Americans listed for LT (in whom HLA-DR3 is rare), no association between HLA-DR3 and PSC was found, but a strong association with HLA-B8 was present.[39]

In addition to HLA, at least 22 other genes have been associated with PSC through genome-wide association studies, with most having roles in the function of innate and adaptive immune responses, particularly T-cell responses.[47,49] Only half of the PSC-associated genes are also associated with UC, Crohn disease, or both. In fact, although the genetic correlation between PSC and IBD is generically strong ($r = 0.56$), the correlation with UC is much weaker ($r = 0.29$), and that with Crohn disease was not found to be statistically significant ($r = 0.04$).[50] In addition, network analysis has not identified any common functional pathways to suggest a specific mechanism that predisposes to both IBD and PSC. Furthermore, many genes associated with PSC are also associated with classic autoimmune diseases (pleiotropy) such as RA and type 1 diabetes mellitus. Despite these advances, less than 10% of the heritability of PSC can be explained by the genes identified to date.

Genetic modifiers of disease progression in PSC are even less well documented. Several studies have investigated HLA haplotypes and clinical outcomes, but the findings have been inconsistent, likely due to the small cohort sizes. An analysis of genome-wide association studies data from 3402 patients did not find an association between time to clinical events and the HLA haplotype. However, there was a significant association with rs853974 on chromosome 6, with the AA genotype being protective compared with the GG and AG genotypes (hazard ratios of 0.46 and 0.55, respectively).[59] The rs853974 polymorphism is located near the R-spondin 3 (*RSPO3*) gene, which is highly expressed in cholangiocytes, suggesting a potential mechanistic role in PSC disease progression. The rs738409 variant (I148M) of the *PNPLA3* gene, which has been associated with severity of several liver diseases, was found to be associated with reduced transplant-free survival among patients with PSC and a dominant stricture.[60]

Immunologic Factors

Despite the strong clinical and genetic evidence of an immunologic basis for PSC, the precise targets and immune responses that lead to PSC or contribute to its progression have yet to be delineated. Whether PSC is similar to classic autoimmune diseases in which there is targeted destruction of tissue directed at a specific self-antigen, or more akin to an autoinflammatory disease such as IBD in which there is an abnormal innate immune response to antigens of the intestinal flora activating an adaptive immune response, is unclear. A popular hypothesis linking IBD with PSC is that PSC is triggered by bacteria or pathogen-associated molecular patterns such as lipopolysaccharide that enter the portal circulation through an inflamed, permeable intestine (leaky gut) (see Chapter 2). Pathogen-associated molecular patterns activate macrophages, dendritic cells, and NK cells through pattern recognition receptors, including Toll-like receptors and CD14, leading to the secretion of cytokines. NK cells are activated in turn by interleukin (IL)-12 and promote recruitment and activation of lymphocytes via TNF-α, IL-1β, and CXCL8. NK cells may be activated by MHC class I chain-related gene products MICA and MICB, which are stress-induced proteins that can promote the cytotoxic function of NK, NKT, and $\gamma\delta$T cells through the NKG2D receptor.

Macrophages uniquely accumulate in the sinusoidal and perisinusoidal spaces in PSC and, as key cells in the transition from innate to adaptive immune responses, may play a major role in PSC. Compared with normal subjects, the liver in patients with PSC has been shown to have a significantly greater number of CD68 and/or myeloperoxidase-positive cells in the portal areas.[61] Genetic studies have linked macrophage stimulating protein 1, a circulating preprotein and suppressor of macrophages, to susceptibility to PSC. GPBAR1 is a cell surface receptor for bile acids on macrophages, biliary epithelial cells (BEC), and intestinal epithelial cells that suppresses macrophage function,[62–64] and variants of the *GPBAR1* gene that reduce or abolish the encoded protein function have also been associated with PSC.[57]

Bone marrow-derived IBA1$^+$CD163^{low} macrophages accumulate near portal tracts and increase with increasing fibrosis.[65] These macrophages also express triggering-receptor-expressed-on-myeloid-cells-2 (Trem2), which inhibits TLR-mediated signaling and protects against cholestatic injury in mouse models of PSC.[66,67] Further, these IBA1$^+$ macrophages express CCL24, whose cognate receptor CCR3 is expressed on cholangiocytes in livers from patients with PSC. Treatment of PSC mouse models with a neutralizing antibody to CCL24 significantly improved inflammation and fibrosis.[68]

Although genetic studies have implicated the adaptive immune response, little is known about the functional abnormalities in PSC. Historically, immunohistochemical studies have defined the infiltrate in PSC livers to consist primarily of nonactivated memory CD8$^+$ T cells that express the gut-homing integrin $\alpha4\beta7$ concentrated around portal tracts. T cells also localize to areas of fibrosis along with mucosal-associated invariant T cells, invariant T cells enriched in the human liver with the capacity to recognize bacterial antigens and produce IL-1 and IL-17, among other cytokines.[69] Notably, PSC peripheral blood mononuclear cells have a significantly greater IL-17 response after stimulation with *Enterococcus faecalis* or *Candida albicans*, and IL-17A-producing cells are prominent in PSC livers.[70] Single-cell sequencing of intrahepatic and peripheral blood T cells suggests that there is a population of tissue-resident naïve-like CD4$^+$ T cell predisposed to polarize toward Th17 cells.[71]

The number of peripheral regulatory T cells (Tregs), which are important mediators of resolution of immune activation, is reduced in patients with PSC compared with healthy controls and patients with PBC or UC, with the most pronounced reductions in patients homozygous for the PSC risk allele in the *IL2RA* gene.[72] The function of peripheral Tregs has also been found to be impaired in patients with PSC compared with controls. The number of Tregs is also reduced in PSC livers compared with PBC livers,[73] although a greater frequency of peripheral CD4$^+$CD25$^+$ T cells has been found in UC patients with PSC compared with UC patients without PSC.[73,74] It should be noted, however, that prior reports have documented a reduced frequency of peripheral and tissue Tregs in both PBC and UC patients relative to healthy and disease controls, suggesting that changes in Tregs may be a generic feature of inflammatory diseases.[75,76]

The gene encoding CD28, a costimulatory molecule for T-cell activation, survival, and proliferation, has been genetically associated with PSC, and CD4$^+$CD28$^-$ T cells are enriched in the liver compared with the periphery in patients with PSC. In addition, CD4$^+$CD28$^-$ T cells were more frequent in PSC livers compared with PBC, NASH, and normal livers.[74] These CD28$^-$ T cells were activated memory cells with intracellular stores of cytotoxic molecules and expressed adhesion molecules and chemokine receptors that promote tissue infiltration and localization to bile ducts and were also able to activate BEC *in vitro*.

Lymphocyte Trafficking

Recognition of the common mechanisms of liver and gut lymphocyte trafficking has led to an improved understanding of the link between IBD and PSC as well as the observation that PSC may develop years after total colectomy. Evidence suggests that adhesion molecules and chemokine receptors that are normally restricted to the gut are expressed in the PSC liver, leading to the recruitment of lymphocytes of intestinal origin,[77–81] though recent studies suggest that this is not specific to PSC.[82] In the intestine, the recruitment of lymphocytes involves activation by dendritic cells in gut-associated lymphatic tissue, resulting in lymphocyte expression of the $\alpha4\beta7$ integrin and the CCR9 chemokine receptor, which are dependent on mucosal addressin in cell adhesion molecule-1 (MAdCAM-1) and chemokine ligand 25 (CCL25), respectively. In PSC, not only were MAdCAM-1 and CCL25 expressed in the portal vein and sinusoidal endothelium,[83] but also CCR9$^+$ liver lymphocytes were specifically increased in patients with PSC compared with those with PBC. Also, approximately 20% of lymphocytes from PSC livers expressed CCR9 compared with less than 2% in normal or PBC livers.[79] The expression of MAdCAM-1 in the liver appears to be mediated by deamination of methylamine by vascular adhesion protein 1, a semicarbazide-sensitive amine oxidase expressed in the human liver.[84] In the presence of TNF-α, methylamine induces the expression of functional MAdCAM-1 on hepatic endothelial cells and is associated with increased adhesion of lymphocytes from patients with PSC to hepatic vessels.

Dysbiosis

The study of intestinal and biliary microbiota in PSC may help to explain the important link between the gut and liver in PSC. Several studies have documented alterations in the composition of intestinal bacteria, bacteriophage, and fungi in UC and Crohn disease, most commonly a decrease in the diversity of the population along with some specific alterations in the members of the population (findings reminiscent of the "hygiene hypothesis" of autoimmunity). Dysbiosis is also frequently found in patients with chronic liver diseases, especially those with advanced cirrhosis. In addition, bile acids can significantly impact the microbiome in PSC and IBD.[85] However, studies to date suggest that the intestinal microbiota of patients with PSC are distinct from those in patients with IBD,[85–93] as well as with IgG4-related sclerosing cholangitis (IgG4-SC).[94] In fact, patients with PSC with IBD tend to have microbiota more closely related to patients with PSC without IBD than to those with IBD alone.

The importance of intestinal microbes to PSC disease progression has been highlighted in studies of the *Mdr2* knockout mouse model. Transfer of *Mdr2*-null intestinal microbiota into healthy control mice induced NLRP3 inflammasome activation, providing evidence that cholestasis induces changes in intestinal microbial communities that contribute to PSC disease progression.[95] Conversely, when raised in a germ-free environment, *Mdr2* knockout mice demonstrate worse fibrosis, ductular reaction, and ductopenia compared to conventionally housed *Mdr2* knockout mice.[96] The lack of intestinal microbes in these mice results in a lack of secondary bile acids to activate the farnesoid X receptor (FXR) and inhibit bile acid synthesis.[97] In addition, loss of short-chain fatty acid–producing bacteria such as *Lachnospiraceae* has been implicated in aggravating liver disease in the *Mdr2* knockout model.[98] Further, in this model, there is an increase in the frequency of intestinal *Lactobacillus* species, and interestingly, *Lactobacillus gasseri* is enriched in the livers from *Mdr2* knockout mice and could induce hepatic γδ TCR$^+$ cells to produce IL-17.[99]

Gnotobiotic studies with stool from patients with UC with or without PSC or healthy controls inoculated into *Mdr2* knockout mice demonstrated that *Klebsiella pneumoniae* in the stool of patients with PSC could translocate to mesenteric lymph nodes, was associated with IL-17-expressing T cells (TH17) in the liver, and enhanced susceptibility to hepatobiliary injury.[100] In addition, the *K. pneumoniae* isolated from PSC patients could induce epithelial damage in a bacterial-organoid coculture system. Further, *Mdr2* knockout mice inoculated with *K. pneumoniae* treated with a cocktail of bacteriophage targeting *K. pneumoniae* mitigated the effects of *K. pneumoniae*.[101] An important issue related to these findings is whether a single or few organisms could be responsible for a large effect in PSC. *K. pneumoniae* is present in up to 82% of patients with PSC in Japan, regardless of IBD status. In contrast, *K. pneumoniae* was not found in a cohort in Germany,[102] and in a Norwegian PSC cohort, fewer than 20% of patients were found to carry *K. pneumoniae* that was associated with more advanced liver disease.[103]

In addition to the intestinal microbiota, the biliary microbiota may also be altered in PSC. The fucosyltransferase-2 gene (*FUT2*) is involved in protein glycosylation, and genetic variants leading to truncated FUT2 proteins, so-called nonsecretors, have been linked to PSC and Crohn disease. Interestingly, microbes in the bile in PSC varied by *FUT2* genotypes, with *Firmicutes* spp. being significantly increased and *Proteobacteria* spp. significantly decreased among nonsecretors. The presence of *Enterococcus* spp. has been associated with poor clinical outcomes in patients with PSC but may reflect colonization in advanced disease rather than having a pathogenic role.[104,105]

Toxic Bile Theory

Although genetic evidence does not support a role for bile as an initiator of PSC, several lines of evidence suggest that bile is important in the progression of PSC. Bile is a complex mixture of bile acids, bilirubin, cholesterol, phospholipids, and proteins for which several protective mechanisms have evolved (see Chapter 66). Changes in the composition of bile, decreased bile flow, and increased biliary pressure in PSC may all disrupt the normal homeostasis and lead to the formation of toxic bile. BEC are protected from bile by dilution and alkalization, the so-called bicarbonate umbrella. In addition, mixed micelles with phosphatidylcholine and cholesterol prevent bile acid toxicity. These mechanisms can be compromised by impairment of transporters responsible for maintaining the bile acid/phospholipid ratio [MDR3 (multidrug resistance protein 3) or BSEP (bile salt export pump)] or bicarbonate excretion and hydration of bile [CFTR or AE2 (anion exchange protein 2)]. Alternatively, bile stasis, a frequent phenomenon in PSC, may lead to formation of toxic bile and exacerbation of bile duct injury.

Support for the toxic bile acid theory comes primarily from the *Mdr2* knockout mouse.[106–108] Targeted disruption of *Mdr2* leads to sclerosing of the biliary tract with extra- and intrahepatic biliary strictures and dilatations, onion-skin type periductal fibrosis, and focal obliteration of bile ducts similar to that seen with primary and SSC in humans.[106] Variants of the human orthologue of *Mdr2* [*MDR3 or ABCB4* (ATP-binding cassette subfamily B, member 4)] in humans are associated with intrahepatic cholestasis of pregnancy and gallbladder disease in an autosomal dominant fashion and progressive familial intrahepatic cholestasis type 3 in a rare autosomal dominant condition (see Chapter 64). In addition, some rare variants have been associated with sclerosing cholangitis,[109,110] but genetic studies have not found any association between genetic variants in *ABCB4* and susceptibility to PSC.[111]

PSC patients with normal serum bilirubin levels have been shown to have normal biliary excretion of bile acids and lipids, suggesting that the toxic bile theory may only play a role in the later stages of PSC.[111,112] In fact, changes in serum bile acid composition have been associated with short-term clinical outcomes, and bile acid synthesis is fully suppressed later in disease.[113,114]

Biliary Epithelial Cells

The role of BEC in the pathogenesis of PSC remains unclear, but an understanding of the function of BEC in the recruitment and activation of immune cells suggests that BEC are active participants rather than innocent bystanders. BEC from patients with PSC were noted to have reduced levels of the bile acid receptor TGR5, which normally promotes secretion, proliferation, and tight junction integrity. In PSC BEC, the reduced level of TGR5 promotes the development of a reactive BEC phenotype.[115] When activated, BEC express a host of receptors, cytokines, and chemokines that can orchestrate several immunologic processes. In addition to MHC class II antigens, BEC express CD1d and can present lipid antigens to NK T cells.[116] CD1d is downregulated in PSC. Toll-like receptors are also expressed on BEC, and IgG found in the sera of some PSC patients and directed against BEC induce the expression of TLR4 and TLR9 on BEC in culture.[117] In fact, treatment of BEC with PSC sera containing anti-BEC antibodies induces secretion of granulocyte-macrophage colony-stimulating factor, IL-1β, and IL-8. However, the target(s) of these anti-BEC antibodies remain unknown. BEC expression of adhesion molecules, such as intracellular adhesion molecule-1, could also play a role in the recruitment of T lymphocytes.[118]

Further, BEC from patients with PSC display a senescence phenotype[119,120]

Clinical, Laboratory, and Imaging Features

PSC and IBD

The relationship between PSC and IBD is striking and incompletely understood. Although early studies suggested that approximately 80% of patients with PSC had concomitant IBD, subsequent data have shown that the frequency of IBD in patients with PSC is 65%–70%.[7,23–25,121] Across all series of patients with PSC and IBD, nearly 80% have UC, with fewer than 20% having Crohn disease.[7,23–25] Conversely, PSC is present in 2.4%–4.0% of all patients with UC and 1.4%–3.4% of those with Crohn disease.[33,122] The association with IBD is stronger with more extensive colonic involvement; the frequency of PSC is approximately 5.5% in those with pancolitis, in contrast to 0.5% in those with only distal colitis.[122] PSC is not thought to occur in association with Crohn disease isolated to the small intestine. Racial differences may exist, with concomitant IBD seen in only 58.8%–60.5% of African Americans with PSC and 21% of Japanese patients with PSC.[39,40,123]

Unlike other extraintestinal manifestations of IBD, such as uveitis and erythema nodosum, PSC typically progresses independently of IBD,[124] and, in fact, PSC may be diagnosed years after total proctocolectomy for UC.[125,126] The colitis of PSC is often extensive, although clinically quiescent, regardless of whether it is classified as UC or Crohn disease.[127–129] Inflammation is more pronounced in or may be limited to the right colon. In addition, PSC patients who have undergone proctocolectomy and ileal pouch-anal anastomosis have a higher frequency of pouchitis.[129–132] Crohn disease associated with PSC is not typically associated with strictures or fistulas but is restricted to the colon.

Although older reports demonstrated no histologic[133] or cholangiographic[134] differences between patients with or without IBD, subsequent studies have shown that the presence and type of IBD affect the outcomes of PSC. Patients with concurrent UC have a much earlier age of onset and much higher rates of hepatobiliary cancer, LT, and death.[31,135]

Some patients without overt symptoms of IBD may have subclinical histologic changes detected in the colon or may develop overt colitis at a later date.[124] Therefore a high index of suspicion for the emergence of IBD is warranted, and colonoscopy with random biopsies of the colonic mucosa is recommended in all patients with a new diagnosis of PSC.[4]

Symptoms

The understanding of the symptom burden of PSC has evolved as subjective data collected from the clinician perspective has moved to more objective data from patient-reported surveys and outcome measures. The initial clinical presentation of PSC can be quite varied and may run the gamut from asymptomatic elevations of serum alkaline phosphatase levels to decompensated cirrhosis with jaundice, ascites, hepatic encephalopathy, or variceal bleeding. The most common symptoms at the time of presentation include jaundice, fatigue, pruritus, and abdominal pain.[136–140] Other associated symptoms may include fever, chills, night sweats, sleep disturbances, and weight loss (Table 70.2). Increasingly, PSC is diagnosed at an asymptomatic or minimally symptomatic stage. Large series have shown that 15%–44% of patients with PSC are asymptomatic at the time of diagnosis,[13,136,138–141] probably because of routine liver biochemical screening in patients with IBD as well as the widespread availability of MRCP and ERCP for the evaluation of elevated serum alkaline phosphatase levels.

Several efforts to develop and validate instruments to capture symptoms have been attempted, but further work on these tools continues.[142–144] Challenges to developing these tools include symptoms that may be confounded by IBD as well as the intermittent nature of pruritus, jaundice, abdominal pain, and fever that are typically interspersed with asymptomatic periods of varying duration.[145]

Physical Examination

Physical findings may be normal in patients with PSC, particularly in early stages. When physical abnormalities are present, the most common are hepatomegaly, jaundice, and splenomegaly (see Table 70.2). Skin findings are common and include cutaneous hyperpigmentation, excoriations resulting from pruritus, and xanthomata. As liver disease progresses, spider telangiectasias, muscle atrophy, peripheral edema, ascites, and other signs of advanced liver disease may appear (see Chapter 76).[136,137]

Laboratory Findings

Chronic elevation of serum alkaline phosphatase levels, typically three to five times the upper limit of normal, is the biochemical hallmark of PSC. A normal alkaline phosphatase level, however, may be found in up to 6% of patients with cholangiography-proven PSC.[146,147] In some cases, an advanced histologic stage has been demonstrated on a liver biopsy specimen despite normal serum alkaline phosphatase levels.[147] Serum aminotransferase levels are typically elevated, although rarely above four to five times the upper limit of normal, except in the pediatric population, in the setting of acute cholangitis, or in overlap with AIH.[19,37,148] The serum bilirubin level may be normal or elevated and often fluctuates. When the serum bilirubin level is elevated, the bilirubin is predominantly conjugated. Reductions in the serum albumin level and prolongation of the prothrombin time may reflect hepatic synthetic dysfunction with advanced liver disease. In addition, malnutrition and underlying IBD may lower serum albumin levels. Vitamin K malabsorption related to cholestasis may play a role in prolonging the prothrombin time. Other nonspecific consequences of cholestasis are elevations in serum copper, serum ceruloplasmin, and hepatic copper levels; increased urinary copper excretion; and elevated serum cholesterol levels.

Several immunologic markers and serum autoantibodies are found in most patients with PSC, although none is specific for the

TABLE 70.2 Most Common Symptoms and Signs at the Time of Diagnosis of PSC[15,136,137,139–141]

Symptom	Frequency (%)
Fatigue	65–75
Abdominal pain	24–72
Pruritus	15–69
Fever/night sweats	13–45
None	15–44
Weight loss	10–34
Sign	
Jaundice	30–73
Hepatomegaly	34–62
Splenomegaly	32–34
Hyperpigmentation	14–25
Ascites	4–7

disease. Hyperglobulinemia is frequent; serum IgM levels are elevated in up to 50% of patients, and IgG and IgA levels may also be elevated.[136] Autoantibodies are commonly detected in patients with PSC.[149] ANA, often in low titer, may be detected in 24%–53% of patients. SMA are found in 13%–20% of patients, but AMA are found in less than 10%.[150] Most commonly found in patients with PSC are ANCA (specifically perinuclear ANCA or pANCA),[151] which are detected in 65%–88% of patients and appear to react to a heterogeneous group of antigens.[152,153] These antigens have been found to represent neutrophil nuclear envelope proteins predominantly, and the corresponding antibodies have been referred to as antineutrophil nuclear antibodies.[154] ANCA are not specific for PSC and are also commonly found in patients with IBD as well as in a large number of patients with AIH.[154] ANCA positivity has been associated with younger age at the diagnosis of PSC, lower frequency of cholangiocarcinoma, and higher prevalence of HLA-B*08 and DDRB1*03 in the Norwegian population.[155] In contrast, antiglycoprotein 2 is associated with a worse prognosis and greater risk of cholangiocarcinoma.[156] Anticardiolipin antibodies are detected in 66% of patients with PSC, and the titer has been reported to correlate with disease severity.[150,155] In children, ANA, pANCA, and SMA are present in roughly 50%, 66%, and 45%, respectively.[37] In general, despite the high frequency of autoantibodies in patients with PSC, a clear association between the presence of these antibodies, pathogenesis of the disease, and prognosis or response to treatment (see later) remains unproved. Measurement of autoantibodies is, therefore, of limited clinical value in patients with PSC.

Imaging

Cholangiography by ERCP, MRCP, or percutaneous transhepatic cholangiography (PTC) is central to a diagnosis of PSC and provides information regarding the distribution and extent of disease. MRI with MRCP is considered the modality of choice for the diagnosis of PSC,[157–159] and recommendations have been published to standardize its use.[160] New methods using machine learning are being developed to assist with the diagnosis of PSC.[161] In addition, MRI can provide prognostic information using semiqualitative scores[162,163] or fully quantitative measures.[164–166]

The characteristic cholangiographic findings are multifocal stricturing and ectasia of the biliary tract. The strictured segments are usually short, annular, or band-like in appearance (Fig. 70.2), Areas of narrowing are interspersed with areas of normal or near-normal caliber and of prestenotic dilatation. The result is a classic "beaded" appearance to the biliary tract.

Both the extrahepatic and intrahepatic bile ducts are abnormal in approximately 75% of cases. Isolated intrahepatic duct involvement may be observed in 15%–20% of cases.[122,162,167] Isolated abnormalities of the extrahepatic biliary tract are rarer, reported in approximately 6% or less of patients.[141,146,162] The cystic duct and gallbladder may be involved in up to 15% of patients but may not be well visualized on routine cholangiography.[168] Nonspecific gallbladder abnormalities are reported in 41% of patients with PSC and include a thickened gallbladder wall, gallbladder distension, cholelithiasis, cholecystitis, and gallbladder mass lesions.[169] Pancreatic duct irregularities similar to those seen in chronic pancreatitis may rarely be noted.[170]

Dominant strictures, defined as strictures on ERCP with a diameter of less than 1.5 mm of the common bile duct or less than 1.0 mm of a hepatic duct within 2 cm of the bifurcation, develop at a cumulative frequency of 36%–57% and often involve the bifurcation of the hepatic duct.[4,157] Analogous to a dominant stricture on ERCP, the MRI equivalent termed *high-grade stricture* is defined as a >75% reduction in the common bile duct or hepatic ducts.[4,171] Due to the limitations of such strict definitions that may not have clinical relevance, the term *relevant stricture* has been introduced to refer to any biliary stricture of the common bile duct or hepatic ducts associated with signs or symptoms of obstructive cholestasis and/or bacterial cholangitis.[4]

Other findings commonly observed on MRI include wall thickening and mural contrast enhancement of the biliary ducts on contrast-enhanced T1w images[172] and as fibrosis progresses, heterogeneity of contrast enhancement of the liver parenchyma as well as focal parenchymal atrophy.[162,173] Periportal lymphadenopathy is common, detected in up to 77% of patients, but it is nonspecific and not indicative of malignancy.[174,175]

MR elastography can be added to MRI with MRCP and allows staging of hepatic fibrosis (see Chapter 76).[176] Vibration-controlled transient elastography has also been studied in PSC, and liver stiffness measurements were found to correlate with the stage of fibrosis, with accuracy for the diagnosis of advanced fibrosis and cirrhosis superior to the AST/platelet ratio, FIB-4 score, and Mayo risk score (see Chapter 76).[177] Optimal liver stiffness cutoff values for fibrosis stages in PSC of greater than or equal to F1, greater than or equal to F2, greater than or equal to F3, and F4 were 7.4, 8.6, 9.6, and 14.4 kPa, respectively.

Histology

Gross and histologic specimens from the extrahepatic bile ducts demonstrate a diffusely thickened, fibrotic duct wall. The fibrosis is accompanied by a mixed inflammatory infiltrate that may involve the epithelium and biliary glands.[178,179] Florid hyperplasia of the biliary glands with accompanying neural proliferation has been described.[180] Examination of PSC explants removed at the time of LT has demonstrated areas of thin-walled saccular dilatation, termed *cholangiectasias*, that correspond to the beaded appearance on cholangiography.[181]

A wide range of liver biopsy findings may be seen in patients with PSC, and histologic findings are not typically diagnostic for PSC. The characteristic bile duct lesion is a fibro-obliterative process that may lead to an "onion-skin" appearance of concentric fibrosis surrounding medium-sized bile ducts (Fig. 70.3); however, this finding is seen in less than half of biopsy specimens.[178,179] The smaller interlobular and septal bile duct branches may be entirely obliterated by this process, resulting in *fibro-obliterative cholangitis*. This finding is present in only 5%–10% of biopsy specimens but is thought to be virtually pathognomonic of PSC.[181] In this process, the biliary epithelium may degenerate and atrophy and be replaced entirely by fibrous cords. Other characteristic histopathologic findings may include bile duct proliferation, periductal inflammation, and ductopenia. The degree of inflammation can be quite variable but is typically a portal-based mixture of lymphocytes, plasma cells, and neutrophils with a periductal focus. Lymphoid follicles or aggregates may also be seen.[180,181]

Many of the histologic findings of PSC are nonspecific and may be seen in other disorders; in particular, distinguishing PSC from PBC may be difficult. In one study, histologic examination could classify only 28% of patients who had 1 of the 2 diseases.[182] When lymphocytic interface hepatitis is prominent, the distinction from AIH may be challenging, especially because hypergammaglobulinemia and autoantibodies may be present in both conditions.[19,183] When severe cholestasis develops, hepatic copper accumulation can be dramatic and may mimic that seen in Wilson disease (see Chapter 78).[184]

Common histologic staging systems used in chronic viral hepatitis, such as the METAVIR and Ishak scoring systems (see Chapters 73 and 82), have not been well studied in PSC. The system most widely used in patients with PSC was described by Ludwig et al.[133] and is essentially the same as a system previously described for staging PBC (see Chapter 93). In stage 1 (*portal stage*), changes are confined to the portal tracts and consist of portal inflammation, connective tissue expansion, and cholangitis. Stage 2 (*periportal stage*) is characterized by the expansion

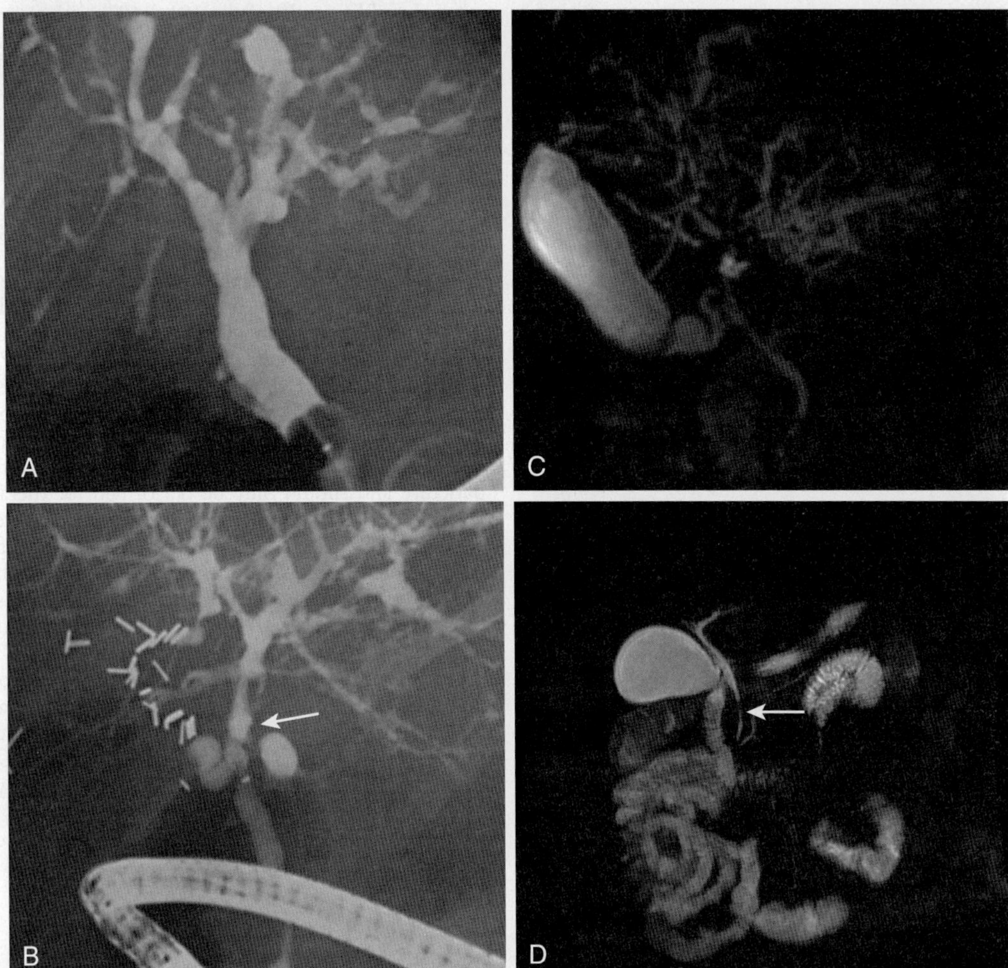

Fig. 70.2 Cholangiograms from ERCP (A and B) and MRCP (C and D) in patients with PSC. (A) ERCP with contrast injected through a balloon catheter (seen in the distal bile duct). The intrahepatic ducts are mainly affected and show diminished arborization (pruning), with diffuse segmental strictures alternating with normal-caliber or mildly dilated duct segments (cholangiectasias), resulting in a beaded appearance. (B) ERCP imaging features include diffuse irregularity of the intrahepatic ducts, multiple short strictures and cholangiectasis, small diverticula in the wall of the common hepatic duct (*arrow*), and clips from a prior cholecystectomy. (C) MRCP imaging demonstrating normal common bile duct with stricture at hilum and diffuse intrahepatic strictures. (D) MRCP demonstrating a high-grade stricture (>75% reduction in lumen) of the common bile duct (*arrowhead*).

of inflammatory and fibrotic processes beyond the confines of the limiting plate, resulting in interface hepatitis (piecemeal necrosis) and periportal fibrosis. Depending on the degree of biliary obstruction, ductular proliferation and cholangitis may be of varying severity. Stage 3 (*septal stage*) is characterized by fibrous septa that bridge one portal tract to the next. Bridging necrosis may occasionally be seen but is uncommon. Stage 4 (*cirrhotic stage*) implies progression to biliary cirrhosis. The degree of inflammatory activity may subside as the stage of the disease progresses, and focal bile ductular proliferation may be striking.

The Ishak system of histologic staging commonly used for chronic viral hepatitis ranges from 0 to 6 and has been studied in PSC in a more limited fashion,[185–188] and even less studied is the use of the METAVIR fibrosis stage.[177] A system for staging PBC proposed by Nakanuma et al.,[189] developed originally for PBC, incorporates bile duct loss and cholestasis measured by orcein-positive granules in addition to fibrosis. The actual Nakanuma stage is the sum of the scores for the last 3 features: stage 1 is a score of 0, stage 2 is 1–3, stage 3 is 4–6, and stage 4 is 7–9. Although the Nakanuma, Ishak, and Ludwig histologic staging systems are all associated with transplant-free survival and time to LT in patients with PSC, the Nakanuma system showed the most robust associations, with the degree of fibrosis and orcein-positive granules deposition being the most discriminative features.[129,187]

Only one study has reported the interobserver agreement in histologic staging in PSC.[187] Among 6 pathologists scoring 119 biopsies using the Ludwig, Ishak, and Nakanuma systems, agreement was substantial, with a kappa index (κ) of 0.62, 0.64, and 0.67 for the Ludwig, Ishak, and Nakanuma fibrosis scores, respectively. Notably, the agreement was only moderate ($\kappa = 0.56$) for the composite Nakanuma score. In addition, Ishak and Ludwig stages were highly correlated ($r = 0.93$, $P < .001$).

The progression of histologic stage over time has been examined in a single observational study and several clinical trials in which liver biopsy findings were included as an endpoint. In the only observational, longitudinal study of histologic progression, Angulo et al. examined 307 liver biopsy specimens from 107 PSC patients with a median time between biopsies of 11 months. Using a Markov model, they estimated the rates of progression for patients with stage 2 disease to be 42%, 66%, and 93% at 1, 2, and 5

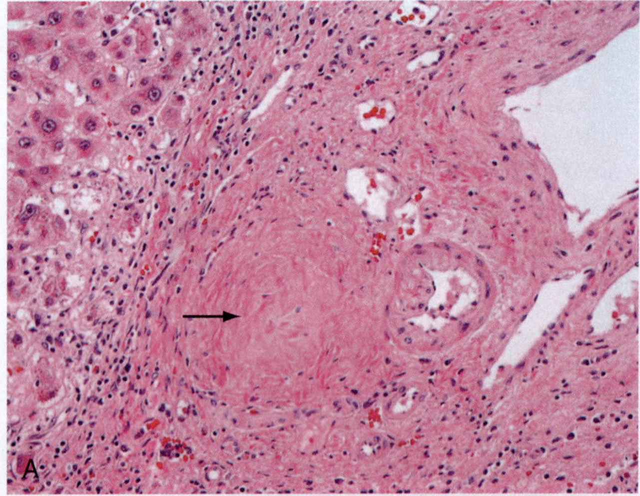

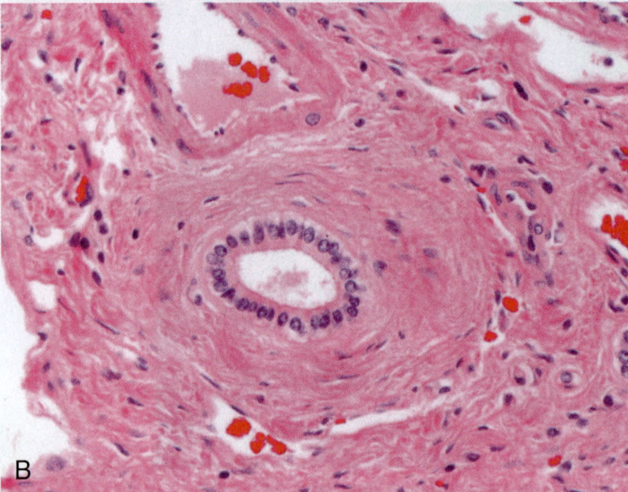

Fig. 70.3 Liver histopathology in PSC. (A) A segmental bile duct is obliterated by fibrosis (*arrow*), demonstrating "fibro-obliterative cholangitis" (H&E, ×200). (B) A medium-sized bile duct is surrounded by concentric fibrosis with an onionskin appearance (H&E, ×400). (Courtesy Matthew Yeh, MD, PhD, Seattle, WA.)

years, respectively.[190] Similarly, progression from stages 2 to 4 (biliary cirrhosis) was estimated to occur in 14%, 25%, and 52% after 1, 2, and 5 years, respectively. Regression of stage was observed in 15% of patients.

Unlike observational studies, clinical trials provide prospectively collected biopsies at defined intervals with less chance of treatment bias. Overall, these studies have not demonstrated significant changes in histologic stage over 1–5 years.[190–192] Even when considering progression, regression, or no change, the majority of patients have no change in histologic stage, with similar proportions demonstrating either progression or regression.[185,193–198] The most detailed assessment of histologic fibrosis progression in PSC comes from a randomized controlled trial of simtuzumab, a monoclonal antibody directed against lysyl oxidase-like 2 (see later). A total of 225 PSC patients were enrolled in a 2-year randomized trial of simtuzumab or placebo with liver biopsies performed at baseline and annually.[186] Mean hepatic collagen content ranged from 4.5% to 6.3% and did not change significantly over the course of 2 years, regardless of treatment assignment. Biopsy specimens were also staged for fibrosis by the Ishak system, and of 216 subjects with evaluable liver biopsy specimens, 74 (34%) had no change, 80 (37%) progressed at least one stage, and 62 (29%) regressed at least one stage. In addition, 30 of the 191 (16%) without cirrhosis at entry progressed to cirrhosis over 2 years.

Diagnosis

No standardized criteria for the diagnosis of PSC have been universally adopted. The diagnosis of PSC generally occurs in the setting of cholestatic liver tests and is based on typical cholangiographic findings (see Imaging section earlier) (Fig. 70.4). Historically, ERCP was considered the standard for establishing a diagnosis of PSC but carries risks of bleeding, perforation, infection, and pancreatitis in up to 10% in patients with PSC.[157,199] A meta-analysis that included six large studies found that MRCP is sufficiently sensitive and specific to replace ERCP as the first-line diagnostic test. ERCP allows therapeutic interventions, but due to its risks, it should only be performed for these purposes and not for simple diagnosis of PSC.[4] PTC may also yield diagnostic images and allow therapeutic intervention but requires percutaneous puncture and should only be performed for therapeutic purposes when ERCP is not technically feasible (see Chapter 72).

Patients with IBD and a cholestatic pattern of liver biochemical test elevations should undergo imaging of the hepatobiliary system by MRCP due to the relatively high pretest probability of PSC (see Chapter 22). In the absence of IBD, secondary causes of sclerosing cholangitis must be excluded. US or CT is insufficient for a diagnosis of PSC. If the MRCP is of good quality and nondiagnostic, then liver biopsy to diagnose small-duct PSC or another liver disease should be considered. Testing for genetic causes of cholestasis, such as variants in *ABCB4*, should be considered in cases of small-duct PSC, particularly in the absence of IBD. ERCP should be used in patients in whom there is concern for malignancy or therapeutic dilation of a stricture is anticipated (Fig. 70.5).

Differential Diagnosis

In a patient with IBD and a cholangiogram characteristic of sclerosing cholangitis, the diagnosis of PSC can be made with confidence. However, secondary causes of sclerosing cholangitis must be excluded, especially in the absence of IBD (Table 70.1). Although differences between the features of PSC and SSC have been described, they are not sufficiently specific to make an accurate diagnosis (see Table 70.3).[157]

Choledocholithiasis and cholangiocarcinoma may both develop in conjunction with, or independent of, PSC. In the presence of extensive choledocholithiasis or diffuse cholangiocarcinoma, identifying underlying PSC may be difficult. Cholangiographic findings in patients with cirrhosis from causes other than PSC may at times be mistaken for PSC; however, cholangiography in cirrhotic patients without PSC typically shows diffuse intrahepatic attenuation of bile ducts without the ductal irregularity or stricturing seen in patients with PSC.

PBC is a chronic cholestatic condition that shares some clinical features with PSC (see Chapter 93); however, PBC predominantly affects middle-aged women, has no association with IBD, and is associated strongly with high titers of AMA. Although liver histologic findings in the two disorders may overlap (see earlier),[182] the distinction between the two is readily apparent on cholangiography. Patients with advanced PBC may demonstrate smooth tapering and narrowing of the intrahepatic bile ducts, but ductal irregularity or strictures are not seen, and extrahepatic biliary strictures do not occur. AMA-negative PBC may be difficult to distinguish from small-duct PSC because serologic profiles and cholangiographic findings may overlap, but the demographic and histologic features of the two disorders are distinct. Furthermore, the presence of PBC-specific ANA, such as anti-gp210 and anti-Sp100, may help diagnose AMA-negative PBC (see Chapter 93).[200] IgG4-

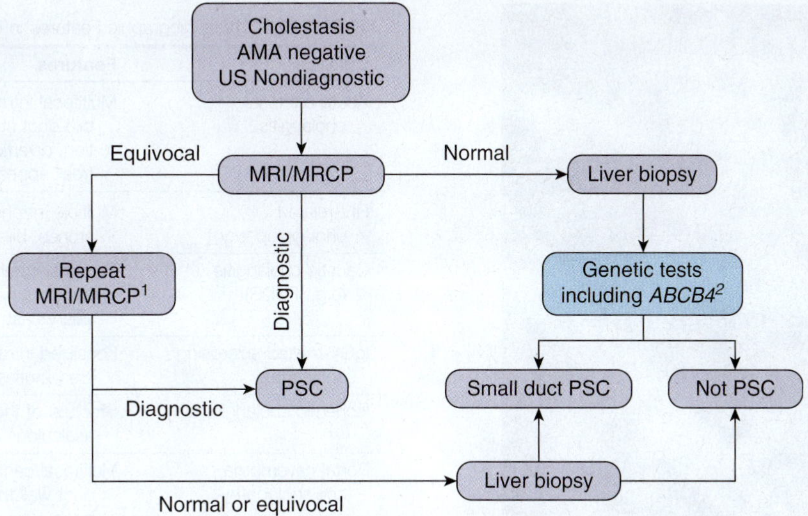

Fig. 70.4 Diagnostic algorithm for PSC. Patients typically present with cholestasis. Common causes of cholestasis can be excluded by US. The absence of AMA generally excludes PBC. In the absence of secondary causes of sclerosing cholangitis, an MRCP may be diagnostic of PSC. If the MRCP is of good quality and nondiagnostic, then liver biopsy should be performed. If histology is consistent with PSC in the presence of IBD, then small-duct PSC can be made. In the absence of IBD, testing for variants in the *ABCB4* gene and others associated with cholestasis should be conducted to exclude a genetic basis of the cholestasis. If the MRCP is equivocal, then a higher quality MRI should be considered or repeat MRI in 1 year. ERCP should not be used for diagnostic purposes.

sclerosing cholangitis, also known as *IgG4-related cholangitis* and sometimes seen with autoimmune pancreatitis, should also be excluded (see later).[201]

Natural History and Prognostic Models

PSC is a heterogeneous disease, with multiple clinically recognized phenotypes, that progresses at variable rates toward one or many possible outcomes. The disease typically progresses from a subclinical phase of normal liver biochemistries and absence of symptoms through periods of abnormal liver tests and development of symptoms and finally to cirrhosis and its complications. In studies of physician-recorded symptoms, patients with PSC who do not have symptoms are reported to make up 15%–44% of cohorts.[138,139] However, in a study of patient-reported symptoms, over half reported experiencing pruritus, abdominal pain, fatigue, or sleep disturbances.[8] Some reports have suggested that asymptomatic patients typically have a benign course of disease, but these must be interpreted with caution given the lack of correlation between physician recording of symptoms and patient experience.

The estimated overall prognosis of PSC has changed over time. Whether this is due to a change in the behavior of the disease, diagnosis of milder cases, or more representative sampling of patients is not clear. For example, a study of 174 patients with PSC in the Netherlands[202] suggested a better overall prognosis, with a median expected survival of 18 years compared with prior studies. The reason for improved survival in this study is not known, but patient data were predominantly from the 1990s, compared with data from the 1970s and 1980s in the other studies described earlier. Although therapeutic advances were not dramatic in the interim, earlier diagnosis in the 1990s may have led to differences in patient selection that appeared to affect outcomes. In agreement with this study, a large population-based study from the Netherlands that included 590 patients estimated median transplant-free survival time to be 21.2 years in nontransplant centers compared with 13.2 years among patients followed at transplant centers, suggesting a strong influence of referral bias.[7] Consistent with these findings is a median transplant-free survival of 14.5 years reported in the large International PSC Study Group registry of over 7000 patients, including those diagnosed several decades earlier and all from specialized centers.[31] By contrast, a patient-reported registry of just over 800 patients estimated the median transplant-free survival to be 21 years.[8] In general, older age at the time of diagnosis, male gender, large-duct PSC (as opposed to small-duct disease), and coexisting UC (in contrast to Crohn disease or no IBD) are associated with an increased likelihood of death or LT.[31]

Small-Duct PSC

Three studies initially examined the extended clinical follow-up in patients with small-duct PSC. A combined cohort of 83 patients was compared with 157 age- and gender-matched controls with large-duct PSC.[16] Twenty-two percent of patients with small-duct PSC progressed to large-duct disease over a median period of 7.4 years. Twenty patients with large-duct PSC developed cholangiocarcinoma, but the only case of this malignancy among patients with small-duct PSC was noted after the subject had progressed to large-duct PSC. In addition, patients with small-duct disease had a longer mean transplant-free survival (13 vs. 10 years). Therefore, in some cases, small-duct PSC may represent an early stage of PSC and progress to large-duct PSC, but it does not seem to be associated with cholangiocarcinoma. Small-duct PSC is associated with better long-term survival than classic PSC.

PSC in Children

PSC has a progressive course in children as well. In a large international study that included 781 children with PSC from 36

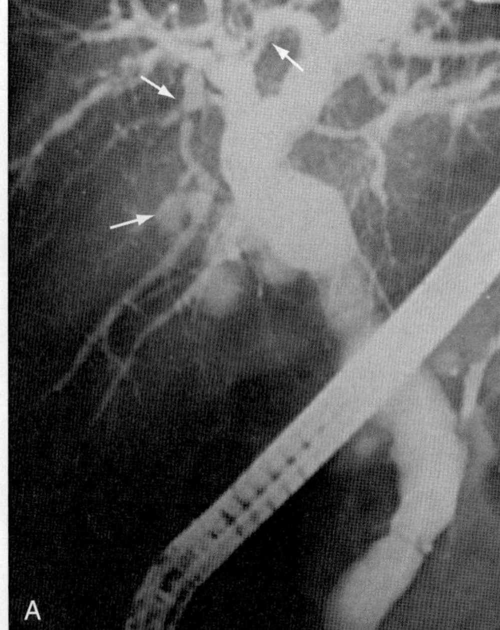

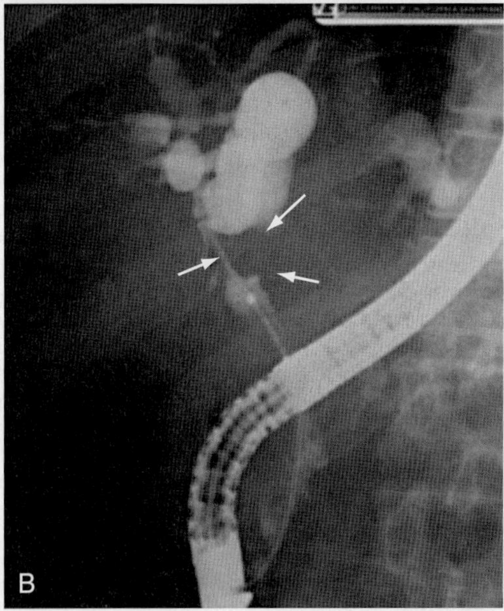

Fig. 70.5 Cholangiographic progression of cholangiocarcinoma complicating PSC. This 43-year-old man with a history of mild UC for 3 years presented with pruritus and an elevated serum alkaline phosphatase level. (A) Initial ERCP showed mild, diffuse changes compatible with uncomplicated PSC. Several short, annular strictures and cholangiectasias are present in the intrahepatic ducts (*arrows*), with a single, short, annular stricture of the bile duct. The cystic duct is not filled. (B) A second ERCP was performed 7 months later after progressive jaundice and weight loss developed rapidly. Now a 2-cm mass is projecting into, and obstructing, the common hepatic duct (*arrows*). A catheter has been passed beyond the obstructing mass. There is marked dilatation of the left main duct proximal to the obstruction; the right main duct is completely occluded.

institutions, the median age at diagnosis was 12 years; 39% were female, and 76% had coexisting IBD.[37] Large-duct PSC was present in 87% and associated with AIH in one-third of the patients. Complications of portal hypertension were present in 5% of patients at the time of diagnosis of PSC and in 38% after 10 years. Transplant-free survival was 88% at 5 years and 70% at 10 years. Interestingly, 8 children developed cholangiocarcinoma at a median of 6 years after their diagnosis.

TABLE 70.3 Cholangiographic Features in PSC and SSC

Disease	Features
Acute bacterial cholangitis	Multifocal intrahepatic and extrahepatic bile duct strictures, slight biliary dilatation, diverticular outpouchings, "pruned tree" appearance
HIV-related cholangiopathy	Multiple intrahepatic bile duct strictures, stones, biliary abscesses
Caustic cholangitis (e.g., FUDR)	Proximal intrahepatic bile duct strictures, bile duct necrosis, bilomas, abscesses, biliary cast
IgG4-related sclerosing cholangitis	Localized intrahepatic bile duct strictures, irregularities of bile duct wall
Ischemic cholangiopathy	Stricture of the distal bile duct, papillitis, acalculous cholecystitis
Portal cavernoma cholangiopathy	Multifocal central bile duct strictures, bile duct wall thickening with visible lumen, pancreatic abnormalities compatible with autoimmune pancreatitis
PSC	Central and extrahepatic bile duct irregularities

FUDR, Floxuridine; *IgG4*, immunoglobulin G4.

Prognostic Models

Natural history studies have provided insight into the specific clinical, biochemical, and histologic features of PSC that may influence prognosis. The first model was presented in Wiesner et al.[136] and was based on age, serum bilirubin level, hemoglobin value, presence or absence of IBD, and histologic stage. With this model, three risk groups (low, intermediate, high) were identified, and predicted survival curves were shown to be similar to observed survival curves. Since then, other models have been developed, including the revised Mayo Risk Score, which is best at estimating transplant-free survival up to 4 years of follow-up.[203] Newer models include the Amsterdam-Oxford Model,[204] UK-PSC Score,[205] PSC Risk Estimate Tool (PREsTo),[206] and for pediatric patients the SCOPE model.[207] Each model is best suited to specific patient populations but generally uses the same variables and has similar performance characteristics (Table 70.4).

A validated prognostic model taking into consideration the cholangiographic aspects of PSC is lacking. Ponsioen et al. incorporated the Amsterdam cholangiography staging system, based on the type and severity of intrahepatic and extrahepatic involvement on ERCP, into a model to calculate a prognostic index.[202] The cholangiographic staging was correlated inversely with survival, confirming the prognostic value for cholangiographic findings. Semiquantitative scores of MRCP images, including the Anali and DiStrict scores, have been created to predict the course of the disease[162,163] The Anali score includes dilatation of the intrahepatic bile ducts, hepatic dysmorphy, and portal hypertension if MRI is performed without gadolinium and hepatic dysmorphy and parenchymal enhancement heterogeneity if gadolinium is used. However, the Anali score has high interobserver variability.[208]In contrast, the DiStrict score includes measures of dilation and stricture of the intrahepatic and extrahepatic ducts and has reported high inter- and intrareader agreements.[163]More sophisticated, quantitative analyses of MRCP

TABLE 70.4 Independent Predictors of Survival and Prognostic Index Formulas Used in Natural History Models of PSC

Revised Mayo Model[203]	Amsterdam-Oxford Model[204]	UK-PSC Score[a,205]	PREsTO[206]	SCOPE[207]
Patient Population	—	—	—	—
Adult	—	—	—	Pediatric
Outcome				
Liver transplant/death	Liver transplant/death	Liver transplant/ death	Hepatic decompensation	Liver transplant listing/death from liver disease
Age	Age	Age	Age	—
—	Age at diagnosis	—	Disease duration	—
—	PSC subtype	Extrahepatic disease	—	Large-duct PSC
Total bilirubin	Total bilirubin	Total bilirubin	Total bilirubin	Total bilirubin
Albumin	Albumin	Albumin	Albumin	—
AST	AST	—	AST	—
—	Alkaline phosphatase	Alkaline phosphatase	Alkaline phosphatase	r-Glutamyl transferase
Variceal bleeding	Platelets	Platelets	—	Platelets
—	—	—	Sodium	—

[a]UK-PSC Score for long-term prognosis.

images have been developed and identified features that are associated with clinical outcomes.[164,166,209]

These models can be useful in the clinical care of patients with PSC but must be used with caution when counseling the individual patient. They may facilitate discussion about the risk and possible timing of LT by comparing predicted survival with readily available post-LT survival rates. The availability of multiple models with differing prognostic variables, however, may be confusing in clinical practice. The models also may not account for other clinical events, such as the development of cholangiocarcinoma, that may affect prognosis in patients with PSC.

Complications

Cholestasis

The complications associated with all causes of chronic cholestasis may develop in patients with PSC (see also Chapter 22 and 93). Pruritus is one of the most common symptoms of PSC and adversely affects quality of life.[8,210–213] Severe excoriations and debilitating symptoms may develop. The pathogenesis of pruritus in chronic cholestasis is poorly understood, and response to therapy is inconsistent (see Chapter 93). The accumulation of bile acids in the plasma and tissue of cholestatic patients has been cited as a potential cause of pruritus, and the pruritus of cholestasis has typically been treated with oral administration of bile acid–binding resins such as cholestyramine. Not all patients with elevated serum bile acid levels itch, however, and there is inconsistent correlation between the degree of bile acid elevation and the intensity of itching. In addition, pruritus is frequently intermittent, despite the relative stability of serum bile acid levels. Several lines of evidence suggest that cholestasis is associated with an increased level of endogenous opioids. In animal models, cholestasis is associated with an increase in plasma levels of endogenous opioids.[214] In humans, cholestatic patients may experience opiate withdrawal-like symptoms after the administration of an opioid antagonist. In addition, the administration of naloxone and naltrexone, which have opioid antagonist properties, has been reported to relieve pruritus in cholestatic patients in small clinical trials.[215,216]

Lysophosphatidic acid is a neurotransmitter potentially involved in the mediation of cholestatic itch. Activity of autotaxin, the enzyme that synthesizes lysophosphatidic acid from lysophosphatidylcholine, correlates with the presence and intensity of cholestatic itching. In some reports, it correlates with reduction in bile acids and effectiveness of therapeutic interventions for itching.[217,218] More recently, IL-31 was identified as a target for the treatment of pruritus from atopic dermatitis, and serum levels have been shown to be elevated in cholestatic liver diseases, including PSC.[219,220]

Nutritional deficiencies may complicate chronic cholestasis in patients with advanced PSC. Intestinal absorption of the fat-soluble vitamins A, D, E, and K is particularly affected and is thought to be related to decreased intestinal concentrations of conjugated bile acids, with one study reporting deficiencies of vitamins A, D, and E in 40%, 14%, and 2% of patients enrolled in a clinical trial and in 82%, 57%, and 43% of patients being evaluated for LT.[221] Concomitant diseases such as IBD, chronic pancreatitis, and celiac disease may also contribute to intestinal malabsorption. Clinical consequences include night blindness (vitamin A deficiency) and coagulopathy (vitamin K deficiency).

The importance of metabolic bone disease, also referred to as *hepatic osteodystrophy*, is often underrecognized in patients with PSC. Two forms of metabolic bone disease may develop: osteomalacia and osteoporosis. With improvements in nutritional management, osteomalacia (decreased bone mineralization) is now relatively rare, and most bone disease in cholestatic patients is osteoporosis. Bone mineral density is significantly lower in patients with PSC than in age- and sex-matched controls[222]; one-third of patients with PSC have bone mineral density below 1.0 standard deviation in the hip or spine, with a relatively high rate of nonvertebral fragility fractures (18%).[223] The pathogenesis of bone density loss in PSC and other chronic cholestatic liver diseases is unknown. Intestinal malabsorption of vitamin D is probably not the primary abnormality, because serum vitamin D levels are often normal, and vitamin D repletion does not usually have a major impact on the severity of osteoporosis. Longstanding concomitant IBD is an independent risk factor for osteoporosis in this population, and the use of glucocorticoids may play a role in exacerbating bone loss.

Biliary Stones

Cholelithiasis and choledocholithiasis are more common in patients with PSC than in the general population. Gallstones, often pigmented calcium bilirubinate stones, are found in approximately 25% of patients with PSC (see Chapter 67).[169] Biliary strictures may predispose to bile stasis and intraductal sludge and stone formation. US has only an intermediate sensitivity for detecting intraductal stones. Therefore patients with PSC and worsening cholestasis or jaundice should undergo diagnostic ERCP (with the anticipation of a therapeutic intervention) to distinguish biliary stone disease from the development of a dominant stricture or cholangiocarcinoma.

Cholangiocarcinoma

Cholangiocarcinoma is a feared complication of PSC arising from bile duct epithelium (see Chapter 71). PSC is a premalignant condition of the biliary tract, analogous to the relationship between UC and carcinoma of the colon. The lifetime risk of developing cholangiocarcinoma in patients with PSC ranges between 5% and 20% with the greatest risk in the first year following the diagnosis of PSC, followed by a 0.5%–1.5% annual frequency.[7,31,224,225] Tumors are most commonly found in the common hepatic duct and perihilar region but may involve only the bile duct, intrahepatic ducts, and cystic duct. Since the introduction of LT, cholangiocarcinoma has become the leading cause of death in patients with PSC. Risk factors for the development of cholangiocarcinoma in patients with PSC include older age, male sex, large-duct PSC, and UC, whereas small-duct PSC and Crohn disease or absence of IBD appear to be protective.[31,224–227] Serum alkaline phosphatase levels at or near normal may also be protective against the development of cholangiocarcinoma.[228,229]

The pathogenesis of cholangiocarcinoma in PSC is poorly understood. Although cholangiocarcinoma may complicate any stage of the disease, chronic inflammation is thought to predispose to epithelial dysplasia and an increased risk of malignant transformation. A role for proinflammatory cytokines in stimulating oxidative DNA damage and inactivation of DNA repair processes has been postulated.

Biliary malignancy should be suspected when a patient with PSC exhibits clinical deterioration with worsening jaundice, weight loss, or abdominal pain; however, a benign dominant stricture without cholangiocarcinoma may present identically. The diagnosis of cholangiocarcinoma presents a particular challenge in patients with PSC. A malignant biliary stricture may be indistinguishable from the underlying PSC on cholangiogram (Fig. 70.5). Because of the tendency of cholangiocarcinoma to grow in sheets as opposed to a discrete mass, cross-sectional imaging with CT or MRI has low sensitivity for detection of cholangiocarcinoma.

Carbohydrate antigen 19-9 (CA19-9) has been the most extensively tested potential serum marker for cholangiocarcinoma. CA19-9 is a glycolipid expressed by many different cancers, and serum levels can be increased during cholestasis. Although an optimal cutoff value of 129 U/mL demonstrated sensitivity of 78% and specificity of 98% in one study, another study using a cutoff of 20 U/mL demonstrated a sensitivity of 78% and specificity of 67%. In addition, CA19-9 requires Lewis blood group antigen expression, which 5%–10% of the population lack. Further, variants of the fucosyltransferase genes *FUT2* and *FUT3* affect serum levels of CA19-9. Adjusting for these genotypes with different cutoff values may improve the sensitivity of CA19-9.[230]

Obtaining an adequate tissue sample presents a particular challenge in the diagnosis of cholangiocarcinoma. Brush cytology by ERCP is highly specific for the diagnosis of cholangiocarcinoma; however, the sensitivity of this approach is less than 60%.[231,232] The introduction of intraductal biopsies was expected to increase the detection of biliary malignancies, but this expectation has not been substantiated. Early studies suggested that combining brush cytology and biopsy increased the sensitivity for the identification of malignancy to 70%.[233] The sensitivity of cytologic examination may be increased by the use of specialized techniques such as fluorescent in situ hybridization, or FISH, to identify aneusomy, an equivalent of aneuploidy.[234,235] The presence of an increased number of copies of chromosomes 3, 7, or 17 and/or deletion of 9p21 increases the sensitivity of cytology to 89%,[236] which may be improved with a specific set of pancreatobiliary FISH probes.[237] An approach that includes cytology, biopsy, and FISH was reported to have an overall sensitivity of 82%, specificity of 100%, positive predictive value of 100%, and negative predictive value of 87%.[238] Other modalities, including EUS, intraductal US, and cholangioscopy, may improve the diagnostic accuracy of tissue sampling (see Chapter 72).

The development of cholangiocarcinoma is ominous, with a median survival of 5 months after diagnosis.[239] Due to the high rate of recurrence of cholangiocarcinoma after LT, few patients with cholangiocarcinoma are considered candidates for LT (see Chapter 71). In addition, up to 10% of patients with PSC who undergo LT may be found to have an occult cholangiocarcinoma.[239]

Screening for cholangiocarcinoma in patients with PSC remains controversial without strong evidence that survival is improved.[240–242] Nevertheless, the incidence of cholangiocarcinoma in patients with PSC is high, and the consequences are significant, and current guidelines recommend annual screening with MRI/MRCP with or without measurement of serum CA19-9 levels.[4,243,244]

Patients with PSC are also at increased risk for the development of gallbladder cancer and, in patients with cirrhosis, HCC. Although prior estimates of the frequency of gallbladder cancer in PSC have been 3%–14%,[245] an analysis of over 7000 patients with PSC from an international consortium found the frequency of gallbladder cancer and HCC in patients with PSC to each be only 0.8%.[31] Still, professional societies in both North America and Europe have recommended annual screening for gallbladder cancer using US (see also Chapters 71 and 98).[4,244]

Colonic Neoplasia

Patients with concomitant PSC and UC are at significantly higher risk for developing colonic neoplasia (dysplasia or carcinoma) than patients with UC alone.[7,246,247] UC alone is known to be associated with an increased risk of colonic dysplasia and carcinoma (see Chapter 118); the duration and extent of disease are the strongest associated risk factors. In a population-based study of 590 cases of PSC in the Netherlands, the cumulative risk of high-grade dysplasia or colorectal cancer after 10, 20, and 30 years from the diagnosis of PSC was 3%, 7%, and 13%, respectively. The risk of colorectal cancer in PSC patients with UC was increased 9-fold compared with an age- and gender-matched population and 10-fold compared with UC controls.[7] Notably, colorectal cancer occurred at a younger age in PSC-IBD patients compared with patients with UC, and surveillance colonoscopy was associated with lower colorectal cancer-related mortality. In a large longitudinal collaborative study from the United States and the Netherlands, 1911 patients with colonic IBD were evaluated for development of advanced colorectal neoplasia. Although the degree of inflammation and the rate of low-grade dysplasia did not differ between groups, patients with PSC-IBD had a twofold increased risk of developing advanced colorectal neoplasia compared with patients without PSC.[247] In addition to PSC, increasing age and active colonic inflammation were independent risk factors for colorectal neoplasia. Additionally, the rate of development of advanced neoplasia following a diagnosis of low-grade dysplasia was 2.5 times higher in patients with PSC-IBD.

Patients with PSC and UC are also more likely than patients with UC alone to have synchronous sites of dysplasia in the colon. A systematic review, including 14 surveillance studies of patients with UC and low-grade dysplasia, confirmed that PSC, invisible dysplasia, distal location, and multifocal low-grade dysplasia are associated with dysplasia progression to colorectal cancer.[248] PSC patients without IBD do not appear to be at increased risk of colorectal cancer.[7]

The mechanisms by which PSC confers an added risk of colonic neoplasia are not well understood. A high colonic concentration of secondary bile acids may play a role because patients with UC and colonic dysplasia or carcinoma have higher fecal bile acid concentrations than patients with UC who do not have dysplasia or carcinoma.[249] This theory is supported by the higher frequency of right-sided colon cancer in patients with UC and PSC than in those with UC alone. Remarkably, the composition of gut microbiota in patients with PSC-IBD differs significantly from that of patients with IBD alone, with decreased diversity of and enrichment in organisms from the *Ruminococcus* and *Fusobacterium* genera.[87,88,92] In contrast to colonic dysplasia in UC, patients with PSC appear to have dysplasia that is characterized by a restricted set of Th17 T cells, suggesting an antigen-driven etiology.[250] Unique correlations between gut microbiota and stool bile acids in patients with PSC-IBD are also described.[85]

Increased colonic secondary bile acid concentrations may also explain the possible chemoprotective effect of UDCA against the development of colonic neoplasia. Two studies have reported that UDCA use is associated with a lower risk of colonic dysplasia or cancer in patients with UC and PSC.[251,252] UDCA may confer protection against colonic neoplasia by reducing colonic concentrations of secondary bile acids, as well as by affecting expression of protein kinase C isoforms, metabolism of arachidonic acid, and expression of COX-2.[253–256] On the other hand, a nested cohort study of patients with PSC enrolled in a double-blind, placebo-controlled trial of high-dose (25–30 mg/kg/day) UDCA found that patients treated with UDCA had a significantly higher risk of developing colorectal neoplasia than did those treated with placebo.[257] Given these conflicting data, UDCA is not currently recommended for chemoprevention of colorectal neoplasia in patients with PSC and IBD.[159]

Patients with PSC who have UC should undergo surveillance for the detection of colonic dysplasia or cancer every 1–2 years,[4] beginning at the time of diagnosis of PSC. As in patients with UC alone, multiple mucosal biopsy specimens should be obtained (see Chapter 118). Although targeted biopsies using chromoendoscopy increase the rate of detection of neoplasia, random biopsies detect an additional 20% of neoplastic sites and should be performed in association with chromoendoscopy.[258] Surveillance should continue even after LT, because these patients remain at increased risk of colonic neoplasia.[259–261] Patients without known IBD should undergo a colonoscopy at the time PSC is diagnosed. In these patients, multiple biopsies should be obtained to exclude microscopic evidence of colitis. If biopsies are negative, a repeat colonoscopy may be considered at 5-year intervals.[4,262]

Peristomal Varices

Varices at the stoma may develop in up to a quarter of PSC patients who have undergone proctocolectomy with ileostomy for IBD.[263] These varices may bleed spontaneously, and the bleeding may be dramatic. Treatment modalities that may initially be effective in achieving hemostasis include injection sclerotherapy, coil embolization, surgical stomal revision, and TIPS placement (see Chapter 94).[264–266] Nevertheless, recurrent bleeding is common, and LT should be considered to relieve portal hypertension and treat the underlying liver disease.

Treatment

Except for LT, no specific therapy has proved effective for treating PSC. The objectives of management prior to liver decompensation should be the treatment of complications, such as bacterial cholangitis and pruritus, prevention of osteoporosis and nutritional deficiencies, and early diagnosis of malignancies, including cholangiocarcinoma, gallbladder cancer, and colon cancer. Once the liver disease is advanced, then evaluation for LT should be initiated.

Medical Treatment of the Underlying Disease

A wide variety of medications have been studied in patients with PSC, with only a few randomized, placebo-controlled trials of significant size with UDCA (Table 70.5). In addition, the defined study endpoints, whether clinical, biochemical, histologic, or a risk score, have varied greatly among published studies. Consensus on the surrogate endpoints continues to evolve but should improve the likelihood of successful drug development.[199,267] Nevertheless, no current medical treatment has been shown to alter the natural course of PSC.

UDCA has been the most extensively studied drug in patients with PSC through several controlled clinical trials.[185,192,194,268–272] The mechanisms by which UDCA is thought to exert a beneficial effect in cholestatic conditions include protection of cholangiocytes against cytotoxic hydrophobic bile acids, stimulation of hepatobiliary secretion, protection of hepatocytes against bile acid–induced apoptosis, and induction of antioxidants (see also Chapter 93).[273,274] Although the majority of clinical trials have demonstrated improvement in serum liver biochemical test levels, none have demonstrated a survival benefit or delay in the requirement for LT. In addition, there have been no beneficial

TABLE 70.5 Randomized Placebo-Controlled Trials of Ursodeoxycholic Acid for PSC*

Year	*N*	UDCA Dose (mg/kg/day)	Duration (months)	Outcome	References
1997	105	13–15	24	No benefit in time to treatment failure (composite of death, LT, cirrhosis, histologic progression >2 stages, decompensated cirrhosis, liver biochemistries, or symptomatic progression) Improved liver biochemistry	[194]
2001	26	20	24	Improved liver biochemistries, reduced histologic, and cholangiographic progression	[185]
2005	219	17–23	60	No benefit in transplant-free survival, liver biochemistries, or quality of life	[271]
2008	31	10 vs. 20 vs. 30	24	Improved liver biochemistries and Mayo Risk Score (high dose only)	[197]
2009	150	28–30	60	No benefit, increased adverse events	[192]

effects of UDCA on fatigue, pruritus, or development of cholangiocarcinoma.

Because of the disappointing results with standard-dose UDCA, several groups studied the use of UDCA up to 30 mg/kg daily, twice the dose recommended for PBC.[185,192,270,271] A large study of 219 Scandinavian patients randomized to 17–23 mg/kg/day of UDCA or placebo for 5 years failed to show any difference in transplant-free survival. The investigators were unable to recruit the number needed to adequately power the study, and only 18 of 219 patients reached the endpoint over 5 years, reflecting the inherent difficulty with PSC clinical trials. The results of a prospective, placebo-controlled randomized trial of UDCA in a dose of 25–30 mg/kg/day for 6 years, however, demonstrated a higher risk of death, need for LT, and development of varices in patients receiving high-dose UDCA compared with those receiving placebo.[275] Nevertheless, post hoc analyses of these studies have suggested that patients in whom liver biochemical test levels improve may obtain some clinical benefit,[229,276] and withdrawal of UDCA has been associated with deterioration in serum biochemical liver test levels and the Mayo Risk Score in addition to increased pruritus.[277]

Several newer bile acid–modulating agents have shown promising initial results in improving liver biochemical test levels. These have included *nor*-UDCA, a C_{23} homolog of UDCA with potent choleretic activity[278] that, in preclinical studies, showed significant anticholestatic, anti-inflammatory, and anti-proliferative properties [279] with less toxicity than UDCA. In a multicenter phase 2 clinical trial in Europe, *nor*-UDCA improved serum alkaline phosphatase levels regardless of prior UDCA use.[280]

The immunologic basis of PSC would appear to make immunosuppressive therapy a reasonable treatment option. Glucocorticoids, administered both orally and via nasobiliary lavage, have not shown a clear benefit in uncontrolled studies.[281] Oral budesonide has been evaluated in an uncontrolled pilot study in 21 patients with PSC but was not effective and resulted in significant loss of bone mass.[282] In a small prospective, controlled trial of methotrexate, no biochemical, histologic, or cholangiographic differences between therapy and placebo were seen after 2 years of treatment.[283] A study of tacrolimus demonstrated significant biochemical improvement after 1 year but no change in cholangiographic or histologic severity.[284] Neither infliximab nor etanercept, both of which are TNF-α inhibitors, showed in clinical trials a benefit in patients with PSC.[198,285] Real-world data has also failed to show any potential benefit of TNF-α inhibitors or anti-integrin agents used for the treatment of IBD in patients with concomitant IBD.[286–288]

Antibiotics have been used with no clear benefit but remain under study. In 14 pediatric patients with PSC treated with oral vancomycin, all had improvement in liver biochemical test levels, especially those without cirrhosis.[289] The same investigators subsequently found that oral vancomycin improved liver histology and imaging findings, while increasing plasma levels of transforming growth factor-β (TGF-β) and peripheral Tregs, thereby suggesting an immunomodulatory mechanism.[290] In adults, oral vancomycin demonstrated a modest reduction in serum alkaline phosphatase levels over 12 weeks of treatment[291] and the only randomized, placebo-controlled trial of 12-week duration ($n = 35$) reported biochemical improvements.[292] Despite these promising results, the potential harm from indiscriminate alterations in gut flora, as illustrated by the *Mdr2*-null mouse raised in a germ-free environment, should temper enthusiasm for their widespread use.[96–98]

Other approaches under study include antifibrotic medications, but to date none has shown significant benefit. Combination therapy targeting several pathways may be needed for effective therapy in PSC. Historically, combinations of various agents, such as azathioprine, glucocorticoids, UDCA, and antibiotics, have been studied in a limited fashion.[196,293,294] The results of these studies have been mixed, with some showing no benefit and others demonstrating histologic improvement in small numbers of patients. Moreover, combination therapy increases the risk of adverse drug reactions.

Several novel clinical approaches are being taken to find an effective treatment for PSC but face significant barriers. Most approaches target cholestasis and include FXR and peroxisome-proliferator-activated receptor (PPAR) agonists. The largest randomized controlled trial in PSC investigated the effects of the nonsteroidal FXR agonist cilofexor on histologic progression but was terminated due to futility.[295] This study, along with the simtuzumab trial described earlier,[186] illustrates the difficulties in clinical trial design for PSC. Although histologic staging is associated with clinical endpoints, there are significant shortcomings to its use in trials. Specifically, fibrosis progression is slow especially in those with early stage disease, and histologic assessments do not reflect dynamic changes in fibrosis activity. In addition, there is a large placebo effect, with more than half of placebo-treated patients showing improvement or no progression. A more dynamic serum measure of fibrosis activity, such as the enhanced liver fibrosis (ELF) test, has been shown to be predictive of transplant-free survival[296,297] and responsive to treatment in a 12-week treatment period.[298] However, questions remain regarding the liver specificity of ELF and the change in ELF required to be clinically meaningful.[299]

As a silver lining, in a 12-week phase 2 placebo-controlled randomized clinical trial including 68 patients, treatment with the PPAR alpha/delta agonist elafibranor was well tolerated and led to significant improvements in liver biochemistries and pruritus. A 96 week open label extension is ongoing.[299a]

Medical Treatment of Complications

An important component in the medical care of patients with PSC is the management of complications of the disease, including pruritus, nutritional deficiencies, and bacterial cholangitis. Pruritus should be managed as in other cholestatic conditions (see Chapter 93), including counseling on the exacerbating effects of heat and other stimuli on pruritus. Anion-exchange resins, such as cholestyramine, colestipol hydrochloride, or colesevelam, are considered first-line therapy, although compliance is a problem due to their relative unpalatability, constipating effects, and interference with the absorption of other medications. Bezafibrate, a fibrate with PPAR and activity, is effective in treating cholestatic pruritus, including in PSC.[300] However, bezafibrate is not currently available in the United States and many other countries. Whether other PPAR agonists such as fenofibrate with activity restricted to PPAR-, have similar effects is unknown. Rifampin may be an effective and safe alternative for patients who do not respond to these measures.[301] Opioid antagonists such as naloxone and naltrexone have also been shown to be effective for cholestatic pruritus, although self-limited episodes of opioid withdrawal-like symptoms may occur.[215,216,302,303] Selective serotonin reuptake inhibitors have shown limited efficacy.[304] Patients with severe pruritus who are unresponsive to these measures and who do not obtain relief from endoscopic or percutaneous drainage (see later) may need to be considered for plasmapheresis or nasobiliary drainage. LT may be considered for intractable pruritus but is unlikely to be a viable option unless a suitable living donor is available.

Patients with PSC should be screened for nutritional deficiencies by measurement of fat-soluble vitamin levels and the INR. In most patients, vitamin supplements are given orally, but a parenteral route may be necessary in patients with severe intestinal fat malabsorption. Along with vitamin D deficiency, osteopenia is frequent in patients with PSC, and the severity is unrelated to the severity of liver disease.[305] Therefore patients with PSC should be screened at diagnosis and every 2–3 years for mineral bone deficiency. If osteopenia is detected, vitamin D (1000 IU/day) and calcium (1–1.5 g/day) repletion should be started, whereas bisphosphonate therapy should be considered in those with osteoporosis.[158] Prolongation of the INR is more likely to be the result of advanced liver disease than of vitamin K deficiency, although a trial of oral vitamin K is warranted in patients with coagulopathy (see Chapter 94).

Bacterial cholangitis is a frequent complication of PSC and occurs in approximately 10% of patients annually. In addition to the risk of spontaneous bacterial cholangitis, patients with PSC are at high risk of cholangitis following biliary instrumentation and should receive antibiotic prophylaxis following any biliary procedure, usually with a 5–7-day course of a fluoroquinolone, cephalosporin, or a beta-lactamase inhibitor. There are no established criteria for the diagnosis of bacterial cholangitis in PSC; established criteria such as the Tokyo Guidelines for acute cholangitis (see Chapter 67) rely on abnormal liver biochemical test levels and are not applicable in PSC. Bacterial cholangitis in patients with PSC can be indolent, and the illness should be suspected in the presence of fever, leukocytosis, RUQ pain, or a worsening of liver biochemical test levels. Although some patients have recurring bouts of bacterial cholangitis that can be debilitating, bacterial cholangitis did not increase the risk of waitlist mortality in a multicenter study of patients with PSC listed for LT.[306] Patients with recurring cholangitis may benefit from long-term suppressive antibiotic prophylaxis with rotating courses of amoxicillin-clavulanic acid, ciprofloxacin, and/or trimethoprim/sulfamethoxazole every 3–4 weeks. Patients with cirrhosis and recurrent episodes of severe cholangitis requiring intensive care may qualify for liver transplantation in the absence of hepatic decompensation.

Endoscopic Management

In select patients, endoscopic therapy for PSC carries the potential to relieve jaundice, pruritus, and abdominal pain; improve biochemical cholestasis; decrease the frequency of episodes of bacterial cholangitis; and improve bile flow. In theory, improved long-term biliary patency could slow the progression of the disease and prevent or delay biliary cirrhosis, but studies of endoscopic intervention in patients with PSC have been small, retrospective, and uncontrolled. Therefore routine endoscopic therapy in PSC is not recommended.

Patients who are most likely to benefit from endoscopic intervention are those with a known or suspected dominant stricture, defined as a stenotic area with diameter less than or equal to 1.5 mm in the bile duct or less than or equal to 1 mm in the hepatic duct,[307] or a relevant stricture, specifically any stricture of the common bile duct, common hepatic duct associated with worsening jaundice or pruritus, cholangitis, or abdominal pain.[4] Dominant strictures are associated with reduced transplant-free survival[225] and multiple studies have reported significant improvements in clinical, biochemical, and cholangiographic endpoints in patients with a dominant stricture treated with endoscopic therapy,[308–312] usually balloon dilation with or without temporary stent placement. Sphincterotomy is controversial because it can result in further sclerosis of the distal biliary tract and increase the risk of bacterial cholangitis. Despite an increased risk of periprocedural bleeding, especially in cirrhotic patients, sphincterotomy may protect against post-ERCP pancreatitis in those who are likely to undergo multiple ERCPs with complex cannulation.

Choledocholithiasis should be considered in patients with worsening cholestasis. In as many as 30% of the cases, small stones may be missed by ERCP and regarded as wall irregularities, consistent with PSC.[313] Use of direct cholangioscopy enables the detection of these stones and the use of lithotripsy, if needed. Direct visualization with cholangioscopy is also useful for the evaluation of dominant strictures and allows targeted biopsies, which may improve overall diagnostic accuracy compared with ERCP.[314]

Placement of a biliary stent after balloon dilation appears to increase the risk of complications compared with balloon dilation alone.[315,316] Professional society guidelines recommend avoiding routine placement of a stent for dominant biliary strictures in PSC, although short-term stenting (<2 weeks) may be required for tight strictures.[157,159] Importantly, patients with PSC should receive antibiotic prophylaxis prior to undergoing ERCP, with continuation of treatment for 3–5 days after the ERCP.

Three studies have suggested that progression of the underlying disease process may be slowed by endoscopic therapy of a dominant stricture. Baluyut et al.[317] performed graduated and balloon dilation, with or without stent placement, in 63 patients with PSC, with a median follow-up of 34 months, and observed a 5-year survival that was significantly better than the survival predicted by the revised Mayo Risk Score (see Table 70.4). Stiehl et al.[307] performed endoscopic balloon dilation and occasional stent placement in 52 patients with PSC in whom a dominant stricture developed while the patients were on therapy with UDCA. Actuarial survival free of LT at 3, 5, and 7 years was significantly better than that predicted from the multicenter model score (see Table 70.4). An extension of this study that included 96 patients suggested that there was an improvement in LT-free survival with dilation.[318] Finally, a retrospective study by Gluck et al.[319] reported that patients who underwent endoscopic therapy had a significantly higher survival rate than predicted by the revised Mayo model score at 3 and 4 years.

Endoscopic therapy in PSC has important limitations, including increased risks of complications of ERCP, such as pancreatitis, cholangitis, worsening cholestasis, and perforation, with an overall rate of 7.3%–10%.[319] Patients with diffuse intrahepatic biliary stricturing and no dominant stricture are less likely to derive benefit from endoscopic intervention and may be at higher risk of post-ERCP cholangitis.[320] If ERCP is performed in expert hands and only for specific indications such as worsening jaundice, pruritus, or cholangitis—that is, for the subgroup of patients who are most likely to benefit from therapy—the risks in patients unlikely to benefit will be minimized (see Chapter 72).[321] In light of the limitations of the studies suggesting a benefit and the risks of biliary manipulation in PSC, routine endoscopic intervention for stricture management remains controversial.

Percutaneous Management

PTC with balloon dilation, stenting, or both can also be undertaken to treat biliary strictures in patients with PSC. This approach is typically recommended only when endoscopic intervention is contraindicated or unsuccessful because of the added risks of bleeding and bile peritonitis, as well as patient discomfort associated with percutaneous intervention (see Chapter 72).

Surgical Management

Biliary Surgery

The role of biliary surgery in PSC has diminished considerably with improvements in endoscopic therapy and the advent of LT. Resection of a dominant stricture of the bile duct or near the hepatic bifurcation followed by hepaticojejunostomy or choledochojejunostomy has been the most commonly performed operations.[322–324] Postoperative mortality is increased significantly in patients with PSC and cirrhosis. In addition, biliary surgery may complicate future LT. Currently, biliary surgery in patients with PSC is rarely indicated and should be reserved for the small subset of patients who have early stage PSC and biliary strictures that are not amenable to endoscopic or percutaneous intervention.

LT

LT is the only therapy that has been shown conclusively to improve the natural history of PSC. In addition, quality of life improves after LT.[325,326] As in other liver diseases, the procedure is recommended for patients with PSC in whom decompensated cirrhosis and complications of portal hypertension develop (see Chapter 99). Recurrent cholangitis, intractable pruritus, and early stage perihilar cholangiocarcinoma are infrequent indications for LT. The percentage of adult liver transplants performed for PSC in the United States has been stable, fluctuating between 4.0% and 4.8%, since 2005.[327] Although early studies suggested that patients undergoing LT for PSC should have a Roux-en-Y bile duct anastomosis, this dogma has been challenged. Several studies now indicate that a duct-to-duct anastomosis is associated with lower rates of posttransplant cholangitis and late-onset nonanastomotic strictures compared with a Roux-en-Y anastomosis, while maintaining similar patient and graft survival rates (see Chapter 99).[328–330]

Patient and graft survival after LT for PSC is excellent.[331–333] A large single-center experience demonstrated 1-, 5-, and 10-year actuarial patient survival rates of 93.7%, 86.4%, and 69.8%, respectively. Corresponding graft survival rates were 83.4%, 79.0%, and 60.5%.[331] Overall, survival rates after LT for PSC are significantly better than those for any other disease except PBC.[334,335] Recipient factors that have been associated with a worse prognosis after LT for PSC are older age, decreased serum albumin level, renal failure, Child-Pugh class C cirrhosis, and advanced UNOS status.[334,336,337]

The presence of cholangiocarcinoma has a major impact on the outcome after LT for PSC. Early studies demonstrated that even in cases in which cholangiocarcinoma was discovered incidentally in the explant, recipient survival was poor, with a 1-year survival rate of 30% in one series.[338] On the basis of such studies, cholangiocarcinoma was generally considered a contraindication to LT. Another report confirmed the poor post-LT outcome in patients with known cholangiocarcinoma but suggested a good survival rate for those who had a small cholangiocarcinoma found incidentally at the time of transplantation.[333] Subsequent studies have demonstrated 1- and 5-year survival rates of 65%–82% and 35%–42%, respectively, after LT in patients with cholangiocarcinoma.[339,340] A collaborative study that included data from 12 centers in the United States showed a 65% rate of recurrence-free survival after 5 years when patients underwent external radiation, brachytherapy, radiosensitizing therapy, and/or chemotherapy prior to LT (see Chapter 71).[341]

Biliary strictures commonly recur after LT for PSC and may represent recurrent PSC. In addition to recurrent PSC, potential causes of biliary strictures after LT include ABO blood group incompatibility, hepatic artery occlusion, chronic ductopenic graft rejection, Roux-en-Y-related cholangitis, and preservation-related ischemia. The diagnosis of recurrent PSC has been proposed to be confined to those patients who have a consistent cholangiographic pattern and compatible liver histology showing fibrous cholangitis, fibro-obliterative lesions, biliary fibrosis, or biliary cirrhosis, and who lack other risk factors for biliary strictures, such as hepatic artery occlusion, ABO incompatibility, or ductopenic graft rejection, or who develop nonanastomotic strictures within 90 days of transplantation.[342] With these stringent criteria, the frequency of recurrent PSC after LT ranges from 5.7% to 59.1% after 2.6 to 9.1 years.[332,333,343–346] Although multiple risk factors have been identified for the development of recurrent PSC, including active IBD prior to transplantation and use of tacrolimus-based immunosuppression, none has been universally confirmed. In addition, several studies suggest that colectomy before LT is associated with reduced rates of recurrent PSC.[344,347,348] Whether live donor LT is a risk factor for recurrent PSC remains controversial.[349,350] Unfortunately, no specific therapy has been shown to treat or prevent recurrent PSC effectively after LT, and there is a substantial increase in the risk of graft failure or death among patients with recurrent PSC.[347,351,352] Following LT, up to one-third of patients with PSC will develop progressive disease leading to death or the need for retransplantation.

The effect of LT on the course of underlying IBD and risk of subsequent colonic neoplasia remains an area of investigation. The clinical course of IBD after LT has varied greatly among studies.[126,332,353–357] A study from Mayo Clinic of 151 patients with PSC-IBD and an intact colon at the time of transplantation found that, despite transplant-related immunosuppression, 37.1% required escalation of therapy for IBD, 57.6% had a stable course, and 5.3% improved during a median follow-up of 10 years.[358] In this study, use of tacrolimus-based immunosuppression was associated with a worsening IBD course, whereas use of azathioprine was protective. Of 84 patients with PSC without IBD at the time of transplantation, 26.2% developed de novo IBD, and use of mycophenolate mofetil appeared to increase this risk. A large single-center study[356] showed that LT was associated with an increased risk of colectomy, although other studies have refuted this finding. The risk of colorectal neoplasia is generally agreed to be increased after LT in patients with UC,[261,262,332,357] although this finding has not been confirmed in all studies. Annual surveillance colonoscopy is recommended after LT for PSC in patients with UC.

SECONDARY SCLEROSING CHOLANGITIS

Several diseases other than PSC may present with biliary features similar to those of PSC and are referred to collectively as SSC (see Table 70.1). Frequently, SSC is caused by ischemia or biliary injury after cholecystectomy or LT. With the initial introduction of laparoscopic cholecystectomy, the rate of iatrogenic biliary injury rose from 0.1% to 0.2% for open cholecystectomy to 0.8%–1.4%.[359] However, as the laparoscopic procedure has gained widespread use, biliary injury has occurred at rates similar to those for open cholecystectomy.[360] At one time, HIV cholangiopathy was a common finding, occurring in up to 26% of HIV-infected patients and usually seen only in patients with a CD4 count below 100/mm^3, but it also has become rare as HIV treatment has improved. *Cryptosporidium*, *Microsporidium*, CMV, and other organisms have been isolated from the bile of affected patients (see Chapter 33).[361–364] By contrast, the frequency of biliary strictures following LT appears to be increasing due to the increased risk associated with the use of marginal donors, deceased donors after cardiac death, and partial LT, including live-donor LT, with anastomotic strictures occurring in 5%–25% and nonanastomotic strictures in 10%–15% of patients.[365]

Other causes of SSC include a number of inflammatory conditions such as sarcoidosis, eosinophilic cholangitis, and IgG4-related sclerosing cholangitis.[233] More recently, cases of SSC have been attributed to severe acute respiratory syndrome CoronaVirus-2 (SARS-CoV2)[366,367] infections and within the spectrum of checkpoint inhibitor-induced liver injury.[368,369] Exposure of the bile ducts to toxins such as intra-arterial floxuridine[370] and formaldehyde administered to treat a hydatid cyst, when the cyst communicates with the biliary tract,[371] can produce the cholangiographic appearance of SSC (see Table 70.3, and Chapters 86 and 90).

Sarcoidosis frequently affects the liver and, in rare cases, has been reported to cause cholestasis and features resembling PSC.[372] Eosinophilic cholangitis is an extremely rare disorder characterized by a dense transmural infiltrate of eosinophils.[373] Mast cell infiltration of the bile ducts is common in a variety of disorders that cause SSC as well as in PSC, and in a case report, it has been associated with systemic mastocytosis.[374]

Toxins and vascular insults can also lead to SSC. In addition to hepatic artery thrombosis after LT,[375] SSC in critically ill patients has been described following burns and sepsis and is believed to have a similar vascular basis.[376] Rare cases of impaired hepatic artery perfusion from polyarteritis nodosa have also been described.[377] Extrinsic compression and vascular injury of the bile ducts by large collateral vessels or cavernous transformation of the portal vein can lead to biliary changes similar to PSC and has been called portal biliopathy or portal cavernoma cholangiopathy.[378,379]

IgG4-Related Sclerosing Cholangitis

IgG4-related sclerosing cholangitis, also known as IgG4-associated cholangitis or IgG4 sclerosing cholangitis, is a phenotype of IgG4-related disease, which is characterized by a lymphoplasmacytic infiltrate of IgG4 plasma cells and eosinophils along with obliterative phlebitis and storiform fibrosis.[380] It is a distinct entity with fecal microbiome and metabolome signatures that differ from PSC.[94,381] The underlying pathogenesis of IgG4-sclerosing cholangitis is believed to be an antigen-driven immune response that drives B cells to produce IgG4 along with secretion of profibrotic cytokines by activated T cells.[382] In one study, long-term exposure to solvents and industrial gases was linked to the development of IgG4-sclerosing cholangitis, suggesting that an environmental agent may lead to the development of a neo-antigen that drives the immune response.[383] A type 2 helper T-cell (Th2) cytokine profile, including IL-4 and IL-13 as well as TGF-β and IL-10 production, has been proposed to be mediated by plasma cell-derived RANKL (receptor activator of nuclear factor kappa-B ligand)-activating myeloid-derived suppressor cells that in turn suppress T-cell proliferation and induce Th2 differentiation.[384,385] Tissue-activated follicular T-helper cells are expanded and drive class switching and proliferation of IgG4-committed B cells.[386] Annexin A11, a protein found in cholangiocytes but not at other sites of IgG4-related diseases, has been proposed to be the target autoantigen driving IgG4-sclerosing cholangitis,[387] with IgG4 antibodies disrupting annexin A11 function, resulting in a cholangiocyte phenotype that is susceptible to bile acid cytotoxicity.[388]

Patients with IgG4-related sclerosing cholangitis are usually over 60 years of age and predominantly male.[389,390] Involvement of the pancreas or other organs, including sialadenitis, is frequent, but there is no association with IBD. The prevalence and incidence of IgG4-sclerosing cholangitis are not known, but the disorder appears to be rare.

The appearance of IgG4-related sclerosing cholangitis can be identical to that of PSC or suggest cholangiocarcinoma, leading to missed diagnosis (see Table 70.3).[157,391–393] The diagnosis of IgG-4-related sclerosing cholangitis should be considered in all cases of suspected PSC or cholangiocarcinoma, especially in older men without IBD, and should be based on histology, imaging, serology, other organ involvement, and response to glucocorticoid therapy, so-called HISORt criteria, which were originally developed for the diagnosis of autoimmune pancreatitis (see Chapter 61).[394] Although serum IgG4 levels are elevated in approximately 10% of patients with PSC (a phenomenon that appears to be linked to specific HLA alleles),[56] the serum IgG4 level tends to be lower in patients with PSC than in those with IgG4-related sclerosing cholangitis, with levels greater than four times the upper limit of normal being 100% specific for IgG-4-related sclerosing cholangitis.[395] Further, serum IgG4 levels are not elevated in up to 30% of cases of IgG4-related sclerosing cholangitis. Confidence in the diagnosis of IgG4-related sclerosing cholangitis can be made if high numbers of IgG4-positive lymphocytes (>20 per high-powered field) are identified in pinch biopsies obtained from the major papilla or bile duct.[201,396,397]

The treatment of IgG4-sclerosing cholangitis is similar to that of autoimmune pancreatitis and includes glucocorticoids, to which more than 95% will respond.[391] However, relapse is frequent and often requires long-term maintenance therapy with azathioprine or other immunosuppressants, including rituximab.[390,398] Development of cirrhosis or cholangiocarcinoma is rare, and the long-term prognosis is excellent.

Recurrent Pyogenic Cholangitis

Recurrent pyogenic cholangitis (RPC) is a form of SSC that was first described by Digby in 1930 and defined by Cook et al. as a syndrome characterized by recurrent bacterial cholangitis, intrahepatic pigment stones, and biliary strictures, possibly leading to chronic liver disease and cholangiocarcinoma.[399,400] RPC has also been called "oriental cholangiohepatitis," "Hong Kong disease," "biliary obstruction syndrome of the Chinese," and hepatolithiasis. Although the prevalence has been decreasing, RPC remains most common in Southeast Asia and can also be found in immigrants to Western countries. Men and women are affected equally, and rural residence and lower socioeconomic status appear to be risk factors,[401,402] suggesting that the changing epidemiology may be related to the adoption of a Western-style diet with a higher protein content, improved hygiene, and reduction in disease burden related to *Clonorchis sinensis* and *Ascaris lumbricoides*, infections often cited as contributors to RPC (see Chapter 86).

Infection with *C. sinensis*, *Opisthorchis* species, and *A. lumbricoides* is endemic in the same geographic region where RPC is prevalent, suggesting an important role of these infections. However, patients with RPC do not appear to have an increased frequency of these infections compared with the general population, and approximately one-half of patients with RPC demonstrate no evidence of infection.[403–405] Furthermore, some parts of Asia with a high prevalence of RPC have low or undetectable rates of infection with *C. sinensis*.[406] Bacterial infections have also been proposed as a cause of RPC, and portal bacteremia, possibly related to GI infection and bacterial translocation, has been associated with low socioeconomic status and malnutrition.[402] Diets low in saturated fat have been implicated due to the potential to reduce gallbladder contractility and promote stone formation.

Clinical Features and Diagnosis

Patients with RPC often present with symptoms of acute bacterial cholangitis, including fever, RUQ pain, and jaundice, also referred to as *Charcot triad* (see Chapter 67).[407] Patients may also present with abdominal pain or pancreatitis. Imaging findings in patients with RPC are characteristic, with the majority of patients (75%–80%) having intrahepatic stones, with predominant involvement of the left hepatic duct (Fig. 70.6). Dilatation of the bile ducts is found almost universally. The central bile ducts are dilated disproportionately, with abrupt tapering and attenuation of more peripheral bile ducts within the liver. The presence of bile duct calculi is usually associated with intrahepatic bile duct dilatation and downstream strictures.[408] Direct cholangiography, whether performed by the percutaneous or endoscopic route, allows localization of intrahepatic stones and strictures and placement of drains or extraction of stones. In a comparison with direct cholangiography, MRCP identified all dilated bile ducts and 98% of focal duct strictures and intraductal stones; however, only 44%–47% of segmental bile duct abnormalities were identified by direct cholangiography. Therefore MRCP is the

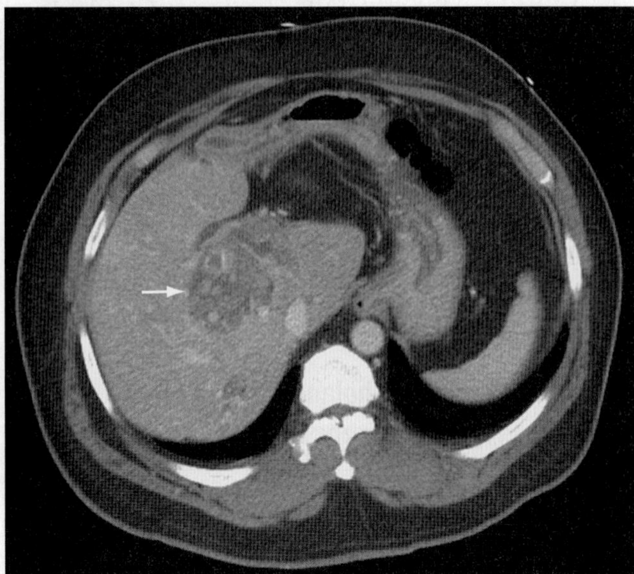

Fig. 70.6 CT in a patient with a history of recurrent pyogenic cholangitis. Note the severe right-sided intrahepatic biliary dilatation with obvious intraductal calculi (*arrow*).

preferred diagnostic test.[409] In 82 patients in whom cholangiocarcinoma was associated with RPC, cholangiocarcinoma tended to be located in atrophic segments associated with biliary calculi and was often accompanied by portal vein occlusion or narrowing.[410]

Patients who present with an initial episode of cholangitis associated with intrahepatic stones and strictures should undergo evaluation for infection with *Clonorchis* and *Opisthorchis* species, particularly if the patient comes from or has traveled to an endemic area. The diagnosis of a parasitic infection is made by the identification of eggs in fecal specimens; concentrated stool may be required. Eggs are present in stool after 4 weeks of infection.[408] Duodenal or biliary fluid may also demonstrate eggs or intact worms. Peripheral eosinophilia may be present in cases of parasitic infection and may be associated with elevated serum IgE levels.[411]

Treatment

Antibiotic therapy should be initiated promptly once cultures of blood and bile (if accessible) have been obtained. In those with parasitic infection, treatment with an anthelminthic agent is indicated in patients with evidence of active parasitic infection (see also Chapter 86).

In patients with evidence of cholangitis and dilated intra- and extrahepatic bile ducts, ERCP is the preferred interventional procedure. ERCP with sphincterotomy, with or without placement of a nasobiliary drain or percutaneous biliary drainage, may be required to remove bile duct stones and traverse strictures (see Chapter 72). Several studies have reviewed the success of various nonoperative interventions for the initial management of patients with RPC presenting acutely. Sperling et al.[407] compared outcomes in 41 patients with RPC based on whether they underwent therapeutic ERCP, hepatobiliary surgery, or no intervention. Symptoms recurred in 62% of patients who underwent only diagnostic ERCP but half as often in those treated with therapeutic ERCP or surgery. Therapeutic ERCP was particularly effective in patients with disease involving the extrahepatic bile ducts and was comparable in efficacy to surgery. Patients with disease involving both the right and left hepatic duct branches tend to undergo more imaging studies, percutaneous cholangiograms, and endoscopic or surgical procedures.[412]

Hepaticojejunostomy has been a commonly used surgical procedure for the treatment of intrahepatic stones in patients with RPC.[413] Laparoscopic biliary bypass surgery has been proposed as a technically feasible and effective option for patients with RPC.[414,415]

Prognosis and Complications

The natural history of RPC has not been well documented. Recurrent cholangitis is common, recurring in 25% at 3 years and 37% at 5 years.[416] Secondary biliary cirrhosis may develop and require LT. Cholangiocarcinoma is associated with RPC with a cumulative frequency of 3%–9% (see Chapter 71).[417] In a study of 310 patients with RPC, acute cholangitis, liver abscesses, cirrhotic complications, and cholangiocarcinoma developed in 41.3%, 19.4%, 9.7%, and 7.4%, respectively, over a mean follow-up of 84 months.[418] The risk of developing cholangiocarcinoma was associated with bilateral hepatic lobe atrophy.

Acknowledgments

The authors acknowledge the contributions of Drs. Andrew S. Ross and Kris V. Kowdley to this chapter in previous editions of the book.

Full references for this chapter can be found at https://ebooks.health.elsevier.com.

71 Tumors of the Bile Ducts, Gallbladder, and Ampulla

Sumera I. Ilyas, Gregory J. Gores

IN THIS CHAPTER

Biliary malignancies comprise the vast majority of biliary neoplasms and are divided into three categories: (1) carcinomas of the intra- and extrahepatic bile ducts (cholangiocarcinomas), (2) carcinoma of the gallbladder, and (3) carcinoma of the ampulla of Vater.[1] Cholangiocarcinomas are further classified into intrahepatic, perihilar, and distal cholangiocarcinoma on the basis of their anatomic location within the biliary tract. In the United States and other Western nations, biliary malignancies are rare. In certain parts of the world, however, their prevalence rates are high, making them leading causes of cancer death in these regions. Biliary cancers are highly aggressive with dismal prognoses.

CHOLANGIOCARCINOMA

Cholangiocarcinoma is an adenocarcinoma with differentiated features of biliary epithelium that arises from the intra- and extrahepatic biliary tract.[2] It is the most common bile duct tumor and second most common primary hepatic malignancy [after HCC (see Chapter 98)]. Since the 1970s, the incidence of cholangiocarcinoma has increased worldwide.[3–6]

On the basis of their location within the biliary tract, cholangiocarcinomas are divided into intrahepatic, perihilar, and distal subtypes. Each anatomic subtype has a distinct epidemiology, pathogenesis, risk factors, management, and prognosis.[7] Intrahepatic cholangiocarcinomas arise within the liver parenchyma and above the second-order bile ducts (see Chapter 64). Perihilar or hilar cholangiocarcinomas arise between second-order bile ducts and the insertion of the cystic duct. Distal cholangiocarcinomas arise below the insertion of the cystic duct (Fig. 71.1A).[2] Perihilar cholangiocarcinomas, also referred to as *Klatskin tumors*, are described clinically according to the Bismuth-Corlette classification as types I to IV (see Fig. 71.1B). Type I cholangiocarcinomas involve the common hepatic duct distal to the union of the right and left hepatic ducts; type II tumors involve the union of the right and left hepatic ducts; type IIIa tumors involve the union of the right and left hepatic ducts and extend up the right hepatic duct; type IIIb tumors involve the union of the right and left hepatic ducts and extend up the left hepatic duct; and type IV tumors are multifocal or involve the biliary confluence and extend up the right and left hepatic ducts. The natural course of cholangiocarcinoma is aggressive, with a median survival of less than 24 months following diagnosis.[8]

Epidemiology

Cholangiocarcinoma is the most common biliary and the second most common primary hepatic malignancy, accounting for approximately 15% of all primary liver tumors.[9,10] It accounts for less than 2% of all malignancies but is the ninth most common GI malignancy. Hepatobiliary malignancies account for 13% and 3% of overall cancer-related mortality in the world and in the United States, respectively; 10%–20% of these deaths are caused by cholangiocarcinoma.[11]

The worldwide incidence of cholangiocarcinoma has increased steadily over the past several decades.[4] Global incidence rates for cholangiocarcinoma are heterogeneous. The highest incidence is observed in Southeast Asia, with age-adjusted incidence rates in males up to 115 per 100,000 population.[13] Moreover, global mortality rates of intrahepatic cholangiocarcinoma have increased progressively, while reported mortality rates for perihilar and distal cholangiocarcinoma have decreased.[12] In the United States, the highest mortality rate is observed in patients of Asian descent, while there has been a significant increase in the mortality rates of cholangiocarcinoma in patients of African descent.[16] The age-adjusted mortality rates of cholangiocarcinoma are higher for males than females, for older patients than younger patients, and higher in Asian countries than in Western countries.[4,9,12] Worldwide, the average age at diagnosis is around 50 years.[9,14] In Western industrialized nations, most cases are diagnosed in patients over the age of 65 years, and cholangiocarcinoma is uncommon before the age of 40 years, except in patients with PSC (see Chapter 70).[9,14]

Although perihilar cholangiocarcinomas account for the majority of cholangiocarcinomas, there has been a progressive increase in the incidence of intrahepatic cholangiocarcinomas.[17] Since the 1980s, an increase in the incidence of intrahepatic cholangiocarcinomas and a concomitant decrease in the incidence of perihilar and distal cholangiocarcinomas have been reported in multiple studies.[19] These trends may, in part, be explained by

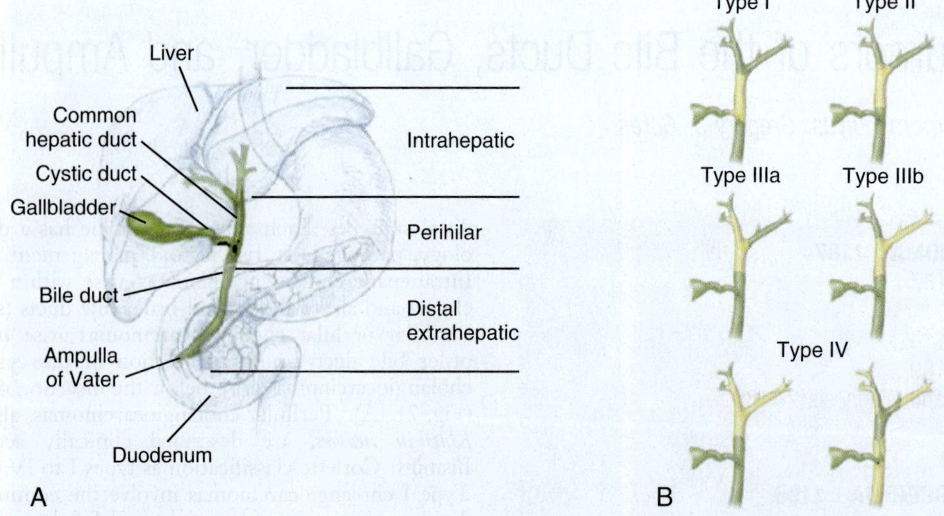

Fig. 71.1 Classification of cholangiocarcinoma. (A) Anatomic classification of intrahepatic, perihilar, and distal cholangiocarcinoma. (B) Bismuth-Corlette classification of hilar cholangiocarcinoma as types I to IV. Tumor is depicted in *yellow* and normal bile ducts in *green*. (Modified from Blechacz BR, Komuta M, Roskams T, Gores GJ. Clinical diagnosis and staging of cholangiocarcinoma. *Nat Rev Gastroenterol Hepatol*. 2011;8:512–522.)

BOX 71.1 Risk Factors for Cholangiocarcinoma

DEFINITE

- Caroli disease
- Choledochal cyst
- Hepatolithiasis
- *Opisthorchis viverrini* infection
- PSC
- Thorotrast

PROBABLE

- Biliary-enteric drainage procedures
- Cirrhosis
- *Clonorchis sinensis* infection
- Heavy alcohol consumption
- Hepatitis C
- Toxins (dioxins, polyvinyl chloride)

misclassification of perihilar tumors as intrahepatic. According to the Surveillance, Epidemiology, and End Results database in the United States, the age-adjusted incidence rate for intrahepatic cholangiocarcinomas increased between 1990 and 2001, whereas the incidence rate for perihilar and distal cholangiocarcinomas decreased over this time period. The second edition of the International Classification of Diseases for Oncology classified Klatskin tumors as intrahepatic. In the third edition, published in 2001, Klatskin tumors were reclassified as extrahepatic.[3,19] The next iteration of International Classification of Diseases for Oncology will have separate codes for intrahepatic, perihilar, and distal cholangiocarcinoma.[20]

Etiology

In the majority of cases, the etiology of cholangiocarcinoma is unknown. Several risk factors have been identified (Box 71.1). These risk factors are characterized by their association with inflammation and cholestasis; however, studies exploring the association of risk factors with cholangiocarcinoma are frequently limited by inter- and intracontinental heterogeneity and inaccuracies of cancer registries, such as classification of cholangiocarcinoma with other biliary malignancies and HCC.

Established Risk Factors

Although there are several known risk factors for cholangiocarcinoma,[21] most cases are sporadic and occur in the absence of a known risk factor. PSC is one of the most common risk factors for cholangiocarcinoma (see Chapter 70); however, only 10% of cholangiocarcinomas are attributed to PSC. In patients with PSC, the annual incidence of cholangiocarcinoma is 0.6%–1.5%, and the 30-year cumulative incidence is 20%.[5] A new diagnosis of PSC should heighten suspicion for cholangiocarcinoma; 27%–37% of biliary tract cancers are detected within the first year of the diagnosis of PSC.[5] Other cholangiopathies have also been found to be risk factors for cholangiocarcinoma.[21] Patients with Caroli disease and choledochal cysts, in particular types I and IV, have an up to 50-fold increased risk of cholangiocarcinoma, with lifetime incidence rates of 6%–30% (see Chapter 64). Cyst excision reduces but does not eliminate the risk for the development of cholangiocarcinoma.[11] Hepatolithiasis with recurrent pyogenic cholangitis carries a 10% risk of cholangiocarcinoma (see Chapter 70).[22] Recurrent bacterial cholangitis in the setting of a biliary-enteric drainage procedure has also been associated with the development of cholangiocarcinoma.[22] Other risk factors for cholangiocarcinoma include biliary infections with *Opisthorchis viverrini* and *Clonorchis sinensis*, which are endemic in East Asia (see Chapter 86).[23] Carcinogens, such as thorotrast (used as a radiologic contrast agent in the past) and dioxins, have been associated with an increased risk of cholangiocarcinoma (see Chapter 91).[24]

Possible Risk Factors

The association between cholangiocarcinoma and IBD (UC or Crohn disease) is controversial and likely influenced by the presence and duration of PSC; therefore it is unclear if the presence of IBD confers additional risk for cholangiocarcinoma in patients with PSC.[9] Intrahepatic cholangiocarcinoma has been associated with HCV and HBV infection and cirrhosis, and perihilar cholangiocarcinoma has been associated only with cirrhosis (see Chapter 98).[6,9,21,25] Obesity, type 2 diabetes mellitus, and NAFLD have been associated with an increased risk of cholangiocarcinoma, but the data are inconsistent. The incidence of these conditions has been increasing in Western industrialized nations, a trend that could account for the increasing incidence of intrahepatic cholangiocarcinomas in these countries. Heavy alcohol consumption has been associated both with intrahepatic and with perihilar and distal cholangiocarcinoma and is thought to be a likely risk factor.[9,21,25,26]

Pathology

Cholangiocarcinoma is a paucicellular, highly desmoplastic tumor. Macroscopically, intrahepatic cholangiocarcinomas can have three subtypes: mass-forming, periductal-infiltrating, and intraductal growth type. The mass-forming type is the most common type of intrahepatic cholangiocarcinoma, accounting for more than 85% of cases.[7,27] Histologically, 90% of cholangiocarcinomas are adenocarcinomas. The two main histological subtypes of intrahepatic cholangiocarcinoma are small bile duct cholangiocarcinoma and large bile duct cholangiocarcinoma.[10,28] Small bile duct intrahepatic cholangiocarcinomas are small tubular or acinar adenocarcinomas that have a nodular growth pattern with invasion of the liver parenchyma. Large bile duct intrahepatic cholangiocarcinomas, on the other hand, originate from the large intrahepatic bile ducts and produce mucin.[10,29,30] Macroscopically, perihilar cholangiocarcinomas have a periductal-infiltrating, nodular, or intraductal growth pattern, with the periductal-infiltrating subtype being the most common. Because perihilar cholangiocarcinomas have a tropism for bile, the initial growth pattern is typically periductal, and with tumor progression, a mass lesion is formed, resulting in a mass-forming and periductal-infiltrating lesion.[31,32] Intraductal-papillary adenocarcinomas spread superficially along the biliary mucosa without deep invasion of the fibromuscular wall layers and have a better prognosis than nonpapillary cancers[33]; metastases to regional and peripancreatic lymph nodes are frequently observed with this type. Other, much less common histologic types include intestinal-type adenocarcinoma, clear cell adenocarcinoma, signet-ring cell carcinoma, adenosquamous carcinoma, squamous cell carcinoma, and small cell carcinoma.[34]

Pathogenesis

The pathogenesis of cholangiocarcinoma is complex and likely related to inflammation in the microenvironment, environmental factors, and genetic aberrations of the tumor cells (both acquired and germline). Most available information relates to genetic aberrations, including analysis of the transcriptome, copy number variations, DNA methylation, microRNA profiling, and somatic mutations.[35–38] The most comprehensive resource on genetic aberrations is *The Cancer Genome Atlas* integrated genomic analysis of cholangiocarcinomas that were predominantly intrahepatic, liver-fluke negative, and hepatitis virus negative.[38] Inactivating mutations in tumor suppressor genes, including *ARID1A*, *ARID1B*, *BAP1*, tumor protein p53 (*TP53*), and phosphatase and tensin homolog (*PTEN*), and gain-of-function mutations in the oncogenes isocitrate dehydrogenase (*IDH*) 1 and 2, *BRAF*, and *KRAS*, were identified in these tumors.[38] Discrete carcinogenic risk factors may impact the pattern of somatic aberrations in cholangiocarcinomas. For instance, liver-fluke–related cholangiocarcinomas have a higher frequency of *TP53* mutations, whereas *IDH1*, *IDH2*, and *BAP1* mutations occur more frequently in non-liver-fluke–related cholangiocarcinomas.[38]

The repertoire of genomic alterations in cholangiocarcinoma varies by anatomic subtype. The frequencies of molecular aberrations in fibroblast growth factor receptor (*FGFR*) 1–3, *IDH 1* and *2*, and *BAP1* are higher in intrahepatic cholangiocarcinoma, whereas the frequencies of mutations of *ARID1B*, *PBRM1*, and protein kinase cyclic AMP-activated catalytic subunit alpha (*PRKACA*) and beta (*PRKACB*) are higher in distal and perihilar cholangiocarcinomas.[36] Inactivating mutations in E74-like ETS transcription factor 3 (*ELF3*) occur preferentially in distal cholangiocarcinoma (Table 71.1).[39]

Deregulation of FGF signaling with consequent carcinogenesis occurs in a spectrum of malignancies, including cholangiocarcinoma. Gene fusions of *FGFR2*, a receptor tyrosine kinase, result in its ligand-independent activation. *FGFR2* gene fusions are present in 11%–14% of intrahepatic cholangiocarcinomas.[40–42] The discovery of these gene fusions is notable because they are often targetable driver mutations. *IDH* mutations are relatively common genetic aberrations in cholangiocarcinoma that are observed in 23%–28% of intrahepatic cholangiocarcinomas.[43,44] IDH1 and IDH2 are enzymes that catalyze the reaction leading to generation of α-ketoglutarate. Point mutations of *IDH* and *IDH2* result in an increase in 2-hydroxyglutarate, an oncometabolite that promotes extensive epigenetic aberrations in malignancy.[44,45]

Clinical Features and Diagnosis

The diagnosis of cholangiocarcinoma is challenging because the presentation is often insidious, and the results of diagnostic studies are frequently nonspecific. A multidisciplinary approach that includes clinical evaluation and laboratory, endoscopic, and imaging studies is required (Figs. 71.2 and 71.3).[46]

Intrahepatic cholangiocarcinomas are diagnosed incidentally in approximately 25%–30% of patients.[47] Intrahepatic cholangiocarcinomas are often asymptomatic during the earlier

TABLE 71.1 Molecular Aberrations in Cholangiocarcinoma

Cholangiocarcinoma Subtype	Molecular Aberration
Intrahepatic	Fibroblast growth factor receptor (*FGFR*) 2 gene fusions
	Isocitrate dehydrogenase (IDH) 1/2 mutations
	Mcl-1 amplification
	MET-hepatocyte growth factor (HGF) overexpression
	BAP1 inactivating mutations
	ARID1A inactivating mutations
	PTPN3-activating mutations
	KRAS-activating mutations
	PIK3CA-activating mutations
Perihilar	*HER2* amplifications
	ERBB2 genetic aberrations
	Protein kinase cyclic AMP-activated catalytic subunit alpha (*PRKACA*) and beta (*PRKACB*) gene fusions
	KRAS-activating mutations
	PIK3CA-activating mutations
Distal	E74-like ETS transcription factor 3 (ELF3) inactivating mutations
	ERBB3 mutations
	KRAS-activating mutations
	PIK3CA-activating mutations

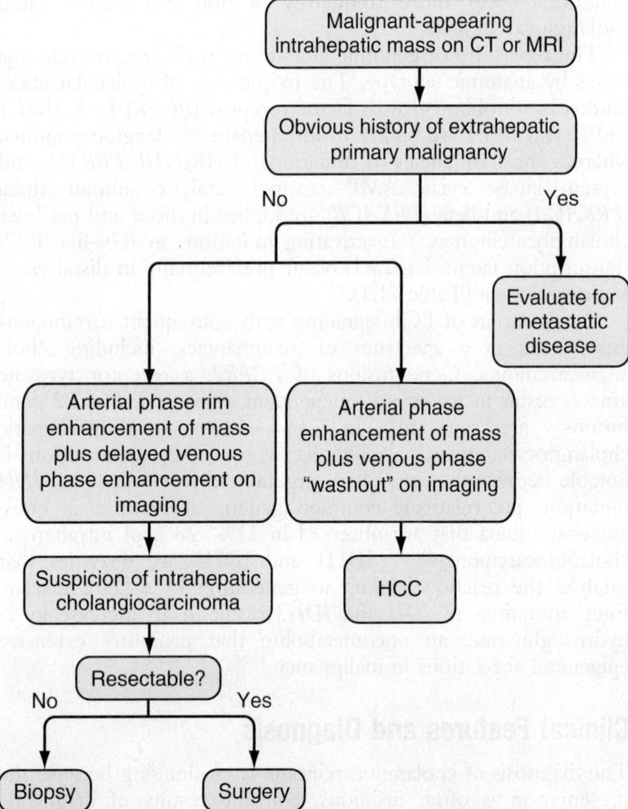

Fig. 71.2 Algorithm for the diagnosis of intrahepatic cholangiocarcinoma. In cases of an intrahepatic mass lesion and in the absence of known extrahepatic primary malignancy, dynamic imaging with either CT or MRI of the liver should be performed. Contrast enhancement of a mass throughout the arterial phase with "washout" in the portal venous phase indicates an HCC. Contrast rim enhancement of a mass throughout the arterial phase and delayed portal venous enhancement should raise the suspicion of an intrahepatic cholangiocarcinoma; in such cases, the resectability of the tumor should be determined. If the lesion is deemed resectable, the patient should be referred for surgical resection without biopsy. If an intrahepatic cholangiocarcinoma is deemed unresectable, a biopsy should be performed to confirm the diagnosis and guide appropriate treatment.

disease stages, and as disease progresses, patients may present with abdominal pain and/or systemic symptoms such as cachexia, malaise, and fatigue. Perihilar and distal cholangiocarcinomas manifest in most cases with painless jaundice due to malignant biliary obstruction. In 10% of patients, bacterial cholangitis is the initial presenting symptom. An "atrophy-hypertrophy" complex can be documented by physical examination as palpable hypertrophy of the contralateral, unaffected lobe of the liver, with atrophy of the affected lobe as a result of vascular encasement and bile ductal obstruction.

Laboratory analysis may reveal evidence of obstructive cholestasis. In cases of indeterminate strictures, immunoglobulin G4 (IgG4) cholangiopathy should be ruled out serologically and with biliary sampling (see Chapters 61 and 70). The most commonly used serum tumor marker in cholangiocarcinoma is CA 19-9. In patients with PSC, the sensitivity and specificity of CA 19-9 for the diagnosis of cholangiocarcinoma are 79% and 98%, respectively, when the cutoff value is 129 U/mL. In patients without PSC, the sensitivity is 53% with a cutoff value of 100 U/mL.[48] High levels of CA 19-9 (>1000 U/mL) have been associated with metastatic cholangiocarcinoma.[48] It is important to note that patients who do not express Lewis antigen on red blood cells or in body fluids (approximately 5%–10% of the general population) have undetectable serum CA 19-9 levels.[49] Significant CA 19-9 elevations can occasionally be observed in patients with bacterial cholangitis and choledocholithiasis (see Chapter 67). Notably, up to one-third of patients with an elevated serum CA 19-9 level do not have cholangiocarcinoma.[50]

Intrahepatic Cholangiocarcinoma

Intrahepatic cholangiocarcinoma often presents as a mass lesion in the liver. In the presence of cirrhosis, it can be challenging to differentiate intrahepatic cholangiocarcinoma from HCC. In the assessment of intrahepatic lesions more than 2 cm in diameter, dynamic CT and MRI (Fig. 71.4) are helpful for distinguishing cholangiocarcinoma from HCC based on progressive contrast enhancement through the venous, arterial, and delayed venous phases in cholangiocarcinomas compared with the washout phenomenon observed in HCCs (see Chapter 98).[51,52] An initial rim or peripheral arterial enhancement pattern in the early phases of dynamic CT or gadolinium-enhanced MRI with progressive centripetal enhancement in delayed phases is characteristic of intrahepatic cholangiocarcinoma.[51,52]

CT is used primarily for preoperative planning; it provides information on vascular and other anatomic structures, and its accuracy in the assessment of resectability is 60%–88%.[53] The sensitivity of CT for detection of nodal N2 metastases (see later) is only 54%.[53] For detection of the primary tumor, PET/CT has limited utility with a sensitivity and specificity of approximately 92% and 51%, respectively. However, PET/CT does appear to have better diagnostic performance for detection of lymph node and distant metastasis.[55] Thus PET/CT may play a role in the staging of intrahepatic cholangiocarcinoma. In intrahepatic cholangiocarcinoma, a tissue diagnosis should be limited to nonresectable cases because differentiation from HCC will affect the choice of therapy.

Perihilar and Distal Cholangiocarcinoma

An essential diagnostic tool for perihilar and distal cholangiocarcinomas is cholangiography, which provides both anatomic information and material for a tissue diagnosis. Several approaches can be used, including ERCP, percutaneous transhepatic cholangiography (THC), and MRCP (Fig. 71.5). The choice of ERCP or percutaneous THC depends on the location of a suspicious biliary stricture, local expertise, and accessibility of the stricture to the technique. Either ERCP or percutaneous THC provides information on intrabiliary tumor extension and allows cytologic sampling and therapeutic intervention for malignant biliary obstruction. Such interventions are not possible with MRCP, but this technique is noninvasive and provides additional information on the extent of the tumor, vascular encasement, the relation of the primary tumor to surrounding structures, and intra- as well as extrahepatic metastases.[56] Cross-sectional imaging should be performed prior to cholangiography to help guide decisions regarding biliary drainage. MRI with MRCP is currently the best imaging technique for estimating the extent of biliary neoplastic invasion in perihilar cholangiocarcinoma, whereas CT is superior in detecting vascular enhancement and assessing resectability.[57] For perihilar cholangiocarcinomas, the sensitivity and specificity of PET are only 69% and 67%, and the sensitivity for the detection of local lymph node metastases is only 13%–38%.[58,59] False-positive PET results can be observed in the setting of inflammation.[54] Therefore its use in perihilar lesions should be limited to cases that are indeterminate with regard to extent and other features (including malignancy) after other studies have been performed. Mass lesions

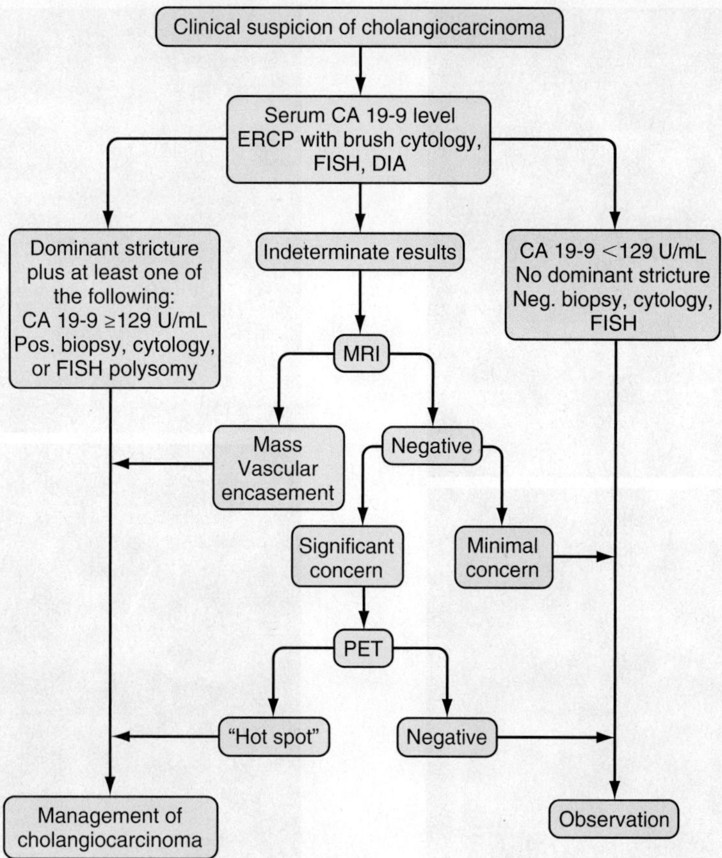

Fig. 71.3 Algorithm for the diagnosis of perihilar cholangiocarcinoma. In cases of clinically suspected perihilar cholangiocarcinoma, a serum CA 19-9 level, ERCP, and conventional as well as molecular cytologic analysis of endoscopically-obtained biliary brushings of malignant-appearing areas should be performed. If the results of these tests are normal or negative, close follow-up of the patient is recommended. Management of cholangiocarcinoma should be prompted by identification of a dominant stricture, a serum CA 19-9 level above 129 U/mL, or a biopsy or cytology result that is positive for carcinoma or polysomy. In indeterminate cases, gadolinium-enhanced MRI of the liver is recommended. If a mass lesion or vascular encasement is identified, management of cholangiocarcinoma should be initiated. If the MRI study is negative but clinical concern about cholangiocarcinoma persists, PET can be performed. If "hot spots" are identified on PET (positive result), treatment for cholangiocarcinoma should be initiated. If the PET result is negative, close follow-up of the patient is recommended. If MRI is negative and cholangiocarcinoma is considered unlikely, the patient can be followed expectantly. *DIA*, Digital image analysis; *FISH*, fluorescence in situ hybridization; *neg.*, negative; *pos.*, positive.

are unusual in distal cholangiocarcinomas, and frequently these tumors are grouped with perihilar cholangiocarcinomas in clinical studies; therefore, the same laboratory and imaging criteria should be applied as for perihilar cholangiocarcinoma.

EUS can contribute additional information about tumor dimension and anatomic location in relation to surrounding structures. Compared with CT or MRI, EUS has a higher tumor detection rate, particularly in distal cholangiocarcinoma.[60] In addition, EUS provides information about regional lymphadenopathy and allows sampling of lymph nodes by FNA. Biopsy of the primary lesion via EUS is highly discouraged, however, because of the potential for tumor cell spread, especially if LT is a therapeutic option.[61]

As for most malignancies, a tissue diagnosis of cholangiocarcinoma is desirable; however, a pathologic diagnosis is challenging because of the tumor's paucicellular character. Tissue is difficult to obtain, and cellular reactive changes resulting from inflammation often complicate the diagnosis. The most common technique for collecting tumor tissue in patients with perihilar and distal cholangiocarcinoma is brush cytology during ERCP.[62] Although conventional cytology has a high specificity (100%), it is limited by low sensitivity (43%).[62] Fluorescence in situ hybridization (FISH) has been demonstrated to increase the sensitivity and specificity of cytology for diagnosing cholangiocarcinoma in patients with and without PSC.[63] Because chromosomal instability is a hallmark of cancer, the FISH assay is used for the assessment of chromosomal aneusomy (gains or losses of chromosomes) via the use of fluorescently labeled DNA probes. An optimized FISH probe set (targeting the 1q21, 7p12, 8q24, 9p21 loci) has enhanced sensitivity and specificity (93% and 100%, respectively) for the detection of pancreaticobiliary malignancies.[64]

Newer techniques for diagnosing cholangiocarcinoma include cholangioscopy, intraductal US, and confocal laser endomicroscopy.[65] A limited number of prospective studies in a small number of patients have demonstrated an improvement in diagnostic accuracy with cholangioscopy-directed biopsy compared with biliary brushings of indeterminate strictures.[65] Therefore these techniques are not yet established in routine practice and should be reserved for cases that remain unconfirmed after use of the aforementioned methods when the level of suspicion for cholangiocarcinoma is high.

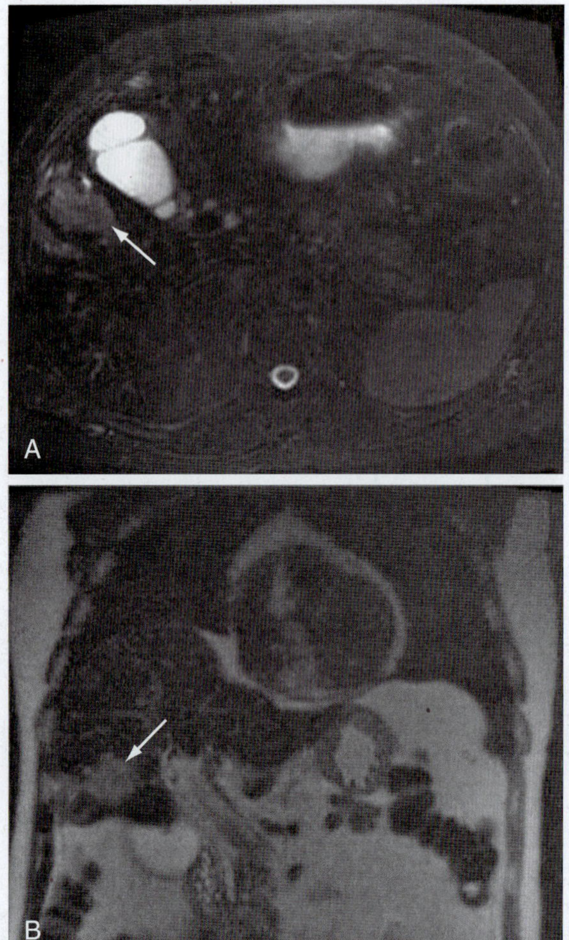

Fig. 71.4 Imaging of intrahepatic cholangiocarcinoma. A gadolinium-enhanced MRI with ferumoxide in a patient with an intrahepatic cholangiocarcinoma is depicted. The *arrows* point to the tumor in the T2-weighted images: (A) axial view and (B) coronal view.

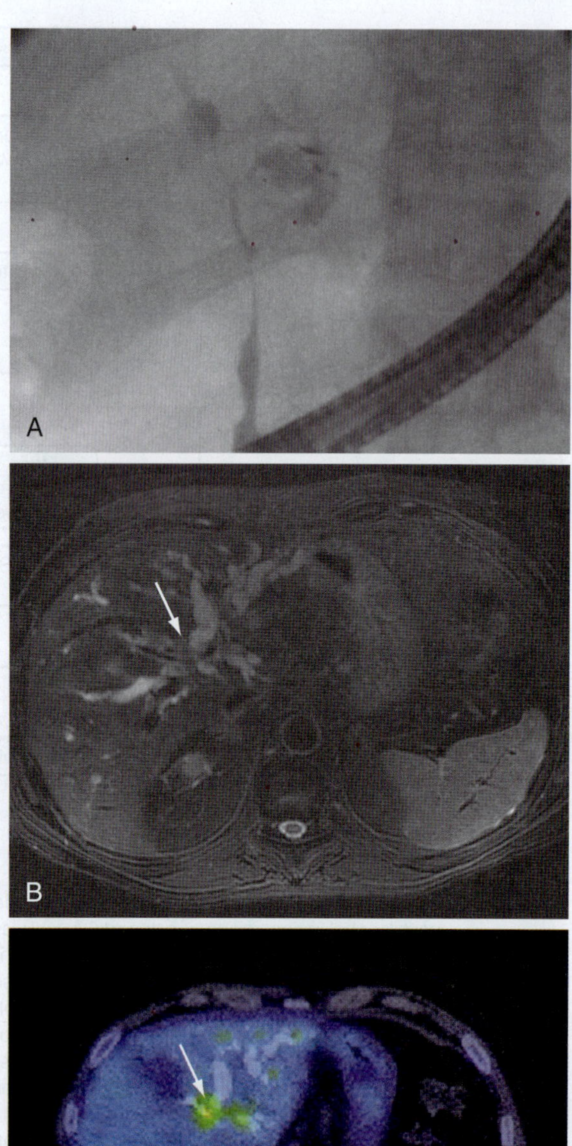

Fig. 71.5 Imaging of perihilar cholangiocarcinoma. (A) Film from an ERCP in a patient with perihilar cholangiocarcinoma demonstrating dominant strictures of the biliary tract consistent with Bismuth-Corlette type IV. (B) Gadolinium-enhanced MRI with ferumoxide in the same patient. The *arrow* points to the biliary tumor seen on a T2-weighted image. (C) PET/CT scan of the same patient. The biliary tumor is seen as an enhancing region (*arrow*).

Staging

Staging systems of malignancies aim to provide guidance in prognostication and treatment. Several staging systems exist for intrahepatic, perihilar, and distal cholangiocarcinomas; unfortunately, none of these has proved to be optimal. A modification was introduced in the American Joint Committee on Cancer (AJCC)/the Union for International Cancer Control (UICC) TNM system in 2009 by assigning a separate staging system to each cholangiocarcinoma type.[58,66]

Independent prognostic factors for intrahepatic cholangiocarcinomas include the number of tumors, vascular invasion, and lymph node metastases.[67] The staging systems for intrahepatic cholangiocarcinoma include the AJCC/UICC TNM staging system and the Liver Cancer Study Group of Japan staging system.[68] These differ primarily in their T staging approach. Moreover, only the AJCC/UICC TNM staging system (Table 71.2) has shown a correlation between stage and survival, but the system is limited by its requirement for a tissue diagnosis for the Tis (carcinoma in situ) and T4 stages.[69]

Independent prognostic factors for perihilar cholangiocarcinomas include tumor differentiation, lymph node metastases, and negative (R0) surgical resection margins. Four major staging systems for perihilar cholangiocarcinoma are the Bismuth-Corlette classification,[70,60] the Memorial Sloan-Kettering Cancer Center (MSKCC) staging system,[71] the AJCC/UICC TNM staging system,[69] and the Mayo Clinic staging system.[72] The Bismuth-Corlette classification was developed for guiding surgical treatment and is not a staging system; it does not provide prognostication and is not designed to correlate with surgical outcomes. Although the MSKCC staging system (Table 71.3) showed a correlation between T stage and R0, N2, and M1 status, it was not able to distinguish resectable from unresectable disease reliably. Unlike the other three systems that use operative

TABLE 71.2 TNM and AJCC/UICC Staging Systems for Intrahepatic Cholangiocarcinoma

TNM Stage	Criteria		
Tx	Primary tumor cannot be assessed		
T0	No evidence of primary tumor		
Tis	Carcinoma in situ (intraductal tumor)		
T1a	Solitary tumor ≤5 cm without vascular invasion		
T1b	Solitary tumor >5 cm without vascular invasion		
T2	Solitary tumor with vascular invasion *OR* multiple tumors, with or without vascular invasion		
T3	Tumor perforating the visceral peritoneum		
T4	Tumor involving the local extrahepatic structures by direct invasion		
Nx	Regional lymph nodes cannot be assessed		
N0	No regional lymph node metastases		
N1	Regional lymph node metastases are present		
M0	No distant metastases		
M1	Distant metastases		
AJCC/UICC Stage	**Tumor**	**Node**	**Metastasis**
0	Tis	N0	M0
IA	T1a	N0	M0
IB	T1b	N0	M0
II	T2	N0	M0
IIIA	T3	N0	M0
IIIB	T4	N0	M0
	Any T	N1	M0
IV	Any T	Any N	M1

AJCC, American Joint Committee on Cancer; *UICC*, Union for International Cancer Control.

TABLE 71.3 MSKCC Staging System for Perihilar Cholangiocarcinoma

Stage	Criteria
T1	Tumor involving biliary confluence ± unilateral extension to secondary radicles
T2	Tumor involving biliary confluence ± unilateral extension to secondary radicles *AND* Ipsilateral portal vein involvement ± ipsilateral hepatic lobe atrophy
T3	Tumor involving biliary confluence + bilateral extension to secondary radicles *OR* Unilateral extension to secondary radicles + contralateral portal vein involvement *OR* Main or bilateral portal vein involvement

MSKCC, Memorial Sloan Kettering Cancer Center.

TABLE 71.4 Mayo Clinic Staging System for Perihilar Cholangiocarcinoma

Stage	Criteria
I	Unicentric mass ≤3 cm ECOG performance status 0 Serum CA 19-9 level (U/mL) <1000 No vascular encasement No metastasis
II	Unicentric mass ≤3 cm ECOG performance status 1-2 Serum CA 19-9 level (U/mL) <1000 Vascular encasement present No metastasis
III	Unicentric mass >3 cm or multicentric ECOG performance status 0-2 Serum CA 19-9 level (U/mL) ≥1000 Lymph node metastasis present
IV	ECOG performance status 3–4 Peritoneal (or other organ) metastasis present

ECOG, Eastern Cooperative Oncology Group.

information, the Mayo Clinic staging system (Table 71.4) is based on nonoperative information at the time of diagnosis. Therefore the Mayo Clinic staging system can be used to predict survival in patients with unresectable disease. Moreover, this system had better prognostic performance, demonstrated by greater concordance statistics, compared with the AJCC/UICC system (Table 71.5).[72] Independent prognostic factors for distal cholangiocarcinomas include the depth of tumor invasion; lymph node metastasis; perineural, microscopic vascular, and pancreatic invasion; and R0 resection. Lymph node metastases are more commonly observed with this type of cholangiocarcinoma than with the others. The AJCC/UICC TNM staging system is the only staging system for distal cholangiocarcinomas (Table 71.6). As outlined earlier, the separation of perihilar from distal cholangiocarcinomas is an improvement over previous versions, as is the redefinition of the T stages. This staging system provides prognostic information, which requires validation but does not guide management.

TABLE 71.5 TNM and AJCC/UICC Staging Systems for Perihilar Cholangiocarcinoma

TNM Stage	Criteria
Tx	Primary tumor cannot be assessed
T0	No evidence of primary tumor
Tis	Carcinoma in situ
T1	Tumor confined to the bile duct, with extension up to the muscle layer of fibrous tissue
T2a	Tumor invades beyond the wall of the bile duct to surrounding adipose tissue
T2b	Tumors invade adjacent hepatic parenchyma
T3	Tumor invades unilateral branches of the portal vein or hepatic artery
T4	Tumor invades main portal vein or its branches bilaterally *OR* Tumor invades the common hepatic artery *OR* Tumor invades unilateral second-order biliary radicles, with contralateral portal vein or hepatic artery involvement
Nx	Regional lymph nodes cannot be assessed
N0	No regional lymph node metastases
N1	Regional lymph node metastases ($\leq$3 lymph nodes) (includes hilar, cystic duct, common bile duct, hepatic artery, posterior pancreatoduodenal, and portal vein lymph nodes)
N2	Regional lymph node metastases ($\geq$4 lymph nodes)
M0	No distant metastases
M1	Distant metastases

AJCC/UICC Stage	Tumor	Node	Metastasis
0	Tis	N0	M0
I	T1	N0	M0
II	T2a-b	N0	M0
IIIA	T3	N0	M0
IIIB	T4	N0	M0
IIIC	Any T	N1	M0
IVA	Any T	N2	M0
IVB	Any T	Any N	M1

AJCC, American Joint Committee on Cancer; *UICC,* Union for International Cancer Control.

Treatment

Intrahepatic Cholangiocarcinoma

Surgical Resection and LT

The only curative treatment option for cholangiocarcinoma is surgical extirpation. Surgical outcomes have improved substantially in the 2000s because of careful patient selection, with lower surgical mortality rates and higher rates of R0 resection.[60] Solitary intrahepatic cholangiocarcinomas can be resected by hepatic segmentectomy or lobectomy. Up to 54% of patients are unresectable at the time of presentation, and approximately 30% of those deemed resectable are found to be unresectable at the time of surgery. Recurrence rates following resection are as high as 62%.[73] Overall, 5-year survival rates after resection of intrahepatic cholangiocarcinoma range from 22% to 42%. R0 resection is achieved in 63% of patients,[74] and 5-year survival rates of 40%−63% have been reported after R0 resection. Surgery-associated morbidity and mortality rates are 35% and 5%, respectively.[18,75] Survival is positively correlated with R0 resection, negative lymph node metastasis status (N0), solitary tumor, younger age, and better performance status.[18,73,74,76] Neoadjuvant therapy has not shown benefit in cholangiocaricnoma. There have been three phase II randomized trials assessing adjuvant therapy in biliary tract cancers (cholangiocarcinoma and gallbladder carcinoma). The BCAT trial assessed gemcitabine,[77] and the PRODIGE-12 trial assessed gemcitabine and oxaliplatin[78] in the adjuvant setting. There was no benefit of adjuvant therapy in either of these trials.[77,78] The BILCAP study investigated adjuvant capecitabine in biliary tract cancers.[79] Although a statistically significant benefit in intention to treat overall survival analysis was not observed, there was a benefit of adjuvant capecitabine in a prespecified sensitivity analysis.[79] Accordingly, guidelines have incorporated adjuvant capecitabine as a standard of care.[80,81]

Intrahepatic cholangiocarcinoma has traditionally been considered a contraindication to LT due to poor outcomes. However, LT may be an option in a subset of cirrhotic patients with "very early" intrahepatic cholangiocarcinoma (single tumors $\leq$2 cm in diameter).[82] In one study, patients with very early intrahepatic cholangiocarcinoma had a 5-year survival of 65%, compared with 45% for patients with advanced disease (single tumor >2 cm or multifocal disease).[83]

Locoregional Therapies

In patients with advanced, unresectable intrahepatic cholangiocarcinoma, locoregional therapies represent an alternative treatment option. Transarterial chemoembolization (TACE) is associated with a median overall survival of 12−15 months in patients with advanced intrahepatic cholangiocarcinoma.[84] The safety and effectiveness of transarterial radioembolization using yttrium-90 microspheres are comparable to those of TACE.[85]

71

TABLE 71.6 TNM and AJCC/UICC Staging Systems for Distal Cholangiocarcinoma

TNM Stage	Criteria		
Tx	Primary tumor cannot be assessed		
Tis	Carcinoma in situ (intraductal tumor)		
T1	Tumor invades the bile duct wall with a depth <5 mm		
T2	Tumor invades the bile duct wall with a depth of 5-12 mm		
T3	Tumor invades the bile duct wall with a depth >12 mm		
T4	Tumor involves the celiac axis, superior mesenteric artery, and/or the common hepatic artery		
Nx	Regional lymph nodes cannot be assessed		
N0	No regional lymph node metastases		
N1	Regional lymph node metastases (≤3 lymph nodes)		
N2	Regional lymph node metastases (≥4 lymph nodes)		
M0	No distant metastases		
M1	Distant metastases		
AJCC/UICC Stage	**Tumor**	**Node**	**Metastasis**
0	Tis	N0	M0
I	T1	N0	M0
IIA	T1	N1	M0
IIA	T2	N0	M0
IIB	T2	N1	M0
IIB	T3	N0-1	M0
IIIA	T1	N2	M0
IIIA	T2-3	N2	M0
IIIB	T4	N0-2	M0
IV	Any T	Any N	M1

AJCC, American Joint Committee on Cancer; *UICC*, Union for International Cancer Control.

Perihilar and Distal Cholangiocarcinoma

Surgical Resection and LT

Surgical resection is also the treatment of choice for perihilar and distal cholangiocarcinomas in the absence of PSC (Box 71.2). Perihilar cholangiocarcinomas are resected by lobar or extended lobar hepatic and biliary duct resection with regional lymphadenectomy and Roux-en-Y hepaticojejunostomy. Occasionally, resectability can be achieved by preoperative portal vein embolization, resulting in compensatory hyperplasia of the contralateral hepatic lobe. This technique allows extended partial hepatectomy because of the increased volume of the remnant liver.[86] Surgical treatment of distal cholangiocarcinoma is performed by a Whipple resection. A total of 5-year survival rates in N0 patients after R0 resection are 20%−67% for perihilar and 27%−37% for distal cholangiocarcinomas; outcomes have improved in the 2000s.[86,87] Unfortunately, R0 resectability rates are generally less than 50%.[76,86] Surgical mortality rates are approximately 10% for perihilar cholangiocarcinomas and 3.0% for distal cholangiocarcinoma.[18,76,87,88] Although neoadjuvant therapy has not shown benefit in perihilar/distal cholangiocarcinoma, guidelines have incorporated adjuvant capecitabine for biliary tract cancers based on the BILCAP trial.[79−81]

In patients with PSC, surgical resection of a cholangiocarcinoma may be complicated by liver failure or a second cholangiocarcinoma, which has a tendency to develop in the area of a biliary-enteric anastomosis.[22,90] Therefore patients with PSC and perihilar cholangiocarcinoma are considered nonresectable and should be considered for LT instead of resection. In the past, LT was not an option for patients with perihilar cholangiocarcinoma, because 5-year survival rates following transplantation were only 23%−26%.[90] Subsequently, new LT protocols were developed, consisting of neoadjuvant external beam radiation therapy with concurrent systemic 5-fluorouracil chemotherapy, followed by brachytherapy and oral maintenance chemotherapy with capecitabine until transplantation. A total of 5- and 10-year recurrence-free survival rates in patients completing this treatment regimen successfully have been 65% and 59%, respectively; posttransplant rates of recurrence and all-cause mortality have been 20% and 22%, respectively.[91] In patients without PSC, the selection criteria include a radial diameter of the perihilar tumor of less than 3 cm, absence of intra- or extrahepatic metastases, and nonresectability.

BOX 71.2 Criteria for Unresectability of Perihilar Cholangiocarcinoma

- Atrophy of one liver lobe with encasement of the contralateral portal vein branch
- Atrophy of one liver lobe with contralateral secondary biliary radicle involvement
- Bilateral portal vein branch encasement
- Bilateral hepatic artery encasement
- Distant lymph node metastases
- Hilar cholangiocarcinoma, Bismuth-Corlette type IV
- Intrahepatic or distant metastases
- PSC
- Significant comorbid conditions

Chemotherapy, Radiation Therapy, and Targeted Therapy

No curative medical therapies for cholangiocarcinoma are available. A variety of chemotherapeutic agents such as gemcitabine, other antimetabolites, taxanes, platinum analogs, anthracyclines, and mitomycin have been evaluated as single or combination therapies. In 2010 the ABC-02 trial[92] showed a statistically significant 3-month overall and progression-free survival benefit for gemcitabine-cisplatin combination therapy compared with gemcitabine alone. The only adverse effect that was more severe in patients in the combination treatment arm was hematologic toxicity; however, patients with cirrhosis were not included in the trial.[92] Gemcitabine and cisplatin subsequently received FDA approval and became the standard of care in the first-line setting for patients with advanced/metastatic cholangiocarcinoma. The combination of cytotoxic chemotherapy and immune checkpoint inhibition is under active investigation. Gemcitabine, cisplatin, and durvalumab were assessed in the phase III TOPAZ-1 trial.[94] In this trial, patients with treatment-naïve advanced-stage biliary tract cancer (cholangiocarcinoma and gallbladder cancer) were randomized to either gemcitabine and cisplatin plus either placebo or durvalumab, an anti–programmed death-ligand 1 (PD-L1) antibody. The combination of gemcitabine and cisplatin plus durvalumab met the primary endpoint of a statistically significant benefit in overall survival compared to gemcitabine and cisplatin plus placebo (median 12.8 vs. 11.5 months in the placebo group).[94] Gemcitabine, cisplatin, and durvalumab have received FDA approval as a first-line treatment option for advanced-stage cholangiocarcinoma. The largest ever phase III trial of biliary tract cancer, KEYNOTE-966, evaluated the combination of gemcitabine and cisplatin plus pembrolizumab, an anti-PD-1 antibody, or placebo in treatment-naïve patients with unresectable, locally advanced, or metastatic biliary tract cancer.[95] Gemcitabine and cisplatin plus pembrolizumab met the primary endpoint of a statistically significant improvement in median overall survival compared to gemcitabine and cisplatin (12.7 vs. 10.9 months).[95] Based on these results, gemcitabine, cisplatin, and pembrolizumab received FDA approval in 2023 for locally advanced unresectable or metastatic CCA.

A number of targeted therapies have also received FDA approval for treatment of cholangiocarcinoma. The *FGFR* inhibitor pemigatinib became the first targeted therapy to receive FDA approval for the treatment of previously treated advanced-stage cholangiocarcinoma with *FGFR2* gene fusions or rearrangements in April 2020.[96,97] Futibatinib, a next-generation *FGFR* inhibitor, had an objective response rate of 41.7% in a phase II study of patients with unresectable or metastatic *FGFR2* fusion positive or *FGFR2* rearrangement positive intrahepatic cholangiocarcinoma. On the basis of this trial, futibatinib received FDA accelerated approval for this indication in 2022.[98] The phase III ClarIDHy trial evaluated ivosidenib, an oral inhibitor of mutant *IDH1*, in previously treated *IDH1*-mutant cholangiocarcinoma.[99] Progression-free survival was significantly improved with ivosidenib compared to plabebo (median progression-free survival of 2.7 vs. 1.4 months, hazard ratio 0.37).[99] These results led to the FDA approval of ivosidenib for treatment of *IDH1*-mutated cholangiocarcinoma in 2021.[100]

No large, randomized controlled trials have evaluated the benefit of radiation therapy in unresectable cholangiocarcinoma. Therefore the use of radiation therapy remains controversial.[2]

Palliative Treatment

Patients with cholangiocarcinoma commonly experience cholestasis, abdominal pain, and cachexia, which limit the quality of life. Therefore palliative treatments are essential in the management of patients with cholangiocarcinoma. Options for restoration of biliary drainage include endoscopic, percutaneous, and surgical techniques. Endoscopic and percutaneous methods are based on placement of biliary stents (see Chapter 72), whereas surgical approaches create a bypass via a choledocho- or hepaticojejunostomy. The efficacies of comparable endoscopic and surgical approaches are similar, but the mortality rate, frequency of procedure-related complications, and duration of hospital stay are higher for surgical palliation.[93] The decision to pursue endoscopic or percutaneous biliary stent deployment is based on the anatomic location of the malignant stricture (see Chapter 72). Although unilateral restoration of bile flow is generally sufficient, bilateral restoration of biliary drainage has been associated with increased survival.[101,102] Cross-sectional imaging is critical before a stent is placed to avoid attempts at endoscopic drainage of an atrophic lobe or a lobe in which adequate drainage is not feasible. Retrograde injection of dye without drainage carries a high risk of iatrogenic bacterial cholangitis, which can be severe. Early intervention in a patient with malignant biliary obstruction is recommended because the time to normalization of the serum bilirubin level doubles from 3 to 6 weeks when the serum total bilirubin level is greater than 10 mg/dL.[103]

External beam radiation and intraoperative or intraductal brachytherapy have been suggested for palliative treatment.[104] No large, prospective randomized controlled trials providing sufficient evidence for the use of these techniques in cholangiocarcinoma, however, have been conducted. Although a few retrospective studies have suggested a survival benefit with TACE, no large, prospective randomized controlled trials providing sufficient evidence of the efficacy of TACE, or other locoregional therapies, in cholangiocarcinoma have been performed.[105]

GALLBLADDER CARCINOMA

Gallbladder carcinoma is the second most common primary biliary malignancy and the fifth most common malignancy of the GI tract. Like other biliary malignancies, gallbladder carcinoma is diagnosed at an advanced stage in the majority of cases. In only one-third of the cases is a diagnosis of gallbladder carcinoma made prior to surgical exploration.[106] The growth kinetics of gallbladder carcinoma are faster than those for cholangiocarcinoma, and, in general, gallbladder carcinoma is diagnosed at a later stage than ampullary carcinoma (see later). Gallbladder carcinoma is not amenable to medical or radiation therapy, and surgical resection is the only potentially curative treatment. Unfortunately, only a minority of patients are surgical candidates at the time of diagnosis. The prognosis of gallbladder carcinoma is dismal, with 5-year survival rates of 0%–10% and a median survival of less than 6 months. More aggressive surgical approaches have been advocated.

Epidemiology

The distribution of gallbladder carcinoma is geographically heterogeneous and is two to three times as common in females as in males.[107,108] The average age at diagnosis is 65 years, and the peak incidence is observed in the seventh and eighth decades of life. The highest incidence of gallbladder cancer globally is in Northern India and South-Central Chile, with age-standardized incidence rates of 27/100,000 in females and 12/100,000 in males.[107] Incidence rates are also high in Asia and certain Eastern European countries such as Poland.[109] Gallbladder carcinoma is rare in Western European countries and the United States, with an age-adjusted incidence rate of 1.4 per 100,000 from 1973 to 2009.[110] In the United States, gallbladder cancer has a significantly higher incidence rate in females than in males (1.7/100,000 vs. 1/100,000).[108] Compared with Caucasians, Native Americans and Alaska Natives have a significantly higher incidence of gallbladder carcinoma (ethnic incidence rate ratio of 4.5 for males and 5.4 for females).[111] Global incidence rates of gallbladder carcinoma parallel the incidence rates of cholelithiasis (see Chapter 67). Overall, the incidence of gallbladder carcinoma in the United States has decreased in most ethnic subgroups (the rate has been steady in African Americans) since 1990.[108,112] Similar trends have been observed across Europe, Canada, and Japan.[113] Although there has been speculation that the declining incidence may be related to an increased number of cholecystectomies during the same period, an association between cholecystectomy rates and the incidence of gallbladder carcinoma has not been found,[114,115] The age-adjusted mortality rate for gallbladder carcinoma in the United States between 2000 and 2005 was 0.7 per 100,000, with an overall decrease since 1990.[8] The highest mortality rate (35 per 100,000) has been reported in Southern Chile.[116]

Etiology

The cause of gallbladder carcinoma is not well understood but is thought to be multifactorial. Several risk factors for gallbladder carcinoma have been described (Box 71.3). The primary risk factor for gallbladder carcinoma is cholelithiasis (see Chapter 67). Gallstones are found in 65%–90% of patients with gallbladder carcinoma. Populations with high rates of cholelithiasis also have high rates of gallbladder carcinoma. Autopsy-based studies from Chile have suggested a sevenfold increased risk of gallbladder carcinoma in patients with cholelithiasis, whereas epidemiologic studies in the United States have observed only a marginally significant threefold increased risk of gallbladder carcinoma in men with cholelithiasis.[115,116] Gallbladder carcinoma actually develops in only 1%–3% of patients with cholelithiasis, and 20% of patients with gallbladder carcinoma do not have evidence of cholelithiasis. Therefore a prophylactic cholecystectomy in an asymptomatic patient with gallstones to prevent gallbladder carcinoma cannot be recommended. A positive correlation between the risk of gallbladder carcinoma and the size and number of gallstones has been reported but likely reflects the duration of cholelithiasis.[117] No differences in the risk of gallbladder carcinoma have been observed with different types of gallstones. Porcelain gallbladder (extensive calcification of the gallbladder wall) is a classic, albeit controversial, risk factor for gallbladder carcinoma.[118] Although an increased risk of gallbladder carcinoma has been reported in patients with a porcelain gallbladder, the risk may be limited to patients with selective mucosal calcification (types II and III porcelain gallbladder) rather than those with diffuse mucosal calcification (type I).[119]

Adenomatous polyps of the gallbladder constitute another risk factor for gallbladder carcinoma (see Chapter 69). The risk correlates positively with the size, type, and growth rate of the polyps. Patients with adenomatous polyps that are greater than 1 cm in size, sessile, and associated with gallstones, exhibit a rapid increase in size, demonstrate arterial flow on Doppler US, or are symptomatic, are at increased risk of malignant transformation, and warrant prophylactic cholecystectomy.[118,120] However, a more recent study has demonstrated that the risk of gallbladder carcinoma is similar amongst patients with or without gallbladder polyps.[121] Pancreaticobiliary malunion, or anomalous union of the pancreaticobiliary ductal system (AUPBD), has been associated with the development of gallbladder carcinoma (see Chapter 57).[122] In this congenital defect, the pancreatic and bile ducts unite outside the duodenal wall in a long common channel. The anomaly is most prevalent in Asia, particularly Japan, and leads to cholestasis and reflux of pancreatic secretions into the gallbladder, with resulting chronic inflammation of the mucosa. The frequency of biliary tract cancer, especially gallbladder carcinoma, is high in patients with AUPBD, with some series reporting a frequency of approximately 50%.[122] However, the frequency can vary from 10% to 38%, depending on the presence or absence of associated bile duct dilatation.[123] Patients with an associated choledochal cyst have a lower frequency of gallbladder carcinoma than those without a choledochal cyst.[123] Patients with AUPBD are usually 10 years younger at the time of diagnosis of gallbladder carcinoma and have a lower frequency of cholelithiasis than those without AUPBD.[123] On the basis of the significantly increased risk of gallbladder carcinoma, several Japanese hepatobiliary oncology associations have recommended prophylactic cholecystectomy in patients with AUPBD.[118,123]

BOX 71.3 Risk Factors for Gallbladder Carcinoma

- Aflatoxin
- Carcinogens*
- Cholangiocarcinoma
- Cholelithiasis (stone size >1 cm)
- Chronic *Salmonella typhi* or *Paratyphi* carrier status
- First-degree relative with gallbladder cancer
- IBD
- Intrahepatic biliary dysplasia
- Lynch syndrome
- Pancreaticobiliary malunion
- Porcelain gallbladder
- PSC
- Segmental adenomyomatosis in patients ≥60 years of age

*Methylcholanthrene, O-aminoazotoluene, nitrosamines, possibly others.

PSC has been associated with gallbladder carcinoma, and studies have reported that adenocarcinoma of the gallbladder develops in up to 20% of patients with PSC and that 40%–60% of gallbladder masses in patients with PSC are malignant.[124] Therefore patients with PSC and a gallbladder mass of any size should undergo cholecystectomy or be monitored closely for gallbladder carcinoma (see Chapters 69 and 70).

Adenomyomatosis of the gallbladder is characterized by microscopic invaginations (Rokitansky-Aschoff sinuses) of the mucosa with cyst formation in the muscularis propria (see Chapter 67). A large Japanese study showed an increased frequency of gallbladder carcinoma in patients 60 years of age or older with segmental adenomyomatosis of the gallbladder.[125] In general, however, adenomyomatosis is viewed as a benign condition.

Other conditions associated with gallbladder carcinoma include IBD, intrahepatic biliary dysplasia, and cholangiocarcinoma.[124] Chronic carriers of *Salmonella typhi* or *paratyphi* have been shown to be at increased risk for the development of gallbladder carcinoma.[126] Other bacteria such as *Escherichia coli* and *Helicobacter pylori* have also been associated with gallbladder carcinoma, but the data are not conclusive. First-degree relatives of patients with gallbladder carcinoma have a relative risk of 13.9 for developing this malignancy.[127] Exposure to aflatoxin, a known liver carcinogen, has been linked to gallbladder carcinoma.[128,129] Patients who have higher plasma levels of aflatoxin adducts have an odds ratio for gallbladder carcinoma development of 7.61 compared with patients who have lower levels.[129,130] Other carcinogens, including methylcholanthrene, *O*-aminoazotoluene, and nitrosamines, have been identified in animal models of gallbladder carcinoma. Other potential carcinogens include mustard oil, products of free radical oxidation, and secondary bile acids. Obesity has been suggested to be a risk factor for gallbladder carcinoma, especially in women,[131] but the independence of obesity from cholelithiasis as a risk factor has not been shown. Menopausal hormonal therapy, including combined formulations of estrogen and progesterone as well as orally administered hormonal therapy, has been linked with an increased risk of gallbladder carcinoma.[132]

Pathology

From 80% to 95% of gallbladder carcinomas are adenocarcinomas; the majority of these are moderately to well differentiated.[133] Adenocarcinomas are further divided into papillary, tubular, and nodular variants, with the papillary adenocarcinomas being the least aggressive form.[134] Less common types, in order of frequency, include undifferentiated or anaplastic carcinoma, squamous cell carcinoma, and adenosquamous carcinoma. Gallbladder squamous cell carcinomas tend to be higher grade and are diagnosed at a later stage compared to gallbladder adenocarcinoma.[135] Rare types include carcinoids, small cell carcinomas, malignant melanomas, lymphomas, and sarcomas.[134] Overall, 60% of gallbladder carcinomas are located in the gallbladder fundus, 30% are found in the body, and 10% are found in the gallbladder neck.[133] Analogous to cholangiocarcinoma, the papillary form of gallbladder carcinoma has a lower potential for invasion and metastatic spread to lymph nodes.[134] Gallbladder carcinoma spreads via direct invasion, lymphatic or hematogenous metastasis, perineural invasion, and intraperitoneal or intraductal invasion. Lymphatic tumor cell spread is determined by the physiologic gallbladder lymphatic plexus, including the first-level lymph nodes along the biliary tract (cystic duct, bile duct, and hepatic duct), followed by pancreaticoduodenal lymph nodes, as well as lymph nodes along the common hepatic artery and celiac axis. Lymph node metastases are described in 54%–64% of patients and correlate with the depth of invasion. Gallbladder carcinoma has a predisposition to involve the liver bed because of venous drainage, predominantly into hepatic segments IVb and V (see Chapter 73), and the anatomic proximity that allows direct hepatic invasion. Perineural spread is observed in 24% and intraductal spread in 19% of cases.

Pathogenesis

Gallbladder carcinoma can develop from foci of mucosal dysplasia or carcinoma in situ that progress to adenocarcinoma or from an adenoma-carcinoma sequence similar to that seen with colon cancer (see Chapter 129).[136–138] Foci of dysplasia and carcinoma in situ are frequently found adjacent to gallbladder carcinoma in surgically resected gallbladder specimens and are thought to be precursors of invasive adenocarcinoma.[109] The time of progression of dysplasia to carcinoma is estimated to be 10–15 years.[137] The major pathogenic factor is inflammation.

Whole-exome and targeted gene sequencing studies have helped define the mutational landscape of gallbladder carcinoma. These analyses indicate that gallbladder carcinomas are genetically distinct from cholangiocarcinomas.[139,140] In one cohort, whole-exome and ultradeep sequencing identified mutations in the *ErbB* family of proteins in 35.8% of cases.[139] Moreover, cases with *ErbB* pathway mutations had a worse outcome. Similarly, molecular characterization of biliary tract cancer, including gallbladder carcinoma, identified frequent activation of the epidermal growth factor receptor (EGFR) family of genes (*EGFR*, *ERBB2*, *ERBB3*) in gallbladder carcinoma, as well as somatic telomerase reverse transcriptase (*TERT*) promoter mutations.[36] Mutations in the tumor suppressor gene *TP53* have been reported in 47.1%–59% of gallbladder carcinomas in different series.[139,140] Activating mutations of *PIK3CA* have been reported in 5.95%–12.5% of gallbladder carcinomas.[140,141] *PIK3CA* mutations lead to activation of the PI3K pathway–AKT pathway, which mediates oncogenesis in a spectrum of malignancies. Other genetic aberrations encountered in gallbladder carcinoma include *CDKN2A/B* loss (5.9%–19%) and mutations in *KRAS* (4%–13%), as well as in *ARID1A* (13%) and *NRAS* (6.3%).[140]

Clinical Features and Diagnosis

In 47%–78% of patients, gallbladder carcinoma is found incidentally during cholecystectomy for presumed benign disease, reflecting the initial clinically silent nature of this malignancy.[142] Incidentally diagnosed gallbladder carcinomas generally are lower in stage than symptomatic carcinomas at the time of diagnosis and are associated with better median survival rates.[142]

Common clinical presentations include biliary or abdominal pain and jaundice secondary to direct invasion of the biliary ducts or metastasis to the hepatoduodenal ligament. Weight loss, abdominal distention, or other symptoms resulting from compression or invasion of adjacent organs indicate more advanced disease.

CEA and CA 19-9 are the most commonly used tumor markers for gallbladder carcinoma.[143] At a cutoff at 4.0 ng/mL, an elevated serum CEA level has a sensitivity and specificity of 50% and 93%. The sensitivity and specificity of an elevated serum CA 19-9 level at a cutoff of 20 U/mL are 79% and 79%.[143,144] These tests aid in diagnosis but should not be relied on because levels can be elevated in inflammatory conditions and other GI and gynecologic malignancies; moreover, a subset of the population does not produce CEA.

Abdominal US is often one of the first imaging studies performed in a patient who presents with the aforementioned symptoms. The sensitivity and accuracy of US for gallbladder carcinoma are 85% and 80%, respectively; early cancers, especially sessile polyps, can be missed. Typical imaging presentations of gallbladder carcinoma include focal or diffuse mural thickening of the gallbladder, an intraluminal mass greater than 2 cm in size that originates in the gallbladder wall, and a subhepatic mass that replaces or obscures the gallbladder and often invades adjacent organs (Fig. 71.6). Findings indicative of the malignant nature of a gallbladder lesion include irregular, asymmetrical mural thickening greater than 1 cm in depth and a nodular or smooth intraluminal mass greater than 1 cm in size, with fixation to the gallbladder wall, that is not displaced by the patient's movements and has no acoustic shadow. In indeterminate cases, Doppler US can be attempted to differentiate a malignant from a benign gallbladder lesion on the basis of the pattern of the color signal, blood flow velocity, and resistive index (a measure of resistance to arterial blood flow).[145]

MRI and CT can be helpful in the diagnosis if the US findings are indeterminate. Helical CT has 83%–86% accuracy in assessing the local extent, with better performance in T2 and higher stages (see later), and is, thus, helpful in preoperative planning.[146,147] The role of PET in gallbladder carcinoma is evolving and not routine.[148] The sensitivity of PET for detecting gallbladder carcinoma is only 75%–78%.[149,150] Its main impact is in the detection of distant metastases that result in a change in management.[54]

Staging

Staging systems for gallbladder carcinoma include the Nevin-Moran classification system and the Japanese Biliary Surgical Society staging system. The most commonly used staging system is the TNM system described by the AJCC and UICC (Table 71.7). The TNM-based staging system correlates with survival. Reported 5-year survival rates for patients with stages 0, I, II, III A, III B, IV A, and IV B gallbladder carcinoma are 80%, 50%, 28%, 8%, 7%, 4%, and 2%, respectively. In the 2018 version of the AJCC/UICC staging system, stage T2 was separated into T2a (tumor location on the peritoneal side of gallbladder) and T2b (tumor location on the hepatic side of the gallbladder).[69] In comparing different prognostic and therapeutic studies, it is important to account for differences in the version of the applied staging system.

Treatment

Surgery is the only potentially curative therapeutic option for gallbladder carcinoma.[151] Only 15%–47% of patients are candidates for surgical resection at the time of diagnosis because the

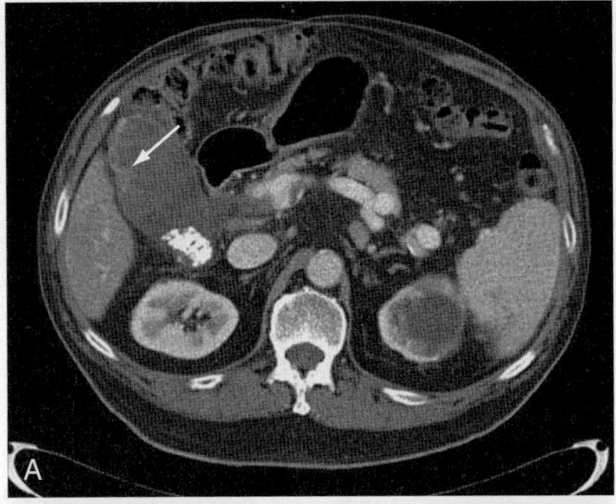

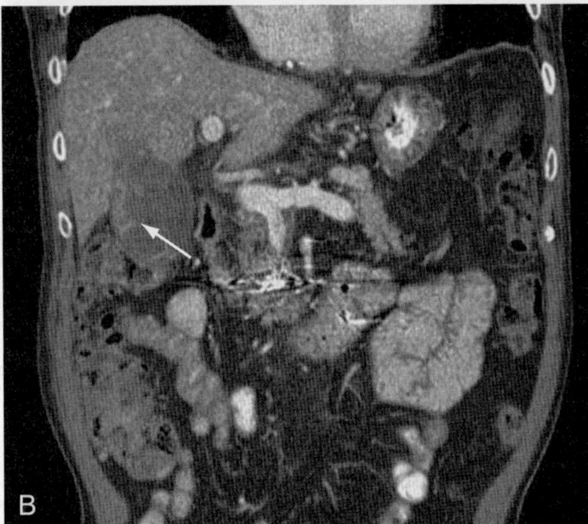

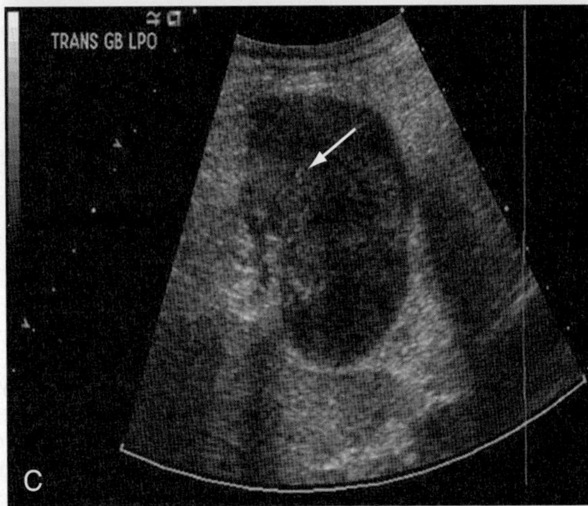

Fig. 71.6 Imaging of gallbladder carcinoma. (A) Axial CT view of the abdomen. Cholelithiasis is seen inferior to the gallbladder mass (*arrow*). (B) Coronal view of the same patient. (C) US in the same patient showing a large mass (*arrow*) originating from the gallbladder wall and protruding into the lumen.

stage of the disease is advanced in most cases. Contraindications to resection include multiple hepatic or distant metastases, gross vascular invasion or encasement of major vessels, malignant ascites, and poor functional status.[133] Direct invasion of the colon, duodenum, or liver is not considered an absolute contraindication to surgical resection. The goal of surgical treatment is an R0 resection, defined as negative margins and nodal dissection one level past microscopically involved lymph nodes. R0 resection in gallbladder carcinoma has been shown to correlate with survival and with significantly increased 5-year survival rates[142,152]; however, R0 resection is achieved in only 36%–49% of patients undergoing surgical exploration or reexploration.[142,152]

Surgical procedures with curative intent include (1) simple cholecystectomy; (2) extended or radical cholecystectomy with additional resection of greater than 2 cm of the gallbladder bed plus lymphadenectomy of the hepatoduodenal ligament behind the second part of the duodenum, head of the pancreas, and celiac axis; (3) extended cholecystectomy with hepatic, segmental, or lobar resection; (4) extended cholecystectomy with extensive para-aortic lymph node resection; and (5) extended cholecystectomy with bile duct resection or pancreaticoduodenectomy. The surgical approach is dictated by the extent of tumor. Less than 10% of patients with gallbladder carcinoma are diagnosed with Tis and T1a tumors. At these stages, gallbladder carcinomas can be treated with simple cholecystectomy, with 5-year survival rates of 85%–100%. A few reports have also favored simple cholecystectomy for stage T1b gallbladder carcinoma and have reported similar survival rates after either simple or radical cholecystectomy.[153,154] Up to 15% of patients with stage T1b gallbladder carcinoma, however, are positive for lymph node metastases, compared with 2.5% of patients with stage T1a gallbladder carcinoma.[155] Also, higher recurrence rates have been observed after simple (vs. radical) cholecystectomy; therefore radical cholecystectomy is recommended for stage 1b gallbladder carcinoma.[155–158]

Invasion of the muscularis propria, as in stage T2 tumors, requires radical cholecystectomy, resulting in 5-year survival rates of 59%–90%, compared with 17%–40% with simple cholecystectomy.[159–161] It is important to note that the risk of tumor invasion and mode of cancer spread in T2 gallbladder carcinoma is influenced by whether the tumor is located on the hepatic or peritoneal side of the gallbladder. Patients with T2 gallbladder carcinoma with tumors on the hepatic side have higher rates of vascular invasion, neural invasion, and nodal metastasis than those with tumors on the peritoneal side (51% vs. 19%, 33% vs. 8%, and 40% vs. 17%, respectively).[162] Therefore the updated AJCC/UICC staging system has divided T2 gallbladder carcinoma into T2a and T2b on the basis of tumor location on the peritoneal or hepatic side of the gallbladder, respectively.[69]

The surgical approach to stage T3 and T4 tumors (tumors invading beyond the serosa) is controversial. Some studies have shown no 5-year survival benefit after radical cholecystectomy for stage T3 and T4 tumors, but other studies have reported 5-year survival rates of 15%–63% and 7%–25%, respectively.[163] Because of the poor prognosis of gallbladder carcinoma and the possibility of a survival benefit, as well as prolongation of survival until recurrence, a radical surgical approach to these advanced-stage gallbladder carcinomas is recommended by many centers.

When gallbladder carcinoma is diagnosed during laparoscopy, the procedure should be converted to an open procedure, and the laparoscopic port sites should be resected because tumor may recur at these sites secondary to iatrogenic dissemination.[164] Further surgical management then depends on the tumor stage, as outlined earlier and in Fig. 71.7. When gallbladder carcinoma is diagnosed postoperatively, further management depends on the tumor stage and the presence or absence of tumor at the margins of the surgical specimen. The likelihood of finding residual disease at reexploration has been reported to be 50%, 61%, 85%, and 100% for stages T1, T2, T3, and T4 tumors, respectively, in the initial specimen.[142] Adjuvant therapy with capecitabine has become standard of care based on the results of the BILCAP trial (see earlier).[79]

TABLE 71.7 TNM and AJCC/UICC Staging Systems for Gallbladder Carcinoma

TNM Stage	Criteria		
Tx	Primary tumor cannot be assessed		
T0	No evidence of primary tumor		
Tis	Carcinoma in situ		
T1a	Tumor invades lamina propria		
T1b	Tumor invades muscularis propria		
T2a	Tumor invades perimuscular connective tissue on the peritoneal side, without involvement of serosa		
T2b	Tumor invades perimuscular connective tissue on the hepatic side, without direct extension into the liver		
T3	Tumor perforates the serosa *AND/OR* Tumor directly invades the liver *AND/OR* Tumor invades one other adjacent organ (i.e., stomach, duodenum, colon, pancreas, omentum, extrahepatic bile ducts)		
T4	Tumor invades the portal vein or hepatic artery *OR* Tumor invades ≥2 extrahepatic organs or structures		
Nx	Regional lymph nodes cannot be assessed		
N0	No regional lymph node metastases		
N1	Regional lymph node metastases (≤3 lymph nodes)		
N2	Regional lymph node metastases (≥4 lymph nodes)		
M0	No distant metastases		
M1	Distant metastases		
AJCC/UICC Stage	**Tumor**	**Node**	**Metastasis**
0	Tis	N0	M0
I	T1	N0	M0
IIA	T2a	N0	M0
IIB	T2b	N0	M0
IIIA	T3	N0	M0
IIIB	T1-3	N1	M0
IVA	T4	N0-1	M0
IVB	Any T	N2	M0
	Any T	Any N	M1

AJCC, American Joint Committee on Cancer; *UICC,* Union for International Cancer Control.

The standard of care for patients with unresectable gallbladder carcinoma has been chemotherapy with gemcitabine combined with cisplatin. This recommendation is based largely on the ABC-02 trial (see earlier), which included 149 patients with gallbladder carcinoma and showed an improvement in overall survival with gemcitabine and cisplatin compared to gemcitabine alone (median overall survival 11.7 vs. 8.1 months, hazard ratio, 0.64), similar to that for cholangiocarcinoma.[92] The combination of gemcitabine, cisplatin, and durvalumab has also received FDA approval for unresectable gallbladder carcinoma based on the results of the TOPAZ-1 trial, although the subgroup analysis for gallbladder patients ($n = 85$) did not demonstrate a statistically significant benefit.[94] Other chemotherapeutic agents and gemcitabine-based combination therapies [with oxaliplatin, 5-fluorouracil (5-FU), or capecitabine] and targeted agents (cetuximab, erlotinib, or bevacizumab) have been assessed in smaller studies but have failed to show outcomes superior to those for the combination of gemcitabine and cisplatin, which, therefore, remains first-line treatment for unresectable gallbladder carcinoma. In general, gallbladder carcinoma is considered radioresistant.[93]

AMPULLARY CARCINOMA

Carcinomas of the ampulla of Vater belong to the family of periampullary carcinomas. This family includes carcinomas of the duodenum, ampulla of Vater, distal bile duct, and pancreas (see Chapter 62). Ampullary carcinomas are the second most common form of periampullary carcinoma (after pancreatic head cancer). The distinction among the different forms is important because ampullary carcinomas are often diagnosed earlier than the others and, therefore, at a resectable stage, thereby resulting in a better prognosis.[165]

Epidemiology

Ampullary carcinomas are rare, accounting for fewer than 1% of all GI cancers and 4%–8% of periampullary carcinomas. The annual incidence has been estimated to be 0.6 per 100,000 population.[165,166] Peak incidence is in the seventh decade of life. There is a slight male predominance, with a male-to-female ratio of 1.48:1.[167] Racial heterogeneity has been observed; the vast

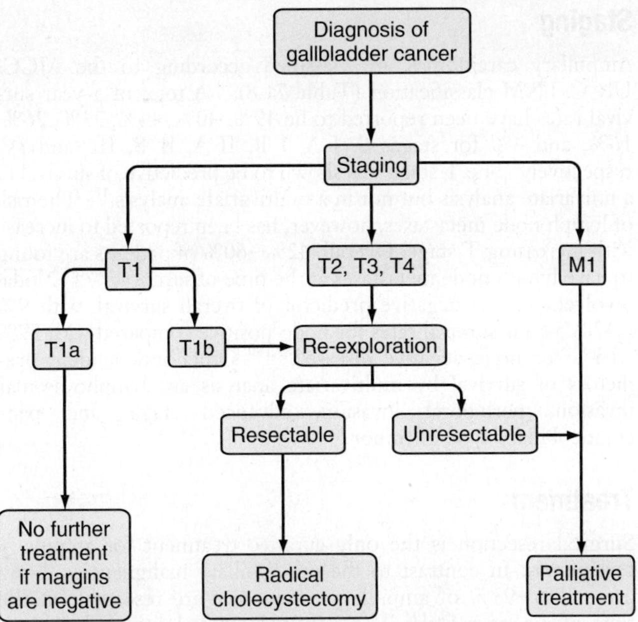

Fig. 71.7 Algorithm for the management of gallbladder carcinoma discovered intra- or postoperatively at laparoscopic cholecystectomy. In cases in which pathologic examination of the cholecystectomy specimen identifies a stage T1a tumor with negative surgical margins, no further treatment is indicated. If the tumor is found to be a stage T1b tumor or the margins of resection are positive for malignant tissue, reexploration for further resection is indicated. Similarly, patients with gallbladder carcinoma found to be stage T2, T3, or T4 should undergo surgical reexploration. If reexploration reveals resectable gallbladder carcinoma, radical cholecystectomy should be performed. If the tumor is deemed unresectable, palliative management is indicated. When postoperative staging reveals metastatic spread, palliative management is indicated. *M*, Metastasis stage; *T*, tumor stage. (Modified from Misra S, Chaturvedi A, Misra NC, Sharma ID. Carcinoma of the gallbladder. *Lancet Oncol*. 2003;4:167–176.)

majority of patients are Caucasian, followed by patients of Hispanic and Asian descent. African Americans have the lowest incidence rates in the United States.[165] The incidence of ampullary carcinoma has increased by 0.9% annually in the United States since the 1970s.[167]

Etiology

Although the etiology of ampullary carcinomas is unknown in the majority of cases, several conditions have been associated with this malignancy, mostly in case reports or small series. Familial adenomatous polyposis (FAP) is an important risk factor for the development of ampullary carcinomas (see Chapter 128).[168] Periampullary carcinoma is the second most common cause of death (after colon cancer) in patients with FAP. Usually, periampullary carcinoma arises later than colorectal carcinoma in this patient group but earlier in comparison with sporadic ampullary carcinomas.[168] Screening for upper GI neoplasms (polyps or carcinoma) at regular intervals of 6 months to 4 years, depending on the degree of duodenal polyposis, is, therefore, recommended in patients with FAP.[168] Similarly, increased rates of ampullary carcinoma have been described in patients with Gardner syndrome, a variant of FAP (see Chapter 128).[169] Lynch syndrome (hereditary nonpolyposis colorectal cancer) does not appear to predispose to ampullary carcinoma (see Chapter 129).[170] Other genetic diseases reported to predispose to the development of ampullary carcinoma include neurofibromatosis type 1 and Muir-Torre syndrome.[171,172] As in cholangiocarcinoma, chronic liver-fluke infection has been reported to be a risk factor for ampullary carcinoma (see Chapter 86).[166]

Pathology

The ampulla of Vater is an anatomically complex area that consists of the papilla, common pancreaticobiliary channel, distal bile duct, and distal main pancreatic duct. Macroscopically, ampullary carcinomas are classified into the following three types: (1) intramural protruding (intra-ampullary), (2) extramural protruding (periampullary), and (3) ulcerating ampullary.[166] The ulcerating type is usually diagnosed at an advanced stage and has the highest rate of lymph node metastasis. Consistent with its anatomic heterogeneity, the ampulla includes several different histologic cell types, such as epithelia of the common pancreaticobiliary channel, bile duct, pancreatic duct, or duodenal mucosa, Brunner glands, and aberrant pancreatic acini in the wall of the bile duct. The most common site of cellular atypia is found in the area of the common pancreaticobiliary channel, followed by the pancreatic duct, duodenal epithelium, and Brunner glands.[173] Overall, 75% of all ampullary neoplasms are adenocarcinomas, 20% are benign adenomas, and 5% are neuroendocrine tumors.[174] Adenocarcinomas account for 90% of ampullary malignancies; the rest include unusual types, such as mucinous, signet-ring cell, and undifferentiated carcinomas.[174] Histopathologically, 90% of ampullary adenocarcinomas can be classified into pancreaticobiliary or intestinal types.[175,176] Histomolecular phenotyping of ampullary carcinomas based on histologic subtype and immunohistochemical expression of caudal-type homeodomain transcription factor 2 (CDX2) and mucin 1 (MUC1) staining may have prognostic value. In two different series, patients with a pancreaticobiliary histomolecular phenotype (CDX2 negative, MUC1 positive) had worse outcomes than patients with an intestinal phenotype (CDX2 positive, MUC1 negative)[177,178]; however, a subsequent study did not identify prognostic differences between the two subtypes.[179]

Pathogenesis

The majority of ampullary carcinomas follow an adenoma-carcinoma sequence. In 30%–91% of ampullary carcinomas, residual adenomatous tissue is found.[166] Although precursor lesions can develop from intestinal as well as pancreaticobiliary-type tissue, carcinomas of the intestinal type typically develop from adenomas, whereas pancreaticobiliary and ulcerating carcinomas often lack a precursor lesion.[166] The intestinal and pancreaticobiliary types have distinct molecular alterations. *KRAS* alterations are more frequent in pancreaticobiliary type, whereas adenomatous polyposis coli (*APC*) gene alterations are a more frequent occurrence in the intestinal type.[180] Other genetic aberrations include *TP53* mutations, *ERBB2* amplification, and *CDKN2A* loss.[180] Based on in-depth genomic analyses of ampullary carcinomas, the frequency of driver gene mutations differs between the intestinal and pancreatobiliary types, although there is significant overlap for common mutations, including *KRAS*, *TP53*, *SMAD4*, and *CTNNB1*.[181] Notably, *ELF3* has been identified as a novel mutated driver tumor suppressor gene in ampullary carcinoma. Inactivating mutations of *ELF3*, a member of the ETS transcription factor family that encodes an E26 transformation-specific transcription factor, are present in 10%–12% of ampullary carcinomas.[39,181] *ELF3* inactivation promotes motility and invasion of epithelial cells.[181]

Clinical Features and Diagnosis

Like the other periampullary and biliary malignancies, ampullary carcinomas present initially with obstructive jaundice in 70% to

82% of cases. Pancreaticobiliary ampullary carcinomas in particular have been reported to present initially with obstructive jaundice.[175] Because of their anatomic location, cholestasis develops at an earlier stage than do other periampullary and biliary malignancies, and the resectability rate is, therefore, higher at the time of diagnosis. Anicteric patients may present with bacterial cholangitis. Rare patients have "silver stools" as a result of the combination of acholic stools that result from bile duct obstruction and bleeding of the tumor. When obstructive cholangitis is suspected, further diagnostic evaluation is similar to that for other biliary malignancies. Immunohistochemical analysis has shown high expression of CEA and CA 19-9 in the tumor.[182] Elevated serum concentrations of CEA and CA 19-9 have been detected in 11%–29% and 41%–63%, respectively, of patients with ampullary carcinomas. Elevations of these serum tumor markers have been associated with tumor recurrence and lower rates of disease-free survival in univariate but not multivariate analyses.[182,183]

Usually, ampullary carcinomas are diagnosed by endoscopy on the basis of their macroscopic appearance and findings on biopsy specimens (Fig. 71.8). Subsequent diagnostic tests are directed toward an assessment of resectability and detection of metastases. As for other biliary and periampullary carcinomas, imaging techniques, such as CT and MRI, are commonly used in this setting.[184] On MRI with MRCP, ampullary carcinoma is usually seen as a discrete, hypodense mass on T2-weighted images. Occasionally, the tumor can present as irregular thickening around the bile duct or bulging into the duodenum. Frequently, the dilatation of both the bile and pancreatic ducts (double-duct sign) or only the bile duct is seen; the dilatation of the pancreatic duct alone is rarely seen.[184] Addition of diffusion-weighted imaging to conventional MR imaging enhances detection of ampullary carcinoma.[185] Often, EUS is used in the preoperative evaluation. Its accuracy for detecting invasion of adjacent organs is 80%–90%, and its sensitivity and specificity for detecting vascular invasion are 73% and 90%, respectively.[186,187] The role of PET in ampullary neoplasms has not been well studied.

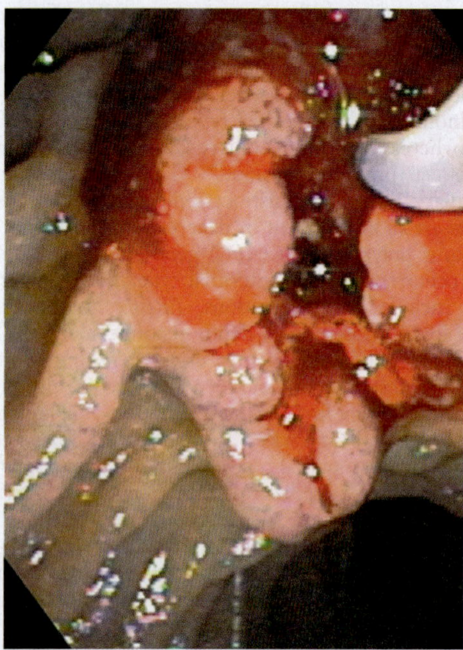

Fig. 71.8 Endoscopic appearance of ampullary carcinoma. A catheter was placed in the ampulla of Vater for biliary drainage after a sphincterotomy was performed.

Staging

Ampullary carcinomas are classified according to the AJCC/UICC TNM classification (Table 71.8).[69] A total of 5-year survival rates have been reported to be 49%, 40%, 44%, 33%, 26%, 16%, and 4% for stages 0, I A, I B, II A, II B, III, and IV, respectively. The T stage was shown to be predictive of survival in a univariate analysis but not in a multivariate analysis.[175] The risk of lymph node metastases, however, has been reported to increase with increasing T stage. Overall, 42%–60% of patients are found to have lymph node metastases at the time of surgery.[188,189] Nodal involvement is a negative predictor of overall survival, with 9%–47% 5-year survival rates for node-positive compared with 59%–63% for node-negative disease.[182,190] Other independent predictors of survival by multivariate analysis are lymphovascular invasion, perineural invasion, advanced stage, and pancreaticobiliary type of tumor.[175,182,191]

Treatment

Surgical resection is the only curative treatment for ampullary carcinomas. In contrast to the other biliary malignancies, however, 77%–93% of ampullary carcinomas are resectable at the time of diagnosis.[188,192] The standard surgical approach is pancreaticoduodenectomy. Outcomes are good in the absence of lymph node metastases, with 5-year survival rates of 59%–78%.[88,193,194] In the presence of lymph node-positive disease, the prognosis worsens significantly, with 5-year survival rates of 16%–25%.[193–195] Extracapsular lymph node involvement results in further worsening of the prognosis, with a 5-year survival rate of only 9%. Node microinvolvement has been reported to be an adverse prognostic factor, and immunohistochemical analysis of resected nodes has been recommended.[196] Limited surgical or endoscopic papillectomy has been reported but is not recommended, because recurrence rates are higher than with pancreaticoduodenectomy.[1] A retrospective analysis of patients who received preoperative chemotherapy with or without radiotherapy did not show a mortality benefit nor an improvement in 5-year overall survival.[197] Therefore further studies are needed to evaluate the role of neoadjuvant therapy in ampullary carcinoma.

Two large, randomized controlled trials have evaluated the benefit of adjuvant chemotherapy and chemoradiation therapy. The Johns Hopkins–Mayo Clinic collaborative study showed a significant improvement in outcome in lymph node-positive patients with adjuvant 5-FU-based chemoradiation, with an increase in the 5-year survival rate from 6% to 28%.[194] Similarly, the European Study Group for Pancreatic Cancer-3 periampullary cancer trial reported a median survival of 58 months in patients who received adjuvant 5-FU plus folinic acid and 71 months in patients who received gemcitabine, compared with 41 months in those who did not receive adjuvant chemotherapy; the benefit of adjuvant chemotherapy reached statistical significance after correction for independent prognostic factors.[198] Subsequent meta-analyses have reported conflicting results, with one demonstrating a significant reduction in the risk of death (hazard ratio 0.75) in patients receiving adjuvant chemoradiotherapy[199] and the other showing no survival benefit for adjuvant therapy.[200] More recent retrospective analyses have shown a benefit of adjuvant chemotherapy in patients with resected ampullary adenocarcinoma.[201,202] In summary, adjuvant chemotherapy or chemoradiation may have a role in a subset of patients with ampullary carcinoma, in particular those with lymph node–positive disease.

The benefit of chemotherapy or radiation therapy for patients with unresectable ampullary carcinoma has not been evaluated in large, randomized controlled trials. Treatment trials have included patients with various types of periampullary cancers, including 20 patients with ampullary carcinoma in the ABC-02

TABLE 71.8 TNM and AJCC/UICC Staging Systems for Ampullary Carcinoma

TNM Stage	Criteria		
Tx	Primary tumor cannot be assessed		
T0	No evidence of primary tumor		
Tis	Carcinoma in situ		
T1a	Tumor limited to ampulla of Vater or sphincter of Oddi		
T1b	Tumor invades beyond the sphincter of Oddi and/or into the duodenal submucosa		
T2	Tumor invades into the duodenal muscularis propria		
T3a	Tumor invades pancreas (≤0.5 cm)		
T3b	Tumor extends >5 cm into the pancreas *OR* Tumor extends into the peripancreatic soft tissue without involvement of the celiac axis or superior mesenteric artery *OR* Tumor invades the duodenal serosa without involvement of the celiac axis or superior mesenteric artery		
T4	Tumor involves the celiac axis, superior mesenteric artery, and/or the common hepatic artery		
Nx	Regional lymph nodes cannot be assessed		
N0	No regional lymph node metastases		
N1	Regional lymph node metastases (≤3 lymph nodes)		
N2	Regional lymph node metastases (≥4 lymph nodes)		
M0	No distant metastases		
M1	Distant metastases		
AJCC/UICC Stage	**Tumor**	**Node**	**Metastasis**
0	Tis	N0	M0
IA	T1a	N0	M0
IB	T1b-2	N0	M0
IIA	T3a	N0	M0
IIB	T3b	N0	M0
IIIA	T1-3	N1	M0
IIIB	T4	Any N	M0
	Any T	N2	M0
IV	Any T	Any N	M1

AJCC, American Joint Committee on Cancer; *UICC*, Union for International Cancer Control.

trial described earlier.[92] In the absence of randomized controlled trials of sufficient numbers of patients with unresectable ampullary carcinoma, the roles of chemotherapy and radiation therapy are not defined.

Palliative treatment should be directed at alleviating tumor-associated complications, with the goal of optimizing the patient's quality of life. Obstructive cholestasis is a major cause of morbidity and can usually be treated palliatively either by endoscopic or percutaneous placement of a biliary stent or by a surgical bypass similar to that carried out for other biliary or periampullary malignancies.

OTHER TUMORS OF THE BILIARY TRACT

Other neoplastic diseases may involve the biliary tract (Box 71.4). Their inclusion in the differential diagnosis of biliary tumors is essential because management differs depending on the tumor type. Tumors of neuroectodermal origin, such as carcinoids (see Chapter 43) and paragangliomas, are rare and typically nonfunctioning.[203] They are most commonly located in the ampulla of Vater. Occasionally, carcinoids develop in the extrahepatic biliary tract, predominantly in the bile duct. Patients are usually female and young. Primary carcinoids of the biliary tract constitute less than 1% of all GI carcinoids and usually are not associated with the carcinoid syndrome.[204,205] Approximately one-third of patients have metastases at diagnosis. The treatment of choice is surgical resection, and the prognosis is generally good.[206–208] Patients with paragangliomas often present with GI bleeding; only 25% present with jaundice. Their malignant potential has been estimated to be 33%, and some investigators recommend pancreaticoduodenectomy as the treatment of choice.[209] Granular cell tumors, which are of neuronal derivation, are extremely rare; only a few cases have been described. Usually, they are located in the extrahepatic biliary tract, particularly at the junction of the cystic duct and the bile duct.[210] Occasionally, they can cause biliary obstruction, as occurs when they are located in the hepatic hilum.[210] Because of their benign character, resection is usually curative.[211] Rarely, neuromas of the extrahepatic biliary tract develop after cholecystectomy.[212] Mesenchymal tumors, such as lipomas, leiomyomas, hemangiomas, and lymphangiomas, have been described in the gallbladder. In general, mesenchymal tumors are extremely rare and restricted to case reports. Lymphangiomas are often asymptomatic and detected incidentally; however, they can increase in size and result in abdominal pain or jaundice. US, CT, and MRI with MRCP aid in the preoperative diagnosis. Usually, lymphangiomas manifest as a multilocular, fluid-filled, cystic mass with thin walls and septa and show enhanced signal density with administration of a contrast agent.[213] Most of the reported cases have been treated successfully with

BOX 71.4 Tumors of the Biliary Tract Other than Adenocarcinoma

GALLBLADDER

Benign

Adenoma
Granular cell tumor
Mesenchymal tumor (lipoma, leiomyoma, hemangioma, lymphangioma)
Paraganglioma

Malignant

Adenosquamous carcinoma
Neuroendocrine tumor (carcinoid)
Small cell carcinoma
Spindle cell sarcomatoid carcinoma
Others (angiosarcoma, carcinosarcoma, Kaposi sarcoma, leiomyosarcoma, malignant fibrous histiocytoma, melanoma, metastatic tumors, non-Hodgkin lymphoma, rhabdomyosarcoma)

Tumor-Like Lesions

Adenomyoma/adenomyomatosis
Cholesterol polyp
Heterotopia (gastric, pancreatic, liver, adrenal, thyroid)
Inflammatory polyp

BILE DUCTS

Benign

Adenofibroma
Adenoma
Adenomyoma
Ciliated hepatic foregut cyst
Cystadenoma and cystadenocarcinoma
Granular cell tumor
Hamartoma
Neuroma
Serous cystadenoma
Solitary or multiple cysts

Malignant

Embryonal (botryoid) rhabdosarcoma
Leukemia
Lymphoma
Melanoma
Metastatic tumor
Neuroendocrine tumor (carcinoid)
Paraganglioma

Precursor Lesions

Dysplasia (intraepithelial neoplasia/atypical hyperplasia)
Intraductal papillary mucinous tumor of the bile duct (biliary papillomatosis)

surgical resection, including cholecystectomy, if the tumor is located within the gallbladder, or endoscopic resection if the tumor is in the area of the ampulla of Vater.[214–217] Hamartomas have also been reported in the area of the ampulla of Vater and have been resected successfully by endoscopy.[218]

Heterotopia of the gallbladder may be caused by gastric, pancreatic, hepatic, adrenal, or thyroid tissue. Clinical complications such as hemorrhage are extremely rare.[219,220] Benign bile duct lesions include adenomas, cystadenomas, adenofibromas, cysts, and granular cell tumors. Adenomyomas are found more commonly in the ampulla of Vater. Cystadenomas are more common in women and manifest primarily with abdominal pain. They are found predominantly in the intrahepatic biliary tract and are characterized on US by papillary extrusions of the wall and septa. They are considered premalignant because of their potential to transform into cystadenocarcinomas; therefore the treatment of choice is complete resection.[221–223]

Malignant tumors of the biliary tract other than cholangiocarcinoma include cystadenocarcinomas, lymphomas, and malignant melanomas. These malignancies arise primarily in the extrahepatic bile ducts. Cystadenocarcinomas can be distinguished morphologically from cholangiocarcinomas by their cystic character.[224] They are rarely located in the gallbladder.[225] Symptoms are nonspecific, and CT and MRI can be helpful in making the diagnosis. The treatment of choice is surgical resection.[225] Malignant melanoma of the biliary tract is uncommon and should prompt investigation for a cutaneous melanoma, because cases of metastatic spread to the bile ducts have been described.[226,227] Lymphomas can occasionally involve the extrahepatic biliary tract and are often mistaken for cholangiocarcinoma.[228,229] In general, biliary lymphomas are very rare and account for less than 1% of lymphomas.[229,230] Few reports exist of follicular lymphomas originating in the extrahepatic biliary tract and gallbladder. Often, these tumors are diagnosed after resection. Embryonal rhabdomyosarcoma of the biliary tract is extremely rare in adults but is the most common malignant tumor at this anatomic location in children.[231] Frequently, it is misdiagnosed preoperatively as a choledochal cyst.[232] Complete surgical resection is rarely possible, and a multidisciplinary approach to treatment is recommended. The prognosis of biliary rhabdosarcomas is good, with reported 5-year survival rates of up to 78%.[233]

Precursor lesions for cholangiocarcinoma include high-grade dysplasia and intraductal papillary mucinous tumor (neoplasm) of the bile duct (IPNB). High-grade dysplasia of the bile ducts may be a harbinger of cholangiocarcinoma, particularly in patients with PSC.[234–237] Patients with high-grade dysplasia are more likely to have FISH polysomy compared with those with low-grade dysplasia or no dysplasia.[235] A metaplasia-dysplasia-carcinoma sequence has been described in PSC-associated cholangiocarcinoma[236]; however, the management of PSC patients with high-grade dysplasia remains a challenge. A conservative approach, which includes observation and intensive surveillance with serial MRCPs and/or ERCPs, is typically used in the United States. In countries with favorable organ allocation, LT has been proposed as the treatment of choice for high-grade dysplasia arising in the setting of PSC.[234]

IPNB encompasses intraductal papillary cholangiocarcinoma and precursor lesions such as biliary papillomatosis and biliary intraductal papillary mucinous neoplasm.[238] Biliary papillomatosis, a rare disease with high malignant potential, is characterized by numerous papillary adenomas in the biliary tract.[239] The clinical presentation of IPNB includes recurrent abdominal pain, jaundice, and acute cholangitis. Because IPNB is a diffuse/multifocal entity, MRCP or ERCP is used to delineate its extent within the biliary tract.[240] Patients with IPNB should be considered for surgical resection due to the high malignant potential of these lesions.[241]

Acknowledgment

This work was supported by NIH K08CA236874 (S.I.I.).

Full references for this chapter can be found at https://ebooks.health.elsevier.com.

72 Endoscopic and Radiologic Treatment of Biliary Disease*

Gregory A. Coté

IN THIS CHAPTER

INTRODUCTION

The basic principles of endoscopic and fluoroscopic interventions for extrahepatic biliary disorders are to diagnose and treat the etiology of pathologic obstruction. Broadly, extrahepatic bile duct pathology includes impaired biliary outflow from benign or malignant strictures, gallstones, intraductal tumors, and parasitic or congenital anomalies such as a choledochocele; the latter are uncommon, particularly in Western countries. Innovations in flexible endoscopes, echoendoscopes, and access or drainage devices reduce the need for laparoscopic or open surgery. Interventional radiologists perform radiologic interventions primarily by a percutaneous and transhepatic approach with fluoroscopic guidance. Endoscopic interventions leverage endoluminal ultrasound (US) [i.e., endoscopic US (EUS)] or combined endoscopic and fluoroscopic imaging [endoscopic retrograde cholangiopancreatography (ERCP)]. Endoscopy reduces the need for external drains and should be able to address most extrahepatic pathology in the first treatment session. Many of the techniques overlap, with percutaneous approaches being unencumbered by postoperative foregut anatomy and often helpful when there is multifocal biliary obstruction at the hepatic confluence.

Keeping these overarching principles in mind, the optimal approach to patients with biliary pathology occurs in three stages: (1) localization and diagnosis using minimally invasive, cross-sectional imaging, then (2) development of a multidisciplinary treatment developed by gastroenterologists, interventional radiologists, surgeons, or some combination, followed by (3) utilization of one or more endoscopic and percutaneous treatments, almost without exception before considering a laparoscopic or open surgical salvage.

STAGE I: CROSS-SECTIONAL IMAGING OF THE BILIARY TRACT

Evaluate patients presenting with suspected biliary pathology with cross-sectional imaging before intervention. Diagnostic EUS is useful for patients with a suspected common bile duct stone or indeterminate bile duct stricture but avoid diagnostic ERCP and percutaneous transhepatic cholangiography (PTC) with biliary drainage (PTBD) without imaging confirmation of a biliary obstruction or leak. Common presenting complaints include right upper quadrant abdominal pain, jaundice, weight loss, and pruritis, among others. Noninvasive imaging modalities include transabdominal US (TUS), contrast-enhanced computed tomography (CECT), and magnetic resonance imaging (MRI) with cholangiopancreatography (MRCP). A brief review of each study's properties is critical to choosing the ideal study(-ies) according to the differential diagnosis (Table 72.1).

Transabdominal US

TUS is widely available, radiation sparing, relatively low cost, and noninvasive. Given its widespread availability—especially in emergency departments—TUS is often performed to evaluate patients with suspected cholecystitis and obstructive jaundice. TUS is excellent for the diagnosis of gallbladder stones, but its sensitivity for choledocholithiasis is poor (<70%) and thus inadequate to rule out a retained common bile duct stone.[1–6] For patients with jaundice or cholestatic biochemistries, TUS is reasonably accurate in distinguishing extrahepatic obstruction from an intrinsic liver etiology but cannot provide sufficient resolution to precisely localize the obstruction (e.g., periampullary or mid-common hepatic duct) or refine the differential diagnosis. Therefore unless TUS serendipitously identifies choledocholithiasis in the appropriate clinical context, TUS usually leads to further imaging when biliary obstruction is inferred by another observation, such as extrahepatic bile duct dilation. While elastography is emerging as a useful tool for the noninvasive assessment of hepatic fibrosis/stiffness, this and other advances in TUS imaging have not found a clear role in the diagnosis of biliary pathology.[7–9]

Contrast-Enhanced Computed Tomography

Cynics would argue that CECT has replaced the abdominal exam given its ubiquitous application in clinical practice; for every 100

*Previous authors: Theodore W. James Todd H. Baron

TABLE 72.1 Overview of Biliary Cross-Sectional Imaging Studies.

Study Type	Strengths	Limitations	Common Biliary Indications
Transabdominal ultrasound	• Low cost • Widely available • High sensitivity for gallbladder stones and cholecystitis	• Low sensitivity for pancreas and common bile duct imaging • Moderately accurate in distinguishing extrahepatic bile duct obstruction from intrinsic etiologies of jaundice • Imaging impaired by truncal obesity	• Suspected acute cholecystitis • "Screening test" for new onset jaundice • Bile leak
CECT	• Widely available • Low interobserver variability in image acquisition and interpretation • Sensitive for pancreas tumors >2 cm	• Radiation equivalent of approximately 3–5 years normal background radiation[1] • Limited sensitivity (70%–80%) for choledocholithiasis • Inability to precisely characterize obstruction involving the hepatic confluence	• Abdominal pain • Obstructive jaundice • Acute pancreatitis
MRCP	• Noninvasive and sensitive imaging of the biliary tree, pancreas, and liver • Excellent anatomic characterization of obstruction involving the hepatic confluence • High (>80%) sensitivity for choledocholithiasis • Radiation sparing	• Cost • Higher interobserver variability than CECT • Inability to intervene in the same setting • Longer time to complete study • Contraindicated in specific patient populations	• Suspected choledocholithiasis • Obstructive jaundice with involvement of the hepatic confluence • Bile leak with possible involvement of intrahepatic ducts • Intrahepatic masses
Endoscopic ultrasound	• High (>80%) sensitivity for pancreatic masses and choledocholithiasis • Ability to pivot to ERCP for immediate intervention • Performance of guided tissue sampling in same session • Increased application as an intervention for biliary obstruction	• Cost • Higher interobserver variability than CECT • Requires sedation and local expertise	• Suspected choledocholithiasis • Obstructive jaundice • Palliation of biliary obstruction when ERCP not possible
ERCP	• Gold standard for treatment of choledocholithiasis and extrahepatic bile duct obstruction or leak • Avoids need for percutaneous drains • Should rarely require repeat intervention for common indications	• High risk, particularly when used solely as a diagnostic test • Dependent upon provider and facility expertise • Technically challenging in certain patients, particularly those with altered foregut anatomy	• Choledocholithiasis • Obstructive jaundice • Bile leak **Therapeutic test in almost all cases*
Percutaneous transhepatic cholangiography	• Ability to proceed with drain placement in same session • Relatively low-risk • Unencumbered by prior foregut surgery • Does not require deep sedation/ general anesthesia, especially for follow-up studies of an existing drain	• Drainage requires a percutaneous tube • More invasive than CECT, MRCP, and transabdominal ultrasound as an imaging test	• Same indications as ERCP, though usually second-line when ERCP not possible • Obstructive jaundice involving the hepatic confluence • Intrahepatic stone disease **Therapeutic test in almost all cases*

CECT, Contrast-enhanced computed tomography; *ERCP*, endoscopic retrograde cholangiopancreatography; *MRCP*, magnetic resonance imaging with cholangiopancreatography.
From Radiology Info for patients RadiologyInfo.org. Available from: https://www.radiologyinfo.org/en/info/safety-xray#safety-benefits-risks [cited 2023 March 9].

beneficiaries of Medicare in the United States, 50 CT scans are performed. More than 70 million CTs are performed each year in the United States,[10,11] so as a subspecialist evaluating patients with abdominal complaints, most will already have an abdominal CT. CECT is faster to obtain, more widely available, and has reduced interobserver variability in image acquisition and interpretation compared with MRI. These are countered by its potentially harmful effects of ionizing radiation and iodinated contrast, particularly in those who will undergo multiple imaging studies or have kidney injury.

Providers performing EUS and ERCP should be comfortable reviewing abdominal CECT images and dialoguing with radiologists as part of their preprocedure planning. It is also important to recognize the limitations of CECT in the evaluation of patients with biliary obstruction. While better than TUS, CECT has two critical limitations. First, its sensitivity for detecting choledocholithiasis is approximately 70%–80%[12]; like TUS, CECT has a high false negative rate for common bile duct stones in patients with an intermediate or high probability by clinical presentation (Fig. 72.1).[13,14] Therefore an inconclusive CECT should

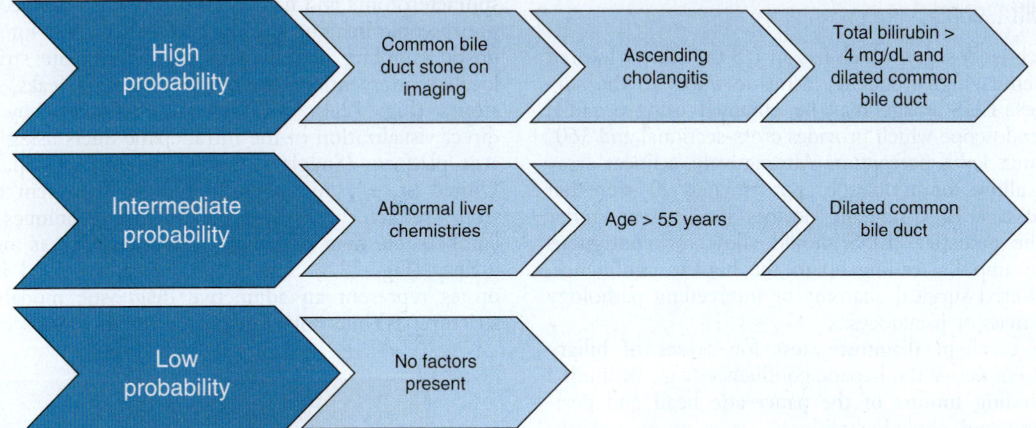

Fig. 72.1 Assessment of risk for choledocholithiasis. Classify patients as high probability or intermediate probability if one or more features are present, respectively. While useful as a clinical tool, strongly consider MRCP, EUS, or IOC before proceeding to ERCP (unless a common bile duct stone is confirmed on another imaging study) since many (>15%) patients classified as high probability will not have a common bile duct stone at ERCP. (Adapted from the American Society for Gastrointestinal Endoscopy Standards of Practice Committee guideline. ASGE Standards of Practice Committee, Buxbaum JL, Abbas Fehmi SM, Sultan S, et al. ASGE guideline on the role of endoscopy in the evaluation and management of choledocholithiasis. *Gastrointest Endosc*. 2019;89(6):1075–1105.e15. doi: 10.1016/j.gie.2018.10.001.)

be followed by a more sensitive test such as MRCP or EUS. Second, CECT is inferior to MRCP in the precise localization of biliary strictures involving the hepatic confluence, especially in the absence of a measurable mass lesion.[15] For these reasons, CECT is not recommended for patients with suspected choledocholithiasis and inferior to MRI/MRCP in the delineation of strictures involving the hepatic confluence (Bismuth-Corlette types II–IV).[15,16]

Magnetic Resonance Imaging With Cholangiopancreatography

MRCP is an MRI study (and thus noninvasive) that is dependent on the high T2-signal characteristics of bile, which produce a high-intensity bright signal on the resulting image. Solid material such as choledocholithiasis will appear as well-defined, dark filling defects within the bile duct. MRCP does not require the administration of oral or IV contrast material. For the detection of choledocholithiasis, MRCP has a sensitivity ranging from 81% to 100%, a specificity ranging from 96% to 100%, and high overall diagnostic accuracy (Fig. 72.2).[17–19] False-positive results may arise from pneumobilia and, in certain cases, filling defects within the biliary tree other than gallstones (e.g., bile duct polyps or polypoid tumors). In addition, MRCP is highly accurate in delineating the presence and location of a stricture.[15,16] In planning for maximal sectoral biliary drainage, MRCP is a useful—arguably mandatory—antecedent diagnostic test before ERCP or PTC evaluation of strictures that involve the hepatic confluence.

MRI intravenous contrast agents are gadolinium chelated to a compound such as gadodiamide (Omniscan, GE Healthcare, United Kingdom) or gadopentetate dimeglumine (Magnevist, Bayer Healthcare, Leverkusen, Germany, or MultiHance, Bracco, Princeton, NJ, United States). These agents work similar to iodine for CECT; for hepatobiliary imaging, the compound enters the liver through the portal vein and hepatic artery before being redistributed into the interstitial space. Its role as a contrast agent is how these compounds amplify adjacent water protons. Importantly, intravenous contrast is not required for MRCP or delineating biliary anatomy.[20] However, IV contrast can be

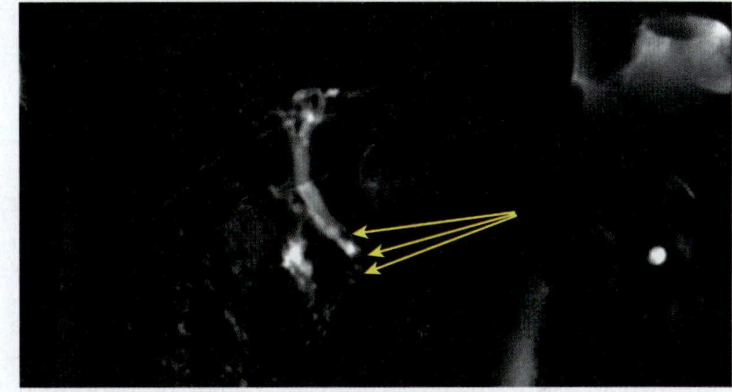

Fig. 72.2 Magnetic resonance imaging with cholangiopancreatography demonstrating choledocholithiasis.

helpful in assessing for an enhancing lesion such as a cholangiocarcinoma, and this may correlate with prognosis.[21]

In contrast to traditional gadolinium derivatives, intravenous hepatobiliary contrast agents such as mangafodipir trisodium (Teslascan, Amersham Health, Princeton, NJ, United States) improve the specificity of MRI for distinguishing focal nodular hyperplasia from adenomas, detect smaller solid liver metastases, and can be useful in more complex biliary pathology such as postoperative (especially posttransplant) bile leaks and strictures.[22–24] In addition, MRI can be performed with an IV contrast agent, such as to detect and characterize mass lesions in the liver, porta hepatis, or pancreas. Contraindications to MRI include a cardiac pacemaker, an automatic implantable cardioverter defibrillator, and some types of cerebral aneurysm clips. A particular concern about gadolinium-based IV contrast agents is that they may precipitate nephrogenic systemic fibrosis, a rare scleroderma-like disease manifested by hardening of the skin and fibrotic changes that affect multiple organs. The cause remains unclear, but reports suggest that patients with preexisting kidney disease (renal failure) are at greatest risk.[25] Avoiding gadolinium and using lower doses in patients with renal insufficiency reduces risk.

Endoscopic Ultrasound

EUS uses an echoendoscope which has an US transducer located at its tip and emits high-frequency acoustic waves to the surrounding tissues. EUS image may be obtained using a radial scanning echoendoscope which provides cross-sectional and 360° views but without depth perception. Alternatively, a linear array echoendoscope allows for an oblique, approximately 90° view that permits the passage of echogenic devices into tissues under endosonographic guidance. EUS should allow for contiguous views from the ampulla leading up to the hepatic confluence, assuming no altered surgical anatomy or interceding pathology such as a large mass or pseudocyst.

EUS is an excellent diagnostic test for causes of biliary obstruction >2 cm below the hepatic confluence (e.g., Bismuth I strictures), including tumors of the pancreatic head and periampullary region and choledocholithiasis. It is more sensitive (>90%) than CECT (5%–77%), TUS (50%–67%), MRI (50%–67%), and ERCP (90%) for the detection of pancreatic tumors (see Chapter 62), particularly when the tumor is <2 cm in greatest diameter.[26] EUS is less invasive than ERCP and has no associated radiation or contrast exposure. EUS combined with fine needle aspiration or biopsy permits tissue diagnosis of masses and lymph nodes; by combining the sensitivity of EUS imaging with the specificity of EUS-guided cytopathology, EUS represents the current gold standard for diagnosing pancreatobiliary cancers.

EUS is also highly sensitive for diagnosing choledocholithiasis. Like TUS except with superior views of the common bile duct, EUS images of choledocholithiasis are characterized by hyperechoic foci with acoustic shadowing (Fig. 72.3).[17,27] If a common bile duct stone is identified, ERCP can be performed during the same anesthetic to remove it.

Endoscopic Retrograde Cholangiopancreatography

At its inception, ERCP was a revolutionary fluoroscopic imaging modality of the pancreatobiliary ducts in an era before MRI, CECT, and EUS. Now, ERCP should be used rarely for the sole purpose of diagnosis given the risks of post-ERCP pancreatitis, infection, and perforation. For example, ERCP should not be performed for suspected choledocholithiasis unless other modalities (MRCP, EUS) are inconclusive or cannot be performed. ERCP may still be needed in cases of suspected primary sclerosing cholangitis (PSC) when MRCP with or without liver biopsy is unconvincing. Even sphincter of Oddi manometry—classically described as a diagnostic maneuver during ERCP for patients with suspected sphincter of Oddi disorders—has been largely abandoned since it does not correlate with response to sphincterotomy and has no clear prognostic value.[28,29] That said, fluoroscopic imaging during ERCP is critical for targeted diagnostic sampling in the case of indeterminate strictures and to localize interventions for the treatment of leaks, strictures, and stones (Fig. 72.4).[30] Intraductal cholangioscopy now permits direct visualization of the intrahepatic ducts using a single operator platform (Spyglass, Boston Scientific Corp., Natick, MA, United States); this is useful for the treatment of large CBD stones refractory to standard extraction techniques and often less cumbersome than advanced techniques such as mechanical lithotripsy (Fig. 72.5). Cholangioscopically guided intraductal biopsies represent an adjunctive diagnostic modality for biliary strictures. While not clearly superior to fluoroscopically guided

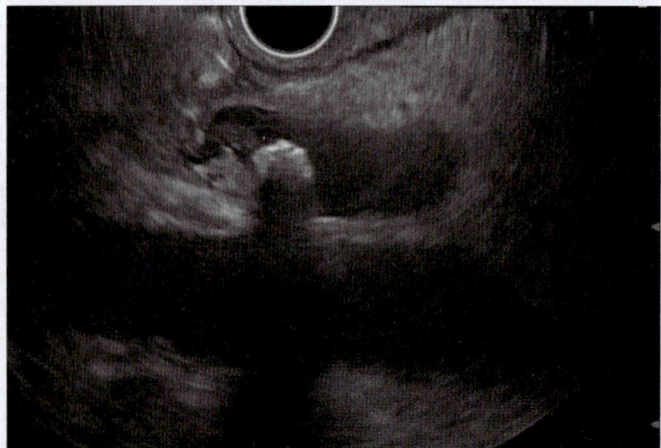

Fig. 72.3 EUS image demonstrating choledocholithiasis. Note a single stone in the middle third of the bile duct. Stones have a hyperechoic interface with the EUS transducer and postacoustic shadowing.

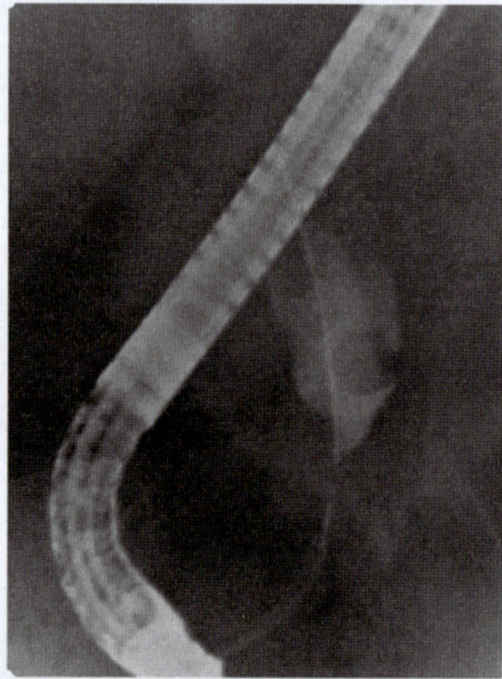

Fig. 72.4 Endoscopic retrograde cholangiopancreatography demonstrating choledocholithiasis lodged at the insertion of the cystic duct (*right*, on the image) into the common hepatic duct (*left*).

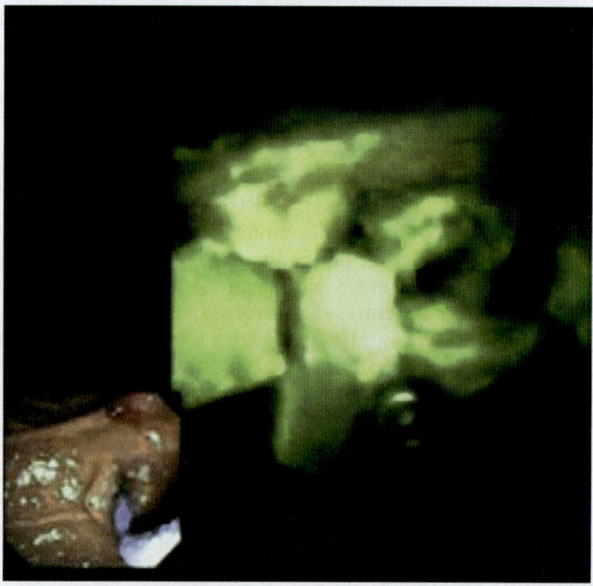

Fig. 72.5 Cholangioscopy with electrohydraulic lithotripsy is used to facilitate extraction of an impacted gallstone in the cystic duct causing biliary obstruction (Mirizzi syndrome).

biopsies in all cases, cholangioscopy permits more precise targeting within the stricture and is relatively easy to perform once the endoscopist has positioned the cholangioscope within or immediately distal to the stricture.[31] Cholangioscopy is not sufficiently accurate to diagnose a malignant stricture; cytopathology remains the gold standard.[32,33]

Percutaneous Transhepatic Cholangiography

Similar to ERCP, PTC is useful as a diagnostic test but principally reserved for planned interventions since it is more invasive than TUS, EUS, CECT, and MRI/MRCP. PTC should be performed once the pathology is localized by one or more of these less invasive modalities. PTC without planned PTBD—planned placement of a transhepatic drainage catheter—should be exceedingly rare. Consider PTC the antegrade variant of ERCP with a few nuances: (1) access may be more challenging when the biliary tree is nondilated (such as a bile leak); (2) access is easier when the ducts are dilated and the patient has altered foregut anatomy (e.g., Roux-en-Y) (Fig. 72.6); (3) PTC is more easily performed with moderate sedation,[34] whereas ERCP is much easier under deep sedation or general anesthesia; (4) palliation of very high-grade strictures may be easier, since the interventional radiologist has more leverage approaching the stricture through a straight catheter as opposed to a retroflexed catheter inserted through a duodenoscope. If retrograde drainage via ERCP fails, the procedure is a technical failure. If antegrade drainage via PTC cannot be achieved, a short-term palliative maneuver is to leave a drain proximal (above) the stricture and drain externally. Often, a second attempt after this type of decompression will be successful. Finally, palliation of biliary obstruction due to a stricture involving both hepatic lobes and multiple intrahepatic radicles (e.g., Bismuth type IV strictures) may only be achievable with a percutaneous approach. PTBD is probably associated with a lower rate of postprocedure pancreatitis, although the literature is sparse on this topic; other serious PTC/PTBD-related adverse events include bleeding, cholangitis, pneumothorax, and bile leak.[35,36]

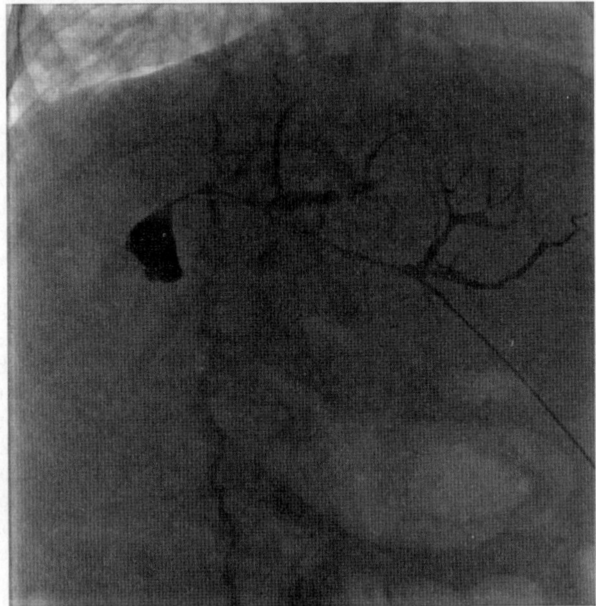

Fig. 72.6 Percutaneous transhepatic cholangiography in a young patient with a prior history of hepaticojejunostomy and evidence of an anastomotic stricture.

Technique

CECT and MRCP localize the biliary obstruction, informing the best percutaneous approach (e.g., left vs. right vs. bilateral) and avoiding key regional structures such as the colon. Dilated bile ducts on the left side may be easily accessible with a minimal number of needle passes with the use of transabdominal US guidance from a subxiphoid approach.[37] A standard right-sided approach is used most frequently, however, and is performed from an intercostal approach, usually via the mid-axillary region below the 10th intercostal space (Fig. 72.7).

From either side, the procedure is initiated by advancing a 22-ga needle under fluoroscopic guidance centrally toward the liver hilum and gently injecting contrast as the needle is withdrawn slowly. The initial use of such a small needle reduces hepatic trauma and bleeding despite the potential need for multiple needle passes to cannulate a bile duct, particularly when the bile ducts are not dilated. US guidance or CT guidance can be used to access nondilated bile ducts.[38,39]

Once a bile duct is cannulated, diagnostic cholangiography follows. Isolated ducts, because of strictures or stones that do not communicate with the rest of the biliary tract, may need to be opacified via additional needle passes. If the procedure is only diagnostic and biliary obstruction is not evident, the needle is withdrawn (this should be uncommon). If the biliary system is obstructed, the next step is to place a transhepatic drain—the equivalent of the endobiliary stent placed via ERCP. The risk of hepatic arterial injury is reduced by using a peripheral intrahepatic bile duct for final access. If the duct cannulated initially is too central (the larger branches of the hepatic artery tend to be more central), a more peripheral duct should be chosen for access into the biliary tract. Frequently, use of a second needle to puncture a more peripheral duct is required, and the initial needle is used to opacify and visualize this new and safer approach. A guidewire is then advanced into the biliary tree, and the access system is "upsized" by the passage of catheters of increasing diameter using the Seldinger technique. Once access is secured, the guidewire and catheter can be manipulated with the goal of traversing the obstruction and the sphincter of Oddi (or choledochojejunal anastomosis if prior surgery has been performed). Over the transhepatic wire, a drain can be placed; usually, this is an external-internal drain initially, meaning that bile can flow through the drain and into the bowel (internal) or out of the drain and into a bag (external). This permits rapid diagnosis of intraductal hemorrhage and early assessment of drainage adequacy. After short-term monitoring, the drain can be capped to external drainage, and all bile flow obligated to the small intestine. Drainage tubes have holes positioned above the level of obstruction; a distal pigtail is configured within the small intestine to minimize dislodgement. The size of the tube usually ranges from 8 to 12 Fr. A larger tube may yield better decompression but oversizing could lead to apposition of the bile duct wall and obstruct drainage from smaller ducts; this is particularly important in the setting of PSC, in which many of the obstructed ducts are not dilated.

A contraindication to PTC is coagulopathy. Generally, the procedure is thought to be safe with an INR of less than 1.8 and platelet count greater than 50,000/mm^3 (see Chapter 94). Any abnormalities are generally corrected immediately before the procedure. Ascites between the liver and puncture site is not an absolute contraindication although its presence is associated with a higher risk of bile leak and secondary peritonitis; in addition, ascites may result in a tortuous tract for the biliary drain, leading to higher rates of spontaneous dislodgement and challenges with drain exchanges later. If ERCP is not an option, a preprocedure, large-volume paracentesis can mitigate some of these issues.

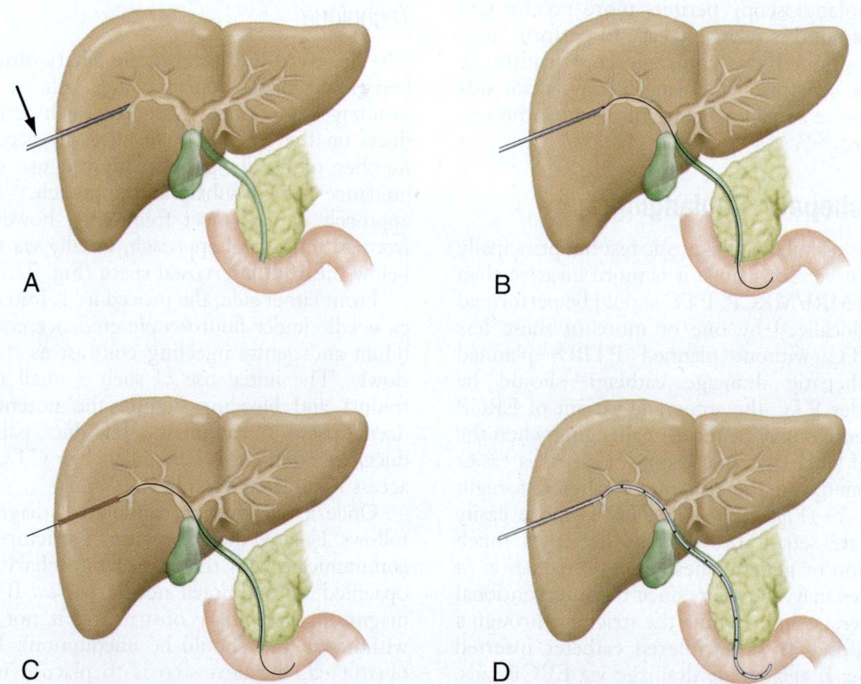

Fig. 72.7 Schematic showing percutaneous transhepatic cholangiography. (A) A peripheral bile duct is identified and entered with a needle (*arrow*), (B) a guidewire is passed through the needle across the obstructing lesion into the duodenum, (C) the needle has been withdrawn, and (D) an internal-external catheter is inserted over the guidewire.

Monitor patients closely for the first 24–48 hours following PTBD and avoid further intervention until fever and sepsis have resolved. A small amount of blood in the biliary drain may be observed in the first 2 days after initial placement or significant manipulation during a follow-up procedure. Brisk bleeding around the catheter site, through the catheter itself, or from the GI tract suggests the possibility of hepatic arterial injury.[40] Hepatic artery pseudoaneurysms may not present for up to 1–2 weeks post-PTBD. One should investigate persistent bleeding that results in a profound fall in the hemoglobin level or hemodynamic instability with hepatic angiography and embolization if an injured vessel is recognized.

STAGE II: DEVELOPMENT OF A DIAGNOSTIC AND TREATMENT PLAN: SPECIAL CONSIDERATIONS

Patients with suspected biliary pathology often consume a multitude of imaging studies as part of their diagnostic and therapeutic evaluation. Every effort should be made to provide high-value care by pivoting to the imaging study that is most likely to result in a definite diagnosis; this usually requires a careful history, physical examination, and biochemistries (Fig. 72.8). For example, acute onset of biliary symptoms in a young person suggests gallstone disease, in which case a transabdominal US can be followed by an MRCP or EUS if choledocholithiasis remains intermediate probability, skipping the CECT. Alternatively, an older patient with painless jaundice should be triaged to a CECT followed by an MRI/MRCP if a more complex (Bismuth II–IV) biliary obstruction is suggested by the former. The findings should direct the team to proceed with EUS ± ERCP, PTC, or some combination. Plans for tissue sampling and drainage should be informed by the likelihood of further treatments: For example, achieving a definitive tissue diagnosis is less important than palliation of obstructive symptoms in an elderly patient with very low performance status who is unlikely to tolerate systemic chemotherapy or surgical resection. Candidates for liver transplant should be treated with particular care, since transluminal or transhepatic biopsies of a primary hepatobiliary lesion may be associated with tumor tracking; centers that offer a transplant protocol for unresectable cholangiocarcinoma may disqualify a patient who has undergone such a maneuver.[41]

Bile Leaks

As discussed previously, bile leaks arise as a result of postsurgical complications and trauma. Bile duct injuries following laparoscopic cholecystectomy occur in 0.06%–0.3% of cases.[42] Most commonly, postcholecystectomy bile leaks arise from either the cystic duct or duct of Luschka (see Chapter 66). Posthepatectomy leaks are more common (4%–13%) and may occur from the cut surface of the liver remnant (e.g., peripheral biliary radicles) or from a larger bile duct.[43] The most challenging leaks occur in the setting of an intrahepatic or complete bile duct transection, where a liver segment is partially or completely disconnected from the bile duct circuitry. During cholecystectomy, this may occur due to misclassifying and severing a hepatic duct during attempts to dissect the cystic duct; some patients are predisposed to a complex injury because of anomalous biliary anatomy, such as a right hepatic duct insertion into the cystic duct. These are uncommon (<0.5%) but should be considered since traditional endoscopic interventions to treat a bile leak will not address a disconnected bile duct sector; retrograde, transpapillary injection will not opacify a completely disconnected intrahepatic sector.

Bile leaks are typically diagnosed by the presence of persistent bile output from an operative drain or presentation with a symptomatic biloma; most postoperative leaks present within 1 week of surgery. Since many leaks will resolve on their own, a HIDA scan may be performed to confirm persistent extravasation

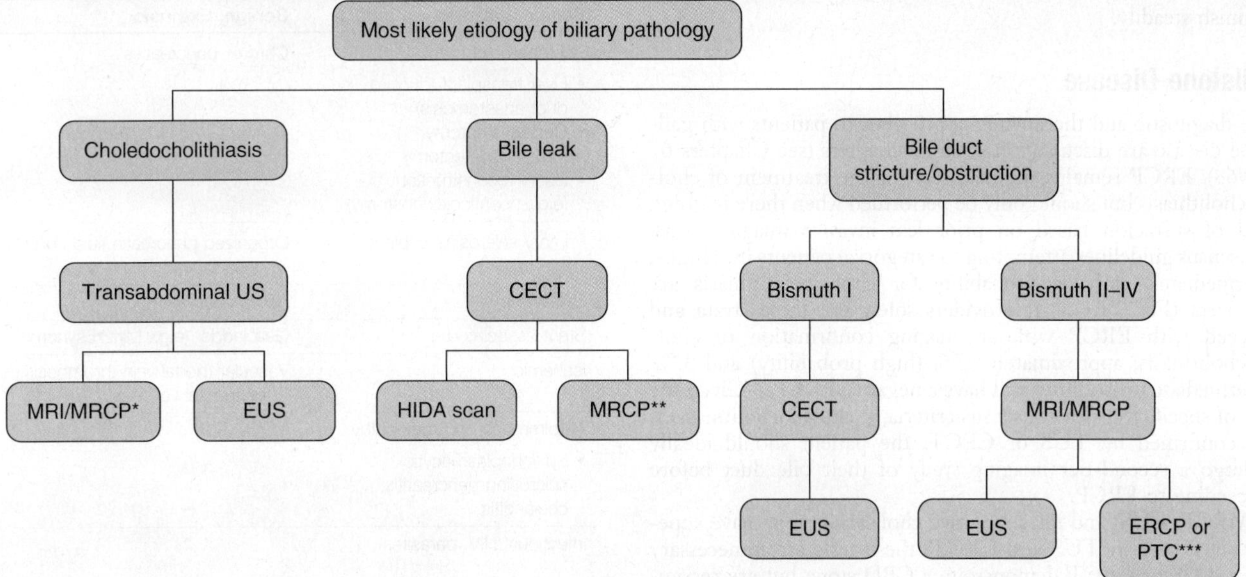
Personalized approach to the evaluation of a patient with suspected biliary pathology
Most likely etiology of biliary pathology
Choledocholithiasis
Bile leak
Bile duct stricture/obstruction
Transabdominal US
CECT
Bismuth I
Bismuth II–IV
MRI/MRCP*
EUS
HIDA scan
MRCP**
CECT
MRI/MRCP
EUS
EUS
ERCP or PTC***
* An MRCP without IV contrast is sufficient to evaluate for suspected choledocholithiasis, unless concomitant pathology is suspected (e.g., pancreatic or hepatobiliary mass)
** An MRCP with biliary contrast may be helpful in the setting of a complex biliary injury, such as after a partial hepatectomy, or when a completely disconnected bile duct is suspected after cholecystectomy
*** The decision to proceed with ERCP or PTC is often based on local expertise and the confidence with which an endoscopist believes that at least 50% of liver volume can be drained via ERCP

Fig. 72.8 Personalized approach to the evaluation of a patient with suspected biliary pathology.

before embarking upon intervention. Persistent bilious output from a postoperative drain, confirmed by a fluid:serum bilirubin ratio >5 when gross examination of the fluid is unclear, is sufficient to diagnose a bile leak.[44]

Once a bile leak has been confirmed clinically or radiographically, ERCP is the first-line approach to therapy unless cross-sectional imaging unequivocally reveals complete transection of the bile duct or an intrahepatic duct sector (Fig. 72.9). Leaks are typically graded dichotomously, with low-grade leaks only evident after retrograde opacification of secondary biliary radicles.[45,46] These low-grade leaks can usually be managed with biliary sphincterotomy alone, placement of a plastic biliary stent (7–10 Fr), or both.[47] Transpapillary drainage is effective because it reduces the pressure gradient required for biliary outflow; thus bile flow is diverted away from the area of leak which can then close by secondary intent. High-grade leaks, such as those at a biliary anastomosis following orthotopic liver transplant, require placement of a larger caliber (10 Fr or greater) plastic stent or a removable, fully covered metallic stent across the leak in combination with biliary sphincterotomy.[48,49]

In more complex bile duct injuries when ERCP is inconclusive—often the case when the leak occurs in discontinuity with the main biliary tree—MRCP with hepatobiliary contrast can localize it and facilitate treatment planning.[24] PTBD is usually unnecessary unless ERCP is technically unsuccessful or the leak involves a disconnected hepatic segment. In these more complex cases, a PTBD placed into the disconnected sector will control the leak and facilitate a subsequent surgical repair. In rare cases, the PTBD can reconstitute communication with the main biliary tree and delay or avoid surgical repair indefinitely.[50,51]

In addition to controlling the bile leak with ERCP or PTBD, a percutaneous biloma drain may be required to treat large, infected, or highly symptomatic bilomas. This is most common when a drain was not left in the gallbladder fossa or adjacent to the site of partial hepatectomy.[159–161] If a persistent bile leak is treated successfully and symptoms improve within 24 hours, percutaneous drainage of the biloma can be deferred. On the other hand, use CECT to evaluate patients with persistently high pain or signs of secondary infection (fever, persistent leukocytosis, positive blood cultures, imaging evidence for an abscess, or some combination)

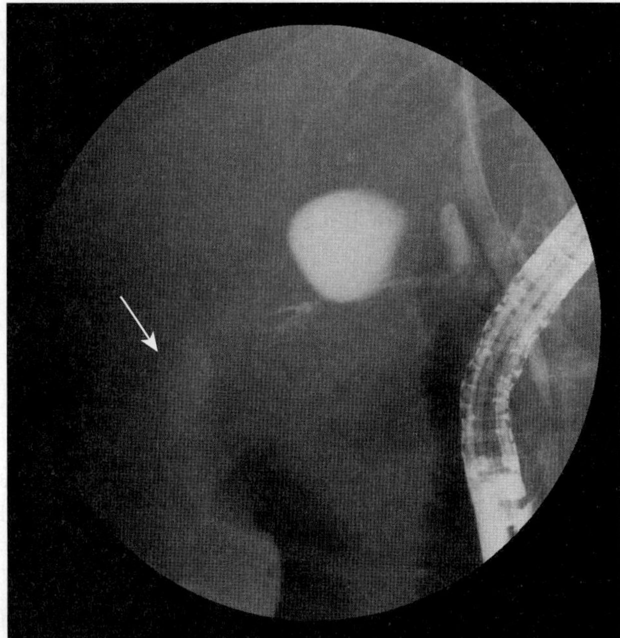

Fig. 72.9 Gallbladder perforation (*arrow*) with bilious ascites.

to identify a drainable biloma. A biloma drain will serve as an indicator for resolution of the bile leak, since output should diminish steadily.

Gallstone Disease

The diagnostic and therapeutic approaches to patients with gallstone disease are discussed in separate chapters (see Chapters 67 and 68). ERCP remains the mainstay for the treatment of choledocholithiasis but should only be performed when there is a high level of suspicion based on prior less invasive imaging tests. Consensus guidelines attempting to categorize patients into high-, intermediate-, and low-probability for choledocholithiasis are imperfect (Fig. 72.1).[13] If providers solely use these strata and proceed with ERCP without imaging confirmation of choledocholithiasis, approximately 15% (high probability) and 33% (intermediate probability) will have a negative ERCP.[52] Given the lack of specificity with consensus criteria, if choledocholithiasis is not confirmed by TUS or CECT, the patient should ideally undergo a second-tier imaging study of their bile duct before proceeding to ERCP.

MRCP, EUS, and intraoperative cholangiography have superior sensitivity to TUS and CECT; these tests are unnecessary when TUS or CECT demonstrate a CBD stone but are recommended when the clinical picture is unclear.[13] In centers with interventional GI expertise, most offer EUS and ERCP in the same anesthetic; this renders a significant operational advantage for EUS over MRCP as a less invasive test for choledocholithiasis: When a CBD stone is visualized, the patient can (and should) proceed to ERCP immediately. PTBD should be reserved for cases in which ERCP cannot be achieved due to uncommon postoperative anatomy (e.g., duodenal switch procedure or long limb hepaticojejunostomy performed for congenital biliary disease) or comorbidity that precludes the use of general anesthesia; even in the setting of bariatric surgery, balloon-assisted enteroscopy and EUS transgastric ERCP (EDGE) permit reasonably high technical success for endoscopic approaches. Laparoscopic (preferred to open) common bile duct exploration remains a reasonable option for patients with choledocholithiasis who also require cholecystectomy. However, many surgical training programs have struggled to maintain volumes to train a surgical workforce to utilize this approach across the United States; this reflects the dominance of ERCP as the preferred modality in Western countries.

Bile Duct Strictures

There is no universal definition for a bile duct stricture—particularly one that is clinically significant. However, generally speaking, one can diagnose a stricture based on a subjective assessment of abnormal narrowing of any segment of the biliary tree visible by cross-sectional imaging. Clinically significant bile duct strictures would be those that present with biochemical or clinical evidence of cholestasis. The approach is best considered by categorizing these into three etiologic groups (benign, malignant, and indeterminate) and two anatomic locations (Bismuth-Corlette type I vs. II–IV). PSC represents a particularly unique set of diagnostic and therapeutic challenges and is discussed elsewhere (see Chapter 70).

Benign Biliary Strictures

Benign bile duct strictures may be intrinsic or extrinsic to the biliary tree (Table 72.2—reuse from Ref. [54]), and their location relative to the hepatic confluence, as defined by the Bismuth-Corlette classification system, informs the best approach to treatment.[54] The short-term goal is to restore normal bile flow through some combination of dilation and stent placement. Since permanent stenting is suboptimal for benign etiologies of biliary obstruction, the long-term goal is to remodel the stricture so that bile flow is restored without the need for re-intervention.

TABLE 72.2 Differential Diagnosis for Benign Bile Duct Strictures

Benign, Intrinsic	Benign, Extrinsic
Postoperative • Liver transplant (duct-to-duct anastomosis) • Cholecystectomy • Partial hepatectomy • Biliary reconstruction (e.g., hepaticojejunostomy)	Chronic pancreatitis
Primary sclerosing cholangitis	Organized pancreatic fluid collection/ pseudocyst
Gallstones	Acute pancreatitis
Stent-associated	Gallbladder (e.g., Mirizzi syndrome)
Ischemic	Vascular (portal vein thrombosis, periductal varices)
Autoimmune cholangiopathy • Lymphoplasmacytic sclerosing pancreatitis/ cholangitis	
Infectious (HIV, parasites)	

Postoperative Bismuth type I strictures have the best prognosis whether treated endoscopically or percutaneously, with >90% long-term resolution rates when treated aggressively (near-complete or complete obliteration of the stricture sustained for at least several months).[55,56] PSC and ischemic cholangiopathy, the latter often after liver transplant or other liver surgery compromising all or a portion of the hepatic artery, often involve the intrahepatic ducts and may be recalcitrant to drainage efforts since the underlying etiology is irreversible. Recurrent, benign bile duct strictures—regardless of etiology or location—have a lower likelihood of achieving durable resolution with a second round of endoscopic or percutaneous therapy.

The endoscopic and percutaneous approaches are very similar: (1) achieve intraductal access across the stricture, (2) dilate the stricture with either graduated catheter or hydrostatic balloon, seeking to eliminate the stricture's waist, and (3) place an endobiliary stent(s) or PTBD to maintain bile flow and allow remodeling of the stricture to a larger diameter. ERCP permits the placement of multiple large-bore plastic stents (10–11.5 Fr) in parallel across the stricture, with variability in stent exchanges for up to 1 year (Fig. 72.10).[57,58] This approach is associated with a lower rate of stricture recurrence. Fully covered, self-expandable metallic stents (fcSEMSs) have several advantages over serial plastic stenting. First, fcSEMSs are larger than plastic alternatives (8–10 mm vs. 7–11.5 Fr). Second, deployment of a SEMS often eliminates the need for dilation since the fcSEMS exerts its own radial force on the stricture (Fig. 72.11). Last, fcSEMSs have longer patency rates and may be left in place for 6–12 months without the need for scheduled exchanges.[59–61] For strictures involving the hepatic confluence, fcSEMSs are contraindicated in most cases since deployment into one hepatic lobe may obstruct the other side. Additionally, fcSEMS should not "oversize the duct" as this may result in stent-induced strictures; this may be relevant in the posttransplant setting, when the recipient or donor duct segment may be <6 mm in diameter. In these uncommon scenarios, it is best to resort to the traditional approach of multiple plastic stents in parallel.

For indeterminate strictures, avoid the use of fcSEMS since these may interfere with subsequent diagnostics (e.g., MRI/

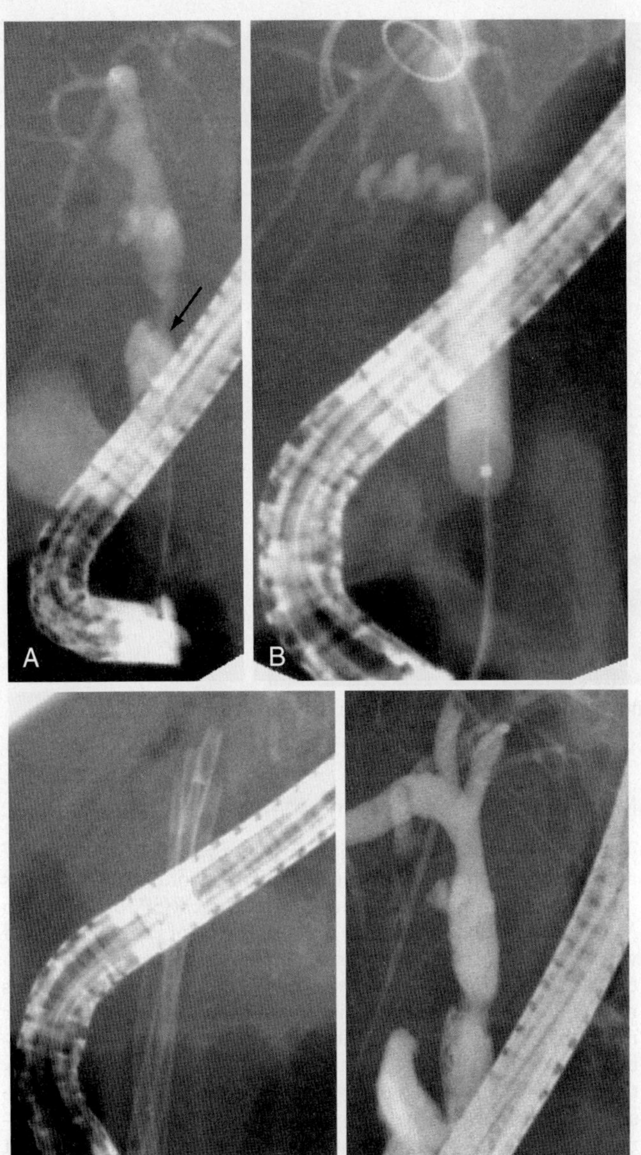

Fig. 72.10 Endoscopic treatment of a choledochocholedochal anastomotic stricture with multiple stents. (A) Cholangiography demonstrating a stricture (*arrow*) at the anastomosis, (B) balloon dilation of the stricture, (C) multiple plastic stents are placed, and (D) follow-up cholangiogram shows improvement.

MRCP and EUS-FNA) and, practically speaking, may have to be removed sooner to facilitate repeat intraductal sampling. Since fcSEMSs are more expensive than plastic stents, removing such a device after limited indwell reduces its efficacy and adds to the overall cost of treatment. Uncovered SEMS causes irreversible tissue hyperplasia and stent embedment, precluding subsequent removal; these are contraindicated for the treatment of benign and indeterminate bile duct strictures. Despite these considerations, there is a growing trend to using fcSEMS as a first-line approach to treating benign, Bismuth type I strictures since they appear to be at least noninferior to serial plastic stenting and require fewer ERCPs.[60,61]

Chronic pancreatitis is the most common extrinsic etiology for distal common bile duct strictures (Fig. 72.12). Stricture recurrence rates are higher (20%–25%) than Bismuth type I postoperative strictures since the extrinsic compression persists during and after intervention.[61,62] These cases require prolonged (up to 1 year) and aggressive stenting, increasingly with fcSEMS as the first-line strategy.

Serial PTBD is the percutaneous alternative to multiple plastic endobiliary stents. The treatment algorithm is similar to traditional ERCP approaches using serial dilation and multiple plastic stents: After a drain tract is achieved, the stricture is dilated using hydrostatic balloon catheters sized to the unaffected bile duct above and below the stricture. A PTBD is left in place between dilation sessions, though the PTBD is limited by the diameter of the drain itself (typically 12 Fr). Still, outcomes from this approach are excellent.[63–67]

A PTBD may be converted to an fcSEMS via antegrade deployment, with the result being identical to endoscopic (retrograde) deployment. However, these fcSEMSs require removal; if removal is required antegrade due to an inaccessible major papilla (for postoperative reasons), a PTBD is usually left in place to facilitate fcSEMS extraction through the tract. With few exceptions, treat benign Bismuth I strictures endoscopically unless endoscopic access to the bile duct is very difficult.

INDETERMINATE BILIARY STRICTURES

A bile duct stricture is indeterminate when a definitive benign or malignant etiology remains elusive after contrast-enhanced cross-sectional imaging (CECT ± MRI/MRCP), EUS, and ERCP with intraductal sampling. Since EUS-FNA has a sensitivity of >80% for distal common bile duct strictures, it is uncommon to have indeterminate strictures below the hepatic confluence. However, ERCP-based techniques have improved marginally for the diagnosis of Bismuth types II–IV strictures (Video 72.1—Reuse from Ref. [67]).[68] Cholangioscopy with white light, artificial intelligence schemes, and expert classification systems do not have sufficient specificity to replace cytopathology for achieving a definitive diagnosis.[31–33,69,70] Other intraductal imaging technologies, such as confocal endomicroscopy and optical coherence tomography, have also fallen short. Intraductal tissue sampling, even with cholangioscopic biopsies, remains imperfect with sensitivities of 50%–70% when multiple modalities are used (intraductal brushings for cytology, intraductal forceps for histology, and intraductal brushings for fluorescence in situ hybridization). Next-generation sequencing has promise, though it is not used widely since panels have not achieved >95%–99% specificity to allow as a surrogate for cytopathologic diagnosis.[71,72]

Malignant Biliary Strictures

Since a malignant bile duct stricture does not require further diagnostics, focus on durable palliation of the biliary obstruction with as few interventions as possible. Malignant strictures below the hepatic confluence are generally treated endoscopically; when transpapillary, ERCP-based techniques are not feasible due to an inaccessible papilla or very high-grade stricture, a trained endoscopist may pivot to interventional EUS for biliary access. Once access is achieved, there are three options: (1) transpapillary, rendezvous with subsequent placement of a transpapillary stent; the end result is the same as ERCP, but interventional EUS can facilitate the procedure; (2) direct choledochoduodenal stent placement proximal to the stricture (above or closer to the hepatic confluence); (3) hepaticogastrostomy. These techniques will be reviewed in greater detail later in this chapter. PTBD is a viable alternative to transpapillary drainage, especially when the malignancy is complicated by gastric outlet obstruction or altered foregut anatomy precluding ERCP and interventional EUS.[35] Consensus guidelines (written by endoscopists) increasingly favor

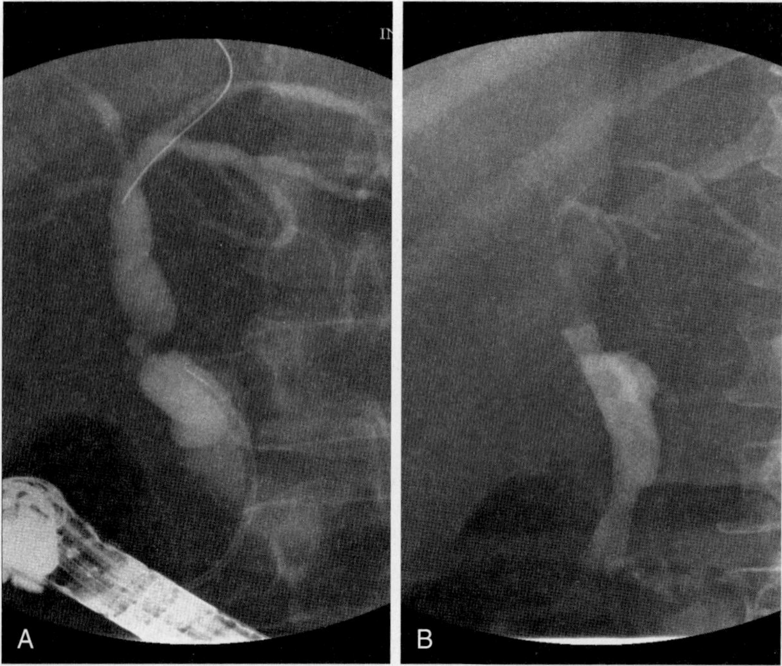

Fig. 72.11 Anastomotic bile duct stricture (A) treated with fully covered self-expandable metallic stent (B).

the use of EUS techniques before pivoting to percutaneous strategies; this reflects some practice bias but also a concerted effort to avoid the morbidity associated with percutaneous drains.[53,73,74]

Empiric biliary drainage of periampullary cancers is not required in the absence of overt biliary obstruction, which is typically defined by a serum bilirubin that precludes full-dose chemotherapy or clinical symptoms.[75] However, nearly all distal bile duct malignant strictures require intervention since these cancers are increasingly treated with neoadjuvant systemic therapy.[76] When malignancy is confirmed, a SEMS (uncovered, partially covered, or fully covered) will achieve more durable biliary drainage than plastic stents.[77] To avoid multiple interventions, endobiliary approaches should lead with this strategy. Even if PTC is used for biliary access due to altered anatomy or technical failure of endoscopy, interventional radiology may be able to place a SEMS antegrade and eliminate the need for temporary PTBD.[78] Regardless of approach to biliary access, deploy a SEMS below the hepatic confluence for optimal drainage and to avoid interfering with biliary reconstruction at the time of pancreaticoduodenectomy.

Single 10 Fr plastic stents have a median patency of 3–4 months, with occlusion caused by the development of a biofilm and sludge within and proximal to the stent. Larger diameter SEMS mitigates this risk, with a median patency of 6–9 months. Partially and fully covered SEMS were developed to address issues of tissue hyperplasia and tumor overgrowth that may cause an uncovered SEMS to occlude. However, comparative effectiveness trials do not show a consistent benefit of these covered variants in terms of median time to reintervention; lower rates of tissue ingrowth are offset by higher rates of stent migration—both cause clinical signs of biliary obstruction and require repeat ERCP to treat.[77,79,80] Acute cholecystitis may occur more frequently with fully covered SEMS, especially when they overlap the cystic duct insertion.[81] SEMS may be replaced (when fully covered) or treated with placement of plastic or additional SEMS within the lumen of the prior stent. Intraductal radiofrequency ablation may palliate tissue ingrowth, with retrospective cohorts suggesting prolonged stent patency.[82–85]

Malignant Strictures Involving the Hepatic Confluence

The success rate of endoscopic drainage of Bismuth type II–IV malignant strictures is lower due to inconsistent technical success in draining enough liver volume. Before ERCP or PTC, an MRCP is helpful in estimating the proportion of liver volume that will be drained after stenting one or more liver segments. Additionally, a hepatobiliary surgeon should determine if the tumor is resectable or if orthotopic liver transplant is an option. For resectable tumors, intrahepatic placement of SEMS may introduce more difficult with hepatectomy. For unresectable tumors that may be amenable to liver transplant, transhepatic tissue sampling (e.g., EUS-guided transgastric liver biopsy or percutaneous liver biopsy) is contraindicated because of concerns about tumor tracking.[41] While acceptable to most liver transplant programs, ERCP is still preferred to PTBD for the same reason.[86]

At least 50% of the liver should be drained at the first intervention; if CECT and MRCP suggest that endobiliary drainage is unlikely to achieve this because of the multifocality, length, or angulation of the malignant stricture(s), consider PTBD as the first-line palliation.[35,87–91] If the imaging is inconclusive, most centers still try for endobiliary drainage first and then pivot to PTBD if the bilirubin fails to drop below 5 mg/dL, which is generally the threshold for systemic therapy.

Placement of a single transpapillary stent (a.k.a., "unilateral" drainage) is technically easier than placement of two or more stents in different hepatic sectors and should be adequate for Bismuth II-III strictures, as long as the larger liver segment is selectively accessed.[92] *Atrophic liver segments should be avoided altogether*. Furthermore, if this can be achieved without opacification of the undrained sectors, the risk of post-ERCP cholangitis declines precipitously.[93]

Unlike Bismuth I malignant strictures, where SEMSs are firmly established, numerous studies have not persuaded the majority of endoscopists to treat higher grade strictures with SEMS during the initial procedure. SEMS at the hepatic confluence should only be considered when tumor resection has been ruled out and when there is high confidence that stent

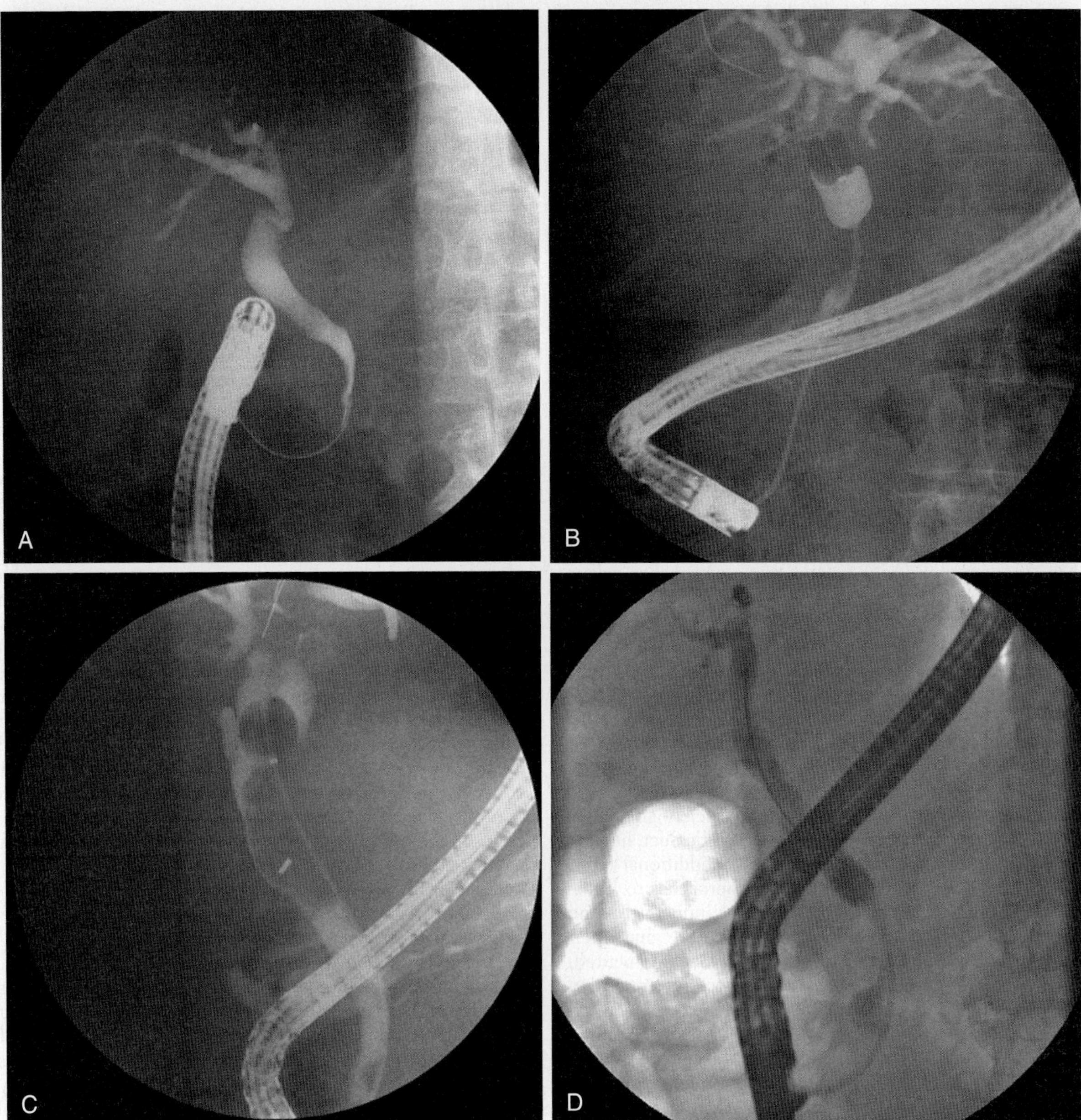

Fig. 72.12 Cholangiography of bile duct strictures due to chronic pancreatitis (A) with smooth tapering of the terminal common bile duct, cholangiocarcinoma (B) with shelf-like defect in the common hepatic duct, superior to the intrapancreatic portion of the bile duct, biliary cystadenocarcinoma (C) with a polypoid filling defect located in the proximal common hepatic duct and extending into the left main hepatic duct, and a distal common bile duct stricture with the appearance of an "apple core," consistent with pancreatic ductal adenocarcinoma (D).

placement will resolve the obstruction. Reintervention through or alongside a hilar SEMS is extraordinarily challenging.[91,94,95] Intraductal therapies such as photodynamic therapy and radiofrequency ablation may prolong stent patency and even survival in patients with unresectable cholangiocarcinoma, but comparative effectiveness studies are lacking.[96–104] Radiofrequency ablation is less expensive and cumbersome for providers and patients, so it is easier to operationalize than photodynamic therapy in practice. Until a comparative effectiveness trial can prove that intraductal ablation prolongs survival or stent patency compared with standard of care, these techniques remain relegated to cases requiring rescue therapy for stents with tissue ingrowth or early stent failure.

STAGE III: ENDOSCOPIC AND PERCUTANEOUS INTERVENTIONS FOR ACCESS AND DRAINAGE: UNIQUE CONSIDERATIONS

Choledocholithiasis

If there is a defining indication for ERCP, it is the extraction of common bile duct stones. Advances in sphincterotomy and lithotripsy have now relegated percutaneous approaches to the most refractory disease (e.g., intrahepatic duct casts or stones due to ischemic cholangiopathy or stone-forming PSC) or anatomic limitations to endoscopic access to the papilla.[105] The standard method for stone removal is a complete or near complete endoscopic biliary sphincterotomy, which facilitates the passage of devices into the bile duct for extraction. The majority (75%–90%) of common bile duct stones <1 cm in diameter should be extracted successfully during the first ERCP and with low rates of repeat intervention.[13,106,107] For most ERCPs indicated for choledocholithiasis, the technically limiting factor is bile duct access; newer literature suggests that pivoting to precut sphincterotomy, whereby an incision is made on the papilla prior to cannulation and/or wire guidance, should be considered earlier in the procedure when traditional cannulation techniques are failing (Video 72.2). These observations are limited to skilled providers in all ERCP techniques.[108–110] When the pancreatic duct is accessed inadvertently, alternative approaches include the use of a second guidewire, placement of a prophylactic pancreatic duct stent (to block the pancreatic duct and lever for a guidewire or catheter to be advanced into the bile duct), and transpancreatic sphincterotomy.[111]

Like the percutaneous, antegrade approach to common bile duct stone extraction, an endoscopist can supplement a sphincterotomy or replace it with balloon sphincteroplasty.[112–114] Without biliary sphincterotomy, a balloon sphincteroplasty preserves the sphincter of Oddi by temporarily dilating the sphincter complex for stone extraction. In patients with altered anatomy, such as Billroth II gastrojejunostomy, sphincteroplasty may be easier than sphincterotomy due to endoscope and device orientation.[115] The largest experience with sphincteroplasty of the intact sphincter is in Asia; the largest studies emphasize the importance of a sufficiently large dilation to avoid impaction of stones during extraction.[114] This may explain earlier observations of sphincteroplasty and their association with post-ERCP pancreatitis.[116] The combination of biliary sphincterotomy and large-diameter balloon dilation (12–20 mm, titrated to the size of the largest stone and the diameter of the bile duct) reduces the need for lithotripsy (Video 72.3).[112]

Large common bile duct stones, defined by society guidelines as >1 cm in diameter, and those located in the cystic duct, hepatic confluence, or intrahepatic ducts, often require additional techniques for extraction.[13,107,117] There are two approaches to lithotripsy, which is intended to reduce the size of individual stone fragments. Mechanical lithotripsy requires capture and then crushing of a stone within a compatible basket. Once fragmented, remove the stones using standard extraction techniques (Video 72.4). Electrohydraulic or laser lithotripsy—techniques adapted from kidney stones—is now much easier with the use of a single operator cholangioscope.[107] Cholangioscopy facilitates direct visualization of the stone, thereby minimizing trauma to the bile duct wall (Video 72.5). If all stones cannot be cleared during the first procedure, particularly in the setting of acute cholangitis, place an endobiliary stent to ensure short-term drainage.

PTC is useful for intrahepatic stone disease or cases in which endoscopic access to the papilla is very difficult. The techniques are identical to those used endoscopically but perform antegrade: sphincteroplasty, lithotripsy (with or without cholangioscopy), and flushing stones through the sphincter of Oddi and into the duodenum.[118] A principal disadvantage to PTC is the need for a mature tract (approximately 6 weeks) to allow for lithotripsy and stone extraction.[119] After stone clearance, the PTBD is typically replaced for a few days postprocedure to ensure no postprocedure cholangitis.

EUS-Guided Biliary Drainage

In tertiary centers, EUS-guided biliary drainage (EUS-BD) is now an alternative method of biliary decompression in patients who fail traditional ERCP or in whom ERCP is not feasible, as may occur because of surgically altered anatomy, gastric outlet obstruction, periampullary diverticulum, or inability to advance a guidewire beyond the obstruction.[74,120–124] Although PTBD has conventionally been performed in cases of failed ERCP, percutaneous drains are associated with high morbidity and reduced quality of life.[125] Endoscopists capable of pivoting from ERCP to interventional EUS may achieve biliary drainage without the need for a second intervention. Many endoscopists consent patients for interventional EUS while obtaining informed consent for ERCP, in the event of technical failure using a retrograde approach. Early observations suggest that these approaches may be noninferior.

Interventional EUS can achieve transmural biliary access via the stomach or duodenum. Once access is achieved, the endoscopist may pivot to a rendezvous technique by placing a guidewire antegrade through the stricture and major papilla, thereby facilitating completion of a traditional ERCP. Alternatively, the endoscopist may decide to place a stent (typically fcSEMS) using direct drainage by EUS-guided choledochoduodenostomy (EUS-CD) or EUS-guided hepaticoenterostomy (EUS-HE).

EUS-RV is used in cases of failed ERCP as a means to aid cannulation and/or guidewire placement on a repeat attempt at ERCP. The procedure consists of EUS-guided puncture of the biliary system from either the stomach or duodenum followed by a cholangiogram and guidewire placement into the biliary system.[120,126] The guidewire is advanced beyond the ampulla and into the duodenum. Following fluoroscopic confirmation of guidewire placement, the echoendoscope and needle are removed, while the guidewire position is maintained. One of two approaches can next be performed. In the first, a duodenoscope is inserted alongside the guidewire and advanced to the ampulla, where the guidewire is found and used to assist in cannulation. Alternatively, the distal end of the guidewire can be grasped using forceps or snare and withdrawn through the mouth, either through the accessory channel or along with the endoscope; a duodenoscope can then be back-loaded over the guidewire and advanced to the ampulla. By either method, the ultimate aim is to achieve retrograde access to the bile duct after rendezvousing with the guidewire placed endosonographically. The technique is most useful when the papilla cannot be discerned due to a large periampullary diverticulum or invasive periampullary cancer.

EUS-CD skips rendezvous and immediately pivots to placement of a transmural bile duct stent over a guidewire.[127] Various biliary access and fistula dilation methods have been described; endoscopists should adopt whichever approach is safest and effective in their hands; a meta-analysis of EUS-CD suggests high technical success rates (94%) but with a modest rate of early adverse events (19%).[120,127,128] fcSEMSs are typically easier to deploy since they require less tract dilation, especially with electrocautery-enhanced lumen-apposing stents now available on the market.

EUS-HE consists of transgastric or transjejunal (in the case of surgically altered anatomy) FNA puncture of a branch of the left intrahepatic bile duct followed by advancement of a guidewire into the biliary system and stent placement (Fig. 72.13).[129] Color Doppler is used to avoid interposing vessels, and biliary puncture is confirmed by aspirating bile and performing a cholangiogram. EUS-HE can be used as definitive therapy, as in palliation of malignant biliary obstruction, for preoperative decompression, or as a portal for downstream therapy, including antegrade stent placement.[130,131]

The choice of EUS-BD modality depends on both patient and provider characteristics and is often determined by the preference of the endoscopist. It has been proposed that EUS-RV should be initially attempted if the ampulla is accessible, followed by EUS-CD or EUS-HE as a salvage procedure if the guidewire cannot be advanced to the desired location.[132] EUS-CD or EUS-HE may be attempted initially if the ampulla is inaccessible. Both strategies appear to be equally effective and safe in patients with failed ERCP. A growing body of evidence suggests that EUS-BD may be equivalent to ERCP as a primary therapy for malignant biliary

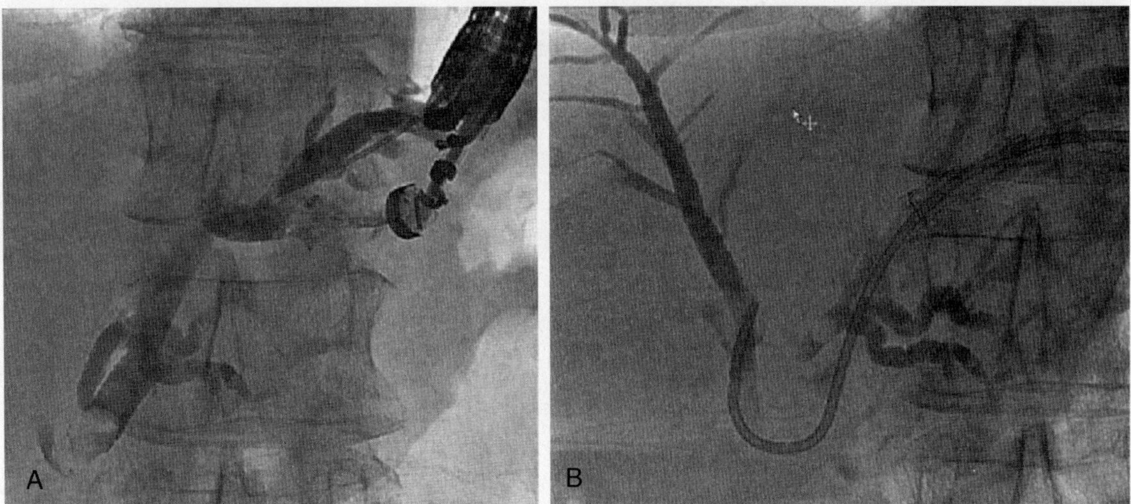

Fig. 72.13 Fluoroscopic images of EUS-guided hepaticogastrostomy (HG) in a patient who had undergone surgical hepaticojejunostomy after a bile duct injury during laparoscopic cholecystectomy. (A) Radiographic image showing injection of contrast material into the biliary tract through a 19-ga needle. An obstructing stone is seen proximal to the hepaticojejunostomy. (B) Radiographic image showing the HG stent in place. Through the HG stent, a 7-Fr plastic stent was placed into the right biliary system across the bifurcation after balloon dilation.

obstruction when performed by an endoscopist with experience in both modalities.[133,134]

Gallbladder Drainage

The standard treatment of acute calculous cholecystitis is cholecystectomy (see Chapter 68). Percutaneous gallbladder drainage is useful for the management of severe acute calculous cholecystitis in poor operative candidates or those in whom the surgeon believes are at high risk for conversion to open cholecystectomy. Another indication is acute acalculous cholecystitis (see Chapter 69), often suspected in patients who are critically ill and unresponsive in the intensive care unit. A percutaneous cholecystostomy drain is a minimally invasive way to treat these patients, can be performed with a local anesthetic or moderate sedation, and facilitates resolution of severe cholecystitis prior to subsequent laparoscopic cholecystectomy.[135–137] Drain placement enables immediate decompression of the gallbladder, with sampling of bile useful to direct antimicrobial therapy. Injection of the drain at placement or in follow-up clarifies cystic duct patency, cholecystolithiasis, and even distal common bile duct obstruction. For those with acalculous cholecystitis who survive their acute illness, recurrence is very low (<5%) after long-term follow-up.[138]

The utility of a percutaneous cholecystostomy drain is counterbalanced by several factors, including patient discomfort, the need to manage an external tube, and associated adverse events such as catheter dislodgement, cellulitis, fistula formation, and infection. For this reason, it should be avoided as a long-term solution.[139] Although the intent of a percutaneous cholecystostomy drain is to bridge a patient to cholecystectomy, the tube may become permanent when operative risk persists. Long-term percutaneous drain placement can result in significant pain, inconvenience, and cosmetic disfigurement, leading to a decrease in quality of life.

An emerging complement to percutaneous cholecystostomy tubes is EUS-guided cholecystoduodenostomy, which may obviate the need for a percutaneous drain altogether or facilitate its removal (Video 72.6). The procedure consists of FNA puncture of the gallbladder neck through the wall of the duodenum followed by guidewire placement into the gallbladder. Over the guidewire, a transmural stent can be deployed (Fig. 72.14). Similar to choledochoduodenostomy, an electrocautery-enhanced, lumen-apposing metal stent facilitates tract dilation and stent delivery simultaneously.[140] A plastic pig-tail stent within the lumen-apposing metal stent may prevent stent occlusion.

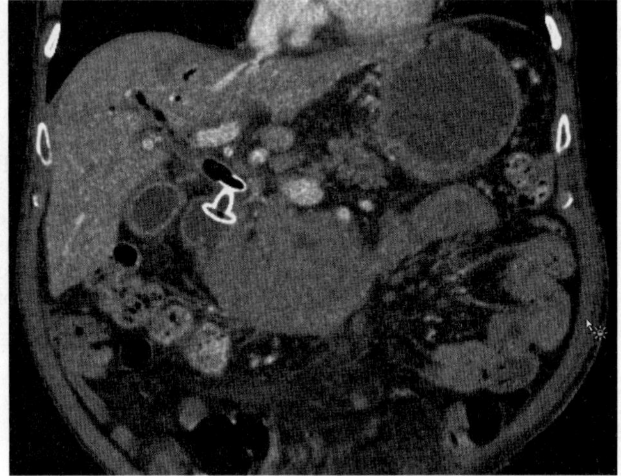

Fig. 72.14 Choledochoduodenostomy with lumen-apposing stent.

Surgically Altered Anatomy

Altered foregut anatomy (e.g., antrectomy with Billroth anastomosis, Whipple procedure, and Roux-en-Y gastric bypass) causes several unique challenges to the execution of ERCP. With few exceptions, PTBD is not encumbered by these prior surgical interventions and was the preferred first-line approach. Balloon-assisted enteroscopy and interventional EUS have resuscitated endoscopic approaches to biliary access and treatment in these cases, although PTBD remains an important component of treatment algorithms.

The most difficult postoperative anatomy is Roux-en-Y gastric bypass (see Chapter 9), since the bariatric jejunal limb precludes papillary access using traditional endoscopes. In such patients, alternative approaches include unique endoscopic techniques,[141] EUS-guided approaches,[142–144] or a combined endoscopic and laparoscopic-assisted approach.[145] The endoscopic approach to the biliary tract in patients with surgically altered anatomy often involves the use of long-length endoscopes, including balloon-assisted and spiral enteroscopes. Disadvantages to this approach include increased procedure duration, lower technical success rates, forward-viewing optics, and a reduced toolset for therapeutic intervention.[146] Additionally, complex papillary access is magnified in cases that are likely to require multiple ERCPs (e.g., large common bile duct stones or benign bile duct strictures).

When a gastric remnant is accessible, laparoscopically assisted ERCP is performed using a standard duodenoscope that is introduced transabdominally through a laparoscopic trocar placed into the gastric remnant. With this approach, the technical success is very similar to standard ERCP and an excellent option when there is another indication for laparoscopy such as cholecystectomy with choledocholithiasis.[147] However, this approach requires the coordination of multiple specialty providers and the need to perform these procedures outside of the endoscopy suite.[148]

EUS can be used to create a gastro-gastric fistula when endoscopic access to the gastric remnant, duodenum, and papilla is indicated. The technique is fairly straightforward, starting with FNA and fluid (often saline mixed with contrast to incorporate fluoroscopic guidance) injection of the gastric remnant. Then, a guidewire is advanced through the FNA tract and coiled in the gastric remnant, akin to a pseudocyst drainage. Over the guidewire, a large diameter (15 or 20 mm) lumen-apposing stent is deployed between the two structures. The stent can be dilated and sutured endoscopically to minimize the risk of spontaneous migration. Depending on the urgency of biliary drainage, ERCP using a standard duodenoscope through the gastro-gastric fistula can be performed that day or approximately 1 week later; some advocate for suturing the stent in place to minimize spontaneous dislodgement during the ERCP.[149] Most endoscopists prefer to leave the stent in place for about 1 month to minimize the risk of gastric leak and peritonitis.[121,142]

COMBINED PERCUTANEOUS AND ENDOSCOPIC APPROACHES

In some situations in which ERCP is unsuccessful but the bile duct still needs to be accessed endoscopically, a percutaneous-endoscopic rendezvous should be considered (Fig. 72.15). An example is a patient with a large duodenal diverticulum and a bile duct stone. If the diverticulum prevents endoscopic biliary access, a guidewire is passed percutaneously into the duodenum; the patient is then brought to the ERCP suite, and an ERCP is repeated. The wire is grasped by forceps, and accessories are passed over the wire, thereby allowing sphincterotomy and stone extraction. A similar method may be performed with EUS guidance for guidewire placement (see earlier). The technique is not needed for most malignant strictures, which can be managed entirely with a percutaneous approach if the endoscopic approach fails.

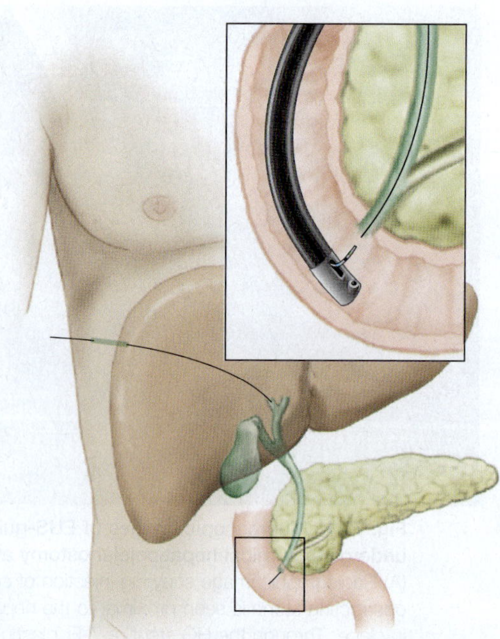

Fig. 72.15 Schematic of a combined percutaneous and endoscopic approach to the biliary tract. The guidewire is passed into the duodenum and identified endoscopically (*inset*), after which it is grasped with a snare and pulled through the endoscope and out through the mouth, thereby providing access to the biliary tract.

ADVERSE EVENTS

Five major types of AEs of ERCP may occur: sedation-related, pancreatitis, bleeding, perforation, and infection.[150] Reported rates of post-ERCP pancreatitis vary because of differences in patient selection and operator technique and experience. Patients at highest risk are young, otherwise healthy women, especially those with known or suspected sphincter of Oddi dysfunction.[151] Older adults and those with chronic pancreatitis or pancreatic cancer have lower rates of pancreatitis. Prophylactic placement of a stent into the main pancreatic duct reduces the risk of pancreatitis in high-risk patients and nearly eliminates the risk of severe pancreatitis. Pancreatic duct stenting is generally recommended when bile duct cannulation is challenging and when the pancreatic duct has been inadvertently cannulated.[152] Rectally administered prophylactic NSAIDs have been shown to reduce the risk of post-ERCP pancreatitis and are now widely recommended for high-risk individuals; many also advocate for use in all patients undergoing an ERCP without a preexisting biliary sphincterotomy.[153–155]

Bleeding may occur after biliary sphincterotomy. Risk factors for postsphincterotomy bleeding include coagulopathy and institution of anticoagulation within 72 hours of sphincterotomy.[156] Perforation of the duodenum occurs in less than 1% of patients and may require surgical management, especially when the lateral duodenal wall is injured.[157] Infection occurs primarily in patients in whom drainage of the biliary tract after ERCP is inadequate. Such patients include those with extensive intrahepatic PSC or advanced perihilar tumors and those who have undergone a failed stent placement for biliary obstruction. A lower ERCP volume by an endoscopist also appears to be associated with a lower success rate and higher AE rate (see also Chapter 40).[158–166] For this reason, efforts are underway to create standardized training in EUS and ERCP, along with methods to assess technical proficiency.[167,168]

SUMMARY

Clinicians responsible for the diagnosis and treatment of biliary disease should be familiar with the performance characteristics of all minimally invasive imaging techniques. ERCP and PTC are nonsurgical interventions that should be preceded by a comprehensive diagnostic work-up. A clear idea of the underlying pathology and treatment plan should be outlined before embarking upon one or both of these procedures. Despite numerous advances in ERCP and EUS techniques, many of these cases still require multidisciplinary collaboration between gastroenterologists, surgeons, and interventional radiologists.

Full references for this chapter can be found at https://ebooks.health.elsevier.com.

Index

Note: Page numbers followed by "f" indicate figures, "t" indicate tables, and "b" indicate boxes.

G

I

O

S

X

Y

Z

Sleisenger and Fordtran's

GASTROINTESTINAL and LIVER DISEASE

PATHOPHYSIOLOGY | DIAGNOSIS | MANAGEMENT

EDITORS

RAYMOND T. CHUNG, MD
Professor of Medicine
Harvard Medical School
Zhou Family Endowed Chair
Chief, Gastroenterology, Hepatology and Endoscopy
Mass General Brigham
Associate Member, Broad Institute
Boston, Massachusetts

DAVID T. RUBIN, MD
Joseph B. Kirsner Professor of Medicine
Chief, Section of Gastroenterology, Hepatology, and Nutrition
Department of Medicine
University of Chicago
Chicago, Illinois

C. MEL WILCOX, MD, MSPH
Chief of Gastroenterology and Hepatology
Director, Pancreatology
Digestive Health Institute
Chair, US Pancreatic Disease Study Group
Orlando Health
Orlando, Florida

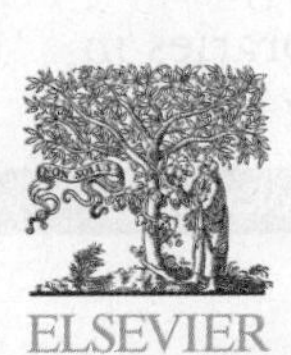

ELSEVIER

Elsevier
1600 John F. Kennedy Blvd.
Ste 1800
Philadelphia, PA 19103-2899

SLEISENGER AND FORDTRAN'S GASTROINTESTINAL AND LIVER DISEASE,
TWELFTH EDITION

ISBN: 978-0-443-11657-5
Volume 1: 978-0-443-11704-6
Volume 2: 978-0-443-11705-3

Executive Content Strategist: Nancy Anastasi Duffy
Content Development Manager: Meghan Andress
Senior Content Development Specialist: Kevin Travers
Publishing Services Manager: Catherine Jackson
Senior Project Manager: Cindy Thoms
Senior Book Designer: Patrick Ferguson

Printed in Canada

Last digit is the print number: 9 8 7 6 5 4 3 2 1

Contributors

Nezam H. Afdhal, MD, DSc
Chief of Gastroenterology and Hepatology
Beth Israel Deaconess Medical Center
Charlotte and Irving Rabb Professor of Medicine
Harvard Medical School
Boston, Massachusetts, United States

Rakesh Aggarwal MD, DM
Professor, Department of Gastroenterology
Sanjay Gandhi Postgraduate Institute of Medical Sciences
Lucknow, UP, India

Sameer Al Diffalha, MD
Associate Professor of Pathology
University of Alabama at Birmingham
Birmingham, Alabama, United States

Jaime Almandoz, MD, MBA, FTOS
Associate Professor of Internal Medicine
Endocrinology
University of Texas Southwestern
Dallas, Texas, United States

Taymeyah Al-Toubah, MPH
Senior Research Project Manager GI Oncology
H. Lee Moffitt Cancer Center
Tampa, Florida, United States

Amin Amin, MB, ChB
Assistant Professor, Internal Medicine: Digestive and Liver Diseases
University of Texas Southwestern
Dallas, Texas, United States

Ashwin N. Ananthakrishnan, MD, MPH
Director of the MGH Crohn's and Colitis Center
Associate Professor of Medicine
Harvard Medical School Division of Gastroenterology
Massachusetts General Hospital
Boston, Massachusetts, United States

Karin L. Andersson, MD, MPH
Assistant Professor of Medicine, Harvard Medical School
Hepatologist, Division of Gastroenterology
Massachusetts General Hospital
Boston, Massachusetts, United States

Louis J. Aronne, MD
Sanford I. Weill Professor of Metabolic Research
Department of Medicine
Weill Cornell Medicine
New York, New York, United States

Jordan E. Axelrad, MD, MPH
Director, Clinical and Translational Research
Inflammatory Bowel Disease Center
NYU Langone Health
Associate Professor
Division of Gastroenterology
NYU Grossman School of Medicine
New York, New York, United States

Fernando Azpiroz, MD, PhD
Chief, Department of Gastroenterology
University Hospital Vall d'Hebron
Professor of Medicine
Universitat Autònoma de Barcelona
Barcelona, Spain

William Balistreri, MD
Pediatric Liver Care Center
Gastroenterology, Hepatology, and Nutrition
Cincinnati Children's Hospital Medical Center
Cincinnati, Ohio, United States

Ji Young Bang, MD, MPH
Director of Clinical Research, Digestive Health Institute
Orlando Health
Orlando, Florida, United States

S. George Barreto, FRACS, PhD
Consultant, HPB and Liver Transplant Unit
Flinders Medical Centre
Deputy Director, Medical Program (MD)
Coordinator | MD Advanced Studies
College of Medicine and Public Health
Flinders University
Bedford Park South Africa

Lee M. Bass, MD
Professor of Pediatrics
Gastroenterology, Hepatology, and Nutrition
Ann and Robert H. Lurie Children's Hospital of Chicago
Chicago, Illinois, United States

Alex S. Befeler, MD
Professor of Internal Medicine and Medical Director Liver Transplantation
Division of Gastroenterology and Hepatology
Saint Louis University
St. Louis, Missouri, United States

Daniel Behin, MD
Assistant Professor of Medicine
Montefiore Medical Center
New York, New York, United States

Mark Benson, MD
Professor of Medicine
Section of Gastroenterology and Hepatology
University of Wisconsin School of Medicine and Public Health
Madison, Wisconsin, United States

Adil E. Bharucha, MBBS, MD
Professor of Medicine
Division of Gastroenterology and Hepatology
Mayo Clinic
Rochester, Minnesota, United States

Divya B. Bhatt, MD, MA
Assistant Professor of Medicine Digestive and Liver Diseases
University of Texas Southwestern Medical Center
Assistant Professor of Gastroenterology
Veterans Affairs North Texas Health Care System
Dallas, Texas, United States

Taft P. Bhuket, MD
Associate Clinical Professor of Medicine
Division of Gastroenterology
University of California, San Francisco
San Francisco, California, United States;
Chief of Gastroenterology and Hepatology, Director of Endoscopy
Alameda Health System
Oakland, California, United States

Yangzom D. Bhutia, DVM, PhD
Assistant Professor, Cell Biology and Biochemistry
Texas Tech University Health Sciences Center
Lubbock, Texas, United States

J. Andrew Bird, MD
Professor, Pediatrics, Division of Allergy and Immunology
University of Texas Southwestern Medical Center
Director, Food Allergy Center
Children's Medical Center
Dallas, Texas, United States

Diego V. Bohórquez, PhD
Associate Professor
Departments of Medicine and Neurobiology
Duke University Medical Center
Durham, North Carolina, United States

Shoma Bommena, MD, MS
Fellow in Gastroenterology and Hepatology, Internal Medicine
University of Arizona College of Medicine
Tucson, Arizona, United States

Jan Bornschein, MD
Nuffield Department of Experimental Medicine
Oxford, United Kingdom

Christopher L. Bowlus, MD
Professor and Chief
Division of Gastroenterology and Hepatology
University of California Davis
Sacramento, California, United States

Lawrence J. Brandt, MD
Professor of Medicine and Surgery
Albert Einstein College of Medicine
Emeritus Chief, Division of Gastroenterology
Montefiore Medical Center
Bronx, New York, United States

Robert Scott Bresalier, MD
Professor of Medicine
Lydia and Birdie J Resoft Distinguished Professor in GI Oncology
Gastroenterology, Hepatology, and Nutrition
The University of Texas MD Anderson Cancer Center
Houston, Texas, United States

Stuart M. Brierley, PhD
Professor, NHMRC Investigator Leadership Fellow
Hopwood Centre for Neurobiology, Lifelong Health Theme
South Australian Health and Medical Research Institute (SAHMRI)
Adelaide, Australia

Simon J.H. Brookes, PhD
Professor, Human Physiology
College of Medicine, Flinders University
Adelaide, South Australia, Australia

Alan L. Buchman, MD, MSPH
Professor of Clinical Surgery
University of Illinois at Chicago
Director, Gastroenterology
Chicago, Illinois, United States,
Elevance Health
Intestinal Rehabilitation and Transplant Center
Indianapolis, Indiana, United States

Callie B. Burgin, MD
Assistant Professor of Clinical Dermatology
Dermatology, Indiana University School of Medicine
Indianapolis, Indiana, United States

Ezra Burstein, MD, PhD
Professor, Departments of Internal Medicine and Molecular Biology
UT Southwestern Medical Center
Dallas, Texas, United States

Allison M. Bush, MD, MPH
Gastroenterology
Uniformed Services University
Bethesda, Maryland, United States

James P. Callaway, MD
Assistant Professor, Department of Gastroenterology
University of Alabama at Birmingham
Birmingham, Alabama, United States

David J. Cangemi, MD
Consultant, Gastroenterology and Hepatology
Mayo Clinic
Jacksonville, Florida, United States

Dustin A. Carlson, MD, MS
Assistant Professor of Medicine
Northwestern University Feinberg School of Medicine
Chicago, Illinois, United States

Andres F. Carrion, MD
Gastroenterologist and Hepatologist
GastroMed
Miami, Florida, United States

Amanda K. Cartee, MD
Assistant Professor, Gastroenterology and Hepatology
University of Alabama at Birmingham
Birmingham, Alabama, United States

Francis K.L. Chan, MBChB(Hons), MD, DSc
Professor of Medicine
Department of Medicine and Therapeutics
Chinese University of Hong Kong
Hong Kong, China

Michael R. Charlton, MD
Professor of Medicine
Chief of Hepatology
Director, Center for Liver Diseases
Medical Director, Transplantation Institute
University of Chicago
Chicago, Illinois, United States

Ellie Chen, MD
Division of Gastroenterology
University of California, Los Angeles
Los Angeles, California, United States

Alice Cheng, MD, PhD
Assistant Professor of Medicine
University of Chicago
Chicago, Illinois, United States

Shivakumar Chitturi, MD
Associate Professor
Australian National University
Senior Staff Hepatologist
The Canberra Hospital
Australian Capital Territory, Australia

Daniel C. Chung, MD
Professor of Medicine
Harvard Medical School
Division of Gastroenterology
Massachusetts General Hospital
Medical Co-Director
Center for Cancer Risk Analysis
Massachusetts General Hospital Cancer Center
Boston, Massachusetts, United States

Raymond T. Chung, MD
Professor of Medicine
Harvard Medical School
Zhou Family Endowed Chair
Chief, Gastroenterology, Hepatology and Endoscopy
Mass General Brigham
Associate Member, Broad Institute
Boston, Massachusetts, United States

Gregory A. Coté, MD, MS
Division Head, Professor, Department of Medicine
Division of Gastroenterology and Hepatology
Oregon Health & Science University
Portland, Oregon, United States

Cary C. Cotton, MD, MPH
Assistant Professor of Medicine
Department of Medicine
Division of Gastroenterology and Hepatology
UNC School of Medicine
Chapel Hill, North Carolina, United States

Marc Roger Couturier, PhD, D(ABMM)
Professor, ARUP Laboratories
University of Utah
Salt Lake City, Utah, United States

Brian G. Czito, MD
Professor, Radiation Oncology
Duke University Medical Center
Durham, North Carolina, United States

Sushila Dalal, MD
Associate Professor of Medicine
Section of Gastroenterology, Hepatology, and Nutrition
University of Chicago
Chicago, Illinois, United States

Paul A. Dawson, PhD
Professor Pediatrics
Gastroenterology, Hepatology, and Nutrition
Emory University
Atlanta, Georgia, United States

Jose Debes, MD, PhD, MS
Professor, Division of Infectious Diseases and International Medicine
Department of Medicine
University of Minnesota
Minneapolis, Minnesota, United States

Roshani J. Desai, MD
Assistant Professor, Gastroenterology and Hepatology
Saint Louis University
Saint Louis, Missouri, United States

Jill K. Deutsch, MD
Assistant Professor, Department of Internal Medicine
Section of Digestive Diseases
Yale New Haven Hospital
Yale University School of Medicine
New Haven, Connecticut, United States

Kenneth R. DeVault, MD
Professor of Medicine and Chair
Mayo Clinic College of Medicine
Jacksonville, Florida, United States

John K. DiBaise, MD
Professor of Medicine
Division of Gastroenterology and Hepatology
Mayo Clinic
Scottsdale, Arizona, United States

Philip G. Dinning, PhD
Senior Hospital Scientist
Department of Gastroenterology and Surgery
Professor, College of Medicine and Public Health
Flinders Medical Centre
Adelaide, South Australia, Australia

Michael Dougan, MD, PhD
Associate Professor of Medicine
Harvard Medical School
Division of Gastroenterology, Hepatology and Endoscopy
Mass General Brigham
Boston, Massachusetts, United States

Douglas A. Drossman, MD
Professor Emeritus of Medicine and Psychiatry
Division of Digestive Disease and Nutrition
University of North Carolina
President, Center for Education and Practice of Biopsychosocial Care
Chapel Hill, North Carolina, United States
President, Drossman Gastroenterology PLLC
Durham, North Carolina, United States

Kerry B. Dunbar, MD, PhD
Section Chief, VA Gastroenterology Section
Department of Medicine–Gastroenterology and Hepatology
VA North Texas Healthcare System–Dallas VA Medical Center
Associate Professor of Medicine
Department of Medicine–Division of Gastroenterology and Hepatology
University of Texas Southwestern Medical School
Dallas, Texas, United States

Steven A. Edmundowicz, MD
Professor of Medicine
Interim Director, Division of Gastroenterology and Hepatology
University of Colorado Anschutz Medical Campus
Aurora, Colorado, United States

Adam Edwards, MD, MS
Assistant Professor, Department of Medicine
University of Alabama at Birmingham
Birmingham, Alabama, United States

David E. Elliott, MD, PhD
University of Iowa Carver College of Medicine
Department of Internal Medicine
Division of Gastroenterology and Hepatology
Iowa City VAHCS, Department of Internal Medicine
Veterans Administration Health Care System
Iowa City, Iowa, United States

B. Joseph Elmunzer, MD, MSc
Peter B. Cotton Professor of Medicine and Endoscopic Innovation
Division of Gastroenterology and Hepatology
Medical University of South Carolina, Charleston
Charleston, South Carolina, United States

Charles O. Elson, MD
Professor of Medicine and Microbiology
Vice Chair for Research in the Department of Medicine
Basil I. Hirschowitz Chair in Gastroenterology
University of Alabama at Birmingham
Birmingham, Alabama, United States

Swathi Eluri, MD, MSCR
Assistant Professor of Medicine
Division of Gastroenterology and Hepatology
University of North Carolina School of Medicine
Chapel Hill, North Carolina, United States

Jill E. Elwing, MD
Assistant Professor of Medicine
Division of Gastroenterology
John T. Milliken Department of Medicine
Washington University in St. Louis
St. Louis, Missouri, United States

Michael B. Fallon, MD
Chair, Professor of Medicine
Gastroenterology, Hepatology, and Nutrition
University of Arizona
Vice Chair, Department of Internal Medicine
University of Arizona—Phoenix
Phoenix, Arizona, United States

Jordan J. Feld, MD, MPH
Professor of Medicine
University of Toronto
Research Director
Toronto Centre for Liver Disease
Senior Scientist
Sandra Rotman Centre for Global Health
Toronto General Hospital
Toronto, Ontario, Canada

Marc Fenster, MD
Division of Gastroenterology
Montefiore Medical Center
Albert Einstein College of Medicine
Bronx, New York, United States

Nielsen Fernandez-Becker, MD
Clinical Associate Professor of Medicine
Division of Gastroenterology and Hepatology
Stanford University
Redwood City, California, United States

Paul Feuerstadt, MD
Attending Physician, Gastroenterology
Gastroenterology Center of Connecticut
Hamden, Connecticut
Associate Clinical Professor of Medicine, Gastroenterology
Yale University School of Medicine
New Haven, Connecticut, United States

Peter Fickert, Prof
Division of Gastroenterology and Hepatology
Medical University of Graz
Graz, Austria

David R. Flum, MD, MPH, FACS
Professor of Surgery
University of Washington,
Seattle, Washington, United States

Lawrence S. Friedman, MD
Professor of Medicine, Harvard Medical School
Professor of Medicine, Tufts University School of Medicine
The Anton R. Fried, MD
Chair, Department of Medicine
Newton-Wellesley Hospital
Newton, Massachusetts Assistant Chief of Medicine
Massachusetts General Hospital
Boston, Massachusetts, United States

Vadivel Ganapathy, PhD
Professor, Cell Biology and Biochemistry
Texas Tech University Health Sciences Center
Lubbock, Texas, United States

Marc G. Ghany, MD, MHSc
Senior Investigator, Liver Diseases Branch
National Institute of Diabetes and Digestive and Kidney Diseases
National Institutes of Health
Bethesda, Maryland, United States

Pere Ginès, MD, PhD
Chairman, Liver Unit, Hospital Clinic Barcelona
Full Professor of Medicine, University of Barcelona
Principal Investigator
Institut d'Investigacions Biomediques August Pi i Sunyer (IDIBAPS)
Barcelona, Spain

Robert E. Glasgow, MD
Professor and Vice Chairman, Surgery
University of Utah
Salt Lake City, Utah, United States

Amit Goel, MBBS, MD, DNB, DM
Professor and Head, Hepatology
Sanjay Gandhi Postgraduate Institute of Medical Sciences
Lucknow, Uttar Pradesh, India

Amanda R. Gomez, MD, MPH
Assistant Professor
Division of Gastroenterology, Hepatology, and Nutrition
Ann & Robert H. Lurie Children's Hospital of Chicago
Chicago, Illinois, United States

Alex J. Gooding, MD, PhD
Medical Resident, Radiation Oncology
Duke University
Durham, North Carolina, United States

Gregory J. Gores, MD
Professor of Medicine
Division of Gastroenterology and Hepatology
Mayo Clinic
Rochester, Minnesota, United States

Peter H.R. Green, MD
Phyllis and Ivan Seidenberg Professor of Medicine
Columbia University Medical Center
New York, New York, United States

Drew Gunnells, MD, FACS
Assistant Professor, GI Surgery
University of Alabama at Birgmingham
Birmingham, Alabama, United States

Malika Gupta, MBBS
Associate Professor of Pediatrics
Department of Pediatrics
University of Texas Southwestern
Dallas, Texas, United States

C. Prakash Gyawali, MD, MRCP
Professor of Medicine
Division of Gastroenterology
Department of Medicine
Washington University in St. Louis
St. Louis, Missouri, United States

Hazem Hammad, MD
Assistant Professor of Medicine
Division of Gastroenterology and Hepatology
University of Colorado Anschutz Medical Campus
Aurora, Colorado, United States

Heinz F. Hammer, MD
Associate Professor of Medicine
Department of Internal Medicine
Medical University
Graz, Austria

David J. Hass, MD
Associate Clinical Professor of Medicine
Division of Digestive Diseases
Yale University School of Medicine
New Haven, Connecticut, United States

Asif Hitawala, MBBS
Liver Disease Branch
NIH/NIDDK
Bethesda, Maryland, United States

Thanh P. Ho, MD
Assistant Professor of Oncology
Department of Oncology
Mayo Clinic
Rochester, Minnesota, United States

David M. Hockenbery, MD
Member, Clinical Research
Fred Hutchinson Cancer Research Center
Professor of Medicine
Division of Gastroenterology
University of Washington
Seattle, Washington, United States

Christoph Högenauer, MD
Associate Professor of Medicine
Department of Internal Medicine
Medical University of Graz
Graz, Austria

Jacinta A. Holmes, MBBS, PhD
Division of Gastroenterology
Massachusetts General Hospital
Boston, Massachusetts, United States
Gastroenterology, St. Vincent's Hospital
University of Melbourne
Fitzroy, Victoria, Australia

Amy E. Hosmer, MD
Clinical Assistant Professor, Medicine
Digestive Health Institute
University Hospitals of Cleveland
Cleveland, Ohio, United States

Colin W. Howden, MD
Professor Emeritus, Hyman Professor of Medicine
Division of Gastroenterology
University of Tennessee Health Science Center
Memphis, Tennessee, United States

Bridget Hron, MD, MMSc
Assistant Professor, Pediatrics
Harvard Medical School
Associate Director, Center for Nutrition
Boston Children's Hospital
Boston, Massachusetts, United States

Christine Hsu, MD
NIH-NIDDK, Liver Disease Branch
National Institute of Digestive and Diabetes and Kidney Diseases
Bethesda, Maryland, United States

Sohail Z. Husain, MD
Professor of Pediatrics
Division of Gastroenterology, Hepatology, and Nutrition
Stanford University School of Medicine
Stanford, California, United States

Neil Hyman, MD
Chief, Section of Colon and Rectal Surgery
Co-Director Digestive Disease Center
Department of Surgery
University of Chicago Medicine
Chicago, Illinois, United States

Sumera I. Ilyas, MBBS
Assistant Professor of Medicine
Division of Gastroenterology and Hepatology
Mayo Clinic
Rochester, Minnesota, United States

M. Nedim Ince, MD
University of Iowa Carver College of Medicine
Department of Internal Medicine
Division of Gastroenterology and Hepatology
Iowa City VAHCS, Department of Internal Medicine
Veterans Administration Health Care System
Department of Internal Medicine
Veterans Administration Health Care System
Iowa City, Iowa, United States

Johanna C. Iturrino Moreda, MD
Assistant Professor of Medicine
Harvard Medical School
Beth Israel Deaconess Medical Center
Boston, Massachusetts, United States

Harry L.A. Janssen, MD, PhD
Professor of Medicine, Gastroenterology and Hepatology
University of Toronto
Toronto, Ontario, Canada
Professor of Medicine, Gastroenterology and Hepatology
Erasmus MC University Medical Center
Rotterdam, Netherlands

Dennis M. Jensen, MD
Professor of Medicine, Gastrointestinal
David Geffen School of Medicine at UCLA
Staff Physician, Medicine-Gastrointestinal
VA Greater Los Angeles Healthcare System
Key Investigator, Director
Human Studies Core and Gastrointestinal Hemostasis Research Unit
CURE Digestive Diseases Research Center
Los Angeles, California, United States

D. Rohan Jeyarajah, MD
Chair of Surgery, Assistant Chair of Clinical Sciences, Head of Surgery
TCU and UNTHSC School of Medicine
Fort Worth, Texas, United States
Director, Gastrointestinal Services, Methodist Richardson Medical Center
Director, HPB/UGI Fellowship
Associate Program Director, General Surgery Residency Program
Methodist Richardson Medical Center
Richardson, Texas, United States

Adrià Juanola, PhD
Clinician, Liver Unit
Hospital Clínic de Barcelona
Institut d'Investigacions Biomèdiques August Pi i Sunyer (IDIBAPS)
Barcelona, Spain

Patrick S. Kamath, MD
Professor of Medicine, Division of Gastroenterology and Hepatology
Consultant, Gastroenterology and Hepatology
Mayo Clinic College of Medicine and Science
Rochester, Minnesota, United States

Nuray Kanbur, MD
Professor of Pediatrics
University of Ottawa
Ottawa, Ontario, Canada

Gilaad G. Kaplan, MD, MPH
Professor of Medicine
University of Calgary
Calgary, Alberta, Canada

Jennifer Katz, MD
Assistant Professor of Medicine
Division of Gastroenterology
Montefiore Medical Center
Bronx, New York, United States

David A. Katzka, MD
Professor of and Consultant in Medicine, Gastroenterology
Mayo Clinic
Rochester, Minnesota, United States

Debra K. Katzman, MD, FRCPC
Professor of Pediatrics, Department of Pediatrics
The Hospital for Sick Children and University of Toronto
Toronto, Ontario, Canada

Jonathan D. Kaunitz, MD
Professor of Medicine and Surgery
UCLA School of Medicine
Attending Gastroenterologist
West Los Angeles Veterans Affairs Medical Center
Los Angeles, California, United States

Laurie Keefer, PhD
Professor Medicine and Psychiatry
Icahn School of Medicine at Mount Sinai
New York, New York, United States

Ciarán P. Kelly, MD
Professor of Medicine, Gastroenterology
Harvard Medical School
J Thomas Lamont Professor of Gastroenterology
Beth Israel Deaconess Medical Center
Boston, Massachusetts, United States

Sahil Khanna, MBBS, MS
Associate Professor of Medicine
Gastroenterology and Hepatology
Mayo Clinic
Rochester, Minnesota, United States

Arthur Yu-shin Kim, MD
Associate Professor of Medicine
Harvard Medical School
Division of Infectious Diseases
Massachusetts General Hospital
Boston, Massachusetts, United States

Kenneth L. Koch, MD
Professor of Medicine, Department of Medicine
Section on Gastroenterology and Hepatology
Wake Forest University School of Medicine
Winston-Salem, North Carolina, United States

Kris V. Kowdley, MD
Director
Liver Institute Northwest
Seattle, Washington, United States

Braden Kuo, MD
Director of the MGH Center for Neurointestinal Health
Gastroenterology
Massachusetts General Hospital
Boston, Massachusetts, United States

Brian E. Lacy, MD, PhD
Professor of Medicine
Division of Gastroenterology
Mayo Clinic
Jacksonville, Florida, United States

Anne M. Larson, MD
Clinical Professor of Medicine
Division of Gastroenterology/Hepatology
University of Washington
Seattle, Washington, United States

Ivan S.F. Lau, MB, BCh, BAO
Clinical Lecturer, Medicine and Therapeutics
The Chinese University of Hong Kong
Sha Tin, Hong Kong

James Y.W. Lau, MD
Professor of Surgery
Department of Surgery
The Chinese University of Hong Kong
Director
Endoscopy Centre
Prince of Wales Hospital
Hong Kong, China

Benjamin Lebwohl, MD, MS
Associate Professor of Medicine and Epidemiology
Columbia University Medical Center
New York, New York, United States

Peter J. Lee, MBChB
Assistant Professor of Clinical Medicine
Gastroenterology, Hepatology and Nutrition
The Ohio State University Wexner Medical Center
Columbus, Ohio, United States

William M. Lee, MD
Professor, Internal Medicine
UT Southwestern Medical Center at Dallas
Dallas, Texas, United States

Anthony J. Lembo, MD
Vice Chair of Research
Digestive Disease and Surgery Institute Cleveland Clinic
Cleveland, Ohio, United States

Cynthia Levy, MD
Professor of Medicine
Division of Digestive Health and Liver Diseases
University of Miami
Miami, Florida, United States

Blair Lewis, MD
Medical Director, Carnegie Hill Endoscopy
Clinical Professor of Medicine
Mount Sinai Medical Center
New York, New York, United States

James H. Lewis, MD
Professor of Medicine, Director of Hepatology
Division of Gastroenterology
Georgetown University Medical Center
Washington, DC, United States

Rodger A. Liddle, MD
Professor of Medicine
Department of Medicine
Duke University Medical Center
Durham, North Carolina, United States

Steven D. Lidofsky, MD, PhD
Professor of Medicine, University of Vermont
Director of Hepatology, University of Vermont Medical Center
Burlington, Vermont, United States

Cara L. Mack, MD
Chief Professor of Pediatrics
Division of Gastroenterology
Medical College of Wisconsin, Children's
Milwaukee, Wisconsin, United States

Matthias Maiwald, MD, PhD
Senior Consultant in Microbiology
Department of Pathology and Laboratory Medicine
KK Women's and Children's Hospital, Singapore
Adjunct Associate Professor
Department of Microbiology and Immunology
Yong Loo Lin School of Medicine, National University of Singapore
Adjunct Associate Professor
Duke-NUS Graduate Medical School
Singapore, Singapore

Lawrence A. Mark, MD, PhD
Associate Professor of Clinical Dermatology
Department of Dermatology
Indiana University School of Medicine
Indianapolis, Indiana, United States

Paul Martin, MD, FRCP, FRCPI
Hepatologist, Karsh Division of Gastroenterology and Hepatology
Cedars Sinai
Los Angeles, California, United States

Joel B. Mason, MD
Professor of Medicine and Nutrition
Divisions of Gastroenterology and Clinical Nutrition
Tufts University
Director, Vitamins and Carcinogenesis Laboratory
USDA Human Nutrition Research Center at Tufts University
Boston, Massachusetts, United States

Blaine A. Mathison, BS, M(ASCP)
Technical Director of Parasitology
Technical Operations, Infectious Diseases
ARUP Laboratories
Salt Lake City, Utah, United States

Jeffrey B. Matthews, MD
Dallas B. Phemister Professor and Chairman
Department of Surgery
The University of Chicago Medicine
Chicago, Illinois, United States

Marlyn J. Mayo, MD
Professor of Internal Medicine
University of Texas Southwestern
Dallas, Texas, United States

Craig J. McClain, MD
Professor of Medicine and Pharmacology and Toxicology
Vice President for Health Affairs and Research
University of Louisville
Director, Gastroenterology
Robley Rex VA Medical Center
Louisville, Kentucky, United States

Stephen A. McClave, MD
Professor and Director of Clinical Nutrition
Department of Medicine
University of Louisville School of Medicine
Louisville, Kentucky, United States

Megha S. Mehta, MD
Assistant Professor of Pediatrics
University of Texas Southwestern Medical Center
Dallas, Texas, United States

Joanna M.P. Melia, MD
Assistant Professor of Medicine
Johns Hopkins University School of Medicine
Baltimore, Maryland, United States

Dejan Micic, MD
Associate Professor of Medicine
Division Chief, Division of Gastroenterology and Nutrition
Loyola University Medical Center
Maywood, Illinois, United States

Frederick H. Millham, MD, MBA
Surgeon-in-Chief, Surgery
South Shore Hospital
Weymouth, Massachusetts
Associate Professor of Surgery (Part Time)
Harvard Medical School
Boston, Massachusetts, United States

Ginat W. Mirowski, DMD, MD
Adjunct Associate Professor
Department of Oral Pathology, Medicine, and Radiology
Indiana University School of Dentistry
Adjunct Clinical Associate Professor
Department of Dermatology
Indiana University School of Medicine
Indianapolis, Indiana, United States

Daniel S. Mishkin, MD, CM
Physician, Gastroenterology
Atrius Health
Lecturer, Harvard Medical School
Boston, Massachusetts, United States

John Magaña Morton, MD, MPH, MHA
Medical Director of Bariatric and Minimally Invasive Surgery
Department of Surgery
Yale School of Medicine
New Haven, Connecticut, United States

Baha Moshiree, MD, MSci
Professor of Medicine, Gastroenterology
Atrium Health, Wake Forest Medical University
Charlotte, North Carolina, United States

William Conan Mustain, MD
Associate Professor of Surgery
Division of Colon and Rectal Surgery
University of Arkansas for Medical Sciences
Little Rock, Arkansas, United States

Mayur Narkhede, MD
Assistant Professor, Department of Internal Medicine
Division of Hematology/Oncology
University of Alabama at Birmingham
Birmingham, Alabama, United States

Rohit Nathani, MBBS
Gestroenterology Fellows
Department of Internal Medicine
The University of Iowa
Iowa City, Iowa, United States

Filipe Gaio Nery, MD
Physician, Departamento de Anestesiologia
Cuidados Intensivos e Emergência
Centro Hospitalar do Porto–Hospital Santo António
Porto, Researcher, EPIUnit, Instituto de Saúde Pública
Universidade do Porto, Porto
Researcher, Ciências Médicas
Instituto de Ciências Biomédicas de Abel Salazar
Porto, Portugal

Siew C. Ng, MBBS (Lond), PhD (Lond)
Professor of Medicine
Department of Medicine and Therapeutics
State Key Laboratory of Digestive Disease
LKS Institute of Health Science
The Chinese University of Hong Kong
Hong Kong, China

Nhi T. Nguyen, MS
Graduate Student, Cell Biology and Biochemistry
Texas Tech University Health Sciences Center
Lubbock, Texas, United States

Long H. Nguyen, MD, MS
Assistant Professor of Medicine
Massachusetts General Hospital and Harvard Medical School
Boston, Massachusetts, United States

Mark L. Norris, BSc (Hon), MD
Professor of Pediatrics, Pediatrics
Children's Hospital of Eastern Ontario
University of Ottawa
Ottawa, Ontario, Canada

Mazen Noureddin, MD, MHSc
Professor of Medicine
Lynda K. and David M. Underwood Center for Digestive Disorders
Houston Methodist Hospital
Houston, Texas, United States

Kinga S. Olortegui, MD, MS
Assistant Professor of Surgery
The University of Chicago Medicine
Chicago, Illinois, United States

Endashaw Omer, MD, MPH, AGAF, FACG, PNS
Associate Professor of Internal Medicine
University of Louisville
Associate Professor of Internal Medicine
VA Medical Center
Lousville, Kentucky, United States

Babak J. Orandi, MD, PhD, MSc, FACS, ABOM Diplomate
Associate Professor of Surgery and Medicine
Departments of Surgery and Medicine
New York University
New York, New York, United States

Tamas Ordog, MD
Professor of Physiology
Department of Physiology and Biomedical Engineering and Division of Gastroenterology and Hepatology
Department of Medicine
Mayo Clinic
Rochester, Minnesota, United States

Stephen J. Pandol, MD
Professor, Medicine
Cedars-Sinai Medical Center
Los Angeles, California, United States

Georgios I. Papachristou, MD, PhD
Professor of Medicine, Gastroenterology
Ohio State University
Powell, Ohio, United States

Darrell S. Pardi, MD, MS
Chair, Division of Gastroenterology and Hepatology
Professor of Medicine
Mayo Clinic
Rochester, Minnesota, United States

Parth Patel, MD
Washington Regional Gastroenterology
Washington Regional/UAMS Internal Medicine Residency GME Faculty
Fayetteville, Arkansas, United States

Mythili Pathipati, AB, MD
Gastroenterology
Massachusetts General Hospital
Boston, Massachusetts, United States

Mark R. Pedersen, MD
Assistant Professor, Internal Medicine, Digestive and Liver Disease
University of Texas Southwestern Medical Center
Dallas, Texas, United States

Vyjeyanthi S. Periyakoil, MD
Director, Palliative Care Education and Training
Department of Medicine
Stanford University School of Medicine
Stanford, California, United States

Patrick R. Pfau, MD
Professor, Chief of Clinical Gastroenterology
Section of Gastroenterology and Hepatology
University of Wisconsin School of Medicine and Public Health
Madison, Wisconsin, United States

Anna Evans Phillips, MD, MS
Assistant Professor of Medicine
Department of Medicine
Division of Gastroenterology, Hepatology, and Nutrition
University of Pittsburgh School of Medicine
Pittsburgh, Pennsylvania, United States

Elisa Pose, MD, PhD
Hepatologist, Liver Unit, Hospital Clínic de Barcelona
Institut d'Investigacions Biomèdiques August Pi i Sunyer (IDIBAPS)
Centro de Investigación Biomédica en Red de Enfermedades Hepáticas y Digestivas (CIBEReHD)
Barcelona, Spain

Daniel S. Pratt, MD
Director, Autoimmune and Cholestatic Liver Center
Division of Gastroenterology
Massachusetts General Hospital
Assistant Professor of Medicine
Harvard Medical School
Boston, Massachusetts, United States

David O. Prichard, MB, BCh, PhD
Gastroenterologist
Gastroenterology and Hepatology
Mayo Clinic
Rochester, Minnesota

Michael Quante, Prof
Universitätsklinikum Freiburg
Klinik für Innere Medizin II
Gastrointestinale Onkologie
Freiburg, Germany

Balakrishnan S. Ramakrishna, MBBS, MD, DM, PhD
Director, Institute of Gastroenterology
SRM Institutes for Medical Science
Chennai, Tamil Nadu, India

Mrinalini C. Rao, PhD
Professor, Department of Physiology and Biophysics
Division of Gastroenterology and Hepatology
University of Illinois at Chicago
Chicago, Illinois, United States

Satish S.C. Rao, MD, PhD
Professor of Medicine
Harold J. Harrison, MD Distinguished University Chair in Gastroenterology, Medicine-Gastroenterology/Hepatology
Augusta University
Augusta, Georgia, United States

Christopher K. Rayner, MBBS, PhD
Professor, Adelaide Medical School, University of Adelaide
Consultant Gastroenterologist
Department of Gastroenterology and Hepatology
Royal Adelaide Hospital
Adelaide, South Australia, Australia

Miguel D. Regueiro, MD
Chair and Professor of Medicine
Department of Gastroenterology and Hepatology
Cleveland Clinic, Digestive Disease and Surgery Institute
Cleveland, Ohio, United States

John F. Reinus, MD
Professor of Medicine
Department of Medicine
Albert Einstein College of Medicine
Medical Director of Liver Transplantation
Montefiore-Einstein Center for Transplantation
Montefiore Medical Center
Bronx, New York, United States

David A. Relman, MD
Thomas C. and Joan M. Merigan Professor, Departments of Medicine and Microbiology and Immunology
Stanford University, Stanford, California
Chief of Infectious Diseases
Veterans Affairs Palo Alto Health Care System
Palo Alto, California, United States

Joel E. Richter, MD
Professor and Director, Division of Digestive Diseases and Nutrition
University of South Florida
Director, Joy McCann Culverhouse Center for Swallowing Disorders
University of South Florida
Tampa, Florida, United States

Mary E. Rinella, MD
Professor of Medicine
University of Chicago
Chicago, Illinois, United States

Eve A. Roberts, MD, PhD
Professor Emerita, Pediatrics, Medicine, and Pharmacology and Toxicology
University of Toronto
Adjunct Scientist, Genetics and Genome Biology Program
Hospital for Sick Children Research Institute
Associate, Division of Gastroenterology, Hepatology, and Nutrition
The Hospital for Sick Children
Toronto, Ontario, Canada
Associate Fellow, History of Science and Technology Program
University of King's College
Halifax, Nova Scotia, Canada

Matthew L. Roberts, MD
Associate Professor of Surgery
Department of Surgery
University of Arkansas for Medical Sciences
Little Rock, Arkansas, United States

Stephanie Romutis, MD
Clinical Assistant Professor of Medicine, Gastroenterology
University of Pittsburgh Medical Center
Clinical Assistant Professor of Medicine, Gastroenterology
VA Pittsburgh Medical Center
Pittsburgh, Pennsylvania, United States

Marc E. Rothenberg, MD, PhD
Professor of Pediatrics, Allergy & Immunology
Cincinnati Children's Hospital Medical Center
Cincinnati, Ohio, United States

Jayanta Roy-Chowdhury, MBBS
Professor, Departments of Medicine and Genetics
Director, Genetic Engineering and Gene Therapy Core Facility
Albert Einstein College of Medicine
New York, New York, United States

Namita Roy-Chowdhury, PhD
Professor, Departments of Medicine and Genetics
Albert Einstein College of Medicine
New York, New York, United States

David T. Rubin, MD
Joseph B. Kirsner Professor of Medicine
Chief, Section of Gastroenterology, Hepatology, and Nutrition
Department of Medicine
University of Chicago
Chicago, Illinois, United States

Gustavo A. Rubio, MD
Associate Medical Director
Colon and Rectal Surgery
Jackson Health System,
Miami, Florida, United States

Jayashree Sarathy, PhD
Professor, Department of Biological Sciences
Director of Graduate Programs, Biological Sciences
Benedictine University
Lisle, Illinois
Visiting Research Professor
Department of Physiology and Biophysics
University of Illinois at Chicago
Chicago, Illinois, United States

Jessica B. Sarthi, PhD
Research Scientist, Pediatrics, Gastroenterology, Hepatology and Nutrition
Palo Alto, California, United States

Thomas J. Savides, MD
Professor of Clinical Medicine
Division of Gastroenterology
University of California San Diego
La Jolla, California, United States

Gregory S. Sayuk, MD, MPH
Professor of Medicine and Psychiatry, Gastroenterology Division
Washington University in St. Louis School of Medicine
Staff Physician, Gastroenterology Section
St. Louis Veterans Affairs Medical Center
St. Louis, Missouri, United States

Zachary M. Sellers, MD, PhD
Assistant Professor of Pediatrics
Pediatrics - Gastroenterology
Stanford University
Palo Alto, California, United States

Vijay H. Shah, MD
Carol M. Gatton Professor of Medicine, Physiology, and Cancer Cell Biology
Kinney Executive Dean of Research,
Chair Department of Medicine
Mayo Clinic College of Medicine and Science
Rochester, Minnesota, United States

Nicholas J. Shaheen, MD, MPH
Professor of Medicine
University of North Carolina
Chapel Hill, North Carolina, United States

Jordan M. Shapiro, MD, MS
Staff Physician, Gastro Health and Nutrition
Houston, Texas, United States

Angela Shih, MD
Assistant in Pathology, Pathology
Massachusetts General Hospital
Assistant Professor, Harvard Medical School
Boston, Massachusetts, United States

Stuti Girish Shroff, MBBS, PhD
Department of Pathology
Mass General Hospital
Mass General Brigham
Watertown, Massachusetts, United States

Vikesh Singh, MD, MSc
Professor of Medicine, Division of Gastroenterology
Director of Endoscopy, Director of Pancreatology
Johns Hopkins University School of Medicine
Baltimore, Maryland, United States

Maria H. Sjogren, MD, MPH
Senior Hepatologist, Department of Medicine
Walter Reed National Medical Center
Bethesda, Maryland, United States

Valeriya Skorobogatko, MD
Resident Appointee
Department of Dermatology
Indiana University School of Medicine
Indianapolis, Indiana, United States

Adam Slivka, MD, PhD
Professor, Medicine
University of Pittsburgh Medical Center
Pittsburgh, Pennsylvania, United States

Phillip D. Smith, MD
Professor of Medicine and Microbiology
University of Alabama at Birmingham
Birmingham, Alabama, United States

Kjetil Soreide, MD, PhD, FRCS (Edin), FACS, FEBS (Hon)
Consultant Surgeon (HPB Unit), Karolinska Institutet
Karolinska University Hospital
Stockholm, Sweden
General and HPB Surgeon, Dept of Gastrointestinal Surgery
Stavanger University Hospital
Professor of Surgery, Department of Clinical Medicine
University of Bergen
Bergen, Norway

Milan J. Sonneveld, MD, PhD
Gastroenterology and Hepatology
Erasmus University Medical Center
Rotterdam, Netherlands

James E. Squires, MD, MS
Associate Professor, Department of Pediatrics
Associate Director of Hepatology
UPMC Children's Hospital of Pittsburgh
Pittsburgh, Pennsylvania, United States

Neil H. Stollman, MD
Associate Clinical Professor, Department of Medicine
Division of Gastroenterology
University of California San Francisco
San Francisco, California
Chief Division of Gastroenterology
Alta Bates Summit Medical Center
Oakland, California, United States

R. Todd Stravitz, MD
Professor of Medicine, Internal Medicine
Virginia Commonwealth University
Richmond, Virginia, United States

Sarah E. Streett, MD
Clinical Associate Professor
Director IBD Education
Division of Gastroenterology and Hepatology
Stanford University
Redwood City, California, United States

Jonathan R. Strosberg, MD
Professor, Gastrointestinal Oncology
Moffitt Cancer Center
Tampa, Florida, United States

Frederick J. Suchy, MD
Senior Research Strategist
Children's Hospital Colorado
Professor of Pediatrics and Associate Dean for Child Health Research, Pediatrics
University of Colorado School of Medicine
Aurora, Colorado, United States

Shelby Sullivan, MD
Director of the Metabolic and Bariatric Program
Division of Gastroenterology and Hepatology
Center for Digestive Health
Dartmouth-Hitchcock Health
Lebanon, New Hampshire

Shahnaz Sultan, MD, MHSc
Doctor of Medicine
University of Minnesota
Minneapolis, Minnesota, United States

Hidekazu Suzuki, MD, PhD
Associate Professor
Division of Gastroenterology and Hepatology
Department of Internal Medicine
Keio University School of Medicine
Tokyo, Japan

Gyongyi Szabo, MD, PhD
Mitchell T. Rabkin, MD Chair, Chief Academic Officer
Beth Israel Deaconess Medical Center and Beth Israel Lahey Health
Faculty Dean for Academic Affairs
Harvard Medical School
Boston, Massachusetts, United States

Nicholas J. Talley, MD, PhD
Pro Vice-Chancellor and Professor, Distinguished Laureate Professor
Faculty of Health and Medicine
University of Newcastle, Australia
Newcastle, New South Wales, Australia

Narci C. Teoh, MD
Professor of Medicine, Australian National University
Senior Staff Hepatologist
The Canberra Hospital
Australian Capital Territory, Australia

June Tome, MD
Gastroenterology and Hepatology
Mayo Clinic
Rochester, Minnesota, United States

Clara Y. Tow, BA, MD
Assistant Professor of Medicine, Internal Medicine/Hepatology
Montefiore Medical Center
Albert Einstein College of Medicine
Bronx, New York, United States

Shannan Tujios, MD
Associate Professor, Internal Medicine
University of Texas Southwestern Medical Center
Dallas, Texas, United States

Kiran Turaga, MD, MPH
Associate Professor
Department of Surgery
The University of Chicago
Chicago, Illinois, United States

Konstantin Umanskiy, MD
Professor of Surgery
University of Chicago
Chicago, Illinois, United States

Michael F. Vaezi, MD, PhD, MS
Professor of Medicine and Otolaryngology
Clinical Director, Division of Gastroenterology and Hepatology
Vanderbilt University Medical Center
Nashville, Tennessee, United States

Dominique Charles Valla, MD
Professor Emeritus of Hepatology, Liver Unit
Hôpital Beaujon, APHP, Clichy-la-Garenne
France
CRI, UMR1149
Inserm and Université de Paris
Paris, France

Shyam M. Varadarajulu, MD
President, Digestive Health Institute
Orlando Health
Winter Park, Florida, United States

Christopher Vélez, MD
Associate Program Director, Advanced Fellowship in Functional and Gastrointestinal Motility Disorders
Center for Neurointestinal Health
Division of Gastroenterology, Department of Medicine
Massachusetts General Hospital
Assistant Professor, Harvard Medical School
Boston, Massachusetts, United States

Axel von Herbay, MD
Professor of Pathology, Faculty of Medicine
University of Heidelberg
Heidelberg Hans Pathologie
Hamburg, Germany

Nikita Wadhwani, MBBS
Resident Physician, General Surgery
University of Alabama at Birmingham
Birmingham, Alabama, United States

David Q.-H. Wang, MD, PhD,[†]
Professor of Medicine, Departments of Medicine and Genetics
Director, Molecular Biology and Next Generation Technology Core
Marion Bessin Liver Research Center
Albert Einstein College of Medicine
Bronx, New York, United States

Sachin Wani, MD
Professor of Medicine, Division of Gastroenterology and Hepatology
Katy O and Paul M Rady Endowed Chair in Esophageal Cancer Research
Executive Director, Katy O and Paul M Rady Esophageal and Gastric Center of Excellence
University of Colorado Anschutz Medical Campus
Aurora, Colorado, United States

Frederick Weber, MD
Clinical Professor, Division of Gastroenterology and Hepatology
University of Alabama Birmingham
Birmingham, Alabama, United States

Barry K. Wershil, MD
Professor, Pediatrics
Northwestern University Feinberg School of Medicine
Chief, Division of Gastroenterology, Hepatology, and Nutrition, Pediatrics
Ann & Robert H. Lurie Children's Hospital of Chicago
Chicago, Illinois, United States

David C. Whitcomb, MD, PhD
Professor, Medicine, Cell Biology and Molecular Physiology, and Human Genetics
University of Pittsburgh and UPMC
Pittsburgh, Pennsylvania, United States

C. Mel Wilcox, MD, MSPH
Chief of Gastroenterology and Hepatology
Director, Pancreatology
Digestive Health Institute
Chair, US Pancreatic Disease Study Group
Orlando Health
Orlando, Florida, United States

Christopher G. Willett, MD
Mark W. Dewhirst Distinguished Professor and Chairman, Radiation Oncology
Duke University
Durham, North Carolina, United States

John A. Windsor, BSc, MD, FRACS, FACS, FRCSEd, FRSNZ
Professor of Surgery and Director of the Surgical and Translational Research Centre
University of Auckland
Honorary Consultant HBP/Upper GI Surgeon
Auckland City Hospital
Auckland, New Zealand

Simin Zhang, MD
Division of Rheumatology, Allergy and Immunology
Department of Internal Medicine
University of Cincinnati College of Medicine
Cincinnati Children's Hospital Medical Center
Cincinnati, Ohio, United States

Irene Y. Zhang, MD, MPH
General Surgery Resident, Department of Surgery
University of Washington
Seattle, Washington, United States

Foreword

We are honored to present the Foreword to the twelfth edition of *Sleisenger and Fordtran's Gastrointestinal and Liver Disease*. For over five decades, this textbook has stood as a foundational reference for clinicians, educators, and researchers in gastroenterology and hepatology. When first published in 1973, by Drs. Marvin H. Sleisenger and John S. Fordtran, the book was heralded for its groundbreaking inclusion of detailed discussions of the pathophysiologic basis of diseases. Each subsequent edition has reflected the dynamic evolution of our field, and this latest volume continues that tradition with a renewed commitment to scientific rigor, clinical relevance, and global inclusivity.

This edition is especially meaningful as we pay tribute to the late Dr. Mark Feldman, whose visionary leadership and editorial excellence helped shape this work into the gold standard it is today. Mark served as an associate editor of the fifth edition and co-editor of the sixth through eleventh editions; sadly, he passed away on March 5, 2024. His contributions to academic medicine and gastroenterology were profound—his scholarship, mentorship, and editorial voice elevated the quality of this text and inspired generations of physicians. A master "tablemaker" with a talent for stylistic clarity and consistency, Mark left an indelible stamp on this book. We are grateful to the editors for allowing the dedication of this edition to his memory and for honoring his enduring legacy.

As we were preparing this Foreword, we also learned of the passing, on February 23, 2025, of the legendary John S. Fordtran, founding co-editor of this textbook and a superb writer, editor, researcher, and educator. As noted in his obituary, John was "more than a brilliant doctor. He was a mentor, a storyteller, a man of integrity, and a rock of quiet strength and humility. He lived a life…marked by kindness and an unshakable love for those around him."*

On a positive note, we are delighted to pass the torch to three outstanding new editors, each of whom served as an associate editor of the eleventh edition. Dr. Raymond T. Chung, a global authority in hepatology, brings deep insight into liver disease and translational research; Dr. David T. Rubin, a pioneer in inflammatory bowel disease and precision medicine, provides a forward-looking perspective on innovation and patient-centered care, and Dr. C. Mel Wilcox, a respected clinician, interventional endoscopist, and educator, contributes a wealth of experience in gastrointestinal disorders and academic leadership. Their collective vision has enriched this edition in both scope and depth, and they have assembled an international array of outstanding authors who are foremost authorities in their fields.

This twelfth edition arrives at a time of remarkable progress in gastroenterology and hepatology. Advances in artificial intelligence and machine learning are transforming diagnostic imaging and endoscopic interpretation. The expansion of multi-omics technologies—genomics, proteomics, and metabolomics—is enabling personalized approaches to complex diseases such as inflammatory bowel disease, colorectal cancer, and metabolic dysfunction-associated steatotic liver disease. Novel biologic agents and small molecules are reshaping therapeutic strategies, while research in intestinal microbiota, gut-brain interactions, and autoimmune mechanisms continues to uncover new pathways of disease pathogenesis and new opportunities for treatment (and new complications of such treatments).

In addition to scientific and clinical advancements, this edition expands coverage of critical issues that shape the practice of medicine today. Areas such as health equity, digital health, palliative care, and the impact of climate change on gastrointestinal health are thoughtfully incorporated, reflecting the broader context in which we care for patients.

This classic textbook remains steadfast in its commitment to the principles that have defined it since its inception: scientific excellence, clinical utility, and educational clarity. We are confident that this edition will continue to serve as a trusted companion for all who seek to understand and improve the care of patients with gastrointestinal and liver diseases.

Lawrence S. Friedman, MD
Newton, MA
Lawrence J. Brandt, MD
Bronx, NY
Former Editors of *Sleisenger and Fordtran's Gastrointestinal and Liver Disease*

*https://obits.dallasnews.com/us/obituaries/dallasmorningnews/name/john-fordtran-obituary?id=57732653, accessed August 15, 2025

The Sleisenger and Fordtran Editors

Mark Feldman, MD

Editions 5-11

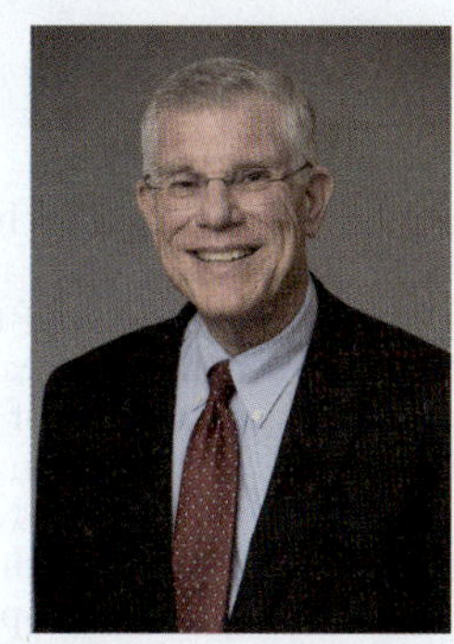

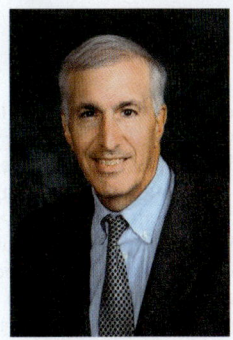

Lawrence S. Friedman, MD

Editions 7-11

Lawrence J. Brandt, MD

Editions 8-11

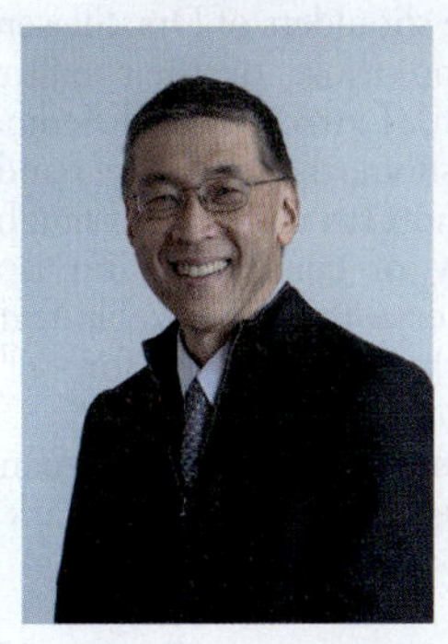

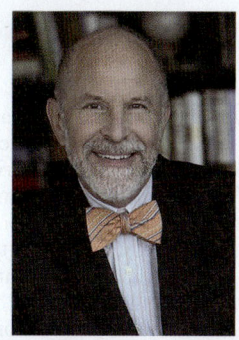

Raymond T. Chung, MD

Editions 11, 12

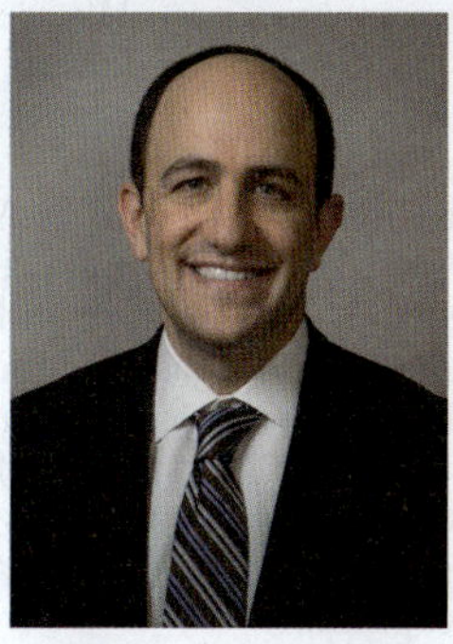

David T. Rubin, MD

Editions 11, 12

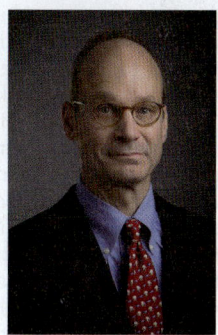

C. Mel Wilcox, MD

Editions 11, 12

Marvin H. Sleisenger, MD

Editions 1-7

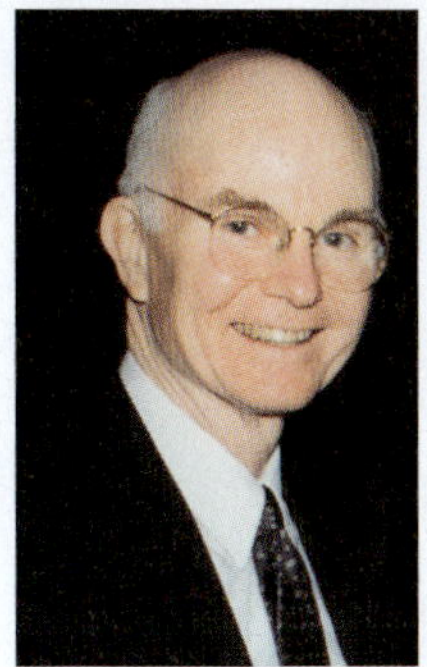

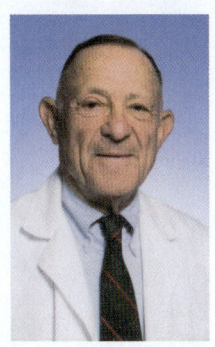

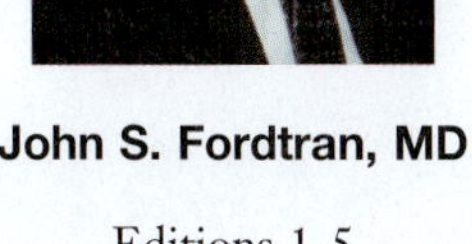

John S. Fordtran, MD

Editions 1-5

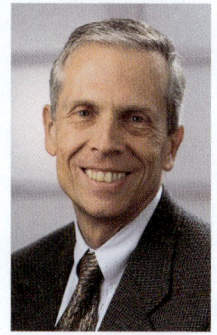

Bruce F. Scharschmidt, MD

Editions 5-6

Preface

Over a half century ago, Drs. Marvin H. Sleisenger and John S. Fordtran embarked on a project to develop a textbook that incorporated pathophysiologic principles underpinning digestive diseases. Their project, the original edition of the textbook that now bears their names, was both novel and extremely well received. Of course, the ultimate testament to the success of their approach has been manifest as international recognition and the publication of ten more editions of this now classic text.

With this, the 12th edition of *Sleisenger & Fordtran's Gastrointestinal and Liver Disease: Pathophysiology/Diagnosis/Management*, we are pleased to honor the approach developed by Drs. Sleisenger and Fordtran by providing updates on the diagnosis and treatment of chronic hepatitis B and C, including curative treatments for HCV; evolution in the management of *Helicobacter pylori* infection and its complications; improvements in techniques for screening and surveillance of gastrointestinal cancer; new approaches to the recognition and treatment of Barrett esophagus; the remarkable expansion and increased incidence and prevalence of IBD across the globe; the development of many advanced therapies, mechanistic targets, and new strategies for the management of IBD; improvements in endoscopic management of pancreaticobiliary disorders and gastrointestinal bleeding; enhanced understanding of the gut microbiome and its role in the pathophysiology of nearly all GI and hepatic disorders (and many non-GI disorders, too!); the rapid pace of our understanding of disorders of gut-brain interaction and their expanding treatment options; recognition of the increasing array of autoimmune diseases affecting the entire GI tract and liver; and continued advances in transplantation of solid organs, including liver, pancreas, and small intestine. In recognition of more recent trends in medicine, we introduce new chapters to describe the GI and hepatic complications of the immune checkpoint inhibitors that have revolutionized cancer therapy; advances in our understanding of the benefits of palliative care applied to GI and hepatology; and, in the aftermath of the COVID-19 pandemic, recognition of the short- and long-term consequences of coronavirus infection. In many of the chapters throughout the text, the possible application of rapid advances in artificial intelligence to the management of GI disorders, particularly in the areas of diagnosis and prognosis, has been introduced. In addition to topical breadth, we have continued the S and F tradition of including diverse authors from around the world, including rising stars in their disciplines.

We are proud to stand on the shoulders of Drs. Sleisenger and Fordtran, and more directly on those of their editorial descendants, Drs. Mark Feldman, Lawrence S. Friedman, and Lawrence J. Brandt. In their wisdom, they mentored and "broke us in" as Associate Editors for the 11th edition and taught us the art of precision writing, clarity of communication, and most importantly stewardship to preserve this remarkable text. As we assume the Editorship of the 12th edition, we are forever grateful for their guidance and trust.

Regretfully, one of those mentors, Dr. Mark Feldman, passed away on March 5, 2024, at the age of 76. We miss Mark greatly. We dedicate the 12th edition to his memory.

Raymond T. Chung
David T. Rubin
C. Mel Wilcox

Acknowledgments

The editors of the 12th edition of *Sleisenger & Fordtran's Gastrointestinal and Liver Disease* express their gratitude to the more than 240 authors from North America, Europe, Asia, and Australia who contributed their deep knowledge and experience to this book. We are indebted to the talented staff at Elsevier, particularly Kevin Travers and Nancy Duffy who assembled the book. Special thanks to Cindy Thoms, who oversaw the highly professional production of the book. We thank our predecessors and mentors Drs. Lawrence Friedman and Lawrence Brandt for their thoughtful Foreword, but more importantly for teaching us the fine art of editing. We remember and fondly acknowledge the mentorship and contributions of our third predecessor, Dr. Mark Feldman, who passed away in 2024. We are thankful for the love and support of our spouses: Rebecca Rubin, and Diane Abraczinskas. Finally, we thank our caregiver and scientist readers who will use this updated edition to improve the care and outcomes of those who suffer from digestive illnesses.

Contents

VOLUME 1

PART XII
Additional Treatments for Patients with Gastrointestinal and Liver Disease

Video Contents

Abbreviation List

AASLD American Association for the Study of Liver Diseases
ACG American College of Gastroenterology
ACTH Corticotropin
AE Angioectasia
AFP Alpha fetoprotein
AGA American Gastroenterological Association
AIDS Acquired immunodeficiency syndrome
ACLF Acute on chronic liver failure
ALD Alcohol-associated liver disease
ALF Acute liver failure
ALT Alanine aminotransferase
AMA Antimitochondrial antibodies
ANA Antinuclear antibodies
ANCA Antineutrophil cytoplasmic antibodies
APACHE Acute physiology and chronic health examination
APC Argon plasma coagulation
ASGE American Society for Gastrointestinal Endoscopy
AST Aspartate aminotransferase
ATP Adenosine triphosphate
BICAP Bipolar electrocoagulation
BMI Body mass index
BRBPR Bright red blood per rectum
CBC Complete blood count
CCK Cholecystokinin
CEA Carcinoembryonic antigen
CDI *Clostridioides difficile* infection
CF Cystic fibrosis
CFTR Cystic fibrosis transmembrane conductance regulator
CMV Cytomegalovirus
CNS Central nervous system
CO_2 Carbon dioxide
COVID-19 Coronavirus disease 2019
COX Cyclooxygenase
CT Computed tomography
CTA Computed tomography angiography
CTP Child-Turcotte-Pugh score
DAA Direct-acting antiviral agent
DIC Disseminated intravascular coagulation
DILI Drug-induced liver injury
DNA Deoxyribonucleic acid
DU Duodenal ulcer
DVT Deep vein thrombosis
EBV Epstein-Barr virus
EGD Esophagogastroduodenoscopy
EGF Epidermal growth factor
EMG Electromyography
ERCP Endoscopic retrograde cholangiopancreatography
ESR Erythrocyte sedimentation rate
EUS Endoscopic ultrasonography
FDA U.S. Food and Drug Administration
FIB-4 Fibrosis-4 index
FNA Fine-needle aspiration
GAVE Gastric antral vascular ectasia
GERD Gastroesophageal reflux disease
GGTP Gamma glutamyl transpeptidase
GI Gastrointestinal
GIST GI stromal tumor
GU Gastric ulcer
H&E Hematoxylin and eosin
H2RA Histamine-2 receptor antagonist
HAV Hepatitis A virus
HBV Hepatitis B virus
HCC Hepatocellular carcinoma
HCG Human chorionic gonadotropin
HCV Hepatitis C virus
HDL High-density lipoprotein
HDV Hepatitis D virus
HELLP Hemolysis, elevated liver enzymes, low platelets
HEV Hepatitis E virus
Hgb Hemoglobin
HHT Hereditary hemorrhagic telangiectasia
HIV Human immunodeficiency virus
HLA Human leukocyte antigen
HPV Human papillomavirus
HSV Herpes simplex virus
Hp *Helicobacter pylori*
IBD Inflammatory bowel disease
IBS Irritable bowel syndrome
ICI Immune checkpoint inhibitor
ICU Intensive care unit
IMA Inferior mesenteric artery
IMT Intestinal microbiota transplantation
INR International normalized ratio
IV Intravenous
IVIG Intravenous immunoglobulin
LDH Lactate dehydrogenase
LDL Low-density lipoprotein
LGI Lower gastrointestinal
LGIB Lower gastrointestinal bleed

LLQ Left lower quadrant
LT Liver transplantation
LUQ Left upper quadrant
MASLD Metabolic dysfunction-associated liver disease
MASH Metabolic dysfunction-associated steatohepatitis
MELD Model for end-stage liver disease
MEN Multiple endocrine neoplasia
MHC Major histocompatibility complex
MRA Magnetic resonance angiography
MRCP Magnetic resonance cholangiopancreatography
MRI Magnetic resonance imaging
NG Nasogastric
NPO Nil per os (nothing by mouth)
NSAID(s) Nonsteroidal anti-inflammatory drug(s)
O_2 Oxygen
PBC Primary biliary cholangitis
PCR Polymerase chain reaction
PET Positron emission tomography
PPI Proton pump inhibitor
PSC Primary sclerosing cholangitis
PSE Portosystemic encephalopathy
PUD Peptic ulcer disease
RA Rheumatoid arthritis
RLQ Right lower quadrant
RNA Ribonucleic acid
RUQ Right upper quadrant
SBO Small bowel obstruction
SBP Spontaneous bacterial peritonitis
SIBO Small intestinal bacterial overgrowth
SLE Systemic lupus erythematosus
SOD Sphincter of Oddi dysfunction
TB Tuberculosis
TG Triglyceride(s)
TIPS Transjugular intrahepatic portosystemic shunt
TNF Tumor necrosis factor
TNM Tumor node metastasis
TPN Total parenteral nutrition
UC Ulcerative colitis
UDCA Ursodeoxycholic acid
UGI Upper gastrointestinal
UGIB Upper gastrointestinal bleed
UGIS Upper gastrointestinal series
UNOS United Network for Organ Sharing
US Ultrasonography
USA United States of America
VLDL Very-low-density lipoprotein
WBC White blood cell
WHO World Health Organization
ZES Zollinger-Ellison syndrome

PART X Liver

73 Embryology, Anatomy, Histology, and Developmental Anomalies of the Liver

Stuti Shroff, Angela R. Shih

IN THIS CHAPTER

EMBRYOLOGY

The liver develops at 3–4 weeks' gestation as an outgrowing diverticulum of proliferating endodermal cells from the ventral wall of the foregut in response to signals from the adjacent developing heart (Fig. 73.1).[1,2] In the fourth week, two buds can be recognized in the hepatic diverticulum: the cranial bud becomes the liver and the hilar biliary tract, whereas the caudal bud develops into a superior bud that forms the gallbladder and cystic duct, and an inferior bud that forms the ventral pancreas.[3,4] Initially, the liver bud is separated from the mesenchyme of the septum transversum by the basement membrane.[1] However, this basement membrane is quickly lost, and; E-cadherin expression is downregulated. Cells delaminate from the bud and invade the septum transversum as cords of bipotential hepatoblasts that differentiate into hepatocytes and cholangiocytes.[2,5,6] As they invade the septum transversum mesenchyme, hepatoblasts intermingle with endothelial cells, an interaction that appears critical for hepatic morphogenesis.[1]

Hepatic differentiation is highly dependent on signals from the cardiogenic mesoderm and septum transversum mesenchyme, which produces fibroblast growth factor and bone morphogenetic protein.[2,5] The control of hepatocytic differentiation is complex and involves several transcription factors at various stages of development. For example, GATA4 and forkhead box A (FoxA) are involved in developmental "competence" because they have the ability to interact with compacted chromatin and act as "pioneer" factors that can mark domains of chromatin as competent to be expressed in response to later developmental cues.[6,7] Prospero homeobox protein 1 (Prox1) may be involved in downregulation of E-cadherin, because mutant hepatoblasts maintain high levels of E-cadherin and fail to degrade the matrix surrounding the liver bud.[6] Terminal differentiation of hepatocytes requires the overlapping interaction of a group of transcription factors including hepatocyte nuclear factor (HNF)1β, FoxA2, HNF1α, HNF4α1, HNF6, and liver receptor homolog (LRH)-1.[6,7] These cross-regulating factors form a dynamic transcriptional network by binding to each other's promoters and to the promoters of other hepatic transcription factors, creating synergistic interdependence as hepatocyte maturation proceeds.[7] The contribution of Wnt signaling and β-catenin is complex and stage-dependent. During early development, canonical Wnt/β-catenin signaling represses hematopoietically-expressed homeobox (Hhex), another early transcription factor in hepatic development; therefore early in the process, Wnt must be suppressed in the anterior endoderm to facilitate commitment of the endoderm to a hepatic fate. After specification, Wnt signaling promotes hepatogenesis.[6,8]

By most accounts, the extrahepatic biliary system develops originally as a solid structure that becomes canalized at the end of the 5th week.[3] However, it may develop *ab initio* as a hollow structure, refuting the concept that biliary atresia results from a failure of the bile duct to canalize.[9] Extrahepatic biliary tract development may require the expression of sex determining region Y-box 17 (SOX17), which is regulated by the homolog of hairy/enhancer-of-split (Hes1).[6] Another transcription factor involved in extrahepatic biliary development is Hhex; in Hhex-null embryos, the bile duct is replaced by tissue resembling duodenum.[6] Either the extrahepatic and intrahepatic biliary systems merge at the hepatic hilum or they maintain luminal continuity from the start.[9]

Intrahepatic biliary development begins at 6 weeks when a subset of hepatoblasts close to the portal mesenchyme strongly express biliary-specific antigens (see Chapter 64).[10] These biliary precursor cells form a continuous single-layered ring around the portal mesenchyme, called the ductal plate. This plate becomes partly bilayered in the next step with the cells closest to the portal mesenchyme maintaining a biliary phenotype and those closest to the parenchyma resembling hepatoblasts, a process known as transient asymmetry.[11,12] A period of remodeling follows in which focal dilatations appear between the two cell layers and eventually form lumens. The parts of the ductal plate not involved in the formation of ducts regress by apoptosis, and around the time of birth, the remaining ducts are incorporated into the portal mesenchyme.[10] Incorporation and elongation of ducts begins in the hilum and extends to the periphery of the liver.[11,12] At birth, the most peripheral small portal tracts require an additional 4 weeks before the ductal plates develop into bile ducts.[9] Similarly, bile canaliculi develop their fully mature appearance during the perinatal and early postnatal period, even though the major bile transporters are expressed at the midgestational age.[9]

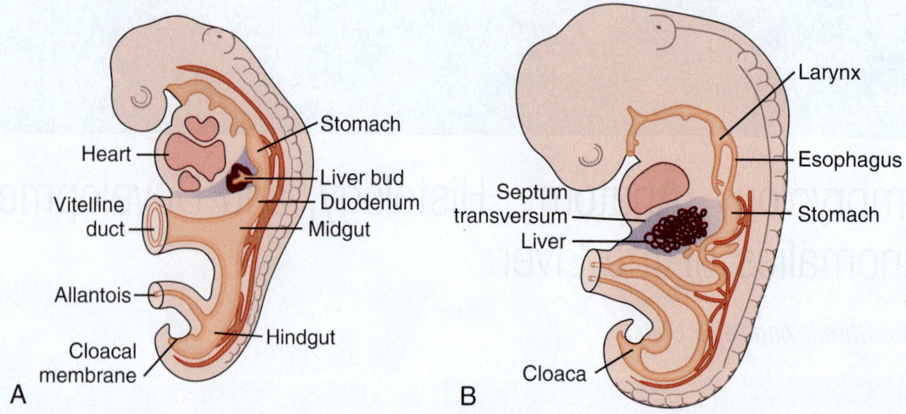

Fig. 73.1 Embryology of the liver. (A) At the 3-mm embryo stage, the liver bud forms in response to signals from the developing heart. (B) At the 5-mm stage, the hepatoblasts penetrate the septum transversum.

The switch in phenotype of hepatoblasts to cholangiocytes requires the coordinated activity of various signaling systems and transcription factors. The earliest sign of biliary differentiation is expression of SOX9, a transcription factor that regulates the timing of biliary duct development.[6] The Wnt/β-catenin signaling system may also play a temporal role in the commitment of hepatoblasts to biliary epithelial cells.[8] HNF6 and HNF1β also regulate biliary differentiation; mice deficient in these factors show cystic dysgenesis of the biliary tract and abnormalities in the hepatic arterial branches.[11] The developing ducts produce vascular endothelial growth factor (VEGF), which cooperates with angiopoietin-1 produced by hepatoblasts to promote arterial vasculogenesis and to recruit mural pericytes to the developing arteries.[11] The maintenance of duct structure during the elongation phase requires that mitoses be aligned uniformly along the axis of the duct, a process called planar cell polarity, which is controlled by noncanonical Wnt signaling and is defective in fibropolycystic liver disease.[11]

Two signaling systems have emerged as critical to biliary differentiation and restriction of biliary differentiation to a periportal location. Transforming growth factor-β (TGF-β) generated by portal mesenchyme stimulates hepatoblasts to switch to a biliary phenotype, and TGF-β signaling is greater near the portal vein and less in the parenchyma.[11,12] The Notch pathway is also involved in bile duct development; Jagged-1 expressed in portal vein mesenchyme interacts with Notch2 on hepatoblasts to induce biliary differentiation at the expense of hepatocyte differentiation.[11–13] Notch signaling is also instrumental in biliary tubulogenesis. In its absence, formation of the ducts beyond the monolayer ductal plate is impaired.[6,8] Mutations in the gene that codes for Jagged-1 are associated with Alagille syndrome (see Chapter 64).

Mesothelial cells and submesothelial cells derived from the septum transversum migrate inward from the liver surface and give rise to stellate cells, portal fibroblasts, and perivascular mesenchymal cells.[14,15] Kupffer cells, the tissue-resident macrophages of the liver, arise from yolk sac-derived erythromyeloid precursors rather than from hematopoietic stem cells (HSCs) in the bone marrow.[16] In mice embryos, erythromyeloid precursors develop in the yolk sac, migrate and colonize the fetal liver, and give rise to fetal erythrocytes, macrophages, granulocytes, and monocytes. Seeding of the liver by monocyte precursors appears to be regulated by sinusoidal endothelial cells.[17] Subsequently, HSC-derived cells replace erythrocytes, granulocytes, and monocytes, but Kupffer cells are only minimally replaced in adult mice. Similarly, the fetal liver is the major site of hematopoiesis in humans before the bone marrow matures.

Hepatic Stem Cells and Maturational Lineages

The existence of hepatic stem cells in the mature liver has been debated, with various cell populations proposed to serve this function. The broader consensus is that the mature liver contains a population of hepatic stem cells that are not equivalent to embryonic stem cells (hepatoblasts) but are similar in that they are self-renewing, proliferative, and bipotential (i.e., capable of generating hepatocytes and cholangiocytes).[18–20]

These stem cells express epithelial cell adhesion molecule, neural cell adhesion molecule, and cytokeratin 19 and weakly express albumin, but not alpha fetoprotein.[18,19] They likely also express the Wnt target gene leucine-rich-repeat-containing G-protein-coupled receptor 5.[21] These stem cells are found in the canals of Hering and generate hepatocytes and cholangiocytes in response to liver injury.[18,19] They decline in number with advancing age.[19] When grown in culture, they produce cords of hepatoblast-like cells that more strongly express albumin; express epithelial cell adhesion molecule, alpha fetoprotein, and intracellular adhesion molecular 1; have reduced cytokeratin 19 expression; and lose neural cell adhesion molecule.[18] In contrast, committed progenitor cells are diploid, unipotent, immature cells that give rise to only one adult cell type. They are either intermediate hepatocytes that express albumin and hepatic enzymes, or small cholangiocytes (oval cells) that line canals of Hering, intrahepatic bile ducts, and bile ductules.[19,20] Diploid adult cells can undergo 6 or 7 rounds of division before reaching subcultivation capacity.[19]

Vascular Development

During early development, there are three major venous systems in the embryo: 2 extraembryonic and 1 intraembryonic. The extraembryonic venous systems are the omphalomesenteric (vitelline) and umbilical (placental) veins, and the intraembryonic system includes the cardinal veins that drain the venous blood of the embryo to the heart.[22] These systems converge into the sinus venosus, a quadrangular cavity that is incorporated into the heart; the vitelline and umbilical veins drain into the sinus venosus via hepatocardiac channels.

The developing liver eventually incorporates the vitelline and umbilical veins, which become enclosed by dividing hepatoblasts and develop asymmetrically.[23] At this time, sinusoids enter from the sinus venosus to form a sinusoidal network. The right umbilical vein regresses, whereas the left umbilical vein forms 2 left-right shunts, 1 with the right vitelline vein (the portal sinus) and 1 with the right hepatocardiac channel (the venous duct).[23] These shunts direct placenta-derived arterial blood from the umbilical vein to the inferior vena cava, bypassing the liver.[22] After formation of these shunts, portal vein branches develop from the intrahepatic portions of the vitelline and umbilical veins. The portal sinus and parts of the left umbilical vein give rise to the left portal vein, whereas the right vitelline vein gives rise to the right portal vein.[23] After birth, the obliterated prehepatic segment of the left umbilical vein becomes the round ligament of the liver (ligamentum teres hepatis) in the free edge of the falciform ligament, and the ductus venosus collapses to become the ligamentum venosum.[22]

The arterial supply of the liver begins as an offshoot of the celiac trunk at around the eighth week of gestation. By the 10th week, the first arterial radicles are visible in the central portion of the liver, and by the 15th week, they reach the periphery of the liver.[22] As discussed earlier, development of the arterial supply is closely coordinated with bile duct development. The processes of vasculogenesis and vascular remodeling are dependent on stage-specific expression of angiogenic growth factors VEGF and angiopoietin-1 (by ductal plate cells and hepatoblasts, respectively), and by their receptors (on developing endothelial and perivascular smooth muscle cells).[24]

Sinusoidal endothelial cells are derived in part from a common endothelial/blood cell progenitor called "hemangioblasts," initially located in the vitelline and umbilical veins, and in part from the endocardium of the sinus venosus.[25] Endothelial cell maturation occurs between the 5th and 12th week of gestation. During that time, sinusoidal endothelial cells between the hepatocyte plates acquire fenestrae, lose expression of typical endothelial markers CD34 and CD31, and become invested by a perisinusoidal matrix rich in tenascin and poor in laminins.[22] These alterations may be necessary to adapt the liver to its hematopoietic function during fetal life.[22]

ANATOMY

Peritoneum covers the liver except for the bare area, where the liver comes in direct contact with the diaphragm and is suspended by fibrous tissue and the hepatic veins.[26] The peritoneal reflections that surround the bare area comprise the superior and inferior coronary ligaments and the right and left triangular ligaments, which attach the liver to the diaphragm; these avascular attachments are not true ligaments but are in continuity with Glisson's capsule.[27]

Traditionally, four lobes are distinguished in the liver based on its external appearance: right, left, caudate, and quadrate. On the anterior surface, the falciform ligament divides the liver into the right and left anatomic lobes. On the inferior surface, the quadrate lobe is defined by the gallbladder fossa, porta hepatis, and ligamentum teres hepatis. The caudate lobe is delineated by the inferior vena cava groove, porta hepatis, and ligamentum venosum fissure.[28] Although these lobes are convenient and well known, they are not true functional lobes.[27]

The true right and left lobes of the liver are of roughly equal size and are divided not by the falciform ligament, but rather by a plane passing through the bed of the gallbladder and the notch of the inferior vena cava. This plane, which has no external indications, is called the Cantlie line.[26,28] Based on arterial blood supply, portal venous blood supply, biliary drainage, and hepatic venous drainage, the liver is divided into right and left functional lobes, each of which is divided into two segments, and these are further subdivided into two subsegments.[26] Several systems of subdivision have been proposed, but the most widely used systems are those of Couinaud, which follows the distribution of portal and hepatic veins, and Healey and Schroy, which follows the distribution of bile ducts.[29] In these systems, the subsegments are numbered from 1 to 8, with the caudate lobe being subsegment 1 and the others following in a clockwise pattern (Fig. 73.2).[28]

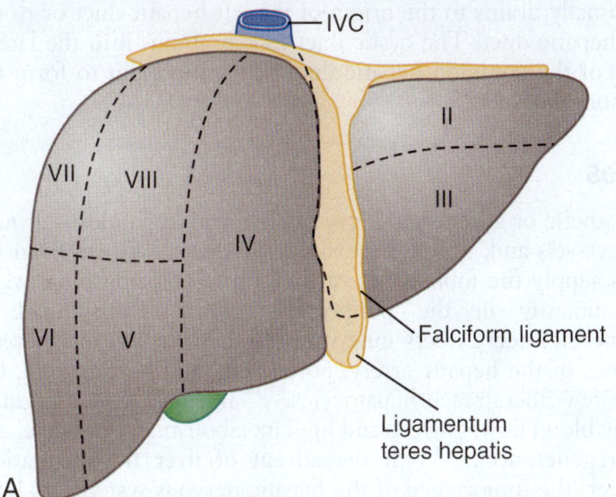

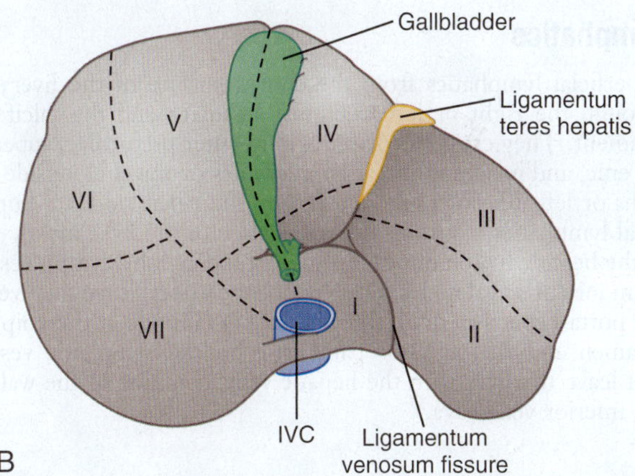

Fig. 73.2 Segmental anatomy of the liver based on the Couinaud terminology. The 8 segments are identified: (A) anterior view and (B) inferior view. *IVC*, Inferior vena cava.

The liver receives approximately 70% of its blood supply and 40% of its oxygen from the portal vein, and 30% of its blood supply and 60% of its oxygen from the hepatic artery.[29] The portal vein is formed from the confluence of the superior mesenteric vein and the splenic vein. At the hilum, the portal vein divides into right and left branches, upon which the right and left lobes of the liver are based.[27,30] Although Couinaud's scheme holds that the right and left portal veins branch to supply eight venous territories, there is a wide variation in the number of second-order branches of the right and left portal veins.[31] The hepatic artery commonly arises from the celiac trunk, although occasionally it arises from the superior mesenteric artery.[30] A common variant is a left hepatic artery that branches from the left gastric artery and a right hepatic artery branch that arises from the superior mesenteric artery.[30] Within the hilum, the hepatic artery lies anterior to the portal vein and to the left of the bile duct. In the liver, arteries, portal veins, and bile ducts are surrounded by a fibrous sheath called the Glissonian sheath, whereas hepatic veins lack this structure.[26] Three major hepatic veins (right, middle, and left) drain into the inferior vena cava, although in 60%–85% of persons, the left and middle veins unite to enter the inferior vena cava as a single vein.[26,27,30]

The extrahepatic biliary tract is composed of the common hepatic duct, cystic duct, gallbladder, and right and left hepatic ducts. The right and left hepatic ducts drain the right and left lobes of the liver, respectively. The fusion of the right and left hepatic ducts gives rise to the common hepatic duct. The caudate lobe usually drains to the origin of the left hepatic duct or to the right hepatic duct. The cystic duct usually drains into the lateral aspect of the common hepatic duct below its origin to form the common bile duct.[32]

Nerves

Sympathetic or adrenergic nerve fibers form a rich plexus around blood vessels and, to a lesser extent, bile ducts.[33] Fibers from the plexus supply the lobules where they run along sinusoidal walls, predominantly in the periportal region.[33] Parasympathetic (cholinergic) nerve fibers innervate extrahepatic and intrahepatic branches of the hepatic artery, portal vein, and hepatic vein, but only a few fibers reach hepatocytes.[33,34] Intrinsic nerves regulate hepatic blood flow, glucose and lipid metabolism, food intake, and liver regeneration.[35] With the advent of liver transplantation, however, the importance of the hepatic nervous system has been questioned, given the adequate functioning of the denervated allograft.[34,36]

Lymphatics

Superficial lymphatics from the convex surface of the liver run through the right or left triangular ligament and the falciform ligament. They cross the diaphragm to enter precardiac, superior phrenic, and juxtaesophageal lymph nodes or travel alongside the right or left inferior phrenic artery to the celiac nodes.[37] Superficial lymphatics from the visceral surface of the liver mostly run to the hepatic lymph nodes. From the caudate lobe, lymph vessels drain into precaval nodes. Deep lymphatic vessels leave the liver at the porta hepatis to drain into the foraminal node at the epiploic foramen and the superior pancreatic nodes. Lymphatic vessels that leave the liver with the hepatic veins continue in the wall of the inferior vena cava.[37]

HISTOLOGY

The liver is a muralium consisting of anastomosing sheets of hepatocytes arranged in thin trabecular plates, separated by a thin sinusoidal plexus. Trabecular plates are typically 1–2 hepatocytes in thickness, recognized as large polygonal cells with eosinophilic cytoplasm, round nuclei of varying sizes, and frequent binucleation (Fig. 73.3). Portal tracts are fibrous structures within the parenchyma that contain branches of the hepatic arteriole, portal vein, and bile duct bundled together as the portal triad (Fig. 73.4). Accompanying small nerves and lymphatic vessels are also present within portal tracts. The basolateral aspect of the hepatocytes faces the sinusoids, which are the vascular spaces between trabecular plates.

Hepatic vascular inflow occurs via the terminal hepatic arterioles and terminal portal venules in portal tracts, which supply blood to the sinusoids. Terminal hepatic arterioles are invested by smooth muscle and are capable of forming presinusoidal sphincters.[36] In contrast, the terminal portal venules do not possess a muscle layer and so have no inlet sphincters at their junction with sinusoids; however, large endothelial cells at that junction bulge their nuclei into the lumen and, by means of contraction, control blood flow into the sinusoids.[36] The sinusoids contain an admixture of arterial and portal blood, and drain to the terminal hepatic venules (also known as central veins), where a similar endothelial-driven sphincter-like activity occurs at the site where the sinusoid connects with the terminal hepatic venule.[36] These terminal hepatic venules drain into sublobular veins, subsequently into hepatic veins, and eventually into the inferior vena cava.

Sinusoidal endothelial cells are specialized endothelial cells that form the barrier between blood and hepatocytes. They are fenestrated and lack a basement membrane, constituting a relatively "leaky" barrier.[25] The size of fenestrae varies across the lobule (with larger fenestrae toward the centrilobular region) and changes dynamically with physiological states. In response to injury, sinusoidal endothelial cells lose their fenestrae and acquire a basement membrane (i.e., "capillarized"). The resulting increase in shear stress activates the transcription factor Kruppel-like factor 2, leading to release of the vasoconstrictive agent endothelin-1.[25] Decreased permeability and increased vasoconstriction lead to increased sinusoidal pressure and contribute to development of portal hypertension (see Chapter 94).

Sinusoidal vascular tone is regulated by endothelial cells via paracrine regulation of stellate cell contractility.[25] Hepatic stellate cells, formerly known as "Ito cells" or perisinusoidal fat-storing cells, are perisinusoidal cells that, in their quiescent state, are the main site of vitamin A storage.[36] They encircle the sinusoidal wall and participate in regulating the width of the lumen. When

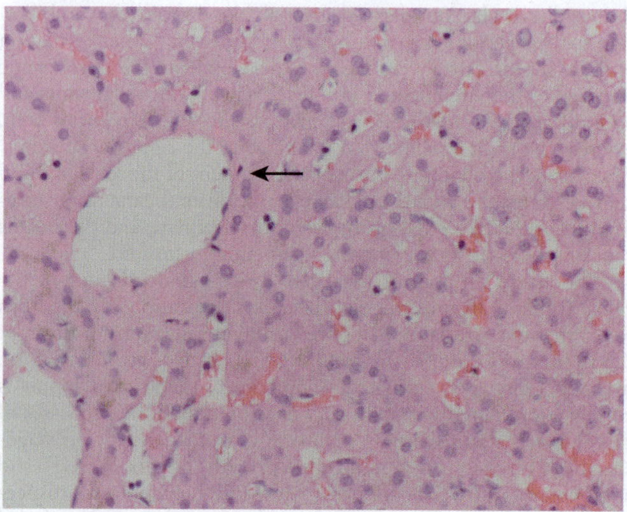

Fig. 73.3 Histology of normal liver parenchyma. Normal liver parenchyma consists of thin trabecular hepatocellular plates approximately 1–2 cells in thickness with interspersed sinusoidal spaces (*center right*); the central vein is also present (*arrow*). Other perisinusoidal cell types are not typically readily identified on routine stains (hematoxylin and eosin, ×400).

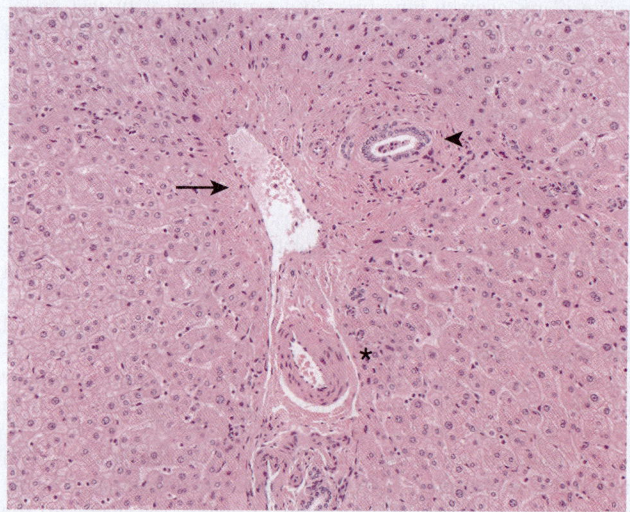

Fig. 73.4 Histology of normal portal tract. Normal portal tracts contain a portal vein (*arrow, left*), small arteriole (*asterisk, bottom*), and native bile duct (*arrowhead, right*) (hematoxylin and eosin, ×200).

hepatic stellate cells are activated in the setting of liver inflammation and injury, they transform into myofibroblasts that express desmin and smooth muscle actin and synthesize extracellular matrix.[38] Activated hepatic stellate cells are the main effectors of liver fibrosis in chronic liver diseases.

A perisinusoidal space, the space of Disse, remains between the sinusoidal lining and the vascular pole of hepatocytes and communicates with the sinusoidal space through multiple fenestrations.[35] This space contains plasma and collagen types I, III, IV, and V, which act as the scaffolding of the organ.[35] The space of Mall is a space between the periportal hepatocytes and portal connective tissue. Lymphatic fluid accumulates in the space of Disse and then passes into the space of Mall before draining into lymphatic vessels.[38,39] Lymphatic vessels form a network in the portal spaces in association with branches of the hepatic artery.[35]

Also lining the sinusoids are Kupffer cells, which are the resident macrophages of the liver and are more numerous, larger, and more phagocytically active in the periportal region.[38] Their major role is clearance of senescent red blood cells and toxic substances (both endogenous and exogenous).[40] Kupffer cells also handle low-density lipoprotein and produce lymphokine mediators that direct hepatocyte protein synthesis, inflammatory mediators, and hepatocyte-protective prostaglandins.[36]

Whereas the basolateral aspect of hepatocytes faces the sinusoid, the apical aspect faces the bile canaliculus. Canaliculi direct bile to the terminal canals of Hering, which are lined partly by hepatocytes and partly by cholangiocytes.[41] The canals of Hering do not stop at the limiting plate of the portal tract but extend into the periportal region of the lobule. The canals of Hering pass into bile ductules, which are lined entirely by cholangiocytes.[41] The ductules in turn connect to the smallest interlobular bile ducts, which lead to septal bile ducts and hepatic bile ducts. Histologically, the smaller ducts are lined by cuboidal cells, whereas the larger ducts are lined by columnar epithelial cells.

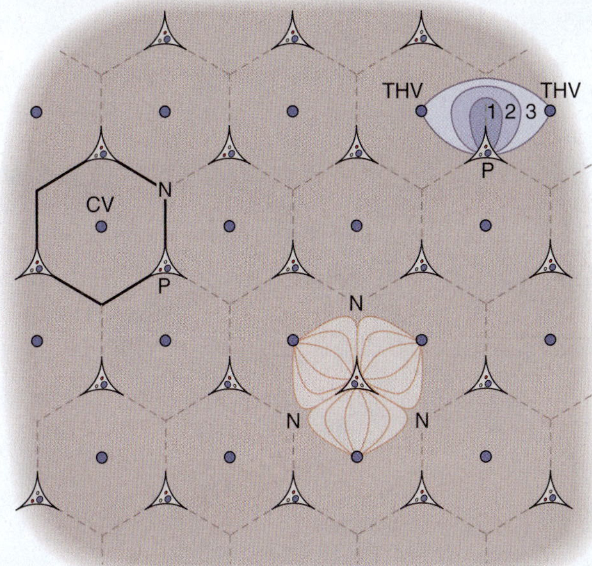

Fig. 73.5 Schematic drawing of liver architecture. At the left is the classic hepatic lobule, with the central vein as its center and portal tracts at 3 corners. Near the middle is the portal unit, with the portal tract at its center and central veins and nodal points at its periphery. At the right is the liver acinus, the center of which is the terminal afferent vessel (in the portal tract) and the periphery of which is drained by the terminal hepatic venule, or central vein. Zones 1, 2, and 3 extending from the portal tract to the terminal hepatic venule are shown. *CV*, Central vein; *N*, nodal point; *THV*, terminal hepatic venule; *P*, portal tract.

Organization of Liver Parenchyma

The physiologic microscopic subunit of the liver parenchyma can be described as either the classic lobule or the liver acinus. The classic lobule of the liver was described in 1833 by Kiernan as a hexagon with a central vein at its center and portal tracts at its vertices and is considered an anatomical construct. Alternatively, the liver acinus was defined in 1954 by Rappaport as the parenchyma around terminal afferent portal and arterial vessels; with a portal tract at its center, the terminal hepatic venules (central veins) are present at the periphery, which follows vascular flow and metabolic physiologic function.[36] In this model of the liver acinus, the parenchyma can be divided into three zones based on oxygenation status: (1) the periportal zone (zone 1), which is supplied by blood with high oxygen content; (2) the intermediate zone (zone 2); and (3) the perivenular zone (zone 3), which receives blood that is relatively low in oxygen content.[36] The acinus represents a functional and structural unit that facilitates the description of lesions such as bridging necrosis and fibrosis (Fig. 73.5).[38]

In 1982, Matsumoto and Kawakami presented a view of liver architecture based on its angioarchitecture.[42] In this concept, the portal and hepatic venous systems are divided into a conducting portion (delivering blood to and draining blood from the parenchyma) and a parenchymal portion, together forming the basis for the primary lobule. The parenchymal portion of the portal and hepatic venous systems consists of minute side branches that originate as orderly rows along the terminal branches of the conducting portion. The portal venous branches divide several times more often than the hepatic venous branches, thereby creating a larger number of portal venous channels for each hepatic venous channel. The terminal divisions of the portal venous system are known as septal branches. The conical cluster of hepatocytes fed by a septal branch and drained by a hepatic vein branch forms a "primary lobule." As 6–8 draining venules combine to form the central vein, several primary lobules together form a classic lobule.

Matsumoto and Kawakami also noted that the sinusoids that arise from the septal branches have a transverse course near the portal tract before turning radially to the central vein, and this bed of transverse sinusoids forms a sickle-shaped "inflow front" for perfusion of the lobule that differs from the linear supply proposed by the acinus model (Fig. 73.6).[42] The convex aspect of the sickle abuts a portal tract, its arms extend along septal branches, and the concave aspect faces the central vein. This arrangement defines two zones: the peripheral part of the classic lobule composed of adjoining sickle-shaped areas and the centrilobular portion bound by these sickle-shaped areas. Immunohistochemical studies of hepatic enzymes highlight the presence of a continuous periportal network around portal tracts and terminal afferent vessels and a distinct concentric perivenous area around the central vein, supporting the idea that liver architecture resembles the classic lobule more than the acinus.[43]

The zonal arrangement of the lobule gives rise to functional heterogeneity of hepatocytes in the lobule, or "metabolic zonation"; that is, hepatocytes in different zones are specialized for different metabolic programs.[44–47] Zonation has been demonstrated for the metabolism of carbohydrates, lipids, amino acids, ammonia, and xenobiotic compounds. For example, gluconeogenesis occurs largely in the periportal region (zone 1), whereas glycolysis occurs predominantly in the centrilobular region (zone 3); similarly, centrilobular regions appear to have a higher degree of cytochrome P450 activity.[45] As such, zonation is likely a more complicated process than traditionally envisioned, with nonmonotonic distribution of some enzymes and complex regulatory mechanisms.[48] A possible key factor in regulatory mechanisms is

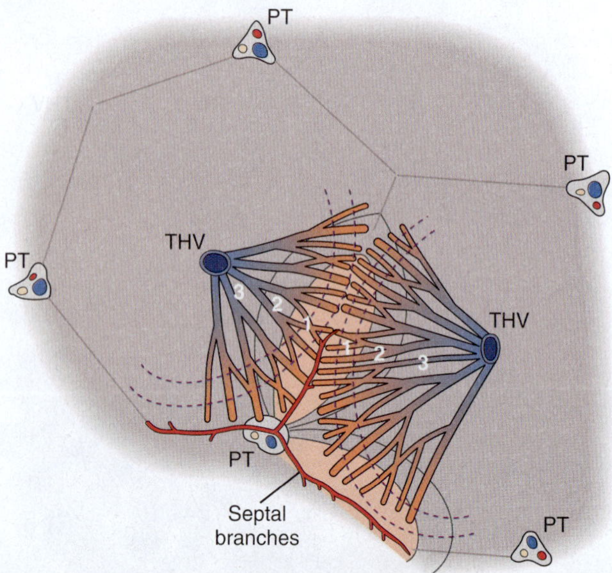

Fig. 73.6 Drawing that compares liver blood flow in the 3 zones of the acinus model with Matsumoto's concept of liver architecture. According to the model by Matsumoto, sinusoids that abut portal tracts and terminal afferent vessels (septal branches) form a hemodynamically equipotential sickle-shaped perfusion front (*dotted lines*). This model conforms to the concept of the classic lobule rather than to the acinus. Zones 1, 2, and 3 of the hepatic acinus are labeled. *PT*, Portal tract; *THV*, terminal hepatic venule.

the oxygen gradient across the lobule, which may lead to differential expression of genes involved in metabolic pathways via oxygen-responsive transcription factors known as hypoxia-inducible factors.[49] The Wnt/β-catenin and Hedgehog signaling pathways also play important roles and exhibit substantial cross-talk with hypoxia-inducible factors.[49,50] The concept of metabolic zonation is important because its dysregulation likely underlies the zonal distribution of some liver diseases in humans, such as metabolic associated steatohepatitis (formerly known as nonalcoholic steatohepatitis), which canonically preferentially affects the centrilobular region.[51]

DEVELOPMENTAL ANOMALIES

Riedel Lobe

Riedel lobe is anatomical variation denoted by a right liver lobe with a prominent anterior edge that extends below the level of the umbilicus. It occurs more often in women than in men and may be mistaken for an abdominal mass. Liver biochemical test levels are normal, and the diagnosis is established by ultrasound.[52] Most patients remain asymptomatic, although in rare cases, extrinsic compression or torsion may occur.[53] The exact etiology remains unclear.

Abernethy Malformation

The Abernethy malformation is a rare vascular anomaly involving a congenital extrahepatic portocaval shunt, of which two types are known to occur. In a type 1 malformation, portal blood is diverted directly into the inferior vena cava, with absence of the portal vein. In a type 2 malformation, an intact portal vein is present but demonstrates a side-to-side anastomosis with the inferior vena cava, leading to shunting.

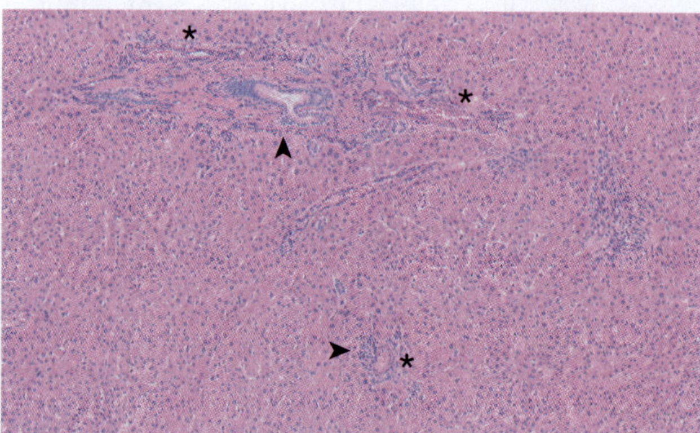

Fig. 73.7 Histology of Abernethy malformation. Abernethy malformations are characterized by the absence of a portal venule within a portal tract. The portal tracts show only a native bile duct (*arrowhead*) and small hepatic arteriole (*asterisk*) (hematoxylin and eosin, ×200).

Type 1 Abernethy malformations occur more often in girls than in boys; are associated with other congenital abnormalities such as cardiac defects, biliary atresia, and polysplenia; may manifest with hypergalactosemia, hyperbilirubinemia, hyperammonemia, or variceal bleeding; and may be complicated by the formation of hepatic tumors.[54] Type 1 Abernethy malformation can be further divided into subtype 1a, in which the superior mesenteric vein and the splenic vein drain separately into a systemic vein; and subtype 1b, in which the superior mesenteric vein and splenic vein form a common trunk that drains into a systemic vein.[54,55] In contrast, a type 2 shunt occurs in both girls and boys and is not associated with other malformations.[54,56] The type of shunt is important in determining treatment.

Patients have variable clinical presentations ranging from asymptomatic to acute decompensation or cirrhosis. Early recognition of a portosystemic shunt is important due to the risk of hepatic neoplasms, including benign focal nodular hyperplasia, hepatocellular adenoma, and regenerative nodules (see Chapter 98).[54] In addition to the presence of associated hepatic neoplasms or markedly regenerative changes in the parenchyma, histology of Abernethy malformations classically shows absence of portal venules within portal tracts (Fig. 73.7).

Biliary Atresia

Biliary atresia is a fibrosing obstructive pediatric cholangiopathy that affects both the extrahepatic and intrahepatic bile ducts and leads to fibrosis, portal hypertension, and liver failure that often necessitates transplantation (see Chapter 64).[57] It is the most common cause of neonatal jaundice. Although there are many possible etiologies for biliary atresia, including viral infections and environmental agents, a subset of biliary atresia cases is related to genetic alterations. Syndromic forms are less frequent and have been linked to PKD1L1 mutations[58] as well as other extrahepatic developmental anomalies, including splenic malformation (referred to as BASM syndrome). Nonsyndromic forms have been linked to common variants in ciliary genes such PCNT, KIF3B, and TC17, as well as a small number of other genes.[59–62]

Histologic findings simulate those of a large duct obstructive cholangiopathy, showing portal expansion, portal edema, and a prominent bile ductular proliferation at the periphery of the portal tracts. Ductular cholestasis is often present as well (Fig. 73.8). Additionally, primitive ductal structures and ductal plate malformations may also be seen, likely as a remnant of failure in the remodeling process of ductal plates during

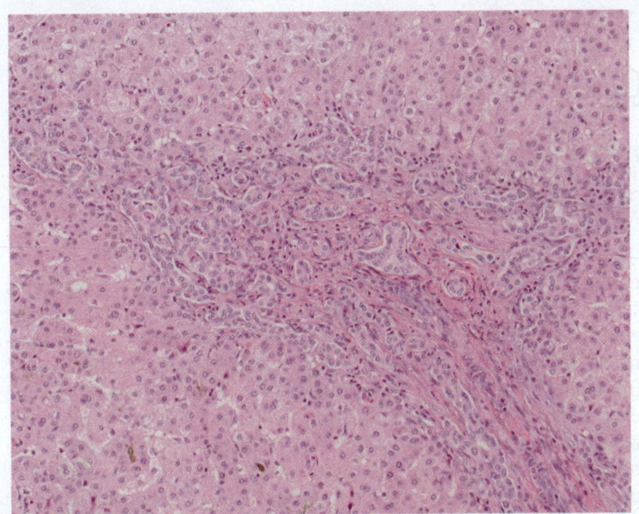

Fig. 73.8 Histology of biliary atresia. Biliary atresia is characterized by a prominent ductular reaction at the periphery of the portal tract. Background liver parenchyma shows canalicular cholestasis (hematoxylin and eosin, ×200.)

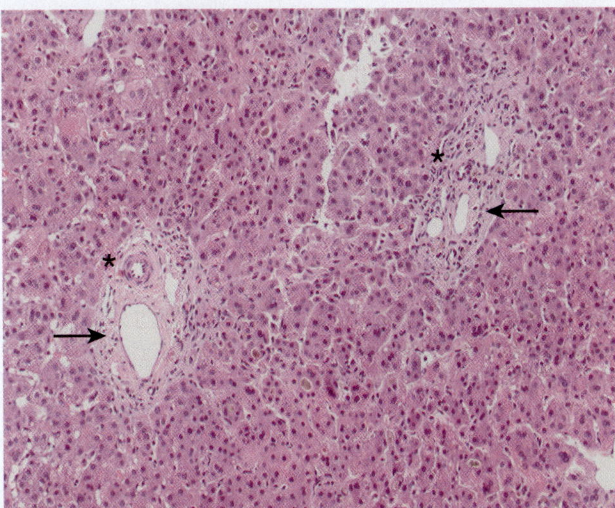

Fig. 73.9 Histology of Alagille syndrome. Alagille syndrome is characterized by native bile duct loss within portal tracts. Both portal tracts contain a small portal venule (*arrow*) and small hepatic arteriole (*asterisk*), with absence of a native bile duct. There is no accompanying ductular reaction. The background liver parenchyma shows canalicular cholestasis (hematoxylin and eosin, ×200).

embryogenesis.[63,64] The fibrotic disease progresses with age from extrahepatic biliary fibrous obliteration to destructive injury of smaller intrahepatic ducts. As such, very early biopsies may show nonspecific findings, but classic histologic findings are typically present by 30 days of age.[63] Secondary lobular features may also be present, including multinucleated giant cell transformation of hepatocytes, extramedullary hematopoiesis, mixed inflammatory infiltrate, and mild lobular architectural disarray with cholestatic injury. Without treatment, patients quickly progress to cirrhosis.

Alagille Syndrome

Alagille syndrome is a rare autosomal dominant disorder with multisystemic manifestations (see Chapter 64). In the liver, it is characterized by abnormal development of intrahepatic bile ducts, resulting in chronic cholestasis that often presents as jaundice in the neonatal period.[65] The syndrome is associated with disruptions in the Notch signaling pathway, most commonly mutations or deletions in JAGGED1 (approximately 90% of cases) and NOTCH2 (smaller minority of cases).[66,67] However, reduced penetrance and variable expression results in a very broad range of clinical features. As Notch signaling is known to be important in a number of cell types during developmental stages, many patients have additional extrahepatic features, including pulmonary artery stenosis, vertebral segmentation anomalies, characteristic facies, and dysplastic kidneys.[68] In the absence of other clinical manifestations, the finding of bile duct loss may be best termed nonsyndromic bile duct paucity, which is associated with a wide range of genetic, infectious, and inflammatory disorders and exposures.[69]

On histology, the vast majority of reported cases show a paucity of bile ducts with associated cholestasis (Fig. 73.9).[70,71] In the newborn, a ductular reaction can occasionally be seen, which may cause confusion with biliary atresia. The process often presents in the neonatal period or first 3 months of life, and appears to be progressive with age, leading to cirrhosis and liver failure in approximately 15% of cases. Interestingly, a small proportion of patients have no manifestation of liver disease.[68,72]

Full references for this chapter can be found at https://ebooks.health.elsevier.com.

74 Liver Physiology and Energy Metabolism

Namita Roy-Chowdhury, Jayanta Roy-Chowdhury

IN THIS CHAPTER

Hepatic parenchymal cells (hepatocytes and cholangiocytes) and nonparenchymal cells [liver sinusoidal endothelial cells (LSECs), stellate cells, Kupffer cells, and pit cells] have distinct functions that are integrated through extensive crosstalk and a specialized extracellular matrix. Liver parenchymal cells are polarized. The distinctive polarization pattern of hepatocytes is unique among glandular epithelial cells and is essential for the wide variety of functions served by the liver. Hepatocyte polarization is maintained by energy-consuming processes. Hepatocytes and LSECs are organized into three functional zones: zone 1 (periportal); zone 2 (midzonal); and zone 3 (pericentral) (see also Chapter 73). Gene expression and differential function of hepatocytes in the different zones are regulated by a gradient of cell signaling molecules. The body-to-liver weight ratio is tightly regulated. Although adult hepatocytes are relatively quiescent, they retain a lifelong capacity for massive regeneration following liver injury or loss of liver mass. Once a body weight-appropriate liver mass is achieved, the cessation of hepatocyte proliferation is mediated by bile acid signaling, which is a part of the bile acid-farnesoid X receptor (FXR)-fibroblast growth factor (FGF) receptor axis. The liver also has key immunoregulatory functions that involve both hepatocytes and nonparenchymal cells. In addition to its synthetic and secretory functions, the liver plays a central role in the body's energy metabolism by orchestrating the synthesis, utilization, and catabolism of carbohydrates, proteins, and lipids. The liver's molecular "clock" synchronizes the body's energy needs to the availability of nutrients.

LIVER CELL TYPES AND ORGANIZATION

Liver cells can be classified into three groups: parenchymal cells, which include hepatocytes and bile duct epithelia; sinusoidal cells, which include LSECs and Kupffer cells (hepatic macrophages); and perisinusoidal cells, which consist of hepatic stellate cells (HSCs) and pit cells. Hepatocytes comprise 60% of the adult liver cell population and represent ~78% of the tissue volume (see Chapter 73).[1]

Hepatocytes

Hepatocytes are large polyhedral cells approximately 20–30 μm in diameter.[2] Consistent with their high synthetic and metabolic activity, hepatocytes are enriched in organelles.

Hepatocyte Nucleus

The nuclei of hepatocytes are relatively large and have prominent nucleoli. At birth, most hepatocytes are diploid, that is, they contain single nuclei with two sets of chromosomes. However, subsequently the percentages of tetraploid and octaploid hepatocytes increase progressively to ~40% in normal human livers and to ~80% in 1-year-old mice. Polyploidy may be nuclear (the presence of multiple nuclei) or cellular (a single nucleus with multiple sets of chromosomes).[3] Furthermore, a significant portion of normal human hepatocytes (25%–40%) are aneuploid, that is, they randomly lack one discrete chromosome (except chromosome 12, which has not found to be absent).[4] The impact of polyploidy and aneuploidy in normal liver physiology is not clearly understood at this time, but the finding of increased polyploidy during hepatic inflammation has led to the postulation of a protective role against the development of liver cancer. Polyploidy results from a mismatch between chromosomal replication and subsequent cytokinesis. The mechanistic pathways and pathophysiological implications of hepatocyte polyploidy have been reviewed recently[5] and are briefly summarized here. Centrosomes limit polyploidy by activating the P53 signaling network via PIDDosome, a multiprotein complex containing the P53-induced protein with a death domain. In addition to the transcriptional pathways, inhibition of cytokinesis involves targeting of the cytokinesis effector transcripts by miR-122, the most abundant microRNA in hepatocytes.[6] In addition to pathways that act on cytokinesis, hepatocyte ploidy is controlled by regulating CDK inhibitors. Yes-associated protein (YAP), a component of the Hippo pathway, sequesters cytoplasmic Skp2, leading to the accumulation of its target p27, thereby causing polyploidization.[7]

The two concentric nuclear membranes are stabilized by networks of intermediate filaments, one inside the inner membrane and one outside the outer membrane.[8] The outer nuclear membrane is in direct continuity with the endoplasmic reticulum (ER) membranes. The perinuclear space between the two nuclear membranes surrounds the nucleus and is continuous with the ER lumen. The nuclear membrane contains pores through which molecules are selectively transported to and from the cytoplasm. The ribonuclear protein network and the perinucleolar chromatin radiate from the nucleolus.

The Nuclear Chromatin Contains the Chromosomes and Associated Proteins. The chromosomes comprise a series of genes, interspersed with intragenic deoxyribonucleic acid (DNA). The DNA is transcribed into ribonucleic acid (RNA), which undergoes multiple processing steps, giving rise to messenger RNA (mRNA) molecules that are translocated across the nuclear pores into the cytoplasm, where they become associated with ribosomes. Nuclear DNA also encodes additional RNA types that have accessory roles in protein synthesis and other functions. Ribosomal RNAs (rRNAs) are encoded by DNA within the nucleolus. Transfer RNA (tRNA) binds to amino acids and provides a necessary link between the nucleic acid code and sequential amino acid incorporation in the growing protein chain during translation. Other RNAs are involved in the processing of mRNA, rRNA, and tRNA molecules. Just before cell division, both the DNA and protein components of chromatin are duplicated. The two copies of each duplicated chromosome are separated and distributed precisely so that the two daughter cells each receive a complete set of genes.

Transport Between the Nucleus and the Cytoplasm of Hepatocytes. Pores of the nuclear envelope are associated with a large number of proteins, organized with an octagonal symmetry.[9] The nuclear pore complex (NPC) is a large macromolecular assembly that protrudes into both the cytoplasm and the nucleoplasm. Bidirectional nucleocytoplasmic transport occurs through the central aqueous channel in NPCs.[10] Histones, DNA and RNA polymerases, transcription factors, and RNA processing proteins are selectively transported into the nucleus from the cytoplasm, where they are synthesized, whereas tRNAs and mRNAs are synthesized in the nucleus and exported to the cytoplasm through the NPCs.

Often, the export and import processes are interrelated. For example, ribosomal proteins are imported into the nucleus from the cytoplasm and, after assembly with rRNA, are exported to the cytoplasm as a ribosomal subunit. Proteins containing nuclear localization motifs that consist of specific cationic amino acid sequences are recognized by pore complex receptors, termed *importins* or *karyopherins*, and are rapidly transported into the nucleus via an energy-consuming process powered by specific adenosine triphosphatase (ATPase)/guanosine triphosphatase (GTPase) enzymes. In other cases, large molecules diffuse slowly through the nuclear pores and are retained in the nucleus by binding to specific intranuclear sites. Molecules that are smaller than 5 kD diffuse freely across the nuclear pores.

Hepatocyte Endoplasmic Reticulum

The ER is the largest intracellular membrane compartment, consisting of membranous tubules or flattened sacs (cisternae) that enclose a continuous lumen or space and extend throughout the cytoplasm.[11] The domain of ER in which active protein synthesis occurs has attached ribosomes and is termed the *rough ER*. The other domain, the *smooth ER*, is devoid of ribosomes and is the site of lipid biosynthesis, detoxification, and calcium regulation. The nuclear envelope is a specialized domain of the ER.[12]

Golgi Complex of Hepatocytes

The Golgi complex consists of a stack of flat, sac-like membranes (cisternae) that are dilated at the margins.[13] Many proteins synthesized in the rough ER are transported to the Golgi apparatus in protein-filled transition vesicles. The aspect of the Golgi complex facing the ER is the *cis* face; the opposite side is termed the *trans* face. Glycoproteins are thought to be transported between the Golgi sacs via shuttle vesicles. The highly mannosylated glycosyl moiety of proteins that are *N*-glycosylated in the ER is processed in the Golgi sacs into mature forms. Some proteins are *O*-glycosylated in the Golgi complex. These proteins are then sorted for transport to appropriate cellular organelles (see later discussion of exocytosis and endocytosis).[14]

Polarity of Hepatocytes

Hepatocytes are polarized epithelial cells. Their plasma membranes have three distinct domains: (1) the sinusoidal surface (~37% of the cell surface) that comes in direct contact with plasma through the fenestrae of the specialized LSECs; (2) the canalicular surface (~13% of the cell surface) that encloses the bile canaliculus (BC); and (3) contiguous surfaces. By analogy with glandular epithelia, the sinusoidal, canalicular, and contiguous plasma membrane domains are also termed basolateral, apical, and lateral surfaces, respectively.[15] The sinusoidal and canalicular surfaces contain microvilli, which greatly extend the surface area of these domains. The unique type of polarization of hepatocytes differs from that of other epithelial cells, such as epithelia of the intestines, bile ducts, or renal tubules that are polarized in the plane of the tissue.[16] In contrast, in hepatocytes, "apical" plasma membranes of two adjacent cells join to enclose the BC, which is the smallest tributary of the bile duct system.

Maintenance of both structural and functional polarity of hepatocytes requires mitochondrial energy production, which is regulated by 5′ adenosine monophosphate-activated protein kinase. Structural polarity is supported by the extracellular matrix, which, in addition to serving as an attachment scaffold, functions as a signaling platform needed for maintenance of the differentiated phenotype of hepatocytes and desmosome (tight junction) proteins, for example, claudin 1 and tight junction protein 2 that delimit the bile canalicular space. Functional polarity of hepatocytes is conferred by distinctive localization of various solute carriers, ion channels, water channels, and ATP-driven pumps in specific plasma membrane domains. Basolateral membrane proteins traffic directly to this domain after their synthesis in the ER and modification in the Golgi apparatus and the *trans*-Golgi network (TGN). Some of these proteins are monotopic, that is, they anchor only to the inner leaflet of the plasma membrane bilayer via glycosylphosphatidylinositol (GPI), while others are termed polytopic because they traverse the membrane bilayer. Canalicular monotopic GPI-terminated proteins, such as 5′ nucleotidase or aminopeptidase, initially traffic from the TGN to the basolateral domain and are transported from there to the canalicular domain via apical recycling endosomes (ARE). In contrast, canalicular polytopic transporters, such as the ATP-binding cassette proteins, traffic from the TGN to the canalicular membrane directly or via ARE. Protein cargo destined for apical and basolateral sites is thought to be sorted at the TGN and possibly at additional sites.[17]

Hepatocyte Plasma Membranes

The plasma membranes consist of lipid bilayers composed of glycerophospholipids, cholesterol, and sphingolipids that provide barrier to water and most polar substances.[18] The inner and outer leaflets of the plasma membrane differ in lipid, protein, and carbohydrate composition, reflecting their functional differences. Protein molecules within the leaflets mediate transport of specific molecules and serve as a link with cytoskeletal structures and the extracellular matrix. Hepatocyte plasma membranes consist of 36% lipid, 54% protein, and 10% carbohydrate by dry weight. Outer leaflets of hepatocyte plasma membranes are enriched in carbohydrates.

Lipid Rafts. Lipid rafts are microdomains (~50 nm diameter) of the outer leaflets of the plasma membrane that are highly enriched in cholesterol and sphingolipids.[19] These are coupled to cholesterol-rich microdomains in the inner leaflet by an unknown mechanism. Raft lipids and associated proteins diffuse together laterally on the membrane surface. Some surface receptors become associated with the rafts on ligand binding, or they can lead to "clustering" of smaller rafts into larger ones. Lipid rafts are important in signal transduction, apoptosis, cell adhesion and migration, cytoskeletal organization, and protein sorting during both exocytosis and endocytosis (see later). Certain viruses enter cells via the lipid rafts.

Membrane proteins perform receptor, enzyme, and transport functions.[20] Integral membrane proteins traverse the lipid bilayer once or multiple times or are buried in the lipid. Additional "extrinsic" protein molecules are associated with plasma membrane. Membrane proteins can rotate or diffuse laterally but usually do not flip-flop from one leaflet to another. Concentration of specific membrane proteins is maintained by a balance between their synthesis and degradation by shedding of membrane vesicles, proteolytic digestion within the membrane, or internalization into the cell. Receptor proteins internalized into the cell may be degraded or recycled to the cell surface.

Space of Disse. The space between the endothelia and the sinusoidal villi is termed the space of Disse. There is bidirectional exchange of liquids and solutes at the sinusoidal surface between the plasma within the space of Disse and hepatocytes. In many cases, the molecular transfer is augmented by proteins that facilitate diffusion along a downhill concentration gradient or use ATP-derived energy to actively pump molecules into the space of Disse. The fluid in the space of Disse drains into hepatic lymphatics, which lead to liver hilum lymphatics, cisterna chili, thoracic duct, and, eventually, into the central venous circulation. Excess fluid in the space of Disse gains access to the Glisson's capsule on the liver surface and "sweat out" forming ascites.

Hepatocyte Cell Junctions. Hepatocytes are organized into sheets (seen as cords in two-dimensional sections) by occluding (tight), communicating (gap), and anchoring junctions (Fig. 74.1). Tight junctions or desmosomes form gasket-like seals around the bile canaliculi, thereby permitting a concentration difference of solutes between the cytoplasm and BC. Desmosomes are specialized membrane structures that anchor intermediate filaments to the plasma membrane and link cells together. Gap junctions are subdomains of contiguous membranes of hepatocytes that comprise ~3% of the total surface membrane. They consist of hexagonal particles with hollow cores, termed connexons, made up of six connexin molecules.[21] Connexons of one cell are joined to those of an adjacent cell to form a radially symmetrical cylinder that can open or close the central channel. Gap junctions are involved in nutrient exchange, synchronization of cellular activities, and conduction of electrical impulses.

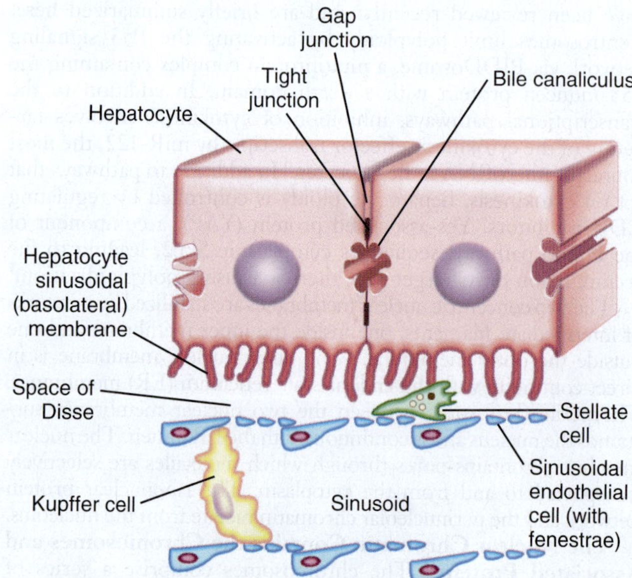

Fig. 74.1 The spatial relationship among the different cell types of the liver. Sinusoidal plasma comes in direct contact with hepatocytes in the space of Disse. The endothelial cells are fenestrated and lack a basement membrane. Kupffer cells are located in the lumen of the sinusoid, where they are in direct contact with the sinusoidal endothelial cells and portal blood. Stellate cells are situated between the endothelial cells and hepatocytes and come in direct contact with both cell types. The hepatocytes are joined with each other by tight junctions and the communicating gap junctions. The canalicular domain of the plasma membrane of two adjacent hepatocytes encloses the bile canaliculus.

Cytoskeleton of Hepatocytes

The hepatocyte cytoskeleton supports the organization of subcellular organelles, cell polarity, intracellular movement of vesicles, and molecular transport.[22,23] It comprises microfilaments, microtubules, and intermediate filaments, as well as the cytoskeleton-associated proteins.[24] Intermediate filaments are polymers of fibrous polypeptides (cytokeratins and lamins) that provide structural support to the cells. In addition, vimentin is expressed by hepatocytes in tissue culture, and neurofilaments appear in injured hepatocytes and form Mallory bodies (also termed Mallory-Denk bodies or Mallory's hyaline). Hepatocytes express two cytokeratins, CK8 and CK18. Bile duct epithelial cells express these proteins and CK19. Plectin is a giant protein that crosslinks intermediate filaments to each other and to the plasma membrane, microtubules, and actin filaments.

Microtubules are hollow tubular structures (with an outer diameter of 24 nm) that consist of polymerized dimers of α and β tubulin and are involved in intracellular transport and cellular organization.[25,26] Microtubules serve as tracks to the movement of cytoplasmic vesicles, mediated by ATPase-powered motor proteins, kinesin, dynein, and dynamin. Depolymerization of the microtubules, for example, by colchicine treatment, inhibits plasma protein secretion without affecting protein synthesis. Microtubules participate in cellular organization by interacting with the Golgi apparatus, intermediate filaments, and F-actin.[27] They also maintain the integrity of the surface membrane during canalicular contraction.[28]

Microfilaments are composed of double-helical F-actin strands, which are polymers of G-actin. Several actin-associated proteins control the polymerization, depolymerization, and splicing of F-actin. Together with myosins, actins maintain the integrity of the cell matrix, facilitate bile canalicular contraction, and control tight junction permeability. Microfilaments are also important in receptor-mediated endocytosis (RME) and various transport processes. Collapse of the cellular structure of hepatocytes during apoptosis and formation of apoptotic bodies may be related to remodeling of the actin cytoskeleton of hepatocytes.[29]

Hepatocyte Lysosomes

Lysosomes consist of a system of membrane-bound sacs and tubules that contain hydrolytic enzymes that are active at pH 4.5–5.[30,31] The ATPase-powered proton pump maintains the acid pH by importing hydrogen ions into the lysosomal lumen.[30] Lysosomal enzymes are glycoproteins with *N*-linked oligosaccharides. Following synthesis in the ER, the carbohydrate moieties are modified in the Golgi apparatus, where their mannose residues are phosphorylated. Recognition of these mannose 6-phosphate (M6P) groups by the M6P receptor in *trans*-Golgi stacks[30] results in their segregation and translocation into late endosomes, which transform into lysosomes.[32,33]

Hepatocyte Mitochondria

Mitochondria constitute about 20% of the cytoplasmic volume of hepatocytes and are responsible for cellular respiration.[34,35] They contain the enzymes of the tricarboxylic acid cycle, fatty acid oxidation, and oxidative phosphorylation.[35,36] Mitochondria conserve the energy generated by oxidation of substrates as high-energy phosphate bonds of ATP. In addition, parts of the urea cycle, gluconeogenesis, fatty acid synthesis, regulation of intracellular calcium concentration, and heme synthesis take place in the mitochondria. Mitochondria play a key role in programmed cell death, or *apoptosis* (see later).[37]

The outer smooth surface membrane of the mitochondrion is functionally different from the inner membrane, which is highly folded to form cristae. Mitochondria are positioned at major sites of ATP utilization by translocation along microtubules. In addition to soluble enzymes, the mitochondrial matrix includes large intramitochondrial granules that store calcium and other ions and smaller granules that contain mitochondrial ribosomes. Mitochondrial DNA, embedded within the matrix, encodes a number of mitochondrial proteins. The remaining mitochondrial proteins are encoded by nuclear genes.

Glycolysis and fatty acid oxidation in the mitochondria generate chemical intermediates that feed into the citric acid cycle of energy-yielding reactions.[38,39] The citric acid cycle breaks down acetyl coenzyme A (acetyl CoA) into three molecules of nicotinamide adenine dinucleotide (NADH), one molecule of flavin adenine dinucleotide ($FADH_2$), and two molecules of carbon dioxide. Electrons derived from NADH and $FADH_2$ drive an electron transport pathway in the inner mitochondrial membrane, leading to ATP production. Passage of electrons across the inner mitochondrial membrane to the space between the inner and outer membranes generates a proton gradient that drives ATP synthesis.[40]

Hepatocyte Peroxisomes

Peroxisomes are spherical-appearing structures that enclose a matrix that contains a lattice or crystalline core.[41] Peroxisomes are abundant in hepatocytes and are thought to be essential for life. Several oxidative catabolic reactions, as well as anabolic reactions, take place in peroxisomes, which provide important links between the metabolism of carbohydrates, lipids, proteins, fats, and nucleic acids.

Exocytosis and Endocytosis by Hepatocytes

Exocytosis and endocytosis are pathways involved in exporting, importing, and intracellular trafficking of molecules. Addition of new proteins and lipids to the plasma membrane by exocytosis and removal of membrane components into cytoplasmic compartments by endocytosis keep the cell surface in a state of dynamic polarization. During exocytosis, secreted proteins, synthesized in the ER, pass sequentially through the *cis*-, *medial*-, and *trans*-Golgi stacks and the TGN and finally appear at the cell surface.[42,43] This vectorial transport through the Golgi stacks occurs via vesicles that are coated by proteins termed coatamers or COPs (COPI and COPII), which are distinct from clathrin (see later).[44,45] Guanosine triphosphate (GTP)-guanosine diphosphate exchange factors and GTP-activating proteins that are specific for each type of vesicle stimulate membrane binding and catalytic activation of small GTPases. Once bound to the membrane, GTPases induce recruitment of COP proteins. In the ER, the first coat protein to be recruited is COPII, and vesicular/tubular clusters are formed. These clusters are thought to coalesce to form a complex tubular network, termed the ER/Golgi intermediate compartment. Acquisition of COPI proteins by the membranes of this tubular network results in the formation of vesicles that carry out bidirectional protein transport to and from the Golgi stacks. Some vesicles that emerge from the exit side of the Golgi apparatus, termed the TGN, can transport multiple protein molecules simultaneously and release them together into the extracellular medium. Other types of vesicles that carry membrane proteins and enzymes destined for specific intracellular organelles also pass through this secretory pathway. These vesicles are sorted at the TGN, and vesicles carrying specific cargo are delivered to appropriate target organelles.[46]

Endocytosis is the import of extracellular macromolecules by processes that include pinocytosis, phagocytosis, RME, and caveolae internalization.[47] Pinocytosis refers to nonselective bulk-phase uptake of extracellular fluid via engulfment by plasma membrane invaginations. Phagocytosis is the ingestion of particles as well as regions of the cell surface. In contrast to these nonspecific modes of uptake, RME is a mechanism of uptake of specific molecules (ligands). After the ligands bind to their specific cell surface receptors, the ligand-receptor complexes concentrate in "pits" that are coated on the cytoplasmic surface by three-pronged structures (triskelions) composed of three heavy chains and three light chains of clathrin. The assembled coats consist of a geometric array of 12 pentagons and a variable number of hexagons, depending on the size of the coat. The coated pits pinch off into the underlying cytoplasm as coated vesicles.[48] In the next step, the vesicles lose their clathrin coat and are termed endosomes. Endosomal vesicles travel along microtubules and can take three distinct pathways. Some endosomes return to the cell surface, and the contained ligand-receptor complexes are secreted out of the cells by a process termed diacytosis. Transferrin is a prototype ligand for diacytosis. Some other ligands, such as immunoglobulin A oligomers, may traverse the cells to be secreted into bile along with the receptor. This process is termed transcytosis.[49]

The best studied type of RME is the classical endocytotic pathway, in which the interior of the endosome is acidified by the action of a proton pump, thereby leading to ligand-receptor uncoupling.[50] By mechanisms that have not been elucidated fully, the dissociated ligands and receptors are sorted into different vesicles. The ligand-containing vesicles proceed to lysosomes, where the ligand is degraded by lysosomal hydrolases. A majority of the ligand-free receptors translocate to the cell surface and replenish the receptor pool. Some receptors, such as the insulin receptor, do not undergo recycling and are rapidly degraded in lysosomes. In addition to the recruitment of clathrin, the initiation of the formation of endocytotic vesicles requires adaptor proteins, particularly AP-2, which localizes between the lipid bilayer and clathrin. Nonscaffold proteins, such as the GTPases and dynamin, are also important in the conversion of a coated pit to a coated vesicle. This function of dynamin requires association with a protein termed amphiphysin. Genetic, cell biological, and biochemical studies are identifying additional proteins that are required for clathrin coat and vesicle formation.[50] In addition to physiological ligands, many viruses use RME to enter cells.

Internalization via caveolae is another pathway by which macromolecules can enter cells. Binding of caveolin to the cytoplasmic aspect of cholesterol-rich lipid rafts on the plasma membrane generates 50- to 60-nm flask-shaped invaginations of the plasma membrane. These invaginations bud off into the cytoplasm to form vesicles, termed caveolae or plasmalemmal vesicles. Caveolae perform various functions, including signal transduction, calcium regulation, nonclathrin-dependent internalization, and transcytosis. GPI-anchored proteins, the β-adrenergic receptor, and tyrosine kinase are concentrated in caveolae.[51]

Functional Zonation of Hepatocytes

Hepatocytes are organized in metabolic zones within the liver cell plates in a manner that optimizes their metabolic function to internalize molecules arriving through the portal vein and hepatic artery and to biotransform, synthesize, and secrete products into the systemic circulation via the hepatic vein and to the intestine through the bile ducts. The functional unit of liver consists of a row of 15–25 hepatocytes extending from the periportal region (zone 1) toward the central vein (zone 3 or pericentral). For example, hepatocytes in zone 1 that are exposed to highly oxygenated blood are enriched in enzymes involved in energy-demanding functions, such as gluconeogenesis and urea production, whereas zone 3 hepatocytes specialize in glycolysis and xenobiotic metabolism. Correspondingly, zone 1 hepatocytes express Ass110, As110, Alb8, and cyp2f29, whereas zone 3 hepatocytes express Glul and Cyp2e19 in nearly mutually exclusive manner. In addition, zone 2 (midzonal) hepatocytes are also enriched in the expression of certain genes, such as Hamp and Hamp2 (encoding hepcidin, a liver hormone that regulates systemic iron levels), Igfbp2, Mup3, and Cyp8b1. Overall, nearly half of all genes expressed in hepatocytes are spatially zonated.[52]

The developmental mechanism of hepatic zonation appears to be based in the spatial separation and functional antagonism between the adenomatous polyposis coli (*APC*) gene product expressed in zone 1 cells and β-catenin in zone 3, which is activated by Wnt signaling from endothelial cells in zone 3. In the absence of Wnt signals, a degradation complex containing the products of the tumor suppressor genes *APC* and axins, and the kinases GSK-3β and CK1 promotes phosphorylation and subsequent degradation of β-catenin. The lack of β-catenin signaling in zone 1 and an ascending gradient of the signaling toward zone 3 is thought to generate and maintain the zonation of gene expression and function of the liver.[53]

Bile Duct Epithelial Cells

Bile duct epithelial cells, or cholangiocytes, consist of large and small subpopulations of cells, the cell volumes of which correlate roughly with the diameter of the intrahepatic bile ducts (see Chapter 64). Large cholangiocytes have a relatively more developed ER and a lower nuclear-to-cytoplasmic ratio than do small cholangiocytes.[54] Low expression of cytochrome P450-dependent monooxygenase activity imparts a survival advantage to the small cholangiocytes against injury by chemicals. For example, cytochrome P450 2E1–mediated formation of toxic intermediates of carbon tetrachloride leads to the loss of large cholangiocyte function after administration of the protoxin, whereas small cholangiocytes are resistant to the toxin.

Secretory and Absorptive Function of Cholangiocytes. Bile ducts are not mere passive conduits for biliary drainage but play an active role in the secretion and absorption of biliary components, as well as regulation of the extracellular matrix composition. Cholangiocytes are highly polarized. A sodium-dependent bile salt transporter (ABAT), located at the apical (luminal) surface of cholangiocytes, mediates the uptake of conjugated bile acids, whereas an alternatively spliced truncated form of the protein (ASBT), located at the basolateral surface, mediates sodium-independent efflux of bile acids. The sodium-dependent glucose transporter (SGLT1), located at the apical domain, and GLUT1, a facilitative glucose transporter on the basolateral domain, are responsible for glucose reabsorption from bile. Aquaporin-1 at the apical and basolateral surfaces constitutes water channels that may mediate hormone-regulated transport of water into bile. The purinergic receptor (P_{2u}) stimulates chloride ion efflux. Activation of apical P_{2u} by ATP, which is secreted into the bile by hepatocytes, mobilizes Ca^{2+} stores, thereby stimulating Cl^- efflux from cholangiocytes. The large, but not the small, cholangiocytes express secretin and somatostatin receptors, the chloride/bicarbonate exchanger, and the cystic fibrosis transmembrane regulator, which may enable this population of cholangiocytes to modulate water and electrolyte secretion in response to secretin and somatostatin (see also Chapter 66).[55]

Primary Cilia of Cholangiocytes. Cholangiocytes are the only liver cells with primary cilia. "Primary bile" secreted by hepatocytes is subsequently modified by cholangiocytes, which modulates its fluidity and alkalinity by secreting Cl^- and HCO_3^-, and by absorbing bile salts, glucose, and amino acids, followed by passive movement of water into or out of the bile duct lumen along osmotic gradients. These functions require sensing the flow rate, osmolality, and composition of bile, which is provided by primary cilia of cholangiocytes. Each cholangiocyte has one primary cilium consisting of a shaft, termed the axoneme, which is composed of nine peripheral microtubule doublets arranged around a hollow central core. The axoneme is attached to a centriole-derived microtubule organizing center, termed the basal body. Axonemes of large cholangiocytes are 7.35 ± 1.32 μm long, whereas those of small cholangiocytes are approximately half as long. The primary cilium extends from the apical (luminal) plasma membrane into the bile duct lumen and is, therefore, positioned strategically to serve as a mechanoreceptor, osmoreceptor, and chemoreceptor that modulates the secretory/absorptive functions of cholangiocytes in response to the pulsatile flow of primary bile.[56]

Liver Sinusoidal Endothelial Cells

LSECs comprise 15%–20% of all liver cells but account for only 3% of the total liver volume. During embryogenesis, LSECs are derived from hemangioblasts and endocardium of the sinus venosus. These cells are distinguished from capillary endothelial cells by the presence of 50–125 nm fenestrae (pores) in their flat, thin extensions that form sieve plates. Unlike capillary endothelial cells, LSECs do not form intracellular junctions and simply overlap each other (see Fig.74.1). During human embryonic development, the structural differentiation of human LSECs from other endothelial cells occurs between gestational weeks 5 and 12, when LSECs progressively loose cell markers of continuous endothelial cells (e.g., CD31, CD34, and 1F10 antigen) and acquire adult LSEC markers, including CD4, CD32, and the intracellular adhesion molecule-1 (ICAM-1). LSEC differentiation is mediated by direct intercellular interactions with hepatoblasts, as well as through vascular endothelial growth factor (VEGF) released by hepatoblasts.

The presence of fenestrae and the absence of a basement membrane make these cells the most permeable of all endothelial cells of the mammalian body and permit plasma to enter the space of Disse and come in direct contact with the sinusoidal surface of hepatocytes, while excluding blood cells.[57] Sieve plates are surrounded by microtubules, and the diameter and number of the fenestrae are actively controlled by the actin-containing components of the cytoskeleton in response to changes in the chemical milieu.[58] By virtue of an abundance of scavenger receptors and mannose receptors, LSECs have a high endocytotic capacity and can clear an array of metabolites and microbial products.[58] LSECs are professional pinocytes that internalize soluble macromolecules as well as small particles. Some molecules endocytosed at the sinusoidal surface of LSECs undergo transcytosis, that is, exocytosis into the space of Disse, which facilitates subsequent uptake through the sinusoidal surface of hepatocytes. Thus LSECs serve as a selective barrier between the blood and the hepatocytes. LSECs can secrete prostaglandins and a wide variety of proteins, including interleukin (IL)-1 and IL-6, interferon, tumor necrosis factor-α (TNF-α), and endothelin. In normal adult liver, LSECs turn over slowly and are replenished by mitosis of mature LSECs under stimulation by VEGF and FGFs. After liver injury or loss of liver mass, for example, following partial liver resection, two additional cell types contribute to LSEC renewal, namely, sinusoidal endothelial progenitor cells resident in the liver and bone marrow-derived sinusoidal endothelial cell progenitors. LSECs are the predominant source of coagulation factor VIII. Von Willebrand factor is not expressed in young individuals but may be expressed in older livers.[57] Normally, LSECs are tolerogenic, and abnormality of these cells is associated with inflammation and liver fibrosis. Reduced porosity of LSECs in patients with cirrhosis or diabetes, as well as in older subjects, may lead to reduced clearance of chylomicron remnants and is proposed to be a cause of atherosclerosis.[57]

Zonation of LSECs. As in the case of hepatocytes, there are zonal differences among LSECs present in the periportal, midzonal, and pericentral regions of the liver lobule. Cozonation of hepatocytes with LSECs is controlled by the expression of specific angiocrine molecules from the portal and central veins.[59] The size and number of the fenestrae of LSECs vary according to their location in the liver lobule, with larger but fewer fenestrae per sieve plate in the periportal region and smaller but more numerous fenestrae in the centrilobular region. Functional zonation can also be demonstrated by immunochemical staining for different marker proteins, as well as transcriptional pattern.

Regulation of Sinusoidal Blood Flow by LSECs. LSECs regulate hepatic vascular tone, which helps in maintaining a low portal pressure despite major increases in hepatic blood flow during digestion. LSECs are the main source of the vasodilatory molecule nitric oxide (NO) through endothelial NO synthase, which is activated by shear stress.[58,60] KLF2 downregulates the vasoconstrictive activity of endothelin-1. LSECs also produce the vasodilatory agent carbon monoxide and metabolites of the cyclooxygenase pathway (thromboxane A2 and prostacyclin).[61] These molecules act on HSCs present in the space of Disse, keeping them quiescent, thereby preventing their vasoconstrictive effect.

LSECs and Liver Regeneration. Following loss of liver mass due to acute liver injury or partial hepatectomy, hepatic VEGF expression increases, which stimulates bone marrow sinusoidal progenitor cell proliferation and their mobilization to the circulation, followed by engraftment in liver sinusoids and differentiation to mature LSECs. VEGF stimulates liver regeneration through hepatocyte growth factor (HGF) production by LSECs, which leads to the proliferation of both hepatocytes and LSECs. Additionally, increased shear stress resulting from portal blood flow into a smaller liver volume stimulates LSECs to produce NO, which, in turn, augments the effect of HGF on hepatocytes. Platelets recruited to the liver after partial hepatectomy adhere to HSECs and stimulate secretion of key molecules in hepatocyte and HSEC proliferation and survival.[58]

Kupffer Cells

Kupffer cells are specialized tissue macrophages that account for 80%–90% of the total population of fixed macrophages in the body. These cells are derived from bone marrow stem cells or monocytes and are highly active in removing particulate matter and toxic or foreign substances that appear in the portal blood from the intestine.[62] Kupffer cells are located in the sinusoidal lumen and are in direct contact with endothelial cells (see Fig. 74.1). They possess bristle-coated micropinocytic vesicles, fuzzy-coated vacuoles, and worm-like structures that are special features of cells that are active in pinocytosis and phagocytosis. An abundance of lysosomes reflects their prominent role in degrading substances taken up from the bloodstream. Kupffer cells secrete a variety of vasoactive toxic mediators, which may be involved in host defense mechanisms and in pathophysiologic processes in some liver diseases. Kupffer cells increase in number and activity in chemical, infectious, or immunologic injury to the liver.[63]

Hepatic Stellate Cells

HSCs are also known as Ito cells, vitamin A–storing cells, fat-storing cells, or lipocytes. These cells are a part of the stellate cell system, which includes similar cells in the pancreas, lung, kidney, and intestine. HSCs are located between the endothelial lining and hepatocytes (see Fig.74.1). These mesenchymal cells represent 5%–8% of all liver cells and are important sources of paracrine, autocrine, juxtacrine, and chemoattractant factors that maintain homeostasis in the microenvironment of the hepatic sinusoid. Microfilament and microtubule-enriched flat cytoplasmic extensions of quiescent stellate cells store vitamin A-enriched lipid droplets and spread out parallel to the endothelial lining, contacting several cells.[64] HSCs express receptors for retinol-binding protein (RBP), which mediates the endocytosis of RBP-retinol complexes.[65]

After chronic liver injury, the slender star-shaped HSCs become activated to elongated myofibroblasts. They lose retinoids and upregulate the synthesis of extracellular matrix components, such as collagen, proteoglycan, and adhesive glycoproteins. Stellate cell activation is the central event in hepatic fibrosis.[66] Activation of HSCs is initiated by paracrine stimulation by neighboring LSECs, Kupffer cells, endothelial cells, and hepatocytes, as well as platelets and leukocytes. Endothelial cells participate in Kupffer cell activation by producing cellular fibronectin and by converting the latent form of TGF-β to its active, profibrogenic form. Binding of TGF-β to its receptor on HSCs plays a critical role in stellate cell activation. Binding of bacterial lipopolysaccharides (LPS) arriving to the liver from the intestine to Toll-like receptor 4 (TLR4) enhances the effect of TGF-β on HSCs by two different mechanisms.[67] First, increased chemokine expression by stellate cells results in chemotaxis of Kupffer cells, which secrete TGF-β. Second, LPS binding to TLR4 activates nuclear factor kappa B (NF-κB) via the adapter protein MyD88 (myeloid differentiation response protein), thereby downregulating the TGF-β pseudoreceptor BAMBI (bone morphogenic protein and the activin membrane-bound inhibitor) and sensitizing the HSCs to TGF-β signaling. The three-dimensional structure of the extracellular matrix modulates the shape, proliferation, and function of HSCs, probably by signal transduction via binding to cell surface integrins, followed by changes in cytoskeleton assembly. Hedgehog proteins secreted by hepatocytes under stress can signal HSCs, leading to their activation, proliferation, and transition to myofibroblasts.[68] HSC activation by continued effect of these stimuli leads to several discrete changes in cell behavior, such as proliferation, contractility, overexpression of extracellular matrix proteins (e.g., collagens I, III, IV, V, and VI; laminin; tenascin; undulin; hyaluronic acid; and proteoglycans), matrix degradation by releasing metalloproteinases, and the release of leukocyte chemoattractants and cytokines. The overall number of HSCs increases during fibrosis because of a change in the balance between proliferation and apoptosis, which is influenced by soluble growth factors and the matrix.

Pit Cells

Pit cells, the natural killer (NK) cells of the liver, are located mainly within the sinusoidal lumen, close to Kupffer cells. They have the appearance of large lymphocytes and are adherent to the sinusoidal wall, often anchored with villous extensions (pseudopods).[69] In the human liver, pit cells have pronounced polarity, abundant cytoplasm containing dense granules, a conspicuous cytocenter, and a locomotory shape characterized by hyaloplasmic pseudopods and a uropod (a tail-like structure that forms on the trailing end of a moving cell). The cytoplasmic granules appear as pits by microscopy, hence the name pit cells. Pit cells are short-lived and are replenished from extrahepatic sources.

In common with circulating NK cells, the pit cells express OX-8 antigen, and some express asialoganglioside gangliotetrasylceramide (asialo-GMr1). Pit cells do not express the pan-T-cell marker, OX-19, which is expressed by circulating NK cells. Although the source of pit cells remains debated, they are antigenically related to NK cells of other viscera. Pit cells have tumor cell-killing activity in the liver and are also thought to remove virus-infected liver cells. Their per-cell cytolytic activity is greater than that of circulating NK cells. Pit cells may also have a role in controlling the growth and differentiation of liver cells and possibly in liver graft rejection.[70]

INTEGRATION OF THE FUNCTIONS OF THE DIFFERENT CELL TYPES

Functional integration of the various groups of liver cells occurs through direct cell-to-cell communication (e.g., via gap junctions), paracrine secretion that affects neighboring cells, cell signaling, interaction with the extracellular matrix, and generalized response to endocrine and metabolic fluxes.[71] Hepatocytes and LSECs lack a continuous basement membrane, and the spatial relationship of the cells is maintained through interaction with the extracellular matrix. Anchoring to the extracellular matrix is important for the survival of hepatocytes. Anchoring also provides traction for movement and permits liver cells to receive signals from matrix components and matrix-bound growth factors. Hepatic extracellular matrix components are produced during development along the migration path of the hepatocytes and exhibit unique patterns of distribution and organization. Stellate cells, hepatocytes, and, to some extent, endothelial cells are major producers of the extracellular matrix in the liver. Excess deposition of connective tissue causes changes in hemodynamic properties and eventually impairs liver function.[66]

Cell-Matrix Interactions

Cell-matrix interactions in the liver are important in maintaining hepatocyte morphology and proliferation. For example, when plated on a flat layer of collagen, hepatocytes synthesize DNA at a level that is fourfold higher than when they are grown on gels composed of basement membrane proteins. The type of matrix determines the level of expression of albumin and other hepatocyte-specific gene products in cultured hepatocytes.[71,72] On the other hand, cell-cell and cell-matrix interactions determine the level of synthesis and deposition of hepatic extracellular matrix proteins by the various types of liver cells. Such interaction also modulates the production of specific enzymes and their inhibitors that mediate remodeling of the extracellular matrix.

Integrin and nonintegrin receptors mediate the interaction of liver cells with extracellular matrix. Integrins bind to extracellular matrix proteins at specialized cell attachment sites that often contain the arginine-glycine-aspartate motif, thereby resulting in attachment of the extracellular matrix to the intracellular cytoskeleton network. This attachment results in changes in cell shape, spreading, and migration. Integrins also influence cell proliferation, differentiation, survival, apoptosis, and gene expression via signal transduction.[73,74] Nonintegrin surface receptors mediate cell attachment by different mechanisms.

Components of the Extracellular Matrix

Components of the extracellular matrix include collagens, noncollagenous glycoproteins, and proteoglycans. The liver contains five types of collagen (I, III, IV, V, and VI) and seven classes of noncollagenous glycoproteins [fibronectin, laminin, entactin/nidogen, tenascin, thrombospondin, SPARC (secreted protein, acidic, and rich in cysteine), and undulin]. Hepatic extracellular matrix also includes a large number of proteoglycans and glycosaminoglycans, such as membrane-associated syndecan, thrombomodulin, and betaglycan, and extracellular matrix-associated versican, biglycan, decorin, fibromodulin, and perlecan.[71,75]

REGENERATION AND APOPTOSIS OF LIVER CELLS

Regeneration

Normal adult hepatocytes divide infrequently, with fewer than 1 in 10,000 hepatocytes undergoing mitosis at any given time—yet the liver possesses a unique capacity to replace tissue mass after liver injury or loss of liver mass. The liver is also unique as it scales with body size so that liver size is adjusted to the needs of the body. The capacity of the liver to regulate its own growth is evident in liver transplantation, where the size of the transplanted organ increases or decreases as appropriate to the size of the recipient. Such finely regulated hyperplasia of the liver is also seen after successful single-lobe liver transplantation in children.[76,64] During homeostasis, the hepatocyte mass is maintained predominantly by division of hepatocytes located in the midzone (zone 2) of the liver lobule, with a major contribution by mitosis of diploid hepatocytes.[77] However, lineage tracing after liver injury showed that periportal and midzonal hepatocytes reconstitute liver after a pericentral (zone 3) injury, whereas pericentral and midzonal hepatocytes reconstitute liver after periportal (zone 1) injury.

Hepatic regeneration has been studied extensively in rodents. Following resection of two-thirds of the liver in rats, the residual liver cells proliferate and restore the liver mass within days to weeks. Although generally termed regeneration, this process is, in fact, restorative hyperplasia because the total liver mass, rather than the lobulated anatomic configuration, is reconstituted. In the rat, DNA synthesis peaks at 24 hours after partial hepatectomy, when approximately 35% of hepatocytes are in cell cycle. Cell division occurs 6–8 hours after DNA synthesis. The time frame of DNA synthesis varies from species to species. For example, in mice, maximum DNA synthesis occurs 36–40 hours after hepatic resection. Because 80%–95% of hepatocytes undergo mitosis, liver mass is restored after one or two cell divisions. All classes of hepatocytes, including diploid, tetraploid, and octoploid, participate in this quasisynchronized proliferation, either by mitosis of mononucleated cells or by cytokinesis of binucleated or tetranucleated hepatocytes, after DNA synthesis in all nuclei. Interestingly, adult hepatocytes, rather than liver progenitor cells, contribute to liver regeneration after partial hepatectomy. Only when the proliferation of adult hepatocytes is inhibited because of certain toxic or physical injuries do progenitor cells, often termed oval cells, proliferate. The oval cells are thought to give rise to both hepatocytes and bile duct epithelial cells.[78]

Hippo-Yap Pathway of Regulation of Hepatocyte Mitosis

The Hippo pathway regulates cell proliferation by contact inhibition of cell proliferation, differentiation, and tissue homeostasis by controlling the stability of the transcriptional coactivators YAP and PDZ-binding domain (TAZ). A phosphorylation cascade, the mammalian Ser/Thr kinase Mst 1 and 2 (Hippo in Drosophila), activate the kinases Lats1 and Lats2, which phosphorylate YAP and TAZ, causing them to be excluded from the nucleus, retained in the cytoplasm, and degraded. Several mechanisms sensing disruption of adherens junctions, loss of epithelial polarity, alteration of cell shape, and mechanical stress inactivate this phosphorylation cascade, thereby permitting the unphosphorylated YAP and TAZ to accumulate in the nucleus, where they interact with the DNA-binding TEAD transcription factors, as well as many other transcription factors, to turn on the expression of growth-promoting and apoptosis-inhibiting genes. Thus the Hippo-Yap pathway is an integrator of several prominent signaling pathways, including the Wnt, G protein-coupled receptor, epidermal growth factor (EGF), bone morphogenetic protein/TGF-β, and Notch pathways involved in cell proliferation following loss of a cell mass and cell quiescence once the tissue volume is reconstituted.[7]

Growth Factors That Mediate Liver Regeneration

After liver injury, early signals for hepatocyte replication come from nonparenchymal cells (see Fig. 74.2B).[79,80] LPS derived from intestinal microbiota, as well as intestine-derived cytokines, stimulate Kupffer cells and hepatic sinusoidal endothelial cells to produce TNF-α and IL-6. Growth factors, such as hepatocyte growth factor (HGF), are released from stores in the hepatic matrix and are secreted by HSCs, whereas EGF is secreted into portal blood by epithelial cells of the proximal small intestine and salivary glands.[79] Hormones, such as triiodothyronine, insulin, and norepinephrine, are important cooperative factors in liver regeneration.[81] Replication of nonparenchymal cells lags behind that of hepatocytes by 24–72 hours. Initially, the newly proliferated hepatocytes form clusters, first in zone 1 and later in other zones of the liver (see Chapter 73). Regenerating LSECs invade these clusters and restore the single-cell thick liver plates.

Wnt/β-Catenin Signaling

After liver injury or loss of hepatocyte mass, Wnt/β-catenin signaling pathway contributes significantly to regeneration and

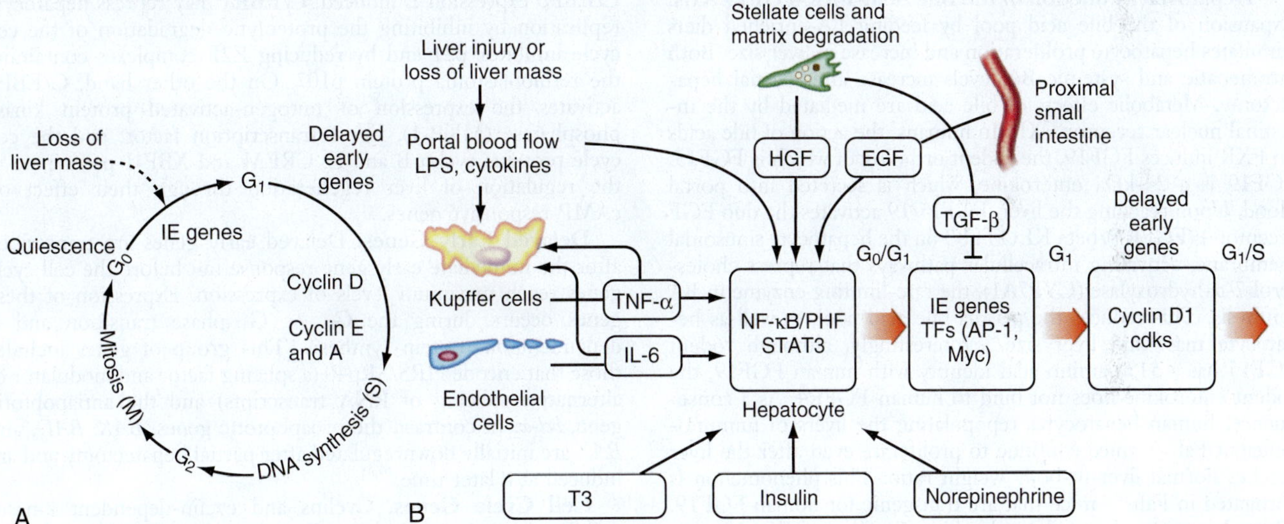

Fig. 74.2 (A) The cell cycle of hepatocytes in response to liver injury or loss of liver mass. Quiescent hepatocytes (G_0) rapidly enter G_1 after loss of liver mass (e.g., partial hepatectomy), along with expression of immediate early genes. This phase is followed sequentially by the expression of delayed early genes and cyclins. DNA synthesis (S phase) reaches a peak in 24 h in rats and 36–40 h in mice. Shortly thereafter, the cell enters G_2 and undergoes mitosis (M). (B) The sequence of signals that leads to liver regeneration following liver damage or partial hepatectomy. Intestine-derived LPS and cytokines in the portal venous blood activate Kupffer cells and endothelial cells, which release TNF-α and IL-6. These signals lead to the activation of NF-κB, also known as PHF, and STAT3 (signal transducer and activator of transcription-3), without the need for new protein synthesis. HGF is released by hepatic stellate cells and also may be derived from storage sites following matrix degradation. EGF, secreted by proximal small intestinal and salivary gland epithelial cells, as well as insulin, T3, and norepinephrine, serve as cooperative factors for transition of hepatocytes through G_1 to the S phase. IE genes and TFs, including AP-1 and Myc, are expressed as the hepatocyte enters the initial phase of G_1. Delayed early genes and cyclins are expressed later in G_1. TGF-β, which inhibits hepatocyte DNA synthesis, is blocked during the proliferative phase. Removal of the block at the end of the cell cycle may be one of the factors that permit the hepatocyte to return to the quiescent state. AP-1, activator protein-1; cdks, cyclin-dependent kinases; *EGF*, epidermal growth factor; *HGF*, hepatocyte growth factor; *IE*, immediate early; *IL-6*, interleukin-6; *LPS*, lipopolysaccharides; *NF-κB*, nuclear factor kappa B; *PHF*, posthepatectomy factor; *TFs*, transcription factors; *TGF-β*, transforming growth factor-β; *TNF-α*, tumor necrosis factor-α; *T3*, triiodothyronine. (Data from Taub R. Liver regeneration: from myth to mechanism. *Nat Rev Mol Cell Biol*. 2004;5:836–847.)

functional recovery of the liver. In the absence of canonical Wnt signaling, β-catenin undergoes phosphorylation, ubiquitination, and proteosomal degradation in a multiprotein "destruction complex." Shortly after liver injury, Wnt is activated in LSECs and macrophages by glycosylation and palmitoylation. The activated hydrophobic Wnt protein binds to Wntless and is transported out of the cells. Activated Wnt ligands then bind to hepatocytes in a paracrine manner via frizzled receptors and low-density lipoproteins (LDL)-related protein-5/6 coreceptors, resulting in stabilization and nuclear translocation of β-catenin. In the nucleus, β-catenin interacts with the T-cell factor family of transcription proteins, resulting in the induction of cyclin D1 for proliferation and other genes that regulate hepatocyte function.[82]

Early as well as late changes occur in the expression of extracellular matrix components and the enzymes that modulate them. The mitotic phase is mostly completed in 3 days, and the liver mass is restituted in about 7 days. Liver cells return to their quiescent state when the liver weight to body weight ratio is restored to within 10% of the original. A balance between mitosis and apoptosis fine-tunes the restoration of hepatic mass.

Signals for Cessation of Growth of the Regenerating Liver

The ability of the liver to regulate its size is dependent on signals from outside the liver, such as hormonal or metabolic signals, as well as internal signals generated within the liver.[78]

"Hepatostat" Function of the Bile Acid-FXR-FGF19 Axis. Expansion of the bile acid pool by feeding BA-enriched diets stimulates hepatocyte proliferation and increase in liver size. Both intrahepatic and systemic BA levels increase after partial hepatectomy. Metabolic effects of bile acid are mediated by the intestinal nuclear receptor FXR. In humans, the action of bile acids on FXR induces FGF19, the rodent ortholog of which is FGF15. FGF19 is a 24-kDa enterokine, which is secreted into portal blood. Upon reaching the liver, FGF15/19 activates the duo FGF receptor 4 (FGFR4)/beta KLOTHO on the hepatocyte sinusoidal membrane, activating intracellular pathways that repress cholesterol 7-α-hydroxylase (CYP7A1), the rate-limiting enzyme in BA synthesis. This reduces the plasma bile acid pool, as well as hepatocyte mass and liver size.[83] Interestingly, although rodent FGF15 has a 51% amino acid identity with human FGF19, the rodent enterokine does not bind to human FGFR4. As a consequence, human hepatocytes repopulating the livers of immunodeficient $Fah^{-/-}$ mice continue to proliferate even after the liver reaches normal liver-to-body weight ratio. This phenomenon is abrogated in $Fah^{-/-}$ mice that are transgenic for human FGF19. This observation has led to the identification of FGF19 as a "hepatostat" and has established the key role of bile acids in initiation and termination of liver regeneration.[83]

Gene Expression During Liver Regeneration

The regenerative process is a cascade of events that move cells from their resting G_0 phase through the G_1 phase, S (DNA synthesis) phase, G_2 phase, and then to M (mitotic cell division) phase (Fig. 74.2A). Expression of a large number of genes is upregulated or downregulated after partial hepatectomy at transcriptional or posttranscriptional levels.[79,81] The sequence of activation of various genes during liver regeneration has been elucidated by studies using partial hepatectomy and gene knockout mice that lack specific cytokines. These genes include cell cycle genes, metabolic genes, genes coding for extracellular matrix proteins, growth factors, cytokines, and transcription factors. Chronologically, these genes can be grouped into immediate early genes, delayed early genes, and cell cycle–associated genes. Expression of these genes is modulated by signal transduction pathways that receive and transduce stimuli for cell replication and tissue remodeling.

Immediate Early Genes. Immediate early genes are activated almost immediately after partial hepatectomy without the need for protein synthesis. More than 70 immediate early genes have been identified, and more are expected to be discovered by microarray analysis of gene expression following partial hepatectomy. Many of these immediate early genes are involved in metabolic processes not directly linked to DNA synthesis. In addition to the protooncogenes, c-*fos*, c-*jun*, c-*myc*, and c-*ets*, the immediate early genes include transcription factors, such as NF-κB, STAT3 (signal transducer and activator of transcription), activator protein-1 (AP-1), C/EBPβ (CCAAT enhancer binding protein β), insulin-like growth factor-binding protein-1, phosphatases, cyclic AMP responsive promoter element modulator gene (CREM), X-box-binding protein 1 (XBP-1), and metabolic genes such as phosphoenolpyruvate carboxykinase (PEPCK) and glucose-6-phosphatase.[81]

In the quiescent liver, NF-κB remains in the cytosol and is inactivated by binding to its inhibitor (IκB). Binding of TNF to its cell surface receptor initiates a signaling cascade that culminates in phosphorylation of IκB, causing the release of NF-κB and its translocation to the nucleus and resulting in transcriptional activation of more than a dozen genes likely to be involved in the immediate early response. IL-6 is one of the target genes of NF-κB. IL-6 is a strong inducer of STAT3 activation and is thought to play an important role in hepatic regeneration. C/EBPα expression is downregulated during liver regeneration, whereas C/EBPβ expression is induced. C/EBPα may repress hepatocyte replication by inhibiting the proteolytic degradation of the cell cycle inhibitor p21 and by reducing E2F complexes containing the retinoblastoma protein p107. On the other hand, C/EBPβ activates the expression of mitogen-activated protein kinase phosphatase (MKP-1), Egr-1 transcription factor, and the cell cycle proteins cyclin B and E. CREM and XBP-1 participate in the regulation of liver regeneration through their effect on cAMP-responsive genes.

Delayed Early Genes. Delayed early genes are transcribed after the immediate early gene response but before the cell cycle genes reach maximum levels of expression. Expression of these genes occurs during the $G_0 \rightarrow G_1$ phase transition and is dependent on protein synthesis. This group of genes includes those that encode HRS/SRp40 (a splicing factor and modulator of alternative splicing of RNA transcripts) and the antiapoptotic gene, *bcl-x*. In contrast, the proapoptotic genes, *BAK*, *BAD*, and *BAX* are initially downregulated after partial hepatectomy and are induced at a later time.[79,81]

Cell Cycle Genes. Cyclins and cyclin-dependent kinases (cdks) are expressed during cell cycle progression from the G_1 through S to M phase. During the G_1 phase, cdks catalyze the phosphorylation of retinoblastoma gene protein (pRb), causing its dissociation from the E2F family of proteins. This dissociation eliminates the repression of gene expression by pRb. In regenerating mouse liver cyclin D1, mRNA is expressed before DNA synthesis, whereas the expression of cyclin E mRNA coincides with DNA synthesis. Cyclin D1 forms a complex with cdk4, which causes phosphorylation of pRb, resulting in E2F activation. Cyclin D1 may also sequester the cell cycle inhibitor p27.[81]

Integration of Cytokine and Growth Factors in Liver Regeneration

The early, reversible phase of liver regeneration, during which hepatocytes can enter the cell cycle by moving from the quiescent G_0 state to early G_1 phase, is termed *priming*.[79] This phase is initiated by the effect of cytokines, the best studied of which include TNF-α and IL-6. Generation of reactive oxygen species as a consequence of the acute metabolic changes and release of

LPS that occur in response to the loss of hepatic functional mass may have a role in triggering the initial cytokine response. During priming, NF-κB and STAT3 are activated, and AP-1 and C/EBP are expressed. Together, these factors lead to the immediate early gene expression response after partial hepatectomy (see earlier). The priming events sensitize hepatocytes to growth factors. In the absence of growth factors, the cells cannot move past a certain "restriction point" in G_1.

The second phase of liver regeneration, termed *progression*, requires HGF and TGF-α as well as cyclins D1 and E. During the progression phase, the cells move past the restriction point in G_1 to S and beyond.

When the peak level of cyclin D1 expression is reached, cells progress autonomously through the cell cycle, without further need for growth factors. Expression of HGF, TGF-α, and probably EGF increases after partial hepatectomy. These factors are the direct mitogens for liver regeneration. EGF binds to both the EGF receptor and the TGF-α receptor, and c-met is the receptor for HGF. Growth hormone, thyroid hormones, and parathyroid hormone are permissive for liver regeneration, whereas insulin and norepinephrine are considered adjuvant factors.[79]

HGF and c-met. Major sources of HGF in the liver are Kupffer cells and HSCs. HGF is produced as a single 87–90-kD proprotein by nonparenchymal cells and is cleaved into ~64- and ~32-kD peptides that form heterodimers.[78,79] HGF mRNA levels are increased 12–24 hours after partial hepatectomy in rats. Elevated levels of HGF have been observed in the serum of patients with fulminant hepatic failure, thus suggesting an important role for HGF in regeneration of human liver. C-met, the HGF receptor, is a heterodimer consisting of a 145-kD β-chain and a 45-kD α-chain, linked by disulfide bonds. The two polypeptide chains of c-met are also derived from proteolytic cleavage of a single precursor protein. The β-chain contains the transmembrane region and the intracellular tyrosine kinase domain. HGF binding to the extracellular domain of c-met activates tyrosine kinase, thereby initiating a signal transduction pathway.

PROGRAMMED CELL DEATH

Programmed cell death, or *apoptosis*, is an integral part of hepatic regeneration. Apoptosis is involved in a fine-tuning and remodeling process that results in reconstruction of the hepatic architecture. Apoptosis results in the removal of damaged, senescent, or supernumerary cells, without altering the cellular microenvironment. Loss of function of proapoptotic proteins, overexpression of antiapoptotic proteins, or loss of apoptotic signaling in cells can lead to the survival of DNA-damaged cells, leading in turn to several forms of cancer.[84]

Apoptotic signals can originate within the cells through mechanisms that sense DNA damage and inappropriate proliferative signals. In other cases, the apoptotic signals come from other cells in at least three ways.[85] First, cells recognized as foreign or as pathogens may receive apoptotic signals from immune mediator cells. Second, the loss of nurturing signals from neighboring cells or extracellular matrix may result in apoptosis of anchor-dependent cells. Third, some cells undergo apoptosis in response to certain growth factors such as TGF-β1.

In contrast to necrosis, apoptosis is an active process that culminates in cell death. During the *latent* phase of apoptosis, the cell undergoes molecular and biochemical change but remains morphologically intact. In the *execution* phase, a series of dramatic structural changes take place that culminate in the fragmentation and condensation of the cell into membrane-enclosed *apoptotic bodies*. Initially, a variety of stimuli, including DNA damage, growth factor withdrawal, toxins, or radiation, trigger the apoptotic pathway. The signal is transduced by a series of defined protein-protein interactions. Finally, cell death is executed by the activation of specific proteases called caspases that cleave multiple substrates, leading to DNA fragmentation, chromatin condensation, cell shrinkage, and membrane blebbing. The apoptotic cell may be phagocytosed or simply lose contact with neighboring cells. Apoptosis does not cause an acute inflammatory reaction. All these morphologic features of apoptosis contrast with those of necrosis, in which the cell swells and releases proinflammatory material into the neighboring space.[84]

The two major apoptotic pathways include activation of cell surface death receptors[85] and mitochondrial permeability transition.[86] At least six different cell surface molecules can function as death receptors. One of the best characterized death receptors is Fas (also known as Apo1 or CD95). Fas belongs to the family of TNF receptors. Binding of Fas to Fas ligand leads to an interaction between the cytoplasmic domain of the Fas receptor and the death domain of the adaptor protein, FADD (Fas-associated protein with death domain), which, in turn, recruits and activates procaspase-8. Once activated, caspase-8 activates downstream caspases such as caspase-3. The second major pathway involves mitochondria and is triggered by various toxic insults. Either Bax or Bak opens channels and thereby releases the electron transport protein cytochrome c and other proteins from the intermembranous space into the cytoplasm. Cytochrome c binds the scaffolding protein Apaf-1. The C-terminal portion of Apaf1 is a negative regulator of apoptosis. The N-terminal region contains a caspase recruitment domain and an ATPase domain. Binding of cytochrome c and deoxyadenosine triphosphate removes the negative regulatory influence of the C-terminus of Apaf-1, thereby permitting binding and autoactivation of caspase-9. Activated caspase-9, in turn, activates caspases-3 and -7, thus initiating cell death. In addition, permeabilization of the mitochondrial outer membrane results in the loss of function of the electron transport chain, which is essential for most mitochondrial functions, including ATP generation.

Expression of Genes Involved in Apoptosis During Liver Regeneration

Liver regeneration is a complex process that involves a balance of cell replication, apoptosis, and remodeling and is orchestrated by several molecular mediators. Genes involved in apoptosis are actively expressed in the regenerating liver. These genes include the inducing genes c-*fos*, c-*jun*, c-*myc*, *TP53*, *Bax*, *Bad*, *Bak*, and *TGF-β*; the apoptosis inhibitory genes, *Bcl-2*, *Bcl-X_L*, *TRPM-2/clusterin*; and the *Rb* gene. Some of these genes are also involved in cell proliferation through regulation of the cell cycle.

PROTEIN SYNTHESIS AND DEGRADATION IN THE LIVER

Hepatic Gene Expression

Compared with most organs, the liver expresses many genes. Over 90% of plasma proteins and about 15% of the total protein mass of the body are produced in the liver.[87] As in all mammalian cells, gene expression is initiated by transcription of the gene into an RNA transcript, mediated by RNA polymerase II. The nascent RNA is modified by capping of the 5′-terminus with 7-methylguanosine, excision of the noncoding intervening sequences (introns), splicing together of the coding sequences (exons), and, in most cases, polyadenylation at the 3′-end. The processed mRNA is actively transported out of the nucleus. In the cytoplasm, the association of the mRNA with the 40S ribosomal subunit and methionine RNA requires several initiation factors, a cap-binding protein, and ATP hydrolysis.

Once this initiation complex is formed, the 60S ribosomal subunit is recruited, and polypeptide chain elongation proceeds as specific tRNAs recognize corresponding codons and sequentially attach appropriate amino acids. Chain elongation requires elongation factors and energy provided by GTP hydrolysis. Cessation of translation at the stop codons requires recognition by a termination factor. In most cases, the nascent protein is processed by cleavage of an amino terminal signal peptide. Many proteins undergo further proteolytic cleavage, cotranslational glycosylation, and modification of the carbohydrate moieties in the Golgi apparatus before being secreted or transported to other intracellular organelles (see earlier).

Gene expression is regulated at multiple levels. Gene transcription is regulated by the state of the chromatin, which determines the accessibility of specific genes to the transcription machinery, and binding of specific transcription factors that promote or repress gene transcription. Posttranscriptional regulation can involve differential splicing, modulation of mRNA stability and efficiency of translation, protein folding, association with self or other proteins, or phosphorylation or other forms of protein modification. Modulation of protein degradation is another important mechanism that regulates net protein content. All of these modes of regulation are active in liver cells and are areas of intensive investigation.

Some genes expressed in hepatocytes, loosely termed "housekeeping genes," are expressed in many other organs as well. In addition, the expression of many other genes occurs preferentially or uniquely in the liver. Expression of these liver-specific genes permits the liver to perform essential functions of the body, including secretion of plasma proteins, gluconeogenesis, glycogen storage, glucose metabolism, cholesterol homeostasis, bile salt production, and detoxification of endogenous metabolites and exogenous substances. A series of *cis*-acting elements in specific genes mediate their hepatocyte-preferred expression.[88] These *cis*-acting DNA elements bind different families of HNFs. Although none of these factors is entirely liver-specific, high levels of liver-preferred gene expression occur only in the presence of combinatorial interaction of these transcription factors. Maintenance of hepatocyte-enriched expression of specific transcription factors involves cross-regulation by other unrelated liver-enriched transcription factors. Some of the transcription factors involved in hepatocyte specificity are also important in hepatic tissue specification during embryogenesis. Many of the transcription factors are normally located in the cytoplasm. Binding of hormones or cytokines to their respective cell surface receptors causes conformational changes in the cytoplasmic domain of these receptors, often through phosphorylation. Such conformational changes lead to a series of events that eventually lead to the translocation of specific transcription factors to the nucleus and their binding to the respective *cis*-acting elements in the regulatory regions of genes. Thus extracellular signals are transduced to a series of intracellular events, culminating in the induction or repression of gene expression.

Regulation of gene transcription is the most important, but not the only, mechanism of modulation of gene expression. Stability of the RNA, translational regulation, and posttranslational modifications can all affect the steady-state concentration, intracellular or extracellular location, and activity of a given gene product. The major plasma proteins synthesized and secreted by the liver are shown in Table 74.1.

TABLE 74.1 Some Serum Proteins Produced by the Liver

Protein	Molecular Weight (Daltons)	Function	Association With Liver Disease	Acute-Phase Response
α_1-Acid glycoprotein (orosomucoid)	40,000	Inhibits proliferative response of peripheral lymphocytes to mitogens	–	Increased
Albumin	66,500	Binding protein, osmotic regulator	Decreased in chronic liver disease	Decreased
Alpha-fetoprotein	66,300	Binding protein	Increased in hepatocellular carcinoma	Decreased
α_1-Antichymotrypsin	68,000	Inhibits chymotrypsin-like serine proteinase	–	Increased
α_1-Antitrypsin (α_1-AT)	54,000	Inhibitor of elastin	Missense mutations associated with liver disease	Increased
Ceruloplasmin	132,000	Ferroxidase	Decreased in Wilson disease	Increased
Complement C3	185,000	Complement pathway	–	Increased
Complement C4	200,000	Complement pathway	–	Increased
C-reactive protein	118,000	Binds pathogens and damaged cells to initiate their elimination	–	Increased
Ferritin	450,000	Intracellular iron storage	Increased in hemochromatosis	Increased
Fibrinogen	340,000	Precursor to fibrin in hemostasis, wound healing	Decreased in chronic liver disease	Increased
Haptoglobin	≈100,000	Binds hemoglobin released by hemolysis	–	Increased
Serum amyloid A	9000	Unknown	–	Increased
Transferrin	79,500	Iron-binding protein	Increased in iron deficiency	Decreased
Coagulation factor VIII	267,009	Coagulation factor	Absent or mutated in hemophilia A	

Data from Katz N, Jungermam K. Metabolic heterogeneity of the liver. In: Tavoloni N, Berk PD, eds. *Hepatic Transport and Bile Secretion: Physiology and Pathophysiology*. New York: Raven Press; 1993:55; Putnan FW. Progress in plasma proteins. In: *The Plasma Proteins: Structure, Function, and Genetic Control*. Orlando: Academic Press; 1984:45.

Nuclear Receptors

Modulation of metabolic pathways and detoxicating mechanisms according to the needs of the body often requires coordinated upregulation or repression of the expression of a set of genes. In many cases, such coordination is mediated by nuclear receptors, such as retinoid X receptor (RXR), liver X-receptor, farnesoid X-receptor (FXR), constitutive androstane receptor (CAR), peroxisome proliferator activator receptor (PPAR), and thyroid hormone receptor (TR).[89] For example, expression of proteins that mediate bilirubin uptake by hepatocytes, intracellular storage of bilirubin, glucuronidation of bilirubin, and bile canalicular excretion of bilirubin glucuronides may all be regulated by CAR. Nuclear receptors mediate induction or repression of genes by small nonprotein molecules. For example, phenobarbital binds to CAR in the cytoplasm, leading to the translocation of CAR to the nucleus and thereby resulting in simultaneous induction of multiple genes that have CAR-binding elements in their *cis*-regulatory regions. Similarly, bile acids bind to FXR, fibrates bind to PPAR, and thyroid hormones bind to TR. In most cases, nuclear receptors function by forming heterodimers with RXR, although some nuclear receptors can function as homodimers.

PROTEIN FOLDING

Proteins that are destined for export to intracellular membranes or secretion into the plasma are translocated into the ER where folding takes place prior to secretion through the Golgi apparatus.[90] The ER contains a number of molecular chaperones and folding catalysts that promote efficient folding. All chaperones enable and promote protein folding and assembly, but their specific functions differ. Many chaperones work in tandem with one other. Some molecular chaperones bind to nascent chains as they emerge from the ribosome and protect aggregation-prone hydrophobic regions. Other chaperones are involved in later stages of folding, particularly for complex proteins that include oligomeric species and multimolecular assemblies.

In addition to promoting proper folding, chaperones play an important role in the "quality control" of proteins through a complex series of glycosylation and deglycosylation processes and prevention of misfolded proteins from being secreted from the cell.[91] The unfolded or misfolded proteins are targeted for degradation through the ubiquitin-proteasome pathway.[92] Up to one-half of all polypeptide chains fail to satisfy the quality control mechanism in the ER, and for some proteins, such as the cystic fibrosis transmembrane conductance regulator, the success rate is even lower. The proportion of molecules that misfold is increased greatly in mutant proteins with amino acid substitutions. Some molecular chaperones are able to rescue misfolded proteins to enable them to have a second chance to fold correctly. Under some circumstances, chaperones can solubilize proteins that have aggregated because of misfolding. In some cases, energy for such active intervention may be derived from ATP hydrolysis. Many molecular chaperones, such as the heat shock protein, are upregulated in stressful situations, when protein misfolding is more prone to occur.

In addition to molecular chaperones, several classes of folding catalysts accelerate steps in the folding process. For example, peptidylprolyl isomerases increase the rate of *cis/trans* isomerization of peptide bonds involving proline residues, and protein disulfide isomerases enhance formation and reorganization of disulfide bonds within proteins.

PROTEIN CATABOLISM

Like protein synthesis, proteolysis is a major process that contributes to the body protein turnover. The autophagic-lysosomal pathway and the ubiquitin/proteasome pathway are the two major mechanisms of protein degradation. The autophagic-lysosomal mechanism is responsible for bulk degradation of endogenous proteins, as well as degradation of other cellular components such as RNA, carbohydrates, and lipids. One function of this pathway may be seen as a cell restructuring mechanism. The autophagy system is regulated physiologically by plasma levels of the amino acids leucine, glutamine, tyrosine, phenylalanine, proline, methionine, tryptophan, and histidine, probably through binding to cell surface receptors and subsequent intracellular signaling. Protein kinase cascades, such as mTOR, Erk, eIF2a, and others, may be involved in the regulation of autophagy. Amino acids may exert their effects through these pathways in combination with insulin.[93] Chaperone-mediated autophagy (CMA) is a selective mechanism for the degradation of altered cytosolic proteins in lysosomes. Synthesis of a lysosomal receptor that is critical for CMA declines in aged animals, thereby leading to the accumulation of altered proteins and eventually leading to the characteristic functional alterations in the aging liver and other organs. In transgenic mice in which the abundance of the lysosomal receptor for CMA is retained until advanced age, less damaged proteins accumulate intracellularly, and liver functions are maintained at youthful levels.[94]

The ubiquitin/proteasome pathway is the principal mechanism for turnover of normally short-lived proteins in mammalian cells.[95] Ubiquitin is a small protein that can link covalently to itself or to other proteins, either as monomers or as chains of polyubiquitin. Ubiquitin is added to a target protein by ubiquitin-activating, ubiquitin-conjugating, and ubiquitin-ligating enzymes. The first function attributed to ubiquitin was the covalent binding to misfolded proteins, thereby directing proteasome-dependent proteolysis. Now, ubiquitin and ubiquitin-related proteins are also known to direct specific proteins through the endocytotic pathway by modifying cargo proteins, as well as by regulating components of the cytoplasmic protein trafficking machinery. By regulating the turnover of mitotic cyclins, ubiquitination plays an important role in cell cycle regulation.[96,97]

Although the ubiquitin/proteasome pathway has been generally considered a separate process from the lysosomal proteolysis mechanism, ubiquitination is sometimes required for lysosomal proteolysis. A subset of endocytosed proteins must be conjugated to ubiquitin as a trigger for internalization from the plasma membrane.[98,99] Thus ubiquitin conjugation appears to be important in several protein trafficking steps, including endocytosis. Primary structure of the protein to be degraded contains amino acid sequences, such as hydrophobic amino acid clusters or N-terminal motifs that specify its stability. The secondary structure may also determine its conformational stability or expose the hydrophobic regions to the environment. At a tertiary level, proteasomes can degrade only soluble proteins, but not protein aggregates. Although most misfolded soluble proteins are degraded by proteasomes, when the proteasomal system is saturated, such proteins can be degraded by micro- and macro-autophagy. Another level of cross-talk between the proteasomal degradation and autophagy is related to the type of ubiquitin, or ubiquitin-like protein, that is attached to the protein to be degraded. Misfolded or damaged proteins are first detected by the chaperone/cochaperone system. Proteins misfolded during synthesis or denatured by heat shock, oxidation, glycation, etc. become attached to cochaperones, such as C-terminus of Hsp70-interacting protein and Bcl-2-associated athanogene proteins function as molecular switches that direct the misfolded proteins to the proteosomal versus autophagic pathways for degradation. Consequence of early identification by chaperone/cochaperone complexes is the attachment of a tag, usually ubiquitin, to the protein to be degraded. The type of ubiquitination may direct the substrate toward one or the other degradative pathway. For example, polyubiquitin chains linked to lysine-48 of a protein may target the substrate to the proteasome, whereas those linked to lysine-63 may target it to the autophagic pathway.[100]

The Liver as an Immunoregulatory Organ

Extensive vascularization, dual blood supply from the portal vein and hepatic artery, slow blood flow, and highly permeable fenestrated LSECs provide liver cells with extensive access to contents of both portal blood and the systemic circulation. From an immunological point of view, the liver sinusoids are lined with various specialized cells, including the LSECs, intravascular resident macrophages (Kupffer cells), and liver dendritic cells (DCs). Eighty percent of all body macrophages are present in the liver. In addition, myeloid cells, such as blood monocytes, scan the liver vasculature and can infiltrate into the liver, giving rise to liver DCs and monocyte-derived macrophages that are distinct from Kupffer cells. Each of these cells can present antigens, as well as produce cytokines and chemokines. Therefore these cells play a key role in initiating and directing liver immune responses toward immune tolerance or inflammatory response. During homeostasis, the liver is constantly exposed to nonself proteins derived from food or resident microbiota that constantly present bacterial endotoxins. Specialized mechanisms have evolved to induce tolerance to these harmless antigens. Liver tolerance is relevant in spontaneous acceptance of liver allografts in some recipients of liver transplants. On the flipside, these tolerance mechanisms may also allow viruses and parasites to chronically persist in the liver. However, mechanisms exist in the liver to rapidly switch to inflammatory immune response. The cellular and molecular mechanisms of tolerance and inflammatory immune response have been reviewed recently[101] and are briefly summarized below.

Some mechanisms are key in guiding the decision between immune homeostasis and triggering of inflammation. Homeostatic immune tolerance is mediated by the resident "reticuloendothelial network" (macrophages and DCs) that samples the antigenic environment of the liver, attenuates the passing lymphocytes through cell-cell interactions, and maintains an immunosuppressive environment by secreting regulatory cytokines such as IL-10, TGF-β, IDO, and PGE2. Cell-contact-dependent immune suppression involves the presentation of MHC-bound protein antigens to T cells, resulting in T-cell depletion or anergy, or production of regulatory T cells (T_{reg}). Homeostatic immunosuppression is triggered by constant low-level exposure to bacterial endotoxins, as well as liver-endogenous immunosuppressive factors such as prostaglandins and HSC-derived retinoic acid. Presentation of unconventional antigens, such as glycolipids, via CD1d to NKT cells and γδ T cells results in the secretion of cytokines such as IL-4, which inhibits classical activation of macrophages to M1 cells and promotes their differentiation into repair macrophages (M2 cells), coupled with secretion of IL-10 and TGF-β, resulting in reduction of inflammatory response. Cell-bound immunosuppression is mediated via surface markers such as PD-L1 and CTLA-4. Interestingly, actively invading $CD8^+$ T cells can be internalized by hepatocytes and degraded in the lysosomes. This process, which is independent of phagocytosis by Kupffer cells, plays a role in removing autoreactive CD^+ T cells.[102]

In contrast to the homeostatic immune tolerance, several triggers can switch the immune response to hepatic inflammation. Such triggers are often initiated by cytopathic effects to the liver. Inflammatory activation of Kupffer cells and chemokine-mediated infiltration of monocytes are key in a variety of inflammatory diseases. The TLR family senses danger signals by recognizing pathogen-associated molecular patterns, such as bacterial proteoglycans (via TLR2 and TLR4) or unconventional RNA or DNA structures (via TLR3, TLR7, and TLR9). TLR-mediated activation occurs as a result of high levels of the cognate ligands or simultaneous activation of several TLRs. Inflammatory immune response can also result from endogenous (nonforeign) stimuli, such as extracellular ATP, bile acids, uric acid, free cholesterol, or oxidized lipids, which are released during nonapoptotic cell death. These danger-associated molecular patterns (DAMPs) are sensed via multiprotein complexes, termed the inflammasomes, which lead to the activation and secretion of IL-1β and IL-18, two key cytokines that initiate innate immunity and activate monocytes, neutrophils, and NK cells. The liver also contains lymphoid cells that are normally found at mucosal sites, such as innate lymphoid cells and mucosa-associated invariant T cells, which respond to PAMPs and DAMPs, which are also termed alarmins.[103] Alarmins include the high mobility group protein B1 and IL-33, which are released from injured hepatocytes. Similarly, accumulation of bile acids outside the bile ducts increases the levels of inflammatory cytokines, for example, IL-1β, chemokines (CXCL1, CXCL9, CXCL10, CXCL11, CCL2, CCL5), growth factors (G-CSF, GM-CSF), and adhesion molecules (ICAM-1 and VCAM-1) that mediate firm adhesion to endothelial cells and diapedesis into the liver tissue. Functional diversity of macrophages and DCs, and the balance between proinflammatory and anti-inflammatory T-cell populations determine the ultimate pattern of hepatic immune response.

Hepatic Nutrient Metabolism

The liver is at the hub of numerous metabolic pathways. In this chapter, we will present a brief description of the role of the liver in energy metabolism. The liver provides energy continuously to the entire body through its ability to store and modulate the availability of systemic nutrients.[104] In turn, the metabolic function of the liver is regulated by hormones secreted by the pancreas, adrenals, thyroid, and adipose tissue, as well as neuronal inputs. A liver-adipose tissue-brain-pancreas axis,[105] as well as a gut-brain-liver axis,[106] orchestrates the management of the energy supply to body tissues. In addition to serving as a store for excess energy as lipids, the adipose tissue, particularly visceral fatty tissue that drains into the portal circulation, plays an active role in hepatic energy metabolism by releasing free fatty acids (FFAs) into plasma and releasing a series of adipokines that either increase or decrease insulin sensitivity in the liver and other tissues.[105] During nutrient absorption (fed state), the liver regulates nutrient flux as the absorbed nutrients are metabolized, modified for storage in the liver and fatty tissue, or made available to other organs as an energy source. During fasting, the energy supply is maintained from the stored fuel and by synthesis. Starvation induces breakdown of triglycerides in adipose tissues into FFAs and glycerol. FFAs reduce insulin sensitivity, thereby affecting glucose metabolism in muscles and the liver. FFAs bind and activate PPARs in liver and other tissues, thereby affecting their gene expression.[107] In the hepatocyte, most of the acetyl CoA produced by oxidation of FFA is used to synthesize ketone bodies (e.g., acetoacetate and β-hydroxybutyrate) that are released into circulation and used as an energy source by many peripheral tissues. The glycerol released by triglyceride hydrolysis is used by the liver for the synthesis of glucose, which is the only source of energy for neurons and red blood cells (RBCs), or of triglyceride. The triglyceride is packaged into very-low-density lipoproteins (VLDL) (see later) and returns to the adipose tissue.[108]

The role of a gut-brain-liver axis in glucose homeostasis has also been established.[106] In rats, lipids arriving in the intestine give rise to long-chain fatty acyl-coenzyme A by the action of acyl-CoA synthase, which sends an afferent signal to the nucleus of the solitary tract in the hindbrain through the vagus nerve. This signal leads to *N*-methyl-D-aspartate ion channel-dependent glutamatergic neurotransmission through the efferent vagal fibers that supply the liver, thereby resulting in a reduction in glucose production by the liver that precedes the actual postabsorptive glucose influx from the intestine. Thus the rapid gut-brain-liver communication helps prevent excessive fluctuation of the blood glucose level. Unfortunately, this mechanism becomes inoperative with continued intake of excessive calories for several days. Detailed reviews of hepatic nutrient metabolism are available elsewhere.[109]

CARBOHYDRATE METABOLISM

Glucose is the primary energy source for the brain, erythrocytes, muscle, and renal cortex. Maintaining adequate circulating levels of glucose is essential for the central nervous system, which normally uses glucose as its major metabolic fuel. After a person fasts for 24–48 hours, the brain can use ketones as a metabolic fuel, thereby reducing its glucose requirement by 50%–70%.[90] The liver is the principal organ that maintains total carbohydrate stores by synthesizing glycogen and generating glucose from precursors.[110] Glucose is synthesized from nonoxidative metabolic products of glucose (pyruvate and lactate) that are generated predominantly by RBCs and from amino acid precursors that are derived predominantly from muscle during prolonged starvation or exercise.

Circadian Rhythm of Gluconeogenesis. Circadian clocks align nutrient availability-related behavior and energy metabolism with the diurnal cycle.[111] The mammalian circadian clock consists of heterodimeric complexes of the transcription factor locomotor output cycles kaput (CLOCK) and the brain and muscle Arnt-like protein 1 (BMAL1), which initiate expression of period (PER)1/2 and cryptochrome (CRY)1/2. CRY1/2 and PER1/2 repress the transcriptional activity of CLOCK by feedback inhibition. In addition, Bmal1 expression is stimulated by retinoid-related orphan receptors and repressed by nuclear hormone receptor REV-ERBa. Degradation of PER and CRY shortens the length of circadian period, while the stabilization of CRY lengthens the period. In addition to repressing CLOCK, CRY1 suppresses hepatic gluconeogenesis by regulating CREB/cAMP signaling via rhythmic repression of glucocorticoid receptor and decreasing levels of nuclear FoxO1 that downregulate expression of gluconeogenic genes. Ubiquitination-mediated proteasomal degradation of CRY1 is known to be regulated by multiple factors. Recent studies on rodents have shown that macroautophagy affects the circadian clock by selectively degrading CRY1. Degradation of CRY1 removes its inhibitory effect on gluconeogenesis at a time of the day when rodents rely on gluconeogenesis, thus synchronizing CRY1 degradation with the need for maintenance of blood glucose when nutrients are not available. High-fat diet accelerates CRY1 autophagy, thereby contributing to obesity-associated hyperglycemia.[112]

Regulation of Glucose Uptake and Efflux From Hepatocytes. Glucose is a critical molecule in the metabolic pathway because it can be converted to amino acids, fatty acids, or glycogen, the major storage form of glucose. Glucose enters hepatocytes via the glucose transporter-2, which facilitates the diffusion of glucose across the sinusoidal membrane.[113] Glucose transporter-2 differs from other members of the glucose transporter family in that it is independent of metabolic conditions or insulin levels. Because of the low-affinity, high-capacity characteristics of glucose transporter-2, intrahepatic glucose concentration is determined by the plasma glucose level, which, in turn, is regulated by glucokinase (GK) activity (see "Formation of Glucose-6-Phosphate" later).[114] Glucose transporter-1, which is present in the brain, RBCs, and hepatocytes, particularly in zone 3, is a low-capacity, high-affinity glucose transporter that permits glucose uptake by hepatocytes when the circulating glucose concentration is low. Increased expression of glucose transporter-1 during fasting enhances glucose uptake by hepatocytes. Hepatocellular glucose homeostasis is maintained by interlinking pathways that are regulated by multiple signals, which prevent competing pathways from operating at the same time.[115] Fig. 74.3 illustrates these pathways and the modulating influences that control the metabolic flux of glucose and other sugars, such as fructose.

Formation of Glucose-6-Phosphate. Rapid conversion of glucose to glucose-6-phosphate (glucose-6-P) modulates the glucose concentration within the hepatocyte, thereby regulating influx or efflux of glucose from the hepatocyte.[110] Glucose-6-P is a nodal branch point compound that can enter three independent metabolic pathways: (1) synthesis of glycogen, which can be mobilized rapidly during fasting; (2) anaerobic glycolysis via the Embden-Meyerhof pathway, which generates pyruvate or lactate as a substrate for the tricarboxylic acid (Krebs) cycle in mitochondria; or (3) the pentose-phosphate shunt, which generates reducing equivalents necessary for anaerobic glycolysis and fatty acid synthesis. The pentose-phosphate shunt is regulated by the activity of mitochondrial glucose-6-P dehydrogenase.[92] Conversion of glucose to glucose-6-P is catalyzed by hexokinase, which accepts several different hexose substrates, and GK (also termed hexokinase type 4 or D), which is expressed predominantly in the liver and pancreas and is specific for glucose.[116]

A low-affinity, high-capacity system, GK is not inhibited by the reaction product, glucose-6-P. Therefore the level of GK activity regulates hepatocellular glucose concentration, which determines the net uptake of glucose by hepatocytes from hepatic sinusoidal plasma. GK is activated by insulin and inhibited by glucagon.[109] Mutations in the GK gene are associated with some rare cases of maturity-onset diabetes of young adults.[116] Fructose-1-phosphate modulates GK activity by regulating the inhibitory activity of a GK regulatory protein.[117] The regulation of GK by fructose is thought to prevent futile cycling between glucose and glucose-6-P that consumes ATP. Starvation decreases GK activity, thereby promoting glucose efflux from the hepatocyte.

Conversion of Glucose-6-Phosphate to Glucose. Conversion of glucose-6-P to glucose is catalyzed by glucose-6-phosphatase (glu-6-Pase), a multisubunit enzyme with its active site located within the ER lumen.[97] Thus glucose-6-P needs to traverse the ER membrane to be dephosphorylated. Inherited deficiency of glu-6-Pase causes glycogen storage disease type Ia.[118] Glucose-6-P transport is mediated by a microsomal transport protein, which, when defective, causes type Ib glycogen storage disease. As expected, glu-6-Pase activity is increased by starvation, resulting in an increase in hepatocellular glucose concentration and consequent efflux of glucose into the sinusoidal space by the bidirectional glucose transporter-2.

Glucose-6-P can enter the pentose monophosphate shunt that generates the reduced form of nicotinamide dinucleotide phosphate (NADPH). The other possible metabolic fate of glucose-6-P is conversion to fructose-6-P, which can enter the fructose 6-P-fructose 1,6-diphosphate (fructose-1,6-P_2) pathway. Fructose-1,6-P_2 modulates the activity of pyruvate kinase (PK), which can affect substrate cycling in the subsequent pyruvate (PYR)-phosphoenol pyruvate (PEP) pathway. These opposing enzyme reactions regulate the formation of gluconeogenesis precursors and glycolysis.

The relative production of fructose 6-P and fructose-1,6-P_2 is regulated by the opposing action of 6-phosphofructo-1-phosphokinase (6-PK-1-K) and fructose-1,6-bisphosphatase (fruc-1,6_2Pase).[91] Within this cycle is a unique enzyme: 6-phosphofructo-2-kinase/fructose-2,6-biphosphatase (6-fru kinase/Pase). This enzyme, which combines the properties of both a 6-PF-2K and its corresponding phosphorylase enzyme activity, produces the regulatory product fructose-2,6-P_2. Fructose-2,6-P_2 is a potent activator of 6-PF-1-K and inhibitor of fruc-1,6_2Pase. Moreover, it favors the formation of the fructose-1,6-P_2 product. The enzyme is regulated by both hormonal and nutrient regulations and serves as another modulator of glucose metabolism. During starvation, when fructose-2,6-P_2 levels are low,

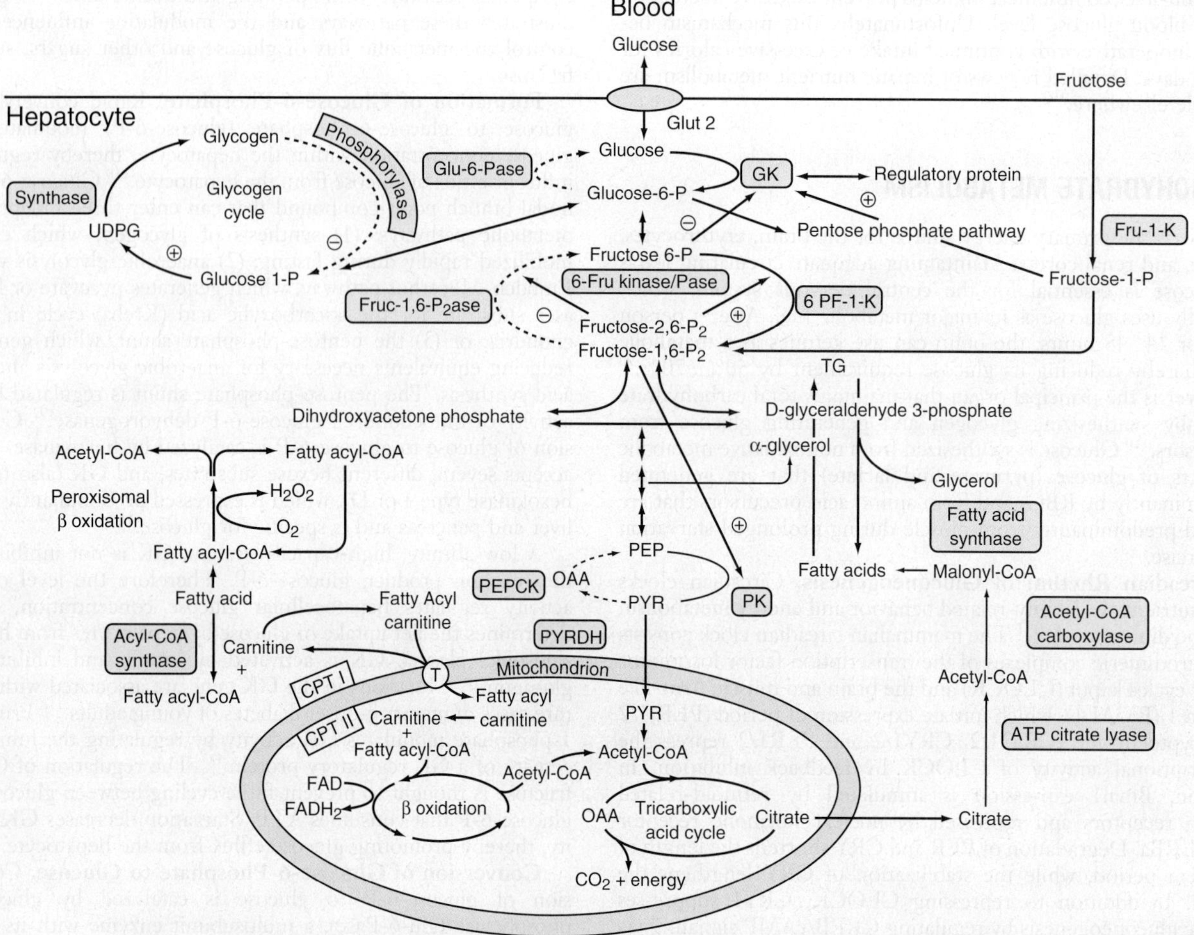

Fig. 74.3 Hepatic carbohydrate and lipid metabolism. Gluconeogenic pathways are identified by *dashed lines*. *6-Fru Kinase/Pase*, 6-Phosphofructo-2-kinase/fructose-2,6-biphosphatase; *6 PF-1-K*, 6-phosphofructo-1-kinase; *ATP*, adenosine triphosphate; *CoA*, coenzyme A; *CPT*, carnitine palmitoyl-transferase; *FAD*, flavine adenine dinucleotide; *$FADH_2$*, reduced flavine adenine dinucleotide; *Fru-1-K*, hepatic fructokinase; *Fruc-1,6-P_2ase*, fructose-1,6-biphosphatase; *Fructose-1-P*, fructose-1-phosphate; *Fructose-1,6-P_2*, fructose-1,6-diphosphate; *Frucose-2,6-P_2*, fructose-2,6-diphosphate; *Fructose 6-P*, fructose-6-phosphate; *GK*, glucokinase; *Glucose-6-P*, glucose-6-phosphate; *Glu-6-Pase*, glucose-6-phosphatase; *Glut 2*, glucose transporter 2; *OAA*, oxaloacetate; *PEP*, phosphoenol pyruvate; *PEPCK*, phosphoenol pyruvate carboxykinase; *PK*, pyruvate kinase; *PYR*, pyruvate; *PYRDH*, pyruvate dehydrogenase; *T*, carnitine:acylcarnitine transferase; *UDPG*, uridine diphosphate glucose. (Data from Piklis SJ, Granner DK. Molecular physiology of the regulation of hepatic gluconeogenesis and glycolysis. *Annu Rev Physiol*. 1992;54:885–909.)

gluconeogenesis is enhanced. On the other hand, high levels of 6-fru kinase/Pase found during refeeding and insulin administration promote glycolysis and fatty acid synthesis. The phosphorylation status of the 6-fru kinase/Pase is regulated by the cAMP-dependent kinase site and phosphatase 2A activity.

From fructose-1,6-P_2, a sequence of four biochemical reactions leads to the formation of PEP with generation of eight molecules of ATP.[104] PEP can then be metabolized into PYR as part of the third regulatory cycle in glucose metabolism. PK, which transforms PEP to PYR, generates two ATP molecules. PYR is another nodal branch point in the metabolic pathway, from which it can undergo further metabolism in mitochondria to form acetyl-CoA. Thereafter, it can undergo aerobic metabolism by the tricarboxylic acid cycle. In this pathway, PYR may be metabolized ultimately to water and carbon dioxide, with the production of 15 molecules of ATP per molecule of PYR. Other products of the tricarboxylic acid cycle are also precursors for fatty acid (citrate) or amino acids by means of oxaloacetate formation. Fructose-1,6-P_2 is also an inducer of PK.[119] In the reverse reaction, PYR is metabolized to oxaloacetate, which is a precursor to the amino acid L-aspartate. Oxaloacetate is converted by the energy-dependent activity of PEPCK, an important regulator of gluconeogenesis. PEPCK expression is inhibited by insulin at the transcriptional level[109,119] and is upregulated during fasting and in diabetes mellitus.

Hepatic Metabolism of Galactose and Fructose. Lactose, a major disaccharide present in human and cow milk, is split into glucose and galactose. Galactose can be converted to glucose-6-P, after which it can be used for glycogen synthesis, or it can be oxidized further to form PYR or acetyl-CoA for additional energy generation or fatty acid synthesis.[104] Galactose is initially phosphorylated by galactokinase to form galactose-1-phosphate (galactose-1-P). In the presence of uridine diphosphoglucose, further metabolism by uridyltransferase forms glucose-1-phosphate (glucose-1-P) and UDP-galactose. UDP-galactose can be epimerized by UDP-glucose-4-epimerase to form UDP-glucose, which is a precursor to glucose-1-P. Glucose-1-P can be converted to glucose-6-P. Thus, like glucose, galactose can participate in the glycolytic pathway.

Fructose, an abundant sugar in the diet, is absorbed by the intestinal epithelium by a sodium-independent carrier distinct from the intestinal glucose transporter. It is converted to fructose-1-phosphate (fructose-1-P) by hepatic fructokinase (Fru-1-K), using either ATP or GTP as a cofactor. Fructose-1-P activates GK activity by removing the inhibitory regulatory protein. Fructose-1-P does not enter the glucogenic pathway but is further metabolized by fructose-1-phosphate aldolase to form two trioses: dihydroxylacetone phosphate and glyceraldehyde-3-phosphate. Dihydroxylacetone phosphate may be isomerized to glyceraldehyde phosphate and enter the glycolytic pathway or may be reduced to glyceraldehyde-3-phosphate and provide the glycerol backbone for triacylglycerol and phospholipids. Glyceraldehyde-3-phosphate may be combined with dihydroxylacetone phosphate by aldolase B ultimately to form fructose-1,6-P_2. Depending on the metabolic requirements of the liver, fructose-1,6-P_2 can be used for gluconeogenesis and glycogen synthesis or may be subjected to glycolysis, ultimately resulting in the formation of lactate. Because fructose enters the carbohydrate cycle at the second regulatory step, fructose is a better substrate for lipogenesis in the liver than glucose. Aldolase B deficiency results in hereditary fructose intolerance as a result of excess fructose-1-P build-up. Treatment consists of avoidance of sucrose and fructose in the diet.

Glycogen Formation. Glycogen stored in the liver is the main source of rapidly available glucose for the glucose-dependent tissues, such as RBCs, retina, renal medulla, and brain.[120] Hepatic glycogen stores contain up to a 2-day supply of glucose before gluconeogenesis occurs, mainly from lactate, a 3-carbon end product of anaerobic glucose metabolism.[104,121] Hepatic gluconeogenesis produces up to 240 mg of glucose a day, which is approximately twice the metabolic need of the RBCs, retina, and brain. The 3-carbon precursors generated by anaerobic metabolism from muscle, intestine, liver, or RBCs may account for up to 50% of the glycogen pool formed during nonabsorptive states. Alanine, another major glucose precursor, is generated by the catabolism of muscle proteins, which is a major cause of muscle wasting during prolonged fasting. Glycogen stored in muscle is used locally and cannot be exported out of the cell because muscles lack glu-6-Pase. The relative contribution of each of the precursors to glycogen synthesis depends on the nutritional status, amount, and route of glucose administration (oral vs. intravenous) and on hormonal regulation.

Rapid switching between glycogen synthesis and breakdown is mediated by a cascade of enzymes that are regulated by local nutrients and hormones.[104] Glycogen phosphorylase, which is activated by phosphorylation, catalyzes the breakdown of glycogen subunits, and glycogen synthase, which is activated by dephosphorylation, catalyzes the addition of UDP-glucose to the expanding glycogen chain. In addition, glucose and glucose-6-P are allosteric activators of the synthase enzyme, whereas glucose binding inactivates the phosphorylase.

Glycogen exists as two distinct populations consisting of proglycogen, with a molecular weight of approximately 4×10^5, and macroglycogen, with a molecular weight of 1×10^7, the concentrations of which depend on the relative activities of enzymes favoring proglycogen formation (phosphorylase and debranching enzymes) and those favoring glycogenin formation (branching enzymes). The ability of glycogenin to initiate the formation of glycogen is important in hepatic carbohydrate metabolism. The existence of these two distinct pools of glycogen permits subtle control of glucose levels, and their relative contributions could have a physiologic role in disease states such as diabetes mellitus.

Regulation of Glycolytic-Gluconeogenic Pathways. The glycolytic-gluconeogenic pathways are regulated by hormonal signals and the relative availability of nutrients. Insulin upregulates the expression of genes that encode the glycolytic enzymes and represses the expression of metabolic enzymes responsible for gluconeogenesis. Glucagon, catecholamines, corticosteroids, and growth hormone increase cellular cAMP levels, thereby augmenting the gluconeogenic pathway. In many cases, posttranscriptional mRNA stabilization or degradation, posttranslational phosphorylation or end-product inhibition, or allosteric modulation contributes to the relative abundance or activity of specific enzymes.[110,119] Glucose and fructose modulate the enzyme activities by direct inhibition or by allosteric modulation of the enzymes. In the fed state, high activity of GK, 6-PF-1-K, and PK induced by insulin favors formation of PYR, with low activity of PEPCK and other gluconeogenic enzymes. During fasting, the fall in plasma insulin levels removes the inhibition of the gluconeogenic enzymes PEPCK and fruc-1,6-P_2ase. Simultaneously, an increase in glucagon and β-adrenergic agonists raises intracellular cAMP levels, leading to inhibition of 6-PK-2 kinase activity and stimulation of fruc-2,6-Pase, thereby reducing fructose-2,6-P_2 concentration and activation of fruc-1,6-P_2ase, with a net increase in gluconeogenesis. After a prolonged fast, gluconeogenesis is further stimulated by an increase in the supply of substrate and alterations in the concentration of various enzymes.

Carbohydrate Metabolism in Cirrhosis. Patients with cirrhosis have an increased frequency of hyperglycemia and relative hyperinsulinemia.[122] The hyperglycemia may be explained by decreased glucose uptake by muscle and reduced glycogen storage in liver and muscle. These changes lead to insulin resistance, which causes an increase in plasma insulin levels. Other causes of relative insulin resistance include increased serum FFA levels that can inhibit glucose uptake by muscle, altered second messenger activity after insulin binds to its receptor, and increased serum concentrations of cytokines that result from elevated serum levels of LPS. Increased levels of glucagon and catecholamines may be contributing factors. The net result is impaired nonoxidative use of glucose with decreased storage of glycogen and impaired uptake of glucose by muscle, thereby causing a relative insulin-resistant state similar to that found in patients with diabetes mellitus and obesity.

LIPID METABOLISM

Fatty acids are an important energy source for the liver and serve as an efficient fuel store within and outside the liver because oxidation of fatty acids yields the highest ATP production of any metabolic fuel.[104] In addition, most organs are capable of using fatty acids as a fuel.[123] The liver plays a central role in regulating the body's total fatty acid needs. Excess glucose can be converted to fatty acid for future use and stored at distal sites such as adipose tissue and delivered by lipoproteins (see "Lipid Transport" later). Triglycerides are stored in the cytoplasm of hepatocytes, where they are enclosed in a monolayer of phospholipids to form lipid droplets, which are important in the energy balance of the cell and the whole organism. Under conditions of excess lipid accumulation in the hepatocyte, for example, in overnutrition, the risk of acquiring insulin resistance increases. Lipid droplet formation may require a family of PPARα-induced ER proteins, termed fat-inducing transcripts 1 and 2 (FIT-1 and FIT-2).[124] Beta oxidation of fatty acids in mitochondria and peroxisomes has different physiologic consequences.[125] Furthermore, fatty acids are structural components of cell membranes and are important in cellular function and cell anchoring. The regulation of fatty acid synthesis and transport of fatty acids to other organs in association with lipoproteins constitutes another critical role of the liver in managing the metabolic needs of the entire body.

Fatty Acid Synthesis. Fatty acid synthesis occurs in the cytosol and is regulated closely by the availability of acetyl-CoA, which forms the basic subunit of the developing fatty acid carbon chain.[104] Acetyl-CoA is synthesized predominantly in mitochondria and is derived mainly from carbohydrate metabolism, with a small fraction coming from amino acids. Acetyl-CoA is condensed with oxaloacetate to form citrate, which is exported from the mitochondria and is then cleaved by the cytosolic ATP citrate lyase to produce oxaloacetate and acetyl-CoA. Conversion of acetyl-CoA to malonyl-CoA by the action of acetyl-CoA carboxylase is the first step in fatty acid synthesis. Acetyl-CoA carboxylase is the key enzyme in regulating fatty acid synthesis because it provides the necessary building blocks for elongation of the fatty acid carbon chain.[126]

Malonyl-CoA is used by a set of enzymatic activities contained within a single-peptide chain that comprises the remarkable fatty acid synthase system.[104] Malonyl-CoA binds to acyl carrier protein (ACP). Catalytic activity is contained within two distinct domains that catalyze sequential condensation, reduction, dehydrogenation, and reduction, which constitute the fatty acid synthetic cycle. Two NADPH molecules are required for each 2-carbon unit that is added to the growing fatty acid chain. After completion of the first cycle, the 4-carbon butyl group is transferred from ACP to a peripheral thiol, thereby allowing it to accept the next malonyl-CoA group to restart the entire cycle. The cycle continues for additional six or seven rounds until a carbon-16 (palmitate) or carbon-18 (stearate) fatty acid is synthesized. Fatty acid-CoA is then released and used for other metabolic pathways.

Further elongation of the fatty acid chain can occur either in the mitochondrion or within the microsomal membrane.[104] In the mitochondrion, the first step is mediated by enoyl-CoA reductase. Microsomal elongation uses malonyl-CoA to increase the size of fatty acyl-CoA in a process that involves four separate enzymatic reactions. The elongation ability of microsomes is tissue dependent and serves the needs of specific organs. The fatty acid chain elongates until an appropriate length has been achieved, and the fatty acid is then esterified with glycerol to form triglycerides. These newly formed triglycerides can be transported by lipoproteins to distal sites for storage and use. In situations of excess carbohydrates, PYR can be converted to acetyl-CoA by the mitochondrial pyruvate dehydrogenase complex to serve as fatty acid precursors, although lipogenesis from carbohydrates consumes about 25% of the energy contained in the carbohydrates.

Beta Oxidation of Fatty Acids. Fatty acid beta oxidation is an important source of energy for many organs, including the liver. Beta oxidation occurs in mitochondria and peroxisomes, and the process requires transport of substrates across the membranes delimiting these organelles.

Mitochondrial Beta Oxidation. Fatty acids are translocated across the mitochondrial membranes by first undergoing fatty acyl-CoA formation by the activity of distinct fatty acyl-CoA synthetases that are specific for short-, medium-, or long-chain fatty acids in the mitochondrial outer membrane.[104,127] In the inner mitochondrial membrane, the conjugation of fatty acyl-CoA with carnitine is catalyzed by carnitine palmitoyltransferase I, with formation of fatty acylcarnitine, which is translocated into the mitochondrion, in exchange for free carnitine, by an integral inner membrane protein, fatty acylcarnitine:carnitine translocase.[128] Inside the mitochondrion, a reverse reaction mediated by carnitine palmitoyltransferase II releases fatty acyl-CoA, which is now a substrate for beta oxidation. The first step that is unique to beta oxidation is formation of *trans*-enol fatty acid, which is generated by acyl-CoA dehydrogenase. Acyl-CoA dehydrogenase transfers two electrons to flavin adenine dinucleotide (FAD), which then transfers them to the electron transport chain in the mitochondrion. 3-Keto fatty acyl-CoA then undergoes a series of sequential reactions to acetyl-CoA and fatty acyl-CoA, which undergo another round of beta oxidation. Acetyl-CoA can enter the tricarboxylic acid cycle, thereby generating 12 ATP, or it can enter the 3-hydroxyl methyl glutaryl-CoA cycle to form ketone bodies. Only mitochondria in the liver are capable of forming ketone bodies. Regulation of mitochondrial beta oxidation lies with fatty acylcarnitine formation, which is catalyzed by carnitine palmitoyltransferase I.[128] Malonyl-CoA, the basic subunit of fatty acid synthesis, is a potent inhibitor of carnitine palmitoyltransferase I and thus prevents beta oxidation and fatty acid synthesis from occurring concurrently.

Peroxisomal Beta Oxidation. Peroxisomes have lesser capacity than mitochondria for beta oxidation of fatty acid. The relative contribution of peroxisomes to beta oxidation depends on the fatty acid chain length and administration of peroxisome proliferators. In contrast to fatty acid oxidation in the mitochondrion, initial fatty acyl-CoA formation within the peroxisome does not require fatty acyl carnitine formation for entry into peroxisomes. During the next metabolic step, in which *trans*-enoyl fatty acyl-CoA is formed, another significant difference occurs in the peroxisomes as compared with mitochondria: Two electrons produced are transferred to FAD to form $FADH_2$, which is then transferred directly to oxygen to form hydrogen peroxide. Hydrogen peroxide is detoxified by catalase to form water and oxygen (in the mitochondrion, electrons are delivered to the mitochondrial electron transport system that ultimately generates water and ATP). The significance of this difference lies in both the lack of ATP production and generation of hydrogen peroxide in the peroxisomes, which, in the presence of transitional metals, can yield toxic hydroxyl radicals and can promote lipid peroxidation and oxidant injury.

NADH generated in subsequent reactions needs to be removed from the peroxisomes, whereas, in mitochondria, NADH can enter the electron transport cycle and generate additional ATP molecules. Peroxisomal enzymes can metabolize only long-chain fatty acids with a minimal chain length of 10 carbons and a maximal length of 24 carbons. As in mitochondria, beta oxidation in peroxisomes proceeds similarly by 2-carbon acetyl-CoA cleavage until octanoyl-CoA is formed. Octanoyl-CoA is then combined with carnitine to form fatty acyl carnitine, which can be transported by the mitochondrial inner membrane transporter and undergo completion of beta oxidation. Acyl-CoA formed in peroxisomes by beta oxidation of fatty acids can diffuse out of the peroxisomes after formation of acetyl carnitine.[128]

The regulation of peroxisomal metabolism of fatty acids appears to be solely at the level of substrate availability, which may be regulated by a family of soluble fatty acid binding proteins (FABPs) present in the cytosol of all cells. The peroxisomal pathway provides a supply of acetyl-CoA that does not require citrate formation and that can be used in fatty acid synthesis. Because the initial electron transfer is not coupled to the mitochondrial electron transport system, peroxisomal fatty acid oxidation is less efficient than mitochondrial beta oxidation and may provide a means of eliminating fatty acids with energy loss. Peroxisomes proliferate on administration of many hypolipidemic agents, such as clofibrate, with a resulting 5–10-fold increase in the relative contribution of peroxisomal fatty acid beta oxidation. Because peroxisomal beta oxidation produces less ATP than does beta oxidation in mitochondria, a relative increase in peroxisomal fatty acid beta oxidation can lead to a reduction in lipid mass and to weight loss. This pathway also provides a means of generating hydrogen peroxide, which can be used by catalase for the oxidation of substrates such as ethanol.

Increased triglyceride synthesis, reduced synthesis of lipid transport proteins (see later), and a decreased level of beta oxidation can result in the accumulation of fat within hepatocytes (steatosis). A classic example of this process is alcoholic steatosis, which occurs when a large percentage of the total caloric intake is derived from ethanol. Alteration in the redox potential with excess NADH produced by ethanol metabolism results in an increased

NADH/NAD ratio, which favors the formation of α-glycerol phosphate, which, in turn, promotes triglyceride formation. In addition, a decrease in NAD content in mitochondria may reduce fatty acid beta oxidation, thereby contributing to fatty acid accumulation.[129]

Lipoproteins. Apolipoproteins (apo), which are synthesized by the liver, in combination with triglycerides, phospholipids, cholesterol, and cholesterol esters, constitute circulating lipoproteins, which mediate the transport of lipids from the liver into the plasma and from the plasma into the liver and other tissues. The liver also expresses cell surface receptors for circulating lipoproteins and modulates plasma levels of these important macromolecules. Lipoprotein trafficking has been reviewed elsewhere[130] and is summarized in the following section.

Types of Lipoproteins. Lipoproteins were originally classified according to their relative density, which is inversely related to their particle size. Listed in increasing order of density, they are chylomicrons, VLDL, intermediate-density lipoproteins (IDL), LDL, and high-density lipoproteins (HDL). Density differences in these particles reflect the type and amount of specific lipids and the proportion of protein present within these lipoprotein fractions.[130] Specific apolipoproteins bind lipids to form lipoproteins, which are modified by enzymes in plasma or endothelial cells and act as ligands for specific lipoprotein receptors that mediate their uptake by target tissues.

The lipid components are in constant dynamic flux because of delivery of lipids and cholesterol to cells, transfer to other lipoproteins (mediated by lipid transfer proteins), and catalysis by lipolytic enzymes. Triglycerides are the major lipids contained in chylomicrons that are generated in the intestinal epithelial cells and VLDL produced in the liver. They are the energy source for peripheral tissues and components of cellular membrane structures. Cholesterol is the major lipid in LDL and HDL. Cholesterol, unlike triglycerides, is not used as a fuel source but as a structural component of membranes and as precursors for steroid hormones. Trafficking of cholesterol is usually in the form of cholesteryl ester, which is generated in the plasma by the activity of lecithin-cholesterol acyltransferase (LCAT) (see later).

Tangier Disease. A rare autosomal recessive disorder characterized by the accumulation of cholesteryl esters in reticuloendothelial cells, including the tonsils, thymus, and lymph nodes, as well as liver, spleen, and gallbladder, in combination with the near absence of serum HDL cholesterol, is now recognized to be caused by mutations in the ATP-binding cassette transporter A1, a member of the ABC supergene family.[110] Affected patients classically present with enlarged, orange-colored tonsils and have a four- to sixfold increased risk of atherosclerotic heart disease. Although the function of the transporter is not completely known, its location at the plasma membrane suggests that it mediates the active transport (flipping) of cholesteryl ester from the inner to the outer leaflet of the plasma membrane, from which it can be transferred to apolipoproteins and secreted.[131]

Apolipoproteins. The major apolipoproteins associated with triglyceride transport are apoB-100, which is synthesized in the liver, and apoB-48, which is synthesized in the intestine.[132] Both proteins are translated from the same mRNA. In human intestinal epithelium, the apoB mRNA undergoes posttranscriptional RNA editing, which generates a stop codon by cytidine deamination that results in the translation of a form of apoB that is approximately 48% of the size of the full-length apoB-100 generated in the liver. The carboxy-terminal domain that is absent in apoB-48 is essential for binding to the LDL receptor. Unlike the apoB-100-containing VLDL, chylomicron remnants, which contain apoB-48, are rapidly cleared from plasma and do not give rise to LDL.[132]

ApoC is synthesized predominately in the liver, with minor expression in the intestine and other organs, and is composed of three different gene products that may inhibit the uptake of chylomicron remnants by the liver. ApoC-1 is a minor component of VLDL, HDL, and IDL and is of unknown function. ApoC-II is present in VLDL, IDL, HDL, and chylomicrons and is an essential activator of lipoprotein lipase (LPL) (see "Intestinal Lipoprotein Metabolism," later). Inherited deficiency of apoC-II causes hypertriglyceridemia. ApoC-III is present in IDL, HDL, and chylomicrons and may be an inhibitor of LPL activity.[133]

ApoE is synthesized in the liver and is found on all lipoproteins. ApoE is important for removal of lipoprotein remnants in the serum, can bind to the LDL receptor and other membrane proteins, and is important in targeting lipoproteins to specific receptors on peripheral cells. Three major alleles of the apoE gene exist (ε2, ε3, and ε4), with the ε3 allele being the most abundant and ε2/ε3 genotype being the most frequent. Each allele possesses a different ability to bind to the LDL receptor. The absence of apoE leads to reduced clearance of chylomicron and VLDL remnants, resulting in elevated plasma levels and a consequent increase in the risk of atherosclerosis.[134] ApoE is also important in lipid transport in the central nervous system, especially after neuronal injury. Inheritance of a single apoε4 allele is associated with a 6- to 8-year earlier onset of Alzheimer's disease than that associated with the ε3/ε3 genotype.[135]

ApoA-I and -II are synthesized in the liver and intestine. ApoA-I is the major component of HDL lipoproteins. In a lipid-poor state, apoA-I accepts cholesterol from the cell membrane. ApoA-I is a key activator of LCAT, which enhances cholesterol esterification in the plasma, and the absence of a specific, conserved region in apoA-I causes loss of its LCAT-activating property. ApoA-II is another component of HDL. ApoA-IV is a minor constituent synthesized in the intestine.[136]

Lysosomal Hydrolysis of Triglycerides via Autophagy. Triglycerides and cholesterol are stored in the cytoplasm as lipid droplets. During nutrient deprivation, triglycerides in the lipid droplets are hydrolyzed, generating FFAs that are oxidized to provide energy. Hydrolysis of the droplet enclosed occurs through autophagy, which is a known cellular response to starvation. By analogy with mitophagy (autophagy of damaged mitochondria), this process was termed "macrolipophagy," which links autophagy with lipid metabolism.[137]

Lipolytic Enzymes (LPL). LPL is synthesized in fat and muscle cells and is located in the luminal surface of the capillary bed of adipose, lung, and muscle tissues.[138] LPL catalyzes lipolysis of triglycerides present in VLDL, chylomicrons, or HDL. LPL is stimulated by fasting, fatty acids, hormones, and catecholamines. Patients who are homozygous for LPL deficiency present with severe hypertriglyceridemia in childhood and pancreatitis.

Hepatic triglyceride lipase (HTGL) is another member of the lipase family. It is synthesized in the liver and binds to the luminal surface of hepatic endothelial cells. It is involved in lipolysis of VLDL or IDL and thus plays a major role in LDL formation. HDL may be another substrate for HTGL activity. Inherited deficiency of LPL leads to accumulation of large particles containing both apoB-100 and apoB-48, with almost complete absence of smaller apoB-containing lipoprotein. In animal studies, inhibition of HTGL results in accumulation of VLDL and IDL, with the enrichment of HDL in triglycerides.

Lipid Transport Proteins. In plasma, lipid exchange between particles is facilitated by the activity of LCAT and cholesteryl ester transfer protein (CETP).[138] LCAT is synthesized in the liver, and apoA-I is a cofactor for LCAT activity. CETP is synthesized predominantly in the liver and circulates in association with HDL. CETP mediates the exchange of cholesteryl esters from HDL with triglycerides from chylomicrons or VLDL. The activity of LCAT in combination with the lipid transfer proteins, CETP and phospholipid transfer protein (PLTP), is essential for the transfer of cholesterol from nonhepatic tissue to the liver.[138]

Intestinal and Hepatic Lipid Transport

The liver functions as the hub for receiving fatty acids and cholesterol from the diet and peripheral tissues, packages them into lipoprotein complexes, and releases the complexes into the circulation (Fig. 74.4). Following absorption by intestinal epithelial cells, fatty acids are formed into triglycerides, and cholesterol is esterified. Both lipids are packaged into nascent chylomicrons composed predominantly of triglycerides (85%–92%), phospholipids (6%–12%), cholesteryl ester (1%–3%), fat-soluble vitamins, and the following apolipoproteins (1%–3%): apoB-48, apoA-I, apoA-II, and apoA-IV.[139] Nascent chylomicrons enter the interstitial space and are carried into the systemic venous circulation via the thoracic duct. In the interstitial space, chylomicrons acquire apoC-II, which activates LPL, thereby promoting triglyceride release. Triglyceride release may be reduced by acquisition of apoC-III, which may inhibit LPL activity. The addition of apoE is critical for targeting the chylomicron remnant, which can then be taken up by hepatocytes through the chylomicron remnant receptor.

Release of triglycerides by LPL and extraction by peripheral tissues increases the relative cholesteryl ester concentration in chylomicron remnants, which are taken up by hepatocytes via a hepatocyte membrane transporter that recognizes a binding domain on apoE. The endocytosed chylomicron remnants are targeted to lysosomes, where they are degraded. Inherited mutations of the binding domain of apoE reduce chylomicron remnant clearance. When chylomicron excretion is delayed, as occurs with mutations of the binding domain of apoE or reduced LPL activity or apoC-II levels, chylomicron remnants that accumulate in the serum may be taken up by endothelial cells or macrophages, which transform into foamy cells. The foamy cells are precursors of fatty streaks and atheromas. Increased VLDL secretion resulting from excess fatty acid absorption can also compete with the chylomicron remnant uptake system.

Fatty acids released from adipocytes by the action of intracellular hormone-sensitive lipase are bound to serum albumin and transported to other tissues, including the liver, where they are used for synthesis of phospholipids and triglycerides.[140] The liver synthesizes cholesterol from low-molecular-weight precursors. Hepatic cholesterol synthesis is regulated by the rate-limiting enzyme 3-hydroxyl-3- methylglutaryl coenzyme A reductase (HMG-CoA reductase). Lipids are exported from the liver as VLDL particles, which are the major carriers of plasma triglycerides during nonabsorptive states.[104] Lipids may be stored temporarily in the liver as fat droplets and cholesteryl esters, excreted directly into bile, or metabolized into bile acids. The liver is the major site of sterol excretion from the body and is the site of bile acid synthesis.

The coordinated input, synthesis, and excretion of sterols require complex regulation of multiple enzymatic pathways. Bile acids returning to the liver via the enterohepatic circulation modulate these enzyme activities. Bile acids recycle 20–30 times per day via the enterohepatic circulation and use specific

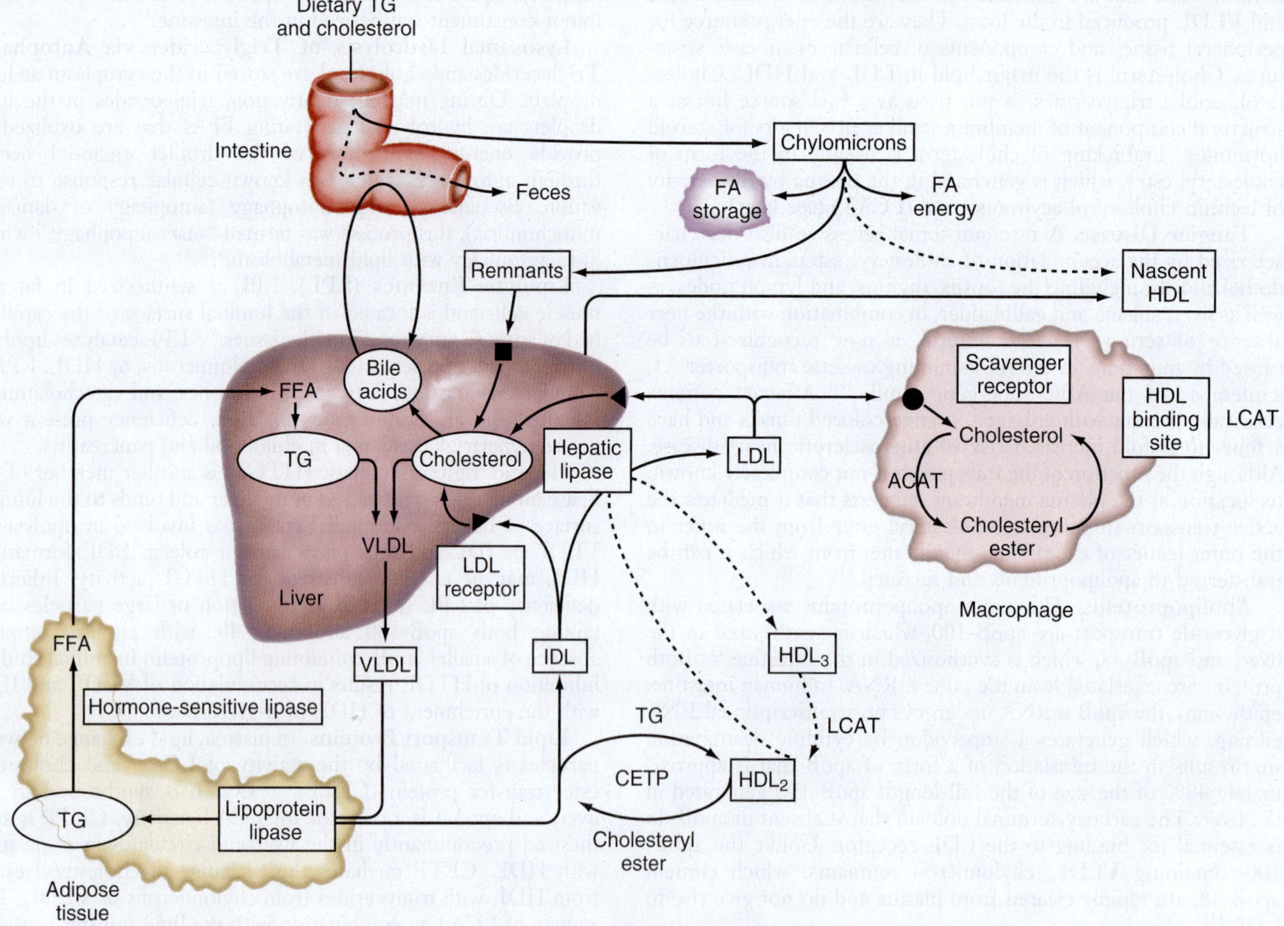

Fig. 74.4 Lipoprotein metabolism. *ACAT*, Acylcholesterol acyltransferase; *CETP*, cholesteryl ester transfer protein; *FA*, fatty acid; *FFA*, free fatty acid; *HDL*, high-density lipoproteins; *LCAT*, lecithin-cholesterol acyltransferase; *LDL*, low-density lipoproteins; *VLDL*, very-low-density lipoproteins. (Modified from Shepherd J. Lipoprotein metabolism: an overview. *Drugs*. 1994;47(suppl 2):1–10.)

transmembrane transporters at apical and basolateral domains of hepatocyte plasma membrane, as well as intracellular binding proteins.[141] In the terminal ileum, a great majority of the bile acid molecules are reabsorbed via a sodium-dependent bile acid transporter. Bile acids are also important in micellization of fats for intestinal absorption and as coactivators of bile acid–dependent lipase activity. FXR, a member of the sterol nuclear receptor family, binds to and is activated by bile salts. Heterodimers of activated FXR and RXR modulate the coordinated regulation of multiple genes that encode key bile salt transporters, such as the sodium-dependent taurocholate pump (NTCP) at the sinusoidal domain of hepatocytes, bile salt export pump at the canalicular domain, intestinal bile acid transporter in the terminal ileum, and cholesterol-7α-hydroxylase in hepatocytes (see Chapter 66).[142]

Transport of ApoB-Containing Lipoproteins

In the fasting state, VLDL, which is synthesized in the liver, replaces chylomicrons as the major transporter of triglycerides and cholesterol. In addition to the full-length apoB-100, VLDL contains triglycerides (taken up from plasma or synthesized in the liver), cholesteryl esters (exogenous or endogenous), and phospholipids.[143] During fasting, fatty acids in VLDL are derived predominantly from the activity of hormone-sensitive lipase in adipocytes, whereas after a meal, dietary fatty acids are the major source. Fatty acids may be taken up by hepatocytes by passive diffusion or via fatty acid transport proteins in the sinusoidal domain of the cell membrane. In hepatocyte cytosol, fatty acids are stored bound to the abundant 12-kD FABP family, which may direct fatty acids to specific subcellular targets, such as the smooth ER for VLDL synthesis or peroxisomes for beta oxidation. FABPs are transcriptionally regulated by peroxisome proliferating agents (e.g., fibrates), suggesting that their role is physiologic in global lipid metabolism.

ApoB-100 is the predominant transport carrier in VLDL; apoC-I, C-II, C-III, and apoE arise from other lipoproteins within the serum. ApoB-100 synthesis and VLDL secretion are regulated by the availability of cotransported lipids and sterols in the smooth ER. ApoB-100 synthesis may change dramatically without alteration in apoB-100 mRNA levels.[144] Following synthesis in the smooth ER, apoB-100 interacts with newly synthesized triglycerides and cholesteryl esters that enter the ER via specific membrane transporters. The apoB-lipid complex is translocated into the lumen, transported through the Golgi apparatus, and secreted into the sinusoidal space as VLDL. When the lipid components are not available, apoB-100 undergoes degradation in the ER. During periods of low plasma triglyceride levels, the liver secretes smaller IDL-like particles or even LDL-type particles.

In the plasma, the activity of LPL and HTGL removes triglycerides from VLDL, generating progressively smaller and denser IDL and LDL particles. Conversion of IDL to LDL requires the activity of apoE. LDL particles become enriched in cholesteryl esters, both by removal of triglycerides and acquisition of cholesteryl esters from other lipoproteins, predominantly HDL, with release of apoC to HDL. LDL is subsequently removed from the circulation by LDL receptors in the liver and peripheral tissues. Subpopulations of VLDL that begin as large VLDL undergo lipolysis and are converted to IDL, which is taken up via the LDL receptor.

Transport of ApoA-Containing High-Density Lipoprotein

HDL, another major class of lipoproteins secreted by the liver, appears to have a protective role against atherosclerosis. HDL is a heterogeneous population of lipoproteins that can be separated by sophisticated analytic centrifugation techniques. Nascent HDL is formed in the liver and intestine by lipolysis of VLDL and chylomicrons, respectively, with modification by peripheral tissue. The major protein constituents of HDL are apoA-I and -II, with minor amounts of apoA-IV, apoC, apoE, and others.[145] In humans, apoA-I is synthesized in the liver and intestine. Nascent apoA-containing lipoprotein complexes that appear as discoid particles can be transformed into HDL particles in the serum by the action of LCAT and the lipid transfer proteins CETP and PLTP.

The HDL_3 subclass is particularly important because these cholesterol-poor particles are able to deliver cholesterol extracted from peripheral membranes and provide a substrate for plasma LCAT activity. Cholesteryl esters formed by LCAT are extremely hydrophobic and move into the core of the lipoprotein complex, thereby providing space on the surface of the lipoprotein for extraction of additional cholesterol from cell membranes. This complex enlarges with increasing amounts of cholesteryl esters, which are able to accommodate apoC-II and C-III, thereby resulting in HDL_2 formation. CETP removes esterified cholesterol from HDL in exchange for triglycerides, which are eventually hydrolyzed by HTGL, thereby regenerating small HDL. Acquisition of apoC-II also promotes LPL activity, thereby increasing lipolysis.[138]

The movement of apolipoproteins between HDL and chylomicrons allows the recycling of lipids and proteins between these two pools. Cholesterol and phospholipids are also transferred to the chylomicrons as triglycerides are released by LPL activity to local tissues. As the remnant is further processed, apoC-II and apoC-III, phospholipids, and cholesterol are transferred back to HDL. Triglycerides that are transferred from VLDL and chylomicrons to HDL are more accessible to lipolysis by endothelial-based lipases because of their smaller size. With the removal of triglycerides, these particles revert to HDL_3 and apoC-II, after which apoC-II and apoE recycle to chylomicrons and VLDL.

Lipoprotein Receptors. The major lipoprotein receptors for LDL, chylomicron remnants, HDL, and the scavenger receptor are members of the larger LDL receptor supergene family.[146] These receptors share four major structural features: (1) cysteine-rich complement-type repeats; (2) EGF precursor-like repeats; (3) a transmembrane domain; and (4) a cytoplasmic domain.[147]

The LDL receptor exists as an oligomeric surface glycoprotein that plays a pivotal role in LDL clearance and cholesterol homeostasis. It binds ligands at the cell surface, after which the ligand-receptor complex is internalized via the classic endocytotic pathway. The ligand dissociates from the receptor in acidic endosomal vesicles. Subsequently, the ligand is delivered to lysosomes for degradation, and the receptor returns to the surface. The LDL receptor is present on all cell types; however, the liver contains approximately 70% of the total body pool of LDL receptors. The LDL receptor recognizes apoE and apoB-100, but not apoB-48. ApoE-containing chylomicron remnants, VLDL, LDL, IDL, and HDL can all be taken up via the LDL receptor. Approximately two-thirds of LDL is cleared by this receptor. Homozygous deficiency of the functional LDL receptor occurs in approximately 1 in 1 million persons and is associated with accelerated atherosclerosis manifesting in childhood (familial hypercholesterolemia). LDL receptors are highly conserved among species.[146]

Very-Low-Density Lipoprotein Receptor. The VLDL receptor has a high-sequence homology with the LDL receptor but is expressed predominantly in extrahepatic tissues such as heart, muscle, and fat. Unlike the LDL receptor, the VLDL receptor does not bind to apoB and may serve specifically to take up triglyceride-rich apoE-containing lipoproteins, such as VLDL or IDL.[146,147]

Chylomicron Remnant Receptor. The chylomicron remnant receptor accepts apoE as a ligand. Chylomicron remnants are removed from the circulation exclusively by the liver, probably because these large complexes can penetrate the unique sinusoidal vascular space. The multifunctional, α_2-macroglobulin/LDL receptor-related protein (LRP) is the chylomicron remnant receptor.[148] LRP is present in liver, brain, and muscle. In cultured cells, LRP can mediate the endocytosis of apoE-containing chylomicron remnants. Mice that lack LRP in the liver do not have hepatic chylomicron remnant uptake, confirming that LRP is the major chylomicron remnant receptor. Unlike the LDL receptor, LRP is able to bind a number of unrelated ligands, such as lipoprotein, proteinase-inhibitor complex, and protein-lipid complex.

Low-Density Lipoprotein Scavenger Receptor. Ligands for the scavenger receptor A include LPS, polyanionic lipids, and LDL, in which some of the free lysine residues have been chemically modified.[149] These receptors exist in two forms as trimeric integral membrane glycoproteins in endothelial cells, macrophages, and Kupffer cells. Oxidized LDL is internalized via the scavenger receptors but is metabolized poorly in macrophages, leading to the accumulation of cholesteryl esters within the cell. Monocytes, which migrate into lipid-enriched atherosclerotic lesions, can also be induced to express the scavenger receptor.

High-Density Lipoprotein Receptor. A high-affinity HDL binding protein has been identified in the plasma membrane of hepatocytes, macrophages, adrenal cells, and adipocytes.[149] These receptors appear to recognize specifically apoA present in HDL particles. The HDL receptor does not mediate endocytosis but allows only selective delivery of lipids to and from the HDL lipoproteins. By mediating the transfer of cholesterol from the plasma membrane to the HDL lipoprotein, the HDL receptor facilitates reverse cholesterol transport. The HDL receptor is a class B scavenger receptor, referred to as SR-B1.[145] This receptor is most abundant in the liver, ovary, and adrenal glands—organs previously shown to be the principal sites of cholesterol uptake from HDL in vivo. HDL is a major source of cholesterol secreted in bile. Overexpression of SR-B1 in mouse liver increases biliary cholesterol secretion and reduces plasma HDL.[150] Conversely, deficiency of this receptor results in decreased biliary cholesterol secretion.[151]

Derangement of Lipid Metabolism in Liver Disease. The most common lipid abnormality in patients with chronic liver disease is hypertriglyceridemia (plasma levels of 250–500 mg/dL), which is found in patients with alcoholic or viral liver disease and tends to resolve when the liver disease improves. Excess ethanol ingestion causes predominantly hypertriglyceridemia, due to increased fatty acid synthesis and decreased beta oxidation of fatty acids, resulting from increased NADH production by alcohol metabolism. Moderate alcohol ingestion is associated with increased HDL_3 levels, which may reduce the risk of atherosclerosis. LDL, HDL, and total serum cholesterol levels decrease progressively with cirrhosis advancing from Child class A to class C (see Chapters 76 and 88). Serum cholesterol level may be a useful prognostic marker in patients with noncholestatic liver diseases.[152]

Cholestatic disorders manifest with a distinct pattern of dyslipoproteinemia because of the retention of cholesterol, phospholipids, and bile salts that are normally secreted in bile.[153] A prolonged increase in total serum cholesterol and lipid levels, as seen in primary biliary cirrhosis, for example, can be associated with formation of xanthoma. Within the LDL fraction of the serum of cholestatic patients, three distinct lipoproteins can be identified, namely, β_2-lipoprotein (triglyceride rich), also known as lipoprotein Y (LP-Y), lipoprotein X (LP-X), and normal LDL. LP-Y appears to be a remnant of a triglyceride-rich lipoprotein that is distinct from IDL. Cholestatic patients with elevated triglyceride levels often have clear (not lipemic) serum because most of the triglycerides are contained in LP-Y and LDL. LP-X is a complex composed of equimolar amounts of excess phospholipid and cholesterol in combination with albumin and certain members of the apoC family. The phospholipid flippase activity of multidrug resistance protein-3 (MDR3), also termed ATP-binding cassette protein B4 (see Chapter 66), is essential for LP-X formation. Mice lacking mdr2 (the murine homolog of MDR3) are unable to form LP-X during cholestasis caused by complete bile duct obstruction.

In patients with chronic parenchymal liver disease, plasma cholesteryl ester levels are often reduced, a finding that suggests that LCAT activity is diminished because of impaired hepatic synthesis. Alternatively, decreased LCAT activity may result from reduced apoC-II levels or release of cholesteryl ester hydrolase from damaged hepatocytes, with conversion of cholesteryl esters to cholesterol. Chronic dyslipoproteinemia in these patients can also lead to alterations in cellular membrane lipids, resulting in formation of abnormal RBCs, such as echinocytes, and altered membrane function with potential pathophysiologic consequences.

Full references for this chapter can be found at https://ebooks.health.elsevier.com.

KEY REFERENCES

Anghel SI, Wahli W. Fat poetry: a kingdom for PPARgamma. *Cell Res.* 2007;17:486–511. (Ref 105).

Bedossa P, Paradis V. Liver extracellular matrix in health and disease. *J Pathol.* 2003;200:504–515. (Ref 71).

Chen Y, Choi SS, Michelotti GA, et al. Hedgehog controls hepatic stellate cell fate by regulating metabolism. *Gastroenterology.* 2012;143: 1319–1329. (Ref 68).

Conner SD, Schmid SL. Regulated portals of entry into the cell. *Nature.* 2003;422:37–44. (Ref 47).

Hazari Y, Bravo-San Pedro JM, Hertz C, et al. Autophagy in hepatic adaptation to stress. *J. Hepatol.* 2020;72:183–196. (Ref 93).

Karpen SJ. Nuclear receptor regulation of hepatic function. *J Hepatol.* 2002;36:832–850. (Ref 89).

Miller JP. Liver disease, alcohol and lipoprotein metabolism. In: Zakim D, Boyer TD, eds. *Hepatology: A Textbook of Liver Diseases.* 4th ed. Philadelphia: WB Saunders; 2003:127 (Ref 130).

Nakielny S, Dreyfuss G. Transport of proteins and RNAs in and out of the nucleus. *Cell.* 1999;99:677–690. (Ref 10).

Newmeyer DD, Ferguson-Miller S. Mitochondria: releasing power for life and unleashing the machineries of death. *Cell.* 2003;112:481–490. (Ref 37).

Nordlie RC, Foster JD, Lange AJ. Regulation of glucose production by the liver. *Annu Rev Nutr.* 1999;19:379–406. (Ref 114).

Sorensen KK, Smedsrod B. Liver sinusoidal endothelial cell: basic biology and pathobiology. In: Arias IM, et al., eds. *The Liver: Biology and Pathobiology.* 6th ed. Hoboken, NJ: John Wiley and sons Inc; 2020: 62–74. (Ref 57).

Taub R. Liver regeneration: from myth to mechanism. *Nat Rev Mol Cell Biol.* 2004;5:836–847. (Ref 79).

Totland MZ, Rasmussen NL, Knudsen LM, et al. Regulation of communication by connexin ubiquitination: physiological and pathophysiological implications. *Cell. Mol. Life Sci.* 2020;77:573–591. (Ref 21).

Yin XM, Ding WX. Death receptor activation-induced hepatocyte apoptosis and liver injury. *Curr Mol Med.* 2003;3:491–508. (Ref 85).

Zegers MMP, Hoekstra D. Mechanisms and functional features of polarized membrane traffic in epithelial and hepatic cells. *Biochem J.* 1998;336:257–269. (Ref 15).

75 Liver Chemistry and Function Tests

Daniel S. Pratt

IN THIS CHAPTER

When appropriately ordered and interpreted, serum liver biochemical tests, the so-called liver function tests or liver chemistries, can be useful in the evaluation and management of patients with liver disorders. The term *liver biochemical tests* is preferable to *liver function tests* because the most commonly used tests—the aminotransferases and alkaline phosphatase (ALP)—do not measure a known function of the liver. These tests have the potential to identify liver disease, distinguish among types of liver disorders, gauge the severity and progression of liver dysfunction, and monitor response to therapy. Understanding the shortcomings of these tests, however, is important. No test can accurately assess the liver's total functional capacity; biochemical tests measure only a few of the thousands of biochemical functions performed by the liver. Furthermore, considered individually, these tests lack sensitivity and specificity for liver injury; a battery of tests must be used to evaluate the liver. The standard battery of tests that is most helpful in assessing liver disease includes total and direct bilirubin, albumin, prothrombin time, and the serum enzymes: alanine aminotransferase (ALT), aspartate aminotransferase (AST), ALP, and occasionally gamma glutamyl transpeptidase (GGTP) and 5′-nucleotidase (5′-NT). Interpretation of these results in concert with careful history taking and a physical examination may suggest a specific type of liver injury, thereby allowing a directed evaluation, risk assessment for surgical procedures, and estimation of prognosis. Other more specialized tests include quantitative tests of liver function and a growing number of options to assess the degree of hepatic fibrosis.

BILIRUBIN

Metabolism

Bilirubin is a breakdown product of heme (ferroprotoporphyrin IX) (see Chapter 2). About 4 mg/kg body weight of bilirubin is produced each day, nearly 80% from the breakdown of hemoglobin in senescent red blood cells and prematurely destroyed erythroid cells in the bone marrow and the remainder from the turnover of hemoproteins such as myoglobin and cytochromes distributed throughout the body.[1] The initial steps of bilirubin metabolism occur in reticuloendothelial cells, predominantly in the spleen. Heme is converted to biliverdin by the microsomal enzyme heme oxygenase. Biliverdin is then converted to bilirubin by the cytosolic enzyme biliverdin reductase.

Bilirubin formed in reticuloendothelial cells is lipid soluble and virtually insoluble in water. To be transported in blood, unconjugated bilirubin must be solubilized. The process is initiated by reversible, noncovalent binding to albumin, which has both high-affinity and lower affinity binding sites for unconjugated bilirubin. The unconjugated bilirubin-albumin complex passes readily through the fenestrations in the endothelium lining the hepatic sinusoids into the space of Disse, where the bilirubin dissociates from albumin and is taken up rapidly by hepatocytes through multiple membrane transporters (see Chapter 22).

After entering the hepatocyte, unconjugated bilirubin is bound in the cytosol to a number of proteins, including proteins in the glutathione *S*-transferase superfamily.[2] These proteins serve to reduce efflux of bilirubin back into the serum and present the bilirubin for conjugation. The enzyme bilirubin uridine diphosphate glucuronosyl transferase (B-UGT) found in the endoplasmic reticulum solubilizes bilirubin by conjugating it to glucuronic acid to produce bilirubin monoglucuronide and diglucuronide.[3] The now hydrophilic bilirubin diffuses to the canalicular membrane for excretion into the bile canaliculi. Conjugated bilirubin is transported across the canalicular membrane by the multidrug resistance–associated protein 2 (MRP2) via an ATP-dependent process.[4] This is the only energy-dependent step in bilirubin metabolism and explains why even patients with ALF have a predominantly conjugated hyperbilirubinemia. Once in the bile, conjugated bilirubin passes undisturbed until it reaches the distal ileum and colon, where bacteria containing β-glucuronidases hydrolyze conjugated bilirubin to unconjugated bilirubin, which is further reduced by bacteria to colorless urobilinogen.[5] The urobilinogen is either excreted unchanged, oxidized, and excreted as urobilin (which has an orange color), or absorbed passively by the intestine into the portal venous system. The majority of the absorbed urobilinogen is reexcreted by the liver. A small percentage filters across the renal glomerulus and is excreted in urine. Unconjugated bilirubin is never found in urine because in the serum it is bound to albumin and not filtered by the glomerulus. The presence of bilirubin in urine indicates conjugated hyperbilirubinemia and hepatobiliary disease.

Measurement

The terms *direct* and *indirect bilirubin*, which correspond roughly to conjugated and unconjugated bilirubin, respectively, derive from the original van den Bergh reaction.[6] Serum bilirubin is still measured in clinical laboratories by some modification of this method.[7] In this assay, bilirubin is exposed to diazotized sulfanilic acid. The conjugated fraction of bilirubin reacts promptly, or "directly," with the diazo reagent without the need for an accelerant and thereby allows measurement of the conjugated bilirubin fraction by photometric analysis within 30–60 seconds. The total bilirubin is measured 30–60 minutes after the addition of an accelerant such as alcohol or caffeine to allow the release of unconjugated bilirubin from albumin binding sites. The unconjugated, or indirect, fraction is then determined by subtracting the direct component from the total bilirubin. An enzymatic method that employs bilirubin oxidase to oxidize conjugated bilirubin to biliverdin has been in use for many years.

More accurate methods of measuring bilirubin, such as high-performance liquid chromatography, are generally not available because they are more difficult to perform and do not add additional information beyond that provided by the diazo method in most clinical situations. These newer methods allow the identification of delta bilirubin—conjugated bilirubin tightly linked to albumin through covalent binding. Delta bilirubin is found in cases of prolonged and severe elevation of serum conjugated bilirubin levels, and because of the strength of the covalent binding, the half-life of delta bilirubin is that of albumin, 14–21 days, which far exceeds the usual serum half-life of bilirubin of 4 hours. The identification of delta bilirubin explains why the decline in serum bilirubin in some patients with prolonged jaundice seems to lag behind clinical recovery and why some patients with conjugated hyperbilirubinemia do not have bilirubinuria.

Using the diazo method, normal values of total serum bilirubin are between 1.0 and 1.5 mg/dL, with 95% of a normal population falling between 0.2 and 0.9 mg/dL.[8] Normal values for the indirect component are between 0.8 and 1.2 mg/dL. The diazo method, however, tends to overestimate the amount of conjugated bilirubin, particularly within the normal range. As a result, "normal" ranges for conjugated bilirubin have crept upward over time. In general, if the direct acting fraction is less than 15% of the total, the bilirubin can be considered to be entirely indirect. The most frequently reported upper limit of normal for conjugated bilirubin is 0.3 mg/dL. The presence of even a mild increase in conjugated bilirubin in the serum should raise the possibility of liver injury. The measurement and fractionation of serum bilirubin in patients with jaundice do not allow differentiation between parenchymal (hepatocellular) and obstructive (cholestatic) jaundice.

The magnitude and duration of hyperbilirubinemia have not been critically assessed as prognostic markers. In general, the higher the serum bilirubin level in patients with viral hepatitis, the greater the hepatocellular damage and the longer the course of disease. Patients may die of ALF, however, with only a modest elevation of serum bilirubin. The total serum bilirubin level correlates with poor outcomes in alcohol-associated hepatitis and is a critical component of the Maddrey discriminant function, which is used to identify patients at high risk of short-term mortality who may benefit from treatment with corticosteroids.[9] The total bilirubin is also part of the MELD score, which is used to estimate survival of patients with end-stage liver disease (see later and Chapter 99). Pretreatment levels of serum bilirubin and bilirubin levels during treatment are associated with prognosis in patients with PBC.[10,11]

Approach to the Patient With an Elevated Level

Hyperbilirubinemia may be the result of overproduction of bilirubin through excessive breakdown of hemoglobin; impaired hepatocellular uptake, conjugation, or excretion of bilirubin; or regurgitation of unconjugated and conjugated bilirubin from damaged hepatocytes or bile ducts. The presence of conjunctival icterus suggests a total serum bilirubin level of at least 3.0 mg/dL but does not allow differentiation between conjugated and unconjugated hyperbilirubinemia. Tea- or cola-colored urine may indicate the presence of bilirubinuria and thus conjugated hyperbilirubinemia.

The evaluation of the patient with an isolated elevation of the serum bilirubin level is quite different from that of the patient with an elevated bilirubin associated with elevated liver enzyme levels; the latter suggests either a hepatocellular or cholestatic process, as discussed later. The first step in the evaluation of a patient with an isolated elevation of the serum bilirubin level is to fractionate the bilirubin to determine if it is conjugated or unconjugated (Fig. 75.1). If less than 15% of the total is conjugated, one can be assured that virtually all the serum bilirubin is unconjugated. Overproduction of bilirubin as a result of excessive breakdown of hemoglobin can occur with any of several inherited or acquired disorders (Table 75.1). The patient's medication history should be reviewed for drugs that can cause impaired hepatocellular uptake of bilirubin. If no cause is identified, a genetic enzyme deficiency that results in impaired conjugation of bilirubin, the most common of which is Gilbert syndrome, is likely.

As discussed in Chapter 22, Gilbert syndrome is common, with a reported frequency of 6%–12% (see Table 21.2). A mutation in

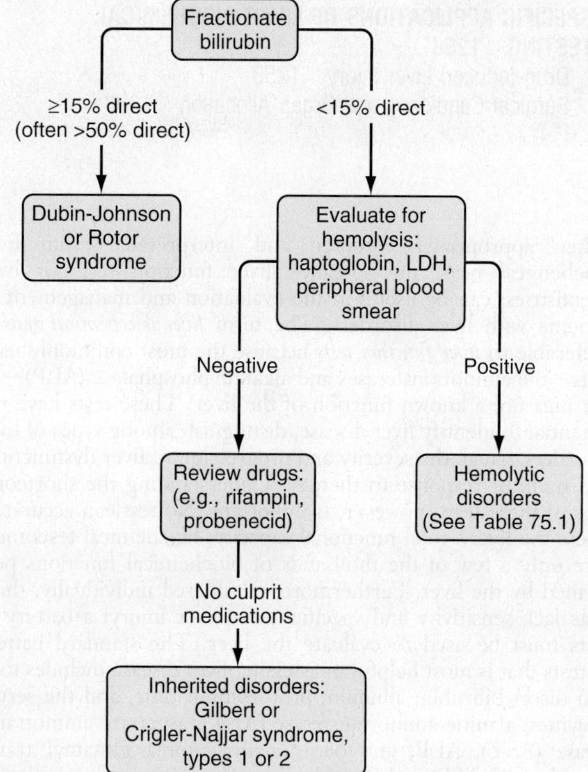

Fig 75.1 Evaluation of an isolated elevation of the serum bilirubin level.

TABLE 75.1 Causes and Mechanisms of Isolated Hyperbilirubinemia in Adults

Cause	Mechanism
INDIRECT HYPERBILIRUBINEMIA	
Hemolytic Disorders	Overproduction of bilirubin
Inherited Red cell enzyme defects (e.g., glucose-6-phosphate dehydrogenase deficiency) Sickle cell disease Spherocytosis and elliptocytosis	
Acquired Drugs and toxins Hypersplenism Immune mediated Paroxysmal nocturnal hemoglobinuria Traumatic: macro- or microvascular injury	
Ineffective Erythropoiesis	Overproduction of bilirubin
Cobalamin deficiency Folate deficiency Profound iron deficiency Thalassemia	
Drugs: Rifampin, Probenecid	Impaired hepatocellular uptake of bilirubin
Inherited Conditions	Impaired conjugation of bilirubin
Crigler-Najjar syndrome types I and II Gilbert syndrome	
Other	
Hematoma and massive blood transfusion	Overproduction of bilirubin
DIRECT HYPERBILIRUBINEMIA	
Inherited Conditions	
Dubin-Johnson syndrome Rotor syndrome	Impaired excretion of conjugated bilirubin

the TATAA element in the 5′ promoter region of the B-UGT gene results in a reduction in enzyme activity to approximately one-third of normal. The mildly elevated indirect serum hyperbilirubinemia seen in Gilbert syndrome is generally of no clinical consequence and may actually have protective effects. This benign clinical course contrasts with those of much rarer conditions, Crigler-Najjar syndrome types I and II (see Table 22.2). The mutations in these conditions result in significantly reduced B-UGT activity: less than 10% in Crigler-Najjar type II and complete absence of enzyme activity in Crigler-Najjar type I, leading to much greater elevations of unconjugated serum bilirubin to levels that carry an increased risk of kernicterus.

When isolated hyperbilirubinemia is associated with a conjugated fraction of over 15%, and typically over 50%, the diagnosis is either the uncommon Dubin-Johnson syndrome or the even rarer Rotor syndrome (see Fig. 75.1; Tables 22.2 and 64.5). The defect in Dubin-Johnson syndrome is in the gene that encodes MRP2. A 2012 study identified the defect in Rotor syndrome as coexisting deficiencies of the organic anion transporting polypeptides OATP1B1 and OATP1B3 (see Chapter 64).[12] In Dubin-Johnson syndrome, excretion of conjugated bilirubin across the bile canalicular membrane is reduced, whereas in Rotor syndrome reuptake of conjugated bilirubin across the sinusoidal membrane is reduced. Both result in an increase in the conjugated serum bilirubin level. Neither syndrome is associated with adverse clinical outcomes. Additional genetic disorders of bile acid transport that may be associated with hyperbilirubinemia are discussed in Chapters 64 and 79.

AMINOTRANSFERASES

The serum aminotransferases (also called *transaminases*), the most sensitive markers of acute hepatocellular injury, have been used to identify liver disease since the 1950s.[13] ALT (formerly serum glutamic pyruvic transaminase) and AST (formerly serum glutamic oxaloacetic transaminase) catalyze the transfer of the α-amino groups of alanine and L-aspartic acid, respectively, to the α-keto group of ketoglutaric acid. AST, found in cytosol and mitochondria, is widely distributed throughout the body; it is found, in order of decreasing concentration, in liver, cardiac muscle, skeletal muscle, kidney, brain, pancreas, lung, leukocytes, and erythrocytes. ALT, a cytosolic enzyme also found in many organs, is present in greatest concentration by far in the liver and is, therefore, a more specific indicator than AST of liver injury. Increases in serum values of the aminotransferases reflect either damage to tissues rich in these enzymes or changes in cell membrane permeability that allow ALT and AST to leak into serum; hepatocyte necrosis is not required for the release of aminotransferases, and the degree of elevation of the aminotransferases in serum does not correlate with the extent of liver injury.[14]

Aminotransferases have no function in serum and act like other serum proteins. They are distributed in plasma and interstitial fluid and have half-lives measured in days. The activity of ALT and AST at any moment reflects the relative rate at which they enter and leave the circulation. They are probably cleared by cells of the reticuloendothelial system, with AST cleared more rapidly than ALT.

Normal values for aminotransferases in serum vary widely among laboratories, but values gaining general acceptance are equal to or below 30 U/L for men and 19 U/L for women.[15] The interlaboratory variation in the normal range is the result of technical issues; no reference standards exist to establish the upper limits of normal for serum ALT and AST levels. Therefore each reference laboratory is responsible for identifying a locally defined reference population or for using a normal range first established in the 1950s.[13] The normal range is defined as the mean of the reference population plus 2 standard deviations; approximately 95% of a uniformly distributed population will fall within this "normal" range. Some investigators have recommended revisions of normal values for the aminotransferases with adjustments for sex and BMI, but others have raised concern about the potential costs and unclear benefits of implementing such a change.[15–19] A longitudinal analysis observed that serum levels of ALT decrease with age, independent of sex, alcohol use, BMI, diabetes mellitus, serum TG levels, and other factors known to affect ALT levels, thereby prompting the investigators to suggest that clinicians consider a patient's age, especially in older adults, when interpreting serum ALT levels.[20] A serum aminotransferase level below the lower limit of normal is of no clinical importance; it has been reported in patients with chronic kidney disease on hemodialysis and is believed to be caused in part by vitamin B_6 deficiency.

Approach to the Patient With an Elevated Level

Serum aminotransferase levels are typically elevated in all forms of liver injury; levels up to 300 U/L are nonspecific. In certain circumstances the degree and pattern of elevation of the aminotransferases, evaluated in the context of a patient's characteristics, symptoms, and physical examination findings, can suggest particular diagnoses and direct the subsequent evaluation (Box 75.1). The differential diagnosis of marked elevations of aminotransferase levels (>1000 U/L) includes acute viral hepatitis (A–E), toxin-induced liver injury, drug-induced liver injury (DILI), ischemic hepatitis, and less commonly, autoimmune hepatitis, acute Budd-Chiari syndrome, ALF caused by Wilson disease, and acute obstruction of the biliary tract.

The ratio of AST to ALT in serum is helpful in a few specific circumstances—perhaps most importantly in the recognition of alcohol-associated liver disease. If the AST level is less than 300 U/L, a ratio of AST to ALT of more than two suggests alcohol-associated liver disease, and a ratio of more than three is highly suggestive of alcohol-associated liver disease.[21] The ratio results from a deficiency of pyridoxal 5′-phosphate in patients with alcohol-associated liver disease; ALT synthesis in the liver requires pyridoxal phosphate more than AST synthesis does.[22] When a patient with chronic alcohol-associated liver disease sustains a superimposed liver injury, particularly acetaminophen hepatotoxicity, the aminotransferase levels can be strikingly elevated, yet the AST/ALT ratio is maintained.

Elevated AST and ALT levels may also be seen in muscle disorders. The degree of elevation is typically less than 300 U/L, but in rare cases, such as rhabdomyolysis, levels typically observed in patients with acute hepatocellular disease can be reached. In cases of acute muscle injury, the AST/ALT ratio may initially be greater than 3:1, but the ratio quickly declines toward 1:1 because of the shorter serum half-life of AST.[23] The ratio typically is close to 1:1 in patients with chronic muscle diseases.

Although the AST/ALT ratio is typically less than 1 in patients with chronic viral hepatitis and metabolic dysfunction-associated steatotic liver disease (MASLD, formerly known as NAFLD), a number of investigators have observed that, as cirrhosis develops, the ratio rises and may become greater than 1. Studies have shown that an AST/ALT ratio of greater than 1 has a high specificity (94%–100%) but a relatively low sensitivity (44%–75%) as an indicator of cirrhosis in patients with chronic hepatitis C.[24] The increase in AST/ALT ratio with the development of cirrhosis is believed to result from impaired functional hepatic blood flow, with a consequent decrease in hepatic sinusoidal uptake of AST.[25]

The majority of patients evaluated for elevated serum aminotransferase levels are asymptomatic and have mild elevations (less than or equal to fivefold) identified during routine screening. The first step in the evaluation of mildly elevated serum aminotransferase levels is to repeat the test to confirm persistence of the elevated value. If the aminotransferase level remains elevated, the recommended evaluation is illustrated in Fig. 75.2. The next step is to take a careful history focused on identifying all of the patient's medications, including over-the-counter (OTC) medications, complementary and alternative medications (CAM), and substances of abuse. Correlating the use of medications temporally with the laboratory abnormalities will sometimes reveal a specific culprit. Almost any medication, including OTC medications, CAM, and substances of abuse, has the potential to elevate serum aminotransferase levels. Relatively common offending agents include NSAIDs, antibiotics, hydroxymethylglutaryl-coenzyme A reductase inhibitors (statins), antiepileptics, and anti-TB medications (see Chapter 90). The association between use of a medication and liver enzyme elevations is readily established by stopping the medication and observing return of the enzyme levels to normal. Rechallenge with the suspect medication followed by a rise in serum aminotransferase levels is confirmatory but often not undertaken. Muscle disease should also be excluded by obtaining serum creatine kinase and aldolase levels.

The next step in the evaluation is to assess the patient for the more common and treatable causes of liver disease, including chronic hepatitis B and C, hemochromatosis, autoimmune hepatitis, Wilson disease, and MASLD. Although autoimmune hepatitis is commonly considered a disease of young to middle-aged women, it is also seen in men and has been reported in all ethnic groups (see Chapter 92). The clinical onset of Wilson disease is usually between 3 and 55 years of age; the diagnosis should be considered initially in all patients aged 40 or younger and those older than age 40 with aminotransferase elevations that remain unexplained after other causes are excluded (see Chapter 78). MASLD is the most common cause of elevated serum aminotransferase levels in the world (see Chapter 89), but there is no specific laboratory test for MASLD.

If testing for the more common causes fails to provide a diagnosis, the less common causes of liver disease, such as α_1-antitrypsin deficiency, and extrahepatic causes of persistently

BOX 75.1 Causes of Elevated Serum Aminotransferase Levels[a]

CHRONIC, MILD ELEVATIONS, ALT > AST (<150 U/L OR 5 × NORMAL)

Hepatic

α_1-Antitrypsin deficiency
Autoimmune hepatitis
Chronic viral hepatitis (B, C, and D)
Hemochromatosis
Medications and toxins
Steatosis and steatohepatitis
Wilson disease

Nonhepatic

Celiac disease
Hyperthyroidism

SEVERE, ACUTE ELEVATIONS, ALT > AST (>1000 U/L OR >20–25 × NORMAL)

Hepatic

Acute bile duct obstruction
Acute Budd-Chiari syndrome
Acute viral hepatitis
Autoimmune hepatitis
Drugs and toxins
Hepatic artery ligation
Ischemic hepatitis
Wilson disease

SEVERE, ACUTE ELEVATIONS, AST > ALT (>1000 U/L OR >20–25 × NORMAL)

Hepatic

Medications or toxins in a patient with underlying alcohol-associated liver injury

Nonhepatic

Acute rhabdomyolysis
Chronic, mild elevations, AST > ALT (<150 U/L, <5 × normal)

Hepatic

Alcohol-associated liver injury (AST/ALT >2:1, AST nearly always <300 U/L)
Cirrhosis

Nonhepatic

Hypothyroidism
Macro-AST
Myopathy
Strenuous exercise

[a]Virtually any liver disease can cause moderate aminotransferase elevations (5–15 × normal).

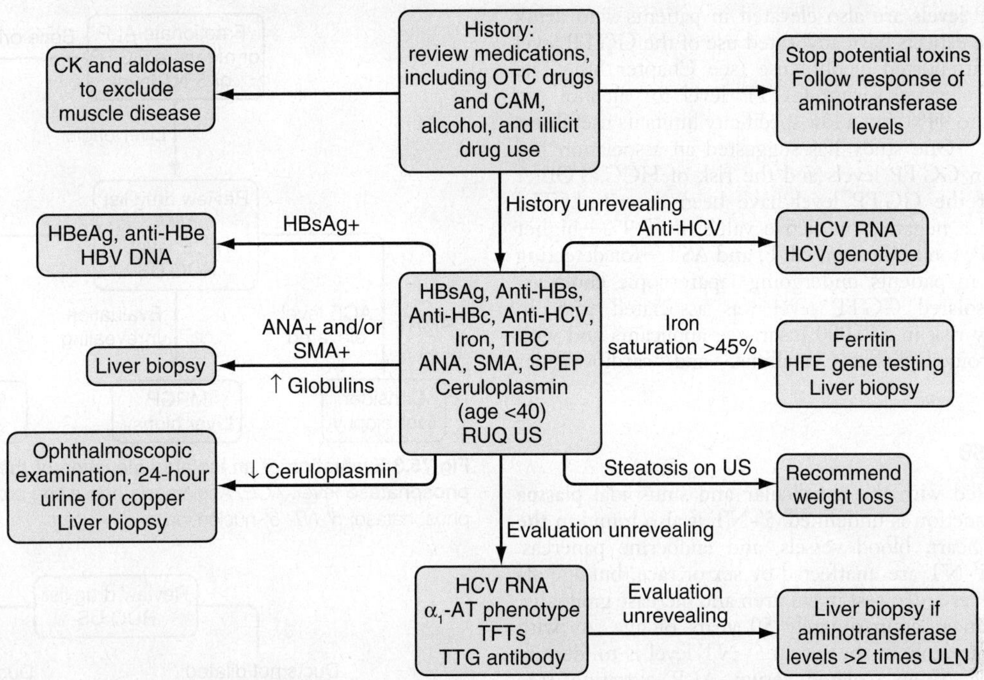

Fig 75.2 Evaluation of asymptomatic elevation of serum aminotransferase levels. *a_1-AT*, a_1-antitrypsin; *ANA*, antinuclear antibodies; *anti-HBc*, antibody to hepatitis B core antigen; *anti-HBe*, antibody to hepatitis B e antigen; *anti-HBs*, antibody to hepatitis B surface antigen; *anti-HCV*, antibody to HCV; *CAM*, complementary and alternative medicines; *CK*, creatine kinase; *HBeAg*, hepatitis B e antigen; *HBsAg*, hepatitis B surface antigen; *HFE*, hemochromatosis; *OTC*, over the counter; *SMA*, smooth muscle antibodies; *SPEP*, serum protein electrophoresis; *TIBC*, total iron binding capacity; *TFTs*, thyroid function tests; *TTG*, tissue transglutaminase; *ULN*, upper limit of normal.

elevated liver enzyme levels, such as thyroid disease and celiac disease, should be sought. A meta-analysis of 11 studies has shown that undetected celiac disease is a potential cause of otherwise unexplained elevated serum aminotransferase levels in 3%–4% of cases (and thus a more common explanation than Wilson disease).[26] If testing for these disorders is negative, the decision to perform a liver biopsy is determined by the degree of aminotransferase elevation, with the recognition that in most cases the results of the biopsy are unlikely to alter management.

ALKALINE PHOSPHATASE

The term *alkaline phosphatase* applies generally to a group of isoenzymes distributed widely throughout the body.[27] The isoenzymes of greatest clinical importance in adults are in the liver and bone because these organs are the major sources of serum ALP. Other isoenzymes originate from the placenta, small intestine, and kidneys. In the liver, ALP is found on the canalicular membrane of hepatocytes; its precise function is undefined. ALP has a serum half-life of approximately 7 days, and although the sites of degradation are unknown, clearance of ALP from serum is independent of either patency of the biliary tract or functional capacity of the liver. Hepatobiliary disease leads to increased serum ALP levels through induced synthesis of the enzyme and leakage into the serum, a process mediated by bile acids.[28]

A number of individual physiologic variations in serum ALP levels have been identified. Patients with blood groups O and B have elevations in serum ALP levels caused by release of intestinal ALP after a fatty meal.[29] This observation is the basis for the recommendation by some authorities that the serum ALP level be checked in the fasting state. An increased serum ALP level of intestinal origin is seen in benign familial elevation of the serum ALP. Serum ALP values vary with age. Male and female adolescents have serum ALP levels twice the level seen in adults; the level correlates with bone growth, and the increase in serum is in bone ALP. Although the level of serum ALP increases after 30 years of age in both men and women, the increase is more pronounced in women than in men; a healthy 65-year-old woman has a serum ALP level 50% higher than that of a healthy 30-year-old woman.[30] The reason for this difference is not known. In a person with isolated elevation of the serum ALP level, the serum GGTP or 5′-NT is used to distinguish a liver from a bone origin of the ALP elevation (see later). A low serum ALP level may occur in patients with Wilson disease, especially those presenting with ALF and hemolysis, possibly because of reduced activity of the enzyme owing to displacement of the cofactor zinc by copper (see Chapter 78).

Gamma Glutamyl Transpeptidase

GGTP is found in the cell membranes of a wide distribution of tissues, including liver (both hepatocytes and cholangiocytes), kidney, pancreas, spleen, heart, brain, and seminal vesicles. It is present in the serum of healthy persons. Serum levels are not different between men and women and do not rise in pregnancy. Although an elevated serum GGTP level has high sensitivity for hepatobiliary disease, its lack of specificity limits its clinical utility. The primary use of serum GGTP levels is to identify the source of an isolated elevation in the serum ALP level; GGTP is not elevated in bone disease (Fig. 75.3).[31] GGTP is elevated in patients taking antiepileptics, including phenytoin, carbamazepine, valproic acid, and barbiturates, as well as some drugs used in antiretroviral therapy, such as nonnucleoside reverse transcriptase inhibitors and the nucleoside reverse transcriptase inhibitor abacavir.[32–34]

Serum GGTP levels are also elevated in patients who drink alcohol, and some experts have advocated use of the GGTP level for identifying unreported alcohol use (see Chapter 88). The sensitivity of an elevated serum GGTP level for alcohol use ranges from 52% to 94%, but a low specificity limits its usefulness for this purpose.[35] One study has suggested an association between high serum GGTP levels and the risk of HCC.[36] Other potential uses of the GGTP level have been described. The GGTP level had a negative predictive value of 97.9%—higher than that for ALP, total bilirubin, ALT, and AST—for detecting bile duct stones in patients undergoing laparoscopic cholecystectomy.[37] An isolated GGTP level was associated with an elevated mortality risk in 560,000 insurance applicants and with metabolic syndrome, diabetes mellitus, and cardiovascular disease.[38]

5′-Nucleotidase

5′-NT is associated with the canalicular and sinusoidal plasma membranes; its function is undefined. 5′-NT is also found in the intestine, brain, heart, blood vessels, and endocrine pancreas. Serum levels of 5′-NT are unaffected by sex or race, but age affects the level; values are lowest in children and increase gradually, reaching a plateau at approximately 50 years of age. As with GGTP, the primary role of the serum 5′-NT level is to identify the organ source of an isolated serum ALP elevation (see Fig. 75.3). The 5′-NT level is not increased in bone disease and is increased primarily in hepatobiliary disease.

Approach to the Patient With an Elevated Level

The first step in the evaluation of a patient with an isolated and asymptomatic elevation of the serum ALP is to identify the tissue source (see Fig. 75.3). The most precise way of doing this is via fractionation through electrophoresis; each isoenzyme of ALP has a different electrophoretic mobility.[39] Tests used in the past that involved heat and urea denaturation of ALP are neither sensitive nor specific. An acceptable alternative method is to check either the serum GGTP or 5′-NT level; elevation of either verifies that the elevated ALP is the result of hepatobiliary disease. A normal 5′-NT level, however, does not rule out the possibility of hepatobiliary disease, because the 5′-NT and ALP do not necessarily increase in parallel in early or mild hepatic injury, thus making GGTP the preferred test.

The primary value of an elevated serum level of ALP of liver origin is to allow the recognition of a cholestatic disorder (i.e., a disorder associated with impaired bile flow, often with jaundice). In general, a serum ALP elevation out of proportion to the level of the aminotransferases suggests a cholestatic disorder (see Chapter 22). A fourfold elevation of the serum ALP is seen in approximately 75% of patients with chronic cholestasis, both intrahepatic and/or extrahepatic, whereas lesser elevations are nonspecific and can occur in a wide range of conditions. Figs. 75.3 and 75.4 illustrate the recommended evaluation of cholestatic liver enzymes—either an isolated ALP elevation (see Fig. 75.3) or a disproportionate elevation of the ALP compared with the aminotransferases (see Fig. 75.4).

Central to the evaluation of an elevated ALP level is imaging of the biliary tract. Absence of dilated intrahepatic bile ducts focuses the search on intrahepatic causes of cholestasis (Box 75.2), whereas dilated ducts should lead to an evaluation of extrahepatic causes of cholestasis (Box 75.3). As with elevated aminotransferase levels, the evaluation of intrahepatic causes of cholestatic liver enzymes begins with a carefully taken history of medication use, including OTC medications, CAM, and drugs of abuse, and temporal correlation of their use with elevation of the liver enzyme levels. Withdrawal of the offending agent and resolution of the liver enzyme elevations is sufficient to confirm the diagnosis, and a liver biopsy is generally not required. The rate of improvement can be slow, and if bile duct destruction has developed (vanishing bile duct syndrome), the changes may be irreversible.

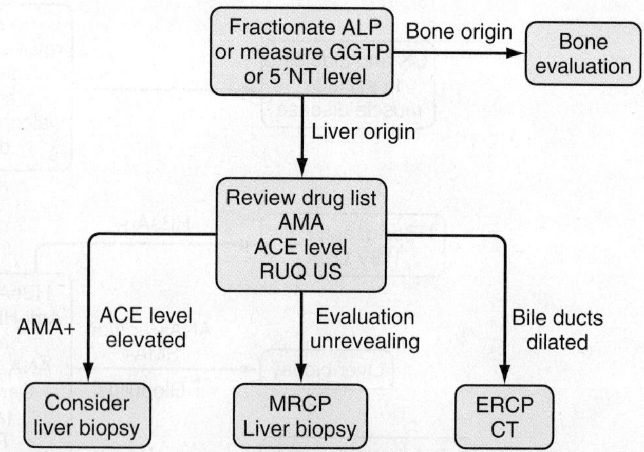

Fig 75.3 Evaluation of an isolated elevation of the serum alkaline phosphatase level. *ACE*, Angiotensin-converting enzyme; *ALP*, alkaline phosphatase; *5′-NT*, 5′-nucleotidase.

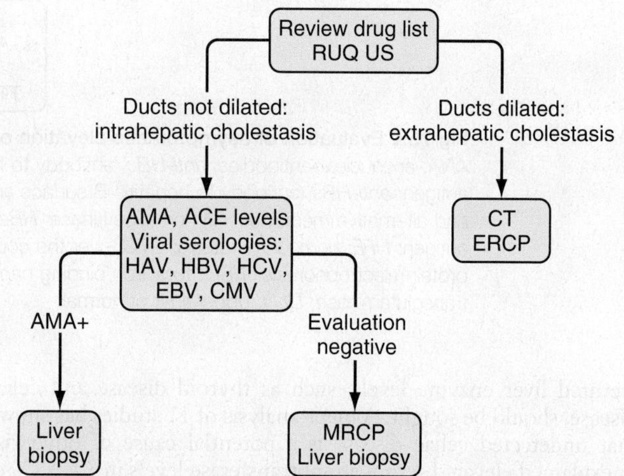

Fig 75.4 Evaluation of cholestatic liver enzyme elevations. *ACE*, Angiotensin-converting enzyme.

PBC is a classic autoimmune disease. The immunologic injury is characterized by T cell–mediated destruction of the intrahepatic bile ducts. Although predominantly a disease of middle-aged women, with a median age at diagnosis of approximately 50 years, 5%–10% of affected patients are men. The reported age range is 22–93 years. AMA is found in serum in 95% of patients and is diagnostic in combination with cholestatic serum liver enzymes; a liver biopsy specimen that demonstrates characteristic histologic findings is confirmatory (see Chapter 93).

PSC is a disease of altered immunity marked by inflammation and fibrosis of the intra- or extrahepatic bile ducts, or both. The disorder is strongly associated with IBD and is found most commonly in younger men. The diagnosis is confirmed by cholangiography, either MRCP or ERCP (see Chapter 70).

Granulomatous liver disease can be caused by several disorders (see Box 75.2). Infectious etiologies must be excluded because the treatment for many of the other causes of granulomatous liver disease is immunosuppressive therapy. Sarcoidosis is the most common etiology. The diagnosis is based on typical extrahepatic manifestations and, in some cases, an elevated angiotensin-converting enzyme level. Hepatic involvement, however, is

BOX 75.2 Intrahepatic Causes of Cholestatic Liver Enzyme Elevations in Adults

Drugs[a]
- *Bland cholestasis*
  - Anabolic steroids
  - Estrogens
- *Cholestatic hepatitis*
  - Angiotensin-converting enzyme inhibitors: captopril, enalapril
  - Azathioprine
  - Chlorpromazine
  - NSAIDs: sulindac, piroxicam
- *Granulomatous hepatitis*
  - Allopurinol
  - Antibiotics: amoxicillin-clavulanic acid, dicloxacillin, flucloxacillin, macrolides, sulfonamides
  - Antifungals: ketoconazole
  - Antiepileptics: carbamazepine, phenytoin
  - Cardiovascular agents: hydralazine, procainamide, quinidine
  - Phenylbutazone
- *Vanishing bile duct syndrome*
  - Phenothiazines: chlorpromazine

PBC

PSC

Granulomatous Liver Disease
- Infections
- Brucellosis
- Fungal: histoplasmosis, coccidioidomycosis
- Leprosy
- Q fever
- Schistosomiasis
- TB, *Mycobacterium avium* complex, bacillus Calmette-Guérin
- Sarcoidosis
- Idiopathic granulomatous hepatitis
- Other
- Crohn disease
- Heavy metal exposure: beryllium, copper
- Hodgkin disease

Viral Hepatitis
- HAV
- HBV and HCV, including fibrosing cholestatic hepatitis
- HDV
- HEV
- EBV
- CMV

Idiopathic Adulthood Ductopenia

Genetic Conditions
- Progressive familial intrahepatic cholestasis
- Type 1 (formerly Byler disease)
- Type 2
- Type 3

Benign recurrent intrahepatic cholestasis
- Type 1
- Type 2

Cystic Fibrosis

Malignancy
- HCC
- Metastatic disease
- Paraneoplastic syndrome
- Non-Hodgkin lymphoma
- Prostate cancer
- Renal cell cancer

Infiltrative Liver Disease
- Amyloidosis
- Lymphoma

Intrahepatic Cholestasis of Pregnancy

TPN

Graft-Versus-Host Disease

Sepsis

[a]Categorized by histologic pattern. Drug lists are not meant to be comprehensive.

BOX 75.3 Extrahepatic Causes of Cholestatic Liver Enzymes in Adults

INTRINSIC

AIDS cholangiopathy
Ampullary cancer
Ascariasis
Autoimmune pancreatitis
Cholangiocarcinoma
Choledocholithiasis
CMV
Cryptosporidiosis
Immune-mediated duct injury
Infections
Malignancy
Microsporidiosis
Parasitic infections
PSC

EXTRINSIC

Gallbladder cancer
Malignancy
Metastases, including portal adenopathy from metastases
Mirizzi syndrome
Pancreatic cancer
Pancreatic pseudocyst
Pancreatitis

uncommonly the impetus for initiating therapy for sarcoidosis (see Chapter 35).

Viral hepatitis, particularly cases caused by EBV and CMV, can manifest with a prominent cholestatic liver enzyme pattern (see Chapter 85). A number of familial conditions produce intrahepatic cholestasis. Progressive forms of these disorders manifest in childhood, whereas the benign forms—benign recurrent intrahepatic cholestasis types 1 and 2—can manifest for the first time in adulthood (see Chapter 79). Other intrahepatic causes of cholestatic liver enzymes are listed in Box 75.2.

If imaging shows intrahepatic ductal dilatation, the evaluation focuses on the extrahepatic biliary tract to identify an intrinsic or extrinsic cause of biliary obstruction (see Box 75.3). The evaluation often includes an ERCP for tissue acquisition and placement of a biliary stent if obstruction is present (see Chapter 72). CT provides assessment for an extrinsic process, and tissue acquisition can be performed with CT or EUS guidance.

TESTS OF HEPATIC SYNTHETIC FUNCTION

Albumin

Quantitatively, the most important plasma protein, albumin, accounts for 75% of the plasma colloid oncotic pressure and is synthesized exclusively by hepatocytes. The average adult produces approximately 15 g/day and has 300–500 g of albumin distributed in body fluids. The liver has the ability to double the rate of synthesis in the setting of rapid albumin loss or a dilutional decrease in the serum albumin concentration.[40] The half-life of albumin is 14–21 days; there are multiple sites of degradation, including skin, muscle, liver, and kidney, as well as leakage in the gut. Albumin synthesis is regulated by changes in nutritional status, osmotic pressure, systemic inflammation, and hormone levels.[41] Therefore the differential diagnosis of serum hypoalbuminemia, in addition to hepatocellular dysfunction, includes malnutrition, excessive loss from protein-losing enteropathy or nephrotic syndrome, chronic systemic inflammatory conditions, and hormonal imbalances.

The long half-life of albumin in serum accounts for its unreliability as a marker of hepatic synthetic function in acute liver injury. Serum albumin levels less than 3 g/dL in a patient with newly diagnosed hepatitis should raise suspicion of a chronic process. Serum albumin is an excellent marker of hepatic synthetic function in patients with chronic liver disease and cirrhosis, with the exception of patients with cirrhosis and ascites, who may have normal or increased albumin production but an increased volume of distribution that results in a low serum albumin level. Albumin has no utility as a screening test in patients for whom there is low suspicion of liver disease; a study in which the serum albumin level was measured in 449 consecutive patients yielded 56 abnormal results, of which only 2 (0.4%) were of clinical importance.[42]

Prothrombin Time

Clotting is the end result of a complex series of enzymatic reactions involving clotting factors, all of which are produced in the liver except factor VIII, which is produced by vascular endothelial cells. The prothrombin time is a measure of the rate at which prothrombin is converted to thrombin, reflecting the extrinsic pathway of coagulation (see Chapter 96). Factors involved in the synthesis of prothrombin include II, V, VII, and X. The INR is used to express the degree of anticoagulation on warfarin therapy. The INR standardizes prothrombin time measurement according to the characteristics of the thromboplastin reagent used in a particular laboratory; the initial measurement is expressed as an international sensitivity index (ISI), which is then used in calculating the INR. Because the ISI is validated only for patients taking a vitamin K antagonist, concern has been raised about the validity of using the ISI (and INR) in patients with chronic liver disease.[43] Two studies have demonstrated, in fact, that the ISI, as currently determined, is not accurate for calculating the INR in patients with cirrhosis, and the investigators have proposed that specific ISI and INR determinations using control patients with liver disease can eliminate interlaboratory variability in calculating the INR in patients with cirrhosis.[44,45]

A prolonged prothrombin time can be caused by a number of conditions besides reduced hepatic synthetic function: congenital deficiency of clotting factors, vitamin K deficiency (vitamin K is required for normal functioning of factors II, VII, IX, and X), and DIC. DIC can be identified by measuring a factor VIII level in serum; the level is decreased in DIC and normal or increased in liver disease. Vitamin K deficiency is identified by demonstrating that IV administration of vitamin K (e.g., 10 mg) leads to improvement in the prothrombin time; a 30% or more improvement in the prothrombin time is consistent with hypovitaminosis K. Oral vitamin K may not be absorbed by the intestine in patients with jaundice (see Chapter 96).

Measurement of the prothrombin time in patients with liver disease is most useful in cases of acute liver disease. Unlike the serum albumin, the prothrombin time allows an assessment of current hepatic synthetic function; factor VII has the shortest serum half-life (6 hours) of all the clotting factors. The prothrombin time has prognostic value in patients with acute acetaminophen- and nonacetaminophen-related liver failure (see Chapter 97), as well as alcohol-associated hepatitis (see Chapter 88). The INR is a component of the MELD score, which is used to allocate donor organs for LT (see Chapter 99). The MELD score accurately predicts survival in patients with decompensated cirrhosis (see later).

The prothrombin time is not an accurate measure of bleeding risk in patients with cirrhosis, because it assesses only the activity of procoagulant clotting factors, not anticoagulant factors such as protein C and antithrombin, the production of which is also reduced in cirrhosis. The partial thromboplastin time (PTT) assesses the intrinsic pathway of the coagulation cascade. The PTT can be prolonged in patients with advanced cirrhosis, but prolongation of the PTT is less sensitive than the PT for detecting coagulopathy.

TESTS TO DETECT HEPATIC FIBROSIS

Although liver biopsy is the standard for the assessment of hepatic fibrosis, noninvasive measures of hepatic fibrosis have been developed and have shown promise (see Chapters 76 and 82).[46] These measures include single serum biochemical markers that potentially reflect the activity level of hepatic fibrogenesis [hyaluronic acid (or hyaluronan) is the best to date] and multiparameter tests aimed at detecting and staging the degree of hepatic fibrosis (>20 such tests are described in the literature).

Hyaluronic acid is a glucosaminoglycan produced in mesenchymal cells and widely distributed in the extracellular space. Typically degraded by hepatic sinusoidal cells, serum levels of hyaluronic acid are elevated in patients with cirrhosis as a result of sinusoidal capillarization (see Chapter 94). A fasting hyaluronic acid level greater than 100 mg/L had a sensitivity of 83% and specificity of 78% for the detection of cirrhosis in patients with a variety of chronic liver diseases.[47] Hyaluronic acid has been shown to be useful for identifying advanced fibrosis in patients with chronic hepatitis C, chronic hepatitis B, alcohol-associated liver disease, and NASH.[48] Preoperative serum hyaluronic acid levels also have been shown to correlate with the development of hepatic dysfunction after hepatectomy.[49]

FibroTest (marketed as FibroSure in the United States) is the best evaluated of the multiparameter blood tests. The test incorporates haptoglobin, bilirubin, GGTP, apolipoprotein A-I, and α_2-macroglobulin and has been found to have high positive and negative predictive values for diagnosing advanced fibrosis in patients with chronic hepatitis C (see Chapter 82). One study showed that use of a higher index cutoff led to a sensitivity of 90%, specificity of 36%, positive predictive value of 88%, and negative predictive value of 40% for the diagnosis of bridging fibrosis in patients with chronic hepatitis C.[50] The test has similar performance characteristics in patients with chronic hepatitis B and alcohol-associated liver disease and has been shown to predict advanced fibrosis in patients taking methotrexate for psoriasis.[51] The FIBROSpect II assay (subsequently FIBROSpect HCV and FIBROSpect NASH) incorporates hyaluronic acid, tissue inhibitor of metalloproteinase 1, and α_2-macroglobulin. In a group of patients with chronic hepatitis C, FIBROSpect II had a sensitivity of 72% and a specificity of 74% for identifying advanced fibrosis.[52] The Enhanced Liver Fibrosis (ELF) test combines measurements of three markers of the hepatic extracellular matrix—procollagen type III N-terminal peptide, tissue inhibitor of metalloproteinase-1, and hyaluronic acid.[53] ELF has been shown to perform well as a marker of fibrosis in viral hepatitis, MASLD, and cholangiopathies.

Vibration-controlled transient elastography, marketed as FibroScan, as well as acoustic radiation force impulse elastography, uses US waves to measure hepatic stiffness noninvasively (see Chapter 76). Central to the development of this technique were the principles that fibrosis leads to increased stiffness of hepatic tissue and that a shear wave will propagate faster through stiff material than through elastic material.[54] The US transducer emits a low-frequency (50 Hz) shear wave, and the amount of time required for the wave to go through a set "window" of tissue is measured.[55] The window of tissue is 1 cm by 4 cm—100 times the area of an average liver biopsy specimen. A meta-analysis showed that transient elastography performed best at differentiating cirrhosis from absence of cirrhosis but was less accurate for the estimation of lesser degrees of fibrosis.[56] Transient elastography has been shown to be accurate for identifying advanced fibrosis in patients with chronic hepatitis C, PBC, hemochromatosis, MASLD, and recurrent chronic hepatitis after LT[57–60] and was approved by the FDA in 2013 for use in patients with liver disease.

Magnetic resonance elastography (MRE) is another noninvasive technique that has been approved by the FDA. The shear elasticity of the liver is measured after low-frequency (65 Hz) waves are transmitted into the right lobe of the liver. In one study,[61] MRE was found to be superior to transient elastography for staging liver fibrosis in patients with a variety of chronic liver diseases, but it is more expensive.

QUANTITATIVE LIVER FUNCTION TESTS

Quantitative function tests have been developed in the hope of evaluating the excretory or detoxification capacity of the liver more specifically than does the serum bilirubin level. Although these tests lead to improved sensitivity, their lack of specificity and often cumbersome methodology have limited their widespread acceptance, except in research settings.

Indocyanine Green Clearance

Indocyanine green (ICG) is a nontoxic dye that is cleared exclusively by the liver; 97% of an administered dose (0.5 mg/kg given as an IV bolus) is excreted unchanged into bile. ICG can be measured directly by spectrophotometry. Noninvasive methods (dichromatic earlobe densitometry and fingertip optical sensors) generate data that appear to correlate well with levels determined by blood sampling. Possible uses of ICG include the assessment of hepatic dysfunction, measurement of hepatic blood flow, and prediction of clinical outcomes in patients with liver disease. Unfortunately, measurement of ICG has proved to be insensitive for detecting hepatic dysfunction and is inaccurate for measuring blood flow in patients with cirrhosis because of decreased ICG extraction by the diseased liver. Although ICG measurement has shown some promise for predicting outcomes in certain clinical populations, such as burn patients, it has not been used widely outside of research protocols.[62]

Galactose Elimination Capacity

The galactose elimination capacity (GEC) has been studied as a measure of functional hepatic mass. Galactose is given as a single IV bolus (0.5 g/kg), and blood samples are collected. Patients with cirrhosis and chronic hepatitis have reduced galactose clearance from serum as compared with healthy controls. In a study of 781 patients with newly diagnosed cirrhosis and a decreased GEC, the GEC was a strong predictor of short- and long-term all-cause and cirrhosis-related mortality.[63]

Caffeine Clearance

Caffeine clearance tests quantify functional hepatic capacity by assessing the activity of cytochrome P450 1A2, *N*-acetyltransferase, and xanthine oxidase. Caffeine is given orally (200–366 mg), and levels are measured in blood, urine, saliva, breath, or scalp hair. The alternative (nonblood measurement) methods correlate well with the plasma clearance method. Tobacco use increases caffeine clearance, and drug interactions can affect results. Increasing age correlates with decreased caffeine clearance. Overnight salivary caffeine clearance has been shown to correlate with ICG measurements and galactose clearance as well as with results of the aminopyrine breath test (ABT) (see later).[64]

Lidocaine Metabolite Formation

Lidocaine is metabolized to its major metabolite monoethylglycinexylidide (MEGX) by the hepatic cytochrome P450 system.[65] Serum samples are taken 15, 30, and 60 minutes after IV administration of lidocaine (1 mg/kg). Neither MEGX formation nor galactose elimination was found to be superior to the Child-Turcotte-Pugh (CTP) (see Chapter 94) or MELD score (see Chapter 99) in predicting prognosis in patients with cirrhosis secondary to viral hepatitis (see later).[66] Other studies have suggested that a decline in MEGX concentration correlates well with histologic worsening in patients with chronic liver disease.[67]

Aminopyrine Breath Test

The ^{15}C and ^{14}C ABTs measure hepatic mixed-function oxidase mass. The radioactive methyl groups of aminopyrine undergo demethylation and eventual conversion to labeled CO_2, which is then exhaled and can be measured. After an overnight fast, a known dose of ^{15}C aminopyrine (1–2 μCi) is administered orally, and breath samples are taken every 30 minutes for 4 hours; some investigators check a single sample at either 1 or 2 hours. Healthy subjects excrete 6.6% ± 1.3% of the administered dose in the breath in 2 hours; patients with hepatocellular injury excrete considerably less. The degree of decrease in excretion of aminopyrine overlaps considerably in patients with all types of severe liver disease, including cirrhosis, chronic hepatitis, alcohol-associated liver disease, and HCC.[68] Although data have been conflicting regarding the ability of this test to predict survival in patients with chronic liver disease, a study in 2012 of 50 patients showed that the ABT accurately predicted the risk of disease progression in patients with HCV-related chronic hepatitis.[69]

BILE ACIDS

Bile acids are synthesized from cholesterol in hepatocytes, conjugated to glycine or taurine, and secreted into bile (see Chapter 66). After passage into the small intestine, most bile acids are actively reabsorbed. The liver efficiently extracts bile acids from the portal blood. In healthy persons, all bile acids in serum emanate from the reabsorption of bile acids in the small intestine. Maintenance of normal serum bile acid concentrations depends on hepatic blood flow, hepatic uptake, secretion of bile acids, and intestinal transit. Serum bile acids are sensitive but nonspecific indicators of hepatic dysfunction and allow some quantification of functional hepatic reserve. Serum bile acid levels correlate moderately well with the results of ABTs in patients with chronic hepatitis.[70] Unfortunately, the correlation between serum bile acid levels and the histologic severity of chronic hepatitis and alcohol-associated liver disease is poor.[71] Serum bile acid levels are elevated in patients with cholestatic liver diseases but normal in patients with Gilbert syndrome and Dubin-Johnson syndrome and can be used to make the distinction. Although decreased serum bile acid levels are highly specific indicators of liver dysfunction, they are not as sensitive as initially hoped.

SPECIFIC APPLICATIONS OF LIVER BIOCHEMICAL TESTING

Liver biochemical tests have been used to monitor for and assess the severity of DILI, assess operative risk, identify candidates for LT, and direct donor organ allocation.

Drug-Induced Liver Injury

Most drugs that are hepatotoxic cause idiosyncratic liver injury, defined as injury that is unpredictable, occurs at therapeutic drug levels, and is infrequent (see Chapter 90). The estimated frequency of idiosyncratic DILI for any particular medication ranges from 1 in 1000 to 1 in 100,000. These reactions are marked by a variable latency period ranging from 5 to 90 days, or even longer.[72] Other drugs produce dose-dependent toxicity. These injuries are predictable, have a high incidence, and generally have a well-understood mechanism. Acetaminophen is the classic example of a drug that causes dose-dependent liver injury. The dose of acetaminophen exceeds 15 g, almost four times the recommended daily dose, in 80% of cases. Acetaminophen doses within the therapeutic range (≤4 g/day) can be sufficient to cause liver injury in susceptible persons, such as those who use ethanol chronically. The King's College criteria identify patients with a poor prognosis from acetaminophen-induced liver injury: those with an arterial pH below 7.3 or those with an INR above 6.5, serum creatinine level above 3.4 g/dL, and stage 3–4 hepatic encephalopathy (see Chapters 90 and 97).[73]

Most occurrences of DILI are mild and respond promptly to drug withdrawal with complete resolution. Isolated elevation of the serum aminotransferase levels, even to values greater than three times the upper limit of normal, is associated with a favorable outcome. When aminotransferase elevations are associated with clinical jaundice (so-called Hy's Law, after the late Dr. Hyman Zimmerman), the risk of mortality is increased to as high as 10% (see Chapter 90).[74]

Surgical Candidacy and Organ Allocation

Patients with acute and chronic liver disease are potentially at increased risk of morbidity and mortality if they undergo surgery. The risk depends on the etiology of the liver disease, severity of the liver disease, and planned operation.[75] Although routine preoperative liver biochemical testing is not recommended in otherwise healthy people, the identification of unexpected elevated liver enzyme levels should prompt a postponement of surgery until the cause of the abnormalities has been identified. A retrospective analysis found that patients with acute viral hepatitis who undergo laparotomy had an operative mortality rate of approximately 9.5%.[76] Elective surgery should be postponed in patients with acute hepatitis. The surgical risk in patients with chronic hepatitis correlates with the severity of histologic inflammation in the liver. Those with only portal inflammation and interface hepatitis have low operative risk, whereas those with panlobular hepatitis have an increased risk. The etiology of chronic hepatitis does not influence outcome.

Examination of histology is also critical in assessing the surgical risk in patients with alcohol-associated liver disease. Hepatic steatosis alone is associated with a low operative risk, whereas alcohol-associated hepatitis is associated with a mortality rate as high as 55% in patients undergoing portosystemic shunt surgery, for example. A period of abstinence of 3–6 months before elective surgery is recommended in these patients. Few data exist for surgical risk in patients with MASLD, but the mortality rate appears to correlate with the severity of steatosis in patients undergoing liver resection. Steatohepatitis may carry a higher risk than that for steatosis.

An estimated 10% of patients with advanced liver disease undergo surgery in the last 2 years of their lives. Cirrhosis is associated with increased operative risk, particularly with certain types of surgery, including hepatic resection, other abdominal operations, and cardiothoracic surgery. The data evaluating the surgical risk in these patients were derived retrospectively but point consistently toward the usefulness of the CTP scoring system for predicting perioperative mortality. Two studies performed more than 10 years apart examined mortality after abdominal surgery in cirrhotic patients and reported nearly identical rates of mortality for patients with Child-Pugh class A, B, and C cirrhosis: 10%, 30%–31%, and 76%–82%, respectively[77,78]; however, lower mortality rates have since been reported with greater use of laparoscopic surgery at an expert center.[79] In general, surgery may be undertaken in patients with Child-Pugh class A cirrhosis, whereas the medical condition of patients with Child-Pugh class B cirrhosis should be optimized prior to planned surgery. The mortality rate in patients with Child-Pugh class C cirrhosis is prohibitive, and surgery should be avoided.

The MELD score was created originally to predict survival in patients with cirrhosis and portal hypertension undergoing placement of a TIPS.[80] The score has subsequently been validated as an accurate predictor of survival in patients with advanced liver disease. The MELD score incorporates 3 objective variables into a mathematical formula: $9.57 \times \log_e(\text{creatinine}) + 3.78 \times \log_e(\text{total bilirubin}) + 11.2 \times \log_e(\text{INR}) + 6.43$. The working range is 6–40, and the score has been shown to correlate with mortality in patients undergoing surgery other than LT, including hepatic resection, other abdominal procedures, and cardiac surgery.[81–83] The MELD score is used most often for prioritizing the allocation of donor organs for LT.[84] After implementation of the MELD score for prioritizing organ allocation, the number of deaths among patients on the wait list decreased (see Chapter 99).

In 2016 the serum sodium was added to the MELD score equation for the purpose of organ allocation: $\text{MELD} + 1.32 \times (137 - \text{Na}) - [0.033 \times \text{MELD} \times (137 - \text{Na})]$. It was shown that doing so increases the predictive accuracy for determining death on the transplant waiting list.[85] Furthermore, investigators showed that implementation of the MELD-Na score would prevent 7% of waiting-list deaths.[86] The use of the MELD-Na score in assessing surgical risk (other than LT) has not been studied.

In 2023 a new model, MELD 3.0, which incorporated female sex, serum albumin, and a creatinine cutoff, was introduced after it was shown to improve mortality prediction compared to the MELD-Na model.[87]

Full references for this chapter can be found at https://ebooks.health.elsevier.com.

76 Overview of Cirrhosis

Patrick S. Kamath, Vijay H. Shah

IN THIS CHAPTER

DEFINITION

Cirrhosis, a final pathway for a wide variety of chronic liver diseases (Box 76.1), is a pathologic entity defined as diffuse hepatic fibrosis with the replacement of the normal liver architecture by nodules. The rate of progression of chronic liver disease to cirrhosis may be quite variable, from weeks in patients with complete biliary obstruction to decades in patients with steatotic liver disease and chronic hepatitis. Cirrhosis has traditionally been classified as *compensated* or *decompensated*. The development of complications of variceal hemorrhage, ascites, and hepatic encephalopathy characterizes decompensated cirrhosis. In compensated cirrhosis, the usually asymptomatic phase of cirrhosis, these complications are absent.[1] An overview of cirrhosis highlighting the natural history, diagnosis, and treatment goals is shown in Fig. 76.1.

GLOBAL BURDEN OF CIRRHOSIS

Cirrhosis is the 11th leading cause of death worldwide, but the 10th leading cause of death in Africa; 9th leading cause in Southeast Asia and Europe; and the 5th leading cause of death in the Eastern Mediterranean. Cirrhosis was the cause of 2.4% of global deaths in 2019.[2] Cirrhosis represents the 12th leading cause of disability-associated life-years in the age range of 25–49 years. In the United States in 2016, liver-related expenditure was $32.5 billion (95% CI, $27.0–$40.4 billion), with two-thirds for inpatient or emergency department care.[3] The cost of care for patients with cirrhosis is increasing by 4% per year, primarily driven by hospital-based services. Patients with cirrhosis are at risk for liver-related morbidity and mortality when they transition to a decompensated state. Hepatic decompensation (see Chapter 96) is more likely when the hepatic venous pressure gradient (HVPG) is ≥10 mm Hg, the threshold for defining clinically significant portal hypertension (CSPH). Globally, there were 10.6 million prevalent cases of decompensated cirrhosis and 112 million prevalent cases of compensated cirrhosis in 2017.[4]

The most common etiologies of cirrhosis worldwide are alcohol-associated liver disease, metabolic dysfunction-associated steatotic liver disease (MASLD, formerly known as nonalcoholic fatty liver disease), and viral hepatitis B and C.[1] Alcohol is the leading cause of cirrhosis globally and is responsible for almost 60% of cirrhosis in Europe, North America, and Latin-America. Alcohol is the etiology of more than 50% of cirrhosis deaths in the United States; globally, in 2019, more than 25% of cirrhosis deaths were associated with alcohol.[5] The amount of alcohol consumed, male sex, older age, obesity, type 2 diabetes mellitus, and gut microbial dysbiosis in genetically susceptible individuals are key factors in the development of cirrhosis and HCC. MASLD is the second leading cause overall of cirrhosis leading to liver transplantation and the leading cause among females in the United States. Viral hepatitis B and C–related disease, largely cirrhosis and its complications, resulted in 1.1 million deaths in 2020.

The progression from chronic liver disease to cirrhosis irrespective of all etiologies likely follows a common pathway involving the stellate cell.

PATHOGENESIS

In normal liver, the hepatic stellate cell is viewed as a pericyte that lies abluminal to the sinusoidal endothelial cell in the space of Disse[1] (see Chapter 73). On activation, a hepatic stellate cell transforms into a myofibroblast (Fig. 76.2).[6] Activation is characterized by increases in the expression of smooth muscle actin, motility, and contractility. Most importantly for the development of liver fibrosis, the stellate cell begins to generate various forms of matrix, which lead to liver fibrosis.[6] Fibronectin is the earliest form of matrix produced by stellate cells, which ultimately produce other forms of matrix, including collagen type 1.[7] Matrix deposition in turn leads to further hepatic stellate cell activation as tissue stiffness promotes hepatic stellate cell activation. Matrix also leads to changes in the hepatic angioarchitecture.[7] The canonical pathways that are most implicated in the activation of the hepatic stellate cell include kinase activation pathways mediated through platelet-derived growth factor, transforming growth factor-β, and integrin signaling pathways.

In addition to the hepatic stellate cell, other cells, including portal fibroblasts,[8] may ultimately culminate in the myofibroblast phenotype that deposits collagen matrix. The portal fibroblast resides closer than hepatic stellate cells to the portal tract and is implicated in the liver fibrosis that develops in response to portal-based cholestatic injury, as in PBC and PSC.[8] It is hypothesized that epithelial cell injury in the periportal region leads to the transformation of portal fibroblasts into myofibroblasts. Other studies suggest that hepatic stellate cells may be responsible for fibrosis even in biliary forms of liver injury.[9]

Cell types other than myofibroblasts are also important in the fibrosis process. For example, epithelial cell injury is the initiating step in most forms of liver injury that lead to fibrosis. Injury to epithelial cells, either through apoptosis, inflammation, or sterile necrosis, culminates in the recruitment and activation of hepatic

BOX 76.1 Causes of Cirrhosis

VIRAL

HBV
HCV
HDV + HBV

IMMUNE-MEDIATED

Autoimmune hepatitis
PBC
PSC

TOXIC

Alcohol
? Arsenic

METABOLIC

α_1 Antitrypsin deficiency
Galactosemia
Glycogen storage disease
Hemochromatosis
MASLD/MASH
Wilson disease

BILIARY

Atresia
Biliary strictures

VASCULAR

Budd-Chiari syndrome
Cardiac cirrhosis

GENETIC

CF
Lysosomal acid lipase deficiency

IATROGENIC

Biliary injury/strictures
Drugs: high-dose vitamin A, methotrexate

stellate cells.[10] The macrophage is also important in fibrosis owing to the release of inflammatory cytokines, which in turn lead to transactivation of hepatic stellate cells into myofibroblasts. Macrophages are a complex target because some subclasses promote fibrosis, whereas others are required for fibrosis resolution.[6] Studies have also indicated an important role for the sinusoidal endothelial cell in fibrosis development. Sinusoidal endothelial cells act through autocrine and paracrine signaling pathways to participate in angiogenesis. Angiogenesis may lead to fibrosis through paracrine release of hepatic stellate cell-activating molecules from angiogenic sinusoidal endothelial cells. Therefore multiple cell types in the liver participate in fibrogenesis, although the hepatic stellate cell is most directly implicated in this process because of its abundant capacity to produce matrix.

DIAGNOSIS

Liver biopsy has long been the gold standard for diagnosing cirrhosis but is associated with costs and procedure-related risks, albeit infrequently. The major concerns regarding the use of a liver biopsy to diagnose cirrhosis include sampling error and interobserver disagreement in the estimation of the extent of fibrosis.[11] Although cirrhosis is strictly speaking a histologic diagnosis (Fig. 76.3), a combination of clinical, laboratory, and imaging features can help confirm a diagnosis of cirrhosis.

It is important to emphasize that physical findings that are typical of cirrhosis are seen only in patients with decompensated cirrhosis. An intense red coloration of the thenar and hypothenar eminences suggests palmar erythema. Terry's nails are characterized by proximal nail bed pallor, which can also involve the entire nail plate, with predominant involvement of the thumb and index finger. Clubbing of the fingernails may result from the presence of arteriovenous shunts in the lung as a result of portal hypertension and may reflect the presence of hepatopulmonary syndrome. Gynecomastia is the enlargement of the male breast with palpable tissue. Spider telangiectasias (or angiomata) are dilated arterioles characterized by a prominent central arteriole with radiating vessels. Compression of the central arteriole with a pinhead results in blanching followed by reformation of the "spider" after release of pressure on the arteriole. In general, more than two to three spider telangiectasias are considered abnormal. Dilated abdominal veins (caput medusae) with flow away from the umbilicus, toward the inferior vena cava in the infraumbilical area and toward the superior vena cava in the supraumbilical area, suggest intrahepatic portal hypertension. On the other hand, dilatation of veins in the flank with blood draining toward the superior vena cava suggests inferior vena caval obstruction. Parotid enlargement is also a feature of cirrhosis, especially alcohol-associated cirrhosis.

Patients with a history of chronic liver disease with gastroesophageal varices, ascites, or hepatic encephalopathy are likely to have cirrhosis, and liver biopsy is not essential in such cases for confirming cirrhosis. In patients with a diagnosis of chronic liver disease without these complications, physical findings of an enlarged left hepatic lobe with splenomegaly, along with the cutaneous stigmata of liver disease described earlier, suggest cirrhosis, especially in the setting of thrombocytopenia (the most common laboratory abnormality that suggests a diagnosis of cirrhosis) and impaired hepatic synthetic function (e.g., hypoalbuminemia and prolongation of the prothrombin time). If physical and laboratory findings are not suggestive of cirrhosis, imaging studies can help make a diagnosis of cirrhosis. A small nodular liver with splenomegaly and intra-abdominal collaterals and the presence of ascites on abdominal US (or other cross-sectional imaging study) suggests cirrhosis (Fig. 76.4).

A number of commercially available tools combine hematologic parameters, liver biochemical tests, and serologic markers to determine the degree of hepatic fibrosis.[12] In general, these tools are useful for discriminating early from late stages of fibrosis but not between individual stages of fibrosis (see Chapters 75 and 82). The best validated, cheap, and easy-to-use serological tests are the Fibrosis-4 index (FIB-4) which utilizes AST, ALT, platelets, and age; and the aspartate aminotransferase (AST)-to-platelets ratio index (APRI)[13] (Chapter 75). The NAFLD Fibrosis Score (NAFLD-FS) is more specific to MASLD. Commercially available biomarkers include FibroTest/FibroSure, Fibrospect NASH, enhanced liver fibrosis (ELF) panel, and NIS4. These panels are expensive but not appreciably more accurate than the FIB-4 and APRI tests. FIB-4 is a better test than APRI for assessment of hepatic fibrosis: a score <1.3 rules out significant fibrosis, whereas a score of ≥ 2.67 suggests F3 or F4 hepatic fibrosis, especially in patients with MASLD/MASH (Table 76.1). In general, noninvasive tests are more accurate in ruling out than in ruling in advanced hepatic fibrosis.

Where available, vibration-controlled transient elastography (or fibroelastography), acoustic radiation force impulse elastography (another form of US elastography),[12] or magnetic resonance elastography (MRE) can help confirm a diagnosis of cirrhosis (Table 76.1). In the US prospective study involving patients with MASLD, there were increased risks of liver-related complications and death with fibrosis stages F3 and F4.[14] It is also recognized that F3 and F4 stages are a continuum rather than distinct. With increasing use of liver stiffness measurement (LSM) by TE to assess degree of hepatic fibrosis without a liver biopsy

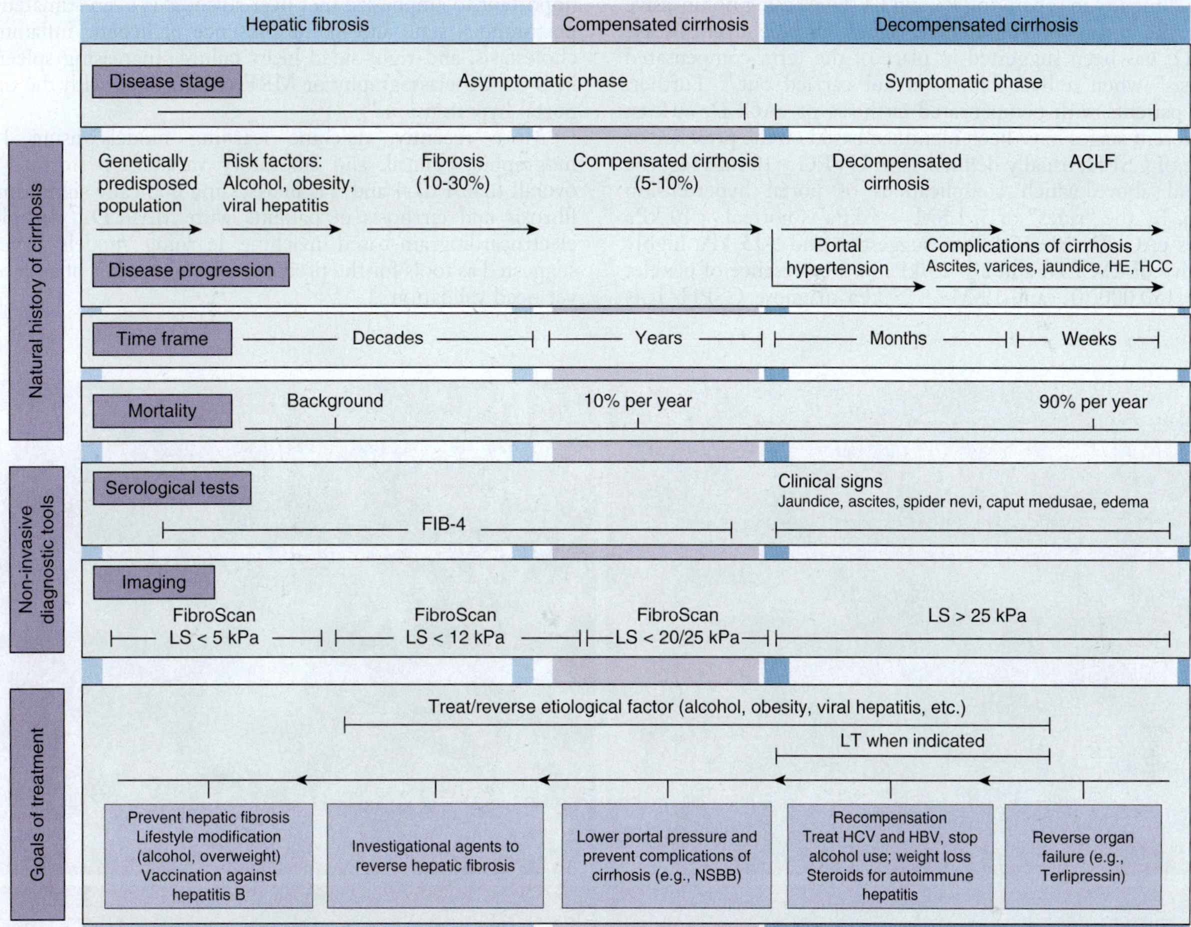

Fig. 76.1 An overview of cirrhosis highlighting the natural history, diagnostic tools, and goals of treatment. (Modified from Gines P, Krag A, Abraldes JG, Sola E, Fabrellas N, Kamath PS. Liver cirrhosis. *Lancet*. 2021;398(10308):1359–1376. https://doi.org/10.1016/S0140-6736(2101374-X).)

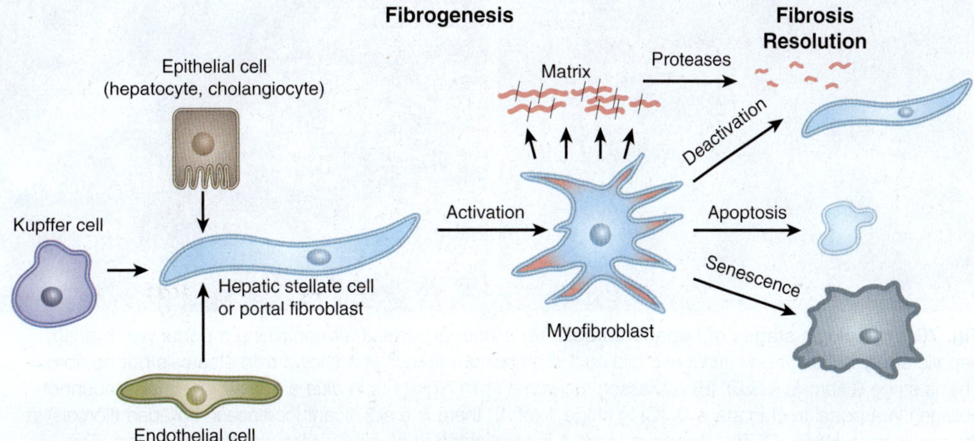

Fig. 76.2 Schematic overview of the pathogenesis of fibrosis and reversal of fibrosis in cirrhosis. Epithelial cell injury in combination with release of cytokines by Kupffer cells and release of paracrine molecules by sinusoidal endothelial cells leads to activation of hepatic stellate cells (or portal fibroblasts) into myofibroblasts. Reversal of fibrosis results from deactivation, apoptosis, or senescence of myofibroblasts. Release of matrix proteases can also lead to resolution of fibrosis (see text for details).

and the difficulty in separating F3 and F4 stages using noninvasive testing, the term compensated advanced chronic liver disease (cACLD) has been suggested in place of the term compensated "cirrhosis" when a liver biopsy is not carried out.[15] Further, among patients with compensated cirrhosis or cACLD, at least two different stages have been identified based on the presence or absence of CSPH, usually defined as an HVPG ≥10 mm Hg, the threshold above which complications of portal hypertension develop. By the "rules" of 5, LSM < 5 kPa is normal; <10 kPa excludes cACLD; 10–15 kPa is suggestive and >15 kPa highly suggestive of cACLD; and 20–25 kPa in the presence of platelet count <150,000/μL, and LSM ≥ 25 kPa diagnose CSPH. It is important to emphasize that liver stiffness is overestimated in the postprandial state and in the presence of hepatic inflammation, cholestasis, and right-sided heart failure. Increasing spleen stiffness on US elastography or MRE is associated with the onset of portal hypertension.[16]

More recently, machine learning models using 17 demographic, clinical, and laboratory variables performed better overall than FIB-4 and TE in assessing clinically significant liver fibrosis and cirrhosis in patients with MASLD.[17] In addition, electrocardiogram-based machine learning models have been suggested as tools for the prediction and diagnosis of cirrhosis but yet need validation.[18]

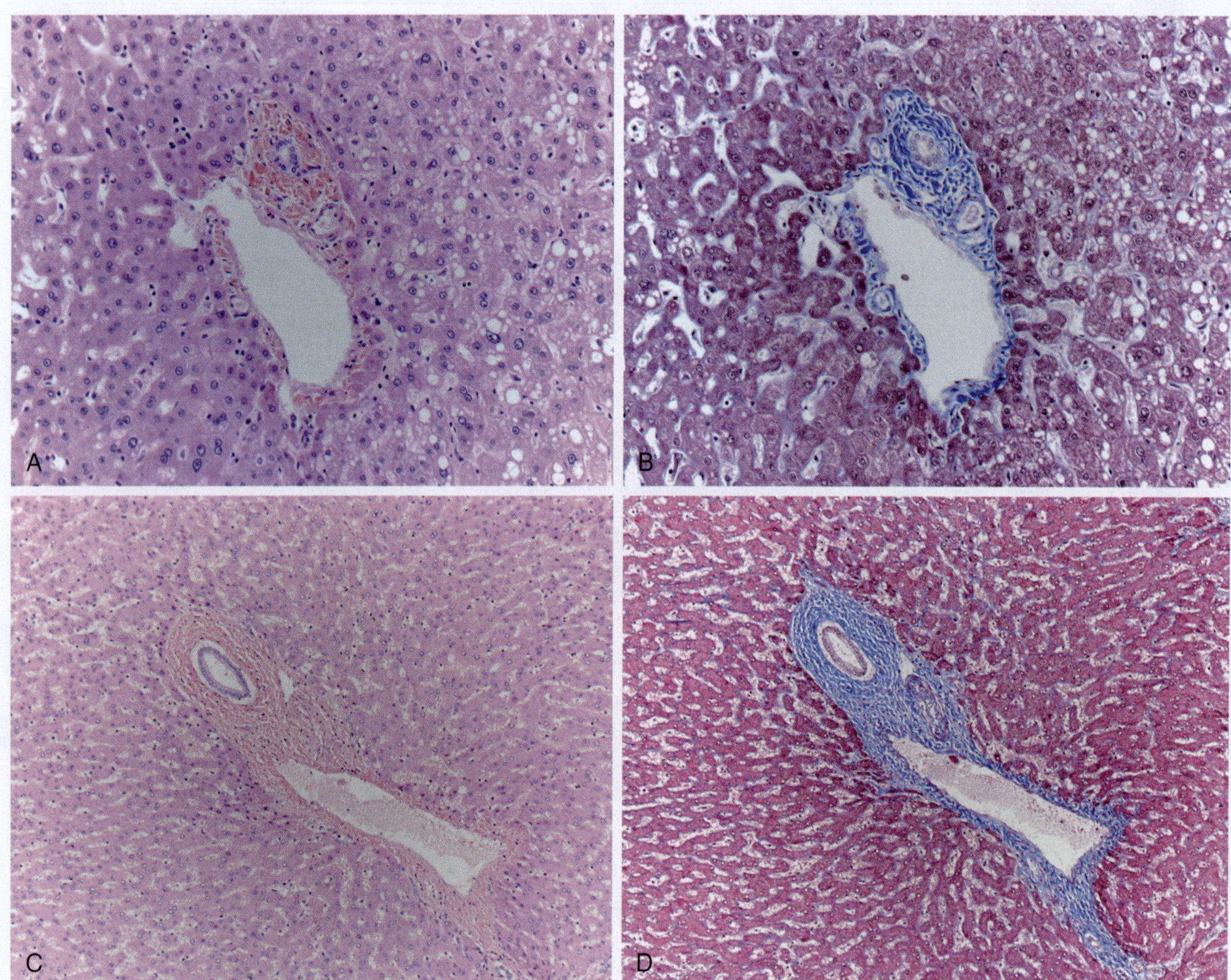

Fig. 76.3 Histologic stages of hepatic fibrosis. (A) A normal portal tract containing a portal vein branch, hepatic artery branch, and interlobular bile duct. The acinar parenchyma shows mild steatosis but no fibrosis. This is stage 0 fibrosis (H&E). (B) A Masson trichrome stain highlights in *blue* a normal (minimal) amount of collagen in a portal tract in stage 0. (C) In stage 1 (of 4), there is a significant increase in collagen (fibrosis) in the portal tract (H&E). (D) The fibrosis in stage 1 is highlighted in *blue* by a Masson trichrome stain. The fibrosis expands the portal tract but does not involve the surrounding periportal acinar parenchyma. (E) Periportal fibrosis characterizes stage 2. Expansion of the portal tract by fibrosis in *blue* is seen. The collagen is not confined to the portal tract but also extends to involve the surrounding periportal acinar parenchyma (*arrows*) (Masson trichrome stain). (F) In stage 3, bridging fibrosis is seen. Multiple portal tracts demonstrate increased fibrosis in *blue* and connect with one another, forming fibrous bridges (*arrows*) (Masson trichrome stain). (G) In cirrhosis (stage 4), the normal liver architecture is completely distorted and replaced by regenerative nodules that are separated by fibrous septa in *blue* (Masson trichrome stain). (Images courtesy Taofic Mounajjed, MD, Rochester, MN.)

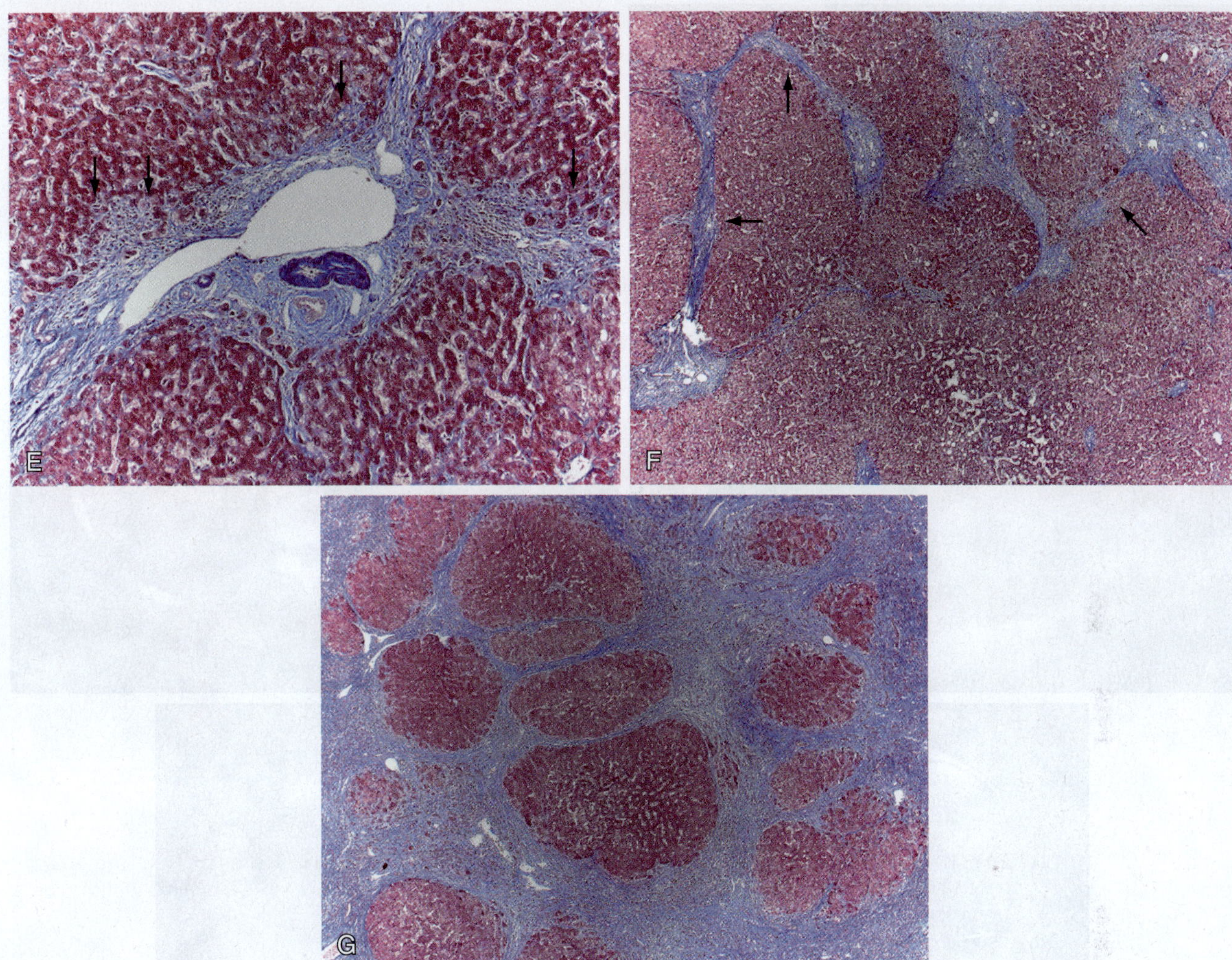

Fig. 76.3 cont'd

PROGNOSIS

Four clinical stages of cirrhosis have been proposed: Stages 1 and 2 represent compensated cirrhosis, and stages 3 and 4 represent decompensated cirrhosis. Stage 1 cirrhosis is characterized by absence of both ascites and varices; stage 2 cirrhosis is characterized by the presence of varices without bleeding and the absence of ascites; stage 3 cirrhosis is characterized by ascites with or without esophageal varices; and stage 4 cirrhosis is characterized by variceal bleeding with or without ascites. In the future, staging of cirrhosis may consider not only clinical and histologic parameters but also hemodynamic and biological data.[19]

As compared to the general population, patients with compensated cirrhosis and decompensated cirrhosis have a 5-fold and 10-fold increased risk of mortality, respectively. The median survival in patients with compensated cirrhosis is 9–12 years, compared with 2 years in those with decompensated cirrhosis. The overall survival for persons with compensated and decompensated cirrhosis, respectively, is 87% versus 75% at 1 year and 67% versus 45% at 5 years.[20] Deaths during the compensated cirrhosis phase are related to cardiovascular disease, malignancy, and chronic kidney disease.[21] However, most deaths in patients with cirrhosis occur later as a result of hepatic decompensation leading to sepsis, hepatic and extrahepatic organ failure. In the Danish study,[22] there was a 1-year survival rate of 83% in those with compensated cirrhosis, 80% in those with variceal bleeding, 71% in those with ascites, 51% in those with ascites and variceal bleeding, and 36% in those with hepatic encephalopathy. Infection is now recognized as a distinct stage in the natural history of cirrhosis and associated with poor survival even after clearance of the infection.[10,23] Infection and renal failure are commonly associated with mortality in patients with cirrhosis (see Chapters 95 and 96). Cirrhotic patients with an infection have a fourfold increase in mortality compared with cirrhotic patients without an infection.[24] Cirrhotic patients with renal failure have a seven- to eightfold increased risk of death compared with cirrhotic patients without renal failure.[25]

An alternative pathway to multiple organ failure and death, acute-on-chronic liver failure (ACLF), often related to infection, has been recognized in patients with cirrhosis (see later).

Prognosis depends not only on the clinical stage of the disease and complications but also on the presence of comorbidities. Generic scores to determine mortality risk include the Child-Turcotte-Pugh score (Child-Pugh class) and the MELD score and its modifications (see Chapters 75 and 99), as well as C-reactive protein and von Willebrand factor levels[26] (see Chapter 96). Measuring the hepatic vein pressure gradient (HVPG) (see Chapter 94) is a useful tool to assess prognosis but is invasive and expensive, making repeated measurements impractical. Machine learning models using a variety of laboratory variables are promising tools to determine prognosis but require wide validation before they can replace current prognostic instruments.[27]

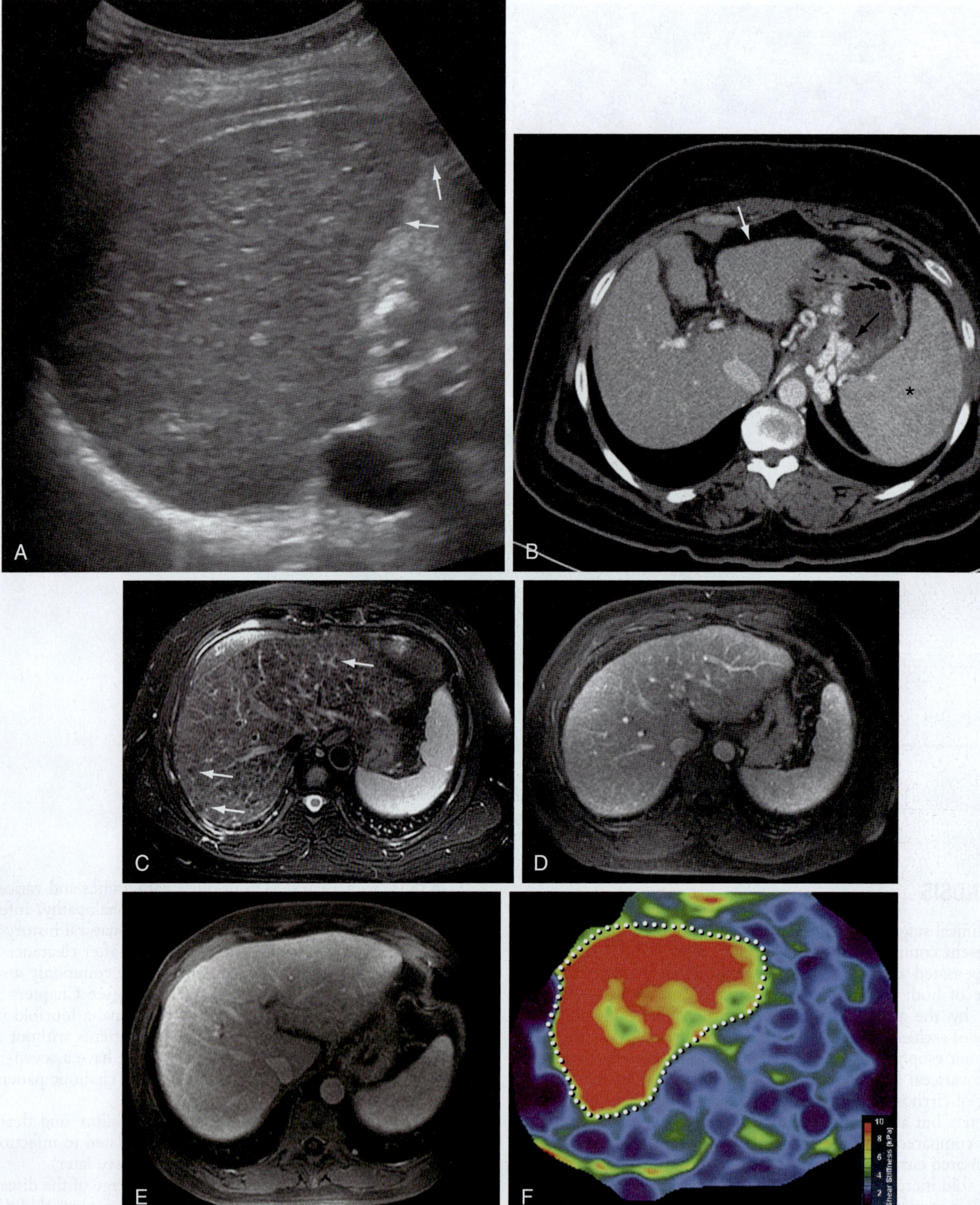

Fig. 76.4 Imaging in cirrhosis. (A) A transverse US image of the right lobe of liver demonstrates the characteristic heterogeneous liver parenchyma with surface nodularity (*arrows*). (B) Axial contrast-enhanced CT image shows a nodular left lobe of the liver (*white arrow*). Note the gastric and esophageal varices (*black arrow*) and splenomegaly (*asterisk*). (C) Images from T2-weighted and (D) contrast-enhanced T1-weighted MRIs show hypointense siderotic nodules (*white arrows*) and an enlarged left lobe and splenomegaly. (E) Contrast-enhanced MRI shows a heterogeneous liver with an enlarged left lobe. (F) A stiffness map from magnetic resonance elastography shows increased stiffness of the liver (*dotted outline*), with a mean stiffness value of 9.2 kPa. The normal liver stiffness value is less than 2.93 kPa. (From Yin M, Talwalkar JA, Glaser KJ, et al. Assessment of hepatic fibrosis with magnetic resonance elastography. *Clin Gastroenterol Hepatol*. 2007;5:1207–1213. Other images courtesy Sudhakar Venkatesh, MD, Rochester, MN.)

TABLE 76.1 Commonly Used Tools for Diagnosing Cirrhosis

NIT	Cut-Off to Rule Out Significant Hepatic Fibrosis	Cut-Off to Rule in Advanced Hepatic Fibrosis
FIB-4	<1.3	>2.67
APRI	<0.3	>1
VCTE	<6 kPa	>10 kPa
MRE	<2.9 kPa	>3.9 kPa

In general, the lower the value for these NITs, the less likely the patient has significant hepatic fibrosis; the higher the value, the more likely advanced hepatic fibrosis is ruled in. Combination of NITs has higher predictive value than single test. *APRI*, Aspartate aminotransferase platelet ratio index; *FIB-4*, Fibrosis-4 score; *MRE*, magnetic resonance elastography; *NIT*, noninvasive test; *VCTE*, vibration-controlled transient elastography.

In the aging cirrhosis population, especially in patients in whom the etiology of cirrhosis is MASLD, the combination of aging and aging-related comorbidities (e.g., diabetes mellitus, sarcopenia, and coronary artery disease) also contributes to negative outcomes. The term *frailty* refers to a state of decreased physiologic reserve and increased vulnerability to health stressors. A key component of frailty is sarcopenia. Frailty negatively impacts morbidity, duration of hospitalization, and days in an ICU, as well as LT wait-list mortality.[12]

Because most deaths in patients with cirrhosis are due to progression to a decompensated state, it is important to determine the risk of progression to decompensated cirrhosis. Decompensation occurs at the rate of 4%–12% per year but varies by underlying disease etiology. For example, the risk of progression from MASLD to cirrhosis is 3% in 15 years; compensated cirrhosis to first decompensation is 33% in 4 years (8%/year); and from first decompensation to ≥2 decompensations is 48% in 2 years.[28] The annual rate of decompensation varies with the etiology of liver disease; it is 4% for patients with HCV-related cirrhosis, 6%–10% in those with alcohol-associated cirrhosis (and even higher if they continue to drink actively), and 10% in those with HBV-related cirrhosis.[29] The 10-year probability of decompensation from a compensated state is 58%. The risk of decompensation is also associated with the serum albumin level, MELD score, and HVPG. An HVPG less than 10 mm Hg (corresponding to LSM <10 kPa) has a 90% negative predictive value for the development of clinical decompensation over 4 years.[30] An increase in MELD score and a decrease in the serum albumin level are also associated with decompensation.

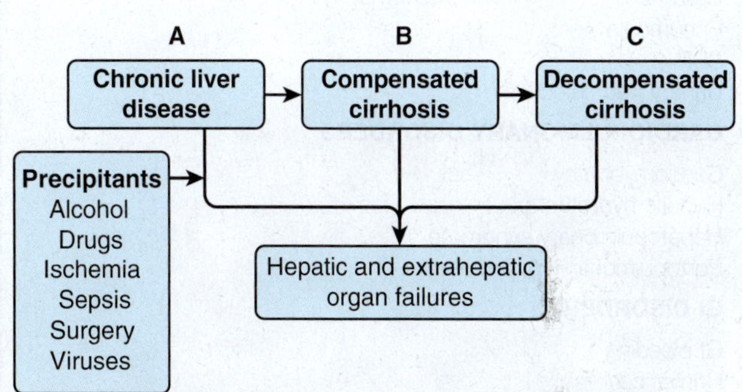

Fig. 76.5 Types (A, B, and C) and precipitants of acute-on-chronic liver failure.

TREATMENT

The major goal in patients with compensated cirrhosis is to prevent hepatic decompensation (Fig. 76.5). This includes surveillance for HCC with US of the liver every 6 months (see Chapter 98), surveillance for esophageal varices by EGD (see Chapter 94), cessation of alcohol use, weight loss, and other lifestyle changes, although the cost-effectiveness of screening for HCC in patients with alcohol-associated cirrhosis has been questioned.[31] Weight loss is associated with a reduction in portal pressure and reduced risk of hepatic decompensation[32]; however, abdominal exercises that increase intra-abdominal pressure and the risk for variceal hemorrhage should be avoided. Immunization against HAV, HBV, pneumococcal pneumonia, COVID-19, and influenza is recommended. Live-attenuated vaccines are not contraindicated in patients with cirrhosis. The progression of compensated cirrhosis to a decompensated state may be delayed or even prevented by treatment of the underlying cause of cirrhosis (e.g., chronic hepatitis B and C),[33] abstinence from alcohol, and weight loss. Patients with chronic viral hepatitis who use statins have a reduced risk of hepatic decompensation and mortality.[16] The use of low-molecular-weight heparin may delay decompensation even in patients without portal vein thrombosis but is currently not recommended (see Chapter 87).

The protean manifestations of cirrhosis are summarized in Box 76.2. The management of patients with decompensated cirrhosis and complications such as ascites (Chapter 95), variceal bleeding (Chapter 94) and hepatic encephalopathy (Chapter 96) is discussed separately. The ultimate goal of treatment in patients with decompensated cirrhosis, albeit achieved infrequently, is "recompensation" defined by all three of the following criteria: (1) adequate treatment of the etiology of cirrhosis (viral elimination for hepatitis C, sustained viral suppression for hepatitis B, sustained alcohol abstinence for alcohol-associated cirrhosis; and significant weight loss); (2) resolution of complications of cirrhosis, namely, ascites, hepatic encephalopathy, and absence of recurrent variceal hemorrhage for at least 1 year without treatment; and (3) normalization of liver biochemistry.[15]

In general, acetaminophen in doses of up to 2 g daily may be used in persons with cirrhosis (see Chapter 90). Aspirin and other NSAIDs should be avoided in patients with decompensated cirrhosis, especially those with ascites. Aminoglycosides are contraindicated, but other antibiotics are acceptable, as are statins for treatment of hyperlipidemia. In patients with diabetes mellitus, oral hypoglycemic agents may be used if the cirrhosis is compensated, but in patients with decompensated cirrhosis, insulin is preferred. Patients with cirrhosis have protein-calorie malnutrition, and frequent high-calorie small meals, as well as bedtime snacks, are recommended. Fat-soluble vitamins and zinc levels should be monitored, with replacement if required.

Problems that occur in patients with cirrhosis for which there are no clear management solutions include fatigue, muscle cramps, and sexual dysfunction. Fatigue is a major factor in reducing a patient's quality of life and may be a manifestation of covert encephalopathy. Fatigue is more common in patients with obesity, depression, and sleep apnea. A search for reversible causes of fatigue, including anemia and thyroid disease, should be conducted. Muscle cramps also impair the patient's quality of life and

BOX 76.2 Principal Complications of Cirrhosis

PORTAL HYPERTENSION

Ascites
Variceal bleeding
Hepatic encephalopathy

MALIGNANCY

Cholangiocarcinoma
HCC

BACTERIAL INFECTIONS

Bacteremia
C. difficile infection
Cellulitis
Pneumonia
SBP
Urinary tract infection

CARDIOPULMONARY DISORDERS

Cardiomyopathy
Hepatic hydrothorax
Hepatopulmonary syndrome
Portopulmonary hypertension

GI DISORDERS

GI bleeding
Nonvariceal
Variceal
Protein-losing enteropathy
Venous thrombosis

RENAL DISORDERS

Hepatorenal syndrome
Other causes of acute kidney injury

METABOLIC DISORDERS

Adrenal insufficiency
Hypogonadism
Malnutrition
Osteoporosis

NEUROPSYCHIATRIC DISORDERS

Depression
Hepatic encephalopathy

HEMATOLOGIC DISORDERS

Anemia
Hypercoagulability
Hypersplenism
Impaired coagulation

UNCLEAR ETIOLOGY

Erectile dysfunction
Fatigue
Muscle cramps

are independent of age, disease severity, and diuretic use. Unfortunately, no effective therapy is available to alleviate muscle cramps, but baclofen and hydroxychloroquine have been used with some success. Erectile dysfunction is a common problem, but agents such as phosphodiesterase inhibitors typically used for the treatment of erectile dysfunction may be ineffective in patients with cirrhosis. Women with cirrhosis infrequently become pregnant. Pregnant women with cirrhosis require coordinated care by a team that includes a high-risk obstetrician, hepatologist, and endoscopist, because of the increased risk of variceal bleeding in the third trimester of pregnancy.[11] Finally, depression occurs in 30%–40% of patients with cirrhosis, especially in those patients with hepatitis C and alcohol-associated cirrhosis, and is associated with obesity, diabetes mellitus, and sleep disorders. Selective serotonin reuptake inhibitors and mirtazapine are safe and effective agents for the treatment of depression in patients with cirrhosis.

REVERSAL OF FIBROSIS

In the future, treatment of cirrhosis will involve reversal of hepatic fibrosis and prevention of hepatic decompensation using a combination of drugs aimed at reducing portal pressure and hepatic inflammation.[34] Evidence to indicate that fibrosis is reversible has come from clinical observations in humans and experimental studies in animal models of liver fibrosis. Human evidence that fibrosis is reversible is based on the observation that fibrosis improves in response to control of the underlying disease process. For example, patients with liver fibrosis secondary to chronic biliary obstruction in whom the obstruction is relieved show improvement in hepatic histology. The same occurs in patients who have undergone successful therapy for chronic viral hepatitis. In animal models, genetic disruption of fibrogenic signaling pathways prevents or reverses liver fibrosis (or both).[35] A number of compounds have also been shown to reverse or prevent liver fibrosis in animal models, such as lanifibranor,[35] but fibrosis is easier to prevent or reverse in animal models than in humans.

Specific factors and pathways that have been studied as mediators of fibrosis or its reversal include statins, angiotensin, nuclear receptors, receptor tyrosine kinases, integrins, angiogenesis, and matrix-degrading proteases.[36] These pathways broadly aim to reverse the myofibroblast state of hepatic stellate cells by inducing senescence, deactivation, or apoptosis (see Fig. 76.2)[36] and have been studied in preclinical models; however, evidence of their clinical utility in humans is as yet lacking. Pan-PPAR agonists may have a human antifibrotic signal but further studies are needed.[37] Early studies show that the pan-PPAR agonist lanifibranor improves portal hypertension and hepatic fibrosis in experimental advanced chronic liver disease.[38]

A number of limitations have precluded successful antifibrosis therapy in humans. One limitation is the lack of effective tools to precisely assess fibrosis noninvasively.[36] Despite advances in US elastography and MRE, most clinical trials still require liver biopsy, which is invasive and unappealing to patients. Resolution of fibrosis may take years to achieve, further complicating trial design. In addition, development of fibrosis is a multifactorial process, and it is challenging to target the correct cell selectively with a specific pharmacologic intervention. Although early stages of fibrosis may be amenable to resolution, advanced stages of fibrosis may not be reversible, owing to fixed angioarchitectural changes. Progress in both study design and efficacy is exemplified by the clinical trial of cenicriviroc for MASH (NASH) fibrosis.[19]

ACUTE-ON-CHRONIC LIVER FAILURE

ACLF has been proposed as an additional pathway in the natural history of patients with chronic liver disease. Following a precipitating event that is not always identifiable, patients may develop hepatic and extrahepatic multiorgan failure leading to death. The key features of ACLF are underlying chronic liver disease, a precipitating event, hepatic and extrahepatic organ failure, and high mortality risk.

Definition

There are considerable differences among the various definitions of ACLF proposed by various professional societies, largely because precipitating events leading to hepatic and extrahepatic organ failure are different in the East (HBV reactivation, HEV superinfection in patients with chronic liver disease, and alcohol-associated hepatitis) and in the West (alcohol-associated hepatitis, bacterial infection).[39] The major reason, however, for a lack of agreement is that the pathophysiology of the process has not been ascertained, and the condition is defined based on the observed clinical presentation. A working definition of ACLF is "a condition in patients with underlying chronic liver disease with or without cirrhosis that is associated with mortality within 3 months in the absence of treatment of the underlying liver disease, liver support, or liver transplantation."[40] The clinical presentation of ACLF may depend on the stage of the underlying liver disease and the precipitating insult to the liver, namely, underlying chronic liver disease without cirrhosis; underlying compensated cirrhosis; or underlying decompensated cirrhosis.[22] An unmet need is to define ACLF as an entity distinguishable from chronic liver disease, compensated cirrhosis, and traditional decompensated cirrhosis by a distinct pathophysiology and identification of a diagnostic symptom, sign, or confirmatory test.

Epidemiology

In the last two decades, the number of hospitalizations for ACLF and for complications of cirrhosis has increased. In a nationwide study, more than 5% of all hospitalizations in patients with cirrhosis were for ACLF, and the number has been rising.[41] More than two-thirds of these patients had an infection, with an in-hospital mortality rate of approximately 50%. Surviving patients are at a significant risk for readmission following discharge from the hospital.[24] Therefore there is an increasing incidence of ACLF, high prevalence of infection, unacceptably high mortality, significant costs, and risk of readmission. In fact, mortality in patients with ACLF is higher than that for patients with acute liver failure (ALF) after the first week of hospitalization. The high mortality risk persists as opposed to the risk of mortality in patients with ALF, which returns to baseline in approximately 3 weeks.[25] In addition, approximately one-half of patients with ACLF listed for LT are either delisted or are deceased within 6 months.[29]

Pathophysiology

The gut microbiome plays an important role in liver disease, especially following an alcohol binge that results in translocation of bacterial products into the circulation.[30] Patients with ACLF have more prominent features of systemic circulatory dysfunction and systemic inflammation than patients with decompensated cirrhosis.[31] Levels of markers of cell death are also more marked.[33] This inflammatory state becomes more pronounced with the progression of the ACLF. The mechanisms of inflammation are unclear but include sterile inflammation secondary to precipitating factors such as excessive alcohol-induced hepatocyte death and inflammation secondary to bacterial infections.

Bacterial infection is a common precipitating factor of ACLF in the West. Host factors, including age, genetic factors, and comorbidities, and pathogen-related factors, including the virulence and load of bacteria and production of pathogen-associated molecular patterns, result in propagation of the inflammatory state (see Chapter 2).[42] Nevertheless, routine use of antibiotics in patients with cirrhosis with the goal of preventing complications of cirrhosis is not currently recommended.[34]

The role of the immune system in the pathogenesis of ACLF is evolving. Patients with ACLF have significant suppression of the innate immune system.[35] It has been hypothesized that the severity of disease is related to failed immune tolerance. There is also a compensatory anti-inflammatory response resulting in immunosuppression with enhanced susceptibility to secondary infections and organ failure.[42]

Clinical Features and Prognosis

Patients have features of the systemic inflammatory response syndrome, with fever, tachycardia, tachypnea, and leukocytosis. They also have manifestations of organ failure that are summarized in Table 76.2. The number of organ failures in turn determines prognosis and is captured in the different scoring systems.[36,43,44] In the simplest terms, the presence of two or more extrahepatic organ failures is associated with a poor prognosis. Renal failure as an extrahepatic organ failure is defined as the need for renal replacement therapy; brain failure as grades 3–4 hepatic encephalopathy; circulatory failure as the need for pressor support; and respiratory failure as the need for ventilatory support (see Chapter 96). Using these definitions, the in-hospital mortality rate with two organ failures is 27%; with three organ failures 65%; and with four organ failures 97%.

Treatment

It is unclear at this time whether ACLF can be prevented. The patient with ACLF is best managed by a multidisciplinary team with expertise in critical care and LT.[45] The various interventions that are carried out once ACLF is diagnosed are summarized in Table 76.3 and are highlighted in two recent guidelines.[40,46]

The goals of management of patients with ACLF include treating precipitating events (e.g., alcohol-associated hepatitis and HBV infection) and aggressive support of the failing organs. The effectiveness of current organ supportive therapy is, however, questionable. For example, patients with hepatorenal syndrome and advanced ACLF may have a poor response to terlipressin (see Chapter 96).[47] Hepatic regenerative therapy and artificial liver support are considered as bridges to LT, but bioartificial liver support has thus far not been proven to be effective (see Chapter

TABLE 76.2 Clinical Manifestations of Organ Failure in Acute-On-Chronic Liver Failure

Organ Failure	Manifestations
Adrenal gland	Hypotension
Bone marrow	Suppression
Brain	Hepatic encephalopathy grade 3–4
Circulatory	Need for vasopressor support
Kidneys	HRS-AKI or need for renal replacement therapy
Liver	Loss of metabolic function with hypoglycemia, lactic acidosis, hyperammonemia, coagulopathy
Lungs	Acute lung injury and/or acute respiratory distress syndrome requiring ventilatory support

Modified from Bernal W, Wendon J. Acute liver failure. *N Engl J Med.* 2014;370:1170–1171.

TABLE 76.3 Management of Acute-On-Chronic Liver Failure

Pathophysiology	Intervention
Liver failure	Hepatic regenerative therapy; artificial and bioartificial liver support and/or LT
Precipitating events:	
Alcohol-associated hepatitis	Glucocorticoids
Extrahepatic organ failure	Organ support
Hepatitis B	Antiviral agents
Infections	Antibiotics

97). Studies specifically targeting patients with ACLF have not demonstrated improvement in mortality with the use of liver support devices.[48,49] Hepatic regenerative therapy is promising; a combination of granulocyte-colony stimulating factor and erythropoietin has been shown in studies in Asia to decrease the risk of mortality in patients with decompensated cirrhosis.[50] This finding has not been validated outside of Asia.[51]

LT offers the only hope of long-term survival to patients with ACLF (see Chapter 99). Patients with multiple organ failures, however, may be too sick for LT.[52] In selected patients (especially those with alcohol-associated hepatitis) in whom LT has been carried out, long-term results have been good.[53] Future directions include a more acceptable and universal definition of ACLF, early diagnosis of sepsis, effective treatment of severe alcohol-associated hepatitis, hepatic regenerative therapies, and short-term as well as long-term artificial and bioartificial liver support.

Full references for this chapter can be found at https://ebooks.health.elsevier.com

77 Hemochromatosis

Kris V. Kowdley, Christine Hsu

IN THIS CHAPTER

INTRODUCTION

Trousseau was the first to describe a case of hemochromatosis in the French pathology literature in 1885.[1] Twenty-five years later, von Recklinghausen was the first to use the term *hemochromatosis* to describe how pigmentation ("chromo") in tissues of such patients was caused by something in their blood ("hemo").[1] Sheldon, a geriatrician, was the first to collect a series of 311 cases and believed that this disorder was genetically inherited and that excess iron deposition led to tissue injury and damage.[1] In 1976 Simon et al. localized the gene for hereditary hemochromatosis (HH) to the HLA region, and then finally in 1996 Feder identified the *HFE* gene on chromosome 6.[1] This discovery enabled genetic testing for the two major mutations (C282Y, H63D) that are responsible for *HFE*-related HH (Table 77.1).[1] The prevalence of *HFE*-related HH is estimated to range from 1 in 200 to 400 persons according to prospective studies.[2] In a multiethnic cohort that was screened for C282Y homozygotes (HEIRS, Hemochromatosis and Iron Overload [IO] Screening Study research investigators), the prevalence was highest in non-Hispanic whites (0.44%) and lowest in those of African and Asian decent (0.014% and 0.00039%, respectively).[3] The majority of HH cases (80% −90%) are type 1, and most patients are homozygous C282Y (type 1a) or compound heterozygote C282Y/H63D (type 1b).[4,5] HH is characterized by increased intestinal iron absorption due to decreased expression of hepcidin, which is an iron regulatory protein.[6] Other mutant alleles, such as *S65C*, occur in <1% of clinically significant HH.[3,5] Other types include type 2A or 2B with hemojuvelin (*HJV*) or hepcidin (*HAMP*) mutation (also known as juvenile hemochromatosis), type 3 with transferrin receptor 2 (*TfR2*) mutation, and type 4 with ferroportin (FPN) (*SLC40A1*) mutation.[2]

Niederau et al. initially showed that life expectancy is reduced in those with HH and particularly in those who have cirrhosis, diabetes, or unable to have adequate iron depletion within 18 months of venesection therapy.[7] Average life expectancy was

TABLE 77.1 Iron Overload Syndromes

Hereditary Hemochromatosis	Gene Mutation
Type 1	*HFE* C282Y homozygous C282Y/H63D heterozygous Other HFE mutations
Type 2A (Juvenile Hemochromatosis)	Hemojuvelin (*HJV*) mutations
Type 2B (Juvenile Hemochromatosis)	Hepcidin antimicrobial Protein (*HAMP*)
Type 3	Transferrin receptor 2 (*TFR2*) mutations
Type 4	Ferroportin (*SLC40A1*) Loss of function—Decreased expression Gain of function—Increased expression
African Iron Overload	
Secondary Iron Overload	
Iron-Loading Anemia	
Myelodysplastic syndrome	
Thalassemia syndromes	
Sickle cell disease	
Sideroblastic anemia	
Aplastic anemia	
Pyruvate kinase deficiency	
Chronic hemolytic anemia	
Diamond-Blackfan syndrome	
Parenteral Iron Overload	
Iron injections	
Long-term dialysis	
Red blood cell transfusions	
Chronic Liver Disease	
Viral hepatitis (hepatitis B and C)	
Alcohol-associated liver disease	
Metabolic dysfunction-associated steatotic liver disease (MASLD)/metabolic dysfunction-associated steatohepatitis (MASH)	
Dietary Iron Overload	
Miscellaneous	
Aceruloplasminemia	
Congenital alloimmune hepatitis (neonatal hemochromatosis)	
Congenital atransferrinemia	

76% at 10 years and 49% at 20 years.[7] With increased awareness, greater screening, and earlier diagnosis with genotype testing, it is now known that the clinical expression of disease is lower than previously expected.[8] While the majority of patients have elevated serum transferrin-iron saturation (TS) and many have elevated serum ferritin (SF), hepatic IO is only seen in ~56% of the patients and hepatic fibrosis/cirrhosis is seen in 16%–25% of patients in population-based studies.[9–11] Overall, 25%–35% of C282Y homozygotes may have normal SF and may not develop IO.[8] Among C282Y homozygotes, cirrhosis has generally been described in 1%–10% of the patients[3,8,12]; a meta-analysis showed a pooled prevalence of ~10% for severe liver disease.[13]

Secondary IO can arise from iatrogenic iron administration, hematological conditions that lead to ineffective erythropoiesis (IE), or repeated blood transfusions. The most common form of secondary IO are the thalassemia syndromes. The most severe forms are β-thalassemia major, α-thalassemia hemoglobin H disease (three out of four α-globin genes have mutations or deletions), and Bart's hydrops fetalis (four of the α-globin genes are missing).[14] Other hematological conditions leading to IO include myelodysplastic syndrome (MDS), primary myelofibrosis, sickle cell disease, Diamond-Blackfan syndrome, sideroblastic (SA) anemia, or aplastic anemia (AA). SA and AA can be genetic or acquired from exposure to viral infections, chemical toxins (e.g., benzene), chemotherapy, or certain drugs.[14] AA may be an iatrogenic complication of drugs such as antiseizure medications, immune checkpoint inhibitors, temozolomide, and nonsteroid anti-inflammatory medications, while SA may be caused by hormonal therapy, isoniazid, copper-chelating agents, and certain antibiotics.[14]

PATHOPHYSIOLOGY

Intestinal Iron Absorption and Hepcidin

Total body iron can range between 3 and 5 g, with approximately 1 g stored in the liver.[15] Erythrocytes account for approximately 2.5 g of iron in the body, while circulating iron (transferrin-bound iron) is extremely low (3–4 mg).[15] Dietary iron can be heme and nonheme.[16] Heme iron is absorbed with mechanisms that are not fully understood.[2] Most dietary iron (or nonheme iron) is ferric iron (Fe^{3+}) and is converted to ferrous iron (Fe^{2+}) by the brush border protein called duodenal cytochrome B (dctyB)[16] (Fig. 77.1). Once iron is converted to the ferrous form, it crosses the enterocyte apical brush border via the divalent metal iron transporter (DMT1).[16] The subsequent fate of absorbed iron depends on the demand for iron.[16] If the iron demand is low, hepcidin (regulator of iron homeostasis) expression is increased, which leads to decreased iron absorption and reduced expression of FPN (iron exporter on the basolateral membrane of the enterocyte)[2,16] (Fig. 77.1). The iron then remains intracellular, bound to the protein ferritin (iron storage protein), and is lost with enterocyte sloughing few days later.[16] If there is a high demand for iron, the iron will be exported via FPN and increased in the circulation[16] (Fig. 77.1). Hephaestin (ferrioxidase) subsequently converts ferrous iron back to ferric iron (Fe^{3+}).[2]

Hepcidin is a 25-amino acid peptide produced in the liver that regulates overall iron homeostasis.[17] If there is low demand for iron, hepcidin prevents iron efflux by binding to FPN via tyrosine phosphorylation of the cytoplasmic domains and allowing for its internalization and degradation.[17,18] Hepcidin

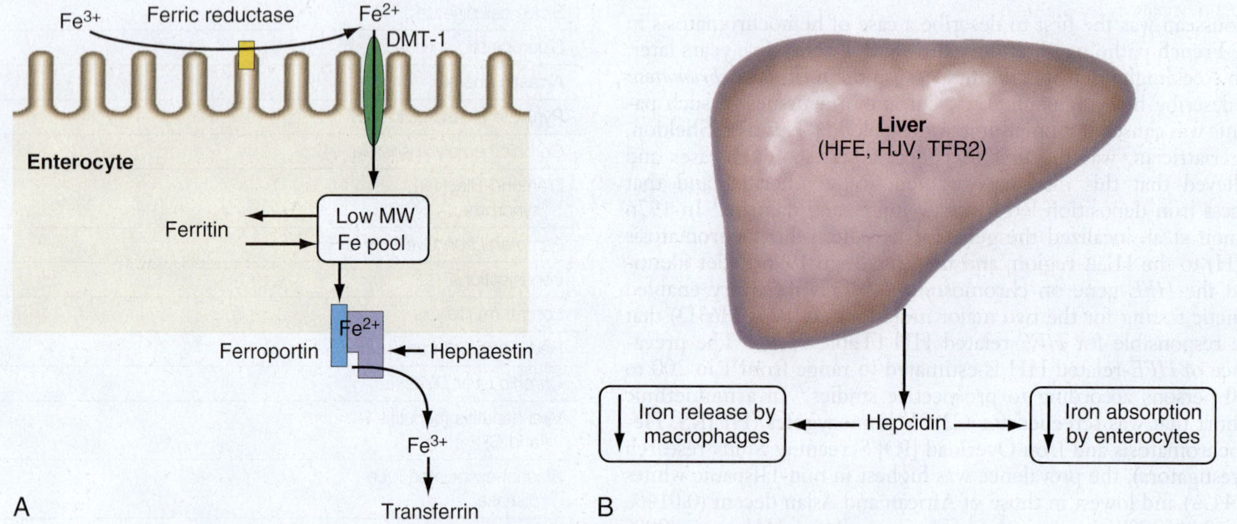

Fig. 77.1 Iron absorption pathway in duodenal enterocytes and the role of hepcidin. (A) Duodenal enterocytes are the major site of iron absorption. Before uptake, dietary ionic iron requires reduction from the ferric (Fe^{3+}) to the ferrous (Fe^{2+}) state. This is accomplished by ferric reductases that are expressed on the luminal surface of enterocytes. Ferrous iron is taken up by the apical divalent metal transporter 1 (DMT-1). Iron may be stored within the cell as ferritin and then lost with the sloughed senescent enterocyte or transferred across the basolateral membrane to the plasma. This latter process occurs via the transporter ferroportin and requires oxidation of iron back to the ferric state by the ferroxidase hephaestin, followed by transport of iron to red blood cells and tissues by transferrin. (B) Hepcidin is produced by the liver and secreted into the blood. HFE protein, hemojuvelin (HJV), and transferrin receptor 2 (TFR2) may participate in the hepatic iron-sensing mechanism that regulates hepcidin expression. Hepcidin reduces iron release by macrophages (and thereby increases macrophage iron stores) and also reduces iron absorption by duodenal enterocytes to decrease the amount of dietary iron in the circulation. In *HFE*-related hereditary hemochromatosis, loss of functional HFE protein leads to aberrant hepatocellular sensing of plasma iron, inappropriately low levels of hepcidin, diminished macrophage iron stores, and greater duodenal iron absorption. *MW*, Molecular weight.

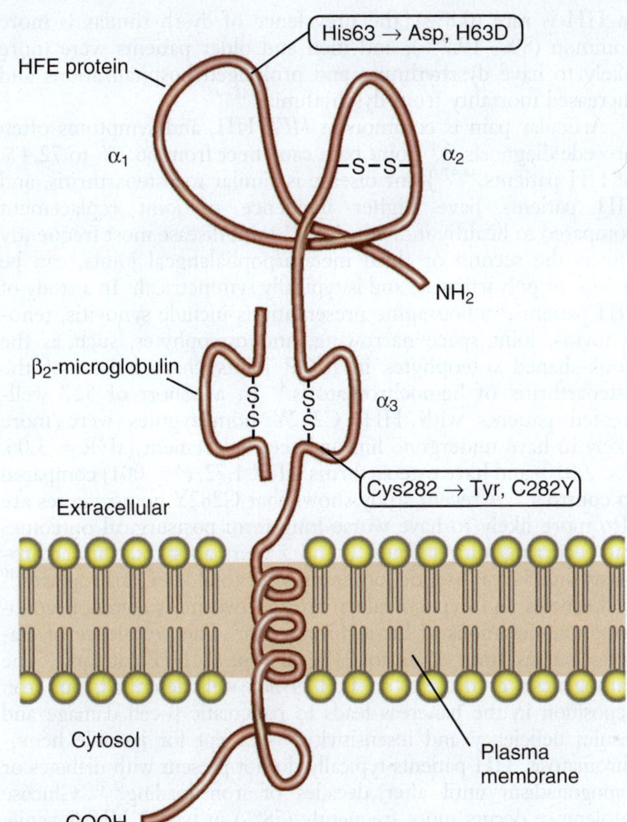

Fig. 77.2 Schematic model of HFE protein in association with β2-microglobulin at the cell surface. The three extracellular domains of HFE protein are designated α1, α2, and α3. β2-Microglobulin is physically associated with the α3 domain. HFE protein also contains a transmembrane domain and a short intracellular domain. Positions of the two common HFE mutations, C282Y and H63D, are shown.

can also bind to macrophages in addition to intestinal absorptive cells to promote decreased enterocyte iron absorption, decreased iron efflux from cells, and decreased iron mobilization from macrophages.[2] This leads to overall decreased iron in the circulation.[2] In type 1 HH, a G to A mutation at the 845 nucleotide of the *HFE* gene leads to a replacement of cystine by tyrosine at amino acid 282 (C282Y)[2] (Fig. 77.2). Subsequently, this mutation leads to decreased overall hepcidin synthesis.[2] However, hepcidin synthesis can also be reduced with other gene mutations. Mutations in *HAMP* or *HJV* genes (type 2 juvenile hemochromatosis) and in *TfR2* (type 3 hemochromatosis) can also lead to reduced hepcidin synthesis.[19] Increased FPN expression leads to increased iron export, especially from macrophages and intestinal cells, which then leads to increased levels of non-transferrin bound iron (NTBI).[19] NTBI is taken up by various organs including hepatic, pancreatic, cardiac, and endocrine cells leading to overall systemic IO.[19]

Mutations in the *FPN1* gene (*SLC40A1*) lead to reduced FPN expression (autosomal recessive type 4A HH), which then leads to increases in intracellular iron because of decreased iron efflux.[2,19] These patients typically present with normal or low levels of TS and plasma iron but elevated SF.[2] Because macrophages have high FPN1 activity, the spleen is the most affected organ in this disease.[2] Autosomal dominant type 4B HH results from FPN1 insensitivity to hepcidin.[19] In contrast to decreased FPN expression (or loss of function), this is a gain of function disease as FPN is insensitive to hepcidin which then leads to increased expression and increased iron efflux and iron circulation.[19]

Chronic elevation in NTBI is harmful and may lead to premature death.[15] TS must exceed 30%–60% for appreciable extracellular iron to be detected.[15] The labile plasma iron (LPI) in NTBI is a toxic chelatable inorganic compound that has been shown to cause hepatic necrosis, cardiovascular collapse, and metabolic acidosis in accidental iron overdose.[20,21] Iron is toxic because of its ability to interchange between Fe^{2+} and Fe^{3+} and generate ROS (reactive oxygen species) which lead to cellular damage.[15] The LPI enters the cell and becomes part of the labile cytosolic transit iron pool (LCI), which is responsible for fundamental biochemical reactions at low level.[21] However, oxidative stress occurs after there is uncontrolled expansion of the LCI pool.[21] Extracellular stresses can also lead to intracellular increases in ROS production, which then results in programmed cell death.[15] Excess iron in solution with oxygen can also lead to generation of free radicals via Fenton and Haber-Weiss chemistry where hydrogen peroxide (H_2O_2) is converted into hydroxyl radical (HO^-).[22] Radical formation promotes lipid peroxidation (LP) of cell membranes and toxic long-lived LP byproducts.[21] These LP byproducts cause DNA and protein damage by adduct formation, cross-linking, or fragmentation.[21] The oxidative stress also leads to mitochondrial dysfunction, lysosomal fragility, and decreased cytochrome activity.[21] This hepatocyte damage and necrosis subsequently lead to inflammation via Kupffer cell (KC) activation and activation of the fibrogenic cascade.[21] The KCs phagocytose iron-laden hepatocytes, which may then lead to hepatic stellate cell and portal myofibroblast activation and hepatic fibrogenesis.[21,23]

CLINICAL MANIFESTATIONS OF PRIMARY IRON OVERLOAD

Primary IO is described as HH, with four main types depending on the mutation pattern; type 1 associated with *HFE* mutations (with subtypes 1a–1c), type 2A or 2B with hemojuvelin (*HJV*) or hepcidin (*HAMP*) mutations, type 3 with *TfR2* mutations, and type 4 with *FPN* (*SLC40A1*) mutations. The vast majority (95%) of HH cases are caused by the C282Y homozygous mutation (type 1a). The prevalence of *HFE*-related HH is similar (1 case in 200–400 persons) in the United States, Europe, and Australia, with the highest prevalence in patients of Irish and Scandinavian origin, and lowest in African-Americans.[2] In the HEIRS study (diverse multiethnic cohort from the United States, Europe, and Canada), the prevalence of C282Y homozygosity was highest in non-Hispanic whites (0.44%), followed by Native Americans (0.11%), Hispanics (0.027%), African-Americans (0.014%), and lowest in Asian-Americans (0.000039%).[24] *HFE* genotype 1b is classified as compound heterozygous with the H63D mutation (C282Y/H63D).[2] The prevalence of this subtype ranges from 2% to 4% in patients with Northern European origin.[2] Although compound heterozygotes may have elevated SF and TS, they rarely present with clinically significant IO disease and the clinical penetrance is quite low (0.5%–3.5%)[25] without concomitant hepatic steatosis, significant alcohol use, or type 2 diabetes.[2,25,26] C282Y/H63D compound heterozygotes have reported similar prevalence of liver disease (7% vs. 3%), hepatomegaly (8% vs. 4%), elevated transaminases (8% vs. 14%), and arthritic symptoms (2% vs. 2%) when compared to the general population.[26] Genotype 1c is classified as S65C.[2] Similarly, S65C heterozygotes may exhibit elevated SF and TS levels and even mild-to-moderate IO, but clinically significant hemochromatosis has only been described in C282Y-containing compound heterozygotes (C282Y/S65C) when compared to wild-type *HFE* patients.[27,28] None of the S65C patients had fibrosis related to hepatic IO.[29]

The other subtypes are not related to the *HFE* gene and have lower prevalence.[2] Mutations in the *HJV* and *HAMP* genes (types 2A and 2B) have led to "juvenile hemochromatosis," a condition where clinical presentation is similar to *HFE* hemochromatosis, but patients present at an earlier age with hypogonadism and cardiac complications at an accelerated rate.[30] *HJV* mutations were first described in 12 families from Greece, France, and Canada.[30] Patients with type 3 HH (TfR2) typically have early onset of symptoms in their third decade of life with weakness, fatigue, arthropathies, skin hyperpigmentation, and hepatomegaly.[31] Type 4 (*FPN* mutations) HH patients can have heterogenous presentations but can have milder disease than other HH types.[32,33] Fibrosis (without cirrhosis) progression has been described in a few, and development of hepatocellular carcinoma (HCC) has been described; however, this was in an elderly man with occult hepatitis B virus (HBV).[34] Type 4A is associated with decreased *FPN* expression "loss of function," intracellular increases in iron, and hyperferritinemia with low or normal TS.[32] Type 4A is associated with macrophage IO and termed "M phenotype."[32] Type 4B is associated with increased *FPN* expression ("gain of function") as *FPN* is insensitive to hepcidin regulation.[32] Type 4B is associated with hepatic IO and elevated TS and is termed "H phenotype."[32]

The clinical manifestations of *HFE* HH are predominantly hepatic, cardiac, and endocrine due to iron deposition in liver, heart, and endocrine glands. Men typically present earlier in life since iron loss via menses leads to reduced body iron stores in women. Elevated ferritin was described in 63%–77% of C282Y homozygotes, elevated liver enzymes in 11%–61% of the patients, hepatic IO in 56%–71% of males and 33%–35% of females, and hepatic fibrosis in 18.4%–43% of males and 0%–5.4% of females.[9–12] Cirrhosis was present in 3.9%–23.4% of the C282Y homozygote patients.[9–11] HCC can occur in those with or without cirrhosis.[2] Hepatic complications are the most life-threatening and account for most of the disease-specific mortality.[35] A study of 527 C282Y homozygotes showed an eightfold (aHR = 8.3, $P < .0001$) increase in HCC risk and fourfold (aHR 3.87, $P < .0001$) increased risk for cirrhosis even in those treated with phlebotomy, with risk more pronounced in men.[35] Phlebotomy has been shown to reverse fibrosis and reduce HCC risk, although complete reversal of cirrhosis is less common.[35,36] SF > 1000 μg/L has been shown in multiple studies to be associated with cirrhosis in HH with a 100% sensitivity and 77% specificity in diagnosing cirrhosis.[10,37,38] Other risk factors for cirrhosis include increasing age, male sex, diabetes, and heavy alcohol ingestion (typically >60 g daily).[10,11,37,39] In patients with heavy alcohol ingestion, advanced fibrosis/cirrhosis can be present in up to 61% of patients.[39] In "juvenile hemochromatosis," liver disease typically develops after hypogonadism and cardiac disease, although a significant proportion of patients have cirrhosis (42%).[30,40]

Other clinical manifestations of HH include cardiac disease, arthropathies, diabetes, and hypogonadotropic hypogonadism.[2] Although cardiac manifestations for *HFE* HH are less common, heart failure is the second leading cause of death in *HFE* HH patients.[41,42] Cardiomyopathy is more frequent than ischemic heart disease and can be restrictive or dilated cardiomyopathy.[43] Iron deposition can lead to diastolic dysfunction, systolic dysfunction, and eventually biventricular failure.[41] Clinical presentation depends on the rate and amount of iron influx; patients with juvenile hemochromatosis have rapid iron loading and tend to have more severe and earlier onset of symptoms.[42] For "juvenile hemochromatosis," the typical clinical presentation is hypogonadotropic hypogonadism in the second decade of life and congestive heart failure by the fourth decade.[30] Iron can also deposit in the atrioventricular node, rather than sinoatrial node, which leads to more frequent supraventricular arrhythmias and paroxysmal atrial fibrillation.[41,42] Overall, while cardiomyopathy in HH is rare (0.8%), the prevalence of dysrhythmias is more common (8%–19.7%), and men and older patients were more likely to have dysrhythmias and prolonged hospitalizations and increased mortality from dysrhythmias.[43–45]

Articular pain is common in *HFE* HH, and symptoms often precede diagnosis.[46,47] Joint pain can affect from 66.7% to 72.4% of HH patients.[46,47] Joint disease is similar to osteoarthritis, and HH patients have higher incidence of joint replacement compared to healthy individuals.[35,48] Joint disease most frequently affects the second or third metacarpophalangeal joints, can be mono- or polyarticular, and is typically symmetrical.[2] In a study of HH patients, radiographic presentations include synovitis, tenosynovitis, joint space narrowing, and osteophytes, such as the hook-shaped osteophytes in MCP joints characteristic of the osteoarthritis of hemochromatosis.[49] In a cohort of 527 well-treated patients with HH, C282Y homozygotes were more likely to have undergone hip or knee replacement (aHR = 3.06, $P < .0010$) and have osteoarthritis (aHR 1.72, $P < .001$) compared to controls.[35] A recent study shows that C282Y homozygotes are also more likely to have worse long-term postsurgical outcomes and recurring joint stiffness 2 and 5 years after total hip arthroplasty and 5-year aseptic loosening after total knee arthroplasty.[50]

Diabetes and hypogonadism are the two most common endocrine manifestations of hemochromatosis.[2] The prevalence of diabetes ranges from 13% to 23% in type 1 HH patients.[2] The pathogenesis of diabetes in HH is not well described, but iron deposition in the pancreas leads to pancreatic β-cell damage and insulin deficiency and insensitivity.[2,51] Except for juvenile hemochromatosis, HH patients typically do not present with diabetes or hypogonadism until after decades of iron loading.[2,51] Glucose intolerance occurs more frequently (58%) in type 2 HH (juvenile hemochromatosis or *HJV* or *HAMP* HH) than in type 1 HH (27%) or type 3 HH (9%).[51] In type 2 HH, there can be up to 75% prevalence of hypogonadism and up to 41% cardiac involvement.[52] Clinical manifestations of hypogonadism typically include loss of libido, impotence, and amenorrhea or more rarely premature menopause in women.[2] HH patients are at increased risk of osteopenia and osteoporosis and approximately 25% and 41% of type 1 HH patients have osteoporosis and osteopenia, respectively.[48,53]

Iron can be deposited in the skin, which can lead to increased melanin production and deposition and the classic "bronze hyperpigmentation."[2] The melanin deposition predisposes to rapid tanning with minimal sun exposure.[54] Hyperpigmentation can be one of the earliest signs of disease and most pronounced in sun-exposed areas such as the face.[54] The color changes can range from brown to gray metallic.[2,54] Other dermatological findings include skin atrophy, ichthyosiform alterations leading to dry scaly skin, koilonychia, and even hair loss.[54]

DIAGNOSTIC TESTING

The initial evaluation in those suspected to have IO disorders includes testing for serum iron level, SF, total iron binding capacity, and TS (Fig. 77.3). If SF is elevated (>300 μg/L in men or >200 μg/L in women) or TS > 45%, then confirmatory genetic testing for C282Y or H63D is recommended. A normal SF and TS < 45% has a 97% negative predictive value for excluding IO.[55] However, an elevated TS and normal SF do not exclude *HFE*-related HH.[5] In the HEIRS study, only 88% of C282Y homozygous men had SF > 300 μg/L, and 57% of women had SF > 200 μg/L[3]; thus many genotypically affected patients had normal SF. H63D is more common than C282Y, with the highest prevalence in Caucasians, with 20% carrying at least one copy of H63D.[2] In a U.S. population study, the prevalence of C282Y homozygosity was 0.26% whereas it was 1.89% for H63D homozygosity and 1.97% for compound heterozygosity.[56] However, the prevalence of patients carrying one C282Y allele did increase

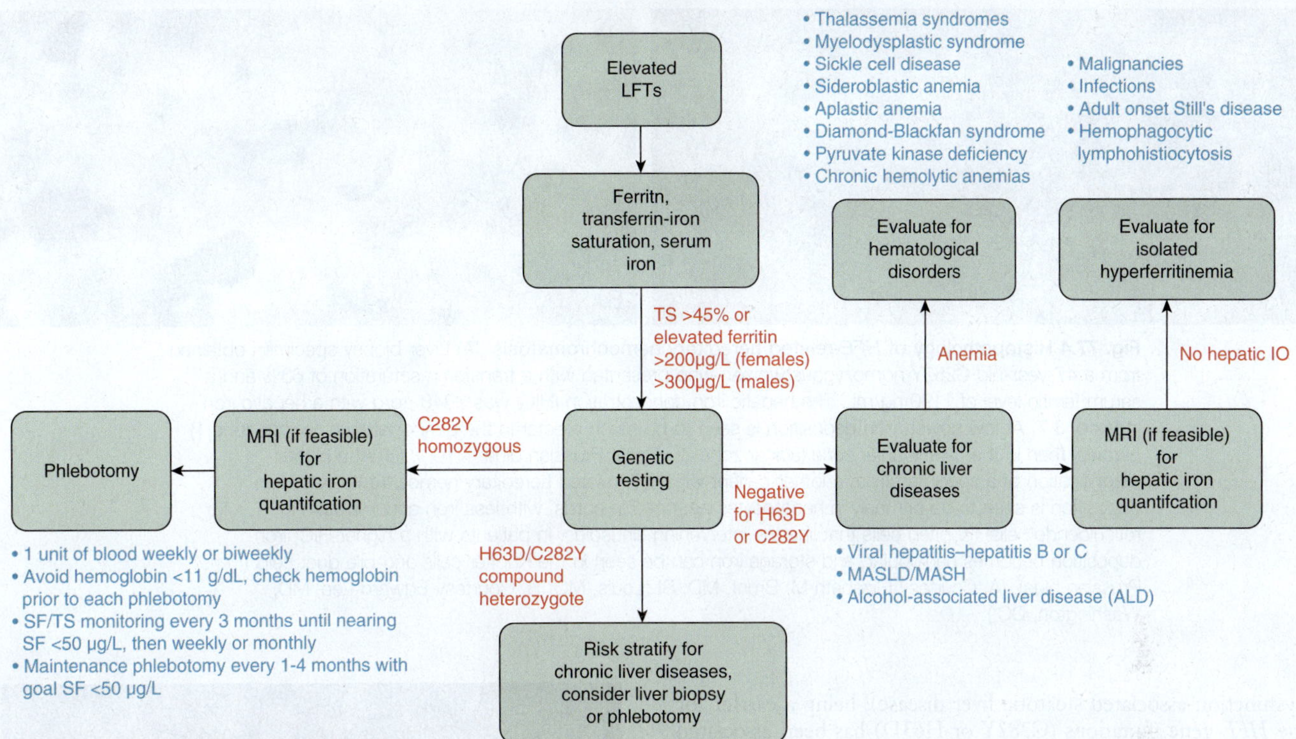

Fig. 77.3 Evaluation and management of patients with elevated iron tests and hereditary hemochromatosis.

to 9.54% among non-Hispanic whites.[56] H63D/C282Y compound heterozygosity or H63D homozygosity may be accompanied by increased SF and TS levels, but are not neccessarily at increased risk of hepatic IO or hemochromatosis-related morbidity.[57,58] Therefore if a patient has elevated TS or SF, and compound heterozygosity or H63D homozygosity, concomitant chronic liver disease (CLD) evaluation should be considered. The utility of testing for the *S65C* mutation is unclear in light of its rarity and unknown clinical significance.

Assessment for hepatic IO with MRI should be considered during evaluation of elevated serum iron tests. Liver biopsy has been historically used to detect and quantify hepatic IO but now its primary utility is for fibrosis staging and to evaluate for concomitant CLD.[2] Hepatic iron will influence relaxation times of hepatic parenchyma in a magnetic field (T2 and T2*) and is proportional to the degree of IO.[59] Hepatic iron decreases the decay time of transverse magnetization with T2 and T2*, leading to reduced signal intensity.[59] Iron assessment by MRI can be subjective (graded mild, moderate, or severe) or quantitative.[59] Various quantitative methods have been developed and include (1) liver to muscle signal intensity ratio, measuring decreasing signal intensity in comparison to reference tissue, such as paraspinal muscle; (2) R2 and T2 relaxometry, which has been validated and approved by FDA and is currently commercialized as FerriScan[60]; and (3) quantitative susceptibility mapping which utilizes the augmentation of magnetic field by hemosiderin or ferritin.[59] R2 and T2 relaxometry utilizes liver proton transverse relaxation rates (R2) and correlates with LIC (liver iron concentration).[60]

Liver biopsy should be considered in a patient with elevated iron tests when evaluating for concomitant liver disease or for fibrosis staging if needed. Liver biopsy provides the opportunity for hepatic iron staining and determination of hepatic iron concentration (HIC) and hepatic iron index (HII)[2] (Fig. 77.4). Hepatic iron staining, HIC, and HII have been used to differentiate C282Y homozygotes from compound heterozygotes, with C282Y homozygotes displaying (1) 4+ stainable iron in hepatocytes in a periportal distribution, and not in KCs; (2) HIC > 71 µmol/g dry weight; and (3) HII > 1.9.[2,61] Several studies have evaluated noninvasive biomarkers to predict advanced fibrosis/cirrhosis. The absence of elevated aspartate aminotransferase, hepatomegaly, and SF > 1000 µg/L predicted almost zero risk of advanced fibrosis or cirrhosis, while conversely, the presence of thrombocytopenia (platelets <200 × 10^9/L), high ferritin (>1000 µg/L), and AST above upper limit of normal leads to correct diagnosis of cirrhosis in 77%–90% of the cases.[38,62] Noninvasive markers such as APRI and FIB-4 have only been validated against liver biopsy in a recent retrospective study. In *HFE* HH patients, an APRI > 0.44 and FIB-4 > 1.1 could detect advanced fibrosis with AUROC of 0.88 and 0.86, respectively.[63] Transient elastography with a cutoff of >9.5 kPa (similarly to hepatitis C) has been shown to predict advanced fibrosis/cirrhosis with 86% sensitivity, 91% specificity, and with a PPV of 75% and NPV of 96% in a small cohort of *HFE* HH patients (n = 77).[64] Further validation with a large multicentered study is still needed. Legros et al. also showed that with a cutoff of <6.4 kPa, none of the *HFE* HH patients evaluated had severe liver fibrosis, and with a cutoff of ≥13.9 kPa, all of the patients had severe liver fibrosis. The study further suggested that liver biopsy be used for fibrosis staging in patients with intermediate values (between 6.4 and 13.9 kPa).[64]

In the setting of elevated iron tests (elevated SF or TS) but without imaging findings of hepatic IO, evaluation for CLDs, secondary IO disorders, hematological disorders, malignancies, infections, and even inflammatory conditions should be considered. In the setting of anemia accompanied by hepatic IO, hematological disorders such as thalassemia syndromes, MDS, and sickle cell disease should be considered.[14] CLD can lead to hepatic IO in alcohol-associated liver disease, viral hepatitis [due to hepatitis C virus (HCV) or HBV], and MASLD (metabolic

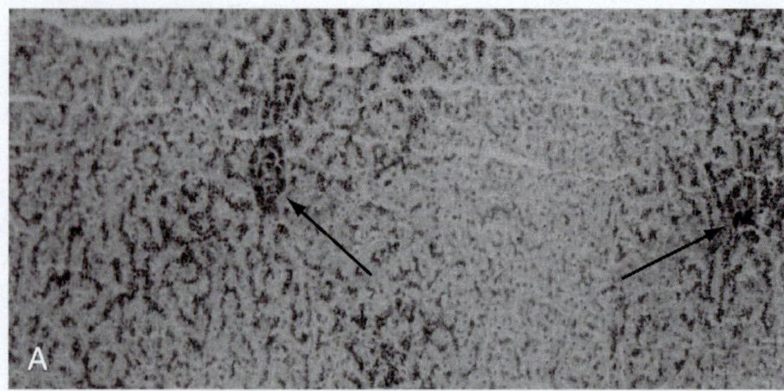

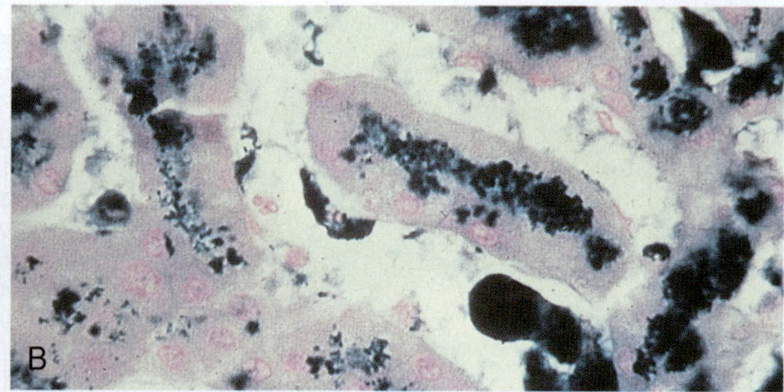

Fig. 77.4 Histopathology of *HFE*-related hereditary hemochromatosis. (A) Liver biopsy specimen obtained from a 47-year-old C282Y homozygous woman who presented with a transferrin saturation of 63% and a serum ferritin level of 1190 ng/mL. The hepatic iron concentration (HIC) was 9840 μg/g with a hepatic iron index of 3.7. At low power, iron deposition is seen to be much greater in the periportal zone (acinar zone 1) (*arrows*) than in the centrilobular zone (acinar zone 3). (Perls' Prussian blue; ×100). (B) At a higher magnification of a specimen from another patient with *HFE*-related hereditary hemochromatosis, iron deposition is seen to be primarily in hepatocytes arranged in cords, with less iron accumulation in reticuloendothelial (Kupffer) cells that line the intervening sinusoids. In patients with a higher HIC, iron deposition becomes panlobular, and storage iron can be seen in the Kupffer cells and bile duct cells (Perls' Prussian blue). (A, Courtesy Elizabeth M. Brunt, MD, St. Louis, MO; B, Courtesy Edward Lee, MD, Washington, DC.)

dysfunction-associated steatotic liver disease); being a carrier for the *HFE* gene mutations (C282Y or H63D) has been associated with increased disease severity in chronic hepatitis C.[14] In special considerations, where ferritin >10,000 μg/L, adult-onset Still's disease or hemophagocytic lymphohistiocytosis should be considered.[14]

TREATMENT AND PROGNOSIS OF HEREDITARY HEMOCHROMATOSIS

C282Y homozygotes with elevated SF (>300 μg/L in men and >200 μg/L in women) and TS (≥ 45%) should be treated (Fig. 77.5). Patients with normal SF and TS should be serially monitored with liver enzymes and iron tests. In the HealthIron Study, a cohort of 202 C282Y homozygotes <15% of the patients with normal SF at baseline developed SF > 1000 μg/L.[65] For men with SF 300–1000 μg/L at baseline, the probability of progressing to SF > 1000 μg/L ranged from 13% to 25%, whereas it was 16% –22% for women.[65] Similarly, in a smaller cohort of C282Y homozygous patients ($n = 22$), 91% of patients with normal SF at baseline remained within normal limits in follow-up.[66] Phlebotomy is the mainstay of therapy for *HFE* HH with elevated SF or TS,[2] and treatment consists of induction therapy followed by maintenance therapy. Most *HFE* HH patients can have up to 20–30 g of total whole body iron stores and may need therapeutic phlebotomy for 2–3 years to remove the excess iron.[5] Each unit of blood contains 200–250 mg of elemental iron, and most patients are able to safely tolerate 1 U of blood removal either weekly or biweekly.[5] A hemoglobin or hematocrit should be checked prior to each phlebotomy to avoid reducing hemoglobin to <11 g/dL.[2,5] The recommendation for the frequency of SF/TS monitoring varies according to guidelines; there appears to be consensus that SF/TS should be monitored approximately every 3 months (or every 10–12 phlebotomies) with extremely high SF levels and increase in frequency to monthly or every 2 weeks when nearing the goal SF of 50 μg/L for induction therapy.[5,67,68] For maintenance therapy, it is advised that patient's SF is closely followed and considered for phlebotomy every 1–4 months to keep SF < 50 μg/L.[68] In patients with advanced cardiac disease with arrhythmias or cardiomyopathy, sudden death is possible in the setting of rapid mobilization of iron.[2,5] Vitamin C can accelerate intestinal iron absorption and should be avoided in HH patients, particularly in patients undergoing phlebotomy.[2,5] Elimination of red meat and other sources of dietary iron is not necessary in those undergoing phlebotomy.[2]

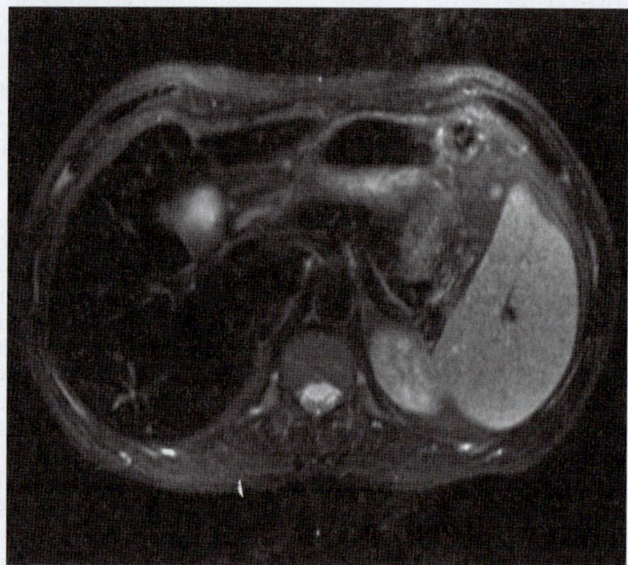

Fig. 77.5 MRI of a patient with hemochromatosis. This T2-weighted image shows low signal intensity in the liver due to the magnetic susceptibility effects of iron, compared with normal signal intensity in the spleen. In secondary iron overload, the spleen would also have low signal intensity due to increased iron deposition in reticuloendothelial cells.

The decision to treat in patients with C282Y/H63D heterozygosity and H63D homozygosity is more complex. A natural history study of 180 nonobese compound heterozygotes (C282Y/H63D) without heavy alcohol intake found similar prevalence of disease as *HFE* wild-type genotype, with similar rates of second or third metacarpal joint involvement (effusion, tenderness, or bony spurs), fatigue, arthritis diagnosis, elevated liver enzymes, liver disease, and hepatomegaly by physical exam.[57] Documented IO (defined as hepatic iron staining of 3+ or 4+, HII > 1.9, or HIC of >90 μg/g) was only observed in 1.2% of the compound heterozygote men and in 0% of the compound heterozygote women.[57] Most of the liver disease in compound heterozygotes is due to concomitant heavy alcohol use, fatty liver disease, or type 2 diabetes.[69] Similarly, in H63D homozygotes, there is a low prevalence of IO disease (3.2%).[70] However, a recent Swedish study of 1345 compound heterozygotes (C282Y/H63D) showed an increased risk of HCC, cirrhosis, and type 2 diabetes when compared to a reference control population.[71] Thus for H63D homozygotes and C282Y/H63D compound heterozygotes, a liver biopsy can be considered for fibrosis staging, and phlebotomy can be considered only if there is evidence of significant IO (HII > 1.9 or iron concentration >70 μg/g of dry weight liver).[2]

Prognosis for *HFE* HH patients is related to degree of IO, and the presence of cirrhosis, cardiomyopathy, or diabetes at baseline. In a study of 251 patients with *HFE* HH, survival of noncirrhotic, nondiabetic patients diagnosed between 1982 and 1991 was similar to a matched control population.[7] However, patients with cirrhosis, diabetes, or clinically significant IO had reduced survival compared to the control population; the most common causes of death were liver cancer (119-fold more frequent), liver cirrhosis (10 times), and diabetes (14 times) than control population.[7] Cumulative survival of the patients in this cohort was 77% at 10 years, 55% at 20 years, and 20% at 30 years.[7] Hepatic fibrosis and cirrhosis correlate with degree of IO and have been shown to regress (by 2 METAVIR stages) in 69% of F3 patients and 35% of F4 patients after phlebotomy.[10,72] Improvement of portal hypertension and of esophageal varices has also been described after phlebotomy.[72] Phlebotomy in cirrhotic patients with end-stage liver disease must be conducted carefully, since many such patients are often anemic at baseline. Phlebotomy does not reverse diabetes, arthropathy, and, in most cases, hypogonadism.[2] Cardiomyopathy and skin hyperpigmentation can slowly regress with phlebotomy.[2]

For those intolerant of phlebotomy, IV or oral iron chelators can be considered. There are currently three FDA-approved IV or oral chelators: (1) deferoxamine (DFO); (2) deferiprone (DFP); and (3) deferasirox (DFX) (Table 77.2).[73] DFO, the oldest drug, is administered parenterally (subcutaneously or intravenously), while DFP and DFX are orally administered.[73] In phases 1 and 2 dose escalation studies, DFX (oral iron chelator) reduced ferritin levels by 64%–75% after 1 year of treatment in HH patients.[74] However, approximately 20%–26% of the patients had increases in creatinine and liver enzymes during treatment, and many had symptoms of nausea, vomiting, and diarrhea.[74] In a follow-up study, 10 patients were treated with 10 ± 5 mg/kg/day and able to achieve >50% reduction in ferritin after median 7.5 months, and fewer experienced side effects, and no increases in creatinine were observed.[75] Therefore in *HFE* HH patients who are intolerant of phlebotomy, iron chelators can be considered, but data are only available in phase 2 clinical trials.

Erythrocytapheresis is an alternative to phlebotomy and can remove larger volumes of RBCs (up to 1000 mL) with each session.[2] It is a method to remove RBCs while returning clotting factors, platelets, and protein.[2] Patients generally can have a session every 2–3 weeks with a goal of keeping post-erythrocytapheresis hemoglobin levels above 10 mg/dL.[2] RBC volume typically removed is between 350 and 800 mL; this technique can be helpful in patients with thrombocytopenia or hypoproteinemia.[2]

Because they reduce the acidic environment that enhances dietary iron absorption, proton pump inhibitors (PPIs) have been evaluated for their ability to reduce the frequency and need for phlebotomy. In a randomized controlled trial of 30 C282Y homozygote patients, those on PPI required a median of only 1.3 procedures versus 2.6 procedures for those not on PPI (P = .005).[2] However, given the small size of these trials, routinely starting PPIs in *HFE* HH patients undergoing phlebotomy is not recommended.[2]

TABLE 77.2 Depiction of Clinical Presentations of Patients with Hereditary Hemochromatosis or C282Y Homozygotes

Study	Olynyk et al.		Powell et al.		Barton et al.	Allen et al.
Country	Australia		Australia		Australia, the United States, Canada	
Number of patients (gender)	16 (7M, 9F)		672 (359M, 313F)		368	203
Clinical presentation (%)						
Elevated ferritin	63		77			67.5
Liver manifestation						
Elevated liver enzymes			30	8.6	61	11.5
Hepatomegaly	43	0	17	4.2		1.9
Hepatic iron overload	71	33	56	35		18.9
Fibrosis	43	0	12.8	3.5		
Cirrhosis	6.3		3.9		23.4[a]	
Arthropathies	38		7	1.9	54.9	11.8
Diabetes			2.5	3.8	12.9	1.5
Skin hyperpigmentation	38					
Cardiac arrhythmia			0.5	0.6		

[a]The cohort from Barton et al. had 30.7% prevalence of fatty liver, and thus cirrhosis prevalence is higher than other depicted cohorts and may be confounded by underlying concomitant chronic liver disease. Only available data are reported.

In those with HCC, end-stage liver disease, or decompensated cirrhosis, liver transplantation (LT) can be considered. Outcomes in *HFE* HH are comparable to a cross-matched CLD cohort using propensity matching; the 1- and 5-year post-LT survival rates were 88.7% [95% confidence interval (CI), 85.4%–91.4%] and 77.5% (95% CI, 72.8%–81.4%), which is similar to a non-HH matched cohort (P value = .96).[76] However, previous cohorts of either C282Y homozygous or compound heterozygote (C282Y/H63D) patients showed worse post-LT survival in patients with *HFE* HH, and IO was a significant risk factor for post-LT infections, particularly fungal infections.[77–80] In these cohorts, sample size remained small (n = 22–41) with estimated 1-year and 5-year survival ranging from 64% to 80.7% and 34% to 74%, respectively.[77–80] However, a subsequent study showed that while there was poor survival in the era of patients transplanted from 1990 to 1996, similar post-LT survival as non-*HFE* HH patients was observed in patients transplanted from 1997 to 2006.[81] In several studies of HH patients who underwent liver transplants, the most common causes of post-LT death were infections, recurrent HCC, or malignancy.[76,79,80]

CAUSES AND CLINICAL MANIFESTATIONS OF SECONDARY IRON OVERLOAD

Secondary IO can result from iatrogenic iron administration, repeated blood transfusions, IE due to a chronic hematological disorder, and from CLD.[14] The most common syndromes of IE and secondary IO are thalassemia syndromes, MDS, but can include myelofibrosis, sickle cell disease, SA or AA, Diamond-Blackfan syndrome, and pyruvate kinase deficiency.[14] Thalassemia and MDS can be classified as transfusion dependent (TD) and independent.[14] Thalassemias are inherited genetic disorders with gene mutations in α-globin or β-globin genes. Hemoglobin H (HbH) disease (mutations of 3 out of 4 α-globin genes) and Bart's hydrops fetalis (absence of all 4 α-globin genes) are the most severe forms in α-thalassemia.[14] The clinical phenotypes for β-thalassemias include β-thalassemia minor (or β-thalassemia trait, with clinically silent, microcytic anemia), β-thalassemia intermedia (TI, with mild-to-moderate anemia associated with IO and IE), and β-thalassemia major (TM, severe with early transfusion dependence).[82] The combination of thalassemia mutations with the structural variant hemoglobin E (HbE) results in a compound heterozygote β-thalassemia (HbE/β-thalassemias). Patients with secondary IO typically present with anemia and IO.[14]

IE can lead to IO via a hepcidin regulator protein hormone called erythroferrone.[14] In animal models of β-thalassemia, bone marrow and spleen erythroid precursors make erythroferrone that inhibits hepcidin production.[83] Growth differentiation factor 15 (GDF-15) has also been implicated in IE and is produced by apoptotic erythroblasts; GDF-15 levels have been most elevated in TDT (TD thalassemia),[84,85] more modestly elevated in TI, and normal in HbH disease,[86] supporting it as a marker of IE, even if its role in suppressing hepcidin production has not been confirmed in patients with β-thalassemia.[14]

While hepatic complications contribute to most of the morbidity and mortality in *HFE* HH, cardiac complications contribute to most of the morbidity and mortality in TDT syndromes or MDS.[14] TDT and transfusion-dependent MDS patients typically have higher mortality rates than nontransfusion-dependent patients and have more cardiac than hepatic or endocrine complications.[14] In β-thalassemia major patients who are TD early in life, congestive heart failure, dysrhythmias, or even sudden death may occur even in their 20s.[87] In a Japanese study of MDS, myelofibrosis, and AA,[88] 24% had cardiac failure, while only 6.7% had liver failure.[88] Similarly, in an Italian MDS cohort, the most common nonleukemic causes of death were cardiac complications (51%) followed by infections (31%), hemorrhage (8%), and cirrhosis (8%).[89] The majority (73%) of MDS patients had a cardiac event in a 3-year follow-up period and had increased risk of diabetes (40.1% vs. 33.3%), hepatic diseases (0.8% vs. 0.2%), and infections (22.5% vs. 6.1%) (P < .01) compared to non-MDS patients.[90] In patients with β-TI, the most threatening complication is pulmonary hypertension, but they also develop clinical complications of thrombotic events, extramedullary hematopoiesis, cholelithiasis, osteoporosis, hypogonadism, leg ulcers, and abnormal liver enzymes.[91]

Despite the lower prevalence of hepatic complications, there is a rising incidence of HCC (estimated annual incidence of 2%[92]) in thalassemia patients[93] as they are being treated with iron chelators earlier in life and living longer. Additionally, many patients have acquired HCV from blood transfusions, and HCV antibody testing can be positive up to 85% of thalassemia patients with 50%–57% of them being HCV viremic.[94,95] In a study of 57 thalassemia patients, 3.5% developed HCC; the incidence was higher in TI patients (P = .032).[94] In this cohort, 33% of the HCC patients had liver siderosis and advanced fibrosis and no viral hepatitis, indicating that these patients are at risk of HCC from the IO alone.[94]

CLD with viral hepatitis (HCV or HBV), alcohol-associated liver disease, and MASLD/MASH (metabolic dysfunction-associated steatotic liver disease/steatohepatitis, formerly NAFLD/NASH) can present with secondary IO.[14] Dysmetabolic IO syndrome (DIOS) is used to describe MASLD associated with IO.[96] The pattern of hepatic IO has been predictive of disease severity in MASLD; stainable iron in reticuloendothelial system (RES) alone pattern is more often associated with MASH and advanced fibrosis rather than a hepatocellular pattern alone or a mixed pattern.[97] In HCV, IO is also associated with more severe histological activity and cirrhosis (17% with IO vs. 3% without IO, P = .004).[98] Conversely, carrying *HFE* mutations is associated with an increased risk of advanced fibrosis/cirrhosis (OR = 18, 95% CI, 1.7–193 after adjusting for disease duration) in patients with chronic hepatitis C.[99] It is more controversial whether or not MASLD patients carrying *HFE* mutations are at greater risk of advanced fibrosis; one study showed that MASH patients with C282Y heterozygosity have an increased risk of having stainable hepatic iron and bridging fibrosis or cirrhosis (44% vs. 21%, P = 0.05), while two other studies showed no association.[100–102]

Similarly, ferritin can be elevated in 63% of alcohol-associated liver disease patients, and stainable iron in hepatic parenchyma and RES has been observed in 52% of patients.[103] In chronic hepatitis B, coinfection with hepatitis D was associated with more grade 3 hepatic iron deposits than in HBV monoinfected patients (27.8% vs. 2.1%, respectively, P < .0001).[104] In that cohort of HBV patients, 41.5% had at least one of the serum iron indices elevated, and 35.1% had hepatic iron deposits although the majority were minimal to mild.[104]

TREATMENT OF SECONDARY IRON OVERLOAD

The mainstay of treatment for secondary IO is iron chelation therapy (ICT), as most patients have anemia and are intolerant of phlebotomy. ICT is typically started after 2–3 years of regular PRBC transfusions, >10 PRBC transfusions, or if SF ≥ 1000 μg/L in thalassemia syndromes.[73] ICT is recommended for patients with SF > 1000 μg/L or LIC of 7 mg Fe/g dw in transfusion-dependent sickle cell disease or other transfusion-dependent chronic anemias.[105,106] NIH guidelines recommend ICT in patients with >120 cm^3 of PRBC/kg of transfusions.[105] As noted, three iron chelators are currently approved for use: DFO, DFP, and DFX.[14] Patients are typically administered one agent and followed serially with MRI iron quantification to assess for efficacy.[14] If MRI iron quantification is not available, ferritin can be used as a surrogate measure.[14] In TDT, thalassemia major patients, ICT is predominantly aimed at preventing cardiac complications[107] and has been shown in multiple studies to improve overall survival.[108] In the large THALASSA study, where nontransfusion-dependent thalassemia patients were randomized to DFX or placebo, ferritin >2000 μg/L has been the proposed cutoff for dose escalation because SF levels of 1700–2000 μg/L have a 100% PPV in predicting LIC > 7 mg Fe/g dw.[109] Ferritin levels <300 μg/L have been proposed as a lower threshold to hold chelation therapy.[109] In the phase 3 study comparing DFO and DFX, thalassemia patients were dosed based on initial LIC concentrations, and those with baseline >7 mg Fe/g dw had statistically significant LIC reduction (5.3 ± 8 mg Fe/g dw, $P < .001$) after 1 year of ICT with DFX, which was noninferior to DFO (4.3 ± 5.8 mg Fe/g dw, $P = .367$).[110] In this trial, patients were given 5 or 10 mg/kg/day for mild IO (<7 mg Fe/ g dw), 20 mg/kg for moderate IO (7–14 mg Fe/g dw), and 30 mg/kg for severe IO (>14 mg Fe/g dw).[110] Similarly, DFO was dosed according to mild (25–35 mg/kg), moderate (35–50 mg/kg), or severe IO (≥ 50 mg/kg) and given 5 days/week.[110] Although patients with <7 mg Fe/g dw did not achieve statistically significant reductions in LIC, they were still able to achieve a LIC reduction of 4 ± 3.8 mg Fe/g dw.[110] Most common side effects include gastrointestinal symptoms (15.2%), mild dose-dependent increases in creatinine (38%), skin rash (10.8%), and more rarely elevated liver enzymes (two patients), neurosensory deafness (0.3% in DFX and 1.7% in DFO).[110] DFO has been linked to auditory toxicities, with highest risk in patients with mild IO treated with high doses of DFO.[111] DFO has also been associated with ophthalmological toxicities such as optic neuropathy, blurred vision, night blindness, and loss of central vision but again typically seen at high doses.[111] Agranulocytosis or cytopenias (another known side effect of DFP) were not reported in this trial.[73,110]

Hepatic fibrosis reversal and stability have been shown to occur in up to 82.6% of the TDT (TD thalassemia) patients treated with ICT.[112] Additionally, combination therapy with DFO-DFP has been shown to be superior in improving cardiac iron, left ventricular ejection fraction, and SF than treatment with DFO alone.[113] In β-TI, and in the OPTIMAL CARE study, blood transfusion with a higher target hemoglobin rather than ICT is associated with improvement in multiple complications: thrombosis, extramedullary hematopoiesis, heart failure, pulmonary hypertension, leg ulcers, and cholelithiasis.[91,107] However, blood transfusion can worsen endocrinopathies, and thus ICT has been used to improve endocrinopathies and pulmonary hypertension.[91] Most TI trials considered ICT when LIC exceeded 5 mg Fe/g dw or when SF > 300 μg/L but the prevalence of sensorineural hearing loss was rather high at 38% and occurred most often in young patients with mild IO and correlated well with mean peak DFO concentrations.[107] Thus the decision to start ICT in TI patients needs to be heavily weighed against the risks of therapy.

In MDS, ICT is controversial due to high rates of adverse events from treatment. In the TELESTO trial (prospective, randomized controlled trial), ICT prolonged event-free survival (EFS) by 1 year [3.9 vs. 3 years for chelated vs. nonchelated with HR 0.64 (CI, 0.42–0.96)].[114] Events were categorized as death, transformation to AML (acute myeloid leukemia), liver dysfunction, or cardiac events. EFS at 3 years was higher (61.5% vs. 47.3%) in treated versus untreated patients, and ICT improved EFS with a hazard ratio of 0.64 (95% CI, 0.42–0.96).[114] Similarly, another study showed that DFX was associated with improved LIC, hemoglobin, platelets, and decreased liver enzymes.[115,116] Despite the benefits, most trials show high rates of DFX discontinuation due to adverse effects (48%–75%).[114,117–119] Most guideline recommendations recommend considering ICT in MDS patients after >20 U of PRBC transfusion or SF 1000–2500 μg/L with a goal to reduce ferritin to <1000 μg/L.[120]

In sickle cell disease, while it has been shown that IO is associated with increased mortality (5% if SF < 100 ng/mL and TS < 50% compared to 64% mortality with SF > 1500 ng/mL and TS > 50%[108,121]), ICT has not been shown to directly improve survival as there was no comparator group of nonchelated patients in the trial.[108] The only RCT compared DFP to DFO and showed similar 5-year survival of >80%–90%.[122] Six deaths occurred in the trial, and half were due to hepatic failure.[122]

In CLD, a small randomized controlled trial in MASLD patients with ferritin ≥250 ng/mL and NAFLD activity score >1 showed that phlebotomy was associated with improved liver enzymes and hepatic steatosis when compared to patients who did not undergo phlebotomy at 2-year follow-up.[123] However, a subsequent randomized controlled trial showed no difference in liver enzymes, hepatic steatosis, or insulin resistance in those who underwent phlebotomy compared to those who did not.[124] Currently, phlebotomy is not recommended for DIOS and MASLD.[14] For HCV during the interferon treatment era, phlebotomy was previously evaluated as an adjuvant therapy to augment the HCV treatment response given prior studies showing an inverse relationship between iron and interferon response.[125] However, in the DAA (direct-acting antiviral) era, DAAs are associated with excellent cure rates (>95%), so phlebotomy is not currently used to augment HCV treatment response rate.[126]

MALIGNANCY RISK

HFE HH patients are at increased risk of HCC.[127] Initial studies from Brisbane and Düsseldorf showed the risk of HCC to be 200-fold in *HFE* HH patients with an incidence of 8%–10% in cohort studies,[127–129] but subsequent studies have shown lower rates. In a Danish study, the SIR (standardized incidence ratio) was noted to be 92.9 (95% CI, 25.0–237.9) for increased HCC risk for *HFE* HH patients when compared to the average population but in a recent Swedish study, the SIR was 21 (95% CI, 16–22).[130,131] Even when compared to CLD patients, *HFE* HH patients were shown to be at increased risk of HCC (OR 1.8, 95% CI, 1.1–2.9).[132] However, this study did not characterize the severity of CLD.[127,132] HCC in noncirrhotic *HFE* HH patients has also been described.[127] Studies evaluating the pathology of HCC in noncirrhotic *HFE* HH show that typically more than half (~54%) have stainable iron on biopsy and that degree of IO often correlated with advanced fibrosis.[133] Given the additional increased HCC risk in advanced fibrosis/cirrhosis, *HFE* HH patients should undergo screening for advanced fibrosis/cirrhosis with noninvasive biomarkers or US elastography and pursue HCC screening for METAVIR F3 and F4 patients per AASLD guidelines.[134]

Studies have yielded conflicting results with regards to the risk of extrahepatic malignancies. In a Danish study, *HFE* HH patients had an increased risk of extrahepatic malignancies (SIR 3.5, 95% CI, 1.9–6.0), particularly esophageal cancer (SIR 42.9, 95% CI, 4.8–154.9) and melanoma (SIR 27.8, 95% CI, 3.1–100.3).[130] In the Melbourne Collaborative Cohort Study (comprised of patients from Ireland, United Kingdom, or Australia) where 28,509 patients were genotyped for *HFE*, C282Y homozygous men were discovered to be at increased risk of colorectal cancer (HR 2.28; 95% CI, 1.22–4.25; $P = .01$), while C282Y homozygous women were at increased risk of breast cancer (HR 2.39; 95% CI, 1.24–4.61; $P = .01$).[135] Compound heterozygotes (C282Y/H63D) were not at increased risk of breast, colorectal, or prostate cancer.[135] Additionally, one U.S. population-based case-control study showed patients carrying any H63D or C282Y mutations had an increased risk of colon cancer (adjusted OR = 1.40, 95% CI, 1.07–1.87) even after adjusting for age, gender, ethnicity, NSAID use, red meat, or iron intake.[136] Although not statistically significant, one study showed that *HFE* HH patients have a nearly doubled prevalence of extrahepatic malignancies (0.9% vs. 0.5%, HR 1.8; 95% CI, 0.8–4) when compared to patients with noniron CLD.[132] In that study, even adjusted for alcohol abuse, smoking, and family history of cancer, the overall risk of cancer was increased in *HFE* HH (HR 1.9; 95% CI, 1.1–3.1) when compared to noniron-related CLD.[132] However, a subsequent Swedish study showed no increased risk of extrahepatic malignancy (SIR 1.2; 95% CI, 1–1.4).[43] First-degree relatives similarly are not at increased risk of extrahepatic malignancy but are at mild increased risk of hepatobiliary malignancies (SIR 1.5, 95% CI, 1–2.4).[43] Regardless, prior epidemiological studies do show an association between increased total body iron stores and carcinogenesis,[127,137,138] and thus there is likely a positive relationship.[127] Although there are no current guidelines to intensify surveillance strategies for cancer screening in *HFE* HH patients, strict adherence to age-appropriate cancer screening should be advised.

In secondary IO, there is an increased incidence of HCC in thalassemia patients, particularly those with TI.[93] Previously, thalassemia patients were more likely to die from cardiac complications but are now living longer because of more effective chelating agents.[93] HCC cases in thalassemia patients were originally reported predominantly in Italy and Greece, with some cases in the United Kingdom, Lebanon, and Iran.[139] Subsequently, one prospective study of ultrasound screening of 105 Italian thalassemia patients showed an incidence of 2% over a 1-year observation period,[92] and of the HCC patients, all had IO, 64% had chronic HCV infection, and the minority (14%) had cirrhosis.[92] TI patients are more affected than TM patients because they are living longer with the combination of IO and chronic viral hepatitis.[93] In one study, 3.5% developed HCC, and incidence was higher in TI patients ($P = .032$).[94] Similarly, in a large study comprised of 55 Italian centers, HCC incidence was higher in TI [1.74% (95% CI, 1.16–2.51)] than TM [0.75% (95% CI, 0.52–1.06)].[140] The overall HCC incidence in that cohort was 1.02% (95% CI, 0.78–1.13)[140] and the outcomes of the HCC patients were poor; ~50% survival at 2 years with median survival of 11.5 months.[140] A minority of patients received curative therapy with resection or transplantation (32%).[140] These observations stress the importance of early HCC screening and detection in thalassemia patients, particularly TI patients. Additionally, although HCV curative treatment can reduce HCC risk, it does not eliminate the risk. In a single-center study, despite 50% of patients achieving HCV cure, HCC incidence was only reduced from 3.36% to 1.47%,[141] underscoring the potential contribution of IO and aging to hepatocarcinogenesis.

FAMILY SCREENING

First-degree relatives of *HFE* HH patients should undergo screening with TS and SF and if C282Y homozygotes and compound heterozygotes (C282Y/H63D) are discovered with clinical signs of IO, then therapeutic phlebotomy should be pursued.[2,5] In children of a proband, testing of the other parent is advised; if the other parent is negative for *HFE* mutations, then the child does not need to undergo testing as they are a heterozygote and not at increased risk of IO.[2,142] One study showed that with spousal testing, 239 children could be spared testing, and all children who were tested in the study were C282Y homozygotes with 39% cost-savings.[142] However, if the other parent cannot be tested, then the child can likely be tested in late teenage years as clinically significant manifestations of IO rarely occur in the first two decades of life.[143]

Full references for this chapter can be found on https://ebooks.health.elsevier.com.

78 Wilson Disease

Eve A. Roberts

IN THIS CHAPTER

Copper, a component of numerous essential enzymes, is toxic to cells when present in excess. Dietary intake of copper generally exceeds the trace amount required physiologically, and mechanisms to control influx and efflux from cells must maintain an appropriate balance. The two main human disorders of copper transport are *Menkes disease*, an X-linked defect in the transport of copper from the intestine that leads to generalized copper deficiency, and *Wilson disease* (WD), an autosomal recessive disorder of copper overload. WD (hepatolenticular degeneration) was first described in 1912 by Kinnier Wilson as a familial disease characterized by progressive, lethal neurological dysfunction with liver cirrhosis.[1] Complementing Wilson's observations, Bramwell reported a family in which three children died of liver disease without experiencing neurological abnormalities, and he speculated that this was an earlier stage of the disorder.[2] In WD, inadequate hepatic copper excretion leads to copper accumulation in the liver, brain, kidney, and cornea. For years, based on somewhat limited data, the estimated prevalence in most populations has been set at approximately 1 in 30,000; recent studies support this prevalence.[3,4] The allele frequency may be greater than that implied by this estimate.[5–7] Accordingly, WD may demonstrate incomplete penetrance, thus making it inherently difficult to determine allele frequency.

COPPER METABOLISM

Dietary copper is absorbed in the proximal small intestine. Loosely bound to albumin and also to histidine and α_2-macroglobulin, copper is distributed throughout a variety of tissues. Portal blood flow directs most copper to the liver. Trace amounts of copper are required for essential enzymes that affect connective tissue and elastin cross-linking (lysyl oxidase), free radical scavenging (superoxide dismutase), electron transfer (cytochrome oxidase), pigment production (tyrosinase), and neurotransmission (dopamine β-monooxygenase). Copper is a key component of cytochrome *c* oxidase, which is complex IV of the electron transport chain in mitochondria. Molecular copper is never free within a cell. Copper in hepatocytes and other cells is bound to metallochaperones, low-molecular-weight proteins that specifically deliver copper to a target molecule. Metallothioneins and glutathione also bind intracellular copper.

In the liver, copper is incorporated into apoceruloplasmin to produce ceruloplasmin (technically: holo-ceruloplasmin). More than 90% of the copper in plasma is an integral part of ceruloplasmin, an α_2-glycoprotein that contains six molecules of copper and has a molecular weight of 132 kD. The normal serum concentration of ceruloplasmin in adults, as measured by immunochemical or enzymatic techniques, is 200–400 mg/L, rising from a very low level at birth to 300–500 mg/L in the first years of life and then settling to adult levels. Because it is an acute-phase reactant, ceruloplasmin levels are elevated by inflammation (including inflammatory hepatic disease), pregnancy, and the use of exogenous estrogen. Most ingested copper is excreted via the bile; a very small fraction is excreted in urine. When intestinal or liver cells are overloaded with copper, metallothioneins, a class of low-molecular-weight cysteine-rich proteins, are induced and sequester copper in a nontoxic form. The normal pathways of copper transport in the body and in the hepatocyte are shown in Figs. 78.1 and 78.2.

MOLECULAR PATHOGENESIS

Our knowledge of the pathogenesis of WD increased dramatically with the identification of the gene associated with Menkes disease and the one associated with WD. The gene that is abnormal in Menkes disease (*ATP7A*), which was cloned by using a chromosomal breakpoint in an affected female patient, was found to be related to bacterial copper-resistance genes. Cloning of the gene in which mutations result in WD (*ATP7B*) was accomplished in the first instance by a combination of linkage analysis, physical mapping of the relevant region of chromosome 13q14, and recognition of its extensive homology with *ATP7A*.[8,9] The coding region of the *ATP7B* gene is 4.1 kb in length, with messenger RNA of about 8 kb; the gene is distributed over 80 kb. The product, ATP7B (nonacronymic: Wilson ATPase), is a membrane-bound copper-transporting P_1-type ATPase that consists of 1443 amino acid residues and has a molecular mass of 160 kD. The structure[10,11] comprises six metal-binding domains (previously referred to as "copper-binding units") in the amino-terminus "tail"; a phosphatase P-domain, an ATP-binding N-domain, and an actuator A-domain; eight transmembrane segments forming a pore; and a partially disordered carboxy terminus that includes a trileucine motif important for intracellular trafficking (Fig. 78.3). All functionally important regions of the gene are conserved between bacteria and yeast. Mutations in the *ATP7B* gene result in retention of copper in the liver. The Long-Evans cinnamon (LEC) rat, the LPP rat derived from the LEC rat, and both versions of the toxic milk (tx) mouse have mutations

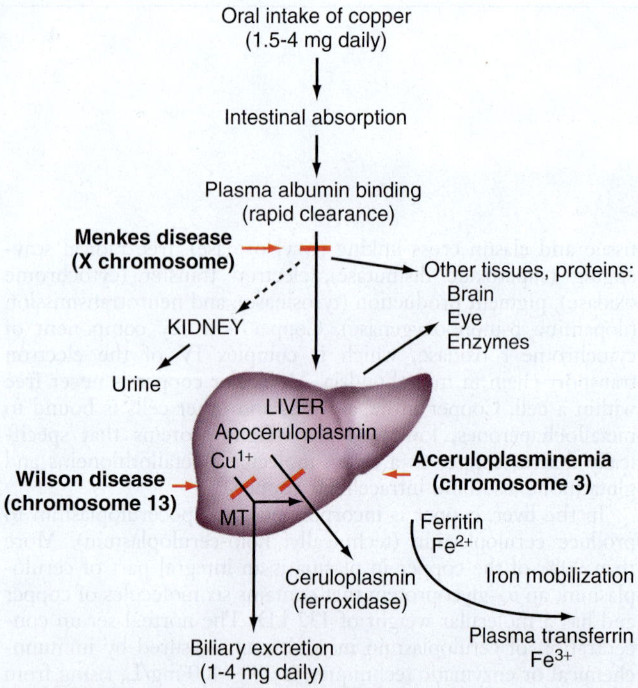

Fig. 78.1 Simplified overview of the pathways for copper ion transport and the steps affected in genetic disorders of copper metabolism. *MT*, Metallothioneins. (Modified from Cox DW. Genes of the copper pathway. *Am J Hum Genet*. 1995;56:828–834.)

in their homologous *ATP7B* genes and are thus suitable models for the study of WD mechanisms and therapies.[12–15] A knockout mouse (Atp7b$^{-/-}$), developed by introducing a mutation in *Atp7b* to exclude exon 2, fails to produce Atp7b, the murine version of the Wilson ATPase.[16] A mouse with a targeted loss of Atp7b expression in the liver has been developed.[17]

Although *ATP7A* is expressed in many tissues, *ATP7B*, abnormal in WD, is expressed predominantly in the liver and kidney, with minor expression in brain, lungs, and placenta.[8] In the liver, the Wilson ATPase (ATP7B) has two principal intracellular functions: synthesis of enzymatically active ceruloplasmin and biliary excretion of copper. It is localized in the *trans*-Golgi network and traffics to cytoplasmic vesicles in the presence of increased copper. Specifically, when intracellular copper concentrations are elevated, ATP7B is found near the apical (bile canalicular) membrane in hepatocytes, consistent with its proposed function of facilitating excretion of copper via bile.[18] Evidently, ATP7B also has an additional function: sensing ambient hepatocellular copper concentration. The role of copper, and indirectly ATP7B, in lipid metabolism is an important area of investigation.[19,20]

Additional proteins are involved in the intracellular disposition of copper. Loosely bound to intracellular metallochaperones (also called *copper chaperones*), copper is transported to specific proteins, such as superoxide dismutase in the cytoplasm and various copper-containing proteins in mitochondria. The metallochaperone antioxidant 1 copper chaperone (ATOX1) transports copper to the Wilson ATPase (ATP7B). Based on initial reports, the interactome for ATP7B includes COMMD1, glutaredoxin, dynactin p62, PLZF (promyelocytic leukemia zinc finger) protein,

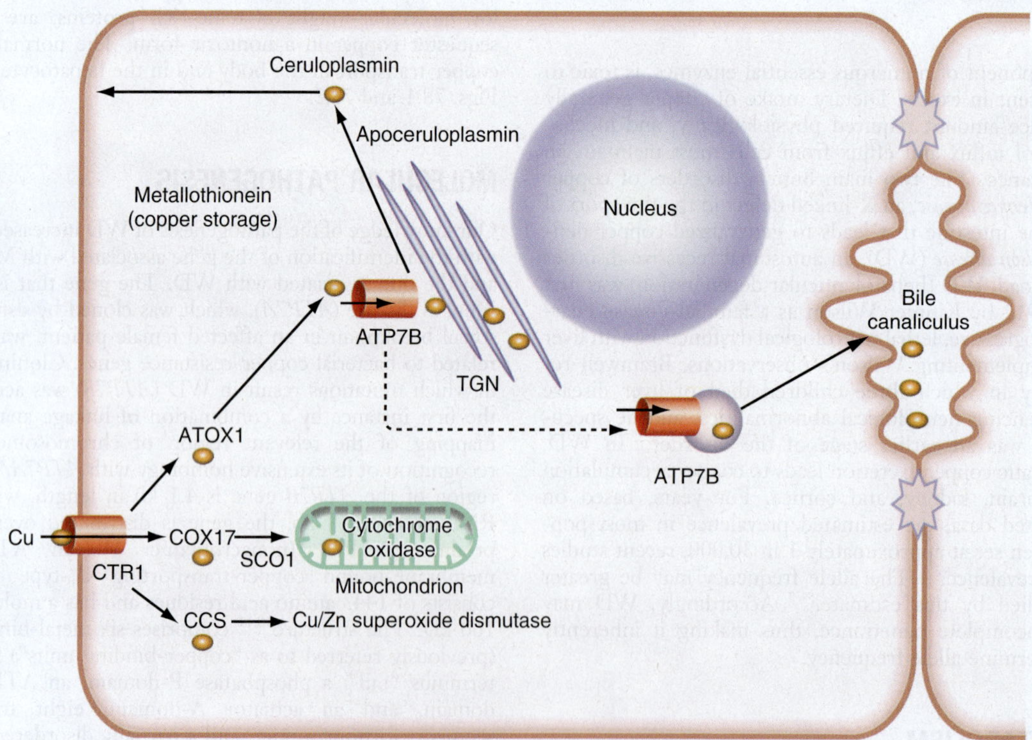

Fig. 78.2 Model of a hepatocyte showing the major proteins in the copper transport pathway. Low-molecular-weight metallochaperones [ATOX1 (antioxidant 1 copper chaperone), COX17 (cytochrome *c* oxidase 17), and CCS (copper chaperone for superoxide dismutase)] deliver copper (Cu) to specific target proteins (ATP7B, cytochrome oxidase, and superoxide dismutase, respectively). SCO1 (synthesis of cytochrome *c* oxidase 1) transports copper across the mitochondrial membrane. ATP7B (shown as a channel) traffics from the *trans*-Golgi network (TGN) to cytoplasmic vesicles that deliver copper to the bile canaliculus.

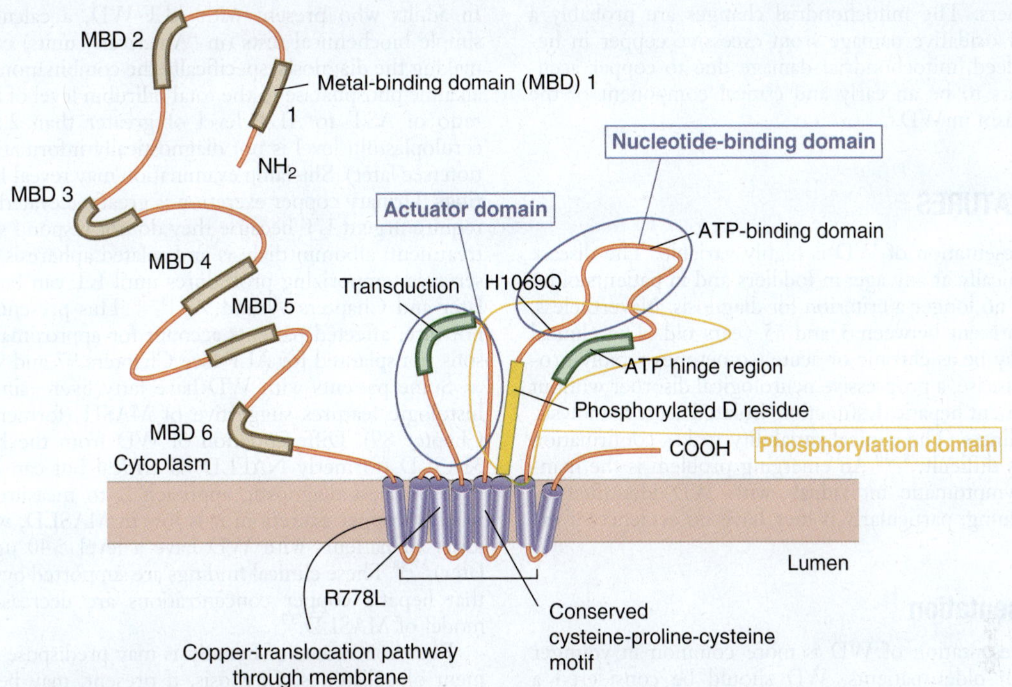

Fig. 78.3 A model of the Wilson ATPase, the product of *ATP7B*. The features conserved in both the Menkes ATPase and the Wilson ATPase include the metal-binding region, which comprises 6 metal-binding domains (MBD 1-6), shown as tan cylinders, and the actuator (*vertical blue ellipse*), phosphorylation (*yellow outline*), and nucleotide-binding (*angled blue ellipse*) domains. These domains are indicated in comparison with previous terminology relating to "transduction" and the "ATP hinge region," which are shown as *green* cylinders. A copper-translocation pathway is shown as eight *purple* cylinders that span the membrane. Movement of copper is from the cytoplasm into the lumen. Numerous mutations occur in functionally important regions. The positions of common missense mutations, H1069Q and R778L, are shown. (Model modified from Bull PC, Cox DW. Wilson disease and Menkes disease: new handles on heavy-metal transport. *Trends Genet*. 1994;10:246–252.)

clusterin (apolipoprotein j), and the Niemann-Pick protein C1, in addition to ATOX1. However, with high-throughput testing, the interactome has proved to be more extensive.[21] The gene *COMMD1* (initially called *MURR1*) was identified through the study of inherited hepatic copper toxicosis in Bedlington terriers. Affected dogs show clinical variability that ranges from death or hepatic disease at 2–3 years of age to less severe chronic disease to simply a high hepatic copper level. The proposed defective canine gene was identified by positional cloning; the gene has a deletion of one exon in some,[22] but not all, affected dogs. Although the genetic mechanism for Bedlington terrier copper toxicosis may be more complicated than simply COMMD1 dysfunction, the disease in Bedlington terriers has highlighted other genes that may be involved in response to excess copper. COMMD1 has been found to interact with the amino-terminal end of ATP7B and play an important role in its vesicular trafficking; COMMD1 may also enhance ATP7B proteolysis. Additionally, COMMD1 interacts with the X-linked inhibitor of apoptosis, which can also bind copper.[23]

PATHOLOGY

In the earliest stages, before cirrhosis develops, histological findings in the liver include steatosis, focal necrosis, glycogenated nuclei in hepatocytes, and sometimes apoptotic bodies. As parenchymal damage progresses, possibly through repeated episodes of lobular necrosis, periportal fibrosis develops. Cirrhosis is usually macronodular.

Early in the course of WD, hepatocellular copper is bound mainly to metallothionein and is distributed diffusely in the cytoplasm of hepatocytes; therefore histochemical stains for copper are negative. As the disease progresses, the copper content exceeds the storage capacity of metallothionein, and copper is deposited in lysosomes. Lysosomal aggregates of copper can be detected by special staining techniques for copper or copper-binding protein (e.g., rubeanic acid and orcein, respectively). In the cirrhotic liver, some areas may have no stainable copper at all. If the clinical presentation mimics autoimmune hepatitis (see later), a liver biopsy specimen may reveal classic histologic features such as interface hepatitis. Inflammation may be severe. Mallory-Denk bodies may be found. In patients who present with classic acute liver failure due to WD (ALF-WD: see later), histologic findings confirm preexisting liver disease, often cirrhosis, and parenchymal copper is located mainly in Kupffer cells rather than hepatocytes.

Changes in hepatocellular mitochondria, identified with electron microscopy, are an important feature in WD.[24] The mitochondria vary in size, and the numbers of dense bodies in mitochondria may be increased. The most striking change is dilatation of the tips of the mitochondrial cristae resulting from separation of the inner and outer membranes of the cristae, with widening of the intercristal space until the appearance is irregularly cystic. The crista resembles a tennis racquet if only the tip is dilated. This finding, although not entirely specific for WD, can be helpful diagnostically, notably in young and minimally affected patients.[25] Involvement of hepatocytes may not be uniform, and abnormalities may be found in some hepatocytes in some lobules and not in others. The mitochondrial changes are probably a consequence of oxidative damage from excessive copper in hepatocytes.[26] Indeed, mitochondrial damage due to copper accumulation appears to be an early and critical component of the disease mechanism in WD.[27]

CLINICAL FEATURES

The clinical presentation of WD is highly variable. The disease can present clinically at any age: in toddlers and in patients older than 60. Age is no longer a criterion for diagnosis. Nevertheless, most patients present between 3 and 55 years old. The clinical presentation may be as chronic or acute (sometimes rapidly progressive) liver disease, a progressive neurological disorder without clinically prominent hepatic dysfunction, isolated acute hemolysis, or psychiatric illness. The clinical variability makes confirmation of the diagnosis difficult.[28–30] An emerging problem is the management of asymptomatic individuals with WD identified by molecular screening, particularly if they have no evidence of organ damage.

Hepatic Presentation

The hepatic presentation of WD is more common in younger patients than in older patients. WD should be considered a possible diagnosis in any child, symptomatic or not, with hepatomegaly, persistently elevated serum aminotransferase levels, or evidence of fatty liver. Symptoms may be vague and nonspecific, such as fatigue, anorexia, or abdominal pain. Occasional patients present with a self-limited clinical illness that resembles acute hepatitis, with malaise, anorexia, nausea, jaundice, elevated serum aminotransferase levels, and abnormal coagulation test results (acute liver injury). Some patients have a history of episodic self-limited jaundice, likely caused by hemolysis due to direct toxicity of copper to the erythrocyte membrane. Patients may present with decompensated chronic liver disease with hepatosplenomegaly, ascites, a low serum albumin level, and persistently abnormal coagulation test results. Rare patients have isolated splenomegaly without hepatomegaly. Many of these findings reflect portal hypertension due to WD, not the metabolic dysfunction itself.

WD may present in children and young adults with clinical liver disease indistinguishable from autoimmune hepatitis (see Chapter 92).[31] As in autoimmune hepatitis, the onset may be acute. Fatigue, malaise, arthropathy, and rashes may occur; laboratory findings include elevated aminotransferase levels, a greatly increased serum immunoglobulin (Ig)G concentration, and detectable nonspecific autoantibodies, such as ANA and smooth muscle (antiactin) antibodies. In patients with apparent autoimmune hepatitis, WD must be specifically ruled out. Treatment of WD differs from that of autoimmune hepatitis. With appropriate treatment, the long-term outlook for patients with WD that resembles autoimmune hepatitis appears to be favorable, even if cirrhosis is present.

WD may present as ALF, with severe coagulopathy and encephalopathy (ALF-WD; see Chapter 97). In some patients, encephalopathy is not initially present but develops within a few days of clinical presentation. Frequently, the ALF has a classic clinical picture, reflecting the role of copper excess in the disease mechanism. In classic ALF-WD, acute, often severe, Coombs-negative intravascular hemolysis is present, and renal failure may develop. In contrast to ALF of other etiologies, ALF-WD typically features disproportionately low aminotransferase levels (usually much less than 1500 U/L) at the onset of clinically apparent disease. The serum alkaline phosphatase level is in the normal range or even low for the patient's age, and the serum bilirubin level is often extremely elevated as a result of hemolysis.

In adults who present with ALF-WD, a calculation based on simple biochemical tests (in "American" units) can be helpful in making the diagnosis, specifically the combination of a ratio of the alkaline phosphatase to the total bilirubin level of less than 4 and a ratio of AST to ALT level of greater than 2.2.[32] The serum ceruloplasmin level is not diagnostically informative in this situation (see later). Slit-lamp examination may reveal Kayser-Fleischer rings. Urinary copper excretion is greatly elevated. These patients require urgent LT because they do not respond well to chelation treatment; albumin dialysis and related apheresis techniques may serve as temporizing procedures until LT can be performed (see later and Chapters 97 and 99).[33–36] This presentation of WD is not rare; affected patients account for approximately 3% of persons transplanted for ALF (see Chapters 97 and 99).

Some patients with WD have fatty liver—simple steatosis or histologic features suggestive of MASH (formerly NASH) (see Chapter 89). Differentiation of WD from the highly prevalent MASLD (formerly NAFLD) is critical but can be problematic. The simplest diagnostic approach is to measure basal 24-hour urinary copper excretion; it is low in MASLD, whereas the majority of patients with WD have a level >40 μg/24 hours (see later).[37,38] These clinical findings are supported by the observation that hepatic copper concentrations are decreased in a mouse model of MASLD.[39]

Recurrent bouts of hemolysis may predispose to the development of gallstones. Cirrhosis, if present, may be a further predisposing factor. Children with unexplained cholelithiasis, particularly bilirubinate stones, should be tested for WD. Occurrence of hepatic neoplasia in WD is controversial. Compared with other chronic liver diseases, WD is infrequently complicated by HCC or cholangiocarcinoma.[40–42] Yet HCC complicating WD has been reported in the pediatric age bracket.[43] Routine screening for HCC in cirrhotic WD patients is mandated, and it may be appropriate for those with regressed cirrhosis.

In patients who have predominantly hepatic disease, evidence of subtle neuropsychiatric involvement can often be found. Clumsiness or cramped, illegible handwriting may be identified by careful direct questioning. A soft whispery voice (hypophonia) is another early feature of neurological involvement. Mood disturbance (mainly depression, but sometimes impulsive behavior or anxiety disorders) or deterioration in school performance may be evident.

Neurological Presentation

The neurological presentation of WD tends to occur in the second and third decades or later but has been reported in children as young as 6–10 years of age. Most patients with a neurological presentation have hepatic involvement, albeit often asymptomatic. Neurological involvement follows two main patterns: a movement disorder or dystonia. A movement disorder tends to occur earlier and includes tremors, poor coordination, and loss of fine motor control. Dystonic disorders generally develop later, with mask-like facies, rigidity, and gait disturbance. Pseudobulbar involvement manifests as dysarthria, drooling, and difficulty swallowing. Dysarthria is overall the most common neurological presentation. Rarely, patients present with peripheral neuropathy or dysautonomia.[44] Seizures are uncommon but may occur, and intellect is not impaired. Recently, restless leg syndrome has been found to occur with WD.[45] Likewise, sleep disorders may be frequent in WD.[46,47]

Imaging of the brain is important for assessing neurologic WD, and results may be abnormal in the absence of overt neurological symptoms. Magnetic resonance imaging is the preferred modality.[48,49] Clinical rating scales (Unified Wilson's Disease Rating Scale and Global Assessment Scale for Wilson's Disease) have been developed at two different centers: they have differing areas of emphasis but are valuable for systematic assessment.[50]

Psychiatric Presentation

As many as 20% of patients may present with purely psychiatric symptoms.[51–53] These symptoms are highly variable, although depression is common. Phobias and compulsive behaviors have been reported; aggressive or antisocial behavior may also be found. Delay in diagnosis is an important issue with psychiatric WD because such delays average 2–3 years.[51]

Although WD is not typically associated with major cognitive deficits or dementia, subtle cognitive disorders may be present. These include problems in executive functioning, abstract thinking, working memory, impulse control, and maintaining attention.[54–56] In asymptomatic patients with WD, formal testing may be required to identify these problems. Correlates to MRI findings have recently been described.[57]

Ocular Signs

The Kayser-Fleischer ring is caused by copper deposition in Descemet's membrane of the cornea. Copper is actually distributed throughout the cornea, but fluid streaming favors accumulation near the limbus, especially at the superior and inferior poles, and eventually circumferentially around the iris. Kayser-Fleischer rings are visible on direct inspection only when iris pigmentation is light and copper deposition is heavy. In general, a careful slit-lamp examination is mandatory. Anterior segment optical coherence tomography is a new alternative test for identifying Kayser-Fleischer rings and characterizing them quantitatively.[58,59] Copper deposition in the lens (sunflower cataract), which does not interfere with vision, may be seen on slit-lamp examination and, like Kayser-Fleischer rings, disappears with chelation therapy. Kayser-Fleischer rings may be absent in 40%–60% of patients with exclusively hepatic involvement and in asymptomatic patients. Most patients with a neurological or psychiatric presentation of WD have Kayser-Fleischer rings; only 5% do not. Kayser-Fleischer rings are not specific for WD; they may be found occasionally in patients with other types of chronic liver disease, usually with a prominent cholestatic component, such as PBC, PSC, or familial cholestatic syndromes. In rare persons with Kayser-Fleischer rings found incidentally, WD should be excluded.

Involvement of Other Systems

WD can be accompanied by various extrahepatic disorders apart from neurological disease. Self-limited episodes of Coombs-negative hemolytic anemia can result from the sudden release of copper into the blood. Renal disease, mainly Fanconi syndrome, may be prominent. Findings include microscopic hematuria, aminoaciduria, phosphaturia, and defective acidification of the urine. Nephrolithiasis has also been reported. Arthritis, mainly affecting the large joints, may be due to synovial copper accumulation. Other musculoskeletal problems include osteoporosis and osteochondritis dissecans. A so-called osseomuscular presentation has been reported mainly in India. Vitamin D–resistant rickets may develop as a result of the renal damage. Copper deposition in skeletal muscle can cause rhabdomyolysis. Copper deposition in the heart can lead to cardiomyopathy or cardiac arrhythmias, including atrial fibrillation.[3,60] Sudden death in WD has been attributed to cardiac involvement. Endocrine disorders can occur. Hypoparathyroidism has been attributed to copper deposition. Amenorrhea and testicular problems appear to result from WD itself, not from cirrhosis. Infertility or repeated spontaneous abortion may signal WD. Pancreatitis, possibly resulting from copper deposition in the pancreas, may also occur.

DIAGNOSIS

The patient with chronic liver disease, tremor or dystonia, and Kayser-Fleischer rings is readily diagnosed on clinical grounds, but such patients are uncommon. A diagnostic scoring system (Leipzig score system)[61] has had limited validation[62,63]; however, it provides guidance as to diagnostic strategy and is valuable for clinical research. Suggestive clinical symptoms are often the main prerequisite for diagnosing WD, and laboratory investigations may provide confirmation. Kayser-Fleischer rings should be sought through a careful slit-lamp examination, repeated if necessary. Lack of Kayser-Fleischer rings does not exclude the diagnosis of WD. Serum aminotransferase levels are usually mildly to moderately elevated. Serum levels of AST may be much higher than those of ALT, possibly reflecting damage to hepatocyte mitochondria.

Tests

A summary of biochemical features in WD in comparison with normal persons is shown in Table 78.1. The classic feature of a low ceruloplasmin concentration has proved less typical than previously thought. Hepatic inflammation may be sufficient to elevate serum ceruloplasmin levels. Also, the normal range for serum ceruloplasmin is increased in very young children. However, the method of measuring ceruloplasmin is likely the most important reason for finding normal ceruloplasmin levels in patients with WD. Immunological methods, which are used in most laboratories, measure both apoceruloplasmin and holoceruloplasmin and typically overestimate the true amount of functional ceruloplasmin in plasma. The oxidase assay, although technically less convenient for laboratories that perform automated testing, provides a more reliable measure of ceruloplasmin for diagnosis because the assay measures enzymatically active, copper-containing ceruloplasmin.[64] This method can also indicate possible early copper deficiency in treated patients.[65]

Serum ceruloplasmin measurement by itself is not an adequate diagnostic test for WD. Some patients with WD have a normal serum ceruloplasmin, in part because it is an acute phase reactant. A low serum level of ceruloplasmin is not unique to WD. Synthesis of ceruloplasmin may be reduced in other types of chronic liver disease and with malnutrition; ceruloplasmin may be lost with intestinal malabsorption or nephrotic syndrome. Furthermore, a subnormal ceruloplasmin concentration is found in at least 10% of heterozygotes for WD. An impressively low ceruloplasmin concentration (<10 mg/dL) strongly suggests WD; it can also point to a mimic disorder (see below). Complete absence of ceruloplasmin is found in hereditary aceruloplasminemia, a rare autosomal recessive condition that is associated with neurological,

TABLE 78.1 Biochemical Parameters in Normal Adults and in Patients with Wilson Disease

	Normal Adults	Wilson Disease[a]
Serum ceruloplasmin (mg/dL) (mg/L)	20–35 200–350	~0–20 ~0–200
Serum copper (μg/dL) (μmol/L)	7–15 11–24	19–64 3–10
Basal 24-hour urinary copper (μg/day) (μmol/day)	≤40 ≤0.6	>40–10,000 >0.6
Liver copper (μg/g dry weight)	20–50	>250 (possibly >70)

[a]For all the assays, results in homozygotes and heterozygotes may overlap.

retinal, and pancreatic degeneration caused by iron accumulation in the brain, retina, and pancreas, respectively.[66] Anemia and an elevated plasma ferritin level are observed. Aceruloplasminemia has confirmed the important function of ceruloplasmin as a ferroxidase that oxidizes iron for transport from ferritin to transferrin. Targeted disruption of the ceruloplasmin gene in a mouse model has confirmed the critical role of ceruloplasmin in transporting iron out of cells.[67] Rarely, patients with WD who undergo rigorous chelation therapy over decades may resemble those with hereditary aceruloplasminemia, if ceruloplasmin oxidase activity is reduced to undetectable levels.[68] The concurrence of WD and genotype-confirmed hereditary hemochromatosis is rare but renders management of both diseases more complex.[69–72]

In patients with WD, the serum copper concentration is low, in parallel with the low serum ceruloplasmin level. A limited amount of copper is not bound within ceruloplasmin and is bioavailable. The nonceruloplasmin-bound copper concentration can be estimated. The usefulness of this calculation, which is highly dependent on the accuracy of the serum copper and ceruloplasmin measurements, is extremely limited[73]; it was not intended as a diagnostic criterion and has little value for assessing treatment efficacy. Methods are being developed to measure nonceruloplasmin-bound copper concentration directly.[74–76] A method for measuring exchangeable copper in the plasma compartment has been developed: exchangeable copper, expressed as the percentage of total serum copper (relative exchangeable copper), may provide accurate diagnostic information.[77,78] The method for measuring exchangeable copper itself may require further refinement. Importantly, despite the linguistic convention, what is measured is not actually "free" copper. Copper in the plasma compartment is always loosely bound to albumin or various amino acids. Conceptually, the point is that some copper is bioavailable. Calling it "exchangeable" copper has merits.

Serum uric acid and phosphate concentrations may be low in patients with untreated WD, reflecting renal tubular dysfunction. Urinalysis may show microscopic hematuria; if possible, aminoaciduria, phosphaturia, and proteinuria should be quantified.

Measuring basal urinary copper excretion, preferably with three separate 24-hour urine collections, has proved useful for diagnosis.[79] Urinary copper excretion reflects the nonceruloplasmin-bound copper concentration in plasma. The collection must be complete, and the volume and total creatinine excretion should be measured; precautions against contamination with copper in the collection process are essential. The basal 24-hour urinary copper excretion is elevated at least two to three times normal in the vast majority of patients. The conventional diagnostic criterion of greater than 100 μg/day (>1.6 μmol/day), although typical, is not sufficiently sensitive. A patient with a basal 24-hour urinary copper excretion of greater than 40 μg/day (>0.6 μmol/day) requires further investigation for WD.[80] Heterozygotes usually have a normal basal 24-hour urinary copper excretion, although the value may be borderline abnormal in some cases.[81] Although a normal person may excrete as much as 20 times the baseline level of copper after administration of D-penicillamine, a patient with symptomatic WD will excrete considerably more. In the standard provocative test with administration of D-penicillamine, urinary copper excretion of 25 μmol (1600 μg) or more per 24 hours is diagnostic of WD; however, the test lacks sensitivity for diagnosing WD and for identifying asymptomatic affected siblings.[82]

Hepatic tissue copper concentration, which usually is measured by neutron activation analysis or atomic absorption spectrometry, may provide important diagnostic information. A hepatic copper content greater than 250 μg/g dry weight of liver is considered diagnostic of WD in the appropriate clinical context. Based on a large series of genetically diagnosed patients, a value of greater than 70 μg/g dry weight was proposed as a better diagnostic threshold, although some specificity is lost.[37] In an adequate sample, hepatic parenchymal concentrations of less than 50 μg/g dry weight constitute strong evidence against a diagnosis of WD in most patients. Liver biopsy samples must be collected without extraneous copper contamination, but in general, ordinary disposable liver biopsy needles can be used. Importantly, the sample submitted must be large enough—at least 1–2 cm in length. In the early stages of WD, when copper is distributed diffusely in the liver cell cytoplasm, this measurement may clearly indicate hepatic copper overload. In later stages of hepatic WD, the measurement of hepatic copper is less reliable because copper is distributed unequally in the liver (see earlier). Moreover, liver biopsy may not be safe in such patients because of coagulopathy or ascites; a transjugular biopsy may be performed, or hepatic copper measurement may be omitted. Some heterozygotes have minor elevations of liver tissue copper. An elevated hepatic copper concentration is not specific for WD; patients with chronic cholestasis or Indian childhood cirrhosis may also have elevated hepatic copper levels.

Mimic Disorders

WD may mimic autoimmune hepatitis and MASLD clinically: it is on the differential diagnosis for these more common disorders. Likewise, various genetic disorders may mimic WD. Specifically, patients with multidrug resistance protein 3 (MDR3) deficiency (PFIC3) may be misdiagnosed as having WD because of severe hepatic copper retention (see Chapter 64)[83–86]; they may fulfill Leipzig score criteria. Congenital disorders of glycosylation (CDGs) may mimic WD by presenting as hepatic disease with low serum ceruloplasmin; however, basal 24-hour urinary copper excretion is typically not increased.[87–91] Genetic disorders of manganese disposition can resemble WD clinically.[92] MEDNIK syndrome has a closely related disease mechanism, but it is quite different clinically.[93]

Approach to Diagnosis

In view of the numerous available diagnostic tests, a methodical approach is required. The classic patient with WD, whether displaying hepatic or neurological findings, may be visualized as someone between 6 and 40 years of age with a serum ceruloplasmin level less than 5 mg/dL (<50 mg/L) and definite Kayser-Fleischer rings. Many patients are not classic. Age is no longer a meaningful diagnostic criterion. In the presence of chronic liver disease (indicated by hepatomegaly or biochemical abnormalities) or typical neurological symptoms, the combination of a low serum ceruloplasmin level (<140 mg/L)[94] and elevated basal 24-hour urinary copper excretion (>40 μg/day) is highly suggestive of WD. Typical ocular findings complete the clinical diagnosis but are not essential. A percutaneous liver biopsy is useful for assessing the severity of liver damage and measuring parenchymal copper concentration, which is regarded by some to be the *sine qua non* for the diagnosis of WD. This procedure, however, may have to be delayed in patients with severe liver dysfunction. Other clinical entities in the differential diagnosis must be appropriately excluded. Ultimately, molecular genetic analysis is the only convincing and reliable diagnostic procedure.

Mutation Analysis

More than 600 pathogenic variants in *ATP7B* have been detected in many different populations since the original mutations were described. Many of these mutations were recorded in the WD Mutation Database.[95] At the present time, various databases, including ClinVar and gnomAD, are available in the public domain. There are several proprietary databases. The usual approach to detection of a mutation is high-throughput sequencing of either selected or all exons of the gene, supplemented by sequencing of the promoter region, close examination of exon/intron boundaries, and exclusion of large deletions by multiplex ligation-dependent probe amplification technology. Although identification of a mutation is technically straightforward, care must be taken that the change detected actually causes disease and is not a rare normal variant, particularly for single amino acid missense mutations. Because of the similarity between yeast and mammalian copper transport systems, yeast and cell assay systems have been developed for the functional assessment of variants.[96–98] Alternatively, structural changes in the Wilson ATPase (ATP7B) due to a gene alteration can be assessed in silico. Of the various algorithms available for this purpose, the SIFT (*s*orting *i*ntolerant *f*rom *t*olerant) score (which predicts whether an amino acid substitution affects function) works best for *ATP7B* and its gene product.[99] Most patients with WD are compound heterozygotes, having a different *ATP7B* disease-causing mutation on each allele. The identification of one mutation may be adequate to confirm the diagnosis, if characteristic clinical symptoms and biochemical features are present and if the one mutation detected is clearly established as a disease-causing mutation. Complete genetic characterization is greatly preferred. With current analytical techniques, two mutations can be found in more than 95% of affected patients.

The majority of mutations in *ATP7B* identified to date are missense mutations. Small deletions, insertions, nonsense, and splice-site mutations occur throughout the gene. Large gene deletions, which are found in about 20% of patients with Menkes disease, occur rarely in persons with WD, and the mutation spectrum for *ATP7A* in Menkes disease is different from that for *ATP7B*.[97] Various ethnic groups have different specific mutations. The histidine1069glutamine (H1069Q) mutation is present, at least in the heterozygous state, in 35%–75% of Europeans with WD.[100] Exon 8 of the *ATP7B* gene is particularly rich in mutations in European populations. The mutation arginine778leucine (R778L) is common in Chinese populations. Mutation detection is more challenging in Japanese and Mediterranean populations, in whom no mutation is present in high frequency. In populations with ethnic homogeneity or in which a limited spectrum of mutations is established, testing strategies can identify the mutations in most patients. A prominent example is Sardinia, where the disease frequency is 1 in 7000 live births[101] and a mutation in the 5′-untranslated region predominates. In populations with a limited number of mutations, use of a customized *ATP7B* microarray[102,103] might be cost-effective. Targeted next-generation sequencing approaches are in development.[104]

Genetic diagnosis is important for identifying simple heterozygotes. Someone who is clinically normal with only mild biochemical signs of copper mishandling could be a simple heterozygote, carrying only one mutated allele. Such heterozygotes have not been known to develop clinical disease or require treatment. Individuals with a late age of onset pose a similar challenge. Current data consistent with incomplete penetrance of *ATP7B* mutations suggest that it is entirely possible that these are atypical presentations of WD. Correct genetic diagnosis is thus critical. Likewise, genetic analysis revealing normal *ATP7B* genotype and a disease-causing genotype for *ABCB4* (MDR3 deficiency), *CP* (aceruloplasminemia), any of the CDG-associated genes, or genes encoding manganese transporters is the most efficient way to sort out these diagnoses.

No granular genotype-phenotype correlations exist in WD. Nevertheless, there may be some high-level genotype-phenotype correlations. *ATP7B* mutations resulting in absent or totally nonfunctional Wilson ATPase/ATP7B are associated with severe, usually hepatic, disease.[105,106] (This is also evident in the comparison of the $Atp^{-/-}$ mouse and the tx-j Jackson toxic milk mouse.) Gene deletions, duplications, nonsense mutations, and splice-site mutations may prevent the formation of the gene product almost completely and thus produce a severe defect. Such truncating mutations have been associated with absent holo-ceruloplasmin production and the early onset of clinical disease[107] or with ALF-WD.[108] The common H1069Q mutation might be associated with neurological disease and young-adult onset[109]; however, this mutation has been reported in homozygotes as young as 9 years of age with hepatic disease. The positions of this and R778L (see earlier) are shown in Fig. 78.3. Many mutations occur in exons 5–10 and exons 13–20,[105,110] which encode metal-binding domain 6, transmembrane segments, and the ATP loop.

With the opportunity of confirming a diagnosis of WD by direct identification of mutations, the spectrum of manifestations of WD has been found to be even wider than previously recognized. No individual biochemical test is reliable for the identification of patients. In some cases, even all combinations of tests prove inadequate for a diagnosis. Characterization of *ATP7B* can be valuable for such patients. Mutation analysis should also be carried out to distinguish asymptomatic patients from heterozygotes, notably in the context of living-donor LT.

Diagnosis of First-Degree Relatives

If *ATP7B* mutations have been identified in a patient, mutational analysis is easily carried out in first-degree relatives (siblings, parents, and offspring) by direct testing for the mutations found in the patient. If mutations have not been identified, accurate diagnosis can be achieved using markers flanking the gene. The most useful genetic markers are stretches of dinucleotides or trinucleotides that show extensive variability in the normal population, so that parents within any one family will carry different alleles of these markers. This variability allows the tracking of the disease gene as it segregates within families, as shown in Fig. 78.4. It is important that informative markers flank the gene, because an erroneous diagnosis could result if markers on only one side of the gene are informative and a recombination event has occurred close to the gene. The combination of markers, or haplotype, reliably indicates the genetic status within the family. According to haplotype analysis or genotypic diagnosis, an occasional person thought likely to be an asymptomatic patient, based on biochemical testing, has been shown to be a simple heterozygote. Therefore confirmation of the genotype is highly recommended before treatment is initiated. Conversely, if the clinical diagnosis of a simple heterozygote is uncertain, genetic diagnosis can be highly informative.

In the absence of genetic analysis, screening should include physical examination, liver biochemical tests, serum copper and ceruloplasmin measurements, a basal 24-hour urinary copper determination, and a careful slit-lamp examination. Children 6 years of age or younger who appear to be unaffected should be rechecked at yearly intervals over the next 5–10 years. Genetic screening with the use of flanking markers (i.e., haplotype analysis) or by direct mutation analysis, however, is the most reliable way to identify an affected first-degree relative when the patient's DNA is available for mutation analysis. For deceased patients, tissue from autopsy or biopsy material can be used.

TREATMENT

Three treatments for WD are generally recognized: D-penicillamine, trientine, and zinc salts (Table 78.2).[111] Chelation with tetrathiomolybdate remains experimental and apparently not close to clinical application (see later). With effective lifelong chelation treatment, most patients live normal, healthy lives. Starting treatment early is critical, and the outcome is best for patients in whom the disease is diagnosed and treatment begun when the patient is asymptomatic. Whether routine institution of chelation or zinc therapy in infancy (<2 years of age) is advantageous

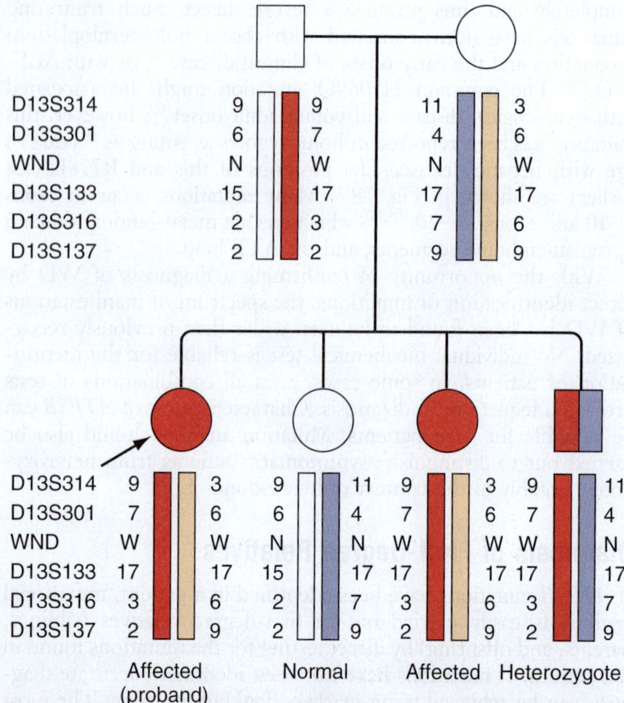

Fig. 78.4 Diagnostic use of polymorphic DNA microsatellite markers for siblings of a confirmed patient with Wilson disease. DNA markers are listed on the left in centromeric to telomeric order. Three markers are usually adequate for an unambiguous result: D13S314, D13S301, and D13S316. Numbers represent alleles of each marker listed. The proband (*arrow*) and asymptomatic sibling confirmed as affected are shown as *filled circles*. WND, original (preliminary) designation for ATP7B.

remains unknown.[112] A cautious approach seems best, given the requirement for copper in early neurological development. The potential role for gene transfer therapy is uncertain; however, success with the adeno-associated vector serotype 8 in the Atp7b$^{-/-}$ mouse has been reported.[113] Dietary treatment alone is ineffective, but patients should eliminate copper-rich foods from the diet. These foods include organ meats, shellfish, nuts, dark chocolate, and mushrooms. Certain foods warrant caution: soy- and nut-based milks, meat-free "veggie burgers." Vegetarians require specific dietary counseling. If the concentration of copper in the patient's drinking water is believed to be high, the water should be analyzed. A copper-removing device may be installed in the plumbing system.

D-Penicillamine, introduced in 1956 by J. M. Walshe, is effective in most patients with WD. Penicillamine, which is the sulfhydryl-containing amino acid cysteine substituted with 2 methyl groups, greatly increases urinary excretion of copper; only the D-penicillamine form is used clinically. Studies in the LEC rat model indicate that D-penicillamine inhibits the accumulation of copper in hepatocellular lysosomes and solubilizes copper for mobilization from these particles, but not from cytoplasmic metallothioneins.[114] In addition to its chelating action, D-penicillamine inhibits collagen cross-linking and has some immunosuppressive properties. The neurological status of patients with mainly neurological symptoms may worsen initially after treatment with D-penicillamine is started[115]; most, but not all, recover with cautious continued use of D-penicillamine. Substituting trientine or zinc reduces this risk of a poor outcome. All these drugs entail some possibility of neurological deterioration. Starting with a low dose of D-penicillamine and increasing the dose slowly over 2–4 weeks is advisable to avoid this adverse effect. A febrile reaction with rash and proteinuria develops in some patients within 7–10 days of beginning treatment. Although D-penicillamine can be restarted slowly along with glucocorticoids, changing to an alternative chelator is preferred.

TABLE 78.2 Recommendations for the Treatment of Wilson Disease

Drug	Dose[a]	Tests for Monitoring Efficacy	Tests for Monitoring Side Effects
D-Penicillamine (+ pyridoxine 25 mg daily)	Initial: 1–1.5 g/day (adults) or 20 mg/kg/day (children) divided into two or three doses	24-hour urinary copper: 200–500 µg (3–8 µmol)/day as target	CBC, urinalysis, and skin examination
	"Start low and go slow"[b]		
	Maintenance: 0.75–1 g/day as needed to maintain cupruresis	24-hour urinary copper: 200–500 µg (3–8 µmol)/day as target	
Trientine[c]	Initial: 1–1.5 g/day divided into two or three doses[d]	24-hour urinary copper: 150–500 µg (2.4–8 µmol)/day as target	CBC and iron studies
	"Start low and go slow"[b]		
	Maintenance: 0.75–1.2 g/day divided into two or three doses	24-hour urinary copper: 150–500 µg (2.4–8 µmol)/day as target	
Zinc	Initial: 50 mg elemental zinc three times daily (adults)[e]	24-hour urinary copper: <100 µg (1.6 µmol)/day as target	Serum zinc level Serum AST and ALT levels
	Maintenance: titrate the dose based on efficacy monitoring data[f]	24-hour urinary copper: <100 µg (1.6 µmol)/day as target	

[a]All medications should be taken 1 hour before or 2 hours after mealtime, if possible, but the timing of the dose may have to be adjusted to enhance consistent adherence to treatment.

[b]"Start low and go slow" means, for D-penicillamine, starting with 250 mg daily for 3–4 days and then increasing by 250-mg increments every 3–4 days until the desired initial dose is reached. For trientine dihydrochloride, the starting dose is 250 mg or 300 mg, depending on formulation, and the increase is by 250-mg or 300-mg increments every 3–4 days to desired full dose.

[c]Requires refrigeration.

[d]The dose of trientine in children is not established (approximately 20 mg/kg/day in divided doses).

[e]The dose of zinc in children is not established. Typical dosing is 25 mg of elemental zinc three times daily until adult stature (≈50 kg body weight) is achieved, when the adult dose of 50 mg of elemental zinc three times daily is used. The dose is not well defined for children younger than 5 years, but 25 mg elemental zinc twice daily has been proposed. The dose in children can also be titrated to achieve optimal 24-hour urinary copper excretion.

[f]The 24-hour urinary copper excretion reflects total body copper load and thus can be used to monitor zinc treatment even though zinc does not cause cupruresis.

D-Penicillamine, although highly effective, can cause serious side effects. Adverse reactions involving the skin include various types of rashes, pemphigus, and elastosis perforans serpiginosa. Hypothyroidism has been reported. Other side effects vary from minor (loss of taste, GI upset, arthralgias) to severe (proteinuria, leukopenia, thrombocytopenia). Aplastic anemia occurs rarely and does not always reverse when D-penicillamine is stopped. Nephrotic syndrome, Goodpasture syndrome, a myasthenia syndrome, and a systemic disease that resembles SLE have all been reported. These severe adverse effects require immediate discontinuation of D-penicillamine and use of a different chelator. Whether lifelong treatment with D-penicillamine is free of adverse consequences is not entirely clear. Patients who have taken D-penicillamine for 30–40 years may have chronic skin changes with loss of elastic tissue. Whether the antifibrotic effect weakens other connective tissues is not known. Theoretically, chronic depletion of other trace metals may occur. In view of these adverse effects, maintenance therapy with D-penicillamine should be at the lowest effective dose.

Trientine, or triethylenetetramine dihydrochloride, is the usual second-line treatment for patients who are intolerant of D-penicillamine. Trientine differs chemically from D-penicillamine in lacking sulfhydryl groups. Copper is chelated by forming a stable complex with the four constituent nitrogens in a planar ring. Trientine increases urinary copper excretion and may interfere with intestinal absorption of copper. Trientine is a less potent chelator than D-penicillamine, but the difference is not clinically important. Trientine produces little significant toxicity in patients with WD. It occasionally causes gastritis, and it may induce iron deficiency, apparently by chelating dietary iron. Bone marrow suppression is rare. Adverse effects of D-penicillamine resolve and do not recur during treatment with trientine.[116] Neurological deterioration after treatment with trientine has been reported. Trientine is highly effective, even in patients with advanced liver fibrosis or as initial treatment in children.[81,117] Recently, a tetrahydrochloride formulation of trientine has been approved after completion of a randomized controlled clinical trial.[118] It is stable at ambient temperatures. The details of converting from trientine dihydrochloride to tetrahydrochloride require further clarification.

Oral zinc, used in Europe since the 1970s,[119] has been investigated extensively as a treatment modality in North America. Its mechanism of action differs from that of the chelators. In pharmacologic doses, zinc interferes with the absorption of copper from the GI tract and increases the excretion of copper in the stool. The postulated mechanism of action is through the induction of metallothionein in enterocytes. The metallothionein has a greater affinity for copper than for zinc and preferentially binds copper from the intestinal contents. Once bound, the copper is not absorbed but is lost in the feces as enterocytes are shed during normal turnover. Zinc may interfere with lipid peroxidation and enhance the availability of glutathione. It may reverse copper-induced downregulation of nuclear receptor farnesoid X receptor and RXR function.[120]

Problems with zinc therapy include gastritis, which is a common side effect, and uncertainty about dosing. Using a zinc salt other than zinc sulfate may minimize gastritis; most zinc salts are equally acceptable for the treatment of WD. Food interferes with the effectiveness of zinc and some investigators recommend that no food be eaten for 1 hour before or 2 hours after a dose of zinc is taken. This dosing regimen tends to increase the severity of gastritis and may be sufficiently inconvenient to compromise adherence, as in adolescents. An alternative approach is to be less rigorous about avoiding zinc at mealtimes and to titrate the dose according to the urinary copper excretion as a measure of effectiveness. Treatment with zinc appears to have few other side effects.[121] Rare patients experience an immediate deterioration in hepatic WD when started on zinc. Long-term studies suggest that zinc is more effective in neurologic WD than in hepatic WD.[115,122] Zinc can serve as primary therapy for WD, but its preferred role is as maintenance therapy.

Long-term treatment requires regular, sometimes close, follow-up. Laboratory tests include a CBC, measures of renal function including urinalysis, and liver biochemical tests. The adequacy of treatment is assessed by measurement of 24-hour urinary copper excretion, which should be high with either oral chelator (D-penicillamine: 200–500 μg/day or 3–8 μmol/day; trientine: 150–500 μg/day or 2.4–8 μmol/day) and low with zinc (20–100 μg/day or 0.32–1.6 μmol/day). Disproportionately low or undetectable copper in a 24-hour urine collection suggests overtreatment. The patient must be asked specifically about general well-being and adherence to the drug regimen. With zinc treatment, adherence can be checked by measurement of 24-hour urinary zinc excretion (>2 mg/day) or serum zinc (>12.5 μg/dL). Elevated serum aminotransferase levels that were previously normal may signal nonadherence and evidence of ongoing hepatic damage. Patients diagnosed while still asymptomatic may be at greater than average risk for lapsing into nonadherence. Nonadherence has a differential diagnosis: intercurrent hepatic disorders such as acute viral hepatitis, intrinsic ineffectiveness of the pharmacologic therapy for an individual patient, or increased intake of copper may produce a similar clinical picture.

For patients who present with decompensated chronic liver disease, combining zinc with a conventional chelator (preferably trientine) has become a popular treatment strategy, despite the absence of extensive validation. The two types of treatments must be temporally dispersed through the day, with at least 4–5 hours between administration of the two drugs, or else they may neutralize each other's effect. This intensive short-term induction regimen is best suited to patients with severe hepatic or neurological disease[123] and remains semi-investigational. Some patients with severe hepatic WD fail on this regimen and require urgent LT; therefore arrangements for LT should be in place.

Ammonium tetrathiomolybdate was investigated as treatment for severe neurologic WD because, unlike D-penicillamine, it is not associated with early neurological deterioration.[124] Tetrathiomolybdate interferes with the absorption of copper from the intestine and also binds to plasma copper with high affinity. In LEC rats, tetrathiomolybdate, unlike D-penicillamine, was found to remove copper from metallothionein at low doses.[125] In the plasma compartment, tetrathiomolybdate forms a highly stable tripartite complex with albumin, effectively trapping the copper.[126] It appears that the copper is excreted via biliary excretion of these complexes. The problem with ammonium tetrathiomolybdate was insufficient chemical stability. A new formulation, bis-choline tetrathiomolybdate, has excellent stability and is pharmacologically equivalent to ammonium tetrathiomolybdate, as shown in the Atp7b$^{-/-}$ mouse.[127] Phase 2 clinical testing suggested that it was effective in WD.[128] Although tetrathiomolybdate is regarded as nontoxic, bone marrow suppression and hepatotoxicity are noteworthy adverse effects. Its role in treating hepatic WD is not established. Addressing such issues is "on hold" since clinical trials have been stopped.

Other potential treatments for WD are on the horizon. One is a peptide produced by *Methylosinus trichosporium*; this methanobactin has high affinity for copper and has been shown to reverse ALF in the LPP rat.[129,130] A different approach involves inhibiting specific mitogen-activated protein kinase pathways in hepatocytes to rescue certain mutant Wilson ATPases (e.g., H1069Q and R778L) that are misfolded and caught in the endoplasmic reticulum.[21] Another innovative therapy involves enhancing liver X receptor action in hepatocytes.[20]

Antioxidants may help prevent tissue damage. Studies in copper-loaded animals and in patients with WD indicate that copper enhances free radical production in tissues and may thereby cause liver damage.[131] Based on anecdotal data, the antioxidant α-tocopherol may be beneficial adjunctive treatment for patients with hepatic decompensation.

For pregnant patients with WD, treatment must be continued throughout pregnancy. Postpartum hepatic decompensation may occur if treatment is stopped completely during pregnancy. Although many pregnancies during treatment with D-penicillamine have been successful, the drug is officially classified as a teratogen. Occasional reports of severe collagen defects in the offspring of a patient treated with D-penicillamine may be caused in part by copper deficiency as a result of prolonged aggressive treatment, as well as the teratogenic effects of D-penicillamine.[132] The safety of trientine during pregnancy is unknown, apart from favorable anecdotal reports. Judicious reduction of the dose of D-penicillamine or trientine by approximately 25%–50% of the prepregnancy dose is advisable, especially if delivery by cesarean section is anticipated. Treatment with zinc may be less likely to produce adverse effects on the fetus. If the patient is switched from chelator to zinc in anticipation of pregnancy, their clinical stability on zinc should be established before the pregnancy commences.

PROGNOSIS

Patients with clinically evident WD are generally regarded as having a good prognosis if the disease is diagnosed promptly and treated consistently. Anyone, for example, an asymptomatic first-degree relative, who is diagnosed on biochemical or genetic grounds and treated before any clinical sign of organ impairment generally has the best long-term outlook. Patients with early hepatic disease have a generally favorable prognosis provided treatment is consistent and tolerated well. Severe neurological disease may not entirely resolve on treatment.

In addition to early and adroit diagnosis of WD, achieving the best 'treated natural history' in a patient involves maintaining good adherence to the medical regimen and recognizing as early as possible apparent treatment failure. Regular medical follow-up with specific attention to adherence is important. The asymptomatic patient identified by screening may not appreciate the potential seriousness of WD; a patient doing well on long-term treatment may become complacent. Financial problems, drug cost/availability, and societal instability may affect adherence. Clear communication with the patient is essential. A team-based approach may help.[133]

Patients with WD who stop taking chelating treatment (or zinc) have a poor prognosis. New neurological abnormalities, such as dysarthria, may develop. Rapidly progressive hepatic decompensation has been observed and occurs on average within 3 years, and as early as 8 months, after treatment is stopped. The liver damage is usually refractory to reinstitution of chelation therapy. Such patients require LT. Ensuring adherence to the medical regimen thus assumes great importance in clinical management.

The role of LT in WD is limited (see Chapters 97 and 99). ALF in a patient with WD necessitates LT. Accruing clinical reports suggest that some sort of apheresis (e.g., plasma exchange and albumin dialysis) may effectively bridge these patients to transplantation or, rarely, obviate the need for LT.[33,35] Patients with severe liver disease unresponsive to drug therapy may also proceed to LT. The outcome is favorable, with 1-year survival rates of 80%–90% and excellent survival beyond 1 year.[134,135] Severe neurological disease may improve after LT, but published experience is inconclusive[28] and LT cannot be recommended for neurologic WD. Patients with neurological or psychiatric manifestations of WD appear to have poor outcomes after LT and adhere poorly to medical regimens.[136] Thus LT should be reserved for WD patients who present with severe, decompensated liver disease that is unresponsive to therapy or with ALF-WD. It may be required for patients who experience treatment failure and develop end-stage liver disease. Live-donor LT, even when the graft is from a family member who is a simple heterozygote, yields adequately functioning grafts.[137,138] If the donor is a first-degree relative (e.g., brother or sister) of the patient, genotypic analysis of their *ATP7B* gene should be performed to exclude asymptomatic WD.

The quality of life of patients with WD may be compromised by drug toxicity. Anecdotal observations suggest that damage to collagen may accrue over decades in patients who are maintained indefinitely on D-penicillamine, but the risk has not been assessed adequately. Deficiencies in trace metals may develop with the use of any chelator, but whether these deficiencies are clinically important is not yet clear. Abnormal iron metabolism, leading to hepatic iron overload and anemia, can be predicted if serum ceruloplasmin oxidase activity is zero. Attention to cardiovascular health is important. Patients should be encouraged to prioritize a healthy lifestyle. They should avoid alcohol use and maintain a normal body weight.

Full references for this chapter can be found at https://ebooks.health.elsevier.com.

79 Other Inherited Metabolic Disorders of the Liver

James E. Squires, William F. Balistreri

IN THIS CHAPTER

Metabolic liver diseases may manifest as acute, life-threatening illnesses in the neonatal period or as chronic liver disease in adolescence or adulthood, with progression to cirrhosis, liver failure, or HCC. Metabolic diseases remain a relatively minor indication for liver transplantation in adults but an increasingly common indication in children.[1] In a 2020 report from the Scientific Registry of Transplant Recipients, 17.3% of all pediatric liver transplants in the United States were performed because of complications resulting from metabolic disease.[2] Nontransplant treatment options have become increasingly available that may, in certain cases, obviate the need for liver transplantation.[3–5]

CLINICAL FEATURES OF METABOLIC LIVER DISEASE

The diverse presenting features of metabolic liver disease are listed in Box 79.1. Certain metabolic liver diseases in young patients may mimic other illnesses, such as acute infections or intoxications. By contrast, the older patient with metabolic liver disease may present with symptoms and signs of chronic liver disease. Because metabolic diseases can resemble multiple other disorders, a high index of suspicion is required. During evaluation of any infant presenting with cholestasis, the differential should include metabolic liver disease. Any presentation with progressive neuromuscular disease, developmental delay, or regression of developmental milestones also should lead to a consideration of a liver-based metabolic cause. Metabolic liver disease should be an immediate consideration in patients of all ages with elevated serum aminotransferase levels and one or more of the presenting features in Box 79.1.

A detailed history can often suggest the possibility of metabolic liver disease. A family history of consanguinity, multiple miscarriages, or early infant deaths may suggest a metabolic derangement. Close relatives with undiagnosed liver disease, progressive neurologic or muscle disease, or undiagnosed developmental delays should also raise suspicion. Introduction of certain foods may correlate with the onset of symptoms, as in patients with urea cycle defects (UCDs), galactosemia, or fructosemia. A history of specific dietary aversions may be revealing.

Recommended initial screening tests are listed in Box 79.2. Notably, the genetic basis for these disorders, combined with the increasing availability of molecular diagnostic testing through targeted gene panels or genome/exome sequencing, allows genotypic evaluation for many diseases when a metabolic etiology is suspected based on initial phenotypic appearance or clinical suspicion. When assessing more routine laboratory investigations, diagnostic studies should be obtained when the patient is experiencing symptoms, as patients with metabolic liver disease can present with acute and recurrent symptoms, and laboratory abnormalities may normalize between episodes. In enigmatic cases, serum and urine samples should be obtained during the acute illness and saved (frozen) for definitive studies, if possible. A liver biopsy can be valuable. In addition to biopsy specimens for standard histology, a frozen specimen should be saved for biochemical assessment, and a sample should be prepared for electron microscopic study to assess subcellular organelles, which may exhibit characteristic changes in some metabolic disorders.

α_1-ANTITRYPSIN DEFICIENCY

Deficiency of α_1-antitrypsin (α_1-AT) is transmitted in an autosomal recessive fashion and leads to an increased risk of lung and liver disease. This deficiency is one of the most common genetic diseases in the world and the second most common metabolic disease affecting the liver after hereditary hemochromatosis (see Chapter 77).[6]

BOX 79.1 Presenting Features of Metabolic Liver Disease

Symptoms	Coma Developmental delay Growth failure Hyperammonemic symptoms Hypoglycemic symptoms Neurologic or motor skill deterioration Recurrent vomiting Seizures
Signs	Ascites Abdominal distention Cardiac dysfunction Cataracts Dysmorphic features Hepatomegaly Hypotonia Jaundice Short stature Splenomegaly Unusual odors
Other findings	Acidosis ALF Cholestasis Ketosis Rickets

BOX 79.2 Screening Laboratory Studies for Metabolic Liver Disease*

Serum	Ammonia Anion gap calculation Bile acids Coagulation profile Electrolytes Ferritin Fractionated bilirubin GGTP Glucose Lactate† Peripheral blood smear Pyruvate† Uric Acid†
Urine	Bile acids Organic acids Orotic acid Reducing substances

*Specimens of serum and urine during acute episodes should be saved for later studies.

†Obtain if the patient is acidotic or has neurologic symptoms.

Pathophysiology

The prototypical member of the serpin family of protease inhibitors (Pis), α_1-AT, binds with and promotes the degradation of serine proteases in the serum and in tissues. The most important serine protease is pulmonary neutrophil elastase, which is inhibited by α_1-AT through formation of a tight 1:1 α_1-AT-to-elastase complex. Therefore the primary role of α_1-AT is to prevent extracellular matrix degradation by neutrophil elastase in the lungs. The pathogenesis of α_1-AT lung disease reflects a *loss of function* mechanism. In persons with the phenotype PiZZ, serum α_1-AT levels are reduced to <15% of the normal serum concentration of 85–250 mg/dL. Consequently, there is relatively uninhibited neutrophil elastase activity and resulting emphysema. The accumulation of small amounts of abnormal α_1-AT Z polymers in the lungs has also been shown to promote inflammation and contribute to interstitial lung disease.[7,8]

Allelic α_1-AT mutant variants produce Pi gene products that can be distinguished from the normal product by electrophoretic methods; the normal allelic representation is designated PiM. The PiZ variant produces a mutant α_1-AT Z protein that contains a single amino acid replacement of glutamine with a lysine residue due to a mutation at position 342 of the α_1-AT *(SERPINA1)* gene. Homozygosity at the PiZ allele is the most common and classic pathologic form of α_1-AT deficiency and is capable of leading to liver and lung disease. Approximately 125 naturally occurring variants of α_1-AT have been described. Although most of these variants are either of no clinical significance or are extremely rare, some variants—PiS(Iiyama), PiKings, PiM(Duarte), and PiM(Malton)—have been reported to be associated with liver injury and cirrhosis.[7,9] Additional variants that have demonstrated liver abnormalities include the PiP(Brescia), PiM(Wurzburg), PiKing's, and PiS alleles, often with compound heterozygosity.[7,9,10]

Under normal circumstances, α_1-AT is produced in the rough endoplasmic reticulum (ER) of hepatocytes and is targeted to the secretory pathway via the Golgi apparatus. Structural misfolding and polymerization of the mutant α_1-AT Z protein cause its aberrant retention in the hepatocyte ER with a resulting *gain-of-function* defect that leads to cirrhosis. Several mechanisms of liver injury in α_1-AT deficiency have been proposed.

The failure of proteins to properly exit the ER results in many diseases. When misfolding occurs, several physiologic responses normally ensue. Often, unfolded or misfolded proteins are tagged for degradation via ER-associated degradation (ERAD), in which chaperones and associated factors recognize and target substrates for retrotranslocation to the cytoplasm, where they are degraded by the ubiquitin-proteasome machinery. If continued accumulation of incorrectly folded proteins occurs, a complementary ER quality control mechanism, the unfolded protein response, is usually triggered.[9,11] Autophagy is a third pathway that reduces ER stress from abnormal protein aggregation. If ERAD efficiency is compromised, autophagy-mediated destruction occurs whereby portions of the ER along with protein aggregates are engulfed in double-membrane structures called autophagosomes and delivered to the lysosome for degradation.[12] Indeed, each of these pathways has been mechanistically linked to the development of α_1-AT-associated liver disease. Studies have demonstrated impaired interaction between abnormal Z-type protein and its ERAD-associated molecular chaperone calnexin, thereby resulting in retention of polymers in the ER.[13,14] Additionally, ERAD defects confounded with other misfolding protein variants, such as the HFE variant H63D, have been reported to increase the risk of liver damage in α_1-AT deficiency.[11] Others have shown that PiZ polymers within the ER are not associated with normal unfolded protein response activation,[11,15] but rather with a secondary ER overload response pathway that results in the proinflammatory release of interleukin-6 and interleukin-8, which are thought to contribute to the development of liver injury in α_1-AT deficiency.[16] Since autophagy is activated by the intracellular accumulation of PiZ, the use of autophagy enhancer drugs has been shown to mitigate the accumulation and proteotoxicity of misfolded PiZ polymers in a *Caenorhabditis elegans* model of α_1-AT deficiency.[17–19]

Clinical Features

Although the prevalence of the classic α_1-AT deficiency allele, PiZ, is highest in populations derived from Northern European ancestry, many racial subgroups are affected worldwide, and millions of persons have combinations of deficiency alleles (i.e., PiSS, PiSZ, or PiZZ).[20–22] In the United States, the overall prevalence of deficiency allele combinations is approximately 1 in 4126 for PiZZ and 1 in 1018 for PiSZ.[20,21] Mounting evidence suggests that heterozygous α_1-AT deficiency states in adults can contribute to the development of cirrhosis, chronic liver failure, and HCC. Furthermore, heterozygosity may exacerbate the chronic liver disease caused by obesity and alcohol abuse in adults, as well as cholestatic liver diseases in children.[4,23,24]

In the most unbiased epidemiologic study of α_1-AT deficiency to date, 200,000 Swedish infants were screened for α_1-AT deficiency; 184 were found to have abnormal allelic forms of α_1-AT (127 PiZZ, 2 PiZnull, 54 PiSZ, and 1 PiSnull); 6 (5 PiZZ and 1 PiSZ) died in early childhood, but only 2 of cirrhosis.[25] About 10% of newborns with α_1-AT deficiency (PiZZ) present with cholestasis, and as many as 50% continue to have elevated serum aminotransferase levels at age 3 months; most were clinically asymptomatic.[25,26] Liver disease does not develop in patients with null α_1-AT phenotypes, whereas early-onset emphysema will develop in all.[27] Nevertheless, investigations using the *C. elegans* model have demonstrated proteotoxic effects from null variants. The investigators concluded that because the mechanism of degradation of null variants is different from that of PiZ polymers, the mechanism of proteotoxicity is likely to be different as well.[28]

Wide variation exists in the severity of liver disease among patients with the classical form of α_1-AT (PiZZ) deficiency, and little is known about the factors that predispose affected persons to severe, progressive hepatic injury.[29] Even children in whom cirrhosis develops can have highly variable progression to end-stage liver disease (ESLD).[30] Moreover, siblings with PiZZ have variable degrees of liver involvement; in a study reported by Hinds and colleagues, five of seven children with PiZZ-associated α_1-AT deficiency who required liver transplantation had siblings with PiZZ who lacked persistent liver involvement.[31] Therefore additional factors must be involved in determining the severity of liver disease in α_1-AT deficiency.[32] ER mannosidase I and sortilin have been identified as possible genetic modifier candidates that contribute to the development of liver disease in PiZZ homozygotes.[33,34] Additional epigenetic signatures, such as those involved in cell methylation, have also demonstrated the potential to stratify patients for liver disease risk.[35]

Of 150 patients with α_1-AT deficiency from Sveger's original study who subsequently underwent evaluation at ages 16 and 18 years, none had physical examination findings of liver disease.[25] Elevated serum aminotransferase or GGTP levels were found in fewer than 20% of patients with a PiZZ phenotype and in fewer than 15% of those with a PiSZ phenotype.[26] By the third decade of life, analysis of this same cohort showed that 6% of PiZZ and 9% of PiSZ patients had a marginal increase in serum ALT levels.[36] A separate analysis of 647 patients with a PiZZ phenotype found that 49% had slight increases in aminotransferase levels when a stricter cutoff for normal levels was used, suggesting ongoing liver injury.[37]

Although liver disease is often mild during infancy and childhood, patients with α_1-AT deficiency have an increased risk of developing cirrhosis and HCC. A study of 57 PiZZ adults with lung disease revealed that 63% had findings of chronic liver disease by conventional liver biochemical testing and liver US.[38] A further analysis of three large U.S. liver transplantation databases revealed that the vast majority, 77.2%, of liver transplants performed in patients with a diagnosis of α_1-AT deficiency occurred in adults. The authors concluded that α_1-AT deficiency-associated liver disease is predominantly an age-dependent degenerative disease and that pediatric cases represent outliers with particularly powerful, as yet unidentified, modifying factors.[39] Therefore the diagnosis of α_1-AT deficiency should be considered in any patient presenting with noninfectious chronic hepatitis, hepatosplenomegaly, cirrhosis, portal hypertension, or HCC.

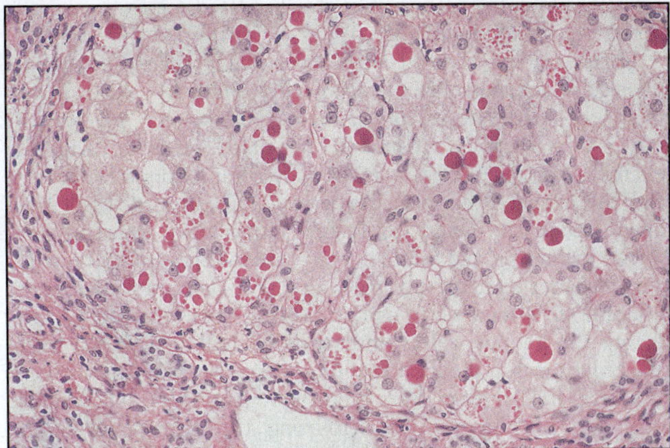

Fig. 79.1 Liver histology in α_1-antitrypsin deficiency. The globules are intensely periodic acid–Schiff (PAS) positive (PAS after diastase digestion). (From Burt A, Portmann B, Ferrell L. *MacSween's Pathology of the Liver*. 6th ed. Philadelphia: Churchill Livingstone Elsevier; 2012.)

Histopathology

Histopathologic features of α_1-AT deficiency change as the patient ages. In infancy, liver biopsy specimens may show bile duct paucity, bile duct proliferation, intracellular cholestasis with or without giant cell transformation, mild inflammatory changes, or steatosis, with few of the characteristic periodic acid–Schiff–positive, diastase-resistant globules.[40] These inclusions, which result from polymerized α_1-AT Z protein, are most prominent in periportal hepatocytes and may also be seen in Kupffer cells. Immunohistochemistry with monoclonal antibody to α_1-AT Z can also be performed to verify the diagnosis. As the patient ages, these changes may resolve completely or progress to chronic injury with fibrosis or cirrhosis.

Diagnosis

α_1-AT is considered a hepatic acute-phase reactant, and its release may be stimulated by stress, injury, pregnancy, or neoplasia. Because these factors can influence α_1-AT production, even in patients with the PiZZ phenotype, the diagnosis of α_1-AT deficiency should be based on phenotype analysis and not solely on the serum α_1-AT level.[41] A liver biopsy specimen, although not generally recommended, can confirm the diagnosis (Fig. 79.1). Commercial tests are available to detect the most common mutant alleles by PCR analysis of genomic DNA. In addition, molecular genetic testing, sequence analysis, and deletion/duplication analysis can be performed to identify common and rare disease variants.[42]

Generalized recommendations to enhance the detection α_1-AT deficiency are available[43,44]; however, targeted approaches have achieved a much higher rate of detection.[45] Adults with chronic lung disease and siblings of affected patients with lung or liver disease should be targeted for screening, and appropriate education and genetic counseling should be offered to patients with α_1-AT deficiency identified by screening.[40]

Treatment

No current disease-specific therapies are available for the hepatic manifestations of α_1-AT deficiency, and the initial management remains monitoring and symptomatic care. The importance of providing fat-soluble vitamin supplementation, when indicated, adequate nutrition, and counseling to avoid obesity, alcohol, smoking, and second-hand smoke cannot be overemphasized. As the pathophysiology is increasingly elucidated, more therapeutic targets are being identified.[46]

Understanding the role of autophagy and other mechanisms involved in the clearance of misfolded proteins has led to assessment of the role of autophagy-enhancer medications (e.g., carbamazepine, rapamycin, nor-ursodeoxycholic acid)[47–49] and the use of viral vectors that can deliver transcription factors that lead to increased autophagic activity.[50] These approaches have demonstrated the ability to reduce intracellular inclusions and fibrosis in animals, and future human-based studies are warranted.[46]

Alternative strategies for treating α_1-AT deficiency may target different steps in the pathogenic process; these include (1) correcting the genetic defect with gene or cell therapy, (2) using chaperones within the ER to promote degradation (e.g., treatment with small molecules or proteostasis modulators), (3) blocking the formation of polymers by stabilizing the immediate folding pathway or the monomer (e.g., treatment with small molecules or intrabodies), or (4) reducing production of the mutant protein through RNA interference (RNAi), which is a naturally occurring cellular mechanism that regulates gene expression.[6]

This latter method was tested in a multicenter, phase 2 open-label trial in adults.[51] Using fazirsiran, an investigational RNAi therapeutic that causes degradation of AAT and Z-AAT messenger RNA, the authors assessed reduction of AAT protein synthesis in the hepatocytes. In two cohorts of adult patients receiving different medication doses, the authors investigated the change in baseline in liver Z-AAT concentrations. Treatment was associated with a reduction in liver Z-AAT accumulation (all patients), a reduction of liver enzyme concentrations (all cohorts), and a regression of fibrosis in 7 of 15 patients. The authors concluded that through an RNAi mechanism, fazirsiran treatment reduced new Z-AAT synthesis, enabling pathways to clear the toxic Z-AAT accumulation. This resulted in a removal of the pathogenic insult driving disease and allowed for native liver restorative processes.[51] Large, placebo-controlled clinical trials of greater treatment duration are required to confirm the effect of fazirsiran on hepatic fibrosis.

Alternatively, targeting pathways to increase the secretion of the misfolded protein products may prove beneficial. Suberoylanilide hydroxamic acid has been shown to promote secretion of the Z protein from epithelial cell lines.[52]

Collectively, these approaches have the potential to decrease hepatocellular accumulation of the misfolded α_1-AT variants and ameliorate the injurious stimuli. Additional technologies, including the use of stem cell technology, likely in combination with gene editing techniques such as clustered regularly interspaced short palindromic repeats (CRISPR), will hopefully play a role in future efforts to better understand and treat α_1-AT deficiency.

α_1-AT deficiency remains the most common genetic liver disease for which liver transplantation is performed. Severe progressive liver disease due to α_1-AT deficiency is most common in adult males, thereby suggesting that the mechanisms of liver injury are similar to those for other age-dependent degenerative diseases and that severe pediatric disease is influenced by powerful modifiers.[39] Liver transplantation not only replaces the injured organ but also corrects the metabolic defect, thereby preventing further progression of systemic disease. This option is a highly effective intervention for those with the most severe phenotypes, with 5-year patient survival rates ranging between 83% and 90% for children and adults.[53,54] Outcomes on the use of technical variant grafts (living-related and split liver) are comparable, and the use of liver allografts from donors heterozygous for α_1-AT deficiency has been shown to be safe and effective.[55] Although data are lacking on the risk of HCC in patients with liver disease due to α_1-AT deficiency, a prudent approach is to follow the American Association for the Study of Liver Diseases (AASLD) guidelines for surveillance: liver US every 6 months in patients with cirrhosis, with or without an accompanying serum AFP determination.[56]

GLYCOGEN STORAGE DISEASES

More than 12 distinct inborn disorders of glycogen metabolism have been described, but only three are associated with serious liver disease: glycogen storage disease (GSD) types I, III, and IV.[57] Other GSDs may cause hepatomegaly or liver histologic changes but generally do not cause clinically important liver disease. The overall incidence of GSD types I, III, and IV is estimated to range from 1 in 50,000 to 1 in 100,000 in the general population.

Glycogen metabolism occurs in many tissues, but the areas of clinical importance are the muscle, liver, and polymorphonuclear neutrophils. The body uses glycogen to store glucose and as a ready reserve when systemic glucose is required (see Chapter 74). Glycogen is composed of long-chain glucose molecules arranged in a linear 1,4 linkage. Overall, 8%–10% of the glucose molecules are attached in a 1,6 linkage to form branching chains, which permit efficient storage of glucose while minimizing the impact on intracellular osmolality. The substrates for glycogen synthesis, glucose-6-phosphate (Glu-6-P) and glucose-1-phosphate, are derived from several pathways, including fructose and galactose metabolic cycles, as well as gluconeogenesis and glycogenolysis (Fig. 79.2).

Type I

GSD type I is the most common inborn error of glycogen metabolism. Clinical and molecular genetic observations have disclosed two subtypes of GSD type I—Ia and Ib, that account for virtually all cases.[58] These result from deficiency of one limb of a two-component enzyme system involved in the transport of Glu-6-P from the cytosol into the ER: 1. GSD type Ib—due to deficient activity of *Glu-6-P translocase* (encoded by the ubiquitously expressed *SLC37A4* gene), and 2. GSD type Ia—due to a subsequent defective cleavage of Glu-6-P by glucose-6-phosphatase (Glu-6-Pase, encoded by the *G6PC1* gene), located on the luminal side of the ER. The clinical phenotype with respect to

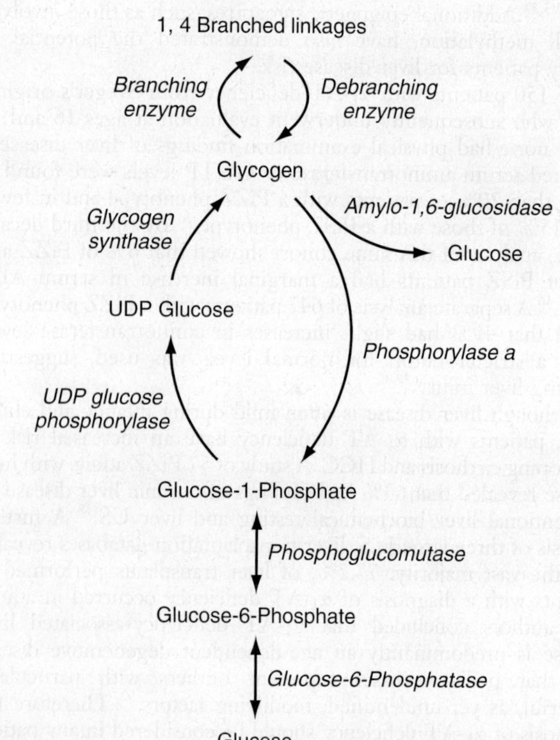

Fig. 79.2 Pathway of glycogen synthesis and glycogenolysis. Enzymes are shown in *italics*. *UDP*, Uridine diphosphate.

liver disease is similar in both forms; however, patients with GSD type Ib often have intermittent severe neutropenia and polymorphonuclear leukocyte (neutrophil) dysfunction, making them prone to recurrent episodes of severe bacterial infections and Crohn-like intestinal disease.[58] Loss of function of an isoform of Glu-6-Pase encoded by the *G6PC3* gene, although also ubiquitously expressed, leads to severe congenital neutropenia type 4, an autosomal recessive condition.[59]

Clinical Features

Most patients with GSD type I present in infancy with symptoms of metabolic derangement, such as lethargy, seizures, or coma as a result of profound hypoglycemia or metabolic acidosis, a protruding abdomen caused by hepatomegaly, muscular hypotonia, and delayed psychomotor development.[58] These features are related to disruption of the function of Glu-6-Pase (type Ia) or Glu-6-P translocase (type Ib) that inhibits the use of glucose in gluconeogenesis, glycogenolysis, and the metabolism of fructose or galactose. This inability to release stored glucose leads to hypoglycemia within 90–180 minutes of the last orally ingested glucose. Lactate and fatty acid metabolism and glycolytic pathways are then used as sources of energy.

Physical signs invariably include hepatomegaly, usually with a normal-sized spleen. Patients in whom the disease is poorly controlled for a long time exhibit short stature and growth failure and may be prone to adiposity. Delayed bone age and reduced postpubertal bone mineral density are common.[60] Patients with GSD type I are susceptible to a wide spectrum of neurologic injury that may result in epilepsy, hearing loss, and abnormal neuroimaging findings, likely a result of recurrent episodes of hypoglycemia.[61]

Other metabolic and extrahepatic comorbidities can be seen. Lactic acid levels can reach four to eight times normal; the accompanying metabolic acidosis may manifest as muscle weakness, hyperventilation, malaise, headache, or recurrent fever. Hyperuricemia is common and may lead to gout, arthritis, or progressive nephropathy. Nephromegaly secondary to increased glycogen deposition is common, and with advancing age, progressive renal disease, hypertension, and renal failure requiring dialysis and transplantation may develop. Because of hypoglycemia, patients have chronically high serum levels of glucagon with depressed levels of insulin. Hypertriglyceridemia and hypercholesterolemia are present in both GSD Ia and GSD Ib (but more prominently in GSD Ia) and may account for xanthoma formation. Xanthomas can appear after puberty and localize to the elbows, knees, buttocks, or nasal septum, the last leading to epistaxis. Hypercalcemia during acute metabolic decompensation has been observed. Bleeding dysfunction, manifesting as recurrent epistaxis, easy bruising, oozing after dental surgeries, and menorrhagia, can be seen secondary to impaired platelet function or acquired von Willebrand–like disease.[58,62]

Patients with GSD type Ib often also have severe intermittent neutropenia and neutrophil dysfunction as well as high platelet counts. Mechanisms for neutropenia include enhanced apoptosis [63] but also dysfunctional differentiation of myeloid progenitor cells that can result from deficiency of G6P translocase.[64] Crohn-like IBD often occurs in patients with GSD type Ib at the time of severe neutropenia, and patients are prone to severe bacterial infections, with abscess formation throughout the body.[65]

Hepatic Involvement

Hepatomegaly in GSD type I results from increased glycogen storage in the liver, as well as a degree of fatty infiltration; the latter likely develops because of a wide array of perturbations in lipid metabolism, including increased free fatty acid flux into the liver.[66] Patients demonstrate mild elevations in serum aminotransferase levels but generally do not develop cirrhosis or liver failure.

Hepatocellular adenomas develop in 22%–75% of patients, as early as 3 years of age but most commonly in the second decade of life, and tend to increase in both size and number as the patient ages (see Chapter 98).[67] In hepatocellular adenomas in GSD type I, β-catenin mutations have been reported in 28% but differ from sporadic adenomas in that hepatic nuclear factor 1α inactivation has not been observed; inflammatory-type adenomas may also occur[68] (see Chapter 98). In rare instances, adenomas can transform to HCC; unfortunately, serum AFP and carcinoembryonic antigen levels, as well as features of the lesions on hepatic imaging, are not predictive of malignant transformation.[69] Mechanisms of HCC/adenoma development are unknown; however, animal models have suggested a possible role for autophagy impairment for these patients.[70] Whether poor metabolic control increases the risk of hepatocellular adenoma formation in patients with GSD type Ia is controversial.[71] In some patients, hepatocellular adenomas have been demonstrated to regress and disappear after adequate nutritional therapy, but the course is unpredictable, especially in nonadherent patients.[67] Because imaging and serum marker levels are unreliable in predicting malignant transformation in this patient population, it is uncertain whether resection of an adenoma or liver transplantation is preferable.[72]

Diagnosis

In suspected cases of GSD type I, mutation analysis is the first choice for diagnosis. Complete *G6PC* sequencing is usually performed first; unless neutropenia is present, in which case *SLC37A4* sequencing should be pursued.[58] Although liver biopsy is no longer necessary when GSD type 1 is suspected, Glu-6-Pase activity can be analyzed on snap-frozen liver tissue. Deficient enzyme activity confirms the diagnosis of GSD type Ia. Targeted mutation analysis is useful for prenatal diagnosis and carrier testing for patients with a known family mutation and may be useful when knowledge of common mutations for specific ethnic groups is available.[58] Multigene panels that include *G6PC*, *SLC37A4*, and other genes of interest are available.[73]

Treatment

GSD type I is a multisystem disorder best managed by a team of health care professionals with experience in managing the multiple aspects of the disease. Management centers on preventing the acute metabolic derangements and potential long-term complications and enabling the patient to attain normal psychological development and a good quality of life. In general, a primary physician with expertise in metabolic disorders should coordinate the patient's care with other specialists, including a metabolic dietician, nephrologist, geneticist, endocrinologist, hepatologist, genetic counselor, neurologist, and cardiologist, depending on the clinical manifestations.[58]

Consensus guidelines for the management of GSD type I have been proposed.[58] Maintaining blood glucose levels at >70 mg/dL is important to achieve good metabolic control. Levels should be kept consistent to avoid hypoglycemia and fluctuations in the blood glucose levels. In infants and children, the avoidance of fasting for more than 3 hours is critical, because hypoglycemia and its accompanying complications often can develop. In older children and adolescents, fasting up to 6 hours may be safe. Regular blood glucose monitoring is the key to establishing an optimal regimen. Offering smaller, more frequent meals and avoiding sucrose, fructose, and galactose are generally recommended. Access via nasogastrostomy or a surgically placed gastrostomy tube is recommended for emergencies and overnight gastric feeds. Raw, uncooked cornstarch is often introduced between 6 and 12 months of age for management. General guidelines for dosing are 1.6 g of cornstarch per kilogram of body weight every 3–4 hours for young children and 1.7–2.5 g of cornstarch per kilogram every 4–5 hours for older children, adolescents, and adults. Some adults may require only one dose of cornstarch at bedtime to maintain their glucose levels.[74] Overnight administration of modified cornstarch has demonstrated the ability to prevent hypoglycemia more effectively than uncooked cornstarch.[75] Because optimal glycemic control is not always possible and the risk of severe hypoglycemia is high if delivery of glucose is interrupted inadvertently, serum lactate levels should be kept at the high end of normal, because lactate is an alternative fuel for the brain. Multivitamins, calcium, and vitamin D supplementation are necessary because of the restricted nature of the diet. Importantly, both undertreatment (resulting in hypoglycemia) and overtreatment (resulting in insulin resistance) can be harmful.[58]

Patients should undergo regular monitoring for the development of liver adenomas, especially after the onset of puberty. Although good metabolic control may lead to regression of the adenomas, there remains the risk of transformation to HCC, particularly when the size or number of lesions increases rapidly or the vascularity increases. An abdominal US should be performed at baseline and then every 12–24 months. Additional imaging modalities such as CT, MRI, or contrast-enhanced US can be considered to characterize suspicious lesions. Percutaneous ethanol injection, radiofrequency ablation, and partial liver resection are treatment options for liver adenomas (see Chapter 98).[58] Monitoring for the development of renal comorbidities in patients with GSD type I should include US assessment to determine kidney size and growth, as well as the presence of nephrolithiasis or nephrocalcinosis. Urinalysis, urine electrolyte determination, and glomerular filtration rate (GFR) determinations should be assessed regularly. Angiotensin-converting enzyme inhibitors can be used in the setting of hyperfiltration (sustained estimated GFR >140 mL/min/1.73 m^2) and when either microalbuminemia or proteinuria occurs.[58]

The presence of anemia should prompt investigation for nutritional causes, adenomas, enterocolitis, and occult blood loss. Severe anemia should trigger an evaluation for adenomas in GSD type Ia and enterocolitis in GSD type Ib. Neutropenic patients with GSD type Ib should be treated with granulocyte colony-stimulating factor (G-CSF), particularly if there is associated fever, infections, or enterocolitis.[58] Additionally, elucidation of the mechanisms driving apoptosis via the accumulation of a phosphorylated glucose analog[63] has identified an alternative treatment option—the use of SGLT2 inhibitors, such as empagliflozin. Real-world experience with empagliflozin has resulted in overall favorable effects on the neutropenia/neutrophil dysfunction-related symptoms in patients with GSD type 1b, with most patients able to either reduce or completely stop their G-CSF medication.[76]

Adenoviral-mediated gene replacement therapy of recombinant Glu-6-Pase in both murine and canine models of GSD type Ia deficiency has led to encouraging results and may be a future option in humans[77]; however, the adenoviral vector genomes have been shown to be gradually lost over the weeks following vector administration.[78] Hepatocyte transplantation has been performed successfully in patients with GSD type I, but long-term outcomes are lacking.[79–81] Liver transplantation has corrected the metabolic error in patients with GSD type I and permitted normalization of fasting tolerance and catch-up growth; however, other extrahepatic comorbidities such as renal disease and neutropenia persist and progress.[82]

Type III

GSD type III results from mutations in the *AGL* gene with resulting deficiency in the glycogen-debranching enzyme (GDE) and leads to the accumulation of limit dextrin units, which restrict subsequent glucose release by phosphorylase. Because deficiency of GDE does not interfere with metabolism of Glu-6-P, patients with GSD type III retain effective mechanisms for gluconeogenesis. Therefore the clinical course is milder than in patients with GSD type I, and patients can fast for longer periods; most survive into adulthood. In infancy, however, GSD type III may be indistinguishable from GSD type I.

GDE possesses two independent catalytic activities, an amylo-1,6-glucosidase and oligo-1,4→1,4 glucan transferase. Both activities are deficient in the two main clinical subtypes of GSD type III, types IIIa and IIIb. Differential expression of the four major GDE mRNA isoforms in liver and muscle tissue distinguishes the two types: type IIIa affects liver and muscle and accounts for 80% of patients, and type IIIb affects the liver only and accounts for 15% of patients. Rare isolated loss of one of the GDE activities has been observed (i.e., glucosidase activity in type IIIc and transferase activity in type IIId).[83,84]

Clinical Features

Persons with GSD type III typically exhibit hypoglycemia, hepatomegaly, and growth failure. Liver enlargement results from increased glycogen deposition, not fatty infiltration. The liver may show fibrotic septa that rarely lead to frank cirrhosis and ESLD. Serum lactate and uric acid levels are normal, and aminotransferase levels are increased only moderately until advanced liver disease occurs. Hyperlipidemia may be present but is not as pronounced as in GSD type I. Patients have normal responses to fructose and galactose loading.

Patients with GSD type III may also display progressive skeletal, cardiac, and bulbar muscle weakness, which worsens with activity, and muscle wasting.[83,85] Nephromegaly is not seen, but ventricular hypertrophy or cardiac arrhythmias may occur; frequent cardiac evaluation and monitoring are recommended. Hepatomegaly and ketotic hypoglycemia accompanied by elevations in serum aminotransferase and creatinine kinase (representing muscle injury) levels are suggestive of GSD type III. Identifying pathogenic *AGL* variants confirms the diagnosis with both targeted single-gene testing and multigene panels available. If genetic testing does not confirm the diagnosis, direct enzyme analysis of peripheral leukocytes, muscle, or liver tissue can be performed.[83] Comorbidities in GSD type III are common, including cardiac complications in 58%–91%, neuromuscular complications in 34%–80%, and hepatic complications in 11% of patients.[86,87]

Treatment

A high-protein, low-carbohydrate diet has been suggested to normalize metabolic activity, ensure normal growth, restore muscle function, and minimize hepatomegaly. This diet provides adequate substrates for gluconeogenesis while reducing the need for glycogen storage. Unlike GSD type I, patients with GSD type III need not avoid fructose and galactose, because these sugars can be used for energy production. Patients with refractory hypoglycemia or persistent hepatomegaly may require a nighttime continuous infusion or cornstarch, as is used for GSD type I. A potential role for dietary lipid manipulation has also been explored with improvements in creatine kinase concentrations and a decrease in cardiac hypertrophy noted in pediatric patients with GSD type III on a high-fat diet. Notably, long-term monitoring for potential complications of a high-fat diet, such as growth restriction, liver inflammation, and HCC development, is warranted, and definitive studies are needed.[88] Liver transplantation has been successful but is usually not necessary for patients with GSD type III, even in those with evidence of cirrhosis, if liver synthetic function remains well preserved. Following

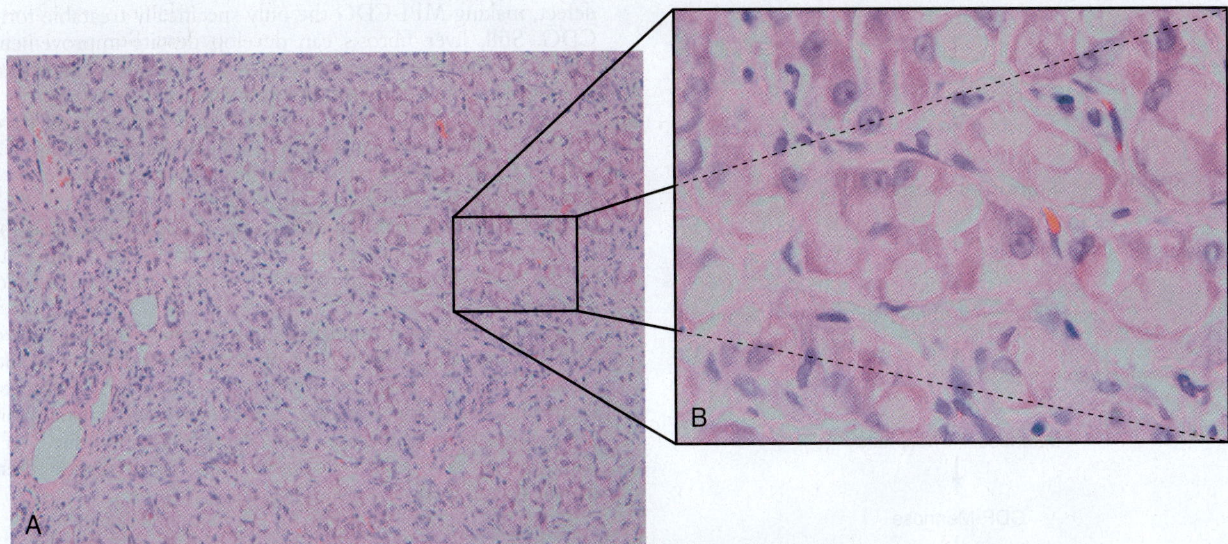

Fig. 79.3 Histopathology of a liver biopsy specimen from a patient with glycogen storage disease type IV. (A) At low power, the loss of the normal trabecular hepatic architecture is seen (H&E, ×20). (B) A higher-power photomicrograph shows the accumulation of "ground-glass" cytoplasmic inclusions within the hepatocytes; this finding is a consequence of abnormal intracellular processing of amylopectin-like material (H&E, ×100).

transplantation, extrahepatic complications such as heart and muscle dysfunction persist.[83,84]

Type IV

Deficiency of the branching enzyme is seen in GSD type IV, a rare syndrome also known as *amylopectinosis*. Glycogen and amylopectin accumulate in hepatocytes, leading to hepatomegaly, abdominal distention, and failure to thrive, most commonly during infancy. Signs of liver disease, when present, predominate later in the disease course. Several variable forms of GSD type IV have been observed: a *fatal perinatal neuromuscular subtype*, which presents in utero with fetal akinesia deformation sequence, polyhydramnios, and hydrops, with fetal death generally occurring in the neonatal period; a *congenital neuromuscular subtype*, which presents in the newborn period with profound hypotonia, respiratory distress, and dilated cardiomyopathy, with death usually in early infancy; a *classic (progressive) hepatic subtype* in which the child appears normal at birth but rapidly develops failure to thrive with hepatomegaly, liver dysfunction, hypotonia, and dilated cardiomyopathy, with death from liver failure usually by 5 years of age; a *nonprogressive hepatic subtype* in which children demonstrate liver dysfunction that does not progress; and a rare *childhood neuromuscular subtype* in which clinical features may not present until the second decade and the clinical course is variable.[89] While consensus guidelines are lacking, expert recommendations for the diagnosis and management have been published with practical steps to confirm a GSD type IV diagnosis and best practices for medical management.[90] Genotype-phenotype analyses of the branching enzyme gene have revealed a high degree of molecular heterogeneity without clear clinical associations.[91,92]

Hypoglycemia is relatively uncommon, and responses to fructose and galactose challenges are normal. Serum lactate and pyruvate levels are normal, and serum aminotransferase levels are typically elevated in the hepatic subtypes. Progressive macronodular cirrhosis is present with an abundance of periodic acid–Schiff–positive deposits (amylopectin) in hepatocytes (Fig. 79.3). Cirrhosis may progress to liver failure, and, rarely, adenomas and HCC may develop.[93] The confirmatory diagnosis of GSD type IV relies on molecular testing of *GBE1* to document biallelic pathogenic variants. Biochemical analysis proving GBE enzyme reduction of deficiency and histopathology of affected tissue(s) is supportive of a GSD type IV diagnosis.[90]

Most patients die within the first 3 years of life. Diets high in protein and low in carbohydrate have been associated with improved growth but have had little effect on liver involvement. Liver transplantation results in correction of the metabolic error and normal growth for most patients; however, persistence of amylopectin deposits in the heart (with progressive cardiomyopathy leading to death) and leukocytes has been described in a small subset of patients.[94]

CONGENITAL DISORDERS OF GLYCOSYLATION

Congenital disorders of glycosylation (CDGs) are inherited metabolic diseases caused by defects in the genes important for the process of protein and lipid glycosylation.[95] These rare genetic disorders disrupt the posttranslational modification of glycoproteins and the synthesis of glycolipids.[96] More than 130 CDGs involving both asparagine *(N)*- and serine/threonine *(O)*-linked protein glycosylation have been reported.[97,98] The CDGs can be divided into four groups: (1) disorders of protein *N*-glycosylation, (2) disorders of protein *O*-glycosylation, (3) disorders of glycosylphosphatidylinositol anchor biosynthesis, and (4) disorders of other glycosylation pathways and of multiple glycosylation pathways.[95] The clinical spectrum is broad, impacting every organ system. Many of these disorders lead to dysfunction of the liver, intestine, or both.[99]

Protein glycosylation is complex and involves multiple enzymatic steps and subcellular compartments.[100] Secretory glycoproteins with altered carbohydrate moieties in patients with CDGs include coagulation factors, albumin and other binding proteins, growth hormone, apolipoproteins, insulin, and thyroxine-binding globulin. Because protein glycosylation occurs in all cells, it is not surprising that patients with a CDG exhibit multisystem abnormalities, often dominated by central nervous system manifestations.[100]

Potential glycosylation disorders can be assessed with biochemical biomarkers. The use of advanced mass spectrometry

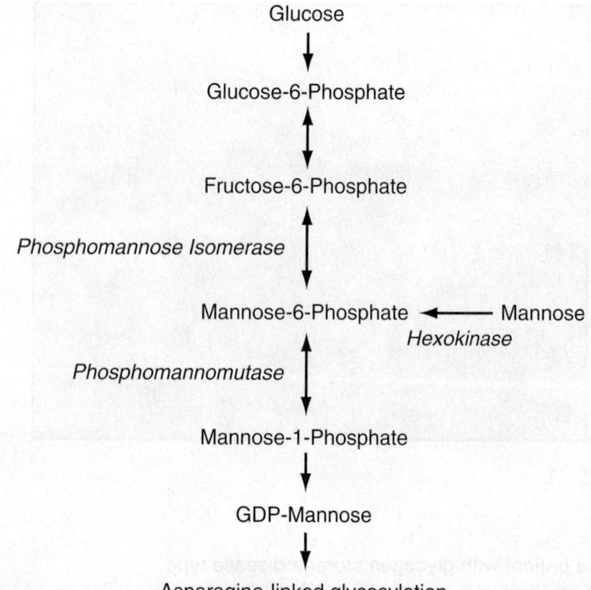

Fig. 79.4 Pathway of mannose metabolism. Enzymes are shown in *italics*. *GDP*, Guanosine diphosphate.

to detect abnormalities in serum transferrin is the best marker for detecting most disorders affecting the *N*-glycosylation pathway.[101] However, markers do not identify the specific genetic defect.

Hepatic dysfunction in patients with CDG is present in about 22% of patients.[102] CDGs cluster into those that present with predominant or isolated liver disease, liver disease with other significant multisystem comorbidities, and isolated aminotransferase elevations.[96] Liver involvement in CDG is mild, with hepatic steatosis and fibrosis typically seen on light microscopy; on electron microscopy, lysosomal vacuoles, termed *myelosomes*, with concentric electron-dense membranes and variable electron-lucent and electron-dense material, are noted. Patients can uncommonly progress to cirrhosis and liver failure.[102]

A simplified nomenclature system uses a nonitalicized gene name followed by CDG. The most frequently encountered CDG is PMM2-CDG caused by defects in phosphomannomutase (PMM), an enzyme that converts mannose-6-phosphate to mannose-1-phosphate (Fig. 79.4). Multiple distinct mutations have been found in the *PMM2* gene; most patients are compound heterozygotes for mutations that likely preserve some residual PMM enzymatic activity, thereby suggesting that complete loss of PMM activity is incompatible with life. Targeted disruption of the *PMM2* gene in the mouse leads to early embryonic lethality.[103] Patients with PMM2-CDG typically have severe neurologic abnormalities, dysmorphisms (inverted nipples, abnormal fat distribution, and esotropia), and congenital hepatic fibrosis and steatosis.[104] The liver phenotype of PMM2-CDG is usually mild, with most patients exhibiting elevated aminotransferase levels that slowly improve and ultimately normalize by around 5 years of age.[96]

Patients with mutations in phosphomannose-isomerase CDG (MPI-CDG) have a defect in phosphomannose isomerase, which converts fructose-6-phosphate to mannose-6-phosphate (see Fig. 79.4). In addition to intractable diarrhea, protein-losing enteropathy, and congenital hepatic fibrosis, recurrent episodes of hyperinsulinemic hypoglycemia and cyclic vomiting have been reported.[105] Neurologic symptoms are usually absent, and dysmorphic features are less common than in PMM2-CDG. Recognizing MPI-CDG is key because it is effectively treated with dietary mannose supplementation to bypass the underlying defect, making MPI-CDG the only specifically treatable form of CDG. Still, liver fibrosis can develop despite improvement in clinical symptoms.[106] Liver transplantation has been shown to be beneficial in a few patients with full clinical recovery.[107]

Transient hepatomegaly, without congenital hepatic fibrosis, has been noted in patients with α-1-3-glucosyltransferase CDG (ALG6-CDG); otherwise, the clinical features of patients with ALG6-CDG are similar to, but milder than, those of PMM2-CDG.[99] Children with untyped cases of CDG have been found to have isolated cryptogenic chronic liver disease, mild coagulopathy, and mild portal fibrosis and focal steatosis on liver biopsy specimens.[108]

Any patient with unexplained congenital hepatic fibrosis, protein-losing enteropathy, or a procoagulant tendency should be evaluated for CDG. Initial screening is with a serum transferrin level with isoelectric focusing, followed by confirmatory enzymatic analysis in fibroblasts, leukocytes, or liver tissue.[99] If the diagnosis of MPI-CDG is confirmed, oral mannose therapy should be initiated.

PORPHYRIAS

The porphyrias are a diverse group of metabolic diseases that result from a deficiency in an enzyme involved in the heme synthetic pathway.

Pathophysiology

The metabolic pathways of heme synthesis are essentially the same in the two tissues in which heme synthesis primarily occurs, the liver (15%–20%) and the bone marrow (75%–80%), although synthetic control may be different in these tissues. The rate-limiting step in hepatic heme synthesis begins with the conversion of glycine and succinyl coenzyme A (CoA) to 5-aminolevulinic acid (ALA) by the action of ALA synthase (Fig. 79.5). ALA synthase activity is decreased by the end product of the pathway, heme, and is increased by substances that induce hepatic cytochrome P450 enzymes. Six additional enzymatic steps convert ALA to protoporphyrin IX (see Fig. 79.5). In the final step of the pathway, protoporphyrin IX is coupled to ferrous iron by ferrochelatase to create heme. Enzyme deficiencies arising from any of the 8 steps of the heme synthetic pathway lead to clinically apparent porphyria.[109]

The porphyrias are commonly classified according to clinical features into two main groups: *acute porphyrias*, which are due to hepatic overproduction of the porphyrin precursors and characterized by dramatic, potentially life-threatening neurologic symptoms, and *cutaneous porphyrias*, which result from overproduction of photosensitizing porphyrins and typically cause few or no neurologic symptoms but give rise to a variety of severe skin lesions (Table 79.1). In five of the porphyrias, the liver is the major site of expression; in two others, both the liver and bone marrow are involved; and in one only the bone marrow is involved.[109]

Acute Porphyrias

The symptoms and signs of the acute neurovisceral attacks that occur in the acute porphyrias vary considerably. Abdominal pain is present in more than 90% of patients, followed in frequency by tachycardia and dark urine in about 80% of patients. Neuropsychiatric features include hysteria, depression, psychosis, confusion, hallucinations, seizures, and coma, although little evidence suggests that chronic psychiatric illness occurs. An inability to concentrate may be the initial presenting complaint.[110] Other features are constipation, extremity pain, paresthesias, nausea, vomiting, urinary retention, hypertension, peripheral sensory

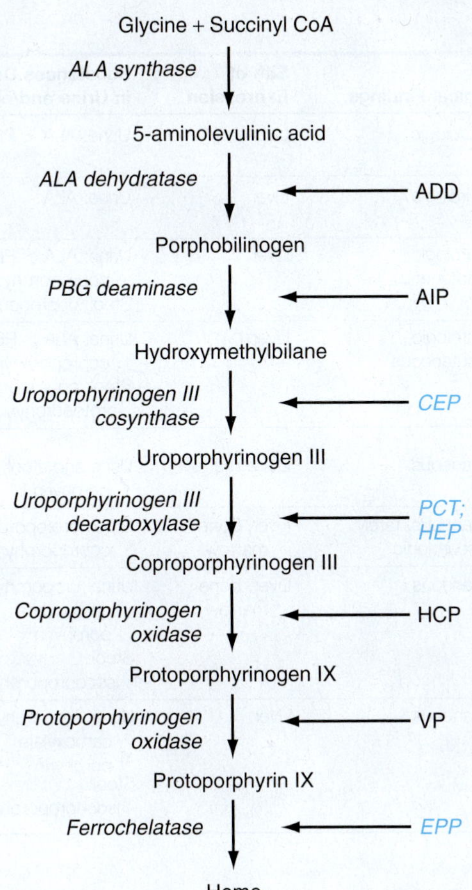

Fig. 79.5 Pathway of heme synthesis. The location of the enzymatic deficiency in the various forms of porphyria is noted. On the *left*, the enzymes are shown in *italics*. On the *right*, abbreviations for the cutaneous porphyrias are shown in *italics* and *blue*, and those for the acute porphyrias are shown in *Roman typeface*. *ADD*, 5-Aminolevulinic acid (ALA) dehydratase deficiency; *AIP*, acute intermittent porphyria; *CEP*, congenital erythropoietic porphyria; *CoA*, coenzyme A; *EPP*, erythropoietic protoporphyria; *HCP*, hereditary coproporphyria; *HEP*, hepatoerythropoietic porphyria; *PBG*, porphobilinogen; *PCT*, porphyria cutanea tarda; *VP*, variegate porphyria.

deficits (often in a "bathing trunk" distribution), and weakness leading to ascending paralysis or quadriplegia. These neurologic attacks appear to be related to the overproduction of ALA and porphobilinogen (PBG), which leads to higher serum and tissue levels of these neurotoxic products.

Acute episodes are approximately fivefold more common in women than men and may be precipitated by many factors, most commonly drugs, alcohol ingestion, and smoking.[111] Other inciting factors are fasting, infections, and pregnancy; some women report greater problems during the luteal phase of their menstrual cycles. The disease is clinically latent in 65%–80% of patients.

ALA dehydratase deficiency is a rare syndrome with autosomal recessive transmission in which the enzyme activity is <3%. The enzyme activity is 50% of normal in carriers, who are asymptomatic. Affected patients have severe, recurrent neurologic attacks that may be life-threatening. They excrete large amounts of ALA in their urine. Liver transplantation was reported to result in complete resolution of symptoms in one patient with ALA dehydratase deficiency.[112]

The three remaining acute porphyrias—acute intermittent porphyria (AIP), hereditary coproporphyria (HCP), and variegate porphyria (VP)—result from partial deficiency of the enzymes PBG deaminase, coproporphyrinogen oxidase, and protoporphyrinogen oxidase, respectively. All are inherited in an autosomal dominant fashion with variable expression. AIP, the most common, with the prevalence of mutations in Western populations of approximately 1 carrier per 2000 persons, manifests primarily as derangements in the autonomic nervous system or as a psychiatric disorder.[109,113] VP is more common in South Africa than elsewhere. Although HCP and VP give rise to neurologic symptoms similar to those of AIP, cutaneous lesions also occur in HCP and predominate in VP.[114]

Cutaneous Porphyrias

The cutaneous porphyrias differ from the acute porphyrias in that affected patients exhibit few or no neurologic symptoms. In these illnesses, excess porphyrins or porphyrinogens are deposited in the upper dermal capillary walls, where these photoreactive compounds cause tissue damage that manifests as cutaneous vesicles and bullae in areas exposed to light or excessive mechanical manipulation. Scarring, infection, pigment changes, and hypertrichosis can follow and lead to severe mutilation.

Porphyria cutanea tarda (PCT), the most common of the porphyrias, typically involves an 80% reduction in activity of the enzyme uroporphyrinogen III decarboxylase (UROD). Patients usually present after 40 years of age. Two types of PCT are recognized: (1) type I PCT affects 80% of patients and is a sporadic (acquired) form in which the enzyme deficiency is restricted to the liver; (2) type II, which affects the other 20% of patients, is familial and inherited in an autosomal dominant fashion with incomplete penetrance; the enzyme deficiency occurs in all tissues.[115] Symptoms develop in fewer than 10% of patients with type II PCT.

Type I PCT is strongly associated with high alcohol intake, estrogen therapy, and systemic illnesses, including systemic lupus erythematosus, diabetes mellitus, chronic kidney disease, and HIV infection. HCV infection, a known susceptibility factor for PCT, increases oxidative stress in hepatocytes, suppresses hepcidin production, and increases iron absorption from the intestine. HCV is associated with 50%–70% of cases of PCT in the United States.[116] The frequency of mutations of the *HFE* gene, which causes hereditary hemochromatosis, is increased in patients with types I and II PCT, and these mutations are susceptibility factors for clinical expression of the PCT phenotype (see Chapter 77).[117] Iron overload enhances oxidation of uroporphyrinogen to uroporphomethene, an inhibitor of UROD activity, thereby explaining the association of increased oxidative stress and the unmasking of the PCT phenotype.[118] This association is consistent with pathologic findings in liver biopsy specimens from patients with PCT, of whom 80% have siderosis, 15% have cirrhosis, and most have evidence of iron overload. Patients usually do not show signs of overt clinical liver disease, apart from elevated serum aminotransferase levels.

Hepatoerythropoietic porphyria (HEP) is a rare form of porphyria with a pathogenesis like that of PCT. HEP results from pathogenic variants in the UROD gene with resulting UROD deficiency, yielding <10% of normal enzyme activity. The cutaneous lesions, which resemble those of PCT and are characterized by blistering skin lesions, hypertrichosis, and scarring, are typically severe and mutilating. The disease usually manifests in the first year of life. As the patient ages, the dermatologic manifestations may subside, but liver disease, characterized by a nonspecific hepatitis, worsens.[119]

Congenital erythropoietic porphyria (CEP), a rare form of porphyria with autosomal recessive transmission, is caused by deficiency of uroporphyrinogen III cosynthase, which mainly affects erythropoietic tissue. Patients typically present in the first year of life with blisters and disfiguring skin lesions in exposed

TABLE 79.1 The Porphyrias

Acute Porphyrias	Enzymatic Defect	Mode of Inheritance	Clinical Findings	Site of Expression	Substances Detected in Urine and/or Stool
Acute intermittent porphyria	PBG deaminase	Autosomal dominant	Neurologic	Liver	Urine: ALA < PBG
ALA dehydratase deficiency	ALA dehydratase	Autosomal recessive	Neurologic	Liver	Urine: ALA
Hereditary coproporphyria	Coproporphyrinogen oxidase	Autosomal dominant	Neurologic, cutaneous	Liver	Urine: ALA > PBG, coproporphyrin Stool: coproporphyrin
Variegate porphyria	Protoporphyrinogen oxidase	Autosomal dominant	Neurologic, cutaneous	Liver	Urine: ALA > PBG, coproporphyrin Stool: coproporphyrin, protoporphyrinogen
CUTANEOUS PORPHYRIAS					
Congenital erythropoietic porphyria	Uroporphyrinogen III cosynthase	Autosomal recessive	Cutaneous	Bone marrow	Urine and stool: coproporphyrin I
Erythropoietic protoporphyria	Ferrochelatase	Various	Cutaneous, rarely neurologic	Liver, bone marrow	Stool: protoporphyrin, coproporphyrin
Hepatoerythropoietic porphyria	Uroporphyrinogen III decarboxylase	Autosomal recessive	Cutaneous	Liver, bone marrow	Urine: uroporphyrin, 7-carboxylate porphyrin Stool: isocoproporphyrin
Porphyria cutanea tarda	Uroporphyrinogen III decarboxylase	Autosomal dominant or acquired	Cutaneous	Liver	Urine: uroporphyrin, 7-carboxylate porphyrin Stool: isocoproporphyrin

ALA, 5-Aminolevulinic acid; *PBG*, porphobilinogen.

areas; pink urine and photosensitivity may be present. As patients age, erythrodontia, a pathognomonic red or brownish discoloration of the teeth, is commonly seen. CEP can be distinguished clinically from HEP by the presence in some cases of a Coombs-negative hemolytic anemia, which can be quite severe. Splenomegaly is common. Gain-of-function mutations in the ALA synthase 2 *(ALAS2)* gene in patients with CEP suggest that *ALAS2* is a modifier gene for CEP disease by increasing the flux of ALA production.[120]

Erythropoietic protoporphyria (EPP) is caused by partial deficiency of the enzyme ferrochelatase, the final step in the heme synthetic pathway. EPP is the second most common type of porphyria and has been thought to be inherited in an autosomal recessive manner.[121,122] Although the bone marrow is the predominant source of excess protoporphyrin, with a variable contribution from the liver and other tissues, the skin is the primary site of deposition of this phototoxic compound in patients with EPP. Therefore the principal clinical manifestation is exquisite photosensitivity, which may present during infancy and can lead to a wide spectrum of symptoms (e.g., itching, burning, pain) and to scars and lichenification of the skin. Vesicles are rare. Patients with EPP may have a mild hypochromic, microcytic anemia.[121]

Clinical liver disease, reported in the patient's medical history or determined by elevated serum aminotransferase levels, has been reported in up to 33% of patients with EPP and results from progressive hepatic accumulation of protoporphyrin.[121,123] Liver disease typically occurs after age 30 but has been described in children. The liver appears black and nodular, with hepatocellular necrosis, portal inflammation, cholestasis, and extensive deposits of dark brown pigment in hepatocytes, Kupffer cells, and biliary structures; birefringence of pigment deposits is seen on polarization microscopy.[124] Biochemically, total erythrocyte protoporphyrin (ePPIX) levels can be measured. Increased levels have been shown to be a significant determinant of disease severity and liver dysfunction. Patients with higher ePPIX levels (>2000 µg/dL) should be monitored more closely for evidence of liver disease.[121]

Hepatic Involvement

Hepatic involvement in porphyria is variable; in general, patients with acute porphyria may have elevated serum aminotransferase and bile acid levels, with further increases during acute episodes. Liver biopsy specimens may show steatosis and iron deposition. Although these changes are minor, patients with acute porphyria are at increased risk for the development of primary liver cancer.[125]

Diagnosis

The approach to the diagnosis of the porphyrias is summarized in Table 79.1. Clinical features alone are usually not specific enough to confirm a diagnosis or distinguish among the various forms of porphyrias. The diagnosis of porphyria should be considered in patients with recurrent bouts of severe abdominal pain, dark urine, constipation, and neuropsychiatric disturbances or in patients with typical dermatologic findings. To differentiate among the different porphyrias, urine, and stool samples should be obtained for porphyrin studies and a urine specimen collected for quantitative ALA and PBG determinations.

In AIP, elevated PBG levels in urine or plasma are specific, reaching up to 150 times the upper limit of normal during an acute flare.[109] Patients with HCP and VP excrete high levels of

ALA and PBG in the urine; in contrast to those with AIP, these patients excrete more ALA than PBG. A "spot" urine test to detect urinary PBG, ALA, and creatinine is recommended to diagnose the acute porphyrias, except for the rare patient with ALA dehydratase deficiency.[126,127] Fecal coproporphyrins are increased in both HCP and VP, whereas the amount of fecal protoporphyrin in VP is also increased.

Once a diagnosis of porphyria is biochemically confirmed, gene sequencing should be performed.[127,128] Many gene mutations have been identified for several acute porphyrias, including AIP, VP, and HCP. Specific gene sequencing can be performed in the setting of a specific biochemical profile, and when results are incomplete or not definitive, multigene panels are available.[128] Given the high degree of genetic heterogeneity, the lack of clear genotype-phenotype correlations, and the failure to find mutations in 5%–10% of families with available techniques, genetic testing is not recommended as a general screening tool.[127–129] If an index case of porphyria is identified, screening of asymptomatic family members, together with appropriate genetic counseling, may be helpful.

Treatment

The overall survival of patients with acute porphyria is good. Consensus guidelines for the treatment of acute porphyria attacks are available.[126,127,130] Generous fluid and glucose administration (preferably 10% dextrose in 0.45% saline) is recommended during acute attacks and can elicit the "glucose effect" that diminishes ALA synthase activity. Antiemetic agents, analgesic agents, and, if indicated, antiseizure medications are administered.[109] IV administration of hematin, a congener of heme, is the only current specific treatment for acute attacks. The medicine is generally effective at a dose of 3–4 mg/kg given once per day, with a notable decrease in PBG levels by the third day of treatment. Resolution of pain and nausea typically follows, and patients can be discharged once weaned from narcotics and tolerating oral intake.[109] Notably, hematin has several shortcomings, including instability in solution, the need for rapid infusion following constitution, the requirement for use of a large vein or central catheter for administration, negative effects on platelet function and coagulation, and the potential for hepatic iron buildup, with resulting iron overload-induced injury.[109] Therefore alternatives to the use of IV hematin are being developed. Both viral vector gene therapy and small interfering RNA approaches are under investigation. A pilot investigation using viral gene therapy demonstrated the therapy to be well tolerated from a safety perspective, but there was no noticeable effect on ALA or PBG levels following delivery of a normal hydroxymethylbilane synthase gene.[131] A phase 3, double-blind placebo-controlled trial investigating the use of subcutaneous givosiran (2.5 mg/kg of body weight), an RNAi therapy targeting ALAS1, resulted in a 74% lower rate in mean annualized attacks in those receiving therapy vs. placebo. Givosiran led to lower levels of urinary ALA and PBG, fewer days of hemin use, and better daily scores for pain than placebo.[132] Subsequent approval by the U.S. Food and Drug Administration and the European Medicines Agency has led to recommendations to consider givosiran as prophylactic therapy in patients with recurrent attacks.[127]

Recommendations for the long-term management of acute hepatic porphyrias are also available.[127,128] A baseline physical examination, including complete dermatologic and neurologic assessments and laboratory testing, should be performed. Iron deficiency, not related to the porphyria, is common and should be treated when present, because it can contribute to chronic symptoms.[133] Patients should be monitored for the development of porphyria-related nephropathy, typically manifesting as chronic tubulointerstitial nephropathy or focal cortical atrophy.[134–136] Important in the overall management of patients with porphyria is the identification, with subsequent avoidance or elimination, of precipitating factors that can trigger or worsen an acute attack. Particular attention should be paid to medications that have been demonstrated to be unsafe or risky in patients with porphyria, and a publicly available drug database is available at http://www.drugs-porphyria.org/. Liver transplantation has been successful in patients with severe, intractable disease that has not responded to traditional therapeutic approaches. Because of the associated increase in morbidity and mortality and because of the risk of reaccumulation of toxic metabolites in the graft, liver transplantation should be considered a treatment of last resort.[127,128,137–140] Because of the increased frequency of HCC, patients with AIP with recurrent attacks or past symptoms should undergo surveillance liver imaging at 6- to12-month intervals after age 50 (see Chapter 96).[127,128]

Patients with AP and advanced renal disease tolerate and benefit from renal transplantation. Some patients with both repeated attacks and end-stage renal disease have undergone combined liver-kidney transplantation.[141]

The dermatologic sequelae of porphyrias are best managed with sunlight avoidance. The wavelengths of light that excite the porphyrins (410 nm) are common to many light sources, and patients affected by porphyria are at risk from exposure not only to sunlight, but also to household, fluorescent, and operating room lights. Furthermore, because this wavelength passes through window glass, patients are also sensitive to indoor sunlight. Patients must therefore use special sunscreen lotions that block rays in the 400–410-nm range. Skin trauma should be minimized as much as possible; early treatment of skin infections can decrease scarring. Special screens may be especially useful for protection against indoor lighting. Some patients have incurred severe or lethal internal burns during surgery, including liver transplantation; therefore appropriate precautions must be taken.[109,142]

Treatment of PCT initially consists of removal of any offending agent. Historically, treatment has included phlebotomy to decrease iron overload and hepatic siderosis. This approach, combined with restriction of alcohol, tobacco, and estrogen, has been shown to produce remission.[109] In patients who cannot tolerate or who have adverse reactions to phlebotomy, chelation therapy has demonstrated some efficacy.[143] An alternative to iron depletion therapy is chloroquine, which complexes within hepatocytes to mobilize porphyrins to facilitate its urinary excretion, but the drug is potentially hepatotoxic, and caution is indicated in patients with cirrhosis or renal insufficiency.[144] The efficacy of chloroquine has been variable in patients with PCT who are homozygous for mutations in the *HFE* gene; for these patients, phlebotomy should be first-line therapy.[109] Importantly, two-thirds of patients with PCT have HCV coinfection and reports have suggested that eradication of HCV can lead to resolution of the skin manifestations of PCT.[145] Treatment strategies for HEP are similar to, but have not been as successful as, those for PCT.

Several therapeutic interventions have been reported to lead to varying degrees of clinical improvement in patients with EPP, but long-term resolution has not been demonstrated. Based on the observation that skin-related symptoms are inversely related to skin pigmentation, agents such as oral β-carotene have been suggested to improve sunlight intolerance; however, systemic reviews have found insufficient evidence to confirm efficacy.[146] Newer agents such as afamelanotide, a congener of α-melanocyte-stimulating hormone, which increases production of eumelanin to darken the skin, have shown benefit in phase 3 controlled studies.[147,148] Liver transplantation has been carried out in patients with EPP and ESLD with mixed results, as the erythropoietic defect persists and the allograft remains at risk for EPP-related damage.[149,150] Afamelanotide is now approved in Europe, the United States, and Australia.[151] A retrospective review of 20 patients with EPP who have undergone liver transplantation in the United States revealed unique perioperative complications, including light-induced tissue damage in 4 patients and neuropathy in 6, as well as recurrent EPP-associated liver disease in 65% of patients who survived more than 2 months. Overall patient and graft survival rates were statistically similar to those for all other patients transplanted in the United States during the same period.[152] Similar results were reported in a European study of 34 liver transplant recipients with EPP-associated liver disease.[150] Therefore liver transplantation must be considered symptomatic therapy, except in patients with ALF, given the high risk of recurrent disease in the graft and the added risk of intraoperative photodynamic injury to internal organs. Hematopoietic stem cell transplantation, which can correct the underlying enzymatic defect, performed after liver transplantation, has been reported to be successful in both children and adults with EPP-induced ESLD.[153,154]

TYROSINEMIA

Four known human diseases are caused by enzymatic deficiencies in the catabolic pathway for the amino acid tyrosine: alkaptonuria and hereditary tyrosinemia (HT) types I, II, and III. Although all the enzymes involved in this pathway are found in the liver, only HT-I leads to progressive liver dysfunction. Formerly known as hepatorenal tyrosinemia, HT-I also affects other organ systems, in particular the kidneys and peripheral nerves. A disease with autosomal recessive transmission, HT-I has a worldwide incidence of about 1 in 100,000. The incidence is higher in Northern Europe (1 per 8000) and in the Saguenay-Lac-St. Jean region of Quebec, Canada (1 per 1846), where a founder effect has been documented.[155] Advances in our understanding of the pathophysiology of the disease process and treatment options that inhibit an early step in the degradation pathway have improved the clinical course of affected persons dramatically.

Pathophysiology

The pathway for tyrosine metabolism is shown in Fig. 79.5. The enzymatic defect in patients with tyrosinemia has been identified in fumarylacetoacetate (FAA) hydrolase (FAH), the final step in the tyrosine degradation process. More than 100 mutations in FAH have been found in patients with HT-I, but no clear correlation between FAH genotype and HT-I phenotype has been appreciated.[156] FAH deficiency leads to accumulation of the upstream metabolites FAA and maleylacetoacetate, which are then converted to the toxic intermediates succinylacetoacetate (SAA) and succinylacetone (SA). FAA has been shown to deplete blood and liver of glutathione, the consequence of which may be augmentation of the mutagenic potential of FAA. SA inhibits renal glucose and amino acid transport and the degradation of ALA to PBG, probably via direct modification of amino acids in enzyme active sites. SA also inhibits DNA ligase activity in fibroblasts isolated from patients with HT-I.[157] Over time, the combined effects of high levels of FAA and SA on the integrity of DNA and cellular repair mechanisms may account for increased chromosomal breakage in fibroblasts isolated from patients with HT-I, as well as an increased risk of HCC.[158]

Clinical and Pathologic Features

Patients with HT-I present either acutely with liver failure or with chronic liver disease, with or without HCC. In the acute form of HT-I, patients manifest liver disease in the first 6 months of life; symptoms include those associated with severe hepatic synthetic dysfunction, such as hypoglycemia, ascites, jaundice, and coagulopathy, as well as anorexia, vomiting, and irritability. Laboratory studies show elevations of serum aminotransferase, GGTP, and bilirubin levels and decreased levels of coagulation factors. Serum tyrosine, methionine, and AFP levels are elevated. Analysis of the urine may reveal phosphaturia, glucosuria, hyperaminoaciduria, renal acidosis, and increased excretion of SA, SAA, ALA, and phenolic acids. The acute form of HT-I, if not promptly treated, is potentially fatal within the first 2 years of life. In a multicenter study, van Spronsen and associates showed that 77% of patients with tyrosinemia presented before the age of 6 months. The 1- and 2-year survival rates were 38% and 29%, respectively, if patients presented between birth and 2 months of age, and 74% and 74%, respectively, if they presented between 2 and 6 months. Survival for both time intervals rose to 96% if the first symptoms appeared after age 6 months. The cause of death was usually recurrent bleeding and liver failure; however, HCC and neurologic crisis accounted for some deaths.[159] Of note, these predate the NTBC treatment era.

Patients with the chronic form of HT-I classically have symptoms that are similar to, but milder than, those with an acute presentation; serum aminotransferase levels as well as plasma tyrosine and methionine levels may be within the normal range. These patients usually present after 1 year of age with hepatomegaly, rickets, nephromegaly, severe hypertension, and growth retardation. They also are likely to have neurologic problems and to develop HCC. The pathologic changes in the liver differ between the acute and chronic forms of the disease. In the acute form, the liver may appear enlarged with a pale nodular pattern or may be shrunken, firm, and brown. Micronodular cirrhosis, fibrotic septa, bile duct proliferation and plugging, steatosis, pseudoacinar and nodular formations, and giant cell transformation may be found on histologic examination. Varying amounts of FAH enzyme activity have been found in liver tissue from patients with HT-I because of spontaneous reversion of FAH gene mutations. Patients with the chronic form of the disease have a higher level of reversion and a lower frequency of liver dysplasia.[159] In the chronic form of tyrosinemia, the liver appears enlarged, coarse, and nodular. In histologic specimens, micronodular and macronodular cirrhosis may be present, as may steatosis, fibrotic septa, and a mild lymphoplasmacytic infiltrate. Cholestasis is less pronounced than in the acute form of HT-I. Large- or small-cell dysplasia may be present, reflecting premalignant changes. Because of the nodular changes, identification of progression to HCC can be difficult. The serum AFP value is elevated before HCC develops, and measurement of AFP is not helpful in the diagnosis. Imaging is required to screen for HCC.

Renal involvement is nearly universal in patients with tyrosinemia. Findings include a decreased GFR, proximal renal tubular dysfunction, nephromegaly, phosphaturia (which is responsible for the development of rickets), glucosuria, and aminoaciduria. The toxic metabolites SA and SAA are thought to have a direct effect on the kidney. Some patients progress to renal failure and require kidney transplantation.[160] One-third of patients develop cardiomyopathy, most commonly interventricular septal hypertrophy, which is reversible with either medical or surgical management of the disease.[161]

The neurologic manifestations may be the most concerning feature in older patients with tyrosinemia; affected patients may experience porphyria-like symptoms with neurologic crises.[162] Further complications include delayed neurodevelopment and attention deficit disorders, which have been reported to occur despite early diagnosis and treatment.[163,164]

Diagnosis

Diagnosis and treatment recommendations are available.[165] The diagnosis of tyrosinemia should be suspected in any child with neonatal liver disease or a bleeding diathesis or in any child older than 1 year with undiagnosed liver disease, rickets, or a hepatic mass. The diagnosis is suggested by increased serum tyrosine, methionine, phenylalanine, and AFP levels. Elevated serum and urine SA and urine ALA levels are regarded as pathognomonic for tyrosinemia. The diagnosis can be confirmed with an assay for FAH in lymphocytes, erythrocytes, skin fibroblasts, or liver tissue. Molecular genetic approaches and targeted mutation analysis are becoming more widely available and are recommended, if possible, for all cases in which SA elevations are detected on newborn screening.

Prenatal diagnosis can be performed by determining SA levels in amniotic fluid or by measuring FAH activity in chorionic villus biopsy specimens. If the specific gene mutation in a family is known, early genetic diagnosis can be made from chorionic villus biopsy specimens as well.[166] Improved newborn screening methodologies measure SA in addition to amino acid levels in dried blood specimens. HT-I is included in both the Secretary of Health and Human Services' Recommended Uniform Screening Panel and the American College of Medical Genetics and Genomics core panel of conditions for which every newborn in the United States should be screened.[165,167]

Treatment

In 1992 Lindstedt and associates published data on the treatment of tyrosinemia with the herbicide 2-(2-nitro-4-trifluoro-methylbenzoyl)-1,3-cyclohexanedione (NTBC).[168] Later, Holme and Lindstedt published the results of a large, long-term study of 220 patients with HT-I who were treated with this agent for up to 7 years.[169] NTBC, known as nitisinone (Orfadin), is a potent inhibitor of 4-hydroxyphenylpyruvate dioxygenase, one of the initial steps in tyrosine metabolism (Fig. 79.6). Blocking the degradation of tyrosine to its downstream toxic metabolites (FAA, SA, and SAA) was postulated to lead to improved hepatic function. Treated patients exhibited improved liver synthetic function, as reflected by a shortening of the prothrombin time, as well as decreased serum aminotransferase levels and a reduction in liver parenchymal heterogeneity and nodules on imaging. In addition, serum AFP and ALA levels decreased, and renal tubular dysfunction reversed.[170] Therefore elevated AFP levels in a patient receiving NTBC therapy should raise concern about the patient's nonadherence to therapy or the development of HCC.[171]

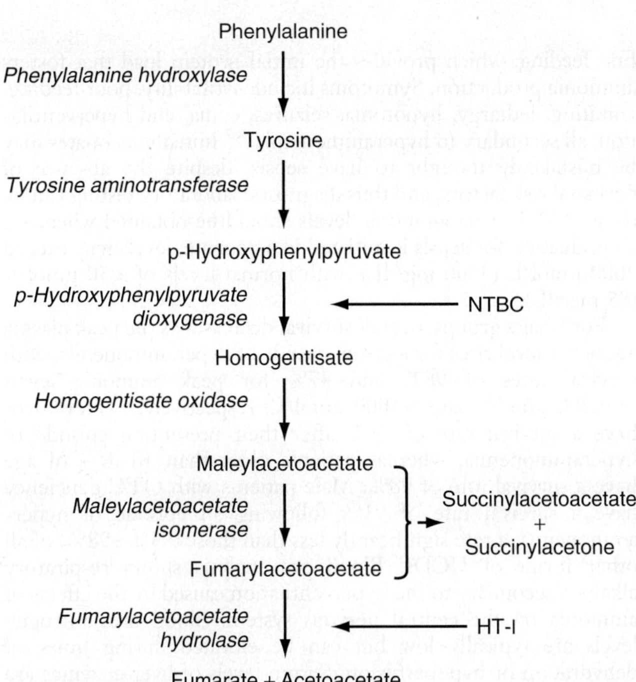

Fig. 79.6 Pathway of tyrosine metabolism. The location of the enzymatic defect in hereditary tyrosinemia type I (HT-I) and the site of action of 2-(2-nitro-4-trifluoro-methylbenzoyl)-1,3-cyclohexanedione (NTBC) are shown. Enzymes are shown in *italics*.

Long-term results have demonstrated continued improvement in all parameters noted in the earlier reports, as well as a reduction in the need for liver transplantation.[172] Cognitive impairment resulting in learning problems may be a complication of long-term use of NTBC in this patient population, possibly from the effects of chronic hypertyrosinemia.[173] NTBC should be started as soon as the diagnosis of HT-I is suspected, starting at 1 mg/kg/day. The total calculated amount of NTBC should be divided into two doses daily in the first year of life. Thereafter, single daily dosing can be considered.[165] Use of NTBC requires careful clinical and biochemical monitoring. A rapid liquid chromatography coupled with negative electrospray ionization tandem mass spectrometry method has been developed and validated for the quantification of NTBC in heparinized human plasma.[174] The minimum dose of NTBC should be used to achieve a blood concentration of 40–60 μmol/L and/or blood SA level within the normal range of the reference laboratory.[165]

Liver transplantation retains a role in the management of HT-I in patients with malignancy or decompensated liver disease refractory to NTBC or in those for whom NTBC is not available.[165] When indicated, liver transplantation provides a metabolic cure. A review of 125 patients with HT-I in the UNOS database who were transplanted before 2008 showed 1- and 5-year survival rates of 90.4%.[175] While novel therapeutic approaches such as viral vector gene therapy[176] and mRNA-based therapy[177] have shown promise in various animal models, human trials will be needed prior to establishing roles in the overall management of tyrosinemia.

UREA CYCLE DEFECTS

The urea cycle consists of five enzymes that process ammonia derived from amino acid metabolism to urea. Genetic defects in each of these enzymes have been reported, and their overall incidence has been estimated to be 1 in 35,000 births, although partial defects may make the number much higher.[178] Although the syndromes related to the UCDs are not associated with serious liver injury, the basic genetic defect is located within the liver, and the manifestations can mimic those of other metabolic liver diseases.

Pathophysiology

The steps of the urea cycle are illustrated in Fig. 79.7. Carbamyl phosphate synthetase (CPS) I forms carbamyl phosphate from ammonium and bicarbonate. This step requires the cofactor *N*-acetyl glutamate, which is synthesized from *N*-acetyl CoA and glutamic acid by *N*-acetyl glutamate synthetase. Ornithine transcarbamylase (OTC) combines carbamyl phosphate with ornithine to form citrulline. A second nitrogen enters the cycle as aspartate, which combines with citrulline by the action of argininosuccinate synthetase (AS) to form argininosuccinate, which is then converted to arginine and fumarate by argininosuccinase, or argininosuccinate lyase (AL). Arginase then catalyzes the breakdown of arginine to urea and ornithine in the final step of the pathway. Several amino acid transporters, such as citrin, an aspartate/glutamate carrier protein that supplies aspartate to the urea cycle, are involved in shuttling metabolites into the urea cycle.[179]

CPS II, through the pyrimidine synthetic pathway, leads to the formation of orotic acid. Excess carbamyl phosphate can be used by this pathway if a block occurs distal to OTC in the metabolic pathway. Excess nitrogen in the form of amino acids can be shunted to alternative pathways of waste-nitrogen excretion by

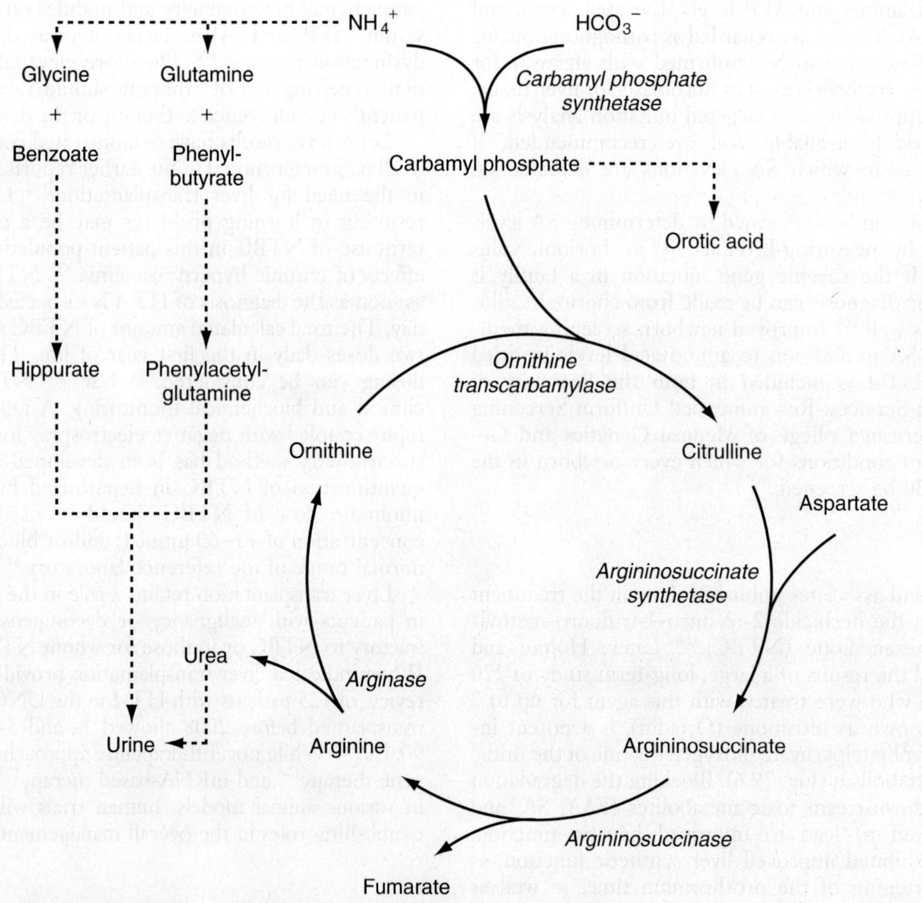

Fig. 79.7 The urea cycle. Alternative pathways that are used therapeutically for waste nitrogen disposal are also illustrated (*dotted lines*). Enzymes are shown in *italics*.

the medicinal use of sodium benzoate and sodium phenylacetate, leading to the generation of hippurate and phenylacetylglutamine, respectively.

Enzymatic defects have been identified in all five steps of the urea cycle. Deficiency of four of the enzymes is transmitted through autosomal recessive inheritance, whereas OTC deficiency is transmitted as an X-linked trait. More than 400 different mutations in the OTC gene give rise to OTC deficiency, the most common UCD.[180] Numerous defects in the other enzymes or amino acid transporters of the cycle (e.g., *N*-acetylglutamate synthetase, citrin) have been characterized as well.[178] Moreover, several mRNA instability mutations have been found in patients with CPS I deficiency.[181]

A UCD has two main biochemical consequences: Arginine becomes an essential amino acid [except in arginase deficiency (see later)], and nitrogen accumulates in a variety of molecules, some of which can have deleterious toxic effects.

Clinical Features

The spectra of clinical presentations in patients with any of the UCDs are virtually identical; in the neonatal period, these disorders classically manifest as acute life-threatening events. Later presentations (>30 days) have been reported in up to two-thirds of patients,[182,183] and late-onset adult presentations have been reported in cases associated with an illness or dietary change[184,185] or with psychiatric symptoms, which may be the initial presenting feature.[186] With the neonatal presentation, affected infants appear normal for the first 24–72 hours until they are exposed to their first feeding, which provides the initial protein load that fosters ammonia production. Symptoms include irritability, poor feeding, vomiting, lethargy, hypotonia, seizures, coma, and hyperventilation, all secondary to hyperammonemia.[187] Initially, neonates may be mistakenly thought to have sepsis, despite the absence of perinatal risk factors, and thus diagnostic laboratory testing can be delayed.[188] Plasma ammonia levels should be obtained whenever an evaluation for sepsis is initiated in a neonate; levels may exceed 2000 μmol/L (3400 mg/dL), with normal levels of <50 μmol/L (85 mg/dL).

For all age groups, overall survival decreases as the peak plasma ammonia level rises for a given episode of hyperammonemia, with survival rates of 98% and 47% for peak ammonia levels of <200 μmol/L and >1000 μmol/L, respectively.[189] Newborns have a survival rate of 73% after their presenting episode of hyperammonemia, whereas patients older than 30 days of age have a survival rate of 98%. Male patients with OTC deficiency have a survival rate of 91% following an episode of hyperammonemia, a rate significantly less than those (93%–98%) of all other forms of UCDs. Blood gas analysis shows respiratory alkalosis secondary to the hyperventilation caused by the effects of ammonia on the central nervous system. Blood urea nitrogen levels are typically low but can be elevated during times of dehydration or hypoperfusion. Serum levels of liver enzymes are usually normal or minimally elevated, although acute liver failure, reflected in severe coagulopathy not corrected by vitamin K, has been reported in up to 50% of patients.[189–191]

OTC deficiency is the most common UCD (57%–62%), followed by argininosuccinic aciduria (AL deficiency, 11.5%

–18%) and citrullinemia (AS deficiency, 13%–19%).[192] Male patients with OTC deficiency have been diagnosed as late as 40 years of age with varied phenotypic presentations. As many as 20% of female carriers of OTC deficiency can have symptoms, which may be severe and fatal, although most female carriers have no symptoms or report only nausea after high-protein meals.[180,193] Late-onset CPS deficiency has also been described,[186] and the adult form of AS deficiency is relatively common in Japan.[194]

Symptoms and signs of late-onset UCDs, especially OTC and CPS deficiencies, include episodic irritability, lethargy, or vomiting; self-induced avoidance of protein such as milk, eggs, and meats; and short stature or growth delays. Neurologic symptoms, which can also be episodic, include ataxia, developmental delays, behavioral abnormalities, combativeness, biting, confusion, hallucinations, headaches, dizziness, visual impairment, diplopia, anorexia, and seizures. Acute hyperammonemic episodes can resemble Reye syndrome (see Chapter 90). Such episodes can be precipitated by high-protein meals, viral or bacterial infections, medications, trauma, or surgery. Infants may present after being weaned from breast milk to infant formulas, which have a higher protein content. Female adult-onset UCD, such as OTC and CPS deficiencies, have been reported to occur during pregnancy and in the postpartum periods secondary to increased physiologic stress and comorbidities such as hyperemesis gravidum.[195,196]

Citrin deficiency, caused by mutations in the *SLC25A13* gene, can manifest in newborns as neonatal intrahepatic cholestasis caused by citrin deficiency (NICCD), in older children as failure to thrive and dyslipidemia caused by citrin deficiency, and in adults as recurrent hyperammonemia and neuropsychiatric symptoms in citrullinemia type II.[197] NICCD is associated with a history of low birth weight with growth restriction and transient intrahepatic cholestasis, hepatomegaly, diffuse fatty liver, and parenchymal cellular infiltration associated with hepatic fibrosis, variable liver dysfunction, hypoproteinemia, decreased coagulation factors, hemolytic anemia, and/or hypoglycemia.[197] Biochemically, NICCD has been shown to have significantly different indices from children with biliary atresia or idiopathic neonatal cholestasis with higher serum bile acid levels, lower aminotransferase levels, and lower direct bilirubin levels compared with disease controls.[198] Other specific findings include increases in blood or plasma concentration of ammonia, plasma or serum concentration of citrulline and arginine, plasma or serum threonine-to-serine ratio, and serum concentration of pancreatic secretory trypsin inhibitor.[197] In most patients with NICCD, all biochemical abnormalities resolve spontaneously or with minimal dietary restrictions (e.g., the use of lactose-free formulas); however, several affected infants have required liver transplantation before 1 year of age. Therefore jaundiced infants with multiple abnormal newborn metabolic screen results must be observed closely because of the risk for development of ESLD caused by NICCD; a chubby face outside the realm of normal may be a diagnostic clue.[199] The diagnosis can be made by sequence analysis of the *SLC25A13* gene.

Diagnosis

Suggested guidelines for the diagnosis and management of the UCDs are available.[187] Ultimately, a high index of suspicion is required for prompt diagnosis of UCDs. Symptoms can mimic those of other acute neonatal problems, such as infections, seizures, and pulmonary or cardiac disease. Later presentations can mimic other behavioral, psychiatric, or developmental disorders. The first clue may be an elevated serum ammonia level with near normal serum aminotransferase levels and without metabolic acidosis. Therefore if a UCD is considered, the following laboratory measurements should be obtained: serum ammonia, arterial blood gases, urine organic acids, serum amino acids, and urinary orotic acid; Table 79.2 reviews the expected results.

Urinary organic acid profiles are typically normal in patients with UCDs; however, the plasma amino acid profiles are distinctive, with abnormal levels of arginine, ornithine, and citrulline. Citrulline levels are barely detectable in OTC or CPS deficiencies but markedly raised in AS and AL deficiencies. AL deficiency can be distinguished from AS deficiency by the finding of argininosuccinic acid in the plasma and urine. OTC deficiency is differentiated from CPS deficiency by excessive urinary excretion of orotic acid. Direct enzyme analysis can be performed and can be useful in patients who have a partial deficiency or who present in adulthood. Early neonatal diagnosis leads to improved survival, so prenatal enzyme and genetic linkage analysis can be carried out in family members of known carriers to aid in early diagnosis.[200]

Treatment

All external protein intake should be discontinued in infants presenting acutely with a suspected or confirmed UCD. An attempt should be made to rapidly restore serum ammonia levels to normal. The use of oral lactulose to lower the nitrogen load has not been studied in this patient population. Given the extremely high ammonia levels often encountered, continuous arteriovenous hemodialysis or hemofiltration is frequently required. Exchange transfusions and peritoneal dialysis are ineffective. Alternative pathways for waste nitrogen disposal should be used, specifically IV administration of sodium benzoate and sodium phenylacetate; however, sodium benzoate should be used with caution in patients with cirrhosis, because a paradoxical rise in blood ammonia levels has been observed.[201] Oral phenylbutyrate can be substituted for phenylacetate to improve palatability.

Levels of serum arginine, carnitine, and long-chain fatty acids are usually low in affected patients and should be supplemented.[187,202] Low-dose arginine (100 mg/kg/day) together with an ammonia scavenger is effective in repleting arginine stores, maintaining low ammonia levels, and minimizing liver enzyme elevations compared with high-dose arginine (500 mg/kg/day), although consensus guidelines recommend an intermediate dose

TABLE 79.2 Laboratory Values in Urea Cycle Defects

Enzyme Deficiency	Ammonia (Plasma)	Citrulline (Serum)	Argininosuccinate (Urine or Serum)	Orotic Acid (Urine)	Arginine/Ornithine (Serum)
Carbamyl phosphate synthetase	↑–↑↑↑	↓	↓	↓	↓
Ornithine transcarbamylase	↑–↑↑↑	↓	↓	↑↑	↓
Argininosuccinate synthetase	↑–↑↑↑	↑↑↑	↓	Normal–↑	↓
Argininosuccinase	↑–↑↑↑	↑↑↑	↑↑↑	Normal–↑	↓
Arginase	↑	↑↑	↑↑	Normal–↑	↑↑

of arginine (250 mg/kg/day).[187,203] Once the patient stabilizes, low levels of dietary protein, 0.5–1 g/kg, may be introduced, with progressive increases as tolerated to provide sufficient protein for growth and tissue repair while minimizing urea production. Further therapy and protein restriction are then tailored to the patient; those with a severe disorder may need essential amino acids to supplement their protein intake. Long-term dietary treatment strategies for UCD vary significantly among conditions and centers. Further studies examining the outcome of treatment compared with the type of dietary therapy and nutritional support received are needed.[204,205]

The outcome for patients who present with hyperammonemic coma and a delayed diagnosis is poor.[189] The level of ammonia at the time of the first hyperammonemic episode is a rough guide to the eventual neurodevelopmental outcome.[206] The sooner the hyperammonemia is treated and the correct diagnosis is made, the better the long-term survival; however, for patients who survive the neonatal period, there remains a high risk of recurrence of severe hyperammonemic crises, often during intercurrent viral infections, which correspond to a high mortality rate.[207]

Patients with a UCD and deterioration or lack of improvement despite therapy have undergone either orthotopic or auxiliary liver transplantation successfully (see Chapter 99), with normalization of enzyme activity and ammonia levels, restored ability to tolerate a normal diet, and survival rates of 93%, 89%, and 87% at 1, 5, and 10 years, respectively.[208] Liver transplantation, if considered, should ideally be done before neurologic damage is permanent, because the patient's neurologic status may not improve after liver transplantation. A possible exception is patients transplanted before the age of 1 year, in whom developmental, and possible neurocognitive, outcomes may improve.[209,210] Hepatocyte transplantation has demonstrated some success in patients with UCDs; however, metabolic cure has not been achieved.[211,212] A phase I/II trial of liver-derived mesenchymal stem cells demonstrated overall safety, and ongoing efforts seek to establish a more definitive role for this strategy.[213]

The importance of identifying the deleterious mutation in a patient with a UCD will likely become increasingly important not only as a means of allowing carrier testing and prenatal diagnosis, but also as an aid to treatment decisions. For example, patients with a mutation that results in the most severe OTC deficiency (e.g., abolished enzyme activity) may benefit preferentially from immediate liver transplantation to prevent severe intellectual disability or death, whereas those with a mutation that leads to milder disease may be better managed medically with dietary restrictions and ammonia scavengers to facilitate growth before possible liver transplantation. Although the use of gene therapy has an ominous history with the UCDs,[214] its use may need to be reconsidered in the future because success in correcting the underlying metabolic abnormalities has been demonstrated in knockout mice.[215]

Arginase Deficiency

At least two forms of arginase activity occur in humans. Arginase I predominates in the liver and red blood cells, and arginase II is found predominantly in kidney and prostate. Arginase deficiency involving arginase I is the least common of the UCDs. Hyperammonemia is unusual in affected persons, but hyperammonemic coma and death have been reported.[216] Clinical features are distinct from those of the other UCDs. The disease is characterized by indolent deterioration of the cerebral cortex and pyramidal tracts, leading to progressive dementia and psychomotor retardation, spastic diplegia progressing to quadriplegia, seizures, and growth failure. The syndrome is often confused with cerebral palsy.[217]

Laboratory studies may reveal elevated blood arginine values, mild hyperammonemia, and a mild increase in urine orotic acid excretion. Many guanidine compounds may accumulate in the blood and cerebrospinal fluid of these patients, which could play an important pathophysiologic role, and guanidinoacetate, a well-known potent epileptogenic compound, has demonstrated usefulness as a target for the therapeutic monitoring of patients with arginase deficiency.[218] Varying amounts of urea are still produced in these patients secondary to the compensatory elevated expression of arginase II in the kidneys that ameliorates the clinical disorder. The diagnosis is confirmed by enzymatic analysis, which can be performed prenatally on cord blood samples. Treatment consists of protein restriction and, when needed, sodium phenylbutyrate.[219]

BILE ACID SYNTHESIS AND TRANSPORT DEFECTS

The pathways for bile acid synthesis and the mechanism of bile acid transport within the hepatobiliary system are complex, involving several enzymes and regulated transport processes located in multiple subcellular fractions of the hepatocyte (see Chapter 66). With advances in molecular biology, genetics, and mass spectrometry, several different inborn errors in bile acid synthesis and transport have been identified as causes of clinical disease. The classification of these disorders has been clarified, particularly in the clinically heterogeneous subset of cases that comprise progressive familial intrahepatic cholestasis (PFIC) syndromes. For some of the disorders, this progress has led to improved diagnosis and life-saving therapy.[220]

PFIC refers to a heterogeneous group of mostly autosomal-recessive disorders that disrupt bile formation and present with cholestasis of hepatocellular origin. Historically, the diagnosis of PFIC has been imprecise; broad criteria have included the presence of chronic, unremitting intrahepatic cholestasis, exclusion of identifiable metabolic or anatomic disorders, and characteristic clinical, biochemical, and histologic features. Other symptoms and signs are severe pruritus, hepatomegaly, wheezing and cough, short stature, delayed sexual development, fat-soluble vitamin deficiency, and cholelithiasis. Affected persons exhibit severe and progressive intrahepatic cholestasis, usually manifesting within the first few months of life and often proceeding to cirrhosis and ESLD by the second decade of life.[221]

Specific types of PFIC due to defective bile acid synthesis or transport have been identified, and each is associated with mutations in enzymes or hepatocellular transport-system genes involved in bile formation. With the discovery of these specific defects and the development of sophisticated biochemical and molecular methodology and gene mutation analysis, precise characterization is now possible using techniques such as mass spectrometry, multigene cholestasis panels, and DNA sequencing by capillary electrophoresis. These complementary tests allow rapid, sensitive, and cost-effective bile acid profiling and mutation screening to aid clinical diagnosis in patients with intrahepatic cholestasis. Patients previously believed to have idiopathic neonatal hepatitis or an undiagnosed familial hepatitis syndrome may now be diagnosed accurately. Table 79.3 lists the known errors of primary and secondary bile acid synthesis and transport.

Bile Acid Synthesis Defects

Defects in bile acid synthesis due to mutations in genes that encode the enzymes responsible for primary bile acid formation may have profound effects on hepatic and GI function and integrity. Disorders in bile acid synthesis and metabolism can be broadly classified as primary or secondary. Primary enzyme defects involve congenital deficiencies in enzymes responsible for

TABLE 79.3 Inborn Errors of Bile Acid Synthesis and Transport

Defects in Bile Acid Synthesis	
Alterations of the enzymes involved in modification of the steroid ring	3β-hydroxy-Δ^5-C_{27}-steroid oxidoreductase deficiency *(HSD3B7)* Δ^4-3-oxosteroid 5β-reductase deficiency *(AKR1D1)* Oxysterol 7α-hydroxylase deficiency *(CYP7B1)* Cholesterol 7α-hydroxylase deficiency *(CYP7A1)* 12α-hydroxylase deficiency *(CYP8B1)*
Alterations of the enzymes involved in modification of the side chain	CTX-sterol 27-hydroxylase deficiency *(CYP27A1)* 2-methylacyl-CoA racemase deficiency *(AMACAR)* Bile acid–CoA: amino acid *N*-acyl-transferase deficiency *(BAAT)* Bile acid–CoA ligase deficiency *(BACL; SLC27A5)* Sterol 25-hydroxylase deficiency *(CH25H)*
Organelle or cell injury	Peroxisomal biogenesis disorders Zellweger syndrome Neonatal adrenoleukodystrophy Infantile Refsum disease Rhizomelic chondrodysplasia punctata Disorders with loss of a single peroxisomal function Generalized hepatic synthetic dysfunction ALF (multiple causes) Neonatal iron storage disease Tyrosinemia Disorders of cholesterol metabolism Smith-Lemli-Opitz syndrome *(DHCR7)*
Defects in Bile Acid or Phospholipid Transport	
	PFIC type I: FIC1 deficiency *(ATP8B1, or FIC1)* Byler disease Benign recurrent intrahepatic cholestasis Greenland familial cholestasis PFIC type II: BSEP deficiency *(ABCB11)* PFIC type III: MDR3 deficiency *(ABCB4)* Farnesoid X receptor *(NR1H4)* Myosin VB *(MYO5B)*
Disorders of Cytoskeleton and Tight Junction Protein	
	PFIC type IV: TJP2 deficiency *(TJP2)* USP53 deficiency *(USP53)* *LSR* *VPS50* *PLEC*

Corresponding genes are shown in *italics*. *BSEP*, Bile salt export pump; *FIC1*, familial intrahepatic cholestasis 1; *MDR*, multidrug resistance protein; *PFIC*, progressive familial intrahepatic cholestasis; *TJP*, tight junction protein.

catalyzing key reactions in the synthesis of cholic acid and chenodeoxycholic acid (CDCA). The primary defects include cholesterol 7α-hydroxylase (CYP7A1) deficiency, 3β-hydroxy-C_{27}-steroid oxidoreductase deficiency, Δ^4-3-oxosteroid 5β-reductase deficiency, oxysterol 7α-hydroxylase deficiency, 27-hydroxylase deficiency or cerebrotendinous xanthomatosis (CTX), 2-methylacyl-CoA racemase deficiency, trihydroxycholestanoic acid CoA oxidase deficiency, amidation defects involving a deficiency in the bile acid–CoA ligase, and a side-chain oxidation defect in the 25-hydroxylation pathway for bile acid resulting in an overproduction of bile alcohols. Secondary metabolic defects that impact primary bile acid synthesis include peroxisomal disorders, such as cerebrohepatorenal syndrome of Zellweger and related disorders, and Smith-Lemli-Opitz syndrome. Typical biochemical abnormalities detected in patients with bile acid synthetic defects include elevated serum aminotransferase and conjugated bilirubin levels with normal GGTP levels; serum cholesterol concentrations are also usually normal.[222]

These disorders respond well to replacement and displacement therapy.[223] Such therapy is based on the principle that inborn errors of bile acid biosynthesis lead to underproduction of normal trophic and choleretic primary bile acids and overproduction of hepatotoxic primitive bile acid metabolites.[224] Replacement therapy with cholic acid is effective; ursodeoxycholic acid (UDCA) may also be effective. The former bypasses the enzymatic block and provides negative feedback to earlier steps in the synthetic pathways, whereas the latter displaces toxic bile acid metabolites and serves as a hepatobiliary cytoprotectant.[225]

Diagnosis

Marked alterations in urinary, serum, and biliary bile acid composition and concentration may be found in infants and children with severe liver disease of any etiology. Therefore determining whether these changes are primary or secondary to the liver dysfunction may be difficult, and a detailed biochemical evaluation is necessary. Initially, defects in bile acid synthesis were discovered with the use of liquid secondary ionization mass spectrometry; specifically, fast atom bombardment ionization mass spectrometry allowed direct analysis of bile acids from a drop of urine. More advanced mass spectrometry approaches, including electrospray ionization tandem mass spectrometry, as well as gene sequencing techniques, have subsequently been applied. The mass spectra generated permit accurate identification of the absence of primary bile acids and presence of atypical bile acids specific to each primary defect.[226]

Disorders of Enzymes Involved in Modification of the Steroid Ring

The most common inborn error of bile acid biosynthesis is *3β-hydroxy-Δ^5-C_{27}-steroid dehydrogenase/isomerase (3β-HSD) deficiency*. This disorder is caused by deficient activity of the second step in the bile acid synthetic pathway, the conversion of 7α-hydroxycholesterol into 7α-hydroxy-4-cholesten-3-one. This reaction is catalyzed by a microsomal 3β-hydroxy-Δ^5-C_{27}-steroid oxidoreductase; deficiency of this enzyme results in the accumulation of 7α-hydroxycholesterol within the hepatocyte. The normal primary bile acids (cholic acid and CDCA) are not formed; instead, C_{24}-bile acids that retain the 3β-hydroxy-Δ^5-structure are synthesized. Affected patients may present with pruritus, jaundice, hepatomegaly, steatorrhea, and fat-soluble vitamin deficiencies.[224,226] Reports of 3β-HSD deficiency in adults not only highlight the clinical utility of homozygosity mapping in diagnosing autosomal recessive metabolic disorders but also illustrate the wide variation in expressivity that occurs in 3β-HSD deficiency and underscore the need to consider a bile acid synthetic defect as a possible cause of liver disease in patients of all ages.[227]

Δ^4-3-Oxosteroid 5β-reductase (AKR1D1) deficiency was first described in monochorionic twins born with marked and progressive cholestasis.[228] This cytosolic enzyme is responsible for the conversion of 7α-hydroxy- and 7α,12α-dihydroxy-4-cholesten-3-one into the corresponding 3-oxo-5β (H) analogs.

Deficiency of Δ^4-3-oxosteroid 5β-reductase usually leads to neonatal cholestasis, which rapidly progresses to synthetic dysfunction and liver failure.[228,229] *Cholesterol 7a-hydroxylase (CYP7A1) deficiency* is associated with hypertriglyceridemia and gallstone disease in adults; it does not present as cholestatic disease.

Disorders of Enzymes Involved in Side-Chain Modification

Aberrant bile acid side-chain hydroxylation and oxidation may manifest as neurologic disease and/or fat-soluble vitamin malabsorption; in general, liver disease is mild in affected patients (see Table 79.3).[230]

CTX, sterol-27-hydroxylase deficiency, is a rare autosomal recessive neurologic disease. Clinical symptoms and signs include adult-onset progressive neurologic dysfunction (i.e., ataxia, dystonia, dementia, epilepsy, psychiatric disorders, peripheral neuropathy, and myopathy) and premature nonneurologic manifestations (i.e., tendon xanthomas, childhood-onset cataracts, infantile-onset diarrhea, premature atherosclerosis, osteoporosis, and respiratory insufficiency).[231] CTX is caused by a mutation in the sterol 27-hydroxylase gene *(CYP27A1)* and has been treated with CDCA (see Chapters 66 and 67).[232] The classical symptoms and signs, namely elevated levels of cholestanol and bile alcohols in serum and urine, abnormal brain MRI, and the mutation in the *CYP27A1* gene confirm the diagnosis of CTX.[231] Prompt diagnosis and initiation of CDCA treatment is important in preventing neurologic damage and deterioration. After significant neurologic pathology is established, the effect of treatment is limited and deterioration may continue.[233]

2-Methylacyl Co-A racemase deficiency has been identified in an infant presenting with mildly elevated liver enzyme levels and low serum 25-hydroxyvitamin D and vitamin E concentrations.[234]

Finally, bile acid synthesis culminates in conjugation with glycine and taurine, and genetic defects in conjugation and amidation have been identified using mass spectrometry analysis of urine, bile, and serum samples and sequence analysis of the genes encoding bile acid–CoA:amino acid *N*-acyltransferase and bile acid–CoA ligase (gene symbol *SLC27A5*).[230] Affected persons exhibit fat-soluble vitamin deficiency and growth failure, indicating the importance of bile acid conjugation in lipid absorption. In some patients, liver disease with features of a cholangiopathy has been present. Oral glycocholic acid therapy has been shown to be safe and effective in improving growth and fat-soluble vitamin absorption in children and adolescents with these disorders.[235]

Peroxisomal Disorders

Peroxisomes are responsible for beta oxidation in the final steps of bile acid synthesis to yield the primary bile acids, cholic acid and CDCA. Defects in peroxisomal assembly and function have a significant impact on bile acid synthesis, because peroxisomes contain multiple enzymes required for the oxidation and conjugation of bile acids. The peroxisomopathies encompass a diverse group of genetic disorders caused by impairment in one or more peroxisomal functions. These disorders are subdivided into three main groups: (1) peroxisome biogenesis disorders (PBDs) that cause multiple abnormalities, (2) single peroxisomal protein (enzyme) deficiencies that result in limited dysfunction, and (3) single peroxisomal substrate transport deficiencies.[236] PBDs comprise a group of disorders that share similar clinical and biochemical features; this group includes Zellweger syndrome (ZS), neonatal adrenoleukodystrophy (NALD), infantile Refsum disease (IRD), and rhizomelic chondrodysplasia punctata, which is characterized by severe rhizomelic shortening of the limbs, severe skeletal abnormalities, cataracts, and facial abnormalities.[236]

PBDs are caused by defects in any of at least 14 different PEX (or peroxin) genes, which encode proteins involved in peroxisome assembly and proliferation. The single peroxisomal enzyme deficiency group consists of D-bifunctional protein and phytanoyl-CoA hydroxylase (adult Refsum disease) deficiencies, among others. The single peroxisomal substrate transport deficiency group consists of only one disease, X-linked adrenoleukodystrophy.[237]

These neurometabolic diseases are highly variable in age of onset and severity, with clinical and biochemical consequences dependent on the specific function of the affected protein in peroxisomal metabolism. The spectrum includes death in infancy, rapid functional decline, slow decline over a long term, and an apparently stable course. Leukoencephalopathy may be detected on cerebral MRI.[238]

Liver histologic changes are frequent in patients with peroxisomal disorders.[239] Collectively, a comparison of different patients (and mouse models of disease) does not provide an unambiguous picture of the histologic findings. Whereas accumulating bile acid intermediates seem to underlie liver damage and failure with some disorders,[234,240] comparable levels do not elicit pathology in other instances.[241–243]

Zellweger spectrum disorders (ZSD) include three separate entities considered different presentations within the same clinical and biochemical spectrum: ZS, NALD, and IRD.[236] The multiple features of ZSD include distinctive dysmorphic features (hypertelorism, large anterior fontanelle, deformed earlobes), neonatal hypotonia, impaired hearing, retinopathy, cataracts, seizures, and skeletal changes. Patients with ZS often die within the first years of life, whereas those with NALD and IRD often reach their teens and even early adulthood.[236] Hepatomegaly is common, and the progressive liver disease that develops in patients with ZS is similar to that identified in other errors of bile acid synthesis.[244] Peroxisome biogenesis involves multiple PEX genes and requires the targeting and importation of cytosolic proteins into the peroxisomal membrane and matrix. Importation of proteins fated for the peroxisomal matrix requires guidance from one of two peroxisome-targeting signals, PTS1 and PTS2. Patients with ZSD display defects in the importation of proteins that use PTS1 and PTS2, whereas patients with rhizomelic chondrodysplasia punctata have a defect in the importation of proteins that use PTS2.[245]

The most common disorder of peroxisomes, adrenoleukodystrophy, is included in the second group of peroxisomopathies. This disorder results from a defect in the peroxisomal adrenoleukodystrophy protein, which is a member of the ATP-binding cassette (ABC) superfamily of membrane transporters (see Chapter 66).[246] NALD, a distinct genetic disorder of autosomal recessive inheritance, must be distinguished from ZS and X-linked adrenoleukodystrophy; all three conditions lead to storage of very-long-chain fatty acids. Clinical features in NALD, present at birth, include hypotonia, severe psychomotor delay, and failure to thrive.

These disorders are associated with multiple clinical abnormalities and a wide range of biochemical abnormalities. They are diagnosed through a combination of biochemical and histologic assessment, such as a search for very-long-chain fatty acids and ultrastructural abnormalities in tissue biopsy specimens, and genetic confirmation of suspected patients can be performed by sequencing candidate genes.[236] DNA testing for PBDs may be used for carrier testing of relatives, early prenatal diagnosis or preimplantation genetic diagnosis, and counseling in families with a risk of recurrence for one of these disorders.

Bile Acid Transport Defects

The study of intrahepatic cholestasis syndromes has enhanced our understanding of hepatic excretory function and bile acid metabolism (see Chapter 66). The spectrum of diseases associated with mutations in genes involved in bile acid transport physiology is large and growing. The precise terminology used to describe these disorders continues to evolve as well (see Table 79.3). Historically, the PFIC family of diseases included a group of rare disorders presumably caused by specific defects in bile secretion. The three classic disorders of bile acid transport defects included familial intrahepatic cholestasis 1 (FIC1) disease (Byler disease, PFIC1), bile salt export pump (BSEP) disease (PFIC2), and multidrug resistance protein 3 (MDR3) disease (PFIC3). However, it was long suspected that additional genetic defects related to bile acid transport may be responsible for a similar phenotype; multiple subsequent genetic diseases associated with low-GGTP intrahepatic cholestasis have been identified, including mutations in the genes for tight junction protein 2 (TJP2), myosin VB, and the nuclear bile acid farnesoid X receptor (FXR).[221,247–250] Diagnosis has been aided by the development of several resequencing chips that efficiently identify the most common disease-causing mutations.

FIC1 disease (also called *PFIC type I*, or PFIC1) encompasses a continuum comprising intermediate phenotypes of at least three disease states: Byler disease, which generally presents in infancy and leads to progressive cholestasis often associated with severe pruritus; benign recurrent intrahepatic cholestasis (BRIC) type I, which gives rise to recurrent episodes of intrahepatic cholestasis beginning in childhood or adulthood that can last days to months and resolve spontaneously without causing detectable lasting liver damage; and intrahepatic cholestasis of pregnancy (ICP) type 1, which is a transient cholestasis limited to pregnancy with complete resolution after delivery. The occurrence of extrahepatic features in patients with FIC1 disease, including chronic diarrhea, deafness, and pancreatic insufficiency, suggests a biological cell function for the FIC1 protein.

In patients with FIC1 disease, serum GGTP and cholesterol levels are normal or mildly elevated, and levels of bile acids are elevated in the serum and low in the bile. Serum aminotransferase and bilirubin levels are mildly elevated as well. Impaired bile acid transport in the intestine may account for the striking malabsorption and diarrhea in some patients. These intestinal clinical features do not resolve after liver transplantation and may worsen as cholestasis is improved and the terminal ileum is exposed to a normal bile acid concentration. Histology of liver tissue from patients with FIC1 disease typically shows bland canalicular cholestasis, with varying degrees of hepatocellular ballooning and giant cell transformation; portal fibrosis and eventually cirrhosis may be seen later in the course of the disease. (The liver histology of patients with BRIC type I and ICP type 1 is classically normal). On electron microscopic evaluation of liver tissue from patients with FIC1 disease, characteristic coarse, granular bile deposits are seen in the canaliculus ("Byler's bile").[221]

FIC1 disease is caused by mutations in the *ATP8B1* gene (initially named the *FIC1* gene) that encodes the FIC1 protein, a P-type adenosine triphosphatase involved in ATP-dependent aminophospholipid transport. FIC1 protein is expressed on the hepatocyte canalicular membrane and in several other organs, including the intestine and pancreas. The mechanisms by which FIC1 protein dysfunction leads to the phenotype of low-GGTP cholestasis remain uncertain. Two pathophysiologic mechanisms have been proposed. The first involves the maintenance of canalicular membrane integrity via the enrichment of phosphatidylserine and phosphatidylethanolamine on the inner leaflet of the plasma membrane, including microvilli formation. In disease states, FIC1 dysfunction results in an abnormal constitution of lipids at the canalicular membrane with resulting disruption of the biliary secretion of bile acids, which explains the reduced biliary bile acid concentrations found in patients with FIC1 disease. The second proposed mechanism stems from the finding that impaired ATP8B1 function can downregulate FXR, a nuclear receptor involved in the regulation of bile acid metabolism, with subsequent downregulation of BSEP protein in the liver and upregulation of bile acid synthesis and of the apical sodium bile salt transporter in the intestine (see Chapter 66).[221]

BSEP disease (PFIC type II, or PFIC2) is caused by a wide spectrum of mutations in the *ABCB11* gene, which encodes an ABC protein that serves as the canalicular BSEP, the major transport protein governing the secretion of bile acids from hepatocytes into bile. BSEP, which is expressed exclusively in hepatocytes, is localized to the canalicular membrane and is therefore responsible for the bile salt-dependent bile flow, governing the transport of monovalent bile acids (see Chapter 64).

Patients with the progressive form of BSEP disease present with high serum bile acid levels but low or low-normal serum GGTP levels and usually have intense pruritus, jaundice, poor weight gain, and hepatosplenomegaly.[221] Genotype-phenotype correlations have been established based on the degree of predicted protein dysfunction and suggest that in patients with the most severe dysfunction, native liver survival and response to therapy may be suboptimal.[251] In addition, genetically distinct forms of BRIC and ICP (type II) are associated with mutations in *ABCB11*. Patients with BRIC type II commonly have cholelithiasis and lack other extrahepatic manifestations.[252]

Early in the course of BSEP disease, nonspecific giant cell hepatitis is found on histologic examination of the liver, and on electron microscopy amorphous bile deposits are seen in the canaliculi. For unclear reasons, patients with clinically severe, nonremitting intrahepatic cholestasis ascribed to *ABCB11* mutations associated with absence or severe deficiency of BSEP expression have an increased risk of developing malignancies of the hepatobiliary system, such as hepatoblastoma, HCC, and cholangiocarcinoma.[251,253] Children who undergo orthotopic liver transplantation for severe BSEP deficiency are at risk for post-transplantation episodes of cholestatic dysfunction that mimics the original disease secondary to the development of BSEP antibodies posttransplantation.[254] This phenomenon has been termed antibody-induced BSEP deficiency, and remission can be achieved by intensifying immunosuppressive therapy or adding antibody-depleting medications to the regimen.[255]

MDR3 disease (PFIC type III, or PFIC3) is caused by mutations in the *ABCB4* gene that encodes the MDR3 glycoprotein, an ABC phosphatidylcholine translocase expressed on the canalicular membrane of hepatocytes.[221] This phospholipid translocator is involved in biliary phospholipid (phosphatidylcholine) excretion.[256] MDR3 deficiency is thought to lead to cholestasis via decreased excretion of cytoprotective biliary phospholipids, leaving an increased pool of cytotoxic, detergent biliary bile acids that are not inactivated by phospholipids and giving rise to bile duct damage and proliferation and release of GGTP into the serum.

Patients with MDR3 disease present with several disease phenotypes as well, ranging from neonatal cholestasis to the later presentation of cirrhosis, intrahepatic and gallbladder lithiasis, ICP, adult-onset ductopenic cholestatic liver disease, drug-induced cholestasis, and some cases of transient neonatal cholestasis, adult idiopathic cirrhosis, and cholangiocarcinoma.[257,258] Patients with MDR3 deficiency present with high serum levels of GGTP and bile acids as well as bile ductular proliferation on routine microscopy. Some female patients with ICP have been shown to be heterozygous carriers of a mutation in *ABCB4*; other nongenetic factors are likely required for full expression of the disease.[253]

Identifying the genetic causes of cholestasis has led to advancements in the understanding of the pathophysiology of liver diseases. Other chronic intrahepatic cholestatic diseases with known genetic components include *North American Indian childhood cirrhosis*, which is caused by a single point mutation in the cirhin gene encoding a nucleolar protein of unknown function,[259] *neonatal icthyosis sclerosing cholangitis* due to mutations in the gene encoding claudin-1,[260] neonatal sclerosing cholangitis due to mutations in the gene encoding *doublecortin domain–containing*

2 protein,[261] and *arthrogryposis-renal dysfunction-cholestasis syndrome* due to mutations in the *VP533B* (vacuolar protein sorting 33B) gene. Yet in many individuals, particularly those with normal-GGTP progressive cholestasis, genetic mutations have not been identified,[262] and novel gene sequencing techniques are being applied to elucidate the genetic causes.

Collectively, these efforts have led to the discovery of new genes for which dysfunction or absence of the encoded protein results in the phenotype of progressive cholestasis. Homozygous, truncating mutations in *TJP2* with resulting absence of the TJP2 (also known as zona-occludens-2) have been reported in children with severe liver disease, often requiring liver transplantation.[250,263] Mutations in *NR1H4*, which encodes FXR, a bile acid-activated nuclear hormone receptor that regulates bile acid metabolism through its promotion of BSEP trafficking to the canalicular membrane, can cause cholestatic liver disease.[247] Clinical features of severe, persistent *NR1H4*-related cholestasis include neonatal onset with rapid progression to ESLD, vitamin K–independent coagulopathy, low-to-normal serum GGTP activity, elevated serum AFP levels, and undetectable liver BSEP expression.[247] In a similar fashion, defects in myosin VB, encoded by *MYO5B*, previously identified as disease-causing mutations in children with microvillus inclusion disease, have been shown to impair the targeting of BSEP to the canalicular membrane, thereby resulting in hampered bile acid secretion and cholestasis. The intractable diarrhea that defines microvillus inclusion disease can be absent or mild, and *MYO5B deficiency* has been hypothesized to underlie up to 20% of previously undiagnosed cases of low-GGTP cholestasis.[248,249] Homozygous loss-of-function variants in the *Ubiquitin-specific protease 53 (USP53)*, a protein thought to colocalize with TJP2 and contribute to tight junction stability, have been identified in patients with early onset cholestasis.[264]

Classically, individuals with genetic mutations resulting in cholestasis have presented in the neonatal period; however, as newer analytic methods are developed, an expanded role for mutations in these genes has been identified as causative of both cryptogenic cholestasis in adults and in ICP.[265]

Treatment

Symptomatic improvement in pruritus, optimization of nutritional status, and management of complications of chronic liver disease constitute the main medical approaches to treatment in patients with disorders of bile acid transport. Supportive treatment requires supplementation of fat-soluble vitamins (A, D, E, and K) and administration of medium-chain TGs, which are absorbed independently of bile acids. Antipruritic agents such as UDCA, rifampin, hydroxyzine, cholestyramine, naloxone, and sertraline have demonstrated varying degrees of success (see Chapter 93). Importantly, while treatment usually includes a combination of the therapies described, their overall effects remain suboptimal. Surgical interruption of the enterohepatic circulation by ileal exclusion or partial biliary diversion has been shown to be well tolerated and generally, although not uniformly, results in improvement in pruritus and cholestasis[266]; however, the presence of cirrhosis at the time of diversion has been associated with poor outcomes, and recurrent, self-limited cholestasis episodes can occur.[267] Development of the family of medications referred to as the ileal bile acid transporter (IBAT) inhibitors has introduced a novel tool in the armamentarium for the medical treatment of PFIC. These compounds induce a pharmacological interruption of the enterohepatic circulation and have been shown in clinical studies to reduce the bile salt pool size, alleviate pruritus, and reduce the need for surgical intervention.[268,269] Several IBAT inhibitors have been approved for pediatric patients with PFIC as well as patients with Alagille syndrome, another cholestatic disease in children that can share many features of the PFIC disorders.[270] Liver transplantation can lead to good overall outcomes, with normalization of bile acid synthesis and growth, even in patients who receive a live-donor organ from a potentially heterozygous parent.[253] Extrahepatic manifestations of FIC1 deficiency, such as diarrhea, can worsen after transplantation. The resulting malnutrition has been linked to the development of fatty infiltration of the liver graft that can progress to the development of cirrhosis and require retransplantation. In these rare cases, internal and external biliary diversions have demonstrated some success in ameliorating the disease process.[271]

CYSTIC FIBROSIS

Defects in the CFTR protein, found on the apical surface of cholangiocytes, lead to a wide spectrum of hepatobiliary conditions collectively referred to as CF-associated liver disease (CFLD).[272] Although the pulmonary manifestations of CF historically have dominated the all-cause mortality, improvements in lung disease management have resulted in an increased frequency of extrapulmonary complications, and CFLD is now the third leading cause of mortality in patients with CF.[273]

Clinical and Pathologic Features

The clinical features of CFLD are varied and have been noted to include liver enzyme elevations, hepatic steatosis, neonatal cholestasis, focal biliary cirrhosis (FBC), multilobular cirrhosis, noncirrhotic portal hypertension, gallbladder abnormalities, and cholangiopathy[272,273]; however, liver involvement in CF is not a universal feature of the disease. Although CF has been identified in fewer than 2% of patients with neonatal cholestasis, the diagnosis should be considered in any infant who presents with neonatal jaundice. Up to 40% of patients may have clinical or symptomatic liver disease after the neonatal period.[274] In subjects with CFLD, disease usually develops early in childhood (approximately 10 years of age) and is more common in boys than in girls.[275]

Hepatobiliary diseases noted in patients with CF can be grouped into three categories (Table 79.4). The pathognomonic lesion of CF is FBC, with and without evidence of portal hypertension; an increasing frequency of noncirrhotic portal hypertension has been reported in patients with CF.[276,277] At autopsy, FBC has been identified with a frequency of 11%–50%.[273] Progression to multilobular biliary cirrhosis occurs in 5%–10% of patients with CF and leads to symptoms associated with portal hypertension, such as splenomegaly and variceal bleeding.[278] Hepatic steatosis also develops in roughly half of patients but does not appear to correlate with outcome. Biliary abnormalities range from microgallbladder, which is largely asymptomatic and is found in up to 20% of patients, to cholelithiasis and cholangiocarcinoma.[279] The presence of liver disease does not necessarily correlate with the severity of pulmonary disease.

Pathophysiology

The pathogenesis of CFLD is complex. The pathognomonic lesion of CF, FBC, presumably results from defective function of the CFTR protein and is thought to result from obstruction of small bile ducts leading to chronic inflammatory changes, bile duct proliferation, and portal fibrosis. CFTR dysfunction has been shown to lead to fibrotic liver disease in a murine model.[280] An additional mechanism by which a defective CFTR protein is thought to induce biliary disease is through a complex relationship among CFTR, Toll-like receptor 4, and the Rous sarcoma oncogene cellular homolog (Src). Under normal physiologic conditions, CFTR acts to regulate Toll-like receptor 4, which in turn inhibits Src activity. When CFTR is defective, however, Src

TABLE 79.4 Hepatobiliary Disease in Patients with CF

Specific to CF	Hepatic Focal biliary cirrhosis with inspissation Multilobular biliary cirrhosis with inspissation Biliary Microgallbladder Mucocele Mucous hyperplasia of the gallbladder
Secondary to extrahepatic disease	Hepatic (associated with cardio-pulmonary disease) Centrilobular necrosis Cirrhosis Pancreatic Fibrosis (leading to bile duct compression/stricture)
Increased in frequency in patients with CF	Hepatic Drug hepatotoxicity Fatty liver Neonatal cholestasis Viral hepatitis Biliary Biliary sludge Cholangiocarcinoma Cholelithiasis Sclerosing cholangitis

Modified from Balistreri WF. Liver disease in infancy and childhood. In: Schiff ER, Sorrell MF, Maddrey WC, eds. *Schiff's Diseases of the Liver*. 9th ed. Philadelphia: Lippincott-Raven; 1999:1379.

can self-activate, leading to increased production of inflammatory cytokines and a loss of epithelial barrier function, thereby resulting in increased biliary epithelial inflammation and permeability.[281]

Although all patients with CF express defective CFTR in cholangiocytes, not all develop CFLD. There is no association between specific CFTR mutations and CFLD.[282] The variable occurrence and clinical course of liver disease in patients with CF suggest that other genetic or environmental factors are involved in disease expression. For example, the α_1-AT Z allele has been shown to be a risk factor for liver disease and portal hypertension in patients with CF,[283] and hepatic expression of certain genes correlates with the severity of fibrosis.[284] Differential expression of a number of genes is associated with hepatic fibrogenesis, including downregulation of collagens, matrix metalloproteinases, and chemokines, thereby providing evidence of a transcriptional basis for the pathogenesis of CFLD.[284]

Diagnosis

A joint National Institutes of Health and Cystic Fibrosis Foundation Clinical Research Workshop on CFLD suggested criteria to diagnose progressive liver disease in patients with CF.[273] If two or more of the following are present, a diagnosis of CFLD is established: (1) hepatomegaly (e.g., liver edge palpable >2 cm below the costal margin) and/or splenomegaly, confirmed by ultrasound; (2) elevations of ALT, AST, and GGTP above the laboratory upper limits of normal for greater than 6 months, after excluding other causes of liver disease; (3) ultrasonographic evidence of coarseness, nodularity, increased echogenicity, or portal hypertension, as described earlier; and (4) liver biopsy specimens showing FBC or multilobular cirrhosis (if liver biopsy is performed). Notably, these criteria are meant to enable identification of patients to include in epidemiological and research studies.

Additional areas of focus and key points of interest in the field include (1) the need for a universal consensus on the definition of CFLD to clarify disease stage and to identify relevant biomarkers to assess disease severity was highlighted; (2) a deeper understanding of the pathophysiology and prognostic factors for the long-term evolution of CFLD; and (3) exploring novel experimental models and new treatment options under investigation.[278]

Treatment

Children with CF should be screened yearly with physical examination, liver biochemical and function tests, and abdominal imaging to assess for CFLD.[285,286] Those with suspected CFLD should be evaluated by a hepatologist to exclude other causes of liver disease. Once a diagnosis of CFLD is established, the inclusion of the liver specialist on a multidisciplinary care team is important for future management and potential interventions. Nutrition is a critical area of focus because fat malabsorption may be exacerbated by the cholestasis of CFLD. Additionally, optimizing overall liver health through avoidance of alcohol, hepatotoxic medicines, herbal and dietary supplements, and vaccinations against hepatotropic viruses should be encouraged. The mainstay of treatment is to mitigate the complications of portal hypertension and cirrhosis. Although UDCA therapy is commonly prescribed, few trials have assessed its effectiveness, and evidence to justify its routine use in CF has overall been insufficient.[287] On the other hand, in patients with mild CFLD, UDCA has shown to exhibit a positive effect on overall survival.[288] Thus the ultimate utility of UDCA in CFLD remains inconclusive.

CFTR modulation therapies have been approved for CF lung disease, but their impact on the development or progression of CFLD remains unknown, in part because advanced liver disease was an exclusion criterion in the CFTR modulator clinical trials.[272] While liver enzyme elevations were reported in 5%–10% of patients receiving modulator therapy in clinical trials, real-world experiences have reported a decrease in aminotransferase levels during the year after starting therapy and no objective progression of liver disease.[289] Additional experience and targeted clinical trials will be needed before the true impact of modulator therapy on CFLD is elucidated.

Because patients with CF rarely have true hepatocellular dysfunction, the role of liver transplantation is often reserved for patients with clinically significant complications related to their portal hypertension. Clarity regarding the appropriateness for candidacy and optimal timing of transplantation is lacking, although updated recommendations have been published.[286]

The published data on liver transplantation reveal discrepancies relating to improved lung function, nutritional status, and quality of life in patients with CFLD.[273] Long-term outcomes following liver transplantation are acceptable but are inferior to the outcomes of transplantation for other diseases. One study suggested that liver transplantation was neither beneficial nor detrimental to pulmonary function in patients with CF.[290] Notably, these studies predate the modulator therapy era. A portosystemic shunt (TIPS) can be an effective treatment in patients with variceal bleeding; long-term outcomes are comparable to those for patients who undergo liver transplantation.[291]

MITOCHONDRIAL LIVER DISEASES

Many diseases associated with liver dysfunction have been attributed to defects in mitochondrial function. In addition to defects in mitochondrial enzymes involved in the urea cycle or energy metabolism, several mitochondrial hepatopathies involve respiratory chain/oxidative phosphorylation/electron transport defects or alterations in mitochondrial DNA (mtDNA) levels.

The mitochondrial genome is especially vulnerable to oxidative injury not only because of its spatial relationship to the respiratory chain but also because of its lack of protective histones and of an adequate excision and recombination repair system. mtDNA is inherited almost entirely from the maternal ovum; therefore many primary mitochondrial deficiencies are inherited in a dominant fashion. Many nuclear genes, however, such as DNA polymerase-γ *(POLG)*, thymidine kinase 2, deoxyguanosine kinase *(DGUOK)*, *SCO1*, *BCS1L*, and *MPV17*, encode proteins critical to maintaining proper amounts of mtDNA and to allowing normal mitochondrial respiratory function. Most mitochondrial diseases with primary involvement of the liver are caused by nuclear rather than mitochondrial gene mutations.[292]

Mitochondrial respiratory chain disorders can affect one in 5000 births, with liver involvement occurring in 10%–20% of patients.[293,294] Striking heterogeneity of clinical features, ranging from single-organ involvement to multisystem disease, can lead to a delayed or missed diagnosis and can confound therapeutic decision-making, for example, with respect to the advisability of liver transplantation. This heterogeneity of clinical presentations is likely due to the observations that mitochondrial quantity and function are uniquely influenced by both nuclear and mtDNA, and cells in various tissues can contain different mixtures of normal and abnormal mitochondrial genomes (heteroplasmy).[293]

The diagnosis of a mitochondrial respiratory chain defect should be considered in a patient with liver disease who has unexplained neuromuscular symptoms, including a seizure disorder; involvement of seemingly unrelated organ systems; a rapidly progressive course; or a chronic course that proves to be a diagnostic dilemma.[293] In about 80% of patients, symptoms appear before age 2. The plasma lactate level and the ratio of lactate to pyruvate are often elevated, especially when the presentation is insidious.[293,295] Given the complex array of tests that are useful for establishing a diagnosis of a mitochondrial hepatopathy, a tiered approach to the diagnostic workup has been proposed.[293] However, as new sequencing approaches such as whole-genome sequencing have become more accessible and cost-effective, the diagnostic approach to patients with suspected mitochondrial hepatopathy has evolved.[292]

Infantile liver failure has been reported in numerous mitochondrial disorders, including cytochrome *c* oxidase deficiency, caused by mutations in the *SCO1* or *BCS1L* genes; succinyl-CoA enzyme deficiency, caused by mutations in the *SUCLG1* genes; mutations in the *TRMU* gene encoding the mitochondrial-specific tRNA-modifying enzyme; and mutations in the *TSFM* gene encoding the mitochondrial translation elongation factor EFTs.[296–298] Although an elevated serum lactate and/or lactate-to-pyruvate ratio is often identified as key feature of these disorders, the clinical use of these markers in the setting of acute liver failure may be less specific.[299] Infants with Alpers-Huttenlocher syndrome (progressive neuronal degeneration in childhood with liver disease ascribed to mitochondrial dysfunction) experience vomiting, hypotonia, seizures, and liver failure, often beginning by 6 months of age. Frequently, the liver disease is unsuspected clinically and becomes evident late in the course of the disease. Alpers-Huttenlocher syndrome has been shown to be caused by mutations in *POLG* and in the *FARS2* gene encoding a mitochondrial phenylalanyl transfer RNA synthetase.[300] Alternatively, in *mtDNA depletion syndrome* (caused by mutations in the *POLG*, *DGUOK*, or *MPV17* genes), hypoglycemia, acidosis, and liver failure develop early in infancy, and neurologic abnormalities are less prominent.[301]

Navajo neurohepatopathy has been shown to be caused by mtDNA depletion and a defect in the *MPV17* gene product, which is involved in mtDNA maintenance and regulation of oxidative phosphorylation.[302,303] Other multisystemic mitochondrial diseases with liver involvement are *Pearson marrow-pancreas syndrome* (caused by large deletions of mtDNA segments) and chronic diarrhea and intestinal pseudo-obstruction with liver involvement.[304]

Liver biopsy specimens in mitochondrial hepatopathy typically show macrovesicular and microvesicular steatosis. Cholestasis may be present, and conditions associated with chronic liver disease can show micronodular cirrhosis. Other findings include hepatocyte hypereosinophilia and hemosiderosis. Immunohistochemical techniques can be used (e.g., to diagnose cytochrome *c* oxidase deficiency). When needed, electron microscopy may show cytoplasmic crowding by atypical mitochondria.[305] Cholestasis may be present, and conditions associated with chronic liver disease can show micronodular cirrhosis. Lactic acidemia may be constant, intermittent, or absent in mitochondrial disorders.[306] Direct measurement of the enzymatic activity of the respiratory chain electron transport protein complexes can be performed on frozen tissue from the organ that expresses the clinical disease, although skin fibroblasts and lymphocytes may also be used. Few academic centers around the world perform the assays for mitochondrial respiration (polarographic studies) or mtDNA analysis.

There is no therapy that has been shown to alter the course of mitochondrial respiratory chain disorders. Strategies proposed to delay the progression of these disorders include the use of antioxidants such as vitamin E or ascorbic acid; electron acceptors and cofactors, such as coenzyme Q10, thiamine, or riboflavin; and supplements proposed to work by other mechanisms, such as carnitine, creatine, or succinate. A Cochrane systematic review, however, failed to show any clear evidence to support their general use in mitochondrial disorders, but specific diseases, such as coenzyme Q deficiency, may respond to treatment.[304,307] Liver transplantation has generally been contraindicated in these patients, but some reports have demonstrated successful outcomes.[295,304,308]

Full references for this chapter can be found at https://ebooks.health.elsevier.com.

80 Hepatitis A

Allison M. Bush, Maria H. Sjogren

IN THIS CHAPTER

Hepatitis A virus (HAV) infection is the most common form of acute viral hepatitis worldwide.[1] It is a self-limited infection caused by a cytopathic, nonenveloped, single-stranded RNA virus that is transmitted by the fecal-oral route by contaminated food or water.[1,2] HAV is endemic in many developing countries, while developed countries more commonly have smaller epidemic outbreaks.[4] HAV was first characterized in 1973 when scientists detected the virus in the stool of human volunteers who were infected with HAV.[3] The ensuing development of sensitive and specific serologic assays for the diagnosis of HAV infection and the isolation of HAV in cell culture permitted an understanding of the epidemiology of HAV infection and the development of vaccines.[4]

VIROLOGY

In 1982 HAV was classified as an enterovirus belonging to the Picornaviridae family. Subsequent determination of the sequence of HAV nucleotides and amino acids led to the creation of a new genus, *Hepatovirus*.[5] HAV has an icosahedral shape, measures 27–28 nm in diameter, and can survive in acidic environments but is inactivated when heated to 85°C for 1 minute. HAV is capable of surviving in seawater (4% survival rate), dried feces at room temperature for 4 weeks (17% survival), and live oysters for 5 days (12% survival).[6] HAV has only one known serotype and no antigenic cross-reactivity with hepatitis B, C, D, or E virus or human pegivirus. The HAV genome consists of a positive-sense RNA that is 7.48 kb long, single-stranded, and linear (Fig. 80.1).

The onset of HAV replication in cell culture systems takes weeks to months. Primate cells, including African green monkey kidney cells, primary human fibroblasts, human diploid cells, and fetal rhesus kidney cells, are favored for the cultivation of HAV in vitro. Two conditions control the outcome of HAV replication in cell culture.[7] The first is the genetic makeup of the virus; HAV strains mutate in distinct regions of the viral genome as they become adapted to cell culture. The second is the metabolic activity of the host cell at the time of infection. Cells in culture, although infected simultaneously, initiate HAV replication asynchronously. This asynchronicity may be caused by differences in the metabolic activity of individual cells, but definitive evidence of cell-cycle dependence of HAV replication is lacking.[8]

An initial step in the lifecycle of a virus is the attachment to a cell surface receptor. The location and function of these receptors determine tissue tropism. Little is known about the mechanism of entry of HAV into cells. Some work has suggested that HAV could infect cells by a surrogate-receptor binding mechanism (involving a nonspecified serum protein). HAV infectivity in tissue culture has been shown to require calcium and to be inhibited by the treatment of the cells with trypsin, phospholipases, and β-galactosidase.[9] A surface glycoprotein, HAVcr-1, on African green monkey kidney cells has been identified as a receptor for HAV. Blocking of HAVcr-1 with specific monoclonal antibodies prevents infection of otherwise susceptible cells. Experimental data suggest that HAVcr-1 not only serves as an attachment receptor but may also facilitate the uncoating of HAV and its entry into hepatocytes.[10]

Once HAV enters a cell, the viral RNA is uncoated, cell host ribosomes bind to viral RNA, and polysomes are formed. HAV is translated into a large polyprotein of 2227 amino acids. This polyprotein is organized into three regions: P1, P2, and P3. The P1 region encodes structural proteins VP1, VP2, VP3, and a putative VP4. The P2 and P3 regions encode nonstructural proteins associated with viral replication (see Fig. 80.1).

The HAV RNA polymerase copies the plus-RNA strand. The RNA transcript, in turn, is used for translation into proteins, which are used for assembly into mature virions. Downregulation of HAV RNA synthesis appears to occur as defective HAV particles appear.[11] In addition, a group of specific RNA-binding proteins has been observed during persistent infection.[12] The origin and nature of these proteins are unknown, but they exert activity on the RNA template and are believed to play a regulatory role in the replication of HAV.[13]

Human HAV strains can be grouped into four different genotypes (I, II, III, and VII), whereas simian strains of HAV belong to genotypes IV, V, and VI.[14] Despite the nucleotide sequence heterogeneity, the antigenic structure of human HAV is highly conserved among strains. The HAV VP1/2A and 2C genes are thought to be responsible for viral virulence, as demonstrated by experiments in which the genotypes and phenotypes of viruses were compared after animals were infected with 1 of 14 chimeric virus genomes derived from 2 infectious cDNA clones that encoded a virulent HAV isolate and an attenuated HAV isolate (HM175 strain), respectively.[15]

Among the many strains of HAV, the HM175 and CR326 human HAV strains were used to produce commercially available vaccines. In 1978 strain HM175 was isolated from the human feces of Australian patients in a small outbreak of hepatitis A. CR326 was isolated from Costa Rican patients infected with HAV. The nucleotide and amino acid sequences showed 95% identity between the two strains. Vaccines prepared from these strains are thought to protect against all relevant human strains of HAV.

Variations in the HAV genome are thought to play a role in the development of acute liver failure (ALF) during acute HAV infection. The 5′untranslated region of the HAV genome was sequenced in serum samples from 84 patients with HAV infection,

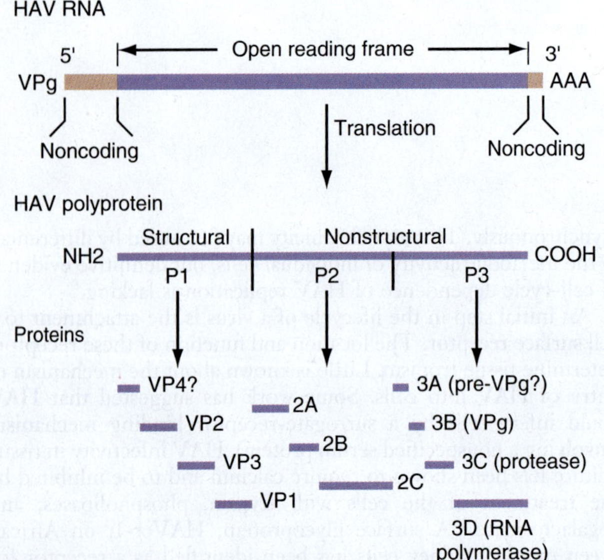

Fig. 80.1 Genomic organization of HAV. *VP*, Viral protein; *VPg*, 5′ terminal protein. (From Levine JE, Bull FG, Millward-Sadler GH, et al. Acute viral hepatitis. In: Millward-Sadler GH, Wright R, Arther MJP, eds. *Wright's Liver and Biliary Disease*. 3rd ed. London: WB Saunders; 1992:679.)

including 12 with ALF.[16] The investigators observed fewer nucleotide substitutions in the HAV genome from patients with ALF than in those from patients without ALF ($P < .001$). The differences were most prominent between nucleotides 200 and 500, suggesting that nucleotide variations in the central portion of the 5′ untranslated region influence the clinical severity of HAV infection.

EPIDEMIOLOGY

Acute hepatitis A is a reportable infectious disease in all 50 states, as well as the District of Columbia and US territories. Since 2002, incidence in the United States has ranged from 0.1 case per 100,000 people to 5.1 cases per 100,000 people.[17,18] Incidence steadily declined by more than 95% from 1995 to 2011. This initial decrease in rates of HAV infection is, in large part, caused by the expanded use of the HAV vaccine (see later). In 2006 the Centers for Disease Control and Prevention (CDC) recommended routine vaccination of children in all 50 states.

Although the impact of HAV vaccination has been profound, coverage rates for the complete HAV vaccination series remain below rates for other routine childhood vaccines. In the United States in 2016, the HAV vaccination rate in adolescents for the first dose was 73.9%, but only 64.4% received a second dose.[19] More than 90% of persons who receive the two-dose vaccination series will have persistent antibodies for 40 years, compared with 11 years if only one dose is received.[20,21] The frequency of HAV antibodies in 32,502 Air Force recruits from 2013 to 2014 was greater than 50% only in recruits from Alaska, Nevada, Utah, Arizona, and New Mexico. The frequency of HAV antibodies in recruits from the remaining 45 states was below 50%, and those from 16 states had rates lower than 35%.[22] This low rate of adult HAV immunity in a low-endemic nation has resulted in susceptibility to infection from sporadic food-associated outbreaks or person-to-person transmission in a large portion of the adult population.

From 2013 to 2016, there were small increases in HAV infections due to foodborne outbreaks; then, from 2016 to 2020, the number of cases of HAV infection in the United States increased owing to multistate increases in HAV outbreaks as a result of person-to-person spread primarily among adults who experience homelessness or use drugs.[23,25] From 2016 to 2022, 37 states reported outbreaks resulting in 44,650 cases, 27,250 hospitalizations, and 415 deaths. The shift from foodborne outbreaks to outbreaks among high-risk populations led to a 2019 recommendation by the Advisory Committee on Immunization Practices (ACIP) for vaccination of persons experiencing homelessness and ongoing recommendations for vaccination for persons who use drugs. In the following years, the number of outbreak-affected states decreased from 37 to 13 in 2022.[24]

Historically, in the United States, the highest rate of disease has been among children 5–14 years of age. A rapid rate of disease decline among children has occurred since the implementation of vaccination. When rates of HAV infection are compared between 2012 and 2016 by age groups, all groups saw an increase except persons 0–9 years of age (0.1 cases per 100,000 in 2016). People ages 20–29 and 30–39 years old had the highest rate (0.9 cases per 100,000), likely explained by a low prevalence of HAV antibodies in these groups. A transition has also occurred in the reported risk-exposure behaviors for persons with HAV infection; international travel was the most common risk factor from 2001 to 2007, whereas food and waterborne outbreaks were the most common in 2018.[25]

Globally, 1.5 million people are infected with HAV annually.[26] The distribution of the virus is dependent upon socioeconomic factors such as housing, sanitation, vaccination programs, and water quality. With improvements in these factors, disease susceptibility has shifted from children to older adults.[27] HAV infection generally follows one of three epidemiologic patterns.[27,28] In countries where sanitary conditions are poor, most children are infected at an early age. Although earlier seroepidemiologic studies routinely showed that 100% of preschool children in these countries had detectable antibodies to HAV (anti-HAV) in serum, presumably reflecting previous subclinical infection, subsequent studies have shown that the average age of infection has risen rapidly to 5 years and older, when symptomatic infection is more likely. The second epidemiologic pattern is seen in industrialized countries where the prevalence of HAV infection is low among children and young adults. The third epidemiologic pattern is observed in closed or semiclosed communities, such as some isolated communities in the South Pacific, where HAV is capable (through epidemics) of infecting the entire population, which then becomes immune. Thereafter, newborns remain susceptible until the virus is reintroduced into the community.[27]

The primary route of transmission of HAV is the fecal-oral route, by either person-to-person contact or ingestion of contaminated food or water. Although rare, the transmission of HAV by a parenteral route has been documented after transfusion of blood[29,30] or blood products.[31] Cyclical outbreaks among people who inject drugs, users of noninjection illicit drugs, and men who have sex with men (up to 10% may become infected in outbreak years) have been reported.[32] Clinical sequelae of HAV infection are more severe in older than younger adults; therefore developed countries with low endemicity and recent outbreaks have experienced high rates of hospitalization and increased costs.[27]

HAV is resistant to warming, freezing, drying, and acidic environments and has prolonged viability in feces, soil, and sewage. In the United States, efforts to provide effective sanitation services and facilities that offer maintenance of healthy personal hygiene habits in populations such as those affected by homelessness have been effective in combating transmission via fecal-oral contact with contaminated food and water or person-to-person contact during outbreaks.[27,33] Successful initiatives that address homelessness and higher rates of completion of childhood vaccination series will have the most profound and durable impact on the frequency of HAV infection and other infectious outbreaks in the United States.[34]

PATHOGENESIS

After HAV is ingested and survives gastric acid, it traverses the small intestinal mucosa, reaches the liver via the portal vein, and is taken up by hepatocytes. In hepatocytes, virus particles replicate, assemble, and are secreted into the biliary canaliculus, from which they pass into the bile duct and back to the small intestine, with eventual excretion in the feces. The enterohepatic cycles of the virus lifecycle continue until neutralizing antibodies and other immune mechanisms interrupt the cycle.[35,36]

The pathogenesis of HAV-associated hepatocyte injury is not completely defined. The lack of injury to cells in culture systems suggests that HAV is not cytopathic. Immunologically mediated cell damage is more likely. The emergence of anti-HAV antibodies could result in hepatic necrosis during immunologically mediated elimination of HAV.

CLINICAL FEATURES

Infection with HAV usually results in an acute self-limited episode of hepatitis. HAV does not result in a chronic infection, but rarely, acute hepatitis A can have a prolonged or relapsing course, which can include profound cholestasis.[37] The incubation period is commonly 2–4 weeks, rarely up to 6 weeks. The mortality rate is low in previously healthy persons. Morbidity can be substantial in older children and adults.

The most common clinical feature of cases of hepatitis A reported to the CDC in 2010 was jaundice in 68.1% of patients. The rates of hospitalization and death were 42.5% and 1%, respectively, possibly reflecting a reporting bias in favor of more severe cases. Adults and older adults are more likely to have profound hepatocellular dysfunction, require hospitalization, and have higher mortality rates.[38] The increased morbidity and mortality in older adults may be caused by the reduced regenerative capacity of the liver with advanced age, increased comorbidity, and a decline in immune function, including decreased antibody affinity to antigens.[39] By contrast, the rate of hospitalization in a younger population of active-duty US Armed Forces members with acute HAV infection from 1991 to 2011 was 1.3 per 100,000 person-years. Because of a 1996 Department of Defense directive to provide HAV vaccine to all active-duty and reserve members, with the goal of immunization of the entire force by the end of 1998, the rate of hospitalization fell to 0.2 to 0.7 per 100,000 patient-years from 2000 to 2011.[40]

Patients with HAV infection usually present with one of the following five clinical patterns: (1) asymptomatic without jaundice; (2) symptomatic with jaundice and self-limited after approximately 8 weeks; (3) cholestatic, with jaundice lasting 10 weeks or more[37]; (4) relapsing, with two or more bouts of acute hepatitis occurring over a 6–10-week period; and (5) ALF. Children younger than 2 years of age are usually asymptomatic; jaundice develops in only 20% of them, whereas symptoms develop in most children (80%) 5 years of age or older. HAV infection with prolonged cholestasis is a rare variant but occasionally leads to invasive diagnostic procedures (inappropriately) because the diagnosis of acute hepatitis may not be readily accepted in patients who have jaundice for several months, even in the presence of detectable anti-HAV of the immunoglobulin (Ig) M class (see later).[37] A relapsing course is observed in 10%–15% of patients with acute hepatitis A within 6 months after the acute illness has resolved; however, this variant (or any other) does not result in the development of chronic HAV infection.[41] There are no known risk factors for relapsing disease. The mechanism of relapsing HAV is unknown, but proposed theories include an immune response to HAV or, alternatively, a persistent HAV infection with intermittent reactivation of symptoms.[82] Serologic testing has shown a recurrence of HAV IgM, and shedding of HAV in stool has been documented during the relapse phase.[42] Neither the cholestatic variant nor relapsing hepatitis A is associated with an increase in mortality.

In a retrospective observational multicenter study of 47 patients with acute HAV infection during the prodrome phase (from 3 to 30 days after infection), the most common symptoms were fever (87%), malaise (74%), and jaundice (62%).[2] Additional prodromal symptoms included fatigue, weakness, anorexia, nausea, vomiting, and abdominal pain. Less common symptoms were headache, arthralgias, myalgias, and diarrhea.[43] Dark urine precedes other symptoms in approximately 90% of infected persons, a symptom that occurs within 1–2 weeks of the onset of prodromal symptoms. Symptoms of hepatitis may last from a few days to 2 weeks and usually decrease with the onset of clinical jaundice. RUQ tenderness and mild liver enlargement are found on physical examination in 85% of patients, and splenomegaly and cervical lymphadenopathy are each present in 15% of patients.

Complete clinical recovery is achieved in 60% of affected persons within 2 months and in nearly everyone by 6 months. The overall prognosis of acute hepatitis A in otherwise healthy adults is excellent. Potentially fatal complications (e.g., ALF) develop in a small minority of patients.[44]

Acute hepatitis A, unlike hepatitis E (see Chapter 84), is not associated with a higher mortality rate in pregnant women; however, in a retrospective review of 13 cases of acute HAV infection during the second and third trimesters of pregnancy, gestational complications including premature contractions, premature rupture of membranes, placental separation, and vaginal bleeding developed in nine patients (69%). In eight of these patients, complications led to preterm labor at a median of 34 gestational weeks (range, 31–37 weeks).[45]

Acute HAV infection must be differentiated by appropriate serologic testing from other causes of acute viral hepatitis, AIH, and other causes of acute nonviral hepatitis. In some cases, the diagnosis may be difficult to make because the patient may harbor another viral infection, such as chronic hepatitis B or chronic hepatitis C, with superimposed acute HAV infection.

ALF Caused by HAV Infection

ALF due to HAV is rarely seen in children, adolescents, or young adults. The case-fatality rate in 2008 was calculated by the CDC to be 0.02 per 100,000 population, with the highest mortality rates in persons older than 75 (0.12 deaths per 100,000 population). Mortality rates were similar between the black population and other people of color, who had rates slightly higher than those of the white population. From 2004 to 2008, the mortality rate of acute hepatitis A was consistently higher among male patients than female patients.[46] In addition to age, risk factors for ALF and mortality include underlying liver disease and chronic viral hepatitis.[47] Clinical predictors of ALF-associated mortality in a 2012 study were a serum creatinine level greater than 2 mg/dL, total bilirubin greater than 9.6 mg/dL, and albumin less than 2.5 g/L. Of these predictors, a serum creatinine level greater than 2 mg/dL had the highest sensitivity and specificity for predicting ALF and mortality.[2] ALF caused by HAV becomes manifest in the first week of illness in approximately 55% of affected patients and during the first 4 weeks in 90%; the onset of ALF rarely occurs after 4 weeks of illness.[44] Late hepatic failure was reported in one patient 79 days after the onset of symptoms of HAV infection, with long-term survival achieved after live-donor LT.[48]

The contribution of HAV infection to ALF has been reported to be greater in populations classified as hyperendemic for HAV. In a report from India, where 276 patients with ALF were seen between 1994 and 1997, 10.6% of the cases among adults were caused by HAV. HAV had been responsible for only 3.5% of cases among 206 patients with ALF seen in the same community from 1978 to 1981.[49] Although two reports since the late 1990s have described a decline in the number of cases of acute viral hepatitis among patients with ALF in the United States,[50,51] this decline is attributable principally to the control of HBV infection.

Extrahepatic Manifestations

Extrahepatic manifestations are less frequent in acute HAV infection than in acute HBV infection and consist most commonly of an evanescent rash (14%) and arthralgias (11%) and, uncommonly, of leukocytoclastic vasculitis, glomerulonephritis, and arthritis, in which immune-complex disease is believed to play a pathogenic role. Cutaneous vasculitis is typically seen on the legs and buttocks; skin biopsies reveal the presence of anti-HAV IgM and complement in blood vessel walls. HAV-associated arthritis also appears to have a predilection for the lower extremities. Both vasculitis and arthritis have been associated with cryoglobulinemia, although cryoglobulinemia in general is more frequently associated with HCV infection. Cryoglobulins in acute hepatitis A have been shown to contain anti-HAV IgM. Other rare extrahepatic manifestations that may be immune-complex related include toxic epidermal necrolysis, myocarditis, renal failure in the absence of liver failure, optic neuritis, transverse myelitis, polyneuritis, and cholecystitis. Hematologic complications include thrombocytopenia, aplastic anemia, and red cell aplasia. Patients with more protracted illness appear to have a higher frequency of extrahepatic manifestations.

Autoimmune Hepatitis After Acute Hepatitis A

Several viruses have been reported to trigger the onset of autoimmune hepatitis (AIH) (see Chapter 92). In rare cases, acute hepatitis A has been followed by the development of type 1 AIH. AIH may also result in the detection of anti-HAV IgM for a prolonged period. Genetic predisposition is thought to play a role.[52–57]

DIAGNOSIS

Acute hepatitis A is clinically indistinguishable from other forms of viral hepatitis. The diagnosis of infection is based on the detection of specific antibodies against HAV (anti-HAV) in serum (Fig. 80.2). A diagnosis of acute hepatitis A requires the demonstration of anti-HAV IgM in serum. The test result is positive from the onset of symptoms[55] and usually remains positive for approximately 4 months.[56] Some patients may have low levels of detectable anti-HAV IgM for more than a year after the initial infection.[56] Anti-HAV IgG is also detectable at the onset of the disease, remains present usually for life, and after clinical recovery is interpreted as a marker of previous HAV infection (as demonstrated by a positive result on a commercial assay for total anti-HAV and a negative result for anti-HAV IgM).

Testing for HAV RNA is limited to research laboratories. HAV RNA has been detected in serum, stool, and liver tissue. Viral RNA can be amplified by PCR methodology.[57] With a PCR assay, HAV RNA has been documented in human sera for up to 21 days after the onset of illness.[32] The use of HCV RNA testing has been described in a report of 76 French patients with acute HAV infection seen between January 1987 and April 2000[58]; 19 had ALF, 10 who required LT, and 1 of whom died while awaiting LT. The HAV RNA status was determined in 39 of the 50 patients in whom sera and clinical data were available, including the 19 with ALF. HAV RNA was detected in 36 of these 50 patients (72%). The presence of low-titer HAV RNA in patients with severe acute hepatitis may signal an ominous prognosis and the need for early referral for LT. As in other studies, the genotype of HAV did not seem to play a role in the severity of clinical manifestations.[59]

PREVENTION AND TREATMENT

Recommendations concerning immunoprophylaxis against HAV were published by the CDC in 1999 for persons in groups at increased risk for hepatitis A or its adverse consequences. In 2006 these recommendations were updated by the ACIP, which specifically recommended routine vaccination of children in the United States.[32] The overall strategy is to protect persons from disease and to lower the incidence of HAV infection in the United States. The currently available monovalent vaccines were initially licensed for use in children older than age 2 but are now licensed for use after age 12 months.[26,60] The decline in incidence rates, not surprisingly, has been greater in children than in adults, effectively removing children as a high-risk population and potentially removing the primary reservoir for the virus in the United States.[19,32] Box 80.1 lists the populations now considered to be at the highest risk of HAV infection. In 2012 the WHO recommended deferring large-scale vaccination programs in highly endemic countries where almost all persons are

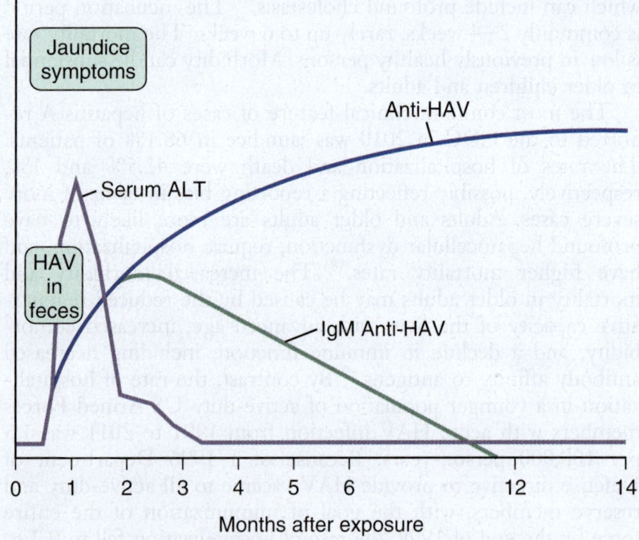

Fig. 80.2 Typical course of a case of acute hepatitis A. *Anti-HAV*, Antibody to HAV; *IgM*, immunoglobulin M. (From Hoofnagle JH, DiBisceglie AM. Serologic diagnosis of acute and chronic viral hepatitis. *Semin Liver Dis*. 1991;11:73–83.)

BOX 80.1 Groups at High Risk of HAV Infection

Healthy persons who:
- Travel to endemic areas
- Work in occupations for which the likelihood of exposure is high
- Have infected family members
- Adopt infants or children from an endemic area

Men who have sex with men
Persons who have tested positive for HIV
Persons with chronic liver disease
Persons with a clotting factor disorder
People who inject drugs or users of noninjection illicit drugs

asymptomatically infected with HAV in childhood, thereby effectively preventing clinical hepatitis A in adolescents and adults. In countries with intermediate HAV endemicity (or in those with high endemicity and rapidly improving socioeconomic status), a relatively large proportion of the adult population is susceptible to HAV infection, and large-scale HAV vaccination is likely to be cost-effective and is recommended. In countries with low or very low endemicity, the WHO has recommended targeted vaccination to provide individual health benefits. Groups for which vaccination should be offered include travelers to areas of intermediate or high endemicity, persons who require lifelong blood product transfusions, men who have sex with men, persons with chronic liver disease, workers in contact with nonhuman primates, and people who inject drugs.[26]

No specific medications are available to treat acute hepatitis A, and symptomatic treatment is recommended. Historically, attention to sanitation and administration of serum immune globulin (IG) have been the mainstay of preventing HAV infection. The availability of excellent HAV vaccines, the high cost of IG, and the short-term protection of IG through passive immunity have significantly limited the use of IG for preexposure prophylaxis. IG is still indicated in susceptible individuals traveling to intermediate or high endemic areas in less than 2 weeks (Table 80.1).[61]

In 2007 the HAV vaccine was approved for use in the postexposure prophylaxis of immunocompetent persons, 12 months–40 years of age, without chronic liver disease.[62] This new indication for the HAV vaccine was based on the results of a study that compared the efficacy of the HAV vaccine with that of IG for postexposure prophylaxis against HAV infection. Clinical hepatitis A developed in 4.4% of subjects in the vaccine group compared with 3.3% of those in the IG group.[63] Analysis revealed no statistical difference between the two groups (95% confidence interval, 0.70–2.67) but likely excluded persons with asymptomatic infection. In the vaccine group, 162 persons with HAV IgM in serum were excluded, compared with 50 persons in the IG group, because of either a lack of symptoms or absence of an elevated serum ALT level of at least two times the upper limit of normal. The possibility exists that several persons with asymptomatic hepatitis A still posed an infectious risk to others. Although both the HAV vaccine and IG appear to be effective when administered within 2 weeks of exposure to HAV, advantages of the HAV vaccine include long-term protection (when a second dose is subsequently administered), a good safety record, and wide availability.[64] Postexposure prophylaxis with IG is still indicated in infants younger than 12 months of age and can be considered in individuals greater than 40 years of age; however, the vaccine is likely also effective in the latter group (see Table 80.1). In 2017 prescribing recommendations for IG [GamaSTAN S/D (manufactured by Grifols Therapeutics, Inc., Clayton, NC), the only IG approved by the FDA for HAV prophylaxis] were updated considering the decreased concentration of HAV IgG (and thus IgG potency) among donors (see Table 80.1).[61]

Taking into consideration data from Canada and the United Kingdom, where the HAV vaccine has been used for postexposure prophylaxis since the early 2000s, the ACIP concluded that the HAV vaccine is safe and comparable to IG in protecting recipients against clinical hepatitis A. The ACIP guidelines allow persons who have recently been exposed to HAV and who have not been vaccinated previously to be given a single dose of a single-antigen HAV vaccine or IG (0.01 mL/kg) as soon as possible within 2 weeks of exposure. The standard vaccine schedule is detailed in Table 80.2.[61,62] Although IG is considered safe, the perception is widespread that it poses a risk because it is a blood-derived product. IG can cause fever and myalgias, just as the vaccine can, but pain at the injection site is usually more pronounced with IG than with the vaccine. Postexposure prophylaxis with IG can be administered at the same time as the initiation of active immunization with the vaccine.[64]

The HAV vaccine was first licensed in the United States in 1995; two inactivated HAV vaccines are commercially available. The extensive use of vaccines in clinical trials and postmarketing surveillance supports the safety and efficacy of these products. HAVRIX is manufactured by GlaxoSmithKline Biologicals, Rixensart, Belgium, and VAQTA is manufactured by Merck & Co Inc., West Point, Pennsylvania. Both vaccines are derived from HAV grown in cell culture. The final products are purified and formalin-inactivated; they contain alum as an adjuvant. The basic difference between the two commercially available vaccines is the HAV strain used for preparation. HAVRIX was prepared with the HM175 strain, whereas VAQTA was prepared with the CR326 strain.[65,66] The difference is of little practical importance because both vaccines are safe and immunogenic. The doses and schedule of immunization are shown in Table 80.2. After vaccination with HAVRIX, anti-HAV is estimated to remain detectable in serum for approximately 40 years; immunity may last longer.[20] Among adults, the most common local side effects have been soreness at the injection site (56%), headache (14%), and malaise (7%). In children, the most common side effects have been soreness at the injection site (15%), feeding problems (8%), headache (4%), and induration at the injection site (4%).[32]

In the United States in November 2012, the Vaccine Adverse Event Reporting System received 20,057 reports of unexplained adverse events after immunization with the HAV vaccine alone or

TABLE 80.1 Dosing Instructions for Immune Globulin for HAV Prophylaxis

Indication	Circumstance(s)	Dose	Simultaneous Administration of HAV Vaccine
Preexposure prophylaxis	1 month of travel[a] to begin in <2 weeks	0.1 mL/kg	Yes[b,c]
	2 months of travel[a] to begin in <2 weeks	0.2 mL/kg	Yes[b,c]
	>2 months of travel[a] to begin in <2 weeks	0.2 mL/kg (repeat every 2 months)	Yes[b,c]
Postexposure prophylaxis	<12 months and >40 years of age Chronic liver disease Contraindication to HAV vaccine Immunocompromised person	0.1 mL/kg	Yes[b,c], but only if >12 months of age

[a]Travel to area of intermediate or high HAV endemicity.
[b]Vaccine should be administered in a separate anatomic site from immune globulin in infants >12 months and adults <40 years of age.
[c]Except when the vaccine is contraindicated (e.g., because of an allergy).

TABLE 80.2 Recommended Vaccines for HAV[a]

Vaccine	Schedule	Age (Years)	Dose	Volume (mL)	Dosing Schedule
HAVRIX	Standard	1–18	720 ELU	0.5	0, 6–12 months
	Standard	>18	1440 ELU	1	0, 6–12 months
	Accelerated	≥1	Single age-appropriate dose	Age appropriate	≥2 weeks prior to travel[b]
	Postexposure prophylaxis	≥1	Single age-appropriate dose	Age appropriate	<2 weeks after exposure[b]
VAQTA	Standard	1–18	25 U	0.5	0, 6–18 months
	Standard	>18	50 U	1	0, 6–18 months
	Accelerated	≥1	Single age-appropriate dose	Age appropriate	≥2 weeks prior to travel[b]
	Postexposure prophylaxis[c]	≥1	Single age-appropriate dose	Age appropriate	<2 weeks after exposure[b]
TWINRIX	Standard	≥18	720 ELU HAV, 20 mg HBV	1	0, 1, 6 months
	Accelerated	≥18	720 ELU HAV, 20 mg HBV	1	0, 7, 21–30 days[b]

[a]Vaccines are injected intramuscularly into the deltoid muscle.
[b]Timing of the booster dose (necessary for long-term protection): VAQTA, 6 months; HAVRIX, 6-12 months; TWINRIX, 12 months.
[c]Not FDA approved.
ELU, Enzyme-linked immunoassay (ELISA) units; *U*, units.

in combination with other vaccines. Of the 20,057 reports, 1230 were considered serious and included Guillain-Barré syndrome, immune thrombocytopenic purpura, elevated serum aminotransferase levels, and seizures in children.[32] No reported serious event, however, could be attributed definitively to the HAV vaccine, and the reported rates did not exceed the expected background rates. For example the general population incidence of Guillain-Barré syndrome ranges from 0.5 to 2.4 cases per 100,000 person-years, and among adult HAV vaccine recipients, the incidence of Guillain-Barré was 0.2 cases per 100,000 person-years.[32]

A combined formulation of hepatitis A and B vaccines (TWINRIX, GlaxoSmithKline Biologicals, Rixensart, Belgium) is available and has an excellent record of efficacy and safety.[67] Although some long-term studies have shown persistence of anti-HAV in children and adolescents, seroconversion rates for TWINRIX are lower in children 1–6 years of age than those for standard monovalent vaccines.[68] Currently, therefore, TWINRIX is approved only for persons 18 years of age and older.

As a result of the reduction in endemic cases of hepatitis A in the United States, a large proportion of patients who now become infected with HAV are nonimmune adults traveling to endemic areas. Even if medical advice is sought before travel, the time is usually insufficient for completing the standard immunization schedule. HAVRIX and VAQTA are approved by the FDA for use in an accelerated vaccination schedule before planned travel. If given at least 2 weeks before travel, a single dose of either monovalent vaccine results in protective anti-HAV titers.[62] IG is still indicated and highly effective for passive immunity for those traveling in less than 2 weeks. In 2008 the FDA also approved an accelerated vaccination schedule for TWINRIX that can be completed within 30 days, with a booster at 12 months, after studies showed equivalent protection when TWINRIX was compared with standard and alternative schedules of the individual monovalent vaccines. After 1 year, HAV seroconversion rates were 100%, and HBV seroconversion rates were 96.4%–100% with TWINRIX.[69,70] The TWINRIX accelerated schedule is being considered for use in new inmates at correctional facilities in the United States, where high-risk activities place the inmates at risk for both HAV and HBV infections.[71] Dosing schedules are shown in Table 80.2.

Another population that may have an increased risk of contracting HAV infection appears to be close contacts of newly arriving international adoptees. In 2009 the CDC provided updated recommendations for use of the HAV vaccine in this population after receiving case reports of new HAV infections among persons in close contact with new international adoptees, including a case of ALF in a nontraveling household contact of an asymptomatic adoptee from Ethiopia. From 1998 to 2008, some 18,000 children were adopted from foreign countries by families in the United States; 99.8% of those children were from countries considered to be of high or intermediate endemicity for HAV. Given this data, the CDC now recommends vaccination of all previously unvaccinated persons who anticipate close personal contact with an international adoptee from a country of high or intermediate endemicity during the first 60 days following the arrival of the adoptee in the United States.[72]

Immunization Against HAV in Patients With Chronic Illnesses

Persons with chronic liver disease are at an increased risk of HAV-related morbidity and mortality if they acquire HAV infection. Therefore preexposure prophylaxis with the HAV vaccine has been recommended for patients with chronic liver disease who are susceptible to HAV.[73] This recommendation should be extended to patients awaiting LT as well as those who have already undergone LT, although the immunogenicity of the HAV vaccine is reduced in such persons.[74]

An episode of acute hepatitis in a patient with underlying chronic liver disease poses the risk of considerable morbidity and mortality. Although current guidelines recommend immunization against HAV for all patients with chronic liver disease,[32] the results of several cost-effectiveness analyses have been conflicting. A report published in 2000 found that saving the life of one patient with HCV infection through HAV vaccination would cost 23 million Canadian dollars,[75] although some of the assumptions in this report have been challenged.[76] Two other studies of patients with chronic hepatitis C showed a decided benefit to immunization against HAV.[77,78] The methods used in these studies were dissimilar, and some analyses may have been insensitive to the incidence of HAV or may have underestimated the economic and societal costs of a case of ALF. Universal immunization against HAV during childhood, before the possible occurrence of chronic liver disease, offers the greatest promise of preventing HAV infection.[79]

Patients infected with HIV should be vaccinated against HAV. The response to vaccination, however, may be reduced because of a blunted immune system. Earlier studies have suggested HAV seroconversion rates above 97% in HIV-infected children on antiretroviral therapy[80]; however, another study found that a $CD4^+$ count of less than 25/mm^3 and an HIV viral load of more than 400 copies/mL predicted a reduced seroconversion rate.[81] Although the discrepancies among studies can be explained in part by different sensitivities of assays for anti-HAV, it appears that the more immunosuppressed a person is, the less likely the person is to respond to vaccination. In this population, consideration should be given to checking postvaccination IgG anti-HAV titers to assess immunity. Small studies have shown limited additional benefit to a third dose of the HAV vaccine in persons who fail to respond to the standard vaccine schedule.[81]

Full references for this chapter can be found at https://ebooks.health.elsevier.com.

81 Hepatitis B

Harry L.A. Janssen, Milan J. Sonneveld

IN THIS CHAPTER

INTRODUCTION

An estimated 296 million persons in the world today are chronically infected with HBV.[1] The majority of these individuals will not experience complications, but if untreated it is estimated that 8%–25% of patients who acquired chronic hepatitis B (CHB) perinatally will die of HBV-related cirrhosis or HCC.[2,3] If infected at an older age, the risk of progression from acute to chronic infection decreases to less than 5% in immunocompetent adults.[3,4] The World Health Organization (WHO) estimated that chronic HBV infection results in over 820,000 deaths per year globally.[1]

Most deaths are related to cirrhosis and liver cancer. This number has increased between 1990 and 2019 but has varied considerably between regions (highest in Western Pacific region and lowest in the Region of the Americas).[5] Globally a decline in cases of acute hepatitis B infection has been observed, but in the United States this decrease seems to have leveled off.[6,7] The decrease is most likely due to broader vaccination and use of antiviral therapy. In the United States, the favorable trends appear to be counterbalanced by a continuing increase in new cases of CHB and HCC in the Western world, mainly due to immigration from high endemic regions.[7]

A small proportion of patients with acute hepatitis B develop acute liver failure (ALF).[8,9] Around 8% of all cases of ALF are caused by hepatitis B, one of the main causes of ALF in developing countries.[10] Liver transplantation (LT) is the definitive treatment for HBV related ALF and acute on chronic liver failure (ACLF) and is associated with 1-year survival rates of 80% –85%.[11–14]

Effective vaccines against HBV have been available since the early 1980s, but perinatal and early life exposure continue to be major sources of infection in much of the developing world because of limited resources that preclude a policy of universal vaccination for newborns. From a global perspective, widespread implementation of early-life vaccination programs in high- and intermediate-risk countries will ultimately have the greatest impact on liver disease-related mortality in future generations. Promiscuous sexual contact and injection drug use account for most new cases of hepatitis B in adults in low-prevalence areas, such as the United States and Western Europe. Even in these areas, however, a further reduction in the incidence of acute infections will remain a challenge in the future because persons in these risk groups greatly underutilize vaccination. The WHO has implemented a strategy to eliminate hepatitis B and C infection globally through increased vaccination, screening, and treatment.[15]

EPIDEMIOLOGY

Geographic Distribution and Sources of Infection

The prevalence of HBV infection varies markedly around the world but is globally estimated around 4%.[1,5] In highly endemic regions, such as Southeast Asia, China, and much of Africa, 6% or more of the population are chronic HBV carriers, and the lifetime risk of infection ranges from 60% to 80%.[5,16] In these high-risk areas, perinatal transmission and horizontal spread among children are the major means of transmission. Regions of intermediate risk include parts of Southern and Eastern Europe, the Middle East, Japan, the Indian subcontinent, much of the former Soviet Union, and Northern Africa. In these areas, the lifetime risk of infection is between 20% and 60%. Horizontal transmission occurs among a broad age range, but neonatal exposure is also presumed to be common. Areas of low prevalence include North America, Western Europe, certain parts of South America, and Australia, where the lifetime risk of HBV infection is less than

20% and transmission is primarily horizontal between young adults.

Perinatal transmission accounts for most new infections in the world and is believed to account for at least half of all hepatitis B surface antigen (HBsAg)-positive carriers. Overall 60%–90% of hepatitis B e antigen (HBeAg)-positive mothers typically have a high-level of viremia (viral load) and transmit the infection to their offspring, whereas mothers who are positive for antibody to HBeAg (anti-HBe) transmit the disease less frequently (5%–15%) (see later). Fortunately, the incidence of new infections and childhood HCC has diminished greatly in countries, such as Taiwan, where universal vaccination has been in place for decades.[17]

Infectivity

HBV is transmitted efficiently by percutaneous and mucous membrane exposure to infectious body fluids. The virus is 50–100 times as infectious as HIV and 10 times as infectious as HCV. A high viral load indicates a higher risk not only of transmission from mother to child but also after needlestick exposure and in the setting of household contact. HBV DNA has been detected by sensitive techniques, such as PCR, in most body fluids, except for stool that has not been contaminated with blood. Although HBV replicates primarily in hepatocytes, the presence of replicative intermediates and virally encoded proteins in other sites, such as the adrenal gland, testis, colon, nerve ganglia, and skin, suggests that a vast extrahepatic reservoir for infectious virus exists.[18] Small amounts of HBV DNA have been demonstrated in peripheral mononuclear cells and liver tissue years after apparent resolution of chronic infection.[19,20] Extrahepatic localization of low levels of replicating virus could result in HBV transmission from a HBsAg-negative, anti-HBc-positive liver transplant donor or in HBV reactivation (HBV-r) after an HBV indicated LT.[21–25] Fortunately, the rate of reactivation after LT has decreased to less than 10% due to the use of antiviral therapy pre- and posttransplant with or without hepatitis B immune globulin (HBIG) (see later).[24]

Prevalence

In several highly endemic countries, the prevalence of hepatitis B is decreasing due to improved socioeconomic status, universal vaccination programs, and, possibly, effective antiviral therapy.[26] The global prevalence is estimated around 4% in all ages and has decreased in all WHO regions.[5] In the United States, an estimated 880,000 persons are living with a chronic HBV infection, of which 70% were not born in the United States, which could explain why most chronic HBV infections in the United States are imported[27,28] (Fig. 81.1).

Furthermore, a decline in acute cases of hepatitis B since the 1990s has been the result of universal vaccination of newborns, adult vaccination programs for high-risk persons, changes in sexual lifestyle, refinements in blood screening procedures, and the availability of virus-inactivated blood components.[29] Health care workers have experienced a striking decline in HBV infection owing to high rates of vaccination.

In much of the developed world, the highest incidence of acute cases continues to be in sexually active young adults. Since 1995 most cases of acute hepatitis B reported to the Centers for Disease Control and Prevention (CDC) were caused by intimate contact among heterosexuals, injection drug use, and sex between men.[30] The proportion of cases attributable to injection drug use has significantly increased due to the opioid abuse epidemic. Rates of new HBV infection are highest among adults 30–49 years of age, reflecting low HBV vaccination coverage among adults at risk.[31] Cases of hepatitis B continue to result from hemodialysis, acupuncture, artificial insemination, and, rarely, blood transfusion, but these cases account for a small contribution to the overall number of newly established acute infections.

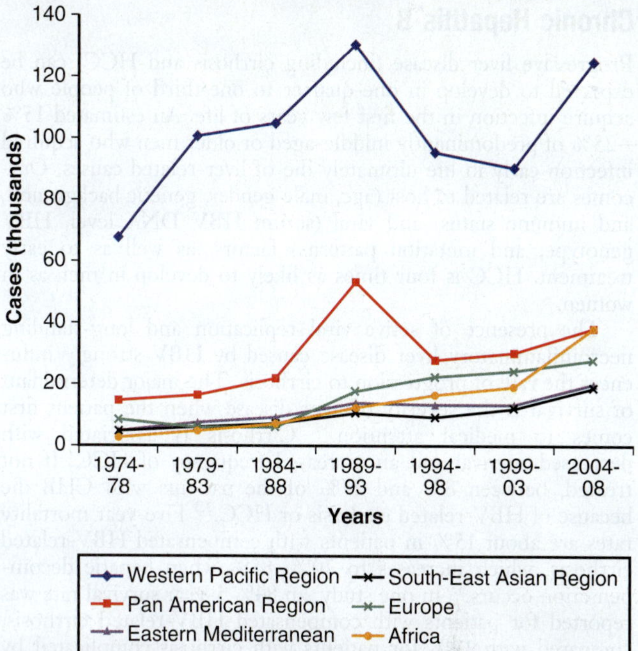

Fig. 81.1 Estimated number of cases of chronic HBV infection imported into the United States by WHO region of origin, from 1974 to 2008. (Modified from Mitchell T, Armstrong GL, Hu DJ, et al. The increasing burden of imported chronic hepatitis B—United States, 1974–2008. *PLoS One*. 2011;6:e27717, with permission of author.)

As mentioned earlier, infant vaccination has been an important milestone for HBV elimination. At the moment, all WHO regions achieved three-dose vaccination rates above 80% before the age of 1 year and nearly a hundred countries are compliant with the 2020 WHO target of 1% HBV prevalence among children aged 5 years.[32] According to new CDC data, infant vaccine coverage levels are up to 97% if born from hepatitis B-infected persons.[33]

CLINICAL OUTCOMES

Acute Hepatitis B

The age at which a person becomes infected with HBV is the principal determinant of the clinical outcome. Perinatal exposure leads to the chronic HBV carrier state in as many as 95% of persons because of immunologic tolerance to the virus (see later). By contrast, children exposed during the first 5 years of life have a 30% chance of developing chronic HBV. Less than 5% of adults with an intact immune system become chronically infected.[3]

Two-thirds of patients with acute hepatitis B have an asymptomatic or subclinical illness that goes unrecognized. In the other third, acute hepatitis, ranging from mild to moderate in severity, develops, with ALF occurring in 1%.[8,9] Although uncommon, hepatitis B accounts for 8% of all cases of ALF (see Chapter 97).[10] Rapid viral elimination may result in clearance of HBsAg from serum by the time of initial presentation. In these cases, the accurate diagnosis of acute hepatitis B may require testing with immunoglobulin M (IgM) anti-HBc (see later).

The rate of spontaneous survival in ALF caused by HBV is only approximately 20%.[34] One-year survival rates after LT for ALF and ACLF ranges between 80% and 85%.[11–14] Recurrent disease in the allograft is uncommon because of the successful application of HBIG and antiviral agents (see later and Chapter 99).

Chronic Hepatitis B

Progressive liver disease (including cirrhosis and HCC) can be expected to develop in one-quarter to one-third of people who acquire infection in the first few years of life. An estimated 15%–25% of predominantly middle-aged or older men who acquired infection early in life ultimately die of liver-related causes. Outcomes are related to host (age, male gender, genetic background, and immune status) and viral (serum HBV DNA level, HBV genotype, and mutation patterns) factors, as well as to early treatment. HCC is four times as likely to develop in men as in women.

The presence of active viral replication and long-standing necroinflammatory liver disease caused by HBV strongly influences the rate of progression to cirrhosis. The major determinant of survival is the severity of liver disease when the patient first comes to medical attention.[35] Cirrhosis is associated with decreased survival and an increased frequency of HCC. If not treated, between 8% and 25% of the patients with CHB die because of HBV-related cirrhosis or HCC.[2,3] Five-year mortality rates are about 15% in patients with compensated HBV-related cirrhosis, which increases to 70%–85% when hepatic decompensation occurs.[35] In one study, an 84% 5-year survival rate was reported for patients with compensated HBV-related cirrhosis, compared with 14% for patients with cirrhosis complicated by ascites, jaundice, encephalopathy, or a history of variceal bleeding (see Chapters 76 and 94).[36] Multivariate analyses in several large cohort studies have identified age, ascites, hyperbilirubinemia, and renal dysfunction as correlating independently with survival in patients with HBV-related cirrhosis. Therefore early hepatic decompensation is an immediate indication for antiviral therapy as well as evaluation for LT (see later). If compensated CHB patients are treated with antiviral therapy, survival outcomes are similar to the general population, and development of HCC may have the biggest impact on survival rates for these patients.[37]

Clearance of HBsAg from serum in patients with early HBV-related cirrhosis has been associated with a good prognosis, including improvement in liver histology and function, a decreased risk of viral reactivation, and improved long-term survival.[35] HBsAg clearance, however, is not an absolute safeguard against the future development of HCC, particularly not in persons who have preexisting cirrhosis.[38]

VIROLOGY

HBV is a small DNA virus that belongs to the Hepadnaviridae family. Other members of this family are HBV-like agents that infect the woodchuck, ground and tree squirrels, woolly monkey, crane, heron, Ross goose, and duck. HBV is a small (3.2 kb) virus with a DNA genome that has a relaxed, circular, partially double-stranded configuration (Fig. 81.2). The genome is composed of four open reading frames (ORFs) and has a compact design in which several genes overlap and use the same DNA to encode different viral proteins. The four viral genes components include the core, surface, X, and polymerase genes. The core gene encodes the core nucleocapsid protein, which is important in viral packaging and production of HBeAg. The surface gene encodes the pre-S1, pre-S2, and S proteins [comprising the large (L), middle (M), and small (S) surface proteins]. The X gene encodes the X protein, which has transactivating properties and may be important in hepatic carcinogenesis. The polymerase gene has a large ORF ($\approx$800 amino acids) and overlaps the entire length of the surface ORF. It encodes a large protein with functions that are critical for packaging and DNA replication (including priming, RNA- and DNA-dependent DNA polymerase, and RNase H activities).

Viral Replication

Although HBV is a DNA virus, replication occurs through an RNA intermediate and requires an active viral reverse transcriptase/polymerase enzyme (Fig. 81.3). The mutation rate is higher for HBV than for other DNA viruses (with an estimated 10^{13}–10^{15} point mutations per day).[39] Complete HBV genomic sequencing has identified a large number of mutations within the HBV genome, many of which are silent or do not alter the amino acid sequence of encoded proteins. Because of genomic overlap, however, some of the silent mutations in one ORF (e.g., the polymerase gene) may result in an amino acid substitution in an overlapping ORF (surface gene), although with uncertain clinical implications.

HBV replication begins with encapsidation of the pregenomic RNA through complex interactions between host and viral proteins.[40] HBV DNA polymerase reverse transcribes the pregenomic RNA into a negative-strand HBV DNA, which in turn serves as the template for positive-strand synthesis to form a partially double-stranded genome. Concurrent with HBV DNA synthesis, the nucleocapsid undergoes maturation and, through an incompletely understood mechanism, interacts with the S protein to initiate viral assembly in the endoplasmic reticulum. S protein is synthesized in the endoplasmic reticulum, where monomer aggregates that exclude host membrane proteins subsequently bud into the lumen as subviral particles. When formed, HBsAg undergoes glycosylation in the endoplasmic reticulum and the Golgi apparatus. Noninfectious subviral particles (spherical and filamentous forms of HBsAg) are secreted in great abundance when compared with mature virions. These subviral HBsAg particles exceed virions in number by a variable factor of 10^2–10^5 and can accumulate up to concentrations of several 100 μg/mL in serum.[41]

HBV Genotypes

A genetic classification based on comparisons of complete genomes has demonstrated 10 genotypes (designated A through J) and numerous subtypes of HBV (Box 81.1).[42] These classifications are defined as a divergence in the entire HBV genomic sequence of 8% or more. Genotype A is the predominant genotype in Northern Europe and the United States. Genotypes B and C are confined to populations in eastern Asia and the Far East, but changes in immigration patterns have resulted in an influx of Asian HBV carriers with these genotypes into the United States.[43,44] Genotype D is found worldwide but is especially prevalent in the Mediterranean area, Middle East, and Southern Asia. Genotype E is indigenous to western areas of sub-Saharan Africa, and genotype F prevails in Central and South America. Cases of genotype G have been reported in the United States and France. Genotype H has been described in Mexico. Genotypes I and J are the most recently discovered and have been observed in Vietnam and the Ryukyu Islands in Japan, respectively.[3,42]

Clinical associations appear to exist with the various genotypes (see Box 81.1).[45] The strongest clinical associations appear to be that (1) HBeAg seroconversion occurs earlier in patients with HBV genotype B than in those with genotype C, and (2) the response to therapy with interferon (IFN) is better with genotypes A and B than with C and D (see later).[46] The viral genotype also has implications for the frequency of precore and core mutations (see later) and may have an effect on the frequency of HCC. There is no compelling evidence that genotypes affect the HBV DNA response to nucleoside analogs (see later).

The clinical associations with the various genotypes have become increasingly clear but have not yet led to specific recommendations for routine testing because genotype classification does not generally lead to a difference in management. One exception to this rule, however, occurs when a patient is being

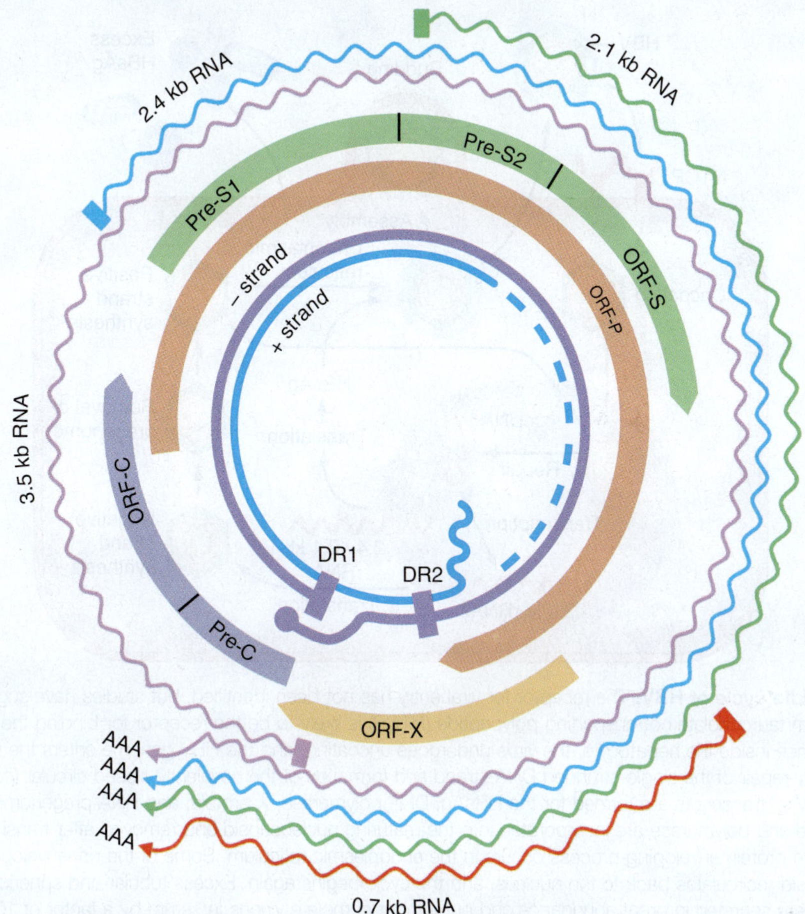

Fig. 81.2 The molecular structure and organization of HBV. Note the overlapping *ORFs* of the viral genome and its major transcripts (*wavy lines*). The genome is partially double stranded with four overlapping *ORFs*, or genes. The S gene encodes the viral surface envelope protein (hepatitis B surface antigen, HBsAg) and is composed of the pre-S1, pre-S2, and S regions. The core gene (C) consists of the precore (Pre-C) and core regions, which give rise to the HBeAg and core protein, respectively. The polymerase (P) gene overlaps the entire S gene, and mutations in this region may, in theory, give rise to changes in the HBsAg protein that affect neutralization by antibody to HBsAg. The fourth gene (X) encodes an incompletely understood protein, hepatitis B X protein (HBX). Two 11-base-pair direct repeats (DR1 and DR2) are required for strand-specific HBV DNA synthesis during viral replication. *AAA*, Polyadenosine tail at 3′ end of RNA.

BOX 81.1 Geographic Distribution and Proposed Clinical Associations of HBV Genotypes (A–J)

GEOGRAPHIC DISTRIBUTION

A: Northwestern Europe, North America, Central Africa
B: Southeast Asia, including China, Japan, and Taiwan (prevalence is increasing in North America)
C: Southeast Asia (prevalence is increasing in North America)
D: Southern Europe, Middle East, India
E: West Africa
F: Central and South America, United States (Native Americans), Polynesia
G: United States, France, Germany
H: Central and South America
I: Vietnam and Laos
J: Ryuku, Japan

PROPOSED CLINICAL ASSOCIATIONS

Shorter time to HBeAg seroconversion and higher probability of HBsAg loss: B > C
Response to treatment with interferon-α: A > B $\geq$ C > D
Precore/core promoter mutant frequency: B and D > A and C
Active liver disease activity and risk of progression: C > B
Evolution to chronic liver disease: non-A > A
HCC risk: B > C in younger age group in Taiwan, but C > B in older age group in Japan

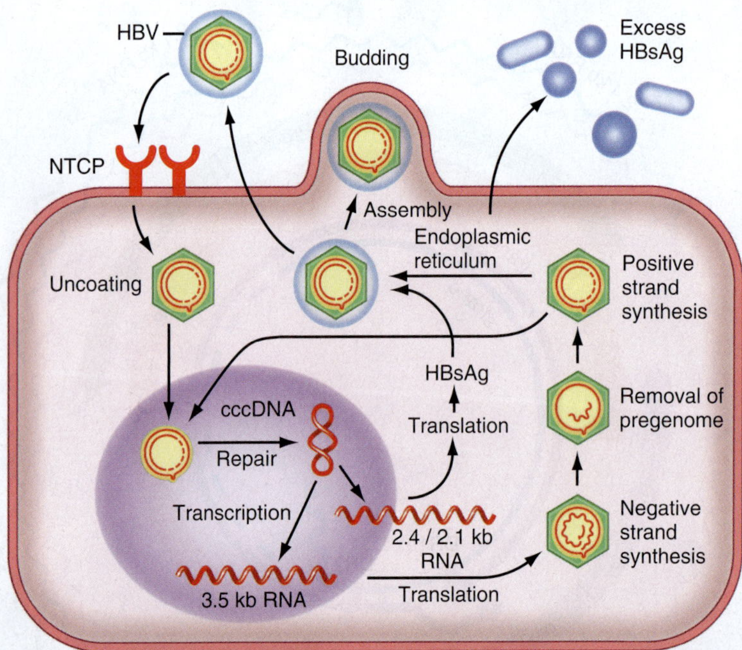

Fig. 81.3 Life cycle of HBV. The receptor for viral entry has not been identified, but studies have suggested that sodium taurocholate cotransporting polypeptide (NTCP) is likely to be the receptor for binding the HBsAg protein. Once inside the hepatocyte, the virus undergoes uncoating, and the HBV genome enters the nucleus, followed by repair of the single-stranded DNA strand and formation of the covalently closed circular (*ccc*) *DNA* template. Viral transcripts are formed for the HBsAg, DNA polymerase, X protein, and RNA pregenome; the pregenome and polymerase are incorporated into the maturing nucleocapsid and removed after translation. The surface protein enveloping process occurs in the endoplasmic reticulum. Some of the nonenveloped nucleocapsid recirculates back to the nucleus, and the cycle begins again. Excess tubular and spherical forms of HBsAg are secreted in great abundance and outnumber complete virions in serum by a factor of 10^3 or more. *HBsAg,* Hepatitis B surface antigen. (Yan H, Zhong G, Xu G, et al. Sodium taurocholate cotransporting polypeptide is a functional receptor for human hepatitis B and D virus. *Elife*. 2012;1:e00049.)

considered for pegylated IFN (PegIFN) therapy. In patients who are suitable candidates based on age and other factors (see later), genotype testing may have clinical value because genotypes A and B are associated with higher rates of sustained virologic response and HBsAg clearance.[47,48] The response to future curative treatments may be dependent on specific genotype profiles.

Mutations

Most mutations in the HBV genome that are identified by comparing nucleotide sequences with those of wild-type HBV are silent or do not alter the amino acid sequence in a particular ORF. Some mutations have potentially important disease associations, however, and are described later.

Hepatitis B Surface Antigen

HBsAg gene mutants result from a primary mutation in the HBsAg gene or a mutation in the overlapping DNA polymerase gene arising during nucleoside antiviral therapy (see later). Once the mutation appears, mutated virions can become selected immunologically as the dominant form of the virus.

Mutations in the HBsAg gene between amino acid positions 124 and 147 are potentially important because this region of the HBsAg gene includes the major "a" epitope that binds to neutralizing antibody to HBsAg (anti-HBs). The mutation can lead to failure to detect HBsAg by commercial assays, which depend on binding to anti-HBs, and to failure of neutralization by HBIG or of vaccination.

Infection with HBsAg gene-mutant HBV is accompanied by detection of anti-HBc. Serum HBV DNA levels can vary to the same extent seen in HBsAg carriers (see later). These mutants need to be distinguished from cases of "occult" hepatitis B, which has been linked to cryptogenic cirrhosis and an increased risk of HCC.[49,50] In occult HBV infection, HBsAg-negative persons have detectable HBV DNA in serum.[49] Some of these persons may lack evidence of other serologic markers of infection (e.g., anti-HBc). Occult HBV infection is thought to result from active suppression of viral replication by the host immune system; as a result, when HBV DNA is detectable in serum, it is present in low levels (<200 IU/mL).

Large-scale vaccination programs in regions endemic for HBV have revealed a 2%–3% frequency of vaccine-escape HBsAg mutants. It remains controversial whether additional mutants will be further selected in the future and increase the risk for widespread vaccine failure, but most available evidence does not support this scenario. The importance of HBsAg gene mutants for HBIG failure after LT is less controversial.

Precore, Basal Core Promoter, and Core Proteins

Mutations in the precore and basal core promoter regions of the HBV genome can influence the production of HBeAg. A precore mutation results in a stop codon at nucleotide 1896 that abolishes the synthesis of HBeAg,[51] whereas mutations in the basal core promoter at nucleotides 1762 and 1764 decrease HBeAg synthesis by approximately 70% while maintaining pregenomic RNA levels.[52] Both types of mutations have been observed in cases of severe hepatitis, which has been attributed to the loss of the immune-tolerizing effects of HBeAg (see later). The presence of core promoter mutations has been linked to an increased risk of HCC, and a higher frequency has been found in patients infected with HBV genotype C.[42] Precore and basal core promoter mutants have been described in the same patients and are particularly common in Asian and South European patients harboring HBV genotypes B, C, and D. A large serosurvey of HBV carriers residing in the United States has found that precore and core promoter mutations are common (frequencies of 27% and 44%, respectively). Both mutant forms of HBV were observed far more commonly in HBeAg-negative patients (precore mutation in 38% of HBeAg-negative vs. 9% of HBeAg-positive patients; core promoter mutation in 51% vs. 36%).[53] In addition to these mutations, upstream mutations in the core gene can influence immunologic responses to HBV. Core gene mutations have been shown to block recognition of HBV by cytotoxic T lymphocytes (CTLs), a key mode of viral clearance. Therefore the mutations contribute to HBV immune escape and possibly influence the response to IFN.[54,55] Core gene mutations within the immunodominant epitopes of the HBV nucleocapsid also can affect CD4$^+$ T-cell reactivity.

In patients with perinatally acquired CHB, a prolonged immune tolerant phase with minimal to absent hepatic necroinflammatory activity is typically seen for the first 20–30 years of HBV infection. Sequencing studies have demonstrated stable core gene sequences during this phase. Precore mutations are also uncommon during this phase. Core gene mutations become more common as patients pass from the immune active phase and undergo HBeAg seroconversion, at which time a growing number of mutations are observed in the region of the core gene that includes many B- and T-cell epitopes. Both precore stop codon mutants and core gene mutants have been associated with a poor response to IFN therapy.[55]

HBV DNA Polymerase

The polymerase gene encodes a DNA polymerase enzyme needed for encapsidation of viral RNA into core particles, conversion of the pregenomic viral RNA into a negative strand of viral DNA (reverse transcription), and conversion of this first HBV DNA strand into a second DNA strand of positive polarity. In general, the HBV reverse transcriptase function of the polymerase gene is highly conserved because major mutations that impair the efficiency of viral replication lead to selection pressure against such variants. As indicated earlier, HBV has low replication fidelity, however, meaning that it has a propensity to mispair nucleotide bases when it reverse transcribes viral RNA to DNA. HBV DNA polymerase also lacks any proofreading activity, so it cannot repair its mistakes. Therefore when a nucleotide base is misplaced, it remains in the growing viral DNA strand as a base mutation, and the new HBV DNA genome has a different sequence from the original (wild-type) genome. The overall error rate of HBV DNA polymerase is estimated to be 1 per 10,000 nucleotides copied, which translates to the potential for 10 million base-pair errors per day in an infected person. All possible single-base mutations can be produced in a 24-hour period, although many such mutations will yield nonviable viruses.[56]

Single or double nucleotide substitutions alter the amino acid sequence in the reverse transcriptase domain of the HBV DNA polymerase enzyme, thereby decreasing binding of drugs to its active site. Mutations in the HBV polymerase gene can lead to clinically apparent resistance to nucleoside analog therapy whenever there is both decreased susceptibility to the antiviral drug and sufficient replication fitness to allow continued propagation in the expanding viral population (quasispecies).

High-levels of viral replication and high mutability of the virus allow the emergence of single and even double polymerase mutants as a minor component of the viral quasispecies even before antiviral therapy is begun. Because of the limitations in sensitivity of currently available molecular assays (e.g., the line probe assay), these mutants are not detectable until they constitute at least 5%–10% of the entire viral population. Ultradeep pyrosequencing is a technique with the ability to detect HBV mutants that constitute less than 1% of the total population.[57] It is expected that next-generation sequencing will further dissect viral genome variability, thereby opening avenues to individualized medicine.[58] Persistent infection with drug-resistant HBV has been associated with progression of disease and blunting of hepatic histologic improvement with antiviral therapy.[59] Severe flares of hepatitis have also been reported in conjunction with the emergence of drug-resistant mutants,[60] and acquisition of these mutants may lead to rapidly progressive liver disease after LT.[61] Horizontal transmission of these mutants also has been described.

PATHOGENESIS

HBV is generally not a cytopathic virus, and the severity of HBV-associated liver disease is considered related to the intensity of the host immunologic response to the virus. Whereas both cellular and humoral immune responses are needed for effective clearance and long-term protection against reinfection, the cellular immune response appears to be the arm principally involved in the pathogenesis of disease. The immunologic response to HBV encompasses both an innate, or nonantigen-specific, response (e.g., natural killer cells and IFNs)[62] and an adaptive immune response, including antibodies to viral antigens, HLA class II-restricted CD4$^+$ T cells, and HLA class I-restricted CD8$^+$ CTLs.[63] Induction of the antigen-specific T-cell response is thought to occur in lymphoid organs, where the host T cells encounter viral peptide antigens (or epitopes) that are presented by antigen-presenting cells, such as dendritic cells, B cells, and macrophages.[64] This process results in the maturation and expansion of T cells that are specific for these viral epitopes and is followed by their migration to the liver, where they perform their effector function.

During acute HBV infection, HBV spreads through the liver without causing clinically overt liver inflammation until it reaches a logarithmic phase of replication.[65] At this point, HBV-specific T cells are detectable and most HBV DNA are cleared from the liver via noncytopathic mechanisms mediated by cytokines that are released by liver-infiltrating HBV-specific CD8$^+$ cells.[66] Cell-mediated immune responses are efficient in self-limited infection because the responses are vigorous, multispecific, and oriented toward type 1 helper T-cell functions. In contrast, persons with chronic HBV infection exhibit infrequent, narrowly focused, and weak HBV-specific T-cell responses that fail to clear HBV from infected hepatocytes.[67] In CHB, the majority of mononuclear cells in liver infiltrates of patients at any given time are nonantigen-specific.[68]

CD8$^+$ CTLs are the primary mediator of HBV clearance[69,70]and higher frequencies of HBV-specific T cells correlate with better control of HBV replication in chronically infected patients.[71,72] However, the antiviral function of CD8$^+$ CTLs can also contribute to immunopathology by inducing chemokines that drive nonspecific mononuclear inflammatory infiltrates observed during hepatitis.[73] To be recognized by the CD8$^+$ CTLs, targeted hepatocytes must present viral epitopes as short peptides that have been endogenously processed and fit within the peptide-binding groove of the class I MHC molecules.[74] The binding of the CTL T-cell receptor to the peptide-MHC complex on the hepatocyte surface can then result in the direct killing of the infected cell and release of potent antiviral cytokines by the activated CTL. Although hepatocytes express MHC-I, there is little evidence that they express MHC-II or are directly recognized by MHC class

II-restricted CD4+ helper T cells. CD4+ T cell activation requires the appropriate presentation of viral peptides in the context of class II MHC molecules, which may occur in lymphoid tissues or liver-resident antigen-presenting cells, such as dendritic cells, Kupffer cells, and endothelial cells. The CD4+ cells produce antiviral cytokines and provide help in stimulating neutralizing antibody production. Antibody neutralization limits intrahepatic spread of virus during primary infection and serves an important role in preventing reinfection.

NATURAL HISTORY

Five phases of CHB have been described: (1) HBeAg-positive chronic HBV infection (immune tolerance), (2) HBeAg-positive CHB (immune clearance), (3) HBeAg-negative chronic HBV infection (inactive carrier state), (4) HBeAg-negative CHB (reactivation), and (5) the HBsAg-negative phase (Fig. 81.4).[75] These consecutive phases are much more likely to be apparent in patients with acquisition of CHB early in life. The newer nomenclature is based on the description of the two main characteristics of chronicity: infection (no inflammation) versus hepatitis (inflammation).[75]

HBeAg-positive chronic HBV infection (immune tolerant phase) is often the earliest phase to be recognized when there is a history of infection at birth or the first few years of life. It is characterized by HBeAg positivity, high levels of HBV DNA ($\geq 10^7$ IU/mL), low or normal levels of serum aminotransferases, and minimal or no necroinflammation or fibrosis in the liver. During this phase, the rates of HBeAg loss are low. Experiments in transgenic mice suggest that HBeAg induces a state of immunologic tolerance to HBV in neonates.[76] Perinatal transmission of HBeAg is considered one of several potential mechanisms underlying the immune tolerant phase.[77]

HBeAg-positive CHB (immune reactive HBeAg-positive phase) often begins after several decades of HBV infection and is characterized by elevated serum aminotransferase levels, lower HBV DNA levels (10^4–10^7 IU/mL) than in HBeAg-positive chronic HBV infection, and histologic evidence of chronic hepatitis. The trigger mechanisms for this apparent immunologic activation against HBV are poorly understood, but CD8+ CTL-mediated lysis of infected hepatocytes has been shown to occur. The duration of this phase varies and frequently lasts many years. Continued pressure by the host immune system against the virus may result in HBeAg seroconversion (loss of HBeAg with the development of anti-HBe in serum). The annual rate of spontaneous HBeAg seroconversion generally ranges from 2% to 15%.[3] However, the rate is lower among Asians, women, and persons of younger age, who have normal ALT levels, and who are immunocompromised.[3,35,78]

HBeAg-negative chronic HBV infection (inactive carrier phase) is the third phase and occurs in most patients who undergo HBeAg seroconversion. This phase is characterized by normalization of serum ALT and low (<2000 IU/mL) or nondetectable serum HBV DNA levels (see Fig. 81.4). Over time, hepatic necroinflammation and fibrosis subside.[79] The inactive phase may last many decades, but reactivation remains a risk.

HBeAg-negative CHB develops after reactivation, which may occur spontaneously because of a loss of immunologic control over viral replication or may be due to immunosuppressive drug therapy (see later). Reactivation is defined by the reappearance of high levels of HBV DNA (>2000 IU/mL) in serum and often a noticeable rise in serum ALT levels. Therefore HBeAg seroconversion does not always indicate quiescent disease. As many as 30% of persons who undergo HBeAg seroconversion enter into a subsequent phase of active disease that is caused by the selection of HBeAg-negative mutants (precore mutation, core promoter mutation, or a combination of both).[80] At least 50% of these persons exhibit fluctuations in HBV DNA and aminotransferase levels, and recognition of active disease and exclusion of the inactive HBsAg carrier state (see later) may require serial assessment of both serum HBV DNA, quantitative HBsAg, and aminotransferase levels.[81]

The HBsAg-negative phase is the last phase and is characterized by a negative test for HBsAg and a positive test for antibody to HBcAg (anti-HBc), with or without detectable antibody to HBsAg (anti-HBs). In rare cases, the absence of HBsAg could be related to the sensitivity of the assay used for detection. Patients in this phase have normal ALT values and almost always undetectable serum HBV DNA. Covalently closed circular HBV DNA (cccDNA) can still be detected in the liver (see later).

If the active hepatitis phases remain untreated, cirrhosis can be anticipated to develop in at least 20% of cases. Various factors have been determined to increase the risk of cirrhosis, and, of these, older age, male gender, the stage of fibrosis at presentation, and ongoing HBV replication are perhaps the most important clinically. Combined infection with HDV (see this chapter), HCV (see Chapter 82), or HIV, as well as concomitant alcohol abuse, and presence of (elements of the) metabolic syndrome and/or of metabolic dysfunction-associated steatotic liver disease (MASLD, formerly NAFLD) has also been linked to a higher rate of development of cirrhosis and HCC.[82,83]

When cirrhosis develops, two major complications may occur: hepatic decompensation and HCC. If untreated, the estimated 5-year risk of developing hepatic decompensation in HBV-associated cirrhosis is 20%; the annual rate of HCC is 2%–5%.[75,84] Factors associated with an increased risk of HCC include male gender, age 45 years or greater, having a first-degree relative with HCC, the presence of cirrhosis, HBeAg positivity, reversion from anti-HBe to HBeAg positivity, and increased HBV DNA levels regardless of the HBeAg state.[85,86] Many of these risk factors are part of the risk scores that have been developed for predicting the occurrence of HCC in persons with CHB, for example the PAGE-B score.[87,88] HCC can still develop in HBsAg-positive persons with none of the identified risk factors, but less frequently. In addition, HCC can occur in cirrhotic patients who have undergone HBsAg seroconversion, and all patients with cirrhosis need continued surveillance [Box 81.2 (see Chapter 98)].[89]

Serum ALT as a Surrogate Marker for Disease Activity

The serum ALT level has been used conventionally as a measure of disease activity in patients with CHB. A serum ALT level within the normal laboratory reference range, however, has been shown to be an imperfect surrogate marker for lack of disease activity. Clinical laboratories base their range of normal values on blood donors without known liver disease, but this population may include persons who are obese, consume alcohol, and have diabetes mellitus, each of which tends to increase the apparent upper limit of normal (ULN). For purposes of guiding management of CHB, a ULN for serum ALT of 35 U/L for males and 25 U/L for females is recommended.[89] Studies in Asia and the United States have shown that as many as 20%–30% of Asian HBV carriers with persistently normal serum ALT levels and serum HBV DNA levels over 2000 IU/mL (roughly equivalent to 10,000 copies/mL) have grade 2 or greater inflammation and stage 2 or greater fibrosis (on scales of 0–4) on a liver biopsy specimen.[90] HBeAg-negative Asian HBV carriers with high-normal serum ALT levels by standard reference ranges tend to be older, have a greater frequency of serum HBV DNA levels in excess of 2000 IU/mL, and have a higher frequency of basal core promoter HBV mutations—all features that can be associated with adverse long-term outcomes.[91] Therefore liver biopsy or a noninvasive determination of hepatic fibrosis can be a useful tool

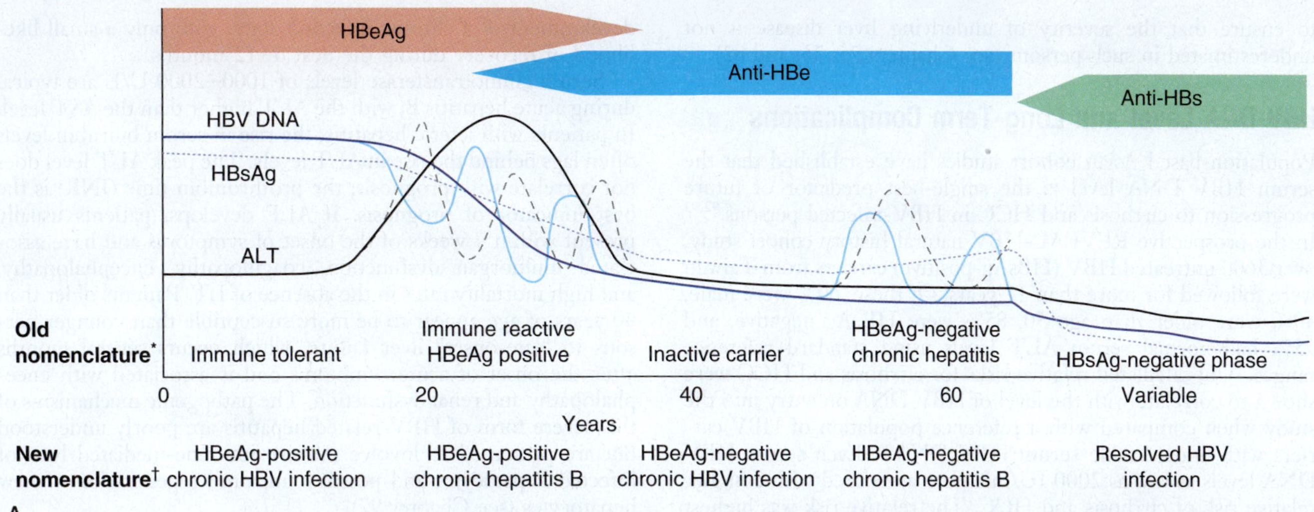

	HBeAg-positive		HBeAg-negative		HBsAg-negative
	Chronic HBV infection	**Chronic hepatitis B**	**Chronic HBV infection**	**Chronic hepatitis B**	**Resolved HBV infection**
HBsAg	High	High/ intermediate	Low	Intermediate	Negative
HBV DNA	≥10^7 IU/mL	10^4-10^7 IU/mL	<2000 IU/mL‡	≥2000 IU/mL	Undetectable
ALT	Normal	Elevated	Normal	Elevated§	Normal
Liver disease	None/minimal	Moderate/severe	None	Moderate/severe	None
Old terminology	Immune tolerant	Immune reactive HBeAg positive	Inactive carrier	HBeAg-negative chronic hepatitis	HBsAg-negative phase

B

Fig. 81.4 Natural history of and new nomenclature for patients with chronic HBV infection. The course is shown graphically in (A), and the criteria for each phase are shown in (B). Particularly in patients who are infected early in life, the first phase is *HBeAg-positive chronic HBV infection* (previously known as the immune tolerant phase). After decades of normal serum ALT and high HBV DNA levels, this phase evolves to *HBeAg-positive chronic hepatitis B* (previously known as the immune reactive phase) of variable duration. In this phase, there is active viral replication (high serum HBV DNA levels) and inflammation (high serum ALT levels) and an indication for antiviral therapy. Ultimately, patients enter a spontaneous or therapeutically induced phase of *HBeAg-negative chronic HBV infection* (previously known as the inactive carrier state), with minimal disease activity, which can last indefinitely. At the time of HBeAg seroconversion, however, immunologic pressure may select for a viral mutant (precore, core promoter, or both), which is incapable of producing HBeAg antigen. Viral and serum ALT levels typically fluctuate during this phase of *HBeAg-negative chronic hepatitis B*, and antiviral treatment is usually indicated. The last phase, which is the *HBsAg-negative phase*, (previously known as the HBsAg-negative phase) is characterized by negative HBsAg in serum and the presence of antibodies to HBcAg (anti-HBc), with or without detectable antibodies to HBsAg (anti-HBs). This phase is considered functional cure of HBV infection. If the patient has not entered this phase and is not treated, late disease complications often occur. The relative time dimensions of each phase are shown; note that there may be significant overlap of features among the various phases. *Anti-HBe,* Antibody to HBeAg; *HBeAg,* hepatitis B e antigen; *HBsAg,* hepatitis B surface antigen. *Data from Lok AS, Zoulim F, Dusheiko G, Ghany MG. Hepatitis B cure: from discovery to regulatory approval. *J Hepatol*. 2017;67:847–861. †European Association for the Study of the Liver. EASL 2017 Clinical Practice Guidelines on the management of hepatitis B virus infection. *J Hepatol*. 2017;67:370–398. ‡HBV DNA levels can be between 2000 and 20,000 IU/mL in some patients without signs of chronic hepatitis. §Persistently or intermittently, based on the traditional upper limit of normal (~40 IU/L).

BOX 81.2 Persons With HBV Infection for Whom HCC Screening is Recommended

African American carriers over 20 years of age
Asian female carriers over 50 years of age
Asian male carriers over 40 years of age
Carriers who have a family history of HCC
Persons who are coinfected with HDV, HCV, or HIV
Persons with HBV cirrhosis (at any age)
Persons with persistent active infection (high serum levels of HBV DNA and evidence of ongoing liver injury)

to ensure that the severity of underlying liver disease is not underestimated in such persons (see Chapters 75, 76, and 82).

HBV DNA Level and Long-Term Complications

Population-based Asian cohort studies have established that the serum HBV DNA level is the single-best predictor of future progression to cirrhosis and HCC in HBV-infected persons.[92,93] In the prospective REVEAL-HBV natural history cohort study, over 3600 untreated HBV (HBsAg-positive) carriers from Taiwan were followed for more than 11 years. Of these, 60% were male, 40% were older than age 50, 85% were HBeAg negative, and 95% had normal serum ALT levels using standard reference ranges. The calculated relative risks for cirrhosis and HCC were shown to correlate with the level of HBV DNA on entry into the study when compared with a reference population of HBV carriers with undetectable serum HBV DNA.[93] Even serum HBV DNA levels as low as 2000 IU/mL were associated with a higher relative risk of cirrhosis and HCC. The relative risk was highest (hazard ratio of 10) in persons with a serum HBV DNA level that was greater than 20,000 IU/mL and intermediate (hazard ratio of 3.8) in persons in whom the serum HBV DNA level decreased spontaneously from greater than 100,000 copies/mL at the time of enrollment to less than 2000 IU/mL at the last point of follow-up. These data can be interpreted to mean that both the duration and level of viremia are important risk factors for the development of HCC. The data also suggest that suppression of serum HBV DNA levels, whether spontaneous or induced by antiviral therapy, lowers the risk of HCC.

Some authorities recommend that Asian men 50 years of age or older with serum HBV DNA levels 20,000 IU/mL or greater receive long-term therapy with a nucleoside (or nucleotide) analog to prevent HCC, even if serum ALT values are normal.[94] Additional support for this recommendation can be found in a landmark study in which more than 600 Asian patients with advanced fibrosis and a serum HBV DNA level greater than 20,000 IU/mL were randomized in a ratio of 2:1 to active treatment with the nucleoside analog lamivudine or placebo.[95] Disease progression and HCC occurred significantly less frequently in the group of patients randomized to lamivudine.

CLINICAL AND PATHOLOGIC FEATURES

Acute Hepatitis B

The incubation period of acute hepatitis B varies from a few weeks to 6 months (average, 60–90 days), depending on the amount of replicating virus in the inoculum. In many patients, particularly in children, acute hepatitis B remains asymptomatic. The disease may be more severe in patients coinfected with other hepatitis viruses and in those with established underlying liver disease.[96] Acute infections are heralded by malaise, nausea, vomiting, and, in 10%–20% of patients, a prodrome of fever, arthralgias or arthritis, and rash that is most commonly maculopapular or urticarial. This prodrome results from circulating HBsAg-anti-HBs complexes that activate complement and are deposited in the synovium and walls of cutaneous blood vessels. These features generally abate before the manifestations of liver disease and peak serum aminotransferase elevations are observed. Jaundice develops in only about 30% of patients.

Clinical symptoms and jaundice generally disappear after 1–3 months. In general, elevated serum ALT levels and serum HBsAg titers decline and disappear together, and in approximately 80% of cases, HBsAg disappears by 12 weeks after the onset of illness. IgM anti-HBc is the best viral biomarker to confirm acute hepatitis B and to distinguish it from chronic infection. Persistence of HBsAg after 6 months implies development of a chronic infection state, with only a small likelihood of recovery during the next 6–12 months.

Serum aminotransferase levels of 1000–2000 U/L are typical during acute hepatitis B, with the ALT higher than the AST level. In patients with icteric hepatitis, the rise in serum bilirubin levels often lags behind the rise in ALT levels. The peak ALT level does not correlate with prognosis; the prothrombin time (INR) is the best indicator of prognosis. If ALF develops, patients usually present within 4 weeks of the onset of symptoms and have associated multiorgan dysfunction, coagulopathy, encephalopathy, and high mortality rates in the absence of LT. Patients older than 40 years of age appear to be more susceptible than younger persons to "late-onset" liver failure, which occurs several months after the onset of acute symptoms and is associated with encephalopathy and renal dysfunction. The pathogenic mechanisms of this severe form of HBV-related hepatitis are poorly understood but are presumed to involve massive immune-mediated lysis of infected hepatocytes and possibly impaired regeneration of new hepatocytes (see Chapter 97).

Chronic Hepatitis B

A history of acute or symptomatic hepatitis is often lacking in patients with chronic HBV infection. When symptoms are present, fatigue tends to predominate over other constitutional symptoms, such as poor appetite and malaise. Patients mostly remain asymptomatic, even during periods of reactivated hepatitis, until the presence of decompensated cirrhosis. Particularly when superimposed on cirrhosis, reactivation of HBV infection may be associated with frank jaundice and signs of liver failure.

Physical examination may be normal, or hepatosplenomegaly may be found. In decompensated cirrhosis, jaundice, ascites, and peripheral edema are common. During exacerbations of disease, serum ALT levels may be as high as 1000 U/L or more, and the clinical and laboratory picture is indistinguishable from that of acute hepatitis B, including the presence in serum of IgM anti-HBc in some cases. Progression to cirrhosis should be suspected whenever hypersplenism, hyperbilirubinemia, hypoalbuminemia (in the absence of nephropathy), or a high INR is found.

Extrahepatic Manifestations

Although uncommon, extrahepatic syndromes can occur with chronic and acute hepatitis B. They are important to recognize because they may occur without clinically apparent liver disease and can be mistaken for independent disease processes in other organ systems. The pathogenesis is not completely understood but likely involves an aberrant immunologic response to extrahepatic viral proteins.[97] Many of the extrahepatic manifestations are observed in association with circulating immune complexes that activate serum complement. Serum complement levels are generally low, and antiviral therapy may be beneficial in reducing the amount of immunologically activating viral antigens.

Arthritis-Dermatitis

The arthritis-dermatitis prodromal manifestations of acute hepatitis B must be distinguished from inflammatory forms of arthritis, because glucocorticoid therapy, if mistakenly given to these patients, can lead to enhanced HBV replication, and abrupt withdrawal of these agents may be associated with a potentially severe flare in disease activity.

Polyarteritis Nodosa

As many as 30% of patients with polyarteritis nodosa are infected with HBV, but the disorder develops in less than 1% of patients with chronic HBV infection. This association has been reported predominantly in North America and Europe but less so in Asia, where HBV is acquired perinatally. Typical features include arthralgias, fever, rash, abdominal pain, renal disease, hypertension, mononeuritis multiplex, and CNS abnormalities. Plasmapheresis may be useful, but the best therapeutic responses have also been observed with antiviral agents, given alone or in combination with plasmapheresis or immunosuppressive therapy.

Glomerulonephritis

Several types of glomerular lesions have been described in patients with chronic HBV infection; membranous nephropathy, polyarthritis nodosa, and membranoproliferative glomerulonephritis are the most common.[98] Renal biopsy specimens have demonstrated immune-complex deposition and cytoplasmic inclusions in the glomerular basement membrane. Nephrotic syndrome is the most common presentation of HBV-associated glomerulonephritis. The diagnosis requires the presence of immune-complex glomerulonephritis in a renal biopsy specimen and the demonstration of glomerular deposits of one or more HBV antigens, such as HBsAg, HBcAg, or HBeAg, by immunohistochemistry. The renal disease typically resolves in months to several years in children. Resolution may occur after HBeAg seroconversion. The natural history of HBV-related glomerulonephritis in adults has not been well defined, but several reports suggest that glomerular disease is often slowly and relentlessly progressive.[99] Successful treatment has been accomplished with nucleoside (or nucleotide) analogs and PEG-IFN-α, and has been linked to long-term control of HBV replication, however, limited data on these treatments is available.[98,100,82]

Cryoglobulinemia

Type II cryoglobulins consist of a polyclonal IgG and monoclonal IgM with rheumatoid factor activity, whereas type III cryoglobulins contain polyclonal IgG and IgM. Type II and type III cryoglobulinemia have been associated with hepatitis B, but the association, unlike that with hepatitis C, is uncommon. Cryoglobulinemia may be associated with systemic vasculitis (purpura, arthralgias, peripheral neuropathy, and glomerulonephritis) but is often asymptomatic. Nucleos(t)ide analog therapy has been used successfully to treat symptomatic cryoglobulinemia.[101]

Histopathologic Features

Chronic HBV infection is characterized by mononuclear cell infiltration in the portal tracts. Periportal inflammation often leads to the disruption of the limiting plate of hepatocytes (interface hepatitis), and inflammatory cells often can be seen at the interface between collagenous extensions from the portal tracts and liver parenchyma (referred to as *active septa*). During reactivated hepatitis B, lobular inflammation is more intense and reminiscent of that seen in acute viral hepatitis. Steatosis is not a feature of CHB, as it is of chronic hepatitis C.

The only histologic feature noted on routine light microscopy that is specific for CHB is the presence of ground-glass hepatocytes (Fig. 81.5). This morphologic finding results from accumulation of HBsAg particles (20–30 nm in diameter) in the dilated endoplasmic reticulum. Ground-glass hepatocytes may also be seen in HBV carriers, in whom they may be detected in up to 5% of cells. When present in abundance, ground-glass hepatocytes often reflect a high level of viral replication. Immunofluorescence and electron microscopic studies have shown HBcAg inside the nuclei of affected hepatocytes. During periods of intense hepatitis activity, cytoplasmic core antigen staining is generally observed. After successful treatment of HBV infection with a nucleos(t)ide analog, the cytoplasmic core antigen staining often disappears, but nuclear core antigen staining due to persistence of the HBV cccDNA transcriptional template may remain.

Acute Flares and Reactivation

CHB is often punctuated by sudden flares of disease activity that are characterized by a precipitous increase in serum aminotransferase levels. Although a uniform biochemical definition of a flare is lacking, it has frequently been described as an increase in serum ALT levels to at least two to three times the baseline value and at least 100 IU/mL. Flares are an important part of the natural history of hepatitis B because they can lead to histologic progression when they occur repeatedly and are moderate or severe. Acute flares in CHB occur in association with a number of circumstances (Table 81.1). Most flares are preceded by an increase in viral replication, which stimulates an enhanced cellular immune response that targets virus-infected hepatocytes. The mechanisms behind the increase in viral replication are unknown in many instances and are presumed to be due to the weakening of immune control over viral replication or to the emergence of replication-fit viral mutants, such as core promoter mutants or drug-resistant mutant HBV (see earlier). Flares following viral

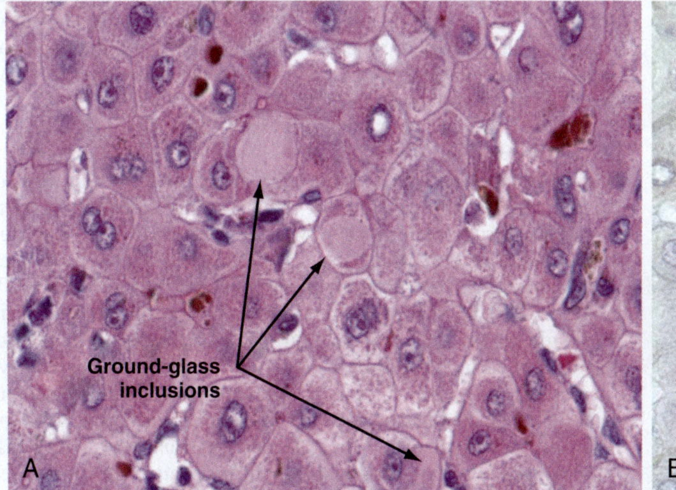

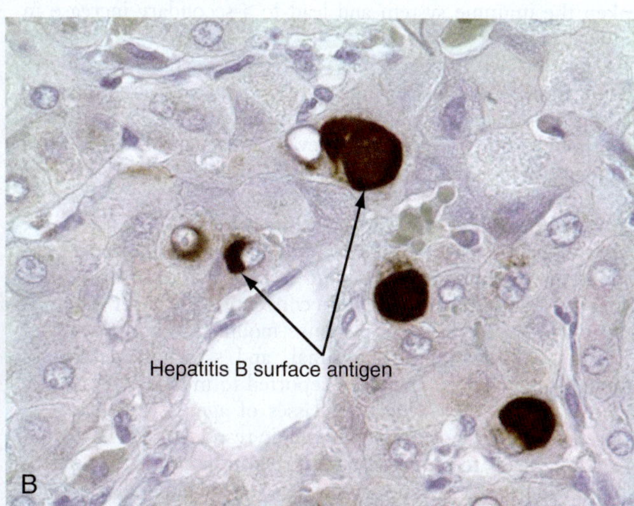

Fig. 81.5 Histopathology of HBV infection. (A) Photomicrograph showing ground-glass inclusions in hepatocytes. These inclusions represent large amounts of hepatitis B surface antigen (HBsAg) in the endoplasmic reticulum (H&E, ×630). (B) Immunohistochemical stain for HBsAg. Note that the brownish inclusions correspond to the ground-glass inclusions seen in (A) (×630). (Courtesy Dr. Gist Farr, New Orleans, LA.)

TABLE 81.1 Differential Diagnosis of Hepatitis Flares in Persons With Chronic Hepatitis B

Cause of Flare	Comment
Spontaneous	Factors that precipitate viral replication and loss of immune control are unclear
Immunosuppressive therapy	Flares are often observed during or shortly after withdrawal of the agent; preemptive antiviral therapy is required
Interferon	Flares may be observed within the first 3 months of initiating therapy in 30% of patients and may herald HBeAg seroconversion in some patients
Nucleos(t)ide analog	–
During treatment	Reinforce patient education to improve medication adherence
Antiviral resistance	Mainly an issue for agents that have a low genetic barrier to resistance, such as lamivudine and telbivudine Confirm genotypic resistance with resistance testing
Off treatment	Flares indicate clinical relapse (re-evaluation of serum ALT levels and re-appearance of HBV DNA in serum in those previously virally suppressed)
HIV coinfection	Flares can occur as a result of the direct toxicity of ART or with immune reconstitution; HBV increases the risk of antiretroviral drug hepatotoxicity
Other liver diseases	Alcohol overuse Autoimmune liver disease Drug and toxin-induced liver injury NAFLD
Precore and core promoter mutants	Fluctuations in serum ALT levels are common in HBeAg-negative patients who harbor these variants
Coinfection with HCV	HBV may be suppressed in HCV-coinfected patients Beware of HBV reactivation in coinfected patients undergoing DAA therapy for HCV infection
Coinfection with HDV	HBV is typically suppressed in HDV coinfected patients Higher risk of liver disease progression requires close monitoring

ART, Antiretroviral therapy; *HBeAg,* hepatitis B e antigen.

relapse after nucleos(t)ide analogs are stopped have been well described. Irrespective of the cause of the increased viral replication, however, the biochemical abnormalities usually occur coincident to or immediately after an increase in serum HBV DNA levels.

Spontaneous Flares

Spontaneous flares have been observed in patients with HBeAg-positive CHB, in whom they occur in 5%–10% of patients annually, and in those with HBeAg-negative CHB, in whom fluctuations of both serum HBV DNA and ALT levels are common. It is not clear if severe physical or emotional stress can weaken the immune system and lead to a secondary increase in viral replication.

In persons who acquire HBV infection early in life, flares become more common during adulthood. In this situation, the flares are almost certainly host-driven rather than virally mediated, and although poorly understood, they are most likely the result of a change in the regulation of viral antigen-specific T cells.[77]

Immunosuppressive Therapy–Induced Flares

Reactivation of hepatitis B with flares of serum aminotransferase levels is a well-recognized complication of cytotoxic or immunosuppressive therapy, including conventional cancer chemotherapy and potent biologic response modifiers that are used to treat rheumatologic, gastrointestinal, and skin disorders.[102,103] Although many drugs have been reported to induce HBVr, they tend to fall into one of several classes of agents (Fig. 81.6).[104] Suppression of the normal immunologic responses to HBV during therapy leads to enhanced viral replication and is thought to result in widespread infection of hepatocytes. In general, the more potent the immunosuppression, the higher the level of viral replication and, thus, the greater the potential for serious clinical consequences. The literature provides ample evidence for HBV-r leading to severe hepatitis, death from ALF, and delay or inability to continue treatment for the underlying disease. When reactivation occurs in the setting of cancer chemotherapy or systemic treatment for a severe autoimmune disorder, the patient may not be eligible for salvage LT. A growing body of evidence shows benefit to screening all patients in need of immunosuppressive drug therapy for HBsAg and anti-HBc and prophylactically treating HBsAg-positive patients with antiviral therapy. Reactivation of hepatitis B is discussed later in the chapter.

Antiviral Therapy–Induced Flares

Antiviral treatment of CHB can be associated with ALT increases and flares of hepatitis in several circumstances. Flares may occur during IFN or nucleos(t)ide analog therapy, after withdrawal of nucleos(t)ide analogs or glucocorticoid therapy, and in association with the emergence of lamivudine-, adefovir-, entecavir (ETV)-, or telbivudine-resistant mutants.

During Interferon Therapy

IFN-induced flares of CHB occur in approximately one-third of treated patients and result from the immunostimulatory properties of the drug. Flares occur with conventional and pegylated formulations of IFN (see later and Chapter 80) and have been reported to occur more frequently in patients infected with HBV genotype A than with other genotypes. This finding may explain the higher rate of sustained virologic response and HBsAg clearance seen in this group of patients.[46] Serum ALT flares have been shown to be a predictor of sustained virologic response and may be especially important in achieving a sustained virologic remission in patients with a high level of viremia.[105,106] Flares that occur in patients with advanced liver fibrosis have been associated with clinical deterioration, and, as a result, IFN should be used cautiously in patients with cirrhosis and should not be used in patients with decompensated cirrhosis.

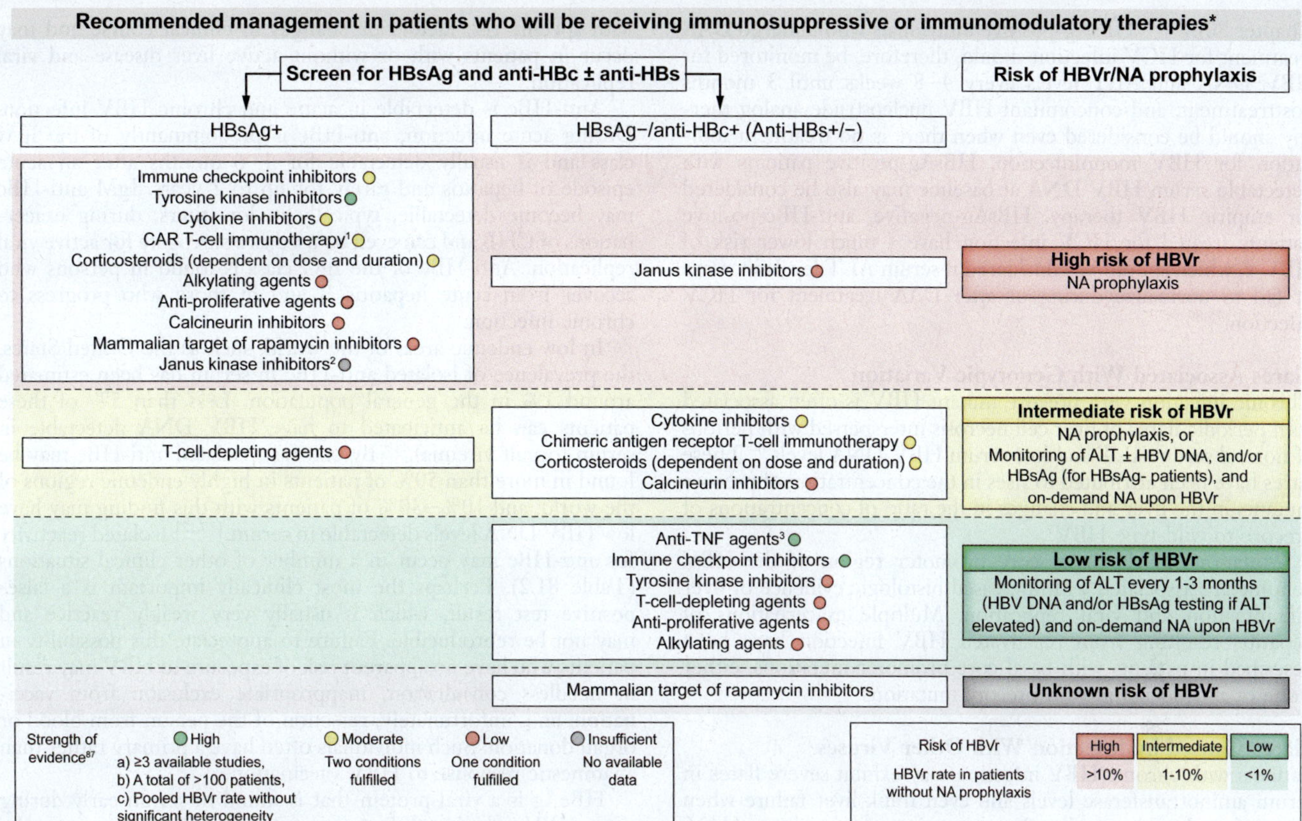

Fig. 81.6 Recommended management in patients who will be receiving immunosuppressive or immunomodulatory therapies. [1]Risk estimation based on 11% HBVr risk in HBsAg+ patients receiving CAR T-cell immunotherapy under NA prophylaxis; [2]Risk estimation based on 14% HBVr risk in HBsAg-/anti-HBc+ patients receiving Janus kinase inhibitors without NA prophylaxis; [3]HBVr risk in HBsAg-/anti-HBc+ patients receiving anti-TNF agents was categorized as low based on data from recent large studies and expert opinions, although it was 1% and could be marginally categorized as intermediate; HBVr risk associated with anti-TNF agents in HBsAg+ patients was not assessed (recent studies and most experts agree showed that this risk is high). Categorization of HBVr risk and recommendations for drug classes with low-quality evidence should be considered provisional. *ALT*, Alanine aminotransferase; *anti-HBC±*, anti-hepatitis B core antibody positive/negative; *anti-HBs±*, anti-hepatitis B surface antibody positive/negative; *HBVr*, HBV reactivation; *NA*, nucleos(t)ide analogue. *Long-term NA therapy is required in HBsAg+ patients who meet hepatitis B treatment indications. (From Papatheodoridis GV, Lekakis V, Voulgaris T, et al. Hepatitis B virus reactivation associated with new classes of immunosuppressants and immunomodulators: a systematic review, metaanalysis, and expert opinion. *J Hepatol*. 2022;77(6):1670–1689.)

During Nucleos(t)ide Analog Therapy

The registration studies for all nucleos(t)ide analogs have detected ALT flares during treatment in less than 10% of patients, and these flares were no more common or severe than those occurring in untreated patients. Whether a reduction in viral burden results in a transient restoration of immune competence is controversial, but the interaction does not appear to be clinically important. Serum aminotransferase increases are generally brief, even with continuation of therapy.[107]

After Withdrawal of a Nucleos(t)ide Analog

Serum ALT flares occur in more than 40% of patients after withdrawal of nucleos(t)ide analog therapy. These flares are thought to be caused by rapid resurgence of HBV, and, although generally well tolerated, they may be associated with serious clinical exacerbations in patients with advanced liver disease. Reinstitution of the original therapy is usually associated with a decline in HBV DNA levels. In selected HBeAg-negative patients, stopping nucleos(t)ide analog therapy may induce a temporary increase in serum HBV DNA levels accompanied by a flare followed by a decline in HBsAg levels and sometimes HBsAg loss.[108,109]

During Other Antiviral Therapy

Serum ALT flares occur in patients coinfected with HIV and HBV who receive dually active antiretroviral therapy (ART).[110] The cause of these flares can be multifactorial. One of the most common causes is immunologic reconstitution due to the effectiveness of ART.[111] Patients with low CD4 counts before ART therapy and high HBV DNA levels are often at greatest risk for this syndrome, and ALF may occasionally result.[112]

HBV infection increases the risk of hepatotoxicity from ART, usually within 6 months after the initiation of treatment, and hepatotoxicity should be suspected if serum aminotransferase elevations occur despite an appropriate decline in HBV DNA levels. Affected HIV-infected patients may also be particularly susceptible to ALT flares because of a higher risk of infection with other hepatitis viruses.

In patients coinfected with HBV and HCV, there is a potential risk for HBV-r and flare after HCV clearance using DAAs (see

Chapter 80).[113,114] HBsAg-positive individuals who undergo DAA treatment for HCV infection should, therefore, be monitored for HBV DNA and ALT levels every 4–8 weeks until 3 months posttreatment, and concomitant HBV nucleos(t)ide analog therapy should be considered even when there is no treatment indication for HBV monoinfection. HBsAg-positive patients with detectable serum HBV DNA at baseline may also be considered for empiric HBV therapy. HBsAg-negative, anti-HBc-positive patients treated for HCV infection have a much lower risk of HBV-r, which should be considered if serum ALT levels increase or fail to normalize during or after DAA treatment for HCV infection.[75,89]

Flares Associated With Genotypic Variation

Chronic infection with precore mutant HBV is often associated with periodic flares of liver cell necrosis interspersed with periods of normal serum ALT and low serum HBV DNA levels.[80] These flares have been attributed to rises in the concentration of precore mutants in the liver and changes in the ratio of concentrations of precore to wild-type HBV.

Mutations in the basal core promoter region of the HBV genome are associated with increased histologic evidence of liver inflammation and viral replication. Multiple exacerbations of hepatitis resulting from reactivated HBV infection have been described in patients with basal core promoter mutations, either alone or in association with precore mutations.

Flares Caused by Infection With Other Viruses

Patients with chronic HBV infection may exhibit severe flares in serum aminotransferase levels and even frank liver failure when superinfected with another hepatotropic virus, such as HAV, HCV, or HDV. Increased mortality has been reported when HDV superinfection is superimposed on CHB, and chronic HDV infection is often associated with frequent fluctuations in serum aminotransferase levels (see this chapter).

Acute hepatitis C superimposed on CHB has been reported to be as clinically severe as HDV superinfection and has been associated with high rates of liver decompensation (34%) and death (10%).[115] In a large study involving 2123 noncirrhotic HBV patients, 1-year mortality of patients who developed a HEV superinfection was 2.4% which increased to 37.5% in patients who also developed cirrhosis during follow-up.[116] In comparison with HAV superinfection, HEV is also associated with higher rates of complications, including liver failure and death.[117]

DIAGNOSIS

HBsAg appears in serum 2–10 weeks after exposure to HBV and before the onset of symptoms or elevation of serum aminotransferase levels. In self-limited acute hepatitis, HBsAg usually becomes undetectable after 4–6 months. Persistence of HBsAg for more than 6 months implies evolution to chronic HBV infection.

The disappearance of HBsAg is followed several weeks later by the appearance of anti-HBs. In most patients, anti-HBs persists for life and provides long-term immunity. In some patients, anti-HBs may not become detectable after disappearance of HBsAg, but these patients do not appear to be susceptible to recurrent HBV infection.[118] Anti-HBs may not be detectable during a window period of several weeks to months after the disappearance of HBsAg. During this period, the diagnosis of acute HBV infection is made by the detection of IgM anti-HBc in serum.

Coexistence of HBsAg and anti-HBs in serum has been reported in approximately 10%–20% of HBV carriers. The mechanisms of this finding are not clear but most likely relate to antibodies formed against minor variants of the HBsAg protein. The presence of these heterotypic antibodies is not associated with specific risk factors or changes in clinical course and may occur in patients with or without active liver disease and viral replication.

Anti-HBc is detectable in acute and chronic HBV infection. During acute infection, anti-HBc is predominantly of the IgM class and is usually detectable for 4–6 months after an acute episode of hepatitis and rarely for up to 2 years. IgM anti-HBc may become detectable, typically in low titers, during exacerbations of CHB and can even be used as a surrogate for active viral replication. Anti-HBc of the IgG class is found in persons who recover from acute hepatitis B and in those who progress to chronic infection.

In low endemic areas of the world, such as the United States, the prevalence of isolated anti-HBc in serum has been estimated around 1% in the general population. Less than 5% of these patients can be anticipated to have HBV DNA detectable in serum (occult viremia).[119] By contrast, isolated anti-HBc may be found in more than 50% of patients in highly endemic regions of the world, and 10%–30% of patients with this finding may have low HBV DNA levels detectable in serum.[120,121] Isolated reactivity for anti-HBc may occur in a number of other clinical situations (Table 81.2). Perhaps the most clinically important is a false-positive test result, which is usually very weakly reactive and may not be reproducible. Failure to appreciate this possibility in patients who have no apparent risk of exposure to HBV may result in needless consultation, inappropriate exclusion from vaccination, and, unfortunately, rejection of the person from blood or organ donation. Such individuals often have a primary rather than anamnestic response to HBV vaccination.

HBeAg is a viral protein that is found in serum early during acute HBV infection. HBeAg reactivity usually disappears at the time of or soon after the peak in serum aminotransferase levels, and persistence of HBeAg 3 or more months after the onset of illness indicates a high likelihood of transition to chronic HBV infection. The finding of HBeAg in the serum of an HBsAg-positive carrier indicates a high-level of viral replication and greater infectivity for intimate contacts. Nearly 90% of patients with HBeAg-positive CHB have been found to have serum HBV DNA levels persistently above 20,000 IU/mL.[122] Serum HBV DNA values can be as high as 10^9 IU/mL[19,20] during the HBeAg-positive chronic infection (immune tolerant phase). By contrast, anti-HBe-positive patients have much lower serum HBV DNA levels, with the highest values being found in those with persistently or intermittently elevated serum ALT levels.

HBV DNA is a crucial component in the evaluation of HBV infection. Most clinical laboratories use a quantitative real-time PCR assay with a sensitivity of 5–10 IU/mL and a dynamic

TABLE 81.2 Possible Interpretations of an Isolated Positive Test Result for Antibody to Hepatitis B Core Antigen (Anti-HBc)

Interpretation	Comments
Resolved or remote infection	Common in persons who come from endemic areas of the world where acquisition of infection is frequent early in life Serum HBV DNA is usually undetectable
False-positive result	Weakly positive anti-HBc Repeat serology in 3–6 months
Window period of acute hepatitis B	IgM anti-HBc is positive during this phase HBsAg and HBV DNA are also positive in this phase
Occult infection	An uncommon variant of chronic hepatitis B associated with progressive liver damage Serum HBV DNA is typically detectable in low levels

HBsAg, Hepatitis B surface antigen; *Ig,* immunoglobulin.

range of at least 7 $\log_{10}$ IU/mL. The quantification of serum HBV DNA is commonly used to evaluate a patient's candidacy for antiviral therapy and to monitor response during treatment. Patients with a high serum HBV DNA level ($>2\times10^8$ IU/mL) at baseline respond less commonly to therapy with PegIFN than do those with lower levels.[123] By contrast, baseline serum HBV DNA levels have not been shown to correlate with response to nucleos(t)ide analog therapy because of the more potent inhibition of viral replication by these agents. Monitoring of HBV DNA levels at key intervals, such as 12 and 24 weeks, of therapy allows prediction of the likelihood of HBeAg clearance with both PegIFN and nucleos(t)ide analog therapy. In the past, reappearance of HBV DNA in serum during treatment predominantly suggested that drug resistance had occurred.[124] This is not the case, however, with high–genetic barrier nucleos(t)ide analog therapy, during which the reemergence of HBV DNA more likely signals poor adherence to therapy.[75]

HBV genotypes A through J have distinct geographical distributions (see earlier) and are of importance in assessing the progression of HBV-related disease, the risk of HCC, and serologic response to both PegIFN and nucleos(t)ide analog therapy. Genotype testing is unfortunately not licensed and, therefore, rarely used in the United States.

Assays for quantification of HBsAg have become commercially available and are licensed in many parts of the world. HBsAg reflects cccDNA activity, the template of viral replication, in HBeAg-positive patients but not in HBeAg-negative patients, in whom HBsAg is also derived from integrated DNA.[41] HBsAg levels vary by HBV genotype and over the different phases of HBV infection. In clinical practice, HBsAg is used in HBeAg-negative patients to distinguish true inactive disease (HBsAg level <1000 IU/mL) from relapsing disease.[81] HBsAg levels also provide prognostic information with regard to the risk of the progression of liver disease and HCC.

Clinical trials in both HBeAg-positive and HBeAg-negative patients have demonstrated a rapid decline in HBsAg concentration during PegIFN therapy and a much slower decline during the first few years of nucleos(t)ide analog therapy.[126] High negative predictive values at Week 12 (>90%) have led to validated stopping rules that would avoid unnecessary extension of PegIFN therapy in both HBeAg-positive and -negative patients and prompt initiation of a different treatment regimen.[127,128] In the setting of nucleos(t)ide analog treatment, a greater than 1 log decline in HBsAg levels has been predictive of HBsAg loss, and HBsAg levels of less than 100 IU/mL have been associated with a sustained off-treatment response following consolidation treatment in HBeAg-negative patients.[41] With current efforts to achieve functional cure (sustained HBsAg loss) of CHB using novel finite treatments, HBsAg levels will become increasingly important to monitor treatment and to be used as endpoint.[129,130]

New serum biomarkers which likely best reflect cccDNA activity are hepatitis B core related antigen (HBcrAg) and hepatitis B virus RNA (HBV RNA). Assays for both biomarkers are currently in development but require further validation and improvements in assay sensitivity. Since kinetics of these biomarkers may differ, combinations of biomarkers may help improve predictive performance.[131,132]

TREATMENT

Eight antiviral agents have been approved for the treatment of CHB in North America. These include IFN-α (standard and PegIFN) and the nucleos(t)ide analogs lamivudine, adefovir, telbivudine, ETV, tenofovir disoproxil fumarate (TDF), and tenofovir alafenamide (TAF). Nucleos(t)ide analogs target HBV replication through inhibition of the reverse transcriptase function of HBV DNA polymerase, whereas PegIFN has both antiviral and immunomodulatory activities. Most patients on treatment receive nucleos(t)ide analogs due to their excellent safety record, oral route of administration, and tolerability compared with PegIFN. First-line nucleos(t)ide analogs include TDF, ETV, or TAF owing to high antiviral potency and a high genetic barrier to resistance.[75,89,133] These agents are particularly useful in the management of patients with advanced liver disease, whereas PegIFN can further decompensate liver function and cause life-threatening infections. PegIFN offers a shorter duration of treatment (6–12 months) but is less desirable for many patients, because it is given by injection only and has unpleasant side effects.

81

Goals

The ultimate goals for treatment of patients with CHB include arrest of progression of liver disease, prevention of late complications, and improvement in survival. Several studies have now documented the long-term benefits of treatment, such as reversal of cirrhosis and reductions in the frequency of HCC and the need for LT.[95,134] Classical endpoints of treatment include suppression of serum HBV DNA, HBeAg seroconversion in HBeAg-positive patients, serum ALT normalization, and histologic improvement. Each of these endpoints may be achieved with long-term suppression of viral replication using PegIFN or nucleos(t)ide analogs. However, the most desirable endpoint is HBsAg loss or seroconversion, which has been associated with improved survival.[135,136] Unfortunately, fewer than 10% of patients treated with PegIFN or an oral agent will achieve HBsAg loss.[137,138] Therefore there remains an urgent need to develop new therapies that can induce a "functional cure" of HBV (sustained HBsAg loss) for the majority of chronic HBV patients. Missed opportunities for HBV screening and confusion regarding the indications for treatment of HBV infection have impeded fulfillment of the goals of treatment.[139–141]

Barriers

The WHO has set a goal of Viral Hepatitis Elimination by 2030. This goal targets a 90% reduction in the incidence of chronic viral hepatitis and 65% reduction in liver-related mortality due to chronic HBV and HCV infection.[142] To fulfill the goal of global hepatitis elimination, most countries will need to improve efforts in HBV screening, diagnosis, and treatment, as a recent study suggests that only 5% of patients eligible for treatment receive antiviral therapy.[32]

Barriers to care for HBV patients include lack of patient awareness of liver disease and the need for lifelong monitoring and treatment in some cases. Many immigrant populations with CHB come from highly endemic countries, and some do not readily seek health care and may be reluctant to start treatment due to cultural, language, and financial barriers. Social stigma remains an important issue for HBV-infected persons, who may be embarrassed or fearful of the diagnosis and worry about spreading infection to other family members.[139,140,143] Another barrier to long-term antiviral treatment is the cost of therapy for many patients who have limited financial resources. In many countries, only a minority of patients has access to private medication insurance, and most patients require public reimbursement or must pay out of pocket for medications.[144] The availability of generic antiviral medications has led to significant cost savings and improved access to treatment for many patients, and low-cost versions of antiviral medications will reduce the need to import drugs for personal use from other countries. Language barriers may impede efforts in patient education, particularly with regard to monitoring of liver disease, the need for treatment, and adherence to long-term treatment.[145] Strategies to combat these impediments include the development of patient-centered education programs delivered in the patient's native language and the creation of language-specific peer-support groups.

Indications

Many factors are involved in the decision to start treatment of CHB, and the decision is often a difficult one. The challenge is to identify persons at risk for the development of complications of CHB. Key factors to be considered include high serum HBV DNA levels, elevated serum ALT levels, and evidence of advanced hepatic fibrosis or cirrhosis.[146] Other potentially relevant factors include the patient's HBeAg status, HBV genotype, age, and medical comorbidities. Before starting long-term antiviral therapy, the patient must be able to afford and be willing to take long-term treatment. For many, treatment may be of indefinite duration, and they must therefore adhere to lifelong monitoring with serial blood samples and periodic abdominal US.

HBV DNA

Several large, long-term prospective studies have correlated serum HBV DNA levels at recruitment with clinical outcomes.[93,147,148] These studies have each concluded that the risks of developing cirrhosis and HCC and of liver-related mortality increase with higher serum HBV DNA levels at recruitment and with persistence of high HBV DNA levels during follow-up. Typical patients in these studies were middle-aged Asian men who were HBeAg-negative, and the proportion of patients under age 30 was small. Therefore, in HBeAg-negative patients over age 30, the serum HBV DNA level is a good predictor of adverse outcomes. This may also be true in older HBeAg-positive patients, but the findings do not apply to younger HBeAg-positive patients with normal serum ALT levels.

ALT

Many studies have shown a correlation between serum ALT levels and outcome, but the association was not as strong as for serum HBV DNA levels. In particular, patients with a serum ALT level within the normal range were also at risk for the development of cirrhosis and HCC if the serum HBV DNA concentration was higher than 2000 IU/mL. The serum ALT level is an imperfect marker of liver disease in persons with CHB. Several studies from East Asia have clearly demonstrated that higher serum ALT levels correlate with worse liver disease outcomes.[149,150] In a study from Hong Kong of 3233 untreated patients with HBV infection, those with normal and even subnormal serum ALT levels were found to have the lowest risk of HBV-related complications.[149] These and other studies suggest that the ULN for serum ALT used in many laboratories may be too high for carriers of CHB. Therefore the 2018 AASLD guidance for CHB endorses the ULN for serum ALT of 35 and 25 U/L for males and females, respectively.[89] HBV-infected patients with normal or near normal serum ALT levels may still be at risk for significant liver disease progression and may warrant treatment, as exemplified by a recent study showing a reduction in fibrosis progression with antiviral therapy among CHB patients with minimally elevated ALT.[151]

Liver Fibrosis

To reduce overtreating patients who may be at lower risk of developing significant liver disease, other markers of severity of liver disease should be considered prior to starting therapy. Approaches can include noninvasive markers of fibrosis such as transient or ultrasound elastography or serum-based fibrosis markers [e.g., FibroSure, FIB-4, APRI, ELF (Enhanced Liver Fibrosis) score] (see Chapters 76 and 82) or liver biopsy evidence of at least more than mild fibrosis and/or inflammation. The diagnostic accuracy of conventional cutoffs for widely used biochemical indices of hepatic fibrosis, such as FIB-4 and APRI, is poor in CHB,[152] and they should be used with caution. FibroTest > 0.8 is thought be a marker of advanced fibrosis (> stage 3 fibrosis), and a liver stiffness score of greater than 10 kPa on transient elastography has been correlated with cirrhosis in HBV-infected patients.[153,154] A transient mild serum ALT elevation may not be associated with significant disease, but persistent or prolonged serum ALT elevations for more than 3–6 months are more likely to be associated with significant liver injury. Therefore some form of fibrosis assessment in patients with normal serum ALT levels is necessary to determine the presence of hepatic fibrosis to make an informed treatment decision.

For both HBeAg-positive and HBeAg-negative patients, treatment should be considered when the HBV DNA is higher than 2000 IU/mL. Older studies suggested that progressive liver damage occurs once the serum HBV DNA level increases above a level of approximately 2000 IU/mL.[155,156] Although liver injury is uncommon if the serum HBV DNA level is below 2000 IU/mL, some patients may have HBV-induced liver disease at low viral loads. In this setting, liver biopsy may be needed to exclude an alternative diagnosis and to confirm viral-induced liver injury. Table 81.1 shows the differential diagnosis of an elevated serum ALT level in patients known to have CHB. Furthermore, serum HBV DNA levels may fluctuate, so that repeated measurements are required. A serum HBV DNA level greater than 2000 IU/mL accompanied by an elevated serum ALT level in an HBeAg-negative CHB patient typically warrants treatment; this form of CHB is associated with more advanced liver disease and rarely remits completely.

Timing

Young adults who are HBeAg-positive usually have high viral loads (>10^7 IU/mL), with variable serum ALT levels.[157,158] Patients with persistently normal ALT levels usually have no or minimal liver disease on liver biopsy specimens. Those who have elevated ALT levels may not always require immediate treatment because they may undergo spontaneous HBeAg seroconversion. It is often difficult to predict, however, which individuals will lose HBeAg with remission of disease prior to the development of significant liver injury. HBeAg-positive patients with a normal serum ALT level and high viral load (immune tolerant phase, or HBeAg-positive chronic infection) generally do not warrant treatment but instead should undergo regular monitoring as per current treatment guidelines. Fig. 81.7 provides an algorithm for identifying individual patients who require antiviral treatment. Nevertheless, it is important to note that high-level viremia is a risk factor for HCC development, and that several potentially carcinogenic processes, including integration of HBV DNA into the host genome is present in "immune tolerant" patients.[159]

Treatment guidelines vary in their ALT and HBV DNA thresholds for initiation of antiviral therapy.[75,89,133] The AASLD recommends starting therapy when the serum ALT level is persistently above 2× ULN (ULN, 35 U/L for men and 25 U/L for women), whereas other guidelines recommend therapy when the serum ALT level is greater than 1× ULN. Serum HBV DNA levels above 2000 IU/mL are thought to be associated with progression of liver disease and serve as the threshold to start therapy, according to European Association for the Study of Liver Disease guidelines. Although liver biopsy is not mandatory to stage fibrosis, treatment is recommended in those with more than mild hepatic fibrosis [>stage 2 fibrosis by METAVIR (see Chapters 76 and 82)]. Noninvasive assessment of fibrosis, such as transient elastography, MR elastography, or serum markers of fibrosis, may be helpful when liver biopsy is either not possible or contraindicated (see earlier).[160] In addition, the new guidelines recognize the potentially increased risk of adverse outcomes in patients with

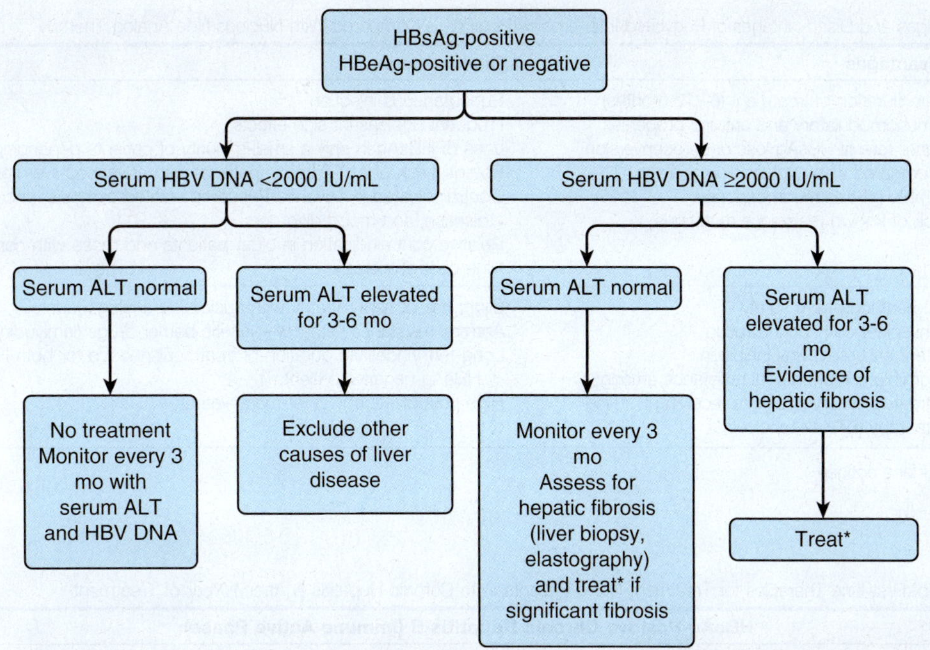

Fig. 81.7 Algorithm for the selection of patients with chronic hepatitis B for antiviral therapy. Indications for antiviral treatment include persistently elevated serum ALT levels greater than the ULN, serum HBV DNA levels greater than or equal to 2000 IU/mL, and some degree of hepatic fibrosis. For patients who have normal serum ALT levels or HBV DNA levels less than 2000 IU/mL, additional assessment, including liver biopsy, to exclude other causes of liver disease may be necessary. *First-line agents for HBeAg-positive patients: PegIFN, TDF, TAF, or ETV; first-line agents for HBeAg-negative patients: TDF, TAF, or ETV. *HBeAg,* Hepatitis B e antigen; *PegIFN,* pegylated interferon; *TAF,* tenofovir alafenamide; *TDF,* tenofovir disoproxil fumarate.

long-standing high level viremia despite normal ALT levels, and suggests that treatment can be considered in patients in the immune tolerant phase aged over 30.[75]

In summary, the decision to treat requires consideration of several factors: the patient's age, serum HBV DNA levels, HBeAg status, and evidence of significant liver disease in the form of persistent or intermittent elevation of the serum ALT level, significant hepatic fibrosis or inflammation on a liver biopsy specimen, or evidence of significant hepatic fibrosis on noninvasive assessment. Ultimately, patient adherence to therapy and follow-up will have a major impact on the success of antiviral treatment for CHB.

Drugs

The last generation of nucleos(t)ide analogs—TDF, TAF, and ETV—are highly potent and have a high−genetic barrier to resistance. They are effective when used as monotherapy in both HBeAg-positive or HBeAg-negative patients. In most treatment guidelines, TDF, TAF, ETV, and PegIFN are recommended as first-line treatment options.[75,89,133] However, in resource-constrained regions of the world, less preferable agents, such as lamivudine and adefovir, are sometimes used due to their lower cost and greater availability.

PegIFN and nucleos(t)ide analogs each have advantages and disadvantages that should be considered when making a treatment decision, as outlined in Table 81.3. One major advantage of PegIFN is that treatment duration is limited to 6−12 months, and virologic responses tend to be durable, especially in patients with HBeAg-positive hepatitis B.[48,161] However, the drug must be administered subcutaneously and has been associated with unpleasant side effects. The shorter duration of treatment may be an important factor for younger patients of childbearing potential who wish to be medication-free during the family planning years. Table 81.4 illustrates the relative potency of the different antiviral agents from various clinical trials in a nonhead-to-head comparison.

Nucleoside and Nucleotide Analogs

Nucleos(t)ide analogs have become the standard of care for treatment of most patients with treatment-naïve and treatment-experienced CHB. The lack of side effects and high efficacy of first-line agents, such as TDF, TAF, and ETV, make them particularly attractive. Approximately 70% and 95% HBeAg-positive and HBeAg-negative patients, respectively, will achieve undetectable HBV DNA during the first year of treatment with TDF.[162] Virologic responses progressively increase with longer duration of therapy, although a small minority of patients may have persistently low-level viremia or viral "blips" after several years of continuous therapy.[163] The most likely explanation for these occurrences is nonadherence to long-term therapy, which occurs in at least 10%−15% of patients.[164,165] The serum HBV DNA level usually declines with education of the patient on the importance of adherence to treatment. Antiviral resistance is distinctly uncommon with TDF, TAF, and ETV. In fact, no antiviral-resistant mutation has been identified in patients on TDF after 10 years of treatment.[166,167] Although low-level viremia may be acceptable in many cases, persistent low-level viremia has been associated with an increased risk of HCC among patients with cirrhosis.[168] Table 81.5 highlights first-line nucleos(t)ide analog therapy in a number of clinical situations.

Lamivudine

Lamivudine was the first HBV antiviral agent to be approved for use. It has an excellent long-term safety record and relatively high antiviral potency. Its major disadvantage is the rapid development

TABLE 81.3 Advantages and Disadvantages of Pegylated Interferon-α (PegIFN-α) Compared With Nucleos(t)ide Analog Therapy

Agent	Advantages	Disadvantages
PegIFN-α	Finite duration of treatment (6–12 months) Immunomodulatory and antiviral properties Higher rate of HBsAg loss or seroconversion compared with nucleos(t)ide analogs Durable off-treatment response Lack of known resistance mutations	Subcutaneous injection Frequent unpleasant side effects Loss of HBsAg in only a small minority of patients depending on HBV genotype Potential risk of ALT flares in patients with advanced liver fibrosis Contraindicated in advanced/decompensated cirrhosis, uncontrolled autoimmune disease, and mood disorders Relative contraindication in older patients and those with comorbid illnesses High cost of therapy
Nucleos(t)ide analogs	Excellent long-term safety Convenient oral administration Potent and rapid viral inhibition Negligible risk of antiviral resistance among treatment-naïve patients receiving first-line therapy (ETV or tenofovir)	Slight risk of nephropathy with nucleotide analogs (adefovir, tenofovir) Antiviral resistance with low–genetic barrier drugs (lamivudine, telbivudine) Long-term/indefinite duration of treatment needed for both HBeAg-positive and HBeAg-negative patients High cost of therapy (over many years)

HBsAg, Hepatitis B surface antigen.

TABLE 81.4 Results of First-Line Therapies for Treatment-Naïve Patients With Chronic Hepatitis B After 1 Year of Treatment

HBeAg-Positive Chronic Hepatitis B (Immune Active Phase)				
Outcome (%)	**PegIFN-α[a]**	**ETV**	**TDF**	**TAF**
Viral suppression	32 (<4 log IU/mL)	67 (<60 IU/mL)	66 (<60 IU/mL)	64 (<29 IU/mL)
HBeAg loss	34	22	21	14
ALT normalization	41	68	68	72
Histologic response	49	72	74	N/A
HBsAg loss	3	2	3	1
HBeAg-Negative Chronic Hepatitis B (Reactivation Phase)				
Outcome (%)	PegIFN-α	ETV	TDF	TAF
Viral suppression	43 (<3 log IU/mL)	90 (<60 IU/mL)	71 (<60 IU/mL)	94 (<29 IU/mL)
ALT normalization	59	78	76	83
Histologic response	55	70	72	N/A
HBsAg loss	4	<1	0	0

[a]End of follow-up at 24 weeks posttreatment

ETV, Entecavir; *N/A,* not available, *PegIFN,* pegylated interferon; *TAF,* tenofovir alafenamide; *TDF,* tenofovir disoproxil fumarate.

of mutations in the YMDD (tyrosine-methionine-aspartic acid-aspartic acid) active site of the HBV polymerase: 20% in Year 1, 35% in Year 2, and greater than 75% in Year 4.[169,170] For this reason, lamivudine is no longer recommended as first-line therapy.

Adefovir Dipivoxil

Adefovir is a nucleotide analog with antiviral activity against both wild-type and lamivudine-resistant HBV. Due to its limited potency, primary treatment failure was observed in 30% of patients.[171] Potentially reversible nephrotoxicity was reported in about one-third of patients after only 1 year of treatment. Moreover, reverse transcriptase (rt) mutations causing resistance to adefovir (rtA181V/T or rtN236T) were documented in nearly 30% of patients by the end of 5 years of continuous therapy.[172] For these reasons, adefovir is not recommended for treatment of HBV infection. Side effects of adefovir include reversible nephrotoxicity and, rarely, Fanconi syndrome.

Emtricitabine

Structurally similar to lamivudine, emtricitabine also inhibits HBV DNA polymerase and HIV reverse transcriptase. Emtricitabine is not FDA-approved for use in hepatitis B but is approved in a combined tablet with tenofovir for HIV infection. Due to its structural similarity to lamivudine, it is cross-resistant and is not an option for lamivudine-resistant salvage therapy.[173]

Entecavir

ETV is a guanosine analog that is more potent than lamivudine and has a very high–genetic barrier to resistance, requiring 2–3 additional HBV polymerase mutations superimposed on the backbone of a preexisting lamivudine-resistant mutation. ETV resistance was found in only 2% of treatment-naïve patients during 5 years of continuous treatment, as opposed to greater than 50% in lamivudine-refractory patients.[174,175] ETV at a dose of 0.5 mg daily is recommended in treatment-naïve patients, whereas a dose of 1 mg is prescribed in patients who have lamivudine-resistant HBV infection; however, ETV is not the preferred option for lamivudine-resistant HBV due to risk for the long-term development of ETV resistance. TDF is preferred in these cases due to its nonoverlapping resistance profile.[75,89,133]

In a long-term real-world cohort study of Chinese patients treated with ETV, 99% of patients maintained suppression of serum HBV DNA, and 98% normalized serum ALT levels.[176]

TABLE 81.5 Choice of Nucleoside or Nucleotide Analog for HBV Infection

Clinical Situation	First-Line Therapy	Second-Line Therapy	Comment
Treatment-naïve	ETV or TDF or TAF		
Prior lamivudine or telbivudine exposure	Switch to TDF or TAF	ETV	ETV
Proven lamivudine resistance	Switch to TDF or TAF		
Proven adefovir resistance	Switch to ETV	TDF or TAF	Adefovirresistance reduces susceptibility to TDF
Primary drug failure with both lamivudine and adefovir[a]	Switch to TDF or TAF ETV	TDF/TAF plus ETV	
Proven ETV resistance	Switch to TDF or TAF		–
Proven telbivudine resistance	Switch to TDF or TAF		–
Persistent low-level viremia during treatment with high –genetic barrier drug	Continue TDF, TAF, or ETV or switch to one of the others	None	Nonadherence should be considered; resistance testing may be necessary Low level viremia may be associated with an increased risk of adverse events in patients with cirrhosis
Treatment-naïve, reduced GFR (<60 mL/min)	ETV or TAF		

[a]See text for definition of primary drug failure.
GFR, Glomerular filtration rate; *TAF*, tenofovir alafenamide; *TDF*, tenofovir disoproxil fumarate.

Resistance to ETV was reported in only 1% of patients during long-term follow-up. Although only 2%–3% patients lost HBsAg, predictors of HBsAg loss included baseline quantitative HBsAg levels less than 100 IU/mL and on-treatment annual HBsAg decline of greater than 0.2 log IU/mL. ETV is safe and well tolerated with rare side effects, which include lactic acidosis observed among a few patients with severe liver dysfunction.[177]

Telbivudine

Telbivudine is a nucleoside analog that is more potent than lamivudine in both HBeAg-positive and HBeAg-negative patients.[178] Unfortunately, genotypic resistance was found in 5% and 11% of patients after 1 and 2 years of telbivudine, respectively, demonstrating a resistance profile that was only slightly better than that of lamivudine.[179] Due to cross-resistance with lamivudine, it cannot be used as salvage therapy in this setting. Telbivudine is not a preferred treatment for HBV infection in North America because of the high rate of resistance and the side effect of myopathy.

Tenofovir Disoproxil Fumarate

TDF is a nucleotide analog inhibitor of reverse transcriptase similar to adefovir, but it is significantly more potent, as shown in randomized clinical studies. TDF has demonstrated efficacy in patients with treatment-naïve HBeAg-positive and HBeAg-negative CHB.[162] Large phase 3 studies reported that HBV DNA suppression to less than 69 IU/mL was achieved in over 99% of HBeAg-positive and -negative patients after 10 years.[167] Serum ALT normalization occurred in 80% of patients, HBeAg loss was reported in 59% of HBeAg-positive patients, and HBsAg loss occurred in 12% of patients after 7 years.[166] At the end of 5 years of treatment, 80% of patients had improvement in liver histology.[180] Seventy-five percent of patients with cirrhosis at baseline had at least a 2-point reduction in Ishak fibrosis score after long-term TDF therapy. Importantly, no confirmed cases of antiviral resistance to TDF have been documented after up to 10 years of continuous treatment.[167,181] Interestingly, HBsAg loss occurred in 10%–15% of mainly Caucasian patients during the same period of treatment. Predictors of HBsAg loss included a decline in HBsAg levels on treatment, HBV genotype A, and a shorter duration of chronic infection (<4 years). TDF (or TAF) is recommended in HBV-HIV coinfection as the backbone of an ART regimen (see later). TDF has been associated with reversible nephrotoxicity and hypophosphatemia in up to 2%–4% patients treated with long-term treatment, and, rarely, Fanconi syndrome has been reported.[182]

Tenofovir Alafenamide

TAF, a novel prodrug of tenofovir, is delivered more efficiently into hepatocytes. In large phase 3 studies of HBeAg-positive and HBeAg-negative treatment-naïve patients, TAF was compared with TDF, followed by 5 years of open-label TAF.[183,184] Although virologic (HBV DNA <29 IU/mL) and serologic responses were similar between the two groups, higher rates of serum ALT normalization were seen after 1 year of treatment in those randomized to TAF. Importantly, TAF is superior to TDF in terms of renal safety as measured by serum creatinine and glomerular filtration rate and bone safety as shown by dual-energy X-ray absorptiometry scans. In patients taking TDF who were switched to TAF, not only was viral suppression maintained, but also improvement in renal function and bone mineral density and higher rates of serum ALT normalization were observed within 6–12 months.[185–187]

Treatment Response and Endpoints

Typically, randomized controlled trials of HBV antiviral therapy have defined biochemical, virologic, and histologic endpoints at 1 year (48 weeks) of treatment to evaluate the response. Biochemical response is defined as normalization of serum ALT levels according to central laboratory values; virologic response is defined as undetectable serum HBV DNA; and histologic response is a 2-point or greater improvement in the necroinflammatory score without worsening fibrosis. Serologic response requires HBeAg loss or seroconversion to anti-HBe for HBeAg-positive patients. The more elusive endpoint is functional cure of HBV, defined as loss of serum HBsAg, with or without appearance of anti-HBs, and undetectable serum HBV DNA. Sterilizing or virologic cure of HBV requires not only undetectable serum HBsAg and HBV DNA but also a loss of cccDNA from the hepatocyte nucleus.[188]

For patients treated with nucleo(s)tide analogues, achievement of undetectable HBV DNA, that is, virological response, is the primary aim of therapy; this endpoint can be achieved for most adherent patients, although this may require prolonged therapy in those with high baseline HBV DNA levels. Achievement of HBeAg loss and/or seroconversion may herald a first step toward achieving immune control and subsequent HBsAg clearance among pretreatment HBeAg-positive patients. Sterilizing cure of HBV is not attainable with NA therapy.

Primary Nonresponse

Primary nonresponse is defined as a 1 log or less reduction in serum HBV DNA levels at 24 weeks of antiviral therapy.[189] The most likely explanation for primary nonresponse is nonadherence. Based on a database of prescription utilization, at least 10%–15% of patients fail to take their medication appropriately and miss one or more doses each month.[165] Antiviral resistance testing is recommended for those receiving agents with a low genetic barrier to resistance to differentiate between resistance and medication nonadherence. Counseling for those found to be nonadherent is recommended. For patients not responding to lamivudine or telbivudine at Week 24, treatment can be switched to a more potent agent, such as TDF, TAF, or ETV (in the absence of lamivudine resistance), and the serum HBV DNA level repeated in 3 months, as suggested by the HBV roadmap concept of response-guided therapy.[190] Primary nonresponse is extremely unusual in those receiving high potency agents, such as TDF, TAF, or ETV, as the first-line therapy. For those who experience virologic breakthrough (increase in serum HBV DNA by 1 log IU/mL from nadir) on TDF, switching to ETV is reasonable (and vice versa).[89]

Viral Breakthrough

A viral breakthrough is defined as an increase in HBV DNA by at least 1 log from the nadir. Among patients treated with low genetic barrier agents this may be due to the development of resistance, whereas nonadherence is the most likely explanation for patients treated with ETV, TDF, or TAF.

Partial Virological Response

Partial virological response to nucleo(s)tide analogues is defined as at least a 1 log decline in HBV DNA from baseline, but failure to achieve undetectable HBV DNA after 1 year of therapy. A limited subset of patients treated with ETV, TDF, and TAF will experience such a partial virological response. The main risk factor is high baseline HBV DNA levels. Prolonged treatment will result in further increase in the number of patients achieving complete viral suppression, and therapy adaptation is not required in most cases.[191] A potential exception are patients with cirrhosis with persistent low level viremia during long-term therapy; these subjects could potentially benefit from treatment adaptation as low level viremia has been linked to an increased risk of adverse outcomes.[168] In patients treated with agents with a low genetic barrier to resistance, therapy adaptation is recommended if HBV DNA suppression is not achieved as outlined in Table 81.5.[75,89,133]

Monitoring

Patients who undergo treatment with a nucleos(t)ide analog should be followed with serial ALT and HBV DNA assessments at 3-month intervals until they achieve undetectable serum HBV DNA levels. Once serum HBV DNA is undetectable or less than 10–20 IU/mL, follow-up intervals can be extended to every 6 months for those receiving treatment with a drug of high genetic barrier to resistance with demonstrated adherence to therapy. Quantitative HBsAg levels, if available, and HBeAg status can be measured every 6 months on therapy to detect HBsAg decline and HBeAg loss or seroconversion in HBeAg-positive patients. Serum creatinine (or glomerular filtration rate) and phosphate levels are recommended every 3–6 months for those receiving treatment with TDF. Bone density assessment using dual-energy x-ray absorptiometry scans is not routinely measured in patients on TDF or TAF, unless the patient has several risk factors for osteoporosis.

Duration of Therapy

Prolonged, and potentially lifelong, antiviral therapy until functional cure (i.e., sustained HBsAg loss and/or seroconversion) is indicated for the majority of patients, given the high risk of virological relapse after cessation of antiviral therapy among HBsAg positive patients.[192] Cessation of treatment after HBsAg loss is associated with a low risk of relapse.[193,194] Unfortunately, HBsAg loss is distinctly uncommon in Asian patients with CHB, irrespective of treatment used. In a long-term study of TDF versus adefovir for HBeAg-positive and HBeAg-negative patients, 15% of Caucasian patients compared with 0% of Asians experienced HBsAg loss.[162] Similarly, a real-world study of 222 patients with CHB in Hong Kong treated with continuous ETV for 7 years reported a 2.5% cumulative rate of HBsAg loss, suggesting that long-term treatment is necessary for the majority of Asian patients with CHB.[176]

Recent studies have therefore focused on exploring outcomes after cessation of nucleo(s)tide analogue therapy in HBsAg positive patients. These studies have shown that some patients may achieve durable disease remission after cessation of nucleo(s)tide analogue therapy despite HBsAg positivity at the time of therapy discontinuation.[109] Several studies, particularly those that included predominantly white patients, have also reported HBsAg loss rates after therapy withdrawal that appear to exceed those that would be expected during prolonged NA therapy.[108] However, cessation of antiviral therapy is associated with recurrence of viremia in the majority of patients, which can potentially result in development of severe hepatitis flares leading to liver failure.[195,196] Careful selection of patients most likely to achieve favorable outcomes after therapy cessation is therefore required. Current European guidelines have identified two subsets of noncirrhotic CHB patients who could be considered for therapy withdrawal: (1) pretreatment HBeAg-positive patients who have achieved sustained HBeAg seroconversion followed by an additional period of at least 12 months of "consolidation" therapy, and pretreatment HBeAg-negative patients with 3 years HBV DNA suppression.[8] Subsequent studies have shown that the majority of patients complying with these criteria will not achieve durable remission or HBsAg loss,[109,197] suggesting that other factors should be taken into consideration when selecting HBsAg-positive patients for finite therapy. Recent studies have identified several predictors of favorable outcomes after therapy withdrawal, including white ethnicity, low end of treatment HBsAg, HBcrAg and hepatitis B virus RNA (HBV RNA) levels, and HBV genotype C. Combining these factors could potentially help optimize patient selection, although decision algorithms remain to be defined.[109,197,198]

Antiviral Resistance

Antiviral resistance in HBV infection has become a minor issue owing to use of agents with a high barrier to resistance, such as TDF, TAF, and ETV. However, lamivudine-resistant HBV is common in some countries, and a working knowledge of antiviral resistance mutations and resistance profiles is required to properly select initial and salvage therapies. When genotypic resistance develops, particularly to lamivudine, secondary mutations may

TABLE 81.6 Characteristics of Antiviral-Resistant HBV Infection

	Nucleos(t)ide Analog to Which HBV is Resistant				
Characteristic	**Lamivudine**	**Adefovir**	**ETV**	**Telbivudine**	**TDF/TAF**
Reverse transcriptase (rt) mutations	rtL180M± rtM204V/I	rtA181V/T± rtN236T	rtL180M± rtM204V/I± rtS202I rtM250V	rtL180M± rtM204V/I	None known
Rate of resistance	Year 1: 20% Year 4: 75%	Year 1: 9% Year 3: 30%	Year 1: 0% Year 3: 1%	Year 1: 10% Year 2: 25%	Year 1: 0%[b] Year 8: 0%[b]
Overlapping resistance to other drugs	Emtricitabine Telbivudine ETV	Tenofovir[a]	Lamivudine Emtricitabine Telbivudine	Lamivudine Telbivudine ETV	None
Drug(s) to switch to	TDF or TAF	ETV, TDF, or TAF	TDF or TAF	TDF or TAF	ETV

[a]Partial resistance to TDF.
[b]Resistance rates for TDF. No resistance to TAF was reported at 2 years.
TAF, Tenofovir alafenamide; *TDF*, tenofovir disoproxil fumarate.

occur that may reduce susceptibility to other antiviral agents.[199] Table 81.6 summarizes specific HBV polymerase resistance mutations, rates of resistance, and management strategies for patients with resistance to common nucleos(t)ide analogs in current use.

Testing

Monitoring for antiviral resistance requires regular assessment of serum HBV DNA levels. Resistance is suspected in case of virological breakthrough (i.e., rise in HBV DNA by at least 1 log IU/mL) occurs in a treatment-adherent patient. Genotypic resistance can be confirmed by various methods, such as population sequencing, reverse hybridization, clonal analysis, and ultradeep sequencing methods. Common polymerase mutations known to confer resistance can be detected by a commercially available reverse hybridization. This method can detect drug-resistant HBV that constitutes at least 10% of the viral population.[189] Ultradeep sequencing has a greater sensitivity and detects minor variants that constitute less than 1% of the total HBV quasispecies.[200]

Clinical Outcomes

Adverse clinical outcomes have been reported in patients in whom antiviral resistance develops. There is considerable evidence that the benefits of viral suppression are lost when resistance occurs.[201,202] Acute flares of hepatitis related to lamivudine- or adefovir-resistant HBV infection can occur, and these flares may be fatal, particularly in cirrhotic patients. Therefore the development of resistance to antiviral agents is a strong indication to change therapy. Early detection of antiviral resistance is important to avoid ALT flares and decompensation of liver disease. Table 81.6 shows the substitutions in the HBV polymerase gene that are associated with resistance to various agents.[203]

Lamivudine Resistance

Resistance to lamivudine monotherapy occurs commonly: 15%−20% at Year 1, 30% at Year 2, 50% at Year 3, and greater than or equal to 75% at Year 4.[170] Adverse clinical outcomes such as loss of initial response, reduced HBeAg seroconversion, hepatic decompensation, and death have been reported in patients in whom lamivudine resistance develops; however, many of the relevant studies were performed before effective salvage therapy, such as tenofovir, was available. A randomized study of 280 patients with chronic HBV with documented lamivudine-resistant mutations (rtL180M ± rtM204V/I) compared TDF versus TDF plus emtricitabine (Truvada) for 5 years.[204] Patients had received a mean of 4 years of lamivudine prior to enrollment, and 10% had evidence of cirrhosis. Rates of virologic suppression were identical between the two groups (83%), and the rate of HBeAg seroconversion was relatively low (15%) after 5 years. HBsAg loss or seroconversion was observed in only 7 patients. Data from this study and others suggest that there is no benefit to combination antiviral treatment compared with TDF monotherapy and that TDF is the treatment of choice for lamivudine-resistant HBV infection.

Entecavir Resistance

ETV resistance requires a lamivudine-resistant backbone (YMDD mutation, see earlier). The YMDD mutation alone decreases ETV potency but is not sufficient to produce resistance. Nevertheless, in the presence of mutations rtM204V and rtL180M, one or more additional mutations (rt169T, rtT184G, rtS202I, and rtM250V) are able to confer resistance to ETV.[205] In the registration studies of ETV in lamivudine-resistant patients, ETV resistance mutations were detected in a small proportion of patients at baseline prior to the introduction of ETV. As a result, genotypic resistance was identified in 7% and viral breakthrough in 1.6% patients at the end of the first year of therapy.[174] This rate increased to more than 30% at the end of the third year of therapy. By contrast, in nucleoside-naïve subjects, resistance to ETV occurred in only 1% patients after 3 years.[206] Therefore preexisting lamivudine-resistant ETV-treated patients are at risk of developing resistance to ETV, and, for this reason, ETV should not be used to rescue patients with lamivudine-resistant HBV.

In a small study of patients in South Korea with lamivudine and ETV resistance, TDF demonstrated similar efficacy compared with TDF plus ETV, with serum HBV DNA levels less than 15 IU/mL in 71% and 73% of patients, respectively.[207] Therefore ETV resistance can be salvaged by TDF and most likely also by TAF.

Tenofovir Resistance

To date, there have been no confirmed cases of TDF or TAF resistance in HBV monoinfected patients after 10 years of continuous TDF and 2 years of TAF therapy.[167,181] In fact, there is no known signature HBV polymerase mutation for tenofovir. A case report documented an rtA194T substitution in an HBV-HIV coinfected patient, but the clinical significance of this mutation in HBV monoinfected patients is unclear. In registration trials of TDF, among 4% of patients who did not achieve undetectable HBV DNA levels, population sequencing failed to reveal any conserved site changes, although resistance surveillance is ongoing.[162]

Although TAF has not been formally studied in antiviral-resistant patients in a dedicated study, a small number of patients in the registration studies were found to have lamivudine, adefovir, or ETV-resistant mutation at baseline. The response to TAF compared with TDF was similar. Based on in vitro studies and case reports, TAF is expected to have significant activity against common antiviral-resistant mutations. One case report has suggested that TAF is a suitable alternative to TDF for multidrug-resistant HBV infection, and switching from TDF to TAF in patients with a history of drug resistance is effective.[208,209]

Multidrug Resistance

The most common form of multidrug resistance in clinical practice is lamivudine and adefovir resistance (rtM204V/I + rtN236T or rtA181T/V). In a small study of lamivudine-resistant HBV-infected patients with persistent viremia on adefovir, 95% achieved rapid viral suppression using TDF as salvage therapy.[210] In a case report, a patient with multidrug resistance was rescued with TAF, which led to virologic suppression within 6 months.[208] In a study of ETV and/or adefovir-resistant HBV-infected patients, virologic suppression was found in the vast majority of those who received a TDF-based rescue regimen,[207] and no resistance mutation to TDF was detected over the 3-year period. Taken together, these data suggest that TDF or TAF is safe and effective for the treatment of multidrug-resistant HBV infection.

Pegylated Interferon-Alpha (IFN-α)

IFN-α has antiviral and immunomodulatory properties and may induce long-term immunologic control. Potential advantages of IFN compared with nucleos(t)ide analogs include a finite duration therapy and lack of antiviral resistance.[161] On the other hand, major disadvantages include unpleasant systemic side effects (fatigue, fever, chills, depression, cytopenias) and the route of administration (subcutaneous injection).

PegIFN-α has supplanted standard IFN in clinical practice because of its once-weekly dosing schedule and evidence of at least equal efficacy.[211] PegIFN-α is approved by the FDA for both HBeAg-positive and HBeAg-negative CHB for 48 weeks in a dose of 180 μg weekly. IFN is contraindicated in pregnant women and in patients with decompensated cirrhosis, although fully compensated cirrhotic patients (normal liver synthetic function and no evidence of portal hypertension) may still be considered for treatment.

HBeAg-Positive Chronic Hepatitis B

HBeAg seroconversion occurs in 25%–40% of IFN-treated patients.[48,212] In long-term follow-up studies of up to 8 years, the durability of IFN-induced HBeAg seroconversion has been high (70%–80%).[213–215] However, HBsAg clearance occurs in only 5%–7% of patients.[48] IFN-induced HBeAg seroconversion is associated with improved overall and complication-free survival.[46,216–218] Several reports have demonstrated that the frequency of HCC is reduced in IFN-treated patients.

HBeAg-Negative Chronic Hepatitis B

PegIFN-α with or without lamivudine for 48 weeks was effective in HBeAg-negative patients.[219] Suppression of serum HBV DNA levels to less than 400 copies/mL (80 IU/mL) at the end of treatment was achieved in 63% of PegIFN-treated patients, whereas only 19% had durable viral suppression 24 weeks after stopping therapy. The combined endpoint of serum ALT normalization and a serum HBV DNA level less than 20,000 copies/mL (~4000 IU/mL) was achieved in 36% of the PegIFN-treated group at 24 weeks of follow-up. HBsAg loss was reported in only 4% of patients at Week 72.

Treatment Endpoints and Durability

A composite endpoint of HBeAg loss and low serum HBV DNA (<20,000 IU/mL) level was used in the definition of a sustained virologic response in several trials of PegIFN, because undetectable HBV DNA occurs less frequently with IFN-based therapy than with nucleos(t)ide analog therapy.[218,219] The durability of the response to PegIFN is related to heightened immune control of HBV infection and is estimated to be approximately 80% of HBeAg-positive patients when evaluated many years later.[48] Unfortunately, a sustained response to IFN has been reported in a limited subset of the HBeAg-negative patients.[220]

Predictors of Response and Stopping Rules

Given the modest response rates and potential systemic side effects associated with PegIFN, predictors of response are needed to select optimal treatment candidates. In addition, robust stopping rules limit therapy in those unlikely to respond and reduce the potential for side effects. Pretreatment predictors of non-response to PegIFN include high viral loads (serum HBV DNA $>2\times10^7$ IU/mL), low serum ALT (<2 × the ULN), age over 40 years, male gender, and presence of cirrhosis. HBV genotypes C and D compared with A and B are associated with lower rates of HBeAg seroconversion. Quantitative HBsAg levels on treatment have been shown to be an on-treatment predictor of response to PegIFN. In a study of over 800 HBeAg-positive patients, a serum HBsAg level greater than 20,000 IU/mL at Week 24 of PegIFN was associated with a 99% negative predictive value for response (defined as HBeAg loss with a serum HBV DNA level <2000 IU/mL) and is a criterion for discontinuation of therapy.[127]

Combination Therapy

Combination antiviral therapy has been shown to be highly effective for the treatment of HIV infection and the eradication of chronic hepatitis C infection. Combination therapy targets different steps in the viral life cycle and reduces the risk of genotypic resistance. However, combination NA treatment does not appear to be superior to TDF or ETV monotherapy for most patients and is not recommended in current treatment guidelines.

Peginterferon Plus Nucleos(t)ide Analogs

Various combinations of PegIFN plus nucleos(t)ide analogs have been studied in which both agents were started simultaneously or PegIFN was added in patients who were virally suppressed on nucleos(t)ide analog therapy or a switch to PegIFN from nucleos(t)ide analog therapy was made.[218,219] Studies combining PEG-IFN with lamivudine did not show a benefit of lamivudine addition.[46] In another large study, over 700 HBeAg-positive or-negative noncirrhotic patients were randomized to receive PegIFN-α2a (180 μg/week, subcutaneously) of two different durations: TDF plus PegIFN for 48 weeks or TDF alone for 120 weeks or PegIFN alone for 48 weeks.[138] The cumulative probability of HBsAg loss at Week 72 was higher for patients allocated to combination therapy versus PegIFN monotherapy. However, not all cases of HBsAg loss were sustained, which makes interpretation of these findings challenging.[221] Based on this study, de novo combination therapy of PegIFN and nucleos(t)ide analogs cannot be recommended in general clinical practice. Given the higher HBsAg loss rates observed with PegIFN versus NA, several studies have addressed the potential of PegIFN add-on therapy for patients on long-term NA therapy. Available evidence suggests that PegIFN add-on may increase the chance of HBeAg loss among patients still HBeAg positive on NA therapy.[222,223] Furthermore, addition of PegIFN may increase HBsAg decline and HBsAg loss among HBeAg-negative patients to a very limited degree.[223,224]

Nucleos(t)ide Analog Combinations

Combination oral nucleos(t)ide analog therapy has been investigated in several studies to explore the potential for improved virologic and/or biochemical outcomes compared with monotherapy. In a single-center study in which combination lamivudine plus adefovir was compared with lamivudine alone, no difference in HBV DNA suppression, HBeAg seroconversion, or serum ALT normalization was observed.[225] However, resistance to lamivudine was significantly lower in the combination group compared with monotherapy. In another study, combination lamivudine plus telbivudine was less effective than telbivudine alone for all endpoints,[226] possibly due to antiviral antagonism.

In a large randomized open-label, multicenter study of ETV plus TDF compared with ETV alone, nucleos(t)ide analog-naïve patients were randomized by HBeAg status to combination therapy versus monotherapy.[227] A similar proportion of individuals achieved the primary endpoint of a serum HBV DNA level less than 50 IU/mL at Week 96 in the ETV plus TDF arm and the ETV alone arm (83.2% vs. 76.4%). However, in the subset of HBeAg-positive patients with a baseline HBV DNA level greater than 8 $\log_{10}$ IU/mL, a greater proportion of those treated with combination therapy achieved a serum HBV DNA level less than 50 IU/mL at Week 96. Rates of HBeAg loss were similar in the two treatment groups. No difference in the overall low rates of HBsAg loss was observed.

In another study, combination antiviral treatment using TDF plus emtricitabine compared with TDF alone for 192 weeks was used to treat HBeAg-positive patients with a high viral load and normal serum ALT levels (immune tolerant).[228] Seventy-six percent of patients in the TDF plus emtricitabine group achieved a serum HBV DNA level less than 69 IU/mL at Week 192 versus 55% in the TDF group ($P = .016$). However, only three patients experienced HBeAg seroconversion, all in the TDF group, and no HBsAg loss occurred during the study. This study clearly demonstrated that antiviral treatment in immune tolerant patients led to a lower than expected rate of HBeAg seroconversion, and its findings support the notion that these patients should be observed rather than receive immediate nucleos(t)ide analog therapy. Future long-term studies in large populations should demonstrate whether treating immune tolerant patients will eventually reduce the frequency of liver cirrhosis or HCC.

Taken together, these data demonstrate no convincing benefit of combination compared with nucleos(t)ide analog monotherapy for routine use in patients with CHB.

Unique Populations

Unique populations of HBV-infected patients include pregnant women, those with severe acute exacerbations of HBV infection, compensated and decompensated cirrhotic patients, and those with viral coinfection (HIV, HCV, and HDV).

Pregnant Women

Mother-to-child transmission of HBV remains the most important route of HBV transmission in endemic countries.[229] Therefore all pregnant women should undergo screening for HBV in the first trimester of pregnancy. The highest risk period for HBV transmission is thought to occur intrapartum, although intrauterine transmission may also occur. Pregnant women found to be HBsAg-positive will require further testing, including full HBV serology, serum HBV DNA, and liver biochemical tests. Infants born to HBsAg-positive mothers must receive immunoprophylaxis with HBIG and the first dose of HBV vaccine within 12 hours of birth. The remaining doses of the HBV vaccine are given to the infant at 2 and 6 months of age (see later). Testing for immunity (anti-HBs) in the infant can be performed after the age of 9–12 months. Failure of immunoprophylaxis has been reported in up to 10%–30% of women who are highly viremic during pregnancy.[230,231]

For women who become pregnant on nucleos(t)ide analog therapy, treatment is continued throughout the pregnancy provided the patient is receiving TDF, telbivudine, or lamivudine. The safety of other agents, such as ETV and adefovir, has not been established, so women of childbearing age who are contemplating pregnancy, especially in those who cannot discontinue therapy with these regimens (advanced liver disease or HBeAg-positive without seroconversion) should be switched to safer agents. An algorithm for the management of HBV during pregnancy is illustrated in Fig. 81.8.

Highly viremic mothers with a serum HBV DNA level greater than 200,000 IU/mL should receive antiviral prophylaxis early in the third trimester of pregnancy starting around Week 30–32 with nucleos(t)ide analogs that are safe in pregnancy (TDF, telbivudine, or lamivudine).[75,89,133] Treatment may be continued until the day of delivery or up to 1 or 3 month(s) postpartum, depending on the guideline.[75,89] Antiviral prophylaxis in pregnancy combined with immunoprophylaxis of the newborn has been shown to reduce the risk of viral transmission from mother to child from approximately 10% with immunoprophylaxis alone to 0%. In a randomized study performed in China, TDF starting at Week 32 until 1 month postpartum was compared with placebo in a group of 200 mother-baby pairs. All infants received standard of care HBIG and HBV vaccination.[231] TDF was generally well tolerated during pregnancy and mother-to-child transmission was significantly lower in the TDF group (0% vs. 7%). In another study, immunoprophylaxis was administered within 1 hour of birth, and a total of four doses of HBV vaccine were given. With this intensive regimen, which cannot practically be initiated in most clinical settings internationally, no benefit of TDF prophylaxis was observed.[232] Based on the excellent safety and high potency of TDF in pregnancy, most guidelines recommend the use of antiviral prophylaxis in pregnancy when the HBV DNA level is above 5 log IU/mL. Other high-risk situations requiring antiviral prophylaxis include previous birth of a HBsAg-positive child, obstetric risk factors, such as premature rupture of membranes, preterm labor, or invasive testing, such as amniocentesis.[233]

HBsAg-positive women not currently on treatment who are found to have elevated liver enzyme levels and a high viral load during pregnancy may start nucleos(t)ide analog treatment before the third trimester. In this setting, the goal is to treat the maternal liver disease and prevent obstetric complications, such as preterm labor or intrauterine growth restriction. Treatment is continued in the postpartum period until the usual endpoints are achieved (see earlier). Postpartum flares of HBV infection may occur in up to 20% of women, and monitoring serum liver enzyme and HBV DNA levels in the first 3–6 months postpartum is recommended.[234]

From a safety perspective, TDF and telbivudine are FDA category B drugs and have not been associated with harmful effects to mother or baby. Use of lamivudine (FDA category C) is also reasonable.[235,236] Data from the U.S. Antiretroviral Pregnancy Registry of mainly HIV-positive women have confirmed the safety of TDF—the rate of congenital anomalies on TDF is no higher than that in the general population.[237] A systematic review and meta-analysis evaluated 26 studies enrolling 3622 pregnant viremic HBV carriers who received antiviral treatment in the second or third trimester of pregnancy.[229] Lamivudine, telbivudine, and TDF effectively reduced mother-to-child transmission by 70%, as reflected by HBsAg and HBV DNA undetectability in the infant at 6–12 months of age. Moreover,

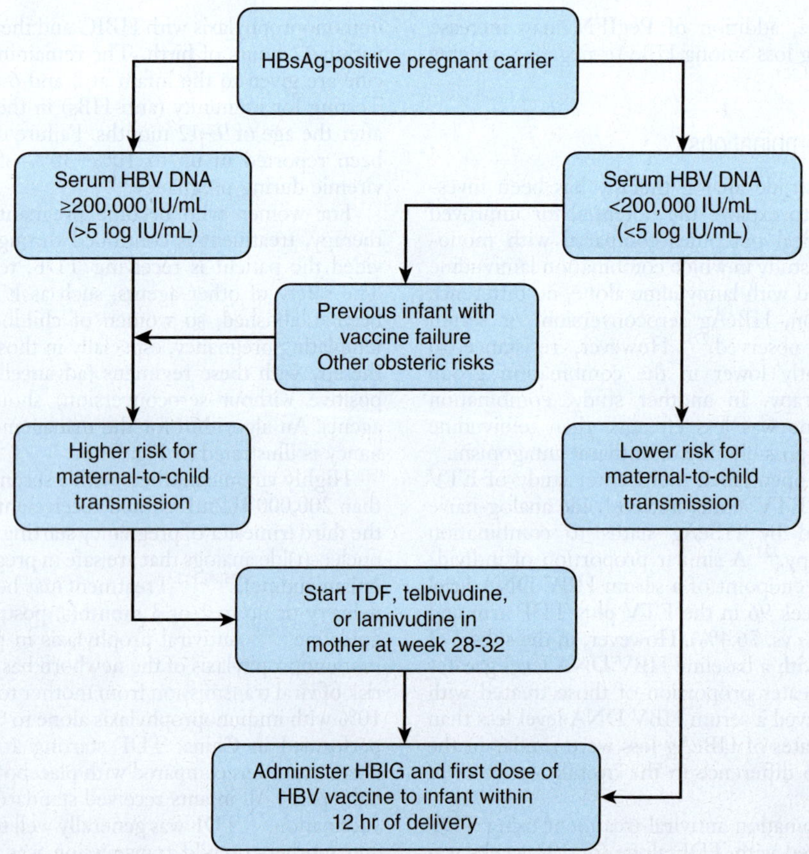

Fig. 81.8 Algorithm for the treatment of HBsAg-positive mothers during pregnancy. The goal of treatment in highly viremic mothers is to lower the serum HBV DNA level by several $\log_{10}$ IU/mL by the time of delivery to minimize the chance of newborn infection. The choice of antiviral agent is limited to those that are safe in pregnancy and include TDF, telbivudine, and lamivudine. These agents can be continued postpartum if necessary, but breastfeeding is not recommended in this setting. See text for further details about drug selection. *HBIG*, Hepatitis B immune globulin; *TDF*, tenofovir disoproxil fumarate. (Modified from Mitchell T, Armstrong GL, Hu DJ, et al. The increasing burden of imported chronic hepatitis B—United States, 1974–2008. *PLoS One*. 2011;6:e27717, with permission of author.)

antiviral therapy did not increase adverse outcomes in mother or baby. PegIFN is contraindicated in pregnancy. Although breastfeeding while on nucleos(t)ide analog therapy is officially contraindicated because small amounts of drug can be detected in breast milk,[238] adverse events have not been observed thus far.

Severe Acute Hepatitis

Symptoms of severe acute hepatitis B include deep jaundice, nausea, vomiting, RUQ abdominal tenderness, and possibly confusion. In general, a high rate (>95%) of virologic clearance (HBsAg loss) occurs in immune competent adults, and nucleos(t)ide analog treatment is not routinely required. For patients who have acute hepatitis B without evidence of liver dysfunction, close monitoring with weekly bloodwork and without immediate treatment is recommended. On the other hand, in those in whom ALF develops (hepatic encephalopathy, INR >1.5, and total bilirubin >3 mg/dL), mortality ranges from 30% to 70% in the absence of LT (see Chapter 95),[239,240] and antiviral treatment may be necessary to stabilize liver function, avoid LT, and improve survival. Nucleos(t)ide analog therapy in this situation is generally safe, and preferred agents include TDF, TAF, ETV, or lamivudine, but PegIFN is contraindicated in patients with abnormal liver function. The optimal duration of therapy is unknown, and the endpoint of therapy is confirmed by HBsAg loss or seroconversion.

Cirrhosis

Nucleos(t)ide analog therapy is safe and effective in patients with cirrhosis and advanced liver disease. In a study of HBV-infected patients in Taiwan with advanced liver disease and a high viral load, those who received lamivudine showed improvement in the Child-Turcotte-Pugh score (see Chapters 74 and 97) and fewer complications, including HCC and hepatic decompensation, compared with those who received placebo.[95] Although the benefit for those with HBV cirrhosis and a lower viral load is unclear, existing guidelines recommend that this group be treated. Preferred agents in patients with cirrhosis are the same as those for noncirrhotic patients (TDF, TAF, or ETV), and the duration of therapy in this group of patients is indefinite. PegIFN should not be considered for those with cirrhosis because of the risk of severe toxicity, including flares leading to liver failure. Long-term antiviral suppression with TDF or ETV has been associated with regression of cirrhosis.[180,241] In a study of 348 patients who underwent liver biopsies at baseline and Year 5 and who responded to long-term therapy with TDF, continuous treatment resulted in regression of cirrhosis in 75% at Year 5.[180] A reduction in fibrosis by at least one stage was observed in over 60% of responders to TDF over 5 years. Although there is no direct evidence from prospective clinical trials demonstrating a reduction in the risk of HCC associated with nucleos(t)ide analog therapy, amassed data from retrospective studies and modeling have found that the risk of HCC is reduced in treated patients compared with historical control groups.[134,231,242]

For patients with decompensated HBV cirrhosis, prompt initiation of nucleos(t)ide analog therapy is essential regardless of the serum HBV DNA level, so long as HBV DNA is detectable. Nucleos(t)ide analog treatment has been shown in several studies to improve liver function and liver-related survival. In an uncontrolled study of patients with decompensated HBV cirrhosis treated with lamivudine for 19 months, 65% had significant improvement in liver function and subsequently did not require LT.[243] In another study, liver transplant-free survival was above 80% in those who received long-term nucleos(t)ide analog therapy.[244] Combination therapy with TDF plus emtricitabine has been compared with TDF monotherapy in a small study of decompensated HBV-infected patients, but combination therapy showed no benefit in terms of antiviral suppression or stabilization of liver disease.[245] Improvement in liver function generally requires 6–9 months of therapy, and lifelong treatment is recommended in the setting of advanced liver disease.

In general, nucleos(t)ide analog therapy is safe and well tolerated in patients with decompensated cirrhosis. Recommended agents include TDF, TAF, and ETV. Renal function is a major predictor of survival in this population, and renal function must be monitored closely in those receiving TDF. If the serum creatinine level rises on TDF treatment, a dose adjustment is required; switching to TAF or ETV are other reasonable options. In a small case series, lactic acidosis was reported in HBV-infected patients with advanced cirrhosis (MELD score >20, see Chapter 99) receiving ETV treatment.[177] Although it is unclear whether the lactic acidosis was indeed related to ETV, this study underscores the need for close monitoring of patients with decompensated cirrhosis to detect changes in liver function and to exclude treatment side effects. Moreover, ultrasound screening for HCC is key in the management of this high-risk patient population, irrespective of response to antiviral treatment (see Chapter 76).

HBV-HIV Coinfection

With improved control of HIV disease with ART, liver disease has emerged as one of the leading causes of death in patients with HIV infection (see Chapter 33).[246] HBV coinfection is estimated in approximately 10% of patients living with HIV infection. Progression of liver disease to cirrhosis and HCC is accelerated in HBV-HIV coinfection. Therefore guidelines from the U.S. Department of Health and Human Services recommend therapy for HBV infection in all HBV-HIV coinfected patients irrespective of the CD4 count with ART that is active against both viruses.[247] Recommended regimens include a tenofovir-based regimen (TDF or TAF) in combination with either lamivudine or emtricitabine to avoid the development of HIV resistance to tenofovir. Switching to such a regimen is recommended in patients on an antiretroviral regimen that does not include an HBV-active drug. Conversely, ART that includes an HBV-active medication, such as TDF or TAF, should not be discontinued due to the risk of HBV relapse. Adding ETV for treatment of HBV infection is reasonable in those in whom HIV is suppressed, although there have been case reports of ETV-resistant HIV polymerase mutations.

HBV-HCV Coinfection

When compared with monoinfected patients, HBV-HCV coinfected patients tend to have more severe liver injury and a higher risk of cirrhosis and HCC.[248,249] Optimal treatment is directed toward the more active infection, which is obvious in most cases (see also Chapter 82). HBV-HCV coinfected patients often exhibit high-level HCV viremia and suppressed HBV DNA or vice versa. Cases of HBVr among HBV-HCV coinfected individuals during or after HCV DAA therapy have been reported.[250] Studies from Asia have shown that patients at highest risk are those who are HBsAg-positive and who have advanced liver fibrosis.[251] Such patients should receive prophylaxis against HBVr when receiving HCV DAA therapy. By contrast, those who are HBsAg-negative but anti-HBc-positive may be monitored with serum HBV DNA levels measured at least once during DAA therapy, with initiation of HBV treatment when the serum HBV DNA level increases by 1 log IU/mL. These studies underscore the importance of screening for HBV prior to treatment of HCV infection and the need for monitoring HBV during HCV DAA therapy.

HBV-HDV Coinfection

HBV-HDV coinfection is believed to be the most severe form of viral hepatitis with a high risk of complications, such as cirrhosis, HCC, and need for LT (see this chapter).[252–254] Coinfection with HDV should be suspected in HBsAg-positive patients from areas endemic for HDV, such as Mongolia, Western Africa, Eastern Europe, and South America, those who have advanced liver disease at an early age (<40 years), and elevated serum ALT levels despite very low or undetectable serum HBV DNA levels.[254] Other risk groups include immunosuppressed patients, men who have sex with men, and persons who inject drugs. HDV infection should also be suspected in patients with CHB on nucleos(t)ide analog therapy who have persistently elevated serum ALT levels despite adequate suppression of HBV. The diagnosis of HDV coinfection is made by detection of anti-HDV in serum, and active disease is confirmed by a positive HDV RNA testing.

Until recently, the only well-studied therapy for HBV-HDV coinfection is PegIFN given for at least 48 weeks. The goals of therapy are ALT normalization, which correlates with serum HDV RNA suppression and histologic improvement in liver necroinflammation and fibrosis. Unfortunately, a sustained response occurs in only 20%–50% patients after 1 year of treatment with PegIFN, and late relapses are common.[255–257] Nucleos(t)ide analog therapy does not directly affect HDV replication. Studies using adefovir alone or in combination with PegIFN failed to show any incremental benefit in HDV RNA suppression.[255] Therefore there is an urgent need to develop more agents for the treatment of HBV-HDV coinfection.

Recently, the entry-inhibitor bulevirtide, which targets the sodium taurocholate cotransporting polypeptide (NTCP), has shown efficacy alone and combined with PEG-IFN. Future studies will have to shed light on durability of response.[258,259] Other new agents under development include prenylation inhibitors (lonafarnib) and nucleic acid polymer REP 2139.[260,261] The potential mechanisms of action of these, and other investigational agents, are shown in Fig. 81.9.

HBV Reactivation (HBVr) During Immunosuppressive Therapy

The definition of HBVr has varied across different studies, and its incidence has, thus, been difficult to estimate. HBVr can be defined as an increase in HBV DNA replication (e.g.,>1 log) from baseline or reappearance of HBV DNA in serum and/or HBsAg seroreversion (reappearance of HBsAg in the serum) in HBsAg-negative persons, sometimes followed by elevation of serum aminotransferase levels, with or without jaundice or other signs of liver failure.[102,262] The risk of HBVr is higher in HBsAg-positive individuals receiving immunosuppressive therapy compared with HBsAg-negative, anti-HBc-positive individuals but also depends on the specific immunosuppressive regimen and the presence of underlying cirrhosis.

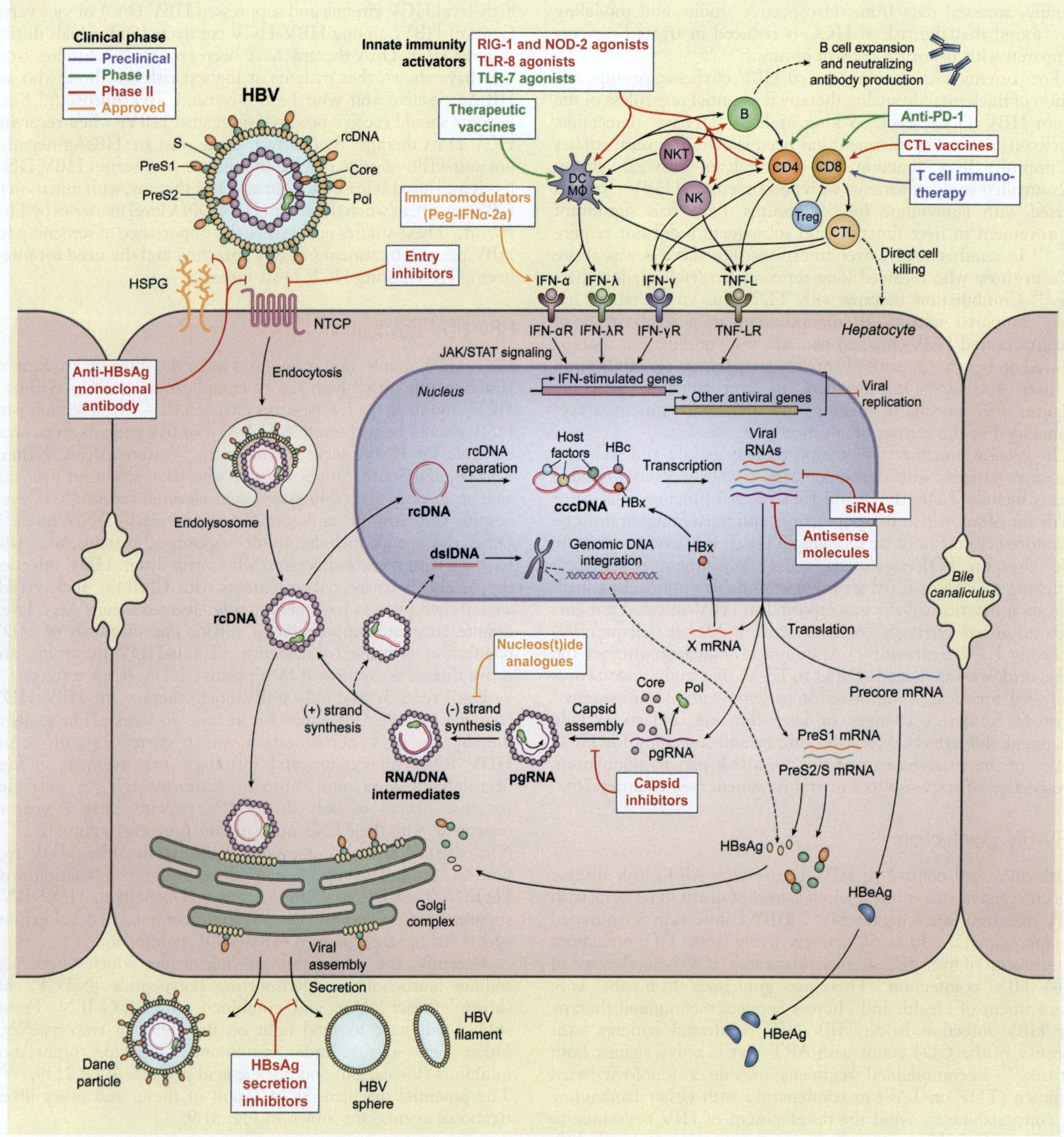

Fig. 81.9 New antiviral and immunomodulating agents in clinical development for cure of HBV. (From Mouzannar K, Liang TJ. Hepatitis B virus—recent therapeutic advances and challenges to cure. *J Hepatol.* 2020;73(3):694–695.)

Screening

Given the high prevalence of hepatitis B in many populations, and the potential for poor clinical outcomes associated with HBVr in patients receiving immunosuppressive therapy, screening for HBV has been recommended by both the American Oncology and Hepatology Societies.[89,263] Recommended serologic screening tests include HBsAg and anti-HBc. In HBsAg-positive patients, testing for serum HBV DNA, HBeAg, and anti-HBe should follow[75,89,133,264] to further characterize the status of underlying HBV infection.

Risk Stratification

The risk of HBVr depends on the baseline serologic status of HBV and on the type of immunosuppressive therapy. In general, the risk of HBVr is highest in HBsAg-positive individuals at baseline and much lower in HBsAg-negative, anti-HBc-positive individuals. Moreover, different immunosuppressive agents are associated with different risks of inducing HBVr. The highest risk is associated with the use of anti-CD20 monoclonal antibodies (e.g., rituximab, ofatumumab, obinutuzumab), and the lowest risk is associated with the use of conventional and weaker immunosuppressants, such as azathioprine or methotrexate.[265]

Immunosuppressive medications and cytotoxic agents that have been associated with HBVr are listed according to their estimated risk category in Fig. 81.6.[104]

In most reports, the rates of HBVr have varied from 10% to 50% in HBsAg-positive patients,[265,266] and 3% to 41% in HBsAg-negative, anti-HBc-positive patients receiving cytotoxic chemotherapy.[267,268] The median time to reactivation was 3 months after the last dose of rituximab, or approximately after six doses of rituximab, although late reactivation beyond 6 months after the last dose of rituximab was reported in 29% of patients.[266] Because of the high risk of HBVr in patients receiving anti-CD20 agents, the FDA issued a black box warning for rituximab.[269]

Glucocorticoids have also been identified as an independent predictor of HBVr in many studies. These agents are thought to increase viral replication by acting on a glucocorticoid-responsive element found in the HBV genome and may be associated with an initial decrease in the serum ALT level. A significant flare in ALT levels is typically seen 4–6 weeks after withdrawal of glucocorticoids.[270] Because glucocorticoids are often used in combination with other immunosuppressive agents, the risk attributable to high-dose glucocorticoids alone remains difficult to determine, but estimates vary from 30% to 70%.[271–273] By contrast, HBVr is less common in patients who have received low-dose glucocorticoids (<20 mg of prednisone per day for less than 4 weeks).[265]

Traditional immunosuppressants, such as methotrexate, azathioprine, and 6-mercaptopurine, have a low risk of HBVr, less than 1% based mainly on case series. Higher risk (18%) has been associated with the use of anthracycline agents, such as doxorubicin, especially in patients with breast cancer.[265,274] There have been increasing reports of HBVr in patients receiving TNF inhibitors, such as infliximab or adalimumab, from 0% to 40% in HBsAg-positive patients,[275,276] compared with only 0%–5% in HBsAg-negative patients.[265,277,278,104] It is important to note that there is still limited data on HBVr risk with novel chemotherapies, immunosuppressants and targeted therapies (including abatacept, ustekinumab, natalizumab, vedolizumab, imatinib, and nilotinib) and caution is advised when using these agents in patients with (past) HBV infection.[104,279]

Antiviral Prophylaxis

Several small randomized controlled trials and large cohort studies have demonstrated the efficacy of antiviral therapy, mainly with lamivudine or ETV, in preventing HBV-r.[280–282] Several meta-analyses and systematic reviews have also reported a significant reduction in HBVr, by 80%–100%, while also decreasing the risk of HBV-associated hepatitis.[283,284] Overall mortality, however, did not decrease, suggesting that overall survival is likely related to the prognosis of the underlying malignancy. Little is known about the effect of interrupting immunosuppressive therapy because of HBVr, but a meta-analysis demonstrated a reduced rate of need to interrupt chemotherapy in patients who received HBV prophylaxis.[285]

Lamivudine has been used widely as prophylaxis because of its relatively low cost, excellent safety profile, and short-term efficacy. However, lamivudine has been associated with a high risk for the development of antiviral resistance mutations (rtM204V/I ± rtL180M) after prolonged use (see earlier).[170] Therefore highly potent antiviral agents with a high barrier to resistance (e.g., TDF or ETV) are the preferred agents suggested by current guidelines.[75,89,133]

In a randomized controlled trial of ETV versus lamivudine in HBsAg-positive patients with diffuse large B-cell lymphoma treated with R-CHOP (rituximab-cyclophosphamide, doxorubicin, vincristine, prednisone) in China, reduced rates of HBVr (6.6% vs. 30%, $P = .001$), HBV-related hepatitis (0% vs. 13%, $P = .003$), and interruption of chemotherapy (1.6% vs. 18.3%, $P = .002$), respectively, were reported.[286] ETV treatment and lower stages of lymphoma were associated with a lower risk of HBVr. No randomized controlled trials have compared TDF with lamivudine, but based on available data, TDF is superior to lamivudine and at least equipotent to ETV. Therefore lamivudine should only be considered in patients receiving a short course of immunosuppressive therapy (<6–12 months) who have a low baseline serum HBV DNA level (<2000 IU/mL). Otherwise, TDF or ETV should serve as the preferred agent for prophylaxis.

Timing and Duration of Prophylaxis

Ideally, antiviral therapy should be initiated prior to the start of immunosuppressive therapy, but the exact time required has not been well established.[103,265] Prophylaxis should be initiated at least 1 week before the start of immunosuppression in HBsAg-positive patients, and the same is likely true for HBsAg-negative, anti-HBc-positive patients who require prophylaxis. Some experts recommend a reduction in serum HBV DNA levels to less than 3 logs IU/mL before immunosuppressive therapy is started, if possible.[75,89,103,133]

The duration of prophylactic antiviral therapy also depends on the type of immunosuppressive therapy, baseline HBV DNA level, and severity of underlying liver disease. In general, antiviral therapy should be continued for at least 6–12 months after withdrawal of immunosuppression; most guidelines extend this duration to more than 12–18 months with B-cell depleting anti-CD20 agents.[75,89,103,133,265] For hematopoietic stem cell or solid organ transplant patients, antiviral therapy may need to continue indefinitely, because these patients will likely remain on chronic immunosuppressive medications, and there have been reports of delayed HBVr (see Chapter 34). In HBsAg-positive patients with a serum HBV DNA level greater than 2000 IU/mL or those with underlying cirrhosis, antiviral therapy should be given for a prolonged duration, according to current treatment guidelines for cirrhotic noncancer patients and until the usual treatment endpoints are reached (see earlier).

Deferred Therapy

In a study of HBsAg-positive patients with lymphoma treated with R-CHOP who were randomized to delayed lamivudine therapy, HBV serology, including serum HBV DNA and HBsAg, was monitored monthly to detect early HBVr.[287] HBVr was detected in 56% of patients in the delayed treatment group compared with 12% of patients in the prophylaxis group. These data confirm the efficacy of prophylaxis but also demonstrate that delayed treatment of HBsAg-positive patients may be an option, provided that very close monitoring is feasible. However, close monitoring is expensive and difficult to obtain in real-world practice and therefore generally not recommended in HBsAg-positive patients treated with immunosuppressive therapy. On the other hand, monitoring alone is an option for HBsAg-negative, anti-HBc-positive patients receiving immunosuppressive agents that have a moderate or low risk of HBVr in whom careful follow-up can be assured.[75,89,103,133,265]

Future Treatments

Available antiviral therapies effectively suppress viral replication, normalize serum liver enzyme levels, improve hepatic fibrosis, and even reduce the risk of complications, such as HCC. However, the vast majority of patients cannot be cured with current treatments, which are unable to eradicate or silence cccDNA.[288] A functional cure of HBV is defined as sustained off treatment HBsAg loss and HBV DNA undetectability. This unfortunately occurs in only 2%–10% of patients with CHB treated with available antiviral agents.[176] Therefore novel antiviral agents, likely in combination and targeting multiple steps in the viral life cycle and the immune system, will be required to achieve cure of HBV infection in most patients. In view of therapeutic advances that have led to a cure for chronic hepatitis C (see Chapter 82), there has been a renewed interest in achieving cure of HBV infection using novel antiviral and immunomodulating agents in clinical development (Fig. 81.9).

Entry Inhibition

HBV and HDV enter the hepatocyte after binding to the receptor NTCP. Therefore blocking or silencing NTCP is a potential strategy to treat CHB. Bulevirtide is a novel entry inhibitor that has been studied in HBV and HBV-HDV coinfected patients. Although a decline in serum HBV DNA levels and normalization of serum ALT levels were observed in some patients, no significant reduction in HBsAg levels was seen in early studies.[289] In HDV infection bulevirtide is effective in producing a decline of HDV RNA and transaminase levels, which has led to licensing in several European countries.

RNA Interference

Because HBV replicates via RNA intermediates, it is susceptible to targeting by RNA targeting agents. A significant drop in serum HBsAg levels has been observed during treatment with RNA targeting using small interfering RNA or antisense oligonucleotides, although the absolute number of patients achieving durable HBsAg clearance was limited.[290] With longer therapy and combination with other antivirals or immune modifying agents, the decrease in HBsAg levels could contribute to higher rates of sustained functional cure.[188]

Capsid Assembly Modulators

Capsid assembly modulators (CAM) are a new class of antiviral agents that target the HBV core protein. Their primary mechanism of action is prevention of HBV encapsidation and blockade of viral replication, thereby resulting in aberrant or empty capsids that contain no viral genome.[290a] A secondary yet unproven antiviral mechanism involves inhibition of de novo cccDNA formation via capsid disassembly, thereby reducing the replenishment of cccDNA inside the hepatocyte. In contrast to nucleos(t)ide analogs, CAM in combination with other classes of antiviral agents show promise in reducing serum HBV DNA but also HBV RNA levels and, with newer generation CAM, reduced HBsAg levels, suggesting inhibition of transcriptionally active cccDNA. Whether this strategy alone will lead to a functional cure is uncertain.[291,292]

HBsAg Release Inhibitors

HBsAg is produced in vast excess in HBV carriers, but the precise reason for overproduction of this viral protein is unclear. Most HBsAg exists in the form of subviral particles, which contain no viral DNA or RNA. HBsAg is thought to act to exhaust T cells, thereby leading to immune tolerance to the virus and evasion of immune attack. Therefore significant reductions in HBsAg levels may restore host immunity to HBV. Although the first studies with HBsAg release inhibitors have been promising, further studies are required to confirm durability of HBsAg responses.[260,293,294]

Immune Modulation

Several approaches to restore HBV specific immune responses are under investigation. Toll-like receptors (TLRs) normally recognize pathogens, such as HBV, and stimulate innate and adaptive immunity through endogenous production of IFN in the liver. TLR agonists upregulate IFN-stimulating genes to inhibit viral replication, whereas HBV attempts to downregulate expression of TLR. A TLR-7 agonist resulted in IFN-stimulated gene expression, but no significant reduction in HBsAg levels was observed.[295] A recent study of Selgantolimod, an oral TLR-8 agonist, showed dose dependent induction of immune responses and limited HBsAg decline in a minority of cases during short-term treatment.

The lack of a T-cell mediated response in chronic HBV is due partly to the expression of coinhibitory receptors and to the expression of immunosuppressive cytokines. Checkpoint inhibitors have been shown to restore antitumor adaptive immunity and are being investigated to revitalize HBV-specific T cells and thus reverse immune exhaustion.[296] Interesting results have been obtained in animal models and human studies. The main concerns of this approach are the potential induction of autoimmunity and in particular uncontrolled hepatitis flares. Several therapeutic vaccines designed to boost $CD8^+$ T-cell responses against HBV have also been evaluated with limited success, but interesting new vaccine formulations are under clinical evaluation.[296]

PREVENTION

Immunoprophylaxis against HBV can be delivered by passive immunization using HBIG or active immunization using HBV vaccine. Active immunization provides long-term immunity, whereas passive immunization confers only immediate and short-lived protection.

Hepatitis B Immune Globulin

HBIG is prepared from plasma that is known to contain high titers of anti-HBs. Numerous clinical trials have established the efficacy of HBIG in preventing HBV infection in high-risk persons, such as hemodialysis patients, sexual partners of persons with CHB, and newborn infants of HBsAg-positive mothers within 12 hours of birth along with simultaneous vaccination. HBIG licensed in the United States has an anti-HBs titer of 1:100,000. In Europe, several preparations of HBIG with different concentrations and pharmacokinetic properties are available. HBIG is safe, although rare anaphylactic reactions can occur. Myalgias, rash, and arthralgias have also been reported and are believed to result from formation of antigen-antibody complexes.

Hepatitis B Vaccine

Currently marketed HBV vaccines use recombinant DNA technology by introducing the S gene encoding HBsAg into the genome of yeast cells. Three vaccines are available in the United States: Recombivax HB (Merck, licensed in 1986), Engerix-B (GlaxoSmithKline, licensed in 1989), HEPLISAV-B (DynaVax, licensed in 2017, and PreHevbrio (VBI, licensed in 2022). No serious side effects of the HBV vaccine have been reported. The HBV vaccine is administered intramuscularly in the deltoid muscle of adults and the anterolateral thigh of neonates and infants.

HBV vaccines typically achieve an anti-HBs titer greater than 100 mIU/mL. Antibody titers greater than 100 mIU/mL confer 100% protection against HBV infection, and a lower antibody titer (up to 10 mIU/mL) is seroprotective in most instances. Peak antibody titers and persistence of antibody levels vary among different persons. The titers drop steadily over the first 2 years after vaccination, sometimes to levels below 10 mIU/mL. Studies in different populations have demonstrated that anti-HBs titers decrease to nonprotective levels in at least 25%–50% of recipients over a period of 5–10 years.[297]

Although protective anti-HBs response rates after HBV vaccination occur in approximately 90% of patients, a number of factors can reduce the antibody response. Five percent to 8% of HBV vaccine recipients do not achieve detectable anti-HBs levels (nonresponders). Smoking, obesity, injection into the buttock, chronic liver disease, presence of HLA-DR3, DR7, and DQ2 alleles, absence of the HLA-A2 allele, and older age may be associated with reduced immunogenicity. Such "hyporesponders" may benefit from a higher dose of vaccine. Response rates are also lower in immunocompromised patients, such as organ transplant recipients, those receiving chemotherapy, and those with end-stage liver disease. In a study of 62 cirrhotic patients on the liver transplant waiting list undergoing 3-dose HBV vaccination, the response rate was only 44% but increased to 62% after additional booster doses were administered. These findings indicate that persons with chronic liver disease should undergo vaccination prior to the development of cirrhosis.[298] Poor vaccine response rates of approximately 60% in hemodialysis patients can likely be increased to around 90% using a new vaccine (HEPLISAV-B) with higher immunogenicity.

Therefore patients with chronic liver and kidney disease should be vaccinated early during their disease course, before progression of the disease, to ensure an optimal response to vaccination.

Although HBV vaccination is recommended for patients with HIV infection, response rates appear to be decreased in this population. In a large randomized study of stable HIV-infected patients on ART, the proportion of patients given a 4-dose HBV vaccine regimen who had a durable response (anti-HBs >10 mIU/mL) was 71%.[299] A high-level response (anti-HBs >100 mIU/mL) was observed in 42% of the patients.

Because HBV vaccination results in strong immunologic memory capable of preventing infection even in patients with low or undetectable antibody titers, a booster vaccine dose in immunocompetent adults and children is not recommended. On the other hand, high-risk patients, such as those undergoing hemodialysis, should receive a booster dose when anti-HBs titers drop below 10 mIU/mL.[300] Data from Taiwan demonstrated a surprisingly high rate of HBsAg positivity in adolescents who were vaccinated at birth, especially those born to HBeAg-positive mothers who did not receive HBIG or who had fewer than four doses of vaccine, suggesting that maternal viral load was very high at the time of birth and that perhaps a booster dose may be needed at age 15 or older in some individuals.[301]

Vaccination Schedule

The typical vaccination schedule is 0, 1, and 6 months after birth. High anti-HBs titers are achieved in over 95% of individuals after the third dose of vaccine. However, the HELPISAV-B vaccine requires only two doses given 1 month apart. Seroprotection rates of 91%–95% were reported by Week 24 after vaccination in adults.[302] In immunocompromised patients and those undergoing hemodialysis, four vaccine doses are recommended, with the fourth dose given to maximize the anti-HBs titer response. If vaccination is interrupted, the second dose should be administered as soon as possible after the first.[303] If the third dose is not given on schedule, it should be given at least 2 months after the second dose.

In the United States and HBV-endemic countries, the HBV vaccine is administered to all infants and children as a part of a universal immunization program. Furthermore, all WHO regions have achieved three-dose vaccination rates above 80% before the age of 1 year.[32]

Combination HBV vaccines with diphtheria-pertussis-tetanus and *Haemophilus influenzae* type B (Hib) (DTPw-HB/Hib) are in use for immunization of infants. The other component antigens do not reduce the immunogenicity against HBV.[304] Adolescents who have not been vaccinated in infancy or childhood should also be vaccinated.

Postexposure and Perinatal Prophylaxis

Table 81.7 lists recommendations for prophylaxis after exposure to a known HBsAg-positive source. Postexposure vaccination should be considered for any percutaneous, ocular, or mucous membrane exposure. The type of immunoprophylaxis is determined by the HBsAg status of the source and the vaccination-response status of the exposed person. If a patient is a known responder to previous vaccination, then no further action is required.

TABLE 81.7 Recommended Postexposure Prophylaxis for HBV According to the Vaccination Status of the Exposed Person

Vaccination Status of Exposed Person	Recommended Prophylaxis
Unvaccinated	HBIG (0.06 mL/kg) and initiate hepatitis B vaccine series
Previously vaccinated:	No action required
Known responder[a]	HBIG × 2 doses (1 month apart)
Known nonresponder	*OR* HBIG × 1 dose and initiate HBV revaccination
Antibody response unknown	Test for anti-HBs Anti-HBs titer ≥10 mIU/mL: no action required Anti-HBs titer <10 mIU/mL: HBIG × 1 dose and administer vaccine booster dose

[a]Anti-HBs ≥10 mIU/mL.
Anti-HBs, Antibody to hepatitis B surface antigen; *HBIG,* hepatitis B immune globulin; *HBsAg,* hepatitis B surface antigen.

Bivalent Vaccine

A combined HAV and HBV vaccine has been licensed commercially (TWINRIX, GlaxoSmithKline, Research Triangle Park, NC) and has been shown to be highly immunogenic and protective against both viruses. This vaccine offers ease of administration for persons at increased risk of both HAV and HBV infection, such as world travelers, men who have sex with men, and those with underlying chronic liver disease.[305]

Recommendations

Recommendations for HBV vaccination from the CDC included universal infant vaccination, revaccination of nonresponder infants, serologic testing of infants whose maternal HBsAg status is unknown, HBV DNA testing in all HBsAg-positive pregnant women, and vaccination of patients with chronic liver disease.[306,6] The CDC also recommends HBV vaccination in adults aged 19 through 59 years, aged above 60 years with risk factors for hepatitis B (e.g., sexual exposure, risk by blood exposure) and unvaccinated children aged <19 years.[33]

HBsAg-Positive Health Care Workers

Although HBV transmission from a health care worker to a patient is considered rare in the United States because of HBV vaccination and strict adherence to universal precautions, the CDC has published recommendations for the management of HBsAg-positive health care workers and students.[307] Health care providers must be aware of their HBV and other bloodborne virus status, and those who lack HBV immunity should receive HBV vaccination followed by routine testing for anti-HBs to verify immunity. If anti-HBs remains undetectable, repeat vaccination is recommended as well as testing for HBsAg and anti-HBc, to identify those with active HBV infection.

The exact threshold for HBV infectivity necessary for transmission from health care worker to patient is unknown, but it is thought to be in the range of 2000–8000 IU/mL, regardless of HBeAg status. Nevertheless, HBsAg-positive health care providers are generally able to maintain their current form of practice, but review by an independent panel is recommended for those who perform exposure-prone procedures. Prenotification of patients of the health care provider's HBV status is not recommended for fear of stigmatization and avoidance by the provider of regular serologic monitoring and appropriate antiviral treatment if needed. CDC guidelines do not prohibit HBsAg-positive health care providers or students from practicing or studying medicine or dentistry if they are otherwise qualified and agree to HBV DNA monitoring in some circumstances.[308]

Exposure-prone procedures are defined as those in which surgical access is difficult or situations in which a needlestick injury is likely to occur. These include procedures that involve digital palpation of a needle tip or other sharp object in a closed cavity in which visualization is poor. For persons who perform exposure-prone procedures, such as surgeons, dentists, obstetricians/gynecologists, and surgical residents, an independent panel of experts must review their practice and HBV DNA results every 6 months. Regular activities can be maintained if serum HBV DNA levels are documented to be less than 1000 IU/mL. If HBV DNA is above this threshold, performance of exposure-prone procedures is temporarily suspended until the HBV DNA level is documented to drop below 1000 IU/mL, either spontaneously or with antiviral therapy. Health care workers who perform exposure-prone procedures may opt to start long-term antiviral treatment to maintain viral suppression that permits regular clinical activities, even though they may not meet the usual criteria for initiation of treatment. On the other hand, for health care workers and students who do not perform exposure-prone procedures, no special oversight by the panel is required.

Acknowledgment

Drs. Edo J. Dongelmans supported revision of this chapter, and Drs. Scott Fung, Jennifer T. Wells, and Robert Perrillo contributed to this chapter in previous editions of the book.

Full references for this chapter can be found at https://ebooks.health.elsevier.com.

82 Hepatitis C

Jacinta A. Holmes, Raymond T. Chung

IN THIS CHAPTER

More than 56 million people worldwide are chronically infected with HCV.[1] In the United States, conservative estimates suggest that more than 2.2 million people live with HCV.[2] Unfortunately, HCV successfully evades the host immune response in 50%–90% of acutely infected persons, thereby leading to chronic infection in the majority of cases. The natural history of hepatitis C varies greatly; reasons for this heterogeneity remain incompletely understood but are related to viral, host, and environmental factors. Chronic HCV infection can lead to cirrhosis and HCC; HCV-related mortality increased dramatically after 1995, plateaued around 2002, and has been rapidly increasing from 2003, owing to the aging HCV population.[3–5] Complications of HCV-related cirrhosis remain a leading indication for LT in the United States and Europe. With the introduction of highly effective DAA therapy, the frequency of these complications has already begun to decline since 2016.[2]

Currently, chronic hepatitis C is the only chronic viral infection that can be cured by antiviral therapy. Importantly, successful antiviral treatment can prevent short- and long-term complications of HCV infection in many patients.[6] Substantial progress in understanding the HCV replication cycle, along with development of the replicon system and crystallization of the HCV proteins, has enabled the development of new therapeutic agents that target discrete steps in the viral life cycle, culminating in highly potent well-tolerated interferon (IFN)-free therapy. Combination therapy with DAAs has altered the treatment landscape dramatically, affording sustained virologic response (SVR) at 12 weeks (SVR12) rates (defined as absence of HCV RNA in serum 12 weeks after discontinuation of treatment) in excess of 95% for most patients. An SVR12 is almost always associated with an SVR at 24 weeks (SVR24, defined as absence of HCV RNA in serum 24 weeks after discontinuation of treatment, which was the prior decision point for determining cure with IFN-based therapy) and durable long-term eradication of the virus.[7–10] The term SVR now implies an SVR12.

VIROLOGY

Structure

The HCV virion is an enveloped virus that is 50 nm in diameter.[11] The two envelope proteins, E1 and E2, heterodimerize, and assemble into tetramers, creating a smooth outer layer, which has a "fishbone" configuration with icosahedral symmetry. The envelope proteins are anchored to a host cell–derived lipid bilayer envelope membrane that surrounds the nucleocapsid. The nucleocapsid is believed to be composed of multiple copies of the core protein and forms an internal icosahedral viral coat that encapsulates the genomic RNA.[12] HCV circulates in various forms in the serum of an infected host, including (1) virions that are bound to VLDL and LDL and appear to represent the infectious fraction; (2) virions bound to immunoglobulin (Ig); and (3) free virions.

Genomic Organization

HCV is a single-stranded positive-sense RNA virus that belongs to the Flaviviridae family and has been classified as the sole member of the genus *Hepacivirus*.[13] The genome of HCV contains approximately 9600 nucleotides with an open reading frame (ORF) that encodes one large viral polypeptide precursor of about 3000 amino acids. The HCV ORF is flanked upstream by a 5′ untranslated region (UTR) that functions as an internal ribosome entry site to direct cap-independent translation (i.e., without the addition of an extra ribonucleotide to the 5′ end of the viral messenger RNA) and downstream by a 3′ UTR that is critical for initiation of new RNA strand synthesis.[14] The 5′ and portions of the 3′ UTR are the most conserved regions of the HCV genome.

Viral Replication and Life Cycle

Although peripheral blood mononuclear cells, B cells, T cells, and dendritic cells have been reported to support HCV replication, hepatocytes are the major site of viral replication.[15,16] HCV entry involves the attachment of envelope proteins E1 and E2 to cell surface molecules (Fig. 82.1).[17] The expression and function of CD81, a member of the tetraspanin superfamily, is essential for HCV entry into hepatocytes.[18] In addition, human scavenger receptor class B type 1 (SR-B1), a selective importer of cholesteryl esters from HDL into cells, has been shown to interact with E2 and is also essential for HCV entry.[19] Whereas CD81 and SR-B1 are required early in the process of viral entry, claudin-1, a tight junction component that is highly expressed on hepatocytes, and occludin are required later in the cell entry process.[20,21] Heparin sulfated proteoglycans and LDL have also been shown to be involved in HCV cell entry.[22,23] Additional cellular factors and receptors suggested to be required for viral entry include EGF[24] and Niemann-Pick C1-like 1, a cholesterol uptake receptor.

Once HCV attaches to the cell, the endocytosis of the bound virion is presumed to occur, as with other flaviviruses. A pH drop in the vesicle causes conformational changes in the glycoproteins that lead to fusion of the viral and cellular membranes[25] and release of viral RNA into the cytoplasm. In the cytosol, the 5′ UTR functions as an internal ribosome entry site, which directs the RNA to its docking site on the endoplasmic reticulum and mediates cap-independent internal initiation of HCV polyprotein translation by recruiting both cellular proteins, including eukaryotic initiation factors 2 and 3, and viral proteins.[26] The large polyprotein is co- and posttranslationally processed proteolytically into at least 11 viral proteins, including both structural [nucleocapsid (C), or p21; envelope 1 (E1), or gp31; and envelope 2 (E2), or gp70] and nonstructural (NS2, NS3, NS4A, NS4B, NS5A, and NS5B) proteins (Fig. 82.2). The functions of these specific nonstructural proteins are described later in the chapter.

After polyprotein processing, NS4B expression causes the membrane alterations that are seen on electron microscopy known as a membranous web.[27] The replication complex associates viral proteins, cellular components, and nascent RNA strands. HCV replication is catalyzed by the NS5B RNA-dependent RNA polymerase (RdRp). The positive-strand genomic RNA serves as a template for the synthesis of a negative-strand intermediate. The negative-strand RNA serves as a template for production of numerous strands of RNA of positive polarity that are used for polyprotein translation and synthesis of new intermediates of replication and that are packaged into new virus particles.[28]

Finally, viral particle formation is initiated by the interaction of the core protein with genomic RNA in the endoplasmic reticulum.[29] By analogy with pestiviruses, HCV packaging and release are likely to be inefficient because much of the virus remains in

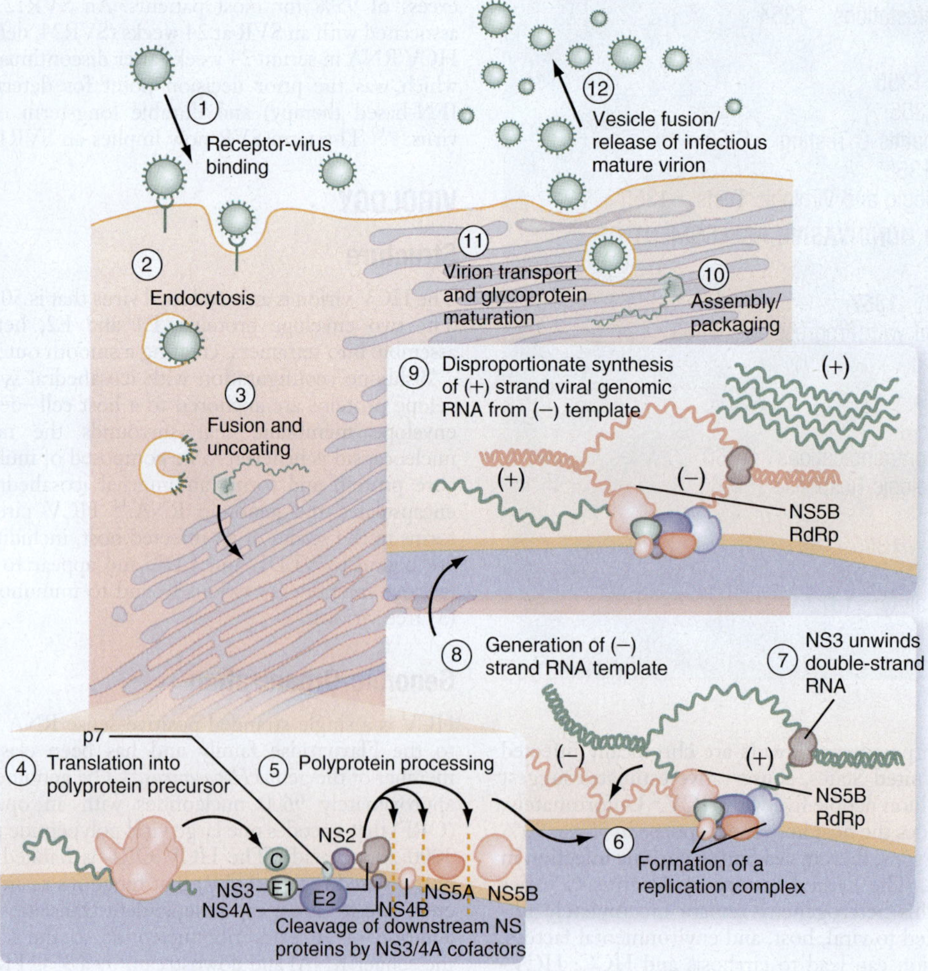

Fig. 82.1 Putative life cycle of HCV (see text for details and Fig. 82.2 for functions of the HCV proteins). *C*, Core; *E*, envelope; *NS*, nonstructural; *RdRp*, RNA-dependent RNA polymerase. (Reproduced with permission from Pawlotsky JM, Chevaliez S, McHutchison JG. The hepatitis C virus life cycle as a target for new antiviral therapies. *Gastroenterology*. 2007;132:1979–1998.)

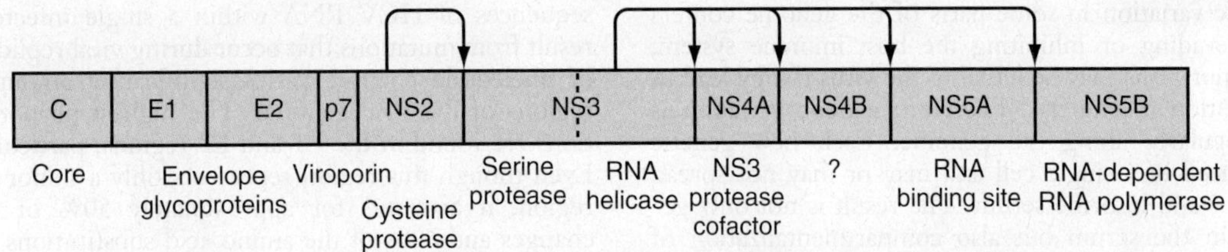

Fig. 82.2 Schematic representation of the HCV polyprotein. The structural proteins *C* (core), *E1*, and *E2* (envelope proteins) are cleaved from the polyprotein by the host signal peptidase. *p7*, a viroporin protein, is cleaved by the endoplasmic reticulum signal peptidase and forms an ion channel that is essential for assembly and release of infectious virions. The NS2 cysteine protease autocatalytically cleaves itself from the polyprotein (first *arrow*). The NS3 protease cleaves the remainder of the nonstructural proteins: *NS3* (serine protease and RNA helicase), *NS4A* (NS3 protease cofactor), *NS4B*, *NS5A* (RNA binding site), and *NS5B* [RNA-dependent RNA polymerase (second, third, fourth, and fifth *arrows*)].

the cell. Following release, viral particles may infect adjacent hepatocytes or enter the circulation, where they are available for infection of another cell or host.

Virus Protein Function

The large polyprotein generated by translation of the HCV genome is cleaved by cellular and viral proteases to form structural and nonstructural proteins. The structural proteins are separated from the nonstructural proteins by the short membrane peptide p7, believed to be a viroporin, a protein that plays a role in viral particle maturation and release.[30] The crystal structures of most of the ORF proteins have been elucidated and have led to an understanding of protein interactions and functions. Although these proteins are most important for viral replication, some also interact with host proteins and may facilitate persistence of the virus by impairing the host immune response.

The core protein is first cleaved from the large polypeptide and then further processed by a host signal peptidase.[28] In infectious HCV virions, the core protein forms the viral nucleocapsid and binds RNA. The core protein has been found attached to lipid rafts and the endoplasmic reticulum, and it translocates into the nucleus. When core protein attaches to lipid rafts, it recruits nonstructural proteins, thereby resulting in the assembly of infectious virions. The core protein can also interact with the host immune system by inactivating the RNA silencing activity of Dicer, a cellular endoribonuclease that produces small interfering RNA to bind and target HCV RNA for destruction by the cell.[31] The core protein can also bind to Janus kinase-1 (JAK1) and JAK2 and alter the activation of signal transducer and activator of transcription (STAT) proteins, leading to impairment of IFN production.[32] Extracellularly, core protein inhibits T-cell activation and proliferation, possibly by downregulating costimulatory molecules on dendritic cells.[33] Specific polymorphisms in core protein have also been associated with intracellular lipid accumulation[34]; this may be the result of facilitation of phosphorylation of insulin receptor substrate-1, thereby leading to insulin resistance.[35] Mutations in core protein have also been associated with an increased risk of HCC in patients; core protein alone can cause HCC in transgenic mice.[36]

E1 and E2 proteins are cleaved from the polypeptide by host signal peptidase.[37] The two proteins form highly glycosylated heterodimers and then tetramers that are essential for viral assembly (see earlier). They also mediate cell entry by binding to surface receptors.[38] Subsequently, they are responsible for fusion between the host cell membrane and the viral envelope. Because E1 and E2 are expressed on the surface of the virion, they are targets of host antibodies. The first 27 amino acids of E2 form hypervariable region 1 (HVR1); alterations in HVR1 are believed to be an attempt by the virus at antibody-mediated immune evasion.

p7 is cleaved by the endoplasmic reticulum signal peptidase and forms an ion channel. This viroporin protein is essential for efficient assembly and release of infectious virions but not for cell entry.

NS2 complexes with NS3 and zinc to form a cysteine protease, with two composite active sites, that autocatalytically cleaves NS2 from NS3.[39] No other function of NS2 has been discovered to date. NS3 has several functions in addition to complexing with NS2 for autocatalytic cleavage of the NS2-NS3 site.[39] Its function as a serine protease is markedly enhanced by its association with NS4A. The enzyme results in cleavage of the polyprotein at the NS3-NS4A, NS4A-NS4B, NS4B-NS5A, and NS5A-NS5B sites.[40,41] The NS3 protease also cleaves and thereby destroys the function of Cardif and TRIF (Toll/interleukin receptor domain-containing adapter-inducing IFN-β), which are intermediates in two separate pathways of host-cell IFN secretion in response to viral infection.[42–44] This property may have a significant effect in impairing the host response to HCV infection. Finally, a portion of the NS3 protein functions as a helicase that unwinds viral RNA as well as host DNA. The helicase function is dependent on ATP, may require dimerization of NS3, and progresses in discrete steps like an inchworm.[45] NS4A complexes with NS3 and functions to stabilize the protease and helicase activities and anchor the complex to the endoplasmic reticulum membrane.[40,46] It also regulates hyperphosphorylation of NS5A.[47] The only known function of NS4B is to induce the formation of the membranous web on which HCV transcription occurs.[48] NS5A binds zinc and forms homodimers that are bound to the endoplasmic reticulum membrane.[46] NS5A is essential for viral replication and is believed to provide an RNA-binding site within the replication complex.[49] In addition, NS5A inhibits apoptosis in infected cells,[50,51] and some mutations confer improved sensitivity to IFN therapy.[52] NS5B is the viral RdRp.[40] The crystal structure elucidates the tunnel of the enzyme that directs single-stranded RNA into the active site.[53] It can synthesize both negative-strand HCV RNA templates and positive-strand HCV RNA genomes.

Genotypes and Quasispecies

HCV has an inherently high mutational rate that results in considerable heterogeneity throughout the genome. This high mutational rate is in part a consequence of the RdRp of HCV, which lacks 3′- to 5′-exonuclease proofreading ability that ordinarily would remove mismatched nucleotides incorporated during replication. An average of one error occurs for every 10^4–10^5 nucleotides copied. This phenomenon is favored by a high viral turnover rate; 10^{10}–10^{12} virions are produced per day.[54] The estimated half-life of HCV in serum is only about 45 minutes.[55] A substantial proportion of newly synthesized viral genomes have alterations. Because of the functional differences in HCV proteins, genetic variation in some parts of the genome confers advantages by evading or inhibiting the host immune system, whereas other mutations may be lethal to the virus if they lead to defective replication machinery. Therefore genetic variation is distributed irregularly along the genome. Each new genetic variant is produced in a single cell and may or may not spread through the liver and into the serum. The result is not only genetic diversity in the serum but also compartmentalization of variant virions in different parts of the liver and perhaps in extrahepatic sites.

Because of the vast genetic variation, a classification scheme was devised whereby viral sequences are given a genotype and subtype. The first division used to describe the genetic heterogeneity of HCV is the viral *genotype*, which refers to genetically distinct groups of HCV isolates that have arisen during the evolution of the virus. Nucleotide sequencing has shown variation of up to 34% between genotypes.[56] The most conserved region (5′ UTR) has a maximum nucleotide sequence divergence of 9% between genotypes, whereas the highly variable regions that encode the envelope proteins (E1 and E2) exhibit a nucleotide sequence divergence of 35%–44% between genotypes. The sequences cluster into 7 major genotypes (designated by numbers), with sequence similarities of 60%–70%, and more than 67 *subtypes* (designated by a lower case letter) within these major genotypes, with sequence similarities of 77%–80%.[57] In this scheme, the first variant, which was cloned by Choo et al., is designated type 1a.[58] The HCV genotype is an intrinsic characteristic of the infecting HCV strain and does not change over time; therefore the genotype only needs to be determined once in an infected person. Mixed-genotype infections may be seen and reflect either coinfection with more than one HCV virus or methodologic problems in genotype testing. In addition, intergenotypic HCV recombinants have been described[59]; these are thought to arise because of recombination among different genotypes in patients with repeated exposure. The recombination events have been reported to occur in or between NS2 and NS3.[60]

Global geographic differences exist in the distribution of HCV genotypes, as well as in the mode of acquisition. In the United States, genotype 1a is the most prevalent, accounting for approximately 46% of HCV infections, followed by genotype 1b in 26%, genotype 2 in 11%, genotype 3 in 9%, and genotypes 4–6, or mixed/other in less than 8%.[61] Racial differences are seen in the prevalence of genotypes; approximately 90% of African Americans are infected with HCV genotype 1, whereas only 70% of whites and 71% of Hispanics are infected with genotype 1.[62] In Europe, the most prevalent genotype is 3 (41%), followed by 1b (40%), 1a (13%), and 1c/other (18%).[61] Genotype 4 is found mainly in Egypt, the Middle East, and Central Africa.[61,63] In Egypt, approximately 6.5%–7% of the population is infected with HCV, and more than 90% have HCV genotype 4.[61,64] Genotype 5, although originally isolated in South Africa, is also seen in specific regions of Europe (France and Belgium) and the Middle East (Lebanon and Syria).[61,65] Genotype 6 is found predominantly in Asia. The distribution of genotypes is ever changing with immigration and alterations in the primary modes of viral transmission. Therefore the frequencies of viral genotypes change over time.

In the era of IFN-based therapy, HCV genotype was an important predictor of response to treatment. Although HCV genotype as a predictor of treatment outcome is less relevant with DAA-based therapy, HCV genotype is still important, because some DAAs only have activity against specific HCV genotypes (see later). HCV genotype may also play a role in disease progression and complications of chronic HCV infection. Specifically, HCV genotype 3 has been associated with faster liver fibrosis progression,[66] as well as with an increased risk of cirrhosis and HCC.[67]

The second component of genetic heterogeneity is *quasispecies* generation.[56] Quasispecies are closely related, yet heterogeneous, sequences of HCV RNA within a single infected person that result from mutations that occur during viral replication. The rate of nucleotide changes varies significantly among the different regions of the viral genome. The highest proportions of mutations are found in the E1 and E2 regions, particularly in HVR1. Even though this region represents only a minor part of the E2 region, it accounts for approximately 50% of the nucleotide changes and 60% of the amino acid substitutions within the envelope region.

The development of quasispecies may be one mechanism by which the virus escapes the host's immune response and establishes persistent infection.[68] During acute infection or during treatment, the lack of diversity in the quasispecies is associated with viral clearance, and the development of numerous quasispecies is associated with viral persistence.[69] In acute disease, patients in whom genetic variation in the HVR1 region develops after antibody seroconversion progress to chronic disease, whereas those in whom such genetic variation does not develop are more likely to achieve viral clearance.[68] Genetic variation before seroconversion does not correlate with outcome, indicating that quasispecies formation results from antibody-mediated immune pressure. Interestingly, no intrinsically IFN-resistant variants of HCV have been defined, indicating that both viral and host factors play important roles in determining whether the virus persists or is cleared. An increased number of quasispecies has also been associated with more rapid progression to cirrhosis and the development of HCC.[70]

EPIDEMIOLOGY

Incidence and Prevalence

The worldwide prevalence of HCV infection, based on detection of HCV RNA in serum, is estimated to be 0.7%, with more than 56 million people infected chronically.[1] The overall worldwide prevalence increased from 1990 to 2010,[61] but has been decreasing since the widespread introduction of DAAs.[1] Marked geographic variation exists, with infection rates ranging from 0.1% in the Netherlands, Fiji, and Samoa, to 0.9% in the United States, 6.3% in Egypt, and 7% in Gabon.[61] In 2002 between 3.2 and 5 million persons were infected with HCV in the United States [71]; however, these estimates were based on HCV seroprevalence (presence of anti-HCV antibody only). More recent studies between 2017 and 2020 estimate the viremic prevalence to be 2.2 million. The prevalence of HCV infection in the United States may be underestimated because the National Health and Nutrition Examination Survey data did not evaluate persons who are homeless, incarcerated, or in the military, all populations previously identified as being at higher risk for hepatitis C infection.[72] In addition, the coronavirus disease 2019 pandemic has significantly adversely affected hepatitis C testing and treatment, with precipitous decreases in the number of hepatitis C tests performed,[73,74] and a parallel decreases in the number of hepatitis C DAA prescriptions. Because the highest seroprevalence in different age groups shifted from 35 to 44 years (2.5%) to 55 to 64 years in 2005 (2.7%).[61] It had been recommended that all persons born between 1945 and 1965 be tested for anti-HCV.[75] However, because of more recent increased incidence of acute HCV infection in young adults who inject drugs (see below).[72,76] In 2020 the Centers for Disease Control and Prevention (CDC) recommended that all adults over age 18 and all pregnant women be tested for anti-HCV unless they are in a setting in which the prevalence of HCV infection is less than 0.1%.[77] The prevalence is higher in males (1.4%) than in females (0.5%), and is similar among black people (4.8%) and white people (5.0%).[72] Risk factors for HCV infection are injection drug use,[78] blood transfusion before the implementation of routine blood product screening in many countries in 1992, more than 50 lifetime sexual partners, family income below the poverty level, occupational exposure, incarceration, and being born in an endemic country.

Worldwide, three different epidemiologic patterns of HCV infection have emerged: (1) previous exposure through health care with a peak prevalence in older persons; (2) exposure through injection drug use, the major risk factor since data first became available in about 1960, with a peak prevalence among young and middle-aged persons; and (3) ongoing high levels of infection in areas where high rates of infection occur in all age groups.

Given the factors that influence viral diversity (see earlier), estimating the site of origin and age of HCV by phylogenetic analysis is difficult. The best estimate is that HCV originated in Western and sub-Saharan Africa.[79] Subsequent global spread probably occurred coincident with trade and human migration. Evolution of the virus led to a geographic distribution of genotypes, so that genotypes 1–3 are most common in North America and Europe, genotype 4 is most common in the Middle East, and genotype 6 is most common in Southeast Asia. In Japan, HCV transmission transitioned from constant to exponential growth in the 1920s, and the prevalence of HCV infection is highest in older persons.[80] In Japan, and later in Southern and Eastern Europe and Egypt, health care–related procedures, particularly reuse of contaminated syringes, played a major role in viral spread. In the United States, Australia, and other developed countries, peak prevalence is in persons 55–64 years of age,[72] and analysis of risk factors suggests that most HCV transmission occurred between the mid-1980s and the mid-1990s, through injection drug use. In Egypt, the spread of HCV increased exponentially from the 1930s to the 1980s because of mass vaccination campaigns with reuse of medical equipment.[63] In Egypt and other developing countries, high rates of infection are observed in all age groups, suggesting that an ongoing risk of HCV acquisition exists.

In the United States, there have been distinct changes in the epidemiology of acute HCV infection. The incidence of acute HCV peaked in 1989, gradually declining over the following 15 years, before stabilizing from 2006 until 2010.[81] The peak incidence was estimated to be 180,000 cases per year in the mid-1980s, but the rate declined to less than 20,000 cases by 2010.[82] Many factors have contributed to the falling incidence of acute hepatitis C. In the 1980s, when blood was purchased from donors, 2%–10% of blood units were infected with HCV, leading to a high rate of transfusion-acquired HCV infection.[83] The institution of volunteer blood donation, creation of recombinant clotting factors, and implementation of HCV blood testing (between 1990 and 1992) dramatically decreased transfusion-acquired HCV infection. However, since 2011, the incidence of acute hepatitis C has steadily increased fourfold, particularly in the 18–39-year-old age group (a 400% increase in 18–29-year-olds and 325% increase in 30–39-year-olds),[84] attributable to the opioid injection drug use epidemic.[85]

An important mechanism of transmission worldwide has been the lack of sterilization of medical instruments such as syringes. Although the incidence of HCV transmission by medical instruments has also decreased markedly, the risk has not been eliminated, even in the United States. New HCV infections in the United States and other developed countries occur primarily as a result of injection drug use.

HCV Elimination

Because of the epidemic of HCV-related liver disease complications, together with the rising incidence of HCV, and the development of highly effective well-tolerated DAAs, the WHO set ambitious targets in 2016 to eliminate hepatitis C as a global health threat by the year 2030, specifically a 90% reduction of new hepatitis C infections, 80% of HCV-positive patients treated, and a 65% reduction in mortality.[86] To achieve HCV elimination, it is imperative that efforts must be made to streamline the complex cascade of care for hepatitis C management; widespread universal screening must occur to increase case finding of hepatitis C infection and streamlined models need to be implemented to link these individuals to treatment and ultimately cure of hepatitis C. Furthermore, treatment as prevention has been shown to be important in HCV elimination as persons who have successfully achieved SVR can no longer transmit virus; even small increases in treatment among persons who inject drugs (PWID) have been shown to decrease both prevalent and incident HCV infection.[87–90]

Transmission

Modes of transmission of HCV can be divided into percutaneous (blood transfusion and needlestick inoculation) and nonpercutaneous (sexual contact and perinatal exposure). Patients are often unwilling to disclose percutaneous risk factors, and therefore apparent nonpercutaneous transmission may represent occult percutaneous exposure.

Percutaneous Transmission

Blood transfusion (before the introduction of screening) and injection drug use are the most clearly documented risk factors for HCV infection. Following the introduction of anti-HCV screening of blood donors between 1990 and 1992, the number of transfusion-related cases of HCV infection declined sharply to the point that less than 1 case occurs per 2,000,000 U transfused, virtually eliminating transmission of HCV by blood transfusion.[91] In many countries, blood products are assayed directly for HCV RNA by "mini-pool" testing, although not all developing countries implement blood product screening; therefore post-transfusion associated HCV infection remains a risk in these regions.

Injection drug use has always been the major route of HCV acquisition in the United States and accounts for the majority of newly acquired HCV cases.[84,85] The frequency of HCV infection in PWID ranges from 57% to 90%.[78,81] Although risk factors for HBV and HIV infection overlap with those for HCV infection, the prevalence of HCV infection in this population is the highest among the three viruses. The majority of PWID become anti-HCV positive within 6 months of initiating injection drug use with shared paraphernalia.

Chronic hemodialysis is also associated with increased rates of HCV infection. The frequency of anti-HCV in patients on hemodialysis ranges from less than 10% in the United States to 55%–85% in Jordan, Saudi Arabia, and Iran.[92] Serologic assays for anti-HCV may underestimate the frequency of HCV infection in this relatively immunocompromised population, and HCV RNA testing may be necessary for accurate diagnosis.[93]

Occupational transmission may occur from infected patients to health care workers. Anti-HCV seroconversion rates are approximately 0.3%–4% in longitudinal studies of health care workers after percutaneous inoculation from anti-HCV-positive sources, although the risk is dependent on the type of needle (hollow vs. solid, infusion vs. withdrawal), volume of inoculum, depth of injury, time the body fluid has spent ex vivo, level of viremia (viral load), and HIV status of the inoculating body fluid.[94–96] Although less common, transmission of HCV may also occur from health care workers to patients.[97] Because acute HCV infection is often subclinical, nosocomial transmission may occur with greater frequency than has been recognized previously. Strict adherence to universal precautions to protect health care workers and patients is critically important. No treatment has been proved effective for postexposure prophylaxis, and no data support such treatment even if it were available.

Nonpercutaneous Transmission

Nonpercutaneous modes of HCV transmission include sexual practices and childbirth. Available evidence indicates that transmission by nonpercutaneous routes occurs but is inefficient. From 10% to 20% of patients with HCV infection report that their only risk factor is sexual exposure to a partner with HCV infection. Most seroepidemiologic studies, however, have demonstrated anti-HCV in only a small proportion of sexual contacts of HCV-infected persons. In a large prospective study of monogamous seronegative partners of HCV-infected patients who denied anal intercourse and intercourse during menstruation, no instances of HCV transmission of a virus with the same gene sequence occurred over a 10-year period of time.[98] Similarly, a study in which 500 anti-HCV-positive persons and their long-term heterosexual partners were followed identified only three couples (0.6%) with concordant viral strains.[99] The calculated maximum HCV transmission rate was 1 per 190,000 sexual contacts (0.07% per year). Therefore many of the cases presumed to be the result of sexual transmission are likely the result of other, perhaps unreported or unrecognized, exposures. If the index sexual partner is infected with HIV or the partners engage in high-risk sexual practices (e.g., anal intercourse); however, the transmissibility of HCV is increased.[100]

The incidence of acute hepatitis C has been reported to have increased in HIV-infected men having sex with men in the 2000s in different regions of the world, including the United States, Australia, and Europe.[101] Permucosal risk factors, including specific sexual practices and mucosally administered drugs, have been suggested to be responsible for the increase in incidence of HCV transmission.

Compared with the high efficiency of perinatal transmission of HBV infection (see Chapter 81), the risk of perinatal transmission of HCV infection is low, averaging 5.1%–6.7% for HCV-monoinfected patients and two to three times higher for HCV-HIV-coinfected patients.[102,103] Mothers with a high serum level of HCV RNA (high viral load) are more likely to transmit HCV to their infants, a finding that may explain why infants born to mothers with HCV-HIV coinfection are at higher risk of HCV infection. The use of antiretroviral therapy (ART) in HCV-HIV-coinfected mothers may decrease the risk of perinatal transmission of both HIV and HCV.[103] Data regarding the risk associated with vaginal delivery as opposed to cesarean delivery are uncontrolled, but evidence for a higher risk of HCV transmission with vaginal delivery is unconvincing. This issue remains controversial, and some authorities recommend elective cesarean section before membrane rupture.[102]

Although little data exist, the risk of HCV transmission from breastfeeding is negligible to small. The CDC and international societies have concluded that breastfeeding by HCV-infected mothers is generally safe.[104,105] Because anti-HCV can be acquired passively by the infant, testing for HCV RNA is required if the diagnosis of HCV infection is suspected. Infants of infected mothers should not undergo serologic testing for anti-HCV before 18 months of age, because maternal antibodies may persist in the infant's serum and lead to diagnostic confusion.

Sporadic HCV Infection

The source of transmission is unknown in up to one-third of cases of HCV infection. Such sporadic HCV infection probably results from an undisclosed or unrecognized percutaneous route of infection. This presumption is supported by the observation that intranasal cocaine use is not considered a major risk factor for HCV transmission (although it was considered a risk factor in the past).[106] HCV infection can be acquired from noncommercial tattooing and body piercing when equipment is reused, shared, or improperly sterilized. Commercial tattooing is now well controlled and likely conveys little risk of HCV infection. Iatrogenic transmission of HCV is well documented in a variety of circumstances, most notably via contaminated multiuse vials and inadequately sterilized multiuse instruments and syringes, as seen with schistosomal treatment campaigns in Egypt.[107]

PATHOGENESIS

Determinants of persistence of HCV include (1) the evasion of immune responses through several viral mechanisms; (2) inadequate induction of the innate immune response; (3) insufficient induction or maintenance of an adaptive immune response; (4) the production of viral quasispecies; and (5) the induction of immunologic tolerance or exhaustion.[108,109] Chronic hepatitis develops in 50%–90% of persons with acute HCV infection. In the minority of patients in whom acute HCV resolves spontaneously, an early and multispecific T-cell response occurs.[110] This response can be detected up to 20 years after resolution of infection[111] and may contribute to protection in the case of subsequent exposures to HCV. Although the immune response is essential in preventing viral persistence, in those without viral clearance the immune response mediates hepatic cell destruction and fibrosis.

Viral Mechanisms

In chronically infected patients, the pathogenesis of liver damage is largely immune mediated. In a small subset of immunocompromised HCV-infected patients among both HIV-infected patients and organ transplant recipients, however, a syndrome termed *fibrosing cholestatic hepatitis* develops (see Chapter 99).[112,113] Such cases are thought to result from direct viral hepatotoxicity of infected cells, because viral levels are typically greater than 30 million copies/mL and hepatocytes contain enormous concentrations of virus and viral proteins.[114] Survival in such patients has been poor.

The majority of patients with HCV infection have a variable immune response that, although inadequate to eradicate acute infection, appears to regulate the vigor of persistent infection and avoid the development of fibrosing cholestatic hepatitis. The immune response to HCV is incompletely understood because animal models that recapitulate human disease and immunology are not readily available,[115] and therefore most studies in humans rely on observations in peripheral blood rather than the hepatic immune environment.

Immune-Mediated Mechanisms

HCV infection elicits an immune response in the host that involves both an initial innate response and a subsequent adaptive response. The innate response is the first line of defense against the virus and includes several arms such as natural killer (NK) cell activation and cellular antiviral mechanisms triggered by pathogen-associated molecular patterns recognized by the cell (see Chapter 2). These processes can lead to apoptosis of infected cells within the first few hours of infection. NK cells, as the effector cells of the innate immune system, also produce TNF-β and IFN-α, cytokines that are critical for dendritic cell maturation and subsequent induction of adaptive immunity. NK cells can also attack virus-infected cells directly, as do other immune cells by different effector molecules.[116] Subsequently, however, the virus initiates a number of mechanisms that undermine the ability of the host to control the infection.

Virus-related disruption of the innate, and later adaptive, immune response occurs at several levels. NK cell function is slowed possibly because NK cell–mediated cytotoxicity and production of cytokines are interrupted when the HCV E2 protein binds its cellular receptor CD81.[117] Expression of TNF-related apoptosis-inducing ligand on NK cells correlates with disease activity in both acute[118] and chronic[119] hepatitis C, thereby suggesting that NK cells have a direct role in the immunopathogenesis of hepatitis C. Pathogen-associated molecular patterns activate several cellular processes, including the JAK-STAT proteins pathway and Toll-like receptor-3, activation of both of which ultimately results in production of cellular IFNs, IFN-stimulated genes (ISGs), and IFN-regulated factors that convey antiviral properties to the cell. NS3/4 protease degrades TRIF, an essential intermediate in this pathway, and cleaves IFN promoter stimulator-1, an intermediate in the signaling cascade, to block activation of IFN when retinoic inducible gene-1 binds viral intermediates.[120] In addition, HCV core protein promotes STAT-1 degradation, inhibits STAT-1 phosphorylation, promotes suppressor of cytokine signaling induction (an inhibitor of JAK-STAT signaling), and impairs ISG factor-3, a heterotrimer of STAT-1, STAT-2, and IFN-β promoter stimulator (IRF-9) from binding to the promoter regions of IFN-stimulated response elements, thereby inhibiting transcription of IFN response genes. Even when IFN response genes are activated, NS5A and E2 both can disrupt protein kinase R function to suppress translation, thereby allowing viral replication to continue.[120] In addition, NS5A inhibits 2′−5′-oligoadenylate synthetase, which is expressed in response to HCV infection and leads to HCV RNA degradation. Taken together, HCV is able to disrupt the innate immune response at several levels, and these strategies appear to be pivotal in establishing the chronicity of infection.

The ability of HCV to impair the innate immune response prevents development of a vigorous adaptive immune response to the infection. NK cells do not adequately activate dendritic cells, and as a result, the priming of $CD8^+$ and $CD4^+$ T cells in HCV-infected patients is inadequate.[121] Even if an adequate T-cell response is created, HCV-infected patients have a large number of regulatory T cells in their portal tracts[122]; intrahepatic immune regulation by these cells has not been demonstrated but is presumed.

HCV-specific T cells are enriched at the site of viral replication, with an increased number in the liver when compared with the peripheral blood.[123] $CD8^+$ lymphocytes predominate, suggesting that cytotoxic T lymphocytes are the main perpetrators of hepatocellular injury. The T-cell immune response in the liver may result in direct lysis of infected cells and inhibition of viral replication by secreted antiviral cytokines.[108]

Whereas the cellular immune response plays a pivotal role in the pathogenesis of HCV infection, the importance of the humoral immune response is less clear. Antibodies to viral proteins are produced and do not appear to correlate with the stage of infection or immune reactivity. Furthermore, administration of high-titer HCV-enriched or HCV-specific Ig has little effect on viral levels or persistence in humans.

In summary, viral products play an integral role in the immune regulation that leads to chronic infection instead of viral clearance. Both the virus and the immune response probably play a role in the development of hepatocellular injury. The mechanisms by which hepatocellular injury leads to hepatic fibrosis are discussed in Chapter 76.

CLINICAL FEATURES

Acute Hepatitis C

HCV accounts for an estimated 20% of cases of acute hepatitis. Acute hepatitis C is rarely seen in clinical practice, however, because nearly all cases are asymptomatic. Within 7−21 days after viral transmission, HCV RNA becomes detectable in serum.[124] Longer incubation periods can occur, especially in cases in which only a small amount of virus has been transmitted. These data suggest that the duration of the incubation period may vary among different transmission routes. HCV RNA levels rise rapidly in serum after infection, followed by a delayed increase in serum ALT levels 4−12 weeks after infection, indicative of hepatic injury. Serum ALT levels frequently reach values more than 10 times the upper limit of normal, with concomitant rises in the serum bilirubin level in some individuals (Fig. 82.3).[125] Some patients also develop clinical symptoms 2−12 weeks after viral transmission, but the majority of patients remain asymptomatic during the acute phase and most infected persons do not become aware of their disease. Therefore it is not easy to study the early phase of HCV infection. Several studies have investigated patients recruited during the acute symptomatic phase of HCV infection, and 80% of the patients have presented with diverse symptoms.[126] Even in symptomatic patients, however, most of the clinical symptoms are nonspecific. Commonly reported symptoms include fatigue, nausea, abdominal pain, loss of appetite, mild fever, itching, and myalgia. Jaundice, which is the most specific liver-related symptom, develops in 50%−84% of patients with clinically overt acute HCV infection. ALF caused by HCV has been reported in only single cases, in contrast to infections with other hepatotropic viruses (see Chapter 97). The presentation may be more apparent and the clinical course more severe when acute HCV infection occurs in patients who drink large amounts of alcohol or have coinfection with HBV or HIV.

The rate of viral persistence after acute infection ranges from 45% to more than 90%. Age and gender clearly influence the risk of chronicity, with younger and female patients having the lowest rates of chronicity. Other factors that may play a role include the source of infection and size of inoculum (chronicity may be less common in PWID than in those who acquire HCV infection by blood transfusion), immune status of the host (chronicity rates are higher in persons with immunodeficiency states such as agammaglobulinemia and HIV infection), and the patient's race (rates of viral persistence are higher in blacks than in whites and Hispanic Americans in the United States).[127] Finally, the rate of spontaneous clearance is higher in symptomatic patients in whom jaundice develops during acute infection than in those who remain asymptomatic.[128]

Single-nucleotide polymorphisms (SNPs) close to the IFN lambda-3, or interleukin 28B, gene (*IFN-λ3, IL28B*) have been found to be associated with the outcome of acute hepatitis C. The *IFN-λ3* gene is located on chromosome 19 and encodes IFN-λ3. Ge et al. reported a significant role for a specific SNP in the *IFN-λ3* gene region (rs12979860 CC) in the response to pegylated IFN-α–based therapy for chronic hepatitis C in 2009.[129] Shortly

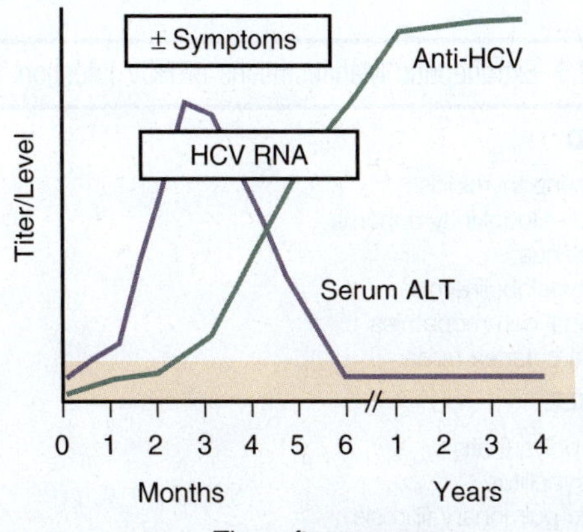

Fig. 82.3 Typical course of acute HCV infection followed by recovery. Symptoms may or may not be present during acute infection. *Anti-HCV*, Antibody to HCV. (Modified from the Centers for Disease Control and Prevention. www.cdc.gov/hepatitis/Resources/Professionals/Training/Serology/training.htm#one.)

thereafter, Thomas et al. identified a major contribution for the same SNP in spontaneous clearance of acute HCV infection.[130] Subsequently, these findings were confirmed by other investigators in different cohorts.[128,131] An association between clearance of acute HCV infection and the *IFN-λ3* genotype may differ, however, between symptomatic and asymptomatic patients, because the CC *IFN-λ3* polymorphism was associated with spontaneous recovery only in nonicteric patients in a cohort of East German women exposed to HCV in a single-source outbreak in the late 1970s.[128]

Chronic Hepatitis C

Serum ALT levels are usually elevated in patients with chronic HCV infection. Because levels commonly fluctuate, however, as many as half of patients may have a normal ALT level at any given time.[132] The ALT level may remain normal for prolonged periods of time in about 20% of cases, although transient elevations occur even in these cases.[132] Persistently normal ALT levels are more common in women, and such cases typically are associated with lower serum HCV RNA levels and less inflammation and fibrosis on liver biopsy specimens.

Most patients with chronic hepatitis C are asymptomatic before the onset of advanced hepatic fibrosis. Patients who have been diagnosed with chronic infection, however, often complain of nonspecific symptoms such as fatigue, vague abdominal pain, or depression, and they consistently score lower than HCV-negative persons in all aspects of health-related quality of life (HRQOL).[133] Whether the decrease in HRQOL is related to viral factors, social factors (e.g., injection drug use), social stigmatization, or worry related to the diagnosis itself is unclear. Nevertheless, HRQOL scores improve if the patient achieves a sustained response to antiviral therapy. Less common symptoms may include arthralgias, paresthesias, myalgias, sicca syndrome, nausea, anorexia, and difficulty with concentration. The severity of these symptoms may be, but is not necessarily, related to the severity of the underlying liver disease.

Extrahepatic Manifestations

Patients with HCV infection may present with extrahepatic conditions, or these manifestations may occur in patients known to have chronic HCV infection. Classification of the extrahepatic manifestations of HCV is shown in Box 82.1 and is based on the strength of available data to prove a correlation. Types 2 and 3 cryoglobulinemia, characterized by polyclonal IgG plus monoclonal IgM and polyclonal IgG plus polyclonal IgM, respectively, can both be caused by HCV infection. Among HCV-infected patients, 19%–50% have cryoglobulins in serum, but clinical manifestations of cryoglobulinemia are reported in only 5%–10% of these patients and are more common in patients with cirrhosis. Symptoms and signs include fatigue, arthralgias, arthritis, purpura, Raynaud phenomenon, vasculitis, peripheral neuropathy, and nephropathy. The diagnosis is clear when a rheumatoid factor is detected, cryoglobulins are present, and complement levels are low in serum; however, the reliability of cryoglobulin measurements is dependent on proper handling and processing of the sample.[134]

BOX 82.1 Extrahepatic Manifestations of HCV Infection

PROVED

Autoimmune thyroiditis
B-cell non-Hodgkin lymphoma
Lichen planus
Mixed cryoglobulinemia
Monoclonal gammopathies
Porphyria cutanea tarda

POSSIBLE

Chronic polyarthritis
Diabetes mellitus
Idiopathic pulmonary fibrosis
Noncryoglobulinemic nephropathies
Sicca syndrome
Thyroid cancer
Renal cell carcinoma
Vitiligo

Glomerular disease generally manifests as cryoglobulinemic nephropathy, membranoproliferative glomerulonephritis, and membranous nephropathy. Cryoglobulinemic nephropathy manifests as hematuria, proteinuria, edema, and renal insufficiency of varying degrees and features of membranoproliferative glomerulonephritis on renal biopsy specimens. At diagnosis, 20% of patients with type 2 cryoglobulinemia have renal involvement, and renal involvement develops in another 35%–60% over time. In about 15% of patients, cryoglobulinemic nephropathy progresses to end-stage kidney disease requiring dialysis.

As HCV infection drives these extrahepatic manifestations, treatment of the underlying HCV infection should be considered in patients with symptomatic cryoglobulinemia. There are increasing data regarding the use of IFN-free DAA regimens to treat extrahepatic manifestations of HCV, particularly cryoglobulinemia.[135,136] Overall, SVR12 rates in real-world studies of these individuals with extrahepatic manifestations are comparable, ranging from 74% to 100%. Clinical response of the extrahepatic manifestations to DAA therapy were observed in over 80% of patients, with partial clinical response in 20% and complete clinical response in 60%.[135] In addition to antiviral therapy for HCV infection, monoclonal antibody therapy targeting B cells (anti-CD20 therapy with rituximab) has been shown to be useful for HCV-related cryoglobulinemia, particularly in patients with severe renal disease, because rituximab reduces B-cell clones that are responsible for producing cyroglobulins.[137,138] Although this approach has been shown to be effective in randomized controlled studies when used alone or in combination with DAAs, rituximab is not licensed for treatment of extrahepatic manifestations of HCV. Prednisone, cyclophosphamide, other chemotherapeutic agents, and plasmapheresis have been used with variable success; however, these approaches do not treat the underlying HCV infection.

Patients with vasculitis due to HCV infection may benefit from low-dose interleukin-2 therapy. This cytokine may promote the survival of immunosuppressive regulatory T cells.[139]

HCV infection is associated with the development of B-cell non-Hodgkin lymphoma and monoclonal gammopathy of uncertain significance.[140] The relative risk of lymphoma is small (1.28) in the United States,[141] but the relative risk may be higher in regions where the HCV prevalence is higher; a large meta-analysis of 9038 cases and 12,224 controls demonstrated an overall relative risk estimation of 2.3.[142] The most prevalent forms of lymphoma found in patients infected with HCV are follicular lymphoma, chronic lymphocytic lymphoma, lymphoplasmacytic lymphoma, and marginal zone lymphoma.[140] Type 2 cryoglobulinemia evolves into lymphoma over time in 8%–10% of patients. Despite the known association of HCV infection with lymphoma, HCV RNA does not integrate into the host genome and therefore HCV cannot be considered a typical oncogenic virus. Rather, HCV shows lymphotropism and may facilitate the development and selection of abnormal B-cell clones by chronic stimulation of the immune system. In addition, genetic rearrangements in B cells, specifically the Bcl2/J_H rearrangement and the t(14;18) translocation, have been found in HCV-infected patients in some,[143] but not all,[144] studies.

Other extrahepatic manifestations of HCV infection include porphyria cutanea tarda, lichen planus, and sicca syndrome. In addition, insulin resistance and diabetes mellitus have been thought to be associated with HCV infection, although the association has been questioned.[145] Although associations between HCV infection and both thyroid cancer and idiopathic pulmonary fibrosis have been described, data about the effect of HCV eradication on disease progression are lacking. A myriad of other conditions has been observed in association with HCV infection, but a true link has not been firmly established for these disorders (see Box 82.1).

Although not associated with disease, seropositivity for autoantibodies (e.g., ANA with a titer greater than 1:40 in 9%, smooth muscle antibodies with a titer greater than 1:40 in 20%, antiliver–kidney microsomal antibodies in 6%) is found in many HCV-infected persons.[146] Therefore the diagnosis of an autoimmune condition in a patient with HCV infection can never be based on serology alone.

The spectrum of extrahepatic manifestations may adversely impact the overall survival of HCV-infected persons. The prospective Taiwanese population-based R.E.V.E.A.L.-HCV (Risk Evaluation of Viral Load Elevation and Associated Liver Disease/Cancer) study, in which almost 24,000 adults 30–65 years of age were followed, demonstrated that HCV-infected persons had not only increased liver-related mortality, but also higher mortality from extrahepatic diseases compared with anti-HCV–negative persons.[147]

DIAGNOSIS

Several immunologic and molecular assays are used to detect and monitor HCV infection. The presence of anti-HCV in high titer in serum [generally an enzyme immunoassay (EIA) ratio >9] indicates exposure to the virus but does not differentiate among acute, chronic, and resolved infection. Anti-HCV usually persists for many years in patients after spontaneous resolution of infection or an SVR following antiviral therapy. Anti-HCV titers may decline over time, however, and can become undetectable 5–20 years after HCV clearance.[111,148] Serologic assays are used initially for diagnosis, whereas virologic nucleic acid assays are required for confirming current active infection, monitoring response to treatment, and evaluating immunocompromised patients.

Indirect Assays

EIAs detect antibodies against different HCV antigens. The time course of the development of symptoms, detection of anti-HCV, and appearance of HCV RNA after acute infection is shown in Fig. 82.3. Three generations of EIAs have been developed. The third-generation EIAs detect antibodies against HCV core, NS3, NS4, and NS5 antigens as early as 7–8 weeks after infection, with sensitivity and specificity rates of 99%.[149] Despite ongoing viral replication, serologic test results can be negative in patients who are on hemodialysis or are immunocompromised. Because the performance characteristics of third-generation EIAs are so good, confirmation with a recombinant immunoblot assay is no longer required. Instead, patients who are anti-HCV positive should undergo HCV RNA testing to determine if they have active viremia or have cleared the infection.

Direct Assays

Quantitative, highly sensitive, "real-time" HCV RNA tests represent the state of the art for determining HCV viremia in anti-HCV-positive persons.[150] The lower limit of detection of most assays varies from 10 to 15 IU/mL.[151] These assays have a linear dynamic range of 1–7 $\log_{10}$ IU/mL and are the preferred testing method in practice. Transcription-mediated amplification is also extremely sensitive, but available assays are not quantitative in the lower dynamic range of the test. The advantages of these very sensitive tests include positivity within 1–3 weeks after acute infection and detection of low-level residual infection during antiviral therapy.

A disadvantage of all quantitative tests is the lack of comparability among different assays. Although conversion to a standard IU/mL concentration attempted to resolve such discrepancies, results are still variable. Reported conversion factors vary from 0.9 to 5.2 copies/mL per IU/mL. For this reason, the same laboratory and assay are recommended during antiviral treatment monitoring.

A cheaper and faster alternative to nucleic acid testing for HCV RNA to confirm HCV viremia is the HCV core antigen assay. Fully automated immunoassays have been developed that detect the HCV core antigen, and the assays have proved to be robust across HCV genotypes and in different patient populations,[152,153] but with major limitations in sensitivity. Therefore the assay cannot be used to monitor response to antiviral therapy and make decisions regarding therapy. If viremia needs just to be confirmed, however, HCV core antigen testing is a reasonable alternative to HCV RNA testing.

Point-of-Care Hepatitis C Testing

More recently a number of point-of-care (POC) tests have become available to rapidly screen individuals for anti-HCV antibodies and HCV RNA from fingerstick, oral and/or dried blood spot samples. Depending on the type of test and technology, results may be available within 1–15 (hepatitis C antibody POC tests) to 60 minutes (hepatitis C nucleic acid POC tests), thereby allowing for rapid hepatitis C diagnosis and linkage to hepatitis C treatment.[154] Such technology is likely to be important for global hepatitis C elimination efforts.

HCV Genotype

Identifying the genotype and subtype of HCV is important because some DAA regimens are only recommended for certain HCV genotypes and subtypes. HCV genotyping can be accomplished by several methods. The most accurate approach uses PCR methodology and direct sequencing of the NS5B or E1 region; however, this approach is not practical in clinical practice. HCV genotyping can be performed by evaluating type-specific antibodies and has a 90% concordance in immunocompetent patients when results are compared with sequence analysis of the HCV genome. Testing can also be accomplished with reverse hybridization to genotype-specific probes, restriction fragment length polymorphism analysis, or PCR amplification of the 5′ noncoding region of the HCV genome. These tests have 92%–96% concordance with the correct genotype; genotype 1 is identified with the highest accuracy. Because of mutations in the regions studied, errors in subtype identification occur in 10%–25% of cases regardless of the technique used. A line-probe assay (INNO-LiPA) using genotype-specific probes for reverse transcription of the 5′ portion of the HCV genome is the most popular commercial assay for HCV genotyping.

Selection of Serologic and Virologic Tests

For patients at low risk for HCV infection, a negative result of an EIA for anti-HCV is sufficient to exclude HCV infection. HCV RNA testing should be performed to confirm active infection if a positive anti-HCV test is returned. In high-risk patients, such as those with an elevated serum ALT level who have a known risk factor for HCV, have experienced recent exposure, or are either immunocompromised or on dialysis, a positive anti-HCV result is sufficient to confirm HCV infection; however, HCV RNA testing should also be performed to confirm that the infection is active. If the anti-HCV result is negative, then HCV RNA testing should be performed in patients with a recent exposure in case the anti-HCV result is falsely negative because of insufficient time for anti-HCV to develop or immunocompromise in the host with failure to produce sufficient anti-HCV.[105]

LIVER BIOPSY AND NONINVASIVE ASSESSMENT OF FIBROSIS

The risk of progressive hepatic injury from HCV infection varies considerably, with some patients showing little or no progression after decades of infection and others progressing rapidly to cirrhosis.[155] The presence or absence of cirrhosis also influences the choice and duration of treatment; therefore an assessment of the degree of liver injury is recommended in all patients with HCV infection. For many years, this assessment was performed by percutaneous liver biopsy (Box 82.2), but noninvasive methods are now used for initial assessment of liver fibrosis stage, with liver biopsy reserved when noninvasive markers are indeterminate, noninvasive test results are incongruent with other noninvasive liver fibrosis markers or with the clinical picture, or other causes of liver disease need to be excluded.

Several histologic scoring systems have been used to quantify hepatic injury into discrete grades of inflammation and stages of fibrosis (Fig. 82.4) (see also Chapters 75 and 76). The first system used was the Histology Activity Index described by Knodell et al. The components of this system include periportal inflammation and necrosis (graded as 0–10), lobular inflammation and necrosis (0–4), portal inflammation (0–4), and fibrosis (0–4). This scoring system combines inflammation and fibrosis into one score. Scheuer created a simplified scoring system that separates grade of inflammation from stage of fibrosis: portal inflammation and interface hepatitis (0–4), lobular activity (0–4), and fibrosis stage (0–4). The Ishak system is a modification of Knodell's system but separates histologic grade from fibrosis stage. Ishak fibrosis scores range from 0 to 6 (1 or 2, portal fibrotic expansion; 3 or 4, bridging fibrosis; and 5 or 6, cirrhosis) (see Fig. 82.4). The higher number of stages of fibrosis has made the Ishak system popular for scoring progression of fibrosis in clinical trials. The METAVIR scoring system is the most popular in practice; it is simpler than all the aforementioned systems. Inflammation is graded from 0 to 4 (none, mild, moderate, and severe) and fibrosis is staged from 0 to 4 [(1) portal fibrotic expansion, (2) portal fibrosis with septa formation, (3) bridging fibrosis, and (4) cirrhosis) (see Fig. 82.4).

BOX 82.2 Reasons to Perform a Liver Biopsy in a Patient with Hepatitis C

- Assessment of the need for surveillance for HCC
- Evaluation for concomitant liver diseases
- Guidance for decisions regarding treatment of hepatitis C
- Staging of fibrosis, including when noninvasive fibrosis markers are incongruent with other methods of noninvasive fibrosis assessment or with the clinical picture

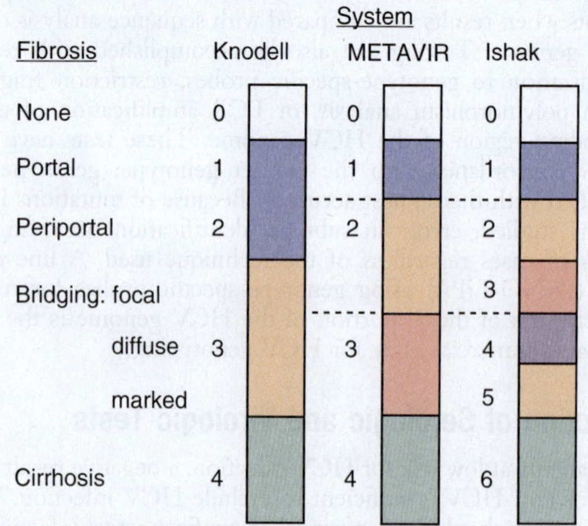

Fig. 82.4 Comparison of the Knodell, METAVIR, and Ishak hepatic fibrosis staging systems. The METAVIR staging system is similar to the Scheuer system. Portal, periportal, bridging, and cirrhosis describe the degree (stage) of fibrosis (see also Fig. 82.5).

Although examination of liver biopsy specimens is still considered the gold standard for establishing the grade of inflammation and stage of fibrosis, limitations of liver biopsy include (1) associated morbidity (pain occurs in as many as 30% in some series, and hemorrhage or bile leak occurs in 0.3% of patients) and mortality (0.03%); (2) cost; (3) poor patient acceptance; (4) intraobserver and interobserver variability in the interpretation of findings (with current scoring systems, intraobserver and interobserver concordance for staging fibrosis among hepatopathologists is ≈90% and 85%, respectively); (5) inaccuracy in the interpretation of findings, particularly for the diagnosis of cirrhosis (with a false-negative rate of 15%); and (6) sampling error (a 33% difference in one stage of fibrosis and 2.4% difference in two stages of fibrosis is seen in simultaneously obtained biopsy specimens from the right and left hepatic lobes).[156,157] Interobserver and intraobserver variability is increased when inexperienced pathologists use a complicated scoring system to evaluate liver tissue. Sampling error is especially common when small biopsy specimens are obtained. A biopsy should be done with at least a 16-ga needle, be 15–20 mm or more in length, and contain at least 6 portal triads, although 11 or greater is considered optimal.[158,159]

Because of the limitations of liver biopsy, several noninvasive tests to estimate fibrosis have been developed (Table 82.1) (see also Chapter 76). FibroSure (or FibroTest) is a noninvasive measure of fibrosis that creates a composite score, adjusted for gender and age, derived from the serum levels of α_2-macroglobulin, haptoglobin, apolipoprotein A-1, GGTP, and total bilirubin.[157] The test accurately categorizes patients with stage 0 and 1 fibrosis and those with cirrhosis; however, it is less useful in patients with intermediate scores. The AST-to-platelet ratio index (APRI) is used primarily to diagnose or exclude cirrhosis.[160] In an initial evaluation, 81% of cirrhotic patients were accurately excluded with an APRI score of 0.5 or less; however, the index does not discriminate among lower levels of fibrosis. The APRI score may be more useful to exclude cirrhosis; an APRI score of <1.0 has a high negative predictive (98%) value for cirrhosis.[160]

Additional techniques and instruments (e.g., transient elastography, acoustic radiation force impulse imaging, and magnetic resonance elastography) are now available to determine liver stiffness (see Chapter 76). The most frequently used system is transient elastography (FibroScan) to assess liver stiffness, which correlates with the amount of hepatic fibrosis. In a meta-analysis, the area under the receiver operating curve (an estimate of accuracy) of FibroScan for predicting cirrhosis was 0.94.[161] Combining transient elastography with serum markers increases the accuracy of predicting fibrosis and cirrhosis and may avoid liver biopsy in many patients.[162,163] Although noninvasive testing has improved dramatically, all available tests have limitations. Most importantly, the degree of hepatic inflammation is not assessed by these tests, and inflammation may significantly alter

TABLE 82.1 Performance of Noninvasive Tests for Predicting Hepatic Fibrosis in Patients With Hepatitis C

Test	Number of Patients Studied	Fibrosis Staging System	Histologic Fibrosis (F) Stages Compared	Sensitivity (%)[a]	Specificity (%)[a]	PPV for Fibrosis-Cirrhosis (%)	Test Accuracy (%)[b]
APRI	270	Ishak	F0-2 vs. F3-6	41	95	88	70
			F0-4 vs. F5-6	89	75	57	77
FibroSure	339	METAVIR	F0-1 vs. F2-4	100	22	50	57
			F0-2 vs. F3-4	70	95	91	84
Transient elastography (FibroScan)	327	METAVIR	F0-1 vs. F2-4	56	91	88	68
			F0-3 vs. F4	86	96	78	94

[a]Sensitivity and specificity for distinguishing higher stages of fibrosis from lower stages of fibrosis.

[b]Accuracy = (sensitivity) (prevalence) + (specificity) (1 − prevalence).

APRI, AST-to-platelets ratio index; *PPV*, positive predictive value.

Data from Wai CT, Greinson JT, Fontana RJ, et al. A simple noninvasive index can predict both significant fibrosis and cirrhosis in patients with chronic hepatitis C. *Hepatology*. 2003;38:518–526; Imbert-Bismut F, Ratziu V, Pieroni L, et al. Biochemical markers of liver fibrosis in patients with hepatitis C virus infection: a prospective study. *Lancet*. 2001;357:1069–1075; Ziol M, Handra-Luca A, Kettaneh A, et al. Noninvasive assessment of liver fibrosis by measurement of stiffness in patients with chronic hepatitis C. *Hepatology*. 2005;41:48–54.

noninvasive test results. Moreover, although cirrhosis is accurately predicted by several noninvasive tests, the finer discrimination of the fibrosis score is not as reliable as examination of liver biopsy specimens.

Regardless of the degree of serum aminotransferase elevations, a determination of the stage of liver fibrosis, either by liver biopsy or noninvasive methods, is recommended in patients undergoing initial assessment of chronic hepatitis C. Liver biopsy is not required when cirrhosis is already suggested by clinical findings (e.g., ascites, splenomegaly, spider telangiectasias, low platelet count, and prolonged prothrombin time) or imaging (e.g., nodularity of the liver, evidence of portal hypertension). It is also not indicated following successful antiviral therapy, although histology generally improves significantly over time following eradication of HCV (see later). Surveillance for HCC and varices is recommended for all patients with cirrhosis, including patients who achieve an SVR12 with antiviral therapy, because these patients remain at increased risk (see Chapters 94 and 98).[164]

NATURAL HISTORY

Once chronic HCV infection is established, spontaneous HCV clearance rarely occurs. Chronic hepatitis C can cause continuous liver damage, resulting in liver cirrhosis and subsequently HCC (Fig. 82.5). The individual course of liver disease is highly variable. Patients may report symptoms such as RUQ discomfort, nausea, fatigue, myalgia, arthralgias, or weight loss. All of these clinical features are nonspecific, however, and are not associated with the severity of liver injury. Most liver-related symptoms are restricted to patients with advanced cirrhosis.

The most feared complication of chronic HCV infection is liver-related mortality due to decompensated liver cirrhosis (see Chapters 76 and 94–96) or development of HCC (see Chapter 98). Studies published since the 1990s have shown remarkably different frequency rates of cirrhosis. Whereas very low rates of cirrhosis were reported in some cohorts like young women infected in the late 1970s through receipt of contaminated anti-D immune globulin,[165] cirrhosis has been described in up to 69% of patients in hospital-based settings.[166] In a meta-analysis, Thein et al. calculated that in a large number of studies that have been published, cirrhosis developed on average in 16% of patients within 20 years after the onset of HCV infection.[167] Cirrhosis was attributable to HCV infection in 27% of cases, with a wide range among studies (14%–62%) that can be explained by regional differences and the presence of cofactors.[127,168]

A key challenge in clinical practice is to identify persons at high risk for disease progression who may require more

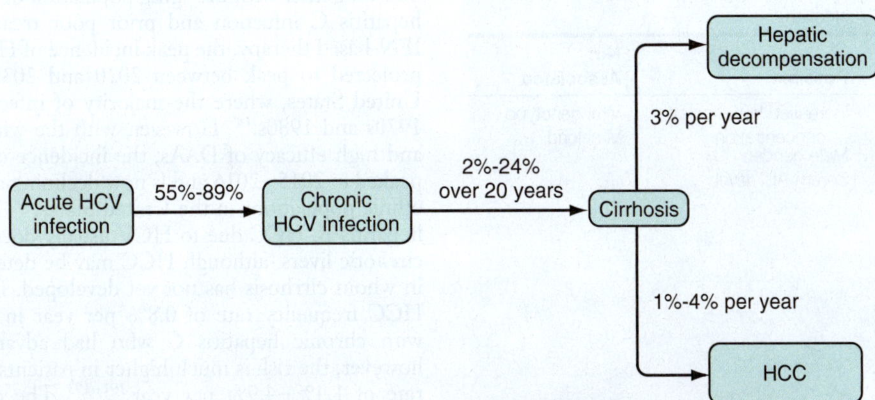

Fig. 82.5 Natural history of HCV infection. Hepatic decompensation includes ascites, hepatic encephalopathy, variceal hemorrhage, hepatorenal syndrome, or hepatic synthetic dysfunction.

immediate antiviral therapy. Several factors reported to influence the liver-related outcomes of chronic hepatitis C remain controversial (Table 82.2; see next section). Still, some of these factors may help estimate the risk of cirrhosis and identify groups of patients who require immediate antiviral treatment.

Factors Associated with Progression

Age is one of the most important risk factors for fibrosis progression in chronic HCV infection (see Table 82.2). A longer duration of infection has also been associated with a higher stage of liver fibrosis, but HCV infection acquired during childhood seems to follow a milder course.[169] Overall, the development of HCV-related cirrhosis seems to be a dynamic process that accelerates exponentially with increasing age. The mechanisms by which progression of fibrosis accelerates with aging are not well defined. Changes in the regenerative capacity of the liver, alterations in the immune system, and telomere shortening may play roles. A higher risk for fibrosis progression in patients older than 40 years has been described in patients with various causes of liver disease.[170] Some studies, but not others, have suggested that older age in general, and more specifically older age at the time of infection, is a risk factor for progression of fibrosis.[171–173] Overall, cirrhosis has been predicted to develop in most patients with hepatitis C by about 65 years of age, irrespective of the age at infection.[174]

Some studies have suggested that the mode of viral transmission may influence the degree of liver damage; however, the role of the route of transmission in fibrosis progression remains controversial. By contrast, female gender seems to be protective, and fibrosis progression is much faster in HCV-infected men, thereby suggesting that hormonal factors may be important in the regulation of liver fibrosis.[175] Genetic factors also play a role in the development of cirrhosis. Histologic activity and the frequency of cirrhosis are lower in African Americans than in Caucasians.[176] Several specific genes have been suggested to be involved in fibrosis progression; these include certain variants of the HLA class I and II antigens.[177] A cirrhosis risk score based on polymorphisms in seven genes has been proposed for patients with HCV infection[178]; this score was able to predict fibrosis progression in patients with initially mild chronic hepatitis C.[179]

Elevated serum aminotransferase levels are used widely as a surrogate for ongoing intrahepatic inflammation, and elevated serum ALT levels during chronic hepatitis C are associated with an increased risk of liver fibrosis progression.[180] Lower progression rates of fibrosis are reported in patients with normal serum ALT levels, but normal levels do not exclude the possibility of fibrosis progression.[132]

TABLE 82.2 Factors Associated With Progression of Hepatic Fibrosis in Patients With Chronic HCV Infection

Established	Possible	Not Associated
Age >40 years	Increased hepatic iron concentration	Viral genotype
Alcohol consumption	Male gender	Viral load
HBV coinfection	Serum ALT level	
HIV coinfection		
Immunosuppressed state		
Insulin resistance		
Marijuana use		
Obesity		
Schistosomiasis		
Severe hepatic necroinflammation		
Smoking		
White race		

Differences in the natural history of hepatitis C have been reported for different HCV genotypes. Several studies have described accelerated disease progression in patients infected with HCV genotype 3,[66] which is consistent with higher reported mortality rates in patients infected with HCV genotype 3.[181] Flares of hepatitis seem to occur more frequently in HCV genotype 2 infection and may result in a more severe course of liver disease.[182] By contrast, viral load is not related to the degree of liver damage or fibrosis.[183]

Hepatic steatosis is a histologic hallmark of chronic hepatitis C. Several studies have shown that steatosis is linked to the stage of liver fibrosis in patients with chronic HCV infection.[66] Some studies suggest that HCV infection itself can trigger hepatic steatosis as well as NASH, and HCV infection may cause insulin resistance. There is also evidence for a direct association between HCV infection and hepatic steatosis. The strongest association exists between HCV genotype 3 infection and steatosis, and a direct molecular effect has been shown in a mouse model in which HCV genotype 3 is expressed.[184]

Mild to moderately increased hepatic iron stores are associated with more advanced liver fibrosis. A consistent relationship between C282Y and H63D heterozygosity (see Chapter 77) and increased progression of fibrosis in patients with HCV infection has not been established, however. A reduction in hepatic iron concentrations does not reduce the risk of progression of fibrosis or improve the response to antiviral treatment.[185]

Excessive alcohol consumption is clearly an independent major cause of cirrhosis, and chronic alcohol intake of more than 50 g/day is associated with a remarkable increase in the risk of cirrhosis in HCV-infected patients. On the other hand, coffee consumption has been reported to have a beneficial effect on overall mortality from HCV infection in population-based studies, and drinking coffee has been associated with a more favorable course of liver disease in general.[186] Freedman et al. have also shown that greater coffee consumption correlates with a lower stage of liver fibrosis, reduced fibrosis progression, less steatosis and insulin resistance, and lower serum ALT levels; the best outcomes occur in persons who drink 3 or more cups per day.[186,187]

HCC

The incidence of HCC has been rising rapidly in the industrial countries since the 1980s (see Chapter 98). In the United States, the incidence of HCC is three times higher than in 1975,[188] and the global HCV epidemic has contributed to the rising incidence of HCC worldwide. Overall, chronic hepatitis C is responsible for approximately 25% of cases of HCC worldwide, with particularly high prevalence rates in East Asia.[80] The development of HCC in HCV-infected patients is an indolent and age-dependent process. This, together with the aging population of individuals living with hepatitis C infection and prior poor treatment responses with IFN-based therapy, the peak incidence of HCV-related HCC was projected to peak between 2020 and 2030 in Europe and the United States, where the majority of infections occurred in the 1970s and 1980s.[189] However, with the widespread introduction and high efficacy of DAAs, the incidence of HCV-related HCC peaked in 2015–2016 and is now declining among most racial and ethnic populations in the United States.[190] In contrast to chronic hepatitis B, HCC due to HCV usually does not develop in noncirrhotic livers, although HCC may be detected in some patients in whom cirrhosis has not yet developed. Lok et al. reported an HCC frequency rate of 0.8% per year in noncirrhotic patients with chronic hepatitis C who had advanced liver fibrosis[191]; however, the risk is much higher in patients with cirrhosis, with a rate of 1.4%–4.9% per year.[191–193] The overall 5-year risk of HCC has been reported to be as high as 7%–30% in patients with HCV-related cirrhosis.[194,195] The appearance of HCC is frequently the first clinical complication of HCV-related cirrhosis and often occurs before hepatic decompensation becomes evident. However, successful hepatitis C eradication with DAAs significantly reduces the risk of HCC by over 70% compared to nonresponders in large cohorts form the United States.[196,197] In Europe, the cumulative incidence rate of HCC at 1 year was 2.6% in those who achieved an SVR compared to 8% in those who did not achieve an SVR, with failure to achieve SVR identified as an independent risk factor for HCC.[198]

Risk factors for the development of HCC in patients with chronic HCV infection are similar to those associated with the development of cirrhosis. For example, older age is related to a higher frequency of HCC, and male gender and substantial alcohol consumption are well-established risk factors. Moreover, type 2 diabetes mellitus has been identified as an important independent risk factor.[199,200] Coinfection with HBV increases the risk of HCC. Importantly, the various risk factors act synergistically to enhance the overall risk of HCC. Genetic factors also contribute to the development of HCC. Kumar et al. performed a genome-wide association study in 721 persons with HCV-related HCC and showed that a SNP (rs2596542) at the gene encoding MICA (major histocompatibility class I polypeptide-related sequence A) was strongly associated with the development of HCC in HCV-infected persons.[201] Conversely, coffee consumption has been associated with a reduced risk of HCC.[202]

TREATMENT

IFN-α monotherapy was approved for the treatment of chronic hepatitis C, then known as *non-A, non-B hepatitis*, before HCV was even identified. Substantial advances in treatment have been made since then with the introduction of prolonged treatment periods, longer acting pegylated formulations of IFN, the oral guanosine analog RBV, and, most recently, the DAAs. The development of the replicon system and crystallization of the HCV nonstructural proteins (see earlier) paved the way for characterization of the HCV life cycle, generation of high throughput models for drug development, and, ultimately, the development of DAAs.[41,203–206] In 2011 the first DAAs, telaprevir and boceprevir, were approved for the treatment of chronic HCV genotype 1 infection, and in 2013, simeprevir (another protease inhibitor) and sofosbuvir (a first-in-class nucleotide polymerase inhibitor) were approved, all initially used in combination with PegIFN and RBV. The development of highly potent, well-tolerated IFN-free all oral DAA regimens, many of which have been approved by the FDA, has resulted in a complete shift in the treatment paradigm of hepatitis C. Treatment has been evolving since the first introduction of DAAs, and the choice of agents has changed from being highly individualized, based on the availability of DAAs, HCV genotype, stage of liver disease, and presence or absence of baseline RAS, to a choice of a two FDC regimens that are applicable to all patients.

Goals

The primary goal of therapy for HCV infection is eradication of the virus. A consequence of achieving this goal is prevention of liver-related deaths associated with the development of decompensated cirrhosis and HCC. SVR—the absence of detectable virus in blood 12 weeks after completion of therapy—is an excellent surrogate marker for the resolution of HCV infection. Late relapses are rare. Long-term follow-up studies confirm sustained responses in more than 99% of cases if the patient is HCV RNA negative in serum 12 weeks after completion of DAA therapy.[7–10] SVR is also associated with a reduction in hepatic

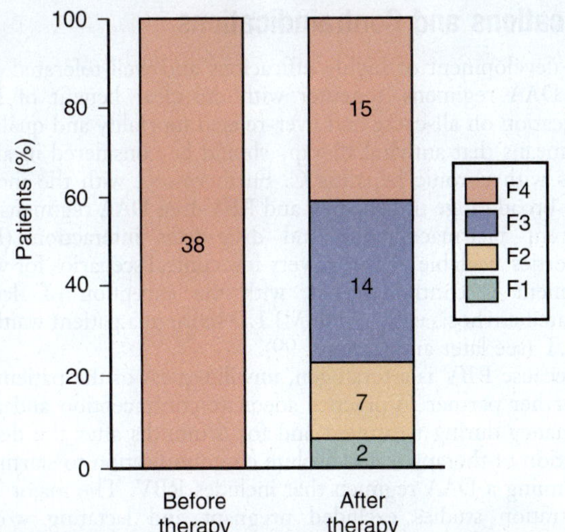

Fig. 82.6 Reversal of cirrhosis in 38 patients with chronic hepatitis C who achieved a sustained virologic response to antiviral therapy. F1 to F4 indicate stages of fibrosis, with F4 being cirrhosis. (Redrawn from D'Ambrosio R, Aghemo A, Rumi MG, et al. A morphometric and immunohistochemical study to assess the benefit of a sustained virological response in hepatitis C virus patients with cirrhosis. *Hepatology*. 2012;56:532–543.)

inflammation and regression of fibrosis during IFN plus RBV therapy (Fig. 82.6).[207,208] Moreover, an improvement in HRQOL has been documented in patients successfully treated with IFN plus RBV.[209,210] Data regarding these endpoints during DAA therapy are limited owing to the more recent implementation of DAAs, lack of longer term follow-up studies, and the more widespread use of noninvasive fibrosis testing to evaluate fibrosis rather than liver biopsy. However, a number of studies have evaluated changes in elastography fibrosis scores and other noninvasive scores of fibrosis (such as FIB-4 and APRI) 6–18 months following DAA therapy.[211] All studies showed an overall improvement in liver fibrosis following successful DAA therapy using these noninvasive scoring systems, although it is unclear if this represents true regression of fibrosis or resolution of hepatic inflammation.[212,213] In addition, the proportion of patients with noninvasive fibrosis scores consistent with cirrhosis reduced during follow-up. Two studies have evaluated liver histology at 6 months following DAA therapy in small cohorts of patients.[214,215] In one study, although inflammation significantly improved, overall, fibrosis stage did not change significantly, with improvement seen in 25%, no change in 55% and worsening fibrosis in 20% at 41 weeks following successful viral eradication with DAAs.[214] Conversely, in a second small study of patients with advanced fibrosis who achieved SVR, METAVIR fibrosis scores improved in 61.9% of patients, with no change in 23.8% and progression in 14.3% of patients.[215]

Antiviral treatment prevents the development of clinical endpoints. An SVR following DAAs has been associated with a reduction in both liver-related and all-cause mortality even after adjustment for multiple confounders.[216,217] In addition to a reduction in HCC risk, reductions in portal hypertension[218,219] and hepatic decompensation,[216] as well as recompensation and improvement in hepatic function[220,221] have been demonstrated following SVR with DAAs. Similar to IFN-based therapy, extrahepatic mortality and morbidity is also reduced following SVR with DAAs, including major adverse cardiovascular events,[222] improvement in glycemic control,[223] and reduction in extrahepatic cancers and HCV-related lymphoma.[224]

Indications and Contraindications

The development of highly efficacious and well-tolerated IFN-free DAA regimens, together with the clear benefit of HCV eradication on all-cause and liver-related mortality and quality of life, means that antiviral therapy should be considered in all patients with chronic hepatitis C. Furthermore, with the increasingly broad range of IFN-free and RBV-free DAA regimens with different pharmacokinetic and drug-drug interaction (DDI) properties available, there are very few clinical scenarios for which treatment is contraindicated, with the exception of decompensated cirrhosis with a high MELD score in a patient waitlisted for LT (see later and Chapter 99).

Because RBV is a teratogen, unwillingness of the patient and his or her partner to practice adequate contraception and avoid pregnancy during treatment and for 6 months after the discontinuation of therapy is an absolute contraindication to starting or continuing a DAA regimen that includes RBV. The major DAA registration studies excluded pregnant and lactating women. There are increasing data from small studies and case series that have not raised any concerns regarding safety. However, as there are no large-scale clinical trials in pregnant women, the guidelines do not recommend routine DAA treatment in pregnant women but suggest that DAA treatment may be considered on a case-by-case basis after considering the risks and benefits.[225]

On-Treatment Virologic Response

During IFN-based therapy, the rate of HCV clearance from the circulation was an important predictor of subsequent SVR24. Predictors of an SVR included a rapid virologic response (RVR, negative HCV RNA level at treatment week 4) and a complete early virologic response (negative HCV RNA level at treatment week 12).[104] However, with the extremely potent DAAs, the majority of patients achieve an RVR during DAA therapy. Furthermore, failure to attain an RVR does not preclude subsequent SVR12 with DAA-based therapy.[226,227]

Drugs

Interferon

IFN-based regimens became the cornerstone of antiviral therapy for HCV infection in the late 1980s. IFNs are naturally occurring glycoproteins that exert a wide array of antiviral, antiproliferative, and immunomodulatory effects. Pegylated IFNs consist of IFN bound to a molecule of polyethylene glycol of varying length. The large size of the molecule increases the half-life of the IFN, thereby allowing once-weekly dosage. Two pegylated IFNs are licensed for use in the United States and elsewhere. The first is 40-kd peginterferon alfa-2a, used in a fixed dose of 180 μg/week. The second is 12-kd peginterferon alfa-2b, prescribed according to the patient's body weight in a dose of 1.5 μg/kg/week. Pegylated IFNs replaced standard IFN, used in the past, and resulted in a significant increase in the SVR.[228] The use of IFN has been succeeded by IFN-free DAA regimens.

Ribavirin

RBV is an oral guanosine analog with activity against DNA and RNA viruses. When RBV is used in combination with IFN, the end-of-treatment response improves and the relapse rate decreases. Several mechanisms to explain the synergistic effect of RBV when administered in combination with IFN have been proposed, including (1) alterations of the cytokine milieu leading to a change from a type 2 T-helper cell (Th2) to a Th1 immune response; (2) depletion of intracellular guanosine triphosphate through inhibition of the host enzyme inosine monophosphate dehydrogenase; (3) inhibition of the action of the HCV RdRp; (4) induction of lethal mutagenesis during HCV RNA replication; and (5) increasing responsiveness to type I IFNs.[229] RBV generally is well tolerated, although it results in a dose-dependent hemolytic anemia. The dose administered is based on the patient's weight, and the patient's Hgb level must be monitored during treatment. Furthermore, in patients with a history of cardiopulmonary disease who cannot tolerate a sudden fall in the Hgb level, RBV must be used with caution, if at all. In addition, RBV is teratogenic; patients taking RBV and their partners are required to avoid pregnancy during therapy and for 6 months after cessation of the drug. RBV has a long cumulative half-life in serum and is excreted by the kidneys; as a result, it can lead to severe side effects, particularly hemolysis, in patients with kidney disease. The dose of RBV must be adjusted for renal function, and the drug should be administered with extreme caution to patients with a creatinine clearance less than 50 mL/min. RBV is not removed by hemodialysis. RBV still may be considered in some IFN-free DAA regimens in more difficult-to-treat patient populations, such as cirrhotic patients with genotype 3 HCV infection, decompensated cirrhosis, and prior DAA failure.

DAAs

Novel DAAs against HCV include compounds that target the HCV NS3/NS4A protease, the HCV NS5A protein, and the HCV NS5B polymerase. These drugs inhibit HCV replication by interfering with the respective steps in the HCV life cycle. An ideal DAA regimen should have activity against all HCV genotypes; have high antiviral potency and good oral bioavailability, allowing once daily dosing; possess few DDIs; be well tolerated with minimal toxicity; and have a high barrier to resistance. In contrast to IFN plus RBV, resistance to DAAs, either baseline resistance or resistance selected during DAA therapy, is a well-known consequence of DAA therapy that has implications for the success of certain treatment regimens and for retreatment following DAA failure. There are two factors to consider regarding the barrier to resistance: the genetic barrier, which is the number of amino acid substitutions required to confer resistance, and the fitness of the resistance-associated substitution (RAS), which is the ability of the RAS to sustain replication and be selected within the quasispecies (Box 82.3).

Many of these DAAs are now available as coformulated fixed-dose combinations (FDCs), allowing for once-daily dosing of a single pill for several of the approved IFN-free DAA regimens. The properties of each DAA class and approved DAAs are listed in Table 82.3.

NS3/4A Protease Inhibitors (-Previrs)

HCV NS3/4A protease inhibitors generally have high antiviral potency but differ in respect to the development of resistance. Most of the compounds show better response rates in HCV genotype 1b than in genotype 1a infection.[230] Boceprevir and telaprevir were the first two DAAs approved by the FDA in 2011; however, these agents were associated with significant toxicity and limited HCV genotype antiviral activity and required twice-daily or three times daily dosing with a large pill burden. Subsequently, the second wave of first-generation protease inhibitors, simeprevir and faldaprevir, were developed with more favorable safety profiles and dosing schedules; simeprevir was approved by the FDA in 2013. These have been superseded by second-generation protease inhibitors in combination with other DAAs that have the added advantage of extended HCV genotype activity. FDA-approved protease inhibitors are simeprevir, paritaprevir (boosted with ritonavir), grazoprevir, glecaprevir, and voxilaprevir; these agents are all used in combination with DAAs from other classes.

TABLE 82.3 Properties of Classes of DAAs

	Genotype Coverage	Potency	Barrier to Resistance	Drug-Drug Interactions	Metabolism	Approved Drugs[a]
NS3/4A protease inhibitors (-previrs)	+ to ++	++ to +++	+ to ++	++ to +++	Hepatic	Simeprevir Grazoprevir Paritaprevir **Glecaprevir** **Voxilaprevir**
NS5A inhibitors (-asvirs)	+ to +++	+++	+ to ++	+ to ++	Hepatic	Daclatasvir Ombitasvir Elbasvir **Ledipasvir** **Velpatasvir** **Pibrentasvir**
Nucleoside NS5B inhibitors (-uvirs)	+++	+++	+++	+	Renal	Sofosbuvir

[a]In order of approval, currently recommended agents in bold.
+, lowest; +++, highest.

NS5A Inhibitors (-Asvirs)

NS5A inhibitors are characterized by very high antiviral potency at picomolar doses. The cross-genotype efficacy of these agents varies, with greater genotypic coverage with the second-generation than first-generation NS5A inhibitors. Approved and second-generation NS5A inhibitors include daclatasvir, ledipasvir, ombitasvir, elbasvir, velpatasvir, and pibrentasvir.

NS5B Polymerase Inhibitors (-Buvirs)

HCV NS5B polymerase inhibitors are categorized as nucleoside or nucleotide analog and nonnucleoside polymerase inhibitors. Nonnucleoside polymerase inhibitors are the weakest class of compounds against HCV because of a low barrier to resistance. Most drugs in this class are active mainly against HCV genotype 1b and to a lesser extent against HCV genotype 1a. Different domains in the polymerase protein can be targeted by nonnucleoside polymerase inhibitors, and theoretically, use of a combination of different nonnucleoside polymerase inhibitors is possible. Importantly, there is also no cross-resistance between drugs targeting different polymerase domains.[231] The only FDA-approved nonnucleoside inhibitor is dasabuvir. In contrast, the nucleos(t)ide analogs are active across all HCV genotypes and have a high barrier to resistance. Nucleos(t)ide analog RAS may emerge but have very low fitness and do not expand rapidly, because they cause a chain termination and thereby block HCV replication. A triphosphorylated agent is usually required for activity. The first compound tested in a large number of patients was mericitabine.[232,233] Unfortunately, the compound had only modest antiviral activity, and relapses after treatment and breakthroughs during treatment were observed frequently in phase 2 trials when mericitabine was used in combination with protease inhibitors. The first approved nucleotide NS5B polymerase inhibitor was sofosbuvir, which has pangenotypic activity and a very high barrier to resistance.[234]

Approved DAAs in Common Use

Sofosbuvir

Sofosbuvir is a pangenotypic NS5B nucleotide inhibitor that is administered as a single 400-mg tablet or as part of an FDC with other DAAs (discussed later), with or without food. Sofosbuvir is predominantly excreted renally (80%), mostly as an active metabolite, but dose reduction is not required even in patients with end-stage renal failure. No dose adjustment is required with severe hepatic impairment, thereby allowing sofosbuvir to be administered in patients with decompensated cirrhosis. Sofosbuvir is well tolerated, and when used in combination with other DAAs, the most common adverse events were fatigue and headache. Although sofosbuvir is not metabolized extensively by the liver, it is transported by P glycoprotein (P-gp); therefore sofosbuvir should not be coadministered with strong inducers of P-gp, such as rifampin, carbamazepine, phenytoin, or St. John's Wort.

Although the precise mechanism is still not fully known, sofosbuvir is contraindicated in patients receiving amiodarone, because severe and life-threatening bradycardia within hours to weeks of coadministration has been reported. If a sofosbuvir-containing DAA regimen is planned for a patient on amiodarone and the amiodarone can be safely discontinued, the DAAs should be delayed for at least 3 months after cessation of amiodarone, due to its long half-life. Caution is recommended with other antiarrhythmics.

Sofosbuvir/Ledipasvir

The combination of sofosbuvir (see earlier) plus the NS5A inhibitor ledipasvir is administered as a two-drug FDC of sofosbuvir 400 mg and ledipasvir 90 mg as a single, once-daily tablet, with or without food. In contrast to sofosbuvir, ledipasvir is metabolized predominantly in the liver and excreted unchanged in bile. However, ledipasvir can be given safely to patients with severe hepatic impairment with no significant effect on plasma ledipasvir levels or pharmacokinetics. Because sofosbuvir is renally excreted, this regimen is not recommended for patients with severe renal impairment (eGFR < 30 mL/min/1.73 m^2). The most frequently reported adverse events were fatigue and headache. Both ledipasvir and sofosbuvir are transported by P-gp and breast cancer resistance protein (BCRP), and therefore potent P-gp/BCRP inducers will lower sofosbuvir and ledipasvir levels. Because this regimen contains sofosbuvir, the same DDIs that exist with sofosbuvir alone apply to this FDC. Rosuvastatin coadministration is not recommended because of inhibition of OATP by ledipasvir, and careful monitoring for statin-related adverse events is required with use of other HMG-CoA reductase inhibitors. Medications that alter gastric pH such as antacids, H2RAs, and PPIs may also affect ledipasvir levels, because ledipasvir becomes less soluble as gastric pH increases. In real-world experiences with this regimen, SVR rates were slightly lower in patients receiving high-dose PPIs.[235] Therefore H2RAa and PPIs should be dosed 12 hours apart from sofosbuvir/ledipasvir, with a maximal daily dose equivalent of 40 mg for famotidine or 20 mg for omeprazole. Sofosbuvir/ledipasvir can be administered with antiretrovirals with the exception of tenofovir and ritonavir/cobicistat–containing regimens due to an increase in tenofovir levels, which require monitoring.

Sofosbuvir/Velpatasvir

Sofosbuvir 400 mg and the next-generation NS5A inhibitor velpatasvir 100 mg are coformulated in a single FDC tablet given once daily, with or without food. The combination has pangenotypic coverage. Velpatasvir undergoes hepatic metabolism by CYP2B6, CYP2C8, and CYP3A4 and is also transported by P-gp, BCRP, and, to a small extent, OATP1B1. Velpatasvir can be administered to patients with severe hepatic impairment without alterations in velpatasvir plasma concentration or pharmacokinetics. The major adverse events reported with this FDC were headache, fatigue, and nausea, and their frequencies were similar to those reported in the placebo arm. Due to CYP metabolism and P-gp/BCRP binding of velpatasvir, potent CYP and P-gp inducers are contraindicated with this regimen (see Table 82.4). As with ledipasvir, the solubility of velpatasvir decreases with increasing gastric pH levels; therefore recommendations regarding use of antacids, H2RAs, and PPIs as outlined for sofosbuvir/ledipasvir therapy should also be followed with sofosbuvir/velpatasvir.

Glecaprevir/Pibrentasvir

The combination of the NS3/4A protease inhibitor glecaprevir 100 mg and the NS5A inhibitor pibrentasvir 40 mg are coformulated as a two-drug FDC tablet given as three tablets once daily with food. This FDC has pangenotypic activity. Both drugs are excreted predominantly in the bile and are inhibitors of the transporter proteins P-gp, BCRP, OATP1B1, and OATP1B3. Because of significantly higher glecaprevir exposure in patients with moderate and severe hepatic impairment, this combination is

TABLE 82.4 Drug-Drug Interactions With DAAs

Coadministered Drug Class	DAA				
	Glecaprevir/ Pibrentasvir	**Sofosbuvir/ Ledipasvir**	**Sofosbuvir**	**Sofosbuvir/ Velpatasvir**	**Sofosbuvir/ Velpatasvir/ Voxilaprevir**
ANESTHETICS, MUSCLE RELAXANTS					
Analgesics	Alfentanil Fentanyl Hydrocodone Metamizole Oxycodone	Buprenorphine Fentanyl	–	Buprenorphine Metamizole	Buprenorphine Metamizole
Antihelminitics	–	–	–	–	–
Antiarrhythmics	Amiodarone Digoxin Dronedarone Quinidine	Amiodarone Digoxin Dronedarone Quinidine	Amiodarone Dronedarone	Amiodarone Digoxin Dronedarone Quinidine	Amiodarone Digoxin Dronedarone Quinidine
Antibiotics	Bedaquiline Clarithromycin Erythromycin Isoniazid Rifabutin Rifampicin Rifapentine Rifaximin Telithromycin Troleandomycin	Bedaquiline Isoniazid Rifabutin Rifampicin Rifapentine Telithromycin	Isoniazid Rifabutin Rifampicin Rifapentine	Isoniazid Rifabutin Rifampicin Rifapentine Troleandomycin	Clarithromycin Erythromycin Isoniazid Rifabutin Rifampicin Rifapentine Rifaximin Telithromycin Troleandromycin
Anticoagulants, antiplatelets, fibrinolytics	Acenocoumarol Apixaban Dabigatran Edoxaban Eltrombopag Fluindione Phenprocoumon Rivaroxaban Ticagrelor Warfarin	Apixaban Dabigatran Edoxaban Phenprocoumon Rivaroxaban Ticagrelor Warfarin	Warfarin	Apixaban Dabigatran Edoxaban Eltrombopag Rivaroxaban Ticagrelor Warfarin	Apixaban Dabigatran Edoxaban Eltrombopag Fluindione Phenprocoumon Rivaroxaban Ticagrelor Warfarin
Anticonvulsants	Carbamazepine Eslicarbamazepine Oxcarbazepine Phenobarbital Phenytoin Primidone Rufinamide	Carbamazepine Eslicarbamazepine Oxcarbazepine Phenobarbital Phenytoin Primidone Rufinamide Zonisamide	Carbamazepine Oxcarbazepine Phenobarbital Phenytoin Primidone Rufinamide	Carbamazepine Eslicarbamazepine Oxcarbazepine Phenobarbital Phenytoin Primidone Rufinamide	Carbamazepine Eslicarbamazepine Oxcarbazepine Phenobarbital Phenytoin Primidone Rufinamide
Antidepressants	–	–	–	–	–
Antidiabetics	Glibenclamide Repaglinide Vildagliptin	Canagliflozin	–	Empagliflozin Repaglinide	Empagliflozin Repaglinide Vildagliptin
Antifungals	Ketoconazole Posaconazole	Miconazole	–	–	–

TABLE 82.4 Drug-Drug Interactions With DAAs—cont'd

Coadministered Drug Class	DAA				
	Glecaprevir/ Pibrentasvir	**Sofosbuvir/ Ledipasvir**	**Sofosbuvir**	**Sofosbuvir/ Velpatasvir**	**Sofosbuvir/ Velpatasvir/ Voxilaprevir**
Antihistamines	Astemizole Bilastine Fexofenadine Terfenadine	Bilastine	–	Bilastine	Bilastine Fexofenadine
Antimigraine agents	Dihydroergotamine Ergotamine Methylergonovine	Dihydroergotamine Ergotamine Methylergonovine	–	–	–
Antiprotozoals	Mefloquine Quinine	Mefloquine Quinine	–	Artemesinin Artesunate Dihydroartemisinin	Artemesinin Artesunate Dihydroartemisinin Mefloquine Quinine
Antipsychotics, neuroleptics	Aripiprazole Clozapine Paliperidone Pimozide Quetiapine Thioridazine	Paliperidone Pimozide	–	–	Paliperidone
Anxiolytics, hypnotics, sedatives	Amobarbital Clotiapine	Amobarbital Clotiapine Midazolam	Amobarbital	Amobarbital	Amobarbital
β Receptor antagonists	Carvedilol	Carvedilol	–	Carvedilol	Carvedilol
Bronchodilators	Theophylline	–	–	–	–
Calcium channel blockers	Diltiazem Verapamil	Amlodipine Diltiazem Felodipine	–	Diltiazem	Diltiazem Verapamil
Cancer therapies	Bosutinib Brentuximab vedotin Doxorubicin Erlotinib Everolimus Imatinib Irinotecan Lapatinib Methotrexate Mitoxantrone Nilotinib Sunitinib Vinblastine Vincristine Vinorelbine	Erlotinib Everolimus Irinotecan Lapatinib Mitoxantrone Temsirolimus Vinorelbine	–	Erlotinib Everolimus Imatinib Irinotecan Lapatinib Methotrexate Mitoxantrone Nilotinib Tamoxifen Temsirolimus Vinblastine Vincristine Vinorelbine	Erlotinib Everolimus Imatinib Irinotecan Lapatinib Methotrexate Mitoxantrone Nilotinib Tamoxifen Temsirolimus Vinblastine Vincristine Vinorelbine
Contraceptives, hormone replacement	Estradiol Ethinylestradiol	–	–	Estradiol	Estradiol Ethinylestradiol
Erectile dysfunction	–	–	–	–	–
GI agents	Cimetidine Cisapride Domperidone Droperidol Esomeprazole Famotidine Lansoprazole Loperamide Omeprazole Pantoprazole Rabeprazole Ranitidine Sulfasalazine	Aluminum hydroxide Antacids Cimetidine Cisapride Esomeprazole Famotidine Lansoprazole Loperamide Omeprazole Pantoprazole Prucalopride Rabeprazole Ranitidine	Aluminium hydroxide Antacids	Aprepitant Cimetidine Esomeprazole Famotidine Lansoprazole Omeprazole Pantoprazole Rabeprazole Ranitidine Sulfasalazine	Aluminium hydroxide Antacids Cimetidine Esomeprazole Famotidine Lansoprazole Loperamide Omeprazole Pantoprazole Rabeprazole Ranitidine Sulfasalazine
Hepatitis nucleos(t)ide analogs	–	TDF	–	TDF	TDF
Herbal, supplements, vitamins	St. John's Wort	St. John's Wort	St. John's Wort	St. John's Wort	St. John's Wort

Continued

TABLE 82.4 Drug-Drug Interactions With DAAs—cont'd

Coadministered Drug Class	DAA				
	Glecaprevir/ Pibrentasvir	**Sofosbuvir/ Ledipasvir**	**Sofosbuvir**	**Sofosbuvir/ Velpatasvir**	**Sofosbuvir/ Velpatasvir/ Voxilaprevir**
HIV entry/integrase inhibitors	Bictegravir/FTC/ TAF	Elvitegravir/cobi/ FTC/TDF	–	Elvitegravir/cobi/FTC/ TDF	Elvitegravir/cobi/FTC/ TDF
HIV NNRTIs	Efavirenz Etravirine Nevirapine	Efavirenz	–	Efavirenz Etravirine Nevirapine	–
HIV NRTIs	–	TDF	–	TDF	TDF
HIV protease inhibitors	ATZ Cobi/ATV/DRV DRV Fosamprenavir Indinavir Lopinavir Nelfinavir Ritonavir Saquinavir Tipranavir	Cobi/ATV/DRV Lopinavir Tipranavir	Nelfinavir Tipranavir	Tipranavir	ATZ Cobi/ATV/DRV DRV Fosamprenavir Indinavir Lopinavir Nelfinavir Ritonavir Saquinavir Tipranavir
Hypertension, heart failure agents	Aliskiren Ambrisentan Bosentan Candesartan Enalapril Eplerenone Irbesartan Isradipine Olmesartan Prazosin Ranolazine Telmisartan	Aliskiren Eplerenone Irbesartan Isradipine Ranolazine	–	Bosentan Prazosin	Aliskiren Ambrisentan Bosentan Candesartan Enalapril Irbesartan Isradipine Olmesartan Prazosin Ranolazine Telmisartan Valsartan
Illicit, recreational	Gamma-hydroxybutyrate	–	–	–	–
Immunosuppressants	Cyclosporine Sirolimus Tacrolimus	–	–	–	Cyclosporine Sirolimus Tacrolimus
Lipid-lowering agents	Atorvastatin Ezetimibe Fluvastatin Gemfibrozil Lovastatin Pitavastatin Pravastatin Rosuvastatin Simvastatin	Atorvastatin Fluvastatin Lovastatin Pitavastatin Pravastatin Rosuvastatin Simvastatin	–	Atorvastatin Fluvastatin Lovastatin Pitavastatin Rosuvastatin Simvastatin	Atorvastatin Ezetimibe Fluvastatin Lovastatin Pitavastatin Pravastatin Rosuvastatin Simvastatin
Miscellaneous agents	Activated charcoal Colchicine Cholestyramine Dexamfetamine Eliglustat Flibanserin Glycerol phenylbutyrate Lofexidine Lumacaftor/ ivacaftor Modafinil Orlistat Strontium ranelate UDCA	Activated charcoal Colchicine Cholestyramine Dexamfetamine Glycerol phenylbutyrate Lofexidine Lumacaftor/ ivacaftor Modafinil Orlistat Sevelamer Strontium ranelate UDCA	Activated charcoal Cholestyramine Lumacaftor/ ivacaftor Modafinil Orlistat Sevelamer Strontium ranelate UDCA	Activated charcoal Colchicine Cholestyramine Dexamfetamine Glycerol phenylbutyrate Lofexidine Lumacaftor/ivacaftor Modafinil Orlistat Sevelamer Strontium ranelate UDCA	Activated charcoal Colchicine Cholestyramine Dexamfetamine Glycerol phenylbutyrate Lofexidine Lumacaftor/ivacaftor Modafinil Orlistat Sevelamer Strontium ranelate UDCA
Oxytocics	Ergometrine (ergonovine)	Ergometrine (ergonovine)	–	–	–
Parkinsonism agents	–	–	–	–	–
Steroids	Dexamethasone	–	–	–	–
Urologic agents	–	–	–	–	–

Blue, Potential weak interaction; *orange*, potential interaction; *red*, significant interaction—do not coadminister. *ATV*, Atazanavir; *cobi*, cobicistat; *DRV*, darunavir; *FTC*, emtricitabine; *NNRTIs*, non-nucleoside reverse transcriptase inhibitors; *NRTIs*, nucleoside reverse transcriptase inhibitors; *PrOD*, paritaprevir/ritonavir/ombitasvir and dasabuvir; *TAF*, tenofovir alafenamide; *TDF*, tenofovir disoproxil fumarate.

contraindicated in those with Child-Pugh class B and C cirrhosis. The regimen is safe in patients with severe renal impairment, including patients with end-stage renal disease (ESRD) with and without dialysis. As with many other DAAs, DDIs include strong inducers of P-gp and CYP3A4, including antiretrovirals (see Table 82.4). The solubility of glecaprevir decreases as gastric pH increases; however, dose modification is not required for doses of PPIs equivalent to omeprazole 40 mg/day; higher doses have not been formally studied.

Elbasvir/Grazoprevir

The combination of the NS5A inhibitor elbasvir 50 mg and the NS3/4A protease inhibitor grazoprevir 100 mg is available as a single FDC tablet administered once daily, with or without food, in patients with HCV genotypes 1 and 4. Both grazoprevir and elbasvir are partially metabolized by CYP3A4 and predominantly excreted in bile and feces. Both are extensively bound to plasma proteins. Grazoprevir exposure is increased greatly with severe hepatic impairment, and therefore, like all protease inhibitors, the drug is contraindicated in patients with decompensated Child-Pugh class B or C cirrhosis. This regimen is safe in patients with severe renal failure. The most common adverse events are headache and fatigue. Relevant DDIs to consider are inducers of CYP3A and P-gp, including some antiretrovirals (see Table 82.4).

Sofosbuvir/Velpatasvir/Voxilaprevir

Sofosbuvir 400 mg, velpatasvir 100 mg, and the NS3/4A protease inhibitor voxilaprevir 100 mg coformulated as a single three-drug FDC tablet is administered once daily with food. This FDC has pangenotypic activity. Voxilaprevir is metabolized extensively in the liver by CYP3A4 and, like velpatasvir, is an inhibitor of P-gp, BCRP, OATP1B1, and OATP1B3. As with all protease inhibitors, voxilaprevir exposure is significantly higher with moderate and severe hepatic impairment, and therefore, the drug is not recommended in patients with decompensated Child-Pugh class B cirrhosis and contraindicated in those with Child-Pugh class C cirrhosis. The most frequently reported adverse events with this triple regimen were headache, diarrhea, and nausea, suggesting increased additional GI toxicity with voxilaprevir. Because these agents are metabolized by CYP3A4 and are inhibitors of transporter proteins, DDIs occur with substrates of these transporters and potent inducers of CYP3A4, including antiretrovirals (see Table 82.4). Rosuvastatin, in particular, is contraindicated because coadministration was associated with 19-fold higher plasma levels of rosuvastatin. Sofosbuvir/velpatasvir/voxilaprevir is contraindicated in women taking ethinylestradiol-based contraception due to the risk of elevations in serum ALT levels. Because this regimen also contains velpatasvir, DDIs with agents that increase gastric pH are also relevant.

Acute Hepatitis C

Although postexposure prophylaxis against HCV is not effective, the treatment of acute HCV infection is effective.[236] With the significant increase in the incidence of acute hepatitis C in the United States and the subsequent recognition of this population as critical to onward transmission of HCV and HCV elimination efforts, treatment is now recommended at diagnosis of acute hepatitis C infection (HCV RNA positive) rather than awaiting possible spontaneous clearance. These individuals should receive the same treatment as individuals with chronic HCV infection; abbreviated treatment courses are not recommended due to inferior SVR rates.[237–240] Treatment of acute hepatitis C in the context of HIV coinfection is similar to that for patients with HCV monoinfection.[238,241,242] IFN-based regimens are no longer recommended.

Chronic Hepatitis C

In contrast to most other chronic viral infections, cure of HCV infection is possible. HCV has an entirely cytoplasmic life cycle; therefore suppression of viral replication in the absence of resistance can cure HCV-infected cells. Owing to the extremely high efficacy and minimal toxicity, universal treatment for individuals with acute and chronic hepatitis C infection is recommended; HCV therapy is not recommended for those with a short life expectancy that is unlikely to be attenuated by DAA therapy, liver transplantation or another specific therapy.

Until 2011 the standard of care for the treatment of HCV infection was the combination of a PegIFN plus RBV. However, IFN-based therapy was associated with poor overall cure rates (54%–56%),[104,105,243] with significant toxicity leading to discontinuation of therapy in 14% of patients. In addition, many patients were either ineligible for or intolerant of IFN, thereby limiting treatment options in these patients.

The first DAAs (telaprevir, boceprevir, simeprevir, and sofosbuvir) were developed as "triple" therapy to be used in combination with PegIFN plus RBV.[244–251] Although SVR rates were higher, limitations included restricted HCV genotypic activity, additional toxicity beyond PegIFN/RBV, poor response in cirrhotic patients and prior null responders, and RAS considerations, as well as a requirement for PegIFN/RBV eligibility. Subsequently, combination IFN-free DAA regimens were developed (see earlier). IFN-based regimens are no longer recommended for the treatment of HCV infection.

Combinations of DAAs that target distinct and complementary steps in the HCV life cycle (see Fig. 82.1) have revolutionized the treatment of HCV infection, yielding SVR rates in excess of 95% with minimal toxicity and widespread eligibility. The first proof-of-concept study showing an SVR in four patients with chronic hepatitis C with an IFN-free DAA combination therapy was published in 2012.[252] The compounds investigated were the HCV NS5A inhibitor daclatasvir and the HCV NS3 protease inhibitor asunaprevir. SVR rates were only 22% (2/9) in HCV genotype 1a patients; however, SVR rates were considerably higher in HCV genotype 1b patients (90% for treatment-naïve patients and 82% for patients who were prior nonresponders to or ineligible for IFN),[253] providing proof-of-concept that IFN-free therapy can cure HCV, but that the efficacy of all-oral combination regimens may differ among HCV genotypes and subtypes. Since this study, many DAAs have undergone clinical development, 13 of which have been approved by the FDA as of early 2024 and include the NS3/4A protease inhibitors simeprevir, paritaprevir (ritonavir boosted), grazoprevir, glecaprevir, and voxilaprevir; the NS5A inhibitors daclatasvir, ombitasvir, ledipasvir, elbasvir, velpatasvir, and pibrentasvir; and the NS5B inhibitors sofosbuvir and dasabuvir (see Table 82.3). The older IFN-free DAA regimens are HCV genotype-specific, whereas the more recently approved IFN-free regimens have pangenotypic coverage. Genotype-specific drugs or FDCs include sofosbuvir/ledipasvir, and elbasvir/grazoprevir. Pangenotypic drugs include sofosbuvir, sofosbuvir/velpatasvir, sofosbuvir/velpatasvir/voxilaprevir, and glecaprevir/pibrentasvir. RBV can be added to some IFN-free DAA regimens in more difficult-to-treat populations, such as HCV genotype 3 cirrhotic patients, decompensated liver disease, and prior DAA failure. Treatment regimens are discussed in the context of DAA treatment history and presence/absence of cirrhosis, as these factors are important considerations when choosing an IFN-free DAA regimen. Special populations, including persons with prior DAA failures, decompensated cirrhosis, pregnancy, children and adolescents, HCV recurrence following LT, and receipt of HCV-positive organs, are discussed under "Unique Populations."

Initial Treatment for Treatment-Naïve Adults Without Cirrhosis and With Compensated (Child-Pugh A) Cirrhosis

All individuals with acute or chronic hepatitis C infection should be offered HCV therapy; however, to be able to implement this recommendation, expanding the settings where treatment can be provided and developing simplified and streamlined treatment algorithms with minimal monitoring are critical. The advent of pangenotypic DAA regimens together with real-world global data demonstrating that a minimal monitoring treatment approach is safe and effective with comparable SVR rates, including in patients with compensated cirrhosis,[254] has made this achievable.[225] For these patients, on-treatment monitoring is not required, but a consultation during treatment may be scheduled for additional support or symptom assessment if required.

Patients eligible for a minimal monitoring simplified treatment algorithm include treatment-naïve patients with any HCV genotype, without cirrhosis or with compensated (Child-Pugh A) cirrhosis, and can include patients with HIV-HCV coinfection, although careful attention to DDIs is required. Patients who are not eligible for minimal monitoring treatment algorithms are patients who have previously received DAA therapy, those coinfected with HBV infection (HBsAg-positive), those with compensated cirrhosis and ESRD (eGFR < 30 mL/min/m^2), decompensated cirrhosis (Child-Pugh B ≥ 7), pregnant, suspected or known hepatocellular carcinoma, liver transplantation, and receipt of HCV-viremic organs.

Several FDA-approved IFN-free all-oral DAA regimens are recommended for the initial treatment of hepatitis C infection in adults that all have similar efficacy. These can be divided into pangenotypic regimens or HCV genotype-specific regimens (Table 82.5). HCV reinfection (HCV RNA positive following prior HCV infection with confirmed SVR12 after a course of DAA therapy) can be considered as a new infection and therefore is considered in the same treatment category as initial HCV infection.

TABLE 82.5 Initial Treatment for Treatment-Naïve Adults Without Cirrhosis and With Compensated (Child-Pugh A) Cirrhosis

	Duration (Weeks)	Fibrosis Stage	SVR12 (%)	Study
Pangenotypic Regimens				
Glecaprevir (300 mg)/Pibrentasvir (120 mg)				
HCV 1	8	F0-3	97-99.7	SURVEYOR-I/II ENDURANCE-1
	8	F4	97.8	EXPEDITION-8
HCV 2	8 8	F0-3 F4	98 100	SURVEYOR-II EXPEDITION-8
HCV 3	8	F0-3	95–97	SURVEYOR-II ENDURANCE-III
	8	F4	95.2	EXPEDITION-8
HCV 4–6	8 8	F0-3 F4	93 100	SURVEYOR-II EXPEDITION-8
Sofosbuvir (400 mg)/Velpatasvir (100 mg)				
HCV 1	12	F0-3	98.4	ASTRAL-1
HCV 1, 4–6	12	F4	99.2	ASTRAL-1
HCV 2	12 12	F0-3 F4	99 100	ASTRAL-2 ASTRAL-2
HCV 3	12 12	F0-3 F4	96.9 91.3	ASTRAL-3 ASTRAL-3
HCV 4	12	F0-3	100	ASTRAL-1
HCV 1, 4–6	12	F4	99.2	ASTRAL-1
HCV 5	12	F0-3	97.1	ASTRAL-1
HCV 1, 4–6	12	F4	99.2	ASTRAL-1
HCV 6	12	F0-3	100	ASTRAL-1
HCV 1, 4–6	12	F4	99.2	ASTRAL-1
Genotype-Specific Regimens				
Sofosbuvir (400 mg)/Ledipasvir (90 mg)				
HCV 1	12 8[a] 12	F0-3 F0-3 F4	100 94.0 97.0	ION-1 ION-3 ION-1
HCV 4	12	F0-4	100	ION-4
HCV 5	12	F0-4	95.1	Abergel 2016
HCV 5	12	F0-4	96.0	Foster NEJM 2015
Elbasvir (50 mg)/Grazoprevir (100 mg)				
HCV 1b	12	F0-4	99	C-EDGE
HCV 4	12	F0-4	96	Asselah 2018
Sofosbuvir (400 mg)/Velpatasvir (100 mg) ± weight-based RBV				
HCV 3[b]	12	F4	96	Foster NEJM 2015

[a]If baseline HCV RNA <6 million IU/mL in HCV monoinfection only.

[b]In patients with baseline Y93H (NS5A) RAS.

F0-3, METAVIR fibrosis stages 0–3; *F4*, METAVIR fibrosis stage 4, compensated (Child-Pugh A); *RAS*, resistance-associated substitutions; *RBV*, ribavirin; *SVR12*, sustained virologic response 12 weeks after completion of therapy.

Pangenotypic Regimens (HCV Genotypes 1–6)

Glecaprevir/Pibrentasvir

Glecaprevir (100 mg) plus pibrentasvir (40 mg) FDC administered as three tablets once daily for 8 weeks is approved for all HCV genotypes (1–6) in noncirrhotic and compensated cirrhotic patients. SVR12 rates of >95% were observed for all HCV genotypes, including in patients with and without cirrhosis (Table 82.5).[255–257] Treatment was tolerated extremely well, with only one treatment-related adverse event, and no treatment discontinuation was observed due to adverse events. The presence of baseline RAS did not significantly impact SVR rates in non-HCV genotype 3 patients in a posthoc analysis[258] of the major phase 3 registration studies.[256,259–261] In HCV genotype 3 patients with the baseline A30K polymorphism and compensated cirrhosis, SVR rates were slightly lower following 8 weeks of glecaprevir/pibrentasvir (78%), although this RAS was uncommon (10%). The Y93H NS5A RAS did not affect SVR rates in this subgroup.

Sofosbuvir/Velpatasvir

The FDC of sofosbuvir (400 mg)/velpatasvir (100 mg) given as one tablet once daily for 12 weeks is also a pangenotypic regimen approved for HCV genotypes 1–6. SVR rates were >95% across all HCV genotypes and in patients with and without compensated cirrhosis (Table 82.5).[262,263] In patients with HCV genotype 3 and the Y93H baseline RAS, SVR rates were observed to be lower (84%) compared to those without this baseline RAS (97%), largely in the compensated cirrhotic patients.[263] The addition of RBV in compensated cirrhotic patients with HCV genotype 3 reduced relapse rates.[264]

Genotype-Specific Regimens

Sofosbuvir/Ledipasvir

Noncirrhotic and Compensated Cirrhotic Patients with HCV Genotypes 1, 4–6. The FDC of sofosbuvir (400 mg)/ledipasvir (90 mg) once daily for 12 weeks is approved for HCV genotypes 1, 4–6 infection in patients with and without compensated cirrhosis based on data from the phase 3 registrations studies, ION-1[265] and ION-3.[266] SVR12 rates were universally high, all >95% across all treatment arms and irrespective of HCV genotype and fibrosis stage. ION-3[266] investigated whether the duration of therapy with sofosbuvir/ledipasvir could be shortened and compared 8 weeks of sofosbuvir/ledipasvir with and without RBV versus 12 weeks of sofosbuvir/ledipasvir in treatment-naïve HCV genotype 1-infected noncirrhotic patients. In an intention-to-treat analysis, there was no difference in SVR12 among the treatment arms (93%–95%), although relapse rates were numerically higher in the 8-week treatment arm irrespective of RBV use. A posthoc analysis of the 8-week RBV-free arm revealed higher relapse rates in patients with high viral loads (>6 million IU/mL) at baseline. Although this was a posthoc analysis, these data led to the recommendation that 8 weeks of sofosbuvir/ledipasvir without RBV is sufficient in noncirrhotic HCV genotype 1 treatment-naïve patients with a baseline HCV RNA level of less than 6 million IU/mL. Real-world clinical experience has confirmed the similar efficacy rates of 8 and 12 weeks of sofosbuvir/ledipasvir for this group of patients.[267]

Elbasvir/Grazoprevir

Noncirrhotic and Compensated Cirrhotic HCV Genotype 1b and 4 Patients Without Baseline NS5A RAS. The FDC of elbasvir (50 mg)/grazoprevir (100 mg) once daily for 12 weeks is also approved for HCV genotype 1b and 4 infection based on data from the phase 3 C-EDGE study.[268] The SVR12 rate in patients with HCV genotype 1b infection was 99% and 96% in the pooled analysis of the phase 2/3 studies in HCV genotype 4 patients.[269] SVR12 rates were significantly lower in HCV genotype 1a patients with baseline NS5A RAS, particularly in HCV genotype1a patients with cirrhosis. Therefore this regimen is only an alternative regimen for HCV genotype 1a patients without baseline NS5A RAS; patients with baseline NS5A RAS should receive another regimen.

Sofosbuvir/Velpatasvir/Voxilaprevir

Compensated Cirrhotic Patients With HCV Genotype 3 Infection and Baseline Y93H RAS. The FDC of sofosbuvir (400 mg)/velpatasvir (100 mg)/voxilaprevir (100 mg) once daily for 12 weeks is approved as an alternative regimen for HCV genotype 3 patients with compensated cirrhosis who have the baseline Y93 RAS on NS5A testing. This is based on data from POLARIS-3,[270] which evaluated 8 weeks of sofosbuvir/velpatasvir/voxilaprevir compared to 12 weeks of sofosbuvir/velpatasvir in compensated cirrhotic DAA-naïve patients with HCV genotype 2 and 3 infection. SVR12 rates were 96% in both arms, but importantly, baseline NS5A RAS did not compromise SVR12 rates, and no patients receiving sofosbuvir/velpatasvir/voxilaprevir developed RAS following virological failure. Although 8 weeks of sofosbuvir/velpatasvir/voxilaprevir was evaluated in this study, 12 weeks of this regimen is the alternative regimen for HCV genotype 3 patients with cirrhosis and the baseline Y93H RAS.

Treatment of Treatment-Experienced Adults Without Cirrhosis and With Compensated Cirrhosis

The vast majority of patients receiving DAA therapy achieve an SVR12; however, there is a small percentage of individuals that are not cured and require retreatment. Retreatment options are based on the prior DAA regimen, and are divided into sofosbuvir-based failure, NS5A inhibitor-containing failure, and multiple DAA failure (Table 82.6). This does not include individuals who have previously received IFN-based therapies or those who received a first-generation protease-inhibitor (NS3/4A inhibitor) together with pegIFN plus RBV, as these populations continue to have equivalent SVR12 rates to treatment-naïve patients with current recommended DAA regimens.[271]

Retreatment of Prior Sofosbuvir-Based DAA Failure

For patients who have failed a sofosbuvir-based regimen, retreatment with the FDC of sofosbuvir (400 mg)/velpatasvir (100 mg)/voxilaprevir (100 mg) once daily for 12 weeks is recommended among all HCV genotypes and in patients with and without compensated cirrhosis. SVR12 rates were between 96% and 98% in the phase 3 registration studies, although few patients with HCV genotype 3 infection were included.[272,273] In subsequent real-world studies of prior sofosbuvir-based DAA failure, SVR12 rates ranged from 90% to 100% but were higher in patients who completed therapy compared to those who did not complete the treatment course.[274–277] Baseline NS5A RAS did not significantly impact SVR12 rates, but SVR12 rates were noted to be lower in patients with compensated cirrhosis and HCV genotype 3 in several of the studies, lowest in patients with HCV genotype 3 infection with compensated cirrhosis (69%).[277] Therefore the addition of weight-based RBV is recommended in compensated cirrhotic patients with HCV genotype 3 infection if there is no contraindication.

An alternative regimen for prior sofosbuvir-based DAA failure is the FDC of glecaprevir (100 mg)/pibrentasvir (40 mg) administered as three tablets daily for 16 weeks.[278–280] In the MAGELLAN-1 Part 2 study for HCV genotype 1, 2, 4–6 patients, SVR12 rates were 91% in patients receiving 16 weeks of glecaprevir/pibrentasvir, compared to 89% following 12 weeks of therapy.[279] Past treatment with one class of DAA (either NS3/4A or NS5A inhibitor) did not impact SVR rates, but prior dual treatment with an NS3/4A inhibitor plus an NS5A inhibitor was associated with significantly lower SVR rates. Similarly, in the phase 3b open-label study of glecaprevir/pibrentasvir with or without RBV for 12 or 16 weeks in HCV genotype 1 patients, SVR rates were higher in the patients receiving 16 weeks of glecaprevir/pibrentasvir (94% for

TABLE 82.6 Treatment of Treatment-Experienced Adults Without Cirrhosis and With Compensated Cirrhosis

	Duration (Weeks)	Fibrosis Stage	SVR12	Study
Retreatment of Prior Sofosbuvir-Based DAA Failure				
Sofosbuvir (400 mg)/Velpatasvir (100 mg)/Voxilaprevir (100 mg)				
HCV 1-6	12	F0-4	96%–100%	References [286–291]
Sofosbuvir (400 mg)/Velpatasvir (100 mg)/Voxilaprevir (100 mg) + weight-based RBV				
HCV 3	12	F4	69% without RBV	Reference [291]
Glecaprevir (300 mg)/Pibrentasvir (120 mg)				
HCV 1, 2, 4-6	16	F0-3, F4	91%–94%	MAGELLAN-1 Part 2 Reference [294]
Retreatment of Prior Glecaprevir/Pibrentasvir DAA Failure				
Glecaprevir (300 mg)/Pibrentasvir (120 mg) + Sofosbuvir (400 mg) + weight-based RBV				
HCV 1-6	16	F0-3, F4	96%	MAGELLAN-3
Sofosbuvir (400 mg)/Velpatasvir (100 mg)/Voxilaprevir (100 mg)				
HCV 1–6[a]	12	F0-3, F4	95%	Reference [296]
Retreatment of Prior Multiple DAA Failures				
Glecaprevir (300 mg)/Pibrentasvir (120 mg) + Sofosbuvir (400 mg) plus weight-based RBV twice daily				
HCV 1, 2, 4–6 naïve to NS3/4A and/or NS5A inhibitor	12	F0-3	100%	MAGELLAN-3
HCV 1, 2, 4–6 prior treatment with NS3/4A or NS5A inhibitor; OR HCV 3	16[b]	F0-3 F4	95%	MAGELLAN-3
Sofosbuvir (400 mg)/Velpatasvir (100 mg)/Voxilaprevir (100 mg) plus weight-based RBV				
Prior sofosbuvir/velpatasvir/voxilaprevir failure	24	F0-3, F4		Reference [239]

[a]RBV is recommended in patients with compensated cirrhosis.

[b]Treatment extension to 24 weeks can be considered in patients with factors that increase the risk of failure of treatment.

16 weeks vs. 90% for 12 weeks) and were similar with and without RBV.[280] This regimen has not been studied in HCV genotype 3 patients with prior sofosbuvir/NS5A inhibitor failure and therefore is not recommended in this population.

Retreatment of Prior Glecaprevir/Pibrentasvir DAA Failure

For patients who have failed prior glecaprevir/pibrentasvir DAA therapy, the multi-DAA combination of glecaprevir (300 mg)/pibrentasvir (120 mg) plus sofosbuvir (400 mg) plus weight-based RBV twice daily for 16 weeks is recommended. This is based on data from the MAGELLAN-3 study in patients with HCV genotypes 1–6 with and without cirrhosis.[281] The majority (91%) had baseline NS5A RAS detected, and despite this, the overall SVR12 rate was 96%.

A second recommended regimen for those who have failed prior glecaprevir/pibrentasvir DAA therapy is sofosbuvir (400 mg)/velpatasvir (100 mg)/voxilaprevir (100 mg) for 12 weeks. The overall SVR12 rate was 94%, despite the presence of baseline NS5A RAS in 90% of subjects.[282] Although not specifically investigated in this study, in patients with compensated cirrhosis, the addition of weight-based RBV is recommended due to slightly lower SVR rates in this subgroup.

Retreatment of Prior Multiple DAA Failures

There is a small proportion of patients that still fail to respond to retreatment with salvage DAA therapies, such as sofosbuvir/velpatasvir/voxilaprevir and sofosbuvir plus glecaprevir/pibrentasvir. There are limited data, mostly retrospective case series, describing retreatment of this group of multiexperienced DAA failure patients. Pibrentasvir is a next-generation NS5A inhibitor and has been demonstrated to have improved and potent activity against common NS5A RAS compared to other NS5A inhibitors.[283] In MAGELLAN-3,[281] a small number of multi-DAA experienced patients, all of whom were retreated with glecaprevir/pibrentasvir but developed virologic failure were then retreated with glecaprevir/pibrentasvir plus sofosbuvir plus weight-based RBV twice daily for 12 weeks if noncirrhotic with non-HCV genotype 3 infection and naïve to a protease inhibitor and/or NS5A inhibitor prior to glecaprevir/pibrentasvir failure, or 16 weeks if HCV genotype 3 infection, compensated cirrhotics, prior NS5A/protease inhibitor prior to first treatment failure with glecaprevir/pibrentasvir. No patients with prior sofosbuvir/velpatasvir/voxilaprevir exposure were included. Overall SVR12 rates were 96%, with no on-treatment virologic failure; 1 patient experienced viral relapse at posttreatment week 4. Based on data from case reports, extension to 24 weeks or longer could be considered in patients with factors that increase the risk of failure of treatment, such as HCV genotype 3 cirrhosis or prior treatment failure with sofosbuvir plus glecaprevir/pibrentasvir.[284–287]

For patients who fail to respond to sofosbuvir/velpatasvir/voxilaprevir, retreatment may be more challenging. Current guidelines recommend 24 weeks of sofosbuvir/velpatasvir/voxilaprevir plus weight-based RBV for 24 weeks in patients with prior sofosbuvir/velpatasvir/voxilaprevir failure.[225] In a small retrospective real-world study of 40 patients from the European Resistance Study Group, retreatment strategies varied; patients received glecaprevir/pibrentasvir alone ($n = 2$) or combined with sofosbuvir ± RBV ($n = 15$), sofosbuvir/velpatasvir/voxilaprevir ± RBV ($n = 4$) or sofosbuvir/velpatasvir + RBV ($n = 1$). Treatment duration varied from 12 to 24 weeks.[286] The overall SVR12 rate was 81%, suggesting that retreatment with multiple targeted therapies can be effective in most patients.

Treatment of Unique Populations

Because of the pharmacokinetic properties and DDIs of many of the DAAs, treatment regimens may differ in unique populations, including patients with decompensated liver disease, acute HCV infection, HCV-HIV coinfection, recurrent HCV infection after LT, receipt of HCV-viremic organs, in pregnancy, children and adolescents, HCV-HBV coinfection, and chronic kidney disease (CKD). Treatment recommendations for unique populations are summarized in Table 82.7.

TABLE 82.7 DAA Regimens for Unique Populations

Decompensated Cirrhosis (Child-Pugh B or Child-Pugh C)				
	Duration (Weeks)	**Fibrosis Stage**	**SVR12 (%)**	**Study**
TREATMENT-NAÏVE DECOMPENSATED CIRRHOSIS (CHILD-PUGH B OR CHILD-PUGH C)				
Sofosbuvir (400 mg)/Velpatasvir (100 mg) + weight-based RBV				
HCV 1-6[a]	12	F4	94%–96%	ASTRAL-4, Reference [313]
Sofosbuvir (400 mg)/Velpatasvir (100 mg)				
HCV 1–6	24	F4	86%	ASTRAL-4, Reference [313]
Sofosbuvir (400 mg)/Ledipasvir (90 mg)				
HCV 1, 4–6	12	F4	75%–87%	SOLAR-1, SOLAR-2
Sofosbuvir (400 mg)/Ledipasvir (90 mg) + RBV				
HCV 1, 4–6	24	F4	77%–89%	SOLAR-1, SOLAR-2
DAA TREATMENT-EXPERIENCED DECOMPENSATED CIRRHOSIS (CHILD-PUGH B OR CHILD-PUGH C)				
Sofosbuvir (400 mg)/Velpatasvir (100 mg) + weight-based RBV				
HCV 1–6[a]	24+	F4	91%–100%	References [305,314,315]
Sofosbuvir (400 mg)/Ledipasvir (90 mg) + weight-based RBV				
HCV 1–6[a]	24+	F4	91%–100%	References [305,314,315]
Acute HCV infection				
As per treatment-naïve HCV infection (Table 82.5)				
HCV-HIV coinfection				
As per treatment-naïve HCV infection (Table 82.5)[b]				
HCV treatment in Children and Adolescents				
Weight	Dose	Duration (weeks)	SVR12	Study
Glecaprevir/Pibrentasvir				
<20 kg	Glecaprevir (150 mg)/Pibrentasvir (60 mg)	8		References [334–340]
≥20 to <30 kg	Glecaprevir (200 mg)/Pibrentasvir (80 mg)			
≥30 to <45 kg	Glecaprevir (250 mg)/Pibrentasvir (100 mg)			
≥45 kg	Glecaprevir (300 mg)/Pibrentasvir (120 mg) [Adult dose]			
Sofosbuvir (400 mg)/Velpatasvir (100 mg)				
<17 kg	Sofosbuvir (150 mg)/Velpatasvir (37.5 mg)	8		References [334–340]
≥17 to <30 kg	Sofosbuvir (200 mg)/Velpatasvir (50 mg)			
≥30 kg	Sofosbuvir (400 mg)/Velpatasvir (100 mg)			

HCV treatment in pregnancy
HCV should be treated prior to pregnancy when possible to minimize any risk of vertical transmission. If this is not possible, then treatment should ideally be initiated in the postpartum period. The AASLD-IDSA HCV Guidance Panel[225] suggest that DAA treatment may be considered during pregnancy on a case-by-case basis after a discussion of potential risks and benefits (Child-Pugh B or Child-Pugh C)

HCV recurrence postliver transplantation Duration (Weeks)	Fibrosis Stage	SVR12 (%)	Study
Glecaprevir (300 mg)/Pibrentasvir (120 mg)			
12	F0-4	96%–98%	MAGELLAN-2, Reference [360]
Sofosbuvir (400 mg)/Velpatasvir (100 mg)			
12	F0-4	96%	Reference [361]
Sofosbuvir (400 mg)/Ledipasvir (90 mg)			
12	F0-4 HCV 1, 4–6	94%–97%	SOLAR-2, Reference [363]

[a]Protease (NS3/4A) inhibitors are contraindicated.
[b]Careful attention must be paid to drug-drug interactions prior to commencement of DAA therapy.
F0-3, METAVIR fibrosis stages 0–3; *F4*, METAVIR fibrosis stage 4, decompensated (Child-Pugh B/C); *RBV*, ribavirin; *SVR12*, sustained virologic response 12 weeks after completion of therapy.
*If Y93H NS5A RAS is present.
†In patients without baseline Y93H RAS.

Treatment-Naïve Patients With Decompensated (Child-Pugh B and Child-Pugh C) Cirrhosis

In the IFN era, treatment of patients with decompensated cirrhosis was extremely challenging, because both IFN and RBV were considered contraindicated due to the risk of hepatic failure, in addition to the poor efficacy and poor safety profile of these agents in decompensated cirrhotic patients. The introduction of IFN-free DAA regimens has simplified HCV treatment in these patients; however, the optimal timing of antiviral therapy while a patient is on the transplant waiting list is still unknown, as there is a trade-off between potentially improving clinical and biochemical parameters by treating HCV infection as most patients with decompensated cirrhosis who achieve SVR12 experience significant biochemical and clinical improvement,[288–294] but prolonging the time on the waiting list or providing insufficient improvement to obviate the need for LT.[295] While defined predictors of benefit or further deterioration with DAAs have not been clearly established, a modeling study suggested that treatment is beneficial at a MELD threshold between 23 and 27, although the cutoff value may vary depending on the UNOS region.[296] Therefore patients with MELD scores greater than 23–27 or severe portal hypertension may benefit more from LT and DAA therapy in the peritransplant period rather than immediate antiviral therapy.[297] Because the HCV protease inhibitors (glecaprevir, voxilaprevir) undergo hepatic elimination, the regimens containing these agents are contraindicated in patients with decompensated cirrhosis.

Recommended DAA regimens for decompensated cirrhotics include the pangenotypic regimen of sofosbuvir (400 mg)/velpatasvir (100 mg) plus weight-based RBV for 12 weeks if RBV eligible, or sofosbuvir (400 mg)/velpatasvir (100 mg) for 24 weeks if RBV ineligible. This is based on data from the ASTRAL-4 study where patients with decompensated cirrhosis were randomized to receive sofosbuvir/velpatasvir for 12 weeks, sofosbuvir/velpatasvir plus RBV for 12 weeks, or sofosbuvir/velpatasvir for 24 weeks. SVR12 rates were 83%, 94%, and 86%, respectively.[298] Patients with HCV genotype 3 infection had superior SVR12 rates in the RBV arm, suggesting that patients with HCV genotype 3 benefit significantly from the addition of RBV. Similar findings were observed in a real-world study of sofosbuvir/velpatasvir plus RBV in decompensated cirrhotics, where the SVR12 rate was 96%.[299] Improvements in Child-Pugh and MELD scores were seen at 84% and 65%, respectively.

Another recommended regimen for decompensated cirrhotics with HCV genotype 1, 4–6, is sofosbuvir (400 mg)/ledipasvir (90 mg) plus RBV for 12 weeks, if RBV eligible, or sofosbuvir (400 mg)/ledipasvir (90 mg) for 24 weeks for those that are not eligible for RBV. These recommendations are based on data from the SOLAR-1 trial of HCV genotype 1 and 4 patients with decompensated cirrhosis.[290] Patients were randomized to sofosbuvir/ledipasvir plus RBV for 12 or 24 weeks. SVR12 rates were 87% and 89% in Child-Pugh B patients receiving 12 and 24 weeks of treatment, respectively. Similarly, in the Child-Pugh C patients, SVR12 rates were 86% and 87% in the 12- and 24-week treatment groups, respectively. Adverse events increased with increasing treatment duration, and most of the serious adverse events were attributable to RBV. This DAA regimen was also evaluated in the multicenter SOLAR-2 study, with a similar design[288] SVR12 rates were 85% and 75% in the Child-Pugh B and C patients receiving 12 weeks of sofosbuvir/ledipasvir plus RBV, respectively, and 90% and 77% in the Child-Pugh B and C patients receiving 24 weeks of therapy.

DAA Treatment-Experienced Patients With Decompensated (Child-Pugh B and Child-Pugh C) Cirrhosis

The retreatment of patients with decompensated cirrhosis who have failed prior DAA therapies remains challenging owing to the inability to use a triple DAA regimen containing an NS3/4A protease inhibitor (glecaprevir or voxilaprevir), which is included in all the salvage regimens. There are no clinical trials on outcomes of patients with decompensated cirrhosis with prior sofosbuvir plus NS5A failure. Retreatment with sofosbuvir/velpatasvir plus weight-based RBV or sofosbuvir/ledipasvir plus low-dose RBV, increasing as tolerated, for 24 weeks is recommended, and showed favorable SVR12 rates of 91%–100% in small studies of patients with compensated cirrhosis[291,300,301]; therefore these treatment recommendations have also been expanded to the decompensated cirrhotic DAA treatment-experienced population.

Acute HCV Infection

As mentioned, the treatment of acute hepatitis C infection is recommended both to prevent progression to and sequelae of chronic liver disease, but also to reduce onward transmission and reduce the prevalence and incidence of hepatitis C infection. Treatment recommendations are the same as for treatment-naïve chronic hepatitis C infection (Table 82.5).

HCV-HIV Coinfection

Owing to their shared transmission routes, HCV-HIV coinfection is not uncommon. Patients with HCV-HIV coinfection are likely to progress more rapidly to cirrhosis than are HCV-monoinfected patients; therefore treatment of HCV infection should always be considered in this group.[302] Patients are at even higher risk of progression of hepatic fibrosis if they are female, are older than 33 years of age, have an increase in the CD4 count of less than 100/mm^3 with ART, continue to have a detectable HIV viral load during ART, or have untreated HCV infection.

In the IFN era, SVR rates were significantly lower in HCV-HIV-coinfected patients compared with HCV-monoinfected patients[303]; however, SVR12 rates are now equivalent in HCV-monoinfected and HCV-HIV-coinfected individuals with the newer IFN-free DAA regimens.[289,295–297,304] DDIs between antiretroviral drugs and HCV protease inhibitors need to be considered (see earlier, Table 82.4, and http://hep-druginteractions.org). Otherwise, contraindications to antiviral therapy for HCV infection in HCV-HIV-coinfected patients do not differ from those for monoinfected patients.

As mentioned above, HCV-HIV-coinfected individuals who are DAA treatment-naïve without cirrhosis or with compensated cirrhosis can be treated similarly to treatment-naïve HCV-monoinfected patients (Table 82.5). This is based on a number of studies demonstrating that the SVR12 rates and adverse events are similar to those with HCV monoinfection.[305–309] However, there can be significant DDIs between DAAs and antiretroviral medications, so caution and attention must be practiced when treating these individuals. A summary of regimens not recommended in patients with HIV/HCV coinfection (Table 82.8).

HCV Treatment in Children and Adolescents

HCV policies and elimination efforts have largely focused on the adult population,[310] despite there being an estimated 3.26 million people under the age of 18 living with HCV infection worldwide.[311] Furthermore, the rising incidence and prevalence of HCV infection in young women of childbearing age[312–314] carries a parallel risk of increased rates of mother-to-child transmission, the main transmission route in children (6% mother-to-child transmission rate).[313–317] However, children were excluded from the DAA registration studies.

Recently, two pangenotypic FDC regimens have been approved by the FDA for the treatment of HCV infection in children as young as 3 years of age,[318,319] the same two pangenotypic regimens recommended in treatment-naïve adults (Table 82.7). SVR12 rates were comparable to those observed in adults.[320–326]

TABLE 82.8 DAA Regimens Not Recommended for Patients With HCV-HIV Coinfection

Regimens Not Recommended for Patients With HIV/HCV Coinfection	
Not Recommended	**Rating**
Antiretroviral treatment interruption to allow HCV therapy is not recommended	III, A
Elbasvir/grazoprevir should not be used with cobicistat, efavirenz, etravirine, nevirapine, or any HIV protease inhibitor	III, B
Glecaprevir/pibrentasvir should not be used with atazanavir, efavirenz, etravirine, nevirapine, or ritonavir-containing antiretroviral regimens	III, B
Sofosbuvir/velpatasvir should not be used with efavirenz, etravirine, or nevirapine	III, B
Sofosbuvir/velpatasvir/voxilaprevir should not be used with efavirenz, etravirine, nevirapine, ritonavir-boosted atazanavir, or ritonavir-boosted lopinavir	III, B
Sofosbuvir-based regimens should not be used with tipranavir	III, B
Ribavirin should not be used with didanosine, stavudine, or zidovudine	III, B

From AASLD/IDSA HCV Guidance: Recommendations for Testing, Managing, and Treating Hepatitis C. Update Dec 2023.

HCV in Pregnancy

In the US, the opioid epidemic has been associated with a threefold increase in the incidence of acute hepatitis C between 2010 and 2015.[327] Importantly, more than a third were among women, and the highest incidence was in women of childbearing age (20–39 years).[328] Globally, it is estimated that up to 8% of pregnant women have markers of hepatitis C infection. In parallel with the increasing incidence and prevalence of hepatitis C infection, the percentage of pregnant women testing positive to hepatitis C infection has also increased from 2.6% in 2011 to 3.6% in 2016.[317] Therefore all pregnant women should be screened for hepatitis C infection during pregnancy.[225,329,330] However, pregnant and lactating women were excluded from the large registration studies of DAA therapy for hepatitis C infection leading to questions regarding the safety of these regimens during conception and pregnancy, as well as ongoing concerns about onward mother-to-child transmission of hepatitis C.

The FDA categorization of drugs for use in pregnancy of all the DAAs is category B, indicating that animal studies have now demonstrated evidence of harm to the fetus but there are no well-controlled studies in pregnant women. It should be noted that ribavirin is category X (teratogenic) and therefore is a contraindication during pregnancy, and women and men should avoid becoming pregnant for 6 months following treatment with ribavirin.

Although there are no large-scale clinical trials to evaluate the safety of DAA therapy during pregnancy, there is an increasing body of data from smaller studies and case series regarding DAA therapy during pregnancy.[331–334] To date, these studies have not demonstrated any significant safety concerns, and SVR12 rates have been comparable. Therefore DAA treatment of hepatitis C infection in pregnant women is not routinely recommended. Given the short duration of treatment with the DAA regimens (8–12 weeks), current recommendations are that HCV should be treated prior to pregnancy when possible to minimize any risk of vertical transmission. If this is not possible, then treatment should ideally be initiated in the postpartum period. The AASLD-IDSA HCV Guidance Panel[225] suggests that DAA treatment may be considered during pregnancy on a case-by-case basis after a discussion of potential risks and benefits.

DAA Treatment of HCV Recurrence Postliver Transplantation

Prior to the widespread availability of DAAs, the sequelae of hepatitis C infection were the leading indication for liver transplantation in the Western world, which had been rising in the years prior to their introduction.[335] Although the proportion of HCV-related liver transplants is now reducing, liver transplantation for HCV-related complications is still occurring (see Chapter 99). Patients who have detectable HCV RNA in serum at the time of LT almost universally experience HCV reinfection of the allograft. The natural history of hepatitis C after LT is characterized by more rapid progression of liver fibrosis. At least 25% of patients will develop cirrhosis within 5–10 years after transplantation.[292,293] Once cirrhosis is established, transplanted patients show an accelerated natural history, with decompensation rates as high as 40% after 12 months. Across different countries and transplantation programs, the 5-year posttransplantation survival rate for patients with hepatitis C has been significantly lower than those of patients who underwent LT for other chronic liver diseases. Factors associated with graft loss in HCV-infected patients include an older donor age, steatosis of the donor organ, specific immunosuppressive regimens, female sex, high necroinflammatory activity in the allograft 1 year after transplantation, and high HCV viral loads.[292,294] Additional factors thought to influence the long-term outcome of graft HCV infection include herpes virus infections,[336] the degree of HLA matching, and the matching of the *IFN-λ3* haplotypes of the donor and recipient.[337–339] Cellular immune responses by both T cells and NK cells are thought to play a major role in the pathogenesis of chronic hepatitis C after transplantation. HCV-specific T-cell responses have been associated with improved histologic and clinical outcomes and also with spontaneous HCV clearance after LT.[340] Reducing serum HCV RNA to undetectable levels before transplantation may prevent reinfection in some cases[341,342]; this was difficult in the IFN era due to the risks of significant morbidity and mortality with IFN-based therapy. The IFN-free DAA regimens have transformed HCV treatment in these patients[343]; however, as mentioned earlier, there is a trade-off between potential improvement in clinical and biochemical parameters and delaying transplantation. Therefore if HCV infection cannot be safely treated or the benefit of treatment prior to transplantation is limited, HCV infection can be treated after LT (see Table 82.3). Treatment of HCV infection early posttransplantation, after recovery from the initial operation, is likely to improve graft survival and long-term outcomes significantly in patients with HCV recurrence after transplantation. Ideally, patients should be on stable immunosuppressive regimens at the time antiviral therapy is initiated.

Immunosuppressive therapies have been suggested to influence the outcome of graft HCV infection. The two approved calcineurin inhibitors (CNIs), cyclosporine and tacrolimus, have been studied extensively in liver transplant recipients with HCV infection.[344] Some earlier studies suggested that immunosuppression with cyclosporine might be associated with a better histologic outcome of graft hepatitis C; however, the vast majority of subsequent studies did not identify major differences between cyclosporine and tacrolimus in the outcome of HCV infection after LT.[344] Conversely, a retrospective study of more than 8000 HCV-positive liver-transplanted persons showed that death, graft failure, liver failure owing to recurrent disease, and acute cellular rejection were slightly more frequent in the cyclosporine-treated group than in the tacrolimus-treated group.[345]

Early treatment with DAAs during the peri-transplantation period allows for the opportunity to clear HCV either before (prevention of recurrence) or after liver transplantation (treatment of recurrence). Treatment should be initiated as soon as possible postliver transplantation to reduce the risk of hepatic fibrosis in the donor liver and to particularly avoid fibrosing cholestatic hepatitis. DDIs are an important consideration prior to considering HCV treatment and should be addressed prior to commencement of DAA therapy. In particular, DDIs between DAA agents and CNIs are complicated and unpredictable; sofosbuvir/velpatasvir/voxilaprevir should not be coadministered with cyclosporin due to significant increases in the AUC of the DAAs, and coadministration of glecaprevir/pibrentasvir and cyclosporine >100 mg/day is also not recommended (Table 82.7).

The current guidelines recommend the pangenotypic FDC of glecaprevir (300 mg)/pibrentasvir (120 mg) or sofosbuvir (400 mg)/velpatasvir (100 mg) both for 12 weeks for patients without cirrhosis and with compensated cirrhosis. The MAGELLAN-2 trail evaluated glecaprevir/pibrentasvir for 12 weeks in liver and kidney transplant recipients, excluding patients with cirrhosis. Patients receiving cyclosporine >100 mg/day and prednisolone >10 mg/day were excluded, but all other stable immunosuppression regimens were included. SVR12 rates were 98%, and treatment was well tolerated.[346] Similarly high SVR12 rates were observed with sofosbuvir/velpatasvir for 12 weeks, where overall SVR12 rates were 96%.[347] Treatment was well tolerated, and no change to immunosuppressed was required for DDIs or concerns about rejection.

Sofosbuvir (400 mg)/ledipasvir (90 mg) for 12 weeks is a further recommended regimen for patients with HCV genotype 1, 4–6 infection. The SOLAR-2 study investigated this regimen for 12 and 24 weeks, and transplant recipients were included.[348] SVR12 rates were 94% and 100% in the 12- and 24-week arms in transplant recipients without cirrhosis, respectively, and 97% in the 12- and 24-week arms in those with compensated cirrhosis. Similar results were observed in a real-world study of sofosbuvir/ledipasvir for 12 or 24 weeks with or without RBV.[349] The cohort included patients with liver or kidney transplantation, and 44% had cirrhosis, 26% with hepatic decompensation, and 54% had prior treatment failure with a non-NS5A inhibitor. SVR12 rates were 97% in the group receiving RBV and 95% in the group not receiving RBV.

HCV Treatment Following Receipt of HCV-Viremic Donor Organs in HCV-Uninfected Recipients

There is still a paucity of organs available for transplantation which is inadequate to meet the waiting list demands. To increase the pool of available organs, the donor organ pool is increasingly being expanded to include more marginal donor organs, including HCV-viremic organs; previously, HCV-viremic organs were discarded. However, the widespread availability and high efficacy of DAAs have significantly changed the framework of organ allocation, and HCV-viremic organs are increasingly being offered to both HCV-infected recipients and HCV-uninfected recipients. This approach has been shown to be safe with successful treatment of HCV in the recipients and, importantly, has been shown to reduce the time to transplantation and reduce waitlist mortality, with comparable graft survival outcomes.[350] Extensive consultation and informed consent are required risks and benefits, including the risks of HCV infection, risks to caregivers, and risks and benefits of DAA treatment. To reduce the likelihood of liver and extrahepatic manifestations and complications of HCV infection, HCV treatment should be commenced as soon as possible upon receiving an HCV-viremic organ in an HCV-uninfected recipients.[351–355]

In a multicenter prospective study of 24 HCV-uninfected recipients receiving HCV-viremic livers (n = 13) and kidneys (n = 11), 96% became viremic following transplantation with a median HCV RNA level at Day 3 of 6.5 $\log_{10}$ IU/mL in the liver transplant recipients and 3.6 $\log_{10}$ IU/mL in the renal transplant recipients. All patients received sofosbuvir (400 mg)/velpatasvir (100 mg) for 12 weeks. SVR12 rate was 100%, and no treatment-related adverse events were observed.

In a second multicenter study of 30 HCV-uninfected recipients receiving HCV-viremic kidney transplants, the pangenotypic FDC of glecaprevir (300 mg)/pibrentasvir (120 mg) for 8 weeks was administered earlier posttransplant, between 2 and 5 days posttransplantation.[352] All patients achieved SVR12, and no severe adverse events were deemed related to DAA therapy.

Owing to the concern of HCV-related complications, further studies have evaluated preventive or preemptive strategies of HCV treatment postreceipt of HCV-viremic organs in HCV-uninfected individuals, starting treatment on Day 0 (preventative/prophylactic strategy) or Day 0–7 (preemptive strategy). The presence of HCV viremia was not required to initiate DAA therapy. In addition to extremely high SVR12 rates, HCV-related complications were significantly lower with this strategy of early HCV treatment.[352] Longer term follow-up data has shown similar or superior graft outcomes that are comparable to HCV-negative donor organs.[356,357]

HCV-HBV Coinfection and HBV Reactivation During DAA Therapy

Because of the shared transmission routes, all HCV-positive individuals should undergo testing for HBV infection. Although HBV reactivation is a well-recognized complication of immunosuppressive therapy, it has been an unexpected sequela of DAA therapy in patients previously exposed to HBV. In the registration studies for each of the approved IFN-free DAA regimens, HCV-HBV-coinfected individuals were excluded. However, since the approval and widespread use of these agents, more than 24 cases of HBV reactivation have been reported to the FDA or published,[302,303,306,307,309,358–361] including ALF in two fatal cases and another case requiring LT, thereby prompting a black box warning from the FDA. Interestingly, HBV reactivation in these reported cases occurred in individuals with current HBV infection (hepatitis B surface antigen positive with or without detectable HBV DNA), occult infection, and, most surprisingly, past infection (hepatitis B surface antigen negative, HBV DNA negative, but antibody to hepatitis B core antigen positive). In contrast to IFN, DAAs target specific HCV proteins involved in the HCV replication cycle and are not known to have direct immunomodulatory properties or have activity against HBV; therefore the mechanism underlying HBV reactivation in this setting is unknown.

A systematic review and meta-analysis of HBV reactivation in HCV-HBV-coinfected individuals following IFN-based and DAA-based IFN-free therapy demonstrated that the frequency of HBV reactivation is similar with IFN-based (14.5%) and DAA-based regimens (12.2%).[302] However, the clinical presentation differed between the two treatment regimens, with HBV reactivation occurring earlier and having a more severe clinical presentation during DAA therapy. Because the true frequency of HBV reactivation is still unknown, prophylactic antiviral therapy for HBV is not recommended; patients with HBV (current or past) infection should be monitored during DAA therapy for HCV. HBV reactivation should be suspected in any patient with a sudden increase in serum aminotransferase levels during DAA therapy.

Anti-HBc-positive individuals were not excluded from the large registration clinical trials, and no cases of HBV reactivation were reported. In a study of 173 HBsAg-negative HCV-viremic individuals where 60% were found to be anti-HBc positive without detectable HBV DNA, no HBV reactivation was observed.[362] In a second study of 124 patients with occult HBV infection (HBsAg negative with measurable HBV DNA) receiving DAAs for HCV infection, no HBV reactivation was observed. Again, reassuringly, no cases of HBV reactivation were observed.[363]

In HBsAg-positive individuals, data from the US Veterans database of more than 62,920 individuals receiving DAA therapy, HBV serology was performed in around 85% of individuals (0.7% HBsAg positivity).[364] HBV reactivation was seen in 9 of the 62,920 patients; 8 were HBsAg positive at baseline (8 of 53,784 patients, 0.01%), including 1 who was on concurrent tenofovir for their hepatitis B, and 1 was isolated anti-HBc positive (1 of 18,462 patients, <0.006%). A hepatitis B flare was seen in 1 patient who was HBsAg positive, with a peak ALT of 1540 U/mL with a peak HBV DNA 22,200,000 IU/mL, although the baseline HBV DNA level was 2361 IU/mL and within HBV treatment initiation guidelines.

Therefore it is recommended that all patients testing positive to HCV also undergo testing for HBV infection. For those who are anti-HBc positive, the risk of HBV reactivation remains extremely low, and these patients do not need to undergo any specific monitoring during DAA therapy. For HBsAg-positive individuals, HBV therapy should be initiated based on HBV current guidelines, and it is reasonable to monitor patients who do not require HBV antiviral therapy during DAA therapy, although this should not delay HCV treatment given the very low risk.

Chronic Kidney Disease

HCV itself can cause CKD as an extrahepatic complication of HCV infection. Furthermore, there is an increased frequency of proteinuria and CKD, accelerated progression of CKD, and higher all-cause mortality on dialysis in HCV-infected persons.[339,365] Therefore timely treatment of HCV infection is important to optimize outcomes in persons with CKD. In the IFN/RBV era, treatment was difficult owing to the toxicities associated with these therapies, particularly anemia. However, the development of IFN- and RBV-free regimens has dramatically simplified antiviral therapy in these patients.

Stages 1, 2, 3, 4, or 5 CKD

Stage 1 CKD (normal renal function) is defined by an eGFR greater than 90 mL/min. Stage 2 CKD (mild renal impairment) is defined by an eGFR of 60–89 mL/min. Stage 3 CKD (moderate renal impairment) is defined by an eGFR of 30–59 mL/min. Stage 4 CKD (severe renal impairment) is defined by an eGFR of 15–29 mL/min. Stage 5 CKD (ESRD) is defined by an eGFR of less than 15 mL/min. In patients with stages 1–5 CKD, no dose modifications are required for any of the approved DAAs, and, therefore, DAA regimens should be chosen based on HCV genotype, fibrosis stage, and treatment history, as discussed earlier.

Monitoring and Safety

Monitoring

Before antiviral therapy is started, baseline liver biochemical test levels, a CBC, and an INR should be obtained. A baseline assessment of liver fibrosis stage is important as this will determine if individuals will require HCC surveillance following DAA therapy (even if SVR12 is achieved, the risk of HCC still persists in patients with pretreatment cirrhosis) or surveillance for portal-hypertensive complications. A pregnancy test is required in women before DAA therapy is initiated. An HCV PCR should be performed to confirm viremia and therefore need for DAA therapy. With the development of pangenotypic DAA regimens, the requirement for HCV genotyping has been reduced. However, HCV genotype is useful in regions where access to pangenotypic regimens is limited and also to evaluate treatment failures to determine if they are due to true virological failure or reinfection. HCV genotype may also be important to determine DAA treatment choice in patients with cirrhosis (see earlier). Pretreatment serum HCV RNA quantification (viral load) only influences treatment choice and duration with shortened therapy with the FDC of sofosbuvir/ledipasvir (see earlier); HCV viral load otherwise does not impact DAA choice or duration. On-treatment viral kinetics do not predict subsequent SVR12 with the newer DAA regimens; therefore HCV RNA testing during therapy is not recommended. An HCV PCR should be performed at least 12 weeks after completion of therapy to determine if a

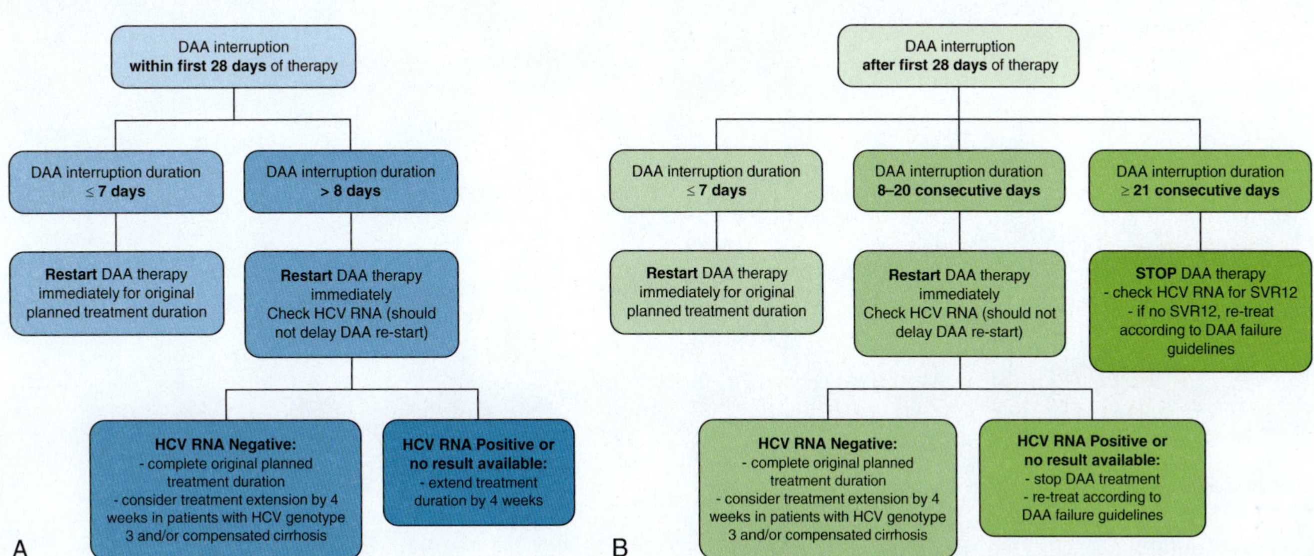

Fig. 82.7 Management of DAA nonadherence if (A) DAA interruption is within the first 28 days of therapy and (B) if DAA interruption is after the first 28 days of therapy. (Data adapted from Bhattacharya D, Aronsohn A, Price J, Lo Re V, AASLD-IDSA HCV Guidance Panel. Hepatitis C guidance 2023 update: AASLD-IDSA recommendations for testing, managing, and treating hepatitis C virus infection. *Clin Infect Dis*. 2023.)

cure has been achieved. As past HCV infection does not provide lasting immunity against HCV reinfection, at least annual HCV testing (or more frequent depending on the clinical scenario) with an HCV PCR is recommended for individuals with ongoing risk factors for hepatitis C acquisition.

In addition, due to the shared transmission routes and risk of HBV reactivation (see earlier), HIV and HBV testing should be performed.

With RBV, anemia, cough, pharyngitis, insomnia, dyspnea, pruritus, rash, nausea, and anorexia are the most common side effects. The most serious side effects are anemia and teratogenicity. Hemolytic anemia is reversible and usually resolves within the first month after therapy is stopped. The full blood count should be monitored during DAA regimens that include RBV. If the patient has significant comorbidities that may be exacerbated by anemia, an RBV-free DAA regimen can be chosen.

Safety

DAAs are well tolerated. The most common adverse events reported are nausea, headache, and fatigue. Specific adverse events relevant to each DAA are discussed earlier. Biochemical abnormalities are uncommon and generally not clinically significant; therefore specific monitoring during DAA therapy is not required.

Medication adherence is not uncommon and may occur in clinical practice, thereby potentially compromising SVR12 rates and contributing to RAS development. Data regarding DAA medication nonadherence is limited; however, studies that have examined this have reported incomplete DAA adherence in 10%–40% of patients.[366–369] In one of these studies, adherence was assessed in 103 participants with hepatitis C infection and recent injecting drug use receiving DAAs and a history of recent injecting drug use.[367] Overall median adherence to DAA therapy (defined as ≥90% adherence) was 94%. Although 32% were considered nonadherent, 61% of these episodes of nonadherence lasted 1–2 days only, and nonadherence increased as the treatment course progressed. Despite this, SVR12 rates did not differ between those who were adherent compared to those who were not considered to be adherent (94% in both groups). Inconsistent timing of DAA ingestion was independently associated with nonadherence.[367] Studies have since demonstrated that early treatment and premature discontinuation significantly reduces SVR12 rates; SVR12 was 50% in those completing <4 weeks DAA therapy, compared to 99% in those receiving ≥4 weeks of therapy.[370] In a second larger study of 1447 patients, factors associated with medical nonadherence were alcohol use, younger age, non-white race, and DAA regimen, but not substance misuse or history of mental health disorders.[369] While large-scale studies evaluating the degree of DAA adherence whereby SVR12 rates become negatively impacted are lacking, these data suggest that both timing and duration of medication nonadherence are important in determining likelihood of subsequent treatment failure; these factors form the basis of current recommendations for the management of DAA nonadherence (Fig. 82.7).

Acknowledgment

The authors acknowledge the contributions of Drs. Heiner Wedemeyer, Jacqueline G. O'Leary, and Gary L. Davis to this chapter in previous editions of the book.

Full references for this chapter can be found at https://ebooks.health.elsevier.com.

83 Hepatitis D

Asif Hitawala, Marc G. Ghany

IN THIS CHAPTER

Hepatitis D virus (HDV) (also known as the delta agent) is the causative agent of hepatitis D and is associated with both acute and chronic hepatitis. It is one of the most severe forms of chronic viral hepatitis. HDV is classified as a satellite virus, because it requires the presence of hepatitis B surface antigen (HBsAg) for its life cycle (see Chapter 81).

EPIDEMIOLOGY

HDV infection occurs worldwide. It is estimated that 5% of HBsAg carriers worldwide are infected with HDV, corresponding to approximately 12–15 million persons.[1] The true global prevalence, however, is difficult to ascertain. This is highlighted by the results of three recent meta-analyses that provided widely varying pooled prevalence estimates ranging from 0.16% to 0.98% among the general population and 4.5%–15.6% among HBsAg-positive individuals worldwide. This translates to an estimated 12–72 million HDV-infected individuals globally.[2–4] Several factors contribute to this uncertainty, such as underreporting from many areas of the world, lack of good-quality prevalence studies, the small scale of most studies, the lack of standardized screening for HDV among hepatitis B virus (HBV) carriers, and lack of gold standard diagnostic testing. The prevalence of HDV infection is reported to be highest in the Mediterranean region, the Middle East, central and northern Asia, west and central Africa, Taiwan, and the Amazon basin (Fig. 83.1).[1] The prevalence is low in North America, Northern Europe, Japan, and Korea.

Although HDV requires HBV to complete its replication cycle, the geographic distribution of HDV does not always mirror that of HBV. For example, the prevalence of HDV infection is relatively low in the Far East, a region endemic for HBV infection. Possible explanations for this discordance may relate to different routes of transmission and virulence of the various HDV genotypes and differences in genetic susceptibility of individuals to infection.

Since the 1980s the prevalence of HDV infection has declined among the local population in certain regions of the world, such as Mediterranean countries, but has remained stable in other regions, for example, Africa and the Amazon basin. In Italy, the frequency of HDV infection in HBV carriers declined from 24.6% to 14.4% between 1983 and 1992.[5] Subsequently, the frequency fell to 8.7% in 1997,[6] but then increased to 11.9% in 2014.[7] In 2020 the overall prevalence was noted to be 9.9%; although it had decreased to 6.4% in the native population, it increased to 26.4% in the nonnative population due to immigration or persons from endemic regions.[8] Similarly, in Spain, the frequency declined from 15% to 7.1% from 1975 to 1992 and subsequently to less than 5% after 2010.[9,10] In Turkey, the frequency declined from 31% to 11% between 1980 and 2005[11] and decreased further to about 3% by 2011.[12] In Taiwan, the frequency decreased from 23.7% to 4.2% between 1983 and 1996 and remained low in the general population (4.4%) through 2012, declining further to 1.2% by 2021.[13–15] The decline in prevalence in these regions has been attributed to widespread administration of the hepatitis B vaccine, greater use of barrier protection to prevent sexually transmitted diseases and improved socioeconomic conditions. However, the frequency of HDV may be on the rise again in the Mediterranean region due to immigration from endemic regions and continued transmission among persons who inject drugs (PWID).[16–18]

Data on the prevalence of HDV infection in the United States vary widely based on the population studied. The National Health and Nutrition Examination Survey, a population-based survey spanning the period 1999–2012, reported an overall prevalence of HDV infection of 0.02%.[19] A higher prevalence rate of 0.11% was reported for the period 2011–2016, corresponding to approximately 357,000 persons with active or past HDV infection.[20] This is probably an underestimate of the true prevalence due to the exclusion of high-risk populations, such as homeless, incarcerated, and institutionalized persons. A retrospective analysis from the Veterans Healthcare Administration of all HBsAg-positive veterans from the period October 1999 to December 2013 reported an HDV frequency of 3.4%; however, only 8.5% of the at-risk population were tested for HDV.[21] By contrast, surveys of PWID in Baltimore and San Francisco have reported a much higher frequency of HDV infection among HBsAg-positive individuals of 50% and 36%, respectively.[22,23]

HDV is highly endemic in the chronic hepatitis B population in the western Amazon region of South America, where the frequency is 32%.[24,25] In Africa, a systematic review of the prevalence of HDV infection among the general population in the sub-Saharan region reported a pooled rate of 7.3% in West Africa, 24.6% in Central Africa, and 0.05% in East and Southern Africa.[26]

Modes of Transmission

HDV is transmitted similarly to HBV (see Chapter 81), primarily the parenteral route through exposure to blood and other

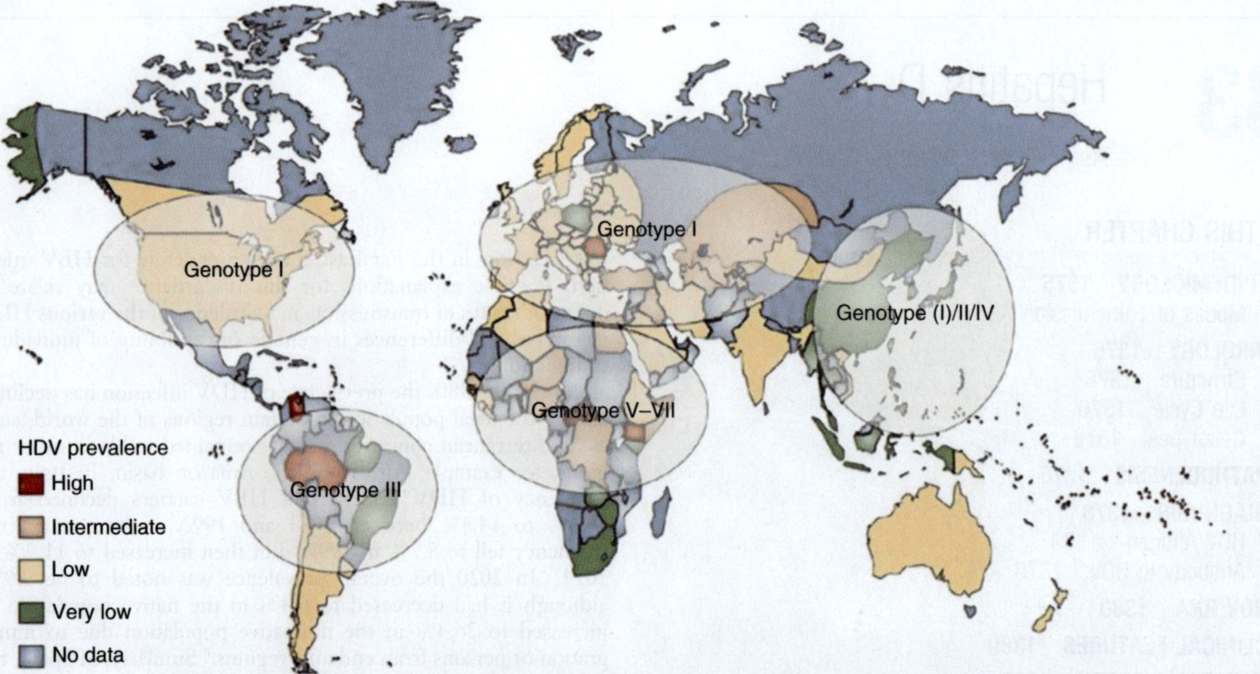

Fig. 83.1 Global prevalence of HDV and distribution of HDV genotypes. Eight HDV genotypes have been reported. HDV genotype 1 is found worldwide, whereas genotype 2 is found in Japan, Taiwan, and the Yakutia region of Russia. Genotype 3 (the most diverse genotype) is found predominantly in the Amazon basin, whereas genotype 4 is found in Taiwan and Japan. HDV genotypes 5–8 are found in individuals of African origin. Map lines delineate study areas and do not necessarily depict accepted national boundaries.

infectious body fluids.[27] Consequently, the primary modes of transmission are through injection drug use and sexual contact, but intrafamilial spread has been reported in endemic regions.[28–32] In contrast to HBV, perinatal transmission is not a major route of spread of HDV.

VIROLOGY

HDV is considered a satellite virus. Satellite viruses are subviral particles that carry their own distinct nucleic acid, usually RNA, that requires a helper virus for transmission and multiplication. HDV is the only member of the Deltaviridae family, *Deltavirus* genus. It is the smallest known infectious agent to infect humans and bears no similarity to other infectious animal pathogens.[33] HDV has been likened to plant viroids because their RNAs share several features that include a circular structure, compact folding due to intramolecular base pairing, and replication via a rolling-circle mechanism.

Structure

The complete infectious virion is a small, spherical particle of about 36 nm in diameter. It is composed of an outer lipoprotein envelope, consisting of small, middle, and large HBsAg antigen, that surrounds an inner ribonucleoprotein (RNP). The RNP consists of the small and large hepatitis delta antigen (HDAg) complexed to the viral genome. The viral genome is a single-stranded, negative-sense RNA of approximately 1700 nucleotides.[34] Its high guanosine-cytosine content results in self-complementization of nearly 74% of the nucleotides, thereby allowing the genome to form a partially double-stranded, rod-like RNA structure.[35]

Life Cycle

Both HBV and HDV share a similar mechanism of entry into the hepatocyte. The HDV virion interacts initially with heparan-sulfate proteoglycans mediated by the pre-S1 domain of the large HBsAg and the antigenic loop of the S domain (Fig. 83.2). On anchoring to the hepatocyte, HDV binds irreversibly to the sodium taurocholate cotransporting polypeptide (NTCP) via the myristoylated N-terminal region of pre-S1 of the large HBsAg and is taken up into the hepatocyte by an ill-defined mechanism.[36] Fusion of the viral membrane to the endosomal membrane is postulated with the release of the RNP into the cytoplasm. The RNP complex is transported to the nucleus via a nuclear localization signal within the HDAg.[37]

Replication of the HDV RNA genome occurs in the nucleus using the hepatocyte RNA polymerases I to III, a process that is dependent on the small HDAg.[38,39] Recently, the host enzymes carbamoyl-phosphate synthetase 2, aspartate transcarbamylase, and dihydroorotase (CAD) and the estrogen receptor alpha were identified as host factors important for HDV replication.[40] Targeting these host factors may have therapeutic potential. HDV employs a double-rolling circle replication strategy, whereby HDV RNA is synthesized first as linear antigenomic RNA that contains multimers of the genome that are cleaved to a uniform 1-U length by a ribozyme encoded in the antigenic strand (see Fig. 83.2).[41] Circularization of the monomers is achieved by the ribozyme and cellular ligases.[42,43] In the second rolling circle replication, the circular monomeric RNAs serve as templates for the production of HDV genomic multimers that are cleaved by a second ribozyme encoded in the genomic strand.

The HDV genome contains a single open reading frame that is located on the antigenomic RNA strand from which a linear

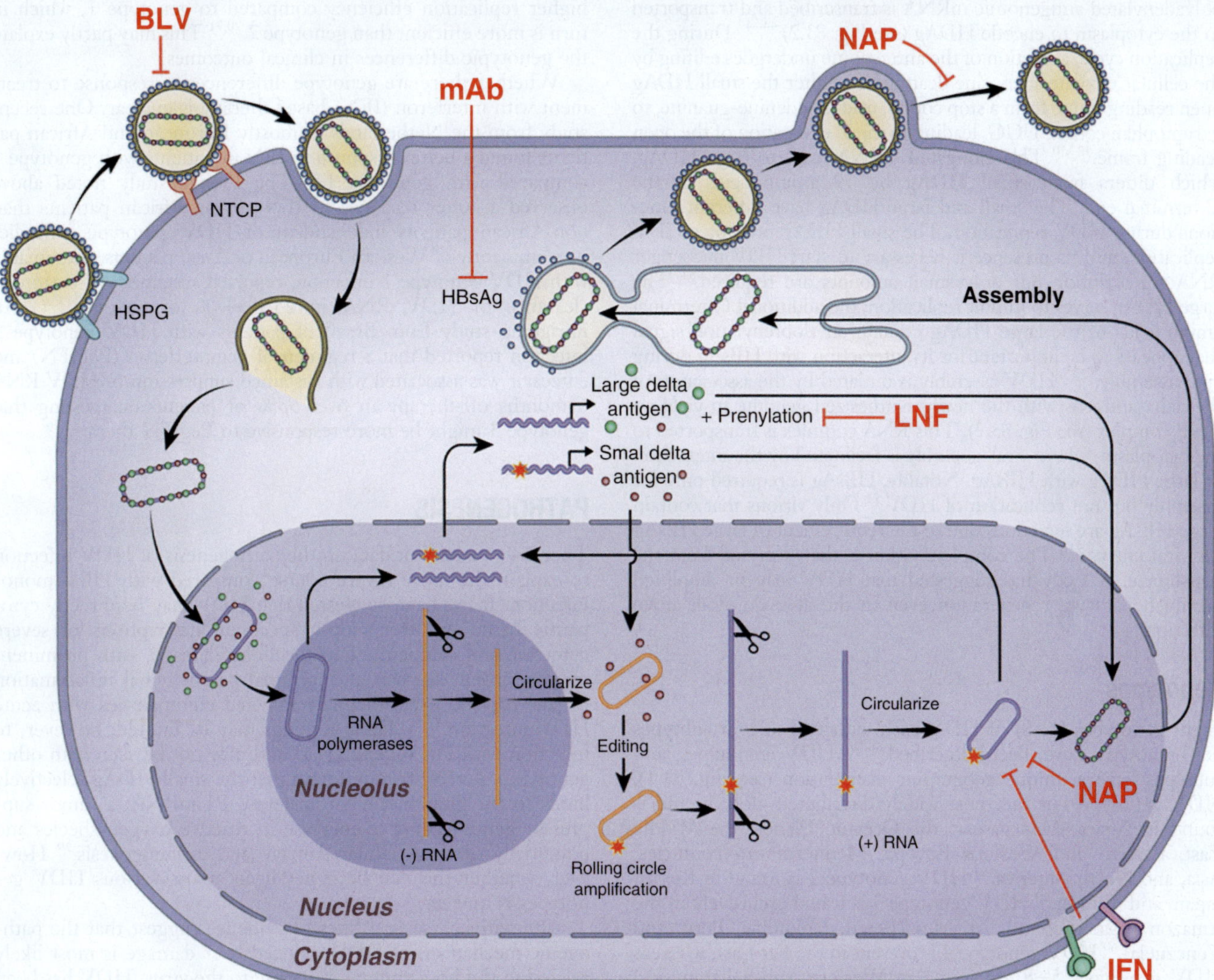

Fig. 83.2 HDV life cycle. The HDV virion interacts initially with heparan-sulfate proteoglycans (HSPG) mediated by the pre-S1 domain of the large hepatitis B surface antigen (HBsAg) and the antigenic loop of the S domain and then binds irreversibly to the sodium taurocholate cotransporting polypeptide (NTCP) via the myristoylated N-terminal region of pre-S1 of the large HBsAg, after which it is taken up into the hepatocyte by an ill-defined mechanism. Fusion of the viral membrane to the endosomal membrane is postulated with release of the ribonucleoprotein (*RNP*) into the cytoplasm. The RNP complex is transported to the nucleus via a nuclear localization signal within the HDAg. Replication of the HDV RNA genome occurs in the nucleus using the hepatocyte RNA polymerases I–III, a process that is dependent on the small HDAg. HDV employs a double-rolling circle replication strategy, whereby HDV RNA is synthesized first as linear antigenomic RNA that contains multimers of the genome that are cleaved to a uniform 1-U length by a ribozyme encoded in the antigenic strand.[41] Circularization of the monomers is achieved by the ribozyme and cellular ligases. In the second rolling circle replication, the circular monomeric RNAs serve as templates for the production of HDV genomic multimers that are cleaved by a second ribozyme encoded in the genomic strand. The HDV genome contains a single open reading frame, which is located on the antigenomic RNA strand from which a linear polyadenylated antigenomic mRNA is transcribed and transported to the cytoplasm to encode HDAg. During the replication cycle, a fraction of the antigenome undergoes editing by the cellular enzyme adenosine deaminase to alter the small HDAg open reading frame from a stop codon to a tryptophan codon, leading to the 3′ elongation of the open reading frame.[48–50] This elongated mRNA leads to large HDAg, which differs from small HDAg by 19 amino acids at the C-terminal end. The small and large HDAg have different functions during HDV replication. The small HDAg promotes HDV replication, whereas the large HDAg serves to inhibit replication and the additional C-terminal amino acids of the large HDAg contain a prenylation signal that appears to be important for interaction with HBsAg during viral assembly. HDV assembly is initiated by the association of the HDV antigens with the newly synthesized genome to yield an RNP complex. This RNA complex is transported to the cytoplasm where viral assembly is facilitated by the interaction of large HDAg with HBsAg. HBsAg is required for assembly, not replication, of HDV. The complete virion is then secreted from the hepatocyte. None are Food and Drug Administration (FDA) approved. Anti-HDV agents and their proposed locus of action. *BLV*, bulevirtide; *IFN-a*, interferon alfa, *LNF*, lonafarnib; *NAP*, nucleic acid polymer.

polyadenylated antigenomic mRNA is transcribed and transported to the cytoplasm to encode HDAg (see Fig. 83.2).[44–47] During the replication cycle, a fraction of the antigenome undergoes editing by the cellular enzyme adenosine deaminase to alter the small HDAg open reading frame from a stop codon, uridine-adenine-guanine, to a tryptophan codon, UGG, leading to the 3′ elongation of the open reading frame.[48–50] This elongated mRNA leads to large HDAg, which differs from small HDAg by 19 amino acids at the C-terminal end. The small and large HDAg have different functions during HDV replication. The small HDAg promotes HDV replication, and its presence is necessary to start HDV messenger RNA transcription but only small amounts are required.[51] The large HDAg serves to inhibit replication; the additional C-terminal amino acids of the large HDAg contain an isoprenylation signal that appears to be important for its interaction with HBsAg during viral assembly.[52,53] HDV assembly is initiated by the association of the delta antigens with the newly synthesized genome to yield an RNP complex (see Fig. 83.2). This RNA complex is transported to the cytoplasm, where viral assembly is facilitated by the interaction of large HDAg with HBsAg. Notably, HBsAg is required only for assembly but not replication of HDV.[54] Only virions that contain large HBsAg are infectious due to the requirement of large HBsAg for viral entry.[55,56] The complete virion is then secreted from the hepatocyte. A study has suggested that HDV may be amplified during hepatocyte regeneration even in the absence of de novo infection.[57]

Genotypes

Eight genotypes (1–8) of HDV each with two to four subtypes per genotype have been described.[58,59] HDV genotypes and subtypes have a unique geographic distribution (see Fig. 83.1). HDV genotype 1 is the most widely distributed globally and is found in Africa, Madagascar, the Oceanic Islands, the Middle East, Eastern and Western Europe, Mediterranean countries, Asia, and North America.[60] HDV genotype 2 is found in Russia, Japan, and Taiwan.[60] HDV genotype 3 is found exclusively in the Amazon basin of South America (Brazil, Colombia, Peru, and Venezuela).[60] HDV genotype 4 is present in the Far East, whereas HDV genotypes 5–8 are found in Western, sub-Saharan, and Central Africa.[60] All HDV genotypes, with the exception of HDV 2–4, originated from Africa. Recent studies suggest that the geographic distribution of HDV genotypes is changing due to human migration. For example, one Canadian study reported the detection of HDV genotypes 2 and 5–7 in addition to genotype 1 amongst their HDV patient population.[61]

Emerging data suggest that the HDV genotype may be associated with clinical outcomes. Typically, HDV genotype 1 is associated with mild-to-severe hepatitis with rapid progression to cirrhosis and an increased risk of HCC.[62,63] By contrast, HDV genotype 2 is associated with milder disease.[64,65] HDV genotype 3 is reported to cause severe outbreaks of acute hepatitis with a high rate of acute liver failure (ALF) and death.[66] HDV genotype 4 has been reported to be associated with severe hepatitis.[67] Infection with genotype 5 was reported to have a more favorable outcome compared with HDV genotype 1.[68] However, a large French study that included predominantly immigrants (86%), originating from sub-Saharan and Northern Africa, Southern and Eastern Europe, the Middle East, Asia, and South America, reported that patients infected with African genotype 5 and European genotype 1 were at greater risk of developing cirrhosis. The 10-year cumulative risk of cirrhosis was lower among patients infected with African genotypes 1, 6, 7, and 8 (26.4%), compared to non-African patients infected with genotype 1 (53.7%).[69] Whether the effect on incidence of cirrhosis was actually due to genotype, race, or perhaps environmental factors remains uncertain. Studies of other genotypes are lacking. Interestingly, efficacy of replication may differ between genotypes, with genotype 3 having a higher replication efficiency compared to genotype 1, which in turn is more efficient than genotype 2.[70,71] This may partly explain the genotypic differences in clinical outcomes.

Whether there are genotype differences in response to treatment with interferon (IFN)-based therapy is unclear. One recent study from the Netherlands of mostly European and African patients found a better response to IFN in patients with genotype 5 compared with genotype 1.[68] The French study noted above observed a better response to IFN among African patients than non-African patients independent of HDV genotype.[72] Studies predominantly of Western European or Asian patients, presumably with HDV genotype 1 infection, reported sustained off-treatment clearance of HDV RNA in 25%–47% of patients.[73–75] An intriguing study from Brazil of patients with HDV genotype 3 infection reported that a regimen of peginterferon (PegIFN) and entecavir was associated with sustained suppression of HDV RNA 6 months off-therapy in over 95% of patients, suggesting that genotype 3 might be more responsive to PegIFN therapy.[76]

PATHOGENESIS

There is a paucity of data on the pathogenesis of HDV infection to explain the more severe course compared with HBV mono-infection. It has been suggested that HDV may be directly cytopathic based on liver biopsy specimen descriptions of severe cytotoxic and cytopathic hepatocellular damage, with prominent microvesicular steatosis and minimal parenchymal inflammation in patients and experimentally infected chimpanzees with acute HDV infection.[77,78] These findings may be limited, however, to infection with HDV genotype 3 and may not be seen with other genotypes. A recent study found that the small HDAg selectively binds to the glutathione *S*-transferase P1 mRNA, a tumor suppressor gene, leading to increase in reactive oxygen species and potentially causing cellular damage and carcinogenesis.[79] However, whether this can be generalized across various HDV genotypes is unclear.

Alternatively, several lines of evidence suggest that the pathogenic mechanism of HDV-induced liver damage is most likely related to the host immune response to the virus. HDV has been shown to induce a strong innate immune response, in a chimeric mouse model, in contrast to HBV infection.[80] In addition, an increased frequency, but not differentiation, of peripheral natural killer cells was shown in untreated patients with chronic HDV infection.[81] One study reported that cytotoxic $CD4^+$ cells, which provide a helper function to $CD8^+$ T and B cells by secretion of cytokines, were found at a higher frequency in patients with HDV infection compared with those with HBV and HCV coinfection.[82] Another study, however, reported that detection of HDAg-specific $CD4^+$ T-cell responses in the peripheral blood of individuals with chronic HDV infection was associated with lower disease activity based on serum ALT levels.[83] The observation that the frequency of activated HDV-specific $CD8^+$ T cells correlated with ALT activity and IFN-gamma production by $CD8^+$ T cells inversely correlated with HDV level, suggests a role for $CD8^+$ T cells in mediating liver injury.[84,85] The limited data available suggest that HDV-associated liver disease is immune-mediated.

DIAGNOSIS

The Centers for Disease Control and Prevention does not recommend routine population screening for HDV because infection and disease occur only in persons with HBV infection. Testing for HDV should be considered in the following clinical scenarios: persons presenting with acute hepatitis B who have additional risk factors for HDV, including a history of injection drug use; persons from endemic regions who present with a severe or protracted hepatitis; patients with chronic hepatitis B and acute hepatitis of undetermined origin; and persons with HBsAg-positive chronic hepatitis B from an endemic region (Box 83.1).

Several tests are available for the diagnosis of hepatitis D (Table 83.1). The only commercially available assays for HDV infection in the United States are anti-HDV antibody—total [immunoglobulin (Ig)M and IgG] and IgM anti-HDV. Other nonapproved tests include HDAg, HDV RNA, and immunohistochemistry for HDAg. Initial testing for diagnosis should begin with total anti-HDV, because anti-HDV invariably appears in the serum of individuals exposed to HDV. Acute HDV coinfection can be differentiated from HDV superinfection by the presence or absence of IgM antibody against hepatitis B core antigen (IgM anti-HBc). In the case of acute HDV coinfection, both IgM anti-HDV and IgM anti-HBc will be present, whereas in acute HDV superinfection, total anti-HDV will be positive but IgM anti-HBc will be negative (see Table 83.1). HDV RNA can be detected in serum early in the course of coinfection, but commercial assays are not readily available. Therefore the diagnosis of acute coinfection depends on the detection of IgM anti-HDV, HBsAg, and IgM anti-HBc and superinfection on the detection of IgM anti-HDV and HBsAg in the appropriate clinical setting.[86] A negative test for total anti-HDV does not necessarily exclude a diagnosis of acute HBV-HDV coinfection.

The diagnosis of chronic HDV infection rests on detection of anti-HDV (IgG and IgM) and should be confirmed by the presence of HDV RNA by a reverse transcription-PCR (RT-PCR) assay or immunohistochemical staining of liver biopsy specimens for HDAg, if available. HDAg may not be detectable in liver biopsy specimens in patients with chronic HDV infection, particularly during the late stages of infection.

HDV Antigen

HDAg is the only protein encoded by HDV. It is a nuclear phosphoprotein that exists in two forms: a 24-kD species, small HDAg, which is required for replication, and a 27-kD species, large HDAg, which is required for virion assembly and inhibits HDV replication.[87] The amino acid sequence of the two forms are identical with the exception of an additional 19 amino acids at the C-terminal end of the large HDAg.[48] Several assays are available for the detection of HDAg in serum, including an enzyme-linked assay and a radioimmunoassay, although none are commercially available or FDA approved in the United States. During acute HDV infection, HDAg is detectable within 1–10 days after the onset of symptoms, but its presence is short-lived. HDAg begins to decline during the acute phase in patients who are destined to clear HDV.[86,88] A similar pattern was observed in chimpanzees experimentally infected with HDV, in which HDAg was detected in the preacute or early acute phase of infection.[89] Because humans are generally not symptomatic until the acute phase of infection, HDAg may not be detected during acute infection.

Detection of HDAg is not a sensitive test for the diagnosis of chronic HDV infection because neutralizing antibodies are present in high titers during chronic infection and can interfere with detection of HDAg. HDAg can be detected, however, in liver biopsy specimens from patients with chronic HDV infection by direct immunofluorescence or immunohistochemical staining.[90] The detection of intrahepatic HDAg has been proposed as the "gold standard" for the diagnosis of chronic HDV infection; however, as many as 50% of liver biopsy specimens from patients who have been infected for 10 or more years may be negative for HDAg, suggesting that the levels of HDV replication may decrease with time.[91] In patients who are negative for HDAg, the diagnosis of chronic HDV infection must rely on the detection of HDV RNA and anti-HDV in high titers in the serum.

BOX 83.1 Persons in Whom HDV Testing Is Recommended

PERSONS WITH ACUTE HEPATITIS B

Risk factors for HDV (e.g., persons who inject drugs, persons from endemic countries, persons who present with a severe or protracted hepatitis)

PERSONS WITH CHRONIC HEPATITIS B

Risk factors for HDV (e.g., persons who inject drugs, persons from endemic countries)

An unexplained acute flare of chronic hepatitis B that is not due to acute hepatitis A or C or reactivation of hepatitis B

HBsAg positive and persistently HBV DNA negative but with active liver disease

HBsAg positive with rapid progression to cirrhosis

HBsAG, Hepatitis B surface antigen.

TABLE 83.1 Patterns of Serologic Markers in HDV Infection

Serologic Marker	Acute HBV-HDV Coinfection	Acute HDV Superinfection	Chronic HDV Infection
HBsAg	Positive	Positive	Positive
IgM anti-HBc	Positive	Negative	Negative
HDAg	Positive (early and transient)	Positive (early and transient)	Negative
Total anti-HDV	Weakly positive (transient, low titers)	Positive (rising titers)	Positive (high sustained titers)
IgM anti-HDV	Weakly positive (transient, low titers; may be the only marker of infection)	Positive (rising titers)	Positive (high sustained titers)
HDV RNA	Positive (early and transient)	Positive (early and persistent)	Positive (usually persistent)

Anti-HDV, Antibody to HDV; *IgM anti-HBc*, immunoglobulin M antibody to hepatitis B core antigen; *HBsAg*, hepatitis B surface antigen; *HDAg*, hepatitis D antigen.

Antibody to HDV

The most reliable marker of HDV infection is anti-HDV. Two antibody tests are commercially available but none are FDA approved, and both can be detected in currently infected patients: IgM anti-HDV and total anti-HDV, which is composed of both IgM and IgG anti-HDV. IgM anti-HDV appears in serum at the time of acute infection, and IgG anti-HDV (indicated by a positive total anti-HDV result and negative IgM anti-HDV result) develops later in the course.[86] In acute self-limited HBV-HDV coinfection, IgM anti-HDV is generally detected first, followed by the development of IgG anti-HDV during recovery. Other patterns have been observed, including the isolated detection of IgM anti-HDV or IgG anti-HDV.[86] By contrast, in acute HDV superinfection of a chronic HBV carrier, both IgM and IgG anti-HDV can be detected during the acute period, increase in levels, and persist during the chronic period. IgM anti-HDV is often detectable in high titers in patients with chronic HDV infection, and levels tend to parallel the activity of liver disease.[92–94] Therefore it is frequently regarded as a marker of serious liver damage.[93] A decline in IgM anti-HDV levels may indicate either a decline in disease activity or resolution of HDV infection.[92,93] In patients in whom HDV infection resolves, IgG anti-HDV may remain detectable in serum, but levels are low. IgG anti-HDV is not a protective antibody.[95] Testing for HDV RNA is the only reliable method to distinguish chronic HDV infection from recovery.

A quantitative microarray antibody capture assay for IgG anti-HDV has been developed. In this assay, recombinant HDAg is immobilized on slides coated with a noncontinuous, nanostructured plasmonic gold film, thereby enabling quantitative fluorescent detection of anti-HDV in a small aliquot of a patient's serum.[96] Quantitative cutoff values of captured anti-HDV have been shown to correlate with positivity on a standard western blot assay or with detection of HDV RNA by a real-time quantitative PCR assay. Potential advantages of this methodology over existing assays include the requirement for only a small volume of a patient's serum and the potential for high-throughput screening.

HDV RNA

Detection of HDV RNA by RT-PCR is considered the gold standard for diagnosis of current HDV infection.[97] Several real-time PCR-based assays allow both detection and quantification of HDV RNA levels.[98–103] However, many of the assays dramatically underestimate HDV RNA levels and even fail to detect HDV RNA[97,104] due to the high genetic diversity of HDV and the use of different primer-probe sets among assays. These results highlight some of the challenges for developing a commercial assay. The availability of a WHO international standard has permitted optimization of quantification assays across various centers and laboratories. In addition to diagnostic uses, development of standardized assays will be required to monitor the response to novel antiviral therapy for HDV infection. RT-PCR assays will also allow sequencing of the HDV genome and identification of the HDV genotype, although the clinical utility of such testing is uncertain.

CLINICAL FEATURES

The clinical features of acute HDV infection are indistinguishable from those of acute hepatitis caused by other hepatotropic viruses (see Chapters 80–82 and 84). The clinical presentation is usually an asymptomatic hepatitis recognized only by elevated serum aminotransferase levels. Approximately 20%–30% of acute infections present with symptomatic hepatitis accompanied by jaundice. Typical symptoms include anorexia, fatigue, low-grade fever, flu-like symptoms, and pain or aching in the RUQ. Rarely, the presentation is as ALF; this presentation may be more commonly associated with HDV genotype 3 than with other genotypes.

Acute HDV infection may occur as a coinfection simultaneously with HBV in an individual without prior exposure to HBV or as a superinfection in a person with chronic HBV infection. HDV coinfection (Fig. 83.3) usually presents with jaundice and tends to run a self-limited course. Some patients may demonstrate a biphasic increase in serum aminotransferase levels separated by a few weeks.[95] The first peak in serum aminotransferase levels is related to HBV replication and the second to HDV replication. Serologic markers for both HBV and HDV are detectable at the time of acute HDV coinfection and include IgM anti-HBc, HBsAg, HBV DNA, IgM anti-HDV, and HDV RNA.[95] Expression of HDAg is usually short-lived in HDV coinfection and may be absent. The acute hepatitis typically resolves

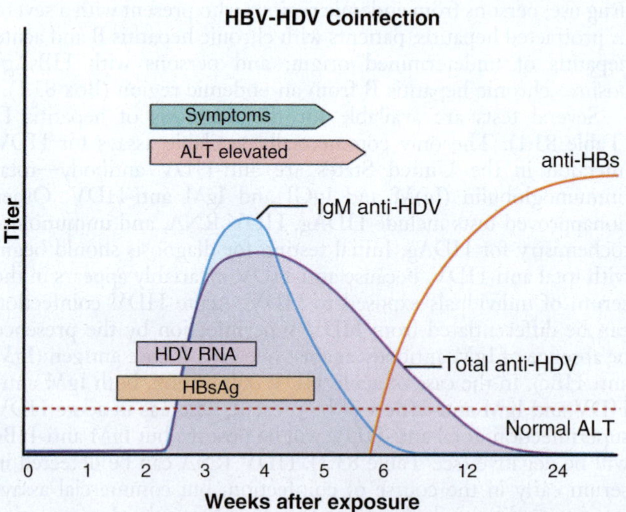

Fig. 83.3 Serologic course of acute HDV coinfection. Serologic markers of HBV are usually detected first, followed later by serologic markers of HDV. The presence of immunoglobulin (Ig)M antibody to hepatitis B core antigen (anti-HBc) is an important finding of acute HDV coinfection and a discriminating marker for distinguishing acute HDV coinfection from superinfection. Early in the course of acute coinfection, hepatitis D antigen (HDAg) is not detectable unless the hepatitis is severe, but within 1–2 weeks, IgM antibody to HDV (anti-HDV) becomes detectable. The appearance of IgG anti-HDV is usually delayed for several weeks after the onset of illness and, in some cases, is present only transiently during the convalescent phase. The late and poor antibody response in acute HDV coinfection makes the diagnosis difficult. Testing for IgM anti-HDV should be repeated to confirm HDV coinfection. HDV RNA can be detected in serum early in the course of coinfection. *HBsAg*, Hepatitis B surface antigen.

in a few weeks, with a gradual return of liver biochemical test levels to normal. As the infection resolves, HBV DNA and HDV RNA levels decline rapidly, and antibody to HBsAg (anti-HBs) appears after the disappearance of HBsAg.[95,105] Occasionally, IgM anti-HDV may persist after anti-HBs appears and serum aminotransferase levels return to normal. Evolution to chronic HDV infection is uncommon and is characterized by the persistence of HBsAg, HBV DNA, HDV RNA, and IgM and/or IgG anti-HDV in serum.

HDV superinfection (Fig. 83.4) manifests clinically as an acute hepatitis in an otherwise stable chronic HBV carrier. Clinically, HDV superinfection can mimic a spontaneous flare of chronic HBV infection. These two diagnostic possibilities can usually be easily differentiated, because patients with HDV superinfection have detectable HDV RNA and IgM anti-HDV in serum as well as a corresponding decline in or low serum HBV DNA levels instead of a high level that is typical of a hepatitis B flare. Also, in contrast to a flare of chronic HBV infection or HDV coinfection, IgM anti-HBc is not detectable in serum.

NATURAL HISTORY

Acute HDV Infection

As previously discussed, acute HDV infection may occur as a coinfection simultaneously with HBV or as a superinfection of a person with chronic HBV infection. In the majority of individuals (>90%) with acute HDV-HBV coinfection, both infections resolve simultaneously within a period of 6 months. The risk of progression to chronic HDV infection is usually less than 5%. ALF is rare but is more common compared to HBV

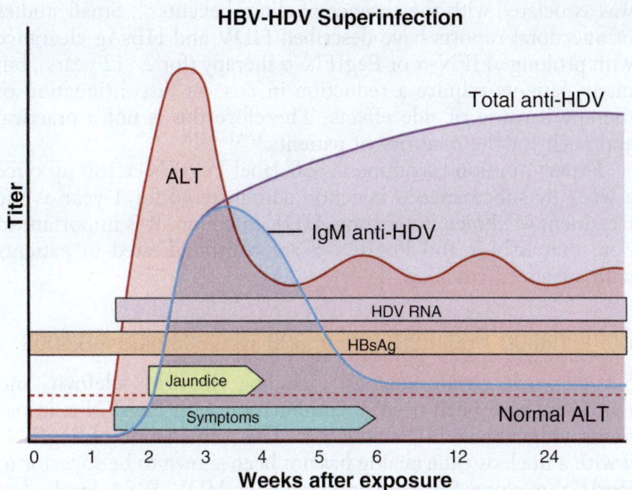

Fig. 83.4 Serologic course of acute HDV superinfection. Acute HDV superinfection occurs in the setting of chronic hepatitis B. Hepatitis D antigen and HDV RNA can be detected early in the course of infection. In contrast to acute HDV coinfection (see Fig. 83.3), immunoglobulin (Ig) M and IgG antibody to HDV (anti-HDV) are both present early during the symptomatic phase of acute HDV superinfection. IgM antibody to hepatitis B core antigen (anti-HBc) is usually absent or present in low levels. The diagnosis of acute HDV superinfection is established by the detection of anti-HDV and HBsAg and absence of IgM anti-HBc. *HBsAg*, Hepatitis B surface antigen.

monoinfection and may be related to the infecting HDV genotype. By contrast, most persons (~90%) with acute HDV superinfection progress to chronic HDV infection due to preexisting HBsAg that is required for HDV entry into the hepatocyte. Acute HDV superinfection can sometimes result in acute-on-chronic liver failure and hepatic decompensation in chronic HBV carriers (see Chapter 97). Less commonly, the HDV infection resolves, while the chronic HBV infection persists, and, rarely, acute HDV superinfection leads to clearance of HBsAg and resolution of both infections. During acute HDV superinfection, serum HDV RNA levels are high because HBsAg, which is necessary for the viral life cycle, is usually present at high levels in chronic HBV carriers.[91] A consequence of the high serum HDV RNA levels is the inhibition of HBV replication and reciprocal low serum levels of HBV DNA.[106]

Chronic HDV Infection

The natural history of chronic HDV infection is variable, ranging from a mild chronic hepatitis to severe hepatitis with rapid progression to cirrhosis and hepatic decompensation. During the early phase of chronic HDV infection, serum HDV RNA levels tend to be high and gradually decline over time.[91] In the late phase of chronic infection, declining serum HDV RNA levels may lead to an increase in serum HBV DNA levels.

Studies from the early 1970s, originating mostly from Southern Europe, reported severe cases of chronic HDV infection with rapid progression to hepatic decompensation among PWID.[6,107–109] In retrospect, many of these patients were shown to be coinfected with HCV or HIV, which may explain the more rapid clinical course.[110–114] In addition, most of the studies originated from tertiary referral centers, which may have biased patient cohorts toward more advanced liver disease. Subsequent data have suggested that only a minority of patients exhibit a rapidly progressive course to cirrhosis and hepatic decompensation. Rather, most patients with chronic HDV infection demonstrate an initial active hepatitis that progresses rapidly to cirrhosis, after which the hepatitis becomes inactive and runs a more indolent course. In one notable longitudinal study from Italy, among 299 patients with chronic HDV infection followed for up to 28 years, the annual frequency of cirrhosis was 4% and that of HCC was 2.8%; spontaneous HBsAg seroconversion occurred in only 0.25%.[115] Similar results were reported in another study from Spain that demonstrated that among 158 patients with chronic HDV infection followed for a median of 13 years, 72% remained stable, 18% developed hepatic decompensation, 3% developed HCC, and 8% cleared HBsAg.[116] In a large study of 1112 patients from France, the majority of whom were foreign-born, 88% of those tested ($n = 748$) were viremic and 28% had cirrhosis at presentation, half of whom had experienced a decompensation event. The 5-year risk of cirrhosis, decompensation, HCC, LT, or death were 49.4%, 23.3%, 8.2%, and 20.2%, respectively.[72] Factors that have been shown to be associated with faster progression to cirrhosis include persistent and high levels of HDV replication and HDV genotype.[72,115,116] In the aforementioned study from France, persistent viremia was associated with a 6.1-fold higher rate of incident cirrhosis. Once cirrhosis develops, either virus may predominate, or spontaneous clearance of both viruses may occur. HDV genotypes 1 and 3 may be associated with faster progression of liver disease compared with HDV genotypes 2 and 4.[63,66] The short-term prognosis following the development of cirrhosis is generally good, with an estimated 5-year survival rate of 81%–90%.[117] Chronic HDV infection is associated with a faster progression to cirrhosis and mortality compared with chronic HBV infection alone.[118,119]

Chronic HDV infection is associated with an increased risk of HCC but there has been some debate whether HDV is directly oncogenic or if the increased HCC risk is due to a higher prevalence of cirrhosis, which is considered a premalignant condition. Data from a European Concerted Action on Viral Hepatitis study of patients with compensated cirrhosis reported that patients with chronic HDV infection had a threefold increased risk of HCC and a twofold increased risk of mortality compared with those in whom cirrhosis was related to chronic HBV infection.[119,120] Similarly, a study from Sweden using the Swedish Hospital Discharge Register and Outpatient Registry reported a sixfold increased rate of HCC among patients with chronic HDV infection compared with those with chronic HBV infection alone.[121] These data would suggest that HDV is a strong risk factor for HCC. Differences in reported rates of HCC among studies likely relate to different populations with different ages at infection, durations of disease, severity of disease, and perhaps HDV genotypes.

TREATMENT

Acute Hepatitis D

Treatment of acute hepatitis D is mainly supportive. No effective antiviral therapy has been approved for the treatment of acute HDV infection. LT is an option for patients who present with ALF (see Chapter 99).

Chronic Hepatitis D

There is no approved treatment for chronic HDV infection in the United States. For patients in whom treatment is considered, off-label IFN-α and pegylated IFN (PegIFN)-α have had limited success. These agents are associated with being poorly tolerated due to numerous side effects and are contraindicated in patients with decompensated cirrhosis, pregnancy, and autoimmune conditions. Therefore the decision to recommend treatment should be individualized, weighing carefully the benefits of treatment against the side effects of the drug. Treatment should be considered in persons with elevated serum ALT levels, high HDV RNA levels, evidence of chronic hepatitis on liver biopsy, and those with compensated cirrhosis. The goals of therapy are to eradicate or maintain long-term suppression of both HDV and HBV, that is, clearance of HDV RNA as measured by a sensitive PCR-based assay and loss of HBsAg, to prevent the development of cirrhosis, decompensated liver disease, HCC, and death from chronic HDV infection. Durable suppression of HDV RNA was shown to be associated with a reduced risk of liver-related complications (hepatic decompensation, HCC, LT, and liver-related death).[75,122]

Interferon-α/Peginterferon-α

IFN-α and PegIFN-α (see Figure 83.2) are the only available drugs in the United States with antiviral activity against HDV. The most effective dose and optimal duration of standard IFN-α have not been established. IFN-α in a dose of 5 million U/m^2 three times a week for 4 months followed by 3 million U/m^2 three times a week for another 8 months was compared with no treatment in a randomized trial involving 61 patients.[123] At the end of treatment, there was no difference in the proportion of subjects who became HDV RNA negative between the treated group [14/31 (45%)] and the untreated group [8/30 (27%)]. Similarly, the proportion of patients who were HDV RNA negative 12 months after completion of treatment was not different between treated and untreated patients. A greater proportion of treated patients achieved a normal serum ALT level at the end of treatment (26% vs. 7%) but at the end of follow-up, only 3% of treated and 0% of untreated patients had a normal serum ALT level.[123] In another study, a high (9 million U three times a week) and low dose (3 million U three times a week) of IFN-α 2a for 48 weeks were compared with no treatment among 41 patients with chronic HDV infection. A complete response (defined as normalization of serum ALT levels and undetectable HDV RNA) at the end of treatment was more frequent in the high-dose group (50%) than in the low-dose (21%) and untreated (0%) groups, but all patients experienced virologic relapse 12 months after stopping treatment.[124] With longer follow-up (12 years), patients in the high-dose IFN group had improved clinical outcomes and survival compared to receiving low-dose IFN or no therapy, even though the majority of patients had active cirrhosis before the onset of therapy.[122] The improvement in clinical outcomes correlated with a sustained reduction of HDV viremia by ≥2 log compared to baseline. A meta-analysis of five trials that compared IFN with no therapy (a total of 169 participants) concluded that IFN was effective in suppressing viral replication and improving liver disease activity in a minority of patients, but this improvement was rarely sustained in the majority of patients.[125] Therefore the results of treatment with IFN-α are mixed, and only a small proportion of patients achieve a beneficial response that correlated with maintained suppression of viral replication. Expert opinion recommends the use of either IFN 9 million U three times a week or 5 million U three times a week for 1 year.

PegIFN-α appears to be more effective than standard IFN-α for therapy of chronic hepatitis D, but data are limited. The few published studies of PegIFN-α 2b administered for 48–72 weeks reported sustained viral suppression in 17%–43% of subjects 6 months after completion of therapy.[74,126–130] A follow-up study of patients treated with PegIFN-α either alone or in combination with adefovir (see below) reported maintained off-treatment viral suppression (HDV RNA negative) in 6/14 (43%) patients after a mean follow-up of 8.9 years. All HDV RNA negative patients were also HBsAg negative suggesting that loss of HBsAg is associated with absence of replication. Interestingly, among 33 viremic patients at the end of treatment, an additional 7 became HDV RNA negative during the follow-up period in the absence of HBsAg loss. Importantly, long-term suppression of HDV RNA was associated with the absence of clinical events.[131] Small studies or anecdotal reports have described HDV and HBsAg clearance with prolonged IFN-α or PegIFN-α therapy (for 2–12 years), but many patients require a reduction in dose or discontinuation of therapy because of side effects. Therefore this is not a practical approach for the majority of patients.[129,132,133]

Expert opinion recommends off-label PegIFN-α 180 μg once a week by subcutaneous injection administered for 1 year as the treatment of choice for chronic HDV infection. It is important to note that IFN-α and PegIFN-α are contraindicated in patients with advanced cirrhosis.

Combination Peginterferon-α and Nucleos(t)ide Analogs

Several nucleos(t)ide analogs, including ribavirin, adefovir, and tenofovir, have been used in combination with PegIFN-α in patients with chronic HDV infection. The combination of PegIFN-α with a nucleos(t)ide analog has not been shown to be superior to PegIFN-α alone for the suppression of HDV RNA levels, but there may be a benefit to combination with adefovir disoproxil fumarate or tenofovir dipivoxil in reducing HBsAg levels (see Chapter 81). In one study, PegIFN-α 2b 1.5 μg/kg once a week plus ribavirin for 48 weeks followed by PegIFN-α 2b 1.5 μg/kg once a week alone for 24 weeks was compared with PegIFN-α 2b 1.5 μg/kg once a week alone for 72 weeks in 38 patients with chronic HDV infection.[127] Serum HDV RNA became negative in 19% of patients who received PegIFN-α 2b compared with 7% of those who received combination therapy, suggesting no benefit of ribavirin on viral clearance.[127] In another study, the combination of PegIFN-α 2a 180 μg once a week and adefovir dipivoxil 10 mg daily was compared with PegIFN-α 2a 180 μg once a week plus placebo or adefovir dipivoxil 10 mg daily alone for 48 weeks.[74] Both PegIFN-α 2a treated groups experienced a higher rate of undetectable HDV RNA levels at the end of treatment, PegIFN-α 2a plus adefovir 23%, PegIFN-α 2a alone 24%, compared to those who received adefovir dipivoxil monotherapy (0%).[74] Twenty-four weeks after stopping treatment, 28% of patients randomized to a PegIFN-α 2a-containing arm were negative for HDV RNA compared with 0% of patients in the adefovir dipivoxil arm. Long-term outcome data were available on 60 of the original 90 patients. After a mean follow-up of 8.9 years, however, more than one-half (57%) of the patients who were negative for HDV RNA experienced virological relapse. Nineteen of 60 patients required retreatment (8/39 in the PegIFN-α 2a-containing arms and 11/21 in the adefovir only arm) and 17/60 developed a clinical complication (liver-related death, liver transplantation, HCC, and hepatic decompensation).[131] Development of a clinical outcome was related to the presence of cirrhosis pretreatment and nonresponse to therapy. Overall, this study demonstrated that there was no additive antiviral effect of combining adefovir dipivoxil to PegIFN-α 2a, sustained virologic responses were uncommon, adefovir monotherapy had minimal-to-no effect on HDV replication, and suppression of viremia was associated with the absence of clinical complications. Another study evaluated a longer duration of PegIFN-α 2a 180 μg once a week for 96 weeks with or without tenofovir disoproxil fumarate.[134] At the end of treatment, 47% of patients who received combination therapy achieved undetectable HDV RNA compared with 33% of patients who received PegIFN-α 2a monotherapy; however, a substantial proportion of patients experienced a posttreatment relapse. Twenty-four weeks after stopping therapy, the proportion who were negative for HDV RNA decreased from 47% to 30% among those who received combination therapy and from 33% to 23% among those who received PegIFN-α 2a monotherapy.[134] A reanalysis of HDV RNA levels from the trial using a more sensitive HDV RNA assay identified that low-level HDV viremia at week 48 or 96 was associated with a high risk for relapse after stopping treatment. In summary, neither extending the duration of

PegIFN-α therapy nor combining PegIFN-α with a nucleos(t)ide analog was shown to be of benefit in treating chronic HDV infection.

Nucleos(t)ide Analogs

Nucleos(t)ide analogs are not effective at inhibiting HDV replication[135] but may have a role in the management of patients with chronic HDV infection who have high HBV DNA levels by controlling HBV-related liver disease (see Chapter 81). It is also conceivable that nucleos(t)ide analogs may be of some benefit in patients with chronic HDV infection by lowering HBsAg levels and limiting HDV replication. The effect of nucleos(t)ide analogs on HBsAg levels tends to be minimal (<1 log IU/mL), however, and there is little evidence to support their use as primary therapy for chronic HDV infection.

LT

Liver transplantation (LT) is the only option for patients with HDV-related decompensated cirrhosis (see Chapter 99). LT may be curative because of the use of hepatitis B immune globulin that binds HBsAg, which is necessary for HDV entry.[136] Indeed, the outcome of LT for chronic HDV infection is better than that for chronic HBV infection and may lead to resolution of both infections.[136–138] Graft reinfection rates are less than 10% with the use of hepatitis B immune globulin.[138] Current recommendations to prevent graft reinfection are the combination of hepatitis B immune globulin and a potent nucleos(t)ide analog. Several recent studies suggest that the hepatitis B immune globulin can be safely discontinued without reappearance of HDV or graft loss with continued use of the nucleos(t)ide analog.[139–141] However, the optimal duration of the hepatitis B immune globulin prior to withdrawal is not known, and such a strategy requires further study before such a practice could be universally adopted.

Novel Therapies

Drug development for HDV is hampered by the lack of suitable viral targets and animal models. Several promising agents that target host factors involved with viral entry and assembly and HBsAg production and secretion are in various stages of development for the treatment of patients with chronic HDV infection. Two therapeutic strategies are being pursued simultaneously. The first and preferred strategy is to achieve loss of HBsAg and unquantifiable HDV RNA with finite duration therapy. This is a high bar to achieve, and therefore an alternate strategy is long-term suppression of HDV RNA, ideally to unquantifiable. If this is not achievable, regulatory authorities have accepted a two-log reduction in HDV RNA and normalization of serum ALT as an endpoint of novel therapy based on the recommendation of an international expert panel.[142]

Entry Inhibitors

As discussed earlier, HDV entry into hepatocytes is dependent on binding of the myristoylated N-terminal region of pre-S1 of the large HBsAg to the hepatocyte-specific NTCP receptor,[143] and to a lesser extent an interaction of the antigenic loop of the S domain with heparan-sulfate proteoglycans. Bulevirtide (BLV), see Figure 83.2 is a synthetic lipopeptide that mimics the receptor binding site of the pre-S1 of the large HBsAg and irreversibly binds to NTCP, thereby blocking HDV infection of uninfected hepatocytes.[144] Bulevirtide 2 mg, administered by subcutaneous injection daily, was approved by the European Medicines Agency (EMA) for treatment of chronic HDV infection. It is currently being evaluated by the Food and Drug Administration for approval in the United States.

An initial randomized pilot study evaluated bulevirtide 2, 5, and 10 mg either alone, or in combination with PegIFN-α 2a compared with PegIFN-α 2a alone,[145] demonstrated that bulevirtide monotherapy was associated with a reduction in HDV RNA levels, and there may be an additional benefit to combining bulevirtide with PegIFN-α 2a. Treatment with bulevirtide was generally well tolerated, although moderate increases in serum levels of conjugated bile acids were observed.[145] Based on these encouraging preliminary data, bulevirtide was further evaluated in three phase 2b multicenter trials either in combination with tenofovir disoproxil fumarate (study MYR202) or PegIFN-α 2a (MYR203) and (MYR204).

In study MYR202, bulevirtide in doses of 2, 5, and 10 mg subcutaneously once a day was studied in combination with tenofovir disoproxil fumarate 300 mg once daily for 24 weeks, followed by tenofovir disoproxil fumarate alone for 24 weeks, and compared with tenofovir disoproxil fumarate alone for 48 weeks among 120 patients with chronic HDV infection, one-half of whom had cirrhosis.[146] After the 24-week bulevirtide dosing period, undetectable or at least a 2-log reduction in HDV RNA levels was observed in 54% of patients who received the 2-mg dose, 50% of those who received the 5-mg dose, and 77% of those who received the 10-mg dose, compared with only 4% of those assigned to tenofovir disoproxil fumarate monotherapy.[147] Serum HDV RNA levels rebounded, however, in the majority of patients after bulevirtide was stopped. Twenty-four weeks after bulevirtide was stopped, only 7% of patients who received the 2-mg dose of bulevirtide, 3% of those who received the 5-mg dose, and 3% of those who received the 10-mg dose and none who received tenofovir disoproxil fumarate maintained undetectable HDV RNA or ≥2-log reduction in HDV RNA and normal ALT levels. Analysis of a subset of 22 patients, receiving bulevirtide plus tenofovir disoproxil fumarate, with paired liver biopsy specimens at baseline and treatment week 24 showed a strong intrahepatic decline in HDV RNA and delta antigen.[148] However, no substantial changes in HBsAg levels were observed in any of the treatment groups. These data demonstrate a dose-dependent antiviral effect of bulevirtide but a high rate of relapse with 24-week duration of therapy. Future studies will address whether sustained HDV RNA suppression is possible, and, if so, the appropriate dose and duration of therapy required to achieve elimination of HDV RNA.

Study MYR203 was a 48-week extension of the pilot study evaluating different doses of bulevirtide either alone or in combination with PegIFN-α 2a.[149] Ninety patients with chronic HDV infection were randomized to one of six treatment arms: 2, 5, and 10 mg of bulevirtide plus PegIFN-α 2a, PegIFN-α 2a alone, 2 mg bulevirtide only, and 10 mg bulevirtide plus tenofovir disoproxil fumarate.[149] The primary efficacy endpoint, HDV RNA below the lower limit of detection (<10 IU/mL) at 24 weeks off-therapy, was achieved in 53%, 27%, and 7% of patients randomized to 2, 5, and 10 mg bulevirtide plus PegIFN-α 2a, respectively, compared to 0% of those who received PegIFN-α 2a alone and 7% of patients who received bulevirtide 2 mg and 33% of those who received 10 mg BLV plus tenofovir disoproxil fumarate. HBsAg loss occurred only among patients who received bulevirtide in combination with PegIFN-α 2a; in 4 (27%) patients treated with bulevirtide 2 mg plus PegIFN-α 2a, and in 1 (7%) treated with bulevirtide 10 mg plus PegIFN-α 2a. The combination of bulevirtide plus PegIFN-α 2a showed strong synergism in terms of on-treatment suppression of HDV RNA, but sustained off-treatment suppression of HDV viremia was observed only in patients who achieved an HBsAg response. Somewhat surprising was the divergent results obtained with low- and high-dose bulevirtide depending on whether combined with tenofovir disoproxil fumarate or PegIFN-α 2a. When bulevirtide was combined with tenofovir disoproxil fumarate, the highest suppression of HDV RNA was achieved with the 10-mg dose of bulevirtide, whereas when combined with PegIFN-α 2a, the 10-mg dose of bulevirtide yielded the lowest rate of viral suppression and vice versa for the 2-mg dose. The reasons for this finding remain unclear and deserve further investigation. The EMA has approved the 2-mg dose despite its lower efficacy compared to the 10-mg dose when used with a nucleos(t)ide analog. The optimal treatment duration is unknown, and therapy can be continued so long as clinical benefit is maintained.

Study MYR204 was designed as a finite duration study to assess the safety and efficacy of bulevirtide 2 or 10 mg subcutaneously once daily in combination with PegIFN-α 2a 180 μg once weekly for 48 weeks followed by bulevirtide monotherapy 2 or 10 mg for 48 weeks compared with PegIFN-α 2a 180 μg once weekly for 48 weeks or bulevirtide 10 mg subcutaneously once daily for 96 weeks.[150] The primary endpoint of HDV RNA undetectable 24 weeks off-treatment was achieved in 17% of patients assigned to PegIFN-α 2a monotherapy, 32% of patients assigned to bulevirtide 2 mg plus PegIFN-α 2a, 46% of patients assigned to bulevirtide 10 mg plus PegIFN-α 2a, and 12% of patients assigned to bulevirtide 10 mg monotherapy. Despite the high rates of undetectable HDV RNA 24 weeks off-treatment, HBsAg loss was observed in only 4%, 8%, 8%, and 1% of the four treatment arms, respectively. The safety profile of bulevirtide 2 or 10 mg in combination with PegIFN-α 2a was similar to PegIFN-α 2a monotherapy. These results suggest that high rates of HDV RNA clearance can be achieved with finite duration therapy in the absence of HBsAg loss. Longer-term follow-up to assess durability of response is awaited.

Recently, week 48 on-treatment interim results of the phase 3 trial evaluating bulevirtide 2 or 10 mg subcutaneously once daily for 144 weeks compared with no therapy for the initial 48 weeks followed by bulevirtide 10 mg subcutaneously once daily for 96 weeks were published.[151] The primary endpoint, defined as undetectable HDV RNA or a ≥2 log decline from baseline and ALT normalization assessed at week 48, was achieved in 44.9% and 48% of the bulevirtide 2 and 10 mg arms, respectively, compared to 2% of untreated controls. Undetectable HDV RNA was achieved in 12.2% and 20% of those receiving bulevirtide 2 and 10 mg, respectively, compared to 0% of untreated patients. The trial is ongoing, and all patients are scheduled to be followed for 96 weeks off-therapy to establish durability of response.

There is emerging evidence that bulevirtide may also benefit patients with compensated and decompensated cirrhosis. In a report of three patients with HDV-related compensated cirrhosis, long-term administration of bulevirtide at an initial dose of 10 mg/day for up to 3 years in a compassionate use program,[152] one subject who stopped therapy at 48 weeks was able to maintain low HDV RNA and normal ALT levels. Two patients who received uninterrupted treatment for 3 years maintained undetectable HDV RNA and normal ALT levels despite dose reduction. Treatment was well tolerated with asymptomatic elevation of bile salts noted. One of the latter two patients experienced resolution of esophageal varices with marked histological improvement on repeat liver biopsy and maintained undetectable HDV RNA with normal ALT levels 72 weeks off-treatment, suggesting the possibility of "cure" without HBsAg loss with long-term maintenance therapy.[153] Bulevirtide treatment may also be beneficial among patients with compensated cirrhosis and clinically significant portal hypertension.[154]

Inhibitors of Viral Assembly

Virion assembly is dependent on the host protein farnesyltransferase, which is required for farnesylation of the large delta antigen.[155,156] Lonafarnib (LNF), see Fig. 83.2, a farnesyltransferase inhibitor, was demonstrated to affect HDV virion release in vitro and in vivo.[156,157] Lonafarnib was evaluated at doses of 100 and 200 mg twice daily, in 14 patients with chronic HDV infection in a proof-of-concept study.[158] The 100-mg dose resulted in an average decline in serum HDV RNA levels of 0.73 log IU/mL, and the 200-mg dose was associated with a mean decline in HDV RNA levels of 1.54 log IU/mL at 28 days compared with baseline.[158] In follow-up, HDV RNA levels returned to baseline within 4 weeks of drug discontinuation. All patients experienced dose-limiting GI side effects, including bloating, nausea, diarrhea, and weight loss.

The LOWR HDV-1 study was designed to explore strategies to optimize the lonafarnib dosing such as split dosing and combination with ritonavir, a cytochrome P450 3A4 inhibitor which permits lower dosing of lonafarnib, while limiting the GI side effects. Patients were intolerant of the higher doses of lonafarnib in combination with PegIFN and did not complete the study. The greatest decline in HDV RNA levels was achieved with the combination of lonafarnib 100 mg twice daily and ritonavir 100 mg once daily for 8 weeks, with a 2.4-log IU/mL decline in HDV RNA levels.[159] Declines in HDV RNA levels were accompanied by a reduction in serum ALT levels, but no changes in HBsAg levels were noted. In posttreatment follow-up, HDV RNA levels returned to baseline levels in all but two patients.[159]

Subsequent studies, LOWR-2, -3, and -4, evaluated the safety and efficacy of different doses of lonafarnib in combination with ritonavir without or with PegIFN-α 2a for 12–24 weeks. LOWR HDV-2 evaluated 10 regimens that could be broadly grouped as five high-dose lonafarnib regimens (≥75 mg twice daily and ritonavir 100–200 mg daily) for 12–24 weeks, four low-dose lonafarnib regimens (lonafarnib 25 or 50 mg bid and ritonavir 200 mg daily) for 24 weeks, and combination low-dose lonafarnib with PegIFN-α (LNF 25 or 50 mg bid and ritonavir 200 mg daily plus PegIFN-α) for 24 weeks. The optimal regimens for achieving the primary endpoint of a ≥2 $\log_{10}$ decline or < lower limit of quantification of HDV-RNA from baseline at the end of treatment were lonafarnib 50 mg bid plus ritonavir 100 mg bid, 39% (5 of 13), and lonafarnib (25 or 50 mg bid) and ritonavir plus PegIFN-α, 89% (8 of 9).[160] LOWR HDV-3 explored three doses of lonafarnib 50, 75, and 100 mg plus ritonavir 100 mg daily for 12 or 24 weeks. After 12 weeks of dosing, the greatest decline in HDV RNA was achieved with the lonafarnib 50 plus ritonavir 100 mg regimen, 1.6 log IU/mL.[161] Overall, 6/21 achieved ≥2 log decline in HDV RNA. LOWR-HDV-4 evaluated dose escalation of lonafarnib from 50 to 100 mg bid plus ritonavir 100 mg bid for 24 weeks as a strategy to achieve higher lonafarnib doses. However, only 10/15 patients were able to tolerate dose escalation. At end of dosing, mean HDV RNA decline from baseline was −1.58 $\log_{10}$ IU/mL.[162] Finally, the LIFT HDV study assessed the combination of lonafarnib 50 mg plus ritonavir 100 mg bid with PegINF-λ 180 μg weekly for 24 weeks.[163] Among 26 patients, 77% achieved ≥2 log HDV RNA decline, and 50% were <lower limit of quantitation after 24 weeks of therapy.[163] Twenty-four weeks off-treatment the virological response was maintained in 5 (19%) patients by intention-to-treat analysis.

A large randomized placebo-controlled phase 3 study to evaluate the safety and efficacy of lonafarnib 50 mg and ritonavir 100 mg twice daily with or without PegIFN-α 2a compared with PegIFN-α 2a 180 μg once weekly alone for 48 weeks or placebo with 24-week posttreatment follow-up.[164] The primary endpoint was a ≥2 $\log_{10}$ IU/mL decline in HDV RNA and ALT normalization at end of dosing (week 48). After 48 weeks, the primary endpoint was achieved in 19.2% assigned to the lonafarnib and ritonavir plus PegIFN-α 2a arm, 10.1% assigned to the lonafarnib and ritonavir arm, and 9.6% assigned to PegIFN-α 2a arm, compared to 1.9% assigned to the placebo arm. At week 48, HDV RNA below the limit of quantification was achieved in 20.8% of patients receiving lonafarnib, ritonavir plus PegIFN-α 2a, 8.4% receiving lonafarnib and ritonavir, 26.9% receiving PegIFN-α 2a, and 3.8% receiving placebo. Among patients with paired liver biopsies, a ≥2 point improvement in histology activity index and no worsening of fibrosis was seen in 53% of patients assigned to lonafarnib and ritonavir plus PegIFN-α 2a, 33% of patients assigned to lonafarnib and ritonavir, 38% of patients assigned to

PegIFN-α 2a, and 27% of patients assigned to placebo. Predictors of the primary endpoint were an HBsAg level <1000 IU/mL, female sex, and age older than 45 years. These data suggest that a proportion of patients may benefit from finite duration therapy and highlight the effect of PegIFN-α 2a monotherapy.

Inhibitors of HBsAg Translation

Another attractive approach to treat chronic HBV infection is to use an siRNA against HBsAg because of the dependence of HDV on HBsAg for viral entry. In a pilot study, REEF-D, 22 patients were randomized to receive an siRNA, JNJ-3989 100 mg every 4 weeks subcutaneously plus a nucleos(t)ide analog daily for up to 144 weeks or placebo plus nucleos(t)ide analog daily for the initial 48 weeks followed by crossover to JNJ-3989 100 mg every 4 weeks subcutaneously plus a nucleos(t)ide analog daily for 48 weeks.165 At Week 48, treatment with JNJ-3989 led to robust reductions in HBsAg (-1.75 log10 IU/mL) and HDV RNA (-1.52 log10 IU/mL) from baseline. However, 12/17 (71%) patients in the active treatment arm and 2/4 (50%) patients in the placebo arm experienced ALT elevations and HDV RNA rebound that eventually led to discontinuation of JNJ-3989. ALT elevations were more frequently observed in patients with high levels of HBsAg and HDV RNA at baseline. The cause for the elevated ALT levels remains unexplained and highlights a potential concern with use of siRNAs in chronic HDV infection. JNJ-3989 is no longer in development.

Another pilot trial, Solstice, evaluated two complementary approaches to inhibit HDV entry an siRNA, VIR-2218, alone, a monoclonal antibody, VIR-3434 (which is directed against a conserved epitope within the a-determinant of HBsAg), alone, and the combination of the two agents.[166] Patients responding to VIR-2218 or VIR-3434 after 12 weeks continued monotherapy at reduced dosing every 8 weeks up to Week 96. Patients not achieving ALT normalization and virologic response at Week 12 with either agent could transition to combination therapy or follow up until Week 96. Preliminary Week 12 data demonstrated that VIR-2218 and VIR-3434 monotherapy every 4 weeks achieved median HDV RNA reductions of -1.4 and -2.0 log10, respectively and median reduction in HBsAg levels of -1.35 log10 IU/mL and -0.18 log10 IU/mL, respectively. Combination therapy achieved the greatest HDV RNA reductions of -4.3 log10 from baseline. ALT elevations occurred in two patients receiving siRNA monotherapy, both with baseline HBsAg > 10,000 IU/mL. In another cohort, 32 treatment-naïve patients initiated both drugs together, VIR-2218 (siRNA) 200mg subcutaneously every 4 weeks and VIR-3434 (monoclonal antibody) 300 mg subcutaneously every 4 weeks for up to 96 weeks. At week 12, 14/27 (52%) and week 24 11/11 (100%) of patients achieved HDV RNA<LLOQ (<63 IU/mL) and ALT normalization at week 24 occurred in 7/11 (64%). Among 14 patients reaching week 24, the median reduction in HBsAg level was 3.3 log10 IU/mL. These data demonstrate that the combination of an siRNA (VIR-2218) and an anti-HBsAg monoclonal antibody was associated with rapid virological and biochemical response and represents a promising therapeutic strategy.[166a]

Inhibitors of Viral Release

Nucleic acid polymers (NAP, see Figure 83.2) are negatively charged oligomers that selectively block assembly and secretion of subviral HBsAg particles. Their precise mechanisms of action are not well understood but may be through an interaction with host chaperones. Nucleic acid polymers are undergoing evaluation in patients with chronic HBV and HDV infection. In an open-label study, 12 patients with chronic HDV infection received the nucleic acid polymer REP 2139 500 mg once a week intravenously for 15 weeks, followed by REP 2139 250 mg weekly in combination with PegIFN-α 2a 180 μg subcutaneously once a week for 15 weeks, followed by PegIFN-α 2a 180 μg once a week for 33 weeks.[167] All patients experienced a reduction in HBsAg levels, with a mean reduction of 3.5 $\log_{10}$ IU/mL, and five patients cleared HBsAg. In parallel with the reduction in HBsAg levels, treatment with REP 2139 resulted in a profound reduction in HDV RNA levels, with a mean decline of 5.3 log IU/mL, and 9 of 12 patients achieved undetectable HDV RNA at end of treatment.[167] Seven patients remained HDV RNA negative after 3.5 years of follow-up. HBsAg loss was persistent in three patients and was achieved by a fourth patient 3.5 years off-treatment.[168] Treatment with REP 2139 was generally safe and well tolerated.

Alternate Interferon Preparations

IFNλ is a type III IFN with similar antiviral activity as type I IFN but better tolerance due to type III IFN receptors being primarily expressed on epithelial cells in the liver and GI tract (see Fig. 83.2). The safety and efficacy of PegIFNλ were evaluated in chronic HDV infection. In an open-label pilot study, 33 patients received PEG-IFNλ 120 or 180 μg subcutaneously once weekly in addition to nucleos(t)ide analogs for 48 weeks. The PEG-IFNλ 180 μg dose achieved greater suppression of HDV RNA at end of treatment compared to the 120-μg dose, −2.14 compared with −1.23 $\log_{10}$ IU/mL.[169] At 24 weeks off-therapy, a greater proportion of patients receiving PEG-IFNλ 180 μg compared to 120 μg achieved HDV RNA < LLOQ 5/14 (36%) versus 3/19 (16%), respectively.[169] Flu-like symptoms and ALT elevations were the most common side effects. Of some concern was hyperbilirubinemia that required drug discontinuation in 8/33 (24%) patients. Of note, an ongoing phase 3 study (LIMT-2) evaluating PEG-IFNλ 180 μg weekly for 48 weeks with 24 weeks follow-up or no treatment for initial 12 weeks followed by PegIFNλ 180 μg weekly with 24 weeks of follow-up was halted due to the occurrence of hepatic decompensation in four patients. As a consequence, the development of PegIFNλ has been discontinued.[170]

In summary, several promising agents with demonstrable antiviral activity are in development for the treatment of chronic HDV infection. The preliminary evidence suggests that they will likely be used in combination with other agents, including PegIFN-α and nucleos(t)ide analogs for finite duration strategies and as monotherapy for long-term maintenance treatment. Safety of extended dosing will need to be demonstrated, and the results of ongoing studies are awaited before further conclusions about their benefit can be determined.

PREVENTION

Primary prevention of HDV infection can be achieved through HBV vaccination of individuals who have not been exposed to HBV because of the dependence of HDV on HBsAg for its life cycle. Persons at higher risk for HDV infection, including PWID and men who have sex with men, should be targeted for vaccination. Experiments in a woodchuck hepatitis model have demonstrated that partial protection against HDV infection through active immunization may be feasible, but further studies are required.[171] In the absence of a specific HDV vaccine, persons with chronic HBV infection should be educated and counseled on behavioral methods to limit exposure to HDV.

Full references for this chapter can be found at https://ebook.health.elsevier.com.

84 Hepatitis E

Rakesh Aggarwal, Amit Goel

IN THIS CHAPTER

Hepatitis E is a form of viral hepatitis caused by hepatitis E virus (HEV). The disease, often acute, self-limited, and associated with icterus, was first recognized in the 1980s, when sera collected during a large epidemic in Delhi, India, in 1955,[1] and during another epidemic in Kashmir, India, in 1978,[2] were found to lack serologic markers of HAV and HBV infection.[3] In retrospect, several hepatitis outbreaks that occurred around the world in the 18th and 19th centuries have had epidemiologic features resembling those of hepatitis E epidemics.[4] HEV was identified in 1983 by immune electron microscopy,[5] and its genome was cloned and sequenced in the early 1990s.[6] HEV infection was initially believed to be limited to humans residing in developing countries and to cause acute liver disease. However, the subsequent discovery of HEV-like genomic sequences in pigs (swine HEV) and other animal species,[7] and close genetic relatedness between the animal-HEV and HEV in some locally acquired human cases (including immunosuppressed persons with chronic hepatitis) and healthy blood donors in developed countries[8] indicate a broader host range and geographic distribution for the virus than was previously thought. In addition, the infection has also been shown to be associated with chronic liver disease and several extrahepatic manifestations.

VIROLOGY

HEV, currently placed in the family Hepeviridae and subfamily Orthohepevirinae,[9] has icosahedral virions that are 27–34 nm in diameter and contain 180 copies of the capsid protein. The virions exist in two forms—nonenveloped virions, primarily excreted in feces, and quasienveloped virions, the main form in blood circulation.[10,11] The enveloped virions are wrapped in a host-derived membrane, which protects them from neutralization by the circulating antibody, and is the form most likely responsible for cell-to-cell spread of virus. The nonenveloped form is most likely derived from the enveloped virions through stripping of the membrane by detergent action of bile.

The virus has an approximately 7.2-kilobase-long, single- and positive-stranded, polyadenylated RNA genome with three open reading frames (ORFs)[12] that encode viral nonstructural proteins (ORF1), the viral capsid protein (ORF2), and a small multifunctional protein (ORF3), respectively (Fig. 84.1). The ORF3-encoded protein is involved in biogenesis of the viral envelope and is found only in the enveloped form of HEV but not in the unenveloped virus.[13] A novel ORF4, placed entirely within the ORF1 sequence but in an alternate reading frame, has been identified in HEV genotype 1 strains[14]; however, it does not appear essential for viral replication and infectiousness.[15] The ORF2-encoded capsid protein consists of three functional domains: S (shell), M (middle), and P (protruding). The protruding domain is involved in the binding of HEV to susceptible cells and contains neutralization epitopes.[16] The virus shows weak growth in vitro, and the mechanisms of its entry into, replication in, and release from host cells remain largely uncertain. Though HEV primarily infects hepatocytes, it also appears to be capable of infecting small intestinal mucosal and neural cells.[17,18]

The members of Hepeviridae family are placed in 2 subfamilies, 5 genera, and 10 species.[9] Subfamily Parahepevirinae members infect salmon and trout, and members of the Orthohepevirinae infect mammals and birds.[9] The latter subfamily consists of four genera: *Avihepevirus* (birds), *Chirohepevirus* (bats), *Rocahepevirus* (rodents), and *Paslahepevirus* (primates including humans). Members of the species *Paslahepevirus balayani* are known to infect humans and several other mammals such as pig, deer, wild boar, rabbit, and camel. Phylogenetic analysis of strains of this species reveals eight distinct genotypes, four of which (genotypes 1 to 4; Table 84.1) are responsible for most of the human disease.[9,19] These four genotypes show distinct geographic distributions and host specificity. Occasional cases of human infection with *Rocahepevirus ratti*, which primarily infects rats, have been reported.[20]

Genotype 1 HEV includes isolates from Asia and Africa, and genotype 2 includes one isolate from Mexico and some isolates from Western Africa; both of these genotypes are restricted to humans and have been associated with waterborne disease outbreaks. By contrast, genotypes 3 and 4 HEV circulate in several animal species, particularly in pigs, wild boars, and deer, and only occasionally cause human infection. HEV genotype 3 causes human disease in Europe, the United States, and South America, and HEV genotype 4 causes disease in Northeast Asia (China, Taiwan, Japan, and Vietnam) and occasional cases in Europe. In geographic regions where human cases of HEV genotype 3 or 4 infections are reported, swine and human isolates of HEV belong to the same genotype. In addition, the swine and human HEV strains in these regions often show greater genetic similarity with each other than with swine and human HEV isolates from other parts of the world, suggesting zoonotic transmission to humans.[21] In India, a highly endemic area, however, human and swine isolates have been found to be genetically dissimilar, belonging to genotypes 1 and 4, respectively.[22,23] Piglets acquire a natural infection with swine HEV by the fecal-oral route, usually at 2–4 months of age, and have a transient viremia and no clinical manifestations, although liver biopsy may show mild hepatitis.[7] Genotypes 5–8 appear to infect only animals, except for an occasional report of human genotype 7 HEV infection acquired from camels.[24] Despite their considerable genomic heterogeneity,

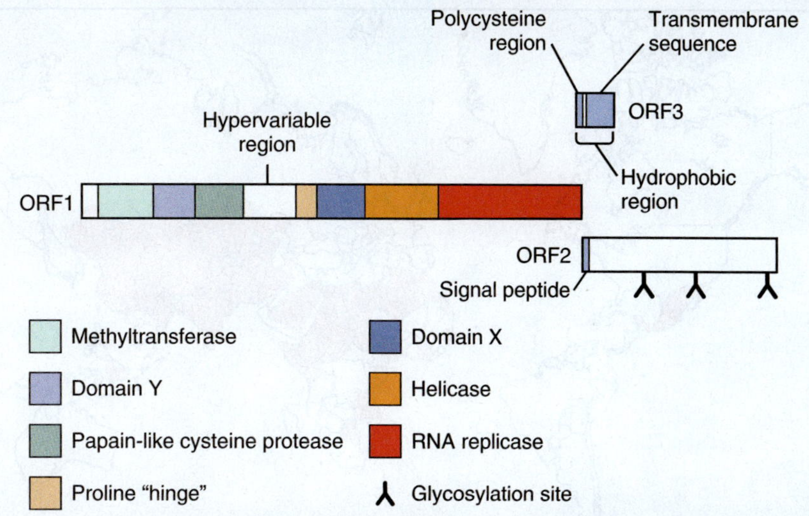

Fig. 84.1 The genome of HEV. The three open reading frames—*ORF1*, *ORF2*, and *ORF3*—are shown.

TABLE 84.1 HEV Genotypes That Cause Human Infection and Their Geographic Distribution

Genotype*	Human Infection	Animal Infection
1	South, Southeast, and Central Asia, Africa	–
2	Mexico, Western Africa	–
3	United States, South America, Europe (France, Spain, United Kingdom, and The Netherlands), and Japan	United States, China, Japan, Southeast Asia, Australia, New Zealand, and South America
4	China, Taiwan, Japan, and Vietnam	India, China, Taiwan, and Japan
7	Middle East (only one case has been reported)	Middle East

*Genotypes 5, 6, and 8 have been reported to cause infection only in animals.

all HEV genotypes show extensive serologic cross-reactivity with a single serotype.

EPIDEMIOLOGY

Two distinct epidemiologic patterns of infection and human disease caused by HEV are observed: (1) genotype 1 or 2 HEV disease in areas of high endemicity; and (2) genotype 3 or 4 disease in areas of lower endemicity (Table 84.2).

Areas of High Endemicity

In developing countries of Asia (Indian subcontinent, Southeast and Central Asia), the Middle East, Africa, parts of South America, and Mexico, HEV disease is highly endemic.[25,26] In these areas, human HEV infection occurs in the form of disease outbreaks[1,2,27,28] and frequent cases of sporadic disease (Fig. 84.2). The outbreaks can be large, causing several hundred to several thousand cases, with overall population incidence rates ranging from 1% to 15%—higher in adults (3%–30%) than in children (0.2%–10%) and in men than in women.

TABLE 84.2 Comparison of Epidemiologic and Clinical Features Associated With HEV Genotypes 1 and 2 Versus 3 and 4

Characteristic	Genotypes 1 and 2	Genotypes 3 and 4
Epidemiologic patterns of human disease	Large epidemics, small outbreaks, and frequent sporadic cases	A small proportion of cases with sporadic acute hepatitis
Persons affected	Young, otherwise healthy persons; males > females	Mostly older adults, often with other comorbid conditions; males > females
Animal-to-human transmission	Not reported	Demonstrated; a likely route is through consumption of undercooked meat or close contact with animals
Waterborne transmission	Well known to occur; most common route	Unknown
Animal reservoir	No	Yes (pigs, wild boars, and deer)
Severity	Variable severity, including ALF; severe disease is particularly more common in pregnant women	Severity and poor outcomes are related to comorbid conditions
Chronic infection	Not known to occur after acute infection	Immunosuppressed persons: transplant recipients receiving immunosuppressive drugs

Characteristically, the rates of disease and mortality are higher in pregnant women. The epidemics vary from single-peaked, short-lived outbreaks to prolonged, multipeaked epidemics lasting more than 1 year. In these areas, hepatitis E accounts for up to 30%–70% of cases of sporadic acute hepatitis; these cases demographically and clinically resemble those observed during outbreaks.

The predominant route of transmission of HEV infection in these areas is fecal-oral. Following HEV infection, viral shedding

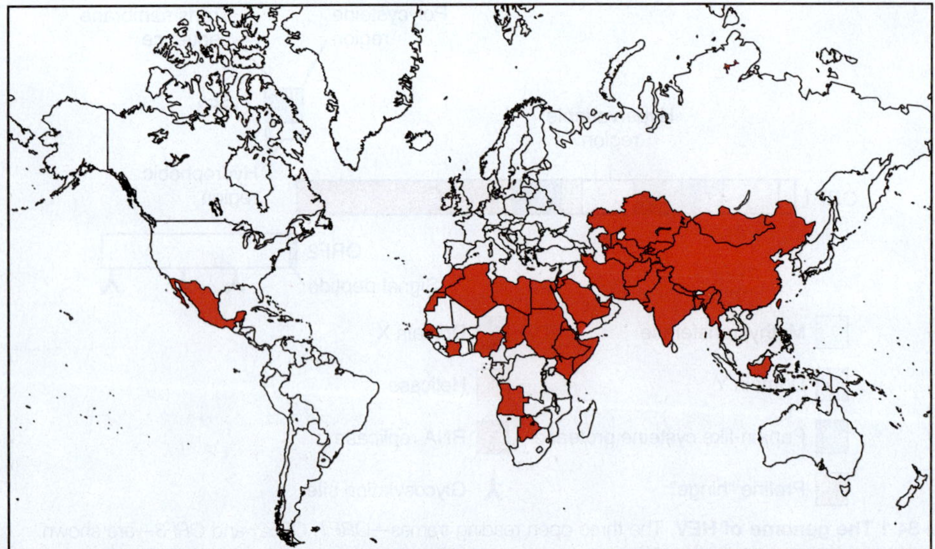

Fig. 84.2 Geographic distribution of areas where HEV genotype 1 and 2 infection is highly endemic (*red areas*). Map lines delineate study areas and do not necessarily depict accepted national boundaries.

in feces may continue for up to 3 weeks after the onset of symptoms.[29] Recently, the excretion of viral nucleic acid and protein has been described in urine; however, the data are limited to HEV genotypes 3 and 4.[30,31] In most outbreaks, epidemiologic investigations have shown an association of disease occurrence with consumption of fecally contaminated drinking water (Box 84.1). In some situations, HEV RNA has been detected in wastewater, sewage, and drinking water. The outbreaks frequently follow heavy rains and floods, but some are related to decreased flow in rivers during summers, with a consequent increase in the concentration of water contaminants. Genotypes 1 and 2 HEV, the prevalent genotypes in human cases of hepatitis E in these regions, appear not to cause either natural or experimental infection in animals; therefore the likely source of water contamination is human feces, from persons with either a clinical disease or subclinical HEV infection. Although data on subclinical HEV infection in humans are limited, viral excretion has been demonstrated during subclinical HEV genotype 1 infection in a macaque model.[32]

Person-to-person transmission of HEV appears to be uncommon during both epidemic and sporadic settings.[33,34] Vertical transmission from pregnant mothers to newborn babies[35] and transmission by blood transfusion[36] are well documented in the HEV genotype 1–predominant regions, but the contribution of these modes to the overall disease burden appears to be low.

Seroprevalence rates in highly endemic areas are generally higher than those in developed countries and increase with age. In India, the seroprevalence rates in adults are around 40%,[37] lower than those expected from the frequent occurrence of outbreaks and sporadic disease and from the nearly universal detection of antibody to HAV by adolescence in the same area. These observations suggest the possibility of a reduction in titer or disappearance of antibody to HEV (anti-HEV) over time. By contrast, in Egypt, where hepatitis E outbreaks have not been reported, anti-HEV is commonly found in children, and its seroprevalence rate in young adults exceeds 70%[38]; these findings are poorly understood, and infection with an attenuated or animal strain of HEV has been proposed.

BOX 84.1 Features of HEV Genotypes 1 and 2

- Cause acute infection with no evidence of chronicity
- Responsible for large outbreaks involving up to several thousand persons in developing countries
- Frequent sporadic cases
- Fecal-oral transmission, usually through contaminated water
- Highest attack rates are among young adults 15–40 years of age; infrequent in children
- Clinical disease is most likely to occur in young adults
- Infrequent person-to-person transmission
- No evidence of sexual transmission
- Greater likelihood of severe disease (ALF) with high (15%–25%) mortality rates in pregnant women, especially in the third trimester
- Mother-to-newborn (transplacental) transmission is known to occur

Areas of Lower Endemicity

In Europe, North America, developed countries in Asia (Japan, Taiwan), Australia, and New Zealand, hepatitis E has been reported in the form of case reports and case series and accounts for fewer than 1% of cases of acute viral hepatitis. Initially, most of these infrequent cases were believed to be related to travel to HEV-endemic regions and caused by the HEV genotype 1. However, several cases caused by autochthonous (locally acquired) HEV infection have been recognized[39,40]; these cases have been related mostly to HEV genotype 3, with a few cases, primarily in Japan, China, and Taiwan, caused by HEV genotype 4.[39,40]

In the United Kingdom,[41] persons with acute hepatitis E have often presented with features of liver disease such as jaundice, but many patients have had an anicteric illness with nonspecific symptoms or asymptomatic serum aminotransferase elevations. The number of cases appears to peak in the spring and summer, and the disease appears to be more common in residents of coastal and estuarine areas. Case series with similar characteristics have been described from other parts of Europe and, less frequently, North America.[39,40]

The source and route of infection in autochthonous hepatitis E in the areas of low endemicity remain unclear. The available evidence strongly suggests that most of such cases are related to zoonotic transmission from pigs (or other animals). Such transmission appears to occur through the consumption of undercooked meat, close contact with infected animals, or contamination of water supplies from animal feces. An instance of definite animal-to-human transmission of HEV was reported from Japan, where hepatitis E developed in members of two families after ingestion of uncooked deer meat; the viral genomic sequences obtained from these cases were similar to those retrieved from leftover meat.[42] Genomic sequences from human cases of hepatitis E in various areas of low endemicity have shown close molecular similarity to swine isolates of HEV from the same area. HEV genomic sequences have been isolated from pig livers and pig-liver sausages in Japan, Europe, and the United States and have been closely related to those from human cases of hepatitis E in these areas.[43,44] Consumption of raw or undercooked shellfish from HEV-contaminated waters has also been implicated.

Recently, zoonotic transmission of the rat HEV has also been reported from Europe,[45] China, and Hong Kong.[20]

Some HEV infections in these areas appear to be related to transmission through infected blood and blood products. HEV RNA has been detected in 1 in 600 to 1 in 15,000 healthy blood donors in various countries of Europe and North America, and transmission of HEV infection has been shown in a subset of recipients of such infected blood and blood components.[46–48]

In areas where autochthonous HEV genotype 3 hepatitis is diagnosed, anti-HEV seroprevalence rates have varied widely among studies, even within the same country; this may be in part because of differences in the assays used but may represent true geographic differences in the rates of infection. Seroprevalence rates among healthy people in the United States,[49] the United Kingdom,[42] and other European countries appear to be higher than would be expected from the relatively infrequent occurrence of clinical disease. These high rates could be related to subclinical infection with HEV genotype 3; alternative explanations include serologic cross-reactivity with other agents, exposure to animal reservoirs of HEV-like viruses, or false-positive results.

In China, outbreaks of disease due to the HEV genotype 1 were common in the past; however, since 2000, no outbreaks have been reported, and sporadic cases have been caused mainly by HEV genotype 4. These findings may represent an epidemiologic transition from a high-endemicity pattern to a low-endemicity pattern.

PATHOGENESIS

The current understanding of virologic, serologic, and pathologic events during acute HEV infection (Fig. 84.3) is based on data from experimentally infected animals, human volunteers, and a few patients. The events that occur between ingestion of HEV and its reaching the liver remain unclear. Recent data show that explanted intestinal cells can support HEV replication with release of quasienveloped virions, mostly on the apical surface but also on their basolateral aspect; the latter may enter the circulation, thereby reaching and infecting the liver cells.[17] The incubation period ranges from 2 to 10 weeks. In humans, HEV can be detected in feces approximately 1 week before the onset of illness. Viremia and fecal shedding of the virus last until about 3 weeks after the onset of illness.[29] In experimentally infected primates, HEV RNA appears in serum, bile, and feces a few days before the elevation of serum ALT levels. HEV antigen expression in hepatocytes is seen within 7 days after inoculation, can involve more than 50% of cells, and declines sharply as serum ALT levels increase.[50] Elevation of serum ALT and appearance of histopathologic changes in the liver generally correspond with the appearance of anti-HEV in serum.

Available evidence suggests that HEV is noncytopathic. This, along with temporal concordance of the HEV-specific immune response with the onset of liver pathology, suggests that liver injury in hepatitis E is immune mediated, as is the case in hepatitis B and C. Data on cellular immune events during HEV infection are relatively limited. Patients with acute hepatitis E show $CD4^+$ and $CD8^+$ T-cell responses to HEV proteins,[22,51–53] although the quality and strength of these responses have varied across studies, which used different techniques. In some studies, the responses have been weaker in patients with ALF than in those without ALF.[54] Also, the HEV-specific T-cell responses appear to decline with time. In addition, changes in natural killer T cells and regulatory T cells have been reported.[55] Gene expression data from experimentally HEV-infected chimpanzees suggest that the infection may induce an innate immune response and that adaptive immunity seems to be less important for viral clearance.[56] Occurrence of chronic HEV infection in immunosuppressed persons suggests a role for T-cell responses in viral clearance.

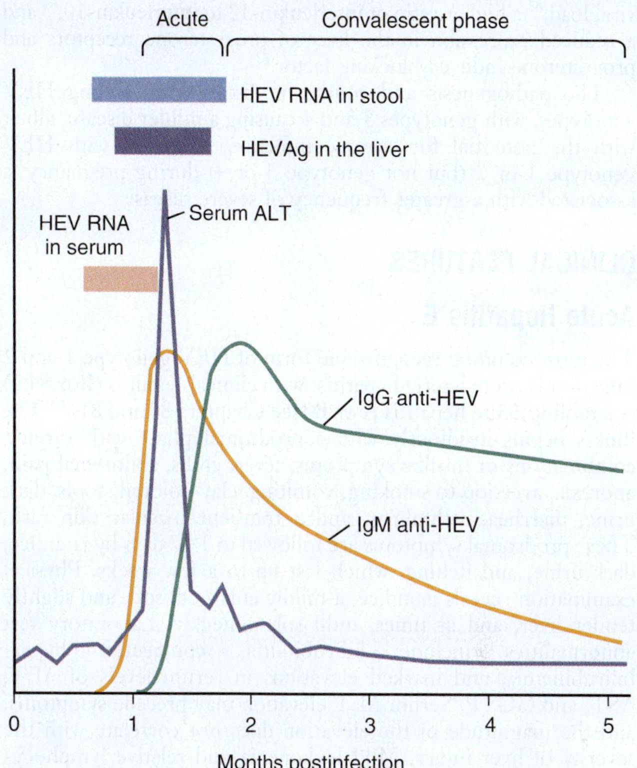

Fig. 84.3 Typical course of HEV infection (based on studies in human subjects and in experimentally infected primates). (*Ag*, Antigen; *anti-HEV*, antibody to HEV; *IgG*, immunoglobulin G; *IgM*, immunoglobulin M.)

Histopathologic changes in acute hepatitis E mirror those of other forms of acute hepatitis and include ballooned hepatocytes, acidophilic bodies, focal parenchymal necrosis, and inflammatory infiltrates in the lobules and expanded portal tracts. Some patients have prominent cholestasis, characterized by canalicular bile stasis and gland-like transformation of parenchymal cells, with less marked hepatocytic changes.[57] The liver shows infiltration with $CD8^+$ T cells.[58] Severe disease is associated with submassive or massive hepatocyte necrosis and collapse of liver parenchyma. Chronic HEV genotype 3 viremia is associated with evidence of prolonged liver inflammation and injury and can progress from chronic hepatitis to cirrhosis over time in immunosuppressed persons.[59]

The reason for severe liver damage during pregnancy, especially during the third trimester, remains unknown, although immune and hormonal factors have been suspected to play a role.[60] These factors have included a bias in helper T cell type 1/type 2 cytokine balance in favor of helper T cell type 2 cytokines,[61] suppression of the p65 subunit of nuclear factor-κB in both peripheral blood mononuclear cells and liver tissue from such patients,[62] a higher viral load,[63] a higher ratio of interleukin-12 to interleukin-10,[64] and a reduced expression in the liver of progesterone receptors and progesterone-induced blocking factor.[63]

The pathogenesis and course of disease vary among HEV genotypes, with genotypes 3 and 4 causing a milder disease, albeit with the potential for chronic infection. Infection with HEV genotype 1 or 2 (but not genotype 3 or 4) during pregnancy is associated with a greater frequency of severe disease.

CLINICAL FEATURES

Acute Hepatitis E

The most common recognizable form of HEV genotype 1 and 2 infection is acute icteric hepatitis, with clinical features (Box 84.2) resembling acute hepatitis A or B (see Chapters 80 and 81).[64] The illness begins insidiously with a prodromal phase with varying combinations of flu-like symptoms, fever, chills, abdominal pain, anorexia, aversion to smoking, vomiting, clay-colored stools, dark urine, diarrhea, arthralgias, and a transient macular skin rash. These prodromal symptoms are followed in 1–7 days by jaundice, dark urine, and itching, which last up to a few weeks. Physical examination reveals jaundice, a mildly enlarged, soft, and slightly tender liver, and at times, mild splenomegaly. Laboratory test abnormalities include bilirubinuria, conjugated hyperbilirubinemia, and marked elevations in serum levels of ALT, AST, and GGTP. Serum ALT elevation may precede symptoms, and the magnitude of the elevation does not correlate with the severity of liver injury. Mild leukopenia and relative lymphocytosis may occur. Ultrasound (US) may show a mildly enlarged liver, increase in hepatic parenchymal echogenicity, gallbladder wall edema, prominence of portal venules, and a slightly enlarged spleen; its main purpose is exclusion of biliary obstruction as the cause of jaundice.

Acute hepatitis E is usually self-limited. A few patients have a prolonged course with marked cholestasis (cholestatic hepatitis), including persistent jaundice lasting from several weeks to a few months, prominent itching, and marked elevation of the serum alkaline phosphatase level, most often with ultimate spontaneous resolution. Case fatality rates in highly endemic areas are generally low—0.5%–4% in hospital-based data and 0.07%–0.6% in population surveys during outbreaks.[27]

Some HEV-infected persons have only nonspecific symptoms resembling those of an acute viral febrile illness, with serum aminotransferase elevations but without jaundice (anicteric hepatitis), and some remain entirely asymptomatic; these forms appear to be more common in children. Anicteric and asymptomatic infections are more frequent than icteric disease, because a large proportion of HEV-seropositive persons in endemic areas do not recall ever having had jaundice. In a small proportion of patients, the disease is severe and associated with acute or subacute hepatic failure.

BOX 84.2 Clinical Features of Acute Hepatitis E

- Incubation period of 2–10 weeks
- Varying clinical manifestations:
  - Inapparent, asymptomatic infection
  - Anicteric hepatitis
  - Icteric hepatitis
  - Severe hepatitis leading to ALF
- Clinical illness similar to that with other types of acute viral hepatitis (except among pregnant women)
- Milder illness in children
- Low mortality rate (0.07%–0.6%) (except in pregnant women; see Table 84.2)

Pregnant women, particularly those in the second or third trimester, are affected more frequently during hepatitis E outbreaks than are others in the population and have a worse outcome, with mortality rates of 5%–25%. In an epidemic in Kashmir, India, clinical hepatitis E developed in 17.3% of pregnant women (8.8%, 19.4%, and 18.6% of those in trimesters 1, 2, and 3, respectively), compared with 2.1% of nonpregnant women and 2.8% of men of similar age[65]; ALF was observed in approximately 22% of the affected pregnant women. In addition, there is an increased frequency of abortions, stillbirths, and neonatal deaths.

Risk of severe disease is also higher among persons with a chronic liver disease, such as cirrhosis. Due to preexisting reduction in liver reserve, acute HEV infection in them is more likely to be associated with liver failure and poorer outcomes, including higher mortality.[66,67]

In geographic areas where HEV genotype 3 infection is observed, the manifestations are generally similar, except that the patients are generally older and more likely to have history of alcohol use and other coexisting illnesses,[8,41] and the liver disease is milder than that with HEV genotype 1. Several cases in these areas may go undiagnosed, as suggested by identification of hepatitis E on retrospective serologic testing among patients who had originally been diagnosed as having drug-induced hepatitis.[68]

Extrahepatic Manifestations

Several extrahepatic manifestations have been reported among persons with an HEV infection, mostly as case reports or small case series. These include a wide variety of neurologic, renal, hematologic, and autoimmune manifestations and acute pancreatitis. Of these, neurologic manifestations have been the most reported. This may reflect a particular affinity of HEV for neural cells, since neural cell lines have been shown to support HEV replication,[18] and brain invasion has been reported in HEV infection.[69] The neurological manifestations have been particularly reported from areas of low endemicity with a predominance of HEV genotype 3.[70] By contrast, acute pancreatitis has been reported more frequently in areas where the HEV genotype 1 predominates. The mechanisms of these manifestations and their viral causation remain uncertain.

Chronic Hepatitis E

Chronic infection with HEV, with persistent viremia and fecal excretion extending beyond 3–6 months to years, can occur[71]; all such cases have been reported from areas of low endemicity and have been associated with HEV genotype 3 and, occasionally, genotype 4 infection. Persistent infection is limited to immunosuppressed persons, including organ transplant recipients, those receiving cancer chemotherapy or immunotherapy, and HIV-infected persons. These patients may be either asymptomatic or have mild, persistent clinical symptoms of liver disease and often have high serum ALT and AST levels, indicating continuing inflammation of the liver. Over time, progressive liver damage and fibrosis may lead to development of cirrhosis[59]; the overall frequency of this complication remains unclear.

The predominant routes of acquisition of infection in such cases appear to be similar to those for autochthonous cases in areas of low endemicity. Transmission via the grafted organ has been considered but appears unlikely.

DIAGNOSIS

Human HEV infection can be diagnosed either directly by detection of HEV RNA or viral capsid antigen in clinical specimens or indirectly by demonstration of a virus-specific host immune response (see Fig. 84.3).[72] Detection of HEV RNA relies mostly on in-house reverse transcription-PCR assays, because commercial assays only became available in some regions in the 2010s. HEV antigen can be detected in the serum using an enzyme immunoassay. Enzyme immunoassays for the detection of immunoglobulin (Ig)M and IgG antibodies to HEV are based on recombinant HEV proteins expressed in *Escherichia coli* or insect cells, synthetic peptides corresponding to immunogenic epitopes of HEV, and protein expressed from a synthetic gene encoding multiple linear-antigenic epitopes from the ORF2 and ORF3 regions.[72]

The presence of IgM anti-HEV in serum strongly suggests acute infection, whereas detection of IgG anti-HEV indicates the acute or convalescent phase or past exposure. IgM anti-HEV appears in the early phase of clinical illness, lasts 4–5 months, and can be detected in 80%–100% of cases during outbreaks of hepatitis E. IgG anti-HEV appears a few days after IgM anti-HEV and remains detectable for at least 1 year to several years. With time, IgG anti-HEV appears to show a decline in titer and may become undetectable; the exact time frame for this is not known.

The several commercial kits for the detection of IgM and IgG anti-HEV available in various countries use different target antigens from different HEV strains and have been produced using different expression systems, making the results of various tests noncomparable. In one study, the sensitivities of 6 IgM anti-HEV assays varied from 72% to 98%, and their specificities varied from 78% to 96%.[73] More recently developed assays appear to perform better, although no consensus on the best assay has been reached. No FDA-approved assay is yet available in the United States.

HEV RNA can be detected in stool and serum during the acute phase of infection and in persons with a chronic infection. HEV antigen can be detected in serum during the initial phases of acute hepatitis E but not in the later phases,[74] as also in those with chronic HEV viremia; antigen assays thus may represent a simpler and cheaper alternative to HEV RNA detection. Recent data show that HEV antigen is also excreted in urine in large quantities,[31] and its detection in urine may have a better sensitivity than serum HEV RNA or antigen.[30]

In disease-endemic areas, clinical diagnosis of HEV infection is usually based on the presence of IgM anti-HEV. By contrast, in areas where the disease is infrequent, the positive predictive value of such a result is not sufficiently high, and detection of HEV RNA is often considered important for reliable diagnosis. Detection of the viral genome is also essential for diagnosis of HEV infection in immunodeficient persons, who may lack an antibody response, and for the diagnosis and assessment of response to treatment in patients with chronic HEV infection (see later). Viral genotyping requires amplification and sequencing of a segment of the viral genome. Duration of detection of HEV antigen in serum may help discriminate between acute and chronic HEV infection.[75]

TREATMENT

Acute hepatitis E is usually self-limited, and only supportive care is needed; antiviral therapy has no role in this condition. Patients with acute or acute-on-chronic liver failure need admission to an ICU, supportive treatment, measures to control cerebral edema, and consideration for liver transplantation (LT) (see Chapters 97 and 99). In pregnant women, termination of pregnancy has not been proved to provide any benefit; postpartum hemorrhage resulting from deranged coagulation may require treatment with fresh frozen plasma.

In chronic HEV infection, withdrawal or reduction in dose of immunosuppressive drugs leads to the disappearance of HEV viremia in about one-third of patients. In a retrospective case series of patients with chronic hepatitis E, treatment with ribavirin in a median dose of 600 mg daily for 3 months showed a high success rate in achieving sustained virologic response (no detectable HEV RNA in serum 3–6 months after treatment is stopped)[76]; however, no controlled trials are available. Among patients who fail to respond, mutations in the HEV genome have been identified.[77] In some patients, administration of pegylated interferon-α induced a sustained virologic response[78]; however, this drug carries a risk of acute rejection in patients with an organ transplant.

PREVENTION

Prevention of hepatitis E in endemic areas depends primarily on the availability of clean drinking water and strict attention to sewage disposal. In an epidemic setting, measures to improve the quality of water—as simple as boiling water—lead to a rapid decline in the number of new cases. Administration of immune globulin manufactured in endemic areas, either pre- or post-exposure, does not appear to provide any protection against HEV infection. In areas of low endemicity, zoonotic transmission can be avoided through emphasis on thorough cooking of pork and avoidance of undercooked meats; these measures may be particularly important for immunosuppressed persons.

Some countries in Europe have introduced universal targeted (only for high-risk recipients, such as immunosuppressed persons) or partial (in selected centers or geographic areas) screening of donated blood for HEV RNA.[79]

Experimental studies in HEV-susceptible primates using different recombinant HEV capsid proteins have shown an evidence of protection against hepatitis and viremia, although viral excretion was not prevented.[80] Two of these vaccines have undergone extensive human trials.[81,82]

The first vaccine to undergo efficacy trials in humans contained a recombinant truncated HEV capsid protein (amino acid 112–607) produced in insect cells as virus-like particles and used aluminum hydroxide as an adjuvant. In a phase 2, double-blind, randomized placebo-controlled trial, nearly 2000 seronegative young adults (>99% male) in Nepal[81] received three doses of either this vaccine or a matched placebo (at 0, 1, and 6 months). Over a 2-year follow-up period, the vaccine showed 95.5% protective efficacy against clinical acute hepatitis E; data on longer-term protection are not available. IgG anti-HEV, although present in high titer at 1 month after the third vaccine dose in all volunteers, was detectable in only 56% by the end of follow-up. This vaccine has not undergone further development.

The second vaccine consists of a 239-amino acid-long (amino acid 368–606) truncated ORF2 protein expressed in *E. coli*, which forms 23-nm virus-like particles. In a randomized field trial in Southern China with more than 110,000 volunteers, administration of 3 intramuscular doses (at 0, 1, and 6 months) showed a protective efficacy against clinical acute hepatitis E of 100% during a 13-month follow-up period and was safe, with only minor local adverse events.[82] In a longer-term follow-up extending up to 4.5 years, the rate of protective efficacy was 87%.[83] The vaccine was safe in a few pregnant women who received it inadvertently. Further studies using this vaccine have shown it to be immunogenic among elderly persons,[84] and when administered as an accelerated schedule (0, 7, and 21 days).[85] This vaccine has been marketed in China since 2012 and in Pakistan since 2021 but is not available elsewhere.

HEV vaccines are likely to be useful for travelers in regions where hepatitis E is highly endemic, for pregnant women and persons with a chronic liver disease who reside in such areas, and for immunosuppressed persons. Data on efficacy of the vaccine in the postexposure setting and against HEV genotype 1 or 3 disease, duration of protective efficacy, and effect on subclinical HEV infection and fecal shedding of the virus should be helpful in promoting more widespread use of this vaccine. Recently, the vaccine has been used in the setting of a disease outbreak in South Sudan.[86]

At least two other vaccines have recently undergone phase 1 trials in China[87] and India.[88] Attempts are also being made to determine whether administration of HEV vaccines to animals can help prevent zoonotic transmission.[89,90]

Full references for this chapter can be found at https://ebooks.health.elsevier.com.

85 Hepatitis Caused by Other Viruses

Jordan J. Feld

IN THIS CHAPTER

In addition to hepatitis A–E, a number of other viruses have been shown to be hepatotropic in that viremia is occasionally associated with elevations in serum aminotransferase levels and viral replication may occur in hepatocytes; however, causality with significant acute or chronic liver disease has been difficult to establish. Such viruses include human pegivirus (HPgV) [formerly known as hepatitis G virus (HGV) and the GB agents], TT virus (TTV), Sanban virus, Yonban virus, SEN virus, and TTV-like minivirus. Other novel agents such as the NV-F virus-like agent, which may exacerbate the severity of chronic hepatitis C, have been reported, but little is known about them.

Other viral diseases may sometimes involve the liver as part of a systemic infection. The agents of such infections include HIV (see Chapter 33), Epstein–Barr virus (EBV), *Cytomegalovirus* (CMV), herpes simplex virus (HSV), varicella-zoster virus (VZV), along with the virus that causes severe acute respiratory syndrome (SARS), and SARS-CoV-2, the virus that causes COVID-19 (coronavirus disease 19), parvovirus B19, and human herpesvirus 6 (HHV-6). Infection with any of these viruses may rarely lead to severe, sometimes fatal, hepatitis.

DISCOVERY OF NOVEL HEPATITIS VIRUSES

During the long search for the cause of transfusion-associated non-A, non-B hepatitis (see Chapter 82), candidate hepatitis viruses were discovered, primarily in individual or small numbers of patients with an acute clinical hepatitis and negative testing for all known viruses. Viral discovery programs with more advanced sequencing technology such as metagenomics continue with the hope of isolating pathogens in individuals with acute hepatitis syndromes who test negative for hepatitis A–E (non–A-E hepatitis). Although a number of viruses have been identified, a causal link with liver disease has been challenging to demonstrate in most instances.

GBV-C/HUMAN PEGIVIRUS

The GB agent (GBV) and HGV were discovered and later shown to be two isolates of the same virus. A 35-year-old surgeon with the initials GB developed an acute icteric hepatitis. When his serum was serially inoculated into healthy tamarins, they too developed hepatitis. Analysis of the tamarins infected with derivations of the GB serum led to the identification of 2 distinct viruses, labeled *GBV-type A (GBV-A)* and *GBV-type B (GBV-B)*.[1] Neither GBV-A or GBV-B infect humans, but a third virus, closely related to the GB agents, was subsequently identified by the same investigators from a human sample and was classified as *GBV-C*.[2] At approximately the same time, another group independently identified a virus from the serum of a patient with cryptogenic non–A-E hepatitis, which they named *HGV*.[3] Subsequent studies revealed 96% homology between the genomes of HGV and GBV-C, indicating that they were actually two strains of the same virus.[4] Because large epidemiologic studies have not demonstrated any association between infection with GBV-C/HGV and acute or chronic hepatitis, the use of the term "HGV" has been questioned. More recently, even the name GBV has been challenged. GBV-A and -B infect only new-world primates, and a more recently discovered related virus called GBV-D infects only bats. In fact, even the index patient (GB) was subsequently shown to be infected with HCV as the cause of his liver disease. As such, in 2011, a new nomenclature was adopted that preserved the name GBV only for the original GBV-B strain and called the other related viruses *Pegivirus* to indicate that they cause persistent (*Pe*) infection and originate from the historically named *G* or *GB* viruses.[5] They are all in the class of GBV-C, which is now known as HPgV. Notably, despite some structural similarities with HCV, HPgV should no longer be classified as a hepatitis virus. Although HPgV is detected in many patients with non-A-to-E acute and chronic hepatitis and may persist for years, it does not appear to cause liver (or any other) disease, even in immunocompromised persons.[6–20] HPgV infection has been established in Old World monkeys, including cynomolgus macaques.[11,21] Interestingly, following acute inoculation and progression to chronicity of HPgV infection, very little sequence evolution was seen, supporting the nonpathogenicity of this viral family. It is primarily, if not exclusively, lymphotropic,[22] and for persons with HIV infection, coinfection with HPgV is associated with a milder course of HIV-related disease and a better response to antiretroviral therapy,[23,24] possibly through direct competition for the same cell-type or through induction of cytokines.[16–20,23–43]

Because HPgV infection is not associated with clinical liver disease, no treatments have targeted HPgV specifically. In HIV-HCV-HPgV coinfected persons, peginterferon and ribavirin treatment led to sustained HPgV clearance in 31% of patients, with no observable subsequent effect on the course of HCV or HIV infection.[44] In patients coinfected with HPgV and HCV who were treated with interferon and ribavirin, HPgV RNA disappeared from serum during therapy but reappeared in all patients following discontinuation of therapy.[45,46] Importantly, no effect of HPgV infection on the response to treatment of HCV or HBV infection was observed.[9,47] Neither the effect of HCV direct-acting antiviral agents (DAAs) on HPgV replication nor the effect of HPgV on the response to DAAs has been reported.

TT VIRUS INFECTION

TTV was first identified in 1977, by the use of representational difference analysis in a patient (with the initials TT) in Japan who had acute posttransfusion non–A-G hepatitis.[48] TTV is also referred to as the transfusion-transmitted and torque teno virus.[49]

Virology

TTV is a nonenveloped, single-stranded, negative-polarity, circular DNA virus. It is closely related to a family of animal viruses known as Circoviridae, which have not been associated with human disease. TTV is the first human single-stranded circular DNA virus to be identified and does not fit precisely into any known virus family. Other TTV-like viruses were subsequently discovered and together make up the human Anellovirus family.[50,51]

TTV is hepatotropic based on the observation that viral levels are higher in the liver than in the serum of infected patients. TTV has also been identified within hepatocytes and shown to replicate by in situ hybridization and PCR; however, no or only minor morphologic changes have been seen in cells with positive hybridization signals.[52] TTV has also been shown to replicate in stimulated peripheral blood mononuclear cells and bone marrow cells.[53]

Epidemiology

TTV is found worldwide and is common. Initial studies documented infection in 1%–40% of healthy blood donors.[54] As more inclusive primers have been used to detect differing genotypes, the reported prevalence among blood donors has increased dramatically, approaching 100% in some studies.[55] The prevalence of TTV infection increases with age but appears to reach a plateau by early childhood.[56] TTV is also found in a variety of nonhuman primate species.

Clinical Features

Although TTV was associated with acute hepatitis in the patient in whom it was first identified, other studies have not supported a causal association between TTV and liver disease.[57–60] In the original study,[48] viremia was detected 6 weeks after exposure and 2 weeks before a rise in serum ALT levels.

Treatment

Formal studies of treatment of TTV infection have not been performed. A small study of HCV-TTV–coinfected patients showed that TTV infection had no effect on the sustained virologic response to therapy with peginterferon and ribavirin for HCV infection. Although TTV viremia cleared after therapy in 6 of 10 patients, 4 of the 6 relapsed within 6 months.[61]

SANBAN, YONBAN, SEN VIRUS, AND TT VIRUS–LIKE MINIVIRUS INFECTIONS

Since the discovery of TTV in 1997,[48] several similar viruses with a small DNA genome have been isolated in Japan and named *Sanban*, *Yonban*, and *TTV-like minivirus*.[49] These viruses have been divided into 29 genotypes, with a sequence divergence of greater than 30%.[46] Like TTV, they are readily transmitted parenterally and can also be passed by the fecal-oral route. None has been clearly associated with human liver disease to date.

In 1999 a novel virus was identified in an HIV-positive person (with the initials SEN) who had posttransfusion hepatitis of unknown etiology. This virus was found with the use of degenerate primers from the prototype TTV. The SEN virus is a small, nonenveloped, single-stranded DNA virus, but unlike that of TTV, the SEN genome is linear. Nucleotide sequencing has shown 50% homology with the prototype TTV, but only 30% of amino acids are homologous. Sequencing of multiple isolates has demonstrated sequence divergence of 15%–50%.[62]

Like TTV, SEN virus is transmitted both parenterally and by the fecal-oral route.[63] Vertical transmission occurs but, in most cases, does not lead to chronic infection. Natural clearance of both perinatally and parenterally acquired SEN virus does not appear to protect against reinfection.[64] The prevalence varies markedly and is highest among patients with parenteral risk factors, particularly those coinfected with HCV.[65] The prevalence among healthy blood donors is approximately 2% in the United States and 10% in Japan.[65–67]

The clinical significance of SEN infection remains controversial. One study of patients with posttransfusion non–A-E hepatitis suggested that SEN was the cause in a majority (11 of 12) of cases. SEN viremia persisted for more than 1 year in 45% of those infected; however, clinical hepatitis did not develop in a majority (86%) of transfused patients who acquired SEN infection. None of the patients with hepatitis had a fulminant course, nor did chronic liver disease or cirrhosis develop during follow-up.[68] Other reports and case series have identified SEN or TTV viremia in patients with both ALF and chronic hepatitis or HCC, but causation has been difficult to establish.[69] Most studies have shown neither an association between SEN or any of the other viruses in this group and human disease, nor an effect of these viruses on the course or response to treatment for chronic viral hepatitis.[63,70]

THE SEARCH FOR OTHER NON–A-E VIRAL HEPATITIS INFECTIONS

Cases of acute hepatitis continue to occur that test negative for both known hepatotropic viruses and systemic infections with liver involvement. Such cases are often referred to as non–A-E hepatitis, but some investigators prefer the term "indeterminate hepatitis" to indicate that a nonviral etiology may be responsible.[71] Advances in technology, such as next-generation metagenomic sequencing, have improved the ability to identify novel viruses or other human pathogens. With the use of this approach, all extracted RNA and DNA are sequenced with no or minimal amplification. Although this approach avoids biases and errors associated with amplification and can detect multiple viruses simultaneously, it leads to lower sensitivity than standard PCR-based methods.[72] A study aimed at viral discovery in a cohort of persons who inject drugs with HIV-HCV coinfection found that a metagenomic approach had a sensitivity of 10,000 copies or

IU/mL for known viruses.[73] However, the approach was successful in documenting a novel HPgV, which has also been referred to as HPgV 2.[73] Although no clinical consequences were apparent as a result of coinfection with this newly discovered virus, the approach highlights the power of this technique to detect new pathogens. With continuing advances, sensitivity is likely to improve.

Although powerful, metagenomic tools have potential pitfalls. Chinese investigators identified viral fragments in a cohort of patients with acute non–A-E hepatitis. After assembly of the complete genome, the new virus was provisionally designated NIH-CQV and was found to have homology to Parvoviridae and Circoviridae families of viruses. Of 90 patients, 63 (70%) had detectable DNA, which was not found in any of 45 controls.[74] However, this virus was subsequently shown to be identical to a virus called parvovirus-like hybrid virus, which was eventually found to be a contaminant of silica-binding columns used for nucleic acid extraction rather than a true human pathogen,[75] thereby highlighting the potential for powerful sequencing technologies to lead to spurious conclusions.

HPgV, SEN virus, TTV, and other pathogens were initially reported as causes of acute viral hepatitis; however, carefully performed studies subsequently showed that the frequency was similar in cases and controls, thus raising doubt about a causal relationship. Well-characterized clinical cases of "indeterminate hepatitis" and appropriate controls will be critical for rigorous independent validation of discoveries and proper assessment of associations between any novel microbes and liver disease.

SYSTEMIC VIRAL INFECTIONS THAT MAY INVOLVE THE LIVER

Epstein–Barr Virus

EBV infection is common and covers a wide spectrum of clinical presentations. Most infected infants and children are either asymptomatic or have mild, nonspecific complaints, whereas adolescents and adults typically present with the triad of pharyngitis, fever, and lymphadenopathy.[76] Although usually subclinical, liver involvement is nearly universal in patients with EBV mononucleosis and ranges from serum aminotransferase elevations to rare cases of acute and even fatal liver failure.[77]

Up to 90% of patients with acute mononucleosis have serum aminotransferase and LDH elevations two to three times the upper limit of normal (ULN). The enzyme levels typically rise over a 1- to 2-week period, and peak levels are usually less than fivefold the ULN, much lower than those normally seen in patients with acute hepatitis A, B, D, or E.[78] Elevated levels of alkaline phosphatase are common, and mild hyperbilirubinemia is observed in as many as 45% of cases.[78,79] In most patients, liver biochemical test levels normalize within 1 month, often before complete resolution of clinical symptoms.[80] As with infectious mononucleosis, EBV hepatitis tends to be more severe in adults older than 30 years of age than in younger adults and children.[81] Older adults occasionally present with jaundice, fever, and RUQ pain that may be confused with extrahepatic biliary obstruction.[82] Although jaundice may be caused by viral-induced cholestasis, autoimmune hemolytic anemia should be excluded in hyperbilirubinemic patients. Cholestatic jaundice with pruritus may be observed in young women with EBV infection who continue taking oral contraceptive pills.

Fatal ALF due to EBV hepatitis has been described in both immunocompetent and immunocompromised persons and appears to be associated with a greater than usual EBV viral burden, particularly in T cells as opposed to B cells.[83] A small minority of patients develop a chronic form of EBV infection at the time of initial infection that resembles infectious mononucleosis, with involvement of liver, lungs, and other organs, but that does not resolve and may be life-threatening. High levels of EBV DNA are found in the blood, with associated fever, hepatitis, and lymphadenopathy.[84] Treatment with immunosuppressive agents may induce remission, but only hematopoietic stem cell transplantation has been reported to be curative.[84] In addition to chronic EBV infection, a hemophagocytic syndrome characterized by fever, hepatosplenomegaly, hepatic synthetic dysfunction, cytopenias, and marked hyperferritinemia (>10,000 μg/L) may develop in patients with EBV infection. The syndrome, also known as *hemophagocytic lymphohistiocytosis*, is caused by natural killer T-cell dysregulation, leading to lymphocyte proliferation and activation with uncontrolled hemophagocytosis and cytokine production. The syndrome is associated with primary or reactivated EBV infection and is also seen in the context of hematologic malignancies and collagen vascular diseases (see Chapter 35).[67] Successful treatment has been reported with immunosuppressive therapy with glucocorticoids or cyclosporine, or both, chemotherapy, and hematopoietic stem cell transplantation. Although rare, the syndrome is usually severe and may be fatal.[85]

EBV hepatitis is a relatively infrequent cause of acute hepatitis in adults, accounting for just 0.85% of 1995 cases of hepatitis reported at a tertiary center. Notably, only a minority (12%) had clinical features of infectious mononucleosis, but all had lymphocytosis and 88% had splenomegaly. Mild thrombocytopenia may also be seen.[86] The monospot test is sensitive for the detection of heterophile antibodies but is not a specific test for EBV infection. Levels of EBV-specific immunoglobulin (Ig)M antibodies peak early in serum and may persist for many months, at which point IgG antibodies appear. Findings on abdominal US are usually nonspecific and may include hepatosplenomegaly, lymphadenopathy, and possibly gallbladder wall thickening, which has been reported to portend more severe liver disease.[87] Liver biopsy is rarely necessary for diagnosis and, if done, shows portal and sinusoidal mononuclear cell infiltration with no disruption of hepatic architecture; multinucleated giant cells are not a feature. In more severe cases, focal hepatic necrosis may be evident. In situ hybridization or PCR testing of biopsy samples may be used to confirm the diagnosis, but immunohistochemistry for EBV proteins is rarely positive.[88]

No specific treatment for EBV hepatitis exists. Acyclovir inhibits EBV replication and reduces viral shedding from the nasopharynx but has no effect on clinical symptoms or outcome.[89] Improvement in acute and chronic EBV hepatitis has been reported with ganciclovir treatment, but this approach has not been well studied.[90] Liver transplantation (LT) has been performed for ALF caused by EBV. EBV rarely causes hepatitis after LT but has been associated with posttransplantation lymphoproliferative disease (see Chapter 34). EBV DNA is commonly found in the blood after LT, but viral titers are not associated with symptoms or complications.[91] Similarly, although EBV DNA can be isolated from the liver in the setting of posttransplant graft hepatitis, it is not associated with graft survival or other outcomes (see Chapter 99).[92] By contrast, high levels of HHV-6 DNA have been associated with graft hepatitis with impaired graft survival.[92] In a patient with chronic EBV hepatitis after kidney transplantation, treatment with rituximab has been reported to lead to improvement in serum liver enzyme levels and hepatic pathology.[93]

Cytomegalovirus

CMV is the largest member of the Herpesviridae family and, like other herpesviruses, persists lifelong in a latent, nonreplicative state after resolution of primary infection. Consequently, clinical disease caused by CMV may occur as a primary infection or, more commonly, as reactivation of latent infection,[94] particularly in immunocompromised persons.

In immunocompetent children and adults, primary CMV infection is usually subclinical but may cause a mononucleosis-like illness. Liver involvement is common and is characterized by mild-to-moderate serum aminotransferase (88%) and alkaline phosphatase (64%) elevations with or without hepatosplenomegaly.[95] Although the clinical course is mild in most patients, rare instances of granulomatous cholestatic CMV hepatitis, with or without jaundice, and even massive, fatal hepatic necrosis have been described.[96] In addition to the congenital CMV syndrome (jaundice, hepatosplenomegaly, thrombocytopenic purpura, and severe neurologic impairment), CMV is a common cause of neonatal hepatitis.[97] A number of case reports also suggest a possible association between CMV infection and acute portal vein thrombosis; however, the mechanism is unclear.[98]

Disseminated, life-threatening CMV infection with multi-organ involvement may develop in patients with impaired cell-mediated immunity (see Chapters 33 and 34). Hepatobiliary involvement by CMV is common in patients with AIDS and may manifest as hepatitis, pancreatitis, or acalculous gangrenous cholecystitis.[99] CMV also may cause AIDS-associated cholangiopathy, which manifests with chronic cholestasis and mimics PSC clinically and radiographically (see Chapter 33).[100] Patients may have papillary stenosis alone or in combination with intra- or extrahepatic (or both) biliary structuring and dilatation (see Figs. 85.1 and 35.8). Antiviral therapy has no effect on this syndrome, but papillotomy, with or without placement of a biliary stent, may lead to symptomatic improvement.[99] Organ transplant recipients are also at risk for aggressive CMV hepatitis, including fibrosing cholestatic hepatitis (see Chapter 99), but for unclear reasons, cholangiopathy does not develop in these patients.[101] CMV hepatitis can be difficult to distinguish from graft rejection in liver transplant recipients.[102]

The diagnosis of CMV infection is based on the results of serologic and nucleic acid studies, liver biopsy, or both. In acute primary CMV infection, IgM antibodies to CMV are present. For patients with reactivation of latent CMV, direct measurement of viremia with PCR is necessary. Because CMV viremia precedes organ involvement, testing for CMV PCR in blood is a useful screening tool in immunocompromised patients.[103] Multinucleated giant cells with mononuclear portal and parenchymal inflammatory infiltrates and cholestasis are commonly seen on liver biopsy specimens. Large nuclear inclusions, sometimes referred to as "owl's eye" inclusions, may be seen in hepatocytes or biliary epithelial cells (Fig. 85.2).

With mild CMV disease in an immunocompetent adult, treatment is unnecessary. In immunocompromised patients, antiviral therapy is indicated. Ganciclovir, a guanosine nucleoside analog with a much longer intracellular half-life than that of acyclovir, has proved to be most effective. The major toxicity is bone marrow suppression, particularly granulocytopenia. Because viremia correlates with disease outcome, ganciclovir should be continued until CMV antigenemia or viremia is undetectable.[104] For patients resistant to or intolerant of ganciclovir, alternative agents include foscarnet and cidofovir.

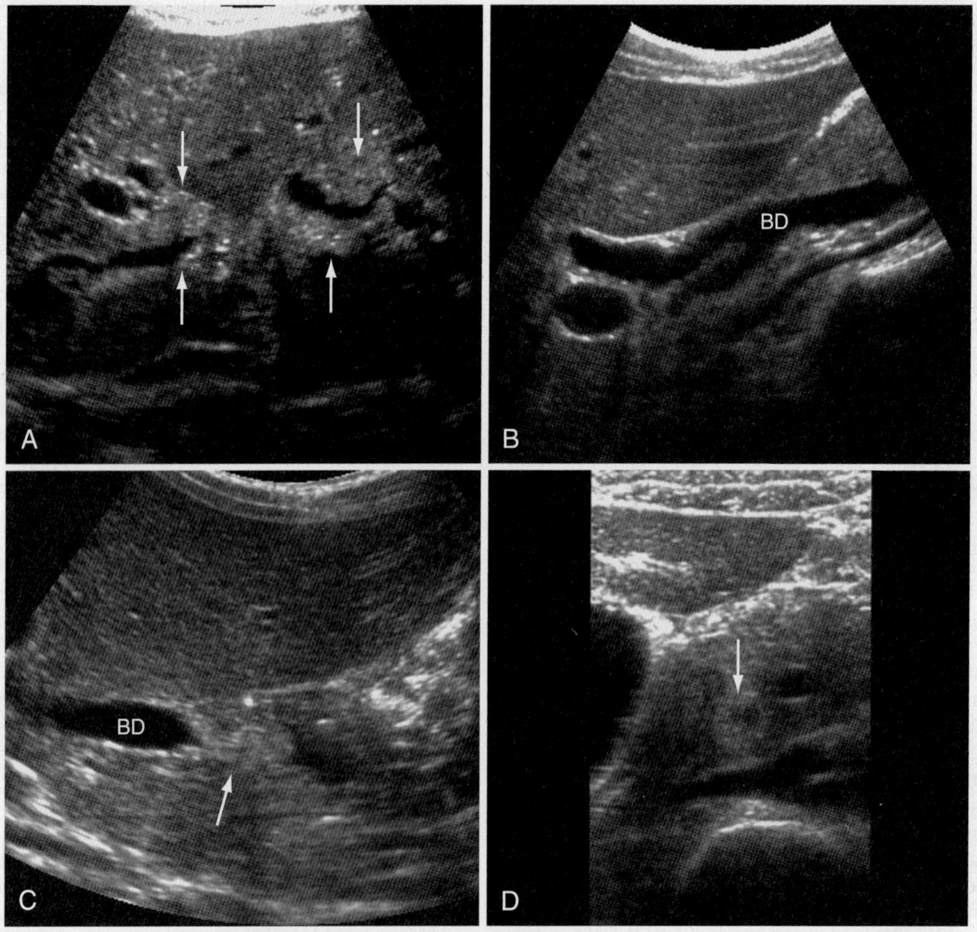

Fig. 85.1 US findings in AIDS cholangiopathy and CMV infection. (A) A thick rind of echogenic tissue (*arrows*) surrounds the central portal triads and causes irregular narrowing of the intrahepatic bile ducts (*BDs*). (B) The *BD* is dilated, and its wall is minimally irregular. (C) The dilated *BD* tapers abruptly at an echogenic, inflamed ampulla (*arrow*), indicative of papillary stenosis. (D) The ampulla (*arrow*) is enlarged and echogenic, as viewed transversely in the caudal aspect of the pancreatic head.

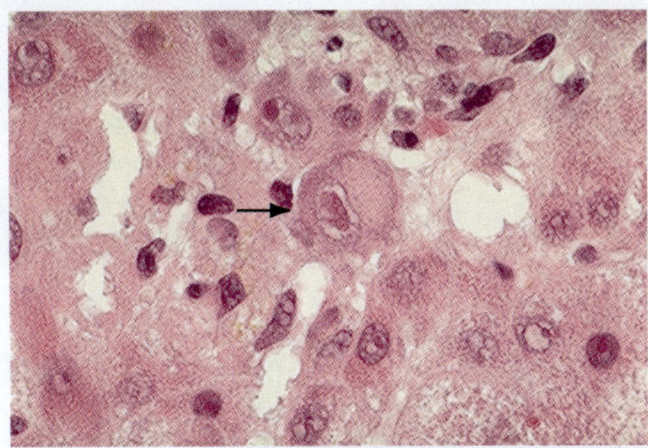

Fig. 85.2 Histopathology of CMV hepatitis. In the center (*arrow*) is a large hepatocyte with a large nucleus that contains an "owl's eye" inclusion (H&E). (Courtesy Dr. Maha Guindi, Toronto, Canada.)

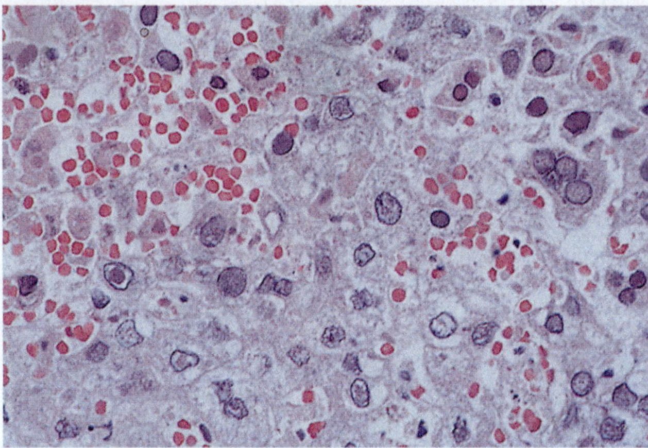

Fig. 85.3 Histopathology of HSV hepatitis. At the edge of a necrotic zone, some hepatocytes are multinucleated, and many nuclei contain eosinophilic viral (Cowdry type A) inclusions (H&E). (From Lucas SB. Other viral and infectious diseases and HIV-related liver disease. In: Burt AD, Portmann BC, Ferrell LD, eds. *Pathology of the Liver*. 5th ed. London: Churchill Livingstone; 2007:446.)

Herpes Simplex Virus

HSV typically causes mucocutaneous vesicular oral or genital lesions; visceral involvement may occur in certain clinical settings. HSV hepatitis is seen in neonates, pregnant women, and immunocompromised persons and can be aggressive and life-threatening, with up to 80% mortality reported in some series.[105] Hepatitis may be caused by HSV-1 or HSV-2.[106] Cases of severe HSV hepatitis in immunocompetent persons have been reported as well.[107] Severe hepatitis with multiorgan involvement and, often, adrenal insufficiency may develop in neonates exposed to infected maternal genital secretions at the time of delivery.[108] Risk factors for severe disease and the need for LT include the lack of skin lesions, positive HSV DNA by PCR testing, thrombocytopenia, and liver synthetic dysfunction.[109] In pregnant women, HSV hepatitis usually has a fulminant course. The disease is most common in late gestation, typically (in 65% of patients) in the third trimester. Mucocutaneous lesions are present in only 50% of cases, and a high index of clinical suspicion is important to ensure timely diagnosis.[110] Maternal and perinatal mortality rates approach 40%, and in the largest series, 25% of patients were diagnosed only at autopsy. Early diagnosis and initiation of antiviral therapy are critical.[111]

Mild, asymptomatic liver enzyme elevations may be seen in 14% of immunocompetent patients with acute genital HSV infection. By contrast, immunocompromised patients may present with ALF.[112] Hepatitis is more common with acute infection than with reactivation and presents with fever, leukopenia, and markedly elevated serum aminotransferase levels. Coagulopathy, including DIC, and jaundice may be seen. Acute and sometimes severe abdominal pain has been reported.[113] Of reported cases, only 50% had a rash at presentation, and 58% were diagnosed at autopsy.[114] Risk factors for progression to death or LT include male gender, age over 40 years, a serum ALT level over 5000 U/L, a platelet count less than 75,000/mm^3, and lack of antiviral therapy.[114]

Liver biopsy is essential for diagnosis, particularly in pregnancy. The transjugular route may be required because liver failure may develop rapidly, precluding percutaneous biopsy. Focal or extensive hemorrhagic or coagulative necrosis, with few inflammatory infiltrates, is seen. Intranuclear (Cowdry A type) inclusions may be identified in hepatocytes at the margins of the necrosis. In addition, some periportal multinucleated hepatocytes show a ground-glass appearance suggestive of viral inclusions (Fig. 85.3).[115] Electron microscopy, immunohistochemical staining, and PCR techniques can be used to confirm the diagnosis.[116] Serum PCR testing has been reported to allow rapid diagnosis with early institution of therapy.[117]

HSV hepatitis constitutes an emergency, and empirical therapy should be instituted pending diagnostic confirmation. High-dose IV acyclovir (at least 10 mg/kg every 8 hours) is effective and appears to be safe in pregnant patients.[118] Prolonged therapy may be required because severe relapse has been reported.[107] Although successful LT has been reported, transplant outcomes for HSV hepatitis have been disappointing, with just a 38% 1-year survival rate in the European transplant registry.[119]

Varicella Zoster Virus

Like HSV infection, VZV infection occasionally can be complicated by hepatitis. Serum liver enzyme levels may be elevated in up to 3.4% of children with chickenpox; however, clinically significant hepatitis has been reported only rarely.[120] Although VZV reactivation in adults usually is limited to the skin, dissemination with liver, lung, and pancreatic involvement may occur.[121] Rarely, visceral involvement has been reported to develop before cutaneous manifestations in bone marrow or solid organ transplant recipients. If visceral involvement is suspected, treatment with high-dose IV acyclovir should be instituted.

Severe Acute Respiratory Syndrome and SARS-CoV-2

During the 2003 outbreak of SARS, elevated serum aminotransferase levels were commonly observed during the acute illness. Subsequently, cases of SARS hepatitis were reported in three patients in whom the coronavirus that causes SARS was demonstrated in the liver by reverse transcriptase-PCR techniques; no viral particles were seen on electron microscopy. All three cases fulfilled the World Health Organization (WHO) criteria for SARS. Examination of liver tissue revealed marked apoptosis, ballooning of hepatocytes, and moderate lobular lymphocytic infiltration.[122]

In late 2019 a related, but distinct, coronavirus (SARS-CoV-2) was identified in China in people presenting with severe viral pneumonia. Spread of SARS-CoV-2 led to the global COVID-19 pandemic that resulted in millions of deaths worldwide. Acute hepatitis has been described as an extra-pulmonary complication of SARS-CoV-2 infection, and underlying chronic liver disease has been shown to be a risk factor for more severe COVID-19.[123] Chronic liver injury in the form of SARS-CoV-2 cholangiopathy has been reported as a rare but potentially severe complication of COVID-19.[124]

Acute Hepatitis From SARS-CoV-2

Liver enzyme elevation, typically with a hepatocellular pattern, has been described in patients with COVID-19. Accurate data are lacking for outpatients with mild COVID-19 but multiple studies have shown that transaminase elevation is common, ranging from 19% to over 60%, and is associated with severe disease in hospitalized COVID-19 patients, including a more severe course of disease, need for ICU care, and death from COVID-19.[125–128] Enzyme levels are usually 2–5× the ULN with normal bilirubin and preserved liver synthetic function, but rarely, ALT levels over 1000 U/L with jaundice have been reported.[125,127] In most patients, enzyme elevations resolve with recovery from COVID-19.[125]

Compelling evidence suggests that SARS-CoV-2 is able to directly infect liver cells. Although ACE2, the primary entry factor for SARS-CoV-2, is expressed primarily on cholangiocytes in a resting state, in the setting of inflammation, the expression of ACE2 and other key entry factors (e.g., TMPRSS2 and procathepsin L) is also present in hepatocytes.[129] SARS-CoV-2 RNA has been documented in hepatocytes using in situ hybridization and infectious virus has been recovered from liver tissue postmortem.[130] Careful transcriptomic and proteomic analyses have also shown activation of interferon responses, JAK-STAT signaling, and metabolic changes, similar to those seen during infection with hepatotropic viruses, suggesting direct infection by SARS-CoV-2 of hepatocytes in at least some patients.[131] Local inflammation, immune dysregulation, and vascular injury, including endotheliopathy, may also directly contribute to liver injury.[132,133] Beyond direct effects of the virus on liver cells, liver injury during COVID-19 may also stem from consequences of systemic infection such as hepatic congestion and thrombosis, as well as from drug-induced liver injury from antiviral or supportive therapies.[133] Multiple histologic patterns have been described in patients undergoing liver biopsy during COVID-19, including micro- and macrovesicular steatosis, portal and lobular inflammation, and vascular pathology, reflective of the multifactorial etiology of liver damage.[130,134,135]

Post-COVID Cholangiopathy

In addition to acute liver injury, chronic hepatic sequelae, particularly COVID-19 cholangiopathy, have been described in patients with SARS-CoV-2 infection. Secondary sclerosing cholangitis may occur in people with severe systemic illness related to an ischemic biliary injury (ICU cholangiopathy); however, cholangiopathy after COVID-19 has been reported more frequently than in similarly ill cohorts of influenza patients with some distinct histologic features, suggesting that it may be a direct consequence of SARS-CoV-2 infection.[136] The precise incidence of post-COVID cholangiopathy is unknown but it appears to be more frequent in patients with underlying liver disease and has only been reported in people with severe COVID-19 requiring ICU care and mechanical ventilation.[137] In one study, 10 of 65 (15.4%) of patients with chronic liver disease who were hospitalized for COVID-19 developed secondary sclerosing cholangitis.[138] The pathophysiology of cholangiopathy is uncertain but may relate to ischemic injury, similar to "ICU cholangiopathy," but other mechanisms have been proposed including direct infection of cholangiocytes by SARS-CoV-2 and immune-mediated injury due to cytokine release and systemic inflammation.[139] Cholangiopathy is associated with ALP (often >1000 U/L) and bilirubin elevation and is confirmed by typical findings on MRCP of beading of intrahepatic bile ducts with strictures and associated dilatation (Fig. 85.4).[137] In a series of 30 reported cases, cholangiopathy was identified a mean of 66 (±36) days after COVID-19 diagnosis and was more common in men (83%), 53% of whom had underlying hypertension.[137] Liver biopsy findings include portal and periportal fibrosis, features of degenerative cholangiocyte injury, and duct paucity or absence.[140] The natural history is not well documented, but some patients develop progressive cholestatic liver injury that may lead to ESLD and death. ERCP has been used for stone/sludge removal, sphincterotomy, and stent placement when required but has not been shown to affect liver-transplant-free survival in small series.[137] Some patients have been treated empirically with ursodeoxycholic acid, as well as with remdesivir without clear evidence of benefit.[137] Reports of plasmapheresis have suggested possible benefit as a bridge to transplant, possibly through removal of pathogenic antibodies; however, the precise mechanisms and clear evidence of benefit are lacking.[141] LT has been successfully used for patients with post-COVID cholangiopathy who are otherwise well enough to undergo the procedure.[137]

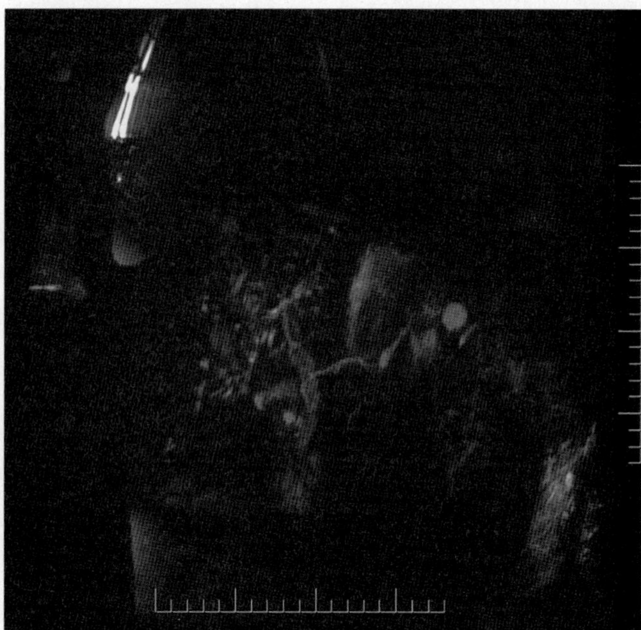

Fig. 85.4 MRCP images of post-COVID-cholangiopathy. The typical beaded appearance of intrahepatic bile ducts is seen in this woman who recovered from severe COVID-19 requiring ICU care and mechanical ventilation and died of complications of end-stage liver disease.

COVID-19 in Patients With Chronic Liver Disease

Underlying chronic liver disease, particularly the presence of cirrhosis, has been consistently shown to be a risk factor for poor outcomes in people with COVID-19.[99,135,142] A large population-based study, including over 220,000 patients with chronic liver disease, reported that hospitalized patients with cirrhosis and SARS-CoV-2 infection had an 8.9% 30-day mortality compared to 3.9% among uninfected patients with cirrhosis. After controlling for other risk factors, the hazard ratio (HR) for death at 30 days with cirrhosis and SARS-CoV-2 infection was 2.38 (95% CI, 2.18–2.59) compared to cirrhosis alone.[143] The presence of cirrhosis is a key determinant of outcome, with an HR of 3.31 for 30-day mortality in patients with cirrhosis and COVID-19 compared to SARS-CoV-2-infected patients with chronic liver disease but without cirrhosis. Factors associated with worse outcome include increasing age, Child-Pugh score, and alcohol-associated liver disease.[144] The most common cause of death among patients with cirrhosis was COVID-19-related lung disease but hepatic decompensation and liver failure were also common.[143]

Alcohol-associated liver disease has been most consistently associated with poor COVID-19 outcomes, possibly related to the consequences of alcohol on immune function.[144,145] Some studies have reported less severe COVID-19 outcomes in patients with cholestatic liver disease, possibly due to the use of ursodeoxycholic acid, which downregulates ACE2 expression and limits SARS-CoV-2 infection into cholangiocytes in vitro.[146] Despite the need for immunosuppression, no increase in complications from COVID-19 has been reported in patients with autoimmune hepatitis.[144] Metabolic risk factors including obesity and diabetes have been consistently associated with more severe COVID-19 and likely explain the early reports that nonalcoholic fatty liver disease was a risk factor for severe disease.[147,148] Follow-up studies have not shown an independent effect of metabolic dysfunction-associated steatotic liver disease (MASLD) on SARS-CoV-2 susceptibility or outcome.[149,150] Despite in vitro evidence that SARS-CoV-2 replication is inhibited by HBV (tenofovir)[151] and HCV (sofosbuvir, daclatasvir)[152] antivirals, no benefit (or harm) of antiviral treatment for viral hepatitis on the course of COVID-19 has been shown.

Flares and *de novo* autoimmune hepatitis have been reported after SARS-CoV-2 vaccination[153]; however, the overall incidence of AIH has not increased, suggesting that this is an infrequent occurrence.[154,155] As has been shown with other vaccines, responses to SARS-CoV-2 vaccines are impaired and wane more quickly in patients with cirrhosis than in those without liver disease.[156,157] However, vaccination is safe and associated with a reduced risk of severe COVID-19 and is therefore recommended in patients with chronic liver disease, particularly those with cirrhosis.

Adenovirus—Severe Acute Hepatitis in Children

In early 2022 cases of severe acute hepatitis in children under 10 years of age were reported first in the United Kingdom and then in multiple countries around the world. A definition for this syndrome was developed by the UK Health Security Agency and subsequently was modified by the WHO to help with surveillance efforts. The WHO developed a probable case definition of children under age 16 with ALT >500 since October 2021 who tested negative for hepatitis A-E and other known causes of acute hepatitis including CMV and EBV. They also tested negative for genetic and metabolic liver diseases.

Of 100 probable cases reported to the WHO between April 2022 and July 2022, the most common presenting symptoms were nausea and vomiting (60%), jaundice (53%), general weakness (52%), and abdominal pain (50%).[158] Similar presenting features were reported in series from the United Kingdom and the United States, with most children presenting under age 6.[159,160] In a UK cohort of 44 children who met the case definition, 6 (14%) developed coagulopathy and went on to require LT, while the other children recovered spontaneously. Of 30 children tested for human adenovirus, 27 tested positive in either blood (93%), respiratory samples (67%), or feces (67%). All samples had similar sequence homology to serotype 41F, a serotype previously associated with gastrointestinal symptoms but not liver disease. Viral loads were higher in children who went on to require LT than in children who recovered spontaneously (no transplant: median viral load 2733 copies/mL vs. transplant: 20,772 copies/mL). Of 39 children tested for SARS-CoV-2 RNA, 11 (28%) tested positive, and 5 of 13 (38%) tested positive for SARS-CoV-2 antibodies. None had been vaccinated for SARS-CoV-2.[159] Similar findings were described in other small cohorts, including variable association with adenovirus and weaker associations with SARS-CoV-2 exposure.[160] While some regions have reported a higher incidence of acute severe hepatitis in children, including those meeting the definition for pediatric ALF in 2022 compared to previous years, other reports have shown no clear increase.[161,162]

Although adenovirus 41F has been implicated, whether other cofactors, either in the host or the same or another pathogen, are necessary to cause disease, remains unclear. A series in Germany found that severe acute hepatitis in children increased across the country starting in 2019 compared to prior years.[163] They confirmed adenoviral infection in only two cases, both of which occurred prior to the 2022 outbreak (2004 and 2016), leading the authors to suggest that adenovirus was a new trigger of a known phenomenon that may have multiple etiologies. They and others have proposed that lack of exposure to common pathogens during the COVID-19 pandemic may in part account for the cases of hepatitis described; however, a clear mechanism is lacking.[162–164]

Ho and colleagues have proposed that adeno-associated virus 2 (AAV2) may be the cause of unexplained episodes of hepatitis.[165] They found evidence of recent AAV2 infection in 26/32 (81%) cases compared to 5/74 (7%) controls in blood and liver samples from children with acute hepatitis. They were able to confirm the presence of AAV2 in ballooned hepatocytes on liver biopsy and notably found that hepatitis was strongly associated with HLA class II DRB01*04:01 (25/27 93% cases vs. 10/64 controls, $P = 5.49\times10E\text{-}12$), which has been previously associated with $CD4^+$ T cell-mediated pathology.[165] Notably, AAV2 requires human adenovirus for replication, which could explain the associations previously seen with adenovirus and severe acute hepatitis. A second report also identified AAV2 but noted that in severe cases, in addition to human adenovirus, human herpes virus 6B was also present.[166] The requirement for a specific HLA-type and potentially coinfections to result in disease may explain the variability in previous association studies where the correlation with adenovirus varied widely.

The incidence of new cases decreased in the fall of 2022 and although the AAV2-adenovirus hypothesis is compelling, the etiology as well as the consequences of this syndrome remain uncertain.

Others

A number of other viruses have been reported to involve the liver, ranging from mild hepatitis to ALF. Parvovirus B19 is a common childhood exanthem that may also precipitate aplastic anemia. Liver enzyme elevations have been described, and rare cases of hepatitis with synthetic dysfunction or even ALF have been reported in both immunocompetent and immunocompromised persons.[167–169] Severe or fulminant cases are more commonly reported in children and adolescents than adults; however, the true incidence is unknown due to probable underrecognition and underreporting.[170] Rare cases of chronic hepatitis caused by parvovirus B19 have been reported.[171] The frequency of parvovirus B19 exposure has been reported to be increased in patients with HBV and HCV infections, and some studies have reported an association with worse hepatic outcomes,[172] but this has not been a universal finding.[173] A diagnosis is made using serologic tests for IgM and IgG parvovirus B19 antibodies or detection of viral DNA in blood or liver tissue by PCR methodology. No specific therapy is available.

HHV-6 has also been associated with hepatitis and ALF, most commonly in the setting of reactivation after LT, including presentation as syncytial giant cell hepatitis.[174–176]

Although a clear association with a specific virus has not been documented, a syndrome characterized by severe acute hepatitis followed by aplastic anemia has been recognized. Some cases have been associated with a known cause of acute viral hepatitis (HAV, HBV, parvovirus B19),[177,178] but in others, all virologic testing has been negative.[179] The syndrome affects children and young adults and is characterized by marked elevation of serum aminotransferase levels and conjugated hyperbilirubinemia with a CD8+ T cell-predominant portal injury and endothelial damage on liver biopsy.[180] Bone marrow failure occurs within weeks to 2 months of initial presentation.[181] Treatment with antithymocyte globulin and cyclosporine or hematopoietic stem cell transplantation has been effective in small series of patients.[177,181]

Nonspecific liver biochemical test abnormalities are common in many viral illnesses, including influenza, Chikungunya, Middle East respiratory syndrome, Ebola virus infection, and rare instances of frank hepatitis may occur.[182]

Full references for this chapter can be found at ebooks.health.elsevier.com.

86 Bacterial, Parasitic, and Fungal Infections of the Liver, Including Liver Abscesses

Arthur Yu-shin Kim

IN THIS CHAPTER

The liver serves as the initial site of filtration of absorbed intestinal luminal contents and is particularly susceptible to contact with microbial antigens of all varieties. In addition to infection by viruses (see Chapters 80-85), the liver can be affected by (1) spread of bacterial or parasitic infection from outside the liver; (2) primary infection by spirochetal, protozoal, helminthic, or fungal organisms; or (3) systemic effects of bacterial or mycobacterial infections.

BACTERIAL INFECTIONS INVOLVING OR AFFECTING THE LIVER

Gram-Positive and Gram-Negative Bacteria

A number of extrahepatic infections can lead to derangements in hepatic function, ranging from mild abnormalities of liver biochemical test results to frank jaundice and, rarely, hepatic failure.

Toxic Shock Syndrome: *Staphylococcus aureus* or Group A Streptococci

Toxic shock syndrome is a multisystem disease caused by toxic shock syndrome toxins, which are superantigens that cause T-cell activation and massive cytokine release. Originally described in association with serious infections caused by *Staphylococcus aureus*, this syndrome is now more frequently a complication of group A streptococcal infections, particularly necrotizing fasciitis.[1] Risk factors for *S. aureus* toxic shock syndrome include tampon use and surgical wound infection. Typical findings include a scarlatiniform rash, mucosal hyperemia, hypotension, vomiting, and diarrhea.[2] Hepatic involvement is almost always present and can range from elevations of serum aminotransferase levels to jaundice and extensive hepatic necrosis. Histologic findings in the liver include microabscesses and granulomas. The diagnosis is confirmed by culture of toxigenic *Streptococcus pyogenes* or *S. aureus* from the wound, blood, or other body sites. For wound infections or necrotizing fasciitis, surgical intervention is critical. Clindamycin, in conjunction with another active agent, is recommended to interfere with bacterial toxin production. Antibiotics effective against *S. aureus* include nafcillin or cefazolin for methicillin-sensitive isolates and vancomycin or linezolid for methicillin-resistant isolates, whereas penicillin remains active against *S. pyogenes*. Treatment with IV immunoglobulin in the setting of toxic shock syndrome is controversial.[3]

Clostridium perfringens

Clostridial myonecrosis involving *Clostridium perfringens* usually is a mixed anaerobic infection that results in the rapid development of local wound pain, abdominal pain, and diarrhea. The skin lesions become discolored and even bullous, and gas gangrene spreads rapidly, leading to a high mortality rate. Jaundice may develop in up to 20% of patients with gas gangrene and is predominantly a consequence of massive intravascular hemolysis caused by an exotoxin elaborated by the bacterium.[4] Evidence of liver involvement may include abscess formation and gas in the portal vein. Hepatic involvement does not appear to affect mortality. The presence of clostridial bacteria portends a poor prognosis in persons with cirrhosis.[5] Surgical débridement with wide excision is essential; penicillin and clindamycin are effective antibiotics.

Actinomyces

Actinomycosis is caused most commonly by *Actinomyces israelii*, a Gram-positive anaerobic bacterium. Although cervicofacial infection is the most frequent manifestation of actinomycotic infection, GI involvement occurs in 13%–60% of patients.[6,7] Hepatic involvement is present in 15% of cases of abdominal actinomycosis and is believed to result from metastatic spread from other abdominal sites. Common presenting manifestations of actinomycotic liver abscess include fever, abdominal pain, and anorexia with weight loss.[8,9] The course is more indolent than that seen with the usual causes of pyogenic hepatic abscess (see later) and thus may be mistaken for a tumor.[8] Fistula formation and invasion of other surrounding tissues such as the pleural space can occur. Leukocytosis, an elevated erythrocyte sedimentation rate or C-reactive protein, and an elevated serum alkaline phosphatase level are frequently observed. Imaging findings are nonspecific and may be mistaken for cancer; multiple abscesses may be seen in both lobes of the liver. Portal or hepatic venous thrombosis has been reported.[6]

The diagnosis is based on the aspiration of an abscess cavity and either visualization of characteristic sulfur granules or positive results on an anaerobic culture. Most abscesses resolve with a prolonged course of IV penicillin or oral tetracycline. Large abscesses can be drained percutaneously or resected surgically.[10]

Listeria

Hepatic invasion in adult human *Listeria monocytogenes* infection is uncommon. One report described 34 cases of listeriosis involving the liver, ranging from solitary to multiple abscesses and acute and granulomatous hepatitis.[11] Hepatic histologic features include multiple abscesses and granulomas. Predisposing conditions include immunosuppression, diabetes mellitus, and underlying liver disease, including cirrhosis, hemochromatosis, and chronic hepatitis. The diagnosis of disseminated listerial infection is based on a positive culture result from blood or from an aspirate in the case of a liver abscess. Cholecystitis with *L. monocytogenes* has also been described.[12] Treatment is with ampicillin or penicillin, often with gentamicin for synergy.[13]

Shigella and *Salmonella*

Several case reports have described cholestatic hepatitis attributable to enteric infection with *Shigella* spp.[14,15] Histologic findings in the liver have included portal and periportal infiltration with polymorphonuclear leukocytes (neutrophils), hepatocyte necrosis, and cholestasis. Severe hepatic dysfunction associated with *Shigella* spp. infection has been reported.[16]

Typhoid fever, caused by *Salmonella typhi*, is a systemic infection that frequently involves the liver. Elevation of serum aminotransferase levels is common, whereas the serum bilirubin level may rise in a minority of cases.[17] Some patients may present with an acute hepatitis-like picture, characterized by fever and tender hepatomegaly.[18] Cholecystitis and liver abscess may complicate hepatic involvement with *S. typhi* infection.[19]

Hepatic damage by *S. typhi* appears to be mediated by bacterial endotoxin, although organisms can be visualized within the liver tissue. Endotoxin may produce focal necrosis, a periportal mononuclear infiltrate, and Kupffer cell hyperplasia in the liver. These changes resemble those seen in Gram-negative sepsis. Characteristic typhoid nodules scattered throughout the liver are the result of profound hypertrophy and proliferation of Kupffer cells. The clinical course can be severe, with a mortality rate approaching 20%, particularly with delayed treatment or in patients with other complications of *Salmonella* infection. Severe typhoid fever with jaundice and encephalopathy may be differentiated from ALF by the presence of an elevated serum alkaline phosphatase level, mild hypoprothrombinemia, thrombocytopenia, hepatomegaly, and an AST level greater than the ALT level.[20] Ceftriaxone is the first-line agent for the treatment of typhoid fever, with ciprofloxacin as an alternative in areas where resistance is uncommon. Extensively drug-resistant strains have emerged, and a carbapenem is recommended in travelers returning from certain countries.[21]

S. paratyphi A and B (*Salmonella enterica* serotypes paratyphi A and B) are the predominant causes of paratyphoid fever. As in typhoid fever, abnormalities in liver biochemical test results, particularly elevated serum aminotransferase levels, with or without hepatomegaly, are common.[22] Liver abscess is a rare complication.[23] Treatment is with a third-generation cephalosporin or, where the prevalence of resistance is low, a fluoroquinolone.

Yersinia

Infection with *Yersinia enterocolitica* manifests as ileocolitis in children and as terminal ileitis or mesenteric adenitis in adults. Arthritis, cellulitis, erythema nodosum, and septicemia may complicate Yersinia infection. Most patients with complicated disease have an underlying comorbid condition, such as diabetes mellitus, cirrhosis, or hemochromatosis. Excess tissue iron, in particular, may be a predisposing factor because growth of the *Yersinia* bacterium is enhanced by iron. Acute liver injury accompanying *Yersinia* infection is considered rare but has been reported.[24]

The subacute septicemic form of the disease resembles typhoid fever or malaria. Multiple abscesses are distributed diffusely in the liver and spleen. In some cases, the occurrence of *Y. enterocolitica* liver abscesses may lead to the detection of underlying hemochromatosis.[25,26] The mortality rate is approximately 50%. Fluoroquinolones may be used for most cases; for septicemia, third-generation cephalosporins are preferred.

Gonococci

In approximately 50% of patients with disseminated gonococcal infection, serum alkaline phosphatase levels are elevated, and in 30%–40% of patients, AST levels are elevated.[27] Jaundice is uncommon.

The most common hepatic complication of gonococcal infection is the Fitz-Hugh-Curtis syndrome, a perihepatitis that is believed to result from direct spread of the infection from the pelvis (see later).[27] Clinically, patients describe a sudden, sharp pain in the RUQ. The pain may be confused with that of acute cholecystitis or pleurisy. Most patients have a history of pelvic inflammatory disease. The syndrome is distinguished from gonococcal bacteremia by a characteristic friction rub over the liver and negative blood culture results. The diagnosis is made by vaginal culture for gonococci. The overall prognosis of gonococcal infection appears to be unaffected by the presence of perihepatitis.[28] Although resistance to various antibiotics is of increasing concern, ceftriaxone remains the antibiotic of choice. Presumed coinfection with *Chlamydia trachomatis* should be treated empirically (see later) with doxycycline.

Legionella

Legionella pneumophila, a fastidious Gram-negative bacterium, is the cause of Legionnaires' disease. Although pneumonia is the predominant clinical manifestation, abnormal liver biochemical test results are frequent, with elevations in serum aminotransferase levels in 50%, alkaline phosphatase levels in 45%, and bilirubin levels in 20% of cases (but usually without jaundice). Involvement of the liver does not influence clinical outcome. Liver histologic changes include microvesicular steatosis and focal necrosis; organisms can be seen occasionally. The diagnosis is confirmed by the detection of a direct fluorescence antibody in the serum or sputum or of antigen in the urine.[29] The antibiotic of choice is azithromycin or a fluoroquinolone.

Burkholderia pseudomallei (Melioidosis)

Burkholderia pseudomallei is a soil-borne and water-borne Gram-negative bacterium that is found predominantly in Southeast Asia. The clinical spectrum of melioidosis ranges from asymptomatic infection to fulminant septicemia with involvement of the lungs, GI tract, and liver. Histologic changes in the liver include inflammatory infiltrates, multiple microabscesses, and focal necrosis. Organisms can be visualized with a Giemsa stain of a liver biopsy specimen. With chronic disease, granulomas may be seen. Some liver abscesses may demonstrate a "honeycombing" appearance on CT.[30] Abscesses may need to be drained or débrided, and ceftazidime or meropenem is the initial drug of choice, followed by a prolonged course of trimethoprim/sulfamethoxazole, with or without doxycycline.[31]

Brucella

Brucellosis may be acquired from infected pigs, cattle, goats, and sheep (*Brucella suis*, *Brucella abortus*, *Brucella melitensis*, and *Brucella ovis*, respectively) and typically manifests as an acute febrile illness. Hepatic abnormalities are seen in a majority of infected persons, and jaundice may be present in severe cases. Typically, multiple noncaseating hepatic granulomas are found in liver biopsy specimens; less often, focal mononuclear infiltration of the portal tracts or lobules is seen.[32] Rarely, brucellosis also may produce hepatosplenic abscesses.[33,34] The diagnosis can be made by the isolation of the organism from a cultured specimen of liver tissue and is confirmed by serologic testing in combination with a history of exposure to animals. Surgical drainage may be required for management of *Brucella* abscesses. The combination of doxycycline with either streptomycin or gentamicin is the most effective antimicrobial therapy.

Coxiella burnetii (Q Fever)

Infection by *Coxiella burnetii*, typically acquired by the inhalation of animal aerosols or dusts, causes the clinical syndrome of Q fever, which is characterized by relapsing fevers, headache, myalgias, malaise, pneumonitis, and culture-negative endocarditis. Liver involvement is common.[35] The predominant abnormality is an elevated serum alkaline phosphatase level, with minimal elevations of AST or bilirubin levels. The histologic hallmark in the liver is the presence of characteristic fibrin ring granulomas. The diagnosis is confirmed by serologic testing via indirect immunofluorescence or for complement-fixing antibodies.[36] Treatment with doxycycline is usually effective.

Bartonellosis (Oroya Fever, Cat-Scratch Fever, and Bacillary Angiomatosis)

Bartonella species are fastidious, Gram-negative bacilli that cause a range of illnesses. *Bartonella bacilliformis* is endemic to Colombia, Ecuador, and Peru. It is transmitted by a sand fly and causes an acute febrile illness known as Oroya fever accompanied by jaundice, hemolysis, hepatosplenomegaly, and lymphadenopathy. Centrilobular necrosis of the liver and splenic infarction may occur. As many as 40% of patients die of sepsis or hemolysis. Prompt treatment prevents fatal complications.[37] First-line treatment is ciprofloxacin, in combination with ceftriaxone for severe cases.

Cat-scratch disease, caused by *Bartonella henselae*, usually affects children and young adults with typical cutaneous and lymph node manifestations but rarely can disseminate with visceral involvement, including necrotizing granuloma in the liver and spleen.[38] Infection is frequently associated with exposure to cats or to their fleas.[39] Mild cat-scratch disease is treated with azithromycin.

Bacillary angiomatosis is an infectious disorder that primarily affects persons with AIDS or other immunodeficiency states, in many cases caused by *B. henselae* but in some cases by *Bartonella quintana*.[40] Bacillary angiomatosis is characterized most commonly by multiple blood-red papular skin lesions but disseminated infection with or without skin involvement has also been described.[41] The causative bacilli can infect liver, lymph nodes, pleura, bronchi, bones, brain, bone marrow, and spleen. Additional manifestations include persistent fever, bacteremia, and sepsis. Hepatic infection should be suspected when serum aminotransferase levels are elevated in the absence of other explanations. Hepatic infection in persons with bacillary angiomatosis may manifest as peliosis hepatis, or blood-filled cysts (see Chapter 87). Histologically, peliosis in patients with AIDS is characterized by an inflammatory myxoid stroma containing clumps of bacilli and dilated capillaries surrounding the blood-filled peliotic cysts. Increasingly, the diagnosis of *Bartonella* infection is by PCR-based methods.[42] Bacillary angiomatosis is treated with doxycycline with either rifampin or gentamicin added for severe manifestations. For visceral infection, prolonged treatment should be administered.[40]

Bacterial Sepsis and Jaundice

Jaundice may complicate systemic sepsis caused by Gram-negative or Gram-positive organisms. Exotoxins and endotoxins liberated in overwhelming infection can directly or indirectly, through cytokines such as TNF-α, inhibit the transport of bile acids and other organic anions across the hepatic sinusoidal and bile canalicular membranes, thereby leading to intrahepatic cholestasis (see Chapter 22).[43] Serum bilirubin levels can reach 15 mg/dL or higher. The magnitude of the jaundice does not correlate with mortality. Results of cultures of liver biopsy specimens are usually negative.

Chlamydia

Fitz-Hugh-Curtis Syndrome

Although perihepatitis was first associated with gonococcal salpingo-oophoritis (see earlier), it is now most frequently associated with *C. trachomatis* infection. The presentation is similar to perihepatitis caused by gonococcal infection, with RUQ pain accompanying a urogenital infection such as pelvic inflammatory disease. The diagnosis can be made by direct visualization at laparoscopy or laparotomy and supported by pathologic demonstration of endometritis, salpingitis, and microbiologic detection of *C. trachomatis* in the genital tract. Liver biochemical test results are generally normal. The treatment of choice should follow guidelines for treatment of *C. trachomatis* or pelvic inflammatory disease.[44]

Rickettsiae

Rocky Mountain Spotted Fever

Mortality from Rocky Mountain spotted fever, a systemic tick-borne rickettsial illness, has decreased considerably as a result of prompt recognition of the classic maculopapular rash in association with fever and an exposure history. A small subset of patients, however, present with multiorgan manifestations and have a high mortality rate.[45] A characteristic severe vasculitis develops in these patients and is believed to be the result of a microbe-induced coagulopathy. Hepatic involvement is frequent in multiorgan disease. In one postmortem study, rickettsiae were identified in the portal tracts of eight of nine fatal cases. Portal tract inflammation, portal vasculitis, and sinusoidal erythrophagocytosis were consistent findings, but hepatic necrosis was negligible. The predominant clinical manifestation was jaundice; elevations of serum aminotransferase and alkaline phosphatase levels varied. Jaundice probably results from a combination of inflammatory bile ductular obstruction and hemolysis and is associated with increased mortality.[35,46]

Ehrlichiae

Ehrlichiae are rickettsiae that parasitize leukocytes. In the United States, human monocytic ehrlichiosis is caused principally by *Ehrlichia chaffeensis* and, less often, by *Ehrlichia canis*. Human granulocytic anaplasmosis (formerly known as human granulocytic ehrlichiosis) is caused by *Anaplasma phagocytophilum*.[35,47] In contrast to Rocky Mountain spotted fever, a rash is often absent. Hepatic involvement is seen in more than 80% of cases, usually in the form of mild, transient serum aminotransferase elevations. More marked aminotransferase elevations may occur occasionally, in association with cholestasis, hepatosplenomegaly, and liver failure. Liver injury is attributable to proliferation of organisms within hepatocytes and provocation of an immune response. Focal necrosis, fibrin ring granulomas, and cholestatic hepatitis can be observed. A mixed portal tract infiltrate and lymphoid sinusoidal infiltrate are usually seen. The disease generally resolves with appropriate antibiotic therapy with doxycycline.[48]

Spirochetes

Leptospirosis

Leptospirosis is one of the most common zoonoses in the world, and the causative organism has a wide range of domestic and wild animal reservoirs. Humans acquire the spirochete by contact with infected urine or contaminated soil or water. In humans, disease can occur as anicteric leptospirosis or as Weil syndrome.

Anicteric leptospirosis accounts for more than 90% of cases and is characterized by a biphasic illness. The first phase begins, often abruptly, with viral illness-like symptoms associated with fever, leptospiremia, and conjunctival suffusion, which serves as an important diagnostic clue. Following a brief period of improvement, the second phase in 95% of cases is characterized by myalgias, nausea, vomiting, abdominal tenderness, and, in some cases, aseptic meningitis.[49] During this phase, a few patients have elevated serum aminotransferase and bilirubin levels with hepatomegaly.

Weil syndrome is a severe icteric form of leptospirosis and constitutes 5%–10% of all cases. The first phase of this illness is often marked by jaundice, which may last for weeks. During the second phase, fever may be high, and hepatic and renal manifestations predominate. Jaundice may be marked, with serum bilirubin levels approaching 30 mg/dL (predominantly conjugated). Serum aminotransferase levels usually do not exceed five times the upper limit of normal.[50] Acute tubular necrosis often develops and can lead to renal failure, which may be fatal. Hemorrhagic complications are frequent and are the result of capillary injury caused by immune complexes.[49] Spirochetes are seen in renal tubules in a majority of autopsy specimens but rarely are found in the liver. Hepatic histologic findings are generally nonspecific and do not include necrosis. Altered mitochondria and disrupted membranes in hepatocytes on electron microscopy suggest the possibility of a toxin-mediated injury.

The diagnosis of leptospirosis is made on clinical grounds in conjunction with a positive result of a blood or urine culture specimen in the first and second phase, respectively. Serologic testing confirms the diagnosis when culture results are unrevealing. Doxycycline is effective if given within the first several days of illness. Most patients recover without residual organ impairment.

Syphilis

Secondary Syphilis

Liver involvement is characteristic of secondary syphilis.[51] The frequency of hepatitis in secondary syphilis ranges from 1% to 50%.[51,52] Symptoms and signs are usually nonspecific, including anorexia, weight loss, fever, malaise, and sore throat. A characteristic pruritic maculopapular rash involves the palms and soles. Jaundice, hepatomegaly, and tenderness in the RUQ are less common. Almost all patients exhibit generalized lymphadenopathy. Biochemical testing generally reveals low-grade elevations of serum aminotransferase and bilirubin levels, with a disproportionate elevation of the serum alkaline phosphatase level; isolated elevation of the alkaline phosphatase is common.[53] Proteinuria may be present.

Histologic examination of the liver in syphilitic hepatitis generally discloses focal necrosis in the periportal and centrilobular regions. The inflammatory infiltrate typically includes neutrophils, plasma cells, lymphocytes, eosinophils, and mast cells.[51] Kupffer cell hyperplasia may be seen, but bile ductule injury is rare. Granulomas may be seen. Spirochetes may be demonstrated by silver staining in as many as 50% of patients. Resolution of these findings without sequelae follows treatment with penicillin.

Tertiary (Late) Syphilis

Tertiary syphilis is now rare. Although hepatic lesions are common in late syphilis, most patients are asymptomatic. Some patients describe anorexia, weight loss, fatigue, fever, or abdominal pain. The characteristic hepatic lesion in tertiary syphilis is the gumma, which can be single or multiple. It is necrotic centrally, with surrounding granulation tissue consisting of a lymphoplasmacytic infiltrate and endarteritis; exuberant deposition of scar tissue may occur, giving the liver a lobulated appearance (hepar lobatum). If hepatic involvement is unrecognized, hepatocellular dysfunction and portal hypertension with jaundice, ascites, and gastroesophageal varices can ensue. Hepatic gummas may resolve after therapy with penicillin.[54]

Lyme Disease

Lyme disease is a multisystem disease caused by the tick-borne spirochete *Borrelia burgdorferi*. Predominant manifestations are dermatologic, cardiac, neurologic, and musculoskeletal. Hepatic involvement has been described. Among 314 patients, abnormal liver biochemical test results with generally increased serum aminotransferase and lactate dehydrogenase levels were seen in 19%.[55] Clinical findings include anorexia, nausea and vomiting, weight loss, RUQ pain, and hepatomegaly, usually within days to weeks of the onset of illness and often accompanied by the sentinel rash, erythema migrans.[56] Coinfection with ehrlichiosis or anaplasmosis should be considered.

In early stages of the illness, the spirochetes are believed to disseminate hematogenously from the skin to other organs, including the liver.[35] Histologic examination of the liver in Lyme hepatitis reveals hepatocyte ballooning, marked mitotic activity, microvesicular fat, Kupffer cell hyperplasia, a mixed sinusoidal infiltrate, and intraparenchymal and sinusoidal spirochetes.[57]

The diagnosis of Lyme disease is confirmed with serologic studies in patients with a typical clinical history. Hepatic involvement tends to be more frequent in disseminated disease but does not appear to affect overall outcome, which is excellent in primary disease after the institution of treatment with oral doxycycline, amoxicillin, clarithromycin, or azithromycin.[58] Ceftriaxone is the drug of choice for late disease.[59]

Mycobacteria

Granulomas are found in liver biopsy specimens in approximately 25% of persons with pulmonary TB and 80% of those with extrapulmonary TB. Tuberculous granulomas can be distinguished from sarcoid granulomas by central caseation, acid-fast bacilli, and the presence of fewer granulomas, with a tendency to coalesce.[60] Multiple granulomas in the liver also may be seen following vaccination with Bacille Calmette-Guérin, especially in persons with an impaired immune response. Patients with multiple granulomas caused by TB rarely have clinically significant liver disease. Occasionally, tender hepatomegaly is found. Jaundice with elevated serum alkaline phosphatase levels may occur in miliary infection. The treatment of tuberculous granulomatous disease of the liver is the same as that for active pulmonary TB.[61] Hepatic involvement in *Mycobacterium avium* complex infection is discussed in Chapter 33.

PARASITES

Protozoa

Malaria

An estimated 300–500 million persons in more than 100 countries are infected with malaria each year (see also Chapter 115). The liver is affected during two stages of the malarial life cycle: first in the preerythrocytic phase and then in the erythrocytic phase, which coincides with clinical illness (Tables 86.1 and 86.2).

TABLE 86.1 Classification of Parasitic Diseases of the Liver and Biliary Tract by Pathologic Process

Pathologic Process	Diseases
LIVER	
Granulomatous hepatitis	Capillariasis Fascioliasis Schistosomiasis Strongyloidiasis Toxocariasis
Portal fibrosis	Schistosomiasis
Hepatic abscess or necrosis	Amebiasis Toxoplasmosis
Cystic liver disease	Echinococcosis
Peliosis hepatis	Bacillary angiomatosis
RETICULOENDOTHELIAL CELLS	
Kupffer cell infection or hyperplasia	Babesiosis Malaria Toxoplasmosis Visceral leishmaniasis
BILIARY TRACT	
Cholangitis	Clonorchiasis/opisthorchiasis Fascioliasis
Biliary hyperplasia	Ascariasis Clonorchiasis Cryptosporidiosis Fascioliasis
Cholangiocarcinoma	Clonorchiasis/opisthorchiasis

The Plasmodium Life Cycle

The life cycle of the prototypical malarial parasite is illustrated in Fig. 86.1. Malarial sporozoites injected by an infected mosquito circulate to the liver and enter hepatocytes. Maturation to schizonts ensues. When the schizont ruptures, merozoites are released into the bloodstream, where they enter erythrocytes. The major species of Plasmodium responsible for malaria differ with respect to the number of merozoites released and the maturation times. Infection by *Plasmodium falciparum* and *Plasmodium malariae* is not associated with a residual liver stage after the release of merozoites, whereas infection by *Plasmodium vivax* and *Plasmodium ovale* is associated with a persistent exoerythrocytic stage, the hypnozoite, which persists in the liver and, when activated, can divide and mature into schizont forms. *Plasmodium knowlesi* has been identified as a fifth species capable of infecting humans and occasionally results in severe manifestations, including jaundice, hepatic dysfunction, and acute kidney injury.[62]

The extent of hepatic injury varies with the malarial species (most severe with *P. falciparum*) and the severity of infection. Unconjugated hyperbilirubinemia is most commonly seen as a result of hemolysis, but hepatocellular dysfunction is also possible, leading to conjugated hyperbilirubinemia. Moderate elevations of serum aminotransferase and 5′-nucleotidase levels may be observed.[63] Synthetic dysfunction (e.g., prolongation of the prothrombin time, hypoalbuminemia) may be seen, as well. In severe falciparum malaria, hypoglycemia and lactic acidosis are late and life-threatening complications.[64] Reversible reductions in portal venous blood flow have been described during the acute phase of falciparum malaria, presumably as a consequence of micro-occlusion of portal venous branches by parasitized erythrocytes.[65]

Histopathologic Features

In acute falciparum malaria in a previously unexposed person, hepatic macrophages hypertrophy, and large quantities of malarial pigment (the result of hemoglobin degradation by the parasite) accumulate in Kupffer cells, which phagocytose parasitized and unparasitized erythrocytes.[66] Histopathologic features include Kupffer cell hyperplasia with pigment deposition and a mononuclear infiltrate. Hepatocyte swelling and centrizonal necrosis may be seen. All abnormalities are reversible with treatment.

86

Clinical Features

Only the erythrocytic stage of malaria is associated with clinical illness. Symptoms and signs of acute infection typically develop 30–60 days following exposure and include fever, which often is hectic, malaise, anorexia, nausea, vomiting, diarrhea, and myalgias. Jaundice caused by hemolysis is common in adults, especially in heavy infection with *P. falciparum*. In general, hepatic failure is seen only in association with concomitant viral hepatitis or with severe *P. falciparum* infection.[67,68] One series identified evidence of hepatic encephalopathy in 15 of 86 patients with falciparum malaria and jaundice; 4 cases were fatal.[67] Tender hepatomegaly with splenomegaly is common. Cytopenias are common in acute infection. The differential diagnosis includes viral hepatitis, gastroenteritis, amebic liver abscess, yellow fever, typhoid, TB, and brucellosis.

Diagnosis

The diagnosis of acute malaria rests on the clinical history, physical examination, and identification of parasites on peripheral thin and thick blood smears. Because the number of parasites in the blood may be small, repeated smear examinations should be performed by an experienced examiner when the index of suspicion is high. *P. knowlesi* may resemble *P. malariae* in morphology, and PCR-based tests may help distinguish these two species.[62] Rapid antigen detection assays are available but have yet to be implemented widely.[69]

Treatment

The treatment of acute malaria depends on the species of parasite and, for falciparum infection, the pattern of chloroquine resistance. Chloroquine generally is effective in areas endemic for chloroquine-sensitive species. Resistant falciparum infections can be treated with mefloquine alone; quinine and either doxycycline or clindamycin; pyrimethamine-sulfadoxine (Fansidar); a combination of atovaquone and proguanil; or artemisinin derivatives, including artemisinin, artemether, and artesunate.[70] For *P. vivax* and *P. ovale* infections, the addition of primaquine (in persons without glucose-6-phosphate dehydrogenase deficiency) to chloroquine or mefloquine is indicated to eliminate the exoerythrocytic hypnozoites in the liver.[71]

Hyperreactive Malarial Splenomegaly (Tropical Splenomegaly Syndrome)

In endemic areas, repeated exposure to malaria may lead to an aberrant immunologic response characterized by overproduction of B lymphocytes, circulating malarial antibody, and increased levels of circulating immune complexes, resulting in dense hepatic sinusoidal lymphocytosis and stimulation of the reticuloendothelial cell system. The clinical picture includes massive splenomegaly, markedly elevated antimalarial antibody levels, and high serum immunoglobulin (Ig)M levels. Severe debilitating anemia caused by hypersplenism, especially in women of childbearing age, can result.[72] Variceal bleeding is uncommon but may result from portal hypertension consequent to markedly increased splenic and portal venous blood flow. Treatment consists of lifelong antimalarial therapy and blood transfusions.

Babesiosis

Babesiosis, caused by *Babesia* species, is a malaria-like illness transmitted by the deer tick *Ixodes scapularis*.[73] The disease is

TABLE 86.2 Parasitic Diseases of the Liver and Biliary Tract

Disease (Cause)	Endemic Areas	Predisposing Factors	Pathophysiology	Manifestations	Diagnosis	Treatment[a]
PROTOZOANS						
Amebiasis (*Entamoeba histolytica*) (see also Chapter 115)	Worldwide, especially Africa, Asia, Mexico, South America	Poor sanitation, sexual exposure	Hematogenous spread and tissue invasion, abscess formation (see Fig. 86.10)	Fever, RUQ pain, peritonitis, elevated right hemidiaphragm, rupture	Cysts in stool, serology (e.g., ELISA, CIE, IHA), hepatic imaging	Metronidazole 750 mg (oral or IV) 3 times daily × 7–10 days or tinidazole 2 g × 3 days, followed by iodoquinol 650 mg 3 times daily × 20 days or diloxanide furoate 500 mg 3 times daily × 10 days or aminosidine (paromomycin) 25–35 mg/kg/day in 3 divided doses × 7–10 days
Malaria (*Plasmodium falciparum, Plasmodium malariae, Plasmodium vivax, Plasmodium ovale, Plasmodium knowlesi*)	Africa, Asia, South America	Blood transfusion, IV drug use	Sporozoite clearance by hepatocytes; exoerythrocytic replication in the liver	Tender hepatomegaly, splenomegaly, rarely hepatic failure (*P. falciparum*)	Identification of the parasite on a blood smear	*P. falciparum*: chloroquine (chloroquine-sensitive), mefloquine, or quinine and either doxycycline or clindamycin; or pyrimethamine-sulfadoxine (Fansidar); or atovaquone/proguanil (chloroquine-resistant); or an artesiminin *P. malariae*: chloroquine *P. vivax, P. ovale, P. knowlesi*: chloroquine and primaquine (chloroquine-sensitive) or mefloquine and primaquine (chloroquine-resistant)[b]
Babesiosis (*Babesia* spp.)	The United States	Exposure to deer tick	Hemolysis with multiorgan involvement	Fever, anemia, hepatosplenomegaly, abnormal liver test results, hemoglobinuria	Identification of the parasite on a blood smear, PCR	Azithromycin 500 mg on day 1, then 250 mg daily and atovaquone 750 mg twice daily × 7-10 days or clindamycin 300-600 mg IV every 6 hr or 600 mg orally every 8 hr and quinine 650 mg every 8 hr × 7–10 days
Visceral leishmaniasis (*Leishmania donovani*)	Eurasia, Central America, South America, Africa	Immunosuppression (AIDS, organ transplantation)	Infection of RE cells	Fever, weight loss, hepatosplenomegaly, secondary bacterial infection, skin hyperpigmentation (kala-azar)	Amastigotes seen in the spleen, liver, or bone marrow	Pentavalent antimonial (stibogluconate sodium and meglumine antimoniate) 20 mg/kg/day × 28 days (no longer available in the United States); or liposomal amphotericin B (IV) 3 mg/kg/day on days 1–5, 14, and 21; or aminosidine (paromomycin) 16–20 mg/kg/day × 21 days; or pentamidine isethionate, 2–4 mg/kg/day for up to 15 days; or miltefosine 2.5 mg/kg/day × 28 days
Toxoplasmosis (*Toxoplasma gondii*)	Worldwide	Congenital infection, immunosuppression (AIDS, organ transplantation)	Replication in the liver leading to inflammation, necrosis	Fever, lymphadenopathy, occasionally hepatosplenomegaly, atypical lymphocytosis	Serology (IF, ELISA), isolation of the organism in the tissue	Pyrimethamine 100 mg loading dose followed by 25–50 mg/day, plus sulfadiazine 2–4 g/day in 4 divided doses; or clindamycin 300 mg 4 times daily, plus folinic acid 10–25 mg daily; or trimethoprim-sulfamethaxazole (160 mg TMP, 800 mg SMX) twice daily for 6 wks
NEMATODES (SEE ALSO CHAPTER 116)						
Toxocariasis (*Toxocara canis, Toxocara cati*)	Worldwide	Exposure to dogs or cats, especially for children <5 years	Migration of larvae to the liver (visceral larva migrans)	Granuloma formation with eosinophilia	Larvae in tissue, serology (ELISA)	Albendazole 10 mg/kg/day × 5 days or mebendazole 100–200 mg twice daily × 5 days
Hepatic capillariasis (*Capillaria hepatica*)	Worldwide	Exposure to rodents	Migration of larvae to the liver; inflammatory reaction to eggs	Acute, subacute hepatitis, tender hepatomegaly, occasionally splenomegaly, eosinophilia	Adult worms or eggs in a liver biopsy specimen (see Fig. 86.2)	Supportive; possibly albendazole, mebendazole, or thiabendazole

Ascariasis (*Ascaris lumbricoides*)	Tropical climates	Ingestion of raw vegetables	Migration of larvae to the liver; invasion of the bile ducts by adult worms	Abdominal pain, fever, jaundice, biliary obstruction, granulomas	Ova or adult in stool or contrast study	Albendazole 400 mg × 1 dose; or mebendazole 100 mg twice daily × 3 days; or pyrantel pamoate 11 mg/kg up to 1 g; or ivermectin 200 μg/kg × 1 dose
Strongyloidiasis (*Strongyloides stercoralis*)	Asia, Africa, South America, Southern Europe, United States	Immunosuppression (AIDS, chemotherapy, organ transplantation) predisposes to hyperinfection	Larval penetration from the intestine to the liver	Hepatomegaly, occasionally jaundice, larvae in the portal tract or lobule	Larvae in the stool or duodenal aspirate	Ivermectin 200 μg/kg/day × 2 days; or albendazole 400 mg/day × 3 days
Trichinosis (*Trichinella spiralis*)	Temperate climates	Ingestion of undercooked pork	Hematogenous dissemination to the liver	Occasionally jaundice, biliary obstruction, larvae in hepatic sinusoids	History, eosinophilia, fever, muscle biopsy	Glucocorticoids for allergic symptoms; albendazole 400 mg twice daily × 10–15 days; or mebendazole 200 mg/day × 10–15 days
TREMATODES (SEE ALSO CHAPTER 116)						
Schistosomiasis (*Schistosoma mansoni*, *S. japonicum*)	Asia, Africa, South America, Caribbean	Travelers exposed to bodies of fresh water	Fibrogenic host immune response to eggs in the portal vein	*Acute:* eosinophilic infiltrate *Chronic:* hepatosplenomegaly, presinusoidal portal hypertension, granulomas	Ova in the stool, rectal or liver biopsy	Praziquantel 40–60 mg/kg in 2–3 divided doses × 1 day; or oxamniquine for *S. mansoni* (not readily available) Acute toxemic schistosomiasis: praziquantel 40–60 mg/kg in 2–3 divided doses × 1 day + glucocorticoids
Fascioliasis (*Fasciola hepatica*)	Worldwide	Cattle or sheep raising; ingestion of contaminated watercress	Migration of larvae through the liver; penetration of the bile ducts or surgery	*Acute:* fever, abdominal pain, jaundice, hemobilia *Chronic:* hepatomegaly	Ova in the stool, flukes in the bile ducts at ERC	Triclabendazole 10 mg/kg × 2 doses
Clonorchiasis and opisthorchiasis (*Clonorchis sinensis*, *Opisthorchis viverrini*, *O. felineus*)	Southeast Asia, China, Japan, Korea, Eastern Europe	Ingestion of raw fresh-water fish	Migration through the ampulla; egg deposition in the bile ducts	Biliary hyperplasia, obstruction, sclerosing cholangitis, stone formation, cholangio carcinoma	Ova in the stool, flukes in the bile ducts at ERC or surgery	Praziquantel 75 mg/kg in 3 divided doses × 2 days
CESTODES						
Echinococcosis (*Echinococcus granulosus*, *Echinococcus multilocularis*)	Worldwide	Cattle or sheep raising (*E. granulosus*)	Migration of larvae to the liver; encystment (hydatid cyst)	Tender hepatomegaly, fever, eosinophilia, cyst rupture, biliary obstruction	Serology (ELISA, IHA), hepatic imaging	Surgical resection or percutaneous drainage. Perioperative albendazole 400 mg twice daily continuing × 8 weeks

[a]All drugs are given orally unless otherwise specified.
[b]For dosing guidelines for malaria, please refer to https://www.cdc.gov/malaria/resources/pdf/treatmenttable.pdf.
CIE, Counterimmunoelectrophoresis; *ELISA*, enzyme-linked immunosorbent assay; *ERC*, endoscopic retrograde cholangiography; *IF*, immunofluorescence; *IHA*, indirect hemagglutination assay; *RE*, reticuloendothelial.

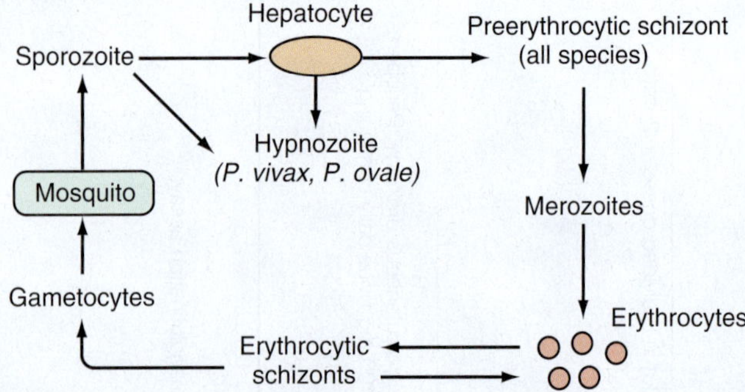

Fig. 86.1 The life cycle of *plasmodium* species.

endemic to coastal areas of the northeast and areas of the midwest in the United States. Clinical features include fever, anemia, mild hepatosplenomegaly, abnormalities on liver biochemical tests, hemoglobinuria, and hemophagocytosis on bone marrow biopsy specimen. The disease is especially severe in asplenic and immunocompromised patients. In rare cases, marked pancytopenia occurs. Hepatic involvement reflects the severity of the systemic illness but generally is not severe. Uncomplicated cases are treated with a combination of the following active agents: (1) oral azithromycin, 500-mg single dose followed by 250 mg once daily, plus atovaquone, 750 mg twice daily, for 7–10 days; or (2) oral clindamycin, 600 mg three times daily, in combination with quinine, 650 mg three times daily, for 7–10 days. In severe cases, partial or complete exchange transfusion should be considered.[73]

Leishmaniasis

Visceral leishmaniasis is caused by *Leishmania donovani* and is endemic in Mediterranean countries, central Asia, the former Soviet Union, the Middle East, China, India, Pakistan, Bangladesh, Africa, Central America, and South America.[74] This entity should be considered in immigrants, returning travelers, and military personnel from these areas. Amastigotes are ingested by the sand fly (*Lutzomyia* in the New World, *Phlebotomus* in the Old World) and become flagellated promastigotes. Following injection into the human host, the promastigotes are phagocytosed by macrophages in the reticuloendothelial system, where they multiply.

Histopathologic Features

In visceral leishmaniasis, organisms usually can be found in mononuclear phagocytes of the liver, spleen, bone marrow, and lymph nodes. Proliferation of Kupffer cells is often seen, and amastigotes (Leishman-Donovan bodies) can be detected within these cells.[75] Occasionally, parasite-bearing cells aggregate within noncaseating granulomas.[76] Hepatocyte necrosis can range in degree from mild to severe. Healing is accompanied by fibrous deposition, and occasionally the liver takes on a cirrhotic appearance. Nevertheless, complications of chronic liver disease are rare.

Clinical Features

Visceral infection caused by *L. donovani* begins with a papular or ulcerative skin lesion at the site of the sand fly bite. Following an incubation period of 2–6 months (sometimes years), intermittent fevers, weight loss, diarrhea (of bacillary, amebic, or leishmanial origin), and progressive painful hepatosplenomegaly develop, often accompanied by pancytopenia and a polyclonal hypergammaglobulinemia. Secondary bacterial infections resulting from suppression of reticuloendothelial cell function are important causes of mortality and include pneumonia, pneumococcal infection, and TB.

Physical findings include hepatomegaly, massive splenomegaly, jaundice or ascites in severe disease, generalized lymphadenopathy, and muscle wasting.[77] Cutaneous gray hyperpigmentation, which prompted the name *kala-azar* (black fever), is characteristically seen in patients in India. Oral and nasopharyngeal nodules resulting from granuloma formation also may be seen.

Diagnosis

The diagnosis is based on the history, physical examination, and microscopic demonstration of amastigotes by a Wright or Giemsa stain of affected tissue samples. The highest yield (90%) comes from the aspiration of the spleen. Liver biopsy is less risky and associated with a yield nearly as great as that of splenic aspiration. The yield of bone marrow aspirates is 80% and may be higher with a longer time of observation[78] and higher than that of lymph node aspirates. Culture requires specialized media and may take several weeks. Serologic testing [enzyme-linked immunosorbent assay (ELISA), immunofluorescence, direct agglutination] can be used to support a presumptive diagnosis of visceral leishmaniasis but is insensitive, particularly in immunocompromised hosts.[79] The leishmanin skin test (Montenegro test) is not helpful in acute visceral disease. PCR-based testing of blood or other tissue may also be useful for diagnosis as well as monitoring.[80]

Treatment

Pentavalent antimonial compounds have been used for all forms of leishmaniasis. Parenteral sodium stibogluconate is no longer available through the Centers for Disease Control and Prevention for treatment of infections in the United States. Liposomal amphotericin B is considered first-line, with alternative parenteral agents available in some parts of the world, such as aminosidine (paromomycin).[81] Miltefosine, a phosphocholine analog administered orally, has a reported initial cure rates of 82%–97% for visceral leishmaniasis but is also limited by GI toxicity and potential for relapse.[82,83] Patients with AIDS and leishmaniasis without immune reconstitution often fail to respond to or relapse following treatment with conventional regimens.[79]

Toxoplasmosis

Toxoplasmosis, caused by *Toxoplasma gondii*, is found worldwide. In the United States, serologic surveys suggest that exposure to *T. gondii* has decreased over time; in women aged 15–44 years, the overall seroprevalence was 7.5%.[84] The infection may be transmitted congenitally or occur as an opportunistic infection that causes cerebral mass lesions in patients with AIDS. Oocysts of *T. gondii* in soil, water, or contaminated meat are ingested and mature in the intestinal tract of humans to become sporozoites, which penetrate the intestinal mucosa, become tachyzoites, and circulate systemically, invading a wide array of cell types.[85] Hepatic involvement has been observed in severe, disseminated infection.

Clinical Features

Although most primary infections are asymptomatic, acquired toxoplasmosis can manifest as a mononucleosis-like illness with fever, chills, headache, and regional lymphadenopathy.[86] Hepatomegaly, splenomegaly, and minimal elevations of serum aminotransferase levels are uncommon findings.[87,88] Infections of immunocompromised hosts can result in pneumonia, myocarditis, encephalitis, and, rarely, hepatitis.[85,89] Toxoplasmosis can produce atypical lymphocytosis, an otherwise unusual feature of parasitic disease.

Diagnosis

The diagnosis is best made by detecting specific IgM or IgG antibody using highly specific indirect immunofluorescence or an enzyme immunoassay.[90] Specialized histologic staining techniques and tissue culture systems can provide adjunctive diagnostic support. PCR analysis of serum and liver also can be helpful in ambiguous cases.[91]

Treatment

Antibiotic therapy should be administered to all persons with severe symptomatic infection and to immunocompromised or pregnant patients with acute uncomplicated infection. Treatment consists of a combination of pyrimethamine and either sulfadiazine or clindamycin, plus folinic acid to minimize hematologic toxicity, for 6 weeks; trimethoprim/sulfamethoxazole is an alternative.[85]

Helminths

Nematodes (Roundworms)

Nematodes are nonsegmented roundworms that have a thick cuticle covering the body (see also Chapter 116). Toxocariasis and capillariasis manifest with major hepatobiliary features, whereas ascariasis, strongyloidiasis, and trichinosis affect the liver less frequently or less severely.

Toxocariasis

Toxocara canis and *Toxocara cati* infect dogs and cats, respectively. Infection occurs worldwide, especially in children, and is acquired when embryonated eggs in soil or contaminated food are ingested. The eggs hatch in the small intestine and release larvae that penetrate the intestinal wall, enter the portal venous circulation, and reach the liver and systemic circulation. Blocked by narrowing vascular channels, the immature worms bore through vessel walls and migrate through the tissues, where they cause hemorrhagic, necrotic, and secondary inflammatory responses. When larvae become trapped in tissue, they provoke granuloma formation with a predominance of eosinophils. Tissue larvae may remain in inflammatory capsules or granulomas for months to years. The liver, brain, and eye are affected most frequently.[92]

Clinical Features

Most infected persons are asymptomatic. Two clinical syndromes are recognized: (1) visceral larva migrans, and (2) "occult" infections associated with nonspecific symptoms, including abdominal pain, anorexia, fever, and wheezing.[92]

Visceral larva migrans is seen most commonly in children with a history of pica. Findings include fever, hepatomegaly, urticaria, leukocytosis with persistent eosinophilia, hypergammaglobulinemia, and elevated blood group isohemagglutinins.[92] Toxocariasis has been implicated in the development of chronic cholestatic hepatitis[93] as well as pyogenic liver abscess.[94] Pulmonary manifestations include asthma and pneumonitis. Neurologic involvement can result in focal or generalized seizures, encephalopathy, and abnormal behavior.[92] Ocular larva migrans is often associated with granulomatous lesions, vitritis, uveitis, visual loss, and strabismus.[95]

Diagnosis

The possibility of toxocariasis should be considered in persons with a history of pica, exposure to dogs or cats, and persistent eosinophilia.[96] Stool studies are not useful for toxocariasis, because these organisms do not produce eggs in humans nor do they remain in the GI tract. A definitive diagnosis is made by the identification of the larvae in affected tissues, although blind biopsies are not routinely recommended.[97] The finding of an eosinophilic granuloma may be specific for visceral larva migrans.[98] A liver biopsy may be necessary to differentiate visceral larva migrans from hepatic capillariasis (see later). A strongly positive result on an ELISA using larval antigens provides support for the diagnosis.[99]

Treatment

Treatment is primarily supportive because visceral larva migrans is generally self-limited. If required, antihelminthic therapy with albendazole, 10 mg/kg/day in two divided doses for 5 days, or mebendazole, 100–200 mg twice daily for 5 days, may be used. Severe pulmonary, cardiac, ophthalmologic, or neurologic manifestations may warrant use of systemic glucocorticoids.[97]

Hepatic Capillariasis

Human infection with *Capillaria hepatica* is rare. Infection with *C. hepatica* is acquired by ingesting soil, food, or water contaminated with embryonated eggs. Larvae released in the cecum penetrate the intestinal mucosa, enter the portal venous circulation, and lodge in the liver. Four weeks after infection, adult worms disintegrate, releasing eggs into the hepatic parenchyma and producing an intense inflammatory reaction with macrophages, eosinophils, and giant cells. Resolution is accompanied by marked peri-egg fibrosis.

Clinical Features

Hepatic capillariasis typically manifests as acute or subacute hepatitis. Findings include fever, nausea, vomiting, diarrhea or constipation, anorexia, myalgias, arthralgias, tender hepatomegaly, and occasionally splenomegaly. Laboratory investigation may reveal leukocytosis with eosinophilia; mild elevations of serum AST, alkaline phosphatase, and bilirubin levels; anemia; and an increased erythrocyte sedimentation rate. A chest x-ray may show pneumonitis.[100]

Diagnosis

The diagnosis is established by detection of adult worms or eggs in the liver (Fig. 86.2). Histologic findings in the liver include necrosis, fibrosis, and granulomas.[101] A finding of *C. hepatica* eggs in stools is not indicative of acute infection and probably reflects passage of undercooked liver from an infected animal.

Treatment

While capillariasis may resolve without specific treatment, hepatic capillariasis is typically treated with albendazole, thiabendazole or mebendazole.

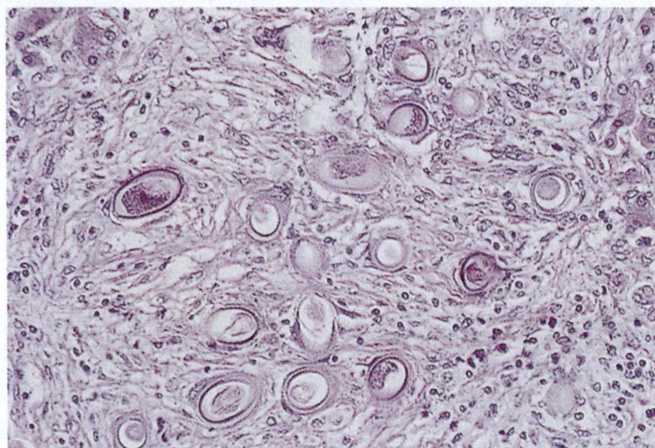

Fig. 86.2 Histopathology of hepatic capillariasis. An intrahepatic granuloma may be seen surrounding numerous eggs (H&E). (From Lucas SB, Zaki SR, Portmann BC. Other viral and infectious diseases and HIV-related liver disease. In: Burt AD, Portmann BC, Ferrell LD, editors. *MacSween's Pathology of the Liver*. 6th ed. London: Churchill Livingstone; 2012:436.)

Ascariasis

Ascaris lumbricoides infects at least 1 billion persons, particularly in areas of lower socioeconomic standing.[102] Humans are infected by ingesting embryonated eggs, usually adherent to raw vegetables. The eggs hatch in the small intestine, and the larvae penetrate the mucosa, enter the portal circulation, and reach the liver, pulmonary artery, and lungs; they grow in the alveolar spaces, are regurgitated and swallowed, and become mature adults in the intestine 2–3 months after ingestion. Then the cycle repeats itself.

Clinical Features

Symptoms generally occur in persons with a large worm burden; most infected persons are asymptomatic. Cough, fever, dyspnea, wheezing, substernal chest discomfort, and hepatomegaly may occur in the first 2 weeks. Chronic infection more frequently is characterized by episodic epigastric or periumbilical pain. If the worm burden is particularly heavy, small bowel complications such as obstruction, intussusception, volvulus, perforation, or appendicitis may occur.[103] Fragments of disintegrating worms within the biliary tract can serve as nidi for the development of biliary calculi.[104] Preexisting disease of the biliary tract or pancreatic duct can predispose the patient to migration of the worm into the bile ducts, with development of obstructive jaundice, cholangitis, or intrahepatic abscesses.[102,105]

Diagnosis

A history of regurgitating a worm or passing a large worm (15–40 cm long) in the stool suggests ascariasis. In the absence of such a history, the diagnosis is made by identification of characteristic eggs in stool specimens. Larvae may also be identified in sputum and gastric washings and in liver and lung biopsy specimens. In patients with biliary or pancreatic symptoms, US, MRCP, or ERCP is performed. ERCP also allows extraction of the worm.[106] A chest x-ray may show an infiltrate, and eosinophilia may be present.

Treatment

One of the following regimens may be used: (1) a single dose of albendazole, 400 mg; (2) mebendazole, 100 mg twice daily for 3 days; (3) pyrantel pamoate, 11 mg/kg to a maximum of 1 g; or (4) a single dose of ivermectin, 200 μg/kg.[107] Intestinal or biliary obstruction may require endoscopic or surgical intervention.

Strongyloidiasis

Strongyloides stercoralis is prevalent in the tropics and subtropics, Southern and Eastern Europe, and the United States. Infection is usually asymptomatic. Humans are infected by the filariform larvae, which penetrate intact skin, are carried to the lungs, migrate through the alveoli, and are swallowed to reach the intestine, where maturation ensues. Autoinfection can occur if the rhabditiform larvae transform into infective filariform larvae in the intestine; reinfection occurs by penetration of the bowel wall or perianal skin. Symptomatic infection results from a heavy infectious burden or infection in an immunocompromised patient. In the latter case, a hyperinfection syndrome may result from dissemination of filariform larvae into tissues that usually are not infected.[108]

Clinical Features

Acute infection can lead to a pruritic eruption, followed by fever, cough, wheezing, abdominal pain, diarrhea, and eosinophilia. In immunocompromised patients, the hyperinfection syndrome may be characterized by invasion of any organ, including the liver, lung, and brain. Hyperinfection should be considered, particularly in the setting of sepsis caused by multiple organisms found in intestinal flora, a consequence of burrowing of larvae through the intestinal mucosa.[109] When the liver is affected, features include jaundice and cholestatic liver biochemical test abnormalities. A liver biopsy specimen may show periportal inflammation, eosinophilic granulomatous hepatitis, or both. Larvae may be observed in intrahepatic bile canaliculi, lymphatic vessels, and small branches of the portal vein.[108]

Diagnosis

Serologic tests include ELISA and decreasing titers can be used for posttreatment response.[110] The diagnosis of active infection is firm when larvae are identified in the stool or intestinal biopsy specimens. An obstructive hepatobiliary picture in a person with known strongyloidiasis should alert the clinician to the possibility of dissemination.

Treatment

For treatment of acute infection, the drug of choice is ivermectin, 200 mg/kg/day for 2 days. Clearance rates are high. An alternative agent is albendazole, 400 mg/day for 3 days for adults and children older than 2 years of age, but retreatment may be necessary, and this drug is less effective for disseminated disease. The hyperinfection syndrome requires longer courses of treatment than those used for the primary acute infection.[111]

Trichinosis

Humans may be infected with *Trichinella spiralis* by eating raw or undercooked pork bearing larvae, which are released in the small intestine, penetrate the mucosa, and disseminate through the systemic circulation. Larvae can be found in the myocardium, cerebrospinal fluid, brain, and, less commonly, liver and gallbladder. The larvae then reenter the circulation and reach striated muscle, where they become encapsulated.

Clinical Features

Clinical manifestations occur when the worm burden is high and include diarrhea, fever, myalgias, periorbital edema, and leukocytosis with marked eosinophilia. Rarely, larvae can be seen invading hepatic sinusoids on examination of a liver biopsy specimen. Jaundice may result from biliary obstruction. Hepatic complications may be associated with fatal cases.[112]

Diagnosis

The diagnosis is suggested by a characteristic history in a patient with fever and eosinophilia. Serologic assays for antibody to *Trichinella* may not be helpful in the acute phase of infection but can be useful after 2 weeks.[113] Muscle biopsy may help us to confirm the diagnosis. DNA-based tests are investigational.

Treatment

Treatment consists of glucocorticoids to relieve allergic symptoms, followed by antihelminthic treatment with albendazole, 400 mg twice daily for 10–15 days, or mebendazole, 200 mg/day for 10–15 days.[113]

Trematodes (Flukes)

Schistosomiasis (Bilharziasis)

About 230 million persons worldwide are infected with trematodes of the genus *Schistosoma*. *Schistosoma mansoni* is found in the Western Hemisphere, Africa, and the Middle East; *Schistosoma haematobium* is found in Africa and the Middle East; *Schistosoma japonicum* and *Schistosoma mekongi* are found in the Far East; and *Schistosoma intercalatum* is found in parts of central Africa. The last two species are much less common than the other three and cause liver disease and colonic disease, respectively.[114]

The Schistosomal Life Cycle

The infectious cycle is initiated by penetration of the skin by free cercariae in fresh water (Fig. 86.3). The cercariae reach the

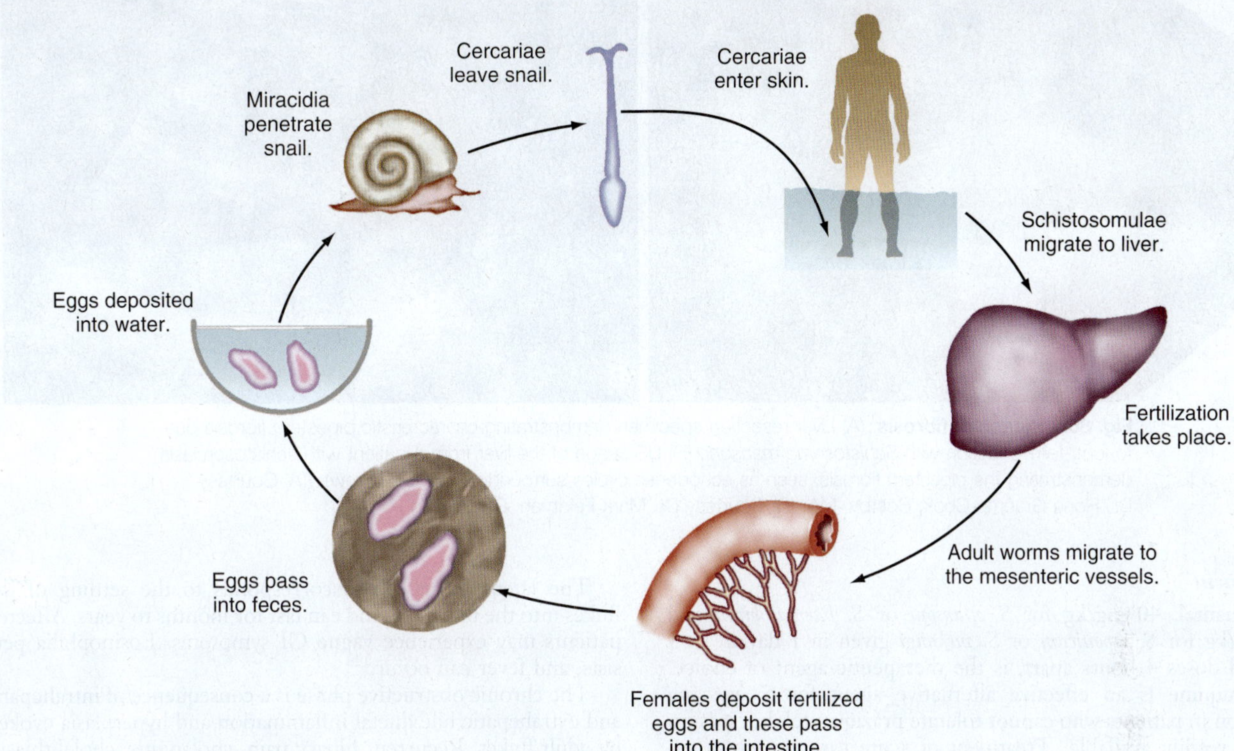

Fig. 86.3 The life cycle of *Schistosoma* species. (From Gitlin N, Strauss R. Atlas of clinical hepatology. Philadelphia: WB Saunders; 1995:72.)

pulmonary vessels within 24 hours, pass through the lungs, and reach the liver, where they lodge, develop into adults, and mate. Adult worms then migrate to their ultimate destinations in the inferior mesenteric venules (*S. mansoni*), superior mesenteric venules (*S. japonicum*), or veins around the bladder (*S. haematobium*). These locations correlate with the clinical complications associated with each species. Each female fluke can lay 300–3000 eggs daily. The eggs are deposited in the terminal venules and eventually migrate into the lumen of the involved organ, after which they are expelled in the stool or urine. Eggs remaining in the organ provoke a robust granulomatous response. Excreted eggs hatch immediately in fresh water and liberate early intermediate miracidia that infect their snail hosts. The miracidia transform into cercariae within the snails and then are released into the water, from which they may again infect humans.[114]

Clinical Features

Acute toxemic schistosomiasis (Katayama syndrome or Katayama fever), presumably a consequence of the host immunologic response to mature worms and eggs, occurs approximately 4–6 weeks after exposure. Manifestations include headache, fever, chills, cough, diarrhea, myalgias, arthralgias, tender hepatomegaly, and eosinophilia.

Untreated acute schistosomiasis invariably progresses to chronic disease. Mesenteric infection leads to hepatic complications, including periportal fibrosis, presinusoidal occlusion, and, ultimately, portal hypertension, as a result of the inflammatory reaction to eggs deposited in the liver. The development of periportal fibrosis appears to be related to production of TNF-α.[115] The lungs and central nervous system may be affected when eggs or adult worms pass through the liver into the systemic circulation, especially in *S. japonicum* infection; pulmonary hypertension and cor pulmonale may result.[116] With severe schistosomal infection, portal hypertension becomes progressive, leading to gastroesophageal varices, splenomegaly, and rarely ascites.

Chronic schistosomal infection may be complicated by increased susceptibility to Salmonella infections.[117] Hepatitis B or hepatitis C viral coinfection is also common in persons living in endemic areas and may accelerate the progression of liver disease and development of hepatocellular carcinoma (HCC).[118] In African intestinal schistosomiasis, pseudopolyps of the colon may develop, leading in some cases to protein-losing colopathy and formation of an inflammatory mass in the descending colon.

Laboratory findings in chronic schistosomiasis include anemia from recurrent luminal GI bleeding or hypersplenism, leukocytosis with eosinophilia, an elevated ESR, and increased serum IgE levels. Results of liver biochemical tests generally are normal until the disease is at an advanced stage.

Diagnosis

The possibility of acute schistosomiasis should be considered in a patient with a history of exposure, abdominal pain, diarrhea, and fever. Multiple stool examinations for ova may be required to confirm the diagnosis because results frequently are negative in the early phase of disease. Serologic testing such as ELISA or Western blot cannot distinguish between past infection and active disease but may be useful in a returned traveler. Sigmoidoscopy or colonoscopy may reveal rectosigmoid or transverse colon involvement and may be useful in chronic disease, when few eggs pass in the feces. US and liver biopsy are useful for demonstrating periportal (pipestem or clay pipestem) fibrosis (Fig. 86.4), but not for diagnosing acute infection because of their insensitivity for detecting schistosomal eggs.[119] CT may show low-attenuation rings around main portal vein branches with marked enhancement with contrast.[120]

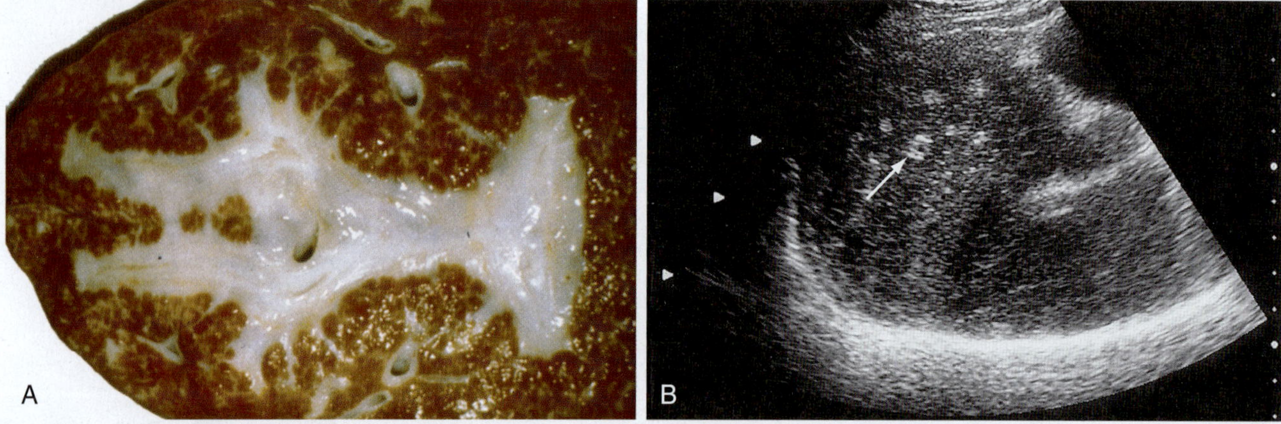

Fig. 86.4 Pipestem fibrosis. (A) Liver resection specimen demonstrating characteristic pipestem fibrosis due to long-term infection with *Schistosoma mansoni*. (B) US image of the liver from a patient with schistosomiasis demonstrating the pipestem fibrosis, seen as echodense circles surrounding vessels (*arrow*). ((A) Courtesy Dr. Fiona Graeme-Cook, Boston, MA; (B) Courtesy Dr. Mark Feldman, Dallas, TX.)

Treatment

Praziquantel, 40 mg/kg for *S. mansoni* or *S. haematobium* and 60 mg/kg for *S. japonicum* or *S. mekongi* given in 1 day in 2–3 divided doses 4 hours apart, is the therapeutic agent of choice. Oxamniquine is an effective alternative agent for *S. mansoni* infection in patients who cannot tolerate praziquantel, but it is no longer readily available. Treatment of acute toxemic schistosomiasis often requires prednisone to suppress immune-mediated helminthicidal or drug reactions, in conjunction with praziquantel at the dose appropriate for the particular species for 3–6 days.[114] Retreatment after 2–3 months is often necessary after Katayama fever.[121]

Band ligation or injection sclerotherapy of varices is effective in controlling variceal bleeding (see Chapter 94). Management of advanced chronic schistosomal liver disease may require placement of a distal splenorenal shunt or esophagogastric devascularization with splenectomy. Fortunately, since the advent of praziquantel, complicated schistosomal liver disease has become uncommon.

Fascioliasis

Fascioliasis is endemic in parts of Europe and Latin America, North Africa, Asia, the Western Pacific, and some parts of the United States. Fascioliasis is caused by the sheep liver fluke *Fasciola hepatica*. Eggs passed in the feces of infected mammals into fresh water give rise to miracidia that penetrate snails and eventually emerge as mobile cercariae, which attach to aquatic plants such as watercress. Hosts become infected when they consume plants containing encysted metacercariae, which then bore into the intestinal wall, enter the abdominal cavity, penetrate the hepatic capsule, and eventually settle in the bile ducts, where they attain maturity. Mature flukes release eggs that are passed in the host's feces to complete the life cycle.[122]

Clinical Features

Three phases (or syndromes) are recognized: acute or invasive, chronic latent, and chronic obstructive.[123] The acute phase corresponds to the migration of young flukes through the liver and is marked by fever, pain in the RUQ, and eosinophilia. Urticaria with dermatographia and nonspecific GI symptoms are common. Physical examination often reveals fever and a tender, enlarged liver. Splenomegaly is seen in as many as 25% of cases, but jaundice is rare and liver biochemical test abnormalities are mild.[124] Eosinophilia can be profound, with eosinophils sometimes exceeding 60% of the differential leukocyte count.[125]

The latent biliary phase corresponds to the settling of the flukes into the bile ducts and can last for months to years. Affected patients may experience vague GI symptoms. Eosinophilia persists, and fever can occur.[124]

The chronic obstructive phase is a consequence of intrahepatic and extrahepatic bile ductal inflammation and hyperplasia evoked by adult flukes. Recurrent biliary pain, cholangitis, cholelithiasis, and biliary obstruction may result. Blood loss from epithelial injury occurs, but overt hemobilia is rare. Liver biochemical testing commonly demonstrates a pattern suggestive of biliary obstruction.[126] Long-term infection may lead to biliary cirrhosis and secondary sclerosing cholangitis, but no convincing association with biliary tract or hepatic malignancy has been demonstrated.[127]

Diagnosis

The diagnosis should be considered in a patient with prolonged fever, abdominal pain, diarrhea, tender hepatomegaly, and eosinophilia. Cross-sectional imaging may reveal multiple hypodense nodular branching subcapsular lesions that enhance after contrast.[128] Because eggs are not passed during the acute phase, diagnosis depends on the detection of antibody, usually by ELISA. In the latent and chronic phases, a definitive diagnosis is based on the detection of eggs in stool, duodenal aspirate specimens, or bile.[122] On occasion, US or ERCP demonstrate flukes in the gallbladder and bile duct.[129] If one member of a family is diagnosed with fascioliasis, all household members should be evaluated.

Hepatic histologic findings include necrosis and granulomas with eosinophilic infiltrates and Charcot-Leyden crystals. Eosinophilic abscesses, epithelial hyperplasia of the bile ducts, and periportal fibrosis may be seen.[130]

Treatment

The drug of choice is triclabendazole, 10 mg/kg given orally daily for 2 days.[131] Praziquantel, mebendazole, and albendazole are not effective for fascioliasis. Nitazoxanide is another medication that may be potentially efficacious.

Clonorchiasis and Opisthorchiasis

Clonorchis sinensis, *Opisthorchis viverrini*, and *Opisthorchis felineus* are trematodes of the family Opisthorchiidae. Infection by *C. sinensis* and *O. viverrini* is widespread in East and Southeast Asia and is linked to lower socioeconomic status. *O. felineus* infects humans and domestic animals in Eastern Europe. All three have similar life cycles and result in similar clinical manifestations. Eggs are passed in the feces into fresh water, consumed by snails, and hatch as free-swimming cercariae, which seek and penetrate fish or crayfish and encyst in skin or muscle as metacercariae. The mammalian host is infected when it consumes raw or undercooked fish. The metacercariae excyst in the small intestine and migrate into the ampulla of Vater and bile ducts, where they mature into adult flukes. Infection can be maintained for two decades or longer.[122]

Clinical Features

In general, acute infection is clinically silent. Occasional symptoms include fever, abdominal pain, and diarrhea. Chronic manifestations correlate with the fluke burden and are dominated by hepatobiliary features: fever, pain in the RUQ, tender hepatomegaly, and eosinophilia. If the worm burden in the bile ducts is heavy, chronic or intermittent biliary obstruction can ensue, with frequent cholelithiasis, cholecystitis, jaundice, and, ultimately, recurrent pyogenic cholangitis (see Chapter 70). Liver biochemical test results, especially serum alkaline phosphatase and bilirubin levels, are elevated. Long-standing infection leads to exuberant inflammation, resulting in periportal fibrosis, marked biliary epithelial hyperplasia and dysplasia, and, ultimately, a substantially increased risk of cholangiocarcinoma.[132] Cholangiocarcinoma resulting from clonorchiasis or opisthorchiasis tends to be multicentric and arises in the secondary biliary radicles of the hilum of the liver. Cholangiocarcinoma should be suspected in infected persons with weight loss, jaundice, epigastric pain, or an abdominal mass and is more common in persons with diabetes (see Chapter 71).

Diagnosis

The diagnosis of clonorchiasis or opisthorchiasis is made by the detection of characteristic fluke eggs in the stool, except late in the disease when biliary obstruction has supervened. In these cases, the diagnosis is made by identifying flukes in the bile ducts or gallbladder at surgery or in bile obtained by postoperative drainage or percutaneous aspiration (Fig. 86.5). Endoscopic or intraoperative cholangiography reveals slender, uniform filling defects within intrahepatic ducts that are alternately dilated and strictured, mimicking sclerosing cholangitis. Serologic methods of diagnosis cannot distinguish between past or current infection.[122]

Treatment

All patients with clonorchiasis or opisthorchiasis should receive praziquantel, which is uniformly effective in a dose of 75 mg/kg/daily in three divided doses for 2 days. Side effects are uncommon and include headache, dizziness, and nausea. After treatment, dead flukes may be seen in the stool or biliary drainage. When the burden of infecting organisms is high, the dead flukes and surrounding debris or stones may cause biliary obstruction, necessitating endoscopic or surgical drainage.[122] Reinfection rates in hyperendemic areas are high, so repeated treatment courses are often necessary.[133]

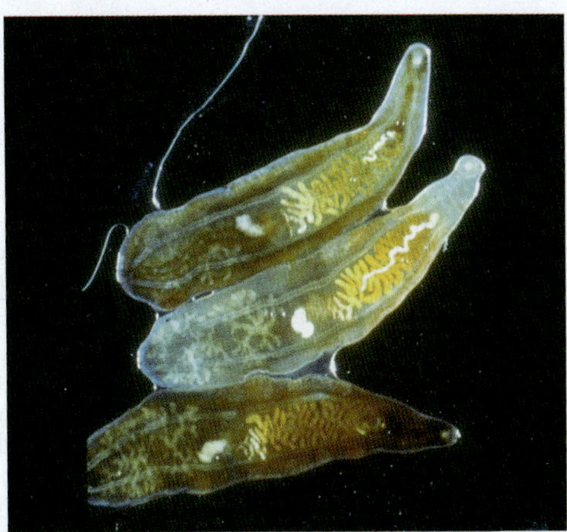

Fig. 86.5 *Clonorchis sinensis*. (Courtesy Dr. Fiona Graeme-Cook, Boston, MA.)

Cestodes (Tapeworms)

Echinococcosis

Infections with *Echinococcus granulosus* can be found worldwide in areas where dogs are used to help raise livestock. *Echinococcus multilocularis* is distributed in northern North America and Eurasia, whereas *Echinococcus vogeli* is found in scattered areas of Central and Latin America.

The Echinococcal Life Cycle

Infection occurs when humans eat vegetables contaminated by dog feces that contain embryonated eggs. The eggs hatch in the small intestine and liberate oncospheres that penetrate the mucosa and migrate via vessels or lymphatics to distant sites. The liver is the most common destination (70%), followed by the lungs (20%), kidney, spleen, brain, and bone. In these organs, a hydatid cyst develops by vesiculation and produces thousands of protoscolices. The cyst wall contains three layers: an outer adventitial layer, which is host-derived and can calcify, and intermediate acellular and inner germinal layers, which are worm-derived. A protoscolex is produced asexually within small secondary cysts that develop from the inner layer. Rupture of the hydatid cyst releases the viable protoscolices, which set up daughter cysts in secondary sites. The adult *Echinococcus* tapeworm consists of a scolex, which contains a rostellum with 20–50 hooklets and 4 suckers, a neck, and an immature, mature, and gravid proglottid. Dogs acquire the infection by consuming organs of sheep, cattle, or other livestock bearing the hydatid cyst.

Clinical Features

Most patients with a hydatid cyst in the liver have no symptoms. As the cysts of *E. granulosus* grow within the liver (Fig. 86.6), they begin to cause low-grade fever, pain, tender hepatomegaly (usually affecting the right hepatic lobe), and eosinophilia. If the cysts grow large enough, they may rupture spontaneously or after trauma into the lungs, thereby leading to dyspnea and hemoptysis. More extensive rupture into the peritoneum or lungs may lead to

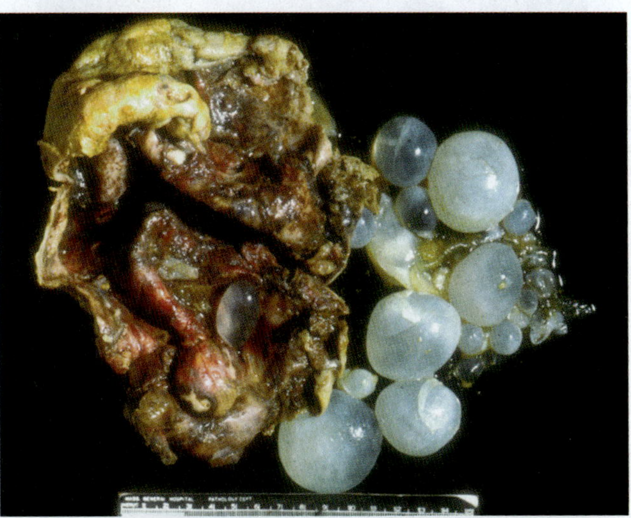

Fig. 86.6 Liver resection specimen of a hydatid cyst caused by *Echinococcus granulosus*. Multiple daughter cysts are seen. (Courtesy Dr. Fiona Graeme-Cook, Boston, MA.)

a life-threatening anaphylactic reaction to the cyst contents. Rupture into the biliary tract can cause cholangitis and obstruction; marked eosinophilia may be present. Superinfection of the hepatic cysts can lead to pyogenic liver abscesses in up to 20% of patients with hepatic disease. Rare complications of hydatid cysts or cyst rupture include pancreatitis, portal hypertension, Budd-Chiari syndrome, and rupture into the pericardial sac.

E. multilocularis is highly invasive; infection leads to formation of solid masses in the liver that are easily confused with cirrhosis or carcinoma. *Alveolar hydatid disease* is the term applied to hepatic nodules that appear on microscopy as alveoli-like microvesicles.[134] Daughter cysts bud from the germinal membrane in an uncontrolled manner, with "invasion" of the surrounding liver parenchyma by the scolices. Infection of bile ducts and vessels and necrosis of parenchyma may result in cholangitis, liver abscess, sepsis, portal hypertension, hepatic vein occlusion, and biliary cirrhosis. Unfortunately, infection generally is not diagnosed until the lesions are inoperable because of extensive invasion or distant metastatic disease, and mortality rates without antiparasitic treatment are high, approaching 90%.[135]

Infection with *E. vogeli* has clinical features intermediate between those of infections caused by the other two species and is characterized by multiple fluid-filled cysts containing daughter cysts and protoscolices. Although not as aggressive as *E. multilocularis* infection, *E. vogeli* infection can spread to contiguous sites.

Diagnosis

A history of exposure in a patient with hepatomegaly and an abdominal mass is highly suggestive of hepatic echinococcosis, but the most important diagnostic tools are imaging and serology. Ring-like calcifications in up to one-fourth of hepatic cysts are visible on plain abdominal films in patients infected with *E. granulosus*. The sensitivity and specificity of both US and CT in confirming the diagnosis are high (Fig. 86.7).[136] Both modalities can demonstrate intracystic septations and daughter cyst formation in about half of the cysts. Contrast-enhanced CT may display avascular cysts with ring enhancement. Percutaneous aspiration of the cyst had traditionally been discouraged because of concern about anaphylactic reactions. Encouraging reports, however, suggest that under carefully controlled conditions, with use of thin needles and concomitant antihelminthic therapy, percutaneous aspiration for diagnosis and therapy may be safe.[137,138] The detection of protoscolices or acid-fast hooklets in the cyst fluid confirms the diagnosis.[139] An ELISA is the best serologic assay for diagnosis, with a sensitivity of 84%–90%.[140] Assays for detecting circulating antigen or DNA-based methods are likely to provide additional diagnostic benefit in the future. The Casoni skin test, used in the past, is nonspecific and no longer recommended.

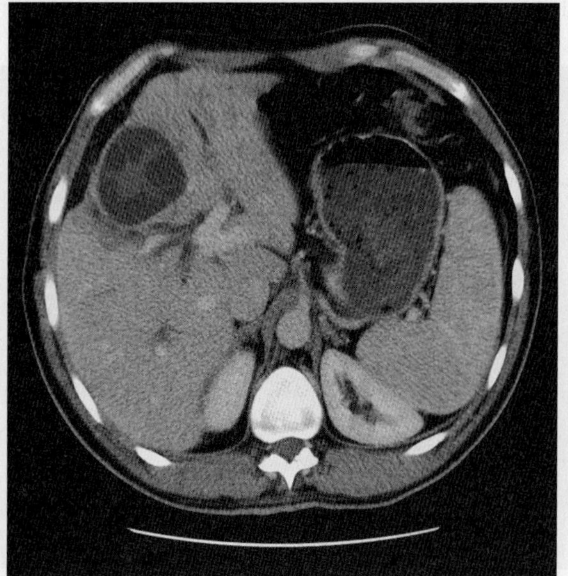

Fig. 86.7 CT showing the typical appearance of a hydatid cyst in the liver. (Courtesy Dr. Mukesh Harisinghani, Boston, MA.)

E. multilocularis infection can be diagnosed with a combination of ELISA and CT, which often shows scattered areas of calcified necrotic tissue. In *E. vogeli* infection, CT demonstrates polycystic lesions in the liver or peritoneal space.

Treatment

In the past, accessible cysts in younger persons were always treated surgically, and surgery is still considered the preferred treatment in many cases. The goal has been removal of the cestode without disruption of cyst contents. Care must be taken to isolate the cyst and to inject cidal agents (such as 20% hypertonic saline) before the cyst is aspirated. Successful approaches have included cystectomy, endocystectomy, omentoplasty, and marsupialization. A laparoscopic approach is feasible in some cases. In complicated cases, hepatic lobectomy or hemihepatectomy may be necessary. Calcified cysts need not be removed.

Promising data indicate that careful percutaneous drainage is a safe and effective alternative to surgery for the treatment of complicated cysts.[141] In addition to surgery or drainage, administration of an antihelminthic, such as albendazole, 10 mg/kg daily for 8 weeks, is recommended.[142] *P*uncture, *a*spiration, *i*njection (of a scolicidal agent), and *r*e-aspiration (PAIR) can be performed safely with long-term control of echinococcal cysts.[138] Injection of hydatid liver cysts with albendazole has also been described.[137] Therefore nonsurgical approaches are now available for management of hydatid cysts. The decision between surgical and nonsurgical techniques depends on the extent and type of lesions.[143] Cysts that cannot be treated surgically or percutaneously should be treated with albendazole, preferably, or mebendazole. Large doses and prolonged treatment are required (e.g., albendazole 10–15 mg/kg/day in two divided doses for at least 28 days).

Surgical resection is curative in up to one-third of cases of *E. multilocularis* infection. In most cases, the disease is advanced when the diagnosis is made. In such cases, palliative drainage procedures or long-term treatment with albendazole or another benzimidazole carbamate may prolong survival.[134,144] Surgery appears to be the most effective approach to the management of *E. vogeli* infection.

FUNGI

Candidiasis

Candida species may cause invasive systemic infection with hepatic involvement in severely immunocompromised persons (see Chapters 33 and 34). The liver can become infected by *C. albicans* and related species in the setting of disseminated multiorgan disease. Most disseminated infections occur in leukemic patients undergoing high-dose chemotherapy and become clinically evident during the period of recovery from severe neutropenia. In several series, hepatic candidiasis was present in 51%–91% of predominantly leukemic patients with disseminated candidiasis.[145,146] Disease is often overwhelming, with a high mortality rate.[146] Fortunately, cases are rarer in the modern era due to antifungal prophylaxis and antifungal therapies applied during periods of fever and neutropenia.[147]

Other, less frequent, presentations in the compromised host include isolated or focal hepatic or hepatosplenic candidiasis.[148] Focal candidiasis is believed to result from colonization of the GI tract by *Candida*, which disseminates locally following the onset of neutropenia and mucosal injury caused by high-dose chemotherapy.[148] Resulting fungemia of the portal vein seeds the liver and leads to formation of hepatic microabscesses and macroabscesses.

In either focal or disseminated candidiasis involving the liver, clinical features include fever, abdominal pain and distention, nausea, vomiting, diarrhea, and tender hepatomegaly. The serum alkaline phosphatase level is almost invariably elevated, with varying elevations in serum aminotransferase and bilirubin levels. CT and MRI of the abdomen are sensitive tests to detect hepatic or splenic abscesses, which often are multicentric (Fig. 86.8).[149,150] In cases diagnosed antemortem, liver biopsy or laparoscopy reveals macroscopic nodules, necrosis with microabscesses, and characteristic yeast or hyphal forms of *Candida*.[151] The results of cultures of blood and/or biopsy material are negative in most cases. PCR methodology has been used to diagnose hepatic candidiasis.[152] The utility of serum beta-D-glucan for diagnosis of hepatic candidiasis has not been established.

Response rates to therapy are better (almost 60%) for focal hepatic candidiasis than for disseminated disease. The success of treatment is far from optimal, however. Intravenously administered echinocandins such as caspofungin, micafungin, or anidulafungin are often used due to fewer toxicities than IV liposomal amphotericin for at least 2 weeks, before step-down therapy to an azole such as fluconazole.[153,154] Unfortunately, widespread use of fluconazole has resulted in a shift toward infections with species of yeast resistant to this agent. Adjunctive glucocorticoids may speed recovery from the inflammatory response that accompanies disseminated candidiasis as neutrophils return.[155]

Histoplasmosis

Infection with *Histoplasma capsulatum* is acquired through the respiratory tract and in most cases is confined to the lungs. Severely immunocompromised persons (e.g., those with AIDS), however, are predisposed to disseminated histoplasmosis (see Chapter 33). The liver can be invaded in both acute and chronic progressive disseminated histoplasmosis. Fever, oropharyngeal ulcers, hepatomegaly, and splenomegaly may be present in patients with chronic disease.[156] In children with acute hepatic disease, which appears to be an extension of primary pulmonary infection, marked hepatosplenomegaly is universal and is associated with high fever and lymphadenopathy. In one series of 111 cases of disseminated histoplasmosis, serum ALT levels were elevated in 39%, AST levels were elevated in 27%, and alkaline phosphatase levels were greater than 200 U/L in 55%.[157] Hepatosplenomegaly is present in approximately 30% of adults with acute disease (often the AIDS-defining illness).

Yeast forms can be identified in liver biopsy specimens with standard H&E staining. The silver methenamine method is superior for detecting yeast forms in areas of caseating necrosis or in granulomas. The organism is difficult to culture and almost never grows from biopsy specimens. Serologic testing for antibodies is therefore helpful in confirming the diagnosis. In immunocompromised persons who may not be capable of mounting an antibody response, the detection of *H. capsulatum* antigens in urine and serum can be useful.[158] Treatment options include therapy with amphotericin B, fluconazole, or itraconazole.[156]

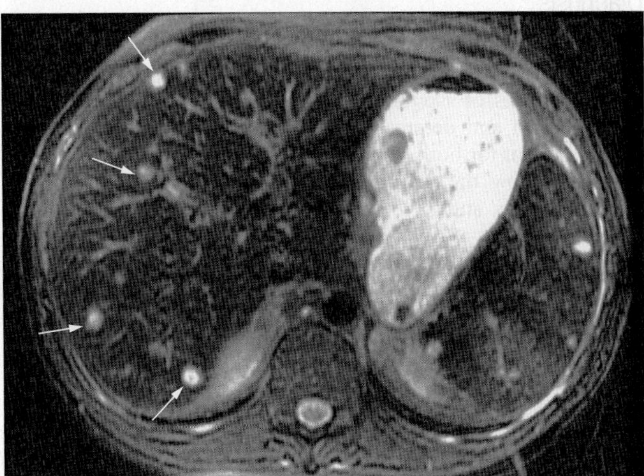

Fig. 86.8 T2-weighted MRI showing the characteristic small high-intensity foci (*arrows*) of hepatosplenic candidiasis. (Courtesy Dr. Mukesh Harisinghani, Boston, MA.)

LIVER ABSCESS

Pyogenic

In the past, most cases of pyogenic liver abscess were a consequence of appendicitis complicated by pylephlebitis (portal vein inflammation) in a young patient. This presentation has become uncommon as a result of earlier diagnosis and effective antibiotic therapy. Most cases now are cryptogenic or occur in older men with underlying biliary tract disease.[159] Predisposing conditions include malignancy, immunosuppression, diabetes mellitus, use of proton pump inhibitors, and previous biliary surgery or interventional endoscopy.

Pathogenesis

Infections of the biliary tract (e.g., cholangitis, cholecystitis) are the most common identifiable source of liver abscess. Infection may spread to the liver from the bile duct, along a penetrating vessel, or from an adjacent septic focus (including pylephlebitis). Pyogenic liver abscess may arise as a late complication of endoscopic sphincterotomy for bile duct stones or within 3–6 weeks of a surgical biliary-intestinal anastomosis.[160] Pyogenic liver abscesses may complicate recurrent pyogenic cholangitis, which is found predominantly in East and Southeast Asia and is characterized by recurring episodes of cholangitis, intrahepatic stone formation, and, in many cases, biliary parasitic infections (see earlier and Chapter 70). Less commonly, liver abscess is a complication of bacteremia arising from underlying abdominal disease, such as diverticulitis, appendicitis, perforated or penetrating peptic ulcer, GI malignancy, IBD, or peritonitis, or rarely from bacterial endocarditis or penetration of a foreign body through the wall of the colon. One population-based study suggested a fourfold higher risk of GI malignancy in patients with pyogenic liver abscesses.[161] The risk of liver abscess may be increased in patients with underlying diabetes mellitus or cirrhosis.[162,163] The use of proton pump inhibitors has been associated with increased risk of pyogenic liver abscesses.[164] Occasionally, a pyogenic liver abscess may be the presentation of a hepatocellular or gallbladder carcinoma or a complication of chemoembolization or percutaneous ablation of a hepatic neoplasm.[159]

In approximately 40% of cases of pyogenic liver abscess, no obvious source of infection can be identified. Oral flora have been proposed to be a potential source in such cases, particularly in patients with severe periodontal disease.[165]

Microbiology

Most pyogenic liver abscesses are polymicrobial. The bacterial organisms that have been cultured from liver abscesses are listed in Box 86.1. The most frequently isolated organisms are *Escherichia coli* and *Klebsiella*, *Proteus*, *Pseudomonas*, and *Streptococcus* species, particularly the *Streptococcus milleri* (*anginosus*) group. Certain virulent strains of *Klebsiella pneumoniae* present in East

BOX 86.1 Organisms That May Be Isolated from the Abscess and the Blood in Patients With a Pyogenic Liver Abscess

GRAM-NEGATIVE AEROBIC BACTERIA

Escherichia coli
Klebsiella pneumoniae
Enterobacter spp.
Pseudomonas spp.
Citrobacter spp.
Morganella spp.
Proteus spp.
Salmonella spp.
*Serratia marcescens**
Yersinia spp.*
*Burkholderia pseudomallei**
*Capnocytophaga canimorsus**
*Pasteurella multocida**
*Achromobacter xylosoxidans**

GRAM-POSITIVE AEROBIC BACTERIA

Enterococcus spp.
Streptococcus pyogenes
Staphylococcus aureus
Streptococcus milleri (anginosus) group
*Listeria monocytogenes**
*Bacillus cereus**

ANAEROBIC BACTERIA

Bacteroides spp.
Fusobacterium spp.
Streptococcus spp.
Peptostreptococcus spp.
Peptococcus spp.
Prevotella spp.*
Clostridium spp.*
Actinomyces spp.*

OTHERS

Candida spp.
Mycobacterium tuberculosis

*Rare

Asia can cause liver abscess in the absence of underlying hepatobiliary disease, often with metastatic infection.[166,167] With improved cultivation methods and earlier diagnosis, the number of cases caused by anaerobic organisms has increased. The most commonly identified anaerobic species are *Bacteroides fragilis* and *Fusobacterium necrophorum*; anaerobic streptococci have also been identified. Pyogenic abscess associated with recurrent pyogenic cholangitis may be caused by *S. typhi*. *Clostridium* and *Actinomyces* species are uncommon causes of liver abscess, and rare cases are caused by *Y. enterocolitica*, *Pasteurella multocida*, *Haemophilus parainfluenzae*, and *Listeria* species. Septic melioidosis also has been described (see earlier). Liver abscesses caused by *S. aureus* infection are most common in children and patients with septicemia or other conditions associated with impaired host resistance, including chronic granulomatous disease.[168] Fungal abscesses of the liver may occur in immunocompromised hosts, particularly those with a hematologic malignancy (see earlier).

Clinical Features

In the preantibiotic era, patients with a pyogenic liver abscess typically presented with acutely spiking fevers, pain in the RUQ, and, in many cases, shock. After the introduction of antibiotics, the presentation of pyogenic liver abscess became less acute. The presentation often is insidious, particularly in older adult patients, and is characterized by malaise, low-grade fever, anorexia, weight loss, and dull abdominal pain that may increase with movement. Symptoms may be present for 1 month or more before a diagnosis is made. Multiple abscesses are typical when biliary disease is the source and are associated with a more acute systemic presentation, often with sepsis and shock, than is the case with solitary abscesses. When an abscess is situated near the dome of the liver, pain may be referred to the right shoulder, or a cough resulting from diaphragmatic irritation or atelectasis may be present.

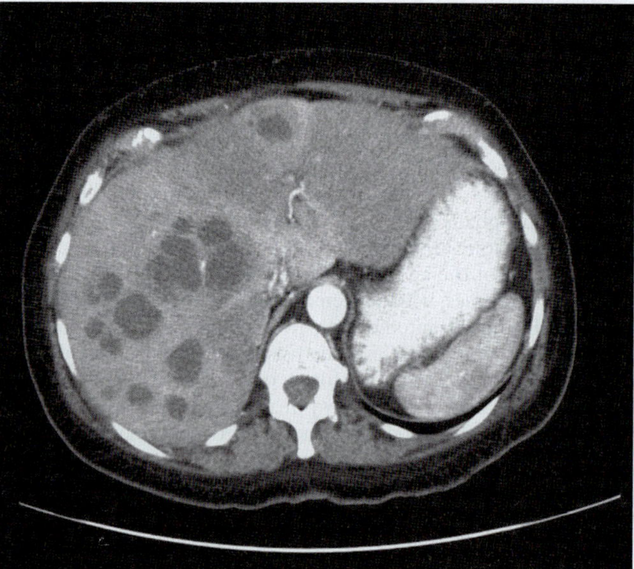

Fig. 86.9 CT showing multiple pyogenic abscesses in the liver. (Courtesy Dr. Mukesh Harisinghani, Boston, MA.)

Physical examination usually discloses fever, hepatomegaly, and liver tenderness, which is accentuated by movement or percussion. Splenomegaly is unusual, except with a chronic abscess. Ascites is rare, and in the absence of cholangitis, jaundice is present only late in the course of the illness. Portal hypertension may follow recovery if the portal vein has been thrombosed. Laboratory findings include anemia, leukocytosis, an elevated ESR, and abnormal liver biochemical test results, especially an elevated serum alkaline phosphatase level.

Diagnosis

Blood culture specimens will identify the causative organism in at least 50% of cases if drawn before antibiotic administration.[169] Direct cultures of aspirated fluid are useful for identification of the organism and determination of antibiotic susceptibility and should be sent for both aerobic and anaerobic culture.[170] Chest x-rays may show the elevation of the right hemidiaphragm and atelectasis. US and CT are the initial imaging modalities of choice. Abscesses as small as 1 cm in diameter can be detected. US is inexpensive and accurate and can guide needle aspiration of the abscess. Culture specimens of aspirated material yield positive results in 90% of cases (although the yield probably is lower if the patient has been receiving antibiotics). CT is also accurate, with a sensitivity approaching 100%, but is more expensive than US. Hepatic abscesses are usually hypodense on a CT and may display a rim of contrast enhancement in less than 20% of cases (Fig. 86.9). CT permits precise localization of an abscess, assessment of its relationship to adjacent structures, and detection of gas in the abscess, which is associated with increased mortality.

An abscess must be distinguished from other mass lesions in the liver, including cystic lesions, benign and malignant neoplasms, soft tissue tumors (neurofibroma, leiomyoma, and malignant fibrous histiocytoma), focal nodular hyperplasia, and hemangiomas (see Chapter 98), as well as inflammatory pseudotumors. MRI is more sensitive than CT for detecting small abscesses, which have low signal intensity on T1-weighted images and high signal intensity on T2-weighted images and enhance with gadolinium. ERCP is indicated in patients with imaging evidence of biliary stones or prominent cholestasis.[171] Rarely, arteriography may be of value in distinguishing an abscess from a tumor.

Inflammatory pseudotumor of the liver (also called *plasma cell granuloma*) is a rare, benign lesion characterized by proliferating fibrous tissue infiltrated by inflammatory cells. The cause is unknown. Affected persons (typically young men) often have a history of recent infection, but a causative infectious agent is rarely isolated from the lesion. Additional associated disorders include chronic inflammatory and autoimmune disorders, particularly ascending cholangitis and PSC, as well as diabetes mellitus, Sjögren syndrome, gout, UC, Crohn disease, HIV infection, EBV infection, and acute myeloblastic leukemia. Patients typically present with intermittent fever, abdominal discomfort, vomiting, diarrhea, weight loss, and malaise and have hepatomegaly, RUQ tenderness, and jaundice on physical examination. Portal hypertension may develop. Laboratory findings are also similar to those associated with liver abscess, including polyclonal hyperglobulinemia in 50% of cases, and imaging studies generally are interpreted as showing a tumor or an abscess. Treatment generally has been by a surgical resection of the lesion, although some patients may recover spontaneously or after treatment with antibiotics or glucocorticoids, once the diagnosis is made based on needle biopsy findings.[172,173]

Prevention and Treatment

Pyogenic liver abscesses are best prevented by the prompt treatment of acute biliary and abdominal infections and by adequate drainage of infected intra-abdominal collections under appropriate antibiotic coverage. Treatment of a hepatic abscess requires antibiotic therapy directed at the causative organism(s) and, in most cases, drainage of the abscess, usually percutaneously with imaging guidance. An indwelling drainage catheter may be placed in the abscess until the cavity has resolved, particularly for lesions greater than 5 cm in size, although intermittent needle aspiration may be as effective as continuous catheter drainage for smaller lesions.[174,175] With multiple abscesses, only the largest abscess may need to be aspirated; smaller lesions often resolve with antibiotic treatment alone, but rarely, each lesion may need drainage. For a small abscess, antibiotic therapy without drainage may suffice. Biliary decompression is essential when a hepatic abscess is associated with biliary tract obstruction or communication and may be accomplished through the endoscopic or transhepatic route (see Chapter 72). Surgical drainage of a hepatic abscess may be necessary in patients with incomplete percutaneous drainage, unresolved jaundice, renal impairment, a multiloculated abscess, or a ruptured abscess.[176] A laparoscopic approach may be feasible in select cases.

Initial antibiotic coverage, pending culture results, should be broad in spectrum, as with a third-generation cephalosporin plus metronidazole, or a combination of a beta-lactam and beta-lactamase inhibitor active against enteric organisms, including anaerobes. If amebiasis is suspected, metronidazole should be started before aspiration is performed (see later). Alternative regimens include carbapenems and fluoroquinolones with metronidazole. After culture results and sensitivity profiles have been obtained, IV antibiotic therapy directed at the specific organism(s) should be administered until a clinical response to therapy is demonstrated, followed by an oral regimen for up to 6 weeks.[177]

The mortality rate for patients with hepatic abscesses treated with antibiotics and percutaneous drainage has improved since the 1980s.[176,178] A worse prognosis is associated with a delay in diagnosis, multiple abscesses, multiple organisms cultured from blood, a fungal cause, shock, jaundice, hypoalbuminemia, a pleural effusion, an underlying biliary malignancy, multiorgan dysfunction, sepsis, or other associated medical diseases.[176,179–183] Complications of pyogenic liver abscess include empyema, pleural or pericardial effusion, portal or splenic vein thrombosis, rupture into the pericardium, thoracic and abdominal fistula formation, and sepsis. Metastatic septic endophthalmitis occurs in as many as 10% of diabetic patients with a liver abscess caused by *K. pneumoniae*.[184]

Amebic

Amebiasis occurs in approximately 50 million persons worldwide annually and is most common in tropical and subtropical regions (see also Chapter 115).[185,186] Endemic areas include Africa, Southeast Asia, India, Mexico, and parts of Central and South America. In the United States, it is a disease of young, often Hispanic adults. Amebic liver abscess is the most common extraintestinal manifestation of amebiasis. Compared with affected persons who reside in an endemic area, persons in whom an amebic liver abscess develops after travel to an endemic area are older and more likely to be male, have marked hepatomegaly, and have a large abscess or multiple abscesses. The occurrence of an amebic liver abscess in a person who has not traveled to or resided in an endemic area should raise the suspicion of underlying immunosuppression, particularly AIDS.[187,188] Other persons at increased risk include inpatients in residential institutions and men who have sex with men. Host factors that contribute to the severity of disease include younger age, pregnancy, malnutrition, alcoholism, glucocorticoid use, and malignancy.

Pathogenesis

During its life cycle, *Entamoeba histolytica* exists as trophozoite or cyst forms (Fig. 86.10). After infection, amebic cysts pass through the GI tract and become trophozoites in the colon, where they invade the mucosa and produce typical "flask-shaped" ulcers. The organism is carried by the portal vein circulation to the liver, where an abscess may develop. Occasionally, organisms travel beyond the liver and can establish abscesses in the lung or brain. Rupture of an amebic liver abscess into the pleural, pericardial, and peritoneal spaces can also occur.

Clinical Features

Amebic liver abscess is 10 times as common in men as in women and is rare in children.[185] An amebic liver abscess is more likely than a pyogenic liver abscess to be associated with an acute presentation. Symptoms are present on average for 2 weeks by the time a diagnosis is made. A latency period between intestinal and subsequent liver infection of up to many years is possible, and less than 10% of patients report an antecedent history of bloody diarrhea with amebic dysentery.

Pain is typically in the RUQ but may be localized to the right chest, epigastrium, or right shoulder. Fever is nearly universal but may be intermittent. Malaise, myalgias, and arthralgias are common. Jaundice is uncommon and signifies a poor prognosis. Pulmonary symptoms and signs may be present, but a pericardial rub and peritonitis are rare. Occasionally a friction rub is heard over the liver. Laboratory features resemble those found in pyogenic abscess and eosinophilia is typically not present. Coinfection with bacterial pathogens is uncommon. Rare complications of amebic abscesses can include intraperitoneal, intrathoracic, and pericardial rupture and multiorgan failure.

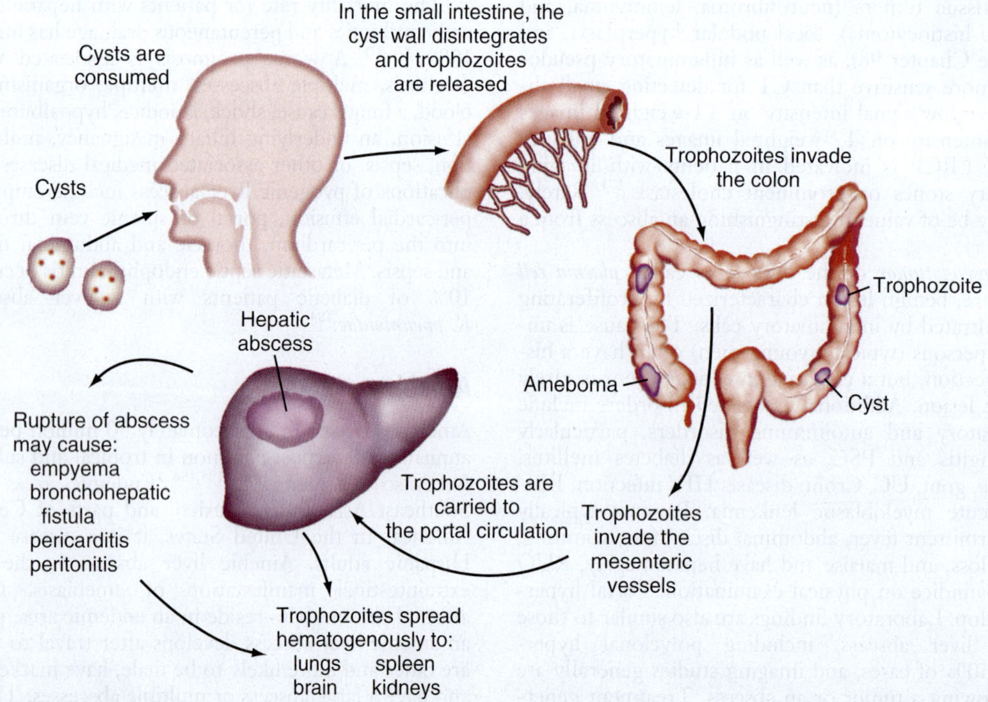

Fig. 86.10 The life cycle of *Entamoeba histolytica* in amebiasis. (From Gitlin N, Strauss R. Atlas of clinical hepatology. Philadelphia: WB Saunders; 1995:64.)

TABLE 86.3 Comparisons of Pyogenic and Amebic Liver Abscess

Parameter	Pyogenic	Amebic
Number	Often multiple	Usually single
Location	Either lobe of liver	Usually right hepatic lobe, near the diaphragm
Presentation	Subacute	Acute
Jaundice	Mild	Moderate
Diagnosis	US or CT ± aspiration	US or CT and serology
Treatment	Drainage (if technically feasible) + IV antibiotics (see text)	Metronidazole, 750 mg 3 times daily for 7–10 days orally or IV; or tinidazole, 2 g orally for 3 days, followed by iodoquinol, 650 mg orally 3 times daily for 20 days; diloxanide furoate, 500 mg orally 3 times daily for 10 days; or aminosidine (paromomycin) 25–35 mg/kg/day orally in 3 divided doses for 7–10 days

Diagnosis

The diagnosis of amebic liver abscess is based on clinical suspicion, hepatic imaging, and serologic testing. As amebic colitis has usually resolved, the organism is isolated from the stool in the minority of patients. Hepatic imaging studies cannot distinguish a pyogenic from an amebic liver abscess (Fig. 86.11). An amebic abscess is commonly localized to the right hepatic lobe, close to the diaphragm, and is usually single (Table 86.3).[189] The most commonly used serologic tests are based on ELISA. Serologic test results must be interpreted in the clinical context because serum antibody levels may remain elevated for years after recovery or cure. The sensitivity of these tests is approximately 95%, and the specificity is more than 95%. False-negative results may occur within the first 10 days of infection.[186] PCR-based tests to detect amebic DNA and an ELISA to detect amebic antigens in specimens are available.[190–192]

Aspiration of an amebic abscess should be performed if the diagnosis remains uncertain. The presence of a reddish-brown pasty aspirate ("anchovy paste" or "chocolate sauce") is typical;

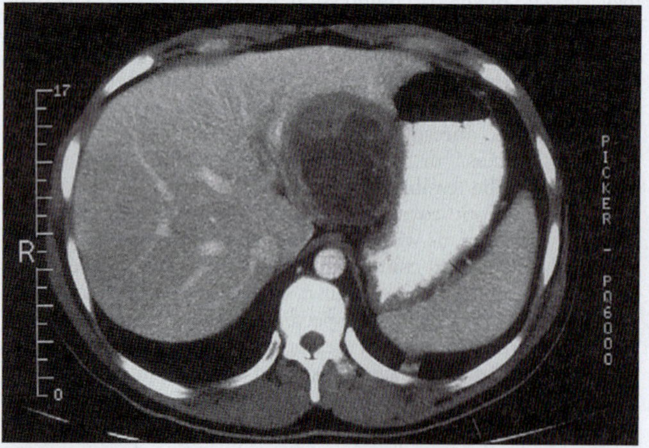

Fig. 86.11 CT showing a large amebic abscess in the left lobe of the liver. (Courtesy Dr. Mark Feldman, Dallas, TX.)

trophozoites rarely are identified. Aspiration also may be considered when no response to antibiotic therapy has occurred after 5–7 days or when an abscess in the left lobe of the liver is close to the pericardium.[193,194]

Treatment

Standard therapy consists of metronidazole, 750 mg three times daily by mouth or, if necessary, IV for 7–10 days. Tinidazole or chloroquine may be substituted for metronidazole. The response to treatment usually occurs within 96 hours. Following a course of metronidazole, most authorities recommend the addition of an oral luminal amebicide—such as iodoquinol, 650 mg three times daily for 20 days; diloxanide furoate, 500 mg three times daily for 10 days; or aminosidine (paromomycin), 25–35 mg/kg daily in three divided doses for 7–10 days—to eradicate residual amebae in the gut.[195] The development of a vaccine against *E. histolytica* has been hampered in part because natural infection does not result in long-term immunity.

Full references for this chapter can be found at https://ebooks.health.elsevier.com.

87 Vascular Diseases of the Liver

Filipe Gaio Nery, Dominique Charles Valla

IN THIS CHAPTER

Vascular disorders of the liver are characterized by a primary alteration in blood or lymphatic vessels, excluding the vascular changes secondary to parenchymal or biliary diseases. Primary alterations consist of obstruction, fistula, aneurysm, or absence (due to agenesis or disappearance) affecting the large or small vessels (or both). This chapter reviews a heterogeneous group of disorders of the hepatic vasculature as well as liver involvement in cardiovascular disease. Vasculitis involving the liver is discussed in Chapter 35.

BUDD-CHIARI SYNDROME

Budd-Chiari syndrome (BCS) is defined as the obstruction of hepatic veins or terminal inferior vena cava (IVC).[1–3] The term *obliterative hepatocavopathy* has been coined to designate obstruction of the IVC or of the hepatic vein ostia in the IVC and has been suggested to be distinct from BCS[4]; however, this distinction has not been widely accepted. Primary BCS arises from a venous anomaly, whereas secondary BCS arises from an initial lesion outside the veins.

Epidemiology

BCS is a rare disease. In Sweden, the incidence in 1990–2001 was estimated to be 1.4 per million population.[5] In northwest Italy, the incidence of hospitalization for BCS between 2002 and 2012 was estimated to be 2 per million in males and 2.2 per million in females,[6] higher than the estimated incidence of 0.68 per million in a survey conducted in 2010 in France.[7] There is a slight female predominance. The median age at diagnosis was 38 in one case series.[8] In China, the overall incidence and prevalence have been estimated to be 0.88 per million and 7.79 per million population, respectively.[9] The scarcity of publications in this field has been reflected in a meta-analysis that only considered 6 studies on the incidence and prevalence of BCS, revealing a pooled annual incidence of 1 per million and prevalence of 11 per million. Geographic variations in the frequency of BCS, probably reflects differing prevalence of related etiologies.[10] BCS accounted for 17% of hospital admissions for liver-related disease in Kathmandu, Nepal, from 1990 to 1992.[11] In the United States, hospital admissions due to BCS-related complications doubled over a 20-year period, from 1998 to 2017.[12]

Risk factors for BCS consistently identified in Western patients are shown in Table 87.1.[3] In a study from 2009, one risk factor was found in 84% of patients and 2 or more risk factors in 46%. A local risk factor (e.g., venous anomaly) was found in only 5% of patients.[8]

Etiology

The causes of BCS are listed in Box 87.1. Myeloproliferative disorders have accounted for up to 41% of patients with primary BCS,[13] a much higher proportion than in patients with non-splanchnic venous thrombosis (see Chapter 35).[14] In patients with BCS and a myeloproliferative disorder, portal hypertension may lead to normalization of the blood cell counts. A primary deficiency in protein C, protein S, or antithrombin is difficult to establish as a cause of BCS, because these coagulation inhibitors are decreased nonspecifically in liver disease.[3] Several genetic polymorphisms in coagulation or fibrinolysis factors have been associated with an increased risk of BCS, but their clinical relevance is still uncertain.[15]

In Asia, a myeloproliferative disorder, paroxysmal nocturnal hemoglobinuria, and oral contraceptive use, are rarely implicated in BCS,[16–19] whereas hyperhomocysteinemia and the C677T polymorphism of methylenetetrahydrofolate reductase are reported to be common in China.[20] In Nepal, as in China, an unexplained association between obstruction of the terminal IVC and extreme poverty has been shown[11,20]; the overwhelming representation of this cause may lead to lack of recognition of other causes. An average of about 7% of the reported cases of BCS have been associated with pregnancy or the puerperium, with large differences among reports.[21]

TABLE 87.1 Frequencies of Acquired and Inherited Risk Factors for Budd-Chiari Syndrome and Acute Portal Vein Thrombosis in European Cohort Studies

Risk Factor[a]	Budd-Chiari Syndrome (n = 163) 6% With Risk Factor	Acute Portal Vein Thrombosis (n = 102) 28% With Risk Factor
Myeloproliferative neoplasms	39	21
Recent oral contraceptive use	33	44
JAK2 mutation V617F	29	16
Antiphospholipid syndrome	25	8
Systemic disease[b]	23	4
Hyperhomocysteinemia	22	11
Paroxysmal nocturnal hemoglobinuria	19	0
Factor V Leiden mutation	12	3
Local factor[c]	6	21
Recent pregnancy	6	1
Protein C deficiency	4	1
Factor II (prothrombin) mutation G20210A	3	14
Protein S deficiency	3	5
Antithrombin deficiency	3	2
>1 risk factor	46	52

[a]Not all patients were assessed for each risk factor.
[b]Including connective tissue disease, IBD, Behçet disease, and HIV infection.
[c]Acute pancreatitis, intra-abdominal focus of infection, or abdominal trauma.
JAK2, Janus kinase 2.

BOX 87.1 Causes of Budd-Chiari Syndrome

HYPERCOAGULABLE STATES

Antiphospholipid syndrome
Antithrombin deficiency
Factor V Leiden mutation
Methylenetetrahydrofolate reductase C677T polymorphism
Myeloproliferative neoplasm*
Oral contraceptives
Paroxysmal nocturnal hemoglobinuria
Postpartum thrombocytopenic purpura
Pregnancy
Protein C deficiency
Protein S deficiency
Prothrombin gene mutation G20210A
Sickle cell disease

INFECTIONS

Aspergillosis
Filariasis
Hydatid cysts (*Echinococcus granulosus* or *E. multilocularis*)
Liver abscess (amebic or pyogenic)
Pelvic cellulitis
Schistosomiasis
Syphilis
TB

MALIGNANCIES

Adrenal carcinoma
HCC
Leiomyosarcoma
Leukemia
Lung cancer
Myxoma
Renal carcinoma
Rhabdomyosarcoma

MISCELLANEOUS

Behçet disease
Celiac disease
Dacarbazine therapy
IBD
Laparoscopic cholecystectomy
Membranous obstruction of the vena cava
Polycystic liver disease
Sarcoidosis
Trauma to abdomen or thorax

*May be associated with *JAK2* (Janus kinase 2) V617F or calreticulin gene mutation.

Secondary BCS is related to several mechanisms: (1) invasion by a malignant tumor or alveolar echinococcosis; (2) compression by cysts or focal nodular hyperplasia, usually without clinically significant liver disease; (3) compression and inflammation due to polycystic liver disease or liver abscesses; or (4) blunt abdominal or thoracic trauma.[3]

Pathogenesis

A territory corresponding to at least two major hepatic veins needs be obstructed before clinical manifestations of BCS develop.[22] The pattern and speed of the occlusive process varies among the major veins and from patient to patient.[4,22] Following initial thrombosis, a vein may transform into a fibrous cord or undergo wall thickening, a process that affects a variable length of the vein and causes varying degrees of narrowing. Short-length stenosis may simulate a membrane. Often, the occlusion predominates at the ostia of a major hepatic vein into the IVC and the adjacent portion of the IVC.[4] A collateral circulation develops, draining into the neighboring patent intra- and extrahepatic veins. When the IVC is obstructed, collaterals form from the lumbar and azygos veins. Such collaterals, coursing subcutaneously, provide a ready clue to the diagnosis. Restoration of hepatic venous drainage through large collaterals may alleviate all symptoms and signs and carries a good prognosis.[22]

Increased hepatic venous and sinusoidal pressures translate into sinusoidal distention and congestion, predominantly in the centrilobular area of hepatic lobules, and cause ascites formation. Outflow tract obstruction reduces the low-pressure portal venous inflow. Due to stasis and an underlying prothrombotic condition, intra- and extrahepatic portal vein thrombosis (PVT) is common.[23] A decrease in hepatic blood flow causes ischemic coagulative necrosis and apoptosis, predominantly in the central parts of hepatic lobules, leading to liver dysfunction or liver failure.[23] Subsequently, the loss of hepatocytes results in so-called parenchymal extinction, with replacement of liver cells with connective tissue.[23]

Regions of the liver with a preserved blood supply undergo hypertrophy, as is commonly the case for segment I (caudate lobe), for which the venous drainage is preserved because its drainage is independent of the major hepatic veins (see Chapter 73). Areas deprived of portal venous inflow but with enhanced arterial inflow undergo regenerative changes, which can be microscopic (regenerative foci or nodular regenerative hyperplasia) or macroscopic (regenerative macronodules or focal nodular hyperplasia).[23] Fibrosis typically bridges together central areas, eventually leading to venocentric cirrhosis. In a model of partial IVC ligation in mice, the development of fibrosis was related to the sinusoidal deposition of fibrin and stretching of sinusoids, which induced hepatic stellate cell activation.[24] Associated portal venous obstruction also induces portoportal or portovenous fibrosis. Asynchronous involvement of the diverse venous and portal structures explains the considerable variation of one area of the liver from another.[23]

Clinical Features

The spectrum of clinical presentation ranges from a completely asymptomatic disease to ALF to chronic liver disease.[8,25] ALF is, however, rare.[26] Major features include ascites, abdominal pain, and fever. All complications of chronic liver disease may occur, including GI bleeding, bacterial infections, hepatorenal syndrome, and encephalopathy.[8,25] Serum aminotransferase, creatinine, bilirubin, and albumin levels, as well as the prothrombin time, are variably altered.[8,25] A moderate increase in serum alkaline phosphatase levels is common. Blood cell counts are influenced by the underlying cause of BCS. In patients with a myeloproliferative disorder, blood cell counts are usually normal or decreased due to marked hypersplenism.[8,27] The contrast between normal blood cell counts and severe portal hypertension suggests that a myeloproliferative disorder is present. In patients with a Janus kinase 2 (*JAK2*) V617F-positive myeloproliferative disorder and BCS, liver dysfunction is more severe than in those without the polymorphism.[27]

Diagnosis and Natural History

Abdominal imaging with Doppler US, CT, or MRI show variable findings in the hepatic veins and IVC (Fig. 87.1), including (1) lack of visibility, (2) dilatation upstream due to a complete or partial obstruction of the terminal portion, (3) diffuse narrowing and irregularity, and (4) transformation into a cord-like remnant. Collateral veins draining peripheral segments of a venous territory into another vein, either hepatic or extrahepatic, are usual. The size, course, and location of these collaterals are diverse.[22] Additional findings are common (see Fig. 87.1): (1) a combination of liver sectorial atrophy and hypertrophy, including segment I enlargement; (2) ascites, portosystemic collaterals, and enlargement of the spleen; (3) patchy enhancement in the arterial and portal phases, which disappears at the late phase, a pattern indicating decreased portal perfusion due to stasis; and (4) a marked nodular enhancement in the arterial phase with disappearance in the portal and late phases, without washout, corresponding to regenerative macronodules, some of which have a central scar (Fig. 87.2),[23] although some regenerative nodules may show washout.[28]

Because of the variable presentation, the diagnosis of BCS should be suspected in any patient with acute or chronic liver disease, particularly when a cause of BCS is present. The diagnosis is based on direct or indirect evidence of hepatic vein or IVC obstruction.[1–3] The differential diagnosis includes sinusoidal obstruction syndrome (SOS; see later), constrictive pericarditis (see later), and cirrhosis (see Chapter 76). As a rule, the accuracy of Doppler US in showing hepatic venous outflow tract obstruction is excellent and depends mostly on the operator's experience and clinical suspicion. MRI and multiphasic CT are excellent alternatives. MRI is particularly useful for the characterization of hepatic nodules (see Fig. 87.2). Liver biopsy is not required for diagnosis, except in a BCS variant in which large hepatic veins and the IVC are patent and small veins are thrombosed and in patients with a presentation that mimics cirrhosis when the hepatic veins are not visible on imaging. Direct (transhepatic) or retrograde (transjugular) hepatic venography is almost never needed for making the diagnosis, but when combined with venous pressure measurements, venography allows percutaneous therapy (see later). Differentiating benign regenerative macronodules from HCC often requires US-guided liver biopsy.[28] Alpha-fetoprotein may be useful in differentiating benign and malignant liver nodules, with a cutoff value of 15 ng/mL having a positive predictive value for HCC of 100% and a negative predictive value of 91%, together with the size of the largest nodule.[28]

The underlying cause of BCS should be identified to determine prognosis and implement appropriate therapy (see Box 87.1). A recommended evaluation for the underlying cause[1,3] should include a general examination for systemic disease, imaging for secondary BCS, a CBC, assessment for the *JAK2* V617F mutation, and calreticulin gene mutations (in a patient with a spleen height >16 cm, platelet count >200,000/mm^3, and undetectable *JAK2* V617F mutation), flow cytometry of blood cells for paroxysmal nocturnal hemoglobinuria, factor V Leiden and prothrombin G20210A gene mutations, and a lupus anticoagulant and anti-β_2-glycoprotein I antibodies for antiphospholipid syndrome.[3,29] Determination of antithrombin, protein C, and protein S levels is warranted only if the prothrombin level is normal. Bone marrow biopsy should be considered when testing for *JAK2*

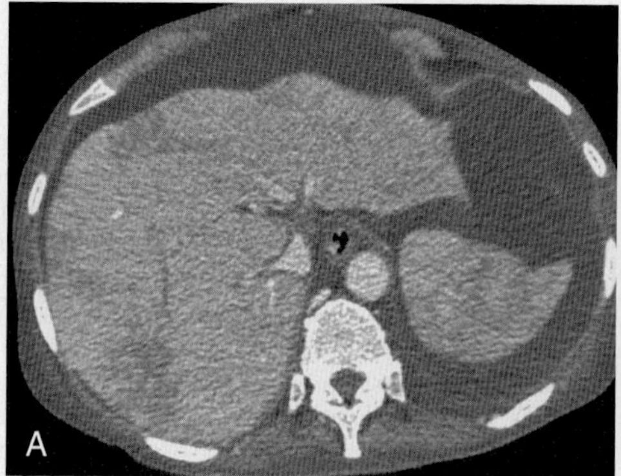

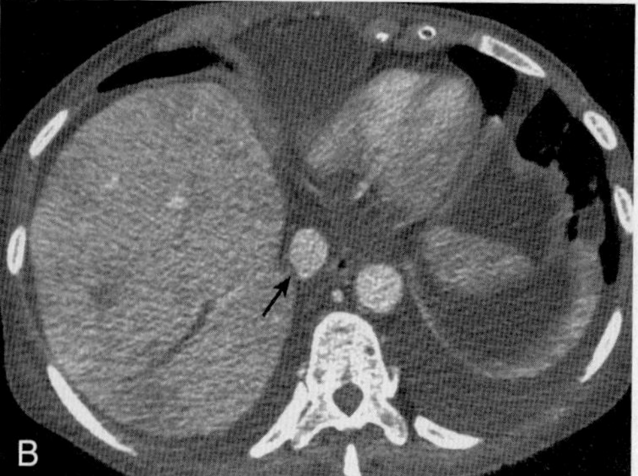

Fig. 87.1 CT in a patient with Budd-Chiari syndrome. The venous phase of vascular enhancement is shown. The liver is dysmorphic (better seen in A) and enhances in an inhomogeneous fashion. Ascites is present. The hepatic veins are visible as slender, unenhanced structures converging toward an enhanced patent inferior vena cava (most prominent in B) (*arrow*).

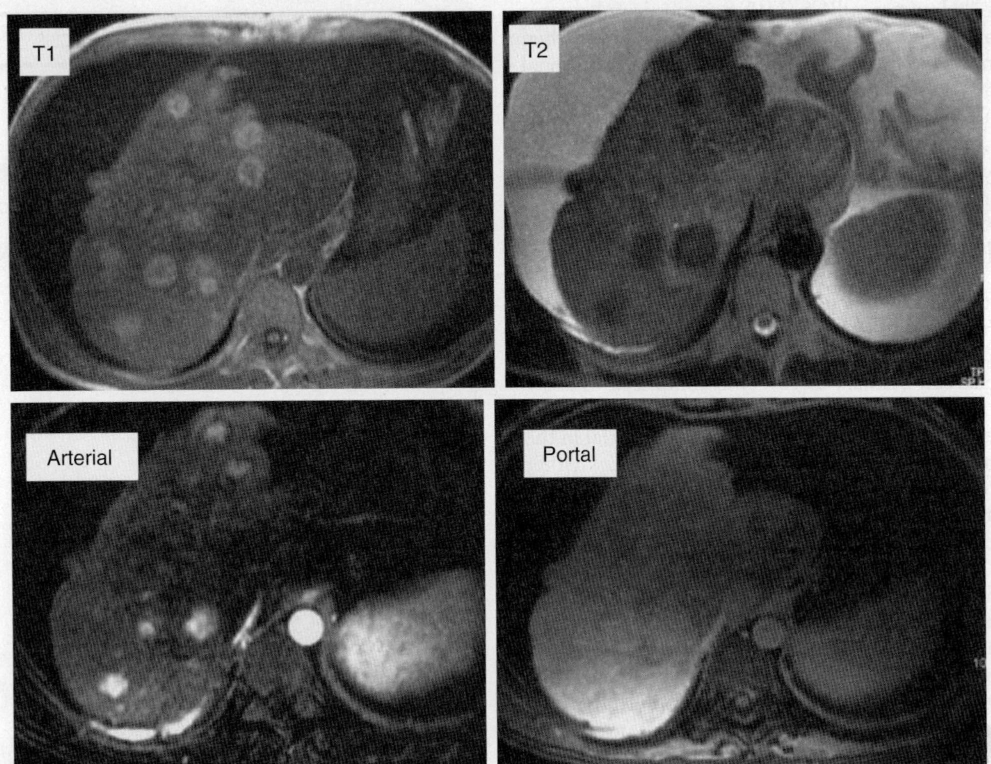

Fig. 87.2 MRI in a patient with Budd-Chiari syndrome. Numerous regenerative macronodules less than 2 cm in diameter are hyperintense in the T1-weighted sequence and hypointense in the T2-weighted sequence. Marked enhancement of the nodules is seen in the arterial phase, with isointensity in the portal venous phase.

V617F and calreticulin gene mutations are negative. Next-generation sequencing may aid in the diagnosis of patients with a negative thrombophilic study, determining high molecular risk variants.[30] Identification of one causative factor should not stop the search for other factors.[3]

The natural history of BCS is not well known in the late phase. Early studies suggested that 90% of the patients would die from liver disease within 3 years of diagnosis. Subsequent data have indicated that patients with asymptomatic disease have an excellent medium- and long-term outcome. Patients with IVC obstruction are at high risk of developing HCC (see Chapter 98).[28]

Treatment

According to a widely accepted treatment algorithm,[1–3] all patients with primary BCS should receive anticoagulation and specific therapy for the underlying disease. The implementation of routine anticoagulation has been accompanied by a marked improvement in outcome.[31] Guidelines for anticoagulation in cases of venous thromboembolism should be followed.[32] Unfractionated heparin should be reserved for patients with creatinine clearance of <30 mL/min and those in whom urgent procedures are expected, as almost one-third of patients may develop heparin-induced thrombocytopenia.[33,34] Patients with manifestations of portal hypertension (ascites, variceal bleeding, and encephalopathy) should receive medical or endoscopic therapy as appropriate, according to standard recommendations for patients with cirrhosis (see Chapters 94 and 96). It is still a matter of debate as to whether asymptomatic patients with a short stenosis of a major hepatic vein or IVC should undergo percutaneous angioplasty. In symptomatic patients, venous lesions amenable to percutaneous angioplasty should be investigated and treated accordingly. When symptoms and signs are not well controlled, or angioplasty is not feasible, a TIPS should be placed, generally through a transcaval approach (see Chapter 94). When the patient does not improve with TIPS, or TIPS proves unfeasible or fails, a surgical portacaval shunt or LT should be considered (see Chapters 94 and 99). Because medical, interventional, and surgical management may prove difficult, patients with BCS should be referred to specialized centers with expertise.[1,3]

Long-term results achieved with this algorithm have been reported.[35] At a median follow-up of 4 years, 20% of the patients had died and 80% were alive; one-fourth had survived on medical therapy, about 5% were alive after percutaneous angioplasty and stenting, about 40% were alive after TIPS, and about 10% were alive after LT. Anticoagulation therapy, given to 85% of patients, was associated with a bleeding rate of 17%. Portal hypertension was the main cause of bleeding, followed by intracranial hemorrhage. The rate of bleeding-related deaths was 2%, similar to that in patients anticoagulated for venous thromboembolism in general. Even though Asian patients with BCS differ from Western patients by the level of obstruction and causal factors, this treatment algorithm has yielded similar results. In India, a response rate of 60.5% was achieved with anticoagulant therapy alone in patients with a Child-Turcotte-Pugh (CTP) score up to nine.[36] In China, percutaneous transluminal angioplasty and stent placement, if appropriate, led to a 73% 10-year survival rate,[37] whereas TIPS placement in a group of 51 patients achieved a 76.9% 3-year survival rate.[38] A 1-year survival rate after TIPS of 94.6% has been found in a meta-analysis of 33 publications.[39]

Prognostic factors include the CTP or MELD scores (see Chapters 94 and 99).[30,34] The Rotterdam score for intervention-free survival and BCS-TIPS prognostic index score for overall survival in patients undergoing TIPS placement have been externally validated in a large European multicenter cohort.[35] These scores are of little utility, however, for guiding management in an individual patient.[40] However, a BCS-TIPS prognostic index score above seven in patients before TIPS placement is of interest when considering the need for liver transplantation.[34] High in-hospital mortality rates (60%) are found in patients with BCS presenting with ALF, but the algorithm can be applied to this group of patients as well.[26] Long-term complications include HCC and consequences of the underlying disease.[1,3,28]

EXTRAHEPATIC PORTAL VEIN OBSTRUCTION

Extrahepatic portal vein obstruction (EHPVO) may or may not extend into the intrahepatic portal veins.[1,41] Secondary EHPVO may be caused by malignant invasion, compression, or encasement of the portal vein. Primary EHPVO is comprised of acute PVT and portal cavernoma. Acute PVT is characterized by the presence of a thrombus, shown on imaging as solid material in the lumen of the portal vein, in the absence of a cavernoma; whether the recent onset of symptoms should be added to these criteria has been debated. The subsequent transformation of an acutely thrombosed portal vein into a portal cavernoma has frequently been referred to as chronic PVT. Portal cavernoma is characterized by the disappearance of the normal portal vein and its replacement by a network of portoportal collaterals. Whether a portal cavernoma is always preceded by thrombosis remains unclear. When a portal cavernoma is found in a child, a congenital malformation should also be considered. Therefore EHPVO is the preferred general designation for all conditions leading to obstruction of the portal vein. The term *chronic PVT* is better reserved for those cases in which the initial stage of acute PVT has been well documented; *portal cavernoma* is otherwise the more appropriate descriptive term.[1,41]

An autopsy study in Sweden estimated the prevalence of EHPVO to be as high as 1.0%.[42] A Swedish study based on hospital discharge diagnoses, however, showed a much lower prevalence (3.7 per 100,000 population),[43] and a recent Italian report was in line with this result, with an incidence of 3.78 and of 1.73 per 100,000 population in males and females, respectively.[44] The difference between these two estimates suggests that EHPVO commonly develops at a late stage of many diseases. Chronic liver disease and abdominal malignancy are each found in about one-third of patients.[42,43]

Acute Portal Vein Thrombosis in the Absence of Cirrhosis

Etiology

According to a prospective study in 2010, one risk factor for venous thrombosis is found in 67% of patients with acute PVT, and two such factors are found in 18%.[45] A local factor (e.g., vascular anomaly or injury) was identified in only 25% of patients. Furthermore, one-third of the patients with a local factor also had a systemic risk factor for thrombosis.[45] Therefore as for primary BCS, acute PVT is usually associated with multiple systemic risk factors, whereas local factors generally are unrecognized; however, they should be pursued. Risk factors for PVT are shown in Table 87.1, and the potential causes are listed in Box 87.2. Unlike BCS, PVT has been associated with similar factors in Western and Asian studies.[3,17,19,27,43,45–47] Myeloproliferative disorders account for 25%–35% of cases.[13] Patients with myeloproliferative disorders and PVT are commonly younger and tend to be women.[48] Calreticulin mutations, which are found more rarely, tend to occur later in life than Jak2 mutations.[49] In contrast to primary BCS, oral contraceptives, paroxysmal nocturnal hemoglobinuria, and factor V Leiden mutation have not been clearly associated with PVT, whereas the prothrombin G20210A gene mutation appears to be particularly frequent.[46] Next-generation sequencing may provide, in the near future, additional information on diagnosis and prognosis in patients with PVT.[30]

BOX 87.2 Causes of Portal Vein Thrombosis

HYPERCOAGULABLE STATES

Antiphospholipid syndrome
Antithrombin deficiency
Factor V Leiden mutation
Methylenetetrahydrofolate reductase C677T polymorphism
Myeloproliferative neoplasm*
Nephrotic syndrome
Oral contraceptives
Paroxysmal nocturnal hemoglobinuria
Pregnancy
Prothrombin gene mutation G20210A
Protein C deficiency
Protein S deficiency
Sickle cell disease

INFECTIONS

Appendicitis
Cholangitis
Cholecystitis
Diverticulitis
Liver abscess (amebic or pyogenic)
Schistosomiasis
Umbilical vein infection

INFLAMMATORY DISEASES

Behçet disease
IBD
Pancreatitis

COMPLICATIONS OF THERAPEUTIC INTERVENTIONS

Alcohol injection
Colectomy
Endoscopic sclerotherapy
Fundoplication
Gastric banding
Hepatic chemoembolization
Hepatobiliary surgery
Islet cell injection
LT
Peritoneal dialysis
Radiofrequency ablation of hepatic tumor(s)
Splenectomy
TIPS procedure
Umbilical vein catheterization

IMPAIRED PORTAL VEIN FLOW

Budd-Chiari syndrome
Cirrhosis
Cholangiocarcinoma
HCC
Nodular regenerative hyperplasia
Pancreatic carcinoma
Sinusoidal obstruction syndrome

MISCELLANEOUS

Central obesity
Bladder cancer
Choledochal cyst
Living at high altitude

*May be associated with *JAK2* (Janus kinase 2) V617F or calreticulin gene mutation.

Pathogenesis

Local factors associated with PVT can be classified into three main categories: (1) inflammatory foci, particularly acute pancreatitis,[50] as well as bacterial cholangitis, appendicitis, and diverticulitis; (2) injury to the portal, splenic, or mesenteric veins (e.g., splenectomy and blunt abdominal trauma); and (3) stasis of blood in the portal venous bed due to cirrhotic or noncirrhotic intrahepatic block.[51] The trigger for the development of PVT usually remains unknown. The thrombotic occlusion is extremely variable in degree (partial or complete) and extent [involving only the portal vein or one of its two branches or the splenic or superior mesenteric vein (or both)]. Independent of the local factor, acute PVT is often associated with a marked systemic inflammatory response syndrome (SIRS). Superinfection with bacteria, however, is uncommon. By contrast, an infected thrombus ab initio is characteristic of septic pylephlebitis. Commonly encountered bacteria include *Bacteroides* spp., *Escherichia coli*, or *Streptococcus* spp.[51,52]

As long as the thrombus does not reach the mesenteric venous arches, the intestine appears to be protected from ischemia.[53] Intestinal ischemia and necrosis, when they develop, may well be related to intense arterial vasoconstriction in response to extensive mesenteric venous thrombosis.[51,53] There is no evidence of ischemic injury to the liver unless the hepatic artery is also obstructed or circulatory shock occurs, in which case a liver infarct develops. Hepatic blood flow is maintained because of increased arterial blood flow and rapid opening of portoportal collaterals that permit blood flow around the obstructed segment of the portal vein.[51] These collaterals can be demonstrated within hours or days of the onset of PVT.

Clinical Features

At the stage of uncomplicated acute PVT, severe abdominal pain is a major feature and is often accompanied by a steady fever. By contrast, physical examination is unremarkable at this stage. A spiking fever with chills suggests septic pylephlebitis. Blood counts may show nonspecific changes, mostly reflecting the SIRS (which may be marked) or the underlying blood disease. Liver biochemical test results usually show no alterations or minor transient changes.

Diagnosis and Natural History

Abdominal imaging usually shows the thrombus as solid material filling the lumen of the portal vein and extending variably into portal vein branches or to the splenic and superior mesenteric veins (Fig. 87.3).[3] Doppler US shows the absence of flow in the portal vein and is preferred to US alone because the thrombus is not always hyperechoic at the early stage. Contrast-enhanced CT is most accurate for disclosing the filling defect in the portal vein lumen. When the thrombus is less than 30 days old, unenhanced images appear as hyperattenuated material. When the thrombus is limited to a branch of the portal vein, there is increased enhancement at the arterial phase in the liver corresponding to the thrombosed branch.[51] Patchy enhancements in the arterial phase "mosaic pattern" may predominate in the peripheral areas of the liver and persist during the portal venous phase, with homogeneous enhancement in the late phase. This pattern reflects portal blood stasis.[51] The collateral vessels that enhance in the portal phase can be demonstrated within days of onset, particularly in the gallbladder wall.[51] MRI, like CT, reveals a luminal filling defect and perfusion changes but may not be available on an emergency basis. A diffusely thickened intestinal wall is usually found in uncomplicated PVT, likely corresponding to congestion induced by intestinal outflow tract

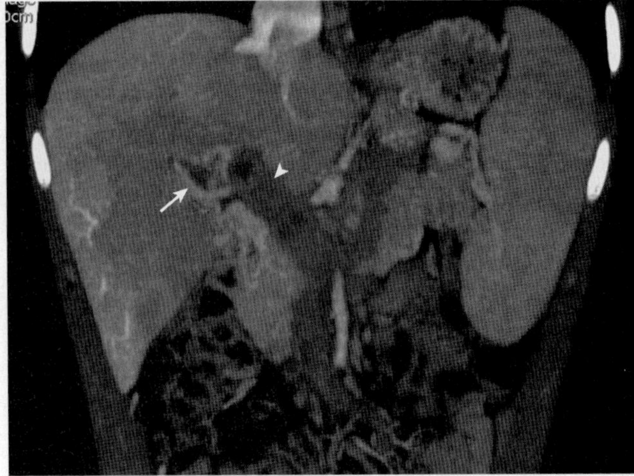

Fig. 87.3 CT in a patient with acute portal vein thrombosis. The portal venous phase is shown and demonstrates vascular enhancement. The portal and mesenteric veins are enlarged and lack enhancement (*arrowhead*). Dilated veins are seen in the porta hepatis, particularly in the gallbladder wall (*arrow*).

obstruction. The intestinal mucosa enhances homogeneously. A small amount of ascites may be detected on imaging in the absence of intestinal ischemia.[45]

The natural history of acute PVT is not known. When noninvasive imaging was not available in the past for the assessment of acute abdominal pain, most cases of acute PVT escaped attention. EHPVO was recognized at the time of a late complication related to portal hypertension.[54] The limited data available show that spontaneous recanalization of the portal vein is unlikely to occur in patients with symptomatic acute PVT.[3,51,55] Whether acute PVT may develop in the absence of symptoms and whether asymptomatic PVT may regress remain unanswered questions.

Intestinal ischemia usually occurs in patients whose pain lasts for several days. The occurrence of ascites or rectal bleeding usually heralds intestinal ischemia. Signs of multiorgan dysfunction, acidosis, or lactic acidemia are major indicators of severe intestinal involvement requiring surgical exploration.[3,51] On abdominal imaging, homogeneous or heterogeneous hypoattenuated or hyperattenuated intestinal wall thickening and intestinal dilatation, abnormal or absent wall enhancement, and mesenteric stranding, as well as ascites, pneumatosis cystoides, and portal venous gas, suggest intestinal ischemia or necrosis.[56] Decreased wall enhancement and dilatation of the lumen have been proposed as criteria for differentiating transmural infarction from nontransmural ischemia.[57] The spontaneous development of ischemic intestinal necrosis appears to be invariably fatal; however, some patients with nontransmural intestinal ischemia may recover spontaneously and are recognized subsequently when presenting with an intestinal stricture.[58] Venous intestinal infarction is a major cause of short bowel syndrome (see Chapters 108 and 120).

Demonstrating solid material in the portal vein lumen is sufficient for establishing a diagnosis of acute PVT, once a malignant cause of portal vein obstruction has been ruled out. Evidence for malignant obstruction includes demonstration of a tumor in the vicinity of the portal vein, enhancement of endoluminal material in the arterial phase, or neoplastic cells on biopsy specimens of the endoluminal material. The enhancement of the gallbladder wall, combined with pain and an SIRS, may suggest an erroneous diagnosis of acute cholecystitis (see Fig. 87.3).

Treatment

Early initiation of anticoagulation is associated with complete and partial recanalization of the portal vein in about 40% and 15% of patients with acute PVT, respectively.[45,55] Extension of thrombosis in the portal venous system is prevented, as are intestinal ischemia and necrosis, with only up to 3% of patients on anticoagulation requiring small bowel resection.[45,55] Complications of anticoagulation therapy appear to be uncommon.[45,54] Even at a later stage of intestinal ischemia, anticoagulation may increase survival.[59,60]

Recanalization of the portal vein is unlikely to occur beyond 6 months of the initiation of anticoagulation, if it has not already been achieved.[45] Splenic or mesenteric veins may continue to recanalize after at least 1 year of anticoagulation.[45] Anticoagulation is recommended for at least 6 months. Extending anticoagulation beyond this period is advocated for patients with an underlying prothrombotic condition, and could be considered out of this context.[34] The extension of the thrombus, and the type of underlying prothrombotic condition, must be taken into account when a decision is made to prolong anticoagulation.[1,3] The recently published RIPORT study showed that for patients without a recognized major risk factor for PVT, anticoagulation could be stopped with D-dimer evaluation at 1 month. If the D-dimer exceeds 500 ng/mL, anticoagulation should be resumed, as thrombosis recurrence risk is high.[61] As with BCS, UFH should only be used in selected patients. Otherwise, anticoagulation shall be started using low-molecular-weight heparin with a switch to vitamin K antagonists or direct-acting oral anticoagulants as long as antiphospholipid syndrome and pregnancy are excluded.[34] Direct-acting oral anticoagulants seem to perform similarly to low-molecular-weight heparin regarding rate of recanalization, with superiority and reduced bleeding complications when compared to vitamin K antagonists,[62] thrombolytic therapy, usually given after anticoagulation has failed, has achieved recanalization rates similar to those for anticoagulation. Rates of adverse events and mortality, however, are particularly high.[55] Therefore the benefit-to-risk ratio of thrombolytic therapy is generally not considered acceptable in patients with acute PVT.[1,3] Indications for surgery for intestinal ischemia are discussed in Chapter 120.

In patients with uncomplicated acute PVT, long-term overall survival is relatively good, whether or not recanalization has occurred.[3,51] The prognosis depends primarily on the underlying disease.[51,63] The presence of ascites (detected on imaging) and splenic vein involvement have been identified as independent predictors of nonrecanalization; no patient with both features has experienced recanalization.[45] In patients with acute intestinal ischemia due to mesenteric venous thrombosis, the overall in-hospital mortality rate has averaged 44%, highlighting the severity of this condition.[64] Intestinal infarction due to venous thrombosis is responsible for short bowel syndrome and a high rate of delayed mortality. Early initiation of anticoagulation therapy is likely critical to preventing this dreaded complication.[45]

Portal Cavernoma

Causes of portal cavernoma (cavernous transformation of the portal vein) and of acute PVT in adults are similar except for a lower proportion of local factors recognized at the stage of portal cavernoma.[54] In adults, therefore, a workup for an underlying cause similar to that for primary BCS is recommended.[1,3] Caution should be taken in interpreting decreased levels of coagulation inhibitors and low levels of anticardiolipin antibodies, because these findings are common and nonspecific in patients with a portal cavernoma.[3,51] In children, prothrombotic conditions are less frequently encountered,[65–68] whereas underlying vascular malformations are common, suggesting that a congenital defect is often a contributing factor, as are prior umbilical cannulation and infection.[67,68] Irrespective of extensive investigation, up to 50% of patients remain without a recognized underlying cause.[69]

A cavernoma does not protect a patient from nor relieve portal hypertension. Portoportal collaterals arise from preexisting veins in the porta hepatis and pancreas. These collaterals can be considerably developed or limited. Collaterals that emanate from the bile duct veins can produce deformity of the bile ducts; a condition termed *portal hypertensive biliopathy* or *portal cholangiopathy*.[70] These biliary changes may rarely be accompanied by evidence of cholestasis. In the absence of preexisting liver disease, liver structure and function remain normal because the cavernoma restores, at least partially, the abolished portal venous inflow to the liver, while hepatic arterial inflow increases.[51] Liver biopsy specimens usually show no abnormalities.[51] In patients with normal liver biochemical test results and normal or near-normal liver biopsy findings, however, a portal cavernoma is associated with atrophy of the peripheral segments of the liver (left liver lobe, segments VI and VII) and hypertrophy of the central segments (segments I and IV) (see Chapter 73), suggesting impaired perfusion of the former.[71] Sinusoidal dilatation of unclear pathogenesis,[72] as well as regenerative hepatocellular changes or minimal portal fibrosis,[73] can be seen on liver biopsy specimens. Plasma levels of coagulation factors and inhibitors are decreased,[74] and these alterations are increased by portosystemic shunting but ameliorated by portal reperfusion.[75] Minimal hepatic encephalopathy is common.[76] Overall, however, the impact of a portal cavernoma on liver function appears to be limited.

Most patients have no symptoms or signs until they present with GI bleeding related to portal hypertension.[63] Otherwise, the diagnosis is usually made fortuitously by finding an enlarged spleen, esophageal varices, or thrombocytopenia. The most conspicuous laboratory findings are related to hypersplenism. Liver biochemical test levels are usually normal or near normal, although plasma levels of coagulation factors and inhibitors can be moderately decreased.[63] Biliary manifestations include pain and cholecystitis related to biliary stones.[77] Mild-to-moderate increases in the serum GGTP and alkaline phosphatase levels are common even in the absence of portal cholangiopathy. Conversely, patients with cholangiopathy often have normal liver biochemical test results. US and CT or MRI, with and without contrast enhancement, show the replacement of the portal vein by a network of convoluted channels (Fig. 87.4).[71,78] Liver findings

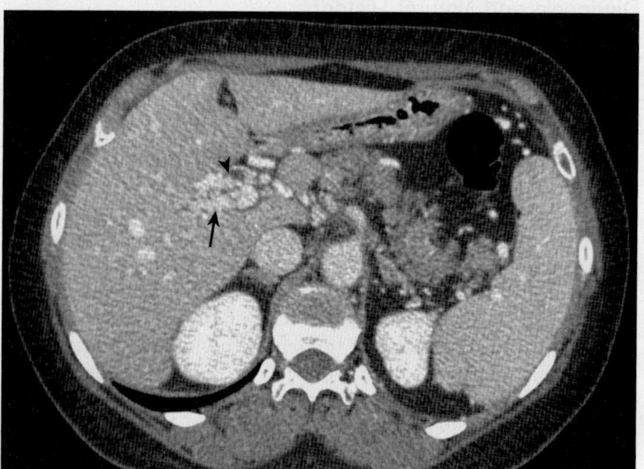

Fig. 87.4 CT in a patient with a portal cavernoma. The portal venous phase with vascular enhancement is shown. The portal vein bifurcation is not visible and is replaced by serpiginous structures that enhance during the portal venous phase and represent the cavernoma (*arrow*). Structures that enhance in the wall of the bile duct correspond to biliary veins (*arrowhead*).

may include atrophy of the periphery and hypertrophy of the central part of the liver and hypervascular nodules in the arterial phase, without washout during the later phases; these findings correspond to benign regenerative nodules.[71,78]

Data on the natural history of portal cavernomas are limited. GI bleeding related to portal hypertension is the most frequent complication, followed by recurrent venous thrombosis, mostly in the portal venous territory.[63] A past history of bleeding and moderate to large esophageal varices are independent risk factors for GI bleeding, and an underlying prothrombotic condition is an independent risk factor for recurrent thrombosis.[63] Ascites and hepatic encephalopathy are uncommon findings.[79] Biliary complications affect about 25% of patients, mostly those with biliary dilatation[77]; however, chronic cholestasis is unusual.

The diagnosis has been made straightforward by modern imaging modalities.[1,3] There are some pitfalls, however, mainly related to an atypical aspect of the cavernoma: some patients have a large portal collateral vein that runs straight in the small omentum and that can be mistaken for a normal portal vein. In rare patients, the appearance is that of a solid mass that causes biliary obstruction. The differential feature is the enhancement of the "pseudotumor" in the portal phase of the study.[80]

The therapeutic challenge is to balance the increased risks of bleeding and thrombosis. Based on limited data, anticoagulation therapy is not associated with an increased risk or severity of GI bleeding, as compared with the absence of anticoagulation therapy.[63] There is circumstantial evidence that anticoagulation therapy effectively prevents recurrent thrombosis.[1,3] Even though the decision regarding long-term anticoagulation must be made on an individual basis, taking into account the prothrombotic potential of the underlying condition and the likelihood of adherence to therapy,[1,3] it should always be considered.[34] Recurrent bleeding related to portal hypertension can be prevented with a nonselective β-adrenergic blocking agent or endoscopic variceal ligation.[81] The feasibility of a surgical portocaval shunt or TIPS is limited, and their long-term patency rates are unknown.[1,3] Yet, when considered, they should be made in experienced centers, since restoration of adequate function is crucial. Portal hypertension can be managed as in patients with cirrhosis (see Chapter 94). When feasible, a meso-Rex shunt has provided excellent results in children, in whom it is the preferred option,[75] but experience in adults is lacking (see Chapter 94).

Mortality in patients with a portal cavernoma is related mostly to the underlying condition, not to the complications of portal hypertension.[3,51] Involvement of the superior mesenteric vein is an independent predictor of a poor long-term outcome.[47,82]

PORTAL VEIN THROMBOSIS IN PATIENTS WITH CIRRHOSIS

PVT in cirrhosis has an increased incidence with increasing severity of liver disease, with a pooled incidence of 10.4% and prevalence of 13.9%.[83] The risk of PVT is independently related to multiple factors: a high MELD or CPT score, a decreased blood flow velocity in the portal vein, large esophageal varices, and, although not consistently found, inherited prothrombotic factors (e.g., prothrombin gene G20210A mutation).[84–87] In contrast to noncirrhotic PVT, the thrombus is usually nonocclusive.[85] These risk factors, particularly those related to an increase in portal hypertension may justify the new findings related to the pathophysiology underlying PVT. It has been found that patients with PVT have an underlying thickened and fibrotic tunica intima, with almost one-half with associated fibrin rich thrombus.[88] Portal cavernoma is uncommon.

The manifestations of PVT must be differentiated from the circumstances that led to its recognition. Many patients have no acute symptoms when PVT is found on routine US. On the other hand, extension to the superior mesenteric vein may induce intestinal ischemia.[87] Nonselective beta-blocker use[89] and pancreatitis or intra-abdominal infection[90] have been related to further progression of PVT, but longitudinal and robust studies are lacking.

PVT in patients with cirrhosis has been associated with a small liver and complications of liver disease.[87,91] A causal role for PVT in these complications, however, is questionable,[91] and the impact of PVT on preliver transplant survival, independent of the severity of liver disease, is minimal or absent.[92] In one-half of patients on the wait list for LT, PVT is recognized only at the time of LT.[93] On the other hand, PVT makes LT more difficult[72] and is associated with decreased posttransplant survival.[93,94]

Differentiating PVT unassociated with HCC from PVT due to malignant invasion is challenging. Features that suggest malignant invasion are a markedly increased diameter of the vein, a contiguous tumor in the liver, endoluminal enhancement in the arterial phase of imaging or arterial signals recorded on Doppler US or contrast-enhanced US, and malignant cells detected on biopsy specimens of the endoluminal material.[3,95]

Two treatment options are available: anticoagulation and TIPS.[85,86,96,97] Controlled clinical trials are lacking, however, and the actual benefit of these two approaches is unclear. In those receiving anticoagulation, there is a threefold greater probability of recanalization, the latter being observed in up to 70% of patients; extension of the thrombus is almost completely prevented; and the risk of bleeding is decreased.[98,99] The type of anticoagulant (low-molecular-weight heparin, an oral vitamin K antagonist, or a direct-acting oral anticoagulant) and the duration of administration to achieve an optimal result remain to be studied.[96,97] Yet, there is increased evidence for efficacy and safety of direct-acting oral anticoagulants. Their use has been shown to be superior to LMWH or oral vitamin K antagonists in achieving complete recanalization,[100] and is now a recommended option in the latest Baveno recommendations.[34] There is evidence for improved recanalization rates with early initiation of anticoagulation therapy.[97] Laboratory targets and the optimal approach to monitoring also remain unclear. TIPS seems to be feasible when intrahepatic portal venous branches are visible on imaging and is followed by recanalization in over 50% of patients in the absence of anticoagulation therapy.[85,86]

A randomized controlled trial in patients with Child-Pugh classes B to C cirrhosis (without PVT) showed that enoxaparin given for 48 weeks was well tolerated, completely prevented the development of PVT, and prevented decompensation and death.[101] These findings lend support to the notion that thrombosis of intrahepatic portal and hepatic venous branches is a determinant of both extrahepatic PVT and decompensation in patients with cirrhosis.[91,102] Confirmation of these findings by other groups is needed before prophylactic anticoagulation in patients with cirrhosis can be recommended.

PORTO-SINUSOIDAL VASCULAR DISORDER

Porto-sinusoidal vascular disorder (PSVD), previously known as idiopathic noncirrhotic portal hypertension, idiopathic portal hypertension, noncirrhotic portal fibrosis or hepatoportal sclerosis, has recently been defined. This entity is associated with a wide spectrum of presentation (with or without portal hypertension). Excluding cirrhosis is a major diagnostic step, as well as documenting particular lesions at histology.[34,103] Well-characterized causes of intrahepatic portal hypertension including schistosomiasis and congenital hepatic fibrosis (see Chapters 64 and 86) and SOS (veno-occlusive disease) (see later), must be ruled out. Yet, PSVD may be present in patients with other causes of liver diseases such as alcohol intake or viral hepatitis. As mentioned above, PSVD overlaps with various entities characterized either by portal hypertension and unusual histopathologic findings (e.g., noncirrhotic portal fibrosis, idiopathic portal hypertension, and hepatoportal sclerosis) or purely by histopathologic features (e.g., obliterative portal venopathy, nodular regenerative hyperplasia, and perisinusoidal fibrosis) in the absence of clinically significant portal hypertension.

Several conditions may be associated with PSVD[103–105]: (1) prolonged exposure to certain drugs and toxins, including purine analogs (e.g., didanosine, azathioprine, and 6-thioguanine) and oxaliplatin; (2) immune disorders, including connective tissue diseases, common variable immunodeficiency, and HIV infection; (3) prothrombotic conditions including antiphospholipid syndrome, and protein C or S deficiency; (4) blood disorders including myeloproliferative disorder, and Hodgkin's lymphoma; (5) infectious diseases such as repeated urinary tract and GI infections; and (6) genetic disorders including Turner syndrome, telomerase disease, Adams-Oliver syndrome, and familial obliterative portal venopathy, the gene for which is located on chromosome 4.[106] The rare familial aggregation also suggests that PSVD may result from a developmental anomaly that could have other genetic bases,[104,105] one of them recently discovered FCHSD1, an uncharacterized gene, that leads to mTOR pathway overactivation.[107]

Liver biopsy specimens may show a variety of lesions.[103,105] A primary alteration may be obstruction of the intrahepatic portal venules, with sinusoidal dilatation, regenerative hepatocellular changes, and perisinusoidal or portal fibrosis as consequences. Alternatively, the primary damage may be to the hepatic sinusoids. It is likely that neither small samples obtained at needle biopsy of the liver nor examination of explanted livers with advanced disease provide sufficient clues to the cause of PSVD.[105] Obliterative portal venopathy is characterized by a complete loss of portal veins in most portal tracts (Fig. 87.5), a marked thickening of the venous wall, replacement of portal venules by numerous small vascular structures, regarded as equivalent to a microscopic cavernoma, and dilated, thin-walled microscopic vessels in an ectopic location in the vicinity of portal tracts.[105,108] Typically, there is little or no lobular or portal inflammation. Slender bridging septa are common and are prominent in the related entity of incomplete septal fibrosis.[104] Frank nodular regenerative hyperplasia is characterized by a widespread distribution of regenerative nodules and atrophic plates of hepatocytes at their periphery (Fig. 87.6). Scattered, less well-defined areas of regenerative changes of hepatocytes are common.[105] It remains to be established that nodular regenerative hyperplasia is always associated with obliterative changes in the portal veins.[108] Calcifications are often seen in extrahepatic portal veins, suggesting a primary disease of the portal venous wall.[109] The frequency of associated extrahepatic PVT is high.[104]

The lesions described constitute a block to intrahepatic portal flow that causes portal hypertension. The hepatic venous pressure gradient (see Chapter 94) is typically normal but may be increased because the site of the block is not always exclusively presinusoidal.[108] As for BCS and EHPVO, an enlarged hepatic artery and regenerative macronodules (focal nodular regenerative hyperplasia-like nodules) are common.[109]

The clinical presentation is similar to that of EHPVO, with pure portal hypertension but without ascites or liver failure. Nevertheless, some patients have come to LT because of advanced liver disease, often with a misdiagnosis of cirrhosis.[104,105] Enlargement of the spleen is often conspicuous. On the other hand, obliterative portal venopathy can be found in patients in whom features of portal hypertension are inconspicuous or lacking.

Laboratory tests usually show a mild to moderate increase in serum aminotransferase, GGTP, and alkaline phosphatase levels. Abnormalities of the serum bilirubin, albumin, and coagulation factor levels are common, but pronounced changes are

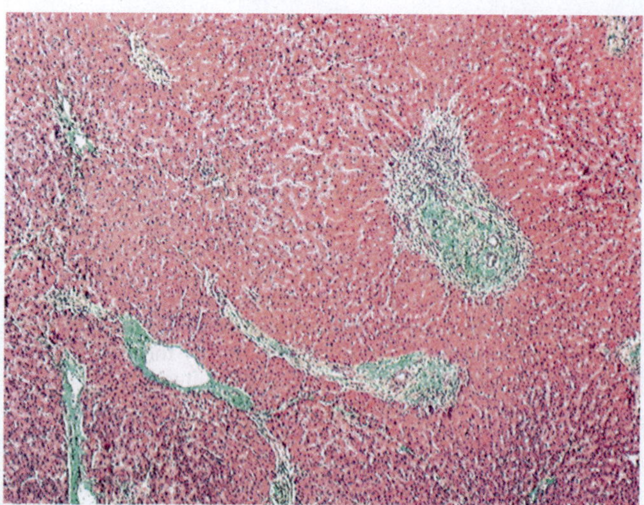

Fig. 87.5 Histopathology of obliterative portal venopathy. Sclerotic portal tracts devoid of patent venules, irregularly distributed in a noncirrhotic parenchyma, are seen (Masson trichrome stain, ×40).

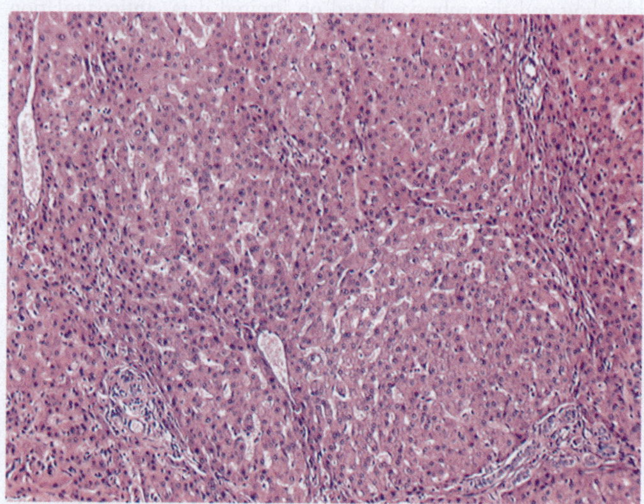

Fig. 87.6 Histopathology of nodular regenerative hyperplasia. Small regenerative nodules within the acini are surrounded by atrophic hepatocytes in a nonfibrous parenchyma (H&E, ×100).

unusual.[104,105,108] Blood counts characteristically show features of marked hypersplenism.

On abdominal imaging, intrahepatic portal tract abnormalities (reduced caliber, occlusive thrombosis, and lack of visibility), focal nodular hyperplasia-like nodules, peripheral parenchymal atrophy with compensatory hypertrophy of central segments are usually found. Atrophy of segment IV and hypertrophy of segment I of the liver are much less common than in patients with cirrhosis. Finally, in MRI with gadoxetic acid enhancement, a periportal hyperintensity in the hepatobiliary phase was found to be specific for PSVD.[110] EHVPO might be found at presentation.[108]

Diagnosis always requires exclusion of cirrhosis, even though common causes of liver diseases may be present (metabolic syndrome, alcohol intake, and viral hepatitis). Patients usually have preserved liver function even in the presence of severe portal hypertension. Liver biopsy is required. An expert pathologist and an adequately sized liver tissue for examination (>20 mm length) are crucial.[103,105] When EHPVO is also present, portal hypertension should not be attributed solely to the infrahepatic block. In the presence of portal hypertension, a low liver stiffness

(<10 kPa) strongly suggests PSVD and, above 20 kPa, the diagnosis becomes unlikely.[111] A plasma metabolic signature may also prove helpful in this regard.[112]

Portal hypertension (manifesting primarily as variceal bleeding) and PVT (a frequent complication) can be managed as in patients with cirrhosis (see earlier and Chapter 94). For patients with severe portal hypertension and normal kidney function, placement of a TIPS may also be an option (see Chapter 94).[113] Treatment of associated conditions is probably of benefit. The rationale for using anticoagulation therapy includes the frequent association with prothrombotic conditions, a high risk of superimposed extrahepatic PVT, anecdotal reports of marked improvement in liver function with therapy, and the extrapolation of data on the prevention of PVT with anticoagulation in patients with cirrhosis.[101] The benefit-to-risk ratio of this approach is unknown, and caution is needed when considering anticoagulation therapy.[104] LT is an option for patients with advanced liver disease, usually with a good outcome.[104] Yet, patients with high bilirubin levels, renal failure or a severe PSVD associated condition must be evaluated for LT with caution, as they have a worse prognosis after LT.[114]

Limited data are available on the outcome and prognosis. Portal hypertension does not appear to be an important cause of mortality.[104] De novo PVT occurs in 20%–40% of patients within 5 years of follow-up; a prothrombotic condition is a risk factor for PVT.[105] The actual impact of PVT on outcome is unknown. Short- and medium-term outcomes appear to be favorable and much better than those in patients with cirrhosis. In the long term, however, advanced liver disease may complicate the course in 10% of patients.[105,108] Baseline prognostic factors are still unknown. The risk of developing HCC is unclear, but it represents a rare indication for LT.[104,114]

SINUSOIDAL OBSTRUCTION SYNDROME (HEPATIC VENO-OCCLUSIVE DISEASE)

SOS is characterized by destruction of sinusoidal endothelial cells predominantly in the central part of the hepatic lobule, with focal obstruction of sinusoidal lumens and resulting congestion.[3,115] In many, but not all, cases, nonthrombotic occlusion of the central hepatic veins is also present (hence the original designation of veno-occlusive disease). In practice, the diagnostic criteria are clinical, rather than histologic, and have therefore produced some confusion (see later).

Etiology

SOS is due almost exclusively to agents that are toxic to both bone marrow progenitor cells and sinusoidal endothelial cells.[3,115] These agents include irradiation of the liver area, chemotherapy, immunosuppressive agents, and plant alkaloids related to pyrrolizidine (see Chapters 34 and 91). The most common settings for SOS are conditioning for hematopoietic cell transplantation (HCT), chemoradiation for abdominal organ malignancy, immunosuppression with thiopurine derivatives, and chemotherapy with oxaliplatin for metastatic colorectal cancer to the liver.[116] Epidemics related to the consumption of flour contaminated with alkaloid-containing plants, as well as sporadic cases related to herbal teas or contaminated herbal remedies, still occur (see Chapter 91).[3,115] Causative agents are transformed in the liver and detoxified by glutathione. Sinusoidal endothelial cells appear to be more sensitive than hepatocytes to the toxic effects of the transformed drugs, possibly related to lower stores of glutathione in sinusoidal endothelial cells.[3,115] Changes similar to SOS have been described in liver transplant recipients in the absence of exposure to azathioprine. Several arguments suggest that endothelialitis related to graft rejection is the cause of this particular entity (see Chapter 99).[117]

In the context of HCT, risk factors for the development of SOS are underlying liver disease (particularly iron overload and viral hepatitis), administration of female sex hormones to prevent uterine bleeding, use of high-intensity regimens (particularly those containing busulfan or cyclophosphamide), and use of gemtuzumab ozogamicin. The frequency of SOS is 20% on average.[3,115]

Pathology

Sinusoidal dilatation and a loss of hepatocytes in the centrilobular area are the two major histopathologic features (Fig. 87.7). Their severity varies greatly from patient to patient.[3,115] Occasionally, sinusoidal congestion is so marked as to mimic peliosis hepatitis (see later). Endothelial damage in the central veins manifests as a rounding of the cells, followed by subendothelial edema and hemorrhage, producing the characteristic eccentric narrowing of the lumen. Central vein damage is more marked in areas where sinusoidal dilatation is more severe. Fibrosis of veins and sinusoids produces varying degrees of occlusion. Characteristically, the periportal area, portal tracts, and portal vessels remain intact.

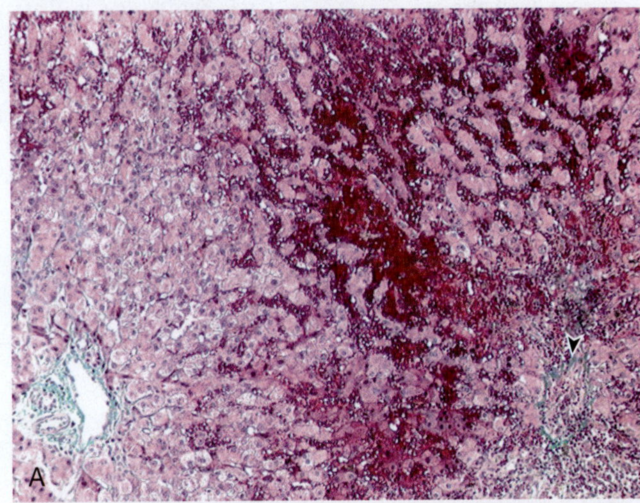

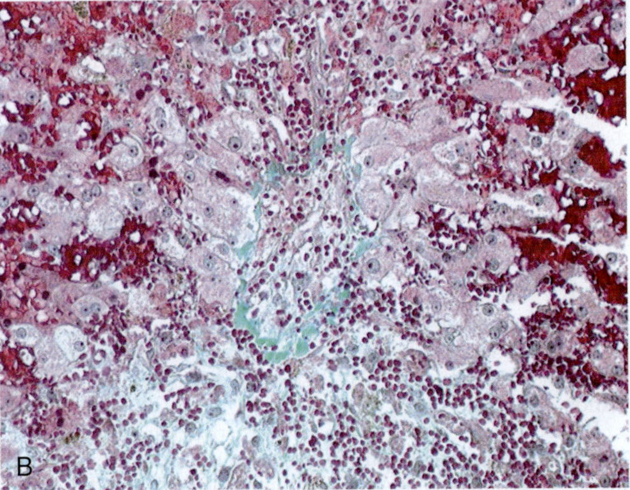

Fig. 87.7 Histopathology of acute sinusoidal obstruction syndrome. (A) Massive centrilobular and mid-lobule congestion with obliteration of a terminal hepatic vein (*arrowhead*) is seen (Masson trichrome stain, ×100). (B) A higher power image shows obliteration of the terminal hepatic vein by subendothelial edema and fine collagen tissue (×250).

Studies in the monocrotaline rat model of SOS have indicated that the earliest lesion occurs in sinusoidal endothelial cells and that repopulation with bone marrow–derived endothelial progenitor cells is instrumental in repairing sinusoidal lesions.[3,115] The acute development of sinusoidal obstruction induces abrupt ischemia, as well as portal hypertension related to a postsinusoidal block.[3,115]

Clinical Features and Diagnosis

Clinical and laboratory manifestations of SOS closely mimic those of BCS, with a range from asymptomatic, to acute with conspicuous ischemic necrosis of the liver, to subacute or chronic with ascites. Liver dysfunction of varying severity is common. On imaging, the liver is enlarged with a mosaic pattern suggestive of altered perfusion similar to that seen in BCS. Gross changes in the flow pattern in the portal and hepatic veins, as well as hepatic arteries, are nonspecific.[3,115] In the setting of HCT, symptoms and signs usually develop within the first 2 months after conditioning, but not more than 100 days after conditioning. Liver biopsy specimens after 100 days may still show features of SOS, albeit in association with another condition (e.g., graft-versus-host disease, viral hepatitis).[3,115] As a rule, the diagnosis of SOS can only be established with liver biopsy, after patency of large hepatic veins and the IVC is shown on imaging. The differential diagnosis of the histopathologic finding includes right-sided heart failure (see later), BCS due to pure small hepatic vein thrombosis, and pure sinusoidal dilatation or peliosis hepatis (see later). In the context of HCT, liver biopsy is difficult to obtain, and clinical diagnostic criteria have been proposed, generally incorporating weight gain or ascites, increased serum bilirubin levels, and the absence of other causes of liver dysfunction, particularly sepsis and graft-versus-host disease.[3,118] The hepatic venous pressure gradient is increased.[3,115] The clinical features are nonspecific, however, and may relate to preexisting liver disease, such as transfusion-related viral hepatitis and iron overload, drug toxicity, hematologic disease, alcohol-associated liver disease, or metabolic syndrome.

Treatment

Treatment options for SOS have been evaluated mainly in the context of HCT. Prevention relies on decreasing the intensity of conditioning regimens.[3,115] Nevertheless, in a retrospective study of prophylactic administration, defibrotide has shown some efficacy to increase SOS free 1-year survival from 28% to 38% in patients undergoing hematopoietic stem cell transplantation, and an increase in 1-year event-free survival, but no improvement of 1-year overall survival.[119] Cost issues regarding the use of defibrotide need to be closely considered. Beyond its benefit in prophylaxis, defibrotide was suggested to increase survival and the rate of complete response in patients with SOS and multiorgan dysfunction, in a phase-3 trial with historical controls.[120] Bevacizumab has been reported to protect against oxaliplatin-related SOS.[116,121] However, this finding is tempered by the observation in an animal model that bevacizumab exacerbated SOS, with overproduction of metalloproteinase 9.[122] A 64% response rate has been reported for a high-dose methylprednisolone administration protocol given as monotherapy.[123]

The occurrence of SOS has a negative impact on overall outcome. Serum bilirubin or aminotransferase elevations are major determinants of immediate prognosis.[118] In HCT recipients, features of SOS have been associated with early mortality rates ranging from 0% to 67%, but the contribution of SOS to mortality is difficult to delineate in these frail patients with multiorgan failure.[3,115] In patients receiving oxaliplatin for metastatic colorectal cancer, the occurrence of SOS increases the incidence of complications after hepatic resection.[121] A favorable benefit-to-risk ratio still exists for preoperative chemotherapy to reduce the size of hepatic metastases but not as adjuvant therapy for resectable metastasis.[121] Patients requiring intensive care, particularly those with increased age and lung and/or renal failure, requiring support, have a higher mortality rate.[124] Long-term sequelae of SOS include pericentral fibrosis, nodular regenerative hyperplasia, and focal nodular hyperplasia.[3,115,125] The latter two appear to be nonspecific consequences of the uneven alterations in intrahepatic perfusion and arterialization.

CONGENITAL PORTOSYSTEMIC SHUNTS

A congenital portosystemic shunt (CPSS) is characterized by a large communication between the portal venous system and the systemic venous circulation in the absence of parenchymal or biliary disease.[3,126,127] This entity has also been referred to as the *Abernethy malformation*, of which two types have been described: type 1 is characterized by the absence of a detectable portal vein (an end-to-side shunt), and type 2 is characterized by a still demonstrable portal vein (side-to-side shunt) (see Chapter 73). The type 2 CPSS is further divided according to the intrahepatic or extrahepatic location of the shunt.[126] The associations that suggest that a type 1 CPSS is a congenital malformation are the female predominance and the frequent occurrence with situs inversus, polysplenia, and congenital heart defects. The etiology of type 2 CPSS is unclear. The prevalence of CPSS has been estimated to be 1 in 30,000.[126] A systematic review was able to find only about 320 reported.[127] A recent multicenter observational study described 66 patients, most asymptomatic at diagnosis, which was established at 21 years of age on average.[128]

Closure of a CPSS is usually followed by reperfusion of the liver with a structure resembling a normal portal vein, thereby suggesting that the term "portal vein agenesis" is inappropriate for characterizing this entity.[126] The clinical expression is related to portosystemic shunting and deprivation of portal blood inflow to the liver. Portosystemic shunting explains why some patients present with hepatic encephalopathy, primary pulmonary arterial hypertension, or hypoxemia due to hepatopulmonary syndrome (see Chapter 96). Portal blood deprivation explains the liver hyperarterialization and regenerative changes, including nodular regenerative hyperplasia and regenerative macronodules, which have been reported as adenomas or focal nodular hyperplasia.[126,127]

Among reported cases of CPSS, one-third have had anomalies related to hyperammonemia or neurologic anomalies. The spectrum of neurologic involvement has ranged from changes in brain imaging and subtle abnormalities on neuropsychological testing to learning disabilities and overt encephalopathy. Such a mode of presentation can occur late in life.[126,127] Liver tumors have accounted for one-fourth of the reported cases. Their characteristics can be typical of benign regenerative macronodules or focal nodular hyperplasia. Completely benign nodules can have a heterogeneous appearance and not remain stable in size or features. Adenomas typically occur at a younger age (median age 18 years old), while HCC are usually diagnosed later (median age 39 years) and almost exclusively in men.[128] Portopulmonary hypertension and hepatopulmonary syndrome occur in a lower proportion of cases.[126,127] Liver dysfunction and ascites are extremely uncommon.

The diagnosis of CPSS is based on their demonstration by abdominal imaging (US, contrast-enhanced CT, or MRI).[3,126] In patients presenting with unexplained brain dysfunction, the demonstration of hyperammonemia or signal intensity of the lesion on MRI is most useful in suggesting portosystemic shunting. The diagnosis of CPSS should be considered in neonates who screen positive for galactosemia. In patients with multiple regenerative macronodules, CPSS should be routinely considered, as should hereditary hemorrhagic telangiectasia (HHT, see later).

Specific treatment for CPSS should be considered in patients with portosystemic encephalopathy, hepatopulmonary syndrome, or portopulmonary hypertension. Shunt closure can be performed with percutaneous interventional radiology techniques or surgically.[126] Even when the portal vein lumen cannot be identified prior to the procedure, portal reperfusion to the liver can be achieved following closure of the shunt.[126] When the preprocedural portal venous pressure is high and the portal vein is not demonstrated, progressive banding of the shunt may be an option. The possibility of closing a shunt should limit the need for LT. In a patient with regenerative macronodules, surgical resection or LT should not be considered unless HCC or marked dysplasia has been demonstrated unequivocally. Moreover, compensatory hypertrophy of the remnant liver following resection may be considerably slower than observed in the absence of a portosystemic shunt.

Outcomes are excellent following closure of a CPSS for encephalopathy, portopulmonary hypertension, or hepatopulmonary syndrome, as well as for large liver nodules, which decrease in size.[126,128] A handful of cases of HCC have been reported in association with CPSS, and monitoring with repeated abdominal imaging is probably warranted.[3,126–128]

ISCHEMIC HEPATITIS

Because *hepatitis* refers to inflammation of the liver, the term *ischemic hepatitis* is a misnomer, because inflammation is typically not present. A more physiologic term would be *hypoxic hepatitis*, because the primary cause of this syndrome is tissue hypoxia, which may be the result of hypoperfusion from cardiac failure or shock of any other etiology, systemic hypoxemia from respiratory failure, or increased oxygen requirements from sepsis.[129] The name *ischemic hepatitis* is used, however, because of clinical similarities to other forms of acute hepatitis and the characteristic pathologic feature of acute centrilobular necrosis. Ischemic hepatitis is probably the most commonly encountered form of vascular liver disease.

Etiology

Of all cases of extreme serum AST elevations (to >3000 U/L), ischemic hepatitis accounts for about half.[130] The most common cause of ischemic hepatitis is cardiovascular disease, which accounts for more than 70% of cases, followed in frequency by respiratory failure and sepsis, each of which accounts for less than 15% of cases.[129] Hypotension is documented as a precipitating factor in more than 50% of patients with ischemic hepatitis but does not need to be evident for ischemic hepatitis to occur. Hypotension often is clinically apparent as a result of acute myocardial infarction, severe heart failure, or sepsis but may be less obvious following a transient arrhythmia or silent coronary ischemic event. Ischemic hepatitis is present in about 2.5% of intensive care unit admissions.[131] The presence of heart failure significantly increases the likelihood that a drop in cardiac output from any cause will result in ischemic hepatitis. More than 80% of cases of ischemic hepatitis occur in the setting of heart failure.[132] Acute trauma, hemorrhage, burns, and heat stroke can also cause ischemic hepatitis, but the likelihood is substantially less in the absence of underlying heart disease.

Clinical Features and Diagnosis

Ischemic hepatitis often is first considered when extreme serum aminotransferase elevations are detected in a patient hospitalized for problems not primarily associated with the liver. Findings on physical examination are usually dominated by the underlying precipitating medical condition. The patient's mental status is often altered because of diminished cerebral perfusion. Laboratory studies show extreme elevations of the aminotransferase levels (>3000 U/L). The serum LDH level is profoundly elevated, often more so than the ALT, and an ALT/LDH ratio of less than 1.5 is more typical of ischemic hepatitis than of viral hepatitis.[133] The prothrombin time may be prolonged by 2 or 3 seconds, and the serum bilirubin level is often mildly increased, with peak levels seen after the aminotransferase levels peak. Serum creatinine and blood urea nitrogen levels are often elevated because of acute tubular necrosis. Characteristically, serum aminotransferase levels peak 1–3 days after the hemodynamic insult and return to normal within 7–10 days.

The differential diagnosis of this type of severe acute injury includes acute hepatitis caused by viral infections, autoimmunity, toxins, and medications (see Chapter 75). Liver biopsy specimens, although usually unnecessary, reveal bland, centrilobular necrosis with preservation of the hepatic architecture (Fig. 87.8). Occasionally, a definitive diagnosis of ischemic hepatitis can be difficult to make, but the typical prompt rise in serum aminotransferase and LDH levels followed by a rapid fall within a few days is more characteristic of ischemic hepatitis than of other causes of severe acute liver injury (Fig. 87.9).[134]

Treatment

Most cases of ischemic hepatitis are transient and self-limited. In the most severely affected patients, ischemic hepatitis is just one manifestation of multiorgan failure and signals a poor prognosis. ALF resulting from ischemic hepatitis is uncommon but is more likely to occur when chronic heart failure or cirrhosis ("acute-on-chronic" liver failure, see Chapter 76) is also present. The overall prognosis depends primarily on the severity of the underlying predisposing condition, not the severity of the liver disease. No specific therapy exists for ischemic hepatitis, and treatment is directed at improving cardiac output and systemic oxygenation. Nevertheless, early hemodynamic restoration is crucial, as only 50% survival rate at discharge is achieved.[131] Also, in patients with cirrhosis admitted with variceal bleeding, *N*-acetylcysteine perfusion over a 72-hour period was shown to decrease the probability of developing ischemic hepatitis, acute kidney injury and death.[135]

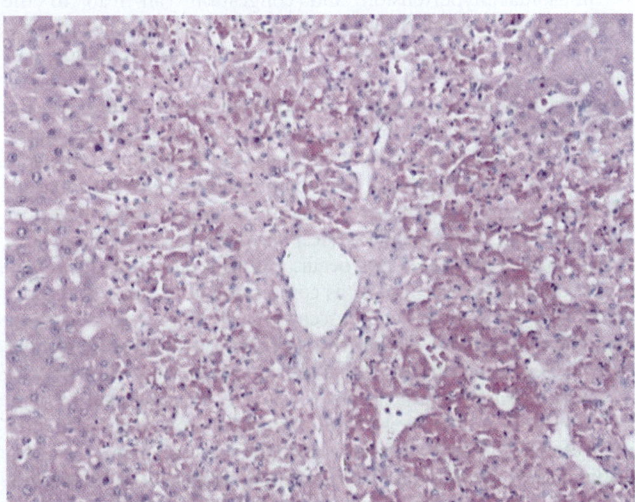

Fig. 87.8 Histopathology of ischemic hepatitis. This low-power photomicrograph demonstrates centrilobular necrosis, loss of hepatocytes, and sinusoidal congestion with red blood cells, but only a scant inflammatory infiltrate. Perivenular fibrosis is evident (H&E). (Courtesy Dr. Pamela Jensen, Dallas, TX.)

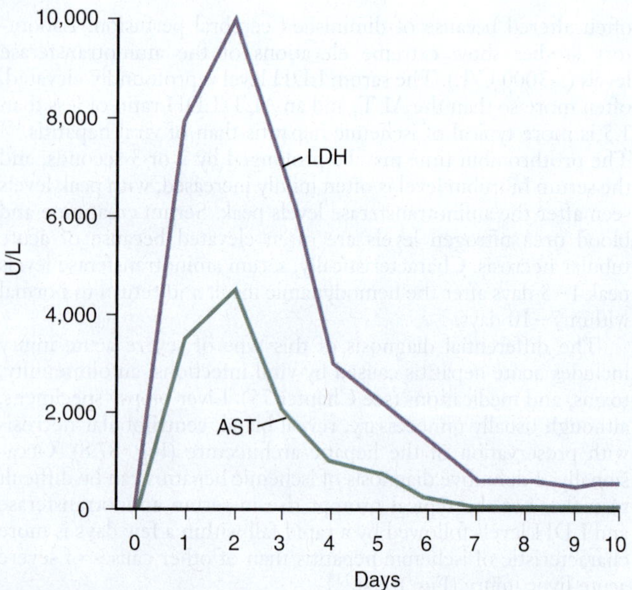

Fig. 87.9 A frequently observed course of serum AST and LDH levels in ischemic hepatitis. (Adapted from Gitlin NG, Serio KM. Ischemic hepatitis: widening horizons. *Am J Gastroenterol*. 1992;7:831–836.)

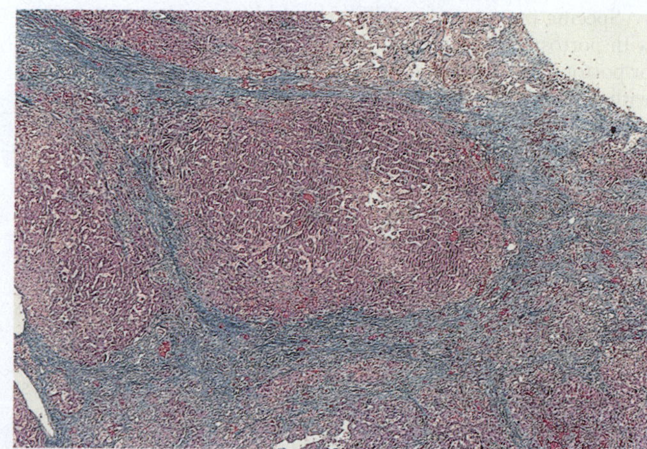

Fig. 87.10 Histopathology of cardiac cirrhosis. This low-power view shows a portal tract in the center of a regenerative nodule and fibrotic bands bridging central veins. The size of the scar and the presence of the nodule attest to the long-term course of the fibrotic process. Even at low power, the bland nature of the cirrhosis is apparent. No inflammatory cells are evident. The sinusoids are dilated and congested (Masson trichrome stain). (Courtesy Dr. Edward Lee, Washington, DC.)

CONGESTIVE HEPATOPATHY

The effects of heart failure on the liver predictably include decreased hepatic blood flow, increased hepatic vein pressure, and decreased arterial oxygen saturation.[136] Right-sided heart failure results in transmission of increased central venous pressure from the heart directly to the hepatic sinusoids. The result is centrilobular congestion and sinusoidal edema that further decrease oxygen delivery. The injurious effects of superimposed ischemic hepatitis are common in these patients (see earlier). The acute and chronic damage results in progressive centrilobular fibrosis. The mechanical force induced by sinusoidal dilatation and the stasis that induces intravascular thrombosis are probably the major determinants explaining fibrosis development.[24]

Sinusoidal hypertension and congestion can lead to the development of ascites, with a characteristically high serum-ascites albumin gradient and a high protein concentration (see Chapter 95).

Clinically, the symptoms and signs of heart failure are the predominant features. Dull RUQ pain in association with hepatomegaly is common. The liver may be pulsatile if tricuspid regurgitation is present, and hepatojugular reflux is often apparent on compression over the liver. Spider telangiectasias and varices are usually not present, and variceal bleeding caused by congestive hepatopathy alone does not occur. Mild elevation of the serum bilirubin level (to <3 mg/dL) is common, and jaundice is seen in fewer than 10% of patients, occurring in those with severe or acute heart failure.[137] The prothrombin time is prolonged in more than 75% of cases and usually is resistant to therapy with vitamin K. Other liver biochemical test levels are often normal or only mildly elevated. Liver test results improve slowly or normalize with effective therapy of the underlying heart failure. Imaging findings are useful when congestive hepatopathy is suspected. Doppler US not only excludes hepatobiliary diseases, but also suggests additional etiologies such as right-sided heart failure or tricuspid insufficiency according to the morphology of the spectral wave of the hepatic veins. CT and MRI are also of interest as the presence of heterogeneous enhancement mainly at the periphery of the liver correlates with parenchymal congestion.[138]

Other typical radiological findings in congestive hepatopathy include hepatomegaly, ascites and dilatation of the IVC and hepatic veins. Liver stiffness has been found to be a surrogate marker of an increased central venous pressure, even better than brain natriuretic peptide, to have a role as a prognostic marker in acute decompensated heart failure, and to monitor decongestion in the same setting.[139] Despite a moderate increase in liver stiffness found in patients with congestive hepatopathy, there is no exact cutoff that can differentiate congestive hepatopathy from liver fibrosis.[140]

The histologic features of congestive hepatopathy include atrophy of hepatocytes, sinusoidal distention, and centrilobular fibrosis. Centrilobular necrosis, consistent with ischemic hepatitis, is frequent in liver biopsy specimens that show congestive hepatopathy and usually correlates with recent hypotension.[141] Bridging fibrosis typically extends between central veins (rather than between portal tracts) to produce a pattern of "reverse lobulation" characteristic of cardiac cirrhosis Fig. 87.10. The distribution of fibrosis throughout the liver is highly variable and correlates with focal sinusoidal thrombosis, with obliteration of central and portal veins that leads in turn to localized ischemia, parenchymal extinction, and fibrosis.[142]

The presence of congestive hepatopathy does not affect the prognosis in patients with heart failure; the mortality rate is determined primarily by the severity of the underlying cardiac disease. Occasionally, paracentesis may be needed to alleviate tense ascites, but therapy is generally directed at improving cardiac disease. Even though HCC incidence seems to be low in congestive hepatopathy, it has been described as high as 13.3% after 30 years of Fontan surgery. Patients evolving to cardiac cirrhosis shall undergo regular screening for HCC, even though treatment options could be limited mainly due to the related cardiac condition.[143]

ISCHEMIC CHOLANGIOPATHY

Ischemic cholangiopathy (IC) is the designation for the biliary changes that result from impaired arterial blood flow.[144] The term *ischemic cholangitis* is also used, although inflammation is not a primary mechanism. Circumstances in which arterial blood supply to the bile ducts is compromised are mostly iatrogenic and include LT, surgery on the liver and bile ducts, arterial chemotherapy, and embolization.[144] The disease may develop in survivors of intensive care for septic shock or trauma.[145] Systemic causes of arterial disease account for a small proportion of cases; polyarteritis nodosa and primary or secondary antiphospholipid syndrome are the most typical examples.[146] Although IC is relatively common in the setting of LT, overall it is a rare condition. Nevertheless, IC occurs more frequently in patients receiving a graft from a donor postcardiac death (DCD), a situation that can be circumvented by administering thrombolytic tissue plasminogen activator in DCD liver transplantation.[147] It has recently been showed that the use of continuous mechanical perfusion of the liver allograft decreases the probability of IC compared to static cold storage but its impact beyond 1 year after liver transplantation is still unclear.[148]

Bile ducts receive blood almost exclusively from arteries, many of which are branches of the common hepatic artery; others (e.g., diaphragmatic branches) penetrate the liver through the capsule, away from porta hepatis. Extensive anastomoses between these arteries open whenever one arterial branch is obstructed, explaining why ligation or embolization of an isolated large artery is generally harmless. The peribiliary arteriolar plexus also acts as a collateral pathway. Ischemia to the bile duct occurs when the collaterals are prevented from providing compensation,[149] as may happen early after LT (due to dissection of the liver) or when the small arterial vessels of the peribiliary plexus are obstructed, as by arteritis, toxic injury from infusion of floxuridine, or embolization with small-sized particles. In HHT, diversion of blood from the peribiliary plexus is thought to cause biliary ischemia (see later). Nonocclusive ischemia to the bile ducts is thought to occur in patients in whom cholangiopathy develops following a stay in the intensive care unit for shock.[144]

The initial stage of IC consists of ischemic necrosis of the biliary mucosa, which leads to biliary cast formation. Subsequently, full-thickness ischemia of the bile duct wall occurs and may result in necrosis with extravasation of bile and formation of collections (bilomas) in the liver parenchyma or porta hepatis. Later, ischemic areas undergo fibrous transformation, resulting in biliary strictures.[144]

Acutely, pain, SIRS, and cholestatic jaundice herald IC. This initial phase, which develops a few days to a few weeks after the ischemic insult, may be unrecognized. Presentation at a later stage is generally with cholestatic features or bacterial cholangitis.[144] Bile duct imaging with MRI or direct cholangiography initially shows finely irregular, dilated bile ducts with filling defects corresponding to the casts. Later, bilomas may develop and may or may not be superinfected. At a late stage, multiple strictures of extra- and intrahepatic ducts mimic those of PSC (see Chapter 70). Strictures are often particularly marked at the termination of right and left bile ducts and proximal portion of the common bile duct.[144]

Diagnosis relies heavily on a setting in which the arterial blood supply to the bile ducts is likely to be impaired and the demonstration of bile duct changes compatible with IC.[144] MR cholangiography is the test of choice for demonstrating biliary casts, bilomas, and biliary strictures. The main differential diagnosis during the initial phase of IC includes biliary stones and abscesses and in the late phase primary or secondary sclerosing cholangitis (see Chapter 70). The diagnosis can be difficult to make when the ischemic insult to the bile ducts escapes attention, as may occur during a stay in an ICU.[145] After LT, monitoring of arterial blood flow with Doppler US is the cornerstone of early diagnosis of hepatic arterial impairment (see Chapter 99).

In the transplant setting, prevention and early correction of impaired arterial blood flow is of utmost importance (see Chapter 99). Early recognition of hepatic arterial impairment allows early correction, either by percutaneous radiologic intervention or surgery. In other settings, the treatment in supportive LT is the only definitive therapy. In the absence of LT, the outcome of diffuse IC is extremely poor.[144] Causes of death are liver failure and sepsis. The outcome of localized ischemic stenosis may be better, except when the main bile duct is involved.

IDIOPATHIC SINUSOIDAL DILATATION AND PELIOSIS HEPATIS

Idiopathic sinusoidal dilatation is characterized by widening of hepatic sinusoidal lumens in the absence of a postsinusoidal block or infiltration of the sinusoids by abnormal cells or substances (Fig. 87.11A).[72,150,151] Peliosis hepatis is similar to idiopathic sinusoidal dilatation and is characterized by a "lake-forming," hemorrhagic dilatation of the sinusoids (see Fig. 87.11B).[152] Peliosis hepatis shares etiologic and clinical features with idiopathic sinusoidal dilation but is less common and more severe.

Conditions reported to be associated with idiopathic sinusoidal dilatation can be separated into the following four categories[72,150,151]: (1) portal venous inflow impairment, including EHVPO, obliterative portal venopathy, CPSS, and sarcoidosis;

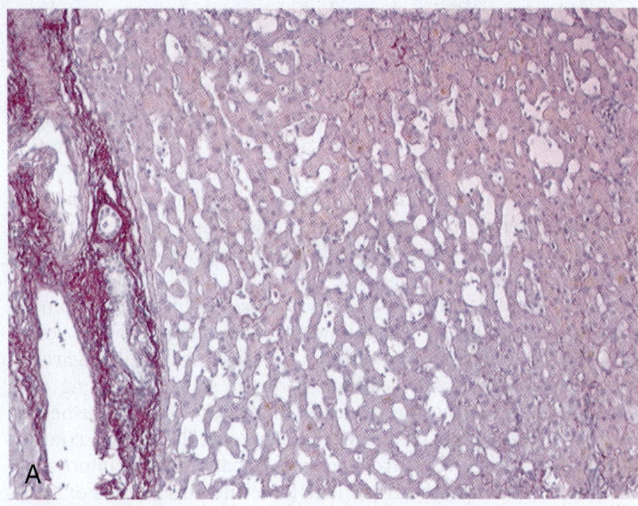

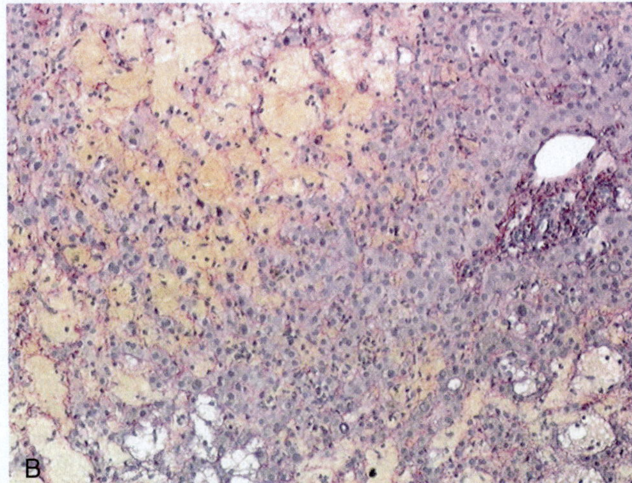

Fig. 87.11 Histopathology of sinusoidal dilatation and peliosis hepatis. (A) Pure noncongestive sinusoidal dilatation with continuous hepatocyte plates and sinusoid walls. (B) Peliosis hepatitis with lobular blood cysts surrounded by interrupted hepatocytes plates and sinusoid walls (Picrosirius-hemalum stain, ×100).

(2) neoplasia, including hepatic metastases, renal cell carcinoma, and Hodgkin disease; (3) nonneoplastic conditions associated with SIRS, including Castleman disease, Crohn disease, RA, Takayasu arteritis, SLE, sarcoidosis, infections with intracellular microbes, acute bacterial pyelonephritis, and *Bartonella henselae* infection; and (4) exposure to certain drugs and toxins, including thiopurines and oxaliplatin. Oral contraceptives have been associated with sinusoidal dilatation, although often in combination with other causative conditions.[150] Overall, the incidence of idiopathic sinusoidal dilatation is low but likely underestimated.

The lumens of the sinusoids are widened and may appear empty or filled with erythrocytes. The endothelial cells have a normal appearance in most cases. The hepatocellular plates bordering the dilated sinusoids are commonly atrophic. Other regions of the liver may demonstrate regenerative hepatocytes or frank nodularity and perisinusoidal fibrosis.[72,150,151] The mechanism underlying sinusoidal dilatation is unknown. A role for interleukin-6 has been suggested but remains unproved.

Clinical manifestations are usually lacking. Whether abdominal pain can be a manifestation of the condition or simply a trigger for the investigation that discloses it is uncertain. Liver biochemical test levels are generally mildly abnormal. Other laboratory features reflect associated conditions.[72,150,151] A particular imaging feature seen on CT or MRI is vague heterogeneity of the liver, particularly in the peripheral subcapsular areas. On the arterial and portal phases, the enhancement follows a mosaic or vaguely nodular pattern. Late-phase images show a homogeneous parenchyma.[153] Imaging findings may be unremarkable.

The mosaic pattern of enhancement following IV injection of a contrast agent appears to be specific for sinusoidal dilatation once other causes of an altered perfusion pattern have been excluded. In contrast-enhanced ultrasonography, a mild heterogeneous arterial hyperenhancement, washout in the very late portal venous phase and a lack of mass effect on B-mode can be seen.[154]

Histologically, peliosis hepatis can be distinguished from sinusoidal dilatation by the following contrasting features: round lake-like blood collections, random locations of the dilated area in the hepatic lobule, and destruction of the sinusoidal lining with erythrocytes found in the space of Disse. SOS is distinguished by the associated lesions of the central veins and the clinical context, although the distinction from peliosis hepatis may be impossible.

There is no specific treatment for either disorder. For sinusoidal dilatation, the outcome of the hepatic disease is excellent, and prognosis is related to any associated condition. For peliosis hepatis, severe complications have occasionally been reported, including portal hypertension, liver failure, liver rupture, and death. Liver transplantation may be indicated as for liver cirrhosis. Peliosis hepatis recurrence after liver transplantation may occur.[155]

HEPATIC ARTERY ANEURYSM AND HEPATIC INFARCTION

A hepatic artery aneurysm (HAA) is characterized by a localized blood-filled balloon-like bulge in the wall of an artery. HAAs are uncommon, but they are the second leading site for visceral artery aneurysms (after splenic artery aneurysms) and account for more than 20% of cases. A true aneurysm is one that involves all three layers of the wall of an artery (intima, media, and adventitia). A majority of true HAAs are isolated, saccular, and extrahepatic lesions involving the full arterial wall. In the past, HAAs were mainly mycotic (infectious) in etiology, but today they typically result from atherosclerosis, mediointimal degeneration, trauma, and, less commonly, infection. Other rare causes of true HAAs are vasculitides (e.g., polyarteritis nodosa, SLE, Takayasu arteritis, and Kawasaki disease) and connective tissue disorders [e.g., Marfan syndrome, Ehlers-Danlos syndrome, and HHT (see later)].[156] Nearly half of HAAs are pseudoaneurysms, or false aneurysms, characterized by blood leaking out of the vessel but confined by the surrounding tissue. Pseudoaneurysms usually result from trauma as a result of a liver biopsy, transhepatic biliary drainage, cholecystectomy, hepatectomy, or LT.[157]

Symptoms of HAA include epigastric or right subchondral pain, but most affected persons are asymptomatic until the aneurysm ruptures. Rarely, a pulsatile RUQ mass or thrill may be detected. Patients may present with rupture into the biliary tract, with hemobilia, epigastric pain, and jaundice; rupture into the portal vein, with portal hypertension and variceal bleeding; or rupture into the peritoneal cavity, with abdominal pain and shock. The mortality rate from rupture of an HAA is more than 30%. Nonatherosclerotic aneurysms and multiple HAAs carry an increased risk of rupture and should be treated. Although the risk of rupture of an aneurysm is independent of its size, atherosclerotic aneurysms greater than 2 cm in diameter should also be treated.[156]

Doppler US studies and CT readily demonstrate HAAs, but angiography is especially useful for defining these lesions, accessing the collateral circulation, and planning treatment. Hepatic artery pseudoaneurysms are treated effectively by angiographic embolization.[157] All symptomatic or vasculopathy- or vasculitis-associated HAA, regardless of their size, must be repaired. For asymptomatic cases, treatment must be considered if >2 cm or annual growth of >0.5 cm. When anatomically feasible and no risk for associated ischemia, an endovascular approach is desirable. Other surgical options must be considered otherwise.[158]

Despite its frequency in the general population, atherosclerosis is rarely a cause of liver disease. Intimal thickening and atherosclerosis in hepatic arteries are less common and occur later in life than is typical for coronary arteries.[159] Hepatic infarction resulting from atherosclerosis alone is rare. The dual blood supply to the liver undoubtedly confers protection from ischemia. Nevertheless, atherosclerosis is the primary cause of approximately one-third of HAAs (see earlier).[160] In addition, because the bile duct derives all its blood supply from the hepatic artery, atherosclerosis can result in IC with biliary strictures and obstruction (see earlier).[161] The presence of atherosclerosis occasionally prevents the use of a donor liver for LT. Atherosclerosis makes arterial anastomoses technically more difficult to secure and may predispose the liver to ischemic injury during transport and reperfusion.

Most cases of *hepatic infarction* result from acute compromise of portal venous flow (see earlier), primarily after LT or hepatobiliary surgery; others result from hepatic artery occlusion or systemic diseases that reduce hepatic artery blood flow. Hepatic artery occlusion can result from atherosclerosis, thrombosis, embolus, PAN, and sickle cell disease. Other causes of hepatic infarction include shock, trauma, a hypercoagulable state, and preeclampsia or other complications of pregnancy. Patients may present with abdominal pain, nausea, vomiting, and elevated serum aminotransferase levels. The infarct may be located peripherally in the liver and appear as a wedge-shaped ill-defined area of hypoechogenicity on US or hypoattenuation on CT or less commonly may be more centrally located and round. An infarct must be distinguished from focal hepatic steatosis, a hepatic abscess, or a neoplasm. Treatment is that of the underlying disease.

HEREDITARY HEMORRHAGIC TELANGIECTASIA (HHT)

HHT, or Osler-Weber-Rendu disease, is a genetic disorder with autosomal-dominant inheritance and is characterized by widespread cutaneous, mucosal, and visceral telangiectasias (see Chapters 21 and 36).[162] HHT is reported to affect 1–2 per 10,000 population. Three major genes cause HHT.[163] Most patients have mutations in the *ENG* gene that encodes endoglin (HHT type 1, HHT1) and *ACVRL1* gene, encoding activin A receptor type II-like 1 (ALK-1) (HHT type 2, HHT2), both of which are involved in the transforming growth factor-β pathway. Mutations in the *SMAD4* gene can cause a rare syndrome that combines juvenile polyposis and HHT. Additional genes have been found on chromosomes 5 and 7.[162] Hepatic vascular malformations (HVMs) are found in 44%−74% of patients with HHT and are more frequent in those with the HHT2 genotype than with the HHT1 genotype.[3] The penetrance increases with age, and the mean age of patients with HVMs is 52 years. Women are more commonly affected than men.[164,165]

The abnormal blood vessels in HHT result in a direct artery-to-vein connection.[161] Vascular malformations affect the liver diffusely, although haphazardly. They encompass a spectrum from microscopic telangiectasias to large arteriovenous shunts.[164,165] Vascular malformations increase in size in about 20% of patients by approximately 4 years.[164] Three types of shunting may occur and coexist[3,164,165]: (1) hepatic artery-to-hepatic vein shunting can induce a decrease in systemic vascular resistance and high cardiac output, eventually evolving to heart failure; (2) hepatic artery-to-portal vein shunting can produce portal hypertension; and (3) portal vein-to-hepatic vein shunting, the rarest form, may lead to hepatic encephalopathy. Shunting of blood may produce IC (see earlier) and mesenteric ischemia.[164,165] There is a marked increase in hepatic arterial blood flow and accordingly in the size of hepatic arteries.[164,165] By causing uneven parenchymal perfusion, shunting of blood and portal venous inflow deprivation are likely responsible for nodular regenerative hyperplasia, regenerative macronodules, and focal nodular hyperplasia that develop in areas with preserved inflow of hyperarterialized blood.[164,165]

High-output heart failure and complications of portal hypertension are the most common manifestations of HVMs. GI bleeding in patients with portal hypertension is more frequently related to intestinal telangiectasias than to ruptured gastroesophageal varices (see Chapter 36).[164] A systolic bruit may be heard in the hepatic area. An acute presentation with severe cholangitis related to IC is uncommon. An exceptional picture of ALF is related to acute ischemic necrosis of large bile ducts (also referred to as "acute disintegration" of the liver).[3] Increased serum alkaline phosphatase and GGTP levels, with a normal serum bilirubin level, are common. These abnormalities are not necessarily associated with large bile duct damage.[164,165]

In patients with HVMs, abdominal imaging usually shows a heterogeneous, enlarged, dysmorphic liver and patchy enhancement during the arterial phase.[164,165] Enhancement of the hepatic veins in the arterial phase indicates severe hepatic artery-to-hepatic vein shunting. The hepatic artery is markedly enlarged. Regenerative macronodules and focal nodular hyperplasia may have a typical massive and homogeneous enhancement during the arterial phase while reaching attenuation similar to that of the surrounding parenchyma during the later phases. Purely benign nodules may occasionally be extremely heterogeneous and even show washout in the late phase.[164,165] Recognizing HHT in patients with hepatic anomalies relies on a comprehensive history and thorough physical examination for telangiectasias. HHT should be considered in patients with multiple focal nodular hyperplasias. Genetic testing is needed to diagnose sporadic cases. Recognizing HVMs in patients with known or suspected HHT is based mostly on indirect evidence of arteriovenous shunting on imaging, with early enhancement of the hepatic veins during the arterial phase and an enlarged hepatic artery. US is the recommended initial examination.[3,164] Liver biopsy, which is hazardous in such patients, is rarely needed once a diagnosis of HHT with liver involvement has been made.[3] The probability that hepatic nodules are benign regenerative nodules or focal nodular hyperplasia is highest in this setting, whereas biliary disease is likely to be IC in HHT-related HVMs.

Asymptomatic patients with HVMs do not require treatment. Management of patients with high-output cardiac failure requires aggressive therapy.[3] In patients with complications of portal hypertension, the guidelines for treatment of patients with cirrhosis may be applied (see Chapter 94).[3] In patients failing to respond to the first-line intensive symptomatic therapy, second-line therapeutic options include bevacizumab therapy,[166] staged embolization, and LT.[3] Of these options, only LT is definitive. Yet, bevacizumab, an antiangiogenic therapy, is currently recommended for the treatment of severe liver arteriovenous shunts, particularly for patients older than 65 years old, for those who are not candidates for LT, or as a bridge to LT.[163] Over 90% of patients with HVMs are asymptomatic. Still, rates of complications and death are 3.6 and 1.1 per 100 person-years, respectively.[164] There is a correlation between a Doppler US-based grading of hepatic involvement and clinical outcome.[164] Cardiac failure and portal hypertension have occurred at a rate of 1.4 and 1.2 per 100 person-years, respectively.[164] Cardiac failure and portal hypertension are each responsible for half of the fatalities related to HVMs.[164] About two-thirds of patients show a complete response to intensive first-line therapy for complicated HVMs and therefore do not need embolization or LT.[164] Survival rates close to 90% have been reported after LT; performance of LT for heart failure achieves better results than for portal hypertension.[167]

DIABETIC HEPATOSCLEROSIS

NASH, Mauriac syndrome, and glycogenic hepatopathy are known liver-related complications of diabetes mellitus.[168] Diabetic hepatosclerosis (DHS) refers to diabetic vascular disease of the liver, with an estimated prevalence of 12%, affecting patients in their fifth−sixth decades, with a longer history of diabetes, need for insulin therapy, and with vascular involvement of other organs, particularly the kidney.[169] The serum alkaline phosphatase level is frequently raised, with otherwise normal or nearly normal aminotransferase levels.[170] No characteristic imaging features have been described. Final diagnosis relies on liver biopsy, with features of perisinusoidal fibrosis and no evidence of steatosis or necroinflammatory activity.[169] Patients with Mauriac syndrome also have severe growth retardation and delayed puberty. It is a form of diabetic microangiopathy that affects the liver in which hyaline thickening of small hepatic artery branches and perisinusoidal basement membrane deposition occurs and is distinct from NASH.[170] DHS appears to be clinically silent and has an unknown prognosis.[168,170]

Full references for this chapter can be found at https://ebooks.health.elsevier.com.

88 Alcohol-Associated Liver Disease

Gyongyi Szabo, Craig J. McClain

IN THIS CHAPTER

Alcohol-associated liver disease (ALD) remains a challenging enigma for basic scientists and clinicians. Despite extensive research and clinical trials since the 1940s, many important facets of this disease have yet to be resolved.[1] Paramount among these important questions are the following: (1) Why does cirrhosis develop in only a small fraction of persons who misuse alcohol? (2) What is the pathogenesis of severe ALD? (3) What are the most effective treatments for patients with ALD, especially those with severe ALD?

EPIDEMIOLOGY

A systematic analysis of the global burden of disease in 2016 evaluated 195 locations around the world and showed that alcohol use was the seventh leading risk factor for both deaths and disability-adjusted life-years.[2] Globally, 32.5% of people between 15 and 95 years of age were current drinkers. Another study found that between 1999 and 2016 in the United States, annual deaths from cirrhosis increased by 65%, and rates of hepatocellular carcinoma (HCC) doubled.[3] Alcohol was a major contributing factor to these events. Mortality trends from chronic liver disease 2007–2016 in the United States also showed that hepatitis C virus (HCV)-related mortality has begun to decline due to the use of direct acting antiviral agents, while ALD continues to increase.[4] During the COVID-19 pandemic, there was a marked increase in social isolation and an increase in alcohol intake. This increased alcohol misuse markedly impacted ALD. For example, in 2020, there was an approximate 20% increase in hospitalizations for ALD.[5,6] Younger patients were disproportionately affected.[5] During COVID, there were also increases in ALD-related mortality and referrals for liver transplantation (LT). In contrast, during the same period, there was a decrease in hospitalization for other GI diseases.[6] In a modeling study, a 1-year increase in alcohol consumption during the COVID-19 pandemic was estimated to result in 8000 additional ALD-related deaths between 2020 and 2040.[7] Patients with alcohol-associated hepatitis (AH) with COVID-19 had an especially ominous prognosis. COVID-19 and AH share several metabolic and biochemical features, including leukocytosis with marked neutrophilia, hypoalbuminemia, elevated serum ferritin levels, and hypercoagulability.[8] Thus there may be overlapping mechanisms of toxicity. Because of the increased risk of mortality, all patients with ALD should take every precaution to avoid COVID infection, including receiving timely vaccination.

Alcohol abuse is the most common etiology of cirrhosis in the developed world. It is the underlying cause of 44% of liver disease deaths in the United States (approximately 13,000 deaths annually), exceeding those for hepatitis C, the second most common fatal liver disease in this country.[9–11] In Europe and the United States combined, ALD and its complications account for approximately 50,000 deaths each year.[12] While addiction and mental disorders have increasingly gained support from medical care and social support systems, it is remarkable that alcohol misuse remains severely stigmatized.[13] Unfortunately, pejorative, stigmatizing language related to individuals with alcohol and substance use disorders can adversely affect treatment seeking, quality of care, and patient outcomes. Therefore several organizations[14–16] have suggested terminology changes as shown in Box 88.1 to do away with pejorative terms such as "alcoholic." In concert with these changes, several societies have collectively changed the terminology related to the spectrum of steatotic-related liver diseases. For example, the correct terminology is "metabolic dysfunction-associated steatohepatitis (MASH)," not "nonalcoholic steatohepatitis (NASH)," as described later.[17]

Several studies have shown that ALD develops in women after a shorter duration of drinking and with a lower daily alcohol intake than in men.[18,19] Population-based surveys have suggested that men usually must drink 40–80 g of alcohol daily and women 20–40 g daily for 10–12 years to experience a significant risk of liver disease.[18–20] The 2020–2025 Dietary Guidelines for Americans (U.S. Department of Health and Human Services and U.S. Department of Agriculture, 2020) put forward the concept of the standard drink and the fact that if alcohol is consumed, it should be in moderation; that is, up to one drink/day for women and two drinks/day for men in adults of legal drinking age (Fig. 88.1). The standard drink contains 14 g of alcohol.[21] People who misuse alcohol frequently consume large amounts of alcohol, which may contribute to the displacement of needed nutrients. Indeed, we and others have reported that patients in alcohol treatment programs or hospitalized with alcohol-asociated hepatitis (AH) may be consuming 1000–20,000 calories/day in "empty calories" (Fig. 88.1). This emphasizes the potential for mechanistic interactions between nutrition and alcohol use disorder (AUD)/ALD. Of interest, in one study in a treatment program, there were no major differences between alcohol intake in subjects hospitalized for severe AH compared to those with or without early liver disease (Fig. 88.1).

SPECTRUM OF DISEASE

Chronic alcohol misuse can result in a spectrum of liver injury that ranges from mild fatty infiltration to steatohepatitis, steatohepatitis with fibrosis, cirrhosis, and HCC (Fig. 88.2).[22–25] Fat accumulation in liver cells, the earliest and most predictable response to alcohol ingestion, is seen in 90%–100% of heavy drinkers.[25,26] Although fatty liver is considered to be a benign condition that reverses quickly with abstinence, cirrhosis can develop within 5 years in 10% of patients who continue to drink heavily.[27] Much more important than steatosis is the development of necroinflammation and fibrosis (AH) that occurs in approximately 10% –35% of heavy drinkers. On liver histology, steatosis, steatohepatitis with or without fibrosis, and alcohol-associated cirrhosis represent the spectrum of ALD. However, it is unclear whether the histological findings always correlate with clinical presentation.[28] For example, on liver biopsy, alcohol-associated steatohepatitis can be present in patients with minimal symptoms (moderate AH) or with severe clinical manifestations of the disease (severe AH). Moderate AH is less often diagnosed because these patients may not seek medical care or only visit emergency departments with nonspecific symptoms of nausea, diarrhea, or fatigue.[29] At this time, there is no specific treatment of moderate AH other than cessation of alcohol use and nutritional counseling. A novel pilot study funded by the NIAAA suggested that treatment with the probiotic, *Lactobacillus* GG, decreased drinking and improved liver disease in moderate AH. This finding supports the potential importance of the microbiome in AUD/ALD, but these results need to be confirmed.[30] AH is an important clinical entity for several reasons: (1) Patients with severe AH have relatively high short-term mortality rates; (2) they also can develop portal hypertension in the absence of cirrhosis; and (3) this entity is a well-documented precursor of cirrhosis, with an elevated long-term risk nine times higher than for patients with fatty liver alone.[27,31] With continued alcohol misuse, a fine mesh-like pattern of fibrosis (micronodular cirrhosis) develops in 8%–20% of heavy drinkers. Over time this lesion can evolve to include broad bands of fibrosis that separate large nodules of liver tissue (macronodular cirrhosis).[24] HCC typically develops in this setting of cirrhosis.[32]

BOX 88.1 New Terminology

Alcohol misuse
Alcohol use disorder (AUD)
Person with AUD
Alcohol-associated liver disease (ALD)
Alcohol-associated hepatitis (AH)

PATHOGENESIS

Ethanol Metabolism and Toxic Metabolites

The liver is the main organ responsible for ethanol metabolism; other organs such as the stomach contribute to much lesser degrees. Ethanol is metabolized by three major systems in the liver:

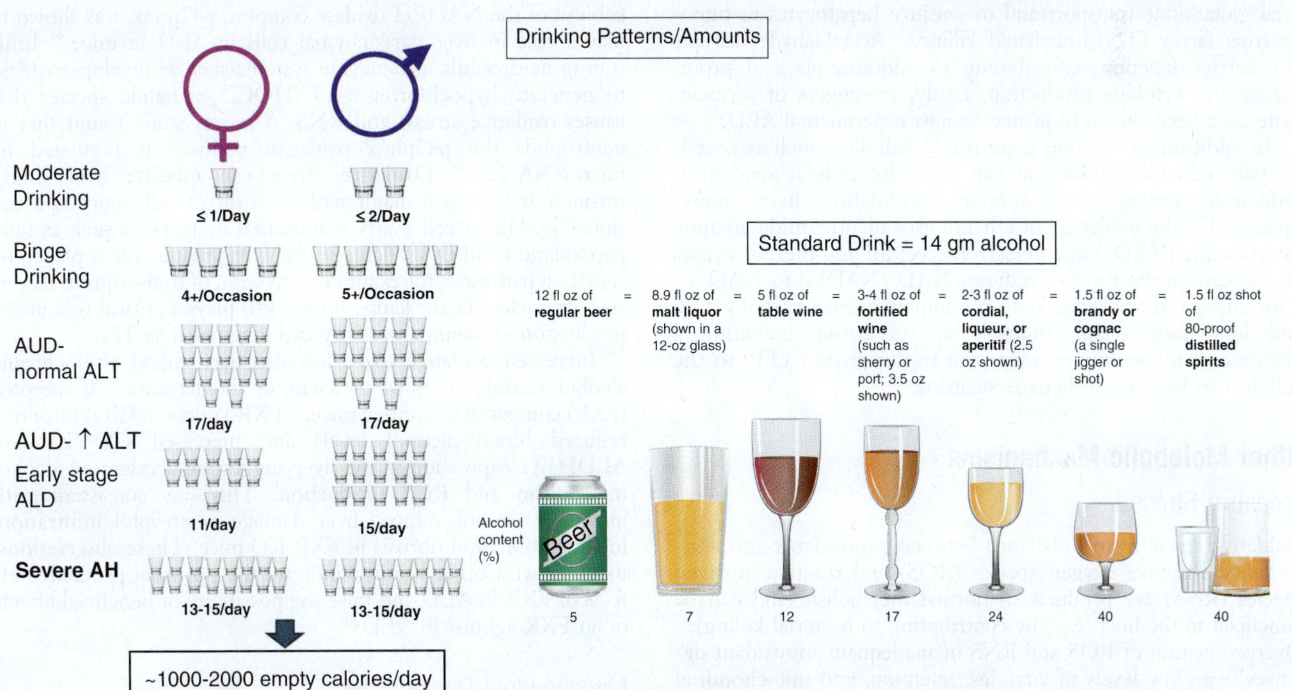

Fig. 88.1 Standard American Drink (from NIAAA) and quantities of alcohol consumed by patients with alcohol use disorder (AUD).

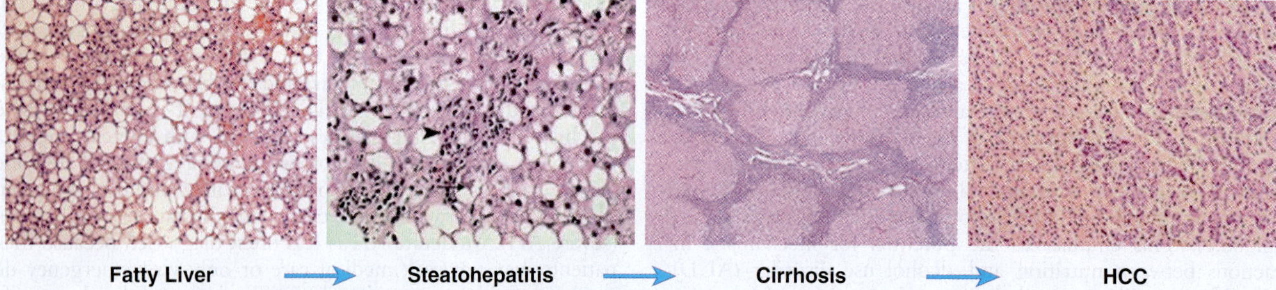

Fig. 88.2 Histologic spectrum of alcohol-associated liver disease.

alcohol dehydrogenase (ADH), cytochrome P450 2E1 (CYP2E1), and, of least importance, catalase.[33] ADH is the primary enzyme system responsible for metabolism of ethanol at low concentrations, whereas CYP2E1 contributes to ethanol metabolism at higher tissue concentrations of ethanol (greater than 10 mM). Furthermore, CYP2E1 activity is upregulated by exposure to ethanol, leading to faster metabolism with chronic excessive alcohol use. Both ADH and CYP2E1 convert ethanol to acetaldehyde, which is then converted to acetate by aldehyde dehydrogenase (ALDH). Acetaldehyde is a highly reactive and potentially toxic compound that is responsible for many of the clinical systemic toxic effects of alcohol, such as nausea, headaches, and flushing.

Acetaldehyde is also postulated to play an etiologic role in ALD by forming adducts with reactive residues on proteins or small molecules (e.g., cysteines). These chemical modifications can alter or interfere with normal biologic processes, exert cellular toxicity, and/or stimulate the host's immune response and cause autoimmune-like manifestations. Antibodies against such oxidatively modified proteins were found in both human and animal models of ALD.[34] An example is the hybrid adduct of malondialdehyde and acetaldehyde, unique to alcohol exposure, which induces an immune reaction in human alcoholics and in animal models.[34] Acetaldehyde also has been shown to impair mitochondrial glutathione transport and to sensitize hepatocytes to tumor necrosis factor (TNF)-mediated killing.[35] Acetaldehyde disrupts gut barrier function, contributing to endotoxemia and proinflammatory cytokine production. Lastly, scavengers of acetaldehyde have been shown to protect against experimental ALD.[36]

In addition to forming cytotoxic metabolites such as acetaldehyde, ethanol metabolism can alter the cellular oxidation-reduction (redox) state, thereby modulating liver injury. Specifically, the oxidation of ethanol uses nicotinamide-adenine dinucleotide (NAD^+) as an electron acceptor and thereby causes an increase in the ratio of reduced NAD (NADH) to NAD^+.[33] This change in the redox state can impair normal carbohydrate and lipid metabolism; multiple effects ensue, including a decrease in the supply of adenosine triphosphate (ATP) to the cell and an increase in hepatic steatosis.

Other Metabolic Mechanisms

Oxidative Stress

Oxidative stress is an imbalance between prooxidants and antioxidants. Reactive oxygen species (ROS) and reactive nitrogen species (RNS) are products of normal metabolism and can be beneficial to the host (e.g., by contributing to bacterial killing).[37] Overproduction of ROS and RNS or inadequate antioxidant defenses (e.g., low levels of vitamins, selenium, and mitochondrial glutathione), or both, can lead to liver injury. Oxidative stress in ALD is usually documented by detection of one of several indirect markers: (1) protein oxidation (e.g., protein thiol or carbonyl products); (2) lipid oxidation (e.g., isoprostanes, malondialdehyde, and cardiolipin oxidation); (3) DNA oxidation (e.g., oxodeoxyguanosine); or (4) depletion or induction of antioxidant defenses (e.g., vitamin E, glutathione, and thioredoxin).[38]

The stimulus for oxidative stress in the liver comes from multiple sources. Alcohol consumption in mice can directly contribute to oxidation of hepatic cardiolipin, facilitating cytochrome *c* release and cellular apoptosis.[39] In hepatocytes, CYP2E1 expression increases after alcohol consumption—in part because of stabilization of messenger RNA (mRNA). The CYP2E1 system leaks electrons to initiate oxidative stress.[37] CYP2E1 is localized in the hepatic lobule in areas of alcohol-induced liver injury. Moreover, overexpression of CYP2E1 in mice and in HepG2 cells (a human hepatoma cell line) in vitro leads to enhanced alcohol hepatotoxicity.[40,41] Nonparenchymal cells and infiltrating inflammatory cells (e.g., polymorphonuclear neutrophils) are another major source of prooxidants that are used for normal cellular processes, such as killing invading organisms. Major enzyme systems for prooxidant production in Kupffer cells and infiltrating monocytes and monocyte-derived macrophages (MoM) in the liver include NAD phosphate oxidase (NADPHox) and inducible nitric oxide synthase (iNOS).[42] Mice deficient in NADPHox or treated with a drug to block NADPH oxidase activity are resistant to ethanol-induced liver injury.[43] A critical subunit of the NADPH oxidase complex, p47phox, was shown to play a role in liver parenchymal cells in ALD in mice.[44] Infiltrating neutrophils use enzyme systems such as myeloperoxidase to generate hypochlorous acid ($HOCl^-$, a halide species that causes oxidative stress) and RNS. A recent study found that in neutrophils the p47phox oxidative pathway is regulated by microRNA-223.[45] Oxidative stress can mediate liver injury through at least two major pathways: direct cell injury and cell signaling. Direct cell injury is indicated by markers such as lipid peroxidation and DNA damage. An even greater role is played by signaling pathways; for example, activation of transcription factors such as nuclear factor kappa B (NF-κB) plays a critical role in the production of proinflammatory cytokines such as TNF.

Increased oxidative stress has also been found after chronic alcohol feeding in mice deficient in the farsenoid X receptor (FXR) compared to control mice.[46] FXR knockout (KO) mice had reduced blood alcohol levels and increased CYP2E1 and ALDH1A1 expression in the liver suggesting accelerated alcohol metabolism and ROS production. This was consistent with increased alcohol-induced liver damage, neutrophil infiltration, inflammation, and fibrosis in FXR KO mice. These observations, together with other reports, indicate the potential protective effects of FXR in ALD and raise the possibility of beneficial effects of an FXR agonist in ALD.[46]

Mitochondrial Dysfunction

Mitochondria are the major consumers of molecular oxygen and major generators of ROS in the liver. Mitochondrial dysfunction is well documented in ALD and contributes to oxidative stress.[47] Mitochondrial abnormalities in ALD include megamitochondria observed on light and electron microscopy and functional mitochondrial abnormalities as documented by an abnormal ^{13}C ketoacid breath test results (ketoacids are metabolized by mitochondria). In ALD, there is a reduction in the amount of mitochondria per hepatocyte that may further compromise energy metabolism.[48] Further, activity of the mitochondrial respiratory chain complexes are significantly reduced in the liver of severe AH patients.[49] Short-term administration of alcohol causes increased hepatic superoxide generation in liver mitochondria, with an increased flow of electrons along the respiratory electron transport chain. The increased NADH/NAD^+ ratio caused by ethanol intake favors superoxide generation.[37] Because hepatic mitochondria lack catalase, glutathione plays a critical role in protecting mitochondria against oxidative stress. Mitochondria do not make glutathione but instead import it from the cytosol. In ALD, the transport of glutathione into mitochondria is impaired, and selective mitochondrial glutathione depletion is observed. Glutathione depletion also sensitizes the liver to the toxic effects of TNF, and TNF also impairs mitochondrial function.

Normal mitochondrial function requires continuous exchange of substrate between the cytosol and the mitochondrial matrix, and this is catalyzed by specific exchangers within the inner mitochondrial membrane. On the other hand, exchange of most water-soluble metabolites between the cytosol and the intermembrane space occurs through the voltage-dependent anion channel (VDAC) in the mitochondrial outer membrane. Alcohol-mediated closure of the VDAC limits free diffusion of metabolites into the intermembrane space and causes mitochondrial dysfunction.[50] This is likely a cause of global alterations in mitochondrial function related to alcohol misuse and ALD. DNA protein kinase activation by alcohol can also contribute to mitochondrial damage, resulting in hepatocellular apoptosis in mice.[39]

Hypoxia

The centrilobular area of the hepatic lobule (the functional unit of the liver) has the lowest oxygen tension and greatest susceptibility to hypoxia. Chronic alcohol intake increases oxygen uptake by the liver and increases the lobular oxygen gradient. A chronic intragastric feeding model in rats has been used to define the mechanisms underlying hepatic hypoxia and the association of these mechanisms with cycling of urinary alcohol levels (UALs).[51] At high UALs, hepatic hypoxia is observed, along with reduced ATP levels; the NADH/NAD^+ ratio is shifted to the reduced state, and hypoxia-inducible factor (HIF) genes are upregulated. When UALs fall, reperfusion injury occurs, resulting in free radical formation and peak liver enzyme release from hepatocytes. Hepatocyte-specific HIF-1α has been shown to be upregulated in alcohol-fed mice and to play a role in hepatic lipid accumulation.[52] The HIF-1α increase in ALD is mediated, in part, by microRNA-122, a negative regulator of HIF-1α.[53] Levels of microRNA-122, the most abundant microRNA in hepatocytes, are increased in the circulation but significantly decreased in the liver in ALD in mice and in humans. The low miR-122 levels in ALD are due to a direct inhibitory effect of alcohol at the transcriptional regulation level of this microRNA.[53] While HIF and HIF-regulated proteins appear to be upregulated in the liver during alcohol feeding, intestinal HIF is markedly downregulated. This appears to play a role in the increased gut permeability with subsequent endotoxemia and liver injury. Indeed, one mechanism of beneficial action for the probiotic *Lactobacillus* GG in experimental ALD appears to be maintaining intestinal HIF.[54,55]

Endoplasmic Reticulum Stress, Impaired Proteasome Function, and Autophagy

Endoplasmic reticulum (ER) stress response is induced by the accumulation of unfolded or misfolded proteins. To deal with the ER stress response, cells activate a series of signaling pathways termed the unfolded protein response (UPR), which can be either protective (usually in the short term) or detrimental (usually in the long term). One of the effects of a prolonged UPR can be increased production of triglycerides and cholesterol, leading to fatty liver. Some potential inducers of the ER stress in ALD include elevated homocysteine levels, acetaldehyde and acrolein adducts, and oxidative stress.[56–58] Moreover, the cascade of ER stress, and activation of the ER-associated molecule, STING, which triggers phosphorylation of interferon regulatory factor 3 (IRF3), has been identified as an important mechanism for alcohol-induced hepatocyte damage. Phosphorylated IRF3 interacts with mitochondrial apoptotic proteins to result in hepatocyte damage, apoptosis and the release of damage associated molecular patterns (DAMPs), such as ATP and uric acid, which then contribute to inflammasome activation.[59]

Of the two major pathways that degrade most cellular proteins in eukaryotic cells, the ubiquitin-proteasome system and autophagy, both are affected in ALD.[60] The 26S ubiquitin-proteasome pathway is the primary proteolytic pathway of eukaryotic cells (see Chapter 74). It controls the levels of numerous proteins involved in gene regulation, cell division, and surface receptor expression, as well as stress response and inflammation. The proteasome system is now considered a cellular defense mechanism because it also removes irregular and damaged proteins generated by mutations, translational errors, or oxidative stress.[61] Animal studies have demonstrated that chronic ethanol feeding results in a significant decrease in proteolytic activity of the proteasome; this decreased activity can lead to abnormal protein accumulation, including accumulation of oxidized proteins.[62] The decrease in proteasome function correlates significantly with the level of hepatic oxidative stress. Hepatocytes from patients with ALD contain large amounts of ubiquitin in the form of cellular inclusions, or Mallory (or Mallory-Denk) bodies, which accumulate because they are not degraded efficiently by the proteasome.[63] When hepatocytes die as a result of proteasome inhibition, they inappropriately release cytokines such as interleukin (IL)-8 and IL-18. IL-8 recruits neutrophils and probably plays a role in neutrophil infiltration in AH, whereas IL-18 sustains inflammation in the liver.[64]

The effects of alcohol on autophagy, a process responsible for degradation of long-lived or aggregated proteins and cellular organelles, are being increasingly recognized. Studies in multiple rodent models indicate that alcohol consumption inhibited multiple key steps in the autophagy process.[65,66]

Alcohol Effects on the Gut Microbiome and the Gut-Liver Axis

It is now generally accepted that the gut flora and gut-derived toxins play a critical role in the development of ALD and its complications (Fig. 88.3).[67] Indeed, more than a half century ago, it was shown that germ-free rodents or rodents treated with antibiotics to "sterilize the gut" were resistant to nutritional and toxin-induced liver injury. Early studies showed that rats fed a choline-deficient diet developed cirrhosis, which could be prevented by oral neomycin.[68] However, when endotoxin was added to the water supply, neomycin no longer prevented the development of liver injury and fibrosis.[68] Subsequently, antibiotics, prebiotics, and probiotics have all been used to prevent experimental alcohol-induced liver injury.[69]

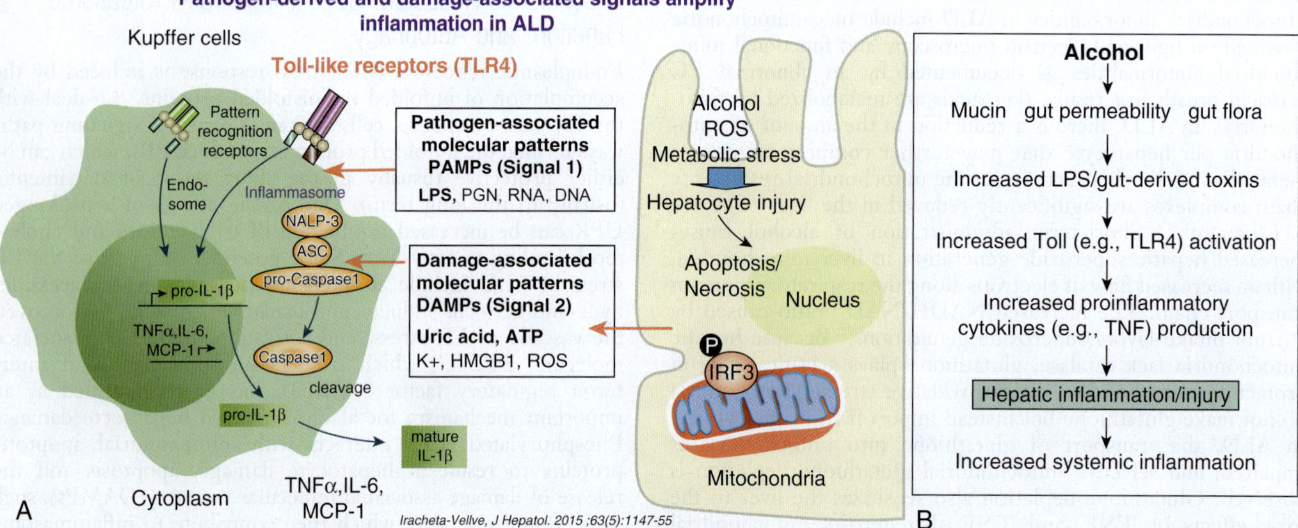

Fig. 88.3 Gut-Liver Axis. (A) Under certain circumstances, gut-derived pathogen-associated molecular patterns (PAMPs), including lipopolysaccharide (LPS), lipopeptides, unmethylated DNA, double-stranded RNA etc., translocate from the gut into the portal vein and to the liver, where they are recognized by specific recognition receptors, the Toll-like receptors (TLRs), resulting in initiation of innate immune response, production of inflammatory mediators, and subsequent liver injury. (B) Alcohol alters gut-barrier function promoting bacteria/LPS translocation, TLR activation, cytokine production, liver injury, and potentially other organ injury. This includes brain inflammation which may stimulate further alcohol consumption.

Alcohol-induced gut barrier dysfunction and endotoxemia are multifactorial events, with altered microflora and impaired intestinal integrity among the causal factors (Fig. 88.3). Recent studies showed that alcohol changes the composition of the bacteria, fungi, and virome in the gut. Alcohol promotes the overgrowth of Gram-negative bacteria in the intestines of patients with chronic alcohol abuse. Studies on gut flora from alcoholics in an inpatient treatment program demonstrated altered microflora composition, with decreased numbers of *bifidobacteria* and *lactobacilli*.[70] A human study found a depletion of *Akkermansia muciniphila* in humans with ALD and showed that replacement of *Akkermansia* can ameliorate alcohol-induced liver disease in mice.[71] Another study found that after a brief 10-day alcohol feeding plus binge, decrease in intestinal *A. muciniphila* was an early change in the gut microbiome related to alcohol.[72] Multiple animal studies have documented altered gut flora with chronic alcohol feeding. Intestinal bacterial overgrowth of both aerobic and anaerobic bacteria after 3 weeks of intragastric alcohol feeding has been demonstrated in an animal model of ALD.[73] Hepatic steatosis and steatohepatitis occurred at a similar time as translocation of live bacteria into the systemic circulation. Importantly, prebiotic therapy attenuated liver injury. In a second study, mice were fed alcohol for 8 weeks.[74] Major changes in gut flora occurred relatively late in the disease process, while changes in gut-barrier function and endotoxemia occurred much earlier. Fecal pH increased in association with altered gut flora, and probiotic therapy for the last 2 weeks effectively treated liver disease (decrease in liver enzymes, reduction in endotoxemia, and correction of intestinal trefoil factor and tight-junction proteins). In both studies, alcohol intake decreased levels of critical gut antimicrobial peptides.

Evidence for alcohol effects on altering the mycobiome, the fungal composition of the gut, has been found both in humans and in mouse models of ALD.[75] In general, alcohol use was associated with a reduction in the diversity of the mycobiome and overgrowth of *Candida*. In humans, increased ASCA antibody levels correlated with poor clinical outcome in patients with alcohol-associated cirrhosis.[75] Finally, emerging evidence suggests that intestinal fungi also contribute to ALD. Alcohol-dependent patients displayed reduced intestinal fungal diversity and overgrowth of *Candida*.[75] Consistent with this, antifungal therapy reduced the alcohol-related intestinal fungal overgrowth and increased serum ß-glucan levels.[75]

The composition of the intestinal virome is also altered by alcohol use,[76] and in experimental models, modulation of the virome with bacteriophage-based therapy offered benefits in ALD.[77]

Alcohol and its metabolite, acetaldehyde, induce intestinal permeability to various macromolecules including LPS in both human subjects and animal models of ALD.[78] Translocation of LPS across the gut epithelial barrier has been attributed to the disruption of intestinal barrier integrity. Indeed, decreased tight junction (ZO-1) protein levels were observed in sigmoid colon biopsies of subjects with AUD compared with healthy controls. This was attributed to an increase in miRNA-212 expression observed in subjects with AUD compared with controls.[79] Alcohol-induced oxidative stress and generation of nitric oxide in the intestines of experimental animals leading to loss of tight junction integrity, gut leakiness, endotoxemia, hepatic inflammation, and liver injury also has been reported.[80] Multiple laboratories have also reported increased intestinal permeability in experimental animal models of ALD due to redistribution and decreased expression of intestinal tight junction proteins.[78] Increased intestinal production of proinflammatory cytokines, such as TNF-α and IL-6, can also contribute to alcohol-induced endotoxemia by altering tight junction morphology and distribution, thereby creating a self-perpetuating vicious cycle that can amplify bacterial translocation.[81]

Similar to its effects in the liver, alcohol induces inflammation in the gut, particularly in the small bowel.[82] A recent study showed that chronic alcohol plus binging in mice results in increased inflammatory cytokine expression in the proximal small intestine and that this correlates with abnormally increased abundance of Paneth cells in this intestinal region.[83] Paneth cells are a major source of antibacterial peptides and therefore likely play a key role in intestinal barrier function and regeneration. Alcohol-induced ER stress and NLRP3 inflammasome activation in Paneth cells resulted in increased IL-18 and IL-17A production; blocking IL-17 could ameliorate these effects and prevent alcohol-induced damage of tight junctions.[82] Interestingly, acute on chronic alcohol was particularly effective at inducing ER stress and NLRP3 inflammasome activation that could be attenuated by a reduction of the intestinal bacterial load via antibiotic treatment.[82]

Altogether, these observations highlight the importance of alcohol-related changes in the gut bacterial, fungal, and viral flora as well as in intestinal barrier function in ALD. Through these mechanisms alcohol use results in translocation of pathogen-associated molecular patterns (PAMP) from the intestine to the liver via the portal circulation where essentially all resident cell types can be activated or primed though sensing PAMPs via their respective pattern recognition receptors such as toll-like receptors (TLRs), NOD-like receptors (NLR), retinoid X receptors (RXRs), and inflammasomes.[84,85]

Immune and Inflammatory Mechanisms

Gut-Liver Axis and Pathogen-Associated Molecular Patterns (PAMPs)

Numerous clinical studies also have demonstrated that plasma endotoxin levels are significantly elevated in patients with different stages of ALD—fatty liver, hepatitis, and cirrhosis—when compared with healthy control subjects. Ethanol-induced endotoxemia observed in experimental rodent models of ALD also provides support for the essential role of LPS in the development of liver injury. Drastic reduction of the gut microbiome with antibiotics in mice resulted in significant attenuation of alcohol-induced inflammation not only in the liver but also in the intestine and in the brain.[86] However, despite prevention of alcohol-induced LPS increases in the circulation and elimination of liver inflammation, alcohol still induced alanine aminotransferase (ALT) elevations in mice, suggesting a direct effect of alcohol in hepatocyte damage.[86]

LPS is a prototype PAMP that represents a strong inflammatory signal for the host through recognition by TLR4, a pattern recognition receptor expressed on immune cells and many other cell types in the liver.[84] With increased gut leakiness, many different PAMPs can translocate to the liver via the portal circulation and contribute to inflammatory cell activation.[87]

Inflammasome Activation and Damage-Associated Molecular Patterns (DAMPs)

Inflammasomes are intracellular multiprotein complexes that sense danger signals from damaged cells and pathogens and assemble to mediate caspase-1 activation that results in proteolytic cleavage of pro-IL-1β and IL-18 into bioactive forms.[85] Inflammasome activation is present in the liver in ALD and the NLRP3 inflammasome seems to play a central role (Fig. 88.3). The levels of DAMPs, including uric acid and ATP, are increased in ALD and inhibition of these sterile danger signals can prevent inflammasome activation in mice.[88] It has been shown that metabolic DAMPs mediate inflammation and crosstalk between damaged hepatocytes and mediate immune cell activation in ALD.[89] Interestingly, inflammasome activation in chronic alcohol use is not limited to the liver, because NLRP3 inflammasome activation and increased IL-1β were also found in the brains of alcohol-fed mice.[90] Inflammasome activation requires two signals in which the first, usually a TLR-mediated signal, induces pro-IL-1β production, and a second, usually DAMP-induced, signal results in inflammasome and capase-1 activation that releases bioactive IL-1β.[91] Secreted IL-1β quickly binds to its receptor, thereby amplifying inflammation, increasing hepatocyte damage and promoting liver fibrosis.[91] Inhibition of IL-1β actions with a recombinant IL-1 receptor antagonist improves ALD in mice and accelerates liver regeneration after chronic alcohol exposure.[92,93] Unfortunately, despite compelling in vitro and animal data, IL-1 inhibition is human AH did not significantly reduce mortality.[94]

A recent study showed that in addition to elevated production of IL-1β and IL-1β release, NLRP3 inflammasome activation in acute AH also results in extracellular release of apoptosis-associated speck-like protein containing a CARD (ASC) by liver monocytes/macrophages and, to a lesser extent, hepatocytes.[95] These extracellular specks can act locally in the liver as well as in the systemic circulation to cleave pro-IL-1β in other cells and thereby amplify IL-1β production even in the absence of alcohol. The cascade of NLRP3-ASC speck-IL-1 activation may contribute to the sustained activation of the inflammatory cascade in acute AH even after a cessation of alcohol intake in patients.[95]

Inflammasome activation can also lead to pyroptosis, a form of cell injury and death.[96] In experimental AH with pyroptosis, it was shown that caspase-11 was upregulated in hepatocytes in AH, and gasdermin D downstream of caspase 11 contributed to pyroptosis.[97] In addition to ATP and uric acid that activate NLRP3, there is experimental evidence for the role of other DAMPs in ALD. For example, high mobility group box-1 (HMGB-1) is highly induced in ALD, whereby hepatocytes were shown to secrete HMGB-1, a normally intracellular and intranuclear protein.[98,99] HMGB-1 is sensed by TLR4 and receptors for advanced glycation end products (RAGE), and its role has been delineated in ALD.[100]

Dysregulated Cytokines

Increased plasma/hepatic concentrations of proinflammatory cytokines (e.g., TNF-α) are consistently observed in rodent models of ALD and are stimulated in large part by gut-derived toxins (Fig. 88.3). TLR-4 activation by endotoxin results in recruitment of the adaptor molecules, MyD88, and Toll/interleukin-1 receptor (TIR) domain–containing adapter inducing interferon-β (TRIF), which each activate separate downstream signaling cascades. Recent data suggest that the MyD88-independent pathway (TRIF) is more important in the development of experimental ALD, whereas MASH appears to signal through the MyD88-dependent pathway.[101]

Dysregulated cytokine metabolism in human ALD has been recognized for over 30 years, with the initial observation that peripheral blood monocytes from patients with AH had significantly increased basal and LPS-stimulated TNF production.[102,103] Serum concentrations of TNF-inducible cytokines and chemokines, such as IL-6, IL-8, IL-18, and monocyte chemoattractant protein-1 (MCP-1), are elevated in patients with AH or cirrhosis, and their levels often correlate with markers of the acute-phase response, reduced liver function, and poor clinical outcomes.[102,104]

This enhanced cytokine response to a physiologic stimulus such as LPS is termed *priming*. Increased serum or urinary levels of neopterin and other markers indicate that monocytes and Kupffer cells are primed in ALD. This priming for LPS-stimulated TNF production has been reproduced in vitro by culturing monocyte cell lines with relevant concentrations of alcohol. This response appears to be mediated, at least in part, by induction of CYP2E1 and oxidative stress.[105] Not only are levels of proinflammatory cytotoxic cytokines increased in ALD, but also monocyte and Kupffer cell production of protective anti-inflammatory cytokines, such as IL-10, is decreased.[106]

Several strategies have been devised to decrease cytokine production or activity in an attempt to block or attenuate liver injury. Examples include antibiotics to modulate intestinal flora and LPS, gadolinium chloride to destroy Kupffer cells, and antioxidants such as glutathione prodrugs to inhibit cytokine production. Each of these strategies has been successful in attenuating alcohol-induced liver injury in rats.[102] Prebiotics, such as oat bran, and probiotics have also been shown to decrease endotoxemia in experimentally induced ALD. Moreover, anti-TNF antibody has been used to prevent liver injury in alcohol-fed rats,[107] and alcohol-related liver injury does not develop in mice that lack the TNF type I receptor.[108] Trials in severe AH with inhibitors of TNF and IL-1 have, unfortunately, not shown benefit. However, some pilot studies of probiotics in early-stage ALD have shown some benefit and need to be confirmed.[40,109]

Neutrophils

On histologic examination, neutrophil infiltration in the liver is a key feature of AH. Neutrophils have pleiotropic functions, as they play a fundamental role in innate immune defense against pathogens but can result in tissue damage when activated.[110] The role of neutrophils in AH is controversial. The neutrophil to lymphocyte ratio has been suggested as a prognostic indicator for poor clinical outcomes in AH.[111] Neutrophils also exhibit activation and increased ROS production with increased susceptibility to infection in AH. Recently, different populations of neutrophils were described in which high density neutrophils showed a highly activated phenotype while a low density neutrophil population in AH displayed a highly exhausted and potentially immune-inhibitory phenotype. It was also shown that in high-density neutrohils alcohol exposure results in neutrophil extracellular trap (NET) release, and surviving neutrophils take on the exhausted low-density neutrophil (LDN) phenotype.[112] The low density neutrophils survive and stay in the liver due to reduced efferocytosis by macrophages in the setting of alcohol exposure; however, the significance of these surviving LDNs remains to be determined. NETs are found in the liver and circulation in mouse as well as in human AH. In vitro experiments showed that even after removal of neutrophils, NETs can activate monocytes to aquire an inflammatory phenotype and directly activate hepatic stellate cells. Furthermore, in a preclinical model, inhibition of NETs with DNAse treatment-attenuated ALD, liver damage and inflammation. These findings suggest that neutrophils play a central role in the inflammation and fibrosis of ALD.

Immune Responses to Altered Hepatocellular Proteins

AH may persist histologically for many months after exposure to ethanol has ceased, suggesting an ongoing immune or autoimmune response. Autoimmune reactions are now well documented in patients with ALD, with autoantibodies directed against phospholipids, ADH, heat shock protein, and other potential antigens. Patients with ALD are at increased risk for the development of immune responses directed at neoantigens generated from the interactions of metabolites of alcohol (e.g., acetaldehyde or hydroxyethyl radicals) with hepatocyte proteins. Some studies also have linked genetic susceptibility and autoimmunity in ALD.[113]

Genetic and Epigenetic Factors

Genetic polymorphisms in alcohol-metabolizing systems such as CYP2E1 and ADH likely play a role in susceptibility to ALD. People with nucleotide substitutions from glutamine to lysine in ALDH have significantly low or absent ALDH activity, leading to acetaldehyde accumulation.[114–118] Cytochrome P450 2E1 is inducible, with its activity increased by 20-fold after alcohol consumption. The C2 variant has higher activity than that of C1, leading to the assumption that it will lead to high levels of acetaldehyde, oxidative stress and liver injury.[119–123] However, none of these polymorphisms explains the spectrum of ALD among different subjects. Polymorphisms in the promoter regions of cytokines TNF and IL-10 also have been reported to predispose affected persons to the development of ALD and are under active study.[124] A sequence variation within the gene coding for patatin-like phospholipase encoding 3 (*PNPLA3*, rs738409) was found to modulate steatosis, necroinflammation, and fibrosis in nonalcoholic fatty liver disease (NAFLD) metabolic dysfunction-associated steatotic liver disease (MASLD) and it is also a genetic risk factor for progressive ALD.[124] A large GWAS study also identified the variants of two genes on chromosome 19—*TM6SF2* and *MBOAT7*—which are significantly associated with alcohol-associated cirrhosis.[125,126]

Epigenetic mechanisms that regulate gene expression primarily involve alterations to the chromatin structure via DNA and histone modifications, without changes to the underlying DNA sequence. In the past decade, it has been clearly demonstrated that alcohol administration to experimental animals results in epigenetic alterations in the liver including posttranslational histone modifications and DNA methylation.[127–129] MECP2 (Methyl-CpG binding protein 2) is a reader that recognizes methyl groups leading to the repression of gene expression and is upregulated in human AH and AC liver tissue.[130] Histone acetylation is a key component in the regulation of gene expression and is associated with enhanced transcriptional activity, whereas deacetylation is typically associated with transcriptional repression. Steady-state levels of acetylation of the core histones result from the balance between the opposing activities of histone acetyltransferases and histone deacetylases (HDACs). Binge EtOH exposure significantly alters mRNA expression of liver Class I, II, and IV HDACs.[131] These data strongly support a major pathogenic role for binge alcohol-induced changes in HDACs as key regulators of the expression of genes that are relevant for hepatic steatosis. Another type of epigenetic effect is through the activity of microRNA (miRNA, small noncoding RNA molecules that regulate gene expression post transcriptionally). Several miRNAs have been linked to both ALD and HCC as either biomarkers or molecular mediators. For example, miRNA-155 has been shown to modulate lipopolysaccharide-induced TNF-α production in Kupffer cells and TNF production in macrophages from patients with ALD.[132] Furthermore, deficiency in miR-155 in a mouse model attenuated alcohol-induced liver steatosis through PPARα and inflammation involving PPARγ regulation. Fibrogenic gene expression was also attenuated in alcohol-fed miR-155 knockout mice compared to controls.[133]

Selected Emerging Mechanisms

Endogenous cannabinoids, which are ubiquitous lipid signaling molecules that mediate their effects through specific cannabinoid receptors, CB1 and CB2, appear to have a role in ALD. Studies have demonstrated that inhibition of CB1 receptors can cause weight loss and attenuate fatty liver and hyperlipidemia in animal models of obesity and steatohepatitis. Moreover, CB1 blockade reduces hepatic fibrosis in a variety of animal models of cirrhosis.[134]

Malnutrition has reemerged as another mechanism of interest. Alterations in micronutrients, such as vitamins A, D, and zinc, as well as macronutrients, such as dietary fat, are increasingly recognized to play a role in the development and progression of ALD.[132] Decreased serum zinc levels, inadequate dietary zinc intake and altered zinc metabolism are well documented in ALD.[135] Zinc plays a critical role in a host of metabolic pathways including functioning of zinc-finger proteins. Oxidative stress can cause zinc to be released from the zinc-finger proteins and cause loss of functional activity. Moreover, a diet rich in omega-6 unsaturated fats markedly enhances, and omega-3 fats protect against, experimental ALD.[136–138] Hypoalbuminemia is a hallmark of end-stage ALD that has long been thought to be due to both malnutrition and reduced liver expression of albumin. More recently, it has been demonstrated that hepatic albumin protein expression is elevated in AH and AC, suggesting that it is being retained in the liver in ALD.[130] Phosphoregulation of albumin is a key regulatory step for its systemic release that is compromised in ALD. Therapies that regulate hepatic albumin release may be potential future treatment for hypoalbuminemia in ALD. Lastly, deficiency of *S*-adenosylmethionine (SAM) is well documented in patients with ALD and in experimental animal models of ALD.[78,139] In models of alcohol-induced hepatotoxicity, SAM has been shown to maintain mitochondrial glutathione levels and to protect against LPS-induced liver injury.[78,139–142] In summary, nutrient modulation may be a way of protecting against or treating ALD as discussed later in this chapter.

Complement activation can regulate the production of ROS and induce oxidative stress in ALD.[143] The role of C1q has been reported in the pathogenesis of alcohol-induced liver injury in mice.[144] In patients with AH, complement factor I and soluble C5b9 have been proposed as diagnostic and prognostic indicators of disease severity and mortality.[145] Given the multifactorial effects of alcohol on many key cellular pathways, it is important to note that the mechanisms identified here likely act together in vivo to culminate in the overall biological effects of alcohol. Furthermore, studies suggest that upon sustained cessation of alcohol exposure/use some of these mechanisms can be reverted. A recent multiomic study in a mouse model of ALD showed that alcohol abstinence restores abnormalities in the liver transcriptome, portal blood metabolome, and gut microbiome.[146]

Extracellular vesicles are membrane coated vesicles that include exosomes (40–150 nm) and microvesicles (200–1000 nm) found in the circulation. In patients with ALD and AH as well as in animal models of ALD, there is an increase in the number of circulating EVs.[147] Exosomes are produced by all cell types in the liver as a result of active sorting mechanisms.[148] Alcohol was shown to regulate exosome production via miR-155-dependent effects on autophagy and lysosomal functions.[66] The cargo of EVs in ALD and AH was also found to be different compared to healthy conrols. Thus circulating exosomes are being exploited for biomarker discovery in ALD and AH. Evidence suggests that exosomes are widely distributed to most organs in the body and serve as means of intercellular or interorgan communication.[149] For example, in ALD, it was shown that alcohol-induced hepatocyte-derived EVs contain miR-122 that can be taken up by macrophages, resulting in their increased susceptibility to LPS stimulation.[150] Alcohol-exposed macrophages also produce exosomes that harbor unique microRNA cargo[148] and can modulate functions of native monocytes and macrophages. Exosome production in hepatocytes and macrophages is linked to cellular autophagy and is at least partially regulated by miR-155.[66] Alcohol-induced disruption of autophagy, a homeostatic mechanism to remove damaged cellular components, is linked to impaired lysosomal function and results in increased exosome release.

Fibrosis

The development of hepatic fibrosis, culminating in cirrhosis, represents a maladaptive wound healing response in ALD. The development of fibrosis is a dynamic state, with constant remodeling of scar tissue[151]; fibrosis may regress with discontinuation of exposure to alcohol. The activated hepatic stellate cell (HSC, myofibroblast) is the major source of collagen production in the liver.[152] It normally exists in a quiescent state and serves as a major depot for vitamin A. With activation, the stellate cell assumes a myofibroblast-like contractile phenotype and produces collagen. The cytokine TGF-β is a major stimulus for stellate cell activation and collagen production. Selected other cytokines implicated in the activation of stellate cells include platelet-derived growth factor and connective tissue growth factor. While the hepatic stellate cell is considered the major origin of myofibroblasts, other resident cells (portal fibroblasts), bone-marrow derived mesenchymal cells, and cells undergoing epithelial-to-mesenchymal transition have been postulated as additional sources of myofibroblasts.[152,153] Importantly, TLR4 signaling plays a major role in stellate cell activation, myofibroblast chemokine secretion, interactions between myofibroblasts and Kupffer cells, and sensitization of myofibroblasts to TGFβ1 signaling.[154]

Macrophages play a critical role in both initiation and progression of fibrosis. Hepatocyte damage and release of DAMPs and chemokines leads to the recruitment of peripheral monocytes to the liver.[152] Kupffer cells and MoM promote HSC activation by secreting cytokines such as TGFβ1, PDGF, TNFα, and IL-1β.[155] MoMs also stimulate HSC migration and recruitment to the liver by releasing chemokines like osteopontin.[156] Additionally, disruption in gut permeability and dysbiosis in ALD lead to increased levels of bacteria and bacterial products in the liver, which results in activation of liver macrophages and fibrosis.[157] A recent report elegantly demonstrated that alcohol-induced NETs present in the liver in AH can directly activate HSCs to become fibrogenic.[157a]. Together, these findings suggest that multiple direct and indirect mechanisms lead to fibrogenic HSC activation in ALD and AH.

Oxidative stress also plays a major role in stellate cell activation,[158] and a variety of antioxidants can block both HSC activation and collagen production in vitro. Serum levels of 4-hydroxy-nonenal, a specific product of lipid peroxidation, are elevated in patients with ALD and upregulate both procollagen type I and tissue inhibitor of metalloproteinase-1 (TIMP-1) gene expression. Matrix metalloproteinase-1 plays a major role in degrading type I collagen. TIMP-1 levels also are elevated in ALD. The result appears to be an increase in HSC activation and collagen production on the one hand and a decrease in matrix degradation on the other hand.[159–161]

The main ECM (extracellular matrix) protein associated with fibrosis is collagen type I, but several other important ECM proteins also accumulate, including fibrin(ogen). The liver is the major organ regulating the fibrin coagulation system. Fibrin metabolism is regulated via two pathways, coagulation and fibrinolysis.[33] Inhibition of fibrinolysis by plasminogen activator inhibitor-1 can cause fibrin ECM to accumulate, even in the absence of enhanced fibrin deposition by the thrombin cascade. Hepatic injury in models of liver disease often involves dysregulation of the coagulation cascade/fibrinolysis, resulting in the formation of fibrin clots in the hepatic sinusoids.[33] Fibrin clots block blood flow within the hepatic parenchyma (i.e., hemostasis), causing microregional hypoxia and subsequent hepatocellular death.[33] In summary, important crosstalk between cell types (e.g., HSC and Kupffer cells) and major metabolic pathways (e.g., wound healing, clotting, and innate immunity) play a critical role in both early and late stages of fibrosis.

DIAGNOSIS OF ALCOHOL MISUSE

Alcohol misuse should be suspected if there is a history of heavy alcohol intake, other organ system damage is present, or a history of an excessive frequency of falls, lacerations, or fractures. Only 10% of patients with drinking problems are identified by primary care providers.[162] Owing to delays in diagnosis and treatment, many patients have cirrhosis by the time they are referred to a gastroenterologist.[163] Underdiagnosis is common in teenagers and older patients and is of particular concern in women of child-bearing age.[164,165] The first step to ensure more timely diagnoses of alcohol misuse is the uniform application of screening tools in various practice settings. Three such tools are now in common use: the 10-item AUDIT (*A*lcohol *U*se *D*isorders *I*dentification

Test), the 3-item AUDIT-C consumption questionnaire, and the four-item CAGE questionnaire.[166,167] An alternative approach is the use of a single question: "How many times in the past year have you had *x* or more drinks a day?" ($x = 5$ for men; 4 for women) to identify individuals with risky drinking.[166] Specific tools also have been developed for use in pregnant women.[165] Regardless of which instrument is chosen, it is important that physicians incorporate systematic screening into their practices.[168]

There is ongoing interest in developing laboratory tests that can reliably identify patients with problem drinking, particularly those suspected of drinking who deny alcohol use. Blood or breath alcohol measurements are the most sensitive and specific indicators of recent alcohol use, particularly among binge drinkers.[169] The major limitation of these tests is the short half-life of ethanol in blood, urine, and breath. As a result, recent efforts have focused on developing biomarkers of alcohol misuse that are detectable over longer periods of time. An early recognized biomarker is the carbohydrate-deficient transferrin (CDT).[170] Even higher sensitivity and specificity for alcohol abuse has been reported by combining CDT with mean corpuscular erythrocyte volume and serum gamma glutamyl transpeptidase levels.[171] Measurement of alcohol metabolites, phosphatidylethanol (PEth), ethyl glucuronide, and ethyl sulfate, also shows promise in detecting recent alcohol use.[172–174] The PEth is used in a variety of clinical situations ranging from the ICU to the posttranplant setting to diagnose recent alcohol misuse.[175] It reflects alcohol intake over time, and it is commercially available.[174,176] An innovative new approach undergoing research is the development of transdermal sensors/wearable devices to continuously monitor alcohol use.[174,176,177]

DIAGNOSIS OF ALCOHOL-ASSOCIATED LIVER DISEASE

The clinical diagnosis of ALD and AH can be accurate, and liver biopsy is not generally performed in the United States.[28] A consensus report from the National Institute on Alcoholism and Alcohol Abuse defined the clinical diagnosis of acute AH.[178] This working definition of AH includes the onset of jaundice within 60 days of heavy consumption (>50 g/day) of alcohol for a minimum of 6 months, a serum bilirubin >3 mg/dL, an elevated AST (50–400 U/L), an AST:ALT ratio >1.5, and no other obvious cause for hepatitis.[178] Patients with a MELD >21 were considered to have severe AH and those with MELD <21 had moderate AH. This consensus statement proposed classifying patients with AH as definite when a liver biopsy was used to establish the diagnosis; probable when the clinical and laboratory features were present without potential confounding factors; and possible when confounding factors were present.

History

Most patients with fatty liver are asymptomatic. Although patients with AH and cirrhosis may be asymptomatic, many present with a variety of complaints including anorexia, nausea and vomiting, weakness, jaundice, weight loss, abdominal pain, fever, and diarrhea.

Physical Examination

The most detailed clinical information on ALD in the United States comes from studies of hospitalized patients who were assigned the diagnosis on the basis of classical histologic features.[179,180] The most common physical finding in patients with fatty liver and AH is hepatomegaly, which is detectable in more than 75% of patients, regardless of disease severity. Patients with AH and cirrhosis also may have hepatic tenderness, rarely an audible bruit over the liver, spider angiomata, splenomegaly, and peripheral edema. Jaundice and ascites, which are found in approximately 60% of patients, are more frequent in patients with severe disease (Table 88.1). Various degrees of hepatic encephalopathy can be seen, usually in the most severely ill patients. Some patients with AH have a fever, with temperatures as high as 104°F.

In patients with compensated cirrhosis, the physical examination can be normal; however, some patients have obvious hepatomegaly and most have splenomegaly. As the disease progresses, the liver decreases in size and has a hard and nodular consistency. Patients with decompensated cirrhosis typically have muscle wasting, ascites, spider angiomata, palmar erythema, and Dupuytren's contractures. Enlarged parotid and lacrimal glands may be seen, and severely ill patients may have Muehrcke's lines or white nails. Patients with hepatopulmonary syndrome often have digital clubbing (see Chapter 96).

Laboratory Tests

Patients with even severe AH have only minimal elevations in serum AST and ALT levels (see Table 88.2).[179,180] Serum AST levels are almost always less than 300–500 U/L and typically are associated with trivial elevation of serum ALT levels, resulting in an AST/ALT ratio greater than 2. A ratio >2 is characteristic of AH, in part because of deficiency of pyridoxal 5′ phosphate (a cofactor for aminotransferase activity) in these patients (see Chapter 75). Importantly, the elevation in AST and ALT do not reflect the degree of liver injury/disease severity.[181,182] Indeed, patients with early stage ALD may have AST and ALT levels higher than those seen in patients with severe AH.[181] Serum alkaline phosphatase levels can range from normal to values greater than 1000 U/L. Serum bilirubin levels range from normal to 20–40 mg/dL, and serum albumin levels may be normal or depressed to a value as low as 1.0–1.5 g/dL. Many patients with ALD are anemic and have some degree of thrombocytopenia. By contrast, the white blood cell count usually is normal or elevated, occasionally to levels consistent with a leukemoid state. Severely ill patients usually have marked prolongation of the prothrombin time—often expressed as the international normalized ratio—and often have elevated serum creatinine values.

A panel of tests are routinely ordered in patients with suspected ALD to exclude other forms of liver disease and to further solidify the diagnosis of ALD (Box 88.2). Utilization of noninvasive tests (NITs) is gaining acceptance across liver diseases, including ALD. While specific NITs for ALD are yet to be

TABLE 88.1 Symptoms and Signs in Hospitalized Patients With Alcohol-associated Liver Disease[a]

Symptom or Sign	Patients Affected (%) Mild Disease ($n = 89$)	Moderate Disease ($n = 58$)	Severe Disease ($n = 37$)	Overall
Hepatomegaly	84.3	94.7	79.4	86.7
Jaundice	17.4	100	100	60.1
Ascites	30.3	79.3	86.5	57.1
Hepatic encephalopathy	27.3	55.2	70.3	44.6
Splenomegaly	18.0	30.9	39.4	26.0
Fever	18.0	31.0	21.6	22.8

[a]Moderate disease was defined by a serum bilirubin level >5 mg/dL, severe disease by a bilirubin level >5 mg/dL and a prolonged prothrombin time >4 seconds.

Data from Mendenhall CL. Alcoholic hepatitis. *Clin Gastroenterol.* 1981;10:417–441.

TABLE 88.2 Laboratory Values in Hospitalized Patients With Alcohol-associated Liver Disease[a]

	Mean Value		
Laboratory Test	**Mild Disease (*n* = 89)**	**Moderate Disease (*n* = 58)**	**Severe Disease (*n* = 37)**
Hematocrit value (%)	38	36	33
MCV (μm^3)	100	102	105
WBC count (per mm^3)	8000	11,000	12,000
Serum AST level (U/L)	84	124	99
Serum ALT level (U/L)	56	56	57
Serum alkaline phosphatase level (U/L)	166	276	225
Serum bilirubin level (mg/dL)	1.6	8.7	13.5
Prolongation of prothrombin time (seconds)	0.9	2.4	6.4
Serum albumin level (g/dL)	3.7	2.7	2.4

[a]Moderate disease was defined by a serum bilirubin level >5 mg/dL, severe disease by a bilirubin level >5 mg/dL and a prolonged prothrombin time >4 seconds.

ALT, Alanine aminotransferase; *AST*, aspartate aminotransferase; *MCV*, mean corpuscular volume; *WBC*, white blood cell.

Data from Mendenhall CL. Alcoholic hepatitis. *Clin Gastroenterol*. 1981;10:417–441.

BOX 88.2 Tests for Differential and Evaluation of Alcohol-associated Liver Disease (ALD)

- AH/ALD: Alcohol consumption in standard drinks.
- Viral hepatitis: Hepatitis B surface antigen and core antibody, hepatitis C virus antibody and/or HCV RNA, hepatitis A antibody IgM, hepatitis E antibody (in an appropriate geographical setting).
- Autoimmune liver disease: ANA, AMA.
- Hereditary causes of liver disease: Hereditary hemochromatosis, Wilson disease, alpha-1-antitrypsin deficiency—iron/TIBC, ferritin, ceruloplasmin.
- Drug-induced liver disease: Careful medication history.
- Hepatic mass or blood flow alterations: Hepatic US with Doppler.
- Diagnosis usually made on clinical, biochemical, and imaging assessment; biopsy not routinely performed in the U.S.

defined, commonly used serum based as well as imaging based NITs are useful to assess the extent of liver disease in ALD.[183] Transient elastography (Fibroscan) can accurately detect advanced fibrosis and cirrhosis; however, it is unreliable in AH where inflammation and swelling of the liver interfere with the test.[183] The controlled attenuation parameter has been developed as part of transient elastography as a novel tool to noninvasively assess liver steatosis. Among blood-based nonproprietary markers, FIB-4 has been most studied and shown to have high sensitivity (80%–90%), but low specificity (60%–70%) in excluding advanced fibrosis (F3-4). The enhanced liver fibrosis score and FibroTest are patented blood-based biomarkers with high specificity (80%–90%), but at higher cost than the easily performed FIB-4.[174] Numerous studies have documented the potential of circulating biomarkers in ALD and in AH. For example, serum cytokeratin-18 has been shown to be diagnostic, prognostic, and therognostic in AH.[181,182,184] The combination of age and serum IL-13 levels correlated with survival in severe AH a recent study.[104] Future clinical studies should validate these and other noninvasive biomarkers, including promising metabolomic biomarkers, for the diagnosis, prognosis, and response to therapy in ALD and AH.[185–187]

Histopathology

The clinical diagnosis of ALD is quite sensitive and specific; therefore liver biopsy is usually not needed to establish the diagnosis. A liver biopsy is useful, however, in selecting patients for clinical trials, for determining the presence of cirrhosis, and for clarifying the diagnosis in atypical cases (Fig. 88.2). Centrilobular and perivenular fatty infiltration is seen in most persons who drink more than 60 g of alcohol daily. Classic histologic features of AH include ballooning degeneration of hepatocytes, alcoholic hyaline (Mallory or Mallory-Denk bodies) within damaged hepatocytes, and a surrounding infiltrate composed of polymorphonuclear leukocytes.[22,23,25] Most patients have moderate to severe fatty infiltration. Varying degrees of fibrosis may be present, and some patients exhibit an unusual perisinusoidal distribution of fibrosis, at times with partial or complete obliteration of the terminal hepatic venules *sclerosing hyaline necrosis*.[25,31] Cirrhosis can be identified by the presence of nodules of hepatic tissue that are completely surrounded by fibrous tissue.

Alcohol-associated cirrhosis typically is micronodular or mixed micro- and macronodular. In patients with coexisting AH, alcohol-related hyaline is almost universal, and sclerosing hyaline necrosis and moderate-to-severe fatty infiltration are common. In patients with alcohol-associated cirrhosis who abstain from alcohol for long periods, a frequent finding is a gradual transformation to macronodular cirrhosis, which is indistinguishable from cirrhosis caused by other forms of liver disease.[24,25,31]

Conditions That May Resemble Alcohol-Associated Liver Disease

Although the clinical diagnosis of ALD usually is quite straightforward, the similarity of clinical and/or histologic features of other disorders to those of ALD sometimes causes diagnostic confusion. The most commonly encountered conditions that have clinical or histologic features in common with ALD are MASLD, hereditary hemochromatosis, and Budd-Chiari syndrome.

Metabolic Dysfunction-Associated Steatotic Liver Disease

MASLD, formerly known as NAFLD, is the most difficult condition to differentiate from ALD. There is essentially complete overlap between its histologic features of MASLD and ALD.[25,188] As a consequence, the differentiation between the two conditions requires careful clinicopathologic correlation. Patients with ALD typically manifest clinical features of more advanced liver disease. Patients with MASLD are more likely to have features of the metabolic syndrome, including peripheral insulin resistance, obesity, hypertension, and dyslipidemia, although these features are not invariably present.[189,190] They also should have weekly alcohol intake of less than 21 drinks for men and 14 for women.[191] When a patient's alcohol intake cannot be reliably quantified, differentiating the two conditions can be difficult, if not impossible. The use of structured questionnaires or PEth to assess alcohol intake is recommended in this situation.[191] Importantly, together with the nomenclature change accompanying MASLD, a new disease category was created—MetALD (Fig. 88.4). This describes a major group of patients with MASLD who drink more

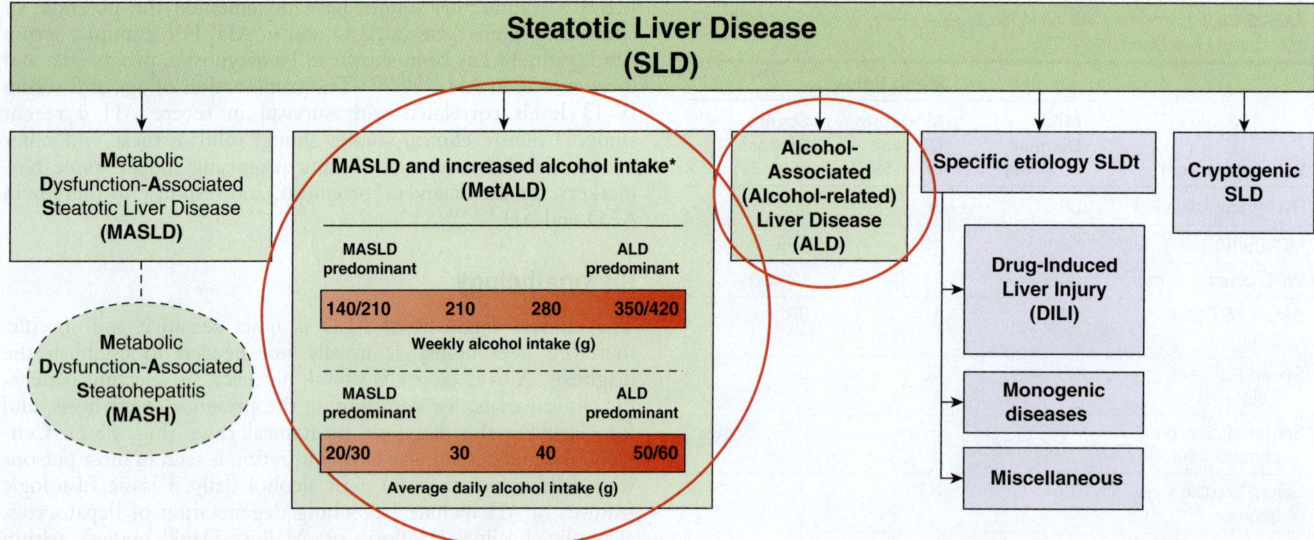

Fig. 88.4 Spectrum of steatotic liver diseases including the new diagnosis of MetALD.

alcohol than the cutoff criteria for MASLD, and in whom alcohol likely combines to drive the liver disease. The calories from alcohol add to the problem of obesity and the metabolic syndrome. It is important to note that patients with MetALD have substantial alcohol consumption, but at levels still much lower than those typically seen with patients with AUD in a treatment program or those hospitalized with AH[192] (Fig. 88.1).

Hereditary Hemochromatosis

On occasion, distinguishing patients with ALD and secondary iron overload from those with liver disease caused by hereditary hemochromatosis can be difficult. Patients with end-stage liver disease from alcohol-associated cirrhosis or severe AH can have elevated serum iron and ferritin levels and increased hepatic iron levels suggestive of hereditary hemochromatosis.[193] To complicate matters further, 15%–40% of patients with hereditary hemochromatosis consume more than 80 g of alcohol daily.[194]

The overlapping clinical features of hereditary hemochromatosis and ALD include hepatomegaly, testicular atrophy, cardiomyopathy, and glucose intolerance. Testing for mutations in the gene for hereditary hemochromatosis and measuring the hepatic iron index are the best methods for differentiating the two conditions. Few patients with alcohol-induced cirrhosis and iron overload are homozygous for *C282Y* or heterozygous for the *C282Y* and *H63D HFE* genes and few have hepatic iron index values greater than 1.9 (see Chapter 77).[193,195]

Drug Induced Liver Disease

Drug-induced liver injury (DILI) can occur in the setting of chronic alcohol consumption/ALD. The interaction between heavy alcohol consumption and acetaminophen toxicity has been well documented for over 40 years.[196] This is discussed subsequently. Other interactions with drugs, such as methotrexate, isoniazid, and certain antiretroviral agents, have also been reported.[197] Moreover, patients with ALD often consume drugs that frequently cause DILI, such as certain antibiotics. Interestingly, a meta-analysis of data from the DILI Network showed that anabolic steroids were the most common cause of DILI in individuals who were heavy alcohol consumers.[197] However, when heavy drinkers were compared to nondrinkers, DILI was not associated with an overall greater proportion of liver-related deaths or LT. Because DILI can have variable presentation, it is important to have a high index of suspicion in patients with AUD/ALD who undergo changes in their liver/metabolic profiles. This includes an increase in AST or ALT above the range expected in ALD.

COFACTORS THAT MAY INFLUENCE PROGRESSION OF ALCOHOL-ASSOCIATED LIVER DISEASE

Many people drink heavily, yet only a limited number (~35%) develop more advanced disease such as AH or cirrhosis. Thus there must be modifying factors that act to slow or accelerate disease activity/progression. These factors can either be fixed (e.g., genetics) or can be modifiable (e.g., smoking and diet). We list 10 disease modifiers of particular importance to ALD in Box 88.3, and we review selected modifiers. Some, such as continued drinking (the most important modifier), and genetics are covered elsewhere in this chapter.

Obesity and smoking are highly associated with ALD. Obesity is also an independent risk factor for disease progression in AH and cirrhosis.[166,168,198,199] Patients with alcohol-associated cirrhosis who are overweight also appear to be at increased risk for developing HCC.[200] Cigarette smoking also has been shown to accelerate the progression of fibrosis and risk for HCC.[166,201,202]

Diet and nutrition play a major role in ALD, and patients with ALD show various degrees of nutritional deficiency.[203] Studies conducted by the Veterans Health Administration (VA) Cooperative Studies Program in patients having AH[204–207] showed that almost every patient with severe AH had some degree of malnutrition.[205] Approximately 50% of patients' energy intake came from alcohol. Although calorie intake was frequently not inadequate, intake of protein and critical micronutrients was often deficient. Dietary fat represents a macronutrient dietary modifier for ALD. Dietary unsaturated fat, enriched in linoleic acid (LA) in particular, promotes alcohol-induced liver damage.[138,208,209] LA is enzymatically converted to bioactive oxidation products, OXLAMs, which are highly inflammatory and hepatotoxic. Deficiency of the micronutrient, zinc, also appears to occur early in alcohol associated liver injury and to play a role in the development/progression of liver injury.[210]

Alcohol and drugs (including prescription medications, over-the-counter agents and illicit drugs) may interact to cause

BOX 88.3 Disease Modifiers

1. Continued drinking
2. Obesity
3. Smoking
4. Diet/nutrition
5. Medications/drugs of abuse
6. Occupational/environmental exposure
7. Age
8. Sex
9. Race
10. Other liver diseases
11. Genetics/epigenetics/family history

hepatotoxicity. For example, subjects with chronic alcohol misuse are more susceptible to acetaminophen hepatotoxicity for multiple reasons. Alcohol misuse can occur in HIV-infected patients, and alcohol abuse can enhance hepatotoxicity of certain ART regimens.[211] Alcohol may also interact with illicit drugs such as 3,4-methylenedioxymethamphetamine (MDMA; ecstasy), commonly used with alcohol.[212]

Exposure to potential toxins in the workplace or environment can cause hepatotoxicity, which can be exacerbated by alcohol. Vinyl chloride (VC) represents an industrial exposure whose toxicity overlaps with alcohol. VC induced histologic steatohepatitis that was indistinguishable from alcohol-induced steatohepatitis, and this is termed toxicant-associated steatohepatitis (TASH).[213] VC is metabolized in a similar fashion as is ethanol, and this could potentially account for the observed similarities between TASH and ALD. With environmental exposures, there are usually multiple contaminants rather than just one compound. Use of a cocktail of 22 clinically relevant contaminants (Northern Contaminant Mixture) showed that both a high-fat diet and alcohol increased fatty liver and liver injury in exposed mice.[214]

Female gender is now a well-accepted risk factor for the development and rapid progression of ALD.[18,19,215] Studies in rats or mice chronically fed alcohol also have demonstrated that women are more susceptible than men to liver injury. Risk factors for the development of liver disease in women appear to include sex hormone levels, endotoxemia, lipid peroxidation, chemokines, and NF-κB activation. These risk factors are critical for determining "safe" levels of alcohol consumption in women. Indeed, many authorities consider any amount of alcohol above 14 g a day (one standard drink) to be a risk factor for the development of liver disease in women.

Race can influence susceptibility to ALD. Research from large multicenter Veterans Affairs studies showed that alcohol-associated cirrhosis was more frequent in Hispanics (73%) than in non-Hispanic white/Caucasians (52%) and black Americans (44%). Moreover, blacks have consistently shown to be more likely to have hepatitis B or hepatitis C as confounders.[216]

Between one-fourth and one-third of patients with ALD also have, or previously had, hepatitis C.[217] Liver disease is more severe, advanced disease develops at a younger age, and survival is shorter in patients with both ALD and HCV infection.[11,166,168,217] In addition, alcohol and HCV act synergistically in the development of HCC (see Chapter 82).[200,218,219] Fortunately, curative direct acting antiviral agents for HCV have recently markedly reduced this interaction.

PROGNOSIS

The prognosis for individual patients with ALD depends on the degree of pathologic injury, the patient's nutritional status, complications of advanced liver disease, the presence of other comorbid conditions such as obesity and HCV infection, and the patient's ability to discontinue destructive patterns of drinking. Patients with fatty liver have the best outcome, those with AH or cirrhosis have an intermediate outcome, and those with cirrhosis combined with AH have the worst outcome (Fig. 88.5).[220] Estimating the prognosis of patients with ALD is particularly important to determine the need for specific therapy in patients with severe AH and LT in those with AH and/or cirrhosis.

Alcohol-Associated Hepatitis

Patients with AH account for almost 1% of hospital admissions in the United States. Almost 7% during their initial hospitalization and 40% of those with severe disease die within 6 months of clinical presentation.[221,222] Clinical features associated with severe disease include hepatic encephalopathy, marked prolongation of prothrombin time, and elevation of serum bilirubin level (often above 25 mg/dL), and development of acute kidney injury.

A number of formulae have been shown to predict short-term prognosis in these often critically ill patients.[223] Maddrey and Boitnott discovered a simple formula called the *discriminant function* (DF), which proved useful in identifying patients with poor short-term survival rates.[224] A modification of the original DF (mDF) calculated as {[4.6 × prothrombin time—control value (seconds)] + serum bilirubin (mg/dL)} has proven useful in identifying patients with a poor prognosis who should be considered for specific therapy.[225] The mDF has been incorporated into the selection criteria for most of the initial therapeutic trials for patients with AH. The prognosis of patients with mDF values >32 can be further stratified by the presence of encephalopathy and development of acute kidney injury.[225,226]

Three other prognostic models, the MELD score, the Glasgow AH score, and the ABIC scores have been shown to predict survival in patients with severe AH more effectively than mDF.[227,228] The original MELD is probably the most widely used formula, and a MELD >21 is used in the definition of severe AH.[166,168,178,229]

Alcohol-Associated Cirrhosis

The 5-year mortality of patients with alcohol-associated cirrhosis ranges from 60% to 85%.[230] Within 15 years 90% of patients can be expected to die if they do not receive LT.[231] Prognosis among individual patients is dependent on the development of complications. One year mortality is 15%–20% in patients with no complications, 20% following variceal bleeding, 30% after developing ascites, 50% in those with variceal bleeding and ascites, and 65% following the development of hepatic encephalopathy.[230] The clinical tool used most widely to determine prognosis in patients with alcohol-associated cirrhosis is the Child-Turcotte-Pugh (CTP) score. Although it has limitations, the CTP score been adopted widely for risk-stratifying patients with cirrhosis because of its simplicity and ease of use. Five-year survival rates for patients with alcohol-associated cirrhosis vary dramatically based on the CTP score at the time of clinical presentation (Fig. 88.6).[232,233] The other major model that has been used to predict prognosis in patients with alcohol-induced cirrhosis is the MELD score. The MELD score (and several modified versions), which is useful for predicting short-term survival in groups of patients with various liver diseases, is the system used for allocation of donor organs in the United States (see Chapter 90).

Acute-On-Chronic Liver Failure

Patients with stable, compensated cirrhosis can gradually develop complications or they can suddenly develop jaundice and

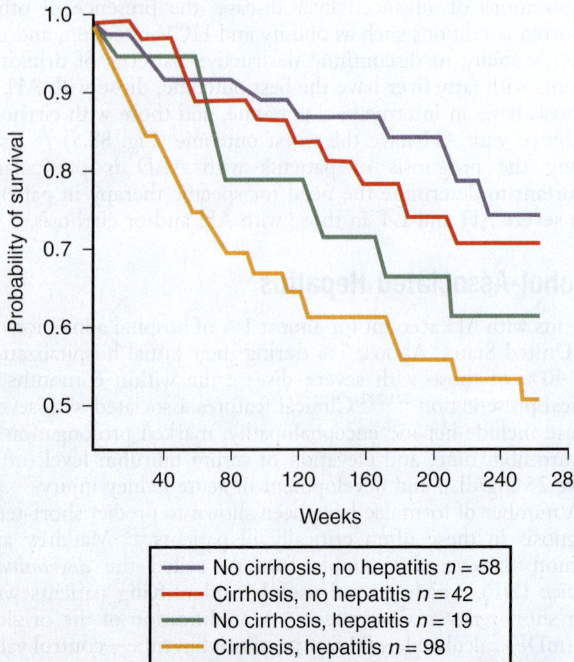

Fig. 88.5 Survival of patients with alcohol-associated liver disease stratified by histologic severity of disease. (From Orrego H, Black JE, Blendis LM, Medline A. Prognosis of alcoholic cirrhosis in the presence or absence of alcoholic hepatitis. *Gastroenterology*. 1987;92:208–214, with permission.)

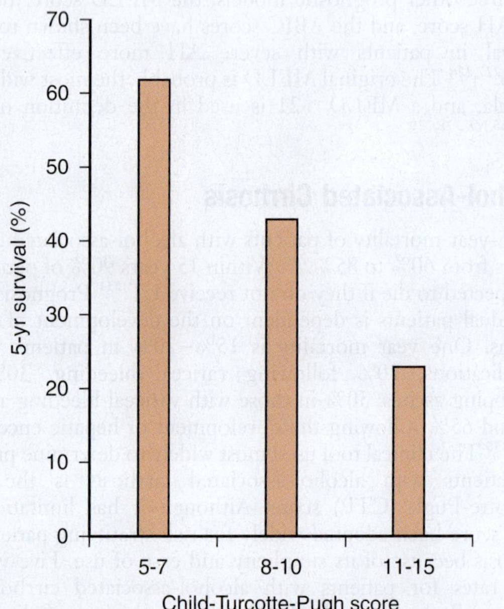

Fig. 88.6 Five-year survival rates in patients with alcohol-associated cirrhosis according to their Child-Turcotte-Pugh scores.

coagulopathy with rapid development of ascites and/or encephalopathy, a syndrome referred to as acute-on-chronic liver failure.[230,234,235] The three most common precipitating factors are superimposed AH due to an increase in alcohol intake, infections, and drug toxicity.[236]

Patients hospitalized with decompensated cirrhosis or acute-on-chronic liver failure are inordinately predisposed to infection and the subsequent development of hepatic encephalopathy, sepsis, acute kidney injury, and multiorgan failure.[237,238] The 90-day mortality of patients who require intensive care unit management for three or more failing organ systems due to these complications exceeds 90%.[239] The prognosis of patients hospitalized in the ICU is more accurately reflected by sequential organ failure assessment scores than by the Child-Pugh or other liver-related scores.[166,239,240]

Acute Viral Illness

Patients with alcohol-associated cirrhosis are vulnerable to sudden decompensation from infection with hepatotropic viruses including hepatitis A, B, and E and nonhepatotropic viruses such as influenza A.[234] The potential for sudden deterioration from these infections underscores the importance of routine immunizations for vaccine-preventable infections.[241]

Hepatotoxic Drugs

Sudden and unexplained clinical deterioration in patients with alcohol-associated cirrhosis can also result from ingestion of hepatotoxic medications and herbal remedies. The morbidity and mortality associated with these conditions are considerable. Because of induction of CYP2E1, drinkers are uniquely susceptible to acetaminophen hepatotoxicity. Subjects with AUD with or without major liver disease who take excessive doses of this drug over a period of days to weeks for relief of a headache, toothache, or other minor pain can experience sudden deterioration of their clinical condition.[242] The clinical features in these patients are indistinguishable from ALD, with one obvious exception: the ALT and AST values are frequently more than 1000 U/L, much higher than expected in patients with ALD. Because liver injury has already occurred by the time of hospitalization, acetaminophen levels are often not helpful for diagnosis or management. Recognition of the cause of the unusually elevated serum aminotransferase levels comes from careful questioning of the patient and family about acetaminophen ingestion in the days before hospitalization. Sudden clinical deterioration in patients with alcohol-associated cirrhosis also can result from idiosyncratic hepatotoxic reactions to a number of other drugs and herbal medications.[243,244]

Hepatocellular Carcinoma

Although many other cancers are decreasing in the United States, HCC has doubled in the last 15 years, and alcohol has been postulated to play a major etiologic role. Some of the potential mechanisms for alcohol in the initiation and promotion of HCC include acetaldehyde-DNA adduct formation, generation of ROS, chronic inflammation, glutathione depletion, hypomethylation of oncogenes, retinoic acid depletion in hepatocytes, liver fibrosis, and decreased natural killer cell function/number.[245] Moreover, alcohol has also been shown to potentiate liver cancer in animal models. However, the true frequency of HCC in patients with alcohol-associated cirrhosis is still somewhat unclear.[246] Although ALD has been long considered to be the leading cause of HCC in the United States and Europe, many of these patients were also infected with hepatitis C. Some research suggests an HCC incidence two to three times higher in HCV coinfected patients than the normal population without evidence of HCV infection.[32] The HCC risk shows a strong correlation with alcohol intake and is roughly doubled with concurrent HCV infection.[219] The risk of HCC is higher in males and increases with age.[200] Given the ongoing risk for HCC, lifetime surveillance with ultrasound imaging every 6 months is recommended for all patients with alcohol-associated cirrhosis.[246] Early detection with surveillance markedly improves prognosis, and multiple new therapies markedly improved the outlook for HCC.[247]

TREATMENT

Therapy for ALD can be viewed as an inverted pyramid, with everyone receiving lifestyle modification, most receiving nutritional intervention, some receiving drug therapy, and only a few being eligible for/receiving LT (Fig. 88.7). Importantly, therapy should be directed, in part, by disease severity.

Abstinence and Lifestyle Modification

Abstinence from continued excessive drinking is the most important predictor of survival in patients with alcohol-associated cirrhosis,[166,168,231,233,248] and this has been a consistent finding in over a half-century of studies. The 3-year survival rate is 70%–80% among patients who abstain or dramatically reduce their excessive drinking, compared with only 20%–30% in those who continue to drink heavily.[248] Reducing, but not completely stopping, alcohol consumption also has been shown to improve survival (Fig. 88.8).[231] The question is how best to effectively achieve these goals. Recognition, diagnosis and early treatment of AUD in patients with AH is the standard in the care of these patients.[249,250] A multidisciplinary approach to the care of ALD and AUD provides optimal team treatment.[251]

The first steps are to identify excessive drinking, to determine the severity of the drinking problem and to assess the patient's motivation for change. Patients may experience risky drinking, alcohol abuse, or dependence.[252] Patients with risky drinking without dependence respond well in primary care settings to brief interventions resulting in reduced consumption and reduction in alcohol-related injury and mortality.[166,253] Brief interventions have also been effective in reducing alcohol intake in pregnant women with subsequent reduction in fetal mortality.[165] Unfortunately, most patients seen in acute care settings by gastroenterologists suffer from alcohol misuse and dependence. Although brief interventions may be very effective in individual patients, the majority need a referral to a qualified alcohol and substance abuse counselor for assessment and specialty treatment if they are to have the best opportunity to achieve long-term remission. Roughly 20%–30% of patients remain abstinent for a year after a single course of treatment and another 10% reduce their intake to the point that they no longer experienced adverse consequences from their drinking.[252]

Three oral medications (disulfiram, acamprosate, and naltrexone) and an extended-release injectable form of naltrexone have been FDA-approved to treat alcohol dependence. Pharmacotherapy with these agents is only modestly effective; however, all have side effects and are underutilized.[166,168,252] *Baclofen*, a gamma aminobutyric acid B-receptor agonist, shows promise to decrease craving and to improve abstinence and decrease the likelihood of relapse in patients with alcohol-associated cirrhosis.[166,254] Baclofen and acamprosate are the only two agents that have been studied in ALD. Given the limited efficacy of the currently available medications to prevent relapse, a number of new approaches are under active investigation.[255] This includes therapy to decrease neuroinflammation, which may be a factor in continued alcohol intake. Involvement in mutual support groups, such as Alcoholics Anonymous (AA), can reduce the risk of relapse, primarily by building social support for sobriety.[252] An excellent guide to various treatment strategies is available at: https://www.niaaa.nih.gov/research/major-initiatives/medications-development-program. The NIAAA Alcohol Treatment Navigator also has a website to provide information on local treatment programs (https://alcoholtreatment.niaaa.nih.gov).

The goal of intervention should be sustained abstinence, as it improves the histological features of alcohol-associated liver injury, reduces portal pressure, and slows progression to cirrhosis.[166,168] In two-thirds of patients significant clinical improvement can be seen within 3 months.[168] Within 2 years many patients achieve complete clinical and biochemical recovery, regain lost muscle mass, and can safely stop diuretics and other liver-related medicines.[256] Although reducing alcohol intake to "safe" levels does reduce mortality and morbidity, only 10% of individuals are able to maintain safe levels of drinking over extended periods of time.[252] Three-quarters of patients have a relapse within a year. Longitudinal care by the treatment program is important. Clinicians can also be helpful by providing regular visits in a nonjudgmental manner and providing ongoing counseling and support of the longer-term treatment goals.[252] It is also important to address obesity and smoking, the two comorbidities associated with progression of ALD.

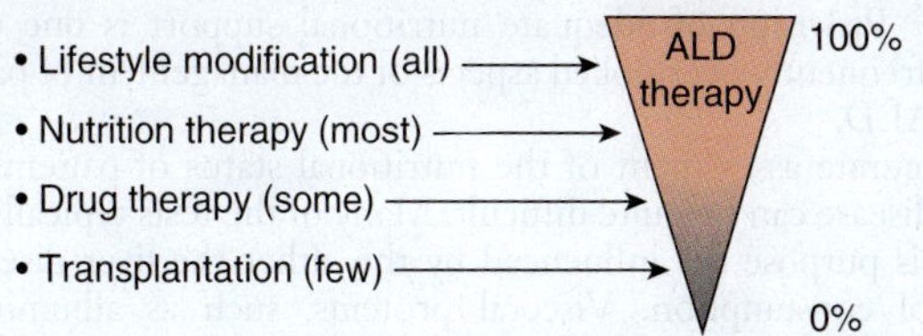

Fig. 88.7 Therapy for the spectrum of alcohol-associated liver disease.

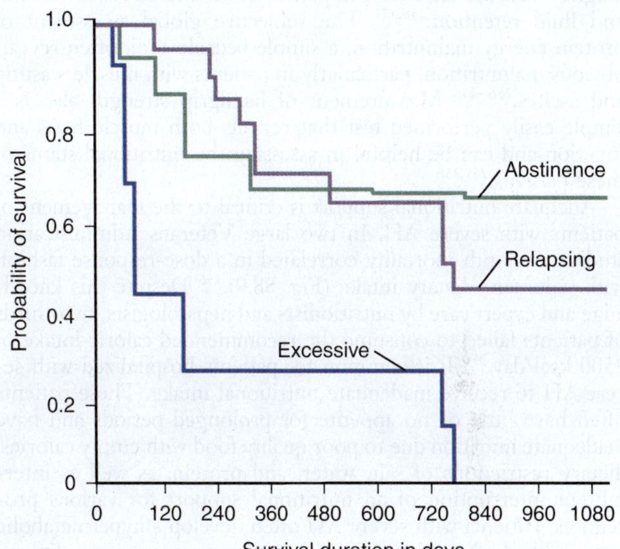

Fig. 88.8 Survival curves in patients with severe alcoholic cirrhosis during the 3 years following hospital discharge according to alcohol consumption during this period: abstinence, patients who were abstinent; relapsing, patients with one or more periods of abstinence alternating with one or more periods of excessive consumption; excessive, patients with excessive consumption of alcohol at the first follow-up point. Survival differed significantly between patients who were abstinent and those who were drinking excessively ($P < .001$). (Modified with permission of Veldt BJ, Laine F, Guillygomarc'h A, et al. Indication of liver transplantation in severe alcoholic liver cirrhosis: qualitative evaluation and optimal timing. *J Hepatol*. 2002;36:93–98.)

Nutritional Support

Malnutrition is a widespread clinical problem among patients with ALD. In a study from the U.S. Veterans Administration, every patient with moderate to severe AH or cirrhosis showed some signs of malnutrition. The presence of malnutrition is associated with higher rates of liver-related complications and mortality. Malnutrition also has been associated with longer ICU stays, longer duration of hospitalization, and higher mortality rates after

LT.[257] Provision of adequate nutritional support is one of the most frequently overlooked aspects of the management of patients with ALD.

Accurate assessment of the nutritional status of patients with liver disease can be quite difficult. Many of the tests typically used for this purpose are influenced by the either the liver disease or alcohol consumption. Visceral proteins, such as albumin and prealbumin, are produced in the liver and correlate better with the severity of liver disease than nutritional status. Anthropometric measurements, such as triceps skin fold, BMI, and the creatinine height index, are unreliable in patients with altered renal function and fluid retention.[256,257] The subjective global assessment of protein energy malnutrition, a simple bedside tool, often reveals obvious malnutrition, particularly in patients with muscle wasting and ascites.[256–258] Measurement of handgrip strength also is a simple easily performed test that reflects both muscle mass and function and can be helpful in assessing the nutritional status of these patients.[257,258]

Adequate nutritional support is critical to the management of patients with severe AH. In two large Veterans Administration studies, 6-month mortality correlated in a dose-response fashion with voluntary dietary intake (Fig. 88.9).[256] Despite this knowledge and expert care by nutritionists and hepatologists, two-thirds of patients failed to consume the recommended caloric intake of 2500 kcal/day.[256] It is common for patients hospitalized with severe AH to receive inadequate nutritional intake. These patients often have little or no appetite for prolonged periods and have inadequate nutrition due to poor quality food with empty calories, dietary restrictions of salt, water, and protein, as well as intermittent interruption of all nutritional support for various procedures. Patients with severe AH often develop a hypermetabolic state with higher than normal resting energy expenditures. Because of the vital need for adequate nutrition in these often critically ill patients, we do not hesitate to place a nasogastric feeding tube if the patient cannot voluntarily ingest at least 2500 calories daily, even when esophageal varices are present.[179,256,259,260] Indeed, in a multicenter study from Europe, hospitalized patients with AH were randomized to glucocorticoid therapy or aggressive enteral feeding. Enteral feeding provided the same 1-month survival benefit, with significantly lower mortality at 1 year. This study further emphasizes the importance of nutrition in these patients.

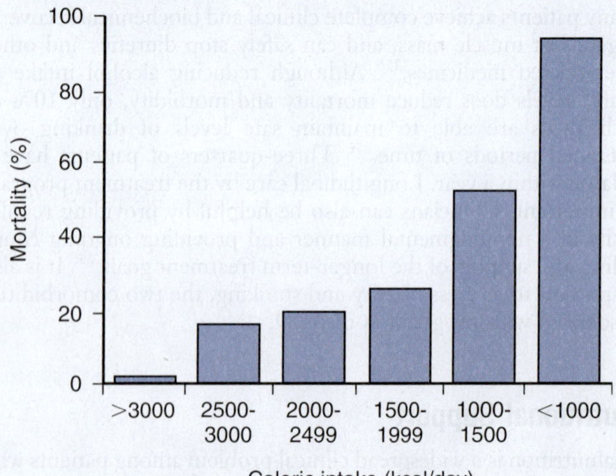

Fig. 88.9 Relation between voluntary dietary intake and survival in patients with severe alcohol-associated hepatitis. (From McClain CJ, Barve SS, Barve A, Marsano L. Alcoholic liver disease and malnutrition. *Alcohol Clin Exp Res*. 2011;35(5):815–820, with permission.)

Patients with stable cirrhosis have nutritional deficiencies almost as severe as those in patients with AH.[256] The frequency of malnutrition increases with the severity of disease. For example, the risk of profound malnutrition increases from 45% in patients with Child's class A to 95% in those with Child's C cirrhosis.[256,257] Patients with cirrhosis who require hospitalization have a substantially higher prevalence of malnutrition compared with general medical inpatients and have significantly longer hospital stays and a 2-fold higher risk of in-hospital mortality.[261] Even in patients with stable, compensated cirrhosis, malnutrition is associated with higher mortality (20% vs. 0%) and complication rates (65% vs. 13%) within a year.[257,258]

Hepatic glycogen stores are depleted in patients with cirrhosis. As a result, these patients move into an early starvation mode after only 12 hours of fasting compared to 48 hours in normal individuals. Thus even short periods of inadequate nutrition can result in muscle proteolysis, which contributes to protein malnutrition. Patients with decompensated cirrhosis also can be hypermetabolic. Not surprisingly, the protein intake recommended for patients with cirrhosis is higher than for healthy adults.[258,259] The positive impact of judicious nutritional supplements in patients with cirrhosis is illustrated by a randomized trial showing that a nighttime snack of 700 kcal each evening resulted in an accrual of 2 kg of lean tissue over 12 months.[262] Thus patients with severe AH/cirrhosis should be given nighttime (9 p.m.) snacks to prevent "starvation" overnight and subsequent muscle breakdown. This is especially important in the outpatient setting.

It needs to be emphasized that protein restriction has no beneficial effect on encephalopathy and can be nutritionally catastrophic.[256,258,263] If, despite appropriate medical therapy, standard enteral formulas lead to encephalopathy, a branched chain amino acid-enriched formula can be given as a supplement to meet nitrogen needs.[256,259]

Patients with ALD also can suffer from a plethora of vitamin and mineral deficiencies.[256,257] In addition to the commonly recognized deficiencies in folate and B vitamins, deficiencies in fat soluble vitamins (A, D, and E) and minerals (magnesium, selenium, and zinc) are common causes of symptoms and physical findings in these patients.[257] Zinc deficiency, for example, may be an important component of the skin lesions, night blindness, mental irritability, confusion and hepatic encephalopathy, anorexia, altered taste and smell, hypogonadism, and altered wound healing that can be seen in patients with ALD.[264] Assessment and judicious corrections of each of these deficiencies is an important aspect of the care of these patients.

The nutritional status of patients at the time of LT also is important. Morbid obesity and severe malnutrition are each predictors of poor outcomes.[265] Among those transplanted in the United States over the past 20 years, extremes of body mass index (BMI <18.5 and >40) were more common in patients with ALD than in patients transplanted for other conditions. Severely malnourished patients had longer lengths of stay, a higher retransplantation rate and diminished survival.[265,266]

Drug Therapy for Alcohol-Associated Hepatitis

Glucocorticoids for Severe AH

Glucocorticoid therapy was first demonstrated to provide a short-term survival benefit for patients with severe AH in a small U.S. prospective randomized multicenter trial nearly 30 years ago.[225] Each of the patients enrolled had a clinical diagnosis of AH and either an mDF > 32, spontaneous hepatic encephalopathy, or both. Treatment consisted of 28 days of 32 mg of methylprednisolone daily followed by a 2-week taper. The 28-day mortality among patients who received prednisolone was only 6%, compared to 35% among the placebo-treated controls. It is now generally accepted that glucocorticoid therapy has a beneficial effect on 1-month survival, as confirmed by many studies over the ensuing years, although this effect is now documented to be relatively modest. Unfortunately, there is no benefit of survival at 3 or 6 months. These data are supported by a recent meta-analysis on glucocorticoid therapy in severe AH.[267]

Glucocorticoids work by binding to receptors (GRs) in the cytoplasm. GRs then translocate to the nucleus and bind to the glucocorticoid response elements in the promoter regions of glucocorticoid responsive genes to switch on expression of certain anti-inflammatory genes and reduce inflammation.[268] Unfortunately, many patients are "steroid resistant" through multiple mechanisms and do not respond to glucocorticoid therapy. Early identification of the subset of resistant patients (25%–30%) is important for implementing treatment strategies. One simple and clinically utilized definition of glucocorticoid resistance in patients with severe AH is the lack of an early change in bilirubin levels at 7 days.[269] The subsequently developed Lille model also allows patients to receive a 7-day course of corticosteroids and then assesses the responsiveness based on an algorithm combining age, renal insufficiency, albumin, prothrombin time, bilirubin, and evolution of bilirubin at Day 4 or 7 (Table 88.3). Patients with a score > 0.45 had a 6-month survival of only about 25% and could be discontinued from corticosteroids. However, those patients with scores <0.45 had an 85% survival and would benefit from continued corticosteroid treatment. This scoring system allows discontinuation of steroids early in patients who will receive no benefit.[270]

TABLE 88.3 Lille Score

Laboratory Values Included	Lille Score Score <0.45	Lille Score Score >0.45
1. Age 2. Albumin	15% mortality at 6 months	75% mortality at 6 months
3. Bilirubin (initial) 4. Bilirubin level (Day 7) 5. Prothrombin time	Score at 7 days indicates response to treatment	

The pivotal study involving current therapy for severe AH was the STOPAH trial which evaluated prednisolone, pentoxifylline (PTX), the combination, or placebo in severe AH.[271] This large, multicenter trial of more than 1000 patients showed a modest beneficial effect of prednisolone at 28 days, but no later beneficial effect on mortality. For all groups, 28- and 90-day mortality were excellent at <20% and <30%, respectively (Fig. 88.10). Unfortunately, the overall 1-year mortality was 56%, and only about 37% of people remained abstinent at 1 year. Thus return to drinking was a major health problem. This study confirms the beneficial effects of glucocorticoids on 1-month survival and suggests that PTX has no impact on survival. Moreover, the combination of PTX and steroids showed no significant benefit. The mortality data from the STOPAH trial were considered to be the benchmark until the publication of a recent NIAAA-sponsored multicenter trial. This study evaluated the efficacy and safety of treating patients with AH (MELD scores 20–35) with the IL-1 receptor antagonist, anakinra, plus zinc, or prednisone.[272] The trial was stopped early after a prespecified interim analysis showed that the prednisone group had higher 90-day overall survival (91% vs. 70%, $P = .0025$) than the anakinra plus zinc group. This is the first study evaluating glucocorticoids in severe AH that utilized the Lille stopping rules. The 90-day mortality of 30% in the anakinra plus zinc arm was as expected from recent trials, such as the STOPAH study (30% 90-day mortality). The 9% mortality is much better than ever previously achieved with glucocorticoids or any drug therapy. All other studies/meta-analyses have reported a moderate 1-month survival benefit with glucocorticoids, but none at later time points. These data need to be replicated, but they emphasize the importance of the stopping rule.

Thus, at the current time, one can utilize glucocorticoids in selected patients with severe AH.[273] One should apply early stopping rules at one week or even earlier (4 days) to ensure using glucocorticoids only in those patients who will benefit (Fig. 88.11). Clearly, new drugs are needed. New approaches also

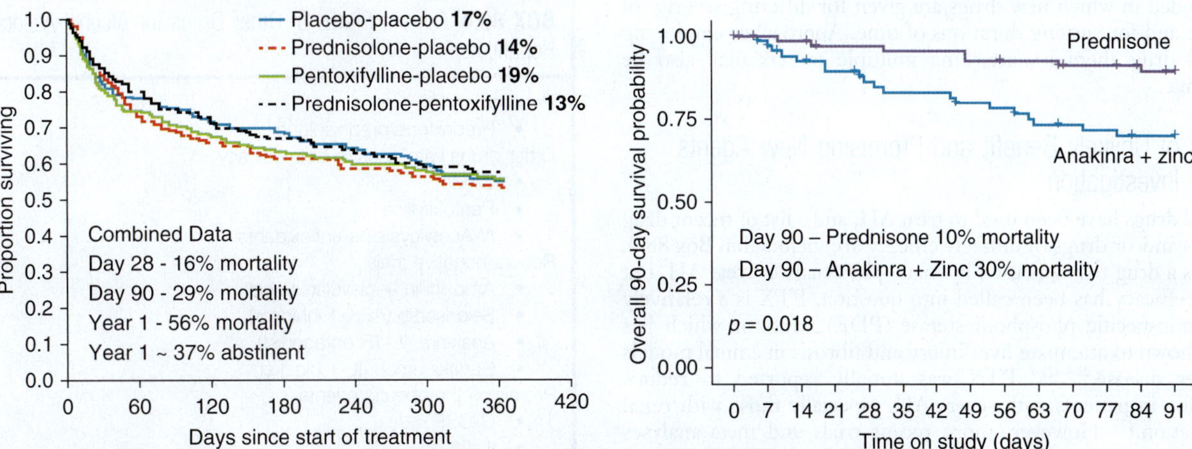

Fig. 88.10 The STOPAH trial and many recent studies show a 90-day mortality of approximately 30%. The recent AlcHepNet trial showed a 90-day mortality of only 10% with prednisolone therapy and use of the Lille stopping rule. (Left, from Thursz MR, Richardson P, Allison M, et al. Prednisolone or pentoxifylline for alcoholic hepatitis. *N Engl J Med*. 2015;372(17):1619–1628; Right, from Gawrieh S, Dasarathy S, Tu W, et al. Randomized trial of anakinra plus zinc vs. prednisone for severe alcohol-associated hepatitis. *J Hepatol*. 2024;80(5):684–693.)

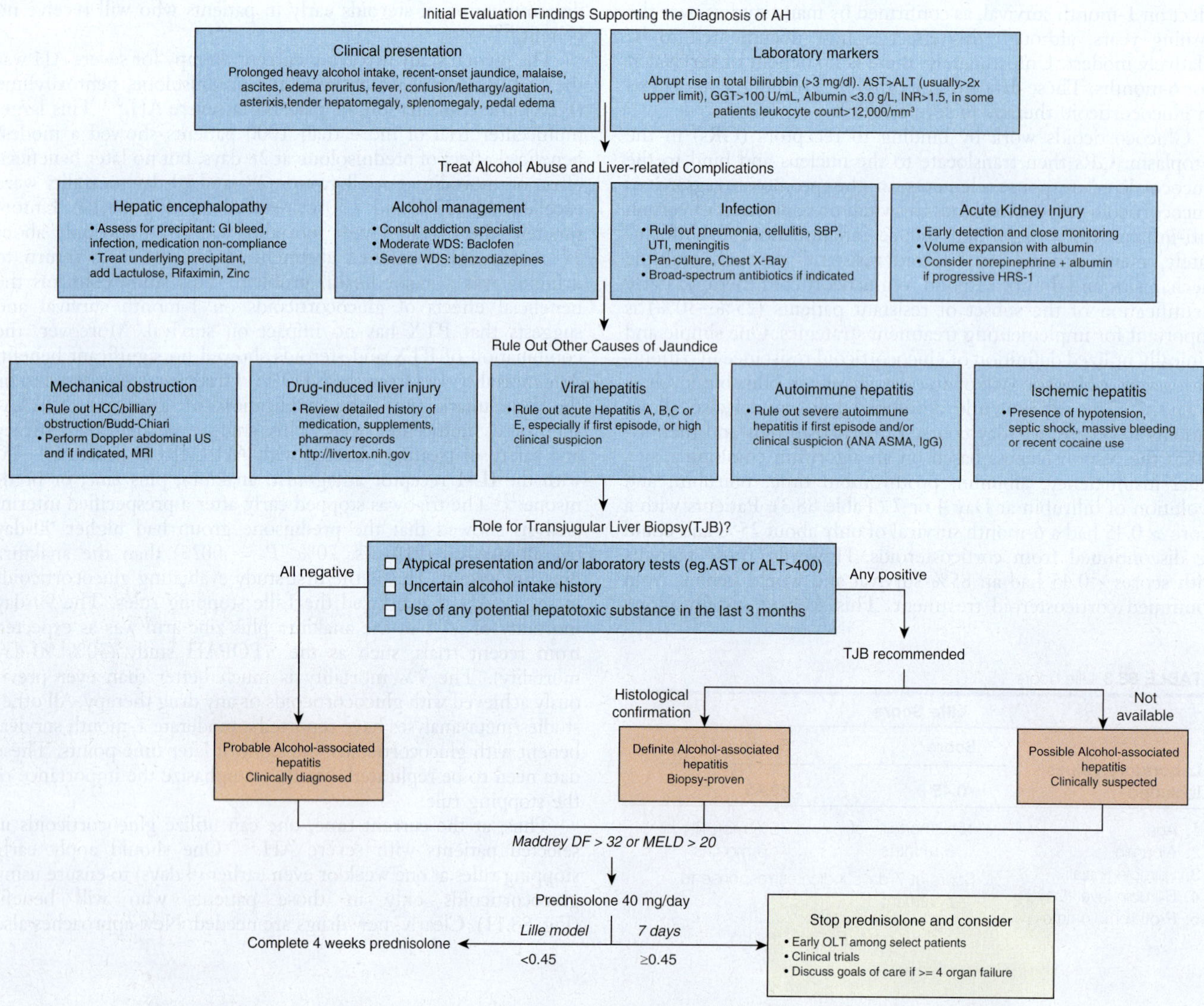
Initial Evaluation Findings Supporting the Diagnosis of AH
Clinical presentation
Prolonged heavy alcohol intake, recent-onset jaundice, malaise, ascites, edema pruritus, fever, confusion/lethargy/agitation, asterixis,tender hepatomegaly, splenomegaly, pedal edema
Laboratory markers
Abrupt rise in total bilirubbin (>3 mg/dl). AST>ALT (usually>2x upper limit), GGT>100 U/mL, Albumin <3.0 g/L, INR>1.5, in some patients leukocyte count>12,000/mm3
Treat Alcohol Abuse and Liver-related Complications
Hepatic encephalopathy
• Assess for precipitant: GI bleed, infection, medication non-compliance
• Treat underlying precipitant, add Lactulose, Rifaximin, Zinc
Alcohol management
• Consult addiction specialist
• Moderate WDS: Baclofen
• Severe WDS: benzodiazepines
Infection
• Rule out pneumonia, cellulitis, SBP, UTI, meningitis
• Pan-culture, Chest X-Ray
• Broad-spectrum antibiotics if indicated
Acute Kidney Injury
• Early detection and close monitoring
• Volume expansion with albumin
• Consider norepinephrine + albumin if progressive HRS-1
Rule Out Other Causes of Jaundice
Mechanical obstruction
• Rule out HCC/billiary obstruction/Budd-Chiari
• Perform Doppler abdominal US and if indicated, MRI
Drug-induced liver injury
• Review detailed history of medication, supplements, pharmacy records
• http://livertox.nih.gov
Viral hepatitis
• Rule out acute Hepatitis A, B,C or E, especially if first episode, or high clinical suspicion
Autoimmune hepatitis
• Rule out severe autoimmune hepatitis if first episode and/or clinical suspicion (ANA ASMA, IgG)
Ischemic hepatitis
• Presence of hypotension, septic shock, massive bleeding or recent cocaine use
Role for Transjugular Liver Biopsy(TJB)?
All negative
Atypical presentation and/or laboratory tests (eg.AST or ALT>400)
Uncertain alcohol intake history
Use of any potential hepatotoxic substance in the last 3 months
Any positive
TJB recommended
Histological confirmation
Not available
Probable Alcohol-associated hepatitis Clinically diagnosed
Definite Alcohol-associated hepatitis Biopsy-proven
Possible Alcohol-associated hepatitis Clinically suspected
Maddrey DF > 32 or MELD > 20
Prednisolone 40 mg/day
Lille model
7 days
Complete 4 weeks prednisolone
<0.45
≥0.45
Stop prednisolone and consider
• Early OLT among select patients
• Clinical trials
• Discuss goals of care if >= 4 organ failure

Fig. 88.11 Algorithm for diagnosis of alcohol use disorder (AUD) using Alcohol Use Disorders Identification Test (AUDIT) tool and management of early alcohol-associated liver disease (ALD).

are needed in which new drugs are given for differing severity of disease and for varying durations of time. Approaches employing several drug therapies attacking multiple targets may also be attractive.

Drugs of Unlikely Benefit and Promising New Agents Under Investigation

Several drugs have been used to treat AH, and a list of recent drug failures and/or drugs of unlikely efficacy are included in Box 88.4. PTX is a drug that was used by many physicians to treat AH, but whose efficacy has been called into question. PTX is a relatively weak nonspecific phosphodiesterase (PDE) inhibitor which has been shown to attenuate liver injury and fibrosis in animal models of liver disease.[274–276] PTX was initially reported to reduce mortality in patients with severe AH, especially those with renal dysfunction.[277] However, more recent trials and meta-analyses failed to show beneficial effects, and the large STOPAH trial showed no benefit of PTX.[271] A major disadvantage of PTX is that it is an oral drug that is taken three times a day. This is required for drug efficacy. Patients with AUD/ALD are well known to be noncompliant with medications. In a recent study, the compliance with PTX in severe AH patients was only 49%

BOX 88.4 Current Status of Other Drugs for Alcohol-Associated Hepatitis

Recommended drug
- Prednisone/prednisolone

Older drugs with questionable efficacy
- SAMe
- Pentoxifylline
- *N*-Acetylcysteine/antioxidants

Recent negative trials
- Amoxicillin + clavulanic acid
- Selonsertib (ASK-1 inhibitor)
- Anakinra (IL-1R antagonist)
- Canakinumab (IL-1 blocker)

Promising therapeutic agents
- G-CSF
- IL-22
- Fecal microbiota transplant
- DUR-928
- FGF-21
- GLP-1

over a 1-month treatment period.[94] Thus, while the concept of PDE inhibition in AH is likely reasonable, better medications with longer durations of action are required. *S*-adenosyl methionine is another drug that showed favorable results in one large trial in AC, but also requires strict t.i.d. therapy and there have been no major published follow-up studies.[278] Lastly, multiple studies have evaluated antioxidant cocktails and individual antioxidants in ALD/AH without benefit.[174,279] There are some data that IV *N*-acetylcysteine may be beneficial as an adjunct to corticosteroid therapy in AH. Indeed, this adjunct therapy was recommended in recent ACG guidelines, but further trials are necessary.[174] Multiple other agents, including androgenic steroids, propylthiouracil and specific antitumor necrosis factor therapy failed to show efficacy. Recent trials targeting the microbiome and IL-1 signaling have also yielded disappointing results.

Several agents have been used in human AH with some reported benefit. Initial trials of granulocyte colony-stimulating factor (G-CSF) showed promise in severe AH.[94] G-CSF is thought to stimulate liver regeneration and improve granulocyte function. Meta-analyses suggest a benefit of G-CSF in patients with severe AH. Interestingly, cumulative data have generally shown a beneficial effect of G-CSF in Asia, but not in Europe or the United States, for reasons that remain unclear.[174] IL-22 is a cytokine with antioxidant and antiapoptotic, antisteatotic and antimicrobial effects.[280] A Phase 2a study has been completed using the drug in patients with moderate and severe AH with good safety and some efficacy effects. Larsucosterol is an endogenous cholesterol derivative which has anti-inflammatory and epigenetic effects. A Phase 2a study showed safety and some efficacy signals and a Phase 2b trial has been completed.[281] GLP-1 agonists and FGF-21 are both in human trials for MASH, and both also appear to reduce alcohol intake in experimental animal models and anecdotally in humans.[282–286] Drugs that target both AUD and ALD are a novel and desirable approach. A nondrug therapy that has received much recent attention in severe AH is fecal transplantation, with very positive results in pilot studies.[278,279] Indeed, fecal transplant has been reported to improve survival in patients with severe AH and to decrease PSE and drinking behavior in patients with cirrhosis.[287] There is a strong link between drinking and the microbiome.[287] These findings are supported by findings from a pilot study of patients with moderate AH who were treated with the probiotic, LGG. Both MELD score and drinking behavior improved in treated subjects.[30]

Current Recommendations

Corticosteroid therapy can result in dramatic improvement in survival in carefully selected patients with severe AH.[225,288] Three factors limit their usefulness: (1) a number of patients are not candidates for therapy because of obvious contraindications (infection, GI bleeding); (2) a substantial portion of patients fail to respond; and, (3) corticosteroids have limited efficacy in patients with chronic renal failure or acute kidney injury and do not appear to prevent the development of hepatorenal syndrome. Therefore in patients who have contraindications to corticosteroid therapy or any degree of renal disease, aggressive standard medical care with attention to factors such as nutrition, infection, and adequate perfusion should be achieved, and opportunities for clinical trials on transplantation should be considered. Fig. 88.11 illustrates the factors that should be taken into account in patients with severe AH.

Specific Therapy for Treatments for Alcohol-Associated Cirrhosis

Abstinence is the only treatment that clearly improves survival in patients with alcoholic cirrhosis. All patients should also receive optimal inpatient and outpatient nutrition support. A variety of treatments for which there is a specific rationale have been investigated over the years. Examples include silymarin, SAM, betaine, colchicine, androgenic steroids, lecithin, vitamin E, and pentoxifylline. None has been shown to improve survival.[9,166] Patients should receive appropriate therapy for disease complications such as ascites or encephalopathy. Often overlooked and misunderstood is the important role of palliative care, which focuses on improving the quality of life of patients with life-limiting illness, as well as their caregivers.[289,290] Palliative care is applicable across the spectrum of cirrhosis, regardless of transplant eligibility. Palliative care is not synonymous with hospice care, which should be considered for patients who have comfort-oriented goals and a prognosis of 6 months or less.

Liver Transplantation

ALD is the most common indication for LT in the United States.[1,291] The outcome following LT is quite favorable (see also Chapter 99).[292]

Important factors that reduce survival after LT are concurrent HCV infection, smoking-related cancers, cardiovascular disease and a return to destructive patterns of drinking.[202,292–295] Although almost half of the transplant recipients drink some alcohol after the operation, very few return to destructive patterns of alcohol misuse.[296] A multidisciplinary approach both before and after the operation that includes addiction specialists, psychiatrists, and transplant professionals appears to offer the best opportunity for patients with ALD to achieve long term high quality of life after LT.[297,298]

Some patients with apparently advanced alcohol-associated cirrhosis can recover to the degree that transplantation is not required if they can abstain from drinking.[248] Because the benefits of abstinence can be dramatic in individual patients, requiring a period of abstinence before proceeding with transplantation is reasonable; however, if patients do not show evidence of significant recovery within 3 months, they are unlikely to survive without transplantation.[291] Referral to a transplant center at this time for further evaluation of their alcohol misuse and candidacy for transplantation, gives patients the best opportunity to be placed on the transplant waiting list after the “traditional six month abstinence period” required by some transplant centers and insurance companies. This “six-month rule” was initiated in 1997 to help ensure maximal hepatic recovery off alcohol and to document sobriety; however, this arbitrary time limit has not been shown to affect long-term survival or sobriety and most centers have adoped a much more personalized and less rigid approach.

It is important to be able to diagnose alcohol consumption accurately as part of the transplant evaluation process and following transplantation. As noted previously, various methods of history taking, unique biomarkers and wearable alcohol sensors have been proposed/used. Recent studies suggest that addiction experts may be better than hepatologists at uncovering alcohol intake posttransplantation,[299] again supporting a role for a team approach in diagnosis and follow-up. Moreover, the PEth level has been reported to be 100% specific and detects more than 90% of moderate-to-heavy drinkers and has been used to detect clandestine drinking post-LT.[2,300]

Patients with severe AH traditionally have not been considered to be appropriate candidates for LT because of recent drinking, the fear that they will return to drinking after the operation, and the assumption that many will recover with abstinence or appropriate medical therapy.[9,168,221] These assumptions were challenged by a multicenter French-Belgian study in which carefully selected patients with severe AH who failed to respond to corticosteroid therapy were shown to have a dramatic improvement in survival with early LT compared to matched controls (Fig. 88.12).[301] These initial results from Europe have

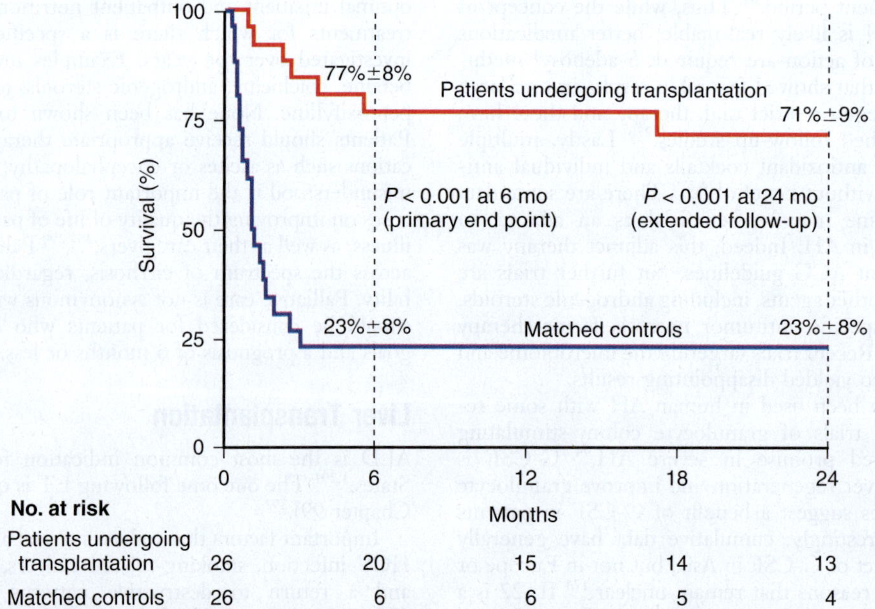

Fig. 88.12 Kaplan-Meier estimates of survival in patients with severe alcohol-associated hepatitis who failed glucocorticoid therapy and underwent early liver transplantation compared with matched controls who did not undergo liver transplantation. (From Mathurin P, Moreno C, Samuel D, et al. Early liver transplantation for severe alcoholic hepatitis. *N Engl J Med*. 2011;365(19):1790–1800, with permission.)

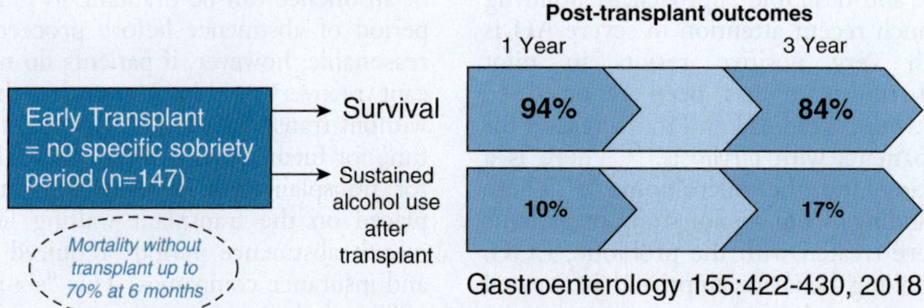

Fig. 88.13 Outcomes of early liver transplantation for patients with severe alcohol-associated hepatitis. (From Lee BP, Mehta N, Platt L, et al. Outcomes of early liver transplantation for patients with severe alcoholic hepatitis. *Gastroenterology*. 2018;155(2):422–430.e1.)

been replicated in a single center pilot program in the United States (100% survival at 6 months)[302] as well as in the ACCELERATE-AH study from the American Consortium of Early Liver Transplantation for Alcoholic Hepatitis—12 centers in 8 UNOS regions.[303] In that study, 1- and 3-year survival were excellent (94% and 84%, respectively), and sustained alcohol use was 17% at 3 years (Fig. 88.13).

Alcohol relapse appears to remain low in longer-term follow-up, although this is still a concern and major efforts are made to predict and prevent relapse.[3,4] Thus we are in an evolving era of LT in ALD, with likely expanded indications and better multidisciplinary approaches.

Optimal Management

Reducing the terrible morbidity and mortality associated with alcohol misuse will only occur if the global medical community makes a major commitment to early diagnosis of alcohol misuse. This will require systematic application of alcohol questionnaires at all points of entry into medical care. Government programs that provide frequent monitoring and swift, certain, and modest sanctions for violations also show promise in reducing arrests for repeat DUIs and domestic violence.[304]

For patients with stable cirrhosis, maintaining abstinence is the most important aspect of management, since there are no drugs that have been shown to improve survival. Nutritional support with evening snacks can be very beneficial. All should receive recommended vaccinations. In addition, they should undergo regular surveillance for HCC and screening for esophageal varices as appropriate(see Chapter 94). In addition, weight control and elimination of smoking are important adjuncts.

Hospitalized patients with AH or cirrhosis should have electrolyte disturbances and vitamin deficiencies corrected and withdrawal symptoms treated when present. During the first few days of admission the patient should be offered a nutritious diet if the mental status is adequate. Patients with severe AH should receive enteral feedings to ensure adequate calorie and protein intake. In patients with severe AH who do not have a systemic infection or gastrointestinal bleeding, a short course of glucocorticoid therapy should be considered. Transfer to a specialized liver/transplant center for participation in a clinical trial should be considered in selected patients, including those who are not candidates for glucocorticoid therapy. Given the extremely poor prognosis of patients hospitalized with multiple organ failure, palliative care teams should be involved within the first few days after admission to provide appropriate support for both patients and families.

LT is very effective in providing prolonged survival with excellent quality of life in carefully selected patients with alcohol-associated cirrhosis and, potentially, in patients with severe AH who fail to respond to medical therapy.

Full references for this chapter can be found at https://ebooks.health.elsevier.com.

KEY REFERENCES

30. Vatsalya V, Feng W, Kong M, et al. The beneficial effects of *Lactobacillus* GG therapy on liver and drinking assessments in patients with moderate alcohol-associated hepatitis. *Am J Gastroenterol.* 2023;118(8):1457–1460. https://doi.org/10.14309/ajg.0000000000002283.
173. Jophlin LL, Singal AK, Bataller R, et al. ACG clinical guideline: alcohol-associated liver disease. *Am J Gastroenterol.* 2024;119(1):30–54. https://doi.org/10.14309/ajg.0000000000002572.
177. Crabb DW, Bataller R, Chalasani NP, et al. Standard definitions and common data elements for clinical trials in patients with alcoholic hepatitis: recommendation from the NIAAA alcoholic hepatitis consortia. *Gastroenterology.* 2016;150(4):785–790. https://doi.org/10.1053/j.gastro.2016.02.042.
250. Shroff H, Gallagher H. Multidisciplinary care of alcohol-related liver disease and alcohol use disorder: a narrative review for hepatology and addiction clinicians. *Clin Ther.* 2023;45(12):1177–1188. https://doi.org/10.1016/j.clinthera.2023.09.016.
256. Plank LD, Gane EJ, Peng S, et al. Nocturnal nutritional supplementation improves total body protein status of patients with liver cirrhosis: a randomized 12-month trial. *Hepatology.* 2008;48(2):557–566. https://doi.org/10.1002/hep.22367 (Comparative Study Randomized Controlled Trial) (In eng).
264. Louvet A, Naveau S, Abdelnour M, et al. The Lille model: a new tool for therapeutic strategy in patients with severe alcoholic hepatitis treated with steroids. *Hepatology.* 2007;45(6):1348–1354. https://doi.org/10.1002/hep.21607 (In eng).
265. Thursz MR, Richardson P, Allison M, et al. Prednisolone or pentoxifylline for alcoholic hepatitis. *N Engl J Med.* 2015;372(17):1619–1628. https://doi.org/10.1056/NEJMoa1412278.
266. Gawrieh S, Dasarathy S, Tu W, et al. Randomized trial of anakinra plus zinc vs. prednisone for severe alcohol-associated hepatitis. *J Hepatol.* 2024;80(5):684–693. https://doi.org/10.1016/j.jhep.2024.01.031.
298. Lee BP, Mehta N, Platt L, et al. Outcomes of early liver transplantation for patients with severe alcoholic hepatitis. *Gastroenterology.* 2018;155(2):422–430.e1. https://doi.org/10.1053/j.gastro.2018.04.009.

89 Metabolic Dysfunction-Associated Steatotic Liver Disease/Nonalcoholic Fatty Liver Disease

Mary E. Rinella, Mazen Noureddin, Michael R. Charlton

IN THIS CHAPTER

ABBREVIATIONS

APRI aspartate aminotransferase-to-platelet ratio index
BMI body mass index
CAP controlled attenuation parameter
CI confidence interval
CVD cardiovascular disease
CPR clinical prediction rule
CSPH clinically significant portal hypertension
cT1 corrected T1
DNL de novo lipogenesis
ELF enhanced liver fibrosis panel
ER endoplasmic reticulum
FAST Fibroscan-aspartate aminotransferase score
FIB-4 fibrosis-4 index
GH growth hormone
GLP glucagon-like peptide
HCC hepatocellular carcinoma
HGP hepatic glucose production
HRT hormone replacement therapy
kPa kilopascals
LSM liver stiffness measurement
MASLD metabolic dysfunction-associated steatotic liver disease
MASH metabolic dysfunction-associated steatohepatitis
MetALD metabolic dysfunction and alcohol-associated liver disease
MEFIB MRE combined with FIB-4
MRE magnetic resonance elastography
MRI-PDFF magnetic resonance imaging–derived proton density fat fraction
NAFLD nonalcoholic fatty liver disease
NAS NAFLD activity score
NASH nonalcoholic steatohepatitis
NIT noninvasive test
NPV negative predictive value
OR odds ratio

PCOS polycystic ovarian syndrome
PDFF proton density fat fraction
PPAR peroxisomal proliferator-activated receptor
PPV positive predictive value
RYGB Roux-en-Y gastric bypass
RR relative risk
SGLT sodium-glucose cotransporter
SLD steatotic liver disease
T2DM type 2 diabetes mellitus
TZD thiazolidinedione
VAT visceral adipose tissue
VCTE vibration-controlled transient elastography

This chapter will review the epidemiology, pathophysiology, histology, diagnosis, and management of metabolic dysfunction-associated steatotic liver disease [metabolic dysfunction-associated steatotic liver disease (MASLD), formerly nonalcoholic fatty liver disease (NAFLD)]. Understanding of and approach to these areas is evolving rapidly. This is especially true of the recommended approach to screening for and evaluating MASLD, which has moved substantially toward decoupling the diagnosis from liver biopsy in most patients. Herein, we focus on aspects of MASLD that are best understood and are most relevant to the evaluation and management of this condition.

EVOLUTION OF NONALCOHOLIC FATTY LIVER DISEASE NOMENCLATURE

Since the term "NASH" was coined by Ludwig in 1980,[1] NAFLD has been used as an umbrella term for all hepatic histological manifestations of intrahepatic fat accumulation unrelated to alcohol use. The term encompassed a spectrum of disease ranging from isolated hepatic steatosis nonalcoholic fatty liver to nonalcoholic steatohepatitis (NASH) with or without progressive fibrosis. This terminology was used for decades with the understanding that the nomenclature and definition had important drawbacks. Namely, it was a diagnosis of exclusion that did not acknowledge the driving factors of the disease and allowed for significant heterogeneity. Further, the stigma associated with the use of the terms "nonalcoholic" and "fatty" in the name became increasingly evident. To address the drawbacks of the established nomenclature, a new nomenclature was developed using a global modified Delphi process. The process was led by the American Association for the Study of Liver Diseases and European Association for Study of the Liver with active collaboration from the Latin American-Association for the Study of the Liver, other gastroenterology, endocrine, and pediatric societies, patient advocacy groups, and content experts representing over 56 countries. The findings from this consensus process were published in 2023 and endorsed by numerous societies.[2–4] The new nomenclature is also intended to allow for the recognition of newly emerging disease subtypes, incorporating new knowledge and addressing the impact of disease heterogeneity, for example, the role of alcohol on the risk and presence of disease progression and response to therapy. The revised nomenclature for NAFLD is summarized in Box 89.1 and Fig. 89.1.

BOX 89.1 Disease definitions

1. **Steatotic liver disease (SLD)** is the broad umbrella term, under which metabolic dysfunction-associated steatotic liver disease (MASLD) (replacing NAFLD), MetALD (representing patients who meet criteria for MASLD but also consume 30–60 g/d of alcohol), and other subtypes, such as drug-induced SLD, genetic SLD (e.g., hypobetalipoproteinemia), and cryptogenic SLD (for those not meeting criteria for any other category) (Fig. 89.1).
2. **Metabolic dysfunction-associated steatotic liver disease (MASLD)** is defined as the presence of hepatic steatosis in an individual consuming less than 20g (females) or 30g (males) in addition to the presence of at least one cardiometabolic risk factor **(41).** If other specific causes of hepatic steatosis are present, they must be noted separately.[215]
3. Within MASLD, **metabolic steatohepatitis (MASH)** will replace NASH, characterized by the specific presence of hepatocellular injury (hepatocyte ballooning and inflammation) in the setting of steatosis and metabolic dysfunction-associated steatotic liver (MASL), in cases where steatosis is present without steatohepatitis, replacing NAFL (Fig. 89.1).

EPIDEMIOLOGY

MASLD (formerly NAFLD) is a condition in which excess lipid accumulates in the liver. It is the most common liver disease in the world.[5] The prevalence of MASLD and metabolic dysfunction-associated steatohepatitis (MASH) (formerly NASH) has been closely linked to the increasing prevalence of obesity and type 2 diabetes (T2DM), which began a sustained upward inflection in the 1970s. The current prevalence of MASLD (hepatic steatosis with or without inflammation and fibrosis) has been estimated to be 25%–30% overall globally.[5–7] The prevalence of MASLD varies widely, corresponding with the prevalence of obesity, metabolic syndrome, genetic risk factors, and social and cultural determinants.[8,9] In the United States, there are approximately 80 patients with MASLD undiagnosed for every patient diagnosed with the disease.[10] Hepatic steatosis was observed in 38% of American adults in a landmark prospective study of patients undergoing routine screening colonoscopy in Texas ($n = 664$), based on highly sensitive and specific magnetic resonance imaging–derived proton density fat fraction (MRI-PDFF).[11] This study, in which biopsies were performed in most patients with increased hepatic fat content/hepatic steatosis on MRI-PDFF, found steatohepatitis in 14%, with significant (stage $\geq$2) fibrosis (also known as at-risk MASH/NASH) in 5.9% of screened patients,[11]

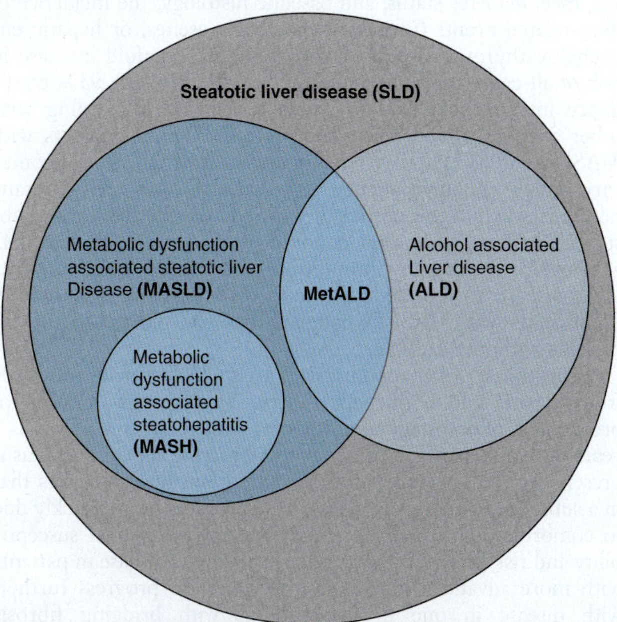

Fig. 89.1 Revised nomenclature of NAFLD: steatotic liver disease.

corresponding to a prevalence of steatohepatitis of 37% in those with MASLD overall. The prevalence of MASLD is much higher among patients with T2DM and metabolic syndrome (>6% for both),[12] with T2DM also being an important predictor of progression of fibrosis.[13] MASLD can also occur in the presence of normal body mass index (BMI) (lean MASLD, <25 kg/m^2 in non-Asian or <23 kg/m^2 in Asian cohorts). The prevalence of lean patients with MASLD is higher in Asian communities and overall varies from 4% to 19%, depending on the study (~4%) and in Asia (~10%).[14–16] Based on the lower, stable prevalence of lean patients with MASLD, this subset of disease is likely to be on the basis of one or more distinct pathophysiologies, for example, genetic susceptibility factors.

The prevalence of MASLD with advanced fibrosis (bridging fibrosis and cirrhosis) has increased in parallel with the increase in obesity and MASLD.[17] The current prevalence of bridging fibrosis and cirrhosis has been estimated to be 0.3%–2.4% (0.6–5 million adults) in the United States, with the prevalence of decompensated cirrhosis being 0.02%–0.04% (50,000–100,000 adults).[17] The prevalence of advanced disease is expected to more than double by 2030.[17] In the context of an accelerating prevalence of BMI >30 kg/m^2 in the United States and Western Europe during the COVID pandemic, these estimates may be conservative.[18]

Understanding of the natural history of MASLD has increased substantially in recent years with the availability of data from longitudinal, often prospective, analyses. One of the most important contributions has been that of the prospective National Institutes of Health-sponsored NASH Clinical Research Network (NASH-CRN), which included 1773 adults with MASLD who were followed for a median of 4 years.[19] As nearly all the liver-related events, including MASLD, occur in patients with advanced fibrosis (cirrhosis and, to a much lesser extent, bridging fibrosis), understanding the frequency of and factors that predict progression to bridging fibrosis and cirrhosis is critical. In the NASH-CRN study, the incidence of liver-related complications per 100 person-years increased 8–30-fold with fibrosis stage (F0–F2 vs. F3 vs. F4). Patients with cirrhosis also had a higher incidence of T2DM (7.53 vs. 4.45 events per 100 person-years) and a decrease of more than 40% in the estimated glomerular filtration rate (2.98 vs. 0.97 events per 100 person-years). Importantly, the incidences of the most common causes of death (cardiac events and nonhepatic cancers) were similar across fibrosis stages. In multivariate analysis, after adjustment for age, sex, race, diabetes status, and baseline histology, the incidence of liver-related events (variceal hemorrhage, ascites, or hepatic encephalopathy) was associated with a nearly sevenfold increase in risk of all-cause mortality (adjusted hazard ratio, 6.8; 95% confidence interval, 2.2–21.3).[19] These results are in keeping with other analyses of morbidity and mortality among patients with MASLD and MASH.[20–22] The natural history and clinical course vary widely among patients with MASLD and are generally nonlinear. While the impact of MASLD on the liver is of substantial interest, comorbid conditions associated with MASLD account for the greatest proportion of morbidity and mortality. Liver disease is only the fourth most common cause of mortality for patients with MASLD, compared to 12th most common for patients without MASLD.[23]

Progression of hepatic fibrosis is a key risk factor for mortality from hepatic and nonhepatic causes. The average duration of progression of one stage of fibrosis for patients with MASLD is 7 years if steatohepatitis is present and 14 years if hepatic steatosis is present without steatohepatitis. An important observation is that in a subset of patients, the disease may progress more quickly due to comorbidities as well as genetic and environmental susceptibility and risk factors.[24] Perhaps unsurprisingly, disease in patients with more advanced fibrosis is most likely to progress further, with disease in one in five patients with bridging fibrosis progressing to cirrhosis and one in five patients with cirrhosis experiencing a liver-related clinical event in <3 years.[25]

Although fibrosis is, by far, the most important determinant of clinical events and portal hypertension, lipotoxicity and inflammation (steatohepatitis) are drivers for fibrosis. While liver biopsies and histological assessments are waning as diagnostic and treatment response tools, prospective longitudinal studies of histology have revealed that patients with steatohepatitis and at least fibrosis stage 2 are at substantial risk of disease progression to liver-related events and overall mortality.[21,26] Further, those defined as "at-risk" NASH/MASH [NAFLD activity score (NAS) ≥4 and fibrosis ≥F2] are at increased risk of liver-related events. MASH, for example, is the most rapidly increasing cause of cirrhosis leading to hepatocellular carcinoma (HCC).[27] While the risk of liver-related events is heavily associated with more advanced fibrosis stages (≥2), all grades and stages of MASLD, including possibly simple steatosis, are associated with increased risk of liver-related mortality and liver cancer.[22]

PATHOGENESIS

An understanding of the pathogenesis of MASLD is essential in developing and applying rational approaches to diagnosis and management. At its core, MASLD and MASH are characterized by the net accumulation of intrahepatic lipids, typically in the context of chronic excessive caloric intake (Fig. 89.2). The consequent inflammatory and progressive fibrotic responses that occur in an important minority of patients with MASLD[17] depends on the net effect of a host of susceptibility and protective factors. Genetics, nutritional content, the microbiome, societal, and behavioral factors all contribute to susceptibility and protection. In addition, the histological and clinical course of MASLD can be influenced by concomitant endocrine comorbidities.

Nutritional Factors

Chronic caloric excess and insulin resistance are hallmarks of MASLD, with variation in the duration and degree of elevation in BMI required before the development of MASLD. Patients of Asian ethnicity, for example, are more susceptible to MASLD at lower BMIs (lean MASLD) than are patients of African or European ethnicities.[28] Susceptible BMI thresholds for MASLD are 25 kg/m^2 for White and 23 kg/m^2 for Asian populations. The accumulation of peripheral and visceral adipose tissue results in increased systemic levels of TNF-alpha and IL-6 and decreased adiponectin levels,[29] with a net effect of a proinflammatory, insulin-resistant state. Insulin resistance, contributed to by cytokines and reduced density of GLUT-4 receptors at the adipocyte cell surface (as they expand with increasing intracellular lipid content), is associated with increased adipocyte release of free fatty acids (FFA), with hepatic uptake of a proportion of FFAs.[30]

Hepatic steatosis, a primary characteristic of MASLD, is caused by the net accumulation of intrahepatic lipids, the combined effect of increased FFA uptake, increased de novo lipogenesis, and concomitant decreased hepatic lipid export, with a proportionately lower increase in hepatic oxidation of lipids. Increased circulating levels of glucose, fructose, and insulin mediate activation of carbohydrate and sterol regulatory-element binding proteins (ChREBP and SREBP-1), the master regulators of hepatic de novo lipogenesis in MASLD.[31] The inevitable increase in circulating insulin levels that occurs with overnutrition, particularly of carbohydrates, decreases hepatic synthesis of apolipoprotein B-100, a rate-determining factor in hepatic lipid export.[32] Approximately 85% of hepatic lipids are derived from increased FFA uptake (~60%) and de novo lipogenesis (~25%).[33] Whereas triglyceride accumulation is sufficient to

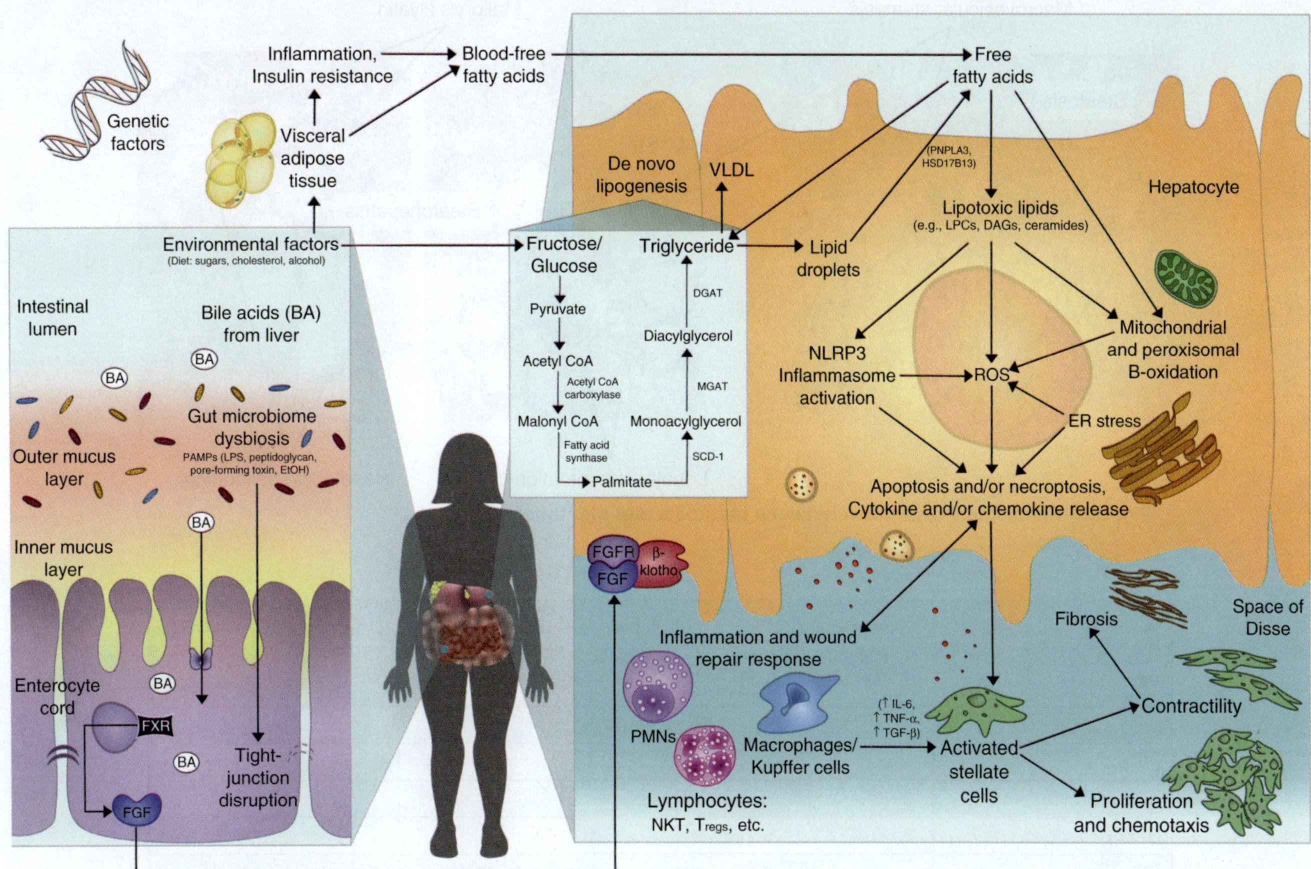

Fig. 89.2 Pathogenesis of MASLD.

cause hepatic steatosis, triglycerides are not inherently lipotoxic. In contrast, dietary cholesterol and saturated fats are important causes of cell injury and fibroinflammatory response and are a prerequisite of nutrition-based animal models of fibrosing MASLD.[34] Hepatic lipotoxicity, characterized by the accumulation of reactive oxygen species, oxidative mitochondrial injury, and unfolded protein response, results in programmed cell death, TNF-alpha activation, and recruitment of resident macrophages (Kupffer cells), hepatocellular injury, and stellate cell activation, with subsequent fibrosis.[35]

Genetic Factors

Genetic heterogeneity is an increasingly recognized important mediator of variance in severity of inflammation and fibrosis progression in MASLD. Among the host of genetic polymorphisms associated with histological phenotype in MASLD, genotypes of *PNPLA3*, *HSD17B13*, *TM6SF2*, and *MBOAT7*, all of which affect lipid metabolism, play important roles in the severity and progression of liver disease.[36–38] Prevalent loss-of-function variants in *HSD17B13*, an enzyme that localizes to hepatic lipid droplets, have been linked to ~35% lower risk of cirrhosis and HCC.[38] Much of the risk of progression of MASLD associated with genetic variants is determined by and/or can be attenuated by the intake of nutritional substrates.[39,40] PNPLA3 rs738409 is not associated with increased fibroinflammatory biomarkers in lean individuals with MASLD.[41] In a multivariate analysis of the interaction between PNPLA3 rs738409 genotype and micro- and macronutrient intake among at risk (BMI $\geq$ 25 kg/m^2) individuals, high-carbohydrate intake was associated with *increased* risk of hepatic fibrosis (fibrosis stage $\geq$2). In contrast, higher intake of *n*-3 polyunsaturated fatty acids (g/d) (Adj. OR: 0.17, $P < .01$), isoflavones (mg/d) (Adj. OR: 0.74, P=0.049), methionine (mg/d) (Adj. OR: 0.32, $P < .01$), and choline (mg/d) (Adj. OR: 0.32, $P < .01$) was associated with *decreased* risk of significant fibrosis.[40] The interaction among nutrients, genes, and fibroinflammatory pathways has important implications for nutritional counseling in patients with MASLD (Fig. 89.2).

HISTOPATHOLOGY

MASH (previously NASH) has long been histologically distinguished from isolated hepatic steatosis by the presence of ballooned hepatocytes and lobular inflammation in the context of macrovesicular hepatic steatosis (Fig. 89.3). The two most common composite diagnostic scoring systems are the NASH-CRN, commonly used in the United States, and the Steatosis, Activity, and Fibrosis score, commonly used in Europe.[42,43] Irrespective of the diagnostic scoring system used, description and quantification of steatosis, inflammatory activity, hepatocyte ballooning, and fibrosis should be included in liver pathology reports.[44] While patients' long-term outcomes are irrefutably linked to the extent of fibrosis, the presence of MASH and the extent of activity drive fibrosis progression.[45] Reflecting this, the two endpoints required for conditional FDA drug approval are (1) resolution of MASH, without worsening of fibrosis, and (2) improvement in fibrosis of $\geq$1 stage, without worsening of MASH. Use of these endpoints is challenging because of high rates of interobserver variability, especially with interpretation of hepatocyte ballooning, in the diagnosis of and resolution of MASH.[46] Fig. 89.3 illustrates variability in the appearance of ballooned cells that likely explains the discordance in histological interpretation. The requirement of

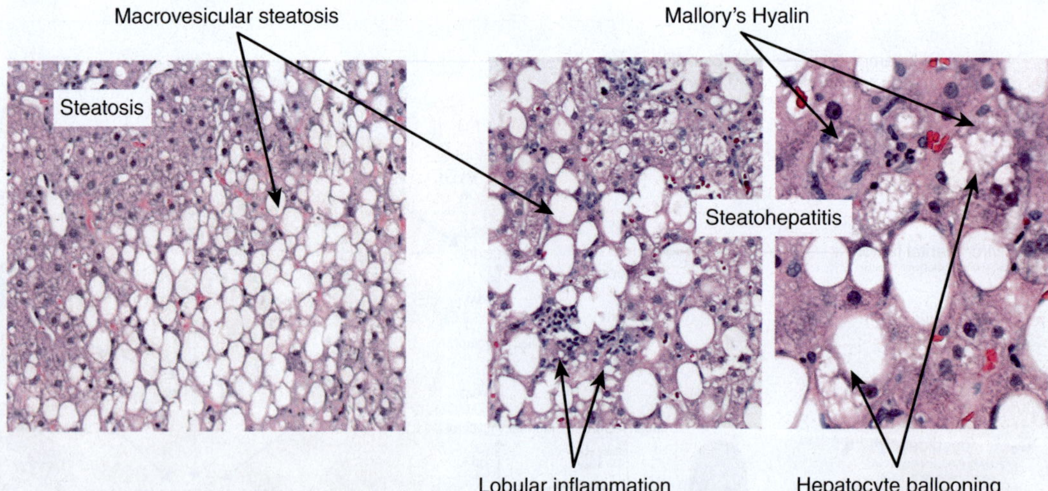

Fig. 89.3 Histological distinction between steatosis and steatohepatitis.

Noninvasive modality	Early disease (F0-1)/exclude advanced fibrosis	'Clinically significant fibrosis' or 'at risk' NASH (NAS≥4, F≥2)	Advanced fibrosis (F3-4)
		Blood based	
FIB4	X		
ELF			X
NIS2+		X	
Pro-C3			X
		Imaging	
Transient elastography	X		X
MRE	X		X
MRI cT1	X	X	
Ultrasound ARFI	X		X
		Combination tests	
FAST		X	X
MAST		X	X
MEFIB		X	
MASEF		X	
AGILE 3			X
AGILE 4			X
Liver histology, trichrome stain	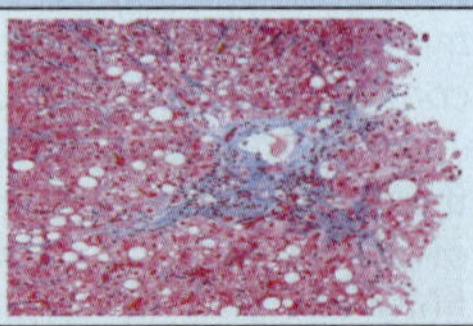	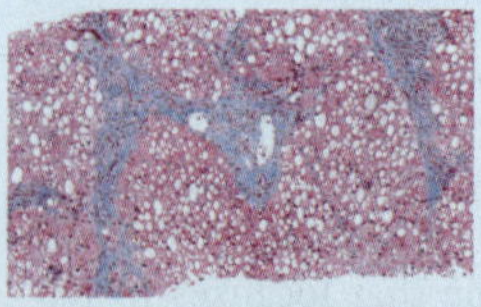	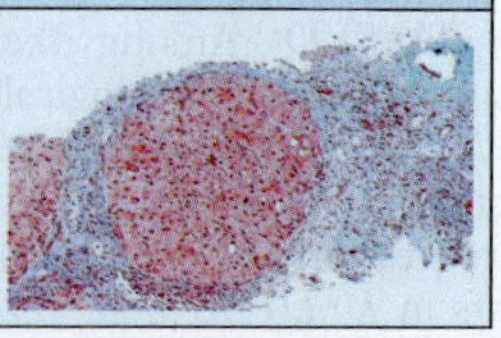

Fig. 89.4 Noninvasive assessment linked to histological fibrosis stage.

at least a 1-point improvement in fibrosis stage has also proved challenging, given the broad range of collagen content within a given stage, in particular stage 3 (bridging fibrosis) or stage 4 (cirrhosis) (Fig. 89.4). Use of artificial intelligence/machine learning and digital quantification of collagen content and distribution may provide the ability to assess disease improvement or progression on a linear scale.[47] Given the high prevalence of MASLD and the inherent limitations of liver biopsy, it is impractical to require liver biopsy to guide management. Use of noninvasive tests (NITs) as substitutes for liver biopsy is appealing. Although NITs can identify or exclude the presence of clinically significant fibrosis (>F2) with reasonable precision, NITs are less accurate in identifying steatohepatitis (*see noninvasive risk stratification and* Fig. 89.4).

COMORBID DISEASE ASSOCIATED WITH METABOLIC DYSFUNCTION-ASSOCIATED STEATOTIC LIVER DISEASE

Obesity

The prevalence of obesity (BMI > 30) has doubled in the United States over the last three decades and largely explains the rise in MASLD, which is four times more prevalent in patients with obesity and affects 80%–90% of patients who undergo bariatric surgery.[48] Indeed, high BMI and waist circumference predict the presence of MASH and advanced hepatic fibrosis.[49] Although obesity is highly associated with MASLD, a portion of MASLD patients are lean, and they present distinct challenges for evaluation and management.[50]

Cardiometabolic Disease

Cardiometabolic comorbidities such as those comprising the metabolic syndrome include abdominal obesity, elevated triglycerides (≥150 mg/dL), reduced high-density lipoprotein (HDL) cholesterol (<40 mg/dL in men and <50 mg/dL in women), elevated blood pressure (systolic ≥130 mmHg or diastolic ≥85 mmHg), and elevated fasting glucose (≥110 mg/dL).[51] The more components of metabolic syndrome there are, the more likely the diagnosis of MASLD is. For this reason, the definition of MASLD now includes metabolic parameters in the context of hepatic steatosis (Box 89.1). Conversely, it has been suggested that MASLD contributes to the development of the metabolic syndrome. An example is increased energy intake, which leads to fat accumulation in the liver, which, in turn, stimulates hepatic gluconeogenesis and initiates insulin resistance.[52]

Type 2 Diabetes

The prevalence of MASLD is patient with T2DM is estimated to be between 30% and 75%[85–87] and around 6%–19% of those with T2DM and MASLD have significant fibrosis.[53–57] In a prospective study[57] in adults aged ≥50 years with T2DM who were recruited from primary care or endocrinology clinics and completed MRI-PDFF, magnetic resonance elastography (MRE), or vibration-controlled transient elastography (VCTE) studies, the prevalence of MASLD was 65%, advanced fibrosis was 14%, and cirrhosis was 6%. In multivariable adjusted models, obesity and insulin use were each associated with increased odds of having advanced fibrosis (odds ratio 2.50; 95% CI 1.38–4.54; $P = .003$ and odds ratio 2.71; 95% CI 1.33–5.50; $P = .006$, respectively). In a population-based study of more than 330 patients with T2DM [90], the presence of MASLD was associated with a twofold increase in all-cause mortality over a mean follow-up period of 11 years. In another study using paired biopsies,[58] the development of T2DM was the strongest predictor of the progression of MASH and hepatic fibrosis. For these reasons, society guidances have recommended screening for the presence of clinically significant fibrosis in this high-risk population.[53,59,60] In addition to patients with T2DM, those with medically complicated obesity or a family history of MASH cirrhosis should undergo primary screening for the presence of advanced fibrosis.[59]

Cardiovascular Disease

The leading cause of death in patients with MASLD is cardiovascular disease (CVD), especially at early stages of steatotic liver disease.[61,62] MASLD has been associated with increases in coronary-artery calcium score, carotid artery intimal media thickness, and arterial wall stiffness.[63] MASLD has also been associated with increased severity of coronary artery disease in patients undergoing cardiac catheterization[64] and in patients with carotid atherosclerosis.[65] MASLD may adversely impact cardiovascular health through numerous mechanisms: MASLD and MASH are associated with an atherogenic lipid profile characterized by elevated triglycerides, low HDL, and increased levels of both total LDL and small dense LDL.[66] In this setting, de novo lipogenesis can increase production of highly atherogenic small dense LDL independent of BMI and insulin resistance.[67]

MASLD is associated with increased risk of atherosclerotic disease, arrhythmias (e.g., atrial fibrillation), and abnormalities in cardiac structure and function.[68–70] While studies of statin medications for the treatment of MASH revealed no histologic improvement in the liver abnormalities,[71] there is no evidence that statin use should be avoided in MASLD patients who have elevated CVD risk. Because of the substantial risk of CVD in patients with MASLD, statins, antihypertensives, and antiplatelet therapies should be utilized when indicated.[72]

Chronic Kidney Disease

MASLD and CKD are closely linked diseases that share numerous cardiometabolic risk factors: metabolic syndrome, T2DM, and obesity. These risk factors increase the risk of MASLD and CKD and exacerbate their severity. Accumulation of fructose and uric acid in the liver contributes to the development and progression of MASLD and CKD.[73,74] Oxidative stress, aging, and intestinal dysbiosis also play a role in the pathogenesis of MASLD and CKD.[74] Platelet activation, regulated by oxidative stress and dyslipidemia, is a key player in the inflammatory pathways that interconnect MASLD and CKD.[75] These mechanisms contribute to end-organ damage and accentuate the burden of both diseases.

Furthermore, the prevalence and severity of CKD positively correlate with increased severity of MASLD, even after adjusting for confounding features.[76,77] In patients with cirrhosis, the progressively higher prevalence of CKD, which is correlated with MASLD severity, becomes a special burden, for whom liver transplantation is often lifesaving.[78] However, preliver transplantation CKD is associated with postliver transplantation mortality, thus highlighting the importance of understanding and appropriately managing CKD in patients with MASLD. Studies of the impact of MASLD on prognosis and adverse clinical outcomes in patients with CKD have yielded conflicting results.[79]

Obstructive Sleep Apnea

There is an increased hepatic fat content in patients with obstructive sleep apnea (OSA), independent of BMI. Also, chronic intermittent hypoxia, a hallmark feature of OSA, has been associated with increased hepatic fibrosis.[80] Findings from animal models suggest that hypoxia can drive fat accumulation and inflammation in the liver via multiple pathways. Hypoxia can increase fasting glucose and systemic triglyceride levels and induce hepatic lipogenesis by altering gene expression. Hypoxia can also increase oxidative stress and reduce β-oxidation, leading to the production of lipotoxic lipids. These hypoxia-induced changes are typically more pronounced in obese subjects than in nonobese subjects. Despite the adverse metabolic effects of OSA-induced hypoxia in the setting of MASLD, preliminary short-term studies have failed to show an association between treatment of OSA with continuous positive airway pressure and improvement in MASLD.[81,82] Larger, long-term prospective trials may help clarify this uncertainty.

ROLE OF SELECTED ENDOCRINOPATHIES

MASLD is associated with a host of endocrine comorbidities. Although identifying causal relationships between individual endocrinopathies and the histological features of MASLD is difficult, endocrine dysregulation can play important roles in the pathophysiology and management of MASLD.

Growth Hormone

Growth hormone is produced by the anterior pituitary gland, stimulating production of insulin-like growth factor-1, reducing visceral and peripheral fat, decreasing lipogenesis, improving insulin sensitivity, and promoting senescence of hepatic stellate cells.[83] Decreases in growth hormone promote increases in visceral adiposity, insulin resistance, and intrahepatic fat accumulation.[84] However, excessive growth hormone is neutral with respect to risk of hepatic steatosis.

There is evidence that individuals with growth hormone deficiency are at increased risk of MASLD.[83,85–87] Thus patients with Alström syndrome, a rare monogenic disease associated with functional growth hormone deficiency, may result in MASH with progressive fibrosis and the metabolic features of MASLD.[88] The liver and metabolic features of Alström syndrome have been reversed by exogenous growth hormone supplementation.[87,89] Deficiency of growth hormone in association with panhypopituitarism can lead to MASLD cirrhosis in the second or third decade of life.[90]

Thyroid Hormone

The liver is profoundly affected by the thyroid hormone axis via thyroid hormone receptor isoforms—α and ß (THRα, THRß), with THRß being the more prevalent isoform in the liver. Thyroid hormones, via the interaction of thyroxine with THRß, stimulate LDL receptor uptake, increase fatty acid oxidation, stimulate mitophagy, and mitochondrial biogenesis.[91,92] In addition to the metabolic effects of THRß activation, the liver is also a conversion site of thyroxine (T4) to triiodothyronine (T3), and it synthesizes thyroxine carrier proteins, thyroxine-binding globulin, transthyretin, and albumin.[93,94]

While there are negative studies,[95] the preponderance of the literature investigating the association between thyroid dysregulation and development of MASLD has reported a positive association between hypothyroidism and risk of MASLD. Supportive findings include correlations between lower T4 and higher TSH levels with more severe MASLD[96] and correlations between MASLD and T4, TSH, and free T3 alone.[97–99] While the link between the thyroid axis and MASLD is complicated by the association of hypothyroidism with increased BMI,[100] biopsy-based studies examining the relationship between hypothyroidism and MASLD have observed a consistent, positive association, including an association between hypothyroidism and more advanced hepatic fibrosis.[101–104] At a tissue level, there is an inverse correlation of THRß mRNA levels with components of the NAS score.[104] Perhaps the strongest indication of a role of the thyroid hormone signaling in MASLD comes from late-stage clinical trials: resmetirom, a THRß agonist with several-fold greater selectivity for THRß than for T3, in a phase 3 clinical trial of more than 950 patients with biopsy-confirmed fibrosing MASH, achieved both primary endpoints, specifically, improvement of at least one stage in fibrosis without worsening of MASH and MASH resolution with ≥2-point NAS reduction with no worsening of fibrosis ($P < .0001$ at both doses). Resmetirom was also associated with potentially clinically meaningful LDL lowering ($P < .0001$) and multiple positive effects on MASH biomarkers and imaging.[105] Based on the results of the phase 3 study, resmetirom was granted accelerated approval by the Food and Drug Administration for treatment of adults with noncirrhotic MASH with moderate to advanced liver fibrosis (consistent with stages F2 to F3 fibrosis). Patient selection and monitoring for disease response were subsequently proposed by expert consensus panel.[261] Verification and description of clinical benefit is ongoing in confirmatory trials.

A phase 2 multicenter, imaging-based study in men with T2DM and hepatic steatosis reported improvement in hepatic steatosis with low doses of levothyroxine,[106] and treatment of hypothyroidism, including subclinical disease, reportedly improved facets of MASLD.[107]

Although recent guidance from the American Association of Clinical Endocrinology does not recommend screening for MASLD in hypothyroidism, testing for hypothyroidism in patients with poorly controlled or progressing MASH is reasonable, especially if symptoms of hypothyroidism are present.

As thyrotoxicosis can cause liver injury, possibly via reactive oxidative species generated by hypermetabolism,[93] it will be important to monitor longer term effects of THRß agonism on hepatic health.

Sex Hormones in Men

Androgens play an important role in hepatic lipid metabolism and content.[108–110] Physiologic levels of androgens protect against obesity and insulin resistance (features of the metabolic syndrome) and MASLD.[111] Men with MASLD have lower mean testosterone levels than do men without MASLD, and low testosterone levels are independently associated with risk of MASLD.[112–119] Androgen deficiency, for example, through androgen receptor knockout, is associated with development of hepatic steatosis, accelerated weight gain, insulin resistance, and impaired glucose tolerance.[120–122] Exogenous supplementation of testosterone decreases hepatic lipid content.[123] Determination of primary and secondary effects of androgens on MASLD is complicated.[124] Men with idiopathic hypogonadotropic hypogonadism have a high prevalence of hepatic steatosis, which may be secondary to increased BMI,[125] and diet-induced obesity in a murine model of MASLD lowers testicular mass and decreases testicular testosterone,[126] suggesting lower terstosterone levels in MASLD may be a secondary event.

Studies reporting the effects of hypogonadism on MASLD in humans are few. In animal studies, before developing obesity, castrated mice had increased hepatic expression and synthesis of de novo lipogenesis genes, which decrease with testosterone restoration.[127] This observation suggests a causative link between androgen deficiency and MASLD.

Male Androgen Supplementation

Despite some favorable effects on hepatic lipid metabolism and body composition, androgenic and anabolic steroids, and in particular the C-17α alkylated testosterones, have been implicated in four distinct forms of liver injury: transient serum enzyme elevations, an acute cholestatic syndrome "bland cholestasis," chronic vascular injury to the liver (peliosis hepatis), and hepatic tumors, including adenomas and HCC.[128–133]

In contrast to the effects of androgen replacement in hypogonadal men, androgen deprivation induced by the treatment of prostate cancer is associated with weight gain and increased prevalence of MASLD.[134,135] Collectively, these findings suggest that the association between lower testosterone and MASLD is mediated by the presence of metabolic risk factors for MASLD, including obesity and insulin resistance, although testosterone levels may also have a direct effect on intrahepatic triglyceride handling. Screening for low testosterone is not recommended for patients with MASLD in the absence of signs or symptoms of hypogonadism, for example, decreased libido. Glucagon-like peptide-1 receptor agonist therapy with semaglutide in the setting of low testosterone has been associated with increasing androgen levels, possibly mediated by weight loss.[136]

Sex Hormones in Women

Unlike the case in men, androgens are associated with disease progression of MASLD in women. Estrogens have a well-established cardiovascular protective effect, and they decrease the incidence and severity of the metabolic syndrome.[137,138] Estrogen deficiency is associated with an increased risk of hepatic steatosis.[139] Elevated androgen levels, as seen in polycystic ovary syndrome, are also associated with increased risk of MASLD, insulin resistance, and obesity.[140–142] Estrogen treatment has decreased hepatic triglyceride content,[143,144] and physiological estrogen deficiency in postmenopausal women has been associated with an increased prevalence of MASLD.[145–147]

Estrogens are key regulators of hepatic lipid metabolism, inhibiting lipogenesis and lipid uptake.[110] Hypogonadism in women upregulates hepatic de novo lipogenesis, resulting in hepatic steatosis.[110] Estrogen replacement therapy in postmenopausal women results in a lower prevalence of MASLD, decreased prevalence and severity of metabolic syndrome, improved elevated liver enzymes, and insulin resistance.[148,149]

Treatment with tamoxifen or nonsteroidal aromatase inhibitors, for example, anastrozole and letrozole, is associated with increased prevalence of hepatic steatosis,[150] possibly through increased de novo lipogenesis due to estrogen inhibition and reduced hepatic mitochondrial beta-oxidation.[151] Serial monitoring of serum liver enzymes is recommended in patients receiving tamoxifen.[152]

HEPATOCELLULAR CARCINOMA

HCC is experiencing a significant global shift (see Chapter 98). Studies in Europe support the growing importance of MASLD as a leading cause of HCC, now accounting for 12%–29% of cases in the 2010s.[153] Italy and Asia are witnessing similar trends, with MASLD projected to become the primary cause of HCC in Italy by 2023.[154,155] South America also reflects this shift, where MASLD has emerged as the main cause of liver disease in HCC cases, now accounting for 37% of cases.[156,157]

The rise of MASLD-related HCC has made it the leading indication of HCC-related liver transplantation.[158] Global trends indicate a growing incidence of primary liver cancer due to MASLD, particularly in older age groups.[159]

Factors influencing the development of HCC in the context of MASLD include the tissue and immune microenvironment, genetic variances related to PNPLA3, HSD17B13, and other genes, and the microbiome.[160–162] MASLD-HCC exhibits distinct molecular and immune characteristics and affects both men and women equally. Overall outcomes in treating MASLD-HCC are similar to those of patients with other etiologies of liver disease.[163]

EXTRAHEPATIC MALIGNANCY

MASLD is also associated with an increased risk of extrahepatic malignancies, including those of the colon, esophagus, stomach, pancreas, kidney, and breast, which are collectively the second leading cause of death in patients with MASLD.[164] Several large population-based studies, primarily from Asia, have found that MASLD is associated with an increased risk of colorectal neoplasms, with a 1.5–1.7-fold increased risk for colonic adenomas and a 1.9–3.1-fold increased risk for colorectal cancer.[165–167]

A population-based study that included 2224 incident cancers found that MASLD is associated with a 90% higher risk of malignancy, with the highest increase in liver cancer (IRR = 2.8; 95% CI, 1.6–5.1), uterine cancer (IRR = 2.3; 95% CI, 1.4–4.1), stomach cancer (IRR = 2.3; 95% CI, 1.3–4.1), pancreatic cancer (IRR = 2.0; 95% CI, 1.2–3.3), and colon cancer (IRR = 1.8; 95% CI, 1.1–2.8).[168]

A recent meta-analysis that included 10 cohort studies with 182,202 middle-aged individuals (24.8% with MASLD) and 8485 incident cases of extrahepatic cancers, with a median follow-up of 5.8 years, found that MASLD is associated with a nearly 1.5–2-fold increased risk of developing gastrointestinal cancers (esophageal, gastric, pancreatic, or colorectal).[169] MASLD is also associated with an approximately 1.2–1.5-fold increased risk of developing lung, breast, gynecological, or urinary system cancers.[164]

Whereas altered screening practices for cancers specific to MASLD are not recommended (except for HCC in MASLD cirrhosis), healthcare providers should adhere to recommended screening and remain vigilant for signs and symptoms of malignancies, particularly in those who have risk factors such as obesity, diabetes, or advanced hepatic fibrosis.

NONINVASIVE ASSESSMENT

Liver biopsy has traditionally been the reference standard for diagnosing MASH. However, due to the invasiveness, risk of complications, cost, and limited availability of liver biopsy, NITs have been developed for diagnosing and monitoring the stages of NAFLD.[170] NITs are derived from three sources: blood-based, demographic (e.g., age or BMI), imaging-based or combinations thereof. Blood-based tests can be further divided into simple scores, which use routine laboratory tests, and proprietary scores, which use complex algorithms and/or proprietary biomarkers (Fig. 89.4).[171] Imaging-based NITs include ultrasound-based methods, such as transient elastography and MRI-based methods. The latter include MRE and PDFF measurement.[171]

It is critical to identify patients with established or high risk for advanced fibrosis (e.g., at risk MASH) as these are the patients at highest risk for adverse liver outcomes. Thus the identification of such patients is an important focus of biomarker development. Combinations that use multiple biomarkers (serum and/or imaging) with or without clinical variables to predict the presence of MASH and significant fibrosis, which is the target group for pharmacological therapies in MASH trials, are becoming increasingly used. While there are numerous NITs under development, here we will focus on those that are the most validated or promising.

Blood-Based Biomarkers

Fibrosis-4 Index

Fibrosis-4 index (FIB-4) is the best studied and validated biomarker for the identification and exclusion of advanced fibrosis. It is widely accessible since it is calculated from routine blood tests; aspartate aminotransferase (AST), alanine aminotransferase (ALT), platelet count, and age.[171,172] Thus it is recommended by several professional societies for the initial assessment of the patient with confirmed or suspected steatosis for risk stratification.[172,173]

The strength of FIB-4 is mostly in its negative predictive value (NPV). Values <1.3 rule out advanced fibrosis in most, whereas values ≥ 2.67 can be used to identify individuals likely to have advanced fibrosis.[173] Patients whose values fall between these 2 cutoff values (indeterminate zone) should undergo secondary testing, such as transient elastography or the enhanced liver fibrosis (ELF) test for further evaluation[172,173] (Fig. 89.5). Paradoxically, in patients with T2DM, who are at highest risk of

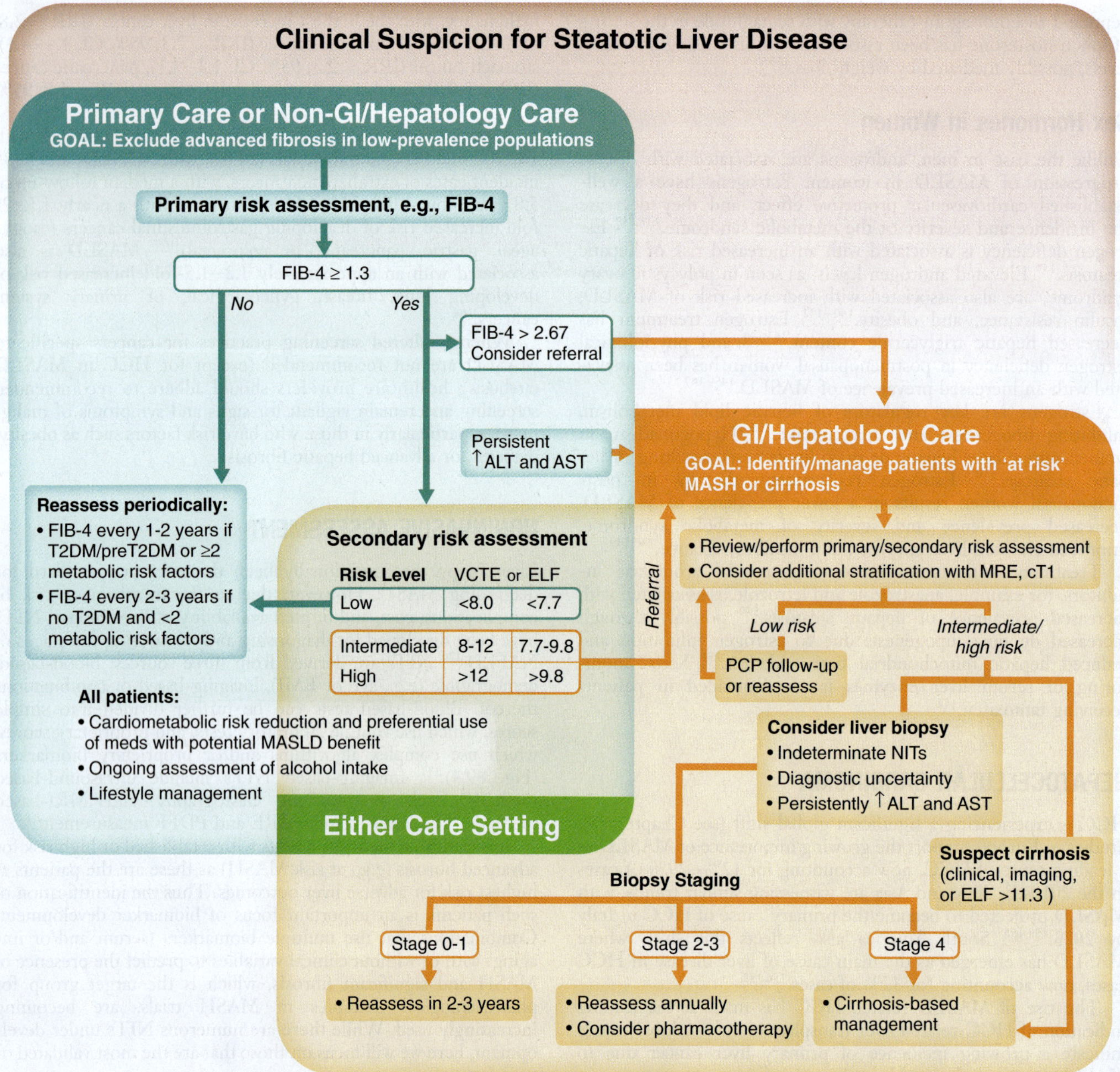

Fig. 89.5 Algorithm for risk stratification. (From Kanwal et al. *Hepatology*; modified from Rinella et al. *Hepatology*. 2023.)

disease progression, the accuracy of FIB-4 is diminished, likely necessitating lower cutoffs in the future, once more data are available. In older age groups, a higher cutoff is required (>2.0, rather than 1.3) as FIB-4 can increase with age independent of aminotransferase levels or platelet count. FIB-4 is not well validated and is not helpful in individuals <35 years of age[174] (Fig. 89.5).

Increasing FIB-4 index may reflect progression of fibrosis, and FIB-4 can predict the occurrence of adverse clinical liver events and disease progression.[175] While FIB-4 is a valuable, noninvasive test for diagnosing the stages of MASLD,[176] caution is needed in interpreting the results and considering follow-up testing.

The Enhanced Liver Fibrosis (ELF) Test

The ELF test is a noninvasive biomarker derived from three markers of fibrogenesis (N-terminal propeptide of type III procollagen, hyaluronic acid, and tissue inhibitor of metalloproteinase-1).[171] In a systematic review and meta-analysis published in 2020 by Vali et al.,[177] largely including studies in populations with a high prevalence of advanced, the ELF test had a sensitivity of 0.93 (95% CI 0.98) for excluding fibrosis at a low cut-off value of 7.7, but the specificity is limited. At a high cut-off value of 9.8, the specificity can be raised to 0.86 (95% CI 0.92), although the sensitivity is lowered. The ELF test's performance can vary based on the prevalence of the target population.

The ELF test can also identify patients at increased risk of progression of MASH to cirrhosis and the development of liver-related adverse events. A score of ≥11.3 is associated with a fivefold increased risk of liver-related events. In contrast, a cutoff value of <9.8 has a high NPV (90%) for excluding liver-related adverse events within 1 year.[178] Though further work is needed, the ELF test may have a role as a dynamic biomarker, such that it can reflect change in response to therapeutic interventions.[176,179]

The test has been approved in the United States for use as a prognostic tool for MASH patients with advanced fibrosis.

Propeptide of Type III Collagen

Fibrogenesis results in the release of extracellular matrix protein fragments, 1 of which is N-terminal propeptide of type III collagen (PRO-C3), into the circulation.[180] Luo et al. established PRO-C3 as a noninvasive, independent diagnostic tool that can distinguish advanced fibrosis (F3–F4) from mild-moderate fibrosis (F1–F2) or no fibrosis (F0) among patients in the MASLD spectrum [odds ratio 1.84 with 95% CI (1.05, 3.23), *P*-value .03.[181] Daniels et al. concluded that PRO-C3 is independently associated with advanced fibrosis (OR 1.054, 95% CI 1.07) and can identify patients with advanced fibrosis, with an AUROC of 0.81 (95% CI 0.76–0.85).[182]

The value of PRO-C3 changes over time with the severity of fibrosis that has been previously noted.[179,183] PRO-C3 has also been incorporated into diagnostic algorithms to stage MASH.[182,184] While promising, PRO-C3 will require further validation. Thus until more data are available, the clinical utility of PRO-C3 in MASH management remains uncertain.

While both PRO-C3 and PIIINP, one of the three components of the ELF score, assess the rate of formation of type III collagen through quantification of the N-terminal propeptide, they are distinct assays. The antibody used in measuring PIIINP is directed to an internal epitope within the N-terminal propeptide, whereas antibodies used in measuring PRO-C3 target the site at which ADAMTS2 cleaves off the propeptide,[185] a more direct measure of fibrogenesis.

Lipidomic- and Proteomic-Based Tests

Leveraging metabolomics may be a rich source for the development of noninvasive diagnostic biomarkers for MASLD.[186] A lipidomic serum-based profiling of triglycerides, developed from 467 patients, distinguished patients with normal livers from those with MASLD as well as from patients with MASH and isolated hepatic steatosis.[187] In the discovery cohort, this BMI-dependent lipidomic test distinguished patients with MASLD from those with normal liver, with an AUROC of 0.90, 0.98 sensitivity, and 0.78 specificity. The test also distinguished patients with MASH from those with MASL,[188] with an AUROC of 0.95, sensitivity 0.83, and specificity 0.94.[187]

Data from a multicenter international cross-sectional study was used to develop a serum-based score, the Metabolomics Advanced Steatohepatitis Fibrosis Score (MASEF), to identify at-risk MASH patients.[189] The MASEF score is a serum-based test that includes 12 lipids, BMI, AST, and ALT. The discovery and validation cohorts have an AUROC of 0.76 and 0.79 that outperformed the FAST score (see below) in the same cohort.[189]

A proteomic approach, using an eight-protein panel, can distinguish MASL/MASH fibrosis stage 0–1 from fibrosis stage 2–4, with an AUROC of 0.87–0.89.[190] The ADAMTSL2 protein alone was able to distinguish MASLL/MASH fibrosis stage 0–1 from fibrosis stage 2–4, with an AUROC of 0.86–0.89.[190]

Imaging-Based Biomarkers

Vibration-Controlled Transient Elastography

VCTE is a noninvasive method that uses the speed of a mechanically induced shear wave in the liver to measure liver stiffness measurement (LSM), which estimates the degree of hepatic fibrosis.[171] In a prospective study, LSM identified patients with fibrosis stage ≥F2, F≥3, and F4, with AUROC of 0.77, 0.80, and 0.89, respectively.[191] The cutoff strata for LSM, which were 8.2 kPa for F≥2, 9.7 kPa for F≥3, and 13.6 kPa for F4, were optimized with Youden criteria to account for clinical priorities.

In addition to LSM, VCTE can quantify hepatic steatosis by measuring the controlled attenuation parameter (CAP). In one study, CAP identified patients with steatosis, with AUROC 0.87, 0.77, and 0.70 for steatosis grade 1 or above, grade 2 or above, and grade 3, respectively.[191] Steatosis grade corresponds to the percentage of fat within the hepatocytes. Cutoff values were also optimized for each steatosis grade. LSM, determined by VCTE, is a predictor of prognosis in MASLD patients. In a longitudinal study, patients with higher levels of fibrosis at baseline had poor overall survival and survival free of death from liver-related complications.[192,193] LSM, determined by VCTE, was found a significant predictor of both all-cause mortality and mortality from liver-related complications.[193] The prognostic value of LSM, determined by VCTE, was also corroborated in the retrospective analysis.[194] Despite its use in clinical trials, the ability of LSM, determined by VCTE, to monitor response to pharmacological agents and correlate with histology has been assessed in few published studies; further studies are underway to assess its potential in these areas.[176,183,195]

Vibration-Controlled Transient Elastography Combination Modalities

Fibroscan-Aspartate Aminotransferase Score

The FibroScan-AST score (FAST score) is an algorithm used to identify at-risk MASH patients by combining LSM, CAP, and AST.[26] The FAST score relies on a dual cutoff approach. In a multicenter study, cutoffs were established at ≤0.35 for a sensitivity of 0.90 or greater (rule-out threshold) and ≥0.67 for a specificity of 0.90 or greater (rule-in threshold). The AUROC for the derivation cohort was 0.80 (95% CI 0.85), which indicates acceptable performance.[26] These cutoffs had a positive predictive value (PPV) of 0.83 and an NPV of 0.85 in the derivation cohort. Similar AUROC values were found in external validation cohorts, with an AUROC of 0.85 (95% CI 0.34). Notably, values for 30%–39% of patients fell into the gray zone between the 2 cutoff values. Therefore sequential testing or even liver biopsy may be indicated in such cases.

Agile 3+ and Agile 4

Although LSM measured by VCTE can accurately exclude F ≥ 3 and F4, with nearly 90% NPV, it inadequately rules in F≥3 and F4, which necessitates confirmatory testing in the case of positivity. Two novel VCTE-based noninvasive scores, Agile 3+ and Agile 4, integrate demographic features (age, gender, and the absence/presence of T2DM), blood tests (AST, ALT, and platelets), and VCTE LSM to better identify F ≥ 3 and F4 and may be superior to LSM determined by VCTE and FIB-4.[196,197] These scores are now clinically applicable, but further studies are needed to determine their role in the longitudinal assessment of disease progression and regression.

Shear Wave Elastography (SWE) and Acoustic Radiation Force Impulse (ARFI)

Comparable cutoff points for shear wave elastography and several other ultrasound-based elastography techniques are gradually emerging as potential alternatives.[198] However, it is important to note that these options still lack sufficient validation when compared to the more robust data available for transient elastography.

Magnetic Resonance Imaging—Derived Proton Density Fat Fraction

Abdominal ultrasound has traditionally been the first-line assessment for hepatic steatosis in patients with suspected

MASLD, but it has many limitations, including its inability to accurately quantify steatosis.[171] On the other hand, MRI-PDFF is a highly accurate tool able to detect even small (<5%) changes in hepatic lipid content.[171,199] In clinical practice, MRI-PDFF can be coupled with MRE, often bundled in the same examination, providing accurate quantification of hepatic steatosis and liver stiffness correlated with fibrosis.

In a proof of concept study, MRI-PDFF correlated with histologically graded steatosis.[199] Steatosis reduction of ≥30% tracked with improvement in histological MASH, but less convincingly with fibrosis.[200] [65] Despite its accuracy and potential utility to assess treatment response, it is not a point-of-care test and carries significantly more cost than transient elastography.

Magnetic Resonance Elastography

The two-dimensional (2D-MRE) has emerged as one of the most accurate tools for assessing fibrosis in MASLD.[171] Data from 117 patients with biopsy-proven MASLD who underwent 2D-MRE demonstrated that 2D-MRE accurately discriminated advanced fibrosis (F3–F4) from F0 to F2 fibrosis. In a meta-analysis, MRE maintained sensitivity and specificity above 80% and AUROC above 0.90 for detecting patients with $F \geq 3$ or $F \geq 4$. The AUROC of MRE for detecting fibrosis stages was 0.87, 0.91, 0.92, and 0.90 for $F \geq 1$, $F \geq 2$, $F \geq 3$, and $F = 4$, respectively.[201] Similar results for MRE were found from a pooled analysis by Liang et al.[202]

In addition to its diagnostic ability, stiffness assessed by MRE is predictive of liver clinical events and outcomes.[203–205] A multicenter, retrospective study was the first demonstrate that values of LSM by MRE correlate with liver-related outcomes.[204] An MRE threshold of 4.39 kPa, with an AUROC of 0.92 (95% CI 0.989), 81.8% sensitivity, and 91.8% specificity, distinguished patients with cirrhosis from those without cirrhosis. Additionally, an MRE cutoff at 6.48 kPa differentiated compensated cirrhosis from decompensated cirrhosis, with an AUROC of 0.71 (95% CI 0.902), 66.7% sensitivity, and 80.8% specificity, and each kPa increase in MRE-measured LSM translates to 3.28 times higher risk of hepatic decompensation (OR 3.28).[204]

Gidener et al., using LSM determined with MRE, found that a baseline LSM of 5 and 8 kPa indicated a 9% and 20% probability of developing decompensation or death within 1 year, respectively.[203] Moreover, with baseline LSM values used, the risk of developing cirrhosis increased per 1 kPa increment with HR 2.93 (95% CI, 1.62) and *c*-statistic of 0.86. Similar correlations were found for liver-related events, with an HR 1.32 (95% CI 1.56) for an increase in baseline LSM by 1 kPa.[203]

MRE has also been found capable of identifying longitudinal changes in fibrosis such that LSM strata of 2–5 kPa at baseline determined the timing of longitudinal monitoring at 5, 3, and 1 year, respectively.[203] Such findings indicate that MRE is a potential noninvasive longitudinal monitoring tool for fibrosis quantification. However, further studies are needed to assess the role of MRE in monitoring disease response to therapies.

Multiparametric Magnetic Resonance Imaging

Iron-corrected T1 mapping (cT1) is an MRI-based biomarker that reproduces regional tissue water content and is a promising quantitative imaging biomarker for MASH and MASLD. In a retrospective analysis of observational MASH studies, Dennis et al.[206] found a correlation between cT1 and NAS (rs = 0.36) and the individual components of steatosis, ballooning, and inflammation (rs = 0.54, 0.36, and 0.17, respectively). cT1 and fibrosis also were moderately correlated (rs = 0). In another study, cT1 predicted clinical liver events, all-cause mortality, and event-free survival; at a threshold of 825 ms or above, 12 of 13 (92%) clinical events and 9 of 10 (90%) deaths were identified in 197 chronic liver disease patients.[207] At a threshold of ≥825 ms, cT1 predicted liver-related clinical outcomes with HR 9.9.[207] Thus multiparametric MRI may be a promising tool in MASLD, but further data are needed for more definitive validation.

Magnetic Resonance Imaging-Based Combination Modalities

MAST Score

The MAST (MRI and AST) score is a noninvasive tool derived from MRI-PDFF, MR elastography, and AST values to predict the presence of at-risk MASH.[208] The MAST score uses dual cutoff values, with a low cutoff threshold of 0.165, indicating 90% sensitivity and 98.1% NPV, and a high cutoff threshold of 0.242, indicating 90% specificity and 50% PPV. The overall AUROC of the MAST score in the validation cohort was 0.93 (95% CI 0.97), which was higher than the NFS, FIB-4 index, and FAST scores. Importantly, the MAST score resulted in fewer patients having indeterminate scores compared with scores in previously established models.[208]

In one study, the MAST score predicted liver clinical events with high accuracy, including a *c*-statistic of 0.92.[209] While the MAST score is being used primarily in research trials for subject recruitment, it has shown potential to reduce the requirement for liver biopsies, especially in the selection of patients for phase II trials.

MEFIB Score

Jung et al. evaluated the diagnostic accuracy of MRE combined with FIB-4 index in a dichotomous score, called MEFIB, to identify MASH patients with significant fibrosis.[210] Here, cutoff thresholds of ≥3.3 kPa for MRE and ≥1.6 for FIB-4 index were used. MEFIB demonstrated a PPV of 97.1% ($P < .02$) and an AUROC of 0.90 (95% CI 0.95) to rule in significant fibrosis.[210] The same diagnostic accuracy was seen in a validation cohort from Japan, with MEFIB maintaining a PPV of 91.0% ($P < .003$) and an AUROC of 0.84 (95% CI 0.57), with the same parameters used for MRE and FIB-4 index. Although these results were not similar in subsequent studies from the same group,[211] MEFIB remains a promising noninvasive screening test to identify MASH patients with significant fibrosis who may benefit from pharmacological treatment of MASLD. Indeed, like MAST, MEFIB has shown excellent ability to predict clinical liver events and outcomes.[205,212]

Future Direction in Noninvasive Biomarkers

While great progress has been made with blood-based and imaging-based tests in achieving accuracy in assessing stages of MASLD and MASH and, to some extent, correlating with clinical outcomes, more data are needed to assess longitudinal changes and response to therapy. With the emerging positive results from the first phase 3 MASH clinical trials, it is expected that these data will continue to build. Future data will likely incorporate genetic risk scores (including PNPLA3) with other tests and scores. Artificial intelligence and machine learning will continue to evolve and aid in the identification of individuals with advanced disease or those at risk for liver-related outcomes.[213,214]

INITIAL ASSESSMENT OF THE PATIENT WITH METABOLIC DYSFUNCTION-ASSOCIATED STEATOTIC LIVER DISEASE

The initial assessment of a patient with suspected MASLD includes an assessment of metabolic comorbidities, exclusion of other causes of hepatic steatosis and disease modifiers, and quantification of alcohol intake, as summarized in Table 89.2. The initial assessment is followed by risk stratification for the presence of advanced fibrosis in patients with confirmed or suspected hepatic steatosis (Fig. 89.5). Subgroups at increased risk for advanced fibrosis (and hence adverse liver-related outcomes) include those with T2DM, medically complicated obesity, moderate or severe alcohol use, or a family history of MASH cirrhosis.[59]

TREATMENT

Healthy Habits to Promote Liver Wellness

"Lifestyle modification" in the form of dietary modification and increased activity level is the foundation of treatment of patients with MASLD. There is a clear link between caloric excess, in particular a diet enriched with simple carbohydrates, sugar-sweetened beverages, and saturated fat, and the development of MASLD. Hence, counseling patients on a liver healthy diet, ideally through a multidisciplinary team, is critical. While caloric restriction may not be appropriate for lean patients with MASLD, who may have a normal BMI and predominantly truncal adipose tissue deposition, changes in macronutrient dietary composition can be impactful.[50] Dietary changes should include a reduction in carbohydrates and saturated fats. For patients with no central adiposity and no evidence of insulin resistance or cardiometabolic risk factors, secondary causes of hepatic steatosis must be excluded.[215]

TABLE 89.1 Cardiometabolic Criteria for the Diagnosis of Metabolic Dysfunction-Associated Steatotic Liver Disease in Adults

One or More of the Following in the Presence of Confirmed or Suspected Hepatic Steatosis

• **Diabetes/prediabetes:** Fasting serum glucose ≥100 mg/dL *or* 2-h postload glucose levels ≥140 mg/dL or HbA1c ≥5.7% *or* type 2 diabetes *or* antidiabetic treatment
• **Central obesity:** BMI >25 kg/m^2 (23 for Asians) or waist circumference >94 cm (M), 80 cm (F) or ethnically adjusted for Asian populations
• **Hypertension:** Blood pressure >130/85 mmHg or use of antihypertensive therapy
• **Metabolic dyslipidemia**
  • Plasma triglycerides ≥150 mg/dL *or* use of lipid-lowering therapy
  • Plasma HDL-cholesterol ≤40 mg/dL (M), or ≤50 mg/dL (F) *or* use of lipid-lowering therapy

BMI, Body mass index; *HDL*, high-density lipoprotein.

Weight Loss

Weight loss in obese individuals, whether achieved through diet, medications, or surgery, improves metabolic health. Weight loss in overweight individuals with MASH typically leads to improvement in or resolution of steatosis, steatohepatitis and even fibrosis, depending on the extent of weight lost.[216,217] However, even within a clinical trial, weight loss via diet and exercise can be difficult to achieve (typically ≤10% succeed) and even more challenging to sustain.[218] Success in achieving and maintaining weight loss depends on many factors: It is critical to consider and address psychosocial, socioeconomic, and other barriers that can impede weight loss. Consistent support via a multidisciplinary team that includes a specialist in nutrition should be central to the management plan.

Dietary Intervention

The advantages of one diet over another with respect to its impact on MASLD are not clear. However, independent of weight loss, a Mediterranean-style diet (MedDiet), rich in fiber and *n*-3 polyunsaturated fatty acids, is sensible, given its positive impact on cardiovascular health and possible independent benefit in MASLD.

A systematic review and metanalysis of dietary patterns and their impact on hepatic fat reduction revealed that low carbohydrate versus low calorie (−27%, $P = .008$, one study, $n = 18$) and MedDiet versus low fat are more effective in reducing liver fat (−4.4%, $P = .030$, one study, $n = 12$).[219] In contrast, in a carefully conducted but small study ($n = 39$) (MEDINA trial), subjects with MASLD and obesity were randomized to either MedDiet or low-fat diet for 12 weeks. The primary outcome measure was reduction in hepatic fat; also, adherence to the assigned diet group was measured with validated instruments, and macronutrient intake was carefully documented. No difference in liver fat reduction was found between groups (−17% vs. 8% relative fat reduction in the low-fat diet and MedDiet groups, respectively), though, notably, those on the low-fat diet lost nearly 5% body weight, whereas those in the MedDiet gained 1.6 kg body weight. This difference suggests that apparent improvements in liver fat on the low-fat diet could be attributed to weight loss, rather than to the macronutrient content. This study also demonstrated a modest hepatic and metabolic benefit from MedDiet, while highlighting the complexities of following dietary recommendations in an ethnically diverse population.[220]

Alternate-day fasting is an increasingly popular dietary approach for achieving weight loss and improving metabolic health. Alternate-day fasting alone or in combination with moderate-intensity exercise (5, 60-minute sessions/week) were more effective than exercise alone or no intervention in reducing

TABLE 89.2 Initial Assessment of the Patient With Hepatic Steatosis or Suspected MASLD

History Elements	Physical Examination	Laboratory Assessment	Imaging
• Assess CMRFs • OSA testing if not previously done • Medications (including recent) • Family history: first degree relative with T2DM, MASLD, or cirrhosis • Alcohol use: quantity, pattern, and duration	• Adipose tissue distribution (gynoid vs. android) • Note signs of insulin resistance (acanthosis nigricans, skin tags, dorsocervical hump) • Note signs of advanced liver disease (gynecomastia, prominent abdominal veins, ascites, firm liver, splenomegaly, spider angiomata, palmar erythema)	• Liver chemistry tests • Renal chemistry • CBC • INR • Fasting lipid profile • HgbA1c • Hepatitis C if not previously tested and exclusion of other causes of liver injury if elevated liver chemistries are present • FIB-4	• As indicated clinically or by FIB-4 testing (see Fig. 89.2)

FIB-4, Fibrosis-4 index; *OSA*, obstructive sleep apnea.

liver fat, measured as absolute % reduction by MRI-PDFF. For those in the combination group, liver fat reduction was −5.48% compared with −1.30% in the exercise group (P = .02) and −0.17%, in the control group (P < .01). Liver fat reduction with the combination of alternate-day fasting and exercise was numerically higher than with alternate-day fasting alone (−2.25%; 95% CI, −4.46% to −0.04%; P = .05).[221] In a meta-analysis of 11 trials (7 RCT), with small numbers and heterogeneity in measurement of fat and other macronutrient content, a low-carbohydrate diet had no benefit over isocaloric low-fat diet in reducing liver fat or liver enzymes.[222] In an open-label RCT comparing a low- carbohydrate, high-fat diet to intermittent calorie restriction (2 sequential days of 500 cal/day or 5:2 diet) to control, the low-carbohydrate diet and the 5:2 diet were equally effective in reducing liver fat and weight, suggesting that dietary recommendations should be tailored to the individual.

The impact of other dietary intake, such as ultra-processed foods on liver wellness, is often overlooked. In a study of 789 subjects, consumption of ultra-processed foods was associated with MetS (OR 1.88, 95% CI 1.31−2.71, P = .001), MASLD, and a higher risk of MASH among those with MASLD (OR 1.89, 1.07−3.38, P = .030).[223] In another study in the same population, the consumption of red meat or processed meat was independently associated with a higher odds of MASLD, even after adjustment for saturated fat, cholesterol, smoking, BMI, alcohol, physical activity, and energy content (OR1.47; 95% CI 1.04−2.09; P = .03).[224]

Coffee

In contrast with the adverse impact of contemporary calorie-dense and processed foods coupled with a more sedentary lifestyle, coffee intake is a regular aspect of many people's lives that can positively impact liver health. Numerous studies demonstrate that coffee intake may protect against liver fibrosis in the context of alcohol, hepatitis C, and MASLD.[225,226] Consuming over 2 eight-ounce cups of coffee daily is linked to a lower risk of liver fibrosis, cirrhosis, HCC, and mortality from chronic liver diseases.[227] Regular coffee consumption, particularly in preparations with longer exposure time with the coffee beans, independently protects against liver fibrosis compared to other caffeine sources.[228]

Exercise

Exercise plays an important role in improving cardiometabolic health, which is of benefit to all patients. While exercise is an important aspect of lifestyle change, exercise advice needs to be individualized and tailored to the person's abilities and interests to optimize the chance of adherence. Both aerobic and strength training are beneficial to MASLD, though the extent to which this is independent of weight loss is less clear.[229] The impact of moderate-intensity exercise (150 minutes/week) or an increase of 60 minutes above baseline activity levels can prevent MASLD.[230] More intense exercise is likely needed to resolve steatohepatitis or improve fibrosis.[231] When possible, diet should be combined with exercise to optimize beneficial impact on MASLD and overall health.[221]

PHARMACOLOGIC THERAPY

Liver-Directed Therapy

In March 2024, the FDA granted accelerated approval for the first drug for noncirrhotic MASH with clinically significant fibrosis. Resmetirom is a thyroid hormone receptor β agonist, (see Fig. 89.6) that was initially developed as a lipid-lowering agent, subsequently demonstrating efficacy in Phase 2 trials of patients with MASH.[183] In the Phase 3 MAESTRO-NASH trial, 966 patients were randomized to placebo, 80 mg, or 100 mg of resmetirom.[232] After 52 weeks of treatment, 25.9% and 29.9% receiving resmetirom 80 and 100 mg, respectively, compared to 9.7% of placebo-treated patients (P < .001 vs. placebo) achieved MASH resolution. Fibrosis improvement was significantly more common in those receiving resmiterom versus placebo; 24.2% and 25.9% of patients receiving resmetirom 80 and 100 mg, respectively, compared to 14.2% of placebo-treated patients (P < .001 vs. placebo). There were additional reductions in lipid levels as expected with this mechanism of action, and, importantly, efficacy was not significantly impacted by the presence of T2DM or concomitant use of glucagon-like peptide-1 (GLP-1) receptor agonists.[232] Treatment initiation criteria included the presence of F2/F3 on biopsy or noninvasive biomarkers consistent with F2/F3. Because of the inherent variance in predicitivity of noninvasive tests, it is recommended that more than one noninvasive test be used to identify patients who are likely to have fibrosis stage 2 or 3. Although participants in MAESTRO-NASH were preselected based on VCTE cutoff of 8.5 kPa and higher, the cohort was already enriched by screening for likelihood of having advanced fibrosis, for example, by ELF score. In data derived from a population more akin to that encountered in clinical practice, a cutoff of 9.8 was shown to have a lower rate of misclassification, leading to a threshold of 10 kPa being recommended for identifying patients who may be appropriate for resmetirom therapy[261] to reduce misclassification of patients as having clinically significant fibrosis, it is recommended that a cutoff of 9.8 be used when ELF is used in isolation (e.g., where VCTE or MRE assessment of liver stiffness is not available). When ELF scores are between 9.2 and 9.7, we recommend an additional NIT to confirm the likelihood of stage 2−3 fibrosis (Table 89.3).

Given the metabolic nature of the pathophysiology that underpins the fibroinflammatory injury of MASH, the required duration of therapy is unclear but is anticipated to be long-term. While most patients on resmetirom therapy who achieve histological response experience improvement in transaminases on therapy, patients who do not achieve transaminase reductions may also experience histological benefit. Currently, there is insufficient evidence to fully assess treatment response or failure using NITs at this time, although data are emerging.

Approved Pharmacotherapies With Potential Metabolic Dysfunction-Associated Steatohepatitis Benefit

Several drugs approved for the management of cardiometabolic conditions are in advanced development for the treatment of MASH. Several society guidelines now recommend preferential use of many of these available medications within their FDA-approved indications for MASLD, given their additional hepatic benefits, while the approval of liver-directed therapies is awaited[172,173] (Table 89.3).

Vitamin E

Vitamin E is an antioxidant with several isoforms of different bioavailability. rrr-Alpha tocopherol has the highest bioavailability and is one of the most studied compounds for the treatment of MASLD. In the PIVENS trial, Vit E was superior to placebo in improving liver enzymes, steatosis, and inflammation, though it appeared to have no impact on fibrosis.[233] Other studies, including metaanalyses, have shown similar effects.[234,235] Despite its lack of effect on fibrosis, a retrospective single-center study compared 90 patients taking 800 IU daily of vitamin E for at least 2 years to propensity-matched controls and found that vitamin E users had improved transplant-free survival (78% vs. 49%, P <

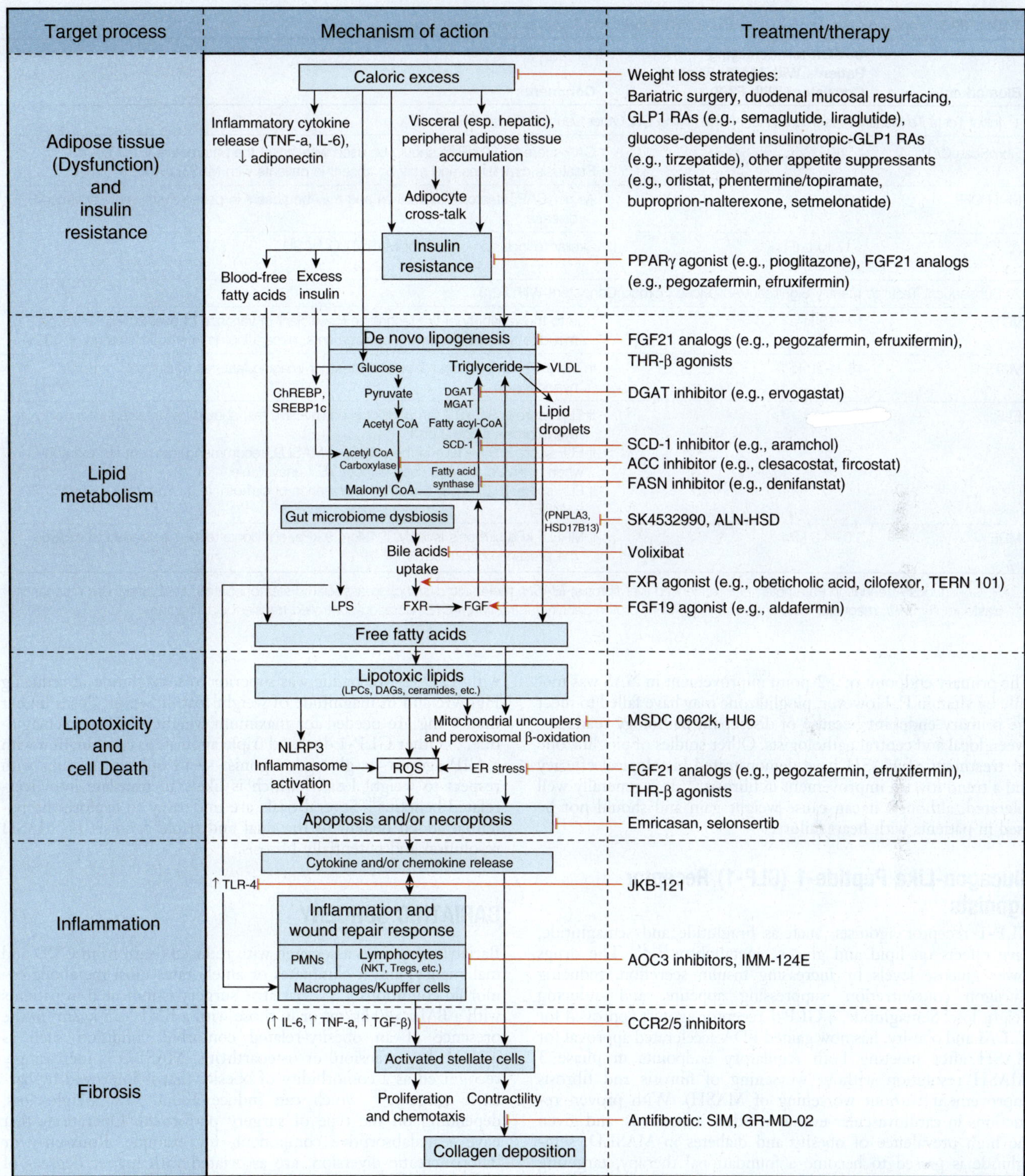

Fig. 89.6 Targets of emerging therapies for MASH.

.01) and lower rates of decompensation, 37% versus 62%, $P = .04$, respectively.[236] These findings may be in part explained by the effect of vitamin E on coagulation, possibly preventing microthrombosis.[237] Vitamin E use has been associated with a higher risk of hemorrhagic stroke but a lower risk of thrombotic stroke,[238] though other studies have found no significant impact on either.[239] Data on overall impact of vitamin E on mortality or cardiovascular outcomes are mixed.[239–241] However, there is a paucity of data on the impact of rrr-alpha tocopherol at doses used in prior studies (800 IU daily) in MASH.[242]

Pioglitazone

The first adequately powered MASH treatment trial was the PIVENS trial, published in 2010.[233] In the trial, vitamin E 800 IU was compared with pioglitazone 30 mg and placebo for 72 weeks.

TABLE 89.3 Proposed Criteria to Identify Patients With MASH and Significant/Advanced Fibrosis

Biomarker	Cut-Off for Identifying Patients With MASH Fibrosis Consistent With F2/3	Comments
1. Initial Tests To Identify Presumed MASH (After Ruling Out Other Causes of Liver Disease)		
FibroScan CAP	≥280 dB/m	CAP score ≥280 dB/m should be used with ≥1 of the parameters listed below Steatosis diminishes and may be absent in patients with MASH cirrhosis
MRI PDFF	≥5%	As per CAP, steatosis diminishes and may be absent in patients with more advanced disease
AST	>17 IU/L (F) >20 IU/L (M)	Similar to inclusion criteria for MAESTRO-NASH
2. Subsequent Tests to Identify Significant/Advanced Fibrosis Consistent With F2/3		
VCTE	10–15 kPa	Due to the variability of the technique (coefficient of variance of over 20%), it is recommended to obtaining >10 measurements, generating an interquartile range of <30%
VCTE	15.1–20 kPa	In the absence of clinical, laboratory test, or imaging features of cirrhosis or portal hypertension
ELF	9.2–10.4	If ELF score is 9.2–9.7, an additional noninvasive test should be obtained to corroborate likely fibrosis stage 2 or 3 If ELF score is 9.8–10.4 in the setting of MASLD, recommend transient elastography when available. Can be used without TE if unavailable If ELF score 10.5–11.3, exclude the presence of cirrhosis (e.g., liver stiffness by VCTE or MRE)
MRE	3.0–4.3 kPa	If MRE 5 kPa cirrhosis is likely, if 4.4–4.9 kPa, additional testing is needed to exclude the presence of cirrhosis

CAP, Continuous Attenuation Parameter; *ELF*, enhanced liver fibrosis; *MASH*, metabolic dysfunction-associated steatohepatitis; *MRE*, magnetic resonance elastography; *MRI*, magnetic resonance imaging; *PDFF*, proton density fat fraction; *VCTE*, vibration-controlled transient elastography.

The primary endpoint of ≥2-point improvement in NAS was met only by vitamin E. However, pioglitazone may have failed to meet the primary endpoint because of discrepant pathology reads between local and central pathologists. Other studies of pioglitazone for treatment of MASH have demonstrated histological efficacy and a trend toward improvement in fibrosis.[243] It is generally well tolerated, although it can cause weight gain and should not be used in patients with heart failure.

Glucagon-Like Peptide-1 (GLP-1) Receptor Agonists

GLP-1 receptor agonists, such as liraglutide and semaglutide, have effects on lipid and glucose metabolism.[244,245] The drugs lower glucose levels by increasing insulin secretion, reducing glucagon concentration, suppressing appetite, and inducing weight loss. Semaglutide, a GLP-1 receptor agonist approved for T2DM and obesity, has now gained FDA accelerated approval for MASH after meeting both regulatory endpoints in phase 3 (MASH resolution without worsening of fibrosis and fibrosis improvement without worsening of MASH). With proven reductions in cardiovascular events in other indications, and given the high prevalence of obesity and diabetes in MASLD, semaglutide is poised to become a foundational therapy, targeting systemic drivers of disease alongside histological efficacy.[262–264] Given the proven benefit of weight loss in the improvement of MASH activity, including fibrosis, drugs such as tirzepatide, a glucose-dependent insulinotropic polypeptide (GIP) and GLP-1 receptor agonist, will likely be beneficial because of the profound weight loss they produce both in diabetic and nondiabetic patients, that is, 20.9% (95% CI, −21.8 to −19.9) with 15-mg doses and −3.1% (95% CI, −4.3 to −1.9) with placebo ($P <$ .001 for all comparisons with placebo). Ninety-one percent of those receiving 15 mg achieved the primary endpoint of >5% weight loss compared with placebo.[246] In a trial comparing tirzepatide 5, 10, and 15 mg with semaglutide up to 1 mg in patients with T2DM, tirzepatide was superior to semaglutide in reducing HgbA1c and in magnitude of weight lost; however, doses higher than 1 mg are needed for maximum weight loss from semaglutide.[247] Other GLP-1 dual and triple agonists as combination with a GIP agonist or glucagon agonist seem quite promising with respect to weight loss,[248] which is likely to translate into liver-related benefit.[249] Several trials are underway to explore the potential added benefit of the dual and triple agonists on MASH resolution and potentially fibrosis.

BARIATRIC SURGERY

Bariatric surgery is associated with reduced death from CVD and malignancy, and it eliminates or ameliorates most metabolic comorbid conditions.[250,251] Bariatric surgery is indicated in patients with a BMI >40 kg/m^2 or in those with a BMI ≥35 kg/m^2 in the presence of an obesity-related comorbid condition such as T2DM, hypertension, or osteoarthritis. MASLD is increasingly recognized as a comorbidity of obesity that is improved by bariatric surgery,[252] which can induce about 30% weight loss, depending on the type of surgery performed. Operations that have a malabsorptive component, for example, Roux-en-y or biliopancreatic diversion, are associated with higher degrees of weight loss, depending on the patient's comorbid conditions and the extent of liver disease. The most often performed bariatric procedure is sleeve gastrectomy. Patients with advanced hepatic fibrosis may not tolerate procedures associated with more rapid weight loss, as this can precipitate liver dysfunction. MASH resolves in 90% of patients one year after bariatric surgery; fibrosis also improves, even in those with stage 3 fibrosis. While nine patients with cirrhosis were included in this study, only four had available paired biopsies, making it not possible to gauge the impact of bariatric surgery in this population.[217] The results of other studies suggest that carefully selected patients with compensated cirrhosis can tolerate bariatric surgery and benefit

TABLE 89.4 Approved Drugs for Common Comorbidities That May Benefit MASLD

Mechanism of Action (Drug)	Population Studied	Clinical Benefits	Potential Side Effects	FDA Indication
PPAR gamma agonists (pioglitazone)[233,243,254]	MASH with and without T2DM	**Hepatic** Improves steatosis, activity, and MASH resolution Fibrosis improvement? **Other** Prevention of diabetes CV risk reduction	Weight gain Heart failure exacerbation Bone loss	T2DM
GLP-1 agonists (e.g., liraglutide, semaglutide)[255,256]	Noncirrhotic MASH	**Hepatic** Improves steatosis and steatohepatitis No proven impact on fibrosis but may slow progression **Other** Insulin sensitizing Weight loss CV risk reduction Renoprotective	**Gastrointestinal** Gallstones Pancreatitis (rare) Loss of lean mass Anhedonia	T2DM Obesity
GLP-1/GIP agonists (e.g., tirzepatide)[257,258]	T2DM or obesity with MASLD	**Hepatic** Reduces steatosis on imaging **Other** Insulin sensitizing Weight loss	**Gastrointestinal** Gallstones Pancreatitis (rare) Loss of lean mass Anhedonia	T2DM Obesity
SGLT2 inhibitors (e.g., empagliflozin, dapagliflozin)[259,260]	T2DM and MASLD	**Hepatic** Reduction in steatosis **Other** Insulin sensitizing Cardiorenal risk reduction Benefit in heart failure Modest weight loss	Genitourinary infections Volume depletion Bone loss	T2DM
Antioxidants Vitamin E (rrr-alpha)[235,242]	MASH without T2DM or cirrhosis	**Hepatic** Improves steatosis and steatohepatitis No proven benefit on fibrosis	Hemorrhagic stroke Possible increased risk of prostate cancer	N/A

GLP-1, Glucagon-like peptide-1; *MASH*, metabolic dysfunction-associated steatohepatitis; *T2DM*, type 2 diabetes.

from an improvement in morbidity. Liver-related risk in this population is the dominant competing risk, and benefit in liver-related outcomes with bariatric surgery has not been demonstrated. In patients with severe obesity likely to undergo transplantation, bariatric surgery may serve as a bridge to transplantation if obesity is a barrier to transplantation.

EMERGING THERAPIES

The complex pathophysiology of MASH supports the potential to leverage numerous pathways, either alone or in combination, to ameliorate disease activity and ultimately reduce fibrosis progression. Given the rapid evolution of individual therapeutics in this space, specifics of early phase trials are better summarized elsewhere. Broadly, the most impactful approaches thus far have targeted lipid metabolism (primarily via interfering with de novo lipogenesis or upregulating β-oxidation), weight loss, alteration of adipocytokine signaling via action on the visceral adipose tissue compartment, improvement in insulin sensitivity, farnesoid x receptor agonism, and THR-β agonism (Fig. 89.6, **Targets for emerging therapeutics**).

Future Directions

Based on the broad experience with hepatitis C and HCC, even with excellent screening tools, widely accepted recommendations for screening, and availability of effective and safe therapies of MASLD, many patients with MASLD are likely to be undiagnosed and untreated. It is anticipated that with the approval of resmetirom, screening for patients with more advanced disease will increase. Meaningful reduction of the impact on MASLD will require screening at a population level using tools that require little or no initial input from providers. The future is likely to see the development of artificial intelligence/machine learning tools that are applied routinely through electronic medical records. Such an approach is already possible with FIB-4 and is emerging for electrocardiograms.[253] Patients identified as being at increased risk of clinically significant MASLD will need to be linked to care that includes rapidly evolving algorithms for more detailed evaluation and, in some instances, therapy.

Therapy of MASH is only in its infancy; the magnitude of effect on fibrosis improvement has been modest, though most drugs are being initially tested as monotherapies. The complex biology of MASH makes it likely that a multifaceted approach will emerge that includes individualized combination pharmacotherapy. Development of combination therapies is, however, challenging. Prediction of the incremental benefit, when compared to monotherapy, of the individual components of a combination regimen is particularly vexing. Regulatory pathways are also constraining, with requirements including data from a full portfolio of clinical trials of individual components to preclinical models and phase 1−3 clinical trials of combination therapies, including complex late-stage therapeutic trials. The emergence of approved therapies will further complicate trial design of combination therapies. In addition to the development of combination therapies, therapeutic strategies that are tailored to individual patient profiles are likely to emerge. For example, RNA-based therapies, which will certainly cost more than oral metabolic agents, may be reserved for patients with more advanced disease or pretreatment biomarkers (e.g., based on genetic profile) with low likelihood of response to oral metabolic therapies. Combination therapies will be highly demanding of patient, investigator, and sponsor resources. Meanwhile, a holistic approach to the health of patients with MASLD that includes a therapeutic strategy tailored to the overlapping presence and impact of comorbidities, such as T2DM and elevated BMI, will be an enduring cornerstone of management.

Acknowledgments

Dana Coons for the excellent work on the figures and illustrations. John Hart for providing histology pictures.

Full references for this chapter can be found at https://ebooks.health.elsevier.com.

90 Liver Disease Caused by Drugs

Shivakumar Chitturi, Narci C. Teoh

IN THIS CHAPTER

HEPATIC DRUG METABOLISM

Role of the Liver in Drug Elimination

The liver, by virtue of the portal circulation, is highly exposed to drugs and toxins absorbed from the intestine. Drugs, many of which are lipophilic compounds, are readily taken up by the liver but cannot be easily excreted unchanged in bile or urine. The liver is well equipped to handle such agents by an adaptable (inducible) series of metabolic pathways. These pathways include those that alter the parent molecule (phase 1); synthesize conjugates of the drug or its metabolite with a more water-soluble moiety, such as a sugar, amino acid, or sulfate molecule (phase 2); and excrete in an energy-dependent manner the parent molecule, its metabolites, or conjugates into bile (phase 3). For any given compound, 1, 2, or all 3 steps may be necessary for drug elimination. Expression and subcellular location of the proteins (enzymes, membrane transporters) that mediate these steps are controlled by a set of nuclear receptors that function as transcriptional regulators and coregulators, thereby accounting for coordinated regulation of the 3 phases of hepatic drug elimination.

Pathways of Drug Metabolism

Phase 1 and Cytochrome P450

Phase 1 pathways of drug metabolism include oxidation, reduction, and hydrolytic reactions. The products can generally be readily conjugated or excreted without further modification.[1,2]

Most phase 1 reactions are catalyzed by microsomal drug oxidases, which contain a hemoprotein of the cytochrome P450 (CYP) gene superfamily as a key component. The apparent promiscuity of drug oxidases toward drugs, environmental toxins, steroid hormones, lipids, and bile acids results from the existence of multiple closely related CYP proteins. More than 20 CYP enzymes are present in the human liver.[2,3]

The reaction cycle involves binding of molecular oxygen to the iron in the heme prosthetic group, with subsequent reduction of oxygen by acceptance of an electron from nicotinamide-adenine dinucleotide phosphate (NADPH) cytochrome P450 reductase, a flavoprotein reductase. The resulting "activated oxygen" is incorporated into the drug or another lipophilic compound. Reduction of oxygen and insertion into a drug substrate (mixed function oxidation) generates chemically reactive intermediates, including free radicals, electrophilic "oxy-intermediates" (e.g., unstable epoxides, quinone imines), and reduced (and therefore *r*eactive) *o*xygen *s*pecies (ROS). The quintessential example is the CYP2E1-catalyzed metabolite of acetaminophen, *N*-acetyl-*p*-benzoquinone imine (NAPQI), an oxidizing and arylating metabolite that is responsible for acetaminophen hepatotoxicity. Other examples of reactive quinone compounds include metabolites of troglitazone, quinine, and methyldopa. Likewise, hepatic metabolism of some plant toxins can generate potentially hepatotoxic epoxide metabolites of diterpenoids (see Chapter 91).[4] ROS contributes significantly to tissue injury, particularly by generating oxidative stress and triggering tissue stress responses and cell death pathways, as discussed later.

The hepatic content of CYP proteins is higher in acinar zone 3 than in zone 1. Localization of CYP2E1 is usually confined to a narrow rim of hepatocytes, one to two cells thick around the terminal hepatic venule. This explains in part the zonality of hepatic lesions produced by drugs and toxins, such as acetaminophen and carbon tetrachloride, which are converted to reactive metabolites.

Genetic and Environmental Determinants of Cytochrome P450 Enzymes

Pharmacogenetics and Polymorphisms of Cytochrome P450 Expression

The hepatic expression of each CYP enzyme is genetically determined. This finding largely explains the fourfold or greater differences in rates of drug metabolism among healthy subjects. Some CYPs, particularly minor forms, are also subject to polymorphic inheritance, with some individuals lacking the encoded protein. One example is CYP2D6, which metabolizes debrisoquine and perhexiline. Poor metabolizers lack CYP2D6 and accumulate perhexiline with usual doses; the lack of CYP2D6 is the critical determinant in serious adverse effects of perhexiline, including chronic hepatitis and cirrhosis.[5] Other examples include CYPs 2C9 and 2C19, which affect the metabolism of *S*-warfarin, omeprazole, and phenytoin and of *S*-mephenytoin, respectively[2]; 3% of white populations and 15% of Asians are poor metabolizers of *S*-mephenytoin.

Developmental Regulation and Constitutive Expression

Expression of several CYPs is developmentally regulated. During adult life, the expression of some CYPs declines slightly (by up to 10%) with advancing age, but this change is minor compared with the effects of genetic variation, environmental influences, and liver disease. Age-related changes that may influence hepatic drug exposure include pseudocapillarization of liver sinusoidal endothelial cells. Gender differences in the expression of CYPs 3A4 and 2E1 may explain the slightly enhanced metabolism of certain drugs (erythromycin, chlordiazepoxide, midazolam) in women, but whether this difference contributes to the increased risk of hepatic drug reactions in women remains unclear.[6]

Nutrition and Disease-Related Changes

A person's nutritional status influences the expression of certain CYPs, both in health and in liver disease.[1,2,7] CYP2E1 expression is increased by obesity, high fat intake, diabetes mellitus, and fasting.[2,6,8] Diseases that alter the expression of hepatic CYPs include hypothyroidism (decreased CYP1A) and hypopituitarism (decreased CYP3A4).[2] Cirrhosis is associated with decreased levels of total cytochrome P450 and also with reduced hepatic perfusion; the result is a decrease in the clearance of drugs such as propranolol that are metabolized rapidly by the liver.[2,8] The effects of cirrhosis vary, however, among individual CYP families (Table 90.1) and with the type of liver disease (e.g., CYP3A4 levels are preserved with cholestatic but reduced with hepatocellular liver disease).[8–10]

Adaptive Response and Enzyme Induction

Exposure to lipophilic substances generates an adaptive response that usually involves transient liver cell injury (discussed later) as well as synthesis of new enzyme protein, a process termed enzyme induction. The molecular basis for genetic regulation of constitutive and inducible expression of CYP3A4, the major human hepatic cytochrome P450, has been determined. Drugs such as rifampin interact with the pregnane X-receptor (PXR), a member of the orphan nuclear receptor family of transcriptional regulators. Activated PXR and the analogous constitutive androstane receptor (CAR) in turn bind to cognate nucleotide sequences upstream to the CYP3A4 structural gene within a xenobiotic-regulatory enhancer module. This interaction regulates the CYP3A4 promoter downstream and, ultimately, the transcription of CYP3A4 protein. Similar control mechanisms apply to several other CYP pathways, particularly those involved in bile acid synthesis.[9]

TABLE 90.1 Cytochrome P450 (CYP) Isoenzymes Involved in Phase I Drug Metabolism in Humans

CYP Isoenzymes	Substrates	Effect of Liver Disease on CYP Activity
CYP1A2	Caffeine, theophylline, clonazepam	↓↓↓
CYP2A6	Halothane, methoxyflurane	↓↓
CYP2C9	Diclofenac, losartan, warfarin	↓
CYP2C19	Citalopram, diazepam, omeprazole	↓↓↓
CYP2D6	Codeine, haloperidol, metoprolol	↔
CYP2E1	Enflurane, halothane, acetaminophen	↓
CYP3A4	Amiodarone, carbamazepine, cyclosporine, terfenadine	↓↓↓

Common examples of environmental agents, inducing microsomal enzymes, include cigarette and cannabis smoking (CYP1A2)[8] and alcohol (CYP2E1 and possibly CYP3A4).[2] Several drugs are potent inducers of CYP enzymes. Isoniazid induces CYP2E1, whereas phenobarbital and phenytoin increase the expression of multiple CYPs.[2] Rifampin is a potent inducer of CYP3A4, as is hypericum, the active ingredient of St. John's Wort, a commonly used herbal medicine, examples illustrating typical interactions between conventional medicines and complementary and alternative medicine (CAM). Regulation of hepatic drug metabolizing enzymes is reviewed elsewhere.[11,12]

The implications for drug-induced liver disease are twofold. First, enzyme induction often extends beyond the CYP system, possibly due to PXR and CAR activation. This induction may influence bile acid metabolism and liver growth and could account for increases in serum alkaline phosphatase and GGTP levels, which reflect "hepatic adaptation" to chronic drug ingestion. Second, the influence of one drug on expression and activity of drug metabolizing enzymes and drug elimination (phase 3) pathways can alter the metabolism or disposition of other agents. Such drug-drug interactions may be relevant to mechanisms of drug-induced liver injury.

Inhibition of Drug Metabolism

Some chemicals inhibit drug metabolism. In individuals taking more than one medication, for example, competition for phase 2 pathways such as glucuronidation and sulfation facilitates the presentation of unconjugated drug to the CYP system. This may explain in part why agents such as zidovudine and phenytoin lower the dose threshold for acetaminophen-induced hepatotoxicity.

Other Pathways of Drug Oxidation

In addition to CYP enzymes, mitochondrial electron transport systems can generate tissue-damaging reactive intermediates during drug metabolism. Examples include nitroradicals from nitrofuran derivatives (nitrofurantoin, cocaine). Subsequent electron transfer by flavoprotein reductases into molecular oxygen generates superoxide and other ROS. Some anticancer drugs (e.g., doxorubicin, imidazole antimicrobials) can participate in other oxidation-reduction (redox) cycling reactions that generate ROS.

Phase 2 (Conjugation)

Phase 2 reactions involve formation of ester links to the parent compound or to a drug metabolite to form hydrophilic conjugates that can be excreted readily in bile or urine. The responsible enzymes include glucuronyl transferases, sulfotransferases, glutathione *S*-transferases, and acetyl and amino acid *N*-transferases. Conjugation reactions are also regulated by CAR and other nuclear transcription factors and can be retarded by depletion of their rate-limiting cofactors, such as glucuronic acid and inorganic sulfate; the relatively low capacity of these enzyme systems restricts the efficacy of drug elimination when substrate concentrations exceed enzyme saturation. In general, drug conjugates are nontoxic, and phase 2 reactions are considered to be detoxification reactions, with exceptions. For example, some glutathione conjugates can undergo cysteine *S*-conjugate beta-lyase–mediated activation to highly reactive intermediates. In general, conjugation reactions are minimally affected by liver disease, with the possible exception of some reduction of enzyme activity and resulting drug clearance in decompensated cirrhosis; this is relevant to selection of major analgesics (morphine rather than pethidine) and hypnotics (oxazepam rather than diazepam).

Phase 3

This phase involves secretion of drugs, drug metabolites, or their conjugates into bile. Several transporters participate in these pathways that involve ATP-binding cassette (ABC) proteins and are powered by energy from ATP hydrolysis (see Chapter 66). ABC transport proteins are widely distributed in nature and include the CF transmembrane conductance regulator and the canalicular and intestinal copper transporters.

Multidrug resistance protein 1 (MDR1, gene symbol *ABCB1*) is highly expressed on the apical (canalicular) plasma membrane of hepatocytes, where it transports cationic drugs, particularly anticancer agents, into bile. Another family of ABC transporters, the multidrug resistance-associated proteins (MRPs), is also expressed in the liver. At least two members of this family excrete drug (and other) conjugates from hepatocytes: MRP-3 (gene symbol *ABCC3*) on the basolateral surface facilitates passage of drug conjugate into the sinusoidal circulation, and MRP-2 (gene symbol *ABCC2*), expressed on the canalicular membrane, pumps endogenous compounds (e.g., bilirubin diglucuronide, leukotriene-glutathionyl conjugates, glutathione) and drug conjugates into bile. The bile salt export pump (BSEP) and MDR3 (gene symbols *ABCB4* in humans and *Mdr2* in mice) are other canalicular transporters involved, respectively, in bile acid and phospholipid secretion into bile. Polymorphisms involving these genes are associated with human cholestatic liver diseases. BSEP interacts with several drugs.[11]

Regulation of the membrane expression and activity of these drug elimination pathways is complex. Altered expression or impaired activity (by competition between agents, changes in membrane lipid composition, or damage from reactive metabolites or covalent binding) could lead to drug accumulation, impairment of bile flow, or cholestatic liver injury. This has been demonstrated for estrogens,[13] troglitazone,[14] terbinafine,[15] and flucloxacillin[16] and has wider mechanistic implications for drug-induced cholestasis and other forms of liver injury.[11]

Effect of Liver Disease on Drug Metabolism

In considering the safety of prescribing medications in patients with liver disease, physicians need to understand the hepatic extraction ratio of the drug (its rate of uptake and metabolism), its disposition (hepatic, renal, other), the pathways involved if it is subject to hepatic drug metabolism, and whether there are potential interactions between drug effects (pharmacodynamics) and disease complications. In light of the complexity of hepatic drug handling, it is fortunate that most drugs are safe to use in most patients with liver disease. The contexts that will give rise to concern are liver disease associated with reduced hepatic blood flow (cirrhosis and portal hypertension), in which hepatic clearance of drugs with high clearance is reduced, and poor metabolic (synthetic) function of the liver. Apart from subjects already awaiting liver transplantation, this category includes patients with alcohol-associated hepatitis and cirrhosis, severe autoimmune hepatitis (AIH), and viral hepatitis with hepatic decompensation. In such patients, oral doses of high-clearance compounds must be reduced substantially because systemic bioavailability may increase 2–10-fold as a result of the reduced "first-pass" hepatic clearance. The best example is propranolol, which is usually prescribed in this context to lower portal venous pressure and reduce the risk of variceal bleeding. Instead of doses used for cardiovascular indications (such as 160–320 mg daily), the usual starting dose in a patient with cirrhosis should be 10–20 mg daily. Other high-clearance compounds affected by severe liver disease include pethidine, tricyclic antidepressants, and salbutamol.

The pathways of hepatic drug metabolism and elimination most affected by liver disease are those involving CYP (see Table 90.1). As mentioned earlier, cholestatic forms of liver disease have little effect on CYP3A4 and therefore minimally affect hepatic metabolism of commonly used drugs, such as glucocorticoids, angiotensin-converting enzyme (ACE) inhibitors, cyclosporine, and HIV protease inhibitors. Drugs that rely on hepatic elimination through biliary excretion are minimally affected by liver disease, with the exception of cancer chemotherapeutic agents. Patients with jaundice are at increased risk of liver injury with such agents. By contrast, liver disease has much less effect on conjugation pathways (phase 2 drug metabolism), a property that can be exploited in the choice of sedatives or major analgesics (see later).

Drugs known to precipitate liver complications should be avoided. Patients with cirrhosis have impaired creatinine clearance and are at risk of developing gentamicin nephrotoxicity. Another challenge is the appropriate choice of a sedative to manage alcohol withdrawal in a patient with alcohol-associated cirrhosis. Diazepam is a poor choice in this setting because it is extensively metabolized by CYPs; its clearance is delayed, and hepatic encephalopathy may be precipitated by its use. An alternative benzodiazepine that is metabolized by conjugation alone (e.g., oxazepam) would be a safer choice. Other adverse effects that are not usually related to hepatic drug metabolism include exaggerated effects on clotting factor synthesis (even though warfarin metabolism is not usually affected by liver disease); sodium and water retention by NSAIDs, which also confer high risk of GI bleeding; metabolic acidosis or profound hypoglycemia by metformin and other oral hypoglycemic agents; and hypotension after administration of an ACE inhibitor or major tranquilizer. Acetaminophen appears to be the safest analgesic agent to use in cirrhosis (see later). In general, however, most commonly used agents (antimicrobials, DAAs, antiepileptics, antidepressants, antihypertensives, statins, and oral contraceptives) are safe to use in patients with liver disease.

LIVER DISEASE CAUSED BY DRUGS

Definitions and Importance

Drugs are a relatively common cause of liver injury, which usually is defined by abnormalities of liver biochemical test levels, particularly an increase in the serum ALT, alkaline phosphatase, or bilirubin level to more than twice the upper limit of normal (ULN). Drug-induced liver injury (DILI) can be difficult to define in clinical practice because the biochemical tests used to detect liver injury may also be elevated as part of a hepatic adaptive response. Indeed, evidence indicates that some forms of hepatic adaptation to drugs follow an earlier transient process of self-limiting liver injury, followed in turn by operation of innate immunity. Further, the severity of DILI varies from minor nonspecific changes in hepatic structure and function to ALF, cirrhosis, and liver cancer.[17]

The term drug-induced liver disease should be confined to cases in which the nature of the liver injury has been characterized histologically. With the exception of acetaminophen, anticancer drugs, and some botanical or industrial hepatotoxins, most cases of DILI represent adverse drug reactions or hepatic drug reactions. These effects are noxious and unintentional and occur at recommended doses. The latent period is longer (typically from 1 week to 3–6 months) than that for direct hepatotoxins (from hours to a few days), and extrahepatic features of drug hypersensitivity may be present.

Although DILI is a relatively uncommon cause of jaundice or acute hepatitis in the community, it is an important cause of more severe acute liver disease, particularly among older people. The overall mortality rate among patients hospitalized for DILI is approximately 10%[18] but varies greatly for individual drugs.[19,20] Reported frequencies of individual hepatic drug reactions are underestimated because of the inadequacy of spontaneous reporting.[19,20] With reliable prospective and epidemiologic techniques, the frequency (or risk) of most types of drug-induced liver disease is between 1 per 10,000 and 1 per 100,000 persons exposed.[21] Because these responses to drug exposure are clearly rare and unpredictable, they are often termed idiosyncratic drug reactions. Their rarity blunts diagnostic acumen because most clinicians will see few, if any, cases and therefore do not have an appropriate level of clinical suspicion. This concern applies especially to CAM preparations (see Chapter 91). Failure to withdraw the causative agent after the onset of symptoms of drug hepatitis or re-exposure to such a drug is a common and avoidable factor in ALF attributable to DILI.[1,22–24] Another challenge is that DILI includes an array of clinical syndromes and pathologic findings that mimic known hepatobiliary diseases. Furthermore, although individual agents (and some drug classes) typically produce a characteristic "signature syndrome," they can also be associated with other and sometimes multiple clinicopathologic syndromes.

DILI is one of the most common reasons for withdrawal of an approved drug. The subject therefore has medicoeconomic, legal, and regulatory ramifications. Because most types of idiosyncratic hepatic drug reactions are infrequent, serious hepatotoxicity is not usually detected until postmarketing surveillance is conducted. Historically, drugs with a reputation for potential hepatotoxicity have usually been replaced by more acceptable alternatives. Examples include troglitazone, the prototypic thiazolidinedione, and bromfenac, an NSAID, both of which were withdrawn due to fatal hepatotoxicity.[1,22,24,25]

The burgeoning number of available conventional medications and CAM preparations now includes many hundreds that are cited as rare causes of drug-induced liver disease. This poses several challenges to clinicians,[1,5,22–25] including concern about what constitutes an adequate level of patient information at the time a drug is prescribed and the reliability of evidence linking an individual agent to a particular type of liver injury.[1,26,27] Another development is the appreciation that in the context of a complex medical setting, drug toxicity can interact with other causes of liver injury. Notable examples of such situations are bone marrow transplantation, cancer chemotherapy, antiretroviral therapy (ART) for HIV infection, use of antituberculosis drugs in patients with chronic viral hepatitis, and rifampin hepatitis in patients with PBC and metabolic dysfunction-associated steatotic liver disease (MASLD), precipitated by tamoxifen.

Epidemiology

Frequency or risk, the number of adverse reactions for a given number of persons exposed, is the best term for expressing how common a drug reaction is. Time-dependent terms such as incidence and prevalence are not appropriate because the frequency is not linearly related to the duration of exposure. For most reactions, the onset occurs within a relatively short exposure time, or latent period, although some forms of chronic liver disease occur months or years later. The frequency of drug-induced liver disease is derived from postmarketing surveillance reports submitted to the manufacturers or adverse drug reaction monitoring bodies. In the United States, following approval by the FDA, drug companies are required to report serious adverse events (any incident resulting in death, a threat to life, hospitalization, or permanent disability [Code of Federal Regulations]). Surveillance becomes a more passive process, however, when a drug is approved for marketing and physicians and pharmacists are encouraged to file voluntary written reports through the MedWatch program. Nevertheless, MedWatch receives reports for fewer than 10% of adverse drug reactions,[19] similar to the rate of reporting in France (<6%).[20] The electronic tool for drug-induced serious hepatotoxicity is a graphic instrument that can help identify participants in clinical trials who may be at risk of severe liver disease. Both at-a-glance laboratory data (especially serum aminotransferase and bilirubin levels) for all participants and time-course data for individual patients can be obtained for further scrutiny.[27]

Case Definition: Which Agent?

Many drugs have been implicated in DILI.[28] The evidence for most drugs, however, is confined to individual or small numbers of case reports, especially in letters to scientific journals or to regulatory authorities, or small observational series. Therefore, for most agents, the evidence that they could cause liver injury is circumstantial and incomplete. Reports often lack pathologic definition, thorough exclusion of other disorders, and logistic imputation of causality, especially with respect to temporal associations (see later).[1,23,25] Of the drugs listed in the LiverTox DILI database in 2022, about one-half had convincing associations with DILI. Approximately 50 new agents are added each year, and between 50 and 150 are updated. In general, agents most commonly used in clinical practice and in the community, including antimicrobials, antineoplastic agents, and NSAIDs, are those that have been implicated in causing DILI. The challenge of identifying the culprit drug among multiple candidates is discussed later.

Frequencies of Hepatic Drug Reactions

Because of incomplete reporting, frequencies of hepatic drug reactions are often underestimated. These estimated frequencies are also crude indicators of risk because of the inherent inaccuracies of case definitions (see later) and because case recognition and reporting depend on the skill and motivation of observers.[25] The increased interest of prescribers when initial cases of drug-induced liver disease have been described, together with inappropriate prescribing (e.g., prolonged use of bromfenac, which was approved only for 7 days of use, and overprescribing of flucloxacillin and amoxicillin-clavulanic acid in some countries), can give rise to apparent "mini-epidemics." More appropriate epidemiologic methods applied to hepatotoxicity have included prescription event monitoring, record linkage, and case-control studies. Prescription event monitoring and record linkage have been used to estimate the frequency of liver injury with some antimicrobials (erythromycins, sulfonamides, tetracyclines, flucloxacillin, and amoxicillin-clavulanate) and NSAIDs.[26]

Epidemiologic studies confirm the rarity of drug-induced liver disease with current drugs. For NSAIDs, the risk of liver injury is between 1 and 10 per 100,000 individuals exposed. Amoxicillin-clavulanic acid has been associated with cholestatic hepatitis in 1–2 per 100,000 exposed persons, and low-dose tetracyclines have caused hepatotoxicity in less than 1 case per million persons exposed.[1,18,21,22] The frequency of liver injury may be higher for agents that exert a metabolic type of hepatotoxicity. For example, isoniazid causes liver injury in up to 2% of persons exposed; the risk depends on the patient's age and gender, concomitant exposure to other agents, and presence of HBV and HCV infections. For some drugs in which other host factors play a pathogenic role, case-control studies have been used to define attributable risk. Examples include the association of aspirin with Reye syndrome and oral contraceptives with liver tumors and hepatic vein thrombosis.

In the 1970s, the late Hyman Zimmerman hypothesized a relationship between the frequency and severity of serum ALT elevations that indicate liver injury and the risk of severe hepatotoxicity.[22] According to "Hy's rule," elevations of serum ALT levels to threefold or more above the ULN with an associated increase in the serum bilirubin concentration ($\geq 2 \times$ ULN) without an elevation of the serum alkaline phosphatase level ($< 2 \times$ ULN) indicate a potential for the drug to cause ALF at a rate of about 10% of the number of cases with jaundice. Therefore if 2 cases of jaundice associated with DILI are observed in a phase 3 clinical trial of 2500 patients, 1 case of ALF would be expected for every 12,500 subjects who received the drug during the marketing phase. Modifications of Hy's rule have been suggested to improve its specificity in identifying cases that may progress to ALF.[29,30] These include using an R ratio (ALT/ULN divided by ALP/ULN) or a modified nR ratio (which uses either ALT or AST depending on whichever parameter produces the higher R ratio) of greater than 5. Applying these approaches to a Spanish DILI cohort improved the specificity from 44% (Hy's rule) to 67% (R ratio) and 63% (nR ratio) with similar sensitivities.[29]

Importance of Drugs as a Cause of Liver Disease

Hepatotoxicity accounts for less than 5% of cases of jaundice or acute hepatitis in the community and for even fewer cases of chronic liver disease.[1,22] However, drugs are an important cause of more severe types of liver disease and for liver disease in older people. They account for 10% of cases of severe hepatitis admitted to the hospital in France[22] and for 43% of cases of hepatitis among patients 50 years of age or older.[23] Drugs account for more than one-half of the cases of ALF referred to a special unit in the United States.[23] The pattern and frequency of agents incriminated vary among countries; for example, herbal and dietary supplements accounted for over a quarter of DILI cases in South Korea (see Chapter 91).

In most cases of DILI, drugs are the sole cause of hepatic damage. In other cases, drugs increase the relative risk for types of liver disease that may occur in the absence of drug exposure. Examples include salicylates in Reye syndrome, oral contraceptive steroids (OCS) in hepatic venous thrombosis, methotrexate in hepatic fibrosis associated with alcohol-associated liver disease and MASLD, and tamoxifen in MASLD and metabolic dysfunction-associated steatohepatitis (MASH). Predisposition of patients with preexisting liver disease to DILI is minimal, but potential interactions between chronic HCV infection and several groups of drugs and between chronic HBV infection and antituberculous chemotherapy are now reasonably established. On the other hand, liver failure may be more likely to develop if the patient with a hepatic drug reaction (e.g., to amoxicillin-clavulanic acid) that usually is associated with a good outcome has underlying chronic liver disease.

Risk Factors

For dose-dependent hepatotoxins such as acetaminophen and methotrexate and for some idiosyncratic reactions that are partly dose dependent (e.g., bromfenac, tetracyclines, dantrolene, tacrine, oxypenicillins), the factors that influence the risk of drug-induced liver disease include the drug dose (DILI is more likely with a drug dose $\geq$50 mg daily),[31] blood level of the drug, and duration of intake. For idiosyncratic reactions, however, host determinants are central to liver injury. The most critical determinant is likely to be genetic predisposition, but other "constitutional" and environmental factors can influence the risk of liver injury (Table 90.2). The most important factors are age, gender, exposure to other substances, a history or family history of previous drug reactions, other risk factors for liver disease, and concomitant medical disorders.[21]

Genetic Factors

Genetic determinants predispose to drug-induced liver disease, as they do for other types of drug reaction, such as penicillin allergy.[32] The contention that atopic patients may be at increased risk of some types of drug hepatitis is unproven, however. Genetic factors determine the activity of drug-activating and antioxidant pathways, encode pathways of canalicular bile secretion, and modulate the immune response, tissue stress responses, and cell death pathways. Documented examples of drugs associated with a familial predisposition to adverse hepatic drug reactions are few and include valproic acid and phenytoin.[33] Inherited mitochondrial diseases are a risk factor for valproic acid–induced hepatotoxicity.[33] Some forms of drug-induced liver disease, particularly drug-induced hepatitis and granulomatous reactions, are associated with the reactive metabolite syndrome (see later). Initial studies showed no or only weak associations between specific HLA haplotypes and some types of drug-induced liver disease. Genome-wide association studies (GWAS) have revealed stronger associations between specific HLA haplotypes and several drugs, including flucloxacillin and amoxicillin-clavulanic acid (Table 90.3).[34]

Age

Most hepatic drug reactions are more common in adults than in children. Exceptions include valproic acid hepatotoxicity, which is most common in children under 3 years of age but rare in adults, and Reye syndrome, in which salicylates play a key role. In adults, the risk of isoniazid-associated hepatotoxicity is greater in persons older than 40 years of age. Similar observations have been made for nitrofurantoin, halothane, etretinate, diclofenac, and troglitazone.[1,18,21] The increased frequency of adverse drug reactions in older subjects is largely the result of increased exposure, polypharmacy, and altered drug disposition. In addition, the clinical severity of hepatotoxicity increases strikingly with age, as exemplified by fatal reactions to isoniazid and halothane.[1,18,21]

Gender

Women are particularly predisposed to drug-induced hepatitis, a difference that cannot be attributed simply to increased exposure. Examples include toxicity caused by halothane, nitrofurantoin, sulfonamides, flucloxacillin, minocycline, and troglitazone.[1,22] Drug-induced chronic hepatitis caused by nitrofurantoin, diclofenac, or minocycline has an even more pronounced female preponderance.[1,22] Conversely, equal sex frequency, or even male preponderance is common for some cholestatic drug reactions (e.g., amoxicillin-clavulanic acid). Azathioprine-induced liver disease occurs more frequently in male renal transplant recipients than in female recipients.[35]

Concomitant Exposure to Other Agents

Patients who are taking multiple drugs are more likely to experience an adverse reaction than those who are taking one agent.[1,25] The mechanisms include enhanced CYP-mediated metabolism of the second drug to a toxic intermediate (see later). Examples include toxicity caused by acetaminophen, isoniazid, valproic acid,

TABLE 90.2 Factors Influencing the Risk of Liver Diseases Caused by Drugs

Factor	Examples of Drugs Affected	Influence
Age	Halothane, isoniazid, nitrofurantoin, troglitazone Valproic acid, salicylates	Age >60 years: increased frequency, increased severity More common in children
Gender	Halothane, minocycline, nitrofurantoin Amoxicillin-clavulanic acid, azathioprine	More common in women, especially those with chronic hepatitis More common in men
Dose	Acetaminophen, aspirin, some herbal, and dietary supplements Oxypenicillins, tacrine, tetracycline Vitamin A	Blood levels are directly related to the risk of hepatotoxicity Idiosyncratic reactions, with partial relationship to dose Total dose, dosing frequency, and duration of exposure are related to the risk of hepatic fibrosis
Genetic factors	Halothane, phenytoin, sulfonamides Abacavir, amoxicillin-clavulanic acid, flucloxacillin Valproic acid	Multiple cases in families Strong HLA association Familial cases, association with mitochondrial enzyme deficiencies
Other drugs	Acetaminophen Valproic acid Anticancer drugs	Isoniazid, phenytoin, and zidovudine lower the dose threshold and increase the severity of hepatotoxicity Other antiepileptic drugs increase the risk of hepatotoxicity Interactive vascular toxicity
History of other drug reactions	Enflurane, halothane, isoflurane Erythromycins Diclofenac, ibuprofen, tiaprofenic acid COX-2 inhibitors, sulfonamides	Instances of cross-sensitivity have been reported among members of each drug class but are rare
Excessive alcohol use	Acetaminophen Isoniazid, methotrexate	Lowered dose threshold, poorer outcome Increased risk of liver injury, hepatic fibrosis
Nutritional Status		
Obesity	Halothane, methotrexate, tamoxifen, troglitazone	Increased risk of liver injury, hepatic fibrosis
Fasting	Acetaminophen	Increased risk of hepatotoxicity
Preexisting liver disease	Hycanthone, pemoline Antituberculosis drugs, ibuprofen	Increased risk of liver injury Increased risk of liver injury with chronic hepatitis B and C
Other Diseases/Conditions		
Diabetes mellitus	Methotrexate	Increased risk of hepatic fibrosis
HIV/AIDS	Sulfonamides	Increased risk of hypersensitivity
Renal failure	Methotrexate, tetracycline	Increased risk of liver injury, hepatic fibrosis
Organ transplantation	Azathioprine, busulfan, thioguanine	Increased risk of vascular toxicity

TABLE 90.3 Genetic Variants Associated With DILI

Drug	Category	Allele(s)	Odds ratio (CI) for DILI
Amoxicillin-clavulanic acid	Antibiotic	**HLA-DRB1*1501;** DRB5*0101; DQB1*0602	2.3 (1.0–5.26)
Diclofenac	NSAID	ABCC2 C-24T [MRP2]	6 (2.4–17)
Flucloxacillin	Antibiotic	HLA-B*5701	80.6 (23–285)
Lapatinib	Tyrosine kinase inhibitor	HLA-DRB1*07:01	6.2 (4.1–9.5)
Lumiracoxib	NSAID	HLA-DQA1*0102; **DRB1* 1501;** DQB1*0602; DRB5*0101	6.3 (4.1–9.6)
Minocycline	Antibiotic	B*35:02	30
Nevirapine	Protease inhibitor	B*58:01	3.5
Sex hormones	Various	ABCB11 V444A [BSEP]	1.7; 4
Terbinafine	Antifungal drug	A*3301	2.3
Ticlopidine	Antiplatelet	HLA A*3303	36.5 (7.3–184)
Trimethoprim-sulfamethoxazole	Antibiotic	HLA B*14:01 (Caucasians) HLA B*35:01 (African Americans)	9.2 2.8
Ximelagatran	Thrombin inhibitor	HLA-DRB1*0701	4.4

*Alleles in bold are the most important in the pathogenesis of DILI for the particular drug.
ABC, ATP-binding cassette; *BSEP*, bile salt export pump; *CI*, confidence intervals; *MRP2*, multidrug resistance-associated protein 2.

other anticonvulsants, and anticancer drugs. Alternatively, drugs may alter the disposition of other agents by reducing bile flow or competing with canalicular pathways for biliary excretion (phase 3 drug elimination). This mechanism may account for interactions between OCS and other drugs to produce cholestasis. Drugs or their metabolites may also interact through mechanisms of cellular toxicity and cell death that involve mitochondrial injury, intracellular signaling pathways, activation of transcription factors, and regulation of hepatic genes involved in controlling the response to stress and injury that triggers proinflammatory and cell death processes.[6,36]

Previous Drug Reactions
A history of an adverse drug reaction generally increases the risk of reactions to the same drug as well as other agents. Nevertheless, instances of cross-sensitivity to related agents in cases of drug-induced liver disease are surprisingly uncommon. Examples of cross-sensitivity between drugs (or drug classes) include the haloalkane anesthetics (see Chapter 91), erythromycins, phenothiazines and tricyclic antidepressants, isoniazid and pyrazinamide, and some NSAIDs. A crucial point is that a previous reaction to the same drug is a major risk factor for an increase in the severity of DILI.[22] A Spanish study examined the risk of DILI in persons with a history of DILI (with a different drug).[37] Recurrent DILI was infrequent (1.2%) and was attributable most commonly to drugs that were structurally similar or had similar targets, whereas others exhibited features consistent with AIH, thereby raising the possibility that immune-mediated processes may be mechanistically involved or that the correct diagnosis was actually AIH.

Alcohol
Chronic excessive alcohol ingestion decreases the dose threshold for and enhances the severity of acetaminophen-induced hepatotoxicity and increases the risk and severity of isoniazid hepatitis, niacin (nicotinic acid, nicotinamide) hepatotoxicity, and methotrexate-induced hepatic fibrosis.

Nutritional Status
Obesity is strongly associated with the risk of halothane hepatitis and is an independent risk factor for MASH and hepatic fibrosis in persons taking methotrexate or tamoxifen. Fasting also predisposes to acetaminophen hepatotoxicity[38] and a role for undernutrition has been proposed in isoniazid hepatotoxicity.[39]

Preexisting Liver Disease
In general, liver diseases, such as alcohol-associated cirrhosis and cholestatic disorders, do not predispose to adverse hepatic reactions.[40] Exceptions include toxicity due to some anticancer drugs, niacin, pemoline, and hycanthone. Preexisting liver disease is a critical determinant of methotrexate-induced hepatic fibrosis. Patients with chronic HBV or HCV infection or HIV/AIDS appear to be at heightened risk of liver injury during antituberculous or ART therapy,[41] after exposure to ibuprofen and possibly other NSAIDs, after myeloablative therapy in preparation for bone marrow transplantation (resulting in sinusoidal obstruction syndrome),[42] and possibly after taking antiandrogens, such as flutamide and cyproterone acetate (CPA).[43] A particularly strong association has been reported between HCV infection and the risk of liver injury during ART; the risk may be increased 2–10-fold.[44,45]

Other Diseases
RA increases the risk of salicylate hepatotoxicity, and a curious, unexplained observation is that sulfasalazine hepatitis is more common in patients with RA than in those with IBD. Diabetes mellitus, obesity, and chronic kidney disease predispose to methotrexate-induced hepatic fibrosis, whereas HIV/AIDS confers a heightened risk of sulfonamide hypersensitivity.[46–48] A retrospective cohort study found that the age- and sex-standardized incidence of drug-induced ALF in patients with diabetes mellitus was 0.08–0.15 per 1000 person-years, irrespective of the therapeutic agent used (the number using troglitazone was small); the incidence was highest (approximately 0.3 per 1000) during the first 6 months of exposure.[47] Renal transplantation is a risk factor for azathioprine-associated vascular injury, whereas kidney disease predisposes to tetracycline-induced fatty liver.[22] Finally, sinusoidal obstruction syndrome induced by anticancer drugs is more common after bone marrow transplantation[41] and in persons with HCV infection.[1,22,24,25]

Pathophysiology

Toxic Mechanisms of Liver Injury

Direct Hepatotoxins and Reactive Metabolites
Highly hepatotoxic chemicals injure key subcellular structures, particularly mitochondria and the plasma membrane. The injury arrests energy generation, dissipates ionic gradients, and disrupts the physical integrity of the cell. This type of overwhelming cellular injury does not apply to currently relevant hepatotoxins, most of which require metabolic activation to mediate damage to liver cells. The resulting reactive metabolites can interact with critical cellular target molecules, particularly those with nucleophilic substituents such as thiol-rich proteins and nucleic acids. Together with ROS, they act as oxidizing species within the hepatocyte to establish oxidative stress, a state of imbalance between pro-oxidants and antioxidants. ROS are also key signaling molecules that mediate biological responses to stress, as discussed later. Alternatively, reactive metabolites bind irreversibly to macromolecules, particularly proteins and lipids. Such covalent binding may produce injury by inactivating key enzymes or by forming protein-drug adducts that could be targets for immunodestructive processes that cause liver injury. Notwithstanding these comments, there is increasing evidence that "direct hepatotoxins," such as acetaminophen, activate innate immune mechanisms in the liver in response to stress with release of danger-activated molecular patterns; the latter (as well as bacterial products such as endotoxin, a pathogen-associated molecular pattern) trigger Toll-like receptors to activate proinflammatory and cell death pathways.[49]

Oxidative Stress and the Glutathione System
The liver is exposed to oxidative stress by the propensity of hepatocytes to reduce oxygen, particularly in mitochondria and in microsomal electron transport systems (such as CYP2E1), and by NADPH-oxidase-catalyzed formation of ROS and nitroradicals in Kupffer cells, endothelial cells, and stimulated polymorphonuclear leukocytes (neutrophils) and macrophages. To combat oxidative stress, the liver is well-endowed with antioxidant mechanisms, including micronutrients, such as vitamin E and vitamin C, thiol-rich proteins (e.g., metallothionein, ubiquinone), metal-sequestering proteins (e.g., ferritin), and enzymes that metabolize reactive metabolites (e.g., epoxide hydrolases), ROS (e.g., catalase, superoxide dismutase), and lipid peroxides (e.g., glutathione peroxidases). Glutathione (L-δ-glutamyl-L-cysteine-glycine) is the most important antioxidant in the mammalian liver.[36]

Hepatocytes are the exclusive site of glutathione synthesis. Hepatic levels of glutathione are high (5–10 mmol/L) and can be increased by enhancing the supply of cysteine for glutathione synthesis; this mechanism is the cornerstone of thiol antidote therapy for acetaminophen poisoning. Hepatocyte glutathione synthesis increases in response to pro-oxidants, as occurs when CYP2E1 is overexpressed as a result of signaling via the redox-sensitive transcription factor Nrf.[6,36,50,51] Glutathione synthesis, via expression of the rate-limiting enzyme glutamate cysteine ligase, is also a response to mitochondrial injury by such agents as acetaminophen. Glutathione in its reduced form (GSH) is a critical cofactor for several antioxidant pathways, including thiol-disulfide exchange reactions and glutathione peroxidase. Glutathione peroxidase has a higher affinity for hydrogen peroxide than does catalase, and it disposes of lipid peroxides, free radicals, and electrophilic drug metabolites. GSH is also a cofactor for conjugation reactions catalyzed by the glutathione *S*-transferases involved with phase 3 transport of drug metabolites into bile. Other reactions proceed nonenzymatically. In turn, the products include glutathione-protein mixed disulfides and oxidized glutathione. The latter can be converted back to glutathione by proton donation catalyzed by glutathione reductase.

Normally, most glutathione within the hepatocyte is in the reduced state, indicating the importance of this pathway for maintenance of the redox capacity of the cell. The reduced form of NADPH is an essential cofactor for glutathione reductase; NADPH formation requires ATP, thereby illustrating a critical link between mitochondrial integrity and the energy-generating capacity of the liver and its ability to withstand oxidative stress. Glutathione is also compartmentalized within the hepatocyte, with the highest concentrations found in the cytosol. Adequate levels of glutathione are essential in mitochondria, where ROS are constantly being formed as a minor byproduct of oxidative respiration and in response to some drugs or metabolites that interfere with the mitochondrial respiratory chain. Mitochondrial glutathione is maintained by active uptake from the cytosol via a transport system that is altered by chronic ethanol exposure and in some forms of lipotoxicity (e.g., with cholesterol) and is therefore another potential target for drug toxicity.[36]

Biochemical Mechanisms of Cellular Injury

Mechanisms once thought to be central to hepatotoxicity, such as covalent binding to cellular enzymes and peroxidation of membrane lipids, are no longer regarded as exclusive pathways of cellular damage. Rather, oxidation of proteins, phospholipid fatty acyl side chains (lipid peroxidation), and nucleosides appears to be a component of the biochemical stress that characterizes toxic liver injury. In one experiment, healthy volunteers were administered a variety of low-molecular-weight heparins, known to cause transient serum ALT elevations.[52] In addition to aminotransferase increases in >90% of cases, markers of subcellular injury (cytosolic, mitochondrial), apoptosis [M30 fragmentation product of cytokeratin (CK) 8/18], microRNA (miRNA)-122, DNA, and high-mobility group box-1 (HMGB1) increased; HMGB1 is a DAMP released in necrosis. The authors concluded that heparins as a class caused self-limited and mild necrosis with secondary activation of an innate immune response. Secondary reactions, including posttranslational modification of proteins via adenosine diphosphate ribosylation or protease activation, cleavage of DNA by activation of endogenous endonucleases, and disruption of lipid membranes by activated phospholipases, may also play a role in DILI.[7] Some of these catabolic reactions could be initiated by a rise in the cytosolic ionic calcium concentration $(Ca^{2+})_i$, as a result of increased Ca^{2+} entry or release from internal stores in the endoplasmic reticulum and mitochondria.[7] The potential role of endoplasmic reticulum stress in DILI is less well defined.[53]

The concept that hepatotoxic chemicals cause hepatocyte cell death by a biochemical final common pathway [e.g., activation of catalytic enzymes by a rise in (Ca^{2+})] has proved inadequate to explain the diverse processes that can result in lethal hepatocellular injury. Rather, a variety of processes can damage key organelles, thereby causing intracellular stress that activates signaling pathways and transcription factors. Mitochondrial injury, particularly that signaled via activation of the c-Jun *N*-terminal kinase (JNK), appears to be critically involved with acetaminophen and most likely several other hepatotoxins.[49,54–56] In turn, the balance between these factors can trigger the onset of cell death or facilitate protection of the cell, as discussed later.

Types of Cell Death

Apoptosis

Apoptosis is an energy-dependent, genetically programmed form of cell death that typically results in controlled deletion of individual cells. In addition to its major roles in developmental biology, tissue regulation, and carcinogenesis, apoptosis is important in toxic, viral, and immune-mediated liver injury.[57–60] The ultrastructural features of apoptosis are cell and nuclear shrinkage, condensation and margination of nuclear chromatin, plasma membrane blebbing, and ultimately fragmentation of the cell into membrane-bound bodies that contain intact mitochondria and other organelles. Engulfment of these apoptotic bodies by surrounding epithelial and mesenchymal cells conserves cell fragments that contain nucleic acid and intact mitochondria. These fragments are then digested by lysosomes and recycled without release of bioactive substances. As a consequence, apoptosis in its purest form (usually found only in vitro) does not incite an inflammatory tissue reaction. The cellular processes that occur in apoptosis are often mediated by caspases, a family of proteolytic enzymes that contain a cysteine at their active site and cleave polypeptides at aspartate residues; noncaspase-mediated programmed cell death has also been described in experimental hepatotoxicity.

Apoptosis rarely, if ever, is the sole form of cell death in common forms of liver injury, such as ischemia-reperfusion injury, cholestasis, and toxic liver injury, all of which are typically associated with at least some necrosis and a hepatic inflammatory response. Whether activation of prodeath signals causes cell death depends on several factors, including prosurvival signals, the rapidity of the process, the availability of glutathione and ATP, and the role of other cell types. Some of these issues are discussed briefly here and are reviewed in more detail elsewhere.[57–60]

The operation of hepatocellular apoptosis can be determined by detection of the caspase-3-cleaved fragmentation product (M30) of CKs 8 and 18 that is specific to hepatocytes. Hepatocytes undergo apoptosis when proapoptotic intracellular signaling pathways are activated, either because of toxic biochemical processes within the cell (intrinsic pathway) or because cell surface receptors are activated to transduce cell death signals (external pathway). Proapoptotic receptors are members of the TNF receptor superfamily, which possess a so-called death domain. These receptors include Fas, for which the cognate ligand is Fasligand (FasL), TNF-R1 receptor (cognate ligand is TNF), and *T*NF-*r*elated *a*poptosis-*i*nducing *l*igand (TRAIL) receptors (cognate ligand is TRAIL). In addition to model hepatotoxins such as the quinone, menadione, and hydrogen peroxide, some drugs (e.g., acetaminophen, plant diterpenoids) have been shown to be converted into pro-oxidant reactive metabolites, thereby initiating the following sequence: CYP-mediated metabolism to form reactive metabolites → glutathione depletion → mitochondrial injury with release of cytochrome *c* and activation of the mitochondrial membrane permeability transition → caspase activation → apoptosis.

Mitochondria play a pivotal role in pathways that provoke or oppose apoptosis.[55,57,58,60] In the external pathway, the activation of the death domain of proapoptotic receptors recruits adapter molecules, Fas-associated death domain and TNF receptor-associated death domain, which bind and activate procaspase 8 to form the death-inducing signaling complex. In turn, caspase 8 cleaves Bid, a proapoptotic member of the B cell lymphoma/leukemia (Bcl-2) family, to tBid. Then, tBid causes translocation of Bax to the mitochondria, where it aggregates with Bak to promote permeability of the mitochondria.[57] Release of cytochrome *c* and other prodeath molecules, including Smac [which binds caspase inhibitor proteins, such as inhibitor of apoptosis proteins (IAPs)] and apoptosis-inducing factor (AIF, also known as Apaf),[58] allows formation of the "apoptosome," which activates caspase 9 and eventually caspase 3 to execute cell death (Fig. 90.1). Intracellular stresses in various sites release other mitochondrial permeabilizing proteins (e.g., Bmf from the cytoskeleton and Bim from the endoplasmic reticulum), whereas members of the Bcl-2 family, Bcl-2 and Bcl-xL, antagonize apoptosis and serve as survival factors by regulating the integrity of mitochondria; the protective mechanism is not yet fully understood but involves myeloid cell leukemia sequence 1 (Mcl-1). Stress-activated protein kinases, particularly JNK, are also proapoptotic,[59] targeting Mcl-1 degradation and phosphorylating and inactivating the mitochondrial protective protein Bcl-xL.

Execution of cell death by apoptosis usually occurs via activation of caspase 3, but more than one caspase-independent pathway of programmed cell death has been described.[60] Stresses to the endoplasmic reticulum can bypass mitochondrial events by activation of caspase 12, which, in turn, activates caspase 9 independently of the apoptosome. The final steps of programmed cell death are energy dependent. Therefore depletion of ATP abrogates the controlled attempt at "cell suicide," resulting instead in necrosis (see later) or an overlapping pattern that has been designated as "apoptotic necrosis" or "necrapoptosis."[61,62] Furthermore, when apoptosis is massive, the capacity for rapid phagocytosis can be exceeded, and "secondary" necrosis can occur.[62]

Intracellular processes and activation of proapoptotic death receptors are not mutually exclusive pathways of cell death in toxic liver injury. In fact, drug toxicity could predispose the injured hepatocyte to apoptosis mediated by TNF-R or Fas-operated pathways by several mechanisms, including blockade of nuclear factor kappa B (NF-κB), which usually is a hepatoprotective transcription factor in hepatocytes, and inhibition of purine and protein synthesis. Furthermore, activation of Kupffer cells (e.g., by endotoxin) and recruitment of activated inflammatory cells can increase production of TNF.

Caspase inhibition is an important protective mechanism against cell death. Such antiapoptotic pathways include chemical blockade of the cysteine thiol group by nitric oxide (NO) or ROS and cellular depletion of glutathione.[7] Protein inhibitors include IAP family members, heat shock proteins, and FLICE (caspase-8)-inhibitory proteins (FLIP).[57–59] FLIP inhibits caspase-8 activation as a decoy for Fas-associated death domain binding. Bcl-2 and Bcl-xL inhibit mitochondrial permeability, whereas

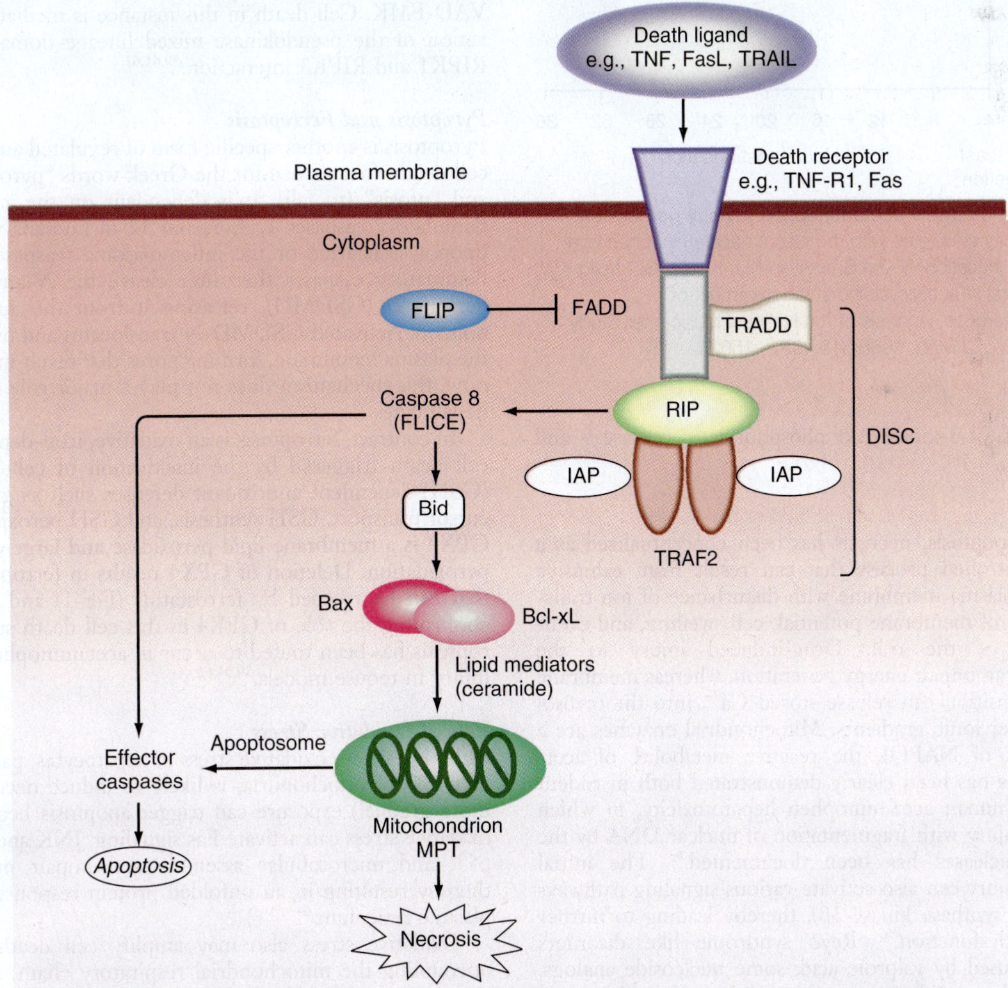

Fig. 90.1 Apoptosis and necrosis pathways in mammalian cells. See text for details. *Bcl*, B-cell lymphoma/leukemia family (Bax, Bid, and Bcl-xL are members); *DISC*, death-inducing signaling complex; *FADD*, Fas-associated death domain; *FLIP*, FLICE-inhibitory proteins; *IAP*, inhibitor of apoptosis proteins; *MPT*, mitochondrial permeability transition; *RIP*, receptor-interacting protein; *TNF*, tumor necrosis factor; *TNF-R1*, TNF receptor-1; *TRADD*, TNF receptor-associated death domain; *TRAF2*, TNF receptor-associated factor-2; *TRAIL*, TNF-related apoptosis ligand.

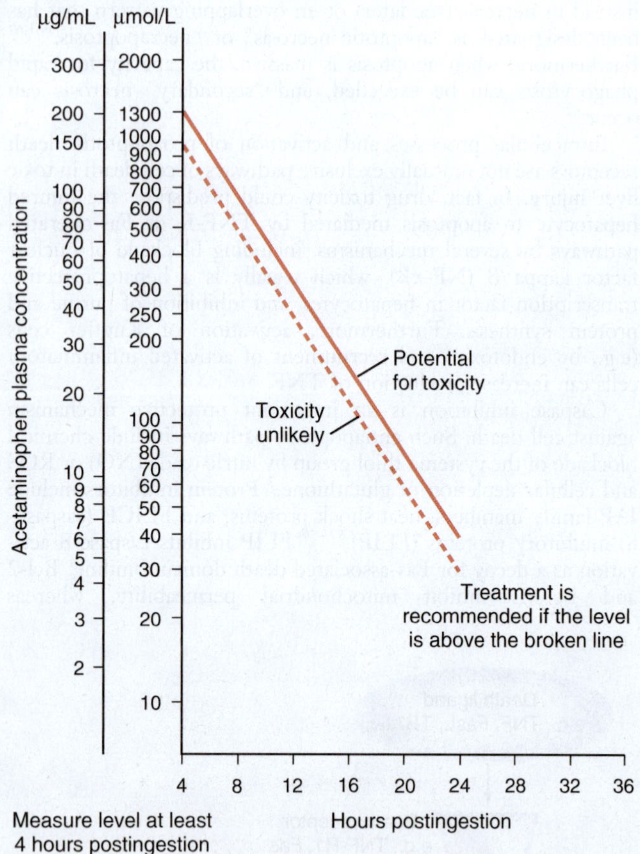

Fig. 90.2 Rumack-Matthew acetaminophen toxicity nomogram. The risk of hepatotoxicity correlates with the plasma acetaminophen level and the time after ingestion. (From Smilkstein MJ, Knapp GL, Kulig KW, et al. Efficacy of oral *N*-acetylcysteine in the treatment of acetaminophen overdose. Analysis of the National Multicenter Study [1976–1985]. *N Engl J Med*. 1988;319:1557–1562.)

phosphatidylinositol 3-kinase/Akt phosphorylates caspase 9 and activates NF-κB.

Necrosis

In contrast to apoptosis, necrosis has been conceptualized as a relatively uncontrolled process that can result from extensive damage to the plasma membrane with disturbance of ion transport, dissolution of membrane potential, cell swelling, and eventually rupture of the cell. Drug-induced injury to the mitochondrion can impair energy generation, whereas membrane permeability transition can release stored Ca^{2+} into the cytosol and perturb other ionic gradients. Mitochondrial enzymes are a particular target of NAPQI, the reactive metabolite of acetaminophen. This has been clearly demonstrated both in rodent models and in human acetaminophen hepatotoxicity, in which mitochondrial injury with fragmentation of nuclear DNA by the released endonucleases has been documented.[63] The initial mitochondrial injury can also activate various signaling pathways (JNK, glycogen synthase kinase-3β), thereby leading to further mitochondrial dysfunction.[55] Reye syndrome–like disorders (e.g., toxicity caused by valproic acid; some nucleoside analogs, such as fialuridine, didanosine, zidovudine, zalcitabine; and possibly "ecstasy") may also result from mitochondrial injury. Mitochondrial injury can result in cell death by either apoptosis or necrosis[61,62]; the type of cell death pathway may depend primarily on the energy state of the cell, as well as the rapidity and severity of the injury process. In the presence of ATP, cell death can proceed by apoptosis, but when mitochondria are de-energized, the mechanism of cell death is necrosis. This apparent dichotomy between cell death processes is probably artificial, and apoptosis and necrosis more likely represent the morphologic and mechanistic ends of a spectrum of overlapping cell death processes.[36,62]

One important way in which necrosis differs from apoptosis is that uncontrolled dissolution of the cell liberates danger-activated molecular patterns (e.g., HMGB1) and macromolecular breakdown products, including lipid peroxides, aldehydes, and eicosanoids. The latter products act as chemoattractants for circulating leukocytes, which then partake in the inflammatory response in the hepatic parenchyma. Even before cell death occurs, oxidative stress produced during drug toxicity can upregulate adhesion molecules and chemokines that are expressed or secreted by endothelial cells. These processes contribute to recruitment of the hepatic inflammatory response, which is prominent in some types of drug-induced liver disease. Lymphocytes, polymorphonuclear leukocytes (neutrophils and eosinophils), and macrophages also may be attracted to the liver as part of a cell-mediated immune reaction.[64]

Necroptosis

This is a different type of regulated necrosis implicated in drug-induced liver injury, triggered by TNF superfamily member receptor activation in the presence of caspase inhibitors such as Z-VAD-FMK. Cell death in this instance is mediated via the activation of the pseudokinase mixed lineage domain (MLKL) by RIPK1 and RIPK3 interaction.[59,61,62]

Pyroptosis and Ferroptosis

Pyroptosis is another specific form of regulated and inflammatory cell death, first named for the Greek words "pyro" (fire or fever) and "ptosis" (to fall). It is dependent on the activation of inflammatory caspases 1, 4, 5, and 12 in humans via intracellular lipopolysaccharide or the inflammasome (caspase-1). These inflammatory caspases thereafter cleave the *N*-terminus of Gasdermin D (GSDMD), releasing it from the autoinhibitory C domain. Activated GSDMD-N translocates and binds to lipids in the plasma membrane, forming pores that result in cell death. For now, this mechanism does not play a major role in cell death in hepatocytes.[59]

In contrast, ferroptosis is an oxidative, iron-dependent form of cell death triggered by the inactivation of cellular glutathione (GSH)-dependent antioxidant defenses such as glutathione precursor transport, GSH synthesis, and GSH peroxidase 4 (GPX4). GPX4 is a membrane lipid peroxidase and largely prevents lipid peroxidation. Deletion of GPX4 results in ferroptotic cell death that can be rescued by ferrostatins (Fer-1) and iron chelators, confirming the role of GPX4 in this cell death subroutine. Ferroptosis has been touted to occur in acetaminophen-related liver injury in mouse models.[59,61,62]

Role of Oxidative Stress

Although severe oxidative stress in hepatocytes, particularly when focused on mitochondria, is likely to induce necrosis, lesser (or more gradual) exposure can trigger apoptosis because ROS and oxidative stress can activate Fas signaling, JNK and other kinases, p53, and microtubular assembly and impair protein folding, thereby resulting in an unfolded protein response by the endoplasmic reticulum.[64]

Oxidative stress also may amplify cell death processes by uncoupling the mitochondrial respiratory chain, releasing cytochrome *c*, or massively oxidizing and exporting glutathione (intact glutathione is required for Fas signaling). Conversely, oxidative stress may protect against apoptosis in some circumstances through inhibition of caspase or activation of NF-κB. As a result of these opposing effects, predicting the consequences of hepatic oxidative stress in terms of liver injury is not straightforward.

Role of Hepatic Nonparenchymal Cells and the Innate Immune Response

In addition to migratory cells, the activation of nonparenchymal liver cell types is likely to play an important role in drug and toxin-induced liver injury. Kupffer cells function as resident macrophages and antigen-presenting cells, whereas dendritic cells and natural killer T cells are also resident in the liver and play a role in antigen processing and innate immunity. Some of the toxic effects of activated Kupffer cells, as well as of recruited leukocytes, may be mediated by release of cytokines, such as TNF-α, interleukin-1β, and Fas-L, which under some circumstances can induce cell death in hepatocytes by apoptosis or necrosis.[62] In addition, activated Kupffer cells release ROS, nitroradicals, leukotrienes, and proteases. It has been suggested, however, that the sterile inflammatory response may aid in clearing cell debris and pave the way for tissue repair.[65]

Endothelial cells of the hepatic sinusoids or terminal hepatic veins are vulnerable to injury by some hepatotoxins because of their low glutathione content. Such hepatotoxins include the pyrrolizidine alkaloids, which are an important cause of the sinusoidal obstruction syndrome (formerly hepatic veno-occlusive disease).[66] Other types of drug-induced vascular injury may be caused primarily by involvement of the sinusoidal endothelial cells.

Hepatic stellate cells are the principal liver cell type involved in matrix deposition in hepatic fibrosis. Stellate cells are activated in methotrexate-induced hepatic fibrosis. The possibility that vitamin A, ROS, or drug metabolites can transform stellate cells into collagen-synthesizing myofibroblasts is of considerable interest.

Immunologic Mechanisms

Adaptation is an important phenomenon, and the mechanisms likely vary among agents.[67] In general, agents with higher intrinsic toxicity are more likely to cause ALT increases during the early phase of therapy; isoniazid is a classic example. Although such agents are associated with DILI in some cases, the frequency of DILI is typically of the order of only 0.01%–1%, compared with a frequency of 3%–30% for serum ALT elevations early in therapy. Therefore the high proportions of cases of transient serum ALT elevations are associated with a process that is terminated and does not progress to clinically important liver injury—adaptation. Older concepts of how adaptation comes about relate to the induction of cellular proteins that are protective against injury from a reactive metabolite, glutathione antioxidant pathways, and induction of conjugating enzymes, excretory pathways, or anticell death proteins. Subsequent concepts have focused on induction of innate immunity as the final pathway by which adaptation occurs. In this sense, drug reactions that can be explained by an immunoallergic mechanism may be regarded as a failure of adaptation.

Immune attack involves liganding of death receptors, as discussed earlier, or porin-mediated introduction of granzyme.[36,68] The hallmarks of drug allergy include (1) delayed onset after initial exposure and accelerated onset after rechallenge, (2) hepatic inflammatory infiltrates with neutrophils and eosinophils, and (3) fever, rash, lymphadenopathy, eosinophilia, and involvement of other organs. In some cases, the liver is implicated as part of a systemic hypersensitivity reaction, as described later for the drug reaction with eosinophilia and systemic symptoms (DRESS) syndrome, also termed drug-induced hypersensitivity syndrome and, formerly, reactive metabolite syndrome. Why the liver is the predominant site of injury in some persons, whereas other organs are involved in other persons, is unclear; genetic factors relevant to tissue-specific gene expression may be involved.

One possible immunopathogenic mechanism for drug-induced liver disease is the altered antigen concept, in which an initial interaction between drug metabolites and cellular proteins results in the formation of neoantigens (haptens) or drug-protein adducts. An example is the formation of trifluoroacetylated adducts after exposure to halothane or other haloalkane anesthetics (see Chapter 91). For these adducts to initiate tissue-damaging immune responses: (1) processing should be presented in an immunogenic form (e.g., by Kupffer cells, in association with MHC molecules); (2) appropriately responsive $CD4^+$ T cells must be present to provide help to induce an immune response; and (3) the drug-derived antigen, together with a class II MHC molecule, must be expressed on the target cells to attract $CD8^+$ (cytotoxic) T cells. That bile duct epithelial cells are more likely to express class II MHC antigens may explain why they are possible targets in drug-induced cholestatic hepatitis.

Although antibodies directed against trifluoroacetylated protein adducts circulate in the majority of patients following recovery from halothane-induced liver injury,[69] the specificity and pathogenicity of these antibodies remain in doubt. Alternatively, circulating drug-induced antibodies could cause immune-mediated lysis of hepatocytes through molecular mimicry of host enzymes.[70] Experimental evidence suggests that for diclofenac, antibody-dependent cell-mediated immunity could operate as a mechanism for drug-induced liver disease.[71] Finally, for drugs that do not act as haptens, immune-related liver injury can still result either through noncovalent direct interactions of the drug with MHC molecules (e.g., ximelagatran with HLA DRB1*07:01)[72] or by drug modification of the MHC binding groove so that endogenous peptides are perceived as nonself and induce an immune response.[73]

A second type of immunopathogenic mechanism is dysregulation of the immune system, termed drug-induced autoimmunity.[74] This mechanism can lead to the formation of drug-induced autoantibodies [e.g., antiliver-kidney microsome (LKM) antibodies] directed against microsomal enzymes. For tienilic acid, CYP2C9 is the target of anti-LKM, whereas for halothane hepatitis, anti-LKM is directed against CYP2E1. Nontissue-specific autoantibodies (e.g., ANA, smooth muscle antibodies) may be detected in patients with nitrofurantoin, methyldopa, or minocycline hepatitis. Like spontaneous autoimmunity, drug-induced autoimmunity results from genetically determined anomalies of immune tolerance.

Clinicopathologic Features

Classification

Hepatic drug reactions mimic other liver diseases, but classification is often difficult because of overlap among categories. Although a classic (signature) syndrome is associated with many individual agents, a given drug can be associated with more than one clinicopathologic syndrome. Furthermore, the clinical and laboratory features of liver disease and the liver histology may be discordant. Therefore although recognition of specific patterns or syndromes is vital, the chronologic relationship between administration of the drug and liver injury is more important in making a diagnosis.

Drugs are often divided into dose dependent, or predictable, hepatotoxins and dose-independent, or unpredictable (idiosyncratic), hepatotoxins. Dose-dependent hepatotoxins generally require metabolic activation to toxic metabolites or interfere with subcellular organelles and biochemical processes at key sites, such as mitochondria or canalicular bile secretion. Liver injury usually occurs rapidly (within hours), is characterized by zonal necrosis or microvesicular steatosis, and is reproducible in other species. By contrast, idiosyncratic hepatotoxins cause a wide range of histologic changes and do not reliably cause injury in other species; in addition, the latent period is variable in duration. The distinction between dose-dependent and idiosyncratic hepatotoxins is blurred with agents such as dantrolene, flucloxacillin, cyclophosphamide, nucleoside analogs, anticancer drugs, and cyclosporine. Liver injury caused by each of these drugs is partly dose dependent, but reactions occur in only a minority of exposed persons.

Two general types of mechanisms account for idiosyncratic hepatotoxicity: metabolic idiosyncrasy and immunoallergy. Metabolic idiosyncrasy refers to the susceptibility of rare persons to hepatotoxicity from a drug that, in conventional doses, is usually safe. Such susceptibility may result from genetic or acquired differences in drug metabolism or canalicular secretion, mitochondrial defects, or cell death receptor signaling. Immunoallergy indicates involvement of the immune system in mediating the response to a drug. These two mechanisms may be interrelated (see the "Metabolic Idiosyncrasy" section). Other pathogenic mechanisms may include indirect mediation of liver injury, as in vascular and possibly hyperthermic changes produced by cocaine, ecstasy, intra-arterial floxuridine, and possibly anesthetics (see Chapter 91).

The most practical classification of drug hepatotoxicity is based on clinical and laboratory features and liver histology, as summarized in Table 90.4. This classification provides a framework for discussing drug-induced hepatic disease but is imperfect because the clinical and pathologic features are not always congruent. Moreover, much overlap between categories exists, particularly in the spectrum from severe necrosis (which may result from dose-dependent or idiosyncratic hepatotoxicity) to focal necrosis with lobular inflammation (hepatitis) to cholestasis. Many drugs produce a spectrum of syndromes from hepatitis to cholestasis, and some authorities include a further category of mixed cholestatic-hepatocellular reactions. Granulomatous hepatitis has a liver biochemical test profile that is indistinguishable from those typical of hepatitis, cholestasis, or mixed reactions.

Drugs can alter liver biochemical test results without causing significant liver injury. Such adaptive responses include hyperbilirubinemia associated with rifampin, cyclosporine, and indinavir and raised serum GGTP and alkaline phosphatase levels associated with phenytoin and warfarin.[1,22] The latter effect is probably attributable to microsomal enzyme induction. For other agents, transient ALT or AST elevations are probably related to hepatocellular necrosis (discussed earlier for heparins), but with

TABLE 90.4 Clinicopathologic Classification of Drug-Induced Liver Disease

Category	Description	Implicated Drugs: Examples
Hepatic adaptation	No symptoms; raised serum GGTP and AP levels (occasionally raised ALT)	Heparins, phenytoin, warfarin
	Hyperbilirubinemia	HIV protease inhibitors, rifampin
Dose-dependent hepatotoxicity	Symptoms of hepatitis; zonal, bridging, and massive necrosis; serum ALT level >5-fold increased, often >2000 U/L	Acetaminophen, amodiaquine, hycanthone, nicotinic acid
Other cytopathic toxicity, acute steatosis	Microvesicular steatosis, diffuse or zonal; partially dose dependent, severe liver injury, features of mitochondrial toxicity (e.g., lactic acidosis)	ART agents, didanosine, fialuridine, L-asparaginase, some herbal and dietary supplements, valproic acid
Acute hepatitis	Symptoms of hepatitis; focal, bridging, and massive necrosis; serum ALT level >5-fold increased; extrahepatic features of drug allergy in some cases	Acebutolol, dantrolene, disulfiram, etretinate, halothane, ipilimumab, isoniazid, ketoconazole, nitrofurantoin, nivolumab, pembrolizumab, phenytoin, sulfonamides, terbinafine, troglitazone
Chronic hepatitis	Duration >3 months; interface hepatitis, bridging necrosis, fibrosis, cirrhosis; clinical and laboratory features of chronic liver disease; autoantibodies with some types of reaction	Diclofenac, etretinate, minocycline, nefazodone, nitrofurantoin (see Table 90.8)
Granulomatous hepatitis	Hepatic granulomas with varying hepatitis and cholestasis; raised serum ALT, AP, and GGTP levels	Allopurinol, carbamazepine, hydralazine, quinidine, quinine (see Table 90.7)
Cholestasis without hepatitis	Cholestasis, no inflammation; serum AP levels > twice normal	Androgens, oral contraceptives
Cholestatic hepatitis	Cholestasis with inflammation; symptoms of hepatitis; raised serum ALT; and AP levels	Amoxicillin-clavulanic acid, chlorpromazine, cyproterone acetate, erythromycins, tricyclic antidepressants
Cholestasis with bile duct injury	Bile duct lesions and cholestatic hepatitis; clinical features of cholangitis	Chlorpromazine, dextropropoxyphene, flucloxacillin
Chronic cholestasis	Duration >3 months	—
VBDS	Paucity of small bile ducts; resembles PBC, but AMA negative	Chlorpromazine, flucloxacillin, trimethoprim sulfamethoxazole
Sclerosing cholangitis	Strictures of large bile ducts	Intraarterial floxuridine, intralesional scolicidals
Steatohepatitis	Steatosis, focal necrosis, Mallory hyaline, pericellular fibrosis, cirrhosis	Amiodarone, perhexiline, tamoxifen
Fibrosis and cirrhosis	Fibrosis, nodular regeneration (other features, such as interface hepatitis, steatohepatitis, paucity of bile ducts, and cholestasis, depend on etiology)	Cyproterone acetate (see also VBDS, chronic hepatitis, steatohepatitis), methotrexate
Vascular disorders	Nodular regenerative hyperplasia, sinusoidal obstruction syndrome, others	Many (see Table 90.10)
Tumors	HCC, adenoma, angiosarcoma, others	Many (see Chapter 98)

AP, Alkaline phosphatase; *ART*, antiretroviral therapy; *VBDS*, vanishing bile duct syndrome.

some agents such as isoniazid, the distinction between adaptation and minor injury is blurred; adaptation in such cases may be a response to oxidative injury. Conversely, liver tumors or hepatic fibrosis may develop insidiously without significant abnormalities of liver biochemical tests—the former in association with sex steroids or vinyl chloride monomer and the latter with methotrexate, arsenic, or hypervitaminosis A.

The duration of the disorder is another consideration in classifying drug-induced liver diseases. In general, chronic liver disease is much less commonly attributable to drugs and toxins than are acute reactions but not to consider drugs as a possible etiology of chronic liver disease can lead to a missed diagnosis, with serious clinical consequences.[24] In contrast to most liver disorders, drugs and toxins constitute the most important cause of hepatic vascular lesions. Drugs also have been associated with chronic cholestasis, chronic hepatitis, steatohepatitis, hepatic fibrosis, cirrhosis, and benign and malignant liver tumors.

Histopathologic Features

Although no pathognomonic hallmarks of DILI have been identified, certain histologic patterns are suggestive.[75] These include zonal necrosis or microvesicular steatosis (accompanying mitochondrial injury) and mixed histologic features of hepatocellular necrosis and cholestasis. Necrotic lesions that are disproportionately severe compared with the clinical picture also indicate a possible drug cause, whereas destructive bile duct lesions, prominent neutrophils, and eosinophils (at least 25% of the inflammatory cells) suggest drug-induced cholestatic hepatitis. Hepatic granuloma formation is another common type of hepatic drug reaction. In cases of steatohepatitis, hepatic fibrosis, or liver tumors, no specific clues to a drug cause have been recognized, although sex steroids increase the vascularity of hepatic tumors and are frequently associated with sinusoidal dilatation or peliosis hepatis. Drug-induced steatohepatitis caused by amiodarone and perhexiline tends to be associated with severe lesions that more closely resemble alcohol-associated hepatitis than MASH.[76] Other drugs (e.g., tamoxifen, methotrexate) cause lesions that are indistinguishable from MASH. Although detection of "signature" lesions can helpful, most patients with DILI are not subject to liver biopsy unless the reaction is severe or unexpected or improvement fails to occur after cessation of the drug. Liver histology is often sought when AIH is a possibility, but the limitations of liver histology should be recognized. In one study, 4 expert hepatopathologists reviewed 35 cases of AIH and 28 cases of DILI. The interobserver agreement based on histology alone was only 46% but improved modestly (up to 71%) by including conventional clinicopathologic criteria. The best results were achieved using a model that combined certain selected histologic characteristics.[77]

Clinical Features

The history and physical examination can provide important clues to the diagnosis of hepatic drug reactions. Most important is the temporal pattern of disease evolution in relation to exposure to drugs or toxins. The identification of specific risk factors for hepatotoxicity (e.g., chronic excessive alcohol intake in a person taking acetaminophen) and the presence of systemic features of drug hypersensitivity may indicate the correct diagnosis. Systemic features include fever, rash, mucositis, eosinophilia, lymphadenopathy, a mononucleosis-like syndrome, bone marrow suppression, vasculitis, acute kidney injury, pneumonitis, and pancreatitis. These features tend to occur in genetically predisposed persons who have been exposed to drug metabolites that act as haptens to initiate an immunodestructive tissue reaction, termed the DRESS syndrome (see earlier). Viral reactivations (notably human herpes virus-6 and -7 and EBV infections) are also implicated in the pathogenesis.[78]

DRESS Syndrome

Drugs implicated as a cause of DRESS include sulfonamides, aminopenicillins, fluoroquinolones, clozapine, anticonvulsants (phenytoin, lamotrigine, phenobarbital, carbamazepine, valproic acid, minocycline), antiretrovirals (nevirapine, abacavir), pentoxifylline, some NSAIDs, and Chinese herbal medicines.[78] Risk factors include a history of an affected first-degree relative (which increases the risk to 1 in 4) and a personal history of drug allergy, including to aspirin. Using drugs such as glucocorticoids or valproic acid at the time the new agent is started increases the risk 4–10-fold. Immune disorders such as SLE and HIV/AIDS increase the risk 10- and 100-fold, respectively.

The illness characteristically begins between 1 and 12 weeks (typically 2–4 weeks) after the drug is started; "sentinel symptoms" include fever, pharyngitis, malaise, periorbital edema, headache or otalgia, rhinorrhea, and mouth ulcers. A severe rash is an essential feature. Erythematous reactions are usual and may evolve to toxic epidermal necrolysis or erythema multiforme, often with mucositis (Stevens-Johnson syndrome). Early changes include neutrophilia and elevated levels of acute-phase reactants; atypical lymphocytosis and eosinophilia may be noted later. Hepatic reactions are found in about 13% of cases. Findings include cholestasis, acute hepatitis, and granulomas. Other features include lymphadenopathy (16%), nephritis (6%), pneumonitis (6%), and more severe hematologic abnormalities (5%). In a 12-year review of 172 cases reported as DRESS or drug hypersensitivity reactions, all affected persons had cutaneous changes, but the features most often associated with "probable" or "definite" cases of DRESS syndrome were eosinophilia, liver involvement (abnormal liver biochemical test results in 59%, hepatomegaly in 12%), fever, and lymphadenopathy.[79]

Latent Period to Onset

For idiosyncratic reactions, a latent period occurs between starting the drug and the onset of clinical and laboratory abnormalities. This period is usually 2–8 weeks for immunoallergic hepatitis (e.g., DRESS syndrome) and 6–20 weeks or longer for agents such as isoniazid, dantrolene, and troglitazone. Occasionally, liver injury may become evident well after the offending drug is stopped, even as long as 2 weeks for oxypenicillins and amoxicillin-clavulanate. In other cases, hepatotoxicity is rare after the first exposure to a drug but more frequent and more severe after subsequent courses. Examples include halothane, nitrofurantoin, and dacarbazine. Therefore a history of a previous reaction to the drug in question (inadvertent rechallenge) is an important key to the diagnosis of DILI.

Dechallenge and Rechallenge

Another aspect of the temporal relationship between ingestion of a drug and hepatotoxicity is the response to discontinuation of the drug, or dechallenge. Dechallenge should be accompanied by discernible and progressive improvement within days to weeks of stopping the incriminated agent. Exceptions occur with ketoconazole, troglitazone, etretinate, and amiodarone; with these agents, reactions may be severe, and clinical recovery may be delayed for months. Although some types of drug-induced cholestasis also can be prolonged, failure of jaundice to resolve in a suspected drug reaction often indicates an alternative diagnosis. Rarely, deliberate rechallenge may be used to confirm the diagnosis or prove involvement of one particular agent when the patient has been exposed to several drugs or the benefits outweigh the risks, particularly if safer alternatives are unavailable.[80] However, this approach is potentially hazardous, with one study reporting that severe hepatocellular injury developed in 18% of rechallenged persons, and two died.[81] Therefore rechallenge should be undertaken only with fully informed written consent and preferably the approval of an institutional ethics committee.

Diagnosis

In the absence of specific tests, the diagnosis requires clinical suspicion, a thorough drug history, consideration of the temporal relationships between drug ingestion and liver disease, and exclusion of other disorders. The objective weighing of evidence for and against an individual agent—causality assessment—is a probabilistic form of diagnosis.[81] Several clinical scales that assess causality have been described.[25,81,82] A liver biopsy may be necessary to exclude other diseases and to provide further clues to a drug etiology. Rechallenge is the standard test for drug-induced liver disease but is hardly ever used in practice. Future strategies include in vitro tests to provide confirmatory evidence for particular drugs[69,81] and toxicogenomic methods, which encompass transcriptomics, metabolomics, and proteomics (measuring circulating mRNA/microRNA, changes in metabolites, and cellular proteins, respectively).[83] In some studies, toxicogenomic changes preceded alterations in serum aminotransferase levels, thereby raising the hope that these changes could serve as biomarkers of early DILI.[84]

Physician Awareness

Physicians should be aware of the many sources of potential hepatotoxins, including prescribed and over-the-counter drugs (e.g., ibuprofen), CAM preparations (see Chapter 91), recreational drugs (e.g., cocaine, ecstasy), self-poisoning, and environmental contaminants in food and water supplies, the home, the workplace, and the community. Unfortunately, patients and physicians do not always heed early nonspecific symptoms of hepatic drug reactions. For example, preventable deaths from liver failure still occur from isoniazid hepatotoxicity.[85] Although ongoing education about potentially hepatotoxic drugs is important, physicians have a professional and legal obligation to inform patients about possible adverse drug reactions.

Drug toxicity should be considered in cases of obscure or poorly explained liver disease, particularly in cases with mixed or atypical patterns of cholestasis and hepatitis; cholestasis in which common causes have been excluded, especially in older adults; and when histologic features suggest a drug etiology. In such cases, the drug history must be addressed as a special investigation, with attention paid to additional sources of information (household members, primary care providers), household drugs, nonprescribed medications, and environmental toxins (see Chapter 91). LiverTox is a web-based searchable database of information relating to liver injury resulting from the use of prescription and nonprescription drugs (see http://www.livertox.nih.gov/).[23]

Exclusion of Other Disorders

Before a diagnosis of DILI is considered, other liver diseases such as viral hepatitis (including hepatitis E),[86] AIH, and vascular and metabolic disorders should be excluded. Some types of drug-induced chronic hepatitis are associated with autoantibodies and superficially resemble AIH. An approach to the correct diagnosis is described later (see nitrofurantoin). Drug-induced cholestasis should be considered if biliary obstruction has been excluded, and a liver biopsy may be necessary.

Extrahepatic Features

The constellation of rash, eosinophilia, and other organ involvement supports a diagnosis of a hepatic adverse drug reaction (DRESS, see earlier). Because these findings are infrequent, especially with drugs that cause nonimmune idiosyncratic liver injury, their absence is not helpful in excluding DILI. Specific diagnostic tests for individual drug-induced liver diseases have been described[69] but are not generally accepted or available. With dose-dependent hepatotoxins (e.g., acetaminophen), blood levels may be helpful.

Chronologic Relationships

For most drugs, the chronologic relationship among drug ingestion, onset, and resolution of liver injury remains the main consideration in diagnosis. The criteria for temporal eligibility include the relationship of drug ingestion to onset, course of the reaction after stopping the drug, and response to drug readministration.[1,22] Inadvertent rechallenge may have already occurred. The rechallenge is regarded as positive if the serum ALT or alkaline phosphatase level increases at least twofold.[23] Deliberate rechallenge (discussed earlier) may be considered in selected cases.

Which Drug?

New and nonproprietary compounds should arouse particular suspicion. For patients who are taking multiple drugs, the most recently introduced drug preceding the onset of liver injury is often responsible. If that agent is an unlikely cause and another well-known hepatotoxin is being taken, the latter is the more likely culprit. When possible, the most likely hepatotoxin or all therapeutic agents should be discontinued. If the patient improves, the drugs that are unlikely to be responsible can be carefully reintroduced.

Indications for Liver Biopsy

Liver biopsy may be helpful in difficult cases, especially when the temporal relationship between the ingestion of a known hepatotoxic agent and the onset of liver injury is unclear. In practice, for example, the onset of jaundice within 2–6 weeks of starting an agent such as amoxicillin-clavulanic acid or of acute hepatitis with other features of DRESS syndrome in a person taking nevirapine as part of ART strongly suggests a drug etiology, and liver biopsy is usually unnecessary. Conversely, substantially abnormal liver biochemical test levels (e.g., a serum ALT level elevated more than fivefold) in a person who has serologic evidence suggestive of AIH and has been taking a statin for 3–6 months is a clinical challenge that often can be resolved only by liver biopsy. The medical community may benefit when new instances or patterns of drug-induced liver disease are adequately defined; this benefit may persuade the clinician (but not always the informed patient) to proceed with a liver biopsy in equivocal cases.

Considerations in Patients With Viral Hepatitis

Patients with chronic hepatitis B or C may be at higher risk of liver injury from antituberculous chemotherapy, ibuprofen, and possibly other NSAIDs, anticancer drugs, and ART compared with persons without viral hepatitis. A more common clinical problem is the finding of a high serum ALT level (>300 U/L) at a routine office visit in a patient with previous levels less than 150 U/L. In patients with hepatitis C, the rise in serum ALT is more likely the result of DILI than a spontaneous change in the activity of the hepatitis C, particularly when the ALT level is greater than 1000 U/L. The most commonly implicated agents are acetaminophen taken in moderate doses under conditions of increased risk (e.g., fasting, alcohol excess, use of other medication) and CAM preparations (see Chapter 91). Clinical suspicion is essential for recognizing DILI so that appropriate advice can be given. Determination of serum acetaminophen levels may be useful in difficult cases, but the results can be difficult to interpret in the context of regular ingestion, as opposed to a single episode of self-poisoning.

Prevention and Management

With the exception of acetaminophen hepatotoxicity, little effective treatment for drug-induced liver disease is available, other than LT for liver failure. Special emphasis, therefore, must be placed on prevention and early detection of liver injury as well as on prompt withdrawal of the offending agent. Safe use of over-the-counter agents such as acetaminophen, NSAIDs, and CAM preparations is important.

Most drugs associated with drug-induced liver disease are idiosyncratic hepatotoxins, for which liver injury occurs rarely. Avoiding overuse of these drugs can minimize the overall frequency of adverse hepatic reactions; antibiotics such as amoxicillin-clavulanic acid and flucloxacillin are pertinent examples. Similarly, polypharmacy should be avoided when possible. Postmarketing surveillance of new drugs is critical, and all physicians should participate in reporting adverse effects to monitoring agencies.

For dose-dependent hepatotoxins, prevention depends on adherence to dosage guidelines or monitoring of blood levels. This approach has virtually abolished some forms of DILI, such as tetracycline-induced fatty liver, aspirin hepatitis, and methotrexate-induced hepatic fibrosis. In cases with specific risk factors, strategies to prevent toxicity are essential (e.g., avoiding valproic acid use with other drugs in the very young; avoiding methotrexate in persons who consume alcohol in excess). Moderate doses of acetaminophen are also contraindicated in heavy drinkers and after fasting,[38] and halothane should not be readministered within 28 days or in persons suspected of the previous sensitivity to a haloalkane anesthetic.

Early detection is also critical. Patients should be warned to report any untoward symptoms, particularly unexplained nausea, malaise, right hypochondrial pain, lethargy, or fever. These nonspecific features may represent the prodrome of drug-induced hepatitis. They are an indication for liver biochemical testing and, if the results suggest liver injury, for cessation of treatment.

A more difficult issue is whether regular (protocol) screening with liver biochemical tests should be performed when a drug is prescribed. Although authors and drug manufacturers often recommend such screening, the efficiency and cost-effectiveness of this approach are unknown. The onset of liver injury is often rapid, rendering once-a-month or every-second-week screening futile. Furthermore, up to 7.5% of persons who receive placebo in clinical trials have persistently raised serum ALT levels. If liver biochemical test levels are monitored, the threshold at which a drug should be discontinued is uncertain, as illustrated by isoniazid, which causes some liver biochemical test abnormality in 30% of exposed subjects. Generally, it is recommended that isoniazid be stopped if serum ALT levels exceed 250 U/L or more than 5 times the ULN, but elevation of the serum bilirubin level, a decrease in the albumin concentration, prolongation of the prothrombin time, or any pertinent symptoms provides a clearer indication to stop the drug. Conversely, a rise in the serum GGTP level or a minor elevation of the serum alkaline phosphatase level usually indicates hepatic adaptation rather than liver injury. We do not routinely recommend protocol screening except for methotrexate, but this approach could be useful for agents such as valproic acid, isoniazid, pyrazinamide, ketoconazole, dantrolene, thiazolidinediones, and synthetic retinoids, either because the liver injury may be delayed and gradual in some cases or because such screening emphasizes the hepatotoxic potential of these drugs to patients and physicians. Evaluation by liver biopsy or by a noninvasive method such as serum biomarkers or elastography may have a role in the assessment of hepatic fibrosis in patients who take methotrexate (see later).

The management of DILI includes removal of the drug, administration of an antidote (if available), and supportive care. Failure to discontinue the offending drug is the single most important factor leading to poor outcomes, such as ALF and chronic liver disease.[24] For ingested toxins such as metals and acetaminophen, removal of the unabsorbed drug through the aspiration of stomach contents may be appropriate. Methods to remove absorbed toxins (charcoal hemodialysis, forced diuresis) are usually ineffective except in selected circumstances (e.g., acetaminophen).

Thiol replacement therapy, usually with *N*-acetylcysteine (NAC), is indicated as an antidote for acetaminophen poisoning. NAC can also be used in ALF, but early referral for LT should be considered (see Chapter 99). UDCA may help in managing drug-induced cholestasis. In general, glucocorticoids are ineffective in treating drug-induced liver disease; however, case reports attest to the occasional effectiveness of glucocorticoids in protracted cases of hepatitis caused by etretinate, allopurinol, diclofenac, or ketoconazole.[1] Glucocorticoids should be reserved for atypical and refractory cases, particularly those associated with vasculitis.

DOSE-DEPENDENT HEPATOTOXICITY

Few dose-dependent hepatotoxins are clinically relevant today. Examples include acetaminophen, some herbal and dietary supplements, plant and fungal toxins, amodiaquine, hycanthone, vitamin A, methotrexate, cyclophosphamide, anticancer drugs, carbon tetrachloride, phosphorus, and metals (especially iron, copper, and mercury).

Acetaminophen

General Nature, Frequency, and Predisposing Factors

Acetaminophen (paracetamol) is safe in recommended doses of 1–4 g daily, but hepatotoxicity produced by self-poisoning with acetaminophen has been recognized since the 1960s. Despite the effectiveness of thiol-based antidotes, acetaminophen remains the most common cause of DILI in most countries and an important cause of ALF.[87] Attempted suicide is the usual reason for overdose. Although controversial,[88] hepatologists and pediatricians see cases of acetaminophen poisoning that have arisen through what Zimmerman and Maddrey termed "therapeutic misadventure."[89] This occurrence is especially common in persons who habitually drink alcohol to excess and has also been recognized after daily ingestion of moderate therapeutic doses (10–20 g over 3 days) of acetaminophen in adults and children who are fasting or malnourished[38] or who are taking drugs that interact with the metabolism of acetaminophen.[89] In a recent French study, over 20% of patients admitted with acetaminophen-related liver injury had taken doses of ≤6 g/day) of the drug. Further, two-thirds of these patients had taken ≤4 g/day, but yet, over half of these patients developed severe liver injury.[90] The main risk factors for acute liver injury were older age (44 vs. 30 years), fasting for a day or more, excessive alcohol use, and repeated acetaminophen ingestion (median, 4 days).

Single doses of acetaminophen that exceed 7–10 g (140 mg/kg body weight in children) may cause liver injury, but this outcome is not inevitable. Severe liver injury (serum ALT > 1000 U/L) or fatal cases usually involve doses of at least 15–25 g, but because of interindividual variability, survival is possible even after ingestion of a massive single dose of acetaminophen (greater than 50 g).[91] Among persons with an untreated acetaminophen overdose, severe liver injury occurred in only 20%, and among those with severe liver injury, the mortality rate was 20%.[90]

Risk factors for acetaminophen-induced hepatotoxicity are summarized in Table 90.5. Children are relatively resistant to acetaminophen-induced hepatotoxicity,[92] possibly because of their tendency to ingest smaller doses, greater likelihood of vomiting,

TABLE 90.5 Risk Factors for Acetaminophen-Induced Hepatotoxicity

Factor	Relevance
Age	Children may be more resistant than adults
Dose	Minimal hepatotoxic dose: 7.5 g (≈100 mg/kg in adults, 150 mg/kg in children) Severe toxicity is possible with doses >15 g
Blood level of acetaminophen	Influenced by dose, time after ingestion, gastric emptying, coingested drugs Best indicator of risk of hepatotoxicity (see text and Fig. 90.2)
Chronic excessive alcohol ingestion	Toxic dose threshold is lowered; worsens prognosis (also related to late presentation); nephrotoxicity is common
Fasting	Toxic dose threshold is lowered—therapeutic misadventure (see text)
Concomitant medication	Toxic dose threshold is lowered—therapeutic misadventure; worsens prognosis (e.g., isoniazid, phenytoin, and zidovudine)
Time of presentation	Late presentation or delayed treatment (>16 hours) predicts worse outcome

or biological resistance; however, liver injury has been reported with intravenous acetaminophen use in children (usually due to dosing errors)[93] and rarely, even in neonates through transplacental drug transfer after maternal overdose.[94] The presence of underlying liver disease does not predispose to acetaminophen hepatotoxicity.

Self-poisoning with acetaminophen is most common in young women, but fatalities are most frequent in men, possibly because of alcoholism and late presentation.[87,91,95] The time of presentation is critical; early thiol therapy (within 12 hours) of acetaminophen poisoning virtually abolishes significant liver injury (see later). Therapeutic misadventure is also associated with a worse outcome.[88] Concomitant use of agents such as phenobarbital, phenytoin, isoniazid, and zidovudine increases the risk of hepatotoxicity. These drugs promote the oxidative metabolism of acetaminophen to NAPQI by inducing CYP2E1 (for isoniazid) or CYP3A4 (for phenytoin) or by competing with glucuronidation pathways (for zidovudine). Alcohol and fasting have dual effects by enhancing expression of CYP2E1 and by depleting hepatic glutathione. Fasting also may impair acetaminophen conjugation by depleting cofactors for the glucuronidation and sulfation pathways.[38]

Acetaminophen hepatotoxicity produces zone 3 hepatic necrosis, with extension to submassive (bridging) or panacinar (massive) necrosis in severe cases. Inflammation is minimal, and recovery is associated with complete resolution without fibrosis. The zonal pattern of acetaminophen-induced necrosis is related to the mechanism of hepatotoxicity, particularly the role of CYP2E1, which is expressed in zone 3, and to lower levels of glutathione in zone 3 hepatocytes than in hepatocytes in the other zones.

Clinical Course, Outcomes, and Prognostic Indicators

In the first 2 days after acetaminophen self-poisoning, features of liver injury are not present. Nausea, vomiting, and drowsiness are often caused by concomitant ingestion of alcohol and other drugs. After 48–72 hours, serum ALT levels may be elevated, and symptoms, such as anorexia, nausea and vomiting, fatigue, and malaise, may occur. Hepatic pain may be pronounced. Repeated vomiting, jaundice, hypoglycemia, and other features of ALF, particularly coagulopathy and hepatic encephalopathy, characterize severe cases. The liver may shrink because of severe necrosis. Serum levels of ALT are often between 2000 and 10,000 U/L. These high levels can clinch the diagnosis in complex settings, as may occur in heavy drinkers and those with viral hepatitis.[89]

Indicators of a poor outcome[87,88,95] include grade 4 hepatic encephalopathy, acidosis, worsening coagulopathy, and renal failure (see also Chapter 97). Renal failure reflects acute tubular necrosis or hepatorenal syndrome. Uncommon accompanying features include myocardial injury[91] and skin and lung involvement in rare cases of acetaminophen hypersensitivity. Death occurs between 4 and 18 days after the overdose and generally results from cerebral edema and sepsis complicating hepatic and multiorgan failure. The majority of patients recover completely. Cases of apparent chronic hepatotoxicity rarely have been attributed to continued ingestion of acetaminophen (2–6 g/day), usually by a susceptible host, such as a heavy drinker or a person with preexisting, unrecognized liver disease.[1,22]

Treatment

In patients who present within 4 hours of an acetaminophen overdose, the stomach should be emptied with a wide-bore NG tube. Oral charcoal is most useful within the first 1–2 hours but can be used up to 4 hours in patients who present with a large overdose, after ingestion of a sustained-release preparation, or have also consumed drugs that impair gastric emptying. Use of activated charcoal is contraindicated if there is airway compromise. The aim of management is to identify patients who should receive thiol-based antidote therapy and, in those with established severe liver injury, assess the patient's candidacy for LT.

Blood levels of acetaminophen should be measured at the time of presentation. After 4 hours, acetaminophen blood levels are a reliable indicator of the risk of liver injury in patients with an acute overdose, except in patients who have taken a *modified release* acetaminophen preparation or after *repeated supratherapeutic* ingestion. Measurement of serum acetaminophen levels may also be misleading in patients ingesting drugs that impair gastric emptying that could delay acetaminophen absorption. In one instance, the liver injury became apparent 38 hours postingestion despite initial drug concentrations below the treatment threshold.[96]

The risk of liver injury is estimated by reference to the Rumack-Matthew nomogram (Fig. 88.2).[91] Indications for antidote therapy include a reliable history of major poisoning (more than 10 g) or blood acetaminophen levels in the moderate- or high-risk bands on the nomogram or both.[91,95] At-risk patients should be hospitalized for monitoring.

Hepatic necrosis occurs only when glutathione concentrations fall below a critical level, thereby allowing NAPQI to produce liver injury. Administration of cysteine donors stimulates hepatic glutathione synthesis. Many cysteine precursors or thiol donors can be used, but NAC has become the agent of choice. Oral administration was initially used in the United States,[87,91] with a loading dose of 140 mg/kg followed by administration of 70 mg/kg every 4 hours for 72 hours. This regimen is highly effective, despite the theoretical disadvantage that delayed gastric emptying and vomiting may reduce intestinal absorption of NAC. In Europe and Australia, NAC is administered by slow bolus intravenous injection followed by infusion (150 mg/kg over 15 minutes in 200 mL of 5% dextrose, with a second dose of 50 mg/kg 4 hours later, if the blood acetaminophen levels indicate a high risk of hepatoxicity, and a total dose over 24 hours of 300 mg/kg).[91] The intravenous regime, now approved by the FDA, is now preferred in many U.S. centers.[97] The intravenous route may be associated with a higher rate of hypersensitivity reactions because of the higher systemic blood levels achieved. Adverse reactions to NAC are common but are usually mild.[98] However, they can be occasionally severe, with rash, angioedema, and shock. Therefore NAC must be administered under close supervision. In patients known to be sensitized to NAC, methionine is probably just as effective but is not available in a commercial preparation; it must be made up fresh and often causes vomiting.[90] Other regimes that have been explored include shorter (12 hour) and simpler (1 or 2 bag versus 3 bag) schedules.[99,100] Although these schedules have been based on retrospective data, they could prove beneficial in simplifying the treatment protocol while reducing the frequency of adverse reactions. Some guidelines have suggested a higher NAC dose when managing patients presenting after a massive overdose (defined by 4-hour acetaminophen levels over twice the treatment threshold),[101] but the need for an increased dose is disputed.[102]

Cases of acetaminophen-induced severe liver injury are virtually abolished if NAC is administered within 16 hours of acetaminophen ingestion.[87,91]After 16 hours, thiol donation is unlikely to prevent liver injury because oxidation of acetaminophen to NAPQI with consequent oxidation of thiol groups is complete, and mitochondrial injury and activation of cell death pathways are likely to be established. Nevertheless, NAC has been shown to decrease the mortality associated with acetaminophen-induced hepatotoxicity when administered 16–36 hours after self-poisoning,[87,91,95] possibly because NAC stabilizes vascular reactivity in patients with liver failure. Therefore NAC is still used in patients with a late presentation after acetaminophen overdose.

In late presentations, where NAC is less effective, newer approaches to treatment are being explored. These include case reports and phase 1 studies showing the potential benefit of drugs that can prevent oxidative stress-induced mitochondrial injury (e.g., calmangafodipir) or inhibit CYP2E1 and JNK (4-methylpyrazole, fomepizole).[103,104] Larger studies are awaited.

Liver transplantation is an option for selected patients in whom liver failure develops after acetaminophen poisoning.[105] Case selection relies on the prognostic indicators discussed earlier and is strongly influenced by the prospects for successful psychological rehabilitation (see Chapter 99).[95] There are issues relating to poor adherence and self-harm posttransplantation that cannot be accurately predicted by pretransplant assessment. In several series, about 60% of listed patients have been transplanted, and survival rates have exceeded 70%.[95]

Prevention

Safe use of acetaminophen involves adherence to the recommended maximum dose and education about risk factors that lower the toxic dose threshold. Acetaminophen doses of more than 2 g a day are contraindicated in heavy drinkers, in those taking other medications (particularly phenytoin, zidovudine, and isoniazid), and during fasting. Prolonged use of acetaminophen requires caution in patients with severe cardiorespiratory disease or advanced cirrhosis. To address and reduce the risk of self-harm, in January 2011, the U.S. FDA restricted the sale of acetaminophen to smaller doses per tablet (325 mg) in combined acetaminophen/opioid formulations and mandated a boxed warning highlighting the potential for liver injury and allergic reactions. This has had a significant impact on reducing the frequency of hospitalizations with acetaminophen and opioid toxicity (by 11%/year) and also the proportion of cases of acute liver failure attributed to acetaminophen (by 21.8%).[105]

Other Causes

Some hepatotoxins are not as clearly dose dependent as acetaminophen but cause cytopathic changes, such as extensive hydropic change, diffuse or zonal microvesicular steatosis, and zonal necrosis.[1,22] Injury likely represents *metabolic idiosyncrasy*, in which the drug or one of its metabolites accumulates and interferes with protein synthesis or intermediary metabolism, or both. The mitochondrion is often the main subcellular target, and other metabolically active tissues can be involved. Pancreatitis and renal tubular injury may accompany severe liver injury caused by valproic acid, tetracycline, and HAART, and metabolic acidosis with a shock-like state is common. This presentation was first recognized with intravenous high dose tetracycline (>2 g/day for more than 4 days) in pregnant women, men taking estrogens, or with patients in renal failure.[22] With appropriate dose limitations, this reaction is entirely preventable.

Niacin (Nicotinic Acid)

Niacin is a dose-dependent hepatotoxin. All niacin formulations have been linked to liver toxicity.[106] Liver injury usually occurs at doses exceeding 2 g/day but also rarely with low-dose (500 mg/day) sustained-release niacin.[107] The clinicopathologic spectrum encompasses mild and transient increases in serum ALT levels, jaundice, acute hepatitis, cholestasis, and acute liver failure. Acute liver failure is reported with ingestion of a single large dose (20 g) of a native niacin supplement.[108] Patients on sulfonylureas and those with preexisting liver disease, particularly alcohol-related hepatitis, are at increased risk. The symptoms can begin as early as 1 week or may be delayed for up to 4 years. Complete resolution occurs after the drug is stopped. Liver histology shows hepatic necrosis, centrilobular cholestasis, or rarely, diffuse microvesicular steatosis, and a hallmark of mitochondrial toxicity.[106] Substituting one niacin preparation for another without a dose adjustment should be avoided; switching from immediate- to sustained-release preparations requires a 50%–70% dose reduction.

Valproic Acid (Sodium Valproate)

Valproic acid-associated hepatic injury occurs almost exclusively in children, particularly those under 3 years of age. Also at risk are persons with a family history of a mitochondrial enzyme deficiency (chiefly involving the urea cycle or long-chain fatty acid metabolism), Friedreich ataxia, or Reye syndrome, or with a sibling affected by valproic acid hepatotoxicity. Another risk factor is multiple drug therapies. Adult cases are rare. Mutations within the mitochondrial polymerase γ gene (POLG) were present in nearly half (8 of 17) of subjects with valproate hepatotoxicity, and these carried a > 20-fold risk of liver injury compared with population-matched controls.[109] The overall risk of liver injury among valproate users varies from 1 per 500 persons exposed among high-risk groups (children under age 3, polypharmacy, genetic defects of mitochondrial enzymes) to less than 1 in 37,000 in low-risk groups.[110]

No relationship exists between valproic acid toxicity and dose, but blood levels of valproic acid tend to be high in one-half of affected persons. The metabolite 4-en-valproic acid, produced by CYP-catalyzed metabolism of valproic acid, is a dose-dependent hepatotoxin in animals and in vitro. The concept has emerged that valproic acid is an occult dose-dependent toxin in which accumulation of a hepatotoxic metabolite (favored by coexposure to CYP-inducing antiepileptic agents) produces mitochondrial injury in a susceptible host (e.g., young children, especially those with partial deficiencies of mitochondrial enzymes).[111] Valproic acid also inhibits the synthesis of carnitine, a cofactor in mitochondrial fatty acid beta oxidation (and also for valproic acid).

Symptoms begin within 4–12 weeks and are often nonspecific, including lethargy, malaise, poor feeding, somnolence, worsening seizures, muscle weakness, and facial swelling. In typical cases, features of hepatotoxicity follow, including anorexia, nausea, vomiting, right upper quadrant abdominal discomfort, and weight loss.[110,111] When jaundice ensues, hypoglycemia, ascites, coagulopathy, and encephalopathy indicate liver failure with imminent coma and death. In some cases, a neurologic syndrome characterized by ataxia, mental confusion, and coma predominates, with little evidence of hepatic involvement. In other cases, fever and tender hepatomegaly suggestive of Reye syndrome may be present; such cases tend to have a better prognosis. Additional extrahepatic features include alopecia, hypofibrinogenemia, thrombocytopenia, and pancreatitis. There are a few reports of DRESS syndrome with valproic acid.[112] The terminal phase is often indicated by renal failure, hypoglycemia, metabolic acidosis, and severe bacterial infection.

Laboratory features include modest elevations of serum bilirubin and aminotransferase levels; the aspartate aminotransferase (AST) level is usually higher than the ALT level. A profound decrease in clotting factor levels, hypoalbuminemia, and hyperammonemia are common. A small echogenic liver suggestive of steatosis or extensive necrosis is seen on hepatic imaging. Histologic examination shows submassive or massive hepatic necrosis in two-thirds of cases with either zonal or generalized microvesicular steatosis.[111] Ultrastructural studies indicate conspicuous mitochondrial abnormalities.

Treatment is supportive. Small nonrandomized studies have shown that intravenous *L*-carnitine supplementation can reduce hyperammonemia and improve survival in severe cases of liver injury[113] and also in patients with psychiatric disorders developing hyperammonemic encephalopathy without liver disease.[114] Liver transplantation has been performed successfully, but poor outcomes have been recorded, particularly in children.[115] Highly selected adult patients can have a good outcome with liver transplantation.[116] Prevention depends on adherence to guidelines, including avoiding valproic acid in combination with other drugs in children less than 3 years and in those with mitochondrial enzyme abnormalities. Pretreatment screening for *POLG* mutations is recommended for high-risk groups.[117] Liver test abnormalities develop in at least 40% and therefore are an unreliable predictor of valproic acid hepatotoxicity. Patients and parents need to be educated about the importance of reporting any adverse symptoms during the first 6 months of treatment.

Antiretroviral Agents

Abnormal liver biochemical test levels and clinical evidence of liver disease are common in patients with HIV/AIDS. Potential causes include HBV, HCV, and other hepatobiliary infections, lymphoma, and other tumors. The frequency of hepatic injury with ART (which often includes three or four agents) is at least 10%.[40,45] Because HIV coinfection with HBV or HCV increases the risk of hepatotoxicity, all patients should be screened for viral hepatitis before starting ART.[118]

Nucleos(t)ide Reverse Transcriptase Inhibitors

NRTIs are weak inhibitors of mitochondrial DNA polymerase gamma in vitro; the order of their potency is as follows: zalcitabine > didanosine > stavudine > lamivudine > zidovudine > abacavir.[118] Oxidative stress may also cause hepatotoxicity, resulting in further mitochondrial DNA deletion and the consequences of impaired oxidative phosphorylation, fatty acyl beta oxidation, and insulin resistance. Abacavir is associated with liver injury that occurs within 6 weeks as part of a systemic hypersensitivity reaction. This complication is linked to HLA haplotype HLA-B*5701; screening and excluding carriers of this polymorphism has significantly reduced abacavir hypersensitivity reactions (0% vs. 2.7% in controls).[119]

Zidovudine, didanosine, and stavudine are most often implicated in liver injury.[118] Risk factors for mitochondrial drug toxicity among persons with HIV infection include obesity, female gender, pregnancy, and coprescription of didanosine and stavudine.[118] Hallmarks of mitochondrial hepatotoxicity include extensive microvesicular or macrovesicular steatosis (or both), lactic acidosis, and liver biochemical test abnormalities with progression to acute liver failure. Asymptomatic hyperlactatemia is common (especially with stavudine) among persons treated with HAART, but life-threatening lactic acidosis with hepatic steatosis is rare, with an estimated risk of 1.3 per 1000 person-years of antiretroviral use. Onset is within 3–17 months (median, 6 months), usually with nonspecific symptoms, including nausea, vomiting, diarrhea, dyspnea, lethargy, and abdominal pain. Extrahepatic manifestations, such as myopathy or peripheral neuropathy, and in severe cases pancreatitis and renal failure, may follow lactic acidosis and liver injury. Discontinuation of the drug is mandatory but does not prevent fatalities. Nevertheless, the overall mortality rate is low. Regular monitoring of liver tests along with HIV and CD4 testing is recommended. Any new aminotransferase elevation should trigger immediate measurement of serum lactate, creatine kinase, and pancreatic enzyme levels.[120]

Over 60 cases of noncirrhotic portal hypertension have been associated with NRTI.[121] Most involved didanosine alone or in combination with stavudine.[122] Features of portal hypertension, such as variceal bleeding, ascites, splenomegaly, are usually present, but hepatic encephalopathy and liver failure are uncommon. Men (75%) are predominantly affected. They have been on treatment for 1–9 years and have achieved virologic suppression. Nodular regenerative hyperplasia and portal vein thrombosis are the main histologic lesions. Postulated mechanisms include sinusoidal endothelial cell injury or thrombophilia. Discontinuation of didanosine does not reverse the portal hypertension.

Nonnucleoside Reverse Transcriptase Inhibitors

Like abacavir, these agents can cause acute hepatitis as part of an early (<6 weeks) hypersensitivity reaction, which often includes skin rash, lymphadenopathy, peripheral, and tissue eosinophilia.[123] Resolution occurs within 4 weeks of discontinuing the drug. Nevirapine has also been implicated in severe hepatotoxicity, when used for postexposure prophylaxis.[123] Nevirapine hepatotoxicity is linked to a specific HLA haplotype (B*58:01 in black Africans, OR 3.5) and increases with CD4 counts[124]; specific CD4 thresholds have been established (>400 and >250 cells/mm^3 for men and women, respectively). Underlying viral hepatitis B or C increases the risk of liver injury.[125] Of 12 reports to the FDA between 1997 and 2000, over half (7 of 12) had acute hepatitis, 1 patient needed a liver transplant, and the rest had asymptomatic elevations of serum aminotransferases. The recommended 2-week dose escalation regimen was not adhered to in some of the cases.[123] Sequential toxicity with nevirapine followed by efavirenz has been reported in an HIV-HCV coinfected person.[126] The newer NNRTI drugs have not been linked (doravirine) or have significantly lower hepatotoxic potential (etravirine, rilpivirine) than efavirenz.[127]

Protease Inhibitors

Elevated aminotransferases are commonly seen with protease inhibitors, but clinical hepatitis is infrequent. Ritonavir and indinavir are most often implicated. The latter also causes unconjugated hyperbilirubinemia in 7% of treated persons, a finding that is of no clinical consequence. Severe acute hepatitis may occur rarely. The association with peripheral or tissue (in liver biopsies) eosinophilia in some cases suggests an immunoallergic basis for liver injury.[128] Acute hepatitis occurs in 2.9%–30% of persons receiving high dose ritonavir (>400 mg/day) but is not an issue with low-dose regimes except when used as part of combination treatment in advanced cirrhosis.[129] In general, the course of the illness is mild, and the liver injury responds favorably to drug withdrawal. Rarely, acute liver failure may develop; in these cases, liver histology has shown severe microvesicular steatosis, cholestasis, and extensive fibrosis.

Several studies have shown that coinfected patients with HIV and chronic viral hepatitis have a higher frequency of hepatotoxicity while on protease inhibitors. However, liver injury was rapidly reversible in most cases, suggesting that the overall effect of protease inhibitors in coinfected persons is not detrimental.[130] These drugs also induce or inhibit CYP3A4, thereby causing important drug-drug interactions. Furthermore, chronic hepatitis B infection may be reactivated following immune reconstitution after HAART.

There are a few case reports of hepatocellular injury with integrase strand transfer inhibitors (dolutegravir), but significant hepatic injury is rare.[131]

Aspirin

On occasion, aspirin can cause major increases in serum ALT levels suggestive of drug hepatitis, but hepatotoxicity occurs only when blood salicylate concentrations exceed 25 mg/100 mL.[132] In addition, individual susceptibility factors include hypoalbuminemia, active juvenile RA, and SLE. Most cases of aspirin-induced hepatotoxicity are identified by biochemical testing rather than clinical features. If present, symptoms usually begin within the first few days or weeks of high-dose aspirin therapy. ALF and fatalities have been rare. Resolution occurs rapidly after drug withdrawal, and salicylates can be reintroduced at a lower dose. All salicylates appear to carry hepatotoxic potential, so there is no advantage to replacing aspirin with another salicylate. Liver histology shows a nonspecific focal hepatitis with hepatocellular degeneration and hydropic changes. The absence of steatosis usually distinguishes aspirin hepatotoxicity from Reye syndrome.

Reye syndrome has been linked with use of aspirin in febrile children. Although Reye syndrome is not simply a form of drug-induced liver disease, aspirin plays an important role in its multifactorial pathogenesis. Reye syndrome usually occurs between 3 and 4 days after an apparently minor viral infection. It is characterized by acute encephalopathy and hepatic injury, the latter documented by a threefold or greater rise in serum aminotransferase levels or hyperammonemia and by characteristic histology. Effective public health campaigns against the use of aspirin in young febrile children have led to a decline in the incidence of Reye syndrome; however, cases still occur. Misdiagnosis of cases that subsequently were diagnosed as inborn errors of metabolism that mimic Reye syndrome may have also contributed to the declining incidence.

Patients with juvenile RA (Still disease) or SLE are at particular risk of Reye syndrome. Features of chronic liver disease or drug allergy are absent. Management requires clinical suspicion and reducing the dose of (or discontinuing) aspirin. Recovery is usually rapid. Aspirin can be used again in lower doses, but alternative NSAIDs are generally used instead.

Others

L-asparaginase is an antileukemic drug that often causes hepatotoxicity, which usually is reversible but can occasionally result in liver failure associated with diffuse microvesicular steatosis.[22] A GWAS has shown an association between elevated serum aminotransferase levels seen after induction with L-asparaginase and a patatin-like phospholipase domain-containing protein 3 (*PNPLA3*) variant [rs738409 (C>G) I148M] that is implicated in MASLD (see Chapter 89).[133] Other implicated genes include *SOD2* and *ABCC1*, involved in antioxidant activity and biliary organic anion and xenobiotic efflux, respectively.[134] L-carnitine, involved in long-chain fatty acid transport into the mitochondria, has shown benefit in some small case series, but this needs to be verified.[135] Antiparasitic drugs, such as amodiaquine and hycanthone, have also been linked to severe and fatal dose-dependent liver injury (~1:15,000 exposed).[136]

DRUG-INDUCED ACUTE HEPATITIS

The term acute hepatitis refers to lesions characterized by the presence of hepatic inflammation with conspicuous hepatocyte cell death or degeneration. More severe lesions include zonal and bridging necrosis or massive (panlobular) hepatic necrosis; these lesions may be associated with fulminant or subfulminant ALF.[1,22] Acute hepatitis accounts for nearly 50% of hepatic adverse drug reactions, and causative agents are numerous.

Two broad types of drug hepatitis are recognized based on the presence (immunoallergic reactions) or absence of clinical and laboratory features consistent with drug allergy (Table 90.6). Those lacking characteristics of drug allergy could be the result of metabolic idiosyncrasy, partial dose dependence, a relationship between hepatitis and metabolism of the drug, or chemical toxicity. Nitrofurantoin and isoniazid are examples of immunoallergy and metabolic idiosyncrasy, respectively. Other relatively frequent examples of drug hepatitis include those associated with granulomatous reactions and chronic hepatitis.

Immunoallergic Reactions

Nitrofurantoin

Nitrofurantoin is a urinary antiseptic that has long been associated with hepatic injury. This reaction occurs at a frequency of 0.3–3 cases per 100,000 exposed persons.[137] The risk increases with age (particularly after 65 years of age). Two-thirds of acute cases occur in women, and the female-to-male ratio is 8:1 for chronic hepatitis.[137] The range of liver diseases includes acute hepatitis, occasionally with features of cholestasis, hepatic granulomas, chronic hepatitis with autoimmune features, ALF, and cirrhosis.[137] Causality has been proved by rechallenge, and no relationship to dose has been observed; cases have been described after ingestion of milk from a nitrofurantoin-treated cow.[138]

The relative frequencies of hepatocellular and cholestatic or mixed reactions and of acute and chronic hepatitis caused by nitrofurantoin have been debated. The nature of the adverse reactions covers a spectrum of biochemical and histologic features that have no apparent relevance to the patient's clinical outcome. Chronicity depends mostly on the duration of drug ingestion, which has been less than 6 weeks in acute cases but more than 6 months in 90% of chronic cases.[137] Patients with chronic hepatitis often have continued taking nitrofurantoin despite symptoms attributable to an adverse drug effect or have been exposed to another course of the drug after previous toxicity. In older series, the mortality rate for chronic nitrofurantoin hepatitis is 20%, compared with 5%–10% for acute hepatitis.[136] In a contemporary case series, the mortality rate and need for liver transplantation death were reported as 7.4% and 4%, respectively.[139]

The latent period between initial exposure to the drug and the onset of liver disease ranges from a few days to 6 weeks. Early symptoms may be nonspecific (e.g., fever, myalgia, arthralgia, fatigue, malaise, anorexia, and weight loss) and are followed by more specific features of hepatitis, such as nausea and vomiting, hepatic discomfort, jaundice, and, occasionally, pruritus. Rash occurs in 20% of affected persons, and lymphadenopathy may be

TABLE 90.6 Drug-Induced Acute Hepatitis: Immunoallergic Reaction Versus Metabolic Idiosyncrasy

Characteristic	Immunoallergic Reaction	Metabolic Idiosyncrasy
Frequency	<1 case per 10,000 persons exposed	1–50 cases per 10,000 persons exposed
Gender predilection	Women, often ≥2:1	Variable, slightly more common in women
Latent period to onset of hepatitis	Fairly constant, 2–10 weeks	More variable, 2–24 weeks, occasionally >1 year
Relationship to dose	None	Usually none, but drugs with daily doses >50 mg/day are overrepresented in cases of DILI
Interactions with other agents	None	Alcohol; occasionally other drugs (e.g., isoniazid with rifampin)
Course after stopping the drug	Prompt improvement [rare exceptions (e.g., minocycline)]	Variable; occasionally slow improvement or deterioration (e.g., troglitazone)
Positive rechallenge	Always; often fever within 3 days	Usual (in two-thirds of cases), abnormal liver biochemical test levels in 2–21 days
Fever	Usual; often initial symptom, part of prodrome	Infrequent, less prominent
Extrahepatic features (rash, lymphadenopathy)	Common	Rare
Eosinophilia:		
Blood	33%–67% of cases	<10% of cases
Tissue	Usual, pronounced	Common, but mild
Autoantibodies	Often present	Rarely present
Examples	Etretinate, methyldopa, minocycline, nitrofurantoin, phenytoin, sulfonamides	Dantrolene, isoniazid, ketoconazole, pyrazinamide, troglitazone

present. Pneumonitis, which can progress to pulmonary fibrosis, is present in 20% of affected persons and is suggested by cough and dyspnea. Rarely, liver failure develops, with ascites, coagulopathy, and encephalopathy. In patients with chronic hepatitis, clinical findings (such as spider telangiectasias, hepatosplenomegaly, muscle wasting, and ascites) may suggest cirrhosis.

Liver biochemical testing shows pronounced elevation of serum ALT levels, but more often the pattern is mixed, with increases in serum alkaline phosphatase levels as well. In other cases, the results suggest cholestasis. Over 70% of patients with chronic hepatitis had AST to ALT ratio >1.[139] Serum bilirubin levels tend to be increased in proportion to the severity of the reaction. In contrast to most types of acute drug hepatitis, hypoalbuminemia is often present. Raised serum globulin levels are seen more often in patients with chronic hepatitis than in those with acute hepatitis.[136] Eosinophilia occurs in 33% of cases. Autoantibodies (ANA and smooth muscle antibodies) are present in some patients with acute hepatitis and in 80% of those with chronic hepatitis. Their presence can make differentiation of nitrofurantoin-induced fulminant hepatitis from AIH challenging.[140] In contrast to AIH, the frequency of HLA-B8 and -DRw3 is not increased.[137] Hepatic histology often shows striking confluent fibrosis, fibrotic bands, and lobar or diffuse liver atrophy.[141]

Treatment is supportive. Glucocorticoids have no role, even in patients with chronic hepatitis with autoimmune features. Recovery is rapid after nitrofurantoin is discontinued. Monitoring liver biochemical test levels is unlikely to be useful or cost-effective.

Others

Methyldopa was among the first drugs associated with immunoallergic drug hepatitis. Cases are now rare because methyldopa is rarely used, other than in pregnancy.[142] Hepatic reactions vary from abnormal liver biochemical test levels in asymptomatic persons, severe acute hepatitis, granuloma formation, and cholestasis to chronic hepatitis with bridging necrosis and cirrhosis. The female predilection, clinical and laboratory changes, course, and extrahepatic features of drug allergy are similar to those for nitrofurantoin.

Phenytoin causes severe acute drug hepatitis in less than 1 per 10,000 persons exposed.[143] Incidence rates are equal in men and women, and cases can occur in childhood. African Americans may be affected more often than Europeans. Rash, fever, eosinophilia, lymphadenopathy, a pseudomononucleosis syndrome, and other allergic features are common and suggest immunoallergy as part of the DRESS syndrome. Some patients with phenytoin reactions have an individual or familial enzymatic defect that causes reduced disposal of phenytoin arene oxide,[143] indicating a possible reactive metabolite in the pathogenesis of phenytoin toxicity. The current mortality rate has been much lower (13%) than in earlier publications (40%). Some deaths are caused by liver failure, whereas others result from severe systemic hypersensitivity, bone marrow suppression, cutaneous and renal vasculitis, or exfoliative dermatitis. Rare hepatic reactions include cholestatic hepatitis and bile duct injury. The most common association with phenytoin therapy is a hepatic adaptive response with microsomal enzyme induction, with raised serum GGTP levels in two-thirds and alkaline phosphatase in one-third of persons who take the drug. Liver histology shows hepatocytes with ground-glass cytoplasm that represents hypertrophied smooth endoplasmic reticulum.

Barbiturates, including phenobarbital, are rarely associated with acute hepatitis. Described cases have resembled phenytoin reactions; fever and rash are usual; and the rate of mortality as a result of liver failure is high. Among *newer antiepileptic drugs*, lamotrigine,[144] felbamate,[145] and topiramate[146] have been associated with ALF. However, a review of the FDA Adverse Events Reporting System database found that the overall risk of hepatotoxicity is insignificant among the majority of the newer antiepileptic drugs.[147]

Sulfonamides can cause acute hepatitis that is relatively common with combination drugs such as trimethoprim/sulfamethoxazole (TMP/SMX).[148] *Trimethoprim* alone has been associated with cholestatic hepatitis; the estimated risk is 1.4 cases per 100,000 exposed persons.[148] Reactions to TMP/SMX resemble those associated with trimethoprim than with sulfonamide; cholestasis or cholestatic hepatitis is more common than hepatitis. Patients with HIV/AIDS are predisposed to sulfonamide hypersensitivity. Some other drugs have a sulfa moiety that differs from that of sulfonamides and that may increase the risk of cross-sensitivity reactions; for example, severe hepatitis with celecoxib developed in two women with previous sulfonamide sensitivity. Certain variants in HLA classes I and II have been associated with an increased risk of hepatotoxicity (see Table 90.3).[149] Likewise, *sulfonylureas* (e.g., gliclazide) have rarely been associated with drug hepatitis with features of immunoallergy.[150]

The latent period between exposure to the drug and the onset of sulfonamide hepatitis is 5−14 days, and clinical features often include fever, rash, mucositis (Stevens-Johnson syndrome), lymphadenopathy, and vasculitis (i.e., features of DRESS syndrome). Reactions may be severe, and deaths have occurred. The liver biochemical test profile is mainly hepatocellular, but mixed or cholestatic reactions can occur. Other presentations include hepatic granulomas and chronic hepatitis.

Sulfasalazine has been associated with cases of often severe acute hepatitis. This complication may be more frequent than appreciated (0.4%).[151] Although toxicity is usually attributed to the sulfonamide moiety, *mesalamine* (mesalazine) can also cause acute hepatitis.[152] This finding incriminates the salicylate moiety, and like salicylate hepatitis (discussed earlier), sulfasalazine hepatotoxicity is more common in patients with RA than in those with IBD. Other presentations include chronic hepatitis with autoimmune features and granulomatous hepatitis.[153]

Among other drugs used to treat IBD, the *anti-TNF antibodies* can cause acute hepatocellular or mixed hepatocellular-cholestatic injury.[154] Infliximab has been implicated most often (1 in 120 recipients), with lower rates for adalimumab and etanercept (1 in 270 and 1 in 430, respectively).[155] The hepatitis presentation is frequently accompanied by characteristics that suggest an autoimmune basis (positive antinuclear and smooth muscle antibodies, plasma cell infiltrate, and hepatocyte rosettes on histology), and short courses of glucocorticoids are often used to hasten resolution.[156] However, unlike true drug-induced AIH, relapses are rare after the anti-TNF agent is withdrawn. A second biologic agent such as adalimumab could be successfully substituted in most cases. Vedolizumab, a humanized antibody directed at $\alpha4\beta7$ integrin, can cause cholestatic liver injury, which can be protracted despite drug withdrawal. Also, vedolizumab as well as natalizumab (from the same drug class) have been associated with a few cases of acute hepatocellular injury.[157,158]

Immune checkpoint inhibitors (ICI) are an emerging group of drugs that have been associated with acute hepatitis. These reactivate T-cell activity against cancer cells by blocking cytotoxic T-lymphocyte-associated antigen 4 (ipilimumab) or the programmed death-1/programmed death ligand-L1 axis (pembrolizumab, nivolumab). The liver injury (seen in 2%−10%) is part of systemic immune-related toxicity affecting the gastrointestinal tract, skin, and other organs. The risk of liver injury is increased (~25%) in patients receiving a combination of ICI from different drug classes or when combined with systemic chemotherapy.[159] Onset is usually within 6 weeks. In a series of 11 patients undergoing liver biopsy, all of whom had received 1−4 doses of ipilimumab, the liver lesions included a panlobular hepatitis, prominent sinusoidal histiocytic infiltrate, central vein endothelialitis, and bridging and confluent necrosis in severe cases.[160] The spectrum includes asymptomatic aminotransferase elevations to severe acute hepatitis, including fatal hepatic failure in 0.2%. Unlike AIH, where $CD4^+/CD20^+$ T cells and plasma cell infiltrates are characteristic, in ICI-related liver injury, $CD8^+$ T cells predominate, and plasma cell infiltration is infrequent. Fibrin-type granulomas are also reported in CTLA4-related drug reactions. Uncommonly, a cholestatic pattern of liver injury may predominate. Liver biopsies are now performed less often, with most reserved for cases where the diagnosis remains uncertain due to competing causes such as liver metastases, viral hepatitis (HBV) reactivation, or where the patients fail to respond to glucocorticoids. The severity of the presentation dictates management, with temporary cessation of the offending drug in mild cases to permanent discontinuation and use of high-dose glucocorticoids and/or immunosuppressive agents such as mycophenolate mofetil in severe cases.[161] Successful reintroduction with the same immune checkpoint inhibitor after resolution of severe liver injury is reported in small case series.[162] Management guidelines have been recently published.[163,164]

Minocycline and low-dose tetracyclines are rare but important causes of severe acute hepatitis, including cases that have required LT. Minocycline is one of the few agents in current use that can lead to drug-induced AIH (see later).

Disulfiram (Antabuse) rarely has been associated with acute hepatitis, occasionally leading to liver failure.[165] Disulfiram hepatitis is usually easy to distinguish from alcohol-associated hepatitis by the 10-fold or greater elevation of serum ALT levels.

Of the newer oral anticoagulants, ximelagatran was withdrawn due to hepatotoxicity. Rivaroxaban and other direct thrombin antagonists have been associated with acute hepatocellular or mixed hepatocellular-cholestatic injury, with resolution in most cases.[166,167] Acute liver failure was also reported. However, there were confounding factors in these cases, and two recent meta-analyses showed that these drugs were less likely to cause liver injury than warfarin or low-molecular-weight heparin.[168] In an Icelandic study, 14.5% of 2300 patients receiving newer oral anticoagulants had elevated liver enzymes, but only 3 cases (all rivaroxaban) were adjudged by causality assessment as being drug-related.[169]

β-Adrenergic blocking agents have rarely been incriminated in hepatotoxicity. Acebutolol, carvedilol, labetalol, and metoprolol have all been associated with acute hepatitis, some of which were severe; some cases were proven by rechallenge. Data are insufficient to determine whether or not immunoallergy is likely. The *calcium channel blockers* nifedipine, verapamil, diltiazem, and amlodipine[170] have good safety records, but rare cases of acute hepatitis with a short incubation period (5 days to 6 weeks) and other features of immunoallergy have been reported.

Of the *angiotensin II receptor blocking agents*, irbesartan has been linked to two reports of cholestasis.[171] In both cases, jaundice developed within 1 month. Liver histology showed marked cholestasis in both cases and an inflammatory infiltrate and eosinophils in one case. Clinical resolution occurred soon after the drug was stopped, but the liver biochemical test levels remained elevated for over 1 year in one patient. Biliary ductopenia is a rare complication. Losartan, valsartan, and candesartan have also been implicated in cases of acute hepatitis or cholestatic hepatitis.[172] Olmesartan's association with sprue-like enteropathy is well documented but there are a few case reports of an AIH-like presentation.[173]

ACE inhibitor-induced liver disease is an important adverse effect of this drug class, with a frequency of 9 per 100,000 persons treated. Reactions to captopril (the oldest and possibly most hepatotoxic member of this class of drugs), enalapril, and ramipril usually manifest as cholestatic hepatitis, but hepatocellular or mixed hepatocellular reactions can occur.[174] Features of hypersensitivity (DRESS syndrome), such as fever, skin rash, and eosinophilia, may accompany captopril hepatotoxicity.[174] Histologic examination of the liver reveals marked centrilobular cholestasis with eosinophilic portal infiltrates. Liver biochemical abnormalities usually resolve after drug withdrawal, but resolution can be delayed up to 6 months in some cases. ALF has been noted with lisinopril,[175] whereas bland cholestasis is seen with fosinopril, and cholestatic hepatitis progressing to biliary ductopenia and cirrhosis has been associated with ramipril and enalapril, respectively.[174]

Hydroxymethylglutaryl-coenzyme A (HMGCo-A) reductase inhibitors (commonly known as statins) are not strongly associated with important hepatic injury, although published reports and data submitted to drug safety surveillance authorities appear to be discordant. A dose-related rise in serum aminotransferase levels develops in 1%–3% of statin users. The usual manifestation of liver injury is a minor (<2-fold) asymptomatic rise in serum ALT and AST levels. These elevations usually reverse rapidly with withdrawal of the statin and also if therapy is *not* interrupted. Lovastatin, pravastatin, atorvastatin, simvastatin, and rosuvastatin have been implicated in a few reports of acute hepatitis or cholestatic hepatitis.[176,177] Older data estimated the risk of statin-related DILI to be less than 1 per million person-years, but more recent data suggest a frequency between 1 per 11,000 and 1.2 per 100,000 users.[178] Atorvastatin is most often implicated (41%), but the overall frequency of DILI is highest for fluvastatin (17 per 100,000 person-years). Most hepatic reactions occur within 3–6 months. One-third of the patients have had jaundice, and 2 deaths occurred from ALF. In 1 patient receiving atorvastatin 40 mg daily for 15 months uneventfully, severe hepatocellular injury developed when the dose was increased to 80 mg daily.[179] Positive rechallenge has been documented. Retreatment with the same statin is not recommended, but an alternative statin has been used successfully (suggesting a lack of class effect). With respect to the pattern of liver injury, cholestatic and mixed reactions were associated more often with atorvastatin (57%) than simvastatin (25%). Small case series have linked statins to AIH, but the level of evidence for causality is unconvincing. Because these drugs are used by about 15% of the population, it is inevitable that a proportion of patients in whom AIH develops will be taking a statin. Instances of resolution of AIH following discontinuation of statins are not conspicuous in existing reports.

Prescribing guidelines invariably warn about the risk of liver injury when statins are prescribed to persons with preexisting liver biochemical abnormalities, but this recommendation is strongly refuted by a controlled trial of high-dose pravastatin that confirmed the safety of statins in this setting.[180] Likewise, in the Dallas Heart Study, statin users were no more likely to exhibit serum ALT elevations than were nonusers.[181] Also, the risk of statin hepatotoxicity is unrelated to the baseline serum ALT level,[182] and statin use reduces the rate of fibrosis progression and the risk of hepatic decompensation.[183] Finally, cardiovascular events are more likely to develop in patients with raised serum ALT levels who are not receiving statins than in those treated with these agents (30% vs. 10%; relative risk reduction of 68%).[184] Monitoring serum aminotransferase levels in persons taking a statin is no longer mandated by the FDA. Other hypolipidemic drugs that cause hepatocellular injury include niacin and fenofibrate; the latter is also implicated in cholestatic and mixed hepatocellular/cholestatic reactions, including chronic hepatitis and ALF.[185]

Unlike vitamin A (see Chapter 91), *synthetic retinoids*, such as etretinate and acitretin, are not predictable hepatotoxins. Etretinate is associated with raised serum aminotransferase levels in 10%–25% of treated patients[186]; levels normalize with dose reduction, thereby suggesting partial dose dependency. Cases of acute hepatitis have been attributed to etretinate, some confirmed by rechallenge.[186] Most patients were women older than age 50; 2 cases were associated with chronicity, and 1 patient responded to glucocorticoids. Etretinate has been superseded by acitretin, which can also cause acute hepatitis, occasionally with bile duct injury, progressive hepatic fibrosis, and, rarely, ALF (after an acitretin overdose).[187]

Gastric acid suppression drugs have an excellent safety record, although rare adverse hepatic reactions and withdrawals of two H2RAs (oxmetidine, ebrotidine) due to hepatotoxicity have been reported. Cimetidine, ranitidine, and famotidine can cause acute hepatitis, mostly mild and often with cholestatic features. Some cases have been proven by rechallenge. Features of immunoallergy were present in some of the cimetidine reactions. Isolated cases of hepatotoxicity have been attributed to the PPIs omeprazole, lansoprazole, and pantoprazole; causality was not established unequivocally in some of the cases.[188]

Zafirlukast, a *leukotriene receptor antagonist*, has been linked to several cases of ALF.[189] Montelukast has been associated with a few cases of acute hepatitis or cholestatic hepatitis leading to biliary ductopenia.[190]

Cystic fibrosis transmembrane conductance regulator modulators (elexacaftor, tezacaftor, and ivacaftor), used alone or in combination, have been associated with increased transaminases, leading to their discontinuation in 1%–2% of participants enrolled in clinical trials.[191] There are a few case reports of acute hepatitis with histology showing zone 3 hepatic necrosis.[191]

Bland cholestasis has been noted with ticlopidine, an *antiplatelet agent*. Other histologic findings include occasional cholestatic hepatitis with bile duct injury and microvesicular steatosis. Japanese subjects carrying the HLA haplotype A*33:03 (see Table 90.3) and certain cytochrome polymorphisms (CYP2B6*1H or *1J) are at an increased risk of ticlopidine hepatotoxicity.[192] Clopidogrel has become preferred over ticlopidine and can also cause hepatocellular or mixed hepatocellular-cholestatic liver injury.[193]

Metabolic Idiosyncrasy

Isoniazid

Isoniazid-induced liver injury has been characterized since the 1970s, but deaths still occur.[194] Hepatitis develops in about 2% of persons exposed to isoniazid; 5%–10% of cases are fatal. The risk and severity of isoniazid hepatitis increase with age; the risk is 0.3% in the third decade of life and increases to 2% or higher after age 50.[194] Overall frequency rates are the same in men and women, but 70% of fatal cases are in women; black and Hispanic women may be at particular risk.[194] The risk of toxicity is not related to the dose or blood level of isoniazid. Direct bioactivation to a reactive metabolite was considered to be the main basis for the liver injury, but the identification of antidrug/anti-CYP antibodies in some cases suggests immune involvement.[195] The role of genetic factors has been controversial. Associations have been described with specific genes that code for enzymes involved in aspects of drug metabolism or detoxification (CYP2E1, *N*-acetyltransferase, glutathione *S*-transferase), but data are conflicting.[196] Chronic excessive alcohol intake increases the frequency and severity of isoniazid hepatotoxicity,[194] as may concomitant use of rifampin, pyrazinamide, and acetaminophen.[197] Some, but not all, studies have shown that persons with chronic HBV infection are at an increased risk of liver injury from isoniazid and other antituberculosis drugs.[198] Malnutrition may play a role in isoniazid hepatotoxicity in some countries. Likewise, in patients with HCV or HIV infection (or both), the risk of significant serum ALT elevations during antituberculosis drug treatment is increased several-fold; successful antiviral treatment of hepatitis C has allowed the safe reintroduction of antituberculosis drugs.

Serum ALT levels increase in 10%–36% of isoniazid recipients in the first 10 weeks. The elevations typically are minor and resolve spontaneously. In persons in whom hepatitis develops, the latent period from exposure to disease ranges from 1 week to more than 6 months (median, 8 weeks), and, in severe cases, 12 weeks.[194] Reexposure to isoniazid may be associated with an accelerated onset, although the experience in India is that gradual reintroduction of isoniazid and rifampin can be achieved in most cases after the hepatitis has resolved. Prodromal symptoms occur in one-third of patients and include malaise, fatigue, and early symptoms of hepatitis, such as anorexia, nausea, and vomiting. Jaundice appears several days later and is the only feature in approximately 10% of cases. Fever, rash, arthralgias, and eosinophilia are uncommon.

Liver biochemical testing indicates hepatocellular injury; serum AST levels exceed serum ALT levels in one-half of patients. Serum bilirubin levels usually are elevated; values that are increased more than 10-fold indicate a poor prognosis. In one study, one-third of patients had a prolonged prothrombin time, and 60% of these cases were fatal.[194] Liver histology shows hepatocellular injury, which is focal in one-half of the cases, often with marked hydropic change in residual hepatocytes. In the remainder, hepatocellular necrosis is zonal, submassive, or massive, with inflammation confined to the portal tracts. Cholestasis and lobular regeneration suggestive of early cirrhosis are rare features.

Fatal cases have been associated with a longer duration of treatment or continued ingestion of isoniazid after the onset of symptoms.[194,199] Therefore most deaths from isoniazid hepatitis are preventable, and recovery is rapid if symptoms are reported early and isoniazid is discontinued before severe liver injury is established.

Treatment is supportive, with LT indicated in severe cases. In the United States, isoniazid hepatotoxicity is second only to acetaminophen as an indication for LT for DILI.[198] Fortunately, outcomes of transplantation have been good (85% 1-year survival).[200] Children are less susceptible than adults, but serious hepatotoxicity can occur in children; over a 10-year period (1987–1997), 8 children were transplanted for isoniazid hepatotoxicity in the United States.[201]

Prevention is the most appropriate way to avoid isoniazid hepatotoxicity, and determining whether the risks of isoniazid prophylaxis outweigh those of latent tuberculosis is critical. New alternative regimes to the 9-month isoniazid course are gaining favor due to their lower hepatotoxicity and better completion rates [rifampin alone for 4 months or isoniazid with rifapentine for 3 months].[202] The optimal approach to monitoring is uncertain; every-other-week or monthly monitoring of serum ALT levels will not always prevent the rapid onset of severe hepatotoxicity. Effective prevention depends on awareness of early symptoms, no matter how nonspecific. Future approaches may include a pharmacogenomic strategy, with a study from Singapore showing that a model combining clinical and genomic information [*N*-acetyltransferase 2 (NAT2) slow acetylator status] was superior to clinical data alone.[203] Further, the development of a rapid assay for pharmacogenomic testing (*NAT2*) could facilitate wider adoption for such testing, individualized dosing, and the prospect of reducing the risk of liver injury.[204]

Other Antituberculosis Drugs

Most cases of liver injury in which rifampin is implicated have occurred in patients who are also taking isoniazid, but a few have occurred when rifampin was used as monotherapy in persons with underlying liver disease.[205] Pyrazinamide (and a related agent, ethionamide) is a dose-dependent hepatotoxin. The drug is now used in lower doses (1.5–2 g/day) because of the emergence of resistant mycobacterial strains. Patients who take combinations that include isoniazid and pyrazinamide can develop particularly severe liver injury. Monitoring of serum ALT levels during therapy is recommended. Cross-sensitivity among isoniazid, pyrazinamide, and ethionamide may occur. In a network meta-analysis of treatment protocols for latent tuberculosis, pyrazinamide-based regimes carried the highest risk of hepatic injury.[205]

Antifungal Drugs

Ketoconazole is associated with raised serum aminotransferase levels in 5%–17% of treated patients,[206,207] but symptomatic hepatitis is less common (0.007%–0.020%). Women (with a female-to-male ratio of 2:1) and persons older than 40 years of age are particularly susceptible to liver injury.[206–208] Concurrent use of drugs (e.g., lovastatin) that share a similar metabolic pathway of elimination (CYP3A4) with ketoconazole can lead to hepatotoxicity.[209] Reactions are usually mild but can be severe, with rare cases of ALF.[210] Persons who have received multiple courses can present with acute hepatitis and even anaphylaxis within 1–3 days when reexposed to this agent.[211] Patients with chronic liver disease are at an increased risk of severe acute liver injury.[212]

The mortality rate is 3%–7%.[206,207] The onset is within 6–12 weeks, and rarely after the drug is stopped. Toxicity is unrelated to the dose of the drug. Continued ingestion of ketoconazole after the onset of symptoms leads to an adverse outcome. Jaundice occurs in 50% of patients in whom acute hepatitis develops, and up to one-third may present with nonspecific symptoms, such as nausea, anorexia, and vomiting. Fever, rash, eosinophilia, and other immunoallergic characteristics are rare. The pattern of liver biochemical test levels is primarily hepatocellular or mixed, but cholestatic hepatitis or bland cholestasis may occur.[206] Jaundice usually resolves within 12 weeks, but resolution may take months.[206,207] Cirrhosis is a rare complication following acute hepatic injury.[213]

Several cases of cholestatic hepatitis attributed to terbinafine have been reported, with a frequency of 2–3 cases per 100,000 persons exposed.[214] Persons with HLA-A*33:01 are at an increased risk of terbinafine-associated DILI, especially with a cholestatic or mixed pattern.[215] The onset is usually within 4–6 weeks. Recovery is usual with discontinuation of the drug, although prolonged cholestasis with ductopenia has been reported. UDCA has been used to hasten recovery when cholestasis is protracted.[216] Other presentations include sinusoidal obstruction syndrome in a liver transplant recipient[217] and 16 reports to the FDA of ALF possibly linked to terbinafine[218]; the frequency of this outcome has been estimated to be 1 per million persons exposed.[219]

Fluconazole and itraconazole appear to be less hepatotoxic than ketoconazole and terbinafine[220]; elevations of liver biochemical test levels occur in fewer than 5% of patients. Rare cases of severe hepatic necrosis have been ascribed to fluconazole, but other causes were not excluded.[221] Instances of ALF associated with itraconazole have been reported.[222] Elevated serum aminotransferase levels are observed in 20% of persons taking voriconazole. Overt clinical hepatitis leading to treatment discontinuation has been documented in patients receiving voriconazole in a liver ICU.[223] Micafungin, an echinocandin, has been frequently associated with liver injury (10%–24%), predominantly of a cholestatic or a mixed cholestatic-hepatocellular type.[224]

Antidiabetic Drugs

Thiazolidinediones

Troglitazone, the first peroxisome proliferator-activated receptor-δ agonist, was withdrawn due to hepatotoxicity. Elevated serum aminotransferase levels were noted in 0.5%–1.9% of recipients in early trials, but serious hepatotoxicity was not identified until the postmarketing period. During this phase, over 75 cases of fatal hepatotoxicity or liver failure requiring LT were reported.[225,226] Most cases occurred in older women and obese persons, the common phenotype of persons with type 2 diabetes mellitus. Evidence that preexisting liver disease or other drugs predispose to troglitazone hepatotoxicity is lacking, although a progressive course in one patient was attributed to concurrent use of simvastatin and troglitazone.[227] Mitochondrial injury is favored as the mechanism of hepatic injury, but other mechanisms (e.g., reactive metabolites, inhibition of BSEP) have been proposed.[228]

The onset of troglitazone hepatotoxicity was often as late as 9–12 months after treatment was started[229,230]; rare cases had an onset soon after the drug was started (8 days).[231] Presenting symptoms included nausea, fatigue, jaundice, vomiting, and symptoms of liver failure. Progression to ALF was often rapid, and in some cases, deterioration continued despite discontinuation of troglitazone.[232] Histologic examination of liver biopsy specimens, explanted livers, or autopsy material showed submassive or massive hepatic necrosis, with postcollapse scarring, bile duct proliferation, and some eosinophils.[233] Severe cholestasis also was reported,[234] as is sometimes observed with other causes of ALF (e.g., valproic acid) and does not necessarily imply a pathogenic mechanism different from that in cases not associated with cholestasis.

Serious liver injury is rare with the second-generation thiazolidinediones, rosiglitazone, and pioglitazone. In clinical trials, less than 0.3% of recipients had raised serum ALT levels (>3 × ULN),[226] and only a few cases of hepatotoxicity associated with rosiglitazone ($n = 6$) and pioglitazone ($n = 5$) have been reported.[235] Pioglitazone has also been associated with two reports of cholestatic hepatitis with bile duct injury.[236] Most patients have recovered after discontinuing pioglitazone. ALF is rare.[237] Although a series of cases compiled by the FDA noted a high case fatality rate (80%),[238] causality was questioned by the manufacturers,[239,240] citing the background incidence of liver complications in patients with diabetes mellitus and other confounding factors. By contrast, a French pharmacovigilance study concluded that the risk of hepatic reactions with these drugs was similar to that reported with other oral hypoglycemic drugs.[241] Before treatment is started, the FDA recommends baseline liver biochemical tests; the pretreatment serum ALT level should be less than 2.5 times the ULN. Monitoring the serum ALT level every 2 months during the first year of therapy and periodically thereafter is advised. If ALT levels remain persistently elevated (>3 × ULN), the drug should be discontinued. Symptoms suggestive of hepatitis should be assessed immediately. Persons in whom jaundice developed with troglitazone should not take other thiazolidinediones.[242]

Other Oral Hypoglycemic Drugs

Hepatocellular injury was common with older sulfonylureas, such as carbutamide, metahexamide, and chlorpropamide.[243] Currently used drugs (tolbutamide, tolazamide, glimepiride, and glibenclamide) may rarely cause cholestasis or cholestatic hepatitis.[244,245] Similar to sulfonamides, with which they share a structural relationship, hypersensitivity phenomena [fever, skin rash, eosinophilia (i.e., DRESS syndrome)] were present in some cases. Most cases were resolved after withdrawal of the drug; however, chronic cholestasis progressing to vanishing bile duct syndrome (VBDS) has been described with tolbutamide and tolazamide. Fatal liver failure has been reported in two cases, including one with underlying cirrhosis. Gliclazide[245] and glibenclamide have also been associated with hepatocellular injury and, with the latter drug, hepatic granulomas.[246] Metformin, acarbose, repaglinide, and human insulin rarely have been associated with liver injury.

Drugs Used for Psychiatric and Neurologic Disorders

Several neuroleptic agents have been associated with drug hepatitis. Some reactions appear to be immunoallergic, whereas others are related to metabolic idiosyncrasy, depending on the drug structure. Such reactions have been reported for commonly used antidepressants, such as fluoxetine,[247,248] paroxetine,[249] venlafaxine,[250] trazodone,[251] tolcapone,[252] and nefazodone.

Antidepressants

Monoamine Oxidase Inhibitors

Iproniazid was one of the first drugs associated with acute hepatitis. Reactions occurred in 1% of recipients and were often severe, with reports of fatal ALF. The hydrazine substituent (which iproniazid shares in part with isoniazid, ethionamide, pyrazinamide, and niacin) was determined to be the hepatotoxic moiety.[253] Phenelzine and isocarboxazid have been associated with occasional instances of hepatocellular injury, but monoamine oxidase inhibitors are now prescribed infrequently.

Tricyclic Antidepressants

Tricyclic antidepressants bear a structural resemblance to the phenothiazines and are occasional causes of cholestatic or, less commonly, hepatocellular injury. Recovery following cessation of the drug is usual, but amitriptyline[254] and imipramine[255] can cause prolonged cholestasis.

Selective Serotonin Reuptake Inhibitors (SSRIs) and Other Modern Antidepressants

Liver enzyme elevations have been observed in asymptomatic persons taking fluoxetine and paroxetine.[247] A few reports of acute and chronic hepatitis have been attributed to the use of SSRIs,[247,248,256] and acute hepatitis with mirtazapine, a tetracyclic antidepressant, and agomelatine, a melatonin (MT1/MT2) receptor agonist and serotonergic (5-HT2c) receptor antagonist.[257,258] Nefazodone (now withdrawn) was associated with cases of subacute liver failure.[259] Liver histology showed centrilobular, submassive, or massive hepatic necrosis. Trazodone has been implicated in causing acute and chronic hepatocellular injury.[260] The onset can be delayed as long as 18 months or can occur within 5 days of the start of the drug.[260] Occasional reports document severe hepatotoxicity with combinations of antidepressants or with antidepressants used in combination with other neuroleptic agents.[261] Drug regulatory authorities have been alerted about cases of acute hepatocellular injury (including ALF) with atomoxetine, a norepinephrine reuptake inhibitor, but only a few of these have been linked conclusively with the drug.[262]

Antipsychotic Drugs

In addition to chlorpromazine (see later), liver injury can occur with other antipsychotic agents, mainly as hepatocellular or mixed (clozapine, olanzapine, quetiapine, and aripiprazole) or cholestatic (risperidone) reactions.[263] Rare cases of ALF have been attributed to clozapine. By promoting weight gain, some of these drugs (clozapine, olanzapine) also promote hepatic steatosis.

Other Neurologic Drugs

Tolcapone, a catechol-*o*-methyl transferase (COMT) inhibitor used in Parkinson disease, has been associated with four cases of ALF.[264] All were women older than 70 years of age who presented with jaundice and high serum ALT levels. Centrilobular hepatic necrosis was noted at autopsy in one case. Postmarketing surveillance has identified three additional patients with acute hepatocellular injury. Overall, tolcapone is considered safe if patients are monitored appropriately.[265] Current FDA guidelines recommend serum ALT testing every 2–4 weeks for the first 6 months. Thereafter, the frequency of testing is left to the discretion of the treating doctor. Patients in whom the serum ALT rises (to at least 1–2 × ULN) should be monitored closely; persistent serum ALT elevations (>2 × ULN) are an indication to discontinue the drug. Another COMT inhibitor, entacapone, has only rarely been associated with significant liver injury.

Alpidem,[266] zolpidem,[267] and bentazepam[268] are sedative hypnotics that have been implicated in hepatotoxicity. With bentazepam, the clinicopathologic pattern resembled chronic hepatitis, but without autoantibodies or other immunologic features.[268]

Tacrine, a reversible choline esterase inhibitor, was formerly used in Alzheimer disease. Elevated serum ALT levels (>3 × ULN, >20 × ULN) are seen in 25% and 2% of patients, respectively, more often in women than in men.[269] These liver enzyme changes resolved after stopping the drug. Symptoms were rare; only nausea and vomiting correlated with major serum ALT elevations. Liver biopsy specimens showed steatosis and mild lobular hepatitis. Minor degrees of hepatocellular injury were noted in up to 50% of cases, but tolerance eventually developed.[269] There were isolated reports of jaundice, indicating a rare potential for more severe hepatotoxicity. The mechanism of liver injury is unclear, but mitochondrial injury was observed in an animal model of tacrine hepatotoxicity.

Dantrolene, a skeletal muscle relaxant, causes hepatitis in about 1% of exposed persons, with a case-fatality rate of approximately 28%.[270] Most of those affected have been older than 30 years of age. One-third of patients are asymptomatic, and the remainder present with jaundice and symptoms of hepatitis. Liver histology shows hepatocellular necrosis, often submassive or massive.[270] Liver biochemical tests are recommended every 2 weeks while a patient is on treatment, and the drug should be discontinued if the levels become elevated.

Other idiosyncratic hepatotoxins include tizanidine (a centrally acting muscle relaxant),[271] alverine (a smooth muscle relaxant),[272] and riluzole.[273] Patients with cirrhosis who take tizanidine are at risk of hypotension; levels of this CYP1A2-metabolized drug are increased as a consequence of diminished cytochrome activity (see Table 90.1).[274] Riluzole is approved for treating amyotrophic lateral sclerosis and was associated with increased serum ALT levels in 1.3%–10% of subjects in clinical trials. Two cases of acute hepatitis with microvesicular steatosis have since been reported, with onset 4 and 8 weeks, respectively, after the drug was started.[273] Rarely, hepatocellular injury may be delayed up to 6 months. Liver biochemical test elevations resolved rapidly after riluzole was discontinued.

NSAIDs

NSAIDs rarely cause DILI, with or without immunoallergic features and with varying degrees of hepatocellular injury and cholestasis. Bromfenac was withdrawn because of hepatotoxicity.[275]

Although COX-2 inhibitors are less likely than conventional NSAIDs to cause UGI toxicity, they are not necessarily safer with respect to the risk of liver injury.[276] A few cases of acute hepatitis (some severe) have been reported with nimesulide and celecoxib, and rofecoxib was associated with cholestatic liver injury.[277] On the other hand, lumiracoxib was withdrawn because it was associated with severe hepatotoxicity.[276] In clinical trials, celecoxib was associated with rates of liver injury similar to those in placebo-treated patients (0.8% vs. 0.9%, respectively).[277] Increases in serum aminotransferase levels were noted with concurrent use of diclofenac. When serious hepatocellular injury was attributed to celecoxib, female gender was a predisposing factor.[278] The onset of symptoms has been between 4 days and 4 weeks after the drug was started. Delayed presentations (5 months to 2 years) may occasionally occur. Liver biochemical and histology were mostly consistent with a pattern of hepatocellular or mixed liver injury, with rare cases of biliary ductopenia and periductal fibrosis.[277] Some patients had eosinophilia and skin rash suggestive of DRESS syndrome. Most patients recovered within 1–4 months after stopping the drug. Of 18 patients with celecoxib-associated liver injury reported to the FDA, the outcomes included resolution in 12 cases, LT in 2, and persistent biochemical abnormalities 6–18 months after the onset in 4.[279] Celecoxib should not be administered to persons with a documented sulfonamide allergy because of cross-reactivity.

Although the overall frequency of liver injury is very small, nimesulide, an NSAID with COX-2 selectivity, has been linked to acute hepatitis and fatal hepatic failure,[280] especially in women over 55 years. The onset is usually between 15 and 90 days (median, 40 days) but can be delayed up to 8 months.[281] Risk factors for liver injury include increased treatment duration (>30 days) and higher doses (OR, 10.7).[282] Hypersensitivity features with peripheral eosinophilia are infrequent. Liver histology shows centrilobular or bridging necrosis and occasionally bland cholestasis. Median time to recovery is 60 days, but in 1 series of 57 patients, acute liver failure was observed in 12 (21%), with 5 deaths and 3 patients requiring liver transplantation.[281]

DRUG-INDUCED GRANULOMATOUS HEPATITIS

Drugs account for 2%–29% of cases of granulomatous hepatitis (see Chapter 35).[150,246,283–285] Over 40 drugs and foreign compounds are associated with hepatic granulomas (Table 90.7); not all these agents are associated with systemic inflammation or with

TABLE 90.7 Drug-Induced Granulomatous Hepatitis: Major Causative Agents, Frequency, Risk Factors, Clinicopathologic Features, and Outcomes

Causative Agent[a]	Frequency	Risk Factors	Clinicopathologic Features	Outcome
Carbamazepine	16:100,000 treatment-years	Age >40 years, no gender predilection	Two-thirds of cases show granulomatous hepatitis; the remainder show acute hepatitis, cholangitis; no drug allergy features	No reported fatalities, rapid recovery
Phenylbutazone	1:5000 exposed	No age or gender predilection	Severe acute hepatitis, cholestasis, and bile duct injury also reported; signs of drug allergy are common; occasionally vasculitis	Mortality rate 25%, particularly in cases with hepatocellular necrosis
Allopurinol	Rare (<40 cases)	Older men, black race, renal failure, thiazide use	Acute hepatitis, cholestatic hepatitis, and bile duct injury are also frequent; rash (exfoliative dermatitis), nephritis, vasculitis	Mortality rate 15%, especially with vasculitis
Hydralazine	Rare	Older patients, possibly slow acetylators	Other types of reaction are also common: acute hepatitis, cholestatic hepatitis, cholangitis; features of drug allergy are uncommon	Reactions severe, but no mortality reported
Quinine	Rare	No recognized risk factors	Acute hepatitis in two-thirds of cases; rash, interstitial pneumonitis, positive Coombs test, thrombocytopenia	Good prognosis

[a]Other drugs that have been reliably reported to cause granulomatous hepatitis include aspirin, glyburide, mesalamine, nitrofurantoin, papaverine, phenytoin, procainamide, quinidine, sulfasalazine, sulfonamides. Single case reports have implicated many other agents, as referred to briefly in the text.

persuasive evidence of causality. Many (e.g., halothane, methyldopa, nitrofurantoin, troglitazone, amiodarone, and amoxicillin-clavulanic acid) are more commonly associated with other patterns of liver injury. Some of these associations may be fortuitous.

The clinical picture is heralded by fever and systemic symptoms (e.g., malaise, headache, and myalgia) from 10 days to 4 months after the start of treatment. Hepatomegaly and hepatic tenderness are common; splenomegaly is present in 25% of patients. Extrahepatic features of drug hypersensitivity are common, as is eosinophilia (30%). Liver biochemical test levels are typically mixed because of the infiltrative nature of hepatic granulomas and the frequent presence of some hepatocellular necrosis or cholestasis. For several drugs that cause granulomatous hepatitis, continued exposure leads to more severe types of liver disease, such as cholestatic hepatitis with or without bile duct injury and hepatic necrosis (see Table 90.7). Small-vessel vasculitis is another potential complication and may involve the kidneys, bone marrow, skin, and lungs; the mortality rate is high.

DRUG-INDUCED CHRONIC HEPATITIS

Chronic hepatitis is defined as hepatitis that continues for more than 6 months. For drug reactions, however, the definition has often been made inappropriately on hepatic histologic features alone. The histologic features include interface hepatitis, bridging necrosis, and fibrosis. Because these features may be present as early as 6 weeks after the onset of severe reactions, they do not confirm chronicity. The diagnosis of chronic hepatitis is more convincing when clinical or biochemical evidence of hepatitis has been present for more than 3 months and when clinical and laboratory features of chronic liver disease or histologic evidence of established hepatic fibrosis are present. Drugs are an uncommon cause of chronic hepatitis (Table 90.8) because the implicated agents such as methyldopa are now rarely used. Nevertheless, recognition of a drug cause remains important for preventing a poor outcome by timely withdrawal of the drug.

Chronic hepatitis is more common in women (~4-fold) and in older patients (as illustrated by nitrofurantoin) but is rare in children. Drugs associated with chronic hepatitis more commonly cause acute hepatitis, and the latent period to recognition tends to be longer in cases of chronic hepatitis; therefore the duration of drug ingestion may be a risk factor for chronic hepatitis. In one study, the mean duration of use of a drug in patients in whom chronic hepatitis or liver-related morbidity and mortality developed after an episode of DILI was significantly greater than the duration in those in whom an adverse outcome did not occur (153 vs. 53 days).[286]

Two syndromes of drug-induced chronic hepatitis occur. In the first, cases are identical to acute hepatitis but more severe, more prolonged, or later in onset, perhaps due to failure of recognition. These cases may appropriately be termed chronic toxicity. Clinical and laboratory features of chronic liver disease are rare, and hallmarks of autoimmunity are absent. Management consists of withdrawal of the drug and treatment of liver failure (see Table 90.8).

The second syndrome more closely resembles AIH based on the presence of stigmata of chronic liver disease such as spider telangiectasias, a firm liver edge, splenomegaly, bruising, ascites, and other complications related to portal hypertension and liver failure. In addition to raised serum ALT and bilirubin levels, hypoalbuminemia and hyperglobulinemia are usual. The prothrombin time is prolonged in severe cases. ANA and/or smooth muscle antibodies are often present, but, unlike idiopathic AIH, other hallmarks of autoimmunity, such as a history of other autoimmune diseases and genetic predisposition indicated by HLA-B8 and -DRw3 alleles, are absent. Immunosuppressive treatment is not indicated; the clinical condition

TABLE 90.8 Drug-Induced Chronic Hepatitis: Causative Agents, Risk Factors, Clinicopathologic Features, and Outcomes

Causative Agent[a]	Risk Factors	Clinicopathologic Features	Outcome
Nitrofurantoin	Age >40 years; 90% of cases occur in women; continued ingestion of drug after onset	Clinical features of chronic hepatitis, liver failure; some cases with cholestasis; 20% with pneumonitis; hyperglobulinemia is usual, ANA, SMA	Mortality rate ~7%; liver transplantation required in 4%
Methyldopa	Age >50 years; mostly in women (80%); repeated courses, continued ingestion of drug in a sensitized patient	Jaundice, diarrhea, liver failure; hyperglobulinemia, ANA, SMA; protracted course	High mortality rate
Diclofenac	Age >65 years; most cases occur in women	Clinical features of chronic hepatitis, liver failure; hyperglobulinemia, ANA, SMA	Response to glucocorticoids in a few cases
Minocycline	Young women; prolonged use of drug	Often part of drug-induced SLE syndrome (arthritis, rash, nephritis); hyperglobulinemia, ANA	Cases may be severe, with a fatal outcome or need for LT; glucocorticoid treatment may be indicated
Isoniazid	Age >50 years; continued ingestion of drug after onset; duration of therapy	Severe and fatal cases with cirrhosis; no immune phenomena	High mortality rate or need for liver transplantation
Dantrolene	Age >30 years; dose, duration of therapy	Jaundice, liver failure; no immune phenomena	High mortality rate
Etretinate	Age >50 years; two-thirds of cases occur in women	Jaundice, weight loss, liver failure; deterioration after drug is stopped	Response to glucocorticoids in two reported cases
Acetaminophen	Regular intake at moderate doses (2–6 g/day); alcohol, fasting, other drugs	No features of chronic liver disease, no autoimmune phenomena; these are cases of chronic toxicity	Rapid normalization of liver biochemical test levels after drug is stopped

[a]Several other agents, including aspirin, cimetidine, fenofibrate, fluoxetine, germander, halothane, methotrexate, sulfonamides, trazodone, have been mentioned as associated with chronic hepatitis, but the evidence of causation is not necessarily convincing. Other causes, including oxyphenisatin and tienilic acid, are now of historical interest.
SMA, Smooth muscle antibodies.

improves spontaneously after withdrawal of the causative drug. In individual cases, however, glucocorticoids occasionally appear to hasten recovery; nevertheless, immunosuppressive therapy can usually be discontinued, in contrast to most cases (65%) of AIH, in whom discontinuation is followed eventually by relapse.[140]

Diclofenac

Diclofenac is widely prescribed and is considered at least as safe as comparable NSAIDs. Among reports to the U.S. Drug-Induced Liver Injury Network, however, diclofenac was the most frequently implicated NSAID.[287] Also, the frequency of diclofenac hepatotoxicity is much higher (11 per 100,000) than previous reports suggested (1–5 per 100,000).[288] In clinical trials, elevations in serum aminotransferase levels (>3 × ULN and >10 × ULN) were noted in 3.1% and 0.5%, respectively, but liver-disease-related hospitalizations were infrequent (0.023%).[289] More than 200 cases of diclofenac hepatitis have been reported,[290] including several proven by inadvertent rechallenge. Only four cases have been fatal, and five cases can reasonably be regarded as chronic hepatitis. Genetic susceptibility to diclofenac hepatotoxicity has been documented.[291] In these cases, polymorphisms have been observed in genes that affect metabolic pathways that lead to formation of reactive metabolites of the drug and affect biliary excretion. Immune responses to drug metabolite-protein adducts have been identified.[291] Diclofenac has also been shown to induce oxidative stress, leading to impaired autophagy and loss of mitochondrial integrity.[292]

The risk of hepatitis is increased in women and with aging. A prodromal illness characterized by anorexia, nausea, vomiting, and malaise heralds the onset of liver injury, which usually occurs within 3 months (range 1–11 months). Fever and rash occur in 25% of patients.[290] Liver biochemical test results reflect acute hepatitis with or without cholestasis. Reactions tend to be severe, with jaundice occurring in 50% of cases. Liver histology shows acute lobular hepatitis and, in severe cases, bridging or confluent necrosis, interface hepatitis, and fibrous expansion of the portal tracts. The prognosis is usually good; resolution occurs after discontinuation of the drug. Cases of drug-induced chronic hepatitis have been described in which the clinical and laboratory features (ascites, hypoalbuminemia, hyperglobulinemia, and jaundice) suggested AIH, although the frequency of autoantibodies is unclear. These cases usually improve spontaneously after discontinuation of the drug, but glucocorticoids have been used successfully in a few protracted cases.[293] Cross-sensitivity with other NSAIDs seems to be rare but has been reported with ibuprofen. The rarity of severe diclofenac-induced hepatotoxicity makes liver biochemical monitoring unrealistic. Patients should be advised to report adverse effects, and clinicians must be aware that diclofenac can cause both acute and chronic hepatitis.

Minocycline

Minocycline has been associated with rare cases of drug-induced SLE (rash, polyarthritis, hyperglobulinemia, and ANA), chronic hepatitis with autoimmune features, and both syndromes in the same patient.[294] Carriers of the HLA B*35:02 allele have a nearly 30-fold increased risk of DILI as compared with population controls.[294] The onset is often well beyond 6 months (median latency, 318 days) after treatment is started, but early presentations can occur (within 3 months).[295] Young women appear to be particularly affected. In the United States, minocycline was the most common drug associated with idiosyncratic drug hepatotoxicity in children. The reactions are severe; some patients have died or required LT. Progression to cirrhosis has been reported.[296] The course may be prolonged after drug withdrawal; several patients have been treated with glucocorticoids.

DRUG-INDUCED ACUTE CHOLESTASIS

Importance, Types of Reactions, and Diagnosis

Cholestatic drug reactions include acute cholestasis with or without hepatitis, cholestatic hepatitis with cholangitis, and chronic cholestasis, either with VBDS resembling PBC (see Chapter 93) or with biliary strictures reminiscent of sclerosing cholangitis (see Chapter 70).[297,298] The clinical and biochemical features of drug-induced cholestasis resemble other hepatobiliary disorders, and clinicians must elicit a thorough drug history from all patients with cholestasis. The timely cessation of a causative drug prevents an adverse outcome and avoids unnecessary invasive investigations or surgery.

Clinical features include pruritus, dark urine, pale stools, and, in more serious cases, jaundice. Liver biochemical test results show a predominant elevation of serum alkaline phosphatase levels, with lesser increases in serum ALT and GGTP levels and conjugated hyperbilirubinemia. The serum ALT level may be elevated up to eightfold, as a result of either the toxic effects of acute bile retention on hepatocellular integrity or concomitant "hepatitis." In such cases, the ratio of the relative increases in serum ALT and alkaline phosphatase levels (based on multiples of the ULN) is typically less than 2:1 in patients with cholestasis.[297] Cases of mixed cholestasis and hepatitis are highly suggestive of a drug reaction.

Hepatobiliary imaging is critical to exclude biliary obstruction and a hepatic or pancreatic mass lesion. In the absence of such findings, drug-induced cholestasis is more likely, and a liver biopsy is often advisable. Certain histologic features suggest a hepatic drug reaction, whereas others (e.g., edema of the portal tracts) suggest biliary obstruction. When the temporal relationship to drug ingestion indicates a high probability of a drug reaction, the incriminated drug should be discontinued and the patient observed for improvement.

Management should focus on symptom relief, with particular attention to pruritus (see Chapter 93).[297–299] Pruritus is often ameliorated with cholestyramine. In intractable cases, UDCA can be helpful.[299,300] Rifampin, phototherapy, plasmapheresis, and opiate receptor antagonists (e.g., naloxone, naltrexone, and nalmefene) have been used as third-line therapies.[299] Glucocorticoids have no role, and antihistamines are usually ineffective or cause oversedation.

Cholestasis Without Hepatitis

Cholestatic reactions are characterized by bile retention within canaliculi, Kupffer cells, and hepatocytes, with minimal inflammation or hepatocellular necrosis; terms to describe this reaction include pure, canalicular, and bland cholestasis. Cholestasis without hepatitis reflects a primary disturbance in bile flow. Sex steroids are typical causative agents. Other drugs generally associated with cholestatic hepatitis occasionally produce bland cholestasis (e.g., amoxicillin-clavulanic acid, sulfonamides, griseofulvin, ketoconazole, tamoxifen, warfarin, and ibuprofen).[297,298] Cyclosporine is associated with liver biochemical test abnormalities; the features resemble those of cholestasis, but hyperbilirubinemia usually is predominant.[1] The reaction is mild and reverses rapidly with a reduction in dose. Tacrolimus can also cause cholestasis,[301] whereas sirolimus has been implicated in cases of mild acute hepatitis.[302]

Steroids

Oral Contraceptive Steroids

The frequency of cholestasis with OCS is 2.5 per 10,000 women exposed. OCS-associated cholestasis is partly dose dependent and less likely with low-dose than high-dose estrogen preparations.[303] Genetic factors contribute to the high frequency of this complication among women in Chile and Scandinavia.[298] Persons with a history of intrahepatic cholestasis of pregnancy are also at risk (50%) (see Chapter 38). The estrogenic component is most likely responsible and impairs functioning of the BSEP or canalicular water transport (or both).[304] Polymorphisms within genes relating to canalicular transport (e.g., *ABCB4*, *MDR3*, and *BSEP*) also underlie some cases of OCS (see Chapter 66).[305,306] Symptoms develop 2–3 months, rarely as late as 9 months, after OCS are started. A mild transient prodrome of nausea and malaise may occur and is followed by pruritus and jaundice. Serum alkaline phosphatase levels are moderately elevated, and serum aminotransferase levels are increased transiently, occasionally to levels exceeding 10 times the ULN. The serum GGTP level is often normal. Recovery is usually prompt, within days to weeks after cessation of the drug. Chronic cholestasis is rare.[298] Acute hepatitis is also an uncommon complication.[307]

Hormonal replacement therapy is safe in patients with liver disease, but jaundiced patients may experience an increase in serum bilirubin levels. Liver biochemical tests should be monitored in hormonal replacement therapy users with liver disease.[298]

Ulipristal acetate, a selective progesterone-receptor modulator, was used initially for emergency contraception but is now for treatment of uterine fibrosis and has been linked to cases of acute hepatocellular injury, including acute liver failure requiring liver transplantation.[308]

Anabolic Steroids

At high doses, anabolic steroids often produce reversible bland cholestasis, usually within 1–6 months after treatment is started. Recovery usually follows drug withdrawal, but protracted cholestasis with biliary ductopenia can occur. Rarely, anabolic steroids may cause acute hepatocellular injury.[309] Recent formulations of anabolic steroids, targeting selective androgenic receptor modulators with the promise of anabolic without the androgenic effects, have been promoted as alternatives to traditional anabolic steroids. These have also been linked with cholestasis and hepatocellular injury.[310] Polymorphisms within *ABCB11* (which codes for bile salt export protein) were noted in 20% of cases, suggesting a genetic predilection to liver injury in at least some cases.[311]

Both OCS and the 17-alkylated anabolic steroids are associated with cholestasis, vascular lesions, and hepatic neoplasms (see later). The strength of these associations with individual lesions varies. Hepatic adenomas are clearly associated with use of OCS, whereas the association of OCS with HCC is controversial.[312] By contrast, HCC is well documented in anabolic steroid users. Likewise, hepatic and portal vein thrombosis is an established adverse effect of OCS but not of anabolic steroids, whereas peliosis hepatis is seen more often with the latter than with OCS.

Cholestasis With Hepatitis

Cholestasis with hepatitis is a common hepatic drug reaction and is characterized by conspicuous cholestasis and hepatocellular necrosis. Liver histology shows lobular and portal tract inflammation, often with neutrophils and eosinophils, as well as mononuclear cells. This type of reaction overlaps with drug-induced acute hepatitis, cholestasis without hepatitis, and cholestasis with bile duct injury. Causative agents include chlorpromazine (see later), antidepressants and other psychotropic agents, erythromycins and other macrolides,[313] and related ketolide antibiotics, clindamycin,[314] sulfonamides, sulfonylureas, oxypenicillins,[315] ketoconazole, sulindac,[316] ibuprofen, piroxicam, cefazolin,[317] captopril, enalapril, flutamide[318] pravastatin, atorvastatin, ticlopidine, ciprofloxacin and other fluoroquinolones,[319] and metformin.[320]

Chlorpromazine

Chlorpromazine hepatitis, the prototypical drug-induced cholestatic hepatitis,[321] has been recognized since the 1950s. The range of hepatic reactions includes asymptomatic liver biochemical test abnormalities in 20%–50% of recipients and rare cases of fulminant hepatic necrosis. The frequency of cholestatic hepatitis varies from 0.2% to 2.0%, depending on the type of study; the lower value probably is representative of the risk in the general population. No relationship to dose or to underlying liver disease has been recognized. Female predominance is evident. Reactions do not appear to be more common with increasing age but are rare in children.

The onset is within 1–6 weeks after the drug is started but can be delayed by 5–14 days after its discontinuation. Accelerated onset occurs with rechallenge. A prodromal illness of fever and nonspecific symptoms is usual and is followed by GI symptoms and jaundice. Pruritus is common and occurs later with chlorpromazine hepatitis than with drug-induced bland cholestasis. In a small proportion of affected patients, RUQ abdominal pain is severe. Rash is infrequent. Serum bilirubin, ALT, and alkaline phosphatase levels are increased. Eosinophilia is present in 10%–40% of patients. Most patients recover completely: one-third within 4 weeks, another third between 4 and 8 weeks, and the remainder after 8 weeks.[300,321] In about 7% of cases, full recovery has not occurred by 6 months.

Amoxicillin-Clavulanic Acid

Over 150 cases of cholestatic hepatitis have been attributed to this antibiotic. The overall frequency is 1.7 cases per 10,000 prescriptions; male gender, increasing age (>55 years), and prolonged duration of use are risk factors.[322] The clavulanic acid component was previously implicated because similar lesions were noted with ticarcillin-clavulanic acid[323]; however, a subsequent study reported similar cholestatic or mixed-type DILI with amoxicillin alone, suggesting the amoxicillin component may also be involved.[324]

The onset of symptoms is within 6 weeks (mean 18 days) but can be delayed up to 6 weeks after the drug is stopped. Features of hypersensitivity, such as fever, skin rash, and eosinophilia, are seen in 30%–60% of patients. Liver histology shows cholestasis with mild portal inflammation. Bile duct injury (usually mild) and perivenular cholestasis with lipofuscin deposits are often present. Other histologic features include hepatic granulomas, biliary ductopenia, and cirrhosis.[325] Most patients recover in 4–16 weeks. Fatalities and the need for LT are rare.[324] Elevated serum aminotransferase levels can persist for more than 6 months in 11% of patients and return to normal in most, but not all, cases.

The pathogenesis involves innate and/or adaptive immune responses or defects in detoxification, as supported by the strong association of liver injury with certain HLA class II (HLA-DRB1*15:01-DRB5*01:01-DQB1*06:02) haplotypes and class I antigens[326] and by studies identifying amoxicillin- and clavulanic acid-specific T cells.[327] Specific HLA genotypes are linked to variations in clinical presentation (hepatocellular or cholestatic/mixed), severity, and age of onset. "Protective" genotypes (HLA-DRB1*07 family) have also been described.[328,329] A role for defective detoxification was suggested by the association with certain genes involved in ameliorating oxidative stress (e.g., glutathione-*S*-transferase)[330] but a larger study has not confirmed this.[331] Finally, clavulanic acid has also been shown to downregulate the expression of key biliary transporter and synthesis genes, and a consequence of this is intrahepatic cholestasis.[332]

Fluoroquinolones

Most fluoroquinolones have been associated with acute hepatocellular, cholestatic, or mixed reactions,[319] with the highest frequencies attributed to levofloxacin and moxifloxacin. Trovafloxacin was withdrawn due to hepatotoxicity. The onset can be rapid (median 8 days; range 1–39 days) or may be delayed for up to 30 days after the antibiotic course is completed. Hypersensitivity features may be present. Resolution usually follows discontinuation of the drug, but instances of ALF, chronic cholestasis, and VBDS have been reported.[319]

Cholestatic Hepatitis With Bile Duct Injury

Bile duct (cholangiolytic) injury is observed with several drugs that cause cholestatic hepatitis, such as chlorpromazine[300] and flucloxacillin.[315] The severity of bile duct injury may be a determinant of the VBDS (see later).[333] The clinical features resemble those of bacterial cholangitis, with upper abdominal pain, fever, rigors, tender hepatomegaly, jaundice, and cholestasis. Liver biochemical test levels are typical of cholestasis. Compounds associated with this syndrome include carbamazepine,[334] dextropropoxyphene,[335] and methylenediamine, an industrial toxin responsible for an outbreak of jaundice (Epping Jaundice) associated with intake of bread made from contaminated flour (see Chapter 91).[298]

Dextropropoxyphene

Dextropropoxyphene is an opioid analgesic used alone or in compound analgesics and has been linked to over 25 cases of cholestasis with bile duct injury,[335] some proven by inadvertent rechallenge. A female predominance has been recognized. The onset of symptoms is usually within 2 weeks. The illness is often heralded by abdominal pain, which may be severe and simulates other causes of cholangitis. Jaundice is usual. ERCP shows normal bile ducts. Liver biopsy specimens demonstrate cholestasis with expansion of the portal tracts by inflammation and mild fibrosis; portal tract edema also may be present. Other features include irregularity and necrosis of the biliary epithelium, together with an infiltrate of neutrophils and eosinophils on the outer surface of bile ducts. Bile ductular proliferation is universal. Recovery is the rule, with liver biochemical test levels returning to normal within 1–3 months.[334]

DRUG-INDUCED CHRONIC CHOLESTASIS

Drug-induced liver disease is considered to be chronic when typical liver biochemical changes last longer than 3 months[298]; earlier definitions required the presence of jaundice for more than 6 months or anicteric cholestasis (raised serum alkaline phosphatase and GGTP levels) for more than 12 months after the implicated agent was stopped.[297] Drug-induced chronic cholestasis is uncommon but has been ascribed to more than 45 compounds.[297–299,321,335–337] Chronicity complicates liver injury with flucloxacillin in 10%–30%,[298] chlorpromazine in 7%,[300] and erythromycin in <5%[337] of cases and in only isolated instances of toxicity caused by other agents, such as tetracycline,[338] amoxicillin-clavulanic acid,[339] ibuprofen,[340] trimethoprim-sulfamethoxazole,[341] and ciprofloxacin.[342]

Chronic cholestasis is always preceded by an episode of an often severe acute cholestatic hepatitis that is occasionally associated with the Stevens-Johnson syndrome.[340] The severity of the bile duct injury during the initial hepatic reaction is a critical determinant of a chronic course.[333] Other possible mechanisms include continuing toxic or immunologic destruction of the biliary epithelium.[336] Liver histology is characterized by a paucity of smaller (septal, interlobular) bile ducts and ductules, often with residual cholestasis, and portal tract inflammation directed against injured bile ducts. This process may lead to an irreversible loss of biliary patency and the VBDS.[343]

The clinical features are those of chronic cholestasis. Pruritus is the dominant symptom and is often severe. Continuing jaundice, dark urine, and pale stools are possible but not invariable findings and may resolve despite persistence of liver biochemical abnormalities. In severe cases, intestinal malabsorption, weight loss, and bruising caused by vitamin K deficiency may occur; xanthelasma, tuberous xanthomata, and other complications of severe hypercholesterolemia also have been noted. Firm hepatomegaly may be found on physical examination, but splenomegaly is unusual unless portal hypertension develops. AMAs are not usually present. Most cases resolve, but there are rare reports of severe biliary ductopenia and biliary cirrhosis[297,298] and the overall mortality may be as high 10%–19%, with poor outcomes linked to the severity of biliary ductopenia,[344] high bilirubin levels, and impaired liver synthetic function.[345]

Flucloxacillin

Flucloxacillin is an important cause of drug-induced hepatitis in Europe, Scandinavia, and Australia.[315,346] Flucloxacillin-induced hepatotoxicity is usually severe, and several deaths have resulted from the systemic features and associated cholestatic hepatitis. The course is prolonged, and a high proportion of cases have resulted in chronic cholestasis and VBDS.[346] The risk of liver injury is 1 per 12,000 exposed, particularly among patients older than 70 years and those receiving repeated courses (39 and 110 per 100,000, respectively). A GWAS showed a strong association (odds ratio, 80.6) between HLA-B*57:01 and the risk of liver injury.[347] A related allele, HLA-B*57:03, was also identified as a risk factor (OR 79.2). There are also occasional reports of cholestasis with other oxypenicillins (cloxacillin and dicloxacillin), including one report of VBDS with cloxacillin.[313,348] Acute hepatocellular injury has been reported with oxacillin.

Fibrotic Bile Duct Strictures

Fibrotic strictures of the larger bile ducts can cause chronic cholestasis. Recognized causes include intralesional formalin therapy of hepatic hydatids and intra-arterial infusion of floxuridine for metastatic colorectal carcinoma. After several months of floxuridine infusion, the frequency of toxic hepatitis or bile duct injury, or both, was as high as 25%–55% but has declined considerably (to ~5%) with the advent of current protocols.[349] Acalculous cholecystitis also may occur. ERCP shows strictures, typically in the common, left, and right hepatic ducts. Unlike PSC, the common bile duct and the smaller intrahepatic bile ducts are spared. Ischemia has been suspected, and toxicity to biliary epithelial cells is another possibility. Recovery may occur after floxuridine is discontinued. Some patients require dilation or stenting of biliary strictures. Sclerosing cholangitis-type appearances have also been reported with intravenous ketamine and as an occasional complication in patients with severe or protracted cholestatic or mixed DILI from a variety of drugs, including atorvastatin, moxifloxacin, amiodarone, amoxicillin-clavulanate, and also herbal dietary supplements.[350]

DRUG-INDUCED STEATOHEPATITIS AND HEPATIC FIBROSIS

Steatohepatitis is a form of chronic liver disease in which steatosis is associated with focal liver cell injury, Mallory hyaline, focal inflammation of mixed cellularity, including neutrophils, and progressive hepatic fibrosis in a pericentral (zone 3) and pericellular distribution (see Chapters 88 and 89).[351] Alcohol is a common etiologic factor. MASH is associated with insulin resistance, diabetes mellitus, obesity, and several drugs (e.g., perhexiline maleate, amiodarone).[351] In addition to causing steatohepatitis or chronic hepatocyte or bile duct injury, some exogenous compounds promote hepatic fibrogenesis directly, through effects on hepatic nonparenchymal cells, especially stellate cells. Compounds that stimulate hepatic fibrosis include arsenic, vitamin A, and methotrexate.

Amiodarone

Amiodarone hepatotoxicity encompasses a spectrum of abnormalities, including abnormal liver biochemical test levels in 15%−80% of patients to clinically significant liver disease, including rare cases of ALF, in 0.6%.[352–354] ALF (seven cases) has been reported with intravenous amiodarone; the vehicle (polysorbate 80) has been implicated because oral amiodarone could be successfully reinstituted in these cases[355]; however, ALF may occur with intravenous amiodarone formulations lacking polysorbate 80.[355] Other investigators have disputed the diagnosis altogether, contending that these cases represent ischemic hepatitis rather than drug toxicity.[356] In longer-term users, steatohepatitis can develop; cirrhosis develops in 15%−50% of patients with hepatoxicity.[353]

A notable feature of amiodarone-induced liver disease is continued progression even after amiodarone is discontinued. Amiodarone is highly concentrated in the liver, and after a few weeks of treatment, the drug accounts for up to 1% of the wet weight of the liver. The iodine content absorbs radiation so that the liver appears opaque on CT.[357] Although odd, this appearance is not clinically significant.

Hepatic storage of amiodarone also produces phospholipidosis, a storage disorder characterized by enlarged lysosomes stuffed with whorled membranous material (myeloid bodies). In animals fed amiodarone, the development of phospholipidosis is time and dose dependent.[354] Phospholipidosis may result from the direct inhibition of phospholipase or from the formation of nondegradable drug-phospholipid complexes and has no relationship to the development of MASH and hepatocyte injury. Other occasional hepatic abnormalities include granuloma formation and ALF, apparently caused by severe acute hepatitis or a Reye syndrome-like illness.[358] Amiodarone is concentrated in mitochondria and may interrupt mitochondrial electron transport.[359] In rodent models, amiodarone produces microvesicular steatosis, augments mitochondrial production of ROS, and causes lipid peroxidation.[359] In addition, induction of hepatic and adipose tissue endoplasmic stress can promote hepatic free fatty acid accumulation and hepatic lipotoxicity.[360]

Chronic liver disease is detected after a year or more (median, 21 months) of treatment. The treatment duration and possibly the total dose,[361] but not the incremental dose, are risk factors for chronic liver disease. Cases of cirrhosis with low-dose amiodarone have also been documented.[362] The other toxic effects, also likely dose-related, are more frequent among patients with liver disease.[361] Clinical features include fatigue, nausea and vomiting, malaise, and weight loss. Hepatomegaly, jaundice, ascites, bruising, and other features of chronic liver disease may be present. Laboratory test results include increased serum aminotransferase levels (up to 5 × ULN) and minor increases in serum alkaline phosphatase levels. The ratio of serum AST to ALT levels is close to unity, in contrast to that seen in alcohol-associated hepatitis. In severe cases, jaundice, hypoalbuminemia, and prolongation of the prothrombin time are evident. Determining the cause of abnormal liver biochemical test results and hepatomegaly is often difficult in patients taking amiodarone, and a liver biopsy may be indicated. Liver histologic findings include phospholipidosis, steatosis, focal necrosis with Mallory hyaline, infiltration with neutrophils, and pericellular fibrosis.[353] Cirrhosis is often present.

Preventing and managing amiodarone-induced liver disease is problematic because abnormal liver biochemical test levels are common in persons taking amiodarone, especially in those with heart failure. Further, patients with and without baseline serum ALT elevations have a similar frequency of amiodarone hepatotoxicity, and amiodarone should not be withheld in patients with an elevated serum ALT level.[363] In asymptomatic or less severe cases, resolution occurs in 2 weeks to 4 months after amiodarone is discontinued. In cases of severe liver disease, the mortality rate is high.[353] Cessation of amiodarone therapy does not always result in clinical improvement, because of prolonged hepatic storage of amiodarone, and in one study, the outcome was worse (usually from fatal arrhythmias) in patients who discontinued amiodarone than in those who did not.[353] Although serial liver biochemical testing is recommended,[361] the efficacy of this strategy in reducing liver injury and the overall mortality rate is unknown.

Tamoxifen and Other Causes of Drug-Induced Steatohepatitis

For agents reported to be associated with steatohepatitis during the 1990s, causality has been difficult to prove,[351] particularly because MASH is frequent among patients with the metabolic syndrome (see Chapter 89). Calcium channel blockers have rarely been associated with steatohepatitis,[364] and methyldopa has been reported to be associated with cirrhosis in obese middle-aged women[365]; however, these associations may have been fortuitous. Other drugs, including estrogens[366] and glucocorticoids,[367] may precipitate MASH in predisposed persons because of their metabolic effects on the risk factors that drive MASH. On the other hand, the association between MASH and tamoxifen is much stronger.

Several forms of liver injury have been attributed to tamoxifen,[368] including cholestasis, hepatocellular carcinoma,[369] peliosis hepatis,[370] acute hepatitis, massive hepatic necrosis,[368] steatosis, and steatohepatitis, occasionally with cirrhosis.[371–373] In one series of 66 women with breast cancer who had taken tamoxifen for 3−5 years, 24 showed imaging evidence of hepatic steatosis.[372] The median time to the development of MASLD is around 2 years.[374] Seven other patients have been diagnosed with MASH after taking tamoxifen for 7−33 months.[371] In a systematic review of 24 studies, the incidence and prevalence rate of fatty liver among tamoxifen users was approximately 12 and 40 per 100 patient-years, respectively. The incidence rate was more than three times that of untreated controls with breast cancer.[375]

The metabolic profile of women with imaging evidence of hepatic steatosis (or histologic proof of steatohepatitis) during tamoxifen therapy appears to be similar to that of most patients with MASH; one-half have been obese, and the increase in body mass index has correlated with hepatic steatosis. Tamoxifen can induce hypertriglyceridemia, another risk factor for MASH. Reduction in the severity of hepatic steatosis has been documented with bezafibrate, a peroxisome proliferator-activated receptor-α agonist.[376] Therefore tamoxifen may play a synergistic role with other metabolic factors in causing steatohepatitis. This hypothesis is supported by an Italian study that showed that tamoxifen-associated MASLD or MASH was mainly observed in overweight or obese women with the metabolic syndrome.[377]

Clinicians need to be aware of the high frequency (~30%) of hepatic steatosis and steatohepatitis in women receiving tamoxifen. Optimizing body weight is desirable. Tamoxifen recipients should be evaluated periodically for evidence of MASLD by physical examination (to detect hepatomegaly), liver biochemical testing, and annual hepatic ultrasound imaging. Liver biopsy is indicated if the liver biochemical test abnormalities do not resolve after tamoxifen is discontinued, or, in some cases, to exclude metastatic breast cancer. Many patients improve after tamoxifen is discontinued, but the decision to discontinue tamoxifen should be made after discussion with the patient's oncologist. Optimizing body weight is desirable because there is an increased (threefold) risk of developing abnormal glucose tolerance.[378] Other aromatase inhibitors (anastrozole, letrozole) have also been associated with hepatic steatosis, with prevalence rates in postmenopausal women more than double that of controls (54% vs. 26%).[375] However, in one comparative study, tamoxifen was associated with a higher 5-year incidence of fatty liver than aromatase inhibitors (adjusted hazard ratio 1.9).[379]

Toremifene, a tamoxifen analog, is associated with a lower frequency of steatosis or steatohepatitis than tamoxifen.[380] A comparative liver ultrasound/CT-based study of Chinese patients receiving tamoxifen or toremifene found both a significantly increased probability of developing fatty liver in the first 16 months of treatment with tamoxifen (~26% vs. 18%), as well as a higher frequency of severe steatosis (~5.8% vs. 2%). Raloxifene, a selective estrogen receptor modulator, has been implicated in one report of steatohepatitis and another with acute hepatocellular injury accompanied by eosinophilia,[381] but causality could not be conclusively established in this case because preexisting liver disease (MASH) was not excluded. Other drugs associated with steatohepatitis include irinotecan (in the setting of metastatic colorectal cancer)[382] and two other agents that are no longer used, perhexiline maleate and Coralgil (4,4′-diethylaminoethoxyhexestrol).[351]

Cyproterone Acetate

Serious DILI occurs in 2%–5% of patients treated with antiandrogens for metastatic prostate cancer, and although the nonsteroidal agents flutamide and bicalutamide have been implicated most frequently, reactions to CPA are often particularly severe. Mean latency is just under 6 months. Doses usually exceed 100 mg/day in severe cases, but low-dose CPA (25 mg), occasionally used in treating acne and hirsutism in young individuals, has also been associated with acute liver failure.[383] The varied histologic patterns include acute hepatitis, submassive necrosis, cholestatic hepatitis, and AIH-like.[384] While 90% of CPA-related instances of DILI resolved slowly (over 6 months), cases of cirrhosis and HCC have been reported. Although liver test monitoring is recommended,[384] there is no evidence to support its efficacy in preventing severe reactions. Patients receiving CPA and other antiandrogens should be warned to report new symptoms that could indicate liver injury.

Methotrexate

Methotrexate is a dose-dependent toxin. In the 1950s, the high-dose methotrexate treatment of acute childhood leukemia was complicated by severe hepatic fibrosis and cirrhosis and a few cases of HCC. In the 1960s, the use of methotrexate for psoriasis was associated with hepatic fibrosis and cirrhosis in up to 25% of cases. Since then, a clearer picture of methotrexate as a dose-dependent promoter of hepatic fibrosis has emerged, particularly in persons who drink alcohol excessively or have preexisting liver disease. Methotrexate is now usually used as a low-dose weekly regimen in managing RA, psoriasis, and other immunologic conditions, including IBD. Avoiding daily dosing and reducing the weekly dose to 5–15 mg have largely overcome the problem of methotrexate hepatotoxicity.[385–387]

Risk Factors

Risk factors for methotrexate-induced hepatic fibrosis are listed in Table 90.9; dose, alcohol intake, and preexisting liver disease are the most important.[386] Total dose, incremental dose, dose interval, and duration of methotrexate therapy each influence the risk of hepatic fibrosis. After the cumulative ingestion of 3 g of methotrexate, the chance of histologic progression is 20%, but only 3% of patients have advanced hepatic fibrosis.[388] Further, the relevance of cumulative dose as a risk factor for liver injury is also disputed by a systematic review that showed a lack of correlation between the total dose and risk of liver injury.[389] Obesity and diabetes mellitus are important risk factors for hepatic fibrosis

TABLE 90.9 Risk Factors for Methotrexate-Induced Hepatic Fibrosis

Risk Factor	Importance	Implications for Prevention
Age	Increased risk with age >60 years, possibly related to reduced renal clearance and/or a biologic effect on fibrogenesis	Care in use of methotrexate in older patients
Dose	Incremental dose Dose frequency Duration of therapy	5–15 mg/week is safe Weekly bolus (pulse) is safer than a daily schedule Formerly, liver biopsy was recommended every 2 years or after a total dose of 4–5 g. Noninvasive evaluation of liver fibrosis (see text) is now preferred to biopsy.
Alcohol consumption	Increased risk with daily alcohol levels >15 g (1–2 drinks)	Avoid methotrexate use if intake is not curbed. Consider pretreatment and interval liver fibrosis assessment (see above)
Obesity, diabetes mellitus	Increased risk	Consider pretreatment liver fibrosis and interval liver fibrosis assessment (see above)
Preexisting liver disease	Greatly increased risk, particularly related to alcohol, MASH	Consider pretreatment liver fibrosis and interval liver fibrosis assessment (see above). Monitor liver biochemical tests during therapy
Systemic disease	Possibly greater risk with psoriasis than RA (depending on preexisting liver disease, alcohol intake)	None
Impaired renal function	Increased risk because of reduced clearance	Reduce the dose; use methotrexate with caution
Other drugs	Arsenic, NSAIDs, and vitamin A may increase the risk	Use methotrexate with caution; monitor liver biochemical test levels Concurrent folate therapy can decrease the risk and should be used
Genetic factors	Increased risk linked to SNPs in genes involved in drug transport across red blood cells and in folate metabolism	Future strategies could involve pretreatment genetic screening

SNP, Single nucleotide polymorphism.

because they predispose to MASH and are associated with induction of CYP2E1. The strong association between MASH and methotrexate in causing liver injury during long-term, low-dose treatment has been highlighted,[390] as has the possibility that methotrexate itself can cause a pattern of injury resembling steatohepatitis. Increasing age, impaired renal function, and concomitant use of certain drugs decrease the elimination of methotrexate or facilitate tissue uptake by displacing methotrexate from plasma-protein binding sites. Pharmacogenetic factors may also contribute. Single nucleotide polymorphisms within genes involving folate metabolism and methotrexate transport into or out of erythrocytes have also been linked to hepatotoxicity.[391]

Psoriasis and RA are associated with hepatic abnormalities that range from abnormal liver biochemical test levels (25%–50% of cases) and minor histologic changes (50%–70%) to fibrosis (11%) and cirrhosis (1%). In patients with psoriasis, alcoholism often is a complicating factor, and in a,[387] alcohol consumption was the most important determinant of advanced hepatic fibrosis in patients treated with methotrexate; the risk of progressive hepatic fibrosis was 73% in persons who drank more than 15 g of alcohol daily, compared with 26% in those who did not.

The possibility that low-dose (5–15 mg) methotrexate given as a single weekly dose can cause hepatic fibrosis has been debated.[385–387] The available data are limited by a lack of controlled studies with pretreatment liver histologic data, a particularly serious deficiency in view of the high frequency of liver abnormalities among patients with RA and psoriasis. The conclusion has been reached that, although contemporary regimens can promote hepatic fibrosis, at the ultrastructural level at least, cases of clinically significant liver disease are now virtually unknown. Indeed, repeat liver biopsies in some series have shown a reduction in fibrosis despite continuation of methotrexate in lower doses.[388] Therefore although methotrexate remains a potential cause of liver disease, advanced hepatic fibrosis is in large part preventable.

Clinicopathologic Features

Liver biochemical test abnormalities are common among patients who take methotrexate, but advanced hepatic fibrosis occasionally may develop in their absence. Likewise, nausea, fatigue, and abdominal pain are common adverse effects, but patients with hepatic fibrosis are typically asymptomatic unless complications of liver failure or portal hypertension develop. A firm liver edge, hepatomegaly, splenomegaly, and ascites may be noted. Liver biochemical test levels are either normal or show nonspecific changes, including minor elevations of serum ALT and GGTP levels. In more advanced cases, hypoalbuminemia and thrombocytopenia are present, but jaundice and coagulation disturbances are rare.

Liver histologic findings have been graded according to the system of Roenigk.[387] In this system, grades I and II indicate a variable amount of steatosis, nuclear pleomorphism, and necroinflammatory activity, but no fibrosis. Higher grades reflect increasing degrees of fibrosis, as follows: grade IIIa, few septa; grade IIIb, bridging fibrosis; and grade IV, cirrhosis. The pattern of hepatic fibrosis includes pericellular fibrosis, a feature of both alcoholic steatohepatitis and MASH. Cases of hepatic fibrosis with a relative paucity (or complete absence) of portal and lobular inflammation have been reported.

Outcome and Prevention

Serious clinical sequelae (portal hypertension, liver failure, and HCC) are now rarely seen. In a meta-analysis of 32 studies involving over 13,000 patients with RA, psoriasis, and IBD, methotrexate was associated with a greater frequency of elevated aminotransferase levels, but there was no increase in the risk of liver failure, cirrhosis, or death.[392] Cases that have come to LT generally have been associated with suboptimal supervision of methotrexate therapy.[393] Cases of severe hepatic fibrosis (Roenigk grades IIIb and IV) are often associated with lack of progression and even improvement after dose reduction or cessation of methotrexate.[388] In less severe cases, a balanced judgment must be made about the appropriateness of continuing or discontinuing methotrexate.

Current approaches to monitoring patients receiving methotrexate have moved away from liver biopsies to careful appraisal of risk factors before treatment and noninvasive assessment of liver fibrosis. Several guidelines exist and differ in certain aspects. All stress the importance of evaluating current or previous alcohol intake, preexisting chronic liver disease, particularly chronic hepatitis B or C and nonalcoholic fatty liver disease, obesity, and diabetes mellitus. Noninvasive evaluation of liver fibrosis involves conventional (e.g., FIB-4) or patented serum tests (e.g., FibroTest/FibroSure) (see Chapter 76). Patients with abnormal test results or risk factors are referred for a gastroenterology/hepatology consultation, with likely further noninvasive fibrosis evaluation (e.g., with vibration-controlled transient elastography or magnetic resonance elastography) and/or liver biopsy. Routine interval liver biopsies, usually considered after a cumulative dose of 3.5–4.0 g is reached, are also no longer routine, and fibrosis progression is assessed mainly with noninvasive serological tests and/or vibration-controlled transient elastography.[394]

To monitor progress during treatment, liver biochemical testing is also recommended but is problematic because of the lack of specificity and sensitivity of the tests. An international panel of rheumatologists proposed these guidelines: gradual dose escalation, coprescription of folic acid, and checking ALT/AST every 1–1.5 months until a stable dose is reached and 1–3 monthly thereafter. If the ALT/AST levels rise to 3 × ULN, methotrexate should be stopped and liver tests rechecked in 2–4 weeks. The drug can be reintroduced at a lower dose if the liver tests normalize. Persistently elevated ALT/AST greater than 3 × ULN over a 12-month period, decreasing serum albumin, or hepatomegaly warrants investigation by consultation by a gastroenterologist, and/or a liver biopsy should be considered. For patients with MASLD, more recently the American College of Rheumatology recommends restricting methotrexate use to patients with normal liver tests without liver fibrosis and more frequent liver tests (every 4–8 weeks).[395]

DRUG-INDUCED VASCULAR TOXICITY

Drugs and chemical toxins are the main causes of hepatic vascular injury,[396] which includes several unusual liver disorders, including sinusoidal obstruction syndrome (formerly veno-occlusive disease, a form of hepatic venous outflow obstruction), peliosis hepatis (dilatation and destruction of hepatic sinusoids), noncirrhotic portal hypertension, and NRH (Table 90.10) (see Chapter 87). The mechanism of injury is primarily dose-dependent toxicity to sinusoidal and other vascular endothelial cells, particularly when drugs are used in combination or concurrently with radiotherapy. Activation of inflammatory cells may also be important. Individual drugs (e.g., azathioprine) may be associated with more than one vascular syndrome, and the various disorders overlap and may evolve from one type to another. Hepatic imaging and measurement of portal pressure can aid in the diagnosis; some disorders, particularly NRH, are difficult to confirm in needle biopsy specimens.

Azathioprine

Hepatic complications of azathioprine, although rare (<0.1%), may be severe, diverse, and often late in onset. Many cases occur in complex medical situations, particularly after organ

TABLE 90.10 Types of Drug-Induced Hepatic Vascular Disorders[a]

Disorder	Clinicopathologic Features	Outcomes	Implicated Etiologic Agents
Sinusoidal obstruction syndrome (veno-occlusive disease)	Abdominal pain, tender hepatomegaly, ascites, liver failure; occasionally chronic liver disease, other signs of portal hypertension	High mortality rate; some cases may evolve into nodular regenerative hyperplasia	Especially in bone marrow transplantation: 6-thioguanine, busulfan; dactinomycin, azathioprine, mitomycin; gemtuzumab; pyrrolizidine alkaloids; oxaliplatin
Nodular regenerative hyperplasia	Portal hypertension, encephalopathy—especially after variceal bleeding; diagnosed by histology	Relatively good prognosis	Anticancer drugs: busulfan, dactinomycin, azathioprine, didanosine, 6-thioguanine, trastuzumab
Noncirrhotic portal hypertension	Splenomegaly, varices, hypersplenism, ascites if associated hepatocellular disease	Prognosis depends on cause and associated liver injury	Vitamin A, methotrexate, azathioprine, arsenic, vinyl chloride, anticancer drugs, didanosine
Peliosis hepatis	Incidental finding, hepatomegaly, hepatic rupture, liver failure; diagnosed from appearances at surgery, vascular imaging	Prognosis depends on cause and complications	Anabolic steroids, azathioprine, 6-thioguanine
Sinusoidal dilatation	Hepatomegaly, abdominal pain	May regress after stopping oral contraceptives	Oral contraceptive steroids

[a]See also Chapter 87.

transplantation, in which immune activation, viral infections, and other agents may increase the risk of hepatotoxicity. The central role of azathioprine has been confirmed by positive rechallenge or resolution after the drug was stopped.[397,398] Disturbances associated with azathioprine include an asymptomatic increase in serum aminotransferase levels (in 5%−15% of persons taking the drug), bland cholestasis, cholestatic hepatitis with bile duct injury,[398,399] zonal necrosis, HCC (with long-term use), and vascular toxicity,[397] which includes sinusoidal obstruction syndrome, peliosis hepatis, NRH, and noncirrhotic portal hypertension.[397,399,400]

Cholestatic hepatitis is the most common presentation. Other lesions include hepatic zone 3 necrosis and congestion, suggesting acute vascular injury, similar to the vascular toxicity of other thiopurines. All hepatic vascular syndromes have been associated with azathioprine, particularly after organ transplantation, whereas only NRH and sinusoidal obstruction syndrome have been noted in patients with IBD.[396]

Earlier studies showed no relationship between toxicity and the dose or duration of therapy, but this observation was refuted in a case series ($n = 11$) in which dose escalation was found to be a risk for liver injury (59% of cases) from both azathioprine and 6-mercaptopurine, suggesting at least partial dose dependency.[401] The majority of affected patients (86%) developed liver injury within 3 months of the last dose increase. Men are almost exclusively involved in cases of hepatic vascular injury following renal transplantation. Cholestatic reactions present within 2 weeks to 22 months, but vascular toxicity is recognized later, typically 3 months to 3 years, and occasionally more than 9 years, after transplantation.[400] Cases later in onset are the result of delayed recognition and tend to present with complications of portal hypertension and liver failure. Recovery can occur in such cases,[398] but the overall mortality rate is high.

Substitution of 6-mercaptopurine for azathioprine has been reported in cases of azathioprine hepatotoxicity, but cross-reactivity can occur.[401] The range of liver injury is similar to that for azathioprine and includes hepatocellular necrosis (occasionally fatal), cholestatic hepatitis, sinusoidal obstruction syndrome, and NRH.[402] A high frequency of NRH (33%−75%) was reported with 6-thioguanine in patients with IBD, but this adverse reaction has been infrequent and of no clinical significance in *low-dose* 6-thioguanine regimens.[403]

LIVER TUMORS

Several associations between pharmacologic and environmental agents and benign and malignant liver tumors have been described, but causality has been difficult to prove because of the rarity of these associations. For some sex steroid-related tumors, as well as for vinyl chloride-induced angiosarcoma, the relative risk attributable to the causative agent has been determined. The major tumors of interest include cavernous hemangioma, hepatic adenoma, HCC, angiosarcoma, and cholangiocarcinoma (see Chapter 98).

Full references for this chapter can be found at https://ebooks.health.elsevier.com.

91 Liver Disease Caused by Anesthetics, Chemicals, Toxins, and Herbal and Dietary Supplements

James H. Lewis

IN THIS CHAPTER

Contemporary inhalational and parenterally administered anesthetics are rarely hepatotoxic.[1] Although halothane hepatitis is now largely of historical interest in Western nations,[2] it remains in use elsewhere, with ongoing reports of acute liver injury.[3,4] In contrast to the largely unpredictable hepatotoxicity seen with more modern anesthetics and most other medicinal agents (see Chapter 90), liver damage caused by occupationally and environmentally encountered chemical compounds and other toxins is often more predictable, dose related, and predominantly cytotoxic.[5–7] Industrial exposure to hepatotoxic chemicals is a far less frequent occupational hazard today than in the past in industrialized nations, but reports of toxicity from chemical agents, as well as metals, pesticides, adulterated cooking oils, and botanical toxins, have not disappeared, especially from developing countries,[8] nor has the risk of hepatic carcinogenesis been eliminated.[9] The use of complementary and alternative medicine (CAM) preparations continues to increase, especially among patients with chronic liver disease,[10] and reports of liver injury from potentially hepatotoxic herbal agents, dietary supplements, and weight-loss products continue to appear.[10–12] Mushroom poisoning appears to be on the rise, with silibinin emerging as a potential antidote.[13,14] Still, a substantial portion of emergency liver transplants for acute liver failure (ALF) is due to mycelism, herbal preparations, and various chemical compounds (see Chapters 90 and 97).[13–16] A valuable resource is the LiverTox database at https://livertox.nih.gov.

ANESTHETIC AGENTS

The volatile inhalational anesthetics in current use are derivatives of some of the most potent chemical hepatotoxins developed for medicinal purposes.[1,2] Chloroform, the original haloalkane anesthetic, has long been abandoned but remains an important experimental hepatotoxin. Halothane (fluothane), introduced in 1956 as a safer, nonexplosive alternative to ether, is a haloalkane compound that produced a well described but rare syndrome of acute hepatotoxicity, usually after repeat exposure.[1,2,17–19] The anesthetics that followed—methoxyflurane, enflurane, and isoflurane—all have been implicated as a cause of similar injury, albeit much less commonly for enflurane and isoflurane than for halothane; even fewer instances have been reported for the newest agents, sevoflurane, and desflurane[20,21] because of their proportionally lower degree of metabolism.[22] Halothane is no longer produced in the United States but continues to be used in other countries, especially Iran,[3,4,23] and is a case study in the elucidation of immunologic-mediated liver injury.[24]

Halothane

The retrospective National Halothane Study, cited in the past as the basis for exonerating halothane as a cause of hepatotoxicity,[25] is now considered seriously flawed.[2] Nearly 1000 cases of halothane hepatotoxicity were reported worldwide during the 1960s and 1970s.[19,26] A fairly uniform clinical picture of postoperative fever, eosinophilia, jaundice, and hepatic necrosis occurred a few days to weeks after an administration of anesthesia, usually after repeat exposure to halothane, and the case-fatality rate was high (Box 91.1). Rare cases of halothane-induced liver injury have been reported after workplace exposure among anesthesiologists, surgeons, nurses, and laboratory staff and after halothane sniffing for recreational use[27]; in affected persons, antibodies to trifluoroacetylated (TFA) proteins were demonstrated, indicating previous exposure.[27] More recently, elevated urinary bromide levels have been reported to indicate exposure to halothane in anesthesiology personnel.[23]

Two types of postoperative liver injury have been associated with halothane. A minor form (type 1) is seen in 10%–30% of patients in whom mild, asymptomatic, self-limited elevations in serum ALT levels develop between the first and 10th postoperative days; the risk of hepatotoxicity after two or more exposures to halothane is higher than that for repeated use of alternative agents such as enflurane, isoflurane, and desflurane.[21] Evidence of immune activation is lacking in these patients,[28] in whom the serum ALT elevations generally reverse rapidly.

The major form of halothane-induced hepatotoxicity (type 2) is a rare, dose-independent, severe hepatic drug reaction with elements of immunoallergy and metabolic idiosyncrasy (see Box 91.1).[2] After an initial exposure to halothane, the frequency of

BOX 91.1 Epidemiologic, Clinical, and Histopathologic Features of Halothane Hepatitis

EPIDEMIOLOGIC FEATURES

- Estimated incidence
  - After first exposure: 0.3–1.5 per 10,000
  - After multiple exposures: 10–15 per 10,000
- Female-to-male ratio 2–3:1
- Latent period to first symptom
  - *After first exposure:* 6 days (11 days to jaundice)
  - *After multiple exposures:* 3 days (6 days to jaundice)

RISK FACTORS

- Older age (>40 year)
- Female gender
- Two or more exposures (documented in 60%–90% of cases)
- Obesity
- Familial predisposition
- Induction of CYP2E1 by phenobarbital, alcohol, or isoniazid

CLINICAL FEATURES

- Jaundice is the presenting symptom in 25% (range of serum bilirubin: 3–50 mg/dL)
- Fever (75%; precedes jaundice in 75%); chills (30%)
- Rash (10%)
- Myalgias (20%)
- Ascites, renal failure, and/or GI hemorrhage (20%–30%)
- Eosinophilia (20%–60%)
- Serum ALT and AST levels: 25–250 × ULN
- Serum alkaline phosphatase level: 1–3 × ULN

HISTOPATHOLOGIC FEATURES

- Zone 3 massive hepatic necrosis (30%); submassive necrosis (70%; autopsy series)
- Inflammation usually less marked than in viral hepatitis
- Eosinophilic infiltrate (20%)
- Granulomatous hepatitis (occasional)

COURSE AND OUTCOME

- Mortality rate (pre-LT era): 10%–80%
- Symptoms can resolve within 5–14 days
- Full recovery can take 12 weeks or longer
- Chronic hepatitis is not well documented

ADVERSE PROGNOSTIC FINDINGS

- Age >40 years
- Obesity
- Short duration to onset of jaundice
- Serum bilirubin level >20 mg/dL
- Coagulopathy

this form of toxicity is only about 1 per 10,000,[29] but the rate increases to approximately 1 per 1000 after 2 or more exposures, especially when the anesthetic agent is readministered within a few weeks.[2] Typically, zone 3 (centrilobular) hepatic necrosis is seen histologically.[29] The case-fatality rate ranged from 14% to 71% in the preliver transplantation (LT) era[2] and remains high in developing countries where halothane is still used.[3,4]

Risk Factors

Host-related risk factors for halothane hepatitis are listed in Box 91.1. The reaction is rare in childhood[21]; patients younger than 10 years of age represent only about 3% of the total, and cases in persons younger than 30 years account for less than 10%.[21,26] In a 2008 Iranian series, 60% of patients were older than 40, and none were younger than 18.[3] The liver injury tends to be more severe in persons older than 40. Two-thirds of cases have been in women, and repeat exposure to halothane (especially within a few weeks or months) was documented in as many as 90% of cases.[2,30] The time between exposures can be as long as 28 years,[31] although after repeat exposure, hepatitis is earlier in onset and more severe. Obesity is another risk factor, possibly because of storage of halothane in body fat. The induction of cytochrome P450 (CYP) enzymes (especially CYP2E1) that metabolize halothane to its toxic intermediate has been produced experimentally with phenobarbital, alcohol, and isoniazid; valproic acid (VPA) inhibits, and phenytoin has no specific effect on halothane hepatotoxicity. Posttransfusion hepatitis (unknown at the time of the National Halothane Study, which did not include blood transfusion as a potential risk factor) has been recently proposed as a possible cause of some of the initially reported cases.[32]

Pathology

In a study of 77 cases of halothane hepatitis reviewed by the Armed Forces Institute of Pathology,[30] various degrees of liver injury were seen, depending on the severity of the reaction. Massive or submassive necrosis involving zone 3 was present in all autopsy specimens, whereas biopsy material revealed a broader range of injury—from spotty necrosis in about one-third of cases to sharply demarcated zone 3 necrosis in two-thirds. The inflammatory response is less severe than in acute viral hepatitis.

Pathogenesis

Approximately one-third of halothane is metabolized via oxidative pathways involving CYP2E1 and CYP2A6, while less than 1% is metabolized via reduction.[4] Hepatic injury occurs by one or more of three potential mechanisms: hypersensitivity, production of hepatotoxic metabolites, and hypoxia, in decreasing order of importance.[2] Evidence for the role of hypersensitivity is found in the increased susceptibility and shortened latency after repeat exposure, hallmark symptoms and signs of drug allergy (fever, rash, eosinophilia, and granuloma formation), and detection of neoantigens and antibodies. Halothane oxidation yields TFA, which is generated by the reaction between lysine and halothane metabolites and which acts on hepatocyte proteins to produce neoantigens that are responsible for the major form of injury.[4] By contrast, reductive pathways produce free radicals that can act as reactive metabolites that may have a role in causing minor injury.[33–35] Zimmerman suggested that halothane injury most likely results from immunologic enhancement of zone 3 necrosis produced by the reductive metabolites.[2] Accordingly, the hepatotoxic potential of halothane depends on the susceptibility of the patient and on factors that promote the production of hepatotoxic or immunogenic metabolites.[2] A murine model of halothane hepatotoxicity demonstrated female susceptibility based on an increase in levels of γ-interferon, possibly mediated through estrogen, and an increase in natural killer cell activity.[36,37]

A more recent mouse model demonstrated that immune tolerance can be overcome by the TFA halothane protein adducts that are formed in the liver. Hepatic injury was associated with increased levels of interleukin-4 and immunoglobulins G1 and E directed against the halothane protein adducts, as well as increased hepatic infiltration by eosinophils and $CD4^+$ T cells that are features of an allergic reaction.[38]

Course and Outcome

Mortality rates for halothane hepatitis were high in early series; since then, success has been achieved with LT, when necessary.[39] When spontaneous recovery occurs, symptoms usually resolve within 5–14 days, and recovery is complete within several weeks.[2]

Immunosuppressive agents have only rarely been reported to improve the outcome.[21] Zimmerman doubted whether halothane causes chronic hepatitis.[2] However, a case series has suggested that chronic injury may develop after repeated exposure (especially to sevoflurane).[40] Adverse prognostic factors for acute halothane hepatitis include age older than 40 years, obesity, severe coagulopathy, serum bilirubin level greater than 20 mg/dL, and a shorter interval to onset of jaundice.[2,3,26]

The best treatment is prevention, specifically avoidance of reexposure, especially when a previous reaction has occurred. A history of a prior reaction to halothane contraindicates repeat use of halothane.[3,39] Attempts to demonstrate a protective role for zinc, disulfiram (which blocks CYP2E1), and other compounds against halothane hepatitis have been reported in animal models,[41] but none has yet been proved to be of value in humans.

Others

The likelihood that individual haloalkane anesthetics will cause liver injury appears to be related to the extent to which they are metabolized by hepatic CYP enzymes: 20%–30% for halothane, greater than 30% for methoxyflurane, 2% for enflurane, less than 1% for sevoflurane, and 0.2% or less for isoflurane and desflurane.[22] Accordingly, the estimated frequency of hepatitis from the newer agents is much less than that for halothane (Table 91.1).

Methoxyflurane caused hepatotoxicity and a high frequency of nephrotoxicity that led to its withdrawal.[42] Enflurane caused a clinical syndrome similar to that for halothane, with the onset of fever within 3 days and jaundice in 3–19 days after anesthesia[43,44] and with an estimated incidence of enflurane-induced liver injury of about 1 in 800,000 exposed patients.[20]

Despite its low rate of metabolism,[22] several instances of isoflurane-associated liver injury have been reported.[45–49] In one case, cross-sensitivity was suspected 22 years after initial exposure to enflurane.[46] TFA liver proteins have been detected in patients with suspected isoflurane hepatotoxicity.[47] In rats, the number of apoptotic hepatocytes seen after multiple exposures to isoflurane was only about 3% in a periacinar distribution. They were seen in only a small number of lobules, indicating a low propensity to cause hepatotoxicity.[50]

The newer haloalkane anesthetics, desflurane and sevoflurane, appear to be nearly free of adverse hepatic effects. Desflurane undergoes minimal biotransformation and is not associated with the development of TFA antibodies in exposed rats.[22] Only isolated reports of liver injury in patients receiving desflurane anesthesia have been published.[51] The biotransformation of sevoflurane is also minimal, and only rare reports have implicated this agent in postoperative hepatic dysfunction, especially after reexposure.[52–54] In rats, sevoflurane produced fewer than 1% apoptotic hepatocytes after repeated exposures.[50]

Ether, nitrous oxide, and cyclopropane apparently are devoid of significant hepatotoxic potential because of their lack of halogen moieties,[2] and ketamine has only rarely been reported to cause hepatic injury.[55] Propofol is considered largely free of hepatotoxic effects, even in patients with cirrhosis.[57] Although propofol has a high affinity for mitochondrial membranes, no significant impairment in mitochondrial function has been shown in animal models.[57]

Jaundice in the Postoperative Period

Between 25% and 75% of patients undergoing surgery experience postoperative hepatic dysfunction, ranging from mild elevations in liver biochemical test levels to hepatic failure, with postoperative jaundice reported in nearly 50% of patients with underlying cirrhosis.[58] Patients undergoing upper abdominal surgical procedures are at the highest risk of postoperative liver dysfunction, as well as pancreatitis, cholecystitis, and bile duct injury, because of impaired blood flow to the liver.[58] Box 91.2 lists causes of postoperative jaundice and hepatic dysfunction, broadly divided into hepatocellular injury, cholestasis, and indirect hyperbilirubinemia. Drugs that may cause hepatotoxicity in this setting include antibiotics (e.g., erythromycin, amoxicillin–clavulanic acid, trimethoprim/sulfamethoxazole, fluoroquinolones) (see Chapter 90) as well as the halogenated anesthetics discussed earlier.

Table 91.2 contrasts the features of halogenated anesthetic-induced hepatitis, ischemic hepatitis (shock liver)[59] (see Chapter 87), and cholestatic injury in the early postoperative period. Bile cast nephropathy is a relatively newly recognized clinical entity that can contribute to hyperbilirubinemia and the development of hepatorenal syndrome (see Chapter 96) in patients with acute-on-chronic liver injury (see Chapter 76), including postoperatively.[60]

CHEMICALS

Commercial and Industrial Agents

Among the tens of thousands of chemical compounds in commercial and industrial use, several hundred are listed as causing liver injury by the National Institute for Occupational Safety and Health.[61] The National Library of Medicine maintains a database of chemical toxins in its Toxicology and Environmental Health Information Program,[62] as do other sources.[63,64] Table 91.3 lists the various chemical classes associated with hepatotoxicity as a primary toxic effect.

Toxic exposure to chemical agents occurs most often from inhalation or absorption by the skin and less often from absorption by the GI tract after oral ingestion or through a parenteral route. Because most chemical toxins are lipid soluble, when absorbed they can easily cross biological membranes to reach their target organ(s), including the liver.[5,6,8] Hepatotoxic chemical exposure [as with carbon tetrachloride (CCl_4) and phosphorus] usually results in an acute cytotoxic injury that typically consists of three distinct phases, similar to those observed after an acetaminophen overdose (see Chapter 97) or ingestion of toxic mushrooms (see later) (Table 91.4).[2,5] Less commonly, acute cholestatic injury may occur.[65] Many chemicals (e.g., vinyl chloride) are also carcinogenic, and hepatic malignancies have been

TABLE 91.1 Hepatotoxic Anesthetics Other Than Halothane

Anesthetic	Percent Metabolized%	Incidence of Hepatotoxicity	Cross-Reactivity With Other Haloalkanes	Other Clinical Features
Methoxyflurane	>30	Low	Yes	Nephrotoxicity
Enflurane	2	1 in 800,000	Yes	Similar to halothane
Isoflurane	0.2	Rare	Yes	Similar to halothane
Desflurane	<0.2	Few reports	Yes	Cardiac toxicity, malignant hyperthermia
Sevoflurane	Minimal	Rare	Uncertain	None reported

BOX 91.2 Causes of Postoperative Hepatic Dysfunction

Hepatocellular injury (predominant serum ALT elevation, with or without hyperbilirubinemia)

- Acute transfusion-associated viral hepatitis
- Hepatic allograft rejection
- Hepatic artery thrombosis
- Inhalational anesthetics—halothane, others
- Ischemic hepatitis (shock liver)
- Other drugs—antihypertensives (e.g., labetalol), heparin
- Unrecognized chronic liver disease—NASH, hepatitis C, other disorders

Cholestatic jaundice (elevated serum alkaline phosphatase ± ALT; direct hyperbilirubinemia)

- Acalculous cholecystitis
- Benign postoperative cholestasis
- Bile duct injury—following cholecystectomy or LT
- Bile duct obstruction—gallstones, pancreatitis
- Cardiac bypass of prolonged duration
- Cholangitis
- Drugs—amoxicillin-clavulanic acid, chlorpromazine, erythromycin, telithromycin, trimethoprim/sulfamethoxazole, warfarin, others
- Hemobilia
- Microlithiasis (biliary sludge)
- Prolonged TPN
- Sepsis

Indirect hyperbilirubinemia (serum alkaline phosphatase and ALT often normal)

- Gilbert syndrome
- Hemolytic anemia (G6PD deficiency, other causes)
- Multiple transfusions
- Resorbing hematoma

part of the clinicopathologic spectrum of chemical injury (see Chapter 98) (Box 91.3).[2,65] Although liver injury is the dominant toxicity for some agents (see Table 91.3), hepatic damage may be only one facet of more generalized toxicity for other agents.[5]

Carbon Tetrachloride and Other Chlorinated Aliphatic Hydrocarbons

CCl_4 is a classic example of a zone 3 hepatotoxin that causes necrosis leading to hepatic failure (see Table 91.4). Injury is mediated by its metabolism to a toxic trichloromethyl radical catalyzed by CYP2E1.[18,66] Alcohol potentiates the injury through induction of this cytochrome.[2] Most cases have been the result of industrial or domestic accidents, such as inhalation of CCl_4-containing dry cleaning fluids that are used as household reagents or ingestion of these compounds by persons with alcohol use disorder who mistake them for potable beverages.[2,67] At the cellular level, direct damage to cellular membranes results in leakage of intracellular enzymes and electrolytes, leading in turn to calcium shifts and lipid peroxidation.[18] Hepatic steatosis develops as a result of triglyceride accumulation caused by haloalkylation-dependent inhibition of lipoprotein micelle transport out of the hepatocyte.[66] CCl_4 is more toxic than other haloalkanes and haloalkenes because toxicity correlates inversely with the level of bond dissociation energy, number of halogen atoms, and chain length (Table 91.5).[2,66] In older series, complete clinical and histologic recovery from CCl_4-induced liver damage was the rule with modest exposures, but supervening acute tubular necrosis and GI hemorrhage were associated with a case-fatality rate of 10%–25%.[2,5] Activation of endonucleases, causing chromosomal damage and mutations, may result in carcinogenesis.

BOX 91.3 Clinicopathologic Spectrum of Liver Injury Caused by Chemical Hepatotoxins

ACUTE

Necrosis

- Carbon tetrachloride and other haloalkanes
- Cocaine, "ecstasy," phencyclidine
- Haloaromatics, nitroaliphatics, nitroaromatics
- Hydrochlorofluorocarbons
- Copper salts, inorganic arsenic, iron, and phosphorus

Microvesicular Steatosis

- Boric acid
- Chlordecone
- Cocaine
- Dimethylformamide
- Hydrazine
- Hypoglycin
- Thallium
- Toluene, xylene

Cholestasis

- Alpha-naphthylisocyanate
- Aniline—rapeseed oil
- Dinitrophenol
- Methylene dianiline
- Paraquat

SUBACUTE

Necrosis

- Trinitrotoluene

Sinusoidal Obstruction Syndrome

- Pyrrolizidine alkaloids, arsenic, and thorium dioxide

Toxic Cirrhosis

- Hexachlorobenzene, polychlorinated biphenyls
- Tetrachlorethane

Peliosis Hepatis

- Dioxin

CHRONIC

Cirrhosis

- Chloroaliphatics, trinitrotoluene, arsenic, and pyrrolizidine alkaloids

Hepatoportal Sclerosis

- Arsenic, vinyl chloride

NEOPLASIA

HCC

- Aflatoxins, arsenic, and thorium dioxide

Angiosarcoma

- Arsenic, thorium dioxide, and vinyl chloride

Hemangioendothelioma

- Arsenic

Chloroform (trichloromethane) remains an important experimental hepatotoxin, although its use as an anesthetic has long been abandoned (see earlier).[2,5,8,67] Hepatic injury, including chronic hepatitis, has been reported with 1,1,1-trichloroethane,[68] which has been used as an inhaled treatment for trigeminal neuralgia, and instances of jaundice and hepatic necrosis are described in as many as 10% of workers exposed to the compound during its manufacture.[8]

TABLE 91.2 Comparative Features of Causes of Acute Postoperative Liver Injury

Feature	Haloalkane Anesthetic Toxicity	Ischemic Hepatitis	Postoperative Cholestasis
Incidence	Rare	Not uncommon	Common
Latency	2–15 days	Within 24 hours	A few days
Fever, rash, eosinophilia	Present	Absent	Absent
Serum ALT/AST (×ULN)	25–200×	Can exceed 200× (AST ≫ ALT)	Minimal or normal
Jaundice	Common	Rare	Common (direct hyperbilirubinemia)
Histology	Zone 3 necrosis	Coagulative necrosis, sinusoidal congestion	Bile plugs, cholestasis
Mortality	High	Varies with diagnosis	Not from liver disease
Recovery time	Up to 12 weeks	10–12 days with supportive care	Variable, may be prolonged
Risk factors:			
Age	Adults, age >40 years	Any	Any
Gender	F > M 2:1	F = M	F = M
Body weight	Obese	Any	Any
Hypotension	May or may not be present	Documented in 50%	Absent

F, Female; *M*, male; *ULN*, upper limit of normal.

TABLE 91.3 Chemical Classes Associated With Hepatotoxicity as a Primary Toxic Effect

Category	Chemical Name	Other Chemical Name(s)
Aliphatic nitro compounds	2-Nitropropane	Dimethylnitromethane, iso-nitropropane
Aromatic amines	4,4′-Methylenedianiline	MDA, diaminodiphenylmethane
Aromatic nitro compounds	2,4,6-Trinitrotoluene	TNT, 1-methyl-2,4,6-trinitrobenzene
Chlorinated hydrocarbons	Hexachloronapthalene	Halowax
Chlorinated solvents	Ethylene dichloride	1,2-Dichloroethane, glycol dichloride
	1,1,2,2-Tetrachloroethane	Acetylene tetrachloride
	Carbon tetrachloride	Tetrachloromethane
	Propylene dichloride	1.2-Dichloropropane
Halogenated solvents	Ethylene dibromide	1.2-Dibromoethane, glycol dibromide
Nitrosamines	*N*-Nitrosodimethylamine	Dimethylnitrosamine, DMNA NDMA
Other solvents	Dimethylformamide	*N,N*-Dimethylformamide, DMA
	Tetrahydrofuran	Diethyl oxide; tetramethylene oxide, THF
	Dimethyl acetamide	DMAC, acetic acid, dimethylacetone amide

Adapted from reference Haz-Map, available at www.haz-map.com/heptox1.htm; accessed April 7, 2018.

Hydrochlorofluorocarbons (HCFCs) have been associated with liver injury in several industrial workers exposed to dichlorotrifluoroethane (HCFC-123) and 1-chlorotetrafluoroethane (HCFC-124), both of which are metabolized to reactive trifluoroacetyl halide intermediates similar to those implicated in halothane toxicity.[57] Zone 3 necrosis is present on liver biopsy specimens, and autoantibodies against CYP2E1 or P58 protein disulfide isomerase isoform are detected in the serum of many affected persons. As with halothane, liver toxicity may be potentiated by ethanol.[70]

Vinyl Chloride and Other Chlorinated Ethylenes

In the past, exposure to vinyl chloride monomer (VCM), or monochloroethylene, occurred in polymerization plants where vinyl chloride was heated to form polyvinyl chloride (PVC) in the manufacture of plastics; the toxic gas containing VCM was inhaled in this process.[8,9] Vinyl chloride is ubiquitous in the environment and was estimated by the Environmental Protection Agency to exist in at least 10% of toxic waste sites.[6] More than 80,000 chemical workers were estimated to have been exposed to vinyl chloride as of 2010.[71] Although PVC appears to be nontoxic, long-term exposure to VCM has led to chronic liver injury, including nodular subcapsular fibrosis, sinusoidal dilatation, peliosis hepatis, and periportal fibrosis associated with portal hypertension.[2,5] Toxicant-associated steatohepatitis was described in 80% of nonobese chemical workers with high exposure levels to VCM, more than half of whom had significant fibrosis; 16% developed angiosarcoma (see Chapter 98).[72] Although biomarkers of steatohepatitis (ALT and cytokeratin 18) were negative in frozen samples from 17 workers exposed to VC in the 1970s, elevated levels of fatty acids and their oxidized metabolites were seen as part of an abnormal plasma metabolome that distinguished them from healthy unexposed volunteers with 94% accuracy.[71]

Vinyl chloride is also carcinogenic[73] and classified as a group I carcinogen by the International Agency for Research on Cancer.[9] Angiosarcoma was first identified as an occupationally related malignancy in 1974, among workers of a tire manufacturing plant in Kentucky.[74] The tumor develops after a mean latency of 25 years after exposure; the risk is related to the duration and extent of contact.[71,73] Alcohol appears to enhance the hepatocarcinogenicity of vinyl chloride in rodents, and possibly in humans, by inducing CYP2E1, which converts vinyl chloride to a toxic or carcinogenic metabolite (2-chloroethylene oxide).[2] A history of vinyl chloride exposure was found in 15%–25% of all cases of hepatic angiosarcoma reported in the late 1970s,[5] and strict hygienic measures

TABLE 91.4 Phases of Illness After Ingestion of Various Hepatotoxins

	Toxin			
Phase	**Acetaminophen**	**Phosphorus**	***Amanita phalloides***	**Carbon Tetrachloride**
I (1–24 hours)				
Onset of toxicity	Immediate	Immediate	Delayed 6–20 hours	Immediate
Anorexia, nausea, vomiting, diarrhea	+	++++	++++	+
Shock	–	+	±	–
Neurologic symptoms	–	+	±	–
II (24–72 hours)				
Asymptomatic latent period	+	±	+	+
III (>72 hours)				
Jaundice	+	+	+	+
Hepatic failure	+	+	+	+
Renal failure	+	+	+	+
Maximum serum AST and ALT (×ULN)	1000	<10–100	500	500
Zonal necrosis	3	1	3	3
Steatosis	–	++++	+	+
Case-fatality rate (%)	5–15	25–50	20–25	20–25

ULN, Upper limit of normal.
Adapted from Zimmerman HJ. Hepatotoxicity. In: *The Adverse Effects of Drugs and Other Chemicals on the Liver*. 2nd ed. Philadelphia: Lippincott Williams & Wilkins; 1999.

TABLE 91.5 Relative Hepatoxicities of Haloalkane Compounds

Compound	**Relative Toxicity**
Carbon tetrachloride	++++
Tetrachlorethane	++++
Chloroform	++
Trichloroethylene	+ to ++
1,1,2-Trichloroethane	+ to ++
Tetrachloroethylene	+
1,1,1-Trichloroethane	+
Dibromomethane	±
Dichloromethane	±
Methylchloride	–

Scale from ++++, maximal injury, to –, trivial or no injury.
From references Zimmerman H. Hepatotoxicity. In: *The Adverse Effects of Drugs and Other Chemicals on the Liver*. 2nd ed. Philadelphia: Lippincott Williams & Wilkins; 1999; Zimmerman H, Lewis J. Chemical- and toxin-induced hepatotoxicity. *Gastroenterol Clin North Am*. 1995;24:1027–1045.

instituted in 1974 resulted in a marked decrease in the frequency of angiosarcoma; however, persons with the highest exposure still had a fourfold increased risk of developing periportal hepatic fibrosis, which may be a precursor to angiosarcoma.[75] While the development of cirrhosis after VCM exposure has been questioned (along with the risk of hepatocellular carcinoma) due to the potential confounding fibrotic effects of underlying alcohol and viral hepatitis in exposed individuals,[76] newer evidence suggests a pathologic role of VCM for both cirrhosis and HCC. The sequential development of HCC and hepatic angiosarcoma in the same person supports the genotoxic effect of VCM[77] and new epidemiologic evidence from a large cohort of 1658 vinyl chloride workers confirms the risk of death from both cirrhosis and HCC.[78] Persons previously exposed to vinyl chloride should undergo regular clinical examinations for an early detection of liver tumors, and those with known chronic liver disease or high levels of exposure should undergo regular hepatic imaging. Persons who work in PVC plants should undergo regular monitoring of liver biochemical test levels, and those with persistent abnormalities should be removed from workplace exposure.[75]

Nonhalogenated Organic Compounds

Benzene has been associated with minor hepatic injury in animals, including abnormal liver enzymes and reductions in glutathione and CYP2E1 levels.[79] Toluene, which led to steatosis and necrosis in a "glue sniffer,"[80] has been associated with acute fatty liver of pregnancy and has caused elevations in serum GGTP levels after industrial exposure.[5] Xylene can cause mild hepatic steatosis, and styrene (vinyl benzene) has led to elevated serum aminotransferase levels after prolonged exposure.[5] Elevated levels of serum cytokeratins[18] and proinflammatory cytokines have been found in workers with suspected toxicant-associated steatohepatitis exposed to acrylonitrile, styrene, and other elastomers or polymers and may serve as potential biomarkers of occupational liver injury.[81]

Trinitrotoluene and Other Nitroaromatic Compounds

Trinitrotoluene (TNT) was first observed to be hepatotoxic during World War I, when severe acute and subacute hepatic necrosis developed in munitions workers in England, Germany, and the United States; the case-fatality rate was more than 25%.[2,5] The frequency of hepatotoxicity during World War II was lower, with approximately 1 in 500 workers affected, but the estimated frequencies of methemoglobinemia and aplastic anemia were 50 times higher.[5] Subacute hepatic necrosis followed 2–4 months of regular exposure to TNT. Percutaneous absorption was the major source of exposure. In some patients, rapidly progressive liver failure and death occurred within days to months, with massive hepatic necrosis at autopsy. In others, the subacute injury progressed over several months to micronodular cirrhosis and portal hypertension. The relatively low frequency of injury suggests that formation of a toxic metabolite was involved.[2] Nitrobenzene and dinitrobenzene were also observed to be hepatotoxic during World War I. As with TNT, excessive exposure led to methemoglobinemia.[5]

Nitroaliphatic Compounds

Nitromethane, nitroethane, and nitropropane cause variable degrees of hepatic injury. 2-Nitropropane has caused fatal massive hepatic necrosis after occupational exposure as a solvent, fuel additive, varnish remover, and rocket propellant. Toxic hepatitis associated with the chronic inhalation of propane and butane has also been reported.[82]

Polychlorinated Biphenyls and Other Halogenated Aromatic Compounds

Polychlorinated biphenyls (PCBs) are synthetic chlorinated aromatic hydrocarbons created from mixtures of trichloro-, tetrachloro-, pentachloro-, and hexachloro-derivatives of biphenyls, naphthalenes, and triphenyls that have been used in the manufacture of electrical transformers, condensers, capacitors, insulating materials for electrical cables, and industrial fluids. More than 100 different congeners have been synthesized.[9] Acute and chronic hepatotoxicity from PCB exposure seen during World War II resembled that caused by TNT.[5,6] Inhalation of toxic fumes released by the melting of PCBs and chloronaphthalene mixtures during soldering of electrical materials was the most common means of exposure.[2] The severity of liver injury correlated with the number of chlorine molecules.[5] Liver damage appeared as early as 7 weeks after ongoing exposure and was accompanied by anorexia, nausea, and edema of the face and hands. Acne-like skin lesions (chloracne) usually preceded hepatic injury. Once jaundice appeared, death occurred within 2 weeks in fulminant cases, which were characterized by massive necrosis (so-called acute yellow atrophy), or after 1–3 months in subacute cases. Cirrhosis developed in some persons who survived the acute injury.[2] Availability of PCBs declined significantly from a peak in the 1970s owing to a ban on production because of their health and environmental hazards,[83] although many are still in use.[9]

Polybrominated biphenyls appear to be even more toxic than PCBs. Consumption of milk and meat from livestock given feed mistakenly contaminated by a polybrominated biphenyl led to hepatomegaly and minor elevations in liver enzyme levels in exposed persons.[5]

Miscellaneous Chemical Compounds

Dimethylformamide is a solvent used in the synthetic resin and leather industries that causes dose-related massive hepatic necrosis in animals[84] and is capable of producing focal hepatic necrosis and microvesicular steatosis in humans.[5] Most persons exposed for more than 1 year have symptomatic disease that slowly resolves when they are removed from the workplace.[5] Disulfiram-like symptoms can occur.[85] Alcohol use, HBV infection, and a high BMI are risk factors.[86] Animal studies have revealed a mechanistic role for CYP2E1[87] and for a variety of dysregulated proteins, lipids, mitochondrial dysfunction, and glutathione depletion contributing to its hepatotoxicity.[88] Dimethylacetamide hepatotoxicity is well described in animals, with only rare reports after human exposure.[89]

Hydrazine and its derivatives used in jet and rocket fuel cells are also experimental hepatotoxins and carcinogens and have been reported to cause hepatic steatosis in animals[2] and reversible injury in humans after inhalation.[90] Bromoalkanes and iodoalkanes, used in insecticides and aircraft fuels, have rarely caused hepatic injury.[5] Ethylene dibromide (dibromoethane) has led to zone 3 hepatic necrosis after ingestion in attempted suicide and to fatal hepatotoxicity associated with nephrotoxicity and cardiotoxicity following occupational exposure or inadvertent poisoning.[91]

Pesticides

Although exposure to insecticides, herbicides, and other pesticides is common, acute liver injury resulting from these compounds, many of which are chlorinated hydrocarbons, is rare.[2,5] Evidence that dichlorodiphenyl-trichloroethane (DDT) and other organochlorines (aldrin, amitrole, chlordane, dieldrin, lindane, and mirex) lead to liver damage or carcinogenicity is limited,[2] but a study in 2012 suggested a possible relationship with HCC.[92] Agent Orange, a defoliant widely used in Vietnam that is composed of a mixture of 2 phenoxyl herbicides, 2,4-dichlorophenoxyacetic acid (2,4-D) and 2,4,5-trichlorophenoxyacetic acid (2,4,5-T), was reported to cause acute hepatitis after chronic exposure, although contaminating dioxins (formed in the production of some chlorinated organic compounds) have been suggested to be responsible for the toxic effects.[93,94] Moreover, chronic liver injury among Vietnam veterans may have been related to viral infections or alcohol rather than to Agent Orange,[91] and hepatocarcinogenesis has been linked to chronic hepatitis B in some persons.[95]

Although a small increased risk has been reported for the development of cirrhosis (OR = 1.08) among Korean veterans of the Vietnam War,[96] the 2018 update from the Committee to Review the Health Effects in Vietnam Veterans of Exposure to Herbicides concluded that there was inadequate or insufficient evidence to determine whether there is an association between exposure to Agent Orange and other herbicides and liver toxicity (as well as a number of other organic toxicities).[97]

Ingestion of or dermal exposure to dichloride dimethyldipyridilium (paraquat) has been implicated in several instances of hepatotoxicity as a result of attempted suicide and homicide.[98] Patients may present with severe vomiting and profuse diarrhea leading to hypokalemia and often have evidence of oral, pharyngeal, and esophageal caustic injury after ingestion. Death results from a combination of renal, respiratory, cardiac, and hepatic failure; mortality rates are as high as 70%, and death often occurs within the first 48 hours. Histopathologic changes include zone 3 necrosis followed by injury to small- and medium-sized interlobular bile ducts.[99] Treatment with charcoal hemoperfusion in conjunction with cyclophosphamide, dexamethasone, furosemide, and vitamins B and C—the so-called "Caribbean scheme"—has been attempted, but persons who ingest more than 45 mL are likely to die with or without this treatment.[98] In animals, *N*-acetylcysteine and silymarin may be protective.[100]

Chlordecone (Kepone) has been shown to impair biliary excretion and lipid transport and storage,[101] but neurologic toxicity appears to dominate the clinical injury.[102] Occupational exposure has led to hepatic steatosis and elevated serum aminotransferase levels. Trivial hepatic enzyme abnormalities have been seen in persons heavily exposed to chloretone.[5] Hexachlorobenzene in contaminated grain has been associated with an epidemic of porphyria cutanea tarda (see Chapter 79) and liver injury.[5]

Inorganic arsenic has long been used as a homicidal or suicidal agent, and toxic exposure in the past followed ingestion of Fowler's solution (arsenic trioxide), which was used as a treatment for psoriasis and asthma.[2,5] Organic arsenic is present in seafood, whereas inorganic forms are found mainly in contaminated ground and well water[9] and homemade alcohol.[2] Doses greater than 3 g can cause death in 1–3 days, but hepatic injury generally is overshadowed by GI, neurologic, and vascular effects, leading ultimately to CNS depression and vascular collapse.[2] A lesion resembling hepatic sinusoidal obstruction syndrome (SOS) can develop (see Chapter 87),[5] and noncirrhotic portal hypertension developed in more than 90% of 248 patients who consumed contaminated drinking water for up to 15 years.[103]

Occupational exposure to inorganic arsenic is still observed among vineyard workers, farmers, and gold miners,[104] although its use as an insecticide has been curtailed since the 1940s. Lumber treated with chromated copper arsenate as a preservative may be an additional source of exposure.[105] The clinical syndrome associated with arsenicosis includes skin lesions (blackfoot disease), anemia, diabetes mellitus, hearing loss, neurobehavioral disorders, and cardiovascular diseases, in addition to benign and malignant liver disease.[106] Chronic hepatic injury, including cirrhosis and noncirrhotic portal hypertension, may be a precursor to hepatic neoplasms, such as angiosarcomas, hemangioendotheliomas, and HCCs, after exposure of more than 10 years.[9,107] Increased serum levels of EGF receptor have been found in patients with liver cancer who overexpress this biomarker following exposure to arsenic.[108] Treatment with thiol chelators has had variable success in cases of prolonged exposure, and coadministration of antioxidants, such as vitamins C and E, contained in many fruits and vegetables, may be of added benefit, especially in developing countries where heavy metal contamination remains prevalent.[109,110]

METALS

Iron

Most of the estimated 5000 cases of accidental iron poisoning in the United States each year occur in young children who mistake iron supplements for candy.[2] Ferrous sulfate tablets contain 20% elemental iron by weight, and the severity of injury correlates with the dose ingested.[5] Ingestion of less than 20 mg/kg of elemental iron is unlikely to produce serious toxicity, whereas doses of more than 200 mg/kg can be fatal.[2] Severe injury has been seen only with serum iron concentrations above 700 mg/dL measured within the first 12 hours after ingestion.[111] Iron per se is not hepatotoxic, but ferric and ferrous ions can act through free radicals and lipid peroxidation to cause membrane disruption and necrosis.[112] Clinically evident liver injury is uncommon, but zone 1 necrosis occurs in the most severe cases.[2] Clinical illness is characterized by sequential phases of GI injury, subsidence of symptoms, and overt hepatotoxicity accompanied by renal failure.[113] Some cases have progressed rapidly to ALF requiring LT.[114] Hyperbaric oxygen treatment of acute iron intoxication has been effective in an animal model[115] and may offer a potential therapy in cases of human poisoning.

Phosphorus

Poisoning by white phosphorus has been rare because its use in firecrackers and matches was outlawed in the mid-20th century.[5] Cases reported since then usually have been the result of ingestion of rat or roach poison.[2] Shortly after ingestion, vomiting, GI bleeding, convulsions, shock, and death occur within 24 hours. Phosphorescence of the vomitus and stools and a typical garlic-like odor on the breath are characteristic, when present. The predominant hepatic lesion is steatosis and necrosis, most prominent in the periportal region. Serum aminotransferase levels generally are no higher than 10 times the upper limit of normal (ULN).[2]

Copper

Acute poisoning by copper leads to a syndrome resembling iron toxicity. Ingestion of toxic amounts (1–10 mg) is usually seen with suicidal intent, especially on the Indian subcontinent.[5,112] Vomiting, diarrhea, and abdominal pain accompanied by a metallic taste are seen during the first few hours after ingestion. GI tract erosions, renal tubular necrosis, and rhabdomyolysis often accompany zone 3 hepatic necrosis by the second or third day. Jaundice results from both hepatic injury and acute hemolysis caused by high blood copper levels.[5] The mortality rate is 15%, with early deaths resulting from shock and circulatory collapse and late deaths resulting from hepatic and renal failure.[2]

Thorium Dioxide

Thorotrast is a colloidal suspension of radioactive thorium dioxide that was used as an IV contrast medium for radiographic procedures in the first half of the 20th century, with more than 50,000 persons having been exposed.[2] Thorotrast was subsequently found to cause hepatic angiosarcomas and cholangiocarcinomas after latency periods of 20–40 years. The long latency is thought to be due in part to the uneven distribution of radionuclides and the limited range of the emitted alpha particles.[116] Histologically, thorium dioxide is found in Kupffer cells and macrophages as dark brown refractile granules, the identity of which can be confirmed by spectrographic analysis.[7] As with arsenic, reports of hepatic SOS and a Budd-Chiari–like syndrome have also appeared (see Chapter 87).[7] Given the extraordinarily long half-life (hundreds of years) of the compound, exposed persons remain at risk for the development of leukemia, in addition to HCC,[117] and require lifelong monitoring because hepatic malignancies have occurred in approximately 20% of those exposed.[118]

Others

Although cadmium produces hepatic necrosis and cirrhosis in laboratory animals,[119] evidence is lacking that exposure to cadmium causes important human injury.[2] Several metals are associated with apoptosis, which may explain their potential for hepatotoxicity.[120] Beryllium has led to midzonal liver necrosis as a result of phagocytosis of insoluble beryllium phosphate by Kupffer cells.[2] Chronic industrial exposure (usually by inhalation of high concentrations of oxide or phosphorus mixtures) is associated with the formation of hepatic (and pulmonary) granulomas.[5] Therapy with chelating agents and antioxidants has been used in animal models of beryllium toxicity.[121] Lead hepatotoxicity may be seen as part of the larger symptom complex of abdominal pain, constipation, and encephalopathy that occurs with chronic ingestion or environmental exposure.[122] Chromium compounds (especially the hexavalent form) can be hepatotoxic in animals as well as humans, the result of mitochondrial injury and other hepatocyte stress.[123]

DRUGS OF ABUSE

Hepatic abnormalities are frequently encountered in substance abusers, especially those using cocaine and methamphetamine derivatives.[124]

Cocaine

Cocaine is a dose-dependent hepatotoxin.[5] Acute cocaine intoxication affects the liver in 60% of patients and produces a range of hepatic effects from asymptomatic elevations in liver biochemical test levels to severe injury with markedly elevated serum ALT levels (>1000 U/L).[125] Associated features include rhabdomyolysis, hypotension, hyperpyrexia, DIC, and renal failure.[2,5] In a series of 39 patients with rhabdomyolysis, 23 had severe hepatotoxicity associated with a high mortality rate.[126] Hepatic injury is probably the result of toxic metabolites (e.g., norcocaine nitroxide) formed by CYP2E1 and CYP2A,[127] and enhanced hepatotoxicity is seen in persons who regularly consume alcohol.[5] Indeed, the simultaneous consumption of alcohol and use of cocaine results in the formation of cocaethylene, a metabolite, which has been studied as a biomarker of chronic excessive alcohol use among cocaine users.[128] In a large cohort study of cocaine use among HIV-positive patients in Miami, Florida, it was found that African American men had a nearly twofold increase in hepatic fibrosis compared to African American women[129] and that HIV-positive cocaine users with cocaethylene in the blood were more than three times as likely to have liver fibrosis than cocaine nonusers.[130] In animals, pretreatment with *N*-acetylcysteine decreases the risk of cocaine hepatotoxicity,[131] although the usefulness of *N*-acetylcysteine for treating human cocaine-induced hepatic injury has not been determined.

Others

"Ecstasy" (3,4-methylenedioxymethamphetamine) is a euphorigenic and psychedelic amphetamine derivative that can lead to hepatic necrosis as part of a heat stroke–like syndrome resulting from exhaustive dancing in hot nightclubs (raves).[132–134] The injury can be fatal and has necessitated LT in some instances.[134–136] The role of CYP enzymes in the toxicity of this and other so-called designer drugs may relate to specific genetic polymorphisms of CYP2D6 or other cytochromes.[137]

Phencyclidine (angel dust) is another stimulant that can lead to hepatic injury as part of a syndrome of malignant hyperthermia that produces zone 3 hepatic necrosis, congestion, and collapse, with high serum AST and ALT levels reminiscent of ischemic hepatitis.[138]

Cannabis (marijuana) has not been associated with acute or chronic liver injury by itself,[121] although daily use was associated with progression of fibrosis in patients with untreated chronic hepatitis C.[139] Synthetic cannabinoids (known popularly as "Spice," "K2," or other street names) have been associated with hepatic steatosis in animals and a few reports of variable liver injury in humans. Although liver failure from hepatic necrosis is mentioned in some case reports, the mechanism is poorly understood, and clinical details to confirm causality are often scant.[140]

Cannabidiol (CBD) oil is one of the major phytocannabinoids in Cannabis sativa, which is being used for the management of several conditions, including chronic pain and seizure activity.[141] CBD oil is the main ingredient in Epidiolex, approved in 2018 by FDA for the management of Lennox-Gastaut and Dravet syndromes, two pediatric conditions in which epilepsy can be refractory to traditional anticonvulsants.[142,143] In human trials, increases in ALT >3X ULN (without any rise in bilirubin) were seen in 10%–20% of patients, often within one month of starting Epidiolex. These elevations usually resolved spontaneously or after discontinuation or dose reduction of the CBD oil or of VPA taken concomitantly. Importantly, no ALT elevations were seen in subjects not receiving VPA.[142,143] In animals, increases in aminotransferases and bilirubin were seen in a dose-related fashion when CBD was administered acutely with doses up to the equivalent of the maximum Epidiolex dose in humans or when given in lower doses over 10 days. This subacute dosing regimen produced severe toxicity in 75% of mice after 3–4 days.[144] These investigators also found that mice given CBD by gavage for 3 days followed by the intraperitoneal administration of acetaminophen (APAP) on Day 4 developed overt toxicity with a high mortality (37.5%). In contrast, no mortality was observed when CBD was given concurrently with APAP.[145] Greater activation of c-Jun N-terminal kinase was seen in the animals given APAP after CBD and was associated with an SOS-like injury on liver histology. The authors suggested that glutathione depletion and oxidative stress from both drugs were heightened in this setting.[145] These potentially serious adverse drug-drug interactions between CBD and APAP and VPA led to an FDA warning detailing their safety concerns with a call for additional study regarding CBD oil.[146]

BOTANICAL AND ENVIRONMENTAL HEPATOTOXINS

Examples of hepatotoxic mushrooms, fruits, and other foodstuffs, including grains and nuts contaminated by fungal mycotoxins or other potentially injurious compounds, including khat, are listed in Table 91.6.

Mushrooms

There are approximately 100 poisonous varieties of mushrooms among the more than 5000 species, but only about one-third have been associated with fatalities. The amatoxin-containing species belong to three genera: *Amanita*, *Galerina*, and *Lepiota*.[146] More than 90% of cases of fatal poisoning are caused by *Amanita phalloides* (death cap) or *Amanita verna* (destroying angel), found in the Pacific Northwest, Northern California, and the Eastern United States.[147,148]

A fatal outcome can follow the ingestion of a single 50 g (2 oz) mushroom because the toxin is one of the most potent and lethal in nature.[149] Alpha-amatoxin is thermostable, can resist drying for years, and is not inactivated by cooking. Rapidly absorbed through the GI tract, the amatoxin reaches hepatocytes through the enterohepatic circulation and inhibits production of messenger RNA and protein synthesis, leading in turn to cell necrosis. A second toxin, phalloidin, is responsible for the severe gastroenteritis that precedes hepatic and CNS injury.[150,151] Phalloidin disrupts cell membranes by interfering with polymerization of actin. A latent period of 6–20 hours after ingestion of a mushroom precedes the first symptoms of intense abdominal pain, vomiting, and diarrhea. Hepatocellular jaundice and renal failure occur over the next 24–48 hours and are followed by confusion, delirium, convulsions, and eventually coma by 72 hours.[2,142,143] The characteristic hepatic lesion is steatosis and zone 3 hepatic necrosis, with nucleolar inclusions seen on electron microscopy.[5]

Towering serum levels of ALT and AST, similar to those in acetaminophen and other chemical poisonings, can be seen.[152] In a case series of eight patients,[153] the mean serum AST level was

TABLE 91.6 Botanical and Environmental Hepatotoxins

Agent	Toxic Component	Type of Injury	Comment
Ackee fruit	Hypoglycin	Microvesicular steatosis	Jamaican vomiting sickness
Aspergillus flavus	Aflatoxin B1	Acute hepatitis, portal hypertension	Hepatocarcinogenic
Aspergillus tamarii	Cyclopiazonic acid	Acute hepatitis	–
Cycasin	Methylazoxymethanol	Acute hepatitis	–
Khat	?	Chronic hepatitis, fibrosis, cirrhosis	Cases may be confounded by a high frequency of chronic hepatitis B and C among users
Toxic mushrooms	Alpha-amatoxin, phalloidin	ALF	Resembles acetaminophen injury

5488 U/L (range, 1486–12,340), ALT 7618 (range, 3065–15,210), and bilirubin 10.5 mg/dL (range, 1.8–52), with peak levels on Days 4 and 5. In another case series of 27 patients from San Francisco,[154] median ALT levels were 2185 IU/L (range 554–4546 IU/L), and peak AST levels were less than 4000 IU/L by 24–48 hours after admission. Acute kidney injury, requiring dialysis in some cases, has been observed.[153,154] Mortality rates traditionally have been high, especially when the serum ALT level exceeds 1000 U/L, and emergency LT is often required.[154,155] In a case series from Southeast Asia, hepatic involvement was present in 23 of 93 patients (24.7%), and 10 of the 23 (43.5%) died; all deaths were associated with serum bilirubin levels greater than 5 mg/dL.[156] The time from ingestion to symptom onset was about 14 hours in a series from China, in which four deaths from ALF were recorded.[157] Mortality rates from non-Amanita poisonings among several large retrospective series from Switzerland and Iran have been much lower (0%–1.6%).[158,159] In an Italian series, mycologists were able to identify the responsible species in nearly 90%, thereby aiding in management.[160] Several websites, including that of the North American Mycological Association (www.namyco.org/mushrooms_poisoning_syndromes.php), contain photographs of the various poisonous species to help identify the type of mushroom ingested. White et al.[161] have proposed a new updated clinical classification of mushroom poisoning syndromes (Table 91.1).

Some patients with amatoxin poisoning survive with conservative management, which includes NG lavage with activated charcoal, IV penicillin G, *N*-acetylcysteine (using a standard oral or IV protocol [see Chapter 88]), along with milk thistle (*Silybum marianum*) (see Chapter 132).[150,150a] However, the use of these therapeutic modalities is not always effective, and in a large review of 2108 cases over a 20-year period in the United States and Europe,[147] penicillin G, either alone or in combination with other therapy, demonstrated limited benefit. No role for glucocorticoids has been found, but plasmapheresis or hemoperfusion has been beneficial in some instances.[150a,162] In a 2012 study, the addition of IV silibinin (isolated from milk thistle, which blocks the enterohepatic recirculation of amatoxin) in a loading dose of 5 mg/kg, followed by 20 mg/kg continuous infusion for 24 hours, given with standard supportive measures, proved effective in reducing mortality to less than 10% in nearly 1500 cases.[14] These results prompted the authors to recommend silibinin as the antidote of choice. When conservative treatment is ineffective, LT has been lifesaving.[150a]

Other Foodstuffs

The unripe fruit of the ackee tree (*Blighia sapida*), native to Jamaica and West Africa, contains hypoglycin A, a hepatotoxin that produces a clinical syndrome of GI distress and microvesicular steatosis known as *Jamaican vomiting sickness*, that resembles Reye syndrome (see Chapter 97).[163,164] In animals, seizure activity and impaired locomotor and memory function have also been described.[165] Cholestatic jaundice has been described after chronic ingestion.[164] As an important example of a public health effort, following the deaths of 16 children reported in Suriname and French Guyana, no new cases of fatal poisoning from unripe ackee were seen after native "witch doctors" were apprised of its dangers.[166]

Cycasin is a potent hepatotoxin and hepatocarcinogen found in the fruit of the cycad tree (*Cycas circinalis*, *Cycas revoluta*). A small epidemic of acute hepatic injury attributable to the ingestion of cycad nuts was reported from Japan. The purported toxin is methylazoxymethanol, which is normally eliminated or rendered inactive in preparing the nuts before ingestion.[5]

Aflatoxins are a family of mycotoxins found in *Aspergillus flavus* and related fungi that are ubiquitous in tropical and subtropical regions. They contaminate peanuts, cashews, soybeans, and grains stored under warm, moist conditions and are well-known hepatotoxins and hepatocarcinogens.[2,5] Aflatoxin B1, a potent inhibitor of RNA synthesis, is the most hepatotoxic member of the

Updated Mushroom Poisoning Classification

Group	Syndrome	Subgroups (Implicated Toxin or Species)
1	Cytotoxic mushroom poisoning	Subgroup 1.1: primarily hepatotoxicity 1A: primary hepatotoxicity (amatoxins) Subgroup 1.2: primary nephrotoxicity 1B: early primary nephrotoxicity (amino hexadienoic acid) 1C: delayed primary nephrotoxicity (orellanines)
2	Neurotoxic mushroom poisoning	Primary neurotoxicity 2A: hallucinogenic mushrooms (psilocybins and related toxins) 2B: autonomic-toxicity mushrooms (muscarines) 2C: CNS-toxicity mushrooms (ibotenic acid/muscimol) 2D: morel neurologic syndrome (*Morchella* spp.)
3	Myotoxic mushroom poisoning	Syndromes with rhabdomyolysis as primary feature 3A: rapid onset (*Russula* spp.) 3B: delayed onset (*Tricholoma* spp.)
4	Metabolic, endocrine and related toxicity mushroom poisoning	Various clinical presentations 4A: GABA-blocking mushroom poisoning (gyromitrins) 4B: disulfiram-like (coprines) 4C: polyporic poisoning (polyporic acid) 4D: trichothecene poisoning (*Podostroma* spp.) 4E: hypoglycemia (*Trogia venenata*) 4F: hyperprolactinemia (*Boletus satanas*) 4G: pancytopenia (*Ganoderma neojaponicum*)
5	Gastrointestinal irritant mushroom poisoning	Various mushrooms causing predominantly GI symptoms (nausea, vomiting, diarrhea, and abdominal pain
6	Miscellaneous adverse reactions to mushrooms	6A: shiitake mushroom dermatitis 6B: erythromelagic mushrooms (*Clitocybe acromelagia*) 6C: *Paxillus* syndrome[a] (*Paxillus involutus*) 6D: encephalopathy syndrome (*Pleurocybella porrigens*)

[a]Hypersensitivity reaction with rapid onset of vomiting, diarrhea, abdominal pain, and hemolytic anemia with reduced urine output and/or AKI and hemoglobinuria.

After White J, Weinstein SA, De Haro L, et al. Mushroom poisoning: a proposed new clinical classification. *Toxicon*. 2019;157:53e65.

family. Reactive metabolites are formed by CYP enzymes, and malnutrition is a possible potentiating factor (perhaps because of the depletion of glutathione). When consumed in large quantities, aflatoxin B1 is responsible for a clinical syndrome characterized by fever, malaise, anorexia, and vomiting, followed by jaundice. Portal hypertension with splenomegaly and ascites may develop over the next few weeks. In large epidemics, mortality rates have approached 25% and correlate with the dose ingested.[5] Zone 3 hepatic necrosis without inflammation is the characteristic lesion. Other histologic findings include cholestasis, microvesicular steatosis, and bile duct proliferation.[167]

The risk of HCC correlates with the amount of aflatoxin consumed, especially in sub-Saharan Africa and Eastern China, where wheat often exceeds rice as a staple in the diet.[168] Alcohol and possibly exposure to DDT (see earlier) may play an enhancing role in hepatocarcinogenesis.[169] An even more important cofactor may be HBV.[170,171] The frequency of a mutation in the *TP53* tumor suppressor gene correlates with the development of HCC in these regions, but this mutation is rare in HCC from Western countries (see Chapter 96).[170]

Chewing fresh khat leaves (*Catha edulis*), predominantly by men from East Africa and Yemen, have been associated with acute and chronic liver injury, including severe fibrosis and cirrhosis, liver failure, and death.[172–175,175a] Injury appears to be dose-dependent, but the hepatotoxic moiety has not been identified.[175a] Although many patients have other risk factors for chronic liver disease (including hepatitis B and C, alcohol, and schistosomiasis),[176] case-control studies have strongly implicated khat as a growing health hazard.[177]

In a mouse model, the antioxidant coenzyme Q appeared able to ameliorate hepatic and renal injury induced by khat,[178] although human studies have not been performed.

VITAMINS

Vitamins, dietary, weight-loss and body-building supplements, herbal remedies, and other nutraceuticals are often the main components of many CAM preparations, and their use continues to increase (see later and Chapter 131).[179] According to results of the 2012 National Health Interview Survey, nearly 42 million Americans (18.6% of the population) used herbal or homeopathic therapies in the previous year for a variety of health conditions,[179] including chronic liver disorders,[10,180] despite the absence of formal controlled clinical trials to assess their safety and efficacy in this setting.[179,181–183] In a population-based survey of 1040 patients with a wide array of chronic liver diseases (including 18% with cirrhosis), concurrent use of a CAM preparation was listed by 27.3%.[180] The most commonly used products were vitamins and other dietary supplements in 18% and herbal remedies in 16.8%. Interestingly, a CAM preparation had been prescribed by a physician in up to 32% of respondents.[180]

According to the CAM Market Report, (accessed at www.grandviewresearch.com/industry-analysis/complementary-alternative-medicine-market), the global CAM market is expected to expand from $82.27 billion in 2020 at a compound annual growth rate of 22.03% from 2021 to 2028, reaching >$400 billion by 2028. Traditional alternative medicines and botanicals are poised to continue the greatest expansion. However, many so-called health foods, dietary and weight-loss supplements, body-building compounds, and herbal products are potent hepatotoxins that can lead to ALF and the need for emergency LT.[15,16,184,185,185a,185b] Safety concerns involving such dietary supplements persist, despite the enactment of the Dietary Supplement Health and Education Act in 1994.[182,186–188]

Vitamin A

Among vitamin supplements, vitamin A remains the most important hepatotoxin when ingested in supratherapeutic doses. Vitamin A (retinol) is a dose- and duration-dependent hepatotoxin capable of causing injury ranging from asymptomatic elevations in serum aminotransferase levels with minor hepatic histologic changes to perisinusoidal fibrosis leading to noncirrhotic portal hypertension and, in some cases, cirrhosis.[189] Approximately one-third of the U.S. population is estimated to take vitamin supplements containing vitamin A, with as many as 3% of products providing a daily dose of at least 25,000 IU. Hypervitaminosis A usually is the result of self-ingestion, rather than intentional overdose, and all age groups have been affected.[190] The average daily dose of vitamin A in reported cases of liver disease has been nearly 100,000 IU, taken over an average duration of 7.2 years, for a mean cumulative dose of 229 million IU. Liver injury has been described with daily doses of 10,000–45,000 IU,[191] and cirrhosis has occurred after a daily intake of 25,000 IU for at least 6 years.[189,191] By contrast, long-term use of low-dose vitamin A supplements (250–5000 retinol equivalents per day) does not appear to be toxic.[192]

Because of the long half-life of vitamin A in the liver (50 days to 1 year),[191,193] the fibrotic process may continue because of the slow release of hepatic vitamin A stores despite discontinuation of oral intake of the vitamin.[194] Genetic factors may play a role, and apparent familial hypervitaminosis A has occurred in four siblings who ingested large doses as treatment for congenital ichthyosis.[195] Vitamin A toxicity has been reported in native Alaskans who ingest large amounts of fresh polar bear liver,[189] which is plentiful in these arctic predators but does not cause them hepatic injury.[196] Water-soluble, emulsified, and solid formulations of vitamin A are up to 10 times as toxic as oil-based preparations because of higher peak plasma levels, greater hepatic concentrations, and less fecal loss with the water-miscible formulations.[197]

Hepatotoxicity from vitamin A has been attributed to activation of hepatic stellate cells, the body's principal storage site of the vitamin. Resulting hyperplasia and hypertrophy produce sinusoidal obstruction and increased collagen synthesis, leading in turn to portal hypertension.[198] Rare cases of peliosis hepatis have also been attributed to hypervitaminosis A. Ethanol interferes with the conversion of beta carotene, a precursor of vitamin A, to retinol, and the combination of ethanol and beta carotene has resulted in hepatotoxicity in various experimental models.[199]

Liver biopsy specimens show increased storage of vitamin A, seen as characteristic greenish autofluorescence after irradiation with ultraviolet light.[189] The excess vitamin A is stored initially in stellate cells that lie in the space of Disse and become hyperplastic and hypertrophic. The enlarged clear stellate cells compress the hepatic sinusoids, giving rise to a "Swiss cheese" or honeycombed appearance.[189] Hepatocellular injury is usually minor, with microvesicular steatosis and focal degeneration and without significant necrosis or inflammation. Hepatic fibrosis in a perisinusoidal distribution can arise from activated stellate cells that transform into myofibroblasts. In a widely cited series,[189] cirrhosis was present in 59%, chronic hepatitis in 34%, microvesicular steatosis in 21%, perisinusoidal fibrosis in 14%, and peliosis in 3% of cases.

In affected persons, hepatomegaly is common, and in severe cases, splenomegaly, ascites, and esophageal variceal bleeding may be features.[2,189] Hypervitaminosis A can also involve the skin and CNS.[2] Liver biochemical test abnormalities, present in two-thirds of cases, are nonspecific, with only modest elevations in serum aminotransferase and alkaline phosphatase levels.

The diagnosis of vitamin A toxicity rests on a dietary and medication history and clinical suspicion. Plasma vitamin A levels may be normal, and the diagnosis is supported by the demonstration of increased hepatic stores of vitamin A and characteristic histologic findings.[200] The diagnosis may be delayed for several years if hepatotoxicity is not recognized or is misdiagnosed.[189,191]

Symptoms resolve and liver enzymes gradually normalize after discontinuation of vitamin A ingestion in less severe cases, but deterioration may continue in cases of severe intoxication, particularly when cirrhosis is already present.[191] Features of liver failure and cirrhosis at the time of diagnosis indicate a poor prognosis, and LT may be required.[2] Alcohol can potentiate hepatotoxicity and should be avoided. Vitamin A supplements generally should be avoided in other types of liver disease because of possible accentuation of hepatic injury and fibrosis.[199] Severe liver injury has rarely been reported with the use of acitretin, a vitamin A metabolite.[201]

Niacin

Nicotinic acid (vitamin B_3, niacin) is used primarily to treat dyslipidemia by increasing HDL and reducing triglyceride synthesis and VLDL and LDL secretion, via inhibition of hepatocyte diacylglycerol acyltransferase 2.[202] Immediate-release (IR) crystalline preparations given in therapeutic doses have rarely been reported to cause hepatic injury[203] but are associated with flushing and other unpleasant side effects.[204,205] When taken in massive supratherapeutic doses (e.g., 20,000 mg), the IR form has been associated with ALF requiring LT.[206] In contrast to the IR formulations, sustained-release (SR) niacin, developed to reduce the vasodilatory effects of niacin, appears to be a significant hepatotoxin, with about 20% of patients developing symptomatic elevations in ALT and AST levels.[203] Several cases have followed a switch from an IR to an SR formulation. Liver injury has been reported to occur after a widely variable latent period ranging from 1 week to as long as 2 years.[203] Symptoms suggesting acute hepatocellular necrosis include nausea, vomiting, and fatigue, followed by jaundice and pruritus, although recovery within 4–8 weeks is the rule and ALF is rarely reported.[204] Importantly, combining niacin with a statin does not increase the risk of hepatotoxicity.[207]

The mechanism underlying niacin liver injury is thought to be the formation of formulation- and dose-dependent hepatotoxic pyrimidine metabolites. Although amidation pathways rapidly convert IR formulations into nicotinuric acid, thereby leading to vasodilatation and flushing through prostaglandin formation, SR preparations allow for reduced amounts of nicotinuric acid but promote the conversion of niacin to hepatotoxic pyrimidine intermediates.[208] As a result, extended (controlled) and SR formulations are contraindicated in patients with liver disease.[209]

HERBAL, DIETARY, WEIGHT-LOSS, AND BODY-BUILDING SUPPLEMENTS

The increasing use of CAM preparations is well described in patients with liver disease (see Chapter 131.[10,180,181] Silymarin (*S. marianum*, milk thistle) is the most commonly used herbal preparation among these patients,[10]and although it appears to be quite safe,[210] if ineffective.[211–213] An increasing number of reports of hepatotoxicity from several other classes of herbal, dietary, weight-reduction, and body-building supplements (collectively referred to as HDS) have paralleled the rise in use of CAM therapies in both the United States and other Western nations.[184,185a,185b,188214–218] Indeed, the percentage of cases of hepatotoxicity due to HDS in DILI registries has risen steadily in the 2000s, increasing from 7% to 20% of cases in the United States DILI Network between 2004 and 2013[214] and exceeding 50% in some Chinese and other Asian series.[219–221] All age groups can be affected, and according to the 2020 annual report of the American Association of Poison Control Centers, HDS accounted for more than 6% of all poisonings in children 5 years of age and younger, an increase over 2019.[222]

Many HDS compounds are listed as potentially hepatotoxic, including several that are no longer sold (including germander and usnic acid-containing products) and others that have undergone reformulations (e.g., Hydroxycut) (Table 91.7).[214–218,223] Other implicated agents lack sufficient evidence to support their hepatotoxicity.[224] Similarly, the LiverTox database compiled by the National Institutes of Health and National Library of Medicine reviews more than 60 of the best known HDS for potential hepatotoxicity and has found that nearly 40% have no evidence to implicate them in clinical hepatotoxicity (level of evidence E) and another 30% had only limited evidence of liver injury (levels D and C) (see Table 91.7). Additionally, although more than 50 traditional Chinese medicines (TCMs) have been associated with hepatic injury,[225] causality has been established for only about half of these compounds.[226] When TCM has been analyzed prospectively for the development of hepatic injury (defined as a serum ALT level > the ULN), fewer than 4% of 21,470 patients without liver disease developed an ALT level greater than 1 time but less than 5 times the ULN, and only 0.12% had an ALT level exceeding five times the ULN, with a return to normal after the agent was discontinued.[227] Similarly, among nearly 6900 inpatients taking herbal medications in Korean hospitals, 5.1% were diagnosed with liver injury (based on elevated liver biochemical test levels on admission), and 3.1% developed liver injury at the time of discharge.[228] Among 354 patients with elevated liver biochemical test levels on admission, only 9 (2.5%) showed a further increase after treatment with an herbal medication, and among nearly 4800 patients with normal liver test levels on admission, only 27 (0.6%) had liver injury at discharge. The authors concluded that herbal medicines rarely aggravate existing liver injury and that de novo injury is uncommon.[228]

Warnings have been issued for several agents, and, in a few instances, the FDA and other health authorities have requested their removal from the marketplace [e.g., kava kava, *Ephedra* (ma huang), LipoKinetix (usnic acid), Hydroxycut, and kratom in the United States,[223,229,230] and germander in France[231] (see later)]. Any patient with liver disease should be questioned about the ingestion of herbal remedies; Estes et al.,[185] for example, documented the use of several commonly promoted herbal agents (including LipoKinetix, skullcap, ma huang, chaparral, and kava kava) in half of 20 patients with ALF over a 2-year period.

Table 91.8 lists the known or potential hepatotoxic components of the most commonly implicated HDS compounds associated with liver injury. The Roussel Uclaf Causality Assessment Method has emerged as the most widely used diagnostic algorithm to diagnose herbal and dietary supplement liver injury in addition to drug-induced liver injury.[232] The purported hepatotoxicity of many HDS products has come under increasing scrutiny and criticism by Teschke et al., who have drawn attention to many pitfalls in the causality assessment of these agents.[233–238] Although some cases have had well-documented hepatic injury, others have been more weakly confirmed and have not considered alternative causes.[238] In addition, several herbal formulations are known to have been contaminated by other hepatotoxic substances, an occurrence that is probably more common than currently appreciated.[239–241] The section on herbal medications in the LiverTox website notes that adulterants, such as skullcap or other contaminants, may be responsible for cases of liver injury attributed to chondroitin, echinacea, Jin Bu huan, and flavocoxid. Indeed, mislabeling of HDS products is not only frequent but potentially dangerous. In an analysis performed by the National Center for Natural Products Research at the University of Mississippi using ultrahigh performance chromatography coupled with mass spectrometry, Navarro et al. studied more than 340 HDS products used by more than 1260 patients, of which 272 had labels listing their ingredients. They found

TABLE 91.7 HDS Products Specifically Discussed in LiverTox With their Level of Evidence for Hepatotoxicity

HDS Product	Level of Evidence[a]
• *Aloe vera*	B
• Apoaequorin	E
• Ashwagandha	C
• *Astragalus*	E
• Bilberry	E
• Black cohosh	A
• *Boswellia*	E
• Butterbur	C
• Cascara	C
• Cat's claw	E
• Chamomile	E
• Chaparral	B
• Chinese and Other Asian Herbal Medicines	
• Ba Jiao Lian	B
• Chi R Yun	C
• Jin Bu Huan	[b]
• Ma Huang [*Ephedra*]	C
• *Polygonum multiflorum*	A
• Sho Saiko To and Dai Saiko To	B
• Chondroitin	C
• Comfrey	C
• Crofelemer	E
• *Echinacea*	D
• *Ephedra*	C
• Eugenol	C
• Fenugreek	E
• Flavocoxid	C
• *Garcinia cambogia*	B
• Germander	A
• Ginkgo	E
• Ginseng	E
• Glucosamine	D
• Greater celandine	B
• Green tea extract	A
• *Hoodia*	E
• Hops	E
• Horny goat weed	E
• Horse chestnut	D
• Horsetail	C

TABLE 91.7 HDS Products Specifically Discussed in LiverTox With their Level of Evidence for Hepatotoxicity—cont'd

HDS Product	Level of Evidence[a]
• Hyssop	E
• Kava kava	A
• Kratom	B
• Lavender	E
• Maca	E
• Margosa oil	C
• Melatonin	E
• Milk thistle	E
• Mistletoe	E
• Noni	C
• Passionflower	E
• Pennyroyal oil	B
• Quercetin	E
• Red yeast rice	C
• Resveratrol	E
• Saw palmetto	D
• Senna	D
• Skullcap	B
• Spirulina	D
• St. John's Wort	E
• *Tribulus*	E
• Turmeric (curcumin)	B
• Usnic acid	B
• Uva ursi	E
• Valerian	C
• Yohimbine	E
• Multiingredient nutritional supplements	
• Herbalife	A
• Hydroxycut	B
• Move free (chondroitin)	C
• OxyELITE Pro	A
• SLIMQUICK	C

[a]LiverTox levels of evidence of hepatotoxicity: A = well-established hepatotoxicity with >50 cases including case-series; B = highly likely hepatotoxicity with a characteristic clinical signature and 12–50 published cases; C = probable hepatotoxicity but reported uncommonly with no established clinical signature and fewer than 12 published cases; D = possibly hepatotoxicity based on single case reports but fewer than three cases in the literature and injury is considered rare; E = unlikely or no evidence for hepatotoxicity despite extensive use.
[b]Unable to be classified due to adulterants.

serious inaccuracies in the product labels of greater than 50% of the HDS tested.[242] These discrepancies included the failure to confirm the true ingredients in 80% of steroidal compounds, more than 50% of nutritional vitamins, and greater than 40% of botanicals. More disturbing was the finding of undisclosed anabolic steroids in half of the body-building supplements and undisclosed potential hepatotoxins (diclofenac and tamoxifen) in other products.[242] Similarly, in a study of herbal and Ayurvedic compounds used by traditional healers in India, Philips et al. found that several heavy metals (arsenic, lead, mercury, antimony, and cadmium) were present in toxic amounts ranging from 10 to 100 times safe levels.[243] Increased mortality was reported in some recipients of these compounds but was not necessarily due to hepatotoxicity.

TABLE 91.8 Features of Selected Well-Described Hepatotoxic Herbal, Dietary, Weight-Loss, and Body-Building Supplements

Agent	Popular Uses	Source	Postulated Hepatotoxic Component	Hepatic Injury
Black cohosh	Menopausal symptoms	*Cimicifuga racemosa*	Uncertain; ?triterpene glycosides	Latency 2–12 weeks; acute hepatocellular jaundice, some cases autoimmune hepatitis; resolution in 2–6 months
Cascara	Laxative	*Cascara sagrada*	Anthracene glycoside	Cholestatic hepatitis
Chaparral leaf (greasewood, creosote bush)	"Liver tonic," burn salve, weight loss	*Larrea tridentata*	Nordihydroguaiaretic acid	Acute viral-like; latency 3–12 weeks; hepatitis, ALF leading to LT reported; positive rechallenge cases
Chaso/onshido	Weight loss	–	*N*-Nitro-fenfluramine	Acute hepatitis, ALF
Comfrey	Herbal tea	*Symphytum* spp.	Pyrrolizidine alkaloids	Acute SOS after latency 1–2 months with acute RUQ pain, nausea, ascites, weight gain, and hepatocellular jaundice that can lead to ALF; a subacute or chronic injury with insidious onset also described
Garcinia	Weight loss	*Garcinia cambogia*	Hydrocitric acid (HCA)	Acute hepatocellular injury after 1–8 weeks latency
Germander	Weight loss, fever	*Teucrium chamaedry*, *Teucrium capitatum*, *Teucrium polium*	Teucrin A (Diterpenoids, epoxides)	Acute viral-like hepatitis after mean 9 weeks. latency with positive rechallenge and rapid recovery, rare reports of ALF; a second form of injury resembles autoimmune hepatitis after 6–9 months latency presenting with arthralgias and fever
Greater celandine	Gallstones, IBS	*Chelidonium majus*	Uncertain; ?isoquinoline alkaloids	Acute cholestatic hepatitis after 1–6 months in about 50% of cases, resolution in 2 –6 months
Green tea leaf extract	Multiple	*Camellia sinensis*	Catechins	Acute viral-like hepatitis within 3 months (range 0.5–7 months); biopsies have shown variable necrosis, eosinophilia; no immunoallergic features; most recover
Herbalife	Nutritional supplement, weight loss	–	Various; ?*Ephedra*	Insidious hepatocellular or mixed injury presenting with fatigue, nausea, abdominal pain and jaundice after 2–9 months latency; no hypersensitivity features; rare instances of ALF
Hydroxycut	Weight loss	*C. sinensis*, among other constituents	Uncertain	Acute hepatitis, ?ALF
Impila	Multiple	*Callilepis laureola*	Potassium atractylate	Hepatic necrosis
Kava kava	Anxiolytic	*Piper methysticum*	?Kava lactone, pipermethystine (vs. other contaminants)	Acute hepatitis or cholestasis after variable latency (2–24 weeks) with occasional hypersensitivity features and reports of positive rechallenge; rare cases of ALF leading to LT; most patients recover within 1–3 months
Kombucha	Weight loss	Lichen alkaloid	Usnic acid	Acute hepatitis (see LipoKinetix)
Kratom	Pain relief and as a substitute for opioids	*Mitragyna speciosa*	Mitragynine, 7-OH-mitragynine (partial agonists of mu-opioid receptor)	Liver toxicity as well as seizures, respiratory depression and death
Limbrel (Flavocoxid)	Osteoarthritis	Plant bioflavonoids	Baicalin, ?epicatechin,? shullcap	Acute mixed hepatocellular-cholestatic injury
LipoKinetix	Weight loss	Lichen alkaloid	Usnic acid	Acute viral-like hepatitis with jaundice; cases of ALF leading to LT
Mistletoe	Asthma, infertility	*Viscum album*	Uncertain	Hepatitis (in combination with skullcap)
OxyELITE Pro	Weight loss, body building	Multiple ingredients	?Aegeline	Acute hepatocellular viral-like hepatitis with jaundice with marked elevations in ALT; liver biopsy showing severe necrosis; no hypersensitivity features; mortality of 10% in cases with jaundice; second injury pattern with subacute or chronic autoimmune features

Continued

TABLE 91.8 Features of Selected Well-Described Hepatotoxic Herbal, Dietary, Weight-Loss, and Body-Building Supplements—cont'd

Agent	Popular Uses	Source	Postulated Hepatotoxic Component	Hepatic Injury
Pennyroyal (squawmint oil)	Abortifacient	*Hedeoma pulegioides, Mentha pulegium*	Pulegone, monoterpenes	Produces an acute acetaminophen-like injury within hours of ingestion resulting in cardiovascular collapse, DIC, and multiorgan failure with liver injury likely due to ischemic hepatitis
Prostata	Prostatism	Multiple	Uncertain	Chronic cholestasis
Sassafras	Herbal tea	*Sassafras albidum*	Safrole	HCC (in animals)
Skullcap	Anxiolytic	*Scutellaria*	Diterpenoids vs. adulterants	Acute hepatocellular jaundice after 6–24 weeks with rapid resolution; rare reports of ALF
Traditional Chinese Medicines				
Jin bu huan	Sleep aid, analgesic	*Lycopodium serratum*	?Levo-tetrahydropalmitine	Acute or chronic hepatitis or cholestasis, steatosis
Ma Huang	Weight loss	*Ephedra* spp.	Ephedrine	Acute viral hepatitis-like injury with fatigue, nausea, abdominal pain, jaundice, ALF requiring LT reported; most recover in 1–6 months
Shou-Wu-Pian, Chinese knotweed	Antiaging, neuroprotection, laxative	*Polygonum multiflorum* (fleece-flower root)	?Anthraquinones	Acute hepatitis or cholestasis HLA allele B*35:01 appears to be a major risk factor
Sho-saiko-to	Multiple	*Scutellaria* root	Diterpenoids	Hepatocellular necrosis, cholestasis, steatosis, granulomas
Valerian	Sedative	*Valeriana officinalis*	Uncertain	Rare instances of mild-moderate hepatocellular or mixed injury with recovery after 2–4 months; reports of ALF have occurred only when taken with other herbal preparations

ALF, Acute liver failure; *HHC*, hepatocellular carcinoma; *LT*, liver transplant; *SOS*, sinusoidal obstruction syndrome.

Green tea extracts (GTEs), derived from *Camellia sinensis*, have long been associated with herbal and dietary supplement hepatotoxicity. The implicated causative agent is epigallocatechin-3-gallate when taken in amounts ranging from 140 to 1000 mg daily, although a significant degree of interindividual susceptibility exists regarding the hepatocellular injury.[244] Navarro et al. studied various HDS for the presence of catechins and found that, when assayed, just over half of 97 products contained at least one catechin.[245] However, nearly 40% of 73 HDS products that contained catechins did not list GTE or catechins on their labels. Weight-loss products were most likely to be mislabeled in this manner. Perhaps not surprisingly, the mislabeling was also seen in reverse (i.e., several products that listed catechins as an ingredient contained either no or only negligible amounts of catechins).[245]

In addition to the potential hepatotoxicity of many HDS products, several investigators have drawn attention to the risk of herbal-drug interactions that may be mediated through the CYP system[246] or *P*-glycoproteins.[247] One of the best known interactions is seen with St. John's wort, a strong inducer of CYP3A4, which while not considered hepatotoxic when taken alone, can reduce the bioavailability (and subsequent effectiveness) of several drugs, including certain DAA regimens for the treatment of chronic hepatitis C (see Chapter 82).[248]

Because the production and review standards for herbal products and dietary supplements are not as strict as for pharmaceutical products[182] and most HDS are considered to be food products rather than pharmaceuticals (and thus assumed to be safe),[188] it should not be surprising that a number of groups have called for increased regulation regarding the manufacture, quality control, safety, and efficacy of these products in the United States and abroad.[183,187,249–252] Additionally, improved methods to screen for the hepatotoxicity of active compounds in TCMs and HDS are being developed[188,253,254] and more accurate causality assessments (including the development of novel HDS biomarkers) have been recommended to improve the quality of case presentations.[255,256]

Two large case series are instructive in defining the presentation and outcome of HDS in Western countries. In an analysis of the Spanish DILI registry,[218] HDS cases were younger (mean age 48 vs. 55) and more likely to be female (63% vs. 49%) compared with DILI cases. Jaundice was present in 78% and was the most frequent symptom that brought a patient to medical attention. Hypersensitivity hallmarks (fever, rash, and eosinophilia) were present in 28%, and a higher percentage of HDS cases progressed to liver failure (6%), compared with 4% of conventional drugs and none of the patients with anabolic steroid injury. In the United States DILI Network registry,[11] body-building HDS resulted in reversible jaundice in young men, whereas the nonbody-building HDS liver injury occurred predominantly in middle-aged women, was hepatocellular in nature, and, as in the Spanish series, more often led to death or LT compared with non-HDS DILI (13% vs. 3%).[11]

Features of Toxicity

The clinicopathologic features of hepatotoxicity caused by the specific HDS and TCM discussed below are derived from the best available evidence.[7,11,12,214–218,223–225]

Pyrrolizidine Alkaloids

Pyrrolizidine alkaloids (PAs) are found in approximately 3% of all flowering plant species throughout the world, and ingestion of such plants, often as medicinal teas or in other formulations, can produce acute and chronic liver disease, including SOS, in humans and livestock.[252] SOS was first reported in the 1950s as a disease of Jamaican children, manifesting with acute abdominal distention, marked hepatomegaly, and ascites—a triad that resembles Budd-Chiari syndrome (see Chapter 87).[5] The disease was linked to consumption of "bush tea," made largely from plants of *Senecio*, *Heliotropium*, *Crotalaria*, and *Symphytum* species. Many were taken as a folk remedy for acute childhood illnesses. The disease was characterized histologically by centrilobular hepatic congestion with occlusion of the hepatic venules, leading to congestive cirrhosis. In Afghanistan, ingestion of PA-contaminated grains and bread led to a large epidemic of SOS, affecting 8000 persons and innumerable sheep.[5] Although it is a dose-dependent hepatotoxin, comfrey (*Symphytum officinale*) remains commercially available on numerous internet sites and can be found in toxic amounts in "medicinal" herbal teas around the world.[258–260]

Hepatotoxic PAs are cyclic diesters, and some forms (e.g., fulvine, monocrotaline) cause both liver and lung injury. The mechanism of injury is postulated to be impairment of nucleic acid synthesis by reactive metabolites of PAs generated by hepatic microsomes, leading in turn to progressive loss of sinusoidal cells and sinusoidal hemorrhage, as well as injury to the endothelium of the terminal hepatic venule, with deposition of fibrin[256,257] alkaloids and dehydroretronecine generated by the action of the CYP system bind to cellular proteins to form pyrrole-protein adducts and have been shown to be cytotoxic to hepatic sinusoidal endothelial cells due to depletion of glutathione.[261] The ability to test for these pyrrole-protein adducts in patients with PA-associated SOS provides an important diagnostic tool, with a positive predictive value of 95.8% and a negative predictive value of 100%.[262] In addition to PAs, PA N-oxides have been found to be hepatotoxic.[263]

SOS causes acute, subacute, and chronic injury. The acute form is characterized by zone 3 necrosis and sinusoidal dilatation, leading to a Budd-Chiari–like syndrome with abdominal pain and the rapid onset of ascites within 3–6 weeks of ingestion.[5] In Jamaica, the course was rapidly fatal in 15%–20% of affected persons. Approximately one-half of the patients with the acute form recovered spontaneously; transition to a more chronic form of injury occurred in the remainder.[2] In the subacute and chronic forms, central fibrosis and bridging between central veins led to a form of cirrhosis similar to that seen with chronic passive hepatic congestion (so-called cardiac cirrhosis). At one time, this form of injury accounted for one-third of the cases of cirrhosis seen in Jamaica, with death often resulting from complications of portal hypertension in as few as 1–3 years.[2] Certain PAs, such as comfrey extracts, are also hepatocarcinogenic and, like aflatoxins, induce mutations of the *TP53* gene.[257]

Germander

The blossoms of plants from the Labiatae family (*Teucrium chamaedrys*) were used for years in herbal teas and in the mid-1980s as capsules predominantly for weight reduction in France, until several dozen cases of liver injury, including fatal hepatic failure, forced its withdrawal from the French market in 1992.[231,264] Most patients were middle-aged women who had ingested germander for 3–18 weeks, with a consequent development of acute hepatocellular injury, often with jaundice. The injury usually resolved within 1.5–6 months after the germander was discontinued, with prompt recurrence after rechallenge in many persons. The cause of germander hepatotoxicity is an interplay between toxic metabolites and immunoallergic mechanisms. Germander is composed of several compounds, including glycosides, flavonoids, and furan-containing diterpenoids, all of which are converted by the CYP system (especially CYP3A) to reactive metabolites.[246] The furanoneoclerodane diterpene teucrin A is thought to be the toxic component.[265,266] Covalent binding to cellular proteins, depletion of hepatic glutathione, apoptosis, and cytoskeleton membrane injury (bleb formation) cause cell disruption in animal models. Epoxide hydrolase on plasma membranes is a target of germander antibodies, which have been found in the sera of patients who have consumed germander teas over long periods of time.[267] Reports of liver injury have also appeared with other species of *Teucrium*, including *Teucrium capitatum*[268] and *Teucrium polium*.[269]

Chaparral

The dried leaf of the desert shrub chaparral (*Larrea tridentata*), also known as greasewood or creosote bush, is ground into a tea or used in capsules or tablets for various ailments. Multiple reports of hepatitis have appeared; most cases have occurred within 1–12 months of use and resolved within a few weeks to months of discontinuation.[270] Among the 13 cases reported to the FDA, acute hepatocellular or cholestatic injury was observed, with 2 cases of ALF requiring LT and 4 cases progressing to cirrhosis. Renal toxicity and rash can accompany liver injury.[270] The active ingredient, nordihydroguaiaretic acid, an inhibitor of COX and lipoxygenase pathways, is the likely cause of hepatic injury, although the mechanism may also involve phytoestrogen-induced effects on the liver.[271] A case of recurrence on rechallenge suggests a possible role for immunoallergy.[261]

Pennyroyal

The leaves of pennyroyal (the common name for two related plant species, *Hedeoma pulegioides* and *Mentha pulegium*) are used to make oils (squawmint oil), tablets, and home-brewed mint teas. The plant contains pulegone and smaller amounts of other monoterpene ketones. Oxidative metabolites of pulegone (e.g., menthofuran) bind to cellular proteins and deplete hepatic glutathione, thereby leading to liver injury.[246,272] Cases of hepatocellular injury, including fatal necrosis, were associated with GI and CNS toxicity within a few hours of ingestion. In animals, inhibition of pulegone metabolism by the CYP system with disulfiram and cimetidine has limited pennyroyal hepatotoxicity.[273] The use of *N*-acetylcysteine may protect against pennyroyal toxicity in human cases.[273]

Traditional Chinese Herbal Medicines (TCM)

TCMs in China are derived from more than 800 patent drugs for use by TCM practitioners.[274] Most TCMs are composed of several different herbal compounds and usually are dominated by one main ingredient referred to as the "king herb."[274] More than 50 different herbs and herbal mixtures were found in a TCM literature review by Teschke et al., although causality was established for only about half of the compounds.[226] The difficulties inherent in determining hepatotoxicity have also been discussed by others.[275] The traditional preparations discussed below are among the best characterized with respect to hepatotoxicity.[225,226]

Jin bu huan (*Lycopodium serratum*) is a traditional herbal remedy that has been used as a sedative and analgesic for more than 1000 years.[271] Numerous cases of hepatic injury have appeared,[276–278] with a mean latency of 20 weeks (range, 7–52 weeks) after the start of Jin bu huan in recommended doses. Associated symptoms and signs included fever, fatigue, nausea, pruritus, abdominal pain, hepatomegaly, and jaundice. Liver biopsy specimens from a small number of patients showed a range of histopathologic changes, including lobular hepatitis with prominent eosinophils, mild hepatitis with microvesicular steatosis, and fibrotic expansion of the portal tracts. The injury resolved within a mean of 8 weeks (range, 2–30 weeks) but could recur on rechallenge.[277] The only predisposing factor was female gender. Serum ALT levels were increased 20–50-fold, with minor increases in the alkaline phosphatase level, except in one patient with cholestasis. Hyperbilirubinemia was prominent in the more severe cases. A case of chronic hepatitis has been described. The mechanism of injury may involve levotetrahydropalmatine, a neuroactive metabolite with structural similarity to PAs. The FDA banned the importation of jin bu huan anodyne tablets into the United States years ago.[271]

Sho-saiko-to (xiao-chai-hu-tang, dai-saiko-to) contains *Scutellaria* root (skullcap), which is a likely hepatotoxin.[279–281] The spectrum of liver injury has included hepatocellular necrosis, microvesicular steatosis, cholestasis, granuloma formation, and a flare of autoimmune hepatitis. While most cases have been transient and reversible, acute liver failure and need for LT have also been reported (LiverTox website). Reversible acute hepatitis or cholestasis has followed the consumption of shou-wu-pian, a product derived from *Polygonum multiflorum*,[282,283] which contains toxic anthraquinones. A genetic predisposition has been found linked to the HLA allele B*35-01, which was present in 88% of 26 cases compared to just 12% of patients with other forms of acute DILI and 5% of controls.[284]

Ma huang, derived from plants of *Ephedra* species, has been reported to cause acute, sometimes severe, hepatitis, including ALF.[185,274,285] The active ingredient, ephedrine, has also been linked to severe adverse cardiovascular and CNS effects, including fatalities, when used as a stimulant and weight-loss aid.[286] The FDA issued a ruling in 2004 that *Ephedra*-containing products present an unreasonable risk and should be avoided.[287]

Weight-Loss Products

Chaso and Onshido are Chinese herbal dietary weight-loss supplements that were reported to cause severe liver injury, with a mean serum ALT level of 1978 U/L (range, 283–4074 U/L), in 12 patients.[288] ALF developed in two persons; one died, and the other survived after undergoing LT. The suspected hepatotoxic ingredient was *N*-nitroso-fenfluramine, a derivative of the appetite suppressant fenfluramine, which was withdrawn from the U.S. market in 1997.[289]

Another dietary supplement used for weight loss, LipoKinetix [composed of norephedrine, sodium usniate (usnic acid), diiodothyronine, yohimbine, and caffeine], was associated with acute hepatitis, including ALF requiring LT.[184,290] In a case series of seven previously healthy patients (four women, three men; mean age, 27 years), acute hepatitis developed after a latent period of less than 4 weeks in five patients and 8–12 weeks in the other two. Mean serum ALT levels were 4501 U/L (range, 438–14,150 U/L), and mean serum bilirubin levels were 6.5 mg/dL (range, 2.2–14.6 mg/dL). No evidence of immunoallergy was evident. All of the patients recovered spontaneously, with normalization of serum ALT and bilirubin levels within 4 months.[290] ALF necessitating emergency LT was reported in a previously healthy 28-year-old nonobese woman who had taken an over-the-counter preparation of usnic acid for weight loss,[291] suggesting that this agent is the likely hepatotoxic component of LipoKinetix. Usnic acid is also a component of kombucha tea, which has been associated with hepatic injury.[271] Usnic acid is a potent inhibitor of CYP2C19 and CYP2C9 and may interact with other medications or supplements to produce hepatotoxic drug-drug interactions.[292]

A number of additional multi-ingredient weight-loss, muscle-building, and nutritional supplements, including Herbalife, Slimquick, Hydroxycut, and OxyELITE Pro, have received attention in both the scientific and lay press for their association with severe hepatotoxicity. Herbalife was linked to severe liver injury, including the need for LT,[293,294] although many different preparations were taken and other causes may have been responsible in most cases, according to an analysis by Teschke et al.[237]

The weight-loss supplement Hydroxycut has been associated with nearly two dozen spontaneous reports of possible hepatotoxicity, with two patients requiring LT and one death. It was recalled from the U.S. market in 2009.[295,296] Two of its active ingredients, GTE (*C. sinensis*) and *Ephedra* (ma huang), have been implicated in liver injury,[297] although the association with GTE has been called into question in some cases.[233] Although the FDA did not identify a specific hepatotoxic component, Hydroxycut was reformulated with caffeine as the principal ingredient and reintroduced into the market, with only a single subsequent report of liver injury.[298]

Slimquick products contain a variety of vitamins, botanicals, and other ingredients, including GTE. Among the published reports of liver injury, GTE was noted to be the common exposure,[299] although the exact mechanism is unclear.[218]

OxyELITE Pro is a body-building, weight-loss, and performance-enhancing supplement that has come under FDA scrutiny for hepatotoxicity. Its unique story reflects many of the regulatory and manufacturing issues the HDS market has faced and is a cautionary tale for the multibillion dollar supplement industry.[300] Beginning in 2012 the FDA received more than 100 adverse drug reports from 33 states, 2 foreign countries, and Puerto Rico linked to OxyELITE Pro dating back to 2010. Nearly 50% of the reports involved liver disease.[301] In 2013 the FDA banned the use of the original active ingredient in OxyELITE Pro Advanced Formula, 1,3-dimethylamylamine, in all nutritional supplements,[301] This stimulant caused hypertension and was linked to heart attacks, seizures, psychiatric disorders, and death.[302] OxyELITE Pro was reformulated, replacing 1,3-dimethylamylamine with aegeline, an alkaloid extract from the leaves of the Asian bael tree (*Aegle marmelos*). Following an initial report of cases of severe hepatitis from Hawaii and among the military in 2013,[303–305] and the subsequent reporting of more than 50 cases from both within and outside Hawaii by the end of October 2013,[300,301] the FDA issued a warning in October 2013 to avoid the use of the reformulated OxyELITE Pro, and the manufacturer was required to cease production and to recall and destroy the retail product.[306]

Numerous reports have documented the OxyELITE Pro history.[300,305–308] The summary by investigators from the Centers for Disease Control and Prevention, FDA, and Department of Military and Emergency Medicine is perhaps the most informative in chronicling the timeline, the involvement of the numerous agencies that sought to identify cases, and the clinical features and outcomes of the patients.[303] Nevertheless, an animal study of the subsequent formulation of OxyELITE Pro-New Formula has documented elevations in serum AST and ALT levels as well as mortality in female mice, suggesting that even this newest version may be hazardous.[309]

Kava Kava

Kava Kava is a natural sedative and antianxiety agent derived from the root of the pepper plant (*Piper methysticum*). This herbal product has been the subject of an FDA consumer alert[271] after it was banned in the European Union and Canada[281] because of severe hepatotoxicity, including fatal liver failure.[185,311] A review of 78 cases of hepatic injury reported to the FDA included 11 cases of liver failure requiring LT and 4 deaths.[312] Other investigators, however, have questioned the validity of the causality assessment used by regulators, and only rare instances of hepatotoxicity have been found when a more accurate liver-specific causality scale was used.[235,313] Although kavalactone has been shown to inhibit CYP enzymes, deplete hepatic glutathione, and possibly inhibit COX,[312] the hepatotoxic component may be the major kava alkaloid pipermethystine. Contamination of the raw material by molds has been cited as an alternative explanation for hepatotoxicity,[240] although no hard evidence for aflatoxicosis was found.[314] Induction of apoptosis and mitochondrial toxicity are the suspected hepatotoxic mechanisms.[315]

Black Cohosh

Black cohosh (*Actaea racemosa* and *Cimicifuga racemosa*), which is used for menopausal symptoms, has been implicated in numerous reports of hepatic injury (LiverTox evidence A),[316] including a case with features of autoimmune hepatitis,[317] although the toxic component has not been identified. However, causality has been questioned,[318] bolstered by a meta-analysis that included 5 studies involving more than 1100 women that found no evidence for an adverse effect of the isopropanolic extract of black cohosh on the liver.[319]

Greater Celandine Extract

Greater celandine (*Chelidonium majus*) is regarded as a likely hepatotoxin on the basis of both animal studies and human reports subjected to accepted liver-specific causality assessments.[320] Its toxic component appears to be isoquinolone alkaloids.[321] Clinical features include reversible hepatocellular or cholestatic injury with jaundice, with recovery after about 2 months. A majority of the patients have been women who were taking the agent for various dyspeptic complaints.[320] Formal causality assessments undertaken by Teschke et al. have confirmed the hepatotoxic potential of the agent.[321]

Flavocoxid

Flavocoxid (Limbrel), a blend of plant-derived bioflavonoids, is a medical food prescribed for osteoarthritis. It is an uncommon cause of hepatotoxicity among cases contained within the United States DILI Network registry.[322] Four middle-aged women developed acute hepatocellular injury within 1–3 months of starting flavocoxid for arthritis-related complaints. Clinical features included abdominal pain, fever, pruritus, and a rash, with a mean peak serum ALT level of 1286 U/L and moderate elevations of alkaline phosphatase (mean peak 510 U/L) with jaundice [mean peak bilirubin 9.4 mg/dL (with a range of 2.0–20.8 mg/dL)]. The injury was of moderate severity with no sign of ALF, and all four individuals started to recover within days of discontinuing the product.[322] The presence of skullcap, catechins, or other potentially hepatotoxic ingredients may underlie the mechanism for the liver injury according to the LiverTox website.

Garcinia cambogia

Garcinia cambogia (GC) is a tropical fruit whose rind contains hydrocitric acid that is used as an appetite suppressant and weight-loss supplement. Its active ingredient reduces synthesis of fatty acids and glycogen storage via inhibition of ATP citrate lyase. Several reports of hepatocellular (and less often cholestatic) injury have been published, with a latent period ranging from 1 to several weeks and a clinical presentation that often includes nausea, vomiting, fatigue, and jaundice, and instances of severe injury and acute liver failure have appeared.[323–328] Crescioli et al. documented four cases of acute liver injury in which causality was established as probable using the Council for International Organization of Medical Sciences scoring.[327] These investigators also applied causality scoring to a literature review and concluded that GC was a likely cause of HDS.

Kratom

Kratom (*M. speciosa*) leaves have traditionally been used to brew a tea to manage pain and for use as a stimulant, but more recently have been taken as a nonsanctioned means to ameliorate opioid withdrawal symptoms in the United States and elsewhere.[329] Its active components are mitragynine and 7 hydroxymitragynine, which act as partial mu and delta opioid receptor agonists, with the former mediating euphoria, analgesia, and respiratory depression.[330,331] The CDC estimated a more than 10-fold increase in kratom use linked to opioid overdoses between 2010 and 2015,[332] with an increasing number of reports of cholestatic injury along with seizures and death associated with its use.[330,333–335] Nearly 3500 cases were reported from U.S. Poison Control Centers between 2014 and 2019 among individuals aged 18 and older; with the number of cases increasing with time.[336] Of note, while most exposures were in persons under the age of 60, adverse reactions occurred nearly twice as often in those over age 60 as compared to younger individuals (21.9% vs. 12.3%). Liver histologic information, while limited, suggests kratom causes acute zone 3 cholestasis with mild portal inflammation and bile duct injury that has mimicked a form of antimitochondrial antibody-negative primary biliary cholangitis.[337,338] The FDA has classified kratom as an opioid, citing its potential for abuse, addiction, and other potentially deadly risks,[339,340] prompting caution from others.[341,342]

Of interest is the finding by one group that the use of kratom in the United States was associated with taking a greater number of concomitant medications, including nonbenzodiazepine sedatives, compared to countries, such as Thailand.[343] These investigators suggested that the coingestion of these other sedative drugs may explain the higher incidence of clinically adverse effects seen in the United States. While the Drug Enforcement Administration initially proposed that kratom be listed as a Schedule one drug under the Controlled Substances Act, this request was later withdrawn, so kratom remains legal in most states.[344]

Hepatoprotection by Herbal Compounds

In contrast to the hepatotoxicity seen with the HDS discussed in this chapter, an entire field of study has been devoted to the hepatoprotective properties of nutraceuticals and other phytomedicines against liver injury induced by various chemicals, drugs, and other hepatotoxins, including acetaminophen and CCl_4 in animal models. This topic has been reviewed elsewhere.[345–349]

Full references for this chapter can be found at https://ebooks.health.elsevier.com

92 Autoimmune Hepatitis

Mark R. Pedersen, Marlyn J. Mayo

IN THIS CHAPTER

AUTOIMMUNE HEPATITIS

Autoimmune hepatitis (AIH) is an immune-mediated liver disease that responds well to immunosuppression when a timely diagnosis is made. Its classical form is characterized by elevated alanine aminotransferase (ALT) levels, hypergammaglobulinemia, plasma-cell-rich interface hepatitis on biopsy, and a robust response to immunosuppression, usually corticosteroids and azathioprine (AZA). However, there is a heterogenous spectrum of disease exemplified by its nebulous pathophysiology, nonspecific serologies, and variable histologic findings.

Historically, AIH was recognized in case reports in the early 1950s with a picture of chronic, active nonviral hepatitis with associated hypergammaglobulinemia and interface hepatitis that improved with cortisone administration.[1] It has had several names through the years, including "Waldenström's hepatitis" due to the elevated gammaglobulins and "lupoid hepatitis" due the presence of an antinuclear antibody (ANA) that is frequently seen.[2,3] The name "autoimmune hepatitis" was first used in 1965.[4] With the discovery of response to cortisone in the 1950s, AIH was one of the first treatable liver diseases, with a timeframe of treatment discovery similar to Wilson's disease (penicillamine, 1956).[5]

Two forms of AIH have been described, types 1 and 2. Type 1 AIH affects both children and adults and is associated with the ANA and antismooth muscle antibody (SMA). Type 2 AIH is predominately a pediatric disease with a median age of presentation of 10 years and is associated with the anti-liver-kidney-microsome-1 (anti-LKM1) and anti-liver-cytosol-1 (anti-LC1). While both forms are discussed in the chapter, most information describes type 1 unless specified.

EPIDEMIOLOGY

AIH has a global distribution and affects patients of all ages from both genders with an incidence range of 0.67–2.0 per 100,000. While the prevalence generally ranges from 3 to 24.5 per 100,000, some populations such as Alaskan Natives are reported to have a much higher prevalence.[6–16] In children, the incidence of AIH ranges from 0.23 to 0.4 per 100,000 and the prevalence from 2.4 to 3.0 per 100,000, though it is higher in certain populations such as indigenous children in Canada.[17–20]

The incidence of AIH appears to be rising, as seen in Denmark (1.37–2.33 cases from 1994 to 2012), Netherlands (rising over a 10-year period), and Spain (increasing from 1990 to 2003),[9,13,14] though it has been has been steady in New Zealand.[11] Similarly, the prevalence of AIH has been observed to be rising in Japan (8.7–23.9 per 100,000 from 2004 to 2016).[16]

There is a strong female predominance (67%–95% female) for AIH seen in numerous studies.[6–14,16–21] AIH is a disease of all ages, and index diagnosis may be seen in toddlers, octogenarians, and all ages in between. The peak of onset appears to be the middle-to-late life (43–70 years old). While once considered to be bimodal, with one peak in childhood and another later in life, most studies have shown a continuous distribution of age (Table 92.1).[11,13,14]

PATHOPHYSIOLOGY

AIH has a complex pathophysiology that is not fully understood but results in the loss of self-tolerance in the liver. Several factors are thought to be at play, including genetic, immunologic, and environmental factors.

Genetic Predisposition

As with other autoimmune diseases, the major histocompatibility complex (MHC) loci are the major genetic association for AIH. The importance of MHC loci in the pathogenesis of AIH has

TABLE 92.1 Incidence and Prevalence of AIH

Location	Incidence per 100,000	Prevalence per 100,000	Female Proportion	Age of Onset (Years)*
Adults				
Southern Israel[12]	0.67	11.0	95%	Mean 47.9
New Zealand[11]	2.0	24.5	71%	Mean 54 Range <20 to >80
Sweden[10]	0.85	10.7	76%	Mean 43 Range 4.5–83.4
Netherlands[14,21]	1.1	18.3	78%	Mean 43M; 48F Range 6–87M; 5–87F
Denmark[13]	1.68	23.9	72%	Median 70
Norway[6]	1.9	16.9	80%	Median 68 Range 26–80
Singapore[7]		3–8	91%	Mean 57 Median 63
Alaskan Natives[8]		42.9	90%	Median 52 Range 15–85
Spain[9]	0.83	11.6	85%	Mean 45.9 Range 28–66
United States[241]		31.2	80%	1% < 18 years 57% < 18–65 years 42% > 65 years
Japan[16]		23.9	81%	
Children				
Canada[17,20]	0.23	2.4	67%	Mean 10.3–10.9
United States[18,19]	0.4	3.0	75%	Mean 9.8–12.9 Range 2.7–18.1

AIH, Autoimmune hepatitis.

been confirmed in several genome-wide association studies. In white European and North American adult patients, HLA-DRB1*0301 and HLA-DRB1*0401 have been associated with type 1 AIH.[22,23] In pediatric patients, HLA-DRB1*1301, HLA-DQB1*0201, and HLA-DRB1*07 have been associated with type 2 AIH.[24,25]

There is variation of the associations around the world (Table 92.2).[25–28] These variations may explain some of the differences seen in disease presentation. For example, the HLA-A1D8-DR3 haplotype is associated with early onset and relapse, while HLA-DRB04:01 is associated with an older age of onset.[23,29]

A propensity for AIH has also been associated with polymorphisms in Fas [cluster of differentiation 95 (*CD95**)],[30,31] cytotoxic T lymphocyte antigen-4 (CTLA-*4*),[32,33] vitamin D receptor,[34,35] tumor necrosis factor-α (*TNF-α*),[33,36] and signal transducer and activator of transcription 4 (*STAT4*).[37] *TGF-β1* and *Fas* polymorphisms are also associated with increased severity of disease.

AIH as part of the autoimmune polyglandular syndrome type 1 (APS-1) is a rare exception to the complex genetic pathophysiology described. APS-1 is caused by mutation of the autoimmune regulator (*AIRE*) gene, which encodes a protein that normally results in the elimination of self-reactive T cells. Overall, 12% of patients with APS-1 have AIH.[38,39] Patients with APS-1 may have any combination of candidiasis, hypoparathyroidism, adrenal insufficiency, ectodermal dystrophy, and several other autoimmune conditions. AIH in these patients is associated with anti-LKM1 directed at cytochrome P450 1A2 (CYP1A2), CYP2A6, and cytochrome P4502D6 (CYP2D6).[40,41]

Environmental Triggers

Genetic predisposition alone is usually not enough to trigger AIH. The additional factor(s) needed remain unknown but may include viral infections and/or intestinal dysbiosis. Patients with AIH have increased intestinal permeability, derangement of the microbiome, and increased bacterial translocation compared to healthy controls.[42] Several viruses have been postulated to trigger AIH as well. Hepatitis A has been associated with the development of AIH in healthy relatives of patients with known AIH.[43] Hepatitis B,[44] hepatitis C,[45] varicella zoster,[46] and Epstein-Barr virus infection[47] have been associated with the development of AIH in reports. Nonetheless, most patients with AIH usually lack markers of prior infection.[48]

Type II AIH is associated with anti-LKM1 and anti-LC1, which target cytochrome P450 2D6 and formiminotransferase cyclodeaminase, respectively.[41,49,50] Infection of mice with an adenovirus expressing CYP2D6 or immunization of mice with human CYP2D6 or human formiminotransferase cyclodeaminase induces histologic features of AIH and the presence of anti-LKM1/anti-LC1.[51,52] While homologies have been noted between CYP2D6 and hepatitis C, herpes simplex virus type 1, and cytomegalovirus,[53–55] none of these viruses have been shown to trigger clinical type II AIH. The possibility of molecular mimicry having a role in the pathogenesis of type II AIH remains an alluring though unproven theory.

Lymphocyte Differentiation and Hepatocyte Loss

Although the identity of the autoantigens in AIH remain largely elusive, antigen-presenting cells (APCs) stimulate CD4$^+$ T lymphocytes to differentiate via cytokine-directed pathways into

TABLE 92.2 HLA Associations in AIH

Study	Location	Population/AIH Type	MHC Class II Associations	Comments
Seki et al. [28]	Japan	Adults Type 1	DR4 DR53 DQ4 DRB1*0405	DR4 most frequently associated with AIH
Strettel et al. [22]	North America	Adults Type 1	DRB1*0301 DRB1*0401	
Goldberg et al. [242]	Brazil	Mixed	DRB1*1301	DRB*1302 may be protective
Lim et al. [26]	South Korea	Adult Type 1	DRB1*0405 DRB1*0401	
van Gerven et al. [23]	Netherlands	Adult Type 1	DRB1*0301 DRB1*0401	
Fortes et al. [243]	Venezuela	Mixed Type 1	DRB1*1301 DRB1*0301	DQB1*04 may be protective
Bittencourt et al. [244]	Brazil	Mixed Type 1 Type 2	DRB1*13 DRB3 DRB1*03 DRB1*07	DQB1*0301 may be protective
Pando et al. [27]	Argentina	Children Adult	DRB1*1301 DRB1*0301 DRB1*0405	DRB1*1302 was protective in children
Fainboim et al. [25]	Argentina	Children Type 1	DR6 DRB1*1301 DQB1*0603	DR6 not described in adult
Djilali-Saiah et al. [24]	Canada France	Children Type 2	DQ*0201 DRB1*07	

AIH, Autoimmune hepatitis; *MHC*, major histocompatibility complex.

$CD8^+$ cytotoxic T cells, plasma cells, and T helper 17 cells (Th17).[56] $CD8^+$ cytotoxic T cells expressing Fas ligand (FasL) bind to Fas receptors on the surface of hepatocytes, initiating extrinsic apoptosis.[57] B lymphocytes mature to plasma cells leading to increased immunoglobulin G (IgG) production.[56] Th17 cells promote ongoing inflammation by producing pro-inflammatory interleukin (IL) 17, increasing IL-6 production, suppressing regulatory T cells (Tregs), and stimulating proliferation of additional Th17 cells.[58,59] Apoptotic bodies can be phagocytosed by Kupffer cells, the resident APCs of the liver, and restart the cycle of inflammation (Fig. 92.1). Kupffer cells generate reactive oxygen species, leading to mitochondrial damage and intrinsic hepatocyte apoptosis.[57] The ongoing hepatic inflammation leads to the activation of stellate cells and transformation into myofibroblasts, which cause progressive hepatic fibrosis.[60,61]

CLINICAL PRESENTATION AND EVALUATION

Clinical Features

AIH may be asymptomatic (29%–45%) with only elevation of transaminases or may cause nonspecific symptoms such as fatigue (85%), nausea, weight loss, arthralgias, or amenorrhea.[62–66] It may also present with an acute form (about 25%), with abrupt onset of symptoms that coincides with the discovery of laboratory abnormalities, with or without features of liver failure.[67–69] Acute forms may represent true sudden onset of new AIH or a sudden worsening of preexisting disease, as can been seen in a person who has had withdrawal of immunosuppression or who had been pregnant in the recent past. Physical exam findings are nonspecific and may include jaundice or signs of chronic liver disease (hepatomegaly, encephalopathy, splenomegaly, spider angioma, palmar erythema, and caput medusa). Some patients may have normal physical exam findings.

Overall, 3%–6% of patients may present with acute severe (fulminant) AIH, now acute liver failure, defined as a recognized disease duration ≤26 weeks with an INR ≥ 1.5 and encephalopathy.[67,70] The definition of acute severe AIH has changed through the years in concert with the changing definition of acute liver failure; currently, even patients with cirrhosis on biopsy are considered severe acute AIH as long as the disease duration has been recognized for ≤26 weeks.[67]

Concurrent autoimmune diseases are present in 14%–44% of patients.[71–75] Of these, autoimmune thyroiditis, Graves disease, and rheumatoid arthritis are the most common (Table 92.3) in type 1 AIH. Autoimmune thyroiditis, type 1 diabetes, and autoimmune skin diseases are more common in type 2 AIH.[76] Celiac disease can be seen in 1.1%–4% of patients[74,77,78] and can have liver histologic features that overlap with AIH. For these reasons, current guidelines from both the American Association for the Study of Liver Diseases and the European Association for the Study of the Liver recommend screening for both thyroid disease and celiac disease in patients diagnosed with AIH.[79,80] In patients with mucosal candidiasis and multiple endocrine failures, the diagnosis of autoimmune polyendocrinopathy-candidiasis-ectodermal dystrophy should be considered, especially if ectodermal dystrophy is also present.

Laboratory Testing and Autoantibodies

Laboratory testing reveals a hepatocellular liver injury pattern with serum transaminase elevations as well as an elevated protein-albumin gap, driven by elevated IgG levels. Transaminase elevation may be as low as one to two times the upper limit of normal (ULN) to over 1000 in acute severe forms. Hyperbilirubinemia may be present but may not always reach the level needed to yield clinical jaundice. While there may be alkaline phosphatase elevation, it is typically less than two times the ULN. Elevations over four times the ULN are infrequent and should prompt

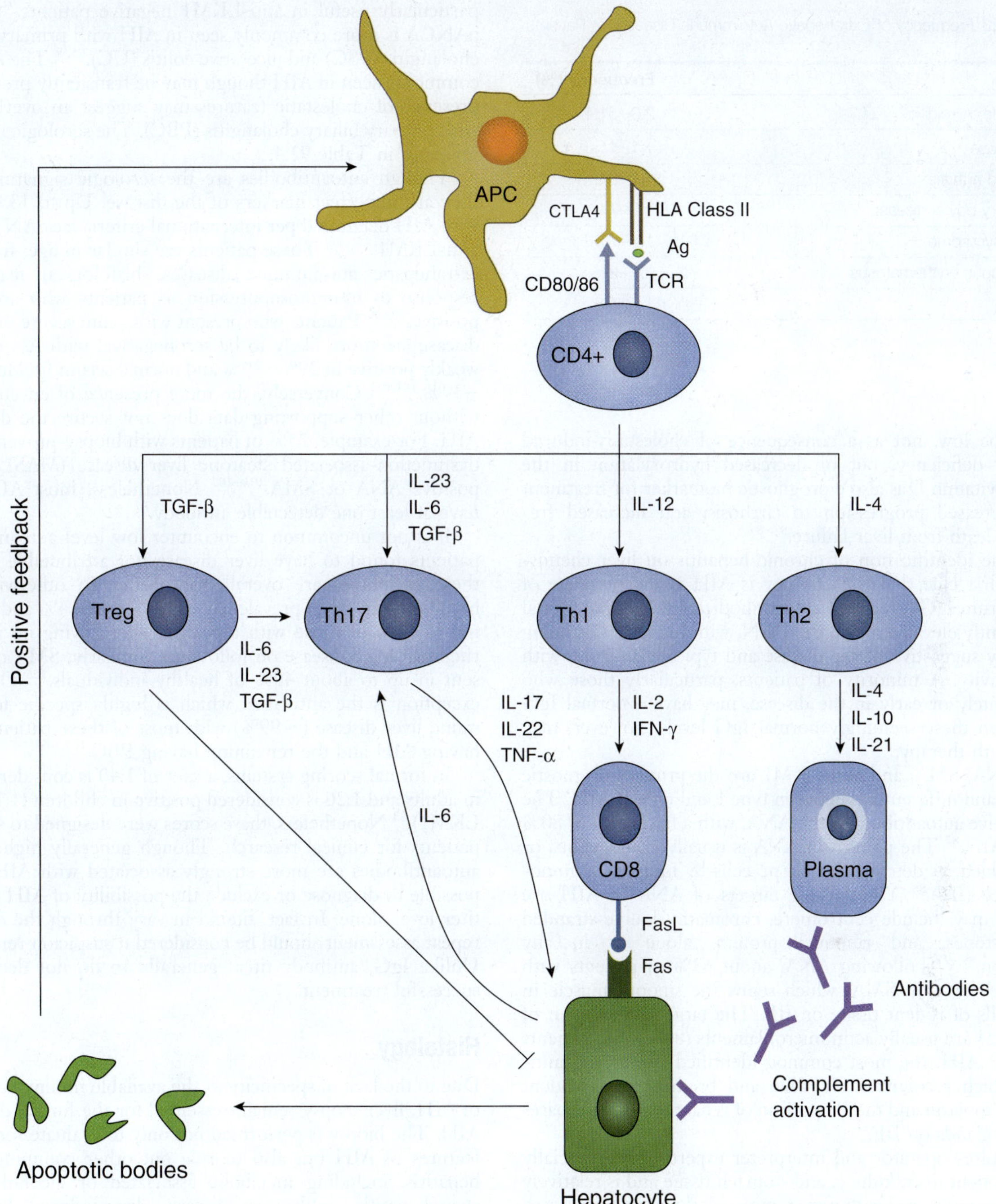

Fig. 92.1 Pathogenesis of autoimmune hepatitis. Antigen-presenting cells (APCs) present autoantigens to self-reactive T cell receptors (TCRs) on CD4$^+$ helper T cells and CD8$^+$ T cells. Costimulation activates the T cells which then proliferate, differentiate, and mature into specific subsets (Th1, Th2, Th17, iTregs) as well as cytotoxic CD8$^+$ T cells (CTLs). Secretion of IL-2 and IFN-γ stimulate CTLs, enhances expression of class I HLA molecules and induces the expression of HLA class II molecules on hepatocytes. CTLs expressing FasL can bind to Fas expressed on hepatocytes and promote apoptosis. Similarly, secretion of IL-4, IL-10, and IL-21 promote maturation of B cells into auto-antibody secreting plasma cells. Th17 cells are pathogenic via the secretion of IL-17, IL-22, and TNF-α. Exposure of normally inflammation moderating Tregs to specific cytokines can transform them into Th17 cells. Apoptotic fragments of hepatocytes can be endocytosed by antigen presenting cells to create a positive feedback loop, initiating the cycle of inflammation again.

investigation into other etiologies of liver injury,[81] including an overlap syndrome.

Other lab abnormalities may be seen as a consequence of the liver injury. An elevated ferritin is often present as part of a general disturbance of iron homeostasis. Elevated ferritin levels in conjunction with an elevated IgG level less than 2 times the ULN has been associated with increase probability of achieving a complete remission.[82] Circulating 25-hydroxyvitamin D levels

TABLE 92.3 Frequency of Extrahepatic Autoimmune Diseases in Patients With AIH[72,73,75]

Disease	Frequency (%)
Autoimmune thyroiditis	2.0–51.4
Celiac disease	1.1–11.8
Rheumatoid arthritis	1.8–8.9
Inflammatory bowel disease	1.0–7.9
Sjogren's syndrome	1.4–7.9
Systemic lupus erythematosus	0.7–2
Vitiligo	1.0–1.8
Diabetes	0.7–1

may also be low, not as a consequence of cholestasis-induced vitamin D deficiency, but of decreased hydroxylation in the liver. Low vitamin D is also a prognostic biomarker for treatment failure, increased progression to cirrhosis, and increased frequency of death from liver failure.[83–85]

After the identification of chronic hepatitis on liver chemistries, the first clue that the etiology is AIH is the presence of elevated serum IgG levels and autoantibodies. IgG are polyclonal and frequently elevated above the ULN, with higher levels being increasingly suggestive of the disease and typically tracking with disease activity. A minority of patients, particularly those who present acutely or early in the disease, may have a normal IgG level.[86] Even these seemingly normal IgG levels, however, may decrease with therapy.

The ANA, SMA, and anti-LKM1 are the primary diagnostic antibodies and differentiate between type I and type II AIH. The most sensitive autoantibody is the ANA, with a frequency of 80% in type 1 AIH.[87] The pattern of ANA is usually homogenous or finely speckled, as detected on HEp2 cells by indirect immunofluorescence (IIF).[88] The specific targets of ANA in AIH are varied and may include centromere, chromatin double-stranded DNA, histones, and ribonucleoprotein, alone or in any combination.[89–91] Following ANA, about 63% of patients with type 1 AIH have an SMA, which stains the smooth muscle in arterial walls of rodent tissue on IIF. The target autoantigen of SMA in AIH are usually actin microfilaments (80%). For patients with type 2 AIH, the most common identified antibody is anti-LKM1, which recognizes CYP2D6 and brightly stains rodent liver cell cytoplasm and the P3 portion of renal tubules, but spares the gastric glands on IIF.[88]

IIF requires operator and interpreter expertise, and specially prepared rodent liver, kidney, and stomach tissue and is relatively cumbersome compared with newer, molecularly based assays such as enzyme-linked immunosorbent assay (ELISA). However, using ELISA to test for the presence of antiactin in place of IIF for SMA will miss the 16%–20% of patients with nonactin SMA.[87,88] ELISA can be particularly helpful in distinguishing anti-LKM1 from antimitochondrial antibody (AMA), both of which stain rodent liver cell cytoplasm and the renal tubules strongly by IIF. The use of ELISA with purified or recombinant antigens of CYP2D6 versus the 2-oxoacid dehydrogenase complex (PDC-E2, BCOADC-E2, and OGDC-E2) should differentiate the two.

The other antibodies seen in AIH carry varying clinical implications. Anti–soluble liver antigen (anti-SLA) is seen in type 1 AIH and portends a more severe course.[92] Anti-LC1, like anti-LKM1, is associated with type 2 AIH and is highly disease specific. As both anti-LKM1 and anti-LC1 target have targets in the hepatocyte cytosol, it is possible to miss anti-LC1 on IIF when anti-LKM1 is present as the staining pattern can be nearly identical (the use of molecular assays can avoid this). It is particularly useful in anti-LKM1 negative patients.[93,94] Atypical pANCA is more commonly seen in AIH with primary sclerosing cholangitis (PSC) and ulcerative colitis (UC).[95,96] The AMA is not commonly seen in AIH though may be transiently present.[94] The presence of cholestatic features may suggest an overlap of AIH with primary biliary cholangitis (PBC). The serologic markers are reviewed in Table 92.4.

Though autoantibodies are the serologic signature of AIH, they are imperfect markers of the disease. Up to 13% of adults with AIH diagnosed per international criteria lack ANA, SMA, or anti-LKM1.[97–100] These patients are similar in age, frequency of extrahepatic autoimmune diseases, histological features, and response to immunosuppression as patients who are antibody positive.[99,100] Patients who present with acute severe or fulminant disease are more likely to be seronegative, with ANA absent or weakly positive in 29%–39% and normal serum IgG level in 25%–39%.[101,102] Conversely, the mere presence of an autoantibody without other supporting data does not secure the diagnosis of AIH. For example, 25% of patients with biopsy-proven metabolic dysfunction-associated steatotic liver disease (MASLD) have a positive ANA or SMA.[103–105] Nonetheless, most AIH patients have at least one detectable antibody.[87]

It is not uncommon to encounter low level autoantibodies in patients found to have liver disease not attributable to AIH as these antibodies are overall nonspecific. In otherwise healthy blood donors, ANA prevalence varies between 4% and 26%, with nearly 75% of those with a positive titer having no identifiable rheumatologic disease on follow-up. Similarly, SMA can be present in up to about 40% of healthy individuals.[106] One notable exception is the anti-SLA, which is highly specific for autoimmune liver disease (~99%) with most of these patients (>90%) having AIH and the remaining having PBC.[107,108]

In formal scoring systems, a titer of 1:40 is considered positive in adults and 1:20 is considered positive in children (1:10 for anti-LKM1).[88] Nonetheless, these scores were designed to standardize patients for clinical research. Though generally higher titers of autoantibodies are more strongly associated with AIH, it is not possible to diagnose or exclude the possibility of AIH based on a titer level alone. In fact, titers can vary through the disease and repeat assessment should be considered if suspicion remains high. Unlike IgG, antibody titers generally to do not decrease with successful treatment.

Histology

Due to the lack of specificity of the available noninvasive markers of AIH, liver biopsy remains essential for the formal diagnosis of AIH. The biopsy is performed not only to evaluate for histologic features of AIH but also to rule out other common causes of hepatitis, including metabolic associated or alcohol-associated steatohepatitis, infiltrative disease, drug-induced liver injury (DILI), and Wilson disease. It is particularly helpful in patients with other autoimmune diseases, such as systemic lupus erythematosus (SLE) or rheumatoid arthritis, who may have elevated transaminases that respond to steroids ("lupoid hepatitis"), but lack the histological features of AIH. As AIH can be a heterogeneous disease, obtaining a quality specimen (at least 2.5 cm in length) is crucial for reliable histologic assessment.

The histologic hallmark of AIH is interface hepatitis. Other features commonly seen are a plasma cell infiltrate in 66% and lobular hepatitis in 47%.[109] Centrilobular necrosis is found in 29% of patients and can be seen in patients with and without cirrhosis.[110–112] Other features include hepatocyte swelling, hepatocyte rosettes, and emperipolesis (the penetration of one intact cell into another intact cell, with both retaining viability). Cirrhosis is present in 28%–33% of adults at the time of presentation.[63,113,114] Features that suggest acute severe (fulminant) AIH include predominant activity in the centrilobular zone,

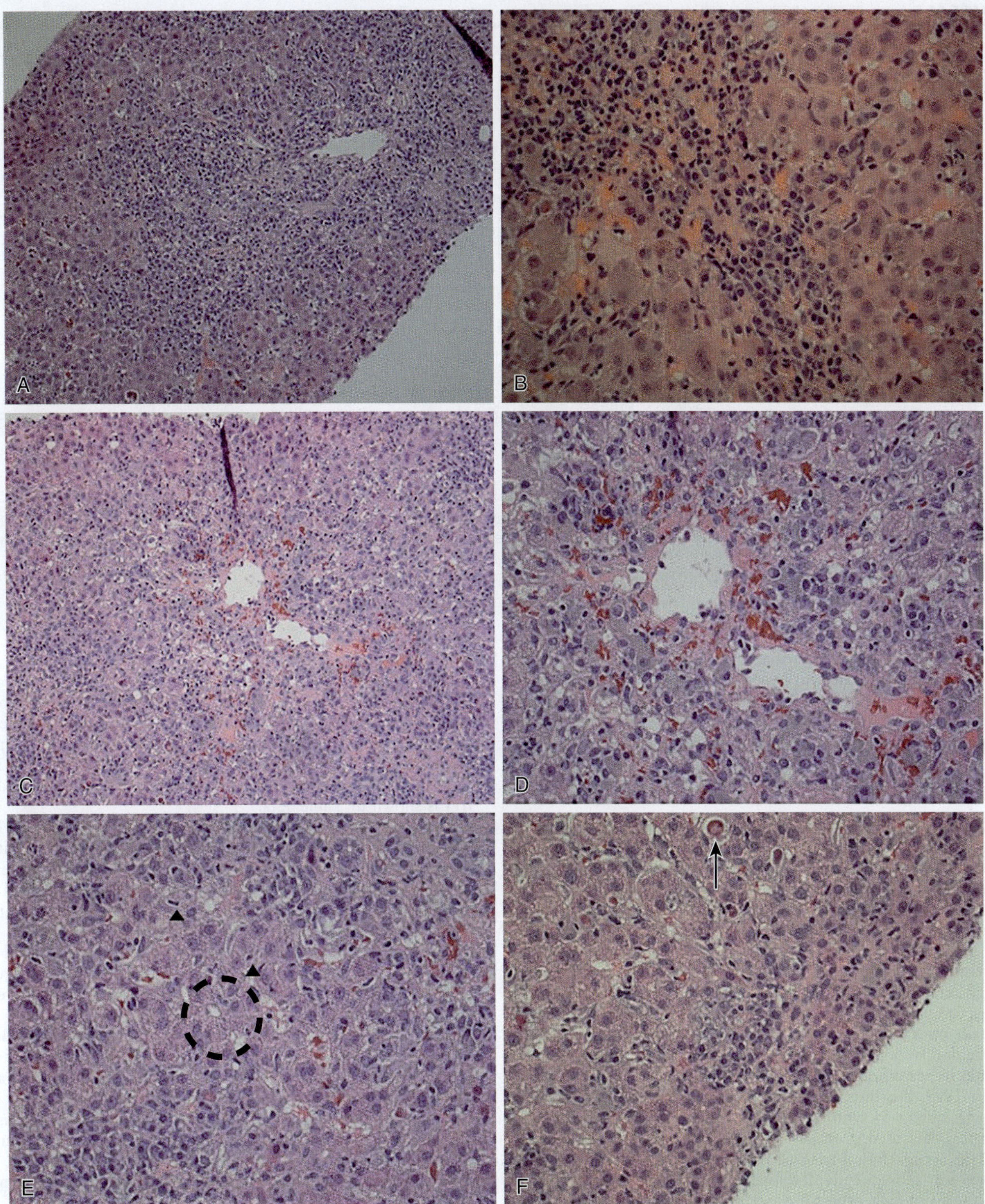

Fig. 92.2 Pathology of autoimmune hepatitis. (A) Portal tract is expanded by severe lymphoplasmacytic infiltration and interface hepatitis. (B) Plasma cell rich infiltrate extending beyond the limiting plate of the portal tract and surrounding hepatocytes (interface hepatitis). (C) Peri-venular hepatocyte drop-out with significant plasma cell inflammation ×200. (D) Peri-venular hepatocyte drop-out with significant plasma cell inflammation ×400. (E) Hepatocyte rosettes (*broken circle*) and emperipolesis (*triangle*) with plasma cell aggregates. (F) Lobular necroinflammatory activity with acidophil body (*arrow*). (Images A, C, D, E, F courtesy Lan Peng, M.D., Department of Pathology, University of Texas Southwestern Medical Center, used with permission. Image B courtesy author MJM.)

TABLE 92.4 Autoantibodies Observed in AIH

Autoantibody	Cell Location	Target	Frequency	Notes
Type 1 AIH				
ANA	Nucleus	Chromatin, ribonucleoproteins[245]	80% type 1 AIH[87]	Diagnostic accuracy: 56% sole marker[246] Pattern is usually homogenous or speckled[88]
SMA	Smooth muscle	Actin (F and G) Nonactin smooth muscle components (14%)[87,247]	63% type 1 AIH[87]	Diagnostic accuracy: 61% sole marker 74% with ANA[246]
Antiactin	Smooth muscle	Actin (F and G)[87]	54% type 1 AIH[87]	Does not detect nonactin smooth muscle components
Anti-SLA	Cytosol	Sep (O-phosphoserine) transfer RNA: Sec (selenocysteine) transfer RNA synthase[248,249]	1%–2% type 1 AIH[248]	High disease specificity[248] Associated with severe AIH and poor outcome[92]
Atypical pANCA	Nucleus	β-Tubulin isotype 5[250,251]	50%–92% type 1 AIH[252]	Associated with PSC and UC
AMA	Mitochondria	E2 subunit of pyruvate dehydrogenase		Associated with PBC
Type 2 AIH				
Anti-LKM-1	Microsome	CYP2D6[55]		Type 2 AIH
Anti-LC-1	Cytosol	Formiminotransferase cyclodeaminase[50]		Type 2 AIH

AIH, Autoimmune hepatitis; *AMA*, antimitochondrial antibody; *ANA*, antinuclear antibody; *CYP2D6*, cytochrome P4502D6; *LKM-1*, liver-kidney microsome-1; *LC-1*, liver cytotosl-1; *PBC*, primary biliary cholangitis; *PSC*, primary sclerosing cholangitis; *SLA*, soluble liver antigen; *SMA*, smooth muscle antibody; *UC*, ulcerative colitis.

including centrilobular necrosis, lymphoplasmacytic infiltration around the central vein with hepatocyte dropout or necrosis, and lymphoid aggregates (Fig. 92.2).[112]

DIAGNOSIS AND CLASSIFICATION

Diagnosis

In spite of the many characteristics associated with AIH, none is pathognomonic, and the diagnosis of AIH requires the careful review of all available clinical, laboratory, and histologic data. Initial evaluation must be careful to evaluate for viral, drug, and metabolic diseases that can mimic AIH.

As the treatment of AIH involves long term immunosuppression, diagnostic certainty is essential. However, certain clinical scenarios, such as acute severe AIH with coagulopathy, may significantly elevate the risk of obtaining a liver biopsy. In these cases, care should be taken to ensure the most accurate diagnosis is made prior to treatment initiation. The histologic features may lag behind laboratory recovery by several months, so liver biopsy should be reconsidered when it becomes safe.[115]

In 1999, the International AIH Group published a detailed scoring system to synthesize the historical, laboratory, and histological data used to make a diagnosis of AIH and standardize patients across clinical trials (Table 92.5).[116] A simplified scoring system was subsequently developed for bedside use that includes only autoantibody expression, serum IgG concentration, histologic features, and viral hepatitis markers (Table 92.6).[117] Both scoring systems are based on autoantibody determinations by IIF, and titer thresholds do not translate well to autoantibodies levels measured with ELISA. Though longer, the comprehensive scoring system performs better for both acute AIH (91% vs. 40%) and fulminant AIH (40% vs. 24%).[118,119] The cutoffs for "definite" and "probable" AIH are somewhat arbitrary and should not replace clinical judgment. Even patients with probable AIH (or a score approaching this) may still have AIH but with simply less pronounced inflammatory changes.[120]

Classification

AIH is frequently classified into two types based on autoantibody profile.[121] There are some differences in outcomes and associations reported. As type 2 tends to be seen predominantly in pediatric populations, elimination of typing has been proposed for adults.[122] A summary of the differences between types 1 and 2 AIH is shown in Table 92.7.

Type 1 AIH is characterized by the presence of an SMA, ANA, or both. It is associated with autoimmune thyroiditis, Graves disease, celiac disease, and UC in addition to several other autoimmune conditions. In patients who present with UC or features of cholestasis that do not improve with therapy, magnetic resonance cholangiopancreatography (MRCP) is indicated to evaluate for concomitant PSC. Type 1 AIH is associated with an abrupt onset of symptoms (fatigue, arthralgia, fever, and jaundice) and may present as acute, severe disease.[123]

Type 2 AIH is characterized typically by an anti-LKM1 and less commonly by anti-LC1. In these patients, IgG levels may be normal and IgA levels may be reduced.[124] Most patients are children (2–14 years old), and it is seen more frequently in Europe than North America.[124] Concurrent autoimmune diseases are seen in up to 18% of patients and include autoimmune thyroiditis, vitiligo, and type 1 diabetes.[124] These patients can be more difficult to treat, and withdrawal of immunosuppression may not be possible.[125]

OVERLAP SYNDROMES AND DRUG-INDUCED LIVER INJURY MIMICKING AIH

Variations of classical AIH exist which require different management and carry a different prognosis. Some of these variants include the "overlap" syndromes, or the presence of more than one liver disease. In addition, some medications and supplements may cause hepatitis that appears very similar to AIH.

TABLE 92.5 Revised Diagnostic Criteria for Autoimmune Hepatitis

Feature	Factor	Score
Gender	Female	+2
Alk P:AST (or ALT) Ratio	>3 <1.5	−2 +2
Globulins or IgG (x upper limit of normal)	>2 1.5–2.0 1.0–1.5 <1.0	+3 +2 +1 0
ANA, ASMA, or anti-LKM1 titers	>1:80 1:80 1:40 <1:40	+3 +2 +1 0
AMAs	Positive	−4
Hepatotoxic drugs	Yes No	−4 +1
Alcohol	<25 g/day >60 g/day	+2 −2
Concurrent immune disease	Any nonhepatic disease of an immune nature	+2
Other autoantibodies	Anti-SLA, antiactin, anti-LC-1, p-ANCA	+2
Histologic features	Interface hepatitis Plasma cells Rosettes None of the above Biliary changes Atypical features	+3 +1 +1 −5 −3 −3
HLA	DR3 or DR4	+1
Treatment response	Remission alone Remission with relapse	+2 +3
PRETREATMENT SCORE		
Definite diagnosis		>15
Probable diagnosis		10–15
POSTTREATMENT SCORE		
Definite diagnosis		>17
Probable diagnosis		12–17

ALT, Alanine aminotransferase; *AMAs*, antimitochondrial antibodies; *ANAs*, antinuclear antibodies; *IgG*, immunoglobulin G; *SMAs*, smooth muscle antibodies.

Reproduced with permission from Alvarez F, Berg PA, Bianchi FB, et al. International Autoimmune Hepatitis Group Report: review of criteria for diagnosis of autoimmune hepatitis. *J Hepatol*. 1999;31:929–938.

TABLE 92.6 Simplified Scoring System for the Diagnosis of AIH

Feature	Factor	Score
ANA, ASMA, or anti-LKM1 titers or anti-LKM-1 titers	1:40 ≥1:80	+1 +2
Anti-LKM1	≥1:40	+2
Anti-SLA	Positive	+2
Globulins or IgG (x upper limit of normal)	>1 >1.1	+1 +2
Absence of viral hepatitis	No viral markers	+2
Histologic features	Compatible with AIH Typical of AIH	+1 +2
PRETREATMENT SCORE		
Definite diagnosis		≥7
Probable diagnosis		6

Note. Typical histology here is defined as the presence of interface hepatitis, lymphoplasmacytic portal tract infiltrates, emperipolesis, and hepatic rosette formation. *ANAs*, Antinuclear antibodies; *IgG*, immunoglobulin G; *SMAs*, smooth muscle antibodies.

Reproduced with permission from Hennes EM, Zeniya M, Czaja AJ, et al. Simplified criteria for the diagnosis of autoimmune hepatitis. *Hepatology*. 2008;48:169–176.

TABLE 92.7 Comparison of Types 1 and 2 AIH

Feature	Type 1 AIH	Type 2 AIH
Population	Children and adults (1–90 years old)[14,21]	Children (2–14 years old)[124]
Antibodies	ANA, and/or SMA Atypical p-ANCA	Anti-LKM1 or anti-LC1
Other associated autoimmune conditions[72–75]	Thyroiditis (12%) Graves disease (6%) Ulcerative colitis (6%) Rheumatoid arthirits Systemic sclerosis Celiac disease Lupus	Autoimmune thyroiditis Type 1 diabetes Vitiligo
Overlap with PSC (ASC in children)	Common in children Atypical p-ANCA positive	Rare
Overlap with PBC	Seen in adults	Not reported
Cirrhosis at presentation	Adults, 28%–33%	Rare
Remission after immunosuppression withdrawal	Possible	Rare

AIH, Autoimmune hepatitis; *ANA*, antinuclear antibody; *SMA*, smooth muscle antibody.

AIH and PBC Overlap

Mild degrees of cholestasis and/or cholangitis can be seen biochemically or histologically in a patient that otherwise has classic AIH, and typically responds to immunosuppression.[115] Persistent or more prominent cholestasis should prompt consideration of an overlapping (coexisting) PBC or PSC. Approximately 2% of patients with AIH and 19% of patients with PBC have a combined AIH and PBC overlap syndrome.[126,127] In these patients, the presence of AIH and PBC should each be substantiated, and the Paris criteria are often used to make the diagnosis (Table 92.8).[128]

The recommended treatment for AIH and PBC overlap is ursodeoxycholic acid (UDCA) 13–15 mg/kg daily in combination with glucocorticoids.[129–131] However, it has also been observed that at least a subset of patients who fulfill the criteria of overlap do well on UDCA alone.[132] One of the difficulties here is that interface hepatitis is also a histological feature of PBC, and transaminase elevations can occur in these patients. Given the rarity of this disease, no trials exist to guide therapy decisions. When one process (either AIH or PBC) appears to be the dominant, it would be reasonable to start treatment of that process followed by close reassessment over 3–6 months. Therapy may be added for the second process depending on the clinical response. If both processes appear to be equally expressed, it would be reasonable to start UDCA, given its benign pharmacologic profile and the possibility of an adequate response.

Immunosuppression for AIH may be added at 3–6 months again depending on the clinical response.

AIH and PSC Overlap

Approximately 6%–11% of adults with AIH and 8%–17% of adults with PSC have an AIH/PSC overlap syndrome.[133–135] A history of inflammatory bowel disease or cholestasis that does not respond to immunosuppression should prompt imaging with MRCP (Fig. 92.3).

Treatment typically begins with conventional AIH therapy (prednisone or prednisolone in combination with AZA) in combination with UDCA. The recommendation for UDCA (13–15 mg/kg/day) is made by several society guidelines, though data supporting its use in PSC alone is tepid.[80,136,137] High dose therapy with UDCA (28–30 mg/kg/day) is not recommended due to increased mortality seen in patients with PSC on this regimen.[138] Patients with AIH and PSC overlap have a higher mortality than patients with AIH alone and those with AIH and PBC overlap.[139]

In children, AIH and PSC overlap may be as frequent as AIH alone, and this specific overlap syndrome is referred to as autoimmune sclerosing cholangitis (ASC). In contrast to classical AIH, about 50% of patients with ASC are male, and 45% have inflammatory bowel disease.[125] The IAIHG scoring system does not discriminate well between these two entities, and therefore MRCP is recommended for all pediatric patients at the onset of their diagnosis with AIH.[137] Patients with ASC respond more favorably to immunosuppression than patients with PSC alone.[140,141] UDCA (13–15 mg/kg/day) is used in these patients though evidence of its role in improving the cholangiopathy is lacking.[125]

TABLE 92.8 Paris Criteria for the Diagnosis of AIH and PBC Overlap[129]

AIH Criteria	PBC Criteria
At least two of the following: • ALT 5 × ULN • IgG 2 × ULN or positive SMA • Moderate to severe interface hepatitis on biopsy	At least two of the following: • Alkaline phosphatase 2 × ULN (or GGT 5 × ULN) • Positive AMA • Histologic destructive cholangitis (florid duct lesion) on biopsy

AIH, Autoimmune hepatitis; *ALT*, alanine aminotransferase; *AMA*, antimitochondrial antibody; *PBC*, primary biliary cholangitis; *SMA*, smooth muscle antibody; *ULN*, upper limit of normal.

Drug-Induced Liver Injury Mimicking AIH

DILI can mimic AIH in an estimated 9% of patients.[142] Minocycline and nitrofurantoin are the most commonly implicated agents that historically accounted for up to 90% of cases.[142–144] Most patients present with an acute onset (median onset from drug exposure 42 days), with jaundice in 69%, but features of hypersensitivity (fever, rash, and eosinophilia) are seen in only 15%–20%.[145] Nonetheless, some patients on chronic therapy with nitrofurantoin or minocycline can have latency periods over 12 months. Similar to classic AIH, histologic features include interface hepatitis with portal and periportal lymphocytes, plasma cells, and eosinophils. Findings that would favor drug-induced etiology include portal neutrophils and intracellular cholestasis, while fibrosis, hepatocyte rosettes, and emperipolesis favor classic AIH.[109] Nonetheless, the two pathologies can be difficult to differentiate even with biopsy. Common causes of DILI that mimic AIH are in Table 92.9.

The key to differentiating DILI from AIH is careful history-taking, making note of the dates and duration of drug exposure and the onset of liver disease. The mainstay of treatment is drug withdrawal. Glucocorticoids are usually administered after drug withdrawal due to an uncertain prognosis and frequently severity of the liver disease (jaundice) at presentation.[142,145] Resolution is expected within 1–3 months of drug withdrawal and treatment.[142] Sustained biochemical remission after the withdrawal of glucocorticoids strengthens the diagnosis of DILI, as 50%–87% of patients with classic AIH will relapse after withdrawal of immunosuppression.[78,146] Ongoing monitoring is recommended for these patients if AIH remains a possibility—while half of patients relapse within the first 3 months, relapse has been reported as late as 22 years after the withdrawal.[147]

The advent of checkpoint inhibitors to manage oncologic conditions has yielded a relatively new category of immune-mediated DILI. These monoclonal antibodies are directed at CTLA-4 (ipilimumab, tremelimumab), which provides needed costimulation for the activation of T cells, and PD-1 (nivolumab,

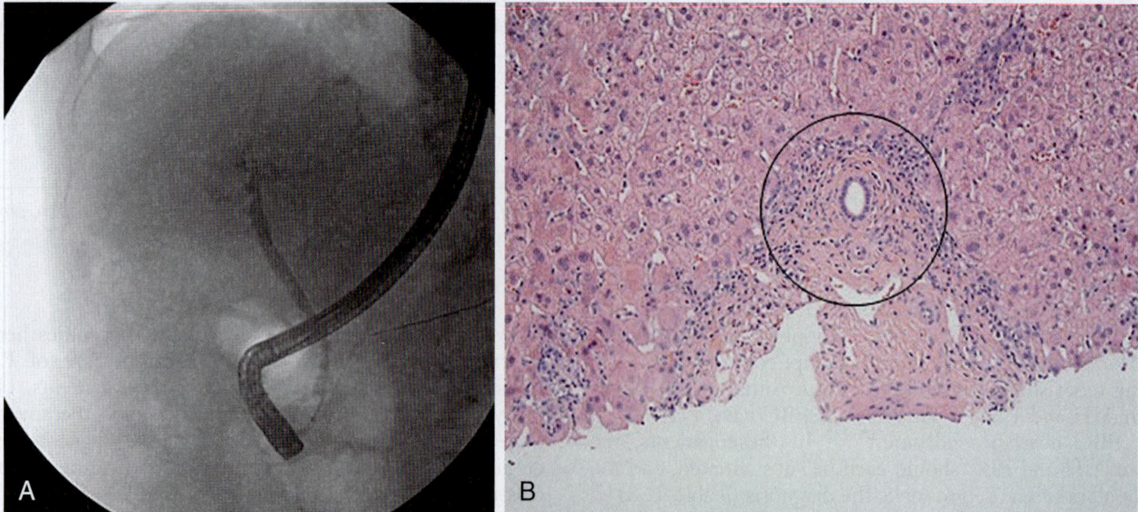

Fig. 92.3 Primary sclerosing cholangitis (PSC) and autoimmune hepatitis overlap. (A) ERCP imaging showing marked beading of the left sided hepatic ducts. (B) Onion-skinning fibrosis, as may be seen in patients with PSC overlap. (Images B courtesy Lan Peng, M.D., Department of Pathology, University of Texas Southwestern Medical Center, used with permission.)

TABLE 92.9 Medications Associated With Drug-Induced AIH

Definite Associations	Probable Associations
Minocycline[144,253]	Propylthiouracil[259]
Nitrofurantoin[143]	Isoniazid[260]
Infliximab, adalimumab[254,255]	Diclofenac[261]
Alpha-methyldopa[256,257]	Etanercept[262]
Halothane[258]	Rosuvastatin, atorvastatin[263–265]
Oxyphenisatin[a]	
Dihydralazine[a]	
Tienilic acid[a]	

[a]Medications no longer available in the United States.
AIH, Autoimmune hepatitis.

pembrolizumab, atezolizumab), which blocks apoptosis of T cells. Though intended to allow the immune system to better recognize and kill malignant cells, these drugs can also allow the recognition of healthy tissue leading to an autoimmune injury. Similar to AIH, checkpoint inhibitor-related hepatitis presents with elevated transaminases, and histology may show interface hepatitis, rosette formation, and portal and periportal inflammatory infiltrates. More commonly, however, biopsies may show lobular hepatitis with milder portal inflammation and fewer plasma cells.[148] Emperipolesis, rosette formation, and fibrosis are not commonly seen.[149] Glucocorticoids are usually sufficient treatment, dosed at 0.5–1 mg/kg/day of prednisone for mild cases and 1–2 mg/kg/day for more severe cases. Resolution is typically expected within 6–12 weeks. For refractory cases, where liver chemistries fail to improve within 3–7 days, the antimetabolite mycophenolate mofetil (MMF) may also be added.[150–153]

Metabolic-Associated Steatotic Liver Disease and AIH

The worldwide prevalence of MASLD is increasing, from 25.5% before 2005 to 37.8% in 2016 or later, though there is considerable heterogeneity between countries ranging from 19.6% in Malaysia to 48.4% in Turkey. Of these patients with MASLD, approximately one-quarter (23%–33%) of patients may have positive autoantibodies (ANA or SMA)[103,154] but less than 8% of these patients have AIH.[103] Conversely, in patients with AIH, the presence of NAFLD is around 17%.[155] There is no noninvasive marker that is well suited to determine which patients with elevated transaminases and positive autoantibodies have NAFLD, which have AIH, and which may have both. Liver biopsy is thus critical to evaluate for histologic features of AIH in patients with suspected MASLD and elevated autoantibodies. Nonetheless, highly active steatohepatitis can have interface hepatitis and make the differentiation of which process is dominant difficult even with liver biopsy.

In patients with NAFLD and AIH overlap, it can be difficult to achieve biochemical remission (normalization of transaminases) as MASLD process may be ongoing and can be worsened by the glucocorticoids used to treat AIH. Liver biopsy can be useful to monitor AIH activity and guide immunosuppression.

TREATMENT OF AIH

All patients with biochemical or histological evidence of liver inflammation should be considered for therapy. In the past, those with mild transaminase elevations were considered for observation, but long-term follow-up studies have demonstrated that even mild inflammation over time will lead to progression to cirrhosis.[156] Thus the treatment goal should be long term complete biochemical and histological remission, defined as normal AST, ALT, IgG, and minimal to no inflammation on liver biopsy, as recommended by current professional society guidelines worldwide.[157]

Since AIH was first described in the 1960s, corticosteroids have successfully been used as the first line therapy. This may have turned out to be the Achilles' heel of AIH, because having an effective therapy that reduces liver enzymes in 80%–90% of patients[158] has also hampered the development of novel therapies that might be more effective or have fewer side effects.

Three randomized, placebo-controlled clinical trials completed in the 1970s demonstrated significant improvements in survival, liver biochemistries, and histology in patients with AIH.[159–161] The response to steroids of transaminases is usually rapid, with 90% of patients achieving complete remission after a mean treatment duration of 3 ± 3 months. Because most patients will relapse if treatment is withdrawn, an extended course of immunosuppression (often lifelong) to maintain remission is required.[162] The prognosis of patients who achieve and maintain clinical remission long term is excellent. In a cumulative observation period of 842 patient years, transplant-free survival was 100%, despite 30% of patients having cirrhosis at treatment initiation.[163] In reality, many patients fail to achieve the ideal treatment goal of complete remission for a lifetime, and overall transplant-free survival in patients with AIH is reduced. Over 20 years of follow up, transplant-free survival is only $48\% \pm 5\%$.[164] Failure to normalize levels of ALT within 12 months, more than four relapses per decade, and cirrhosis at any time are all associated with AIH-related death or need for liver transplantation.[164] Despite best effort treatment, relapses (defined by IAHG as doubling of the transaminase levels and above normal with symptoms or transaminase levels to more than three times the ULN with or without symptoms) occurs in 51% and de novo cirrhosis develops in approximately 34% of patients after 20 years.[156]

Despite their excellent efficacy at achieving remission of disease, corticosteroids are associated with severe long term systemic adverse effects (osteoporosis, fatty liver, diabetes, and hypertension) and are not well tolerated by patients (insomnia, psychosis, acne, and weight gain), leading to high rates of discontinuation and noncompliance. In the 1980s, AZA was introduced as a potential steroid-sparing agent in AIH, and in 1995 King's College in London reported the ability to remove steroids completely and maintain remission with AZA alone.[165] Current therapeutic strategies consist of a steroid-based induction with transition to a steroid-sparing agent for long term remission.

Pretreatment Considerations

AZA is better tolerated long term than steroids but also associated with some potential adverse effects. Acute side effects may include nausea/vomiting, rash, diarrhea, weakness, headaches, and bone marrow suppression. Long-term side effects include a small but increased risk of squamous cell skin carcinoma (OR 1.56, CI 1.11–2.18)[166] and lymphoma (OR 2.40, 95% CI 1.13, 5.11).[167]

AZA is a prodrug that is converted to 6-mercaptopurine (6-MP), which is then metabolized by thiopurine methyl transferase (TPMT) into its active, immunosuppressant metabolite, 6-thioguanine (6-TG) and an inactive, but potentially hepatotoxic metabolite, 6-methylmercaptopurine (6-MMP). Polymorphisms in the TPMT enzyme influence the amount of TPMT produced, which has a direct influence on the proportion of active versus inactive metabolite that is produced. Slow metabolizers with low TPMT levels will accumulate higher levels of 6-TG that can result in profound neutropenia.

Patients with AIH have similar distribution of TPMT phenotypes as compared to the general population: 1%, 9%, and 90%

patients have low (< 5 U/mL), intermediate (5–13.7 U/mL), and high (>=13.8 U/mL) TPMT levels, respectively.[168,169] Blood tests to assess TPMT activity and genetic polymorphisms are commercially available and widely used to predict the risk of severe neutropenia prior to initiation of AZA. Cross-sectional studies have shown that TPMT activity correlates with ability to tolerate AZA in AIH, although there is a significant discordance that ranges from 25%[168] to 50%.[170] None of the studies have specifically accounted for hypersplenism, which would logically reduce the ability to tolerate modest neutropenia. Although no study has prospectively shown the ability of pretreatment testing to reduce side effects of AZA in a population of patients with AIH, including cytopenias, guidelines recommend pretesting for TPMT activity, particularly to identify the rare individuals with very low or absent TPMT activity who are at extreme risk.[80]

Patients who are immunosuppressed are at risk for reactivation of chronic hepatitis B (HBV). Although the HBV reactivation rate specifically in AIH patients is not known, hepatitis B surface antigen, surface antibody, and core antibody should be checked prior to initiation of steroids to estimate the potential of HBV reactivation. Prophylactic therapy with antiviral medication (tenofovir or entecavir) need only be started in high-risk patients (Table 92.10). Therapy with conventional AIH doses of moderate- or low-dose prednisone and AZA is considered medium to low risk and only close monitoring with serial HBV DNA is recommended.[171]

Whenever possible, patients who are hepatitis B surface antigen, surface antibody, and core antibody negative should receive vaccination for hepatitis B, either with a 3-dose recombinant HBV vaccine, or, if available, the 2-dose TLR-9 agonist-adjuvant recombinant HBV vaccine, which has higher response rates in hyporesponsive populations.[172]

Prophylaxis for opportunistic *Pneumocystis jirovecii* pneumonia has not been specifically studied in AIH patients, but some suggest prophylactic treatment with TMP-SMZ may be indicated for any patient who is dually immunosuppressed, for example, those taking prednisone >20 mg for >4 weeks and a second immunosuppressive agent or condition.[173]

Treatment Initiation and Induction of Remission

Initial therapy is directed at achieving a swift biochemical remission. Steroids are the mainstay of therapy for induction due to their proven effectiveness. AZA is useful as a steroid sparing agent during initial therapy but is not successful at inducing complete remission as a single agent. Unfortunately, studies directly comparing different steroid and AZA dose regimens have not been performed. Rather, treatment regimens have been refined over decades of case-series and expert consensuses.[80] Prednisone, prednisolone, or budesonide, alone or in combination with AZA, are all considered effective initial therapy. Different dosing options are provided in Table 92.11.

With combination therapy, AZA may be started at the same time as steroids, although most centers recommend delaying the start of AZA for 2 weeks to confirm steroid responsiveness and evaluate TPMT and HBV status.

Budesonide, a steroid with high (>90%) first pass metabolism and resultant low systemic exposure, has been shown to be highly effective at inducing of remission when given in combination with AZA, and with lower systemic side effects, including moon face, striae, acne, and buffalo hump. In a large multicenter European trial, noncirrhotic patients with AIH were randomized to initial combination therapy with either budesonide 9 mg with AZA 1–2 mg/kg or prednisone 40 mg with AZA 1–2 mg/kg. The budesonide arm achieved higher rates of AST and ALT normalization (47% vs. 18%) with fewer steroid side effects (26% vs. 52%) at 6 months.[174] The budesonide dose was reduced from 3 mg TID to 3 mg BID upon biochemical remission. The dose of prednisone was tapered in a fixed dose taper to 10 mg over the first 6 months, which some argue may have undertreated some patients in the prednisone arm (as opposed to a response-guided taper). A similar randomized trial was performed in children and found budesonide was equivalent to prednisone at inducing remission but was associated with less weight gain.[175] Budesonide is a preferred first line option in AIH patients with diabetes, osteoporosis, obesity, hypertension, and other health conditions that may be exacerbated by systemic steroid exposure. However, budesonide is not recommended for use in cirrhotic patients because the benefit of first pass metabolism is lost in cirrhosis due to a combination of shunting around the liver and decreased hepatic metabolism to 6-MP in the liver.[176] Budesonide has not been shown to be harmful in cirrhosis, but the higher cost and lack of robust data specifically addressing its effectiveness in AIH cirrhosis make it an inadvisable choice in this group.

Use of steroids to treat patients with severe acute (jaundice and INR ≥ 1.5 without cirrhosis or encephalopathy) or fulminant (INR ≥ 1.5 with hepatic encephalopathy) liver failure mandates a careful consideration of overall risks and benefits. For patients who are potential liver transplant candidates, the risk of infection and/or delay in transplantation may supersede the possibility of a response to steroids.[177] There is a wide range of response to steroids in this group, ranging from 20% to 100%.[178] The presence of encephalopathy and MELD > 40 are predictors of poor response to steroids.[179] In the retrospective U.S. Acute Liver

TABLE 92.10 Risk Assessment HBV Reactivation With AIH Immunosuppression[266]

	Surface Antigen (+)	Surface Antigen (−) Core Antibody (+)
High dose steroids (>40 mg short term or >20 mg for >4 weeks)	High	Medium
Moderate dose steroids (20–40 mg short term or 10–20 mg for >4 weeks)	Medium	Low
Low dose/short term steroids; AZA	Low	Very low

AIH, Autoimmune hepatitis; *AZA*, azathioprine; *HBV*, hepatitis B.
Adapted from Loomba R, Liang TJ. Hepatitis B reactivation associated with immune suppressive and biological modifier therapies: current concepts, management strategies, and future directions. *Gastroenterology*. 2017;152:1297–1309.

TABLE 92.11 Options for Initial AIH Treatment

Adults	Children
MONOTHERAPY	
Prednisone 40–60 mg/day	Prednisone 1–2 mg/kg/day (max 60 mg)
Prednisone 1 mg/kg/day	
Prednisolone 0.5–1 mg/kg/day	
COMBINATION THERAPY	
Prednisone 20–40 mg/day + Azathioprine 50–150 mg/day or 1–2 mg/kg/day	Prednisone 1–2 mg/kg/day (max 40 mg) + Azathioprine 1–2 mg/kg daily
Budesonide 9 mg + Azathioprine 1–2 mg/kg/day	

AIH, Autoimmune hepatitis.

Failure Study Group (ALFSG), treatment with steroids did not improve survival and was associated with increase mortality in patients with MELD > 40.[179] On the other hand, other small series have demonstrated decent response rates and no increase in infections for patients with severe acute AIH treated with steroids.[178] One proposed approach in this group is to monitor closely for infection and discontinue steroids after 1–2 weeks if the response is not robust.[80]

AZA may be administered at fixed (50–150 mg/day) or weight-based (1–2 mg/kg/day) dosing. Treating to obtain specific 6-TG metabolite levels has not been shown to be superior strategy for induction of remission. 6-TG levels are similar between adult AIH patients with normalized AST and ALT and those with partial improvement.[180] The "normal" range of 230–400 pmol/8 × 10^8 RBC provided with most laboratory results was developed to guide treatment of inflammatory bowel disease and does not necessarily pertain to AIH. Nevertheless, it is common practice in pediatric hepatology to aim for 6-TG levels of 100–300 pmol/8 × 10^8.[181] Measurement of AZA metabolites is most useful in the assessment of the patient who is failing to achieve biochemical remission. Absent or very low levels of both 6-TG and 6-MMP suggest nonadherence. High 6-MMP levels (>5600 pmol/8 × 10^8 RBC) have been associated with hepatotoxicity and may require lowering of the dosage or the addition of allopurinol in conjunction with dosage reduction to boost 6-TG levels and reduce 6-MMP levels.

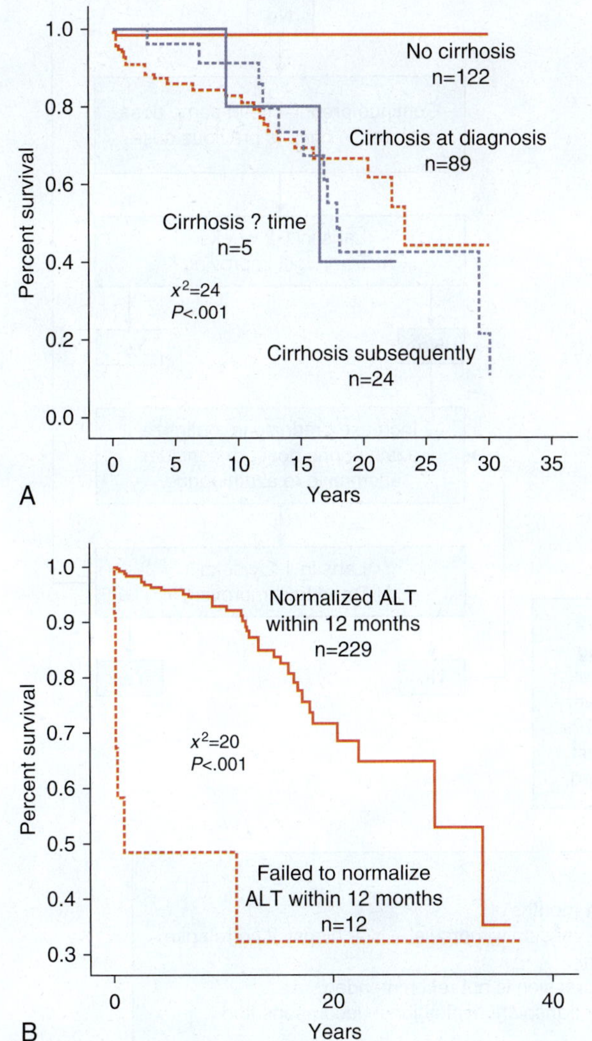

Fig. 92.4 Prognosis of autoimmune hepatitis. The association of liver-related death or need for LT with (A) cirrhosis diagnosed at any time point and (B) normalization of ALT within 12 months. Time = unknown time of onset. (Reproduced with permission from Hoeroldt B, McFarlane E, Dube A, et al. Long-term outcomes of patients with autoimmune hepatitis managed at a nontransplant center. *Gastroenterology*. 2011;140:1980–1989.)

The dose of predniso(lo)ne may not need to be maintained at the full initiation dose until complete biochemical remission is obtained but can potentially be very slowly decreased in a response-guided fashion as long as enzymes are continuing a clear and rapid downward trajectory toward normalization. Enzymes should be checked every 1–2 weeks during the induction period to guide any dose reductions rather than prescribing a fixed dose taper. The optimal downtitration regimen is not known but tends to be slower than is typically used in other diseases such as COPD exacerbation, IBD management, or lupus flares. For example, one strategy is to attempt to reduce 5 mg/week until a dose of 10 mg is obtained.[174] Other consensus guidelines recommend waiting until full normalization of AST, ALT, and IgG is achieved, and then reduce gradually to 20 mg daily, followed by further reductions of 2.5–5 mg every 2–4 weeks.[80] Budesonide is available in 3 mg increments and can be gradually reduced to 3 mg daily.[80] Doses below 10 mg prednisone or 3 mg budesonide are usually not sufficient to induce remission, so reductions below this level are usually deferred until the maintenance phase. A proposed treatment algorithm is illustrated in Fig. 92.5.

Maintenance of Remission

Once biochemical remission (defined as normal AST, ALT, and IgG) is achieved, it may be possible to withdraw the steroid completely and maintain remission with AZA alone. This is a goal that should be sought in all patients to minimize long-term steroid side effects. In the 1995 King's College study of steroid withdrawal in AIH, the investigators waited until the patient had been in complete biochemical remission for 1 year on 5–15 mg/day of prednisolone as a consolidation period, and then the AZA dose was increased to 2.0 mg/kg. After that, the prednisolone was gradually removed 2.5 mg every 2 weeks.[165] The justification for a prolonged consolidation period is rooted in the observation that histological remission lags behind biochemical remission by 3–8 months,[115] and the presence of portal plasma cells is a strong predictor of relapse.[113,182] In addition, the mechanism of action of AZA is to deplete cells by inhibiting purine synthesis. It takes 6–8 weeks for 6-TG levels to achieve steady state and may take several months before the target cell population is effectively reduced. In the original study, histological remission was confirmed with liver biopsy prior to withdrawal of steroids in a subset of patients but was not helpful.

Patients who repeatedly flare their liver enzymes during attempted steroid withdrawal despite adequate and prolonged doses of AZA, or who do not tolerate AZA or other immunomodulators (discussed below under nonresponse) may be continued on steroids for maintenance, at the lowest effective dose, which is typically 2.5–15 mg/day predniso(lo)ne.

Incomplete Response and Second-Line Therapies

Approximately 15% of patients will not be able to achieve complete remission with first line induction therapy of steroids with or without AZA. Those who are unable to reach complete remission after 3 years are at increased risk for progression to cirrhosis and need for liver transplantation.[183] Thus partial or nonresponders should be considered for alternate therapy.

In patients with severe liver dysfunction, the potential benefits of steroids in inducing remission must be weighed carefully against the risk of infection that may impede a life-saving liver

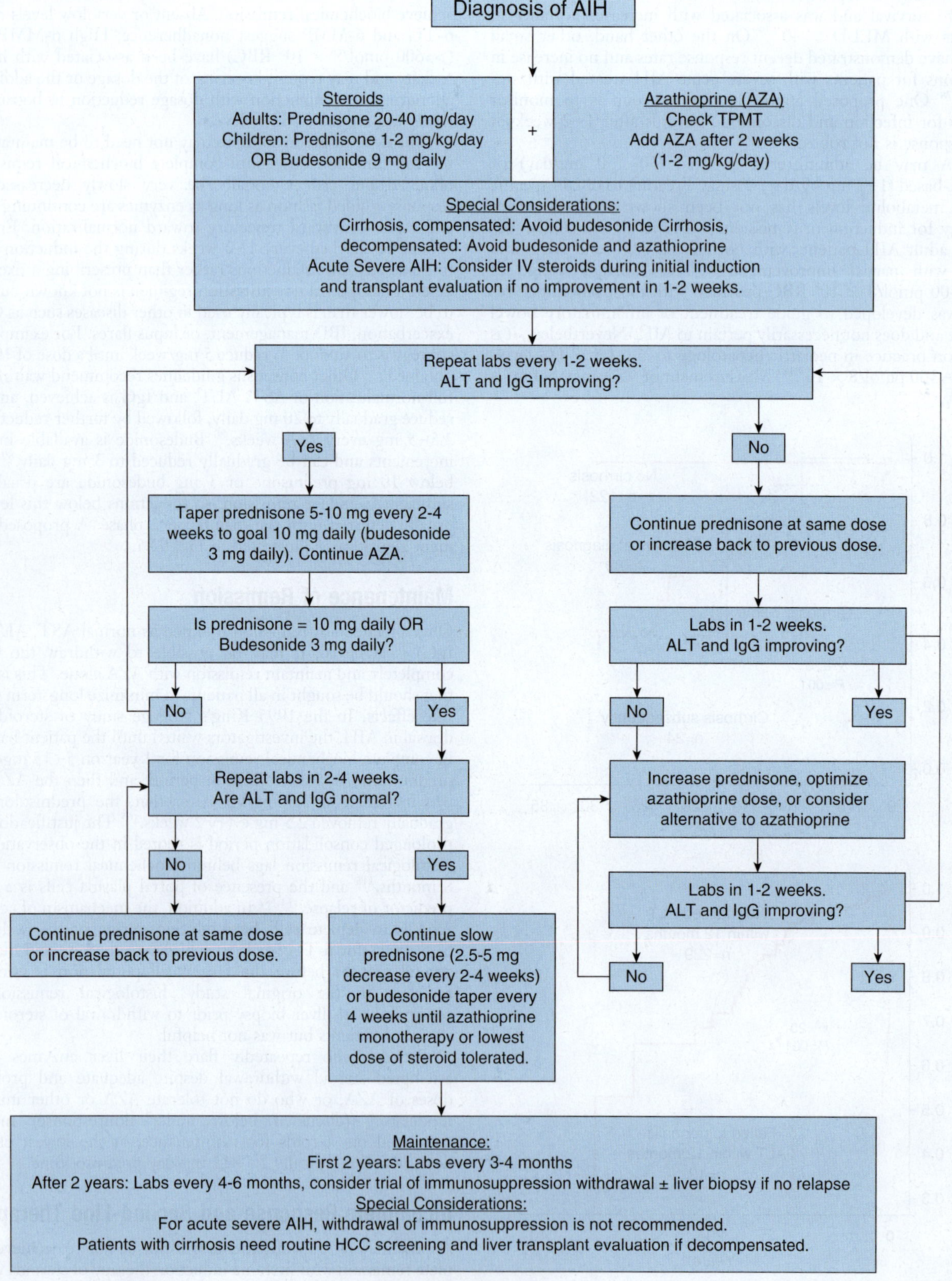

Fig. 92.5 Proposed treatment algorithm for autoimmune hepatitis.

transplant. The French Network for Rare Liver Diseases (FILFOIE) consortium developed the SURFASA (survival and prognostic factors for acute severe AIH) score (see Fig. 92.6) for patients present with severe AIH defined as having a bilirubin >11.7 mg/dL. In the cohort, mean INR was 1.8 and only 19% had hepatic encephalopathy of any grade (mostly grades I–II). Liver transplant-free survival was 92% in patients with a SURFASA score <−0.9 and only 23% for those greater. Similarly, the

$$-6.80 + 1.92*(D_0INR)+1.94*\left(\frac{D_3Bilirubin - D_0Bilirubin}{D_0Bilirubin}\right)$$

D_0INR = Day 0 INR value
$D_0Bilirubin$ = Day 0 bilirubin value
$D_3Bilirubin$ = Day 3 bilirubin value

Fig. 92.6 SURFASA Score.

score correctly classified as 86% of patients correctly being either a responder (<−0.9) or nonresponder (>−0.9) to corticosteroids.

The ALFSG has published prognostic factors in patients who meet criteria for acute liver failure (INR ≥ 2.0 and hepatic encephalopathy without a preestablished history of AIH). In these patients, higher bilirubin, INR, and coma grade were associated with worse outcome. The ALFSG Prognostic Index provides excellent prognostication for patients with acute liver failure related to AIH and is available as a smart phone application. Taken together, patients who have a low (<0.9) SURFASA score at Day 3, worsening or advanced encephalopathy (grades III–IV), or a poor ALFSG prognostic index score should be considered for steroid cessation and early liver transplant evaluation.

For those without immediate severity there are several medication adjustments that may be able to bring the patient into remission. If the initial steroid treatment choice was budesonide, switching to predniso(lo)ne is sometimes effective. Budesonide has less systemic delivery, but it is not known whether exposure to corticosteroids is beneficial only in the liver parenchyma or also in the surrounding hepatic lymph nodes. The stronger effect of prednisone as compared to budesonide in AIH is supported by multiple case reports of patients who were stably controlled on prednisolone therapy, but then flared when switched to budesonide, necessitating the return to prednisolone.[184] If the initial steroid choice was already predniso(lo)ne, a higher dose (e.g., 60 mg) may be considered. If a fixed dose of AZA was initially used, then the dose may be increased to 2 mg/kg.

The most well-studied alternative to AZA is MMF. A systematic review and meta-analysis found that prednisone with MMF was actually superior to prednisone with AZA at inducing complete biochemical remission.[185] However, MMF is not yet recommended in place of AZA for first line treatment[80] due to the relatively limited number of studies and duration of clinical experience, as well as the inherent risk of teratogenicity of MMF in fertile females. However, it is the recommended alternative for patients who fail to respond to, or do not tolerate, AZA.[80] A meta-analysis involving 309 patients who were either AZA intolerant or unresponsive showed that the pooled overall MMF response rate was 82% for AZA intolerance and 32% for AZA nonresponse.[186]

The calcineurin inhibitors, tacrolimus and cyclosporin (CsA), offer a different mechanism of immunosuppression from corticosteroids and purine synthesis inhibitors and have been used with moderately high success in AIH. As a first line agent, CsA, given to achieve trough levels of 150–200 ng/mL, is effective at inducing remission in children, and 50–70 ng/mL is usually adequate to maintain remission.[116,187] Tacrolimus has been studied primarily as an add-on therapy to steroids and/or purine synthesis inhibitors in refractory cases. The rate of improvement or normalization of serum aminotransferases in studies ranges from 75% to 94%.[188,189] An international study of 80 AIH patients treated with tacrolimus for either AZA intolerance or incomplete response documented normalization of serum aminotransferases in 94% of patients with AZA intolerance and 57% with incomplete AZA response.[190] The tacrolimus trough levels varied from 1 to 10 ng/mL.

Other salvage therapies reported in small numbers of patients have included TNF-inhibitors and B cell depletion, although both are associated with a high rate of infectious complications. Infliximab was able to induce biochemical remission in 6/11 patients with refractory AIH, although infectious complications occurred in 7/11.[191] Rituximab was given as second or third line therapy to six patients, with a reported success rate of biochemical remission in 67%.[192] Methotrexate was tried in a series of 11 patients refractory or steroid dependent AIH, and 55% achieved biochemical remission.[193]

Duration of Treatment, Relapse, and Treatment Withdrawal

AIH is a lifelong disease, characterized by periods of flare and remission. Similar to other autoimmune diseases such as multiple sclerosis, each flare in disease activity has the potential to cause more lasting damage, that is, cumulative fibrosis in the liver. Long-term maintenance therapy aims to avoid periods of disease activity, but relapse is commonplace and usually occurs when immunosuppression is withdrawn, often because either steroids were tapered too rapidly or because the patient did not continue the prescribed therapy. Half of all relapses occur within 3 months of drug withdrawal, but the risk continues at a rate of about 3% per year over the next 3 years. Some relapses have even been reported decades after stopping therapy.[147]

Numerous studies have examined the predictors of AIH relapse. The most important variable is the duration and completeness of disease inactivity prior to reduction in immunotherapy.[113,194,195] Delayed biochemical remission (≥5 months),[113] elevated serum ALT and IgG levels,[113,196] prior history of relapse,[197] and persistence of portal plasma cells in the liver tissue[113,198] all predict a higher rate of relapse. The presence of cirrhosis is an inconsistent predictor of future relapse,[199] but patients who progress to cirrhosis during treatment will invariably relapse off treatment.[197]

Repeating the original induction regimen is almost always successful at bringing the disease under control again.[78,197] Some patients may have prolonged periods of disease quiescence with maintenance therapy, raising the possibility of whether immunosuppressive therapy might be purposely completely discontinued, at least for prolonged periods of time. There is no consensus on the criteria for treatment withdrawal, so this decision should be an individualized, shared decision between patient and physician that takes into account the duration and depth of remission, stage of disease, and patient tolerance of medication.

In one retrospective study, 28/288 (10%) of AIH patients were eligible for treatment withdrawal based upon normal ALT and IgG and monotherapy for at least 2-year duration. After a median of 2-year follow-up, 54% remained in remission and did not require retreatment. Higher ALT and IgG levels, even in the upper half of the normal range, were associated with time to relapse.[195] Another retrospective study of 28 AIH patients withdrawn from immunosuppressive therapy found that prewithdrawal remission duration greater than 4 years was associated with significantly lower relapse rates compared to 2–4 or 1–2 years (67% vs. 17% vs. 10%, respectively).[158]

Performing a liver biopsy prior to consideration of treatment withdrawal can provide valuable information regarding the potential risk of relapse and is an important tool in the decision process, although biopsy is not a prerequisite for treatment withdrawal.[194] The relapse rate is 28% in those with normal liver histology, compared to 76% in those with ongoing inflammation.[200] Discontinuation of therapy in patients with cirrhosis should be undertaken cautiously. The risk of relapse off therapy for patients with cirrhosis remains high (82%) even if the cirrhosis has become inactive,[200] and a severe flare could push these patients into a state of decompensated liver failure. Taken together, these data paint the picture of the ideal candidate for withdrawal of all immunosuppression as a person without cirrhosis or history of relapse who has achieved a deep biochemical and histological remission for >4 years, defined as ALT level <50% ULN, serum IgG level <1200 mg/dL, and no inflammation on biopsy.

NONINVASIVE MARKERS OF FIBROSIS

After the index diagnosis, noninvasive markers of fibrosis are becoming a useful adjunct to monitor the development of fibrosis in patients with AIH. One systematic review included 16 studies with 861 patients with AIH examining various noninvasive markers of fibrosis: aspartate aminotransferase to platelet ratio index, fibrosis-4 index (FIB-4), aspartate aminotransferase/ALT ratio, and transient elastography (TE) (Table 92.12).[201]

The optimal staging cutoff values for vibration-controlled TE (VCTE, FibroScan) in AIH are 5.8 kPa for $F \geq 2$, 10.5 kPa for $\geq F3$ and 16 kPa for $\geq F4$. Because histological inflammation increases stiffness of the liver, VCTE obtained prior to initiating treatment usually reflects primarily the grade of inflammation. To estimate fibrosis, it is recommended to defer VCTE until after at least 6 months of successful treatment.[202]

A novel and proprietary method of processing MRI images has shown promise at estimating the grade of inflammation in AIH noninvasively. This method uses iron-corrected T1 relaxation maps (cT1) and is commercially available in the United States. cT1 correlates tightly with transaminases in AIH, even when transaminases are within the normal range.[203] A higher cT1 at baseline predicts future loss of biochemical remission, and failure to maintain remission is associated with rises in cT1 over follow up.[204] Thus its potential future role may be to indicate when it is "safe" to reduce immunosuppression, but randomized prospective trials utilizing cT1 to guide treatment decisions are needed.

HEALTH MAINTENANCE

Patients with AIH are often at increased risk of developing osteoporosis. This risk is not due to the disease per se, but due to coincident risk factors such as long-term steroid therapy, age (women > 65 years and men >75 years), postmenopausal state, and a high rate of vitamin D deficiency. Those on long-term steroids are also at risk for avascular necrosis (AVN) of the hip, and complaints of hip pain in this population should prompt X-ray evaluation for AVN. Bi-annual bone densitometry is recommended for AIH patients with any risk factors.[80] Vitamin D deficiency is very common in patients with AIH, including children. Patients with more inflammation and fibrosis in the liver and a poorer response to treatment are more likely to have low serum vitamin D levels.[205,206] Vitamin D has antiinflammatory and antifibrotic properties[207] and may even play a role in the progression of AIH, in addition to influencing bone health. For all these reasons, vitamin D monitoring and supplementation is well justified in patients with AIH. The American Gastroenterological Association recommends that all patients on steroids receive concomitant daily calcium with vitamin D supplementation (1000–1200 mg calcium with 400–800 IU Vitamin D).[208]

Another risk of steroid therapy is worsening or unmasking of metabolic syndrome (MetS). MetS is the cluster of features associated with developing type 2 diabetes and cardiovascular disease and includes hypertension, central obesity, hypertriglyceridemia, low HDL, and fasting hyperglycemia. It is estimated that 43% of patients with MetS also have MASLD.[209] Steroid therapy should be minimized as much as possible in patients with MetS, and vigilance for signs of developing MetS is prudent. Patients who did not have MASLD on baseline biopsy may develop it throughout the course of steroid therapy. Repeat biopsy to differentiate MASLD from AIH as the cause of persistently elevated transaminase levels is sometimes necessary.

Malignancy is a rare but potential complication of AIH or its therapies. Primary liver cancer, hepatocellular carcinoma (HCC), can arise within a cirrhotic liver from AIH, but almost never arises in noncirrhotic AIH. The overall incidence of HCC in AIH cirrhosis is close to 1% annually.[210] Current guidelines recommend screening for HCC in patients with any cirrhosis, including AIH, with ultrasonogram and serum alpha fetoprotein testing every 6 months.[80] Nonmelanoma skin cancer and non-Hodgkins lymphoma are also found more frequently in AIH patients (1.5% and 1%, respectively) compared to the general population. This risk is associated with but not exclusive to long term use of AZA.[210]

AIH is a lifelong disease that usually requires continuous immunosuppression. As such, vaccinations are important to help avoid serious preventable diseases that could have a worse outcome in persons with suppressed immune responses. Live vaccines may lead to disease, and that risk is closely related to the level of therapeutic immunosuppression.

The United States Centers for Disease Control considers a dose of ≥2 mg/kg or ≥20 mg daily of prednisone given for ≥14 days to be "high dose immunosuppression" and to avoid live vaccines at these doses. Per the CDC, live vaccines are not usually contraindicated at lower doses, but the CDC recommends waiting at least 1 month after administering high dose immunosuppression to give live vaccines[211] and waiting at least 1 month after live vaccination to start immunosuppression. The threshold for "high dose immunosuppression" for AZA is 3 mg/kg/day. Table 92.13 summarizes recommendations for vaccination of patients with chronic inflammatory disease on immunosuppressive medications.

SPECIAL POPULATIONS

Transplant Recipients

Liver transplantation is appropriate therapy for patients with end stage liver disease or fulminant liver failure from AIH. In the United States, approximately 5% of liver transplants are

TABLE 92.12 Noninvasive Methods of Fibrosis Assessment

	AUROC (95% CI)		
Test	**≥*F2***	**≥*F3* (Bridging Fibrosis or Cirrhosis)**	**≥*F4* (Cirrhosis)**
Transient Elastography	0.90 (0.87–0.92)	0.91 (0.89–0.93)	0.89 (0.86–0.92)
APRI	–	0.74 (0.70–0.78)	0.75 (0.72–0.79)
FIB 4	–	0.76 (0.72–0.79)	0.66 (0.62–0.70)
AST/ALT Ratio	–	0.73 (0.69–0.76)	–
MRE			

Note. While not a direct comparison, TE and magnetic resonance elastography (MRE) performed. *ALT*, Alanine aminotransferase.

performed for AIH.[212] The reported patient and graft survival rates are very good (Table 92.14), but the rates of acute and chronic rejection as well as recurrence of disease in the graft are higher than is reported for other chronic liver conditions. The median time to disease recurrence ranges from 2 months to 12 years, with a median time of 2 years posttransplant in adults and 4 years in children.[213] Due to the high rate of rejection and disease recurrence, it has been the policy at many institutions to continue corticosteroids longer than the typical immediate posttransplant period, sometimes indefinitely. However, a systematic review and meta-analysis in 2020 found no significant difference in recurrent AIH, rejection, graft loss, re-transplantation, graft survival or patient survival with this strategy.[214]

Occasionally, AIH may develop in a liver graft where the patient was originally transplanted for a different liver disease. This is referred to as "de novo AIH" and has been reported to occur in 1%–7% of adult and pediatric liver transplant recipients.[215,216] De novo AIH is characterized by elevated serum transaminases, elevated serum IgG, and the presence of autoantibodies, such as ANA, SMA and/or anti-LKM1. Liver biopsy typically shows lymphoplasmacytic infiltrates with interface hepatitis.[215]

TABLE 92.13 Recommended Vaccinations

Vaccine	Degree of IS	
	Low Level IS	**High Level IS**
Haemophilus influenza B conjugate	R	R
Hepatitis A	R	R
Hepatitis B	R	R
DTaP, Td, Tdap	R	R
Human papillomavirus	R, ages 11–26	R, ages 11–26
Influenza (inactivated)	R	R
Influenza (live attenuated)	NR	X
Measles, mumps, rubella (live)	NR	X
Meningococcal conjugate	R	R
Pneumococcal conjugate (PCV13)	R	R
Pneumococcal polysaccharide (PPSV23)	R, ages ≥2	R, ages ≥2
Polio (inactivated)	R	R
Rotavirus (live)	NR	X
Varicella (live)	NR	X
Zoster (live)	NR	X
Zoster (recombinant)	R, ages ≥18	R, ages ≥18
COVID-19 (mRNA)	R, ages >6 months	R, ages >6 months

IS, Immunosuppression; *R*, recommended; *NR*, not recommended; *X*, contraindicated; *DTaP*, diphtheria toxoid.

There is biochemical and histological overlap between de novo AIH and acute rejection, which can sometimes make the diagnosis challenging. In general, the presence of rejection should be excluded before assigning a diagnosis of de novo AIH. One particular form of acute rejection, which is characterized by an abundance of plasma cells, lymphocytic cholangitis and perivenulitis, has been called plasma cell hepatitis, plasma cell rejection, or plasma cell-rich rejection, and can be mistaken for de novo AIH. The outcomes of de novo AIH are dependent upon prompt recognition and institution of additional immunosuppressive therapy to avoid progression to fibrosis and cirrhosis. Approximately 7%–29% will require re-transplantation due to loss of graft function.[216,217]

Pregnant Patients

Very active AIH impairs fertility. In fact, one of the earliest descriptions by Professor Jan Waldenström in the 1950s of what would later come to be called AIH, was that of young women with amenorrhea, jaundice, and elevated globulins that progressed to cirrhosis.[218] However, when the inflammation is not severe, regular menses and fertility usually return. Antiphospholipid antibody syndrome may be associated with AIH, and this can also be a source of infertility/early fetal loss.[219] Because AIH often affects women in their childbearing years, pregnancy in patients with AIH is a relatively common occurrence, even in those with established cirrhosis.

The most common complication of pregnancy in AIH is a disease flare, which is often associated with medication reduction or discontinuation. Disease flare may happen during the pregnancy (7%–12%) but is especially common postpartum (11%–81%) when the maternal immune system, which was suppressed during gestation to ensure that the fetus is not treated as a foreign body, undergoes a process of immune reconstitution.[220]

Pregnancy outcomes are influenced by the state of the liver disease, both the degree of inflammation and the presence or absence of cirrhosis. Overall, the rate of stillbirth/fetal loss is 27% and preterm delivery is 20%, which are rates similar to other chronic inflammatory diseases.[220] The strongest predictor of flare-free pregnancy is biochemical remission in the year prior. Thus deferring pregnancy until AIH has been in complete remission for at least a year is optimal for family planning.

Because preterm birth and fetal loss may be precipitated by disease flare, it is important to continue immunosuppressive medications throughout the pregnancy, except for MMF which is teratogenic and abortifacient. MMF should be immediately stopped and replaced with another immunosuppressive agent. Highly effective birth control should be started 4 weeks prior to initiation of MMF, and MMF should be stopped at least 12 weeks before a planned conception. These recommendations from the U.S. Food and Drug Administration apply to both women and men of child-bearing potential, as MMF is excreted in semen. Older literature linked high dose steroid use in asthmatic mothers with an increased risk of cleft abnormalities, but that risk has been disproven for doses lower than 30 mg daily.[221] Similarly, high dose animal studies originally raised concern over possible teratogenicity from AZA, but data from over 3000 patients treated

TABLE 92.14 Outcomes of Patients With AIH Who Undergo Liver Transplantation[212,213,267–272]

Age Group	Graft Survival (%)		Patient Survival (%)		Acute Rejection (%)	Chronic Rejection (%)	Recurrence (%)	Recurrence (%)
	1 Year	5 Year	1 Year	5 Year			1 Year	5 Year
Adult	84	74	88	80–90	81	16	8–12	36–68
Child	91	83	95	91	72	4	10–20	20–83

with AZA for inflammatory bowel disease failed to show any increased risk of birth defects.[222]

Cirrhosis from AIH in pregnant women is managed in the same manner as cirrhosis from other etiologies.[223] Briefly, there is a large increase in circulating blood volume during pregnancy and progesterone causes an increase in splanchnic blood flow. This worsens portal hypertension and may worsen or precipitate new ascites or variceal bleeding. Ascites can usually be managed with loop diuretics alone; spironolactone may cause feminization of a male fetus. The risk of variceal bleeding is highest during second trimester, during the most rapid rise in blood volume, and in the second stage of labor with repeated valsalva maneuvers. Ideally the presence of varices would be assessed within the year prior to pregnancy and bleeding prophylaxis with nonselective beta blockers or band ligation completed before pregnancy. Alternatively, an endoscopy can be performed in the second trimester to assess the presence of varices, and prophylaxis can be started at that time. Measures to avoid extensive valsalva during labor, such as induction and forceps/vacuum-assisted delivery, may be helpful; cesarean delivery is not recommended for this purpose (only for obstetrical reasons), and patients with varices often have abdominal wall collaterals.

Children

AIH that presents in childhood often has a more aggressive course than AIH that presents in adulthood.[224] Type 1 AIH (ANA and/or SMA positive) accounts for about 2/3 of AIH in children and often presents around puberty, whereas the median age for Type 2 AIH (anti-LKM1 and/or anti-LC1 positive) is younger, age 7. In one prospective study, routine cholangiograms found evidence of ASC in 50% of patients with AIH,[125] indicating that this overlap syndrome is very common in children. ASC is found equally in boys and girls, and it is often associated with UC. Cholangiography is recommended in all pediatric AIH patients at diagnosis because ASC may not be evident from biochemistries or liver biopsy.[137]

The treatment of AIH in children is similar to the treatment for adults, namely corticosteroids with or without AZA. Budesonide does not appear to be more effective at inducing remission in children compared to predniso(lo)ne, but it does cause less weight gain.[225] Calcineurin inhibitors (cyclosporine or tacrolimus) have been used in small pediatric studies as either first or second line treatment with good success.[226–229] MMF (20 mg/kg BID) is almost as effective as calcineurin inhibitors for refractory disease and is usually preferred as a second line agent due to less toxicity.[137,230]

Withdrawal of all immunosuppression may be possible in carefully selected children with disease in deep remission. Approximately 20%–40% of children with type 1 AIH can be successfully withdrawn from treatment without flare, provided they meet the following criteria: (1) completed 2–3 years of therapy, (2) normal transaminases and IgG, (3) ANA and SMA <1:20, and (4) liver biopsy without residual inflammation.[125,137] Type 2 (anti-LKM1 positive) AIH, however, will usually relapse if treatment is withdrawn. The presence of cirrhosis and/or extrahepatic autoimmune disorders are negative predictors of the ability to withdraw immunosuppression.[231] Data for withdrawal of therapy in ASC are limited and concomitant IBD often dictates the need for continued immunomodulation in these children.

Liver transplantation for children with AIH is usually successful and has excellent outcomes (Table 92.14). The largest series of children transplanted for AIH to date was reported from the North American Studies in Pediatric Liver Transplantation registry. In that series, AIH accounted for 113/1524 (7%) of pediatric liver transplants, of which 40% were for fulminant AIH and 60% for chronic disease. The 5-year survival was 86%, which was similar to non-AIH transplants. Late (>3 months) but not chronic rejection was more common in transplants performed for AIH but responded well to steroid treatment without any measurable changes in infections or long-term outcomes.[232]

QUALITY OF LIFE AND TREATMENT ADHERENCE

Health-related quality of life has been observed to be lower in patients with AIH. While no AIH-specific inventory is available, standardized forms such as the Short Form-36 Health Survey (SF-36), the Patient Health Questionnaire-9, and the Chronic Liver Disease Questionnaire have all shown worse quality of life scores in AIH as compared with patients with other chronic liver diseases and healthy controls. Specifically, rates of anxiety, worry, depression, and fatigue have all been observed to be higher. One quality of life study in 103 German adult patients with AIH found increased rates of anxiety and depression which were unrelated to disease severity. Anxiety was driven by concerns about anticipated lifespan, the presence of cirrhosis, and whether offspring would also have AIH. Major depressive symptoms were five times more frequent compared to the general population and correlated with corticosteroid use.[233] Complete biochemical remission has been associated with a relatively higher quality of life in this patient population.[234,236–238]

As treatable as AIH can be, significant barriers exist to do so successfully. Medications such as prednisone and AZA have wide ranging side effects, including weight gain, bone mineral density loss, rashes, acne, diabetes, and gastrointestinal side effect as already discussed. Frequent lab and clinic visits require time and insurance or financial support which is not universally available in all countries. Quality of life issues such as depression and fatigue can lower a patient's motivation to surmount these barriers.[235] All these factors contribute to adherence concerns in AIH. While one study of 52 patients with AIH demonstrated excellent adherence (>80% reported taking their medication >80% of the time), other real-world studies of other rheumatologic conditions such as SLE has shown much lower rates of adherence (25% –57%).[235,239]

While the problem is clearly identified, no specific intervention has been proven to consistently increase adherence or improve many quality-of-life issues. Anxiety and depression may be addressed with traditional mental health interventions (e.g., antidepressants and therapy), though no specific treatment exists for other common issues such as fatigue. For adherence, some of the more frequently used interventions include enhancing social support, involving other allied health professionals (such as pharmacists) to help with medications or counseling, and more recently the use of technology for education and reminders.[240] Nonetheless, interventions to increase adherence should be targeted locally as needed to either specific patients or populations. A strong physician-patient relationship with emphasis on communication and education should be a high priority for the care of patients with AIH.

Full references for this chapter can be found at https://ebooks.health.elsevier.com.

93 Primary Biliary Cholangitis

Cynthia Levy, Christopher L. Bowlus

IN THIS CHAPTER

INTRODUCTION

Primary biliary cholangitis (PBC) is an autoimmune liver disease that generally affects middle-aged women and is the most common chronic cholestatic liver disease in adults in the United States of America (USA). PBC is characterized by progressive intrahepatic bile duct destruction, leading to chronic cholestasis and biliary cirrhosis. In 2015, the nomenclature of *primary biliary cirrhosis* was discarded in favor of *primary biliary cholangitis*, because most affected persons do not have "cirrhosis" at the time of their diagnosis.[1] Fatigue and pruritus are the most common presenting symptoms of PBC, and represent a significant burden to people living with the disease. Ursodeoxycholic acid (UDCA), the only medication shown to improve liver transplant-free survival, does not improve symptoms. Furthermore, nearly 40% of treated patients show an incomplete response to UDCA and remain at risk for disease progression. Obeticholic acid (OCA) was approved for patients who do not have an adequate biochemical response or are intolerant to UDCA and is efficacious in nearly half of treated patients, but can exacerbate pruritus. In the post-UDCA era, liver transplantation is becoming less common as a rescue therapy, but continues to offer a life-extending alternative for patients with end-stage PBC. Quality of life is severely impacted by presence of pruritus and/or fatigue, thus long-term care should focus not only on improving liver chemistries, but also on proper management of these symptoms and other extrahepatic complications of longstanding cholestasis.

EPIDEMIOLOGY

PBC occurs worldwide and predominantly in women, with a female-to-male ratio of 9:1.[2] The diagnosis of PBC is usually made between the ages of 40 and 60 years.[2] PBC is increasingly diagnosed at an earlier disease stage, largely due to increased disease awareness and widespread availability of specialty laboratory testing for PBC-specific antibodies.[3]

PBC affects men and women of all races and ethnicities. In a large, geographically diverse cohort of patients with PBC in the USA, 64% of affected persons were Caucasian, 21% Hispanic, 8% African American, and 7% Asian American/Pacific Islander or American Indian.[4] In the USA, the age-adjusted reported incidence of PBC per 100,000 person-years is 4.5 for women and 0.7 for men (2.7 overall), and the reported prevalence per 100,000 population is 65.4 for women and 12.1 for per men (40.2 overall).[2] However, incidence and prevalence of PBC vary worldwide, with annual incidence estimates from North America, Europe, and Asia of 2.75, 1.86, and 0.84 per 100,000 population, and a noticeable north-south gradient.[5]

Temporal trends suggest an increase in global incidence until the year 2000, with subsequent plateauing.[6] Interestingly, the female-to-male incidence ratios have been decreasing in studies from Italy, Denmark, and Japan,[5,7] and a large study from the Fibrotic Liver Disease Consortium in the USA also indicated lower ratios, with PBC incidence being approximately three times higher for women than men.[8] However, this increased detection of PBC cases in men may have occurred as a result of study methodology using administrative databases, possibly leading to misclassification. In contrast to incidence trends, PBC prevalence has been consistently increasing worldwide, including in North America, Europe, China, and Australia.[6] In the USA, prevalence increased from 21.7 to 39.2 per 100,000: It increased from 33.5 to

57.8 per 100,000 for women (72% increase) and from 7.2 to 15.4 per 100,000 for men (114% increase).[8] Notably, similar increases were observed across different age and race groups. Data suggest that in the last decade patients have had lower serum alkaline phosphatase (ALP) levels and milder fibrosis stage at the time of diagnosis, with improved response rates to UDCA and prolonged transplant-free survival.[3,7]

PATHOGENESIS

Although the etiology of PBC remains elusive, it is likely an immune-mediated process that occurs as a result of complex interactions between the environment and genetically susceptible persons. Several lines of evidence suggest an autoimmune pathogenesis for PBC, including the intense innate, humoral, and cellular responses,[9] loss of tolerance to mitochondrial autoantigens manifested by the presence of highly specific antimitochondrial antibodies (AMA),[10] involvement of T lymphocytes in the destruction of bile ducts,[11] and numerous defects in immunologic regulation.[12] Like other autoimmune diseases, PBC has a clear female predominance and is associated with an increased incidence of other autoimmune diseases in both persons with PBC and their first-degree relatives.[13,14]

Cellular Response

PBC seems to be triggered by an immune-mediated response to one or more allo- or autoantigens, which leads to progressive destruction of bile ducts, chronic cholestasis, and eventual biliary cirrhosis. Indeed, lymphocyte recruitment and homing to the liver through a variety of chemokines appears to be an important step in the pathogenesis of PBC.[15] Immunohistochemical phenotyping of inflammatory cells surrounding the bile ducts shows a combination of $CD4^+$ and $CD8^+$ T lymphocytes, accompanied by B lymphocytes and natural killer cells.[9,16,17] Bile duct destruction is induced directly by the cytotoxicity of $CD4^+$ and $CD8^+$ T cells in contact with biliary epithelium. Although B lymphocytes are relatively uncommon in the inflammatory reaction, they can sometimes be seen in clusters. Intracellular adhesion molecules [e.g., intracellular adhesion molecule-1 (ICAM-1)] are strongly expressed on many epithelial cells, particularly in areas of lymphocyte damage; these molecules may facilitate the interaction between destructive lymphocytes and their targets, and have been found in cholangiocytes of patients with PBC.[18] In the early biliary lesions of PBC, eosinophilic infiltration and granulomas are often seen. While PBC is primarily a disease of the small intrahepatic bile ducts, with progressive loss of the biliary epithelial cells (BEC) lining these ducts and resulting cholestatic damage, PBC is not restricted to the liver; this autoimmune epithelitis also affects salivary and lacrimal glands, with associated cellular phenotypic changes like those seen in the BECs.[19]

Autoantibodies

AMA were described for the first time in patients with PBC in the 1960s and continue to be regarded as the most sensitive and specific immunologic hallmark of the disease.[20] AMA are directed to the E2 component of the pyruvate dehydrogenase complex (PDC-E2), the E2 unit of the branched-chain 2-oxo-acid dehydrogenase complex (BCOADC-E2), and the E2 subunit of the 2-oxo-glutarate dehydrogenase complex (OGDC-E2).[21–23] Other AMA recognize the E1a subunit of PDC (PDC E1a) and the dihydrolipoamide dehydrogenase-binding protein (E3BP) of PDC.[24] These molecules are located on the inner mitochondrial membrane, and all contain a highly preserved sequence motif thought to be essential for antigen recognition.[25] At least one of these components usually reacts with AMA in a patient with PBC. The most frequent antigen against which AMA are directed is PDC-E2; PDC-E2-reacting antibodies are present in up to 95% of sera from persons with PBC.[20,26]

AMA do not appear to be cytotoxic: (1) they persist after liver transplantation even in the absence of disease recurrence; (2) disease severity is unrelated to antibody titer; (3) they are not always present in PBC; (4) they develop in animal models after the injection of recombinant PDC-E2 protein, but without resulting bile duct destruction or inflammation; and (5) AMA positivity is not always associated with PBC.[27–30] Further, the different types and numbers of mitochondrial antigens recognized by Western immunoblot analysis at the time of a patient's presentation is independent of the stage of the liver disease and not associated with specific clinical, biochemical, histologic, and immunologic features or with the Mayo risk score (see later).[31] Although AMA are predominantly of the immunoglobulin (Ig)G1 and IgG3 classes, most patients who have PBC exhibit polyclonal elevation of serum IgM levels; the IgM is not directed at mitochondrial or nuclear antigens. This phenomenon is suggestive of polyclonal activation of the B-cell compartment with an associated failure of isotype switching, representing aberrant B-cell activation.[32]

Antinuclear antibodies (ANA) are present in nearly one half of patients with PBC and in up to 85% of patients with AMA-negative PBC.[33] The most relevant immunofluorescent reactivities of ANA in patients with PBC are the antimultiple nuclear dots antibodies, with the molecular target being a 100-kd soluble protein called *Sp100*, and the antinuclear envelope antibodies.[34] The immunofluorescence pattern of the antinuclear envelope antibodies is characterized as being rim-like and membranous; its molecular targets are structural components of the nuclear pore complex, such as gp210 and nucleoprotein p62, and of the nuclear membrane, such as lamin B receptors.[35] These antibodies are specific for PBC and aid in the diagnosis of AMA-negative patients (see section on diagnosis).[33]

In addition to anti-gp210 and anti-Sp100, other PBC-specific autoantibodies have been identified. These include anti-hexokinase-1 and anti-kelch-like 12 protein, present in 45.7% and 24.9% of AMA-positive PBC patients, and in 24.7% and 19.2% of AMA-negative PBC patients, respectively.[36,37] Whether these PBC-specific ANA have any pathogenic role in disease development is yet to be determined.

Genetic Factors

The occurrence of PBC in relatives of affected persons, abnormalities of cell-mediated immunity in first-degree relatives of patients with PBC, and risk loci involved in key immunoregulatory pathways that have been associated with other autoimmune conditions, such as multiple sclerosis and celiac disease, all suggest a genetic association. Indeed, the concordance of PBC among those with a family history is 5% and is much higher among monozygotic (60%) than dizygotic twins (0%).[38,39] Moreover, AMA are frequently detected among first-degree relatives of patients with PBC (20% of sisters, 15% of mothers, and 10% of daughters).[40,41]

The strongest and most consistent genetic associations come from the HLA locus class II domain, particularly the HLA-DRB1*08 family. The products of HLA genes are essential for antigen presentation and maintenance of immune tolerance. DRB1*0801 and DRB1*0803 are associated with disease susceptibility in North American/European and Japanese populations, respectively. By contrast, DRB1*11 and DRB*13 have been found to be protective in European populations.[42]

Despite these observations, 80%–90% of patients with PBC lack the most common HLA susceptibility alleles, which suggests that non-HLA loci are important. Indeed, genome-wide association studies (GWASs) have identified over 40 non-HLA susceptibility loci in a total of 22 genes.[12] Such loci appear to be involved in key immunoregulatory roles such as T-cell differentiation, toll-like receptors, TNF signaling, interleukin-12, and other cytokine signaling pathways.[41–45] The implicated genes identified to date are estimated to explain roughly 15% of the heritability.[46,47] Consequently, epigenetics is believed to play an important role in the etiopathogenesis. An epigenetic modification has the potential to create phenotypic changes without altering the underlying DNA. Indeed, DNA methylation, histone modifications, and microRNAs have all been implicated in the development of PBC through various mechanisms.[48,49] Studies linking genetic variability to response to therapy and prognosis are lacking.

X Monosomy

Women with PBC have a higher frequency of X chromosome inactivation in peripheral leukocytes compared to healthy controls.[50] It is possible that haploinsufficiency of specific X-linked genes is associated with autoimmunity and female predisposition in PBC. Recently, the first chromosome X-wide association study included data from five GWAS from Italy, UK, Canada, China, and Japan, and identified several genes (TIMM17B, PQPBP1, PIM2, SLC35A2, OTUD5, and GRIPAP1) and a control element (superenhancer GH0XJ048933) possibly contributing to PBC pathogenesis.[51] While epigenetic alterations of the X chromosome involving aberrant DNA methylation and microRNAs have been described in PBC,[52] more in-depth functional investigations are needed.

Biliary Epithelial Cell Apoptosis

Clearance of apoptotic cell debris is tightly controlled by the immune system. Dysregulation in apoptosis may lead to loss of tolerance and the development of autoimmune diseases by three possible mechanisms. First, impaired or enhanced clearance of apoptotic cells can lead to an enhanced inflammatory response or an accumulation of autoimmunogenic fragments. Second, genetic defects in apoptosis can result in autoimmunity by interfering with tolerogenic deletion of lymphocytes. Finally, apoptosis is a common event that can occasionally lead to an abnormal autoantigen presentation resulting in autoimmunity.[53]

During apoptosis, cholangiocytes (unlike other epithelial cells) translocate intact, immunologically active PDC-E2 to apoptotic blebs called apoptopes.[54] When these biliary apoptopes are cultured with macrophages from patients with PBC in the presence of AMA, an inflammatory reaction ensues that may result in apoptosis of surrounding cells.[55] In addition to stimulating the innate immune system, PDC-E2 can react with circulating immune complexes that are processed by antigen-presenting cells, which present the epitope(s) to T cells, thereby leading to specific T and B cell activation.[56] This may help explain the selectivity of PBC for small- and medium-sized bile ducts.

Importantly, BECs are not innocent bystanders. Some BECs become activated and proliferate in the presence of insults, while other BECs undergo senescence and become resistant to apoptosis, acquiring a secretory phenotype that helps mediate peribiliary inflammation.[57] BECs can also act as antigen presenting cells, further enhancing inflammation and contributing to disease progression.

One important function of the BECs is secretion of bicarbonate into bile; bicarbonate acts as a protective barrier against hydrophobic bile acids.[58] Reduced bicarbonate secretion, as seen in PBC, can sensitize BECs to bile salt-induced apoptosis through activation of adenylyl cyclase, a bicarbonate sensor that regulates apoptosis.[59] Indeed, in vitro inhibition of adenylyl cyclase prevents apoptosis.[60] These findings could partly explain the mechanisms whereby UDCA, an agent that has been shown to suppress apoptosis, can delay progression of PBC (see later).

Thus immune-mediated BEC injury is followed by impairment of cholangiocyte function, with progressive cholestasis and reduction of bicarbonate secretion, leading to bile acid–mediated injury. In turn, this sensitizes BECs to apoptosis as well as senescence; subsequent immune activation ensues, generating a self-perpetuating vicious cycle that eventually leads to biliary cirrhosis.

Molecular Mimicry

Molecular mimicry between host autoantigens and unrelated exogenous substances is one of the hypotheses advanced to explain how autoantibodies to self-proteins arise, break tolerance, and lead to autoimmune disease. Molecular mimicry of an extrinsic protein produced by an infectious agent has long been suggested as a possible initiating event in PBC.[61] Microorganisms produce many foreign antigens that collectively constitute the major determinants recognized by the immune system. These antigens potentially include several carbohydrates, lipids, and proteins that can be recognized by specific receptors on inflammatory cells. PDC-E2, particularly its inner lipoyl domain, is highly conserved among bacteria, yeasts, and mammals. Infectious agents implicated in the immune response in PBC include *Escherichia coli*[62] and *Novosphingobium aromaticivorans*.[63] T cell clones reactive to a specific sequence motif in PDC-E2 are found in the peripheral blood of patients with PBC, and T cells reacting to the *E. coli* PDC E2 also cross-react with peptides in human mitochondrial autoantigens. Multiple studies have suggested an association between urinary tract infections and PBC.[45,64]

Notably, molecular mimicry also occurs between mitochondrial and nuclear antigens, such as gp210 and Sp100, which could be of interest to explain disease development in AMA-negative patients with PBC.[65]

Xenobiotics and Other Implicated Agents

Xenobiotics are foreign compounds that may alter self-proteins by inducing a change in the molecular structure of the native protein sufficient to induce an immune response. The immune response may then result in the recognition of both the modified and the native proteins. PBC sera have been shown to react strongly against PDC-E2 modified with synthetic chemicals such as 2-octynoic acid and 2-nonynoic acid and have been shown to induce PBC-like liver lesions when injected in animals.[66–68] In addition, anti-PDC-E2 autoantibodies from persons with PBC cross-react with xenobiotics, including 2-octynoic acid and 6,8-bis (acetylthio) octanoic acid; they also recognize lipoic acid, which is covalently bound to PDC-E2.[69] 2-Octynoic acid is commonly found in cosmetics, possibly explaining increased risk of PBC among frequent users of nail polish and hair dye.[64] Several epidemiologic studies have found an association between smoking and PBC.[45] A study of 223 persons with PBC demonstrated an independent association between smoking and advanced liver fibrosis (Metavir stages F3–F4). In addition, each pack-year of smoking was associated with a 5% increase in the likelihood of advanced fibrosis.[70] This finding was recently confirmed in a meta-analysis including 544 patients with PBC, which indicated a 3.0 pooled OR for advanced liver fibrosis among patients with PBC who were smokers compared to nonsmokers.[71] Consequently, patients with PBC should be counseled about this added risk.

Recently, the role of gut dysbiosis in the pathogenesis of PBC is also being investigated. Bacterial diversity is lower in patients with PBC compared to healthy subjects, with associated loss of beneficial commensals like *Clostridiales*.[72] Such dysbiosis as well as impairment of intestinal barrier functions found in patients with PBC can lead to increased exposure of cholangiocytes to microorganisms, potentially triggering an amplified inflammatory response and eventual fibrosis.[73]

Further environmental risk is demonstrated by clustering of cases around superfund toxic waste areas in New York[74] and in industrialized urban areas in the United Kingdom.[75] In addition, clusters of PBC have been demonstrated near coal mines in the Northeast of England.[76]

CLINICAL PRESENTATION

Subclinical Disease

Widespread use of screening laboratory tests has led to diagnosis of PBC at an asymptomatic stage in over 60% of persons with this condition.[77] Some asymptomatic persons with positive AMA and normal results of liver biochemical tests are found on liver biopsy specimens to have features that are diagnostic of or consistent with PBC; symptoms, signs, and laboratory evidence of chronic cholestasis may develop in these individuals.[78] However, most persons found on screening to have AMA with normal liver biochemical test levels do not ultimately prove to have PBC; the rate of PBC development in these individuals is low, roughly 10–16% after 5 years.[27,79,80] Similarly, the risk of developing PBC in AMA-positive first-degree relatives of patients with PBC is very low.[81]

In a recent study from Switzerland including 30 patients with positive AMA and normal ALP, 24 (80%) had histological features of PBC. Although most had early stage (Nakanuma stages 1–2), two patients had Nakanuma stage 3 disease. Fourteen patients had elevated gamma glutamyl transferase (GGT) levels at baseline, but that did not correlate with histological findings.[82] These data suggest that patients with positive AMA and normal ALP deserve careful and individualized evaluation for evidence of ongoing liver injury.

Clinical Features

A large population-based study from Northeast England found that about 50% of initially asymptomatic patients had developed symptoms of PBC within 5 years of diagnosis, and 95% within 20 years.[77] Symptoms commonly observed in patients with PBC include pruritus, fatigue, dry eyes, dry mouth, and right upper quadrant abdominal pain, as well as symptoms of other autoimmune diseases that can coexist with PBC (Table 93.1). Symptoms may also relate to fat-soluble vitamin deficiency and bone pain, with or without spontaneous fractures. Patients with more advanced disease can present with signs and symptoms of cirrhosis and portal hypertension, including jaundice, lower extremity edema, ascites, GI bleeding, and hepatic encephalopathy. Interestingly, male patients with PBC may have fewer PBC-related symptoms (fatigue and pruritus) compared to female patients; men also tend to present later, with more advanced disease, and higher rates of hepatocellular carcinoma (HCC).[83,84] On physical examination, the most common signs are skin hyperpigmentation (caused by deposition of melanin), hepatosplenomegaly, xanthelasma, and, in more advanced disease, jaundice. Patients with PBC have significantly reduced quality of life, in large part due to the burden of symptoms.

Fatigue

Fatigue, although relatively nonspecific, is considered the most disabling symptom of PBC by many patients.[85] Whereas a clear understanding of the pathogenesis of fatigue is lacking, it appears to result from a combination of peripheral muscle involvement, central nervous system abnormalities, and loss of cerebral autoregulation.[86] Approximately half of patients with fatigue also report cognitive symptoms and have a greater perception of quality-of-life impairment. These patients with fatigue and cognitive impairment are younger, and score higher for depression, anxiety, daytime somnolence and vasomotor autonomic dysfunction, possibly suggesting a more central process.[86] Nonetheless, major brain structural abnormalities have not been found in patients with PBC and fatigue.[87]

Fatigue is often associated with social and emotional dysfunction; thus maintaining social networks may be critical to minimize the impact of fatigue. There is, however, great difference on the reported impact of fatigue in different countries; fatigue was more significant among British study participants compared to those from Japan, Italy, and Spain.[88] Why latitude matters for symptom perception is uncertain, and the role of genetics, cultural differences, and sun exposure requires further evaluation.

Fatigue is unrelated to response to treatment with UDCA. In addition, the etiology of fatigue is often multifactorial, with other factors potentially contributing to fatigue, including sleep disturbance, medications, anemia, and others.[89] Noncirrhotic patients with PBC do exhibit altered sleep patterns compared with healthy controls.[90] Fatigue often persists throughout the disease course, and higher fatigue levels have been associated with an increased risk of death and need for LT.[91,92] Unfortunately, nearly half of patients with PBC who undergo LT still complain of moderate to severe fatigue 2 years later.[93]

Pruritus

Pruritus affects up to 80% of patients with PBC; it may occur at any point, early or late, or intermittently in the course of the disease.[94,95] Occasionally, pruritus precedes the diagnosis of PBC by years. Pruritus is generally intermittent during the day and is most troublesome in the evening and at night. It typically affects the palms and soles, although pruritus can be generalized.[96] In a population-based study of 770 patients with PBC from England, the cumulative risk of developing pruritus in previously asymptomatic patients was 19%, 45%, and 57% at 1, 5, and 10 years, respectively.[97] In contrast, it may fade in more advanced disease stages.[98]

Several factors may contribute to the pathogenesis of cholestatic pruritus; these include presence of pruritogenic substances in bile, liver or systemic circulation. It is well established that use of anion exchange resins, and now of inhibitors of the ileal bile acid transporter, can improve itching in patients with cholestatic diseases, suggesting a pruritogenic substance present in bile and

TABLE 93.1 Extrahepatic Diseases Associated With PBC

Disease	Frequency (%)
Hashimoto's thyroiditis	9–20
Graves' disease	1.5–3.2
Keratoconjunctivitis sicca or Sjögren syndrome	3.5–100
Systemic sclerosis and its variants	2.9–19
Rheumatoid arthritis	1.8–8.1
Raynaud phenomenon	8–30
Cutaneous disorders: psoriasis, vitiligo, lichen planus, lichen sclerosus, urticaria, pemphigus	2.3–3.6
Distal tubular acidosis	Up to 33
Tubulointerstitial nephritis, Fanconi syndrome	Rare
Celiac disease	1–7
Inflammatory bowel disease	1.3

involved in the enterohepatic circulation.[98,99] Moreover, the recently discovered itch-mediating nociceptor Mas-related G-protein-coupled receptor family X4 (MRGPRX4) is activated by bilirubin and certain bile acids.[100,101]

It is also possible that pruritogenic substances are formed or biotransformed in the liver, as suggested by successful resolution of itching with the pregnane X receptor (PXR) agonist rifampin[102] and with the peroxisome proliferator-activated receptor (PPAR) agonist bezafibrate.[103]

An increased tone of endogenous opioids has been described in patients with PBC.[104] Although there is no correlation between itching and opioid metabolites,[105] μ-opioid antagonists and κ-opioid agonists have well-documented antipruritic effect. In addition, increased concentrations and activity of autotaxin, the enzyme involved in generation of lysophosphatidic acid, correlate with the severity of pruritus and decrease with successful treatments.[106] Thus lysophosphatidic acid is considered a potential itching neurotransmitter in cholestatic diseases. Finally, the serum interleukin IL-31 has also been found to correlate with cholestatic pruritus[107] and may represent a measurable biomarker in this setting; the therapeutic implications of this finding are yet to be evaluated.

Chronic pruritus can significantly impact quality of life of patients with PBC independent of fatigue.[108] In some patients, pruritus becomes refractory to all available therapies, leading to social isolation, depression, sleep deprivation, and greater levels of fatigue and emotional distress.[95] This resistant and clinically significant pruritus has been accepted as an indication for liver transplantation.[109–111]

Associated Diseases

Patients with PBC often suffer from other coexisting autoimmune diseases (see Table 93.1). One retrospective study involving 20 centers from Europe, Canada, and the USA found that nearly 30% of patients had at least one of 35 different extrahepatic autoimmune disorders.[13] Hashimoto thyroiditis (9.1%) and Sjögren disease (8.3%) were the most common; others included systemic sclerosis (scleroderma), rheumatoid arthritis, systemic lupus erythematosus, celiac disease, inflammatory bowel disease, some cutaneous disorders such as psoriasis and lichen sclerosus, as well as hematological and renal diseases. Extrahepatic autoimmune diseases were more common in women and in those with seropositivity for AMA, ANA, and/or smooth muscle antibody. PBC severity, response to UDCA and long-term outcomes were not affected by the presence of an extrahepatic autoimmune disease.

The frequency of extrahepatic malignancy does not seem to be increased in patients with PBC. A large study including a total of 758 PBC patients from two European centers (Padova and Barcelona) compared the rates of extrahepatic malignancies between patients with PBC and the standardized incidence ratio derived from local cancer registries. The overall incidence of these malignancies was similar to the expected incidence for the general population.[112] It is possible that more advanced histological disease and presence of an associated extrahepatic autoimmune disease increase the risk of extrahepatic malignancies, although this requires further validation. HCC is an important malignancy associated with PBC, and the risk is nearly 19-fold higher than that in the general population (see later).[113]

DIAGNOSIS

The diagnosis of PBC is established when two out of three of the following criteria are met: chronic cholestatic liver test elevation [typically with ALP ≥ 1.5 times the upper limit of normal (ULN)], positive AMA (titers ≥1:40) or PBC-specific ANA, or histology showing chronic destructive nonsuppurative cholangitis, consistent with PBC (Fig. 93.1). Since AMA is found in 90%–95% of patients with PBC, and PBC-specific ANA became commercially available for widespread use, a liver biopsy is only rarely required to make the diagnosis of PBC. However, it is invaluable in seronegative cases, and in the evaluation of overlapping features of autoimmune hepatitis (AIH, see later).[110,111]

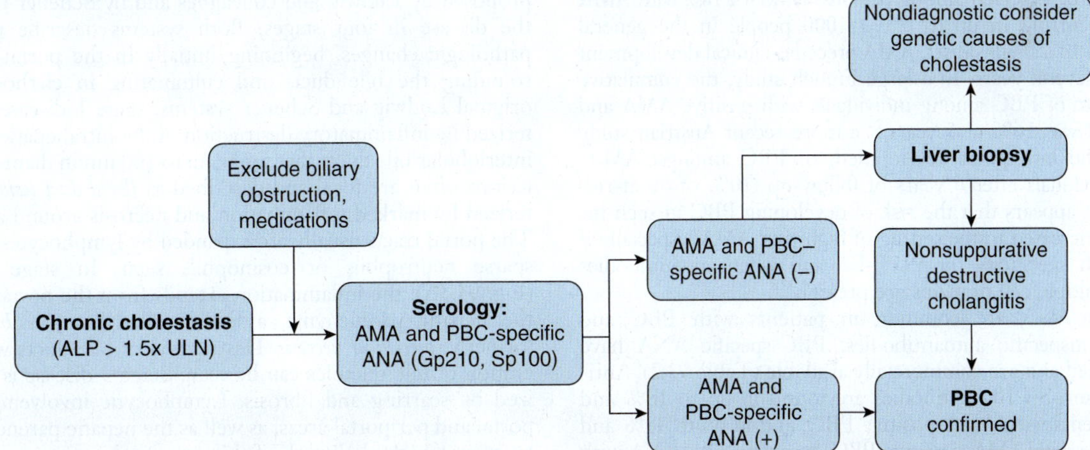

Fig. 93.1 Diagnostic evaluation in primary biliary cholangitis (PBC). In a patient with chronic cholestasis, that is, persistent alkaline phosphatase (ALP) elevation >11.5× ULN, it is important to obtain an ultrasound of the liver and exclude extrahepatic causes of cholestasis. For evaluation of intrahepatic causes, the first step is measurement of autoantibodies including antimitochondrial (AMA) and PBC-specific antinuclear antibodies (ANA). If these are positive and no other obvious cause of ALP elevation is present (i.e., drugs, metabolic syndrome raising suspicion for steatotic liver disease, etc.), then a definite diagnosis of PBC can be made without the need for a liver biopsy. For cases where the PBC-specific autoantibodies are negative and/or there is suspicion for a coexisting or alternative diagnosis, a liver biopsy is indicated. In that setting, evidence of nonsuppurative destructive cholangitis is diagnostic of PBC. If liver biopsy is nondiagnostic, testing for genetic causes of cholestasis is appropriate.

Biochemical Features

Liver biochemical test results show a cholestatic picture. Almost all patients have increased serum levels of ALP and GGT. Serum aminotransferase (AST, ALT) levels are mildly elevated (usually less than three times the ULN); marked elevations (more than five times the ULN) are unusual and may suggest overlapping features of AIH or coexisting diagnosis of viral hepatitis, steatotic liver disease or other. Serum bilirubin levels are usually normal in early stages and increase slowly over the course of the disease. As with other chronic liver diseases, a high serum bilirubin level, low serum albumin, and prolonged prothrombin time indicate advanced disease and a poor prognosis. Serum Ig levels, especially IgM, are increased, as are serum levels of bile acids.[110,111]

Dyslipidemia is evident in ~75% of patients with PBC.[114] In addition, cholesterol composition is abnormal, with two distinct patterns observed in early versus late stage PBC.[115] In early stage PBC, patients exhibit mild elevations of very low-density lipoprotein (VLDL) and LDL cholesterol, associated with an increase in high-density lipoprotein (HDL). In contrast, in late-stage disease there is marked LDL elevation with increased concentration of lipoprotein X, and decreased HDL concentration. Lipoprotein X is an abnormal cholesterol- and phospholipid-rich lipoprotein that lacks apolipoprotein B (ApoB) and has cardioprotective actions.[116] Because of this LDL enrichment with lipoprotein X, it is preferable to follow ApoB levels over LDL cholesterol as a better predictor of risk.

Serology

Indirect immunofluorescence (IIF), immunoblotting, and enzyme-linked immunosorbent assay can detect AMA. IIF is by far the most commonly used method and detects AMA in 90%–95% of patients with PBC[117] (Table 93.2); however, IIF testing requires interpretation by a skilled observer, and the result may be interpreted erroneously as negative for AMA in some patients with PBC. Immunoblotting and enzyme-linked immunosorbent assay have sensitivity and specificity rates higher than 95% for the detection of AMA and can detect AMA in persons with PBC who are AMA-negative by IIF.

AMA can be detected among persons without PBC, with AMA positivity occurring in up to 0.5–1/1000 people in the general population.[27] In a small subset, AMA precedes clinical development of PBC by several years. In a large French study, the cumulative incidence rate of PBC among individuals with positive AMA and normal ALP was 16% at 5 years,[79] a more recent Austrian study confirmed the infrequent development of PBC amongst AMA-positive individuals after 6 years of follow-up (10% of 59 at-risk patients).[80] It appears that the risk of developing PBC in such individuals is increased in the setting of high titer AMA, especially if there is high specificity for PDC-E2, and when autoantibodies targeting multiple cell domains are present.[118]

Although ANA are common in patients with PBC and generally nonspecific autoantibodies, PBC-specific ANA have been identified and are commercially available (Table 93.2). Anti-gp210 and anti-Sp 100 antibodies are found in up to 18% and 31% of patients with AMA-positive PBC, and in up to 45% and 54% of those with AMA-negative PBC, respectively.[33] ANA with the multiple nuclear dots and rim-like and membranous patterns are strongly associated with PBC and are strong markers of PBC in AMA-negative patients.[34,119,120] The specificity of anti-gp210 for PBC when detected by immunoblotting is greater than 99%. Anti-gp210 and possibly anti-p62 also offer prognostic information as they seem to be associated with aggressive disease with worse outcomes, although further studies are needed in this area.[119,121–124]

Other nonspecific autoantibodies found in persons with PBC include rheumatoid factor (65%),[125] smooth muscle antibodies

TABLE 93.2 Frequency of Autoantibodies in PBC

Antibody	Frequency (%)
Antimitochondrial	80–95
Antinuclear (All)	30–50
Nonspecific Autoantibodies	9–30
Anticentromere	28–63
Anti-Ro/SSA or anti-La/SSB	20–65
Rheumatoid factor or CCP-Ab	
PBC-Specific Autoantibodies	24–40
Anti-Sp100	16–18
Anti-Gp210	39–56
Anti-Hexokinase-1	19–25
Anti-Kelch-like 12	

(6%),[14] anticentromere antibodies (30%),[126] and antithyroid (antimicrosomal, antithyroglobulin) antibodies (41%).[127] In addition, autoantibodies related to associated extrahepatic autoimmune diseases can be present, including Sjögren syndrome-related antigen A and Sjögren syndrome-related antigen B, double-stranded DNA, endomysial antibodies, and others.[128,129]

Histopathology

One of the earliest histologic changes associated with PBC may be a loss of the canals of Hering, which can be demonstrated by biliary cytokeratin 19 staining.[130] Damage to the epithelial cells of the small bile ducts can also be appreciated early in the disease course (Figs. 93.2 and 93.3A,B). The most important and only diagnostic clue in many cases is *ductopenia*, defined as the absence of interlobular bile ducts in greater than 50% of portal tracts. The florid duct lesion, in which the epithelium of the interlobular and segmental bile ducts degenerates segmentally, with formation of poorly defined, noncaseating epithelioid granulomas, is nearly diagnostic of PBC but is found in a relatively small number of cases, mainly in early stages.[131]

The two most popular histologic staging systems are those proposed by Ludwig and colleagues and by Scheuer that classify the disease in four stages. Both systems describe progressive pathologic changes, beginning initially in the portal areas surrounding the bile ducts and culminating in cirrhosis. In the original Ludwig and Scheuer systems, stage 1 disease is characterized by inflammatory destruction of the intrahepatic septal and interlobular bile ducts that range up to 100 μm in diameter. These lesions often are focal and described as *florid duct lesions*, characterized by marked inflammation and necrosis around a bile duct. The portal tracts usually are expanded by lymphocytes, with only sparse neutrophils or eosinophils seen. In stage 2 disease (Fig. 93.3A), the inflammation extends from the portal tract into the hepatic parenchyma, a lesion called *interface hepatitis*, or formerly, *piecemeal necrosis*. Destruction of bile ducts with proliferation of bile ductules can be seen. Stage 3 disease is characterized by scarring and fibrosis. Lymphocytic involvement of the portal and periportal areas, as well as the hepatic parenchyma, can be seen, but the hallmark of this stage is the presence of fibrosis without regenerative nodules. Stage 4 disease is characterized by cirrhosis with fibrous septa and regenerative nodules (see Fig. 93.3B and Chapter 73).[132] Subsequently, the Ludwig-Batts staging system, known as the modified Scheuer, emphasized the role of inflammation and separated the inflammatory activity from fibrosis. Portal inflammation (grade 1), periportal hepatitis (grades 2–3 depending on severity), and bridging necrosis (grade 4) are scored separately from the fibrosis stages: portal fibrosis (stage 1), periportal fibrosis (stage 2), bridging fibrosis (stage 3), and cirrhosis (stage 4). Another staging system proposed by

Nakanuma et al. includes a more comprehensive grading of chronic cholangitis activity and hepatitic activity, and staging based on scoring for fibrosis, bile duct loss, and deposition of orcein-positive granules.[133] Despite being more cumbersome, the Nakanuma's staging system appears to predict outcomes more accurately when compared to Ludwig's and Scheuer's classification systems.[134,135]

Stage 1

Stage 2

Stage 3

Stage 4

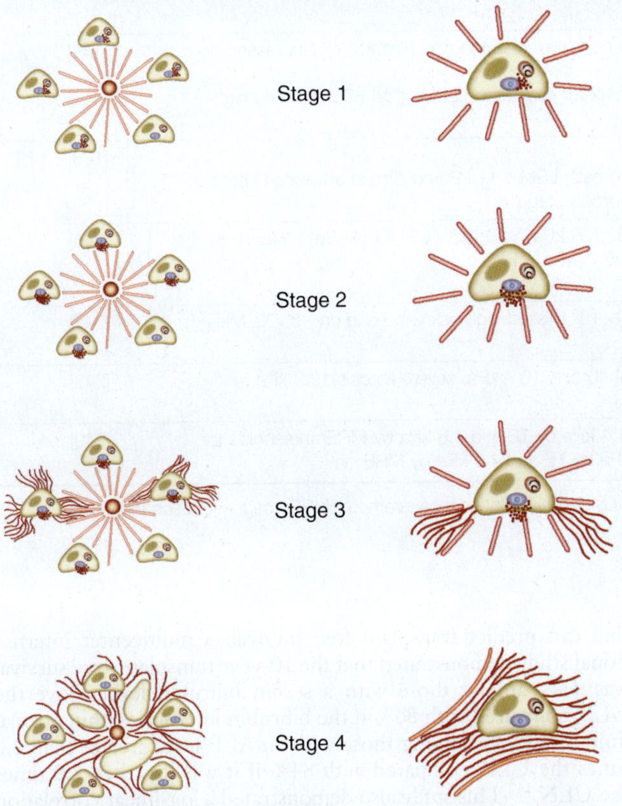

Fig. 93.2 Schematic representation of the staging system of primary biliary cholangitis (Ludwig's classification). The left side of the schematic shows 5 portal tracts surrounding a central vein at each stage. The right side shows a larger single portal tract at each stage (the bile ductule is *blue*). In stage 1, the inflammation is confined to the portal tract and is focused on the bile duct. In stage 2, the inflammation extends into the hepatic parenchyma (interface hepatitis or piecemeal necrosis). In stage 3, fibrosis is present. In stage 4, cirrhosis is present.

In the setting of a positive AMA, the combination of a serum ALP level greater than 1.5 times the ULN and a serum AST level less than five times the ULN is highly predictive for a diagnosis of PBC.[136] Therefore a liver biopsy is not necessary in the majority of patients and should be reserved for AMA-negative and PBC-specific ANA-negative patients (see later), or if an alternative diagnosis such as small duct PSC or overlap with AIH (see Chapters 70 and 92) is being considered.[110,111]

Imaging

Cross-sectional imaging with ultrasound (US), computerized tomography, or magnetic resonance imaging (MRI) is useful for excluding biliary obstruction and plays a key role in the diagnostic evaluation of persons who present with cholestatic liver biochemical test elevations and those who require surveillance for HCC because of cirrhosis. Aside from increased liver echogenicity and signs of portal hypertension, several imaging findings appear to be common in persons with PBC. Nearly two thirds can have a periportal "halo" sign (T1-and T2-weighted hypointensity centered around portal venous branches) on MRI and intra-abdominal lymphadenopathy.[137] Stable periportal adenopathy is important to recognize to avoid undue concern about underlying malignancy; however, large, bulky adenopathy should raise the question of associated malignancy.

US and MR elastography are increasingly used for the noninvasive assessment of hepatic fibrosis (see Chapters 75 and 76). Liver stiffness measurement (LSM) by vibration-controlled transient elastography correlates well with both fibrosis and histological stage in PBC. It is generally accepted that LSM $\geq$7–8, $\geq$10–11, and $\geq$14–17 kPa indicate significant fibrosis, advanced fibrosis, and cirrhosis, respectively (Table 93.3).[138,139] To that end, EASL recently recommended using a cut-off value of 10 kPa to identify patients with PBC and severe fibrosis/compensated advanced liver disease.[140] In addition, LSM has been shown to be an independent prognostic factor in PBC.[141]

NATURAL HISTORY AND PROGNOSIS

PBC is a progressive disease. In early observational studies, most patients had advanced disease at the time of initial presentation,[97,142] with esophageal varices developing in a third of patients

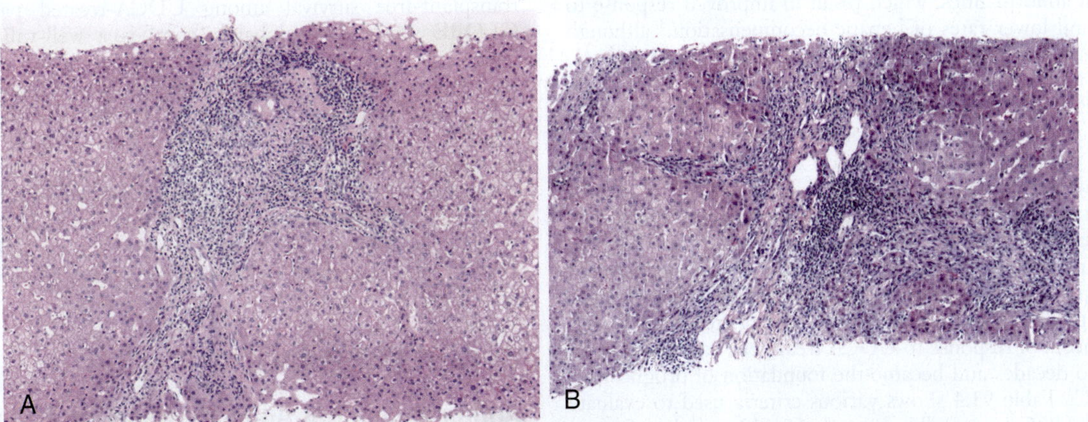

Fig. 93.3 (A), Photomicrograph of stage 2 primary biliary cholangitis (PBC). Mononuclear inflammatory cells expand the portal tracts with some disruption of the limiting plates (interface hepatitis). The bile ducts are surrounded by inflammatory cells, and no fibrosis is evident (H&E, ×100). (B) Stage 4 PBC. Cirrhosis, with areas of fibrosis surrounding the hepatic parenchyma, is present. A dense mononuclear inflammatory infiltrate is still seen in the portal tract, with interface hepatitis (H&E, ×100).

TABLE 93.3 Representative Studies of Elastography in Patients With PBC

Technique	N	Findings	References
TE	103	LSM 7.1 kPa correlates with ≥F1; LSM 8.8 kPa with ≥F2; LSM 10.7 kPa with ≥F3 and LSM 16.9 kPa with = F4	[153]
TE	150	Progression >2.1 kPa/year associated with 8.4-fold increase in risk of decompensation, liver transplantation or death	[153]
TE	3985	LSM is independently associated with poor clinical outcomes; Hazard ratio increases between 5 and 30 kPa LSM< 8kPa identifies patients at low risk for events and LSM ≥ 15 kPa identifies high-risk individuals	[141]
TE	167	All were treatment-naïve patients LSM ≤ 6.5 kPa excluded advanced fibrosis; LSM >11 kPa confirmed advanced fibrosis; only parameter affecting LSM was fibrosis stage	[139]
2D-SWE	53	LSM 5.6 (5.1–6.1) kPa ≥ F0; 7.0 (5.8–7.7) kPa ≥ F1; 9.1 (7.3–11.5) kPa ≥ F2; 10.8 (9.9–12.2) kPa ≥ F3; 14.5 (11.9–25.7) kPa = F4 Portal inflammation accounted for 32% of LSM variation	[246]
2D-SWE	231	LS < 25 kPa and platelet count >110×10^9 missed high-risk varices in only 3.7%. Miss rate for all-size varices was 8.4%	[247]
2D-SWE	157	Cut-off values discriminating significant fibrosis 10.7 kPa, severe fibrosis 12.2 kPa, and cirrhosis 14.1 kPa	[248]
TE or MRE	TE = 286, MRE = 332	Thresholds for predicting stage F4: 14.4 kPa by TE and 4.6 kPa by MRE; thresholds for predicting decompensation: 10.2 kPa by TE and 4.3 kPa by MRE	[249]

2D-SWE, Two-dimensional shear wave elastography; *ALP*, alkaline phosphatase; *LSM*, liver stiffness measurement; *MRE*, magnetic resonance elastography; *N*, number of patients studied; *TE*, transient elastography.

over a 5.6-year follow-up period, and nearly half of those experiencing at least one episode of variceal bleeding.[143] Prior to the introduction of UDCA, the rate of histological progression was roughly 1 stage every 1.5 years,[144] and the median time from diagnosis to death or liver transplantation ranged from 6 to 10 years.[142,144]

The availability of UDCA for treatment of PBC has markedly changed the course of the disease, as UDCA has been shown to delay histological progression,[145] delay development of varices,[146] and improve transplant-free survival.[147] As an example, the adjusted 10-year risk of hepatic decompensation (ascites, variceal hemorrhage, or hepatic encephalopathy), HCC, and liver-related deaths was 19%, 10% and 35%, respectively, in the 1970s, and improved to 6%, 2%, and 6%, respectively, in the 2000s.[3]

The widespread availability of accurate noninvasive diagnostic tests has facilitated the earlier diagnosis of PBC. Most patients are now diagnosed at an earlier disease stage and with milder biochemical abnormalities, which result in improved response to treatment and lower rates of hepatic decompensation,[3] although lead time bias may also have contributed to this finding.

Several independent predictors of prognosis have been identified in PBC. The original Mayo Risk Score was developed to assist clinicians in determining the timing for liver transplantation; it incorporates biochemical and clinical variables to generate survival estimates at 6, 12, and 24 months.[148] However, the above-mentioned shifts toward a milder initial clinical presentation and slower disease progression in the setting of UDCA treatment resulted in different needs for prognostication. It became imperative to monitor patients with earlier disease stage to identify those at risk for progression despite treatment.

The concept of response to UDCA treatment has evolved over the past two decades and became the foundation of prognostication in PBC. Table 93.4 shows various criteria used to evaluate response to UDCA, typically assessed after 12 months of treatment initiation (see later). These criteria are often utilized as endpoints in clinical trials. In clinical practice, however, monitoring of serum bilirubin and ALP levels will suffice. Both the serum bilirubin and ALP levels are important surrogate markers that can predict transplant-free survival: a multicenter international study demonstrated that the 10-year transplant-free survival was 41% among those with a serum bilirubin level above the ULN compared with 86% if the bilirubin level was within normal limits, and 62% among those with an ALP level greater than 2.0 times the ULN compared with 84% if it was less than 2.0 times the ULN.[147] This study also demonstrated a log-linear correlation between serum ALP levels and the hazards of liver transplantation or death, suggesting that the closer to normal the ALP is, the better the prognosis.[149,150]

In addition to serum ALP and bilirubin, other independent predictors of prognosis in the UDCA era include serum GGT greater than 3.2 times the ULN,[151] the enhanced liver fibrosis score (ELF) greater than 9.8,[152] advanced fibrosis stage at diagnosis and LSM greater than 9.6 kPa at baseline.[153] Beyond these dichotomous predictors, mathematical models have been developed to generate more individualized and accurate predictions for transplant-free survival among UDCA-treated patients. The GLOBE score (www.globalpbc.com) is a well-validated prognostic score that uses the patient's age and ALP, total bilirubin, albumin, and platelet count to predict transplant-free survival after 1 year of UDCA, allowing practitioners to risk stratify patients after a trial of UDCA therapy.[154] As an example, the 10-year transplant-free survival with a GLOBE score greater than 0.30 is 60%, compared with 92% with a GLOBE score less than or equal to 0.30. Similarly, the UK-PBC risk score includes the baseline serum albumin and platelet count, and serum bilirubin, ALP, and aminotransferases after 1 year of UDCA treatment to estimate the risk of liver failure within 5,10, and 15 years.[155]

VARIANT SYNDROMES

Antimitochondrial Antibody-Negative Primary Biliary Cholangitis

AMA-negative PBC is the designation for those patients who clinically, biochemically, and histologically appear to have the classic features of PBC but are found not to have AMA in serum

TABLE 93.4 Criteria Defining Biochemical Response to Ursodeoxycholic Acid and Prognosis

Criteria	Duration of Treatment	Definition
Binary response criteria		
Barcelona[178]	1 Year	Normal ALP or ALP reduction >40%
Paris-I[179]	1 Year	ALP < 3× ULN, AST<2× ULN, normal bilirubin
Rotterdam[176]	1 Year	Normal bilirubin, normal albumin
Toronto[184]	2 Years	ALP ≤ 1.67× ULN
Ehime[186]	6 Months	Normal GGT or GGT reduction ≥70%
Paris-II[183]	1 Year	ALP < 1.5× ULN, AST < 1.5× ULN, normal bilirubin
Rochester[185]	1 Year	ALP ≤ 1.67× ULN, bilirubin ≤1 mg/dL
International (Global PBC)[147]	1 Year	ALP < 2× ULN, normal bilirubin
Continuous risk scores		
GLOBE score[154]	1 Year	Bilirubin, ALP, albumin platelet count at 1 year, age at baseline
UK-PBC score[155]	1 Year	ALP, AST/ALT, bilirubin at 1 year, albumin, platelet count at baseline

ALP, Alkaline phosphatase; *AST*, aspartate aminotransferase; *GGT*, gamma glutamyl transferase; *ULN*, upper limit of normal.

by IIF or immunoblotting techniques. Of persons who have PBC by all other criteria, 5% are confirmed AMA negative.[26]

Most persons with AMA-negative PBC have antinuclear (perinuclear/rim-like or multiple nuclear dots pattern) or smooth muscle antibodies (or both).[33] Although these patients may be distinguished by the lack of AMA in serum, the specific AMA antigen PDC-E2 is expressed on the apical region of their biliary epithelium, as occurs in AMA-positive patients—an observation suggesting that the pathogenesis of both conditions may be identical. In fact, AMA-negative and -positive patients have similar clinical, laboratory, and histologic features. When regulatory T cells and the subgroup of T cells suggested to have a role in the genesis of autoimmune disease were examined in patients with PBC, no difference was found between those who had and those who did not have AMA.[156]

The absence of AMA makes liver biopsy mandatory to look for features of PBC and exclude other liver diseases, unless PBC-specific ANA are present. For the AMA-negative, PBC-specific ANA-negative patient, imaging by MRCP is essential to identify other cholangiopathies such as PSC. Liver biopsy and MRCP, along with select laboratory tests, will allow the exclusion of conditions that should be considered in the differential diagnosis, such as celiac disease, hepatitis C, sarcoidosis, small-duct PSC, and IgG4-associated autoimmune cholangitis. Gene testing may be necessary to rule out a genetic cholestatic syndrome.

Patents with AMA-negative PBC tend to follow the same clinical course, and to demonstrate a similar therapeutic response to UDCA, compared to AMA-positive patients.[156,157] Furthermore, a recent study including 521 veterans with PBC cirrhosis showed that AMA-negative patients had similar rates of decompensation, HCC and overall or liver-related death compared to AMA-positive patients.[158]

Primary Biliary Cholangitis with Overlapping Features of Autoimmune Hepatitis (PBC-AIH)

Some patients present either concurrently or sequentially with fluctuating or persistent features of AIH, including elevation of transaminases, high serum IgG levels, positive ANA, positive ASMA and more significant interface hepatitis on histology.[159] This variant presentation, called "PBC with overlapping features of AIH", should not be diagnosed based only on the presence of autoantibodies, nor using the international AIH group criteria for AIH[159] (see Chapter 92). In turn, the Paris criteria are the most widely accepted criteria to diagnose PBC-AIH, stating that in the presence of PBC, two of the following are required: (1) ALT greater than 5 times the ULN, (2) IgG at least 2 times the ULN and/or positive anti-smooth muscle antibody, and/or (3) liver biopsy with moderate or severe interface hepatitis.[160] The sensitivity and specificity of the Paris criteria for PBC-AIH were reported to be 92% and 97%, respectively,[161] and patients who meet these criteria may benefit from corticosteroid treatment in addition to UDCA.[111] Notably, current guidelines emphasize that presence of interface hepatitis of at least moderate severity is required for this diagnosis, given that mild interface hepatitis is frequently observed in patients with classic PBC.[111,159] In addition, mild to moderate transaminase elevation can be seen in PBC and tend to respond well to treatment with UDCA, suggesting that a trial of UDCA should be attempted first, prior to initiation of immunosuppression.

Although limited data suggest patients with PBC-AIH may have worse clinical outcomes compared to those with classic PBC, with increased rates of hepatic decompensation, liver transplantation, or death, this has not been a universal finding.[162–164] Therefore management of patients with PBC and overlapping features of AIH require an individualized approach, often with a trial of UDCA monotherapy prior to initiating immunosuppression.

Ductopenic Variant

Although jaundice is typically a very late event in patients with PBC, appearing only during cirrhotic stage, precirrhotic jaundice has been described in a subgroup of patients with accelerated loss of intrahepatic bile ducts and extreme ductopenia (<10%).[165] It is hypothesized that an aggressive form of immune-mediated biliary injury leads to rapid development of severe ductopenia, with fibrogenesis initially lagging behind and eventually progressing. In such cases, UDCA is rarely effective, and liver transplantation may need to be considered given a markedly negative impact of severe cholestasis on quality of life and nutritional status.

MANAGEMENT: PHARMACOLOGICAL TREATMENT AND DISEASE MONITORING

Ursodeoxycholic Acid

UDCA, the 7-β epimer of chenodeoxycholic acid, occurs naturally in small quantities in human bile (less than 4% of total bile acids). The most efficacious dose of UDCA in patients with PBC is 13–15 mg/kg/day, which can be given in divided doses taken with meals. Increasing the dose beyond this threshold has not proven useful.[166]

Several mechanisms have been proposed to explain the protective actions of UDCA, including: (1) stimulation of hepatic and biliary secretion of bile acids and other organic anions, with increased expression of hepatobiliary transporters, (2) enrichment of the bile acid pool with hydrophilic, less hepatotoxic bile salts through increased hepatocellular secretion of bile acids, inhibition of the intestinal absorption of endogenous hydrophobic bile salts, and replacement of endogenous bile acids with the

BOX 93.1 Impact of UDCA Treatment in PBC

- Improvement in liver chemistries
- Decrease in histologic severity: inflammation, cholestasis, interface hepatitis, bile duct paucity, bile duct proliferation
- Slows the rate of fibrosis progression/progression to cirrhosis
- Reduces rates of hepatic decompensation (development of esophageal varices/ascites)
- Improves survival free of liver transplantation

nonhepatotoxic UDCA, (3) cytoprotection, with stabilization of hepatocyte membranes against toxic bile salts, inhibition of apoptosis and fibrosis, and (4) various immunomodulatory and anti-inflammatory effects.[167] During UDCA therapy, the proportion of UDCA in serum and bile increases to approximately 50% of total bile acids, and the proportion of endogenous bile acids, such as cholic, chenodeoxycholic, deoxycholic, and lithocholic acids, consequently declines.

Treatment with UDCA leads to rapid and long-lasting improvements in liver biochemistries and a decrease in the histologic severity of interface hepatitis, inflammation, cholestasis, bile duct paucity, and bile duct proliferation (Box 93.1).[168–170] UDCA significantly decreases the risk of development of gastroesophageal varices,[146] HCC,[171] and ascites,[172] and delays progression to cirrhosis.[173] The predicted probability that cirrhosis will develop after 5 years of therapy with UDCA for patients with stage 1, 2, or 3 PBC at diagnosis is 4%, 12%, and 59%, respectively; at 10 years of therapy with UDCA, the probability of cirrhosis is 17%, 27%, and 76%, respectively.[173]

UDCA has clearly been shown to improve survival for patients with PBC. Many recent studies have corroborated findings from an early meta-analysis suggesting that long-term use of UDCA improved survival free of LT.[174] For instance, in a racially diverse national cohort with nearly 3500 patients with PBC, UDCA treatment was associated with a 43% reduction in all-cause mortality.[8] Moreover, in a similarly large international cohort, use of UDCA was associated with a 2.2-fold relative reduction in the risk of death or transplantation.[175] The degree of risk reduction is, of course, dependent on baseline characteristics including age, fibrosis stage and severity of ALP elevation.

Approximately 20%–40% of patients do not respond completely to UDCA.[176] Insufficient response to UDCA is associated with a reduced transplant-free survival and increased risk of disease-related complications, including HCC.[177–180] Men and patients who are diagnosed at an earlier age appear to be less likely to respond to UDCA—patients diagnosed before age 30 have a 30% response rate compared with a 90% response rate for those diagnosed after age 70.[181] Similarly, patients of Hispanic ethnicity may be less likely to respond to UDCA.[182]

As mentioned above, a variety of criteria have been proposed to assess responsiveness to UDCA based on liver biochemistries and predict clinical outcomes (Table 93.4).[147,176,178,179,183–186] As such, various optimal cut-off levels for ALP have been suggested, with ALP levels below 1.5–2× ULN currently recommended by practice guidelines.[110,111] However, normalization of ALP may be associated with the best outcomes, especially amongst the highest risk patients.[150] Identification of incomplete responders to UDCA is important so that new or adjunctive therapies can be considered.

Obeticholic Acid

OCA is a first-in-class farnesoid X receptor (FXR) agonist. FXR is a nuclear receptor expressed in the liver, kidneys, adrenal glands and intestine, and plays a key role in bile acid metabolism, liver regeneration, and inflammation.[187] OCA is 100 times more potent than the natural FXR ligand chenodeoxycholic acid. Preclinical data has suggested that OCA has antifibrotic and choleretic properties.

OCA is the only FDA-approved drug for use in patients with PBC who are incomplete responders to, or intolerant of, UDCA. In the pivotal phase 3 trial (POISE trial) 46%–47% of patients treated with OCA met the primary endpoint, compared to only 10% of placebo-treated patients.[188] This primary endpoint was a composite of serum ALP < 1.67 times the ULN, with a reduction in ALP from baseline of at least 15%, while maintaining normal total bilirubin levels. Over the years, this composite endpoint came to be known as "the POISE criteria" and has since been demonstrated to correlate with clinically meaningful outcomes in PBC. Ever since, the POISE criteria have been used as the primary endpoint in most clinical trials for PBC. After 3 additional years of exposure to OCA in an open-label extension study, patients showed sustained reductions in ALP and TB.[189] Further, in a subanalysis of 17 patients who had before and after liver biopsy, continued use of OCA for 3 years was associated with improvement or stabilization of relevant histological findings such as fibrosis, bile duct loss/ductopenia, ductular reaction, interface hepatitis, and lobular hepatitis.[190] In the rare patient intolerant to UDCA, OCA monotherapy also appears effective at improving liver biochemical test levels.[191] However, response rates in cirrhotic patients may be lower than in noncirrhotic patients, with higher dropout rates.[192–196] Although we lack controlled data showing the impact of OCA on survival rates, it is encouraging that a real-world study comparing outcomes of 209 patients treated with OCA for 6 years to thousands of propensity-matched patients not on OCA found that OCA-treated patients had significantly lower rates of hepatic decompensation, liver transplantation, and death.[197]

Pruritus is a common side effect of OCA (56%– 68% compared with 38% for placebo); starting at a lower dose attenuates this side effect. Reductions in serum HDL cholesterol levels have also been observed, and the long-term impact on cardiovascular risk is unclear.[188] Thus OCA should be started at 5 mg/day, with possible increase to 10 mg/day after 3 months based on response and tolerability. Due to reports of hepatic decompensation in patients with cirrhosis, OCA is not recommended for those with advanced cirrhosis, defined as any evidence of portal hypertension (https://www.fda.gov/drugs/fda-drug-safety-podcasts/due-risk-serious-liver-injury-fda-restricts-use-obeticholic-acid-ocaliva-primary-biliary-cholangitis).

In summary, treatment with OCA fills an important unmet need in incomplete responders to UDCA and is associated with significant improvement in liver biochemical test levels and histological stabilization. Real-world data point at improved survival without liver transplantation, although this has not yet been demonstrated in the setting of randomized controlled studies. Safety in patients with advanced liver disease still needs further evaluation.

Fibrates

Fibrates are PPAR agonists. Activation of this nuclear receptor can regulate bile acid homeostasis as well as inflammatory and fibrotic pathways.[198–200] Fenofibrate (PPAR-alpha) and bezafibrate (pan-PPAR) have both been examined in the treatment of PBC. Several meta-analysis suggest that both fenofibrate and bezafibrate can improve liver biochemistries in patients with PBC.[201,202] In the largest randomized, placebo-controlled trial of bezafibrate including 100 patients with PBC and incomplete response to UDCA, treatment with bezafibrate 400 mg/day caused normalization of serum ALP, AST, ALT, and total bilirubin levels and INR in significantly more patients than

TABLE 93.5 Medical Therapy for Cholestatic Pruritus

Drug	Oral Regimen	Adverse Effect(s)	Advice
Cholestyramine	4–16 g, in divided doses. Take 1 hour before or 3 hours after meals, 2–3 hours apart from UDCA, OCA, and other medications that can bind cholestyramine	Fat malabsorption, nausea, decreased intestinal absorption of other medications, constipation	Change to alternative treatment if no improvement is noticed in 2 weeks
Bezafibrate	400 mg daily	Increase in creatinine, myalgias, transient ALT elevation	Not available in the US; fenofibrate appears to be less effective. Monitoring of liver enzymes recommended at 2, 6, and 12 weeks after treatment initiation, then every 12 weeks
Rifampin	Start 150 mg daily May increase to 450–600 mg divided in two doses	Inducer of hepatic enzymes involved in drug metabolism, potential hepatotoxicity (5%), red-orange discoloration of urine and secretions	Monitor liver enzymes at 2, 6, and 12 weeks after treatment initiation, then every 12 weeks
Naltrexone	12.5–50 mg daily	Opiate withdrawal symptoms, increase pain sensation, confuson	For hospitalized patients, may consider IV naloxone 0.002–0.2 µg/kg/min
Sertraline	50–100 mg daily	Hyponatremia, QT prolongation, nausea, vomiting, change in appetite	Monitor sodium levels regularly

ALT, Alanine aminotransferase; *IV*, intravenous; *OCA*, obeticholic acid; *UDCA*, ursodeoxycholic acid; *US*, United States.

treatment with placebo (31% vs 0%).[203] Improvements in pruritus and LSMs were also observed. Real-world studies suggest that fibrates lead to a 50% reduction in ALP from baseline; however, fewer patients achieve normalization of transaminases in comparison to OCA.[195] In a large observational study from Japan, improved transplant-free survival rates were observed in bezafibrate-treated patients compared to UDCA monotherapy.[204]

The most common side effects in patients taking fibrates are GI and musculoskeletal complaints.[205] Elevations in aminotransferases are usually mild and transient, but cases of acute and chronic liver injury have also been reported.

The use of fibrates as an alternative second-line therapy for patients with PBC and incomplete response to UDCA is endorsed by practice guidelines worldwide and is especially valuable in countries where OCA is not approved or available. Further evaluation is needed to assess safety of fibrates in patients with advanced liver disease and its use in decompensated cirrhosis is not currently recommended.

Budesonide

Budesonide is a glucocorticoid structurally related to 16α-hydroxyprednisolone, with extensive first-pass hepatic metabolism and minimal systemic availability. Two prior randomized controlled studies reported improvement in histology and markers of inflammation for patients with noncirrhotic PBC and incomplete response to UDCA treated with budesonide.[206,207] However, a recent 3-year randomized controlled trial failed to show higher rates of histological improvement in these patients.[208] The trial did show reductions in markers of inflammation and improvement in relevant surrogates of disease activity (i.e., ALP $\leq$ 1.67× ULN with $\geq$15% reduction from baseline, and ALP normalization rates) in budesonide-treated patients in comparison to placebo. Reduction in lumbar spine bone density was observed, emphasizing the need for more frequent monitoring in patients receiving budesonide for long duration. Pruritus was unchanged by addition of budesonide.

Collectively, the data suggest that budesonide may rarely be of benefit for patients with early-stage PBC but is associated with important systemic glucocorticoid-related adverse events. Budesonide should be avoided for patients with cirrhosis due to increased risk of these side effects as well as portal vein thrombosis.

Ineffective Medications

Methotrexate

Patients with PBC who experienced biochemical and histologic improvement with methotrexate therapy have been described in observational studies. However, in a large randomized trial evaluating UDCA plus methotrexate versus UDCA plus placebo, with a median time of 7.6 years from randomization to study closure, the hazard ratio for death with or without liver transplantation was no better in the methotrexate-UDCA combination group than in the UDCA-placebo group.[209] Therefore methotrexate should not be recommended as monotherapy or as an adjuvant to UDCA.

Other medications including D-penicillamine, abatacept, azathioprine, chlorambucil, cyclosporine, malotilate, tetracycline, tacrolimus, thalidomide, ustekinumab, rituximab, and silymarin have been evaluated for the treatment of PBC, but no convincing evidence of efficacy was reported for any of these agents, and some were associated with serious adverse events. None of these medications can be recommended for the treatment of PBC. Ten trials of varying methodologic quality have examined the use of colchicine in PBC. These trials were systematically reviewed, and no effects on mortality, LT, histologic progression, or liver biochemical test levels were found.[210]

Future Therapies

Several drugs are currently under investigation in phase 2/3 clinical trials including bile acid therapies [apical sodium-dependent bile acid transporter inhibitors (ASBT), for pruritus], PPAR agonists (seladelpar, elafibranor, saroglitazar), NOX1/4 inhibitors (setanaxib), and immunomodulatory agents (e.g., CNP-104, a biodegradable nanoparticle encapsulating PDC-E2). The ASBT blockers and PPAR agonists, in particular, are fairly advanced in the drug development process and results of pivotal studies are eagerly awaited. Preliminary results of phase 2b/3 trials of PPAR agonists in PBC suggest at least similar efficacy to FDA-approved OCA, without worsening pruritus.[211] In fact, PPAR agonists tend to improve pruritus.[103,212]

MANAGEMENT OF COMPLICATIONS OF CHRONIC CHOLESTASIS

In addition to treating the underlying disease, a key component of caring for patients with PBC is the recognition, prevention, and treatment of disease-related complications.

Pruritus

The cause of pruritus in patients with PBC is not fully understood, which limits our ability to effectively manage this symptom. A number of agents may provide symptomatic relief (Table 93.5), and a stepwise approach is recommended.[110] Occasionally, treatment with UDCA alleviates pruritus, although pruritus may actually worsen with initiation of UDCA. UDCA is not regarded as appropriate treatment for cholestatic itching. Bezafibrate, on the other hand, is currently accepted as second-line therapy for incomplete responders to UDCA and has been shown to ameliorate cholestatic pruritus in open label and controlled studies alike.[103,203,213] However bezafibrate is not available in the US.

Some basic principles may help mitigate pruritus. In warm countries, exposure to ultraviolet light without sunblock can alleviate pruritus, and not surprisingly, the pruritus of PBC subsides during the summer months. However, excess heat (e.g., sauna, hot showers) can exacerbate itching and should be avoided. It is recommended to avoid tight clothing in favor of soft cotton-based garments, and to keep the skin moisturized.

The bile acid-binding resin cholestyramine was the first medication described to alleviate this symptom, and is currently considered first line for the treatment of cholestatic pruritus.[110] Therapy with cholestyramine is successful in most patients who can tolerate the unpleasant side effects of bad taste, bloating, nausea, and occasional constipation. The recommended total dose is 4–16 g/day orally, divided in 1–4 daily doses. All drugs that can potentially bind to cholestyramine (including UDCA and OCA) should be taken at least 1 h before or 3 h after cholestyramine. Colesevelam has a higher bile acid-binding capacity and fewer side effects than cholestyramine; however, a small randomized controlled trial demonstrated that despite a significant reduction in serum bile acid levels, colesevelam was not more effective than placebo at improving pruritus.[214]

Not all patients with pruritus are helped by cholestyramine. The antibiotic rifampin, a PXR agonist which can lower autotaxin levels, is also effective in relieving the pruritus of PBC.[102] Most patients respond to rifampin, and benefit occurs within 1 week of the start of therapy. The starting dose is 150 mg twice daily orally; occasionally, higher doses are needed. Rifampin induces drug-metabolizing enzymes, so caution is needed when concurrent drugs are administered. Among other side effects, rifampin has been associated with reversible liver injury in approximately 5%[215] of patients; thus regular monitoring of liver enzymes is recommended at 2, 6, and 12 weeks after starting the drug.[98]

Given the current understanding that activation of μ opiate receptors promote itching while activation of κ receptors mitigate itching, several drugs known to modulate opioid activity have been evaluated for the treatment of pruritus. Intravenous administration of the μ opiate receptor antagonist naloxone has shown a clear benefit in a double-blind trial. Oral opiate receptor antagonists such as nalmefene and naltrexone have also led to amelioration of pruritus in patients with PBC,[216] and can be used as second- or third-line choices.[110] The κ agonist nalfurafine is licensed in Japan for the management of cholestatic pruritus, but it is not approved in the USA and Europe. In patients with pruritus associated with various liver diseases, the serotonin reuptake inhibitor sertraline (75–100 mg orally) was associated with relief of pruritus as assessed by a visual analog scale and healing of excoriations.[217]

Cholestatic pruritus is at least partially relieved by plasma filtration such as plasmapheresis,[218] plasma separation and anion adsorption,[219] and albumin dialysis.[220] Finally, pruritus of PBC is almost always cured by liver transplantation, which is a viable consideration for patients with severe intractable pruritus. In addition, new therapies targeting the apical sodium-bile acid transporters (ASBT) in the gut are currently in development for the management of cholestatic pruritus, having shown very promising results in phase 2 trials.[99]

Bone Disease

Osteopenic bone disease with a predisposition to spontaneous fracturing is a common complication of chronic cholestatic liver disease. Women with PBC lose bone mass at a rate approximately twice that seen in age-matched controls, and this accelerated bone loss is the result of decreased formation rather than increased resorption of bone.[221] Osteoporosis in patients with PBC denotes perturbations of bone remodeling, and the cause is multifactorial and poorly understood. Factors reportedly involved include insulin growth factor-1 deficiency, hypogonadism, cholestasis, genetic susceptibility such as vitamin D receptor gene polymorphisms, decreased vitamin D levels, and use of concurrent medications such as immunosuppressive therapy in the post-transplant setting.

Dual-energy x-ray absorptiometry and dual-photon absorptiometry are noninvasive techniques that quantify bone mass accurately. Approximately 14%–52% of patients with PBC have osteoporosis, as defined by a *T*-score below −2.5 in either the lumbar spine or the femoral neck, and approximately 10% have severe bone disease, as defined by a *Z*-score below −2 (the *T-score* is the number of standard deviations below the mean peak value in young gender-matched normal subjects, whereas the *Z-score* is the number of standard deviations below mean normal values corrected for age and gender).[222] The risk of osteoporosis (*T*-score below −2.5) is eight times higher in patients with PBC than in a gender-matched population, whereas the risk of severe bone disease (*Z*-score below −2) is four times higher in patients with PBC than in a healthy gender- and age-matched population.[223] The likelihood of osteoporosis increases as liver disease advances; bone mass in patients with stage 1 or 2 PBC is similar to that in a normal age- and gender-matched population, but bone mass is significantly lower in patients with stage 3 or 4 disease.[223] In addition, sarcopenia is recognized as an important risk factor for osteoporosis among patients with PBC.[224] The reported cumulative frequency of all fractures and vertebral fractures in patients with PBC is as high as 21% and 11%, respectively, and remains relevant in more contemporary studies.[225,226] Furthermore, the risk of dying after an osteoporotic fracture is >2 times higher in patients with PBC, compared to the general population.[225] Testing for osteoporosis is indicated at the time of diagnosis of PBC, in the setting of a fragility fracture or prolonged (greater than 3 months) course of glucocorticoids, and before liver transplantation. Repeat testing every 2–3 years in at-risk individuals has been recommended.[110]

Treatment of the bone disease includes adequate exercise and supplemental calcium (1200–1500 mg daily orally) and vitamin D (600–800 IU daily orally or, if deficiency is present, 25,000–50,000 IU orally once or twice per week). Bisphosphonates have dramatically changed the management of osteoporosis in the general population. Alendronate was found to improve bone mass significantly in patients with PBC when compared with placebo,[227] and more so than etidronate.[228] Parenteral bisphosphonates (zoledronic acid, pamidronate, and ibandronate) have been evaluated and were found to be safe and effective in patients with PBC in a small retrospective study and should be considered for patients with a contraindication (e.g., esophageal varices) to oral bisphosphonate therapy.[229]

Fat-Soluble Vitamin Deficiency

Most patients with PBC and fat-soluble vitamin deficiency have advanced liver disease with jaundice. Fat-soluble vitamin deficiency is almost always caused by intestinal malabsorption resulting from decreased amounts of bile salts in the intestinal lumen. Vitamin A and D levels and the prothrombin time should be checked annually in patients with PBC and a bilirubin greater than 2 mg/dL.[110,230]

Vitamin D deficiency can be excluded in patients with PBC by measurement of 25-hydroxyvitamin D, a major metabolite of vitamin D. When vitamin D deficiency is encountered, vitamin D in a dose of 25,000–50,000 IU, given once or twice per week, usually is sufficient to achieve a normal serum vitamin D level. Because 25-hydroxylation of vitamin D is preserved in patients with PBC, vitamin D (rather than the more expensive 25-hydroxyvitamin D or 1,25-hydroxyvitamin D) can be prescribed.

Vitamin A deficiency, which can cause reduced night vision, can occur in patients with PBC. When blood levels of vitamin A are low and the patient is symptomatic, replacement therapy with oral vitamin A, 100,000 IU daily for 3 days, and then 50,000 IU daily for 14 days, should be instituted. If patients are deficient but asymptomatic, a dose of 25,000–50,000 IU 2 or 3 times per week is adequate. The adequacy of replacement therapy is assessed by repeating serum vitamin A assays and evaluating the patient for darkness adaptation, if indicated.

Vitamin K deficiency occurs with severe cholestasis and is manifested by a prolonged prothrombin time. A trial of oral vitamin K, 5–10 mg daily, should be given to determine if the prothrombin time improves. If it does, the patient should be maintained on a water-soluble vitamin K, 5 mg/day.

Deficiency of vitamin E has been reported in a few patients with PBC. Typically, vitamin E deficiency causes a neurologic abnormality that primarily affects the posterior columns and is characterized by areflexia, loss of proprioception, and ataxia. In patients with chronic cholestasis and low serum levels of vitamin E, oral replacement therapy with high-dose vitamin E (100 mg daily) may halt progression of neuropathy.

Hyperlipidemia

Whether or not dyslipidemia in patients with PBC is associated with increased risk of cardiovascular events remains a subject of debate, with most studies failing to indicate a definitive increase in risk.[231] Hypertension, however, appears to increase the risk of cardiovascular events and mortality among patients with PBC and dyslipidemia.[232] Thus risk should be individualized, especially with increasing rates of metabolic syndrome and associated steatotic liver disease worldwide; approximately 30% of patients with PBC also have metabolic syndrome.[233]

Given the controversy surrounding risk of cardiovascular events, one recommended approach in PBC is to regularly assess for presence of cardiovascular risk factors and check a lipid panel that includes ApoB-100 (as a surrogate for true LDL-C) for risk stratification. Lipid lowering treatment is suggested for patients with ApoB > 120 mg/dL in the absence of known risk cardiovascular risk factors or Apo B > 90 if a risk factor is present.[231]

Among patients with PBC who would benefit from lipid-lowering therapy, the use of statins appears to be safe and has not been associated with deterioration of liver function.[234] Therapy with UDCA has been shown to lower the LDL levels in patients with PBC and has been useful in some patients with xanthelasmas. Surgical removal of xanthelasmas is seldom successful, and such attempts should be avoided.

Steatorrhea

Steatorrhea can occur in patients with advanced PBC.[235] Several causes have been described. The most important cause is decreased bile acid delivery with insufficient micellar concentration of bile acids in the small intestine. Occasionally, exocrine pancreatic insufficiency can be found as part of a widespread glandular dysfunction seen in some patients with PBC. Coexisting celiac disease has been reported in a small number of patients with PBC, and SIBO may be the cause of steatorrhea in some patients with PBC and systemic sclerosis.[13,14] Because each of these causes has specific and different treatments, determining the exact cause of steatorrhea is important. Patients with decreased intestinal bile acid concentrations usually benefit from substitution of medium-chain triglycerides for long-chain triglycerides in their diets and a decrease in total fat intake. Those with exocrine pancreatic insufficiency will benefit from pancreatic replacement therapy, while patients with celiac disease require gluten withdrawal from the diet. Small intestinal bacterial overgrowth is managed with intermittent broad-spectrum oral antibiotic therapy.

Fatigue

It is recommended to evaluate for and treat comorbidities that can contribute to fatigue, including anemia, hypothyroidism, obstructive sleep apnea, restless leg syndrome, and depression. Importantly, appropriate management of nocturnal pruritus will lead to improved sleep, which in turn also mitigates fatigue. In addition, certain medications have been associated with fatigue and should discontinued if possible—these include beta blockers, muscle relaxants, benzodiazepines and calcium-channel blockers. As there is no approved therapy for fatigue, management relies primarily on these lifestyle adjustments and development of coping mechanisms.[236] Moreover, mental wellness is increased by mindfulness and physical exercises.[237] Physician awareness of the negative impact of fatigue on patients' overall health is paramount; empathy goes a long way in the long-term management of those with debilitating fatigue.

LIVER TRANSPLANTATION

The best therapeutic alternative for patients with end-stage PBC is liver transplantation. The major manifestations of chronic liver disease that should prompt an evaluation for liver transplantation in patients with other causes of chronic liver disease apply to patients with PBC. Although the development of complications associated with chronic cholestasis, such as a poor quality of life secondary to disabling fatigue, intractable pruritus, and severe muscle wasting, as well as persistent increases in the serum bilirubin level often prompts clinicians to consider referral for liver transplantation even in the absence of cirrhosis, it is notable that these complications are not currently accepted by the National Liver Review Board as standard indications for MELD exception points.[238] Importantly, while patients with PBC experience immediate relief of pruritus after transplantation, fatigue does not usually resolve.[93]

The number of patients waitlisted for PBC has declined by 50% in the United Kingdom and USA since 1995[239] and data from UNOS show a clear trend toward decreased rates of LT for PBC in the USA.[238,240] From 1995 to 2006, the absolute number of liver transplants in the USA increased an average of 249 cases per year, but the absolute number of transplants performed for PBC decreased by an average of 5.4 cases per year.[240] This trend has also been observed in Europe.[241] Because UDCA is now prescribed nearly universally to patients with PBC, the decline in the number of liver transplants for PBC is likely related to a reduction in disease progression from UDCA.

Liver transplantation clearly improves survival, as well as quality of life, for patients with PBC. One-year patient survival rates after liver transplantation are higher than 90%, with 5-year patient survival rates of 80% or higher in most transplant centers.[238] Outcomes following live-donor liver transplantation appear to be comparable to those for 5-year deceased-donor liver transplantation, with low rates of PBC recurrence.[242]

PBC may recur after liver transplantation. The frequency of recurrent PBC varies among centers, with a range of 0%–61%.[238] Recurrent PBC is typically diagnosed between 3 and 5.5 years after transplantation, and the risk increases with time. Diagnosis can be challenging as liver biochemical test levels in patients with recurrent PBC can be normal or mildly elevated, and AMA positivity may persist after LT. Therefore the diagnosis of recurrent PBC relies heavily on the histologic features. Tacrolimus-based immunosuppression has been the most consistently identified risk factor for disease recurrence.[238,243] A recent large international cohort study indicated that recurrent PBC following liver transplantation is associated with increased rates of graft loss and lower patient survival.[243] Preventive treatment with UDCA posttransplantation may decrease the risk of recurrent PBC, graft loss, and both liver-related and all-cause mortality, although confirmation in prospective trials is lacking.[244] Given the excellent safety profile of UDCA and its potential protective role in this setting, many transplant centers routinely prescribe preemptive use of UDCA after liver transplantation for PBC. As expected, UDCA may also play a role in the treatment of recurrent PBC, and its use has been associated with improvement in liver biochemical test levels.[245]

Acknowledgments

The authors thank Keith D. Lindor, John Eaton, Jayant A. Talwalkar, and the late Paul Angulo for their contributions to previous versions of this chapter.

Full references for this chapter can be found at https://ebooks.health.elsevier.com.

94 Portal Hypertension and Variceal Bleeding

Vijay H. Shah, Patrick S. Kamath

IN THIS CHAPTER

Variceal hemorrhage, hepatic encephalopathy, and ascites—the major complications of cirrhosis of the liver (see Chapters 76, 95, and 96)—result from portal hypertension, defined as an increase to 6 mm Hg or greater in hepatic venous pressure gradient (HVPG), a surrogate for hepatic sinusoidal pressure. Portosystemic collaterals are formed in an effort to decompress the hypertensive hepatic sinusoids and give rise to varices at the gastroesophageal junction and elsewhere. The risk of portal hypertension related complications increases when the HVPG is ≥10 mm Hg, the threshold for clinically significant portal hypertension (CSPH).

NORMAL PORTAL CIRCULATION

The portal venous system carries capillary blood from the esophagus, stomach, small and large intestine, pancreas, gallbladder, and spleen to the liver. The portal vein is formed by the confluence of the splenic vein and the superior mesenteric vein behind the neck of the pancreas. The inferior mesenteric vein usually drains into the splenic vein. The left gastric vein, also called the left coronary vein, typically drains into the portal vein at the confluence of the splenic vein and superior mesenteric vein (Fig. 94.1). The portal vein is approximately 7.5 cm in length and runs dorsal to the hepatic artery and bile duct into the hilum of the liver. The uppermost 5 cm of the portal vein does not receive any tributaries. In the hilum of the liver, the portal vein divides into the left and right portal vein branches, which supply the left and right sides of the liver, respectively. The umbilical vein drains into the left portal vein, and the cystic vein from the gallbladder drains into the right portal vein. The portal venules drain into hepatic sinusoids that, in turn, are drained by the hepatic veins into the inferior vena cava. The left and middle hepatic veins usually join and drain into the inferior vena cava separately but adjacent to the confluence of the right hepatic vein with the inferior vena cava. The caudate lobe drains separately into the inferior vena cava (see Chapter 73).

The circulatory system of the normal liver is a high-compliance, low-resistance system that is able to accommodate a large blood volume, as occurs after a meal, without substantially increasing portal pressure. The liver receives a dual-blood supply from the portal vein and the hepatic artery that constitutes nearly 30% of total cardiac output. Portal venous blood derived from the mesenteric venous circulation constitutes approximately 75% of total hepatic blood flow, whereas the remainder of blood to the liver is derived from the hepatic artery, which provides highly oxygenated blood directly from the celiac trunk of the aorta. In the fasting state, the contribution to the liver of oxygenated blood by the portal vein and hepatic artery is about equal. Portal vein–derived and hepatic artery–derived blood flow converge in high-compliance, specialized vascular channels termed *hepatic sinusoids*. A dynamic and compensatory interplay occurs between hepatic blood flow derived from the portal vein and that from the hepatic artery. When portal venous blood flow to the liver is diminished, as occurs in portal vein thrombosis, arterial inflow increases in an attempt to maintain total hepatic blood flow at a constant level. Similarly, after hepatic artery occlusion, portal venous inflow increases in a compensatory manner. This autoregulatory mechanism, aimed at maintaining total hepatic blood flow at a constant level, is termed the *hepatic arterial buffer response*.

The sinusoids are highly permeable and thus facilitate the transport of macromolecules to the parenchymal hepatocytes that reside on the extraluminal side of the endothelial cells. The hepatic sinusoids are highly permeable because they lack a proper basement membrane and because the endothelial cells that line the sinusoids contain fenestrae. Other unique aspects of the hepatic sinusoids are the space of Disse, a virtual space located extraluminal to the endothelial cell and adjacent to the hepatocyte, and its cellular constituents, the hepatic stellate cell (HSC) and the

Kupffer cell (Fig. 94.2; see also Chapters 73 and 76). These two cell types play an important role, in concert with the endothelial cell, in regulating sinusoidal hemodynamics and homeostasis and may contribute to the sinusoidal derangements that occur in portal hypertension. Under basal conditions, HSCs maintain a quiescent phenotype and accumulate vitamin A. On activation, however, as occurs in cirrhosis, these cells develop contractile abilities that permit them to function as sinusoidal pericytes. Kupffer cells contribute to vascular homeostasis by generating cytokines with potent cellular and vasoregulatory actions. While Kupffer cells are resident hepatic macrophages, infiltrating macrophages derived from bone marrow in response to liver injury are also important. Endothelial cells and smooth muscle cells in nonsinusoidal hepatic vessels such as the portal venule and the terminal hepatic venule are important in hepatic vasoregulation, particularly in the normal liver, where HSCs are quiescent, not activated, and presumably less contractile.

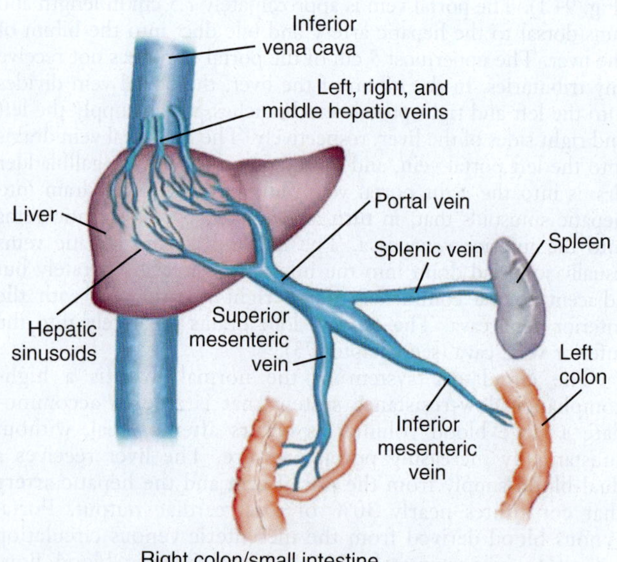

Fig. 94.1 Anatomy of the portal circulation. Blood vessels that constitute the portal circulation and hepatic outflow tracts are depicted.

HEMODYNAMIC PRINCIPLES OF PORTAL HYPERTENSION

In cirrhosis, as well as in most noncirrhotic causes of portal hypertension, portal hypertension results from increases in portal resistance in combination with increases in portal inflow. The influence of flow and resistance on pressure can be represented by the formula for Ohm's law as follows:

$$\Delta P = F \times R$$

in which the pressure gradient in the portal circulation (ΔP) is a function of portal flow (F) and resistance to flow (R). Increases in portal resistance or portal flow can contribute to increased pressure. Portal hypertension almost always results from increases in both portal resistance and portal flow (Fig. 94.3). One exception is an arteriovenous fistula (AVF), which in the initial stages causes portal hypertension largely through an increase in portal flow in the absence of an increase in resistance. The mechanism of the increase in portal resistance depends on the site and cause of portal hypertension; in the Western world, the most common cause is cirrhosis (see later). Because of the increase in hepatic resistance and the decrease in hepatic compliance, small changes in flow that do not increase pressure in the normal liver can have a prominent stimulatory effect on portal pressure in the cirrhotic liver. The increase in portal venous inflow is part of a generalized systemic derangement termed the *hyperdynamic circulatory state*. Collateral vessels that dilate and new vascular sprouts that form connect the high-pressure portal venous system with lower pressure systemic veins. Unfortunately, this process of angiogenesis and collateralization is insufficient for normalizing portal pressure and actually leads to complications of portal hypertension, such as esophageal varices.[1]

The changes in portal flow and resistance also can be viewed as originating from mechanical and vascular factors. Mechanical factors include the fibrosis and nodularity of the cirrhotic liver, with the distortion of the vascular architecture and the remodeling that is recognized to occur in the systemic and splanchnic vasculature in response to the chronic increases in flow and shear stress that characterize the hyperdynamic circulatory state. Vascular factors include intrahepatic vasoconstriction, which contributes to increased intrahepatic resistance, and the

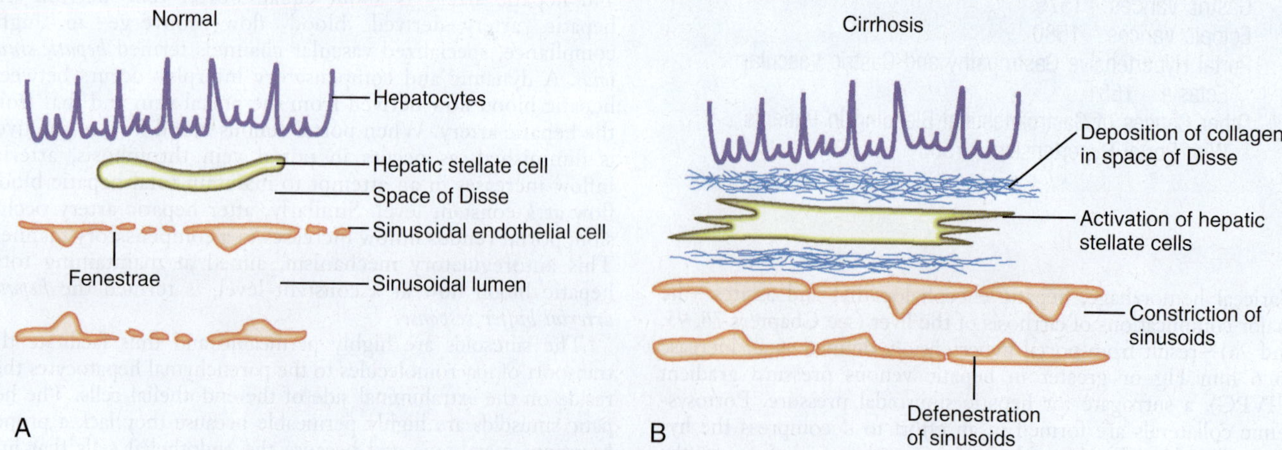

Fig. 94.2 Anatomy of the hepatic microvasculature. (A) Normal sinusoidal microanatomy is depicted. The sinusoidal lumen is lined by fenestrated sinusoidal endothelial cells that allow the transport of macromolecules to the abluminal space of Disse. Quiescent hepatic stellate cells (HSCs) reside within this space, adjacent to hepatocytes and endothelial cells. (B) In cirrhosis, a number of changes occur in the hepatic microcirculation, including loss of fenestrae in endothelial cells (defenestration), constriction of sinusoids, and activation of HSCs with ensuing deposition of collagen and increased contractility.

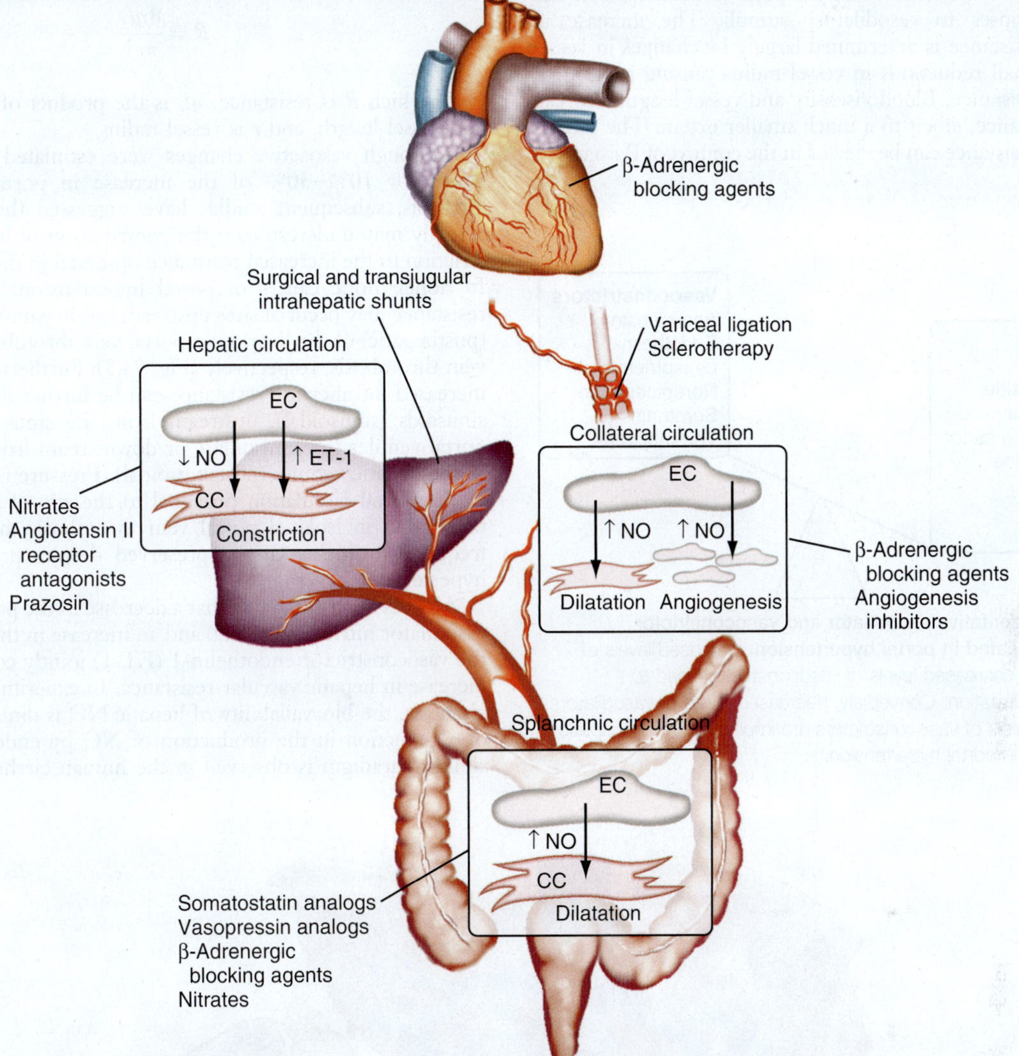

Fig. 94.3 Vascular disturbances in portal hypertension and sites of action of portal pressure-reducing therapies. Portal hypertension typically results from increased resistance, usually from within the liver, in combination with increased portal venous flow. The increase in hepatic resistance results from mechanical factors in combination with dynamic vasoconstriction mediated by decreased nitric oxide (NO) production and increased endothelin-1 (ET-1) production. The increase in portal venous flow occurs as a result of vasodilatation in the splanchnic circulation that is mediated by increased NO production. A collateral circulation, including esophageal varices, develops between the hypertensive portal vasculature and systemic venous system; however, these collaterals are inadequate to decompress the hypertensive portal circulation fully. Collateral vessel development is mediated by dilatation of existing collateral vessels, as well as the development of new blood vessels and sprouts (angiogenesis). Therapies aimed at the different sites of hemodynamic disturbances are shown. *CC*, Contractile cell (e.g., hepatic stellate cell, vascular smooth muscle cell); *EC*, endothelial cell.

splanchnic and systemic vasodilatation that accompanies the hyperdynamic circulatory state. The vascular factors that contribute to portal hypertension are particularly important because they are reversible and dynamic and therefore compelling targets for experimental therapies (Fig. 94.4). Conversely, effective therapies for the fixed, mechanical component of portal hypertension caused by scar, regenerative nodules, and vascular remodeling are currently lacking. Indeed, most available therapies for portal hypertension focus on the correction of hemodynamic alterations in the portal circulation. Other agents reduce the increased intrahepatic resistance (see later).

Increased Intrahepatic Resistance

In cirrhosis, increased portal resistance occurs in great part as a result of mechanical factors that reduce vessel diameter. In addition to regenerative nodules and fibrotic bands, these mechanical factors include capillarization of the sinusoids and swelling of cells, including hepatocytes and Kupffer cells. As discussed earlier, however, reduced hepatic vessel diameter resulting in increased portal resistance, even when caused by cirrhosis, is not a purely mechanical phenomenon.[2] Hemodynamic changes in the hepatic circulation also contribute to increased intrahepatic resistance.

These changes are characterized by hepatic vasoconstriction and impaired responses to vasodilatory stimuli. The increase in intrahepatic resistance is determined largely by changes in vessel radius, with small reductions in vessel radius causing prominent increases in resistance. Blood viscosity and vessel length also can influence resistance, albeit to a much smaller extent. The factors that regulate resistance can be viewed in the context of Poiseuille's law as follows:

$$R = \frac{8\eta L}{\pi r^4}$$

in which R is resistance, ηL is the product of blood viscosity and vessel length, and r is vessel radius.

Although vasoactive changes were estimated initially to account for 10%–30% of the increase in portal resistance in cirrhosis, subsequent studies have suggested that these figures actually may underestimate the contribution of hepatic vasoconstriction to the increased resistance observed in the cirrhotic liver. In noncirrhotic causes of portal hypertension, the increase in resistance may occur at sites upstream (prehepatic) or downstream (posthepatic) of the liver, as in portal vein thrombosis and hepatic vein thrombosis, respectively (Fig. 94.5). Furthermore, the site of increased intrahepatic resistance can be further delineated as the sinusoids (sinusoidal), upstream from the sinusoids within the portal venules (presinusoidal), or downstream from the sinusoids in the hepatic venules (postsinusoidal). Pressure is increased only in the portal circulation proximal to the site of increased resistance, and in isolated portal vein thrombosis, hepatic function frequently remains largely preserved despite prominent portal hypertension.

Most evidence suggests that a decrease in the production of the vasodilator nitric oxide (NO) and an increase in the production of the vasoconstrictor endothelin-1 (ET-1) jointly contribute to the increase in hepatic vascular resistance. In experimental models of cirrhosis, the bioavailability of hepatic NO is diminished because of a reduction in the production of NO by endothelial cells. A similar paradigm is observed in the human cirrhotic liver. Most

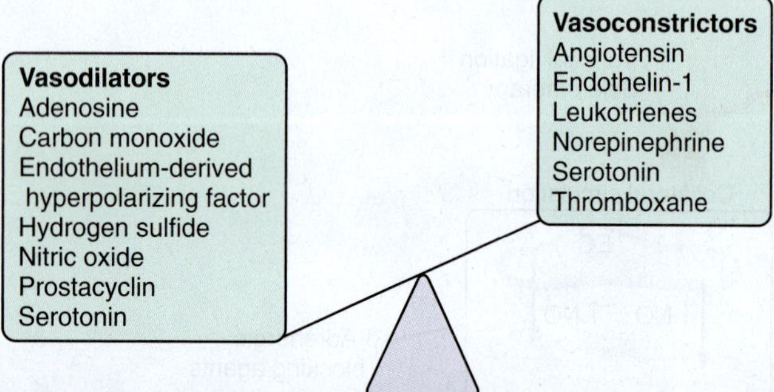

Fig. 94.4 Representative vasodilator and vasoconstrictor molecules implicated in portal hypertension. Increased levels of vasodilators and decreased levels of vasoconstrictors lead to splanchnic vasodilatation. Conversely, decreased levels of vasodilators and increased levels of vasoconstrictors are implicated in intrahepatic vasoconstriction in portal hypertension.

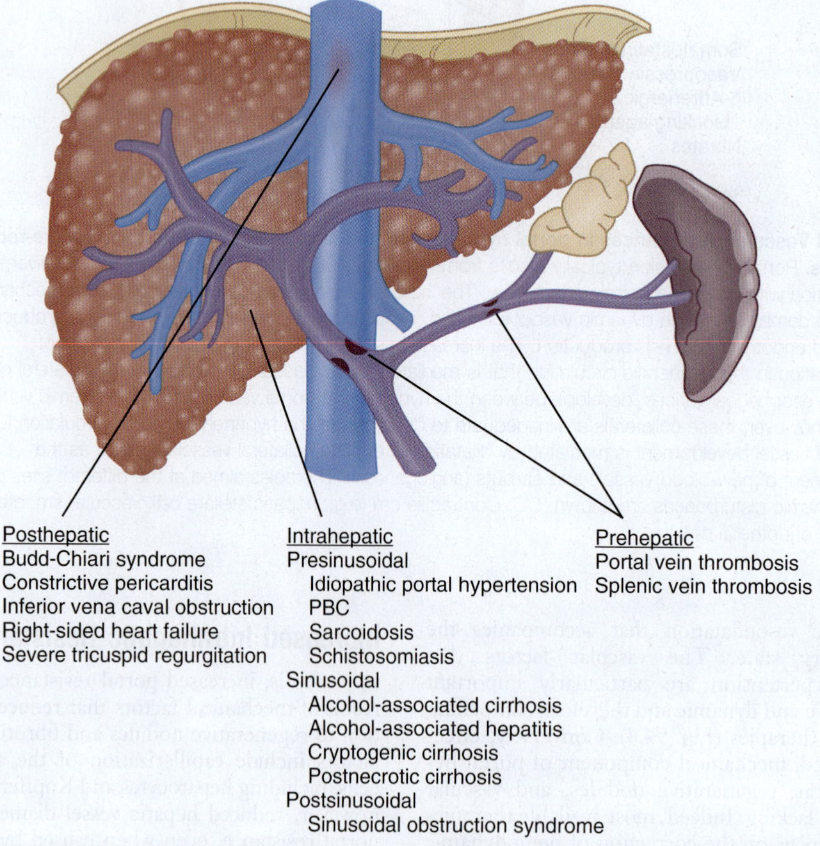

Fig. 94.5 Classification of portal hypertension. The different sites of increased resistance to portal flow (posthepatic, intrahepatic, and prehepatic) and associated diseases are shown. Many diseases cause a mixed pattern. Portal hypertension rarely can occur exclusively as a result of increased portal blood flow, as occurs with an arteriovenous shunt (not shown).

relevant studies indicate that the reduction in NO production occurs not through a reduction in hepatic eNOS levels but through defects in the steps necessary to activate existing eNOS. The lack of availability of NO is thought to allow HSCs, which are activated and highly contractile in cirrhosis, to constrict the sinusoids that they envelop, thereby increasing portal pressure. In clinical practice, NO can be delivered by NO donor agents such as mononitrates. NO donor agents exert their beneficial effects in part by relaxing the actively contractile stellate cells. The systemic actions of these agents, however, tend to cause side effects and exacerbate the hyperdynamic circulatory state.[3,4]

A number of new therapies that target increased intrahepatic resistance are under varying stages of evaluation and development.[5] Human and experimental studies suggest that statins may reduce portal hypertension through multiple mechanisms.[3,6,7] Receptor tyrosine kinase inhibitors that block vascular endothelial growth factor (VEGF), such as sorafenib, are also under evaluation.[8–10] Attempts to reduce portal pressure using pharmacologic agents that inhibit angiotensin activation of HSC contraction have met with mixed results.[3] Carvedilol is of notable interest because it is a nonselective β-receptor blocking agent (beta-blocker) (discussed later) that also improves hepatic sinusoidal perfusion through α-1 adrenergic receptor blockade. FXR agonists are also shown to reduce portal hypertension through multiple mechanisms.[11–13] Enoxaparin reduces sinusoidal microthrombosis and may be beneficial.[14,15] At the preclinical level, new targets include angiocrine signaling, such as endothelial derived chemokines, and inhibition of macrophage and neutrophil activation (NETS).[16,17]

Hyperdynamic Circulation

In addition to the increases in portal resistance discussed earlier, a major factor in the development and perpetuation of portal hypertension is an increase in portal venous flow, or the hyperdynamic circulation. The term *portal venous inflow* indicates the total blood that drains into the portal circulation, not the blood flow in the portal vein itself, which may actually be diminished in portal hypertension because of portosystemic collateral shunts. The hyperdynamic circulation is characterized by peripheral and splanchnic vasodilatation, reduced mean arterial pressure, and increased cardiac output. Vasodilatation, particularly in the splanchnic bed, permits an increase in inflow of systemic blood into the portal circulation.

Splanchnic vasodilatation is caused in large part by relaxation of splanchnic arterioles and ensuing splanchnic hyperemia. Studies of experimental portal hypertension have demonstrated that splanchnic vascular endothelial cells are primarily responsible for mediating splanchnic vasodilatation and enhanced portal venous inflow through excess generation of NO. This excess generation of NO and ensuing vasodilatation, hyperdynamic circulation, and hyperemia in the splanchnic and systemic circulation contrast with the hepatic circulation, in which NO deficiency contributes to increased intrahepatic resistance.

Some of the increase in NO production probably occurs from shear stress–dependent and shear stress–independent increases in the expression of eNOS, which can be corrected in part by beta blockers. Activation of existing eNOS by cytokines or mechanical factors also seems to contribute to excess systemic and splanchnic NO generation through pathways that include eNOS phosphorylation and protein interactions. The physiologic stimuli that mediate this process are not well understood but may include ET-1, which is increased in the serum of patients with portal hypertension, and the cytokine TNF-α. Inhibitors of TNF-α improve portal pressure and the splanchnic circulatory disturbances in both human and experimental portal hypertension; however, TNF-α inhibitors are not safe for use in patients with advanced liver disease and high MELD scores (see later and Chapter 99).[18] TNF-α may be derived from intestinal endotoxin, and intestinal decontamination appears to correct the hyperdynamic circulation in humans, thereby suggesting a link with intestinal inflammation.[19] Studies have linked intestinal microbes and lipopolysaccharide with portal hypertensive hemodynamics.[20] VEGF has also been implicated in this process by excessively activating eNOS.[21,22]

Some evidence also supports a primary defect in smooth muscle cells in portal hypertension, perhaps because of defects in potassium channels. In fact, many pharmacologic therapies for portal hypertension target the splanchnic arteriolar smooth muscle cells, rather than endothelial cells, to reduce splanchnic vasodilatation. For example, octreotide, a synthetic analog of somatostatin, causes marked but transient reductions in portal pressure by contracting splanchnic smooth muscle cells, thereby limiting portal venous inflow, especially after meals. Nonselective beta blockers and vasopressin also reduce portal pressure by constricting splanchnic arterioles and thereby reducing portal venous inflow. Because intrahepatic resistance persists, therapies that target the increase in portal venous inflow usually do not normalize portal pressure entirely but often blunt the prominent increases in portal venous inflow that occur in response to a meal. Combination therapy with an agent that reduces increased intrahepatic resistance, such as a nitrate, and an agent that reduces portal venous inflow, such as a beta-blocker, is more effective in reducing portal pressure than is either agent alone. Carvedilol as a single agent has combined effects of beta blockade and relaxation of intrahepatic sinusoidal vessels.[23] New therapies under evaluation here include antiangiogenic drugs, antibiotics such as rifaximin, and terlipressin.

Collateral Circulation and Varices

The portal vein–systemic collateral circulation develops and expands in response to elevation of the portal pressure. Blood flow in the low volumes that normally perfuse these collaterals and flow toward the portal circulation is reversed in portal hypertension because the increased portal pressure exceeds systemic venous pressure. Therefore flow is reversed in these collateral vessels, and blood flows out of the portal circulation toward the systemic venous circulation. The sites of collateral formation are the distal esophagus and proximal stomach, where gastroesophageal varices are the major collaterals formed between the portal venous system and systemic venous system; the umbilicus, where the vestigial umbilical vein communicates with the left portal vein and gives rise to prominent collaterals around the umbilicus (caput medusae); the retroperitoneum, where in women, collaterals communicate between the ovarian vessels and iliac veins; and the rectum, where the inferior mesenteric vein connects with the pudendal vein and rectal varices develop.

The veins draining the esophagus are divided into intrinsic, extrinsic, and the venae comitantes accompanying the vagus nerve. The intrinsic veins run the length of the esophagus and comprise four distinct zones of venous drainage at the gastroesophageal junction.[64] The gastric zone, which extends for 2–3 cm below the gastroesophageal junction, consists of veins that are longitudinal and located in the submucosa and lamina propria. They coalesce at the upper end of the cardia of the stomach and drain into short gastric and left gastric veins. The palisade zone extends 2–3 cm proximal to the gastric zone into the lower esophagus. Veins in this zone run longitudinally and in parallel in four groups corresponding to the esophageal mucosal folds. These veins anastomose with veins in the lamina propria. The perforating veins in the palisade zone do not communicate with extrinsic (periesophageal) veins in the distal esophagus. The palisade zone is the dominant watershed area between the portal and systemic circulations. More proximal to the palisade zone in the esophagus is the perforating zone, where there is a network of veins. These veins are less likely to be longitudinal and are termed *perforating veins* because they connect the intrinsic veins in the esophageal submucosa and the external veins. The truncal zone, the longest zone, is approximately 10 cm in length, located proximal to the perforating zone in the esophagus, and usually characterized by four longitudinal veins in the lamina propria. Intrinsic veins drain via the perforating veins unidirectionally into the extrinsic veins due to the presence of valves. However, the incompetence of the valves as occurs in portal hypertension may allow reversal of blood flow from the extrinsic to intrinsic veins with resulting increase in size of varices.

Veins in the palisade zone in the esophagus are most prone to bleeding because there are no perforating veins at this level to connect the veins in the submucosa with the periesophageal veins. Varices in the truncal zone are unlikely to bleed, because the perforating vessels communicate with the periesophageal veins, allowing the varices in the truncal zone to decompress. The periesophageal veins drain into the azygos system, and as a result, an increase in azygos blood flow is a hallmark of portal hypertension. The venous drainage of the lower end of the esophagus is through the coronary vein, which also drains the cardia of the stomach, into the portal vein.

The fundus of the stomach drains through short gastric veins into the splenic vein. In the presence of portal hypertension, varices may therefore form in the fundus of the stomach. Splenic vein thrombosis usually results in isolated gastric fundal varices. Because of the proximity of the splenic vein to the renal vein, spontaneous spleno-gastro-renal shunts may develop and are more common in patients with gastric varices than in those with esophageal varices.[24]

The predominant collateral flow pattern in intrahepatic portal hypertension is through the right and left coronary veins, with only a small portion of flow through the short gastric veins. Therefore most patients with an intrahepatic cause of portal hypertension have esophageal varices or gastric varices in continuity with esophageal varices. Unfortunately, portal hypertension caused by cirrhosis generally persists and progresses despite the development of even an extensive collateral circulation. Progression of portal hypertension results from (1) the prominent obstructive resistance in the liver; (2) resistance within the collaterals themselves; and (3) continued increase in portal vein inflow. The collateral circulatory bed develops through a combination of angiogenesis and dilatation and increased flow through preexisting collaterals.[1,25] VEGF, a key NO stimulatory growth factor, may contribute to both the angiogenic and collateral vessel responses.[22,26] Inhibition of VEGF or NO may attenuate the collateral vessel propagation by inhibiting angiogenic responses in experimental models of portal hypertension and collateralization.[25–28] Beta blockers and octreotide may act in part by constricting collateral vessels.[29–32] Attempts to inhibit VEGF and angiogenesis have focused on targeted kinase inhibitors.[21]

The development of gastroesophageal varices requires a portal pressure gradient of at least 10 mm Hg. Furthermore, a portal pressure gradient of at least 12 mm Hg is thought to be required for esophageal varices to bleed; other local factors that increase variceal wall tension are also needed[33] because not all patients with a portal pressure gradient of greater than 12 mm Hg bleed. Factors that influence variceal wall tension can be viewed in the context of Laplace's law as follows:

$$T = \frac{Pr}{w}$$

where T is variceal wall tension, P is the transmural pressure gradient between the variceal lumen and esophageal lumen, r is the variceal radius, and w is the variceal wall thickness. When the varix increases in diameter and pressure, the variceal wall thins, the tolerated wall tension is exceeded, and the varix ruptures. These physiologic observations are manifested clinically by the observation that patients with larger varices (r) in sites of limited soft-tissue support (w), with elevated portal pressure (P), tend to be at greatest risk for variceal rupture from variceal wall tension (T) that becomes excessive. One notable site in which soft-tissue support is limited is at the gastroesophageal junction. The lack of tissue support and high vessel density may contribute to the greater frequency of bleeding from varices at the gastroesophageal junction. Laplace's law also has implications for the relevance of pharmacologic therapies aimed at reducing portal pressure. A reduction in portal pressure reduces the variceal transmural pressure gradient and vessel diameter, thereby reducing the risk that variceal wall tension will become excessive and that varices will rupture. The changes in portal pressure and local variceal factors, however, are dynamic and influenced by several physiologic (an increase in intra-abdominal pressure, meal-induced increases in portal pressure), diurnal (circadian changes in portal pressure), and pathophysiologic (acute alcohol use) factors; moreover, portal pressure and esophageal variceal pressure may vary at different times.

MEASUREMENT OF PORTAL PRESSURE

Portal pressure may be measured indirectly or directly. The most used method of measuring portal pressure is the determination of the HVPG, which is an indirect method. Measurement of splenic pulp pressure and direct measurement of the portal vein pressure are infrequently used approaches because they are invasive and cumbersome. Variceal pressure also can be measured directly but is rarely performed in clinical practice. Measurement of liver stiffness using transient elastography (or other ultrasound-based approaches) or magnetic resonance elastography may indicate the presence of portal hypertension and is currently used as a broad surrogate for portal pressure (see Chapters 75 and 76).

Hepatic Vein Pressure Gradient

The HVPG is the difference between the wedged hepatic venous pressure (WHVP) and free hepatic vein pressure (FHVP) and represents the gradient between the pressure in the portal vein and the intra-abdominal inferior vena caval pressure (FHVP). The HVPG has been validated as the best predictor for the development of complications of portal hypertension.

Measurement of the HVPG requires a passage of a catheter into the hepatic vein under radiologic guidance until the catheter can be passed no further, that is, until the catheter has been "wedged" in the hepatic vein. The catheter can be passed into the hepatic vein through the femoral vein but is usually passed using a transjugular venous approach. The purpose of wedging the catheter is to form a column of fluid that is continuous between the hepatic sinusoids and the catheter. Therefore the measured pressure of fluid within the catheter reflects hepatic sinusoidal pressure. One of the drawbacks of using a catheter that is wedged in the hepatic vein is that the WHVP measured in a more fibrotic area of liver may be higher than the pressure measured in a less fibrotic area because of regional variation in the degree of fibrosis. Using a balloon-occluding catheter in the right hepatic vein to create a stagnant column of fluid in continuity with the hepatic sinusoids significantly reduces this variation in measurement of WHVP because the balloon catheter measures the WHVP averaged over a wider segment of the liver.[34] The pressure in the hepatic vein following deflation of the balloon is the FHVP.

HVPG measurement does not detect presinusoidal causes of portal hypertension. For example, in portal hypertension secondary to portal vein thrombosis, the HVPG is normal. Moreover, the HVPG may underestimate sinusoidal pressure in PBC and presinusoidal causes of portal hypertension, and some patients with MASH (formerly NASH) cirrhosis.[35] Therefore the HVPG is accurate for detecting only sinusoidal and postsinusoidal causes of portal hypertension. In experienced hands, the measurement of the HVPG is highly reproducible, accurate, and safe.[36] An elevation in intra-abdominal pressure increases both WHVP and FHVP equally, so that the HVPG is unchanged. By contrast, using the right atrial pressure as a reference for intra-abdominal pressure gives an erroneous estimation of hepatic sinusoidal pressure.[37] The advantage of the HVPG is that variations in the "zero" reference point have no impact on the HVPG.[38] The HVPG is measured at least three times to demonstrate that the values are reproducible. Total occlusion of the hepatic vein by the inflated balloon to confirm that the balloon is in a wedged position is demonstrated by injecting contrast into the hepatic vein. A sinusoidal pattern should be seen, with no collateral circulation to other hepatic veins. The contrast washes out promptly with a deflation of the balloon. Correct positioning of the balloon is also demonstrated by a sharp increase in the recorded pressure on inflation of the balloon. The pressure then becomes steady until the balloon is deflated, when the pressure drops sharply.

HVPG represents hepatic sinusoidal pressure and is normally $\leq$5 mm Hg; HVPG > 5 mm Hg is diagnostic of portal hypertension. However, varices or ascites do not develop till the HVPG is $\geq$10 mm, the threshold for defining CSPH which is, therefore, defined as HVPG $\geq$ 10 mm Hg. CSPH is predictive of development of varices, ascites, and hepatocellular carcinoma (HCC). Variceal bleeding defining severe portal hypertension occurs with HVPG $\geq$ 12 mm Hg.

Measurement of the HVPG has been proposed for the following indications: (1) to monitor portal pressure in patients taking drugs used to prevent variceal bleeding; (2) as a prognostic marker[39]; (3) as an end point in trials using pharmacologic agents for the treatment of portal hypertension; (4) to assess the risk of hepatic resection in patients with cirrhosis; and (5) to delineate the cause of portal hypertension [i.e., presinusoidal, sinusoidal, or postsinusoidal (Table 94.1)], usually in combination with venography, right-sided heart pressure measurements, and transjugular liver biopsy. Although the indication for HVPG measurement with the most potential for widespread use is to monitor the efficacy of therapies to reduce portal pressure, HVPG monitoring is not done routinely in clinical practice because controlled trials have yet to demonstrate its usefulness. Given the additional drawbacks of HVPG measurement of costs and invasive nature, liver stiffness measurement (LSM) by noninvasive methods is increasingly used for broad categorization of severity of portal hypertension.

Splenic Pulp Pressure

Determination of splenic pulp pressure is an indirect method of measuring portal pressure and involves puncture of the splenic pulp with a needle catheter. Splenic pulp pressure is elevated in presinusoidal portal hypertension, when the HVPG is normal. Because of the potential risk of complications, especially bleeding, associated with splenic puncture, the procedure is seldom used.

Portal Vein Pressure

Direct measurement of the pressure in the portal vein is rarely used but can be carried out through a percutaneous transhepatic route; transvenous approach; via endoscopic ultrasound; or intratraoperatively (although anesthesia can affect portal pressure). The transhepatic route requires portal vein puncture performed under US guidance. A catheter is then threaded over a guidewire into the main portal vein. With increasing use of transjugular intrahepatic portosystemic shunts (TIPS) (see later), radiologists have gained expertise in puncturing the portal vein and measuring portal vein pressure by a transjugular route. Direct portal pressure measurements are carried out when HVPG cannot be measured accurately, as in patients with occluded hepatic veins caused by the Budd-Chiari syndrome (see Chapter 87) in whom a surgical portosystemic shunt is being contemplated or in patients with intrahepatic, presinusoidal causes of portal hypertension, such as idiopathic portal hypertension (IPH), in which the HVPG may be normal.

Endoscopic Variceal Pressure

Varices rupture and bleed when the expanding force of intravariceal pressure exceeds variceal wall tension (see earlier). Measurement of the difference between intravariceal pressure and pressure within the esophageal lumen (the transmural pressure gradient across the varices) is potentially a more important indicator of bleeding risk than measurement of HVPG,[40] especially in patients with portal vein thrombosis and other causes of portal hypertension associated with a normal HVPG.

Variceal pressure can be measured in various ways: by the insertion of a needle connected to a pressure transducer, with use of a miniature pneumatic pressure sensitivity gauge at the tip of an endoscope, or by manometry using an endoscopic balloon. Patients with previous variceal bleeding have been demonstrated to have higher variceal pressures than those in patients without previous bleeding. A variceal pressure greater than 18 mm Hg during a bleeding episode is associated with failure to control bleeding and predicts early rebleeding. Moreover, patients on pharmacologic therapy who show a decrease in variceal pressure of greater than 20% from baseline have a low probability of bleeding, as compared with patients who do not demonstrate a greater than 20% decrease in variceal pressure, in whom the risk of variceal bleeding is 46%. In general, techniques for measuring variceal pressure are cumbersome and have not been found to be suitable or safe for routine clinical use.

TABLE 94.1 Use of Hepatic Vein Pressure Gradient in the Differential Diagnosis of Portal Hypertension

Type of Portal Hypertension	WHVP	FHVP	HVPG
Prehepatic	Normal	Normal	Normal
Presinusoidal	Normal	Normal	Normal
Sinusoidal	Increased	Normal	Increased
Postsinusoidal	Increased	Normal	Increased
Posthepatic			
Heart failure	Increased	Increased	Normal
Budd-Chiari syndrome	–	Hepatic vein cannot be cannulated	–

FHVP, Free hepatic vein pressure; *HVPG*, hepatic vein pressure gradient; *WHVP*, wedged hepatic venous pressure.

Broad Categorization of Portal Hypertension Using Liver Stiffness Measurement

Current data do not support the use of serological markers, such as platelet count, APRI, or FIB-4 alone to exclude CSPH. LSM < 15 kPa with platelets >150/μL essentially rules out the presence of CSPH. A diagnosis of CSPH is strongly supported with high specificity when LSM is >25 kPa; or between 20 and 25 kPa with platelets <150/μL; or between 15 and 20 kPa with platelet count <110/μL. In patients who do not fit these criteria and are in the "gray zone," liver stiffness-spleen size-to-platelet ratio score >2.65 may be a surrogate for CSPH. Spleen stiffness measurements (SSM) by TE correlates better with HVPG than LSM. SSM ≤40 kPa rules out the presence of varices requiring treatment, but the cut-off requires validation because the dedicated spleen probe has not been widely used.[218]

DETECTION OF VARICES

Esophagogastroduodenoscopy

Esophagogastroduodenoscopy (EGD) is recommended to detect esophageal varices in patients with cirrhosis falling in the "gray-zone" where a combination of LSM, platelet count, and SSM cannot confidently rule in or rule out CSPH. Where TE is not available to diagnose CSPH, and in the absence of radiological evidence of CSPH, endoscopic surveillance for high-risk varices is recommended. Surveillance endoscopy is not necessary in patients already on nonselective beta-blocker therapy; patients on a selective beta-blocker may be switched to a nonselective beta-blocker if appropriate, thus avoiding the need for endoscopy as surveillance for high-risk varices. Patients with decompensated cirrhosis should undergo annual endoscopic surveillance for high-risk varices. On the other hand, patients with compensated cirrhosis or cACLD without varices on screening endoscopy should have endoscopy repeated every 2 years when liver injury is persistent (example untreated HCV disease, continued alcohol use), or every 3 years (if liver injury is quiescent, as following elimination of HCV). If high-risk varices are detected, nonselective beta blockers or endoscopic band ligation (EBL) are recommended to prevent the first variceal bleed (primary prophylaxis). If patients are detected to have high-risk varices and started on nonselective beta blockers, and have not had any further bleeding, follow-up endoscopy is not required. EGD is safe in patients with large varices, and even transesophageal echocardiography is not associated with precipitating variceal bleeding.[41]

Endoscopic grading of esophageal varices is subjective. Various criteria have been used to try to standardize the reporting of esophageal varices. The best known criteria are those compiled by the Japanese Research Society for Portal Hypertension. The descriptors include red color signs, color of the varix, form (size) of the varix, and location of the varix.[42] Red color signs include red "wale" markings, which are longitudinal whip-like marks on the varix; cherry-red spots, which usually are 2–3 mm or less in diameter; hematocystic spots, which are blood-filled blisters 4 mm or greater in diameter; and diffuse redness. The color of the varix can be white or blue. The form of the varix at endoscopy is described most. Esophageal varices may be small and straight (grade I), tortuous and occupying less than one-third of the esophageal lumen (grade II), or large and occupying more than one-third of the esophageal lumen (grade III). Varices can be in the lower third, middle third, and upper third of the esophagus. Of all the descriptors, the size of the varices in the lower third of the esophagus is the most important. The size of the varices in the lower third of the esophagus is determined during withdrawal of the endoscope (Fig. 94.6). Small varices are 5 mm or less in diameter, whereas large varices are greater than 5 mm in diameter.[42] As a point of reference, any varix larger in diameter than an open pinch biopsy forceps is likely to be greater than 5 mm in diameter. Large esophageal varices and varices with red color signs are considered "high-risk varices." The increase in bleeding risk attributable to the presence of red color signs, however, is not independent of the risk associated with large variceal size. Therefore prophylactic treatment to prevent variceal bleeding is recommended in all patients with esophageal varices with red color signs and large esophageal varices irrespective of the presence or absence of red color signs (see later).

US

US examination of the liver with Doppler study of the vessels has been used widely to assess patients with portal hypertension. Features suggestive of portal hypertension on US include

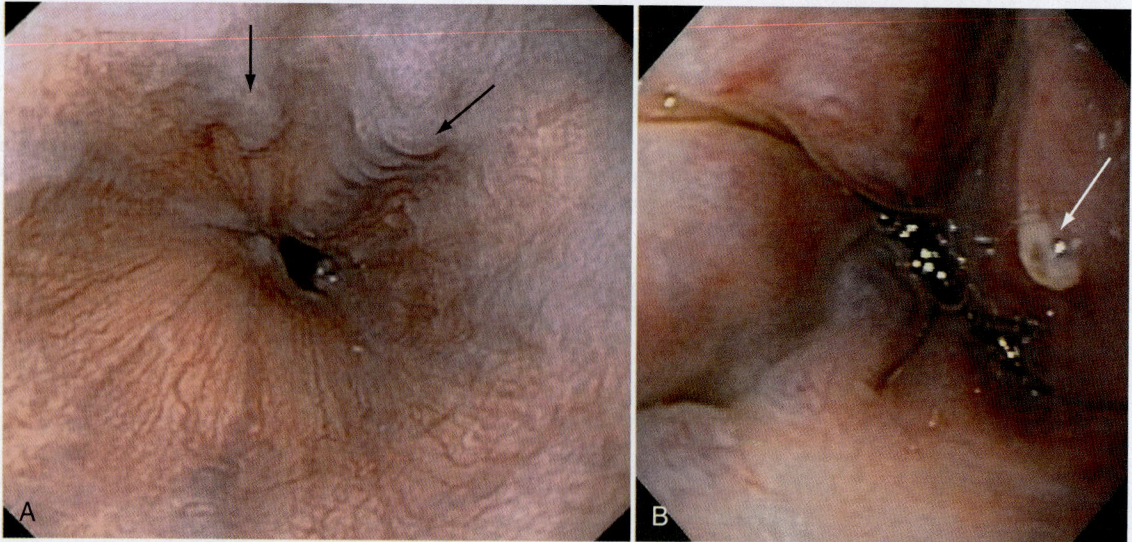

Fig. 94.6 Endoscopic appearances of esophageal varices. (A) Esophagogastroduodenoscopy (EGD) demonstrating dilated and straight veins (small esophageal varices) in the distal esophagus (*arrows*). (B) EGD demonstrating large esophageal varices, greater than 5 mm in diameter, with a fibrin plug (*arrow*) indicating the site of a recent bleed.

splenomegaly, portosystemic collateral vessels, and reversal of the direction of flow in the portal vein (hepatofugal flow). Some studies have demonstrated that a portal vein diameter greater than 13 mm and the absence of respiratory variations in the splenic and mesenteric veins are sensitive but nonspecific markers of portal hypertension. These criteria are not used routinely in clinical practice in most centers. US examination can detect thrombosis of the portal vein, which appears as nonvisualization or cavernous transformation (a cavernoma) of the portal vein; the latter finding indicates an extensive collateral network in place of the thrombosed portal vein. Splenic vein thrombosis also can be demonstrated. Although Doppler US is clinically useful in the initial evaluation of portal hypertension, the technique is not widely used to provide quantitative assessments of the degree of portal hypertension. Shear-wave transient or acoustic radiation force impulse (ARFI) elastography of the liver and spleen may be useful in stratifying patients with or without CSPH but is not sufficiently sensitive to recommend as a modality to monitor decreases in portal pressure in patients on pharmacotherapy (see Chapters 73 and 74).

CT

CT is useful for demonstrating many features of portal hypertension, including abnormal configuration of the liver, ascites, splenomegaly, collateral vessels, and portosystemic shunts (Figs. 94.7 and 94.8). Detection of varices may be an emerging indication for CT. The detection of fundal varices by multidetector CT is at least as accurate as EUS (see later). CT is especially helpful in distinguishing submucosal from perigastric fundal varices[43] and is considered a less invasive alternative to conventional angiographic portography in assessing portosystemic collaterals. In the detection of esophageal varices and high-risk varices in cirrhotic patients, CT imaging is superior to LSM and MRI.[44] Nevertheless, CT is not yet a recommended screening method for detecting large esophageal varices but may ultimately be confirmed as a cost-effective method of screening for varices and preferable to endoscopy by patients.[45]

MRI

Gadolinium-enhanced MRI is also a potentially useful method of detecting esophageal varices.[46] In addition, MRI can be used to measure portal and azygos blood flow, which is increased in patients with portal hypertension.[47] MRI provides excellent detail of the vascular structures of the liver and can detect portal vein thrombosis and spleen stiffness in patients with portal hypertension. Unlike shear-wave transient elastography, MR elastography can accurately assess the stiffness of even fatty livers.[48] However, the role of MR elastography in the assessment of changes in portal pressure in response to pharmacologic agents has not been demonstrated.[49]

EUS

EUS examination (endosonography) using radial or linear array echo-endoscopes or EUS miniprobes passed through the working channel of a diagnostic endoscope has been applied to the

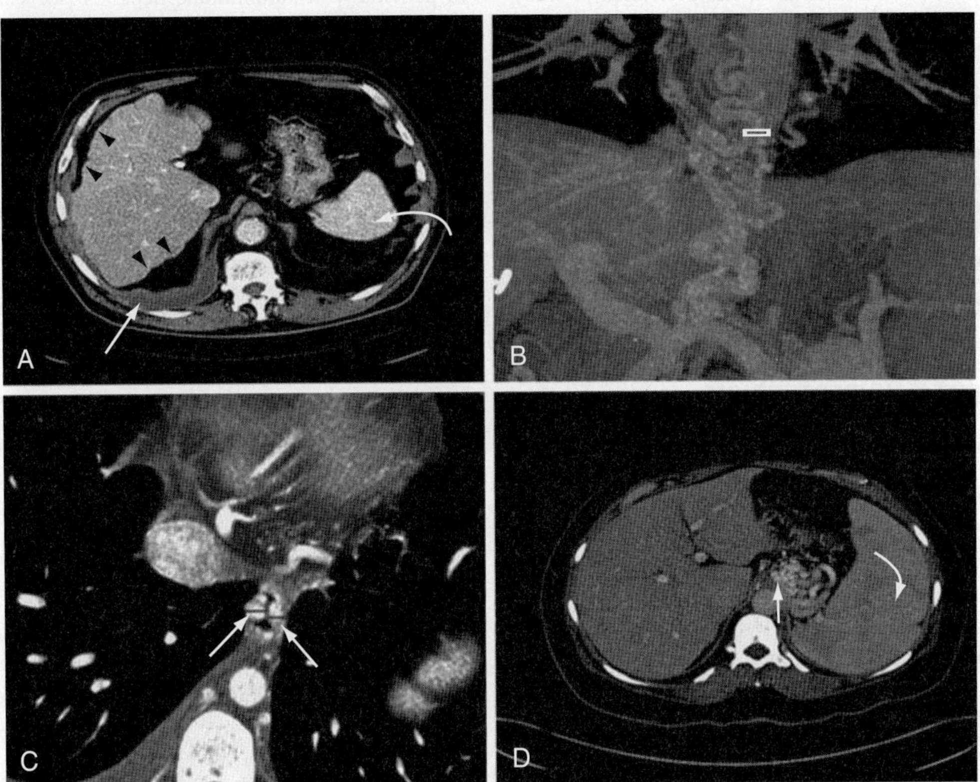

Fig. 94.7 Abdominal CT in patients with portal hypertension. (A) Image showing an irregular contour of the liver (*arrowheads*) typical of cirrhosis. A small right pleural effusion is evident (*straight arrow*). The liver is hypointense relative to the spleen (*curved arrow*), typical of fatty infiltration of the liver in alcohol-associated cirrhosis. (B) Coronal section of a CT showing contrast-enhanced esophageal varices (*cursor*). (C) Image showing two large esophageal varices (*arrows*) 5 and 6 mm in diameter. Varices are almost opposed to each other. (D) Image showing a tuft of gastroesophageal collaterals (*straight arrow*). The enlarged spleen is also seen (*curved arrow*).

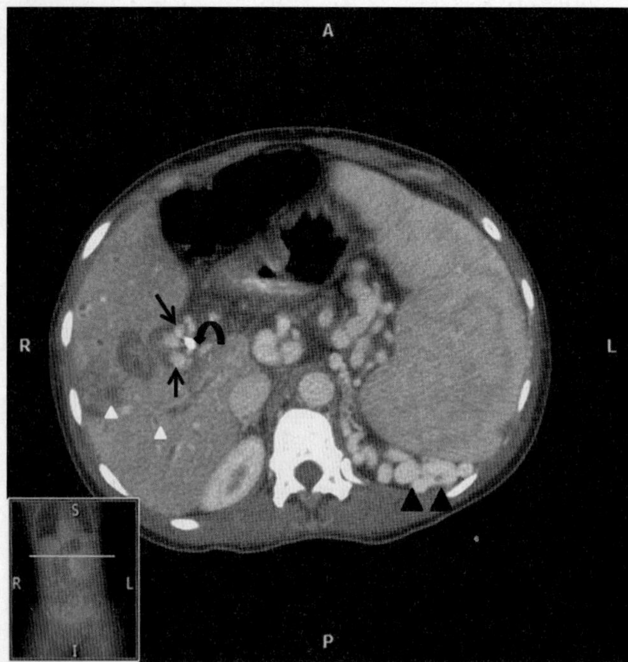

Fig. 94.8 CT showing choledochal varices (*straight arrows*) surrounding a stent in the bile duct (*curved arrow*). Dilated bile ducts (*white arrowheads*) and perisplenic varices (*black arrowheads*) are also seen.

evaluation of patients with varices. EUS has been used to study several aspects of esophageal varices, including the cross-sectional area of varices to identify patients at increased risk of bleeding[33]; size of and flow in the left gastric vein, azygos vein, and para-esophageal collaterals; changes after endoscopic therapy; and recurrence of esophageal varices following variceal ligation (see later).[50] Endosonography can be combined with endoscopic measurement of transmural variceal pressure to allow estimation of variceal wall tension, which is a predictor of variceal bleeding (see earlier).[50,51] Endosonography may be used to target varices for sclerotherapy or glue injection (see later).[52] EUS-guided portosystemic pressure measurement and liver biopsy can be carried out as a combined procedure.[53]

CAUSES OF PORTAL HYPERTENSION

The usual classification of causes of portal hypertension is based on the site of increased resistance to portal blood flow—namely, prehepatic, intrahepatic, and posthepatic—and is outlined in Fig. 94.5. Intrahepatic sites of increased resistance can be presinusoidal, sinusoidal, or postsinusoidal. Many causes of portal hypertension are associated with an increase in resistance at more than one site. For example, alcohol-associated cirrhosis may be associated with increased resistance at the presinusoidal, sinusoidal, and postsinusoidal levels. Therefore classification based on the site of resistance may not be possible for all diseases that cause portal hypertension. A more useful classification is clinically based and considers common and less common causes of portal hypertension (Box 94.1).

Common

Cirrhosis

Complications related to portal hypertension are the usual clinical manifestations of cirrhosis (see Chapter 74). Although all causes of cirrhosis are associated with portal hypertension, some features are disease specific. In alcohol-associated liver disease, elevation of the portal pressure is accurately reflected by the HVPG; moreover, portal hypertension may occur in the absence of cirrhosis but is more marked when cirrhosis is present. Perivenular lesions implicated in the pathogenesis of noncirrhotic alcohol-associated liver injury account for the postsinusoidal component of portal hypertension in these patients (see Chapter 88). Autoimmune hepatitis also may be associated with portal hypertension in the absence of cirrhosis; however, the risk of variceal bleeding is low in patients with autoimmune hepatitis (see Chapter 92). In patients with hemochromatosis, portal hypertension may be seen even before cirrhosis; the severity of portal hypertension increases with increasing fibrosis. Patients with hemochromatosis may bleed from varices despite an HVPG less than 12 mm Hg, indicating a presinusoidal component of portal hypertension. Phlebotomy therapy in patients with hemochromatosis may result in a decrease in portal hypertension (see Chapter 77).[54] In patients with PBC as well, portal hypertension may occur before cirrhosis has developed. The risk of variceal bleeding increases with an increase in the histologic stage of the disease.[55] In earlier stages of PBC, portal hypertension is predominantly presinusoidal and HVPG may underestimate portal pressure in patients with PBC.[35] As the disease progresses, a sinusoidal component develops. Treatment of PBC with UDCA may result in a decrease in portal pressure (see Chapter 93). Portal hypertension occurs in patients with PSC (see Chapter 70) and in those with biliary strictures (see Chapter 72). Although a long duration of biliary obstruction is typically required, portal hypertension has been known to develop even in a few months in patients with chronic bile duct obstruction caused by chronic alcohol-associated pancreatitis (see Chapter 61). Portal hypertension in patients with biliary obstruction regresses following relief of the biliary obstruction. Signs of portal hypertension are present in 25% of patients at the time of diagnosis of MASLD with advanced fibrosis or cirrhosis; however, portal hypertension may occur even in the absence of fibrosis if steatosis is extensive (see Chapter 89).[56]

BOX 94.1 Causes of Portal Hypertension

COMMON
- Cirrhosis
- Schistosomiasis
- Extrahepatic portal vein thrombosis
- Idiopathic portal hypertension
- Cardiac fibrosis

LESS COMMON
- Nodular regenerative hyperplasia
- Partial nodular transformation of the liver
- Fibropolycystic liver disease
- Sarcoidosis
- Malignancy
- Splanchnic arteriovenous fistula
- HHT

Schistosomiasis

Schistosomiasis is a common cause of portal hypertension worldwide (see Chapter 86). Bleeding from esophageal varices is a major cause of death in patients with hepatosplenic schistosomiasis. Portal hypertension results from presinusoidal obstruction caused by a deposition of eggs of *Schistosoma mansoni* or *Schistosoma japonicum* in the presinusoidal portal venules. The host reaction results in granulomatous inflammation, which causes presinusoidal and periportal fibrosis. The fibrosis that results is sometimes called "clay pipestem" or simply "pipestem" fibrosis and is associated with sustained heavy infection. The periportal collagen deposition leads to progressive obstruction of portal blood flow, portal hypertension, and variceal bleeding, along with splenomegaly and hypersplenism.[57] Lobular architecture usually is preserved. Coinfection with HBV or HCV in patients with hepatic schistosomiasis can result in more rapid progression of fibrosis, hepatic failure, and an increased risk of HCC.[58]

The HVPG is typically normal owing to the presinusoidal nature of the obstruction. Some patients with schistosomiasis and portal hypertension may also have portal vein thrombosis. Patients with schistosomiasis may undergo portosystemic shunt surgery to treat variceal bleeding, but TIPS is also associated with excellent long-term outcomes.[59]

Extrahepatic Portal Vein Thrombosis

Extrahepatic portal vein thrombosis is a prehepatic, presinusoidal cause of portal hypertension and a common cause of portal hypertension in children (see Chapter 85). The most common causes of portal vein thrombosis in adults include hematologic disorders, such as polycythemia vera, or other myeloproliferative neoplasms.[60,61] Other causes include a prothrombotic state, such as antithrombin, protein C, or protein S deficiency; antiphospholipid syndrome (or antiphospholipid antibody syndrome); paroxysmal nocturnal hemoglobinuria; oral contraceptive use; a neoplasm, usually intra-abdominal; an inflammatory disease, such as pancreatitis, IBD, or diverticulitis; central obesity; abdominal trauma; and postoperative states, especially postsplenectomy. Isolated splenic vein thrombosis caused by a pancreatic neoplasm or pancreatitis usually is not associated with a thrombophilia; the risk of variceal bleeding is also low, and the benefit of anticoagulation in recanalizing the splenic vein is minimal.[62] Umbilical vein sepsis may be an etiologic factor in children with portal vein thrombosis, but even in these cases, an associated prothrombotic state may be an additional predisposing factor.

Acute and subacute portal vein thrombosis usually does not manifest with variceal bleeding. Chronic portal vein thrombosis is suggested by nonvisualization of the portal or splenic vein and an extensive collateral circulation on imaging studies. Patients may present with nonspecific symptoms or with variceal bleeding and hypersplenism. Bleeding is usually from gastroesophageal varices but may be from duodenal varices and, rarely, other ectopic sites. Gallbladder varices have also been described in patients with portal vein thrombosis.

Portal vein thrombosis occurs in patients with cirrhosis at an annual frequency of 2%–10% per year and is associated with severity of liver disease.[63] CT or MRI is recommended in these patients to rule out HCC, which may be associated with tumor thrombus that is recognized as an arterialized thrombus.

The treatment of chronic portal vein thrombosis is symptomatic, with the aim of controlling variceal bleeding or preventing recurrent variceal bleeding.[61] Patients with a thrombophilia, even in the presence of large esophageal varices, are best managed with anticoagulation because in these patients the benefits of anticoagulation outweigh the risks.[60,61] Anticoagulation in patients with cirrhosis is safe and is associated with a high rate of recanalization of the portal vein and reduced rates of complications of cirrhosis.[64] Comorbidity has a greater impact on outcome of GI bleeding in patients on anticoagulants than does the anticoagulation itself.[65] Local or systemic thrombolytic therapy is seldom required and is generally reserved for patients in whom an acute portal vein thrombus extends into the superior mesenteric vein, with danger of impending intestinal ischemia. Endoscopic therapy is used to control acute variceal bleeding and to prevent recurrent bleeding. Use of pharmacologic agents, such as beta blockers, to prevent variceal bleeding is probably also effective in patients with portal vein thrombosis, but this approach has not been well studied. Patients with portal vein thrombosis have lower mortality and morbidity rates from variceal bleeding than those reported in patients with cirrhosis and variceal bleeding, owing to the lack of coagulopathy and synthetic liver dysfunction. Surgical portosystemic shunt procedures are carried out in patients in whom bleeding cannot be controlled by conservative measures. If a suitable vein is not available for anastomosis, a large collateral vein may be anastomosed to a systemic vein. The mesenterico–left portal venous bypass discussed later is especially effective because it preserves portal blood flow and avoids hepatic encephalopathy while decompressing the portal venous system.[66] Placement of a TIPS is possible in many patients with chronic portal vein thrombosis and cirrhosis, with excellent long-term patency.[67]

Fig. 94.9 provides an algorithmic approach to management of portal vein thrombosis in patients with cirrhosis.

Idiopathic Portal Hypertension

IPH is uncommon in Western countries but is common in parts of Asia, such as India and Japan. This disorder is diagnosed when portal pressure is elevated in the absence of significant histologic changes in the liver or extrahepatic portal vein obstruction.[68] A liver biopsy specimen from affected patients may be entirely normal. Various terms used (rather loosely) to describe IPH include *hepatoportal sclerosis*, *noncirrhotic portal hypertension*, *noncirrhotic portal fibrosis*, and *Banti syndrome*. Some authors include nodular regenerative hyperplasia and incomplete septal fibrosis under the broad term IPH. Use of the term IPH is probably best restricted to portal hypertension in patients in whom no specific hepatic lesion is found on light microscopy and the portal venous system is patent. The term *hepatoportal sclerosis* is used when there is obliterative portal venopathy with subendothelial thickening of the intrahepatic portal veins; thrombosis and recanalization of these veins may follow. Fibrosis of the portal tracts is prominent later in the course (see Chapter 87). Recently, the term *porto-sinusoidal vascular disorder* (*PSVD*) has been used to describe a group of vascular diseases of the liver featuring lesions involving the portal venules and sinusoids; liver biopsy is required to make a diagnosis of PSVD. The histological findings in this PSVD include nodular regenerative hyperplasia, obliterative portal venopathy/portal vein stenosis and incomplete septal fibrosis/cirrhosis. Long-term outcomes in patients diagnosed to have PSVD but without portal hypertension are unknown. A diagnosis of IPH can be strongly considered in the absence of a liver biopsy based on history, physical examination, laboratory testing, abdominal imaging, and transient elastography. Thrombocytopenia with a normal bone-marrow examination in the presence of esophageal varices, otherwise unexplained splenomegaly, and absence of stigmata of chronic liver disease suggests the diagnosis of IPH. MR elastography is particularly relevant in making a diagnosis. On MRE, the normal liver stiffness is $\leq$2.9 kPa, and cirrhosis is diagnosed when the liver stiffness is $\geq$5 kPa.[48] The normal splenic stiffness is $<$3.6 kPa; in the presence of esophageal varices in patients with cirrhosis the spleen stiffness is $>$10.5 kPa.[69] Measuring both spleen stiffness (SSM) and liver stiffness (LSM) can be helpful in distinguishing cirrhosis as a cause of portal hypertension from noncirrhotic causes of portal hypertension. Liver stiffness by MRE is higher in patients with cirrhosis than with noncirrhotic causes of portal hypertension.[70] In IPH, SSM is typically higher than LSM. Using a proposed algorithm on MRE of LSM $<$ 4.7 kPa and an SSM/LSM cutoff of $>$1.23 yields a 97.6% sensitivity, 100% specificity, and an AUROC of 0.99 for diagnosis of NCPH, with only rare cases of NCPH classified as cirrhosis.[70,71] On transient elastography in patients with portal hypertension, LSM $<$ 10 kPa strongly suggests PSVD; when

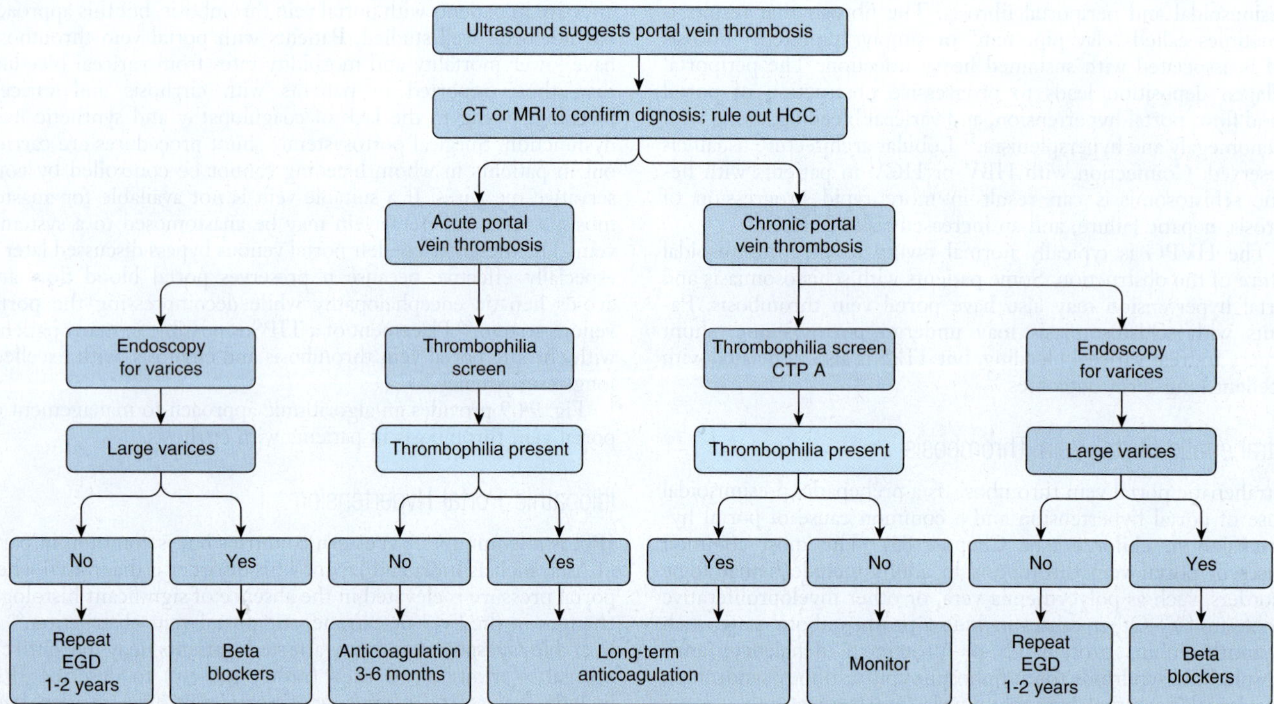

Fig. 94.9 Algorithm for the management of portal vein thrombosis in patients with cirrhosis. *C-P*, Child-Pugh class.

TE-LSM is >20 kPa, PSVD is essentially ruled out.[72] Small studies have shown that ARFI elastography, an ultrasound technique, can also distinguish IPH from cirrhosis. A spleen-liver stiffness ratio value >1.7 strongly suggests IPH.[73]

The cause of IPH is unclear in most patients, although chronic arsenic intoxication, exposure to vinyl chloride, and hypervitaminosis A have been implicated (see Chapter 91). These etiologic factors are present in only a minority of patients. The dominant clinical features of IPH are variceal bleeding and hypersplenism related to a markedly enlarged spleen. A family history of portal hypertension, especially in the presence of premature graying of hair and bone marrow failure supports the presence of telomere shortening disorders as a cause of IPH.[74]

Liver biochemical test levels are usually normal, although the serum alkaline phosphatase level may be mildly elevated. Ascites is uncommon. The HVPG in this disorder is usually normal because the site of increased resistance is presinusoidal.[75] Surgical portosystemic shunts are well tolerated in these patients, although hepatic encephalopathy may occur on long-term follow-up. TIPS is also an excellent option to treat variceal bleeding refractory to endoscopic and pharmacologic therapy,[76] but patients with IPH may have reduced survival and LT may be required in some patients.[77] Hypersplenism in IPH is seldom severe enough to require a splenectomy.

Less Common

Nodular Regenerative Hyperplasia

Nodular regenerative hyperplasia is a histopathologic diagnosis characterized by an atrophy of zone 3 hepatocytes and hypertrophy of zone 1 hepatocytes, without significant fibrosis (see Chapters 35 and 98), and is included in the spectrum of IPH and PSVD.[78] This disorder which is really not a specific clinical entity has been recognized increasingly in patients with portal hypertension and may even occur after LT.[79] Similar histologic changes may be seen in well-established Budd-Chiari syndrome.[80] The nodular hyperplasia may not be apparent on histologic examination unless a reticulin stain is carried out to demonstrate the micronodules. The changes are believed to result from an imbalance between hyperperfused areas of the liver, with resulting regenerative nodules, and poorly perfused areas, with resulting atrophy. Nodular regenerative hyperplasia is associated with a variety of conditions, predominantly IPH, hematologic and rheumatologic conditions, common variable immunodeficiency, and drugs such as chemotherapeutic agents, antiretroviral agents, and thiopurines[81] (see Chapter 35). Mild elevation of the serum aminotransferase levels is seen. Portal hypertension manifesting as variceal bleeding is the predominant clinical presentation. Ascites also may develop in these patients, suggesting that an increase in sinusoidal pressure also occurs.[82] Hepatopulmonary syndrome may also be seen. Hepatic malignancies are rare in patients with NRH and routine surveillance for HCC is not recommended.[83]

Cardiac Cirrhosis

Cardiac cirrhosis has been recognized in patients with long-standing passive congestion of the liver due to heart failure and increasingly in patients with complex congenital heart disease who have had corrective surgery in childhood and live beyond the second decade of life[84] (see Chapter 87). Cirrhosis occurs especially in patients who have undergone a Fontan procedure, which allows systemic venous blood flow to enter the pulmonary artery and bypass the right ventricle. Sequelae of chronic passive congestion of the liver secondary to the procedure are termed *Fontan-associated liver disease*; long-term sequelae include complications of portal hypertension and HCC, and variceal bleeding may occur.[85]

Partial Nodular Transformation of the Liver

Partial nodular transformation of the liver is an uncommon lesion that is characterized by large nodules in the perihilar region.[86] These nodules may be visible on imaging studies of the liver. The rest of the liver may be normal or may show changes of nodular regenerative hyperplasia. Liver biochemical test levels usually are normal. Like nodular regenerative hyperplasia, partial nodular transformation of the liver is believed to be related to an imbalance in portal perfusion of the liver, but the abnormality is restricted to the hilar branches, whereas in nodular regenerative hyperplasia the abnormality is more diffuse. Variceal bleeding is the predominant presentation, although patients with large nodules may experience abdominal pain. HCC may rarely develop in a regenerative nodule. Treatment with a surgical portosystemic shunt is associated with good long-term results.

Fibropolycystic Liver Disease

Fibropolycystic liver disease is a term that encompasses Caroli disease; Caroli syndrome (or complex) when Caroli disease and congenital hepatic fibrosis occur together; congenital hepatic fibrosis alone; and polycystic liver disease (see Chapters 62 and 96). Congenital hepatic fibrosis usually occurs in association with Caroli disease of the liver, polycystic disease of the kidney, and medullary sponge kidney[87] (see Chapter 64). The major manifestation of congenital hepatic fibrosis is variceal bleeding. A portosystemic shunt may be placed in affected patients to treat refractory variceal bleeding, with a low long-term risk of hepatic encephalopathy. Patients with polycystic liver disease, whether associated with polycystic kidney disease or not, can present rarely with portal hypertension because of extensive compression of the portal venous system by the cysts[88] (see Chapter 98); portal hypertension may decrease after treatment of the cysts.[89]

Sarcoidosis

Portal hypertension is an uncommon manifestation of hepatic sarcoidosis[90] (see Chapter 35). The site of increased intrahepatic resistance in patients with sarcoidosis seems to be postsinusoidal, in view of the elevated HVPG. In early disease, however, the resistance is predominantly at a presinusoidal level. Treatment with glucocorticoids may decrease portal hypertension in some patients with hepatic sarcoidosis.

Malignancy

Portal hypertension has been associated with leukemias, lymphomas, and systemic mastocytosis (see Chapters 35 and 41). TIPS has been used as therapy for complications of portal hypertension in patients with myeloproliferative neoplasms, but with a higher risk of stent thrombosis than in other settings.[91] Portal hypertension may also occur in patients with HCC independent of the presence of cirrhosis (see Chapter 98). The pathogenesis of portal hypertension in patients with HCC is thought to be multifactorial; contributing factors include portal vein thrombosis, pressure by the tumor on the portal vein, and, in some cases, a hepatic artery–portal vein fistula.[92] In patients with HCC and tumor thrombosis treated with combination of atezolizumab and bevacizumab, there is an increased risk of variceal bleeding.[93]

Management of acute variceal hemorrhage in patients with HCC is similar to that for patients without HCC. Nonselective beta blockers are recommended for primary prophylaxis.[94] The presence of portal hypertension does not preclude locoregional therapies but TIPS placement may be challenging in patients with HCC. Esophageal varices may be seen in patients with hepatic metastases, although variceal bleeding is unusual.

Splanchnic Arteriovenous Fistula

A splanchnic AVF should be suspected when the onset of ascites and variceal bleeding is acute, especially in the presence of an abdominal bruit. When a splanchnic artery ruptures into a mesenteric vein, the portal pressure increases acutely, reaching levels of systemic arterial pressure.[95] The result may be acute portal hypertension with a development of ascites and variceal bleeding. A bruit may be heard in the LUQ of the abdomen with a splenic AVF and in the RUQ with a hepatic artery–portal vein fistula. With a longstanding fistula, secondary perisinusoidal hepatic fibrosis related to an increase in portal venous inflow may develop. Embolization or ligation of the fistula usually ameliorates the portal hypertension.

HHT

HHT, or Osler-Weber-Rendu disease, is an unusual cause of portal hypertension (see also Chapters 21, 35, and 87). Diagnostic criteria include mucocutaneous telangiectasias, epistaxis, AVFs of the viscera (usually lung or liver), and a family history of the disorder.[96] Hepatic manifestations of HHT depend on the site of fistula formation. A fistula between the hepatic artery and hepatic vein manifests predominantly as biliary disease, mainly biliary strictures and cholangitis, and high-output cardiac failure. A fistula between the hepatic artery and portal vein results in portal hypertension and biliary strictures, whereas a fistula between the portal vein and hepatic vein, which is rare, results in hepatic encephalopathy.[97] Nodular regenerative hyperplasia, which develops in some patients with HHT, may worsen portal hypertension. Treatment with bevacizumab may ameliorate epistaxis as well as gastrointestinal bleeding.[98,99]

CLINICAL ASSESSMENT

Patients with esophageal or gastric variceal bleeding present acutely with hematemesis or melena (or both). Chronic blood loss is a more common presentation of portal hypertensive gastropathy (PHG) or GI vascular ectasia. The classic presentation of patients with variceal bleeding is with effortless and recurrent hematemesis; the vomitus is described as dark red in color (see Chapter 21).

Portal hypertension should be suspected in all patients with GI bleeding and peripheral stigmata of liver disease (see Chapter 76)—namely, jaundice, spider telangiectasias, palmar erythema, Dupuytren contractures, parotid enlargement, testicular atrophy, loss of secondary sexual characteristics, ascites, and encephalopathy. Splenomegaly is an important clue to the presence of portal hypertension, and the presence of ascites makes the presence of esophageal varices even more likely. A bruit may be heard in the left or RUQ in a patient with a splanchnic AVF. A venous hum may be heard in the epigastrium in a patient with portal hypertension and represents high flow through the recanalized umbilical vein (*Cruveilhier–Baumgarten bruit*). The presence of variceal bleeding in a patient with splenomegaly, but without jaundice, ascites, or hepatic encephalopathy and with normal or near normal liver biochemistry, raises the possibility of IPH if other causes of liver disease have been ruled out.

Laboratory studies frequently reveal evidence of hepatic synthetic dysfunction in patients with cirrhosis, including prolongation of the prothrombin time, hypoalbuminemia, and hyperbilirubinemia, as well as anemia. Thrombocytopenia and leukopenia, reflecting hypersplenism and, in patients with alcohol use disorder, bone marrow suppression, may be noted. Patients with severe bleeding may present with hypovolemic shock and renal insufficiency. Abdominal imaging studies frequently reveal splenomegaly, collateral vessels, abnormal liver echotexture and contour, and ascites.

TREATMENT

The treatment of portal hypertension is aimed at either reducing portal blood flow with pharmacologic agents, such as beta-blockers or vasopressin and its analogs; or decreasing intrahepatic resistance with pharmacologic agents, such as nitrates, or by creation of a portosystemic shunt, either radiologic or surgical. Treatment also may be directed at the varices with use of endoscopic or radiologic techniques.

Pharmacologic Therapy

The pharmacologic agents used in the treatment of portal hypertension are divided into two groups: those that decrease splanchnic blood flow and comprise the vast majority of available agents, and those that decrease intrahepatic vascular resistance (Box 94.2). The agents that decrease splanchnic blood flow acutely are vasopressin and its analogs and somatostatin and its analogs. β-Adrenergic blocking agents decrease portal blood flow but are used only to prevent variceal bleeding and rebleeding, not control acute bleeding. Agents that target intrahepatic vascular resistance include α-adrenergic blocking agents, angiotensin receptor blocking agents, and nitrates, but only carvedilol is considered for clinical use. Diuretics, by decreasing plasma volume, may reduce portal pressure but are not recommended if the patient does not have ascites. Prokinetic agents may decrease intravariceal pressure by contracting the lower esophageal sphincter but have not been evaluated in clinical trials.

Vasopressin and Its Analogs

Vasopressin is an endogenous peptide hormone that causes splanchnic vasoconstriction, reduces portal venous inflow, and decreases portal pressure. This drug is associated with serious systemic side effects, however. By causing constriction of systemic vessels, vasopressin may result in necrosis of the bowel. In addition, vasopressin has direct negative inotropic and chronotropic effects on the myocardium that lead to reduced cardiac output and bradycardia, respectively. An increase in cardiac afterload can result in myocardial infarction, and antidiuresis, resulting from the action of vasopressin on the kidney, can result in hyponatremia.

Terlipressin, or triglycyl-lysine-vasopressin, has largely supplanted vasopressin in treatment of variceal hemorrhage and is a semisynthetic analog of vasopressin that is cleaved by endothelial peptidases to release lysine vasopressin. Compared with vasopressin, terlipressin is associated with lower circulatory levels of the vasopressin analog and a lower rate of systemic side effects. Terlipressin is preferred over vasopressin because of its superior safety profile. In addition, an increase in survival has been demonstrated in patients with variceal bleeding treated with terlipressin. For the initial 24–48 hours, terlipressin is administered in a dose of 2 mg intravenously every 4–6 hours; it is then administered in a dose of 1 mg every 4–6 hours for 2–5 days.

BOX 94.2 Drugs Used in the Treatment of Portal Hypertension

DRUGS THAT DECREASE PORTAL BLOOD FLOW

Nonselective β-adrenergic blocking agents (e.g., propranolol, nadolol; also carvedilol)
Somatostatin and its analogs
Vasopressin and terlipressin

DRUGS THAT DECREASE INTRAHEPATIC RESISTANCE

α_1-Adrenergic blocking agents (e.g., prazosin; also carvedilol)
Angiotensin receptor blocking agents
Nitrates

Somatostatin and Its Analogs

Somatostatin is a 14–amino acid peptide. Five somatostatin receptors—SRTR 1–SRTR 5—are recognized, but the actual distribution of the receptors in humans is not clear. Following IV injection, somatostatin has a half-life in the circulation of 1–3 minutes; therefore longer acting analogs of somatostatin, octreotide, lanreotide, and vapreotide have been synthesized.[100] Somatostatin decreases portal pressure and collateral blood flow by inhibiting release of glucagon.[101] The optimal dose and duration of use of somatostatin have not been adequately studied. Following a single 250-μg bolus injection of somatostatin, there is a decrease in portal and azygos blood flow for only a few minutes.[102] Use of higher doses is associated with a more impressive decrease in HVPG. Somatostatin also decreases portal pressure by decreasing postprandial splanchnic blood flow.[103] Following a variceal bleed, blood in the GI tract acts like a meal, leading to an increase in portal flow and elevation in the portal pressure; this elevation in pressure is ameliorated using somatostatin.

The analog octreotide has a half-life in the circulation of 80–120 minutes following IV administration. Its effect on portal pressure is not prolonged, however. Moreover, continuous infusion of octreotide may not decrease portal pressure despite decreasing the postprandial increase in portal pressure.[104] Octreotide is administered as an initial IV bolus of 50 mcg followed by continued infusion at a rate of 25–50 mcg/hour for up to 5 days. Long-acting octreotide does not reliably reduce portal pressure, and side effects with higher doses preclude use of this agent for the treatment of portal hypertension.[105]

Some randomized controlled trials support the view that somatostatin or octreotide may be equivalent in efficacy to terlipressin or sclerotherapy (see later) for controlling acute variceal bleeding. Moreover, early administration of vapreotide may be associated with improved control of bleeding, but without a significant reduction in mortality rate.[106] In clinical practice, somatostatin or octreotide administration should be combined with endoscopic management of variceal bleeding (see later).

β-Adrenergic Blocking Agents

Nonselective β-adrenergic blocking agents have been used extensively since the landmark study of Lebrec et al. demonstrated the efficacy of these agents in preventing variceal rebleeding.[107] Blockade of β_1-adrenergic receptors in the heart decreases cardiac output. Blockade of β_2-adrenergic receptors, which cause vasodilatation in the mesenteric circulation, allows unopposed action of α_1-adrenergic receptors and results in decreased portal flow. The combination of decreased cardiac output and decreased portal flow leads to a decrease in portal pressure. Long-term treatment with beta blockers may increase decompensation-free survival in patients with compensated cirrhosis and CSPH by reducing the incidence of ascites.[108] Among nonselective beta-blockers, nadolol has advantages over propranolol in that it is excreted predominantly by the kidney, has low lipid solubility, and is associated with a lower risk of CNS side effects such as depression. The effectiveness of beta blockers is assessed most accurately by monitoring the HVPG, but this approach is not widely used in clinical practice. An acute hemodynamic response (decrease in HVPG to <12 mm Hg, or by 10%) 20 minutes after administration of IV propranolol may predict the long-term reduction in bleeding risk.[109] The benefit of beta blockers is reduced when hepatic function worsens.[110] The usual method in clinical practice of monitoring the efficacy of beta blockers is to observe a decrease in the heart rate, which is a measure of β_1-adrenergic receptor blockade. Despite adequate β_1-adrenergic receptor blockade, some patients may benefit from a further increase in the dose of beta-blocker to increase the degree of β_2-adrenergic blockade. Raising the dose, however, results in more side effects and the likelihood that treatment will need to be withdrawn.[111] HVPG monitoring, when used in patients on beta-blockers, may be associated with improved survival by facilitating a greater reduction in portal pressure and thus a lower bleeding risk.[112] Patients taking beta blockers prophylactically do not have poorer survival during the episode of acute variceal bleeding.[113] In patients with refractory ascites, beta-blocker use has been reported to be associated with increased mortality. A meta-analysis, however, concluded that use of nonselective beta blockers was not associated with a significant increase in all-cause mortality in patients with cirrhosis and either controlled ascites or refractory ascites. The meta-analysis does not support the position that nonselective beta-blockers should routinely be withheld from all patients with ascites.[114] Rather, they should be discontinued in patients with ascites when they have worsening renal function; premature discontinuation may be detrimental[115] (see Chapter 93).

Combined α- and β-Adrenergic Blocking Agents

Carvedilol decreases cardiac output (β-1 blockade), splanchnic arterial vasoconstriction (β-2 blockade), and intrinsic antialpha-1-adrenergic activity that facilitates the release of NO, inducing intrahepatic vasodilation and further reducing portal pressure. Carvedilol allows for a significantly more pronounced decrease in HVPG than traditional NSBBs (such as propranolol and nadolol). Carvedilol has antioxidant as well as antiproliferative actions and may be superior to endoscopic variceal ligation in the prevention of a first variceal bleed.[23] In addition, carvedilol may delay progression of small esophageal varices to large esophageal varices in patients with cirrhosis.[116] In a competing-risk meta-analysis, carvedilol reduced the risk of hepatic decompensation as well as mortality in patients with compensated cirrhosis[117] and is thus recommended in patients with CSPH.[118] Addition of simvastatin to carvedilol does not improve hemodynamic response over carvedilol monotherapy.[119] Carvedilol may be associated with hypotension and renal sodium retention and should be used cautiously in patients with Child-Pugh class C cirrhosis.

Carvedilol is started at a dose of 3.125 mg twice daily or 6.25 mg at bedtime, and the dose is increased stepwise to a maximum of 25 mg daily. Dose increases are usually limited by arterial hypotension.[120]

Nitrates

Short-acting (nitroglycerin) or long-acting (isosorbide mononitrate) nitrates result in vasodilatation. The vasodilatation results from a decrease in intracellular calcium in vascular smooth muscle cells. Nitrates cause venodilatation, rather than arterial dilatation, and decrease portal pressure predominantly by decreasing portal venous blood flow. The effect on intrahepatic resistance is less impressive than generally has been believed. The combination of vasopressin and nitroglycerin is seldom used now to control acute variceal bleeding. It is unusual for patients to tolerate nitrates for any length of time because of side effects, especially hypotension and headaches. Nitrates are no longer recommended, either alone or in combination with a beta-blocker, for primary or secondary prophylaxis to prevent variceal bleeds.

Other Drugs That Decrease Intrahepatic Vascular Resistance

The ideal agent for treatment of portal hypertension is a drug that selectively decreases intrahepatic vascular resistance without worsening systemic vasodilatation. Besides carvedilol and nitrates, agents that may decrease intrahepatic resistance include α_1-adrenergic blocking agents, such as prazosin, but long-term administration of prazosin causes worsening of the systemic hyperdynamic circulation associated with portal hypertension and consequent sodium retention and ascites.[121] The addition of propranolol to prazosin may ameliorate the adverse effects of prazosin on the systemic circulation. Losartan, an angiotensin II receptor type I antagonist, causes a reduction in portal pressure without significant effects on the systemic circulation.[122] In randomized controlled trials of losartan or another angiotensin II receptor antagonist irbesartan, however, portal pressure was not reduced significantly. In fact, renal function worsened in patients given losartan or irbesartan.[123,124] ET-receptor blockers and liver-selective NO donors are promising investigational agents for therapies that target intrahepatic vascular resistance. Simvastatin may decrease intrahepatic resistance and maintain hepatic blood flow while decreasing portal pressure.[125] Unfortunately, in a randomized controlled trial, the addition of simvastatin to standard therapy did not reduce the rate of rebleeding. In a subgroup analysis, simvastatin was associated with a survival benefit for patients with Child-Pugh class A and B cirrhosis but with an increased risk of rhabdomyolysis.[4] The use of statins to prevent hepatic decompensation is the focus of ongoing trials.[126]

Endoscopic Therapy

Endoscopic therapy is the only treatment modality that is widely accepted for the prevention of variceal bleeding, control of acute variceal bleeding, and prevention of variceal rebleeding. Endoscopic variceal therapy includes band ligation mainly with the occasional use of variceal sclerotherapy. Use of endoscopic hemostatic sprays and EUS-guided angiotherapy are investigational methods of controlling variceal bleeding.[127]

Variceal Ligation

Endoscopic variceal ligation is the preferred endoscopic modality for control of acute esophageal variceal bleeding and prevention of rebleeding; however, the utility of band ligation in the treatment of gastric varices is limited. Variceal ligation is simpler to perform than injection sclerotherapy (Video 94.1). The procedure involves suctioning of the varix into a cap fitted on the tip of an endoscope and deploying a band around the varix. The band strangulates the varix, thereby causing thrombosis. Multiband devices can be used to apply several bands without requiring withdrawal and reinsertion of the endoscope. Varices at the gastroesophageal junction are banded initially, and then more proximal varices are banded in a spiral manner at intervals of approximately 2 cm; the endoscope is then withdrawn. Varices in the mid- or proximal esophagus do not need to be banded. Endoscopic variceal ligation is associated with fewer complications than sclerotherapy and requires fewer sessions to achieve variceal obliteration. Moreover, esophageal variceal ligation during an acute bleed is not associated with a sustained elevation in HVPG, as occurs with sclerotherapy.[128]

Endoscopic variceal ligation can cause local complications, including esophageal ulcers (Fig. 94.10), strictures, and dysmotility, albeit less frequently than does sclerotherapy (Box 94.3). Banding-induced ulcers can be large and potentially serious if gastric fundal varices are banded. A PPI is usually recommended after variceal ligation, even though data to support PPI use are limited.

Sclerotherapy

Endoscopic sclerotherapy has largely been supplanted by EBL, except when poor visualization precludes effective band ligation of bleeding varices. Available evidence does not support emergency sclerotherapy as first-line treatment of variceal bleeding.[129] The technique involves injection of a sclerosant into (intravariceal) or adjacent to (paravariceal) a varix. Some paravariceal injection

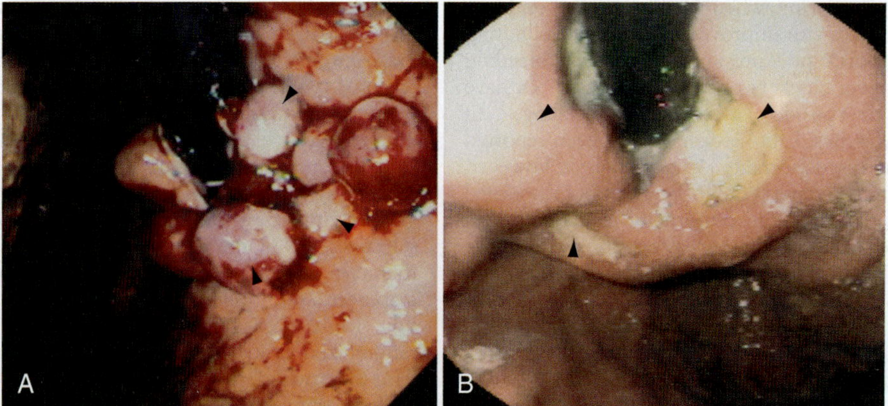

Fig. 94.10 Endoscopic views of gastric varices and esophageal variceal ligation-related ulcers. (A) The gastroesophageal junction is seen on a retroflexed view following ligation of multiple gastric varices (*arrowheads*), which resemble polyps. (B) Esophagogastroduodenoscopy in the same patient 4 weeks later demonstrates ulcers at the sites of earlier variceal ligation (*arrowheads*).

BOX 94.3 Complications of Endoscopic Variceal Therapy*

DURING PROCEDURE

Aspiration pneumonia
Retrosternal chest pain

FOLLOWING PROCEDURE

Bleeding
Esophageal dysmotility
Esophageal stricture
Esophageal ulcers
Mediastinitis
Perforation

SYSTEMIC (USUALLY WITH SCLEROTHERAPY)

Mesenteric venous thrombosis
Pulmonary embolism
Sepsis

*Sclerotherapy and band ligation.

usually takes place during attempted intravariceal therapy. The sclerosants used include sodium tetradecyl sulfate, sodium morrhuate, ethanolamine oleate, and absolute alcohol; the choice of a sclerosant is based on availability, rather than on superior efficacy of one agent over another.

Complications of endoscopic sclerotherapy may arise during or after the procedure. During injection, the patient may experience some degree of retrosternal discomfort, which may persist after the procedure. More serious complications include sclerosant-induced esophageal ulcer-related bleeding, strictures, and perforation. The risk of ulcers caused by sclerotherapy may be reduced by use of oral sucralfate or a PPI after sclerotherapy.

Hemostatic Sprays

Hemostatic powder (Hemospray, Cook Medical, Winston-Salem, North Carolina, United States) forms an adhesive mechanical barrier when in contact with blood leading to rapid control of bleeding. After approximately 24 hours, the adherent layer sloughs off into the lumen. A special delivery system is required using an introducer handle with a built-in carbon dioxide canister to propel the hemostatic powder out of the catheter. In a recent randomized trial of 86 patients with acute variceal bleeding, patients in the study arm had Hemospray application within 2 hours, whereas standard endoscopic treatment was carried out in the control group. At 24 hours, there was failure of endoscopic therapy in only 5/43 patients in the Hemospray group compared to 13/43 in the control arm (12% vs. 30%, $P = .034$). Six-week survival was significantly improved in the study group (7% vs. 30%, $P = .006$).[130] These promising results need validation.

Detachable Snares and Clips

There is only limited experience with detachable snares, generally used to treat large polyps in the colon, in the treatment of gastric varices. The "tails" on the detachable snare can interfere with visualization at endoscopy. Furthermore, traction on the varix during detachment of the snare may tear the varix. The snares are technically difficult to apply, thereby limiting their widespread use in the treatment of gastric varices. Clips have also been used to treat large varices, especially at ectopic sites, but experience is limited (see Chapter 21).

Balloon Tamponade and Stents

About 10%–15% of patients with an acute variceal bleeding are refractory to pharmacologic and endoscopic treatment. Balloon tamponade is used as a temporizing measure until TIPS can be carried out. Varices are easily compressed because they are superficial and thin-walled and the flow of blood is via submucosal vessels. The Sengstaken-Blakemore tube is a triple-lumen tube: one tube is for aspirating gastric contents, another allows the inflation of a gastric balloon to 200–400 mL in volume, and the third inflates an esophageal balloon. The Minnesota tube is a modified Sengstaken-Blakemore tube, with the modifications being a larger gastric balloon (500 mL) and provision of an additional lumen for esophageal aspiration. Inflation of the gastric balloon alone initially is preferred with both the Sengstaken-Blakemore and Minnesota tubes. If bleeding cannot be controlled after inflating the gastric balloon, it is important to reinflate and reposition the gastric balloon before deciding to inflate the esophageal balloon. The Linton-Nachlas tube has a single 600-mL gastric balloon with lumens for aspirating both the stomach and esophagus and is better for tamponading bleeding gastric varices. Balloon tamponade can control bleeding for up to 24 hours in approximately 80%–90% of patients. The risk of pulmonary aspiration is reduced by placement of an endotracheal tube.

Because of the risks and complexity associated with a placement of tamponade balloons, self-expandable metallic covered stents have been used to tamponade esophageal varices. These stents may be left in place for up to 2 weeks and then removed. Esophageal stents are more effective in the control of esophageal variceal bleeding than balloon tamponade, with fewer complications.[131] Esophageal stents may be most beneficial in patients who are not candidates for TIPS.[132] Therefore esophageal stents may be preferred in patients with advanced liver disease with variceal bleeding not controlled by medical and other endoscopic treatment.

Transjugular Intrahepatic Portosystemic Shunts

A TIPS reduces elevated portal pressure by creating a communication between the hepatic vein and an intrahepatic branch of the portal vein. A percutaneous transjugular approach is used to insert the shunt. A TIPS functions as a side-to-side portacaval shunt and has been used to treat complications of portal hypertension, mainly variceal bleeding and refractory ascites, as well as Budd-Chiari syndrome and hepatic hydrothorax (see Chapters 87, 93, and 96).[133,134] A platelet count greater than 60,000/mm^3 and an INR less than 1.5 are sometimes recommended but are not essential in an emergency. Broad-spectrum antibiotic coverage is recommended when TIPS placement is carried out in a patient with PSC and as an emergency procedure.

For TIPS placement, the hepatic vein is cannulated through a transjugular approach with the patient under sedation, and using a Rosch needle, the portal vein is cannulated. A guidewire is then passed to connect the hepatic vein and a branch of the portal vein. Following dilation of the tract, a stent is placed and dilated as required to reduce the portacaval pressure gradient (the pressure difference between the portal vein and the inferior vena cava at the confluence of the hepatic vein) to below 12 mm Hg (Fig. 94.11). Coated stents have an uncoated portion that anchors the stent to the portal vein and a polytetrafluoroethylene-coated portion that lines the tract in the liver parenchyma and the draining hepatic vein. The frequency of shunt stenosis is reduced when coated stents are used instead of uncoated stents.[135]

A TIPS can be placed successfully by an experienced operator in greater than 95% of cases with a mortality rate of less than 1% –2%.[136] The porto-caval gradient 24 hours after the procedure in the awake patient predicts the long-term gradient, but is not typically measured.[137]

Complications following the procedure are classified as procedure related, early (occurring within 30 days), or late (after 30 days) (Table 94.2). The prevention and treatment of procedure-related, early, and late post-TIPS complications are outlined in Table 94.3.

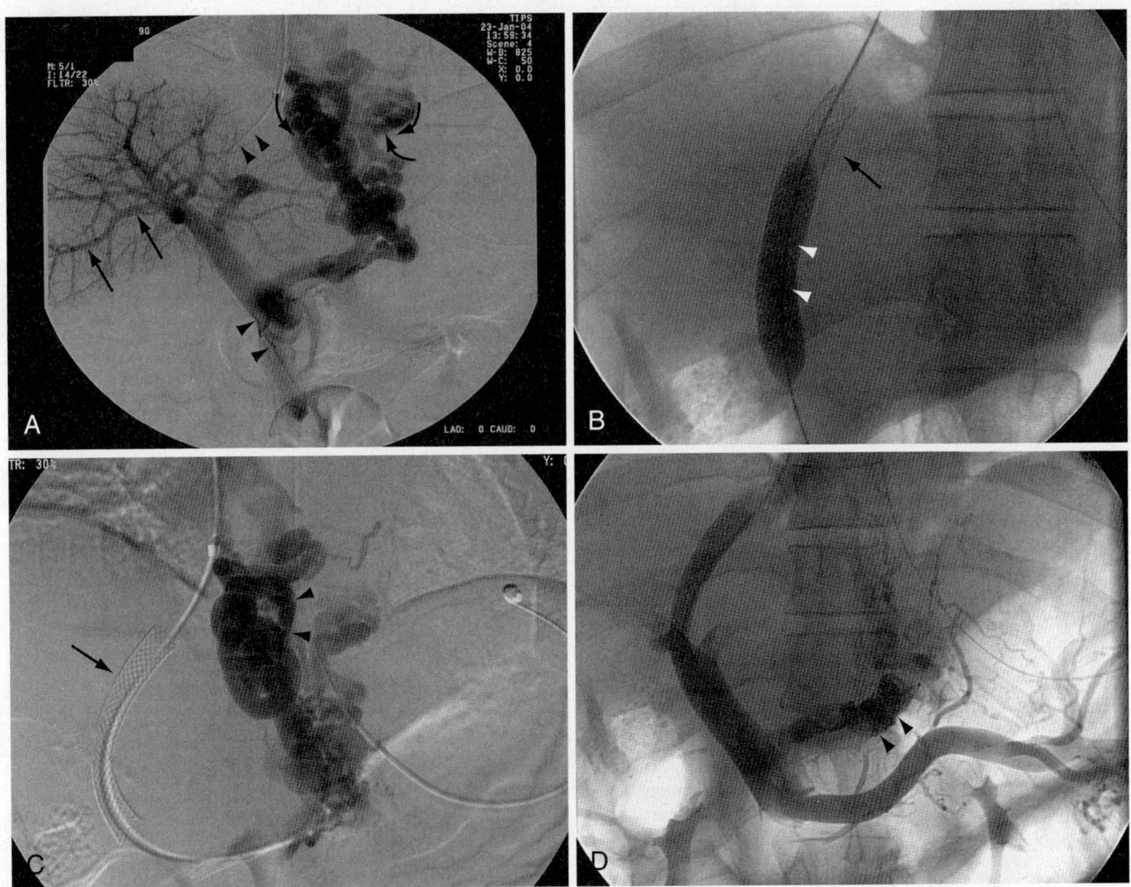

Fig. 94.11 Creation of a transjugular intrahepatic portosystemic shunt. (A) Portogram with a catheter in the portal venous system (*arrowheads*). The portal venous system is clearly outlined (*straight arrows*). Gastroesophageal collaterals are also demonstrated (*curved arrows*). (B) A stent (*arrow*) has been placed to bridge the hepatic vein and the portal vein. A balloon (*arrowheads*) is being used to dilate the parenchymal tract within the liver. (C) Following expansion of the stent (*arrow*), injection into the portal vein demonstrates persistence of the gastroesophageal varices (*arrowheads*). (D) Following embolization of the varices with steel coils (*arrowheads*), the intrahepatic portal vasculature is no longer demonstrated, indicating hepatofugal flow of portal blood through the shunt.

TABLE 94.2 Complications of Transjugular Intrahepatic Portosystemic Shunts (TIPS) Placement

Timing of Complication	Complication
Procedure-related (life-threatening)	Cardiopulmonary failure
	Carotid artery puncture injury
	Intraperitoneal hemorrhage
	Sepsis
Early postprocedure (1–30 days)	Cardiac arrhythmia
	Fever
	Hematoma at puncture site
	Hemolytic anemia
	Hepatic encephalopathy
	Pain at puncture site
	Progressive hepatic failure
	Shunt thrombosis
	Stent migration
	Reaction to contrast media
Late postprocedure (>30 days)	Hepatic encephalopathy
	Liver failure
	Portal vein thrombosis
	Progressive hepatic failure
	Pulmonary artery hypertension
	Shunt stenosis or thrombosis

Modified from Kamath PS, McKusick M. Transjugular portosystemic shunt (TIPS). *Baillieres Clin Gastroenterol*. 1997;11:327–349.

TIPS has been used to *control acute variceal bleeding* when pharmacologic and endoscopic therapies have failed, especially in patients with Child-Pugh class B or C cirrhosis, in whom bleeding is more likely to be refractory to therapy than in patients with Child-Pugh class A cirrhosis. When bleeding from varices cannot be controlled after two sessions of endoscopic therapy within a 24-hour period, TIPS placement is the usual salvage treatment with control of hemorrhage in more than 90% of patients. The mortality rate in such patients is, however, high—greater than 60% within 90 days. TIPS is also used to treat bleeding from isolated gastric fundal varices, for both control of bleeding and prevention of rebleeding.[138]

The use of early or preemptive TIPS (within 72 hours of control of variceal bleeding) in patients at high risk of rebleeding is associated with a reduced rate of treatment failure and mortality, without an increased risk of hepatic encephalopathy, compared with continued pharmacologic and endoscopic therapy.[139] In a meta-analysis of data from 1327 patients with cirrhosis meeting the aforementioned criteria, 1-year survival in the preemptive TIPS group was higher than in patients treated with a combination of drugs and endoscopy.[140] Hepatic encephalopathy is not a contraindication to preemptive TIPS.[141]

In a meta-analysis of randomized controlled trials that compared TIPS with endoscopic therapy for *prevention of rebleeding*, the rate of rebleeding was lower with TIPS, but the frequency of encephalopathy was higher and no effect on survival was observed. Covered TIPS is superior to a combination of variceal ligation and beta blockers to prevent variceal rebleeding but does not improve survival and is associated with higher rates of early hepatic encephalopathy.[142,143] Covered stents may also be associated with better patency and with increased survival in patients with refractory ascites.[144] The best outcomes following TIPS are seen in centers that perform at least 20 TIPS procedures a year.[145] Therefore TIPS is reserved for patients in experienced centers who have failed endoscopic or pharmacologic

TABLE 94.3 Prevention and Treatment of Transjugular Intrahepatic Portosystemic Shunts (TIPS)-Related Complications

Complication	Prevention	Treatment
Inadvertent injury to carotid artery during jugular vein access	Perform with US guidance to facilitate venous access	Manual compression of the carotid puncture site to prevent hematoma
Hepatic capsular laceration during portal vein access	Avoid atrophic lobes and limit needle passes to 3–4 cm of excursion	Usually requires no treatment For severe hemorrhage, transfuse with blood products until stable; obtain an abdominal CT and surgical consultation
Extrahepatic puncture of portal venous system	Delineate the bifurcation of portal vein on preprocedure CT	Leave the catheter in place for a portogram; use as a guide for intrahepatic portal vein puncture Work quickly to establish a functioning shunt, then remove the errant catheter
Intrahepatic arterial or biliary puncture	Work centrally within the liver	Usually no treatment is required; remove the catheter and continue If a fistula develops, embolize the arterial feeder with steel coils
Sepsis after shunt placement	Give prophylactic antibiotics Adhere to strict sterile technique	Broad-spectrum antibiotics
Early shunt thrombosis	Avoid sharp angles when placing the stent Ends of the stent should not abut against the intima of the vein	Shunt venogram and clot lysis using a lytic agent delivered by the pulse-spray technique Extend the shunt to ensure stent coverage of the intrahepatic tract and to ensure an adequate length in hepatic and portal veins
Uncontrollable encephalopathy after shunt placement	Use a narrow shunt in high-risk patients	Reduce the diameter of the shunt
Shunt stenosis	Use a wider or covered stent Avoid bile duct injury	Dilation or atherectomy of the shunt Place an additional stent if necessary
Postshunt liver failure	Avoid the procedure in patients with a MELD score ≥24	Consider early LT

Modified from Kamath PS, McKusick M. Transjugular portosystemic shunt (TIPS). *Baillieres Clin Gastroenterol*. 1997;11:327–349.

therapy of variceal bleeding. Adding variceal embolization to TIPS may not significantly reduce the incidence of variceal rebleeding.[146] Embolization of concurrent large spontaneous portosystemic shunts, however, reduces the risk for overt HE.[147]

Follow-Up Evaluation

The frequency of stenosis of noncovered TIPS was high, ranging from 20% to 78%, depending on the surveillance technique used and the definition of stenosis. This risk is reduced to about 15% nowadays with the use of a covered stent. Neither the optimal interval nor the most costeffective method of surveillance for TIPS stenosis has been determined. Doppler US evaluation is generally used to identify TIPS stenosis, but the negative predictive value of this approach is low and the positive predictive value is only acceptable. The best indicator that a TIPS has stenosed is recurrence of the problem that necessitated the TIPS. The only certain method of demonstrating shunt patency is by means of a TIPS venogram and measurement of the portacaval pressure gradient. An increase in the gradient to greater than 12 mm Hg warrants the dilation of the stent or placement of an additional stent to reduce the gradient.

Selection of Patients

TIPS may worsen liver function by depriving the liver of portal venous blood, thereby increasing the risk of hepatic encephalopathy, with decreased survival in some patients. Therefore the procedure should be used selectively. Age, alcohol related liver disease etiology, hepatic encephalopathy, serum bilirubin, AST and creatinine levels, INR, and emergency TIPS are independent risk factors for liver-related death.[148] In patients in whom TIPS placement has been carried out to prevent variceal rebleeding, 30-day mortality rates may be as high as 44%. Patients with a high Child-Turcotte-Pugh score (Table 94.4) also have reduced survival. The MELD score is a mathematical model originally comprising the serum creatinine level, INR, serum bilirubin level, and etiology of liver disease as variables (see http://www.mayoclinic.org/gi-rst/mayomodel6.html and Chapter 99).[149]

Subsequently, the MELD formula was modified to include only the first three parameters (creatinine, INR, and bilirubin),[150] [and later to include the serum sodium concentration, MELD-Na (see Chapter 99)] The MELD score has been widely validated for predicting survival in patients with cirrhosis, including patients who have undergone TIPS placement, and is more accurate for this purpose than the Child-Pugh classification.

The probability of mortality following TIPS placement can be calculated with use of an online formula (https://www.mayoclinic.org/medical-professionals/model-end-stage-liver-disease/probability-mortality-following-transjugular-intrahepatic-portosystemic-shunts). Patients with a MELD score of 14 or less have an excellent survival rate after TIPS placement; therefore, TIPS may be carried out routinely in such patients when indicated. Patients with a MELD score higher than 24 have reduced survival following TIPS placement, with a mortality rate approaching 30% at 3 months. This high risk should be discussed with the patient before the procedure is undertaken. In the intermediate group with a MELD score ranging from 15 to 24, TIPS placement can be carried out depending on the patient's preference, physician's judgment, and likelihood of LT in the future. This approach has been validated independently. The predictive accuracy of the MELD-Na score (see Chapter 97) has not been well studied in patients undergoing TIPS placement but is likely to be greater than that of the conventional MELD score in patients with a low MELD score and hyponatremia in whom a TIPS is placed for refractory ascites. Age, bilirubin, albumin, and creatinine are components of the Freiburg index of post-TIPS survival (FIPS) that can also identify patients at high risk of postprocedure mortality.[151] The addition of lactate to the MELD score may improve survival predictive accuracy.[152] Society guidelines recommend against TIPS when the Child-Pugh score is >13 or MELD ≥19 in patients bleeding from esophageal or gastric varices.[153]

Balloon-Occluded Retrograde Transvenous Obliteration

Balloon-occluded retrograde transvenous obliteration (BRTO) of varices may be used to occlude gastric varices when a large splenorenal shunt is seen on abdominal cross-sectional imaging. The left renal vein is approached via the femoral vein, and the splenorenal shunt is then catheterized. Other approaches to the gastric varices are via an existing TIPS or via a transjugular approach to the splenic vein. Following occlusion of the shunt with a balloon, the gastric varices are embolized with coils. Although ascites and splenomegaly can be aggravated following this procedure, these complications are easily managed. The long-term durability of the occlusion is uncertain. BRTO has been used for both the prevention and control of gastric variceal bleeding.

A recent meta-analysis suggests BRTO is associated with lower rates of rebleeding, postprocedure hepatic encephalopathy, and mortality at 1 year as compared with TIPS.[154] BRTO may also be more effective than cyanoacrylate injection in preventing gastric variceal rebleeding with similar mortality.[155]

Surgical Therapy

Surgical treatment of portal hypertension is seldom carried out nowadays and falls into three groups: nonshunt procedures, portosystemic shunt procedures, and LT. Surgical procedures (other than LT) may be used as salvage therapy when standard management with

TABLE 94.4 Child-Turcotte-Pugh Scoring System and Child-Pugh Classification

	Numerical Score		
Parameter	**1**	**2**	**3**
Ascites	None	Slight	Moderate/severe
Encephalopathy	None	Slight/moderate	Moderate/severe
Bilirubin (mg/dL)	<2	2–3	>3
Albumin (g/dL)	>3.5	2.8–3.5	<2.8
Prothrombin time (seconds increased)	1–3	4–6	>6
Total Numerical Score	**Child-Pugh Class**		
5–6	A		
7–9	B		
10–15	C		

pharmacologic and endoscopic therapy fails in patients with noncirrhotic causes of portal hypertension, especially in the presence of portal vein thrombosis. Surgical treatment was traditionally considered in patients with excellent liver function who lived at a great distance from centers that can manage variceal bleeding adequately or in whom the cross-matching of blood products was likely to be difficult. LT should be considered in all patients with cirrhosis and variceal bleeding (see Chapter 99).

Nonshunt Procedures

Nonshunt procedures include esophageal transection and gastroesophageal devascularization. With the advent of TIPS, esophageal transection is no longer recommended.

Devascularization Procedures

Devascularization procedures typically have been used to prevent recurrent variceal bleeding in patients with extensive splenic and portal vein thrombosis when a suitable vein is not available for creation of a portosystemic shunt. In the original operation described by Sugiura and Futagawa, both a thoracotomy and a laparotomy were carried out.[156] The operation is now carried out through an abdominal approach and combined with a splenectomy, but the combination procedure may also be carried out laparoscopically.[157] The procedure consists of total devascularization of the greater curve of the stomach combined with devascularization of the upper two-thirds of the lesser curve of the stomach and circumferential devascularization of the lower 7.5 cm of the esophagus. The rate of recurrent bleeding following this procedure is variable but may be as high as 40%, depending on the population being treated and duration of follow-up.

Portosystemic Shunts

With the increasing availability of TIPS, emergency surgical shunts for refractory variceal bleeding are seldom carried out. Surgical shunts are carried out almost exclusively for refractory bleeding due to noncirrhotic portal hypertension, such as congenital hepatic fibrosis and portal vein thrombosis.[66] Surgical portosystemic shunts are categorized as selective shunts such as a distal splenorenal shunt, partial shunts such as a side-to-side calibrated portacaval shunt, and total portosystemic shunts such as a side-to-side portacaval shunt or end-to-side portacaval shunt.

Selective Shunts

The most widely used selective shunt is the distal splenorenal shunt, originally described by Warren et al.[158] With this shunt, only varices at the gastroesophageal junction and spleen are decompressed, and portal hypertension is maintained in the superior mesenteric vein and portal vein; therefore, variceal bleeding is controlled, but the risk of ascites persists. The shunt procedure involves a portal-azygos disconnection and subsequent anastomosis between the splenic vein and left renal vein in an end-to-side fashion (Fig. 94.12). The entire length of the pancreas must be mobilized, and the left adrenal vein must be ligated. The distal splenorenal shunt has been associated with control of variceal bleeding in approximately 90% of patients and a lower rate of hepatic encephalopathy than that reported for total shunts.

Partial Portosystemic Shunts

A partial portosystemic shunt is carried out using a synthetic interposition graft between the portal vein and the inferior vena

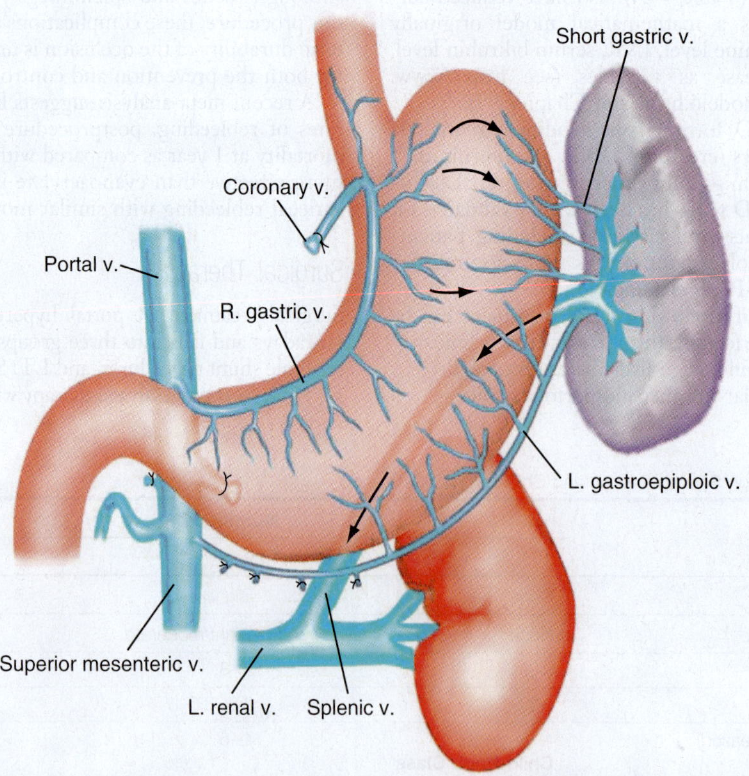

Fig. 94.12 Distal splenorenal shunt. The anatomy following completion of a distal splenorenal shunt is depicted. For this procedure, the splenic vein (v.) is disconnected from the superior mesenteric vein and is separated from the pancreas; all its collaterals are ligated. The portal system is thus disconnected from the azygos system so that all flow from the gastroesophageal junction is through the short gastric veins into the splenic vein. The splenic vein is then anastomosed to the left renal vein in an end-to-side fashion. *L.*, Left; *R.*, right.

cava. When the shunt diameter is 8 mm, portal pressure is reduced below 12 mm Hg, and antegrade flow to the liver is maintained in most patients. Rates of preventing variceal rebleeding and encephalopathy following this shunt are similar to those seen with a distal splenorenal shunt. As in patients who have had a distal splenorenal shunt, ascites may occur in approximately 20% of patients who have had a partial portosystemic shunt, because hepatic sinusoidal pressure is not reduced.[159]

Portacaval Shunts

Any side-to-side portacaval shunt that is greater than 12 mm in diameter is likely to result in a total shunting of portal blood. Therefore a shunt with a diameter less than 12 mm is created with an interposition graft, or alternatively a direct vein-to-vein anastomosis may be constructed. Variceal bleeding, as well as ascites, are well controlled because the hepatic sinusoids are decompressed. Variceal rebleeding following a total shunt was seen in less than 10% of patients, but hepatic encephalopathy occurred in 30%–40% of patients.

LT in patients who have had a portacaval shunt is associated with increased operative morbidity and intraoperative transfusion requirements. The outcome of LT is not otherwise significantly different, however, from that for patients who have not had a portacaval shunt. Nevertheless, surgical portacaval shunts should be avoided in patients who are potential candidates for LT.

Mesenterico–Left Portal Venous Bypass

The mesenterico–left portal venous bypass, or Rex shunt, is carried out in patients with extrahepatic portal vein thrombosis if the intrahepatic portion of the left portal vein is patent.[160] Portal blood flow is restored to the liver, thereby reducing the risk of hepatic encephalopathy or long-term learning disability in children. A jugular vein graft may be used to bridge the superior mesenteric vein to the intrahepatic portion of the left portal vein in the Rex recessus. (The Rex recessus is the location where the left portal vein divides to supply segments III and IV of the liver.) This surgery is the treatment of choice in children with extrahepatic portal vein thrombosis who have complications related to portal hypertension and in adults in whom portal vein thrombosis has developed late after LT.[66] The Rex bypass is recommended for secondary prophylaxis of variceal bleeding in patients with extrahepatic portal vein obstruction when surgical expertise is available.[161]

MANAGEMENT OF SPECIFIC CAUSES OF PORTAL HYPERTENSION-RELATED BLEEDING

Esophageal Varices

Natural History

Esophageal varices are present in approximately 40% of patients with cirrhosis and in as many as 60% of patients with cirrhosis and ascites. In cirrhotic patients who do not have esophageal varices at initial endoscopy, new varices will develop at a rate of approximately 5% per year. In patients with small varices at initial endoscopy, progression to large varices occurs at a rate of about 10% per year and is related predominantly to the degree of liver dysfunction. On the other hand, improvement in liver function in patients with alcohol-associated liver disease who abstain from alcohol is associated with a decreased risk, and sometimes even disappearance, of varices.

Up to 25% of adult patients with newly diagnosed varices will experience variceal bleeding within 2 years. The best clinical predictor of bleeding appears to be variceal size. The risk of bleeding in patients with varices less than 5 mm in diameter is 7% by 2 years, and the risk in patients with varices greater than 5 mm in diameter is 30% by 2 years. Even more important, however, is the HVPG, because the risk of esophageal variceal bleeding is virtually absent when the HVPG is below 12 mm Hg.[40] The risk of variceal bleeding in the pediatric age group has been studied in children with biliary atresia and is <10% at 1 year.[162]

Initial treatment in adults is associated with cessation of variceal bleeding in approximately 80%–90% of patients. Approximately half of patients with a variceal bleed stop bleeding spontaneously because hypovolemia leads to splanchnic vasoconstriction, which results in a decrease in portal pressure. Excessive transfusions may, in fact, increase the chance of rebleeding. Active bleeding at endoscopy, a lower initial hematocrit value, higher serum aminotransferase levels, higher Child-Pugh class, MELD score >20, bacterial infection, an HVPG above 20 mm Hg, and portal vein thrombosis are associated with failure to control bleeding at 5 days. Of patients who have stopped bleeding, approximately one third will rebleed within the next 6 weeks. Of all rebleeding episodes, approximately 40% will take place within 5 days of the initial bleed. Predictors of rebleeding include active bleeding at emergency endoscopy, bleeding from gastric varices, hypoalbuminemia, renal insufficiency, and an HVPG greater than 20 mm Hg. The risk of death associated with acute variceal bleeding is 5%–8% at 1 week and about 20% at 6 weeks. The highest risk of death is among patients who rebleed early, have a MELD score >18, require more than four units of packed RBC transfusions,[163] and in whom renal failure develops. Alcohol as the cause of cirrhosis, a higher serum bilirubin level, a lower serum albumin level, hepatic encephalopathy, and HCC are additional factors associated with an increased 6-week mortality rate. In the United States, the 6-week mortality rate for variceal bleeding in children is 8.8%, with Black or Hispanic children at higher risk of dying.[164]

Treatment of esophageal variceal bleeding is classified as either primary prophylaxis (i.e., prevention of variceal hemorrhage in patients who have never bled), control of acute variceal bleeding, or secondary prevention of rebleeding in patients who have survived an initial bleeding episode.

Prevention of Bleeding: Primary Prophylaxis

Pharmacologic

The utility of preprimary prophylaxis—that is, the efficacy of beta blockers to prevent the formation of varices—has not been demonstrated.[34] Use of nonselective beta blockers in patients with cirrhosis without CSPH is not currently recommended for prevention of variceal bleeding. Rather, the underlying liver disease should be treated to prevent progression to CSPH. In patients with compensated cirrhosis and CSPH, the goal of therapy is to prevent hepatic decompensation and treatment with carvedilol should be considered. In addition, patients characterized to have CSPH using LSM with or without platelet counts should be considered for treatment with NSBB without the need for endoscopy.

Patients not already on beta blockers and with high-risk varices (moderate/large varices or any size varices with red wale marks, or patient with CTP class C should undergo primary prophylaxis to prevent variceal bleeding. If the high-risk varices are small, NSBB are administered. If the high-risk varices are large, both NSBB and EVL may be used, though EVL may be associated with a higher risk of serious complications and higher mortality than NSBB. The absolute risk reduction with beta-blockers is approximately 10%, and the number needed to treat to prevent 1 variceal bleed is approximately 10 patients. The mortality rate is reduced from 28.4% in control patients to 23.9% in patients taking a beta-blocker; the absolute mortality risk reduction is 4.5%. The number of patients needed to be treated to prevent 1 death is approximately 22. In patients who do not bleed during therapy and who do not experience side effects, treatment should be continued indefinitely because withdrawal of a beta-blocker can result in an increased risk of bleeding. Patients who have an initial bleed while on a beta-blocker have an increased risk of future bleeds and death even if variceal ligation is performed.[165]

The side effects of beta-blocker treatment are probably overemphasized because only approximately 15% of patients need to discontinue the drug. A baseline heart rate and blood pressure recording will help determine whether a patient is a candidate for pharmacologic treatment with a beta-blocker. A resting systolic blood pressure less than 90 mm Hg indicates that the patient is likely to be intolerant of beta blockers. Whenever possible, the HVPG should be measured at baseline (Fig. 94.13). Carvedilol is recommended as the preferred nonselective beta-blocker for the treatment of portal hypertension in patients with cirrhosis because of its greater reduction of portal pressure compared with traditional NSBBs, better tolerance, ease of administration, reduced risk of ascites, and possible survival advantage. The initial dose of 3.125 mg twice daily or 6.25 mg daily may be increased after 2 days; the usual maintenance dose is 6.25–12.5 mg given daily as a single bedtime dose. The dose of carvedilol may be higher in patients with hypertension or cardiovascular disease which is more prevalent in patients with NASH related cirrhosis.

When carvedilol is not available, a long-acting preparation of propranolol or nadolol may be started; the usual starting dose of long-acting propranolol is 60 mg once daily and that of nadolol is 20 mg once daily. Because the risk of bleeding is greatest at night, the beta-blocker should probably be administered in the evening.[47] The dose of propranolol or nadolol can be increased gradually every 3–5 days until the target heart rate of 25% below baseline, or 55–60 bpm, or the maximum tolerated dose is reached, provided that the systolic blood pressure remains above 90 mm Hg. The daily dose of long-acting nadolol or propranolol

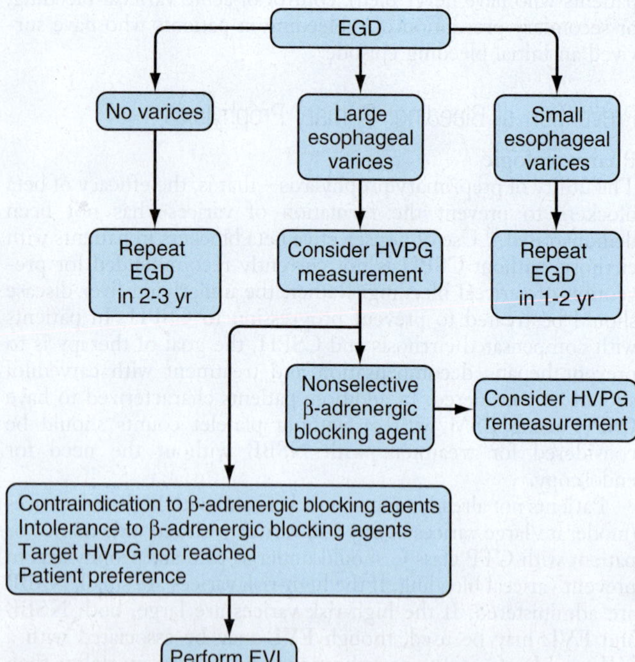

Fig. 94.13 Algorithm for the primary prophylaxis of esophageal variceal bleeding in patients with cirrhosis. The hepatic vein pressure gradient (HVPG) may be measured in patients with large varices before a nonselective β-adrenergic blocking agent (beta blocker) is started and may be remeasured 1 month after the maximum tolerated dose of the beta blocker is reached. The goal of treatment is to reduce the HVPG to <12 mm Hg or by ≥20%. *EVL*, Endoscopic variceal ligation; *HVPG*, hepatic venous pressure gradient.

required to reach the target heart rate ranges from 40 to 160 mg. Patients with a decrease in systolic blood pressure below 90 mm Hg are most likely to experience side effects. Among patients with moderate ascites, propranolol has been associated with poorer control of ascites and increased risk of both AKI and mortality.[166]

In patients on pharmacologic therapy, follow-up endoscopy is unnecessary unless GI bleeding occurs. In patients in whom the HVPG has decreased to less than 12 mm Hg, the risk of esophageal variceal bleeding is virtually eliminated. Patients in whom the HVPG decreases by at least 20% have a risk of variceal bleeding of less than 10%. Unfortunately, only 30%–40% of patients respond to a beta-blocker; those with better liver function show the best response. Moreover, patients who do not achieve a decrease in the HVPG to less than 12 mm Hg, or of greater than 20%, on a beta-blocker may not respond well to endoscopic variceal ligation either.

Endoscopic

The preferred method of endoscopic treatment is variceal band ligation. Primary prophylaxis with endoscopic variceal ligation is considered in patients with high-risk varices who have contraindications or intolerance to or are unwilling to risk side-effects, such as erectile dysfunction, associated with nonselective beta-blockers. Variceal ligation is carried out at 2–4 week intervals until varices are obliterated. Follow-up endoscopy is carried out at 6 months; if varices are obliterated, surveillance endoscopy is then carried out every 12 months to determine need for additional treatment.

Prophylactic sclerotherapy for the prevention of variceal bleeding is not currently recommended. Meta-analysis of the trials that compared endoscopic variceal ligation with a beta-blocker demonstrated a lower bleeding risk with endoscopic variceal ligation, with no difference in mortality rates.[167] A subsequent study has suggested that nonbleeding-related mortality may actually be reduced by beta blockers.[168] Side effects with beta blockers are more frequent than with variceal ligation, but complications of variceal ligation, unlike with beta blockers can be potentially life threatening.

Nineteen randomized trials compared endoscopic variceal ligation and nonselective beta blockers for the primary prevention of variceal bleeding in adults. Variceal band ligation was superior to beta blockers in reducing the risk of GI bleeding and variceal bleeding (RR, 0.69 and 0.67, respectively). This benefit was lost, however, when only high-quality trials were included in the analysis. Bleeding-related mortality is not different, suggesting that beta blockers may have benefits other than a reduction in bleeding risk.

The risks and benefits of the options should be discussed with the patient and treatment individualized. Beta blockers are cheaper and more convenient to use and may potentially reduce the risk of bleeding from gastric varices and PHG. Band ligation is the only option for patients with high-risk varices who have contraindications to beta blockers or who have not responded to or are intolerant of beta blockers. Combined use of a nonselective beta-blocker and endoscopic variceal ligation, or use of TIPS is not recommended for primary prophylaxis for variceal hemorrhage.

Control of Acute Bleeding

Acute esophageal variceal bleeding constitutes a life-threatening emergency and requires management by a well-trained team of hepatologists, endoscopists, intensive care personnel, and radiologists. Treatment is aimed at resuscitating the patient, controlling the bleeding, and preventing complications (see Chapter 21). Volume resuscitation, vasoactive and endoscopic therapy, and antibiotics are the mainstay of management.

Two large-bore IV access lines should be inserted immediately. RBCs should be transfused with the goal of maintaining the hematocrit value around 25%. A restrictive strategy of transfusing RBCs only when the Hgb level drops below 7 g/dL is associated with improved survival in patients with Child-Pugh class A and B cirrhosis, as compared with a strategy of transfusing when the Hgb level drops below 9 g/dL.[169] Isotonic crystalloids may be infused intravenously until packed RBCs are available for transfusion. Excessive RBC transfusions may be associated with risks of massive transfusion, including an increased risk of hypocoagulability; on the other hand, excessive use of saline is associated with ascites and the risk of abdominal compartment control.[170] Fresh frozen plasma and platelet transfusions should not be administered based on specific INR or platelet count targets in acute variceal hemorrhage. FFP administration may be associated with volume overload and increased bleeding risk. The addition of treatment with recombinant factor VIIa to standard therapy has not been shown to improve control of bleeding.[171] A TEG-guided strategy has been suggested to guide blood product transfusions.[172]

In patients with active bleeding, the airway needs to be protected, and endotracheal intubation is advised. Antibiotics should be administered to all patients to prevent bacteremia and spontaneous bacterial peritonitis (see Chapter 95). Norfloxacin, 400 mg orally twice daily for 7 days, has been the preferred choice. When norfloxacin is not available (as in the United States), ciprofloxacin 500 mg orally twice daily for 7 days may be administered.[173] When oral intake is not possible, IV ceftriaxone, 1 g every 24 hours for 7 days; ciprofloxacin, 400 mg every 12 hours; or levofloxacin, 500 mg every 24 hours is recommended. Failure to control infection is associated with a significantly increased risk of mortality and rebleeding.[174] Bacterial infections, most frequently respiratory, may develop in 20% of patients despite antibiotic prophylaxis. Respiratory infections are more common with the use of nasogastric tube, orotracheal intubation and esophageal balloon tamponade.[175]

A combination of endoscopic therapy and vasoactive pharmacologic therapy is superior to pharmacologic treatment alone in controlling variceal bleeding.[176] Pharmacologic agents should be started as early as possible; in some centers, they are started while the patient is being transferred by ambulance to the hospital. Somatostatin, octreotide, vapreotide, or terlipressin are the options for pharmacologic therapy. Vasoactive agents are associated with improved hemostasis and a shorter length of hospitalization. None of the agents studied seems to have a clear benefit over the others, though terlipressin is the first choice in many countries because it has been associated with improved survival. In the United States, octreotide had been the agent used most when terlipressin was not available. Pharmacologic treatment should be continued for up to 5 days to prevent early rebleeding; however, a 24-hour course and a 72-hour course of terlipressin are possibly equally effective when used in conjunction with variceal ligation.[177]

Endoscopic therapy is carried out as soon as the patient is hemodynamically stabilized, and usually within 12 hours of admission. At EGD, esophageal varices as the source of bleeding is diagnosed if active bleeding from the varices is seen; signs of recent hemorrhage, such as a white fibrin plug or a red blood clot over a varix, are present; varices with risk signs for bleeding, such as a cherry-red spot, hematocystic spot, or red wale sign, are seen; or esophageal varices are seen in the absence of any other lesion that could give rise to GI bleeding. Endoscopic treatment, preferably endoscopic variceal ligation, is recommended at the time of initial endoscopy.

At EGD, the actively bleeding varix is ligated (Fig. 94.14). Ligation initially should be at or immediately below the site of

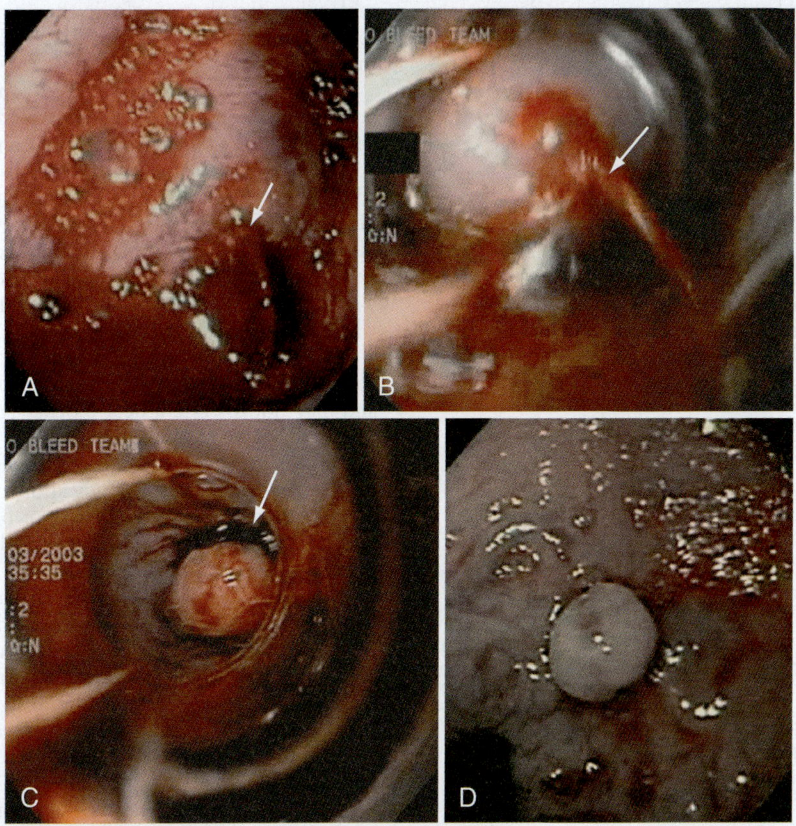

Fig. 94.14 Band ligation for control of esophageal variceal bleeding. (A) On esophagogastroduodenoscopy, an actively bleeding varix can be seen in the distal esophagus (*arrow*). (B) With the variceal banding device in position, the varix is suctioned into the device at the site of active bleeding (*arrow*). (C) After the band is in place (*arrow*) and the varix has been ligated, the bleeding has stopped. (D) Visualization of the varix with the band in place, with complete control of bleeding. (Images courtesy Dr. Louis M. Wong Kee Song, Rochester, MN.)

bleeding on the varix. Other large varices also should be banded during the same session. If active bleeding is not seen, ligation should be carried out beginning with varices at the gastroesophageal junction and proceeding proximally at intervals of 2 cm in a spiral fashion. If bleeding obscures the varices, then multiple bands are placed at the gastroesophageal junction circumferentially until bleeding can be controlled, but the long-term risks of esophageal stricture are increased in such cases. Bleeding can be controlled in up to 85%–90% of patients with a combination of pharmacologic and endoscopic treatment.

Bleeding cannot be controlled in approximately 10%–15% of patients, as defined by any of the following three criteria: (1) transfusion of 4 U of RBCs or more to maintain the hematocrit value above 25%, (2) inability to increase the systolic blood pressure by 20 mm Hg or to greater than 70 mm Hg, or (3) persistence of a heart rate greater than 100 bpm. Rebleeding is defined as recurrence of bleeding after initial control for 24 hours during which the vital signs and Hgb level are stable. When two sessions of endoscopic treatment within a 24-hour period have failed to control variceal bleeding, salvage therapies, such as TIPS, should be carried out (salvage TIPS) (Fig. 94.15), although the mortality rate in this group of patients is high. TIPS is also considered when patients rebleed despite vasoactive therapy and EVL ("rescue" TIPS). Esophageal stents may be used to stabilize the patient until TIPS can be carried out; balloon tamponade may be carried out when esophageal stents are not available.

In the group of patients at high risk of treatment failure (Child-Pugh class C, Child-Pugh class B with active bleeding, or MELD score >18 and requirement for transfusion of >4 U of RBCs), TIPS carried out within 72 hours of the control of bleeding (preemptive TIPS) is associated with reduced rates of mortality and treatment failure.[139] Early TIPS may not be feasible in many centers however, and larger studies are needed to confirm the findings.[178] TIPS placed between 72 hours and 28 days may be associated with similar short- and long-term survival benefits as TIPS placed within 72 hours.[179] TIPS is also considered if patients have refractory ascites in addition. Emergency surgical

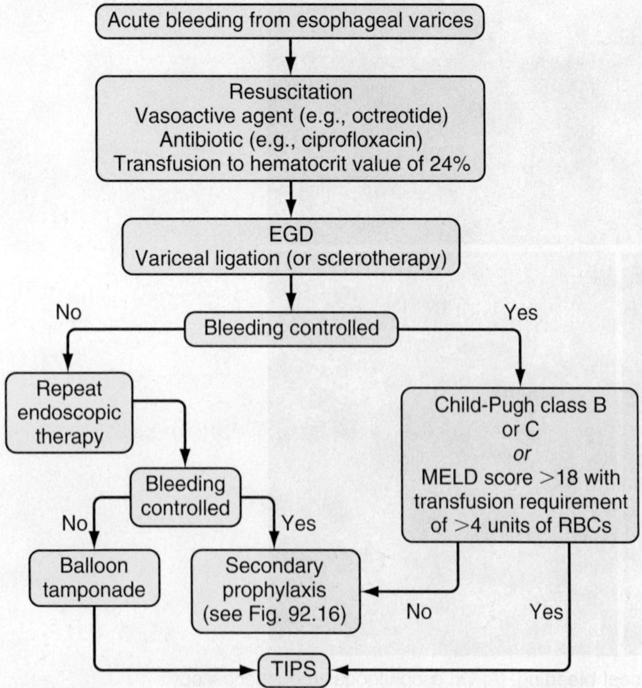

Fig. 94.15 Algorithm for the management of bleeding esophageal varices. *RBC*, Red blood cell.

portosystemic shunts, although extremely effective in controlling variceal bleeding, have been abandoned because of high mortality rates.

When bleeding has been controlled, in patients not undergoing TIPS, NSBB should be initiated when vasoactive therapy is discontinued. Enteral feeding should be started when the bleeding has been controlled and the patient hemodynamically stable for 24 hours. A feeding tube can be placed even if the patient has undergone variceal ligation, but only by experienced personnel. Proton pump inhibitors are often started before the endoscopy but should be discontinued if variceal hemorrhage has been confirmed so as to avoid the increased risk of infections associated with PPI therapy.

The overall adjusted mortality from variceal bleeding has decreased over the past few decades to currently <15%. Racial and ethnic mortality comparison show that, compared with White patients, Black patients have greater odds of mortality [adjusted odds ratio (aOR), 1.53; 95% CI, 1.06–2.21; $P = .02$), and Hispanic patients have lower mortality (aOR, 0.73; 95% CI, 0.54–0.98; $P = .04$). Fewer early (within 24 hours) endoscopic procedures, and more advanced disease on hospital admission may explain the higher mortality in Black patients.[180]

Prevention of Rebleeding: Secondary Prophylaxis

All patients who have had a variceal bleed should receive prophylactic therapy (secondary prophylaxis) to reduce the risk of rebleeding, which otherwise occurs in up to 80% of untreated patients at 2 years. A MELD score at time of bleeding less than 11 is associated with a 5% risk of 6-week mortality, whereas a MELD score >20 is associated with 20% mortality risk.[181,182] Patients with cirrhosis and variceal bleeding should therefore be evaluated for LT (see Chapter 99). Options for preventing variceal rebleeding are pharmacologic therapy, endoscopic therapy, portosystemic shunt (almost invariably TIPS), or combinations of these therapies.

Combined therapy with endoscopic variceal ligation and a nonselective beta-blocker is the preferred initial option, and carvedilol or long-acting propranolol or nadolol may be used. Carvedilol use is associated with survival benefit and fewer hospital admissions.[183] Ideally, the hemodynamic response to a beta-blocker should be monitored, with the goal of reducing the HVPG by greater than 20% or to less than 12 mm Hg. The beneficial effect of long-term pharmacologic therapy in patients with alcohol-associated cirrhosis is largely restricted to patients who remain abstinent.[184]

Endoscopic variceal ligation alone may be performed to prevent variceal rebleeding in patients who have poor liver function and may not tolerate a beta-blocker (Fig. 94.16). In practice, the first endoscopic session is carried out 7–14 days after the initial variceal ligation to control bleeding. One-week ligation intervals may lead to more rapid eradication of varices than 2-week intervals but without a reduced risk of bleeding.[185] If the HVPG is monitored, a reduction in HVPG to less than 12 mm Hg or by greater than 20% should obviate the need for variceal ligation. For patients who bleed during pharmacologic treatment, variceal ligation should be carried out. Conversely, for patients who have undergone variceal ligation alone and experience recurrent bleeding, a beta-blocker should be started, although in patients with a noncirrhotic cause of portal hypertension the addition of propranolol and isosorbide mononitrate to endoscopic variceal ligation may not reduce the risk of bleeding compared with variceal ligation alone.[186]

Compared with a beta-blocker alone, variceal ligation plus a beta-blocker reduces the risk of rebleeding in Child-Pugh class A but not Child-Pugh class B or C patients. Mortality is not reduced in either group. However, when compared with variceal ligation alone, the combination of a beta-blocker and variceal ligation

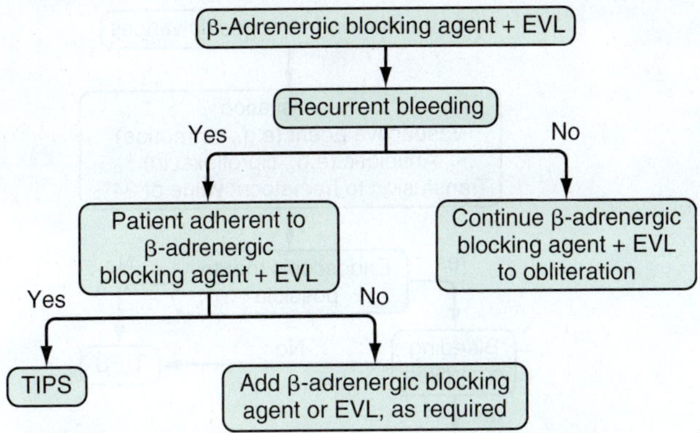

Fig. 94.16 Algorithm for the prevention of recurrent esophageal variceal bleeding (secondary prophylaxis). *EVL*, Endoscopic variceal ligation.

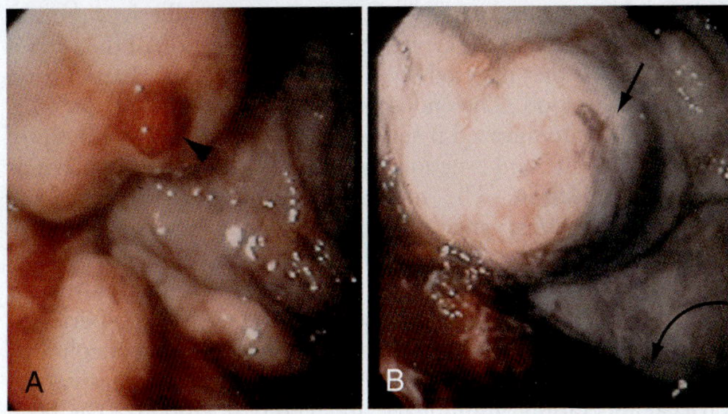

Fig. 94.17 Gastric variceal bleeding. (A) Active bleeding from a gastric varix (*arrowhead*) can be seen. (B) Bleeding from the varix (*straight arrow*) is controlled following injection of sodium tetradecyl sulfate. Pooling of blood in the stomach is indicated by the *curved arrow*.

reduces the risk of rebleeding in all patients with cirrhosis and reduces mortality in those with Child-Pugh class B and C cirrhosis.[187] These results have not been confirmed in the United States. Patients who have variceal rebleeding despite optimal pharmacologic and endoscopic treatment require a portosystemic shunt. Even in patients with Child-Pugh class A cirrhosis, a TIPS may be as effective as a distal splenorenal shunt, and therefore, remains the therapy of choice.

Gastric Varices

The most widely used classification of gastric varices is the Sarin classification.[188] According to this classification, type 1 gastroesophageal varices (GOV1) extend 2–5 cm below the gastroesophageal junction and are in continuity with esophageal varices; type 2 gastroesophageal varices (GOV2) are in the cardia and fundus of the stomach and in continuity with esophageal varices; varices that occur in the fundus of the stomach in the absence of esophageal varices are called isolated gastric varices type 1 (IGV1), whereas varices that occur in the gastric body, antrum, or pylorus are called isolated gastric varices type 2 (IGV2).

Approximately 25% of patients with portal hypertension have gastric varices, most commonly GOV1, which comprise approximately 70% of all gastric varices. Intrahepatic causes of portal hypertension may be associated with both GOV1 and GOV2. Splenic vein thrombosis usually results in IGV1, but the most common cause of fundal gastric varices may be cirrhosis.[189]

Natural History

Gastric varices typically occur in association with advanced portal hypertension. Bleeding is thought to be more common in patients with GOV2 and IGV1 than in those with other types of gastric varices; that is, gastric variceal bleeding is more common from fundal varices than from varices at the gastroesophageal junction. Whereas intraesophageal pressure is negative, intra-abdominal pressure is positive, and the transmural pressure gradient across gastric varices is lower than that across esophageal varices. Gastric varices are supported by gastric mucosa, whereas esophageal varices tend to be unsupported in the lower third of the esophagus. Gastric varices, however, tend to be larger in diameter than esophageal varices. Gastric varices are likely to bleed only when they are large, as demonstrated in a study in which larger gastric varices (>20 mm in diameter) in patients with a MELD score above 17 were more likely than smaller ones to bleed.[190] In contrast to esophageal varices, bleeding from gastric varices has been described with an HVPG less than 12 mm Hg.[191] Gastric varices in continuity with esophageal varices may regress following treatment of the esophageal varices. When gastric varices persist despite obliteration of esophageal varices, the prognosis is poorer, which is probably a reflection of the severity of liver disease.

Prevention of Bleeding

Unfortunately, there is a paucity of studies that have evaluated pharmacologic or endoscopic treatment for primary prophylaxis of gastric variceal hemorrhage, and recommendations are still based primarily on the guidelines for managing esophageal varices. Because these gastric varices usually are associated with esophageal varices, pharmacologic treatment with a nonselective beta-blocker may be initiated to prevent variceal hemorrhage. Cyanoacrylate glue injection may be more effective than beta-blocker therapy in preventing gastric variceal bleeding.[190] Thus patients with GOV2 or IGV1 varices ≥10 mm, especially when associated with red wale signs, and CTP class B/C, are sometimes considered for primary prophylaxis with endoscopic cyanoacrylate glue injection.

TIPS is also not recommended for the primary prevention of gastric variceal bleeding. BRTO has been used in uncontrolled studies to prevent bleeding from gastric varices, with some success.

Control of Acute Bleeding

Initial management of bleeding gastric or ectopic varices should be identical to the management of bleeding esophageal varices, including vasoactive therapy, antibiotics, conservative transfusion strategy, and endoscopic evaluation within 12 hours.

EGD is carried out after patients have been volume resuscitated and stabilized and often following endotracheal intubation to protect the airway. The endoscopic diagnosis of gastric variceal bleeding may be difficult because of pooling of blood in the fundus. A diagnosis of gastric variceal hemorrhage is made if bleeding is noted from a gastric varix (Fig. 94.17); blood emanates from the gastroesophageal junction or the gastric fundus; blood is found in the stomach and gastric varices with a "white nipple sign" (indicating a fibrin-platelet plug) are seen in the absence of other causes of bleeding; or gastric varices are noted in the absence of other lesions in the esophagus and stomach.

Because controlled studies evaluating pharmacologic therapy for gastric variceal bleeding are lacking, the agents used are based on extension of the data relating to esophageal varices. Medical management with vasoactive agents should be started as early as possible, preferably at least 30 minutes before endoscopic therapy is carried out. The preferred endoscopic therapy for fundal gastric variceal bleeding is injection of polymers of cyanoacrylate, usually

N-butyl-2-cyanoacrylate,[192,193] but these tissue adhesives are not currently available in the United States. Obliteration of the varices occurs when the injected cyanoacrylate adhesive hardens on contact with blood. The endoscope may be damaged by the glue, but the risk is minimized if silicone gel is used to cover the tip of the instrument and suction is avoided for 15–20 seconds following injection. The mucosa overlying the varix injected eventually sloughs, and the hardened polymer is extruded. Fortunately, the resulting ulcers occur late, and the risk of bleeding is lower than that associated with sclerotherapy-related ulcers. Cyanoacrylate injection has been found to be superior to both variceal band ligation and sclerotherapy using alcohol.[193] Complications of cyanoacrylate injection include bacteremia and variceal ulceration. Pulmonary and cerebral emboli have been reported on occasion, usually in patients with spontaneous large portosystemic or intrapulmonary shunts. Embolization probably occurs via spontaneous splenorenal shunts. Therefore a combined approach using interventional radiology to occlude the shunt and endoscopic variceal glue injection is probably a safer strategy.[194]

For injection of GOV2 or IGV1, a retroflexed endoscopic approach is recommended. Sclerosants, such as sodium tetradecyl sulfate, ethanolamine oleate, and sodium morrhuate, are not particularly effective for control of gastric variceal bleeding. When sclerotherapy is carried out for gastric varices, the volume of sclerosant required is larger than that used for esophageal varices, and fever and retrosternal pain are more common. It is much easier to obliterate GOV1 than GOV2 or IGV1. IGV1 are the most difficult gastric varices to obliterate and, when present, should prompt early consideration of definitive treatment, such as TIPS, if cyanoacrylate is not available.

Although some investigators recommend ligation of gastric varices up to 20 mm in diameter,[195] this recommendation is not supported by our experience. Band ligation of varices greater than 10 mm in diameter is usually unsafe. Ligation is safest if the varices are in the cardia of the stomach. Because gastric fundal varices are covered by mucosa, drawing the entire varix into the ligation device is often not possible. Application of bands results in creation of a large ulcer on the varix, sometimes with disastrous results (see Fig. 94.10).

If endoscopic and pharmacologic therapies fail to control gastric variceal bleeding, then a Linton-Nachlas tube may be passed as a temporizing measure. Most patients in whom endoscopic and pharmacologic treatment fails to control gastric variceal bleeding will require a TIPS, which can control bleeding in greater than 90% of patients—a rate of efficacy equivalent to that for TIPS in controlling esophageal variceal bleeding (Fig. 94.18).[138]

Prevention of Rebleeding

Cyanoacrylate glue injection may be superior to nonselective beta blockers in preventing gastric variceal rebleeding.[196] In a small study, the 2-octyl-cyanoacrylate polymer (Dermabond) was used to prevent gastric variceal rebleeding, with excellent results.[197] Following an episode of gastric variceal bleeding, if glue therapy has not been carried out, TIPS or BRTO should be considered. If cyanoacrylate glue injection has been carried out, nonselective beta blockers may be administered to prevent rebleeding. Follow-up endoscopy is carried out after a month, and if required, additional glue therapy applied. An average of 1 or 2 additional sessions is usually required for obturation of gastric varices. Surveillance endoscopy is then carried out every year.

In a meta-analysis of nine RCTs with 647 patients with gastric variceal bleeding, BRTO was associated with a lower risk of rebleeding when compared with beta blockers and endoscopic therapy, including cyanoacrylate glue therapy. Beta blockers were associated with a higher risk of rebleeding as well as mortality and

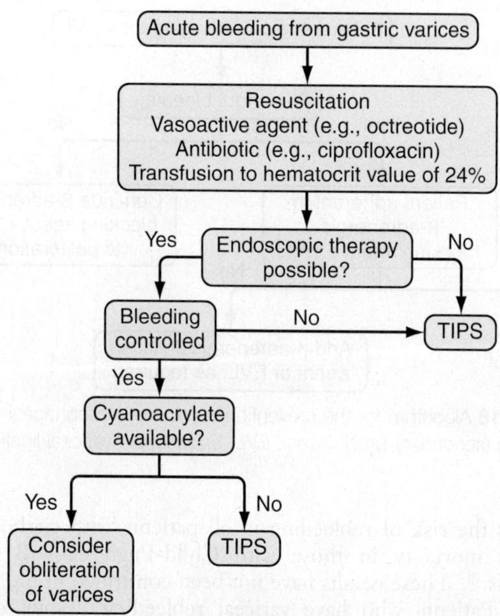

Fig. 94.18 Algorithm for the management of bleeding gastric varices in patients with portal hypertension.

should not be used as the sole therapy to prevent rebleeding in patients who have not undergone glue injection.[198]

Patients who have bled from gastric varices should undergo abdominal cross-sectional imaging to determine the presence or absence of portal and splenic vein thrombosis.

Patients with bleeding gastric varices due to isolated splenic vein thrombosis should be recommended splenectomy.

TIPS is effective in preventing gastric variceal rebleeding. Because TIPS for this indication does not always result in a decrease in the size of gastric varices, the target HVPG is uncertain in these patients. Patients with an HVPG less than 12 mm Hg after TIPS are protected from esophageal variceal bleeding but have been known to bleed from gastric varices. Therefore if the HVPG is reduced to a level below 12 mm Hg but gastric fundal varices are still prominent when contrast is injected into the portal vein (especially if the patient has bled from gastric fundal varices), the gastric varices may be embolized.

Limited data are available regarding use of surgical portosystemic shunts for the treatment of gastric varices in patients with cirrhosis. Two studies performed in patients with good liver function, most of whom had extrahepatic portal vein thrombosis, demonstrated excellent results, with a low long-term risk of bleeding and encephalopathy.[199,200]

Ectopic Varices

Varices that occur at a site other than the esophagus and stomach are termed *ectopic varices* and account for less than 5% of all varix-related bleeding episodes. Ectopic varices most commonly manifest with melena or hematemesis. They also may manifest with hemobilia, hematuria, hemoperitoneum, or retroperitoneal bleeding. The duodenum is a common site of ectopic varices, and varices typically are associated with portal vein obstruction, but in the West, the usual cause of duodenal varices is cirrhosis. The common occurrence of duodenal varices in patients with portal vein obstruction probably relates to the formation of collateral vessels around the thrombosed portal vein that connect pancreaticoduodenal veins to retroduodenal veins, which drain into the inferior vena cava. In some of those patients with extrahepatic portal vein obstruction, varices form around the gallbladder and bile duct, giving rise to portal hypertensive cholangiopathy and biliary strictures (see Fig. 94.8).

The other common site of ectopic varices is peristomal in patients with IBD and PSC who have undergone a proctocolectomy with creation of an ileostomy. Varices develop at the level of the mucocutaneous border of the stoma and are termed *stomal varices*. They are recognized by a bluish halo surrounding the stoma and by a dusky appearance and friable consistency of the stomal tissue; no obvious variceal lesions are seen. Bleeding from stomal varices is readily apparent on presentation.

Anorectal varices are reported in 10%–40% of cirrhotic patients who undergo colonoscopy and must be distinguished from hemorrhoids (Fig. 94.19). Rectal varices are dilated superior and middle hemorrhoidal veins, whereas hemorrhoids are dilated vascular channels above the dentate line.

Ectopic variceal bleeding should be considered in all patients with portal hypertension and overt GI bleeding without an obvious bleeding source on endoscopy, or when there is a drop in the Hgb level associated with abdominal pain and increasing abdominal girth. CT of the abdomen demonstrates layering of free fluid in the peritoneal cavity in patients who have intra-abdominal hemorrhage, typical of fresh blood mixed with ascitic fluid. The diagnosis of intra-abdominal hemorrhage secondary to ectopic variceal bleeding is confirmed by a paracentesis that yields bloody ascitic fluid with clots.

Treatment

At present, no recommendations support primary prophylaxis to prevent bleeding from ectopic varices. In patients suspected of having ectopic variceal bleeding, vasoactive drugs may be administered initially to control the bleeding. If the bleeding ectopic varix is visualized at endoscopy, as typically is the case with duodenal or colonic varices, then endoscopic therapy can be carried out.[200] Endoscopic glue injection or band ligation is the preferred approach for bleeding duodenal varices. Colonic varices tend to be larger in diameter and may require application of hemostatic clips. Patients with bleeding stomal varices can be trained to compress the site locally if bleeding is obvious. Percutaneous sclerotherapy of the stomal varices may be carried out under US guidance. Because bleeding from stomal varices is visible and detected early, the mortality rate for bleeding stomal varices is low.[201]

To prevent rebleeding from ectopic varices, pharmacologic treatment with a beta-blocker is usually tried, although no studies are available to support this approach. If the portal vein is patent, then transhepatic embolization of stomal varices can be carried out with control of bleeding in most patients (Fig. 94.20). The rate of rebleeding is high, however, because portal hypertension persists. In patients in whom embolization fails to prevent rebleeding, TIPS placement may be considered.[202]

A surgical portosystemic shunt is recommended in patients with portal hypertension from extrahepatic portal vein thrombosis when a vein suitable for a shunt is available and TIPS is not feasible. In the rare situations that a surgical shunt is considered for treatment of stomal varices, only a nonselective portosystemic shunt, such as a portacaval shunt, mesocaval shunt, or proximal splenorenal shunt, should be carried out.

Patients with ectopic varices who present with intraperitoneal hemorrhage have a poor outcome because the diagnosis usually is not considered and is often made at laparotomy. Acute bleeding may be controlled by transhepatic obliteration or surgical ligation of the varices. In patients who are critically ill, a TIPS should be placed, followed by embolization of the bleeding varix.

Portal Hypertensive Gastropathy and Gastric Vascular Ectasia

Mucosal changes in the stomach in patients with portal hypertension include PHG and gastric vascular ectasia (GVE). In all likelihood, these lesions are distinct, as demonstrated by histologic

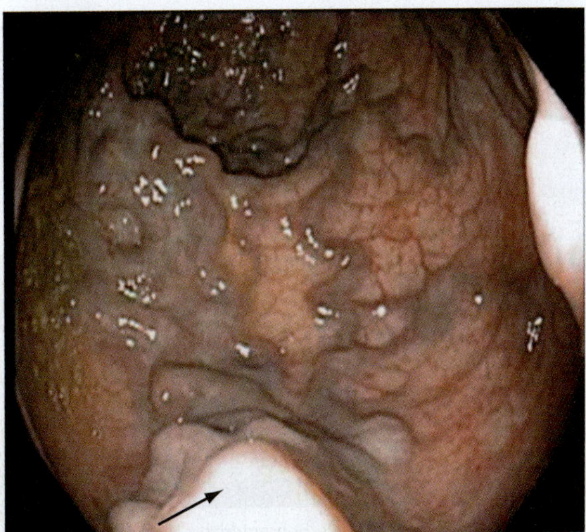

Fig. 94.19 Endoscopic image of a colonic varix (*arrow*).

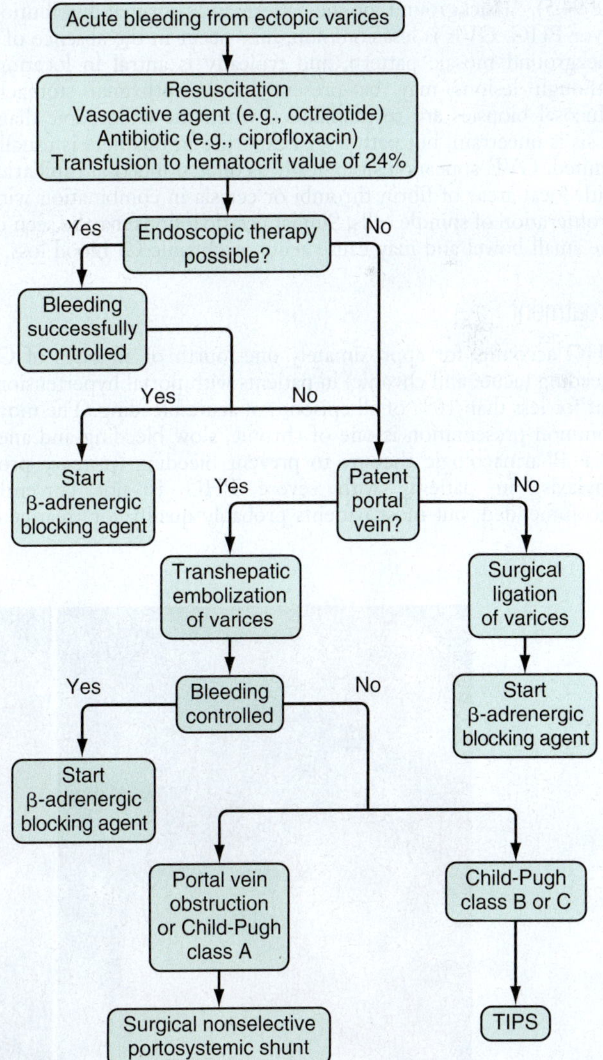

Fig. 94.20 Algorithm for the management of bleeding from ectopic varices in patients with portal hypertension.

features and differences in the response to a TIPS. An appearance in the colon analogous to PHG is termed *portal hypertensive colopathy*[203] (see Chapter 36).

The diagnosis of PHG is based on the presence of a characteristic mosaic-like pattern of the gastric mucosa on endoscopic examination. This pattern is characterized by small polygonal areas with a depressed border. Superimposed on this mosaic-like pattern may be red point lesions that are usually greater than 2 mm in diameter. PHG is considered mild when only a mosaic-like pattern is present and severe when superimposed discrete red spots are also seen (Fig. 94.21).[204] The cause and pathogenesis of PHG are poorly understood. Development of PHG correlates with the duration of cirrhosis but not necessarily the degree of liver dysfunction. It should be emphasized that the diagnosis of PHG should be made on endoscopy and not histology alone since there is limited correlation between histology and endoscopic appearance.[205]

In GVE, aggregates of ectatic vessels can be seen on endoscopic examination as red spots without a mosaic background. When the aggregates are confined to the antrum of the stomach, the term *gastric antral vascular ectasia* (GAVE) is used (see Chapters 21 and 36). If aggregates in the antrum are linear, the term *watermelon stomach* is used to describe the lesion (Fig. 94.22). When the red spots are distributed diffusely, in both the distal and the proximal stomach, the term *diffuse* GVE is preferred.[206]

Distinguishing PHG from GVE is sometimes difficult (Table 94.5). A background mosaic pattern and proximal distribution favor PHG. GVE is less common, may occur in the absence of a background mosaic pattern, and typically is antral in location, although lesions may be present in the proximal stomach. Mucosal biopsies are recommended when the endoscopic diagnosis is uncertain, but pathologist expertise in this field is usually limited. GVE appears histologically as dilated mucosal capillaries with focal areas of fibrin thrombi or ectasia in combination with proliferation of spindle cells. Similar ectatic lesions may be seen in the small bowel and may cause acute or chronic GI blood loss.

Treatment

PHG accounts for approximately one-fourth of all cases of GI bleeding (acute and chronic) in patients with portal hypertension, but for less than 10% of all episodes of acute bleeding. The more common presentation is one of chronic, slow bleeding and anemia. Pharmacologic therapy to prevent bleeding (primary prophylaxis) in patients with severe PHG is not currently recommended, but most patients probably qualify for treatment with nonselective beta blockers since they have CSPH. Small studies have suggested that octreotide may be useful for controlling acute bleeding. Beta blockers are recommended for

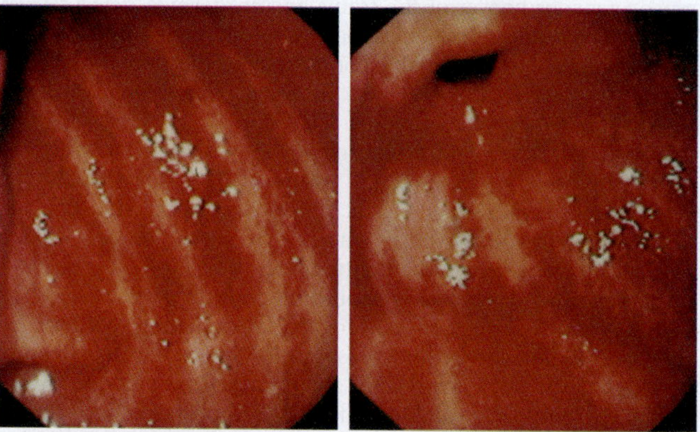

Fig. 94.22 Endoscopic images of severe gastric antral vascular ectasia (watermelon stomach).

TABLE 94.5 Comparison of Portal Hypertensive Gastropathy (PHG) and Gastric Antral Vascular Ectasia (GAVE)

Feature	PHG	GAVE
Distribution	Proximal stomach	Distal stomach
Mosaic pattern	Present	Absent
Red color signs	Present	Present
Findings on gastric mucosal biopsy:		
Thrombi	–	+++
Spindle cell proliferation	+	++
Fibrohyalinosis	–	+++
Treatment	β-Adrenergic blocking agent ?APC TIPS	Endoscopic therapy ?Antrectomy ?LT

APC, Argon plasma coagulation; *TIPS*, transjugular intrahepatic portosystemic shunts.

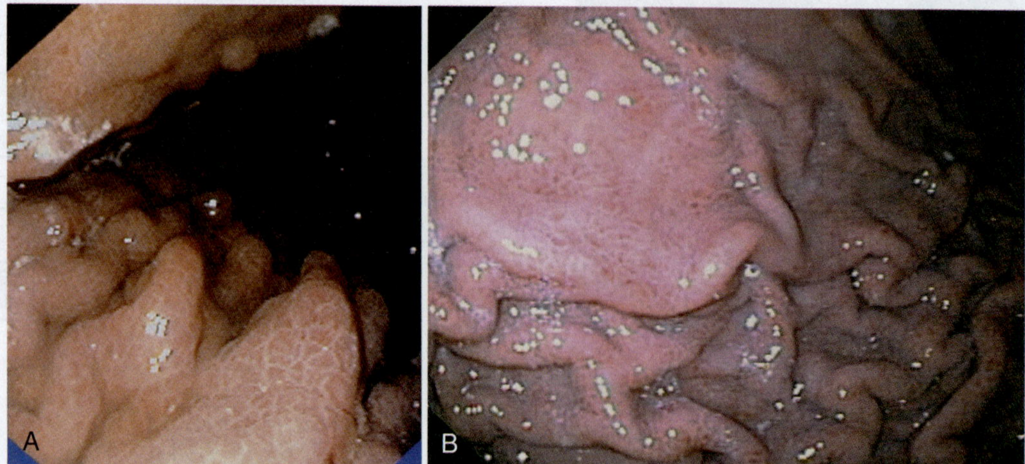

Fig. 94.21 Endoscopic views of portal hypertensive gastropathy (PHG). (A) Mild PHG is characterized by a mosaic appearance without red color signs. (B) Severe PHG is characterized by superimposed red spots.

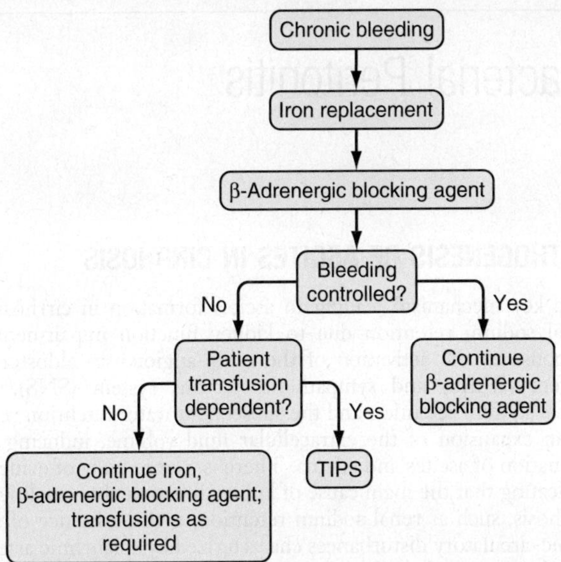

Fig. 94.23 Algorithm for the management of chronic bleeding from portal hypertensive gastropathy.

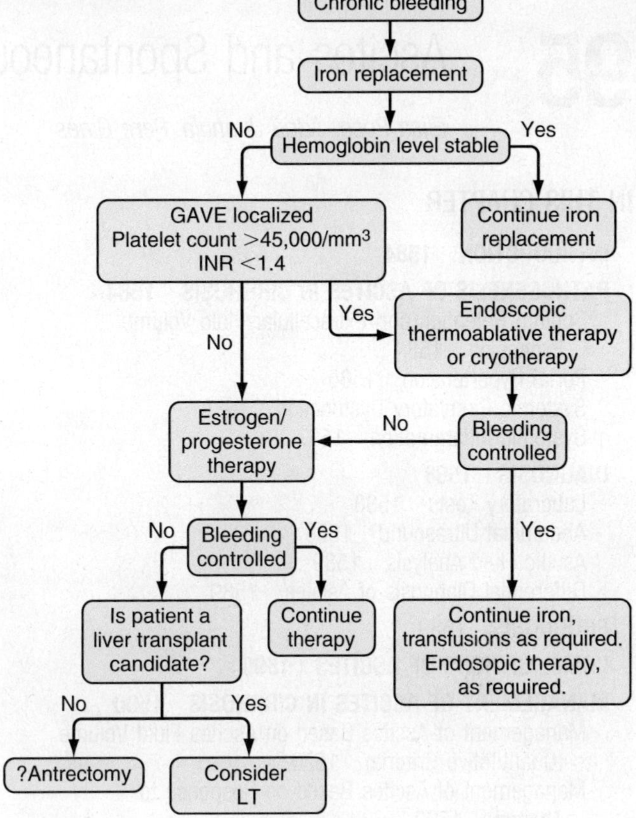

Fig. 94.24 Algorithm for the management of chronic bleeding from gastric antral vascular ectasia (GAVE).

preventing chronic blood loss in patients who have bled from severe PHG. When patients are transfusion dependent despite beta blockade and iron supplementation, a TIPS may be inserted (Fig. 94.23). A TIPS decreases transfusion requirements and results in reversal of the mucosal lesions on endoscopic examination.[206]

Management of GVE is more problematic. Initial treatment involves repletion of iron and RBC transfusions to treat symptomatic anemia. If lesions are localized, thermoablative therapy, as with argon plasma coagulation, may be helpful (Fig. 94.24). The usual settings for argon plasma coagulation are an energy level of 45–60 W and a gas flow rate of 1–2 L/min. If the coagulation parameters are suboptimal, thermal coagulation is associated with an increase in mucosal bleeding in many patients. EBL of vascular ectasia has also been suggested. Usually, 2–3 treatment sessions are required and over 80% of patients respond to treatment.[207] Meta-analysis suggests that EBL therapy may be superior to argon plasma coagulation.[208]

When the vascular ectasias are diffuse and extensive in the stomach, cryotherapy using liquid nitrogen or CO_2 may be tried.[209] If endoscopic treatment fails, therapy with an oral estrogen-progesterone combination (estradiol 35 μg plus norethindrone 1 mg daily) may help reduce transfusion requirements.[210] In women, because the medication is taken daily, no risk of breakthrough vaginal bleeding exists. Rarely, painful gynecomastia may limit use of this combination in men. Bevacizumab may be beneficial in patients who have failed endoscopic and other pharmacologic therapy[99]; surgical antral resection is seldom necessary. TIPS does not reduce the bleeding risk in patients with GVE and is associated with a substantial risk of hepatic encephalopathy[206]; therefore, TIPS placement is not recommended as therapy for GVE. By contrast, GVE is reversed with LT, even in the presence of persistent portal hypertension from portal vein thrombosis, suggesting that GVE is more related to liver failure than to portal hypertension.[211,212]

Other Causes of Gastrointestinal Bleeding in Patients With Portal Hypertension

Other causes of GI bleeding include peptic ulcers, Dieulafoy lesions, Mallory-Weiss tears, hemorrhoids, and portal hypertensive colopathy. Mortality during the bleeding episode in patients with cirrhosis is related to degree of liver dysfunction and severity of bleeding rather than the cause of bleeding (i.e., an ulcer or esophageal varices).[213] The most common findings reported in patients with cirrhosis and LGI bleeding are portal hypertensive colopathy, rectal varices, and hemorrhoids, with diverticulosis a less common cause.[214] Patients with cirrhosis, especially alcohol-associated cirrhosis,[215] are at increased risk of peptic ulcer bleeding,[216] but the risk of ulcer bleeding appears to decline with age.[217]

Full references for this chapter can be found at https://ebooks.health.elsevier.com.

95 Ascites and Spontaneous Bacterial Peritonitis

Elisa Pose, Adrià Juanola, Pere Ginès

IN THIS CHAPTER

INTRODUCTION

Ascites is defined as the abnormal accumulation of fluid in the peritoneal cavity. In Western countries, cirrhosis is the most common cause of ascites, representing up to 80% of cases. In the remaining cases, ascites may be caused by other conditions such as heart failure, malignancies, tuberculosis, or pancreatic diseases.[1–3] Considering its high frequency, this chapter will be focused on the pathophysiology, evaluation, and management of ascites in cirrhosis and its complications.

Ascites is the most frequent complication of patients with cirrhosis, as approximately 50%–60% of patients with compensated cirrhosis will develop ascites within 10 years after the diagnosis of the disease.[4] The development of ascites is associated with impairment of health-related quality of life, increased risk of developing other complications of the disease such as spontaneous bacterial peritonitis (SBP), hyponatremia, and acute kidney injury (AKI), and diminished prognosis.[5–7] The 5-year probability of survival of patients with cirrhosis and ascites is approximately 30%, compared to 80% survival of patients with compensated cirrhosis.[2,8]

PATHOGENESIS OF ASCITES IN CIRRHOSIS

The key mechanism leading to ascites formation in cirrhosis is renal sodium retention due to kidney function impairment in response to the activation of the renin-angiotensin aldosterone system (RAAS) and sympathetic nervous system (SNS).[6,9–12] Renal sodium retention and the subsequent water retention result in an expansion of the extracellular fluid volume, inducing the formation of ascites and edema. There is a large body of evidence indicating that the main cause of kidney function abnormalities in cirrhosis, such as renal sodium retention, is the existence of systemic circulatory disturbances characterized by splanchnic arterial vasodilation as described by the so-called arterial vasodilation theory.[9,10] The most common functional renal abnormalities in patients with cirrhosis include an impaired ability to excrete sodium, an impaired ability to excrete solute-free water, and a reduction of glomerular filtration rate (GFR) due to renal vasoconstriction. Sodium retention is a key factor in the development of ascites and edema, while solute-free water retention is responsible for the development of dilutional hyponatremia, and renal vasoconstriction leads to the occurrence of hepatorenal syndrome (HRS). Chronologically, sodium retention is the earliest alteration of kidney function observed in the natural history of patients with cirrhosis, and dilutional hyponatremia and HRS appear in more advanced stages of the disease.[6,9–13]

Besides these hemodynamics abnormalities, accumulating data from the last decades show that patients with advanced cirrhosis show a chronic systemic inflammatory state that also contributes to the development or further impairment of circulatory dysfunction and may also be involved in direct kidney and multiorgan failure, particularly in patients with advanced cirrhosis[11,14] Fig. 95.1 summarizes the mechanisms involved in the pathophysiology of ascites in cirrhosis.

Sodium Retention and Extracellular Fluid Volume Expansion

Sodium is retained isosmotically together with water, and, therefore, sodium retention is associated with extracellular fluid volume expansion. The amount of sodium retained depends on the balance between the intake of sodium in the diet and the sodium excreted into the urine. If the urinary sodium excreted is lower than that ingested, patients will accumulate ascites and edema. The key role of sodium retention in the pathogenesis of ascites is underscored by the fact that ascites can disappear in some patients with the reduction of dietary sodium intake or by the increase of sodium excretion by the administration of diuretics.[8,10,13,15] In fact, the achievement of a negative sodium balance, by increasing urinary sodium excretion, is the goal of pharmacological therapy of ascites in cirrhosis.

The severity of sodium retention in patients with cirrhosis and ascites is highly variable from patient to patient. In baseline conditions (i.e., without diuretic therapy), some patients have relatively high urinary sodium excretion, while urine sodium excretion is very low in others (Fig. 95.2). Most patients who require hospitalization because of severe or difficult-to-treat ascites have marked sodium retention (<10 mEq/day excreted), and

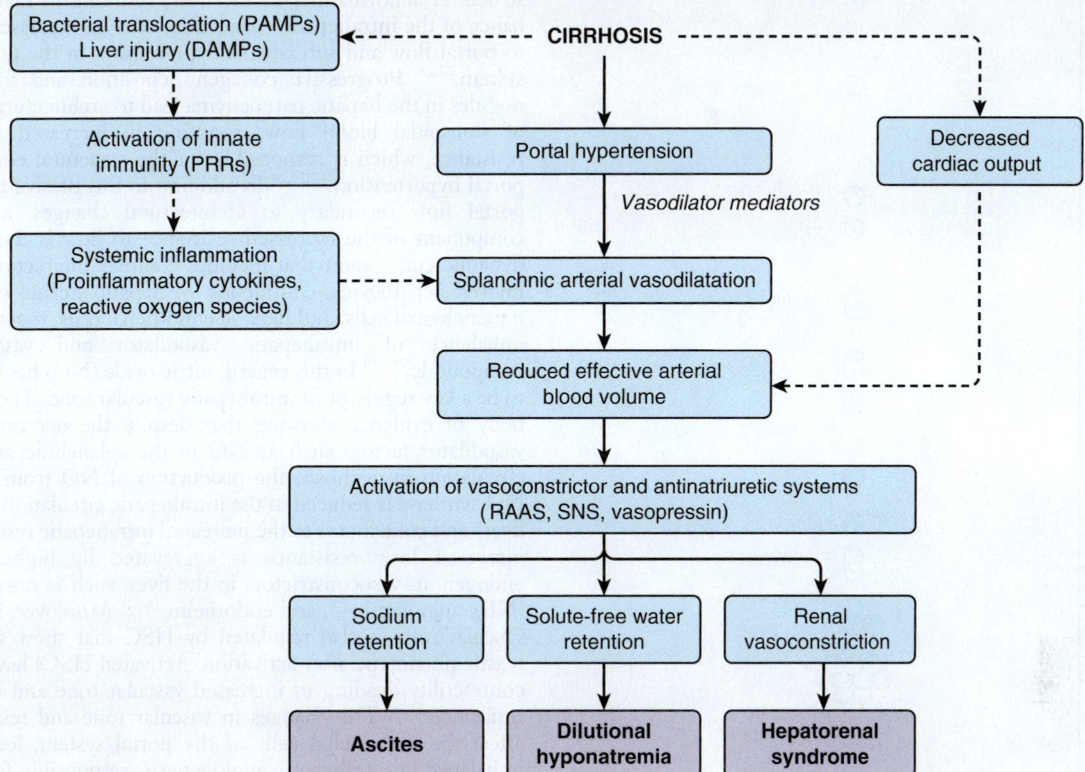

Fig. 95.1 Pathophysiology of ascites and other renal function abnormalities in patients with advanced cirrhosis. Systemic circulatory dysfunction, characterized by splanchnic arterial vasodilation, is the key mechanism leading to renal function abnormalities. The development of effective arterial hypovolemia triggers the activation of vasoconstrictor and antinatriuretic systems aimed at maintaining arterial pressure within normal limits. However, the activation of these systems has deleterious effects in the kidney, such as renal sodium retention, impairment of solute-free water excretion, and kidney vasoconstriction that subsequently leading to the development of ascites, dilutional hyponatremia, and hepatorenal syndrome. At advanced stages of the disease, there is a decrease in cardiac output that also contributes to the decrease in effective blood volume. Finally, patients with advanced cirrhosis have systemic inflammation triggered by PAMPs derived from bacterial translocation and DAMPs from the injured liver. The release of inflammatory mediators contributes to further impairment of circulatory function. *RAAS*, Renin-angiotensin-aldosterone system; *SNS*, sympathetic nervous system; *PAMPs*, pathogen-associated molecular patterns; *DAMPs*, damage-associated molecular patterns; *PRRs*, pattern recognition receptors.

sodium retention is particularly intense in patients with refractory ascites. In contrast, in patients with cirrhosis and mild or moderate ascites, the proportion of patients with marked sodium retention is low, and most patients excrete more than 10 mEq/day (without diuretic therapy). In addition, response to diuretic treatment is usually better in patients with moderate sodium retention than in those with marked sodium retention.[3,8,13,16]

In healthy subjects, approximately 95% of filtered sodium is reabsorbed in the renal tubules (approximately 60%−70% in the proximal tubules, 20%−30% in the thick ascending limb, and 5%−10% in the collecting ducts).[8,9] In most cases, sodium retention in cirrhosis is due to increased tubular reabsorption of sodium because it occurs in the presence of normal or only moderately reduced GFR.[3,8,9,13,16] The contribution of the different segments of the nephron to the increased sodium reabsorption in patients with cirrhosis is not completely known, as experimental and clinical studies have shown discrepant findings. Studies using lithium clearance, which estimates sodium reabsorption in the proximal tubule, suggest that patients with cirrhosis and ascites show a marked increase in proximal sodium reabsorption.[17] On the other hand, clinical studies using spironolactone to antagonize the mineralocorticoid receptor indicate that this agent induces natriuresis in a large proportion of patients with cirrhosis and ascites without renal failure, suggesting a major role for increased sodium reabsorption in distal sites of the nephron.[15,18−21]

Overall, data suggest that in patients with cirrhosis without renal failure, sodium retention is caused by an enhanced reabsorption of sodium in both proximal and distal tubules. As described above, the increased activity of the RAAS and SNS plays a major role in the increased renal sodium reabsorption.[8−10,13] Sodium retention is usually more marked in patients with renal failure than in those without renal failure because of both a reduction in filtered sodium and a more marked activation of sodium-retaining systems.

Portal Hypertension

Portal hypertension represents the triggering factor for the development of circulatory dysfunction and ascites in patients with advanced cirrhosis.[10,11] Cirrhosis is the result of a long process, usually for more than 20 years, of progressive liver inflammation and fibrosis in response to chronic injury (i.e., alcohol consumption, chronic viral hepatitis, and metabolic syndrome). The development of cirrhosis causes remarkable

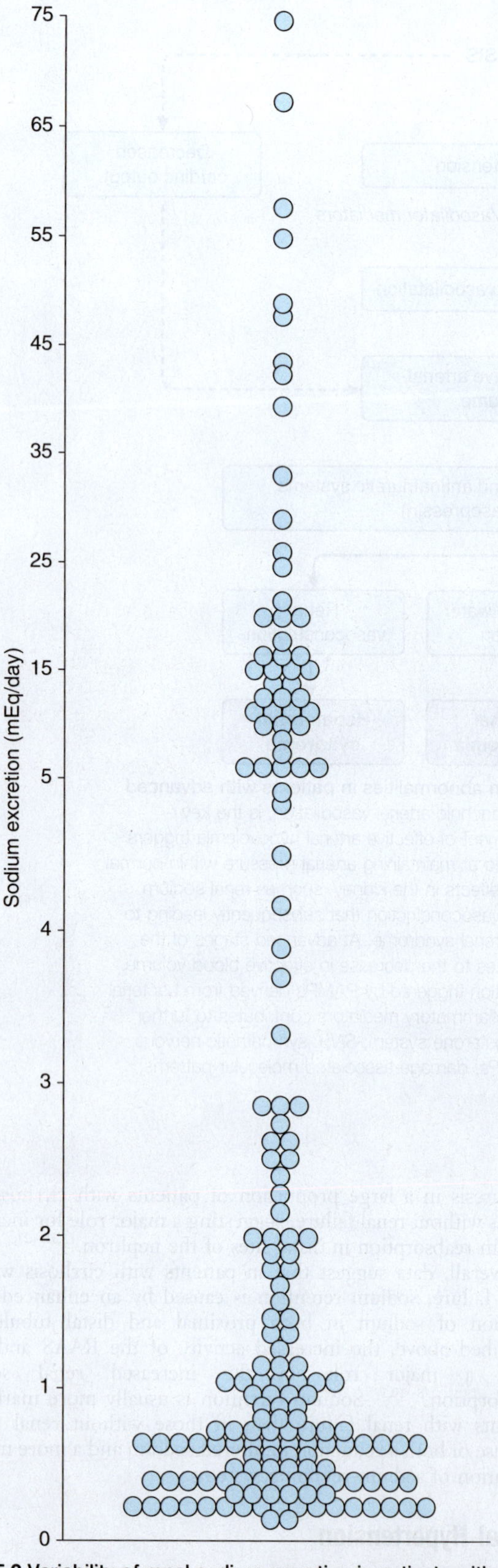

Fig. 95.2 Variability of renal sodium excretion in patients with cirrhosis and ascites. This figure shows individual values of urine sodium excretion in a series of 204 patients with cirrhosis and ascites (urinalysis was performed on a low-sodium diet and without diuretic treatment). The intensity of renal sodium retention is very variable in patients with cirrhosis and ascites and depends on the severity of circulatory dysfunction. Patients who require hospitalization for the management of ascites usually show marked renal sodium retention, particularly those with refractory ascites.

structural abnormalities in the liver, resulting in marked disturbance of the intrahepatic circulation, causing increased resistance to portal flow and subsequent hypertension in the portal venous system.[22,23] Progressive collagen deposition and formation of nodules in the hepatic parenchyma lead to architectural distortion of sinusoidal blood flow, resulting in increased intrahepatic resistance, which is responsible for the structural component of portal hypertension.[10,23,24] In addition to this passive resistance to portal flow secondary to architectural changes, a significant component of the increased resistance to flow is the result of a dynamic component that includes complex interactions between injured hepatocytes, contraction of hepatic stellate cells (HSC), mesenchymal cells, and hepatic endothelial cells, together with an imbalance of intrahepatic vasodilator and vasoconstrictor compounds.[25–28] In this regard, nitric oxide (NO) has been shown to be a key regulator of intrahepatic vascular tone. There is a large body of evidence showing that despite the overproduction of vasodilator factors such as NO in the splanchnic and systemic circulation in cirrhosis, the production of NO from endothelial NO synthase is reduced in the intrahepatic circulation of cirrhotic livers and contributes to the increased intrahepatic resistance. The increased liver resistance is aggravated by higher levels of endogenous vasoconstrictors in the liver, such as norepinephrine (NE), angiotensin-2, and endothelin.[26–29] Moreover, intrahepatic vascular tone is also regulated by HSC that show a myofibroblastic phenotype after activation. Activated HSCs have increased contractility, leading to increased vascular tone and intrahepatic resistance.[23,30] The changes in vascular tone and resistance also affect the endothelial cells of the portal system, leading to an imbalance in intrahepatic angiogenesis, responsible for the sinusoidal remodeling that takes place in the setting of chronic liver disease and that also aggravates portal hypertension.[31] Finally, intrahepatic inflammation has also been reported to play a role in the increased vascular resistance leading to portal hypertension. In advanced cirrhosis, Kupffer cells (KC) are involved in the development of hepatic inflammation and oxidative stress, leading to increased intrahepatic vascular resistance. In response to pathogen-associated molecular patterns (PAMPs) and through toll-like receptor signaling, KC induces the production of proinflammatory cytokines, reactive oxygen species, and vasoactive mediators that lead to hepatic and systemic inflammation and increased intrahepatic vascular tone.[27,31]

In clinical practice, portal hypertension can be assessed by the measurement of the hepatic venous pressure gradient (HVPG), defined as the difference between wedged and free hepatic venous pressure, which is measured through a hepatic catheterization. While 3–5 mm Hg is considered to be the normal portal pressure gradient, clinically significant portal hypertension is defined as an HVPG above 10–12 mm Hg because this is the threshold for clinical manifestations of portal hypertension to appear (i.e., ascites).[32] However, most data are derived from historical cohorts where hepatitis C infection was the predominant etiology of liver disease. More recent data, with an increased prevalence of cirrhosis due to metabolic dysfunction-associated steatotic liver disease (MASLD, formerly known as NAFLD), suggest that liver-related complications such as ascites can occur at lower values of HVPG.[33] This needs to be confirmed in further studies. Moreover, the severity of portal hypertension is associated with prognosis, as an HVPG above 16 mm Hg detects a population at high risk for mortality[34] and an HVPG above 20 mm Hg is associated with treatment failure and mortality in patients with cirrhosis and acute variceal bleeding.[35]

Systemic Circulatory Dysfunction

A large body of evidence indicates that impairment in circulatory function is the main cause of renal dysfunction in cirrhosis, which leads to the development of the major complications of the disease, such as ascites, hyponatremia, and HRS.[6,9–11,36] The arterial vasodilation theory, proposed in 1988, describes the hemodynamic disturbances occurring in patients with decompensated cirrhosis that are mainly characterized by systemic arterial vasodilation, particularly in the splanchnic area.[9] As mentioned before, portal hypertension is the initial event, resulting in splanchnic arterial vasodilation due to the release of several vasodilator factors, particularly NO, but also carbon monoxide (CO) and endogenous endocannabinoids.[37] Splanchnic arterial vasodilation leads to decreased vascular resistance and, as a consequence, to reduction in effective arterial blood volume and arterial pressure.[9–11,37]

In early stages of cirrhosis, when patients are asymptomatic, the increase in hepatic vascular resistance and, therefore, in portal pressure, is moderate. In this setting, there is a slight reduction in systemic vascular resistance due to moderate splanchnic arterial vasodilation, which can be counterbalanced by an increase in cardiac output, allowing the maintenance of arterial blood volume and arterial pressure within normal limits.[9–11] In advanced stages of cirrhosis, when patients have developed complications of the disease, there is an intense splanchnic arterial vasodilation leading to a marked reduction of systemic vascular resistance that cannot be compensated for by further increase in cardiac output. At this stage, effective arterial hypovolemia develops due to the disparity between intravascular blood volume and the enlarged intravascular arterial circulation due to vasodilation.[9–11] As a consequence, there is an activation of vasoconstrictor systems, as a homeostatic response to maintain arterial pressure within normal limits, such as the RAAS, SNS, and, at later stages of the disease, vasopressin (AVP). The activation of these systems helps maintain effective arterial blood volume and arterial pressure within normal limits, but they have important detrimental effects on kidney function, particularly sodium and solute free-water retention, leading to ascites and edema and dilutional hypovolemia, respectively. At late stages of the disease, if the activation of these systems is extreme, patients develop marked renal vasoconstriction that leads to reduction of GFR and development of HRS[2,9–11] (Fig. 95.1). Moreover, there are data indicating that at this stage, there is an associated decrease in cardiac output that also contributes to the arterial underfilling.[38]

The Renin-Angiotensin-Aldosterone System

Of all potential factors involved in the pathogenesis of sodium retention in cirrhosis, aldosterone has been the most extensively studied. Plasma aldosterone levels are increased in most patients with cirrhosis and ascites and marked sodium retention.[3,39–44] The important role of aldosterone in the pathogenesis of sodium retention and ascites is supported by data showing that there is an inverse correlation between urinary sodium excretion and plasma aldosterone levels,[3,39–44] and that the administration of spironolactone, a specific aldosterone antagonist, is able to reverse sodium retention in the great majority of patients with ascites without renal failure.[18–21] The fact that sodium retention may occur in patients with cirrhosis in the absence of increased plasma aldosterone levels has raised the suggestion that factors other than aldosterone may contribute to increased sodium retention in cirrhosis.[44] Nevertheless, it has also been suggested that patients with cirrhosis may have an increased tubular sensitivity to aldosterone.[3,44] This may explain the natriuretic response to spironolactone in patients with normal aldosterone levels.

The increased plasma aldosterone concentration in patients with cirrhosis and ascites is due to a stimulation of aldosterone secretion[9,41,45–47] that can most likely be explained by an increased activity of RAAS. Plasma renin activity (PRA), which estimates the activity of the RAAS, is increased in most patients with ascites and correlates closely with plasma aldosterone concentration.[42,48–50] The administration of angiotensin II receptor antagonists or converting-enzyme inhibitors to patients with cirrhosis and ascites and increased PRA induces a marked reduction in arterial pressure and systemic vascular resistance, which suggests that the activation of RAAS is a homeostatic response to maintain arterial pressure in these patients.[50,51]

Sympathetic Nervous System

The plasma concentration of NE in the systemic circulation, a marker of activation of the SNS, is increased in most patients with ascites, while it is normal or only slightly elevated in patients without ascites.[52–55] The increased plasma NE levels are due to an increased activity of the SNS rather than to an impaired elimination of NE, as the total spillover of NE to plasma is markedly increased in patients with cirrhosis and ascites, but plasma clearance of NE is normal.[56,57] Measurements of NE release have shown that the activity of the SNS is increased in many vascular territories, including the kidneys, splanchnic organs, heart, and muscle and skin, supporting the concept of a generalized activation of the SNS.[57]

There is a large amount of evidence suggesting that the SNS is involved in sodium and water retention in cirrhosis. The activity of the SNS correlates with sodium and water retention.[52,53,55] In addition, a study in a limited number of patients with ascites showed that the administration of diuretics together with clonidine to inhibit SNS activity is more effective than diuretics alone.[58] The cause of the increased activity of the SNS in cirrhosis with ascites is not completely understood; however, the most likely explanation is based on a baroreceptor-mediated response to decreased effective arterial blood volume due to arterial vasodilation.[56,59] This is supported by a large amount of data showing that the activity of the SNS can be suppressed by increasing effective arterial blood volume, such as with the administration of vasopressin analogs and albumin, the insertion of a peritoneovenous shunt or transjugular intrahepatic portosystemic shunt (TIPS).[60–63]

Systemic Inflammation

In the last decade, evidence has accumulated indicating that decompensated cirrhosis is associated with chronic systemic inflammation that may play a role in the progression of cirrhosis and development of complications.[11,30,64–66] Decompensated cirrhosis is associated with increased serum inflammatory markers, such as C-reactive protein and leukocyte count, which increase in parallel with disease severity and independently of the presence of bacterial infections.[11,67] Moreover, patients with advanced cirrhosis show increased serum levels of pro-inflammatory cytokines such as interleukins (IL-6, IL-8) or tumor necrosis alpha (TNF) among others.[67,68]

Patients with cirrhosis and ascites frequently have bacterial translocation (BT), which is the passage of bacteria or bacterial products from the gut to mesenteric lymph nodes, mainly due to increase in gut permeability[68] (reviewed in detail later; see SBP section). The hypothesis has been raised that these bacterial products, known as PAMPs, may activate pattern recognition receptors (PRRs) present in circulating innate immune cells, leading to the activation of immune cells, the release of pro-inflammatory mediators and reactive oxygen species, and the consequent development of an inflammatory response. In addition, damage-associated molecular patterns derived from the injured liver due to local inflammation and cell death may also contribute to the activation of PRRs. The systemic release of these inflammatory mediators would contribute to further impairment of circulatory dysfunction[11,14,30,66] (Fig. 95.1).

DIAGNOSIS

As mentioned above, cirrhosis is the main cause of ascites in the Western world. The evaluation of a patient with the first episode of ascites should be targeted to confirm the diagnosis of chronic liver disease and rule out other causes of ascites, such as malignancies, tuberculosis, or pancreatic diseases. The evaluation of patients should include clinical history, physical examination, laboratory tests to assess liver and kidney function, serum and urine electrolytes, abdominal ultrasound, and ascitic fluid analysis[1,2,6,10,69] (Table 95.1).

According to the International Club of Ascites, ascites may be classified either based on semiquantitative parameters depending on the amount of ascites or based on response to treatment. According to the semiquantitative parameters, grade 1 ascites is defined as mild ascites that is only detectable by ultrasound; grade 2 ascites is defined as moderate ascites detectable by physical examination; and grade 3 ascites is defined as large ascites with marked abdomen distention. According to the classification based on response to treatment, ascites can be classified as uncomplicated, including diuretic-responsive ascites and recurrent ascites, which is ascites that recurs at least three times within a 1-year period despite appropriate treatment; and complicated ascites, which include refractory ascites, which can only be treated with large-volume paracentesis (LVP) (see section "Management of ascites in cirrhosis").[70,71]

Laboratory Tests

Liver function should be evaluated using standard liver function tests and coagulation parameters. Assessment of renal function should include serum creatinine and serum and urine electrolytes. Urine tests should also include a 24-hour urine analysis, including sodium and proteins. These laboratory tests should be performed before initiating diuretic treatment, because results can be modified under diuretic treatment.[1,6,10]

Assessment of Renal Sodium Excretion

The assessment of the urinary excretion of sodium is useful for the management of patients with cirrhosis and ascites because it allows the quantification of sodium retention. Ideally, urine should be collected under conditions of controlled sodium intake (low-sodium diet of approximately 90 mEq/day during the previous 5–7 days), as sodium intake may influence sodium excretion. Although the measurement of sodium concentration in a spot of urine provides an estimate of sodium excretion, the assessment of sodium excretion in a 24-hour period is preferable because it is more representative of sodium excretion throughout the day. Moreover, sodium excretion should be measured without diuretic therapy in patients with the first episode or when there is worsening of ascites (e.g., marked increase in ascites despite treatment).[1,8,10] The measurement of sodium excretion in patients under diuretic therapy may be useful to monitor the response to treatment.

In addition, baseline sodium excretion is also useful because it is a predictive factor of response to diuretic treatment, and it is an excellent marker of prognosis. Patients with moderate sodium retention (urine sodium >10 mEq/day) are more likely to respond to lower doses of diuretics than those with marked sodium retention. Finally, the intensity of sodium retention also provides prognostic information in patients with cirrhotic ascites. Patients with baseline urine sodium lower than 10 mEq/day have a median survival time of only 1.5 years compared with 4.5 years in patients with urine sodium >10 mEq/day (Fig. 95.3).[72,73]

TABLE 95.1 Evaluation of Patients With Cirrhosis and a First Episode of Ascites

Evaluation of Liver Disease
Standard blood tests: liver function, coagulation parameters, complete blood count
Abdominal ultrasound
Upper gastrointestinal endoscopy
Liver biopsy (selected cases)
Evaluation of Kidney Function
Serum creatinine
Serum sodium and potassium
Urine sodium (preferably 24-h urine)
Urine protein (preferably 24-h urine)
Ascitic Fluid Analysis
Neutrophil count
Protein concentration
Bacterial culture (in blood culture flasks)
Other parameters based on clinical presentation (i.e., glucose, lactate dehydrogenase, amylase, triglycerides, cytologic exam, and mycobacteria culture)

Abdominal Ultrasound

An abdominal ultrasound should be performed in all patients with the first episode of ascites to confirm the diagnosis of cirrhosis by evaluating characteristics of liver parenchyma, investigating the presence of signs of portal hypertension, and also assessing portal vein and suprahepatic vein patency and exclude the presence of liver tumors. Abdominal ultrasound is the imaging technique of choice as it is simple and cost-effective. In addition to all patients with the first episode of ascites, abdominal ultrasound should also be performed in patients with previous ascites experiencing impaired response to treatment.[1,8]

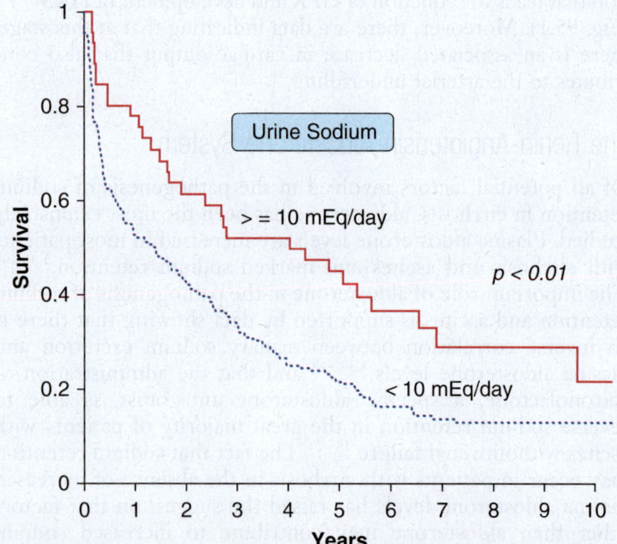

Fig. 95.3 Prognosis of patients with cirrhosis and ascites according to renal sodium excretion. This figure shows the probability of survival in a series of 204 patients with cirrhosis and ascites categorized according to renal sodium excretion. Renal sodium excretion is associated with prognosis in patients with cirrhosis and ascites, with patients with marked renal sodium retention (≤10 mEq/L) showing significantly lower probability of survival compared to patients with renal sodium excretion >10 mEq/L. Other prognostic factors in patients with cirrhosis and ascites are arterial pressure, serum sodium concentration, and serum creatinine. (Adapted from Ginès P, Cárdenas A, Solà E, Schrier RW. Liver disease and the kidney. In: Schrier RW, Coffman TM, Falk RJ, Molitoris BA, Neilson EG, eds. *Schrier's Diseases of the Kidney*. 9th ed. Philadelphia: Lippincott Williams & Wilkins; 2012.)

Ascitic Fluid Analysis

The analysis of ascitic fluid is essential to detect ascitic fluid infection, as well as rule out causes of ascites other than cirrhosis, in cases where the diagnosis of cirrhosis is not clear. A diagnostic paracentesis should be performed in all patients presenting with their first episode of grade 2 or 3 ascites, as well as in those admitted to hospital for any intercurrent complication. Parameters that should always be assessed are neutrophil count and total protein and albumin concentration.

Ascitic fluid protein concentration correlates with the prognosis of patients with ascites. Moreover, low ascitic fluid protein (less than 1.5 g/dL) is also associated with higher risk of developing SBP, especially in patients with impaired liver or kidney function.[74] A neutrophil count higher than 250 cells/µL is diagnostic of SBP (see later; SBP section).[74] Ascitic fluid culture should be performed by inoculating at least 10 mL of ascitic fluid into blood culture flasks.[1,2,10,74,75] Culture is very helpful for treatment guidance in the event that ascitic fluid infection is confirmed. The most common cause of ascitic fluid infection is SBP, and, in this case, the culture is expected to be monomicrobial. In the case of polymicrobial culture results, secondary bacterial peritonitis should be suspected.

The serum-ascites albumin gradient (SAAG) is a sensitive and specific measurement to determine whether ascites is related to portal hypertension.[1,76] The calculation of the SAAG involves measuring albumin concentration in serum and ascitic fluid and simply subtracting the ascitic fluid value from the serum value. If SAAG is 1.1 g/dL (11 g/L) or greater, the patient can be considered to have portal hypertension with an accuracy of approximately 97%. By contrast, if the SAAG is less than 1.1 g/dL (11 g/L), the patient is unlikely to have portal hypertension.[76] The SAAG does not confirm the diagnosis of the cause of ascites but it is an indirect index of portal hypertension. The SAAG is useful when the cause of ascites is not clear after initial routine assessments such as medical history, physical examination, standard blood tests, and abdominal ultrasonography.

The assessment of other tests should be performed at clinical presentation or when causes of ascites other than cirrhosis need to be ruled out.[1,69] If ascitic fluid is infected and secondary bacterial peritonitis rather than SBP is suspected, the measurement of glucose, amylase, lipase, lactate dehydrogenase (LDH), and adenosine deaminase (ADA) in ascitic fluid may be useful in the differential diagnos of ascites infection. Glucose is a small molecule that can easily diffuse into extravascular fluid. Therefore ascitic fluid glucose levels are usually similar to those in plasma, unless glucose is being consumed by leukocytes or bacteria. In the setting of secondary bacterial peritonitis, glucose levels are markedly low and may be close to 0 mg/dL due to significantly increased numbers of leukocytes and bacteria in ascites. In addition, ascites LDH levels markedly increase in secondary bacterial peritonitis due to their release from neutrophils and are typically several fold higher than serum levels.[1,77–79] ADA may be found at high levels in cases of abdominal tuberculosis.[80] Finally, the assessment of Gram stain in ascitic fluid may be useful in the setting of secondary bacterial peritonitis to demonstrate polymicrobial ascites which is typical of this condition.[79] Pancreatic enzymes or mycobacterial culture should be performed when pancreatic disease or tuberculosis, respectively, need to be ruled out. Finally, ascitic fluid cytology should be performed if peritoneal carcinomatosis is suspected as the cause of ascites.

Differential Diagnosis of Ascites

As described earlier, 20% of cases of ascites may be due to causes other than cirrhosis.[1,6] Cirrhosis should be easily diagnosed after medical history and physical examination, together with standard liver tests and abdominal ultrasonography. However, when cirrhosis cannot clearly be diagnosed, other causes of ascites should be sought.

Heart failure may be responsible for approximately 5% of overall cases of ascites. Clinically, heart failure may mimic cirrhosis, as patients present with ascites and may also develop gastroesophageal varices. However, patients with ascites of cardiac origin usually have dyspnea, which persists even when ascites has been removed by LVP. Moreover, in contrast to cirrhosis, cardiac ascites is characterized by high ascitic fluid protein concentration and SAAG <11 g/L.[81,82] Patients with cirrhosis frequently have low hematocrit and low platelet count, which usually is not present in patients with cardiac ascites. In patients with heart failure, chest x-ray may show cardiomegaly. Although ascitic fluid analysis findings may suggest cardiac ascites, diagnosis should be confirmed by echocardiography or cardiac catheterization.[81,82] It is important to emphasize that some patients with persistent ascites of unknown origin may have constrictive pericarditis that may be difficult to diagnose on clinical grounds due to a paucity of symptoms. A good clinical sign to suspect constrictive pericarditis is marked jugular vein distention at physical examination.

Malignancies represent less than 10% of cases of ascites. Cytology of the ascitic fluid has a relatively high sensitivity but low specificity, with detection of malignant cells in 40%–70% of malignant ascites.[83–85] Therefore other parameters have been investigated for the diagnosis of malignant ascites. Marked elevations of ascitic fluid cholesterol have been reported in patients with peritoneal carcinomatosis compared to those in patients with cirrhosis and ascites; this suggests that cholesterol is useful in the differential diagnosis. Available data indicate that a diagnostic sequence based on ascitic fluid cholesterol measurement, followed by cytologic exam and carcinoembryonic antigen determination in samples with cholesterol >45 mg/dL, would be cost-efficient in differentiating malignant versus nonmalignant ascites.[84,86]

Peritoneal tuberculosis is a rare cause of ascites in Western countries, but most patients with peritoneal tuberculosis will develop ascites. Risk factors for developing tuberculosis include HIV infection, immunosuppressive treatments, and also cirrhosis, although the incidence in patients with cirrhosis is very low. Peritoneal tuberculosis should be clinically suspected in patients with ascites and persistent fever, weight loss, and positive epidemiological risk factors. The diagnosis of tuberculosis ascites may be definitely established by the demonstration of *Mycobacterium tuberculosis* in ascitic fluid.[87] Ascitic fluid in patients with peritoneal tuberculosis shows high protein concentration. ADA in ascitic fluid is also helpful, and high levels can be found in patients with peritoneal tuberculosis; however, its sensitivity is low.[87,88] Finally, if the diagnosis is strongly suspected and cannot be confirmed with these previous methods, abdominal laparoscopy with histological analysis of the peritoneum should be considered.[88]

Pancreatic ascites is also an uncommon condition that may appear in patients with severe acute pancreatitis or history of chronic pancreatitis. Ascitic fluid amylase and lipase levels are very high in these patients and should be measured when pancreatic ascites is suspected.[89]

Chylous ascites is an ascitic fluid with milky appearance that has triglyceride levels >200 mg/dL and usually >1000 mg/dL.[90] The mechanism for the development of chylous ascites is the rupture of intra-abdominal lymphatic vessels. Cirrhosis is the most common cause of chylous ascites, and the high lymphatic flow and pressure due to portal hypertension and splanchnic arterial vasodilation are presumed to be the reason for its development. Besides cirrhosis, retroperitoneal surgery or radical surgery in patients with cancer may lead to the development of chylous ascites.[3,90]

PROGNOSIS

The development of ascites in patients with cirrhosis is associated with impaired prognosis, with median 1-year survival of approximately 50%.[5,8,91,92] Therefore patients with ascites should be considered candidates for liver transplantation, particularly those with refractory ascites.[5,8]

In patients with cirrhosis and ascites, independent predictive factors for mortality include low arterial pressure, hyponatremia, low GFR, and low renal sodium excretion.[73] A number of studies have demonstrated the prognostic value of serum sodium concentration in patients with cirrhosis; hence, this parameter was added to MELD score.[93–95] Therefore currently in most cases, the calculation of MELD score includes serum creatinine, serum bilirubin, INR, and serum sodium concentration.

COMPLICATIONS OF ASCITES

The occurrence of ascites is a risk factor for the development of other complications.[4,8] The most common and severe complications of ascites include SBP, refractory ascites, and HRS.[2,8,10] Considering their importance and specific management, refractory ascites and SBP are discussed later in this chapter in separate sections. HRS is discussed in Chapter 96. Other ascites-related complications that deserve specific comment are pleural effusion or hepatic hydrothorax and abdominal wall hernias.

Hepatic hydrothorax is defined as the accumulation of fluid in the pleural space of patients with decompensated cirrhosis and ascites, in the absence of pulmonary, cardiac, or pleural disease. The development of hepatic hydrothorax is due to small diaphragmatic defects that allow the passage of ascites to the pleural space because of the negative thoracic pressure induced by inspiration.[95,96] The risks of hepatic hydrothorax are the development of respiratory failure or spontaneous bacterial infection of the pleural fluid [spontaneous bacterial empyema, (SBE)]. When patients develop pleural effusion, cardiopulmonary and pleural diseases should be ruled out. A diagnostic thoracocentesis should be performed to assess the characteristics of pleural fluid and rule out fluid infection. The diagnostic criteria of SBE are different from those for SBP (see later). Typically, pleural fluid in patients with hepatic hydrothorax has low protein concentration. The development of hepatic hydrothorax is associated with impaired prognosis, with median survival of approximately 1 year, and, therefore, these patients should be considered for liver transplantation.[95,96] As occurs with patients with ascites, MELD score underestimates the prognosis of these patients.[93]

Abdominal wall hernias are common in patients with cirrhosis and ascites, particularly in those with refractory ascites, with a prevalence of up to 20%. They are usually umbilical hernias and, occasionally, inguinal.[97,98] In addition to impaired quality of life, the major risk of abdominal wall hernias is that they can incarcerate and cause intestinal perforation. Despite the increased surgical risk of patients with cirrhosis and ascites, elective surgery should be considered and individualized in all patients with hernias.[99,100] In candidates for transplantation, clinical experience shows that most liver and transplant surgeons prefer to avoid surgery and postpone it until the time of liver transplantation. An elastic abdominal binder can be used in the meantime as a measure to reduce pain and hernia enlargement. Nonetheless, surgical repair of a hernia should be performed urgently in patients with persistent pain, skin ulceration, crusting, or black discoloration.[99–101]

MANAGEMENT OF ASCITES IN CIRRHOSIS

As previously mentioned, patients with cirrhosis and ascites are at high risk of developing other complications of the disease, such as refractory ascites, SBP, or HRS. The absence of these complications defines ascites as uncomplicated.[1,2] According to the International Club of Ascites and current international guidelines, the decision regarding therapy of choice for uncomplicated ascites is based on quantitative criteria and/or on criteria of response to therapy.

Management of Ascites Based on Ascites Fluid Volume (Quantitative Criteria)

Grade 1 Ascites

Until very recently, there was no available data on the natural history of patients with grade 1 ascites, that is, ascites only detectable by ultrasound examination. A recent study showed that grade 1 ascites is associated with systemic inflammation, higher risk of complications, and poor prognosis compared to patients with compensated cirrhosis. Although current guidelines recommend no treatment for patients with grade 1 ascites,[1,2] close monitoring of these patients should be pursued due to the increased risk of death and complications.[92]

Grade 2 Ascites

Patients with grade 2 ascites have moderate renal sodium retention, with baseline urine sodium excretion >20 mEq/L in most cases. Moreover, patients usually have normal GFR without impairment of solute-free water excretion. In this context, a negative sodium balance with loss of ascites can easily be obtained in most cases by reducing dietary sodium intake and increasing renal sodium excretion with diuretics.[1,2] There is no evidence that maintaining supine position for prolonged periods of time improves the management of ascites, and, therefore, prolonged bed rest is not currently recommended. In addition, fluid restriction is not recommended, unless patients have associated hyponatremia.[1,2,10]

Sodium Restriction

Dietary salt restriction is not indicated as a prophylactic strategy in patients who have never developed ascites. By contrast, dietary salt restriction alone may lead to the resolution of ascites in some patients with grade 2 ascites, particularly in those with the first episode of ascites.

Dietary sodium intake should be moderately restricted to 80–120 mEq/day which corresponds to approximately 4.6–6.9 g of salt per day and is generally equivalent to no added salt to the diet with the avoidance of preprepared meals and food with high sodium content. A more severe restriction in sodium intake is not recommended because it is usually poorly tolerated, and it may impair patients' nutritional status.[1,10,13,102,103] Moreover, excessive sodium restriction can be associated with the development of diuretic-induced hyponatremia. Correct nutritional education of these patients and their caregivers is essential to ensure adherence to diet and avoid treatment-related complications.

Diuretic Treatment

Diuretics indicated for the management of ascites are antimineralocorticoids and loop diuretics.[1,2,10] Considering that hyperaldosteronism plays a key role in renal sodium retention in cirrhosis, antimineralocorticoids (particularly spironolactone or eplerenone) represent the first line of treatment for the management of ascites in cirrhosis.[1,2,104] Antimineralocorticoids have a slow mechanism of action and this is the reason why dosage of these diuretics should not be increased earlier than 72 hours after their last dose change. Since proximal tubular sodium reabsorption is also involved in the pathophysiology of renal sodium retention, particularly in patients with long history of ascites, loop diuretics are also indicated in this setting. However, they should not be used alone, but in combination with antimineralocorticoids.[1,2]

Whether treatment of grade 2 ascites should be initiated with antimineralocorticoids alone or in combination with loop diuretics has been controversial. There are two studies that investigated the effect of diuretic regimen based on treatment with initially antimineralocorticoid alone at stepwise increasing dosages with furosemide added in nonresponders compared to a regimen based on antimineralocorticoid and furosemide combined from the beginning of treatment.[20,105] Results from both studies are conflicting. While in one study, the effect of both regimens was similar; the other study showed that the combination regimen was more effective in removing ascites within a shorter period of time. The reason for these different results may be explained by differences in the population of patients included; in one study, most of the population were patients with their first episode of ascites, while in the other, most patients had recurrent ascites. In the view of these results, current guidelines recommend that patients with their first episode of ascites should be treated initially with antimineralocorticoids alone (i.e., spironolactone 100 mg/day), as they will probably show a positive response with low frequency of side effects. In case of no response, dose should be increased in a stepwise manner every 72 hours (in 100 mg steps) to a maximum of 400 mg/day. In patients who do not respond to treatment, defined as body weight reduction below 2 kg/week, or in those who develop hyperkalemia, furosemide should be added at an initial dose of 40 mg/day with sequential increasing to 160 mg/day (40 mg steps).[1,2,10] By contrast, the best approach for patients with recurrent ascites is combined diuretic treatment with antimineralocorticoids and loop diuretics with increasing dose in an stepwise manner according to the response, as described above.[1,2,10] In both cases, diuretic dose should be titrated to achieve a weight loss of up to a maximum of 0.5 kg/day in patients without peripheral edema and up to 1 kg/day in patients with ascites and edema.[1,2,10] Once ascites has been mobilized, diuretic dose should be reduced to the minimum dose necessary to maintain patients without ascites to avoid adverse events, such as AKI, hepatic encephalopathy, or hyponatremia. Table 95.2 summarizes the management of grade 2 ascites.

TABLE 95.2 Management of Grade 2 or Moderate Ascites

Diet

Low-sodium diet (80–120 mEq/day)

Diuretic Treatment

First episode of ascites:

- Start with spironolactone (100 mg/day) and increase in a stepwise manner every 72 h according to treatment response (maximum dose 400 mg/day)
- In case of no response or development of hyperkalemia: add furosemide (initial dose 40 mg/day) increasing in a stepwise manner to a maximum dose of 160 mg/day

Recurrent ascites:

- Combined diuretic treatment with spironolactone and furosemide (same doses as above)

Monitoring:

- Body weight should be monitored daily (recommended body weight loss is up to 0.5 kg/day in patients without leg edema and 0.5–1 kg/day in patients with ascites and leg edema)
- Once ascites has been mobilized: keep the minimum diuretic dose necessary to avoid accumulation of ascites, together with low-sodium diet

TABLE 95.3 Management of Grade 3 or Tense Ascites

Diet

Low-sodium diet (80–120 mEq/day)

Large-Volume Paracentesis

Intravenous albumin should be administered (8 g/L of ascites removed)

Diuretic Treatment

- The minimum diuretic dose necessary to avoid re-accumulation of ascites should be maintained together with low-sodium diet
- If patient did not received previous diuretic treatment: start with spironolactone 100 mg/day and furosemide 40 mg/day
- If patient was already receiving diuretics: restart with a higher dose and if there is no response to treatment: assess correct sodium intake and increase diuretic dose progressively to a maximum of spironolactone 400 mg/day and furosemide 160 mg/day

Grade 3 Ascites

The treatment of choice for patients with grade 3 or large ascites is LVP[1,2,10] (Table 95.3). This is a safe procedure that is associated with very low risk of complications.[1,2,106] Coagulopathy is not a contraindication to perform LVP, as the risk of bleeding is low, even in patients with INR>1.5 and platelet count <50,000/μL. Although the use of fresh frozen plasma or platelet transfusion is a common practice in some centers, there are no data to support their use in this setting. LVP should only be contraindicated in case of severe coagulopathy (disseminated intravascular coagulation) or presence of other risk factors such as abdominal skin infection at the puncture site or severe bowel distention.

The removal of a large volume of ascites without plasma volume expansion is associated with the development of post-paracentesis circulatory dysfunction (PPCD) syndrome, which is characterized by a further reduction of effective arterial blood volume already present in patients with ascites and marked activation of endogenous vasoconstrictor systems, particularly renin-angiotensin-aldosterone system.[1,10,107] This syndrome is characterized by rapid re-accumulation of ascites, high risk of developing HRS and hyponatremia, and increased mortality.[1,10,108] Plasma volume expansion should be performed together with LVP to prevent the development of PPCD. When more than 5 L of ascites are removed, the administration of 20% intravenous albumin is more effective in the prevention of PPCD than other plasma expanders, such as dextran-70, saline or polygeline. In contrast, when LVP is less than 5 L, the risk of PPCD is low, and the efficacy of albumin is similar to that of other plasma expanders.[1,108] However, polygeline is not used in many countries due to the potential risk of transmission of prions. A meta-analysis performed with randomized clinical trials showed that the administration of albumin after LVP is more effective not only in the prevention of PPCD but also in the reduction of hyponatremia and mortality.[109] Finally, the administration of albumin after LVP is more cost-effective than other plasma expanders, because the albumin is associated with reduction of complications of cirrhosis within the first month.[110] On this background, current international guidelines recommend that after LVP of more than 5 L, plasma volume expansion should be performed with IV 20% albumin (8 g/L of ascites removed).[1,2] In addition, European guidelines also recommend the use of 20% albumin (8 g/L of ascites removed) in patients undergoing LVP of less than 5 L because it reduces the risk of PPCD when compared with the administration of other plasma expanders. After LVP, patients should continue with diuretic treatment with the minimum dose necessary to prevent the re-accumulation of ascites.[1,10,111]

Complications of Diuretic Therapy and Treatment Monitoring

The most common complications associated with diuretic therapy are AKI, hepatic encephalopathy, and electrolyte disturbances, particularly hyponatremia and hypo/hyperkalemia.[1,2] Circulatory dysfunction present in patients with cirrhosis and ascites is associated with an increased risk to develop rapid reductions of extracellular fluid volume and AKI due to kidney hypoperfusion.[9,10] Loop diuretics can lead to potassium and magnesium depletion, while antimineralocorticoids may lead to hyperkalemia. Hyponatremia is also a common diuretic-related complication, and while it is more frequently associated with loop diuretics, it can also occur in the setting of treatment with antimineralocorticoids. Hyponatremia may be explained by the inhibition of Na–K–Cl transporter by loop diuretics. However, plasma volume contraction due to diuretic treatment can also trigger the release of arginine-vasopressin leading to solute-free water reabsorption and development of hyponatremia. Painful gynecomastia is one of the most frequent side effects of antimineralocorticoids; pain usually improves after dose reduction, although in few patients, treatment should be discontinued. Finally, muscle cramps may also develop as diuretic-related side effects and are associated with impairment of patients' health-related quality of life. Albumin infusion, baclofen, and sips of pickle juice appear to be beneficial for the management of muscle cramps.[112–114]

International guidelines recommend withdrawal of diuretics in case of severe hyponatremia (serum sodium concentration <125 mEq/L), AKI, hepatic encephalopathy, or incapacitating muscle cramps. Moreover, furosemide should be discontinued if severe hypokalemia develops (<3 mEq/L) and antimineralocorticoids should be stopped in case of hyperkalemia (>6 mEq/L).[1,2]

Considering the potential development of several treatment-related side effects, particularly during the first weeks of therapy, patients should be monitored with repeated kidney function tests (serum creatinine, sodium, potassium) and clinical visits for early detection of treatment-related complications.[1,2] In this regard, patients may benefit from visits with a nurse expert in cirrhosis who should also be available for telephone consultations.

Management of Ascites Based on Response to Therapy

Diuretic-Responsive/Recurrent Ascites

Patients with ascites without other complications of cirrhosis can be managed in an outpatient setting. Treatment of ascites is aimed at achieving a negative sodium balance, and, therefore, treatment strategy is based on reducing sodium intake together with increasing renal sodium excretion with diuretic treatment. Fig. 95.4 summarizes the recommended therapy for each type of ascites based on response to diuretic therapy. Patients with ascites that respond to low-sodium diet and diuretic therapy are classified as diuretic-responsive ascites. However, in some patients, ascites recurs despite adequate treatment at least three times within a 1-year period, varying between grade 2 and grade 3 ascites; these patients are considered to have recurrent ascites, and treatment usually includes low-sodium diet, diuretic therapy, and LVP. Prognosis of recurrent ascites is not worse than that of diuretic-responsive ascites, which means that occurrence of recurrent ascites is not necessarily a sign of increased risk of mortality.[92]

Refractory Ascites

Refractory ascites is defined as ascites that cannot be mobilized or the early recurrence of which cannot be prevented by medical therapy because of lack of response to maximum diuretic treatment or development of complications related to diuretic therapy that preclude the use of an effective diuretic dosage.[2] Diagnostic criteria of refractory ascites are shown in Table 95.4. Approximately 10% of patients with cirrhosis and ascites develop refractory ascites during their lifespan. Refractory ascites is associated with poor short-term prognosis, with a median survival of approximately 6 months.[115] Due to this blunt survival expectancy, all patients with refractory ascites should be considered for liver transplantation.[1,2] Treatment options for the management of refractory ascites are described later.

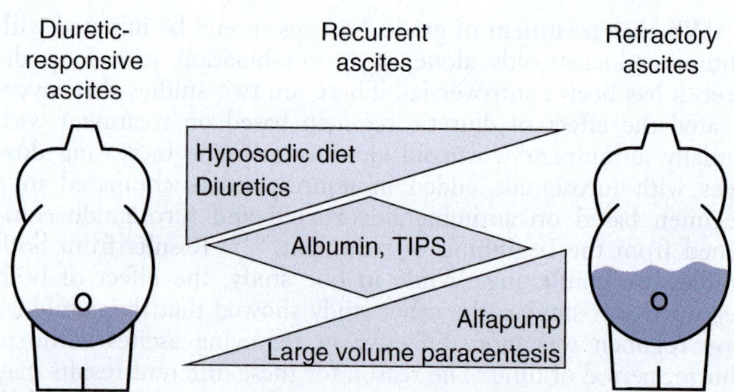

Fig. 95.4 Summarizes the recommended therapy for each type of ascites based on response to diuretic therapy.

TABLE 95.4 Diagnostic Criteria for Refractory Ascites

- Diuretic resistant ascites
  Ascites that cannot be mobilized or the early recurrence of which cannot be prevented because of a lack of response to sodium restriction and diuretic treatment
- Diuretic intractable ascites
  Ascites that cannot be mobilized or the early recurrence of which cannot be prevented because of the development of diuretic-induced complications that preclude the use of an effective diuretic dosage

Definitions:

- Treatment duration: Patients should be on intensive diuretic therapy (spironolactone 400 mg/day and furosemide 160 mg/day) for at least 1 week and on a salt-restricted diet of less than 80 mEq/day
- Lack of response: Mean weight loss of <0.8 kg over 4 days and urinary sodium output less than the sodium intake
- Early ascites recurrence: Reappearance of grade 2 or 3 ascites within 4 weeks of initial mobilization
- Diuretic-induced complications: Diuretic-induced hepatic encephalopathy is the development of encephalopathy in the absence of any other precipitating factor. Diuretic-induced renal impairment is an increase of serum creatinine by >100% to a value >2 mg/dL in patients with ascites responding to treatment

Large-Volume Paracentesis

Repeated LVP associated with plasma volume expansion with intravenous albumin is considered first-line treatment for patients with refractory ascites.[1,2,10]

Diuretics

Once patients develop refractory ascites, it is recommended to stop diuretic treatment to prevent adverse events, because no beneficial effects of diuretics have been demonstrated in these patients. However, in patients who maintain a daily urinary sodium excretion greater than 30 mEq/day under diuretics, diuretic therapy can be maintained, if tolerated, to delay ascites formation and prolong the interval between LVP.[2,10]

Transjugular Intrahepatic Portosystemic Shunt

TIPS is a shunt that communicates an intrahepatic portal branch with the outflow of the hepatic vein, leading to the decompression of the portal system and, thus, to the reduction of portal hypertension.[116] TIPS insertion is associated with an improvement of effective arterial blood volume and kidney hemodynamics that results in increased renal blood flow and increased urinary sodium excretion, leading to better control of ascites.[117–119] Nevertheless, it should be noted that a frequent complication of TIPS, when using uncovered stents, is the development of HE, in up to 50% of patients.[120] However, the incidence of HE is lower with the use of covered stents. In this regard, a recent randomized controlled trial (RCT) comparing TIPS (using covered stents) and repeated LVP for the management of recurrent ascites showed an increase in 1-year transplant-free survival in patients treated with TIPS, without a significant increase in the incidence of hepatic encephalopathy.[121] A recent study, in which TIPS was used for the prevention of variceal bleeding rather than for the management of ascites, reported an incidence of HE of 18% using 8 mm PTFE-covered stents.[122]

Data from six RCTs that investigated the effect of uncovered TIPS for the management of recurrent or refractory ascites,[123–128] and seven meta-analyses based on these previous RCTs,[129–135] show that TIPS is more effective than LVP for the management of recurrent or refractory ascites. However, TIPS was associated with a higher incidence of HE. Studies using covered stents are limited but also showed better control of ascites with TIPS as compared to LVP.

In terms of survival, these trials showed conflicting findings but overall suggest that in patients with recurrent ascites, TIPS insertion is associated with improved survival as compared to LVP. In contrast, in patients with refractory ascites, TIPS does not appear to confer survival benefit. On this background, current international guidelines recommend that patients with recurrent ascites should be evaluated for TIPS insertion, because TIPS improves survival and ascites control. However, in patients with refractory ascites, the treatment of choice is repeated LVP plus albumin, and only a small proportion should be considered for TIPS placement. The use of small-diameter-covered stents is recommended to reduce TIPS dysfunction and the incidence of hepatic encephalopathy.[2,136] After TIPS insertion, diuretic treatment, and dietary sodium restriction should be maintained until ascites resolution, and a close follow-up is recommended for early detection of potential complications.

A relevant drawback of all the previous studies that assessed the efficacy of TIPS for the treatment of ascites and that may explain the controversial results with respect to the effects of TIPS on survival and risk of adverse events is the fact that patients with recurrent and refractory ascites were mixed in different proportions. More research is needed to investigate the effect and applicability of TIPS in the population of patients with recurrent and/or with refractory ascites.

It should be noted that a careful selection of patients for TIPS is essential, because TIPS can be detrimental for patients with advanced cirrhosis. In fact, most trials evaluating the effect of TIPS for the management of ascites excluded patients with advanced cirrhosis and severe cardiopulmonary diseases. Overall, TIPS is not recommended in patients with bilirubin >3 mg/dL, platelet count <75 × 10^9/L, current HE > grade 2 or chronic HE, concomitant active infection, progressive renal failure, severe systolic or diastolic cardiac dysfunction, or pulmonary hypertension.[2]

Pharmacological Therapies

Besides diuretics, other drugs aimed at modifying the pathophysiology of ascites by improving circulatory function have been evaluated. Midodrine is an alpha-1 adrenergic agonist that has been shown to improve circulatory and kidney function in patients with cirrhosis and ascites.[137] With respect to other vasoconstrictors, midodrine has the advantage that it is active orally and, therefore, could be easily used as a chronic treatment in the outpatient setting. Small, randomized control trials and pilot studies have evaluated the effect of midodrine alone or midodrine in combination with other drugs (i.e., clonidine, V2-selective antagonists, octreotide, and albumin) for the management of ascites.[138–140] These studies showed that the administration of midodrine was associated with an improvement of systemic hemodynamics and better control of ascites in short-term follow-up. In contrast, a recent RCT that investigated the effect of midodrine together with albumin in the prevention of complications in patients with cirrhosis in the waiting list for liver transplantation showed no beneficial effect.[141] Overall, results on the efficacy of midodrine are controversial and will require further investigation before it can be recommended in clinical practice for the management of ascites.

Long-term intravenous administration of albumin has been also suggested as a therapy for the management of patients with decompensated cirrhosis. A recent randomized study showed that long-term administration of albumin (up to 18 months) together with diuretics was associated with improved control of ascites and increased survival.[142] However, given the limited information and the controversial results between this study and the previously cited RCT using midodrine and albumin, to date, albumin administration is still not recommended in the international guidelines as a long-term treatment for the management of patients with decompensated cirrhosis.[1,2]

Vaptans are selective antagonists of the kidney vasopressin V2 receptors that are active orally and induce an increase in the excretion of solute-free water.[143] Therefore the administration of vaptans results in an increase in serum sodium concentration in patients with hyponatremia. As described before, patients with advanced cirrhosis usually have increased levels of vasopressin that also contribute to fluid retention. On this background, vaptans were mainly investigated for the management of hypervolemic hyponatremia, but they were also evaluated for the management of ascites.[144,145] Results from phase 2 studies showed that the combination of satavaptan plus diuretics was effective in the control of ascites, as indicated by a decrease in body weight and delay in ascites recurrence after LVP.[145] However, phase 3 studies did not show beneficial effects of satavaptan in the control of ascites, either diuretic-responsive ascites or refractory ascites. Moreover, patients treated with satavaptan had increased morbidity and mortality compared to the placebo group.[146] Therefore satavaptan was withdrawn from development. As far as other vaptans, such as tolvaptan, there is no strong evidence that it is effective in the management of ascites.

Alfapump System

The Alfapump system was developed 10 years ago as a potential new treatment option for refractory ascites.[147] The Alfapump system is an automated pump that moves ascites from the peritoneal cavity to the urinary bladder where it is eliminated spontaneously with the urine. Therefore as LVP, it represents a symptomatic treatment for refractory ascites that does not modify pathogenetic mechanisms responsible for ascites formation.

The system is implanted subcutaneously in the abdominal wall with a surgical procedure under local or general anesthesia. The device consists of a battery-powered pump which is connected to a peritoneal catheter that collects ascitic fluid from the peritoneal cavity. Ascitic fluid is moved by the pump through another catheter that is implanted in the urinary bladder. In contrast to LVP, the system produces a continuous elimination of ascites from the peritoneal cavity to the bladder, the daily amount of which can be programmed externally through a wireless system. Based on the rationale of the continuous elimination of fluid, the administration of albumin has not been recommended to patients treated with this procedure.

To date, there are several prospective studies that have evaluated the efficacy and safety of the Alfapump system for the management of recurrent or refractory ascites.[147–150] The results of these studies show that the Alfapump system significantly reduces the number and volume of LVP in patients with cirrhosis and recurrent or refractory ascites compared to patients treated with standard of care.[147–150] However, the major concern is that treatment was associated with a high number of adverse events, including device-related adverse events and complications of cirrhosis, particularly AKI. Moreover, a single-center study evaluating kidney and circulatory function of a series of 10 patients treated with the Alfapump system showed a high incidence of AKI during follow-up together with an impairment of circulatory function, with a marked increase in PRA and plasma noradrenaline concentration.[149] Therefore although the Alfapump is effective for the removal of ascites, the high frequency of side effects, particularly AKI, casts doubts about its use as a procedure for the management of refractory ascites.

The Alfapump system is only recommended in patients in whom TIPS is not indicated and should only be performed in experienced centers. Moreover, considering the high incidence of side effects, close monitoring of these patients with serial assessment of kidney function is recommended.[2]

Management of Hepatic Hydrothorax

Liver transplantation represents the definitive treatment for patients with hepatic hydrothorax if there are no contraindications to the procedure.[1,2,151,152] The first-line medical treatment for the management of hepatic hydrothorax is diuretic therapy. However, hepatic hydrothorax usually persists despite appropriate diuretic treatment. Therapeutic thoracentesis is indicated as symptomatic treatment to improve dyspnea.[1,2] However, the effect of thoracentesis is transient, and patients usually require repeated therapeutic thoracenteses which increases the risk of side effects related to this technique. There are data showing that TIPS is effective in some patients with hepatic hydrothorax as definitive treatment or as a bridge to liver transplantation. Pleurodesis with different agents (e.g., talc and tetracycline) has shown efficacy, but it is also associated with high incidence of adverse events; therefore it is not recommented.[153]

Drugs Contraindicated in Patients With Cirrhosis and Ascites

The impaired systemic hemodynamics and labile kidney function characteristic of patients with cirrhosis and ascites make them prone to development of AKI.[10] Therefore the use of some drugs that may alter the homeostatic mechanisms operative in patients with cirrhosis and ascites may lead to development of adverse events, particularly AKI.

Nonsteroidal Anti-inflammatory Drugs

Nonsteroidal anti-inflammatory drugs (NSAIDs) are contraindicated in patients with cirrhosis and ascites. NSAIDs inhibit renal prostaglandin synthesis, and patients with cirrhosis and ascites show increased vasodilating renal prostaglandin synthesis to compensate the vasoconstrictor effect of angiotensin-II. Therefore the administration of NSAIDs leads to decreased PG synthesis, renal vasoconstriction, and development of AKI.[154] Because metamizole (dipyrone) also affects PG synthesis, its use is also not recommended in patients with decompensated cirrhosis.

Hypotensive Drugs

As described before, the activation of the renin-angiotensin-aldosterone system helps maintain arterial pressure within normal limits in patients with cirrhosis and ascites. Therefore the administrations of hypotensive drugs such as angiotensin-converting enzyme inhibitors, angiotensin II receptor antagonists, and α1-adrenergic blockers are also contraindicated in patients with cirrhosis and ascites, as they may lead to hypotension and, consequently, AKI.[155,156]

Aminoglycosides

Antibiotics with a high incidence of nephrotoxicity, such as aminoglycosides, should also be avoided in patients with cirrhosis and ascites except in selected cases in which other options are not available.[157]

Nonselective Beta-Blockers

Nonselective beta-blockers (NSBB) are drugs widely used for the primary and secondary prophylaxis of variceal bleeding in patients with cirrhosis.[158] These drugs have recently shown beneficial effects by reducing the incidence of decompensations, especially of ascites, and also long-term survival, in patients with compensated cirrhosis and portal hypertension.[159] However, in recent years, a great controversy has arisen regarding the safety of beta-blockers in patients with advanced cirrhosis, particularly those with refractory ascites and/or SBP. A study from France was the first to raise a warning, showing increased mortality and higher risk of post-paracentesis circulatory dysfunction (PPCD) in patients with refractory ascites under therapy with NSBB. The hypothesis raised by this study was that NSBB may induce arterial hypotension leading to further increased hyperdynamic circulation and impaired organ perfusion and development of complications, such as HRS.[160] Later studies did not confirm these findings, and even some of them reported increased survival in patients with decompensated cirrhosis under NSBB treatment.[161–164] Reasons for the beneficial effects of NSBB on survival in patients with decompensated cirrhosis may go beyond their hemodynamic effects and be related to the beneficial effects of NSBB reducing BT, intestinal permeability, and inflammation.[165,166] However, a recent study evaluated the effect of NSBB on systemic hemodynamics and cardiac and renal function in patients with refractory ascites. This study revealed that the administration of NSBB in patients with refractory ascites hampers cardiac output, decreases renal perfusion pressure, and leads to impairment of renal function.[167] In summary, whether the use of NSBB induces negative effects in patients with decompensated cirrhosis and particularly those with refractory ascites will need to be confirmed in future RCTs. Meanwhile, the recent Baveno VII consensus and the new EASL guidelines for the management of patients with decompensated cirrhosis recommend that in patients with progressive hypotension (systolic blood pressure <90 mm Hg or mean arterial pressure <65 mm Hg), or patients who develop intercurrent complications such as bleeding, sepsis, SBP or AKI, NSBB should be discontinued. After recovery of these complications, NSBB can be reinitiated. However, if contraindications persist or patients have no tolerance to these drugs, bleeding prophylaxis should be managed with non-pharmacological methods, particularly band ligation.[2,158]

SPONTANEOUS BACTERIAL PERITONITIS

Bacterial infections are a very common complication in patients with advanced cirrhosis and are associated with the development of other cirrhosis-related complications (i.e., AKI, HE) and poor prognosis.[168–171] Patients with cirrhosis are at high risk of developing bacterial infections; there is data showing that patients with cirrhosis have a risk of sepsis 2.6-fold higher than patients without underlying chronic liver disease.[172,173] The prevalence of bacterial infections in patients with cirrhosis admitted to the hospital ranges from 25% to 46%.[173–175]

As previously described, SBP is one of the major complications of patients with cirrhosis and ascites. SBP is defined as the bacterial infection of ascitic fluid, without any identifiable intra-abdominal treatable source of infection.[74,170] Together with urinary tract infection, SBP represents the most common type of infection in patients with advanced cirrhosis, followed by pneumonia, skin infections, and spontaneous bacteremia. Although the prognosis of SBP has improved in recent decades with increased awareness, early diagnosis, and appropriate management, mortality remains at approximately 20%.[173,176]

The clinical presentation of SBP is very heterogeneous. It can present with local symptoms, such as abdominal pain, vomiting, or diarrhea, together with other systemic signs such as markers of systemic inflammation (i.e., fever, high leukocyte count, high C-reactive protein, tachycardia), impairment of liver function, HE, AKI, or septic shock. It should be highlighted that some patients may only present with systemic signs without local abdominal symptoms. Moreover, patients with SBP can also be asymptomatic. Because of this heterogeneous and unpredictable clinical presentation, diagnostic paracentesis should always be performed in all patients with cirrhosis and ascites at hospital admission and whenever patients develop any complications, particularly bleeding, HE, and AKI, to rule out SBP.[1,2,74,168–171] Early diagnosis of SBP is essential to improve outcomes, as a delay in antibiotic treatment is associated with increased mortality.[177–179]

Pathophysiology

The increased risk of bacterial infections in patients with cirrhosis is related to multiple factors, particularly impairment in the gut-liver axis characterized by gut dysbiosis, increased intestinal permeability, and BT, together with immune dysfunction characteristic of patients with cirrhosis.[74,170,171] In the specific case of SBP, it is likely that local peritoneal factors may also play a role. Genetic factors may also contribute to the increased risk of infections in patients with cirrhosis. It has been described that patients with variants in the *NOD2* gene have an increased risk of SBP and impaired prognosis.[180]

Impairment of the Gut-Liver Axis

Cirrhosis is characterized by alterations at different levels of the gut-liver axis that result in pathological BT and spillover of endotoxins into the systemic circulation, thus facilitating the development of bacterial infections.[68] First, increased intestinal permeability exists in patients with cirrhosis that may be caused by several factors, including structural changes in the intestinal mucosa (e.g., congestion and edema), oxidative stress, and local inflammation.[68,181] Moreover, intestinal bacterial overgrowth has also been reported to facilitate BT and is the result, at least in part, of delayed intestinal transit time in patients with cirrhosis. Autonomic dysfunction, increased NO synthesis, and oxidative stress have been suggested to play a role in decreased gut motility in these patients.[68]

Finally, recent data suggest that the existence of rectal colonization by multidrug-resistant bacteria is associated with increased risk of infection by the colonizing resistant strains.[182] It is unknown whether these patients should be treated with conventional prophylactic strategies or, alternatively, whether new treatment algorithms should be recommended in this population. Further studies are needed.

Cirrhosis-Associated Immune Dysfunction

Advanced cirrhosis is associated with the development of abnormalities that lead to an impaired immune response, which represents a key factor in the high susceptibility of these patients to bacterial infections.[66] Liver damage leads to the impairment of the immune surveillance capacity of the organ. Moreover, there is a reduced hepatic synthesis of proteins involved in innate immunity and pattern recognition, thus causing decreased bactericidal capacity of phagocytic cells. Cirrhosis progression is also associated with impairment of circulating immune cell function. As described above, decompensated cirrhosis is associated with systemic inflammation which is characterized by persistent activation of circulating immune cells showing increased markers of activity, together with impaired phagocytic capacity.[66] As disease progresses, the immune dysfunction is characterized by features of immunodeficiency, which are associated with increased risk of bacterial infections in patients with more advanced liver disease and, particularly, in those with acute-on-chronic liver failure (ACLF).[174] ACLF is a recently described syndrome characterized by acute decompensation of cirrhosis associated with one or more organ failures; bacterial infections have been reported to be the main trigger of ACLF.[174]

Local Factors

Besides systemic factors, it is possible that local peritoneal factors may also influence the susceptibility of ascitic fluid infection in patients with cirrhosis. Although there is some conflicting data, it is generally believed that a low ascitic fluid protein concentration (<10–15 g/L) is associated with an increased risk of SBP.[74,183,184] In addition, there are few reports suggesting that peritoneal macrophages from patients with cirrhosis and ascites may have functional impairment, leading to decreased bacterial clearance capacity and, thus, increasing susceptibility to bacterial infections.[185,186] However, to date, information on local factors is limited.

Diagnosis

The diagnosis of SBP is based on neutrophil count in ascitic fluid. Peritoneal infection causes a local inflammatory reaction that increases the neutrophil count in ascites. The cutoff with the best sensitivity for the diagnosis of SBP is 250 cells/mm^3.[1,2,74] Although the gold standard technique for neutrophil count is considered to be the manual microscopy count, this is time-consuming and associated with interobserver variability. Therefore in most centers, this has been substituted by automated count, which has a high correlation with manual count. The use of reagent strips for the rapid diagnosis of SBP is not recommended due to its low sensitivity.[187]

Ascitic fluid culture should always be performed in blood culture bottles. It should be noted that a positive culture is not required for the diagnosis of SBP; however, if positive, ascitic fluid culture is very useful to guide antibiotic treatment. Despite the improvement in methods, ascitic fluid culture may be negative in up to 60% of patients with SBP. Patients with culture-negative SBP should be managed identically as those with culture-positive SBP.[1,2,168–171]

In some cases, patients may have positive ascitic fluid culture but neutrophil count is lower than 250 cells/mm^3. This condition is known as bacterascites. In most patients, bacterascites is due to spontaneous bacterial colonization of ascites, and it can be either asymptomatic or associated with symptoms such as abdominal pain or signs of systemic inflammation. Although in some patients, bacterascites may indicate a transient colonization and resolves spontaneously, in others, it may lead to development of SBP.[1,2,74]

Not infrequently (approximately 5%), patients with cirrhosis and ascites may also develop secondary bacterial peritonitis due to intestinal perforation, intra-abdominal infection, or other conditions. As described before, secondary bacterial peritonitis should be included in the differential diagnosis of ascites/SBP. Patients with secondary bacterial peritonitis usually have abdominal pain and the ascitic fluid shows very high neutrophil count, high protein concentration, and multiple organisms are isolated in the ascitic fluid culture. If there is suspicion of secondary bacterial peritonitis, an abdominal CT scan should be performed to confirm the diagnosis and surgery should be considered.[1,2,168–171]

Spontaneous Bacterial Empyema

Spontaneous infection of hepatic hydrothorax, known as SBE, is uncommon but should be considered in patients with pleural effusion and signs of infection. A retrospective analysis of 3390 patients with cirrhosis treated in a tertiary care university hospital during a 4-year follow-up reported an incidence of 16% of SBE among patients who already had hydrothorax at inclusion, with a mortality rate approaching 38%.[188] Diagnosis of this condition is based on a positive culture of the pleural fluid together with more than 250 neutrophils/mm^3, or negative culture with more than 500 neutrophils/mm^3 in the absence of lung infection.[2] Patients with spontaneous bacterial pleural empyema should be managed similarly to patients with SBP.

Management of Spontaneous Bacterial Peritonitis

General Management

After the diagnosis of SBP, it is essential to start antibiotic treatment as soon as possible because delayed appropriate antibiotic treatment is associated with increased mortality and increased risk of septic shock.[1,2,168–171] In fact, several studies have shown that the inefficacy of antibiotic treatment is one of the strongest predictors of mortality in patients with cirrhosis and bacterial infections.[175,178,179]

Vital signs should be assessed regularly in patients with SBP for early detection of circulatory impairment and septic shock. Patients with cirrhosis and bacterial infections have increased risk of developing other complications of the disease, particularly AKI and ACLF.[174,189] Therefore patients with SBP should be closely monitored, and kidney and liver function tests should be assessed frequently, daily, or every 2–3 days until SBP resolution.

Antibiotic Treatment

Considering that selecting the appropriate antibiotic treatment is essential to improve survival, the selection of the empirical antibiotic treatment should be based on: (1) risk of multidrug-resistant (MDR) bacteria; (2) severity of the infection; and (3) local epidemiology.[1,2,170,171,190] Moreover, it is important to implement strategies aimed at optimizing the antibiotics' pharmacokinetics/pharmacodynamics, such as the use of high doses within the first 48–72 hours and of continuous/extended infusions for β-lactams.

Overall, for community-acquired infections, the most common bacteria causing SBP are Gram-negative bacteria.[74,170] In this context, the empiric antibiotic treatment of choice for patients with community-acquired SBP is third-generation cephalosporins.[74,170] Alternative options included amoxicillin/clavulanic acid and quinolones.[1,170,171] However, quinolones are not recommended in patients who are taking these antibiotics for prophylaxis of SBP, due to high rate of quinolone-resistant bacteria.

Over the last several decades, there has been a marked increase in the number of infections caused by MDR bacteria, which are defined as bacteria with acquired nonsusceptibility to at least one agent in three or more antimicrobial categories. The major risk factors for development of infections caused by MDR include repeated hospitalizations or repeated contact with the health care environment, noninvasive procedures, and recent antibiotic treatment.[171,176] Patients with cirrhosis are at high risk of MDR bacterial infections as they usually have the described risk factors. Health care-associated (HCA) infections are defined as infections that developed in a hospital or other health care facility that first appear 48 hours or more after hospital admission, or within 30 days after having received health care,[191] represent a high risk for infection by MDR bacteria. In addition, MDR bacteria increase the mortality of SBP up to fourfold P.[176,178,179] Finally, the epidemiology of MDR bacteria is highly variable among different geographic areas.

Piperacillin/tazobactam is recommended as the first-line treatment in patients with HCA and nosocomial SBP in areas with low prevalence of MDR bacteria. By contrast, in patients with severe HCA SBP, defined by the existance of sepsis or septic shock, or in areas with high prevalence of MDR bacteria, the recommended empirical antibiotic treatment is meropenem alone or in combination with glycopeptides (IV teicoplanin) or daptomycin or linezolid.[1,171,190,192] Fig. 95.5 summarizes the management of SBP according to current guidelines for empirical antibiotic recommendations. It should be noted that narrowing antibiotic coverage according to bacterial susceptibility from positive cultures is recommended to avoid the spread of MDR bacteria.

New criteria have been validated in patients with cirrhosis and bacterial infections to assess the severity of the infection. Recently the Sepsis-3 criteria provided a new definition of sepsis for the general population: a life-threatening organ dysfunction caused by a dysregulated host response to infection. Organ dysfunction was defined as an acute change in the sequential organ failure assessment (SOFA) score $\geq$2 points.[192] Moreover, a new score, the quick SOFA (in which at least two of the following are present: alteration in mental status, systolic blood pressure $\leq$100 mm Hg, or respiratory rate $\geq$22/min) was suggested to screen for sepsis. These criteria have been validated in patients with cirrhosis and bacterial infections and were shown to be more accurate in predicting mortality than the previously used SIRS criteria.[193] Fig. 95.6 shows an algorithm for assessment of severity of SBP in patients with cirrhosis using these new criteria.

The efficacy of antibiotic treatment should be monitored by performing a control diagnostic paracentesis 48 hours after the initiation of treatment.[1,2,170,171] If at this point ascitic fluid neutrophil count has not decreased at least 25% with respect to pretreatment value, there is a high probability of failure to respond to therapy and, thus, poor outcome. If antibiotic treatment is not showing efficacy, it is likely that SBP may be caused by bacteria resistant to the current antibiotic, and therefore treatment should be modified according to culture results or empirically to treat MDR bacteria.[1,2,170,171] Recent studies describe an increase of the so-called extensively drug-resistant (XDR) bacteria, defined as nonsusceptibility to at least one agent in all but two or fewer antimicrobial categories, or pandrug-resistance (PDR) bacteria defined as a nonsusceptibility to all agents in all antimicrobial categories. An increase in these bacteria may reduce the efficacy of the broad-spectrum antibiotics currently recommended for patients with SBP.[176] Until very recently, treatment of infections caused by XDR or PDR bacteria previously required the use of antibiotics such as vancomycin, aminoglycosides or colistin, which are known to have a high risk of nephrotoxicity, especially in patients with cirrhosis and ascites. However, new antibiotic regimens are now available, such as ceftazidime-avibactam, which combines a third-generation cephalosporine with a β-lactamase inhibitor which inactivates the KPC carbapenemases and most OXA-48, or ceftolozane-tazobactam, a new combination of β-lactam/β-lactamase inhibitor with high affinity for *Pseudomonas aeruginosa*'s penicillin-binding proteins. New antibiotics are currently under evaluation and development. Overall, it should be pointed out that the earlier recommendations are based on current epidemiology and current international guidelines.

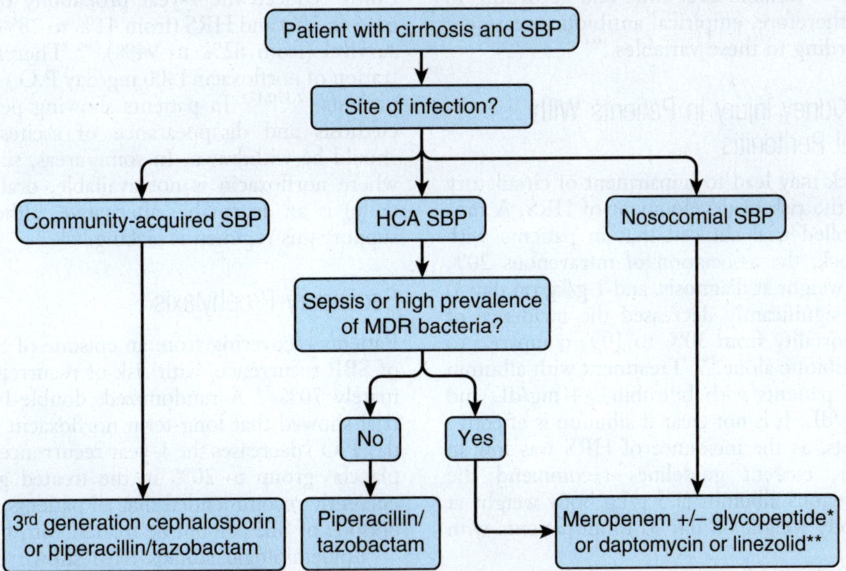

Fig. 95.5 Management of spontaneous bacterial peritonitis (SBP). This is an algorithm showing the current recommendations for empirical antibiotic treatment for patients with SBP. The selection of empirical antibiotic treatment should be based on the site of acquisition of infection and the severity of the episode of SBP (see Fig. 5). *SBP*, Spontaneous bacterial peritonitis; *HCA*, health care-associated infections; *MDR*, multidrug resistant. *Intravenous vancomycin in areas with a high prevalence of methicillin-resistant *Staphylococcus aureus* (MRSA) and vancomycin-susceptible enterococci. **Daptomycin or linezolid should be used in areas with a high prevalence of vancomycin-resistant enterococci. (Adapted from EASL Clinical Practice Guidelines for the management of patients with decompensated cirrhosis. *J Hepatol*. 2018. doi: 10.1016/j.jhep.2018.03.024; Piano S, Brocca A, Mareso S, Angeli P. Infections complicating cirrhosis. *Liver Int*. 2018;38(suppl 1):126–133.)

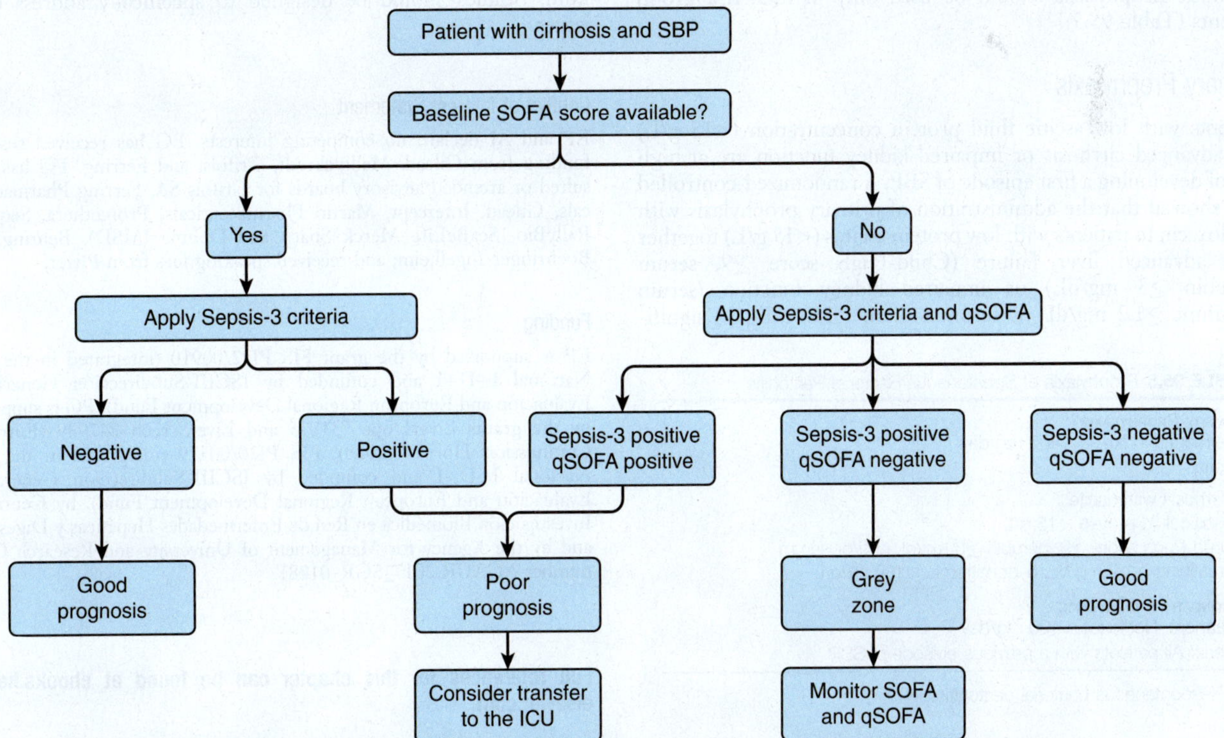

Fig. 95.6 Algorithm to assess the severity of bacterial infections in patients with cirrhosis using the Sepsis-3 and qSOFA criteria. These criteria have been described in the general population and have been recently validated in patients with cirrhosis and bacterial infections. *SBP*, Spontaneous bacterial peritonitis; *SOFA*, sequential organ failure assessment score; *qSOFA*, quick SOFA score; *ICU*, intensive care unit. (Adapted from EASL Clinical Practice Guidelines for the management of patients with decompensated cirrhosis. *J Hepatol*. 2018. doi: 10.1016/j.jhep.2018.03.024; Piano S, Brocca A, Mareso S, Angeli P. Infections complicating cirrhosis. *Liver Int*. 2018;38(suppl 1):126–133.)

However, epidemiology is variable over time and according to geographic areas, and, therefore, empirical antibiotic treatment should be adapted according to these variables.[194]

Prevention of Acute Kidney Injury in Patients With Spontaneous Bacterial Peritonitis

SBP without septic shock may lead to impairment of circulatory dysfunction, increasing the risk of development of HRS. A randomized placebo-controlled trial showed that in patients with SBP without septic shock, the association of intravenous 20% albumin (1.5 g/kg body weight at diagnosis, and 1 g/kg on day 3) to antibiotic treatment significantly decreased the incidence of HRS and the risk of mortality from 30% to 10% compared to patients treated with antibiotic alone.[195] Treatment with albumin is particularly useful in patients with bilirubin >4 mg/dL and serum creatinine >1 mg/dL. It is not clear if albumin is effective in the remaining patients, as the incidence of HRS was low in both groups. However, current guidelines recommend the administration of intravenous albumin (1.5 g/kg body weight at diagnosis and 1 g/kg body weight on day 3) to all patients with SBP.[1,2]

Prophylaxis

The goal of SBP prophylaxis is to reduce the incidence of the SBP in patients at high risk of infection. Considering that the translocation of gram-negative bacteria from the gut plays a key role in the pathophysiology of SBP, prophylaxis is aimed at achieving a selective intestinal decontamination by reducing Gram-negative bacteria. Currently, norfloxacin is the treatment of choice.[1,2,170,171] Although clear beneficial effects of prophylaxis strategies have been described, long-term antibiotic administration may lead to the emergence of MDR bacteria. Therefore antibiotic prophylaxis should be used only in high-risk group patients (Table 95.5).

Primary Prophylaxis

Patients with low ascitic fluid protein concentration (<15 g/L) and advanced cirrhosis or impaired kidney function are at high risk of developing a first episode of SBP. A randomized-controlled trial showed that the administration of primary prophylaxis with norfloxacin to patients with low protein ascites (<15 g/L) together with advanced liver failure (Child-Pugh score ≥9, serum bilirubin ≥3 mg/dL) or impaired kidney function (serum creatinine ≥1.2 mg/dL or serum sodium <130 mEq/L) significantly reduced the 1-year probability of developing SBP (from 61% to 7%) and HRS (from 41% to 28%) and improved 3-month survival (from 62% to 94%).[196] Therefore long-term administration of norfloxacin (400 mg/day P.O.) is recommended in these patients.[1,2,170,171] In patients showing persistent improvement of cirrhosis and disappearance of ascites, antibiotic prophylaxis should be withdrawn. In some areas, such as the United States, where norfloxacin is not available, oral ciprofloxacin (500 mg/daily) is an acceptable alternative, although direct evidence to support this regimen is lacking.[1,74]

TABLE 95.5 Prophylaxis of Spontaneous Bacterial Peritonitis

Primary Prophylaxis
Treatment: Norfloxacin 400 mg/day
Criteria:

- Cirrhosis with ascites
- Ascitic fluid protein <15 g/L
- Child Pugh score ≥9, bilirubin ≥3 mg/dL and/or serum creatinine ≥1.2 mg/dL, hyponatremia <130 mEq/L

Secondary Prophylaxis
Treatment: Norfloxacin 400 mg/day
Criteria: All patients with a previous episode of SBP

SBP, Spontaneous bacterial peritonitis.

Secondary Prophylaxis

Patients recovering from an episode of SBP are at very high risk of SBP recurrence, with risk of recurrence at 1 year of approximately 70%.[74] A randomized, double-blind, placebo-controlled trial showed that long-term norfloxacin administration (400 mg/day P.O.) decreases the 1-year recurrence of SBP from 68% in the placebo group to 20% in the treated group.[197] Therefore it is currently recommended that all patients who have developed one episode of SBP should be treated with norfloxacin.[1,2]

Epidemiologic studies have shown that long-term administration of norfloxacin increases 2.7-fold the risk of developing infections caused by MDR bacteria.[176] Rifaximin has been proposed as a potential alternative prophylactic treatment. A case-control study described a significant benefit of rifaximin in the prevention of SBP when used in patients for HE prevention.[198] Rifaximin could be theoretically effective in preventing the development of SBP. However, to date, data specifically assessing the efficacy and safety of rifaximin in primary and secondary prophylaxis of SBP are not available.[2,171] In addition, it is not known whether patients at risk of SBP under rifaximin treatment should be started on norfloxacin to prevent SBP, or if norfloxacin should be stopped in patients who require treatment with rifaximin. Studies should be designed to specifically address these issues.

Conflict of Interest Statement

EP and AJ declare no competing interests. PG has received research funding from Gilead, Mallinckrodt, Grifols, and Ferring. PG has consulted or attended advisory boards for Grifols SA, Ferring Pharmaceuticals, Gilead, Intercept, Martin Pharmaceuticals, Promethera, Sequana, RallyBio, SeaBeLife Merck Sharp and Dohme (MSD), Behring, and Boehringer-Ingelheim; and received speaking fees from Pfizer.

Funding

EP is supported by the grant FIS PI22/00910 (integrated in the Plan Nacional I+D+I and cofunded by ISCIII-Subdirección General de Evaluación and European Regional Development Fund). PG is supported by the grants LiverHope 731875 and LiverScreen 847989 (European Commission Horizon 2020), FIS PI20/00579 (integrated in the Plan Nacional I+D+I and cofunded by ISCIII-Subdirección General de Evaluación and European Regional Development Fund), by Centro de Investigación Biomédica en Red de Enfermedades Hepáticas y Digestivas, and by the Agency for Management of University and Research Grant number AGAUR 2017_SGR_01281.

Full references for this chapter can be found at ebooks.health.elsevier.com.

96 Hepatic Encephalopathy, Hepatorenal Syndrome, Hepatopulmonary Syndrome, and Other Systemic Complications of Liver Disease

Shoma Bommena, Rohit Nathani, Michael B. Fallon

IN THIS CHAPTER

Chronic liver disease and acute liver failure (ALF) disrupt normal homeostasis and cause systemic manifestations that may dominate the clinical features of liver disease. Most of these extrahepatic syndromes are reversible with liver transplantation (LT).

HEPATIC ENCEPHALOPATHY

The term *hepatic encephalopathy* (HE) encompasses a wide array of transient and subtle reversible neurologic and psychiatric manifestations usually found in patients with chronic liver disease and portal hypertension but also seen in patients with ALF. HE develops in 50%–70% of patients with cirrhosis and is a major cause of health care utilization and socioeconomic burden in patients and their caregivers.[1] The occurrence of HE is a poor prognostic indicator, with projected 1- and 3-year survival rates of 42% and 23%, respectively, without LT.[2] Symptoms may range from mild neurocognitive disturbances to overt coma.[3,4] HE is often triggered by an inciting event that increases the serum ammonia level. The precise underlying pathophysiologic mechanisms are not well understood, and the mainstay of therapy is the elimination of the precipitating event and excess ammonia.[5] LT generally reverses HE.

Pathophysiology

A number of factors, occurring alone or in combination, have been implicated in the development of HE. These factors may differ in acute and chronic liver disease and include the production of neurotoxins, abnormal neurotransmission, and altered permeability of the blood-brain barrier (Fig. 96.1). The best described neurotoxin involved in HE is ammonia, which is produced primarily in the colon, where bacteria metabolize proteins and other nitrogen-based products into ammonia. In addition, enterocytes, which have high glutaminase activity, synthesize ammonia from the intestinal breakdown of the amino acid glutamine.[5–7] Once produced, ammonia enters the portal circulation and, under normal conditions with an intact urea cycle, is metabolized and cleared by hepatocytes. Reduced hepatocyte function and portosystemic shunting in cirrhosis and portal hypertension contribute to increased circulating ammonia levels. Arterial hyperammonemia is observed in up to 90% of patients with HE, although the serum level is neither a sensitive nor specific indicator of its presence.[8–10] Acute hyperammonemia appears to have a direct effect on brain edema, astrocyte swelling, and the transport of neuronally active compounds such as myoinositol, thereby contributing to HE.[11–13] Ammonia may also directly induce an inflammatory response in astrocytes, leading to swelling and cytotoxic brain edema.[14] Finally, distinct allelic mutations in the glutaminase gene increase the risk for overt HE, independent of the hepatic synthetic function, or the presence of minimal HE. This risk may be mediated by enhanced glutaminase transcriptional activity that results in increased levels of ammonia and glutamate.[15]

Alterations in other CNS neurotransmitters, receptors, and neurotoxins may also contribute to HE. Although CNS benzodiazepine levels and γ-aminobutyric acid (GABA) receptor concentrations are unchanged in experimental models, increased sensitivity of the astrocyte (peripheral-type) benzodiazepine receptor, potentiated by neurosteroids, enhances activation of the GABA-benzodiazepine system and causes neuroinhibition.[16] The GABA receptor-modulating steroid antagonists are under clinical investigation as potential HE treatment.[16] In addition, a potential role for bile acid-mediated neuroinflammation in HE has been found in experimental models, although whether modulating bile acid levels or composition influences HE is unknown.[17] Manganese deposition in basal ganglia resulting from impaired biliary excretion and portosystemic shunting in cirrhosis has also been implicated in the psychomotor impairment of HE.[16,18] However, the specific mechanisms of manganese neurotoxicity remain unknown. Hyponatremia is also common in cirrhosis and may alter cognition and exacerbate HE through osmotic effects.[19] Recurrent episodes of overt HE might cause residual neurocognitive impairment, possibly related to neuronal cell death.[16]

Bacterial translocation-driven systemic inflammation and oxidative stress contribute to the severity of HE by compromising the blood-brain barrier and increasing ammonia influx. Increased blood-brain barrier permeability has been shown to increase the uptake and extraction of ammonia by the cerebellum and basal ganglia.[8–10]

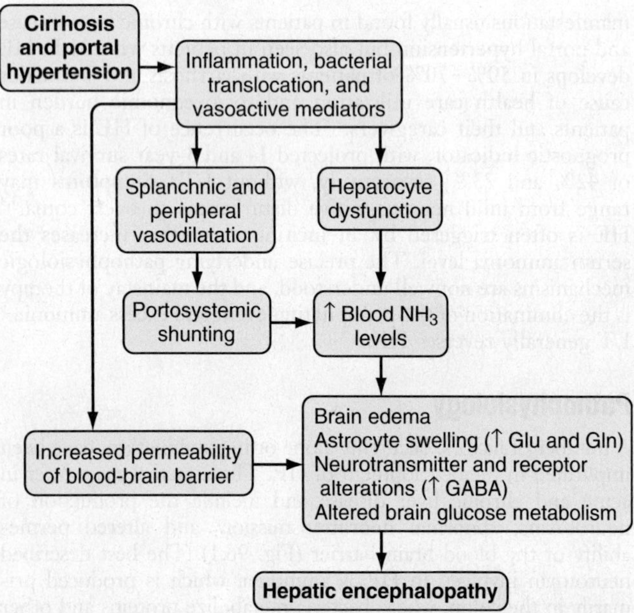

Fig. 96.1 Proposed pathophysiology of hepatic encephalopathy. *GABA,* γ-Aminobutyric acid; *Gln,* glutamine; *Glu,* glutamate; *NH_3,* ammonia.

Clinical Features and Classification

HE may present as a spectrum of reversible neurocognitive symptoms and signs that range from mild changes in cognition to profound coma in patients with acute or chronic liver disease. HE is often precipitated by an inciting event (e.g., gastrointestinal bleeding, electrolyte abnormalities, infections, medications, and dehydration). In addition, patients with sarcopenia are at increased risk of HE.[20] The diagnosis of HE requires careful consideration in the appropriate clinical situation. Occasionally, HE may be the initial presentation of chronic liver disease. Subtle findings in HE may include forgetfulness, alterations in handwriting, difficulty with driving, and reversal of the sleep-wake cycle.[21,22] As HE worsens, findings may include asterixis, agitation, disinhibited behavior, seizures, and coma. Other etiologies of altered mental status, including hypoglycemia, hyponatremia, medication ingestion, and structural intracranial abnormalities resulting from coagulopathy or trauma, should be considered. Unless focal neurologic deficits are present, the likelihood of intracranial hemorrhage is low.[23]

HE is classified according to four factors: the type of underlying disease, the severity of manifestations, time course, and precipitating factors.[24] There are three major categories of underlying disease associated with HE: type A, associated with ALF; type B, associated with portosystemic shunts without liver disease; and type C, associated with chronic and end-stage liver disease and portal hypertension.[4] Type C HE is the most common type and has historically been graded from 0 to 4 based on the West Haven criteria (Table 96.1).[25] The SONIC (spectrum of neurocognitive impairment in cirrhosis) nomenclature expands the delineation of the severity of HE to reflect the wide spectrum of clinical findings and allows more precise clinical and investigative classification. Based on the SONIC classification, cirrhotic

TABLE 96.1 Clinical Stages of Hepatic Encephalopathy: The West Haven Criteria and the SONIC Classification

West Haven Criteria			SONIC Classification			
Grade	**Intellectual Function**	**Neuromuscular Function**	**Classification**	**Mental Status**	**Special Tests**	**Asterixis**
0	Normal	Normal	Unimpaired	Unimpaired	Normal	Absent
Minimal	Normal examination findings; subtle changes in work or driving	Minor abnormalities of visual perception or on psychometric or number tests	Covert HE	Unimpaired	Abnormal	Absent
1	Personality changes, attention deficits, irritability, depressed state	Tremor and incoordination				
2	Changes in sleep-wake cycle, lethargy, mood and behavioral changes, cognitive dysfunction	Asterixis, ataxic gait, speech abnormalities (slow and slurred)	Overt HE	Impaired	Abnormal	Present (absent in coma)
3	Altered level of consciousness (somnolence), confusion, disorientation, and amnesia	Muscular rigidity, nystagmus, clonus, Babinski sign, hyporeflexia				
4	Stupor and coma	Oculocephalic reflex, unresponsiveness to noxious stimuli				

SONIC, Spectrum of neurocognitive impairment in cirrhosis.
From Ferenci P, Lockwood A, Mullen K, et al. Hepatic encephalopathy—definition, nomenclature, diagnosis, and quantification: final report of the working party at the 11th World Congresses of Gastroenterology, Vienna, 1998. *Hepatology*. 2002;35:716–721; Bajaj JS, Cordoba J, Mullen KD, et al. The design of clinical trials in hepatic encephalopathy—an International Society for Hepatic Encephalopathy and Nitrogen Metabolism (ISHEN) consensus statement. *Aliment Pharmacol Ther*. 2011;33:739–747.

patients are divided into (1) unimpaired, (2) covert (or minimal) HE, and (3) overt HE.[26] Unimpaired patients have no clinical, neurophysiologic, or neuropsychometric abnormalities; patients with covert or minimal HE (clinically normal patients with abnormal cognition or neurophysiologic test results) align with grade 1 HE by the West Haven criteria; and patients with overt HE have grade 2 HE or higher by the West Haven criteria (see Table 96.1). This classification eliminates the need to distinguish minimal HE from grade 1 HE and takes advantage of the recognition that disorientation, specifically to time, is a distinct clinical feature that distinguishes grade 1 from grade 2 HE and covert from overt HE.[3,27] HE is also subdivided by time course into (1) episodic, recurrent HE (multiple episodes within a time interval of 6 months) and (2) persistent (altered behavior always present with relapses of overt HE). Finally, HE is divided into spontaneous or secondary based on the presence or absence of precipitating factors such as infections, gastrointestinal bleeding, medications, and others.[24,28] The clinical, pathophysiological, and prognostic features of HE are not homogeneous among all overt HE patients, with marked differences in those with and without acute-on-chronic liver failure (ACLF).[29] Typically, patients with ACLF and HE have higher ammonia levels, more systemic inflammation, more distinct astrocytic swelling in the brain, and worse survival than those without ACLF.[16,30]

BOX 96.1 Differential Diagnosis of Hyperammonemia

- ALF
- Chronic kidney disease
- Cigarette smoking
- Cirrhosis
- GI bleeding
- Inborn errors of metabolism
  - Proline metabolism disorders
  - Urea cycle defects (e.g., carbamoyl phosphate synthetase I deficiency, ornithine transcarbamylase deficiency, argininosuccinate lyase deficiency, *N*-acetylglutamate synthetase deficiency)
- Medications/toxins
  - Alcohol
  - Diuretics (e.g., acetazolamide)
  - Narcotics
  - Valproic acid
- Muscle exertion and ischemia
- Portosystemic shunts
- Technique and conditions of blood sampling
  - High body temperature
  - High protein diet
  - Tourniquet use

Diagnosis

No specific laboratory findings definitively indicate the presence of HE. Serum ammonia levels are commonly measured in patients with cirrhosis and portal hypertension but are not sensitive or specific for the presence of HE. They may, however, be useful in patients with cirrhosis and suspected delirium, where a normal serum ammonia level does not favor the diagnosis of HE.[31] In patients with ALF, higher arterial ammonia levels are associated with the risk of developing intracranial hypertension and cerebral edema, hence a helpful indicator.[16,32] Other factors such as GI bleeding, ingestion of certain medications (e.g., diuretics, alcohol, narcotics, and valproic acid), use of a tourniquet when blood is drawn, and delayed processing and cooling of a blood sample may raise the blood ammonia level irrespective of the presence of HE.[33,34] Measurement of arterial ammonia offers no advantage over venous ammonia levels in patients with chronic liver disease.[13,35–37] Serum ammonia levels may be a helpful indicator of HE in the absence of cirrhosis and portal hypertension, such as in patients with metabolic disorders that influence ammonia generation or metabolism, including urea cycle disorders and disorders of proline metabolism (Box 96.1).[38,39]

The development of standardized neuropsychometric and neurocognitive tests has led to the recognition that routine evaluation is insensitive in diagnosing clinically relevant HE.[40–44] Simple tests such as the psychometric HE score and the Stroop test (an evaluation of cognitive flexibility and psychomotor speed using either paper-and-pencil or an electronic format, EncephalApp) evaluate attention, concentration, fine motor skills, and orientation and are specific for the diagnosis of HE.[40,45,46] These tests are particularly useful for detecting and documenting the adverse effects of minimal HE on quality of life, driving ability, and the risk of developing overt HE. Treatment of minimal HE improves these adverse effects.[22,47,48] A smartphone-based application (EncephalApp) is a streamlined version of the Stroop test validated for use in detecting covert/minimal HE.[49]

Several other novel imaging and functional tests for diagnosing HE have also been studied. Magnetic resonance (MR) spectroscopy and MR T1 mapping with partial inversion recovery have been used to measure clinically relevant parameters of brain dysfunction.[40,41] In one study, abnormal signal intensity in basal ganglia correlated with neuropsychiatric dysfunction in patients with cirrhosis.[50] Patients with ACLF have MRI evidence of cytotoxic and interstitial brain edema.[51] PET studies reveal brain findings of HE mechanisms, including increased ammonia uptake, alterations in cerebral blood flow, neuroinflammation, and increased expression of peripheral benzodiazepine binding sites by glial cells.[52,53] The critical flicker frequency test, a simple light-based test that assesses cerebral cortex function, is a reliable marker of minimal HE. Whether these functional tests will become useful in clinical practice is still unknown, and brain imaging is currently used clinically to exclude other causes of cerebral dysfunction.[41–43]

Treatment

The treatment of HE is directed primarily toward eliminating or correcting precipitating factors (e.g., bleeding, infection, hypokalemia, medications, and dehydration), reducing blood ammonia levels, and avoiding the toxic effects of ammonia on the central nervous system. In the past, dietary protein restriction was considered an important component of treating HE. Subsequent work has suggested that limiting protein-calorie intake is not beneficial in patients with HE.[54–56] Vegetable and dairy proteins may be preferable to animal proteins because of a more favorable calorie-to-nitrogen ratio. Branched-chain amino acid supplementation may benefit HE but has not been shown to affect mortality or quality of life.[57]

Nonabsorbable disaccharides have been the cornerstone of treatment for HE. Oral lactulose or lactitol (the latter is unavailable in the United States) is metabolized by colonic bacteria into byproducts that appear to have beneficial effects by causing catharsis and reducing intestinal pH, thereby inhibiting ammonia absorption.[58] A systematic review of 38 RCTs showed that nonabsorbable disaccharides benefit HE and reduce liver failure, hepatorenal syndrome (HRS), and variceal bleeding compared to no intervention.[59] Side effects are common and include abdominal cramping, flatulence, diarrhea, and electrolyte imbalance. Lactulose may be administered per rectum (as a retention enema) to patients at increased risk of aspiration, although the efficacy of administration by enema has not been evaluated and is less preferred due to inconvenience. Kristalose is powdered lactulose for reconstitution prior to use. It is an option in patients with noncompliance with liquid lactulose, as it is better tolerated relative to the liquid form.[60]

Oral antibiotics have also been used to treat HE, aiming to modify intestinal flora and lower stool pH to enhance the excretion of ammonia. Antibiotics are generally used as second-line agents after lactulose or in patients intolerant of nonabsorbable disaccharides. Rifaximin, given orally at a dose of 550 mg twice daily, was approved in 2010 for the treatment of chronic HE and reduction in the risk of recurrence of overt HE in patients with advanced liver disease.[61,62] Evidence on the use of rifaximin as monotherapy is limited. The combination of lactulose and rifaximin was more effective than lactulose alone in a double-blinded RCT of 126 patients with overt HE.[63] The tolerability and side-effect profile of rifaximin are superior to those of lactulose, albeit at a greater financial cost.[64–68] Other antibiotics, including neomycin, metronidazole, and vancomycin, have been studied in small trials and case series, but their effectiveness in patients with chronic HE is not established.

A single-center RCT conducted among 50 patients compared the efficacy of a single dose of polyethylene glycol 3350-electrolyte solution (PEG) versus standard treatment with lactulose in patients with cirrhosis admitted for overt HE. Results showed that PEG significantly improved HE grade in the first 24 hours, caused more rapid HE resolution, and shortened the length of stay.[69] A recent systematic review and meta-analysis of 4 single-center RCTs found similar results.[70] However, more multicenter studies are needed before recommending its widespread use. Several other agents that may modify intestinal flora and modulate the generation or intestinal absorption of ammonia have been evaluated as potential treatments for HE. Acarbose, an intestinal α-glucosidase inhibitor used to treat type 2 diabetes mellitus, inhibits the intestinal absorption of carbohydrates and glucose and results in their enhanced delivery to the colon. As a result, the ratio of saccharolytic to proteolytic bacterial flora is increased, and blood ammonia levels are decreased. A randomized controlled, double-blind crossover trial has demonstrated that acarbose improves mild HE in patients with cirrhosis and adult-onset diabetes mellitus.[71] However, rare cases of acute hepatitis have been reported with acarbose use.[72,73] Probiotic regimens have been used to modify intestinal flora and diminish ammonia generation. Several studies have suggested that these agents may benefit humans with mild HE.[74–80] A Cochrane database review found that probiotics likely improve recovery, overt HE, quality of life, and plasma ammonia levels, but not mortality; however, the quality of evidence was low.[81]

Another Cochrane review showed improvement in HE with branched chained amino acids without improving mortality or quality of life.[57] A recent double-blind RCT of 146 patients with overt HE showed the combination of L-ornithine L-aspartate (LOLA), which activates the urea cycle and enhances ammonia clearance, given as continuous intravenous infusion with oral lactulose and rifaximin to be superior to lactulose and rifaximin alone in reducing HE grade and 28-day mortality.[82] Oral LOLA has not been shown to be effective for HE treatment.[24] Strategies to enhance ammonia clearance may also be helpful in the treatment of HE. A combination preparation of sodium benzoate-sodium phenylacetate, sodium phenylbutyrate, and carglumic acid is approved by the FDA for treating hyperammonemia resulting from urea cycle enzyme defects and may improve HE in patients with cirrhosis. Administration of sodium benzoate, however, results in a high sodium load, and the efficacy of this agent is not established.[83] Oral zinc supplementation has been used because zinc deficiency is common in patients with cirrhosis and because zinc increases the activity of ornithine transcarbamylase, an enzyme in the urea cycle, which may also improve HE. However, clear efficacy has not been established.[84–86] The benefit of fecal microbiota transplantation (FMT) to improve cognition and gut dysbiosis in patients with cirrhosis and recurrent HE has also been reported in an RCT.[87] Similarly, a systematic review on the effect of FMT as a treatment for HE showed a beneficial effect of FMT with the limitation of a small number of included studies and a lack of long-term follow-up.[88] Another randomized, single-blind, placebo-controlled clinical trial showed the safety and tolerability of oral FMT capsules, which was associated with improved mucosal and stool microbial composition and improvement in EncephalApp performance in patients with cirrhosis and recurrent HE.[89] More extensive controlled studies with longer follow-up periods are needed. Finally, although shunt embolization is helpful in patients with poorly controlled HE with spontaneous portosystemic shunts, it should be considered a bridge to transplantation due to greater chances of developing portal hypertensive complications.[16,90]

HEPATORENAL SYNDROME

The term HRS was first used in 1939 to describe acute kidney injury (AKI), mainly acute tubular necrosis (ATN) or interstitial nephritis, in a group of patients who had undergone biliary tract surgery.[91] As pathophysiologic mechanisms became better elucidated, HRS was recognized as part of a cascade of events associated with intense dilatation of the splanchnic arterial vasculature in the setting of cirrhosis or acute liver injury resulting in profound renal arterial vasoconstriction and progressive renal failure. Experimental models of renal ischemia demonstrate that secondary structural injury and renal tubular damage develop.[92,93] Serum biomarkers of renal tubular injury[92,94] and urinary biomarkers of tubular damage (urinary neutrophil gelatin-associated lipocalin, uNGAL) were found to be increased in patients with HRS, although to a lesser degree than in ATN.[95,96] Hence, the previous concept of HRS being a purely functional disorder with normal kidney histology has evolved to include an additional component of renal parenchymal injury.[95] Function may be restored by correction of portal hypertension, LT, and, in some cases, medical therapy.[97–99]

Acute renal dysfunction occurs in 15%–25% of hospitalized patients with cirrhosis (see also Chapter 95),[100,101] and HRS is found in 10%–30% of such patients. It appears to be an extension of the pathophysiology of prerenal azotemia and, therefore, potentially reversible.[101,102] The annual frequency of HRS in cirrhotic patients with ascites is roughly 8% and, in some reports, as high as 40%.[103–105] HRS develops in approximately 30% of cirrhotic patients who are admitted with spontaneous bacterial peritonitis (SBP) or other infections, 25% who are hospitalized with severe alcohol associated hepatitis, and 10% who require serial large-volume paracenteses (see Chapter 95).[106] No significant gender and racial differences in HRS were found in a nationwide inpatient sample study.[107,108] The observation that morbidity and mortality remain high once the syndrome is established has led to a focus on the prevention, early diagnosis, and therapy of renal dysfunction in cirrhosis.[103]

Pathophysiology

The pathophysiology of HRS is complex, and our understanding has evolved over several decades. The important components contributing to initiating and perpetuating altered renal perfusion involve systemic and renal hemodynamic and inflammatory alterations that trigger renal vasoconstriction and tubular damage (Fig. 96.2).

Splanchnic Arterial Vasodilatation

Splanchnic and systemic arterial vasodilatation is a hallmark of the progression of portal hypertension in patients with cirrhosis and leads to decreased effective circulating blood volume and,

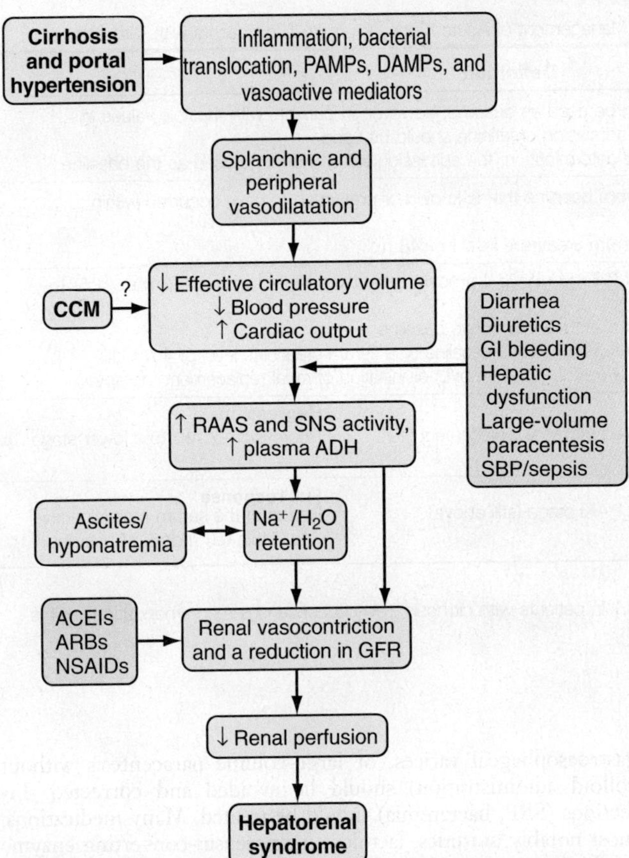

Fig. 96.2 Proposed pathophysiology and triggers of hepatorenal syndrome. *ACEIs,* Angiotensin-converting enzyme inhibitors; *ADH,* antidiuretic hormone; *ARBs,* angiotensin receptor blockers; *CCM,* cirrhotic cardiomyopathy; *DAMPs,* danger-associated molecular patterns; *RAAS,* renin-angiotensin-aldosterone system; *GFR,* glomerular filtration rate; *PAMPs* pathogen-associated molecular patterns*; RAAS,* renin-angiotensin-aldosterone system; *SNS,* sympathetic nervous system.

ultimately, a decrease in blood pressure. This process is mediated by several endogenous substances, including nitric oxide (NO), carbon monoxide (CO), glucagon, prostacyclin, adrenomedullin, and endogenous opiates that are released or act locally in the vasculature in response to mechanical and inflammatory signals.[103,109–111] In the early stages of portal hypertension, increases in heart rate and cardiac output compensate for the decrease in effective circulatory volume and create hyperdynamic circulation.[112] As liver disease and splanchnic vasodilatation progress, additional compensatory mechanisms are activated.

Renal Arterial Vasoconstriction

Splanchnic and systemic vasodilatation leads to compensatory renal vasoconstriction and renal sodium and water retention, leading to hyponatremia and ascites formation. These responses are mediated by stimulation of the sympathetic nervous system, activation of the renin-angiotensin-aldosterone system, nonosmotic release and activity of arginine vasopressin, and altered levels of intrarenal vasoactive mediators.[105,113,114] Ultimately, the balance between vasoconstrictive responses in the kidney and systemic and splanchnic vasodilatation is lost, leading to a prominent increase in renal vascular resistance, a decrease in renal perfusion, and a reduction in the glomerular filtration rate (GFR).[99,112] Finally, the functional syndrome of HRS induced by intense renal vasoconstriction may progress to tubular damage and structural injury.

Cardiac Dysfunction

Impaired cardiac function has also been implicated in renal hypoperfusion in patients with HRS.[115] In one prospective study, the development of HRS in cirrhotic patients correlated with more severe arterial vasodilatation and lower cardiac output.[116] In another study of patients being treated with effective therapy for SBP, renal dysfunction was more common in those with lower cardiac output and lower arterial pressure measurements.[117] These data identify impaired cardiac output as a contributor to HRS risk in patients with cirrhosis.[118]

Systemic Inflammation

Activation of innate host immunity in response to bacterial translocation and cellular injury in cirrhosis, particularly through pathogen-associated molecular patterns (PAMPs) and damage-associated molecular patterns (DAMPs) and subsequent cytokine activation, is recognized to contribute to hemodynamic alterations in AKI.[95,119] In addition to the impact on renal hemodynamics from systemic circulatory dysfunction, activation of PAMPs and DAMPs, specifically toll-like receptor 4, may cause direct renal tubular damage.[120] Cholestasis and elevated bile acid levels may also cause renal inflammation and bile cast nephropathy-related tubular damage in the setting of AKI.[121]

Clinical Features and Diagnosis

HRS is a functional disorder; therefore laboratory and imaging studies alone are insufficient for diagnosis. A high index of clinical suspicion and exclusion of other potential causes of kidney injury is required. The majority of patients with HRS have no renal symptoms, although some may report decreased urine output. AKI causes a decrease in GFR and increases the blood urea nitrogen level and may result in HE as the initial clinical presentation of HRS.

Early diagnostic criteria for HRS included an increase in the serum creatinine level by 50% above baseline to a level higher than 1.5 mg/dL (133 μmol/L).[103] Although this definition provided standardization, a subset of patients with cirrhosis and end-stage liver disease have a profound decrease in muscle mass and urea synthesis. This, in turn, results in reduced serum creatinine and blood urea nitrogen levels, thereby potentially delaying the recognition of HRS.[106,122] Therefore in a 2015 position paper, the International Club of Ascites (ICA) developed updated diagnostic criteria in which new definitions of AKI were incorporated[123]: (1) cirrhosis with ascites; (2) diagnosis of AKI according to ICA-AKI criteria (Table 96.2); (3) lack of response after at least two days of diuretic withdrawal and volume expansion with albumin (1 g/kg of body weight/day, to a maximum of 100 g/day); (4) absence of shock; (5) lack of current or recent treatment with nephrotoxic drugs; and (6) absence of parenchymal kidney disease as indicated by proteinuria of more than 500 mg/day, microhematuria (>50 red blood cells/high-power field), urinary injury biomarkers if available, or abnormal renal US findings (Box 96.2). The new proposed HRS classification includes HRS-AKI, defined as an absolute increase in serum creatinine ≥0.3 mg/dL within 48 hours or ≥50% from baseline, in addition to meeting all other IAC criteria as above. Under this classification, no minimum creatinine value is needed for diagnosis, as opposed to the original HRS-1 definition that was characterized by advanced stage 2 or 3 AKI (see Table 96.2).[95] The previously described Type 2 HRS is an HRS-NAKI (non-AKI) that includes (1) HRS-AKD, defined as a subacute renal impairment that fulfills the criteria of HRS but not of AKI with GFR<60 mL/min per 1.73 m^2 lasts for <3 months, and (2) HRS-CKD as previously proposed, which is GFR<60 mL/min per 1.73 m^2 for >3 months in the absence of other causes (Table 96.3).[124]

TABLE 96.2 International Club of Ascites New Definitions for the Diagnosis and Management of Acute Kidney Injury (AKI) in Patients with Cirrhosis

Feature	Definition		
Baseline serum creatinine level	A value obtained in the previous 3 months can be used as baseline; however, in patients with multiple values in previous 3 months the value closest to the admission creatinine should be used In patients without a previous serum creatinine determination, the admission value should be used as the baseline		
AKI	A 50% increase in the serum creatinine level from baseline that is known or presumed to have occurred within the 7 days prior *OR* A rise of 0.3 mg/dL (26.4 μmol/L) in the serum creatinine level in <48 h		
Staging of AKI	**Stage 1:** A rise in the serum creatinine level of 0.3 mg/dL (26.4 μmol/L) or an increase in serum creatinine ≥1.5- to 2-fold above baseline **Stage 2:** A rise in the serum creatinine level of >2- to 3-fold above baseline **Stage 3:** A rise in the serum creatinine level of >3-fold above baseline or a serum creatinine level of 4 mg/dL (353.6 μmol/L) with an acute increase of ≥0.3 mg/dL (26.4 μmol/L) or initiation of renal replacement therapy		
Progression of AKI	**Progression** Progression of AKI to a higher stage and/or need for renal replacement therapy		**Regression** Regression of AKI to a lower stage
Response to treatment	**No response** No regression of AKI	**Partial response** Reduction of at least 1 AKI stage (still above baseline)	**Full response** Return of the serum creatinine level to within 0.3 md/dL of baseline

AKI, Acute kidney injury.
Adapted from Angeli P, Gines P. Diagnosis and management of acute kidney injury in patients with cirrhosis: revised consensus recommendations of the International Club of Ascites. *J Hepatol*. 2015;62:968–974.

BOX 96.2 Diagnostic Criteria for Hepatorenal Syndrome*

Cirrhosis with ascites
Diagnosis of AKI according to International Club of Ascites-AKI criteria (see Table 96.2)
No or insufficient response in 48 h after diuretic withdrawal and adequate volume expansion with IV albumin
Absence of shock
No evidence of recent use of nephrotoxic agents
Absence of intrinsic renal disease

*As defined by the International Club of Ascites revised consensus recommendations (Angeli P, Ginès P, Wong F, et al. Diagnosis and management of acute kidney injury in patients with cirrhosis. *J Hepatol*. 2015;62:968-74.)
AKI, Acute kidney injury.

HRS-AKI is a clinical diagnosis. Identifying the phenotypes of AKI in cirrhosis, including ATN-AKI, prerenal AKI and HRS-AKI, and postrenal AKI, is essential in the diagnosis.[95] Urinary biomarkers, including NGAL (cut-off values>220 μg/g of creatinine measured on Day 3),[125] albumin, and IL-8, if available, help distinguish ATN-AKI, in which they are significantly elevated, compared to HRS-AKI. However, no markers differentiate HRS-AKI from prerenal-AKI. In addition, fractional excretion of sodium (FENa), with the new cut-off value of <0.2%, may be helpful to differentiate ATN-AKI (FENa is typically high) from other forms of AKI.[95,126] Although obvious symptoms and signs may not accompany SBP, HRS may develop in as many as 20% of affected patients.[123,127] Therefore a low threshold for evaluating cirrhotic patients with ascites for the presence of SBP is required (see Chapter 95).

Prevention and Treatment

The high mortality rate of HRS underscores the importance of prevention. Intravascular volume depletion (resulting from overdiuresis, diarrhea caused by lactulose, GI bleeding from gastroesophageal varices, or large-volume paracentesis without colloid administration) should be avoided and corrected. Infections (SBP, bacteremia) should be treated. Many medications, most notably diuretics, lactulose, angiotensin-converting enzyme inhibitors, angiotensin receptor blockers, and NSAIDs, may influence intravascular volume status and renal perfusion and should be discontinued expeditiously in the setting of acute renal dysfunction. Specific guidelines for the primary and secondary prophylaxis of variceal bleeding, administration of colloid (albumin) to patients with a rising serum creatinine level after a large-volume paracentesis or with SBP, prophylactic administration of antibiotics to patients at high risk of SBP or other infections, and those hospitalized for GI bleeding have been published (see Chapters 94 and 95).[127–130]

The concept that specific treatment of HRS is possible and may improve survival has emerged since 2000. Current options include medical therapies, transjugular intrahepatic portosystemic shunt (TIPS) placement, and LT. Medical therapies for HRS are directed toward reversing the underlying splanchnic and systemic vasodilatation with vasoconstricting agents and increasing the effective circulatory volume with the use of colloid. Such treatment is used as a temporizing measure until definitive treatment for liver disease (LT) or portal hypertension (TIPS) is undertaken or until an acute process (SBP, GI bleeding) has been reversed (Box 96.3).[131,132]

Medical Therapy

The use of vasoconstrictors with or without colloid administration in patients with HRS was initially reported in the 1960s. Since then, three vasoconstrictor regimens have been studied. They include (1) terlipressin and albumin, (2) midodrine, octreotide, and albumin, and (3) norepinephrine and albumin. Pooled analysis of published trials has confirmed that a goal-directed approach using vasoconstrictors improves kidney function in patients with HRS.[133,134]

Terlipressin is an intravenously administered, selective vasopressin V1 receptor agonist vasoconstrictor used widely in Europe and is the first FDA-approved therapy[135] for adults in the United States hospitalized with Type 1 HRS with rapid kidney

TABLE 96.3 New Classification of Hepatorenal Syndrome

New Classification		Criteria
HRS-AKI (Old classification HRS-1)[a]		• A 50% increase in the serum creatinine level from baseline, (Using the last available outpatient serum creatinine within 3 months) *OR* • A rise of 0.3 mg/dL (26.4 µmol/L) in the serum creatinine level within 48 h
HRS-NAKI (Old classification HRS-2)[a]	HRS-AKD	• Estimated GFR < 60 mL/min per 1.73 m^2 lasts for <3 months in the absence of other causes of kidney disease • A <50% increase in the serum creatinine level from baseline (Using the last available outpatient serum creatinine within 3 months)
	HRS-CKD	• Estimated GFR < 60 mL/min per 1.73 m^2 lasts for ≥3 months in the absence of other causes of kidney disease

[a]Follows all criteria of the new International Ascites Club criteria for the diagnosis of HRS, Box 96.2.
AKI, Acute kidney injury; *HRS*, hepatorenal syndrome.
Adapted from Angeli P, Garcia-Tsao G, Nadim MK, Parikh CR. News in pathophysiology, definition and classification of hepatorenal syndrome: a step beyond the International Club of Ascites (ICA) consensus document. *J Hepatol*. 2019;71(4):811–822.

BOX 96.3 Management of Hepatorenal Syndrome (HRS)

PREVENT VARICEAL BLEEDING

Measures to prevent variceal bleeding (e.g., β-receptor blocking agent, band ligation)
Treatment of severe alcohol-associated hepatitis (see Chapter 88)
Prevention of HRS
  Avoidance of intravascular volume depletion (diuretics, lactulose, GI bleeding, large-volume paracentesis without adequate volume repletion)
Avoidance of nephrotoxins (e.g., NSAIDs and antibiotics)
Prompt diagnosis and treatment of infections (SBP, sepsis)
SBP prophylaxis (see Chapter 95)

TREATMENT OF HRS

Discontinuation of all nephrotoxic agents (ACEIs, ARBs, NSAIDs, diuretics)
Antibiotics for infections
Albumin—bolus of 1 g/kg/day on presentation (maximum dose, 100 g daily). Continue at a dose of 20–60 g daily as required to maintain the central venous pressure between 10 and 15 cm H_2O
Vasopressor therapy (in addition to albumin):
Terlipressin—start at 1 mg IV every 6 h and increase up to 2 mg IV every 6 h if the baseline serum creatinine level does not improve by 25% at Day 3 of therapy
OR
Midodrine and octreotide—begin midodrine at 2.5–5 mg orally three times daily and increase to a maximum dose of 15 mg three times daily. Titrate to a MAP increase of at least 15 mm Hg; begin octreotide at 100 µg subcutaneously three times daily and increase to a maximum dose of 200 µg subcutaneously three times daily, or begin octreotide with a 25 µg IV bolus and continue at a rate of 25 µg/h
OR
Norepinephrine—0.1–0.7 µg/kg/min as an IV infusion. Increase by 0.05 µg/kg/min every 4 h and titrate to an MAP increase of at least 10 mm Hg
The duration of vasopressor treatment is generally a maximum of 2 weeks until HRS reverses or LT is performed
Evaluation of patient for LT
*1 vial = 0.85 mg terlipressin (North American FDA label) = 1 mg terlipressin acetate[135a]

decline. In the double-blind, randomized, placebo-controlled CONFIRM trial, patients treated with intravenous terlipressin every 6 hours along with albumin, relative to controls treated with placebo with albumin for ten days, had a significantly higher reversal of HRS without renal replacement therapy (RRT) compared to the placebo group (32% vs. 17%, $P = .006$).[104] The incidence of pulmonary edema and respiratory failure was higher in the terlipressin group. Hence, baseline echocardiography should be performed to exclude reduced ejection fraction (EF) and 6–8 hourly pulse oximeter monitoring during terlipressin treatment to detect SpO_2 <90%. Treatment should be discontinued if pulmonary edema is suspected and the patient requires oxygen supplementation.[136] Terlipressin is used with caution in those with advanced liver disease, acute or chronic liver failure grade 3, and a history of severe cardiovascular and ischemic conditions. Initiation of therapy early in the course of HRS (creatinine <3 mg/dL) improves outcomes, and those patients with a serum creatinine of >5 mg/dL at the time of treatment initiation are unlikely to benefit.[137] Treatment with terlipressin should be discontinued after 14 days when there is partial or no response.[95]

The volume expansion, antioxidant, and immune-modulating properties of albumin are also used for HRS diagnosis and treatment. To distinguish prerenal azotemia from HRS, 1 g/kg body weight, with a maximum dose of 100 g/day for up to 48 hours, is used. A lower dose of 20–40 g/day is used in combination with vasopressor agents for treatment.[138] Midodrine, an orally administered α_1-adrenergic agonist, and octreotide, a somatostatin analog that inhibits endogenous vasodilators, have been combined with albumin for Type 1 HRS.[139,140] Although this regimen has a relatively favorable safety profile and ease of administration,[94,141,142] it is less efficacious when compared to terlipressin and albumin in inducing renal recovery (70.4% vs. 28.6%, $P = .01$).[143,144]

Norepinephrine (noradrenaline), a widely available IV-administered α_1-adrenergic agonist, in combination with albumin, has been used as a less expensive alternative to terlipressin.[145,146] In several randomized clinical trials and meta-analyses, norepinephrine and albumin had similar to somewhat less efficacy than terlipressin regimens.[147,148] However, the need for administration through a central line and concerns for significant cardiovascular side effects have made its use less feasible.[149]

Radiologic and Surgical Therapy

Transjugular Intrahepatic Portosystemic Shunt

TIPS is effective for treating diuretic-resistant ascites, a precursor to HRS-NAKI (see Chapter 95).[150,151] However, TIPS does not appear to be efficacious in HRS-AKI, and the coexistence of severe liver dysfunction limits its use.

Renal Replacement Therapy

RRT, as a sole therapy for HRS-AKI, generally does not offer survival benefits. It can be used as a bridge to LT in patients with treatment-refractory HRS or supportive treatment for volume overload and electrolyte imbalances in situations where liver injury may improve or reverse.[95,121]

Liver Transplantation

LT is the only therapeutic modality that has the potential to reverse both liver dysfunction and HRS and should be considered in any patient found to have HRS.[97,109,128,152] The mean serum creatinine after LT, rates of postoperative complications, and in-hospital mortality are higher in patients transplanted with HRS than those without HRS, and up to 35% of patients with HRS require long-term RRT.[97,110,152] The duration, degree, and cause (HRS or ATN) of renal dysfunction preoperatively are predictors of survival, and patients who require hemodialysis carry a mortality risk that is 1.77 times higher than that of patients who do not need dialysis.[152–155] This increased mortality forms the basis for simultaneous liver-kidney (SLK) transplantation in patients with HRS-AKI. OPTN criteria for eligibility for SLK include sustained AKI, defined as a need for dialysis or a GFR of less than or equal to 25 mL/min for a minimum of 6 consecutive weeks.[156]

HEPATOPULMONARY SYNDROME AND PORTOPULMONARY HYPERTENSION

Cirrhosis and portal hypertension are accompanied by vascular alterations in multiple organs. Two distinct clinical entities, hepatopulmonary syndrome (HPS) and portopulmonary hypertension (POPH), have been recognized in the pulmonary circulation. HPS occurs when pulmonary microvascular alterations impair gas exchange,[157–159] and POPH occurs when vasoconstriction and remodeling in resistance vessels increase pulmonary arterial pressures. The mechanisms whereby these two entities develop are incompletely characterized, although they occur in similar clinical settings and may share pathogenic pathways. The presence of HPS or POPH increases mortality in affected patients.[160,161]

Hepatopulmonary Syndrome

Epidemiology and Natural History

HPS, characterized by intrapulmonary vascular dilatations (IPVDs) associated with impaired gas exchange in patients with cirrhosis or portal hypertension, has a 10%–30% prevalence in patients undergoing LT evaluation.[162] The presence and severity of HPS do not correlate closely with the severity of the liver disease, although MELD scores are, on average, higher in patients with HPS than those with cirrhosis and no HPS.[163,164] A recent study showed that patients with HPS have an increased cardiac index compared with liver disease controls, suggesting a more advanced hyperdynamic state in HPS.[165] The presence of HPS negatively impacts quality of life and increases mortality.[166] Mortality increases as the severity of HPS increases, and death occurs due to cirrhosis and portal hypertension-related complications.[167] There is no effective medical therapy for HPS, but LT improves survival and is generally curative.

Pathophysiology

HPS is characterized by alveolar microvascular alterations and dilatation in the precapillary and capillary pulmonary arterial circulation. These changes result in V/Q mismatch, diffusion limitation, and direct AV communications, ultimately contributing to impaired gas exchange and hypoxemia in HPS.[162] The putative underlying pathophysiological processes responsible for the microvascular changes are predominantly derived from experimental HPS induced by common bile duct ligation, which shares some features of human HPS (Fig. 96.3). They include (1) increased circulating endothelin-1 induced pulmonary vascular dilatation[168]; (2) bacterial translocation-related endotoxemia causing pulmonary infiltration of monocytes, which produce vasodilatory and angiogenic mediators[169]; (3) pulmonary angiogenesis and shunt formation, possibly modulated by single-nucleotide polymorphisms in the angiogenesis-regulating genes, endoglin and vWF, found in some patients with HPS[170,171]; and (4) alveolar dysfunction from decreased surfactant protein levels due to alveolar type II cell dysfunction resulting in restrictive ventilation defects.[162,172]

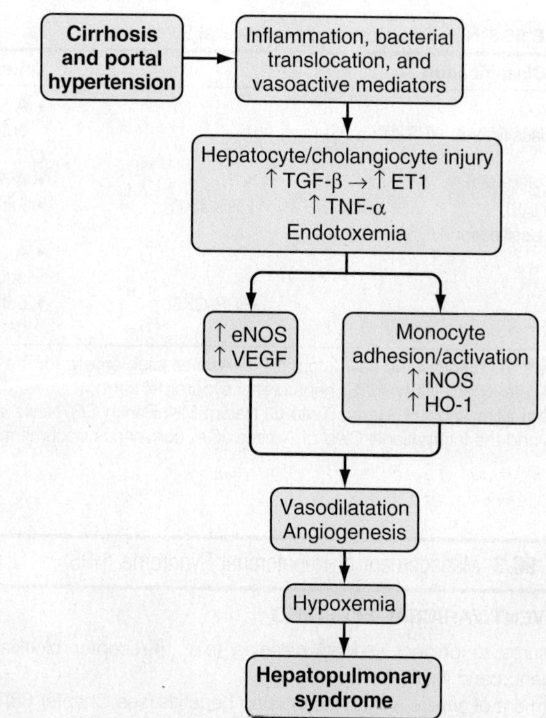

Fig. 96.3 Proposed pathophysiology of hepatopulmonary syndrome. *eNOS*, Endothelial nitric oxide synthase; *ET1*, endothelin-1; *HO-1*, heme oxygenase; *iNOS*, inducible nitric oxide synthase; *TGF-β*, transforming growth factor-β; *VEGF*, vascular endothelial growth factor.

Clinical Features and Diagnosis

The diagnostic criteria for HPS comprise a triad of (1) the presence of IPVD with intrapulmonary shunting of blood identified by the delayed presence of microbubbles in the left atrium on contrast-enhanced echocardiography; (2) a widened age-corrected alveolar-arterial oxygen gradient ($P(A\text{-}a)O_2$ gradient of $\geq$15 mm Hg or >20 mm Hg in patients $\geq$65 years of age) on an arterial blood gas (ABG); and (3) the presence of cirrhosis, portal hypertension, or congenital portosystemic shunts.[173] A task force consensus statement has graded HPS based on the degree of hypoxemia: mild ($PaO_2 \geq 80$ mm Hg), moderate ($PaO_2 > 60–80$ mm Hg), severe ($PaO_2 = 50–60$ mm Hg), and very severe ($PaO_2 < 50$ mm Hg).[174] The presence of HPS significantly increases mortality in patients with cirrhosis,[166] and LT is generally effective in reversing HPS and improving survival. Those with very severe HPS with a $PaO_2 < 45$ may be at higher risk of mortality after LT, though excellent outcomes have been reported even in these advanced cases likely related to advances in surgical technique and peri-operative care.[175–179]

Patients with HPS present most commonly with respiratory complaints in the setting of chronic liver disease. Occasionally, HPS may be the initial manifestation of cirrhosis and may also be found in noncirrhotic and posthepatic portal hypertension, ischemic hepatitis, and chronic hepatitis in the absence of confirmed cirrhosis. A syndrome similar to HPS has been described in children with congenital abnormalities that divert hepatic blood from the pulmonary circulation.[178,180,181]

Classic clinical manifestations of HPS include platypnea (dyspnea worsened by an erect position and improved by a supine position) and orthodeoxia (exacerbation of hypoxia and hypoxemia in an upright position), both of which are relatively uncommon, and the insidious onset and slow progression of dyspnea, clubbing, and distal cyanosis.[157,160,182] Although clubbing and hypoxemia (PaO_2 <60 mm Hg) in patients with liver disease without intrinsic cardiopulmonary disease are highly suggestive of HPS, other clinical features are unreliable for detecting HPS. Many patients, particularly those with early HPS, are asymptomatic or have symptoms only on exertion, underscoring the need to screen patients being evaluated for LT. Cough has also been described as a presenting symptom of HPS.[160,183] The severity of HPS appears to worsen over time, and marked nocturnal desaturation has been reported even in patients with moderate wake-time hypoxemia.[184,185]

Diagnosing HPS requires a high degree of clinical suspicion, measurement of ABGs, detection of intrapulmonary shunting, and exclusion of intrinsic cardiopulmonary disease as a contributor to hypoxemia. However, a recent analysis in a large integrated health system found that diagnostic criteria for HPS were met in less than 25% of patients given the diagnosis, highlighting the need for better screening algorithms.[186] The most sensitive test for the diagnosis of intrapulmonary shunting is contrast echocardiography,[187] which is performed by peripheral intravenous injection of agitated saline to produce microbubbles (>10 μm diameter) that are visualized during transthoracic echocardiography. Usually, microbubbles are absorbed in alveolar regions and do not pass through the pulmonary capillary bed (<8–15 μm diameter). In patients with intracardiac shunting, microbubbles reach the left ventricle early (within 1–3 cardiac cycles after injection); in patients with intrapulmonary shunting, microbubbles reach the left ventricle in a delayed fashion (3–6 cardiac cycles after injection). Up to 60% of patients with cirrhosis have intrapulmonary vasodilatation detected by contrast-enhanced echocardiography. However, only a subset of patients has sufficient vasodilatation to cause abnormal ABG results and HPS.[162]

Intrinsic cardiopulmonary disease should be excluded in patients with pulmonary symptoms, hypoxemia, and intrapulmonary shunting. Chest radiography or CT and pulmonary function tests are generally performed in patients considered for LT to detect the coexistence of chronic obstructive pulmonary disease, asthma, and pulmonary fibrosis. If potentially reversible cardiopulmonary disorders are detected, treatment is initiated, and the assessment of oxygenation is repeated.[188] Cases of coexistence of POPH with HPS and cases of unmasked POPH after LT and resolution of HPS have also been reported.[189] In the small subset of patients found to have severe hypoxemia (PaO_2 <60 mm Hg), intrapulmonary shunting, and significant cardiopulmonary disease, an abnormal technetium-labeled macroaggregated albumin scan (MAA) that demonstrates a greater than 6% shunt fraction may confirm that HPS is contributing to the gas exchange abnormalities.[187,190,191] However, there is a lack of standardization in technique, and the MAA scan cannot differentiate between intrapulmonary and intracardiac shunting.[187] Screening for HPS using pulse oximetry is not sufficiently sensitive, and ABG is mandatory to detect a widened $P(A\text{-}a)O_2$ gradient and mild-to-moderate hypoxemia (Fig. 96.4).[192]

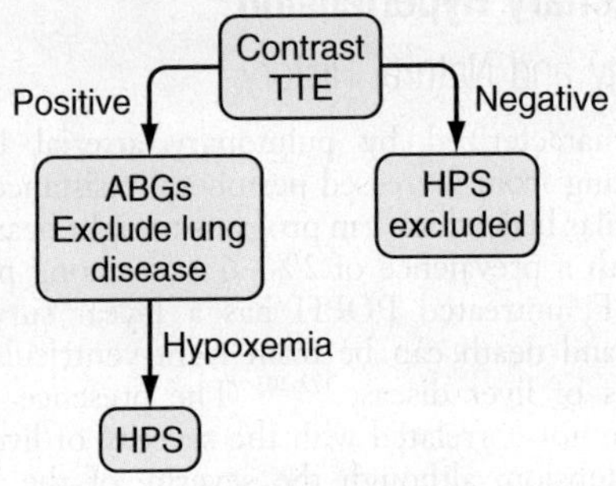

Fig. 96.4 Algorithm for the approach to screening for hepatopulmonary syndrome *(HPS)* in potential candidates for LT. *ABGs,* Arterial blood gases; *TTE,* transthoracic echocardiography.

Treatment

Medical Therapy

Treatment options for HPS are limited. No medical therapies have generally proved effective. Case reports and small case series on treatment with methylene blue, indomethacin, pentoxifylline, and mycophenolate mofetil showed no clear benefit.[162] Several case series and small controlled trials suggest that garlic extracts may improve oxygenation in HPS.[193,194] Most patients with well-preserved hepatic synthetic function and mild-to-moderate hypoxemia are treated symptomatically until oxygenation worsens sufficiently to permit listing for LT based on MELD exception criteria (see Chapter 99). LT reverses HPS in most affected patients, and 5-year post-LT survival in patients with HPS is comparable to those without HPS.

Supportive Care

Early continuous oxygen supplementation is recommended in patients with severe HPS and resting hypoxemia (PaO_2 <60 mm Hg), as chronic hypoxemia could contribute to a high mortality rate in HPS.

Radiologic Therapy

Two radiologic techniques, TIPS to lower portal pressure and pulmonary angiography with embolization to occlude areas of intrapulmonary shunting, have been used as palliative treatment for HPS. Neither approach has been established to be effective in controlled studies. In general, using either technique as primary treatment for HPS is not supported, though TIPS may be effective in treating other complications of portal hypertension in those with HPS.[195]

Liver Transplantation

LT reverses HPS in ± 95% of affected patients within 6–12 months with good post-LT survival.[196] Based on the progressive nature of hypoxemia in HPS, the relationship between increased severity of hypoxemia and poor outcomes post-LT, and the lack of correlation between the severity of HPS and liver disease, a MELD exception is available in patients with severe HPS (resting PaO_2 less than 60 mmHg) to increase priority for transplantation.[177,197,198] Including the MELD exception for HPS has improved survival in HPS patients undergoing LT. The exception point allocation for HPS has been modified to balance outcomes relative to those awaiting LT for other indications.[196,199] Higher post-LT mortality is seen in HPS patients with a PaO_2 <45 mmHg, compared with patients with PaO_2 >45 to <50 mmHg[175] and those needing 100% inhaled oxygen to maintain saturation of ≥85% after LT.[199,200] Advancements in postoperative management algorithms for HPS appear to be important in optimizing outcomes in patients with severe disease.[162,201]

Portopulmonary Hypertension

Epidemiology and Natural History

POPH is characterized by pulmonary arterial hypertension (PAH) resulting from increased peripheral resistance in the pulmonary vascular bed, which can progress to right heart failure and death.[173] With a prevalence of 2%–6%[202] among patients evaluated for LT, untreated POPH has a 1-year survival rate of 35%–46%, and death can be from right ventricular failure or complications of liver disease.[173,203] The presence and severity of POPH are not correlated with the severity of liver disease or portal hypertension, although the severity of the liver disease impacts the outcome in those with POPH.[173,204,205] Female sex and autoimmune hepatitis are risk factors for POPH.[206] Females with POPH appear to have higher PVR, lower MELD, and higher waitlist mortality than affected males.[206] In addition, large spontaneous portosystemic shunts have been associated with moderate-to-severe POPH.[207] A multicenter cross-sectional survey across US LT centers showed marked variability in provider beliefs and clinical practice in managing POPH, highlighting evidence gaps in managing this complex condition.[208] Medical therapies that improve pulmonary hemodynamics in patients with POPH have become available. However, the specific role and timing of LT in POPH are not clearly defined because of the relative impact of POPH and liver disease severity on outcomes in those treated with vasomodulator therapy. In addition, there is an inconsistent resolution of POPH after LT.[209]

Pathogenesis

POPH is characterized by obstruction to blood flow in the pulmonary arterial bed. The mechanisms whereby POPH develops are poorly understood. Histologically, POPH shares the characteristic features of other PAH forms, including medial proliferation and hypertrophy in arteries, plexiform arteriopathy, and in situ vascular thrombosis.[210–212] Altered estrogen metabolism resulting in increased circulating levels related to variations in aromatase genes has been postulated to contribute to POPH.[213–215] Also, increased circulating levels of endothelin-1 in the setting of altered hepatic metabolism may drive pulmonary arterial vasoconstriction and vascular remodeling.[216] Finally, a reduction in bone morphogenic protein (BMP-9) produced by the liver, which generally maintains homeostasis in the pulmonary vasculature by signaling through specific receptors, has been found in patients with POPH and may contribute to pulmonary vascular remodeling.[217,218]

Clinical Features and Diagnosis

POPH is defined as the development of PAH in the setting of portal hypertension. It is included in the Group 1 WHO category. The diagnostic criteria for POPH include the presence of PAH as defined by the WHO: mean pulmonary arterial pressure (mPAP) above 20 mm Hg; pulmonary capillary wedge pressure below 15 mm Hg; and pulmonary vascular resistance more than 240 dynes s/cm^5 occurring in the setting of pre-, intra-, and post-hepatic portal hypertension (as evidenced by splenomegaly, thrombocytopenia, portosystemic shunts, or portal vein hemodynamic abnormalities).[158,219–221] POPH has been found in up to 6% of cirrhotic patients evaluated for LT, and outcomes are worse compared to cirrhotic patients without POPH. POPH is generally graded according to the degree of elevation in mPAP, which correlates with the mortality risk associated with LT and influences decisions regarding therapy.[191] Mild POPH (mPAP ≤35 mm Hg) is not associated with an increased operative risk for LT and may not require medical therapy. Moderate POPH (mPAP = 35–50 mm Hg) is associated with an increased operative risk for LT and is an indication for medical therapy. Severe POPH (mPAP >50 mm Hg) is associated with a prohibitive operative mortality risk and is generally managed with medical therapy. If medical therapy significantly improves POPH, LT can be considered. The most common symptom associated with POPH is exertional dyspnea; other nonspecific symptoms, such as orthopnea, fatigue, chest pressure, syncope, edema, and lightheadedness, may also occur.[220] Characteristic physical examination features of PAH, including an elevated jugular venous pressure, loud second pulmonic heart sound, a murmur of tricuspid regurgitation (TR), and lower extremity edema, have been reported but are not sufficiently sensitive nor specific to be useful diagnostically. In cirrhotic patients, peripheral edema out of proportion to the degree of ascites should prompt consideration of right ventricular dysfunction secondary to pulmonary hypertension. In a number of studies, the majority of cirrhotic patients with significant POPH were asymptomatic.[222,223]

The diagnosis of POPH warrants a high degree of clinical suspicion, and all patients considered for LT or TIPS and patients with suggestive symptoms or physical findings should be evaluated for POPH. Transthoracic echocardiography is the recommended screening test because it evaluates the right-sided cardiac function and allows an estimation of right ventricular systolic pressure by evaluating the tricuspid regurgitant jet.[224] Composite echocardiographic parameters, including tricuspid annular plane systolic excursion/TR gradient (TRG) ratio, that detail right ventricular dysfunction might improve PAH diagnosis in milder forms with TRG ≤46 mm Hg.[225,226] Other causes of elevated right-sided cardiac pressures (e.g., secondary pulmonary hypertension, volume overload, and hyperdynamic circulation) should be assessed. Methods for estimating right ventricular systolic pressure vary among centers, but in general, in the absence of significant pulmonary artery stenosis, an estimated right ventricular systolic pressure higher than 40 mm Hg or the presence of right ventricular abnormalities on echocardiography supports further evaluation for POPH. The absence of both these findings essentially excludes POPH.[223] In all patients with echocardiographic features suggestive of POPH, right heart catheterization should be performed to establish the diagnosis and assess the severity of POPH. Findings on right heart catheterization are useful for distinguishing volume overload and hyperdynamic circulation from POPH.

Treatment

Treatment of POPH has changed substantially since the early 2000s due to the availability of multiple effective oral vasodilators to treat PAH. LT is generally contraindicated in patients with moderate-to-severe POPH because of increased perioperative mortality from poor right-sided cardiac function. The ability to decrease pulmonary vascular resistance and lower PAP with medications has reduced perioperative complications and allows LT to be considered in a larger subset of patients with POPH.

Medical Therapy

Supportive therapy in POPH generally includes diuretics for volume overload and supplemental oxygen if hypoxemia is present. Anticoagulation is often avoided but may be appropriate in the subset of patients with POPH who do not have hepatic decompensation, marked coagulopathy, or gastroesophageal varices. β-Adrenergic blocking agents may reduce right-sided cardiac function, and some clinicians advocate controlling esophageal varices with band ligation and avoiding or withdrawing β-blockers in patients with POPH.[227] Caution should be exerted in placing TIPS in patients with POPH as the post-TIPS hemodynamic changes may be poorly tolerated due to elevated right ventricular pressure and volume. Severe pulmonary hypertension (mPAP ≥45 mm Hg) is an absolute contraindication to TIPS, and moderate POPH (35≤ mPAP <45 mm Hg) is considered a relative contraindication unless POPH can be controlled with vasomodulators.[228]

The pulmonary artery-targeted therapies used in POPH are those used in other group 1 PAH etiologies and are not specific to cirrhosis.[229,230] Targeted PAH lowering therapies can be classified into three groups, (1) prostacyclin analogues, (2) phosphodiesterase subtype 5 inhibitors, and (3) endothelin receptor antagonists. Prostacyclin analogs possess vasodilator, antithrombotic, and antiproliferative properties.[173] Epoprostenol requires complicated IV administration and is reserved for severe disease. Newer agents are effective (iloprost, treprostinil) and easier to administer.[203,222,231,232] An oral prostacyclin receptor agonist (selexipag) is available and shows promise as an effective and simple therapy.[233]

Oral endothelin receptor antagonists, including ambrisentan and macitentan (semiselective endothelin-A receptor antagonists), are increasingly used in POPH.[234–237] PORTICO, the first multicenter randomized controlled trial in POPH, demonstrated the effectiveness of macitentan in improving PVR without adverse effects on liver disease in patients with Child-Pugh class A or B cirrhosis.[229,230] Peripheral edema was a common side effect during macitentan treatment. Oral phosphodiesterase-5 inhibitors, including sildenafil, which potentiate NO signaling by inhibiting cyclic GMP breakdown, have generally been well tolerated in patients with POPH, although the magnitude of improvement in pulmonary arterial pressures has been modest. Long-acting phosphodiesterase-5 inhibitors (tadalafil and vardenafil) are under study and increasingly used.[238–242] A direct cyclic GMP analog (riociguat) has also been approved for treating PAH and appears to benefit POPH.[243,244]

Liver Transplantation

Unlike HPS, LT does not reliably cure POPH despite using PA-targeted therapies. Hence, the role of LT in POPH is evolving. Traditionally, moderate to severe POPH has been a contraindication to LT due to high perioperative mortality, mainly when the mPAP is >35 mm Hg. Using potent vasodilators to decrease pulmonary vascular resistance and pulmonary arterial pressures prior to LT forms the basis for MELD exception criteria for POPH. Pre-LT MPAP of <35 mm Hg and a PVR of <400 dynes s/cm^5, or a PVR of less than 240 dynes s/cm^5 in those with pre-LT MPAP of 35–45 mm Hg is defined as an adequate hemodynamic response to treatment.[245–247] However, several aspects of LT for POPH are not fully defined. First, most studies suggest that only 40%–50% of POPH patients treated with vasomodulator therapy, who are otherwise LT candidates, will have an adequate pulmonary vascular response and can be considered for LT with MELD exception.[247] As medical therapies become increasingly available, the number of patients who respond to medical therapy may increase. Second, current data support that only approximately 50% of patients who undergo LT for POPH have a resolution of PH and can have POPH medications discontinued.[247,248] Although historical OPTN data support that overall LT outcomes in POPH are similar to non-POPH patients, rejection is more frequent in those transplanted with POPH, and no studies have characterized the clinical features and long-term outcomes in patients with POPH who do or do not have a resolution of PH. Finally, recent work, including a large-scale meta-analysis, supports that LT in POPH appears to have the greatest survival benefit in those with more advanced liver disease. At present, it is reasonable to initiate vasomodulator therapy for POPH in patients who are candidates for therapy and consider LT in those who respond and have or develop progressive liver dysfunction.[247,248]

CIRRHOTIC CARDIOMYOPATHY

Cardiac Alterations in Etiologies of Cirrhosis

Systemic hemodynamic changes, including the hyperdynamic circulation characterized by decreased arterial blood pressure, decreased peripheral resistance, and increased cardiac output, have been observed in patients with cirrhosis since the early 1900s.[249] Subsequently, in patients with alcoholic cirrhosis, cardiomyopathy with a distinct pathogenesis called alcoholic cardiomyopathy was identified.[250,251] Alcoholic cardiomyopathy is an acquired dilated cardiomyopathy characterized by left ventricular dilatation with reduced EF caused by chronic heavy alcohol consumption in the absence of ischemic, hypertensive, valvular, and other causes of dilated cardiomyopathy.[252] Cardiac involvement in other causes of cirrhosis has also been observed, including nonalcoholic fatty liver disease, where coronary atherosclerosis, congestive heart failure (CHF) with preserved EF, arrhythmias, and cardiac conduction defects linked to metabolic abnormalities and inflammation are found.[251,253] Patients with Wilson disease have an increased risk of CHF and atrial fibrillation related to altered copper metabolism,[254,255] and patients with hereditary hemochromatosis may develop restrictive or dilated cardiomyopathy from cardiac iron overload.[256,257] These conditions are distinct from cardiac dysfunction independent of the etiology of the liver disease termed *cirrhotic cardiomyopathy* (CCM).[250]

Cirrhotic Cardiomyopathy: Definition

A consensus group during the 2005 Montreal World Congress of Gastroenterology (WGO) proposed a working definition of CCM, which is characterized by (1) systolic dysfunction defined as an EF <55% and a blunted increase in cardiac output in response to exercise and pharmacological stimuli; (2) diastolic dysfunction defined as E/A ratio <1, deceleration time >200 ms, and isovolumetric relaxation time of >80 ms; (3) supportive criteria of cardiac electrophysiologic abnormalities such as prolonged QTc interval (Fig. 96.5).[258–262] Over the past decade, echocardiographic imaging, functional studies, and biomarker development

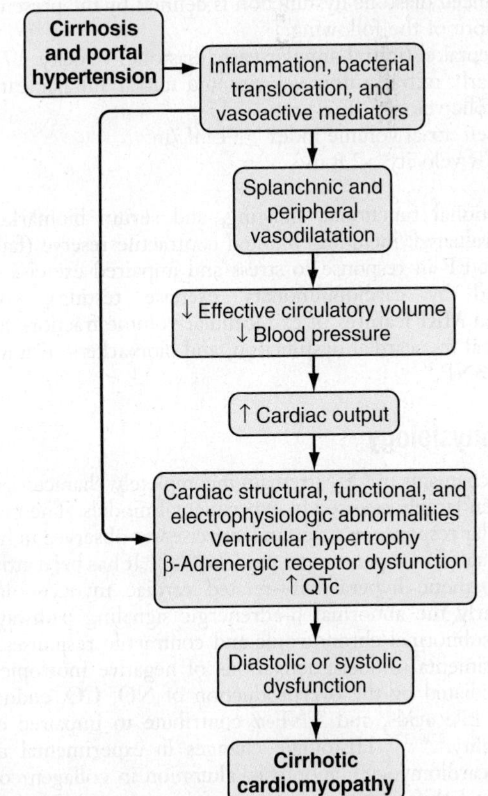

Fig. 96.5 Algorithm for the proposed pathophysiology of cirrhotic cardiomyopathy. *QTc*, Rate-corrected QT interval.

TABLE 96.4 Comparision of Old and New Diagnostic Criteria for Cirrhotic Cardiomyopathy

Definition	Old World Congress of Gastroenterology Criteria (2005)	New Criteria per the Cirrhotic Cardiomyopathy Consortium (2020)
Systolic dysfunction	• Blunted contractile response on stress testing Or • LVEF<55%	LVEF ≤50% Or Absolute global longitudinal strain (GLS) <18% or >22%
Diastolic dysfunction	• Deceleration time >200 ms or • Isovolumetric relaxation time >80 ms or • E/A <1	≥3 of the following • Septal e′ (mitral annular early diastolic) velocity <7 cm/s • Early mitral inflow velocity and mitral annular early diastolic velocity (E/e′) ratio ≥15 • LAVI >34 mL/m² • TR velocity >2.8 m/s
Supportive criteria	• Electrophysiological abnormalities • Abnormal chronotropic response • Electromechanical uncoupling • Prolonged QTc interval • Enlarged left atrium • Increased myocardial mass • Increased BNP • Increased proBNP • Increased troponin I	• Abnormal chronotropic or inotropic response on exercise stress testing, dobutamine stress testing, or at rest on CMRI • Electrocardiographic changes • Electromechanical uncoupling • Myocardial mass change • Serum biomarkers • Chamber enlargement • CMRI

LAVI, Left atrial volume index; *TR*, tricuspid regurgitation.
Adapted from Izzy M, VanWagner LB, Lin G, et al. Redefining cirrhotic cardiomyopathy for the modern Era. *Hepatology*. 2020;71(1):334–345.

have evolved, resulting in more precise diagnostic criteria for CCM in 2019 (Table 96.4), which include:

1. Systolic dysfunction is defined as any of the following:
   - EF ≤50%
   - Absolute global longitudinal strain <18% or >22%
2. Advanced diastolic dysfunction is defined by the presence of 3 or more of the following:
   - Septal e′ (mitral annular early diastolic) velocity <7 cm/s
   - Early mitral inflow velocity and mitral annular early diastolic velocity (E/e′) ratio ≥15
   - Left atrial volume index >34 mL/m²
   - TR velocity >2.8 m/s

Additional functional, imaging, and serum biomarkers are being evaluated, including blunted contractile reserve (failure to augment EF in response to stress and impaired exercise testing measured by cardiopulmonary exercise testing), contrast-enhanced MRI features of extracellular volume fraction, fibrosis, subclinical myocardial dysfunction, and biomarkers such as BNP and proBNP.[263]

Pathophysiology

The mechanisms of CCM remain incompletely characterized and have been largely assessed in experimental models. The impaired ventricular response to stress and exercise was observed in humans and evaluated in experimental models.[264–266] It has been attributed to sympathetic hyperactivity-related cardiac myocyte damage, particularly the abnormal β-adrenergic signaling pathways that lead to subnormal chronotropic and contractile responses.[267–269] In experimental models, activations of negative inotropic pathways mediated by the overproduction of NO, CO, endocannabinoids, bile acids, and TNF-α contribute to impaired cardiac contractility.[270–276] Histologic changes in experimental models include cardiomyocyte apoptosis, alteration in collagen configuration, and shift of the more powerful α-subtype myosin heavy chain to the weaker β-isoform. Derangements of plasma membrane fluidity and membrane ion channel and receptor function may contribute to electrophysiologic abnormalities, including prolongation of the corrected QT interval (QTc) observed in experimental models and patients with CCM.[259,277–279]

Clinical Features and Diagnosis

Early studies found that as many as 50% of cirrhotic patients may have imaging or electrocardiographic features of CCM based on the 2005 WGO criteria.[260] However, many patients have no symptoms, and the long-term clinical consequences of the early cardiac findings are not well defined. A subset of patients develop overt cardiac dysfunction typically in situations that increase cardiac demand, including TIPS placement, bacterial infections such as SBP, and LT.[259] The prevalence of CCM based on the newest consensus criteria (CCMC) in retrospective studies is variable, ranging from 34.8% (driven by diastolic dysfunction[280,281]) to 85.6% (mainly driven by systolic dysfunction[282]). Compared to prior criteria, individuals with diastolic dysfunction identified by the new CCMC criteria have a higher risk of pre-LT mortality, HE, and AKI.[282] Also, those with CCMC-diagnosed cardiomyopathy have an increased risk of postliver transplant-related cardiovascular events.[281] However, prospective multicenter studies are needed to define CCM prevalence and implications for clinical care.

Prevalence and Predictors of Cardiac Decompensation in Cirrhotic Cardiomyopathy

The prevalence of post-TIPS cardiac decompensation requiring hospitalization within 1 year ranges from 10% to 20%.[283] Elevated pre-TIPS right atrial pressure, prolonged QT interval, elevated BNP, and echocardiogram features suggestive of diastolic dysfunction are factors associated with post-TIPS cardiac decompensation.[284] The prevalence of post-LT systolic heart failure is markedly varied and depends on how CHF is defined and its duration in the posttransplant course. New-onset post-LT CHF prevalence can range from 24% 6 months after LT to 10% in the first 5 years.[47] While the pre-LT history of CHF and multiple packed red blood cell transfusion were identified as risk factors for early post-LT systolic CHF,[48] metabolic conditions such as HTN, diabetes mellitus, pretransplant prolonged QT interval>450 ms, echocardiographic features of diastolic dysfunction, and right heart catheterization findings of mPAP >30 mm Hg, and PCWP of >15 mm Hg were predictors of late systolic CHF.[48]

Cirrhotic Cardiomyopathy Detection

The CCM consortium recommends screening for CCM in patients with cirrhosis, particularly those undergoing LT evaluation, using echocardiography with tissue Doppler and strain imaging.[263] Serum biomarkers, ECG assessments, stress testing, markers of right ventricular dysfunction, and advanced cardiac imaging may be of clinical relevance. Whether they improve CCM detection needs to be further evaluated per the CCMC.[263] In patients listed for LT with any degree of systolic or diastolic dysfunction, echocardiography at 6-month intervals is recommended to identify deterioration in cardiac function.[263] For patients with pre-LT CCM, post-LT surveillance with an echocardiogram at 6, 12, and 24 months after LT is recommended. In cirrhotic patients with evidence of heart failure, alternative causes of cardiac dysfunction, including coronary artery disease, valvular abnormalities, and other causes of cardiomyopathy, should be considered.

Treatment

Therapy for CCM remains largely empiric and supportive. Treatment of volume overload includes standard supportive measures and diuresis.[285] Aldosterone antagonists are included based on the potential to reduce cardiac remodeling and portal pressures. Preload and after load reducing agents must be used cautiously, and angiotensin-converting enzyme inhibitors are avoided because of adverse effects on blood pressure and renal perfusion.[264] The role of noncardioselective β-adrenergic blocking agents in CCM, particularly effects on QTc prolongation and hyperdynamic load, is not fully defined.[285,286] While one RCT assessing the effect of 6-month therapy with β-blocker-showed no significant improvement in cardiac function,[287] poor outcomes with β-blocker use in cirrhotic patients with compromised cardiac function assessed by left ventricular stroke work index, a measure of global cardiac performance have been shown.[288] Optimizing volume status and cardiac function is particularly important when considering invasive procedures such as TIPS, where worsening cardiac function may develop. Moreover, in those with risk factors or a diagnosis of posttransplant cardiomyopathy, implementing early interventions, including adherence to strict systolic blood pressure goals (<120 mm Hg) and selection of antihypertensives with the potential for halting cardiac remodeling, should be considered.[263]

ENDOCRINE DYSFUNCTION

Cirrhosis has been linked to abnormalities in the endocrine system, including adrenal insufficiency (AI), abnormal sex hormone metabolism, thyroid disease, and osteoporosis.

Adrenal Insufficiency

The recognition that AI worsens outcomes in sepsis, a syndrome characterized by physiologic abnormalities also seen in liver failure, has led to the evaluation of adrenal dysfunction in patients with liver disease. In cirrhosis, AI exists along a spectrum, ranging from relative AI (RAI), characterized by an inadequate adrenal response to stress and physiological demands, to the other extreme of absolute AI, which is a nonsituational reduction in adrenal steroids.[289,290] The prevalence of RAI (which comprises the majority of AI in cirrhosis) in decompensated cirrhosis ranges from 23% to 68% in the outpatient setting to 26%–59% in noncritically ill hospitalized patients to 51%–82% in critically ill hospitalized patients.[289,291,292] The proposed pathophysiologic mechanisms for RAI include (1) impaired adrenal cortisol synthesis from cholesterol during stress, (2) increased circulating levels of endotoxins and proinflammatory cytokines, and (3) chronic adrenal hypoperfusion.[293,294]

The wide range in frequency reflects the difficulty in diagnosing RAI due to the overlap of common symptoms of AI with neurohumoral changes of portal hypertension and the lack of standardization in stimulation testing in cirrhosis.[289] Currently, standard dose ACTH stimulation testing with measurement of total cortisol levels (increase in total cortisol <250 nmol/L) is recommended for diagnosis.[290] The presence of RAI has been associated with greater hemodynamic instability and increased mortality in cirrhosis,[295,296] although studies on therapeutic corticosteroid administration are conflicting, showing either improved survival or increased mortality due to complications associated with treatment.[297–299] Thus in cirrhosis, glucocorticoids are considered in critically ill patients, though the optimal duration and specific subpopulations that benefit the most are yet to be defined. Likewise, treating RAI in noncritically ill patients is poorly defined, and corticosteroid administration should be considered cautiously. RAI, when present, does appear to resolve within 1–3 months post-LT.[290]

Gonadal Dysfunction

Historical data suggest a high frequency (70%–90%) of central and peripheral hypogonadism and reduced testosterone levels in cirrhotic patients. The mechanisms of hypogonadism may include toxic/metabolic injury of the gonads and the pituitary from alcohol or iron,[300,301] impaired sex hormone clearance, and excessive peripheral androgen to estrogen conversion leading to hyperestrogenism[72] and altered sex hormone–binding globulin (SHBG) levels shifting hormone balance to estrogens. In men, these changes can result in testicular atrophy, decreased libido, infertility, gynecomastia, and sarcopenia.[302,303] Spironolactone, which displaces androgen from its receptor and binding protein, can cause or exacerbate painful gynecomastia.[304] Low testosterone is also associated with increased mortality, independent of the MELD score.[305] While oral testosterone therapy has not been shown to improve survival in men with alcoholic cirrhosis,[306] intramuscular testosterone therapy improves muscle mass and bone mineral density in males with cirrhosis and low testosterone levels.[307] In women with cirrhosis, amenorrhea is the most common menstrual abnormality seen, with a prevalence ranging from 30% to 50%[308,309] and may be the initial manifestation of liver disease in up to 18%. In contrast, women with primary biliary cholangitis are at increased risk of needing hysterectomy for menorrhagia.[310] Although women with chronic liver disease have low fertility, the prevalence of pregnancies in women with cirrhosis has increased over recent years with improved care.[311,312] Postmenopausal women with liver cirrhosis have higher estrogen and lower SHBG and FSH levels, though the clinical consequences of these changes are not fully defined.[313] Most women experience improved menstruation and fertility a few months after successful LT.[308] Both male hypogonadism and greater than 6 months of secondary amenorrhea in females are risk factors for osteoporosis.[314] The impact of gender-affirming hormone therapy in those with cirrhosis is not fully characterized, although testosterone treatment among transmasculine persons may cause transaminase elevations; more studies are needed in this area.[315] LT has been shown to improve sex hormone disturbances.[316,317]

Thyroid Dysfunction

A number of thyroid abnormalities, including increased thyroid volume and decreased serum levels of free triiodothyronine, have been found in patients with cirrhosis. These alterations appear to correlate with the severity of liver disease, and the presence of thyroid disease may predict decreased survival.[318–321] Lower free T3 levels are an independent risk factor for liver fat content and fibrosis.[322,323] In patients with hepatitis C or autoimmune liver disease, the frequency of hypothyroidism and autoimmune thyroid disease increases.[324–326] Whether routine screening for thyroid disease influences survival or quality of life is unknown.

BONE DISEASE

The frequency of osteoporosis among patients with all causes of chronic liver disease ranges from 12% to 55%,[327] negatively impacting the quality of life. Potential risk factors include cholestasis, previous fragility fracture, progression of liver disease, alcohol consumption, hemochromatosis, lower BMI, oral glucocorticoid use for more than 3 months, post-LT status, older age, postmenopausal, and smoking status.[314] Although the pathogenesis in liver disease is complex, key mechanisms involved include a reduction in vitamin D due to cholestasis-related vitamin D malabsorption and decreased production from hepatic dysfunction, sex hormone dysregulation, and cytokine-mediated bone resorption.[314] Women with PBC have a four-fold higher risk of developing osteoporosis and a two-fold higher risk of bone fractures than age-matched controls (see Chapter 93).[328] Treatment with UDCA does not influence bone density in patients with PBC, but avoidance of glucocorticoids and improved nutrition appear to decrease the frequency of osteoporosis.[329,330] Cirrhosis of any etiology is also associated with an increased risk of pathological fractures.[314] Although guidelines specific to cirrhosis are lacking, bone mineral density is an appropriate screening tool for osteoporosis particularly in those with PBC and PSC and those who require more than 3 months of glucocorticoid therapy.[328,330–332] Many transplant centers also screen patients during the evaluation process. Treatment of osteoporosis in patients with chronic liver disease is based on studies of postmenopausal women and is an area of an ongoing investigation. Using calcium, vitamin D, and therapeutic bisphosphonates improves bone mineral density.[332,333] The parenteral route of bisphosphonates is preferred in patients with esophageal varices. Treatment of bone disease before LT is important as osteoporosis worsens early after LT, with accelerated bone loss and a high risk of fractures within 6–12 months of LT.[327,333,334]

COAGULATION DISORDERS

In cirrhosis, the complex interplay among abnormalities in both pro- and anticoagulant factors results in dysfunction of hemostasis, coagulation, and fibrinolysis, resulting in an increased risk for bleeding and hypercoagulability.[335–337] The precise mechanisms for these clinical events are not fully characterized.[338]

Prolongation of Prothrombin Time and Hemostasis

The progressive loss of hepatocytes in cirrhosis leads to decreased synthesis of procoagulant factors, including vitamin K-dependent factors (II, VII, IX, X), factor V, and factor XI. There is also a concurrent decrease in natural anticoagulants such as antithrombin, protein C, and protein S resulting in relative deficiencies of both pro- and anticoagulant pathways and a rebalancing of coagulation.[339] However, this rebalanced hemostasis is fragile relative to healthy individuals and may result in a shift toward bleeding or thrombosis, depending on the situation.[339,340] The prothrombin time (PT) and the international normalized ratio (INR) (where the PT is expressed relative to a normal PT in a particular laboratory) measure the amount of plasma thrombin, the final enzyme in the coagulation cascade produced by procoagulant factors in plasma samples.[109] However, they do not measure the inhibition of thrombin function by anticoagulant factors. Hence, bleeding assessment using only the PT, activated partial thromboplastin time, and INR reflects isolated procoagulant pathways in vitro, not the coagulation balance in vivo.[341] Moreover, the PT and INR were not developed nor calibrated for patients with cirrhosis, and the INR is limited by substantial interlaboratory variability due to the use of differing reagents. INR as a factor is a variable reflection of the degree of hepatic synthetic dysfunction as a component of the MELD score and is less relevant to coagulation and bleeding risk assessment.[342,343]

Therefore assessing bleeding risk using INR is problematic and has been challenged.[341] Administering fresh frozen plasma (FFP), vitamin K, and, occasionally, recombinant factor VIIa to correct coagulopathy in patients with chronic liver disease, particularly in the setting of bleeding or prior to invasive procedures, is not supported by robust data.[344–347] Moreover, the volume of FFP required to achieve clinically significant reductions in the PT in patients with cirrhosis has been associated with a substantial increase in the risk of acute lung injury and volume overload.[348,349] Patients with stable cirrhosis undergoing gastrointestinal procedures, including paracentesis, thoracentesis, liver biopsy, variceal banding, colonic polypectomy, and ERCP, do not require frequent coagulation-related laboratory checks and prophylactic blood product transfusions.[350] Viscoelastic tests (see below) may reflect the in vivo coagulation status and are increasingly used to guide treatment to reduce bleeding.

Thrombocytopenia

Thrombocytopenia is a common feature in cirrhosis with portal hypertension and is generally associated with hypersplenism. Decreased hepatic thrombopoietin synthesis and direct bone marrow toxicity (e.g., from alcohol or HCV) may also lower the platelet count.[351] In addition to quantitative abnormalities, the generation of platelet thrombin appears to be impaired in patients with cirrhosis, particularly when the platelet count is below 50,000/mL, which may contribute to reduced clot formation.[352] On the other hand, cirrhotic patients have higher serum levels of von Willebrand factor (vWf) and lower levels of vWf-cleaving protease ADAMTS13 (a disintegrin and metalloproteinase with thrombospondin type 1 motif member 13), which may promote platelet adhesion to the endothelium at the site of vascular injury.[353,354] Although platelet function, as assessed by measurement of the bleeding time, is commonly impaired in patients with cirrhosis, neither the prolongation of the bleeding time nor its correction with the administration of desmopressin influences the risk of bleeding.[355,356] As a general concept, thrombocytopenia does not appear to increase the risk of bleeding in patients with cirrhosis, and whether the administration of platelets influences bleeding risk in patients who undergo invasive procedures or decreases transfusion requirements in patients with variceal hemorrhage is uncertain. Nevertheless, common clinical practice is to administer platelet transfusions to achieve a minimum platelet count of approximately 50,000/mm^3 prior to an invasive procedure and in the setting of active bleeding.[348,349]

Dysfibrinogenemia

Dysfibrinogenemia, manifested either by hyper- or hypofibrinolysis, is common in patients with cirrhosis. Hyperfibrinolysis, reflected by elevated circulating levels of D-dimer and fibrinogen degradation products and by prolongation of the clot lysis time, is seen in up to 46% of cirrhotic patients.[357,358] These abnormalities result from altered production of activators and inhibitors of fibrinolysis, activation of the coagulation cascade by endotoxemia, and decreased clearance of fibrinolytic proteins in the setting of hepatic synthetic dysfunction. One hypothesis is that hyperfibrinolysis becomes more severe as liver disease progresses, eventually resulting in overt DIC, further increasing the risk of bleeding. Chronic liver disease, however, has also been associated with hypofibrinolysis, including reduced plasminogen levels and increased plasminogen activator inhibitor levels.[359–361] Moreover, results of tests for individual pro- and antifibrinolytic factors are variable, and their measurement in patients with chronic liver disease has not been standardized or uniformly accepted. These findings highlight the complexity and uncertainty of assessing the clinical consequences of dysfibrinogenemia in patients with cirrhosis.[359] Antihyperfibrinolytic therapy with compounds such as ε-aminocaproic acid or tranexamic acid has been used to prevent blood loss or treat bleeding in cirrhotic patients and during LT, but evidence to support the benefits of such an approach is limited.[362,363]

Endogenous Anticoagulants

In addition to decreased production of procoagulant proteins, hepatic synthetic dysfunction in cirrhosis also impairs the production of endogenous anticoagulant proteins, including protein C, protein S, antithrombin, tissue plasminogen activator, and thrombomodulin.[364] These abnormalities may result in hypercoagulability and contribute to[339] an increased risk of portal vein thrombosis, deep venous thrombosis, and pulmonary embolism compared with nonliver disease controls.[365–367] The prevalence of PVT increases with increased liver disease severity and may also be influenced by decreased portal flow and vessel abnormalities, inherited hypercoagulable states (including factor V Leiden, prothrombin 20210A gene mutations, JAK2 mutations), and factors related to obesity, immobility, and malignancy.[350,368–371] In addition, microthrombi formation and thrombin-mediated effects may also contribute to the worsening of hepatic fibrosis[339,372,373] (see also Chapter 87).

Anticoagulation use for standard venous thromboembolism (VTE) prophylaxis is recommended in hospitalized patients with cirrhosis who meet the criteria for VTE prophylaxis.[350] Treatment of PVT with anticoagulation has a low risk of bleeding complications and has the potential benefits of reducing portal hypertensive complications and preventing complete thrombosis and increased surgical risk.[350] Guidelines for managing portal vein thrombosis are available, although the level of supporting evidence is low.[374] Esophageal varices should be treated prior to starting anticoagulation.[350]

Viscoelastic Testing

Viscoelastic tests, including thromboelastography (TEG) and rotational thromboelastometry, are simple point-of-care tests that assess multiple components of in vivo hemostasis, including the cellular and plasmatic components of clot formation, strength, and stability. Studies using TEG suggest that despite thrombocytopenia and evidence of prolonged coagulation on standard laboratory-based assays, many patients with liver disease have a balanced homeostatic milieu in which coagulation may be normal or even enhanced.[375] These observations have driven studies in which TEG has been used to predict the risk of rebleeding from esophageal varices,[376] the need for massive transfusion of blood products during LT,[377] and the length of stay and risk of allograft dysfunction following transplantation.[378]

TEG is also being implemented slowly in clinical practice to guide the need for blood products during invasive procedures in patients with cirrhosis and coagulopathy. A recent systematic review and meta-analysis of the use of VET to guide blood product administration prior to nonsurgical procedures that included paracentesis, thoracentesis, TIPS, percutaneous liver biopsy and endoscopy for variceal bleeding, and control of nonvariceal gastrointestinal bleeding found a significant decrease in blood product use and no increase in postprocedure bleeding.[379] Another systematic review on the use of VET in patients undergoing nonsurgical procedures, similar to those stated above, and invasive procedures, including LT, showed similar results.[380] Although TEG, similar to all blood-based assays, is limited by not accounting for the endothelial-derived coagulation components, it adds significantly to the assessment of coagulation in cirrhosis.[381] It will likely replace traditional strategies for optimizing coagulation prior to invasive procedures, although more data are required.

Full references for this chapter can be found at https://ebooks.health.elsevier.com.

97 Acute Liver Failure

William M. Lee, Shannan Tujios, R. Todd Stravitz

IN THIS CHAPTER

INTRODUCTION AND DEFINITIONS

Acute liver failure (ALF) is the name applied to a condition of rapid loss of hepatocyte function that may result from a variety of etiologies, from viral hepatitis to drug-induced liver injury (DILI) and acetaminophen (APAP) toxicity, among others. It is relatively rare with an estimated 2–4000 incidence annually in North America.[1] Other names for this condition have included fulminant hepatic failure or fulminant hepatitis. The accepted hallmark features are (1) any degree of altered mentation [hepatic encephalopathy (HE)], and (2) coagulopathy with a prolonged prothrombin time measured as international normalized ratio (INR) ≥1.5, in the absence of preexisting cirrhosis, hence the designation "acute".[2] Disease evolution occurs rapidly, with progression from onset of first symptoms to encephalopathy in as few as 2–3 days or as long as several months, but most often in less than 3 weeks. Under certain circumstances, patients presenting acutely without prior knowledge of cirrhosis may be considered for inclusion if the diagnosis of cirrhosis had not been made previously. Wilson Disease (WD), for example, presents with a very specific and unique pattern of rapid onset of hemolysis and kidney injury with a nearly uniform fatal outcome without liver transplantation (LT).[3] Underlying cirrhosis in WD is nearly always present during this unique acute presentation. Likewise, autoimmune hepatitis (AIH) may remain subclinical after onset, without jaundice or obvious symptoms for several months, leading to underlying early cirrhosis in a small number of patients who present with a severe, acute hepatitis.[4] Otherwise, all other etiologies present with short-duration illness but severe hepatocyte insult, typically severe necrosis or apoptosis of cells without a matching degree of cellular regeneration. ALF should be distinguished from acute-on-chronic liver failure (ACLF),[5] in which cirrhosis precedes deterioration as the name implies (see also Chapters 95 and 96). Eventually, loss of hepatocyte function involves nearly all organ systems, including kidneys, lungs, and central nervous system. Outcomes prior to the present era and the widespread availability of LT were very poor with, in one early study, 92% mortality.[6] Currently, with better intensive care and the availability of LT, overall mortality is stillc.30% with up to 45% requiring LT and 25%–40% transplant free survival (TFS).[7,8]

Over the past four decades, research in ALF has been limited somewhat by its rarity and acuity, since controlled clinical treatment trials are difficult to perform for these reasons, as well as the multiplicity of etiologies and the availability of LT as a rescue of these very sick patients.[9] The ALF Study Group, an NIH-sponsored research network, began to enroll patients in 1998, and over the next 22 years, admitted 3364 patients to its registry at 32 tertiary care centers across North America. Combining data and providing biosamples to interested investigators has provided some insights and the ability to overcome the problem of dealing with a rare condition as indicated by the group's publication list at acuteliverfailure.org. As a natural history study, the ALF Study Group has allowed further characterization of the specific presentations of the different etiologies and their unique outcome patterns, as well as allowing the conduct of several clinical trials across the ALF spectrum.[10–13] To broaden slightly the spectrum of disease, we have included a separate category of severe liver injury that is slightly less ominous and that has been termed "acute liver injury," (ALI), wherein INR is ≥2.0 (higher than for ALF) but no HE is present.[14] Outcomes for ALI patients are improved from those with ALF as might be expected, with only 10% evolving to ALF after study enrollment in the ALF Study Group Registry.

EPIDEMIOLOGY

Data from the ALF Study Group Registry over the past 22 years has indicated that the most prevalent etiology for this entire period was APAP (referred to as paracetamol in Europe and the United Kingdom) in 46% of all patients enrolled with little increase or decrease over this time period (Fig. 97.1).[8] Next most frequent is idiosyncratic DILI at 11%,[15,16] followed by AIH[4,17] and acute hepatitis B virus (HBV) infection.[18] Patients who cannot be characterized with regard to etiology are considered indeterminate (IND),[19] although this may be due to lack of adequate etiologic workup (indeterminable) when, for example, specific

TABLE 97.1 Phenotypes of Etiologies

	Acetaminophen (n = 1261)	Ischemia (n = 221)	Drug-Induced Liver Injury (n = 284)	Autoimmunity (n = 193)	Hepatitis B Virus (n = 187)	Hepatitis A Virus (n = 41)	Pregnancy (n = 39)	All other causes (n = 405)
Age (median, years)	37	53	46	44	45	50	30	43
Women (%)	75	58	69	77	47	49	100	61
Jaundice coma (median, days)	1	2	13	15	8	4	6	9
Hepatic encephalopathy grade 3 or higher (%)	50	55	32	28	49	54	54	38
Alanine aminotransferase (median, IU/L)	3779	2334	635	449	1402	2229	60	582
Bilirubin (median, mg/dL)	4.3	3.8	21.6	22.8	19.9	12.0	11.2	18.6
Listed for Transplant (%)	23	5	56	69	56	59	33	48
Transplanted[a] (%)	9	3	41	59	40	32	18	35
Transplant-free survival[a] (%)	69	67	31	17	24	59	67	23
Overall survival[a] (%)	77	68	70	71	59	88	82	56

[a]Represents outcomes 21 days after admission to Acute Liver Failure Study Group Registry.
Data were collected between Jan 1, 1998 and Dec 2, 2022. Total number of ALF patients = 2631
Reprinted with permission from Stravitz RT, Lee WM. Seminar: acute liver failure. *Lancet*. 2019;394:869–881.

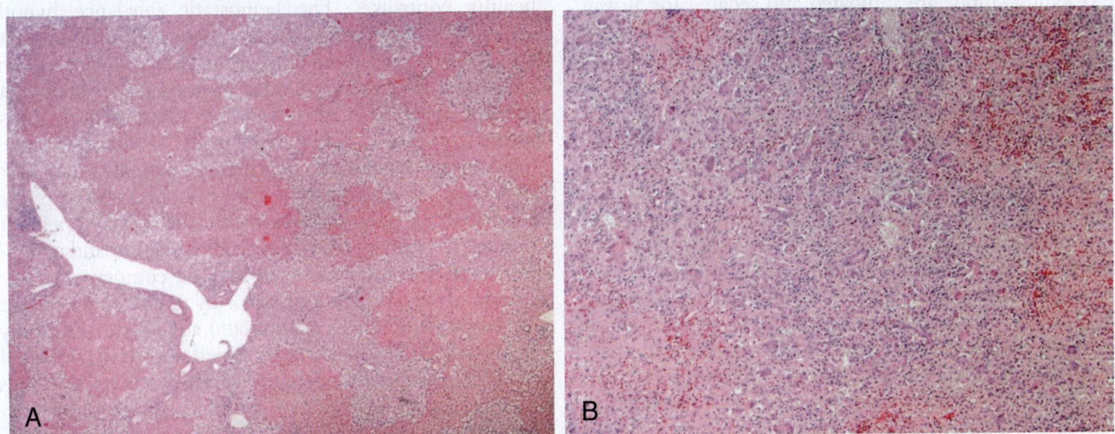

Fig. 97.3 Histopathology of acute liver failure (ALF). (A) Zonal necrosis due to acetaminophen toxicity. There is coagulative necrosis in zone 3 with preserved zone 1 hepatocytes showing steatosis. Only minimal inflammation is present. (H&E, 40×) (B) Fulminant hepatic necrosis due to acute hepatitis B. There is near complete necrosis of hepatocytes with ductular reaction and lymphoplasmacellular inflammation (H&E, 100×). (From Stravitz RT, Fontana RJ, Karvellas C, et al. Future directions in acute liver failure. *Hepatology*. 2023. doi: 10.1097/HEP.0000000000000458. Epub ahead of print. Courtesy of David Kleiner, MD, National Cancer Institute, Bethesda, MD.)

diagnosis is not always straightforward, particularly in comatose patients who cannot give a history.[32]

Ischemic liver injury secondary to poor perfusion or lack of oxygenated blood to perfuse the liver occurs in nearly 10% of ALF cases and is resolved by resuscitation and identification of the underlying cause: cardiac failure, systemic hypoxia due to lung disease, or hypovolemia leading to poor hepatic blood flow.[33]

Idiosyncratic DILI results when a prescription drug, herbal, or dietary supplement causes liver injury and is responsible for 11% of ALF cases in a North American population but up to 50% in Asia where herbal products are more frequently present.[8,15,16] Overall, 20% of North American DILI is related to nonregulated nutritional products and supplements. Onset of DILI ALF always involves latency, thought to represent metabolism of the agent, and immune-mediated reaction to metabolites displayed on the hepatocyte surface.[34] No specific tests are available to determine if the drug has caused the illness observed, so causality tools are available to help sort this out.[35]

AIH and HBV each account for c.~8%–10% of North American cases of ALF and are typically diagnosed by serological testing and, in the case of AIH, liver biopsy.[4,17] Care must be taken to distinguish between acute HBV and those individuals with chronic hepatitis B who receive chemotherapy or other immunosuppressives and develop reactivation.[36]

Space does not permit a detailed review of other minor etiologies. Many have specific tests to determine the diagnosis and specific therapies, such as Budd-Chiari syndrome, where ALF represents simply the most severe and acute manifestation of hepatic vein thrombosis.[37] Likewise, heat stroke is readily identified and resembles ischemic liver injury but requires its own specific management.[38] Other etiologies in the miscellaneous category include pregnancy-associated liver disease,[39] a small number of cancers that result in ALF,[40] and other viruses that cause a small number of cases: hepatitis A virus (HAV), herpes viruses, and rarely in the West, HEV.[41–43]

CLINICAL FEATURES

Hepatic Encephalopathy and Cerebral Edema

By definition, patients with ALF must have HE, the neurocognitive condition ranging from trivial alterations in cognition in its minimal stage to coma in its most severe stage. The earliest manifestations of HE (lack of awareness, distractibility) are tremendously subjective and differentiating between severe ALI (no HE) and ALF, with low-grade HE, is inherently flawed. The difference between grade 1 and 2 HE is also subtle and usually relies on the presence of asterixis in the latter. Moreover, distinguishing grades 3 (stupor) from 4 (coma) is often impossible since those reaching stupor are intubated and sedated for airway protection. Therefore it is more reasonable to grade HE in ALF as low- (grades 1 and 2 by West Haven Criteria) and high-grade (grades 3 and 4) HE.

The clinical presentation and pathogenesis of HE in ALF bears similarities to HE in patients with cirrhosis but is distinct, leading to the subclassification of HE in ALF as "Type A."[44] HE in ALF represents a pure loss of hepatocyte mass, whereas patients with cirrhosis develop HE due to portosystemic shunting as well as hepatocyte insufficiency. In distinction to cirrhosis where serum ammonia concentration correlates poorly with severity of HE, the ammonia concentration in ALF has important prognostic implications because of its relationship with HE grade, risk of cerebral edema, and the development of intracranial hypertension.[45,46] The association of serum ammonia concentration with risk of cerebral edema in ALF supports a role for the generation of osmotically active glutamine from ammonia and glutamate in the pathogenesis of astrocyte swelling and increase in brain volume. Cerebral edema is a prominent feature of HE in ALF but is rarely encountered in cirrhosis due to the severity and rapidity of accumulation of ammonia and other neurotoxins in the former, in whom compensatory mechanisms to counter hyperosmolality (e.g., export of potassium and myo-inositol) are overwhelmed.[47] Other mechanisms of HE and cerebral edema have also been identified in patients with ALF, including neuroinflammation, alterations in gene expression of cell volume-regulating genes, altered neurotransmission, and increased cerebral perfusion due to proinflammatory cytokines and loss of cerebrovascular autoregulation.[48]

The progression to high-grade HE in patients with ALF accompanies systemic inflammation and often infection,[49] and heralds the increasing risk of cerebral edema and intracranial hypertension. Although a serum ammonia of >150 μM was a recognized as a threshold above which the incidence of cerebral edema increased,[45] more refined analysis has shown the risk increases when ammonia >100 μM,[46] particularly if persistent.[50] Physical signs of cerebral edema vary in individual patients but include hyperreflexia, pupillary changes, delirium, asterixis, clonus, seizures, extensor posturing, and finally coma.[51] Head CT scans are often used in anticipation of placing an intracranial pressure (ICP) monitor. Unfortunately, signs of cerebral edema on head CT scan (effacement of sulci, loss of gray/white matter interface, and compression of ventricles; Fig. 97.4) are often absent, and correlation with ICP on insertion of an ICP monitor is only 40%.[52] Intracranial hypertension, the result of brain swelling within the confines of the rigid skull, in late stages often results in downward pressure of the brainstem through the foramen magnum, and tonsillar herniation. Patients exhibit signs of these late complications of cerebral edema in the form of further pupillary changes, hyperventilation, and posturing. It is important to note that the presence of cerebral edema on head CT scan or neurologic signs of intracranial hypertension, for example, decerebrate posturing, and can be seen in patients who survive ALF and have full neurologic recovery.[53]

Disordered Hemostasis

By definition, patients with ALF also have coagulopathy (INR of ≥1.5), frequently accompanied by mild-to-moderate thrombocytopenia.[54] Early series of ALF reported a high incidence and mortality (~30%) from bleeding complications.[55] Two large series from the U.S. ALF Study Group[56] and King's College,[57] however, suggest that bleeding complications are much less common in more recent experience (~10%). The explanation for this decline has not been well-defined.

In patients with ALF, hemostasis is usually "rebalanced,"[58] a term coined in patients with cirrhosis whereby thrombin generation under specific in vitro conditions was similar to normal healthy controls.[59] The hemostatic rebalance hypothesis was explained by the fact that many pro- and antihemostatic factors are liver-derived, and therefore, both decreased in tandem because of liver failure. Under the same experimental conditions, patients with ALF also have thrombin generation similar to normal controls (i.e., rebalanced).[60] Multiple compensatory mechanisms have been identified in patients with ALF for each phase of coagulation.[22] For example, patients with ALF commonly develop mild-moderate thrombocytopenia in proportion to the severity of systemic inflammation and complications.[54] However, thrombocytopenia may be compensated by increased release of von Willebrand factor by endothelial cells, resulting in increased platelet aggregation and adhesion.[61] Fibrinolysis in patients with ALF appears to be tipped toward hypercoagulability, as whole-blood clot lysis is unmeasurably prolonged in most patients with ALF.[61] The result of multiple compensatory schemes has been studied by rotational thromboelastometry (ROTEM) in nearly 200 patients with ALF, an assay of global hemostasis in whole blood.[12] Many patients were shown to have multiple defects in coagulation; by contrast, almost none had defective fibrinolysis.

The sum total of these hemostatic abnormalities suggests that hemostasis in patients with ALF achieves a fragile degree of compensation in which overt, significant bleeding is uncommon. Clinically, in nearly 1800 patients with ALF, few experienced clinically significant bleeding complications, 16% of whom needed a blood transfusion for the bleed, and only 2% experienced bleeding as the proximate cause of death.[56] The most common presentation of bleeding in this population was self-limited upper gastrointestinal bleeding, a presumptive diagnosis of stress-induced gastric mucosal disease as most did not undergo upper endoscopy. A similar number of patients experienced postprocedural bleeding complications (10%). However, most received transfusions of prohemostatic blood products before

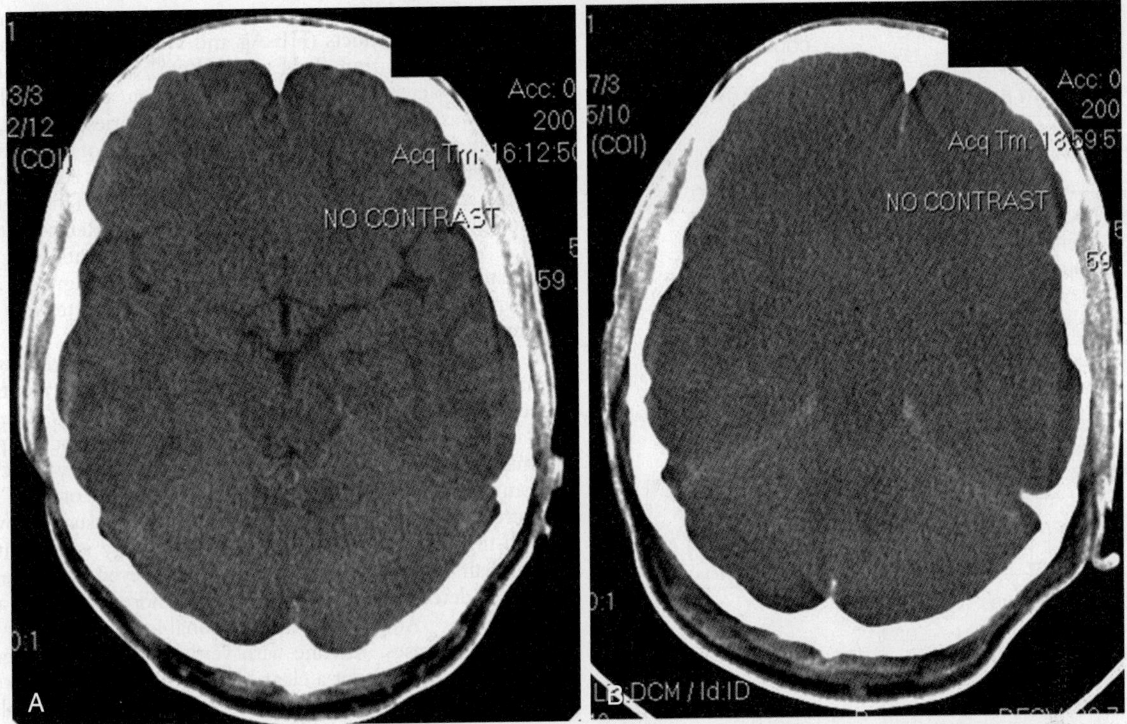

Fig. 97.4 Head CT scans of the same patient with indeterminate acute liver failure (ALF). (A) Head CT on admission to the hospital. (B) Head CT 48 hours after admission to the hospital, showing effacement of sulci, loss of gray/white matter interface, and compression of ventricles. (Reproduced with permission from Lippincott Williams and Wilkins; Civetta, Taylor, and Kirby's Critical Care, Chapter 154, Fourth Ed.)

their procedure, and rare instances of life-threatening bleeding were observed primarily after insertion of an ICP monitor.

Differential Diagnosis

A patient with altered mentation and evidence of liver injury must first be determined to have ALF. ACLF, a more common diagnosis than ALF, may be the most difficult entity to rule out. ACLF presents as acutely decompensated cirrhosis leading to failure of one or more organ systems.[62] Patients with ACLF present similarly to those with ALF, with jaundice, HE, coagulopathy, and evidence of extrahepatic organ system dysfunction. However, the presence of cirrhosis in the former population should be obvious after physical exam and initial laboratories which suggest chronicity (ascites, hypoalbuminemia, sarcopenia, spider angiomata, umbilical hernias, and other findings). Precipitating events of ACLF differ from those of ALF, and include upper GI bleeding, infection, or alcohol-associated hepatitis; these are not typical presenting features of ALF. The laboratories of the patient with ALF also differ from those with ACLF, in that the former have higher aminotransferases, INR and platelet count than the latter. The differential diagnosis of ALF also includes biliary sepsis and alcohol-associated hepatitis. Patients with biliary sepsis should be readily identifiable by evidence of infection on presentation rather than as a late complication, which is more typical of ALF. Evidence of biliary tract disease should be sought by liver ultrasound. Patients with alcohol-associated hepatitis seldom exhibit aminotransferases more than a few hundred units/L with AST>ALT, and often have evidence of underlying cirrhosis, distinctly different than patients with ALF. There are a few etiologies of ALF which present with AST>ALT and might challenge the clinician in this regard, including an early APAP overdose, ischemic liver injury, and herpes simplex virus (HSV) hepatitis.[63]

INITIAL MANAGEMENT

Immediate management decisions are often made in the emergency department and are critical to the outcome of ALF (Fig. 97.5). These include the need for endotracheal intubation for airway protection, central venous access, and NAC. Most patients should receive intravenous NAC in the emergency department on recognition of the ALF syndrome regardless of etiology, a recommendation backed by inconclusive data except in the case of APAP overdose (see below). Relying on an APAP level to make the decision to administer NAC is no longer reasonable. If possible, patients should be admitted to an intensive care unit (ICU), for, regardless of the apparent stability of a patient on admission, abrupt deterioration often occurs. Next, the clinician should consider contacting a tertiary care center with LT capabilities for urgent transfer or activate the LT team within their own center. The question of suitability for LT is never the purview of the intensivist or emergency physician but must be considered by a multidisciplinary LT team.

Initial management in the ICU usually includes ensuring patient comfort, hemodynamic stability, and initiating the assessment for underlying etiology. The head of the bed should be elevated 30 degrees and neck position neutral, which may promote intracranial venous drainage, thereby lowering ICP.

Determining Etiology of ALF and Administration of Treatment for the Liver Injury

The etiology of liver injury may be the single most important parameter predicting outcome and the need for LT for a patient with ALF.[63] Table 97.2 outlines screening and confirmatory tests for each etiology. Some are notably less accurate in the ALF setting than they are in patients with chronic liver disease. For example, HBV serologies may be undetectable in ALF since an

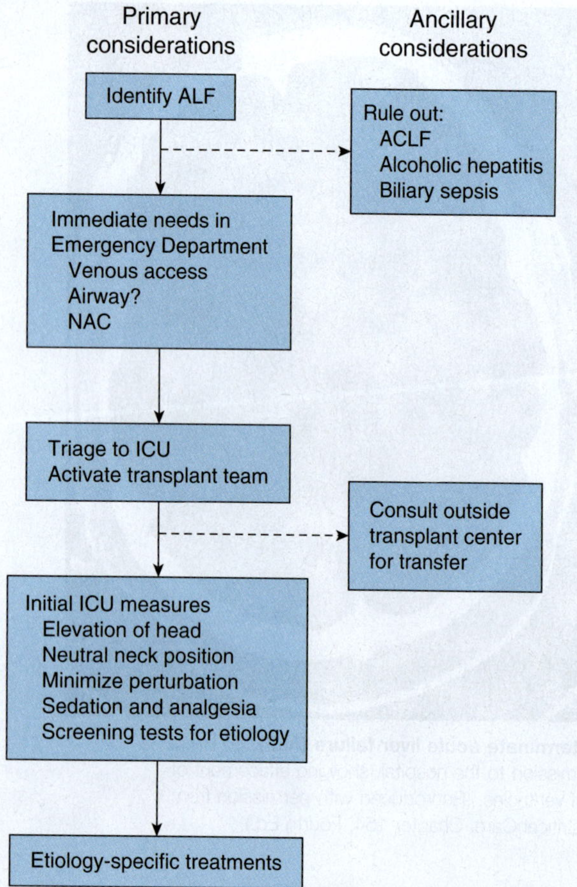

Fig. 97.5 Initial management of acute liver failure (ALF). *ACLF*, Acute-on-chronic liver failure; *NAC*, *N*-acetylcysteine.

overwhelming host immune response may truncate the appearance of viral products (HBsAg and HBV DNA) and markers of immune recognition (IgM anti-HBc).[64] Screening patients with suspected acute WD should not rely on a low ceruloplasmin, which was only ~20% sensitive in one series; instead, standard liver chemistries are helpful.[3] The prevalence of autoantibodies or hypergammaglobulinemia in AIH presenting as ALF is lower than in the chronic setting, only ~50%–60%.[17] Thus determining etiology on admission for ALF has pitfalls. Retrospectively, the ALF Study Group showed that 50% of patients with "indeterminate etiology" could be given a known diagnosis after case review by experts in the field and selective retesting of stored sera.[19]

A history of ingestion of APAP in a patient with liver injury may be unreliable or unobtainable due to altered mentation and lack of forthrightness, especially in suicidal cases. Clues to the diagnosis of APAP-induced ALF include a distinctive pattern of aminotransferase elevation, usually very high with early predominance of AST, and later predominance of ALT, as both decrease with time.[63] Total bilirubin is usually low (rarely >10 mg/dL) unless more than one etiology is present.[65] More than half of patients with ALF or ALI believed to be due to APAP have undetectable serum APAP levels, more often so in accidental overdoses.[30] At present, it is reasonable to administer NAC in ambiguous cases. Anyone with very high aminotransferases and low bilirubin, without a clear history of ischemic injury or APAP exposure, should still be considered for an empiric trial of NAC since unrecognized APAP is quite common.[31]

The optimal regimen of NAC in APAP ALF is not well defined and varies between institutions.[66] Intravenous administration is preferred as it ensures delivery and avoids gastrointestinal side effects, including vomiting which may accompany oral administration. A loading dose followed by two maintenance infusions of NAC are commonly recommended, although lower doses with shorter infusion times may be equally efficacious.[67] The original 20 hours 15 minutes intravenous infusion protocol

TABLE 97.2 Screening and Confirmatory Tests to Consider on Admission for Acute Liver Failure (ALF)

Etiology	Screening Test	Confirmatory Test
Acetaminophen	APAP level	APAP-hepatocyte protein adduct (in development)
Ischemia	Hemodynamic data, TTE	Cardiac catheterization
HAV	IgM anti-HAV	
HBV	IgM anti-HBc, total anti-HBc, HBsAg, anti-HDV	HBV DNA, HDV RNA
HEV	IgM anti-HEV	HEV RNA
DILI	History	Liver biopsy
Autoimmune	ANA, ASMA, anti-LKM, immunoglobulins	Liver biopsy
Budd-Chiari Syndrome	Doppler ultrasound	Hepatic venogram
Wilson Disease	Serum Cu >200 µg/dL, AP/TB < 4, AST/ALT > 2.2, hemolytic anemia, slit-lamp exam of eyes	24 hours urinary Cu, quantitative liver Cu
Pregnancy (AFLP/HELLP)	Third trimester of pregnancy, preeclampsia, β-hCG	Ultrasound
HSV	IgM anti-HSV 1/2	HSV DNA
Malignant infiltration	CT or MRI	Liver biopsy

ANA, Antinuclear antibodies; *AP*, alkaline phosphatase; *APAP*, acetaminophen; *ASMA*, antismooth muscle antibodies; *Cu*, copper; *DILI*, idiosyncratic drug-induced liver injury; *HAV*, hepatitis A virus; *HBV*, hepatitis B virus; *HEV*, hepatitis E virus; *hCG*, human chorionic gonadotropin; *HSV*, herpes simplex virus; *LKM*, liver-kidney microsomal antibodies; *TB*, total bilirubin; *TTE*, transthoracic echocardiogram.

administered a total of 300 mg/kg NAC, infused as 150 mg/kg over 15 minutes (600 mg/kg/h), followed by 50 mg/kg over 4 hours (12.5 mg/kg/h), followed by 100 mg/kg over 16 hours (6.25 mg/kg/h). A Cochrane Review concluded that data regarding the administration of NAC in APAP overdose are of low quality and studies comparing specific regimens were statistically underpowered, although NAC overall appeared superior to placebo.[68]

Based upon literature supporting NAC as a treatment for APAP liver injury, several studies have investigated the efficacy of NAC in non-APAP ALF in adults.[10,69] NAC has a number of potentially beneficial hemodynamic and oxygen delivery properties in ALF in addition to repletion of glutathione stores.[70] Benefit in other etiologies is inferred, but clinical trials in non-APAP cases are of low scientific rigor. The largest study of 173 patients randomized patients to intravenous NAC or placebo for 72 hours.[10] The study did not meet its primary endpoint of an improvement in overall survival. In subgroup analysis, however, patients with low-grade HE who received NAC were shown to have improved TFS compared to those with the same clinical characteristics who received placebo. Other studies have reached similar conclusions on the efficacy of NAC in non-APAP ALF but were nonrandomized, showing improved transplant-free but not overall survival. A Cochrane Review concluded that there were no scientifically rigorous data to support the practice.[71] However, since there are data that support the efficacy of NAC in the most rigorously performed study, since clinicians often cannot be completely confident of the etiology, more than one etiology (including APAP) can exist, and NAC is relatively innocuous, the administration of NAC to all patients with ALF seems reasonable regardless of perceived etiology.

Specific treatments for other etiologies of ALF are even less well substantiated (Table 97.3). Fulminant HBV is often treated with nucleos(t)ide DNA polymerase inhibitors that are extremely effective in halting viral replication and improving clinical course in patients with chronic HBV. As noted above, however, the rationale for using these drugs in patients with ALF is less compelling, since the robust immune response against HBV in patients with ALF usually clears the virus rapidly. Indeed, the only randomized, placebo-controlled study of lamivudine in patients with severe, acute HBV found no benefit in clearance of HBV DNA or outcome.[72] The study included patients without ALF and was probably underpowered, but does not support the use of these agents in acute HBV of any severity. Not surprisingly, a Cochrane Review identified studies of various agents to quell the liver injury of acute HBV, but concluded the studies were heterogeneous and their quality scientifically poor, and found no evidence to support their use.[73] There is, however, an important rationale to start a nucleos(t)ide antagonist in patients with fulminant HBV: preparation for LT to prevent graft infection.

The use of corticosteroids (CS) in patients with autoimmune ALF (AI-ALF) might also be considered an etiology-specific treatment of liver injury. Cases of suspected AI-ALF should be considered for transjugular liver biopsy, which can be useful to guide therapy.[17,74] CS appear to benefit patients with chronic and severe acute AIH.[75] Unfortunately, the data supporting their efficacy in patients with full-blown ALF are scant and also of poor scientific quality. There are also toxicities of CS to consider in patients who are likely to need LT, principally infection. These considerations have led to a few practical guidelines when treating suspected AIH-ALF.[75] CS (e.g., methylprednisolone 60 mg daily IV) should be started as soon as AIH-ALF is suspected, assuming that there are no contraindications. Since AIH-ALF has a very poor TFS (20%–25%), evaluation for LT should be started. If there are no significant improvements in daily laboratories (in bilirubin or INR) in roughly 7 days, CS should be stopped as the avoidance of LT is remote, and the risk of CS increases. A recent study has shown the lack of response at 3 days may be predictive of treatment failure.[76] Finally, a patient with high-grade HE and suspected AIH-ALF should probably be evaluated for LT and the administration of CS forgone as futile.

ALF in pregnant women presents a difficult management challenge to clinicians but may not result in worse outcome than ALF in nonpregnant women due to meticulous supportive care and an early termination of the pregnancy.[77] There are few evidence-based studies on managing the two pregnancy-specific etiologies of ALF, acute fatty liver of pregnancy (AFLP), and the hemolysis-elevated liver chemistry-low platelet (HELLP) syndrome. Early termination of the pregnancy has consistently been reported to improve maternal morbidity and mortality.[78] A meta-analysis of management of the pregnancy in AFLP found a significant improvement in maternal morbidity and mortality after Cesarian-section versus vaginal delivery.[79] In contrast to AFLP, HELLP syndrome, a complication of severe preeclampsia, may occur following delivery. The management of HELLP syndrome differs from that of AFLP and depends upon the age of gestation but also relies on early delivery.[80]

The efficacy of other etiology-specific treatments of ALF are recorded in Table 97.2 as anecdotes in the literature. These include acyclovir for ALF due to HSV,[81] molecular adsorbent recirculating system (MARS) for fulminant WD,[82] silibinin for *Amanita* mushroom poisoning,[83] and thrombolysis/intrahepatic portosystemic shunt placement in acute Budd-Chiari Syndrome.[37]

TABLE 97.3 Interventions for Specific Etiologies of Acute Liver Failure (ALF). NAC Should Be Considered for All Etiologies Except Pregnancy

Etiology	Intervention	Efficacy	Reference
HBV	Nucleos(t)ide DNA polymerase inhibitors	Negative randomized trial in severe acute HBV; consider before LT	Kumar[72]
Autoimmune	Corticosteroids	Anecdotal response with caveats	Rahim[75]
Amanita Sp.	Silibinin, penicillin	Anecdotal responses	Dluholucký[83]
HSV	Acyclovir	Inconsistent responses	Norvell[81]
Pregnancy	Delivery	Effective but may progress after delivery in HELLP syndrome	Knight[78] Haram[80]
Wilson Disease	MARS	Anecdotal responses	Rustom[82]
Budd-Chiari Syndrome	Anticoagulation, thrombolysis, TIPS	Anecdotal responses; may be a bridge to LT	Parekh[37]

HELLP, Hemolysis-elevated liver chemistries-low platelet syndrome; *LT*, liver transplantation; *MARS*, molecular absorbent recirculating system; *TIPS*, transjugular intrahepatic portosystemic shunt.

MANAGEMENT OF SYSTEMIC COMPLICATIONS

General Considerations

There are few data comparing management strategies in patients with ALF head-to-head. However, management practices appear to be converging across centers as clinicians have compiled and analyzed their experience with input from intensivists.[84,85] Extrapolation of management practices from other similar patient populations (for example, those with ACLF) has also helped define reasoned protocols.[86]

Fluids, Electrolytes, and Hemodynamics

Patients who present with ALF are often volume-depleted, related to altered mentation and the circumstances of their discovery. Hypotension also results from a hyperdynamic vasodilated state, a hallmark of ALF due to systemic inflammation (Fig. 97.6). Assessment of volume status in this vasodilated state is difficult, and bedside echocardiography has generally replaced pulmonary catheter methods.[86] There are few data to support the use of one fluid over another for volume resuscitation in ALF. Generally, normal saline boluses with a goal mean arterial pressure (MAP) >65 mm Hg are recommended.[86] Hypotension despite volume repletion should trigger a search for infection and consideration of empiric broad-spectrum antibiotics, as well as vasopressors, the use of which portends a poor prognosis.[87] Norepinephrine is the initial vasopressor of choice.[86] A vasopressin infusion should be added in patients with persistent hypotension despite volume resuscitation and maximal norepinephrine infusion. Stress-dose CS should be considered for persistent hypotension, as relative adrenal insufficiency has been documented in a significant minority of patients with ALF.[88] Hypotension with end-organ hypoperfusion despite these measures indicates very severe systemic inflammation. A randomized, controlled study of 182 patients with ALF suggested that high-volume plasma exchange was effective treatment for refractory hypotension presumably by removing vasoactive inflammatory mediators.[89] Subsequent studies of "standard" and "low-volume" plasma exchange appear to be similarly effective in reversing hypotension.[90,91]

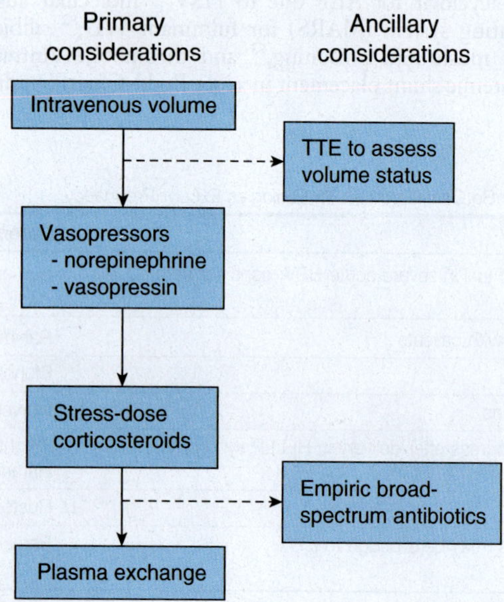

Fig. 97.6 Management of hypotension. *TTE*, Transthoracic echocardiogram.

Electrolyte abnormalities are common in patients with ALF and can be particularly hazardous. Hyponatremia exacerbates cerebral edema and should be cautiously corrected to avoid the demyelination of rapid sodium rise. Prophylaxis against hyponatremia has been shown to decrease ICP in patients with ALF in a randomized study of hypertonic saline (HTS)-induced mild hypernatremia (serum sodium 145–155 mEq/L), as compared to management at normal serum sodium concentrations (135 mEq/L),[92] and may be one of the primary reasons that the incidence of intracranial hypertension has decreased dramatically in recent years.[8,57] Hypokalemia exacerbates HE by increasing renal ammoniagenesis, reducing urea synthesis, and increasing ammonia entry into the brain across the blood-brain barrier, and thus requires prompt repletion.[93] Acute kidney injury (AKI) resulting in hyperkalemia should be treated with renal replacement therapy (RRT) as it may precipitate cardiac arrythmias. Serum phosphate must also be regularly assessed, as hepatic regeneration can result in rapid and profound decrease in phosphate, which is a harbinger of recovery of the native liver.[94]

Renal Failure

AKI complicates the course of ALF in ~70% of affected individuals.[95,96] The systemic inflammatory response syndrome (SIRS) is strongly associated with development of AKI; other risk factors include infection, hypovolemia, and nephrotoxic drugs, including APAP. AKI is more strongly associated with SIRS than the severity of ALF as assessed by the King's College Criteria (KCC), suggesting that it is a complication of systemic inflammation rather than due to liver failure per se. Two types of AKI complicate ALF. Hepatotoxins with intrinsic nephrotoxicity (APAP, other drugs, *Amanita* toxins) can cause acute tubular necrosis relatively early after presentation. Later, a syndrome resembling the functional renal failure of cirrhosis may develop. The pathogenesis of this "hepatorenal syndrome-like" AKI in patients with ALF is associated with portal hypertension and is more often observed in subacute ALF.[97] The functional renal failure of ALF resolves if the native liver recovers or is transplanted.

In the last few years, the indications for RRT in patients with ALF have changed. In contrast to traditional indications for RRT (to treat electrolyte abnormalities, azotemia, acidosis), recent data have shown that that early RRT not only decreases serum ammonia concentrations but also improves outcome.[98,99] Continuous RRT (CRRT) is preferred over intermittent hemodialysis as the former has been associated with greater hemodynamic stability than the latter in patients with ALF, and a lower propensity to exacerbate intracranial hypertension and lower cerebral perfusion.[100] The following indications for instituting CRRT in ALF should be strongly considered: progression to high-grade HE, a serum ammonia concentration of >150 μM,[45] the presence of the SIRS, and infection. These criteria may be met in the absence of azotemia, AKI criteria, or other traditional indications. Serum ammonia concentration is not an absolute criterion for initiating CRRT, but clinicians must recognize that the risk of cerebral edema increases above 100 μM.[46] The choice of dialysate and anticoagulants (including heparin and citrate) to maintain circuit patency do not appear to be major concerns in patients with ALF. A CRRT method of maintaining and weaning high target sodium for patients with ALF and cerebral edema has been described.[101] The use of MARS may also be considered.[102]

Cerebral Edema and Intracranial Hypertension

The incidence of cerebral edema and intracranial hypertension in patients with ALF has decreased by roughly 50% in the last 10 years due to an improved understanding of its pathogenesis and effective prophylaxis (Fig. 97.7). The use of ICP monitors has also

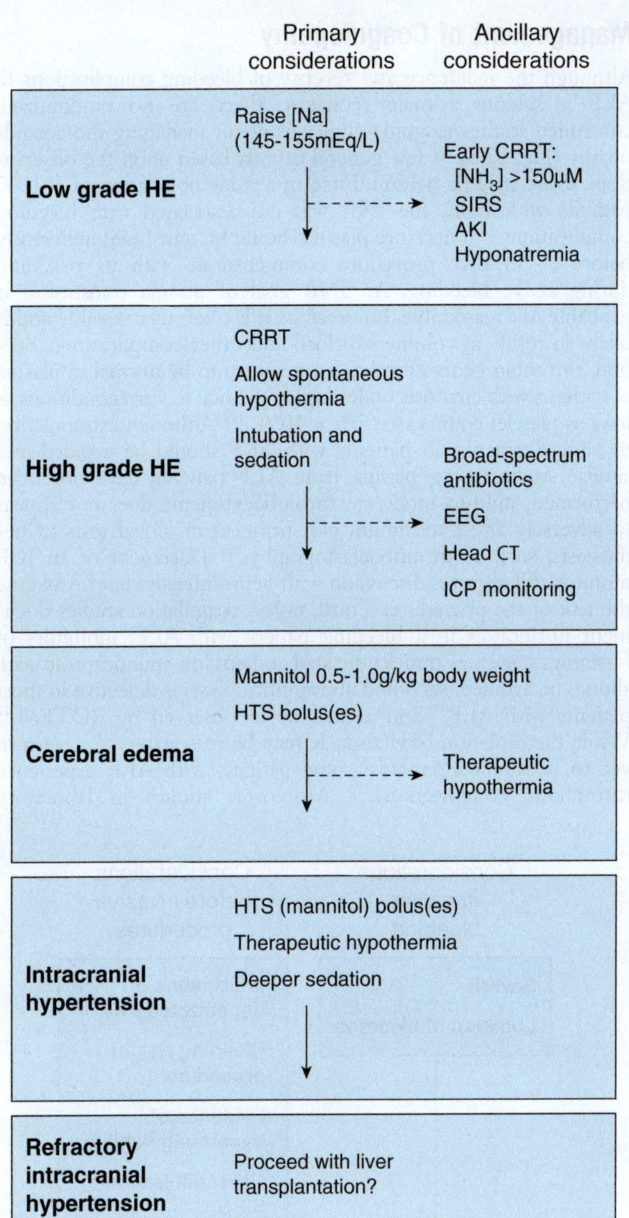

Fig. 97.7 Management of hepatic encephalopathy and cerebral edema. *AKI*, Acute kidney injury; *CRRT*, continuous renal replacement therapy; *EEG*, electroencephalogram; *HE*, hepatic encephalopathy; *HTS*, hypertonic saline; *ICP*, intracranial pressure; *(Na)*, serum sodium concentration; *(NH_3)*, serum ammonia concentration; *SIRS*, systemic inflammatory response syndrome.

decreased for these reasons as well as the consistent finding across nonrandomized series that they do not improve outcome, although are associated with increased maneuvers to manage ICP.[103,104]

There are no studies documenting efficacy of cathartics (lactulose) or nonabsorbable antibiotics (neomycin or rifaximin) in patients with ALF. The administration of a cathartic agent to effect evacuation of the bowel is reasonable on admission, but not as a scheduled therapy thereafter, and may exacerbate ileus and complicate LT surgery due to bowel distension. Prophylactic measures to prevent cerebral edema include maintaining serum sodium at slightly hypernatremic levels (145–155 mEq/L) and the early initiation of RRT.[92,99] Induced hypernatremia acts to osmotically draw water out of astrocytes similarly to mannitol boluses. CRRT has multiple potential effects on preventing cerebral edema by correcting hypoosmolality and removing ammonia.[98,99] Practical guidelines regarding the application of CRRT in patients with ALF have been suggested.[105] A randomized, controlled study of prophylactic hypothermia, lowering core temperature to 34°C, did not improve outcome as compared to patients managed at normal body temperature (36°C–37°C).[106] Temperature management in patients with ALF, therefore, should leave spontaneous hypothermia (such as commonly seen in critically ill patients on CRRT) uncorrected but not induced.

Once cerebral edema is established despite these prophylactic measurements, medical treatments uncommonly sustain normal ICP, and LT is often the only permanent solution. Temporizing measures as a bridge to LT include administering mannitol or HTS boluses, the use of which raise the dilemma of inserting an ICP monitor. Despite more widespread application in cerebral edema from other neurologic disorders (e.g., traumatic brain injury), noninvasive ICP monitoring has not been adopted widely for use in patients with ALF and has not been found to correlate accurately with ICP obtained by invasive monitoring.[107] Insertion of an ICP monitor is highly center- and clinician-dependent but should be considered in patients with high-grade HE who are being considered for LT, in which case the ICP may be as important to identify a patient who should not be transplanted due to long-standing (>2 hours), severe (>40 mm Hg) intracranial hypertension, as to improve its medical management.[53] The ICP goal in patients with ALF is a stable pressure of <20–25 mm Hg, with a cerebral perfusion pressure (CPP = MAP-ICP) of >50–60 mm Hg using vasopressors to a MAP >65 mm Hg.[86] The CPP must be monitored to ensure adequate cerebral perfusion and avoid anoxic brain injury. Once the ICP has increased >25 mm Hg, osmotic treatment is indicated. Mannitol administered intravenously (0.5–1.0 g/kg body weight) has long been the treatment of choice and serves to increase blood osmolality to reduce brain volume. The earliest experience with mannitol in small numbers of patients with ALF[108] established important principles. First, mannitol is modestly effective at achieving a goal ICP <20 mm Hg if a patient has mild-to-moderate intracranial hypertension to start (20–40 mm Hg), but relatively ineffective reaching this goal in patients with more severe intracranial hypertension. Second, the administration of mannitol usually requires repeated dosing, in which case blood osmolality should be monitored to avoid hyperosmolarity (redose only if <320 mOsm/L). Mannitol-treated patients with intracranial hypertension were thus found to have better TFS than those who did not receive mannitol but were still poor. Although contemporary management of intracranial hypertension in ALF continues to rely on mannitol,[85] HTS boluses are increasingly advocated as they are more easily dosed in a patient receiving CRRT. In one small study, mannitol and induced-hypernatremia with HTS were therapeutically equivalent.[109] Ammonia scavenging agents, such as ornithine phenylacetate may be useful in the future, but require further study.[11] The possibility of subclinical seizure activity should be considered, and continuous monitoring by electroencephalogram has been advocated.[110] Prophylactic phenytoin was found to improve outcome in one randomized study[110] but not in another,[111] however.

Once mannitol boluses have either reached the point of maximal therapeutic benefit or the patient's serum osmolality exceeds 320 mosm/L, rescue measures are often considered but seldom prevent herniation. Therapeutic hypothermia, cooling a patient to a core temperature of 32°C–34°C, has been used as a bridge to LT in a small number of patients with ALF who otherwise would likely have herniated, and appears to lower ICP reliably.[112] However, unless a liver graft is en route, prolonged hypothermia is likely to result in complications.[113] A sustained ICP before a LT of >40 mm Hg usually signifies impending neurologic death.[53] However, there are no absolute ICP criteria beyond which LT should be contraindicated. Neurologic recovery has been poor when ICP exceeds 40 mm Hg hours for >2 hours but is still possible in a patient who meets these criteria and undergoes successful LT.

Respiratory Failure

Acute lung injury with failure of oxygenation occurs in a third of patients with ALF and is associated with the development of cerebral edema and circulatory collapse.[114] These associations in the presence of normal left ventricular filling pressures suggest that the pathogenesis is driven by cytokines and/or endogenous vasodilators. There are two general indications for endotracheal intubation in a patient with ALF: airway protection from aspiration and failure of ventilation and oxygenation. Of the two, the former is more common, as patients are routinely intubated as they evolve from low- to high-grade HE. The latter indication is an independent predictor of mortality and is frequently associated with chest and bloodstream infections.[115] Ventilator management in a patient with ALF should be consistent with standard ICU protocol, with low tidal volumes recommended and positive end-expiratory pressure kept low (5–10 mm Hg), as higher levels may exacerbate cerebral edema by impairing intracranial venous drainage.[86] Surveillance tracheal aspirates and chest X-rays should be performed daily to surveille for pneumonia in ventilated ALF patients.

Infection

Patients with ALF are susceptible to infection due to many defects in immunity (Table 97.4).[116,117] Accordingly, infection and sepsis are major reasons for the inability to transplant a patient with ALF. Sepsis may be difficult to distinguish from the ALF syndrome as the two share clinical features of hypotension and the SIRS.[118] A high index of suspicion must be maintained at all times, and daily surveillance cultures of blood, sputum, and urine should be considered, particularly in patients with indwelling catheters, who are intubated, and/or are awaiting LT. Unfortunately, studies of prophylactic antibiotics have not shown improved outcome.[119,120] Indications for the empiric administration of broad-spectrum antibiotics include hypotension resistant to volume repletion, the presence of the SIRS, progression to high-grade HE, and being listed for LT. The latter indication is a center-specific practice but is often invoked as the consequences of infection while awaiting a liver offer are often fatal. Antifungal agents should also be strongly considered,[121] and the identification of an offending organism on surveillance cultures should lead to narrowing antibiotic coverage.

TABLE 97.4 Management of Infectious Diathesis and Established Infection

- Minimize invasive procedures where possible
- Prophylactic antibiotics not recommended
- Surveillance cultures recommended
- Indications for empiric, broad-spectrum antibiotics
  - Hypotension refractory to volume resuscitation
  - High number of SIRS
  - Progression to high-grade HE
  - Additional considerations:
    - Patient listed for liver transplantation?
    - Antifungal agents?
- Deescalation recommended after pathogens identified by surveillance/diagnostic cultures

Management of Coagulopathy

Although the incidence and severity of bleeding complications in ALF is seldom a major concern, there are no randomized, controlled studies to guide clinicians about managing the coagulopathy (Fig. 97.8). A few general caveats based upon the observations above may be helpful. First, in a study population of ~1800 patients with ALF, the INR was not associated with bleeding complications.[56] Therefore plasma should be transfused judiciously before an invasive procedure commensurate with its risk, and during active bleeding. An INR goal of plasma transfusion is probably not reasonable, however, as it is often unattainable and is likely to result in volume overload and other complications. Second, thrombin generation has been shown to be normal in plasma of patients with cirrhosis under highly defined in vitro conditions as long as platelet counts are $>56 \times 10^9$/L.[122] Although extrapolation to clinical practice in patients with ALF should be avoided and similar studies using plasma from ALF patients have not been performed, mild-to-moderate thrombocytopenia does not appear to adversely affect maximum clot firmness in global tests of hemostasis, such as thromboelastography.[123] Placement of an ICP monitor still requires discussion with neurointensivists who assume the risk of the procedure. Third, unless coagulation studies document fibrinolysis in a bleeding patient with ALF, inhibitors of fibrinolysis, such as tranexamic acid and epsilon aminocaproic acid, should be avoided. As noted above, fibrinolysis is defective in most patients with ALF[61] and almost never observed by ROTEM.[12] While the repletion of vitamin K may be reasonable,[125] a concern yet to be studied remains: some patients with ALF experience thrombotic complications.[123] Moreover, studies in laboratory

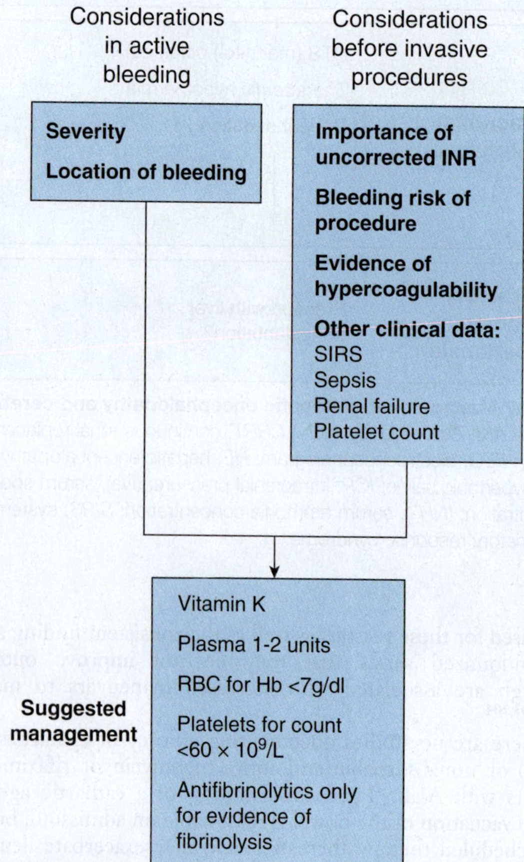

Fig. 97.8 Management of coagulopathy. *Hb*, Hemoglobin; *SIRS*, systemic inflammatory response syndrome.

animals with APAP ALF suggest that intrahepatic microthrombosis may exacerbate APAP-induced liver injury.[124] Finally, blood product transfusions are associated with poorer outcome in patients with ALF,[56] suggesting that blood product transfusion may have adverse effects in ALF. Finally, over the 20 years of collecting data, the ALF Study Group observed progressively fewer blood product transfusions as the incidence of bleeding complications remained stable, suggesting that withholding blood products may be safe.[56]

ASSESSING PROGNOSIS

While advances in critical care management have dramatically improved the survival in patients with ALF from 16% in the 1980s to over 60% in the 21st century, some patients ultimately will require life-saving LT.[57] The challenge remains in determining who might spontaneously recover with few sequelae despite fulminant organ failure from those who will perish without emergent LT. To assist in this difficult decision-making, several prognostic models have been developed to predict immediate outcomes, both mortality and transplant-free survival (Table 97.5). Scoring systems attempt to balance sensitivity of detecting patients who are most likely to die without LT with specificity, the unnecessary application of LT using readily available clinical data in the first 48–72 hours of presentation.

Although no model performs perfectly, the cornerstone of prognosticating outcomes in ALF lies on the correct identification of etiology, the most important determinant. APAP

TABLE 97.5 Prognostic Indices and Scores for Predicting Mortality and Need for Liver Transplantation in Patients With Acute Liver Failure (ALF). Several Additional Bio-Mmarkers Have Been Suggested and Are Discussed in the Text

Test or Index	Etiology	Threshold for Poor Prognosis, Need for Liver Transplantation	Reference
King's College Criteria	Acetaminophen	Arterial pH < 7.30 **or** all of the following: 1. PT > 100 seconds (INR > 6.5) 2. Creatinine >3.4 mg/dL 3. Grade 3/4 encephalopathy sensitivity 58%, specificity 94%	O'Grady[126]
	Nonacetaminophen	PT >100 seconds (INR >6.5) **or** any three of the following: 1. Non-A, non-B hepatitis, drug, or halothane etiology 2. Jaundice to encephalopathy >7 day 3. Age <10 or >40 years 4. PT >50 seconds (INR > 3.5) 5. Bilirubin >17.4 mg/dL sensitivity 68%, specificity 82%	
Factor V (Clichy criteria)	Viral	Age <30 years: factor V <20% **or** Any age: factor V <30% ***and*** grade 3/4 encephalopathy sensitivity 69%, specificity 50%	Bernuau[133]
SOFA score	Acetaminophen	Score ≥12; sensitivity 67%, specificity 80%	Cholongitas[128]
MELD score	Acetaminophen Nonacetaminophen	Score ≥33; sensitivity 60%, specificity 69% Score ≥30; sensitivity 76%, specificity 67% Meta-analysis sensitivity 74%, specificity 67%	Schmidt[129] Yantorno[130] McPhail[131]
ALFSG Initial Index	All etiologies	Coma grade, INR, bilirubin, phosphate, M-30 sensitivity 86%, specificity 65%	Rutherford [137] Craig[138]
ALFSG Prognostic Index[a]	All etiologies	Continuous variables (bilirubin and INR); favorable/unfavorable etiology; encephalopathy grade; use of vasopressors	Koch[87]
BiLE score	All etiologies	Score >6.9; sensitivity 79%, specificity 84%	Hadem[135]
Creatinine-lactate score	Nonacetaminophen	Creatinine-lactate; sensitivity 87%, specificity 71%	Figuera[136]
^{13}C-Methacetin Breath Test	All etiologies	Oral dosing of ^{13}C-methacetin	Fontana[13]
Volumetric CT	Nonacetaminophen	Liver volume <1000 cm^3 sensitivity 46%, specificity 93%	Zabron[158]
Liver biopsy	All etiologies	Hepatocyte necrosis >70%–75% sensitivity 69%, specificity 50%	Donaldson[154] Singhal[155]

[a]The ALFSG Prognostic Index, in contrast to the other indices listed, is designed to predict transplant-free survival rather than death/need for liver transplantation (see text).

ALFSG, Acute liver failure Study Group; *BiLE*, bilirubin-lactate-etiology score; *CT*, computerized tomography; mixed, mixed etiologies; *MELD*, model for end-stage liver disease, *SOFA*, sequential organ failure assessment.

hepatotoxicity presents with markedly elevated transaminases, rapidly rising INR and hyperammonemia with highest risk of cerebral edema but also has the highest probability of spontaneous survival; most other etiologies have a more subacute course with poorer prognosis.[8] The KCC published in 1989 divided APAP etiology from all others and predict mortality in a population of patients with ALF in the pretransplant era.[126] While the KCC have high specificity (94% in APAP; 84% in non-APAP), they lack sensitivity in the modern era even with medication to incorporate lactate to identify patients who are likely to die of multisystem organ failure.[127] When compared to the sequential organ failure assessment (SOFA) score and model for end-stage liver disease (MELD) score in APAP ALF, SOFA performed better than both KCC and MELD.[128] MELD has been applied to both APAP and non-APAP ALF with lower TFS noted in patients with MELD $\geq$33 and $\geq$30, respectively.[129,130] A meta-analysis comparing the accuracy of MELD versus KCC determined KCC predicted the need for transplant better in APAP cases whereas MELD was superior in non-APAP cases.[131] The original KCC have since been replaced with the United Kingdom revised criteria for emergency transplant listing (Table 97.6).[132]

A number of more specific ALF prognostic scores have been developed (Table 97.5). The Clichy criteria were derived from a French acute HBV population noting worse outcomes with factor V levels <20% in patients <30 years of age and <30% in older patients. These results have not been replicated in APAP ALF and are not widely used, however.[133,134] In a German study, bilirubin, lactate, and etiology compose the BiLE score, and creatinine-lactate score may better predict mortality in non-APAP ALF but have yet to be validated.[135,136] The first iteration of the ALF Study Group prognostic index used coma grade, INR, bilirubin, phosphorus, and levels of an apoptosis biomarker, M30, and correctly identified those who were transplanted or died with sensitivity of 86%.[137] However, the score is limited in clinical practice by the availability of the M30 assay and did not outperform SOFA score in further analysis.[138]

More recently, the ALF Study Group developed a mathematical model available as a web-based application which utilizes five readily available clinical features to determine spontaneous survival rather than mortality: etiology (favorable: APAP, ischemia, pregnancy, and HAV, vs. unfavorable: IND, drug, AIH, HBV, and WD), encephalopathy (grade 1–2 vs. grade 3–4), INR and bilirubin as continuous variables, and vasopressor use. The index outperformed KCC and MELD score in predicting 21-day TFS.[87] However, the model may overestimate the need for transplant in favorable etiologies with severe coma grade.

Given the rapidly evolving clinical status of patients with ALF, dynamic modeling has also been employed to better predict outcomes. The ALF "early dynamic model" uses changes in ammonia, bilirubin, INR, and stage of HE on admission and Day 2 to improve prognostic accuracy and has been predominantly applied to ALF due to viral hepatitis.[139] Sequential monitoring of INR and lactate also have been employed by the King's College to discriminate between spontaneously recovering APAP ALF patients and those in need of LT.[140] Recognizing the importance of initial liver injury as well as the regenerative response after injury, serial monitoring of hepatic metabolic function with the ^{13}C-methacetin breath test has also shown promise, but requires further study.[13]

Numerous biomarkers have been investigated to improve the performance of established clinical prognostic models or to provide additional information on severity of liver injury as well as regeneration. Most have been limited by inadequate use in clinical trials, and poor reproducibility and accessibility. The ALF Study Group has evaluated 15 potential biomarkers, including alphafetoprotein,[141] apoptosis markers,[142] Gc-globulin,[143] fatty acid binding protein,[144,145] and others.[146] Most of the studies assess the utility of the biomarkers at a single point in time, while performance may be enhanced with serial monitoring and application to specific etiologies. More recently, patterns of microRNA expression have been identified which are associated with hepatic regeneration and spontaneous survival.[147–149] Genomics have also been explored to identify susceptibility to ALF but have only provided weak associations except in the case of human leukocyte antigen genotypes with some cases of idiosyncratic drug induced liver injury.[150–153]

Histology, when available, may also provide important information on prognosis with >75% necrosis associated with the need for LT or death in cases of viral, autoimmune, or DILI ALF.[154–156] In more subacute cases of DILI, ineffective hepatocyte regeneration manifests as ductular reaction with cholestasis, microvesicular steatosis or fibrosis, findings which portend the need for LT or death, while granulomas and eosinophils are associated with survival.[157] Likewise, cross-sectional imaging of the liver by computed tomography or contrast-enhanced Doppler ultrasound using a threshold volume <1000 cm^3 represents substantial hepatic necrosis predictive of poor outcomes.[158,159]

EXTRACORPOREAL LIVER SUPPORT

Since most patients with ALF retain some capacity for recovery of their native liver, attempts to bridge a patient through the regeneration process with liver support devices has long been an unattainable feat dating back to the 1970s.[84,160] In other patients, such extracorporeal liver support (ECLS) devices, would theoretically bridge a patient to LT. ECLS devices comprise both artificial and bioartificial systems. Artificial devices rely on albumin molecules to bind toxins followed by membrane filtration to remove water-soluble substances and are commercially available as MARS (Gambro, Lund, Sweden), fractionated plasma

TABLE 97.6 United Kingdom Criteria for Emergency Liver Transplant Listing in Acute Liver Failure (ALF)[132]

Criteria for Liver Transplantation in Acetaminophen-Induced ALF	Criteria for Liver Transplantation in Nonacetaminophen-Induced ALF
pH <7.3 following fluid resuscitation and >24 hours since acetaminophen ingestion *or* lactate >3 mg/dL following fluid resuscitation *or* all of the following in a 24-hour period: • INR > 6.5 (PT > 100 seconds) • Cr > 300 µmol/L (3.4 mg/dL) • grade 3 or 4 encephalopathy	INR > 6.5 (PT > 100 seconds) *or* Any three of the following variables: • age <10 or >40 years • etiology: non-A/B hepatitis or drug induced • duration of jaundice to encephalopathy >7 days • INR > 3.5 (PT > 50 seconds) • serum bilirubin >300 µmol/L (17.54 mg/dL) Wilson disease or Budd-Chiari Syndrome: • Any degree of encephalopathy

separation and adsorption device (Prometheus), and single pass albumin dialysis (Fig. 97.9).[161] Bioartificial ECLS devices pass the patient's plasma through porcine hepatocyte or human cell line bioreactors in the HepatAssist (Alliqua Inc., Langhorne, PA) and Extracorporeal Liver Assist Device (Vital Therapies Inc., San Diego, CA) systems, respectively.[162]

While survival benefit has been touted in case series, randomized controlled trials failed to replicate initial findings. A trend toward increased TFS was reported with MARS using a large population of historical controls but was nonrandomized.[102] A randomized, controlled trial of over 100 patients in France showed no benefit of MARS compared to standard-of-care but was confounded by short interval to transplant.[163] Recent meta-analyses of ECLS trials in both ALF and ACLF suggested an improvement in mortality and HE without an increase in adverse events.[164–166] However, these analyses were limited by pooling data from different ECLS modalities across decades of evolving medical care. Although ongoing technological developments, such as bioreactors of hepatocyte spheroids, may advance the field,[167] no form of ECLS has shown adequate efficacy and availability to be widely applied in patients with ALF.

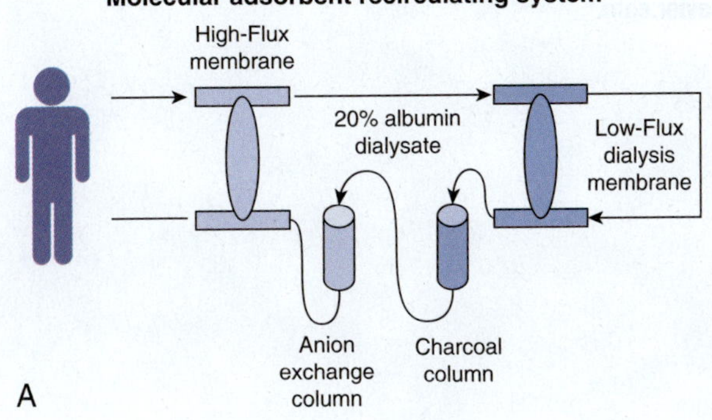

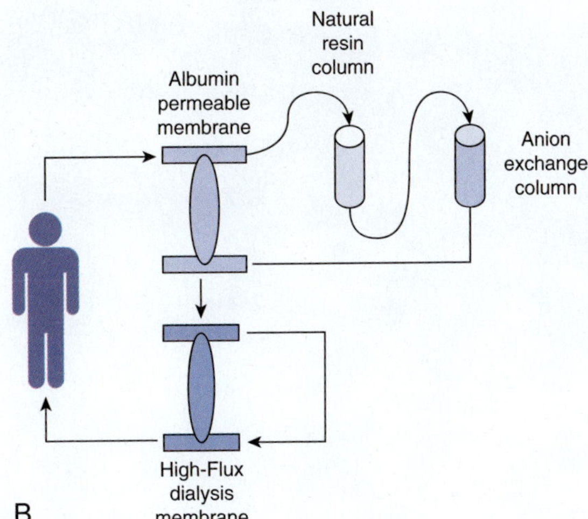

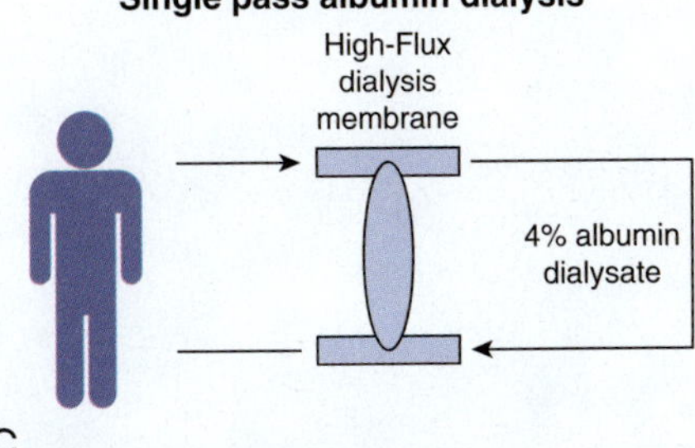

Fig. 97.9 Schematic diagram of extracorporeal liver support devices. (A) Molecular adsorbent recirculating system (MARS). (B) Fractionated plasma separation and adsorption device (Prometheus). (C) Single pass albumin dialysis (SPAD). (From Matar A, Subramanian R. Extracorporeal liver support: a bridge to somewhere. *Clin Liver Dis.* 2021;18:274–279. For permission, PERMISSIONS@WILEY.COM.)

LIVER TRANSPLANTATION

Despite best supportive care, emergent LT is required for survival in a large minority of patients with ALF. Early transfer of patients to a transplant center is paramount as outcomes are determined by Day 4, particularly for patients with APAP ALF. Although APAP ALF often presents with the highest acuity of illness, only a minority are listed for LT. Paradoxically, up to 40% listed for LT improve with supportive care compared to 11% of non-APAP listed patients.[9] However, APAP etiology is an independent risk factor for death while on the transplant waitlist.[168,169]

In subacute ALF, the appearance of even low-grade HE often heralds a dramatic decline and increases urgency for LT. In an ALFSG expert review panel, patients with the longest jaundice-to-HE interval, commonly seen with AIH and DILI etiologies, may derive the most survival benefit from transplant because the pathogenesis of their liver injury persists with time and they often do not achieve adequate regeneration.[19] Indeed, with less than 30% TFS, nearly half of non-APAP ALF patients will ultimately receive LT.[8,170]

Transplant Outcomes

The availability of emergency LT has increased overall survival in ALF from a dismal 16% in 1973 to over 60% by 2008.[57] Posttransplant outcomes are satisfactory with 3-year survival 90%.[168] The highest risk of death is during the index hospitalization due to infection, neurologic compromise, and multisystem organ failure.[171] Risk factors for posttransplant death in a large European registry included male gender, donor age, recipient age, ABO incompatible graft, and small graft.[170] Obesity, creatinine >2 mg/dL and need for life support were noted to be additional risk factors for poor outcomes in the United Network for Organ Sharing (UNOS) database.[171] While APAP etiology was 10 times more likely to result in noncompliance and graft loss in the European cohort, this has not been replicated in the UNOS database perhaps reflective of differing psychosocial listing practices.[169,170]

Given the overall excellent outcomes in this very ill patient population, few absolute contraindications to LT exist. Irreversible neurologic status secondary to cerebral edema with bilateral nonreactive dilated pupils and uncal herniation precludes meaningful recovery posttransplant. Increasing vasopressor requirements, severe adult respiratory distress syndrome, and markedly low cardiac output are also relative contraindications. Bacteremia is not uncommon and should not be a contraindication provided response to therapy.[84]

In the United States, United Kingdom, and many other countries, ALF garners high priority listing for cadaveric LT recognizing the high likelihood of death without a graft. However, the emergent nature of ALF, decreased organ availability and continued deaths on the waitlist highlight the need for additional strategies for successful transplant. Marginal donors and ABO incompatibility are associated with less favorable outcomes and time constraints prevent desensitization.[172] It remains to be determined if ex vivo normothermic perfusion can significantly expand the donor pool in this patient population.

Living Donor Transplant

Living donor transplantation comprises a minority of LT in Western countries but in countries where cadaveric donors are rare, which has been used in ALF with comparable outcomes.[173,174] Ethical concerns have been expressed given the expedited nature unique to ALF and in the United States adult to adult living donor transplant group, less than 1% of donors were to ALF recipients with 1 year survival 70%.[175]

Auxiliary Liver Transplantation

Auxiliary LT implants a partial graft leaving the native liver in place to provide hepatic support during regeneration with the goal of removing the graft once normal function is restored. However, this procedure was associated with more technical complications, and a significant number of patients still required immunosuppression, making this a less desirable approach than conventional LT. The procedure of auxiliary LT is reserved only for the very young, hyperacute patients who also have the best likelihood of TFS.[176,177]

Cell-Based Transplantation

Mesenchymal stem cells, which differentiate into hepatocytes and immune cells, have been used in patients with ALF with improved short-term survival.[178] Liver organoids are being developed for clinical study while additional cell-based therapies are being investigated in hopes of aiding regeneration.[179,180]

Full references for this chapter can be found at https://ebooks.health.elsevier.com.

and tenofovir).[20] Indirect carcinogenic effects are the result of the chronic necroinflammatory hepatic disease, in particular cirrhosis, induced by the virus. The increased hepatocyte turnover rate resulting from continuous or recurring cycles of cell necrosis and regeneration acts as a potent tumor promoter. In addition, the distorted architecture characteristic of cirrhosis contributes to the loss of control of hepatocyte growth, and hepatic inflammation generates mutagenic reactive oxygen species. Data from the REVEAL (Risk Evaluation of Viral Load Elevation and Associated Liver Disease/Cancer)-HBV study in Taiwan have shown that genotype C of HBV and specific mutations of the basal core promoter and precore regions of the HBV genome are associated with a higher risk of HCC,[15] whereas in Alaska, genotype F has been more strongly associated with HCC.[21] The transgenic mouse model of Chisari and coworkers has provided indirect support for the role of prolonged hepatocyte injury in hepatocarcinogenesis.[22] The REACH-B (Risk Estimation for Hepatocellular Carcinoma in Chronic Hepatitis B) score provides a simple-to-use tool for risk estimation for HCC among individuals with chronic HBV infection and includes gender, age, serum ALT level, hepatitis B e antigen status, and serum HBV DNA level.[23]

HCV

Approximately 71 million people in the world today are chronically infected with HCV and are at increased risk for the development of HCC. In Japan, Italy, and Spain, HCV is the single most common etiologic factor for HCC, and in other industrialized countries, HCV infection, often in combination with alcohol abuse, has emerged as a major cause of the malignancy.[7,19] Patients with HCV-induced HCC generally are older than those with HBV-related tumors, and the HCV infection is likely acquired mainly in adult life.

Almost all HCV-induced HCCs arise in cirrhotic livers, and most of the exceptions are in livers with chronic hepatitis and fibrosis. This observation strongly suggests that chronic hepatic parenchymal disease plays a key role in the genesis of HCV-related tumors. Because the HCV genome does not integrate into host DNA, the virus would have to exert a direct carcinogenic effect by other means.

Long-term follow-up of a large group of patients with chronic hepatitis C and cirrhosis or bridging fibrosis found a cumulative 5-year frequency of HCC of just over 5%. The rate was higher among those with cirrhosis (7.0%) than those with bridging fibrosis at baseline (4.1%).[24] A multivariate analysis model showed that older age, black race, lower platelet count, presence of esophageal varices, and smoking were additional risk factors.

It has become apparent that successful treatment of chronic HCV infection, with a sustained virologic response (see Chapter 82), is associated with regression of hepatic fibrosis and a lower-than-expected rate of HCC, approximately 50%–80% reduction.[4,24,25,26] Modern DAAs have increased the rate of viral cure, although HCC may still occur in a cirrhotic patient after treatment has eliminated HCV.[20,27]

Cirrhosis

In all parts of the world, HCC frequently occurs against a background of cirrhosis.[27] All causative forms of cirrhosis may be complicated by tumor formation. A long-term follow-up study of 2126 U.S. military veterans with cirrhosis found that HCC developed in 100 (4.7%) over an average period of 3.6 years.[28,29] The calculated rate was 1.3/100 patient-years. Risk factors for HCC included obesity, a low platelet count, and the presence of antibody to hepatitis B core antigen. A similar study from Italy found an incidence of HCC of 3.7/100 patient-years among cirrhotic persons with HCV infection and 2.0/100 patient-years among persons with HBV infection. Older age and male gender were confirmed as risk factors among patients with cirrhosis.[30] By contrast, a study from Denmark of more than 8000 patients with alcohol-associated cirrhosis found a 5-year cumulative risk of HCC of 1.0, suggesting that perhaps patients with this form of cirrhosis were at lower risk of HCC than, for example, those with HCV-related cirrhosis.[31]

Aflatoxin B_1

Dietary exposure to aflatoxin B_1, derived from the fungi *Aspergillus flavus* and *Aspergillus parasiticus*, is an important risk factor for HCC in parts of Africa and Asia. These molds are ubiquitous in nature and contaminate staple foodstuffs, particularly corn and nuts, in tropical and subtropical regions (see Chapter 91). Multiple epidemiologic studies have shown a strong correlation between the dietary intake of aflatoxin B_1 and incidence of HCC. By meta-analysis HBV increases the risk HCC 11-fold and aflatoxin 6-fold, but the combination increases risk by 73-fold.[32,4] Heavy dietary exposure to aflatoxin B_1 may contribute to hepatocarcinogenesis through an inactivating mutation of the third base of codon 249 of the *TP53* tumor suppressor gene.[33,34]

Other Conditions

HCC develops in as many as 45% of patients with untreated hemochromatosis (see Chapter 77).[35] Malignant transformation was previously thought to occur only in the presence of cirrhosis (and is certainly more likely to do so), but this complication also has been reported in patients without cirrhosis.[36] Excessive free iron in tissues may be carcinogenic, perhaps by generating mutagenic reactive oxygen species.[37] Further support for this theory comes from the observations that black Africans with dietary iron overload are at increased risk of HCC[38] and that rats fed a diet high in iron develop iron-free dysplastic foci and HCC in the absence of cirrhosis.[39] HCC occasionally develops in patients with Wilson disease, but only in the presence of cirrhosis (see Chapter 78).[40] Malignant transformation has been attributed to the cirrhosis but may also result from oxidant stress secondary to the accumulation of copper in the liver.[41] HCC also may develop in patients with other inherited metabolic disorders that are complicated by cirrhosis, such as α_1-antitrypsin deficiency and type 1 hereditary tyrosinemia, and in patients with certain inherited diseases in the absence of cirrhosis—for example, type 1 glycogen storage disease (see Chapter 79). HCC develops in approximately 40% of patients with membranous obstruction of the inferior vena cava, a rare congenital or acquired anomaly (see Chapter 87).

The roles of obesity, diabetes mellitus, and nonalcoholic fatty liver disease (NAFLD) have come to be recognized in the causation of HCC,[42–45] although the mechanisms whereby these overlapping conditions contribute to the development of HCC are unknown. Cirrhosis caused by metabolic-associated steatohepatitis (MASH, previously referred to as NASH) appears to give rise to HCC less frequently than cirrhosis caused by HCV but, nevertheless, appears to carry significant risk.[46] Diabetes mellitus is also a strong risk factor for HCC although it is not clear if the risk is independent of metabolic-associated fatty liver disease [metabolic-associated steatotic liver disease (MASLD), previously referred to as NAFLD].[44,45] An additional 20%–30 % of MASLD-associated HCC occurs in the absence of cirrhosis.[44,45,4]

A statistically significant correlation between the use of oral contraceptive steroids and the occurrence of HCC has been demonstrated in countries in which the incidence of HCC is low and no overriding risk factor for the development of the tumor is present. There is sufficient evidence of an epidemiological link between cigarette smoking and the occurrence of HCC with an estimated increased risk of 60%–70% in smoker.[47] The incidence of HCC is increased in patients with HIV infection compared with controls in the general population, presumably because of the increased rate of chronic viral hepatitis in the HIV-positive population.[48]

Although the aforementioned risk factors have been identified, the precise mechanisms whereby they lead to HCC still require elucidation. Several cellular pathways are involved in causing unconstrained proliferation of hepatocytes and increased angiogenesis against a background of chronic liver disease. These pathways have become the targets for newer molecular therapies against HCC (Box 98.2) (see later).[49]

Clinical Features

Although the typical clinical features of HCC are well recognized (including abdominal pain and weight loss in patients with cirrhosis), many patients are now diagnosed at an early stage when they have no specific symptoms or signs. This trend toward earlier diagnosis is probably the result of surveillance programs in patients with chronic liver disease (see later). In advanced disease, patients with HCC usually present with typical symptoms and signs, and diagnosis is straightforward. In addition, HCC often coexists with cirrhosis,[50] and the onset of HCC is marked by a sudden unexplained change in the patient's condition.

Patients with HCC often are unaware of its presence until the tumor has reached an advanced stage. The most common (and frequently first) symptom is right hypochondrial or epigastric pain. Other symptoms are listed in Table 98.1.

BOX 98.2 Key Molecular Pathways Involved in Hepatocarcinogenesis

- Angiogenic signaling
- Epigenetic promoter methylation and histone acetylation
- Growth factor-stimulated receptor tyrosine kinase
- JAK/STAT signaling
- PI3-kinase/AKT/mTOR
- p53 and cell cycle regulation
- Ubiquitin-proteasome
- Wnt/β-catenin

Adapted from Roberts L. Emerging experimental therapies for hepatocellular carcinoma: what if you can't cure?. In: McCullough A, ed. *AASLD Postgraduate Course.* Boston: AASLD; 2007:185.

TABLE 98.1 Symptoms and Signs of HCC

Symptom	Frequency (%)
Abdominal pain	59–95
Weight loss	34–71
Weakness	22–53
Abdominal swelling	28–43
Nonspecific GI symptoms	25–28
Jaundice	5–26
SIGN	
Hepatomegaly	54–98
Ascites	35–61
Fever	11–54
Splenomegaly	27–42
Wasting	25–41
Jaundice	4–35
Hepatic bruit	6–25

Physical findings vary with the stage of disease (see Table 98.1). Early in the course, evidence of cirrhosis alone may be present, or abnormal findings may be absent. When the tumor is advanced at the time of the patient's first medical visit, the liver is almost always enlarged, sometimes massively. Hepatic tenderness is common and may be profound, especially in the later stages. The surface of the enlarged liver is smooth, irregular, or frankly nodular. An arterial bruit may be heard over the tumor[51]; the bruit is heard in systole, rough in character, and not affected by changing the position of the patient. Although not pathognomonic, a bruit is a useful clue to the diagnosis of HCC. Less often, a friction rub may be heard over the tumor, but this sign is more characteristic of hepatic metastases or abscesses.

Ascites may be present when the patient is first seen or may appear with the progression of the tumor. In most patients, ascites is the result of long-standing cirrhosis and portal hypertension (see Chapter 94), but in some cases, it is caused by invasion of the peritoneum by the primary tumor or metastases or obstruction of the hepatic veins or inferior vena cava.[52] The ascitic fluid may be blood stained. Splenomegaly, if present, reflects coexisting cirrhosis and portal hypertension.

Physical evidence of cirrhosis may also be noted. Severe pitting edema of the lower extremities extending up to the groin occurs when HCC has invaded the hepatic veins and propagates into and obstructs the inferior vena cava.[52] A Virchow-Trosier (supraclavicular) node, Sister Mary Joseph's (periumbilical) nodule, or enlarged axillary lymph node is rarely present.

Paraneoplastic Manifestations

Some of the deleterious effects of HCC are not caused by local effects of the tumor or metastases (Box 98.3). Each of the paraneoplastic syndromes in HCC is rare or uncommon. One of the more important is type B hypoglycemia, which occurs in less than 5% of patients, manifests as severe hypoglycemia early in the course of the disease,[52] and is believed to result from the defective processing by malignant hepatocytes of the precursor to insulin-like growth factor II (pre-IGF II).[53] By contrast, type A hypoglycemia is a milder form of glycopenia that occurs in the terminal stages of HCC (and other malignant tumors of the liver). It results from the inability of a liver extensively infiltrated by tumor, and often cirrhotic, to satisfy the demands for glucose by a large, often rapidly growing tumor and by the other tissues of the body.

Another important paraneoplastic syndrome is polycythemia (erythrocytosis), which occurs in less than 10% of patients with HCC.[54] This syndrome appears to be caused by the synthesis of erythropoietin or an erythropoietin-like substance by malignant hepatocytes.

BOX 98.3 Paraneoplastic Manifestations Associated with HCC

- Carcinoid syndrome
- Hypercalcemia
- Hypertension
- Hypertrophic osteoarthropathy
- Hypoglycemia
- Neuropathy
- Osteoporosis
- Polycythemia (erythrocytosis)
- Polymyositis
- Porphyria
- Sexual changes—isosexual precocity, gynecomastia, feminization
- Thyrotoxicosis
- Thrombophlebitis migrans
- Watery diarrhea syndrome

Patients with HCC, especially the sclerosing variety, may present with hypercalcemia in the absence of osteolytic metastases. When hypercalcemia is severe, it may result in the typical complications of hypercalcemia, including drowsiness and lethargy. The probable cause is secretion of parathyroid hormone–related protein by the tumor.[55]

Cutaneous paraneoplastic manifestations of HCC are rare except for pityriasis rotunda (circumscripta), which may be a useful marker of the tumor in black Africans. The rash consists of single or multiple, round or oval, hyperpigmented, scaly lesions on the trunk and thighs that range in diameter from 0.5 to 25 cm.[56]

Diagnosis

The gold standard for the diagnosis of HCC is pathology. However, for practical purposes (i.e., to apply treatment), HCC can be diagnosed in the presence of an abnormality on imaging of the liver. Dysplastic nodules and even regenerative cirrhotic nodules can be seen on imaging studies and are potentially confused with HCC. Although enhancement patterns with dynamic imaging of dysplastic nodules and HCC are fairly specific (see later), some overlap occurs.[57,58] Nevertheless, there is a growing consensus that, based on guidelines from the major European and American hepatology societies and now backed by published experience, the diagnosis of HCC can be made in the appropriate clinical setting on the basis of specific imaging characteristics, with or without an elevated serum AFP level.[59,60]

Serum Tumor Markers

Serum tumor markers generally are not diagnostic for HCC by themselves but can be used in conjunction with imaging findings to diagnose HCC. Additionally, they may raise the suspicion of HCC and lead to more sensitive and serial imaging of the liver. Conventional liver biochemical tests do not distinguish HCC from other hepatic mass lesions or cirrhosis.

Many of the substances synthesized and secreted by HCC are not biologically active. Nevertheless, a few are produced by a sufficiently large proportion of tumors to warrant their use as serum markers for HCC. The most helpful of these markers is AFP.

AFP

AFP is an α_1-globulin normally present in high concentrations in fetal serum but in only minute amounts thereafter. Reappearance of high serum levels of AFP strongly suggests the presence of HCC [or hepatoblastoma (see later)],[61] especially in populations at risk for HCC.

Measurement of AFP can potentially be used for the diagnosis of HCC, surveillance, and prognostication. With regard to diagnosis, existing guidelines are based on biopsy or liver imaging and do not require use of AFP. Clearly, markedly elevated AFP levels (>10,000 ng/mL to >1,000,000 ng/mL) can be considered diagnostic for HCC in an appropriate clinical context. Although there is no specific diagnostic cutoff, values above 400 ng/mL in association with a liver mass can be considered diagnostic in most cases.[62]

In the context of surveillance for HCC, the tumor must be detected at an early stage when potentially curative treatment can still be applied. Measurement of AFP has been used for early diagnosis but with sometimes disappointing results. For example, Marrero and colleagues studied a large group of patients with HCC and matched controls and found that the optimal cutoff value of serum AFP level that resulted in the greatest sensitivity was 10.9 ng/mL; still, the sensitivity of the test using this value was only 66%.[63] Therefore routine use of AFP as part of a surveillance program for HCC remains controversial.[64]

Serum AFP levels appear to have some prognostic utility, particularly with regard to liver transplantation (LT), for which levels above 1000 ng/mL have been associated with poorer outcomes and higher rates of tumor recurrence. An AFP level higher than about 500 ng/mL predicts worse outcomes with LT compared with lower levels.[65] Attempts to correlate the degree of differentiation of HCC with the production of AFP have produced conflicting results.

False-positive AFP results (for HCC) also may occur in patients with tumors of endodermal origin, nonseminomatous germ cell tumors, pregnancy, and regenerating livers in the setting of ALF. A progressively rising serum AFP concentration is highly suggestive of HCC. Because both false-positive and false-negative results are obtained when AFP is used as a serum marker for HCC, the search for an ideal marker continues; however, alternative markers have not proved to be more useful than AFP.

Fucosylated AFP

AFP is heterogeneous in structure. Its microheterogeneity results from differences in the oligosaccharide side chain and accounts for the differential affinity of the glycoprotein for lectins. AFP secreted by malignant hepatocytes contains unusual and complex sugar chains that are not found in AFP produced by nontransformed hepatocytes. One variant, *Lens culinaris* agglutinin reactive fraction (AFP-L3), has been suggested to improve the specificity of AFP, particularly AFP serum levels from 10 to 200 ng/mL.[66,67] The recommended cutoff value for AFP-L3 to diagnose HCC is higher than 10% although the specificity varies depending on the absolute level of AFP. Studies have not confirmed that AFP-L3 has greater sensitivity or specificity than AFP alone for the diagnosis of early HCC.[63,66] Therefore AFP-L3 is not sufficiently validated to confirm the diagnosis of HCC without other supporting findings, such as suggestive imaging.

Des-γ-Carboxy Prothrombin

Serum concentrations of des-γ-carboxy prothrombin (DCP) (also known as prothrombin produced by vitamin K absence or antagonist II) are raised in most patients with HCC.[68] DCP is an abnormal prothrombin that is thought to result from a defect in the posttranslational carboxylation of the prothrombin precursor in malignant cells.[69] DCP has been suggested to be a better marker than, or at least complementary to, AFP.[70–72] A large study in Western patients with HCV–related cirrhosis, however, did not confirm this finding.[73] Therefore because appropriate diagnostic cutoff values are not well established, the precise role of DCP in the diagnosis of HCC still requires validation.

Combinations of Markers

Combinations of markers such as the GALAD score, which utilizes AFP, AFP-L3, and DCP along with age and gender, appear to have modestly improved performance for early HCC detection, though they are not well established as clinical tools.[74] The combination of DNA methylation markers (HOXA1, TSPYL5, and B3GALT6) from blood with AFP and gender may increase sensitivity over individual biomarkers for HCC detection.[75] A validation study in the setting of an HCC surveillance program has completed enrollment.

Other Markers

Multiple other potential serum markers for HCC have been identified although none of them has an established high–through put method of measurement, as required for a clinical test. The roles in the diagnosis of HCC for markers such as glypican-3 (GPC3), Golgi protein 73, hepatocyte growth factor, IGF 1, and transforming growth factor-β1 await further study.

Imaging

The diagnosis of HCC generally requires imaging evidence of a focal lesion in the liver, although large infiltrating lesions can also be diagnostic. Arterial hyperenhancement, particularly seen on dynamic contrast imaging of the liver, is observed because the blood supply of HCC comes from newly formed abnormal arteries (neoangiogenesis).[57,76,77] As a nodule transforms from low- to high-grade dysplasia and then to HCC, the primary blood supply shifts from portal to arterial; new abnormal arterial branches produce characteristic findings on dynamic contrast imaging of the liver and subsequent hypoenhancement in the portal venous and delayed phases "washout."[78,79] European and American liver societies recommend that a noninvasive diagnosis of HCC can be made in a nodule greater than 1 cm in diameter that demonstrates arterial hyperenhancement and portal venous or delayed washout and capsular enhancement.[59,60]

The American College of Radiology created and updated the Liver Imaging Reporting and Data System (LI-RADS), which attempts to classify liver nodules based on size and imaging characteristics on CT or MRI (American College of Radiology. CT/MRI LI-RADS v2018 CORE https://www.acr.org/-/media/ACR/Files/RADS/LI-RADS/LI-RADS-2018-Core.pdf Accessed 1/22/23) and has been adapted as the terminology to be used for patients on the UNOS transplant list and by American and European liver societies.[59,60] The LI-RAD categories assist the clinician in assessing the risk that a nodule is HCC, with LI-RAD 3 being intermediate risk, LI-RAD 4 probable HCC, LI-RAD 5 definite HCC and LI-RAD M malignant. The individual criteria for LI-RADS have been validated in prospective and retrospective cohort studies.[79,80]

Systematic reviews show that HCC is eventually diagnosed in 38% of patients with LI-RAD 3 lesions, 74% of patients with LI-RAD 4, and 94% of patients with LI-RAD 5 lesions.[80]

US

US detects most HCCs but may not distinguish this tumor from other solid lesions in the liver. Therefore US is a more effective as a tool for screening than for diagnosis. As with all imaging methods, the sensitivity increases with increasing size of the lesion. A systematic review of 8 studies using histologic reviews of liver explants has shown that US has fair sensitivity [pooled estimate, 48%; 95% confidence interval (CI), 34% to 62%] with good specificity (97%; 95% CI, 95%–98%).[58] Advantages of US include safety, availability, and cost-effectiveness. Drawbacks include lack of standardization, examiner dependence, and limited sensitivity with certain body habituses, particularly obesity, and with fatty infiltration of the liver. There are LI-RADS criteria for ultrasound that categorize findings as negative, subthreshold, and positive and rate the quality of the images for surveillance as no or minimal, moderate or severe limitations. (US LI-RADS v2017 CORE https://www.acr.org/-/media/ACR/Files/RADS/LI-RADS/LI-RADS-US-Algorithm-Portrait-2017.pdf accessed 1/22/2023).

The US appearance of HCC is variable because it is influenced by the presence of fat, hemorrhage, and necrosis. Smaller tumors (<5 cm) are most often hypoechoic and may demonstrate a thin peripheral fibrous capsule. Small HCCs can also be uniformly hyperechoic and therefore indistinguishable from focal fat or a hemangioma. With increased size, there is generally increased complexity of the nodule.[81] Tumors located immediately under the right hemidiaphragm may be difficult to detect. US with Doppler technology is useful for assessing the patency of the inferior vena cava, portal vein and its larger branches, hepatic veins, and biliary tract.

Dynamic contrast-enhanced Doppler US with IV infusion of CO_2 microbubbles viewed with grayscale imaging and color Doppler US are refinements that, by characterizing hepatic arterial and portal venous flow in tumorous nodules, facilitate the diagnosis of malignant and benign hepatic nodules.[82] These techniques are generally not performed in the United States, owing to lack of approval by the FDA of the contrast for noncardiac studies.

CT

Multiphase (also called dynamic) multidetector CT is the most frequently utilized imaging technique for the diagnosis of HCC.[58,81,82] To rely on CT or MRI for the diagnosis of HCC, certain technical specifications for imaging equipment, image acquisition, and dynamic contrast timing are necessary.[83,84] Dynamic contrast-enhanced CT can include noncontrast, arterial, portal venous, and delayed phases. The classic and most diagnostic pattern for HCC is a combination of nonperipheral hyperenhancement in the arterial phase (with the uninvolved liver lacking enhancement), loss of central nodule enhancement compared with the enhancing uninvolved liver (washout), and capsular enhancement in the portal venous and delayed phases (Fig. 98.2).[83,85] When the lesion is larger than 2 cm in diameter, this pattern has almost 100% specificity for HCC.[86–88] When the nodule is 1–2 cm, a diagnosis of HCC or high-grade dysplastic nodule can be made with a specificity greater than 95%.[83,89–91] CT often finds so-called hypervascular-only lesions, which enhance in the arterial phase and become isodense to the surrounding liver in the portal venous and delayed phases. These lesions may be dysplastic nodules, arterial-portal shunts, atypical hemangiomas, HCC, intrahepatic cholangiocarcinoma (ICC), confluent fibrosis, or aberrant venous drainage. Only about 30% of nodules less than 2 cm in diameter are HCCs. Both HCCs and cholangiocarcinomas grow over time, whereas other nodules disappear or remain stable on follow-up studies. HCC may also have other patterns on CT, such as washout only on delayed imaging, a hypovascular nodule, or a fat-containing nodule.[78,92] Guidelines recommend considering biopsy of lesions larger than 1 cm without diagnostic features of HCC if management will be altered versus short interval follow-up (repeat cross-sectional imaging in 3 months) and serial imaging for lesions smaller than 1 cm that do not have characteristic arterial enhancement and washout.[59] Overall, the pooled estimates of sensitivity and specificity of CT for detecting HCC are 67.5% (95% CI, 55%–80%) and 92.5% (95% CI, 89%–96%), respectively. Dynamic CT is also useful for detecting invasion into the portal or hepatic veins and identifying the location and number of tumors; these findings are critical for planning treatment (see later).

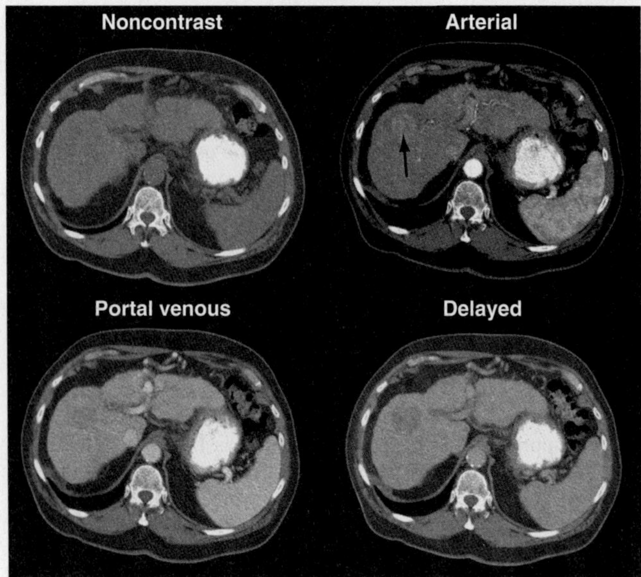

Fig. 98.2 Dynamic CT of a patient with HCC showing no lesion in the noncontrast phase, an enhancing lesion in the right lobe of the liver in the arterial phase of contrast administration *(arrow)*, and a faint lesion in the portal venous phase, seen better in the delayed phase.

MRI

Dynamic MRI using gadolinium contrast agents (extracellular) provides another way of distinguishing HCC from normal or nonmalignant liver tissue. The performance of MRI and the findings on multiphase contrast enhancement are similar or perhaps slightly superior to those described for CT (Fig. 98.3). Hyperintensity of a nodule on T2-weighted images is specific for HCC.[78,81] The pooled estimates of sensitivity and specificity of MRI for detecting HCC are 80.6% (95% CI, 70%–91%) and 84.8% (95% CI, 77%–93%), respectively.[58] Although MRI may be slightly superior overall to CT, especially with regard to sensitivity, local expertise and patient factors (ability to hold breath in a confined space, presence of large amount of ascites, and renal function) should dictate the choice of imaging technique.[93] Close attention to technical specifications is essential.[84] Findings using newer techniques that may improve the specificity of MRI for HCC, particularly those with atypical vascular-enhancement patterns, include hyperintensity on diffusion-weighted images and lack of enhancement on late images using a hepatobiliary-specific contrast agent (gadoxetic acid).[93] LI-RADS is widely used as a way of categorizing nodules recognized on CT or MRI, in patients at high risk of HCC, as definitely benign, probably benign, having an intermediate probability of being HCC, probably HCC, and definitely HCC (corresponding to LI-RADS categories 1–5, respectively) (see earlier).[94]

PET

Whole-body fluorine-18-fluorodeoxyglucose PET combined with CT (PET-CT) may have a role in the evaluation of some patients with HCC. The sensitivities of dynamic CT and MRI are superior to that of PET-CT. Several retrospective case series have shown that high avidity in the primary hepatic lesion predicts an increased risk of recurrence after potentially curative treatment. Once a diagnosis of HCC is made, staging involves imaging of the chest, usually with noncontrast CT, and imaging of other areas of the body based on clinical symptoms. Particularly if the tumor within the liver is beyond the Milan criteria (see later), either a bone scan or PET-CT can sometimes identify an unrecognized extrahepatic metastasis that would change the treatment plan though at the expense of some false-positives requiring biopsy and delaying treatment.[95] The use of PET-CT in HCC needs further study.

Hepatic Angiography

Since the advent of CT and MRI, the role of diagnostic hepatic angiography has been limited. Digital subtraction angiography is helpful for recognizing small hypervascular HCCs but may miss hypovascular tumors. Findings in HCC include arteries that are irregular in caliber and do not taper in the usual way, with smaller branches showing a bizarre pattern and delay in capillary emptying, which is seen as a blush. Angiography is essential for delineating the hepatic arterial anatomy in planning bland embolization, chemoembolization, and radioembolization of the tumor or infusion of cytotoxic drugs directly into the hepatic artery or its branches (see later).

Laparoscopy

Laparoscopy is now rarely performed for this purpose but can be used to detect peritoneal and other extrahepatic spread, ascertain whether the nontumorous part of the liver is cirrhotic, and obtain biopsies under direct vision.

Pathology

Definitive diagnosis of HCC depends on demonstrating the typical histologic features. Suitable samples generally can be obtained by percutaneous biopsy or FNA. The yield and safety of the procedure can be increased by directing the needle under US

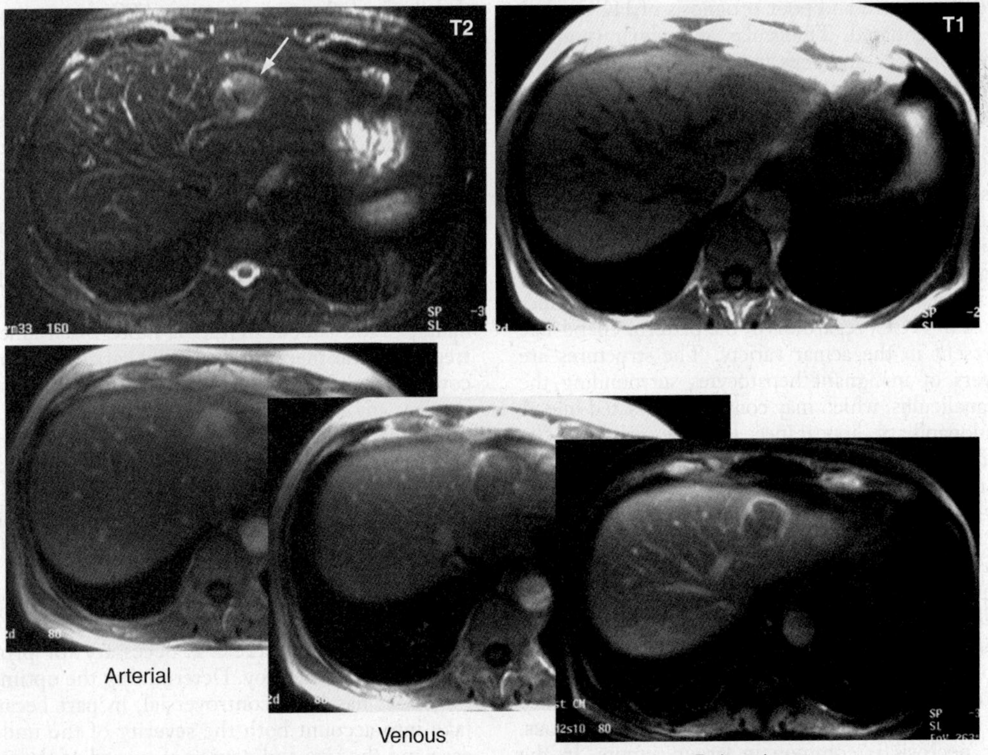

Fig. 98.3 Multiphase MRI of the liver showing HCC with characteristic features, including hyperintensity (*arrow*) on a *T2*-weighted image (*top left panel*) but not on a *T1*-weighted image (*top right panel*), enhancement during the arterial phase of contrast administration (*bottom left panel*), with central washout of contrast and capsular enhancement during the venous and delayed phases (*bottom middle and right panels*).

or CT guidance. Laparoscopically directed biopsy is an alternative approach. Needle biopsy of the tumor carries a small but definite risk of spread along the needle track. Pathologic diagnosis of HCC is based on the recommendations of the International Consensus Panel. Immunostaining for GPC3, heat shock protein HSP70, and glutamine synthetase or gene expression profiling [*GPC3*, *LYVE1* (encoding lymphatic vessel endothelial hyaluronan receptor-1), *BIRC5* (encoding baculoviral inhibitor of apoptosis repeat-containing-5, or surviving)], or both is recommended to differentiate high-grade dysplastic nodules from early HCC.[96]

Gross Appearance

HCC may take one of three forms: nodular, massive, or diffusely infiltrating. The nodular variety of HCC is most common and usually coexists with cirrhosis. It is characterized by numerous round or irregular nodules of various sizes scattered throughout the liver; some of the nodules are confluent. The massive type is characterized by a large circumscribed mass, often with small satellite nodules. This type of tumor is most prone to rupture and is more common in younger patients with a noncirrhotic liver. In the rare diffusely infiltrating variety, a large part of the liver is infiltrated homogeneously by indistinct minute tumor nodules, which may be difficult to distinguish from the regenerative nodules of cirrhosis that are almost invariably present. The portal vein and its branches are infiltrated by tumor in up to 70% of cases seen at autopsy; the hepatic veins and bile ducts are invaded less often.

Microscopic Appearance

HCC is classified histologically into well-differentiated, moderately differentiated, and undifferentiated (pleomorphic) forms, as well as progenitor cell HCC and fibrolamellar HCC (see later).

Well Differentiated

Despite the aggressive nature and poor prognosis of HCC, most tumors are well differentiated. Trabecular and acinar (pseudoglandular) varieties occur, sometimes in a single tumor. In the trabecular variety, the malignant hepatocytes grow in irregular anastomosing plates separated by often inconspicuous sinusoids lined by flat cells resembling Kupffer cells. The trabeculae resemble those of normal adult liver but often are thicker and may be composed of several layers of cells. Scanty collagen fibers may be seen adjacent to the sinusoid walls. The malignant hepatocytes are polygonal, with abundant, slightly granular cytoplasm that is less eosinophilic than that of normal hepatocytes. The nuclei are large and hyperchromatic with prominent nucleoli. Bile production is the hallmark of HCC, regardless of the pattern. Gland-like structures are present in the acinar variety. The structures are composed of layers of malignant hepatocytes surrounding the lumen of a bile canaliculus, which may contain inspissated bile. A tubular or pseudopapillary appearance may be produced by degeneration and loss of cells, or cystic spaces may form in otherwise solid trabeculae. The individual cells may be more elongated and cylindrical than in the trabecular variety.

Moderately Differentiated

Solid, sarcomatous, scirrhous, and clear cell varieties of HCC are described, as well as HCC with lymphoid stroma.[97] In the solid variety, the cells usually are small, although they vary considerably in shape. Pleomorphic multinucleated giant cells are occasionally present. The tumor grows in solid masses or cell nests. Evidence of bile secretion is rare, and connective tissue is inconspicuous. Central ischemic necrosis is common in larger tumors. In the scirrhous variety, the malignant hepatocytes grow in narrow bundles separated by abundant fibrous stroma. Duct-like structures are occasionally present. In most tumors, the cells resemble hepatocytes. In an occasional tumor, the malignant hepatocytes are predominantly or exclusively clear cells. More often, tumors contain areas of clear cells. The appearance of these cells results from a high glycogen or, in some cases, fat content.

Undifferentiated

In undifferentiated HCC, cells are pleomorphic and vary greatly in size and shape. The nuclei are also extremely variable. Large numbers of bizarre-looking giant cells are present and may be spindle shaped, resembling those of sarcomas. Globular hyaline structures may be seen in all types of HCC. These structures reflect the presence of AFP, α1-antitrypsin, or other proteins. Mallory's hyaline is occasionally present.

Progenitor Cell HCC

A class of HCC appears to have its origins in progenitor cells, the stem cells of the liver, located in association with the canals of Hering (see Chapter 73). Progenitor cell activation is seen in association with chronic viral hepatitis and cirrhosis, presumably related to senescence of hepatocytes. These tumors may appear morphologically like typical HCC or mixed cholangiohepatocellular carcinoma. Tumor cells stain positively for cytokeratin (CK) 19, and the tumor appears to have a more aggressive course than typical HCC.[98]

Metastases

Extrahepatic metastases are present at autopsy in 40%–57% of patients with HCCs.[99,100] The most common sites are the lungs (up to 50% in some reports) and regional lymph nodes (≈20%). The adrenal glands are also frequently involved.

Fibrolamellar HCC

Fibrolamellar HCC is a distinct variant of HCC that typically occurs in young patients, has an approximately equal gender distribution, does not secrete AFP, is not caused by chronic hepatitis B or C, and almost always arises in a noncirrhotic liver.[101–103] The hepatocytes are characteristically plump, deeply eosinophilic, and encompassed by abundant fibrous stroma composed of thin, parallel fibrous bands that separate the cells into trabeculae or nodules. The cytoplasm is packed with swollen mitochondria and, in approximately half of the tumors, contains pale or hyaline bodies. Nuclei are prominent, and mitoses are rare. Fibrolamellar HCC has different immunohistochemical characteristics than usual HCC, occurring either with or without cirrhosis; therefore fibrolamellar HCC is much less likely to stain positively for GPC3, although expression of CK7 is more abundant.[104] Fibrolamellar HCC is more often amenable to surgical treatment and therefore generally carries a better prognosis than conventional HCC. It does not, however, respond to chemotherapy any better than other forms of HCC. A mixed form of fibrolamellar HCC has been described, in which some areas of the tumor have the histologic appearance of usual HCC and others resemble fibrolamellar HCC. This mixed type seems to behave more like usual HCC and has a poorer prognosis than typical fibrolamellar HCC.[101]

Staging

Accurate staging of HCC is necessary for prognostication and for selection of therapy. Determining the optimal staging system for HCC has been controversial, in part because staging must take into account both the severity of the underlying liver disease and the size and degree of spread of the tumor. As with all cancers, the TNM system can be used to stage HCC, but this system does not account for the underlying liver disease. A study[105] comparing the usefulness of seven staging systems, including the Okuda, TNM, Cancer of the Liver Italian

Program, barcelona clinic liver cancer (BCLC), Chinese University Prognostic Index, Japanese Integrated Staging, and Group d'Etude et Traitement du Carcinome Hépatocellulaire systems in a cohort of patients from the United States, found that the BCLC staging system (Fig. 98.4) had the best independent predictive power for survival. The BCLC system has been adopted by the AASLD for use in its practice guidelines on management of HCC.[59] This staging classification also includes a treatment schedule based on stage which has been updated multiple times.[59] In addition to staging of the cancer, several systems are in use to stage the degree of liver damage, which is often a limiting factor in applying potentially curative treatments. The Child-Pugh classification has been widely used (see Chapter 94), and the albumin-bilirubin grade is an objective score that can also assist in treatment planning.[106]

Natural History and Prognosis

Symptomatic HCC carries a grave prognosis; in fact, the annual incidence and mortality rates for the tumor are almost identical. The main reasons for the poor outcome are the extent of tumor burden when the patient is first seen and the frequent presence of coexisting cirrhosis and hepatic dysfunction. The natural history of HCC in its florid form is one of rapid progression, with increasing hepatomegaly, abdominal pain, wasting, and deepening jaundice, and with death ensuing in 2–4 months. In industrialized countries, however, the tumor appears to run a more indolent course with longer survival times.[107] Rare cases of spontaneous tumor regression have been reported (see later). When HCC is detected at an early stage, several options for treatment are available and often lead to prolonged survival.

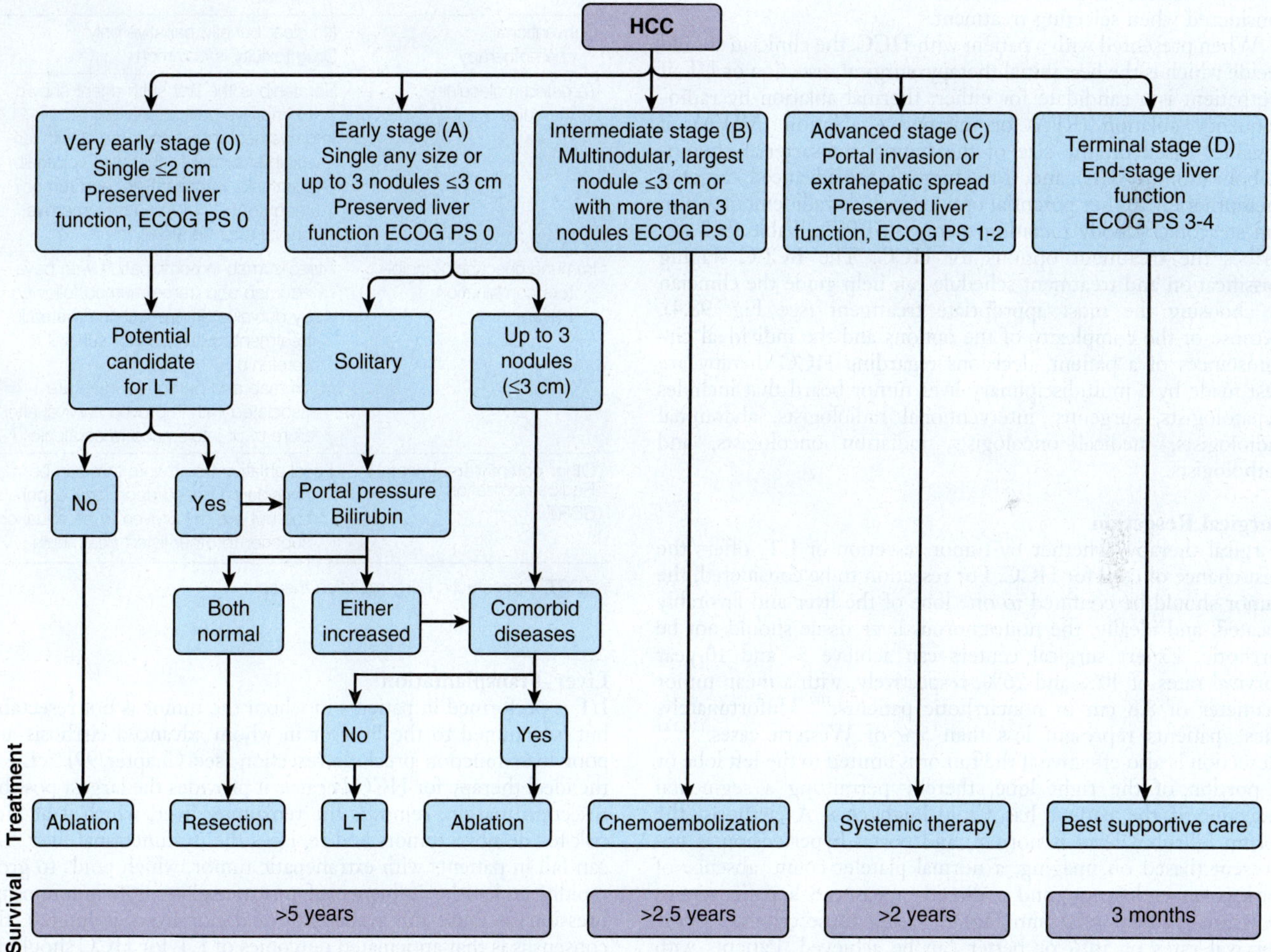

Fig. 98.4 BCLC staging classification and treatment schedule with associated expected survival. Staging is based on tumor size and spread, the patient's Eastern Cooperative Oncology Group (ECOG) performance status (PS) on a scale of 0 (good) to greater than 2 (poor), and liver function as assessed by the Child-Pugh class (see Chapter 92). Patients with very early (*stage 0*) HCC are optimal candidates for surgical resection. Patients with early (*stage A*) HCC are candidates for radical therapy (resection, deceased-donor LT, or live-donor LT, or local ablation via percutaneous ethanol injection or radiofrequency ablation). Patients with intermediate (*stage B*) HCC benefit from transarterial chemoembolization. Patients with advanced HCC, defined as the presence of macroscopic vascular invasion, extrahepatic spread, or cancer-related symptoms (PS 1 or 2) (*stage C*), benefit from first-line immunotherapy combinations or if do not qualify then sorafenib or lenvantanib and regorafenib or nivolumab as second-line therapy. Patients with end-stage disease (*stage D*) should receive symptomatic treatment. The treatment strategy will transition from one stage to another when treatment fails or is contraindicated. (Adapted from Reig M, Forner A, Rimola J et al. *J Hepatology* 2022;76:681–693.)

Treatment

Important advances in the treatment of HCC have occurred since the 1980s and have resulted in improvement of the US population-based 5-year survival rate to 24.5%[108]; these advances include randomized controlled trials that support the benefits of certain treatments such as chemoembolization and the development of a multitude of targeted chemotherapies for advanced HCC, including the multikinase inhibitors (sorafenib, regorafenib, lenvatinib, cabozantenib) and combinations of monoclonal antibody VEGF inhibitors (ramucirimab, bevacizumab) and immune checkpoint inhibitors (ICIs) (nivolumab, atezolizumab, durvalumab, ipilimumab, tremelimumab). Overwhelming evidence supports the superiority of LT over other therapies for patients with portal hypertension and cirrhosis (see Chapter 99). Because HCC is usually a combination of two diseases—the underlying liver disease (usually cirrhosis with varying degrees of decompensation) and the cancer itself—both factors must be considered when selecting treatment.

When presented with a patient with HCC, the clinician should decide which is the best initial therapy: surgical resection or LT, if the patient is a candidate for either; thermal ablation by radiofrequency ablation (RFA) or microwave ablation (MWA), if possible, based on the size of the tumor; transarterial chemoembolization (TACE); and, if the tumor is too advanced, targeted chemotherapy. Other potential options include radioembolization and stereotactic body radiation therapy (SBRT). Table 98.2 describes the treatment options for HCC. The BCLC staging classification and treatment schedule can help guide the clinician in choosing the most appropriate treatment (see Fig. 98.4). Because of the complexity of the options and the individual circumstances of a patient, decisions regarding HCC therapy are best made by a multidisciplinary liver tumor board that includes hepatologists, surgeons, interventional radiologists, abdominal radiologists, medical oncologists, radiation oncologists, and pathologists.

Surgical Resection

Surgical therapy, whether by tumor resection or LT, offers the best chance of cure for HCC. For resection to be considered, the tumor should be confined to one lobe of the liver and favorably located, and ideally, the nontumorous liver tissue should not be cirrhotic. Expert surgical centers can achieve 5- and 10-year survival rates of 40% and 26%, respectively, with a mean tumor diameter of 8.8 cm in noncirrhotic patients.[109] Unfortunately, these patients represent less than 5% of Western cases.[110,111] Resection is also effective if the tumor is limited to the left lobe or a portion of the right lobe, thereby permitting a segmental resection if the patient has Child-Pugh class A cirrhosis, the serum bilirubin level is normal, and portal hypertension is not present (based on imaging, a normal platelet count, absence of varices on endoscopy, and a directly measured hepatic venous pressure gradient <10 mm Hg).[110] Using these criteria, 5-year survival rates of 50% or better can be achieved. Patients with smaller and solitary tumors have better outcomes. In parts of the world where LT is not available, surgical resection is a viable option, particularly for Child-Pugh class A patients without portal hypertension and with a MELD score of 9 or less (see Chapter 99). All the tumor nodules need to be removed, with a negative margin of resection, and the patient needs to be left with enough functional liver volume (usually defined as ≥40% in a patient with cirrhosis) to survive the postoperative period.[112–114] Overall, resection is feasible in only approximately 15% of patients. Resection performed at expert surgical centers carries an operative mortality rate of less than 5%, but at low-volume centers the mortality rate is almost three times greater.[115] Unfortunately, the rate of recurrence after resection is more than 50% in the long term, and salvage LT is rarely possible.[116]

TABLE 98.2 Treatment Options for HCC

Modality	Comments
Surgical resection	Curative but limited to noncirrhotic patients and cirrhotic patients without portal hypertension May be technically difficult High recurrence rate
LT	Successful in selected patients (Milan criteria; see text and Chapter 97) Requires lifelong immunosuppression Expensive and not available worldwide
Radiofrequency ablation or microwave ablation	Potentially curative for small tumors, including multiple tumors High recurrence rate
Transarterial chemoembolization	Prolongs survival in unresectable tumors if hepatic function is preserved; not curative
Conventional chemotherapy	No clear benefit; palliative only Drug toxicity is common
Targeted molecular therapies	Sorafenib is the first such agent shown to improve patient survival Improvement in patient survival with lenvatinib is similar to that with sorafenib Regorafenib, cabozantinib, and ramucirumab (if AFP >400 ng/mL) improve survival after sorafenib failure
Immune checkpoint inhibitors combination therapy	Atezolizumab in combination with bevacizumab and tremelimumab followed by durvalumab are first-line systemic treatments with superior survival to sorafenib Nivolumab and pembrolizumab are associated with improved survival after failure of or intolerance to sorafenib
Other potential treatments Radioembolization SBRT	Local ablative treatments that can be considered based upon local expertise but are not proven to be equal or superior to other listed treatments

SBRT, Stereotactic body radiation therapy.

Liver Transplantation

LT is performed in patients in whom the tumor is not resectable but is confined to the liver or in whom advanced cirrhosis and poor liver function preclude resection (see Chapter 99).[83] LT is the ideal therapy for HCC because it provides the largest possible resection margin, removes the remaining liver, which is at high risk for de novo tumors and replaces the dysfunctional liver. LT can fail in patients with extrahepatic tumor, which tends to grow rapidly under the influence of posttransplantation immunosuppression. Because the availability of donor livers is limited, the consensus is that anticipated outcomes of LT for HCC should be similar to those for other indications for LT and superior to those for other treatments for HCC. Several large series have demonstrated that if one selects candidates based on the Milan criteria—a single tumor up to 5 cm in size or 2–3 lesions, each up to 3 cm in size, with no large-vessel vascular invasion or metastasis—the 5-year survival rate is 70%–75%, and the tumor recurrence rate is 10%–15%.[110,117–119] These criteria led to the HCC MELD exception pathway, which was adopted in the United States in 2002. Because of the change, the frequency of HCC as an indication for LT rose from 4.6% to 26% of the total adult liver transplant population. Additionally, progression of the tumor beyond the Milan criteria before a patient undergoes LT has largely been reduced.[65,120] Bridging therapy with RFA or TACE is usually performed as waiting times are most often greater than 6 months. Bridging therapy theoretically prevents tumor growth beyond Milan criteria, and good response to treatment is correlated with lower recurrence and better survival after LT in some analyses but not others[121,122] (see later). In other parts of the world, waiting times before transplantation remain critical, and when the waiting time increases to 1 year, as many as half of patients will not receive a transplant.[110] An analysis of 4-year survival rates for all patients transplanted in the United States has confirmed that overall outcomes for those transplanted with HCC are only minimally worse than for those transplanted for other indications.[65] Certain subgroups of patients do worse, including those with nodules 3–5 cm in diameter, a MELD score of 20 or greater, and a serum AFP level of 455 ng/mL or higher. High AFP levels, particularly those greater than 1000 ng/mL that do not drop substantially after local regional therapy, are currently a contraindication to LT in the United States.[64]

Most authorities now advocate expansion of the Milan criteria up to five tumors, none greater than 4.5 cm and sum of tumor diameters less than 8 cm, provided that the tumor shrinks to within Milan criteria and remains stable for 3 months after application of locoregional therapy, based on prospective outcomes from small, single-center series.[123,124] These modified criteria have been accepted as a MELD exception pathway in the United States.

Local Ablation

Local ablative therapies are potentially curative treatments for patients with small tumors (usually <3–5 cm in diameter) that are not amenable to resection or LT because of patient preference, the number and location of lesions, or significant hepatic dysfunction (Child-Pugh class B or C; see Fig. 98.4).[64] The first of these techniques available was percutaneous ethanol injection (PEI), a relatively effective, safe, and inexpensive method that is now rarely used in more developed countries. It is most effective for lesions smaller than 2 cm and effective in those up to 3 cm in diameter.[125] PEI requires multiple sessions and, in patients with small tumors and preserved hepatic function, can lead to survival rates similar to those for surgical resection although no randomized studies have been performed to demonstrate equivalent outcomes.[125] Complications are rare and include tumor seeding of the needle track. RFA has generally supplanted PEI because it is more effective, particularly with larger tumors (most effective in lesions up to 3 cm and effective in those up to 5 cm), requires fewer sessions, has similar complication rates, and has superior survival.[126] RFA can be performed percutaneously or by a laparoscopic or open surgical approach. Survival rates are similar to those for surgical resection, although recurrence rates are higher and complications are uncommon.[127,128] MWA is a more recently developed thermal ablation technique for HCC that has the potential advantage over RFA of less heat sink loss to adjacent vessels and faster treatment times with similar clinical outcomes. It has become more common due to its efficiency, but choice should be determined by local expertise.[64] Another emerging option for local ablation is SBRT, which noninvasively delivers high doses of highly conformal radiation in up to five sessions.[129] SBRT results in DNA strand breaks and vascular injury resulting in tumor hypoxemia, apoptosis, death, and immune system activation against tumor antigens.[129] Local control and survival appear to be similar between SBRT and other local ablative therapies based on retrospective and prospective analyses, but randomized comparisons are lacking.[129] Current UNOS rules require a 6-month waiting period to obtain MELD exception points for HCC, and, therefore, local ablative therapy is commonly applied even though benefit has not been well established by randomized trials.[122]

Chemoembolization

TACE is a palliative treatment reserved for patients with relatively intact hepatic function (Child-Pugh class A or B with a total bilirubin level <3 mg/dL), good performance status (lack of or mild tumor-related symptoms), and a tumor that is not amenable to local ablative treatments because of size, number, or location (see Fig. 98.4).[83] Six randomized trials and a meta-analysis have compared embolization or chemoembolization with supportive care and showed overall improved survival with treatment.[130–135] TACE protocols vary greatly (e.g., in chemotherapeutic agents used, number of treatments, and use of embolic agents) in clinical trials and clinical practice across the world. A subsequent meta-analysis that included two additional randomized trials called into question the survival benefit, but the meta-analysis was underpowered to detect a difference.[135] More recently, doxorubicin-eluting bead TACE has supplanted conventional TACE because of equal or better efficacy and a better side-effect profile.[136] Modern TACE protocols produce a median survival of 30 months (range 20–37 months) in Child A patients based on the placebo arms of randomized trials comparing TACE to other therapies.[137] In small randomized and mostly cohort studies in Asia, where patients tend to have HBV-associated liver disease with more hepatic reserve, the combination of TACE and RFA has shown acceptable tolerability with improved survival over either alone.[138] It is prudent to await large randomized clinical trials demonstrating a clear advantage with combination approaches before incorporating them into standard clinical practice. The effectiveness of TACE before LT has not been fully elucidated, but TACE is frequently performed because the waiting time in the United States is greater than 6 months.[139,140] Theoretically, TACE can be used to reduce the size of the tumor to make resection or transplantation possible (downstaging) or to allow a more conservative resection, although study results are mixed as to whether this approach is effective.[141,142]

Chemotherapy

A large number of anticancer drugs, including alkylating agents, antitumor antibiotics, antimetabolites, plant alkaloids, platinum derivatives, procarbazine, estrogen receptor modulators, and somatostatin, have been tried alone and in various combinations and by different routes of administration for the treatment of HCC, but response rates have invariably been less than 20% and no survival advantage has been demonstrated.[132,143] Several small-molecule, targeted anticancer agents have been developed and studied for the treatment of HCC. Sorafenib, an inhibitor of Raf kinase and the tyrosine kinase activity of VEGF receptors and platelet-derived growth factor receptor, is the first of these new agents to show modest improvement in survival compared with supportive care.[144] Lenvatinib, a multikinase inhibitor, has been shown to be non-inferior to sorafenib in the first-line treatment of advanced HCC.[145] Regorafenib and cabozantinib are both multikinase inhibitors that have been shown to provide a modest improvement in survival for patients with Child-Pugh class A cirrhosis and advanced HCC who have had tumor progression after receiving sorafenib and thus are used as second-line therapies.[86,146] Ramucinumab, an antibody to VEGF, also produced modest survival benefit after sorafenib failure in HCC with AFP >400 ng/mL.[147] More recently, ICI-based treatment for HCC has supplanted multikinase inhibitors as first-line treatment in advanced HCC and should be considered for patients with intact hepatic function (Child-Pugh class A or early class B) and portal vein thrombosis, extrahepatic tumor, or failure of other therapies (see Fig. 98.4). Atezolizumab, a monoclonal antibody to the programmed cell death receptor ligand-1 (PD-L1), in combination with bevacizumab, a monoclonal antibody to VEGF, showed improved overall survival (median 19.2 vs. 13.4 months) versus sorafenib with acceptable toxicity.[148] Tremelimumab, an antibody to cytotoxic T lymphocyte–associated antigen 4, followed by durvalumab, an antibody to PD-L1, showed improved overall survival (median 16.4 vs. 13.8 months) versus sorafenib with acceptable toxicity.[149] These combinations have not been assessed in patients with autoimmune disease, coinfection with hepatitis B and C and with untreated varices. Additional Phase 3 studies are ongoing with combinations of ICI and targeted molecular therapies or TACE. Patients with advanced hepatic dysfunction (Child-Pugh class C) or advanced tumor symptoms (Eastern Cooperative Oncology Group performance status >2) have such a poor prognosis that only supportive care should be offered (see Fig. 98.4).[64,150]

Alternative Techniques and Combinations of Therapies

Newer local ablative techniques, including cryoablation, laser ablation, and proton beam radiation, are being studied in HCC, but these techniques have not been adequately compared with PEI, RFA, and MWA; their use should be limited to clinical trials. The role of radioembolization with yttrium (Y)-90 microspheres, which can be used in patients with tumor thrombus, has not been clearly established and awaits ongoing randomized trials, particularly in comparison with TACE. Similar survival following radioembolization with Y-90 microspheres and TACE, with prolonged time to tumor progression, was shown in one randomized controlled trial in which most patients were "bridged" to LT.[151] Two randomized trials of patients with HCC who failed prior locoregional therapies showed similar survival in patients treated with radioembolization with Y-90 microspheres compared with those who received sorafenib.[152,153] Sorafenib as adjuvant therapy after potentially curative resection or thermal ablation is not effective.[154] Adding sorafenib to TACE did not improve time to tumor progression or survival in a medium-sized randomized trial.[155]

Surveillance

Because symptomatic HCC is seldom amenable to surgical cure and responds poorly to conservative treatment, a pressing need exists to prevent the tumor or detect it at a presymptomatic stage when surgical intervention is still possible. An AASLD practice guideline published in 2005 and updated in 2011 and 2018 provides recommendations for surveillance (Table 98.3).[156,59] Patients at high risk for developing HCC should be entered into a surveillance program in which surveillance for HCC is performed using US at 6-month intervals. The role of AFP testing is not well established because of a high false-positive rate, particularly in patients with an elevated serum ALT level. Other serum markers for HCC are unproved in the setting of screening, and their use should be limited to clinical studies. Although CT and MRI are effective imaging modalities for the diagnosis of HCC, they are not recommended for routine use in surveillance but may be considered if adequate US images cannot be obtained because of the patient's body habitus. Growing evidence suggests that surveillance for HCC in patients with cirrhosis improves outcome by detecting HCC at an earlier stage and permitting the application of curative therapies.[157]

TABLE 98.3 Groups of Persons in Whom Surveillance for HCC may be Recommended

Group	Annual Incidence of HCC (%)
HBV carrier with cirrhosis	3–8
HCV-related cirrhosis	3–5
PBC and stage 4 fibrosis	3–5
Hemochromatosis and cirrhosis	Unknown, probably >1.5
α_1-Antitrypsin deficiency and cirrhosis	Unknown, probably >1.5
HBV carrier, Asian men >40 years	0.4–0.6
HBV carrier, Asian women >50 years	0.3–0.6
HBV carrier, family history of HCC	Unknown (higher than without family history)
HBV carrier, born in Africa	At least 0.5 (HCC occurs at a younger age)
HCV infection and stage 3 fibrosis[a]	<1.5
HBV carrier, <40 years (men) and <50 years (women)[a]	<0.2
Other causes of cirrhosis	Unknown

[a]The benefit of surveillance in this group is uncertain.
Adapted from Bruix J, Sherman M. Management of hepatocellular carcinoma: an update. *Hepatology*. 2011;53:1020–1022.

Prevention

Although great progress has been achieved in the primary prevention of HBV-induced HCC with universal infant HBV vaccination in many countries, the full impact of universal HBV vaccination on the occurrence of the tumor will not be realized for many years. A substantial reduction in the frequency of childhood HCC has been well demonstrated in Taiwan, where universal infant vaccination was adopted in the mid-1980s.[158] Similarly, in Alaska, the introduction of universal infant HBV vaccination in 1984 has eliminated HCC in Alaskan Native children.[159] In the meantime, huge numbers of existing HBV carriers worldwide remain at risk for HCC, and little progress has been made in preventing malignant transformation in persons with chronic viral hepatitis. Additionally, a vaccine against HCV will not be available in the near future, and prevention of aflatoxin-induced tumors is far from becoming a reality, despite ongoing trials of chemopreventive agents.

Considerable interest has been expressed in the impact of antiviral therapy against HBV and HCV in reducing the incidence of HCC. One randomized controlled trial of long-term therapy of the nucleoside analog lamivudine compared with placebo in patients with chronic hepatitis B showed a significant decrease in the frequency of clinical events in the treated group, including a decrease in the frequency of HCC (see Chapter 81).[14] Several large retrospective studies have shown a decrease in the frequency of HCC in patients treated successfully for chronic hepatitis C with interferon-based regimens and with DAAs (see Chapter 82).[25,160,161]

Intrahepatic Cholangiocarcinoma

Cholangiocarcinoma is a malignant neoplasm arising from the biliary duct epithelium. It often carries different names based on the particular portion of the biliary tract involved—small intrahepatic bile ducts (peripheral cholangiocarcinoma) proximal to the second-order bile ducts, hepatic duct bifurcation (perihilar cholangiocarcinoma, or Klatskin tumor) between the second-order bile ducts and the cystic duct, and extrahepatic bile ducts (bile duct carcinoma) distal to the cystic duct. The location of the tumor has a major impact on the presenting symptoms and treatment approach. In the past, perihilar cholangiocarcinoma was classified with the intrahepatic group based on *International Classification of Diseases*, 9th revision, codes even though it is extrahepatic in origin and is the most common form.[162,163] This section will be limited to a discussion of true ICC; extrahepatic cholangiocarcinoma, including the perihilar type, is discussed in Chapter 71.

Epidemiology

ICC represents approximately 10%–20% of all primary liver cancers and up to 20% of cholangiocarcinomas. The geographic variation in prevalence rates is marked, ranging from 0.2 to 96/100,000 in men and from 0.1 to 38/100,000 in women, because of differences in the frequencies of known risk factors in various populations.[164] The highest incidence rates are found in parts of

Asia, most notably certain regions of Thailand, Hong Kong, China, Japan, and Korea. Chronic infestation of the biliary tract with one of the liver flukes is thought to be the cause of these high rates (see Chapter 86).[165] The overall incidence rate in the United States is 0.85/100,000, with a 1.5-fold higher rate in men than women. The rate in whites is about equal to that in African Americans and about half that in Asians. ICC is rare before 40 years of age, and historically, the worldwide approximate average age at presentation is 50 years. Epidemiologic data indicate that the age at presentation has shifted to more than 65 years. Additionally, the incidence and mortality rates appear to be increasing worldwide.[162] Surveillance, Epidemiology, and End Results registry data from the United States showed a 165% increase between the late 1970s and the late 1990s.[164] This increase may have been a result, in part, of the increased prevalence of cirrhosis, particularly HCV-associated cirrhosis and more recently (MASLD, also referred to as NAFLD) and alcohol-associated liver disease.[166] In addition, there appears to be significant misclassification of perihilar cholangiocarcinoma as ICC in registry data due to a lack of distinctive categories in ICD-9 and ICD-10 coding between the three types of cholangiocarcinoma, leading to an overestimation of the number of cases.[167]

Etiology and Pathogenesis

Although the underlying predisposing factor for most cases of cholangiocarcinoma is unknown, several risk factors have been recognized. The strongest association is with *Opisthorchis viverrini*, a liver fluke endemic in parts of Southeast Asia and acquired by ingestion of raw or uncooked fish.[164,168] The association with *Clonorchis sinensis*, a related liver fluke, is weaker (see Chapter 86).[169] An association with the radiographic contrast agent thorium dioxide (Thorotrast), which was banned in the 1950s, has been well established.[170] PSC is linked to a diagnosis of cholangiocarcinoma at a young age, with a lifetime risk of 8%–20% (see Chapter 70).[171–173] Congenital and acquired abnormalities of the biliary tract that may result in bile stasis, chronic inflammation, and infection [as in biliary atresia,[174] von Meyenburg complexes,[175] Caroli disease,[176] choledochal cyst,[176] and intrahepatic lithiasis (hepatolithiasis)] have been associated with the development of cholangiocarcinoma (see Chapter 64). The previously discussed risk factors are most important for perihilar and extrahepatic bile duct cancer, although they probably also play a role in ICC. Diabetes mellitus also seems to add to the risk for both types.[177] Cirrhosis, particularly caused by HCV and perhaps alcohol and MASLD, has also been associated with cholangiocarcinoma.[164,166]

Malignant transformation of the bile duct cells generally occurs in an environment of inflammation or cholestasis (or both), usually in the setting of one of the known risk factors, though most cases in the West have no known risk factor. The proposal has been made that a combination of these environmental factors and genetic predisposition (e.g., defects in oncogenes or bile salt transporters) leads to an accumulation of genetic defects that results in carcinoma.[162,178] A polymorphism in the gene for the natural killer cell receptor G2D has been associated with an increased risk of cholangiocarcinoma in patients with PSC.[178] At the molecular level, numerous changes have been described, including mutations of the *K-ras* gene, the gene for interleukin (IL)-6, and allelic loss or mutations of *TP53* and *p16*, as well as many others (see Chapter 71).

Clinical Features

Peripheral cholangiocarcinoma seldom produces symptoms until the tumor is advanced. The clinical features are then similar to those of HCC, including malaise, weight loss, abdominal pain, and jaundice, which may be more frequent and prominent than with HCC.[176,179]

Diagnosis

In patients with peripheral cholangiocarcinoma, often only the serum alkaline phosphatase level is elevated. CA19-9 is the most frequently used serum tumor marker for cholangiocarcinoma but has significant limitations because CA19-9 levels are also elevated in pancreatic, colorectal, gastric, and gynecologic cancers and in acute bacterial cholangitis (see Chapters 62 and 71).[180] In addition, CA19-9 is always undetectable in the 7% of the population that is Lewis blood group negative. In patients with unexplained biliary obstruction without PSC, the sensitivity of CA19-9 is 53%, and the negative predictive value is 72%–92%, for a cutoff value of 100 U/mL. In patients with PSC, the sensitivity ranges from 38% to 89% and specificity from 50% to 98%. The addition of CEA probably does not improve the performance of CA19-9 in the setting of PSC (see Chapter 70). Elevated CA19-9 predicts worse survival independent of the TNM stage.[181]

Initial imaging with US helps identify biliary obstruction. Dynamic contrast-enhanced CT or MRI further aids in localizing the lesion and determining the possibility of resection.[162,182] MRI with MRCP is a superior modality because of a higher sensitivity than CT for detecting lesions and localizing biliary obstruction. The tumor is hypointense on T1-weighted images and moderately intense on T2-weighted images. With dynamic contrast, the tumor generally has progressive enhancement in arterial, portal venous, and delayed phases, thereby helping to distinguish it from HCC, which usually displays washout in the later two phases (see earlier). EUS with FNA of a lesion in patients without PSC has the advantage of improving sensitivity and specificity for the diagnosis of the primary lesion and nodal metastasis but the disadvantage of causing peritoneal seeding and, therefore, should be avoided if surgical resection is contemplated. Percutaneous biopsies also carry the risk of peritoneal seeding and are generally avoided if the tumor is potentially resectable.

Pathology

Peripheral cholangiocarcinoma usually is a large and solitary tumor, but it may be multinodular.[183] It is grayish-white, firm, and occasionally umbilicated and usually produces a focal hepatic mass; rarely, the tumor can grow alongside and infiltrate the bile ducts or occur as an intraductal papillary lesion.[182] The tumor is poorly vascularized and rarely bleeds internally or ruptures. Metastatic nodules may be distributed irregularly throughout the liver. The bile ducts peripheral to the tumor may be dilated, resulting in some cases in biliary cirrhosis. Metastases in regional lymph nodes occur in about 50% of cases.

Microscopically, cholangiocarcinoma exhibits acinar or tubular structures that resemble those of other adenocarcinomas.[184] Most tumors are well to moderately differentiated. Secretion of mucus may be demonstrable, but bile production is not seen. The tumor cells provoke a variable desmoplastic reaction, and in many tumors, the collagenized stroma may be the most prominent feature. Distinguishing the tumor from metastatic adenocarcinoma may be difficult, and some experts have advocated assuming that an adenocarcinoma in the liver is cholangiocarcinoma if no primary tumor can be found elsewhere.[183] Immunohistochemistry may be helpful, with CK7 usually staining strongly and CK20 staining negative or weakly. A panel of immunohistochemical stains is usually used to exclude common sites of metastatic adenocarcinoma although metastasis from gallbladder, pancreas, and upper GI tract cancers needs to be excluded based on imaging and endoscopy, if indicated.[185]

Treatment and Prognosis

Early diagnosis of ICC is unusual, and the annual mortality rate is almost identical to the annual incidence of the tumor.[176,179] Long-term survival after diagnosis in the United States based on the Surveillance, Epidemiology, and End Results database is dismal, with a 1-year survival rate of 28% and a 5-year survival rate less than 5%. The 5-year survival rate has not improved since the late 1980s.[164]

In a person with suspected or proved ICC, staging is recommended to determine surgical resectability, which is the only opportunity for cure. The staging evaluation usually includes dynamic MRI of the abdomen and MRCP (or dynamic helical CT, if MRI is unavailable or if there is concern of vascular invasion) and a chest x-ray or chest CT.[162] PET has been assessed in small series and does not clearly add to other modalities. EUS with FNA of suspicious lymph nodes may detect otherwise unrecognized metastasis in up to 20% of cases, but transduodenal or transgastric biopsy of the primary lesion should be avoided because of a significant risk of needle track seeding.[182] Surgical resectability of ICC should be determined in conjunction with an experienced hepatobiliary surgeon and requires the ability to achieve clear surgical margins, which usually necessitates a major hepatectomy. Criteria for resection include absence of all the following: evidence of extrahepatic metastasis, main portal vein or hepatic artery invasion or encasement, bilateral segmental bile duct involvement, and contralateral hepatic lobar atrophy. Large tumor diameter, multiple lesions, lymph node metastasis, and underlying cirrhosis predict poor outcome after surgery.[186,187] Additionally, the patient must be medically fit to undergo surgery and have sufficient hepatic reserve. Patients well selected for surgical resection achieve a 1- to 2-year median survival and a 29%–36% 5-year survival rate. LT alone or in combination with neoadjuvant and adjuvant chemotherapy results in unacceptably high recurrence rates and less than a 50% 5-year survival though incidental cholangiocarcinoma </= 2 cm can have acceptable 5-year survival.

Small series and comparative studies show about a 1-year median survival with either conventional TACE or TACE with drug eluting beads for unresectable ICC.[186] There is an emerging role for LT as an effective treatment in highly selected < 3 cm ICC in the setting of cirrhosis. Case series of radioembolization with Y-90 microspheres have reported rates similar to those for TACE, although there have been no randomized comparisons with TACE, chemotherapy, or supportive care.[186] The rates of response and survival following chemotherapy are modest but improving. A randomized trial showed a survival benefit of 3.6 months for locally advanced or metastatic biliary tract cancer with the combination of cisplatin and gemcitabine.[188] The addition of durvalumab, a PD-L1 inhibitor, to cisplatin and gemcitabine more than doubled estimated survival at 24 months to 24.9 % in a randomized trial.[189] There is preliminary evidence that patients with cholangiocarcinoma and targetable mutations may benefit from chemotherapy active against their mutation.[167] Small series using external beam radiation for unresectable locally advanced ICC have shown good local control and an approximately 2-year median survival.[186] There are multiple ongoing clinical trials to better define the potential efficacy of chemotherapy, immunotherapy, targeted therapy, and combinations with local regional therapy, but as yet there are no well-defined treatment pathways for ICC if resection is not an option.

Hepatoblastoma

Epidemiology

In children, hepatoblastoma is the third most common liver tumor and the most common malignant liver tumor.[190] It occurs almost exclusively in the first 3 years of life, although cases occurring in older children and adults have been reported; boys are affected twice as often as girls.[1,191,192] While rare (incidence of 1.2–2.1 cases per million population/year), over the past several decades, there has been a statistically significant increase in the incidence of hepatoblastoma in both genders {NCCR website}.[193]

Etiology and Pathogenesis

Hepatoblastoma may occur sporadically or in association with hereditary syndromes such as familial adenomatous polyposis (FAP) (see Chapter 128) and Beckwith-Wiedemann syndrome (characterized by macroglossia, macrosomia, midline abdominal wall defects, ear creases or pits, and neonatal hypoglycemia), suggesting a possible role for chromosomes 5 and 11, respectively, in the genesis of the tumor. Hepatoblastoma is also the most common tumor seen in patients with Trisomy 18, accounting for approximately 66% of malignancies in these patients.[194–197]

When occurring sporadically, the pathogenesis of hepatoblastoma is unknown; however, a study from the Children's Oncology Group has identified a link between parental occupational exposures and hepatoblastoma.[198] Most patients (67%–89%) with sporadic hepatoblastoma have mutations of the FAP tumor suppressor gene, which downregulates β-catenin, and a similar number have activating mutations of the β-catenin gene, raising the possibility that the Wnt signaling pathway plays a role in the development of the tumor (see Chapter 1).[199]

Low birth weight, specifically under 1500 g, carries a higher risk and is recognized as an independent risk factor for the development of hepatoblastoma.[200,201] While this association is clearly established, the mechanism is not well understood at this time. However, it is thought that NICU exposure to radiation, total parental nutrition, and oxygen therapy increases oxidative DNA damage.[200]

Clinical Features

Most children with hepatoblastoma come to medical attention because of abdominal swelling and palpable abdominal mass.[202] Other reasons include failure to thrive, weight loss, poor appetite, abdominal pain, irritability, and intermittent vomiting and diarrhea. The tumorous liver is almost always enlarged and firm and may be tender. Its surface is smooth or nodular. Hepatoblastomas rarely rupture. Distant metastases are evident, usually in the lung, in 20% of patients at presentation.[203] Approximately 15% of children with newly diagnosed hepatoblastoma may present with bone pain due to fractures in the ribs and spine.[204] The tumor occasionally causes isosexual precocity in boys as a result of the ectopic production of human chorionic gonadotropin.[205]

Diagnosis

Diagnosis is often made through a combination of serologies, pathology, and radiography. AFP is present in high concentrations in the serum of 80%–90% of patients with hepatoblastoma and is a useful clue to the diagnosis.[206] The few patients with a low serum AFP level appear to have a worse prognosis.[207] If AFP is found to be elevated, it can be helpful in monitoring response to treatment as it will typically normalize with resolution of the malignancy and increase with recurrence. In addition, anemia is common, as is thrombocytosis, which is attributed to raised serum thrombopoietin levels.

Radiographically, pulmonary metastases and, rarely, mottled calcification in the tumor may be seen on a plain film. US is the most widely used initial imaging technique, although the findings are not specific. CT and MRI are used to define the extent of the tumor and plan definitive surgery. The tumor is seen as an avascular mass on hepatic arteriography.[208]

Pathology

Hepatoblastomas are the malignant derivatives of incompletely differentiated hepatocyte precursors. Their constituents are diverse, reflecting both the multipotentiality of their mesodermal origin and the progressive stages of embryonic and fetal development. Hepatoblastomas can be characterized as either epithelial or mixed (epithelial and mesenchymal) types and can be further stratified into different subtypes based on their histopathologic appearance. Each hepatoblastoma subtype has a distinct clinical course, which allows for histopathology to be used as a parameter in the risk stratification of prognosis. The pure fetal type has an excellent prognosis, whereas the aggressive small-cell undifferentiated tumor type has the worst prognosis and is usually assigned the most intensive therapeutic interventions.[200]

The tumors are usually solitary, ranging in diameter from 5 to 25 cm, and always well circumscribed (about half are encapsulated). They vary in color, ranging from tan to grayish-white, and contain foci of hemorrhage, necrosis, and calcification. Vascular channels may be prominent on the capsular surface. Epithelial hepatoblastomas are solid, whereas tumors of the mixed variety often are separated into lobules by white bands of collagen tissue.

Two types of epithelial cells are present in the tumor.[209] Cells of the first type resemble fetal hepatocytes and are arranged in irregular plates, usually two cells thick, with bile canaliculi between individual cells and sinusoids between plates. Cells of the second type are embryonal and are less differentiated than the fetal type. Mixed hepatoblastomas contain mesenchymal tissue consisting of areas of a highly cellular primitive type of mesenchyme intimately admixed with epithelial elements. Cartilage and striated muscle may be present. Hepatoblastomas may show foci of squamous cells, with or without keratinization, and foreign body–type giant cells. Vascular invasion may be evident. Metastases most commonly involve lung, abdominal lymph nodes, and brain.

Treatment and Prognosis

Treatment of hepatoblastoma is based upon the extent of the tumor. If the tumor is localized to 1–2 segments of the liver, it can be treated with surgical resection. However, if the tumor involves three or more areas of the liver, complete hepatectomy and LT need to be considered. In addition, other factors, such as vascular invasion and extrahepatic disease, play a role in determining treatment options.[210] If the lesion is solitary and sufficiently localized to be resected, surgery is often curative, with 5-year survival rates as high as 75%.[202] When the tumor is judged to be inoperable, neoadjuvant chemotherapy may reduce the size of the tumor sufficiently to permit resection. LT plays an increasing role because of technical success with live donor and split LT (see Chapter 99).

Cisplatin alone or in combination with other chemotherapeutic agents is effective against hepatoblastoma and is associated with 90% survival in selected patients.[211] If surgery is not possible or the tumor recurs after surgery, the prognosis is generally poor.

Angiosarcoma

Epidemiology

Although rare with an estimated frequency of 0.14 to 0.25 per million, angiosarcoma is the most common malignant mesenchymal tumor of the liver.[212,213] It occurs almost exclusively in adults and is most prevalent in the sixth and seventh decades of life.[214,215] Men are affected four times as often as women.

Etiology and Pathogenesis

Despite its rarity, hepatic angiosarcoma is of special interest because specific risk factors have been identified. Angiosarcoma has been commonly associated with several environmental carcinogens, including thorium dioxide (the radioactive compound in thorotrast), vinyl chloride, and arsenic compounds.[216–219] In addition, the use of anabolic steroids has also been associated with hepatic angiosarcoma.[220]

In early reports, the tumor became evident approximately 20 years after exposure to thorium dioxide (see Chapter 91).[221] The mechanism is thought to be related to the storage of α-particles that are emitted from thorium dioxide, which are then stored lifelong in the reticuloendothelial system, including the liver.[212]

Arsenic has also been linked to hepatic carcinogenesis. Angiosarcoma has been reported in German vintners who used arsenic-containing insecticides and drank wine adulterated with arsenic.[219] In addition, a few patients with angiosarcoma had taken potassium arsenite (Fowler's solution) for many years to treat psoriasis.[222] While the association between arsenic and angiosarcoma is apparent, the mechanism of action remains unclear.[223]

Hepatic angiosarcoma was first reported in workers exposed to vinyl chloride monomer (VCM) in 1974.[217,214,218] The monomer is converted by enzymes of the endoplasmic reticulum to reactive metabolites that form DNA adducts and guanosine-to-adenine transitions in the *K-ras* and *TP53* genes. Angiosarcomas have occurred after exposures of 11–37 years (or after shorter periods with a heavy initial exposure).[212] The mean age of patients at diagnosis is 48 years. In addition to angiosarcoma, persons exposed to VCM may be at increased risk of HCC and soft tissue sarcoma.

Clinical Features

The most common presenting symptom is upper abdominal pain. Other frequent complaints are abdominal swelling, rapidly progressing liver failure, malaise, weight loss, poor appetite, and nausea.[213,214] Vomiting occurs occasionally. The duration of symptoms generally ranges from 1 week to 6 months, but a few patients have had symptoms for as long as 2 years before seeking medical attention.

The liver is almost always enlarged and usually tender. Its surface may be irregular, or a definite mass may be felt. An arterial bruit is occasionally heard over the enlarged liver. Splenomegaly may be present and is attributed to the hepatic fibrosis and consequent portal hypertension that may also complicate exposure to VCM. Ascites is frequent, and the fluid may be blood stained. The patient often has jaundice. Fever and dependent edema are less common. Approximately 15% of patients present with acute hemoperitoneum following tumor rupture. Metastases are seen in approximately 60% of patients. The most common locations for metastases are lung, spleen, and bone marrow.[215,224,225]

Diagnosis

A rising serum bilirubin level and other evidence of progressive hepatic dysfunction may be present, especially in the later stages of the tumor. Patients can also be found to have thrombocytopenia, the result of platelet sequestration within the poorly organized tumor vasculature. Because of this localized coagulopathy, systemic DIC may occur as well.[225–227] In addition, hemolytic anemia has been reported in patients with hepatic angiosarcoma.[225,228]

Radiographically, radiopaque deposits of the material may be evident in the liver and spleen in patients exposed to thorium dioxide.[221] One or more mass lesions may be demonstrated on US, CT, or MRI, but diffusely infiltrating tumor may not be visualized. Hepatic arteriography reveals a characteristic appearance.[229] The hepatic arteries are displaced by the tumor, which shows a blush and "puddling" during the middle of the arterial phase that persists for many seconds, except in the central area, which may be hypovascular.

Pathology

Angiosarcomas are usually multicentric.[230] Their hallmark is the presence of blood-filled cysts, although solid growth also is seen.

The lesions are fairly well circumscribed but not encapsulated. Larger masses are spongy and bulge beneath Glisson's capsule.

The earliest microscopic change is the presence of hypertrophic sinusoidal lining cells with hyperchromatic nuclei in ill-defined loci throughout the liver. With the progression of the lesion, sinusoidal dilatation and disruption of hepatic plates occur, and the malignant cells become supported by collagen tissue. Enlarging vascular spaces lined by malignant cells causes the tumor to become cavernous. The malignant endothelial cells usually are multilayered and may project into the cavity in intricate fronds and tufts supported by fibrous tissue. The fronds commonly are elongated with ill-defined borders. The cytoplasm is clear and faintly eosinophilic. Nuclei are hyperchromatic and vary greatly in size and shape; some cells are multinucleated. Evidence of phagocytosis may be seen. Foci of extramedullary hematopoiesis are common, and invasion of the portal and central veins occurs in most cases. Distant metastases are present in 60% of tumors.

Complications and Prognosis

Hepatic angiosarcomas grow rapidly, and the prognosis is poor; mean overall survival is approximately 8 months.[231] In addition, patients may have thrombocytopenia resulting from entrapment of platelets within the tumor (Kasabach-Merritt syndrome), DIC with secondary fibrinolysis,[227] or microangiopathic hemolytic anemia as a result of fragmentation of erythrocytes within the tumor circulation.[228]

Treatment

Operative treatment is usually precluded by the advanced stage of the tumor. Even when surgery is undertaken, the patient commonly survives only 1–3 years, although long-term survival may be achieved in the few patients with a solitary tumor, especially if the tumor size is less than 10 cm.[213,231] Unfortunately, the results of radiation and chemotherapy are poor.

Epithelioid Hemangioendothelioma

Epidemiology

Epithelioid hemangioendothelioma is a rare, low-grade vascular tumor with an estimated incidence of less than 0.1 per 100,000.[212] A series of 137 cases has been collected at a specialized referral center.[232] Two-thirds of patients were female, and the tumor occurred at all ages in adulthood.

Clinical Features

The clinical presentation is variable, ranging between being asymptomatic and hepatic failure.[233] Most commonly, patients present with nonspecific symptoms such as abdominal pain, weakness, and weight loss.

Diagnosis

Imaging studies show a characteristically highly vascular mass that may infiltrate throughout the liver. Case reports indicate that the tumor can be visualized on PET scan. Correct diagnosis requires histologic examination of tissue obtained by biopsy with appropriate immunostaining. Epithelioid hemangioendothelioma should be distinguished from infantile hemangioendothelioma, a not uncommon liver tumor of infancy that may be associated with abdominal distention, failure to thrive, heart failure, bronchiolitis, and even sudden infant death (see later). Type II infantile hemangioendothelioma tends to be more aggressive and may be indistinguishable from hepatic angiosarcoma in some cases.[234,235]

Pathology

Tumors are often multinodular and bilobar.[233] Histologically, they are characterized by the presence of dendritic and epithelioid cells that contain vacuoles, representing intracellular lumina. These cells stain positively for endothelial markers, such as factor VIII–related antigen, CD34, or CD31.

Complications and Prognosis

The tumor has low-grade malignant potential and must be distinguished from angiosarcoma, because it has a much better prognosis if treated appropriately and aggressively. Epithelioid hemangioendothelioma may metastasize, both within and beyond the liver.

Treatment

Due to the rare nature of this tumor, there is no standardized protocol. The primary treatment modality for epithelioid hemangioendothelioma is surgical, including resection or LT. Transplantation appears to be effective for this tumor, even in the presence of advanced or metastatic disease. Furthermore, disease-free survival does not appear to be influenced by factors such as treatments received prior to LT, lymph node status, or the limited presence of extrahepatic disease, though vascular invasion does correlate with decreased long term survival after LT.[233] The tumor does not appear to be sensitive to radiation or chemotherapy.

Others

Undifferentiated (embryonal) sarcoma is a rare primary malignancy of the liver that occurs in both children and adults.[236,237] The tumor tends to be aggressive, but long-term survival can be achieved with radical surgery and chemotherapy.[238] Other rare neoplasms arising in the liver include liposarcoma,[239] primary lymphoma (see Chapter 41),[213,240] and rhabdomyosarcoma.[237]

Hepatic Metastases

Epidemiology and Etiology

The liver is the most frequent target for metastatic spread of tumors. Hepatic metastases occur in 40%–50% of adult patients with extrahepatic primary malignancies.[241] Foremost among the reasons for the high frequency of hepatic metastases are the double blood supply of the liver and the presence of fenestrations in the sinusoidal endothelium that facilitate penetration of malignant cells into the hepatic parenchyma.[242] Hepatic metastases commonly originate from primary sites in the distribution of the portal venous system, including the pancreas, stomach, and colon. Outside this distribution, tumors of the lung and breast are the most common origins of hepatic metastases.

Clinical Features

Symptoms resulting from hepatic metastases are often absent or overshadowed by those of the primary tumor. Occasionally, the symptoms and signs attributable to metastases are the presenting manifestations of an asymptomatic primary tumor. In such cases, the likely symptoms are malaise, weight loss, and upper abdominal pain. Jaundice, when present, is seldom attributable to replacement of hepatic tissue by metastases. Depending on the extent of the metastatic disease, the liver may be enlarged, sometimes markedly. Its surface may be irregular, and umbilicated nodules may be felt by the examiner. A friction rub may be heard over hepatic metastases.

cyst, or torsion of a pedunculated cyst. Jaundice is evident in approximately 5% of patients and is caused by compression of the major intrahepatic or extrahepatic bile ducts. Ascites, if present, is the result of portal hypertension, which generally is caused by associated congenital hepatic fibrosis but occasionally by compression of the hepatic veins by the cysts. Gastroesophageal variceal bleeding has rarely been reported.[359]

Diagnosis

Liver biochemical test results generally are normal, with intact hepatic function, although serum alkaline phosphatase and GGTP levels may be increased. The cysts contain high levels of the tumor marker CA 19-9, and serum levels of CA 19-9 may be elevated. A raised right hemidiaphragm may be evident on a plain film of the chest in patients with severe PCLD. The diagnosis of PCLD is confirmed by US, CT, or MRI (see Fig. 98.9).

Treatment

On the rare occasions when cysts require treatment, fenestration (unroofing) should be performed.[341,360] Cyst fenestration originally was done at laparotomy but is now performed laparoscopically, thereby reducing morbidity.[361] A high recurrence rate is observed for cysts treated with fenestration, although symptomatic relief is usually durable. Cysts have also been treated by percutaneous injection of a sclerosing substance such as alcohol or doxycycline, but most patients have too many small cysts, so percutaneous injection should be reserved for those with one or a few dominant cysts or excessive risk for surgery. Patients who fail to respond to cyst fenestration may be considered for partial hepatic resection combined with cyst fenestration if sufficient relatively uninvolved liver remains after surgery. The morbidity of this approach is substantial, and future LT may be more difficult after resection.[361] LT (sometimes combined with renal transplantation) is associated with excellent outcomes and long-term survival but, because of the organ donor shortage, is generally reserved for patients with severe symptoms that interfere with the patient's quality of life and at least one of the following: hepatic failure, renal failure, or moderate-to-severe protein calorie malnutrition.[361] Several small randomized clinical trials have demonstrated a modest reduction in cyst size and improvement in quality of life with treatment with a long-acting somatostatin analog, but the length of follow-up has been short.[362] Cyst infection is rare, usually diagnosed on clinical grounds (fever, elevated WBC, pain, positive blood cultures), and imaging is sometimes helpful. Antibiotics to cover gut bacterial pathogens should be given for 4–6 weeks as untreated infections can lead to sepsis.[363] Estrogen-containing medications should be stopped in persons with all types of PCLD as they promote cyst growth.[363]

Autosomal Recessive Polycystic Kidney Disease

Fibrocystic liver disease may present in childhood as an autosomal recessive disorder that is usually rapidly fatal as a consequence of associated ARPKD.[341,342] A proportion of patients maintain renal function into adulthood, however, and complications of the associated liver disease then predominate. The liver cysts are microscopic rather than macroscopic and present a clinical picture of congenital hepatic fibrosis. Complications of portal hypertension are the usual hepatic manifestations of the disease. The genes responsible for this disease are *PKHD1* and *DZIP1L*. Fibrocystin, the protein produced by PKHD1, is a transmembrane receptor involved in the regulation of proliferation and morphogenesis.[353] *DZIP1L* mutations are associated with ductal plate malformations in mice.[353] Some carriers of ARPKD may manifest a similar PCLD.[358]

von Meyenburg Complexes

von Meyenburg complexes (also known as biliary microhamartomas) are common and do not produce symptoms; they are small and usually multiple. Each complex is composed of cystically dilated intra- and interlobular bile ducts embedded in a fibrous stroma.[364,365] The cysts are lined by cuboidal or flat epithelium. They occur in almost all patients with congenital hepatic fibrosis and may coexist with Caroli syndrome or ARPKD. von Meyenburg complexes are found in or adjacent to portal tracts and are believed to arise as a result of malformation of the ductal plate (see Chapter 64); they may be complicated by the development of peripheral cholangiocarcinoma.[366]

Caroli Disease

Caroli disease is a rare disorder characterized by congenital nonobstructive gross dilatation of the segmental intrahepatic bile ducts.[340] The disease has been included in the classification of choledochal cysts (as Type V)[340,341] and may occur in association with medullary sponge kidney (in 60%–80% of patients) or congenital hepatic fibrosis (see Chapter 64). Caroli disease is believed to be caused by an intrauterine event that arrests ductal plate remodeling at the level of the larger intrahepatic bile ducts.[367] The resulting bile duct ectasia may be diffuse or localized. Both autosomal recessive and autosomal dominant modes of inheritance have been proposed, and it has been associated with mutations in PKHD1.[363] Caroli disease affects men and women equally and usually becomes symptomatic in early adulthood; more than 80% of patients present with symptoms before 30 years of age.

Patients typically present with recurrent episodes of fever and abdominal pain caused by cholangitis. The liver is often enlarged. Ductal ectasia predisposes to bile stagnation, which in turn may lead to cholangitis, abscess formation, and septicemia.[368] Gallstones form in the ectatic ducts in one-third of patients. The result of these complications may be cholangiocarcinoma, which develops in less than 10% of patients but carries a high mortality rate even with treatment.[369]

Caroli disease is usually discovered when the liver is imaged during the investigation of suspected cholangitis. Irregular dilatations of the larger intrahepatic bile ducts are seen.

Attacks of cholangitis require treatment with antibiotics. Endoscopic retrograde cannulation of the biliary system may be used to facilitate removal of sludge or stones from the accessible part of the biliary system, and the cysts may be drained by an endoscopic or percutaneous route. Liver resection for unilobar Caroli disease and LT for diffuse Caroli disease with recurrent cholangitis are associated with excellent long-term patient survival and a low rate of complications.[370] Annual MRI to provide surveillance for cholangiocarcinoma is reasonable but unproven for patients not undergoing definitive surgical treatment.[363]

APPROACH TO THE PATIENT WITH A HEPATIC MASS

The approach to the diagnosis of a mass in the liver will be influenced by the age and gender of the patient and the presence or absence of symptoms (Fig. 98.10). Making a definitive diagnosis of a mass in the liver solely on clinical grounds is seldom possible. Nevertheless, detailed history taking will provide important clues about the probable benign or malignant nature of the lesion. The approach to a mass in the liver differs depending on whether or not cirrhosis is present.[371] In a noncirrhotic liver, masses may be found in the liver incidentally or because of symptoms; the main concern is cancer metastatic from elsewhere. Initial imaging studies such as US, CT, or MRI will indicate if the

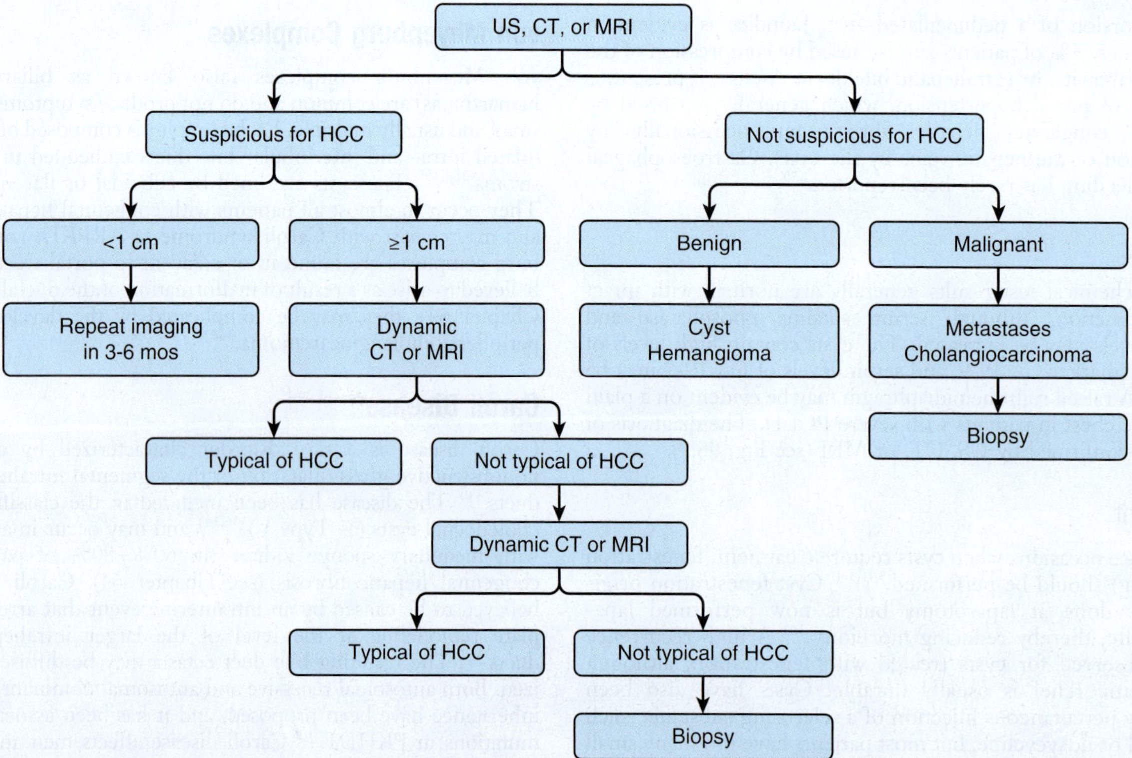

Fig. 98.10 Algorithm for the approach to the patient with a hepatic mass based on the suspicion for HCC.

lesion is cystic. Cystic lesions should be investigated further and treated only if symptomatic or an echinococcal cyst or biliary cystadenoma is suspected, usually based on the complexity of the cyst wall, including calcification, septations, and daughter cysts (see Chapters 71 and 86).

Noncystic lesions in a noncirrhotic liver include a hemangioma, which can be confirmed by contrast-enhanced MRI. Hemangiomas generally show peripheral nodular enhancement in the arterial phase, with progressive centripetal filling in the portal venous and delayed phases. FNH shows intense homogenous enhancement on arterial phase, with a characteristic enhancing scar on delayed phase, by CT or MRI. By contrast, hepatocellular adenoma has less intense arterial enhancement and no central scar. Dynamic MRI with a hepatocyte-specific contrast agent and delayed imaging is helpful for distinguishing FNH from a hepatocellular adenoma because adenomas are hypointense on delayed phase images, whereas FNH are hyper- or isointense. If primary or metastatic malignancy is suspected because of the presence of underlying chronic liver disease, a prior or current malignancy, systemic symptoms or signs (e.g., weight loss), or an elevated serum tumor marker level (AFP, CA 19-9), then a biopsy (under ultrasound or CT guidance) should be considered. Most metastases are less vascular than HCC. A metastasis and peripheral cholangiocarcinoma often have peripheral rim enhancement on the arterial phase. If a biopsy is not performed or not diagnostic, then interval follow-up imaging studies are prudent unless the imaging findings are classic in appearance for FNH or hemangioma.

In a patient known to have cirrhosis, the presence of a nodule or mass should be presumed to be HCC until proved otherwise. AASLD practice guidelines provide criteria for the noninvasive diagnosis of HCC based on the vascularity of the tumor (see earlier). Contrast enhancement during the arterial phase of a multiphase CT or MRI study, with subsequent washout during the portal venous or delayed phase, is considered diagnostic of HCC if the lesion is larger than 1 cm in diameter. If the vascular enhancement pattern is atypical, a biopsy of the lesion should be considered. A high serum AFP level is strongly suggestive of HCC but may rarely occur with other GI malignancies, and its usefulness has been questioned. For a lesion smaller than 1 cm, interval imaging at 3–6 months is recommended. If determining whether a patient has underlying cirrhosis is impossible on clinical and imaging grounds, a biopsy of the nontumorous liver may be done. Although characteristic imaging features of HCC, hemangioma, and FNH have high diagnostic accuracy and can be relied on for treatment decisions, definitive diagnosis often depends on demonstrating the typical histologic features of the tumor.

Full references for this chapter can be found at ebooks.health.elsevier.com.

99 Liver Transplantation

Andres F. Carrion, Paul Martin

IN THIS CHAPTER

Although specific treatments for certain chronic liver diseases may favorably alter their natural history by diminishing, halting, or permitting regression of hepatic fibrosis, once major complications of cirrhosis such as ascites or hepatic encephalopathy develop, treatment options are limited and typically do not extend survival or significantly improve quality of life. Interventions such as variceal band ligation and placement of a TIPS can effectively control life-threatening bleeding but do not abort progression of underlying cirrhosis (see Chapters 76, and 94). With some notable exceptions, as occur with abstinence from alcohol in decompensated alcohol-associated liver disease and antiviral therapy in advanced liver disease due to HBV or HCV infection, the course of clinically overt cirrhosis is almost invariably progressive. Even a patient with previously well-compensated cirrhosis who experiences an index complication of liver disease can develop precipitous deterioration with "acute-on-chronic liver failure," leading to multiorgan involvement, frequently with sepsis and renal failure (see Chapter 76). The major indications for liver transplantation (LT) include decompensated cirrhosis, unresectable primary hepatic malignancies, and ALF, which account for the majority of adult cases.[1]

Both short- and long-term outcomes postliver transplant continue to improve. Graft failure occurs in only 7.9% of deceased donor liver transplant recipients by 1 year, and 5-year graft survival exceeds 75% for most recipients, except those ≥65 years of age (74%), whose model for end-stage liver disease (MELD) score is >40 (74.5%), and who receive donation after circulatory death (DCD) allografts (74.2%). Patient survival largely mirrors that of graft survival, reflecting major advances in surgical techniques, postoperative intensive care, and immunosuppression, as well as better selection of potential candidates. Recurrent disease remains an ongoing concern during long-term follow-up of liver transplant recipients and may result in diminished patient and/or graft survival after an otherwise successful procedure. The advent of interferon-free antiviral regimens with DAAs for HCV infection now permits treatment of recurrent or even de novo (in cases of HCV infected livers transplanted into a previously noninfected recipient) infection in liver transplant recipients with efficacy and safety rates comparable to those for nontransplant populations.[2] Similarly, oral antiviral agents in combination with hepatitis B immunoglobulin permit LT with a low likelihood of recurrent HBV infection posttransplant.[3] Recurrence or development of de novo nonviral liver disease, particularly metabolic dysfunction-associated steatotic liver disease [MASLD, formerly nonalcoholic fatty liver disease (NAFLD)], post-LT is also recognized and presents major future challenges. Effective immunosuppression has made graft rejection less of a threat.[4,5] Recognition that excessive immunosuppression is deleterious and that variable degrees of immune tolerance may develop in selected liver transplant recipients has led to more individualized immunosuppressive regimens.[6]

Although the number of deceased liver donors continues to increase and pretransplant mortality for patients on the waiting list continues to decrease, the shortage of donor organs remains the greatest challenge in LT. Deaths on the transplant waiting list (12.2 per 100 waiting list-years) reflect in large part the sizable and ongoing disparity between the number of individuals in need of transplantation and that of available donor organs. Efforts to expand the deceased-donor supply by public education programs have succeeded, although many potential organ donors remain unidentified. Although living-donor LT (LDLT) in adult recipients can potentially increase the available donor organ pool, potential risks to the donor have limited its widespread application.[7] Other innovations such as splitting of a deceased-donor graft to share between two recipients and use of "extended-criteria" grafts, including those from older and nonheart-beating donors, have also expanded the organ supply, albeit modestly; however, there is an increased frequency of biliary complications with these allografts. Utilization of HCV-infected grafts is one of the more recent strategies aimed at increasing the donor organ pool.[8] Prior to licensure of DAAs that permit safe and effective treatment of HCV infection in liver transplant recipients, this was not adopted because of the risk of HCV acquisition and markedly diminished graft and patient survival. A consequence of the ongoing opioid epidemic in young adults has been expansion of the deceased donor pool due to accidental drug overdoses.[9] Although the shortage of donor organs will undoubtedly persist, and recurrence of the original disease remains a threat, the prospects for long-term survival appear to be excellent for most liver transplant recipients who otherwise would succumb to their underlying liver disease. The predicted 1-year survival rate for patients with decompensated cirrhosis is less than 10% without LT; by contrast, survival is 91% at 1 year and >75% at 5 years post-LT for most indications.[10]

Access to LT has transformed the management of advanced liver disease but has resulted in an expanding cohort of potential recipients with decompensated cirrhosis who require detailed medical attention.[11] The best outcomes following LT are obtained in recipients who have not already experienced multiple complications of liver disease[12]; therefore referral is appropriate when a patient with cirrhosis has had an index complication, such as the new onset of ascites. For at least some potential recipients, access to LDLT may avoid a lengthy waiting period attended by potentially life-threatening complications of liver disease.

In parallel with the evolution of LT, the care of transplant candidates with complex disease and transplant recipients has become an area of special expertise. The transplant hepatologist must combine the skills necessary to practice gastroenterology, multidisciplinary internal medicine, and intensive care.[13]

INDICATIONS

The major indications for LT in adults reflect the most frequent causes of cirrhosis (see Chapter 76), notably alcohol-associated liver disease, MASLD, HCV infection, and to a lesser extent, primary biliary cholangitis (PBC), PSC, autoimmune hepatitis, HBV infection, and hemochromatosis (Fig. 99.1; see Chapters 70, 77, 81, 82, 88, 89, 92, and 93). HCC is the leading indication for LT in the United States, reflecting the high risk for this primary hepatic malignancy in individuals with cirrhosis.[14] Alcohol-associated liver disease remains another major indication for LT in the United States, with temporal trends demonstrating that the frequency of LT for this indication has steadily increased and has become the leading nonneoplastic indication for LT. Many candidates for LT previously described as having "cryptogenic" cirrhosis are now considered to have MASLD (see Chapter 89), which currently follows alcohol-associated liver disease as the second leading nonneoplastic indication for LT in the United States.[15,16] The number of patients with HCV-related chronic liver disease listed for LT in the United States has declined steeply following licensure of DAAs.[17,18] An uncommon but important indication is ALF, which has a high mortality rate in the absence of LT (see Chapter 97). Cholangiocarcinoma, the other major primary adult hepatic malignancy apart from HCC, had been regarded as a contraindication to LT because of its rapid and almost invariable recurrence, leading to dismal recipient survival rates; however, acceptable outcomes can be achieved in a subset of patients with perihilar tumors who receive neoadjuvant external beam radiation and chemosensitization (see Chapter 71).[19] The major indication for pediatric LT is biliary atresia following a failed Kasai procedure (portoenterostomy) or delayed recognition of the diagnosis (see Chapter 64). Other major pediatric indications include α_1-antitrypsin deficiency and other metabolic disorders (see Chapter 79).

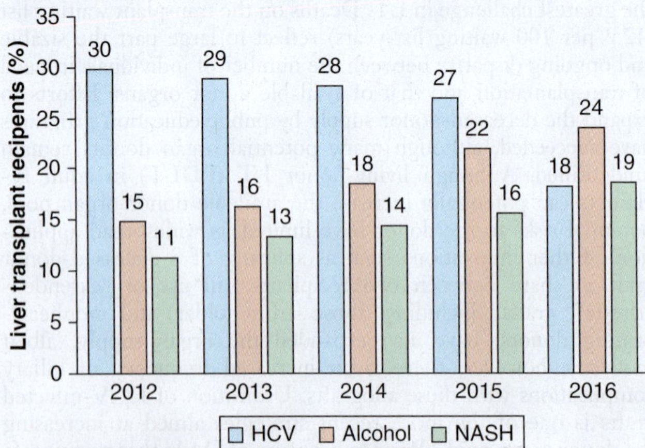

Fig. 99.1 Leading indications for liver transplantation in adults in the United States, 2012–2016. (From Cholankeril G, Ahmed A. Alcoholic liver disease replaces hepatitis C virus infection as the leading indication for liver transplantation in the United States. *Clin Gastroenterol Hepatol.* 2018;16:1356–1358.)

A diagnosis of cirrhosis per se is not an indication for LT, although a key issue in managing patients with cirrhosis is assessing whether this intervention will be needed in the future and when referral for transplant evaluation is appropriate (Box 99.1). Other important aspects of care are the anticipation of complications such as variceal bleeding (see Chapter 94) and surveillance for HCC (see Chapter 98).[11] LT should normally be recommended only when the limits of medical therapy for complications of cirrhosis have been reached. The risk of surgery must always be weighed against a realistic assessment of the potential recipient's prognosis in the absence of LT. For example, in a patient with decompensated cirrhosis caused by HBV infection, effective antiviral therapy may result in significant clinical improvement, delaying or even obviating the need for LT (see Chapter 81). Similarly, alcohol abstinence can result in dramatic improvement with a resolution of signs of hepatic decompensation in a patient with alcohol-associated liver disease (see Chapter 88). However, evaluation for LT should not be deferred even when a potentially reversible component of hepatic decompensation is identified, because clinical improvement does not occur invariably and the course of chronic liver disease remains unpredictable. Although recognition of cirrhosis implies a risk for major complications and diminished life expectancy, the natural history of cirrhosis is a dynamic process, and multiple variables such as the treatment of the underlying cause of liver disease or the presence of comorbid conditions may affect the course.

The development of disease-specific predictive models based on the natural history of PBC (see Chapter 93) and PSC (see Chapter 70) can help clinical decision making for patients with these cholestatic disorders, which tend to progress in a fairly stereotypical fashion.[20] Before introduction of the MELD score (see later), analogous models had not been available for noncholestatic forms of cirrhosis, and the decision to refer a patient for LT was generally based on an estimate of disease severity using objective parameters such as the serum albumin and bilirubin levels, the prothrombin time, as well as more subjective variables such as the presence of hepatic encephalopathy and the severity of ascites, as in the Child-Turcotte-Pugh score (see Chapter 94).

Important indications for LT remain severe hepatocellular dysfunction, reflected by the presence of coagulopathy and jaundice, complications of portal hypertension such as refractory ascites and recurrent variceal bleeding, or the combination of portosystemic shunting and diminished hepatocellular function, as in hepatic encephalopathy (see Box 99.1). Deterioration of a patient's quality of life is not reflected adequately in predictive models, including the MELD score. Disabling symptoms and complications, such as intractable pruritus, severe fatigue, and incapacitating daytime sleepiness in patients with PBC, and recurrent bacterial cholangitis in those with PSC, are also important considerations. MELD "exceptions"—the addition of points to the "biological" MELD score—can be requested on a

BOX 99.1 Indications for LT

ALF
Complications of cirrhosis
- Ascites
- Chronic GI blood loss due to portal hypertensive gastropathy
- Encephalopathy
- Liver cancer
- Refractory variceal hemorrhage
- Synthetic dysfunction

Liver-based metabolic conditions with systemic manifestations
- α_1-Antitrypsin deficiency
- Familial amyloidosis
- Glycogen storage disease
- Primary oxaluria
- Tyrosinemia
- Urea cycle enzyme deficiencies
- Wilson disease

Systemic complications of chronic liver disease
- Hepatopulmonary syndrome
- Portopulmonary hypertension

case-by-case basis from the local UNOS Regional Review Board to facilitate LT for individual patients (see later). The awarding of extra points recognizes that although the MELD score has been a major advance in organ allocation, at least some patients may be disadvantaged by the use of purely objective parameters and exclusion of factors that were incorporated into older allocation schemes (e.g., intractable ascites and encephalopathy) or disabling symptoms that are disease specific. Ideally, LT should occur before a protracted period of disability reduces the likelihood that the recipient will return to full employment and normal social functioning.

LISTING CRITERIA AND POLICIES OF THE UNITED NETWORK FOR ORGAN SHARING

Organ allocation within the United States is administered by UNOS, which uses disease severity (not waiting time, as in the past) to assign a graft to a recipient. Prior to 2002, organ allocation was based on the Child-Turcotte-Pugh score (see Chapter 94). The MELD score [available at www.unos.org (https://optn.transplant.hrsa.gov/resources/allocation-calculators/meld-calculator/)] is a formula that incorporates the serum bilirubin level, creatinine level, and INR. It provides a numerical value (based on a log-transformed equation) that predicts the 3-month mortality rate without LT (e.g., 1.9% with a score <9; 71.3% with a score of 40).[21] The MELD score also overcomes some of the inherent limitations of the Child-Turcotte-Pugh score, including limited discriminatory ability, subjective interpretation of components such as the presence or absence of ascites on the basis of the physical examination, and the "ceiling effect" of the Child-Turcotte-Pugh score (e.g., no greater weight is given to a serum bilirubin level of 35 mg/dL than to a level of 3.5 mg/dL, even though a patient with the markedly higher bilirubin level clearly has more advanced liver disease). Inclusion of the serum creatinine level reflects prognostic implication of renal dysfunction in patients with advanced liver disease. An important modification of the MELD incorporates the serum sodium concentration into the formula "MELD-Na." Its inclusion reflects the adverse effects of hyponatremia in cirrhosis and increases prognostic accuracy. Adjustment to MELD to include (1) female sex and serum albumin as additional variables, (2) interactions between bilirubin and

BOX 99.2 Absolute Contraindications to LT

ALF with a sustained ICP > 50 mm Hg or CPP < 40 mm Hg
AIDS
Active alcoholism or substance abuse
Advanced cardiac or pulmonary disease
Anatomic abnormality that precludes LT
Angiosarcoma
Cholangiocarcinoma (with few exceptions described in the text)
Extrahepatic malignancy
Persistent nonadherence
Uncontrolled sepsis

sodium and between albumin and creatinine, and (3) an upper bound for creatinine at 3.0 mg/dL results in an improved model (MELD 3.0) that predicts short-term mortality more accurately than MELD-Na and addresses the existing sex disparity on the LT waiting list.[174]

An analogous predictive model has been developed and validated for children younger than 12 years of age with chronic liver disease [pediatric end-stage liver disease (PELD) score]. The main difference between the MELD and PELD scores is that the pediatric model does not incorporate serum creatinine but instead uses age, growth failure (≤2 standard deviations below the mean value for that age), and serum albumin level [also available at www.unos.org (https://optn.transplant.hrsa.gov/resources/allocation-calculators/peld-calculator/)].

CONTRAINDICATIONS

Contraindications to LT have changed with advances in medical care. Effective oral antiviral therapy allows LT for HBV-related liver disease with a low likelihood of recurrence.[22] Similarly, antiviral therapy for HCV infection with all-oral DAAs is well tolerated and highly effective in liver transplant recipients, and retransplantation can be considered for recipients with a failing graft caused by recurrent HCV infection.[23] The introduction of antiretroviral therapy permits LT in HIV-infected recipients with decompensated liver disease, typically caused by either HCV or HBV coinfection.[24] Still, absolute and relative contraindications remain (Box 99.2). An absolute contraindication to LT implies that a successful outcome is so unlikely that transplantation should not be offered. A relative contraindication implies that the likelihood of a good outcome is suboptimal, although LT may still be considered in some patients. The role of LT in the management of HCC has become better defined with recognition that a large tumor burden is associated with a high probability of metastatic spread postoperatively.[25] Despite the sophistication of current imaging techniques, tumor characteristics predictive of a poor outcome, most notably vascular invasion, may only be apparent once the explant is available. Although results of LT for cholangiocarcinoma had been poor because of a high rate of tumor recurrence, a subset of patients with perihilar tumors may benefit from multimodal therapy, including neoadjuvant chemotherapy along with concurrent external beam radiation, followed by LT in selected candidates in whom surgical exploration demonstrates stage I or II disease (see Chapter 71).[19] Outcomes of LT remain poor for angiosarcoma, which is an absolute contraindication. By contrast, at least some patients with epithelioid hemangioendothelioma have been transplanted successfully despite an extensive tumor burden, with documented regression of extrahepatic metastases (see Chapter 98).

For transplant candidates with a prior extrahepatic malignancy, therapy of the malignancy must have been curative, with objective evidence on surveillance that implies low likelihood of metastatic spread and/or recurrent disease. A 2-year recurrence-free interval prior to LT is adequate for most nonhepatic malignancies, but a longer period following resection may be desirable for breast cancer, colon cancer, and melanoma.[26] Myeloproliferative disorders frequently underlie Budd-Chiari syndrome (see Chapter 87), but fortunately evolution to acute leukemia is not accelerated following LT.[27]

Ongoing recreational drug use remains an absolute contraindication to LT. If continued abuse is a concern, random toxicology screening tests are appropriate as will be discussed later. Patients with alcohol-related liver disease need a strategy in place to manage the underlying alcohol use disorder. Although medicinal marijuana may be used legitimately for palliation, most transplant programs discourage its use because of concerns about the adherence of users to other therapies and possible pulmonary complications as well as evidence of accelerated fibrosis in HCV-induced liver disease.[28] Cigarette smoking is prohibited in transplant candidates because of its multiple adverse effects, including an association with hepatic artery thrombosis and malignancy postoperatively.[29] A history of prescription narcotic abuse is also a cause for concern because it may contribute to difficulties with pain management postoperatively. Nonnarcotic alternatives should be encouraged for the management of chronic pain. NSAIDs are contraindicated in patients with cirrhosis because of potential renal and gastrointestinal adverse events. With increasing use of herbal compounds and other complementary and alternative medicines, a discussion of their unproved efficacy and unknown toxicities—with caution against their use after transplant because of potential for drug interactions—is appropriate (see Chapters 91 and 132).[30]

The pretransplant evaluation frequently uncovers important comorbidities—typically cardiac and pulmonary. Patients with decompensated cirrhosis were previously considered to have a diminished risk of coronary artery disease (CAD) because of low afterload (reflecting peripheral vasodilatation), decreased hepatic synthesis of cholesterol, and increased circulating estrogen levels. However, subsequent studies have shown that the prevalence of CAD in this population is at least equal to that of an age-matched control population.[31] Risk factors for CAD in patients with cirrhosis include diabetes mellitus and the other components of the metabolic syndrome, which are prevalent among patients with MASLD. Additional risk factors for CAD in the post-LT period include immunosuppressive drugs that contribute to systemic hypertension, hyperlipidemia, and obesity (see later). Clinical assessment of cardiac risk with exercise stress testing may be difficult in patients with cirrhosis because of poor physical stamina, frailty, volume overload, hepatic encephalopathy, and pulmonary complications. IV administration of dobutamine mimics the physiologic effects of exercise and is used in stress echocardiography to exclude clinically significant CAD in liver transplant candidates. Patients who reach 85% of their maximal predicted heart rate without wall-motion abnormalities on stress echocardiography have a low likelihood of peri- and postoperative ischemic cardiac events.[32] CT coronary angiography (CTCA) can provide noninvasive measurement of coronary calcium scores, which correlate well with obstructive CAD. Studies of CTCA in liver transplant candidates are limited and restricted by small sample size. Although the negative predictive value of CTCA for excluding significant CAD (>50% obstruction) in liver transplant candidates was 100% in one small study, its specificity (44%) and positive predictive value (25%) were poor.[33] Cardiac catheterization and coronary angiography should be performed if CAD cannot be confidently excluded by noninvasive testing; however, this intervention is associated with an increased risk of bleeding and higher transfusion requirements for blood products in patients with coagulopathy and thrombocytopenia due to advanced chronic liver disease.[34] Coronary artery stenoses can be managed by pre-LT angioplasty and stenting; however, antiplatelet therapy prescribed following endovascular interventions may pose an important risk for bleeding. Although coronary artery bypass grafting is usually contraindicated because of a risk of perioperative morbidity and mortality in a patient with decompensated cirrhosis, successful bypass surgery may render a patient an acceptable candidate for LT.[35] The pretransplant evaluation may overestimate cardiac performance, and impaired cardiac function may become apparent only after the protective effect of decreased systemic vascular resistance (typical of cirrhosis) is lost following LT, when afterload increases, because of the hypertensive effects of the primary immunosuppressive agents or excessive volume repletion.[36] Specific causes of cirrhosis may be associated with additional cardiovascular events that diminish long-term survival. A large study using the Organ Procurement and Transplantation Network database showed that liver transplant recipients with MASLD have the highest frequency of CAD (7.4%), compared with those with alcohol-associated liver disease (2.9%), HCV infection (2.7%), HBV infection (2.3%), and PBC (1.7%).[37] Fatal cardiac arrhythmias may result in poorer survival in LT recipients with hemochromatosis or amyloidosis.[38]

Pulmonary evaluation in the liver transplant candidate may reveal abnormal arterial oxygenation (see Chapter 96). Although severe chronic obstructive pulmonary disease or pulmonary fibrosis precludes LT, respiratory restriction because of ascites or diminished mass and strength of respiratory muscles caused by chronic illness is reversible and is not a contraindication to LT. Even patients who undergo LT for α_1-antitrypsin deficiency may show improvement in pulmonary function tests postoperatively.[39] Pulmonary artery hypertension [hemodynamically defined as mean pulmonary artery pressure (MPAP) $\geq$25 mm Hg and pulmonary vascular resistance $\geq$240 dynes s cm^{-5} by right heart catheterization] in a patient with established portal hypertension is known as *portopulmonary hypertension*. Importantly, moderate and severe portopulmonary hypertension (MPAP $\geq$35 mm Hg and MPAP $\geq$45 mm Hg, respectively) increases the mortality rate beyond that predicted by the MELD score and, if not improved by medical therapy, is a contraindication to LT (see Chapter 96).[40,41]

The *hepatopulmonary syndrome* (HPS) is characterized by the triad of chronic liver disease, pulmonary vascular dilatations (with right-to-left shunting), and hypoxemia.[42] The diagnosis is suggested by an arterial oxygen tension (PaO_2) less than 80 mm Hg on arterial blood gas obtained with the patient sitting upright or an alveolar-arterial (A-a) oxygen gradient of 15 mm Hg or greater when breathing ambient air; in patients older than 65 years of age, a PaO_2 of 70 mm Hg or less and an A-a gradient of 20 mm Hg or greater are commonly used thresholds (see Chapter 96). Liver transplant candidates should be screened for HPS with pulse oximetry, using a threshold saturation of peripheral oxygen (SpO_2) value less than 96% at sea level (corresponding to a PaO_2 <70 mm Hg). The sensitivity and specificity of pulse oximetry for diagnosing HPS are 100% and 88%, respectively; therefore confirmatory evaluation should be performed in patients with a low SpO_2.[43] Definitive diagnosis is made by the demonstration of intrapulmonary vascular dilatations by contrast-enhanced echocardiography (which is the most sensitive technique), perfusion lung scanning with ^{99m}Tc-labeled macroaggregated albumin, or right heart catheterization with pulmonary arteriography. Contrast-enhanced echocardiography is the imaging test of choice for the diagnosis of HPS. Detection of contrast in the left side of the heart within 3–8 beats after its appearance in the right atrium indicates intrapulmonary shunting. Predictors of potential reversibility of HPS after LT include younger age, a lesser degree of preoperative hypoxemia, and adequate correction of hypoxemia with inspiration of 100% oxygen.[44] In the majority of patients with HPS, hypoxemia resolves within several months after LT, although protracted ventilatory support may be required. Because of the potential for improvement with LT, extra MELD points may be allocated to a patient with HPS.

HPS must be distinguished from portopulmonary hypertension because the latter is associated with high perioperative mortality and frequently unchanged pulmonary hemodynamics despite LT. Specifically, an MPAP greater than 35 mm Hg, pulmonary vascular resistance greater than 300 dynes s cm^{-5}, and cardiac output less than 8 L/min predict a high perioperative risk because the patient will be unable to increase cardiac output appropriately in response to altered intra- and postoperative hemodynamics. Vasodilator therapy may reduce pulmonary arterial pressure and permit LT (see Chapter 96).[45]

Hepatic hydrothorax is accumulation of transudative fluid in the pleural cavity, usually on the right side and often with relatively small volume ascites remaining in the abdominal cavity, as a result of portal hypertension (see Chapter 95). It can be difficult to manage, often requiring repeated thoracentesis or placement of a TIPS prior to LT.[46] Insertion of an indwelling pleural drainage catheter is usually discouraged, because it can lead to infection in the pleural cavity. Similarly, interventions such as pleurodesis or pleural decortication should be avoided prior to LT.

Active uncontrolled extrahepatic infection is an absolute contraindication to LT. In patients with decompensated cirrhosis, unexplained clinical deterioration, such as the onset of altered mental status or systemic hypotension in the absence of gastrointestinal bleeding, should be presumed to reflect sepsis and is an indication to start antibiotics empirically. LT, however, may be the only option for patients with recurrent bacterial cholangitis complicating PSC (see Chapter 70). Recurrent SBP needs to be adequately controlled by antibiotic therapy prior to LT (see Chapter 95). A particularly ominous development is fungemia, which is typically impossible to eradicate in a debilitated patient with decompensated cirrhosis and precludes LT. HIV infection is not a contraindication to LT per se; however, the HIV viral load must be undetectable at the time of transplantation, and the $CD4^+$ T-cell count should be greater than 100/μL in candidates who have never had an opportunistic infection and greater than 200/μL in those who have had an opportunistic infection.[47] Chronic cryptosporidiosis, primary central nervous system lymphoma, and multifocal leukoencephalopathy remain contraindications for LT. Overall, survival rates for HIV-infected liver transplant recipients are similar to those for non-HIV-infected recipients but have historically been worsened by HCV coinfection, inability of the patient to tolerate antiretroviral medications, and low $CD4^+$ T-cell counts.[48] However, oral DAA therapy effectively prevents graft loss due to recurrent HCV infection.

An important consideration in the liver transplant candidate is the presence of vascular abnormalities that may increase the complexity of surgery. With increased surgical experience, such abnormalities, most notably portal vein thrombosis, are less likely to be an obstacle to LT. More extensive vascular thrombosis with involvement of the superior mesenteric vein may necessitate extensive vascular reconstruction, or consideration for multivisceral transplantation.[49] The presence of a prior portosystemic shunt, particularly a nonselective (side-to-side or end-to-side) portocaval shunt, increases the technical complexity of LT (because the shunts need to be taken down during the surgery) but is not a contraindication. A TIPS inserted to control complications of portal hypertension, including variceal hemorrhage, intractable ascites, or hydrothorax, is now the most frequently encountered shunt and does not usually present an operative challenge unless the stent extends into the inferior vena cava or the superior mesenteric vein.[50]

Age restrictions have been relaxed for liver transplant candidates, although close attention must be paid to comorbid conditions in older patients. The presence of comorbidities not only increases perioperative mortality but may also diminish the likelihood that the recipient will be able to return to an active lifestyle, particularly because severe liver disease may result in more frailty in older than in younger patients.[51] Because a subset of robust older recipients have good outcomes, candidates in their late 60s or even older who are otherwise in good health should not be precluded a priori from LT. The proportion of liver transplant recipients aged 65 or more increased from 9% in 2002 to 20% in 2017 in the United States. However, increasing age is an independent risk factor for increased wait list mortality and decreased likelihood of transplantation.[175]

Renal dysfunction in patients with decompensated cirrhosis typically reflects a variety of insults, including sepsis, hypotension, and use of nephrotoxic medications.[176] The differential diagnosis of renal insufficiency in patients with advanced liver disease also includes hepatorenal syndrome, which is potentially reversible (see Chapter 96). Renal insufficiency has a detrimental effect on survival in cirrhotic patients and remains an important predictor of poor outcomes after LT.[52] Assessment of the potential for renal function to recover following LT is critical and simultaneous liver-kidney transplants (SLK) should be considered for patients in whom recovery is unlikely. According to UNOS policy (UNOS policy 9.9, available at www.unos.org), approval for SLK transplantation should be granted to patients with any of the following criteria: (1) chronic kidney disease (CKD), (2) sustained acute kidney injury, or (3) metabolic disease. CKD is defined by an estimated glomerular filtration rate (eGFR) of 60 mL/min or less for greater than 90 consecutive days before listing; to qualify for SLK transplantation, patients should also meet at least one of the following criteria: (1) regular dialysis has been started as standard treatment for end-stage renal disease; (2) an eGFR equal to or less than 30 mL/min at the time of listing; (3) an eGFR equal to or less than 30 mL/min on a date after listing on the kidney transplant waiting list. Sustained acute kidney injury is defined as the requirement for hemodialysis and an eGFR less than 25 mL/min for at least 6 consecutive weeks, and candidates for SLK transplantation must also meet at least one of the following criteria: (1) the candidate has been on dialysis at least once every 7 days or (2) an eGFR $\leq$ 25 mL/min at least once every 7 days. Metabolic diseases that are indications for SLK transplantation include hyperoxaluria, atypical hemolytic-uremic syndrome from mutations in complement factors H or I, familial nonneuropathic systemic amyloidosis, and methylmalonic aciduria.

An important reflection of impaired free water handling in patients with decompensated cirrhosis is dilutional hyponatremia. Consequences of marked hyponatremia include altered mental status and an increased risk of calcineurin inhibitor–induced neurotoxicity after LT (see later). Incorporation of the serum sodium level into the MELD formula (MELD-Na) increases the prognostic accuracy of the MELD score, particularly in patients with relatively low MELD scores, and is now used for organ allocation.[53,54]

Other consequences of decompensated cirrhosis include malnutrition and sarcopenia, which result in frailty. Loss of muscle mass increases the likelihood of perioperative morbidity, with the need for more protracted ventilatory support and poorer patient survival. Peripheral edema and ascites result in changes in body weight or anthropometric measurements such as the BMI, making them unreliable for assessing nutritional status in patients with advanced cirrhosis. More profound nutritional deficiencies may reflect the specific cause of cirrhosis, as with deficiency of multiple vitamins and electrolytes in a malnourished individual with alcohol use disorder or depletion of fat-soluble vitamins in a person with cholestatic liver disease due to malabsorption. Evaluation by a dietitian is an integral part of the pretransplant evaluation. Attempts to improve the nutritional status of liver transplant candidates have included enteral and parenteral nutritional support, which may result in improvement of clinical outcomes, albeit modest.[55] An increasingly growing pool of obese liver transplant candidates is of concern, particularly those with sarcopenic obesity (excessive visceral fat associated with sarcopenia), not only because of the higher prevalence of cardiovascular and metabolic comorbidities, but also because of increased risk for recurrent or de novo MASLD and postoperative complications such as wound infections.[56] Frailty is increasingly recognized in cirrhosis, particularly in patients listed for LT (17%). Importantly, frailty has been identified as a strong predictor of wait-list mortality in liver transplant candidates, even after adjusting for severity of liver disease and other important variables.[57]

TRANSPLANT EVALUATION AND LISTING

Although details of the evaluation process vary by center, key elements include confirmation that LT is indicated for the management of the potential recipient's liver disease, exclusion of comorbidities severe enough to preclude transplantation, and identification of adequate emotional and social resources for the patient to undergo a major surgical procedure and continue long-term immunosuppression thereafter (Table 99.1). Approval for liver transplant evaluation is obtained from the patient's insurance carrier before extensive testing is undertaken. The patient is typically seen during the pretransplant evaluation by a transplant surgeon, hepatologist, psychiatrist, dietitian, and social worker, with additional consultations as clinically indicated. As increasingly frailer and older candidates are evaluated, identifying potential causes of perioperative morbidity, such as sarcopenia or carotid artery stenosis, is imperative. Detailed abdominal imaging is performed not only to screen for HCC but also to uncover vascular abnormalities such as portal vein thrombosis that may make surgery technically challenging. Disease-specific issues need to be addressed, such as the likelihood of recidivism in a patient with alcohol use disorder or management of a large tumor burden in a patient with HCC. The appropriateness of LT is then discussed formally at a meeting of the patient selection committee. If the patient's candidacy is deemed to be appropriate, formal listing is undertaken with UNOS, followed by matching of recipients by blood type and weight with potential deceased donors. Once listed, a patient's priority for organ allocation is determined by the MELD-Na score, either the "biological" score or with additional points awarded in specific circumstances such as HCC. With the seemingly intractable shortage of deceased-donor organs, the challenge has been to develop an equitable system of organ allocation and to ensure that hepatic allografts are not allocated to recipients whose prognosis without LT remains good. Patients with a MELD score of less than 15 appear to have better survival without rather than with transplantation.[58] As shown in Fig. 99.2, the MELD score has been found to correlate with the 3-month survival rate. Patients with a MELD score of less than 10 are ineligible for active listing with UNOS unless they receive extra points for additional complications of liver disease, such as HCC or HPS (UNOS policy 9.5, available at www.unos.org).

Once the evaluation process is complete and the patient is accepted for LT, financial clearance is sought from the patient's insurer. Unfortunately, criteria for LT coverage vary among insurers; however, in the United States, if Medicare, the major federal payor, funds a particular indication, other insurance carriers generally follow suit.

DISEASE-SPECIFIC INDICATIONS

Hepatic Malignancy

HCC is the most common primary hepatic malignancy in adults and is currently the leading indication for LT and placement on the waiting list in the United States.[14] It typically occurs in patients with cirrhosis; a notable exception is chronic HBV infection, in which HCC can arise in the absence of cirrhosis (see Chapters 81 and 98). There is also increasing evidence that HCC can complicate MASLD without cirrhosis. The likelihood of HCC post-LT increases markedly with greater tumor burden,

TABLE 99.1 Transplantation Evaluation Process

Step	Comment
Financial screening	Secure approval for the evaluation
Medical evaluation	As discussed in the text
Hepatology evaluation	Confirm the diagnosis and optimize management
Laboratory testing	Assess hepatic synthetic function, serum electrolytes, renal function, viral serologies, markers of other causes of liver disease, tumor markers, ABO-Rh blood typing; 24-hour urine for creatinine clearance; urinalysis and urine drug screen
Cardiac evaluation	Electrocardiography and two-dimensional echocardiography; stress testing and cardiology consult if risk factors are present and/or the patient is ≥40 years of age
Hepatic imaging	US with Doppler to document portal vein patency, triple-phase CT or MRI with gadolinium for tumor screening
General health assessment	Chest x-ray, colonoscopy if the patient is ≥50 years of age or has PSC, Pap smear and mammogram (women), consider prostate-specific antigen level (men)
Transplantation surgery evaluation	Assess technical issues and discuss the risks of the procedure
Anesthesia evaluation	Required if operative risk is unusually high (e.g., the patient has portopulmonary hypertension, hypertrophic obstructive cardiomyopathy, previous anesthesia complications)
Psychiatry or psychology consultation	If there is a history of substance use disorder, psychiatric illness, or adjustment difficulties
Social work evaluation	Address potential psychosocial issues and the possible effect of transplantation on the patient's personal and social supports
Financial and insurance counseling	Itemize the costs of transplantation and posttransplantation care; help develop a financial management plan
Nutritional evaluation	Assess the patient's nutritional status and provide patient education

Adapted from O'Leary JG, Lepe R, Davis GL. Indications for liver transplantation. *Gastroenterology*. 2008;134:1764–1776, with permission.

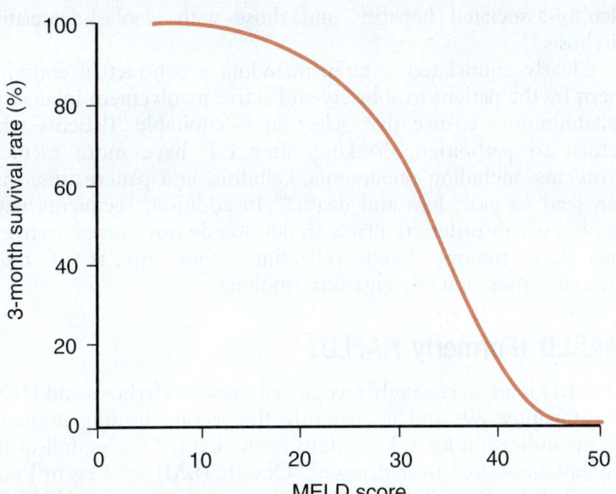

Fig. 99.2 Relationship between the 3-month survival rate and the model for end-stage liver disease score in patients with cirrhosis.

vascular invasion, the presence of multiple lesions, alphafetoprotein (AFP) levels greater than 1000 ng/mL, and certain histologic features such as high nuclear grade, microsatellitosis, and presence of giant or bizarre cells.[59,60] LT remains the definitive treatment of choice for HCC in patients with cirrhosis that are not candidates for resection; indeed, it accounts for approximately 20%–40% of adult LT performed at most centers worldwide, reflecting the frequency of HCC in patients with cirrhosis and the awarding of extra MELD points for this neoplasm.[61]

Improved outcome of LT for HCC reflects better patient selection rather than posttransplant adjuvant therapies.[62] The preoperative workup includes chest CT and bone scan, in addition to abdominal imaging. Portal vein occlusion in a patient with HCC is typically considered evidence of metastatic spread, which precludes LT. PET-based imaging is not accurate for staging early HCC. Generally accepted criteria for LT in patients with HCC include a tumor diameter of less than 5 cm, if the tumor is solitary, or no more than 3 lesions, with the diameter of the largest lesion measuring no greater than 3 cm—the so-called Milan criteria, based on an initial Italian report. Patients who meet the Milan criteria have a posttransplant survival rate comparable to that for patients undergoing LDLT for decompensated cirrhosis in the absence of complicating HCC: 75% at 4 years.[63] Whether the Milan criteria are excessively restrictive, excluding potential recipients who might have done well with a low risk of tumor recurrence, remains controversial.[62] Expanded criteria have been proposed from multiple groups including the University of California, San Francisco to increase the limits of tumor size and number while preserving patient survival rates: specifically, a solitary tumor measuring 6.5 cm or less in diameter or no more than 3 lesions, with the largest lesion measuring 4.5 cm or less and a total tumor diameter of 8 cm or less.[64,65] A meta-analysis, however, supports restriction of LT for HCC to patients who meet the Milan criteria rather than exceed them, although significant heterogeneity among included studies limits the strength of this conclusion.[66] With LDLT, recipients with HCC beyond Milan criteria had comparable survival to those meeting the criteria.[66] The comparable survival between patients undergoing LDLT for HCC under the Milan criteria and those undergoing LT under the expanded criteria reflects a reduction in waiting time for LDLT. An international consensus statement, however, concluded that the Milan criteria remain the benchmark for selection of potential LT candidates with HCC.[67]

As a result of awarding exception points, proportionally more patients with HCC receive LT than their "biological" MELD score would permit.[68] Candidates with T2 HCC lesions are eligible for a standardized MELD exception if the AFP is less than or equal to 1000 ng/mL and the tumor is either a single lesion measuring at least 2 cm and less than 5 cm in diameter, or two or three lesions each greater than or equal to 1 cm and less than or equal to 3 cm in diameter. Candidates with AFP levels greater than 1000 ng/mL and lesions within the previously mentioned criteria (T2) may be treated with locoregional therapies and may be eligible for standardized MELD exception as long as the AFP level remains below 500 ng/mL following treatment.

The MELD exception points for HCC are based upon the median MELD score at transplant (MMaT) of all recipients at least 12 years of age transplanted within a specified geographic area in relationship to the candidate's listing transplant center within 1 year. Candidates are initially listed for LT with their "biological" or calculated MELD score for 6 months. After that, exception points are added with the maximum being limited to the MMaT minus 3 points, and each approved MELD exception extension is valid for an additional 90 days.

Strategies to expand criteria for LT in HCC include downstaging the tumor with the use of locoregional therapies so that the Milan criteria are met; whether this approach will ultimately improve patient survival remains to be determined (see Chapter 98).[65] Candidates are eligible for MELD exception if before completing loco-regional therapies for downstaging the lesion(s) meet the following criteria: (1) one lesion greater than 5 cm but less than or equal to 8 cm; (2) two or three lesions greater than 3 cm but less than or equal to 5 cm and a total diameter of all lesions less than or equal to 8 cm; and (3) four or five lesions each less than 3 cm and a total diameter of all lesions less than or equal to 8 cm. Furthermore, following completion of downstaging therapy, residual lesion(s) must meet the requirement for T2 lesions.[69]

Confounding the management of LT candidates with HCC is the frequent observation that the tumor burden in the explant is significantly underestimated by preoperative imaging. The use of locoregional therapies for HCC reduces waiting list dropout rates. A Markov model has suggested that these interventions could be cost effective when the time on the waiting list exceeds 6 months, which is usually the case for most candidates with HCC but without decompensated cirrhosis.[70,71]

One class of immunosuppressive agents, the mammalian target of rapamycin (mTOR) inhibitors (e.g., sirolimus and everolimus), has antineoplastic properties, and uncontrolled pilot studies had suggested lower tumor recurrence rates and improved survival in liver transplant recipients with HCC treated with sirolimus.[72,73] These results, however, have not been confirmed in randomized controlled trials, and therefore, current recommendations do not endorse the routine use of mTOR inhibitors to reduce the risk of HCC recurrence after LT.[67] Adjuvant systemic chemotherapy for HCC has theoretical benefits that have been noted in some uncontrolled studies but not enough evidence is currently available to recommend this approach outside of clinical trials.[74–76] Nivolumab is licensed for treatment of HCC in nontransplant populations, and scant data from a small series suggest an increased risk for irreversible acute graft rejection when this agent is used in LT recipients.[77]

Patients with the fibrolamellar variant of HCC, which is more common in younger adults without underlying cirrhosis, often present when the tumor burden is already large (see Chapter 98). Extensive resection can be tolerated because cirrhosis is absent, and LT may be performed in patients in whom tumor recurs after resection. Tumor recurrence after LT may be relatively indolent, and although not as infrequent as was once thought, survival rates are acceptable.[78]

Hepatoblastoma is a rare pediatric tumor that also occurs in the absence of underlying parenchymal liver disease. Initial management consists of surgical resection. Adjuvant chemotherapy is indicated for metastatic disease, and LT is an option when the tumor cannot be resected (see Chapter 98).

Cholangiocarcinoma remains the only major primary hepatic tumor for which a definitive role for LT has been difficult to establish. Outcomes following LT for intrahepatic cholangiocarcinoma diagnosed preoperatively had been so poor that its recognition has been regarded as a contraindication to LT, and even tumors discovered only incidentally in the explant have a high recurrence rate. However, a subset of patients with a perihilar tumor and absence of nodal involvement have acceptable 5-year survival rates. The tumor burden, however, is frequently more extensive than suspected on imaging. Some transplant centers follow a specific UNOS-approved protocol that includes preoperative irradiation and chemotherapy, with careful pretransplant operative tumor staging followed by LT (see Chapter 71). A retrospective report evaluating the efficacy of neoadjuvant chemoradiation followed by LT for treatment of perihilar cholangiocarcinoma showed a 65% recurrence-free survival rate at 5 years, with the size of the tumor being an important determinant of recurrent disease (32% and 69% recurrence-free survival rates for patients with tumors measuring 3 cm or less and greater than 3 cm, respectively).[79]

Alcohol-Associated Liver Disease

Alcohol-associated liver disease remains the most frequent cause of decompensated chronic liver disease and is the leading nonneoplastic indication for LT in adults in the United States (see Chapter 88).[80,81] Concerns related to LT for alcohol-associated liver disease had included recidivism following LT, as well as potentially poor patient adherence; however, these fears have not been confirmed.[82] Excellent graft and patient survival rates are the norm following LT for alcohol-associated liver disease.

Key factors in determining candidacy for LT include recognition by the patient of the key role alcohol has played in their liver disease, participation in some form of alcohol rehabilitation such as attendance at Alcoholics Anonymous, stable social support, and a defined period of abstinence prior to LT. Conventionally this period of abstinence has been 6 months, although rigorous studies have failed to confirm that this duration of abstinence confers a high likelihood of continued sobriety but have emphasized the importance of adverse factors such as social isolation or depression. Up to 25% of patients with alcohol-associated liver disease listed for LT deemed to be abstinent continue to use alcohol; therefore monitoring for continued abstinence is prudent.[83] Nevertheless, despite these strategies, as many as 40% of transplant recipients resume alcohol use during long-term follow-up.[84] Surprisingly, graft loss or early death attributable to posttransplant alcohol abuse has been uncommon. A higher rate of return to alcohol use is elicited by use of anonymous questionnaires or random toxicology screening than by direct questioning of patients.

Particularly difficult dilemmas arise in individuals with severely decompensated liver disease and recent alcohol use, in whom the likelihood of surviving without prompt LT is low, and in those with severe alcohol-associated hepatitis (defined by a Maddrey's discriminant function score ≥32) that is nonresponsive to medical therapy with glucocorticoids (Lille score ≥0.45 after 7 days of medical therapy or continuous rise in the MELD score; see Chapter 88). Whether to offer LT to individuals with severe acute alcohol-associated hepatitis not responding to medical therapy is a major quandary, as data from clinical trials have demonstrated a higher rate of survival 6 months after LT compared with those who continue medical therapy (77% and 23%, respectively).[82] In addition, posttransplant outcomes are similar in patients with alcohol-associated hepatitis and those with alcohol-associated cirrhosis.[85]

Clearly enunciated criteria, including a contractual commitment by the patient to sobriety and active involvement in alcohol rehabilitation, ensure that selection is equitable. Patients who return to pathologic drinking after LT have more medical problems, including pneumonia, cellulitis, and pancreatitis, that can lead to graft loss and death.[86] In addition, recipients with alcohol use disorder are prone to develop de novo oropharyngeal and lung tumors, likely reflecting other aspects of their lifestyle—most notably cigarette smoking.[87]

MASLD (Formerly NAFLD)

MASLD is an increasingly recognized cause of cirrhosis and HCC (see Chapter 89) and is currently the second leading nonneoplastic indication for LT in adults in the United States, following alcohol-associated liver disease.[16] Obesity (BMI ≥30 kg/m^2) and type 2 diabetes mellitus are common in patients with MASLD; these two diseases have been recognized as risk factors for HCC, irrespective of the presence or etiology of cirrhosis.[88] Although BMI is not necessarily a reliable indicator of adiposity in patients with end-stage liver disease, particularly in those with fluid retention and ascites, it is commonly used by many LT centers during the patient selection process. Morbid obesity (BMI ≥ 40 kg/m^2 without significant obesity-related comorbidities or BMI ≥35 kg/m^2 associated with obesity-related comorbidities) is commonly regarded as a relative contraindication to LT; however, data from the Organ Procurement and Transplantation Network demonstrate that 16.5% and 5% of patients who underwent LT in 2016 had a BMI greater than or equal to 35 kg/m^2 and greater than or equal to 40 kg/m^2, respectively.[81]

Analysis of data from the UNOS registry has suggested that the risk of primary graft nonfunction is increased and short- and long-term survival is poorer in morbidly obese liver transplant recipients with various causes of end-stage liver disease.[89] However, when analyzed as an entire cohort and not stratified by BMI, patients with MASLD have patient and graft survival rates that are comparable to those for other indications for LT.[90,91] Many of the key precipitants of MASLD (obesity, hyperlipidemia, and insulin resistance) are exacerbated by immunosuppression.[92] Recurrence of MASLD after LT causes graft injury, although graft loss does not typically occur. De novo MASLD after LT is also increasingly common. In the absence of specific therapy for MASLD, therapeutic efforts after LT should center on weight control, optimal glycemic management, and use of a lipid-lowering agent, if indicated. Intensive noninvasive weight loss interventions pre-LT appear to be successful (reduction of BMI to <35 kg/m^2) in a large proportion of patients (84%) enrolled in carefully monitored multidisciplinary protocols; however, 60% of patients regained weight to a BMI ≥35 kg/m^2 post-LT.[93] Although bariatric surgery is feasible in selected patients with MASLD, this intervention is typically reserved for patients with early stages of liver disease and, as is the case for many other abdominal surgical procedures, is contraindicated in those with decompensated cirrhosis because of high morbidity and mortality. A strategy of combining LT with sleeve gastrectomy during the same operation has only been evaluated in small prospective series.[93,94] The mean surgical time was not significantly increased with combined LT/sleeve gastrectomy and the mean BMI reduction with the combined surgical approach was 20 kg/m^2. Metabolic complications, such as posttransplant diabetes mellitus, as well as the steatosis of the graft noted by US were significantly less frequent in patients undergoing LT/sleeve gastrectomy compared with patients who lost weight noninvasively pre-LT.[93] The safety and efficacy of this combined surgical approach and other combinations of less invasive weight loss interventions, such as endoscopic techniques, pre-LT must be confirmed by large prospective studies before they can be recommended. Bariatric interventions are still an option post-LT; however, the procedure should be performed by an experienced surgeon, and the role of less invasive endoscopic techniques post-LT is still under investigation.[95]

Hepatitis C

HCV infection was previously the most frequent indication for LT in the United States and many other Western countries; however, data following licensure of curative DAAs demonstrated a marked decline in the yearly number of wait-listed and transplanted patients with HCV-related liver disease.[17,18] HCV has become the third commonest nonneoplastic indication for LT in adults in the United States, after alcohol-associated liver disease and MASLD. Recurrent HCV infection post-LT had been a major concern, because, if left untreated, it leads to accelerated fibrosis and progression to cirrhosis, resulting in inferior graft and patient outcomes compared with LT for other major causes of cirrhosis. Treatment of recurrent HCV infection in LT recipients changed dramatically with the availability of DAAs that permit use of interferon-free regimens that are highly effective, safe, and associated with a low rate of drug-drug interactions.

Biopsy of the graft helps identify recipients with recurrent HCV infection at increased risk of rapidly progressive disease. Less than 10% of patients with histologically mild recurrent HCV infection at 1 year after LT progress to cirrhosis of the graft within 5 years, whereas two thirds of those with at least moderately severe HCV infection at 1 year after LT develop cirrhosis.[96] Concern has been raised, however, that with longer follow-up, some patients with initially mild recurrent HCV infection will also progress. A prospective study using serial protocol liver biopsy specimens to assess the histologic outcomes of 57 HCV genotype 1b–infected liver transplant recipients with an initially mild histologic recurrence, defined as no or minimal hepatic fibrosis (fibrosis stage F0 or F1) during the first 3 years after LT (see Chapter 82), found that some degree of fibrosis at baseline appears to predict accelerated recurrent HCV infection.[97] However, effective antiviral therapy with DAAs resulting in sustained virological response typically aborts progression of hepatic fibrosis.

A particularly ominous manifestation of recurrent HCV infection had been fibrosing cholestatic hepatitis (FCH). The frequency of FCH in some series had been as frequent as 5%–10%. Infection with HCV genotype 1, and recipient interleukin-28B (interferon lambda-3) genotypes CT or TT (see Chapter 82) were implicated in the development of FCH, as was excessive immunosuppression.[98,99] Histologically, FCH is characterized by extensive dense portal fibrosis with immature fibrous bands extending into sinusoidal spaces, ductal proliferation with hypercellularity, marked canalicular and cellular cholestasis, and moderate inflammation with mononuclear cells.[100] These histologic features, however, lack specificity and may also be observed in acute cellular rejection and chronic graft rejection. Recognition of FCH should prompt a reduction in immunosuppression and initiation of antiviral therapy.[100a] Fortunately, this entity is now rare.

Reported predictors of severe recurrent HCV infection have included several viral and nonviral factors (Box 99.3). Higher serum levels of HCV RNA before and immediately after LT, as well as the possibility of more rapid evolution of HCV quasispecies, have been implicated in aggressive recurrent HCV infection (see Chapter 82).[97] Older deceased-donor age is also an important risk factor. Episodes of acute cellular rejection, particularly if multiple, increase the severity of recurrent HCV infection. A major challenge is to distinguish recurrent HCV infection from graft rejection, because many of the histologic hallmarks of acute rejection, including bile duct injury, are also consistent with recurrent HCV infection. Examination of serial liver biopsy specimens may help clarify this issue and help avoid inappropriate additional immunosuppression in the recipient with recurrent HCV infection, rather than graft rejection. Nevertheless, the replacement of interferon-based regimens with DAAs now allows early initiation of antiviral therapy even if rejection remains in the differential for graft injury.

Once recurrent HCV infection of the graft progresses to cirrhosis, hepatic decompensation, had been frequent until DAAs, which permit treatment of HCV infection even in patients with decompensated cirrhosis prior to LT, became available.[4] Strategies for the treatment of HCV infection in individuals being considered for LT generally fall into two broad categories: (1) pre-LT antiviral therapy, with some restrictions of specific antiviral agents in individuals with decompensated cirrhosis, and (2) post-LT antiviral therapy, generally with initiation of antiviral therapy within 6 months after LT. Results of a simulated model have shown that treating HCV infection pre-LT in candidates with a high MELD score ($\geq$27) may not offer a meaningful benefit and, in fact, may be associated with decreased life expectancy in some cases.[101] Importantly, the decision to treat HCV pre- versus post-LT should be made in conjunction with the transplant center, because many centers now consider transplanting HCV-positive grafts into individuals with HCV infection with administration of antiviral therapy following transplantation. This approach is supported by the International LT Society, which has endorsed antiviral treatment pre-LT for liver transplant candidates with a MELD score less than 20 (in the absence of refractory portal hypertension or other condition requiring more immediate LT) or with HCC who are not expected to undergo LT within 3–6 months.[2]

Hepatic function commonly improves during and after successful antiviral therapy with DAAs, even in individuals with severe hepatic decompensation, as reflected mainly by reductions in the serum bilirubin level and the prothrombin time, thereby resulting in lower MELD scores.[102,103] Nevertheless, despite reductions in the MELD score, some patients may continue to experience a poor quality of life and severe complications of cirrhosis. This has been termed "MELD limbo" or "MELD purgatory" and should be considered before antiviral therapy is started in a patient with decompensated cirrhosis and a MELD score approaching the range in which LT is a realistic option,[104] particularly if manifestations of hepatic decompensation, such as intractable ascites, which is not captured by the MELD score, are present. DAAs are highly effective and now commonly used to treat recurrent HCV infection post-LT with excellent safety

BOX 99.3 Factors Associated With Severe HCV Recurrence Following LT

VIRAL FACTORS

Absence of pretransplantation HBV coinfection
CMV coinfection
HCV genotype 1b
High serum HCV RNA levels before transplantation and within 2 week after transplantation

IMMUNOSUPPRESSION

Multiple episodes of rejection (indicating a high cumulative prednisone dose)

OTHER FACTORS

High TNF-α production in the graft
Impaired HCV-specific CD4$^+$ T-cell responses
Ischemic-preservation injury
Nonwhite recipient

profiles and high virologic efficacy. The efficacy and safety of DAAs post-LT also permits successful transplantation of HCV-positive organs to HCV-negative recipients.[177] Drug-drug interactions must be anticipated and appropriate dose adjustments and close monitoring of immunosuppression during and after antiviral therapy is advised (see also Chapter 82).

Hepatitis B

The availability of the HBV vaccine and public health interventions to promote universal immunization of newborns and high-risk individuals, along with access to potent oral antiviral agents with low rates of resistance, have resulted in a steady decline in the need for LT in patients with decompensated cirrhosis due to HBV infection.[105,106] In addition, suppression of HBV prior to LT leads to a lower rate of recurrent HBV infection of the graft and improved survival after LT.[107] HBV recurrence was frequent and resulted in reduced patient and graft survival rates during the 1980s. Long-term administration of high-dose hepatitis B immune globulin (HBIG) was the initial step in improving posttransplant outcomes. Subsequently, HBIG administered in combination with the nucleoside analog lamivudine further decreased the rate of HBV recurrence. Lamivudine monotherapy for prevention of recurrent post-LT HBV infection was limited by frequent mutations in the HBV polymerase gene, with resulting resistance and graft reinfection (see Chapter 81).[108] Some groups have titrated HBIG doses according to trough serum levels of antibody to hepatitis B surface antigen (anti-HBs). Intramuscular administration of HBIG has been confirmed as an efficacious and less expensive alternative to intravenous HBIG regimens when used in combination with lamivudine. In addition, novel formulations of HBIG for subcutaneous administration are being evaluated.[109,110] Use of HBIG, however, is being replaced by newer oral antiviral agents with a low risk of HBV resistance and a further decrease in post-LT HBV recurrence rates.[111] Emerging data support the efficacy of entecavir and tenofovir in preventing recurrence of hepatitis B after LT, and the use of these potent antiviral agents may obviate the need for HBIG.[112,113,178] The results of prospective studies evaluating the efficacy of entecavir, tenofovir, or a combination of emtricitabine and tenofovir in preventing post-LT recurrence of HBV after discontinuation of HBIG have supported this approach.[114,115]

Cholestatic Liver Disease

PBC and PSC are less common indications for LT. Despite a steady increase in the incidence and prevalence of PBC, there has been a decline in the absolute number of patients requiring LT due to end-stage liver disease, primarily because of earlier diagnosis and the efficacy of bile acid therapy in delaying disease progression.[116] PBC and PSC played a key role in the development of prognostic models, and PBC is a benchmark for patient and graft survival. The Mayo disease models to predict the course of cholestatic disorders (Table 99.2) have aided in determining the optimal timing of referral for LT (see Chapters 70 and 93). A patient with PBC or PSC should be referred for LT evaluation if his or her Mayo risk score predicts a 1-year survival rate of less than 95%. The models, however, do not take into account prominent and frequently disabling complications of cholestatic liver diseases, such as pruritus, fatigue, osteopenia, or, in PSC, recurrent bouts of bacterial cholangitis, and have now been superseded by the MELD score. Indications for LT in patients with cholestatic liver diseases are similar to those for patients with other chronic liver diseases. Per current UNOS/OPTN policy, additional MELD points may be requested for patients with PSC with both of the following criteria: (1) two or more admissions to the intensive care unit over a 3 month period of time for hemodynamic instability requiring vasopressors; (2) the candidate must have cirrhosis. In addition, the candidate for MELD exception points must have one of the following criteria: (1) biliary tract stricture(s) not responsive to treatment by ERCP or percutaneous approaches, (2) diagnosis with a highly-resistant infectious organism (e.g., vancomycin resistant enterococcus, extended spectrum beta-lactamase producing Gram-negative organisms, carbapenem-resistant Enterobacteriaceae, and multidrug-resistant Acinetobacter).[117]

TABLE 99.2 Components of the Mayo Predictive Models for Survival in PBC and PSC

PBC	PSC
Serum bilirubin level	Serum bilirubin level
Serum albumin level	Serum albumin level
Patient's age	Patient's age
Prothrombin time	Serum AST level
Peripheral edema	History of variceal bleeding

Adapted from Murtaugh PA, Dickson ER, Van Dam GM, et al. Primary biliary cirrhosis: prediction of short-term survival based on repeated patient visits. *Hepatology*. 1994;20:126–134; Kim WR, Therneau TM, Wiesner RH, et al. A revised natural history model for primary sclerosing cholangitis. *Mayo Clin Proc*. 2000;75:688–694.

Despite generally excellent outcomes of LT for cholestatic disorders, PBC and PSC recur in approximately 25% of recipients at 10 years posttransplantation.[118,119]

The type of reconstructive biliary anastomosis for patients with PSC undergoing LT has been a matter of debate: Roux-en-Y hepatico- or choledochojejunostomy versus a duct-to-duct anastomosis. Roux-en-Y hepatico- or choledochojejunostomy has been the favored technique of many surgeons because of concern about the development of nonanastomotic biliary strictures post-LT and risk of cholangiocarcinoma in the remnant recipient bile duct. However, data suggest that a duct-to-duct anastomosis is safe, technically feasible in PSC patients, and associated with lower frequencies of post-LT cholangitis and nonanastomotic strictures compared with Roux-en-Y hepatico- or choledochojejunostomy. Published series have shown no difference in recurrence of PSC or survival with these two surgical techniques.[120,121] From a therapeutic perspective, one of the main advantages of a duct-to-duct anastomosis is that it permits easier endoscopic access for treatment of anastomotic strictures or other posttransplant biliary complications (see Chapter 72).

Biliary stricturing can be identified in a minority of recipients following LT for PSC. Differentiation of recurrent disease from other causes of graft injury, such as chronic rejection or ischemia, may be difficult. Recurrent PSC results in nonanastomotic stricturing of the intrahepatic biliary tract. Although some improvement in symptoms can be obtained by balloon dilation and stent placement, long-term graft viability is reduced. Graft loss caused by recurrent PBC appears to be less frequent than that for PSC. A controversial issue is whether colectomy reduces the risk of recurrent PSC in liver transplant recipients with PSC and IBD (see Chapter 70).[122]

Management of recurrent PBC entails exclusion of other causes of hepatic dysfunction. Primary immunosuppression with tacrolimus has been implicated in the recurrence of PBC by some but not all investigators. Data from a retrospective study have suggested that preemptive administration of UDCA to individuals who have undergone LT for PBC may diminish the risk of recurrent PBC posttransplantation.[123] There are as yet no data about the role of obeticholic acid, elafibranor, or seladelpar for prevention of recurrent PBC posttransplantation (see Chapter 93).

Autoimmune Hepatitis

Failure of immunosuppression to arrest progression of autoimmune hepatitis and subsequent overt hepatic decompensation is an indication for LT (see Chapter 92).[124] In addition, the initial presentation of autoimmune hepatitis can be fulminant, requiring prompt LT. In patients with autoimmune hepatitis (AIH) and ALF with a MELD score >40, glucocorticoid therapy may result in increased mortality. Excellent long-term survival is usual after LT for autoimmune hepatitis, although acute cellular rejection may occur more frequently than in recipients with other causes of cirrhosis. In addition, recurrent autoimmune hepatitis has been recognized increasingly and may require higher maintenance doses of immunosuppression. Recurrent disease mimics the features of the disease in the native liver, with associated hypergammaglobulinemia and autoantibodies, and is generally responsive to glucocorticoids. Graft survival is generally not reduced by recurrent autoimmune hepatitis.[125]

ALF

ALF is an uncommon but important indication for LT, given its high mortality with a low likelihood of spontaneous recovery. ALF is defined by the onset of hepatic encephalopathy within 26 weeks of the initial recognition of acute liver disease (see Chapter 97). Despite an abrupt onset, antecedent chronic liver disease is absent, and hepatic recovery is possible. In the past, LT for ALF resulted in poorer patient survival rates than those for benchmark indications such as PBC. Subsequent experience, however, has shown that excellent patient survival rates are possible if ALF is identified early in its course and transplantation occurs before irreversible complications, especially neurologic, supervene.[126] The absence of papilledema on funduscopy and of typical findings on CT do not preclude the presence of cerebral edema complicating worsening encephalopathy; therefore direct intracranial pressure monitoring may be useful to detect and manage this frequently lethal complication of ALF. Direct intracranial pressure monitoring can only be recommended, however, if local neurosurgical expertise and interest are available, because a high rate of complications has tempered enthusiasm for its use. Patients with ALF, regardless of etiology, should be referred promptly for urgent LT evaluation. Specific criteria to identify patients with ALF who are unlikely to recover spontaneously are shown in Box 99.4. The challenge in managing patients with ALF is to avoid unnecessary LT in those who will recover spontaneously or who will not recover with LT, while not delaying it in patients in whom it is their only option for survival. The role of liver assist devices in managing ALF, either as definitive therapy or as a "bridge to transplantation," remains to be defined (see Chapter 97).

Metabolic Disorders

Metabolic disorders amenable to LT (see Chapters 77–79) fall into two broad categories: diseases dominated clinically by obvious hepatocellular disease (e.g., Wilson disease, hemochromatosis, and α_1-antitrypsin deficiency) and those without clinical evidence of liver disease (e.g., primary hyperoxaluria, familial hypercholesterolemia). Metabolic disorders in general are more common in pediatric patients. Adult indications for LT include Wilson disease and hemochromatosis. Substantial improvement can occur following LT for Wilson disease in patients who present with neurologic involvement. A Wilsonian crisis with severe hemolysis is an indication for urgent LT because chelation therapy is ineffective. Compared with other forms of cirrhosis, hemochromatosis was previously associated with poorer survival following LT; however, a more recent study analyzing outcomes for transplants performed between 1997 and 2006 demonstrated survival comparable with that for other indications for LT.[127] Iron reaccumulation in the graft of patients transplanted for hemochromatosis is a theoretical concern, but iron depletion is not typically required.[128] LT has also been performed as a curative procedure in combination with renal transplantation for primary hyperoxaluria, in which end-organ damage is confined to the kidney but the metabolic defect is hepatic. LT may be indicated in cases of multiple hepatic adenomas associated with glycogen storage disease and not only eliminates the risk of progression to HCC but also corrects the underlying metabolic disorder (see Chapter 79).

BOX 99.4 Criteria for LT in ALF

CRITERIA OF KING'S COLLEGE, LONDON

Acetaminophen Cases

Arterial pH <7.30 more than 24 hour after drug ingestion*
All of the following:
- Prothrombin time >100 second or INR >6.5
- Serum creatinine level >3.4 mg/dL (300 μmol/L) or anuria
- Grade 3 to 4 encephalopathy

Nonacetaminophen Cases

Prothrombin time >100 second or INR >6.7
Any 3 of the following:
- Unfavorable etiology (seronegative hepatitis or drug reaction)
- Age <10 or >40 year
- Acute or subacute category (duration of jaundice >7 days)
- Serum bilirubin level >17.5 mg/dL (300 μmol/L)
- Prothrombin time >50 second or INR >3.5

CRITERIA OF HÔPITAL PAUL-BROUSSE, VILLEJUIF

Hepatic encephalopathy *and*
Factor V level <20% in patients age <30 year OR
Factor V level <30% in patients age ≥30 year

*Subsequent modification: arterial pH <7.30 or serum lactate >3.0 mmol/L after adequate fluid resuscitation.

From Keeffe EB. Liver transplantation: current status and novel approaches to liver replacement. *Gastroenterology*. 2001;120:749–762, with permission.

Vascular Disorders

Budd-Chiari syndrome, characterized by hepatic venous outflow obstruction, often mimics decompensated cirrhosis (see Chapter 87).[129] Good long-term results have been described in patients who undergo prompt TIPS or portosystemic shunt surgery, although LT is typically required if advanced fibrosis is present on a liver biopsy specimen. Despite the frequency of an underlying myeloproliferative disorder, accelerated progression to leukemia or bone marrow failure does not seem to occur after LT. Long-term anticoagulation is indicated in transplant recipients with Budd-Chiari syndrome.

Sinusoidal obstruction syndrome (SOS) is a vascular disorder manifested by necrosis of zone 3 hepatocytes and fibrous obliteration of the lumen of central venules. Most commonly seen after hematopoietic stem cell transplantation (HSCT), SOS may lead to hepatic failure and death in up to 25% of patients, despite an otherwise successful procedure. Although experience with LT for hepatic complications of HSCT is limited, LT appears to be the only intervention that consistently alters the course of advanced SOS.[130] Similarly, LT has been shown to be effective in the management of severe post-HSCT graft-versus-host disease with predominantly hepatic involvement (see Chapter 34). Patients with hypocoagulable (e.g., hemophilia A and B) as well as hypercoagulable (e.g., protein C and S deficiencies) hematologic disorders who undergo LT for other indications have been cured of these disorders owing to production of normal clotting factors by the graft and its vascular tissue.

Others

Several other diagnoses are potential indications for LT (see Box 99.1). Adult polycystic disease with marked abdominal distention resulting from multiple hepatic cysts that are not amenable to resection has been treated successfully by LT (see Chapter 98). If CKD is present, combined liver-kidney transplantation is indicated. Cerebral imaging is indicated to exclude intracranial aneurysms, which are a feature of this disease.[131] Diseases with multiorgan involvement for which LT has been performed include Alagille syndrome, sarcoidosis, and amyloidosis (see Chapters 35 and 64). LT successfully arrests systemic manifestations of familial amyloid polyneuropathy. In addition, the explant, which is the source of the abnormal protein, is available for use in a "domino" fashion in an older recipient who will not live long enough for neurologic injury to develop.[132] Biliary cirrhosis associated with CF also has been managed successfully with LT, although patients remain at risk for infectious and other complications of this systemic disorder (see Chapters 59 and 79).

SURGICAL ASPECTS

Once a potential organ donor is identified, the local organ procurement organization coordinates harvesting and provides pertinent donor medical information to centers with suitable potential recipients listed with UNOS. In contrast to other types of organ transplantation, including kidney transplantation and HSCT, absence of HLA compatibility does not appear to affect liver graft survival. Donor-recipient matching is based primarily on ABO blood compatibility and recipient weight[133]. In addition to screening serologic studies and routine liver biochemical testing, particular attention is paid to the donor's medical history, including cardiovascular instability and the need for vasopressor support before determination of brain death.

The typical deceased donor has had a catastrophic head injury or an intracerebral bleed, with brain death but without multisystem organ failure. Electrolyte imbalance and hepatic steatosis in the donor are predictors of graft nonfunction. A "donor risk index" has been derived to assess the likelihood of good graft function.[134] Key adverse factors include older donor age (especially >60 years of age), use of a split or partial graft, and a nonheart-beating donor, from which the organs are harvested after the donor's cardiac output ceases, in contrast to the more typical deceased donation in which the organs are harvested prior to cardiovascular collapse. Use of nonheart-beating donors DCD is associated with reduced rates of long-term graft survival and increased risk of biliary complications, which correlate with the duration of "warm ischemia" after cardiovascular collapse and before retrieval of the organ.[134a] With the critical shortage of deceased organ donors, the expansion of the donor pool has included acceptance of donors 70 years of age and older for selected recipients.

Prior to hepatectomy, the harvesting team makes a visual and, if necessary, histologic assessment of the donor organ. Particular attention is paid to anatomic variants in the hepatic artery that may complicate the graft arterial anastomosis in the recipient. Once donor circulation is interrupted, the organ is rapidly infused with a cold preservation solution (e.g., University of Wisconsin, histidine-tryptophan-ketoglutarate, or Institut Georges Lopez solution). Static cold preservation has been the standard of care for preservation of the donor organ but data about dynamic preservation techniques including normothermic and hypothermic machine perfusion have shown encouraging results for DCD and extended criteria donor organs, although with significant economic and technical implications.[179,180] Donor iliac arteries and veins are also retrieved in case vascular grafting is required. After its arrival at the recipient institution, further vascular dissection, with arterial reconstruction if necessary, is performed before implantation.

Splitting deceased donor livers either in situ during harvesting or ex vivo on return to the transplant center allows two recipients to receive portions of the organ if graft volume and quality are sufficient. An adult deceased donor liver can be divided into two functioning grafts; the left lateral segment (segments II and III) is used for a pediatric recipient, and segments IV to VIII (the so-called right trisegment) are used for an adult recipient. Acceptable graft and patient survival rates can be obtained with split grafts, although high-risk unstable recipients may have poorer outcomes. Fig. 99.3 shows the segmental anatomy of the liver, which is the basis of dissection for both split and LDLT.

Native Hepatectomy

Removal of the native liver is the most technically challenging aspect of deceased-donor LT. Previous abdominal surgery and severe portal hypertension add to its complexity. Hilar dissection is performed to access the major hepatic vessels and devascularize the liver. Clamping of the portal vein during hepatectomy results in increased bleeding during dissection, mesenteric congestion, and production of lactate, whereas clamping of the inferior vena cava aggravates venous stasis and causes renal hypertension, with diminished venous return to the heart. To circumvent these problems, venovenous bypass is achieved by cannulation of the portal vein and inferior vena cava via the femoral vein and return of blood via the axillary vein to the right side of the heart. This

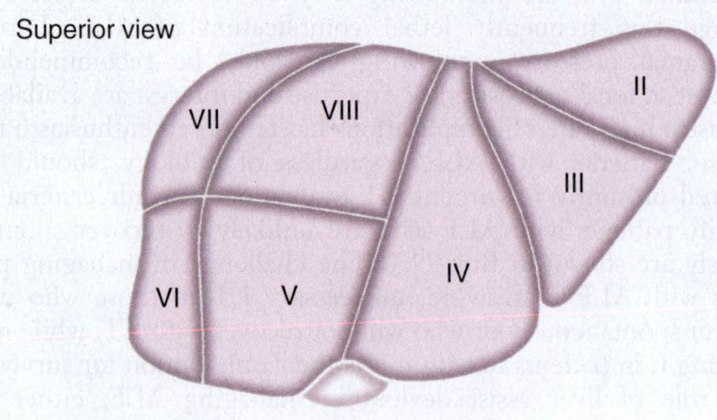

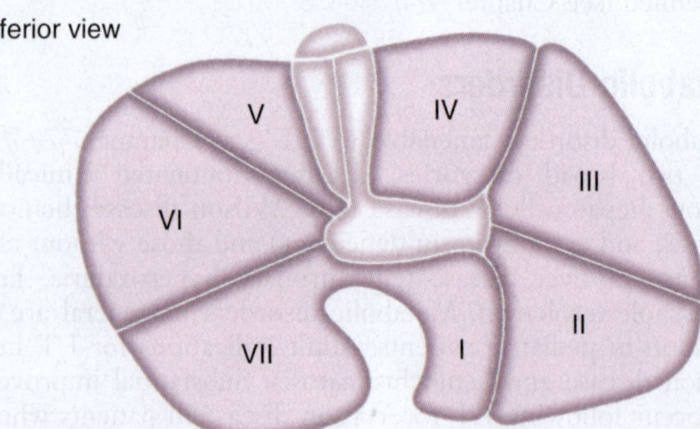

Fig. 99.3 Superior and inferior views of the segmental anatomy of the liver. Segment VIII is visible only on the superior view, and segment I (caudate lobe) is visible only on the inferior view. (From Keeffe EB. Liver transplantation: current status and novel approaches to liver replacement. *Gastroenterology*. 2001;120:749–762, with permission.)

technique can be performed in adults and older pediatric recipients. In some recipients, only a suprahepatic anastomosis to the vena cava is performed, the "piggyback" technique, in contrast to the more usual circumstance in which anastomosis to the vena cava is performed above and below the graft. The piggyback technique may be applicable if uninterrupted caval flow during LT is particularly beneficial, as in a recipient with cardiac instability; a prior portosystemic shunt obviates the need for portal bypass; or the recipient is a pediatric patient in whom venovenous bypass may not be possible. The portal venous anastomosis is performed after portal bypass is terminated and is followed by the hepatic arterial anastomosis. Bile duct continuity is generally fashioned directly as a "duct-to-duct" anastomosis between the graft and recipient. Hepatico- or choledochojejunostomy has been the preferred anastomosis if there is intrinsic bile duct disease, such as PSC, or a major discrepancy in donor and recipient bile duct diameters; however, as previously mentioned, studies have demonstrated that duct-to-duct anastomosis is technically feasible and safe in PSC.[121] Vascular anatomic variations increase the complexity of surgery further. In the past, a direct duct-to-duct anastomosis was typically stented by placement of a T-tube, with the added advantage of easy assessment of bile flow and its quality, as well as potential access for cholangiography postoperatively. The risk of a bile leak during subsequent removal of the T-tube, however, has led to its abandonment.

The use of a living donor organ involves implantation of only a portion of the donor graft and is technically more challenging than using a whole cadaveric organ (see later). In contrast to orthotopic LT, in which the native liver is removed, auxiliary cadaveric LT is the placement of a graft without removal of the native liver. This technique has usually been performed in critically ill patients such as those with ALF who are too unstable to tolerate native hepatectomy.

Irrespective of the type of graft used, after the anastomoses are complete, the newly implanted graft is reperfused, with restoration of normal blood flow. The resulting release of vasoactive agents from pooled blood in the lower half of the body, however, can lead to cardiovascular instability and tachyarrhythmias. Prompt bile production should occur if graft function is adequate. Hyperacute rejection is rare but devastating after LT and leads to rapid graft necrosis within hours and the need for urgent retransplantation.

Living-Donor LT

Extension of LDLT from pediatric recipients to adult recipients has remained controversial because of the risk to the donor in light of the large volume of donor liver required. Data from UNOS demonstrate that LDLT accounted for only 4.7% of all liver transplants performed in the United States in 2020. By contrast, LDLT accounts for 76.5% of transplants in Korea and more than 96% of all liver transplants in Japan because of minimal deceased donation due to cultural considerations in these countries.[135] The potential donor is a healthy adult, typically a family member or close friend of the recipient, who volunteers to be evaluated. A series of checks and balances is necessary to ensure that the potential donor undergoes an adequate medical assessment and is not proceeding under duress. The potential recipient cannot be privy to details of the potential donor's evaluation. In most centers, a hepatologist not involved in the care of the recipient performs an assessment of the donor. Often an independent advocate is also appointed to safeguard the donor's interests. At each stage of the process, the potential donor is given the opportunity to withdraw from consideration.[136] Preoperative evaluation of the donor is best performed in four stages over a period of 1–3 months, with more invasive testing such as liver biopsy undertaken later in the evaluation (Box 99.5). After undergoing complete evaluation, only a relatively small proportion of potential donors are acceptable. One consequence of the evaluation of many potential donors has been the recognition that anatomic aberrations of the biliary and vascular system and unsuspected abnormalities on liver biopsy specimens are common in apparently healthy persons.

BOX 99.5 Protocol for the Evaluation of Potential Living-Related Donors

STAGE 1

Complete history and physical examination

Liver biochemical test levels, blood chemistries, CBC, coagulation profile, urinalysis, AFP, CEA, and serologic tests for HAV, HBV, HCV, CMV, EBV, and HIV

Abdominal US examination, chest x-ray

STAGE 2

Complete psychiatric and social evaluation

CT of the abdomen and pelvis

Pulmonary function tests, echocardiography

STAGE 3

Liver biopsy

Celiac and superior mesenteric CTA with portal phase

STAGE 4

MR cholangiography

Informed consent

Adapted from Ghobrial RM, Amersi F, Busuttil RW. Surgical advances in liver transplantation. Living related and split donors. *Clin Liver Dis*. 2000;4:553–565, with permission.

Right lobes (segments V–VIII), extended right grafts (segments IV–VIII), or left hepatic grafts (segments II–IV) have been used successfully in adult-to-adult LDLT. Adult LDLT allows a reduction in waiting time and potentially mortality for recipients. An expected reduction in the risk of graft rejection because of receipt of a graft from a relative has not been confirmed, and a meta-analysis comparing recipients of deceased- and live-donor grafts has shown similar patient and graft survival.[137]

The overriding concern about LDLT are the consequences to the donor, including immediate perioperative morbidity and mortality, time lost from work, concern about medical insurance after this major procedure, and a lack of long-term follow-up data to ensure that hepatic resection and subsequent regeneration do not result in biliary or other abnormalities. The estimated mortality for live liver donors is different during the early post-donation period and long-term follow-up. For example, the risk of death for live liver donors within the first 90 days after donation has been estimated to be 1.7 per 1000, which is higher than the risk of death for healthy age-matched persons but not significantly different from the risk of death in live kidney donors. Cumulative long-term mortality estimates, however, are not different between live liver donors, live kidney donors, and healthy matched persons up to 11 years after donation.[138] Up to 38% of donors experience complications related to hepatic donation during the first 2 years that follow, including bile leaks, bacterial infections, incisional hernias, pleural effusions, neurapraxia, surgical site infections, and intra-abdominal abscesses.[139]

IMMUNOSUPPRESSION

Immunosuppression is divided into induction (initial) and maintenance (long-term) phases. The goal of immunosuppression is to prevent graft rejection while avoiding morbidity due to its side effects.[140] Episodes of acute cellular and chronic ductopenic rejection require additional immunosuppression (see Chapter 36).[141]

The principal immunosuppressive agents, with route of administration, monitoring, and common adverse effects, are shown in Table 99.3, and drug-drug interactions are shown in Box 99.6. The calcineurin inhibitor tacrolimus is the basis for common induction and maintenance immunosuppressive regimens but has significant side effects. Cyclosporine was used prior to licensure of tacrolimus and patients may be converted from a cyclosporine- to a tacrolimus-based regimen for glucocorticoid-refractory rejection (see later), late rejection (occurring >6 months post-LT), chronic ductopenic rejection, severe cholestasis, intestinal malabsorption of cyclosporine, or cyclosporine toxicity (hirsutism, gingivitis, severe hypertension). In chronic rejection, tacrolimus is less effective once the serum bilirubin levels rise above 10 mg/dL, underscoring the importance of early recognition. The antimetabolite mycophenolate mofetil, and its active metabolite mycophenolic acid, are licensed for prophylaxis of rejection in LT recipients. Either agent, along with a calcineurin inhibitor (typically tacrolimus), is the most common maintenance immunosuppressive regimen used post-LT. Although implicated in hepatic artery thrombosis as well as delayed wound healing and infections, sirolimus has been used as a calcineurin-sparing strategy in liver transplant recipients.[142] Similar to sirolimus, everolimus is also an mTOR inhibitor licensed for immunosuppression in liver transplant recipients. Several clinical trials have demonstrated that the use of everolimus permits important dose reductions of tacrolimus with consequent clinically relevant benefits in renal function.[143–145] Basiliximab is a monoclonal antibody directed against the alpha subunit of the interleukin-2 (IL-2) receptor (CD25) and is licensed for rejection prophylaxis in kidney transplant recipients, but it can be used selectively (off label) as an alternative to glucocorticoids as an induction agent in LT.[146] Preliminary data support the efficacy of alemtuzumab (an anti-CD52 monoclonal antibody) as a glucocorticoid-sparing induction agent; however, an increase in the frequency of infectious complications has been reported with its use.[147] Glucocorticoids are also commonly used during the induction phase of immunosuppression, tapered slowly, and discontinued in most cases to avoid toxicity, except for some center-specific protocols for autoimmune hepatitis in which liver transplant recipients may continue on low doses during the maintenance phase.[141]

POSTOPERATIVE COURSE

Initial Phase to Discharge From the Hospital

Because of the complexity of LT and the often markedly decompensated state of recipients, invasive monitoring (with

BOX 99.6 Clinically Relevant Drug Interactions With Immunosuppressive Drugs

Drugs that increase blood levels of cyclosporine and tacrolimus:
- Antifungals: fluconazole, ketoconazole, itraconazole
- Antibiotics: clarithromycin, erythromycin
- Calcium channel blockers: diltiazem, verapamil
- Others: allopurinol, bromocriptine, metoclopramide

Drugs that decrease blood levels of cyclosporine and tacrolimus:
- Anticonvulsants: phenobarbital, phenytoin
- Antibiotics: nafcillin, rifampin

Drugs that increase nephrotoxicity of cyclosporine and tacrolimus:
- Gentamicin, ketoconazole, NSAIDs

Drugs that interact with mycophenolate mofetil:
- Acyclovir, ganciclovir (increase blood levels)
- Antacids (inhibit absorption)
- Bile salt sequestrants: cholestyramine, colestipol, colesevelam (inhibit absorption)

Drugs that interact with azathioprine:
- Allopurinol, angiotensin-converting enzyme (ACE) inhibitors (increase hematologic toxicity)
- Warfarin (decreased anticoagulant effect)

TABLE 99.3 Immunosuppressive Agents Used in LT

Agent	Mode of Action	Monitoring	Side Effects
Cyclosporine	Calcineurin inhibitor: suppresses IL-2–dependent T-cell proliferation	Blood level	Renal, neurologic, hyperlipidemia, hypertension, hirsutism
Tacrolimus	Same as cyclosporine	Blood level	Renal, neurologic, diabetes mellitus
Prednisone	Cytokine inhibitor (IL-1, IL-2, IL-6, TNF, and IFN-γ)	None	Hypertension, diabetes mellitus, obesity, osteoporosis, infection, depression, psychosis
Azathioprine	Inhibition of T- and B-cell proliferation by interference with purine synthesis	WBC count	Bone marrow suppression, hepatotoxicity
Mycophenolate mofetil	Selective inhibition of T- and B-cell proliferation by interference with purine synthesis	WBC count	Diarrhea, bone marrow suppression
Sirolimus	Inhibition of late T-cell functions	Blood level	Neutropenia, thrombocytopenia, edema, pleural and pericardial effusions, delayed wound healing, hyperlipidemia
Everolimus	Inhibition of T- and B-cell activation and proliferation via mTOR inhibition	Blood level	Edema, pleural and pericardial effusions, pneumonitis, delayed wound healing, hyperlipidemia
Basiliximab	Competitive inhibition of the IL-2 receptor on activated lymphocytes	None	Hypersensitivity reactions

IFN, Interferon; *IL*, interleukin; *mTOR*, mammalian (or mechanistic) target of rapamycin.
Adapted from Everson GT, Karn I. Immediate postoperative care. In: Maddrey WC, Schiff ER, Sorrell MF, eds. *Transplantation of the Liver*. 3rd ed. Philadelphia: Lippincott Williams & Wilkins; 2001:131.

arterial and occasionally pulmonary venous lines) is necessary in the first few postoperative days. In the past, when a T-tube was placed, dark copious bile provided evidence of satisfactory graft function. The patient's overall status, including neurologic recovery from anesthesia, urinary output, and cardiovascular stability, also reflects graft function. Routine antimicrobial prophylaxis includes bowel decontamination with oral nonabsorbable antibiotics, perioperative systemic broad-spectrum antibiotics, antifungal agents, and ganciclovir to prevent CMV infection. Markedly abnormal liver biochemical test levels are typical during the initial 48–72 postoperative hours and reflect several insults to the graft, including ischemia following harvesting and during preservation and subsequent reperfusion injury. The overall trend in serum aminotransferase levels should be downward, with a corresponding improvement in coagulopathy and a falling serum bilirubin level. Thrombocytopenia in the immediate postoperative period reflects a variety of processes, including residual splenomegaly, the effects of medications, and (importantly) reduced graft function.

Worrisome clinical features include metabolic acidosis, depressed mentation, and the need for continued vasopressor support with worsening liver biochemical test levels. Hepatic artery thrombosis needs to be excluded promptly by Doppler US because it is an indication for urgent retransplantation. Hepatic artery thrombosis is more common in pediatric recipients because of the smaller size of the vessels. Antiplatelet therapy is administered to prevent hepatic artery thrombosis.[148] Primary nonfunction of the graft is also an indication for urgent retransplantation and is suggested by sluggish mentation, diminished urine output, cardiovascular instability, and coagulopathy. Donor characteristics associated with an increased likelihood of primary nonfunction include marked hepatic steatosis and profound hyponatremia. If graft function is adequate, however, vasopressor support can be tapered and extubation attempted, although the recipient who is markedly debilitated from advanced cirrhosis may require several days of ventilatory support. Poor graft function and renal insufficiency can also impede weaning.

During the first postoperative week, liver biochemical and coagulation test levels should steadily improve as ischemia and reperfusion injury resolve. Acute cellular rejection with graft dysfunction occurs at 1 week and beyond, with a rise in serum aminotransferase, alkaline phosphatase, and bilirubin levels. Because the biochemical features are nonspecific, liver biopsy is indicated to evaluate other diagnostic possibilities such as slowly resolving reperfusion injury, biliary tract obstruction, and cholestasis related to sepsis. Histologic features of acute cellular rejection are bile duct injury, portal inflammation with eosinophils, and, with more severe injury, endotheliitis (Fig. 99.4). Baseline maintenance immunosuppression must be optimized in all patients with acute cellular rejection, which may be sufficient for patients with mild acute cellular rejection [defined by a rejection activity index (RAI) $\leq$ 4]. Moderate to severe acute cellular rejection (RAI $\geq$ 5) requires treatment with high doses of glucocorticoids (500–1000 mg of IV methylprednisolone or its equivalent daily for 3 doses) followed by a taper (most commonly with oral prednisone or prednisolone) extending over several days. A response is suggested by a return of liver biochemical test levels toward normal.

For the occasional patient with presumed acute cellular rejection who fails to respond to glucocorticoids, additional immunosuppression with antithymocyte globulin or monoclonal antibodies may be necessary. Liver biopsy should be repeated before initiating more intensive therapy to confirm the lack of a histologic response and to exclude other important causes of graft dysfunction, such as ischemia. The ability of recurrent HCV infection to mimic the histologic features of acute cellular rejection led to reevaluation of the need to treat apparent acute cellular rejection aggressively under all circumstances. Routine (protocol) liver biopsies have also fallen out of favor because histologic evidence of acute cellular rejection can be noted in the absence of worsening graft function, with no apparent clinical significance.

In the first 3–4 weeks after LT, infections are typically bacterial and related to surgical complications such as intra-abdominal bleeding, bile leak, or wound infection. A meta-analysis has suggested that administration of probiotics before, or on the day of, LT reduces the rate of postsurgical infectious complications such as urinary tract infections and intra-abdominal infections (from 35% to 7%) but does not affect mortality rates.[149] The timing of various infectious complications following LT is shown in Fig. 99.5.

Other issues encountered during the first weeks following LT are listed in Box 99.7. Neurologic dysfunction can present as an acute confusional state or seizures, with a differential diagnosis that includes lingering effects of hepatic encephalopathy, electrolyte imbalance, poor graft function, sepsis, uremia, and side effects of medications. Of particular concern is the development of neurologic toxicity caused by the major immunosuppressive agents.

Management includes correcting electrolyte imbalances and reducing the dose of calcineurin inhibitors, which can be

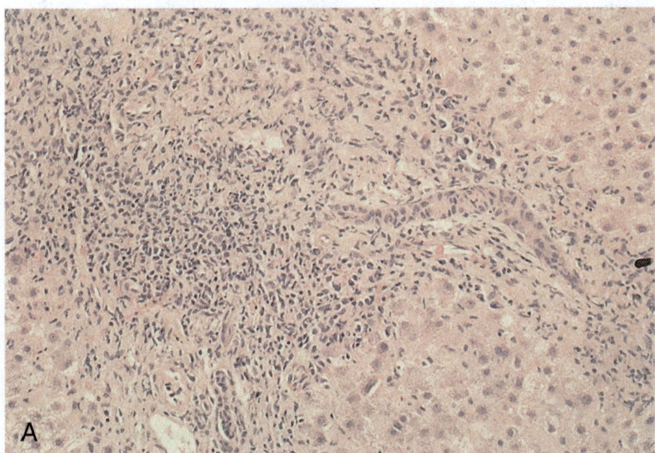

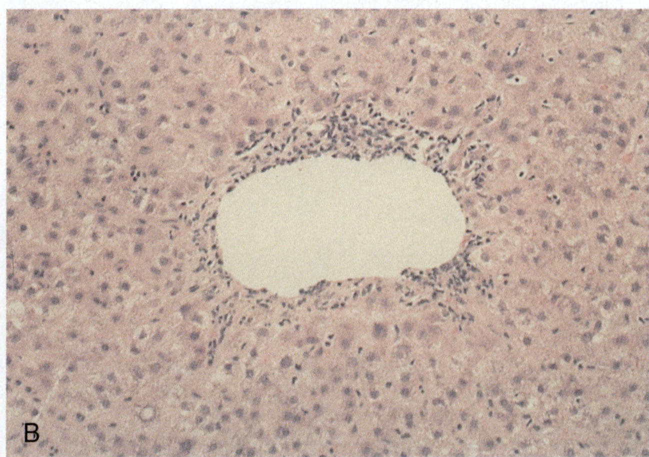

Fig. 99.4 Histopathology of acute cellular rejection of a liver graft. (A) The portal tract shows a lymphocytic and plasma cell infiltrate that spills over into the periportal hepatocytes and bile duct. (B) The central vein shows attachment of lymphocytes to the endothelium (endotheliitis). (From Cotran RS, Kumar V, Collins T, eds. *Robbins' Pathologic Basis of Disease*. 6th ed. CD-ROM. Philadelphia: WB Saunders; 1999, with permission.)

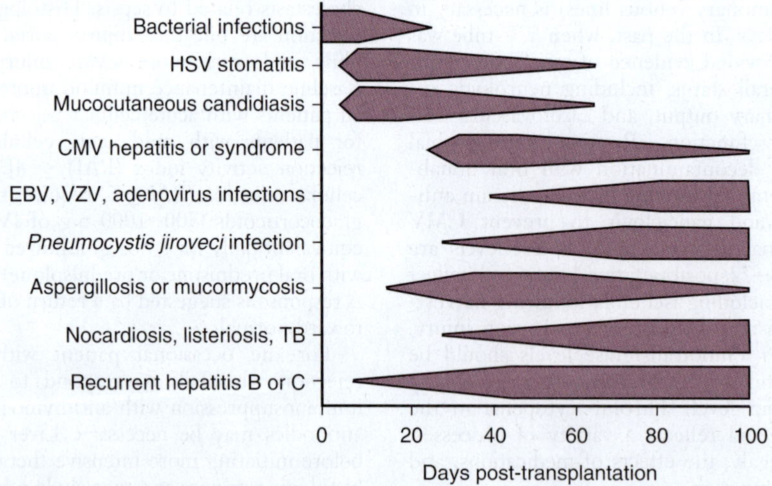

Fig. 99.5 Time course of various infectious complications in liver transplant recipients. *VZV*, Varicella-zoster virus. (Adapted from Everson GT, Kam I. Immediate postoperative care. In: Maddrey WC, Schiff ER, Sorrell MF, eds. *Transplantation of the Liver*. 3rd ed. Philadelphia: Lippincott Williams & Wilkins; 2001:131.)

BOX 99.7 Medical Complications in the Immediate Posttransplantation Period

- Infections
  - Bacterial
  - Viral
  - CMV
  - EBV
  - Fungal
  - Aspergillosis, mucormycosis
  - Candidiasis, torulopsosis
  - *Pneumocystis jiroveci* pneumonia
- Respiratory Complications
  - Acute respiratory distress syndrome
  - Hepatopulmonary syndrome
  - Pneumonia
  - Portopulmonary hypertension
  - Pulmonary edema
- Acute Kidney Injury
- Cardiovascular Diseases
  - Cardiomyopathy
  - Hemochromatosis
  - Hypertrophic cardiomyopathy
  - Hypertension
  - Myocardial ischemia
  - Valvular heart disease
- Neurologic Complications
  - CNS hemorrhage
  - Central pontine myelinolysis
  - Ischemic events
  - Seizures
- Coagulopathies
  - DIC
  - Thrombocytopenia
- Diabetes Mellitus

From Everson GT, Karn I. Immediate postoperative care. In: Maddrey WC, Schiff ER, Sorrell MF, eds. *Transplantation of the Liver*. 3rd ed. Philadelphia: Lippincott Williams & Wilkins; 2001, with permission.

facilitated by the use of mycophenolate mofetil.[150] Overly rapid correction of hyponatremia perioperatively has been implicated in the genesis of central pontine myelinolysis, with evidence of osmotic demyelination on MRI. Diabetes mellitus can present for the first time postoperatively, and HCV infection increases the risk of diabetes mellitus in liver transplant recipients.[151,152] Posttransplant renal impairment can reflect a number of insults, including slowly resolving pre-LT hepatorenal syndrome or renal failure due to other causes, intraoperative hypotension resulting in acute tubular necrosis, and (importantly) the nephrotoxic effects of cyclosporine and tacrolimus, which cause renal afferent arteriolar vasoconstriction with a reduction in glomerular filtration. Adjunctive therapy with mycophenolate mofetil or mycophenolic acid allows a reduction in the doses of cyclosporine and tacrolimus while providing adequate immunosuppression. Short-term renal replacement therapy may be necessary until renal recovery occurs.

Following Discharge From the Hospital

If the initial postoperative course has been smooth, planning for discharge is possible by the end of the first or second week after LT. Recovery is often more protracted, particularly in debilitated recipients. Once discharged, patients are seen at frequent intervals during the first postoperative month. Liver biochemical test levels should normalize within a few weeks. Graft dysfunction is an indication for prompt liver biopsy to exclude acute cellular rejection. CMV becomes an important infectious consideration 3 or more weeks posttransplant.[153] Histologic features suggestive of CMV hepatitis include "owl's eye" inclusion bodies in the hepatocytes, as well as neutrophilic abscesses with focal necrosis of the parenchyma (see Chapter 85). Recipients who are CMV naïve are at increased risk of CMV infection, particularly if they receive a graft from a CMV-seropositive donor. These patients are candidates for more intensive antiviral prophylaxis. Oral valacyclovir or valganciclovir for 3–6 months following LT is recommended for CMV prophylaxis.[154]

A distinction is made between asymptomatic CMV viremia, which may not require additional antiviral therapy, and CMV disease with systemic complaints such as fever, graft hepatitis, and diarrhea. CMV viremia is detected by PCR-based quantitative nucleic acid testing or by identification of CMV pp65 antigenemia.[154] Reactivation of CMV in a previously infected recipient tends to be less clinically severe than de novo infection. The diagnosis of tissue-invasive CMV disease requires confirmation by immunohistochemistry or in situ DNA hybridization techniques, because CMV viremia is not a reliable diagnostic finding in these cases.[154] High-dose IV ganciclovir is effective for treating CMV infection; however, viral resistance has been described. Oral valganciclovir is also a therapeutic option for milder CMV disease. Intravenous ganciclovir is the preferred antiviral agent for patients with severe CMV infection or GI involvement (which may limit the bioavailability of oral antiviral agents). Treatment of CMV infection should be continued for at least 2 weeks and until complete resolution of symptoms with viral eradication is achieved.[154] Not only is CMV infection an important cause of morbidity and mortality in liver transplant recipients, but it also had been implicated in other complications—notably chronic graft rejection and severe recurrent HCV infection. Following an episode of CMV infection, secondary prophylaxis with antiviral agents is not routinely recommended and is not associated with fewer relapses.[154]

Trimethoprim/sulfamethoxazole is prescribed to prevent *Pneumocystis jiroveci* infection. Patients intolerant of sulfa drugs may receive atovaquone, dapsone tablets, or inhaled pentamidine, although these agents are less effective than trimethoprim/sulfamethoxazole and have a narrower spectrum of protection against other opportunistic pathogens.[155] Prophylaxis needs to be continued for at least 1 year following LT.

Fungal infections pose a major threat to liver transplant recipients, particularly for marked debilitated patients, those receiving intensive immunosuppression for rejection, or those undergoing retransplantation. For high-risk recipients with two or more risk factors (prolonged or repeat operation, retransplantation, renal failure, high transfusion requirement, choledochojejunostomy, *Candida* colonization in the preoperative period), antifungal prophylaxis against invasive candidiasis with fluconazole for up to 4 weeks after LT is recommended; alternatives include liposomal amphotericin B or caspofungin.[156,157] Sites of infection are mucocutaneous (oral and esophageal), pulmonary, and intracerebral. Despite prolonged therapy with amphotericin, voriconazole, or itraconazole, a fatal outcome is usual with invasive fungal infection. A diagnosis of brain abscess due to *Aspergillus* spp. implies a dismal prognosis. Superficial skin infections and simple colonization must be distinguished from invasive fungal infections, because topical antifungal agents such as nystatin or clotrimazole can eradicate the former. Similarly, bladder irrigation with amphotericin can cure candida cystitis without the need for systemic antifungal therapy.

Although opportunistic infections are always a concern in liver transplant recipients, nonopportunistic infections also occur. Standard antibiotic therapy is appropriate for community-acquired respiratory infections, but a more extensive workup is indicated when symptoms are unusually severe or fail to resolve rapidly with treatment. Invasive diagnostic testing such as bronchoscopy or lumbar puncture with cultures may be necessary if clinically indicated. Enteric bacteremia may be an initial clue to hepatic artery thrombosis in an otherwise stable recipient. Reactivation of TB may present in an atypical fashion after LT.

Early recurrence of HCV infection may also become apparent during initial follow-up. As noted earlier, it is crucial to recognize that recurrent HCV infection may mimic several histologic features of acute cellular rejection, such as bile duct inflammation and endotheliitis (Table 99.4).

If a liver biopsy specimen shows features suggestive of biliary obstruction or if graft dysfunction is associated with clinical features of cholangitis such as fever and abdominal pain, MRCP is necessary because of its noninvasive nature and high degree of accuracy, irrespective of the type of biliary anastomosis.[158] A stricture at the choledochocholedochal anastomosis is usually easily managed by endoscopic balloon dilation and temporary biliary stenting (see Chapter 72). Surgical intervention is reserved for patients who do not respond to this approach, in which case conversion to a choledocho- or hepaticojejunostomy is usual.

A critical issue is distinguishing anastomotic from nonanastomotic biliary strictures caused by ischemia or other insult to the graft. The bile duct in the transplant recipient is prone to ischemia because of its relatively tenuous arterial blood supply, and the development of a biliary stricture (unless it is obviously anastomotic) may reflect hepatic artery thrombosis. Ischemic stricturing is generally diffuse but can be predominantly hilar. Although temporizing measures such as balloon dilation and stenting may be attempted, such efforts are generally futile if hepatic artery thrombosis is present or stricturing is widespread, and retransplantation will be required. Other causes of nonanastomotic stricturing include the use of an ABO-incompatible graft and protracted cold ischemia after harvesting. Biliary strictures can also be a feature of recurrent PSC.

LONG-TERM MANAGEMENT

General Preventive Measures

Long-term survival after LT is dependent on good general medical care of common disorders, including hypertension, hyperlipidemia, and diabetes mellitus.[159] Once a recipient has stable graft and renal function, serial blood work including blood cell counts and serum liver biochemical tests, creatinine, and calcineurin inhibitor levels are obtained every few months for review by the transplant center.

TABLE 99.4 Histologic Features of Recurrent HCV Infection Compared With Acute Cellular Rejection

Feature	Recurrent HCV Infection	Rejection
Time of onset after LT	Any time; onset usually within the first year	Usually within the first 2 months
Portal inflammation	Most cases	Always
Lymphocytes	Bland, uniform	Activated
Lymphoid aggregates	Usually	Occasionally
Lymphoid follicles	50% of cases	Rarely
Eosinophils	Inconspicuous	Almost always
Steatosis	Often	Never
Acidophilic bodies	Common	Uncommon
Bile ductule damage	About 50% of cases	Common
Atypical features	Cholestasis, ballooning degeneration without significant inflammation, marked ductular proliferation mimicking obstruction, granulomas	Prominent periportal and lobular necroinflammatory activity without subendothelial venular inflammation

From Rosen HR, Martin P. Liver transplantation. In: Schiff ER, Sorrell MF, Maddrey WC, eds. *Schiff's Diseases of the Liver*. 8th ed. Philadelphia: Lippincott-Raven; 1999:1589.

Systemic hypertension is a frequent problem encountered in liver transplant recipients and is related to calcineurin inhibitor–induced renal vasoconstriction, as well as to the effects of other drugs such as glucocorticoids. Unfortunately, a reduction in immunosuppression is generally ineffective in ameliorating hypertension. Another contributing factor is mild renal insufficiency, which is frequent after LT. Initial antihypertensive therapy usually consists of a calcium channel blocker. Angiotensin-converting enzyme inhibitors and potassium-sparing diuretics are relatively contraindicated because of their propensity to accentuate hyperkalemia, which is frequent in liver transplant recipients, who often have renal tubular acidosis caused by the calcineurin inhibitor. Because cyclosporine and tacrolimus levels are increased by verapamil and diltiazem, nifedipine is the agent of choice. β-Adrenergic blocking agents are second-line antihypertensive agents; thiazide and loop diuretics are generally avoided because of concern about exacerbating renal insufficiency and electrolyte imbalance in the liver transplant recipient. Furosemide, however, is the diuretic of choice if fluid overload is present. In the minority of patients in whom hypertension is not controlled, a centrally acting agent such as clonidine is an option. For the occasional patient with intractable hypertension on cyclosporine-based immunosuppression, substitution of tacrolimus for cyclosporine may improve blood pressure control. Both cyclosporine and tacrolimus are nephrotoxic and accentuate impairment of renal function that may have existed perioperatively. Although acute nephrotoxicity may respond to interruption of or a reduction in the dose of these drugs, chronic renal impairment is usually irreversible. Drastic dose reductions of a calcineurin inhibitor may precipitate graft rejection and should be avoided. Cofactors implicated in advanced CKD after LT include recurrent HCV infection with associated glomerulonephritis, diabetes mellitus, and systemic hypertension.[160] Renal transplantation may be considered in liver transplant recipients who become dialysis dependent after an otherwise successful LT.

Hyperlipidemia is observed in up to half of liver transplant recipients and reflects a number of factors including diabetes mellitus, obesity, renal dysfunction, and immunosuppressive agents, especially cyclosporine.[161] Pharmacologic therapy is indicated if hypercholesterolemia fails to improve with weight reduction and tight glycemic control. Pravastatin and fluvastatin are well tolerated in liver transplant recipients and have fewer interactions than other statins with cytochrome P450 3A4 and consequently lesser risk for altering metabolism of immunosuppressants.[162] Diabetes mellitus is common in liver transplant recipients and occurs de novo in approximately one-third of patients after LT. The pathogenesis is multifactorial; immunosuppressive therapy is a major factor because of the hyperglycemic effects of prednisone, cyclosporine, tacrolimus, azathioprine, and mycophenolate mofetil. HCV infection is also implicated. In most diabetic recipients, therapy with insulin is required. The high frequency of diabetes mellitus following LT has prompted the development of glucocorticoid-sparing immunosuppressive regimens (see earlier).

A related problem is *obesity*, which is frequent even in LT recipients who were profoundly malnourished preoperatively. Risk factors include glucocorticoid use, increased caloric intake, and decreased physical activity during recuperation from surgery. Immunosuppression with tacrolimus has been reported to result in less weight gain than occurs with cyclosporine; to a large extent, this difference may reflect the lower glucocorticoid doses used with tacrolimus. Management of obesity in this population includes a reduction in glucocorticoid doses and even complete withdrawal, if possible. Use of mycophenolate mofetil may permit maintenance immunosuppression without glucocorticoids. Pharmacotherapy for obesity may also be considered in selected LT recipients. The glucagon-like peptide 1 analogues lack hepatic metabolism and have limited drug-drug interactions; however, these agents do slow gastric emptying, potentially impairing immunosuppression absorption. There are no data from high-quality studies available evaluating the safety and efficacy of these agents in the management of obesity or PTMD in this population.

Excessive alcohol consumption (>20 g/day for women and >30 g/day for men) is associated with poorer long-term survival after LT, regardless of the primary indication for transplantation.[163] Given the lack of data about the safety of more moderate alcohol consumption in liver transplant recipients, complete abstinence should be encouraged as a conservative approach. Multimodal management should be considered for LT recipients with alcohol use disorder. The following therapies/interventions may be implemented in concert: (1) medication-assisted treatment (MAT), (2) motivational enhancement therapy, and (3) individual therapy and group support.[181] There are several agents that can be considered for MAT, including baclofen and naltrexone, among others. Patients with ALD treated with baclofen were significantly more likely to achieve sustained abstinence and reduced craving compared to those treated with placebo in a randomized clinical trial (71% vs. 21%, respectively).[182] Long-acting injectable naltrexone has been found to be more effective than the oral formulation and avoids hepatic first-pass metabolism.

Bone mineral density disorders are frequently encountered in liver transplant recipients.[164] Although hepatic osteodystrophy is typically associated with cholestatic liver diseases, it is also common in patients with cirrhosis related to other etiologies. Factors implicated in the pathogenesis of hepatic osteodystrophy include poor nutritional status, immobility, the calciuric effect of many diuretics, hypogonadism, and glucocorticoid use in patients with autoimmune hepatitis. In the initial several months after LT, osteopenia is accelerated further by high-dose glucocorticoid therapy as well as the other major immunosuppressive agents. Atraumatic fractures may occur in trabecular bone such as vertebrae or ribs. Bone mass increases after doses of immunosuppressive agents are reduced and mobility increases. Supplemental calcium and vitamin D are prescribed to patients with osteopenia, and bisphosphonates or denosumab can be safely used in patients with osteoporosis.[183]

De novo *malignancies* are increased in frequency following LT.[165] Recipients need ongoing age-appropriate surveillance for common tumors such as breast, cervical, and colon cancer.[166] In the absence of specific recommendations, screening for prostatic carcinoma by yearly digital rectal examination and/or prostate-specific antigen testing in male liver transplant recipients older than age 40 is appropriate. The incidence of prostate cancer in liver transplant recipients appears to be slightly higher to that in nontransplanted men.[167] Screening for colorectal cancer by colonoscopy should also be performed every 5 years after age 45 in asymptomatic recipients; in patients with a history of PSC and UC, yearly colonoscopy with surveillance mucosal biopsies is recommended (see Chapters 70 and 118). Adherence to cervical cancer screening guidelines for the general population and screening female recipients older than age 40 for breast cancer by yearly mammography seem appropriate.[166] Other malignancies that are increased in frequency in organ transplant recipients include those of the skin, lung, liver, female genital tract, and GI tract. Patients with alcohol use disorder may be particularly prone to malignancies of the oropharynx (see Chapter 88).[168] Patients should be encouraged to use sunscreen regularly and have periodic examinations by a dermatologist.

Posttransplantation lymphoproliferative disorder (*PTLD*) varies from a low-grade indolent process to an aggressive neoplasm.[169] Uncontrolled proliferation of B cells after LT, typically in response to primary EBV infection, can be polyclonal or monoclonal. Pediatric recipients are at particular risk because of the absence of prior EBV infection. Intensive immunosuppression for severe rejection increases the risk of PTLD, which can present as a mononucleosis-like syndrome, lymphoproliferation, or malignant lymphoma.

Clinical features suggestive of PTLD include lymphadenopathy, unexplained fever, and systemic symptoms such as weight loss. The majority of patients with PTLD present with extranodal masses, primarily involving the GI tract (stomach or intestine), lungs, skin, central nervous system, or hepatic allograft.[168] The WHO classifies PTLD into four main categories based on clinical, morphologic, immunophenotypic, and genetic features: benign polyclonal lymphoproliferation (early lesions), polymorphic PTLD, monomorphic PTLD, and classic Hodgkin's lymphoma–like PTLD. Management includes a reduction in immunosuppression and antiviral therapy directed against EBV, if present, with ganciclovir. Systemic chemotherapy, including the anti-CD20 monoclonal antibody rituximab, may be required in patients with malignant lymphoma.[168] The higher frequency of PTLD in pediatric recipients has led to surveillance by PCR for EBV viremia with reduction in the level of immunosuppression in patients with a positive result before clinical features of PTLD occur. In addition, antiviral prophylaxis is prescribed for high-risk recipients, including those who are seronegative for EBV and received a graft from a seropositive donor. Chronic graft rejection is increased in frequency in survivors of PTLD because of the reduction in the level of immunosuppression, which may be increased cautiously after PTLD is contained.

Immunizations and Antibiotic Prophylaxis

Immunization against HAV and HBV, influenza, pneumococcus, tetanus, and diphtheria is part of the standard pre-LT management. A substantial proportion of patients may be unable to mount adequate antibody responses because of the immunosuppression associated with end-stage liver disease. Vaccines based on live or attenuated microorganisms (e.g., measles, mumps, rubella, oral polio, Bacille Calmette-Guerin, vaccinia, and varicella-zoster) are contraindicated because of the risk of reactivation. Prophylactic antibiotics are usually recommended for any dental procedure, although this recommendation is not evidence-based.[170]

Hepatic Retransplantation

Although improved immunosuppressive regimens have led to a lower rate of graft loss from chronic rejection, recurrence of the underlying liver disease has been recognized increasingly as a cause of graft failure, as illustrated most strikingly in HCV-infected recipients prior to the availability of DAAs that permit curative antiviral therapy in liver transplant recipients.[171] Understanding the full effect of recurrent disease, especially nonviral disease, on patient and graft survival will require studies with long-term follow-up. For example, although the rate of histologic recurrence of viral hepatitis is greatest in the first year following LT, recurrent PBC or PSC develops in less than 5% of patients by the first year, whereas more than 20% demonstrate histologic recurrence 10 years after LT.[172,173] As patients enter their second and third decades following LT, the number of patients who require retransplantation may deplete the donor pool further. This issue is compounded by the observation that patients who undergo retransplantation experience an approximate 20% overall reduction in the rate of survival but consume an increased amount of resources when compared with primary liver transplant recipients.

Major challenges remain in LT, including the shortage of donor organs, threat of recurrent disease, and morbidity associated with lifelong therapeutic immunosuppression. Nevertheless, the availability of LT has transformed the lives of patients with advanced liver disease and their health care providers from an ultimately futile effort to manage the complications of cirrhosis into a life-prolonging and life-enhancing intervention.

Full references for this chapter can be found at https://ebooks.health.elsevier.com.

100 Anatomy, Histology, Embryology, and Developmental Anomalies of the Small and Large Intestine

Lee M. Bass, Barry K. Wershil, Amanda R. Gomez

IN THIS CHAPTER

ANATOMY

Macroscopic Features

Small Intestine

The small intestine is a specialized tubular structure within the abdominal cavity in continuity with the stomach proximally and the colon distally. The small bowel increases in length from about 250 cm in the term newborn to about 600–800 cm in the adult. The caliber of the small intestine gradually diminishes from proximal to distal, and there is a fourfold reduction in surface area from the distal duodenum to the terminal ileum.

The duodenum is the most proximal portion of the small intestine. It begins with the duodenal bulb, travels in the retroperitoneal space around the head of the pancreas, and ends on its return to the peritoneal cavity at the ligament of Treitz. The biliary and pancreatic ducts usually join together 1–2 cm from the outer margin of the duodenal wall and drain into the medial wall of the second portion of the duodenum through the ampulla of Vater. In 5%–10% of individuals, an accessory pancreatic duct, also known as the *duct of Santorini*, enters separately through the minor papilla 1–2 cm proximal to the ampulla of Vater. The remainder of the small intestine is suspended within the peritoneal cavity by a thin broad-based mesentery that is attached to the posterior abdominal wall and allows relatively free but tethered movement of the small intestine within the abdominal cavity. The proximal 40% of the mobile small intestine is the jejunum, which occupies the left upper portion of the abdomen. The remaining 60% of small intestine is the ileum, and it is normally situated in the right side of the abdomen and upper part of the pelvis. There is no distinct anatomic demarcation between the jejunum and ileum, but the jejunum tends to be thicker, is more vascular, and has a greater diameter than the ileum.

The luminal surface of the small intestine has visible mucosal folds called the *plicae circularis* or folds of Kerckring. They are more numerous in the proximal jejunum, decrease in number distally, and are absent in the terminal ileum. Microscopic aggregates of lymphoid cells are scattered throughout the small intestine and make up the GI-associated lymphoid tissue. Macroscopic lymphoid aggregates, or Peyer patches, are more concentrated in the ileum and can be seen extending through to the serosa. Peyer patches are more prominent in infancy and childhood and regress in size and number with advancing age.

The jejunum and ileum are freely mobile in the abdominal cavity and are attached to the posterior abdominal wall by the intestinal mesentery. The entire length of jejunum and ileum is suspended in this mesentery, except for the distal terminal ileum at the cecum, which is retroperitoneal. The mesentery is formed by a fan-shaped anterior reflection of the posterior peritoneum that extends from the left side of the body toward the right sacroiliac joint. The mesentery envelops a number of important structures, including the jejunum, ileum, jejunal, and ileal branches of the superior mesenteric artery (SMA) and superior mesenteric vein (SMV), nerves, lacteals, lymph nodes, and a variable amount of fat.

The small bowel transitions to the colon at the ileocecal (IC) valve, which consists of two semilunar lips that protrude into the cecum. The IC valve functions like a flutter valve, allowing antegrade flow when a peristaltic wave is strong enough to overcome its resistance but preventing retrograde flow of colonic contents into the small intestine. The angulation between the ileum and cecum, supported by the superior and inferior IC ligaments, is important to the function of the IC valve. The IC valve typically contracts when the cecum is overdistended to prevent ceco-ileal reflux. This explains why during colonoscopy, excessive distention of the cecum with air should be avoided, because this may lead to IC valve contraction, which can then hinder successful intubation of the ileum and also lead to high intracolonic pressure with resultant barotrauma.

Colon and Rectum

The colon is a tubular structure about 30–40 cm in length at birth and measuring some 150 cm in the adult, or about one-quarter the length of the small intestine. The colon begins at the IC valve and ends distally at the anal verge (Fig. 100.1). It consists of four

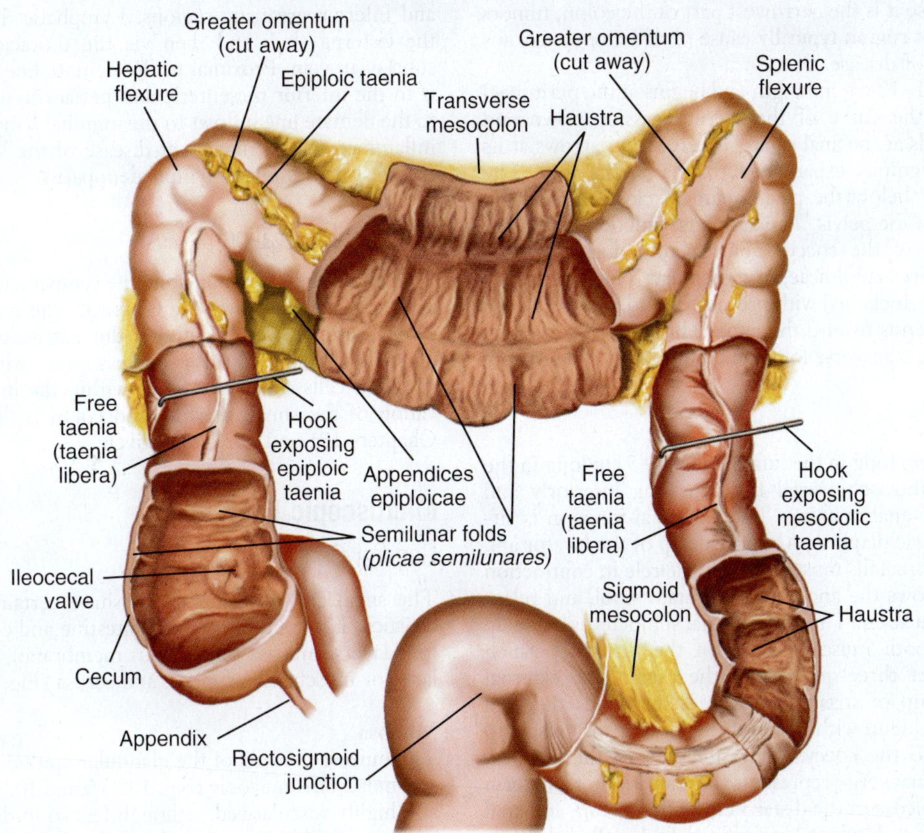

Fig. 100.1 Macroscopic characteristics of the colon. Note the taeniae, haustra between the taeniae, the semilunar folds, and the appendices epiploicae. (Netter illustration from www.netterimages.com.)

segments: cecum and vermiform appendix, colon (ascending, transverse, and descending portions), rectum, and anal canal. The diameter of the colon is greatest in the cecum (7.5 cm) and narrowest in the sigmoid (2.5 cm) until it balloons out in the rectum just proximal to the anal canal.

The colon is distinguished from the small intestine by several features. It is larger in caliber, mostly fixed in position, and has outer longitudinal muscle fibers that coalesce into three discrete bands called *taeniae*: the taenia liberis (free tenia), taenia omentalis (omental tenia), and taenia mesocolica (mesenteric tenia). Taeniae are located at 120-degree intervals around the colonic circumference and extend from the cecum to the proximal rectum. Outpouchings, or haustra, occur between the taeniae, and their mucosal surface is sectioned by semilunar folds to give the serosa a sacculated and puckered appearance. Small sacs of peritoneum filled with adipose tissue, the appendices epiploicae, are found on the external surface of the colon. The mesentery fully suspends the transverse colon and sigmoid colon, while the remainder of the colon has mesentery only on its free anterior surface. The appendix has a short mesentery called the *mesoappendix*.

The cecum is the most proximal portion of the colon. It is about 6–8 cm in length and breadth and lies in the right iliac fossa, projecting downward as a blind pouch below the entrance of the ileum. The large diameter of the cecum makes it susceptible to rupture with distal obstruction and permits tumors to grow to substantial size before producing symptoms of obstruction. The cecum is normally nonmobile because it is fixed in position by a small mesocecum; anomalous fixation, however, occurs in 10%–20% of the population, predominantly women, predisposing them to cecal volvulus.

The IC valve passes perpendicularly through the posteromedial wall of the cecum and consists of a superior and inferior fold arranged in an elliptical manner at the IC orifice. The appendiceal orifice is roughly 2.5 cm inferior to the IC valve, and the vermiform appendix is a blind outpouching extending from the cecum in a direction that varies from person to person. Appendiceal anatomy is discussed further in Chapter 122.

The ascending colon is narrower than the cecum and extends about 12–20 cm from the level of the IC valve to the inferior surface of the posterior lobe of the liver, where it angulates left and forward, forming the hepatic flexure. The ascending colon is covered with peritoneum in about 75% of individuals and thus is usually considered to reside in the retroperitoneum.

At the hepatic flexure, the colon turns medially and anteriorly to emerge into the peritoneal cavity as the transverse colon, fully enveloped in mesentery. The transverse is the longest (40–50 cm) and most mobile segment of the colon. It lies between the hepatic and splenic flexures and drapes itself across the anterior abdomen and anterior to the stomach. The phrenicocolic ligament anchors the colon at the splenic flexure, but the transverse colon is so mobile that in the upright position, it may actually dip down into the pelvis. Abdominal or pelvic surgery that results in adhesion formation can fix the position of the normally mobile transverse colon.

The descending colon is about 25–45 cm in length and travels posteriorly and then inferiorly in the retroperitoneal compartment to the pelvic brim. It emerges from the retroperitoneum into the peritoneal cavity as the sigmoid colon, an S-shaped redundant segment of variable length, tortuosity, and mobility. The mobility of the sigmoid colon renders it susceptible to volvulus, and because it is the narrowest part of the colon, tumors and strictures of this region typically cause obstructive symptoms early in the course of disease.

The rectum is 10–12 cm in length and begins at the peritoneal reflection, follows the curve of the sacrum passing down and posteriorly, and ends at the anal canal. The rectum narrows at its junction with the sigmoid, expanding proximal to the anus. The rectum lies entirely below the peritoneum in close relationship with the structure of the pelvis. The anorectal junction is 2–3 cm anterior to the tip of the coccyx. The rectum does not have sacculation, appendices epiploicae, or mesentery. The outer rectal wall is progressively thickened with prominent and anterior bands of muscle as it descends toward the anus. The luminal surface of the rectum has three transverse folds called the valves of Houston.

Anal Canal

The anal canal is 2 cm long in the infant and 4.5–5 cm long in the adult. It occupies the ischiorectal fossa, passing inferiorly and outward toward the anal opening. The anorectal junction is situated within the pelvic diaphragm and made up of the levator ani, coccygeus, and puborectalis muscles which encircle it; contraction of these muscles allows the anorectum to retain stool, and relaxation allows for defecation. The internal anal sphincter is made up of the circular smooth muscular layer of the intestine, which surrounds the upper three-quarters of the canal. The external sphincter is made up of striated muscle; it surrounds the anal canal, and its fibers blend with those of the levator ani muscle to attach posteriorly to the coccyx and anteriorly to the perineal body. Distally, the anal verge represents the transition of anoderm to true skin. The mucosa of the distal 3 cm of the rectum and anal canal contains 6–12 redundant longitudinal folds called the columns of Morgagni, which terminate in the anal papillae. These columns are joined together by mucosal folds called the anal valves, which are situated at the dentate line. The *zona alba* is a white zone that demarcates the transition to typical squamous epithelium. The anatomy and function of these muscles are described in more detail in Chapter 131.

Vasculature

The proximal duodenum receives arterial blood from the right gastric artery, supraduodenal artery, right gastroepiploic artery, and superior and inferior pancreaticoduodenal arteries. Venous drainage is via the SMV and the splenic and portal veins. The SMA delivers oxygenated blood to the distal duodenum, jejunum, ileum, ascending colon, and proximal two-thirds of the transverse colon. Branches of the inferior mesenteric artery supply the remainder of the colon. The arterial supply of the anal area is from the superior, middle, and inferior hemorrhoidal arteries, which are branches of the inferior mesenteric, hypogastric, and internal pudendal arteries, respectively. Venous drainage of the anus is by both the systemic and portal systems. The internal hemorrhoidal plexus drains into the superior rectal veins and then into the inferior mesenteric vein, which, with the SMV, joins the splenic vein to form the portal vein. The vascularity of the distal anus drains by the external hemorrhoidal plexus through the middle rectal and pudendal veins into the internal iliac vein. (See Chapter 120 for discussion of the intestinal blood supply and its disorders.)

Lymphatic Drainage

Lymphatic drainage courses through the mesentery from villus lacteals and lymphatic follicles and converges at preaortic lymph nodes around the SMA and celiac artery. The lymphatic drainage of both the small intestine and colon follows their respective blood supplies to lymph nodes in the celiac, superior preaortic, and inferior preaortic regions. Lymphatic drainage proceeds to the cisterna chyli and then via the thoracic duct into the left subclavian vein. Proximal to the dentate line, lymphatic drainage is to the inferior mesenteric and periaortic nodes, whereas distal to the dentate line it flows to the inguinal lymph nodes. Therefore inflammatory and malignant disease of the lower anal canal can manifest with inguinal lymphadenopathy.

Extrinsic Innervation

The autonomic nervous system—sympathetic, parasympathetic, and enteric—innervates the GI tract. The sympathetic and parasympathetic nerves constitute the extrinsic nerve supply and connect with the intrinsic nerve supply, which is composed of ganglion cells and nerve fibers within the intestinal wall. Innervation of the small intestine and colon is discussed in detail in Chapters 101 and 102, respectively.

Microscopic Features

General Considerations

The small and large intestines share certain histologic characteristics. The wall of the small intestine and colon is composed of four layers: mucosa (or mucous membrane), submucosa, muscularis (or muscularis propria), and serosa (Fig. 100.2).

Mucosa

The mucosa consists of the glandular epithelium, lamina propria, and muscularis mucosae (Fig. 100.3A and B). The mucosa is thick and highly vascularized, although less so in distal portions. It has concentric folds (*plicae circulares*) that are also referred to as the valves of Kerckring. The surfaces of the mucosal folds are studded with villus projections, and these features combine to produce a 400–500-fold increase in mucosal surface area. An intestinal villus will typically project 0.5–1.5 mm into the lumen, and the height of the villus decreases from proximal to distal small intestine. Villi are wider and more leaf-shaped in the duodenal bulb and proximal duodenum, becoming more finger-like in the distal duodenum, proximal jejunum, and remainder of intestine. The villi are covered with mature absorbing enterocytes interspersed with

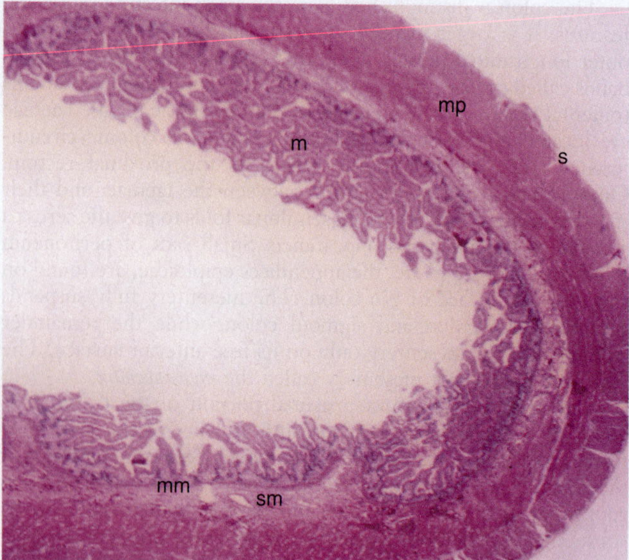

Fig. 100.2 Photomicrograph of small intestine showing its general microscopic architecture. *m*, Mucosa; *mm*, muscularis mucosae; *mp*, muscularis propria; *s*, serosa; *sm*, submucosa (H&E, ×25).

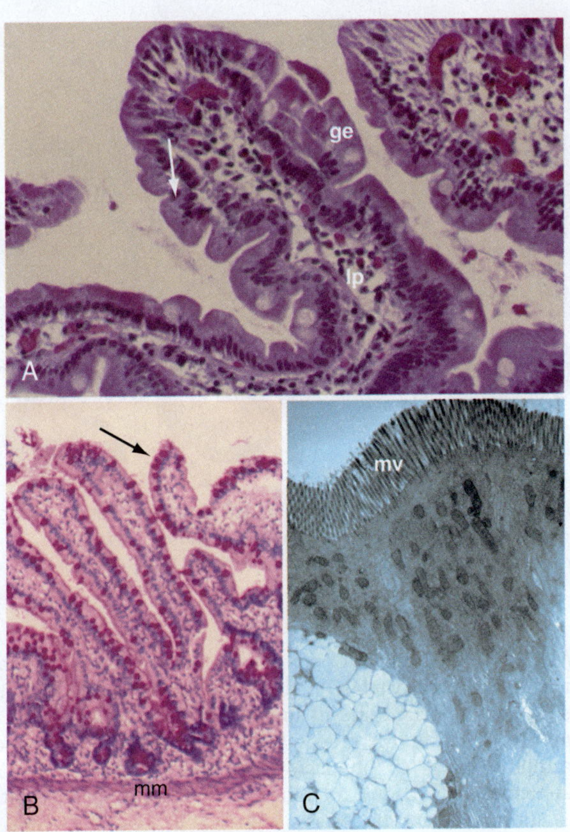

Fig. 100.3 Histologic and electron microscopic photographs of small intestine. (A) Components of the mucosa: *ge*, glandular epithelium; *lp*, lamina propria. Note the absorptive cells that appear as high columnar cells with eosinophilic cytoplasm (*arrow*) (H&E, ×250). (B) Goblet cells (*arrow*) and brush border are stained red. *mm*, Muscularis mucosae (periodic acid–Schiff stain, ×150). (C) Microvilli (*mv*) are seen as delicate finger-like projections on electron microscopic examination, ×9000. ((C) Courtesy S. Teichberg, PhD, Manhasset, New York.)

mucus-secreting goblet cells. Each villus contains an artery, vein, and central lacteal. A capillary bed forms along the epithelium, allowing for rapid clearance of absorbed nutrients, fluids, and electrolytes into the systemic circulation. To facilitate the absorptive process, capillary walls are fenestrated with diaphragmatic covers. The core of the villus also contains nerve fibers, plasma cells, macrophages, eosinophils, and fibroblasts. The villi are surrounded by cylindrical structures called the crypts of Lieberkühn, which extend through the lamina propria down to the muscularis mucosae. The crypts are lined with more immature epithelium that primarily functions as a secretory rather than an absorptive epithelium.

The epithelium of the small intestine is composed of various cell types: absorptive cells (columnar cells), secretory cells (goblet cells), undifferentiated cells, tuft cells, M cells, cup-like cells, and enteroendocrine cells. Crypts contain a similar cell population as the villi, with the addition of Paneth cells and stem cells.

The lamina propria is a layer of reticular connective tissue that provides the structural support for the mucosa, but it also contains many cellular elements important for absorption and immunity. The lamina propria is rich in arterioles, venules lacteals, nerve fibrils, fibroblasts, lymphocytes, macrophages, neutrophils, eosinophils, and mast cells. The muscularis mucosae consists of a thin layer of smooth muscle only 3–10 cells thick at the boundary of the mucosa and submucosa.

Stem cells are pluripotential cells located at the bases of the intestinal crypts. With intense mitotic activity, stem cells give rise to all types of mature intestinal epithelial cells and at the same time replenish themselves through self-renewal. Mucosal epithelial cells turn over every 5–7 days. Intestinal epithelial cells are mature by the time they reach the upper third of the villus. Paneth cells are the only cells that do not migrate. Undifferentiated cells have fewer intracellular organelles and microvilli than absorptive cells. The absorptive cells (see Fig. 100.3A) are high columnar cells with oval basal nuclei, eosinophilic cytoplasm, and a periodic acid–Schiff (PAS)-positive free surface, the brush border (see Fig. 100.3B). On electron microscopic examination, the brush border is seen to be composed of microvilli (see Fig. 100.3C), which are more numerous in the small intestinal than in the colonic epithelium. Enterocyte microvilli are estimated to increase the luminal surface area of the cell 14–40-fold.

Goblet cells are mucin-producing cells that are scattered among intestinal villi but are more common in the distal ileum and large intestine. Goblet cells are oval or round with flattened basal nuclei (Fig. 100.4A); their cytoplasm is basophilic, metachromatic (see Fig. 100.4B), and PAS-positive (see Fig. 100.4C) and consists mostly of mucin-secreting granules. Mucin is secreted by two pathways: in a neutrally mediated continuous manner, and by the active exocytosis of granules in response to extracellular stimuli.

Paneth cells are flask shaped with an eosinophilic granular cytoplasm and a broad base that is positioned against the basement membrane (Fig. 100.5). In the small intestine, Paneth cells are located exclusively in the crypts of Lieberkühn and secrete α-defensins, antimicrobial proteins, lysozyme, and phospholipase A, thought to be important in protection from infectious pathogens and function to maintain enteric homeostasis.[1]

Cup cells and tuft cells are two intestinal epithelial cell types with unidentified functions. Cup cells are present in villi and crypts largely limited to the ileum. Tuft cells are marked by a tuft of long microvilli projecting from the apical surface of the cell.

The mucosa also contains specialized cells called enteroendocrine or neuroendocrine cells (Fig. 100.6A) with specific endocrine functions. Intestinal endocrine cells are sparsely distributed and consist of 11 different cell types (Table 100.1). These are tall columnar cells present in both the crypts and villi and contain prominent secretory granules. The neuroendocrine cells have been divided histologically into argentaffin (i.e., their granules are able to reduce silver nitrate) or enterochromaffin cells and argyrophilic cells (i.e., granules reduce silver nitrate only in the presence of a chemical reducer). These chemical properties subdivide the cell types, but a unifying concept derived from their common origin and functional capacity has led to the term APUD cells. The *a*mine *p*recursor, *u*ptake, and *d*ecarboxylation concept characterize the cells as having a common embryonic origin from the neural crest and displaying similar cytochemical and electron microscopic features.[2]

Ultrastructurally, enteroendocrine cells contain membrane-bound granules with variably sized electrodense cores (see Fig. 100.6B) that consist of large dense-core vesicles and smaller synaptic-type microvesicles. Neurosecretory granules can be demonstrated as dark granules with nonspecific agents [e.g., Grimelius stain (see Fig. 100.6C)], or more specific immunohistochemical stains can be used (e.g., neuron-specific enolase, chromogranin, and synaptophysin). Chromogranin enables identification of the large dense-core vesicles, and synaptophysin targets the small synaptic-like microvesicles (see Fig. 100.6D). With specific immunohistochemical staining agents, it is possible to identify the individual chemical and protein components of neuroendocrine cells. The differential expression of certain proteins also makes it possible to subdivide neuroendocrine cell populations. For example, vesicular monoamine transporter (VMAT) has two isoforms: VMAT1 is restricted to serotonin-

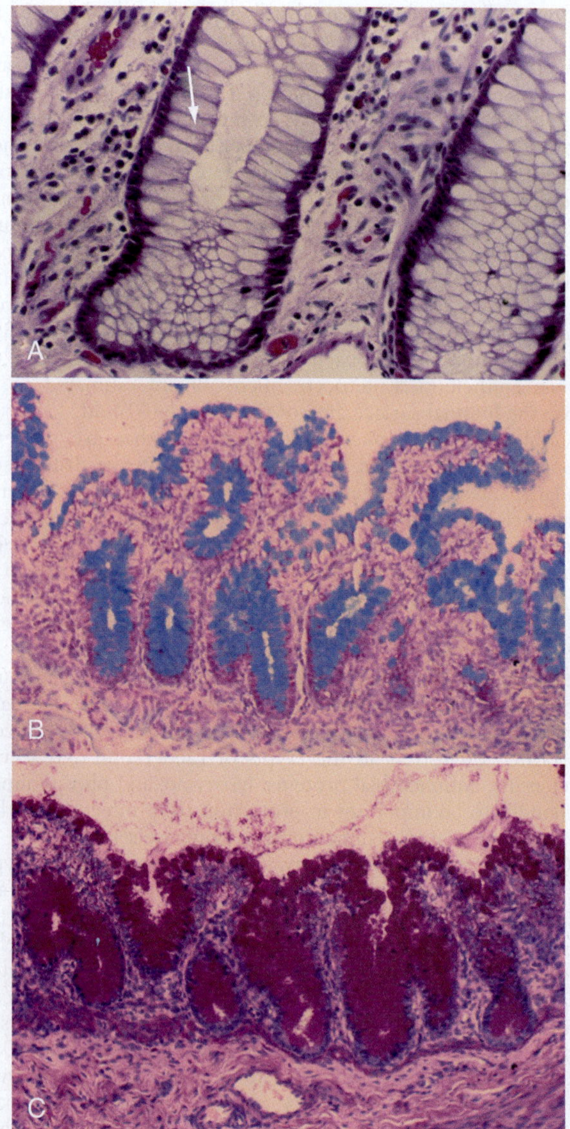

Fig. 100.4 Photomicrographs of large and small intestine demonstrating goblet cells. (A) Clear, empty-looking cytoplasm (*arrow*) and basal nuclei are seen with use of H&E, ×250. (B) Metachromatic staining of the cytoplasm results with use of the alcian blue stain, ×50. (C) The cells demonstrate red staining with use of periodic acid–Schiff stain, ×150.

producing enterochromaffin cells, and VMAT2 is expressed by histamine-producing cells, enterochromaffin-like cells, and pancreatic islet cells.[3]

The hormone products of these cells are discharged into the extracellular space on the basal and basolateral surfaces and have paracrine effects on absorption, secretion, motility, mucosal cell proliferation, possibly immunobarrier control, and even some endocrine effects upon systemic absorption.

The preferred designation of neuroendocrine cells is by their stored peptide. Serotonin-producing enterochromaffin cells, vasoactive intestinal polypeptide cells, and somatostatin D cells are distributed throughout the small and large intestines. Cells that produce gastrin, ghrelin, gastric inhibitory peptide, secretin, and CCK are found predominantly in the stomach and proximal small intestine. Cells that secrete peptide YY, glucagon-like peptide-1, glucagon-like peptide-2, and neurotensin are found in the ileum.[4]

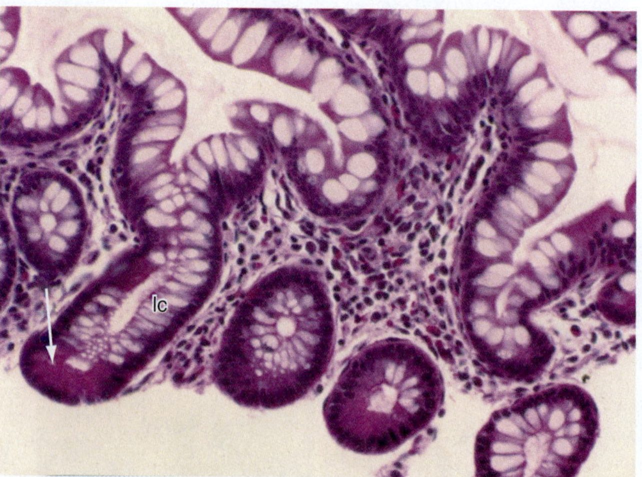

Fig. 100.5 Photomicrograph of small intestinal mucosa demonstrating the crypts of Lieberkühn (*lc*) and Paneth cells (*arrow*), which are characterized by granular eosinophilic cytoplasm (H&E, ×250).

M cells are specialized epithelial cells overlying lymphoid follicles and Peyer patches in the small intestine and colon. M cells are an important site of luminal antigen sampling for immune processing by the mucosal lymphoid system. This process of sampling plays an important role in the development and maintenance of immune tolerance, host defense against pathogens, and intestinal homeostasis.

The interstitial cells of Cajal (ICCs) are found in both the small intestine and colon and are located in the myenteric plexuses within the muscularis propria and the submucosa [Fig. 100.7 (see Chapters 101 and 102)]. The ICCs are important in the regulation of intestinal peristalsis and function as the pacemaker cells of the intestine. They influence the frequency of smooth muscle contraction, amplify neuronal signals, mediate neurotransmission from enteric motor neurons to smooth muscle cells, and set the smooth muscle membrane potential gradient. The ICCs are spindle-shaped or stellate cells with long, ramified processes and express c-Kit (CD117), a tyrosine kinase receptor critical for their survival.[5]

Submucosa

The submucosa is a fibrous connective tissue layer that lies between the muscularis mucosae and the muscularis propria. It contains lymphocytes, fibroblasts, mast cells, blood, and lymphatic vessels, and a nerve fiber plexus—Meissner plexus—composed of nonmyelinated postganglionic sympathetic fibers and parasympathetic ganglion cells. The submucosa supports the mucosa in specialized functions of nutrient, fluid, and electrolyte absorption by conveying a rich network of blood vessels, lymphatics, and nerves that ensure efficient handling of absorbates.

Brunner glands are submucosal glands (see Fig. 100.9B) found primarily in the first portion of the duodenum and in decreased numbers in the distal duodenum; in children, these glands may also be present in the proximal jejunum.

The function of Brunner glands is to secrete a bicarbonate-rich alkaline secretion that helps neutralize gastric chyme, a mucinous secretion that helps lubricate the mucosa; EGF; a variety of trefoil peptides, bactericidal factors, proteinase inhibitors, and surface-active lipids. The secretions that drain into the base of the duodenal crypts contribute to increased luminal pH by promoting pancreatic secretion and gallbladder contraction. The mucous layer protects the epithelial surface from peptic digestion; this protection is thought to be due to glycoprotein class III mucin glycoproteins.[6]

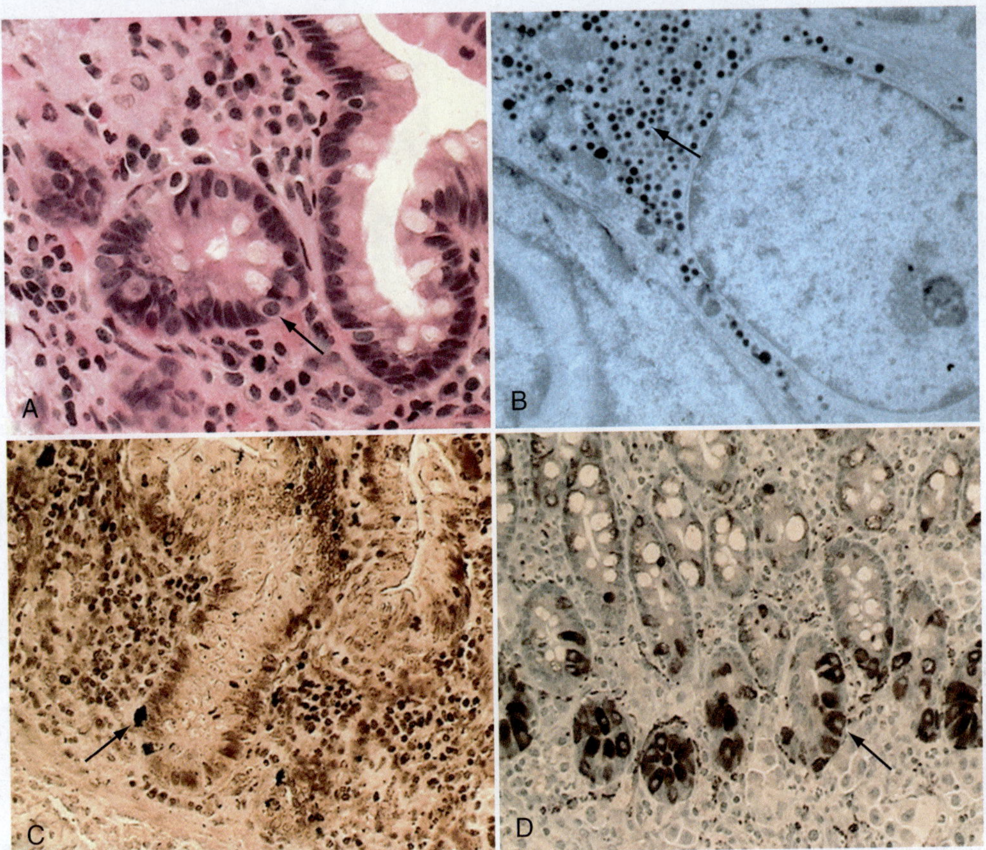

Fig. 100.6 Microscopic characteristics of neuroendocrine cells of the small intestine. (A) Features include clear cytoplasm and a round nucleus (*arrow*) (H&E, ×250). (B) Neurosecretory granules are seen as electron-dense, round black bodies (*arrow*) on electron microscopic examination, ×20,000. (C) Granules in neuroendocrine cells are stained black with the Grimelius stain (*arrow*), ×150. (D) Cells stained with synaptophysin have brown cytoplasm (*arrow*), ×250. ((B) Courtesy S. Teichberg, PhD, Manhasset, New York.)

TABLE 100.1 Enteroendocrine Cells of the Intestinal Tract: Cell Types and Products, Vesicle Markers, and Distribution

		Vesicle Markers							
Cell Type	**Cell Product**	**LDCV**	**SLMV**	**Duod**	**Jej**	**Ileum**	**App**	**Colon**	**Rec**
P/D1	Ghrelin	CgA, VMAT2		f	f	f			
EC	5-HT	CgA, VMAT1	Syn	+	+	+	+	+	+
D	Somatostatin	CgA	Syn	+	+	f	f	f	f
L	GLI/PYY	SgII > CgA	Syn	f	+	+	+	+	+
PP	PP	CgA, SgII, VMAT2	Syn	e					
G	Gastrin	CgA	Syn	+					
CCK	Cholecystokinin			+	+	f			
S	Secretin, 5-HT	CgA		+	+				
GIP	GIP/Xenin	CgA		+	+	f			
M	Motilin			+	+	f			
N	Neurotensin	CgA		f	+	+			

App, Appendix; *CgA*, chromogranin A; *Duod*, duodenum; *e*, presence of cells in fetus and newborn; *EC*, enterochromaffin cell; *f*, presence of few cells; *GIP*, gastric inhibitory polypeptide; *GLI*, glucagon-like immunoreactants (glicentin, glucagon-37, glucagon-29, GLP[glucagon-like peptide]-1, GLP-2); *5-HT*, 5-hydroxytryptamine (serotonin); *Jej*, jejunum; *LDCV*, large dense-core vesicles; *PP*, pancreatic polypeptide; *PYY*, PP-like peptide with *N*-terminal tyrosine amide; *Rec*, rectum; *SgII*, secretogranin II (also known as *chromogranin C*); *SLMV*, synaptic-like microvesicles; *Syn*, synaptophysin; *VMAT1*, *VMAT2*, vesicular monoamine transporter 1, 2; +, presence of cells; >, heavier staining than.

Adapted from Solcia E, Capela C, Fiocca R, et al. Disorders of the endocrine system. In: Ming SC, Goldman H, eds. *Pathology of the Gastrointestinal Tract*. Philadelphia: Williams & Wilkins; 1998:295.

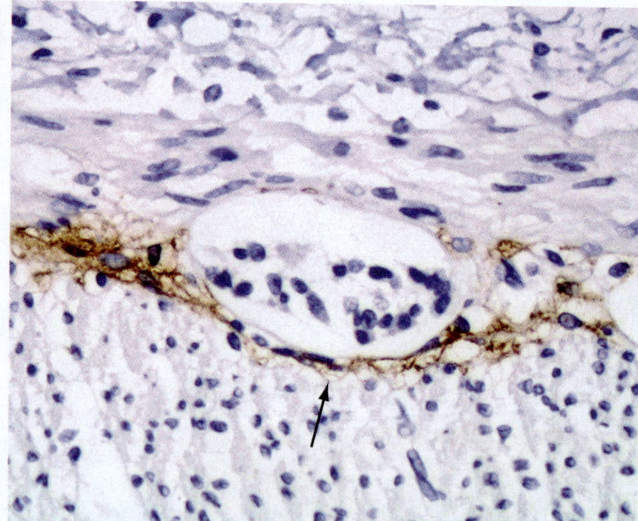

Fig. 100.7 Photomicrograph showing interstitial cells of Cajal in the small intestine. Brown-staining, elongated cells are evident around the myenteric plexus (*arrow*) (CD117 immunostain, ×250).

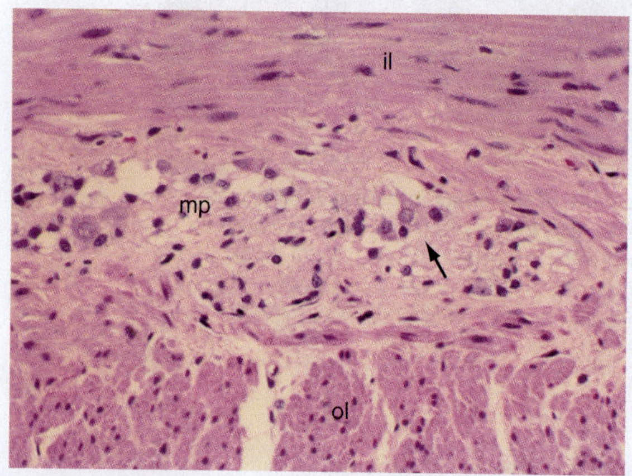

Fig. 100.8 Photomicrograph of muscularis propria of small intestine. The myenteric plexus (*mp*) is seen as a pale area with ganglion cells between the inner and outer layers (*il, ol*) of the muscularis propria (*arrow*) (H&E, ×250).

Muscularis Propria

The muscularis propria is mainly responsible for contractility and peristaltic movement of luminal contents through the GI tract. It consists of two layers of smooth muscle: an inner circular coat and an outer longitudinal coat arranged in a helicoidal pattern. A prominent nerve fiber plexus called the *myenteric* or *Auerbach plexus* is located in the plane between these two muscle layers (Fig. 100.8). The ganglia in the myenteric plexus are more prominent than their submucosal counterpart. Parasympathetic and postganglionic sympathetic fibers terminate in parasympathetic ganglion cells, and postganglionic parasympathetic fibers terminate in smooth muscle.

Serosa

The serosa is the outermost layer of the intestinal wall and is composed of a thin layer of mesothelial cells, representing an extension of the visceral peritoneum and mesentery as it envelops the intestine.

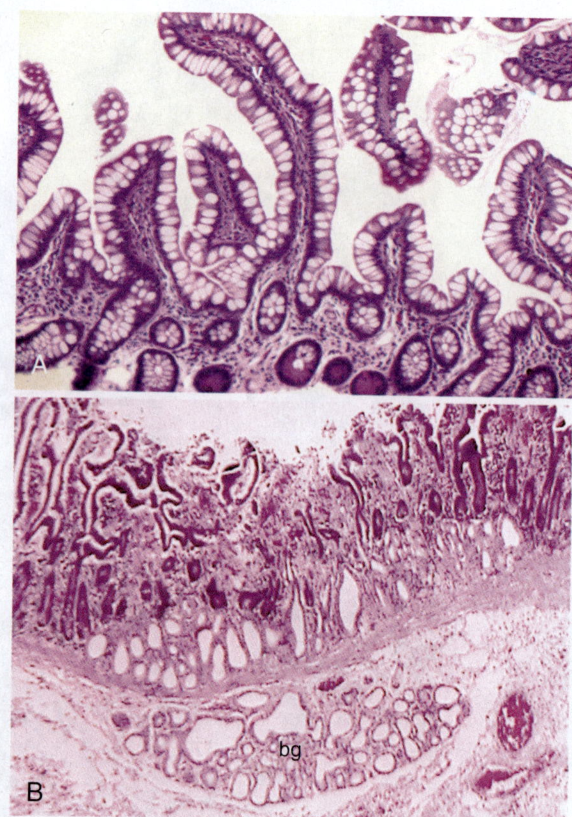

Fig. 100.9 Photomicrographs of duodenal mucosa. (A) Villi are seen as finger-like projections. (B) Brunner glands (*bg*) are found below the mucosa (H&E. A, ×250; B, ×150).

Microscopic Organization

Small Intestine

The mucosa of the small intestine is characterized by folds (*plicae circulares*, or valves of Kerckring) and villi. The mucosal folds actually comprise mucosa and submucosa. Villi are mucosal folds that decrease in size from the proximal to distal small intestine and are of different shapes in the various segments of the small intestine. They may be broad, short, or leaf-like in the duodenum, tongue-like in the jejunum, and finger-like more distally (Fig. 100.9A). The villous pattern may vary in different ethnic groups; biopsy specimens from Africans, Indians, South Vietnamese, and Haitians have shorter and thicker villi, an increased number of leaf-shaped villi, and more mononuclear cells in comparison with specimens from North Americans. The implications of these changes with regard to symptoms and subclinical GI infection are discussed in Chapter 110.

The height of the normal villus is 0.5–1.5 mm; villus height should be more than half the total thickness of the mucosa and three to five times the length of the crypts. Villi are lined by enterocytes, goblet cells, and enteroendocrine cells.

Enterocytes are tall columnar cells, each with a basally located, clear, oval-shaped nucleus, and several nucleoli. The cells are tightly cemented to the basal lamina and adjoined to adjacent enterocytes at the apical pole by intracellular tight junctions. The luminal surface has microvilli that contain necessary enzymes for nutrient absorption; a central core cytoskeleton is made of actin, villin, fimbrin, brush border myosin, and spectrin. The apical surface of the epithelium carries brush border transporters, Na^+/H^+ exchangers, and anion exchangers (see Chapter 103). The junction complexes are made up of three components: the proximal tight junction (*zonula occludens*), the intermediate junction (*zonula adherens*), and the deep junction, which includes the spot desmosome and the macular adherens zone (see Chapter 103). Movement through junctions is by paracellular transport and is the dominant pathway for passive ion and fluid flow. Tight junctions consist of claudins, occludens, and junctional adhesion molecules that bind and prevent passage of molecules between them in a regulated manner. They are leakier and have a lower resistance in the proximal small intestine and tighter in the distal intestine. The *zonula adherens* is less adherent and involved in cell signaling. Spot desmosomes are thought to augment transmembrane linkages spanning the intercellular gap and are involved in cell wall communications. The basolateral membrane is responsible for carriers to facilitate diffusion of organic solutes not coupled to ion movements. Gap junctions allow for communication and intercellular passage of ions and low molecular weight nutrients and intracellular messengers such as cyclic adenosine monophosphate.[6–8]

Two types of glands are present in the small intestine: Brunner glands (see previously) and crypts of Lieberkühn (intestinal crypts). The crypts of Lieberkühn are tubular glands that extend to the muscularis mucosae (see Fig. 100.5); they are occupied mainly by undifferentiated cells and Paneth cells. Cells are generated at the crypt base and migrate up the villus. During this migration, these cells mature and differentiate into a secretory lineage (goblet cells, enteroendocrine cells) and enterocytes. The commitment of the stem cells to differentiate is acquired in the upper third of the crypt where cells lose their ability to divide. The constant renewal of enterocytes is regulated by human acyl-coenzyme A synthetase.[9]

Paneth and columnar cells predominate in the base of the crypt. Above the base are absorptive cells and oligomucin cells; the latter originate from undifferentiated cells and differentiate into goblet cells. Goblet cells predominate in the upper half of the crypt. Enteroendocrine cells are admixed with goblet cells. A certain number of $CD3^{+}$ intraepithelial T lymphocytes (up to 30 per 100 epithelial cells) are normally present in the villi. Smooth muscle is found in the lamina propria of the small intestinal villus, extending vertically up from the muscularis mucosae. Plasma cells containing primarily immunoglobulin A and mast cells are also present. Lymphoid tissue is prominent in the lamina propria as both solitary nodules and confluent masses—Peyer patches—and is seen in the submucosa. Peyer patches are distributed along the antimesenteric border and are most numerous in the terminal ileum; their numbers decrease with age.

Most types of enteroendocrine cells are present in the duodenum. Cells that produce ghrelin, gastrin, CCK, motilin, neurotensin, gastric inhibitory peptide, and secretin are restricted to the small intestine.[2]

The proportions of cells differ in the villi and crypts as well as in different segments of the intestine. Overall, 90% of the villus epithelial cells are absorptive cells intermingled with goblet and enteroendocrine cells. The proportion of goblet to absorptive cells is increased in the ileum. The ICCs are more abundant in the myenteric plexus of the small intestine than in the colon.[5]

Colon

The colonic walls are similar to those of the small intestine. The outer layer forms the *taeniae coli*, which run in parallel to the long axis of the colon throughout its entire length. The width of the taeniae extends from 6 to 12 mm, and thickness gradually increases from the cecum to the sigmoid colon. The epithelial layer is smooth with crescentic folds corresponding to external sacculations. The surface epithelium is simple columnar type and is interspersed with vascular cells and goblet cells. The epithelial surface and upper third of the crypts are mostly lined with tall, slender absorptive columnar cells called principal cells. Goblet cells are the second most abundant cells on the surface of the colonic epithelium; they produce mucin, which aids in the passage of feces. Colonic epithelial cells are generated from stem cells at the base of the crypts and migrate toward the intestinal lumen 3–5 days after initiation of apoptosis. Most epithelial cells undergo apoptosis when they lose contact with the extracellular matrix and are shed into the lumen through caspase (cysteine-aspartic protease) activation. Caspase activation is responsible for the cleavage of essential intracellular proteins that lead to apoptosis and, therefore, loss of anchorage.[10]

The mucosa of the large intestine is characterized by the crypts of Lieberkühn, which dip to the muscularis mucosae and contain goblet cells, absorptive and enteroendocrine cells, and undifferentiated cells that are restricted to the lower third of the crypts. Glucagon-like immunoreactant pancreatic polypeptide-like peptide (PYY) with *N*-terminal tyrosine amide–producing L-cells predominate in the large intestine. Paneth cells are scarce and normally are noted only in the proximal colon. The lamina propria of the large intestine contains solitary lymphoid follicles that extend into the submucosa. Lymphoid follicles are more developed in the rectum and decrease in number with age. Confluent lymphoid tissue is present in the appendix. Macrophages (muciphages) predominate in the subepithelial portion of the lamina propria, are weakly PAS-positive, and are associated with stainable lipids.

Anal Canal

Microscopically, the anal canal is divided into three zones: proximal, intermediate or pectinate, and distal or anal skin. The proximal zone is lined by stratified cuboidal epithelium, and the transition with the rectal mucosa, which is lined by high columnar mucus-producing cells, is called the anorectal histologic junction (Fig. 100.10A). The intermediate or pectinate zone is lined by stratified squamous epithelium but without adnexae (e.g., hair and sebaceous glands) and is also referred to as anoderm. Its proximal margin, in contact with the proximal zone, is called the dentate line; its distal margin, in contact with the anal skin, constitutes the pectinate line, also referred to as the mucocutaneous junction (see Fig. 100.10B). Some authors use the terms pectinate line and dentate line interchangeably. The anal skin is lined by squamous stratified epithelium and contains hair and sebaceous glands.

Vasculature

Large arterial branches enter the muscularis propria through the serosa and pass to the submucosa, where they branch to form large plexuses. In the small intestine, two types of branches arise from the submucosal plexuses: some arteries branch on the inner surface of the muscularis mucosae and break into a capillary network that surrounds the crypts of Lieberkühn; other arteries are destined for villi, each villus receiving 1–2 arteries, to set up the anatomic arrangement that allows a countercurrent mechanism, thus aiding absorption. One or several veins originate at the tip of each villus from the superficial capillary plexus, anastomose with the glandular venous plexus, and then enter the submucosa to join the submucosal venous plexus.

In the colon, branches from the submucosal arterial plexus extend to the surface, giving rise to capillaries that supply the submucosa, and their branch to form a capillary meshwork around the crypts of Lieberkühn. From the periglandular capillary meshwork, veins form a venous plexus between the base of the crypts and the muscularis mucosae. From this plexus, branches extend into the submucosa and form another venous plexus from which large veins follow the distribution of the arteries and pass through the muscularis propria into the serosa.

Lymph Vessels

The lymphatics of the small intestine are called lacteals and become filled with milky-white lymph called chyle after eating. Each villus contains one central lacteal, except in the duodenum,

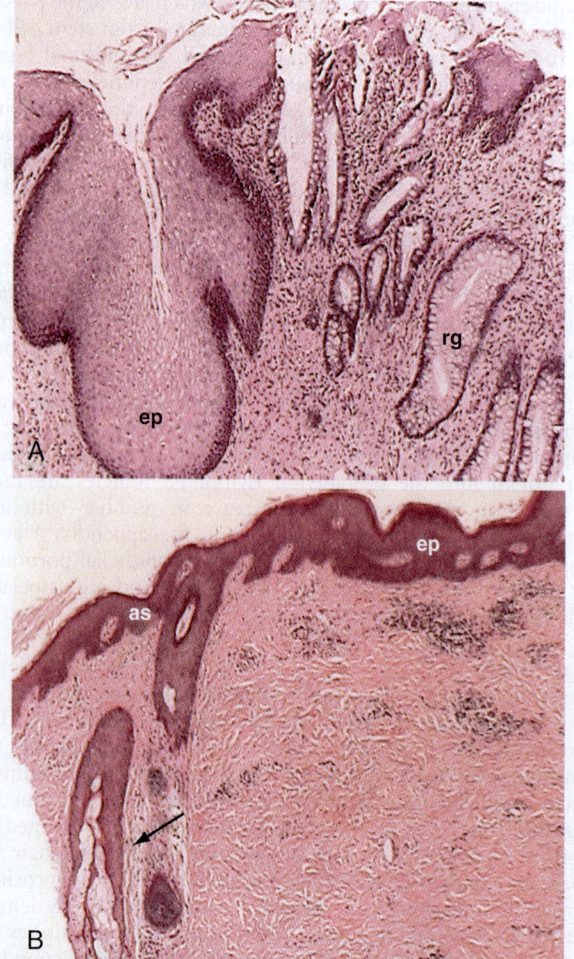

Fig. 100.10 Photomicrograph of anal canal. (A) Anorectal histologic junction. Transition from rectal glandular mucosa (*rg*) to proximal anal mucosa lined by stratified squamous epithelium (*ep*) is evident. (B) Pectinate line is characterized by anal mucosa with stratified squamous epithelium (*ep*) and anal skin (*as*) containing adnexae (*arrow*) (A and B, H&E, ×150).

where two or more lacteals per villus may be present. The wall of the lacteal consists of endothelial cells, reticulum fibers, and smooth muscle cells. At the base of the villus, the central lacteals anastomose with the lymphatic capillaries between the crypts of Lieberkühn. They also form a plexus on the inner surface of the muscularis mucosae. Branches of this plexus extend through the muscularis mucosae to form a submucosal plexus. Branches from the submucosal plexus penetrate the muscularis propria, where they receive branches from plexuses between the inner and outer layers. Lymphatic vessels are absent in the colonic mucosa, but the distribution of lymphatics in the remaining colonic layers is similar to that in the small intestine.

Nerves

The intrinsic nervous system [enteric nervous system (ENS)] consists of subserosal, muscular, and submucosal plexuses. The subserosal plexus contains a network of thin nerve fibers without ganglia that connects the extrinsic nerves with the intrinsic plexus. The myenteric plexus, or Auerbach plexus, is situated between the outer and inner layers of the muscularis propria (see Fig. 100.8); it consists of ganglia and bundles of unmyelinated axons that connect with the ganglia to form a meshwork. These axons originate from processes of the ganglion cells and extrinsic vagus and

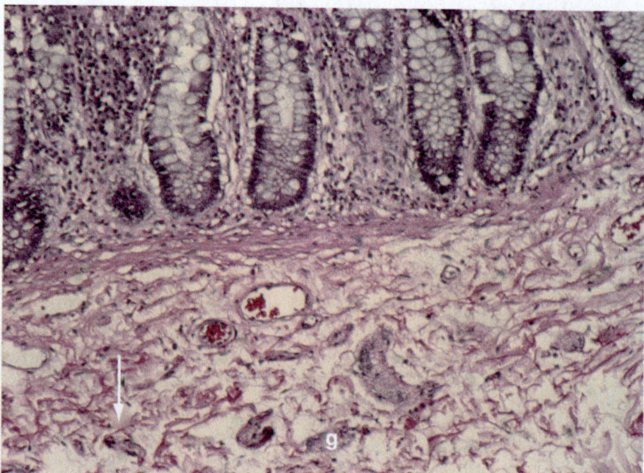

Fig. 100.11 Photomicrograph showing a normal submucosal plexus of the colon. Ganglia (*g*) are identified by their oval structure, and nerve trunks are thin (*arrow*) (H&E, ×150).

sympathetic ganglia. The deep muscular plexus, or Schabadasch plexus, is situated on the mucosal aspect of the circular muscular layer of the muscularis propria. It does not contain ganglia; it innervates the muscularis propria and connects with the myenteric plexus. The submucosal plexus, or Meissner plexus, consists of ganglia and nerve bundles. The nerve fibers of this plexus innervate the muscularis mucosae and smooth muscle in the core of the villi. Fibers from this plexus also form a mucosal plexus that is situated in the lamina propria and provides branches to the intestinal crypts and villi. The ganglion cells of the submucosal plexus are distributed in two layers; one is adjacent to the circular muscular layer of the muscularis propria, and the other is contiguous to the muscularis mucosae. Ganglion cells are large cells, isolated or grouped in small clusters called ganglia (Fig. 100.11). Ganglion cells have an abundant basophilic cytoplasm, a large vesicular round nucleus, and a prominent nucleolus. Ganglion cells are scarce in the physiologically hypoganglionic segment 1 cm above the anal verge.

EMBRYOLOGY

Intestinal Development

The embryo is a bilaminar germ disk at 3 weeks' gestation. Through a process called gastrulation, this disk becomes trilaminar and gives rise to the three primary germ layers: ectoderm, mesoderm, and endoderm. It also establishes bilateral symmetry, a dorsal-ventral orientation, and an anterior-posterior (A-P) axis.

The surface facing the yolk sac becomes endoderm, the surface facing the amniotic sac becomes ectoderm, and the middle layer becomes mesoderm. The oral opening is marked by the buccopharyngeal membrane; the future openings of the urogenital and digestive tracts become identifiable as the cloacal membrane. At 4 weeks' gestation, the alimentary tract is divided into three parts: foregut, midgut, and hindgut, the endoderm connecting with the yolk sac (Fig. 100.12).

These segments form a tube by growth and folding. The folding process brings together the endodermal, mesodermal, and ectodermal layers with the corresponding layers on the opposite side, converting the flat endodermal layer into the intestinal tube. Initially, the foregut and hindgut are blind-ending tubes separated by a midgut that is open to the yolk sac. As the lateral edges of the midgut fuse to become a tube, there is a narrowing of the communication between the yolk sac and endoderm, producing

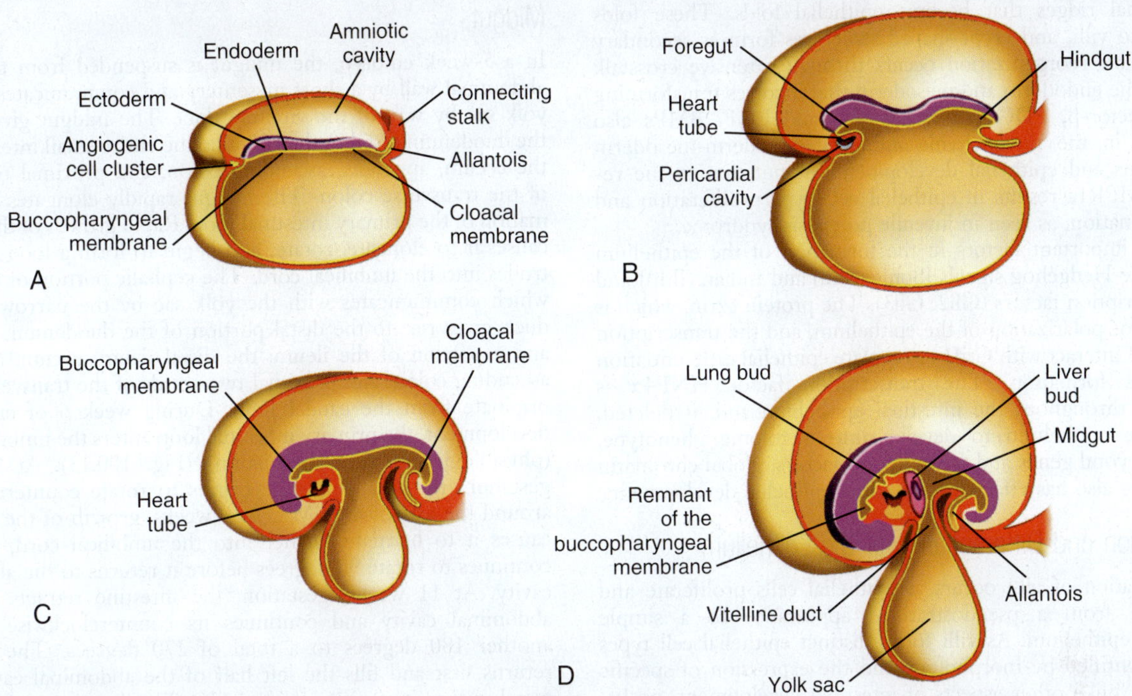

Fig. 100.12 Formation of foregut, midgut, and hindgut (see text for details). (From Sadler YW, ed. *Langman's Medical Embryology*. 10th ed. Philadelphia: Lippincott Williams & Wilkins; 2006.)

the vitelline duct (see Fig. 100.12). With folding of the embryo during week 4 of development, the mesodermal layer splits. The portion that adheres to endoderm forms the visceral peritoneum, whereas the part that adheres to ectoderm forms the parietal peritoneum. The space between the two layers becomes the peritoneal cavity.

The primitive intestine results from incorporation of the endoderm-lined yolk sac cavity into the embryo following embryonal cephalocaudal and lateral folding. The endoderm gives rise to the epithelial lining of the GI tract; muscle, connective tissue, and peritoneum originate from the splanchnic mesoderm. During the ninth week of development, the epithelium begins to differentiate from the endoderm, with villus formation and differentiation of epithelial cell types. Organogenesis is complete by 12 weeks' gestation.

Initially, the foregut, midgut, and hindgut are in broad contact with the mesenchyma of the posterior abdominal wall. The intraembryonic cavity is in open communication with the extra-embryonic cavity. Subsequently, the intraembryonic cavity loses its wide connection with the extra-embryonic cavity. By week 5 of embryonic development, splanchnic mesoderm layers are fused in the midline and form a double-layered membrane, the dorsal mesentery, between the right and left halves of the body cavity. The mesoderm surrounds the intestinal tube and suspends it from the posterior body wall, allowing it to hang into the body cavity. The caudal portions of the foregut, midgut, and most of the hindgut are suspended from the abdominal wall by the dorsal mesentery, which extends from the duodenum to the cloaca. The dorsal mesentery forms the mesoduodenum in the region of the duodenum, the dorsal mesocolon in the region of the colon, and the mesentery proper in the region of the jejunum and ileum.[11]

Molecular Regulation of Intestinal Morphogenesis

Molecular regulation of intestine formation is a complex network of carefully orchestrated gene expression, activation of signal transduction pathways, and cell-cell interactions that work in a cooperative manner; the balance of signals often determines the developmental pathways that follow. Only selected molecular elements are presented here, but comprehensive reviews are available.[12–14]

Intestinal Tube Formation

Development of the intestinal tube requires simultaneous inductive and patterning steps. The transforming growth factor-β superfamily member Nodal is required for the mesoderm and endoderm specification in all vertebrate species and plays a secondary role in A–P patterning. Crosstalk and inductive cues exchanged between the mesoderm and endoderm are thought to play a critical role in gastrulation. The interruption of Fox factors (Fox A2, FoxH1), GATA factors, Sox17, Mixl1, or Smad signaling will result in a failure of tube formation, primarily by altering endoderm development and specification.[1,2,13,14] The Wnt signaling pathway also plays a critical role in intestinal tube formation.

Genes expressed during A–P patterning include *Hhex*, *FoxA2*, and *Sox2* in the anterior gut, while *Cdx* is expressed posteriorly. *Hox* genes play an important role in patterning of the mesoderm and ectoderm, while *Cdx2* is a critical gene in hindgut formation and intestinal specification and patterning, particularly in cecal development. Other genes and factors that play a role in A–P patterning of the endoderm include *FGF*, *Wnt*, *BMP*, and retinoic acid signaling. Intestinal elongation is also controlled by a number of genes. Deletion of *Wnt5a* results in an 80% reduction in small intestine and a 63% reduction in colonic length.[13] The absence of any one of a family of proteins that interact with Wnt5a (secreted frizzled-related proteins) also adversely affect bowel length.[13]

Epithelial Cells and Villus Formation

The endoderm transitions from simple epithelium to columnar epithelium in a rostral-caudal (proximal-distal) manner, including in the colon, which initially has villus-like structures until it undergoes reorganization. The mesenchyme invaginates to form longitudinal ridges that become epithelial folds. These folds evolve into villi, and crypt-shaped structures form as secondary lumina. This reorganization occurs through extensive crosstalk between the endoderm and mesoderm that involves transforming growth factor-β, PDGF, FGF, WNT, and EGF. BMPs also expressed in the mesenchyme influence endoderm-mesoderm interactions and epithelial development. A mutation in the receptor BMPR1a results in epithelial cell hyperproliferation and polyp formation, as seen in juvenile polyposis syndrome.[13]

Other important factors in the formation of the epithelium include the Hedgehog signals [Sonic (Shh) and Indian (Ihh)] and Gli transcription factors (Gli2, Gli3). The protein ezrin, which is required for polarization of the epithelium, and the transcription factor Elf3 interact with Crif1 to regulate epithelial differentiation and villus formation. The transcription factor HNF4α is expressed throughout the intestinal epithelium and, if deleted, causes the epithelium to develop into a colonic phenotype. Finally, beyond genes and transcription factors, global chromatin remodeling also has effects on intestinal epithelial development.

Proliferation and Differentiation of the Epithelium

The formation of villi occurs as epithelial cells proliferate and reorganize from a pseudostratified appearance to a simple columnar epithelium. As villi form, distinct epithelial cell types can be identified by morphology and the expression of specific markers. Unlike other aspects of intestinal development, proliferation and differentiation of the epithelium remain important processes that must be maintained throughout adult life. Two major signaling pathways involved in these processes are Wnt/β-catenin and Notch. Wnt/β-catenin is important in crypt formation, for maintaining the stem cell compartment, proliferation and differentiation in the embryonic and adult intestine, and for Paneth cell maturation. Notch proteins are transmembrane receptors that are important in both proliferation and differentiation of the developing intestine. Evidence suggests that Notch activity regulates factors that influence whether undifferentiated cells will become absorptive or secretory epithelial cells. There also are factors downstream of Wnt/β-catenin and Notch that affect specific lineages: Neurogenin[3] is required for the formation of enteroendocrine cells; SPDEF directs terminal differentiation of goblet cells; Sox9 regulates Paneth and goblet cell formation; and Klf4 regulates colonic goblet cell differentiation.

Specific Structures and Systems

Duodenum

The duodenum originates from the terminal portion of the foregut and cephalic part of the midgut. Early during week 4 of gestation, the caudal foregut begins to expand to initiate formation of the stomach. The liver and pancreas arise at the junction of the midgut and foregut. With rotation of the stomach, the duodenum becomes C-shaped and rotates to the right; the fourth portion becomes fixed in the left upper abdominal cavity. The mesoduodenum fuses with the adjacent peritoneum; both layers disappear, and the duodenum becomes fixed in its retroperitoneal location. The lumen of the duodenum is obliterated during the second month of development by proliferation of its cells; this phenomenon is shortly followed by recanalization. Small intestinal villus and crypt formation occur in a proximal-to-distal progression. The villi appear during week 8 of gestation, along with the microvillus enzymes. At 12 weeks' gestation, crypts are present and grow between the 10th and 14th week of gestation. At 14 weeks, the intestinal enzymes are at an adult level of activity.

Because the foregut is supplied by the celiac artery and the midgut by the SMA, the duodenum is supplied by both arteries and therefore is relatively protected from ischemic injury.[11]

Midgut

In a 5-week embryo, the midgut is suspended from the dorsal abdominal wall by a short mesentery and communicates with the yolk sac by way of the vitelline duct. The midgut gives rise to the duodenum distal to the ampulla, the entire small intestine, and the cecum, appendix, ascending colon, and proximal two-thirds of the transverse colon. The midgut rapidly elongates with formation of the primary intestinal loop. Rapid growth of the midgut causes it to elongate, rotate, and begin to form a loop that protrudes into the umbilical cord. The cephalic portion of this loop, which communicates with the yolk sac by the narrow vitelline duct, gives rise to the distal portion of the duodenum, jejunum, and a portion of the ileum; the distal ileum, cecum, appendix, ascending colon, and proximal two-thirds of the transverse colon originate from the caudal limb. During week 6 of embryonic development, the primary intestinal loop enters the umbilical cord (physiologic umbilical herniation) (Fig. 100.13). At 7 weeks' gestation, the small intestine begins to rotate counterclockwise around the axis of the SMA. At 9 weeks, growth of the intestine causes it to herniate further into the umbilical cord, where it continues to rotate 90 degrees before it returns to the abdominal cavity. At 11 weeks' gestation, the intestine retracts into the abdominal cavity and continues its counterclockwise rotation another 180 degrees to a total of 270 degrees. The jejunum returns first and fills the left half of the abdominal cavity ultimately taking its position in the LUQ. The ileum returns next and fills the right half of the abdominal cavity ultimately assuming its final position in the RLQ. The colon enters last, with fixation of the cecum close to the iliac crest and the ascending and descending colon attaching to the posterior abdominal wall. Elongation of the bowel continues, and the jejunum and ileum form a number of coiled loops within the peritoneal cavity.[11]

The cecum originates as a small dilatation or bud of the caudal limb of the primary intestinal loop by approximately 6 weeks of development. Initially, after returning to the abdominal cavity, it lies in the RUQ, then it descends to the right iliac fossa, placing the ascending colon and hepatic flexure in the right side of the abdominal cavity. The appendix originates from the distal end of the cecal bud. Because the appendix develops during descent of the colon, its final position is frequently retrocecal or retrocolic (Fig. 100.14).

Mesentery

As the caudal limb of the primitive intestine moves to the right side of the abdominal cavity, the dorsal mesentery twists around the origin of the SMA. After the ascending and descending portions of the colon reach their final destinations, their mesenteries fuse with the peritoneum of the posterior abdominal wall, and they become retroperitoneal organs. The appendix, cecum, and descending colon retain their free mesentery. The transverse mesocolon fuses with the posterior wall of the greater omentum. The mesentery of the jejunum and ileum is at first in continuity with the ascending mesocolon; after the ascending colon becomes retroperitoneal, the mesentery only extends from the duodenum to the IC junction.[11]

Hindgut

The distal third of the transverse colon, the descending colon and sigmoid, the rectum, and the upper part of the anal canal originate from the hindgut. The fetal colon develops over 30 weeks in three stages. Primitive stratified epithelium similar to that in the small intestine appears between 8 and 10 weeks. Conversion to villus architecture with developing crypts occurs at 12–14 weeks. Remodeling to the adult-type crypt epithelium with loss of the villi occurs at 30 weeks. Initially the urinary, genital, and rectal

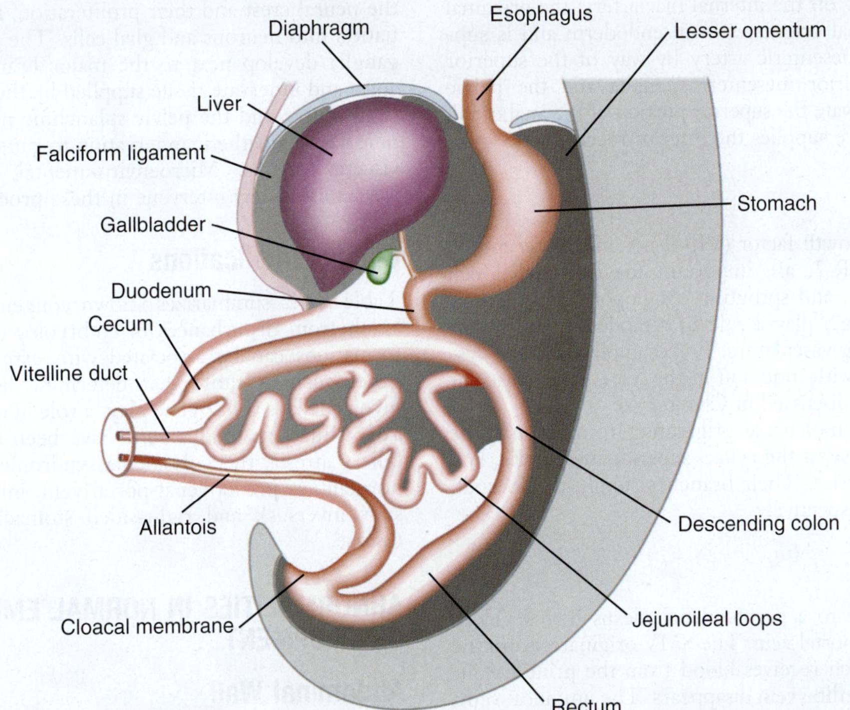

Fig. 100.13 Physiologic umbilical herniation of the intestinal loop during normal development. Coiling of small intestinal loops and formation of cecum occur during herniation. The first 90 degrees of rotation occur during herniation; the remaining 180 degrees occur during return of intestine to abdominal cavity. (From Sadler YW, ed. *Langman's Medical Embryology*. 10th ed. Philadelphia: Lippincott Williams & Wilkins; 2006:219, Fig. 14.26.)

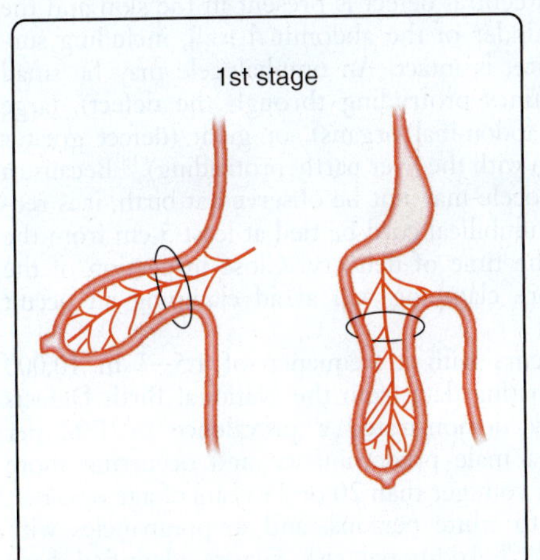

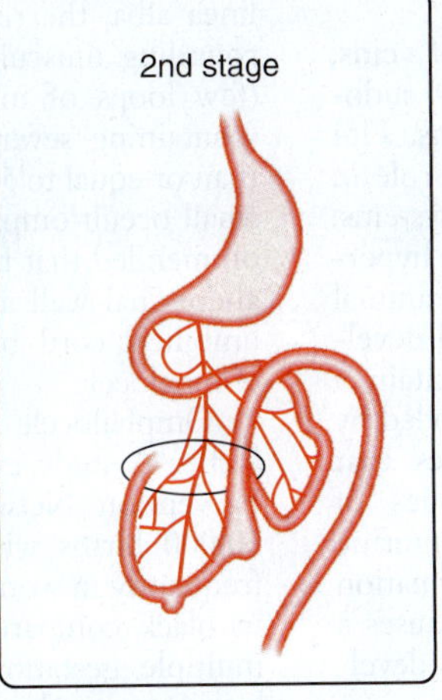

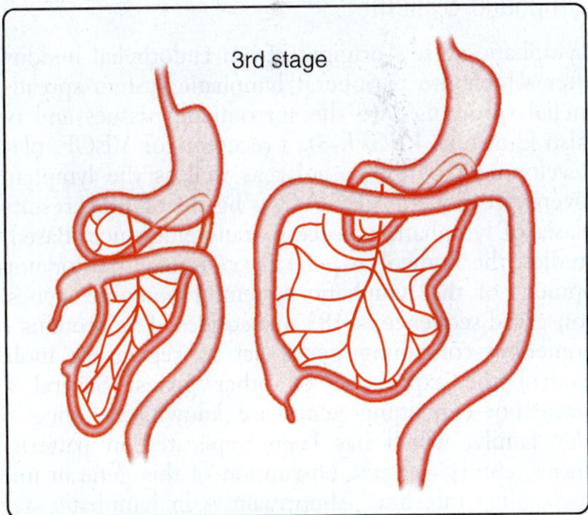

Fig. 100.14 The three stages of normal intestinal rotation (see text for details). (From Gosche JR, Touloukian RJ. Congenital anomalies of the midgut. In: Wyllie R, Hyams JS, eds. *Pediatric Gastrointestinal Disease. Pathophysiology, Diagnosis, Management*. 2nd ed. Philadelphia: WB Saunders; 1999.)

tracts empty into a common channel, the cloaca. They become separated by the caudal descent of the urorectal septum into an anterior urogenital sinus and a posterior intestinal canal. The lateral fold of the cloaca moves to the midline, and the caudal extension of the urorectal septum develops into the perineal body. In a man, the lateral genital ridges coalesce to form the urethra and scrotum; in a woman, no fusion occurs, and the labia minora and majora evolve. The cloaca is lined by endoderm and covered anteriorly by ectoderm. The most distal portion of the hindgut enters into the posterior region of the cloaca, the primitive anorectal canal. The boundary between the endoderm and the ectoderm forms the cloacal membrane. This membrane ruptures by week 7 of embryonic development, creating the anal opening for the hindgut. The anal membrane separates the endoderm and ectodermal portions of the anorectal canal. The anal membrane marks the pectinate line. The pectinate line marks separation of vascular supply of the upper and lower parts of the anal canal. This portion is obliterated by ectoderm but recanalizes by week 9. Thus the distal portion of the anal canal originates from ectoderm and is supplied by the inferior rectal artery, which arises from the internal pudendal artery off the internal iliac artery; the proximal portion of the anal canal originates from endoderm and is supplied by the inferior mesenteric artery by way of the superior rectal artery. The inferior mesenteric ganglia and the pelvic splanchnic nerves innervate the superior portion of the anal canal. The inferior rectal nerve supplies the inferior rectal canal.

Arterial System

Vascular endothelial growth factor (VEGF)-A and its receptors, VEGFR-1 and VEGFR-2, are important for endothelial cell proliferation, migration, and sprouting. Angiopoietins and their receptors, Tie1 and Tie2, play a role in remodeling and maturation of the developing vasculature. For example, vascular dysmorphogenesis is seen with mutation in the Tie2 gene. Vascular malformation is briefly discussed in Chapter 36.

Arteries of the dorsal mesentery, originating from fusion of the vitelline arteries, give rise to the celiac, superior mesenteric, and inferior mesenteric arteries. Their branches supply the foregut, midgut, and hindgut, respectively.

Venous System

Vitelline veins give rise to a periduodenal plexus that develops into a single vessel, the portal vein. The SMV originates from the right vitelline vein, which receives blood from the primitive intestinal loop; the left vitelline vein disappears. The umbilical veins join with the hepatic sinusoids, after which the right umbilical vein disappears and the left umbilical vein joins the inferior vena cava; ultimately the umbilical vein is obliterated and forms the ligamentum teres. The cardinal veins and the proximal portion of the right vitelline vein are involved with forming the inferior vena cava.

Lymphatic System

Lymphatic vessels originate from endothelial budding of veins, after which the peripheral lymphatic system spreads by endothelial sprouting into the surrounding tissues and organs. Flt4 (also known as *VEGFR-3*), a receptor for VEGF, plays a role in development of the vascular as well as the lymphatic systems. Overexpression of VEGF-C, a ligand of Flt4, results in hyperplasia of lymphatic vessels in transgenic mice. Based on animal studies, the homeobox gene *Prox1* is essential for normal development of the lymphatic system. Homeobox genes contain a conserved sequence of 183 nucleotides. The proteins encoded by homeobox-containing genes act as regulatory molecules that control the expression of other genes. Several families of homeobox-containing genes are known, including the murine *Hox* family, which has been implicated in pattern formation during embryogenesis. Disruption of this gene in mice causes a chyle-filled intestine. Abnormalities in lymphatic system development can result in lymphangiectasia (see Chapter 31).

Enteric Nervous System

The ENS originates from vagal, truncal, and sacral neural crest cells. Most of the ENS cells derive from the truncal and vagal neural crest, enter the foregut mesenchyma, and colonize the developing intestine in a cephalocaudal direction. The truncal neural crest gives rise to ganglia of the proximal stomach, whereas the vagal neural crest supplies ganglia to the entire intestine, including the rectum; this colonization is complete by 13 weeks of embryonic development. A small component of the ENS originates from sacral neural crest cells. These cells form extra-intestinal pelvic ganglia that colonize the hindgut mesenchyma before arrival of the vagal-derived neural crest cells.[15] Normal ENS development depends on the survival of cells derived from the neural crest and their proliferation, movement, and differentiation into neurons and glial cells. The prevertebral sympathetic ganglia develop next to the major branches of the descending aorta and innervate tissue supplied by the respective arteries. The vagus nerve and the pelvic splanchnic nerves provide preganglionic parasympathetic innervation to ganglia embedded in walls of visceral organs. Microenvironmental, genetic, or molecular mechanisms may intervene in these processes.

Clinical Implications

Table 100.2 summarizes known congenital clinical entities that result from disturbances in embryologic development. GI malformations can be associated with extraintestinal defects when genes such as those that determine left-right asymmetry are involved. The *CFC1* gene plays a role in establishing the left-right axis. Mutations of this gene have been reported in extrahepatic biliary atresia, the polysplenia syndrome (inferior vena cava abnormalities, preduodenal portal vein, intestinal malrotation, and situs inversus), and right-sided stomach and congenital heart disease.[16,17]

ABNORMALITIES IN NORMAL EMBRYOLOGIC DEVELOPMENT

Abdominal Wall

Omphalocele

Omphalocele, also known as *exomphalos*, is a congenital hernia of the ventral abdominal wall involving the umbilicus. It is covered by an avascular sac composed of fused layers of amnion and peritoneum (Fig. 100.15). The umbilical cord is usually inserted into the apex of the sac, and the blood vessels radiate within the sac wall. Although a central defect is present in the skin and the linea alba, the remainder of the abdominal wall, including surrounding musculature, is intact. An omphalocele may be small (few loops of intestines protruding through the defect), large (containing several abdominal organs), or giant (defect greater than or equal to 5 cm with the liver partly protruding).[18] Because a small occult omphalocele may not be observed at birth, it is recommended that the umbilical cord be tied at least 5 cm from the abdominal wall at the time of delivery. Close inspection of the umbilical cord before clamping will avoid clamping an occult omphalocele.

Omphalocele occurs with a frequency of 1.5–3 in 10,000 births. A study evaluating data from the National Birth Defects Prevention Network demonstrated a prevalence of 1.92 per 10,000 births with a male predominance and occurring more frequently in women younger than 20 or 35 years of age or older, in black compared to white persons, and in pregnancies with multiple gestations.[19,20] Additional risk factors identified have been maternal smoking, alcohol consumption, and usage of medications such as aspirin and selective serotonin reuptake inhibitors.[21] Associated anomalies (e.g., sternal defects) result from failure of closure of the cephalic folds; failure of caudal fold development results in exstrophy of the bladder and, in extreme cases, exstrophy of the cloaca. Additional cranial fold abnormalities (i.e., anterior diaphragmatic hernia, sternal clefts, pericardial defects, and cardiac defects) in the setting of omphalocele are known as the pentalogy of Cantrell.[22]

With a large omphalocele, the liver and spleen are frequently outside the abdominal cavity. Associated anomalies occur in about 75% of children with omphalocele and include chromosomal abnormalities (e.g., trisomy 13 or 18), nonchromosomal syndromes like Beckwith-Wiedemann syndrome (mental retardation, hepatomegaly, large body stature, and hypoglycemia), fetal valproate syndrome, exstrophy of the bladder or cloaca, and

TABLE 100.2 Abnormalities in Normal Embryologic Development

Location	Defect
Body Wall	
Omphalocele	Failure of intestine to return to the abdominal cavity after its physiologic herniation
Gastroschisis	Weakening of abdominal wall
Mesentery	
Mobile cecum	Persistence of mesocolon
Volvulus	Failure of fusion of mesocolon with posterior abdominal wall
Vitelline Duct	
Meckel diverticulum	Persistence of vitelline duct (see Fig. 100.17)
Omphalomesenteric cyst	Focal failure of vitelline duct obliteration
Patent omphalomesenteric duct	Complete failure of vitelline duct obliteration
Rotation	
Malrotation	Failure of rotation of the proximal midgut; distal midgut rotates 90 degrees clockwise
Nonrotation	Failure of stage 2 rotation (see Fig. 100.18)
Reverse rotation	Rotation of 90 degrees instead of 270 degrees
Proliferation	
Duplication	Abnormal proliferation of intestinal parenchyma
Intestinal Atresia and Stenosis	
"Apple-peel" atresia	Coiling of proximal jejunum distal to the atresia around the mesenteric remnant
Duodenum	Lack of recanalization
Small and large intestine	Vascular "accident"
Anorectum	Disturbance in hindgut development
Enteric Nervous System	
Hirschsprung disease	Failure of migration of ganglion cells; microenvironment changes
Intestinal neuronal dysplasia	Controversial
Pseudo-obstruction	Multifactorial (see Chapter 126)
Miscellaneous	
Intestinal epithelial dysplasia	Abnormalities of the basement membrane
Microvillus inclusion disease	Defective protein trafficking and abnormal cytoskeletal and microfilament function
Other Genetic Defects	
Congenital chloride diarrhea	Abnormal Cl^--HCO_3^- exchange in ileum and colon (see Chapter 103)
Congenital glucose or galactose malabsorption	Absence of Na^+-glucose cotransporter for glucose and galactose (see Chapter 104)
Congenital lactase deficiency	Decrease in lactase-phlorizin hydrolase (see Chapter 103)
Congenital sodium diarrhea	Defective sodium-proton exchange (see Chapter 103)
Congenital sucrase/isomaltase deficiency	Abnormal intracellular transport, aberrant processing, and defective function of sucrase or isomaltase (see Chapter 104)
Cystic fibrosis (CF)	Defective CF transmembrane conductance regulator (see Chapter 59)

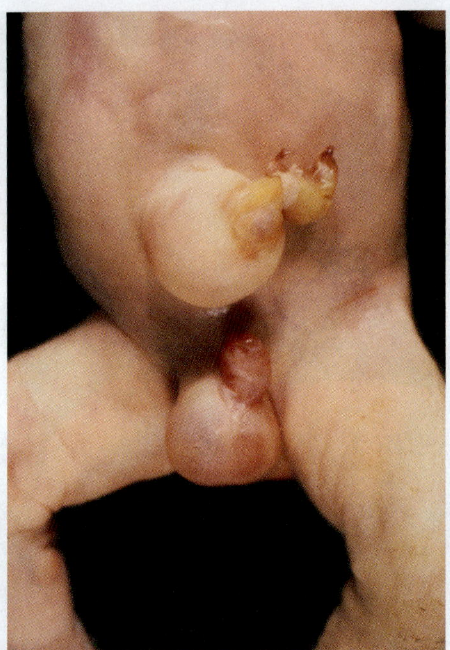

Fig. 100.15 Newborn with omphalocele. Note the translucent saclike structure with its attached umbilical cord.

*O*mphalocele, *E*xstrophy of the bladder, *I*mperforate anus, and *S*pinal (OEIS) defect. Musculoskeletal, cardiovascular, and CNS malformations can also occur.[23,24]

Prenatally, increased levels of maternal serum AFP suggest the possible presence of an omphalocele. US during pregnancy allows the diagnosis of this abdominal wall defect in most infants by the end of the first trimester, which may allow for karyotyping or amniocentesis if required.[25,26] A fetus with omphalocele is at high risk for intrauterine growth restriction, premature delivery, and fetal death.[27] The best survival has been shown to be in isolated cases, and the worst in those with associated chromosomal abnormalities.[19]

Fetal management, including possible termination of pregnancy in cases of severe chromosomal defects, is determined by the physician in consultation with the family. If pregnancy is continued, mode of delivery and provision for care of a child with possibly coexisting anomalies should be considered before labor and delivery. Operative treatment is required in all patients with omphalocele. The size of the omphalocele determines whether a primary repair or delayed primary closure is selected. Negative pressure wound therapy has a low complication and may be an effective therapy for giant omphalocele.[28] Reoperation is necessary in up to 25% of cases of omphalocele, either for stoma reclosure or for subsequent bowel obstruction.

Gastroschisis

Gastroschisis is an abdominal wall defect most commonly located to the right of an intact umbilical cord (Fig. 100.16); rarely, the defect is to the left of the umbilical cord.[29] Incidence of gastroschisis is estimated at 3.1 per 10,000 pregnancies but is higher in mothers younger than age 20.[30] Gastroschisis occurs more frequently in whites and in Hispanic infants than in other races or ethnicities. The cause of gastroschisis is unknown, although several theories have been proposed, including abnormal body wall folding, disruption of the right vitelline artery, and failure of mesoderm formation.[31] In gastroschisis, a sac is absent, and the exposure of the viscera to amniotic fluid and a compromised blood

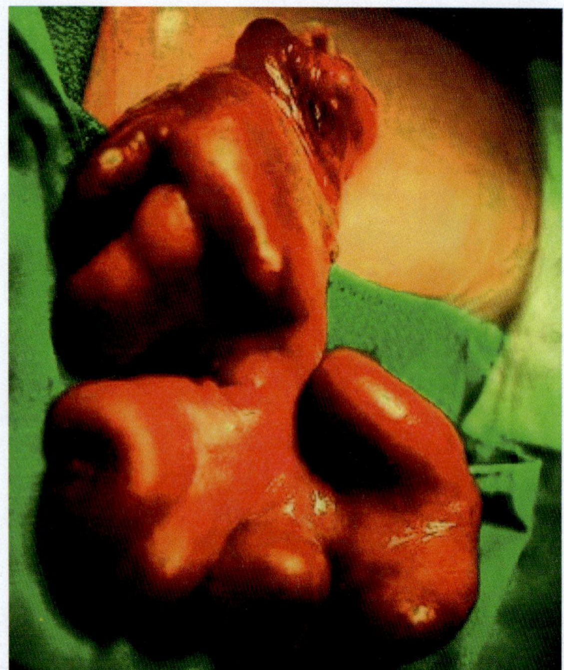

Fig. 100.16 Gastroschisis. In this newborn, there is full-thickness disruption of the abdominal wall and protruding viscera without accompanying peritoneum. (From Feldman's Online Gastro Atlas, Current Medicine.)

supply results in bowel that is edematous, thickened, shortened, and covered in fibrinous exudate.[25] Histologically, the bowel is usually normal. Some affected infants may have an inflammatory peel, or serositis, of the bowel that may make individual bowel loops difficult to distinguish. Some 10%–20% of infants with gastroschisis have associated anomalies (e.g., atresia), and almost all infants with gastroschisis also exhibit malrotation. Other congenital anomalies have been reported in a small number of patients.[23] Prematurity is more common in children born with gastroschisis than it is in children with omphalocele, and extraintestinal anomalies are much more common with omphalocele than they are with gastroschisis. Morbidity and mortality in patients with gastroschisis are largely related to intestinal atresia. Gastroschisis may be complicated by necrotizing enterocolitis, with all its attendant short- and long-term complications.

Increased maternal levels of AFP are suggestive of gastroschisis and omphalocele. Intrauterine growth restriction is frequently observed. In the fetus antenatally diagnosed with gastroschisis, serial US nonstress tests and delivery as close to term as possible are recommended. Early US markers during pregnancy may be able to be used for prognosis of patients with gastroschisis, including likelihood of an atresia.[32]

Gastroschisis requires immediate operation to cover the viscera and prevent desiccation of the tissues. It is necessary to examine the entire bowel in cases of gastroschisis, owing to the intestinal atresias associated with this defect. In most children, the gastroschisis can be closed primarily, but if this is not possible, a silo can be used to provide a protected and moist environment while waiting for the viscera to reduce. For the child with significant intestinal atresia as an associated complication of gastroschisis, bowel exteriorization and secondary closure are often preferred. Most infants require special management and careful serial inspection of the bowel soon after delivery. Use of a spring-loaded silo to cover the bowel may assist with bowel decompression, as well as continuous inspection of blood flow.[33] It is crucial to conserve intestinal length in these children. Adhesive SBO is a frequent and serious complication, especially in the first year of life.[34] A multicenter cohort study demonstrated a 97.8% survival with sepsis as the only independent predictor of mortality.[35] A longitudinal cohort study with median follow-up of 18 years found comparable health-related quality of life among adolescents and adults with history of gastroschisis compared to healthy controls. Common gastrointestinal complaints included weekly abdominal pain (14%), gas bloat (36%), difficulty completing a meal (21%), and gastroesophageal reflux (43%).[36]

Omphalomesenteric (Vitelline) Duct Abnormalities

Between 5 and 7 weeks' gestation, the omphalomesenteric or vitelline duct (which connects the embryo to the yolk sac) attenuates, involutes, and separates from the intestine. Before this separation, the epithelium of the yolk sac develops an appearance similar to that of the gastric mucosa. Under normal circumstances, the omphalomesenteric duct becomes a thin fibrous band that fragments and is absorbed spontaneously during the 5th–10th week of gestation. Persistence of the ductal communication between the intestine and yolk sac beyond the embryonic stage may result in several anomalies of the omphalomesenteric duct (Fig. 100.17): (1) a blind omphalomesenteric duct, or Meckel diverticulum (Md); (2) an omphalomesenteric or vitelline cyst, in which the duct is closed at both ends but patent centrally with a cystic dilatation; (3) an umbilical-intestinal fistula (see Fig. 100.17A), resulting from the duct remaining patent throughout its length; and (4) complete obliteration of the duct, resulting in a fibrous cord or ligament that extends from the ileum to the umbilicus as an omphalomesenteric band.[37] In 1%–4% of all infants, some remnant of the embryonic yolk sac is retained, making the omphalomesenteric or vitelline duct the most common site of congenital GI anomaly; lack of expression of the homeobox gene *CDX2* has been implicated in the pathogenesis of these anomalies.[38]

Meckel Diverticulum

Md is an antimesenteric outpouching of the ileum that is usually found within 2 feet of the IC junction (see Fig. 100.17B). It occurs in 1.2%–2% of the population and has a male-to-female ratio of 3:1.[39] Md accounts for 67% of all omphalomesenteric duct remnants.[37] Md is a true diverticulum, containing all three layers of bowel wall: mucosa, muscularis, and serosa.[40] The length of the Md varies from 1 to 10 cm. Ectopic GI mucosa—duodenal, gastric, biliary, colonic, or pancreatic tissue—is present in about 50% of Md, although 1 study of a series of Md demonstrated 27% had ectopic pancreatic or GI tissue.[41] Gastric mucosa accounts for 80%–85% of all Md-associated ectopic tissue (see Fig. 100.17C).

Painless bleeding per rectum is the most common manifestation of Md. Blood in the stool is usually maroon, even in patients with massive bleeding and hypovolemic shock. BRBPR, as might be seen with bleeding from the left colon, is almost never encountered, but melena may be seen in patients with intermittent, less severe bleeding. The cause of bleeding is peptic ulceration secondary to acid production by the ectopic gastric mucosa within the Md; a "marginal" ulcer often develops at the junction of the gastric and ileal mucosae. Although *Helicobacter pylori* has been observed in the gastric mucosa within an Md, a relationship between bleeding from an Md and presence of this organism is unlikely. Despite massive bleeding, death seldom occurs in children because hypovolemia leads to contraction of the splanchnic blood vessels, causing the bleeding to diminish or cease. Also, children rarely have comorbid conditions that compromise their ability to compensate.

Intestinal obstruction is the next most common manifestation of Md and is caused either by intussusception with the diverticulum as the lead point or by herniation through or volvulus around a persistent fibrous cord remnant of the vestigial vitelline

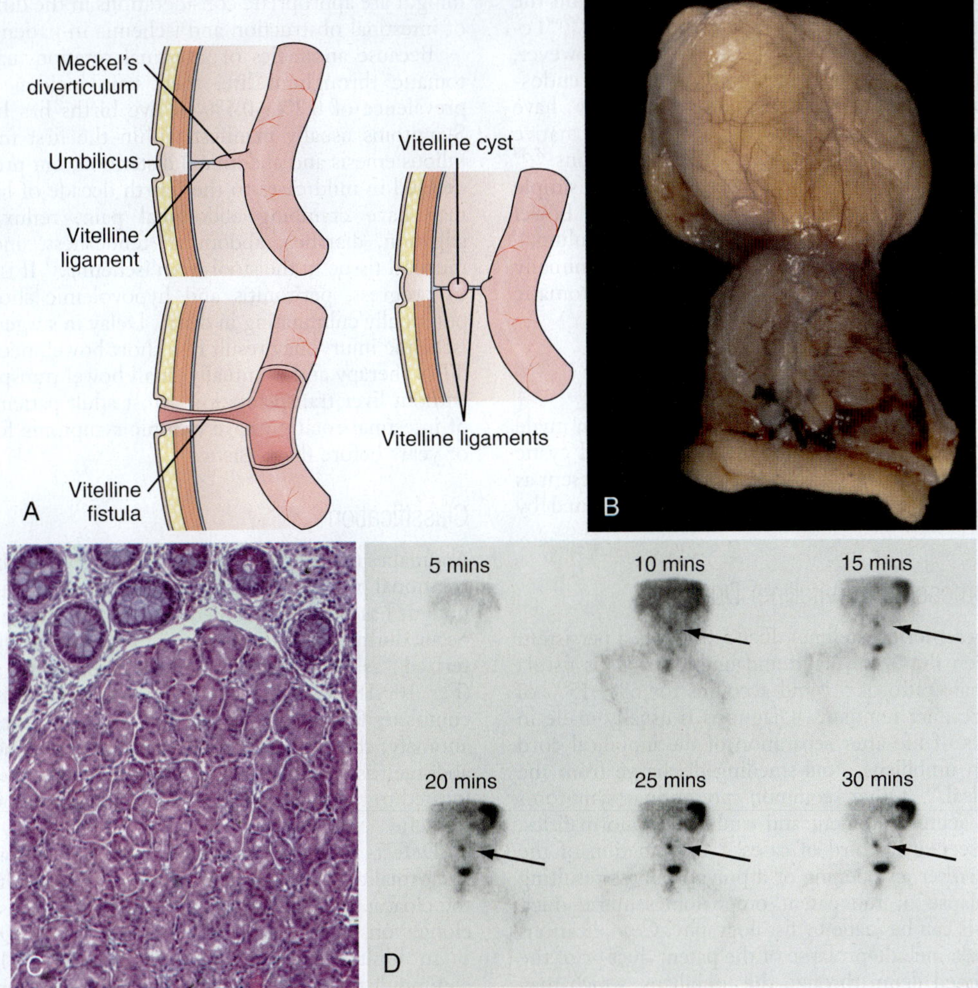

Fig. 100.17 Vitelline duct abnormalities and features of Meckel diverticulum. (A) Schematic representations of a Meckel diverticulum, vitelline cyst, and vitelline fistula. (B) Surgical specimen revealing an outpouching of the ileum (Meckel diverticulum). (C) Photomicrograph showing replacement of small intestinal mucosa by ectopic gastric oxyntic mucosa that lined a Meckel diverticulum (H&E, ×150). (D) Meckel diverticulum scan demonstrating initial uptake of ^{99m}technetium-pertechnetate (*arrows*) by the diverticulum at 10 minutes. ((D), Courtesy Dr. I. Zanzi.)

duct. In children older than age 4, intussusception is almost always secondary to an Md, although Md-related intestinal obstruction may occur at almost any age; volvulus around a vitelline cord has been described in the neonatal period; as with other causes of obstruction, bilious vomiting, and abdominal distention are usually the initial signs.

Diverticulitis of an Md occurs as a result of acute inflammation and is often accompanied by fever, nausea or vomiting, and right lower abdominal pain. Most commonly, affected patients are presumed to have acute appendicitis, and the diagnosis of Meckel diverticulitis is made at exploratory laparotomy. Perforation occurs in about a third of patients with Meckel diverticulitis and may result from peptic ulceration.[42] A chronic form of Meckel diverticulitis (Meckel ileitis) may mimic Crohn disease of the ileum. Rarely, Md has been reported as a predisposing factor to small intestinal malignancy.[43,44]

Md may be an incidental finding.[39] The presence of an Md should always be considered in an infant or child with significant painless rectal bleeding although preoperative identification of a Meckel's diverticulum can be challenging. Standard abdominal plain films, barium contrast studies, and US are seldom helpful in making the diagnosis; rarely, an enterolith (which is often indistinguishable from an appendicolith) or dilated bowel loops with air–fluid level within the Md may be seen on these conventional studies.[45] On CT scan, the Md may present as a tubular blind-ending structure arising from the antimesenteric border of the terminal ileum, although it may be mistaken for a normal small bowel loop.[45] CT enterography has further increased the ability to detect Md.[46] Because bleeding is almost always from ectopic gastric mucosa within the diverticulum, a Meckel scan, which allows imaging of the gastric mucosa, should be the initial diagnostic study (see Fig. 100.17D). Uptake of ^{99m}Tc-pertechnetate is by the mucus-secreting cells of the gastric mucosa, not the parietal cells. The sensitivity and specificity of Md scintigraphy can be improved by administration of pentagastrin, glucagon, or pretreatment with an H_2RA. Pentagastrin increases the metabolism of mucus-producing cells, but this is not the preferred enhancement test because of an associated risk of inducing perforation. Glucagon enhances the study by inhibiting peristaltic dilution and washout of the radionuclide. H_2RAs decrease peptic secretion but not radionuclide uptake, retarding the release of ^{99m}Tc-pertechnetate from the mucus-producing cells. Unfortunately, even an enhanced Meckel study has only 85% sensitivity and 95% specificity, so a negative scan does not necessarily rule out an Md.

When the diagnosis of a bleeding Md is entertained and the Meckel scan is negative, splanchnic angiography and ^{99m}Tc-labeled red blood cell studies may be used; diagnosis, however, is usually made at surgery. Small bowel wireless capsule endoscopy and, in some cases, double balloon enteroscopy have detected an Md in some children with GI bleeding or alternative source of bleeding given Md can coexist with other lesions.[47,48] Once identified, surgical excision can be performed with simple diverticulectomy, wedge-shaped excision, or segmental bowel resection depending on the anatomy of the diverticulum.[49] Balloon-assisted enteroscopy provides alternative minimally invasive endoscopic approaches for treatment of symptomatic Md.[50]

Omphalomesenteric (Vitelline) Cyst

Omphalomesenteric (vitelline) cyst is more common in male subjects and is characterized by a mucosa-lined intestinal cystic mass within the center of a fibrous cord.[37] The cyst may present as a palpable nodule within the umbilicus and be complicated by infection.

Patent Omphalomesenteric (Vitelline) Duct

Patent omphalomesenteric (vitelline) duct represents a persistent connection between the distal ileum and umbilicus. This fistula has a male-to-female ratio of 5:1 and accounts for 6%–15% of omphalomesenteric duct remnants. Diagnosis is usually made in the first few weeks of life after separation of the umbilical cord from the newborn umbilicus. Foul-smelling discharge from the umbilicus is typical.[51] Other common presenting symptoms include SBO, an acute abdomen, and umbilical abnormalities. Ectopic tissue is seen in a third of cases.[52] Examination of the umbilicus reveals either an opening or a polypoid mass resulting from limited prolapse of the patent omphalomesenteric duct. Definitive diagnosis can be made by fistulography. Complications of this type of fistula include prolapse of the patent duct or of the duct and the attached ileum through the umbilicus, which may lead to partial SBO. Prolapse should not be mistaken for an umbilical polyp, because excision of involved tissue might result in perforation. Resection is warranted.[51]

Omphalomesenteric Band

Omphalomesenteric band is diagnosed when the solid cord connecting the ileum to the umbilicus remains intact. This cord may result in SBO from an internal hernia or volvulus.

Vitelline Blood Vessel Remnants

Failure of involution of vitelline blood vessel remnants results in complications similar to those seen with a retained fibrous cord within the peritoneal cavity. Intestinal obstruction occurs when a portion of the small intestine wraps itself around the band. Treatment of all vitelline duct abnormalities is surgical.

Malrotations

Rotation defects result from errors in the normal embryonic development of the midgut, which gives rise to the distal duodenum, jejunum, ileum, cecum, and appendix, as well as the ascending colon and proximal two-thirds of the transverse colon. Aberrations in midgut development may result in a variety of anatomic anomalies, including disorders of rotation and fixation, atresias and stenoses, duplications, and persistence of embryonic structures. Such congenital anomalies may cause symptoms not only in the newborn or neonatal period, but also later in childhood and adulthood. Therefore congenital anomalies of the midgut are appropriate considerations in the differential diagnosis of intestinal obstruction and ischemia in patients of all ages.

Because anomalies of intestinal rotation may remain asymptomatic throughout life, their true incidence is unknown; a prevalence of 0.2%–0.5% of live births has been reported.[53,54] Symptoms usually manifest within the first month of life with bilious emesis and abdominal distention, but presentation may be delayed in mild cases to the fourth decade of life. Older patients may have cramping abdominal pain, reflux, vomiting, constipation, diarrhea, abdominal tenderness, and blood or even mucosal tissue in the stool from ischemia.[55] If ischemia is allowed to progress, peritonitis and hypovolemic shock may develop, potentially culminating in death. Delay in surgery in patients with ischemic injury may result in a short bowel, necessitating chronic TPN therapy and eventually small bowel transplantation, with or without liver transplantation. Most adult patients with anomalies of intestinal rotation have chronic symptoms for several months or years before diagnosis.

Classification

Anomalies of rotation are usually characterized by the stage in the rotational process at which normal embryonic development of the midgut has been interrupted. Most anomalies of midgut rotation occur during the second stage of rotation and have been characterized as nonrotation, reverse rotation, and malrotation (Fig. 100.18). Of these, nonrotation is most common and reflects complete failure of the second stage of rotation. With this anomaly, the intestinal tract occupies the same position in the abdomen as it does in an 8-week-old embryo; the small intestine is located to the right of the midline, and the colon is positioned to the left.

Defects in the first and third stages of rotation are uncommon. Abnormalities in the first stage are associated with extroversion of the cloaca; abnormalities of the third stage cause failure of cecal elongation, and the cecum remains in the RUQ.

In adults, reverse rotation of the midgut loop is the most commonly diagnosed defect of the midgut. Reverse rotation of the midgut loop is rare, however, and accounts for only 4% of all rotational anomalies. In reverse rotation, the midgut rotates 180 degrees *clockwise* during the second stage of rotation, resulting in a net 90 degrees of clockwise rotation. This may produce either the retro-arterial colon type, in which the colon is located behind the SMA, or the liver and entire colon are on the right side of the abdomen, a so-called ipsilateral type of reverse rotation.

Malrotation of the midgut loop, a developmental anomaly of intestinal fixation and rotation, occurs when the proximal midgut fails to rotate around the mesenteric vessels during the second stage of rotation. The distal midgut still does rotate 90 degrees in a counterclockwise direction in the first stage of rotation at about 5 weeks of gestation, however, with the result that the jejunum and ileum remain to the right of the SMA, and the cecum is situated in the subpyloric region. In this position, the small intestine and cecum now have the potential to twist around the SMA and each other.[54] This is the rotation anomaly in adults most frequently associated with ischemic damage, mandating surgical correction.

Associated Abnormalities

Associated anomalies are seen in 30%–60% of patients with defects in intestinal rotation. Nonrotation of the midgut is a significant finding in patients with omphalocele, gastroschisis, and diaphragmatic hernia. Rotation defects are seen in about 30%–50% of infants with duodenal or jejunal atresia and in 10%–15% of children with intestinal pseudo-obstruction. They are also associated with a variety of other conditions, including Hirschsprung disease (HD), esophageal atresia, biliary atresia,

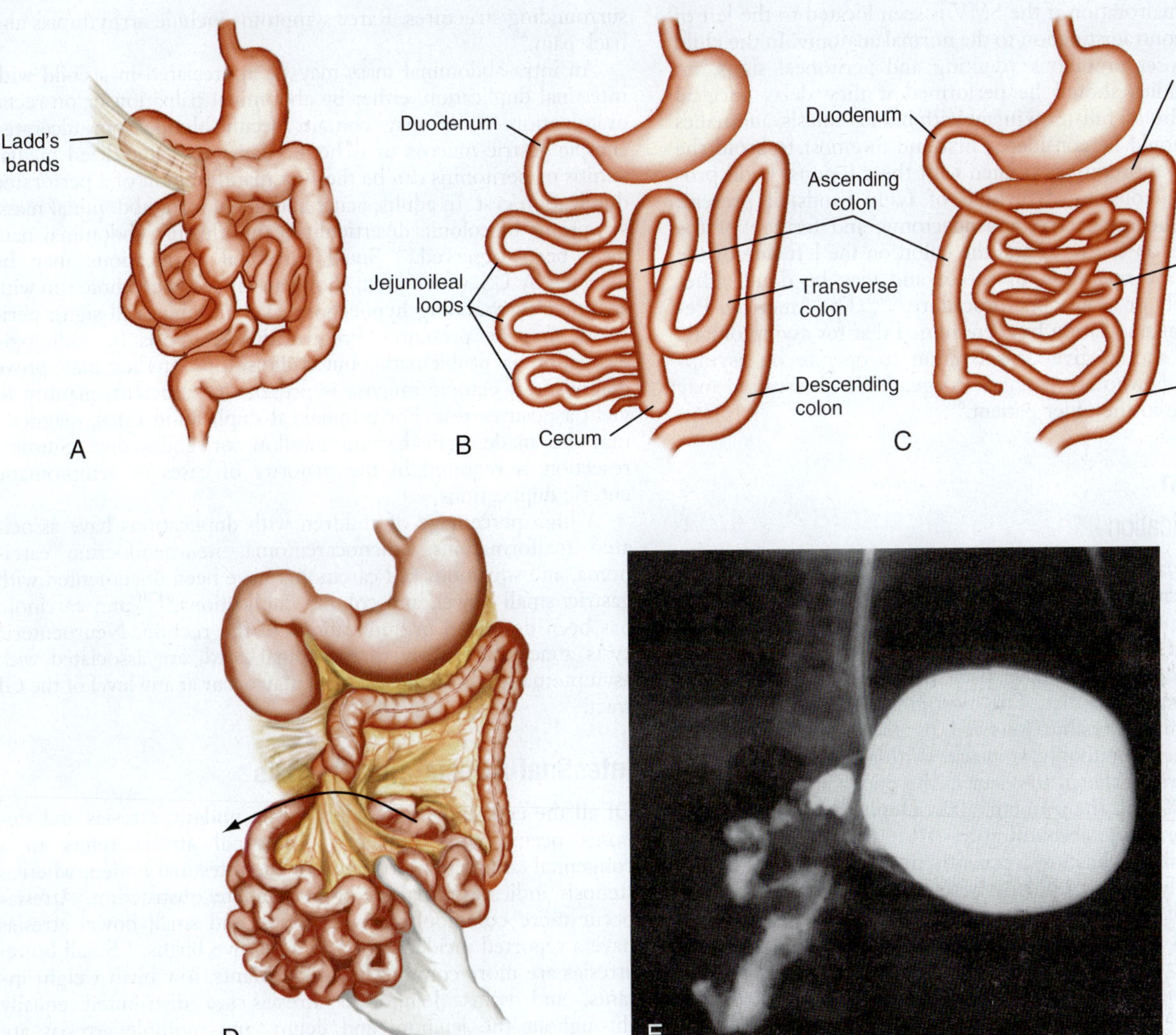

Fig. 100.18 Rotation defects. (A and B) Two examples of nonrotation. (A) Ladd bands are seen crossing the duodenum; some authors would refer to this as a "mixed rotation." (B) In nonrotation, the small intestine is located to the right of the midline, and the colon is to the left of the midline. (C) Reverse rotation. The transverse colon passes behind the duodenum. (D) Malrotation with volvulus characterized by a clockwise twist of the mesentery and strangulation. (E) Radiologic appearance of malrotation depicting the duodenum to the right of the spine, with a volvulus. ((A–C) From Gosche JR, Touloukian J. Congenital anomalies of the midgut. In: Wyllie R, Hyams JS, eds. *Pediatric Gastrointestinal Disease. Pathophysiology, Diagnosis, Management*. 2nd ed. Philadelphia: WB Saunders; 1999. (D) Netter illustration from www.netterimages.com. © Elsevier Inc. All rights reserved. (E) Courtesy Dr. J. Levenbrown.)

annular pancreas, meconium ileus, intestinal duplications, mesenteric cysts, Md, urologic anomalies, and imperforate anus.[56] One recent study demonstrated that patients with omphalocele have a greater risk of developing midgut volvulus.[57] Another study showed that while malrotation occurs with the same frequency among patients with anorectal malformations as in the general population, it is more common in severe malformations (cloaca, covered cloacal extrophy in females, rectoprostatic and recto-bladder neck fistula in males).[58]

Anomalies of rotation can cause acute or chronic intermittent obstruction due to volvulus (see Fig. 100.18D and E). Venous and lymphatic obstruction secondary to volvulus can lead to malabsorption and abnormalities in intestinal motility. Venous obstruction may also lead to ischemic injury of the bowel. Patients may fail to thrive and present with chylous ascites and other symptoms and signs of lymphangiectasia resulting from chronic lymphatic obstruction.

Duodenal obstruction can result from midgut volvulus and peritoneal bands between a malpositioned cecum in the subpyloric region and the peritoneum. These bands, called *Ladd bands*, cross the second or third portion of the duodenum and cause obstruction by intestinal compression or kinking. Ladd bands are an anomaly of peritoneal embryogenesis and persist throughout life.

Diagnosis and Management

If time allows, diagnosis can be made by UGI contrast examination or contrast-enhanced computed tomography and delineation of the site of the duodenojejunal junction. Radiographic findings may suggest malrotation if the SMV is seen located to the left of the SMA, in contradistinction to the normal anatomy. In the child with acute onset of bilious vomiting and peritoneal signs, no diagnostic studies should be performed if they delay surgical intervention. In the full-term infant with bilious emesis, anomalies of rotation should be considered first and foremost to avoid the morbidity and mortality associated with these lesions. Ladd procedure, which consists of division of Ladd bands, if present; widening of the mesentery; appendectomy; and fixation of the small intestine on the right and the colon on the left side of the abdomen, is the operation of choice and may be done either laparoscopically or as an open procedure.[59,60] The American Pediatric Surgical association has determined that for asymptomatic patients, one should give consideration to operate on asymptomatic patients who are younger in age, while observation may be appropriate in the older patient.[61]

Proliferation

Enteric Duplication

Enteric duplications are rare, with an incidence of 1 in 4500 births. The term *duplication* was introduced by Ladd in 1937. Male individuals appear to be more commonly affected, at 60%–80% of cases, and about one-third have associated congenital anomalies. Enteric duplications have been described throughout the entire gastrointestinal tract. The most common GI duplications are in the small intestine followed by the esophagus, colon, rectum, and least commonly, stomach. Within the small intestine, duplications are estimated to occur in the duodenum, 2%–12%; the ileum, 44%; and the jejunum, 50%. Duplication of the colon is a rare abnormality, accounting for 4%–18% of all GI duplications. Colonic duplication frequently involves the entire colon but occasionally, several segments of the colon are affected leaving "skip areas" of normal colon; they often involve the cecum.[62,63] Duplication of the rectum is the most common of the large bowel duplications.

Duplications consist of an epithelial lining from some portion of the GI tract and a smooth muscle wall.[40] Enteric duplications are either tubular or spherical; the tubular type communicates with the normal intestinal tract, whereas the spherical type does not. Tubular duplications may join the intestine at one or at both ends of the duplication. Most duplications do not communicate with the adjacent bowel. With the exception of duodenal duplications, duplications occur on the mesenteric side of the bowel, and a common blood supply and muscular coat are shared by the duplicated segment and the adjacent bowel. Duplication cysts may be completely isolated and have their own blood supply. Small intestinal duplications often contain ectopic pancreatic tissue or gastric mucosa; the latter can be diagnosed by ^{99m}Tc radioisotopic imaging.[64]

The etiology of duplications is unclear but may involve a defect in intestinal recanalization. Duplications may present at any age with 60%–80% manifesting in the first 2 years of life. The clinical presentation varies based on size, location, and possible mass effect of the duplication. Small cystic duplications can be the lead point of an intussusception. Larger tubular duplications can accumulate secretions, dilate, and cause obstructive-type symptoms. Duplications that contain gastric epithelium may secrete acid which can result in ulceration and present with GI bleeding[65] or perforation; rarely heterotopic gastric mucosa contains *H. pylori*. Other modes of presentation include chronic abdominal pain, nausea and vomiting, jaundice, pancreatitis, and an abdominal mass.[40,66,67] Duplication of the rectum may be associated with constipation or diarrhea. Esophageal duplication cysts are usually asymptomatic though they may present with stridor, cough, dysphagia, vomiting, or chest pain due to compression of surrounding structures. Rarer symptoms include arrhythmias and back pain.[68]

An intra-abdominal mass may be appreciated in a child with intestinal duplication, either by abdominal palpation or on rectal examination. Stool may contain occult blood from ulcerated ectopic gastric mucosa or ischemic damage. Generalized mediastinitis or peritonitis can be the first manifestation of a perforated duplication cyst. In adults, acute abdomen, intra-abdominal mass, symptoms of colonic diverticulitis, and chronic abdominal pain have been observed.[69] Small intestinal duplications may be detected by US, which often shows an inner hyperechoic rim with an outer surrounding hypoechoic layer (double-wall sign); peristalsis may be present.[40] Preoperative diagnosis by radiologic evaluation is problematic, but radioisotope studies may prove diagnostic if ectopic mucosa is present in sufficient quantity to yield a positive test. For esophageal duplication cysts, diagnosis may be made with barium swallow or endoscopy. Surgical resection is required in the majority of cases of symptomatic enteric duplications.

A high percentage of children with duplications have associated malformations. Adenocarcinoma, neuroendocrine carcinoma, and squamous cell carcinoma have been documented with gastric, small bowel, and colonic duplications,[64,70] and carcinoid has been described in duplications of the rectum. Neuroenteric cysts attach posteriorly to the spinal cord, are associated with asymptomatic hemivertebrae, and may occur at any level of the GI tract.

Intestinal Atresia and Stenosis

Of all the congenital anomalies of the midgut, atresias and stenoses occur most frequently. Intestinal atresia refers to a congenital complete obstruction of the intestinal lumen, whereas stenosis indicates a partial or incomplete obstruction. Atresias occur more commonly than stenoses, and small bowel atresias have a reported incidence of 1 in 1500 live births.[71] Small bowel atresias are more common in black infants, low birth weight infants, and twins. Jejunoileal atresias are distributed equally throughout the jejunum and ileum, and multiple atresias are found in up to 20% of children. Colonic atresia occurs infrequently and accounts for less than 10% of all atresias.

In the duodenum, atresia results from failure of recanalization of the solid stage of duodenal development, whereas in the remaining small intestine and colon, atresia is the result of intestinal ischemia. Evidence of a vascular "accident" is noted in 30%–40% of infants with atresia; proposed mechanisms include volvulus, constriction of the mesentery in a tight abdominal wall defect like gastroschisis, internal hernia, intussusception, and obstruction with perforation. Jejunoileal atresia may follow maternal use of ergotamine or cocaine taken during pregnancy and is also associated with congenital rubella. Atresias may also result from low-flow states and placental insufficiency[71]; in such cases, evidence of a vascular accident will be absent. Absence of fibroblastic growth factor 10 may also result in intestinal atresia.[72] In familial cases of jejunoileal atresia, there is probably a disruption of a normal embryonic pathway, making this type of atresia a true embryologic malformation rather than an acquired lesion.[73]

Duodenal obstruction may result from atresia (40%–60%), stenosis (35%–40%), or an intestinal web (5%–15%); 80% of these atresias are contiguous with or distal to the ampulla of Vater, and virtually all webs are within a few millimeters of the ampulla. Atresias may be multiple. The incidence of duodenal obstruction varies, ranging from 1 in 10,000 to 20,000 live births. About 25% of patients with duodenal atresia are born preterm. Stenosis most often results from extrinsic duodenal obstruction from an annular pancreas. Other anomalies that may cause duodenal obstruction in children with malrotation are Ladd

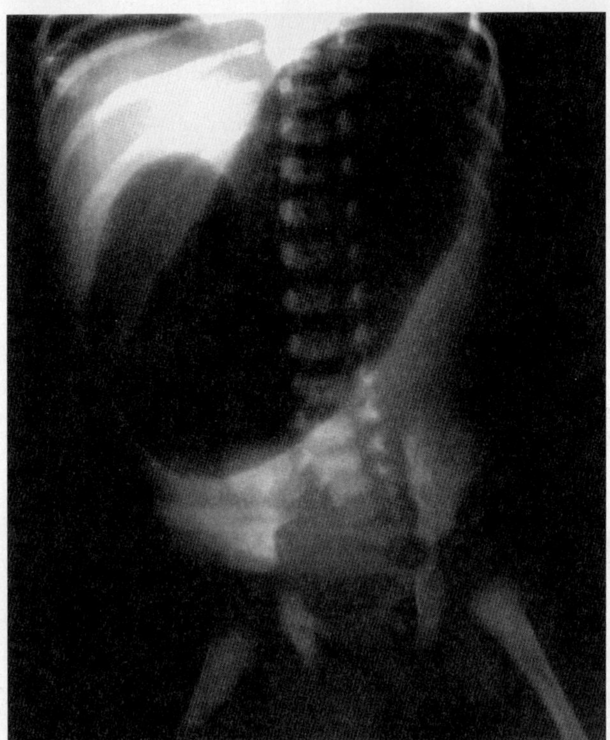

Fig. 100.19 Plain film of the abdomen showing a "double bubble," typical of duodenal atresia. The larger bubble is the gastric bubble; the smaller is the duodenal bubble. (Courtesy Dr. J. Levenbrown, Manhasset, New York.)

bands, an anterior or preduodenal portal vein, or aberrant intramural pancreatic tissue.

Clinically, the presentation is that of a proximal intestinal obstruction with bilious vomiting on the first day of life, usually without abdominal distention. With gastric dilatation, the epigastrium may appear to be full by inspection and palpation. Excessive retention of gastric bile-stained fluid is typical. Duodenal obstruction is easily diagnosed by abdominal films revealing a typical "double bubble" sign with a paucity of small intestinal air (Fig. 100.19). Mothers of infants with duodenal obstruction often have polyhydramnios, and US of the uterus may even demonstrate a double bubble in the unborn fetus. Vomiting, abdominal distention, delayed meconium passage, and jaundice are more frequent with jejunoileal than duodenal atresia.[74] UGI series may reveal the classic windsock sign which may be seen when a duodenal web results in an intraluminal diverticulum.[40]

The classification system of Grosfeld and colleagues comprises five different types of jejunoileal and colonic atresias (Fig. 100.20).[75] In the "apple-peel" atresia or "Christmas tree" deformity (type IIIb), proximal atresia with wide separation of the bowel loops is associated with absence of the distal SMA. The distal ileum receives its blood supply by retrograde perfusion through the ileocolic artery. Type IIIb atresias account for less than 5% of all atresias. Atresias are far more common than stenoses, with a frequency ratio of 15:1. With the exception of multiple atresias and perhaps the apple-peel atresia, heredity appears to be of little significance in most cases.

Roughly 50% of children with duodenal atresia have associated malformations. Of this group, 30% have Down syndrome.[74] Major anomalies occur less frequently with jejunoileal atresias and colonic atresias than with duodenal atresia. The most common anomalies are malrotation, volvulus, and gastroschisis, all of which can cause intestinal ischemia in utero.[76] Extragastrointestinal anomalies associated with atresias include cardiovascular, pulmonary, and renal malformations and skeletal deformities. Prematurity is common, ranging in incidence from 25% with ileal atresias to 40% with jejunal lesions; 50% of babies with multiple atresias are born prematurely. If the obstruction occurs beyond the ampulla of Vater, bilious or feculent vomiting with abdominal distention is seen. The presence of meconium in the colon is uncommon at surgery, but variable amounts may be noted. With distal obstruction, abdominal films may demonstrate multiple dilated air-filled bowel loops. If perforation has occurred in utero, extraluminal air, and intraperitoneal calcifications or calcifications within the scrotal sac may be present, suggesting meconium peritonitis. A "soap-bubble" appearance of the ileum may suggest meconium ileus (cystic fibrosis). Air-fluid levels are rarely seen in meconium ileus. Prenatal US findings in jejunoileal atresia include dilated bowel and polyhydramnios.[77]

Considerations in the differential diagnosis of distal bowel obstruction include small intestinal and colonic atresias, meconium ileus, HD, and meconium plug with or without small left colon syndrome. In small left colon syndrome, the descending and sigmoid colon are narrowed, usually with a caliber transition at or near the splenic flexure. Typically, neonates with small left colon syndrome are born to mothers with gestational diabetes and may experience resolution of obstruction without operation. Contrast studies of the colon are helpful in making a proper diagnosis. An upper GI contrast study may provide additional important information.

Surgery is required to relieve the intestinal obstruction in the atretic or narrowed segment. Postoperative complications include fluid and electrolyte disorders, sepsis, anastomotic leak, adhesive bowel obstruction, nutritional and feeding problems from diarrhea due to short bowel and small bowel failure, and failure to thrive.

Anorectum

Anorectal malformations comprise a wide spectrum of diseases that can involve the male and female anus and rectum as well as the urinary and genital tracts.[78] Anorectal malformations occur in 1 in 4000–5000 newborns and are more common among boys and in children with Down syndrome.[79]

During normal development, after appearance of the urorectal septum, migration of the primitive anus down the posterior wall of the cloaca may occur. Some experts postulate that a craniocaudal fusion of the lateral urorectal ridges occurs from the walls of the cloaca. Migration of the anus is completed when the urorectal septum reaches the perineum. Anorectal malformations during the 4th–12th weeks of gestation are believed to result from failure of migration of the anus and excessive fusion. Vascular accidents, maternal diabetes, and maternal ingestion of thalidomide, phenytoin, and trimethadione have all been proposed causes. Defective development of the dorsal cloaca has also been implicated,[80] and distal 6q deletions have been reported in sacral or anorectal malformations.[81] Alteration in Shh signaling may also play a role in producing abnormal notochord development and sacral or anorectal malformations.[82,83] Anorectal malformations may occur with higher frequency in infants born after in vitro fertilization.[84]

Different types of anorectal malformations are illustrated in Fig. 100.21. Anorectal malformations are divided into low (infra- or translevator), high (supralevator), and intermediate categories. A functional and practical classification of these malformations, the Wingspread classification, is summarized in Table 100.3A. The classification in Table 100.3B is designed, according to Pena,[85] to increase the physician's awareness of the possibility that these lesions are present as well as to establish therapeutic priorities (e.g., need for colostomy).

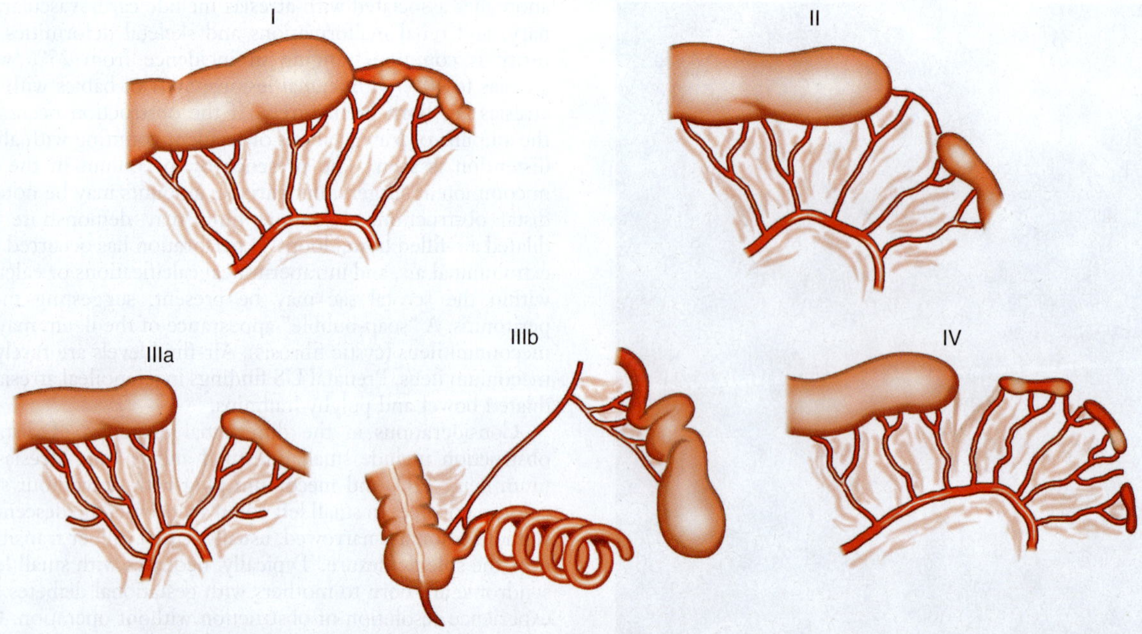

Fig. 100.20 Classification of jejunoileal atresias. *Type I,* Mucosa and submucosa form a web or intraluminal diaphragm, resulting in obstruction. A defect in the mesentery is not present, and the intestine is not shortened. *Type II,* The dilated proximal intestine has a bulbous blind end connected by a short fibrous cord to the blind end of the distal intestine. The mesentery is intact, and the overall length of the small bowel is not usually shortened. *Type IIIa,* The defect in type IIIa is similar to that in type II in that both types have blind proximal and distal ends. In type IIIa, however, complete disconnection exists. In addition, a V-shaped mesenteric defect is present. The proximal blind end is usually markedly dilated and not peristaltic. The compromised intestine undergoes intrauterine absorption, and, as a result, the intestine is shortened. *Type IIIb,* In addition to a large defect of the mesentery, the intestine is significantly shortened. This lesion is also known as *Christmas tree deformity* because the bowel wraps around a single perfusing vessel like the tinsel coil wrapped around a Christmas tree; it is also called an *apple-peel deformity*. The distal ileum receives its blood supply from a single ileocolic or right colic artery, because most of the superior mesenteric artery is absent. *Type IV,* Multiple small intestinal atresias are present in any combination of types I to III. This defect often takes on the appearance of a string of sausages because of the multiple lesions. (From Grosfeld JL, Ballantine TVN, Shoemaker R. Operative management of intestinal atresia and stenosis based on pathologic findings. *J Pediatr Surg*. 1979;14:368–375.)

Anocutaneous Fistula

In anocutaneous (or perineal) fistula, the rectum traverses normally through most of the anal sphincter, but its lower portion deviates anteriorly and ends as a perineal cutaneous fistula anterior to the center of the external anal sphincter. This anomaly is similar in the male and female child and is the least severe of all anorectal defects; associated urologic defects are uncommon (10%). All patients achieve bowel control after proper surgical treatment. Examination of the perineum may demonstrate features indicative of a perineal fistula, including a prominent midline skin ridge ("bucket-handle" malformation) and a subepithelial midline raphe fistula having the appearance of a black ribbon owing to its meconium content. Surgery consists of a simple anoplasty, usually done without a protective colostomy.

Rectourethral Fistula

In rectourethral fistula, by far the most frequent anorectal malformation in male children, the rectum descends through a portion of the pelvic floor musculature but focally deviates anteriorly and communicates with the posterior urethra. This fistula may end in either the lower posterior (bulbar) or upper posterior (prostatic) urethra.[85] Prenatal echogenic calcifications within the bowel (due to a mixture of meconium and urine) should suggest an anorectal malformation with rectourinary fistula and bladder outlet obstruction.[86] Children with prostatic urethral fistulas more commonly have sacral and urologic defects (60%) than children with bulbar prostatic fistulas (30%). About 85% of children with rectourethral bulbar fistula achieve fecal continence after repair, compared with 60% of children with rectoprostatic fistula.

Rectovesical Fistula

In rectovesical fistula, the most proximal anorectal defect in male children, the rectum opens into the bladder neck. These malformations are associated with significant urologic defects (90%), and only 15% of children achieve bowel control after surgical repair.

Vestibular Fistula

In vestibular fistula, the most common anorectal defect of female children, the rectum opens into the vestibular bulb of the clitoris. The vestibular bulbs are erectile structures situated on either side of the vulvovaginal orifice. The rectum and vagina share a thin common wall. About 30% of affected children have associated urologic defects, and 90% of these achieve bowel control after surgery. In the case of vaginal fistula, the rectum opens in the lower or, less frequently, the upper half of the vagina.

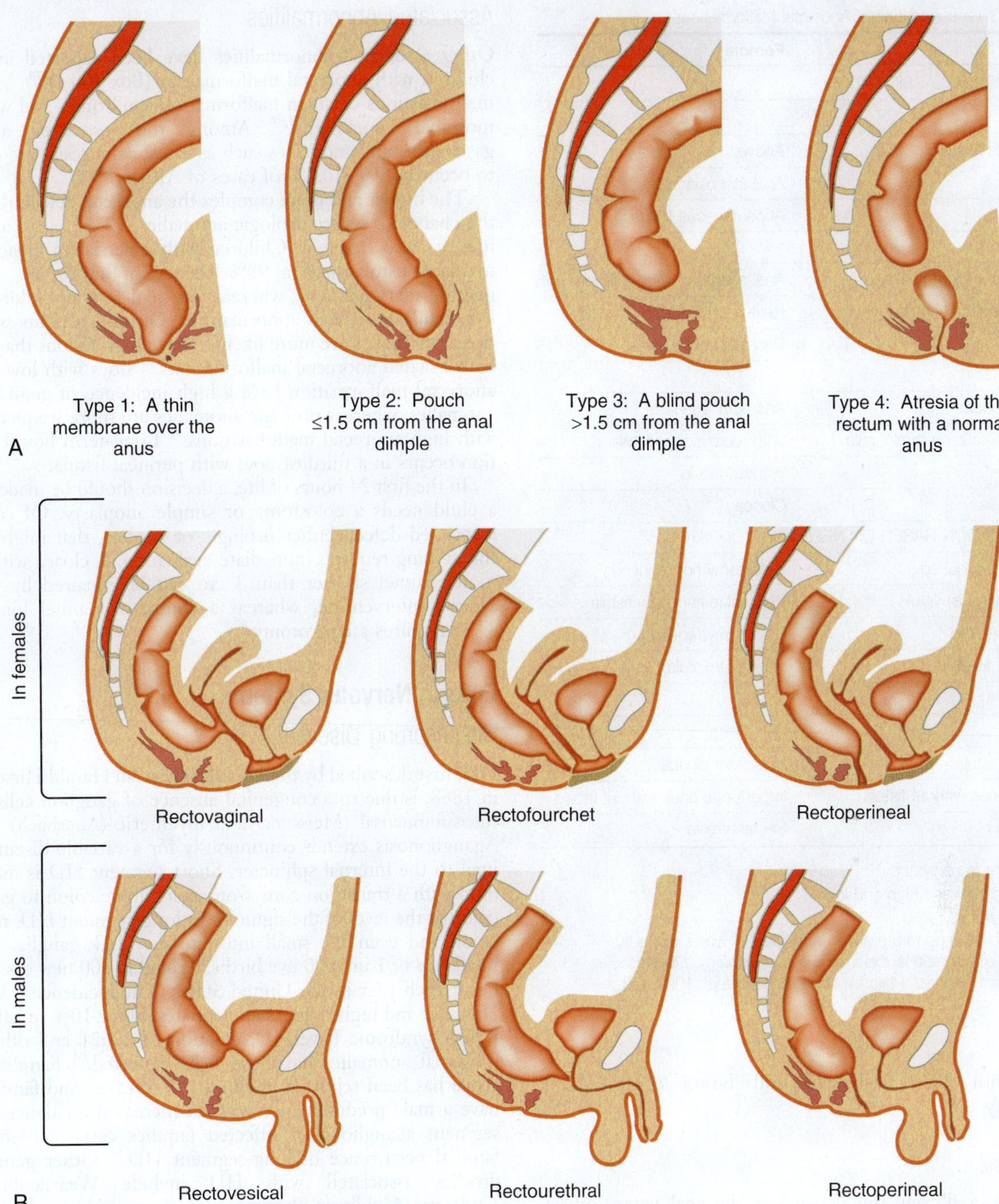

Fig. 100.21 Anorectal malformations. (A) Types of imperforate anus. (B) Types of associated fistulas. (Netter illustration from www.netterimages.com.

Anorectal Agenesis (Imperforate Anus) Without Fistula

In anorectal agenesis, the rectum ends blindly without a fistula approximately 1–2 cm above the perineum. Sphincter function is usually preserved, with 80% of these patients achieving bowel control after surgery. Some 50% of children with imperforate anus have Down syndrome. Conversely, 95% of children with Down syndrome who have anorectal malformations will have this specific type of defect.

Rectal Agenesis (Atresia)

Rectal agenesis occurs more frequently in female than in male children and consists of complete (atresia) or partial (stenosis) interruption of the rectal lumen between the anal canal and the rectum. On inspection of the perineum, the anus appears normal, but an obstruction can be found 1–2 cm above the mucocutaneous junction of the anus. Sphincter function is normal in these patients, and associated urologic defects are rare. Prognosis is

TABLE 100.3 Classifications of Anorectal Malformations

Male	Female
A. WINGSPREAD CLASSIFICATION	
Low[a]	
Anocutaneous fistula	Anovestibular fistula
Anal stenosis	Anal stenosis
	Anocutaneous fistula
Intermediate[b]	
Anal agenesis without fistula	Anal agenesis without fistula
Rectobulbar urethral fistula	Rectovaginal fistula
	Rectovestibular fistula
High[c]	
Anorectal agenesis	Anorectal agenesis
With rectoprostatic urethral fistula	With rectovaginal fistula
Without fistula	Without fistula
Rectal agenesis	Cloaca
B. CLASSIFICATION BASED ON NEED FOR COLOSTOMY[85]	
Colostomy not required	Colostomy not required
Perineal (cutaneous) fistula	Perineal (cutaneous) fistula
Colostomy required	Colostomy required
Rectourethral fistula	Vestibular fistula
Bulbar	
Prostatic	
Rectovesical fistula	Persistent cloaca
Imperforate anus without fistula	Imperforate anus without fistula
Rectal atresia	Rectal atresia

[a]Low: infra-, or translevator.
[b]Intermediate: between high and low.
[c]High: supralevator.
(B) From Pena A. Imperforate anus. In: Wyllie R, Hyams JS, eds. *Pediatric Gastrointestinal Disease. Pathophysiology, Diagnosis, Management*. 2nd ed. Philadelphia: WB Saunders; 1999:499.

excellent, with 100% achieving full bowel control after anorectoplasty.

Anal Stenosis

Anal stenosis, a fibrous ring located at the anal verge, causes constipation and gives the stool a ribbon-like appearance. Response to dilation or surgical disruption is excellent.

Persistent Cloaca

In the complex defect of persistent cloaca, the rectum, vagina, and urethra are fused into a single common channel that opens into one perineal orifice situated at the site of what should be the opening of the normal urethra. Prognosis depends on the intactness of the sacrum and the length of the common channel. Prognosis is better in children with a shorter common channel (<3 cm) than in those with a common channel longer than 3 cm; the latter have a higher incidence of urologic anomalies.[87] Associated urologic problems are an important consideration with persistent cloaca; urologic emergencies from obstructive uropathy are common, and hydrocolpos may compress the opening of the ureters, resulting in bilateral megaureters and massive vesicoureteral reflux.

Associated Abnormalities

Other associated abnormalities have been reported in 70% of children with anorectal malformation (Box 100.1).[78,79] Anorectal malformations occur in malformation syndromes and with chromosomal anomalies.[79,88] Among the associated anomalies, gastrointestinal anomalies such as intestinal atresias are estimated to occur in 5%–10.7% of cases of ARMs. [89–91]

The higher and more complex the anorectal defect, the greater the chance of severe urologic anomalies (72%); sacral abnormalities are also frequent. Children with a persistent cloaca or rectovesical fistula have a 99% chance of having an associated genitourinary anomaly, whereas less than 10% of children with a low fistula have such abnormalities. Overall, patients with additional anomalies are more likely to have high lesions than patients with isolated anorectal malformations.[79] Boys with low and high anorectal malformation have a high incidence of genital and GI anomalies, whereas urologic anomalies are more frequent in girls with high anorectal malformations.[92] Long-term bowel dysfunction occurs in a third of boys with perineal fistula.

In the first 24 hours of life, a decision should be made whether a child needs a colostomy or simple anoplasty. Of course, an associated defect, either urologic or cardiac, that might be life-threatening requires immediate evaluation. A cloaca with a common channel shorter than 3 cm can be repaired by posterior sagittal intervention, whereas a common channel longer than 3 cm requires a laparotomy.[87]

Enteric Nervous System

Hirschsprung Disease

HD, first described by the Danish physician Harald Hirschsprung in 1888, is due to a congenital absence of ganglion cells in both the submucosal (Meissner) and myenteric (Auerbach) plexuses. Aganglionosis extends continuously for a variable distance proximal to the internal sphincter. Short-segment HD is most common with a transition zone from aganglionic colon to ganglionic colon at the level of the sigmoid. In long-segment HD, the entire colon and even the small intestine may lack ganglia. With an incidence of 1 in 5000 live births,[93] roughly 700 new cases of HD occur each year in the United States. The incidence is lowest in Hispanic and highest in Asian neonates. Some 10% of babies with Down syndrome have HD; deletion of 17q21 and other chromosomal anomalies have also been reported.[94] Familial occurrence has been reported in about 7% of cases, and familial cases have a male predominance with an increased incidence of long-segment aganglionosis. Affected families carry a high risk of familial occurrence of long-segment HD.[95] Other genetic syndromes associated with HD include Waardenburg-Shah syndrome, Goldberg-Shprintzen syndrome, Mowat-Wilson syndrome, and Bardet-Biedl syndrome.[96] Known factors that influence familial recurrence include the occurrence of HD in a genetic syndrome, the presence of HD in one or more family members, and characteristics of the proband, including the length of involved GI segment, the proband's gender, and the gender of the at-risk baby. Four subcategories of HD are recognized: In 80% of individuals, aganglionosis is restricted to the rectosigmoid; in 15%–20%, the aganglionosis extends proximal to the sigmoid; in 5%, aganglionosis affects the entire colon; and rarely, aganglionosis extends into the small bowel and sometimes even causes total intestinal aganglionosis.[97] HD is seen most commonly in full-term infants but on occasion does occur in premature births. Approximately 90% of patients with HD are diagnosed in the neonatal period with diagnosis beyond 3 years of age being rare.[98–100] In the short-segment type, a 4:1 male preponderance is observed, and in the long-segment type, the ratio is reduced to about 2:1. Short-segment HD accounts for nearly 90% of cases in

BOX 100.1 Common Abnormalities Associated With Anorectal Malformations

CARDIOVASCULAR

Atrial septal defect
Dextrocardia
Pulmonary stenosis
Tetralogy of Fallot
Ventricular septal defect

CENTRAL NERVOUS SYSTEM

Aqueductal stenosis
Cerebral atrophy
Microcephaly
Myelomeningocele
Teratoma

CHROMOSOMAL ABNORMALITIES

Trisomy 13
Trisomy 18
Trisomy 21

CRANIOFACIAL

Cleft palate
Epicanthal folds
Low-set ears
Potter facies
Simian creases

GASTROINTESTINAL

Duodenal atresia
Esophageal atresia
Malrotation
Tracheoesophageal fistula

GENITOURINARY

Ambiguous genitalia
Cryptorchidism
Multicystic dysplastic kidney
Renal agenesis

MALFORMATION ASSOCIATIONS

VATER complex (*V*ertebral defects, *A*nal atresia, *T*racheoesophageal fistula with *E*sophageal atresia, *R*adial and renal anomalies)
VATERL complex (*V*ertebral, *A*nal, cardiac, *T*racheal, *E*sophageal, *R*enal, and *L*imb anomalies)

MALFORMATION SEQUENCES

Caudal regression syndrome

MALFORMATION SYNDROMES

Cat's-eye syndrome
Opitz syndrome
Potter syndrome type 1

MUSCULOSKELETAL

Abnormal rib number
Deformed or reduced number of sacral vertebrae
Dislocated hip
Hemisacrum
Hemivertebra
Micrognathia
Omphalocele
Polydactyly

RESPIRATORY

Choanal atresia
Diaphragmatic hernia
Hypoplastic lungs
Subglottic stenosis

Data adapted from Cho S, Moore SP, Fangman T. One hundred three consecutive patients with anorectal malformations and their associated anomalies. *Arch Pediatr Adolesc Med*. 2001;155:587–591.

childhood, long-segment HD accounting for the remainder. It is rare that ultrashort-segment HD manifests in the pediatric population, but it does explain certain cases of chronic constipation that come to attention in adulthood (Table 100.4).

Pathogenesis

Two pathogenetic mechanisms have been proposed for HD: failure of migration of neural cells and alteration of the colonic microenvironment. Genetic, vascular, and infectious factors, including the intestinal microbiome, are invoked to explain these alterations.

Failure of Migration

Between the 5th and 12th weeks of gestation, premature arrest of the craniocaudal migration of vagal neural cells will result in HD. Recent work has demonstrated that abnormal proliferation, differentiation, and migration of the neural-crest-derived cells underlie the development of HD.[101,102]

Colonic Microenvironment Changes

A basic defect in the microenvironment necessary for migration, development, and survival of ganglion cells has been postulated. Levels of various substances such as laminin, nicotinamide adenine dinucleotide phosphate-diaphorase, and neural cell adhesion molecules, as well as other polypeptides, have been shown to be reduced in the aganglionic segment. Some investigators have postulated that an alteration in the extracellular matrix with decreased concentrations of laminin and collagen IV constitutes a barrier to neurotrophin 3, thereby impairing neuroblastic migration and colonization. Neurotrophin 3 promotes survival of sympathetic and sensory neurons in vitro and supports growth and survival of differing subsets of neurons. Nitric oxide synthase is reduced in the aganglionic segment in HD, explaining the failure of relaxation of the affected colonic segment. Potassium voltage channels have been noted to be deficient in HD.[103] ENS progenitor cells have been isolated in the aganglionic gut region of HD patients.[104]

Genetics

The genetics of HD have now been characterized.[15] Inheritance of the disease can be autosomal dominant, autosomal recessive, or polygenic. Penetration of mutations is generally low and depends on the extent of aganglionosis in affected family members. *RET* (*RE*-arranged during *T*ransfection) and *EDNRB* (endothelin receptor type B) are two common genes that regulate survival, differentiation, migration, and proliferation of neural crest-derived cells and have been implicated in causation of HD.[105] Mutations in more than 10 genes have been identified, but nearly all patients have a coding or noncoding mutation in the *RET* gene.[93] *RET* mutation penetrance is incomplete and sex dependent. It appears that the mutation, although increasing the odds of a child having HD, is not predictive of any specific abnormality.

TABLE 100.4 Genes Involved in Hirschsprung Disease

Gene	Chromosome Location	Inheritance	Phenotype	Penetrance of HD Trait
RET	10q11.2	AD	HD	70% (male), 50% (female)
GDNF	5p13	AD	HD	Low
NTN	19p13	AD	HD	Low
SOX10	22q19	AD	WS4	80%
EDNRB	13q22	AR/AD	WS4/HD	Low
EDN3	20q13	AD	WS4/HD	5%
ECE1	1p36	AD	HD, CFD, CD	Low
ZFHX1B (SIP1)	2q22	AD	MCA-MR	60%
PHOX2B	4p12	AD	CCHS	20%
TCF4	18q21	AD	Epileptic encephalopathy	Low

AD, Autosomal dominant; *AR*, autosomal recessive; *CCHS*, congenital central hypoventilation syndrome; *CD*, cardiac defect; *CFD*, craniofacial defect; *HD*, Hirschsprung disease; *MCA-MR*, multiple congenital anomalies–mental retardation syndrome; WS4/HD, combination of Shah-Waardenburg syndrome with Hirschsprung disease (see Box 100.2).

Data from Amiel J, Sproat-Emison E, Garcia-Barcelo M, et al. Hirschsprung disease, associated syndromes and genetics: a review. *J Med Genet*. 2008;45:1–14.

RET, a proto-oncogene that codes for a receptor tyrosine kinase protein, is a major susceptibility gene in HD and maps to chromosome 10q11.2. More than 100 mutations of this gene have been identified in patients with HD.[94] Identified gene mutations currently account for only about half of all cases of HD, but it is recommended that *RET* exon 10 mutation analysis be done in all children with HD[15]; germline *RET* mutations can also cause multiple endocrine neoplasia type IIA (MEN-IIA). Although test results will be negative in the vast majority of cases, the significance of identifying MEN-IIA mutation carrier status for that individual and family appears to justify such testing.[94]

Congenital birth defects are found in 5%–33% of patients with HD.[94] Although HD usually occurs as an isolated event, in 30% of patients, it may be part of a syndrome (Box 100.2). Current recommendations for genetic screening include consideration of testing of RET among patients with nonsyndromic HD and referral for screening for specific genes associated with the syndromic phenotype of HD.[99]

Clinical Features

Most children with HD should be diagnosed in the newborn nursery. Any full-term infant who does not pass meconium within the first 48 hours of life should be suspected of having this disorder. Frequently, such infants will have abdominal distention and feeding difficulties. They also may have bilious emesis from partial bowel obstruction. Dilation of the empty rectum by the first examiner usually results in explosive expulsion of retained fecal material and decompression of the proximal normal bowel. HD-associated enterocolitis (HAEC) occurs more frequently in the first 3 months of life, in patients with delayed diagnosis, in children with trisomy 21, in children with long-segment involvement, and in patients who have had prior episodes of HAEC; girls and children with a positive familial history are also more frequently affected. Enterocolitis due to ischemia from colonic distention proximal to the aganglionic segment may develop, with secondary infection from colonic bacteria; *Clostridioides difficile* has been isolated in children with this enterocolitis. Cases have also been reported of HD-associated enterocolitis in the aganglionic segment. Mortality rates of up to 30% have been reported for enterocolitis, which remains the major cause of death in HD. Colonic perforation, most frequently involving the cecum and rarely the appendix, may occur even in utero.

BOX 100.2 Some Congenital Anomalies and Syndromes Associated With Hirschsprung Disease

CONGENITAL ANOMALIES

Cardiac (5% of cases)
- Septal defects

Central nervous system (4% of cases)

Distal limbs

Gastrointestinal (4% of cases)
- Meckel diverticulum
- Pyloric stenosis
- Small bowel atresia

Genital (2%–3% of cases)
- Hypospadias

Renal (4% of cases)
- Dysplasia
- Agenesis

Sensorineural

Skin

Syndromes Bardet-Biedl (central obesity, rod-cone dystrophy, polydactyly, mental retardation, hypogonadism, and renal dysfunction)

Congenital central hypoventilation

Goldberg-Shprintzen (distinctive facial features, skeletal and neurologic abnormalities, craniostosis)

MEN-II (medullary thyroid cancer, pheochromocytoma, parathyroid hyperplasia)

Movat-Wilson (characteristic facies, microcephaly, mental retardation)

Piebaldism (hypopigmentation of skin and hair)

Shah-Waardenburg (regional hyperpigmentation, white forelock, bicolored irides, sensorineural deafness)

Smith-Lemli-Opitz (anteverted nostrils, ptosis of eyelids, syndactyly of second and third toes, hypospadias and cryptorchidism in males)

Syndromes with limb abnormalities (metaphyseal dysplasia, McKusick-type—mild bowing of legs, irregular metaphyses, fine sparse hair)

MEN, Multiple endocrine neoplasia.

Data from Amiel J, Sproat-Emison E, Garcia-Barcelo M, et al. Hirschsprung disease, associated syndromes and genetics: a review. *J Med Genet*. 2008;45:1–14.

Most commonly, infants younger than 6 months of age with HD will continue to have variable but significant constipation, punctuated by recurrent obstructive crises or bouts of fecal impaction, often with failure to thrive. The abdomen may be distended with fecal masses, and peristaltic waves may be visible. Anemia and hypoalbuminemia are common. Blood-flecked diarrhea should suggest the presence of enterocolitis, and immediate evaluation should be undertaken. As the child with HD grows older, problems continue and fecal soiling occasionally may occur. An infant with HD who is breastfed may have fewer difficulties with defecation, because the high concentration of lactose in breast milk causes watery stools that are passed more easily. Once breast milk is discontinued, symptoms of HD may worsen.

Diagnosis

The child with symptomatic HD usually demonstrates signs and symptoms of bowel obstruction. The diagnosis may be made by one or a combination of the following tests: contrast enema, rectal biopsy, and anal manometry. Flexible sigmoidoscopy plays a complementary role in diagnosis.

A contrast enema performed on an unprepared colon will show the distal narrowed hypertonic segment of bowel (usually seen best in a lateral projection). The transition zone between the narrowed distal and dilated proximal intestine will be seen in the most common form of HD—the rectosigmoid form (Fig. 100.22A)—but may not be seen with long- or ultrashort-segment intestinal involvement. In ultrashort-segment HD, a radiologic picture indistinguishable from that of functional constipation with dilated bowel extending to the anus is usually seen. The transition zone may not be evident in rectosigmoid HD if the patient has undergone cleansing enemas or colonic irrigation before the study. Although it has been suggested that the transition zone may not be evident in the first 6 weeks of life, it almost always is noted in the neonate with partial bowel obstruction. Contrast enema for the diagnosis of HD among children >1 year of age demonstrates an 83.3% sensitivity and an 82% specificity.[106]

Flexible sigmoidoscopy typically reveals a normal but empty rectum. The dilated proximal bowel, if within reach of the scope, is traversed easily unless there is abundance of feces in the lumen; occasionally stercoral ulcers may be seen.

Anal manometry is a reliable method by which the gastroenterologist can make the diagnosis of ultrashort-segment HD. The normal physiologic response to rectal distention is relaxation of the internal anal sphincter, which is smooth muscle. In HD, however, rectal distention fails to induce internal sphincter relaxation (see Fig. 100.22B). Sufficient volumes of air must be used to stimulate rectal distention for a reliable study. A false-positive result is most commonly due to a capacious rectum in a child with constipation or megacolon, in whom balloon distention may not stimulate the reflex. Up to 20% of normal children have a falsely absent reflex, especially if they are premature or of low birth weight. Internal sphincter relaxation in response to rectal distention is strong evidence against HD.

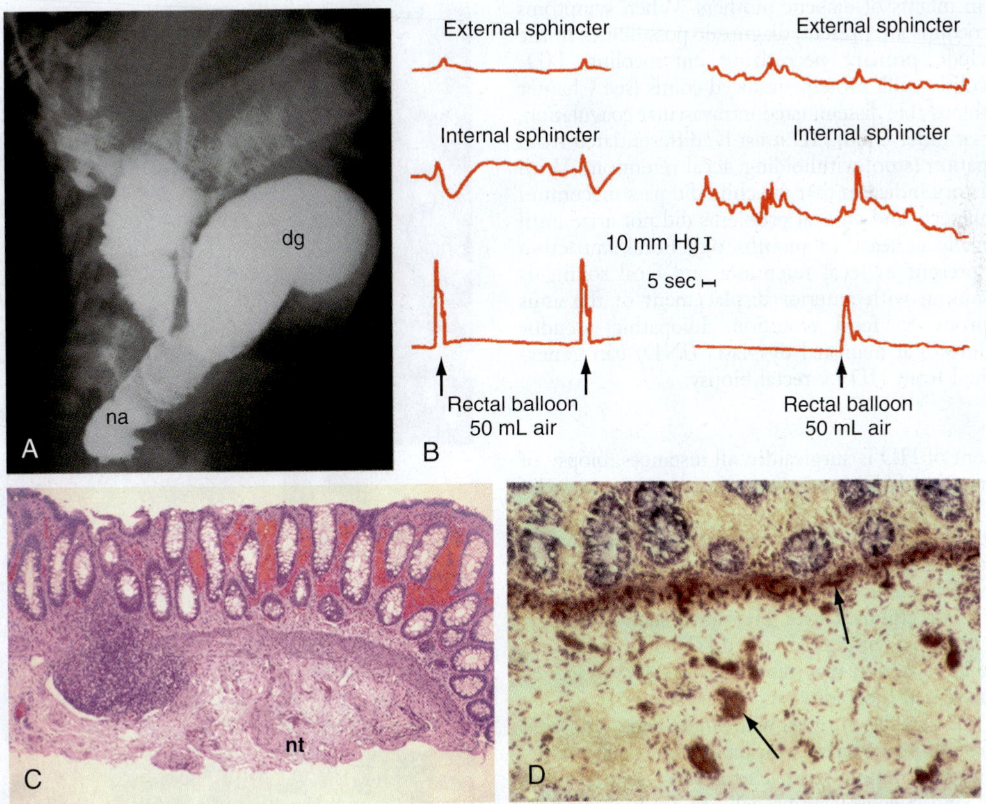

Fig. 100.22 Hirschsprung disease. (A) Film from a barium enema examination showing transition zone between narrowed distal aganglionic segment (*na*) and proximal dilated ganglionic segment (*dg*). (B) Anal manometry. Left tracing illustrates normal function. In the right tracing, note lack of relaxation of the internal sphincter on rectal distention in a patient with Hirschsprung disease. (C) Photomicrograph of a rectal suction biopsy specimen showing the absence of ganglion cells and presence of thickened nerve trunks (*nt*) characteristic of Hirschsprung disease (H&E, ×125). (D) Acetylcholinesterase-positive fibers stained brown (*arrows*) in the muscularis mucosae and lamina propria, ×250. ((A) Courtesy Dr. J. Levenbrown. (B), From Markowitz J. Gastrointestinal motility. In: Silverberg M, Daum F, eds. *Textbook of Pediatric Gastroenterology*. 2nd ed. Chicago: Year Book Medical Publishers; 1988.)

Suction biopsy of the rectal mucosa is the most reliable method of diagnosis, except in patients with ultrashort-segment HD. The biopsy capsule should be placed at least 2 cm above the mucocutaneous junction in infants and 3 cm above the junction in older children to avoid the physiologic hypoganglionic zone. To be certain of the absence of ganglion cells in the submucosal plexus, an experienced pathologist may need to review many serial sections. Hyperplastic sympathetic nerve fibers and proliferating Schwann cells are associated findings (see Fig. 100.22C) but can be absent in total aganglionosis.

Controversy exists regarding the type of stains necessary to make a diagnosis of HD. Because acetylcholinesterase (AChE) is increased in the muscularis mucosae and lamina propria in the aganglionic segment (see Fig. 100.22D), staining for this enzyme has been used for many years. This technique requires fresh, non-formalin-fixed tissue and technical expertise; at best, this stain is confirmatory. False-positive and false-negative reports have been documented in total colonic aganglionosis.[107] Calretinin immunohistochemistry, showing absent calretinin immunoreactive fibers in the submucosa and lamina propria, is replacing the traditional AChE histochemical stain.[108] Calretinin is a calcium-binding protein involved in calcium signaling, which plays an important role in the organization and functioning of the central nervous system. When calretinin immunohistochemistry is positive for HD, it demonstrates a specific staining pattern on formalin-fixed rectal biopsy.

In the neonate, considerations in the differential diagnosis of HD include other causes of intestinal obstruction, such as meconium ileus, ileal atresia, meconium plug syndrome, and the microcolon seen in infants of diabetic mothers. When symptoms and signs of enterocolitis are present, diagnostic possibilities in the neonate also include primary necrotizing enterocolitis, HD-associated enterocolitis, milk protein–induced colitis (see Chapter 11), and sepsis with possible disseminated intravascular coagulation.

In the toddler or older child, HD must be differentiated from functional constipation (stool withholding, fecal retention). With fecal retention, history indicates that the child did pass meconium in the newborn nursery, and clinical problems did not arise until the child was usually at least 18 months old. Fecal impaction almost always is present in fecal retention, and fecal soiling is characteristic. Children with anterior displacement of the anus may be more prone to fecal retention. Idiopathic pseudo-obstruction and intestinal neuronal dysplasia (IND) can generally be distinguished from HD by rectal biopsy.

Management

Definitive treatment of HD is surgical. In all instances, biopsy of the muscularis propria of the bowel is indicated at the time of surgery to assess for the presence of ganglion cells in the myenteric plexus and to delineate the proximal extension of aganglionosis. All full-term babies with a meconium plug in the newborn nursery should be evaluated for HD before discharge, because approximately 15% of children with HD have such a history. Discharge of any newborn with undiagnosed HD and consequent delay in operative intervention may result in a greater frequency of enterocolitis, increased morbidity, and even mortality.

Treatment of HD remains surgical with single-stage transanal endorectal pullthrough procedures, with or without laparoscopy, representing the most common approach for short-segment disease. Both Soave and Swenson transanal procedures are performed with no significant difference in outcomes observed.[109] In a meta-analysis of transanal pullthrough procedures, 14% experienced persistent bowel dysfunction, including 53% with constipation, 29% with HD-associated enterocolitis, and 18% with incontinence or soiling.[110] A recent longer term study of transanal endorectal pullthroughs with 15-year follow-up found that 54% of patients had soiling and 44% developed postoperative HD-associated enterocolitis.[111] Additional studies are being performed to better characterize the urinary, sexual function, and fertility outcomes after pull-through surgery.[112] Overall, long-term prognosis of HD may depend on the length of the aganglionic segment. The exact reasons for these continuing problems remain unclear, but the mechanism may involve an intrinsic abnormality in what is described as normal colon or in the pacemaker system of the colon. Management options among patients with HD and fecal retention or encopresis are often based on patient preference. These may include a combination of oral laxatives, dietary modifications as well as retrograde enema or anterograde continent enema procedures with appendicostomy or cecostomy.[113] Redo surgery may need to be considered in patients with postsurgical recalcitrant strictures, rolled muscle cuff, rectal spur, or aganglionic/transition zone pull-through leading to obstructive symptoms or severe fecal incontinence or constipation.[99,114] ENS progenitors have been isolated from the aganglionic gut region of HD patients, raising the possibility of new treatment targets and hope that ganglion cells may be able to be transferred into aganglionic tissue.[104]

Intestinal Neuronal Dysplasia

IND is a motility disorder that manifests with intestinal obstruction or severe chronic constipation and has a reported incidence of 1 in 7500 newborns.[115] Characteristic biopsy findings include an increased number of enlarged ganglia, neural hypertrophy (Fig. 100.23A),[116] and increased AChE activity in the

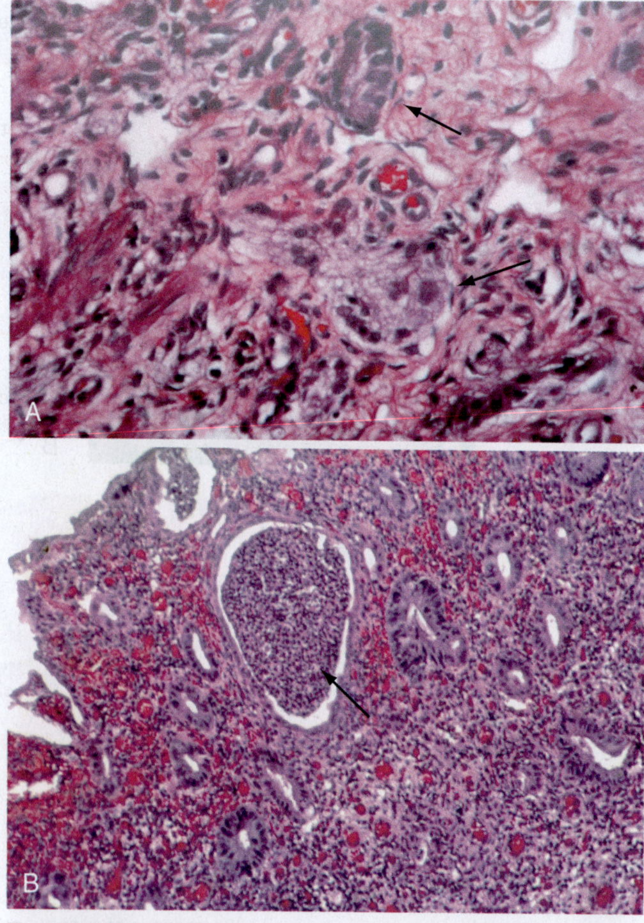

Fig. 100.23 Photomicrographs of a rectal biopsy specimen from a patient with intestinal neuronal dysplasia. (A) Increased number of enlarged ganglia *(arrows)*. (B) Active inflammation of rectal mucosa with a crypt abscess *(arrow)* (A and B, H&E, ×250).

lamina propria and muscularis mucosae. Full-thickness surgical biopsy is often necessary to diagnose IND. IND has been reported as an isolated lesion that especially affects premature infants or infants with a history of formula protein intolerance, ileal stenosis, or small left colon-meconium plug syndrome. Three types of IND have been defined. IND type A usually manifests acutely in the neonatal period with severe constipation and enterocolitis. Biopsy features include mucosal inflammation (see Fig. 100.23B), ulceration with hyperplastic neural changes that are limited to the myenteric plexus, and increased AChE activity in the lamina propria and muscularis mucosae. The submucosal plexus in this type of IND is histologically normal. IND type B, which comprises more than 95% of IND cases, presents as chronic constipation usually during childhood and usually is seen in children between 6 months and 6 years of age who have chronic constipation and megacolon.[93] The diagnosis is made by biopsy showing histopathologic findings, including hyperplastic submucosal ganglia with increased AChE-positive fibers in the muscularis mucosae and lamina propria.[117] Ectopic ganglion cells in the muscularis mucosae and lamina propria have also been described. No changes are seen in the myenteric plexus. Some reports have speculated that some of the morphologic features described in type B are normal age-related phenomena. A third, mixed type of IND has an acute presentation and involves both the submucosal and the myenteric plexuses.

The pathogenesis of IND is controversial. In some patients, it is a congenital malformation, whereas, in others, it is an acquired phenomenon. IND is also seen in association with other syndromes such as neurofibromatosis or MEN-IIB, proximal-segment HD, and congenital anomalies, predominantly of the GI tract.[118] Other associated conditions include cystic fibrosis, microvillus inclusion disease (MID), congenital anomalies, lipoblastomatosis, IBD, anorectal malformations, intestinal malrotation, megacystis-microcolon–intestinal hypoperistalsis syndrome (MMIHS, Berdon syndrome), congenital short bowel syndrome, hypertrophic pyloric stenosis, necrotizing enterocolitis, and Down syndrome.[116] In 1 series of patients, a de novo duplication was detected on chromosome 12 in 1 patient. Therefore IND may not represent a well-defined entity but rather a secondary phenomenon related to age, obstruction, or inflammation.[119] IND can resolve with age. Treatment is similar to that of chronic constipation, with some severe cases requiring surgery, including sphincterotomy, diverting colostomy, or colectomy.[93]

There has been a study comparing the clinical features of HD and IND which demonstrated that patients with HD were more likely to present with symptoms in the neonatal period, have delayed meconium clearance, fail to thrive, and have other acute complications such as entercolitis or acute abdominal obstruction. In contrast, patients with IND were more likely to be diagnosed at a significantly older age with chronic constipation as the predominant symptom.[120]

Chronic Intestinal Pseudo-Obstruction

Chronic intestinal pseudo-obstruction (CIPO) is a rare and severe motility disorder characterized by recurrent or continuous symptoms of intestinal obstruction in the absence of a fixed obstructive lesion (see Chapter 126). CIPO accounts for 15% of cases of chronic intestinal failure in children. Most cases are idiopathic although congenital forms may represent new mutations, and some occur secondary to systemic disease, including myxedema, Duchenne muscular dystrophy, hypothyroidism, hypoparathyroidism, celiac disease, Chagas disease, and mitochondrial disorders.[93]

The pathophysiology of primary CIPO can be neuropathic or myopathic, depending on whether the abnormality lies with the enteric neurons, ICC, or smooth muscle, respectively. Neuropathic CIPO is often due to degenerative loss of enteric neurons or to an inflammatory neuropathy within the enteric ganglia and/or nerve processes.

In any age group, the clinical picture tends to be dominated by abdominal pain and distension (80%), which are particularly severe during acute episodes of pseudo-obstruction. The diagnostic work-up for CIPO consists of ruling out mechanical causes of bowel obstruction, identifying any underlying diseases, excluding drug-induced CIPO-like conditions, and understanding the pathophysiologic features which may provide prognostic information or direct management. Intestinal manometry can be useful to delineate the pathophysiologic (neuromuscular) mechanisms involved in CIPO and to differentiate mechanical from functional causes.[121]

Patients with CIPO are often malnourished from malabsorption and insufficient food intake. Patients who can tolerate oral nutrition should be encouraged to take small, frequent meals (5–6 per day), with an emphasis on liquid calories and protein intake. In the most severe cases, TPN is necessary to maintain nutritional support and an adequate level of hydration. Pyridostigmine, an acetyl cholinesterase inhibitor, increases acetylcholine at the neuromuscular junction promoting intestinal contractions and may be beneficial in CIPO.[122]

Miscellaneous and Genetic Defects

Microvillus Inclusion Disease

Congenital microvillus atrophy, also known as MID, is an autosomal recessive disorder that may manifest with severe diarrhea shortly after birth and is characterized by atrophy of the intestinal villi, with characteristic electron microscopic findings (see later).[123] Although its prevalence is unknown, MID is reported to be the most common cause of familial intractable diarrhea.[124] A female gender predominance has been observed, and consanguinity is reported in 20% of cases. The incidence of MID may be higher among Navajo Indians and persons from the Middle East; in Navajo Indians, a mutation in MYO5B has been implicated.[125] Defective protein trafficking and abnormal cytoskeletal and microfilament function have been proposed as possible etiologies.[126] A blockage in the transport pathway from the Golgi apparatus leads to fusion of small vesicles and formation of microvillus inclusions.[127] Secretory diarrhea is severe, with intolerance to oral feeding and unresponsiveness to most therapeutic modalities. Three variants of MID are recognized: congenital, the most frequent and severe, manifesting within the first week of life; late-onset, starting at 6–8 weeks; and atypical, with either early or late onset. MVID may occur with a less clinically severe presentation.[128]

The wall of the small intestine is paper-thin in MID. The mucosa of the duodenum and small bowel is characterized by villus atrophy, hypoplastic or normal crypts, and normal or decreased cellularity of the lamina propria (Fig. 100.24A). Absence of the brush border membrane is demonstrated by lack of linear staining with PAS, CEA, Rab11, and CD10.[129,130] These stains also visualize the microvillus inclusions on light microscopy. Gastric biopsies have shown focal disruption of the gastric glandular architecture. Colonic biopsies show characteristic cytoplasmic vacuoles and PAS/villin-positive cytoplasmic inclusions.[131]

Evaluation by electron microscopy reveals characteristic ultrastructural abnormalities of the microvillus membrane, including disruption or absence of the brush border membrane, shortening and absence of the microvilli, and microvillus inclusions (see Fig. 100.24B). Although these lesions are most commonly noted in biopsy specimens of the small intestine, microvillus inclusions may also be seen in specimens from the rectum and colon.

TPN must be used to prolong survival. Secretory diarrhea persists but becomes less voluminous. Small bowel transplantation is the only hope to improve the quality of life and long-term prognosis in children with MID.[132,133]

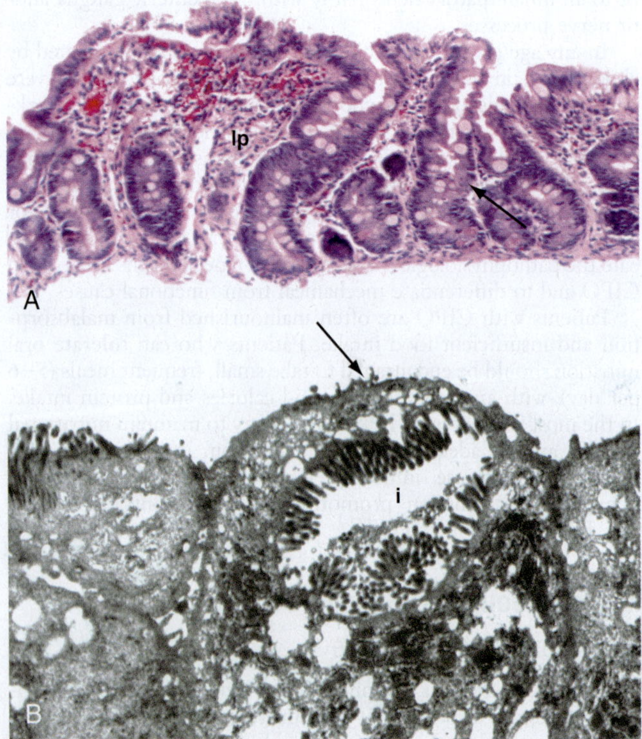

Fig. 100.24 Photomicrographs of duodenum from a patient with microvillus inclusion disease. (A) Villus atrophy with crypt hyperplasia (*arrow*) and decreased cellularity of the lamina propria (*lp*) (H&E, ×250). (B) On electron microscopy, lack of or shortened microvilli (*arrow*) and a cytoplasmic inclusion (*i*) composed of a vesicle lined by microvilli can be seen (×15,000.). (Courtesy S. Teichberg, PhD, Manhasset, New York.)

Intestinal Epithelial Dysplasia

Intestinal epithelial dysplasia (IED), also known as tufting enteropathy, is a congenital enteropathy with early onset, severe intractable diarrhea, and characteristic microscopic findings.[134] In IED, there is a variable degree of villus atrophy. Surface epithelial cells are arranged in tufts with a round apex. Tufts can also be seen in the colonic mucosa. In the basement membrane, heparin sulfate proteoglycan is increased, and laminin is faint and irregular.[134] Tufts result from nonapoptotic epithelial cells that are no longer in contact with the basement membrane. These epithelial cells have an abnormal expression of E-cadherin and do not contain inclusions on electron microscopic examination. Epithelial cell adhesion molecule (EpCAM) stabilizes claudin-7 in IECs, and HAI-2 regulates the cell surface serine protease matriptase, a known modifier of intestinal epithelial physiology.[135] Both EpCAM and SPINT mutations have been strongly associated with IED.[136,137] Lack of staining for EpCAM is noted on intestinal biopsies of patients with IED.[138,139]

The diarrhea is secretory, malabsorption is intractable, and growth is impaired. Several cases of IED have been associated with congenital anomalies.[134] Nonspecific punctate keratitis is observed in more than 60% of patients with IED. Small bowel transplantation is the recommended therapy for IED.

Congenital Glucose and Galactose Malabsorption

Familial glucose and galactose malabsorption is transmitted as an autosomal recessive trait. Mutations in the *SLC5A1* gene, encoding the sodium-glucose cotransporter located in the brush border of enterocytes, have been shown to cause the disease (see Chapter 104). More than 300 subjects of diverse origin have been reported worldwide, most of whom are a result of a consanguineous union.[140] Ingestion of any formula that contains glucose or galactose in the newborn period results in severe, life-threatening watery diarrhea. Stools are strongly positive for reducing substances. Neither blood nor white blood cells are present in the stool. Biopsy specimens of the small intestine and colon are normal. Discontinuation of formula containing glucose, galactose, or lactose (lactose is metabolized to glucose and galactose) and institution of a fructose-containing formula with resultant therapeutic benefit are usually sufficient to make a clinical diagnosis of glucose or galactose malabsorption. Diarrhea abruptly ceases and the newborn begins to thrive when fructose-containing formula feedings are substituted for those containing glucose or galactose. Some reports indicate that the severity of the diarrhea from glucose or galactose malabsorption diminishes with age because of the increased capacity of the intestinal flora to metabolize glucose.

Congenital Sucrase and Isomaltase Deficiency

Because sucrose is not a common dietary carbohydrate during the first 6 months of life, watery stools generally do not develop in children with this disorder until sucrose is administered in baby food. An exception to this rule is in the newborn receiving a formula (usually with soy protein or casein hydrolysate) with sucrose as the carbohydrate. Confirmation is by disaccharidase assay of duodenal or jejunal mucosa obtained endoscopically. Congenital sucrase or isomaltase (SI) deficiency, although extremely rare, is the most common congenital disaccharidase deficiency. The condition is known to be highly prevalent (about 5%–10%) in several Inuit populations.[141] SI gene variants coding for disaccharidases with defective or reduced enzymatic activity predispose to IBS.[142] Sacrosidase is an effective and well-tolerated treatment for patients with congenital SI deficiency. Gene testing and clinical trial of sacrosidase may become an alternative to endoscopic biopsies for diagnosis.[143]

Congenital Lactase Deficiency

Congenital absence of lactase is extremely rare. Affected babies receiving a lactose-containing formula develop severe watery diarrhea, which resolves with the institution of a non–lactose-containing formula. Biopsy specimens of the small intestine are histologically normal, but assay for disaccharidases reveals diminished or absent lactase. The onset of severe forms of congenital lactase deficiency is elicited by mutations in the lactase gene that occur in either a compound heterozygous or homozygous pattern of inheritance.[144] Lymphocytic colitis has been demonstrated to be associated with lactase deficiency and may improve with lactase supplementation alone.[145]

Congenital Chloride Diarrhea (Chloridorrhea)

Congenital chloride (CL^-) diarrhea (CCD) is an autosomal recessive disorder of intestinal $Cl^-HCO_3^-$ exchange caused by mutations of the *SLC26A3* gene.[146] Most disease-causing mutations cause folding defects resulting in impaired trafficking of these membrane glycoproteins from the endoplasmic reticulum to the cell surface which may directly affect transport function.[147] The $Cl^-HCO_3^-$ exchange mechanism in the ileum and colon is reversed, and Cl^- is actively secreted, resulting in a Cl^--rich diarrhea (i.e., chloridorrhea). In utero manifestations may include polyhydramnios and bowel dilatation. The baby with CCD is often premature and may present with an ileus or absence of meconium passage. Watery diarrhea with a high stool Cl^- content and low stool pH starts within a few days of birth and is life-long;

dehydration may result, and increased absorption of HCO_3^- may lead to hypochloremic metabolic alkalemia, hyponatremia, and marked hypokalemia. The stool contains no blood, no white blood cells, and no reducing substances. Urinary Cl^- is low. Biopsy specimens of the small intestine and colon are normal. Extraintestinal complications may include chronic kidney disease, hyperuricemia, and spermatoceles as dysfunctional SLC26A3 may be present in various other tissues.[126] Treatment of CCD is fluid and electrolyte replacement. Acid reduction with PPIs has been tried, with variable results. Butyrate and cholestyramine have also been proposed as a possible therapy for CCD.[148]

Congenital Sodium Diarrhea

Congenital sodium (Na^+) diarrhea (CSD) is caused by defective Na^+ or proton exchange.[149] Patients have acidemia and hyponatremia. The stool concentration of bicarbonate and Na^+ are increased. CSD is clinically and genetically heterogeneous.[150] GUCY2C mutations lead to elevated intracellular cyclic guanosine monophosphate levels and could explain the chronic diarrhea as a result of decreased intestinal Na^+ and water absorption and increased chloride secretion indicating a role in the pathogenesis of CSD.[151] A mutation in the *SPINT2* gene encoding the serine protease inhibitor hepatocyte growth factor inhibitor HAI-2 is also associated with a syndromic form of CSD.[152] The mainstay of treatment has included electrolyte, fluid, and nutritional support with TPN through the first year of life; however, more recently, the ability to maintain electrolyte levels through enteral means and avoiding long-term intravenous access has been demonstrated.[153]

Cystic Fibrosis

CF is an autosomal recessive disorder of cyclic adenosine monophosphate chloride transport that is due to a defect in the cystic fibrosis transmembrane regulator (see Chapter 59).

About 10%–15% of newborns with CF present with neonatal meconium ileus or its complications. Meconium ileus occurs when inspissated meconium obstructs the small bowel at the terminal ileum. Meconium plug syndrome may also occur, resulting in colonic obstruction rather than SBO, as is seen with meconium ileus. Antenatally, small intestinal ischemia and perforation may occur, resulting in meconium cyst, intestinal atresia, or meconium peritonitis with intra-abdominal or scrotal calcifications.

Full references for this chapter can be found at https://ebooks.health.elsevier.com.

101 Small Intestinal Motor and Sensory Function and Dysfunction

Christopher K. Rayner, Stuart M. Brierley

IN THIS CHAPTER

Efficient absorption of nutrients and maintenance of orderly aboral movement of chyme and indigestible residues are the most important goals of small intestinal motor and sensory function. Small intestinal motility is also critically important in preventing SIBO (see Chapter 107). This is achieved by the net aboral flow of luminal contents during both the fed and fasting states, probably with the assistance of the gatekeeper function of the ileocecal junction, which prevents backflow of cecal contents.

Optimal progression of luminal contents allows mixing of digested food with intestinal secretions, and contact of the luminal contents with the epithelium. This contact is important for both the sensing of nutrients within the lumen and their absorption, both of which exert feedback control on gastric and small intestinal motor function. This interplay optimizes the rate at which additional nutrients are presented to the absorptive epithelium and minimizes the amount of nutrients lost to the colon. Thus while the net movement of luminal contents along the small intestine is antegrade, retrograde flow also occurs in normal physiological situations over short distances and over longer distances in the setting of emesis. This coordinated motor pattern underscores the versatile modulation of small intestinal motility according to precise physiological needs.

The motor function of the small intestine depends directly on smooth muscle in the intestinal wall, which contains the basic control mechanisms that initiate contractions and regulate their frequency. Overlying these basic control mechanisms are the enteric nervous system (ENS) and the autonomic nervous system (ANS), which also receive input from extrinsic sensory afferents. In addition, a number of hormones modulate the frequency and coordination of small intestinal contractions. Each of these factors plays a role in the motility of the small intestine in health, and dysfunction of each of these components in certain diseases has helped define their discrete roles.

ANATOMY

In adult humans, the small intestine is approximately 3–7 m long and extends from the duodenal side of the pylorus to the ileocecal valve. It is divided into three regions based on structural and functional considerations: duodenum at the oral end, followed by jejunum, and ending with the ileum. These regions exhibit similar motor characteristics, despite some structural and functional differences. Physiologic sphincters, namely, the pylorus and ileocecal valve, have distinctly different motor patterns, permitting them to act as controllers of flow between the antrum and duodenum and between the ileum and colon, respectively. The motor function of the pylorus and stomach are discussed in Chapter 52, motility of the ileocecal region is discussed in Chapter 102, and general anatomy of the small intestine is discussed in Chapter 100. The duodenum is a fixed, largely retroperitoneal structure located in the upper abdomen, and the distal ileum generally is anchored in the right iliac fossa by its attachments to the cecum. The small intestine is mobile within the peritoneal cavity outside of these regions.

NORMAL SMALL INTESTINAL MOTOR AND SENSORY FUNCTION

Smooth Muscle

The wall of the small intestine comprises mucosa (which consists of the epithelium and lamina propria) submucosa, muscularis, and serosa (Fig. 101.1). On its exterior surface the small intestine receives blood, lymphatic and extrinsic nerve supplies via the mesentery. The muscularis is composed of two distinct muscle layers, comprising the inner circular and outer longitudinal layers of smooth muscle that are present in continuity along the entire length of small intestine. Coordinated circular and longitudinal contractions within these layers are responsible for gross small intestinal motility. Another much thinner muscular layer, the muscularis mucosae, is present between the mucosa and submucosa and plays a role in mucosal or villous motility.[1] The muscularis mucosae does not contribute to gross motility and is not considered further in this chapter.

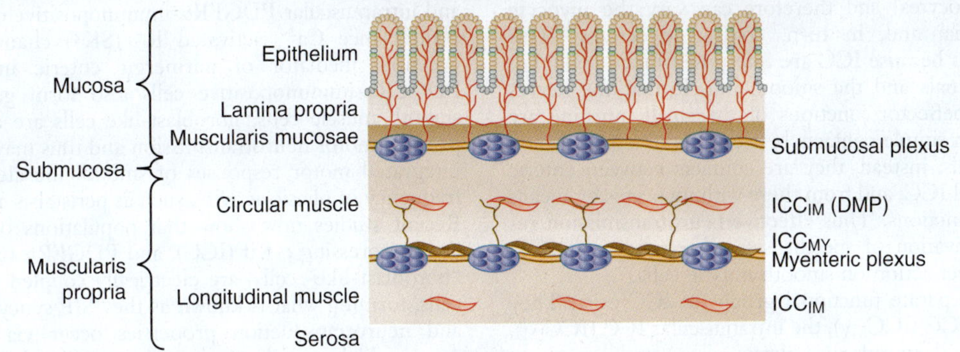

Fig. 101.1 Diagram showing layers and components of the small intestinal wall. *DMP*, Deep muscular plexus; *ICC$_{IM}$*, intramuscular interstitial cells of Cajal; *ICC$_{MY}$*, myenteric interstitial cells of Cajal. (Advice from Dr. Elizabeth Beckett is acknowledged.)

Smooth muscle cells within each muscle layer form a syncytium. Myocytes communicate electrically with each other through physically specialized areas of cell-to-cell contact called *gap junctions*, which are visible by electron microscopy. This intimate contact between adjacent myocytes gives low-resistance electrical contact or coupling among them, enabling them to be excited as a unit. Mechanical connections among myocytes in each layer enable them to function as a contractile unit. Mechanical connections are provided by intermediate junctions at the cellular level and by the dense extracellular stroma of collagen filaments between bundles of smooth muscle cells at the tissue level. Smooth muscle cell bodies are arranged in parallel within each layer, such that the circular muscle layer encircles the lumen, and the longitudinal layer extends axially along the small intestine. Cell bodies in each layer may be controlled independently, and therefore luminal diameter can decrease (circular contraction) and small intestinal length can shorten (longitudinal contraction), alone or in combination.

The myocytes themselves are spindle-shaped cells that derive their contractile properties from specialized cytoplasmic filaments (actin and myosin) and from the attachment of these filaments to cytoskeletal elements. Electron microscopy reveals condensations of electron-dense, amorphous material around the inner aspect of the cell membrane (dense bands) and throughout the cytoplasm (dense bodies). The contractile filaments are arranged in a similar manner to that in skeletal muscle and insert onto the dense bands and bodies approximately in parallel with the long axis of the cell. Thus cell shortening results when the contractile filaments are activated to slide over each other. Most of the Ca^{2+} required for activating the contractile apparatus enters the cells via L-type Ca^{2+} channels (Fig. 101.2). Ca^{2+} entry also can be supplemented to a varying extent by release of Ca^{2+} from the sarcoplasmic reticulum membrane via IP_3 receptor-operated Ca^{2+} channels. IP_3 is generated by phospholipase C, which in turn is activated by G proteins coupled to receptors for excitatory transmitters, G protein-coupled receptors, which are key regulators of intestinal function.[1]

The increased cytoplasmic Ca^{2+} binds to the Ca^{2+} binding protein calmodulin, enabling it to activate myosin light chain kinase, which phosphorylates the 20-kd light chain of myosin (MLC20). Phosphorylation of MLC20 facilitates actin binding to myosin and initiates cross-bridge cycling and development of mechanical force. Phosphorylation of MLC20 is reduced by MLC phosphatase. De-phosphorylation of MLC20 reduces cross-bridge cycling and leads to muscle relaxation. The de-phosphorylation process is under a complex system of hierarchical control, which is important in setting the gain of smooth muscle contractility.[2]

Muscle cells are also nonspecialized mechanosensitive cells and can modify their function in response to forces. They can utilize

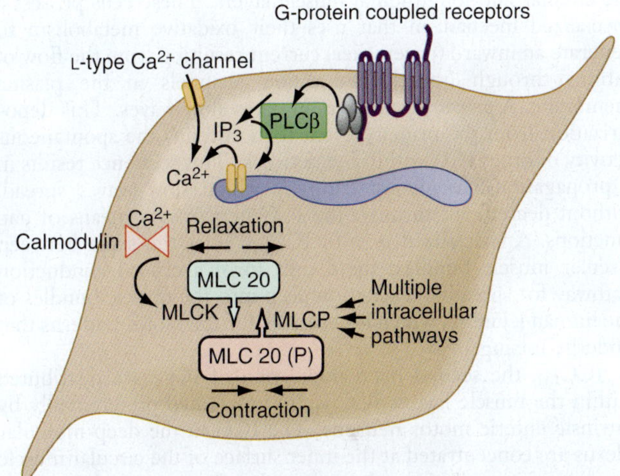

Fig. 101.2 Diagram of a smooth muscle cell showing pathways that lead to contraction and relaxation. See text for details. *MLC20*, 20-kd myosin light chain; *MLCK*, myosin light chain kinase; *MLCP*, myosin light chain phosphatase; *P*, phosphorylated; *PLC*, phospholipase C. (Modified from Sanders KM. Regulation of smooth muscle excitation and contraction. *Neurogastroenterol Motil*. 2008;20(suppl 1):39–53.)

various mechanoreceptors (membrane proteins that detect and convert force into electrical and biochemical signals), and mechanotransducers (membrane proteins that amplify and direct mechanoreceptor responses) to vary their contractile responses.[2] Mechanoreceptors in human jejunal circular muscle cells include the L-type calcium channel $Ca_V1.2$ and the voltage gated sodium channel $Na_V1.5$.[3,4] In mouse small intestine, variants of the transient receptor potential family, TRPC4, TRPC6, and TRPC7 contribute with nonselective cation currents in response to mechanical stimuli, which regulates overall cell excitability.[5,6]

Interstitial Cells of Cajal

Interstitial cells of Cajal (ICC) are specialized cells within the smooth muscle layer that are vital for normal small intestinal motor function. ICC are pleomorphic mesenchymal cells that form an interconnecting network via long, tapering cytoplasmic processes. ICC lie in close proximity to both nerve axons and myocytes, with which they form electrical gap junctions.[3] ICC serve two roles in the control of small intestinal motility: First, they act as pacemakers and generate the electrical slow wave that determines the basic rhythmicity of small intestinal contractions.[4] Second, they transduce both inhibitory and excitatory neural signals to the myocytes[5] and therefore can vary the myocyte membrane potential and, in turn, contractile activity. This transduction occurs because ICC are interposed functionally between nerve terminals and the smooth muscle that the nerves supply. The neuroeffector junctions of the small intestine are more complex than simple contacts between nerve terminals and smooth muscle cells; instead, they are contacts between enteric nerve terminals and ICC, and from there with myocytes by means of electrical gap junctions. Thus effective neurotransmission results from the activation of specific sets of receptors on ICC, rather than by direct action on smooth muscle cells.

At least three separate functional groups of ICC exist. They are the myenteric ICC (ICC_{MY}), the intramuscular ICC (ICC_{IM}), and the ICC in the deep muscular plexus.

ICC_{MY} are the pacemaker cells in the small intestine that trigger the generation of slow waves in the smooth muscle. ICC_{MY} cells form a dense, electrically coupled network within the intermuscular space at the level of the myenteric plexus between the circular and longitudinal muscle layers. These cells possess a specialized mechanism that uses their oxidative metabolism to generate an inward (pacemaker) current resulting from the flow of cations through nonselective cation channels in the plasma membrane. A *primary pacemaker* initiates slow waves. This depolarization from the primary event then entrains the spontaneous activity of other ICC within the network. This sequence results in a propagation-like phenomenon by which slow waves spread, without decrement, through the ICC network by means of gap junctions. A specialized type of ICC_{MY} lines the septa between circular muscle bundles; these cells form a crucial conduction pathway for spreading excitation deep into the muscle bundles of the human jejunum, which is necessary for the motor patterns that underlie mixing.[6]

ICC_{IM}, the second main population of ICC, are distributed within the muscle layers. ICC_{IM} are innervated preferentially by intrinsic enteric motor neurons. The ICC in the deep muscular plexus are concentrated at the inner surface of the circular muscle layer at the region of the deep muscular plexus; they also receive preferential innervation and may be a specialized type of ICC_{IM} in the small intestine.

Both inhibitory and excitatory enteric motor nerve terminals selectively target ICC_{IM}. Their responses are transduced in turn to smooth muscle cells through gap junctions. Inputs from enteric excitatory motor neurons are mediated by muscarinic acetylcholine (ACh) receptors (M_2 and M_3) and NK1 substance P-receptors that result in increased inward currents, thereby causing depolarization. When depolarization reaches the level of the smooth muscle, it increases the opening of L-type Ca^{2+} channels during slow waves, resulting in greater Ca^{2+} entry and more forceful phasic contractions. Inputs from inhibitory enteric motor neurons are mediated by neurotransmitters, including nitric oxide (NO) and vasoactive intestinal polypeptide (VIP), which activate both receptor and nonreceptor mechanisms in ICC_{IM}. The result of these inputs is an increased opening of K^+ channels that, in turn, has a stabilizing effect on membrane potential, reduces Ca^{2+} channel opening, and results in less forceful contractions of the smooth muscle. Therefore the mechanical response of small intestinal muscle to the ongoing slow wave activity depends strongly upon regulation of its excitability by the ENS via ICC_{IM}.

ICC in general play broadly similar roles in the small intestine and colon (for colon, see Chapter 102).[4,5] Absence or inactivity of ICC has been implicated in a number of clinical disorders that manifest as disturbed intestinal motility (see Chapter 126). Recent focus has also centered on involvement of "fibroblast-like cells," which have similar anatomic distributions as ICC, but represent a discrete population of cells. These fibroblast-like cells can be identified by staining with antibodies for platelet-derived growth factor receptor α (PDGFRα), which demonstrates that they are closely associated with both ICC and nerve varicosities. Myenteric and intramuscular PDGFRα-immunopositive cells express small-conductance Ca^{2+} activated K^+ (SK3) channels, which are a potential mediator of purinergic enteric inhibition. Because PDGFRα-immunopositive cells also form gap junctions with smooth muscle cells, fibroblast-like cells are also likely participants in motor neurotransmission and thus may contribute to the integrated motor responses of smooth muscle and possibly the frequency of phasic activity, such as peristalsis and segmentation.[3] Recent studies now show that populations of interstitial cells, those expressing c-Kit (ICC), and PDGFRα (formerly known as "fibroblast-like" cells) are electrically coupled to smooth muscle cells, forming what is known as the "SIP syncytium." Pacemaker and neurotransduction properties occur via ICCs expressing Ano1, which encodes Ca^{2+}-activated Cl^- channels. When activated, Ano1 produces inward currents causing excitatory effects in the SIP syncytium.[7] Altered expression of Ano1 variants in gastric muscles has been linked to human diabetic gastroparesis.[8] The $PDGFR\alpha^+$ cells express the potassium channel Kcnn3, which encodes Ca^{2+}-activated K^+ channels, which when activated result in outward currents and membrane-stabilizing effects in the SIP syncytium. Inputs from enteric and sympathetic neurons regulate Ca^{2+} transients in both ICC and PDGFRα cell types which regulate smooth muscle cells and contractile responses.[7] The transcriptomes of ICCs[9] and PDGFRα cells[10–12] have recently been identified and indicate ICC-specific genes, including *Thbs4*, *Prkcq*, *Kit*, and *Ano1*. In PDGFRα cells the low voltage-dependent T-type Ca^{2+} channel, encoded by the *Cacna1g* gene, has been linked to hyperplasic PDGFRα cells in the intestinal serosa in mouse models of small intestinal obstruction.[11]

Neurons

Neurons that supply the intestine are generally designated either *afferent* or *efferent* functions, depending on the direction in which they conduct information. Information is conducted centrally by *afferent* neurons and peripherally by *efferent* neurons. The small intestine is richly innervated with both intrinsic (enteric) and extrinsic neurons. Enteric neurons have their cell bodies located within the wall of the small intestine and constitute the ENS. Most of these intrinsic enteric neurons have their peripheral terminals within the intestinal wall. However, a separate class of neurons termed *intestinofugal neurons* have cell bodies within the myenteric plexus but have projections from the intestinal wall to prevertebral ganglia (PVG) via extrinsic nerve trunks. Intestinofugal neurons sense and receive information regarding mechanical distension of the intestine and transmit this information to postganglionic sympathetic neurons in the PVG. Overall, these various types of intrinsic enteric neurons greatly outnumber the neurons of the extrinsic supply, which have their cell bodies outside the intestinal wall but projections that end within the intestinal wall. Extrinsic sensory afferent neurons can be classified anatomically according to the location of their cell bodies. Vagal afferents have cell bodies within cranial ganglia and travel via vagal nerves to the CNS, whilst spinal afferents have cell bodies within the dorsal root ganglia and travel via spinal nerve pathways to the CNS (Fig. 101.3). Importantly, the extrinsic *sensory* afferent neurons innervating the small intestine do not belong to either the ANS or ENS. It should be noted that in most texts, the term *afferent* is used interchangeably with *sensory*. However, most sensory information from the small intestine is not perceived at a conscious level. Examples of perceived sensory information include bloating, discomfort, and pain. Extrinsic motor neurons (efferents) do belong to the ANS and connect the CNS with the ENS and, from there, the small intestinal smooth muscle through the ICC. Furthermore, some extrinsic efferent motor neurons terminate directly in the muscle layers. The terms *efferent* and *motor* regarding neural supply are used to describe pathways that conduct signals toward the "effector," in this case the small

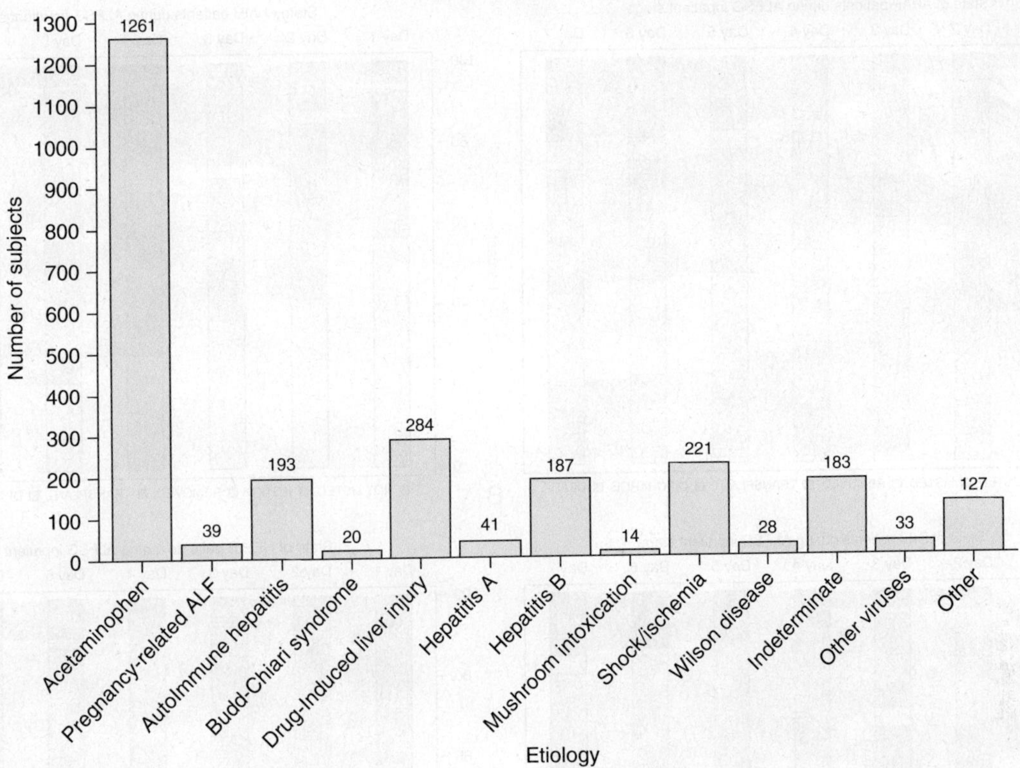

Fig. 97.1 Prevalence of various etiologies of acute liver failure (ALF) in the United States according to enrollment in the ALF Study Group Registry. (Reprinted with permission from Stravitz RT, Lee WM. Seminar: acute liver failure. *Lancet*. 2019;394:869–881.)

screening tests were not included on presentation with ALF. A number of additional etiologies account for small numbers of patients overall (Fig. 97.1) but still present interesting variations on evolution of disease and options for management. Etiologies vary worldwide with APAP being prevalent both in North America and northern Europe, while HBV and hepatitis E virus (HEV) predominate in much of Asia and the developing world, where fewer prescription drugs are available, the use of APAP is infrequent, and herbal supplements are more commonly used.[20]

PHENOTYPES

Early efforts to classify ALF included length of illness as a determining factor. For example, "hyperacute" patients evolved from onset of jaundice to HE in <7 days, "acute" in 7–21 days, and "subacute" in >21 days to 6 months. Each time interval is thought to have a characteristic disease pattern.[21] However, it may be more practical in the current era to group these entities as hyperacute and acute/subacute. Hyperacute etiologies that evolve from start to finish in fewer than 7 days are unique and principally due to APAP overdose and ischemic hepatic injury. Both follow a similar trajectory of very severe aminotransferase elevations, from 2000 IU/L to as high as 40,000 IU/L, associated with low total bilirubin levels, over a 2–3-day illness that peaks in severity by 72–96 hours after onset and subsides in the next 3 days (Fig. 97.2A). Compared to subacute phenotypes, hyperacute etiologies (APAP and ischemia) have better short-term prognosis, with APAP resolving without LT or death in 65% and ischemia in as many as 95% of patients once cardiovascular resuscitation occurs (Table 97.1). By contrast, ALF due to AIH, DILI, and HBV evolve over an average of 2–3 weeks and are associated with much lower aminotransferases and much higher bilirubin levels (Table 97.1, Fig. 97.2B). Liver weights of explants at the time of transplantation are, if anything, increased in APAP from normal weight of 1400–1600 g, to 1700 g or more. By contrast, AIH, DILI, and many HBV explants decreased to 1000 g or less. TFS among subacute etiologies are all <50% and usually <35% if any degree of HE is present.[8,9]

PATHOGENESIS

The cause of severe hepatocyte injury varies by etiology. Several unique cell injury patterns have emerged.[22] APAP and ischemia would appear to involve direct "toxic" hepatocyte injury evoking a secondary inflammatory response. Injury in both APAP and hypoxic injury is centrilobular in location, extending toward portal tracts depending on the severity of injury. Hepatocyte regeneration appears to be rapid and unimpeded except in the most severe cases. Liver failure is associated with >60%–75% necrosis of hepatocytes. By this paradigm, nearly all with less than 50% necrosis should survive. In contrast to APAP and ischemia, liver injury in most other etiologies is slower, and histologically more inflammatory (Fig. 97.3), with disease evolution over 2–4 weeks.[9] Outcomes are poorer overall for the acute/subacute etiologies, including IND ALF (Table 97.1), with many more patients requiring LT.[9] At the time of LT for acute/subacute etiologies, livers frequently are small and shrunken as sufficient regeneration has not taken place. At the same time, the slower evolution allows more time for transplant evaluation, listing, and obtaining an organ offer, so acute/subacute etiologies also have a higher likelihood of successful LT.[9] Precise mechanisms for the hepatocyte damage in acute/subacute ALF have not been definitively identified and are etiology-dependent. This is an area of vigorous research currently in the pursuit of novel therapies that would negate the need for LT.[22]

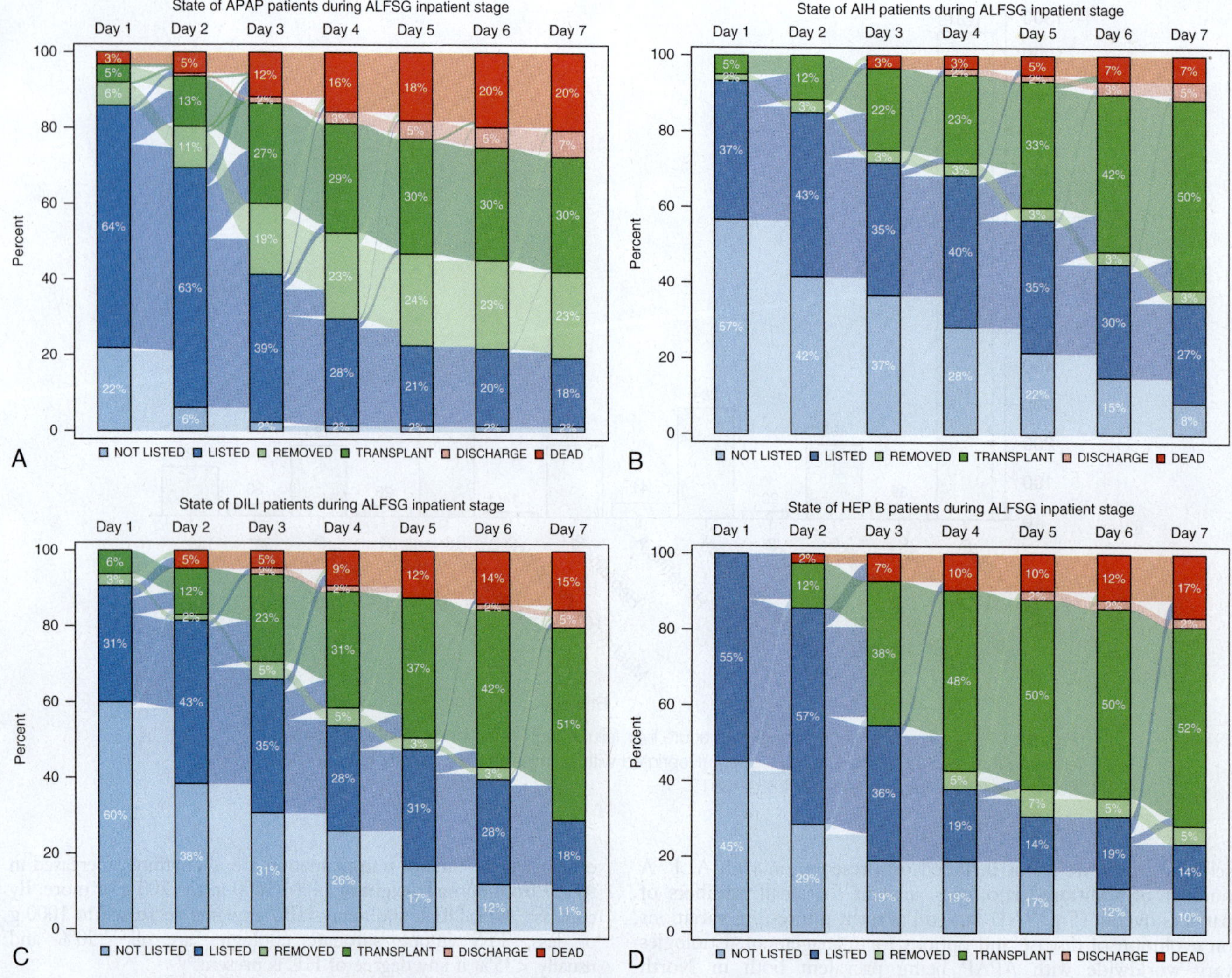

Fig. 97.2 Diagrammatic representation of events by day after registry enrollment/listing according to acute liver failure (ALF) etiology group. (A) Acetaminophen (APAP). (B) Autoimmune hepatitis (AIH). (C) Drug-induced liver injury (DILI). (D) Hepatitis B. Most of the deaths and transplants in the APAP group (A) took place within the first 48 hours, while both deaths and transplants evolved more slowly in the three non-APAP categories (B–D). The figure is restricted to only those patients with a date of listing. (From Reddy KR, Ellerbe C, Schilsky M, et al. Determinants of outcome among patients with acute liver failure listed for liver transplantation in the US. *Liver Transpl.* 2016;22:505–515.)

ETIOLOGIES

APAP remains consistently the most common cause of ALF in North America and most of Europe.[23,24] APAP, approved in Europe and North America as an analgesic and antipyretic in the 1960s and 1970s, is a dose-related hepatotoxin with a narrow therapeutic window, the LD_{50} being about 12 g. While attention was first drawn to intentional (suicidal) overdoses in the United Kingdom and elsewhere, nearly half of all reported incidents of ALF are the result of unintentional overdoses in the pursuit of pain relief or cold symptom management, sometimes referred to as "therapeutic misadventures."[25] There are more than 100,000 calls to U.S. Poison Control Centers and around 4–500 deaths annually due to APAP overdoses. Numerous studies suggest that the bulk of intentional overdoses represent suicide gestures in which the patient admits to the overdose, arrives at an emergency room, and receives *N*-acetylcysteine (NAC), an effective antidote if given within 12–24 hours. By contrast, the unintentional overdose often occurs in the setting of alcohol use disorder and involves ingestion of narcotic/APAP combination medications. Due to the Food and Drug Administration's institution of limits for combination products to no more than 325 mg of APAP/pill in 2014, the incidence of combination overdoses has declined.[26,27] Overall, however, there has not been a major decline in the incidence of APAP ALF over the past two decades.[8]

The development of a definitive test for APAP hepatotoxicity known as the APAP-CYS adduct assay is likely to represent a major advance in identifying patients with APAP ALF. Using high pressure liquid chromatography, APAP hepatotoxicity is proven based on the presence of hepatocyte protein adducts in serum, which represent the reactive APAP metabolite bound to hepatocyte proteins and released into the circulation. While APAP itself has a very short half-life in serum (about 6 hours) and is often undetectable when patients have evolved to ALF, APAP-CYS adducts can be identified in serum up to 9 days after a toxic ingestion.[28–31] A point-of-care assay that would be available in emergency departments should soon be available, since the

98 Hepatic Tumors and Cysts

Alex S. Befeler, Roshani J. Desai

IN THIS CHAPTER

Hepatic mass lesions include tumors, tumor-like lesions, abscesses, cysts, hematomas, and confluent granulomas. Hepatic tumors may originate in the liver—from hepatocytes, bile duct epithelium, or mesenchymal tissue—or spread to the liver from primary tumors in remote or adjacent organs. In adults in most parts of the world, hepatic metastases are more common than primary malignant tumors of the liver, whereas in children, primary malignant tumors outnumber both metastases and benign tumors of the liver. Except for cavernous hemangiomas, benign hepatic tumors are rare in all geographic regions and in all age groups.

MALIGNANT TUMORS

Hepatocellular Carcinoma[1]

Epidemiology

Hepatocellular carcinoma (HCC) is the most common primary malignant tumor of the liver representing 75%–85% of primary liver cancer. It is the fifth most common cancer in men and the ninth most common in women, and it ranks fifth in annual cancer mortality rates.[2]

Information on incidence is derived from an increasing but still limited number of cancer registries, and it is possible to classify countries into broad risk categories only. Moreover, in low human development index countries, especially in sub-Saharan Africa, HCC is underdiagnosed and underreported, in some cases by as much as 50%. Despite these sources of inaccuracy, HCC clearly has an unusual geographic distribution (Fig. 98.1). The incidence of HCC increased considerably in Japan starting in the 1980s, and lesser increases have been recorded in developed Western countries, including North America and Western Europe.[3] Since about 2000, there appear to be declining rates of HCC in Japan, Italy, and France, presumably because of the aging of the cohort of persons infected with HCV and possibly the application of highly effective treatments for HCV.[4] Other European countries continue to have increasing rates of HCC.[4] In contrast, in the United States, HCC is the cancer that has been increasing in incidence most rapidly since 2000, at a time when the incidence of other major cancers such as cancers of the lung, breast, prostate, and colon is decreasing.[5] More recently, the rise in incidence in the United States may be plateauing with the aging of the HCV cohort.[4] Considerable racial and ethnic variation exists in the incidence of HCC in the United States. The incidence among Asians is the highest, almost double that of white Hispanics and more than four times higher than that of non-Hispanic whites.[4]

Migrants from countries with a low incidence to areas with a high incidence of HCC usually retain the low risk of their country of origin, even after several generations in the new environment. The consequences for migrants from countries with a high incidence to those with a low incidence differ, depending on the major risk factors for the tumor in their country of origin and whether chronic HBV infection, if this is the major risk factor, is acquired predominantly by the perinatal or horizontal route (see later and Chapter 81).[6–8]

Men are generally more susceptible than women to HCC. Male predominance is high in the range of two–four-fold in the U.S. and Europe but in some countries in South America and Africa, the male-to-female ratio is closer to 1.[4]

The incidence of HCC increases progressively with advancing age in all populations, although it tends to level off in the oldest age groups after about 75 years of age.[9,6,4] In Chinese and particularly in black African populations, however, the mean age of patients with the tumor is appreciably younger than in other populations. HCC is rare in children.[10,11]

Etiology and Pathogenesis

In contrast to many other malignancies, for which risk factors can only sometimes be identified, the immediate cause of HCC can usually be identified and is most commonly chronic viral hepatitis and other liver diseases that lead to cirrhosis. HCC is multifactorial in cause and complex in pathogenesis. Four major causative factors have been identified (Box 98.1). The differing blend of risk factors in various parts of the world may explain, in part, the diverse biological characteristics of HCC in various populations.[12]

HBV

Some 387 million carriers of HBV exist in the world today, and HCC will develop in as many as 25% of them (see Chapter 81). Chronic HBV infection accounts for up to 80% of HCCs, which occur with high frequency in East Asian and African

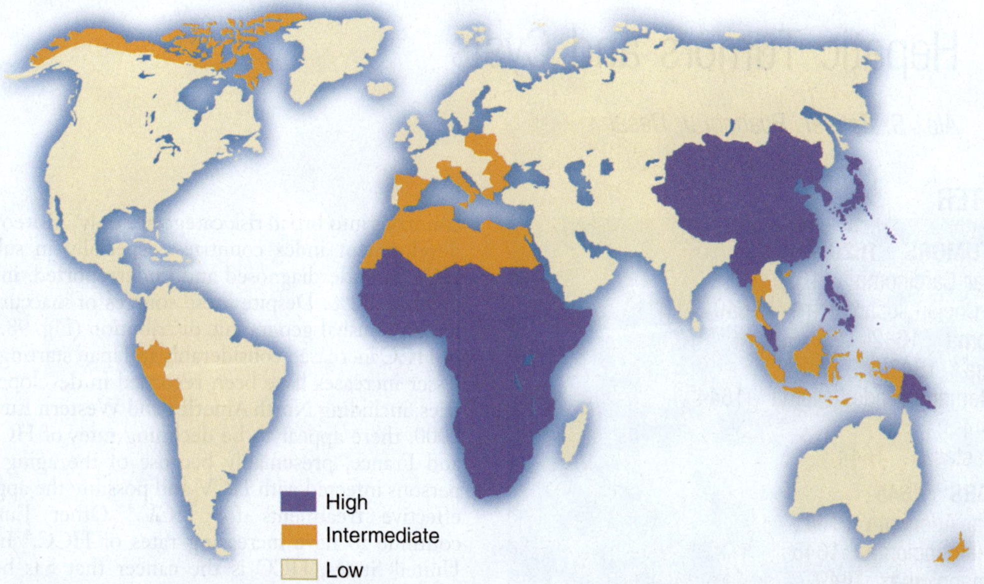

Fig. 98.1 Incidence of HCC in different parts of the world. *High*, age-adjusted rate of more than 15 cases/100,000 population/year; *intermediate*, age-adjusted rate of 5–15 cases/100,000/year; *low*, age-adjusted rate of fewer than 5 cases/100,000/year. Map lines delineate study areas and do not necessarily depict accepted national boundaries.

BOX 98.1 Risk Factors for HCC

MAJOR RISK FACTORS

Chronic HBV infection
Chronic HCV infection
Cirrhosis
NAFLD

OTHER LIVER CONDITIONS

α_1-Antitrypsin deficiency
Hemochromatosis
Membranous obstruction of the inferior vena cava
Type 1 and Type 2 glycogen storage disease
Type 1 hereditary tyrosinemia
Wilson disease

INHERITED CONDITIONS NOT ASSOCIATED WITH LIVER DISEASE

Ataxia-telangiectasia
Hypercitrullinemia

OTHER FACTORS

Cigarette smoking
Diabetes mellitus
Dietary exposure to aflatoxin B_1
Oral contraceptive steroid use

populations.[12,13] Persistent HBV infection antedates the development of HCC by several to many years, an interval commensurate with a cause-and-effect relationship between the virus and the tumor. Indeed, in at-risk populations, the HBV carrier state is largely established in early childhood by perinatal or horizontal infection.[14,15] Nearly 90% of children infected at this stage of life become chronic carriers of the virus, and these early onset carriers face a lifetime relative risk for developing HCC of more than 100 compared with uninfected controls.[16,17]

An effective vaccine against HBV has been available since the early 1980s, and in countries where this vaccine has been included in the expanded program of immunization for a sufficient length of time, the HBV carrier rate among children has decreased by 10-fold or more. Studies in Taiwan, where universal immunization was started in 1984 and where the rate of HBV carriage among children has decreased by more than 10-fold, have shown an 80% reduction in the mortality rate from HCC in the vaccinated age groups.[18] This finding gives promise for the ultimate eradication of HBV-induced HCC and provides further evidence of the causal role of the virus in the development of this tumor.

The precise mechanism by which HBV results in HCC is not known; however, the virus appears to be both directly and indirectly carcinogenic.[19] HBV DNA is integrated into cellular DNA in approximately 90% of HBV-related HCCs.[11] The sites of chromosomal insertion appear to be random, and whether viral integration is essential for hepatocarcinogenesis is still uncertain. Possible direct carcinogenic effects include *cis*-activation of cellular genes as a result of viral integration, changes in the DNA sequences flanking the integrated viral DNA, transcriptional activation of remote cellular genes by HBV-encoded proteins (particularly the X protein), and effects resulting from viral mutations. The transcriptional activity of the HBV X protein may be mediated by interaction with specific transcription factors, activation of the mitogen-activated protein kinase and Janus kinase/signal transducer and activator of transcription (JAK/STAT) pathways, an effect on apoptosis, and modulation of DNA repair. Studies have shown a clear link between the amount of HBV replication [measured as serum level of HBV DNA (viral load)] and subsequent risk of HCC. The long-term risk of HCC increases markedly in patients with serum HBV DNA levels higher than 10^4 copies/mL.[13] A randomized controlled trial of antiviral therapy has also shown a reduction in the incidence of HCC in association with reductions in serum levels of HBV DNA during therapy (see later), although other studies have not been able to confirm this benefit.[14] Multiple cohort studies demonstrate reduced HCC incidence after about 5 years of antiviral therapy for HBV compared to prediction models with no differences in the effectiveness between the currently utilized agents (entecavir

Diagnosis

CT is the most useful imaging technique in the diagnosis of metastatic disease to the liver.[243] Multiphase helical CT and CT during arterial portography are more sensitive than conventional CT. Multislice CT has a sensitivity ranging from 75% to 96%.[150] While routine ultrasound examination may have a limited role, contrast-enhanced ultrasound is useful in the diagnosis of hepatic metastasis, with one study showing contrast-enhanced ultrasound to have 83% sensitivity and 84% specificity in the detection of metastatic disease to the liver.[81,244] T1-weighted MRI may also be helpful, and iron oxide–enhanced MRI is even better. Fluorine-18-fluorodeoxyglucose PET-CT is helpful in identifying a liver mass as malignant and, more importantly, in locating extrahepatic disease that may influence treatment.

Pathology

Macroscopic Appearance

Hepatic metastases usually are multiple.[241] Their pathologic features vary, depending on the site of origin. Metastases are expansive, when they are discrete, or infiltrative. Individual metastases may reach a large size, and with multiple metastases, the liver may be greatly enlarged. Metastases are commonly gray-white and may show scattered hemorrhages or central necrosis. Individual metastases may be surrounded by a zone of venous stasis. Subcapsular lesions are often umbilicated. The dictum that cirrhotic livers are less likely than noncirrhotic livers to harbor metastatic deposits remains to be verified.

Microscopic Appearance

The microscopic features, including the degree of stromal growth, of most hepatic metastases duplicate those of the tumor of origin. Metastatic deposits usually are easily delineated from the surrounding liver tissue. Invasion of portal or hepatic veins may be seen, although less often than with HCC.[241] It may be difficult to distinguish metastatic adenocarcinoma from primary cholangiocarcinoma (see earlier).[183]

Treatment and Prognosis

The extent of replacement of liver tissue by metastases generally determines the patient's prognosis. The greater the tumor burden, the worse the outlook, with only approximately 50% of patients surviving 3 months after the onset of symptoms and less than 10% surviving more than 1 year.[245] Improved imaging modalities, advances in surgical techniques for resection, and new chemotherapeutic agents and regional therapies have made it possible to achieve long-term survival in individual patients. In colorectal cancer, long-term survival of 25%–30% has been achieved most often by resection of hepatic metastases in patients with colorectal cancer, a substantial number of whom have been cured or have obtained disease-free survival for up to 20 years.[245–248] Survival for 5 years can be achieved in up to 60% of those who undergo resection of a solitary colon cancer metastasis to the liver.[17] If the primary tumor has been removed completely and metastases are confined to the liver, resection of hepatic metastases should be considered.[249] Multiple case series suggest benefit with the potential for long-term survival in patients with a solitary breast cancer metastasis to the liver that responds to preoperative chemotherapy.[249] Case series also suggest potential benefit for resection of low-volume (<25% of liver volume) symptomatic liver metastases of neuroendocrine tumors.[249]

LT, with or without chemotherapy, has been limited to a few patients with rare slow-growing malignancies such as neuroendocrine tumors but is generally contraindicated in other types of metastatic disease. LT in combination with chemotherapy is an emerging therapy for unresectable colorectal metastasis. RFA is a valid therapy for colorectal metastases in patients who are unable to tolerate or refuse surgical resection. Other invasive methods of destroying metastases, such as ethanol injection, freezing with cryoprobes, and laser vaporization, warrant further study. Radiation therapy and intra-arterial infusion of cytotoxic drugs have limited roles.

BENIGN TUMORS

Hepatocellular Adenoma

Epidemiology

Hepatocellular adenomas [also termed hepatic adenomas and telangiectatic focal nodular hyperplasia (FNH) or adenomas] are rare benign epithelial tumors of the liver that occur predominantly in women in the second to fifth decades of life. They are commonly associated with the use of estrogen, including exogenous estrogens in oral contraceptive pills (OCPs), and can also be seen in the absence of exogenous estrogens and in men. The annual incidence of hepatocellular adenoma in OCP users is 30–40 per million compared with 1–1.3 per million in non-users.[250] OCP use for more than 5 years, older age, and use of high-potency hormones all appear to increase the risk. Cessation of estrogens often leads to regression of an adenoma, adding support to their role in the pathogenesis. The role of low-dose estrogen hormone replacement therapy in causing hepatocellular adenoma remains uncertain, and this treatment should be used with caution in an individual known to have an adenoma. Hepatocellular adenomas have also been associated with anabolic androgenic steroid use and FAP coli.

Hepatocellular adenomas are common in patients with glycogen storage disease type I, with a frequency of 22%–75%, and type III, with a frequency of 25%. In this setting, there is a male predominance, and the diagnosis is usually made during childhood (see Chapter 79).[251]

The designation *liver adenomatosis* is usually applied to cases with multiple (arbitrarily >10) hepatocellular adenomas and has been associated with germline and somatic mutations in hepatocyte nuclear factor-1α (HNF-1α) and with MASLD (formerly NAFLD) in the adjacent liver parenchyma. It is not clear whether liver adenomatosis is a distinct entity, but it may be more difficult to manage clinically than a single or a few adenomas because of the high number of lesions.[252,253]

Etiology and Pathogenesis

Multiple genetic alterations have been identified in hepatocellular adenomas. Investigators in Bordeaux, France, proposed—and other groups have validated—a phenotypic-genotypic classification that divides hepatocellular adenomas into 6 groups[254–256] (Fig. 98.5). These groups have now been adapted by the WHO Classification of Tumours of the Digestive System. Each group has varying risks for transformation to HCC and implications for management. Biallelic mutations of the *TCF1* gene that encodes HNF-1α have been identified in 35%–45% of patients with hepatocellular adenoma, and this group of tumors is designated HNF-1α inactivated.[252,254,255] HNF-1α is implicated in liver development by affecting hepatocyte differentiation and also helps control glucose and lipid metabolism.[252,257] Most of the mutations are somatic, although germline mutations associated with mature-onset diabetes of the young type 3, an autosomal dominant form of nonketotic diabetes mellitus presenting before age 25, are common in patients with liver adenomatosis (see earlier).[258] A second pathway, the Wnt pathway, which has also been implicated in 10%–25% of HCCs, is activated in 15%–19% of hepatocellular adenomas that have mutations in the gene *CTNNB1* which codes the protein β-catenin.[254,255,259] β-Catenin activation confers a higher

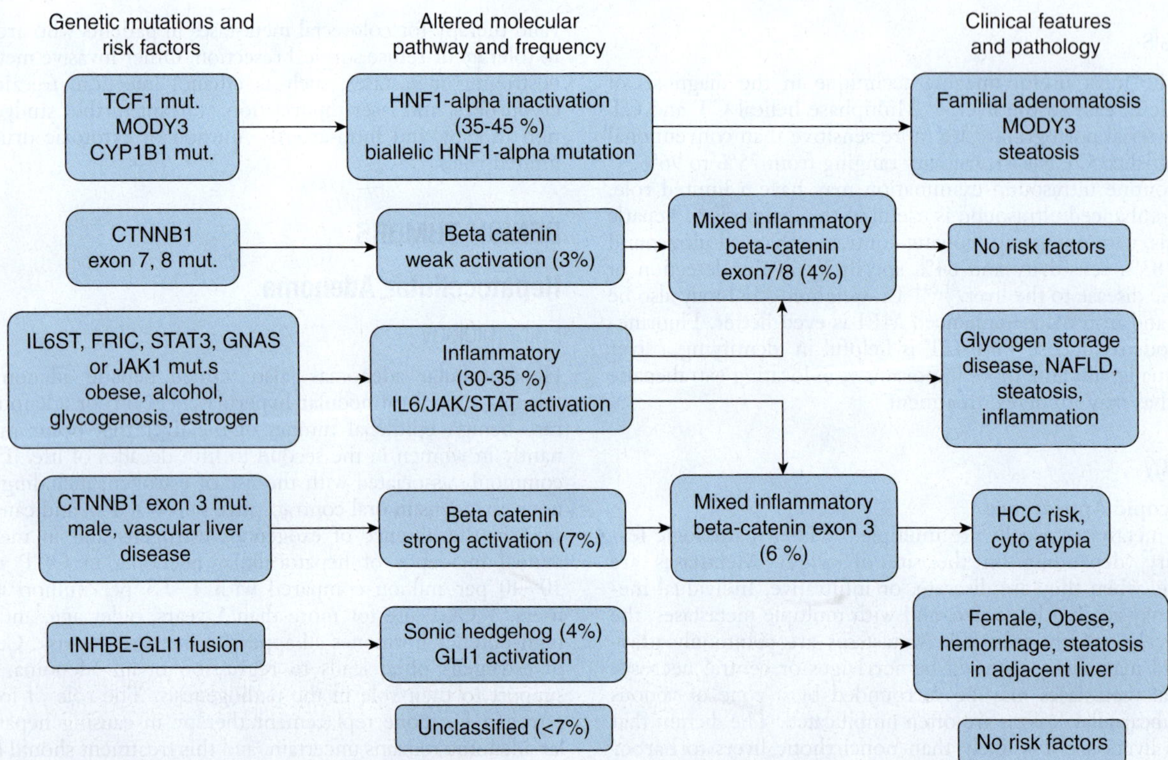

Fig. 98.5 Schematic representation of the principal molecular pathways altered in hepatocellular adenoma. *Left,* Main risk factors and known genetic predispositions. *Center,* Altered molecular pathways and their frequencies. *Right,* Principal clinical and pathologic features of the types of adenomas. *Arrows* indicate the significant relationships. *Some tumors may be simultaneously β-catenin-activated and inflammatory. *CYP1B1,* cytochrome P450 1B1; *HNF-1α,* hepatocyte nuclear factor 1α (gene symbol *TCF1*); *MODY3,* maturity-onset diabetes of the young type 3; *mut,* mutation. (Adapted from Nault JC, Paradis V, Cherqui D et al. Molecular classification of hepatocellular adenoma in clinical practice. *J Hepatol.* 2017;67:1074e–1083e.)

risk of malignant transformation and can be associated with glycogen storage disease and adenomas in male patients.[254,260] The third identified pathway for formation of hepatocellular adenomas includes acute inflammatory responses demonstrable by histologic examination of the tumor,[254,260] and associated with obesity and alcohol (see Fig. 98.5). This group often has activation of the IL-6 inflammatory signaling pathway, via mutations of genes in the IL6/JAK/STAT3 pathway, including FRK and GNAS complex locus, and is termed inflammatory hepatocellular adenomas.[257] A small percentage of this group also exhibits β-catenin activation via *CTNNB1* mutations and can be considered a fourth group. Mutations in *CTNNB1* exon 7/8 have increased risk of hemorrhage, while exon 3 mutations may lead to increased risk for malignancy. A fifth category has recently been identified with constitutive activation of the Sonic hedgehog pathway and seems to be at increased risk for tumor-related bleeding.[261] The sixth group has no identifiable specific associated mutations and is designated unclassified adenoma.[256]

Clinical Features

Hepatocellular adenomas manifest in a number of ways. Often, they may be found incidentally on abdominal imaging and produce no symptoms. Rarely, if large, they can be discovered during routine physical examination. Some patients experience pain in the right hypochondrium or epigastrium. The pain is usually mild and ill-defined but may be severe as a result of bleeding into or infarction of the tumor. If the liver is enlarged, the surface is usually smooth, and the liver may be slightly tender. The most alarming presentation is with severe abdominal pain and hypotension from acute hemoperitoneum following rupture of an adenoma. This complication is linked to OCP use and carries an appreciable mortality rate.[262,263] Tumors that rupture are generally large (>5 cm) and solitary, although the most important determinant of rupture is a superficial location. Often, the affected woman is menstruating at the time; rupture may also occur during pregnancy.[264] The risk of malignant transformation is strongly associated with male gender, β-catenin activation, and a tumor diameter larger than 5 cm.

Diagnosis

Serum AFP concentrations are normal. The serum C-reactive protein (CRP) level and WBC count may be elevated with inflammatory adenomas. Historically, fine-needle biopsy has been useless because hepatocellular adenomas mimic normal hepatocytes microscopically. Core needle biopsy has also been of limited diagnostic value, although a definitive diagnosis can often be made at expert centers with the use of immunohistochemical markers (see later).[265] Dynamic MRI with a hepatobiliary contrast agent such as gadobenate dimeglumine or gadoxetic acid, which are taken up by hepatocytes and excreted into the biliary tree, is the preferred imaging modality for diagnosis because it is most able to distinguish a hepatocellular adenoma from other benign or malignant masses in the liver; dynamic CT can also be helpful.[266,267]

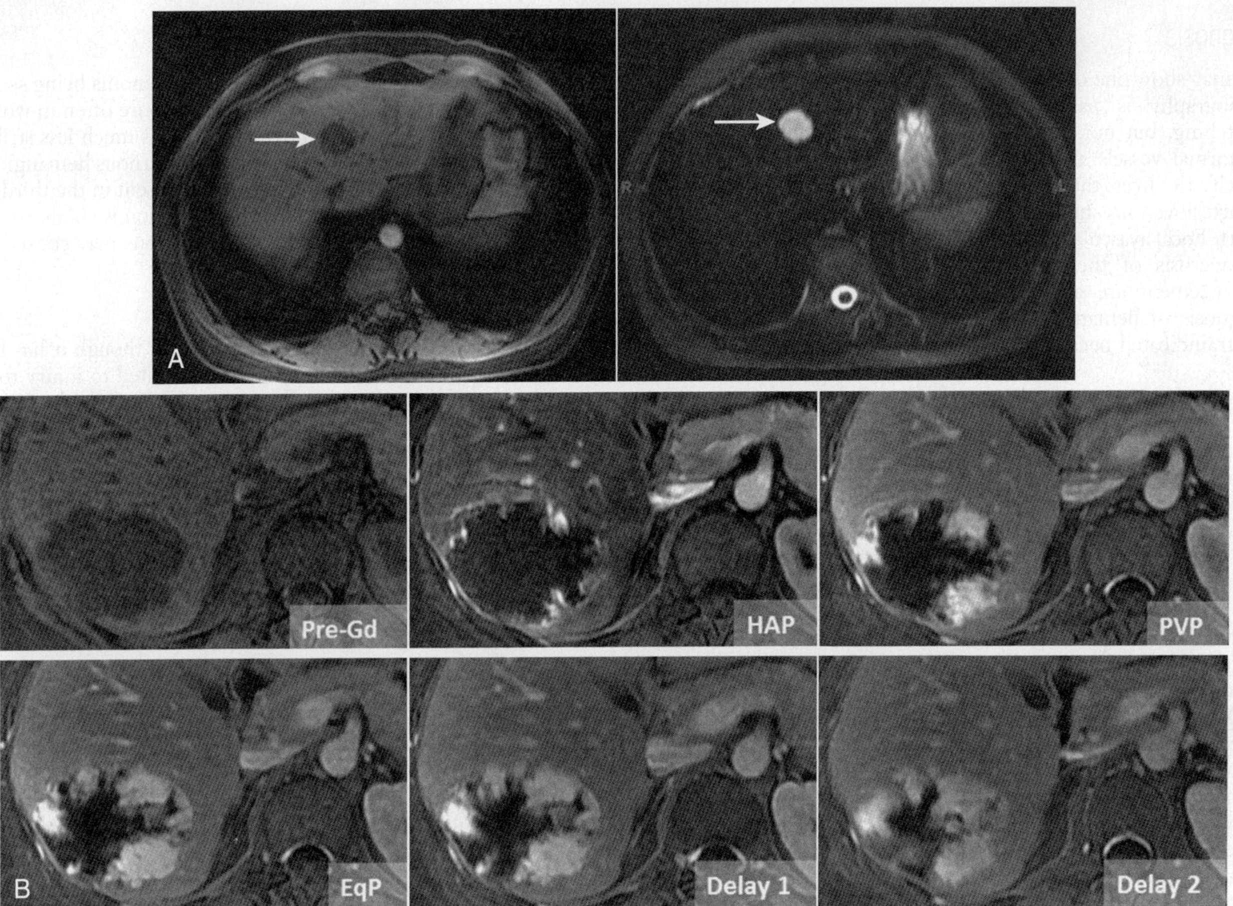

Fig. 98.7 MRI showing a hemangioma of the liver (*arrow*). *Panel* (A) shows T1-weighted image on the left with a dark area where the hemangioma and a T2-weighted image on the right showing the same area of the liver with a very bright signal. *Panel* (B) shows progressive contrast enhancement with gadolinium from the periphery to the center of a hepatic hemangioma. From top left corner, clockwise the phases of the MRI are pregadolinium (Pre-Gd), hepatic arterial phase (HAP), portal venous phase (PVP), and equilibrium phase (EqP), followed by two very delayed phases (Delay 1 and 2). (*Source*: Images courtesy of Jeffrey J. Brown, MD, St. Louis, MO.)

Infantile Hemangioma

Epidemiology

Infantile hemangiomas are the most common tumor of the liver in infants. They can form after birth (infantile hepatic hemangiomas [IHH]) or can be fully formed at the time of birth (congenital hemangioma).[301] Infantile hemangioma is also known as infantile hemangioendothelioma, though the use of this term has been discouraged, due to confusion with epithelioid hemangioendothelioma, a malignant tumor discussed previously. Infantile hemangioma is a benign tumor that is characterized by proliferation of the tumor during gestation or early in the infancy period followed by involution during childhood.[302,1] A majority of these lesions present within the first 6 months of life, up to a third presenting within the first month, and tend to have a 2:1 female predominance.[302,1] The importance of infantile hemangiomas stems from the high incidence of heart failure in infants with this tumor and the resulting high mortality rate.

Clinical Features

IHH can be classified into three categories (focal, multifocal, and diffuse). Focal lesions are single and typically asymptomatic. In contrast, multifocal infantile hemangiomas present as several lesions. Infants with multifocal lesions are often asymptomatic but can develop high-output heart failure associated with arteriovenous shunting. Diffuse IHH presents as diffuse neonatal hemangiomas that significantly displace liver parenchyma, leading to compression of nearby structures, resulting abdominal compartment syndrome, respiratory failure, and multiorgan failure.[301] In addition, diffuse IHH has been associated with profound hypothyroidism due to overproduction of type III iodothyronine deiodinase leading to deactivation of thyronine.[301]

Small hemangioendotheliomas are usually asymptomatic. The presence of a large lesion is recognized clinically by the diagnostic triad of an enlarged liver, high-output heart failure, and multiple cutaneous hemangiomas.[303,304] The liver is larger than expected on the basis of the severity of the heart failure, and hepatomegaly persists after the heart failure has been treated successfully. Approximately one-third of patients have jaundice. Patients may be anemic in up to 50% of cases partly because of the dilutional effect of the increased circulating plasma volume that develops with large peripheral arteriovenous fistulas.[302] A microangiopathic hemolytic anemia may contribute. In addition, thrombocytopenia may be present (Kasabach-Merritt syndrome). Malignant change is a rare complication.

Diagnosis

US may show one or more echogenic masses in the liver. Hepatic angiography is particularly helpful in diagnosis and shows stretching, but not displacement, of the intrahepatic arteries.[305] Abnormal vessels arise from the hepatic arteries and promptly opacify the liver, thereby giving rise to the characteristic blush of an arteriovenous shunt. The circulation time through the liver is short. Focal avascular areas may be evident when hemorrhage into or necrosis of the tumor has occurred. CT and MRI with enhancement are as specific as hepatic arteriography for the diagnosis of hemangioendotheliomas.[306] Percutaneous biopsy is contraindicated because of the danger of bleeding.

Pathology

Multifocal infantile hemangiomas appear as spherical masses separated by segments of normal hepatic parenchyma, whereas diffuse infantile hemangiomas have near-total replacement of hepatic parenchyma.[307] Infantile hemangiomas that are multifocal or diffuse produce nodular deformity of the entire liver. The nodules range in size from a few millimeters to many centimeters and are well demarcated but not encapsulated. At laparotomy, the nodules can be seen to pulsate. They are reddish purple, although large tumors are gray to tan. They may show hemorrhages, fibrosis, or calcification.

Microscopically, infantile hemangioma is composed of a single layer of benign plump endothelial cells that line small, intercommunicating vascular channels. Multifocal and diffuse infantile hemangiomas also stain positive for glucose transporter-1 (Gluc-1), which is one of the most specific histologic markers to help differentiate this lesion from other vascular tumors.[307] In some areas of the tumor, solid masses of mesoblastic primordial cells that differentiate early into vascular structures are observed. Fibrous septa may be prominent, and extramedullary hematopoiesis occurs frequently. Thrombosis may be followed by scarring and calcification.

Treatment and Prognosis

The course of infantile hemangioma is characterized by tumor growth during the early months of life, followed by gradual involution.[303] Life-threatening aspects of the disorder are intractable heart failure and, to a lesser extent, consumptive coagulopathy or rupture of the tumor. Heart failure should be treated by conventional means initially, but if these measures fail, more aggressive treatment of the tumor, such as embolization, ligation of the hepatic artery, surgical resection of the tumor, or LT should be considered.[308,309] Use of glucocorticoids has been successful in many (but not all) patients,[310] whereas irradiation has seldom been beneficial. As in cases of cutaneous hemangiomas, there does appear to be a role for propranolol in treatment of symptomatic IHH.[302,311] When the tumor is confined to one lobe, surgical resection is curative, even in the presence of cardiac failure.[303]

Others

Other rare benign tumors of the liver include angiomyolipoma,[312] bile duct adenoma,[313] biliary cystadenoma, and biliary adenofibroma.[314,315]

TUMOR-LIKE HEPATIC LESIONS

Focal Nodular Hyperplasia

FNH is a well-circumscribed, unencapsulated usually solitary lesion composed of nodules of benign hyperplastic hepatocytes surrounding a central stellate scar.[316,304]

Epidemiology

FNH is more common than hepatocellular adenoma being seen in up to 3% of autopsies.[280] The lesion occurs more often in women than in men, although the gender difference is much less striking than that for hepatocellular adenoma and cavernous hemangioma. FNH occurs at all ages, but most patients present in the third and fourth decades of life.[260,304] The age distribution is similar to that of hepatocellular adenomas, and the two lesions may coexist.

Pathogenesis

The cause of FNH is not completely known, though it has been thought that the development of FNH is related to injury to the portal tract resulting in formation and enlargement of arteriovenous shunting leading to hyperperfusion to local arteries. This results in hepatocellular hyperplasia and oxidative stress causing the hepatic stellate cells to produce the central scar.[260,317] Given the female predominance of FNH, a hormonal relationship has been considered in the development of the lesion. However, studies fail to consistently show that there is significant growth of FNH during pregnancy or regression in size if OCPs are discontinued.[318–320]

Clinical Features

Most of these lesions do not produce symptoms and are often discovered during upper abdominal imaging for other reasons or because an enlarged liver is felt on routine examination or found during abdominal surgery or at autopsy.[304,321,322] Patients may experience mild pain, particularly with bleeding into or necrosis of the lesion. Conditions and complications associated with FNH are listed in Box 98.4.

Diagnosis

Serum AFP levels are normal. The mass lesion seen on US and CT is not specific for FNH[323,324] unless the central scar and feeding artery are seen (Fig. 98.8). MRI may be useful for the diagnosis of FNH, and advances in the use of contrast agents for MRI have substantially improved the utility of this technique to diagnose FNH definitively. Liver-specific gadolinium-based MR contrast agents show FNH to be iso- to hyperintense relative to the liver parenchyma during the hepatobiliary phase of imaging and rarely hypointense, with proved sensitivity greater than 90% for distinguishing FNH from hepatocellular adenomas. Gadoxetic acid is thought to be the best choice of contrast agent for the diagnosis of FNH.[325]

BOX 98.4 Associations with and Complications of Focal Nodular Hyperplasia

ASSOCIATIONS

- Cavernous hemangioma
- Cavernous transformation of the portal vein
- Congenital absence of the portal vein
- Epithelioid hemangioendothelioma
- HHT
- LT (detection in graft)
- Neonatal hepatic hemangioma
- Spinal and pulmonary arteriovenous malformations

COMPLICATIONS

- Budd-Chiari syndrome
- Compression of the inferior vena cava

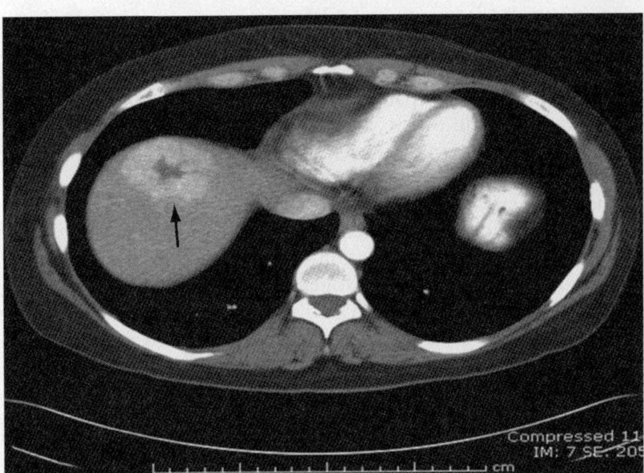

Fig. 98.8 Contrast-enhanced CT of the liver during the arterial phase showing a typical focal nodular hyperplasia (*arrow*) with contrast enhancement of the mass lesion and the central stellate scar that is apparent by its lack of enhancement.

Pathology

FNH manifests as a firm, coarsely nodular, light brown, or yellowish-gray mass of variable size, with a dense central stellate scar and radiating fibrous septa that divide the lesion into lobules.[326] The nodule may be small, resembling a cirrhotic nodule, or extremely large. The lesion of FNH usually occupies a subcapsular position and may be pedunculated. It generally is solitary. Larger lesions may show foci of hemorrhage or necrosis, although these features are seen less frequently than in hepatocellular adenomas. The fibrous septa sometimes are poorly developed, and the central scar may be absent. The lesion is sharply demarcated from the surrounding liver tissue, which is normal, but a true capsule is absent. FNH is associated with hepatic hemangiomas in as many as 20% of cases.

Microscopically, FNH closely resembles a focal form of inactive cirrhosis. Individual hepatocytes are indistinguishable from those of normal liver but lack the usual cord arrangement in relation to sinusoids, central veins, and portal tracts. Kupffer cells are present. Characteristically, the fibrous septa contain numerous bile ductules and vessels. Other features include heavy infiltrations of lymphocytes and, to a lesser extent, plasma cells and histiocytes. Bile duct proliferation in portal tracts may also be evident. Branches of the hepatic artery and portal vein show various combinations of intimal and smooth muscle hyperplasia, subintimal fibrosis, thickening of the wall, occlusive luminal lesions, and thrombosis at times. Whether these vascular changes are primary or secondary is not known. Peliosis hepatis may be an associated lesion (see Chapter 85). The histologic features almost always make it possible to distinguish FNH from hepatocellular adenoma, although the distinction may be difficult to make, particularly in small biopsy specimens.

Treatment

Studies of the natural history of FNH indicate that most lesions remain stable or even regress or disappear after a long follow-up period.[327] If lesions are asymptomatic, FNH should be left alone, given the infrequency of complications. Large symptomatic or complicated lesions can be resected, usually by segmental resection or enucleation. Recurrence after resection is rare. These lesions may also be treated with arterial embolization, arterial chemoembolization, or RFA if patients are not considered surgical candidates.[328–330] Periodic US should be performed if a firm diagnosis of FNH has not been made, and a lesion that increases substantially in size should be considered for resection. The available evidence argues against the notion that FNH is a premalignant condition.

Others

Nodular regenerative hyperplasia is characterized by nodularity of the liver in the absence of significant fibrosis[331] and may be associated with a number of diseases, such as immunological (such as RA and Felty syndrome—see Chapter 35) or hematological disorders (common variable immunodeficiency), certain drugs/toxins (thiopurines, chemotherapy agents, antiretrovirals), neoplasia, or organ transplantation.[332–334] Although generally diffuse, the nodularity is occasionally focal, in which case the lesion may be mistaken for a tumor. Patients with nodular regenerative hyperplasia typically present clinically with non-cirrhotic portal hypertension. Treatment should be geared towards the underlying etiology along with treatment of portal hypertension symptoms. Partial nodular transformation is characterized by nodules that are limited to the perihilar region of the liver. These patients also present with portal hypertension.

Macroregenerative nodules may occur in advanced cirrhosis or after massive hepatic necrosis. In the presence of cirrhosis, they are believed to be premalignant and may, in addition, be mistaken for hepatic tumors during hepatic imaging.[335]

Inflammatory pseudotumor is a rare entity, resulting from focal infection, that may be mistaken for a hepatic tumor (see Chapter 86).[336] It occurs particularly in young men who present with intermittent fever, abdominal pain, jaundice, vomiting, and diarrhea. Leukocytosis, an elevated ESR, and polyclonal hyperglobulinemia are present in approximately 50% of patients. The lesion may be solitary or multiple and shows a mixture of chronic inflammatory cells, with plasma cells predominating. Focal fatty infiltration, or focal fatty sparing in the presence of diffuse fatty infiltration, may also be mistaken for a hepatic tumor (see Chapter 89).[337]

HEPATIC CYSTS

Hepatic cysts are abnormal fluid-filled spaces in the hepatic parenchyma and biliary tract. They are categorized into three main types: fibrocystic diseases of the liver, cystadenomas and cystadenocarcinomas, and hydatid cysts. Cystadenomas and cystadenocarcinomas are discussed in Chapter 71. Hydatid cysts are discussed in Chapter 86.

Fibrocystic diseases of the liver originate from abnormal persistence or defect in the progressive remodeling of the ductal plate during development, resulting in dilated fluid-filled spaces, including hepatic and choledochal cysts, portal fibrosis, and ductal plate malformations (see Chapter 64).[288,289] Fibrocystic disorders of the liver described here include simple hepatic cysts, polycystic liver disease (PCLD), fibrocystic disease associated with autosomal recessive polycystic kidney disease (ARPKD), von Meyenburg complexes, and Caroli disease (type V choledochal cyst). (The other diseases are congenital hepatic fibrosis and Type IV choledochal cysts; see Chapter 64.)

Simple Cysts

Simple hepatic cysts are thought to be congenital in origin and have a frequency of about 2.5% of the population.[338] They are generally smaller than 5 cm in diameter and can number up to 10 before being considered part of PCLD. The cysts are usually asymptomatic and discovered incidentally during upper abdominal imaging. They occur more often in women than in men, and their prevalence increases with age. If symptomatic, hepatic cysts can compress adjacent organs, resulting in symptoms of early satiety, epigastric fullness, or abdominal pain. Although uncommon, patients can also be symptomatic in the setting of internal hemorrhage, infection, rapid enlargement, or rupture. Typically, initial imaging with US, CT, or MRI provides an accurate diagnosis and distinguishes a simple cyst from a hydatid cyst and cystadenoma. Septations, papillary projections, or calcification should raise suspicion of an alternative diagnosis.[339] Asymptomatic solitary hepatic cysts require no further follow-up or intervention. If intervention is required because of symptoms, percutaneous aspiration and sclerosis with alcohol or doxycycline will almost always ablate the cyst, but recurrence is frequent.[340] An alternative approach is laparoscopic (or, rarely, open surgical) fenestration, allowing the cyst to drain into the peritoneal cavity, which is seldom followed by recurrence but has greater morbidity.

Polycystic Liver Disease

PCLD is a rare condition in which multiple cysts, 10 or more, form in the hepatic parenchyma; usually it comes to clinical attention in adulthood (Fig. 98.9). PCLD usually presents in association with autosomal dominant polycystic kidney disease (ADPKD)[341,342] but can appear as isolated PCLD.[343,344]

The cysts range in diameter from a few millimeters to 10 cm or more. They contain clear, colorless, or straw-colored fluid and are lined by a single layer of cuboidal or columnar epithelium, resembling that of bile ducts.[341–345] Rarely, the cysts may be lined by squamous epithelium; these cysts may be complicated by the development of squamous cell carcinoma. In addition to the nature of the lining epithelium, evidence for a biliary origin of these cysts is suggested by the composition of the cystic fluid, which has a low glucose content and contains secretory immunoglobulin (Ig) A and GGTP. The cysts are thought to arise as a result of a ductal plate malformation. This process gives rise to von Meyenburg complexes (see later), which become disconnected from the biliary tract during development and growth and dilate progressively to form cysts.

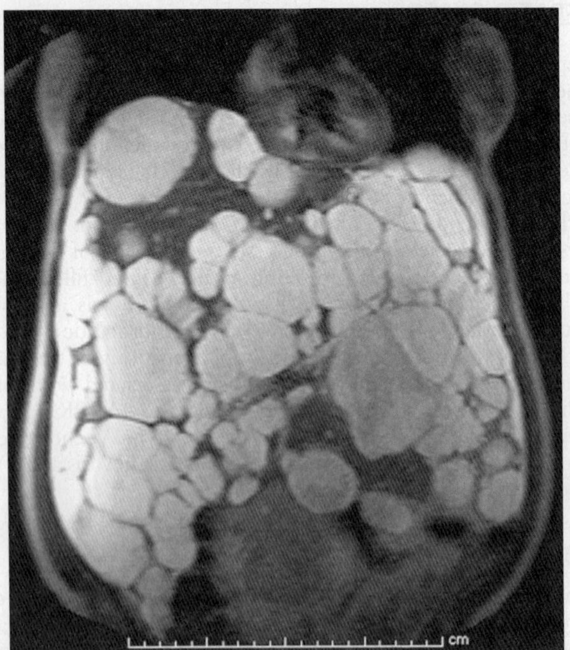

Fig. 98.9 MRI of the abdomen in a patient with severe polycystic liver disease. This coronal T2-weighted image shows a massively enlarged liver with numerous bright fluid-filled cysts. (*Source*: Courtesy Dr. N. Cem Balci, St. Louis, MO.)

Epidemiology

PCLD is relatively common in patients with ADPKD. It occurs in approximately 24% of patients in the third decade of life to 80% in the sixth decade of life, but the kidney disease usually dominates the clinical course.[346] Cysts may also be present in the pancreas, spleen, and (less often) other organs. Symptomatic liver disease correlates with advancing age, severity of renal cysts, and renal dysfunction.[347] Women tend to have larger and more numerous cysts, and a correlation with the number of pregnancies has been found. The use of exogenous female sex hormones may accelerate the rate of growth and size of the cysts. PCLD may coexist with other fibrocystic liver diseases, such as congenital hepatic fibrosis (in which the patient is likely to present with portal hypertension), Caroli disease, or von Meyenburg complexes.[341–345] PCLD is also associated with other conditions such as berry aneurysms, mitral valve prolapse, diverticular disease, and inguinal hernias.

Isolated PCLD not associated with ADPKD is rare, representing 7% of all PCLD in autopsy series.[341–345] It is usually asymptomatic.[348] Like ADPKD-associated PCLD, isolated PCLD is associated with pregnancy and appears to be more symptomatic in women than men.

Etiology and Pathogenesis

ADPKD is a common genetic disease with a frequency of 1:1000 in whites.[349] Two genes are responsible. The gene affected in ADPKD1 is *PKD-1*, which is located on chromosome 16q13-q23 and expresses a ubiquitous protein, polycystin-1.[350,351] The gene responsible for ADPKD2 is *PKD-2*, which is located on chromosome 4 and expresses polycystin-2. The two polycystins are transmembrane glycoproteins that complex and localize in the primary cilium, a microtubule-based structure found on renal and biliary tubule epithelium and thought to act as a flow sensor and regulator of Ca^{2+} influx.[352] Mutations in a small portion of additional genes, including GANAB, LRP5, DNAJB11, and ALG9 which mostly produce endoplasmic reticulum proteins involved with protein trafficking and maturation, can lead to ADPKD-associated PCLD.[353] Although the mutation is inherited as an autosomal dominant trait, a second somatic mutation is thought to be necessary to produce the monoclonally derived cysts.[354]

Isolated PCLD has been shown in North American and Finnish families to be linked to the gene *PRKCSH* (also known as protein kinase C substrate 80K-H) on chromosome 19p13.2–13.1 and to *SEC63* on chromosome 6q21.[350,355,356] The gene products hepatocystin and SEC63p are thought to be involved in the folding and quality control of glycoproteins and protein translocation in the endoplasmic reticulum, respectively.[357] The genes appear to be autosomal dominant, and a second somatic mutation is thought to be needed to cause disease. Five additional genes, *ALG8*, *GANAB*, *SEC61B*, LRP5, and PKHD1, have been identified and linked to isolated PCLD, and their gene products are mostly endoplasmic reticulum proteins necessary for maturation and trafficking of polycystin-1.[358,353]

Clinical Features

The hepatic cysts in PCLD, whether or not they occur in association with renal cysts, rarely cause morbidity, and many affected persons are asymptomatic.[341–345] Symptoms occur in patients with more numerous and larger cysts (10%–15% of patients, usually women), generally with markedly enlarged livers. Abdominal discomfort or pain, postprandial fullness, awareness of an upper abdominal mass, a protuberant abdomen, inability to bend over, and shortness of breath may be present. Severe pain may be experienced with rupture or infection of a cyst, bleeding into a

Because of the complexities associated with the differential diagnosis and the rarity of hepatocellular adenoma, imaging should be conducted at a center with expertise in diagnosing focal liver lesions. The tumor has a clearly defined margin and often has nearly parallel vessels entering it from the periphery ("spoke-wheel" appearance). Alternatively, the lesion may contain tortuous vessels coursing irregularly through it. On arterial-phase images, the tumor enhances irregularly, with areas of increased enhancement and focal avascularity as a result of hemorrhage or necrosis. On portal venous and delayed images, enhancement tends to decrease, and the lesion can be isointense or hypointense "washout." On late images (hepatobiliary phase) using a hepatobiliary contrast agent, almost all hepatocellular adenomas are hypointense compared with FNHs, which show homogenous diffuse hyperintensity or isointensity (see later). Some inflammatory hepatocellular adenomas may show patchy hyperintensity on hepatobiliary phase imaging, but other imaging (see later) and clinical features (obesity, metabolic syndrome, heavy alcohol use) can often help inform the correct diagnosis.[268] HNF-1α–inactivated hepatocellular adenomas show diffuse signal dropout in the lesion on T1-weighted chemical shift sequences because of steatosis.[269] Inflammatory hepatocellular adenomas have marked hyperintensity on T2-weighted sequences, especially in the outer part of the lesions, as a result of sinusoidal dilatation and persistent enhancement in the delayed phases. The uninvolved liver in the inflammatory type often has evidence of steatosis.[269] β-Catenin–activated hepatocellular adenomas can have a poorly delineated scar and may show isointense or increased uptake in the hepatobiliary phase suggesting FNH, so other imaging features and clinical context need to be considered. If there is still uncertainty, a core biopsy evaluated by an expert pathologist is recommended.[270] Surgical excision remains the gold standard for diagnosis (see later).

Pathology

Hepatocellular adenoma generally occurs as a solitary, relatively soft, light brown to yellow tumor. It is sharply circumscribed but does not have a true capsule, although a pseudocapsule is formed by compression of the surrounding liver tissue (Fig. 98.6A).[271] Hepatocellular adenomas arise in an otherwise normal liver, although hepatic steatosis and MASLD are often seen in association with the inflammatory and Sonic hedgehog types. Most tumors are solitary, but multiple tumors can occur. Adenomas range in diameter from 1 to 30 cm. They are larger on average in women taking OCPs than in those not taking them; the lesions usually occupy a subcapsular position and project slightly from the surface of the liver. A pedunculated variety is occasionally seen. The cut surface of the tumor may show ill-defined lobulation but is never nodular or fibrotic. Foci of hemorrhage or necrosis are frequent, and bile staining may be evident.

Microscopically, hepatocellular adenoma may mimic normal liver tissue to an astonishing degree (see Fig. 98.6B).[271] The tumor is composed of sheets or cords of normal-looking or slightly atypical hepatocytes that show no features of malignancy. Few or no portal tracts or central veins are present, and bile ducts are conspicuously absent. Only an infrequent fibrous or vascular septum traverses the lesion. An essentially normal reticulin pattern is demonstrable throughout the adenoma. The HNF-1α–inactivated type often has intratumor steatosis and lacks inflammation. On immunohistochemistry, they do not stain with liver fatty acid–binding protein, in contrast to the surrounding liver and the other types of adenoma.[254] The inflammatory type has scattered inflammatory infiltrates, thick-walled arteries with sinusoidal dilatation (peliosis), mild steatosis, and hemorrhage; in the past, this type was called "telangiectatic FNH." The lesion stains with serum amyloid A (SAA) and with CRP.[254] The β-catenin–activated type has no steatosis, peliosis, or portal tract elements and forms pseudoglands with cytologic abnormalities.

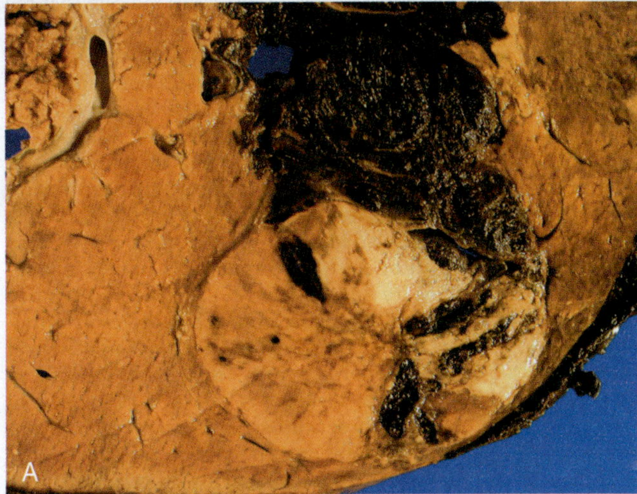

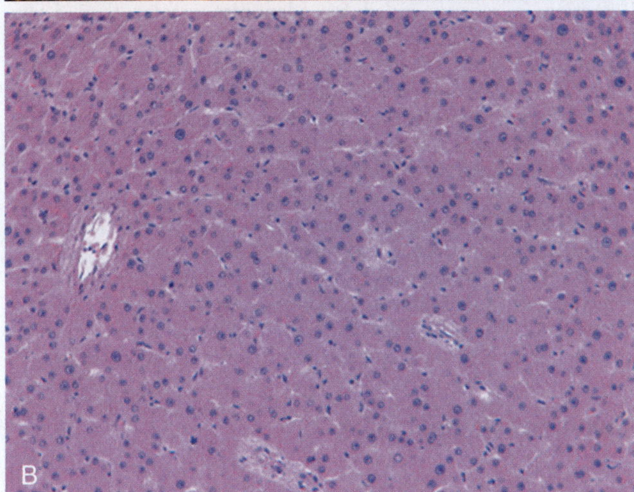

Fig. 98.6 (A) Surgical specimen of a large hepatocellular adenoma. The tumor is yellowish and slightly lobular, with a pseudocapsule and areas of necrosis and hemorrhage. (B) Histopathology of a hepatocellular adenoma showing the resemblance to normal liver tissue, with cords of normal-looking, although generally slightly larger, hepatocytes, as well as Kupffer cells (but fewer in number than normal) lining the sinusoids. Bile ducts and central veins are not seen, but the presence of abnormal vascular structures is evident (H&E). (*Source*: (A) Courtesy Elizabeth Brunt, MD, St. Louis, MO. (B) Courtesy Professor A.C. Paterson, Johannesburg, South Africa.)

On immunohistochemistry, the hepatocyte nuclei stain used for staining with glutamine synthetase is preferred for diagnosis.[255] Molecular analysis for β-catenin is recommended for equivocal staining with glutamine synthetase.[257] Sonic hedgehog-type adenomas are associated with MAFLD in the surrounding liver, intralesional hemorrhage, and increased staining for argininosuccinate synthase 1 in lesion versus surrounding liver.[256] The unclassified type of hepatocellular adenomas does not stain for CRP, SAA, β-catenin, or glutamine synthetase and has normal liver fatty acid–binding protein staining.[254,255]

Treatment and Prognosis

Historically, because of the danger that a hepatocellular adenoma may rupture and bleed, surgical resection was always recommended.[271,272] Resection is usually feasible in an uncomplicated case, but with rupture and hemorrhage, arterial embolization is generally used to control hemorrhage, and resection is considered later for residual adenoma.[262] More recent series indicate that the risk of rupture is related to a size larger than 5 cm, although a few cases of hemorrhage have been reported in smaller lesions.[273] Therefore resection is now recommended for lesions larger than 5 cm or those with evidence of hemorrhage or other symptoms. If the adenoma is not resected, pregnancy and exogenous estrogens should be avoided, although pregnancy without complications can be successful with careful monitoring for growth of the tumor, particularly for those smaller than 5 cm in diameter.[274] Transformation of a hepatocellular adenoma to HCC is a potential risk, with rates estimated to be 4.4%, predominantly limited to adenomas larger than 5 cm in diameter (96%) and more often associated with β-catenin activation from *CTNNB1* exon 3 mutation, male gender, glycogen storage disease, or vascular liver disease.[275,256] The initial approach to a female patient with an asymptomatic hepatocellular adenoma is cessation of exogenous estrogens, weight loss for those who are obese, and interval imaging in 6–12 months.[276,277] If there is no growth and the lesion is less than 5 cm, subsequent annual imaging is recommended. Resection is recommended for adenomas greater than 5 cm, symptomatic patients, males, evidence of prior hemorrhage, and patients with a known β-catenin or Sonic hedgehog mutation. Advances in MRI and core needle biopsy typing of hepatocellular adenomas may improve the management of patients in the future and further reduce the need for resection.

The management of hepatic adenomatosis is problematic.[278] Often in these cases, the number of tumors is large, and they cannot be resected entirely. The size and gender risk factors for malignant transformation and rupture, however, seem to apply to patients with adenomatosis as well. Therefore serial imaging and consideration for biopsy or resection of evolving lesions are recommended. The role of LT for adenomatosis is best reserved for unresectable HCC or recurrent life-threatening hemorrhage.[279]

Cavernous Hemangioma

Epidemiology

Cavernous hemangioma is the most common benign tumor of the liver and is found in as many as 20% of autopsies.[212,280] The lesion is thought to be a congenital malformation or hamartoma that increases in size, initially with growth of the liver and thereafter by ectasia. Cavernous hemangiomas affect persons of all ages, although they manifest most often in the third, fourth, and fifth decades of life. Women are predominantly affected (4:1–6:1) and often present at a younger age and with larger tumors in comparison with men. Cavernous hemangiomas may increase in size with pregnancy or the administration of estrogens and are more common in multiparous than in nulliparous women.

Clinical Features

The great majority of cavernous hemangiomas are small and asymptomatic and are discovered incidentally during imaging of the liver for another reason, at autopsy, or at laparotomy. If symptomatic, patients present with larger or multiple lesions.[281] Those larger than 5 cm in diameter are called giant cavernous hemangiomas, which may be as large as 27 cm. Upper abdominal pain is the most common complaint associated with giant cavernous hemangiomas and results from partial infarction of the lesion or pressure on adjacent tissues. Early satiety, nausea, and vomiting also may occur due to compression on surrounding abdominal structures. Cavernous hemangiomas occasionally rupture. Typically, the only physical finding may be an enlarged liver. Occasionally, an arterial bruit is heard over the tumor. Arteriovenous shunting has been described with cavernous hemangiomas.

Kasabach-Merritt syndrome, a potentially life-threatening syndrome of thrombocytopenia and consumptive coagulopathy, can be seen in patients with large cavernous hemangiomas (>5 cm). This constellation of symptoms is seen occasionally in infants but rarely in adults.[281,282] Malignant transformation has not been reported.

Diagnosis

Cavernous hemangiomas are often detected initially by US. The typical US appearance is an echogenic mass of uniform echodensity that lies in the posterior segment of the right lobe of the liver and is less than 3 cm in diameter.[212,283] Almost all cavernous hemangiomas can be diagnosed by contrast-enhanced US, CT, or MRI with sequential scans.[284] In early imaging sequences, the center of the lesion remains hypodense, whereas the peripheral zone, which varies in thickness and may have a corrugated inner margin, is enhanced. On delayed phases of imaging, there is central enhancement.[285] MRI has a high degree of specificity and a central role in the diagnosis of small hemangiomas (Fig. 98.7).[286,287] With small hemangiomas, the contrast material may assume a ring-shaped or C-shaped configuration, with an avascular center resulting from fibrous obliteration; this appearance is pathognomonic. The radiographic appearance of rapidly filling hemangiomas and giant hemangiomas may not have the typical appearance as described above. However, both types are easily diagnosed by MRI.[29,288,289] Hemangiomas exhibit homogenous hyperintensity on T2-weighted images. MRI has >90% sensitivity and specificity in diagnosing cavernous hemangiomas.[290] Because of the risk of severe bleeding, percutaneous needle biopsy should not be performed if a cavernous hemangioma is suspected. Moreover, a needle biopsy is of limited diagnostic value. Blunt abdominal trauma may sometimes result in rupture of a giant cavernous hemangioma.[291]

Pathology

Cavernous hemangiomas are usually solitary lesions, although multiple tumors occur in 10% of patients.[271] Reddish-purple or bluish masses are seen under Glisson's capsule or deep in the substance of the liver. The larger lesions may be pedunculated. Cavernous hemangiomas are well circumscribed but seldom encapsulated. They may show central necrosis, and in some cases, the whole tumor is firm in consistency and grayish-white in appearance. Microscopically, hemangiomas are composed of multiple vascular channels of varying sizes lined by a single layer of flat epithelium and supported by fibrous septa.[212] The vascular spaces may contain thrombi. The demonstration of mast cells within hemangiomas suggests that mast cells may have a role in pathogenesis.[292] Sclerosing cavernous hemangiomas may sometimes be seen and probably represent natural involution of these lesions.

Occasionally, cavernous hemangiomas are associated with hemangiomas in other organs. They also may coexist with cysts in the liver or pancreas,[293] von Meyenburg complexes (see later and Chapter 64),[294] or FNH (see later).[295]

Treatment

The great majority of cavernous hemangiomas can safely be left untreated. Some controversy exists about allowing pregnancy or use of estrogen-containing medications in patients with cavernous hemangioma, but most authorities consider these to be safe.[213,296] Resection is not commonly recommended. However, in cases of Kasabach-Merritt Syndrome or large localized hemangiomas causing incapacitating symptoms, they should be resected.[281,297] If resection is not feasible, reduction in the size of the tumor with relief of symptoms is rarely achieved with irradiation, arterial ligation, arteriographic embolization, or systemic glucocorticoids.[298,299] RFA has been used with some success. LT is rarely needed but has been reported.[300] If a cavernous hemangioma has ruptured, it may be necessary to embolize or clamp the hepatic artery to stop bleeding before proceeding with resection, although rupture is exceedingly rare.